DRUG INFORMATION HANDBOOK

A Comprehensive Resource for all Clinicians and Healthcare Professionals

American Pharmacists Association®
Improving medication use. Advancing patient care.
APhA

Lexi-Comp is the official drug reference for the American Pharmacists Association

18th Edition

2009-2010

Senior Editors:

Charles F. Lacy, RPh, MS, PharmD, FCSHP
Lora L. Armstrong, RPh, PharmD, BCPS
Morton P. Goldman, RPh, PharmD, BCPS, FCCP
Leonard L. Lance, RPh, BSPharm

LEXI-COMP

DRUG INFORMATION HANDBOOK

A Comprehensive Resource for all Clinicians and Healthcare Professionals

Charles F. Lacy, RPh, MS, PharmD, FCSHP
Senior Editor
Vice President for Executive Affairs
Professor, Pharmacy Practice
Professor, Business Leadership
University of Southern Nevada
Las Vegas, Nevada

Lora L. Armstrong, RPh, PharmD, BCPS
Senior Editor
Vice President, Clinical Affairs
Pharmacy & Therapeutics Formulary Process
Clinical Program Oversight
CaremarkRx
Northbrook, Illinois

Morton P. Goldman, RPh, PharmD, BCPS, FCCP
Senior Editor
Director of Pharmacotherapy Services
Department of Pharmacy
Cleveland Clinic Foundation
Cleveland, Ohio

Leonard L. Lance, RPh, BSPharm
Senior Editor
Pharmacist
Lexi-Comp, Inc.
Hudson, Ohio

LEXI-COMP INC

APhA

NOTICE

This data is intended to serve the user as a handy reference and not as a complete drug information resource. It does not include information on every therapeutic agent available. The publication covers over 1400 commonly used drugs and is specifically designed to present important aspects of drug data in a more concise format than is typically found in medical literature or product material supplied by manufacturers.

The nature of drug information is that it is constantly evolving because of ongoing research and clinical experience and is often subject to interpretation. While great care has been taken to ensure the accuracy of the information and recommendations presented, the reader is advised that the authors, editors, reviewers, contributors, and publishers cannot be responsible for the continued currency of the information or for any errors, omissions, or the application of this information, or for any consequences arising therefrom. Therefore, the author(s) and/or the publisher shall have no liability to any person or entity with regard to claims, loss, or damage caused, or alleged to be caused, directly or indirectly, by the use of information contained herein. Because of the dynamic nature of drug information, readers are advised that decisions regarding drug therapy must be based on the independent judgment of the clinician, changing information about a drug (eg, as reflected in the literature and manufacturer's most current product information), and changing medical practices. Therefore, this data is designed to be used in conjunction with other necessary information and is not designed to be solely relied upon by any user. The user of this data hereby and forever releases the authors and publishers of this data from any and all liability of any kind that might arise out of the use of this data. The editors are not responsible for any inaccuracy of quotation or for any false or misleading implication that may arise due to the text or formulas as used or due to the quotation of revisions no longer official.

Certain of the authors, editors, and contributors have written this book in their private capacities. No official support or endorsement by any federal or state agency or pharmaceutical company is intended or inferred.

The publishers have made every effort to trace any third party copyright holders, if any, for borrowed material. If they have inadvertently overlooked any, they will be pleased to make the necessary arrangements at the first opportunity.

If you have any suggestions or questions regarding any information presented in this data, please contact our drug information pharmacists at (330) 650-6506.

This manual was produced using Lexi-Comp's Information Management System™ (LIMS) — a complete publishing service of Lexi-Comp Inc.

ISBN 978-1-59195-254-1 (North American Edition)

TABLE OF CONTENTS

ABOUT THE AUTHORS

Charles F. Lacy, RPh, MS, PharmD, FCSHP

Dr Lacy is the co-founder and the current Vice President of Executive Affairs at the University of Southern Nevada. In this capacity, Dr Lacy fosters, develops, and maintains new opportunities for the university in the areas of business partnerships, foundational development, external programs development and outreach project design and coordination. Dr Lacy is Professor of Pharmacy Practice in the Nevada College of Pharmacy and Guest Professor in the MBA program and the College of Nursing.

Prior to his promotion to Executive Affairs, Dr Lacy was Vice President for Information Technologies at the University and the Facilitative Officer for Clinical Programs where he managed the clinical curriculum, clinical faculty activities, student experiential programs, pharmacy residency programs, and the college continuing education programs.

Additionally, he spent 20 years at Cedars-Sinai Medical Center, where he was the Department of Pharmacy's Clinical Coordinator. With over 20 years of clinical experience at one of the nation's largest teaching hospitals, he developed a reputation as an acknowledged expert in drug information, pharmacotherapy, and critical care drug interventions.

Dr Lacy received his doctorate from the University of Southern California School of Pharmacy. Presently, Dr Lacy holds teaching affiliations with the Nevada College of Pharmacy, the University of Southern Nevada, Showa University in Tokyo Japan, the University of Alberta at Edmonton School of Pharmacy and Health Sciences, and the Hokkaido College of Pharmacy in Sapporo Japan. He also received his master's degree from Phillips Graduate Institute in Psychology with an emphasis in Marriage and Family Therapy.

Dr Lacy is an active member of numerous professional associations including the American Society of Health-System Pharmacists (ASHP), the American College of Clinical Pharmacy (ACCP), the American Association of Colleges of Pharmacy (AACP), the American Society of Consultant Pharmacists (ASCP), the American Association of Colleges of Pharmacy (AACP), American Pharmaceutical Association (APhA), the Federation of International Pharmacy (FIP), the Japanese Pharmaceutical Association (JPA), the Nevada Pharmacy Alliance (NPA), and the California Society of Hospital Pharmacists (CSHP), through which he has chaired many committees and subcommittees. He is also an active member of the California Association of Marriage and Family Therapists (CAMFT), American Association of Marriage and Family Therapists (AAMFT), the North American Congress of Clinical Toxicology (NACCT) and the European Congress of Clinical Toxicology (ECCT).

Lora Armstrong, RPh, PharmD, BCPS

Dr Armstrong received her bachelor's degree in pharmacy from Ferris State University and her Doctor of Pharmacy degree from Midwestern University. Dr Armstrong is a Board-Certified Pharmacotherapy Specialist (BCPS).

In her current position, Dr Armstrong serves as Vice President of Clinical Affairs with responsibility for the National Pharmacy & Therapeutics Committee process, Clinical Program Oversight process, and Pharmaceutical Pipeline Services at CVS Caremark. Prior to joining Caremark, Inc, Dr Armstrong served as the Director of Drug Information Services at the University of Chicago Hospitals. She obtained experience in a variety of clinical settings including critical care, hematology, oncology, infectious diseases, and clinical pharmacokinetics. Dr Armstrong played an active role in the education and training of medical, pharmacy, and nursing staff. She coordinated the Drug Information Center, the medical center's Adverse Drug Reaction Monitoring Program, and the continuing Education Program for pharmacists. She also maintained the hospital's strict formulary program and was the editor of the University of Chicago Hospitals' *Formulary of Accepted Drugs* and the drug information center's monthly newsletter *Topics in Drug Therapy.*

Dr Armstrong is an active member of the Academy of Managed Care Pharmacy (AMCP), the American Society of Health-Systems Pharmacists (ASHP), the American Pharmaceutical Association (APhA), the American College of Clinical Pharmacy (ACCP), and the Pharmacy & Therapeutics Society (P & T Society). Dr Armstrong wrote the chapter entitled "Drugs and Hormones Used in Endocrinology" in the 4th edition of the textbook *Endocrinology.* She is an Adjunct Clinical Instructor of Pharmacy Practice at Midwestern University. Dr Armstrong currently serves on the Drug Information Advisory Board for the American Pharmaceutical Association Scientific Review Panel for Evaluations of Drug Interactions (EDI).

Morton P. Goldman, RPh, PharmD, BCPS, FCCP

Dr Goldman received his bachelor's degree in pharmacy from the University of Pittsburgh, College of Pharmacy and his Doctor of Pharmacy degree from the University of Cincinnati, Division of Graduate Studies and Research. He completed his concurrent 2-year hospital pharmacy residency at the VA Medical Center in Cincinnati. Dr Goldman is presently the Director of Pharmacotherapy Services for the Department of Pharmacy at the Cleveland Clinic Foundation (CCF) after having spent over 4 years at CCF as an Infectious Disease pharmacist and 10 years as Clinical Manager/Assistant Director. He holds faculty appointments from The University of Toledo and Ohio Northern University, Colleges of Pharmacy and Case Western Reserve University, College of Medicine and is the Pharmacology Curriculum Director for the Cleveland Clinic Lerner College of Medicine. Dr Goldman is a Board-Certified Pharmacotherapy Specialist (BCPS) with added qualifications in infectious diseases.

In his capacity as Director of Pharmacotherapy Services at CCF, Dr Goldman remains actively involved in patient care and clinical research with the Department of Infectious Disease, as well as the continuing education of the medical and pharmacy staff. He is an editor of CCF's *Guidelines for Antibiotic Use* and participates in their annual Antimicrobial Review retreat. He is a member of the Pharmacy and Therapeutics Committee and many of its subcommittees. Dr Goldman has authored numerous journal articles and lectures locally and nationally on infectious diseases topics and current drug therapies. He is currently coauthor of the *Infectious Diseases Handbook* produced by Lexi-Comp, Inc and provides technical support to Lexi-Comp's Clinical Reference Library™ publications.

Dr Goldman is an active member of the Ohio College of Clinical Pharmacy, the Society of Infectious Disease Pharmacists, the American College of Clinical Pharmacy (and is a Fellow of the College), and the American Society of Health-Systems Pharmacists.

Leonard L. Lance, RPh, BSPharm

Leonard L. (Bud) Lance has been directly involved in the pharmaceutical industry since receiving his bachelor's degree in pharmacy from Ohio Northern University in 1970. Upon graduation from ONU, Mr Lance spent four years as a navy pharmacist in various military assignments and was instrumental in the development and operation of the first whole hospital I.V. admixture program in a military (Portsmouth Naval Hospital) facility.

After completing his military service, he entered the retail pharmacy field and has managed both an independent and a home I.V. franchise pharmacy operation. Since the late 1970s, Mr Lance has focused much of his interest on using computers to improve pharmacy service. The independent pharmacy he worked for was one of the first retail pharmacies in the State of Ohio to computerize (1977).

His love for computers and pharmacy lead him to Lexi-Comp, Inc. in 1988. He was the first pharmacist at Lexi-Comp and helped develop Lexi-Comp's first drug database in 1989 and was involved in the editing and publishing of Lexi-Comp's first *Drug Information Handbook* in 1990.

As a result of his strong publishing interest, he presently serves in the capacity of pharmacy editor and technical advisor as well as pharmacy (information) database coordinator for Lexi-Comp. Along with authoring the *Drug Information Handbook for the Allied Health Professional* and *Lippincott Williams & Wilkins Quick Look Drug Book*, he provides technical support to Lexi-Comp's reference publications. Mr Lance also assists over 300 major hospitals in producing their own formulary (pharmacy) publications through Lexi-Comp's custom publishing service. Mr Lance is also Manager of the Dosage Forms database in the Medical Sciences Division at Lexi-Comp.

Mr Lance is past president (1984) of the Summit Pharmaceutical Association (SPA). He is a member of the Ohio Pharmacists Association (OPA), the American Pharmaceutical Association (APhA), and the American Society of Health-System Pharmacists (ASHP).

EDITORIAL ADVISORY PANEL

Harold L. Crossley, DDS, PhD
Associate Professor of Pharmacology
Baltimore College of Dental Surgery
Dental School
University of Maryland Baltimore
Baltimore, Maryland

Melanie Cucchi, PharmD
Pharmacotherapy Specialist
Lexi-Comp, Inc
Hudson, Ohio

Laura Cummings, PharmD, BCPS
Clinical Pharmacy Specialist, Pediatrics
The Children's Hospital at MetroHealth
Cleveland, Ohio

Julie A. Dopheide, PharmD, BCPP
Associate Professor of Clinical Pharmacy, Psychiatry and the Behavioral Sciences
University of Southern California
Schools of Pharmacy and Medicine
Los Angeles, California

Michael S. Edwards, PharmD, MBA, BCOP
Chief, Oncology Pharmacy
Director, Oncology Pharmacy Residency Program
Walter Reed Army Medical Center
Washington, D.C.

Vicki L. Ellingrod, PharmD, BCPP
Associate Professor
University of Iowa
Iowa City, Iowa

Kelley K. Engle, BSPharm
Pharmacotherapy Specialist
Lexi-Comp, Inc
Hudson, Ohio

Erin Fabian, PharmD, RPh
Pharmacotherapy Specialist
Lexi-Comp, Inc
Hudson, Ohio

Margaret A. Fitzgerald, MS, APRN, BC, NP-C, FAANP
President
Fitzgerald Health Education Associates, Inc.
North Andover, Massachusetts
Family Nurse Practitioner
Greater Lawrence Family Health Center
Lawrence, Massachusetts

Lawrence A. Frazee, PharmD
Pharmacotherapy Specialist in Internal Medicine
Akron General Medical Center
Akron, Ohio

Matthew A. Fuller, PharmD, BCPS, BCPP, FASHP
Clinical Pharmacy Specialist, Psychiatry
Cleveland Department of Veterans Affairs Medical Center
Brecksville, Ohio
Associate Clinical Professor of Psychiatry
Clinical Instructor of Psychology
Case Western Reserve University
Cleveland, Ohio
Adjunct Associate Professor of Clinical Pharmacy
University of Toledo
Toledo, Ohio

Morton P. Goldman, RPh, PharmD, BCPS, FCCP
Director of Pharmacotherapy Services
The Cleveland Clinic Foundation
Cleveland, Ohio

Sandra Knowles, RPh, BScPhm
Drug Safety Pharmacist
Sunnybrook and Women's College HSC
Toronto, Ontario

Jill M. Kolesar, PharmD, FCCP, BCPS
Associate Professor
School of Pharmacy
Associate Professor
University of Wisconsin Paul P. Carbone Comprehensive Cancer Center
University of Wisconsin
Madison, Wisconsin

Donna M. Kraus, PharmD, FAPhA
Associate Professor of Pharmacy Practice
Departments of Pharmacy Practice and Pediatrics
Pediatric Clinical Pharmacist
University of Illinois
Chicago, Illinois

Daniel L. Krinsky RPh, MS
Manager, MTM Services
Giant Eagle Pharmacy
Ravenna, Ohio
Assistant Professor
Department of Pharmacy Practice
College of Pharmacy NEOUCOM
Rootstown, Ohio

Kay Kyllonen, PharmD
Clinical Specialist
The Cleveland Clinic Children's Hospital
Cleveland, Ohio

Charles Lacy, MS, PharmD, FCSHP
Vice President for Executive Affairs
Professor, Pharmacy Practice
Professor, Business Leadership
University of Southern Nevada
Las Vegas, Nevada

Brenda R. Lance, RN, MSN
Program Development Director
Northcoast HealthCare Management Company
Northcoast Infusion Network
Beachwood, Ohio

Leonard L. Lance, RPh, BSPharm
Clinical Pharmacist
Lexi-Comp, Inc
Hudson, Ohio

Jeffrey D. Lewis, PharmD
Pharmacotherapy Specialist
Giant Eagle
Canal Fulton, Ohio

Laurie S. Mauro, BS, PharmD
Professor of Clinical Pharmacy
College of Pharmacy
Adjunct Associate Professor of Medicine
College of Medicine
The University of Toledo
Toledo, Ohio

Vincent F. Mauro, BS, PharmD, FCCP
Professor of Clinical Pharmacy
College of Pharmacy
Adjunct Professor of Medicine
College of Medicine
The University of Toledo
Toledo, Ohio

Barrie McCombs, MD, FCFP
Medical Information Service Coordinator
The Alberta Rural Physician Action Plan
Calgary, Alberta, Canada

Joe Snoke, RPh, BCPS
Manager
Core Pharmacology Group
Lexi-Comp, Inc
Hudson, Ohio

Dominic A. Solimando, Jr, MA, FAPhA, FASHP, BCOP
Oncology Pharmacist
President, Oncology Pharmacy Services, Inc
Arlington, Virginia

Joni Lombardi Stahura, BS, PharmD, RPh
Pharmacotherapy Specialist
Lexi-Comp, Inc
Hudson, Ohio

Dan Streetman, PharmD, RPh
Pharmacotherapy Specialist
Lexi-Comp, Inc
Hudson, Ohio

Darcie-Ann Streetman, PharmD, RPh
Pharmacotherapy Specialist
Lexi-Comp, Inc
Hudson, Ohio

Carol K. Taketomo, PharmD
Director of Pharmacy and Nutrition Services
Children's Hospital Los Angeles
Los Angeles, California

Mary Temple, PharmD
Pediatric Clinical Research Specialist
Hillcrest Hospital
Mayfield Heights, Ohio

Elizabeth A. Tomsik, PharmD, BCPS
Manager
Adverse Drug Reactions Group
Lexi-Comp, Inc
Hudson, Ohio

Dana Travis, RPh
Pharmacotherapy Specialist
Lexi-Comp, Inc
Hudson, Ohio

Jennifer Trofe, PharmD
Clinical Transplant Pharmacist
Hospital of The University of Pennsylvania
Philadelphia, Pennsylvania

Beatrice B. Turkoski, RN, PhD
Associate Professor, Graduate Faculty,
Pharmacology for Advanced Practice Nurses
College of Nursing
Kent State University
Kent, Ohio

Amy Van Orman, PharmD
Pharmacotherapy Specialist
Lexi-Comp, Inc
Hudson, Ohio

Christine Weinstein, BS, RPh
Pharmacotherapy Specialist
Lexi-Comp, Inc
Hudson, Ohio

David M. Weinstein, PhD, RPh
Manager
Metabolism, Interactions, and Genomics Group
Lexi-Comp, Inc
Hudson, Ohio

DESCRIPTION OF SECTIONS AND FIELDS USED IN THIS HANDBOOK

The *Drug Information Handbook, 18th Edition* is divided into four sections.

The first section is a compilation of introductory text pertinent to the use of this book.

The drug information section of the handbook, in which all drugs are listed alphabetically, details information pertinent to each drug. Extensive cross-referencing is provided by U.S. brand names, Canadian brand names, and index terms. Many combination monographs have been added to this edition; however, they have been condensed with only brand names and forms available. For more information on these products, see the individual components.

The third section is an invaluable appendix which offers a compilation of tables, guidelines, nomograms, algorithms, and conversion information which can be helpful when considering patient care.

The last section of this handbook contains a Pharmacologic Category Index which lists all drugs in this handbook in their unique pharmacologic class.

The **Alphabetical Listing of Drugs** is presented in a consistent format and provides the following fields of information:

Generic Name	U.S. adopted name
Pronunciation	Phonetic pronunciation guide
U.S. Brand Names	Trade names (manufacturer-specific) found in the United States. The symbol [DSC] appears after trade names that have been recently discontinued.
Canadian Brand Names	Trade names found in Canada
Index Terms	Includes names or accepted abbreviations of the generic drug; may include common brand names no longer available; this field is used to create cross-references to monographs
Pharmacologic Category	Unique systematic classification of medications
Additional Appendix Information	Cross-reference to other pertinent drug information found in the appendix section of this handbook
Use	Information pertaining to appropriate FDA-approved indications of the drug.
Unlabeled/Investigational Use	Information pertaining to non-FDA approved and investigational indications of the drug.
Restrictions	The controlled substance classification from the Drug Enforcement Agency (DEA). U.S. schedules are I-V. Schedules vary by country and sometimes state (ie, Massachusetts uses I-VI)
Pregnancy Risk Factor	Five categories established by the FDA to indicate the potential of a systemically absorbed drug for causing birth defects.
Pregnancy Considerations	Information pertinent to or associated with the use of the drug as it relates to clinical effects on the fetus and clinical effects on the infant
Lactation	Information describing characteristics of using the drug listed in the monograph while breast-feeding (where recommendation of American Academy of Pediatrics differs, notation is made).
Medication Safety Issues	In an effort to promote the safe use of medications, this field is intended to highlight possible sources of medication errors such as look-alike/sound-alike drugs or highly concentrated formulations which require vigilance on the part of healthcare professionals. In addition, medications which have been associated with severe consequences in the event of a medication error are also identified in this field.
Contraindications	Information pertaining to inappropriate use of the drug
Warnings/Precautions	Precautionary considerations, hazardous conditions related to use of the drug, and disease states or patient populations in which the drug should be cautiously used. Boxed warnings, when present, are clearly identified and are adapted from the FDA approved labeling. Consult the product labeling for the exact black box warning through the manufacturer's or the FDA website.
Adverse Reactions	Side effects are grouped by percentage of incidence (if known) and/or body system; in the interest of saving space, <1% effects are grouped only by percentage
Drug Interactions	
Metabolism/Transport Effects	If a drug has demonstrated involvement with cytochrome P450 enzymes, or other metabolism or transport proteins, this field will identify the drug as an inhibitor, inducer, or substrate of the specific enzyme(s) (eg, CYP1A2 or UGT1A1). CYP450 isoenzymes are identified as substrates (minor or major), inhibitors (weak, moderate, or strong), and inducers (weak or strong).
Avoid Concomitant Use	Designates drug combinations which should not be used concomitantly, due to an unacceptable risk: benefit assessment. Frequently, the concurrent use of the agents is explicitly prohibited or contraindicated by the product labeling.
Increased Effect/Toxicity	Drug combinations that result in a increased or toxic therapeutic effect between the drug listed in the monograph and other drugs or drug classes.
Decreased Effect	Drug combinations that result in a decreased therapeutic effect between the drug listed in the monograph and other drugs or drug classes.
Ethanol/Nutrition/Herb Interactions	Information regarding potential interactions with food, nutritionals, herbal products, vitamins, or ethanol.

Stability	Information regarding storage of product or steps for reconstitution. Provides the time and conditions for which a solution or mixture will maintain full potency. For example, some solutions may require refrigeration after reconstitution while stored at room temperature prior to preparation. Also includes compatibility information. **Note:** Professional judgment of the individual pharmacist in application of this information is imperative. While drug products may exhibit stability over longer durations of time, it may not be appropriate to utilize the drug product due to concerns in sterility.
Mechanism of Action	How the drug works in the body to elicit a response
Pharmacodynamics/ Kinetics	The magnitude of a drug's effect depends on the drug concentration at the site of action. The pharmacodynamics are expressed in terms of onset of action and duration of action. Pharmacokinetics are expressed in terms of absorption, distribution (including appearance in breast milk and crossing of the placenta), protein binding, metabolism, bioavailability, half-life, time to peak serum concentration, and elimination.
Dosage	The amount of the drug to be typically given or taken during therapy for children and adults; also includes any dosing adjustment/comments for renal impairment or hepatic impairment and other suggested dosing adjustments (eg, hematological toxicity)
Dietary Considerations	Includes information on how the medication should be taken relative to meals or food.
Administration	Information regarding the recommended final concentrations, rates of administration for parenteral drugs, or other guidelines when giving the medication
Monitoring Parameters	Laboratory tests and patient physical parameters that should be monitored for safety and efficacy of drug therapy
Reference Range	Therapeutic and toxic serum concentrations listed including peak and trough levels
Test Interactions	Listing of assay interferences when relevant; (B) = Blood; (S) = Serum; (U) = Urine
Additional Information	Information about sodium content and/or pertinent information about specific brands
Product Availability	Provides availability information on products that have been approved by the FDA, but not yet available for use. Estimates for when a product may be available are included, when this information is known. May also provide any unique or critical drug availability issues (eg, drug shortage of a critical drug).
Dosage Forms	Information with regard to form, strength, and availability of the drug. *Note:* Additional formulation information (eg, excipients, preservatives) is included when available. Please consult labeling for further information.
Extemporaneous Preparations	Directions for preparing liquid formulations from solid drug products. May include stability information and references.

FDA PREGNANCY CATEGORIES

Throughout this book there is a field labeled Pregnancy Risk Factor and the letter A, B, C, D, or X immediately following which signifies a category. The FDA has established these five categories to indicate the potential of a systemically absorbed drug for causing birth defects. The key differentiation among the categories rests upon the reliability of documentation and the risk:benefit ratio. Pregnancy Category X is particularly notable in that if any data exists that may implicate a drug as a teratogen and the risk: benefit ratio is clearly negative, the drug is contraindicated during pregnancy.

These categories are summarized as follows:

A	Controlled studies in pregnant women fail to demonstrate a risk to the fetus in the first trimester with no evidence of risk in later trimesters. The possibility of fetal harm appears remote.
B	Either animal-reproduction studies have not demonstrated a fetal risk but there are no controlled studies in pregnant women, or animal-reproduction studies have shown an adverse effect (other than a decrease in fertility) that was not confirmed in controlled studies in women in the first trimester and there is no evidence of a risk in later trimesters.
C	Either studies in animals have revealed adverse effects on the fetus (teratogenic or embryocidal effects or other) and there are no controlled studies in women, or studies in women and animals are not available. Drugs should be given only if the potential benefits justify the potential risk to the fetus.
D	There is positive evidence of human fetal risk, but the benefits from use in pregnant women may be acceptable despite the risk (eg, if the drug is needed in a life-threatening situation or for a serious disease for which safer drugs cannot be used or are ineffective).
X	Studies in animals or human beings have demonstrated fetal abnormalities or there is evidence of fetal risk based on human experience, or both, and the risk of the use of the drug in pregnant women clearly outweighs any possible benefit. The drug is contraindicated in women who are or may become pregnant.

SAFE WRITING

Health professionals and their support personnel frequently produce handwritten copies of information they see in print; therefore, such information is subjected to even greater possibilities for error or misinterpretation on the part of others. Thus, particular care must be given to how drug names and strengths are expressed when creating written healthcare documents.

The following are a few examples of safe writing rules suggested by the Institute for Safe Medication Practices, Inc.[1]

1. There should be a space between a number and its units as it is easier to read. There should be no periods after the abbreviations mg or mL.

Correct	**Incorrect**
10 mg	10mg
100 mg	100mg

2. Never place a decimal and a zero after a whole number (2 mg is correct and 2.0 mg is **incorrect**). If the decimal point is not seen because it falls on a line or because individuals are working from copies where the decimal point is not seen, this causes a tenfold overdose.
3. Just the opposite is true for numbers less than one. Always place a zero before a naked decimal (0.5 mL is correct, .5 mL is **incorrect**).
4. Never abbreviate the word unit. The handwritten U or u, looks like a 0 (zero), and may cause a tenfold overdose error to be made.
5. IU is not a safe abbreviation for international units. The handwritten IU looks like IV. Write out international units or use int. units.
6. Q.D. is not a safe abbreviation for once daily, as when the Q is followed by a sloppy dot, it looks like QID which means four times daily.
7. O.D. is not a safe abbreviation for once daily, as it is properly interpreted as meaning "right eye" and has caused liquid medications such as saturated solution of potassium iodide and Lugol's solution to be administered incorrectly. There is no safe abbreviation for once daily. It must be written out in full.
8. Do not use chemical names such as 6-mercaptopurine or 6-thioguanine, as sixfold overdoses have been given when these were not recognized as chemical names. The proper names of these drugs are mercaptopurine or thioguanine.
9. Do not abbreviate drug names (5FC, 6MP, 5-ASA, MTX, HCTZ, CPZ, PBZ, etc) as they are misinterpreted and cause error.
10. Do not use the apothecary system or symbols.
11. Do not abbreviate microgram as µg; instead use mcg as there is less likelihood of misinterpretation.
12. When writing an outpatient prescription, write a complete prescription. A complete prescription can prevent the prescriber, the pharmacist, and/or the patient from making a mistake and can eliminate the need for further clarification. The legible prescriptions should contain:
    a. patient's full name
    b. for pediatric or geriatric patients: their age (or weight where applicable)
    c. drug name, dosage form and strength; if a drug is new or rarely prescribed, print this information
    d. number or amount to be dispensed
    e. complete instructions for the patient, including the purpose of the medication
    f. when there are recognized contraindications for a prescribed drug, indicate to the pharmacist that you are aware of this fact (ie, when prescribing a potassium salt for a patient receiving an ACE inhibitor, write "K serum level being monitored")

[1]From "Safe Writing" by Davis NM, PharmD and Cohen MR, MS, Lecturers and Consultants for Safe Medication Practices, 1143 Wright Drive, Huntington Valley, PA 19006. Phone: (215) 947-7566.

FDA NAME DIFFERENTIATION PROJECT - THE USE OF TALL-MAN LETTERS

Confusion between similar drug names is an important cause of medication errors. For years, The Institute For Safe Medication Practices (ISMP), has urged generic manufacturers to use a combination of large and small letters as well as bolding (ie, chlorpro**MAZINE** and chlorpro**PAMIDE**) to help distinguish drugs with look-alike names, especially when they share similar strengths. Recently the FDA's Division of Generic Drugs began to issue recommendation letters to manufacturers suggesting this novel way to label their products to help reduce this drug name confusion. Although this project has had marginal success, the method has successfully eliminated problems with products such as diphenhydr**AMINE** and dimenhy**DRINATE**. Hospitals should also follow suit by making similar changes in their own labels, preprinted order forms, computer screens and printouts, and drug storage location labels.

Lexi-Comp Medical Publishing will use "Tall-Man" letters for the drugs suggested by the FDA or recommended by ISMP.

The following is a list of generic product names and recommended revisions.

Drug Product	Recommended Revision
acetazolamide	aceta**ZOLAMIDE**
acetohexamide	aceto**HEXAMIDE**
alprazolam	**ALPRAZ**olam
amiloride	a**MIL**oride
amlodipine	am**LODIP**ine
azacitidine	aza**CITID**ine
azathioprine	aza**THIO**prine
bupropion	bu**PROP**ion
buspirone	bus**PIR**one
carbamazepine	car**BAM**azepine
carboplatin	**CARBO**platin
cefazolin	ce**FAZ**olin
ceftriaxone	cef**TRIAX**one
chlordiazepoxide	chlordiaze**POXIDE**
chlorpromazine	chlorpro**MAZINE**
chlorpropamide	chlorpro**PAMIDE**
cisplatin	**CIS**platin
clomiphene	clomi**PHENE**
clomipramine	clomi**PRAMINE**
clonazepam	clonaze**PAM**
clonidine	clo**NID**ine
cycloserine	cyclo**SERINE**
cyclosporine	cyclo**SPORINE**
dactinomycin	**DACTIN**omycin
daptomycin	**DAPTO**mycin
daunorubicin	**DAUNO**rubicin
dimenhydrinate	dimenhy**DRINATE**
diphenhydramine	diphenhydr**AMINE**
dobutamine	**DOBUT**amine
dopamine	**DOP**amine
doxorubicin	**DOXO**rubicin
duloxetine	**DUL**oxetine
ephedrine	e**PHED**rine
epinephrine	**EPINEPH**rine
fentanyl	fenta**NYL**
fluoxetine	**FLU**oxetine
glipizide	glipi**ZIDE**

Drug Product	Recommended Revision
glyburide	gly**BURIDE**
guaifenesin	guai**FEN**esin
guanfacine	guan**FACINE**
hydralazine	hydr**ALAZINE**
hydrocodone	**HYDRO**codone
hydromorphone	**HYDRO**morphone
hydroxyzine	hydr**OXY**zine
idarubicin	**IDA**rubicin
infliximab	in**FLIX**imab
lamivudine	lami**VUD**ine
lamotrigine	lamo**TRI**gine
lorazepam	**LOR**azepam
medroxyprogesterone	medroxy**PROGESTER**one
metformin	met**FORMIN**
methylprednisolone	methyl**PREDNIS**olone
methyltestosterone	methyl**TESTOSTER**one
metronidazole	metro**NIDAZOLE**
nicardipine	ni**CAR**dipine
nifedipine	**NIFE**dipine
nimodipine	ni**MOD**ipine
olanzapine	**OLANZ**apine
oxcarbazepine	**OX**carbazepine
oxycodone	oxy**CODONE**
paroxetine	**PAR**oxetine
pentobarbital	**PENT**obarbital
phenobarbital	**PHEN**obarbital
prednisolone	predniso**LONE**
prednisone	predni**SONE**
quetiapine	**QUE**tiapine
quinidine	qui**NID**ine
quinine	qui**NINE**
rituximab	ri**TUX**imab
sitagliptin	sita**GLIP**tin
sufentanil	**SUF**entanil
sulfadiazine	sulf**ADIAZINE**
sulfisoxazole	sulfi**SOXAZOLE**
sumatriptan	**SUMA**triptan
tiagabine	tia**GAB**ine
tizanidine	ti**ZAN**idine
tolazamide	**TOLAZ**amide
tolbutamide	**TOLBUT**amide
tramadol	tra**MAD**ol
trazodone	tra**ZOD**one
vinblastine	vin**BLAS**tine
vincristine	vin**CRIS**tine

Institute for Safe Medication Practices. "New Tall-Man Lettering Will Reduce Mix-Ups Due to Generic Drug Name Confusion," *ISMP Medication Safety Alert*, September 19, 2001. Available at: http://www.ismp.org.

Institute for Safe Medication Practices. "Prescription Mapping, Can Improve Efficiency While Minimizing Errors With Look-Alike Products," *ISMP Medication Safety Alert*, October 6, 1999. Available at: http://www.ismp.org.

Institute for Safe Medication Practices. "Use of Tall Man Letters Is Gaining Wide Acceptance," *ISMP Medication Safety Alert*, July 31, 2008. Available at: http://www.ismp.org.

U.S. Pharmacopeia, "USP Quality Review: Use Caution-Avoid Confusion," March 2001, No. 76. Available at: http://www.usp.org.

ALPHABETICAL LISTING OF DRUGS

◆ **A200® Lice [OTC]** *see* Permethrin *on page 1176*

◆ **A-200® Lice Treatment Kit [OTC]** *see* Pyrethrins and Piperonyl Butoxide *on page 1271*

◆ **A-200® Maximum Strength [OTC]** *see* Pyrethrins and Piperonyl Butoxide *on page 1271*

◆ **A and D® Original [OTC]** *see* Vitamin A and Vitamin D *on page 1565*

Abacavir (a BAK a veer)

U.S. Brand Names Ziagen®

Canadian Brand Names Ziagen®

Index Terms Abacavir Sulfate; ABC

Pharmacologic Category Antiretroviral Agent, Reverse Transcriptase Inhibitor (Nucleoside)

Additional Appendix Information

Antiretroviral Therapy for HIV Infection: Adults and Adolescents *on page 1758*

Management of Healthcare Worker Exposures to HBV, HCV, and HIV *on page 1719*

Perinatal HIV Guidelines *on page 1730*

Use Treatment of HIV infections in combination with other antiretroviral agents

Restrictions An FDA-approved medication guide and warning card (summarizing symptoms of hypersensitivity) must be distributed when dispensing an outpatient prescription (new or refill) where this medication is to be used without direct supervision of a healthcare provider. Medication guides are available at http://www.fda.gov/cder/Offices/ODS/medication_guides.htm.

Pregnancy Risk Factor C

Pregnancy Considerations It is not known if abacavir crosses the human placenta. No increased risk of overall birth defects has been observed following 1st trimester exposure according to data collected by the antiretroviral pregnancy registry. Cases of lactic acidosis/hepatic steatosis syndrome have been reported in pregnant women receiving nucleoside analogues. It is not known if pregnancy itself potentiates this known side effect; however, pregnant women may be at increased risk of lactic acidosis and liver damage. Hepatic enzymes and electrolytes should be monitored frequently during the 3rd trimester of pregnancy in women receiving nucleoside analogues. Dose adjustment is not needed for pregnancy. The Perinatal HIV Guidelines Working Group considers abacavir to be an alternative NRTI in dual nucleoside combination regimens. Health professionals are encouraged to contact the antiretroviral pregnancy registry to monitor outcomes of pregnant women exposed to antiretroviral medications (1-800-258-4263 or www.APRegistry.com).

Lactation Excretion in breast milk unknown/contraindicated

Contraindications Hypersensitivity to abacavir or any component of the formulation (do not rechallenge patients who have experienced hypersensitivity to abacavir); moderate-to-severe hepatic impairment

Warnings/Precautions Abacavir should always be used as a component of a multidrug regimen. **[U.S. Boxed Warning]: Serious and sometimes fatal hypersensitivity reactions have occurred.** Patients testing positive for the presence of the *HLA-B*5701* allele are at an increased risk for hypersensitivity reactions. Screening for *HLA-B*5701* allele status is recommended prior to initiating therapy or reinitiating therapy in patients of unknown status, including patients who previously tolerated therapy. Therapy is **not** recommended in patients testing positive for the *HLA-B*5701* allele. Patients exhibiting symptoms from two or more of the following: Fever, skin rash, constitutional symptoms (malaise, fatigue, aches), respiratory symptoms (eg, pharyngitis, dyspnea, cough), and GI symptoms (eg, abdominal pain, diarrhea, nausea, vomiting) should discontinue therapy immediately and call for medical attention. Abacavir should be permanently discontinued if hypersensitivity cannot be ruled out, even when other diagnoses are possible and regardless of *HLA-B*5701* status. Abacavir SHOULD NOT be restarted because more severe symptoms may occur within hours, including LIFE-THREATENING HYPOTENSION AND DEATH. Fatal hypersensitivity reactions have occurred following the reintroduction of abacavir in patients whose therapy was interrupted (ie, interruption in drug supply, temporary discontinuation while treating other conditions). Reactions occurred within hours. In some cases, signs of hypersensitivity may have been previously present, but attributed to other medical conditions (eg, acute onset respiratory diseases, gastroenteritis, reactions to other medications). If abacavir is restarted following an interruption in therapy, evaluate the patient for previously unsuspected symptoms of hypersensitivity. Do not restart if hypersensitivity is suspected or if hypersensitivity cannot be ruled out. To report these events on abacavir hypersensitivity, a registry has been established (1-800-270-0425).

[U.S. Boxed Warning]: Lactic acidosis and severe hepatomegaly with steatosis (sometimes fatal) have occurred with antiretroviral nucleoside analogues. Female gender, prior liver disease, obesity, and prolonged treatment may increase the risk of hepatotoxicity. May be associated with fat redistribution. Immune reconstitution syndrome may develop; further evaluation and treatment may be required. Use caution in patients with risks for coronary heart disease; modifiable risk factors (eg, hypertension, hyperlipidemia, diabetes mellitus, and smoking) should be minimized prior to use. Safety and efficacy in children <3 months of age have not been established.

Adverse Reactions Hypersensitivity reactions (which may be fatal) occur in ~5% of patients (see Warnings/Precautions). Symptoms may include anaphylaxis, fever, rash (including erythema multiforme), fatigue, diarrhea, abdominal pain; respiratory symptoms (eg, pharyngitis, dyspnea, cough, adult respiratory distress syndrome, or respiratory failure); headache, malaise, lethargy, myalgia, myolysis, arthralgia, edema, paresthesia, nausea and vomiting, mouth ulcerations, conjunctivitis, lymphadenopathy, hepatic failure, and renal failure.

Note: Rates of adverse reactions were defined during combination therapy with other antiretrovirals (lamivudine and efavirenz **or** lamivudine and zidovudine). Only reactions which occurred at a higher frequency in adults (except where noted) than in the comparator group are noted. Adverse reaction rates attributable to abacavir alone are not available.

>10%:

Central nervous system: Headache (7% to 13%)

Gastrointestinal: Nausea (7% to 19%, children 9%)

1% to 10%:

Central nervous system: Depression (6%), fever/chills (6%, children 9%), anxiety (5%)

Dermatologic: Rash (5% to 6%, children 7%)

Endocrine & metabolic: Triglycerides increased (2% to 6%)

Gastrointestinal: Diarrhea (7%), vomiting (children 9%), amylase increased (2%)

Hematologic: Thrombocytopenia (1%)

Hepatic: AST increased (6%)

Neuromuscular & skeletal: Musculoskeletal pain (5% to 6%)

Miscellaneous: Hypersensitivity reactions (2% to 9%; may include reactions to other components of antiretroviral regimen), infection (EENT 5%)

<1% (Limited to important or life-threatening): Erythema multiforme, fat redistribution, GGT increased, hepatic

steatosis, hepatomegaly, hepatotoxicity, lactic acidosis, MI, pancreatitis, Stevens-Johnson syndrome, toxic epidermal necrolysis

Drug Interactions

Avoid Concomitant Use There are no known interactions where it is recommended to avoid concomitant use.

Increased Effect/Toxicity

The levels/effects of Abacavir may be increased by: Ganciclovir-Valganciclovir; Ribavirin

Decreased Effect

The levels/effects of Abacavir may be decreased by: Protease Inhibitors

Ethanol/Nutrition/Herb Interactions Ethanol: Ethanol may increase the risk of toxicity.

Stability Store oral solution and tablets at controlled room temperature of 20°C to 25°C (68°F to 77°F). Oral solution may be refrigerated; do not freeze.

Mechanism of Action Nucleoside reverse transcriptase inhibitor. Abacavir is a guanosine analogue which is phosphorylated to carbovir triphosphate which interferes with HIV viral RNA-dependent DNA polymerase resulting in inhibition of viral replication.

Pharmacodynamics/Kinetics

Absorption: Rapid and extensive absorption

Distribution: V_d: 0.86 L/kg

Protein binding: 50%

Metabolism: Hepatic via alcohol dehydrogenase and glucuronyl transferase to inactive carboxylate and glucuronide metabolites

Bioavailability: 83%

Half-life elimination: 1.5 hours

Time to peak: 0.7-1.7 hours

Excretion: Primarily urine (as metabolites, 1.2% as unchanged drug); feces (16% total dose)

Dosage Oral:

Children: 3 months to 16 years: 8 mg/kg body weight twice daily (maximum: 300 mg twice daily) in combination with other antiretroviral agents

Adults: 300 mg twice daily or 600 mg once daily in combination with other antiretroviral agents

Dosage adjustment in hepatic impairment:

Mild dysfunction (Child-Pugh score 5-6): 200 mg twice daily (oral solution is recommended)

Moderate-to-severe dysfunction: Use is contraindicated by the manufacturer

Dietary Considerations May be taken with or without food.

Administration May be administered with or without food.

Monitoring Parameters CBC with differential, serum creatine kinase, CD4 count, HIV RNA plasma levels, serum transaminases, triglycerides, serum amylase; *HLA-B*5701* genotype status prior to initiation of therapy and prior to reinitiation of therapy in patients of unknown *HLA-B*5701* status; signs and symptoms of hypersensitivity, particularly in patients untested for the *HLA-B*5701* allele

Additional Information A high rate of early virologic nonresponse was observed when abacavir, lamivudine, and tenofovir were used as the initial regimen in treatment-naive patients. Use of this combination is not recommended; patients currently on this regimen should be closely monitored for modification of therapy.

Hypersensitivity testing (*HLA-B*5701*): Prevalence of hypersensitivity reactions has been estimated at 5% to 8% in Caucasians and 2% to 3% in African-Americans. Pretherapy identification of *HLA-B*5701*-positive patients, and subsequent avoidance of abacavir therapy in these patients has been shown to reduce the occurrence of abacavir-mediated hypersensitivity reactions. A skin patch test is in development for clinical screening purposes; however, only PCR-mediated genotyping methods are currently in clinical practice use for documentation of this susceptibility marker.

Dosage Forms Excipient information presented when available (limited, particularly for generics); consult specific product labeling.

Solution, oral:

Ziagen®: 20 mg/mL (240 mL) [strawberry-banana flavor]

Tablet:

Ziagen®: 300 mg

Abacavir and Lamivudine

(a BAK a veer & la MI vyoo deen)

U.S. Brand Names Epzicom®

Canadian Brand Names Kivexa™

Index Terms Abacavir Sulfate and Lamivudine; Lamivudine and Abacavir

Pharmacologic Category Antiretroviral Agent, Reverse Transcriptase Inhibitor (Nucleoside)

Additional Appendix Information

Antiretroviral Therapy for HIV Infection: Adults and Adolescents *on page 1758*

Management of Healthcare Worker Exposures to HBV, HCV, and HIV *on page 1719*

Use Treatment of HIV infections in combination with other antiretroviral agents

Restrictions An FDA-approved medication guide and warning card (summarizing symptoms of hypersensitivity) must be distributed when dispensing an outpatient prescription (new or refill) where this medication is to be used without direct supervision of a healthcare provider. Medication guides are available at http://www.fda.gov/cder/Offices/ODS/medication_guides.htm.

Pregnancy Risk Factor C

Dosage Oral: Adults: HIV: One tablet (abacavir 600 mg and lamivudine 300 mg) once daily

Dosage adjustment in renal impairment: Cl_{cr} <50 mL/minute: Use not recommended

Dosage adjustment in hepatic impairment: Use contraindicated.

Additional Information Complete prescribing information for this medication should be consulted for additional detail.

Dosage Forms Excipient information presented when available (limited, particularly for generics); consult specific product labeling.

Tablet:

Epzicom®: Abacavir 600 mg and lamivudine 300 mg

Abacavir, Lamivudine, and Zidovudine

(a BAK a veer, la MI vyoo deen, & zye DOE vyoo deen)

U.S. Brand Names Trizivir®

Index Terms 3TC, Abacavir, and Zidovudine; Azidothymidine, Abacavir, and Lamivudine; AZT, Abacavir, and Lamivudine; Compound S, Abacavir, and Lamivudine; Lamivudine, Abacavir, and Zidovudine; ZDV, Abacavir, and Lamivudine; Zidovudine, Abacavir, and Lamivudine

Pharmacologic Category Antiretroviral Agent, Reverse Transcriptase Inhibitor (Nucleoside)

Additional Appendix Information

Antiretroviral Therapy for HIV Infection: Adults and Adolescents *on page 1758*

Management of Healthcare Worker Exposures to HBV, HCV, and HIV *on page 1719*

Use Treatment of HIV infection (either alone or in combination with other antiretroviral agents) in patients whose regimen would otherwise contain the components of Trizivir®

Restrictions An FDA-approved medication guide and warning card (summarizing symptoms of hypersensitivity) must be distributed when dispensing an outpatient prescription (new or refill) where this medication is to be used without direct supervision of a healthcare provider.

Medication guides are available at http://www.fda.gov/cder/Offices/ODS/medication_guides.htm.

Pregnancy Risk Factor C

Dosage Oral:

Adolescents ≥40 kg and Adults: 1 tablet twice daily

Elderly: Use with caution

Dosage adjustment in renal impairment: Because lamivudine and zidovudine require dosage adjustment in renal impairment, Trizivir® should not be used in patients with Cl_{cr} ≤50 mL/minute

Dosage adjustment in hepatic impairment: Use contraindicated.

Additional Information Complete prescribing information for this medication should be consulted for additional detail.

Dosage Forms Excipient information presented when available (limited, particularly for generics); consult specific product labeling.

Tablet:

Trizivir®: Abacavir 300 mg, lamivudine 150 mg, and zidovudine 300 mg

◆ **Abacavir Sulfate** *see* Abacavir *on page 18*

◆ **Abacavir Sulfate and Lamivudine** *see* Abacavir and Lamivudine *on page 19*

Abatacept (ab a TA sept)

U.S. Brand Names Orencia®

Canadian Brand Names Orencia®

Index Terms CTLA-4Ig

Pharmacologic Category Antirheumatic, Disease Modifying

Use

Treatment of moderately- to severely-active adult rheumatoid arthritis (RA); may be used as monotherapy or in combination with other DMARDs

Treatment of moderately- to severely-active juvenile idiopathic arthritis (JIA); may be used as monotherapy or in combination with methotrexate

Note: Abatacept should **not** be used in combination with anakinra or TNF-blocking agents

Pregnancy Risk Factor C

Pregnancy Considerations Teratogenic effects were not observed in animal studies. There are no adequate and well-controlled studies in pregnant women. Due to the potential risk for development of autoimmune disease in the fetus, use during pregnancy only if clearly needed. A pregnancy registry has been established to monitor outcomes of women exposed to abatacept during pregnancy (1-877-311-8972).

Lactation Excretion in breast milk unknown/not recommended

Medication Safety Issues

Sound-alike/look-alike issues:

Orencia® may be confused with Oracea™

Contraindications There are no contraindications listed within the FDA-approved labeling.

Warnings/Precautions Caution should be exercised when considering the use of abatacept in patients with a history of recurrent infections, with conditions that predispose them to infections, or with chronic, latent, or localized infections. Patients who develop a new infection while undergoing treatment should be monitored closely. If a patient develops a serious infection, abatacept should be discontinued. Screen patients for latent tuberculosis infection prior to initiating abatacept; safety in tuberculosis-positive patients has not been established. Treat patients testing positive according to standard therapy prior to initiating abatacept. Adult patients receiving abatacept in combination with TNF-blocking agents had higher rates of infections (including serious infections) than patients on TNF-blocking agents alone. The manufacturer does not recommend concurrent use with anakinra or TNF-blocking agents. Monitor for signs and symptoms of infection when transitioning from TNF-blocking agents to abatacept. Due to the affect of T-cell inhibition on host defenses, abatacept may affect immune responses against infections and malignancies; impact on the development and course of malignancies is not fully defined.

Use caution with chronic obstructive pulmonary disease (COPD), higher incidences of adverse effects (COPD exacerbation, cough, rhonchi, dyspnea) have been observed; monitor closely. Rare cases of hypersensitivity, anaphylaxis, or anaphylactoid reactions have been reported; medications for the treatment of hypersensitivity reactions should be available for immediate use. Patients should be screened for viral hepatitis prior to use; antirheumatic therapy may cause reactivation of hepatitis B. Patients should be brought up to date with all immunizations before initiating therapy. Live vaccines should not be given concurrently or within 3 months of discontinuation of therapy; there is no data available concerning secondary transmission of live vaccines in patients receiving therapy. May contain maltose, which may result in falsely-elevated serum glucose readings on the day of infusion. Higher incidences of infection and malignancy were observed in the elderly; use with caution. Not FDA approved for use in children <6 years of age.

Adverse Reactions Note: Percentages not always reported; COPD patients experienced a higher frequency of COPD-related adverse reactions (COPD exacerbation, cough, dyspnea, pneumonia, rhonchi)

>10%:

Central nervous system: Headache (≤18%)

Gastrointestinal: Nausea

Respiratory: Nasopharyngitis (12%), upper respiratory tract infection

Miscellaneous: Infection (adults 54%; children 36%), antibody formation (2% to 41%)

1% to 10%:

Cardiovascular: Hypertension (7%)

Central nervous system: Dizziness (9%), fever

Dermatologic: Rash (4%)

Gastrointestinal: Dyspepsia (6%), abdominal pain, diarrhea

Genitourinary: Urinary tract infection (6%)

Neuromuscular & skeletal: Back pain (7%), limb pain (3%)

Respiratory: Cough (8%), bronchitis, pneumonia, rhinitis, sinusitis

Miscellaneous: Infusion-related reactions (2% to 9%), herpes simplex, influenza

<1% (Limited to important or life-threatening): Acute lymphocytic leukemia, anaphylaxis, anaphylactoid reactions, cellulitis, COPD exacerbation, disease flare, diverticulitis, dyspnea, flushing, hypersensitivity, hypotension, joint wear, lung cancer, lymphoma; malignancies (including bile duct, bladder, breast, cervical, melanoma, myelodysplastic syndrome, prostate, renal, skin, thyroid and uterine); ovarian cyst, pruritus, pyelonephritis, rhonchi, urticaria, varicella infection, wheezing

Drug Interactions

Avoid Concomitant Use

Avoid concomitant use of Abatacept with any of the following: Natalizumab; Vaccines (Live)

Increased Effect/Toxicity

Abatacept may increase the levels/effects of: Natalizumab; Vaccines (Live)

The levels/effects of Abatacept may be increased by: Anti-TNF Agents; Trastuzumab

Decreased Effect

Abatacept may decrease the levels/effects of: Vaccines (Inactivated)

The levels/effects of Abatacept may be decreased by: Echinacea

Ethanol/Nutrition/Herb Interactions Herb/Nutraceutical: Avoid echinacea (has immunostimulant properties; consider therapy modifications).

Stability Prior to reconstitution, store at 2°C to 8°C (36°F to 46°F); protect from light. Reconstitute each vial with 10 mL SWFI using the provided silicone-free disposable syringe (discard solutions accidentally reconstituted with siliconized syringe as they may develop translucent particles). Inject SWFI down the side of the vial to avoid foaming. The reconstituted solution contains 25 mg/mL abatacept. Further dilute (using a silicone-free syringe) in 100 mL NS to a final concentration of ≤10 mg/mL. Prior to adding abatacept to the 100 mL bag, the manufacturer recommends withdrawing a volume of NS equal to the abatacept volume required, resulting in a final volume of 100 mL. Mix gently; do not shake.

After dilution, may be stored for up to 24 hours at room temperature or refrigerated at 2°C to 8°C (36°F to 46°F). Must be used within 24 hours of reconstitution.

Mechanism of Action Selective costimulation modulator; inhibits T-cell (T-lymphocyte) activation by binding to CD80 and CD86 on antigen presenting cells (APC), thus blocking the required CD28 interaction between APCs and T cells. Activated T lymphocytes are found in the synovium of rheumatoid arthritis patients.

Pharmacodynamics/Kinetics

Distribution: V_{ss}: 0.02-0.13 L/kg

Half-life elimination: 8-25 days

Dosage I.V.:

Children 6-17 years: JIA:

<75 kg: 10 mg/kg, repeat dose at 2 and 4 weeks after initial infusion, and every 4 weeks thereafter

≥75 kg: Refer to adult dosing; maximum dose: 1000 mg

Adults: RA: Dosing is according to body weight: Repeat dose at 2 weeks and 4 weeks after initial dose, and every 4 weeks thereafter:

<60 kg: 500 mg

60-100 kg: 750 mg

>100 kg: 1000 mg

Elderly: Refer to adult dosing; due to potential for higher rates of infections and malignancies, use caution.

Dosage adjustment for toxicity: Withhold therapy for patients with serious infections.

Administration Infuse over 30 minutes. Administer through a 0.2-1.2 micron low protein-binding filter

Monitoring Parameters Signs and symptoms of infection, signs and symptoms of infusion reaction; hepatitis and TB screening prior to therapy initiation

Test Interactions Contains maltose; may result in falsely elevated blood glucose levels with dehydrogenase pyrroloquinolinequinone or glucose-dye-oxidoreductase testing methods on the day of infusion. Glucose monitoring methods which utilize glucose dehydrogenase nicotine adenine dinucleotide (GDH-NAD), glucose oxidase, or glucose hexokinase are recommended.

Dosage Forms Excipient information presented when available (limited, particularly for generics); consult specific product labeling.

Injection, powder for reconstitution [preservative free]:

Orencia®: 250 mg [contains maltose]

◆ **Abbokinase** *see* Urokinase *on page 1533*

◆ **Abbott-43818** *see* Leuprolide *on page 868*

◆ **ABC** *see* Abacavir *on page 18*

◆ **ABCD** *see* Amphotericin B Cholesteryl Sulfate Complex *on page 103*

Abciximab (ab SIK si mab)

U.S. Brand Names ReoPro®

Canadian Brand Names Reopro®

Index Terms 7E3; C7E3

Pharmacologic Category Antiplatelet Agent, Glycoprotein IIb/IIIa Inhibitor

Additional Appendix Information

Glycoprotein Antagonists *on page 1656*

Use Prevention of cardiac ischemic complications in patients undergoing percutaneous coronary intervention (PCI); prevention of cardiac ischemic complications in patients with unstable angina not responding to conventional therapy when PCI is scheduled within 24 hours

Note: Intended for use with aspirin and heparin, at a minimum.

Unlabeled/Investigational Use ST-elevation MI: Combination regimen of abciximab (full dose), tenecteplase (half dose), and heparin (unlabeled dose)

Pregnancy Risk Factor C

Pregnancy Considerations Animal reproduction studies have not been conducted. *In vitro* studies have shown only small amounts of abciximab to cross the placenta. It is not known whether abciximab can cause fetal harm when administered to a pregnant woman or can affect reproduction capacity.

Lactation Excretion in breast milk unknown/use caution

Medication Safety Issues

High alert medication: The Institute for Safe Medication Practices (ISMP) includes this medication among its list of drugs which have a heightened risk of causing significant patient harm when used in error.

Contraindications Hypersensitivity to abciximab, to murine proteins, or any component of the formulation; active internal hemorrhage or recent (within 6 weeks) clinically-significant GI or GU bleeding; history of cerebrovascular accident within 2 years or cerebrovascular accident with significant neurological deficit; clotting abnormalities or administration of oral anticoagulants within 7 days unless prothrombin time (PT) is ≤1.2 times control PT value; thrombocytopenia (<100,000 cells/µL); recent (within 6 weeks) major surgery or trauma; intracranial tumor, arteriovenous malformation, or aneurysm; severe uncontrolled hypertension; history of vasculitis; use of dextran before PTCA or intent to use dextran during PTCA; concomitant use of another parenteral GP IIb/IIIa inhibitor

Warnings/Precautions Administration of abciximab is associated with increased frequency of major bleeding complications, including retroperitoneal bleeding, pulmonary bleeding, spontaneous GI or GU bleeding, and bleeding at the arterial access. Risk may be increased with patients weighing <75 kg, elderly patients (>65 years of age), history of previous GI disease, and recent thrombolytic therapy. Avoid the creation of venous access at noncompressible sites.

The risk of major bleeds may increase with concurrent use of thrombolytics. Anticoagulation, such as with heparin, may contribute to the risk of bleeding. In serious, uncontrolled bleeding, abciximab and heparin should be stopped. Increased risk of hemorrhage during or following angioplasty is associated with unsuccessful PTCA, PTCA procedure >70 minutes duration, or PTCA performed within 12 hours of symptom onset for acute myocardial infarction. Prior to pulling the sheath, heparin should be discontinued for 3-4 hours and ACT ≤175 seconds or aPTT ≤50 seconds. Use standard compression techniques after sheath removal. Watch the site closely afterwards for further bleeding.

Administration of abciximab may result in human anti-chimeric antibody formation that can cause hypersensitivity reactions (including anaphylaxis), thrombocytopenia, or diminished efficacy. Readministration of abciximab within 30 days or in patients with human antichimeric antibodies (HACA) increases the incidence and severity of thrombocytopenia. Safety and efficacy have not been established in children.

Adverse Reactions As with all drugs which may affect hemostasis, bleeding is associated with abciximab. Hemorrhage may occur at virtually any site. Risk is dependent on multiple variables, including the concurrent use of multiple agents which alter hemostasis and patient susceptibility.

>10%:

Cardiovascular: Hypotension (14.4%), chest pain (11.4%)

Gastrointestinal: Nausea (13.6%)

Hematologic: Minor bleeding (4.0% to 16.8%)

Neuromuscular & skeletal: Back pain (17.6%)

1% to 10%:

Cardiovascular: Bradycardia (4.5%), peripheral edema (1.6%)

Central nervous system: Headache (6.45)

Gastrointestinal: Vomiting (7.3%), abdominal pain (3.1%)

Hematologic: Major bleeding (1.1% to 14%), thrombocytopenia: <100,000 cells/mm^3 (2.5% to 5.6%); <50,000 cells/mm^3 (0.4% to 1.7%)

Local: Injection site pain (3.6%)

<1% (Limited to important or life-threatening): Abnormal thinking, allergic reactions/anaphylaxis (possible), AV block, bronchospasm, bullous eruption, coma, confusion, diabetes mellitus, embolism, hyperkalemia, ileus, inflammation, intracranial hemorrhage, myalgia, nodal arrhythmia, pleural effusion, pulmonary embolism, prostatitis, pruritus, stroke, urinary retention, ventricular tachycardia, xerostomia

Drug Interactions

Avoid Concomitant Use

Avoid concomitant use of Abciximab with any of the following: Dextran

Increased Effect/Toxicity

Abciximab may increase the levels/effects of: Anticoagulants; Antiplatelet Agents; Drotrecogin Alfa; Ibritumomab; Monoclonal Antibodies; Salicylates; Thrombolytic Agents; Tositumomab and Iodine I 131 Tositumomab

The levels/effects of Abciximab may be increased by: Dasatinib; Dextran; Herbs (Anticoagulant/Antiplatelet Properties); Nonsteroidal Anti-Inflammatory Agents; Omega-3-Acid Ethyl Esters; Pentosan Polysulfate Sodium; Prostacyclin Analogues

Decreased Effect

The levels/effects of Abciximab may be decreased by: Nonsteroidal Anti-Inflammatory Agents

Stability Vials should be stored at 2°C to 8°C; do not freeze or shake. After admixture, the prepared solution is stable for 12 hours.

Mechanism of Action Fab antibody fragment of the chimeric human-murine monoclonal antibody 7E3; this agent binds to platelet IIb/IIIa receptors, resulting in steric hindrance, thus inhibiting platelet aggregation

Pharmacodynamics/Kinetics Half-life elimination: ~30 minutes

Dosage

Percutaneous coronary intervention (PCI): I.V.: 0.25 mg/kg bolus administered 10-60 minutes prior to start of PCI followed by an infusion of 0.125 mcg/kg/minute (maximum: 10 mcg/minute) for 12 hours

Patients with unstable angina not responding to conventional medical therapy with planned PCI within 24 hours: 0.25 mg/kg bolus followed by an 18- to 24-hour infusion of 10 mcg/minute, concluding 1 hour after PCI.

ST-elevation MI combination regimen (unlabeled): Half-dose tenecteplase (15-25 mg based on weight), abciximab 0.25 mg/kg bolus then 0.125 mcg/kg/minute (maximum: 10 mcg/minute) for 12 hours and heparin dosing as follows: Concurrent bolus of 40 units/kg (maximum: 3000 units), then 7 units/kg/hour (maximum: 800 units/hour) as continuous infusion. Adjust to aPTT target of 50-70 seconds.

Administration Abciximab is intended for coadministration with aspirin postangioplasty and heparin infused and weight adjusted to maintain a therapeutic bleeding time (eg, ACT 300-500 seconds). Solution must be filtered prior to administration. Do not shake the vial.

Bolus dose: Aseptically withdraw the necessary amount of abciximab for the bolus dose into a syringe using a 0.2 or 5 micron low protein-binding syringe filter (or equivalent); the bolus should be administered 10-60 minutes before the procedure.

Continuous infusion: Aseptically withdraw amount required of abciximab for the infusion through a 0.2 or 5 micron low protein-binding syringe filter into a syringe; inject this into 250 mL of NS or D_5W to make solution. If a syringe filter was not used when preparing the infusion, administer using an in-line 0.2 or 0.22 micron low protein-binding filter. **Note:** Alternatively, a standard concentration of 7.2 mg in 250 mL of NS or D_5W may also be prepared for all patients and administered at the standard dose (0.125 mcg/kg/minute; maximum: 10 mcg/minute) with a variable rate in mL/hour. Infuse for 12-24 hours via pump after bolus dose; length of therapy dependent on indication.

Monitoring Parameters Prothrombin time, activated partial thromboplastin time (aPTT), hemoglobin, hematocrit, platelet count, fibrinogen, fibrin split products, transfusion requirements, signs of hypersensitivity reactions, guaiac stools, Hemastix® urine. Platelet count should be monitored at baseline, 2-4 hours following bolus infusion, and at 24 hours (or prior to discharge, if before 24 hours). To minimize risk of bleeding:

Abciximab initiated 18-24 hours prior to PCI: Maintain aPTT between 60-85 seconds during the heparin/abciximab infusion period

During PCI: Maintain ACT between 200-300 seconds

Following PCI (if anticoagulation is maintained): Maintain aPTT between 50-75 seconds

Sheath removal should not occur until aPTT is ≤50 seconds or ACT ≤175 seconds.

Maintain bleeding precautions, avoid unnecessary arterial and venous punctures, use saline or heparin lock for blood drawing, assess sheath insertion site and distal pulses of affected leg every 15 minutes for the first hour and then every 1 hour for the next 6 hours. Arterial access site care is important to prevent bleeding. Care should be taken when attempting vascular access that only the anterior wall of the femoral artery is punctured, avoiding a Seldinger (through and through) technique for obtaining sheath access. Femoral vein sheath placement should be avoided unless needed. While the vascular sheath is in place, patients should be maintained on complete bedrest with the head of the bed at a 30° angle and the affected limb restrained in a straight position.

Observe patient for mental status changes, hemorrhage; assess nose and mouth mucous membranes, puncture sites for oozing, ecchymosis, and hematoma formation; and examine urine, stool, and emesis for presence of occult or frank blood; gentle care should be provided when removing dressings.

Dosage Forms Excipient information presented when available (limited, particularly for generics); consult specific product labeling.

Injection, solution:

ReoPro®: 2 mg/mL (5 mL)

- **Abelcet®** *see* Amphotericin B (Lipid Complex) *on page 106*
- **Abenol® (Can)** *see* Acetaminophen *on page 25*
- **ABI-007** *see* Paclitaxel (Protein Bound) *on page 1129*
- **Abilify®** *see* Aripiprazole *on page 134*
- **Abilify® Discmelt™** *see* Aripiprazole *on page 134*
- **ABLC** *see* Amphotericin B (Lipid Complex) *on page 106*
- **A/B Otic** *see* Antipyrine and Benzocaine *on page 124*
- **Abraxane®** *see* Paclitaxel (Protein Bound) *on page 1129*
- **Abraxane® For Injectable Suspension (Can)** *see* Paclitaxel *on page 1127*
- **Abreva® [OTC]** *see* Docosanol *on page 473*
- **ABT-335** *see* Fenofibric Acid *on page 609*
- **ABX-EGF** *see* Panitumumab *on page 1138*
- **AC 2993** *see* Exenatide *on page 595*
- **ACAM2000™** *see* Smallpox Vaccine *on page 1377*

Acamprosate (a kam PROE sate)

U.S. Brand Names Campral®

Canadian Brand Names Campral®

Index Terms Acamprosate Calcium; Calcium Acetylhomotaurinate

Pharmacologic Category GABA Agonist/Glutamate Antagonist

Use Maintenance of alcohol abstinence

Pregnancy Risk Factor C

Pregnancy Considerations Teratogenic in animal studies. No adequate or well-controlled studies in pregnant women; use only if potential benefit outweighs possible risk to the fetus.

Lactation Excretion in breast milk unknown/use caution

Contraindications Hypersensitivity to acamprosate or any component of the formulation; severe renal impairment (Cl_{cr} <30 mL/minute)

Warnings/Precautions Should be used as part of a comprehensive program to treat alcohol dependence. Treatment should be initiated as soon as possible following the period of alcohol withdrawal, when the patient has achieved abstinence. Acamprosate does not eliminate or diminish the symptoms of alcohol withdrawal. Use caution in moderate renal impairment (Cl_{cr} 30-50 mL/minute). Suicidal ideation, attempted and completed suicides have occurred in acamprosate-treated patients; monitor for depression and/or suicidal thinking. Traces of sulfites may be present in the formulation. Safety and efficacy have not been established in pediatric patients.

Adverse Reactions

Note: Many adverse effects associated with treatment may be related to alcohol abstinence; reported frequency range may overlap with placebo.

>10%: Gastrointestinal: Diarrhea (10% to 17%)

1% to 10%:

Cardiovascular: Syncope, palpitation, edema (peripheral)

Central nervous system: Insomnia (6% to 9%), anxiety (5% to 8%), depression (4% to 8%), dizziness (3% to 4%), pain (2% to 4%), paresthesia (2% to 3%), headache, somnolence, amnesia, tremor, chills

Dermatologic: Pruritus (3% to 4%), rash

Endocrine & metabolic: Weight gain, libido decreased

Gastrointestinal: Anorexia (2% to 5%), flatulence (1% to 3%), nausea (3% to 4%), abdominal pain, dry mouth (1% to 3%), vomiting, dyspepsia, constipation, appetite increased, taste perversion

Genitourinary: Impotence

Neuromuscular & skeletal: Weakness (5% to 7%), back pain, myalgia, arthralgia

Ocular: Abnormal vision

Respiratory: Rhinitis, dyspnea, pharyngitis, bronchitis

Miscellaneous: Diaphoresis (2% to 3%), suicide attempt

<1%, postmarketing, and/or case reports (limited to important or life-threatening): Angina, asthma, exfoliative dermatitis, gastrointestinal hemorrhage, hallucinations, hypothyroidism, MI, ophthalmitis, pancreatitis, photosensitivity, psychosis, pulmonary embolus, renal calculus, renal failure, seizure, suicidal ideation, suicide attempts, suicide completion

Drug Interactions

Avoid Concomitant Use There are no known interactions where it is recommended to avoid concomitant use.

Increased Effect/Toxicity There are no known significant interactions involving an increase in effect.

Decreased Effect There are no known significant interactions involving a decrease in effect.

Ethanol/Nutrition/Herb Interactions

Ethanol: Abstinence is required during treatment. Ethanol does not affect the pharmacokinetics of acamprosate; however, the continued use of ethanol will decrease desired efficacy of acamprosate.

Food: Food decreases absorption of acamprosate (not clinically significant).

Stability Store at 25°C (77°F); excursions permitted to 15°C to 30°C (59°F to 86°F).

Mechanism of Action Mechanism not fully defined. Structurally similar to gamma-amino butyric acid (GABA), acamprosate appears to increase the activity of the GABA-ergic system, and decreases activity of glutamate within the CNS, including a decrease in activity at N-methyl D-aspartate (NMDA) receptors; may also affect CNS calcium channels. Restores balance to GABA and glutamate activities which appear to be disrupted in alcohol dependence. During therapeutic use, reduces alcohol intake, but does not cause a disulfiram-like reaction following alcohol ingestion.

Pharmacodynamics/Kinetics

Distribution: V_d: 1 L/kg

Protein binding: Negligible

Metabolism: Not metabolized

Bioavailability: 11%

Half-life elimination: 20-33 hours

Excretion: Urine (as unchanged drug)

Dosage Oral: Adults: Alcohol abstinence: 666 mg 3 times/day (a lower dose may be effective in some patients)

Adjustment in patients with low body weight (unlabeled): A lower dose (4 tablets/day) may be considered in patients with low body weight (eg, <60 kg).

Note: Treatment should be initiated as soon as possible (following the period of alcohol withdrawal) when the patient has achieved abstinence.

Dosage adjustment in renal impairment:

Cl_{cr} 30-50 mL/minute: Initial dose should be reduced to 333 mg 3 times/day.

Cl_{cr} <30 mL/minute: Contraindicated in severe renal impairment.

Dietary Considerations May be taken without regard to meals. Each 333 mg tablet contains 33 mg of elemental calcium.

Administration May be administered without regard to meals. Tablet should be swallowed whole; do not crush or chew.

Dosage Forms Excipient information presented when available (limited, particularly for generics); consult specific product labeling.

Tablet, enteric coated, delayed release, as calcium:

Campral®: 333 mg [contains calcium 33 mg and sulfites]

- **Acamprosate Calcium** *see* Acamprosate *on page 23*

Acarbose (AY car bose)

U.S. Brand Names Precose®

Canadian Brand Names Glucobay™

Pharmacologic Category Antidiabetic Agent, Alpha-Glucosidase Inhibitor

Additional Appendix Information

Diabetes Mellitus Management, Adults *on page 1801*

Use Adjunct to diet and exercise to lower blood glucose in patients with type 2 diabetes mellitus (noninsulin dependent, NIDDM)

Pregnancy Risk Factor B

Pregnancy Considerations Adverse events have not been reported in animal reproduction studies; therefore, acarbose is classified as pregnancy category B. Low amounts of acarbose are absorbed systemically which should limit fetal exposure. Maternal hyperglycemia can be associated with adverse effects in the fetus, including macrosomia, neonatal hyperglycemia, and hyperbilirubinemia; the risk of congenital malformations is increased when the Hb A_{1c} is above the normal range. Diabetes can also be associated with adverse effects in the mother. Poorly-treated diabetes may cause end-organ damage that may in turn negatively affect obstetric outcomes. Physiologic glucose levels should be maintained prior to and during pregnancy to decrease the risk of adverse events in the mother and the fetus. Acarbose has been studied for its potential role in treating GDM; however, only limited information is available describing pregnancy outcomes. Until additional safety and efficacy data are obtained, the use of oral agents is generally not recommended as routine management of GDM or type 2 diabetes mellitus during pregnancy. Insulin is the drug of choice for the control of diabetes mellitus during pregnancy.

Lactation Excretion in breast milk unknown/not recommended

Medication Safety Issues

Sound-alike/look-alike issues:

Precose® may be confused with PreCare®

International issues:

Precose® may be confused with Precosa® which is a brand name for *Saccharomyces boulardii* in Denmark, Finland, Norway, and Sweden

Contraindications Hypersensitivity to acarbose or any component of the formulation; patients with diabetic ketoacidosis or cirrhosis; patients with inflammatory bowel disease, colonic ulceration, partial intestinal obstruction, or in patients predisposed to intestinal obstruction; patients who have chronic intestinal diseases associated with marked disorders of digestion or absorption, and in patients who have conditions that may deteriorate as a result of increased gas formation in the intestine

Warnings/Precautions Acarbose given in combination with a sulfonylurea or insulin will cause a further lowering of blood glucose and may increase the hypoglycemic potential of the sulfonylurea or insulin. Treatment-emergent elevations of serum transaminases (AST and/or ALT) occurred in up to 14% of acarbose-treated patients in long-term studies. These serum transaminase elevations appear to be dose related and were asymptomatic, reversible, more common in females, and, in general, were not associated with other evidence of liver dysfunction. Fulminant hepatitis has been reported rarely. It may be necessary to discontinue acarbose and administer insulin if the patient is exposed to stress (ie, fever, trauma, infection, surgery). Use not recommended in patients with significant impairment (S_{cr} >2 mg/dL); use with caution in other patients with renal impairment. Safety and efficacy have not been established in children.

Adverse Reactions

>10%:

Gastrointestinal: Diarrhea (31%) and abdominal pain (19%) tend to return to pretreatment levels over time; frequency and intensity of flatulence (74%) tend to abate with time

Hepatic: Transaminases increased (≤4%)

Postmarketing and/or case reports: Edema, erythema, exanthema, hepatitis, ileus/subileus, jaundice, liver damage, rash, urticaria

Drug Interactions

Avoid Concomitant Use There are no known interactions where it is recommended to avoid concomitant use.

Increased Effect/Toxicity

The levels/effects of Acarbose may be increased by: Herbs (Hypoglycemic Properties); Pegvisomant

Decreased Effect

Acarbose may decrease the levels/effects of: Digoxin

The levels/effects of Acarbose may be decreased by: Corticosteroids (Orally Inhaled); Corticosteroids (Systemic); Luteinizing Hormone-Releasing Hormone Analogs; Somatropin

Ethanol/Nutrition/Herb Interactions Ethanol: Limit ethanol.

Stability Store at <25°C (77°F). Protect from moisture.

Mechanism of Action Competitive inhibitor of pancreatic α-amylase and intestinal brush border α-glucosidases, resulting in delayed hydrolysis of ingested complex carbohydrates and disaccharides and absorption of glucose; dose-dependent reduction in postprandial serum insulin and glucose peaks; inhibits the metabolism of sucrose to glucose and fructose

Pharmacodynamics/Kinetics

Absorption: <2% as active drug; ~35% as metabolites

Metabolism: Exclusively via GI tract, principally by intestinal bacteria and digestive enzymes; 13 metabolites identified (major metabolites are sulfate, methyl, and glucuronide conjugates)

Bioavailability: Low systemic bioavailability of parent compound; acts locally in GI tract

Half-life elimination: ~2 hours

Time to peak: Active drug: ~1 hour

Excretion: Urine (~34% as inactive metabolites, <2% parent drug and active metabolite); feces (~51% as unabsorbed drug)

Dosage Oral:

Adults: Dosage must be individualized on the basis of effectiveness and tolerance while not exceeding the maximum recommended dose

Initial dose: 25 mg 3 times/day with the first bite of each main meal; to reduce GI effects, some patients may benefit from initiating at 25 mg once daily with gradual titration to 25 mg 3 times/day as tolerated

Maintenance dose: Should be adjusted at 4- to 8-week intervals based on 1-hour postprandial glucose levels and tolerance until maintenance dose is reached. Dosage may be increased from 25 mg 3 times/day to 50 mg 3 times/day. Some patients may benefit from increasing the dose to 100 mg 3 times/day.

Maintenance dose ranges: 50-100 mg 3 times/day.

Maximum dose:

≤60 kg: 50 mg 3 times/day

>60 kg: 100 mg 3 times/day

Patients receiving sulfonylureas or insulin: Acarbose given in combination with a sulfonylurea or insulin will cause a further lowering of blood glucose and may increase the hypoglycemic potential of the sulfonylurea or insulin. If hypoglycemia occurs, appropriate adjustments in the dosage of these agents should be made.

Dosing adjustment in renal impairment:

Cl_{cr} <25 mL/minute: Peak plasma concentrations were 5 times higher and AUCs were 6 times larger than in volunteers with normal renal function.

Significant renal dysfunction (S_{cr} >2 mg/dL): Use is not recommended.

Dietary Considerations Take with food (first bite of meal).

Administration Should be administered with the first bite of each main meal.

Monitoring Parameters Postprandial glucose, glycosylated hemoglobin levels, serum transaminase levels should be checked every 3 months during the first year of treatment and periodically thereafter, renal function (serum creatinine); blood pressure

Reference Range Recommendations for glycemic control in adults with diabetes:

Hb A_{1c}: <7%

Preprandial capillary plasma glucose: 70-130 mg/dL

Peak postprandial capillary blood glucose: <180 mg/dL

Dosage Forms Excipient information presented when available (limited, particularly for generics); consult specific product labeling.

Tablet: 25 mg, 50 mg, 100 mg

Precose®: 25 mg, 50 mg, 100 mg

- **A-Caro-25** *see* Beta-Carotene *on page 188*
- **Accolate®** *see* Zafirlukast *on page 1575*
- **AccuHist®** *see* Brompheniramine and Pseudoephedrine *on page 214*
- **AccuNeb®** *see* Albuterol *on page 51*
- **Accupril®** *see* Quinapril *on page 1278*
- **Accuretic®** *see* Quinapril and Hydrochlorothiazide *on page 1280*
- **Accutane®** *see* Isotretinoin *on page 825*
- **Accuzyme®** *see* Papain and Urea *on page 1142*
- **Accuzyme® SE** *see* Papain and Urea *on page 1142*
- **ACE** *see* Captopril *on page 249*

Acebutolol (a se BYOO toe lole)

U.S. Brand Names Sectral®

Canadian Brand Names Apo-Acebutolol®; Gen-Acebutolol; Monitan®; Novo-Acebutolol; Nu-Acebutolol; Rhotral; Rhoxal-acebutolol; Sandoz-Acebutolol; Sectral®

Index Terms Acebutolol Hydrochloride

Pharmacologic Category Antiarrhythmic Agent, Class II; Beta Blocker With Intrinsic Sympathomimetic Activity

Additional Appendix Information

Beta-Blockers *on page 1648*

Use Treatment of hypertension; management of ventricular arrhythmias

Unlabeled/Investigational Use Treatment of chronic stable angina

Pregnancy Risk Factor B (manufacturer); D (2nd and 3rd trimesters - expert analysis)

Medication Safety Issues

Sound-alike/look-alike issues:

Sectral® may be confused with Factrel®, Seconal®, Septra®

Dosage Oral:

Adults:

Ventricular arrhythmias: Initial: 400 mg/day in divided doses; maintenance: 600-1200 mg/day in divided doses; maximum: 1200 mg/day

Hypertension: 400-800 mg/day (larger doses may be divided); maximum: 1200 mg/day; usual dose range (JNC 7): 200-800 mg/day in 2 divided doses

Chronic stable angina (unlabeled use): 400 mg/day in divided doses; maintenance: 600-1200 mg/day in divided doses; maximum: 1200 mg/day

Elderly: Initial: 200-400 mg/day; dose reduction due to age-related decrease in Cl_{cr} will be necessary; do not exceed 800 mg/day

Dosing adjustment in renal impairment:

Cl_{cr} 25-49 mL/minute: Reduce dose by 50%.

Cl_{cr} <25 mL/minute: Reduce dose by 75%.

Dosing adjustment in hepatic impairment: Use with caution.

Additional Information Complete prescribing information for this medication should be consulted for additional detail.

Dosage Forms Excipient information presented when available (limited, particularly for generics); consult specific product labeling.

Capsule, as hydrochloride: 200 mg, 400 mg

Sectral®: 200 mg, 400 mg

- **Acebutolol Hydrochloride** *see* Acebutolol *on page 25*
- **Aceon®** *see* Perindopril Erbumine *on page 1174*
- **Acephen™ [OTC]** *see* Acetaminophen *on page 25*
- **Acerola [OTC]** *see* Ascorbic Acid *on page 139*
- **Acetadote®** *see* Acetylcysteine *on page 36*
- **Aceta-Gesic [OTC]** *see* Acetaminophen and Phenyltoloxamine *on page 29*

Acetaminophen (a seet a MIN oh fen)

U.S. Brand Names Acephen™ [OTC]; Apra Children's [OTC]; Aspirin Free Anacin® Maximum Strength [OTC]; Cetafen Extra® [OTC]; Cetafen® [OTC]; Comtrex® Sore Throat Maximum Strength [OTC]; FeverALL® [OTC]; Genapap™ Children [OTC]; Genapap™ Extra Strength [OTC]; Genapap™ Infant [OTC]; Genapap™ [OTC]; Genebs Extra Strength [OTC]; Genebs [OTC]; Infantaire [OTC]; Little Fevers™ [OTC]; Mapap Children's [OTC]; Mapap Extra Strength [OTC]; Mapap Infants [OTC]; Mapap [OTC]; Nortemp Children's [OTC]; Pain Eze [OTC]; Silapap® Children's [OTC]; Silapap® Infants [OTC]; Tycolene Maximum Strength [OTC]; Tycolene [OTC]; Tylenol® 8 Hour [OTC]; Tylenol® Arthritis Pain [OTC]; Tylenol® Children's with Flavor Creator [OTC]; Tylenol® Children's [OTC]; Tylenol® Extra Strength [OTC]; Tylenol® Infants [OTC]; Tylenol® Junior [OTC]; Tylenol® [OTC]; Valorin Extra [OTC]; Valorin [OTC]

Canadian Brand Names Abenol®; Apo-Acetaminophen®; Atasol®; Novo-Gesic; Pediatrix; Tempra®; Tylenol®

Index Terms APAP; N-Acetyl-P-Aminophenol; Paracetamol

Pharmacologic Category Analgesic, Miscellaneous

Use Treatment of mild-to-moderate pain and fever (antipyretic/analgesic); does not have antirheumatic or anti-inflammatory effects

Pregnancy Risk Factor B

Pregnancy Considerations Acetaminophen crosses the placenta. It is generally considered to be safe for use during pregnancy when used at therapeutic doses for short periods of time.

Lactation Enters breast milk/compatible

Medication Safety Issues

Sound-alike/look-alike issues:

Acephen® may be confused with AcipHex®

FeverALL® may be confused with Fiberall®

Tylenol® may be confused with atenolol, timolol, Tuinal®, Tylox®

International issues:

Paralen® [Czech Republic] may be confused with Aralen® which is a brand name for chloroquine in the U.S.

Duorol® may be confused with Diuril® which is a brand name for chlorothiazide in the U.S.

Duplicate therapy issues: This product contains acetaminophen, which may be a component of combination products. Do not exceed the maximum recommended daily dose of acetaminophen.

Contraindications Hypersensitivity to acetaminophen or any component of the formulation

Warnings/Precautions Limit dose to <4 g/day. May cause severe hepatic toxicity on acute overdose; in addition, chronic daily dosing in adults has resulted in liver damage in some patients. Use with caution in patients with alcoholic liver disease; consuming ≥3 alcoholic drinks/day may increase the risk of liver damage. Use caution in patients with known G6PD deficiency.

OTC labeling: When used for self-medication, patients should be instructed to contact healthcare provider if used for fever lasting >3 days or for pain lasting >10 days in adults or >5 days in children.

Adverse Reactions Frequency not defined.

Dermatologic: Rash

Endocrine & metabolic: May increase chloride, uric acid, glucose; may decrease sodium, bicarbonate, calcium

Hematologic: Anemia, blood dyscrasias (neutropenia, pancytopenia, leukopenia)

Hepatic: Bilirubin increased, alkaline phosphatase increased

Renal: Ammonia increased, nephrotoxicity with chronic overdose, analgesic nephropathy

Miscellaneous: Hypersensitivity reactions (rare)

Drug Interactions

Metabolism/Transport Effects **Substrate** (minor) of CYP1A2, 2A6, 2C9, 2D6, 2E1, 3A4; **Inhibits** CYP3A4 (weak)

Avoid Concomitant Use There are no known interactions where it is recommended to avoid concomitant use.

Increased Effect/Toxicity

Acetaminophen may increase the levels/effects of: Vitamin K Antagonists

The levels/effects of Acetaminophen may be increased by: Imatinib; Isoniazid

Decreased Effect

The levels/effects of Acetaminophen may be decreased by: Anticonvulsants (Hydantoin); Barbiturates; CarBAMazepine; Cholestyramine Resin

Ethanol/Nutrition/Herb Interactions

Ethanol: Excessive intake of ethanol may increase the risk of acetaminophen-induced hepatotoxicity. Avoid ethanol or limit to <3 drinks/day.

Food: Rate of absorption may be decreased when given with food.

Herb/Nutraceutical: St John's wort may decrease acetaminophen levels.

Stability Do not freeze suppositories.

Mechanism of Action Inhibits the synthesis of prostaglandins in the central nervous system and peripherally blocks pain impulse generation; produces antipyresis from inhibition of hypothalamic heat-regulating center

Pharmacodynamics/Kinetics

Onset of action: <1 hour

Duration: 4-6 hours

Absorption: Incomplete; varies by dosage form

Protein binding: 8% to 43% at toxic doses

Metabolism: At normal therapeutic dosages, hepatic to sulfate and glucuronide metabolites, while a small amount is metabolized by CYP to a highly reactive intermediate (acetylimidoquinone) which is conjugated with glutathione and inactivated; at toxic doses (as little as 4 g daily) glutathione conjugation becomes insufficient to meet the metabolic demand causing an increase in acetylimidoquinone concentration, which may cause hepatic cell necrosis

Half-life elimination: Prolonged following toxic doses

Neonates: 2-5 hours

Adults: 1-3 hours (may be increased in elderly; however, this should not affect dosing)

Time to peak, serum: Oral: 10-60 minutes; may be delayed in acute overdoses

Excretion: Urine (2% to 5% unchanged; 55% as glucuronide metabolites; 30% as sulphate metabolites)

Dosage Oral, rectal:

Children <12 years: 10-15 mg/kg/dose every 4-6 hours as needed; do **not** exceed 5 doses (2.6 g) in 24 hours; alternatively, the following age-based doses may be used; see table.

Acetaminophen Dosing

Age	Dosage (mg)	Age	Dosage (mg)
0-3 mo	40	4-5 y	240
4-11 mo	80	6-8 y	320
1-2 y	120	9-10 y	400
2-3 y	160	11 y	480

Note: Higher rectal doses have been studied for use in preoperative pain control in children. However, specific guidelines are not available and dosing may be product dependent. The safety and efficacy of alternating acetaminophen and ibuprofen dosing has not been established.

Adults: 325-650 mg every 4-6 hours or 1000 mg 3-4 times/day; do **not** exceed 4 g/day

Dosing interval in renal impairment:

Cl_{cr} 10-50 mL/minute: Administer every 6 hours

Cl_{cr} <10 mL/minute: Administer every 8 hours (metabolites accumulate)

Hemodialysis: Moderately dialyzable (20% to 50%)

Dosing adjustment/comments in hepatic impairment: Use with caution. Limited, low-dose therapy is usually well tolerated in hepatic disease/cirrhosis. However, cases of hepatotoxicity at daily acetaminophen dosages <4 g/day have been reported. Avoid chronic use in hepatic impairment.

Dietary Considerations Chewable tablets may contain phenylalanine (amount varies, ranges between 3-12 mg/tablet); consult individual product labeling.

Administration

Suppositories: Do not freeze.

Suspension, oral: Shake well before pouring a dose.

Monitoring Parameters Relief of pain or fever

Reference Range

Therapeutic concentration (analgesic/antipyretic): 10-30 mcg/mL

Toxic concentration (acute ingestion) with probable hepatotoxicity: >200 mcg/mL at 4 hours or 50 mcg/mL at 12 hours after ingestion

Test Interactions Increased chloride, bilirubin, uric acid, glucose, ammonia (B), chloride (S), uric acid (S), alkaline phosphatase (S), chloride (S); decreased sodium, bicarbonate, calcium (S)

Dosage Forms Excipient information presented when available (limited, particularly for generics); consult specific product labeling. [DSC] = Discontinued product

Caplet: 500 mg

Cetafen Extra® Strength, Genapap™ Extra Strength, Genebs Extra Strength, Mapap Extra Strength, Tycolene Maximum Strength, Tylenol® Extra Strength: 500 mg

Caplet, extended release:

Tylenol® 8 Hour, Tylenol® Arthritis Pain: 650 mg

Capsule: 500 mg

Elixir: 160 mg/5 mL (120 mL, 480 mL, 3780 mL [DSC])

Apra Children's: 160 mg/5 mL (120 mL, 480 mL, 3780 mL [DSC]) [alcohol free; contains benzoic acid; cherry and grape flavors]

Mapap Children's: 160 mg/5 mL (120 mL) [alcohol free; contains benzoic acid and sodium benzoate; cherry flavor]
Gelcap:
Mapap Extra Strength, Tylenol® Extra Strength: 500 mg
Geltab:
Tylenol® Extra Strength: 500 mg
Liquid, oral: 500 mg/15 mL (240 mL)
Comtrex® Sore Throat Maximum Strength: 500 mg/15 mL (240 mL) [contains sodium benzoate; honey lemon flavor]
Genapap™ Children: 160 mg/5 mL (120 mL) [contains sodium benzoate; cherry and grape flavors]
Silapap®: 160 mg/5 mL (120 mL, 240 mL, 480 mL) [sugar free; contains sodium benzoate; cherry flavor]
Tylenol® Extra Strength: 500 mg/15 mL (240 mL) [contains sodium benzoate; cherry flavor]
Solution, oral: 160 mg/5 mL (120 mL, 480 mL)
Solution, oral [drops]: 80 mg/0.8 mL (15 mL) [droppers are marked at 0.4 mL (40 mg) and at 0.8 mL (80 mg)]
Genapap™ Infant: 80 mg/0.8 mL (15 mL) [fruit flavor]
Infantaire: 80 mg/0.8mL (15 mL, 30 mL)
Little Fevers™: 80 mg/1 mL (30 mL) [alcohol free; contains propylene glycol, sodium benzoate; berry flavor; packaged with dropper and forehead thermometer]
Silapap® Infant's: 80 mg/0.8 mL (15 mL, 30 mL) [contains sodium benzoate; cherry flavor]
Suppository, rectal: 120 mg, 325 mg, 650 mg
Acephen™: 120 mg, 325 mg, 650 mg
FeverALL®: 80 mg, 120 mg, 325 mg, 650 mg
Mapap: 125 mg, 650 mg
Suspension, oral: 160 mg/5 mL (5 mL, 10 mL, 20 mL)
Mapap Children's: 160 mg/5 mL (120 mL) [contains sodium benzoate; cherry flavor]
Nortemp Children's: 160 mg/5 mL (120 mL) [alcohol free; contains sodium benzoate; cotton candy flavor]
Tylenol® Children's: 160 mg/5 mL (120 mL, 240 mL) [contains sodium benzoate; bubble gum yum, cherry blast, dye free cherry, grape splash, and very berry strawberry flavors]
Tylenol® Children's with Flavor Creator: 160 mg/5 mL (120 mL) [contains sodium 2 mg/5 mL and sodium benzoate; cherry blast flavor; packaged with apple (4), bubblegum (8), chocolate (4), & strawberry (4) sugar free flavor packets]
Suspension, oral [drops]:
Mapap Infants: 80 mg/0.8 mL (15 mL, 30 mL) [contains sodium benzoate; cherry flavor]
Tylenol® Infants: 80 mg/0.8 mL (15 mL, 30 mL) [contains sodium benzoate; cherry, dye free cherry, and grape flavors]
Tablet: 325 mg, 500 mg
Aspirin Free Anacin® Extra Strength, Genapap™ Extra Strength, Genebs Extra Strength, Mapap Extra Strength, Pain Eze, Tylenol® Extra Strength, Valorin Extra: 500 mg
Cetafen®, Genapap™, Genebs, Mapap, Tycolene, Tylenol®, Valorin: 325 mg
Tablet, chewable: 80 mg
Genapap™ Children: 80 mg [contains phenylalanine 6 mg/tablet; grape flavors] [DSC]
Mapap Children's: 80 mg [contains phenylalanine 3 mg/tablet; bubble gum, fruit, and grape flavors]
Mapap Junior Strength: 160 mg [contains phenylalanine 12 mg/tablet; grape flavor]
Tablet, orally disintegrating: 80 mg, 160 mg
Tylenol® Children's Meltaways: 80 mg [bubble gum, grape, and watermelon flavors]
Tylenol® Junior Meltaways: 160 mg [bubble gum and grape flavors]

◆ **Acetaminophen and Butalbital** *see* Butalbital and Acetaminophen *on page 230*

◆ **Acetaminophen and Chlorpheniramine** *see* Chlorpheniramine and Acetaminophen *on page 309*

Acetaminophen and Codeine

(a seet a MIN oh fen & KOE deen)

U.S. Brand Names Capital® and Codeine; Tylenol® With Codeine

Canadian Brand Names ratio-Emtec; ratio-Lenoltec; Triatec-30; Triatec-8; Triatec-8 Strong; Tylenol Elixir with Codeine; Tylenol No. 1; Tylenol No. 1 Forte; Tylenol No. 2 with Codeine; Tylenol No. 3 with Codeine; Tylenol No. 4 with Codeine

Index Terms Codeine and Acetaminophen

Pharmacologic Category Analgesic, Opioid

Use Relief of mild-to-moderate pain

Restrictions C-III; C-V

Note: In countries outside of the U.S., some formulations of Tylenol® with Codeine (eg, Tylenol® No. 3) include caffeine.

Pregnancy Risk Factor C

Medication Safety Issues

Sound-alike/look-alike issues:
Capital® may be confused with Capitrol®
Tylenol® may be confused with atenolol, timolol, Tuinal®, Tylox®

T3 is an error-prone abbreviation (mistaken as liothyronine)

High alert medication: The Institute for Safe Medication Practices (ISMP) includes this medication among its list of drug classes which have a heightened risk of causing significant patient harm when used in error.

Duplicate therapy issues: This product contains acetaminophen, which may be a component of other combination products. Do not exceed the maximum recommended daily dose of acetaminophen.

Dosage Doses should be adjusted according to severity of pain and response of the patient. Adult doses ≥60 mg codeine fail to give commensurate relief of pain but merely prolong analgesia and are associated with an appreciably increased incidence of side effects. Oral:

Children: Analgesic:
Codeine: 0.5-1 mg codeine/kg/dose every 4-6 hours
Acetaminophen: 10-15 mg/kg/dose every 4 hours up to a maximum of 2.6 g/24 hours for children <12 years; **alternatively, the following can be used:**
3-6 years: 5 mL 3-4 times/day as needed of elixir
7-12 years: 10 mL 3-4 times/day as needed of elixir
>12 years: 15 mL every 4 hours as needed of elixir
Adults:
Antitussive: Based on codeine (15-30 mg/dose) every 4-6 hours (maximum: 360 mg/24 hours based on codeine component)
Analgesic: Based on codeine (30-60 mg/dose) every 4-6 hours (maximum: 4000 mg/24 hours based on acetaminophen component)
1-2 tablets every 4 hours to a maximum of 12 tablets/24 hours

Dosing adjustment in renal impairment: See individual agents.

Dosing adjustment in hepatic impairment: Use with caution. Limited, low-dose therapy is usually well tolerated in hepatic disease/cirrhosis; however, cases of hepatotoxicity at daily acetaminophen dosages <4 g/day have been reported. Avoid chronic use in hepatic impairment.

Additional Information Complete prescribing information for this medication should be consulted for additional detail.

Dosage Forms Excipient information presented when available (limited, particularly for generics); consult specific product labeling. [DSC] = Discontinued product; [CAN] = Canadian brand name

Caplet:

ratio-Lenoltec No. 1 [CAN], Tylenol No. 1 [CAN]: Acetaminophen 300 mg, codeine phosphate 8 mg, and caffeine 15 mg [not available in the U.S.]

Tylenol No. 1 Forte [CAN]: Acetaminophen 500 mg, codeine phosphate 8 mg, and caffeine 15 mg [not available in the U.S.]

Elixir, oral [C-V]: Acetaminophen 120 mg and codeine phosphate 12 mg per 5 mL (5 mL, 10 mL, 12.5 mL, 15 mL, 120 mL, 480 mL) [contains alcohol 7%]

Tylenol® with Codeine [DSC]: Acetaminophen 120 mg and codeine phosphate 12 mg per 5 mL (480 mL) [contains alcohol 7%; cherry flavor]

Tylenol Elixir with Codeine [CAN]: Acetaminophen 160 mg and codeine phosphate 8 mg per 5 mL (500 mL) [contains alcohol 7%, sucrose 31%; cherry flavor; not available in the U.S.]

Suspension, oral [C-V] (Capital® and Codeine): Acetaminophen 120 mg and codeine phosphate 12 mg per 5 mL (480 mL) [alcohol free; fruit punch flavor]

Tablet [C-III]: Acetaminophen 300 mg and codeine phosphate 15 mg; acetaminophen 300 mg and codeine phosphate 30 mg; acetaminophen 300 mg and codeine phosphate 60 mg

ratio-Emtec [CAN], Triatec-30 [CAN]: Acetaminophen 300 mg and codeine phosphate 30 mg [not available in the U.S.]

ratio-Lenoltec No. 1 [CAN]: Acetaminophen 300 mg, codeine phosphate 8 mg, and caffeine 15 mg [not available in the U.S.]

ratio-Lenoltec No. 2 [CAN], Tylenol No. 2 with Codeine [CAN]: Acetaminophen 300 mg, codeine phosphate 15 mg, and caffeine 15 mg [not available in the U.S.]

ratio-Lenoltec No. 3 [CAN], Tylenol No. 3 with Codeine [CAN]: Acetaminophen 300 mg, codeine phosphate 30 mg, and caffeine 15 mg [not available in the U.S.]

ratio-Lenoltec No. 4 [CAN], Tylenol No. 4 with Codeine [CAN]: Acetaminophen 300 mg and codeine phosphate 60 mg [not available in the U.S.]

Triatec-8 [CAN]: Acetaminophen 325 mg, codeine phosphate 8 mg, and caffeine 30 mg [not available in the U.S.]

Triatec-8 Strong [CAN]: Acetaminophen 500 mg, codeine phosphate 8 mg, and caffeine 30 mg [not available in the U.S.]

Tylenol® with Codeine No. 3: Acetaminophen 300 mg and codeine phosphate 30 mg [contains sodium metabisulfite]

Tylenol® with Codeine No. 4: Acetaminophen 300 mg and codeine phosphate 60 mg [contains sodium metabisulfite]

Acetaminophen and Diphenhydramine

(a seet a MIN oh fen & dye fen HYE dra meen)

U.S. Brand Names Excedrin® P.M. [OTC]; Goody's PM® [OTC]; Legatrin PM® [OTC]; Percogesic® Extra Strength [OTC]; Tylenol® PM [OTC]; Tylenol® Severe Allergy [OTC]

Index Terms Diphenhydramine and Acetaminophen

Pharmacologic Category Analgesic, Miscellaneous

Use Aid in the relief of insomnia accompanied by minor pain

Medication Safety Issues

Sound-alike/look-alike issues:

Excedrin® may be confused with Dexatrim®, Dexedrine®

Percogesic® may be confused with paregoric, Percodan®

Tylenol® may be confused with atenolol, timolol, Tuinal®, Tylox®

Duplicate therapy issues: This product contains acetaminophen, which may be a component of other combination products. Do not exceed the maximum recommended daily dose of acetaminophen.

Dosage Oral: Adults: 50 mg of diphenhydramine HCl (76 mg diphenhydramine citrate) at bedtime or as directed by physician; do not exceed recommended dosage; not for use in children <12 years of age

Dosing adjustment in hepatic impairment: Use with caution. Limited, low-dose therapy is usually well tolerated in hepatic disease/cirrhosis; however, cases of hepatotoxicity at daily acetaminophen dosages <4 g/day have been reported. Avoid chronic use in hepatic impairment.

Additional Information Complete prescribing information for this medication should be consulted for additional detail.

Dosage Forms Excipient information presented when available (limited, particularly for generics); consult specific product labeling.

Caplet: Acetaminophen 500 mg and diphenhydramine hydrochloride 25 mg

Excedrin® P.M.: Acetaminophen 500 mg and diphenhydramine citrate 38 mg

Legatrin PM®: Acetaminophen 500 mg and diphenhydramine hydrochloride 50 mg

Percogesic® Extra Strength: Acetaminophen 500 mg and diphenhydramine hydrochloride 25 mg

Tylenol® PM: Acetaminophen 500 mg and diphenhydramine hydrochloride 25 mg [also available in vanilla caplets]

Tylenol® Severe Allergy: Acetaminophen 500 mg and diphenhydramine hydrochloride 12.5 mg

Gelcap:

Tylenol® PM: Acetaminophen 500 mg and diphenhydramine hydrochloride 25 mg

Geltab: Acetaminophen 500 mg and diphenhydramine hydrochloride 25 mg

Excedrin® P.M.: Acetaminophen 500 mg and diphenhydramine citrate 38 mg

Tylenol® PM: Acetaminophen 500 mg and diphenhydramine hydrochloride 25 mg

Liquid:

Tylenol® PM: Acetaminophen 500 mg and diphenhydramine hydrochloride 25 mg per 15 mL (240 mL) [contains sodium benzoate; vanilla flavor]

Powder for oral solution:

Goody's PM®: Acetaminophen 500 mg and diphenhydramine citrate 38 mg [contains potassium 41.9 mg and sodium 3.15 mg per powder]

Tablet: Acetaminophen 500 mg and diphenhydramine hydrochloride 25 mg

Excedrin® P.M.: Acetaminophen 500 mg and diphenhydramine citrate 38 mg

◆ **Acetaminophen and Hydrocodone** *see* Hydrocodone and Acetaminophen *on page 740*

◆ **Acetaminophen and Oxycodone** *see* Oxycodone and Acetaminophen *on page 1122*

Acetaminophen and Pamabrom

(a seet a MIN oh fen & PAM a brom)

U.S. Brand Names Cramp Tabs [OTC]; Midol Teen Formula [OTC]; Tylenol® Women's Menstrual Relief [OTC]

Index Terms Pamabrom and Acetaminophen

Pharmacologic Category Analgesic, Miscellaneous; Diuretic, Combination

Use Temporary relief of symptoms associated with premenstrual and menstrual symptoms (eg, cramps, bloating, water-weight gain, headache, backache, muscle aches)

Medication Safety Issues

Duplicate therapy issues: This product contains acetaminophen, which may be a component of other combination products. Do not exceed the maximum recommended daily dose of acetaminophen.

Dosage Oral: Children ≥12 years and Adults: Acetaminophen 650-1000 mg and pamabrom 50 mg every 4-6 hours as needed (maximum: 8 caplets/tablets/24 hours)

Additional Information Complete prescribing information for this medication should be consulted for additional detail.

Dosage Forms Excipient information presented when available (limited, particularly for generics); consult specific product labeling.

Caplet:

Midol Teen Formula: Acetaminophen 500 mg and pamabrom 25 mg

Tylenol® Women's Menstrual Relief: Acetaminophen 500 mg and pamabrom 25 mg

Tablet:

Cramp Tabs: Acetaminophen 325 mg and pamabrom 25 mg

Acetaminophen and Phenylephrine

(a seet a MIN oh fen & fen il EF rin)

U.S. Brand Names Alka-Seltzer Plus® Sinus Formula [OTC]; Contac® Cold + Flu Maximum Strength Non-Drowsy [OTC]; Mapap® Sinus Congestion and Pain Daytime [OTC]; Sinutab® Sinus [OTC]; Sudafed PE® Sinus Headache [OTC]; Tylenol® Sinus Congestion & Pain Daytime [OTC]

Index Terms Phenylephrine Hydrochloride and Acetaminophen

Pharmacologic Category Analgesic, Miscellaneous; Decongestant

Use Temporary relief of sinus/nasal congestion and pressure, headache, and minor aches and pains

Medication Safety Issues

Duplicate therapy issues: This product contains acetaminophen, which may be a component of combination products. Do not exceed the maximum recommended daily dose of acetaminophen.

Dosage Oral: Children ≥12 years and Adults: General dosing guidelines, refer to specific product labeling: Sinus pain/pressure: Acetaminophen 325 mg and phenylephrine 5 mg/caplet: Take 2 caplets every 4 hours as needed; maximum: 12 caplets/24 hours

Additional Information Complete prescribing information for this medication should be consulted for additional detail.

Dosage Forms Excipient information presented when available (limited, particularly for generics); consult specific product labeling.

Caplet, oral:

Contac® Cold + Flu Maximum Strength Non Drowsy: Acetaminophen 500 mg and phenylephrine hydrochloride 5 mg

Mapap® Sinus Congestion and Pain Daytime, Sinutab® Sinus, Sudafed PE® Sinus Headache: Acetaminophen 325 mg and phenylephrine hydrochloride 5 mg

Tylenol® Sinus Congestion & Pain Daytime: Acetaminophen 325 mg and phenylephrine hydrochloride 5 mg [Cool Burst™ flavor]

Gelcap, oral:

Tylenol® Sinus Congestion & Pain Daytime: Acetaminophen 325 mg and phenylephrine hydrochloride 5 mg

Gelcap, rapid release, oral:

Tylenol® Sinus Congestion & Pain Datyime: Acetaminophen 325 mg and phenylephrine hydrochloride 5 mg

Tablet for solution, oral [effervescent]:

Alka-Seltzer Plus® Sinus Formula: Acetaminophen 250 mg and phenylephrine hydrochloride 5 mg [contains sodium 477 mg/tablet and phenylalanine 4.2 mg/tablet; lemon zest flavor]

Acetaminophen and Phenyltoloxamine

(a seet a MIN oh fen & fen il to LOKS a meen)

U.S. Brand Names Aceta-Gesic [OTC]; Alpain; BeFlex; Dologesic®; Flextra 650; Flextra-DS; Genasec™ [OTC]; Hyflex-DS® [DSC]; Lagesic™; Percogesic® [OTC]; Phenagesic [OTC]; Phenylgesic [OTC]; RhinoFlex 650; RhinoFlex™; Staflex; Vistra 650; Zgesic

Index Terms Phenyltoloxamine Citrate and Acetaminophen

Pharmacologic Category Analgesic, Miscellaneous

Use Relief of mild-to-moderate pain

Pregnancy Risk Factor C

Medication Safety Issues

Sound-alike/look-alike issues:

Percogesic® may be confused with paregoric, Percodan®

Duplicate therapy issues: This product contains acetaminophen, which may be a component of other combination products. Do not exceed the maximum recommended daily dose of acetaminophen.

Dosage Oral:

Analgesic: Based on acetaminophen component:

Children: 10-15 mg/kg/dose every 4-6 hours as needed (maximum: 5 doses/24 hours

Adults: 325-650 mg every 4-6 hours as needed (maximum: 4 g/day)

Product-specific labeling:

Dologesic®:

Children <12 years: 1 caplet/capsule **or** 5 mL every 4 hours

Children ≥12 years and Adults: 1-2 caplets/capsules **or** 15-30 mL every 4 hours (maximum: 8 caplets/24 hours **or** 120 mL/24 hours)

Flextra-650:

Children 6 to <12 years: 1/2 tablet every 6 hours (maximum: 2 tablets/day)

Children ≥12 years and Adults: 1/2-1 tablet every 6 hours (maximum: 4 tablets/day)

Flextra-DS, RhinoFlex™, RhinoFlex™-650:

Children 6 to <12 years: 1/2 tablet every 4 hours (maximum: 2.5 tablets/day)

Children ≥12 years and Adults: 1/2-1 tablet every 4 hours (maximum: 5 tablets/day)

Lagesic™:

Children 6-12 years: 1/2 every 12 hours (maximum: 2 caplets/24 hours)

Children ≥12 years and Adults: 1-2 caplets every 8-12 hours (maximum: 6 caplets/24 hours)

Percogesic®:

Children 6-12 years: 1 tablet every 4 hours (maximum: 4 tablets/24 hours)

Adults: 1-2 tablets every 4 hours (maximum: 8 tablets/24 hours)

Zgesic: Children >12 years and Adults: 1-2 tablets every 8-12 hours (maximum: 6 tablets/24 hours)

Dosing adjustment in renal impairment: Specific dosing adjustment not available; monitor renal function with severe impairment

Dosing adjustment in hepatic impairment: Use with caution. Limited, low-dose therapy is usually well tolerated in hepatic disease/cirrhosis; however, cases of hepatotoxicity at daily acetaminophen dosages <4 g/day have been reported. Avoid chronic use in hepatic impairment.

Additional Information Complete prescribing information for this medication should be consulted for additional detail.

Dosage Forms Excipient information presented when available (limited, particularly for generics); consult specific product labeling. [DSC] = Discontinued product

Caplet:
- Alpain: Acetaminophen 500 mg and phenyltoloxamine citrate 60 mg
- BeFlex: Acetaminophen 500 mg and phenyltoloxamine citrate 55 mg
- Dologesic®: Acetaminophen 500 mg and phenyltoloxamine citrate 30 mg
- Staflex: Acetaminophen 500 mg and phenyltoloxamine citrate 55 mg

Caplet, extended release [scored]:
- Lagesic™: Acetaminophen 600 mg and phenyltoloxamine citrate 66 mg

Capsule:
- Dologesic®: Acetaminophen 500 mg and phenyltoloxamine citrate 30 mg

Liquid:
- Dologesic®: Acetaminophen 500 mg and phenyltoloxamine citrate 30 mg per 15 mL (180 mL)

Tablet: Acetaminophen 325 mg and phenyltoloxamine citrate 30 mg
- Aceta-Gesic, Genasec™, Percogesic®, Phenagesic, Phenylgesic: Acetaminophen 325 mg and phenyltoloxamine citrate 30 mg
- Flextra-650, Vistra 650: Acetaminophen 650 mg and phenyltoloxamine citrate 60 mg
- Flextra-DS, Hyflex-DS® [DSC], RhinoFlex™: Acetaminophen 500 mg and phenyltoloxamine citrate 50 mg
- RhinoFlex™-650: Acetaminophen 650 mg and phenyltoloxamine citrate 50 mg

Tablet, prolonged release, oral:
- Zgesic: Acetaminophen 600 mg and phenyltoloxamine citrate 66 mg

◆ **Acetaminophen and Propoxyphene** *see* Propoxyphene and Acetaminophen *on page 1258*

Acetaminophen and Pseudoephedrine
(a seet a MIN oh fen & soo doe e FED rin)

U.S. Brand Names Allerest® Allergy and Sinus Relief [OTC]; Genapap™ Sinus Maximum Strength [OTC] [DSC]; Mapap Sinus Maximum Strength [OTC]; Medi-Synal [OTC]; Oranyl Plus [OTC]; Ornex® Maximum Strength [OTC]; Ornex® [OTC]; Sudafed® Multi-Symptom Sinus and Cold [OTC]; Tylenol® Cold Daytime, Children's [OTC]; Tylenol® Cold, Infants [OTC] [DSC]; Tylenol® Sinus Daytime [OTC]

Canadian Brand Names Contac® Cold and Sore Throat, Non Drowsy, Extra Strength; Dristan® N.D.; Dristan® N.D., Extra Strength; Sinutab® Non Drowsy; Sudafed® Head Cold and Sinus Extra Strength; Tylenol® Decongestant; Tylenol® Sinus

Index Terms Pseudoephedrine and Acetaminophen

Pharmacologic Category Alpha/Beta Agonist; Analgesic, Miscellaneous

Use Relief of mild-to-moderate pain; relief of congestion

Medication Safety Issues

Sound-alike/look-alike issues:
- Ornex® may be confused with Orexin®, Orinase®
- Sudafed® may be confused with Sufenta®
- Tylenol® may be confused with atenolol, timolol, Tuinal®, Tylox®

Duplicate therapy issues: This product contains acetaminophen, which may be a component of other combination products. Do not exceed the maximum recommended daily dose of acetaminophen.

Dosage Oral:

Analgesic: Based on acetaminophen component:
- Children: 10-15 mg/kg/dose every 4-6 hours as needed; do **not** exceed 5 doses in 24 hours
- Adults: 325-650 mg every 4-6 hours as needed; do **not** exceed 4 g/day

Decongestant: Based on pseudoephedrine component:
- Children:
  - 2-6 years: 15 mg every 4 hours; do **not** exceed 90 mg/day
  - 6-12 years: 30 mg every 4 hours; do **not** exceed 180 mg/day
- Children >12 years and Adults: 60 mg every 4 hours; do **not** exceed 360 mg/day

Product labeling:

Children's Tylenol® Cold Daytime: Children:
- 2-5 years (24-47 lb): 1 teaspoonful every 4-6 hours (maximum: 4 doses/24 hours)
- 6-11 years (48-95 lb): 2 teaspoonfuls every 4-6 hours (maximum: 4 doses/24 hours)

Sudafed® Multi-Symptom Sinus and Cold: Children ≥12 years and Adults: 2 capsules every 4-6 hours (maximum: 8 capsules/24 hours)

Tylenol® Sinus Daytime: Children ≥12 years and Adults: 2 caplets or gelcaps every 4-6 hours (maximum: 8 caplets or gelcaps/24 hours)

Dosing adjustment in hepatic impairment: Use with caution. Limited, low-dose therapy is usually well tolerated in hepatic disease/cirrhosis; however, cases of hepatotoxicity at daily acetaminophen dosages <4 g/day have been reported. Avoid chronic use in hepatic impairment.

Additional Information Complete prescribing information for this medication should be consulted for additional detail.

Dosage Forms Excipient information presented when available (limited, particularly for generics); consult specific product labeling. [DSC] = Discontinued product

Caplet:
- Allerest® Allergy and Sinus Relief, Ornex®: Acetaminophen 325 mg and pseudoephedrine hydrochloride 30 mg
- Genapap™ Sinus Maximum Strength [DSC], Mapap Sinus Maximum Strength, Ornex® Maximum Strength, Tylenol® Sinus Daytime: Acetaminophen 500 mg and pseudoephedrine hydrochloride 30 mg

Capsule, liquid:
- Sudafed® Multi-Symptom Sinus and Cold: Acetaminophen 325 mg and pseudoephedrine hydrochloride 30 mg [contains sodium 16 mg]

Gelcap:
- Tylenol® Sinus Daytime: Acetaminophen 500 mg and pseudoephedrine hydrochloride 30 mg

Liquid:
- Childrens Tylenol® Cold Daytime: Acetaminophen 160 mg and pseudoephedrine hydrochloride 15 mg per 5 mL (120 mL) [contains sodium benzoate; fruit flavor]

Liquid, oral [drops]:
- Infants Tylenol® Cold: Acetaminophen 80 mg and pseudoephedrine 7.5 mg per 0.8 mL [contains sodium benzoate; bubble gum flavor] [DSC]

Tablet:
- Medi-Synal: Acetaminophen 325 mg and pseudoephedrine hydrochloride 30 mg
- Oranyl Plus: Acetaminophen 500 mg and pseudoephedrine hydrochloride 30 mg

Acetaminophen and Tramadol
(a seet a MIN oh fen & TRA ma dole)

U.S. Brand Names Ultracet®

Canadian Brand Names Tramacet

Index Terms APAP and Tramadol; Tramadol Hydrochloride and Acetaminophen

Pharmacologic Category Analgesic, Miscellaneous; Analgesic, Opioid

Use Short-term (≤5 days) management of acute pain

Pregnancy Risk Factor C

Medication Safety Issues

Sound-alike/look-alike issues:

Ultracet® may be confused with Ultane®, Ultram®

Duplicate therapy issues: This product contains acetaminophen, which may be a component of other combination products. Do not exceed the maximum recommended daily dose of acetaminophen.

Dosage Oral: Adults: Acute pain: Two tablets every 4-6 hours as needed for pain relief (maximum: 8 tablets/day); treatment should not exceed 5 days

Dosage adjustment in renal impairment: Cl_{cr} <30 mL/minute: Maximum of 2 tablets every 12 hours; treatment should not exceed 5 days

Dosage adjustment in hepatic impairment: Use is not recommended.

Additional Information Complete prescribing information for this medication should be consulted for additional detail.

Dosage Forms Excipient information presented when available (limited, particularly for generics); consult specific product labeling.

Tablet: Acetaminophen 325 mg and tramadol hydrochloride 37.5 mg

Acetaminophen, Aspirin, and Caffeine

(a seet a MIN oh fen, AS pir in, & KAF een)

U.S. Brand Names Excedrin® Extra Strength [OTC]; Excedrin® Migraine [OTC]; Fem-Prin® [OTC]; Genaced™ [OTC]; Goody's® Extra Strength Headache Powder [OTC]; Goody's® Extra Strength Pain Relief [OTC]; Pain-Off [OTC]; Vanquish® Extra Strength Pain Reliever [OTC]

Index Terms Aspirin, Acetaminophen, and Caffeine; Aspirin, Caffeine and Acetaminophen; Caffeine, Acetaminophen, and Aspirin; Caffeine, Aspirin, and Acetaminophen

Pharmacologic Category Analgesic, Miscellaneous

Use Relief of mild-to-moderate pain; mild-to-moderate pain associated with migraine headache

Pregnancy Risk Factor D

Medication Safety Issues

Sound-alike/look-alike issues:

Excedrin® may be confused with Dexatrim®, Dexedrine®

Duplicate therapy issues: This product contains acetaminophen, which may be a component of other combination products. Do not exceed the maximum recommended daily dose of acetaminophen.

Dosage Oral: Adults:

Analgesic:

Based on **acetaminophen** component:

Mild-to-moderate pain: 325-650 mg every 4-6 hours as needed; do **not** exceed 4 g/day

Mild-to-moderate pain associated with migraine headache: 500 mg/dose (in combination with 500 mg aspirin and 130 mg caffeine) every 6 hours while symptoms persist; do not use for longer than 48 hours

Based on **aspirin** component:

Mild-to-moderate pain: 325-650 mg every 4-6 hours as needed; do **not** exceed 4 g/day

Mild-to-moderate pain associated with migraine headache: 500 mg/dose (in combination with 500 mg acetaminophen and 130 mg caffeine) every 6 hours while symptoms persist; do not use for longer than 48 hours

Product labeling:

Excedrin® Extra Strength, Excedrin® Migraine: Children >12 years and Adults: 2 doses every 6 hours (maximum: 8 doses/24 hours)

Note: When used for migraine, do not use for longer than 48 hours

Goody's® Extra Strength Headache Powder: Children >12 years and Adults: 1 powder, placed on tongue or dissolved in water, every 4-6 hours (maximum: 4 powders/24 hours)

Goody's® Extra Strength Pain Relief Tablets: Children >12 years and Adults: 2 tablets every 4-6 hours (maximum: 8 tablets/24 hours)

Vanquish® Extra Strength Pain Reliever: Children >12 years and Adults: 2 tablets every 4 hours (maximum: 12 tablets/24 hours)

Dosing adjustment in hepatic impairment: Use with caution. Limited, low-dose therapy is usually well tolerated in hepatic disease/cirrhosis; however, cases of hepatotoxicity at daily acetaminophen dosages <4 g/day have been reported. Avoid chronic use in hepatic impairment.

Additional Information Complete prescribing information for this medication should be consulted for additional detail.

Dosage Forms Excipient information presented when available (limited, particularly for generics); consult specific product labeling.

Caplet:

Excedrin® Extra Strength, Excedrin® Migraine: Acetaminophen 250 mg, aspirin 250 mg, and caffeine 65 mg

Vanquish® Extra Strength Pain Reliever: Acetaminophen 194 mg, aspirin 227 mg, and caffeine 33 mg

Geltab (Excedrin® Extra Strength, Excedrin® Migraine): Acetaminophen 250 mg, aspirin 250 mg, and caffeine 65 mg

Powder (Goody's® Extra Strength Headache Powder): Acetaminophen 260 mg, aspirin 520 mg, and caffeine 32.5 mg [contains lactose]

Tablet:

Excedrin® Extra Strength, Excedrin® Migraine, Genaced™, Pain-Off: Acetaminophen 250 mg, aspirin 250 mg, and caffeine 65 mg

Fem-Prin®: Acetaminophen 194.4 mg, aspirin 226.8 mg, and caffeine 32.4 mg

Goody's® Extra Strength Pain Relief: Acetaminophen 130 mg, aspirin 260 mg, and caffeine 16.25 mg

◆ **Acetaminophen, Butalbital, and Caffeine** *see* Butalbital, Acetaminophen, and Caffeine *on page* 229

Acetaminophen, Chlorpheniramine, and Pseudoephedrine

(a seet a MIN oh fen, klor fen IR a meen, & soo doe e FED rin)

U.S. Brand Names Actifed® Cold and Sinus [OTC]; Comtrex® Flu Therapy Nighttime [OTC]; Drinex [OTC]; Kolephrin® [OTC]; Sinutab® Sinus Allergy Maximum Strength [OTC]; Tylenol® Children's Plus Cold Nighttime [OTC] [DSC]

Canadian Brand Names Sinutab® Sinus & Allergy; Tylenol® Allergy Sinus

Index Terms Acetaminophen, Pseudoephedrine, and Chlorpheniramine; Chlorpheniramine, Acetaminophen, and Pseudoephedrine; Chlorpheniramine, Pseudoephedrine, and Acetaminophen; Pseudoephedrine, Acetaminophen, and Chlorpheniramine; Pseudoephedrine, Chlorpheniramine, and Acetaminophen

Pharmacologic Category Alpha/Beta Agonist; Analgesic, Miscellaneous; Histamine H_1 Antagonist; Histamine H_1 Antagonist, First Generation

Use Temporary relief of sinus symptoms

Pregnancy Risk Factor B

Medication Safety Issues

Sound-alike/look-alike issues:

Thera-Flu® may be confused with Tamiflu®, Thera-Flur-N®

Tylenol® may be confused with atenolol, timolol, Tuinal®, Tylox®

Duplicate therapy issues: This product contains acetaminophen, which may be a component of other combination products. Do not exceed the maximum recommended daily dose of acetaminophen.

Dosage Oral:

Analgesic: Based on **acetaminophen** component:

Children: 10-15 mg/kg/dose every 4-6 hours as needed; do **not** exceed 5 doses in 24 hours

Adults: 325-650 mg every 4-6 hours as needed; do **not** exceed 4 g/day

Antihistamine: Based on **chlorpheniramine maleate** component:

Children:

2-6 years: 1 mg every 4-6 hours (maximum: 6 mg/24 hours)

6-12 years: 2 mg every 4-6 hours (maximum: 12 mg/24 hours)

Children >12 years and Adults: 4 mg every 4-6 hours (maximum: 24 mg/24 hours)

Decongestant: Based on **pseudoephedrine** component:

Children:

2-6 years: 15 mg every 4 hours (maximum: 90 mg/24 hours)

6-12 years: 30 mg every 4 hours (maximum: 180 mg/24 hours)

Children >12 years and Adults: 60 mg every 4 hours (maximum: 360 mg/24 hours)

Product labeling:

Sinutab® Sinus Allergy Maximum Strength: Children >12 years and Adults: 2 tablets/caplets every 6 hours (maximum: 8 doses/24 hours)

Dosing adjustment in hepatic impairment: Use with caution. Limited, low-dose therapy is usually well tolerated in hepatic disease/cirrhosis; however, cases of hepatotoxicity at daily acetaminophen dosages <4 g/day have been reported. Avoid chronic use in hepatic impairment.

Additional Information Complete prescribing information for this medication should be consulted for additional detail.

Dosage Forms Excipient information presented when available (limited, particularly for generics); consult specific product labeling. [DSC] = Discontinued product

Caplet: Acetaminophen 325 mg, chlorpheniramine maleate 2 mg, and pseudoephedrine hydrochloride 30 mg

Actifed® Cold and Sinus, Sinutab® Sinus Allergy Maximum Strength: Acetaminophen 500 mg, chlorpheniramine maleate 2 mg, and pseudoephedrine hydrochloride 30 mg

Kolephrin®: Acetaminophen 325 mg, chlorpheniramine maleate 2 mg, and pseudoephedrine hydrochloride 30 mg

Liquid:

Comtrex® Flu Therapy Nighttime: Acetaminophen 100 mg, chlorpheniramine maleate 4 mg, and pseudoephedrine hydrochloride 60 mg per 30 mL (240 mL) [contains alcohol; cherry flavor]

Tylenol® Children's Plus Cold Nighttime: Acetaminophen 160 mg, chlorpheniramine maleate 1 mg, and pseudoephedrine hydrochloride 15 mg per 5 mL (120 mL) [contains sodium benzoate; grape flavor] [DSC]

Tablet:

Drinex: Acetaminophen 650 mg, chlorpheniramine maleate 4 mg, and pseudoephedrine hydrochloride 60 mg

Acetaminophen, Dextromethorphan, and Phenylephrine

(a seet a MIN oh fen, deks troe meth OR fan, & fen il EF rin)

U.S. Brand Names Alka-Seltzer Plus® Day Cold [OTC]; Little Colds® Multi-Symptom Cold Formula [OTC] [DSC]; Mapap® Multi-Symptom Cold [OTC]; Tylenol® Cold Head Congestion Daytime [OTC]; Tylenol® Cold Multi-Symptom Daytime [OTC]; Tylenol® Plus Infants Cold & Cough [OTC] [DSC]; Vicks® DayQuil® Cold/Flu Multi-Symptom Relief [OTC]

Index Terms Dextromethorphan Hydrobromide, Acetaminophen, and Phenylephrine Hydrochloride; Phenylephrine, Acetaminophen, and Dextromethorphan; Phenylephrine, Dextromethorphan, and Acetaminophen

Pharmacologic Category Analgesic, Miscellaneous; Antitussive; Decongestant

Use Temporary relief of common cold and flu symptoms (eg, pain, fever, cough, congestion)

Medication Safety Issues

Duplicate therapy issues: This product contains acetaminophen, which may be a component of other combination products. Do not exceed the maximum recommended daily dose of acetaminophen.

Dosage Product labeling: Oral:

Alka-Seltzer Plus® Day Cold: Children ≥12 years and Adults: 2 capsules or 20 mL every 4 hours (maximum: 6 doses/24 hours)

Tylenol® Cold Head Congestion Daytime: Children ≥12 years and Adults: 2 caplets every 4 hours (maximum: 6 doses/24 hours)

Tylenol® Cold Multi-Symptom Daytime: Children ≥12 years and Adults: 2 caplets/gelcaps or 30 mL every 4 hours (maximum: 6 doses/24 hours)

Vicks® DayQuil® Cold/Flu Multi-Symptom Relief Liqui-Caps: Children ≥12 years and Adults: 2 capsules every 4 hours (maximum: 6 doses/24 hours)

Vicks® DayQuil® Cold/Flu Multi-Symptom Relief Liquid:

Children 6-11 years: 15 mL every 4 hours, up to 5 doses/day (maximum: 75 mL/24 hours)

Children ≥12 years and Adults: 30 mL every 4 hours (maximum: 6 doses/24 hours)

Dosing adjustment in hepatic impairment: Use with caution. Limited, low-dose therapy is usually well tolerated in hepatic disease/cirrhosis; however, cases of hepatotoxicity at daily acetaminophen dosages <4 g/day have been reported. Avoid chronic use in hepatic impairment.

Additional Information Complete prescribing information for this medication should be consulted for additional detail.

Dosage Forms Excipient information presented when available (limited, particularly for generics); consult specific product labeling. [DSC] = Discontinued product

Caplet:

Mapap® Multi-Symptom Cold: Acetaminophen 325 mg, dextromethorphan hydrobromide 10 mg, and phenylephrine hydrochloride 5 mg

Tylenol® Cold Head Congestion Daytime: Acetaminophen 325 mg, dextromethorphan hydrobromide 10 mg, and phenylephrine hydrochloride 5 mg [Cool Burst™ flavor]

Tylenol® Cold Multi-Symptom Daytime: Acetaminophen 325 mg, dextromethorphan hydrobromide 10 mg, and phenylephrine hydrochloride 5 mg [Cool Burst™ flavor]

Capsule, liquid gel:
Alka-Seltzer Plus® Day Cold: Acetaminophen 325 mg, dextromethorphan hydrobromide 10 mg, and phenylephrine hydrochloride 5 mg
Capsule, liquicap:
Vicks® DayQuil® Cold/Flu Multi-Symptom Relief: Acetaminophen 325 mg, dextromethorphan hydrobromide 10 mg, and phenylephrine hydrochloride 5 mg
Gelcap:
Tylenol® Cold Multi-Symptom Daytime: Acetaminophen 325 mg, dextromethorphan hydrobromide 10 mg, and phenylephrine hydrochloride 5 mg
Liquid:
Alka-Seltzer Plus® Day Cold: Acetaminophen 162.5 mg, dextromethorphan hydrobromide 5 mg, and phenylephrine hydrochloride 2.5 mg per 5 mL (180 mL) [alcohol free; contains sodium 3 mg/5 mL, propylene glycol, and sodium benzoate; berry flavor]
Tylenol® Cold Multi-Symptom Daytime: Acetaminophen 325 mg, dextromethorphan hydrobromide 10 mg, and phenylephrine hydrochloride 5 mg per 15 mL (240 mL) [contains sodium 5 mg/15 mL, sodium benzoate, and propylene glycol; Citrus Burst™ flavor]
Vicks® DayQuil® Cold/Flu Multi-Symptom Relief: Acetaminophen 325 mg, dextromethorphan hydrobromide 10 mg, and phenylephrine hydrochloride 5 mg per 15 mL (180 mL, 300 mL) [contains sodium 71 mg/15 mL and propylene glycol]
Liquid [drops]:
Little Colds® Multi-Symptom Cold Formula: Acetaminophen 80 mg, dextromethorphan hydrobromide 2.5 mg, and phenylephrine hydrochloride 1.25 mg per 1 mL (15 mL) [alcohol free, dye free; contains propylene glycol and sodium benzoate; berry flavor] [DSC]
Tylenol® Plus Infants Cold & Cough: Acetaminophen 80 mg, dextromethorphan hydrobromide 2.5 mg, and phenylephrine hydrochloride 1.25 mg per 0.8 mL (15 mL) [contains sodium benzoate; cherry flavor] [DSC]

Acetaminophen, Dextromethorphan, and Pseudoephedrine

(a seet a MIN oh fen, deks troe meth OR fan, & soo doe e FED rin)

U.S. Brand Names Tylenol® Cold Day Non-Drowsy [OTC]; Tylenol® Flu Non-Drowsy Maximum Strength [OTC]

Canadian Brand Names Contac® Complete; Contac® Cough, Cold and Flu Day & Night™; Sudafed® Cold & Cough Extra Strength; Tylenol® Cold Daytime

Index Terms Dextromethorphan, Acetaminophen, and Pseudoephedrine; Pseudoephedrine, Acetaminophen, and Dextromethorphan; Pseudoephedrine, Dextromethorphan, and Acetaminophen

Pharmacologic Category Alpha/Beta Agonist; Analgesic, Miscellaneous; Antitussive

Use Treatment of mild-to-moderate pain and fever; symptomatic relief of cough and congestion

Medication Safety Issues

Sound-alike/look-alike issues:
Sudafed® may be confused with Sufenta®
Thera-Flu® may be confused with Tamiflu®, Thera-Flur-N®
Tylenol® may be confused with atenolol, timolol, Tuinal®, Tylox®

Duplicate therapy issues: This product contains acetaminophen, which may be a component of other combination products. Do not exceed the maximum recommended daily dose of acetaminophen.

Dosage Oral:

Analgesic: Based on acetaminophen component:
Children: 10-15 mg/kg/dose every 4-6 hours as needed; do **not** exceed 5 doses/24 hours
Adults: 325-650 mg every 4-6 hours as needed; do **not** exceed 4 g/day

Cough suppressant: Based on dextromethorphan component:
Children 6-12 years: 15 mg every 6-8 hours; do **not** exceed 60 mg/24 hours
Children >12 years and Adults: 10-20 mg every 4-8 hours **or** 30 mg every 8 hours; do **not** exceed 120 mg/24 hours

Decongestant: Based on pseudoephedrine component:
Children:
2-6 years: 15 mg every 4 hours (maximum: 90 mg/24 hours)
6-12 years: 30 mg every 4 hours (maximum: 180 mg/24 hours)
Children >12 years and Adults: 60 mg every 4 hours (maximum: 360 mg/24 hours)

Product labeling:
Tylenol® Cold Non-Drowsy:
Children 6-11 years: 1 dose every 6 hours (maximum: 4 doses/24 hours)
Children ≥12 years and Adults: 2 doses every 6 hours (maximum: 8 doses/24 hours)
Tylenol® Flu Non-Drowsy Maximum Strength: Children >12 years and Adults: 2 doses every 6 hours (maximum: 8 doses/24 hours)

Dosing adjustment in hepatic impairment: Use with caution. Limited, low-dose therapy is usually well tolerated in hepatic disease/cirrhosis; however, cases of hepatotoxicity at daily acetaminophen dosages <4 g/day have been reported. Avoid chronic use in hepatic impairment.

Additional Information Complete prescribing information for this medication should be consulted for additional detail.

Dosage Forms Excipient information presented when available (limited, particularly for generics); consult specific product labeling.

Caplet:
Tylenol® Cold Day Non-Drowsy: Acetaminophen 325 mg dextromethorphan hydrobromide 15 mg, and pseudoephedrine hydrochloride 30 mg
Gelcap:
Tylenol® Flu Non-Drowsy Maximum Strength: Acetaminophen 500 mg, dextromethorphan hydrobromide 15 mg, and pseudoephedrine hydrochloride 30 mg

◆ **Acetaminophen, Dichloralphenazone, and Isometheptene** *see* Acetaminophen, Isometheptene, and Dichloralphenazone *on page 34*

Acetaminophen, Diphenhydramine, and Phenylephrine

(a seet a MIN oh fen, dye fen HYE dra meen, & fen il EF rin)

U.S. Brand Names Benadryl® Allergy and Cold [OTC]; Benadryl® Allergy and Sinus Headache [OTC]; Children's Tylenol® Plus Cold and Allergy [OTC]; Sudafed PE® Nighttime Cold [OTC]; Sudafed PE® Severe Cold [OTC]; Tylenol® Allergy Multi-Symptom Nighttime [OTC]

Index Terms Acetaminophen, Phenylephrine, and Diphenhydramine; Diphenhydramine, Phenylephrine Hydrochloride, and Acetaminophen; Phenylephrine Hydrochloride, Acetaminophen, and Diphenhydramine

Pharmacologic Category Analgesic, Miscellaneous; Decongestant; Histamine H_1 Antagonist

Use Temporary relief of symptoms of hay fever and the common cold, including: sinus/nasal congestion and pain/pressure, headache, sneezing, runny nose, itchy/watery eyes, sore throat, cough, and minor aches and pains

Medication Safety Issues

Duplicate therapy issues: This product contains acetaminophen, which may be a component of combination products. Do not exceed the maximum recommended daily dose of acetaminophen.

Dosage Oral: General dosing guidelines; refer to specific product labeling:

Hay fever/cold symptoms:

Children 6-11 years (Benadryl® Allergy and Cold, Benadryl® Allergy and Sinus Headache, Sudafed PE® Severe Cold): One caplet every 4 hours as needed; maximum: 5 caplets/24 hours

Children 6-11 years; 48-95 lbs (Children's Tylenol® Plus Cold and Allergy): 10 mL every 4 hours as needed; maximum: 5 doses/24 hours

Children ≥12 years and Adults (Benadryl® Allergy and Cold, Benadryl® Allergy and Sinus Headache, Sudafed PE® Nighttime Cold, Sudafed PE® Severe Cold, Tylenol® Allergy Multi-Symptom Nighttime): Two caplets every 4 hours as needed; maximum: 12 caplets/24 hours

Additional Information Complete prescribing information for this medication should be consulted for additional detail.

Dosage Forms Excipient information presented when available (limited, particularly for generics); consult specific product labeling.

Caplet:

Benadryl® Allergy and Cold, Benadryl® Allergy and Sinus Headache, Sudafed PE® Severe Cold: Acetaminophen 325 mg, diphenhydramine hydrochloride 12.5 mg and phenylephrine hydrochloride 5 mg

Sudafed PE® Nighttime Cold: Acetaminophen 325 mg, diphenhydramine hydrochloride 25 mg and phenylephrine hydrochloride 5 mg

Tylenol® Allergy Multi-Symptom Nighttime: Acetaminophen 325 mg, diphenhydramine hydrochloride 25 mg and phenylephrine hydrochloride 5 mg [Cool Burst™ flavor]

Liquid:

Children's Tylenol® Plus Cold and Allergy: Acetaminophen 160 mg, Diphenhydramine 12.5 mg, and phenylephrine 2.5 mg per 5 mL (120 mL) [contains sodium benzoate; bubble gum flavor]

Acetaminophen, Isometheptene, and Dichloralphenazone

(a seet a MIN oh fen, eye soe me THEP teen, & dye KLOR al FEN a zone)

U.S. Brand Names Amidrine [DSC]; Duradrin® [DSC]; Midrin®; Migquin [DSC]; Migratine; Migrazone® [DSC]; Migrin-A [DSC]

Index Terms Acetaminophen, Dichloralphenazone, and Isometheptene; Dichloralphenazone, Acetaminophen, and Isometheptene; Dichloralphenazone, Isometheptene, and Acetaminophen; Isometheptene, Acetaminophen, and Dichloralphenazone; Isometheptene, Dichloralphenazone, and Acetaminophen

Pharmacologic Category Analgesic, Miscellaneous

Use Relief of migraine and tension headache

Restrictions C-IV

Medication Safety Issues

Sound-alike/look-alike issues:

Midrin® may be confused with Mydfrin®

Duplicate therapy issues: This product contains acetaminophen, which may be a component of other combination products. Do not exceed the maximum recommended daily dose of acetaminophen.

Dosage Oral: Adults:

Migraine headache: 2 capsules to start, followed by 1 capsule every hour until relief is obtained (maximum: 5 capsules/12 hours)

Tension headache: 1-2 capsules every 4 hours (maximum: 8 capsules/24 hours)

Dosing adjustment in hepatic impairment: Use with caution. Limited, low-dose therapy is usually well tolerated in hepatic disease/cirrhosis; however, cases of hepatotoxicity at daily acetaminophen dosages <4 g/day have been reported. Avoid chronic use in hepatic impairment.

Additional Information Complete prescribing information for this medication should be consulted for additional detail.

Dosage Forms Excipient information presented when available (limited, particularly for generics); consult specific product labeling. [DSC] = Discontinued product

Capsule: Acetaminophen 325 mg, isometheptene mucate 65 mg, dichloralphenazone 100 mg [DSC]

Amidrine [DSC], Duradrin® [DSC], Midrin®, Migquin [DSC], Migrazone® [DSC], Migratine, Migrin-A [DSC]: Acetaminophen 325 mg, isometheptene mucate 65 mg, and dichloralphenazone 100 mg

- **Acetaminophen, Phenylephrine, and Diphenhydramine** *see* Acetaminophen, Diphenhydramine, and Phenylephrine *on page 33*
- **Acetaminophen, Pseudoephedrine, and Chlorpheniramine** *see* Acetaminophen, Chlorpheniramine, and Pseudoephedrine *on page 31*
- **Acetasol® HC** *see* Acetic Acid, Propylene Glycol Diacetate, and Hydrocortisone *on page 35*

AcetaZOLAMIDE (a set a ZOLE a mide)

U.S. Brand Names Diamox® Sequels®

Canadian Brand Names Apo-Acetazolamide®; Diamox®

Pharmacologic Category Anticonvulsant, Miscellaneous; Carbonic Anhydrase Inhibitor; Diuretic, Carbonic Anhydrase Inhibitor; Ophthalmic Agent, Antiglaucoma

Additional Appendix Information

Glaucoma Drug Therapy *on page 1808*

Sulfonamide Derivatives *on page 1671*

Use Treatment of glaucoma (chronic simple open-angle, secondary glaucoma, preoperatively in acute angle-closure); drug-induced edema or edema due to congestive heart failure (adjunctive therapy); centrencephalic epilepsies (immediate release dosage form); prevention or amelioration of symptoms associated with acute mountain sickness

Unlabeled/Investigational Use Metabolic alkalosis; respiratory stimulant in COPD; urine alkalinization

Pregnancy Risk Factor C

Medication Safety Issues

Sound-alike/look-alike issues:

AcetaZOLAMIDE may be confused with acetoHEXAMIDE

Diamox® Sequels® may be confused with Diabinese®, Dobutrex®, Trimox®

Dosage Note: I.M. administration is not recommended because of pain secondary to the alkaline pH

Children:

Glaucoma:

Oral: 8-30 mg/kg/day or 300-900 mg/m^2/day divided every 8 hours

I.V.: 20-40 mg/kg/24 hours divided every 6 hours, not to exceed 1 g/day

Edema: Oral, I.V.: 5 mg/kg or 150 mg/m^2 once every day

Epilepsy: Oral: 8-30 mg/kg/day in 1-4 divided doses, not to exceed 1 g/day; extended release capsule is not recommended for treatment of epilepsy

Adults:

Glaucoma:

Chronic simple (open-angle): Oral: 250 mg 1-4 times/day or 500 mg extended release capsule twice daily

Secondary, acute (closed-angle): I.V.: 250-500 mg, may repeat in 2-4 hours to a maximum of 1 g/day

Edema: Oral, I.V.: 250-375 mg once daily

Epilepsy: Oral: 8-30 mg/kg/day in 1-4 divided doses; not to exceed 1 g/day; **extended release capsule is not recommended for treatment of epilepsy**

Metabolic alkalosis (unlabeled use): I.V. 250 mg every 6 hours for 4 doses or 500 mg single dose; reassess need based upon acid-base status

Mountain sickness: Oral: 250 mg every 8-12 hours (or 500 mg extended release capsules every 12-24 hours)

Therapy should begin 24-48 hours before and continue during ascent and for at least 48 hours after arrival at the high altitude

Note: In situations of rapid ascent (such as rescue or military operations), 1000 mg/day is recommended.

Urine alkalinization (unlabeled use): Oral: 5 mg/kg/dose repeated 2-3 times over 24 hours

Respiratory stimulant in COPD (unlabeled use): Oral, I.V.: 250 mg twice daily

Elderly: Oral: Initial: 250 mg twice daily; use lowest effective dose

Dosing adjustment in renal impairment:

Cl_{cr} 10-50 mL/minute: Administer every 12 hours

Cl_{cr} <10 mL/minute: Avoid use (ineffective)

Hemodialysis: Moderately dialyzable (20% to 50%)

Peritoneal dialysis: Supplemental dose is not necessary

Additional Information Complete prescribing information for this medication should be consulted for additional detail.

Dosage Forms Excipient information presented when available (limited, particularly for generics); consult specific product labeling.

Capsule, extended release:

Diamox® Sequels®: 500 mg

Injection, powder for reconstitution: 500 mg

Tablet: 125 mg, 250 mg

Acetic Acid (a SEE tik AS id)

Index Terms Ethanoic Acid

Pharmacologic Category Otic Agent, Anti-infective; Topical Skin Product

Use Irrigation of the bladder; treatment of superficial bacterial infections of the external auditory canal

Pregnancy Risk Factor C

Medication Safety Issues

Sound-alike/look-alike issues:

VoSol® may be confused with Vexol®

Dosage

Irrigation (**Note:** Dosage of an irrigating solution depends on the capacity or surface area of the structure being irrigated):

For continuous irrigation of the urinary bladder with 0.25% acetic acid irrigation, the rate of administration will approximate the rate of urine flow; usually 500-1500 mL/24 hours

For periodic irrigation of an indwelling urinary catheter to maintain patency, about 50 mL of 0.25% acetic acid irrigation is required

Otic: Insert saturated wick; keep moist 24 hours; remove wick and instill 5 drops 3-4 times/day

Additional Information Complete prescribing information for this medication should be consulted for additional detail.

Dosage Forms Excipient information presented when available (limited, particularly for generics); consult specific product labeling.

Solution for irrigation: 0.25% (250 mL, 500 mL, 1000 mL)

Solution, otic: 2% (15 mL)

◆ **Acetic Acid, Hydrocortisone, and Propylene Glycol Diacetate** *see* Acetic Acid, Propylene Glycol Diacetate, and Hydrocortisone *on page 35*

Acetic Acid, Propylene Glycol Diacetate, and Hydrocortisone

(a SEE tik AS id, PRO pa leen GLY kole dye AS e tate, & hye droe KOR ti sone)

U.S. Brand Names Acetasol® HC; VoSol® HC

Index Terms Acetic Acid, Hydrocortisone, and Propylene Glycol Diacetate; Hydrocortisone, Acetic Acid, and Propylene Glycol Diacetate; Propylene Glycol Diacetate, Acetic Acid, and Hydrocortisone

Pharmacologic Category Otic Agent, Anti-infective

Use Treatment of superficial infections of the external auditory canal caused by organisms susceptible to the action of the antimicrobial, complicated by swelling

Medication Safety Issues

Sound-alike/look-alike issues:

VoSol® may be confused with Vexol®

Dosage Children ≥3 years and Adults: Otic: Instill 3-5 drops in ear(s) every 4-6 hours

Additional Information Complete prescribing information for this medication should be consulted for additional detail.

Dosage Forms Excipient information presented when available (limited, particularly for generics); consult specific product labeling.

Solution, otic [drops]:

Acetasol® HC, VoSol® HC: Acetic acid 2%, propylene glycol diacetate 3%, and hydrocortisone 1% (10 mL)

◆ **Acetoxymethylprogesterone** *see* MedroxyPROGESTERone *on page 930*

Acetylcholine (a se teel KOE leen)

U.S. Brand Names Miochol®-E

Canadian Brand Names Miochol®-E

Index Terms Acetylcholine Chloride

Pharmacologic Category Cholinergic Agonist; Ophthalmic Agent, Miotic

Use Produces complete miosis in cataract surgery, keratoplasty, iridectomy, and other anterior segment surgery where rapid miosis is required

Pregnancy Risk Factor C

Pregnancy Considerations Acetylcholine is used primarily in the eye and there are no reports of its use in pregnancy. Because it is ionized at physiologic pH, transplacental passage would not be expected.

Medication Safety Issues

Sound-alike/look-alike issues:

Acetylcholine may be confused with acetylcysteine

Contraindications Hypersensitivity to acetylcholine chloride or any component of the formulation; acute iritis and acute inflammatory disease of the anterior chamber

Warnings/Precautions During cataract surgery, use only after lens is in place. Systemic effects rarely occur but can cause problems for patients with acute cardiac failure, bronchial asthma, peptic ulcer, hyperthyroidism, GI spasm, urinary tract obstruction, and Parkinson's disease; open under aseptic conditions only. Safety and efficacy have not been established in children.

Adverse Reactions Frequency not defined.

Cardiovascular: Bradycardia, flushing, hypotension

Central nervous system: Headache
Ocular: Clouding, corneal edema, decompensation
Respiratory: Dyspnea
Miscellaneous: Diaphoresis

Drug Interactions

Avoid Concomitant Use There are no known interactions where it is recommended to avoid concomitant use.

Increased Effect/Toxicity

The levels/effects of Acetylcholine may be increased by:
Acetylcholinesterase Inhibitors

Decreased Effect There are no known significant interactions involving a decrease in effect.

Stability Store unopened vial at 4°C to 25°C (39°F to 77°F); prevent from freezing. Prepare solution immediately before use and discard unused portion. Acetylcholine solutions are unstable; reconstitute immediately before use.

Mechanism of Action Causes contraction of the sphincter muscles of the iris, resulting in miosis and contraction of the ciliary muscle, leading to accommodation spasm

Pharmacodynamics/Kinetics

Onset of action: Rapid
Duration: ~10 minutes

Dosage Adults: Intraocular: 0.5-2 mL of 1% injection (5-20 mg) instilled into anterior chamber before or after securing one or more sutures

Administration Open under aseptic conditions only. Attach filter before irrigating eye.

Dosage Forms Excipient information presented when available (limited, particularly for generics); consult specific product labeling.

Powder for solution, intraocular, as chloride:
Miochol®-E: 1:100 [20 mg; packaged with diluent (2 mL)]

◆ **Acetylcholine Chloride** *see* Acetylcholine *on page 35*

Acetylcysteine (a se teel SIS teen)

U.S. Brand Names Acetadote®

Canadian Brand Names Acetylcysteine Solution; Mucomyst®; Parvolex®

Index Terms *N*-Acetyl-L-cysteine; *N*-Acetylcysteine; Acetylcysteine Sodium; Mercapturic Acid; Mucomyst; NAC

Pharmacologic Category Antidote; Mucolytic Agent

Use Antidote for acute acetaminophen toxicity, adjunctive mucolytic therapy in patients with abnormal or viscid mucous secretions in acute and chronic bronchopulmonary diseases; pulmonary complications of surgery and cystic fibrosis; diagnostic bronchial studies

Unlabeled/Investigational Use Prevention of contrast-induced renal dysfunction (oral, I.V.); distal intestinal obstruction syndrome (DIOS, previously referred to as meconium ileus equivalent)

Pregnancy Risk Factor B

Pregnancy Considerations Based on limited reports using acetylcysteine to treat acetaminophen overdose in pregnant women, acetylcysteine has been shown to cross the placenta and may provide protective levels in the fetus.

Lactation Excretion in breast milk unknown/use caution

Medication Safety Issues

Sound-alike/look-alike issues:
Acetylcysteine may be confused with acetylcholine
Mucomyst® may be confused with Mucinex®

Contraindications Hypersensitivity to acetylcysteine or any component of the formulation

Warnings/Precautions

Inhalation: Since increased bronchial secretions may develop after inhalation, percussion, postural drainage, and suctioning should follow. If bronchospasm occurs, administer a bronchodilator; discontinue acetylcysteine if bronchospasm progresses.

Intravenous: Acute flushing and erythema have been reported; usually occurs within 30-60 minutes and may resolve spontaneously. Serious anaphylactoid reactions have also been reported. Acetylcysteine infusion may be interrupted until treatment of allergic symptoms is initiated; the infusion can then be carefully restarted. Treatment for anaphylactic reactions should be immediately available. Use caution with asthma or history of bronchospasm.

Acetaminophen overdose: The modified Rumack-Matthew nomogram allows for stratification of patients into risk categories based on the relationship between the serum acetaminophen level and time after ingestion. There are several situations where the nomogram is of limited use. Serum acetaminophen levels obtained prior to 4-hour postingestion are not interpretable; patients presenting late may have undetectable serum concentrations, but have received a lethal dose. The nomogram is less predictive in a chronic ingestion or in an overdose with an extended release product. Acetylcysteine should be administered for any signs of hepatotoxicity even if acetaminophen serum level is low or undetectable. The nomogram also does not take into account patients at higher risk of acetaminophen toxicity (eg, alcoholics, malnourished patients).

Adverse Reactions

Inhalation: Frequency not defined.

Central nervous system: Drowsiness, chills, fever
Gastrointestinal: Vomiting, nausea, stomatitis
Local: Irritation, stickiness on face following nebulization
Respiratory: Bronchospasm, rhinorrhea, hemoptysis
Miscellaneous: Acquired sensitization (rare), clamminess, unpleasant odor during administration

Intravenous:

>10%: Miscellaneous: Anaphylactoid reaction (~17%; reported as severe in 1% or moderate in 10% of patients within 15 minutes of first infusion; severe in 1% or mild to moderate in 6% to 7% of patients after 60-minute infusion)

1% to 10%:

Cardiovascular: Angioedema (2% to 8%), vasodilation (1% to 6%), hypotension (1% to 4%), tachycardia (1% to 4%), syncope (1% to 3%), chest tightness (1%), flushing (1%)
Central nervous system: Dysphoria (<1% to 2%)
Dermatologic: Urticaria (2% to 7%), rash (1% to 5%), facial erythema (≤1%), palmar erythema (≤1%), pruritus (≤1% to 3%), pruritus with rash and vasodilation (2% to 9%)
Gastrointestinal: Vomiting (<1% to 10%), nausea (1% to 10%), dyspepsia (≤1%)
Neuromuscular & skeletal: Gait disturbance (<1% to 2%)
Ocular: Eye pain (<1% to 3%)
Otic: Ear pain (1%)
Respiratory: Bronchospasm (1% to 6%), cough (1% to 4%), dyspnea (<1% to 3%), pharyngitis (1%), rhinorrhea (1%), rhonchi (1%), throat tightness (1%)
Miscellaneous: Diaphoresis (≤1%)

Drug Interactions

Avoid Concomitant Use There are no known interactions where it is recommended to avoid concomitant use.

Increased Effect/Toxicity There are no known significant interactions involving an increase in effect.

Decreased Effect There are no known significant interactions involving a decrease in effect.

Stability

Solution for injection (Acetadote®): Store vials at room temperature, 20°C to 25°C (68°F to 77°F). Following reconstitution with D_5W, solution is stable for 24 hours at room temperature. A color change may occur in opened vials (light purple) and does not affect the safety or efficacy.

Loading dose: Dilute 150 mg/kg in D_5W 200 mL.

Initial maintenance dose: Dilute 50 mg/kg in D_5W 500 mL.

Second maintenance dose: Dilute 100 mg/kg in D_5W 1000 mL.

Note: To avoid fluid overload in patients <40 kg and those requiring fluid restriction, decrease volume of D_5W proportionally. Discard unused portion.

Solution for inhalation (Mucomyst®): Store unopened vials at room temperature; once opened, store under refrigeration and use within 96 hours. The 20% solution may be diluted with sodium chloride or sterile water; the 10% solution may be used undiluted. A color change may occur in opened vials (light purple) and does not affect the safety or efficacy.

Intravenous administration of solution for inhalation (unlabeled route): Using D_5W, dilute acetylcysteine 20% oral solution to a 3% solution.

Mechanism of Action Exerts mucolytic action through its free sulfhydryl group which opens up the disulfide bonds in the mucoproteins thus lowering mucous viscosity. The exact mechanism of action in acetaminophen toxicity is unknown; thought to act by providing substrate for conjugation with the toxic metabolite. The presumed mechanism in preventing contrast-induced nephropathy is its ability to scavenge oxygen-derived free radicals and improve endothelium-dependent vasodilation.

Pharmacodynamics/Kinetics

Onset of action: Inhalation: 5-10 minutes

Duration: Inhalation: >1 hour

Distribution: 0.47 L/kg

Protein binding, plasma: 83%

Half-life elimination:

Reduced acetylcysteine: 2 hours

Total acetylcysteine: Adults: 5.5 hours; Newborns: 11 hours

Time to peak, plasma: Oral: 1-2 hours

Excretion: Urine

Dosage

Acetaminophen poisoning: Children and Adults:

Oral: 140 mg/kg; followed by 17 doses of 70 mg/kg every 4 hours; repeat dose if emesis occurs within 1 hour of administration; therapy should continue until acetaminophen levels are undetectable and there is no evidence of hepatotoxicity.

I.V. (Acetadote®): Loading dose: 150 mg/kg over 60 minutes; **Note:** Extended infusion time recommended by manufacturer as of February, 2006. Loading dose is followed by 2 additional infusions: Initial maintenance dose of 50 mg/kg infused over 4 hours, followed by a second maintenance dose of 100 mg/kg infused over 16 hours. Total dosage: 300 mg/kg administered over 21 hours.

Patients <40 kg: Reduce fluid volume according to the following table.

Acetadote® Dosing / Fluid Volume Guidelines for Patients <40 kg

Body Weight (kg)	Loading Dose 150 mg/kg over 1 h		Second Dose 50 mg/kg over 4 h		Third Dose 100 mg/kg over 16 h	
	Acetadote® (mL)	D_5W (mL)	Acetadote® (mL)	D_5W (mL)	Acetadote® (mL)	D_5W (mL)
30	22.5	100	7.5	250	15	500
25	18.75	100	6.25	250	12.5	500
20	15	60	5	140	10	280
15	11.25	45	3.75	105	7.5	210
10	7.5	30	2.5	70	5	140

Note: If commercial I.V. form is unavailable, the following dose has been reported using solution for oral inhalation (unlabeled): Loading dose: 140 mg/kg, followed by 70 mg/kg every 4 hours, for a total of 13 doses (loading dose and 48 hours of treatment); infuse each dose over 1 hour through a 0.2 micron Millipore filter (in-line).

Shorter treatment courses have been proposed (Woo, 2000), however, only the full course of therapy is currently FDA approved

Adjuvant therapy in respiratory conditions: **Note:** Patients should receive an aerosolized bronchodilator 10-15 minutes prior to acetylcysteine.

Inhalation, nebulization (face mask, mouth piece, tracheostomy): Acetylcysteine 10% and 20% solution (dilute 20% solution with sodium chloride or sterile water for inhalation); 10% solution may be used undiluted

Infants: 1-2 mL of 20% solution or 2-4 mL of 10% solution until nebulized given 3-4 times/day

Children and Adults: 3-5 mL of 20% solution or 6-10 mL of 10% solution until nebulized given 3-4 times/day; dosing range: 1-10 mL of 20% solution or 2-20 mL of 10% solution every 2-6 hours

Inhalation, nebulization (tent, croupette): Children and Adults: Dose must be individualized; may require up to 300 mL solution/treatment

Direct instillation: Adults:

Into tracheostomy: 1-2 mL of 10% to 20% solution every 1-4 hours

Through percutaneous intratracheal catheter: 1-2 mL of 20% or 2-4 mL of 10% solution every 1-4 hours via syringe attached to catheter

Diagnostic bronchogram: Nebulization or intratracheal: Adults: 1-2 mL of 20% solution or 2-4 mL of 10% solution administered 2-3 times prior to procedure

Prevention of contrast-induced nephropathy (CIN) (unlabeled use): Adults: Oral: 600-1200 mg twice daily for 2 days (beginning the day before the procedure); may be given as powder in capsules (some centers use solution, diluted in cola beverage or juice)

Prevention of CIN in acute MI patients requiring emergent cardiac catheterization (unlabeled use): Adults: I.V.: 1200 mg over 5-10 minutes prior to cardiac catheterization, followed by 1200 mg **orally** twice daily for 48 hours

Administration

Inhalation: Acetylcysteine is incompatible with tetracyclines, erythromycin, amphotericin B, iodized oil, chymotrypsin, trypsin, and hydrogen peroxide. Administer separately. Intermittent aerosol treatments are commonly given when patient arises, before meals, and just before retiring at bedtime.

Oral: For treatment of acetaminophen overdosage, administer orally as a 5% solution. Dilute the 20% solution 1:3 with a cola, orange juice, or other soft drink. Use within 1 hour of preparation. Unpleasant odor becomes less noticeable as treatment progresses. If patient vomits within 1 hour of dose, readminister.

I.V.: Intravenous formulation (Acetadote®): Administer loading dose of 150 mg/kg over 60 minutes (see **"Note"**), followed by 2 separate maintenance infusions: 50 mg/kg over 4 hours followed by 100 mg/kg over 16 hours. If not using commercially available I.V. formulation, use a 0.2-µ millipore filter (in-line).

Note: Extended infusion time recommended by manufacturer as of February, 2006.

For use with CIN prevention for emergent cardiac catheterization (unlabeled use): Intravenous formulation (Acetadote®): Administer 1200 mg I.V. push over 5-10 minutes prior to contrast administration.

Monitoring Parameters Acetaminophen overdose: AST, ALT, bilirubin, PT, serum creatinine, BUN, serum glucose, and electrolytes. Acetaminophen levels at ~4 hours postingestion (every 4-6 hours if extended release acetaminophen; plot on the nomogram) and every 4-6 hours to assess serum levels, and LFTs for possible hepatotoxicity. Assess patient for nausea, vomiting, and skin rash following oral administration for treatment of acetaminophen poisoning. If administered I.V., monitor for anaphylaxis/anaphylactoid reactions.

Reference Range Determine acetaminophen level as soon as possible, but no sooner than 4 hours after ingestion (to ensure peak levels have been obtained); administer for acetaminophen level >150 mcg/mL at 4 hours following ingestion; toxic concentration with probable hepatotoxicity: >200 mcg/mL at 4 hours or 50 mcg at 12 hours

Dosage Forms Excipient information presented when available (limited, particularly for generics); consult specific product labeling.

Injection, solution:

Acetadote®: 20% (30 mL) [200 mg/mL; contains disodium edetate]

Solution, inhalation/oral: 10% (4 mL, 10 mL, 30 mL) [100 mg/mL]; 20% (4 mL, 10 mL, 30 mL) [200 mg/mL]

◆ **Acetylcysteine Sodium** *see* Acetylcysteine *on page 36*

◆ **Acetylcysteine Solution (Can)** *see* Acetylcysteine *on page 36*

◆ **Acetylsalicylic Acid** *see* Aspirin *on page 142*

◆ **Achromycin** *see* Tetracycline *on page 1451*

◆ **Aciclovir** *see* Acyclovir *on page 40*

◆ **Acid Gone [OTC]** *see* Aluminum Hydroxide and Magnesium Carbonate *on page 75*

◆ **Acid Gone Extra Strength [OTC]** *see* Aluminum Hydroxide and Magnesium Carbonate *on page 75*

◆ **Acid Reducer (Can)** *see* Ranitidine *on page 1295*

◆ **Acid Reducer Maximum Strength Non Prescription (Can)** *see* Ranitidine *on page 1295*

◆ **Acidulated Phosphate Fluoride** *see* Fluoride *on page 635*

◆ **Acilac (Can)** *see* Lactulose *on page 847*

◆ **AcipHex®** *see* Rabeprazole *on page 1285*

◆ **Acitfed® Cold & Allergy [OTC]** ***[reformulation]*** *see* Chlorpheniramine and Phenylephrine *on page 309*

Acitretin (a si TRE tin)

U.S. Brand Names Soriatane® CK Convenience Kit™; Soriatane® [DSC]

Canadian Brand Names Soriatane®

Pharmacologic Category Retinoid-Like Compound

Use Treatment of severe psoriasis

Restrictions An FDA-approved medication guide must be distributed when dispensing an outpatient prescription (new or refill) where this medication is to be used without direct supervision of a healthcare provider. Medication guides are available at http://www.fda.gov/cder/Offices/ODS/medication_guides.htm.

Pregnancy Risk Factor X

Pregnancy Considerations Acitretin is teratogenic in humans. Severe birth defects have been reported when conception occurred during treatment or after therapy was complete. **[U.S. Boxed Warning]: Not for use by women who want to become pregnant;** patient should not get pregnant for at least 3 years after discontinuation. In addition, because ethanol forms a teratogenic metabolite and would increase the duration of teratogenic potential, ethanol should not be consumed during treatment or for 2 months after discontinuation. Limited amounts of acitretin are found in seminal fluid; although it appears this poses little risk to a fetus, the actual risk of teratogenicity is not known. Any pregnancy which occurs during treatment, or within 3 years after treatment is discontinued, should be reported to the manufacturer at 1-888-500-3376 or to the FDA at 1-800-FDA-1088.

Lactation Enters breast milk/not recommended

Medication Safety Issues

Sound-alike/look-alike issues:

Soriatane® may be confused with Loxitane®

Contraindications Hypersensitivity to acitretin, other retinoids, or any component of the formulation; patients who are pregnant or intend on becoming pregnant; ethanol ingestion; severe hepatic or renal dysfunction; chronically-elevated blood lipid levels; concomitant use with methotrexate or tetracyclines

Acitretin is contraindicated in females of childbearing potential unless all of the following conditions apply.

1) Patient has severe psoriasis unresponsive to other therapy or if clinical condition contraindicates other treatments.
2) Patient must have two negative urine or serum pregnancy tests prior to therapy.
3) Patient must have pregnancy test repeated monthly during therapy. After discontinuation of therapy, a pregnancy test must be repeated every 3 months for at least 3 years.
4) Patient must commit to using two effective forms of birth control starting 1 month prior to acitretin treatment and for 3 years after discontinuation. Prescriber must counsel patient about contraception every month during therapy and every 3 months following discontinuation for at least 3 years.
5) Patient is reliable in understanding and carrying out instructions.
6) Patient has received, and acknowledged, understanding of a careful oral and printed explanation of the hazards of fetal exposure to acitretin and the risk of possible contraception failure; this explanation may include showing a line drawing to the patient of an infant with the characteristic external deformities resulting from retinoid exposure during pregnancy. Patient must sign an agreement/informed consent document stating that she understands these risks and that she should not consume ethanol during therapy or for 2 months after discontinuation.
7) All patients (male and female) should not donate blood during and for 3 years following treatment with acitretin.

Warnings/Precautions [U.S. Boxed Warning]: Not for use by women who want to become pregnant; patient should not get pregnant for at least 3 years after discontinuation. The Do Your P.A.R.T. (Pregnancy Prevention Actively Required During and After Treatment) program explains teratogenic risks and requirements expected of females of childbearing potential to prevent pregnancies from occurring during use and 3 years following discontinuation; this should be used to educate patients and healthcare providers. **[U.S. Boxed Warning]: All patients (male and female) should abstain from ethanol or ethanol-containing products during therapy and for 2 months after discontinuation. [U.S. Boxed Warning]: All patients should be advised not to donate blood during therapy or for 3 years following completion of therapy. [U.S. Boxed Warning]: Changes in transaminases occur in up to 1/3 of patients.** Monitor for hepatotoxicity; discontinue if significant elevations of liver enzymes occur. Use with caution in patients at risk of hypertriglyceridemias. Lipid changes including, increased triglycerides, increased cholesterol, and decreased HDL are common (up to 66%). Rarely associated with pseudotumor cerebri. Discontinue if visual changes occur. May cause a decrease in night vision or decreased tolerance to contact lenses. Patients receiving long-term treatment should be periodically examined for bony abnormalities. Depression, including thoughts of self-harm have been reported. May be photosensitizing; minimize sun or other UV exposure to treated areas. **[U.S. Boxed**

Warning]: All patients must be provided with a medication guide each time acitretin is dispensed. Female patients must also sign an informed consent prior to therapy. Safety and efficacy for pediatric patients have not been established; growth potential may be affected.

Adverse Reactions

>10%:

Central nervous system: Hyperesthesia (10% to 25%)

Dermatologic: Cheilitis (>75%), alopecia (50% to 75%), skin peeling (50% to 75%), dry skin (25% to 50%), nail disorder (25% to 50%), pruritus (25% to 50%), erythematous rash (10% to 25%), skin atrophy (10% to 25%), sticky skin (10% to 25%), paronychia (10% to 25%)

Endocrine & metabolic: Hypercholesterolemia (25% to 50%), hypertriglyceridemia (50% to 75%), HDL decreased (25% to 50%), phosphorus increased (10% to 25%), potassium increased (10% to 25%), sodium increased (10% to 25%), magnesium increased/decreased (10% to 25%), fasting blood sugar increased (25% to 50%), fasting blood sugar decreased (10% to 25%)

Gastrointestinal: Xerostomia (10% to 25%)

Hematologic: Reticulocytes increased (25% to 50%), hematocrit decreased (10% to 25%), hemoglobin decreased (10% to 25%), WBC increased/decreased (10% to 25%), haptoglobin increased (10% to 25%), neutrophils increased (10% to 25%)

Hepatic: Liver function tests increased (25% to 50%), alkaline phosphatase increased (10% to 25%), direct bilirubin increased (10% to 25%), GGTP increased (10% to 25%)

Neuromuscular & skeletal: Paresthesia (10% to 25%), arthralgia (10% to 25%), rigors (10% to 25%), CPK increased (25% to 50%), spinal hyperostosis progression (10% to 25%)

Ocular: Xerophthalmia (10% to 25%),

Renal: Uric acid increased (10% to 25%), acetonuria (10% to 25%), hematuria (10% to 25%), RBC in urine (10% to 25%)

Respiratory: Rhinitis (25% to 50%), epistaxis (10% to 25%)

1% to 10%:

Cardiovascular: Flushing, edema

Central nervous system: Headache, pain, depression, insomnia, somnolence, fatigue

Dermatologic: Skin odor, hair texture change, bullous eruption, dermatitis, diaphoresis increased, psoriasiform rash, purpura, pyogenic granuloma, rash, seborrhea, ulcers, fissures, sunburn

Endocrine & metabolic: Hot flashes, potassium decreased, phosphorus decreased, sodium decreased, calcium increased or decreased, chloride increased or decreased

Gastrointestinal: Gingival bleeding, gingivitis, saliva increased, stomatitis, thirst, ulcerative stomatitis, abdominal pain, diarrhea, nausea, taste disturbance, anorexia, appetite increased, tongue disorder

Hepatic: Total bilirubin increased

Neuromuscular & skeletal: Arthritis, back pain, hypertonia, myalgia, osteodynia, peripheral joint hyperostosis, Bell's palsy

Ocular: Blurred vision, blepharitis, conjunctivitis, night blindness, photophobia, corneal epithelial abnormality, eye pain, eyebrow or eyelash loss, diplopia, cataract

Otic: Earache, tinnitus

Renal: BUN increased, creatinine increased, glycosuria, proteinuria

Respiratory: Sinusitis

<1% (Limited to important or life-threatening): Anxiety, bleeding time increased, chest pain, cirrhosis, conjunctival hemorrhage, constipation, corneal ulceration, cyanosis, deafness, diplopia, dizziness, dyspepsia, dysphonia, dysuria, eczema, esophagitis, fever, furunculosis, gastritis, glossitis, gum hyperplasia, hair discoloration, healing impaired, hemorrhage, hepatic dysfunction, hepatitis, hyperkeratosis, hypertrichosis, hypoesthesia, intermittent claudication, itchy eyes, jaundice, leukorrhea, malaise, melena, MI, moniliasis, myopathy, nervousness, neuritis, pancreatitis, papilledema, peripheral ischemia, photosensitivity, pseudotumor cerebri, scleroderma, skin fragility or thinning, spinal hyperostosis (new lesion), stroke, taste loss, tendonitis, thromboembolism

Drug Interactions

Avoid Concomitant Use

Avoid concomitant use of Acitretin with any of the following: Alcohol (Ethyl); Contraceptive (Progestins); Methotrexate; Tetracycline Derivatives

Increased Effect/Toxicity

Acitretin may increase the levels/effects of: Methotrexate

The levels/effects of Acitretin may be increased by: Alcohol (Ethyl); Tetracycline Derivatives; Vitamin A

Decreased Effect

Acitretin may decrease the levels/effects of: Contraceptive (Progestins); Oral Contraceptive (Estrogens); Oral Contraceptive (Progestins)

Ethanol/Nutrition/Herb Interactions Ethanol: Use leads to formation of etretinate, a teratogenic metabolite with a prolonged half-life; concomitant use of ethanol or ethanol-containing products is contraindicated.

Stability Store between 15°C to 25°C (59°F to 77°F); avoid high temperatures and humidity. Protect from light.

Pharmacodynamics/Kinetics Etretinate has been detected in serum for up to 3 years following therapy, possibly due to storage in adipose tissue.

Onset of action: May take 2-3 months for full effect; improvement may be seen within 8 weeks.

Absorption: Oral: ~72% absorbed when given with food

Protein binding: >99% bound, primarily to albumin

Metabolism: Metabolized to *cis*-acitretin; both compounds are further metabolized. Concomitant ethanol use leads to the formation of etretinate (active).

Half-life elimination: Acitretin: 49 hours (range: 33-96); *cis*-acitretin: 63 hours (range: 28-157); etretinate: 120 days (range: 84-168 days)

Excretion: Feces (34% to 54%); urine (16% to 53%)

Dosage Oral: Adults: Individualization of dosage is required to achieve maximum therapeutic response while minimizing side effects

Initial therapy: Therapy should be initiated at 25-50 mg/day, given as a single dose with the main meal

Maintenance doses of 25-50 mg/day may be given after initial response to treatment; the maintenance dose should be based on clinical efficacy and tolerability

Dietary Considerations Administer with food. Avoid ingestion of additional sources of exogenous vitamin A (in excess of RDA); use of ethanol and ethanol-containing products is contraindicated.

Monitoring Parameters Lipid profile (baseline and at 1- to 2-week intervals for 4-8 weeks); liver function tests (baseline, and at 1- to 2-week intervals until stable, then as clinically indicated); blood glucose in patients with diabetes; bone abnormalities (with long-term use)

Additional Information Female patients are required to use two forms of birth control, at least one of which is a primary form, unless they have undergone a hysterectomy or are postmenopausal. Both forms of birth control must be used simultaneously for at least 1 month prior to therapy and for at least 3 years after discontinuation. Primary forms of birth control include tubal ligation, partner's vasectomy, IUD, or hormonal birth control products. Microdosed progestin products, referred to as "mini-pills," have been shown to be less effective when used with acitretin, and are not recommended. Secondary forms of contraception include diaphragms, latex condoms and cervical caps, all if used with a spermicide.

Dosage Forms Excipient information presented when available (limited, particularly for generics); consult specific product labeling. [DSC] = Discontinued product

Capsule:

Soriatane®: 10 mg [DSC], 25 mg [DSC]

Soriatane® CK Convenience Kit™: 10 mg, 25 mg [packaged with VersaFoam-EF™]

- **Aclaro PD™** *see* Hydroquinone *on page 749*
- **Aclasta® (Can)** *see* Zoledronic Acid *on page 1587*
- **Aclovate®** *see* Alclometasone *on page 53*

Acrivastine and Pseudoephedrine

(AK ri vas teen & soo doe e FED rin)

U.S. Brand Names Semprex®-D

Index Terms Pseudoephedrine Hydrochloride and Acrivastine

Pharmacologic Category Alpha/Beta Agonist; Histamine H_1 Antagonist; Histamine H_1 Antagonist, Second Generation

Use Temporary relief of nasal congestion, decongest sinus openings, running nose, itching of nose or throat, and itchy, watery eyes due to hay fever or other upper respiratory allergies

Pregnancy Risk Factor B

Dosage Oral: Adults: 1 capsule 3-4 times/day

Dosing comments in renal impairment: Do not use

Additional Information Complete prescribing information for this medication should be consulted for additional detail.

Dosage Forms Excipient information presented when available (limited, particularly for generics); consult specific product labeling.

Capsule:

Semprex®-D: Acrivastine 8 mg and pseudoephedrine hydrochloride 60 mg

- **ACT** *see* DACTINomycin *on page 390*
- **ACT® [OTC]** *see* Fluoride *on page 635*
- **Act-D** *see* DACTINomycin *on page 390*
- **ActHIB®** *see Haemophilus* b Conjugate Vaccine *on page 718*
- **Acthrel®** *see* Corticorelin *on page 370*
- **Acticin®** *see* Permethrin *on page 1176*
- **Actidose-Aqua® [OTC]** *see* Charcoal *on page 299*
- **Actidose® with Sorbitol [OTC]** *see* Charcoal *on page 299*
- **Actifed® (Can)** *see* Triprolidine and Pseudoephedrine *on page 1522*
- **Actifed® Cold and Sinus [OTC]** *see* Acetaminophen, Chlorpheniramine, and Pseudoephedrine *on page 31*
- **Actigall®** *see* Ursodiol *on page 1534*
- **Actimmune®** *see* Interferon Gamma-1b *on page 809*
- **Actinomycin** *see* DACTINomycin *on page 390*
- **Actinomycin D** *see* DACTINomycin *on page 390*
- **Actinomycin CI** *see* DACTINomycin *on page 390*
- **Actiq®** *see* FentaNYL *on page 610*
- **Activase®** *see* Alteplase *on page 72*
- **Activase® rt-PA (Can)** *see* Alteplase *on page 72*
- **Activated Carbon** *see* Charcoal *on page 299*
- **Activated Charcoal** *see* Charcoal *on page 299*
- **Activated Ergosterol** *see* Ergocalciferol *on page 538*
- **Activated Protein C, Human, Recombinant** *see* Drotrecogin Alfa *on page 496*
- **Activella®** *see* Estradiol and Norethindrone *on page 558*
- **Actonel®** *see* Risedronate *on page 1321*
- **Actonel® and Calcium** *see* Risedronate and Calcium *on page 1323*
- **Actoplus Met™** *see* Pioglitazone and Metformin *on page 1198*
- **Actos®** *see* Pioglitazone *on page 1195*
- **ACT® Plus [OTC]** *see* Fluoride *on page 635*
- **ACT® x2™ [OTC]** *see* Fluoride *on page 635*
- **Acular®** *see* Ketorolac *on page 841*
- **Acular LS™** *see* Ketorolac *on page 841*
- **Acular® PF** *see* Ketorolac *on page 841*
- **ACV** *see* Acyclovir *on page 40*
- **Acycloguanosine** *see* Acyclovir *on page 40*

Acyclovir

(ay SYE kloe veer)

U.S. Brand Names Zovirax®

Canadian Brand Names Apo-Acyclovir®; Gen-Acyclovir; Nu-Acyclovir; ratio-Acyclovir; Zovirax®

Index Terms Aciclovir; ACV; Acycloguanosine

Pharmacologic Category Antiviral Agent; Antiviral Agent, Topical

Additional Appendix Information

Guidelines for the Prevention of Opportunistic Infections in HIV Infected Persons *on page 1740*

Treatment of Sexually Transmitted Infections *on page 1773*

Use Treatment of genital herpes simplex virus (HSV), herpes labialis (cold sores), herpes zoster (shingles), HSV encephalitis, neonatal HSV, mucocutaneous HSV in immunocompromised patients, varicella-zoster (chickenpox)

Unlabeled/Investigational Use Prevention of HSV reactivation in HIV-positive patients; prevention of HSV reactivation in hematopoietic stem cell transplant (HSCT); prevention of HSV reactivation during periods of neutropenia in patients with acute leukemia

Pregnancy Risk Factor B

Pregnancy Considerations Teratogenic effects were not observed in animal studies. Acyclovir has been shown to cross the human placenta. There are no adequate and well-controlled studies in pregnant women. Results from a pregnancy registry, established in 1984 and closed in 1999, did not find an increase in the number of birth defects with exposure to acyclovir when compared to those expected in the general population. However, due to the small size of the registry and lack of long-term data, the manufacturer recommends using during pregnancy with caution and only when clearly needed. Data from the pregnancy registry may be obtained from GlaxoSmithKline.

Lactation Enters breast milk/use with caution (AAP rates "compatible")

Medication Safety Issues

Sound-alike/look-alike issues:

Zovirax® may be confused with Zostrix®, Zyvox®

International issues:

Opthavir® [Mexico] may be confused with Optivar® which is a brand name for azelastine in the U.S.

Contraindications Hypersensitivity to acyclovir, valacyclovir, or any component of the formulation

Warnings/Precautions Use with caution in immunocompromised patients; thrombocytopenic purpura/hemolytic uremic syndrome (TTP/HUS) has been reported. Use caution in the elderly, pre-existing renal disease, or in those receiving other nephrotoxic drugs. Renal failure (sometimes fatal) has been reported. Maintain adequate hydration during oral or intravenous therapy. Use I.V.

preparation with caution in patients with underlying neurologic abnormalities, serious hepatic or electrolyte abnormalities, or substantial hypoxia.

Safety and efficacy of oral formulations have not been established in pediatric patients <2 years of age.

Varicella-zoster: Treatment should begin within 24 hours of appearance of rash; oral route not recommended for routine use in otherwise healthy children with varicella, but may be effective in patients at increased risk of moderate to severe infection (>12 years of age, chronic cutaneous or pulmonary disorders, long-term salicylate therapy, corticosteroid therapy).

Genital herpes: Physical contact should be avoided when lesions are present; transmission may also occur in the absence of symptoms. Treatment should begin with the first signs or symptoms.

Herpes labialis: For external use only to the lips and face; do not apply to eye or inside the mouth or nose. Treatment should begin with the first signs or symptoms.

Herpes zoster: Acyclovir should be started within 72 hours of appearance of rash to be effective.

Adverse Reactions

Systemic: Oral:

>10%: Central nervous system: Malaise (12%)

1% to 10%:

Central nervous system: Headache (2%)

Gastrointestinal: Nausea (2% to 5%), vomiting (3%), diarrhea (2% to 3%)

Systemic: Parenteral:

1% to 10%:

Dermatologic: Hives (2%), itching (2%), rash (2%)

Gastrointestinal: Nausea/vomiting (7%)

Hepatic: Liver function tests increased (1% to 2%)

Local: Inflammation at injection site or phlebitis (9%)

Renal: BUN increased (5% to 10%), creatinine increased (5% to 10%), acute renal failure

Topical:

>10%: Dermatologic: Mild pain, burning, or stinging (ointment 30%)

1% to 10%: Dermatologic: Pruritus (ointment 4%), itching

All forms: <1% (Limited to important or life-threatening): Abdominal pain, aggression, agitation, alopecia, anaphylaxis, anemia, angioedema, anorexia, ataxia, coma, confusion, consciousness decreased, delirium, desquamation, diarrhea, disseminated intravascular coagulopathy (DIC), dizziness, dry lips, dysarthria, encephalopathy, erythema multiforme, fatigue, fever, gastrointestinal distress, hallucinations, hematuria, hemolysis, hepatitis, hyperbilirubinemia, hypotension, insomnia, jaundice, leukocytoclastic vasculitis, leukocytosis, leukopenia, local tissue necrosis (following extravasation), lymphadenopathy, mental depression, myalgia, neutrophilia, paresthesia, peripheral edema, photosensitization, pruritus, psychosis, renal failure, seizure, somnolence, sore throat, Stevens-Johnson syndrome, thrombocytopenia, thrombocytopenic purpura/hemolytic uremic syndrome (TTP/HUS), thrombocytosis, toxic epidermal necrolysis, tremor, urticaria, visual disturbances

Drug Interactions

Avoid Concomitant Use

Avoid concomitant use of Acyclovir with any of the following: Zoster Vaccine

Increased Effect/Toxicity

Acyclovir may increase the levels/effects of: Mycophenolate; Tenofovir; Zidovudine

The levels/effects of Acyclovir may be increased by: Mycophenolate

Decreased Effect

Acyclovir may decrease the levels/effects of: Zoster Vaccine

Ethanol/Nutrition/Herb Interactions Food: Does not affect absorption of oral acyclovir.

Stability

Capsule, tablet: Store at controlled room temperature of 15°C to 25°C (59°F to 77°F); protect from moisture.

Cream, suspension: Store at controlled room temperature of 15°C to 25°C (59°F to 77°F).

Ointment: Store at controlled room temperature of 15°C to 25°C (59°F to 77°F) in a dry place.

Injection: Store powder at controlled room temperature of 15°C to 25°C (59°F to 77°F). Reconstitute acyclovir 500 mg with SWFI 10 mL; do not use bacteriostatic water containing benzyl alcohol or parabens. For intravenous infusion, dilute to a final concentration ≤7 mg/mL. Concentrations >10 mg/mL increase the risk of phlebitis. Reconstituted solutions remain stable for 12 hours at room temperature. Do not refrigerate reconstituted solutions as they may precipitate. Once diluted for infusion, use within 24 hours.

Mechanism of Action Acyclovir is converted to acyclovir monophosphate by virus-specific thymidine kinase then further converted to acyclovir triphosphate by other cellular enzymes. Acyclovir triphosphate inhibits DNA synthesis and viral replication by competing with deoxyguanosine triphosphate for viral DNA polymerase and being incorporated into viral DNA.

Pharmacodynamics/Kinetics

Absorption: Oral: 15% to 30%

Distribution: V_d: 0.8 L/kg (63.6 L): Widely (eg, brain, kidney, lungs, liver, spleen, muscle, uterus, vagina, CSF)

Protein binding: 9% to 33%

Metabolism: Converted by viral enzymes to acyclovir monophosphate, and further converted to diphosphate then triphosphate (active form) by cellular enzymes

Bioavailability: Oral: 10% to 20% with normal renal function (bioavailability decreases with increased dose)

Half-life elimination: Terminal: Neonates: 4 hours; Children 1-12 years: 2-3 hours; Adults: 3 hours

Time to peak, serum: Oral: Within 1.5-2 hours

Excretion: Urine (62% to 90% as unchanged drug and metabolite)

Dosage Note: Obese patients should be dosed using ideal body weight

Genital HSV:

I.V.: Children ≥12 years and Adults (immunocompetent): Initial episode, severe: 5 mg/kg every 8 hours for 5-7 days

Oral:

Children:

Initial episode (unlabeled use): 40-80 mg/kg/day divided into 3-4 doses for 5-10 days (maximum: 1 g/day)

Chronic suppression (unlabeled use; limited data): 80 mg/kg/day in 3 divided doses (maximum: 1 g/day), re-evaluate after 12 months of treatment

Adults:

Initial episode: 200 mg every 4 hours while awake (5 times/day) for 10 days (per manufacturer's labeling); 400 mg 3 times/day for 5-10 days has also been reported

Recurrence: 200 mg every 4 hours while awake (5 times/day) for 5 days (per manufacturer's labeling; begin at earliest signs of disease); 400 mg 3 times/day for 5 days has also been reported

Chronic suppression: 400 mg twice daily or 200 mg 3-5 times/day, for up to 12 months followed by re-evaluation (per manufacturer's labeling); 400-1200 mg/day in 2-3 divided doses has also been reported

Topical: Adults (immunocompromised): Ointment: Initial episode: 1/2" ribbon of ointment for a 4" square surface area every 3 hours (6 times/day) for 7 days

Herpes labialis (cold sores): Topical: Children ≥12 years and Adults: Cream: Apply 5 times/day for 4 days

Herpes zoster (shingles):
Oral: Adults (immunocompetent): 800 mg every 4 hours (5 times/day) for 7-10 days
I.V.:
Children <12 years (immunocompromised): 20 mg/kg/dose every 8 hours for 7 days
Children ≥12 years and Adults (immunocompromised): 10 mg/kg/dose or 500 mg/m^2/dose every 8 hours for 7 days

HSV encephalitis: I.V.:
Children 3 months to 12 years: 20 mg/kg/dose every 8 hours for 10 days (per manufacturer's labeling); dosing for 14-21 days also reported
Children ≥12 years and Adults: 10 mg/kg/dose every 8 hours for 10 days (per manufacturer's labeling); 10-15 mg/kg/dose every 8 hours for 14-21 days also reported

Mucocutaneous HSV:
I.V.:
Children <12 years (immunocompromised): 10 mg/kg/dose every 8 hours for 7 days
Children ≥12 years and Adults (immunocompromised): 5 mg/kg/dose every 8 hours for 7 days (per manufacturer's labeling); dosing for up to 14 days also reported
Oral: Adults (immunocompromised, unlabeled use): 400 mg 5 times a day for 7-14 days
Topical: Ointment: Adults (non-life-threatening, immunocompromised): 1/2" ribbon of ointment for a 4" square surface area every 3 hours (6 times/day) for 7 days

Neonatal HSV: I.V.: Neonate: Birth to 3 months: 10 mg/kg/dose every 8 hours for 10 days (manufacturer's labeling); 15 mg/kg/dose or 20 mg/kg/dose every 8 hours for 14-21 days has also been reported

Varicella-zoster (chickenpox): Begin treatment within the first 24 hours of rash onset:
Oral:
Children ≥2 years and ≤40 kg (immunocompetent): 20 mg/kg/dose (up to 800 mg/dose) 4 times/day for 5 days
Children >40 kg and Adults (immunocompetent): 800 mg/dose 4 times a day for 5 days
I.V.:
Children <1 year (immunocompromised, unlabeled use): 10 mg/kg/dose every 8 hours for 7-10 days
Children ≥1 year and Adults (immunocompromised, unlabeled use): 1500 mg/m^2/day divided every 8 hours or 10 mg/kg/dose every 8 hours for 7-10 days

Prevention of HSV reactivation in HIV-positive patients, for use only when recurrences are frequent or severe (unlabeled use): Oral:
Children: 80 mg/kg/day in 3-4 divided doses
Adults: 200 mg 3 times/day or 400 mg 2 times/day

Prevention of HSV reactivation in HSCT (unlabeled use): Note: Start at the beginning of conditioning therapy and continue until engraftment or until mucositis resolves (~30 days)
Oral: Adults: 200 mg 3 times/day
I.V.:
Children: 250 mg/m^2/dose every 8 hours or 125 mg/m^2/dose every 6 hours
Adults: 250 mg/m^2/dose every 12 hours

Bone marrow transplant recipients (unlabeled use): I.V.: Children and Adults: Allogeneic patients who are HSV and CMV seropositive: 500 mg/m^2/dose (10 mg/kg) every 8 hours; for clinically-symptomatic CMV infection, consider replacing acyclovir with ganciclovir

Dosing adjustment in renal impairment:
Oral:
Cl_{cr} 10-25 mL/minute/1.73 m^2: Normal dosing regimen 800 mg every 4 hours: Administer 800 mg every 8 hours
Cl_{cr} <10 mL/minute/1.73 m^2:
Normal dosing regimen 200 mg every 4 hours, 200 mg every 8 hours, or 400 mg every 12 hours: Administer 200 mg every 12 hours
Normal dosing regimen 800 mg every 4 hours: Administer 800 mg every 12 hours
I.V.:
Cl_{cr} 25-50 mL/minute/1.73 m^2: Administer recommended dose every 12 hours
Cl_{cr} 10-25 mL/minute/1.73 m^2: Administer recommended dose every 24 hours
Cl_{cr} <10 mL/minute/1.73 m^2: Administer 50% of recommended dose every 24 hours
Hemodialysis: Administer dose after dialysis
Continuous ambulatory peritoneal dialysis (CAPD): Administer 50% of normal dose once daily; no supplemental dose needed
Continuous renal replacement therapy (CRRT): Drug clearance is highly dependent on the method of renal replacement, filter type, and flow rate. Appropriate dosing requires close monitoring of pharmacologic response, signs of adverse reactions due to drug accumulation, as well as drug levels in relation to target trough (if appropriate). The following are general recommendations only (based on dialysate flow/ultrafiltration rates of 1 L/hour) and should not supersede clinical judgment:
CVVH or CVVHD/CVVHDF: 5-7.5 mg/kg every 24 hours
Note: The higher dose of 7.5 mg/kg is recommended for infections with CNS involvement (Trotman, 2005).

Dietary Considerations May be taken with or without food. Acyclovir 500 mg injection contains sodium ~50 mg (~2 mEq).

Administration
Oral: May be administered with or without food.
I.V.: Avoid rapid infusion; infuse over 1 hour to prevent renal damage; maintain adequate hydration of patient; check for phlebitis and rotate infusion sites
Topical: Not for use in the eye. Apply using a finger cot or rubber glove to avoid transmission to other parts of the body or to other persons.

Monitoring Parameters Urinalysis, BUN, serum creatinine, liver enzymes, CBC

Dosage Forms Excipient information presented when available (limited, particularly for generics); consult specific product labeling.
Capsule: 200 mg
Zovirax®: 200 mg
Cream, topical:
Zovirax®: 5% (2 g, 5 g)
Injection, powder for reconstitution, as sodium: 500 mg, 1000 mg
Injection, solution, as sodium [preservative free]: 50 mg/mL (10 mL, 20 mL)
Ointment, topical:
Zovirax®: 5% (15 g)
Suspension, oral: 200 mg/5 mL (480 mL)
Zovirax®: 200 mg/5 mL (480 mL) [banana flavor]
Tablet: 400 mg, 800 mg
Zovirax®: 400 mg, 800 mg

◆ **Aczone®** *see* Dapsone *on page* 396

◆ **AD3L** *see* Valrubicin *on page* 1542

◆ **Adacel®** *see* Diphtheria and Tetanus Toxoids, and Acellular Pertussis Vaccine *on page* 463

◆ **Adagen®** *see* Pegademase Bovine *on page 1150*

◆ **Adalat® XL® (Can)** *see* NIFEdipine *on page 1064*

◆ **Adalat® CC** *see* NIFEdipine *on page 1064*

Adalimumab (a da LIM yoo mab)

U.S. Brand Names Humira®

Canadian Brand Names Humira®

Index Terms Antitumor Necrosis Factor Apha (Human); D2E7; Human Antitumor Necrosis Factor Alpha

Pharmacologic Category Antirheumatic, Disease Modifying; Gastrointestinal Agent, Miscellaneous; Monoclonal Antibody; Tumor Necrosis Factor (TNF) Blocking Agent

Use

Treatment of active rheumatoid arthritis (moderate-to-severe) and active psoriatic arthritis; may be used alone or in combination with disease-modifying antirheumatic drugs (DMARDs); treatment of ankylosing spondylitis

Treatment of moderately- to severely-active Crohn's disease in patients with inadequate response to conventional treatment, or patients who have lost response to or are intolerant of infliximab

Treatment of moderate-to-severe plaque psoriasis

Treatment of moderately- to severely-active juvenile idiopathic arthritis

Restrictions An FDA-approved medication guide must be distributed when dispensing an outpatient prescription (new or refill) where this medication is to be used without direct supervision of a healthcare provider. Medication guides are available at http://www.fda.gov/cder/Offices/ODS/medication_guides.htm.

Pregnancy Risk Factor B

Pregnancy Considerations Teratogenic effects were not observed in animal studies, however, there are no adequate and well-controlled studies in pregnant women. Use during pregnancy only if clearly needed. A pregnancy registry has been established to monitor outcomes of women exposed to adalimumab during pregnancy (877-311-8972).

Lactation Excretion in breast milk unknown/not recommended

Medication Safety Issues

Sound-alike/look-alike issues:

Humira® may be confused with Humulin®, Humalog®

Humira® Pen may be confused with HumaPen® Memoir®

Contraindications There are no contraindications listed within the FDA-approved labeling.

Canada labeling: Additional contraindications (not in U.S. labeling): Hypersensitivity to adalimumab or any component of the formulation; severe infection (eg, sepsis, tuberculosis, opportunistic infection)

Warnings/Precautions **[U.S. Boxed Warnings]: Patients should be evaluated for latent tuberculosis infection with a tuberculin skin test prior to therapy. Treatment of latent tuberculosis should be initiated before adalimumab is used. Tuberculosis (disseminated or extrapulmonary) has been reactivated while on adalimumab.** Most cases have been reported within the first 8 months of treatment. Doses higher than recommended are associated with an increased risk for tuberculosis reactivation. **Patients with initial negative tuberculin skin tests should receive continued monitoring for tuberculosis throughout treatment; active tuberculosis has developed in this population during treatment.** Rare reactivation of hepatitis B virus (HBV) has occurred in chronic virus carriers; evaluate prior to initiation, during, and for several months after treatment. Evaluate patients at risk for HBV infection prior to therapy to determine HBV status. Adalimumab may affect defenses against infections and malignancies.

[U.S. Boxed Warning]: Serious and potential fatal infections (including invasive fungal and other opportunistic infections) have been reported in patients receiving TNF-blocking agents, including adalimumab. Cases of unrecognized invasive fungal infections (eg, histoplasmosis, blastomycosis, coccidioidomycosis) have also been reported with anti-TNF agent use. Use caution with chronic infection, history of recurrent infection, or predisposition to infection (eg, diabetes or residence/travel from areas of endemic mycoses). Do not give to patients with an active chronic or localized infection. Many of the serious infections have occurred in patients on concomitant immunosuppressive therapy. Other opportunistic infections included *Aspergillus* and *Nocardia*. Use caution in patients who have resided in regions where histoplasmosis and tuberculosis are endemic. Patients who develop a new infection while undergoing treatment with adalimumab should be monitored closely. If a patient develops a serious infection or sepsis, adalimumab should be discontinued. Rare cases of lymphoma have also been reported in association with adalimumab. A higher incidence of nonmelanoma skin cancers was noted in adalimumab treated patients, when compared to the control group. Impact on the development and course of malignancies is not fully defined.

May exacerbate pre-existing or recent-onset demyelinating CNS disorders. Worsening and new-onset heart failure (HF) has been reported; use caution in patients with decreased left ventricular function. Use caution in patients with HF. Patients should be brought up to date with all immunizations before initiating therapy. No data are available concerning the effects of adalimumab on vaccination. Live vaccines should not be given concurrently. No data are available concerning secondary transmission of live vaccines in patients receiving adalimumab. Rare cases of pancytopenia (including aplastic anemia) have been reported with TNF-blocking agents; with significant hematologic abnormalities, consider discontinuing therapy. Positive antinuclear antibody titers have been detected in patients (with negative baselines) treated with adalimumab. Rare cases of autoimmune disorder, including lupus-like syndrome, have been reported; monitor and discontinue adalimumab if symptoms develop. May cause hypersensitivity reactions, including anaphylaxis; monitor. The packaging (needle cover of prefilled syringe) may contain latex. Product may contain polysorbate 80.

Adverse Reactions

>10%:

Central nervous system: Headache (12%)

Dermatologic: Rash (6% to 12%)

Local: Injection site reaction (12% to 20%; includes erythema, itching, hemorrhage, pain, swelling)

Neuromuscular & skeletal: CPK increased (15%)

Respiratory: Upper respiratory tract infection (17%), sinusitis (11%)

Miscellaneous: Antibodies to adalimumab (3% to 26%; significance unknown), positive ANA (12%)

5% to 10%:

Cardiovascular: Hypertension (5%)

Endocrine & metabolic: Hyperlipidemia (7%), hypercholesterolemia (6%)

Gastrointestinal: Nausea (9%), abdominal pain (7%)

Genitourinary: Urinary tract infection (8%)

Hepatic: Alkaline phosphatase increased (5%)

Local: Injection site reaction (8%; other than erythema, itching, hemorrhage, pain, swelling)

Neuromuscular & skeletal: Back pain (6%)

Renal: Hematuria (5%)

Miscellaneous: Accidental injury (10%), flu-like syndrome (7%)

<5%:

Cardiovascular: Arrhythmia, atrial fibrillation, chest pain, CHF, coronary artery disorder, heart arrest, MI, palpitation, pericardial effusion, pericarditis, peripheral edema, syncope, tachycardia, thrombosis (leg), vascular disorder

Central nervous system: Confusion, fever, hypertensive encephalopathy, multiple sclerosis, subdural hematoma

Dermatologic: Cellulitis, erysipelas

Endocrine & metabolic: Dehydration, menstrual disorder, parathyroid disorder

Gastrointestinal: Diverticulitis, esophagitis, gastroenteritis, gastrointestinal hemorrhage, vomiting

Genitourinary: Cystitis, pelvic pain

Hematologic: Agranulocytosis, granulocytopenia, leukopenia, pancytopenia, paraproteinemia, polycythemia

Hepatic: Cholecystitis, cholelithiasis, hepatic necrosis

Neuromuscular & skeletal: Arthralgia, arthritis, bone fracture, bone necrosis, joint disorder, muscle cramps, myasthenia, pain in extremity, paresthesia, pyogenic arthritis, synovitis, tendon disorder, tremor

Ocular: Cataract

Renal: Kidney calculus, pyelonephritis

Respiratory: Asthma, bronchospasm, dyspnea, lung function decreased, pleural effusion, pneumonia

Miscellaneous: Adenoma, allergic reactions (1%), carcinoma (including breast, gastrointestinal, skin, urogenital), healing abnormality, herpes zoster, ketosis, lupus erythematosus syndrome, lymphoma, melanoma, postsurgical infection, sepsis, tuberculosis (reactivation of latent infection; miliary, lymphatic, peritoneal and pulmonary)

Postmarketing and/or case reports: Anaphylactoid reaction, anaphylaxis, angioneurotic edema, aplastic anemia, cutaneous vasculitis, cytopenia, erythema multiforme, fixed drug eruption, Guillain-Barré syndrome, infections (bacterial, viral, fungal and protozoal), interstitial lung disease (eg, pulmonary fibrosis), intestinal perforation, septic arthritis, thrombocytopenia, transaminases increased, urticaria

Drug Interactions

Avoid Concomitant Use

Avoid concomitant use of Adalimumab with any of the following: Anakinra; Natalizumab; Rilonacept; Vaccines (Live)

Increased Effect/Toxicity

Adalimumab may increase the levels/effects of: Abatacept; Anakinra; Natalizumab; Rilonacept; Vaccines (Live)

The levels/effects of Adalimumab may be increased by: Abciximab; Trastuzumab

Decreased Effect

Adalimumab may decrease the levels/effects of: Vaccines (Inactivated)

The levels/effects of Adalimumab may be decreased by: Echinacea

Ethanol/Nutrition/Herb Interactions Herb/nutraceutical: Echinacea may decrease the therapeutic effects of adalimumab; avoid concurrent use.

Stability Store under refrigeration at 2°C to 8°C (36°F to 46°F); do not freeze. Protect from light.

Mechanism of Action Adalimumab is a recombinant monoclonal antibody that binds to human tumor necrosis factor alpha (TNF-alpha), thereby interfering with binding to TNFα receptor sites and subsequent cytokine-driven inflammatory processes. Elevated TNF levels in the synovial fluid are involved in the pathologic pain and joint destruction in immune-mediated arthritis. Adalimumab decreases signs and symptoms of psoriatic arthritis, rheumatoid arthritis, and ankylosing spondylitis. It inhibits progression of structural damage of rheumatoid and psoriatic arthritis. Reduces signs and symptoms and maintains clinical remission in Crohn's disease; reduces epidermal thickness and inflammatory cell infiltration in plaque psoriasis.

Pharmacodynamics/Kinetics

Distribution: V_d: 4.7-6 L; Synovial fluid concentrations: 31% to 96% of serum

Bioavailability: Absolute: 64%

Half-life elimination: Terminal: ~2 weeks (range 10-20 days)

Time to peak, serum: SubQ: 131 ± 56 hours

Excretion: Clearance increased in the presence of antiadalimumab antibodies; decreased in patients 40 years and older

Dosage SubQ:

Children ≥4 years: Juvenile idiopathic arthritis:

15 kg to <30 kg: 20 mg every other week

≥30 kg: 40 mg every other week

Adults:

Rheumatoid arthritis: 40 mg every other week; may be administered with other DMARDs; patients not taking methotrexate may increase dose to 40 mg every week

Ankylosing spondylitis, psoriatic arthritis: 40 mg every other week

Crohn's disease: Initial: 160 mg given as 4 injections on day 1 or over 2 days, then 80 mg 2 weeks later (day 15); Maintenance: 40 mg every other week beginning day 29

Plaque psoriasis: Initial: 80 mg as a single dose; maintenance: 40 mg every other week beginning 1 week after initial dose

Administration For SubQ injection; rotate injection sites. Do not use if solution is discolored. Do not administer to skin which is red, tender, bruised, or hard; rotate injection sites. Needle cap of the prefilled syringe may contain latex.

Monitoring Parameters Place and read PPD before initiation. Monitor improvement of symptoms and physical function assessments; CBC; signs of infection, bleeding or bruising.

Dosage Forms Excipient information presented when available (limited, particularly for generics); consult specific product labeling.

Injection, solution [pediatric; preservative free]:

Humira®: 20 mg/0.4 mL (0.4 mL) [contains polysorbate 80]

Injection, solution [preservative free]:

Humira®: 40 mg/0.8 mL (0.8 mL) [contains polysorbate 80]

◆ **Adamantanamine Hydrochloride** *see* Amantadine *on page 78*

Adapalene (a DAP a leen)

U.S. Brand Names Differin®

Canadian Brand Names Differin®; Differin® XP

Pharmacologic Category Acne Products; Topical Skin Product, Acne

Use Treatment of acne vulgaris

Pregnancy Risk Factor C

Dosage Topical: Children >12 years and Adults: Apply once daily at bedtime; therapeutic results should be noticed after 8-12 weeks of treatment

Additional Information Complete prescribing information for this medication should be consulted for additional detail.

Dosage Forms Excipient information presented when available (limited, particularly for generics); consult specific product labeling.

Cream, topical:

Differin®: 0.1% (15 g, 45 g)

Gel, topical:

Differin®: 0.1% (15 g, 45 g) [alcohol free]; 0.3% (45 g) [alcohol free]

- ◆ **ADD 234037** *see* Lacosamide *on page 847*
- ◆ **Addaprin [OTC]** *see* Ibuprofen *on page 760*
- ◆ **Adderall®** *see* Dextroamphetamine and Amphetamine *on page 432*
- ◆ **Adderall XR®** *see* Dextroamphetamine and Amphetamine *on page 432*

Adefovir (a DEF o veer)

U.S. Brand Names Hepsera™

Canadian Brand Names Hepsera™

Index Terms Adefovir Dipivoxil; Bis-POM PMEA

Pharmacologic Category Antiretroviral Agent, Reverse Transcriptase Inhibitor (Nucleoside)

Use Treatment of chronic hepatitis B with evidence of active viral replication (based on persistent elevation of ALT/AST or histologic evidence), including patients with lamivudine-resistant hepatitis B

Pregnancy Risk Factor C

Pregnancy Considerations Teratogenic effects were not observed in animal studies. There are no adequate and well-controlled studies in pregnant women. Use in pregnancy only when clearly needed. Pregnant women exposed to adefovir should be registered with the pregnancy registry (800-258-4263).

Lactation Excretion in breast milk unknown/not recommended

Contraindications Hypersensitivity to adefovir or any component of the formulation

Warnings/Precautions [U.S. Boxed Warning]: Use with caution in patients with renal dysfunction or in patients at risk of renal toxicity (including concurrent nephrotoxic agents or NSAIDs). Chronic administration may result in nephrotoxicity. Dosage adjustment is required in adult patients with renal dysfunction or in patients who develop renal dysfunction during therapy; no data available for use in children ≥12 years or adolescents with renal impairment. In patients with lamivudine-resistant HBV, switching to adefovir was associated with a higher risk of adefovir-resistance compared to adding adefovir to lamivudine therapy. Consider alternative therapy in patients who do not respond to adefovir monotherapy treatment. **[U.S. Boxed Warning]: May cause the development of HIV resistance in patients with unrecognized or untreated HIV infection.** Determine HIV status prior to initiating treatment with adefovir. **[U.S. Boxed Warning]: Lactic acidosis and severe hepatomegaly with steatosis (sometimes fatal) have occurred with antiretroviral nucleoside analogues.** Female gender, obesity, and prolonged treatment may increase the risk of hepatotoxicity. Treatment should be discontinued in patients with lactic acidosis or signs/symptoms of hepatotoxicity (which may occur without marked transaminase elevations). **[U.S. Boxed Warning]: Acute exacerbations of hepatitis may occur (in up to 25% of patients) when antihepatitis therapy is discontinued.** Exacerbations typically occur within 12 weeks and may be self-limited or resolve upon resuming treatment; risk may be increased with advanced liver disease or cirrhosis. Monitor patients following discontinuation of therapy. Safety and efficacy in children <12 years of age have not been established.

Adverse Reactions

>10%:

Central nervous system: Headache (24% to 25%)

Gastrointestinal: Abdominal pain (15% to 18%), diarrhea (up to 13%)

Hepatic: Hepatitis exacerbation (up to 25% within 12 weeks of adefovir discontinuation)

Neuromuscular & skeletal: Weakness (13% to 25%)

Renal: Hematuria (grade ≥3: 11%)

1% to 10%:

Dermatologic: Rash, pruritus

Endocrine & metabolic: Hypophosphatemia (<2 mg/dL: 1% and 3% in pre-/post-liver transplant patients, respectively)

Gastrointestinal: Flatulence (up to 8%), dyspepsia (5% to 9%), nausea, vomiting

Renal: Serum creatinine increased (≥0.5 mg/dL: 2% to 3% in compensated liver disease; incidence may be higher in patients with decompensated cirrhosis or in liver transplant recipients), renal failure

Note: In liver transplant patients with baseline renal dysfunction, frequency of increased serum creatinine has been observed to be as high as 32% to 51% at 48 and 96 weeks post-transplantation, respectively; considering the concomitant use of other potentially nephrotoxic medications, baseline renal insufficiency, and predisposing comorbidities, the role of adefovir in these changes could not be established.

Respiratory: Cough (6% to 8%), rhinitis (up to 5%)

Postmarketing and/or case reports: Fanconi syndrome, hepatitis, myopathy, nephrotoxicity, osteomalacia

Drug Interactions

Avoid Concomitant Use There are no known interactions where it is recommended to avoid concomitant use.

Increased Effect/Toxicity

The levels/effects of Adefovir may be increased by: Ganciclovir-Valganciclovir; Ribavirin; Tenofovir

Decreased Effect

Adefovir may decrease the levels/effects of: Tenofovir

Ethanol/Nutrition/Herb Interactions

Ethanol: Should be avoided in hepatitis B infection due to potential hepatic toxicity.

Food: Does not have a significant effect on adefovir absorption.

Stability Store controlled room temperature of 25°C (77°F).

Mechanism of Action Acyclic nucleotide reverse transcriptase inhibitor (adenosine analog) which interferes with HBV viral RNA-dependent DNA polymerase resulting in inhibition of viral replication.

Pharmacodynamics/Kinetics

Distribution: 0.35-0.39 L/kg

Protein binding: ≤4%

Metabolism: Prodrug; rapidly converted to adefovir (active metabolite) in intestine

Bioavailability: 59%

Half-life elimination: 7.5 hours; prolonged in renal impairment

Time to peak: 1.75 hours

Excretion: Urine (45% as active metabolite within 24 hours)

Dosage Oral: Children ≥12 years and Adults: 10 mg once daily. **Note:** Usual treatment duration is at least 1 year and varies with HBeAg status, consult current guidelines and literature.

Dosage adjustment in renal impairment: Adult recommendations only (no dosage adjustment recommendations available for patients <18 years with renal impairment):

Cl_{cr} ≥50 mL/minute: No dosage adjustment necessary

Cl_{cr} 30-49 mL/minute: 10 mg every 48 hours

Cl_{cr} 10-29 mL/minute: 10 mg every 72 hours

Hemodialysis: 10 mg every 7 days (following dialysis)

Dosage adjustment in hepatic impairment: No adjustment required

Dietary Considerations May be taken without regard to food.

Administration May be administered without regard to food.

Monitoring Parameters HIV status (prior to initiation of therapy); serum creatinine (prior to initiation and during therapy; every 3 months in patients with medical conditions which predispose to renal insufficiency and in all patients treated for >1 year; more frequent monitoring required if preexisting real insufficiency detected [Lok, 2007]); viral load; LFTs for several months following discontinuation of adefovir

Additional Information Adefovir dipivoxil is a prodrug, rapidly converted to the active component (adefovir). It was previously investigated as a treatment for HIV infections (at dosages substantially higher than the approved dose for hepatitis B). The NDA was withdrawn, and no further studies in the treatment of HIV are anticipated (per manufacturer).

Dosage Forms Excipient information presented when available (limited, particularly for generics); consult specific product labeling.

Tablet, as dipivoxil:
Hepsera®: 10 mg

◆ **Adefovir Dipivoxil** *see* Adefovir *on page* 45
◆ **Adenocard®** *see* Adenosine *on page* 46
◆ **Adenoscan®** *see* Adenosine *on page* 46

Adenosine (a DEN oh seen)

U.S. Brand Names Adenocard®; Adenoscan®

Canadian Brand Names Adenocard®; Adenoscan®; Adenosine Injection, USP

Index Terms 9-Beta-D-Ribofuranosyladenine

Pharmacologic Category Antiarrhythmic Agent, Class IV; Diagnostic Agent

Use

Adenocard®: Treatment of paroxysmal supraventricular tachycardia (PSVT) including that associated with accessory bypass tracts (Wolff-Parkinson-White syndrome); when clinically advisable, appropriate vagal maneuvers should be attempted prior to adenosine administration; **not effective in atrial flutter, atrial fibrillation, or ventricular tachycardia**

Adenoscan®: Pharmacologic stress agent used in myocardial perfusion thallium-201 scintigraphy

Unlabeled/Investigational Use Adenoscan®: Acute vasodilator testing in pulmonary artery hypertension

Pregnancy Risk Factor C

Pregnancy Considerations Reports of administration during pregnancy have indicated no adverse effects on fetus or newborn attributable to adenosine.

Lactation Excretion in breast milk unknown

Medication Safety Issues

High alert medication: The Institute for Safe Medication Practices (ISMP) includes this medication among its list of drugs which have a heightened risk of causing significant patient harm when used in error.

Contraindications Hypersensitivity to adenosine or any component of the formulation; second- or third-degree AV block or sick sinus syndrome (except in patients with a functioning artificial pacemaker), atrial flutter, atrial fibrillation, and ventricular tachycardia (this drug is not effective in converting these arrhythmias to sinus rhythm). The manufacturer states that Adenoscan® should be avoided in patients with known or suspected bronchoconstrictive or bronchospastic lung disease.

Warnings/Precautions Adenosine decreases conduction through the AV node and may produce first-, second-, or third-degree heart block. Patients with pre-existing S-A nodal dysfunction may experience prolonged sinus pauses after adenosine; use caution in patients with first-degree AV block or bundle branch block; avoid use of adenosine for pharmacologic stress testing in patients with high-grade AV block or sinus node dysfunction (unless a functional pacemaker is in place). There have been reports of atrial fibrillation/flutter in patients with PSVT associated with accessory conduction pathways after adenosine. Rare, prolonged episodes of asystole have been reported, with fatal outcomes in some cases. Watch for proarrhythmic effects; monitor and adjust dose to prevent QT_c prolongation. Use caution in patients receiving other drugs which slow AV conduction (eg, digoxin, verapamil). Drugs which affect adenosine (theophylline, caffeine) should be withheld for five half-lives prior to adenosine use. Avoid dietary caffeine for 12-24 hours prior to pharmacologic stress testing.

Adenosine may also produce profound vasodilation with subsequent hypotension. When used as a bolus dose (PSVT), effects are generally self-limiting (due to the short half-life of adenosine). However, when used as a continuous infusion (pharmacologic stress testing), effects may be more pronounced and persistent, corresponding to continued exposure. Adenosine infusions should be used with caution in patients with autonomic dysfunction, stenotic valvular heart disease, pericarditis, pleural effusion, carotid stenosis (with cerebrovascular insufficiency), or uncorrected hypovolemia. Use caution in elderly patients; may be at increased risk of hemodynamic effects, bradycardia, and/or AV block.

A limited number of patients with asthma have received adenosine and have not experienced exacerbation of their asthma. Adenosine may cause bronchoconstriction in patients with asthma, and should be used cautiously in patients with obstructive lung disease not associated with bronchoconstriction (eg, emphysema, bronchitis).

Adenocard®: Transient AV block is expected. When used in PSVT, at the time of conversion to normal sinus rhythm, a variety of new rhythms may appear on the ECG. Administer as a rapid bolus, either directly into a vein or (if administered into an I.V. line), as close to the patient as possible (followed by saline flush).

Adverse Reactions Note: Frequency varies based on use; higher frequency of infusion-related effects, such as flushing and lightheadedness, were reported with continuous infusion (Adenoscan®).

>10%:
Cardiovascular: Facial flushing (18% to 44%)
Central nervous system: Headache (2% to 18%), lightheadedness (2% to 12%)
Neuromuscular & skeletal: Discomfort of neck, throat, jaw (<1% to 15%)
Respiratory: Dyspnea (12% to 28%), chest pressure/discomfort (7% to 40%)

1% to 10%:
Cardiovascular: Hypotension (<1% to 2%), AV block (infusion 6%; third degree <1%), ST segment depression (3%), palpitation, chest pain
Central nervous system: Dizziness, nervousness (2%), apprehension
Gastrointestinal: Nausea (3%)
Neuromuscular & skeletal: Upper extremity discomfort (up to 4%), numbness (up to 2%), paresthesia (up to 2%)
Respiratory: Hyperventilation
Miscellaneous: Diaphoresis

<1% (Limited to important or life-threatening): Asystole (prolonged), atrial fibrillation, back discomfort, bradycardia, bronchospasm, blurred vision, burning sensation, hypertension (transient), injection site reaction, intracranial pressure increased, metallic taste, pressure in groin, respiratory arrest, seizure, torsade de pointes, ventricular fibrillation, ventricular tachycardia

Drug Interactions

Avoid Concomitant Use There are no known interactions where it is recommended to avoid concomitant use.

Increased Effect/Toxicity

The levels/effects of Adenosine may be increased by: Dipyridamole; Nicotine

Decreased Effect

The levels/effects of Adenosine may be decreased by: Theophylline Derivatives

Ethanol/Nutrition/Herb Interactions Food: Avoid food or drugs with caffeine. Adenosine's therapeutic effect may be decreased if used concurrently with caffeine. Avoid dietary caffeine for 12-24 hours prior to pharmacologic stress testing.

Stability Store at controlled room temperature of 15°C to 30°C (59°F to 86°F). Do **not** refrigerate; precipitation may occur (may dissolve by warming to room temperature).

Mechanism of Action Slows conduction time through the AV node, interrupting the re-entry pathways through the AV node, restoring normal sinus rhythm

Pharmacodynamics/Kinetics

Onset of action: Rapid

Duration: Very brief

Metabolism: Blood and tissue to inosine then to adenosine monophosphate (AMP) and hypoxanthine

Half-life elimination: <10 seconds

Dosage

Adenocard®: **Rapid I.V. push (over 1-2 seconds) via peripheral line:**

Infants and Children:

Manufacturer's recommendation:

<50 kg: 0.05-0.1 mg/kg. If conversion of PSVT does not occur within 1-2 minutes, may increase dose by 0.05-0.1 mg/kg. May repeat until sinus rhythm is established or to a maximum single dose of 0.3 mg/kg or 12 mg. Follow each dose with normal saline flush.

≥50 kg: Refer to Adult dosing

Pediatric advanced life support (PALS): Treatment of SVT: I.V., I.O.: 0.1 mg/kg; if not effective, administer 0.2 mg/kg; maximum single dose: 12 mg. Follow each dose with normal saline flush.

Adults: 6 mg; if not effective within 1-2 minutes, 12 mg may be given; may repeat 12 mg bolus if needed

Maximum single dose: 12 mg

Follow each I.V. bolus of adenosine with normal saline flush

Note: Preliminary results in adults suggest adenosine may be administered via a central line at lower doses (ie, initial adult dose: 3 mg).

Adenoscan®:

Stress testing: Continuous I.V. infusion via peripheral line: 140 mcg/kg/minute for 6 minutes using syringe or columetric infusion pump; total dose: 0.84 mg/kg. Thallium-201 is injected at midpoint (3 minutes) of infusion.

Acute vasodilator testing (unlabeled use): I.V.: Initial: 50 mcg/kg/minute increased by 50 mcg/kg/minute every 2 minutes to a maximum dose of 500 mcg/kg/minute; acutely assess vasodilator response

Hemodialysis: Significant drug removal is unlikely based on physiochemical characteristics.

Peritoneal dialysis: Significant drug removal is unlikely based on physiochemical characteristics.

Note: Higher doses may be needed for administration via peripheral versus central vein.

Dietary Considerations Avoid dietary caffeine for 12-24 hours prior to pharmacologic stress testing.

Administration For rapid bolus I.V. use only; administer I.V. push over 1-2 seconds at a peripheral I.V. site as proximal as possible to trunk (not in lower arm, hand, lower leg, or foot); follow each bolus with normal saline flush. **Note:** Preliminary results in adults suggest adenosine may be administered via central line at lower doses (eg, adults initial dose: 3 mg)

Monitoring Parameters ECG monitoring, heart rate, blood pressure

Dosage Forms Excipient information presented when available (limited, particularly for generics); consult specific product labeling.

Injection, solution [preservative free]: 3 mg/mL (2 mL, 4 mL)

Adenocard®: 3 mg/mL (2 mL, 4 mL)

Adenoscan®: 3 mg/mL (20 mL, 30 mL)

- ◆ **Adenosine Injection, USP (Can)** *see* Adenosine *on page 46*
- ◆ **Adept®** *see* Icodextrin *on page 764*
- ◆ **ADH** *see* Vasopressin *on page 1552*
- ◆ **Adipex-P®** *see* Phentermine *on page 1181*
- ◆ **ADL-2698** *see* Alvimopan *on page 77*
- ◆ **Adoxa®** *see* Doxycycline *on page 491*
- ◆ **Adrenalin®** *see* EPINEPHrine *on page 525*
- ◆ **Adrenaline** *see* EPINEPHrine *on page 525*
- ◆ **ADR (error-prone abbreviation)** *see* DOXOrubicin *on page 486*
- ◆ **AdreView™** *see* Iobenguane I 123 *on page 810*
- ◆ **Adria** *see* DOXOrubicin *on page 486*
- ◆ **Adriamycin®** *see* DOXOrubicin *on page 486*
- ◆ **Adrucil®** *see* Fluorouracil *on page 636*
- ◆ **Adsorbent Charcoal** *see* Charcoal *on page 299*
- ◆ **Advagraf™ (Can)** *see* Tacrolimus *on page 1419*
- ◆ **Advair® (Can)** *see* Fluticasone and Salmeterol *on page 648*
- ◆ **Advair Diskus®** *see* Fluticasone and Salmeterol *on page 648*
- ◆ **Advair® HFA** *see* Fluticasone and Salmeterol *on page 648*
- ◆ **Advantage-S® [OTC]** *see* Nonoxynol 9 *on page 1077*
- ◆ **Advate** *see* Antihemophilic Factor (Recombinant) *on page 121*
- ◆ **Advicor®** *see* Niacin and Lovastatin *on page 1059*
- ◆ **Advil® [OTC]** *see* Ibuprofen *on page 760*
- ◆ **Advil® (Can)** *see* Ibuprofen *on page 760*
- ◆ **Advil® Children's [OTC]** *see* Ibuprofen *on page 760*
- ◆ **Advil® Cold, Children's [OTC] [DSC]** *see* Pseudoephedrine and Ibuprofen *on page 1267*
- ◆ **Advil® Cold & Sinus [OTC]** *see* Pseudoephedrine and Ibuprofen *on page 1267*
- ◆ **Advil® Cold & Sinus (Can)** *see* Pseudoephedrine and Ibuprofen *on page 1267*
- ◆ **Advil® Infants' [OTC]** *see* Ibuprofen *on page 760*
- ◆ **Advil® Junior [OTC] [DSC]** *see* Ibuprofen *on page 760*
- ◆ **Advil® Migraine [OTC]** *see* Ibuprofen *on page 760*
- ◆ **Aerius® (Can)** *see* Desloratadine *on page 420*
- ◆ **AeroBid®** *see* Flunisolide *on page 632*
- ◆ **AeroBid®-M** *see* Flunisolide *on page 632*
- ◆ **aerohist plus™** *see* Chlorpheniramine, Phenylephrine, and Methscopolamine *on page 313*
- ◆ **aeroKid™** *see* Chlorpheniramine, Phenylephrine, and Methscopolamine *on page 313*
- ◆ **Afeditab™ CR** *see* NIFEdipine *on page 1064*
- ◆ **Afluria®** *see* Influenza Virus Vaccine *on page 788*

Agalsidase Beta (aye GAL si days BAY ta)

U.S. Brand Names Fabrazyme®

Canadian Brand Names Fabrazyme®

Index Terms Alpha-Galactosidase-A (Recombinant); r-h α-GAL

Pharmacologic Category Enzyme
Use Replacement therapy for Fabry disease
Pregnancy Risk Factor B
Medication Safety Issues
Sound-alike/look-alike issues:
Agalsidase beta may be confused with agalsidase alfa, alglucerase, alglucosidase alfa

International issues:
Agalsidase beta may be confused with agalsidase alfa, which is available in international markets

Dosage I.V.: Children ≥8 years and Adults: 1 mg/kg every 2 weeks
Dosage adjustment in toxicity: Patient with IgE antibodies to agalsidase beta (rechallenge): 0.5 mg/kg every 2 weeks at an initial maximum infusion rate of 0.01 mg/minute; may gradually escalate dose (to maximum of 1 mg/kg every 2 weeks) and/or infusion rate (doubling the infusion rate every 30 minutes to a maximum rate of 0.25 mg/minute) as tolerated.
Dosage adjustment in renal impairment: No dosage adjustment required
Additional Information Complete prescribing information for this medication should be consulted for additional detail.
Dosage Forms Excipient information presented when available (limited, particularly for generics); consult specific product labeling.
Injection, powder for reconstitution:
Fabrazyme®: 5 mg [contains mannitol 33 mg; derived from Chinese hamster cells]; 35 mg [contains mannitol 222 mg; derived from Chinese hamster cells]

◆ **Agenerase® [DSC]** *see* Amprenavir *on page 113*
◆ **Agenerase® (Can)** *see* Amprenavir *on page 113*
◆ **Aggrastat®** *see* Tirofiban *on page 1478*
◆ **Aggrenox®** *see* Aspirin and Dipyridamole *on page 145*
◆ **AGN 1135** *see* Rasagiline *on page 1298*
◆ **$AgNO_3$** *see* Silver Nitrate *on page 1370*
◆ **Agrylin®** *see* Anagrelide *on page 115*
◆ **AH-Chew®** *see* Chlorpheniramine, Phenylephrine, and Methscopolamine *on page 313*
◆ **AH-Chew™ Ultra** *see* Chlorpheniramine, Phenylephrine, and Methscopolamine *on page 313*
◆ **AHF (Human)** *see* Antihemophilic Factor (Human) *on page 120*
◆ **AHF (Human)** *see* Antihemophilic Factor/von Willebrand Factor Complex (Human) *on page 122*
◆ **AHF (Recombinant)** *see* Antihemophilic Factor (Recombinant) *on page 121*
◆ **A-hydroCort** *see* Hydrocortisone *on page 743*
◆ **AICC** *see* Anti-inhibitor Coagulant Complex *on page 123*
◆ **Airomir (Can)** *see* Albuterol *on page 51*
◆ **AK-Con™** *see* Naphazoline *on page 1040*
◆ **AK-Dilate®** *see* Phenylephrine *on page 1183*
◆ **AK-Fluor®** *see* Fluorescein *on page 634*
◆ **Akne-Mycin®** *see* Erythromycin *on page 544*
◆ **AK-Pentolate™** *see* Cyclopentolate *on page 376*
◆ **AK-Poly-Bac™** *see* Bacitracin and Polymyxin B *on page 171*
◆ **Akten™** *see* Lidocaine *on page 884*
◆ **AKTob®** *see* Tobramycin *on page 1481*
◆ **AK-Trol® [DSC]** *see* Neomycin, Polymyxin B, and Dexamethasone *on page 1052*
◆ **Alamag [OTC]** *see* Aluminum Hydroxide and Magnesium Hydroxide *on page 76*
◆ **Alamag Plus [OTC]** *see* Aluminum Hydroxide, Magnesium Hydroxide, and Simethicone *on page 76*
◆ **Alamast®** *see* Pemirolast *on page 1161*
◆ **Alavert™ [OTC]** *see* Loratadine *on page 904*
◆ **Alavert™ Allergy and Sinus [OTC]** *see* Loratadine and Pseudoephedrine *on page 905*
◆ **Alavert™ Allergy Relief 24-Hour [OTC]** *see* Loratadine *on page 904*
◆ **Alaway™ [OTC]** *see* Ketotifen *on page 844*
◆ **Albalon® [DSC]** *see* Naphazoline *on page 1040*

Albendazole (al BEN da zole)

U.S. Brand Names Albenza®
Pharmacologic Category Anthelmintic
Use Treatment of parenchymal neurocysticercosis caused by *Taenia solium* and cystic hydatid disease of the liver, lung, and peritoneum caused by *Echinococcus granulosus*
Unlabeled/Investigational Use Albendazole has activity against *Ascaris lumbricoides* (roundworm); *Ancylostoma caninum*; *Ancylostoma duodenale* and *Necator americanus* (hookworms); cutaneous larva migrans; *Enterobius vermicularis* (pinworm); *Gnathostoma spinigerum*; *Gongylonema* sp; *Mansonella perstans* (filariasis); *Opisthorchis sinensis* (liver fluke); visceral larva migrans (toxocariasis); activity has also been shown against the liver fluke *Clonorchis sinensis*, *Giardia lamblia*, *Cysticercus cellulosae*, and *Echinococcus multilocularis*. Albendazole has also been used for the treatment of intestinal microsporidiosis (*Encephalitozoon intestinalis*), disseminated microsporidiosis (*E. hellem*, *E. cuniculi*, *E. intestinalis*, *Pleistophora* sp, *Trachipleistophora* sp, *Brachiola vesicularum*), and ocular microsporidiosis (*E. hellem*, *E. cuniculi*, *Vittaforma corneae*).
Pregnancy Risk Factor C
Pregnancy Considerations Albendazole has been shown to be teratogenic in laboratory animals and should not be used during pregnancy, if at all possible. Women should be advised to avoid pregnancy for at least 1 month following therapy. Discontinue if pregnancy occurs during treatment.
Lactation Excretion in breast milk unknown/not recommended
Medication Safety Issues
International issues:
Albenza® may be confused with Avanza® which is a brand name for mirtazapine in Australia
Contraindications Hypersensitivity to albendazole, benzimidazoles, or any component of the formulation
Warnings/Precautions Reversible elevations in hepatic enzymes have been reported; patients with abnormal LFTs and hepatic echinococcosis are at an increased risk of hepatotoxicity. Discontinue therapy if LFT elevations are >2 times the upper limit of normal; may consider restarting treatment with frequent monitoring of LFTs when hepatic enzymes return to pretreatment values. Agranulocytosis, aplastic anemia, granulocytopenia, leukopenia, and pancytopenia have occurred leading to fatalities (rare); use with caution in patients with hepatic impairment (more susceptible to hematologic toxicity). Discontinue therapy in all patients who develop clinically significant decreases in blood cell counts.

Neurocysticercosis: Corticosteroids should be administered before or upon initiation of albendazole therapy to minimize inflammatory reactions and prevent cerebral hypertension. Anticonvulsant therapy should be used concurrently during the first week of therapy to prevent seizures. If retinal lesions exist, weigh risk of further retinal damage due to albendazole-induced changes to the retinal lesion vs benefit of disease treatment.

Adverse Reactions

>10%:

Central nervous system: Headache (11% neurocysticercosis; 1% hydatid)

Hepatic: LFTs increased (16% hydatid; <1% neurocysticercosis)

1% to 10%:

Central nervous system: Intracranial pressure increased (up to 2%), dizziness (≤1%), fever (≤1%), vertigo (≤1%), meningeal signs (1%)

Dermatologic: Alopecia (<1% to 2%)

Gastrointestinal: Abdominal pain (up to 6%), nausea/vomiting (4% to 6%)

<1% (Limited to important or life-threatening symptoms): Acute liver failure, acute renal failure, aplastic anemia, agranulocytosis, erythema multiforme, granulocytopenia, hepatitis, hypersensitivity reaction, leukopenia, neutropenia, pancytopenia, rash, Stevens-Johnson syndrome, thrombocytopenia, urticaria

Drug Interactions

Metabolism/Transport Effects **Substrate** (minor) of CYP1A2, 3A4; **Inhibits** CYP1A2 (weak)

Avoid Concomitant Use There are no known interactions where it is recommended to avoid concomitant use.

Increased Effect/Toxicity There are no known significant interactions involving an increase in effect.

Decreased Effect

The levels/effects of Albendazole may be decreased by: Aminoquinolines (Antimalarial)

Ethanol/Nutrition/Herb Interactions Food: Albendazole serum levels may be increased if taken with a fatty meal (increases the oral bioavailability by up to 5 times).

Stability Store between 20°C and 25°C (68°F to 77°F)

Mechanism of Action Active metabolite, albendazole sulfoxide, causes selective degeneration of cytoplasmic microtubules in intestinal and tegmental cells of intestinal helminths and larvae; glycogen is depleted, glucose uptake and cholinesterase secretion are impaired, and desecratory substances accumulate intracellulary. ATP production decreases causing energy depletion, immobilization, and worm death.

Pharmacodynamics/Kinetics

Absorption: Poor; may increase up to 5 times when administered with a fatty meal

Distribution: Well inside hydatid cysts and CSF

Protein binding: 70%

Metabolism: Hepatic; extensive first-pass effect; pathways include rapid sulfoxidation to active metabolite (albendazole sulfoxide [major]), hydrolysis, and oxidation

Half-life elimination: 8-12 hours

Time to peak, serum: 2-5 hours

Excretion: Urine (<1% as active metabolite); feces

Dosage Oral:

Children:

Cysticercus cellulosae (unlabeled use): 15 mg/kg/day (maximum: 800 mg/day) in 2 divided doses for 8-30 days; may be repeated as necessary

Echinococcus granulosus (tapeworm) (unlabeled use): 15 mg/kg/day (maximum: 800 mg) divided twice daily for 1-6 months

Children and Adults:

Neurocysticercosis:

<60 kg: 15 mg/kg/day in 2 divided doses (maximum: 800 mg/day) for 8-30 days

≥60 kg: 800 mg/day in 2 divided doses for 8-30 days

Note: Give concurrent anticonvulsant and steroid therapy during first week.

Hydatid:

<60 kg: 15 mg/kg/day in 2 divided doses (maximum: 800 mg/day)

≥60 kg: 800 mg/day in 2 divided doses

Note: Administer dose for three 28-day cycles with a 14-day drug-free interval in between. The manufacturer recommends a total of 3 cycles.

Ancylostoma caninum, *Ascaris lumbricoides* (roundworm), *Ancylostoma duodenale* (hookworm), and *Necator americanus* (hookworm) (unlabeled use): 400 mg as a single dose

Clonorchis sinensis (Chinese liver fluke) (unlabeled use): 10 mg/kg for 7 days

Cutaneous larva migrans (unlabeled use): 400 mg once daily for 3 days

Enterobius vermicularis (pinworm) (unlabeled use): 400 mg as a single dose; may repeat in 2 weeks

Gnathostoma spinigerum (unlabeled use): 800 mg/day in 2 divided doses for 21 days

Gongylonemiasis (unlabeled use): 10 mg/kg/day for 3 days

Mansonella perstans (unlabeled use): 800 mg/day in 2 divided doses for 10 days

Visceral larva migrans (toxocariasis) (unlabeled use): 800 mg/day in 2 divided doses for 5 days

Adults:

Cysticercus cellulosae (unlabeled use): 800 mg/day in 2 divided doses for 8-30 days; may be repeated as necessary

Disseminated microsporidiosis (unlabeled use): 800 mg/day in 2 divided doses

Echinococcus granulosus (tapeworm) (unlabeled use): 800 mg/day in 2 divided doses for 1-6 months

Intestinal microsporidiosis (unlabeled use): 800 mg/day in 2 divided doses for 21 days

Ocular microsporidiosis (unlabeled use): 800 mg/day in 2 divided doses, in combination with fumagillin

Dietary Considerations Should be taken with a high-fat meal.

Administration Should be administered with a high-fat meal. Administer anticonvulsant and steroid therapy during first week of neurocysticercosis therapy. If patients have difficulty swallowing, tablets may be crushed or chewed, then swallowed with a drink of water.

Monitoring Parameters Monitor fecal specimens for ova and parasites for 3 weeks after treatment; if positive, retreat; LFTs and CBC with differential at start of each 28-day cycle and every 2 weeks during therapy (more frequent monitoring for patients with liver disease); pregnancy test

Dosage Forms Excipient information presented when available (limited, particularly for generics); consult specific product labeling.

Tablet:

Albenza®: 200 mg

◆ **Albenza®** *see* Albendazole *on page 48*

◆ **Albert® Glyburide (Can)** *see* GlyBURIDE *on page 701*

◆ **Albert® Pentoxifylline (Can)** *see* Pentoxifylline *on page 1173*

◆ **Albumarc®** *see* Albumin *on page 49*

Albumin (al BYOO min)

U.S. Brand Names Albumarc®; Albuminar®; AlbuRx™; Albutein®; Buminate®; Flexbumin; Plasbumin®

Canadian Brand Names Plasbumin®-25; Plasbumin®-5

Index Terms Albumin (Human); Normal Human Serum Albumin; Normal Serum Albumin (Human); Salt Poor Albumin; SPA

Pharmacologic Category Blood Product Derivative; Plasma Volume Expander, Colloid

Use Plasma volume expansion and maintenance of cardiac output in the treatment of certain types of shock or impending shock; may be useful for burn patients, ARDS, and cardiopulmonary bypass; other uses considered by some investigators (but not proven) are retroperitoneal surgery, peritonitis, and ascites; unless the condition responsible for hypoproteinemia can be corrected, albumin can provide only symptomatic relief or supportive treatment

Unlabeled/Investigational Use In cirrhotics, administered with diuretics to help facilitate diuresis; large volume paracentesis; volume expansion in dehydrated, mildly-hypotensive cirrhotics

Pregnancy Risk Factor C

Lactation Excretion in breast milk unknown/compatible

Medication Safety Issues

Sound-alike/look-alike issues:

Albutein® may be confused with albuterol

Buminate® may be confused with bumetanide

Contraindications Hypersensitivity to albumin or any component of the formulation; patients with severe anemia or cardiac failure

Warnings/Precautions Use with caution in patients with hepatic or renal failure because of added protein load; rapid infusion of albumin solutions may cause vascular overload. All patients should be observed for signs of hypervolemia such as pulmonary edema. Use with caution in those patients for whom sodium restriction is necessary. Avoid 25% concentration in preterm infants due to risk of intraventricular hemorrhage. Nutritional supplementation is not an appropriate indication for albumin.

Adverse Reactions Frequency not defined.

Cardiovascular: CHF precipitation, edema, hyper-/hypotension, hypervolemia, tachycardia

Central nervous system: Chills, fever, headache

Dermatologic: Pruritus, rash, urticaria

Gastrointestinal: Nausea, vomiting

Respiratory: Bronchospasm, pulmonary edema

Miscellaneous: Anaphylaxis

Drug Interactions

Avoid Concomitant Use There are no known interactions where it is recommended to avoid concomitant use.

Increased Effect/Toxicity There are no known significant interactions involving an increase in effect.

Decreased Effect There are no known significant interactions involving a decrease in effect.

Stability Store at a temperature ≤30°C (86°F); do not freeze. Do not use solution if it is turbid or contains a deposit; use within 4 hours after opening vial; discard unused portion.

If 5% human albumin is unavailable, it may be prepared by diluting 25% human albumin with 0.9% sodium chloride or 5% dextrose in water. Do not use sterile water to dilute albumin solutions, as this has been associated with hypotonic-associated hemolysis.

Mechanism of Action Provides increase in intravascular oncotic pressure and causes mobilization of fluids from interstitial into intravascular space

Dosage I.V.:

5% should be used in hypovolemic patients or intravascularly-depleted patients

25% should be used in patients in whom fluid and sodium intake must be minimized

Dose depends on condition of patient:

Children: Hypovolemia: 0.5-1 g/kg/dose (10-20 mL/kg/dose of albumin 5%); maximum dose: 6 g/kg/day

Adults: Usual dose: 25 g; initial dose may be repeated in 15-30 minutes if response is inadequate; no more than 250 g should be administered within 48 hours

Hypoproteinemia: 0.5-1 g/kg/dose; repeat every 1-2 days as calculated to replace ongoing losses

Hypovolemia: 5% albumin: 0.5-1 g/kg/dose; repeat as needed. **Note:** May be considered after inadequate response to crystalloid therapy and when nonprotein colloids are contraindicated. The volume administered and the speed of infusion should be adapted to individual response.

Dietary Considerations

Albumarc®, Albuminar®, Albutein®, Buminate®, Flexbumin: 5% [50 mg/mL] and 25% [250 mg/mL] contain sodium 130-160 mEq/L

Plasbumin®: 5% [50 mg/mL] and 25% [250 mg/mL] contain sodium ~145 mEq/L

Administration For I.V. administration only. Use within 4 hours after opening vial; discard unused portion. In emergencies, may administer as rapidly as necessary to improve clinical condition. After initial volume replacement:

5%: Do not exceed 2-4 mL/minute in patients with normal plasma volume; 5-10 mL/minute in patients with hypoproteinemia

25%: Do not exceed 1 mL/minute in patients with normal plasma volume; 2-3 mL/minute in patients with hypoproteinemia

Do not dilute 5% solution. Rapid infusion may cause vascular overload. Albumin 25% may be given undiluted or diluted in normal saline. May give in combination or through the same administration set as saline or carbohydrates. Do not use with ethanol or protein hydrolysates, precipitation may form.

Monitoring Parameters Blood pressure, pulmonary edema, hematocrit

Additional Information Albumin 5% and 25% solutions contain 130-160 mEq/L sodium and are considered isotonic with plasma. Dilution of albumin 25% solution with sterile water produces a hypotonic solution; administration of such can cause hemolysis and/or renal failure. An albumin 5% solution is osmotically equivalent to an equal volume of plasma, whereas a 25% solution is osmotically equivalent to 5 times its volume of plasma. Albumin solutions are heated to 60°C for 10 hours, decreasing any possible risk of viral hepatitis transmission. To date, there have been no reports of viral transmission using these products.

Dosage Forms Excipient information presented when available (limited, particularly for generics); consult specific product labeling.

Injection, solution [preservative free; human]: 5% (250 mL, 500 mL); 25% (50 mL, 100 mL)

Albuminar®: 5% (50 mL, 250 mL, 500 mL) [50 mg/mL; contains sodium 130-160 mEq/L and potassium ≤1 mEq/L; packaging contains dry natural rubber]; 25% (20 mL, 50 mL, 100 mL) [250 mg/mL; contains sodium 130-160 mEq/L and potassium ≤1 mEq/L; packaging contains dry natural rubber]

AlbuRx™: 5% (250 mL, 500 mL) [50 mg/mL; contains sodium 130-160 mEq/L and potassium ≤2 mEq/L]; 25% (50 mL, 100 mL) [250 mg/mL; contains sodium 130-160 mEq/L and potassium ≤2 mEq/L]

Albutein®: 5% (250 mL, 500 mL) [50 mg/mL; contains sodium 130-160 mEq/L and potassium ≤2 mEq/L]

Buminate®: 5% (250 mL, 500 mL) [50 mg/mL; contains sodium 130-160 mEq/L and potassium ≤2 mEq/L; packaging contains dry natural rubber]; 25% (20 mL, 50 mL, 100 mL) [250 mg/mL; contains sodium 130-160 mEq/L and potassium ≤2 mEq/L; packaging contains dry natural rubber]

Flexbumin: 25% (50 mL, 100 mL) [250 mg/mL; contains sodium 130-160 mEq/L and potassium ≤2 mEq/L]

Human Albumin Grifols®: 25% (50 mL, 100 mL) [250 mg/mL; contains sodium 130-160 mEq/L and potassium ≤2 mEq/L]

Plasbumin®: 5% (50 mL, 250 mL) [50 mg/mL; contains sodium ~145 mEq/L and potassium ≤2 mEq/L]; 25% (20 mL, 50 mL, 100 mL) [250 mg/mL; contains sodium ~145 mEq/L and potassium ≤2 mEq/L]

◆ **Albuminar®** *see* Albumin *on page* 49

Albuterol (al BYOO ter ole)

U.S. Brand Names AccuNeb®; ProAir™ HFA; Proventil® HFA; Proventil® [DSC]; Ventolin® HFA; VoSpire ER®

Canadian Brand Names Airomir; Alti-Salbutamol; Apo-Salvent®; Apo-Salvent® CFC Free; Apo-Salvent® Respirator Solution; Apo-Salvent® Sterules; Gen-Salbutamol; PMS-Salbutamol; ratio-Inspra-Sal; ratio-Salbutamol; Rhoxal-salbutamol; Salbu-2; Salbu-4; Ventolin®; Ventolin® Diskus; Ventolin® HFA; Ventolin® I.V. Infusion; Ventrodisk

Index Terms Albuterol Sulfate; Salbutamol; Salbutamol Sulphate

Pharmacologic Category Beta$_2$-Adrenergic Agonist

Additional Appendix Information

Bronchodilators *on page 1650*

Use Bronchodilator in reversible airway obstruction due to asthma or COPD; prevention of exercise-induced bronchospasm

Unlabeled/Investigational Use As tocolytic agent (injectable form; not available in U.S.)

Pregnancy Risk Factor C

Pregnancy Considerations Albuterol crosses the placenta; tocolytic effects, fetal tachycardia, fetal hypoglycemia secondary to maternal hyperglycemia with oral or intravenous routes reported. Available evidence suggests safe use as an inhalation during pregnancy, and albuterol is the preferred short-acting beta agonist for use in asthma according to the NHLBI 2007 Guidelines for the Diagnosis and Management of Asthma.

Use of the parenteral formulation (not available in the U.S.) as a tocolytic agent has been associated with myocardial ischemia. Patients with a history of cardiac disease should be referred to a cardiologist for evaluation prior to initiating therapy in premature labor. If therapy is initiated, patients should be carefully monitored for ECG changes as well as for changes in fluid balance and cardiopulmonary function. Maternal pulse rate should not exceed 140 beats per minute during I.V. infusion of salbutamol. Consider discontinuing therapy with the development of signs of pulmonary edema or myocardial ischemia. Cautious use of parenteral salbutamol, as with other beta$_2$-agonists, is also warranted when used during labor and delivery for the relief of bronchospasm.

Lactation Excretion in breast milk unknown/use caution

Medication Safety Issues

Sound-alike/look-alike issues:

Albuterol may be confused with Albutein®, atenolol

Proventil® may be confused with Bentyl®, Prilosec® Prinivil®

Salbutamol may be confused with salmeterol

Ventolin® may be confused with phentolamine, Benylin®, Vantin®

Volmax® may be confused with Flomax®

Contraindications Hypersensitivity to albuterol, adrenergic amines, or any component of the formulation

Injection formulation (not available in U.S.): Patients with tachyarrhythmias; risk of abortion during first or second trimester

Warnings/Precautions Optimize anti-inflammatory treatment before initiating maintenance treatment with albuterol. Do not use as a component of chronic therapy without an anti-inflammatory agent. Only the mildest forms of asthma (Step 1 and/or exercise-induced) would not require concurrent use based upon asthma guidelines. Patient must be instructed to seek medical attention in cases where acute symptoms are not relieved or a previous level of response is diminished. The need to increase frequency of use may indicate deterioration of asthma, and treatment must not be delayed.

Use caution in patients with cardiovascular disease (arrhythmia or hypertension or HF), convulsive disorders, diabetes, glaucoma, hyperthyroidism, or hypokalemia. Beta-agonists may cause elevation in blood pressure, heart rate, and result in CNS stimulation/excitation. Beta$_2$-agonists may increase risk of arrhythmia, increase serum glucose, or decrease serum potassium.

Immediate hypersensitivity reactions (urticaria, angioedema, rash, bronchospasm) have been reported. Do not exceed recommended dose; serious adverse events, including fatalities, have been associated with excessive use of inhaled sympathomimetics. Rarely, paradoxical bronchospasm may occur with use of inhaled bronchodilating agents; this should be distinguished from inadequate response. All patients should utilize a spacer device or valved holding chamber when using a metered-dose inhaler; in addition, face masks should be used in children <4 years of age.

Patient response may vary between inhalers that contain chlorofluorocarbons and those which are chlorofluorocarbon-free.

Adverse Reactions Incidence of adverse effects is dependent upon age of patient, dose, and route of administration.

Cardiovascular: Angina, atrial fibrillation, arrhythmias, chest discomfort, chest pain, extrasystoles, flushing, hyper-/hypotension, palpitation, supraventricular tachycardia, tachycardia

Central nervous system: CNS stimulation, dizziness, drowsiness, headache, insomnia, irritability, lightheadedness, migraine, nervousness, nightmares, restlessness, seizure

Dermatologic: Angioedema, rash, urticaria

Endocrine & metabolic: Hyperglycemia, hypokalemia, lactic acidosis

Gastrointestinal: Diarrhea, dry mouth, dyspepsia, gastroenteritis, nausea, unusual taste, vomiting

Genitourinary: Micturition difficulty

Local: Injection: Pain, stinging

Neuromuscular & skeletal: Muscle cramps, musculoskeletal pain, tremor, weakness

Otic: Otitis media, vertigo

Respiratory: Asthma exacerbation, bronchospasm, cough, epistaxis, laryngitis, oropharyngeal drying/irritation, oropharyngeal edema, pharyngitis, rhinitis, upper respiratory inflammation, viral respiratory infection

Miscellaneous: Allergic reaction, anaphylaxis, diaphoresis, lymphadenopathy

Postmarketing and/or case reports: Anxiety, glossitis, hoarseness, myocardial ischemia, pulmonary edema, throat irritation, tongue ulceration

Drug Interactions

Avoid Concomitant Use

Avoid concomitant use of Albuterol with any of the following: Iobenguane I 123

Increased Effect/Toxicity

Albuterol may increase the levels/effects of: Sympathomimetics

The levels/effects of Albuterol may be increased by: Atomoxetine; Cannabinoids; MAO Inhibitors; Tricyclic Antidepressants

Decreased Effect

Albuterol may decrease the levels/effects of: Iobenguane I 123

The levels/effects of Albuterol may be decreased by: Alpha-/Beta-Blockers; Beta-Blockers (Beta1 Selective); Beta-Blockers (Nonselective); Betahistine

Ethanol/Nutrition/Herb Interactions

Food: Avoid or limit caffeine (may cause CNS stimulation).

Herb/Nutraceutical: Avoid ephedra, yohimbe (may cause CNS stimulation). Avoid St John's wort (may decrease the levels/effects of albuterol).

Stability

HFA aerosols: Store at 15°C to 25°C (59°F to 77°F).

Ventolin® HFA: Discard after using 200 actuations or 3 months after removal from protective pouch, whichever comes first. Store with mouthpiece down.

Infusion solution (not available in U.S.): Ventolin® I.V.: Store at 15°C to 30°C (59°F to 86°F). Protect from light. After dilution, discard after 24 hours.

Inhalation solution:

Solution for nebulization (0.5%): Store at 2°C to 30°C (36°F to 86°F). To prepare a 2.5 mg dose, dilute 0.5 mL of solution to a total of 3 mL with normal saline; also compatible with cromolyn or ipratropium nebulizer solutions.

AccuNeb®: Store at 2°C to 25°C (36°F to 77°F). Do not use if solution changes color or becomes cloudy. Use within 1 week of opening foil pouch.

Syrup: Store at 2°C to 30°C (36°F to 86°F).

Tablet: Store at 2°C to 30°C (36°F to 86°F).

Tablet, extended release: Store at 20°C to 25°C (68°F to 77°F)

Mechanism of Action Relaxes bronchial smooth muscle by action on beta$_2$-receptors with little effect on heart rate

Pharmacodynamics/Kinetics

Onset of action: Peak effect:

Nebulization/oral inhalation: 0.5-2 hours

CFC-propelled albuterol: 10 minutes

Ventolin® HFA: 25 minutes

Oral: 2-3 hours

Duration: Nebulization/oral inhalation: 3-4 hours; Oral: 4-6 hours

Metabolism: Hepatic to an inactive sulfate

Half-life elimination: Inhalation: 3.8 hours; Oral: 3.7-5 hours

Excretion: Urine (30% as unchanged drug)

Dosage

Oral:

Children: Bronchospasm:

2-6 years: 0.1-0.2 mg/kg/dose 3 times/day; maximum dose not to exceed 12 mg/day (divided doses)

6-12 years: 2 mg/dose 3-4 times/day; maximum dose not to exceed 24 mg/day (divided doses)

Extended release: 4 mg every 12 hours; maximum dose not to exceed 24 mg/day (divided doses)

Children >12 years and Adults: Bronchospasm (treatment): 2-4 mg/dose 3-4 times/day; maximum dose not to exceed 32 mg/day (divided doses)

Extended release: 8 mg every 12 hours; maximum dose not to exceed 32 mg/day (divided doses). A 4 mg dose every 12 hours may be sufficient in some patients, such as adults of low body weight.

Elderly: Bronchospasm (treatment): 2 mg 3-4 times/day; maximum: 8 mg 4 times/day

Metered-dose inhaler (90 mcg/puff):

Children ≤4 years *(NIH Guidelines, 2007)*:

Quick relief: 1-2 puffs every 4-6 hours as needed

Exacerbation of asthma (acute, severe): 4-8 puffs every 20 minutes for 3 doses, then every 1-4 hours as needed

Exercise-induced bronchospasm (prevention): 1-2 puffs 5 minutes prior to exercise

Children 5-11 years *(NIH Guidelines, 2007)*:

Bronchospasm, quick relief: 2 puffs every 4-6 hours as needed

Exacerbation of asthma (acute, severe): 4-8 puffs every 20 minutes for 3 doses, then every 1-4 hours as needed

Exercise-induced bronchospasm (prevention): 2 puffs 5-30 minutes prior to exercise

Children ≥12 years and Adults:

Bronchospasm, quick relief *(NIH Guidelines, 2007)*: 2 puffs every 4-6 hours as needed

Exacerbation of asthma (acute, severe) *(NIH Guidelines, 2007)*: 4-8 puffs every 20 minutes for up to 4 hours, then every 1-4 hours as needed

Exercise-induced bronchospasm (prevention) *(NIH Guidelines, 2007)*: 2 puffs 5-30 minutes prior to exercise

Solution for nebulization:

Children 2-12 years (AccuNeb®): Bronchospasm: 0.63-1.25 mg every 4-6 hours as needed

Children ≤4 years *(NIH Guidelines, 2007)*:

Quick relief: 0.63-2.5 mg every 4-6 hours as needed

Exacerbation of asthma (acute, severe): 0.15 mg/kg (minimum: 2.5 mg) every 20 minutes for 3 doses, then 0.15-0.3 mg/kg (maximum: 10 mg) every 1-4 hours as needed **or** 0.5 mg/kg/hour by continuous nebulization

Children 5-11 years *(NIH Guidelines, 2007)*:

Quick relief: 1.25-5 mg every 4-8 hours as needed

Exacerbation of asthma (acute, severe): 0.15 mg/kg (minimum: 2.5 mg) every 20 minutes for 3 doses, then 0.15-0.3 mg/kg (maximum: 10 mg) every 1-4 hours as needed **or** 0.5 mg/kg/hour by continuous nebulization

Children ≥12 years and Adults:

Bronchospasm: 2.5 mg every 4-8 hours as needed

Quick relief *(NIH Guidelines, 2007)*: 1.25-5 mg every 4-8 hours as needed

Exacerbation of asthma (acute, severe) *(NIH Guidelines, 2007)*: 2.5-5 mg every 20 minutes for 3 doses then 2.5-10 mg every 1-4 hours as needed, **or** 10-15 mg/hour by continuous nebulization

I.V. continuous infusion: Adults (Ventolin® I.V. solution [not available in U.S.]): Severe bronchospasm and status asthmaticus: Initial: 5 mcg/minute; may increase up to 10-20 mcg/minute at 15- to 30-minute intervals if needed

Hemodialysis: Not removed

Peritoneal dialysis: Significant drug removal is unlikely based on physiochemical characteristics

Dietary Considerations Oral forms should be administered with water 1 hour before or 2 hours after meals.

Administration

Metered-dose inhaler: Shake well before use; prime prior to first use, and whenever inhaler has not been used for >2 weeks or when it has been dropped, by releasing 3-4 test sprays into the air (away from face). A spacer device or valved holding chamber is recommended for use with metered-dose inhalers.

Solution for nebulization: Concentrated solution should be diluted prior to use. Blow-by administration is not recommended, use a mask device if patient unable to hold mouthpiece in mouth for administration.

Infusion solution (Ventolin® I.V.): Do not inject undiluted. Reduce concentration by at least 50% before infusing. Administer as a continuous infusion via infusion pump. Discard unused portion of infusion within 24 hours of preparation.

Oral: Do not crush or chew extended release tablets.

Monitoring Parameters FEV$_1$, peak flow, and/or other pulmonary function tests; blood pressure, heart rate; CNS stimulation; serum glucose, serum potassium; asthma symptoms; arterial or capillary blood gases (if patients condition warrants)

Test Interactions Increased renin (S), increased aldosterone (S)

Additional Information The 2007 National Heart, Lung, and Blood Institute Guidelines for the Diagnosis and Management of Asthma do not recommend the use of oral systemic albuterol as a quick-relief medication and do not recommend regularly scheduled daily, chronic use of inhaled beta-agonists for long-term control of asthma.

Dosage Forms Excipient information presented when available (limited, particularly for generics); consult specific product labeling. [DSC] = Discontinued product; [CAN] = Canadian brand name

Aerosol, for oral inhalation: 90 mcg/metered inhalation (17 g) [200 metered inhalations; contains chlorofluorocarbons]

Proventil®: 90 mcg/metered inhalation (17 g) [200 metered inhalations; contains chlorofluorocarbons] [DSC]

Aerosol, for oral inhalation:

ProAir™ HFA: 90 mcg/metered inhalation (8.5 g) [200 metered inhalations; chlorofluorocarbon free]

Proventil® HFA: 90 mcg/metered inhalation (6.7 g) [200 metered inhalations; chlorofluorocarbon free]

Ventolin® HFA: 90 mcg/metered inhalation (8 g) [60 metered inhalation; chlorofluorocarbon free]; (18 g) [200 metered inhalations; chlorofluorocarbon free]

Injection, solution, as sulphate:

Ventolin® I.V. [CAN]: 1 mg/1mL (5 mL) [not available in U.S.]

Solution for nebulization: 0.042% (3 mL); 0.083% (3 mL); 0.5% (0.5 mL, 20 mL)

AccuNeb® [preservative free]: 0.63 mg/3 mL (3 mL) [0.021%]; 1.25 mg/3 mL (3 mL) [0.042%]

Proventil®: 0.083% (3 mL) [DSC] [preservative free]

Syrup, as sulfate: 2 mg/5 mL (480 mL)

Tablet: 2 mg, 4 mg

Tablet, extended release: 4 mg, 8 mg

VoSpire ER®: 4 mg, 8 mg

◆ **Albuterol and Ipratropium** *see* Ipratropium and Albuterol *on page 812*

◆ **Albuterol Sulfate** *see* Albuterol *on page 51*

◆ **Alcaine®** *see* Proparacaine *on page 1253*

◆ **Alcalak [OTC]** *see* Calcium Carbonate *on page 238*

Alclometasone (al kloe MET a sone)

U.S. Brand Names Aclovate®

Index Terms Alclometasone Dipropionate

Pharmacologic Category Corticosteroid, Topical

Additional Appendix Information

Corticosteroids *on page 1652*

Use Treatment of inflammation of corticosteroid-responsive dermatosis (low to medium potency topical corticosteroid)

Pregnancy Risk Factor C

Medication Safety Issues

Sound-alike/look-alike issues:

Aclovate® may be confused with Accolate®

Dosage Note: Therapy should be discontinued when control is achieved; if no improvement is seen within 2 weeks, reassessment of diagnosis may be necessary.

Topical:

Children ≥1 year: Apply thin film to affected area 2-3 times/day; do not use for >3 weeks

Adults: Apply a thin film to the affected area 2-3 times/day

Additional Information Complete prescribing information for this medication should be consulted for additional detail.

Dosage Forms Excipient information presented when available (limited, particularly for generics); consult specific product labeling.

Cream, as dipropionate: 0.05% (15 g, 45 g, 60 g)

Aclovate®: 0.05% (15 g, 60 g)

Ointment, as dipropionate: 0.05% (15 g, 45 g, 60 g)

Aclovate®: 0.05% (15 g, 45 g, 60 g)

◆ **Alclometasone Dipropionate** *see* Alclometasone *on page 53*

◆ **Alcomicin® (Can)** *see* Gentamicin *on page 692*

◆ **Alcortin™** *see* Iodoquinol and Hydrocortisone *on page 810*

◆ **Aldactazide®** *see* Hydrochlorothiazide and Spironolactone *on page 739*

◆ **Aldactazide 25® (Can)** *see* Hydrochlorothiazide and Spironolactone *on page 739*

◆ **Aldactazide 50® (Can)** *see* Hydrochlorothiazide and Spironolactone *on page 739*

◆ **Aldactone®** *see* Spironolactone *on page 1397*

◆ **Aldara®** *see* Imiquimod *on page 775*

Aldesleukin (al des LOO kin)

U.S. Brand Names Proleukin®

Canadian Brand Names Proleukin®

Index Terms Epidermal Thymocyte Activating Factor; IL-2; Interleukin-2; Lymphocyte Mitogenic Factor; NSC-373364; T-Cell Growth Factor; TCGF; Thymocyte Stimulating Factor

Pharmacologic Category Antineoplastic Agent, Miscellaneous; Biological Response Modulator

Use Treatment of metastatic renal cell cancer, metastatic melanoma

Unlabeled/Investigational Use HIV infection, and AIDS; non-Hodgkin's lymphoma

Pregnancy Risk Factor C

Pregnancy Considerations Maternal toxicity and embryocidal effects were noted in animal studies. There are no adequate and well-controlled studies in pregnant women; use during pregnancy only if benefits to the mother outweigh potential risk to the fetus. Contraception is recommended for fertile males or females using this medication.

Lactation Excretion unknown/not recommended

Medication Safety Issues

Sound-alike/look-alike issues:

Aldesleukin may be confused with oprelvekin

Proleukin® may be confused with oprelvekin

High alert medication: The Institute for Safe Medication Practices (ISMP) includes this medication among its list of drug classes which have a heightened risk of causing significant patient harm when used in error.

Contraindications Hypersensitivity to aldesleukin or any component of the formulation; patients with abnormal thallium stress or pulmonary function tests; patients who have had an organ allograft; retreatment in patients who have experienced sustained ventricular tachycardia (≥5 beats), refractory cardiac rhythm disturbances, recurrent chest pain with ECG changes consistent with angina or myocardial infarction, intubation ≥72 hours, pericardial tamponade, renal dialysis for ≥72 hours, coma or toxic psychosis lasting ≥48 hours, repetitive or refractory seizures, bowel ischemia/perforation, GI bleeding requiring surgery

Warnings/Precautions Hazardous agent - use appropriate precautions for handling and disposal. **[U.S. Boxed Warning]: High-dose aldesleukin therapy has been associated with capillary leak syndrome (CLS) resulting in hypotension and reduced organ perfusion which may be severe and can result in death. Therapy should be restricted to patients with normal cardiac and pulmonary functions as defined by thallium stress and formal pulmonary function testing.** Extreme caution should be used in patients with a history of prior cardiac or pulmonary disease. Patients must have a serum creatinine ≤1.5 mg/dL prior to treatment.

[U.S. Boxed Warning]: Should be administered under the supervision of an experienced cancer chemotherapy physician in a facility with cardiopulmonary or intensive specialists and intensive care facilities available. Adverse effects are frequent and sometimes fatal. May exacerbate pre-existing or initial presentation of autoimmune diseases and inflammatory disorders. Patients should be evaluated and treated for CNS metastases and have a negative scan prior to treatment. Mental status changes (irritability, confusion, depression) can occur and may indicate bacteremia, hypoperfusion, CNS malignancy, or CNS toxicity.

[U.S. Boxed Warning]: Impaired neutrophil function is associated with treatment; patients are at risk for sepsis, bacterial endocarditis, and central line-related gram-positive infections. Antibiotic prophylaxis which has been associated with a reduced incidence of staphylococcal infections in aldesleukin studies includes the use of oxacillin, nafcillin, ciprofloxacin, or vancomycin.

[U.S. Boxed Warning]: Withhold treatment for patients developing moderate-to-severe lethargy or somnolence; continued treatment may result in coma. Standard prophylactic supportive care during high-dose aldesleukin treatment includes acetaminophen to relieve constitutional symptoms and an H_2 antagonist to reduce the risk of GI ulceration and/or bleeding. Safety and efficacy have not been established in children.

Adverse Reactions

>10%:

- Cardiovascular: Hypotension (71%; grade 4: 3%), peripheral edema (28%), tachycardia (23%), edema (15%), vasodilation (13%), cardiovascular disorder (11%; includes blood pressure changes, CHF and ECG changes)
- Central nervous system: Chills (52%), confusion (34%), fever (29%; grade 4: 1%), malaise (27%), somnolence (22%), anxiety (12%), pain (12%), dizziness (11%)
- Dermatologic: Rash (42%), pruritus (24%), exfoliative dermatitis (18%)
- Endocrine & metabolic: Acidosis (12%), hypomagnesemia (12%), hypocalcemia (11%)
- Gastrointestinal: Diarrhea (67%), vomiting (19% to 50%), nausea (19% to 35%), stomatitis (22%), anorexia (20%), weight gain (18%), abdominal pain (11%)
- Hematologic: Thrombocytopenia (37%; grade 4: 1%), anemia (29%), leukopenia (16%)
- Hepatic: Hyperbilirubinemia (40%), AST increased (23%)
- Neuromuscular & skeletal: Weakness (23%)
- Renal: Oliguria (63%; grade 4: 6%), creatinine increased (33%)
- Respiratory: Dyspnea (43%), lung disorder (24%; includes pulmonary congestion, rales, and rhonchi), cough (11%), respiratory disorder (11%; includes acute respiratory distress syndrome, infiltrates and pulmonary changes)
- Miscellaneous: Infection (13%; grade 4: 1%)

1% to 10%:

- Cardiovascular: Arrhythmia (10%), cardiac arrest (grade 4: 1%), MI (grade 4: 1%), supraventricular tachycardia (grade 4: 1%), ventricular tachycardia (grade 4: 1%)
- Gastrointestinal: Abdomen enlarged (10%)
- Hematologic: Coagulation disorder (grade 4: 1%)
- Hepatic: Alkaline phosphatase increased (10%)
- Renal: Anuria (grade 4: 5%), acute renal failure (grade 4: 1%)
- Respiratory: Rhinitis (10%), apnea (grade 4: 1%)
- Miscellaneous: Sepsis (grade 4: 1%)

<1% (Limited to important or life-threatening): Acute tubular necrosis, allergic interstitial nephritis, allergic reactions, anaphylaxis, atrial arrhythmia, AV block, blindness (transient or permanent), bowel necrosis, bradycardia, bullous pemphigoid, BUN increased, cardiomyopathy, cellulitis, cerebral edema, cerebral lesions, cerebral vasculitis, CHF, cholecystitis, colitis, coma, crescentic IgA glomuleronephritis, Crohn's disease exacerbation, depression (severe; leading to suicide), diabetes mellitus, duodenal ulcer, encephalitis, endocarditis, extrapyramidal syndrome, gastrointestinal hemorrhage, hematemesis, hemoptysis, hemorrhage, hepatic failure, hepatitis, hepatosplenomegaly, hypertension, hyperuricemia, hyperventilation, hypothermia, hyperthyroidism, hypoventilation, hypoxia, inflammatory arthritis, injection site necrosis, intestinal obstruction, intestinal perforation, leukocytosis, malignant hyperthermia, meningitis, myocardial ischemia, myocarditis, myopathy, myositis, neuritis, neuropathy, neutropenia, oculobulbar myasthenia gravis, optic neuritis, pancreatitis, pericardial effusion, pericarditis, peripheral gangrene, phlebitis, pneumonia, pneumothorax, pulmonary edema, pulmonary embolus, renal failure, respiratory acidosis, respiratory arrest, respiratory failure, retroperitoneal hemorrhage, rhabdomyolysis, scleroderma, seizure (including grand mal), shock, Stevens-Johnson syndrome, stroke, syncope, thrombosis, thyroiditis, tracheoesophageal fistula, transient ischemic attack, urticaria, ventricular extrasystoles

Drug Interactions

Avoid Concomitant Use There are no known interactions where it is recommended to avoid concomitant use.

Increased Effect/Toxicity

The levels/effects of Aldesleukin may be increased by: Contrast Media (Non-ionic); Interferons (Alfa)

Decreased Effect There are no known significant interactions involving a decrease in effect.

Ethanol/Nutrition/Herb Interactions Ethanol: May increase CNS adverse effects.

Stability Store vials of lyophilized injection in a refrigerator at 2°C to 8°C (36°F to 46°F). Reconstitute vials with 1.2 mL SWFI to a concentration of 18 million units/1 mL (sterile water should be injected towards the side of the vial). Gently swirl; do not shake. Further dilute with 50 mL of D_5W. Smaller volumes of D_5W should be used for doses <1.5 mg; avoid concentrations <30 mcg/mL and >70 mcg/mL (an increased variability in drug delivery has been seen). Reconstituted vials and solutions diluted for infusion are stable for 48 hours at room temperature or refrigerated, per the manufacturer. Solution diluted with D_5W to a concentration of 220 mg/mL and repackaged into tuberculin syringes was reported to be stable for 14 days refrigerated.

Note: Filtration will result in significant loss of bioactivity

Recommendations for aldesleukin dilution: See table on next page.

Mechanism of Action Aldesleukin promotes proliferation, differentiation, and recruitment of T and B cells, natural killer (NK) cells, and thymocytes; causes cytolytic activity in a subset of lymphocytes and subsequent interactions between the immune system and malignant cells; can stimulate lymphokine-activated killer (LAK) cells and tumor-infiltrating lymphocytes (TIL) cells.

Pharmacodynamics/Kinetics

Distribution: V_d: 4-7 L; primarily in plasma and then in the lymphocytes

Half-life elimination: I.V.: Initial: 6-13 minutes; Terminal: 80-120 minutes

Final Dilution Concentration (mcg/mL)	Final Dilution Concentration (10^6 int. units/mL)	Stability
<30	<0.49	Albumin must be added to bag **prior to addition** of aldesleukin at a final concentration of 0.1% (1 mg/mL) albumin; stable at room temperature or at ≥32°C (89°F) for 6 days[1,2]
≥30 to ≤70	≥0.49 to ≤1.1	Stable at room temperature at 6 days without albumin added or at ≥32°C (89°F) for 6 days only if albumin is added (0.1%)[1,2]
70-100	1.2-1.6	Unstable; avoid use
>100-500	1.7-8.2	Stable at room temperature and at ≥32°C (89°F) for 6 days[1,2]

[1]These solutions do not contain a preservative; use for more than 24 hours may not be advisable.

[2]Continuous infusion via ambulatory infusion device raises aldesleukin to this temperature.

Dosage Refer to individual protocols.

I.V.:

Renal cell carcinoma: 600,000 int. units/kg every 8 hours for a maximum of 14 doses; repeat after 9 days for a total of 28 doses per course. Retreat if needed 7 weeks after previous course.

Melanoma:

Single-agent use: 600,000 int. units/kg every 8 hours for a maximum of 14 doses; repeat after 9 days for a total of 28 doses per course. Retreat if needed 7 weeks after previous course.

In combination with cytotoxic agents (unlabeled use): 24 million int. units/m^2 days 12-16 and 19-23

SubQ (unlabeled route):

Single-agent doses: 3-18 million int. units/day for 5 days each week, up to 6 weeks

In combination with interferon:

5 million int. units/m^2 3 times/week

1.8 million int. units/m^2 twice daily 5 days/week for 6 weeks

Investigational regimen: SubQ: 11 million int. units (flat dose) daily for 4 days per week for 4 consecutive weeks; repeat every 6 weeks

Dosage adjustment in renal impairment: No specific recommendations by manufacturer. Use with caution.

Administration Administer as I.V. infusion over 15 minutes (do not administer with an inline filter). Flush before and after with D_5W, particularly if maintenance I.V. line contains sodium chloride. May also be administered by SubQ injection (unlabeled route)

Management of symptoms related to vascular leak syndrome:

If actual body weight increases >10% above baseline, or rales or rhonchi are audible:

Administer furosemide at dosage determined by patient response

Administer dopamine hydrochloride 1-5 mcg/kg/minute to maintain renal blood flow and urine output

If patient has dyspnea at rest: Administer supplemental oxygen by face mask

If patient has severe respiratory distress: Intubate patient and provide mechanical ventilation; administer ranitidine (as the hydrochloride salt) 50 mg I.V. every 8-12 hours as prophylaxis against stress ulcers

Monitoring Parameters

The following clinical evaluations are recommended for all patients prior to beginning treatment and then frequently during drug administration:

CBC with differential, blood chemistries including electrolytes, renal and hepatic function tests

Chest x-rays

Monitoring during therapy should include vital signs (temperature, pulse, blood pressure, and respiration rate) and weight; in a patient with a decreased blood pressure, especially <90 mm Hg, cardiac monitoring for rhythm should be conducted. If an abnormal complex or rhythm is seen, an ECG should be performed; vital signs in these hypotension patients should be taken hourly and central venous pressure (CVP) checked; monitor for change in mental status.

Pulmonary function (baseline and periodic) basis.

Additional Information

1 Cetus unit = 6 int. units

1.1 mg = 18 x 10^6 int. units (or 3 x 10^6 Cetus units)

1 Roche unit (Teceleukin) = 3 int. units

Dosage Forms Excipient information presented when available (limited, particularly for generics); consult specific product labeling.

Injection, powder for reconstitution:

Proleukin®: 22 x 10^6 int. units [18 million int. units/mL = 1.1 mg/mL when reconstituted]

- **Aldex™** *see* Guaifenesin and Phenylephrine *on page 712*
- **Aldex® CT** *see* Diphenhydramine and Phenylephrine *on page 458*
- **Aldomet** *see* Methyldopa *on page 970*
- **Aldoril®** *see* Methyldopa and Hydrochlorothiazide *on page 971*
- **Aldroxicon I [OTC]** *see* Aluminum Hydroxide, Magnesium Hydroxide, and Simethicone *on page 76*
- **Aldroxicon II [OTC]** *see* Aluminum Hydroxide, Magnesium Hydroxide, and Simethicone *on page 76*
- **Aldurazyme®** *see* Laronidase *on page 857*

Alefacept (a LE fa sept)

U.S. Brand Names Amevive®

Canadian Brand Names Amevive®

Index Terms B 9273; BG 9273; Human LFA-3/IgG(1) Fusion Protein; LFA-3/IgG(1) Fusion Protein, Human

Pharmacologic Category Monoclonal Antibody

Use Treatment of moderate to severe chronic plaque psoriasis in adults who are candidates for systemic therapy or phototherapy

Restrictions Alefacept will be distributed directly to physician offices or to a specialty pharmacy; injections are intended to be administered in the physician's office

Pregnancy Risk Factor B

Pregnancy Considerations Effects in pregnancy are not known. Teratogenic effects have not been observed in animal studies. Patients who become pregnant during therapy or within 8 weeks of treatment are advised to enroll in pregnancy registry (866-263-8483).

Lactation Excretion in breast milk unknown/not recommended

Contraindications Hypersensitivity to alefacept or any component of the formulation; history of severe malignancy; patients with HIV infection or other clinically-important infections

Warnings/Precautions Has been associated with hypersensitivity reactions; rare anaphylaxis also reported. Alefacept induces a decline in circulating T-lymphocytes ($CD4^+$ and $CD8^+$); $CD4^+$ lymphocyte counts should be monitored every 2 weeks throughout therapy. Do not initiate in pre-existing depression of $CD4^+$ lymphocytes and withhold treatment in any patient who develops a depressed $CD4^+$ lymphocyte count (<250 cells/μL) during treatment; permanently discontinue if $CD4^+$ lymphocyte counts remain <250 cells/μL for 1 month.

Alefacept may increase the risk of malignancies; use caution in patients at high risk for malignancy. Discontinue if malignancy develops during therapy. Alefacept may increase the risk of infection and may reactivate latent infection; monitor for new infections. Avoid use in patients receiving other immunosuppressant drugs or phototherapy. In post-marketing reports, significant transaminase elevations, as well as rare cases of hepatitis, fatty liver, decompensation of cirrhosis, and acute hepatic failure (a causal relationship not established). Discontinue if signs and symptoms of hepatic injury occur. Safety and efficacy of live or attenuated vaccines have not been evaluated. Safety and efficacy have not been established in pediatric patients.

Adverse Reactions

≥10%:

Hematologic: Lymphopenia (up to 10% of patients required temporary discontinuation, up to 17% during a second course of therapy)

Local: Injection site reactions (up to 16% of patients; includes pain, inflammation, bleeding, edema, or other reaction)

1% to 10%:

Central nervous system: Chills (6%; primarily during intravenous administration), dizziness (≥2%)

Dermatologic: Pruritus (≥2%)

Gastrointestinal: Nausea (≥2%)

Neuromuscular & skeletal: Myalgia (≥2%)

Respiratory: Pharyngitis (≥2%), cough increased (≥2%)

Miscellaneous: Malignancies (1% vs 0.5% in placebo), antibodies to alefacept (3%; significance unknown), infection (1% requiring hospitalization)

<1% (Limited to important or life-threatening): Anaphylaxis, allergic reaction, angioedema, headache, hepatitis, hepatic failure, MI, transaminases increased (≥3 times ULN), urticaria

Drug Interactions

Avoid Concomitant Use There are no known interactions where it is recommended to avoid concomitant use.

Increased Effect/Toxicity There are no known significant interactions involving an increase in effect.

Decreased Effect There are no known significant interactions involving a decrease in effect.

Ethanol/Nutrition/Herb Interactions Ethanol: Avoid ethanol (may increase risk of liver toxicity).

Stability Store under refrigeration at 2°C to 8°C (36°F to 46°F); protect from light. Reconstitute 15 mg vial for I.M. solution with 0.6 mL of SWFI (supplied); 0.5 mL of reconstituted solution contains 15 mg of alefacept. Gently swirl to avoid foaming. Do not filter reconstituted solutions. Following reconstitution, may be stored for up to 4 hours at 2°C to 8°C (36°F to 46°F). Discard any unused solution after 4 hours.

Mechanism of Action Binds to CD2, a receptor on the surface of lymphocytes, inhibiting their interaction with leukocyte functional antigen 3 (LFA-3). Interaction between CD2 and LFA-3 is important for the activation of T lymphocytes in psoriasis. Activated T lymphocytes secrete a number of inflammatory mediators, including interferon gamma, which are involved in psoriasis. Since CD2 is primarily expressed on T lymphocytes, treatment results in a reduction in $CD4^+$ and $CD8^+$ T lymphocytes, with lesser effects on other cell populations (NK and B lymphocytes).

Pharmacodynamics/Kinetics

Distribution: V_d: 0.094 L/kg

Bioavailability: 63% (following I.M. administration)

Half-life: 270 hours (following I.V. administration)

Excretion: Clearance: 0.25 mL/hour/kg

Dosage Adults:

I.M.: 15 mg once weekly; usual duration of treatment: 12 weeks

A second course of treatment may be initiated at least 12 weeks after completion of the initial course of treatment, provided $CD4^+$ T-lymphocyte counts are within the normal range.

Note: $CD4^+$ T-lymphocyte counts should be monitored before initiation of treatment and every 2 weeks during therapy. Dosing should be withheld if $CD4^+$ counts are <250 cells/μL, and dosing should be permanently discontinued if $CD4^+$ lymphocyte counts remain at <250 cells/μL for longer than 1 month.

Elderly: Refer to adult dosing

Dosage adjustment in renal impairment: No dosage adjustment required

Administration I.M. injections should be administered at least 1 inch from previous administration sites.

Monitoring Parameters Baseline $CD4^+$ T-lymphocyte counts prior to initiation and every 2 weeks during treatment course; severity of psoriatic lesions; signs and symptoms of infection

Dosage Forms Excipient information presented when available (limited, particularly for generics); consult specific product labeling.

Injection, powder for reconstitution:

Amevive®: 15 mg [for I.M. administration; contains sucrose 12.5 mg; supplied with SWFI]

Alemtuzumab (ay lem TU zoo mab)

U.S. Brand Names Campath®

Canadian Brand Names MabCampath®

Index Terms C1H; Campath-1H; Humanized IgG1 Anti-CD52 Monoclonal Antibody; NSC-715969

Pharmacologic Category Antineoplastic Agent, Monoclonal Antibody

Use Treatment of B-cell chronic lymphocytic leukemia (B-CLL)

Unlabeled/Investigational Use Treatment of refractory T-cell prolymphocytic leukemia (T-PLL); rheumatoid arthritis; graft-versus-host disease; multiple myeloma; preconditioning regimen for stem cell transplantation and renal and liver transplantation; post-transplant rejection (renal); treatment of autoimmune cytopenias

Pregnancy Risk Factor C

Pregnancy Considerations Human IgG is known to cross the placental barrier; therefore, alemtuzumab may also cross the barrier and cause fetal B- and T-lymphocyte depletion. Well-controlled human trials have not been done. Use during pregnancy only if the benefit to the mother outweighs the potential risk to the fetus. Effective contraception is recommended during and for 6 months after treatment for women of childbearing potential and men of reproductive potential.

Lactation Excretion in breast milk unknown/not recommended

Medication Safety Issues

High alert medication: The Institute for Safe Medication Practices (ISMP) includes this medication among its list of drugs which have a heightened risk of causing significant patient harm when used in error.

Contraindications There are no contraindications listed in the manufacturer's labeling

Warnings/Precautions Hazardous agent - use appropriate precautions for handling and disposal. **[U.S. Boxed Warning]: Serious infections (bacterial, viral, fungal, and protozoan) have been reported. Prophylactic therapy against PCP pneumonia and herpes viral infections is recommended upon initiation of therapy**

and for at least 2 months following last dose or until $CD4^+$ counts are ≥200 cells/μL (whichever is later). $CD4^+$ and $CD8^+$ lymphocyte counts may not return to baseline levels for more than 1 year. Withhold treatment during serious infections; may be reinitiated upon resolution of infection.

[U.S. Boxed Warning]: Serious and potentially fatal infusion-related reactions (acute respiratory distress syndrome, bronchospasm, cardiac arrest, cardiac arrhythmias, chills, fever, hypotension, myocardial infarction, pulmonary infiltrates, rash, rigors, shortness of breath, syncope) may occur, especially during the first week of treatment. Premedication with acetaminophen and an oral antihistamine is recommended. Withhold infusion for grade 3 or 4 infusion reaction. Use caution and carefully monitor blood pressure in patients with ischemic heart disease and patients on antihypertensive therapy. Gradual escalation to the recommended maintenance dose is required at initiation and after interruption of therapy for ≥7 days to minimize infusion-related reactions.

[U.S. Boxed Warning]: Severe, prolonged myelosuppression, autoimmune anemia, and autoimmune thrombocytopenia have occurred. Single doses >30 mg and cumulative weekly doses >90 mg are associated with an increased incidence of pancytopenia and should not be administered. Hemolytic anemia, pure red cell aplasia, bone marrow aplasia, and hypoplasia have also been reported. Median duration of neutropenia and thrombocytopenia is 21 days. Discontinue therapy during serious hematologic or other serious toxicity (except lymphopenia) until the event resolves. Permanently discontinue if autoimmune anemia or autoimmune thrombocytopenia occurs. Patients receiving blood products should only receive irradiated blood products due to the potential for GVHD during lymphopenia.

Patients should not be immunized with live, viral vaccines during or recently after treatment. The ability to respond to any vaccine following therapy is unknown. Women of childbearing potential and men of reproductive potential should use effective contraceptive methods during treatment and for a minimum of 6 months following therapy. Safety and efficacy have not been established in pediatric patients.

Adverse Reactions

>10%:

Cardiovascular: Hypotension (15% to 32%), peripheral edema (13%), hypertension (11% to 15%), dysrhythmia/tachycardia/SVT (10% to 14%)

Central nervous system: Fever (69% to 85%), chills (53%), fatigue (22% to 34%), headache (13% to 24%), dysthesias (15%), dizziness (12%)

Dermatologic: Rash (13% to 40%), urticaria (16% to 30%), pruritus (14% to 24%)

Gastrointestinal: Nausea (47% to 54%), vomiting (33% to 41%), anorexia (20%), diarrhea (10% to 22%), stomatitis/mucositis (14%), abdominal pain (11%)

Hematologic: Lymphopenia (grades 3/4: 97%), neutropenia (77% to 85%; grade 3/4: 42% to 70%; median duration: 28 days), anemia (76% to 80%; grade 3/4: 13% to 47%), thrombocytopenia (71% to 72%; grade 3/4: 13% to 52%; median duration: 21 days)

Local: Injection site reaction (SubQ administration: 90%)

Neuromuscular & skeletal: Rigors (86% to 89%), skeletal pain (24%), weakness (13%), myalgia (11%)

Respiratory: Dyspnea (14% to 26%), cough (25%), bronchitis/pneumonitis (21%), pneumonia (16%), pharyngitis (12%)

Miscellaneous: Infection (43% to 74%; grades 3/4: 21% to 37%; incidence is lower if prophylactic anti-infectives are utilized), CMV viremia (55%), infusion reactions (grades 3/4: 10% to 35%), diaphoresis (19%), CMV infection (16%), sepsis (15%), herpes viral infections (1% to 11%)

1% to 10%:

Cardiovascular: Chest pain (10%)

Central nervous system: Insomnia (10%), malaise (9%), anxiety (8%), depression (7%), temperature change sensation (5%), somnolence (5%)

Dermatologic: Purpura (8%), erythema (4%)

Gastrointestinal: Dyspepsia (10%), constipation (9%)

Hematologic: Neutropenic fever (10%), pancytopenia/marrow hypoplasia (5% to 6%; grade 3/4: 3%), positive Coombs' test without hemolysis (2%), autoimmune thrombocytopenia (2%), autoimmune hemolytic anemia (1%)

Neuromuscular & skeletal: Back pain (10%), tremor (3% to 7%)

Respiratory: Bronchospasm (9%), epistaxis (7%), rhinitis (7%)

Miscellaneous: Moniliasis (8%)

<1% (Limited to important or life-threatening): Acidosis, acute renal failure, acute respiratory distress syndrome, agranulocytosis, alkaline phosphatase increased, allergic reactions, anaphylactoid reactions, angina pectoris, angioedema, anuria, aphasia, aplastic anemia, arrhythmia, ascites, asthma, atrial fibrillation, bacterial infection, biliary pain, bone marrow aplasia, bullous eruption, capillary fragility, cardiac arrest, cardiac failure, cardiac insufficiency, cardiomyopathy, cellulitis, cerebral hemorrhage, cerebrovascular disorder, chronic inflammatory demyelinating polyradiculoneuropathy, coagulation abnormality, colitis, coma, COPD, coronary artery disorder, cyanosis, deep vein thrombosis, dehydration, diabetes mellitus exacerbation, disseminated intravascular coagulation (DIC), duodenal ulcer, ejection fraction decreased, endophthalmitis, Epstein-Barr virus associated lymphoproliferative disorder, esophagitis, fluid overload, flu-like syndrome, gastrointestinal hemorrhage, Goodpasture's syndrome, Graves' disease, Guillain-Barré syndrome, hallucinations, hematemesis, hematoma, hematuria, hemolysis, hemolytic anemia, hemoptysis, hepatic failure, hepatocellular damage, hyperbilirubinemia, hyper-/hypoglycemia, hyper-/hypokalemia, hyperthyroidism, hypoalbuminemia, hyponatremia, hypovolemia, hypoxia, idiopathic thrombocytopenic purpura (ITP), interstitial pneumonitis, intestinal obstruction, intestinal perforation, intracranial hemorrhage, *Legionella* pneumonia, *Listeria* meningitis, lymphadenopathy, marrow depression, melena, MI, mouth edema, myositis, optic neuropathy, osteomyelitis, pancreatitis, paralysis, paralytic ileus, paroxysmal nocturnal hemoglobinuria-like monocytes, peptic ulcer, pericarditis, peritonitis, plasma cell dyscrasia, phlebitis, pleural effusion, pleurisy, *Pneumocystis jiroveci* pneumonia, pneumothorax, polymyositis, progressive multifocal leukoencephalopathy, pseudomembranous colitis, pulmonary edema, pulmonary embolism, pulmonary fibrosis, pulmonary infiltration, pure red cell aplasia, purpuric rash, renal dysfunction, respiratory alkalosis, respiratory arrest, respiratory depression, respiratory insufficiency, seizure (grand mal), serum sickness, splenic infarction, splenomegaly, stridor, subarachnoid hemorrhage, syncope, toxic nephropathy, thrombocythemia, thrombophlebitis, throat tightness, tuberculosis, tumor lysis syndrome, ureteric obstruction, urinary retention, urinary tract infection, ventricular arrhythmia, ventricular tachycardia, viral meningitis

Drug Interactions

Avoid Concomitant Use

Avoid concomitant use of Alemtuzumab with any of the following: Natalizumab; Vaccines (Live)

Increased Effect/Toxicity

Alemtuzumab may increase the levels/effects of: Natalizumab; Vaccines (Live)

The levels/effects of Alemtuzumab may be increased by: Abciximab; Trastuzumab

Decreased Effect

Alemtuzumab may decrease the levels/effects of: Vaccines (Inactivated)

The levels/effects of Alemtuzumab may be decreased by: Echinacea

Ethanol/Nutrition/Herb Interactions Herb/Nutraceutical: Echinacea may diminish the therapeutic effect of alemtuzumab.

Stability Prior to dilution, store at 2°C to 8°C (36°F to 46°F); do not freeze (if accidentally frozen, thaw in refrigerator prior to administration). Do not shake; protect from light. Following dilution, store at room temperature or refrigerate; protect from light; use within 8 hours. Dilute with 100 mL NS or D_5W. Gently invert the bag to mix the solution. Do not shake prior to use.

Mechanism of Action Binds to CD52, a nonmodulating antigen present on the surface of B and T lymphocytes, a majority of monocytes, macrophages, NK cells, and a subpopulation of granulocytes. After binding to $CD52^+$ cells, an antibody-dependent lysis of leukemic cells occurs.

Pharmacodynamics/Kinetics

Distribution: V_d: 0.1-0.4 L/kg

Metabolism: Clearance decreases with repeated dosing (due to loss of CD52 receptors in periphery), resulting in a sevenfold increase in AUC.

Half-life elimination: 11 hours (following first 30 mg dose; range: 2-32 hours); 6 days (following the last 30 mg dose; range: 1-14 days)

Dosage Note: **Dose escalation is required;** usually accomplished in 3-7 days. Do not exceed single doses >30 mg or cumulative doses >90 mg/week. Pretreatment (with acetaminophen and an oral antihistamine) is recommended prior to the first dose, with dose escalations, and as clinically indicated; I.V. hydrocortisone may be used for severe infusion-related reactions.

I.V. infusion, SubQ (unlabeled route): Adults: B-CLL:

Initial: 3 mg/day beginning on day 1; when tolerated (no grade 3 or 4 infusion reactions), increase to maintenance dose of 30 mg/dose 3 times/week on alternate days for a total duration of therapy of up to 12 weeks

Maximum dose/day: 30 mg; maximum cumulative dose/week: 90 mg

Dosage adjustment for hematologic toxicity (severe neutropenia or thrombocytopenia, not autoimmune): **Note:** If delay between dosing is ≥7 days, restart at 3 mg/day and escalate as tolerated.

First occurrence: ANC <250/µL and/or platelet count ≤25,000/µL: Hold therapy; resume at 30 mg/dose when ANC ≥500/µL and platelet count ≥50,000/µL

Second occurrence: ANC <250/µL and/or platelet count ≤25,000/µL: Hold therapy; resume at 10 mg/dose when ANC ≥500/µL and platelet count ≥50,000/µL

Third occurrence: ANC <250/µL and/or platelet count ≤25,000/µL: Permanently discontinue therapy

Patients with a baseline ANC ≤250/µL and/or a baseline platelet count ≤25,000/µL at initiation of therapy: If ANC and/or platelet counts decrease to ≤50% of the baseline value, hold therapy

First occurrence: When ANC and/or platelet count return to baseline, resume therapy at 30 mg/dose

Second occurrence: When ANC and/or platelet count return to baseline, resume therapy at 10 mg/dose

Third occurrence: Permanently discontinue therapy

Administration Administer by I.V. infusion over 2 hours. Consider premedicating with diphenhydramine 50 mg and acetaminophen 500-1000 mg 30 minutes before initiation of infusion. Hydrocortisone 200 mg has been effective in decreasing severe infusion-related events. Start anti-infective prophylaxis. Other drugs should not be added to or simultaneously infused through the same I.V. line. Do not give I.V. push.

SubQ (unlabeled route): A longer dose escalation time (1-2 weeks) may be needed due to injection site reactions. Premedication and anti-infective prophylaxis regimens should be given as are recommended with I.V. administration.

Monitoring Parameters Vital signs; carefully monitor BP especially in patient with ischemic heart disease or on antihypertensive medications; CBC with differential and platelets (weekly); signs and symptoms of infection; $CD4^+$ lymphocyte counts (after treatment until recovery). Monitor closely for infusion reactions (including hypotension, rigors, fever, shortness of breath, bronchospasm, chills, and/or rash).

Test Interactions May interfere with diagnostic serum tests that utilize antibodies.

Dosage Forms Excipient information presented when available (limited, particularly for generics); consult specific product labeling.

Injection, solution [preservative free]:

Campath®: 30 mg/mL (1 mL) [contains polysorbate 80; disodium edetate]

Alendronate (a LEN droe nate)

U.S. Brand Names Fosamax®

Canadian Brand Names Apo-Alendronate®; CO Alendronate; Dom-Alendronate; Fosamax®; Gen-Alendronate; Novo-Alendronate; PHL-Alendronate; PHL-Alendronate-FC; PMS-Alendronate; PMS-Alendronate-FC; ratio-Alendronate; Riva-Alendronate; Sandoz Alendronate

Index Terms Alendronate Sodium

Pharmacologic Category Bisphosphonate Derivative

Use Treatment and prevention of osteoporosis in postmenopausal females; treatment of osteoporosis in males; Paget's disease of the bone in patients who are symptomatic, at risk for future complications, or with alkaline phosphatase ≥2 times the upper limit of normal; treatment of glucocorticoid-induced osteoporosis in males and females with low bone mineral density who are receiving a daily dosage ≥7.5 mg of prednisone (or equivalent)

Pregnancy Risk Factor C

Pregnancy Considerations Safety and efficacy have not been established in pregnant women. Animal studies have shown delays in delivery and fetal/neonatal death (secondary to hypocalcemia). Bisphosphonates are incorporated into the bone matrix and gradually released over time. Theoretically, there may be a risk of fetal harm when pregnancy follows the completion of therapy. Based on limited case reports with pamidronate, serum calcium levels in the newborn may be altered if administered during pregnancy.

Lactation Excretion in breast milk unknown/use caution

Medication Safety Issues

Sound-alike/look-alike issues:

Fosamax® may be confused with Flomax®

International issues:

Fosamax® may be confused with Fisamox® which is a brand name for amoxicillin in Australia

Contraindications Hypersensitivity to alendronate, other bisphosphonates, or any component of the formulation; hypocalcemia; abnormalities of the esophagus which delay esophageal emptying such as stricture or achalasia; inability to stand or sit upright for at least 30 minutes; oral solution should not be used in patients at risk of aspiration

Warnings/Precautions Use caution in patients with renal impairment (not recommended for use in patients with Cl_{cr} <35 mL/minute); hypocalcemia must be corrected before therapy initiation; ensure adequate calcium and vitamin D intake. May cause irritation to upper gastrointestinal mucosa. Esophagitis, esophageal ulcers, esophageal erosions, and esophageal stricture (rare) have been reported; risk increases in patients unable to comply with dosing instructions. Use with caution in patients with dysphagia, esophageal disease, gastritis, duodenitis, or ulcers (may worsen underlying condition).

Bisphosphonate therapy has been associated with osteonecrosis, primarily of the jaw; this has been observed mostly in cancer patients, but also in patients with postmenopausal osteoporosis and other diagnoses. Dental exams and preventative dentistry should be performed prior to placing patients with risk factors on chronic bisphosphonate therapy. Invasive dental procedures should be avoided during treatment.

Severe (and occasionally debilitating) bone, joint, and/or muscle pain have been reported during bisphosphonate treatment. The onset of pain ranged from a single day to several months. Symptoms usually resolve upon discontinuation. Some patients experienced recurrence when rechallenged with same drug or another bisphosphonate; avoid use in patients with a history of these symptoms in association with bisphosphonate therapy. Discontinue use if severe symptoms occur.

Safety and efficacy in children have not been established.

Adverse Reactions **Note:** Incidence of adverse effects (mostly GI) increases significantly in patients treated for Paget's disease at 40 mg/day.

>10%: Endocrine & metabolic: Hypocalcemia (transient, mild, 18%); hypophosphatemia (transient, mild, 10%)

1% to 10%:

Cardiovascular: Atrial fibrillation (1% to 2%)

Central nervous system: Headache (up to 3%)

Gastrointestinal: Abdominal pain (1% to 7%), acid reflux (1% to 4%), dyspepsia (1% to 4%), nausea (1% to 4%), flatulence (up to 4%), diarrhea (1% to 3%), gastroesophageal reflux disease (1% to 3%), constipation (up to 3%), esophageal ulcer (up to 2%), abdominal distension (up to 1%), gastritis (up to 1%), vomiting (up to 1%), dysphagia (up to 1%), gastric ulcer (1%), melena (1%)

Neuromuscular & skeletal: Musculoskeletal pain (up to 6%), muscle cramps (up to 1%)

<1% (Limited to important or life-threatening): Alopecia, anastomotic ulcer, angioedema; bone, muscle, or joint pain (occasionally severe, considered incapacitating in rare cases); dizziness, duodenal ulcer, episcleritis, erythema, esophageal erosions, esophageal perforation, esophageal stricture, esophagitis, fever, flu-like syndrome, hypersensitivity reactions, hypocalcemia (symptomatic), joint swelling, lymphocytopenia, malaise, myalgia, oropharyngeal ulceration, osteonecrosis (jaw), peripheral edema, photosensitivity (rare), pruritus, rash, scleritis (rare), Stevens-Johnson syndrome, taste perversion, toxic epidermal necrolysis, urticaria, uveitis (rare), vertigo, weakness

Drug Interactions

Avoid Concomitant Use There are no known interactions where it is recommended to avoid concomitant use.

Increased Effect/Toxicity

Alendronate may increase the levels/effects of: Phosphate Supplements

The levels/effects of Alendronate may be increased by: Aminoglycosides; Aspirin; Nonsteroidal Anti-Inflammatory Agents

Decreased Effect

The levels/effects of Alendronate may be decreased by: Antacids; Calcium Salts; Iron Salts; Magnesium Salts

Ethanol/Nutrition/Herb Interactions

Ethanol: Avoid ethanol (may increase risk of osteoporosis and gastric irritation).

Food: All food and beverages interfere with absorption. Coadministration with caffeine may reduce alendronate efficacy. Coadministration with dairy products may decrease alendronate absorption. Beverages (especially orange juice and coffee) and food may reduce the absorption of alendronate as much as 60%.

Stability Store tablets and oral solution at room temperature of 15°C to 30°C (59°F to 86°F). Keep in well-closed container.

Mechanism of Action A bisphosphonate which inhibits bone resorption via actions on osteoclasts or on osteoclast precursors; decreases the rate of bone resorption, leading to an indirect increase in bone mineral density. In Paget's disease, characterized by disordered resorption and formation of bone, inhibition of resorption leads to an indirect decrease in bone formation; but the newly-formed bone has a more normal architecture.

Pharmacodynamics/Kinetics

Distribution: 28 L (exclusive of bone)

Protein binding: ~78%

Metabolism: None

Bioavailability: Fasting: 0.6%; reduced 60% with food or drink

Half-life elimination: Exceeds 10 years

Excretion: Urine; feces (as unabsorbed drug)

Dosage Oral: Adults: **Note:** Patients treated with glucocorticoids and those with Paget's disease should receive adequate amounts of calcium and vitamin D.

Osteoporosis in postmenopausal females:

Prophylaxis: 5 mg once daily **or** 35 mg once weekly

Treatment: 10 mg once daily **or** 70 mg once weekly

Osteoporosis in males: 10 mg once daily **or** 70 mg once weekly

Osteoporosis secondary to glucocorticoids in males and females: Treatment: 5 mg once daily; a dose of 10 mg once daily should be used in postmenopausal females who are not receiving estrogen.

Paget's disease of bone in males and females: 40 mg once daily for 6 months

Retreatment: Relapses during the 12 months following therapy occurred in 9% of patients who responded to treatment. Specific retreatment data are not available. Following a 6-month post-treatment evaluation period, retreatment with alendronate may be considered in patients who have relapsed based on increases in serum alkaline phosphatase, which should be measured periodically. Retreatment may also be considered in those who failed to normalize their serum alkaline phosphatase.

Elderly: No dosage adjustment is necessary

Dosage adjustment in renal impairment:

Cl_{cr} 35-60 mL/minute: None necessary

Cl_{cr} <35 mL/minute: Alendronate is not recommended due to lack of experience

Dosage adjustment in hepatic impairment: None necessary

Dietary Considerations Ensure adequate calcium and vitamin D intake; however, wait at least 30 minutes after taking alendronate before taking any supplement. Alendronate must be taken with plain water first thing in the morning and at least 30 minutes before the first food or beverage of the day.

Administration Alendronate must be taken with plain water (tablets 6-8 oz; oral solution follow with 2 oz) first thing in the morning and ≥30 minutes before the first food, beverage, or other medication of the day. Do not take with mineral water or with other beverages. Patients should be instructed to stay upright (not to lie down) for at least 30 minutes **and** until after first food of the day (to reduce esophageal irritation). Patients should receive supplemental calcium and vitamin D if dietary intake is inadequate.

Monitoring Parameters Alkaline phosphatase should be periodically measured; serum calcium and phosphorus; monitor pain and fracture rate; hormonal status (male and female) prior to therapy; bone mineral density (should be done prior to initiation of therapy and after 6-12 months of combined glucocorticoid and alendronate treatment)

Reference Range Calcium (total): Adults: 9.0-11.0 mg/dL (2.05-2.54 mmol/L), may slightly decrease with aging; phosphorus: 2.5-4.5 mg/dL (0.81-1.45 mmol/L)

Test Interactions Bisphosphonates may interfere with diagnostic imaging agents such as technetium-99m-diphosphonate in bone scans.

Dosage Forms Excipient information presented when available (limited, particularly for generics); consult specific product labeling.

Solution, oral:

Fosamax®: 70 mg/75 mL [contains parabens; raspberry flavor]

Tablet: 5 mg, 10 mg, 35 mg, 40 mg, 70 mg

Fosamax®: 5 mg, 10 mg, 35 mg, 40 mg, 70 mg

Alendronate and Cholecalciferol

(a LEN droe nate & kole e kal SI fer ole)

U.S. Brand Names Fosamax Plus D™

Canadian Brand Names Fosavance

Index Terms Alendronate Sodium and Cholecalciferol; Cholecalciferol and Alendronate; Vitamin D_3 and Alendronate

Pharmacologic Category Bisphosphonate Derivative; Vitamin D Analog

Use Treatment of osteoporosis in postmenopausal females; increase bone mass in males with osteoporosis

Pregnancy Risk Factor C

Dosage Oral: Adults: One tablet (alendronate 70 mg/cholecalciferol 2800 int. units **or** alendronate 70 mg/cholecalciferol 5600 int. units) once weekly. Appropriate dose in most osteoporotic women or men: Alendronate 70 mg/cholecalciferol 5600 int. units once weekly.

Dosage adjustment in renal impairment:

Cl_{cr} 35-60 mL/minute: No adjustment needed

Cl_{cr} <35 mL/minute: Not recommended

Dosage adjustment in hepatic impairment: Alendronate: None necessary. Cholecalciferol: May not be adequately absorbed in patients who have malabsorption due to inadequate bile production.

Additional Information Complete prescribing information for this medication should be consulted for additional detail.

Dosage Forms Excipient information presented when available (limited, particularly for generics); consult specific product labeling.

Tablet:

Fosamax Plus D™ 70/2800: Alendronate 70 mg and cholecalciferol 2800 int. units

Fosamax Plus D™ 70/5600: Alendronate 70 mg and cholecalciferol 5600 int. units

◆ **Alendronate Sodium** *see* Alendronate *on page* 58

◆ **Alendronate Sodium and Cholecalciferol** *see* Alendronate and Cholecalciferol *on page* 60

◆ **Alenic Alka [OTC]** *see* Aluminum Hydroxide and Magnesium Carbonate *on page* 75

◆ **Alenic Alka Tablet [OTC]** *see* Aluminum Hydroxide and Magnesium Trisilicate *on page* 76

◆ **Aler-Cap [OTC]** *see* DiphenhydrAMINE *on page* 456

◆ **Aler-Dryl [OTC]** *see* DiphenhydrAMINE *on page* 456

◆ **Aler-Tab [OTC]** *see* DiphenhydrAMINE *on page* 456

◆ **Alertec® (Can)** *see* Modafinil *on page* 1009

◆ **Alesse®** *see* Ethinyl Estradiol and Levonorgestrel *on page* 577

◆ **Aleve® [OTC]** *see* Naproxen *on page* 1041

◆ **Aleve®-D Sinus & Cold [OTC]** *see* Naproxen and Pseudoephedrine *on page* 1043

◆ **Aleve®-D Sinus & Headache [OTC]** *see* Naproxen and Pseudoephedrine *on page* 1043

◆ **Aleve® Cold & Sinus [OTC] [DSC]** *see* Naproxen and Pseudoephedrine *on page* 1043

◆ **Aleve® Sinus & Headache [OTC] [DSC]** *see* Naproxen and Pseudoephedrine *on page* 1043

◆ **Alfenta®** *see* Alfentanil *on page* 60

Alfentanil (al FEN ta nil)

U.S. Brand Names Alfenta®

Canadian Brand Names Alfentanil Injection, USP; Alfenta®

Index Terms Alfentanil Hydrochloride

Pharmacologic Category Analgesic, Opioid; Anilidopiperidine Opioid

Use Analgesic adjunct given by continuous infusion or in incremental doses in maintenance of anesthesia with barbiturate or N_2O or a primary anesthetic agent for the induction of anesthesia in patients undergoing general surgery in which endotracheal intubation and mechanical ventilation are required

Restrictions C-II

Pregnancy Risk Factor C

Medication Safety Issues

Sound-alike/look-alike issues:

Alfentanil may be confused with Anafranil®, fentanyl, remifentanil, sufentanil

Alfenta® may be confused with Sufenta®

High alert medication: The Institute for Safe Medication Practices (ISMP) includes this medication among its list of drug classes which have a heightened risk of causing significant patient harm when used in error.

Contraindications Hypersensitivity to alfentanil hydrochloride, to narcotics, or any component of the formulation; increased intracranial pressure, severe respiratory depression

Warnings/Precautions Use with caution in patients with drug dependence, head injury, morbid obesity, acute asthma and respiratory conditions; hypotension has occurred in neonates with respiratory distress syndrome; use caution when administering to patients with bradyarrhythmias; inject slowly over 3-5 minutes (apid I.V. infusion may result in skeletal muscle and chest wall rigidity, impaired ventilation, or respiratory distress/arrest); use of a nondepolarizing skeletal muscle relaxant may be required. Alfentanil may produce more hypotension compared to fentanyl, therefore, administer slowly and ensure patient has adequate hydration. Shares the toxic potentials of opiate agonists, and precautions of opiate agonist therapy should be observed. Should be administered by trained individuals. Safety and efficacy have not been established in children <12 years old.

Adverse Reactions

>10%:

Cardiovascular: Bradycardia, peripheral vasodilation

Central nervous system: Drowsiness, sedation, intracranial pressure increased

Endocrine & metabolic: Antidiuretic hormone release

Gastrointestinal: Nausea, vomiting, constipation

Ocular: Miosis

1% to 10%:

Cardiovascular: Cardiac arrhythmia, orthostatic hypotension

Central nervous system: Confusion, CNS depression

Ocular: Blurred vision

<1% (Limited to important or life-threatening): Convulsions, mental depression, paradoxical CNS excitation or delirium, dizziness, dysesthesia, rash, urticaria, itching, biliary tract spasm, urinary tract spasm, respiratory depression, bronchospasm, laryngospasm, physical and psychological dependence with prolonged use; cold, clammy skin

Drug Interactions

Metabolism/Transport Effects Substrate of CYP3A4 (major)

Avoid Concomitant Use There are no known interactions where it is recommended to avoid concomitant use.

Increased Effect/Toxicity

Alfentanil may increase the levels/effects of: Alcohol (Ethyl); Alvimopan; Beta-Blockers; Calcium Channel Blockers (Nondihydropyridine); CNS Depressants; Desmopressin; Fospropofol; MAO Inhibitors; Propofol; Selective Serotonin Reuptake Inhibitors

The levels/effects of Alfentanil may be increased by: Amphetamines; Antifungal Agents (Azole Derivatives, Systemic); Antipsychotic Agents (Phenothiazines); Cimetidine; CYP3A4 Inhibitors (Moderate); CYP3A4 Inhibitors (Strong); Dasatinib; Diltiazem; Fluconazole; Macrolide Antibiotics; Succinylcholine

Decreased Effect

Alfentanil may decrease the levels/effects of: Pegvisomant

The levels/effects of Alfentanil may be decreased by: Ammonium Chloride; Rifamycin Derivatives

Stability Store unopened ampuls at 20°C to 25°C (68°F to 77°F). Protect from light. For infusion, dilute in D_5W, NS, LR, or D_5NS to a concentration of 25-80 mcg/mL.

Mechanism of Action Binds with stereospecific receptors at many sites within the CNS, increases pain threshold, alters pain perception, inhibits ascending pain pathways; is an ultra short-acting narcotic

Pharmacodynamics/Kinetics

Onset of action: Rapid

Duration (dose dependent): 30-60 minutes

Distribution: V_d: Newborns, premature: 1 L/kg; Children: 0.163-0.48 L/kg; Adults: 0.46 L/kg

Half-life elimination: Newborns, premature: 5.33-8.75 hours; Children: 40-60 minutes; Adults: 83-97 minutes

Dosage Doses should be titrated to appropriate effects; wide range of doses is dependent upon desired degree of analgesia/anesthesia

Children <12 years: Dose not established

Adults: Dose should be based on ideal body weight as follows (see table).

Administration Administer I.V. slowly over 3-5 minutes or by I.V. continuous infusion.

Monitoring Parameters Respiratory rate, blood pressure, heart rate

Reference Range 100-340 ng/mL (depending upon procedure)

Additional Information Alfentanil may produce more muscle rigidity compared to fentanyl; therefore, be sure to administer slowly.

Dosage Forms Excipient information presented when available (limited, particularly for generics); consult specific product labeling.

Injection, solution [preservative free]: 500 mcg/mL (2 mL, 5 mL)

Alfenta®: 500 mcg/mL (2 mL, 5 mL, 10 mL, 20 mL)

Alfentanil

Indication	Approx Duration of Anesthesia (min)	Induction Period (Initial Dose) (mcg/kg)	Maintenance Period (Increments/ Infusion)	Total Dose (mcg/kg)	Effects
Incremental injection	≤30	8-20	3-5 mcg/kg or 0.5-1 mcg/kg/min	8-40	Spontaneously breathing or assisted ventilation when required.
	30-60	20-50	5-15 mcg/kg	Up to 75	Assisted or controlled ventilation required. Attenuation of response to laryngoscopy and intubation.
Continuous infusion	>45	50-75	0.5-3 mcg/kg/min; average infusion rate 1-1.5 mcg/kg/min	Dependent on duration of procedure	Assisted or controlled ventilation required. Some attenuation of response to intubation and incision, with intraoperative stability.
Anesthetic induction	>45	130-245	0.5-1.5 mcg/kg/min or general anesthetic	Dependent on duration of procedure	Assisted or controlled ventilation required. Administer slowly (over 3 minutes). Concentration of inhalation agents reduced by 30% to 50% for initial hour.

◆ **Alfentanil Hydrochloride** *see* Alfentanil *on page* 60

◆ **Alfentanil Injection, USP (Can)** *see* Alfentanil *on page* 60

◆ **Alferon® N** *see* Interferon Alfa-n3 *on page* 806

Alfuzosin (al FYOO zoe sin)

U.S. Brand Names Uroxatral®

Canadian Brand Names Apo-Alfuzosin; Xatral

Index Terms Alfuzosin Hydrochloride

Pharmacologic Category Alpha$_1$ Blocker

Use Treatment of the functional symptoms of benign prostatic hyperplasia (BPH)

Pregnancy Risk Factor B

Pregnancy Considerations Teratogenic effects were not observed in animal studies; however, alfuzosin is not indicated for use in women.

Lactation Not indicated for use in women

Contraindications Hypersensitivity to alfuzosin or any component of the formulation; moderate or severe hepatic insufficiency (Child-Pugh class B and C); concurrent use with potent CYP3A4 inhibitors (eg, itraconazole, ketoconazole, ritonavir)

Warnings/Precautions Not intended for use as an antihypertensive drug. May cause significant orthostatic hypotension and syncope, especially with first dose; anticipate a similar effect if therapy is interrupted for a few days, if dosage is rapidly increased, or used with antihypertensives (particularly vasodilators), PDE-5 inhibitors, nitrates or other medications which may result in hypotension. Discontinue if symptoms of angina occur or worsen. Alfuzosin has been shown to prolong the QT interval alone (minimal) and with other drugs with comparable effects on the QT interval (additive); use with caution in patients with known QT prolongation (congenital or acquired). Patients should be cautioned about performing hazardous tasks when starting new therapy or adjusting dosage upward. Discontinue if symptoms of angina occur or worsen. Rule out prostatic carcinoma before beginning therapy. Use caution with renal or mild hepatic impairment; contraindicated in moderate to severe hepatic impairment. Intraoperative floppy iris syndrome has been observed in cataract surgery patients who were on or were previously treated with alpha$_1$-blockers. Causality has not been established and there appears to be no benefit in discontinuing alpha-blocker therapy prior to surgery. Not indicated for use in children.

Adverse Reactions

1% to 10%:

Central nervous system: Dizziness (6%), fatigue (3%), headache (3%), pain (1% to 2%)

Gastrointestinal: Abdominal pain (1% to 2%), constipation (1% to 2%), dyspepsia (1% to 2%), nausea (1% to 2%)

Genitourinary: Impotence (1% to 2%)

Respiratory: Upper respiratory tract infection (3%), bronchitis (1% to 2%), pharyngitis (1% to 2%), sinusitis (1% to 2%)

<1% (Limited to important or life-threatening): Angina pectoris (pre-existing CAD), angioedema, chest pain, cholestatic liver injury, diarrhea, edema, flushing, hepatocellular injury, intraoperative floppy iris syndrome (with cataract surgery), jaundice, priapism, pruritus, rash, rhinitis, tachycardia, urticaria

Drug Interactions

Metabolism/Transport Effects Substrate of CYP3A4 (major)

Avoid Concomitant Use

Avoid concomitant use of Alfuzosin with any of the following: Alpha1-Blockers; CYP3A4 Inhibitors (Strong); Silodosin; Tamsulosin

Increased Effect/Toxicity

Alfuzosin may increase the levels/effects of: Alpha1-Blockers; Calcium Channel Blockers; QTc-Prolonging Agents; Silodosin; Tamsulosin

The levels/effects of Alfuzosin may be increased by: Alpha1-Blockers; Beta-Blockers; CYP3A4 Inhibitors (Moderate); CYP3A4 Inhibitors (Strong); Dasatinib; Phosphodiesterase 5 Inhibitors; Silodosin; Tamsulosin

Decreased Effect

The levels/effects of Alfuzosin may be decreased by: CYP3A4 Inducers (Strong); Deferasirox; Herbs (CYP3A4 Inducers)

Ethanol/Nutrition/Herb Interactions

Food: Food increases the extent of absorption.

Herb/Nutraceutical: Avoid St John's wort (may decrease alfuzosin levels).

Stability Store at room temperature of 25°C (77°F); excursions permitted to 15°C to 30°C (59°F to 86°F). Protect from light and moisture.

Mechanism of Action An antagonist of alpha$_1$-adrenoreceptors in the lower urinary tract. Smooth muscle tone is mediated by the sympathetic nervous stimulation of alpha$_1$-adrenoreceptors, which are abundant in the prostate, prostatic capsule, prostatic urethra, and bladder neck. Blockade of these adrenoreceptors can cause smooth muscles in the bladder neck and prostate to relax, resulting in an improvement in urine flow rate and a reduction in BPH symptoms.

Pharmacodynamics/Kinetics

Absorption: Decreased 50% under fasting conditions

Distribution: V_d: 3.2 L/kg

Protein binding: 82% to 90%

Metabolism: Hepatic, primarily via CYP3A4; metabolism includes oxidation, O-demethylation, and N-dealkylation; forms metabolites (inactive)

Bioavailability: 49% following a meal

Half-life elimination: 10 hours

Time to peak, plasma: 8 hours following a meal

Excretion: Feces (69%); urine (24%; 11% as unchanged drug)

Dosage Oral: Adults: 10 mg once daily

Dosage adjustment in renal impairment: Bioavailability and maximum serum concentrations are increased by ~50% with mild, moderate, or severe renal impairment

Note: Safety has not been evaluated in patients with creatinine clearances <30 mL/minute.

Dosage adjustment in hepatic impairment:

Mild hepatic impairment: Use has not been studied

Moderate or severe hepatic impairment (Child-Pugh class B and C): Clearance is decreased 1/3 to 1/4 and serum concentration is increased three- to fourfold; use is contraindicated

Dietary Considerations Take following a meal at the same time each day.

Administration Tablet should be swallowed whole; do not crush or chew. Administer once daily (with a meal); should be taken at the same time each day.

Monitoring Parameters Urine flow; blood pressure

Dosage Forms Excipient information presented when available (limited, particularly for generics); consult specific product labeling.

Tablet, extended release, as hydrochloride:

Uroxatral®: 10 mg

◆ **Alfuzosin Hydrochloride** *see* Alfuzosin *on page* 61

Alglucerase (al GLOO ser ase)

U.S. Brand Names Ceredase®

Index Terms Glucocerebrosidase

Pharmacologic Category Enzyme

Use Replacement therapy for Gaucher's disease (type 1)

Pregnancy Risk Factor C

Medication Safety Issues

Sound-alike/look-alike issues:

Alglucerase may be confused with agalsidase alfa, agalsidase beta, alglucosidase alfa

Ceredase® may be confused with Cerezyme®

Dosage I.V.: Children and Adults: Initial: 30-60 units/kg every 2 weeks; dosing is individualized based on disease severity; average dose: 60 units/kg every 2 weeks. Range: 2.5 units/kg 3 times/week to 60 units/kg once weekly to every 4 weeks. Once patient response is well established, dose may be reduced every 3-6 months to determine maintenance therapy.

Additional Information Complete prescribing information for this medication should be consulted for additional detail.

Dosage Forms Excipient information presented when available (limited, particularly for generics); consult specific product labeling.

Injection, solution [preservative free]:

Ceredase®: 80 units/mL (5 mL) [contains human albumin 1%]

◆ **Alglucosidase** *see* Alglucosidase Alfa *on page* 62

Alglucosidase Alfa (al gloo KOSE i dase AL fa)

U.S. Brand Names Myozyme®

Index Terms Alglucosidase; GAA; rhGAA

Pharmacologic Category Enzyme

Use Replacement therapy for Pompe disease (infantile onset)

Pregnancy Risk Factor B

Medication Safety Issues

Sound-alike/look-alike issues:

Alglucosidase alfa may be confused with agalsidase alfa, agalsidase beta, alglucerase

Dosage I.V.: Children 1 month to 3.5 years (at first infusion): 20 mg/kg over ~4 hours every 2 weeks

Additional Information Complete prescribing information for this medication should be consulted for additional detail.

Dosage Forms Excipient information presented when available (limited, particularly for generics); consult specific product labeling.

Injection, powder for reconstitution [preservative free]:

Myozyme®: 50 mg [contains mannitol 210 mg; polysorbate 80; derived from Chinese hamster ovary cells]

◆ **Alimta®** *see* Pemetrexed *on page 1159*

◆ **Alinia®** *see* Nitazoxanide *on page 1071*

Aliskiren (a lis KYE ren)

U.S. Brand Names Tekturna®

Canadian Brand Names Rasilez®

Index Terms Aliskiren Hemifumarate; SPP100

Pharmacologic Category Renin Inhibitor

Additional Appendix Information

Angiotensin Agents *on page 1632*

Use Treatment of hypertension, alone or in combination with other antihypertensive agents

Unlabeled/Investigational Use Treatment of persistent proteinuria in patients with type 2 diabetes mellitus, hypertension, and nephropathy despite administration of optimized recommended renoprotective therapy (eg, angiotensin II receptor blocker)

Pregnancy Risk Factor C (1st trimester); D (2nd and 3rd trimesters)

Pregnancy Considerations Medications which act on the renin-angiotensin system are reported to have the following fetal/neonatal effects: Hypotension, neonatal skull hypoplasia, anuria, renal failure, and death; oligohydramnios is also reported. These effects are reported to occur with exposure during the second and third trimesters. There are no adequate and well-controlled studies in pregnant women. **[U.S. Boxed Warning]: Based on human data, drugs that act on the renin-angiotensin system can cause injury and death to the developing fetus when used in the second and third trimesters. Aliskiren should be discontinued as soon as possible once pregnancy is detected.**

Lactation Excretion in breast milk unknown/not recommended

Medication Safety Issues

International issues:

Aliskiren may be confused with Aliseum which is a brand name for diazepam in Italy

Contraindications

U.S. labeling: There are no contraindications listed in manufacturer's labeling.

Canada labeling: Hypersensitivity to aliskiren or any component of the formulation

Warnings/Precautions **[U.S. Boxed Warning]: Based on human data, drugs that act on the angiotensin system can cause injury and death to the developing fetus when used in the second and third trimesters. Aliskiren should be discontinued as soon as possible once pregnancy is detected.** Since the effect of aliskiren on bradykinin levels is unknown, the risk of kinin-mediated etiologies of angioedema occurring is also unknown. Use caution in any patient with a history of angioedema (of any etiology) as angioedema has been observed (rarely) with aliskiren use. Discontinue immediately following any signs and symptoms of angioedema. Prolonged frequent monitoring may be required especially if tongue, glottis, or larynx are involved as they are associated with airway obstruction. Patients with a history of airway surgery may have a higher risk of airway obstruction. Aggressive early and appropriate management is critical. Hyperkalemia may occur (rarely) during monotherapy; risk may increase in patients with predisposing factors (eg, renal dysfunction, diabetes mellitus or concomitant use with ACE inhibitors, potassium-sparing diuretics, potassium supplements, and/or potassium-containing salts). Symptomatic hypotension may occur (rarely) during the initiation of therapy, particularly in patients with an activated renin-angiotensin system (ie, volume or salt-depleted patients). Use with caution in patients with severe renal impairment; not studied in patients with severe renal impairment [GFR <30 mL/minute and/or S_{cr} >1.7 mg/dL (women); S_{cr} >2 mg/dL (men)], history of dialysis, nephrotic syndrome, or renovascular hypertension. Use with caution or avoid in patients with deteriorating renal function or renal artery stenosis (bilateral or unilateral). Safety and efficacy have not been established in children.

Adverse Reactions

1% to 10%:

Central nervous system: Dizziness (2%)

Dermatologic: Rash (1%)

Endocrine & metabolic: Hyperkalemia (monotherapy ≤1%; concurrent with ACE inhibitor in patients with diabetes 6%)

Gastrointestinal: Diarrhea (1% to 2%)

Hematologic: Creatine kinase increased (>300%: 1%)

Renal: BUN increased (≤7%), serum creatinine increased (≤7%)

Respiratory: Cough (1%)

<1% (Limited to important or life-threatening): Abdominal pain, anemia, angina, angioedema, dyspepsia, gastroesophageal reflux, gout, hypotension (severe), myositis, renal stone formation, rhabdomyolysis, seizure, uric acid increased

Drug Interactions

Metabolism/Transport Effects **Substrate** of CYP3A4 (minor)

Avoid Concomitant Use

Avoid concomitant use of Aliskiren with any of the following: CycloSPORINE

Increased Effect/Toxicity

Aliskiren may increase the levels/effects of: Amifostine; RiTUXimab

The levels/effects of Aliskiren may be increased by: Atorvastatin; CycloSPORINE; Diazoxide; Herbs (Hypotensive Properties); Ketoconazole; P-Glycoprotein Inhibitors; Prostacyclin Analogues

Decreased Effect

Aliskiren may decrease the levels/effects of: Furosemide

The levels/effects of Aliskiren may be decreased by: Herbs (Hypertensive Properties); Methylphenidate; P-Glycoprotein Inducers; Yohimbine

Ethanol/Nutrition/Herb Interactions Food: High-fat meals decrease absorption.

Stability Store at 15°C to 30°C (59°F to 86°F). Protect from moisture.

Mechanism of Action Aliskerin is a direct renin inhibitor, resulting in blockade of the conversion of angiotensinogen to angiotensin I. Angiotensin I suppression decreases the formation of angiotensin II (Ang II), a potent blood pressure-elevating peptide (via direct vasoconstriction, aldosterone release, and sodium retention). Ang II also functions within the Renin-Angiotensin-Aldosterone System (RAAS) as a negative inhibitory feedback mediator within the renal parenchyma to suppress the further release of renin. Thus, reductions in Ang II levels suppress this feedback loop, leading to further increased plasma renin concentrations (PRC) and subsequent activity (PRA). This disinhibition effect can be potentially problematic for ACE inhibitor and ARB therapy, as increased PRA could partially overcome the pharmacologic inhibition of the RAAS. As aliskiren is a direct inhibitor of renin activity, blunting of PRA despite the increased PRC (from loss of the negative feedback) may be clinically advantageous. The effect of aliskiren on bradykinin levels is unknown.

Pharmacodynamics/Kinetics

Onset of action: Maximum antihypertensive effect: Within 2 weeks

Absorption: Poor; absorption decreased by high-fat meal. Aliskiren is a substrate of P-glycoprotein; concurrent use of P-glycoprotein inhibitors may increase absorption.

Metabolism: Extent of metabolism unknown; *in vitro* studies indicate metabolism via CYP3A4

Bioavailability: ~3%

Half-life elimination: ~24 hours (range: 16-32 hours)

Time to peak, plasma: 1-3 hours

Excretion: Urine (~25% of absorbed dose excreted unchanged in urine); feces (unchanged via biliary excretion)

Dosage Oral:

Adults: Initial: 150 mg once daily; may increase to 300 mg once daily (maximum: 300 mg/day). **Note:** Prior to initiation, correct hypovolemia and/or closely monitor volume status in patients on concurrent diuretics during treatment initiation.

Elderly: No initial dosage adjustment required

Dosage adjustment in renal impairment

Mild-to-moderate impairment [GFR >30 mL/minute and/or S_{cr} <1.7 mg/dL (women); S_{cr} <2 mg/dL (men)]: No dose adjustment required

Severe impairment [GFR<30 mL/minute and/or S_{cr} >1.7 mg/dL (women); S_{cr} >2 mg/dL (men)]: Use caution; not studied in severe renal impairment

Dosage adjustment in hepatic impairment No dosage adjustment required

Dietary Considerations May be taken with or without food; however, a high-fat meal reduces absorption

Administration Administer at the same time daily; may take with or without a meal, but consistent administration with regards to meals is recommended. Avoid taking with high-fat meals.

Monitoring Parameters Blood pressure; serum potassium, BUN, serum creatinine

Dosage Forms Excipient information presented when available (limited, particularly for generics); consult specific product labeling.

Tablet:

Tekturna®: 150 mg, 300 mg

Aliskiren and Hydrochlorothiazide

(a lis KYE ren & hye droe klor oh THYE a zide)

U.S. Brand Names Tekturna HCT®

Index Terms Aliskiren Hemifumarate and Hydrochlorothiazide; Hydrochlorothiazide and Aliskiren

Pharmacologic Category Diuretic, Thiazide; Renin Inhibitor

Use Treatment of hypertension (not recommended for initial treatment)

Pregnancy Risk Factor D

Dosage Oral: Adults: One tablet daily; dosage must be individualized (see below). May be substituted for previously titrated dosages of the individual components. Titrate at 2- to 4-week intervals as necessary.

Patients not controlled with single-agent therapy: Initiate by adding the lowest available dose of the alternative component (aliskiren 150 mg or hydrochlorothiazide 12.5 mg); titrate to effect (maximum daily aliskiren dose: 300 mg; maximum daily hydrochlorothiazide dose: 25 mg)

Dosage adjustment in renal impairment: Not recommended in patients with Cl_{cr} <30 mL/minute

Dosage adjustment in hepatic impairment: Dosage adjustment not required

Additional Information Complete prescribing information for this medication should be consulted for additional detail.

Dosage Forms Excipient information presented when available (limited, particularly for generics); consult specific product labeling.

Tablet:

Tekturna HCT®:

150/12.5: Aliskiren 150 mg and hydrochlorothiazide 12.5 mg

150/25: Aliskiren 150 mg and hydrochlorothiazide 25 mg

300/12.5: Aliskiren 300 mg and hydrochlorothiazide 12.5 mg

300/25: Aliskiren 300 mg and hydrochlorothiazide 25 mg

◆ **Aliskiren Hemifumarate** *see* Aliskiren *on page 63*

◆ **Aliskiren Hemifumarate and Hydrochlorothiazide** *see* Aliskiren and Hydrochlorothiazide *on page 64*

Alitretinoin (a li TRET i noyn)

U.S. Brand Names Panretin®

Canadian Brand Names Panretin®

Pharmacologic Category Antineoplastic Agent, Miscellaneous; Retinoic Acid Derivative

Use Orphan drug: Topical treatment of cutaneous lesions in AIDS-related Kaposi's sarcoma

Unlabeled/Investigational Use Cutaneous T-cell lymphomas

Pregnancy Risk Factor D

Pregnancy Considerations Potentially teratogenic and/or embryotoxic; limb, craniofacial, or skeletal defects have been observed in animal models. If used during pregnancy or if the patient becomes pregnant while using alitretinoin, the woman should be advised of potential harm to the fetus. Women of childbearing potential should avoid becoming pregnant.

Lactation Excretion in breast milk unknown/not recommended

Medication Safety Issues

Sound-álike/look-alike issues:

Panretin® may be confused with pancreatin

High alert medication: The Institute for Safe Medication Practices (ISMP) includes this medication among its list of drugs which have a heightened risk of causing significant patient harm when used in error.

Contraindications Hypersensitivity to alitretinoin, other retinoids, or any component of the formulation; pregnancy

Warnings/Precautions Hazardous agent - use appropriate precautions for handling and disposal. May cause fetal harm if absorbed by a woman who is pregnant. May be photosensitizing (based on experience with other retinoids); minimize sun or other UV exposure of treated areas. Do not use concurrently with topical products containing DEET. Safety in pediatric patients or geriatric patients has not been established.

Adverse Reactions

>10%:

Central nervous system: Pain (0% to 34%)

Dermatologic: Rash (25% to 77%), pruritus (8% to 11%)

Neuromuscular & skeletal: Paresthesia (3% to 22%)

5% to 10%:

Cardiovascular: Edema (3% to 8%)

Dermatologic: Exfoliative dermatitis (3% to 9%), skin disorder (0% to 8%)

Drug Interactions

Avoid Concomitant Use There are no known interactions where it is recommended to avoid concomitant use.

Increased Effect/Toxicity There are no known significant interactions involving an increase in effect.

Decreased Effect There are no known significant interactions involving a decrease in effect.

Stability Store at room temperature.

Mechanism of Action Binds to retinoid receptors to inhibit growth of Kaposi's sarcoma

Pharmacodynamics/Kinetics Absorption: Not extensive

Dosage Topical: Apply gel twice daily to cutaneous lesions

Administration Do not use occlusive dressings.

Dosage Forms Excipient information presented when available (limited, particularly for generics); consult specific product labeling.

Gel:

Panretin®: 0.1% (60 g)

- **Alka-Mints® [OTC]** *see* Calcium Carbonate *on page 238*
- **Alka-Seltzer Plus® Day Cold [OTC]** *see* Acetaminophen, Dextromethorphan, and Phenylephrine *on page 32*
- **Alka-Seltzer Plus® Sinus Formula [OTC]** *see* Acetaminophen and Phenylephrine *on page 29*
- **Alka-Seltzer® P.M. [OTC]** *see* Aspirin and Diphenhydramine *on page 145*
- **Alkeran®** *see* Melphalan *on page 936*
- **Allanderm-T™** *see* Trypsin, Balsam Peru, and Castor Oil *on page 1526*
- **AllanEnzyme** *see* Papain and Urea *on page 1142*
- **Allanfil 405** *see* Chlorophyllin, Papain, and Urea *on page 306*
- **Allanfil Spray** *see* Chlorophyllin, Papain, and Urea *on page 306*
- **AllanFol RX [DSC]** *see* Folic Acid, Cyanocobalamin, and Pyridoxine *on page 655*
- **AllanTan Pediatric [DSC]** *see* Chlorpheniramine and Phenylephrine *on page 309*
- **Allegra®** *see* Fexofenadine *on page 618*
- **Allegra-D® (Can)** *see* Fexofenadine and Pseudoephedrine *on page 619*
- **Allegra-D® 12 Hour** *see* Fexofenadine and Pseudoephedrine *on page 619*
- **Allegra-D® 24 Hour** *see* Fexofenadine and Pseudoephedrine *on page 619*
- **Allegra® ODT** *see* Fexofenadine *on page 618*
- **Allerdryl® (Can)** *see* DiphenhydrAMINE *on page 456*
- **AllerDur™** *see* Dexchlorpheniramine and Pseudoephedrine *on page 428*
- **Allerest® Allergy and Sinus Relief [OTC]** *see* Acetaminophen and Pseudoephedrine *on page 30*
- **Allerest® Maximum Strength Allergy and Hay Fever [OTC]** *see* Chlorpheniramine and Pseudoephedrine *on page 310*
- **Allerfrim [OTC]** *see* Triprolidine and Pseudoephedrine *on page 1522*
- **Allergen®** *see* Antipyrine and Benzocaine *on page 124*
- **Allergy Relief [OTC]** *see* Loratadine *on page 904*
- **AllerMax® [OTC]** *see* DiphenhydrAMINE *on page 456*
- **Allernix (Can)** *see* DiphenhydrAMINE *on page 456*
- **AllerTan™** *see* Chlorpheniramine, Pyrilamine, and Phenylephrine *on page 315*
- **AlleRx™-D** *see* Pseudoephedrine and Methscopolamine *on page 1267*
- **AlleRx™ Suspension** *see* Chlorpheniramine and Phenylephrine *on page 309*
- **Allfen-DM** *see* Guaifenesin and Dextromethorphan *on page 710*
- **Allfen Jr** *see* GuaiFENesin *on page 709*
- **Alli™ [OTC]** *see* Orlistat *on page 1107*
- **Alloprin® (Can)** *see* Allopurinol *on page 65*

Allopurinol (al oh PURE i nole)

U.S. Brand Names Aloprim™; Zyloprim®

Canadian Brand Names Alloprin®; Apo-Allopurinol®; Novo-Purol; Zyloprim®

Index Terms Allopurinol Sodium

Pharmacologic Category Xanthine Oxidase Inhibitor

Additional Appendix Information

Desensitization Protocols *on page 1691*

Use

Oral: Prevention of attack of gouty arthritis and nephropathy; treatment of secondary hyperuricemia which may occur during treatment of tumors or leukemia; prevention of recurrent calcium oxalate calculi

I.V.: Treatment of elevated serum and urinary uric acid levels when oral therapy is not tolerated in patients with leukemia, lymphoma, and solid tumor malignancies who are receiving cancer chemotherapy

Pregnancy Risk Factor C

Pregnancy Considerations There are few reports describing the use of allopurinol during pregnancy; no adverse fetal outcomes attributable to allopurinol have been reported in humans; use only if potential benefit outweighs the potential risk to the fetus.

Lactation Enters breast milk/use caution (AAP rates "compatible")

Medication Safety Issues

Sound-alike/look-alike issues:

Allopurinol may be confused with Apresoline

Zyloprim® may be confused with Xylo-Pfan®, ZORprin®, Zovirax®

Contraindications Hypersensitivity to allopurinol or any component of the formulation

Warnings/Precautions Do not use to treat asymptomatic hyperuricemia. Has been associated with a number of hypersensitivity reactions, including severe reactions (vasculitis and Stevens-Johnson syndrome); discontinue at first sign of rash. Reversible hepatotoxicity has been reported; use with caution in patients with pre-existing hepatic impairment. Bone marrow suppression has been reported; use caution with other drugs causing myelosuppression. Caution in renal impairment, dosage adjustments needed. Use with caution in patients taking diuretics concurrently. Risk of skin rash may be increased in patients receiving amoxicillin or ampicillin. The risk of hypersensitivity may be increased in patients receiving thiazides, and possibly ACE inhibitors. Use caution with mercaptopurine or azathioprine; dosage adjustment necessary.

Adverse Reactions

>1%:

Dermatologic: Rash (increased with ampicillin or amoxicillin use, 1.5% per manufacturer, >10% in some reports)

Gastrointestinal: Nausea (1.3%), vomiting (1.2%)

Renal: Renal failure/impairment (1.2%)

<1% (Limited to important or life-threatening): Acute tubular necrosis, agranulocytosis, angioedema, aplastic anemia, bronchospasm, cataracts, exfoliative dermatitis, granuloma annulare, granulomatous hepatitis, hypersensitivity syndrome, interstitial nephritis, macular retinitis, nephrolithiasis, neuritis, pancreatitis, paresthesia, peripheral neuropathy, Stevens-Johnson syndrome, toxic epidermal necrolysis, toxic pustuloderma, vasculitis

Drug Interactions

Avoid Concomitant Use There are no known interactions where it is recommended to avoid concomitant use.

Increased Effect/Toxicity

Allopurinol may increase the levels/effects of: Amoxicillin; Ampicillin; AzaTHIOprine; CarBAMazepine;

ChlorproPAMIDE; Cyclophosphamide; Didanosine; Mercaptopurine; Pivampicillin; Theophylline Derivatives; Vitamin K Antagonists

The levels/effects of Allopurinol may be increased by: ACE Inhibitors; Loop Diuretics; Thiazide Diuretics

Decreased Effect

The levels/effects of Allopurinol may be decreased by: Antacids

Ethanol/Nutrition/Herb Interactions

Ethanol: May decrease effectiveness.

Iron supplements: Hepatic iron uptake may be increased.

Vitamin C: Large amounts of vitamin C may acidify urine and increase kidney stone formation.

Stability

Powder for injection: Store at controlled room temperature of 15°C to 30°C (59°F to 86°F). Further dilution with NS or D_5W (50-100 mL) to ≤6 mg/mL is recommended. Following reconstitution, intravenous solutions should be stored at 20°C to 25°C (68°F to 77°F). Do not refrigerate reconstituted and/or diluted product. Must be administered within 10 hours of solution preparation.

Tablet: Store at controlled room temperature of 15°C to 25°C (59°F to 77°F).

Mechanism of Action Allopurinol inhibits xanthine oxidase, the enzyme responsible for the conversion of hypoxanthine to xanthine to uric acid. Allopurinol is metabolized to oxypurinol which is also an inhibitor of xanthine oxidase; allopurinol acts on purine catabolism, reducing the production of uric acid without disrupting the biosynthesis of vital purines.

Pharmacodynamics/Kinetics

Onset of action: Peak effect: 1-2 weeks

Absorption: Oral: ~80%; Rectal: Poor and erratic

Distribution: V_d: ~1.6 L/kg; V_{ss}: 0.84-0.87 L/kg; enters breast milk

Protein binding: <1%

Metabolism: ~75% to active metabolites, chiefly oxypurinol

Bioavailability: 49% to 53%

Half-life elimination:

Normal renal function: Parent drug: 1-3 hours; Oxypurinol: 18-30 hours

End-stage renal disease: Prolonged

Time to peak, plasma: Oral: 30-120 minutes

Excretion: Urine (76% as oxypurinol, 12% as unchanged drug)

Allopurinol and oxypurinol are dialyzable

Dosage

Oral: Doses >300 mg should be given in divided doses.

Children ≤10 years: Secondary hyperuricemia associated with chemotherapy: 10 mg/kg/day in 2-3 divided doses **or** 200-300 mg/m²/day in 2-4 divided doses, maximum: 800 mg/24 hours

Alternative (manufacturer labeling): <6 years: 150 mg/day in 3 divided doses; 6-10 years: 300 mg/day in 2-3 divided doses

Children >10 years and Adults:

Secondary hyperuricemia associated with chemotherapy: 600-800 mg/day in 2-3 divided doses for prevention of acute uric acid nephropathy for 2-3 days starting 1-2 days before chemotherapy

Gout: Mild: 200-300 mg/day; Severe: 400-600 mg/day; to reduce the possibility of acute gouty attacks, initiate dose at 100 mg/day and increase weekly to recommended dosage. Maximum daily dose: 800 mg/day.

Recurrent calcium oxalate stones: 200-300 mg/day in single or divided doses

Elderly: Initial: 100 mg/day, increase until desired uric acid level is obtained

I.V.: Hyperuricemia secondary to chemotherapy: Intravenous daily dose can be given as a single infusion or in equally divided doses at 6-, 8-, or 12-hour intervals. A fluid intake sufficient to yield a daily urinary output of at least 2 L in adults and the maintenance of a neutral or, preferably, slightly alkaline urine are desirable.

Children ≤10 years: Starting dose: 200 mg/m²/day

Children >10 years and Adults: 200-400 mg/m²/day (maximum: 600 mg/day)

Dosing adjustment in renal impairment: Must be adjusted due to accumulation of allopurinol and metabolites:

Oral: Removed by hemodialysis; adult maintenance doses of allopurinol (mg) based on creatinine clearance (mL/minute): See table.

Adult Maintenance Doses of Allopurinol[1]

Creatinine Clearance (mL/min)	Maintenance Dose of Allopurinol (mg)
140	400 daily
120	350 daily
100	300 daily
80	250 daily
60	200 daily
40	150 daily
20	100 daily
10	100 every 2 days
0	100 every 3 days

[1]This table is based on a standard maintenance dose of 300 mg of allopurinol per day for a patient with a creatinine clearance of 100 mL/min.

I.V.:

Cl_{cr} 10-20 mL/minute: 200 mg/day

Cl_{cr} 3-10 mL/minute: 100 mg/day

Cl_{cr} <3 mL/minute: 100 mg/day at extended intervals

Hemodialysis: Administer dose posthemodialysis or administer 50% supplemental dose

Dietary Considerations Should administer oral forms after meals with plenty of fluid. Fluid intake should be administered to yield neutral or slightly alkaline urine and an output of ~2 L (in adults).

Administration

Oral: Should administer oral forms after meals with plenty of fluid.

I.V.: Infuse over 15-60 minutes. The rate of infusion depends on the volume of the infusion. Whenever possible, therapy should be initiated at 24-48 hours before the start of chemotherapy known to cause tumor lysis (including adrenocorticosteroids). I.V. daily dose can be administered as a single infusion or in equally divided doses at 6-, 8-, or 12-hour interval.

Monitoring Parameters CBC, serum uric acid levels, I & O, hepatic and renal function, especially at start of therapy

Reference Range Uric acid, serum: An increase occurs during childhood

Adults:

Male: 3.4-7 mg/dL or slightly more

Female: 2.4-6 mg/dL or slightly more

Values >7 mg/dL are sometimes arbitrarily regarded as hyperuricemia, but there is no sharp line between normals on the one hand, and the serum uric acid of those with clinical gout. Normal ranges cannot be adjusted for purine ingestion, but high purine diet increases uric acid. Uric acid may be increased with body size, exercise, and stress.

Dosage Forms Excipient information presented when available (limited, particularly for generics); consult specific product labeling.

Injection, powder for reconstitution, as sodium: 500 mg

Aloprim™: 500 mg

Tablet: 100 mg, 300 mg

Zyloprim®: 100 mg, 300 mg

Extemporaneous Preparations Crush tablets to make a 5 mg/mL suspension in simple syrup; stable 14 days under refrigeration

Nahata MC and Hipple TF, *Pediatric Drug Formulations*, 1st ed, Harvey Whitney Books Co, 1990.

◆ **Allopurinol Sodium** *see* Allopurinol *on page 65*

◆ **All-*trans*-Retinoic Acid** *see* Tretinoin (Oral) *on page 1508*

◆ **Almacone® [OTC]** *see* Aluminum Hydroxide, Magnesium Hydroxide, and Simethicone *on page 76*

◆ **Almacone Double Strength® [OTC]** *see* Aluminum Hydroxide, Magnesium Hydroxide, and Simethicone *on page 76*

◆ **Almora® [OTC]** *see* Magnesium Gluconate *on page 915*

Almotriptan (al moh TRIP tan)

U.S. Brand Names Axert™

Canadian Brand Names Axert™

Index Terms Almotriptan Malate

Pharmacologic Category Antimigraine Agent; Serotonin 5-$HT_{1B,\ 1D}$ Receptor Agonist

Additional Appendix Information

Antimigraine Drugs: 5-HT_1 Receptor Agonists *on page 1642*

Use Acute treatment of migraine with or without aura

Pregnancy Risk Factor C

Pregnancy Considerations There are no adequate and well-controlled studies in pregnant women. Use in pregnancy should be limited to situations where benefit outweighs risk to fetus. In some (but not all) animal studies, administration was associated with embryolethality, fetal malformations, and decreased pup weight.

Lactation Excretion in breast milk unknown/use caution

Medication Safety Issues

Sound-alike/look-alike issues:

Axert™ may be confused with Antivert®

Contraindications Hypersensitivity to almotriptan or any component of the formulation; use as prophylactic therapy for migraine; hemiplegic or basilar migraine; cluster headache; known or suspected ischemic heart disease (angina pectoris, MI, documented silent ischemia, coronary artery vasospasm, Prinzmetal's variant angina); peripheral vascular syndromes (including ischemic bowel disease); uncontrolled hypertension; use within 24 hours of another 5-HT_1 agonist; use within 24 hours of ergotamine derivative; concurrent administration or within 2 weeks of discontinuing an MAO inhibitor (specifically MAO type A inhibitors)

Warnings/Precautions Almotriptan is indicated only in patients ≥18 years of age with a clear diagnosis of migraine headache. If a patient does not respond to the first dose, the diagnosis of migraine should be reconsidered. Do not give to patients with risk factors for CAD until a cardiovascular evaluation has been performed; if evaluation is satisfactory, the healthcare provider should administer the first dose and cardiovascular status should be periodically re-evaluated. Cardiac events (coronary artery vasospasm, transient ischemia, myocardial infarction, ventricular tachycardia/fibrillation, cardiac arrest, and death), cerebral/subarachnoid hemorrhage, stroke, peripheral vascular ischemia, and colonic ischemia have been reported with 5-HT_1 agonist administration. Significant elevation in blood pressure, including hypertensive crisis, has also been reported on rare occasions in patients with and without a history of hypertension. Use with caution in liver or renal dysfunction. Symptoms of agitation, confusion, hallucinations, hyper-reflexia, myoclonus, shivering, and tachycardia (serotonin syndrome) may occur with concomitant proserotonergic drugs (ie, SSRIs/SNRIs or triptans) or agents which reduce almotriptan's metabolism. Safety and efficacy in pediatric patients have not been established.

Adverse Reactions

1% to 10%:

Central nervous system: Headache (>1%), dizziness (>1%), somnolence (>1%)

Gastrointestinal: Nausea (1% to 2%), xerostomia (1%)

Neuromuscular & skeletal: Paresthesia (1%)

<1% (Limited to important or life-threatening): Colitis, coronary artery vasospasm, hypertension, myocardial ischemia, MI, neuropathy, rash, syncope, tachycardia, ventricular fibrillation, ventricular tachycardia, vertigo

Drug Interactions

Metabolism/Transport Effects **Substrate** (minor) of CYP2D6, 3A4

Avoid Concomitant Use

Avoid concomitant use of Almotriptan with any of the following: Ergot Derivatives; MAO Inhibitors; Sibutramine

Increased Effect/Toxicity

Almotriptan may increase the levels/effects of: Ergot Derivatives; Serotonin Modulators

The levels/effects of Almotriptan may be increased by: Ergot Derivatives; Ketoconazole; MAO Inhibitors; Sibutramine

Decreased Effect There are no known significant interactions involving a decrease in effect.

Stability Store at 15°C to 30°C (59°F to 86°F).

Mechanism of Action Selective agonist for serotonin (5-HT_{1B}, 5-HT_{1D}, 5-HT_{1F} receptors) in cranial arteries; causes vasoconstriction and reduce sterile inflammation associated with antidromic neuronal transmission correlating with relief of migraine

Pharmacodynamics/Kinetics

Absorption: Well absorbed

Distribution: V_d: 180-200 L

Protein binding: ~35%

Metabolism: MAO type A oxidative deamination (~27% of dose); via CYP3A4 and 2D6 (~12% of dose) to inactive metabolites

Bioavailability: 70%

Half-life elimination: 3-4 hours

Time to peak: 1-3 hours

Excretion: Urine (40% as unchanged drug); feces (13% unchanged and metabolized)

Dosage Oral: Adults: Migraine: Initial: 6.25-12.5 mg in a single dose; if the headache returns, repeat the dose after 2 hours; no more than 2 doses in 24-hour period

Note: If the first dose is ineffective, diagnosis needs to be re-evaluated. Safety of treating more than 4 migraines/month has not been established.

Dosage adjustment in renal impairment: Initial: 6.25 mg in a single dose; maximum daily dose: ≤12.5 mg

Dosage adjustment in hepatic impairment: Initial: 6.25 mg in a single dose; maximum daily dose: ≤12.5 mg

Dietary Considerations May be taken without regard to meals

Dosage Forms Excipient information presented when available (limited, particularly for generics); consult specific product labeling.

Tablet, as malate:

Axert™: 6.25 mg, 12.5 mg

◆ **Almotriptan Malate** *see* Almotriptan *on page 67*

◆ **Alocril®** *see* Nedocromil *on page 1047*

◆ **Aloe Vesta® 2-n-1 Antifungal [OTC]** *see* Miconazole *on page 989*

◆ **Alomide®** *see* Lodoxamide *on page 898*

◆ **Alophen® [OTC]** *see* Bisacodyl *on page 198*

- **Aloprim™** *see* Allopurinol *on page 65*
- **Alora®** *see* Estradiol *on page 554*
- **Aloxi®** *see* Palonosetron *on page 1132*
- **Alpain** *see* Acetaminophen and Phenyltoloxamine *on page 29*

Alpha-Galactosidase (AL fa ga lak TOE si days)

U.S. Brand Names beano® [OTC]

Index Terms *Aspergillus niger*

Pharmacologic Category Enzyme

Use Prevention of flatulence and bloating attributed to a variety of grains, cereals, nuts, and vegetables containing the sugars raffinose, stachyose, and/or verbascose

Dosage Oral: Children ≥12 years and Adults:

Drops: Take 5 drops per serving of problem food; adjust according to number of problem foods per meal; usual dose/meal: 10-15 drops

Tablet: One tablet per serving of problem food; adjust according to number of problem foods per meal; usual dose/meal: 2-3 tablets

Additional Information Complete prescribing information for this medication should be consulted for additional detail.

Dosage Forms Excipient information presented when available (limited, particularly for generics); consult specific product labeling.

Liquid, oral [drops]:

beano®: 150 galactosidase units/5 drops [contains sodium 5 mg/5 drops]

Tablet, oral:

beano®: 150 galactosidase units/tablet

- **Alpha-Galactosidase-A (Recombinant)** *see* Agalsidase Beta *on page 47*
- **Alphagan® (Can)** *see* Brimonidine *on page 212*
- **Alphagan® P** *see* Brimonidine *on page 212*
- **Alphanate®** ***[new formulation]*** *see* Antihemophilic Factor/von Willebrand Factor Complex (Human) *on page 122*
- **AlphaNine® SD** *see* Factor IX *on page 599*
- **Alphaquin HP®** *see* Hydroquinone *on page 749*
- **Alph-E [OTC]** *see* Vitamin E *on page 1566*
- **Alph-E-Mixed [OTC]** *see* Vitamin E *on page 1566*

ALPRAZolam (al PRAY zoe lam)

U.S. Brand Names Alprazolam Intensol®; Niravam™; Xanax XR®; Xanax®

Canadian Brand Names Alti-Alprazolam; Apo-Alpraz®; Apo-Alpraz® TS; Gen-Alprazolam; Novo-Alprazol; Nu-Alprax; Xanax TS™; Xanax®

Pharmacologic Category Benzodiazepine

Additional Appendix Information

Benzodiazepines *on page 1646*

Use Treatment of anxiety disorder (GAD); panic disorder, with or without agoraphobia; anxiety associated with depression

Unlabeled/Investigational Use Anxiety in children

Restrictions C-IV

Pregnancy Risk Factor D

Pregnancy Considerations Benzodiazepines have the potential to cause harm to the fetus, particularly when administered during the first trimester. In addition, withdrawal symptoms may occur in the neonate following *in utero* exposure. Use during pregnancy should be avoided.

Lactation Enters breast milk/not recommended (AAP rates "of concern")

Medication Safety Issues

Sound-alike/look-alike issues:

ALPRAZolam may be confused with alprostadil, LORazepam, triazolam

Xanax® may be confused with Lanoxin®, Tenex®, Tylox®, Xopenex®, Zantac®, Zyrtec®

Contraindications Hypersensitivity to alprazolam or any component of the formulation (cross-sensitivity with other benzodiazepines may exist); narrow-angle glaucoma; concurrent use with ketoconazole or itraconazole; pregnancy

Warnings/Precautions Rebound or withdrawal symptoms, including seizures, may occur 18 hours to 3 days following abrupt discontinuation or large decreases in dose (more common in patients receiving >4 mg/day or prolonged treatment). Breakthrough anxiety may occur at the end of dosing interval. Use with caution in patients receiving concurrent CYP3A4 inhibitors. Use with caution in renal impairment or predisposition to urate nephropathy. Use with caution in elderly or debilitated patients, patients with hepatic disease (including alcoholics), renal impairment, or obese patients.

Causes CNS depression (dose related) which may impair physical and mental capabilities. Patients must be cautioned about performing tasks that require mental alertness (eg, operating machinery or driving). Effects with other sedative drugs or ethanol may be potentiated. Benzodiazepines have been associated with falls and traumatic injury and should be used with extreme caution in patients who are at risk of these events (especially the elderly). Use with caution in patients with respiratory disease or impaired gag reflex.

Use caution in patients with depression, particularly if suicidal risk may be present. Episodes of mania or hypomania have occurred in depressed patients treated with alprazolam. May cause physical or psychological dependence. Acute withdrawal may be precipitated in patients after administration of flumazenil.

Benzodiazepines have been associated with anterograde amnesia. Paradoxical reactions have been reported with benzodiazepines, particularly in adolescent/pediatric or psychiatric patients. Does not have analgesic, antidepressant, or antipsychotic properties.

Adverse Reactions

>10%:

Central nervous system: Abnormal coordination, cognitive disorder, depression, drowsiness, fatigue, irritability, lightheadedness, memory impairment, sedation, somnolence

Gastrointestinal: Appetite increased/decreased, constipation, salivation decreased, weight gain/loss, xerostomia

Genitourinary: Micturition difficulty

Neuromuscular & skeletal: Dysarthria

1% to 10%:

Cardiovascular: Hypotension

Central nervous system: Agitation, attention disturbance, confusion, depersonalization, derealization, disorientation, disinhibition, dizziness, dream abnormalities, fear, hallucinations, hypersomnia, nightmares, seizure, talkativeness

Dermatologic: Dermatitis, pruritus, rash

Endocrine & metabolic: Libido decreased/increased, menstrual disorders

Gastrointestinal: Salivation increased

Genitourinary: Incontinence

Hepatic: Bilirubin increased, jaundice, liver enzymes increased

Neuromuscular & skeletal: Arthralgia, ataxia, myalgia, paresthesia

Ocular: Diplopia

Respiratory: Allergic rhinitis, dyspnea

<1% (Limited to important or life-threatening): Amnesia, falls, galactorrhea, gynecomastia, hepatic failure, hepatitis, hyperprolactinemia, Stevens-Johnson syndrome

Drug Interactions

Metabolism/Transport Effects Substrate of CYP3A4 (major)

Avoid Concomitant Use There are no known interactions where it is recommended to avoid concomitant use.

Increased Effect/Toxicity

ALPRAZolam may increase the levels/effects of: Alcohol (Ethyl); Clozapine; CNS Depressants

The levels/effects of ALPRAZolam may be increased by: Antifungal Agents (Azole Derivatives, Systemic); Aprepitant; Calcium Channel Blockers (Nondihydropyridine); Cimetidine; CYP3A4 Inhibitors (Moderate); CYP3A4 Inhibitors (Strong); Dasatinib; Disulfiram; Fluconazole; Fosaprepitant; Grapefruit Juice; Isoniazid; Macrolide Antibiotics; Nefazodone; Oral Contraceptive (Estrogens); Oral Contraceptive (Progestins); Protease Inhibitors; Proton Pump Inhibitors; Selective Serotonin Reuptake Inhibitors

Decreased Effect

The levels/effects of ALPRAZolam may be decreased by: CarBAMazepine; CYP3A4 Inducers (Strong); Deferasirox; Rifamycin Derivatives; St Johns Wort; Theophylline Derivatives; Yohimbine

Ethanol/Nutrition/Herb Interactions

Cigarette smoking: May decrease alprazolam concentrations up to 50%.

Ethanol: Avoid ethanol (may increase CNS depression).

Food: Alprazolam serum concentration is unlikely to be increased by grapefruit juice because of alprazolam's high oral bioavailability. The C_{max} of the extended release formulation is increased by 25% when a high-fat meal is given 2 hours before dosing. T_{max} is decreased 30% when food is given immediately prior to dose. T_{max} is increased by 30% when food is given ≥1 hour after dose.

Herb/Nutraceutical: St John's wort may decrease alprazolam levels. Avoid valerian, St John's wort, kava kava, gotu kola (may increase CNS depression).

Stability Orally-disintegrating tablet: Store at room temperature of 20°C to 25°C (68°F to 77°F). Protect from moisture. Seal bottle tightly and discard any cotton packaged inside bottle.

Mechanism of Action Binds to stereospecific benzodiazepine receptors on the postsynaptic GABA neuron at several sites within the central nervous system, including the limbic system, reticular formation. Enhancement of the inhibitory effect of GABA on neuronal excitability results by increased neuronal membrane permeability to chloride ions. This shift in chloride ions results in hyperpolarization (a less excitable state) and stabilization.

Pharmacodynamics/Kinetics

Onset of action: Immediate release and extended release formulations: 1 hour

Duration: Immediate release: 5.1 ± 1.7 hours; Extended release: 11.3 ± 4.2 hours

Absorption: Extended release: Slower relative to immediate release formulation resulting in a concentration that is maintained 5-11 hours after dosing

Distribution: V_d: 0.9-1.2 L/kg; enters breast milk

Protein binding: 80%; primarily to albumin

Metabolism: Hepatic via CYP3A4; forms two active metabolites (4-hydroxyalprazolam and α-hydroxyalprazolam)

Bioavailability: 90%

Half-life elimination:

Adults: 11.2 hours (immediate release range: 6.3-26.9; extended release range: 10.7-15.8)

Elderly: 16.3 hours (range: 9-26.9 hours)

Alcoholic liver disease: 19.7 hours (range: 5.8-65.3 hours)

Obesity: 21.8 hours (range: 9.9-40.4 hours)

Time to peak, serum: Immediate release: 1-2 hours; Extended release: ~9 hours; decreased by 1 hour following bedtime dosing compared to morning dosing

Excretion: Urine (as unchanged drug and metabolites)

Dosage Oral: **Note:** Treatment >4 months should be re-evaluated to determine the patient's continued need for the drug

Children: Anxiety (unlabeled use): Immediate release: Initial: 0.005 mg/kg/dose or 0.125 mg/dose 3 times/day; increase in increments of 0.125-0.25 mg, up to a maximum of 0.02 mg/kg/dose or 0.06 mg/kg/day (0.375-3 mg/day). See "Dose Reduction" comment below.

Adults:

Anxiety: Immediate release: Effective doses are 0.5-4 mg/day in divided doses; the manufacturer recommends starting at 0.25-0.5 mg 3 times/day; titrate dose upward; usual maximum: 4 mg/day. Patients requiring doses >4 mg/day should be increased cautiously. Periodic reassessment and consideration of dosage reduction is recommended.

Anxiety associated with depression: Immediate release: Average dose required: 2.5-3 mg/day in divided doses

Ethanol withdrawal (unlabeled use): Immediate release: Usual dose: 2-2.5 mg/day in divided doses

Panic disorder:

Immediate release: Initial: 0.5 mg 3 times/day; dose may be increased every 3-4 days in increments ≤1 mg/day. Mean effective dosage: 5-6 mg/day; many patients obtain relief at 2 mg/day, as much as 10 mg/day may be required

Extended release: 0.5-1 mg once daily; may increase dose every 3-4 days in increments ≤1 mg/day (range: 3-6 mg/day)

Switching from immediate release to extended release: Patients may be switched to extended release tablets by taking the total daily dose of the immediate release tablets and giving it once daily using the extended release preparation.

Preoperative sedation: 0.5 mg in evening at bedtime and 0.5 mg 1 hour before procedure

Dose reduction: Abrupt discontinuation should be avoided. Daily dose may be decreased by 0.5 mg every 3 days, however, some patients may require a slower reduction. If withdrawal symptoms occur, resume previous dose and discontinue on a less rapid schedule.

Elderly: Initial: 0.125-0.25 mg twice daily; increase by 0.125 mg/day as needed. The smallest effective dose should be used. **Note:** Elderly patients may be more sensitive to the effects of alprazolam including ataxia and oversedation. The elderly may also have impaired renal function leading to decreased clearance. Titrate gradually, if needed.

Immediate release: Initial: 0.25 mg 2-3 times/day

Extended release: Initial: 0.5 mg once daily

Dosing adjustment in renal impairment: No guidelines for adjustment; use caution

Dosing adjustment in hepatic impairment: Reduce dose by 50% to 60% or avoid in cirrhosis

Administration

Immediate release preparations: Can be administered sublingually with comparable onset and completeness of absorption.

Extended release tablet: Should be taken once daily in the morning; do not crush, break, or chew.

Orally-disintegrating tablets: Using dry hands, place tablet on top of tongue. If using one-half of tablet, immediately discard remaining half (may not remain stable). Administration with water is not necessary.

Monitoring Parameters Respiratory and cardiovascular status

Additional Information Not intended for management of anxieties and minor distresses associated with everyday life. Treatment longer than 4 months should be re-evaluated to determine the patient's need for the drug. Patients who become physically dependent on alprazolam tend to have a difficult time discontinuing it; withdrawal symptoms may be severe. To minimize withdrawal symptoms, taper dosage slowly; do not discontinue abruptly. Abrupt discontinuation after sustained use (generally >10 days) may cause withdrawal symptoms.

Dosage Forms Excipient information presented when available (limited, particularly for generics); consult specific product labeling.

Solution, oral [concentrate]:
  Alprazolam Intensol®: 1 mg/mL (30 mL) [alcohol free, dye free, sugar free; contains propylene glycol]
Tablet: 0.25 mg, 0.5 mg, 1 mg, 2 mg
  Xanax®: 0.25 mg, 0.5 mg, 1 mg, 2 mg
Tablet, extended release: 0.5 mg, 1 mg, 2 mg, 3 mg
  Xanax XR®: 0.5 mg, 1 mg, 2 mg, 3 mg
Tablet, orally disintegrating [scored]:
  Niravam™: 0.25 mg, 0.5 mg, 1 mg, 2 mg [orange flavor]

◆ **Alprazolam Intensol®** *see* ALPRAZolam *on page 68*

Alprostadil (al PROS ta dill)

U.S. Brand Names Caverject Impulse®; Caverject®; Edex®; Muse®; Prostin VR Pediatric®

Canadian Brand Names Caverject®; Muse® Pellet; Prostin® VR

Index Terms PGE_1; Prostaglandin E_1

Pharmacologic Category Prostaglandin; Vasodilator

Use

Prostin VR Pediatric®: Temporary maintenance of patency of ductus arteriosus in neonates with ductal-dependent congenital heart disease until surgery can be performed. These defects include cyanotic (eg, pulmonary atresia, pulmonary stenosis, tricuspid atresia, Fallot's tetralogy, transposition of the great vessels) and acyanotic (eg, interruption of aortic arch, coarctation of aorta, hypoplastic left ventricle) heart disease.

Caverject®: Treatment of erectile dysfunction of vasculogenic, psychogenic, or neurogenic etiology; adjunct in the diagnosis of erectile dysfunction

Edex®, Muse®: Treatment of erectile dysfunction of vasculogenic, psychogenic, or neurogenic etiology

Unlabeled/Investigational Use Investigational: Treatment of pulmonary hypertension in infants and children with congenital heart defects with left-to-right shunts

Pregnancy Risk Factor X/C (Muse®)

Pregnancy Considerations Alprostadil is embryotoxic in animal studies. It is not indicated for use in women. The manufacturer of Muse® recommends a condom barrier when being used during sexual intercourse with a pregnant women.

Lactation Not indicated for use in women

Medication Safety Issues

Sound-alike/look-alike issues:
  Alprostadil may be confused with alPRAZolam

Contraindications Hypersensitivity to alprostadil or any component of the formulation; hyaline membrane disease or persistent fetal circulation and when a dominant left-to-right shunt is present; respiratory distress syndrome; conditions predisposing patients to priapism (sickle cell anemia, multiple myeloma, leukemia); patients with anatomical deformation of the penis, penile implants; use in men for whom sexual activity is inadvisable or contraindicated; pregnancy

Warnings/Precautions Use cautiously in neonates with bleeding tendencies. **[U.S. Boxed Warning]: Apnea may occur in 10% to 12% of neonates with congenital heart defects, especially in those weighing <2 kg at birth.** Apnea usually appears during the first hour of drug infusion. When used for patency of ductus arteriosus infuse for the shortest time at the lowest dose consistent with good patient care. Use for >120 hours has been associated with antral hyperplasia and gastric outlet obstruction.

When used in erectile dysfunction, priapism may occur; treat proloonged priapism (erection persisting for >4 hours) immediately to avoid penile tissue damage and permanent loss of potency; discontinue therapy if signs of penile fibrosis develop (penile angulation, cavernosal fibrosis, or Peyronie's disease). When used in erectile dysfunction (Muse®), syncope occurring within 1 hour of administration has been reported. The potential for drug-drug interactions may occur when Muse® is prescribed concomitantly with antihypertensives.

Adverse Reactions

Intraurethral:

>10%: Genitourinary: Penile pain, urethral burning
2% to 10%:
  Central nervous system: Headache, dizziness, pain
  Genitourinary: Vaginal itching (female partner), testicular pain, urethral bleeding (minor)
<2% (Limited to important or life-threatening): Tachycardia, perineal pain, leg pain

Intracavernosal injection:

>10%: Genitourinary: Penile pain
1% to 10%:
  Cardiovascular: Hypertension
  Central nervous system: Headache, dizziness
  Genitourinary: Prolonged erection (>4 hours, 4%), penile fibrosis, penis disorder, penile rash, penile edema
  Local: Injection site hematoma and/or bruising
<1% (Limited to important or life-threatening): Balanitis, injection site hemorrhage, priapism (0.4%)

Intravenous:

>10%:
  Cardiovascular: Flushing
  Central nervous system: Fever
  Respiratory: Apnea
1% to 10%:
  Cardiovascular: Bradycardia, hyper-/hypotension, tachycardia, cardiac arrest, edema
  Central nervous system: Seizure, headache, dizziness
  Endocrine & metabolic: Hypokalemia
  Gastrointestinal: Diarrhea
  Hematologic: Disseminated intravascular coagulation
  Neuromuscular & skeletal: Back pain
  Respiratory: Upper respiratory infection, flu syndrome, sinusitis, nasal congestion, cough
  Miscellaneous: Sepsis, localized pain in structures other than the injection site
<1% (Limited to important or life-threatening): Anemia, anuria, bleeding, bradypnea, bronchial wheezing, cerebral bleeding, CHF, gastric regurgitation, hematuria, hyperbilirubinemia, hyperemia, hyperext1nsion of neck, hyperirritability, hyperkalemia, hypoglycemia, hypothermia, jitteriness, lethargy, peritonitis, second-degree heart block, shock, stiffness, supraventricular tachycardia, thrombocytopenia, ventricular fibrillation

Drug Interactions

Avoid Concomitant Use There are no known interactions where it is recommended to avoid concomitant use.

Increased Effect/Toxicity There are no known significant interactions involving an increase in effect.

Decreased Effect There are no known significant interactions involving a decrease in effect.

Ethanol/Nutrition/Herb Interactions Ethanol: Avoid concurrent use (vasodilating effect).

Stability

Caverject® Impulse™: Store at controlled room temperature of 15°C to 30°C (59°F to 86°F). Provided as a dual-chamber syringe with diluent in one chamber. To mix, hold syringe with needle pointing upward and turn plunger clockwise; turn upside down several times to mix. Device can be set to deliver specified dose, each device can be set at various increments. Following reconstitution, use within 24 hours and discard any unused solution.

Caverject® powder: The 5 mcg, 10 mcg, and 20 mcg vials should be stored at or below 25°C (77°F). The 40 mcg vial should be stored at 2°C to 8°C until dispensed. After dispensing, stable for up to 3 months at or below 25°C. Use only the supplied diluent for reconstitution (ie, bacteriostatic/sterile water with benzyl alcohol 0.945%). Following reconstitution, all strengths should be stored at or below 25°C (77°F); do not refrigerate or freeze; use within 24 hours.

Caverject® solution: Prior to dispensing, store frozen at -20°C to -10°C (-4°F to -14°F); once dispensed, may be stored frozen for up to 3 months, or under refrigeration at 2°C to 8°C (36°F to 46°F) for up to 7 days. Do not refreeze. Once removed from foil wrap, solution may be allowed to warm to room temperature prior to use. If not used immediately, solution should be discarded. Shake well prior to use.

Edex®: Store at controlled room temperature of 15°C to 30°C (59°F to 86°F); following reconstitution with NS, use immediately and discard any unused solution.

Muse®: Refrigerate at 2°C to 8°C (36°F to 46°F); may be stored at room temperature for up to 14 days.

Prostin VR Pediatric®: Refrigerate at 2°C to 8°C (36°F to 46°F); prior to infusion, dilute with D_5W or NS; use within 24 hours.

Mechanism of Action Causes vasodilation by means of direct effect on vascular and ductus arteriosus smooth muscle; relaxes trabecular smooth muscle by dilation of cavernosal arteries when injected along the penile shaft, allowing blood flow to and entrapment in the lacunar spaces of the penis (ie, corporeal veno-occlusive mechanism)

Pharmacodynamics/Kinetics

Onset of action: Rapid

Duration: <1 hour

Distribution: Insignificant following penile injection

Protein binding, plasma: 81% to albumin

Metabolism: ~75% by oxidation in one pass via lungs

Half-life elimination: 5-10 minutes

Excretion: Urine (90% as metabolites) within 24 hours

Dosage

Patent ductus arteriosus (Prostin VR Pediatric®):

I.V. continuous infusion into a large vein, or alternatively through an umbilical artery catheter placed at the ductal opening: 0.05-0.1 mcg/kg/minute with therapeutic response, rate is reduced to lowest effective dosage; with unsatisfactory response, rate is increased gradually; maintenance: 0.01-0.4 mcg/kg/minute

PGE_1 is usually given at an infusion rate of 0.1 mcg/kg/minute, but it is often possible to reduce the dosage to 1/2 or even 1/10 without losing the therapeutic effect. The mixing schedule is as follows. See table.

Alprostadil

Add 1 Ampul (500 mcg) to:	Concentration (mcg/mL)	Infusion Rate	
		mL/min/kg Needed to Infuse 0.1 mcg/kg/min	mL/kg/24 h
250 mL	2	0.05	72
100 mL	5	0.02	28.8
50 mL	10	0.01	14.4
25 mL	20	0.005	7.2

Therapeutic response is indicated by increased pH in those with acidosis or by an increase in oxygenation (PO_2) usually evident within 30 minutes

Erectile dysfunction:

Caverject®, Edex®: Intracavernous: Individualize dose by careful titration; doses >40 mcg (Edex®) or >60 mcg (Caverject®) are not recommended: Initial dose must be titrated in physician's office. Patient must stay in the physician's office until complete detumescence occurs; if there is no response, then the next higher dose may be given within 1 hour; if there is still no response, a 1-day interval before giving the next dose is recommended; increasing the dose or concentration in the treatment of impotence results in increasing pain and discomfort

Vasculogenic, psychogenic, or mixed etiology: Initiate dosage titration at 2.5 mcg, increasing by 2.5 mcg to a dose of 5 mcg and then in increments of 5-10 mcg depending on the erectile response until the dose produces an erection suitable for intercourse, not lasting >1 hour; if there is absolutely no response to initial 2.5 mcg dose, the second dose may be increased to 7.5 mcg, followed by increments of 5-10 mcg

Neurogenic etiology (eg, spinal cord injury): Initiate dosage titration at 1.25 mcg, increasing to a dose of 2.5 mcg and then 5 mcg; increase further in increments 5 mcg until the dose is reached that produces an erection suitable for intercourse, not lasting >1 hour

Maintenance: Once appropriate dose has been determined, patient may self-administer injections at a frequency of no more than 3 times/week with at least 24 hours between doses

Muse® Pellet: Intraurethral:

Initial: 125-250 mcg

Maintenance: Administer as needed to achieve an erection; duration of action is about 30-60 minutes; use only two systems per 24-hour period

Elderly: Elderly patients may have a greater frequency of renal dysfunction; lowest effective dose should be used. In clinical studies with Edex®, higher minimally effective doses and a higher rate of lack of effect were noted.

Administration Erectile dysfunction: Use a 1/2 inch, 27- to 30-gauge needle. Inject into the dorsolateral aspect of the proximal third of the penis, avoiding visible veins; alternate side of the penis for injections.

Monitoring Parameters Arterial pressure, respiratory rate, heart rate, temperature, degree of penile pain, length of erection, signs of infection

Dosage Forms Excipient information presented when available (limited, particularly for generics); consult specific product labeling. [DSC] = Discontinued product

Injection, powder for reconstitution:

Caverject®: 20 mcg, 40 mcg [contains lactose; diluent contains benzyl alcohol]

Caverject Impulse®: 10 mcg, 20 mcg [prefilled injection system; contains lactose; diluent contains benzyl alcohol]

Edex®: 10 mcg, 20 mcg, 40 mcg [contains lactose; packaged in kits containing diluent, syringe, and alcohol swab]

Injection, solution: 500 mcg/mL (1 mL)

Prostin VR Pediatric®: 500 mcg/mL (1 mL) [contains dehydrated alcohol]

Pellet, urethral:

Muse®: 125 mcg (6s) [DSC], 250 mcg (6s), 500 mcg (6s), 1000 mcg (6s)

◆ **Alrex®** *see* Loteprednol *on page 909*

◆ **Altabax™** *see* Retapamulin *on page 1306*

◆ **Altace®** *see* Ramipril *on page 1292*

◆ **Altachlore [OTC]** *see* Sodium Chloride *on page 1381*

◆ **Altafrin** *see* Phenylephrine *on page 1183*

◆ **Altamist [OTC]** *see* Sodium Chloride *on page 1381*

◆ **Altarussin DM [OTC]** *see* Guaifenesin and Dextromethorphan *on page 710*

◆ **Altaryl [OTC]** *see* DiphenhydrAMINE *on page 456*

Alteplase (AL te plase)

U.S. Brand Names Activase®; Cathflo® Activase®

Canadian Brand Names Activase® rt-PA; Cathflo® Activase®

Index Terms Alteplase, Recombinant; Alteplase, Tissue Plasminogen Activator, Recombinant; tPA

Pharmacologic Category Thrombolytic Agent

Use Management of ST-elevation myocardial infarction (STEMI) for the lysis of thrombi in coronary arteries; management of acute ischemic stroke (AIS); management of acute pulmonary embolism

Recommended criteria for treatment:

STEMI: Chest pain ≥20 minutes duration, onset of chest pain within 12 hours of treatment (or within prior 12-24 hours in patients with continuing ischemic symptoms), and ST-segment elevation >0.1 mV in at least two contiguous precordial leads or two adjacent limb leads on ECG or new or presumably new left bundle branch block (LBBB)

AIS: Onset of stroke symptoms within 3 hours of treatment

Acute pulmonary embolism: Age ≤75 years: Documented massive pulmonary embolism by pulmonary angiography or echocardiography or high probability lung scan with clinical shock

Cathflo® Activase®: Restoration of central venous catheter function

Unlabeled/Investigational Use Acute ischemic stroke with symptom onset within 3-4.5 hours of treatment; acute peripheral arterial occlusive disease

Pregnancy Risk Factor C

Lactation Excretion in breast milk unknown/use caution

Medication Safety Issues

Sound-alike/look-alike issues:

Alteplase may be confused with Altace®

"tPA" abbreviation should not be used when writing orders for this medication; has been misread as TNKase (tenecteplase)

High alert medication: The Institute for Safe Medication Practices (ISMP) includes this medication (I.V.) among its list of drugs which have a heightened risk of causing significant patient harm when used in error.

Contraindications Hypersensitivity to alteplase or any component of the formulation

Treatment of STEMI or PE: Active internal bleeding; history of CVA; recent intracranial or intraspinal surgery or trauma; intracranial neoplasm; arteriovenous malformation or aneurysm; known bleeding diathesis; severe uncontrolled hypertension

Treatment of acute ischemic stroke: Evidence of intracranial hemorrhage or suspicion of subarachnoid hemorrhage on pretreatment evaluation; recent (within 3 months) intracranial or intraspinal surgery; prolonged external cardiac massage; suspected aortic dissection; serious head trauma or previous stroke; history of intracranial hemorrhage; uncontrolled hypertension at time of treatment (eg, >185 mm Hg systolic or >110 mm Hg diastolic); seizure at the onset of stroke; active internal bleeding; intracranial neoplasm; arteriovenous malformation or aneurysm; known bleeding diathesis including but not limited to: current use of anticoagulants or an INR >1.7, administration of heparin within 48 hours preceding the onset of stroke and an elevated aPTT at presentation, platelet count <100,000/mm^3.

Other exclusion criteria (NINDS recombinant tPA study): Stroke or serious head injury within 3 months, major surgery or serious trauma within 2 weeks, GI or urinary tract hemorrhage within 3 weeks, aggressive treatment required to lower blood pressure, glucose level <50 mg/dL or >400 mg/dL, arterial puncture at a noncompressible site or lumbar puncture within 1 week, clinical presentation suggesting post-MI pericarditis, pregnancy, breast-feeding.

Warnings/Precautions Concurrent heparin anticoagulation may contribute to bleeding. Monitor all potential bleeding sites. Doses >150 mg are associated with increased risk of intracranial hemorrhage. Intramuscular injections and nonessential handling of the patient should be avoided. Venipunctures should be performed carefully and only when necessary. If arterial puncture is necessary, use an upper extremity vessel that can be manually compressed. If serious bleeding occurs, the infusion of alteplase and heparin should be stopped. Avoid aspirin for 24 hours following administration of alteplase; administration within 24 hours increases the risk of hemorrhagic transformation.

For the following conditions, the risk of bleeding is higher with use of thrombolytics and should be weighed against the benefits of therapy: Recent major surgery (eg, CABG, obstetrical delivery, organ biopsy, previous puncture of noncompressible vessels), cerebrovascular disease, recent gastrointestinal or genitourinary bleeding, recent trauma, hypertension (systolic BP >175 mm Hg and/or diastolic BP >110 mm Hg), high likelihood of left heart thrombus (eg, mitral stenosis with atrial fibrillation), acute pericarditis, subacute bacterial endocarditis, hemostatic defects including ones caused by severe renal or hepatic dysfunction, significant hepatic dysfunction, pregnancy, diabetic hemorrhagic retinopathy or other hemorrhagic ophthalmic conditions, septic thrombophlebitis or occluded AV cannula at seriously infected site, advanced age (eg, >75 years), patients receiving oral anticoagulants, any other condition in which bleeding constitutes a significant hazard or would be particularly difficult to manage because of location.

Coronary thrombolysis may result in reperfusion arrhythmias. Treatment of patients with acute ischemic stroke more than 3 hours after symptom onset is not recommended. Treatment of patients with minor neurological deficit or with rapidly improving symptoms is not recommended. Follow standard management for STEMI while infusing alteplase.

Cathflo® Activase®: When used to restore catheter function, use Cathflo® cautiously in those patients with known or suspected catheter infections. Evaluate catheter for other causes of dysfunction before use. Avoid excessive pressure when instilling into catheter.

Adverse Reactions As with all drugs which may affect hemostasis, bleeding is the major adverse effect associated with alteplase. Hemorrhage may occur at virtually any site. Risk is dependent on multiple variables, including the dosage administered, concurrent use of multiple agents which alter hemostasis, and patient predisposition. Rapid lysis of coronary artery thrombi by thrombolytic agents may be associated with reperfusion-related atrial and/or ventricular arrhythmia. **Note:** Lowest rate of bleeding complications expected with dose used to restore catheter function.

1% to 10%:

Cardiovascular: Hypotension

Central nervous system: Fever

Dermatologic: Bruising (1%)

Gastrointestinal: GI hemorrhage (5%), nausea, vomiting

Genitourinary: GU hemorrhage (4%)

Hematologic: Bleeding (0.5% major, 7% minor: GUSTO trial)

Local: Bleeding at catheter puncture site (15.3%, accelerated administration)

<1% (Limited to important or life-threatening): Allergic reactions: Anaphylaxis, anaphylactoid reactions, laryngeal edema, rash, and urticaria (<0.02%); epistaxis; gingival hemorrhage; intracranial hemorrhage (0.4% to 0.87% when dose is ≤100 mg); pericardial hemorrhage; retroperitoneal hemorrhage

Additional cardiovascular events associated **with use in STEMI:** AV block, cardiogenic shock, heart failure, cardiac arrest, recurrent ischemia/infarction, myocardial rupture, electromechanical dissociation, pericardial effusion, pericarditis, mitral regurgitation, cardiac tamponade, thromboembolism, pulmonary edema, asystole, ventricular tachycardia, bradycardia, ruptured intracranial AV malformation, seizure, hemorrhagic bursitis, cholesterol crystal embolization

Additional events associated **with use in pulmonary embolism:** Pulmonary re-embolization, pulmonary edema, pleural effusion, thromboembolism

Additional events associated **with use in stroke:** Cerebral edema, cerebral herniation, seizure, new ischemic stroke

Drug Interactions

Avoid Concomitant Use There are no known interactions where it is recommended to avoid concomitant use.

Increased Effect/Toxicity

Alteplase may increase the levels/effects of: Anticoagulants; Drotrecogin Alfa

The levels/effects of Alteplase may be increased by: Antiplatelet Agents; Herbs (Anticoagulant/Antiplatelet Properties); Nonsteroidal Anti-Inflammatory Agents; Salicylates

Decreased Effect

The levels/effects of Alteplase may be decreased by: Aprotinin; Nitroglycerin

Ethanol/Nutrition/Herb Interactions Herb/Nutraceutical: Avoid cat's claw, dong quai, evening primrose, feverfew, red clover, horse chestnut, garlic, green tea, ginseng, ginkgo (all have additional antiplatelet activity).

Stability

Activase®: The lyophilized product may be stored at room temperature (not to exceed 30°C/86°F), or under refrigeration. Once reconstituted it should be used within 8 hours. Reconstitution:

50 mg vial: Use accompanying diluent (50 mL sterile water for injection); do not shake. Final concentration: 1 mg/mL.

100 mg vial: Use transfer set with accompanying diluent (100 mL vial of sterile water for injection); no vacuum is present in 100 mg vial; final concentration: 1 mg/mL.

Cathflo® Activase®: Store lyophilized product under refrigeration. Reconstitution: Add 2.2 mL SWFI to vial; do not shake. Final concentration: 1 mg/mL. Once reconstituted, store at 2°C to 30°C (36°F to 86°F) and use within 8 hours. Do not mix other medications into infusion solution.

Mechanism of Action Initiates local fibrinolysis by binding to fibrin in a thrombus (clot) and converts entrapped plasminogen to plasmin

Pharmacodynamics/Kinetics

Duration: >50% present in plasma cleared ~5 minutes after infusion terminated, ~80% cleared within 10 minutes

Excretion: Clearance: Rapidly from circulating plasma (550-650 mL/minute), primarily hepatic; >50% present in plasma is cleared within 5 minutes after the infusion is terminated, ~80% cleared within 10 minutes

Dosage

I.V. (Activase®):

ST-elevation myocardial infarction (STEMI): Front loading dose (weight-based):

Patients >67 kg: Total dose: 100 mg over 1.5 hours; infuse 15 mg over 1-2 minutes. Infuse 50 mg over 30 minutes. Infuse remaining 35 mg of alteplase over the next hour. See "Note."

Patients ≤67 kg: Infuse 15 mg I.V. bolus over 1-2 minutes, then infuse 0.75 mg/kg (not to exceed 50 mg) over next 30 minutes, followed by 0.5 mg/kg over next 60 minutes (not to exceed 35 mg). See **"Note."**

Note: All patients should receive 162-325 mg of chewable nonenteric coated aspirin as soon as possible and then daily. Administer concurrently with heparin 60 units/kg bolus (maximum: 4000 units) followed by continuous infusion of 12 units/kg/hour (maximum: 1000 units/hour) and adjust to aPTT target of 50-70 seconds (or 1.5-2 times the upper limit of control).

Acute pulmonary embolism: 100 mg over 2 hours.

Acute ischemic stroke: Doses should be given within the first 3 hours of the onset of symptoms; **Note:** Initiation of anticoagulants (eg, heparin) or antiplatelet agents (eg, aspirin) within 24 hours after starting alteplase is not recommended; however, initiation of aspirin between 24-48 hours after stroke onset is recommended (Adams, 2007).

Recommended total dose: 0.9 mg/kg (maximum total dose: 90 mg)

Patients ≤100 kg: Load with 0.09 mg/kg (10% of 0.9 mg/kg dose) as an I.V. bolus over 1 minute, followed by 0.81 mg/kg (90% of 0.9 mg/kg dose) as a continuous infusion over 60 minutes.

Patients >100 kg: Load with 9 mg (10% of 90 mg) as an I.V. bolus over 1 minute, followed by 81 mg (90% of 90 mg) as a continuous infusion over 60 minutes.

Unlabeled use: Administration of alteplase may be of benefit for select patients with acute ischemic stroke who present between 3 and 4.5 hours after onset of symptoms (Hacke, 2008)

Intracatheter: Central venous catheter clearance (Cathflo® Activase® 1 mg/mL):

Patients <30 kg: 110% of the internal lumen volume of the catheter, not to exceed 2 mg/2 mL; retain in catheter for 0.5-2 hours; may instill a second dose if catheter remains occluded

Patients ≥30 kg: 2 mg (2 mL); retain in catheter for 0.5-2 hours; may instill a second dose if catheter remains occluded

Intra-arterial: Acute peripheral arterial occlusive disease (unlabeled use): 0.02-0.1 mg/kg/hour for up to 36 hours

Advisory Panel to the Society for Cardiovascular and Interventional Radiology on Thrombolytic Therapy recommendation: ≤2 mg/hour and subtherapeutic heparin (aPTT <1.5 times baseline)

Administration

Activase®: ST-elevation MI: Accelerated infusion: Bolus dose may be prepared by one of three methods:

1) Removal of 15 mL reconstituted (1 mg/mL) solution from vial
2) Removal of 15 mL from a port on the infusion line after priming
3) Programming an infusion pump to deliver a 15 mL bolus at the initiation of infusion

Activase®: Acute ischemic stroke: Bolus dose (10% of total dose) may be prepared by one of three methods:

1) Removal of the appropriate volume from reconstituted solution (1 mg/mL)
2) Removal of the appropriate volume from a port on the infusion line after priming

3) Programming an infusion pump to deliver the appropriate volume at the initiation of infusion

Note: Remaining dose for STEMI, AIS, or total dose for acute pulmonary embolism may be administered as follows: Any quantity of drug not to be administered to the patient must be removed from vial(s) prior to administration of remaining dose.

50 mg vial: Either PVC bag or glass vial and infusion set

100 mg vial: Insert spike end of the infusion set through the same puncture site created by transfer device and infuse from vial

If further dilution is desired, may be diluted in equal volume of 0.9% sodium chloride or D_5W to yield a final concentration of 0.5 mg/mL.

Cathflo® Activase®: Intracatheter: Instill dose into occluded catheter. Do not force solution into catheter. After a 30-minute dwell time, assess catheter function by attempting to aspirate blood. If catheter is functional, aspirate 4-5 mL of blood in patients ≥10 kg or 3 mL in patients <10 kg to remove Cathflo® Activase® and residual clots. Gently irrigate the catheter with NS. If catheter remains nonfunctional, let Cathflo® Activase® dwell for another 90 minutes (total dwell time: 120 minutes) and reassess function. If catheter function is not restored, a second dose may be instilled.

Monitoring Parameters

Acute ischemic stroke: In addition to monitoring for bleeding complications, the 2007 AHA/ASA Guidelines for the early management of acute ischemic stroke recommends the following:

Perform neurological assessments every 15 minutes during infusion and every 30 minutes thereafter for the next 6 hours, then hourly until 24 hours after treatment.

If severe headache, acute hypertension, nausea, or vomiting occurs, discontinue the infusion and obtain emergency CT scan.

Measure BP every 15 minutes for the first 2 hours then every 30 minutes for the next 6 hours, then hourly until 24 hours after initiation of alteplase. Increase frequency if a systolic BP is ≥180 mm Hg or if a diastolic BP is ≥105 mm Hg; administer antihypertensive medications to maintain BP at or below these levels.

Obtain a follow-up CT scan at 24 hours before starting anticoagulants or antiplatelet agents.

Central venous catheter clearance: Assess catheter function by attempting to aspirate blood.

ST-elevation MI: Assess for evidence of cardiac reperfusion through resolution of chest pain, resolution of baseline ECG changes, preserved left ventricular function, cardiac enzyme washout phenomenon, and/or the appearance of reperfusion arrhythmias; assess for bleeding potential through clinical evidence of GI bleeding, hematuria, gingival bleeding, fibrinogen levels, fibrinogen degradation products, prothrombin times, and partial thromboplastin times.

Reference Range

Not routinely measured; literature supports therapeutic levels of 0.52-1.8 mcg/mL

Fibrinogen: 200-400 mg/dL

Activated partial thromboplastin time (aPTT): 22.5-38.7 seconds

Prothrombin time (PT): 10.9-12.2 seconds

Test Interactions Altered results of coagulation and fibrinolytic agents

Dosage Forms Excipient information presented when available (limited, particularly for generics); consult specific product labeling.

Injection, powder for reconstitution, recombinant:

Activase®: 50 mg [29 million int. units; contains polysorbate 80; packaged with diluent]; 100 mg [58 million int. units; contains polysorbate 80; packaged with diluent and transfer device]

Cathflo® Activase®: 2 mg [contains polysorbate 80]

- ◆ **Alteplase, Recombinant** *see* Alteplase *on page 72*
- ◆ **Alteplase, Tissue Plasminogen Activator, Recombinant** *see* Alteplase *on page 72*
- ◆ **ALternaGel® [OTC]** *see* Aluminum Hydroxide *on page 75*
- ◆ **Alti-Alprazolam (Can)** *see* ALPRAZolam *on page 68*
- ◆ **Alti-Amiodarone (Can)** *see* Amiodarone *on page 87*
- ◆ **Alti-Amoxi-Clav (Can)** *see* Amoxicillin and Clavulanate Potassium *on page 100*
- ◆ **Alti-Azathioprine (Can)** *see* AzaTHIOprine *on page 163*
- ◆ **Alti-Captopril (Can)** *see* Captopril *on page 249*
- ◆ **Alti-Clindamycin (Can)** *see* Clindamycin *on page 344*
- ◆ **Alti-Clonazepam (Can)** *see* ClonazePAM *on page 352*
- ◆ **Alti-Desipramine (Can)** *see* Desipramine *on page 418*
- ◆ **Alti-Diltiazem CD (Can)** *see* Diltiazem *on page 450*
- ◆ **Alti-Divalproex (Can)** *see* Valproic Acid and Derivatives *on page 1538*
- ◆ **Alti-Doxazosin (Can)** *see* Doxazosin *on page 483*
- ◆ **Alti-Flunisolide (Can)** *see* Flunisolide *on page 632*
- ◆ **Alti-Flurbiprofen (Can)** *see* Flurbiprofen *on page 643*
- ◆ **Alti-Fluvoxamine (Can)** *see* Fluvoxamine *on page 652*
- ◆ **Alti-Ipratropium (Can)** *see* Ipratropium *on page 811*
- ◆ **Alti-Minocycline (Can)** *see* Minocycline *on page 999*
- ◆ **Alti-MPA (Can)** *see* MedroxyPROGESTERone *on page 930*
- ◆ **Alti-Nadolol (Can)** *see* Nadolol *on page 1031*
- ◆ **Alti-Nortriptyline (Can)** *see* Nortriptyline *on page 1081*
- ◆ **Alti-Ranitidine (Can)** *see* Ranitidine *on page 1295*
- ◆ **Alti-Salbutamol (Can)** *see* Albuterol *on page 51*
- ◆ **Alti-Sulfasalazine (Can)** *see* Sulfasalazine *on page 1409*
- ◆ **Alti-Terazosin (Can)** *see* Terazosin *on page 1440*
- ◆ **Alti-Ticlopidine (Can)** *see* Ticlopidine *on page 1468*
- ◆ **Alti-Timolol (Can)** *see* Timolol *on page 1472*
- ◆ **Alti-Trazodone (Can)** *see* TraZODone *on page 1505*
- ◆ **Altoprev®** *see* Lovastatin *on page 910*

Altretamine (al TRET a meen)

U.S. Brand Names Hexalen®

Canadian Brand Names Hexalen®

Index Terms Hexamethylmelamine; HEXM; HMM; HXM; NSC-13875

Pharmacologic Category Antineoplastic Agent, Miscellaneous

Use Palliative treatment of persistent or recurrent ovarian cancer

Pregnancy Risk Factor D

Pregnancy Considerations Teratogenic effects were noted in animal studies. There are no adequate and well-controlled studies in pregnant women. Women of child-bearing potential should avoid becoming pregnant while on therapy.

Lactation Excretion in breast milk unknown/not recommended

Medication Safety Issues

High alert medication: The Institute for Safe Medication Practices (ISMP) includes this medication among its list of drugs which have a heightened risk of causing significant patient harm when used in error.

International issues:

Hexalen®: Brand name for hexetidine in Greece

Contraindications Hypersensitivity to altretamine or any component of the formulation; pre-existing severe bone marrow suppression or severe neurologic toxicity; pregnancy

Warnings/Precautions Hazardous agent - use appropriate precautions for handling and disposal. **[U.S. Boxed Warning]: Peripheral blood counts and neurologic examinations should be done routinely before and after drug therapy.** Myelosuppression and neurotoxicity are common; use with caution in patients previously treated with other myelosuppressive drugs or with preexisting neurotoxicity. Use with caution in patients with renal or hepatic dysfunction. **[U.S. Boxed Warning]: Should be administered under the supervision of an experienced cancer chemotherapy physician.** Safety and efficacy in children have not been established.

Adverse Reactions

>10%:

Central nervous system: Peripheral sensory neuropathy (31%; moderate-to-severe 9%), neurotoxicity (21%; may be progressive and dose limiting)

Gastrointestinal: Nausea/vomiting (33% to 70%; severe 1%), diarrhea (48%)

Hematologic: Anemia (33%), leukopenia (5% to 15%; grade 4: 1%), neutropenia

1% to 10%:

Central nervous system: Fatigue (1%), seizure (1%)

Gastrointestinal: Stomach cramps, anorexia (1%)

Hematologic: Thrombocytopenia (9%)

Hepatic: Alkaline phosphatase increased (9%)

<1% (Limited to important or life-threatening): Alopecia, ataxia, depression, dizziness, hepatotoxicity, mood disorders, pruritus, rash, tremor, vertigo

Drug Interactions

Avoid Concomitant Use

Avoid concomitant use of Altretamine with any of the following: Natalizumab; Vaccines (Live)

Increased Effect/Toxicity

Altretamine may increase the levels/effects of: MAO Inhibitors; Natalizumab; Tricyclic Antidepressants; Vaccines (Live)

The levels/effects of Altretamine may be increased by: Trastuzumab

Decreased Effect

Altretamine may decrease the levels/effects of: Vaccines (Inactivated)

The levels/effects of Altretamine may be decreased by: Echinacea; Pyridoxine

Stability Store at 15°C to 30°C (59°F to 86°F).

Mechanism of Action Although altretamine's clinical antitumor spectrum resembles that of alkylating agents, the drug has demonstrated activity in alkylator-resistant patients. The drug selectively inhibits the incorporation of radioactive thymidine and uridine into DNA and RNA, inhibiting DNA and RNA synthesis; reactive intermediates covalently bind to microsomal proteins and DNA; can spontaneously degrade to demethylated melamines and formaldehyde which are also cytotoxic.

Pharmacodynamics/Kinetics

Absorption: Well absorbed (75% to 89%)

Distribution: Highly concentrated hepatically and renally; low in other organs

Protein binding: 50% to 94%

Metabolism: Hepatic; rapid and extensive demethylation to active metabolites (pentamethylmelamine and tetramethylmelamine)

Half-life elimination: 13 hours

Time to peak, plasma: 0.5-3 hours

Excretion: Urine (90%, <1% as unchanged drug)

Dosage Refer to individual protocols. Oral: Adults:

Ovarian cancer: 260 mg/m^2/day in 4 divided doses for 14 or 21 days of a 28-day cycle

Alternatively (unlabeled use): 4-12 mg/kg/day in 3-4 divided doses for 21-90 days

Alternatively (unlabeled use): 240-320 mg/m^2/day in 3-4 divided doses for 21 days, repeated every 6 weeks

Alternatively (unlabeled use): 150 mg/m^2/day in 3-4 divided doses for 14 days of a 28-day cycle

Dosage adjustment for toxicity: Temporarily withhold for 14 days or longer, and resume dose at 200 mg/m^2/day for any of the following:

Platelet count <75,000/mm^3

White blood cell count <2000/mm^3 or granulocyte count <1000/mm^3

Progressive neurotoxicity

Gastrointestinal intolerance not responsive to antiemetic regimens

Dietary Considerations Should be taken after meals at bedtime.

Administration Administer total daily dose as 3-4 divided doses after meals and at bedtime.

Monitoring Parameters CBC with differential, liver function tests; neurologic examination

Dosage Forms Excipient information presented when available (limited, particularly for generics); consult specific product labeling.

Gelcap:

Hexalen®: 50 mg

Aluminum Hydroxide

(a LOO mi num hye DROKS ide)

U.S. Brand Names ALternaGel® [OTC]; Dermagran® [OTC]

Canadian Brand Names Amphojel®; Basaljel®

Pharmacologic Category Antacid; Antidote; Protectant, Topical

Use Treatment of hyperacidity; hyperphosphatemia; temporary protection of minor cuts, scrapes, and burns

Pregnancy Risk Factor C

Dosage

Oral:

Hyperphosphatemia:

Children: 50-150 mg/kg/24 hours in divided doses every 4-6 hours, titrate dosage to maintain serum phosphorus within normal range

Adults: Initial: 300-600 mg 3 times/day with meals

Antacid: Adults: 600-1200 mg between meals and at bedtime

Topical: Apply to affected area as needed; reapply at least every 12 hours

Dosage adjustment in renal impairment: Aluminum may accumulate in renal impairment.

Additional Information Complete prescribing information for this medication should be consulted for additional detail.

Dosage Forms Excipient information presented when available (limited, particularly for generics); consult specific product labeling.

Ointment:

Dermagran®: 0.275% (120 g)

Suspension, oral: 320 mg/5 mL (473 mL)

ALternaGel®: 600 mg/5 mL (360 mL)

Aluminum Hydroxide and Magnesium Carbonate

(a LOO mi num hye DROKS ide & mag NEE zhum KAR bun nate)

U.S. Brand Names Acid Gone Extra Strength [OTC]; Acid Gone [OTC]; Alenic Alka [OTC]; Gaviscon® Extra Strength [OTC]; Gaviscon® Liquid [OTC]; Genaton™ [OTC]

Index Terms Magnesium Carbonate and Aluminum Hydroxide

Pharmacologic Category Antacid

Use Temporary relief of symptoms associated with gastric acidity

Dosage Oral: Adults:

Liquid:

Gaviscon® Regular Strength: 15-30 mL 4 times/day after meals and at bedtime

Gaviscon® Extra Strength: 15-30 mL 4 times/day after meals

Tablet (Gaviscon® Extra Strength): Chew 2-4 tablets 4 times/day

Dosage adjustment in renal impairment: Aluminum and/or magnesium may accumulate in renal impairment.

Additional Information Complete prescribing information for this medication should be consulted for additional detail.

Dosage Forms Excipient information presented when available (limited, particularly for generics); consult specific product labeling.

Liquid:

Acid Gone: Aluminum hydroxide 31.7 mg and magnesium carbonate 119.3 mg per 5 mL (360 mL)

Alenic Alka: Aluminum hydroxide 31.7 mg and magnesium carbonate 119.3 mg per 5 mL (355 mL) [contains magnesium 35 mg/5 mL, sodium 13 mg/5 mL, and benzyl alcohol; cool mint flavor]

Gaviscon®: Aluminum hydroxide 31.7 mg and magnesium carbonate 119.3 mg per 5 mL (355 mL) [contains sodium 0.57 mEq/5 mL and benzyl alcohol; cool mint flavor]

Gaviscon® Extra Strength: Aluminum hydroxide 84.6 mg and magnesium carbonate 79.1 mg per 5 mL (355 mL) [contains sodium 0.9 mEq/5 mL and benzyl alcohol; cool mint flavor]

Genaton™: Aluminum hydroxide 31.7 mg and magnesium carbonate 119.3 mg per 5 mL (360 mL)

Tablet, chewable:

Acid Gone Extra Strength: Aluminum hydroxide 160 mg and magnesium carbonate 105 mg

Gaviscon® Extra Strength: Aluminum hydroxide 160 mg and magnesium carbonate 105 mg [contains sodium 19 mg/tablet (1.3 mEq/tablet); cherry and original flavors]

Aluminum Hydroxide and Magnesium Hydroxide

(a LOO mi num hye DROKS ide & mag NEE zhum hye DROK side)

U.S. Brand Names Alamag [OTC]; Rulox No. 1 [DSC]; Rulox [OTC]

Canadian Brand Names Diovol®; Diovol® Ex; Gelusil® Extra Strength; Mylanta™

Index Terms Magnesium Hydroxide and Aluminum Hydroxide

Pharmacologic Category Antacid

Use Antacid, hyperphosphatemia in renal failure

Pregnancy Risk Factor C

Medication Safety Issues

Sound-alike/look-alike issues:

Maalox® may be confused with Maox®, Monodox®

Dosage Oral: 5-10 mL 4-6 times/day, between meals and at bedtime; may be used every hour for severe symptoms

Dosage adjustment in renal impairment: Aluminum and/or magnesium may accumulate in renal impairment.

Additional Information Complete prescribing information for this medication should be consulted for additional detail.

Dosage Forms Excipient information presented when available (limited, particularly for generics); consult specific product labeling. [DSC] = Discontinued product

Suspension: Aluminum hydroxide 225 mg and magnesium hydroxide 200 mg per 5 mL (360 mL)

Alamag, Rulox: Aluminum hydroxide 225 mg and magnesium hydroxide 200 mg per 5 mL (360 mL)

Tablet, chewable:

Alamag: Aluminum hydroxide 300 mg and magnesium hydroxide 150 mg

Rulox No. 1: Aluminum hydroxide 200 mg and magnesium hydroxide 200 mg [DSC]

Aluminum Hydroxide and Magnesium Trisilicate

(a LOO mi num hye DROKS ide & mag NEE zhum trye SIL i kate)

U.S. Brand Names Alenic Alka Tablet [OTC]; Gaviscon® Tablet [OTC]; Genaton Tablet [OTC]

Index Terms Magnesium Trisilicate and Aluminum Hydroxide

Pharmacologic Category Antacid

Use Temporary relief of hyperacidity

Pregnancy Risk Factor C

Dosage Oral: Adults: Chew 2-4 tablets 4 times/day or as directed by healthcare provider

Dosage adjustment in renal impairment: Aluminum and/or magnesium may accumulate in renal impairment.

Additional Information Complete prescribing information for this medication should be consulted for additional detail.

Dosage Forms Excipient information presented when available (limited, particularly for generics); consult specific product labeling.

Tablet, chewable: Aluminum hydroxide 80 mg and magnesium trisilicate 20 mg

Alenic Alka: Aluminum hydroxide 80 mg and magnesium trisilicate 20 mg [butterscotch flavor]

Gaviscon®: Aluminum hydroxide 80 mg and magnesium trisilicate 20 mg [contains sodium 0.8 mEq/tablet; butterscotch flavor]

Genaton: Aluminum hydroxide 80 mg and magnesium trisilicate 20 mg

Aluminum Hydroxide, Magnesium Hydroxide, and Simethicone

(a LOO mi num hye DROKS ide, mag NEE zhum hye DROKS ide, & sye METH i kone)

U.S. Brand Names Alamag Plus [OTC]; Aldroxicon I [OTC]; Aldroxicon II [OTC]; Almacone Double Strength® [OTC]; Almacone® [OTC]; Gelusil® [OTC]; Maalox® Max [OTC]; Maalox® [OTC]; Mi-Acid Maximum Strength [OTC]; Mi-Acid [OTC]; Mintox Extra Strength [OTC]; Mintox Plus [OTC]; Mylanta® Liquid [OTC]; Mylanta® Maximum Strength Liquid [OTC]

Canadian Brand Names Diovol Plus®; Gelusil®; Mylanta® Double Strength; Mylanta® Extra Strength; Mylanta® Regular Strength

Index Terms Magnesium Hydroxide, Aluminum Hydroxide, and Simethicone; Simethicone, Aluminum Hydroxide, and Magnesium Hydroxide

Pharmacologic Category Antacid; Antiflatulent

Use Temporary relief of hyperacidity associated with gas; may also be used for indications associated with other antacids

Pregnancy Risk Factor C

Medication Safety Issues

Sound-alike/look-alike issues:

Maalox® may be confused with Maox®, Monodox®

Mylanta® may be confused with Mynatal®

Maalox® is a different formulation than Maalox® Total Stomach Relief®

Dosage Oral: Adults: 10-20 mL or 2-4 tablets 4-6 times/day between meals and at bedtime; may be used every hour for severe symptoms

Dosage adjustment in renal impairment: Aluminum and/or magnesium may accumulate in renal impairment.

Additional Information Complete prescribing information for this medication should be consulted for additional detail.

Dosage Forms Excipient information presented when available (limited, particularly for generics); consult specific product labeling.

Liquid: Aluminum hydroxide 200 mg, magnesium hydroxide 200 mg, and simethicone 20 mg per 5 mL (360 mL); aluminum hydroxide 400 mg, magnesium hydroxide 400 mg, and simethicone 40 mg per 5 mL (360 mL)

Aldroxicon I: Aluminum hydroxide 200 mg, magnesium hydroxide 200 mg, and simethicone 20 mg per 5 mL (30 mL)

Aldroxicon II: Aluminum hydroxide 400 mg, magnesium hydroxide 400 mg, and simethicone 40 mg per 5 mL (30 mL)

Almacone®: Aluminum hydroxide 200 mg, magnesium hydroxide 200 mg, and simethicone 20 mg per 5 mL (360 mL)

Almacone Double Strength®: Aluminum hydroxide 400 mg, magnesium hydroxide 400 mg, and simethicone 40 mg per 5 mL (360 mL)

Maalox®: Aluminum hydroxide 200 mg, magnesium hydroxide 200 mg, and simethicone 20 mg per 5 mL (360 mL, 770 mL) [lemon and mint flavors]

Maalox® Max: Aluminum hydroxide 400 mg, magnesium hydroxide 400 mg, and simethicone 40 mg per 5 mL (360 mL, 770 mL) [cherry, vanilla creme, and wild berry flavors]

Mi-Acid: Aluminum hydroxide 200 mg, magnesium hydroxide 200 mg, and simethicone 20 mg per 5 mL (360 mL)

Mi-Acid Maximum Strength: Aluminum hydroxide 400 mg, magnesium hydroxide 400 mg, and simethicone 40 mg per 5 mL (360 mL)

Mintox Extra Strength: Aluminum hydroxide 500 mg, magnesium hydroxide 450 mg, and simethicone 40 mg per 5 mL (360 mL) [lemon creme flavor]

Mylanta®: Aluminum hydroxide 200 mg, magnesium hydroxide 200 mg, and simethicone 20 mg per 5 mL (180 mL, 360 mL, 720 mL) [original, cherry, and mint flavors]

Mylanta® Maximum Strength: Aluminum hydroxide 400 mg, magnesium hydroxide 400 mg, and simethicone 40 mg per 5 mL (180 mL, 360 mL, 720 mL) [original, cherry, orange creme, and mint flavors]

Suspension (Alamag Plus): Aluminum hydroxide 225 mg, magnesium hydroxide 200 mg, and simethicone 25 mg per 5 mL (360 mL)

Tablet, chewable: Aluminum hydroxide 200 mg, magnesium hydroxide 200 mg, and simethicone 25 mg

Alamag Plus: Aluminum hydroxide 200 mg, magnesium hydroxide 200 mg, and simethicone 25 mg [cherry flavor]

Almacone®: Aluminum hydroxide 200 mg, magnesium hydroxide 200 mg, and simethicone 20 mg [peppermint flavor]

Gelusil®: Aluminum hydroxide 200 mg, magnesium hydroxide 200 mg, and simethicone 25 mg [peppermint flavor]

Mintox Plus: Aluminum hydroxide 200 mg, magnesium hydroxide 200 mg, and simethicone 25 mg

◆ **Aluminum Sucrose Sulfate, Basic** *see* Sucralfate *on page 1404*

Aluminum Sulfate and Calcium Acetate

(a LOO mi num SUL fate & KAL see um AS e tate)

U.S. Brand Names Domeboro® [OTC]; Gordon Boro-Packs [OTC]; Pedi-Boro® [OTC]

Index Terms Calcium Acetate and Aluminum Sulfate

Pharmacologic Category Topical Skin Product

Use Astringent wet dressing for relief of inflammatory conditions of the skin; reduce weeping that may occur in dermatitis

Dosage Topical: Soak affected area in the solution 2-4 times/day for 15-30 minutes or apply wet dressing soaked in the solution for more extended periods; rewet dressing with solution 2-4 times/day every 15-30 minutes

Additional Information Complete prescribing information for this medication should be consulted for additional detail.

Dosage Forms Excipient information presented when available (limited, particularly for generics); consult specific product labeling.

Powder, for topical solution:

Domeboro®: Aluminum sulfate 1191 mg and calcium acetate 839 mg per packet (12s, 100s)

Gordon Boro-Packs: Aluminum sulfate 49% and calcium acetate 51% per packet (100s)

Pedi-Boro®: Aluminum sulfate 1191 mg and calcium acetate 839 mg per packet (12s, 100s)

◆ **Alupent® [DSC]** *see* Metaproterenol *on page 952*

◆ **Alvesco®** *see* Ciclesonide *on page 322*

Alvimopan (al vi MOE pan)

U.S. Brand Names Entereg®

Index Terms ADL-2698; LY246736

Pharmacologic Category Gastrointestinal Agent, Miscellaneous; Opioid Antagonist, Peripherally-Acting

Use Accelerate the time to upper and lower GI recovery following partial large or small bowel resection surgery with primary anastomosis

Restrictions Only hospitals enrolled in the ENTEREG Access Support and Education (E.A.S.E.™) Program may administer this medication. Hospital staff must be educated on need to limit to short-term (no more than 15 doses) and inpatient use. Hospitals may contact the E.A.S.E.™ program at 1-866-423-6567 (1-866-4ADOLOR).

Pregnancy Risk Factor B

Pregnancy Considerations Animal studies have not shown teratogenic effects to the fetus. However, there are no adequate and well-controlled studies in pregnant women; use during pregnancy only if clearly needed.

Lactation Excretion in breast milk unknown/use caution

Medication Safety Issues

Sound-alike/look-alike issues:

Alvimopan may be confused with almotriptan

Contraindications Patients who have taken therapeutic doses of opioids for more than 7 consecutive days immediately prior to alvimopan

Warnings/Precautions **[U.S. Boxed Warning]: For short-term (≤15 doses) hospital use only. Only hospitals that have registered through the ENTEREG Access Support and Education (E.A.S.E.™) Program and met all requirements may use.** It will not be dispensed to patients who have been discharged from the hospital. Use not recommended in patients with complete bowel obstruction. Use with caution in patients with hepatic or renal impairment; use not recommended in patients with severe hepatic impairment or ESRD. Use with caution is patients recently exposed to opioids; may be more sensitive to gastrointestinal adverse effects (eg, abdominal pain, diarrhea, nausea and vomiting). Contraindicated in patients who have received therapeutic opioids for >7 consecutive days immediately prior to use. A trend towards an increased incidence of MI was observed in alvimopan (low dose) treated patients compared to placebo in a 12-month study in patients treated with opioids for chronic pain. MI was generally observed more frequently in the initial 1-4 months of treatment. Other studies have not observed this trend and a causal relationship has not been found. Safety and efficacy have not been established in children.

Adverse Reactions Note: Incidence reported limited to bowel resection patients only. 1% to 10%:

Endocrine & metabolic: Hypokalemia (10%)
Gastrointestinal: Dyspepsia (7%)
Genitourinary: Urinary retention (3%)
Hematologic: Anemia (5%)
Neuromuscular & skeletal: Back pain (3%)

Drug Interactions

Metabolism/Transport Effects Substrate of P-glycoprotein

Avoid Concomitant Use There are no known interactions where it is recommended to avoid concomitant use.

Increased Effect/Toxicity

The levels/effects of Alvimopan may be increased by: Analgesics (Opioid)

Decreased Effect There are no known significant interactions involving a decrease in effect.

Ethanol/Nutrition/Herb Interactions Food: When administered with a high-fat meal, extent and rate of absorption may be reduced (C_{max} and AUC decreased by ~38% and 21%, respectively).

Stability Store at controlled room temperature of 25°C (77°F).

Mechanism of Action An opioid receptor antagonist which blocks opioid binding at the mu receptor; alvimopan has restricted ability to cross the blood-brain barrier at therapeutic doses. It selectively and competitively binds to the GI tract mu opioid receptors and antagonizes the peripheral effects of opioids on gastrointestinal motility and secretion. Does not affect opioid analgesic effects or induce opioid withdrawal symptoms.

Pharmacodynamics/Kinetics

Distribution: V_d: 20-40 L
Protein binding: Parent drug: 80%; metabolite: 94% (both primarily to albumin)
Metabolism: Hydrolyzed to an amide hydrolysis compound (active metabolite) by gut microflora; further metabolism of active metabolite to glucuronide conjugates and other minor metabolites.
Bioavailability: ~6% (range: 1% to 19%)
Half-life elimination: 10-18 hours
Time to peak, plasma: ~2 hours
Excretion: Urine (35% as unchanged drug and metabolites); feces (via biliary excretion)

Dosage Note: For hospital use only

Oral: Adults:

Initial: 12 mg administered 30 minutes to 5 hours prior to surgery

Maintenance: 12 mg twice daily beginning the day after surgery for a maximum of 7 days or until discharged from hospital (maximum total treatment doses: 15 doses)

Dosage adjustment in renal impairment:

Mild-to-severe impairment: No adjustment needed; use caution

ESRD: Use not recommended

Dosage adjustment in hepatic impairment:

Mild-to-moderate impairment (Child-Pugh class A and B): No adjustment needed; use caution

Severe impairment (Child-Pugh class C): Use not recommended

Dietary Considerations Take with or without food; high-fat meals may decrease the rate and extent of absorption

Administration Patient must be hospitalized. Initial dose should be administered 30 minutes to 5 hours prior to surgery.

Dosage Forms Excipient information presented when available (limited, particularly for generics); consult specific product labeling.

Capsule:

Entereg®: 12 mg

Amantadine (a MAN ta deen)

U.S. Brand Names Symmetrel®

Canadian Brand Names Endantadine®; PMS-Amantadine; Symmetrel®

Index Terms Adamantanamine Hydrochloride; Amantadine Hydrochloride

Pharmacologic Category Anti-Parkinson's Agent, Dopamine Agonist; Antiviral Agent, Adamantane

Additional Appendix Information

Antiparkinsonian Agents *on page 1643*
Community-Acquired Pneumonia in Adults *on page 1766*
Guidelines for the Prevention of Opportunistic Infections in HIV Infected Persons *on page 1740*

Use Prophylaxis and treatment of influenza A viral infection (per manufacturer labeling; also refer to current ACIP guidelines for recommendations during current flu season); treatment of parkinsonism; treatment of drug-induced extrapyramidal symptoms

Note: In certain circumstances, the ACIP recommends use of amantadine in combination with oseltamivir for the treatment or prophylaxis of influenza A infection when resistance to oseltamivir is suspected.

Pregnancy Risk Factor C

Pregnancy Considerations Teratogenic effects were observed in animal studies; limited data in humans. Impaired fertility has also been reported during animal studies and during human *in vitro* fertilization.

Lactation Enters breast milk/not recommended

Medication Safety Issues

Sound-alike/look-alike issues:

Amantadine may be confused with ranitidine, rimantadine
Symmetrel® may be confused with Synthroid®

International issues:

Symmetrel® may be confused with Somatrel® which is a brand name for somatorelin in Denmark

Contraindications Hypersensitivity to amantadine, rimantadine, or any component of the formulation

Warnings/Precautions May cause CNS depression, which may impair physical or mental abilities; patients must be cautioned about performing tasks which require mental alertness (eg, operating machinery or driving). There have been reports of suicidal ideation/attempt in patients with and without a history of psychiatric illness. Use with caution in patients with liver disease, a history of recurrent and eczematoid dermatitis, uncontrolled psychosis or severe psychoneurosis, seizures and in those receiving CNS stimulant drugs; reduce dose in renal disease; when treating Parkinson's disease, do not discontinue abruptly. In many patients, the therapeutic benefits of amantadine are limited to a few months. Elderly patients may be more susceptible to the CNS effects (using 2 divided daily doses may minimize this effect). Use with caution in patients with CHF, peripheral edema, or orthostatic hypotension. Avoid in untreated angle closure glaucoma.

Dopamine agonists have been associated with compulsive behaviors and/or loss of impulse control, which has manifested as pathological gambling, libido increases (hypersexuality), and/or binge eating. Causality has not been established, and controversy exists as to whether this phenomenon is related to the underlying disease, prior behaviors/addictions and/or drug therapy. Dose reduction or discontinuation of therapy has been reported to reverse these behaviors in some, but not all cases.

Due to increased resistance, the ACIP has recommended that rimantadine and amantadine no longer be used for the treatment or prophylaxis of influenza A in the United States until susceptibility has been re-established; consult current guidelines. Safety and efficacy have not been established in children <1 year of age.

Adverse Reactions

1% to 10%:

Cardiovascular: Orthostatic hypotension, peripheral edema

Central nervous system: Agitation, anxiety, ataxia, confusion, delirium, depression, dizziness, dream abnormality, fatigue, hallucinations, headache, insomnia, irritability, nervousness, somnolence

Dermatologic: Livedo reticularis

Gastrointestinal: Anorexia, constipation, diarrhea, nausea, xerostomia

Respiratory: Dry nose

<1% (Limited to important or life-threatening): Aggressive behavior, agranulocytosis, alkaline phosphatase increased, allergic reaction, ALT increased, AST increased, amnesia, anaphylaxis, arrhythmia, bilirubin increased, BUN increased, cardiac arrest, CHF, coma, CPK increased, creatinine increased, delirium, delusions, diaphoresis, dysphagia, dyspnea, eczematoid dermatitis, euphoria, GGT increased, hyperkinesis, LDH increased, leukopenia, mania, neutropenia, neuroleptic malignant syndrome (NMS; associated with dosage reduction or abrupt withdrawal of amantadine), oculogyric episodes, paresthesia, photosensitivity, psychosis, pulmonary edema, rash, respiratory failure (acute), seizures, suicidal ideation, suicide, urinary retention, withdrawal reactions (may include delirium, hallucinations, and psychosis), visual disturbances

Reported with dopamine agonists: Impulsive/compulsive behaviors (eg, pathological gambling, hypersexuality, binge eating)

Drug Interactions

Avoid Concomitant Use There are no known interactions where it is recommended to avoid concomitant use.

Increased Effect/Toxicity

Amantadine may increase the levels/effects of: Trimethoprim

The levels/effects of Amantadine may be increased by: Trimethoprim

Decreased Effect

Amantadine may decrease the levels/effects of: Influenza Virus Vaccine

The levels/effects of Amantadine may be decreased by: Antipsychotics (Atypical); Antipsychotics (Typical); Metoclopramide

Ethanol/Nutrition/Herb Interactions Ethanol: Avoid ethanol (may increase CNS adverse effects).

Stability Store at 25°C (77°F).

Mechanism of Action As an antiviral, blocks the uncoating of influenza A virus preventing penetration of virus into host; antiparkinsonian activity may be due to its blocking the reuptake of dopamine into presynaptic neurons or by increasing dopamine release from presynaptic fibers

Pharmacodynamics/Kinetics

Onset of action: Antidyskinetic: Within 48 hours

Absorption: Well absorbed

Distribution: V_d: Normal: 1.5-6.1 L/kg; Renal failure: 5.1 ± 0.2 L/kg; in saliva, tear film, and nasal secretions; in animals, tissue (especially lung) concentrations higher than serum concentrations; crosses blood-brain barrier

Protein binding: Normal renal function: ~67%; Hemodialysis: ~59%

Metabolism: Not appreciable; small amounts of an acetyl metabolite identified

Bioavailability: 86% to 90%

Half-life elimination: Normal renal function: 16 ± 6 hours (9-31 hours); End-stage renal disease: 7-10 days

Excretion: Urine (80% to 90% unchanged) by glomerular filtration and tubular secretion

Total clearance: 2.5-10.5 L/hour

Dosage Oral:

Children:

Influenza A treatment:

1-9 years: 5 mg/kg/day in 2 divided doses (manufacturers range: 4.4-8.8 mg/kg/day); maximum dose: 150 mg/day

≥10 years and <40 kg: 5 mg/kg/day; maximum dose: 150 mg/day

≥10 years and ≥40 kg: 100 mg twice daily

Note: Initiate within 24-48 hours after onset of symptoms; discontinue as soon as possible based on clinical response (generally within 3-5 days or within 24-48 hours after symptoms disappear)

Influenza A prophylaxis: Refer to "Influenza A treatment" dosing

Note: Continue treatment throughout the peak influenza activity in the community or throughout the entire influenza season in patients who cannot be vaccinated. Development of immunity following vaccination takes ~2 weeks; amantadine therapy should be considered for high-risk patients from the time of vaccination until immunity has developed. For children <9 years receiving influenza vaccine for the first time, amantadine prophylaxis should continue for 6 weeks (4 weeks after the first dose and 2 weeks after the second dose).

Adults:

Drug-induced extrapyramidal symptoms: 100 mg twice daily; may increase to 300-400 mg/day, if needed

Parkinson's disease or Creutzfeldt-Jakob disease (unlabeled use): 100 mg twice daily as sole therapy; may increase to 400 mg/day if needed with close monitoring; initial dose: 100 mg/day if with other serious illness or with high doses of other anti-Parkinson drugs

Influenza A viral infection: 100 mg twice daily; initiate within 24-48 hours after onset of symptoms; discontinue as soon as possible based on clinical response (generally within 3-5 days or within 24-48 hours after symptoms disappear)

Influenza A prophylaxis: 100 mg twice daily

Note: Continue treatment throughout the peak influenza activity in the community or throughout the entire influenza season in patients who cannot be vaccinated. Development of immunity following vaccination takes ~2 weeks; amantadine therapy should be considered for high-risk patients from the time of vaccination until immunity has developed.

Elderly: Adjust dose based on renal function; some patients tolerate the drug better when it is given in 2 divided daily doses (to avoid adverse neurologic reactions).

Influenza A prophylaxis or treatment: ≤100 mg/day in patients ≥65 years

Dosing interval in renal impairment:

Cl_{cr} 30-50 mL/minute: Administer 200 mg on day 1, then 100 mg/day

Cl_{cr} 15-29 mL/minute: Administer 200 mg on day 1, then 100 mg on alternate days

Cl_{cr} <15 mL/minute: Administer 200 mg every 7 days

Hemodialysis: Administer 200 mg every 7 days

Peritoneal dialysis: No supplemental dose is needed

Continuous arteriovenous or venous-venous hemofiltration: No supplemental dose is needed

Monitoring Parameters Renal function, Parkinson's symptoms, mental status, influenza symptoms, blood pressure

Additional Information Patients with intolerable CNS side effects often do better with rimantadine.

Dosage Forms Excipient information presented when available (limited, particularly for generics); consult specific product labeling.

Capsule, as hydrochloride: 100 mg
Capsule, softgel, as hydrochloride: 100 mg
Solution, oral, as hydrochloride: 50 mg/5 mL (473 mL)
Syrup, oral, as hydrochloride: 50 mg/5 mL (10 mL, 480 mL)
Tablet, as hydrochloride: 100 mg
Symmetrel®: 100 mg

- **Amantadine Hydrochloride** *see* Amantadine *on page 78*
- **Amaryl®** *see* Glimepiride *on page 696*
- **Amatine® (Can)** *see* Midodrine *on page 993*
- **Ambien®** *see* Zolpidem *on page 1591*
- **Ambien CR®** *see* Zolpidem *on page 1591*
- **Ambifed-G** *see* Guaifenesin and Pseudoephedrine *on page 713*
- **Ambifed-G DM** *see* Guaifenesin, Pseudoephedrine, and Dextromethorphan *on page 715*
- **AmBisome®** *see* Amphotericin B (Liposomal) *on page 107*

Ambrisentan (am bri SEN tan)

U.S. Brand Names Letairis™
Canadian Brand Names Volibris™
Index Terms BSF208075
Pharmacologic Category Endothelin Antagonist; Vasodilator
Use Treatment of pulmonary artery hypertension (PAH) World Health Organization (WHO) Group I in patients with WHO Class II or III symptoms to improve exercise capacity and decrease the rate of clinical deterioration

Restrictions
Ambrisentan (Letairis™) is only available through the limited distribution program (Letairis Education and Access Program [LEAP]). Only prescribers and pharmacies registered with LEAP may prescribe and dispense ambrisentan. Further information may be obtained from the manufacturer, Gilead Sciences, Inc (1-866-664-5327). FDA-approved medication guides are available at http://www.fda.gov/cder/Offices/ODS/medication_guides.htm.

Pregnancy Risk Factor X

Pregnancy Considerations **[U.S. Boxed Warning]: Use in pregnancy is contraindicated.** Based on animal studies, ambrisentan is likely to produce major birth defects if used by pregnant women. Pregnancy must be excluded prior to initiation of therapy and follow-up pregnancy tests should be obtained monthly. Two reliable methods of contraception must be used throughout treatment unless the patient has undergone a tubal ligation or the insertion of an intrauterine device (Copper T 380A or LNg 20). No other contraceptive measures are required for these patients.

Lactation Excretion in breast milk unknown/not recommended

Contraindications Pregnancy
Canadian labeling: Additional contraindications (not in U.S. labeling): Hypersensitivity to ambrisentan or any component of the formulation

Warnings/Precautions **[U.S. Boxed Warning]: Avoid use in moderate-to-severe hepatic impairment.** Has been associated with significant transaminase (ALT or AST) elevations which are dose dependent. Avoid use in patients with elevated serum transaminases (>3 times upper limit of normal [ULN]) at baseline. Monitor hepatic function closely (at least monthly) for the duration of treatment. Reduce dose or interrupt therapy if transaminases >3 times ULN and ≤5 times ULN and discontinue therapy with levels >5 times ULN and ≤8 times ULN. Treatment should be stopped in patients with transaminases >8 times ULN, elevated transaminases accompanied by symptoms of hepatic injury (unusual fatigue, jaundice, nausea, vomiting, abdominal pain, and/or fever), or those with elevated serum bilirubin >2 times ULN. Safety of reintroduction is unknown.

[U.S. Boxed Warning]: Use in pregnancy is contraindicated; exclude pregnancy prior to initiation of therapy and monthly thereafter. Two reliable methods of contraception must be used during therapy except in patients with tubal ligation or an implanted IUD (Copper T 380A or LNg 20). No other contraceptive measures are required for these patients. A missed menses should be reported to healthcare provider and prompt immediate pregnancy testing.

Use caution in patients with low hemoglobin levels. May cause decreases in hemoglobin and hematocrit (monitoring of hemoglobin is recommended. Development of peripheral edema due to treatment and/or disease state (pulmonary arterial hypertension) may occur; a higher incidence is seen in elderly patients. There have also been postmarketing reports of fluid retention requiring treatment (eg, diuretics, fluid management, hospitalization). Further evaluation may be necessary to determine cause and appropriate treatment or discontinuation of therapy. Use caution when concomitantly administered with CYP3A4 and CYP2C19 inhibitors, and with UGT inhibitors/inducers. Safety and efficacy have not been established in patients <18 years of age.

Adverse Reactions
>10%:
Cardiovascular: Peripheral edema (17%)
Central nervous system: Headache (15%)
1% to 10%:
Cardiovascular: Palpitation (5%), flushing (4%)
Gastrointestinal: Constipation (4%), abdominal pain (3%)
Hematologic: Hemoglobin decreased (7% to 10%)
Hepatic: Liver enzymes increased (1% to 3%)
Respiratory: Nasal congestion (6%), dyspnea (4%), nasopharyngitis (3%), sinusitis (3%)
Postmarketing and/or case reports: Fluid retention

Drug Interactions
Metabolism/Transport Effects Substrate of CYP3A4 (major), 2C19 (major), P-glycoprotein
Avoid Concomitant Use There are no known interactions where it is recommended to avoid concomitant use.
Increased Effect/Toxicity
The levels/effects of Ambrisentan may be increased by: CycloSPORINE; CYP2C19 Inhibitors (Moderate); CYP2C19 Inhibitors (Strong); CYP3A4 Inhibitors (Moderate); CYP3A4 Inhibitors (Strong); Dasatinib
Decreased Effect
The levels/effects of Ambrisentan may be decreased by: CYP2C19 Inducers (Strong); CYP3A4 Inducers (Strong); Deferasirox; Herbs (CYP3A4 Inducers)

Ethanol/Nutrition/Herb Interactions
Food: Grapefruit/grapefruit juice may increase levels/effects of ambrisentan.
Herb/Nutraceutical: Avoid St John's wort (concurrent use may decrease levels/effects of ambrisentan).

Stability Store at controlled room temperature of 25°C (77°F).

Mechanism of Action Blocks endothelin receptor subtypes ET_A and ET_B on vascular endothelium and smooth muscle. Stimulation of these receptors in smooth muscle cells is associated with vasoconstriction. Simulation of ET_B receptors in endothelial cells is associated with vasodilation and antiproliferative effects. Although ambrisentan blocks both ET_A and ET_B receptors, the affinity is greater for the A subtype. Improvement in symptoms of pulmonary artery hypertension and a decrease in the rate of clinical deterioration have been demonstrated in clinical trials.

Pharmacodynamics/Kinetics

Absorption: Rapid

Protein binding: 99%

Metabolism: Hepatic via CYP3A4, CYP2C19, and uridine 5'-diphosphate glucuronosyltransferases (UGTs) 1A9S, 2B7S, and 1A3S; *in vitro* studies also suggest it is a substrate of organic anion transport protein (OATP) and P-glycoprotein (P-gp)

Half-life elimination: 9 hours

Time to peak, plasma: 2 hours

Excretion: Primarily nonrenal

Dosage Oral: Adults: Initial: 5 mg once daily; if tolerated, may increase to maximum 10 mg once daily

Modifications based on transaminase elevation:

If any elevation, regardless of degree, is accompanied by clinical symptoms of hepatic injury (unusual fatigue, nausea, vomiting, abdominal pain, fever, or jaundice) or a serum bilirubin >2 times ULN, treatment should be stopped and not reintroduced.

AST/ALT >3 but ≤5 times ULN: Confirm with additional test; if confirmed, reduce dose or interrupt treatment. Monitor transaminase levels at least every 2 weeks until levels are <3 times ULN. Reinitiate treatment as appropriate with return to pretreatment values and with more frequent checks of transaminase levels.

AST/ALT >5 but ≤8 times ULN: Confirm with additional test; if confirmed, stop treatment. Monitor transaminase levels until they are <3 times ULN. May reintroduce treatment, as appropriate, at starting dose, following return to pretreatment values. More frequent checks of transaminase levels are required after resuming therapy.

AST/ALT >8 times ULN: Stop treatment and do not reintroduce.

Dosage adjustment in renal impairment: No dosage adjustment is required in mild-to-moderate renal impairment. No data available for use in severe renal impairment.

Dosage adjustment in hepatic impairment: Avoid use in patients with moderate-to-severe hepatic insufficiency. Dose reductions may be required in patients with mild hepatic insufficiency.

Dietary Considerations May be taken with or without food. Avoid grapefruit and grapefruit juice.

Administration Swallow tablet whole. Do not split, crush, or chew tablets. May be administered with or without food.

Monitoring Parameters Serum transaminase (AST and ALT) and bilirubin should be determined prior to the initiation of therapy (baseline) and at monthly intervals thereafter. Monitor for clinical signs and symptoms of liver injury (eg, abdominal pain, fatigue, fever, jaundice, nausea, vomiting). Reduce dose or interrupt therapy if transaminases >3 times ULN and ≤5 times ULN and discontinue therapy with levels >5 times ULN and ≤8 times ULN. Monitor levels every 2 weeks until they are <3 times ULN. Therapy may be resumed with more frequent monitoring of levels. Discontinue therapy in patients with transaminases >8 times ULN, elevated transaminases with accompanying symptoms of hepatic injury, or bilirubin >2 times ULN. Monitor for significant peripheral edema and evaluate etiology if it occurs.

A woman of childbearing potential must have a negative pregnancy test prior to the initiation of therapy and monthly thereafter. Hemoglobin and hematocrit should be measured at baseline, at 1 month, and periodically thereafter (generally stabilizes after the first few weeks of treatment).

Dosage Forms Excipient information presented when available (limited, particularly for generics); consult specific product labeling.

Tablet:

Letairis™: 5 mg, 10 mg

Amcinonide (am SIN oh nide)

Canadian Brand Names Amcort®; Cyclocort®; ratio-Amcinonide; Taro-Amcinonide

Pharmacologic Category Corticosteroid, Topical

Additional Appendix Information

Corticosteroids *on page 1652*

Use Relief of the inflammatory and pruritic manifestations of corticosteroid-responsive dermatoses (high potency corticosteroid)

Pregnancy Risk Factor C

Contraindications Hypersensitivity to amcinonide or any component of the formulation; use on the face, groin, or axilla

Warnings/Precautions Systemic absorption of topical corticosteroids may cause hypothalamic-pituitary-adrenal (HPA) axis suppression (reversible) particularly in younger children. HPA axis suppression may lead to adrenal crisis. Risk is increased when used over large surface areas, for prolonged periods, or with occlusive dressings. Adverse systemic effects including hyperglycemia, glycosuria, fluid and electrolyte changes, and HPA suppression may occur when used on large surface areas, for prolonged periods, or with an occlusive dressing. Prolonged treatment with corticosteroids has been associated with the development of Kaposi's sarcoma (case reports); if noted, discontinuation of therapy should be considered. Allergic contact dermatitis can occur, it is usually diagnosed by failure to heal rather than clinical exacerbation. Occlusive dressings should not be used in presence of infection or weeping lesions. Chronic use of corticosteroids in children may interfere with growth and development.

Adverse Reactions Frequency not defined.

Dermatologic: Acne, hypopigmentation, allergic dermatitis, maceration of the skin, miliaria, skin atrophy, striae, telangiectasia

Endocrine & metabolic: Cushing's syndrome, growth retardation (long-term use), HPA suppression, hyperglycemia; these reactions occur more frequently with occlusive dressings

Local: Burning, dryness, folliculitis, hypertrichosis, itching, irritation

Miscellaneous: Secondary infection

Drug Interactions

Avoid Concomitant Use There are no known interactions where it is recommended to avoid concomitant use.

Increased Effect/Toxicity There are no known significant interactions involving an increase in effect.

Decreased Effect

Amcinonide may decrease the levels/effects of: Corticorelin

Mechanism of Action Stimulates the synthesis of enzymes needed to decrease inflammation, suppress mitotic activity, and cause vasoconstriction

Pharmacodynamics/Kinetics

Absorption: Adequate through intact skin; increases with skin inflammation or occlusion

Metabolism: Hepatic

Excretion: Urine and feces

Dosage Topical: Adults: Apply in a thin film 2-3 times/day. Therapy should be discontinued when control is achieved; if no improvement is seen, reassessment of diagnosis may be necessary.

Dosage Forms Excipient information presented when available (limited, particularly for generics); consult specific product labeling.

Cream: 0.1% (15 g, 30 g, 60 g) [contains benzyl alcohol]

Lotion: 0.1% (60 mL)

Ointment: 0.1% (30 g, 60 g) [contains benzyl alcohol]

Amifostine (am i FOS teen)

U.S. Brand Names Ethyol®

Canadian Brand Names Ethyol®

Index Terms Ethiofos; Gammaphos; WR-2721; YM-08310

Pharmacologic Category Adjuvant, Chemoprotective Agent (Cytoprotective); Antidote

Use Reduce the incidence of moderate to severe xerostomia in patients undergoing postoperative radiation treatment for head and neck cancer, where the radiation port includes a substantial portion of the parotid glands; reduce the cumulative renal toxicity associated with repeated administration of cisplatin

Unlabeled/Investigational Use Prevention of radiation proctitis in patients with rectal cancer

Pregnancy Risk Factor C

Pregnancy Considerations Animal studies have demonstrated embryotoxicity. There are no adequate and well-controlled studies in pregnant women.

Lactation Excretion in breast milk unknown/not recommended

Medication Safety Issues

Sound-alike/look-alike issues:

Ethyol® may be confused with ethanol

Contraindications Hypersensitivity to aminothiol compounds or any component of the formulation

Warnings/Precautions Patients who are hypotensive or dehydrated should not receive amifostine. Interrupt antihypertensive therapy for 24 hours before treatment; patients who cannot safely stop their antihypertensives 24 hours before, should not receive amifostine. Adequately hydrated prior to treatment and keep in a supine position during infusion. Monitor blood pressure every 5 minutes during the infusion. If hypotension requiring interruption of therapy occurs, patients should be placed in the Trendelenburg position and given an infusion of normal saline using a separate I.V. line; subsequent infusions may require a dose reduction. Infusions >15 minutes are associated with a higher incidence of adverse effects. Use caution in patients with cardiovascular and cerebrovascular disease and any other patients in whom the adverse effects of hypotension may have serious adverse events.

Serious cutaneous reactions, including erythema multiforme, Stevens-Johnson syndrome, toxic epidermal necrolysis, toxoderma and exfoliative dermatitis have been reported with amifostine. May be delayed, developing up to weeks after treatment initiation. Cutaneous reactions have been reported more frequently when used as a radioprotectant. Discontinue treatment for severe/serious cutaneous reaction, or with fever. Withhold treatment and obtain dermatologic consultation for rash involving lips or mucosa (of unknown etiology outside of radiation port) and for bullous, edematous or erythematous lesions on hands, feet, or trunk; reinitiate only after careful evaluation.

It is recommended that antiemetic medication, including dexamethasone 20 mg I.V. and a serotonin 5-HT_3 receptor antagonist be administered prior to and in conjunction with amifostine. Rare hypersensitivity reactions, including anaphylaxis and allergic reaction, have been reported; discontinue if allergic reaction occurs; do not rechallenge. Medications for the treatment of hypersensitivity reactions should be available.

Reports of clinically-relevant hypocalcemia are rare, but serum calcium levels should be monitored in patients at risk of hypocalcemia, such as those with nephrotic syndrome; may require calcium supplementation. Should not be used (in patients receiving chemotherapy for malignancies other than ovarian cancer) where chemotherapy is expected to provide significant survival benefit or in patients receiving definitive radiotherapy, unless within the context of a clinical trial. Safety and efficacy in children have not been established.

Adverse Reactions

>10%:

Cardiovascular: Hypotension (15% to 61%; grades 3/4: 3% to 8%; dose dependent)

Gastrointestinal: Nausea/vomiting (53% to 96%; grades 3/4: 8% to 30%; dose dependent)

1% to 10%: Endocrine & metabolic: Hypocalcemia (clinically significant: 1%)

<1% (Limited to important or life-threatening): Apnea, anaphylactoid reactions, anaphylaxis, arrhythmia, atrial fibrillation, atrial flutter, back pain, bradycardia, cardiac arrest, chest pain, chest tightness, chills, cutaneous eruptions, dizziness, erythema multiforme, exfoliative dermatitis, extrasystoles, dyspnea, fever, flushing, hiccups, hypersensitivity reactions (fever, rash, hypoxia, dyspnea, laryngeal edema), hypertension (transient), hypoxia, malaise, MI, myocardial ischemia, pruritus, rash (mild), renal failure, respiratory arrest, rigors, seizure, sneezing, somnolence, Stevens-Johnson syndrome, supraventricular tachycardia, syncope, tachycardia, toxic epidermal necrolysis, toxoderma, urticaria

Drug Interactions

Avoid Concomitant Use There are no known interactions where it is recommended to avoid concomitant use.

Increased Effect/Toxicity

The levels/effects of Amifostine may be increased by: Antihypertensives

Decreased Effect There are no known significant interactions involving a decrease in effect.

Stability Store intact vials of lyophilized powder at room temperature of 20°C to 25°C (68°F to 77°F). For I.V. infusion, reconstitute intact vials with 9.7 mL 0.9% sodium chloride injection and dilute in 0.9% sodium chloride to a final concentration of 5-40 mg/mL. For SubQ administration, reconstitute with 2.5 mL NS or SWFI. Reconstituted solutions (500 mg/10 mL) and solutions for infusion are chemically stable for up to 5 hours at room temperature (25°C) or up to 24 hours under refrigeration (2°C to 8°C).

Mechanism of Action Prodrug that is dephosphorylated by alkaline phosphatase in tissues to a pharmacologically-active free thiol metabolite. The free thiol is available to bind to, and detoxify, reactive metabolites of cisplatin; and can also act as a scavenger of free radicals that may be generated (by cisplatin or radiation therapy) in tissues.

Pharmacodynamics/Kinetics

Distribution: V_d: 3.5 L

Metabolism: Hepatic dephosphorylation to two metabolites (active-free thiol and disulfide)

Half-life elimination: ~8-9 minutes

Excretion: Urine

Clearance, plasma: 2.17 L/minute

Dosage Note: Antiemetic medication, including dexamethasone 20 mg I.V. and a serotonin 5-HT_3 receptor antagonist, is recommended prior to and in conjunction with amifostine.

Adults:

Cisplatin-induced renal toxicity, reduction: I.V.: 910 mg/m^2 over 15 minutes once daily 30 minutes prior to cisplatin

For 910 mg/m^2 doses, the manufacturer suggests the following blood pressure-based adjustment schedule:

The infusion of amifostine should be interrupted if the systolic blood pressure decreases significantly from baseline, as defined below:

Decrease of 20 mm Hg if baseline systolic blood pressure <100

Decrease of 25 mm Hg if baseline systolic blood pressure 100-119

Decrease of 30 mm Hg if baseline systolic blood pressure 120-139

Decrease of 40 mm Hg if baseline systolic blood pressure 140-179

Decrease of 50 mm Hg if baseline systolic blood pressure ≥180

If blood pressure returns to normal within 5 minutes (assisted by fluid administration and postural management) and the patient is asymptomatic, the infusion may be restarted so that the full dose of amifostine may be administered. If the full dose of amifostine cannot be administered, the dose of amifostine for subsequent cycles should be 740 mg/m^2.

Xerostomia from head and neck cancer, reduction:

I.V.: 200 mg/m^2 over 3 minutes once daily 15-30 minutes prior to radiation therapy **or**

SubQ (unlabeled route): 500 mg once daily prior to radiation therapy

Prevention of radiation proctitis in rectal cancer (unlabeled use): I.V.: 340 mg/m^2 once daily prior to radiation therapy (Keefe, 2007; Peterson, 2008)

Administration I.V.: Administer over 3 minutes (prior to radiation therapy) or 15 minutes (prior to cisplatin); administration as a longer infusion is associated with a higher incidence of side effects. Patients should be kept in supine position during infusion. **Note:** SubQ administration (unlabeled) has been used.

Monitoring Parameters Blood pressure should be monitored every 5 minutes during the infusion and after administration if clinically indicated; serum calcium levels (in patients at risk for hypocalcemia). Evaluate for cutaneous reactions prior to each dose.

Additional Information Oncology Comment: The American Society of Clinical Oncology (ASCO) guidelines for the use of protectants for chemotherapy and radiation (Hensley, 2008) recommend the use of amifostine for prevention of nephrotoxicity due to cisplatin-based chemotherapy and to decrease the incidence of acute and delayed radiation therapy-induced xerostomia. The ASCO guidelines do not recommend the use of amifostine to reduce the incidence of neutropenia or thrombocytopenia associated with chemotherapy or radiation therapy, neurotoxicity or ototoxicity associated with platinum-based chemotherapy, radiation therapy-induced mucositis associated with head and neck cancer, or esophagitis due to chemotherapy in patients with nonsmall cell lung cancer. Additionally, the guidelines do not support the use of amifostine in patients with head and neck cancer receiving concurrent platinum-based chemotherapy.

Dosage Forms Excipient information presented when available (limited, particularly for generics); consult specific product labeling.

Injection, powder for reconstitution: 500 mg

Ethyol®: 500 mg

- **Amigesic® [DSC]** *see* Salsalate *on page 1352*
- **Amigesic® (Can)** *see* Salsalate *on page 1352*

Amikacin (am i KAY sin)

Canadian Brand Names Amikacin Sulfate Injection, USP; Amikin®

Index Terms Amikacin Sulfate

Pharmacologic Category Antibiotic, Aminoglycoside

Additional Appendix Information

Aminoglycoside Dosing and Monitoring *on page 1630*

Antimicrobial Drugs of Choice *on page 1752*

Tuberculosis *on page 1776*

Use Treatment of serious infections (bone infections, respiratory tract infections, endocarditis, and septicemia) due to organisms resistant to gentamicin and tobramycin, including *Pseudomonas*, *Proteus*, *Serratia*, and other gram-negative bacilli; documented infection of mycobacterial organisms susceptible to amikacin

Unlabeled/Investigational Use Bacterial endophthalmitis

Pregnancy Risk Factor D

Pregnancy Considerations

Amikacin crosses the placenta, produces detectable serum levels in the fetus, and concentrates in the fetal kidneys. Because of several reports of total irreversible bilateral congenital deafness in children whose mothers received streptomycin during pregnancy, the manufacturer classifies amikacin as pregnancy risk factor D. Renal toxicity has been observed in animals, but fetal toxicity in humans has not been reported. No adequate and well-controlled studies have been conducted in pregnant women and it is not known whether amikacin can cause fetal harm. Although the manufacturer considers amikacin pregnancy risk factor D, amikacin-specific clinical data would suggest pregnancy risk factor C.

Due to pregnancy-induced physiologic changes, some pharmacokinetic parameters of amikacin may be altered. Pregnant women have an average-to-larger volume of distribution which may result in lower peak serum levels than for the same dose in nonpregnant women. Serum half-life is also shorter.

Lactation Enters breast milk/compatible

Medication Safety Issues

Sound-alike/look-alike issues:

Amikacin may be confused with Amicar®, anakinra

Amikin® may be confused with Amicar®

Contraindications Hypersensitivity to amikacin sulfate or any component of the formulation; cross-sensitivity may exist with other aminoglycosides

Warnings/Precautions [U.S. Boxed Warning]: Amikacin may cause neurotoxicity, nephrotoxicity, and/or neuromuscular blockade and respiratory paralysis; usual risk factors include pre-existing renal impairment, concomitant neuro-/nephrotoxic medications, advanced age and dehydration. Dose and/or frequency of administration must be monitored and modified in patients with renal impairment. Drug should be discontinued if signs of ototoxicity, nephrotoxicity, or hypersensitivity occur. Ototoxicity is proportional to the amount of drug given and the duration of treatment. Tinnitus or vertigo may be indications of vestibular injury and impending bilateral irreversible damage. Renal damage is usually reversible. Use with caution in patients with neuromuscular disorders, hearing loss and hypocalcemia. Prolonged use may result in fungal or bacterial superinfection, including *C. difficile*-associated diarrhea (CDAD) and pseudomembranous colitis; CDAD has been observed >2 months postantibiotic treatment. Solution contains sodium metabisulfate; use caution in patients with sulfite allergy.

Adverse Reactions

1% to 10%:

Central nervous system: Neurotoxicity

Otic: Ototoxicity (auditory), ototoxicity (vestibular)

Renal: Nephrotoxicity

<1% (Limited to important or life-threatening): Allergic reaction, dyspnea, eosinophilia

Drug Interactions

Avoid Concomitant Use

Avoid concomitant use of Amikacin with any of the following: Gallium Nitrate

Increased Effect/Toxicity

Amikacin may increase the levels/effects of: Bisphosphonate Derivatives; Botulinum Toxin Type A; Botulinum Toxin Type B; CARBOplatin; Colistimethate; CycloSPORINE; Gallium Nitrate; Neuromuscular-Blocking Agents

The levels/effects of Amikacin may be increased by: Amphotericin B; Capreomycin; CISplatin; Loop Diuretics; Nonsteroidal Anti-Inflammatory Agents; Vancomycin

Decreased Effect

Amikacin may decrease the levels/effects of: Typhoid Vaccine

The levels/effects of Amikacin may be decreased by: Penicillins

Stability Store at controlled room temperature. Following admixture at concentrations of 0.25-5 mg/mL, amikcain is stable for 24 hours at room temperature and 2 days at refrigeration when mixed in D_5W, NS, and LR.

Mechanism of Action Inhibits protein synthesis in susceptible bacteria by binding to 30S ribosomal subunits

Pharmacodynamics/Kinetics

Absorption:

I.M.: Rapid

Oral: Poorly absorbed

Distribution: Primarily into extracellular fluid (highly hydrophilic); penetrates blood-brain barrier when meninges inflamed

Relative diffusion of antimicrobial agents from blood into CSF: Good only with inflammation (exceeds usual MICs)

CSF:blood level ratio: Normal meninges: 10% to 20%; Inflamed meninges: 15% to 24%

Protein-binding: 0% to 11%

Half-life elimination (renal function and age dependent):

Infants: Low birth weight (1-3 days): 7-9 hours; Full-term >7 days: 4-5 hours

Children: 1.6-2.5 hours

Adults: Normal renal function: 1.4-2.3 hours; Anuria/end-stage renal disease: 28-86 hours

Time to peak, serum: I.M.: 45-120 minutes

Excretion: Urine (94% to 98%)

Dosage Note: Individualization is critical because of the low therapeutic index

Use of ideal body weight (IBW) for determining the mg/kg/dose appears to be more accurate than dosing on the basis of total body weight (TBW)

In morbid obesity, dosage requirement may best be estimated using a dosing weight of IBW + 0.4 (TBW - IBW)

Initial and periodic peak and trough plasma drug levels should be determined, particularly in critically-ill patients with serious infections or in disease states known to significantly alter aminoglycoside pharmacokinetics (eg, cystic fibrosis, burns, or major surgery)

Usual dosage range:

Infants and Children: I.M., I.V.: 5-7.5 mg/kg/dose every 8 hours

Adults: I.M., I.V.: 5-7.5 mg/kg/dose every 8 hours

Note: Some clinicians suggest a daily dose of 15-20 mg/kg for all patients with normal renal function. This dose is at least as efficacious with similar, if not less, toxicity than conventional dosing.

Indication-specific dosing:

Adults:

Endophthalmitis, bacterial (unlabeled use): Intravitreal: 0.4 mg/0.1 mL NS in combination with vancomycin

Hospital-acquired pneumonia (HAP): I.V.: 20 mg/kg/day with antipseudomonal beta-lactam or carbapenem (American Thoracic Society/ATS guidelines)

Meningitis *(Pseudomonas aeruginosa)*: I.V.: 5 mg/kg every 8 hours (administered with another bacteriocidal drug)

Mycobacterium fortuitum, M. chelonae, or M. abscessus: I.V.: 10-15 mg/kg daily for at least 2 weeks with high dose cefoxitin

Dosing interval in renal impairment: Some patients may require larger or more frequent doses if serum levels document the need (ie, cystic fibrosis or febrile granulocytopenic patients).

Cl_{cr} ≥60 mL/minute: Administer every 8 hours

Cl_{cr} 40-60 mL/minute: Administer every 12 hours

Cl_{cr} 20-40 mL/minute: Administer every 24 hours

Cl_{cr} <20 mL/minute: Loading dose, then monitor levels

Hemodialysis: Dialyzable (50% to 100%); administer dose postdialysis or administer 2/3 normal dose as a supplemental dose postdialysis and follow levels

Peritoneal dialysis: Dose as Cl_{cr} <20 mL/minute: Follow levels

Continuous arteriovenous or venovenous hemodiafiltration effects: Dose as for Cl_{cr} 10-40 mL/minute and follow levels

Dietary Considerations Sodium content of 1 g: 29.9 mg (1.3 mEq)

Administration Administer around-the-clock to promote less variation in peak and trough serum levels. Do not mix with other drugs, administer separately.

I.M.: Administer I.M. injection in large muscle mass.

I.V.: Infuse over 30-60 minutes.

Some penicillins (eg, carbenicillin, ticarcillin, and piperacillin) have been shown to inactivate *in vitro*. This has been observed to a greater extent with tobramycin and gentamicin, while amikacin has shown greater stability against inactivation. Concurrent use of these agents may pose a risk of reduced antibacterial efficacy *in vivo*, particularly in the setting of profound renal impairment. However, definitive clinical evidence is lacking. If combination penicillin/aminoglycoside therapy is desired in a patient with renal dysfunction, separation of doses (if feasible), and routine monitoring of aminoglycoside levels, CBC, and clinical response should be considered.

Monitoring Parameters Urinalysis, BUN, serum creatinine, appropriately timed peak and trough concentrations, vital signs, temperature, weight, I & O, hearing parameters

Some penicillin derivatives may accelerate the degradation of aminoglycosides *in vitro*. This may be clinically-significant for certain penicillin (ticarcillin, piperacillin, carbenicillin) and aminoglycoside (gentamicin, tobramycin) combination therapy in patients with significant renal impairment. Close monitoring of aminoglycoside levels is warranted.

Reference Range

Sample size: 0.5-2 mL blood (red top tube) or 0.1-1 mL serum (separated)

Therapeutic levels:

Peak:

Life-threatening infections: 25-40 mcg/mL

Serious infections: 20-25 mcg/mL
Urinary tract infections: 15-20 mcg/mL
Trough: <8 mcg/mL
The American Thoracic Society (ATS) recommends trough levels of <4-5 mcg/mL for patients with hospital-acquired pneumonia.
Toxic concentration: Peak: >40 mcg/mL; Trough: >10 mcg/mL
Timing of serum samples: Draw peak 30 minutes after completion of 30-minute infusion or at 1 hour following initiation of infusion or I.M. injection; draw trough within 30 minutes prior to next dose

Test Interactions Some penicillin derivatives may accelerate the degradation of aminoglycosides *in vitro*, leading to a potential underestimation of aminoglycoside serum concentration.

Additional Information Aminoglycoside levels measured from blood taken from Silastic® central catheters can sometimes give falsely high readings (draw levels from alternate lumen or peripheral stick, if possible).

Dosage Forms Excipient information presented when available (limited, particularly for generics); consult specific product labeling.
Injection, solution, as sulfate: 50 mg/mL (2 mL); 250 mg/mL (2 mL, 4 mL)

◆ **Amikacin Sulfate** *see* Amikacin *on page 83*
◆ **Amikacin Sulfate Injection, USP (Can)** *see* Amikacin *on page 83*
◆ **Amikin® (Can)** *see* Amikacin *on page 83*

AMILoride (a MIL oh ride)

Canadian Brand Names Apo-Amiloride®
Index Terms Amiloride Hydrochloride
Pharmacologic Category Diuretic, Potassium-Sparing
Use Counteracts potassium loss induced by other diuretics in the treatment of hypertension or edematous conditions including CHF, hepatic cirrhosis, and hypoaldosteronism; usually used in conjunction with more potent diuretics such as thiazides or loop diuretics
Unlabeled/Investigational Use Investigational: Cystic fibrosis; reduction of lithium-induced polyuria; pediatric hypertension
Pregnancy Risk Factor B
Medication Safety Issues
Sound-alike/look-alike issues:
AMILoride may be confused with amiodarone, amLODIPine, amrinone
Dosage Oral:
Children 1-17 years: Hypertension (unlabeled use): 0.4-0.625 mg/kg/day (maximum: 20 mg/day)
Adults: 5-10 mg/day (up to 20 mg)
Hypertension (JNC 7): 5-10 mg/day in 1-2 divided doses
Elderly: Initial: 5 mg once daily or every other day
Dosing adjustment in renal impairment:
Cl_{cr} 10-50 mL/minute: Administer at 50% of normal dose.
Cl_{cr} <10 mL/minute: Avoid use.
Additional Information Complete prescribing information for this medication should be consulted for additional detail.
Dosage Forms Excipient information presented when available (limited, particularly for generics); consult specific product labeling.
Tablet, as hydrochloride: 5 mg

Amiloride and Hydrochlorothiazide
(a MIL oh ride & hye droe klor oh THYE a zide)

Canadian Brand Names Apo-Amilzide®; Gen-Amilazide; Moduret; Novamilor; Nu-Amilzide
Index Terms Hydrochlorothiazide and Amiloride
Pharmacologic Category Diuretic, Combination
Use Potassium-sparing diuretic; antihypertensive
Pregnancy Risk Factor B
Dosage Adults: Oral: Start with 1 tablet/day; may be increased to 2 tablets/day if needed; usually given in a single dose
Elderly: Initial: 1/2 to 1 tablet/day
Dosage adjustment in renal impairment: See individual agents.
Additional Information Complete prescribing information for this medication should be consulted for additional detail.
Dosage Forms Excipient information presented when available (limited, particularly for generics); consult specific product labeling.
Tablet: 5/50: Amiloride hydrochloride 5 mg and hydrochlorothiazide 50 mg

◆ **Amiloride Hydrochloride** *see* AMILoride *on page 85*
◆ **2-Amino-6-Mercaptopurine** *see* Thioguanine *on page 1459*
◆ **2-Amino-6-Methoxypurine Arabinoside** *see* Nelarabine *on page 1047*
◆ **2-Amino-6-Trifluoromethoxy-benzothiazole** *see* Riluzole *on page 1319*
◆ **Aminobenzylpenicillin** *see* Ampicillin *on page 109*

Aminocaproic Acid (a mee noe ka PROE ik AS id)

U.S. Brand Names Amicar®
Index Terms EACA; Epsilon Aminocaproic Acid
Pharmacologic Category Antifibrinolytic Agent; Hemostatic Agent
Use To enhance hemostasis when fibrinolysis contributes to bleeding (causes may include cardiac surgery, hematologic disorders, neoplastic disorders, abruption placentae, hepatic cirrhosis, and urinary fibrinolysis)
Unlabeled/Investigational Use Treatment of traumatic hyphema; control bleeding in thrombocytopenia; control oral bleeding in congenital and acquired coagulation disorders; topical treatment (mouth rinse) of bleeding associated with dental procedures in patients on oral anticoagulant therapy; prevention of perioperative bleeding associated with cardiac surgery
Pregnancy Risk Factor C
Medication Safety Issues
Sound-alike/look-alike issues:
Amicar® may be confused with amikacin, Amikin®, Omacor®
Dosage
Acute bleeding syndrome:
Children (unlabeled use): Oral, I.V.: Loading dose: 100-200 mg/kg during the first hour, followed by continuous infusion at 33.3 mg/kg/hour (I.V.) or 100 mg/kg (oral or I.V.) every 6 hours
Adults: Oral, I.V.: Loading dose: 4-5 g during the first hour, followed by 1 g/hour for 8 hours or until bleeding controlled (maximum daily dose: 30 g)
Control of bleeding in thrombocytopenia (unlabeled use):
Adults:
Initial: I.V.: 100 mg/kg over 30-60 minutes
Maintenance: Oral: 1-3 g every 6 hours
Control of oral bleeding in congenital and acquired coagulation disorder (unlabeled use): Adults: Oral: 50-60 mg/kg every 4 hours
Prevention of dental procedure bleeding in patients on oral anticoagulant therapy (unlabeled use): Oral rinse: Hold 4 g/10 mL in mouth for 2 minutes then spit out. Repeat every 6 hours for 2 days after procedure (Souto, 1996). Concentration and frequency may vary by institution and product availability.

Prevention of perioperative bleeding associated with cardiac surgery (unlabeled use): I.V.:

Children: 100 mg/kg given over 20-30 minutes after induction and prior to incision, 100 mg/kg during cardiopulmonary bypass, and 100 mg/kg after protamine reversal of heparin

Adults: 10 g over 20-30 minutes prior to skin incision, followed by 1-2.5 g/hour (usual dose 2 g/hour) until the end of operation (may continue infusion for 4 hours after protamine reversal of heparin). May add 10 g to cardiopulmonary bypass circuit priming solution.

or

10 g over 20-30 minutes prior to skin incision, followed by 10 g after heparin administration then 10 g at discontinuation of cardiopulmonary bypass prior to protamine reversal of heparin

Traumatic hyphema (unlabeled use): Children and Adults: Oral: 100 mg/kg/dose every 4 hours (maximum daily dose: 30 g)

Dosing adjustment in renal impairment: May accumulate in patients with decreased renal function.

Additional Information Complete prescribing information for this medication should be consulted for additional detail.

Dosage Forms Excipient information presented when available (limited, particularly for generics); consult specific product labeling.

Injection, solution: 250 mg/mL (20 mL)

Amicar®: 250 mg/mL (20 mL) [contains benzyl alcohol]

Solution, oral: 1.25 g/5 mL (240 mL, 480 mL)

Syrup:

Amicar®: 1.25 g/5 mL (480 mL) [raspberry flavor]

Tablet [scored]: 500 mg

Amicar®: 500 mg, 1000 mg

Aminoglutethimide (a mee noe gloo TETH i mide)

U.S. Brand Names Cytadren®

Index Terms BA-16038; Elipten

Pharmacologic Category Antineoplastic Agent, Aromatase Inhibitor; Enzyme Inhibitor; Hormone Antagonist, Anti-Adrenal; Nonsteroidal Aromatase Inhibitor

Use Suppression of adrenal function in selected patients with Cushing's syndrome

Unlabeled/Investigational Use Treatment of prostate cancer (androgen synthesis inhibitor)

Pregnancy Risk Factor D

Medication Safety Issues

Sound-alike/look-alike issues:

Cytadren® may be confused with cytarabine

Dosage Oral: Adults: **Note:** Glucocorticoid and mineralocorticoid replacement therapy may be necessary.

Adrenal suppression: 250 mg every 6 hours may be increased in increments of 250 mg/day at 1- to 2-week intervals to a total of 2 g/day

Prostate cancer (unlabeled use): 250 mg 3 times/day for 3 weeks, then increase to 4 times/day

Additional Information Complete prescribing information for this medication should be consulted for additional detail.

Dosage Forms Excipient information presented when available (limited, particularly for generics); consult specific product labeling.

Tablet [scored]:

Cytadren®: 250 mg

Aminolevulinic Acid (a MEE noh lev yoo lin ik AS id)

U.S. Brand Names Levulan® Kerastick®

Canadian Brand Names Levulan®

Index Terms Aminolevulinic Acid Hydrochloride

Pharmacologic Category Photosensitizing Agent, Topical; Topical Skin Product

Use Treatment of minimally to moderately thick actinic keratoses (grade 1 or 2) of the face or scalp; to be used in conjunction with blue light illumination

Pregnancy Risk Factor C

Dosage Adults: Topical: Apply to actinic keratoses (**not** perilesional skin) followed 14-18 hours later by blue light illumination. Application/treatment may be repeated at a treatment site after 8 weeks.

Additional Information Complete prescribing information for this medication should be consulted for additional detail.

Dosage Forms Excipient information presented when available (limited, particularly for generics); consult specific product labeling.

Powder for topical solution:

Levulan® Kerastick®: 20% (6s) [2-component system containing aminolevulinic acid hydrochloride 354 mg (powder) and diluent containing ethanol 48% (1.5 mL) packaged together in an applicator tube]

◆ **Aminolevulinic Acid Hydrochloride** *see* Aminolevulinic Acid *on page 86*

◆ **Aminosalicylate Sodium** *see* Aminosalicylic Acid *on page 86*

Aminosalicylic Acid (a mee noe sal i SIL ik AS id)

U.S. Brand Names Paser®

Index Terms 4-Aminosalicylic Acid; Aminosalicylate Sodium; Para-Aminosalicylate Sodium; PAS; Sodium PAS

Pharmacologic Category Salicylate

Use Adjunctive treatment of tuberculosis used in combination with other antitubercular agents

Unlabeled/Investigational Use Crohn's disease

Pregnancy Risk Factor C

Pregnancy Considerations Teratogenic effects have been reported in animals, however, adequate studies have not been done in humans. Use during pregnancy only if clearly needed.

Lactation Enters breast milk/not recommended

Contraindications Hypersensitivity to aminosalicylic acid or any component of the formulation

Warnings/Precautions Use with caution in patients with hepatic or renal dysfunction and patients with gastric ulcer. Patients with sensitivity to tartrazine dyes, nasal polyps, and asthma may have an increased risk of salicylate sensitivity.

Adverse Reactions Frequency not defined.

Cardiovascular: Pericarditis, vasculitis

Central nervous system: Encephalopathy, fever

Dermatologic: Skin eruptions

Endocrine & metabolic: Goiter (with or without myxedema), hypoglycemia

Gastrointestinal: Abdominal pain, diarrhea, nausea, vomiting

Hematologic: Agranulocytosis, anemia (hemolytic), leukopenia, thrombocytopenia

Hepatic: Hepatitis, jaundice

Ocular: Optic neuritis

Respiratory: Eosinophilic pneumonia

Drug Interactions

Avoid Concomitant Use There are no known interactions where it is recommended to avoid concomitant use.

Increased Effect/Toxicity

Aminosalicylic Acid may increase the levels/effects of: Anticoagulants; Carbonic Anhydrase Inhibitors; Corticosteroids (Systemic); Drotrecogin Alfa; Methotrexate; Salicylates; Sulfonylureas; Thrombolytic Agents; Valproic Acid; Varicella Virus-Containing Vaccines; Vitamin K Antagonists

The levels/effects of Aminosalicylic Acid may be increased by: Antiplatelet Agents; Calcium Channel Blockers (Nondihydropyridine); Ginkgo Biloba; Herbs (Anticoagulant/Antiplatelet Properties); NSAID (Nonselective); Treprostinil

Decreased Effect

Aminosalicylic Acid may decrease the levels/effects of: ACE Inhibitors; NSAID (Nonselective); Uricosuric Agents

The levels/effects of Aminosalicylic Acid may be decreased by: Corticosteroids (Systemic); NSAID (Nonselective)

Stability Prior to dispensing, store granules below 15°C (59°F). Once dispensed, packets may be stored at room temperature for short periods of time. Do not use if packet is swollen or if granules are dark brown or purple.

Mechanism of Action Aminosalicylic acid (PAS) is a highly-specific bacteriostatic agent active against *M. tuberculosis*. Structurally related to para-aminobenzoic acid (PABA) and its mechanism of action is thought to be similar to the sulfonamides, a competitive antagonism with PABA; disrupts plate biosynthesis in sensitive organisms.

Pharmacodynamics/Kinetics

Absorption: Readily, >90%

Protein binding: 50% to 60%

Metabolism: Hepatic (>50%) via acetylation

Half-life elimination: Reduced with renal impairment

Time to peak, serum: 6 hours

Excretion: Urine (>80% as unchanged drug and metabolites)

Dosage Oral:

Children: Tuberculosis: 200-300 mg/kg/day in 3-4 equally divided doses

Adults:

Tuberculosis: 150 mg/kg/day in 2-3 equally divided doses

Crohn's disease (unlabeled use): 1.5 g/day

Dosing adjustment in renal impairment:

Cl_{cr} 10-50 mL/minute: Administer 50% to 75% of dose

Cl_{cr} <10 mL/minute: Administer 50% of dose

Administer after hemodialysis: Administer 50% of dose

Continuous arteriovenous hemofiltration: Dose for Cl_{cr} <10 mL/minute

Dosing adjustment in hepatic impairment: Use with caution.

Dietary Considerations May be taken with food.

Administration Do not use granules if packet is swollen or if granules are discolored (ie, brown or purple). Granules may be sprinkled on applesauce or yogurt (do not chew) or suspended in tomato or orange juice.

Dosage Forms Excipient information presented when available (limited, particularly for generics); consult specific product labeling.

Granules, delayed release:

Paser®: 4 g/packet (30s) [sugar free]

◆ **4-Aminosalicylic Acid** *see* Aminosalicylic Acid *on page 86*

◆ **5-Aminosalicylic Acid** *see* Mesalamine *on page 949*

◆ **Aminoxin [OTC]** *see* Pyridoxine *on page 1273*

Amiodarone (a MEE oh da rone)

U.S. Brand Names Cordarone®; Pacerone®

Canadian Brand Names Alti-Amiodarone; Amiodarone Hydrochloride for Injection®; Apo-Amiodarone®; Cordarone®; Dom-Amiodarone; Gen-Amiodarone; Novo-Amiodarone; PHL-Amiodarone; PMS-Amiodarone; PRO-Amiodarone; Ratio-Amiodarone; Ratio-Amiodarone I.V.; RIVA-Amiodarone; Sandoz-Amiodarone

Index Terms Amiodarone Hydrochloride

Pharmacologic Category Antiarrhythmic Agent, Class III

Use Management of life-threatening recurrent ventricular fibrillation (VF) or hemodynamically-unstable ventricular tachycardia (VT) refractory to other antiarrhythmic agents or in patients intolerant of other agents used for these conditions

Unlabeled/Investigational Use

Cardiac arrest with persistent ventricular tachycardia (VT) or ventricular fibrillation (VF) if defibrillation, CPR, and vasopressor administration have failed (ACLS/PALS guidelines)

Control of hemodynamically-stable VT, polymorphic VT with a normal QT interval, or wide-complex tachycardia of uncertain origin (ACLS/PALS guidelines)

Control of rapid ventricular rate due to accessory pathway conduction in pre-excited atrial arrhythmias (ACLS guidelines)

Heart rate control in patients with atrial fibrillation and heart failure [no accessory pathway] (ACC/AHA/ESC Practice Guidelines)

Paroxysmal supraventricular tachycardia (SVT)

Prevention of postoperative atrial fibrillation during cardiothoracic surgery

Pharmacologic adjunct to ICD therapy to suppress symptomatic ventricular tachyarrhythmias in otherwise optimally-treated patients with heart failure (ACC/AHA/ESC Practice Guidelines)

Pharmacologic conversion of atrial fibrillation to normal sinus rhythm; maintenance of normal sinus rhythm

Restrictions An FDA-approved medication guide must be distributed when dispensing an outpatient prescription (new or refill) where this medication is to be used without direct supervision of a healthcare provider. Medication guides are available at http://www.fda.gov/cder/Offices/ODS/medication_guides.htm.

Pregnancy Risk Factor D

Pregnancy Considerations May cause fetal harm when administered to a pregnant woman, leading to congenital goiter and hypo- or hyperthyroidism.

Lactation Enters breast milk/not recommended (AAP rates "of concern")

Medication Safety Issues

Sound-alike/look-alike issues:

Amiodarone may be confused with aMILoride, amrinone

Cordarone® may be confused with Cardura®, Cordran®

High alert medication: The Institute for Safe Medication Practices (ISMP) includes this medication among its list of drugs which have a heightened risk of causing significant patient harm when used in error.

Contraindications Hypersensitivity to amiodarone, iodine, or any component of the formulation; severe sinus-node dysfunction; second- and third-degree heart block (except in patients with a functioning artificial pacemaker); bradycardia causing syncope (except in patients with a functioning artificial pacemaker); cardiogenic shock; pregnancy

Warnings/Precautions **[U.S. Boxed Warning]: Only indicated for patients with life-threatening arrhythmias because of risk of toxicity. Alternative therapies should be tried first before using amiodarone. Patients should be hospitalized when amiodarone is initiated.** Currently, the 2005 ACLS guidelines recommend I.V. amiodarone as the preferred antiarrhythmic for the treatment of pulseless VT/VF, both life-threatening arrhythmias. In patients with non-life-threatening arrhythmias (eg, atrial fibrillation), amiodarone should be used only if the use of other antiarrhythmics has proven ineffective or are contraindicated.

[U.S. Boxed Warning]: Lung damage (abnormal diffusion capacity) may occur without symptoms. Monitor for pulmonary toxicity. Evaluate new respiratory symptoms; pre-existing pulmonary disease does not increase risk of developing pulmonary toxicity, but if pulmonary toxicity develops then the prognosis is worse. The lowest effective dose should be used as appropriate for the acuity/severity of the arrhythmia being treated. **[U.S. Boxed Warning]: Liver toxicity is common, but usually mild with evidence of increased liver enzymes. Severe liver toxicity can occur and has been fatal in a few cases.**

[U.S. Boxed Warning]: Amiodarone can exacerbate arrhythmias, by making them more difficult to tolerate or reverse; other types of arrhythmias have occurred, including significant heart block, sinus bradycardia new ventricular fibrillation, incessant ventricular tachycardia, increased resistance to cardioversion, and polymorphic ventricular tachycardia associated with QT_c prolongation (torsade de pointes [TdP]). Risk may be increased with concomitant use of other antiarrhythmic agents or drugs that prolong the QT_c interval. Proarrhythmic effects may be prolonged.

Monitor pacing or defibrillation thresholds in patients with implantable cardiac devices (eg, pacemakers, defibrillators). Use very cautiously and with close monitoring in patients with thyroid or liver disease. May cause hyper- or hypothyroidism. Hyperthyroidism may result in thyrotoxicosis and may aggravate or cause breakthrough arrhythmias. If any new signs of arrhythmia appear, hyperthyroidism should be considered. Thyroid function should be monitored prior to treatment and periodically thereafter. May cause optic neuropathy and/or optic neuritis, usually resulting in visual impairment. Corneal microdeposits occur in a majority of patients, and may cause visual disturbances in some patients (blurred vision, halos); these are not generally considered a reason to discontinue treatment. Corneal refractive laser surgery is generally contraindicated in amiodarone users. Avoid excessive exposure to sunlight; may cause photosensitivity.

Amiodarone is a potent inhibitor of CYP enzymes and transport proteins (including p-glycoprotein), which may lead to increased serum concentrations/toxicity of a number of medications. Particular caution must be used when a drug with QT_c-prolonging potential relies on metabolism via these enzymes, since the effect of elevated concentrations may be additive with the effect of amiodarone. Carefully assess risk:benefit of coadministration of other drugs which may prolong QT_c interval. Patients may still be at risk for amiodarone–related drug interactions after the drug has been discontinued. The pharmacokinetics are complex (due to prolonged duration of action and half-life) and difficult to predict. Correct electrolyte disturbances, especially hypokalemia or hypomagnesemia, prior to use and throughout therapy.

May cause hypotension and bradycardia (infusion-rate related). Caution in surgical patients; may enhance hemodynamic effect of anesthetics; associated with increased risk of adult respiratory distress syndrome (ARDS) postoperatively. Injection contains benzyl alcohol, which has been associated with "gasping syndrome" in neonates. Safety and efficacy of amiodarone in children has not been fully established.

Adverse Reactions In a recent meta-analysis, patients taking lower doses of amiodarone (152-330 mg daily for at least 12 months) were more likely to develop thyroid, neurologic, skin, ocular, and bradycardic abnormalities than those taking placebo (Vorperian, 1997). Pulmonary toxicity was similar in both the low dose amiodarone group and in the placebo group but there was a trend towards increased toxicity in the amiodarone group. Gastrointestinal and hepatic events were seen to a similar extent in both the low dose amiodarone group and placebo group. As the frequency of adverse events varies considerably across studies as a function of route and dose, a consolidation of adverse event rates is provided by Goldschlager, 2000.

Cardiovascular: Hypotension (I.V. 16%, refractory in rare cases)
Central nervous system (3% to 40%): Abnormal gait/ataxia, dizziness, fatigue, headache, malaise, impaired memory, involuntary movement, insomnia, poor coordination, peripheral neuropathy, sleep disturbances, tremor
Dermatologic: Photosensitivity (10% to 75%)
Endocrine & Metabolic: Hypothyroidism (1% to 22%)
Gastrointestinal: Nausea, vomiting, anorexia, and constipation (10% to 33%)
Hepatic: AST or ALT level >2x normal (15% to 50%)
Ocular: Corneal microdeposits (>90%; causes visual disturbance in <10%)

1% to 10%:

Cardiovascular: CHF (3%), bradycardia (3% to 5%), AV block (5%), conduction abnormalities, SA node dysfunction (1% to 3%), cardiac arrhythmia, flushing, edema. Additional effects associated with I.V. administration include asystole, cardiac arrest, electromechanical dissociation, ventricular tachycardia, and cardiogenic shock.
Dermatologic: Slate blue skin discoloration (<10%)
Endocrine & metabolic: Hyperthyroidism (3% to 10%; more common in iodine-deficient regions of the world), libido decreased
Gastrointestinal: Abdominal pain, abnormal salivation, abnormal taste (oral)
Hematologic: Coagulation abnormalities
Hepatic: Hepatitis and cirrhosis (<3%)
Local: Phlebitis (I.V., with concentrations >3 mg/mL)
Ocular: Visual disturbances (2% to 9%), halo vision (<5% occurring especially at night), optic neuritis (1%)
Respiratory: Pulmonary toxicity has been estimated to occur at a frequency between 2% and 7% of patients (some reports indicate a frequency as high as 17%). Toxicity may present as hypersensitivity pneumonitis; pulmonary fibrosis (cough, fever, malaise); pulmonary inflammation; interstitial pneumonitis; or alveolar pneumonitis. ARDS has been reported in up to 2% of patients receiving amiodarone, and postoperatively in patients receiving oral amiodarone.
Miscellaneous: Abnormal smell (oral)

<1% (Limited to important or life-threatening): Acute intracranial hypertension (I.V.), acute renal failure, agranulocytosis, alopecia, anaphylactic shock, angioedema, aplastic anemia, bone marrow granuloma, bronchiolitis obliterans organizing pneumonia (BOOP), bronchospasm, confusion, disorientation, dyspnea, encephalopathy, epididymitis (noninfectious), erectile dysfunction, erythema multiforme, exfoliative dermatitis, hallucination, hemolytic anemia, hemoptysis, hyperglycemia, hypertriglyceridemia, hypotension (oral), hypoxia, impotence, injection site reactions, leukocytoclastic vasculitis, muscle weakness, myopathy, neutropenia, optic neuropathy, pancreatitis, pancytopenia, parkinsonian symptoms, photophobia, pleuritis, proarrhythmia, pruritus, pseudotumor cerebri, pulmonary alveolar hemorrhage, pulmonary edema, pulmonary mass, QT interval increased, rash, renal impairment, renal insufficiency, respiratory failure, rhabdomyolysis, SIADH, sinus arrest, spontaneous ecchymosis, Stevens-Johnson syndrome, thrombocytopenia, thyroid nodules, thyroid cancer, thyrotoxicosis, orsade de pointes (rare), toxic epidermal necrolysis, vasculitis, ventricular fibrillation, wheezing

Drug Interactions

Metabolism/Transport Effects Substrate of CYP1A2 (minor), 2C8 (major at low concentration), 2C19 (minor), 2D6 (minor), 3A4 (major); **Inhibits** CYP1A2 (weak), 2A6 (moderate), 2B6 (weak), 2C9 (moderate), 2C19 (weak), 2D6 (moderate), 3A4 (moderate)

Avoid Concomitant Use

Avoid concomitant use of Amiodarone with any of the following: Nilotinib; Protease Inhibitors; Rivaroxaban; Silodosin; Tetrabenazine; Thioridazine; Topotecan; Ziprasidone

Increased Effect/Toxicity

Amiodarone may increase the levels/effects of: Beta-Blockers; Cardiac Glycosides; CycloSPORINE; CYP2A6 Substrates; CYP2C9 Substrates (High risk); CYP2D6 Substrates; CYP3A4 Substrates; Dabigatran Etexilate; Eplerenone; FentaNYL; Fesoterodine; Flecainide; HMG-CoA Reductase Inhibitors; Lidocaine; Maraviroc; P-Glycoprotein Substrates; Phenytoin; Pimecrolimus; QTc-Prolonging Agents; Ranolazine; Rivaroxaban; Salmeterol; Silodosin; Tamoxifen; Tetrabenazine; Thioridazine; Topotecan; Vitamin K Antagonists; Ziprasidone

The levels/effects of Amiodarone may be increased by: Alfuzosin; Antiarrhythmic Agents (Class Ia); Azithromycin; Calcium Channel Blockers (Nondihydropyridine); Cimetidine; Ciprofloxacin; CYP2C8 Inhibitors (Moderate); CYP2C8 Inhibitors (Strong); CYP3A4 Inhibitors (Moderate); CYP3A4 Inhibitors (Strong); Dasatinib; Gadobutrol; Nilotinib; P-Glycoprotein Inhibitors; Protease Inhibitors

Decreased Effect

Amiodarone may decrease the levels/effects of: Antiarrhythmic Agents (Class Ia); Codeine; Sodium Iodide I131; TraMADol

The levels/effects of Amiodarone may be decreased by: Bile Acid Sequestrants; CYP2C8 Inducers (Highly Effective); CYP3A4 Inducers (Strong); Deferasirox; Grapefruit Juice; Herbs (CYP3A4 Inducers); Orlistat; P-Glycoprotein Inducers; Phenytoin; Rifamycin Derivatives

Ethanol/Nutrition/Herb Interactions

Food: Increases the rate and extent of absorption of amiodarone. Grapefruit juice increases bioavailability of oral amiodarone by 50% and decreases the conversion of amiodarone to N-DEA (active metabolite); altered effects are possible; use should be avoided during therapy.

Herb/Nutraceutical: St John's wort may decrease amiodarone levels or enhance photosensitization. Avoid ephedra (may worsen arrhythmia). Avoid dong quai.

Stability Store at room temperature; protect from light. When admixed in D_5W to a final concentration of 1-6 mg/mL, the solution is stable at room temperature for 24 hours in polyolefin or glass, or for 2 hours in PVC. Infusions >2 hours must be administered in glass or polyolefin bottles. Do not use evacuated glass containers; buffer may cause precipitation.

Mechanism of Action Class III antiarrhythmic agent which inhibits adrenergic stimulation (alpha- and beta-blocking properties), affects sodium, potassium, and calcium channels, prolongs the action potential and refractory period in myocardial tissue; decreases AV conduction and sinus node function

Pharmacodynamics/Kinetics

Onset of action: Oral: 2 days to 3 weeks; I.V.: May be more rapid

Peak effect: 1 week to 5 months

Duration after discontinuing therapy: 7-50 days

Note: Mean onset of effect and duration after discontinuation may be shorter in children than adults

Distribution: V_d: 66 L/kg (range: 18-148 L/kg); crosses placenta; enters breast milk in concentrations higher than maternal plasma concentrations

Protein binding: 96%

Metabolism: Hepatic via CYP2C8 and 3A4 to active N-desethylamiodarone metabolite; possible enterohepatic recirculation

Bioavailability: Oral: ~50%

Half-life elimination: Terminal: 40-55 days (range: 26-107 days); shorter in children than adults

Excretion: Feces; urine (<1% as unchanged drug)

Dosage Note: Lower loading and maintenance doses are preferable in women and all patients with low body weight.

Oral:

Children: Arrhythmias (unlabeled use):

Loading dose: 10-20 mg/kg/day in 1-2 doses for 4-14 days or until adequate control of arrhythmia or prominent adverse effects occur; alternative loading dose in children <1 year: 600-800 mg/1.73 m^2/day in 1-2 divided doses/day

Maintenance dose: Dose may be reduced to 5 mg/kg/day for several weeks (or 200-400 mg/1.73 m^2/day given once daily); if no recurrence of arrhythmia, dose may be further reduced to 2.5 mg/kg/day; maintenance doses may be given 5-7 days/week

Adults:

Ventricular arrhythmias: 800-1600 mg/day in 1-2 doses for 1-3 weeks, then when adequate arrhythmia control is achieved, decrease to 600-800 mg/day in 1-2 doses for 1 month; maintenance: 400 mg/day. Lower doses are recommended for supraventricular arrhythmias.

Atrial fibrillation: Prophylaxis following open heart surgery (unlabeled use): Starting in postop recovery: 400 mg twice daily for up to 7 days. Alternative regimen of amiodarone: 600 mg/day for 7 days prior to surgery, followed by 200 mg/day until hospital discharge, has also been shown to decrease the risk of postoperative atrial fibrillation. **Note:** A variety of regimens have been used in clinical trials.

Atrial fibrillation: Pharmacologic cardioversion (unlabeled use): ACC/AHA/ESC Practice Guidelines: Inpatient: 1.2-1.8 g/day in divided doses until 10 g total, then 200-400 mg/day maintenance. **Note:** Other regimens have been described and may be used clinically (Roy, 2000):

400 mg 3 times/day for 5-7 days, then 400 mg/day for 1 month, then 200 mg/day

or

10 mg/kg/day for 14 days, followed by 300 mg/day for 4 weeks, followed by maintenance dosage of 100-200 mg/day

I.V.:

Children:

Arrhythmias (unlabeled use, dosing based on limited data): Loading dose: 5 mg/kg over 30 minutes; may repeat up to 3 times if no response. Maintenance dose: 2-20 mg/kg/day (5-15 mcg/kg/minute) by continuous infusion

Note: I.V. administration at low flow rates (potentially associated with use in pediatrics) may result in leaching of plasticizers (DEHP) from intravenous tubing. DEHP may adversely affect male reproductive tract development. Alternative means of dosing and administration (1 mg/kg aliquots) may need to be considered.

Pulseless VF or VT (PALS dosing): 5 mg/kg (maximum 300 mg/dose) rapid I.V. bolus or I.O.; repeat up to a maximum daily dose of 15 mg/kg. (**Note:** Maximum recommended daily dose in adolescents is 2.2 g.)

Perfusing tachycardias (PALS dosing): Loading dose: 5 mg/kg (maximum 300 mg/dose) I.V. over 20-60 minutes or I.O.; may repeat up to maximum dose of 15 mg/kg/day. (**Note:** Maximum recommended daily dose in adolescents is 2.2 g.)

Adults:

Atrial fibrillation: Prophylaxis following open heart surgery (unlabeled use): Starting at postop recovery, 1000 mg infused over 24 hours for 2 days has been shown to reduce the risk of postoperative atrial fibrillation. **Note:** A variety of regimens have been used in clinical trials.

Atrial fibrillation: Pharmacologic cardioversion (ACC/AHA/ESC Practice Guidelines) (unlabeled use): 5-7 mg/kg over 30-60 minutes, then 1.2-1.8 g/day continuous infusion or in divided oral doses until 10 g total. Maintenance: See oral dosing.

Ventricular arrhythmias:

Breakthrough VF or VT: 150 mg supplemental doses in 100 mL D_5W over 10 minutes

Pulseless VF or VT: I.V. push: Initial: 300 mg in 20-30 mL NS or D_5W; if VF or VT recurs, supplemental dose of 150 mg followed by infusion of 1 mg/minute for 6 hours, then 0.5 mg/minute (maximum daily dose: 2.1 g)

Stable VT or SVT (unlabeled use): First 24 hours: 1050 mg according to following regimen

Step 1: 150 mg (100 mL) over first 10 minutes (mix 3 mL in 100 mL D_5W)

Step 2: 360 mg (200 mL) over next 6 hours (mix 18 mL in 500 mL D_5W): 1 mg/minute

Step 3: 540 mg (300 mL) over next 18 hours: 0.5 mg/minute

Note: After the first 24 hours: 0.5 mg/minute utilizing concentration of 1-6 mg/mL

I.V. to oral therapy conversion: Use the following as a guide:

<1 week I.V. infusion: 800-1600 mg/day

1- to 3-week I.V. infusion: 600-800 mg/day

>3-week I.V. infusion: 400 mg/day

Recommendations for conversion to intravenous amiodarone after oral administration: During long-term amiodarone therapy (ie, ≥4 months), the mean plasma-elimination half-life of the active metabolite of amiodarone is 61 days. Replacement therapy may not be necessary in such patients if oral therapy is discontinued for a period <2 weeks, since any changes in serum amiodarone concentrations during this period may **not** be clinically significant.

Elderly: No specific guidelines available. Dose selection should be cautious, at low end of dosage range, and titration should be slower to evaluate response.

Hemodialysis: Not dialyzable (0% to 5%); supplemental dose is not necessary.

Peritoneal dialysis effects: Not dialyzable (0% to 5%); supplemental dose is not necessary.

Dosing adjustment in hepatic impairment: Dosage adjustment is probably necessary in substantial hepatic impairment. No specific guidelines available. If hepatic enzymes exceed 3 times normal or double in a patient with an elevated baseline, consider decreasing the dose or discontinuing amiodarone.

Dietary Considerations Administer consistently with regard to meals. Amiodarone is a potential source of large amounts of inorganic iodine; ~3 mg of inorganic iodine per 100 mg of amiodarone is released into the systemic circulation. Recommended daily allowance for iodine in adults is 150 mcg.

Grapefruit juice is not recommended.

Administration

Oral: Administer consistently with regard to meals. Take in divided doses with meals if high daily dose or if GI upset occurs. If GI intolerance occurs with single-dose therapy, use twice daily dosing.

I.V.: For infusions >1 hour, use concentrations ≤2 mg/mL unless a central venous catheter is used. Use only volumetric infusion pump; use of drop counting may lead to underdosing. Administer through I.V. line with in-line filter.

Adjust administration rate to urgency (give more slowly when perfusing arrhythmia present). Slow the infusion rate if hypotension or bradycardia develops. Infusions >2 hours must be administered in glass or polyolefin bottles.

Note: I.V. administration at lower flow rates (potentially associated with use in pediatrics) and higher concentrations than recommended may result in leaching of plasticizers (DEHP) from intravenous tubing. DEHP may adversely affect male reproductive tract development. Alternative means of dosing and administration (1 mg/kg aliquots) may need to be considered.

Monitoring Parameters Blood pressure, heart rate (ECG) and rhythm throughout therapy; assess patient for signs of lethargy, edema of the hands or feet, weight loss, and pulmonary toxicity (baseline pulmonary function tests); liver function tests; monitor serum electrolytes, especially potassium and magnesium. Assess thyroid function tests before initiation of treatment and then periodically thereafter (some experts suggest every 3-6 months). If signs or symptoms of thyroid disease or arrhythmia breakthrough/exacerbation occur then immediate re-evaluation is necessary. Amiodarone partially inhibits the peripheral conversion of thyroxine (T_4) to triiodothyronine (T_3); serum T_4 and reverse triiodothyronine (rT_3) concentrations may be increased and serum T_3 may be decreased; most patients remain clinically euthyroid, however, clinical hypothyroidism or hyperthyroidism may occur.

Perform regular ophthalmic exams.

Patients with implantable cardiac devices: Monitor pacing or defibrillation thresholds with initiation of amiodarone and during treatment.

Reference Range Therapeutic: 0.5-2.5 mg/L (SI: 1-4 µmol/L) (parent); desethyl metabolite is active and is present in equal concentration to parent drug

Dosage Forms Excipient information presented when available (limited, particularly for generics); consult specific product labeling.

Injection, solution, as hydrochloride: 50 mg/mL (3 mL, 9 mL, 18 mL) [contains benzyl alcohol and polysorbate 80]

Tablet, as hydrochloride [scored]: 200 mg, 400 mg

Cordarone®: 200 mg

Pacerone®: 100 mg [not scored], 200 mg, 400 mg

Extemporaneous Preparations A 5 mg/mL oral suspension has been made from tablets and has an expected stability of 91 days under refrigeration; three 200 mg tablets are crushed in a mortar, 90 mL of methylcellulose 1%, and 10 mL of syrup (syrup NF (85% sucrose in water) or flavored syrup) are added in small amounts and triturated until uniform; purified water USP is used to make a quantity sufficient to 120 mL

Nahata MC and Hipple TF, *Pediatric Drug Formulations*, 2nd ed, Cincinnati, OH: Harvey Whitney Books Co, 1992.

◆ **Amiodarone Hydrochloride** *see* Amiodarone *on page 87*

◆ **Amiodarone Hydrochloride for Injection® (Can)** *see* Amiodarone *on page 87*

◆ **Amitiza®** *see* Lubiprostone *on page 912*

Amitriptyline (a mee TRIP ti leen)

Canadian Brand Names Apo-Amitriptyline®; Levate®; Novo-Triptyn; PMS-Amitriptyline

Index Terms Amitriptyline Hydrochloride; Elavil

Pharmacologic Category Antidepressant, Tricyclic (Tertiary Amine)

Additional Appendix Information

Antidepressant Agents *on page 1638*

Use Relief of symptoms of depression

Unlabeled/Investigational Use Analgesic for certain chronic and neuropathic pain; prophylaxis against migraine headaches; treatment of depressive disorders in children

Restrictions An FDA-approved medication guide concerning the use of antidepressants in children, adolescents, and young adults must be distributed when dispensing an outpatient prescription (new or refill) where this medication is to be used without direct supervision of a healthcare provider. Medication guides are available at http://www.fda.gov/cder/Offices/ODS/medication_guides.htm. Dispense to parents or guardians of children and adolescents receiving this medication.

Pregnancy Risk Factor C

Pregnancy Considerations Teratogenic effects have been observed in animal studies. Amitriptyline crosses the human placenta; CNS effects, limb deformities and developmental delay have been noted in case reports.

Lactation Enters breast milk/not recommended (AAP rates "of concern")

Medication Safety Issues

Sound-alike/look-alike issues:

Amitriptyline may be confused with aminophylline, imipramine, nortriptyline

Elavil® may be confused with Aldoril®, Eldepryl®, enalapril, Equanil®, Mellaril®, Oruvail®, Plavix®

Contraindications Hypersensitivity to amitriptyline or any component of the formulation (cross-sensitivity with other tricyclics may occur); use of MAO inhibitors within past 14 days; acute recovery phase following myocardial infarction; concurrent use of cisapride

Warnings/Precautions [U.S. Boxed Warning]: Antidepressants increase the risk of suicidal thinking and behavior in children, adolescents, and young adults (18-24 years of age) with major depressive disorder (MDD) and other psychiatric disorders; consider risk prior to prescribing. Short-term studies did not show an increased risk in patients >24 years of age and showed a decreased risk in patients ≥65 years. Closely monitor for clinical worsening, suicidality, or unusual changes in behavior; the patient's family or caregiver should be instructed to closely observe the patient and communicate condition with healthcare provider. Such observation would generally include at least weekly face-to-face contact with patients or their family members or caregivers during the first 4 weeks of treatment, then every other week visits for the next 4 weeks, then at 12 weeks, and as clinically indicated beyond 12 weeks. Additional contact by telephone may be appropriate between face-to-face visits. Adults treated with antidepressants should be observed similarly for clinical worsening and suicidality, especially during the initial few months of a course of drug therapy, or at times of dose changes, either increases or decreases. A medication guide should be dispensed with each prescription. **Amitriptyline is not FDA-approved for use in children <12 years of age.**

The possibility of a suicide attempt is inherent in major depression and may persist until remission occurs. Monitor for worsening of depression or suicidality, especially during initiation of therapy (generally first 1-2 months) or with dose increases or decreases. Worsening depression and severe abrupt suicidality that are not part of the presenting symptoms may require discontinuation or modification of drug therapy. The patient's family or caregiver should be alerted to monitor patients for the emergence of suicidality and associated behaviors (such as agitation, irritability, hostility, impulsivity, and hypomania) and notify healthcare provider.

May worsen psychosis in some patients or precipitate a shift to mania or hypomania in patients with bipolar disorder. Patients presenting with depressive symptoms should be screened for bipolar disorder. Monotherapy in patients with bipolar disorder should be avoided. **Amitriptyline is not FDA approved for bipolar depression.**

The degree of sedation, anticholinergic effects, orthostasis, and conduction abnormalities are high relative to other antidepressants. Amitriptyline often causes drowsiness/sedation, resulting in impaired performance of tasks requiring alertness (eg, operating machinery or driving). Sedative effects may be additive with other CNS depressants and/or ethanol. Use with caution in patients with a history of cardiovascular disease (including previous MI, stroke, tachycardia, or conduction abnormalities). Use with caution in patients with urinary retention, benign prostatic hyperplasia, narrow-angle glaucoma, xerostomia, visual problems, constipation, or a history of bowel obstruction.

TCAs may rarely cause bone marrow suppression; monitor for any signs of infection and obtain CBC if symptoms (eg, fever, sore throat) evident. May alter glucose control - use with caution in patients with diabetes. Consider discontinuing, when possible, prior to elective surgery. Therapy should not be abruptly discontinued in patients receiving high doses for prolonged periods. May lower seizure threshold - use caution in patients with a previous seizure disorder or condition predisposing to seizures such as brain damage, alcoholism, or concurrent therapy with other drugs which lower the seizure threshold. Hyperpyrexia has been observed with TCAs in combination with anticholinergics and/or neuroleptics, particularly during hot weather. May increase the risks associated with electroconvulsive therapy. Use with caution in hyperthyroid patients or those receiving thyroid supplementation. Use with caution in patients with hepatic or renal dysfunction and in elderly patients.

Adverse Reactions Anticholinergic effects may be pronounced; moderate to marked sedation can occur (tolerance to these effects usually occurs).

Frequency not defined.

Cardiovascular: Orthostatic hypotension, tachycardia, ECG changes (nonspecific), AV conduction changes, cardiomyopathy (rare), MI, stroke, heart block, arrhythmia, syncope, hypertension, palpitation

Central nervous system: Restlessness, dizziness, insomnia, sedation, fatigue, anxiety, cognitive function impaired, seizure, extrapyramidal symptoms, coma, hallucinations, confusion, disorientation, coordination impaired, ataxia, headache, nightmares, hyperpyrexia

Dermatologic: Allergic rash, urticaria, photosensitivity, alopecia

Endocrine & metabolic: Syndrome of inappropriate ADH secretion

Gastrointestinal: Weight gain, xerostomia, constipation, paralytic ileus, nausea, vomiting, anorexia, stomatitis, peculiar taste, diarrhea, black tongue

Genitourinary: Urinary retention

Hematologic: Bone marrow depression, purpura, eosinophilia

Neuromuscular & skeletal: Numbness, paresthesia, peripheral neuropathy, tremor, weakness

Ocular: Blurred vision, mydriasis, ocular pressure increased

Otic: Tinnitus

Miscellaneous: Diaphoresis, withdrawal reactions (nausea, headache, malaise)

Postmarketing and/or case reports: Neuroleptic malignant syndrome (rare), serotonin syndrome (rare)

Drug Interactions

Metabolism/Transport Effects Substrate of CYP1A2 (minor), 2B6 (minor), 2C9 (minor), 2C19 (minor), 2D6 (major), 3A4 (minor); **Inhibits** CYP1A2 (weak), 2C9 (weak), 2C19 (weak), 2D6 (weak), 2E1 (weak)

Avoid Concomitant Use

Avoid concomitant use of Amitriptyline with any of the following: Cisapride; Iobenguane I 123; MAO Inhibitors;

Nilotinib; Sibutramine; Tetrabenazine; Thioridazine; Ziprasidone

Increased Effect/Toxicity

Amitriptyline may increase the levels/effects of: Alcohol (Ethyl); Alpha-/Beta-Agonists (Direct-Acting); Alpha1-Agonists; Amphetamines; Anticholinergics; Aspirin; Beta2-Agonists; Cisapride; CNS Depressants; Desmopressin; NSAID (COX-2 Inhibitor); NSAID (Nonselective); QTc-Prolonging Agents; QuiNIDine; Serotonin Modulators; Sulfonylureas; Tetrabenazine; Thioridazine; TraMADol; Vitamin K Antagonists; Yohimbine; Ziprasidone

The levels/effects of Amitriptyline may be increased by: Alfuzosin; Altretamine; BuPROPion; Cimetidine; Cinacalcet; Ciprofloxacin; CYP2D6 Inhibitors (Moderate); CYP2D6 Inhibitors (Strong); Darunavir; Dexmethylphenidate; DULoxetine; Gadobutrol; Lithium; MAO Inhibitors; Methylphenidate; Nilotinib; Pramlintide; Propoxyphene; Protease Inhibitors; QuiNIDine; Selective Serotonin Reuptake Inhibitors; Sibutramine; Terbinafine; Valproic Acid

Decreased Effect

Amitriptyline may decrease the levels/effects of: Acetylcholinesterase Inhibitors (Central); Alpha2-Agonists; Iobenguane I 123

The levels/effects of Amitriptyline may be decreased by: Acetylcholinesterase Inhibitors (Central); Barbiturates; CarBAMazepine; St Johns Wort

Ethanol/Nutrition/Herb Interactions

Ethanol: Avoid ethanol (may increase CNS depression).

Food: Grapefruit juice may inhibit the metabolism of some TCAs and clinical toxicity may result.

Herb/Nutraceutical: St John's wort may decrease amitriptyline levels. Avoid valerian, St John's wort, kava kava, gotu kola (may increase CNS depression).

Stability Protect Elavil® 10 mg tablets from light.

Mechanism of Action Increases the synaptic concentration of serotonin and/or norepinephrine in the central nervous system by inhibition of their reuptake by the presynaptic neuronal membrane

Pharmacodynamics/Kinetics

Onset of action: Migraine prophylaxis: 6 weeks, higher dosage may be required in heavy smokers because of increased metabolism; Depression: 4-6 weeks, reduce dosage to lowest effective level

Distribution: Crosses placenta; enters breast milk

Metabolism: Hepatic to nortriptyline (active), hydroxy and conjugated derivatives; may be impaired in the elderly

Half-life elimination: Adults: 9-27 hours (average: 15 hours)

Time to peak, serum: ~4 hours

Excretion: Urine (18% as unchanged drug); feces (small amounts)

Dosage

Children:

Chronic pain management (unlabeled use): Oral: Initial: 0.1 mg/kg at bedtime, may advance as tolerated over 2-3 weeks to 0.5-2 mg/kg at bedtime

Depressive disorders (unlabeled use): Oral: Initial doses of 1 mg/kg/day given in 3 divided doses with increases to 1.5 mg/kg/day have been reported in a small number of children (n=9) 9-12 years of age; clinically, doses up to 3 mg/kg/day (5 mg/kg/day if monitored closely) have been proposed

Migraine prophylaxis (unlabeled use): Oral: Initial: 0.25 mg/kg/day, given at bedtime; increase dose by 0.25 mg/kg/day to maximum 1 mg/kg/day. Reported dosing ranges: 0.1-2 mg/kg/day; maximum suggested dose: 10 mg.

Adolescents: Depressive disorders: Oral: Initial: 25-50 mg/day; may administer in divided doses; increase gradually to 100 mg/day in divided doses

Adults:

Depression:

Oral: 50-150 mg/day single dose at bedtime or in divided doses; dose may be gradually increased up to 300 mg/day

Chronic pain management (unlabeled use): Oral: Initial: 25 mg at bedtime; may increase as tolerated to 100 mg/day

Migraine prophylaxis (unlabeled use): Oral: Initial: 10-25 mg at bedtime; usual dose: 150 mg; reported dosing ranges: 10-400 mg/day

Elderly: Depression: Oral: Initial: 10-25 mg at bedtime; dose should be increased in 10-25 mg increments every week if tolerated; dose range: 25-150 mg/day

Dosing interval in hepatic impairment: Use with caution and monitor plasma levels and patient response

Hemodialysis: Nondialyzable

Monitoring Parameters Monitor blood pressure and pulse rate prior to and during initial therapy; evaluate mental status, suicidal ideation (especially at the beginning of therapy or when doses are increased or decreased); monitor weight; ECG in older adults and patients with cardiac disease

Reference Range Therapeutic: Amitriptyline and nortriptyline 100-250 ng/mL (SI: 360-900 nmol/L); nortriptyline 50-150 ng/mL (SI: 190-570 nmol/L); Toxic: >0.5 mcg/mL; plasma levels do not always correlate with clinical effectiveness

Test Interactions May cause false-positive reaction to EMIT immunoassay for imipramine

Dosage Forms Excipient information presented when available (limited, particularly for generics); consult specific product labeling.

Tablet, as hydrochloride: 10 mg, 25 mg, 50 mg, 75 mg, 100 mg, 150 mg

Amitriptyline and Chlordiazepoxide

(a mee TRIP ti leen & klor dye az e POKS ide)

U.S. Brand Names Limbitrol®; Limbitrol® DS

Canadian Brand Names Limbitrol®

Index Terms Chlordiazepoxide and Amitriptyline Hydrochloride

Pharmacologic Category Antidepressant, Tricyclic (Tertiary Amine); Benzodiazepine

Use Treatment of moderate to severe anxiety and/or agitation and depression

Restrictions C-IV

An FDA-approved medication guide concerning the use of antidepressants in children, adolescents, and young adults must be distributed when dispensing an outpatient prescription (new or refill) where this medication is to be used without direct supervision of a healthcare provider. Medication guides are available at http://www.fda.gov/cder/Offices/ODS/medication_guides.htm. Dispense to parents or guardians of children and adolescents receiving this medication.

Pregnancy Risk Factor D

Dosage Initial: 3-4 tablets in divided doses; this may be increased to 6 tablets/day as required; some patients respond to smaller doses and can be maintained on 2 tablets

Additional Information Complete prescribing information for this medication should be consulted for additional detail.

Dosage Forms Excipient information presented when available (limited, particularly for generics); consult specific product labeling.

Tablet: 12.5/5: Amitriptyline hydrochloride 12.5 mg and chlordiazepoxide 5 mg; 25/10: Amitriptyline hydrochloride 25 mg and chlordiazepoxide 10 mg

Limbitrol®: 12.5/5: Amitriptyline hydrochloride 12.5 mg and chlordiazepoxide 5 mg

Limbitrol® DS: 25/10: Amitriptyline hydrochloride 25 mg and chlordiazepoxide 10 mg

Amitriptyline and Perphenazine
(a mee TRIP ti leen & per FEN a zeen)

Canadian Brand Names Etrafon®

Index Terms Perphenazine and Amitriptyline Hydrochloride

Pharmacologic Category Antidepressant, Tricyclic (Tertiary Amine); Antipsychotic Agent, Typical, Phenothiazine

Use Treatment of patients with moderate to severe anxiety and depression

Unlabeled/Investigational Use Depression with psychotic features

Restrictions An FDA-approved medication guide concerning the use of antidepressants in children, adolescents, and young adults must be distributed when dispensing an outpatient prescription (new or refill) where this medication is to be used without direct supervision of a healthcare provider. Medication guides are available at http://www.fda.gov/cder/Offices/ODS/medication_guides.htm. Dispense to parents or guardians of children and adolescents receiving this medication.

Pregnancy Risk Factor D

Dosage Oral: 1 tablet 2-4 times/day

Dosage adjustment in hepatic impairment: Avoid use in severe hepatic failure

Additional Information Complete prescribing information for this medication should be consulted for additional detail.

Dosage Forms Excipient information presented when available (limited, particularly for generics); consult specific product labeling.

Tablet:

2-10: Amitriptyline hydrochloride 10 mg and perphenazine 2 mg

2-25: Amitriptyline hydrochloride 25 mg and perphenazine 2 mg

4-10: Amitriptyline hydrochloride 10 mg and perphenazine 4 mg

4-25: Amitriptyline hydrochloride 25 mg and perphenazine 4 mg

4-50: Amitriptyline hydrochloride 50 mg and perphenazine 4 mg

◆ **Amitriptyline Hydrochloride** *see* Amitriptyline *on page 90*

◆ **AMJ 9701** *see* Palifermin *on page 1129*

Amlexanox (am LEKS an oks)

U.S. Brand Names Aphthasol®

Pharmacologic Category Anti-inflammatory, Locally Applied

Use Treatment of aphthous ulcers (ie, canker sores)

Unlabeled/Investigational Use Allergic disorders

Pregnancy Risk Factor B

Dosage Topical: Administer ~1/4 inch (0.5 cm) directly on ulcers 4 times/day following oral hygiene, after meals, and at bedtime

Additional Information Complete prescribing information for this medication should be consulted for additional detail.

Dosage Forms Excipient information presented when available (limited, particularly for generics); consult specific product labeling.

Paste, oral:

Aphthasol®: 5% (3 g) [contains benzyl alcohol]

AmLODIPine (am LOE di peen)

U.S. Brand Names Norvasc®

Canadian Brand Names Norvasc®

Index Terms Amlodipine Besylate

Pharmacologic Category Calcium Channel Blocker

Additional Appendix Information

Calcium Channel Blockers *on page 1651*

Use Treatment of hypertension; treatment of symptomatic chronic stable angina, vasospastic (Prinzmetal's) angina (confirmed or suspected); prevention of hospitalization due to angina with documented CAD (limited to patients without heart failure or ejection fraction <40%)

Pregnancy Risk Factor C

Pregnancy Considerations Embryotoxic effects have been demonstrated in small animals. No well-controlled studies have been conducted in pregnant women. Use in pregnancy only when clearly needed and when the benefits outweigh the potential hazard to the fetus.

Lactation Excretion in breast milk unknown/not recommended

Medication Safety Issues

Sound-alike/look-alike issues:

AmLODIPine may be confused with aMILoride

Norvasc® may be confused with Navane®, Norvir®, Vascor®

Contraindications Hypersensitivity to amlodipine or any component of the formulation

Warnings/Precautions Increased angina and/or MI has occurred with initiation or dosage titration of calcium channel blockers. Symptomatic hypotension with or without syncope can rarely occur; blood pressure must be lowered at a rate appropriate for the patient's clinical condition. Use caution in severe aortic stenosis and/or hypertrophic cardiomyopathy. Use caution in patients with hepatic impairment. The most common side effect is peripheral edema; occurs within 2-3 weeks of starting therapy. Reflex tachycardia may occur with use. Dosage titration should occur after 7-14 days on a given dose. Initiate at a lower dose in the elderly. Safety and efficacy have not been established in children <6 years of age.

Adverse Reactions

>10%: Cardiovascular: Peripheral edema (2% to 15% dose related)

1% to 10%:

Cardiovascular: Flushing (1% to 3%), palpitation (1% to 4%)

Central nervous system: Headache (7%; similar to placebo 8%), dizziness (1% to 3%), fatigue (4%), somnolence (1% to 2%)

Dermatologic: Rash (1% to 2%), pruritus (1% to 2%)

Endocrine & metabolic: Male sexual dysfunction (1% to 2%)

Gastrointestinal: Nausea (3%), abdominal pain (1% to 2%), dyspepsia (1% to 2%), gingival hyperplasia

Neuromuscular & skeletal: Muscle cramps (1% to 2%), weakness (1% to 2%)

Respiratory: Dyspnea (1% to 2%), pulmonary edema (15% from PRAISE trial, CHF population)

<1% (Limited to important or life-threatening): Abnormal dreams, agitation alopecia, amnesia, anxiety, apathy, arrhythmia, ataxia, bradycardia, cardiac failure, cholestasis, depersonalization, depression, erythema multiforme, exfoliative dermatitis, extrapyramidal symptoms, gastritis, gynecomastia, hepatitis, hypotension, jaundice, leukocytoclastic vasculitis, migraine, nonthrombocytopenic purpura, paresthesia, peripheral ischemia, photosensitivity, postural hypotension, purpura, rash, skin discoloration, Stevens-Johnson syndrome, syncope, thrombocytopenia, tinnitus, transaminases increased, urticaria, weight loss, vertigo, xerophthalmia

Drug Interactions

Metabolism/Transport Effects Substrate of CYP3A4 (major); **Inhibits** CYP1A2 (moderate), 2A6 (weak), 2B6 (weak), 2C8 (weak), 2C9 (weak), 2D6 (weak), 3A4 (weak)

Avoid Concomitant Use There are no known interactions where it is recommended to avoid concomitant use.

Increased Effect/Toxicity

AmLODIPine may increase the levels/effects of: Amifostine; CYP1A2 Substrates; Magnesium Salts; Neuromuscular-Blocking Agents (Nondepolarizing); Nitroprusside; Phenytoin; RiTUXimab; Tacrolimus

The levels/effects of AmLODIPine may be increased by: Alpha1-Blockers; Antifungal Agents (Azole Derivatives, Systemic); Calcium Channel Blockers (Nondihydropyridine); CycloSPORINE; CYP3A4 Inhibitors (Moderate); CYP3A4 Inhibitors (Strong); Dasatinib; Diazoxide; Fluconazole; Grapefruit Juice; Herbs (Hypotensive Properties); Macrolide Antibiotics; Magnesium Salts; Prostacyclin Analogues; Protease Inhibitors; Quinupristin

Decreased Effect

AmLODIPine may decrease the levels/effects of: Clopidogrel; QuiNIDine

The levels/effects of AmLODIPine may be decreased by: Barbiturates; Calcium Salts; CarBAMazepine; CYP3A4 Inducers (Strong); Deferasirox; Herbs (CYP3A4 Inducers); Herbs (Hypertensive Properties); Methylphenidate; Nafcillin; Rifamycin Derivatives; Yohimbine

Ethanol/Nutrition/Herb Interactions

Food: Grapefruit juice may modestly increase amlodipine levels.

Herb/Nutraceutical: St John's wort may decrease amlodipine levels. Avoid dong quai if using for hypertension (has estrogenic activity). Avoid ephedra, yohimbe, ginseng (may worsen hypertension). Avoid garlic (may have increased antihypertensive effects).

Stability Store at room temperature of 15°C to 30°C (59°F to 86°F).

Mechanism of Action Inhibits calcium ion from entering the "slow channels" or select voltage-sensitive areas of vascular smooth muscle and myocardium during depolarization, producing a relaxation of coronary vascular smooth muscle and coronary vasodilation; increases myocardial oxygen delivery in patients with vasospastic angina

Pharmacodynamics/Kinetics

Onset of action: Antihypertensive: 30-50 minutes

Duration of antihypertensive effect: 24 hours

Absorption: Oral: Well absorbed

Distribution: V_d: 21 L/kg

Protein binding: 93% to 98%

Metabolism: Hepatic (>90%) to inactive metabolite

Bioavailability: 64% to 90%

Half-life elimination: 30-50 hours; increased with hepatic dysfunction

Time to peak, plasma: 6-12 hours

Excretion: Urine (10% as parent, 60% as metabolite)

Dosage Oral:

Children 6-17 years: Hypertension: 2.5-5 mg once daily

Adults:

Hypertension: Initial dose: 5 mg once daily; maximum dose: 10 mg once daily. In general, titrate in 2.5 mg increments over 7-14 days. Usual dosage range (JNC 7): 2.5-10 mg once daily.

Angina: Usual dose: 5-10 mg; lower dose suggested in elderly or hepatic impairment; most patients require 10 mg for adequate effect

Elderly: Dosing should start at the lower end of dosing range due to possible increased incidence of hepatic, renal, or cardiac impairment. Elderly patients also show decreased clearance of amlodipine.

Hypertension: 2.5 mg once daily

Angina: 5 mg once daily

Dosage adjustmnent in renal impairment: Dialysis: Hemodialysis and peritoneal dialysis do not enhance elimination. Supplemental dose is not necessary.

Dosage adjustment in hepatic impairment:

Angina: Administer 5 mg once daily.

Hypertension: Administer 2.5 mg once daily.

Dietary Considerations May be taken without regard to meals.

Administration May be administered without regard to meals.

Monitoring Parameters Heart rate, blood pressure, peripheral edema

Dosage Forms Excipient information presented when available (limited, particularly for generics); consult specific product labeling.

Tablet: 2.5 mg, 5 mg, 10 mg

Norvasc®: 2.5 mg, 5 mg, 10 mg

Extemporaneous Preparations A 1 mg/mL suspension was stable for 91 days when refrigerated or 56 days when kept at room temperature when compounded as follows: Triturate fifty 5 mg tablets in a mortar, reduce to a fine powder. In a graduate, mix Ora-Sweet® 125 mL and Ora-Plus® 125 mL together. Add small amount of this mixture to the powder to make a paste. Add the remainder in small quantities while mixing. Shake well before using.

Nahata MC, Morosco RS, and Hipple TF, 4th ed, *Pediatric Drug Formulations*, Cincinnati, OH: Harvey Whitney Books Co, 2000.

Amlodipine and Atorvastatin

(am LOW di peen & a TORE va sta tin)

U.S. Brand Names Caduet®

Canadian Brand Names Caduet®

Index Terms Atorvastatin Calcium and Amlodipine Besylate

Pharmacologic Category Antilipemic Agent, HMG-CoA Reductase Inhibitor; Calcium Channel Blocker

Use For use when treatment with both amlodipine and atorvastatin is appropriate:

Amlodipine: Treatment of hypertension; treatment of symptomatic chronic stable angina, vasospastic (Prinzmetal's) angina (confirmed or suspected); prevention of hospitalization due to angina with documented CAD (limited to patients without heart failure or ejection fraction <40%)

Atorvastatin: Treatment of dyslipidemias or primary prevention of cardiovascular disease (atherosclerotic) as detailed here:

Primary prevention of cardiovascular disease (high-risk for CVD): To reduce the risk of MI or stroke in patients without evidence of heart disease who have multiple CVD risk factors or type 2 diabetes. Treatment reduces the risk for angina or revascularization procedures in patients with multiple risk factors.

Treatment of dyslipidemias: To reduce elevations in total cholesterol, LDL-C, apolipoprotein B, and triglycerides in patients with elevations of one or more components, and/or to increase HDL-C as present in heterozygous hypercholesterolemia (Fredrickson type IIa hyperlipidemias); treatment of primary dysbetalipoproteinemia (Fredrickson type III), elevated serum TG levels (Fredrickson type IV), and homozygous familial hypercholesterolemia

Treatment of heterozygous familial hypercholesterolemia (HeFH) in adolescent patients (10-17 years of age, females >1 year postmenarche) having LDL-C ≥190 mg/dL or LDL-C ≥160 mg/dL with positive family history of premature cardiovascular disease (CVD) or with two or more CVD risk factors.

Pregnancy Risk Factor X

Dosage Oral:

Amlodipine:

Children >10 years: Hypertension: 2.5-5 mg once daily. **Note:** Use in ages >10 years because of atorvastatin content.

Adults:

Hypertension: Initial dose: 5 mg once daily; maximum dose: 10 mg once daily; in general, titrate in 2.5 mg increments over 7-14 days. Usual dosage range (JNC 7): 2.5-10 mg once daily

Angina: Usual dose: 5-10 mg; lower dose suggested in elderly or hepatic impairment; most patients require 10 mg for adequate effect

Elderly: Dosing should start at the lower end of dosing range due to possible increased incidence of hepatic, renal, or cardiac impairment. Elderly patients also show decreased clearance of amlodipine.

Hypertension: 2.5 mg once daily

Angina: 5 mg once daily

Atorvastatin:

Children 10-17 years (females >1 year postmenarche): HeFH: 10 mg once daily (maximum: 20 mg/day)

Adults:

Hyperlipidemias: Initial: 10-20 mg once daily; patients requiring >45% reduction in LDL-C may be started at 40 mg once daily; range: 10-80 mg once daily

Primary prevention of CVD: 10 mg once daily

Dosage adjustment in renal impairment: No dosage adjustment is necessary.

Dosage adjustment in hepatic impairment: Do not use in active liver disease.

Additional Information Complete prescribing information for this medication should be consulted for additional detail.

Dosage Forms Excipient information presented when available (limited, particularly for generics); consult specific product labeling.

Tablet:

Caduet®

2.5/10: Amlodipine 2.5 mg and atorvastatin 10 mg
2.5/20: Amlodipine 2.5 mg and atorvastatin 20 mg
2.5/40: Amlodipine 2.5 mg and atorvastatin 40 mg
5/10: Amlodipine 5 mg and atorvastatin 10 mg
5/20: Amlodipine 5 mg and atorvastatin 20 mg
5/40: Amlodipine 5 mg and atorvastatin 40 mg
5/80: Amlodipine 5 mg and atorvastatin 80 mg
10/10: Amlodipine 10 mg and atorvastatin 10 mg
10/20: Amlodipine 10 mg and atorvastatin 20 mg
10/40: Amlodipine 10 mg and atorvastatin 40 mg
10/80: Amlodipine 10 mg and atorvastatin 80 mg

Amlodipine and Benazepril

(am LOE di peen & ben AY ze pril)

U.S. Brand Names Lotrel®

Index Terms Benazepril Hydrochloride and Amlodipine Besylate

Pharmacologic Category Angiotensin-Converting Enzyme (ACE) Inhibitor; Calcium Channel Blocker

Use Treatment of hypertension

Pregnancy Risk Factor C/D (2nd and 3rd trimesters)

Dosage Oral:

Adults: 2.5-10 mg (amlodipine) and 10-40 mg (benazepril) once daily; maximum: Amlodipine: 10 mg/day; benazepril: 40 mg/day

Elderly: Initial dose: 2.5 mg based on amlodipine component

Dosage adjustment in renal impairment: Cl_{cr} ≤30 mL/minute: Use of combination product is not recommended.

Dosage adjustment in hepatic impairment: Initial dose: 2.5 mg based on amlodipine component

Additional Information Complete prescribing information for this medication should be consulted for additional detail.

Dosage Forms Excipient information presented when available (limited, particularly for generics); consult specific product labeling.

Capsule:

2.5/10: Amlodipine 2.5 mg and benazepril hydrochloride 10 mg

5/10: Amlodipine 5 mg and benazepril hydrochloride 10 mg

5/20: Amlodipine 5 mg and benazepril hydrochloride 20 mg

10/20: Amlodipine 10 mg and benazepril hydrochloride 20 mg

Lotrel® 2.5/10: Amlodipine 2.5 mg and benazepril hydrochloride 10 mg

Lotrel® 5/10: Amlodipine 5 mg and benazepril hydrochloride 10 mg

Lotrel® 5/20: Amlodipine 5 mg and benazepril hydrochloride 20 mg

Lotrel® 5/40: Amlodipine 5 mg and benazepril hydrochloride 40 mg

Lotrel® 10/20: Amlodipine 10 mg and benazepril hydrochloride 20 mg

Lotrel® 10/40: Amlodipine 10 mg and benazepril hydrochloride 40 mg

Amlodipine and Olmesartan

(am LOE di peen & olme SAR tan)

U.S. Brand Names Azor™

Index Terms Amlodipine Besylate and Olmesartan Medoxomil; Olmesartan and Amlodipine

Pharmacologic Category Angiotensin II Receptor Blocker; Calcium Channel Blocker

Use Treatment of hypertension

Pregnancy Risk Factor C/D (2nd and 3rd trimesters)

Dosage Oral: Dose is individualized; combination product may be substituted for individual components in patients currently maintained on both agents separately or in patients not adequately controlled with monotherapy (using one of the agents or an agent the within same antihypertensive class).

Adults: Hypertension: Amlodipine 5-10 mg and olmesartan 20 mg once daily; dose may be titrated after 2 weeks of therapy. Maximum recommended doses: Amlodipine 10 mg/day; olmesartan 40 mg/day.

Elderly: Initiate at lower end of dosing range

Dosing adjustment in renal impairment: No specific guidelines for dosage adjustment

Dosing adjustment in hepatic impairment: Use caution in hepatic impairment; amlodipine and olmesartan exposure increased in presence of hepatic impairment

Additional Information Complete prescribing information for this medication should be consulted for additional detail.

Dosage Forms Excipient information presented when available (limited, particularly for generics); consult specific product labeling.

Tablet:

Azor™:

5/20: Amlodipine besylate 5 mg and olmesartan medoxomil 20 mg

5/40: Amlodipine besylate 5 mg and olmesartan medoxomil 40 mg

10/20: Amlodipine besylate 10 mg and olmesartan medoxomil 20 mg

10/40: Amlodipine besylate 10 mg and olmesartan medoxomil 40 mg

Amlodipine and Valsartan

(am LOE di peen & val SAR tan)

U.S. Brand Names Exforge®

Index Terms Amlodipine Besylate and Valsartan; Valsartan and Amlodipine

Pharmacologic Category Angiotensin II Receptor Blocker; Calcium Channel Blocker

Use Treatment of hypertension

Pregnancy Risk Factor D

Dosage Oral: Dose is individualized; combination product may be used as initial therapy or substituted for individual components in patients currently maintained on both agents separately or in patients not adequately controlled with monotherapy (using one of the agents or an agent within same antihypertensive class).

Adults: Hypertension:

Initial therapy: Amlodipine 5 mg and valsartan 160 mg once daily, dose may be titrated after 1-2 weeks of therapy. Maximum recommended doses: Amlodipine 10 mg/day; valsartan 320 mg/day

Add-on/replacement therapy: Amlodipine 5-10 mg and valsartan 160-320 mg once daily; dose may be titrated after 3-4 weeks of therapy. Maximum recommended doses: Amlodipine 10 mg/day; valsartan 320 mg/day

Elderly: Initiate amlodipine at 2.5 mg/day due to decreased clearance

Dosing adjustment in renal impairment:

Cl_{cr} >10 mL/minute: No dosage adjustment necessary

Cl_{cr} ≤10 mL/minute: Use caution; titrate slowly

Dosing adjustment in hepatic impairment: Mild-to-moderate hepatic impairment: No initial dosage adjustment required, titrate slowly. Amlodipine and valsartan exposure increased in presence of hepatic impairment.

Amlodipine: Use caution in severe hepatic impairment; lower initial doses may be required

Valsartan: Mild-to-moderate hepatic impairment: No dosage adjustment required; however, patients with mild-to-moderate chronic disease have twice the exposure as healthy volunteers.

Additional Information Complete prescribing information for this medication should be consulted for additional detail.

Dosage Forms Excipient information presented when available (limited, particularly for generics); consult specific product labeling.

Tablet:

Exforge®:

5/160: Amlodipine 5 mg and valsartan 160 mg

5/320 mg: Amlodipine 5 mg and valsartan 320 mg

10/160: Amlodipine 10 mg and valsartan 160 mg

10/320: Amlodipine 10 mg and valsartan 320 mg

◆ **Amlodipine Besylate** *see* AmLODIPine *on page* 93

◆ **Amlodipine Besylate and Olmesartan Medoxomil** *see* Amlodipine and Olmesartan *on page* 95

◆ **Amlodipine Besylate and Valsartan** *see* Amlodipine and Valsartan *on page* 96

◆ **Ammens® Medicated Deodorant [OTC]** *see* Zinc Oxide *on page* 1584

◆ **Ammonapse** *see* Sodium Phenylbutyrate *on page* 1385

Ammonium Chloride

(a MOE nee um KLOR ide)

Pharmacologic Category Electrolyte Supplement, Parenteral

Use Treatment of hypochloremic states or metabolic alkalosis

Pregnancy Risk Factor C

Dosage Metabolic alkalosis: The following equations represent different methods of correction utilizing either the serum HCO_3^-, the serum chloride, or the base excess

Dosing of mEq NH_4Cl via the chloride-deficit method (hypochloremia):

Dose of mEq NH_4Cl = [0.2 L/kg x body weight (kg)] x [103-observed serum chloride]; administer 50% of dose over 12 hours, then re-evaluate

Note: 0.2 L/kg is the estimated chloride volume of distribution and 103 is the average normal serum chloride concentration (mEq/L)

Dosing of mEq NH_4Cl via the bicarbonate-excess method (refractory hypochloremic metabolic alkalosis):

Dose of NH_4Cl = [0.5 L/kg x body weight (kg)] x (observed serum HCO_3^- - 24); administer 50% of dose over 12 hours, then re-evaluate

Note: 0.5 L/kg is the estimated bicarbonate volume of distribution and 24 is the average normal serum bicarbonate concentration (mEq/L)

These equations will yield different requirements of ammonium chloride

Additional Information Complete prescribing information for this medication should be consulted for additional detail.

Dosage Forms Excipient information presented when available (limited, particularly for generics); consult specific product labeling.

Injection, solution: Ammonium 5 mEq/mL and chloride 5 mEq/mL (20 mL) [equivalent to ammonium chloride 267.5 mg/mL]

◆ **Ammonul®** *see* Sodium Phenylacetate and Sodium Benzoate *on page* 1384

◆ **AMN107** *see* Nilotinib *on page* 1066

◆ **Amnesteem™** *see* Isotretinoin *on page* 825

Amobarbital

(am oh BAR bi tal)

U.S. Brand Names Amytal®

Canadian Brand Names Amytal®

Index Terms Amobarbital Sodium; Amylobarbitone

Pharmacologic Category Barbiturate; General Anesthetic; Hypnotic; Sedative

Use Hypnotic in short-term treatment of insomnia; reduce anxiety and provide sedation preoperatively

Unlabeled/Investigational Use Therapeutic or diagnostic "Amytal® Interviewing"; Wada test

Restrictions C-II

Pregnancy Risk Factor D

Dosage

Children:

Sedative: I.M., I.V.: 6-12 years: Manufacturer's dosing range: 65-500 mg

Hypnotic (unlabeled use): I.M.: 2-3 mg/kg (maximum: 500 mg)

Adults:

Hypnotic: I.M., I.V.: 65-200 mg at bedtime (maximum single dose: 1000 mg)

Sedative: I.M., I.V.: 30-50 mg 2-3 times/day (maximum single dose: 1000 mg)

"Amytal® interview" (unlabeled use): I.V.: 50-100 mg/minute for total dose of 200-1000 mg or until patient experiences drowsiness, impaired attention, slurred speech, or nystagmus

Wada test (unlabeled use): Intra-arterial: 100 mg over 4-5 seconds via percutaneous transfemoral catheter

Dosing adjustment in renal/hepatic impairment: Dosing should be reduced; specific recommendations not available.

Additional Information Complete prescribing information for this medication should be consulted for additional detail.

Dosage Forms Excipient information presented when available (limited, particularly for generics); consult specific product labeling.

Injection, powder for reconstitution, as sodium:

Amytal®: 500 mg

◆ **Amobarbital Sodium** *see* Amobarbital *on page 96*

◆ **Amoclan** *see* Amoxicillin and Clavulanate Potassium *on page 100*

Amoxapine (a MOKS a peen)

Index Terms Asendin [DSC]

Pharmacologic Category Antidepressant, Tricyclic (Secondary Amine)

Additional Appendix Information

Antidepressant Agents *on page 1638*

Use Treatment of depression, psychotic depression, depression accompanied by anxiety or agitation

Restrictions An FDA-approved medication guide concerning the use of antidepressants in children, adolescents, and young adults must be distributed when dispensing an outpatient prescription (new or refill) where this medication is to be used without direct supervision of a healthcare provider. Medication guides are available at http://www.fda.gov/cder/Offices/ODS/medication_guides.htm. Dispense to parents or guardians of children and adolescents receiving this medication.

Pregnancy Risk Factor C

Lactation Enters breast milk/contraindicated (AAP rates "of concern")

Medication Safety Issues

Sound-alike/look-alike issues:

Amoxapine may be confused with amoxicillin, Amoxil®

Asendin may be confused with aspirin

Contraindications Hypersensitivity to amoxapine or any component of the formulation; use of MAO inhibitors within past 14 days; acute recovery phase following myocardial infarction

Warnings/Precautions [U.S. Boxed Warning]: Antidepressants increase the risk of suicidal thinking and behavior in children, adolescents, and young adults (18-24 years of age) with major depressive disorder (MDD) and other psychiatric disorders; consider risk prior to prescribing. Short-term studies did not show an increased risk in patients >24 years of age and showed a decreased risk in patients ≥65 years. Closely monitor for clinical worsening, suicidality, or unusual changes in behavior; the patient's family or caregiver should be instructed to closely observe the patient and communicate condition with healthcare provider. A medication guide should be dispensed with each prescription. **Amoxapine is not FDA approved for use in patients <16 years of age.**

The possibility of a suicide attempt is inherent in major depression and may persist until remission occurs. Monitor for worsening of depression or suicidality, especially during initiation of therapy (generally first 1-2 months) or with dose increases or decreases. Use caution in high-risk patients. Worsening depression and severe abrupt suicidality that are not part of the presenting symptoms may require discontinuation or modification of drug therapy. The patient's family or caregiver should be alerted to monitor patients for the emergence of suicidality and associated behaviors (such as agitation, irritability, hostility, impulsivity, and hypomania) and notify the healthcare provider.

May worsen psychosis in some patients or precipitate a shift to mania or hypomania in patients with bipolar disorder. Patients presenting with depressive symptoms should be screened for bipolar disorder. Monotherapy in patients with bipolar disorder should be avoided. **Amoxapine is not FDA approved for bipolar depression.** May cause extrapyramidal symptoms, including pseudoparkinsonism, acute dystonic reactions, akathisia, and tardive dyskinesia (risk of these reactions is low). May be associated with neuroleptic malignant syndrome.

The degree of sedation, anticholinergic effects, orthostasis, and conduction abnormalities are moderate relative to other antidepressants. May cause drowsiness/sedation, resulting in impaired performance of tasks requiring alertness (eg, operating machinery or driving). Sedative effects may be additive with other CNS depressants and/or ethanol. Use with caution in patients with a history of cardiovascular disease (including previous MI, stroke, tachycardia, or conduction abnormalities). Use with caution in patients with urinary retention, benign prostatic hyperplasia, narrow-angle glaucoma, xerostomia, visual problems, constipation, or a history of bowel obstruction.

Consider discontinuing, when possible, prior to elective surgery. Therapy should not be abruptly discontinued in patients receiving high doses for prolonged periods. May lower seizure threshold - use caution in patients with a previous seizure disorder or condition predisposing to seizures such as brain damage, alcoholism, or concurrent therapy with other drugs which lower the seizure threshold. May increase the risks associated with electroconvulsive therapy. Use with caution in hyperthyroid patients or those receiving thyroid supplementation. Use with caution in patients with hepatic or renal dysfunction and in elderly patients.

Adverse Reactions

>10%:

Central nervous system: Drowsiness

Gastrointestinal: Xerostomia, constipation

1% to 10%:

Central nervous system: Anxiety, ataxia, confusion, dizziness, excitement, headache, insomnia, nervousness, restlessness

Dermatologic: Edema, skin rash

Endocrine: Prolactin levels increased

Gastrointestinal: Nausea

Neuromuscular & skeletal: Tremor, weakness

Ocular: Blurred vision

Miscellaneous: Diaphoresis

<1% (Limited to important or life-threatening): Agranulocytosis, allergic reactions, diarrhea, extrapyramidal symptoms, galactorrhea, hypertension, impotence, incoordination, intraocular pressure increased, leukopenia, menstrual irregularity, mydriasis, neuroleptic malignant syndrome, numbness, painful ejaculation, paresthesia, photosensitivity, seizure, SIADH, syncope, tardive dyskinesia, testicular edema, tinnitus, urinary retention, vomiting

Drug Interactions

Metabolism/Transport Effects Substrate of CYP2D6 (major)

Avoid Concomitant Use

Avoid concomitant use of Amoxapine with any of the following: Iobenguane I 123; MAO Inhibitors; Nilotinib; Sibutramine; Tetrabenazine; Thioridazine; Ziprasidone

Increased Effect/Toxicity

Amoxapine may increase the levels/effects of: Alcohol (Ethyl); Alpha-/Beta-Agonists (Direct-Acting); Alpha1-Agonists; Amphetamines; Anticholinergics; Beta2-Agonists; CNS Depressants; Desmopressin; QTc-Prolonging Agents; QuiNIDine; Serotonin Modulators; Sulfonylureas; Tetrabenazine; Thioridazine; TraMADol; Vitamin K Antagonists; Yohimbine; Ziprasidone

The levels/effects of Amoxapine may be increased by: Alfuzosin; Altretamine; Cimetidine; Cinacalcet; Ciprofloxacin; CYP2D6 Inhibitors (Moderate); CYP2D6 Inhibitors (Strong); Darunavir; Dexmethylphenidate; DULoxetine; Gadobutrol; Lithium; MAO Inhibitors; Methylphenidate; Nilotinib; Pramlintide; Propoxyphene; Protease Inhibitors; QuiNIDine; Selective Serotonin Reuptake Inhibitors; Sibutramine; Terbinafine; Valproic Acid

Decreased Effect

Amoxapine may decrease the levels/effects of: Acetylcholinesterase Inhibitors (Central); Alpha2-Agonists; Iobenguane I 123

The levels/effects of Amoxapine may be decreased by: Acetylcholinesterase Inhibitors (Central); Barbiturates; CarBAMazepine; St Johns Wort

Ethanol/Nutrition/Herb Interactions

Ethanol: Avoid ethanol (may increase CNS depression).

Food: Grapefruit juice may inhibit the metabolism of some TCAs and clinical toxicity may result.

Herb/Nutraceutical: Avoid valerian, St John's wort, SAMe, kava kava.

Mechanism of Action Reduces the reuptake of serotonin and norepinephrine. The metabolite, 7-OH-amoxapine has significant dopamine receptor blocking activity similar to haloperidol.

Pharmacodynamics/Kinetics

Onset of antidepressant effect: Usually occurs after 1-2 weeks, but may require 4-6 weeks

Absorption: Rapid and well absorbed

Distribution: V_d: 0.9-1.2 L/kg; enters breast milk

Protein binding: 80%

Metabolism: Primarily hepatic

Half-life elimination: Parent drug: 11-16 hours; Active metabolite (8-hydroxy): Adults: 30 hours

Time to peak, serum: 1-2 hours

Excretion: Urine (as unchanged drug and metabolites)

Dosage Once symptoms are controlled, decrease gradually to lowest effective dose. Maintenance dose is usually given at bedtime to reduce daytime sedation. Oral:

Children: Not established in children <16 years of age.

Adolescents: Initial: 25-50 mg/day; increase gradually to 100 mg/day; may administer as divided doses or as a single dose at bedtime

Adults: Initial: 25 mg 2-3 times/day, if tolerated, dosage may be increased to 100 mg 2-3 times/day; may be given in a single bedtime dose when dosage <300 mg/day

Elderly: Initial: 25 mg at bedtime increased by 25 mg weekly for outpatients and every 3 days for inpatients if tolerated; usual dose: 50-150 mg/day, but doses up to 300 mg may be necessary

Maximum daily dose:

Inpatient: 600 mg

Outpatient: 400 mg

Administration May be administered with food to decrease GI distress.

Monitoring Parameters Monitor blood pressure and pulse rate prior to and during initial therapy evaluate mental status, suicidal ideation (especially at the beginning of therapy or when doses are increased or decreased); monitor weight; ECG in older adults

Reference Range Therapeutic: Amoxapine: 20-100 ng/mL (SI: 64-319 nmol/L); 8-OH amoxapine: 150-400 ng/mL (SI: 478-1275 nmol/L); both: 200-500 ng/mL (SI: 637-1594 nmol/L)

Test Interactions Increased glucose, liver function tests; decreased WBC

Additional Information Extrapyramidal reactions and tardive dyskinesia may occur.

Dosage Forms Excipient information presented when available (limited, particularly for generics); consult specific product labeling.

Tablet: 25 mg, 50 mg, 100 mg, 150 mg

Amoxicillin (a moks i SIL in)

U.S. Brand Names Amoxil®; Moxatag®

Canadian Brand Names Apo-Amoxi®; Gen-Amoxicillin; Lin-Amox; Novamoxin®; Nu-Amoxi; PHL-Amoxicillin; PMS-Amoxicillin

Index Terms *p*-Hydroxyampicillin; Amoxicillin Trihydrate; Amoxycillin

Pharmacologic Category Antibiotic, Penicillin

Additional Appendix Information

Animal and Human Bites *on page 1747*

Antimicrobial Drugs of Choice *on page 1752*

Community-Acquired Pneumonia in Adults *on page 1766*

Helicobacter pylori Treatment *on page 1813*

Prevention of Infective Endocarditis *on page 1736*

Treatment of Sexually Transmitted Infections *on page 1773*

Use Treatment of otitis media, sinusitis, and infections caused by susceptible organisms involving the upper and lower respiratory tract, skin, and urinary tract; prophylaxis of infective endocarditis in patients undergoing surgical or dental procedures; as part of a multidrug regimen for *H. pylori* eradication

Unlabeled/Investigational Use Postexposure prophylaxis for anthrax exposure with documented susceptible organisms

Pregnancy Risk Factor B

Pregnancy Considerations Adverse events have not been observed in animal studies; therefore, amoxicillin is classified as pregnancy category B. There is no documented increased risk of adverse pregnancy outcome or teratogenic affects caused by amoxicillin. It is the drug of choice for the treatment of chlamydial infections in pregnancy and for anthrax prophylaxis when penicillin susceptibility is documented.

Due to pregnancy-induced physiologic changes, amoxicillin clearance is increased during pregnancy resulting in lower concentrations and smaller AUCs. Oral ampicillin-class antibiotics are poorly-absorbed during labor.

Lactation Enters breast milk/compatible

Medication Safety Issues

Sound-alike/look-alike issues:

Amoxicillin may be confused with amoxapine, Amoxil®, Atarax®

Amoxil® may be confused with amoxapine, amoxicillin

International issues:

Fisamox® [Australia] may be confused with Fosamax® which is a brand name for alendronate in the U.S.

Fisamox® [Australia] may be confused with Vigamox™ which is a brand name for moxifloxacin in the U.S.

Contraindications Hypersensitivity to amoxicillin, penicillin, other beta-lactams, or any component of the formulation

Warnings/Precautions In patients with renal impairment, doses and/or frequency of administration should be modified in response to the degree of renal impairment; in addition, use of certain dosage forms (eg, extended-release 775 mg tablet and immediate-release 875 mg tablet) should be avoided in patients with Cl_{cr} <30 mL/minute or patients requiring hemodialysis. A high percentage of patients with infectious mononucleosis have developed rash during therapy with amoxicillin; ampicillin-class antibiotics not recommended in these patients. Serious and occasionally severe or fatal hypersensitivity (anaphylactoid) reactions have been reported in patients on penicillin therapy, especially with a history of beta-lactam hypersensitivity, history of sensitivity to multiple allergens, or previous IgE-mediated reactions (eg, anaphylaxis, angioedema, urticaria). Use with caution in asthmatic patients. Prolonged use may result in fungal or bacterial superinfection, including *C. difficile*-associated diarrhea (CDAD) and pseudomembranous colitis; CDAD has been observed >2 months postantibiotic treatment. Chewable tablets contain phenylalanine.

Adverse Reactions Frequency not defined.

Central nervous system: Agitation, anxiety, behavioral changes, confusion, dizziness, headache, hyperactivity (reversible), insomnia, seizure

Dermatologic: Acute exanthematous pustulosis, erythematous maculopapular rash, erythema multiforme, exfoliative dermatitis, hypersensitivity vasculitis, mucocutaneous candidiasis, Stevens-Johnson syndrome, toxic epidermal necrolysis, urticaria

Gastrointestinal: Black hairy tongue, diarrhea, hemorrhagic colitis, nausea, pseudomembranous colitis, tooth discoloration (brown, yellow, or gray; rare), vomiting

Hematologic: Agranulocytosis, anemia, eosinophilia, hemolytic anemia, leukopenia,thrombocytopenia, thrombocytopenia purpura

Hepatic: Acute cytolytic hepatitis, ALT increased, AST increased, cholestatic jaundice, hepatic cholestasis

Renal: Crystalluria

Miscellaneous: Anaphylaxis, serum sickness-like reaction

Drug Interactions

Avoid Concomitant Use There are no known interactions where it is recommended to avoid concomitant use.

Increased Effect/Toxicity

Amoxicillin may increase the levels/effects of: Methotrexate

The levels/effects of Amoxicillin may be increased by: Allopurinol; Uricosuric Agents

Decreased Effect

Amoxicillin may decrease the levels/effects of: Typhoid Vaccine

The levels/effects of Amoxicillin may be decreased by: Fusidic Acid; Tetracycline Derivatives

Stability

Amoxil®: Oral suspension remains stable for 14 days at room temperature or if refrigerated (refrigeration preferred). Unit-dose antibiotic oral syringes are stable for 48 hours.

Moxatag®: Store at 25°C (77°F); excursions permitted to 15°C to 30°C (59°F to 86°F).

Mechanism of Action Inhibits bacterial cell wall synthesis by binding to one or more of the penicillin-binding proteins (PBPs) which in turn inhibits the final transpeptidation step of peptidoglycan synthesis in bacterial cell walls, thus inhibiting cell wall biosynthesis. Bacteria eventually lyse due to ongoing activity of cell wall autolytic enzymes (autolysins and murein hydrolases) while cell wall assembly is arrested.

Pharmacodynamics/Kinetics

Absorption: Oral: Rapid and nearly complete; food does not interfere

Extended-release tablet: Rate of absorption is slower compared to immediate-release formulations; food decreases the rate but not extent of absorption

Distribution: Widely to most body fluids and bone; poor penetration into cells, eyes, and across normal meninges

Pleural fluids, lungs, and peritoneal fluid; high urine concentrations are attained; also into synovial fluid, liver, prostate, muscle, and gallbladder; penetrates into middle ear effusions, maxillary sinus secretions, tonsils, sputum, and bronchial secretions

CSF:blood level ratio: Normal meninges: <1%; Inflamed meninges: 8% to 90%

Protein binding: 17% to 20%

Metabolism: Partially hepatic

Half-life elimination:

Neonates, full-term: 3.7 hours

Infants and Children: 1-2 hours

Adults: Normal renal function: 0.7-1.4 hours

Cl_{cr} <10 mL/minute: 7-21 hours

Time to peak: Capsule: 2 hours; Extended-release tablet: 3.1 hours; Suspension: 1 hour

Excretion: Urine (60% as unchanged drug); lower in neonates**Note:** Extended-release tablets: In healthy volunteers, serum drug concentrations were below 0.25 mcg/mL and undetectable at 16 hours following dosing.

Dosage

Usual dosage range:

Children ≤3 months: Oral: 20-30 mg/kg/day divided every 12 hours

Children >3 months and <40 kg: Oral: 20-50 mg/kg/day in divided doses every 8-12 hours

Children ≥12 years: Oral: Extended-release tablet: 775 mg once daily

Adults: Oral: 250-500 mg every 8 hours or 500-875 mg twice daily

Extended-release tablet: 775 mg once daily

Indication-specific dosing:

Children >3 months and <40 kg: Oral:

Acute otitis media: 80-90 mg/kg/day divided every 12 hours

Anthrax exposure (CDC guidelines): Note: Post-exposure prophylaxis only with documented susceptible organisms: 80 mg/kg/day in divided doses every 8 hours (maximum: 500 mg/dose)

Community-acquired pneumonia:

4 months to <5 years: 80-100 mg/kg/day divided every 8 hours

5-15 years: 100 mg/kg/day divided every 8 hours; **Note:** Treatment with a macrolide or doxycycline (if age >8 years) is preferred due to higher prevalence of atypical pathogens in this age group

Ear, nose, throat, genitourinary tract, or skin/skin structure infections:

Mild to moderate: 25 mg/kg/day in divided doses every 12 hours **or** 20 mg/kg/day in divided doses every 8 hours

Severe: 45 mg/kg/day in divided doses every 12 hours **or** 40 mg/kg/day in divided doses every 8 hours

Tonsillitis and/or pharyngitis: Children ≥12 years: Extended-release tablet: 775 mg once daily

Lower respiratory tract infections: 45 mg/kg/day in divided doses every 12 hours **or** 40 mg/kg/day in divided doses every 8 hours

Lyme disease: 25-50 mg/kg/day divided every 8 hours (maximum: 500 mg)

Prophylaxis against infective endocarditis: 50 mg/kg 1 hour before procedure. **Note:** American Heart Association (AHA) guidelines now recommend prophylaxis only in patients undergoing invasive procedures and in whom underlying cardiac conditions may predispose to a higher risk of adverse outcomes should infection occur. As of April 2007, routine prophylaxis for GI/GU procedures is no longer recommended by the AHA.

Adults: Oral:

Anthrax exposure (CDC guidelines): Note: Post-exposure prophylaxis in pregnant or nursing women only with documented susceptible organisms: 500 mg every 8 hours

Ear, nose, throat, genitourinary tract, or skin/skin structure infections:

Mild to moderate: 500 mg every 12 hours **or** 250 mg every 8 hours

Severe: 875 mg every 12 hours **or** 500 mg every 8 hours

Tonsillitis and/or pharyngitis: Extended-release tablet: 775 mg once daily

***Helicobacter pylori* eradication:** 1000 mg twice daily; requires combination therapy with at least one other antibiotic and an acid-suppressing agent (proton pump inhibitor or H_2 blocker)

Lower respiratory tract infections: 875 mg every 12 hours **or** 500 mg every 8 hours

Lyme disease: 500 mg every 6-8 hours (depending on size of patient) for 21-30 days

Prophylaxis against infective endocarditis: 2 g 30-60 minutes before procedure. **Note:** American Heart Association (AHA) guidelines now recommend prophylaxis only in patients undergoing invasive procedures and in whom underlying cardiac conditions may predispose to a higher risk of adverse outcomes should infection occur. As of April 2007, routine prophylaxis for GI/GU procedures is no longer recommended by the AHA.

Prophylaxis in total joint replacement patients undergoing dental procedures which produce bacteremia: 2 g 1 hour prior to procedure

Dosing interval in renal impairment: Use of certain dosage forms (eg, extended-release 775 mg tablet and immediate-release 875 mg tablet) should be avoided in patients with Cl_{cr} <30 mL/minute or patients requiring hemodialysis.

Cl_{cr} 10-30 mL/minute: 250-500 mg every 12 hours

Cl_{cr} <10 mL/minute: 250-500 mg every 24 hours

Dialysis: Moderately dialyzable (20% to 50%) by hemo- or peritoneal dialysis; approximately 50 mg of amoxicillin per liter of filtrate is removed by continuous arteriovenous or venovenous hemofiltration; dose as per Cl_{cr} <10 mL/minute guidelines

Dietary Considerations May be taken with food. Amoxil® chewable contains phenylalanine 1.82 mg per 200 mg tablet, phenylalanine 3.64 mg per 400 mg tablet.

Moxatag®: Take within 1 hour of finishing a meal.

Administration Administer around-the-clock to promote less variation in peak and trough serum levels. The appropriate amount of suspension may be mixed with formula, milk, fruit juice, water, ginger ale, or cold drinks; administer dose immediately after mixing.

Moxatag® extended release tablet: Administer within 1 hour of finishing a meal.

Some penicillins (eg, carbenicillin, ticarcillin, and piperacillin) have been shown to inactivate aminoglycosides *in vitro*. This has been observed to a greater extent with tobramycin and gentamicin, while amikacin has shown greater stability against inactivation. Concurrent use of these agents may pose a risk of reduced antibacterial efficacy *in vivo*, particularly in the setting of profound renal impairment. However, definitive clinical evidence is lacking. If combination penicillin/aminoglycoside therapy is desired in a patient with renal dysfunction, separation of doses (if feasible), and routine monitoring of aminoglycoside levels, CBC, and clinical response should be considered.

Monitoring Parameters With prolonged therapy, monitor renal, hepatic, and hematologic function periodically; assess patient at beginning and throughout therapy for infection; monitor for signs of anaphylaxis during first dose

Test Interactions May interfere with urinary glucose tests using cupric sulfate (Benedict's solution, Clinitest®)

Some penicillin derivatives may accelerate the degradation of aminoglycosides *in vitro*, leading to a potential underestimation of aminoglycoside serum concentration.

Product Availability Moxatag®: FDA approved January 2009; availability anticipated in March 2009

Moxatag® is an extended-release tablet of amoxicillin intended for once-daily administration.

Dosage Forms Excipient information presented when available (limited, particularly for generics); consult specific product labeling. [DSC] = Discontinued product

Capsule: 250 mg, 500 mg

Amoxil®: 500 mg

Powder for oral suspension: 125 mg/5 mL (80 mL, 100 mL, 150 mL); 200 mg/5 mL (50 mL, 75 mL, 100 mL); 250 mg/5 mL (80 mL, 100 mL, 150 mL); 400 mg/5 mL (50 mL, 75 mL, 100 mL)

Amoxil®: 200 mg/5 mL (50 mL, 75 mL, 100 mL) [contains sodium benzoate; bubble gum flavor] [DSC]; 250 mg/5 mL (100 mL, 150 mL) [contains sodium benzoate; bubble gum flavor]; 400 mg/5 mL (5 mL [DSC], 50 mL [DSC], 75 mL [DSC], 100 mL) [contains sodium benzoate; bubble gum flavor]

Powder for oral suspension [drops]:

Amoxil®: 50 mg/mL (30 mL) [contains sodium benzoate; bubble gum flavor]

Tablet: 500 mg, 875 mg

Amoxil®: 500 mg, 875 mg [DSC]

Tablet, chewable: 125 mg, 200 mg, 250 mg, 400 mg

Amoxil®: 200 mg [contains phenylalanine 1.82 mg/tablet; cherry banana peppermint flavor] [DSC]; 400 mg [contains phenylalanine 3.64 mg/tablet; cherry banana peppermint flavor] [DSC]

Tablet, extended release, as trihydrate:

Moxatag®: 775 mg

Amoxicillin and Clavulanate Potassium

(a moks i SIL in & klav yoo LAN ate poe TASS ee um)

U.S. Brand Names Amoclan; Augmentin ES-600®; Augmentin XR®; Augmentin®

Canadian Brand Names Alti-Amoxi-Clav; Apo-Amoxi-Clav®; Augmentin®; Clavulin®; Novo-Clavamoxin; ratio-Aclavulanate

Index Terms Amoxicillin and Clavulanic Acid; Clavulanic Acid and Amoxicillin

Pharmacologic Category Antibiotic, Penicillin

Additional Appendix Information

Animal and Human Bites *on page 1747*

Antimicrobial Drugs of Choice *on page 1752*

Community-Acquired Pneumonia in Adults *on page 1766*

Use Treatment of otitis media, sinusitis, and infections caused by susceptible organisms involving the lower respiratory tract, skin and skin structure, and urinary tract; spectrum same as amoxicillin with additional coverage of beta-lactamase producing *B. catarrhalis*, *H. influenzae*, *N. gonorrhoeae*, and *S. aureus* (not MRSA). The expanded coverage of this combination makes it a useful alternative when amoxicillin resistance is present and patients cannot tolerate alternative treatments.

Pregnancy Risk Factor B

Pregnancy Considerations Adverse events have not been observed in animal studies; therefore, amoxicillin/clavulanate is classified as pregnancy category B. Both amoxicillin and clavulanic acid cross the placenta. There is no documented increased risk of teratogenic affects caused by amoxicillin/clavulanate. A potential increased risk of necrotizing enterocolitis in the newborn has been noted after maternal use of amoxicillin/clavulanate for preterm labor or premature prolonged rupture of membranes. When used during pregnancy, pharmacokinetic changes have been observed with amoxicillin alone (refer to the Amoxicillin monograph for details).

Lactation Enters breast milk/use caution

Medication Safety Issues

Sound-alike/look-alike issues:

Augmentin® may be confused with Azulfidine®

Contraindications Hypersensitivity to amoxicillin, clavulanic acid, penicillin, or any component of the formulation; history of cholestatic jaundice or hepatic dysfunction with amoxicillin/clavulanate potassium therapy; Augmentin XR™: severe renal impairment (Cl_{cr} <30 mL/minute) and hemodialysis patients

Warnings/Precautions Hypersensitivity reactions, including anaphylaxis (some fatal), have been reported. Prolonged use may result in fungal or bacterial superinfection, including *C. difficile*-associated diarrhea (CDAD) and pseudomembranous colitis; CDAD has been observed >2 months postantibiotic treatment. In patients with renal impairment, doses and/or frequency of administration should be modified in response to the degree of renal impairment. High percentage of patients with infectious mononucleosis have developed rash during therapy; ampicillin-class antibiotics not recommended in these patients. Incidence of diarrhea is higher than with amoxicillin alone. Due to differing content of clavulanic acid, not all formulations are interchangeable. Low incidence of cross-allergy with cephalosporins exists. Some products contain phenylalanine.

Adverse Reactions

>10%: Gastrointestinal: Diarrhea (3% to 34%; incidence varies upon dose and regimen used)

1% to 10%:

Dermatologic: Diaper rash, skin rash, urticaria

Gastrointestinal: Abdominal discomfort, loose stools, nausea, vomiting

Genitourinary: Vaginitis, vaginal mycosis

Miscellaneous: Moniliasis

<1% (Limited to important or life-threatening): Alkaline phosphatase increased, cholestatic jaundice, flatulence, headache, hepatic dysfunction, hepatitis, liver function tests increased, prothrombin time increased, thrombocytosis, vasculitis (hypersensitivity)

Additional adverse reactions seen with **ampicillin-class antibiotics:** Agitation, agranulocytosis, alkaline phosphatase increased, anaphylaxis, anemia, angioedema, anxiety, behavioral changes, bilirubin increased, black "hairy" tongue, confusion, convulsions, crystalluria, dizziness, enterocolitis, eosinophilia, erythema multiforme, exanthematous pustulosis, exfoliative dermatitis, gastritis, glossitis, hematuria, hemolytic anemia, hemorrhagic colitis, indigestion, insomnia, hyperactivity, interstitial nephritis, leukopenia, mucocutaneous candidiasis, pruritus, pseudomembranous colitis, serum sickness-like reaction, Stevens-Johnson syndrome, stomatitis, transaminases increased, thrombocytopenia, thrombocytopenic purpura, tooth discoloration, toxic epidermal necrolysis

Drug Interactions

Avoid Concomitant Use There are no known interactions where it is recommended to avoid concomitant use.

Increased Effect/Toxicity

Amoxicillin and Clavulanate Potassium may increase the levels/effects of: Methotrexate

The levels/effects of Amoxicillin and Clavulanate Potassium may be increased by: Allopurinol; Uricosuric Agents

Decreased Effect

Amoxicillin and Clavulanate Potassium may decrease the levels/effects of: Typhoid Vaccine

The levels/effects of Amoxicillin and Clavulanate Potassium may be decreased by: Fusidic Acid; Tetracycline Derivatives

Stability

Powder for oral suspension: Store dry powder at room temperature of 25°C (77°F). Reconstitute powder for oral suspension with appropriate amount of water as specified on the bottle. Shake vigorously until suspended. Reconstituted oral suspension should be kept in refrigerator. Discard unused suspension after 10 days. Unit-dose antibiotic oral syringes are stable for 48 hours.

Tablet: Store at room temperature of 25°C (77°F).

Mechanism of Action Clavulanic acid binds and inhibits beta-lactamases that inactivate amoxicillin resulting in amoxicillin having an expanded spectrum of activity. Amoxicillin inhibits bacterial cell wall synthesis by binding to one or more of the penicillin-binding proteins (PBPs) which in turn inhibits the final transpeptidation step of peptidoglycan synthesis in bacterial cell walls, thus inhibiting cell wall biosynthesis. Bacteria eventually lyse due to ongoing activity of cell wall autolytic enzymes (autolysins and murein hydrolases) while cell wall assembly is arrested.

Pharmacodynamics/Kinetics Amoxicillin pharmacokinetics are not affected by clavulanic acid.

Amoxicillin: See Amoxicillin monograph.

Clavulanic acid:

Protein binding: ~25%

Metabolism: Hepatic

Half-life elimination: 1 hour

Time to peak: 1 hour

Excretion: Urine (30% to 40% as unchanged drug)

Dosage Note: Dose is based on the amoxicillin component; see "Augmentin® Product-Specific Considerations" table on next page.

Usual dosage range:

Infants <3 months: Oral: 30 mg/kg/day divided every 12 hours using the 125 mg/5 mL suspension

Children ≥3 months and <40 kg: Oral: 20-90 mg/kg/day divided every 8-12 hours

Children >40 kg and Adults: Oral: 250-500 mg every 8 hours or 875 mg every 12 hours

Indication-specific dosing:

Children ≥3 months and <40 kg: Oral:

Lower respiratory tract infections, severe infections, sinusitis: 45 mg/kg/day divided every 12 hours **or** 40 mg/kg/day divided every 8 hours

Mild-to-moderate infections: 25 mg/kg/day divided every 12 hours or 20 mg/kg/day divided every 8 hours

Otitis media (Augmentin® ES-600): 90 mg/kg/day divided every 12 hours for 10 days in children with severe illness and when coverage for β-lactamase-positive *H. influenzae* and *M. catarrhalis* is needed.

Children ≥16 years and Adults: Oral:

Acute bacterial sinusitis: Extended release tablet: Two 1000 mg tablets every 12 hours for 10 days

Bite wounds (animal/human): 875 mg every 12 hours **or** 500 mg every 8 hours

Chronic obstructive pulmonary disease: 875 mg every 12 hours **or** 500 mg every 8 hours

Diabetic foot: Extended release tablet: Two 1000 mg tablets every 12 hours for 7-14 days

Diverticulitis, perirectal abscess: Extended release tablet: Two 1000 mg tablets every 12 hours for 7-10 days

Erysipelas: 875 mg every 12 hours **or** 500 mg every 8 hours

Febrile neutropenia: 875 mg every 12 hours

Pneumonia:

Aspiration: 875 mg every 12 hours

Community-acquired: Extended release tablet: Two 1000 mg tablets every 12 hours for 7-10 days

Pyelonephritis (acute, uncomplicated): 875 mg every 12 hours **or** 500 mg every 8 hours

Skin abscess: 875 mg every 12 hours

Dosing interval in renal impairment:

Cl_{cr} <30 mL/minute: Do not use 875 mg tablet or extended release tablets

Cl_{cr} 10-30 mL/minute: 250-500 mg every 12 hours

Cl_{cr} <10 mL/minute: 250-500 every 24 hours

Hemodialysis: Moderately dialyzable (20% to 50%)

250-500 mg every 24 hours; administer dose during and after dialysis. Do not use extended release tablets.

Peritoneal dialysis: Moderately dialyzable (20% to 50%)

Amoxicillin: Administer 250 mg every 12 hours

Clavulanic acid: Dose for Cl_{cr} <10 mL/minute

Continuous arteriovenous or venovenous hemofiltration effects:

Amoxicillin: ~50 mg of amoxicillin/L of filtrate is removed

Clavulanic acid: Dose for Cl_{cr} <10 mL/minute

Augmentin® Product-Specific Considerations

Strength	Form	Consideration
125 mg	CT, S	q8h dosing
	S	For adults having difficulty swallowing tablets, 125 mg/5 mL suspension may be substituted for 500 mg tablet.
200 mg	CT, S	q12h dosing
	CT	Contains phenylalanine
	S	For adults having difficulty swallowing tablets, 200 mg/5 mL suspension may be substituted for 875 mg tablet.
250 mg	CT, S, T	q8h dosing
	CT	Contains phenylalanine
	T	Not for use in patients <40 kg
	CT, T	Tablet and chewable tablet are not interchangeable due to differences in clavulanic acid.
	S	For adults having difficulty swallowing tablets, 250 mg/5 mL suspension may be substituted for 500 mg tablet.
400 mg	CT, S	q12h dosing
	CT	Contains phenylalanine
	S	For adults having difficulty swallowing tablets, 400 mg/5 mL suspension may be substituted for 875 mg tablet.
500 mg	T	q8h or q12h dosing
600 mg	S	q12h dosing
		Contains phenylalanine
		Not for use in adults or children ≥40 kg
		600 mg/5 mL suspension is not equivalent to or interchangeable with 200 mg/5 mL or 400 mg/5 mL due to differences in clavulanic acid.
875 mg	T	q12h dosing; not for use in Cl_{cr} <30 mL/minute
1000 mg	XR	q12h dosing
		Not for use in children <16 years of age
		Not interchangeable with two 500 mg tablets
		Not for use if Cl_{cr} <30 mL/minute or hemodialysis

Legend: CT = chewable tablet, S = suspension, T = tablet, XR = extended release.

Dietary Considerations May be taken with meals or on an empty stomach; take with meals to increase absorption and decrease GI intolerance; may mix with milk, formula, or juice. Extended release tablets should be taken with food. Some products contain phenylalanine. If you have phenylketonuria or PKU, avoid use. All dosage forms contain potassium.

Administration Administer around-the-clock to promote less variation in peak and trough serum levels. Administer with food to decrease stomach upset; shake suspension well before use. Extended release tablets should be administered with food.

Some penicillins (eg, carbenicillin, ticarcillin, and piperacillin) have been shown to inactivate aminoglycosides *in vitro*. This has been observed to a greater extent with tobramycin and gentamicin, while amikacin has shown greater stability against inactivation. Concurrent use of these agents may pose a risk of reduced antibacterial efficacy *in vivo*, particularly in the setting of profound renal impairment. However, definitive clinical evidence is lacking. If combination penicillin/aminoglycoside therapy is desired in a patient with renal dysfunction, separation of doses (if feasible), and routine monitoring of aminoglycoside levels, CBC, and clinical response should be considered.

Monitoring Parameters Assess patient at beginning and throughout therapy for infection; with prolonged therapy, monitor renal, hepatic, and hematologic function periodically; monitor for signs of anaphylaxis during first dose

Test Interactions May interfere with urinary glucose tests using cupric sulfate (Benedict's solution, Clinitest®, Fehling's solution); may inactivate aminoglycosides *in vitro*.

Some penicillin derivatives may accelerate the degradation of aminoglycosides *in vitro*, leading to a potential underestimation of aminoglycoside serum concentration.

Additional Information Two 250 mg tablets are not equivalent to a 500 mg tablet (both tablet sizes contain equivalent clavulanate). Two 500 mg tablets are not equivalent to a single 1000 mg extended release tablet.

Dosage Forms Excipient information presented when available (limited, particularly for generics); consult specific product labeling. [DSC] = Discontinued product

Powder for oral suspension: 200: Amoxicillin 200 mg and clavulanate potassium 28.5 mg per 5 mL (50 mL, 75 mL, 100 mL) [contains phenylalanine]; 400: Amoxicillin 400 mg and clavulanate potassium 57 mg per 5 mL (50 mL, 75 mL, 100 mL) [contains phenylalanine]; 600: Amoxicillin 600 mg and clavulanate potassium 42.9 mg per 5 mL (75 mL, 125 mL, 200 mL) [contains phenylalanine]

Amoclan:

200: Amoxicillin 200 mg and clavulanate potassium 28.5 mg per 5 mL (50 mL, 75 mL, 100 mL) [contains phenylalanine 7 mg/5 mL and potassium 0.14 mEq/5 mL; fruit flavor]

400: Amoxicillin 400 mg and clavulanate potassium 57 mg per 5 mL (50 mL, 75 mL, 100 mL) [contains phenylalanine 7 mg/5 mL and potassium 0.29 mEq/5 mL; fruit flavor]

Augmentin®:

125: Amoxicillin 125 mg and clavulanate potassium 31.25 mg per 5 mL (75 mL, 100 mL, 150 mL) [contains potassium 0.16 mEq/5 mL; banana flavor]

200: Amoxicillin 200 mg and clavulanate potassium 28.5 mg per 5 mL (50 mL, 75 mL, 100 mL) [contains phenylalanine 7 mg/5 mL and potassium 0.14 mEq/5 mL; orange flavor] [DSC]

250: Amoxicillin 250 mg and clavulanate potassium 62.5 mg per 5 mL (75 mL, 100 mL, 150 mL) [contains potassium 0.32 mEq/5 mL; orange flavor]

400: Amoxicillin 400 mg and clavulanate potassium 57 mg per 5 mL (50 mL [DSC], 75 mL [DSC], 100 mL) [contains phenylalanine 7 mg/5 mL and potassium 0.29 mEq/5 mL; orange flavor]

Augmentin ES-600®: Amoxicillin 600 mg and clavulanate potassium 42.9 mg per 5 mL (75 mL, 125 mL, 200 mL) [contains phenylalanine 7 mg/5 mL and potassium 0.23 mEq/5 mL; strawberry cream flavor]

Tablet: 250: Amoxicillin 250 mg and clavulanate potassium 125 mg; 500: Amoxicillin 500 mg and clavulanate potassium 125 mg; 875: Amoxicillin 875 mg and clavulanate potassium 125 mg

Augmentin®:

250: Amoxicillin 250 mg and clavulanate potassium 125 mg [contains potassium 0.63 mEq/tablet]

500: Amoxicillin 500 mg and clavulanate potassium 125 mg [contains potassium 0.63 mEq/tablet]

875: Amoxicillin 875 mg and clavulanate potassium 125 mg [contains potassium 0.63 mEq/tablet]

Tablet, chewable: 200: Amoxicillin 200 mg and clavulanate potassium 28.5 mg [contains phenylalanine]; 400: Amoxicillin 400 mg and clavulanate potassium 57 mg [contains phenylalanine]

Augmentin®:

125: Amoxicillin 125 mg and clavulanate potassium 31.25 mg [contains potassium 0.16 mEq/tablet; lemon-lime flavor] [DSC]

200: Amoxicillin 200 mg and clavulanate potassium 28.5 mg [contains phenylalanine 2.1 mg/tablet and potassium 0.14 mEq/tablet; cherry-banana flavor] [DSC]
250: Amoxicillin 250 mg and clavulanate potassium 62.5 mg [contains potassium 0.32 mEq/tablet; lemon-lime flavor]
400: Amoxicillin 400 mg and clavulanate potassium 57 mg [contains phenylalanine 4.2 mg/tablet and potassium 0.29 mEq/tablet; cherry-banana flavor] [DSC]

Tablet, extended release:
Augmentin XR®: Amoxicillin 1000 mg and clavulanate acid 62.5 mg [contains potassium 12.6 mg (0.32 mEq) and sodium 29.3 mg (1.27 mEq) per tablet; packaged in either a 7-day or 10-day package]

◆ **Amoxicillin and Clavulanic Acid** *see* Amoxicillin and Clavulanate Potassium *on page 100*

◆ **Amoxicillin, Lansoprazole, and Clarithromycin** *see* Lansoprazole, Amoxicillin, and Clarithromycin *on page 855*

◆ **Amoxicillin Trihydrate** *see* Amoxicillin *on page 98*

◆ **Amoxil®** *see* Amoxicillin *on page 98*

◆ **Amoxycillin** *see* Amoxicillin *on page 98*

◆ **Amphetamine and Dextroamphetamine** *see* Dextroamphetamine and Amphetamine *on page 432*

◆ **Amphocin® [DSC]** *see* Amphotericin B (Conventional) *on page 104*

◆ **Amphojel® (Can)** *see* Aluminum Hydroxide *on page 75*

◆ **Amphotec®** *see* Amphotericin B Cholesteryl Sulfate Complex *on page 103*

◆ **Amphotec® (Can)** *see* Amphotericin B (Lipid Complex) *on page 106*

Amphotericin B Cholesteryl Sulfate Complex

(am foe TER i sin bee kole LES te ril SUL fate KOM plecks)

U.S. Brand Names Amphotec®

Canadian Brand Names Amphotec®

Index Terms ABCD; Amphotericin B Colloidal Dispersion

Pharmacologic Category Antifungal Agent, Parenteral

Use Treatment of invasive aspergillosis in patients who have failed amphotericin B deoxycholate treatment, or who have renal impairment or experience unacceptable toxicity which precludes treatment with amphotericin B deoxycholate in effective doses.

Unlabeled/Investigational Use Effective in patients with serious *Candida* species infections

Pregnancy Risk Factor B

Lactation Excretion in breast milk unknown/contraindicated

Medication Safety Issues

Safety issues:

Lipid-based amphotericin formulations (Amphotec®) may be confused with conventional formulations (Amphocin®, Fungizone®)

Large overdoses have occurred when conventional formulations were dispensed inadvertently for lipid-based products. Single daily doses of conventional amphotericin formulation never exceed 1.5 mg/kg.

High alert medication: The Institute for Safe Medication Practices (ISMP) includes this medication among its list of drugs which have a heightened risk of causing significant patient harm when used in error.

Contraindications Hypersensitivity to amphotericin B or any component of the formulation

Warnings/Precautions Anaphylaxis has been reported with amphotericin B-containing drugs. If severe respiratory distress occurs, the infusion should be immediately discontinued. During the initial dosing, the drug should be administered under close clinical observation. Infusion reactions, sometimes severe, usually subside with continued therapy - manage with decreased rate of infusion and pretreatment with antihistamines/corticosteroids.

Adverse Reactions

>10%: Central nervous system: Chills, fever

1% to 10%:

Cardiovascular: Hypotension, tachycardia
Central nervous system: Headache
Dermatologic: Rash
Endocrine & metabolic: Hypokalemia, hypomagnesemia
Gastrointestinal: Nausea, diarrhea, abdominal pain
Hematologic: Thrombocytopenia
Hepatic: LFT change
Neuromuscular & skeletal: Rigors
Renal: Creatinine increased
Respiratory: Dyspnea

Note: Amphotericin B colloidal dispersion has an improved therapeutic index compared to conventional amphotericin B, and has been used safely in patients with amphotericin B-related nephrotoxicity; however, continued decline of renal function has occurred in some patients.

Drug Interactions

Avoid Concomitant Use

Avoid concomitant use of Amphotericin B Cholesteryl Sulfate Complex with any of the following: Gallium Nitrate

Increased Effect/Toxicity

Amphotericin B Cholesteryl Sulfate Complex may increase the levels/effects of: Aminoglycosides; Colistimethate; CycloSPORINE; Flucytosine; Gallium Nitrate

The levels/effects of Amphotericin B Cholesteryl Sulfate Complex may be increased by: Corticosteroids (Orally Inhaled); Corticosteroids (Systemic)

Decreased Effect

Amphotericin B Cholesteryl Sulfate Complex may decrease the levels/effects of: Saccharomyces boulardii

The levels/effects of Amphotericin B Cholesteryl Sulfate Complex may be decreased by: Antifungal Agents (Azole Derivatives, Systemic)

Stability

Store intact vials under refrigeration.

Reconstitute 50 mg and 100 mg vials with 10 mL and 20 mL of SWI, respectively. The reconstituted vials contain 5 mg/mL of amphotericin B. Shake the vial gently by hand until all solid particles have dissolved. After reconstitution, the solution should be refrigerated at 2°C to 8°C (36°F to 46°F) and used within 24 hours.

Further dilute amphotericin B colloidal dispersion with dextrose 5% in water. Concentrations of 0.1-2 mg/mL in dextrose 5% in water are stable for 14 days at 4°C and 23°C if protected from light, however, due to the occasional formation of subvisual particles, solutions should be used within 48 hours.

Mechanism of Action Binds to ergosterol altering cell membrane permeability in susceptible fungi and causing leakage of cell components with subsequent cell death. Proposed mechanism suggests that amphotericin causes an oxidation-dependent stimulation of macrophages (Lyman, 1992).

Pharmacodynamics/Kinetics

Distribution: V_d: Total volume increases with higher doses, reflects increasing uptake by tissues (with 4 mg/kg/day = 4 L/kg); predominantly distributed in the liver; concentrations in kidneys and other tissues are lower than observed with conventional amphotericin B

Half-life elimination: 28-29 hours; prolonged with higher doses

Dosage Children and Adults: I.V.:

Premedication: For patients who experience chills, fever,

hypotension, nausea, or other nonanaphylactic infusion-related immediate reactions, premedicate with the following drugs 30-60 minutes prior to drug administration: A nonsteroidal (eg, ibuprofen, choline magnesium trisalicylate) with or without diphenhydramine **or** acetaminophen with diphenhydramine **or** hydrocortisone 50-100 mg. If the patient experiences rigors during the infusion, meperidine may be administered.

Range: 3-4 mg/kg/day (infusion of 1 mg/kg/hour); maximum: 7.5 mg/kg/day

Administration Avoid injection faster than 1 mg/kg/hour. For a patient who experiences chills, fever, hypotension, nausea, or other nonanaphylactic infusion-related reactions, premedicate with the following drugs 30-60 minutes prior to drug administration: A nonsteroidal (eg, ibuprofen, choline magnesium trisalicylate) with or without diphenhydramine **or** acetaminophen with diphenhydramine **or** hydrocortisone 50-100 mg. If the patient experiences rigors during the infusion, meperidine may be administered. If severe respiratory distress occurs, the infusion should be immediately discontinued.

Monitoring Parameters Liver function tests, electrolytes, BUN, Cr, temperature, CBC, I/O, signs of hypokalemia (muscle weakness, cramping, drowsiness, ECG changes)

Additional Information Controlled trials which compare the original formulation of amphotericin B to the newer liposomal formulations (ie, Amphotec®) are lacking. Thus, comparative data discussing differences among the formulations should be interpreted cautiously. Although the risk of nephrotoxicity and infusion-related adverse effects may be less with Amphotec®, the efficacy profiles of Amphotec® and the original amphotericin formulation are comparable. Consequently, Amphotec® should be restricted to those patients who cannot tolerate or fail a standard amphotericin B formulation.

Dosage Forms Excipient information presented when available (limited, particularly for generics); consult specific product labeling.

Injection, powder for reconstitution:

Amphotec®: 50 mg, 100 mg

◆ **Amphotericin B Colloidal Dispersion** *see* Amphotericin B Cholesteryl Sulfate Complex *on page 103*

Amphotericin B (Conventional)

(am foe TER i sin bee con VEN sha nal)

U.S. Brand Names Amphocin® [DSC]

Canadian Brand Names Fungizone®

Index Terms Amphotericin B Desoxycholate

Pharmacologic Category Antifungal Agent, Parenteral

Additional Appendix Information

Antifungal Agents *on page 1640*

Desensitization Protocols *on page 1691*

Guidelines for the Prevention of Opportunistic Infections in HIV Infected Persons *on page 1740*

Use Treatment of severe systemic and central nervous system infections caused by susceptible fungi such as *Candida* species, *Histoplasma capsulatum*, *Cryptococcus neoformans*, *Aspergillus* species, *Blastomyces dermatitidis*, *Torulopsis glabrata*, and *Coccidioides immitis*; fungal peritonitis; irrigant for bladder fungal infections; used in fungal infection in patients with bone marrow transplantation, amebic meningoencephalitis, ocular aspergillosis (intraocular injection), candidal cystitis (bladder irrigation), chemoprophylaxis (low-dose I.V.), immunocompromised patients at risk of aspergillosis (intranasal/nebulized), refractory meningitis (intrathecal), coccidioidal arthritis (intra-articular/I.M.).

Low-dose amphotericin B has been administered after bone marrow transplantation to reduce the risk of invasive fungal disease.

Pregnancy Risk Factor B

Lactation Excretion in breast milk unknown/contraindicated

Medication Safety Issues

Safety issues:

Conventional amphotericin formulations (Amphocin®, Fungizone®) may be confused with lipid-based formulations (AmBisome®, Abelcet®, Amphotec®).

Large overdoses have occurred when conventional formulations were dispensed inadvertently for lipid-based products. Single daily doses of conventional amphotericin formulation never exceed 1.5 mg/kg.

High alert medication: The Institute for Safe Medication Practices (ISMP) includes this medication (intrathecal administration) among its list of drugs which have a heightened risk of causing significant patient harm when used in error.

Contraindications Hypersensitivity to amphotericin or any component of the formulation

Warnings/Precautions Anaphylaxis has been reported with amphotericin B-containing drugs. During the initial dosing, the drug should be administered under close clinical observation. Avoid use with other nephrotoxic drugs; drug-induced renal toxicity usually improves with interrupting therapy, decreasing dosage, or increasing dosing interval. Infusion reactions are most common 1-3 hours after starting the infusion and diminish with continued therapy.

Adverse Reactions

Systemic:

>10%:

Cardiovascular: Hypotension, tachypnea

Central nervous system: Fever, chills, headache (less frequent with I.T.), malaise

Endocrine & metabolic: Hypokalemia, hypomagnesemia

Gastrointestinal: Anorexia, nausea (less frequent with I.T.), vomiting (less frequent with I.T.), diarrhea, heartburn, cramping epigastric pain

Hematologic: Normochromic-normocytic anemia

Local: Pain at injection site with or without phlebitis or thrombophlebitis (incidence may increase with peripheral infusion of admixtures)

Neuromuscular & skeletal: Generalized pain, including muscle and joint pains (less frequent with I.T.)

Renal: Decreased renal function and renal function abnormalities including azotemia, renal tubular acidosis, nephrocalcinosis (>0.1 mg/mL)

1% to 10%:

Cardiovascular: Hypertension, flushing

Central nervous system: Delirium, arachnoiditis, pain along lumbar nerves (especially I.T. therapy)

Genitourinary: Urinary retention

Hematologic: Leukocytosis

Neuromuscular & skeletal: Paresthesia (especially with I.T. therapy)

<1% (Limited to important or life-threatening): Acute liver failure, agranulocytosis, anuria, bone marrow suppression, cardiac arrest, coagulation defects, convulsions, dyspnea, hearing loss, leukopenia, maculopapular rash, renal failure, renal tubular acidosis, thrombocytopenia, vision changes

Drug Interactions

Avoid Concomitant Use

Avoid concomitant use of Amphotericin B (Conventional) with any of the following: Gallium Nitrate

Increased Effect/Toxicity

Amphotericin B (Conventional) may increase the levels/effects of: Aminoglycosides; Colistimethate; CycloSPORINE; Flucytosine; Gallium Nitrate

The levels/effects of Amphotericin B (Conventional) may be increased by: Corticosteroids (Orally Inhaled); Corticosteroids (Systemic)

Decreased Effect

Amphotericin B (Conventional) may decrease the levels/effects of: Saccharomyces boulardii

The levels/effects of Amphotericin B (Conventional) may be decreased by: Antifungal Agents (Azole Derivatives, Systemic)

Stability Store intact vials under refrigeration; protect from light. Add 10 mL of SWFI (without a bacteriostatic agent) to each vial of amphotericin B. Further dilute with 250-500 mL D_5W; final concentration should not exceed 0.1 mg/mL (peripheral infusion) or 0.25 mg/mL (central infusion).

Reconstituted vials are stable, protected from light, for 24 hours at room temperature and 1 week when refrigerated. Parenteral admixtures are stable, protected from light, for 24 hours at room temperature and 2 days under refrigeration. Short-term exposure (<24 hours) to light during I.V. infusion does **not** appreciably affect potency.

Mechanism of Action Binds to ergosterol altering cell membrane permeability in susceptible fungi and causing leakage of cell components with subsequent cell death. Proposed mechanism suggests that amphotericin causes an oxidation-dependent stimulation of macrophages (Lyman, 1992).

Pharmacodynamics/Kinetics

Distribution: Minimal amounts enter the aqueous humor, bile, CSF (inflamed or noninflamed meninges), amniotic fluid, pericardial fluid, pleural fluid, and synovial fluid

Protein binding, plasma: 90%

Half-life elimination: Biphasic: Initial: 15-48 hours; Terminal: 15 days

Time to peak: Within 1 hour following a 4- to 6-hour dose

Excretion: Urine (2% to 5% as biologically active form); ~40% eliminated over a 7-day period and may be detected in urine for at least 7 weeks after discontinued use

Dosage

Premedication: For patients who experience infusion-related immediate reactions, premedicate with the following drugs 30-60 minutes prior to drug administration: NSAID (with or without diphenhydramine) **or** acetaminophen with diphenhydramine **or** hydrocortisone 50-100 mg. If the patient experiences rigors during the infusion, meperidine may be administered.

Usual dosage ranges:

Infants and Children:

Test dose: I.V.: 0.1 mg/kg/dose to a maximum of 1 mg; infuse over 30-60 minutes. Many clinicians believe a test dose is unnecessary.

Maintenance dose: 0.25-1 mg/kg/day given once daily; infuse over 2-6 hours. Once therapy has been established, amphotericin B can be administered on an every-other-day basis at 1-1.5 mg/kg/dose; cumulative dose: 1.5-2 g over 6-10 weeks.

Duration of therapy: Varies with nature of infection, usual duration is 4-12 weeks or cumulative dose of 1-4 g

Adults:

Test dose: 1 mg infused over 20-30 minutes. Many clinicians believe a test dose is unnecessary.

Maintenance dose: Usual: 0.05-1.5 mg/kg/day; 1-1.5 mg/kg over 4-6 hours every other day may be given once therapy is established; aspergillosis, rhinocerebral mucormycosis, often require 1-1.5 mg/kg/day; do not exceed 1.5 mg/kg/day

Indication-specific dosing:

Children: Meningitis, coccidioidal or cryptococcal: I.T.: 25-100 mcg every 48-72 hours; increase to 500 mcg as tolerated

Adults:

Aspergillosis, disseminated: I.V.: 0.6-0.7 mg/kg/day for 3-6 months

Bone marrow transplantation (prophylaxis): I.V.: Low-dose amphotericin B 0.1-0.25 mg/kg/day has been administered after bone marrow transplantation to reduce the risk of invasive fungal disease.

Candidemia (neutropenic or non-neutropenic): I.V.: 0.6-1 mg/kg/day until 14 days after last positive blood culture and resolution of signs and symptoms

Candidiasis, chronic, disseminated: I.V.: 0.6-0.7 mg/kg/day for 3-6 months and resolution of radiologic lesions

Cystitis: Candidal: Bladder irrigation: Irrigate with 50 mcg/mL solution instilled periodically or continuously for 5-10 days or until cultures are clear

Dematiaceous fungi: I.V.: 0.7 mg/kg/day in combination with an azole

Endocarditis: I.V.: 0.6-1 mg/kg/day (with or without flucytosine) for 1 week, then 0.8 mg/kg/day every other day for 6-8 weeks postoperatively

Endophthalmitis, fungal:

Intravitreal (unlabeled use): 10 mcg in 0.1 mL (in conjunction with systemic therapy)

I.V.: 0.7-1 mg/kg/day (with or without flucytosine) for at least 4 weeks

Esophagitis: I.V.: 0.3-0.7 mg/kg/day for 14-21 after clinical improvement

Histoplasmosis: Chronic, severe pulmonary or disseminated: I.V.: 0.5-1 mg/kg/day for 7 days, then 0.8 mg/kg every other day (or 3 times/week) until total dose of 10-15 mg/kg; may continue itraconazole as suppressive therapy (lifelong for immunocompromised patients)

Meningitis:

Candidal: I.V.: 0.7-1 mg/kg/day (with or without flucytosine) for at least 4 weeks

Cryptococcal or *Coccidioides*: I.T.: Initial: 25-300 mcg every 48-72 hours; increase to 500 mcg to 1 mg as tolerated; maximum total dose: 15 mg has been suggested

Histoplasma: I.V.: 0.5-1 mg/kg/day for 7 days, then 0.8 mg/kg every other day (or 3 times/week) for 3 months total duration; follow with fluconazole suppressive therapy for up to 12 months

Meningoencephalitis, cryptococcal: I.V.:

HIV positive: 0.7-1 mg/kg/day (plus flucytosine 100 mg/kg/day) for 2 weeks, then change to oral fluconazole for at least 10 weeks; alternatively, amphotericin and flucytosine may be continued uninterrupted for 6-10 weeks

HIV negative: 0.5-0.7 mg/kg/day (plus flucytosine) for 2 weeks

Osteomyelitis: Candidal: I.V.: 0.5-1 mg/kg/day for 6-10 weeks

Penicillium marneffei: I.V.: 0.6 mg/kg/day for 2 weeks

Pneumonia: Cryptococcal (mild to moderate): I.V.:

HIV positive: 0.5-1 mg/kg/day

HIV negative: 0.5-0.7 mg/kg/day (plus flucytosine) for 2 weeks

Sporotrichosis: Pulmonary, meningeal, osteoarticular, or disseminated: I.V.: Total dose of 1-2 g, then change to oral itraconazole or fluconazole for suppressive therapy

Dosing adjustment in renal impairment: If renal dysfunction is due to the drug, the daily total can be decreased by 50% or the dose can be given every other day; I.V. therapy may take several months

Dialysis: Poorly dialyzed; no supplemental dosage necessary when using hemo- or peritoneal dialysis or continuous renal replacement therapy (CRRT)

Administration in dialysate: Children and Adults: 1-2 mg/L of peritoneal dialysis fluid either with or without low-dose I.V. amphotericin B (a total dose of 2-10 mg/kg given over

7-14 days). Precipitate may form in ionic dialysate solutions.

Administration May be infused over 4-6 hours. For a patient who experiences chills, fever, hypotension, nausea, or other nonanaphylactic infusion-related reactions, premedicate with the following drugs 30-60 minutes prior to drug administration: A nonsteroidal (eg, ibuprofen, choline magnesium trisalicylate) with or without diphenhydramine **or** acetaminophen with diphenhydramine **or** hydrocortisone 50-100 mg. If the patient experiences rigors during the infusion, meperidine may be administered. Bolus infusion of normal saline immediately preceding, or immediately preceding and following amphotericin B may reduce drug-induced nephrotoxicity. Risk of nephrotoxicity increases with amphotericin B doses >1 mg/kg/day. Infusion of admixtures more concentrated than 0.25 mg/mL should be limited to patients absolutely requiring volume contraction.

Monitoring Parameters Renal function (monitor frequently during therapy), electrolytes (especially potassium and magnesium), liver function tests, temperature, PT/PTT, CBC; monitor input and output; monitor for signs of hypokalemia (muscle weakness, cramping, drowsiness, ECG changes, etc)

Reference Range Therapeutic: 1-2 mcg/mL (SI: 1-2.2 µmol/L)

Test Interactions Increased BUN (S), serum creatinine, alkaline phosphate, bilirubin; decreased magnesium, potassium (S)

Additional Information Premedication with diphenhydramine and acetaminophen may reduce the severity of acute infusion-related reactions. Meperidine reduces the duration of amphotericin B-induced rigors and chilling. Hydrocortisone may be used in patients with severe or refractory infusion-related reactions. Bolus infusion of normal saline immediately preceding, or immediately preceding and following amphotericin B may reduce drug-induced nephrotoxicity. Risk of nephrotoxicity increases with amphotericin B doses >1 mg/kg/day. Infusion of admixtures more concentrated than 0.25 mg/mL should be limited to patients absolutely requiring volume restriction. Amphotericin B does not have a bacteriostatic constituent, subsequently admixture expiration is determined by sterility more than chemical stability.

Dosage Forms Excipient information presented when available (limited, particularly for generics); consult specific product labeling. [DSC] = Discontinued product

Injection, powder for reconstitution, as desoxycholate: 50 mg

Amphocin®: 50 mg [DSC]

◆ **Amphotericin B Desoxycholate** *see* Amphotericin B (Conventional) *on page 104*

Amphotericin B (Lipid Complex)

(am foe TER i sin bee LIP id KOM pleks)

U.S. Brand Names Abelcet®

Canadian Brand Names Abelcet®; Amphotec®

Index Terms ABLC

Pharmacologic Category Antifungal Agent, Parenteral

Use Treatment of aspergillosis or any type of progressive fungal infection in patients who are refractory to or intolerant of conventional amphotericin B therapy

Unlabeled/Investigational Use Effective in patients with serious *Candida* species infections

Pregnancy Risk Factor B

Lactation Enters breast milk/contraindicated

Medication Safety Issues

Safety issues:

Lipid-based amphotericin formulations (Abelcet®) may be confused with conventional formulations (Amphocin®, Fungizone®)

Large overdoses have occurred when conventional formulations were dispensed inadvertently for lipid-based products. Single daily doses of conventional amphotericin formulation never exceed 1.5 mg/kg.

High alert medication: The Institute for Safe Medication Practices (ISMP) includes this medication among its list of drugs which have a heightened risk of causing significant patient harm when used in error.

Contraindications Hypersensitivity to amphotericin or any component of the formulation

Warnings/Precautions Anaphylaxis has been reported with amphotericin B-containing drugs. If severe respiratory distress occurs, the infusion should be immediately discontinued. During the initial dosing, the drug should be administered under close clinical observation. Acute reactions (including fever and chills) may occur 1-2 hours after starting an intravenous infusion. These reactions are usually more common with the first few doses and generally diminish with subsequent doses.

Adverse Reactions Nephrotoxicity and infusion-related hyperpyrexia, rigor, and chilling are reduced relative to amphotericin deoxycholate.

>10%:

Central nervous system: Chills, fever

Renal: Serum creatinine increased

Miscellaneous: Multiple organ failure

1% to 10%:

Cardiovascular: Hypotension, cardiac arrest

Central nervous system: Headache, pain

Dermatologic: Rash

Endocrine & metabolic: Bilirubinemia, hypokalemia, acidosis

Gastrointestinal: Nausea, vomiting, diarrhea, gastrointestinal hemorrhage, abdominal pain

Renal: Renal failure

Respiratory: Respiratory failure, dyspnea, pneumonia

Drug Interactions

Avoid Concomitant Use

Avoid concomitant use of Amphotericin B (Lipid Complex) with any of the following: Gallium Nitrate

Increased Effect/Toxicity

Amphotericin B (Lipid Complex) may increase the levels/effects of: Aminoglycosides; Colistimethate; CycloSPORINE; Flucytosine; Gallium Nitrate

The levels/effects of Amphotericin B (Lipid Complex) may be increased by: Corticosteroids (Orally Inhaled); Corticosteroids (Systemic)

Decreased Effect

Amphotericin B (Lipid Complex) may decrease the levels/effects of: Saccharomyces boulardii

The levels/effects of Amphotericin B (Lipid Complex) may be decreased by: Antifungal Agents (Azole Derivatives, Systemic)

Stability Intact vials should be stored at 2°C to 8°C (35°F to 46°F) and protected from exposure to light; do not freeze intact vials. Solutions for infusion are stable for 48 hours under refrigeration and for 6 hours at room temperature. Shake the vial gently until there is no evidence of any yellow sediment at the bottom. Dilute with D_5W to 1-2 mg/mL. Protect from light.

Do not dilute with saline solutions or mix with other drugs or electrolytes - compatibility has not been established

Do not use an in-line filter during administration.

Mechanism of Action Binds to ergosterol altering cell membrane permeability in susceptible fungi and causing leakage of cell components with subsequent cell death. Proposed mechanism suggests that amphotericin causes an oxidation-dependent stimulation of macrophages.

Pharmacodynamics/Kinetics

Distribution: V_d: Increases with higher doses; reflects increased uptake by tissues (131 L/kg with 5 mg/kg/day)

Half-life elimination: ~24 hours

Excretion: Clearance: Increases with higher doses (5 mg/kg/day): 400 mL/hour/kg

Dosage Children and Adults: I.V.:

Premedication: For patients who experience infusion-related immediate reactions, premedicate with the following drugs 30-60 minutes prior to drug administration: A nonsteroidal anti-inflammatory agent ± diphenhydramine **or** acetaminophen with diphenhydramine **or** hydrocortisone 50-100 mg. If the patient experiences rigors during the infusion, meperidine may be administered.

Range: 2.5-5 mg/kg/day as a single infusion

Dosing adjustment in renal impairment: None necessary; effects of renal impairment are not currently known

Hemodialysis: No supplemental dosage necessary

Peritoneal dialysis: No supplemental dosage necessary

Continuous renal replacement therapy (CRRT): No supplemental dosage necessary

Administration For patients who experience nonanaphylactic infusion-related reactions, premedicate 30-60 minutes prior to drug administration with a nonsteroidal anti-inflammatory agent ± diphenhydramine **or** acetaminophen with diphenhydramine **or** hydrocortisone 50-100 mg. If the patient experiences rigors during the infusion, meperidine may be administered.

Invert infusion container several times prior to administration and every 2 hours during infusion.

Monitoring Parameters Renal function (monitor frequently during therapy), electrolytes (especially potassium and magnesium), liver function tests, temperature, PT/PTT, CBC; monitor input and output; monitor for signs of hypokalemia (muscle weakness, cramping, drowsiness, ECG changes, etc)

Test Interactions Increased BUN (S), serum creatinine, alkaline phosphate, bilirubin; decreased magnesium, potassium (S)

Additional Information As a modification of dimyristoyl phosphatidylcholine:dimyristoyl phosphatidylglycerol 7:3 (DMPC:DMPG) liposome, amphotericin B lipid-complex has a higher drug to lipid ratio and the concentration of amphotericin B is 33 M. ABLC is a ribbon-like structure, not a liposome.

Controlled trials which compare the original formulation of amphotericin B to the newer liposomal formulations (ie, Abelcet®) are lacking. Thus, comparative data discussing differences among the formulations should be interpreted cautiously. Although the risk of nephrotoxicity and infusion-related adverse effects may be less with Abelcet®, the efficacy profiles of Abelcet® and the original amphotericin formulation are comparable. Consequently, Abelcet® should be restricted to those patients who cannot tolerate or fail a standard amphotericin B formulation.

Dosage Forms Excipient information presented when available (limited, particularly for generics); consult specific product labeling.

Injection, suspension [preservative free]:

Abelcet®: 5 mg/mL (20 mL)

Amphotericin B (Liposomal)

(am foe TER i sin bee lye po SO mal)

U.S. Brand Names AmBisome®

Canadian Brand Names AmBisome®

Index Terms L-AmB

Pharmacologic Category Antifungal Agent, Parenteral

Use Empirical therapy for presumed fungal infection in febrile, neutropenic patients; treatment of patients with *Aspergillus* species, *Candida* species, and/or *Cryptococcus* species infections refractory to amphotericin B desoxycholate (conventional amphotericin), or in patients where renal impairment or unacceptable toxicity precludes the use of amphotericin B desoxycholate; treatment of cryptococcal meningitis in HIV-infected patients; treatment of visceral leishmaniasis

Unlabeled/Investigational Use Treatment of systemic *Histoplasmosis* infection

Pregnancy Risk Factor B

Pregnancy Considerations Animal studies did not demonstrate teratogenicity. There are no adequate and well-controlled studies in pregnant women. Conventional amphotericin B has been used successfully to treat systemic fungal infection in a limited number (case reports) of pregnant women.

Lactation Excretion in breast milk unknown/not recommended

Medication Safety Issues

Safety issues:

Lipid-based amphotericin formulations (AmBisome®) may be confused with conventional formulations (Amphocin®, Fungizone®) or with other lipid-based amphotericin formulations (Abelcet®, Amphotec®)

Large overdoses have occurred when conventional formulations were dispensed inadvertently for lipid-based products. Single daily doses of conventional amphotericin formulation never exceed 1.5 mg/kg.

High alert medication: The Institute for Safe Medication Practices (ISMP) includes this medication among its list of drugs which have a heightened risk of causing significant patient harm when used in error.

Contraindications Hypersensitivity to amphotericin B deoxycholate or any component of the formulation

Warnings/Precautions Patients should be under close clinical observation during initial dosing. As with other amphotericin B-containing products, anaphylaxis has been reported. Facilities for cardiopulmonary resuscitation should be available during administration. Acute infusion reactions (including fever and chills) may occur 1-2 hours after starting infusions; reactions are more common with the first few doses and generally diminish with subsequent doses. Immediately discontinue infusion if severe respiratory distress occurs; the patient should not receive further infusions. Concurrent use of amphotericin B with other nephrotoxic drugs may enhance the potential for drug-induced renal toxicity. Concurrent use with antineoplastic agents may enhance the potential for renal toxicity, bronchospasm or hypotension. Acute pulmonary toxicity has been reported in patients receiving simultaneous leukocyte transfusions and amphotericin B. Safety and efficacy have not been established in patients <1 month of age.

Adverse Reactions Percentage of adverse reactions is dependent upon population studied and may vary with respect to premedications and underlying illness. Incidence of decreased renal function and infusion-related events are lower than rates observed with amphotericin B deoxycholate.

>10%:

Cardiovascular: Peripheral edema (15%), edema (12% to 14%), tachycardia (9% to 19%), hypotension (7% to 14%), hypertension (8% to 20%), chest pain (8% to 12%), hypervolemia (8% to 12%)

Central nervous system: Chills (29% to 48%), insomnia (17% to 22%), headache (9% to 20%), anxiety (7% to 14%), pain (14%), confusion (9% to 13%)

Dermatologic: Rash (5% to 25%), pruritus (11%)

Endocrine & metabolic: Hypokalemia (31% to 51%), hypomagnesemia (15% to 50%), hyperglycemia (8% to 23%), hypocalcemia (5% to 18%), hyponatremia (9% to 12%)

Gastrointestinal: Nausea (16% to 40%), vomiting (11% to 32%), diarrhea (11% to 30%), abdominal pain (7% to 20%), constipation (15%), anorexia (10% to 14%)
Hematologic: Anemia (27% to 48%), blood transfusion reaction (9% to 18%), leukopenia (15% to 17%), thrombocytopenia (6% to 13%)
Hepatic: Alkaline phosphatase increased (7% to 22%), bilirubinemia (≤18%), ALT increased (15%), AST increased (13%), liver function tests abnormal (not specified) (4% to 13%)
Local: Phlebitis (9% to 11%)
Neuromuscular & skeletal: Weakness (6% to 13%), back pain (12%)
Renal: Nephrotoxicity (14% to 47%), creatinine increased (18% to 40%), BUN increased (7% to 21%), hematuria (14%)
Respiratory: Dyspnea (18% to 23%), lung disorder (14% to 18%), cough (2% to 18%), epistaxis (9% to 15%), pleural effusion (13%), rhinitis (11%)
Miscellaneous: Infusion reactions (4% to 21%), sepsis (7% to 14%), infection (11% to 13%)

2% to 10%:
Cardiovascular: Arrhythmia, atrial fibrillation, bradycardia, cardiac arrest, cardiomegaly, facial swelling, flushing, postural hypotension, valvular heart disease, vascular disorder, vasodilation
Central nervous system: Agitation, abnormal thinking, coma, depression, dysesthesia, dizziness (7% to 9%), hallucinations, malaise, nervousness, seizure, somnolence
Dermatologic: Alopecia, bruising, cellulitis, dry skin, maculopapular rash, petechia, purpura, skin discoloration, skin disorder, skin ulcer, urticaria, vesiculobullous rash
Endocrine & metabolic: Acidosis, fluid overload, hypernatremia (4%), hyperchloremia, hyperkalemia, hypermagnesemia, hyperphosphatemia, hypophosphatemia, hypoproteinemia, lactate dehydrogenase increased, nonprotein nitrogen increased
Gastrointestinal: Abdomen enlarged, amylase increased, dyspepsia, dysphagia, eructation, fecal incontinence, flatulence, gastrointestinal hemorrhage (10%), hematemesis, hemorrhoids, gum/oral hemorrhage, ileus, mucositis, rectal disorder, stomatitis, ulcerative stomatitis, xerostomia
Genitourinary: Vaginal hemorrhage
Hematologic: Coagulation disorder, hemorrhage, prothrombin decreased
Hepatic: Hepatocellular damage, hepatomegaly, veno-occlusive liver disease
Local: Injection site inflammation
Neuromuscular & skeletal: Arthralgia, bone pain, dystonia, myalgia, neck pain, paresthesia, rigors, tremor
Ocular: Conjunctivitis, dry eyes, eye hemorrhage
Renal: Abnormal renal function, acute renal failure, dysuria, renal failure, toxic nephropathy, urinary incontinence
Respiratory: Asthma, atelectasis, dry nose, hemoptysis, hyperventilation, pharyngitis, pneumonia, pulmonary edema, respiratory alkalosis, respiratory insufficiency, respiratory failure, sinusitis, hypoxia (6% to 8%)
Miscellaneous: Allergic reaction, cell-mediated immunological reaction, flu-like syndrome, graft-versus-host disease, herpes simplex, hiccup, procedural complication (8% to 10%), diaphoresis (7%)

Postmarketing and/or case reports: Agranulocytosis, angioedema, bronchospasm, cyanosis/hypoventilation, erythema, hemorrhagic cystitis

Drug Interactions

Avoid Concomitant Use

Avoid concomitant use of Amphotericin B (Liposomal) with any of the following: Gallium Nitrate

Increased Effect/Toxicity

Amphotericin B (Liposomal) may increase the levels/effects of: Aminoglycosides; Colistimethate; CycloSPORINE; Flucytosine; Gallium Nitrate

The levels/effects of Amphotericin B (Liposomal) may be increased by: Corticosteroids (Orally Inhaled); Corticosteroids (Systemic)

Decreased Effect

Amphotericin B (Liposomal) may decrease the levels/effects of: Saccharomyces boulardii

The levels/effects of Amphotericin B (Liposomal) may be decreased by: Antifungal Agents (Azole Derivatives, Systemic)

Stability Store intact vials at ≤25°C (≤77°F). Reconstituted vials are stable refrigerated at 2°C to 8°C (36°F to 46°F) for 24 hours. Do not freeze. Manufacturer's labeling states infusion should begin within 6 hours of dilution with D_5W; data on file with Astellas Pharma shows extended formulation stability when admixed in D_5W at 0.2-2 mg/mL (in polyolefin or PVC bags) for up to 11 days when stored refrigerated at 2°C to 8°C (36°F to 46°F).

Reconstitution: Reconstitute with 12 mL SWFI to a concentration of 4 mg/mL. The use of any solution other than those recommended, or the presence of a bacteriostatic agent in the solution, may cause precipitation. **Shake the vial vigorously** for 30 seconds, until dispersed into a translucent yellow suspension.

Filtration and dilution: The 5-micron filter should be on the syringe used to remove the reconstituted AmBisome®. Dilute to a final concentration of 1-2 mg/mL (0.2-0.5 mg/mL for infants and small children).

Mechanism of Action Binds to ergosterol altering cell membrane permeability in susceptible fungi and causing leakage of cell components with subsequent cell death. Proposed mechanism suggests that amphotericin causes an oxidation-dependent stimulation of macrophages (Lyman, 1992).

Pharmacodynamics/Kinetics

Distribution: V_d: 131 L/kg
Half-life elimination: Terminal: 174 hours

Dosage

Usual dosage range:

Children ≥1 month: I.V.: 3-6 mg/kg/day
Adults: I.V.: 3-6 mg/kg/day; **Note:** Higher doses (15 mg/kg/day) have been used clinically (Walsh, 2001)
Note: Premedication: For patients who experience nonanaphylactic infusion-related immediate reactions, premedicate with the following drugs 30-60 minutes prior to drug administration: A nonsteroidal anti-inflammatory agent ± diphenhydramine; **or** acetaminophen with diphenhydramine; **or** hydrocortisone 50-100 mg. If the patient experiences rigors during the infusion, meperidine may be administered.

Indication-specific dosing:

Children ≥1 month: I.V.:
Cryptococcal meningitis (HIV-positive): 6 mg/kg/day (may consider addition of oral flucytosine 25 mg/kg 4 times daily [unlabeled combination; AIDS*info* guidelines, 2008])
Empiric therapy: 3 mg/kg/day
Systemic fungal infections *(Aspergillus, Candida, Cryptococcus, Histoplasmosis)*: 3-5 mg/kg/day
General invasive Candidal disease: 3-5 mg/kg/day (may consider addition of oral flucytosine 25-37.5 mg/kg 4 times daily [unlabeled combination; AIDS*info* guidelines, 2008])
Candidal meningitis: 5 mg/kg/day; (may consider addition of oral flucytosine 25-37.5 mg/kg 4 times daily [unlabeled combination; AIDS*info* guidelines, 2008])

Histoplasmosis (unlabeled use): 3-5 mg/kg/day (AIDS*info* guidelines, 2008)

Visceral leishmaniasis:

Immunocompetent: 3 mg/kg/day on days 1-5, and 3 mg/kg/day on days 14 and 21; a repeat course may be given in patients who do not achieve parasitic clearance

Note: Alternate regimen of 10 mg/kg/day for 2 days has been reportedly effective.

Immunocompromised: 4 mg/kg/day on days 1-5, and 4 mg/kg/day on days 10, 17, 24, 31, and 38

Adults: I.V.:

Cryptococcal meningitis (HIV-positive): 6 mg/kg/day or 4-6 mg/kg/day in combination with addition of oral flucytosine 25 mg/kg 4 times daily (unlabeled combination; AIDS*info* guidelines, 2008)

Empiric therapy: 3 mg/kg/day

Fungal sinusitis: Limited data in immunocompromised patients have shown efficacy with 3-10 mg/kg/day (Pagano, 2004; Rokicka, 2006; Barron, 2005). **Note:** An azole antifungal is recommended if causative organism is *Aspergillus* spp or *Pseudallescheria boydii* (*Scedosporium* sp).

Systemic fungal infections *(Aspergillus, Candida, Cryptococcus, Histoplasmosis)*: 3-5 mg/kg/day

General invasive Candidal disease: 3-5 mg/kg/day with oral flucytosine 25 mg/kg 4 times daily (unlabeled combination; Pappas, 2004)

Candidal meningitis: 5 mg/kg/day with oral flucytosine 25 mg/kg 4 times daily (unlabeled combination; Pappas, 2004)

Histoplasmosis (unlabeled use): 3-5 mg/kg/day (AIDS*info* guidelines, 2008)

Visceral leishmaniasis:

Immunocompetent: 3 mg/kg/day on days 1-5, and 3 mg/kg/day on days 14 and 21; a repeat course may be given in patients who do not achieve parasitic clearance

Note: Alternate regimen of 2 mg/kg/day for 5 days has been reportedly effective.

Immunocompromised: 4 mg/kg/day on days 1-5, and 4 mg/kg/day on days 10, 17, 24, 31, and 38

Dosing adjustment in renal impairment: None necessary; effects of renal impairment are not currently known

Hemodialysis: No supplemental dosage necessary

Peritoneal dialysis effects: No supplemental dosage necessary

Continuous renal replacement therapy (CRRT): No supplemental dosage necessary

Administration Administer via intravenous infusion, over a period of approximately 2 hours. Infusion time may be reduced to approximately 1 hour in patients in whom the treatment is well-tolerated. If the patient experiences discomfort during infusion, the duration of infusion may be increased. Administer at a rate of 2.5 mg/kg/hour. Existing intravenous line should be flushed with D_5W prior to infusion (if not feasible, administer through a separate line). An in-line membrane filter (not less than 1 micron) may be used.

For a patient who experiences chills, fever, hypotension, nausea, or other nonanaphylactic infusion-related reactions, premedicate with the following drugs, 30-60 minutes prior to drug administration: A nonsteroidal (eg, ibuprofen, choline magnesium trisalicylate) with or without diphenhydramine **or** acetaminophen with diphenhydramine **or** hydrocortisone 50-100 mg. If the patient experiences rigors during the infusion, meperidine may be administered.

Monitoring Parameters Renal function (monitor frequently during therapy), electrolytes (especially potassium and magnesium), liver function tests, temperature, PT/PTT, CBC; monitor input and output; monitor for signs of hypokalemia (muscle weakness, cramping, drowsiness, ECG changes, etc); monitor cardiac function if used concurrently with corticosteroids

Additional Information Amphotericin B (liposomal) is a true single bilayer liposomal drug delivery system. Liposomes are closed, spherical vesicles created by mixing specific proportions of amphophilic substances such as phospholipids and cholesterol so that they arrange themselves into multiple concentric bilayer membranes when hydrated in aqueous solutions. Single bilayer liposomes are then formed by microemulsification of multilamellar vesicles using a homogenizer. Amphotericin B (liposomal) consists of these unilamellar bilayer liposomes with amphotericin B intercalated within the membrane. Due to the nature and quantity of amphophilic substances used, and the lipophilic moiety in the amphotericin B molecule, the drug is an integral part of the overall structure of the amphotericin B liposomal liposomes. Amphotericin B (liposomal) contains true liposomes that are <100 nm in diameter.

Dosage Forms Excipient information presented when available (limited, particularly for generics); consult specific product labeling.

Injection, powder for reconstitution:

AmBisome®: 50 mg [contains soy and sucrose]

Ampicillin (am pi SIL in)

Canadian Brand Names Apo-Ampi®; Novo-Ampicillin; Nu-Ampi

Index Terms Aminobenzylpenicillin; Ampicillin Sodium; Ampicillin Trihydrate

Pharmacologic Category Antibiotic, Penicillin

Additional Appendix Information

Animal and Human Bites *on page 1747*

Antibiotic Treatment of Adults With Infective Endocarditis *on page 1748*

Antimicrobial Drugs of Choice *on page 1752*

Community-Acquired Pneumonia in Adults *on page 1766*

Desensitization Protocols *on page 1691*

Prevention of Infective Endocarditis *on page 1736*

Use Treatment of susceptible bacterial infections (nonbeta-lactamase-producing organisms); treatment or prophylaxis of infective endocarditis; susceptible bacterial infections caused by streptococci, pneumococci, nonpenicillinase-producing staphylococci, *Listeria*, meningococci; some strains of *H. influenzae*, *Salmonella*, *Shigella*, *E. coli*, *Enterobacter*, and *Klebsiella*

Pregnancy Risk Factor B

Pregnancy Considerations Adverse events have not been observed in animal studies; therefore, ampicillin is classified as pregnancy category B. Ampicillin crosses the human placenta, providing detectable concentrations in the cord serum and amniotic fluid. Most studies have not identified a teratogenic potential for ampicillin use during pregnancy. Two possible associations (congenital heart disease and cleft palate) have been noted; each of these was observed in a single study, was not substantiated by other studies, and may have been chance associations. Ampicillin is recommended for use in pregnant women for the management of premature rupture of membranes. Ampicillin is considered an acceptable alternative to penicillin for the prevention of early-onset Group B Streptococcal (GBS) disease in newborns.

The volume of distribution of ampicillin is increased during pregnancy and the half-life is decreased. As a result, serum concentrations in pregnant patients are approximately 50% of those in nonpregnant patients receiving the same dose. Higher doses may be needed during pregnancy. Although oral absorption is not altered during pregnancy, oral ampicillin is poorly-absorbed during labor.

Lactation Enters breast milk/use caution

Medication Safety Issues

Sound-alike/look-alike issues:

Ampicillin may be confused with aminophylline

Contraindications Hypersensitivity to ampicillin, any component of the formulation, or other penicillins

Warnings/Precautions Dosage adjustment may be necessary in patients with renal impairment. Serious and occasionally severe or fatal hypersensitivity (anaphylactoid) reactions have been reported in patients on penicillin therapy, especially with a history of beta-lactam hypersensitivity, history of sensitivity to multiple allergens, or previous IgE-mediated reactions (eg, anaphylaxis, angioedema, urticaria). Use with caution in asthmatic patients. High percentage of patients with infectious mononucleosis have developed rash during therapy with ampicillin; ampicillin-class antibiotics not recommended in these patients. Appearance of a rash should be carefully evaluated to differentiate a nonallergic ampicillin rash from a hypersensitivity reaction. Ampicillin rash occurs in 5% to 10% of children receiving ampicillin and is a generalized dull red, maculopapular rash, generally appearing 3-14 days after the start of therapy. It normally begins on the trunk and spreads over most of the body. It may be most intense at pressure areas, elbows, and knees. Prolonged use may result in fungal or bacterial superinfection, including *C. difficile*-associated diarrhea (CDAD) and pseudomembranous colitis; CDAD has been observed >2 months postantibiotic treatment.

Adverse Reactions Frequency not defined.

Central nervous system: Fever, penicillin encephalopathy, seizure

Dermatologic: Erythema multiforme, exfoliative dermatitis, rash, urticaria

Note: Appearance of a rash should be carefully evaluated to differentiate (if possible) nonallergic ampicillin rash from hypersensitivity reaction. Incidence is higher in patients with viral infection, *Salmonella* infection, lymphocytic leukemia, or patients that have hyperuricemia.

Gastrointestinal: Black hairy tongue, diarrhea, enterocolitis, glossitis, nausea, pseudomembranous colitis, sore mouth or tongue, stomatitis, vomiting, oral candidiasis

Hematologic: Agranulocytosis, anemia, hemolytic anemia, eosinophilia, leukopenia, thrombocytopenia purpura

Hepatic: AST increased

Renal: Interstitial nephritis (rare)

Respiratory: Laryngeal stridor

Miscellaneous: Anaphylaxis, serum sickness-like reaction

Drug Interactions

Avoid Concomitant Use There are no known interactions where it is recommended to avoid concomitant use.

Increased Effect/Toxicity

Ampicillin may increase the levels/effects of: Methotrexate

The levels/effects of Ampicillin may be increased by: Allopurinol; Uricosuric Agents

Decreased Effect

Ampicillin may decrease the levels/effects of: Atenolol; Typhoid Vaccine

The levels/effects of Ampicillin may be decreased by: Fusidic Acid; Tetracycline Derivatives

Ethanol/Nutrition/Herb Interactions Food: Food decreases ampicillin absorption rate; may decrease ampicillin serum concentration.

Stability

Oral: Oral suspension is stable for 7 days at room temperature or for 14 days under refrigeration.

I.V.:

I.V. minimum volume: Concentration should not exceed 30 mg/mL due to concentration-dependent stability restrictions. Solutions for I.M. or direct I.V. should be used within 1 hour. Solutions for I.V. infusion will be inactivated by dextrose at room temperature. If dextrose-containing solutions are to be used, the resultant solution will only be stable for 2 hours versus 8 hours in the 0.9% sodium chloride injection. D_5W has limited stability.

Stability of parenteral admixture in NS at room temperature (25°C) is 8 hours.

Stability of parenteral admixture in NS at refrigeration temperature (4°C) is 2 days.

Standard diluent: 500 mg/50 mL NS; 1 g/50 mL NS; 2 g/100 mL NS

Mechanism of Action Inhibits bacterial cell wall synthesis by binding to one or more of the penicillin-binding proteins (PBPs) which in turn inhibits the final transpeptidation step of peptidoglycan synthesis in bacterial cell walls, thus inhibiting cell wall biosynthesis. Bacteria eventually lyse due to ongoing activity of cell wall autolytic enzymes (autolysins and murein hydrolases) while cell wall assembly is arrested.

Pharmacodynamics/Kinetics

Absorption: Oral: 50%

Distribution: Bile, blister, and tissue fluids; penetration into CSF occurs with inflamed meninges only, good only with inflammation (exceeds usual MICs)

Normal meninges: Nil; Inflamed meninges: 5% to 10%

Protein binding: 15% to 25%

Half-life elimination:

Children and Adults: 1-1.8 hours

Anuria/end-stage renal disease: 7-20 hours

Time to peak: Oral: Within 1-2 hours

Excretion: Urine (~90% as unchanged drug) within 24 hours

Dosage

Usual dosage range:

Infants and Children:

Oral: 50-100 mg/kg/day in doses divided every 6 hours (maximum: 2-4 g/day)

I.M., I.V.: 100-400 mg/kg/day in divided doses every 6 hours (maximum: 12 g/day)

Adults: Oral, I.M., I.V.: 250-500 mg every 6 hours

Indication-specific dosing:

Infants and Children:

Prophylaxis against infective endocarditis:

Dental, oral, or respiratory tract procedures: I.M., I.V.: 50 mg/kg within 30-60 minutes prior to procedure in patients not allergic to penicillin and unable to take oral amoxicillin. Intramuscular injections should be avoided in patients who are receiving anticoagulant therapy. In these circumstances, orally administered regimens should be given whenever possible. Intravenously administered antibiotics should be used for patients who are unable to tolerate or absorb oral medications.

Note: American Heart Association (AHA) guidelines now recommend prophylaxis only in patients undergoing invasive procedures and in whom underlying cardiac conditions may predispose to a higher risk of adverse outcomes should infection occur.

Genitourinary and gastrointestinal tract procedures: I.M., I.V.:

High-risk patients: 50 mg/kg (maximum: 2 g) within 30 minutes prior to procedure, followed by ampicillin 25 mg/kg (or amoxicillin 25 mg/kg orally) 6 hours later; must be used in combination with gentamicin. **Note:** As of April 2007, routine prophylaxis for GI/GU procedures is no longer recommended by the AHA.

Moderate-risk patients: 50 mg/kg within 30 minutes prior to procedure

Mild-to-moderate infections:

Oral: 50-100 mg/kg/day in doses divided every 6 hours (maximum: 2-4 g/day)

I.M., I.V.: 100-150 mg/kg/day in divided doses every 6 hours (maximum: 2-4 g/day)

Severe infections, meningitis: I.M., I.V.: 200-400 mg/kg/day in divided doses every 6 hours (maximum: 6-12 g/day)

Adults:

Actinomycosis: I.V.: 50 mg/kg/day for 4-6 weeks then oral amoxicillin

Cholangitis (acute): I.V.: 2 g every 4 hours with gentamicin

Diverticulitis: I.M., I.V.: 2 g every 6 hours with metronidazole

Endocarditis:

Infective: I.V.: 12 g/day via continuous infusion or divided every 4 hours

Prophylaxis: Dental, oral, or respiratory tract: I.M., I.V.: 2 g within 30-60 minutes prior to procedure in patients not allergic to penicillin and unable to take oral amoxicillin. Intramuscular injections should be avoided in patients who are receiving anticoagulant therapy. In these circumstances, orally administered regimens should be given whenever possible. Intravenously administered antibiotics should be used for patients who are unable to tolerate or absorb oral medications.

Note: American Heart Association (AHA) guidelines now recommend prophylaxis only in patients undergoing invasive procedures and in whom underlying cardiac conditions may predispose to a higher risk of adverse outcomes should infection occur.

Prophylaxis in total joint replacement patient: I.M., I.V.: 2 g 1 hour prior to the procedure

Genitourinary and gastrointestinal tract procedures:

High-risk patients: I.M., I.V.: 2 g within 30 minutes prior to procedure, followed by ampicillin 1 g (or amoxicillin 1g orally) 6 hours later; must be used in combination with gentamicin. **Note:** As of April 2007, routine prophylaxis for GI/GU procedures is no longer recommended by the AHA.

Moderate-risk patients: I.M., I.V.: 2 g within 30 minutes prior to procedure

Group B strep prophylaxis (intrapartum): I.V.: 2 g initial dose, then 1 g every 4 hours until delivery

***Listeria* infections:** I.V.: 2 g every 4 hours (consider addition of aminoglycoside)

Sepsis/meningitis: I.M., I.V.: 150-250 mg/kg/day divided every 3-4 hours (range: 6-12 g/day)

Urinary tract infections (enterococcus suspected): I.V.: 1-2 g every 6 hours with gentamicin

Dosing interval in renal impairment:

Cl_{cr} >50 mL/minute: Administer every 6 hours

Cl_{cr} 10-50 mL/minute: Administer every 6-12 hours

Cl_{cr} <10 mL/minute: Administer every 12-24 hours

Hemodialysis: Moderately dialyzable (20% to 50%); administer dose after dialysis

Peritoneal dialysis: Moderately dialyzable (20% to 50%) Administer 250 mg every 12 hours

Continuous arteriovenous or venovenous hemofiltration effects: Dose as for Cl_{cr} 10-50 mL/minute; ~50 mg of ampicillin per liter of filtrate is removed

Dietary Considerations Take on an empty stomach 1 hour before or 2 hours after meals.

Sodium content of 5 mL suspension (250 mg/5 mL): 10 mg (0.4 mEq)

Sodium content of 1 g: 66.7 mg (3 mEq)

Administration Administer around-the-clock to promote less variation in peak and trough serum levels.

Oral: Administer on an empty stomach (ie, 1 hour prior to, or 2 hours after meals) to increase total absorption.

I.V.: Administer over 3-5 minutes (125-500 mg) or over 10-15 minutes (1-2 g). More rapid infusion may cause seizures. Ampicillin and gentamicin should not be mixed in the same I.V. tubing.

Some penicillins (eg, carbenicillin, ticarcillin, and piperacillin) have been shown to inactivate aminoglycosides *in vitro*. This has been observed to a greater extent with tobramycin and gentamicin, while amikacin has shown greater stability against inactivation. Concurrent use of these agents may pose a risk of reduced antibacterial efficacy *in vivo*, particularly in the setting of profound renal impairment. However, definitive clinical evidence is lacking. If combination penicillin/aminoglycoside therapy is desired in a patient with renal dysfunction, separation of doses (if feasible), and routine monitoring of aminoglycoside levels, CBC, and clinical response should be considered.

Monitoring Parameters With prolonged therapy, monitor renal, hepatic, and hematologic function periodically; observe signs and symptoms of anaphylaxis during first dose

Test Interactions May interfere with urinary glucose tests using cupric sulfate (Benedict's solution, Clinitest®)

Some penicillin derivatives may accelerate the degradation of aminoglycosides *in vitro*, leading to a potential underestimation of aminoglycoside serum concentration.

Dosage Forms Excipient information presented when available (limited, particularly for generics); consult specific product labeling.

Capsule: 250 mg, 500 mg

Injection, powder for reconstitution, as sodium: 125 mg, 250 mg, 500 mg, 1 g, 2 g, 10 g

Powder for oral suspension: 125 mg/5 mL (100 mL, 200 mL); 250 mg/5 mL (100 mL, 200 mL)

Ampicillin and Sulbactam

(am pi SIL in & SUL bak tam)

U.S. Brand Names Unasyn®

Canadian Brand Names Unasyn®

Index Terms Sulbactam and Ampicillin

Pharmacologic Category Antibiotic, Penicillin

Additional Appendix Information

Antibiotic Treatment of Adults With Infective Endocarditis *on page 1748*

Antimicrobial Drugs of Choice *on page 1752*

Community-Acquired Pneumonia in Adults *on page 1766*

Treatment of Sexually Transmitted Infections *on page 1773*

Use Treatment of susceptible bacterial infections involved with skin and skin structure, intra-abdominal infections, gynecological infections; spectrum is that of ampicillin plus organisms producing beta-lactamases such as *S. aureus*, *H. influenzae*, *E. coli*, *Klebsiella*, *Acinetobacter*, *Enterobacter*, and anaerobes

Pregnancy Risk Factor B

Pregnancy Considerations Adverse events have not been observed in animal studies; therefore, ampicillin/sulbactam is classified as pregnancy category B. Both ampicillin and sulbactam cross the placenta. When used during pregnancy, pharmacokinetic changes have been observed with ampicillin alone (refer to the Ampicillin monograph for details).

Lactation Enters breast milk/use caution

Contraindications Hypersensitivity to ampicillin, sulbactam, penicillins, or any component of the formulations

Warnings/Precautions Dosage adjustment may be necessary in patients with renal impairment. Serious and occasionally severe or fatal hypersensitivity (anaphylactoid) reactions have been reported in patients on penicillin therapy, especially with a history of beta-lactam hypersensitivity, history of sensitivity to multiple allergens, or previous IgE-mediated reactions (eg, anaphylaxis, angioedema, urticaria). Use with caution in asthmatic patients.

High percentage of patients with infectious mononucleosis have developed rash during therapy with ampicillin; ampicillin-class antibiotics not recommended in these patients. Appearance of a rash should be carefully evaluated to differentiate a nonallergic ampicillin rash from a hypersensitivity reaction. Prolonged use may result in fungal or bacterial superinfection, including *C. difficile*-associated diarrhea (CDAD) and pseudomembranous colitis; CDAD has been observed >2 months postantibiotic treatment. Safety and efficacy have not been established in children <1 year of age.

Adverse Reactions Also see Ampicillin.

>10%: Local: Pain at injection site (I.M.)

1% to 10%:

Dermatologic: Rash

Gastrointestinal: Diarrhea

Local: Pain at injection site (I.V.), thrombophlebitis

Miscellaneous: Allergic reaction (may include serum sickness, urticaria, bronchospasm, hypotension, etc)

<1% (Limited to important or life-threatening): Abdominal distension, candidiasis, chest pain, chills, dysuria, edema, epistaxis, erythema, facial swelling, fatigue, flatulence, glossitis, hairy tongue, headache, interstitial nephritis, itching, liver enzymes increased, malaise, mucosal bleeding, nausea, pseudomembranous colitis, seizure, substernal pain, throat tightness, thrombocytopenia, urine retention, vomiting

Drug Interactions

Avoid Concomitant Use There are no known interactions where it is recommended to avoid concomitant use.

Increased Effect/Toxicity

Ampicillin and Sulbactam may increase the levels/effects of: Methotrexate

The levels/effects of Ampicillin and Sulbactam may be increased by: Allopurinol; Uricosuric Agents

Decreased Effect

Ampicillin and Sulbactam may decrease the levels/effects of: Atenolol; Typhoid Vaccine

The levels/effects of Ampicillin and Sulbactam may be decreased by: Fusidic Acid; Tetracycline Derivatives

Stability Prior to reconstitution, store at ≤30°C (86°F).

I.M. and direct I.V. administration: Use within 1 hour after preparation. Reconstitute with sterile water for injection or 0.5% or 2% lidocaine hydrochloride injection (I.M.). Sodium chloride 0.9% (NS) is the diluent of choice for I.V. piggyback use. Solutions made in NS are stable up to 72 hours when refrigerated whereas dextrose solutions (same concentration) are stable for only 4 hours.

Mechanism of Action The addition of sulbactam, a beta-lactamase inhibitor, to ampicillin extends the spectrum of ampicillin to include some beta-lactamase-producing organisms; inhibits bacterial cell wall synthesis by binding to one or more of the penicillin-binding proteins (PBPs) which in turn inhibits the final transpeptidation step of peptidoglycan synthesis in bacterial cell walls, thus inhibiting cell wall biosynthesis. Bacteria eventually lyse due to ongoing activity of cell wall autolytic enzymes (autolysins and murein hydrolases) while cell wall assembly is arrested.

Pharmacodynamics/Kinetics

Ampicillin: See Ampicillin.

Sulbactam:

Distribution: Bile, blister, and tissue fluids

Protein binding: 38%

Half-life elimination: Normal renal function: 1-1.3 hours

Excretion: Urine (~75% to 85% as unchanged drug) within 8 hours

Dosage Note: Unasyn® (ampicillin/sulbactam) is a combination product. Dosage recommendations for Unasyn® are based on the ampicillin component.

Usual dosage range:

Children ≥1 year: I.V.: 100-400 mg ampicillin/kg/day divided every 6 hours (maximum: 8 g ampicillin/day, 12 g Unasyn®). **Note:** The American Academy of Pediatrics recommends a dose of up to 300 mg/kg/day for severe infection in infants >1 month of age.

Adults: I.M., I.V.: 1-2 g ampicillin (1.5-3 g Unasyn®) every 6 hours (maximum: 8 g ampicillin/day, 12 g Unasyn®)

Indication-specific dosing:

Children:

Epiglottitis: I.V.: 100-200 mg ampicillin/kg/day divided in 4 doses

Mild-to-moderate infections: I.M., I.V.: 100-200 mg ampicillin/kg/day (150-300 mg Unasyn®) divided every 6 hours (maximum: 8 g ampicillin/day, 12 g Unasyn®)

Peritonsillar and retropharyngeal abscess: I.V.: 50 mg ampicillin/kg/dose every 6 hours

Severe infections: I.M., I.V.: 200-400 mg ampicillin/kg/day divided every 6 hours (maximum: 8 g ampicillin/day, 12 g Unasyn®)

Adults: Doses expressed as ampicillin/sulbactam combination:

Amnionitis, cholangitis, diverticulitis, endometritis, endophthalmitis, epididymitis/orchitis, liver abscess, osteomyelitis (diabetic foot), peritonitis: I.V.: 3 g every 6 hours

Endocarditis: I.V.: 3 g every 6 hours with gentamicin or vancomycin for 4-6 weeks

Orbital cellulitis: I.V.: 1.5 g every 6 hours

Parapharyngeal space infections: I.V.: 3 g every 6 hours

Pasteurella multocida **(human, canine/feline bites):** I.V.: 1.5-3 g every 6 hours

Pelvic inflammatory disease: I.V.: 3 g every 6 hours with doxycycline

Peritonitis (CAPD): Intraperitoneal:

Anuric, intermittent: 3 g every 12 hours

Anuric, continuous: Loading dose: 1.5 g; maintenance dose: 150 mg

Pneumonia:

Aspiration, community-acquired: I.V.: 1.5-3 g every 6 hours

Hospital-acquired: I.V.: 3 g every 6 hours

Urinary tract infections, pyelonephritis: I.V.: 3 g every 6 hours for 14 days

Dosing interval in renal impairment:

Cl_{cr} 15-29 mL/minute: Administer every 12 hours

Cl_{cr} 5-14 mL/minute and hemodialysis: Administer every 24 hours; give dose after dialysis

Continuous ambulatory peritoneal dialysis (CAPD): 3 g every 24 hours

Continuous renal replacement therapy (CRRT): Drug clearance is highly dependent on the method of renal replacement, filter type, and flow rate. Appropriate dosing requires close monitoring of pharmacologic response, signs of adverse reactions due to drug accumulation, as well as drug levels in relation to target trough (if appropriate). The following are general recommendations only (based on dialysate flow/ultrafiltration rates of 1 L/hour) and should not supersede clinical judgment:

CVVH: 3 g every 12 hours

CVVHD/CVVHDF: 3 g every 8 hours

Dietary Considerations Sodium content of 1.5 g injection: 115 mg (5 mEq)

Administration Administer around-the-clock to promote less variation in peak and trough serum levels. Administer by slow injection over 10-15 minutes or I.V. over 15-30 minutes. Ampicillin and gentamicin should not be mixed in the same I.V. tubing.

Some penicillins (eg, carbenicillin, ticarcillin, and piperacillin) have been shown to inactivate aminoglycosides *in vitro*. This has been observed to a greater extent with tobramycin and gentamicin, while amikacin has shown greater stability against inactivation. Concurrent use of these agents may pose a risk of reduced antibacterial efficacy *in vivo*, particularly in the setting of profound renal impairment. However, definitive clinical evidence is lacking. If combination penicillin/aminoglycoside therapy is desired in a patient with renal dysfunction, separation of doses (if feasible), and routine monitoring of aminoglycoside levels, CBC, and clinical response should be considered.

Monitoring Parameters With prolonged therapy, monitor hematologic, renal, and hepatic function; monitor for signs of anaphylaxis during first dose

Test Interactions May interfere with urinary glucose tests using cupric sulfate (Benedict's solution, Clinitest®).

Some penicillin derivatives may accelerate the degradation of aminoglycosides *in vitro*, leading to a potential underestimation of aminoglycoside serum concentration.

Dosage Forms Excipient information presented when available (limited, particularly for generics); consult specific product labeling.

Injection, powder for reconstitution: 1.5 g: Ampicillin 1 g and sulbactam 0.5 g [contains sodium 115 mg (5 mEq)/1.5 g)]; 3 g: Ampicillin 2 g and sulbactam 1 g [contains sodium 115 mg (5 mEq)/1.5 g)]; 15 g: Ampicillin 10 g and sulbactam 5 g [bulk package; contains sodium 115 mg (5 mEq)/1.5 g]

Unasyn®:

1.5 g: Ampicillin 1 g and sulbactam 0.5 g [contains sodium 115 mg (5 mEq)/1.5 g)]

3 g: Ampicillin 2 g and sulbactam 1 g [contains sodium 115 mg (5 mEq)/1.5 g)]

15 g: Ampicillin 10 g and sulbactam 5 g [bulk package; contains sodium 115 mg (5 mEq)/1.5 g)]

◆ **Ampicillin Sodium** *see* Ampicillin *on page 109*

◆ **Ampicillin Trihydrate** *see* Ampicillin *on page 109*

Amprenavir (am PREN a veer)

U.S. Brand Names Agenerase® [DSC]

Canadian Brand Names Agenerase®

Pharmacologic Category Antiretroviral Agent, Protease Inhibitor

Additional Appendix Information

Antiretroviral Therapy for HIV Infection: Adults and Adolescents *on page 1758*

Perinatal HIV Guidelines *on page 1730*

Use Treatment of HIV infections in combination with at least two other antiretroviral agents; oral solution should only be used when capsules or other protease inhibitors are not therapeutic options

Pregnancy Risk Factor C

Pregnancy Considerations It is not known if amprenavir crosses the human placenta and there are no clinical studies currently underway to evaluate its use in pregnant women. Use of oral solution is contraindicated during pregnancy. Pregnancy and protease inhibitors are both associated with an increased risk of hyperglycemia. Glucose levels should be closely monitored. Health professionals are encouraged to contact the antiretroviral pregnancy registry to monitor outcomes of pregnant women exposed to antiretroviral medications (1-800-258-4263 or www.APRegistry.com).

Lactation Excretion in breast milk unknown/contraindicated

Contraindications Hypersensitivity to amprenavir or any component of the formulation; concurrent therapy with cisapride, ergot derivatives, midazolam, pimozide, and triazolam; severe previous allergic reaction to sulfonamides; oral solution is contraindicated in infants or children <4 years of age, pregnant women, patients with renal or hepatic failure, and patients receiving concurrent metronidazole or disulfiram

Warnings/Precautions Use with caution in patients taking strong CYP3A4 inhibitors, moderate or strong CYP3A4 inducers and major CYP3A4 substrates (see Drug Interactions); consider alternative agents that avoid or lessen the potential for CYP-mediated interactions. New onset or worsening diabetes mellitus and hyperglycemia have been reported, including cases of diabetic ketoacidosis; use with caution in patients with impaired glucose control. Use with caution in patients with sulfonamide allergy, hepatic impairment, or hemophilia. Redistribution of fat may occur (eg, buffalo hump, peripheral wasting, cushingoid appearance). Immune reconstitution syndrome may develop resulting in the occurrence of an inflammatory response to an indolent or residual opportunistic infection; further evaluation and treatment may be required.

Protease inhibitors have been associated with a variety of hypersensitivity events (some severe), including rash, anaphylaxis (rare), angioedema, bronchospasm, erythema multiforme, and/or Stevens-Johnson syndrome (rare). It is generally recommended to discontinue treatment if severe rash or moderate symptoms accompanied by other systemic symptoms occur.

Amprenavir formulations contain vitamin E; additional vitamin E supplements should be avoided. **[U.S. Boxed Warning]: Certain ethnic populations (Asians, Eskimos, Native Americans) may be at increased risk of propylene glycol-associated adverse effects; therefore, use of the oral solution of amprenavir should be avoided.** Use oral solution only when capsules or other protease inhibitors are not options. Safety and efficacy in children <4 years of age have not been established.

Adverse Reactions

>10%:

Central nervous system: Depression/mood disorder (9% to 16%), paresthesia (peripheral 10% to 14%)

Dermatologic: Rash (20% to 27%)

Endocrine & metabolic: Hyperglycemia (>160 mg/dL: 37% to 41%), hypertriglyceridemia (>399 mg/dL: 36% to 47%; >750 mg/dL: 8% to 13%)

Gastrointestinal: Nausea (43% to 74%), vomiting (24% to 34%), diarrhea (39% to 60%), abdominal symptoms

Miscellaneous: Perioral tingling/numbness (26% to 31%)

1% to 10%:

Central nervous system: Headache, fatigue

Dermatologic: Stevens-Johnson syndrome (1% of total, 4% of patients who develop a rash)

Endocrine & metabolic: Hypercholesterolemia (>260 mg/dL: 4% to 9%), hyperglycemia (>251 mg/dL: 2% to 3%), fat redistribution

Gastrointestinal: Taste disorders (2% to 10%), amylase increased (3% to 4%)

Hepatic: AST increased (3% to 5%), ALT increased (4%)

<1% (Limited to important or life-threatening): New-onset diabetes

Drug Interactions

Metabolism/Transport Effects **Substrate** of CYP2C9 (minor), 3A4 (major); **Inhibits** CYP2C19 (weak), 3A4 (strong)

Avoid Concomitant Use

Avoid concomitant use of Amprenavir with any of the following: Alcohol (Ethyl); Alfuzosin; Amiodarone; Cisapride; Delavirdine; Disulfiram; Eplerenone; Ergot Derivatives; MetroNIDAZOLE; Nilotinib; Nisoldipine; Pimozide; QuiNIDine; Ranolazine; Rivaroxaban; Salmeterol; Silodosin; St Johns Wort

Increased Effect/Toxicity

Amprenavir may increase the levels/effects of: Alfuzosin; Alosetron; Amiodarone; Antifungal Agents (Azole Derivatives, Systemic); Benzodiazepines (metabolized by oxidation); Calcium Channel Blockers (Dihydropyridine); Calcium Channel Blockers (Nondihydropyridine); CarBAMazepine; Ciclesonide; Cisapride; Clarithromycin; Corticosteroids (Orally Inhaled); CycloSPORINE; CYP3A4 Substrates; Digoxin; Enfuvirtide; Eplerenone; Ergot Derivatives; FentaNYL; Fesoterodine; Fusidic Acid; HMG-CoA Reductase Inhibitors; Ixabepilone; Maraviroc; Meperidine; Methadone; Nefazodone; Nilotinib; Nisoldipine; Phosphodiesterase 5 Inhibitors; Pimecrolimus; Pimozide; Protease Inhibitors; QuiNIDine; Ranolazine; Rifamycin Derivatives; Rivaroxaban; Salmeterol; Silodosin; Sirolimus; Sorafenib; Tacrolimus; Temsirolimus; Tenofovir; TraZODone; Tricyclic Antidepressants

The levels/effects of Amprenavir may be increased by: Alcohol (Ethyl); Antifungal Agents (Azole Derivatives, Systemic); Clarithromycin; CycloSPORINE; CYP3A4 Inhibitors (Moderate); CYP3A4 Inhibitors (Strong); Dasatinib; Delavirdine; Disulfiram; Efavirenz; Enfuvirtide; Fusidic Acid; MetroNIDAZOLE; P-Glycoprotein Inhibitors; Phenytoin

Decreased Effect

Amprenavir may decrease the levels/effects of: Abacavir; Clarithromycin; Delavirdine; Meperidine; Oral Contraceptive (Estrogens); PARoxetine; Phenytoin; Valproic Acid; Zidovudine

The levels/effects of Amprenavir may be decreased by: Antacids; CarBAMazepine; CYP3A4 Inducers (Strong); Deferasirox; Efavirenz; Garlic; Nevirapine; Oral Contraceptive (Estrogens); P-Glycoprotein Inducers; Rifamycin Derivatives; St Johns Wort; Tenofovir

Ethanol/Nutrition/Herb Interactions

Ethanol: Avoid ethanol with amprenavir oral solution.

Food: Levels increased sixfold with high-fat meals.

Herb/Nutraceutical: Amprenavir serum concentration may be decreased by St John's wort; avoid concurrent use. Formulations contain vitamin E; avoid additional supplements.

Mechanism of Action Binds to the protease activity site and inhibits the activity of the enzyme. HIV protease is required for the cleavage of viral polyprotein precursors into individual functional proteins found in infectious HIV. Inhibition prevents cleavage of these polyproteins, resulting in the formation of immature, noninfectious viral particles.

Pharmacodynamics/Kinetics

Absorption: 63%

Distribution: 430 L

Protein binding: 90%

Metabolism: Hepatic via CYP (primarily CYP3A4)

Bioavailability: Not established; increased sixfold with high-fat meal; oral solution: 86% relative to capsule formulation (14% less bioavailable than capsule)

Half-life elimination: 7.1-10.6 hours

Time to peak: 1-2 hours

Excretion: Feces (75%, ~68% as metabolites); urine (14% as metabolites)

Dosage Oral: **Note:** Capsule and oral solution are **not** interchangeable on a mg-per-mg basis.

Capsule:

Children 4-12 years **or** 13-16 years (<50 kg): 20 mg/kg twice daily or 15 mg/kg 3 times daily; maximum: 2400 mg/day

Children >13 years (≥50 kg) and Adults: 1200 mg twice daily

Note: Dosage adjustments for amprenavir when administered in combination therapy:

Efavirenz: Adjustments necessary for both agents:

Amprenavir 1200 mg 3 times/day (single protease inhibitor) **or**

Amprenavir 1200 mg twice daily plus ritonavir 200 mg twice daily

Ritonavir: Adjustments necessary for both agents:

Amprenavir 1200 mg plus ritonavir 200 mg once daily **or**

Amprenavir 600 mg plus ritonavir 100 mg twice daily

Note: Oral solution of ritonavir and amprenavir should not be coadministered.

Solution:

Children 4-12 years **or** 13-16 years (<50 kg): 22.5 mg/kg twice daily or 17 mg/kg 3 times daily; maximum: 2800 mg/day

Children >13 years (≥50 kg) and Adults: 1400 mg twice daily

Dosage adjustment in renal impairment: Oral solution is contraindicated in renal failure.

Dosage adjustment in hepatic impairment:

Child-Pugh score between 5-8:

Capsule: 450 mg twice daily

Solution: 513 mg twice daily; contraindicated in hepatic failure

Child-Pugh score between 9-12:

Capsule: 300 mg twice daily

Solution: 342 mg twice daily; contraindicated in hepatic failure

Dietary Considerations May be taken with or without food; do not take with high-fat meal. The 50 mg capsules contain 36.3 int. units of vitamin E per capsule; oral solution contains 46 int. units of vitamin E per mL; avoid additional vitamin E-containing supplements.

Additional Information Propylene glycol is included in the oral solution; a dose of 22.5 mg/kg twice daily corresponds to an intake of 1650 mg/kg of propylene glycol. Capsule and oral solution are not interchangeable on a mg-per-mg basis.

Dosage Forms Excipient information presented when available (limited, particularly for generics); consult specific product labeling. [DSC] = Discontinued product

Capsule:

Agenerase®: 50 mg [contains vitamin E 36.3 int. units (as TPGS)] [DSC]

Solution, oral:

Agenerase®: 15 mg/mL (240 mL) [contains propylene glycol 550 mg/mL and vitamin E 46 int. units/mL; grape-bubble gum-peppermint flavor] [DSC]

◆ **AMPT** *see* Metyrosine *on page* 986

◆ **Amrinone Lactate** *see* Inamrinone *on page* 781

◆ **Amrix®** *see* Cyclobenzaprine *on page* 375

Amyl Nitrite (AM il NYE trite)

Index Terms Isoamyl Nitrite

Pharmacologic Category Antidote; Vasodilator

Use Coronary vasodilator in angina pectoris; adjunct in treatment of cyanide poisoning; produce changes in the intensity of heart murmurs

Pregnancy Risk Factor C

Dosage Nasal inhalation:

Cyanide poisoning: Children and Adults: Inhale the vapor from a 0.3 mL crushed ampul every minute for 15-30 seconds until I.V. sodium nitrite infusion is available

Angina: Adults: 1-6 inhalations from 1 crushed ampul; may repeat in 3-5 minutes

Additional Information Complete prescribing information for this medication should be consulted for additional detail.

Dosage Forms Excipient information presented when available (limited, particularly for generics); consult specific product labeling.

Vapor for inhalation [crushable covered glass capsules]: Amyl nitrite USP (0.3 mL)

- **Amylobarbitone** *see* Amobarbital *on page 96*
- **Amytal®** *see* Amobarbital *on page 96*
- **AN100226** *see* Natalizumab *on page 1044*
- **Anadrol®-50** *see* Oxymetholone *on page 1123*
- **Anafranil®** *see* ClomiPRAMINE *on page 350*

Anagrelide (an AG gre lide)

U.S. Brand Names Agrylin®

Canadian Brand Names Agrylin®; Dom-Anagrelide; Gen-Anagrelide; PHL-Anagrelide; PMS-Anagrelide; Sandoz-Anagrelide

Index Terms Anagrelide Hydrochloride; BL4162A; NSC-724577

Pharmacologic Category Phospholipase A_2 Inhibitor

Use Treatment of thrombocythemia associated with myeloproliferative disorders

Unlabeled/Investigational Use Treatment of essential thrombocythemia (ET)

Pregnancy Risk Factor C

Dosage Note: Maintain for ≥1 week, then adjust to the lowest effective dose to reduce and maintain platelet count <600,000/μL ideally to the normal range; the dose must not be increased by >0.5 mg/day in any 1 week; maximum dose: 10 mg/day or 2.5 mg/dose

Oral: Thrombocythemia:

Children: Initial: 0.5 mg/day (range: 0.5 mg 1-4 times/day)

Adults: 0.5 mg 4 times/day or 1 mg twice daily (most patients will experience adequate response at dose ranges of 1.5-3 mg/day)

Elderly: There are no special requirements for dosing in the elderly

Dosage adjustment in hepatic impairment:

Moderate impairment: Initial: 0.5 mg once daily; maintain for at least 1 week with careful monitoring of cardiovascular status; the dose must not be increased by >0.5 mg/day in any 1 week.

Severe impairment: Contraindicated

Additional Information Complete prescribing information for this medication should be consulted for additional detail.

Dosage Forms Excipient information presented when available (limited, particularly for generics); consult specific product labeling.

Capsule: 0.5 mg, 1 mg

Agrylin®: 0.5 mg

- **Anagrelide Hydrochloride** *see* Anagrelide *on page 115*

Anakinra (an a KIN ra)

U.S. Brand Names Kineret®

Canadian Brand Names Kineret®

Index Terms IL-1Ra; Interleukin-1 Receptor Antagonist

Pharmacologic Category Antirheumatic, Disease Modifying; Interleukin-1 Receptor Antagonist

Use Treatment of moderately- to severely-active rheumatoid arthritis in adult patients who have failed one or more disease-modifying antirheumatic drugs (DMARDs); may be used alone or in combination with DMARDs (other than tumor necrosis factor-blocking agents)

Pregnancy Risk Factor B

Pregnancy Considerations No evidence of impaired fertility or harm to fetus in animal models; however, there are no controlled trials in pregnant women. Women exposed to anakinra during pregnancy may contact the Organization of Teratology Information Services (OTIS), Rheumatoid Arthritis and Pregnancy Study at 1-877-311-8972.

Lactation Excretion in breast milk unknown/use caution

Medication Safety Issues

Sound-alike/look-alike issues:

Anakinra may be confused with amikacin

Contraindications Hypersensitivity to *E. coli*-derived proteins, anakinra, or any component of the formulation; patients with active infections (including chronic or local infection)

Warnings/Precautions Anakinra may affect defenses against infections and malignancies. Safety and efficacy in patients with immunosuppression or chronic infections have not been evaluated. Discontinue administration if patient develops a serious infection. Do not start drug administration in patients with an active infection. Patients with asthma may be at an increased risk of serious infections. Should not be used in combination with tumor necrosis factor antagonists, unless no satisfactory alternatives exist, and then only with extreme caution. Impact on the development and course of malignancies is not fully defined. As compared to the general population, an increased risk of lymphoma has been noted in clinical trials; however, rheumatoid arthritis has been previously associated with an increased rate of lymphoma.

Use caution in patients with a history of significant hematologic abnormalities; has been associated with uncommon, but significant decreases in hematologic parameters (particularly neutrophil counts). Patients must be advised to seek medical attention if they develop signs and symptoms suggestive of blood dyscrasias. Discontinue if significant hematologic abnormalities are confirmed.

Patients should be brought up to date with all immunizations before initiating therapy. Live vaccines should not be given concurrently. Patients with a significant exposure to varicella virus should temporarily discontinue anakinra. Hypersensitivity reactions may occur. Impact on the development and course of malignancies is not fully defined. Use caution in patients with renal impairment; consider increased dosing intervals for severe renal dysfunction (Cl_{cr} <30 mL/minute). Use caution in the elderly due to the potential for higher risk of infections. Efficacy has not been established in children; use is not recommended. The packaging (needle cover) contains latex.

Adverse Reactions

>10%:

Central nervous system: Headache (12%)

Local: Injection site reaction (majority mild, typically lasting 14-28 days, characterized by erythema, ecchymosis, inflammation, and pain; up to 71%)

Miscellaneous: Infection (39% versus 37% in placebo; serious infection 2% to 3%)

1% to 10%:

Gastrointestinal: Nausea (8%), diarrhea (7%), abdominal pain (5%)

Hematologic: Neutropenia (8%; grades 3/4: 0.4%)

Respiratory: Sinusitis (7%)

Miscellaneous: Flu-like syndrome (6%)

<1% (Limited to important or life-threatening): Cellulitis, leukopenia, opportunistic infection, malignancies (including lymphoma, melanoma), thrombocytopenia

Drug Interactions

Avoid Concomitant Use

Avoid concomitant use of Anakinra with any of the following: Anti-TNF Agents; Natalizumab; Vaccines (Live)

Increased Effect/Toxicity

Anakinra may increase the levels/effects of: Natalizumab; Vaccines (Live)

The levels/effects of Anakinra may be increased by: Anti-TNF Agents; Trastuzumab

Decreased Effect

Anakinra may decrease the levels/effects of: Vaccines (Inactivated)

The levels/effects of Anakinra may be decreased by: Echinacea

Stability Store in refrigerator at 2°C to 8°C (36°F to 46°F); do not freeze. Do not shake. Protect from light.

Mechanism of Action Antagonist of the interleukin-1 (IL-1) receptor. Endogenous IL-1 is induced by inflammatory stimuli and mediates a variety of immunological responses, including degradation of cartilage (loss of proteoglycans) and stimulation of bone resorption.

Pharmacodynamics/Kinetics

Bioavailability: SubQ: 95%

Half-life elimination: Terminal: 4-6 hours

Time to peak: SubQ: 3-7 hours

Dosage Adults: SubQ: Rheumatoid arthritis: 100 mg once daily (administer at approximately the same time each day)

Dosage adjustment in renal impairment: Cl_{cr} <30 mL/minute and/or end-stage renal disease: 100 mg every other day

Administration Rotate injection sites (thigh, abdomen, upper arm); injection should be given at least 1 inch away from previous injection site. Do not shake. Provided in single-use, preservative free syringes with 27-gauge needles; discard any unused portion.

Monitoring Parameters CBC with differential (baseline, then monthly for 3 months, then every 3 months); serum creatinine

Additional Information Anakinra is produced by recombinant DNA/*E. coli* technology.

Dosage Forms Excipient information presented when available (limited, particularly for generics); consult specific product labeling.

Injection, solution [preservative free]:

Kineret®: 100 mg/0.67 mL (1 mL) [prefilled syringe; needle cover contains latex]

◆ **Analpram-HC®** *see* Pramoxine and Hydrocortisone *on page* 1227

◆ **Anandron® (Can)** *see* Nilutamide *on page* 1068

◆ **Anaprox®** *see* Naproxen *on page* 1041

◆ **Anaprox® DS** *see* Naproxen *on page* 1041

◆ **Anaspaz®** *see* Hyoscyamine *on page* 756

Anastrozole (an AS troe zole)

U.S. Brand Names Arimidex®

Canadian Brand Names Arimidex®

Index Terms ICI-D1033; NSC-719344; ZD1033

Pharmacologic Category Antineoplastic Agent, Aromatase Inhibitor

Use Treatment of locally-advanced or metastatic breast cancer (ER-positive or hormone receptor unknown) in postmenopausal women; treatment of advanced breast cancer in postmenopausal women with disease progression following tamoxifen therapy; adjuvant treatment of early ER-positive breast cancer in postmenopausal women

Pregnancy Risk Factor D

Pregnancy Considerations Fetotoxicity was observed in animal studies. Safety and efficacy have not been established in premenopausal women; exclude pregnancy prior to treatment.

Lactation Excretion in breast milk unknown/use caution

Medication Safety Issues

Sound-alike/look-alike issues:

Anastrozole may be confused with letrozole

Contraindications Hypersensitivity to anastrozole or any component of the formulation; pregnancy

Warnings/Precautions Hazardous agent - use appropriate precautions for handling and disposal. Use with caution in patients with hyperlipidemias; total cholesterol and LDL-cholesterol increase in patients receiving anastrozole; exclude pregnancy before initiating therapy. Anastrozole may be associated with a reduction in bone mineral density. Safety and efficacy in premenopausal women or pediatric patients have not been established.

Adverse Reactions

>10%:

Cardiovascular: Vasodilatation (25% to 36%), hypertension (2% to 13%)

Central nervous system: Mood disturbance (19%), fatigue (19%), pain (11% to 17%), headache (9% to 13%), depression (5% to 13%)

Dermatologic: Rash (6% to 11%)

Endocrine & metabolic: Hot flashes (12% to 36%)

Gastrointestinal: Nausea (11% to 19%), vomiting (8% to 13%)

Neuromuscular & skeletal: Weakness (16% to 19%), arthritis (17%), arthralgia (2% to 15%), back pain (10% to 12%), bone pain (6% to 11%), osteoporosis (11%)

Respiratory: Pharyngitis (6% to 14%), cough increased (8% to 11%)

1% to 10%:

Cardiovascular: Peripheral edema (5% to 10%), chest pain (5% to 7%), ischemic cardiovascular disease (4%), venous thromboembolic events (3% to 4%), ischemic cerebrovascular events (2%), angina (2%)

Central nervous system: Insomnia (2% to 10%), dizziness (6% to 8%), anxiety (2% to 6%), fever (2% to 5%), malaise (2% to 5%), confusion (2% to 5%), nervousness (2% to 5%), somnolence (2% to 5%), lethargy (1%)

Dermatologic: Alopecia (2% to 5%), pruritus (2% to 5%)

Endocrine & metabolic: Hypercholesterolemia (9%), breast pain (2% to 8%)

Gastrointestinal: Constipation (7% to 9%), abdominal pain (7% to 9%), diarrhea (8% to 9%), anorexia (5% to 7%), xerostomia (6%), dyspepsia (7%), weight gain (2% to 9%), weight loss (2% to 5%)

Genitourinary: Urinary tract infection (2% to 8%), vulvovaginitis (6%), pelvic pain (5%), vaginal bleeding (1% to 5%), vaginitis (4%), vaginal discharge (4%), vaginal hemorrhage (2% to 4%), leukorrhea (2% to 3%), vaginal dryness (2%)

Hematologic: Anemia (2% to 5%), leukopenia (2% to 5%)

Hepatic: Liver function tests increased (2% to 5%), alkaline phosphatase increased (2% to 5%), gamma GT increased (2% to 5%)

Local: Thrombophlebitis (2% to 5%)

Neuromuscular & skeletal: Fracture (2% to 10%), arthrosis (7%), paresthesia (5% to 7%), joint disorder (6%), myalgia (2% to 6%), neck pain (2% to 5%), hypertonia (3%)

Ocular: Cataracts (6%)

Respiratory: Dyspnea (8% to 10%), sinusitis (2% to 6%), bronchitis (2% to 5%), rhinitis (2% to 5%)

Miscellaneous: Lymph edema (10%), infection (2% to 9%), flu-like syndrome (2% to 7%), diaphoresis (2% to 5%), cyst (5%), tumor flare (3%)

<1% (Limited to important or life-threatening): Anaphylaxis, angioedema, CVA, cerebral ischemia, cerebral infarct, endometrial cancer, erythema multiforme, joint pain, joint stiffness, MI, myocardial ischemia, pulmonary embolus, retinal vein thrombosis, Stevens-Johnson syndrome, urticaria

Drug Interactions

Metabolism/Transport Effects Inhibits CYP1A2 (weak), 2C8 (weak), 2C9 (weak), 3A4 (weak)

Avoid Concomitant Use There are no known interactions where it is recommended to avoid concomitant use.

Increased Effect/Toxicity There are no known significant interactions involving an increase in effect.

Decreased Effect

The levels/effects of Anastrozole may be decreased by: Tamoxifen

Ethanol/Nutrition/Herb Interactions Herb/Nutraceutical: Avoid black cohosh, hops, licorice, red clover, thyme, and dong quai.

Stability Store at 20°C to 25°C (68°F to 77°F).

Mechanism of Action Potent and selective nonsteroidal aromatase inhibitor. By inhibiting aromatase, the conversion of androstenedione to estrone, and testosterone to estradiol, is prevented. Anastrozole causes an 85% decrease in estrone sulfate levels.

Pharmacodynamics/Kinetics

Onset of estradiol reduction: 70% reduction after 24 hours; 80% after 2 weeks therapy

Duration of estradiol reduction: 6 days

Absorption: Well absorbed; not affected by food

Protein binding, plasma: 40%

Metabolism: Extensively hepatic (~85%) via N-dealkylation, hydroxylation, and glucuronidation; primary metabolite inactive

Half-life elimination: ~50 hours

Excretion: Urine (10% as unchanged drug; 60% as metabolites)

Dosage Breast cancer: Adults: Oral (refer to individual protocols): 1 mg once daily

Dosage adjustment in renal impairment: Dosage adjustment not necessary

Dosage adjustment in hepatic impairment: Mild-to-moderate impairment: Plasma concentrations in subjects with stable hepatic cirrhosis were within the range concentrations in normal subjects across all clinical trials; therefore, no dosage adjustment required; however, patients should be monitored for side effects. Safety and efficacy in severe hepatic impairment have not been established.

Monitoring Parameters Bone mineral density; total cholesterol and LDL

Test Interactions Lab test abnormalities: GGT, AST, ALT, alkaline phosphatase, total cholesterol, and LDL increased; threefold elevations of mean serum GGT levels have been observed among patients with liver metastases. These changes were likely related to the progression of liver metastases in these patients, although other contributing factors could not be ruled out. Mean serum total cholesterol levels increased by 0.5 mmol/L among patients.

Dosage Forms Excipient information presented when available (limited, particularly for generics); consult specific product labeling.

Tablet:

Arimidex®: 1 mg

- **Anbesol® [OTC]** *see* Benzocaine *on page 183*
- **Anbesol® Baby [OTC]** *see* Benzocaine *on page 183*
- **Anbesol® Baby (Can)** *see* Benzocaine *on page 183*
- **Anbesol® Cold Sore Therapy [OTC]** *see* Benzocaine *on page 183*
- **Anbesol® Jr. [OTC]** *see* Benzocaine *on page 183*
- **Anbesol® Maximum Strength [OTC]** *see* Benzocaine *on page 183*
- **Ancef** *see* CeFAZolin *on page 269*
- **Ancobon®** *see* Flucytosine *on page 627*
- **Andehist NR Drops [DSC]** *see* Carbinoxamine and Pseudoephedrine *on page 258*
- **Andehist NR Syrup** *see* Brompheniramine and Pseudoephedrine *on page 214*
- **Andriol® (Can)** *see* Testosterone *on page 1445*
- **Androderm®** *see* Testosterone *on page 1445*
- **AndroGel®** *see* Testosterone *on page 1445*
- **Android®** *see* MethylTESTOSTERone *on page 979*
- **Andropository (Can)** *see* Testosterone *on page 1445*
- **Androxy™** *see* Fluoxymesterone *on page 641*
- **Anectine®** *see* Succinylcholine *on page 1402*
- **Anestacon®** *see* Lidocaine *on page 884*
- **Anestafoam™ [OTC]** *see* Lidocaine *on page 884*
- **Aneurine Hydrochloride** *see* Thiamine *on page 1458*
- **Anexate® (Can)** *see* Flumazenil *on page 631*
- **Angiofluor™** *see* Fluorescein *on page 634*
- **Angiofluor™ Lite** *see* Fluorescein *on page 634*
- **Angiomax®** *see* Bivalirudin *on page 201*

Anidulafungin (ay nid yoo la FUN jin)

U.S. Brand Names Eraxis™

Canadian Brand Names Eraxis™

Index Terms LY303366

Pharmacologic Category Antifungal Agent, Parenteral; Echinocandin

Additional Appendix Information

Antifungal Agents *on page 1640*

Use Treatment of candidemia and other forms of *Candida* infections (including those of intra-abdominal, peritoneal, and esophageal locus)

Unlabeled/Investigational Use Treatment of infections due to *Aspergillus* spp.

Pregnancy Risk Factor C

Pregnancy Considerations Skeletal teratogenic effects were noted in animal studies. There are no adequate and well-controlled studies in pregnant women. Use only if benefit outweighs risk.

Lactation Excretion in breast milk unknown/use caution

Contraindications Hypersensitivity to anidulafungin, other echinocandins, or any component of the formulation

Warnings/Precautions Histamine-mediated reactions (eg, urticaria, flushing, hypotension) have been observed; these may be related to infusion rate. Elevated liver function tests, hepatitis, and worsening hepatic failure have been reported. Monitor for progressive hepatic impairment if increased transaminase enzymes noted. Safety and efficacy in pediatric patients, neutropenic patients, or other *Candida* infections (eg, endocarditis, osteomyelitis, meningitis) have not been established.

Adverse Reactions

2% to 10%:

Endocrine & metabolic: Hypokalemia (3%)

Gastrointestinal: Diarrhea (3%)

Hepatic: Transaminase increased (<1% to 2%)

<2% (Limited to important or life-threatening): Abdominal pain, alkaline phosphatase increased, amylase increased, angioneurotic edema, atrial fibrillation, back pain, bilirubin increased, bundle branch block (right), candidiasis, cholestasis, clostridial infection, coagulopathy, constipation, cough, CPK increased, creatinine increased, diaphoresis, diarrhea, dizziness, DVT, dyspepsia, ECG abnormality (including QT prolongation), erythema, eye pain, fecal incontinence, flushing, fungemia, GGT increased, headache, hepatic necrosis, hepatitis, hepatic dysfunction, hot flushes, hypercalcemia, hyperglycemia, hyperkalemia, hypernatremia, hyper-/hypotension, hypomagnesemia, infusion-related

reaction, leukopenia (0.7%), lipase increased, nausea, neutropenia (1%), peripheral edema, phlebitis, platelet count increased, prothrombin time prolonged, pruritus, pyrexia, rash, rigors, seizure, sinus arrhythmia, thrombocytopenia, thrombophlebitis, urea increased, urticaria, ventricular extrasystoles, vision blurred, visual disturbance, vomiting

Drug Interactions

Avoid Concomitant Use There are no known interactions where it is recommended to avoid concomitant use.

Increased Effect/Toxicity There are no known significant interactions involving an increase in effect.

Decreased Effect

Anidulafungin may decrease the levels/effects of: Saccharomyces boulardii

Stability Store between 15°C to 30°C (59°F to 86°F). Aseptically add 15 mL (50 mg vial) or 30 mL (100 mg vial) of companion diluent (20% w/w dehydrated alcohol in water for injection) to each vial. Swirl to dissolve; do not shake. Further dilute 50 mg, 100 mg, or 200 mg in 100 mL, 250 mL, or 500 mL, respectively, of D_5W or NS. Reconstituted and diluted solutions are stable for 24 hours at room temperature. Do not refrigerate or freeze.

Mechanism of Action Noncompetitive inhibitor of 1,3-beta-D-glucan synthase resulting in reduced formation of 1,3-beta-D-glucan, an essential polysaccharide comprising 30% to 60% of *Candida* cell walls (absent in mammalian cells); decreased glucan content leads to osmotic instability and cellular lysis

Pharmacodynamics/Kinetics

Distribution: 30-50 L

Protein binding: 84%

Metabolism: No hepatic metabolism observed; undergoes slow chemical hydrolysis to open-ring peptide-lacking antifungal activity

Half-life elimination: 27 hours

Excretion: Feces (30%, 10% as unchanged drug); urine (<1%)

Dosage I.V.: Adults:

Candidemia, intra-abdominal or peritoneal candidiasis: 200 mg loading dose on day 1, followed by 100 mg daily for at least 14 days after last positive culture

Esophageal candidiasis: 100 mg loading dose on day 1, followed by 50 mg daily for at least 14 days and for at least 7 days after symptom resolution

Dosage adjustment in renal impairment: No adjustment necessary, including dialysis patients

Dosage adjustment in hepatic impairment: No adjustment necessary

Administration For intravenous use only; infusion rate should not exceed 1.1 mg/minute

Monitoring Parameters Liver function tests

Dosage Forms Excipient information presented when available (limited, particularly for generics); consult specific product labeling.

Injection, powder for reconstitution:

Eraxis™: 50 mg [contains polysorbate 80; packaged with dehydrated alcohol as diluent]; 100 mg [contains polysorbate 80; packaged with dehydrated alcohol as diluent]

◆ **Anolor 300** *see* Butalbital, Acetaminophen, and Caffeine *on page* 229

◆ **Ansaid® (Can)** *see* Flurbiprofen *on page* 643

◆ **Ansamycin** *see* Rifabutin *on page* 1314

◆ **Antabuse®** *see* Disulfiram *on page* 469

◆ **Antagon** *see* Ganirelix *on page* 682

◆ **Antara®** *see* Fenofibrate *on page* 607

◆ **Anthraforte® (Can)** *see* Anthralin *on page* 118

Anthralin (AN thra lin)

U.S. Brand Names Dritho-Scalp®; Psoriatec™

Canadian Brand Names Anthraforte®; Anthranol®; Anthrascalp®; Micanol®

Index Terms Dithranol

Pharmacologic Category Antipsoriatic Agent; Keratolytic Agent

Use Treatment of psoriasis (quiescent or chronic psoriasis)

Pregnancy Risk Factor C

Dosage Children (unlabeled) and Adults: Topical: Generally, apply once a day or as directed. The irritant potential of anthralin is directly related to the strength being used and each patient's individual tolerance. Always commence treatment using a short, daily contact time (5-10 minutes) for at least 1 week using the lowest strength possible. Contact time may be gradually increased (to 20-30 minutes) as tolerated.

Skin application: Apply sparingly only to psoriatic lesions and rub gently and carefully into the skin until absorbed. Avoid applying an excessive quantity which may cause unnecessary soiling and staining of the clothing or bed linen.

Scalp application: Comb hair to remove scalar debris, wet hair and, after suitably parting, rub cream well into the lesions, taking care to prevent the cream from spreading onto the forehead.

Remove by washing or showering; optimal period of contact will vary according to the strength used and the patient's response to treatment. Continue treatment until the skin is entirely clear (ie, when there is nothing to feel with the fingers and the texture is normal).

Additional Information Complete prescribing information for this medication should be consulted for additional detail.

Dosage Forms Excipient information presented when available (limited, particularly for generics); consult specific product labeling.

Cream:

Dritho-Scalp®: 0.5% (50 g)

Psoriatec™: 1% (50 g)

◆ **Anthranol® (Can)** *see* Anthralin *on page* 118

◆ **Anthrascalp® (Can)** *see* Anthralin *on page* 118

Anthrax Vaccine Adsorbed
(AN thraks vak SEEN ad SORBED)

U.S. Brand Names BioThrax®

Index Terms AVA

Pharmacologic Category Vaccine, Inactivated (Bacterial)

Use Immunization against *Bacillus anthracis* in persons at high risk for exposure.

The Advisory Committee on Immunization Practices (ACIP) recommends routine vaccination for the following:

- Persons who work directly with the organism in the laboratory
- Persons who may come in contact with animal products which come from anthrax endemic areas and may be contaminated with *Bacillus anthracis* spores, such as veterinarians who travel to other countries or persons who work with imported animal hides/furs from areas where standards are insufficient to prevent anthrax spores.
- Military personnel deployed to areas with high risk of exposure

Routine immunization for the general population is not recommended.

Unlabeled/Investigational Use Postexposure prophylaxis in combination with antibiotics

Restrictions Not commercially available in the U.S.; presently, all anthrax vaccine lots are owned by the U.S. Department of Defense. The Centers for Disease Control (CDC) does not currently recommend routine vaccination of the general public.

Pregnancy Risk Factor D

Pregnancy Considerations Adverse events were not observed in animal developemental toxicity studies. Use during pregnancy only if clearly needed. Data from the Department of Defense suggest the vaccine may be linked with a slightly increased number of birth defects when given during the first trimester of pregnancy. Male fertility is not affected by vaccine administration.

Lactation Excretion in breast milk unknown/use caution

Contraindications Hypersensitivity to anthrax vaccine or any component of the formulation; history of anthrax

Warnings/Precautions Immediate treatment for anaphylactic/anaphylactoid reaction should be available during vaccine use. Defer dosing during acute respiratory disease or other active infection; defer dosing during short-term corticosteroid therapy, chemotherapy, or radiation; additional dose required in patients on long-term corticosteroid therapy; immune response may be decreased with immunodeficiency. Persons with a history of anthrax disease may have an increased risk for adverse reactions from the vaccine. Use with caution in patients with a history of bleeding disorders (including thrombocytopenia) and/or patients on anticoagulant therapy; bleeding/hematoma may occur from I.M. administration. For patients at risk of hemorrhage following intramuscular injection, the vaccine can be administered SubQ. In order to maximize vaccination rates, the ACIP recommends simultaneous administration of all age-appropriate vaccines (live or inactivated) for which a person is eligible at a single clinic visit, unless contraindications exist. Packaging may contain natural latex rubber. Safety and efficacy in children <18 years of age or adults >65 years of age have not been established

Adverse Reactions All serious adverse reactions must be reported to the U.S. Department of Health and Human Services (DHHS) Vaccine Adverse Event Reporting System (VAERS) 1-800-822-7967 or online at https://secure.vaers.org.

Note: Percentages reported with I.M. administration:

>10%:

Central nervous system: Headache (4% to 64%), fatigue (5% to 62%)

Local: Tenderness (10% to 61%), erythema (8% to 31%), pain (4% to 23%), edema (1% to 16%), limitation of arm motion (1% to 16%), induration (3% to 14%), warmth (1% to 11%)

Neuromuscular & skeletal: Myalgia (2% to 72%)

Respiratory: Nasopharyngitis (12% to 15%), pharyngolaryngeal pain (12%)

1% to 10%:

Dermatologic: Pruritus (≤2%), rash (≤2%)

Endocrine & metabolic: Dysmenorrhea (7%)

Gastrointestinal: Diarrhea (6% to 8%), nausea (6%)

Local: Itching (≤9%), bruising (3% to 6%), nodule (1% to 6%)

Neuromuscular & skeletal: Back pain (7% to 9%), neck pain (3%), joint sprain (≤2%), rigors (1% to 2%)

Respiratory: Sinusitis (5% to 7%), upper respiratory tract infection (2% to 3%), sinus headache (1% to 3%)

Miscellaneous: Hypersensitivity (2% to 4%), lymphadenopathy (2% to 3%), flu-like illness (2%), tender/painful axillary adenopathy (≤1%)

Postmarketing and/or case reports: Allergic reactions, alopecia, anaphylactoid reaction, arthralgia, arthropathy, erythema multiforme, injection site reactions (cellulitis), paresthesia, pyrexia, rhabdomyolysis, Stevens-Johnson syndrome, syncope, tremor, ulnar nerve neuropathy

Drug Interactions

Avoid Concomitant Use There are no known interactions where it is recommended to avoid concomitant use.

Increased Effect/Toxicity There are no known significant interactions involving an increase in effect.

Decreased Effect

The levels/effects of Anthrax Vaccine Adsorbed may be decreased by: Immunosuppressants

Stability Store under refrigeration at 2°C to 8°C (36°F to 46°F); do not freeze.

Mechanism of Action Active immunization against *Bacillus anthracis*. The vaccine is prepared from a cell-free filtrate of *B. anthracis*, but no dead or live bacteria. Completion of the entire vaccination series is required for full protection.

Dosage I.M.:

Children <18 years: Safety and efficacy have not been established

Adults:

Primary immunization: Five injections of 0.5 mL each given at 0- and 4 weeks, then 6-, 12-, and 18 months

Subsequent booster injections: 0.5 mL at 1-year intervals are recommended for immunity to be maintained in persons who remain at risk

Elderly: Safety and efficacy have not been established for patients >65 years of age

Administration Shake well before use. Do not use if discolored or contains particulate matter. Do not use the same site for more than one injection. Do not mix with other injections. For I.M. administration; do not inject I.V. or intradermally. For patients at risk of hemorrhage following intramuscular injection, the vaccine can be administered SubQ.

Administration with other vaccines:

Anthrax vaccine with other inactivated vaccines: May be given simultaneously or at any interval between doses.

Anthrax vaccine with live vaccines: May be given simultaneously or at any interval between doses.

Vaccine administration with antibody-containing products: Anthrax vaccine and antibody-containing products may be given simultaneously at different sites or at any interval between doses. Examples of antibody-containing products include I.M. and I.V. immune globulin, hepatitis B immune globulin, tetanus immune globulin, varicella zoster immune globulin, rabies immune globulin, whole blood, packed red cells, plasma, and platelet products.

Monitoring Parameters Monitor for local reactions, chills, fever, anaphylaxis; syncope for ≥15 minutes following vaccination

Additional Information Not commercially available in the U.S.

Federal law requires that the date of administration, the vaccine manufacturer, lot number of vaccine, and the administering person's name, title and address be entered into the patient's permanent medical record.

Dosage Forms Excipient information presented when available (limited, particularly for generics); consult specific product labeling.

Injection, suspension:

BioThrax®: *Bacillus anthracis* proteins (5 mL) [contains aluminum, natural rubber/natural latex in packaging]

◆ **Anti-4 Alpha Integrin** *see* Natalizumab *on page 1044*

◆ **131 I Anti-B1 Antibody** *see* Tositumomab and Iodine I 131 Tositumomab *on page 1495*

◆ **131 I-Anti-B1 Monoclonal Antibody** *see* Tositumomab and Iodine I 131 Tositumomab *on page 1495*

◆ **Anti-CD11a** *see* Efalizumab *on page 507*

◆ **Anti-CD20 Monoclonal Antibody** *see* RiTUXimab *on page 1328*

◆ **Anti-CD20-Murine Monoclonal Antibody I-131** *see* Tositumomab and Iodine I 131 Tositumomab *on page 1495*

◆ **Antidigoxin Fab Fragments, Ovine** *see* Digoxin Immune Fab *on page 446*

◆ **Antidiuretic Hormone** *see* Vasopressin *on page 1552*

Antihemophilic Factor (Human)

(an tee hee moe FIL ik FAK tor HYU man)

U.S. Brand Names Hemofil M; Koāte®-DVI; Monarc-M™; Monoclate-P®

Canadian Brand Names Hemofil M

Index Terms AHF (Human); Factor VIII (Human)

Pharmacologic Category Antihemophilic Agent; Blood Product Derivative

Use Prevention and treatment of hemorrhagic episodes in patients with hemophilia A (classic hemophilia); perioperative management of hemophilia A; can be of significant therapeutic value in patients with acquired factor VIII inhibitors not exceeding 10 Bethesda units/mL

Pregnancy Risk Factor C

Pregnancy Considerations Reproduction studies have not been conducted. Safety and efficacy in pregnant women have not been established. Use during pregnancy only if clearly needed. Parvovirus B19 or hepatitis A, which may be present in plasma-derived products, may affect a pregnant woman more seriously than nonpregnant women.

Lactation Excretion in breast milk unknown/use caution

Contraindications Hypersensitivity to any component of the formulation

Warnings/Precautions Risk of viral transmission is not totally eradicated. Because antihemophilic factor is prepared from pooled plasma, it may contain the causative agent of viral hepatitis and other viral diseases. Hepatitis B vaccination is recommended for all patients. Hepatitis A vaccination is also recommended for seronegative patients. Antihemophilic factor contains trace amounts of blood groups A and B isohemagglutinins and when large or frequently repeated doses are given to individuals with blood groups A, B, and AB, the patient should be monitored for signs of progressive anemia and the possibility of intravascular hemolysis should be considered. The dosage requirement will vary in patients with factor VIII inhibitors; optimal treatment should be determined by clinical response. Natural rubber latex is a component of Hemofil M and Monarc-M™ packaging. Hemofil M, Monoclate-P®, and Monarc-M™ contain trace amounts of mouse protein. Products contain naturally-occurring von Willebrand factor for stabilization, however efficacy has not been established for the treatment of von Willebrand disease. Products vary by preparation method; final formulations contain human albumin.

Adverse Reactions <1% (Limited to important or life-threatening): Acute hemolytic anemia, AHF inhibitor development, allergic reactions (rare), anaphylaxis (rare), bleeding tendency increased, blurred vision, chest tightness, chills, fever, headache, hyperfibrinogenemia, jittery feeling, lethargy, nausea, somnolence, stinging at the infusion site, stomach discomfort, tingling, urticaria, vasomotor reactions with rapid infusion, vomiting

Drug Interactions

Avoid Concomitant Use There are no known interactions where it is recommended to avoid concomitant use.

Increased Effect/Toxicity There are no known significant interactions involving an increase in effect.

Decreased Effect There are no known significant interactions involving a decrease in effect.

Stability Store under refrigeration, 2°C to 8°C (36°F to 46°F); avoid freezing. If refrigerated, the dried concentrate and diluent should be warmed to room temperature before reconstitution. Gently swirl or rotate vial after adding diluent; do not shake vigorously. Use within 3 hours of reconstitution. Do not refrigerate after reconstitution, precipitation may occur.

Hemofil M, Monarc-M™: May also be stored at room temperature not to exceed 30°C (86°F).

Koāte®-DVI; Monoclate-P®: May also be stored at room temperature of 25°C (77°F) for ≤6 months.

Mechanism of Action Protein (factor VIII) in normal plasma which is necessary for clot formation and maintenance of hemostasis; activates factor X in conjunction with activated factor IX; activated factor X converts prothrombin to thrombin, which converts fibrinogen to fibrin, and with factor XIII forms a stable clot

Pharmacodynamics/Kinetics Half-life elimination: Mean: 8-27 hours

Dosage Children and Adults: I.V.: Individualize dosage based on coagulation studies performed prior to treatment and at regular intervals during treatment. In general, administration of factor VIII 1 int. unit/kg will increase circulating factor VIII levels by ~2 int. units/dL. (General guidelines presented; consult individual product labeling for specific dosing recommendations.)

Dosage based on desired factor VIII increase (%):

To calculate dosage needed based on desired factor VIII increase (%):

Body weight (kg) x 0.5 int. units/kg x desired factor VIII increase (%) = int. units factor VIII required

For example:

50 kg x 0.5 int. units/kg x 30 (% increase) = 750 int. units factor VIII

Dosage based on expected factor VIII increase (%):

It is also possible to calculate the **expected** % factor VIII increase:

(# int. units administered x 2%/int. units/kg) divided by body weight (kg) = expected % factor VIII increase

For example:

(1400 int. units x 2%/int. units/kg) divided by 70 kg = 40%

General guidelines:

Minor hemorrhage: 10-20 int. units/kg as a single dose to achieve FVIII plasma level ~20% to 40% of normal. Mild superficial or early hemorrhages may respond to a single dose; may repeat dose every 12-24 hours for 1-3 days until bleeding is resolved or healing achieved.

Moderate hemorrhage/minor surgery: 15-25 int. units/kg to achieve FVIII plasma level 30% to 50% of normal. If needed, may continue with a maintenance dose of 10-15 int. units/kg every 8-12 hours.

Major to life-threatening hemorrhage: Initial dose 40-50 int. units/kg, followed by a maintenance dose of 20-25 int. units/kg every 8-12 hours until threat is resolved, to achieve FVIII plasma level 80% to 100% of normal.

Major surgery: 50 int. units/kg given preoperatively to raise factor VIII level to 100% before surgery begins. May repeat as necessary after 6-12 hours initially and for a total of 10-14 days until healing is complete. Intensity of therapy may depend on type of surgery and postoperative regimen.

Bleeding prophylaxis: May be administered on a regular basis for bleeding prophylaxis. Doses of 24-40 int. units/kg 3 times/week have been reported in patients with severe hemophilia to prevent joint bleeding.

If bleeding is not controlled with adequate dose, test for presence of inhibitor. It may not be possible or practical to control bleeding if inhibitor titers are >10 Bethesda units/mL.

Elderly: Response in the elderly is not expected to differ from that of younger patients; dosage should be individualized

Administration Administer I.V. over 5-10 minutes (maximum: 10 mL/minute). Infuse Monoclate-P® at 2 mL/minute.

Monitoring Parameters Heart rate and blood pressure (before and during I.V. administration); AHF levels prior to and during treatment; in patients with circulating inhibitors, the inhibitor level should be monitored; hematocrit; monitor for signs and symptoms of intravascular hemolysis; bleeding

Reference Range Classification of hemophilia; normal is defined as 1 int. unit/mL of factor VIII

Severe: Factor level <1% of normal

Moderate: Factor level 1% to 5% of normal

Mild: Factor level >5% to <40% of normal

Dosage Forms Excipient information presented when available (limited, particularly for generics); consult specific product labeling.

Injection, powder for reconstitution:

Hemofil M: Vial labeled with international units [contains albumin; derived from mouse proteins; packaging may contain natural rubber latex]

Koate®-DVI: ~250 int. units, ~500 int. units, ~1000 int. units [contains albumin]

Monarc-M™: Vial labeled with international units [contains albumin; derived from mouse proteins; packaging may contain natural rubber latex]

Monoclate-P®: ~250 int. units, ~500 int. units, ~1000 int. units, ~1500 int. units [contains albumin; derived from mouse proteins]

Antihemophilic Factor (Recombinant)

(an tee hee moe FIL ik FAK tor ree KOM be nant)

U.S. Brand Names Advate; Helixate® FS; Kogenate® FS; Recombinate; ReFacto®; Xyntha™

Canadian Brand Names Helixate® FS; Kogenate®; Kogenate® FS; Recombinate; ReFacto®

Index Terms AHF (Recombinant); Factor VIII (Recombinant); rAHF

Pharmacologic Category Antihemophilic Agent

Use Prevention and treatment of hemorrhagic episodes in patients with hemophilia A (classic hemophilia or congenital factor VIII deficiency); perioperative management of hemophilia A; can be of significant therapeutic value in patients with acquired factor VIII inhibitors ≤10 Bethesda units/mL; prophylaxis of joint bleeding and to reduce risk of joint damage in children with hemophilia A with no preexisting joint damage

Pregnancy Risk Factor C

Pregnancy Considerations Animal reproduction studies have not been conducted. Safety and efficacy in pregnant women has not been established. Use during pregnancy only if clearly needed.

Lactation Excretion in breast milk unknown/use caution

Medication Safety Issues Confusion may occur due to the omitting of "Factor VIII" from some product labeling. Review product contents carefully prior to dispensing any antihemophilic factor.

Contraindications Hypersensitivity to any component of the formulation

Warnings/Precautions Monitor for signs of formation of antibodies to factor VIII; may occur at anytime but more common in young children with severe hemophilia. The dosage requirement will vary in patients with factor VIII inhibitors; optimal treatment should be determined by clinical response. Allergic hypersensitivity reactions (including anaphylaxis) may occur; monitor. Products vary by preparation method. Recombinate is stabilized using human albumin. Helixate® FS and Kogenate® FS are stabilized with sucrose. Advate, Helixate® FS, Kogenate® FS, ReFacto®, and Xyntha™ may contain trace amounts of mouse or hamster protein. Recombinate may contain mouse, hamster or bovine protein. Products may contain von Willebrand factor for stabilization; however, efficacy has not been established for the treatment of von Willebrand's disease.

Adverse Reactions Actual frequency may vary by product.

>1%:

Central nervous system: Chills, dizziness, fever, headache, pain

Dermatologic: Pruritus, rash, urticaria

Gastrointestinal: Diarrhea, nausea, taste perversion, vomiting

Hematologic: Hemorrhage

Local: Injection site pain, injection site inflammation, infusion site reaction

Neuromuscular & skeletal: Arthralgia, weakness

Respiratory: Cough, dyspnea, nasopharyngitis, pharyngolaryngeal pain

Miscellaneous: Catheter thrombosis, factor VIII inhibitor formation

≤1% (Limited to important or life-threatening): Abdominal pain, adenopathy, allergic reactions, anaphylaxis, anemia, anorexia, arthralgia, AST increased, chest discomfort, chest pain, constipation, depersonalization, diaphoresis, edema, epistaxis, facial edema, facial flushing, factor VIII decreased, fatigue, fever, GI hemorrhage, hives, hot flashes, hypersensitivity reaction, hyper-/hypotension (slight), infection, joint swelling, lethargy, otitis media, pallor, paresthesia, restlessness, rhinitis, rigors, somnolence, tachycardia, urinary tract infection, vasodilation, venous catheter access complications

Drug Interactions

Avoid Concomitant Use There are no known interactions where it is recommended to avoid concomitant use.

Increased Effect/Toxicity There are no known significant interactions involving an increase in effect.

Decreased Effect There are no known significant interactions involving a decrease in effect.

Stability Store under refrigeration, 2°C to 8°C (36°F to 46°F); avoid freezing. Use within 3 hours of reconstitution. Gently agitate or rotate vial after adding diluent, do not shake vigorously. Do not refrigerate after reconstitution, a precipitation may occur.

Advate: May also be stored at room temperature for up to 6 months.

Helixate® FS, Kogenate® FS, ReFacto®, Xyntha™: May also be stored at room temperature (not to exceed 25°C [36°F]) up to 3 months; avoid prolonged exposure to light during storage.

Recombinate: May also be stored at room temperature, not to exceed 30°C (86°F).

If refrigerated, the dried concentrate and diluent should be warmed to room temperature before reconstitution.

Mechanism of Action Factor VIII replacement, necessary for clot formation and maintenance of hemostasis. It activates factor X in conjunction with activated factor IX; activated factor X converts prothrombin to thrombin, which converts fibrinogen to fibrin, and with factor XIII forms a stable clot.

Pharmacodynamics/Kinetics

Distribution: V_{ss}: 0.36-0.57 dL/kg

Half-life elimination: Mean: 8-19 hours

Dosage I.V.:

Hemophilia: Children and Adults: Individualize dosage based on coagulation studies performed prior to treatment and at regular intervals during treatment. In general, administration of factor VIII 1 int. unit/kg will increase circulating factor VIII levels by ~2 int. units/dL. (General guidelines presented; consult individual product labeling for specific dosing recommendations.)

Joint bleeding prophylaxis (Kogenate® FS): Children: 25 int. units/kg every other day

Dosage based on desired factor VIII increase (%):

To calculate dosage needed based on desired factor VIII increase (%):

[Body weight (kg) x desired factor VIII increase (%)] divided by 2%/int. units/kg = int. units factor VIII required

For example:

50 kg x 30 (% increase) divided by 2%/int. units/kg = 750 int. units factor VIII

Dosage based on expected factor VIII increase (%):

It is also possible to calculate the **expected** % factor VIII increase:

(# int. units administered x 2%/int. units/kg) divided by body weight (kg) = expected % factor VIII increase

For example:

(1400 int. units x 2%/int. units/kg) divided by 70 kg = 40%

General guidelines:

Minor hemorrhage: 10-20 int. units/kg as a single dose to achieve FVIII plasma level ~20% to 40% of normal. Mild superficial or early hemorrhages may respond to a single dose; may repeat dose every 12-24 hours for 1-3 days until bleeding is resolved or healing achieved.

Moderate hemorrhage/minor surgery: 15-30 int. units/kg to achieve FVIII plasma level 30% to 60% of normal. May repeat 1 dose at 12-24 hours if needed. Some products suggest continuing for ≥3 days until pain and disability are resolved

Major to life-threatening hemorrhage: Initial dose 40-50 int. units/kg followed by a maintenance dose of 20-25 int. units/kg every 8-24 hours until threat is resolved, to achieve FVIII plasma level 60% to 100% of normal.

Major surgery: 50 int. units/kg given preoperatively to raise factor VIII level to 100% before surgery begins. May repeat as necessary after 6-12 hours initially and for a total of 10-14 days until healing is complete. Intensity of therapy may depend on type of surgery and postoperative regimen.

Bleeding prophylaxis: May be administered on a regular basis for bleeding prophylaxis. Doses of 24-40 int. units/kg 3 times/week have been reported in patients with severe hemophilia to prevent joint bleeding.

If bleeding is not controlled with adequate dose, test for presence of inhibitor. It may not be possible or practical to control bleeding if inhibitor titers >10 Bethesda units/mL.

Elderly: Response in the elderly is not expected to differ from that of younger patients; dosage should be individualized

Dietary Considerations Advate contains sodium 108 mEq/L; Helixate® FS and Kogenate® FS contain sodium 27-36 mEq/L; Recombinate contains sodium 180 mEq/L

Administration I.V. infusion over 5-10 minutes (maximum: 10 mL/minute).

Advate: Infuse over ≤5 minutes (maximum: 10 mL/minute)

Kogenate® FS: Infuse over 1-15 minutes; based on patient tolerability

Xyntha™: Infuse over several minutes; adjust based on patient comfort. Do not admix or administer in same tubing as other medications.

Monitoring Parameters Heart rate and blood pressure (before and during I.V. administration); plasma factor VIII activity prior to and during treatment; development of factor VIII inhibitors; signs of bleeding

Reference Range Classification of hemophilia; normal is defined as 1 int. unit/mL of factor VIII

Severe: Factor level <1% of normal

Moderate: Factor level 1% to 5% of normal

Mild: Factor level >5% to <40% of normal

Product Availability Xyntha™: FDA approved February 2008; availability anticipated in September 2008

Wyeth is replacing ReFacto® with Xyntha™.

Dosage Forms Excipient information presented when available (limited, particularly for generics); consult specific product labeling.

Injection, powder for reconstitution, recombinant [preservative free]:

Advate: 250 int. units, 500 int. units, 1000 int. units, 1500 int. units, 2000 int. units, 3000 int. units [plasma/albumin free; contains sodium 108 mEq/L, mannitol; derived from hamster or mouse proteins]

Helixate® FS: 250 int. units, 500 int. units, 1000 int. units [albumin free; contains sucrose 28 mg/vial, sodium 27-36 mEq/L, polysorbate 80; derived from hamster or mouse protein]

Kogenate® FS: 250 int. units, 500 int. units, 1000 int. units, 2000 int. units [albumin free; contains sucrose 28-56 mg/vial, sodium 27-36 mEq/L; derived from hamster or mouse protein]

Recombinate: 250 int. units, 500 int. units, 1000 int. units [contains human albumin, sodium 180 mEq/L; derived from bovine, hamster or mouse proteins; packaging contains natural rubber latex]

ReFacto®: 250 int. units, 500 int. units, 1000 int. units, 2000 int. units [contains sucrose; derived from hamster or mouse proteins]

Xyntha™: 250 int. units, 500 int. units, 1000 int. units, 2000 int. units [albumin free; contains sucrose, polysorbate 80; derived from hamster proteins]

Antihemophilic Factor/von Willebrand Factor Complex (Human)

(an tee hee moe FIL ik FAK tor von WILL le brand FAK tor KOM plex HYU man)

U.S. Brand Names Alphanate® *[new formulation]*; Humate-P®

Canadian Brand Names Humate-P®

Index Terms AHF (Human); Factor VIII (Human); FVIII/vWF; vWF:RCof

Pharmacologic Category Antihemophilic Agent; Blood Product Derivative

Use

Prevention and treatment of hemorrhagic episodes in patients with hemophilia A (classical hemophilia) (Alphanate®, Humate-P®) or acquired factor VIII deficiency (Alphanate®)

Prophylaxis with surgical and/or invasive procedures in patients with von Willebrand disease (vWD) when desmopressin is either ineffective or contraindicated (Alphanate®)

Treatment of spontaneous or trauma-induced bleeding, as well as prevention of excessive bleeding during and after surgery, in patients with vWD (mild, moderate, or severe) where use of desmopressin is known or suspected to be inadequate (Humate-P®)

Pregnancy Risk Factor C

Dosage

Hemophilia A: General guidelines (consult specific product labeling): Children and Adults: I.V.:

Individualize dosage based on coagulation studies performed prior to treatment and at regular intervals during treatment; in general, administration of factor VIII 1 int. unit/kg will increase circulating factor VIII levels by ~2 int. units/dL.

Minor hemorrhage: Loading dose: FVIII:C 15 int. units/kg to achieve FVIII:C plasma level ~30% of normal. If second infusion is needed, half the loading dose may be given once or twice daily for 1-2 days.

Moderate hemorrhage: Loading dose: FVIII:C 25 int. units/kg to achieve FVIII:C plasma level ~50% of normal; Maintenance: FVIII:C 15 int. units/kg every 8-12 hours for 1-2 days in order to maintain FVIII:C plasma levels at 30% of normal. Repeat the same dose once or twice daily for up to 7 days or until adequate wound healing.

Life-threatening hemorrhage/major surgery: Loading dose: FVIII:C 40-50 int. units/kg; Maintenance: FVIII:C 20-25 int. units/kg every 8 hours to maintain FVIII:C plasma levels at 80% to 100% of normal for 7 days. Continue same dose once or twice daily for another 7 days in order to maintain FVIII:C levels at 30% to 50% of normal.

von Willebrand disease (vWD): Treatment (Humate-P®): Children and Adults: I.V.: Individualize dosage based on coagulation studies performed prior to treatment and at regular intervals during treatment; in general, administration of factor VIII 1 int. unit/kg would be expected to raise circulating vWF:RCof ~5 int. units/dL

Type 1, mild (if desmopressin is not appropriate): Major hemorrhage:

Loading dose: vWF:RCof 40-60 int. units/kg

Maintenance dose: vWF:RCof 40-50 int. units/kg every 8-12 hours for 3 days, keeping vWF:RCof nadir >50%; follow with 40-50 int. units/kg daily for up to 7 days

Type 1, moderate or severe:

Minor hemorrhage: vWF:RCof 40-50 int. units/kg for 1-2 doses

Major hemorrhage:

Loading dose: vWF:RCof 50-75 int. units/kg

Maintenance dose: vWF:RCof 40-60 int. units/kg every 8-12 hours for 3 days to keep the vWF:RCof nadir >50%, then 40-60 int. units/kg daily for a total of up to 7 days

Types 2 and 3:

Minor hemorrhage: vWF:RCof 40-50 int. units/kg for 1-2 doses

Major hemorrhage:

Loading dose: vWF:RCof 60-80 int. units/kg

Maintenance dose: vWF:RCof 40-60 int. units/kg every 8-12 hours for 3 days, keeping the vWF:RCof nadir >50%; follow with 40-60 int. units/kg daily for a total of up to 7 days

von Willebrand disease (vWD): Surgery/procedure prophylaxis (except patients with type 3 undergoing major surgery) (Alphanate®):

Children: I.V.:

Preoperative dose: vWF:RCof 75 int. units /kg 1 hour prior to surgery

Maintenance dose: vWF:RCof 50-75 int. units/kg every 8-12 hours as clinically needed. May reduce dose after third postoperative day; continue treatment until healing is complete.

Adults: I.V.:

Preoperative dose: vWF:RCof 60 int. units /kg 1 hour prior to surgery

Maintenance dose: vWF:RCof 40-60 int. units/kg every 8-12 hours as clinically needed. May reduce dose after third postoperative day; continue treatment until healing is complete. For minor procedures, maintain vWF of 40% to 50% during postoperative days 1-3; for major procedures maintain vWF of 40% to 50% for ≥3-7 days.

von Willebrand disease (vWD): Surgery/procedure prevention of bleeding (Humate-P®): Children and Adults: I.V.:

Emergency surgery: Administer vWF:RCof 50-60 int units/kg; monitor trough coagulation factor levels for subsequent doses

Surgical management (nonemergency):

Loading dose calculation based on baseline target vWF:RCo: (Target peak vWF:RCof - Baseline vWF: RCof) x weight (in kg) / IVR = int. units vWF:RCof required. Administer loading dose 1-2 hours prior to surgery. **Note:** If IVR not available, assume 2 int. units/dL per int. units/kg of vWF:RCof product administered.

Target concentrations for vWF:RCof following loading dose:

Major surgery: 100 int. units/dL

Minor surgery: 50-60 int. units/dL

Maintenance dose: Initial: 1/2 loading dose followed by dosing determined by target tough concentrations, generally every 8-12 hours. Patients with shorter half-lives may require dosing every 6 hours.

Target maintenance trough vWF:RCof concentrations:

Major surgery: >50 int. units/dL for up to 3 days, followed by >30 int. units/dL for a minimum total treatment of 72 hours

Minor surgery: ≥30 int. units/dL for a minimum duration of 48 hours

Oral surgery: ≥30 int. units/dL for a minimum duration of 8-12 hours

Elderly: Response in the elderly is not expected to differ from that of younger patients; dosage should be individualized

Additional Information Complete prescribing information for this medication should be consulted for additional detail.

Dosage Forms Excipient information presented when available (limited, particularly for generics); consult specific product labeling.

Injection, powder for reconstitution [human derived]:

Alphanate®:

250 int. units [Factor VIII and vWF:RCof ratio varies by lot; contains sodium ≥10 mEq/vial, albumin and polysorbate 80; packaged with diluent]

500 int. units [Factor VIII and vWF:RCof ratio varies by lot; contains sodium ≥10 mEq/vial, albumin and polysorbate 80; packaged with diluent]

1000 int. units [Factor VIII and vWF: RCof ratio varies by lot; contains sodium ≥10 mEq/vial, albumin and polysorbate 80; packaged with diluent]

1500 int. units [Factor VIII and vWF:RCof ratio varies by lot; contains sodium ≥10 mEq/vial, albumin and polysorbate 80; packaged with diluent]

Humate-P®:

FVIII 250 int. units and vWF:RCof 600 int. units [contains albumin; packaged with diluent]

FVIII 500 int. units and vWF:RCof 1200 int. units [contains albumin; packaged with diluent]

FVIII 1000 int. units and vWF:RCof 2400 int. units [contains albumin; packaged with diluent]

Anti-inhibitor Coagulant Complex

(an tee-in HI bi tor coe AG yoo lant KOM pleks)

U.S. Brand Names Autoplex® T [DSC]; Feiba VH

Canadian Brand Names Feiba VH Immuno

Index Terms AICC; Coagulant Complex Inhibitor

Pharmacologic Category Activated Prothrombin Complex Concentrate (aPCC); Antihemophilic Agent; Blood Product Derivative

Use Hemophilia A & B patients with factor VIII inhibitors who are to undergo surgery or those who are bleeding

Pregnancy Risk Factor C

Dosage I.V.: Children and Adults:

Autoplex® T: Dosage range: 25-100 factor VIII correctional units per kg depending on the severity of hemorrhage; may repeat in ~6 hours if needed. Adjust dose based on patient response.

Feiba VH: General dosing guidelines: 50-100 units/kg (maximum 200 units/kg)

Joint hemorrhage: 50 units/kg every 12 hours; may increase to 100 units/kg; continue until signs of clinical improvement occur

Mucous membrane bleeding: 50 units/kg every 6 hours; may increase to 100 units/kg (maximum: 2 administrations/day or 200 units/kg/day

Soft tissue hemorrhage: 100 units/kg every 12 hours (maximum: 200 units/kg/day)

Other severe hemorrhage: 100 units/kg every 12 hours; may be used every 6 hours if needed; continue until clinical improvement

Additional Information Complete prescribing information for this medication should be consulted for additional detail.

Dosage Forms Excipient information presented when available (limited, particularly for generics); consult specific product labeling.

Injection, powder for reconstitution:

Autoplex® T: Each bottle is labeled with correctional units of factor VIII [contains heparin 2 units/mL and sodium 162-192 mEq/L; packaging contains natural rubber latex] [DSC]

Feiba VH: Each bottle is labeled with Immuno units of factor VIII [heparin free; contains sodium 8 mg/mL; packaging contains natural rubber latex]

Antipyrine and Benzocaine

(an tee PYE reen & BEN zoe kane)

U.S. Brand Names A/B Otic; Allergen®; Aurodex

Canadian Brand Names Auralgan®

Index Terms Benzocaine and Antipyrine

Pharmacologic Category Otic Agent, Analgesic; Otic Agent, Cerumenolytic

Use Temporary relief of pain and reduction of swelling associated with acute congestive and serous otitis media, swimmer's ear, otitis externa; facilitates ear wax removal

Pregnancy Risk Factor C

Dosage Otic: Children and Adults:

Otitis media: Fill ear canal with solution; moisten cotton pledget with solution, place in external ear, repeat every 1-2 hours until pain and congestion are relieved

Ear wax removal instill drops 3-4 times/day for 2-3 days

Additional Information Complete prescribing information for this medication should be consulted for additional detail.

Dosage Forms Excipient information presented when available (limited, particularly for generics); consult specific product labeling.

Solution, otic [drops]: Antipyrine 5.4% and benzocaine 1.4% (10 mL)

A/B Otic, Allergen®, Aurodex: Antipyrine 5.4% and benzocaine 1.4% (15 mL)

Antithrombin III (an tee THROM bin three)

U.S. Brand Names Thrombate III®

Canadian Brand Names Thrombate III®

Index Terms AT-III; Heparin Cofactor I

Pharmacologic Category Anticoagulant; Blood Product Derivative

Use Treatment of hereditary antithrombin III deficiency in connection with surgical procedures, obstetrical procedures, or thromboembolism

Unlabeled/Investigational Use Acquired antithrombin III deficiencies related to disseminated intravascular coagulation (DIC)

Pregnancy Risk Factor B

Dosage Adults:

Initial dose: Dosing is individualized based on pretherapy AT-III levels. The initial dose should raise antithrombin III levels (AT-III) to 120% and may be calculated based on the following formula:

[desired AT-III level % - baseline AT-III level %] x body weight (kg)
divided by 1.4%/int. units/kg

For example, if a 70 kg adult patient had a baseline AT-III level of 57%, the initial dose would be

[(120% - 57%) x 70] divided by 1.4 = 3150 int. units

Maintenance dose: Subsequent dosing should be targeted to keep levels between 80% to 120% which may be achieved by administering 60% of the initial dose every 24 hours. Adjustments may be made by adjusting dose or interval. Maintain level within normal range for 2-8 days depending on type of procedure.

Additional Information Complete prescribing information for this medication should be consulted for additional detail.

Dosage Forms Excipient information presented when available (limited, particularly for generics); consult specific product labeling.

Injection, powder for reconstitution [preservative free]:

Thrombate III®: 500 int. units, 1000 int. units [contains heparin, sodium chloride 110-210 mEq/L; packaged with diluent]

Antithymocyte Globulin (Equine)

(an te THY moe site GLOB yu lin, E kwine)

U.S. Brand Names Atgam®

Canadian Brand Names Atgam®

Index Terms Antithymocyte Immunoglobulin; ATG; Horse Antihuman Thymocyte Gamma Globulin; Lymphocyte Immune Globulin

Pharmacologic Category Immune Globulin; Immunosuppressant Agent

Use Prevention and treatment of acute renal allograft rejection; treatment of moderate to severe aplastic anemia in patients not considered suitable candidates for bone marrow transplantation

Unlabeled/Investigational Use Prevention and treatment of other solid organ allograft rejection; prevention of graft-versus-host disease following bone marrow transplantation

Pregnancy Risk Factor C

Pregnancy Considerations Reproduction studies have not been conducted; use during pregnancy is not recommended. Women exposed to Atgam® during pregnancy may be enrolled in the National Transplantation Pregnancy Registry (877-955-6877).

Lactation Excretion in breast milk unknown/use caution

Medication Safety Issues

Sound-alike/look-alike issues:

Atgam® may be confused with Ativan®

Contraindications Hypersensitivity to lymphocytic immune globulin, any component of the formulation, or other equine gamma globulins

Warnings/Precautions For I.V. use only. Must be administered via central line due to chemical phlebitis. **[U.S. Boxed Warning]: Should only be used by physicians experienced in immunosuppressive therapy or management of solid organ or bone marrow transplant patients. Adequate laboratory and supportive medical resources must be readily available in the facility for patient management.** Hypersensitivity and anaphylactic reactions can occur; immediate treatment (including epinephrine 1:1000) should be available. Rash, dyspnea, hypotension, or anaphylaxis precludes further administration of the drug. Discontinue if severe and unremitting thrombocytopenia and/or leukopenia occur. Dose must be administered over at least 4 hours. Patient may need to be pretreated with an antipyretic, antihistamine, and/or corticosteroid. Intradermal skin testing is recommended prior to first-dose administration.

Adverse Reactions

>10%:

Central nervous system: Fever, chills

Dermatologic: Pruritus, rash, urticaria
Hematologic: Leukopenia, thrombocytopenia

1% to 10%:

Cardiovascular: Bradycardia, chest pain, CHF, edema, encephalitis, hyper-/hypotension, myocarditis, tachycardia
Central nervous system: Agitation, headache, lethargy, lightheadedness, listlessness, seizure
Gastrointestinal: Diarrhea, nausea, stomatitis, vomiting
Hepatic: Hepatosplenomegaly, liver function tests abnormal
Local: Pain at injection site, phlebitis, thrombophlebitis, burning soles/palms
Neuromuscular & skeletal: Arthralgia, back pain, myalgia
Ocular: Periorbital edema
Renal: Abnormal renal function tests
Respiratory: Dyspnea, respiratory distress
Miscellaneous: Anaphylaxis, diaphoresis, lymphadenopathy, night sweats, serum sickness, viral infection

<1% (Limited to important or life-threatening): Acute renal failure, anemia, aplasia, confusion, cough, deep vein thrombosis, disorientation, dizziness, epigastric pain, faintness, GI bleeding, granulocytopenia, hemolysis, herpes simplex reactivation, hiccups, hyperglycemia, iliac vein obstruction, infection, kidney enlarged, laryngospasm, malaise, neutropenia, nosebleed, pancytopenia, paresthesia, pulmonary edema, renal artery thrombosis, serum sickness, toxic epidermal necrosis, vasculitis, weakness, wound dehiscence

Drug Interactions

Avoid Concomitant Use There are no known interactions where it is recommended to avoid concomitant use.

Increased Effect/Toxicity There are no known significant interactions involving an increase in effect.

Decreased Effect

Antithymocyte Globulin (Equine) may decrease the levels/effects of: Vaccines (Live)

Stability Ampuls must be refrigerated; do not freeze. Dilute into inverted bottle of sterile vehicle to ensure that undiluted lymphocyte immune globulin does not contact air. Gently rotate or swirl to mix. Final concentration should be 4 mg/mL. May be diluted in NS, $D_5$1/4NS, $D_5$1/2NS. Diluted solution is stable for 24 hours (including infusion time) at refrigeration.

Mechanism of Action May involve elimination of antigen-reactive T lymphocytes (killer cells) in peripheral blood or alteration of T-cell function

Pharmacodynamics/Kinetics

Distribution: Poorly into lymphoid tissues; binds to circulating lymphocytes, granulocytes, platelets, bone marrow cells
Half-life elimination, plasma: 1.5-12 days
Excretion: Urine (~1%)

Dosage An intradermal skin test is recommended prior to administration of the initial dose of ATG; use 0.1 mL of a 1:1000 dilution of ATG in normal saline. A positive skin reaction consists of a wheal ≥10 mm in diameter. If a positive skin test occurs, the first infusion should be administered in a controlled environment with intensive life support immediately available. A systemic reaction precludes further administration of the drug. The absence of a reaction does **not** preclude the possibility of an immediate sensitivity reaction.

Premedication with diphenhydramine, hydrocortisone, and acetaminophen is recommended prior to first dose.

Children: I.V.:

Aplastic anemia protocol: 10-20 mg/kg/day for 8-14 days; then administer every other day for 7 more doses; addition doses may be given every other day for 21 total doses in 28 days
Renal allograft: 5-25 mg/kg/day

Adults: I.V.:

Aplastic anemia protocol: 10-20 mg/kg/day for 8-14 days, then administer every other day for 7 more doses, for a total of 21 doses in 28 days
Renal allograft:
Rejection prophylaxis: 15 mg/kg/day for 14 days followed by 14 days of alternative day therapy at the same dose; the first dose should be administered within 24 hours before or after transplantation
Rejection treatment: 10-15 mg/kg/day for 14 days, then administer every other day for 10-14 days up to 21 doses in 28 days

Administration Infuse dose over at least 4 hours. Any severe systemic reaction to the skin test, such as generalized rash, tachycardia, dyspnea, hypotension, or anaphylaxis, should preclude further therapy. Epinephrine and resuscitative equipment should be nearby. Patient may need to be pretreated with an antipyretic, antihistamine, and/or corticosteroid. Mild itching and erythema can be treated with antihistamines. Infuse into a vascular shunt, arterial venous fistula, or high-flow central vein through a 0.2-1 micron in-line filter.

First dose: Premedicate with diphenhydramine orally 30 minutes prior to and hydrocortisone I.V. 15 minutes prior to infusion and acetaminophen 2 hours after start of infusion.

Monitoring Parameters Lymphocyte profile, CBC with differential and platelet count, vital signs during administration

Dosage Forms Excipient information presented when available (limited, particularly for generics); consult specific product labeling.

Injection, solution:
Atgam®: 50 mg/mL (5 mL)

Antithymocyte Globulin (Rabbit)

(an te THY moe site GLOB yu lin RAB bit)

U.S. Brand Names Thymoglobulin®

Index Terms Antithymocyte Immunoglobulin; rATG

Pharmacologic Category Immune Globulin; Immunosuppressant Agent

Use Treatment of acute rejection of renal transplant; used in conjunction with concomitant immunosuppression

Unlabeled/Investigational Use Induction therapy in renal transplant

Pregnancy Risk Factor C

Pregnancy Considerations Reproduction studies have not been conducted.

Lactation Excretion in breast milk unknown/use caution

Contraindications Hypersensitivity to antithymocyte globulin, rabbit proteins, or any component of the formulation; acute viral illness

Warnings/Precautions [U.S. Boxed Warning]: Should only be used by physicians experienced in immunosuppressive therapy for the treatment of renal transplant patients. Medical surveillance is required during the infusion. Initial dose must be administered over at least 6 hours into a high flow vein; patient may need pretreatment with an antipyretic, antihistamine, and/or corticosteroid. Hypersensitivity and anaphylactic reactions can occur; immediate treatment (including epinephrine 1:1000) should be available. An increased incidence of lymphoma, post-transplant lymphoproliferative disease (PTLD), other malignancies, or severe infections may develop following concomitant use of immunosuppressants and prolonged use or overdose of antithymocyte globulin. Appropriate antiviral, antibacterial, antiprotozoal, and/or antifungal prophylaxis is recommended. Reversible neutropenia or thrombocytopenia may result from the development of cross-reactive antibodies.

Adverse Reactions

>10%:

Cardiovascular: Hypertension, peripheral edema, tachycardia

Central nervous system: Chills, fever, headache, pain, malaise

Endocrine & metabolic: Hyperkalemia

Gastrointestinal: Abdominal pain, diarrhea, nausea

Genitourinary: Urinary tract infection

Hematologic: Leukopenia, thrombocytopenia

Neuromuscular & skeletal: Weakness

Respiratory: Dyspnea

Miscellaneous: Antirabbit antibody development, sepsis, systemic infection

1% to 10%:

Central nervous system: Dizziness

Gastrointestinal: Gastritis, gastrointestinal moniliasis

Miscellaneous: Herpes simplex infection, moniliasis

Postmarketing and/or case reports: Anaphylaxis, cytokine release syndrome, PTLD, neutropenia, serum sickness (delayed)

Drug Interactions

Avoid Concomitant Use There are no known interactions where it is recommended to avoid concomitant use.

Increased Effect/Toxicity There are no known significant interactions involving an increase in effect.

Decreased Effect There are no known significant interactions involving a decrease in effect.

Stability Store powder under refrigeration at 2°C to 8°C (36°F to 46°F); do not freeze. Protect from light. Allow vials to reach room temperature, then reconstitute each vial with SWFI 5 mL. Rotate vial gently until dissolved. Prior to administration, further dilute one vial in 50 mL saline or dextrose (total volume is usually 50-500 mL depending on total number of vials needed per dose). Mix by gently inverting infusion bag once or twice. Use immediately following reconstitution.

Mechanism of Action Polyclonal antibody which appears to cause immunosuppression by acting on T-cell surface antigens and depleting CD4 lymphocytes

Pharmacodynamics/Kinetics

Duration: Lymphopenia may persist ≥1 year

Half-life elimination, plasma: 2-3 days

Dosage I.V.: Children and Adults: Treatment of acute rejection: 1.5 mg/kg/day for 7-14 days

Dosage adjustment for toxicity:

WBC count 2000-3000 cells/mm^3 or platelet count 50,000-75,000 cells/mm^3: Reduce dose by 50%

WBC count <2000 cells/mm^3 or platelet count <50,000 cells/mm^3: Consider discontinuing treatment

Administration The first dose should be infused over at least 6 hours through a high-flow vein. Subsequent doses should be administered over at least 4 hours. Administer through an in-line 0.22 micron filter. Premedication with corticosteroids, acetaminophen, and/or an antihistamine may reduce infusion-related reactions.

Monitoring Parameters Lymphocyte profile, CBC with differential and platelet count; vital signs during administration; signs and symptoms of infection

Dosage Forms Excipient information presented when available (limited, particularly for generics); consult specific product labeling.

Injection, powder for reconstitution:

Thymoglobulin®: 25 mg

- **Antithymocyte Immunoglobulin** *see* Antithymocyte Globulin (Equine) *on page 124*
- **Antithymocyte Immunoglobulin** *see* Antithymocyte Globulin (Rabbit) *on page 125*
- **Antitumor Necrosis Factor Apha (Human)** *see* Adalimumab *on page 43*
- **Anti-VEGF Monoclonal Antibody** *see* Bevacizumab *on page 193*
- **Antivert®** *see* Meclizine *on page 928*
- **Antizol®** *see* Fomepizole *on page 659*
- **Anucort-HC®** *see* Hydrocortisone *on page 743*
- **Anu-Med [OTC]** *see* Phenylephrine *on page 1183*
- **Anusol-HC®** *see* Hydrocortisone *on page 743*
- **Anusol® HC-1 [OTC]** *see* Hydrocortisone *on page 743*
- **Anuzinc (Can)** *see* Zinc Sulfate *on page 1584*
- **Anzemet®** *see* Dolasetron *on page 476*
- **APAP** *see* Acetaminophen *on page 25*
- **APAP and Tramadol** *see* Acetaminophen and Tramadol *on page 30*
- **ApexiCon™** *see* Diflorasone *on page 443*
- **ApexiCon™ E** *see* Diflorasone *on page 443*
- **Aphthasol®** *see* Amlexanox *on page 93*
- **Apidra®** *see* Insulin Glulisine *on page 794*
- **Aplisol®** *see* Tuberculin Tests *on page 1527*
- **Aplonidine** *see* Apraclonidine *on page 129*
- **Apo-Acebutolol® (Can)** *see* Acebutolol *on page 25*
- **Apo-Acetaminophen® (Can)** *see* Acetaminophen *on page 25*
- **Apo-Acetazolamide® (Can)** *see* AcetaZOLAMIDE *on page 34*
- **Apo-Acyclovir® (Can)** *see* Acyclovir *on page 40*
- **Apo-Alendronate® (Can)** *see* Alendronate *on page 58*
- **Apo-Alfuzosin (Can)** *see* Alfuzosin *on page 61*
- **Apo-Allopurinol® (Can)** *see* Allopurinol *on page 65*
- **Apo-Alpraz® (Can)** *see* ALPRAZolam *on page 68*
- **Apo-Alpraz® TS (Can)** *see* ALPRAZolam *on page 68*
- **Apo-Amiloride® (Can)** *see* AMILoride *on page 85*
- **Apo-Amilzide® (Can)** *see* Amiloride and Hydrochlorothiazide *on page 85*
- **Apo-Amiodarone® (Can)** *see* Amiodarone *on page 87*
- **Apo-Amitriptyline® (Can)** *see* Amitriptyline *on page 90*
- **Apo-Amoxi® (Can)** *see* Amoxicillin *on page 98*
- **Apo-Amoxi-Clav® (Can)** *see* Amoxicillin and Clavulanate Potassium *on page 100*
- **Apo-Ampi® (Can)** *see* Ampicillin *on page 109*
- **Apo-Atenidone® (Can)** *see* Atenolol and Chlorthalidone *on page 150*
- **Apo-Atenol® (Can)** *see* Atenolol *on page 149*
- **Apo-Azathioprine® (Can)** *see* AzaTHIOprine *on page 163*
- **Apo-Azithromycin® (Can)** *see* Azithromycin *on page 166*
- **Apo-Baclofen® (Can)** *see* Baclofen *on page 172*
- **Apo-Beclomethasone® (Can)** *see* Beclomethasone *on page 176*
- **Apo-Benazepril® (Can)** *see* Benazepril *on page 179*
- **Apo-Benztropine® (Can)** *see* Benztropine *on page 186*
- **Apo-Bisacodyl® (Can)** *see* Bisacodyl *on page 198*
- **Apo-Bisoprolol® (Can)** *see* Bisoprolol *on page 200*
- **Apo-Brimonidine® (Can)** *see* Brimonidine *on page 212*
- **Apo-Brimonidine P (Can)** *see* Brimonidine *on page 212*
- **Apo-Bromocriptine® (Can)** *see* Bromocriptine *on page 213*
- **Apo-Buspirone® (Can)** *see* BusPIRone *on page 226*
- **Apo-Butorphanol® (Can)** *see* Butorphanol *on page 231*
- **Apo-Cal® (Can)** *see* Calcium Carbonate *on page 238*

Apraclonidine (a pra KLOE ni deen)

U.S. Brand Names Iopidine®

Canadian Brand Names Iopidine®

Index Terms Aplonidine; Apraclonidine Hydrochloride; p-Aminoclonidine

Pharmacologic Category Alpha$_2$ Agonist, Ophthalmic

Additional Appendix Information

Glaucoma Drug Therapy *on page 1808*

Use Prevention and treatment of postsurgical intraocular pressure (IOP) elevation; short-term, adjunctive therapy in patients who require additional reduction of IOP

Pregnancy Risk Factor C

Medication Safety Issues

Sound-alike/look-alike issues:

Iopidine® may be confused with indapamide, iodine, Lodine®

Dosage Adults: Ophthalmic:

0.5%: Instill 1-2 drops in the affected eye(s) 3 times/day

1%: Instill 1 drop in operative eye 1 hour prior to anterior segment laser surgery, second drop in eye immediately upon completion of procedure

Dosing adjustment in renal impairment: Although the topical use of apraclonidine has not been studied in renal failure patients, structurally-related clonidine undergoes a significant increase in half-life in patients with severe renal impairment; close monitoring of cardiovascular parameters in patients with impaired renal function is advised.

Dosing adjustment in hepatic impairment: Close monitoring of cardiovascular parameters in patients with impaired liver function is advised because the systemic dosage form of clonidine is partially metabolized in the liver.

Additional Information Complete prescribing information for this medication should be consulted for additional detail.

Dosage Forms Excipient information presented when available (limited, particularly for generics); consult specific product labeling.

Solution, ophthalmic:

Iopidine®: 0.5% (5 mL, 10 mL); 1% (0.1 mL) [contains benzalkonium chloride]

Aprepitant (ap RE pi tant)

U.S. Brand Names Emend®

Canadian Brand Names Emend®

Index Terms L 754030; MK 869

Pharmacologic Category Antiemetic; Substance P/Neurokinin 1 Receptor Antagonist

Use Prevention of acute and delayed nausea and vomiting associated with moderately- and highly-emetogenic chemotherapy (in combination with other antiemetics); prevention of postoperative nausea and vomiting (PONV)

Pregnancy Risk Factor B

Pregnancy Considerations Teratogenic effects were not observed in animal studies. There are no adequate and well-controlled studies in pregnant women; use only if clearly needed.

Lactation Excretion in breast milk unknown/not recommended

Medication Safety Issues

Sound-alike/look-alike issues:

Aprepitant may be confused with fosaprepitant

Emend® (aprepitant) oral capsule formulation may be confused with Emend® for injection (fosaprepitant).

Contraindications Hypersensitivity to aprepitant or any component of the formulation; use with cisapride or pimozide

Warnings/Precautions Use caution with agents primarily metabolized via CYP3A4; aprepitant is a 3A4 inhibitor. Effect on orally administered 3A4 substrates is greater than those administered intravenously. Use caution with hepatic impairment; has not been studied in patients with severe hepatic impairment (Child-Pugh Class C). Not intended for treatment of existing nausea and vomiting or for chronic continuous therapy.

Adverse Reactions Note: Adverse reactions reported as part of a combination chemotherapy regimen or with general anesthesia.

>10%:

Central nervous system: Fatigue (18% to 22%)

Gastrointestinal: Nausea (7% to 13%), constipation (9% to 12%)

Neuromuscular & skeletal: Weakness (3% to 18%)

Miscellaneous: Hiccups (11%)

1% to 10%:

Cardiovascular: Hypotension (≤6%), bradycardia (4%)

Central nervous system: Dizziness (≤7%)

Endocrine & metabolic: Dehydration (6%), hot flushing (3%)

Gastrointestinal: Diarrhea (6% to 10%), dyspepsia (8%), abdominal pain (5%), stomatitis (5%), epigastric discomfort (4%), gastritis (4%), throat pain (3%), vomiting (3%)

Hematologic: Neutropenia (3% to 9%), leukopenia (9%), hemoglobin decreased (2% to 5%)

Hepatic: ALT increased (1% to 6%), AST increased (3%)

Renal: BUN increased (5%), proteinuria (7%), serum creatinine increased (4%)

>0.5% (Limited to important or life-threatening): Acid reflux, acne, albumin decreased, alkaline phosphatase increased, anemia, anxiety, appetite decreased, arthralgia, back pain, bilirubin increased, candidiasis, confusion, conjunctivitis, cough, deglutition disorder, depression, diabetes mellitus, diaphoresis, dry mouth, DVT, dysarthria, dysgeusia, dysphagia, dyspnea, dysuria, edema, eructation, erythrocyturia, febrile neutropenia, flatulence, flushing, herpes simplex, hyperglycemia, hypertension, hypokalemia, hyponatremia, hypovolemia, hypoxia, glucosuria, leukocytes increased, leukocyturia, malaise, MI, muscular weakness, musculoskeletal pain, myalgia, nasal secretion, obstipation, palpitation, pelvic pain, peripheral neuropathy, pharyngitis, pneumonitis, pulmonary embolism, rash, renal insufficiency, respiratory infection, respiratory insufficiency, rigors, salivation increased, sensory disturbance, sensory neuropathy, septic shock, syncope, tachycardia, taste disturbance, thrombocytopenia, tremor, urinary tract infection, visual acuity decreased, vocal disturbance, weight loss, wheezing

Drug Interactions

Metabolism/Transport Effects Substrate of CYP1A2 (minor), 2C19 (minor), 3A4 (major); **Inhibits** CYP2C9 (weak), 2C19 (weak), 3A4 (moderate); **Induces** CYP2C9 (weak), 3A4 (weak)

Avoid Concomitant Use

Avoid concomitant use of Aprepitant with any of the following: Cisapride; Pimozide

Increased Effect/Toxicity

Aprepitant may increase the levels/effects of: Benzodiazepines (metabolized by oxidation); Cisapride; Corticosteroids (Systemic); CYP3A4 Substrates; Diltiazem; Eplerenone; FentaNYL; Maraviroc; Pimecrolimus; Pimozide; Ranolazine; Salmeterol

The levels/effects of Aprepitant may be increased by: Antifungal Agents (Azole Derivatives, Systemic); CYP3A4 Inhibitors (Moderate); CYP3A4 Inhibitors (Strong); Dasatinib; Diltiazem

Decreased Effect

Aprepitant may decrease the levels/effects of: Contraceptive (Progestins); Maraviroc; Oral Contraceptive (Estrogens); Warfarin

The levels/effects of Aprepitant may be decreased by: CYP3A4 Inducers (Strong); Deferasirox; Herbs (CYP3A4 Inducers); Rifamycin Derivatives

Ethanol/Nutrition/Herb Interactions

Food: Aprepitant serum concentration may be increased when taken with grapefruit juice; avoid concurrent use.

Herb/Nutraceutical: Avoid St John's wort (may decrease aprepitant levels).

Stability Store at controlled room temperature of 20°C to 25°C (68°F to 77°F).

Mechanism of Action Prevents acute and delayed vomiting by inhibiting the substance P/neurokinin 1 (NK_1) receptor; augments the antiemetic activity of the 5-HT_3 receptor antagonist and corticosteroid activity and inhibits both acute and delayed phases of chemotherapy-induced emesis.

Pharmacodynamics/Kinetics

Distribution: V_d: ~70 L; crosses the blood brain barrier

Protein binding: >95%

Metabolism: Extensively hepatic via CYP3A4 (major); CYP1A2 and CYP2C19 (minor); forms 7 metabolites (weakly active)

Bioavailability: 60% to 65%

Half-life elimination: Terminal: ~9-13 hours

Time to peak, plasma: ~3-4 hours

Dosage Oral: Adults:

Prevention of chemotherapy-induced nausea/vomiting: 125 mg on day 1, followed by 80 mg on days 2 and 3 in combination with other antiemetics

Prevention of PONV: 40 mg within 3 hours prior to induction

Dosage adjustment in renal impairment: No dose adjustment necessary in patients with renal disease or end-stage renal disease maintained on hemodialysis.

Dosage adjustment in hepatic impairment:

Mild-to-moderate impairment (Child-Pugh Class A and B): No adjustment necessary

Severe impairment (Child-Pugh Class C): No data available

Dietary Considerations May be taken with or without food.

Administration Administer with or without food.

Chemotherapy induced nausea/vomiting: First dose should be given 1 hour prior to antineoplastic therapy; subsequent doses should be given in the morning.

PONV: Administer within 3 hours of induction

Additional Information Oncology Comment: Aprepitant is recommended in the American Society of Clinical Oncology (ASCO) oncology antiemetic guidelines for use in combination with a serotonin receptor antagonist and dexamethasone for chemotherapy with high emetic risk and for chemotherapy regimens of moderate emetic risk which contain an anthracycline and cyclophosphamide (Kris, 2006). The National Comprehensive Cancer Network (NCCN) Clinical Practice Guidelines in Oncology for Antiemesis recommend the same use of aprepitant as is in the ASCO recommendation. The NCCN guidelines however, also suggest that aprepitant may be used for select moderately emetogenic regimens (carboplatin, cisplatin, doxorubicin, epirubicin, ifosfamide, irinotecan, and methotrexate).

Dosage Forms Excipient information presented when available (limited, particularly for generics); consult specific product labeling.

Capsule:
Emend®: 40 mg, 80 mg, 125 mg
Combination package [each package contains]:
Emend®:
Capsule: 80 mg (2s)
Capsule: 125 mg (1s)

- **Aprepitant Injection** *see* Fosaprepitant *on page 666*
- **Apresazide [DSC]** *see* Hydralazine and Hydrochlorothiazide *on page 737*
- **Apresoline [DSC]** *see* HydrALAZINE *on page 736*
- **Apresoline® (Can)** *see* HydrALAZINE *on page 736*
- **Apri®** *see* Ethinyl Estradiol and Desogestrel *on page 575*
- **Apriso™** *see* Mesalamine *on page 949*
- **Aprodine® [OTC]** *see* Triprolidine and Pseudoephedrine *on page 1522*

Aprotinin (a proe TYE nin)

U.S. Brand Names Trasylol®

Canadian Brand Names Trasylol®

Pharmacologic Category Blood Product Derivative; Hemostatic Agent

Use Prevention of perioperative blood loss in patients who are at increased risk for blood loss and blood transfusions in association with cardiopulmonary bypass in coronary artery bypass graft surgery

Restrictions Available in U.S. under an investigational new drug (IND) process. The program will provide aprotinin for the treatment of adult patients undergoing coronary artery bypass graft (CABG) surgery requiring cardiopulmonary bypass (CPB) who are at increased risk of bleeding and transfusion during CABG surgery with no acceptable therapeutic alternative. Healthcare providers using aprotinin for this situation must also ensure that the benefits outweigh the risks for their patient. U.S. healthcare providers with patients who may qualify can access information and forms for enrollment at http://www.trasylol.com/main.htm or contact Bayer Medical Communications at (888) 842-2937.

Pregnancy Risk Factor B

Dosage Adults: Test dose: **All** patients should receive a 1 mL (1.4 mg) I.V. test dose at least 10 minutes prior to the loading dose to assess the potential for allergic reactions.

Notes:

The loading dose should be given after induction of anesthesia but prior to sternotomy. In patients with previous exposure to aprotinin, administer loading dose just prior to cannulation. A constant infusion is continued until surgery is complete.

To avoid physical incompatibility with heparin when adding to pump-prime solution, each agent should be added during recirculation to assure adequate dilution.

Regimen A (standard dose):
2 million KIU (280 mg; 200 mL) loading dose I.V. over 20-30 minutes
2 million KIU (280 mg; 200 mL) into pump prime volume
500,000 KIU/hour (70 mg/hour; 50 mL/hour) I.V. during operation

Regimen B (low dose):
1 million KIU (140 mg; 100 mL) loading dose I.V. over 20-30 minutes
1 million KIU (140 mg; 100 mL) into pump prime volume
250,000 KIU/hour (35 mg/hour; 25 mL/hour) I.V. during operation

Dosage adjustment in renal impairment: No adjustment required, but increased risk of worsening renal dysfunction with use; monitor closely

Dosage adjustment in hepatic impairment: No information available

Additional Information Complete prescribing information for this medication should be consulted for additional detail.

Dosage Forms Excipient information presented when available (limited, particularly for generics); consult specific product labeling.

Injection, solution:
Trasylol®: 1.4 mg/mL [10,000 KIU/mL] (100 mL, 200 mL) [bovine derived]

- **Aptivus®** *see* Tipranavir *on page 1477*
- **Aquacare® [OTC]** *see* Urea *on page 1530*
- **Aquachloral® Supprettes® [DSC]** *see* Chloral Hydrate *on page 300*
- **Aquacort® (Can)** *see* Hydrocortisone *on page 743*
- **AquaMEPHYTON® (Can)** *see* Phytonadione *on page 1191*
- **Aquanil™ HC [OTC]** *see* Hydrocortisone *on page 743*
- **Aquaphilic® With Carbamide [OTC]** *see* Urea *on page 1530*
- **Aquasol A®** *see* Vitamin A *on page 1565*
- **Aquasol E® [OTC]** *see* Vitamin E *on page 1566*
- **Aquatensen® (Can)** *see* Methyclothiazide *on page 970*
- **Aquavan** *see* Fospropofol *on page 673*
- **Aquavit-E [OTC]** *see* Vitamin E *on page 1566*
- **Aqueous Procaine Penicillin G** *see* Penicillin G Procaine *on page 1166*
- **Ara-C** *see* Cytarabine *on page 384*
- **Arabinosylcytosine** *see* Cytarabine *on page 384*
- **Aralen®** *see* Chloroquine *on page 307*
- **Aranelle™** *see* Ethinyl Estradiol and Norethindrone *on page 581*
- **Aranesp®** *see* Darbepoetin Alfa *on page 398*
- **Arava®** *see* Leflunomide *on page 859*
- **Arcalyst™** *see* Rilonacept *on page 1318*
- **Aredia®** *see* Pamidronate *on page 1134*

Arformoterol (ar for MOE ter ol)

U.S. Brand Names Brovana®

Index Terms (R,R)-Formoterol L-Tartrate; Arformoterol Tartrate

Pharmacologic Category $Beta_2$-Adrenergic Agonist

Additional Appendix Information

Bronchodilators *on page 1650*

Use Long-term maintenance treatment of bronchoconstriction in chronic obstructive pulmonary disease (COPD), including chronic bronchitis and emphysema

Restrictions An FDA-approved medication guide must be distributed when dispensing an outpatient prescription (new or refill) where this medication is to be used without direct supervision of a healthcare provider. Medication guides are available at http://www.fda.gov/cder/Offices/ODS/medication_guides.htm.

Pregnancy Risk Factor C

Dosage Nebulization: Adults: COPD: 15 mcg twice daily; maximum: 30 mcg/day

Dosage adjustment in renal impairment: No adjustment required

Dosage adjustment in hepatic impairment: No dosage adjustment required, but use caution; systemic drug exposure prolonged (1.3- to 2.4-fold)

Additional Information Complete prescribing information for this medication should be consulted for additional detail.

Dosage Forms Excipient information presented when available (limited, particularly for generics); consult specific product labeling.

Solution for nebulization:

Brovana®: 15 mcg/2 mL (30s, 60s)

◆ **Arformoterol Tartrate** *see* Arformoterol *on page 131*

Argatroban (ar GA troh ban)

Pharmacologic Category Anticoagulant, Thrombin Inhibitor

Use Prophylaxis or treatment of thrombosis in patients with heparin-induced thrombocytopenia (HIT); adjunct to percutaneous coronary intervention (PCI) in patients who have or are at risk of thrombosis associated with HIT

Unlabeled/Investigational Use To maintain extracorporeal circuit patency (prefilter administration) of continuous renal replacement therapy (CRRT) in critically-ill patients with HIT

Pregnancy Risk Factor B

Pregnancy Considerations Adverse events were not observed in animal studies. There are no adequate and well-controlled studies in pregnant women. Argatroban should be used in pregnant women only if clearly needed.

Lactation Excretion in breast milk unknown/not recommended

Medication Safety Issues

Sound-alike/look-alike issues:

Argatroban may be confused with Aggrastat®, Orgaran®

High alert medication: The Institute for Safe Medication Practices (ISMP) includes this medication among its list of drugs which have a heightened risk of causing significant patient harm when used in error.

Contraindications Hypersensitivity to argatroban or any component of the formulation; overt major bleeding

Warnings/Precautions Hemorrhage can occur at any site in the body. Extreme caution should be used when there is an increased danger of hemorrhage, such as severe hypertension, immediately following lumbar puncture, spinal anesthesia, major surgery (including brain, spinal cord, or eye surgery), congenital or acquired bleeding disorders, and gastrointestinal ulcers. Use caution in critically-ill patients; reduced clearance may require dosage reduction. Use caution with hepatic dysfunction. Argatroban prolongs the PT/INR. Concomitant use with warfarin will cause increased prolongation of the PT and INR greater than that of warfarin alone. If warfarin is initiated concurrently with argatroban, initial PT/INR goals while on argatroban may require modification; alternative guidelines for monitoring therapy should be followed. Safety and efficacy for use with other thrombolytic agents has not been established. Discontinue all parenteral anticoagulants prior to starting therapy. Allow reversal of heparin's effects before initiation. Patients with hepatic dysfunction may require >4 hours to achieve full reversal of argatroban's anticoagulant effect following treatment. Avoid use during PCI in patients with elevations of ALT/AST (>3 times ULN); the use of argatroban in these patients has not been evaluated. Limited pharmacokinetic and dosing information is available from use in critically-ill children with heparin-induced thrombocytopenia.

Adverse Reactions As with all anticoagulants, bleeding is the major adverse effect of argatroban. Hemorrhage may occur at virtually any site. Risk is dependent on multiple variables, including the intensity of anticoagulation and patient susceptibility.

>10%:

Cardiovascular: Chest pain (PCI related: <1% to 15%), hypotension (7% to 11%)

Gastrointestinal: Gastrointestinal bleed (major: <1% to 3%; minor: 3% to 14%)

Genitourinary: Genitourinary bleed and hematuria (major: <1%; minor: 2% to 12%)

1% to 10%:

Cardiovascular: Vasodilation (1% to 10%), cardiac arrest (6%), ventricular tachycardia (5%), bradycardia (5%), myocardial infarction (PCI: 4%), atrial fibrillation (3%), angina (2%), CABG-related bleeding (minor, 2%), myocardial ischemia (2%), cerebrovascular disorder (<1% to 2%), thrombosis (<1% to 2%)

Central nervous system: Fever (<1% to 7%), headache (5%), pain (5%), intracranial bleeding (1% to 4%)

Dermatologic: Skin reactions (bullous eruption, rash; 1% to <10%)

Gastrointestinal: Nausea (5% to 7%), diarrhea (6%), vomiting (4% to 6%), abdominal pain (3% to 4%)

Genitourinary: Urinary tract infection (5%)

Hematologic: Hemoglobin decreased (<2 g/dL), hematocrit decreased (minor: 2% to 10%; major: <1%)

Local: Bleeding at injection or access site (minor: 2% to 5%)

Neuromuscular & skeletal: Back pain (PCI related: 8%)

Renal: Abnormal renal function (3%)

Respiratory: Dyspnea (8% to 10%), cough (3% to 10%), hemoptysis (minor: <1% to 3%), pneumonia (3%)

Miscellaneous: Sepsis (6%), infection (4%)

<1% (Limited to important or life-threatening): Allergic reactions, GERD, limb and below-the-knee stump bleed, multisystem hemorrhage and DIC, pulmonary edema, retroperitoneal bleeding

Drug Interactions

Metabolism/Transport Effects **Substrate** of CYP3A4 (minor)

Avoid Concomitant Use There are no known interactions where it is recommended to avoid concomitant use.

Increased Effect/Toxicity

Argatroban may increase the levels/effects of: Anticoagulants; Ibritumomab; Tositumomab and Iodine I 131 Tositumomab

The levels/effects of Argatroban may be increased by: Antiplatelet Agents; Dasatinib; Herbs (Anticoagulant/Antiplatelet Properties); Nonsteroidal Anti-Inflammatory Agents; Pentosan Polysulfate Sodium; Prostacyclin Analogues; Salicylates; Thrombolytic Agents

Decreased Effect There are no known significant interactions involving a decrease in effect.

Stability Prior to use, store at 15°C to 30°C (59°F to 86°F). Protect from light. The prepared solution is stable for 24 hours at 15°C to 30°C (59°F to 86°F) in ambient indoor light. Do not expose to direct sunlight. May be mixed with 0.9% sodium chloride injection, 5% dextrose injection, or lactated Ringer's injection. Do not mix with other medications.

To prepare solution for I.V. administration, dilute each 250 mg vial with 250 mL of diluent. Mix by repeated inversion for 1 minute. Once mixed, final concentration should be 1 mg/mL. A slight but brief haziness may occur prior to mixing. Prepared solutions that are protected from light and kept at controlled room temperature of 20°C to 25°C (68°F to 77°F) or under refrigeration at 2°C to 8°C (36°F to 46°F) are stable for up to 96 hours.

Mechanism of Action A direct, highly-selective thrombin inhibitor. Reversibly binds to the active thrombin site of free and clot-associated thrombin. Inhibits fibrin formation; activation of coagulation factors V, VIII, and XIII; activation of protein C; and platelet aggregation.

Pharmacodynamics/Kinetics

Onset of action: Immediate

Distribution: 174 mL/kg

Protein binding: Albumin: 20%; α_1-acid glycoprotein: 35%

Metabolism: Hepatic via hydroxylation and aromatization. Metabolism via CYP3A4/5 to four known metabolites plays a minor role. Unchanged argatroban is the major plasma component. Plasma concentration of metabolite M1 is 0% to 20% of the parent drug and is three- to fivefold weaker.

Half-life elimination: 39-51 minutes; Hepatic impairment: ≤181 minutes

Time to peak: Steady-state: 1-3 hours

Excretion: Feces (65%); urine (22%); low quantities of metabolites M2-4 in urine

Clearance is decreased in critically-ill pediatric patients

Dosage I.V.:

Children: **Heparin-induced thrombocytopenia** (dosing based on limited data from critically-ill patients):

Initial dose: 0.75 mcg/kg/minute

Maintenance dose: Patient may not be at steady-state but measure aPTT after 2 hours; adjust dose until the steady-state aPTT is 1.5-3.0 times the initial baseline value, not exceeding 100 seconds; dosage may be adjusted in increments of 0.1-0.25 mcg/kg/minute. **Note:** Frequent dosage adjustments may be required to maintain desired anticoagulant activity.

Adults:

Heparin-induced thrombocytopenia:

Initial dose: 2 mcg/kg/minute

Maintenance dose: Patient may not be at steady-state but measure aPTT after 2 hours; adjust dose until the steady-state aPTT is 1.5-3.0 times the initial baseline value, not exceeding 100 seconds; dosage should not exceed 10 mcg/kg/minute

Note: Critically-ill patients with normal hepatic function became excessively anticoagulated with FDA-approved or lower starting doses of argatroban. Doses between 0.15-1.3 mcg/kg/minute were required to maintain aPTTs in the target range (Reichert, 2003). In a prospective observational study of critically-ill patients with MODS and suspected or proven HIT, an initial infusion dose of 0.2 mcg/kg/minute was found to be sufficient and safe in this population (Beiderlinden, 2007). Consider reducing starting dose to 0.2 mcg/kg/minute in critically-ill patients with multiple organ dysfunction (MODS) defined as a minimum number of two organ failures. Another report of a cardiac patient with anasarca secondary to acute renal failure had a reduction in argatroban clearance similar to patients with hepatic dysfunction. Reduced clearance may have been due to reduced liver perfusion (de Denus, 2003). The American College of Chest Physicians has recommended an initial infusion rate of 0.5-1.2 mcg/kg/minute for patients with heart failure, MODS, severe anasarca, or postcardiac surgery (Hirsch, 2008).

Conversion to oral anticoagulant: Because there may be a combined effect on the INR when argatroban is combined with warfarin, loading doses of warfarin should not be used. Warfarin therapy should be started at the expected daily dose.

Patients receiving ≤2 mcg/kg/minute of argatroban: Argatroban therapy can be stopped when the combined INR on warfarin and argatroban is >4; repeat INR measurement in 4-6 hours; if INR is below therapeutic level, argatroban therapy may be restarted. Repeat procedure daily until desired INR on warfarin alone is obtained.

Patients receiving >2 mcg/kg/minute of argatroban: In order to predict the INR on warfarin alone, reduce dose of argatroban to 2 mcg/kg/minute; measure INR for argatroban and warfarin 4-6 hours after dose reduction; argatroban therapy can be stopped when the combined INR on warfarin and argatroban is >4. Repeat INR measurement in 4-6 hours; if INR is below therapeutic level, argatroban therapy may be restarted. Repeat procedure daily until desired INR on warfarin alone is obtained.

Prefilter administration for continuous renal replacement therapy (CRRT) in critically-ill patients with HIT (unlabeled use; Link, 2008): 0.1 – 1.5 mcg/kg/min Note: Loading dose of 100 mcg/kg was administered during clinical trial; however, this may be unnecessary.

Percutaneous coronary intervention (PCI):

Initial: Begin infusion of 25 mcg/kg/minute and administer bolus dose of 350 mcg/kg (over 3-5 minutes). ACT should be checked 5-10 minutes after bolus infusion; proceed with procedure if ACT >300 seconds. Following initial bolus:

ACT <300 seconds: Give an additional 150 mcg/kg bolus, and increase infusion rate to 30 mcg/kg/minute (recheck ACT in 5-10 minutes)

ACT >450 seconds: Decrease infusion rate to 15 mcg/kg/minute (recheck ACT in 5-10 minutes)

Once a therapeutic ACT (300-450 seconds) is achieved, infusion should be continued at this dose for the duration of the procedure.

If dissection, impending abrupt closure, thrombus formation during PCI, or inability to achieve ACT >300 seconds: An additional bolus of 150 mcg/kg, followed by an increase in infusion rate to 40 mcg/kg/minute may be administered.

Note: Post-PCI anticoagulation, if required, may be achieved by continuing infusion at a reduced dose of 2-10 mcg/kg/minute, with close monitoring of aPTT.

Elderly: No adjustment is necessary for patients with normal liver function

Dosage adjustment in renal impairment: Removal during hemodialysis and continuous venovenous hemofiltration is clinically insignificant. No dosage adjustment required.

Dosage adjustment in hepatic impairment: Decreased clearance and increased elimination half-life are seen with hepatic impairment; dose should be reduced.

Children: Initial dose: 0.2 mcg/kg/minute; adjust dose in increments of ≤0.05 mcg/kg/minute

Adults: Initial dose for moderate hepatic impairment is 0.5 mcg/kg/minute. **Note:** During PCI, avoid use in patients with elevations of ALT/AST (>3 times ULN); the use of argatroban in these patients has not been evaluated.

Administration Solution **must be diluted to 1 mg/mL** prior to administration.

Monitoring Parameters Obtain baseline aPTT prior to start of therapy. Patient may not be at steady-state but check aPTT 2 hours after start of therapy to adjust dose, keeping the steady-state aPTT 1.5-3 times the initial baseline value (not exceeding 100 seconds). Monitor hemoglobin, hematocrit, signs and symptoms of bleeding.

PCI: Monitor ACT before dosing, 5-10 minutes after bolus dosing, and after any change in infusion rate and at the end of the procedure. Additional ACT assessments should be made every 20-30 minutes during extended PCI procedures.

Test Interactions PT/INR levels may become elevated in the absence of warfarin. If warfarin is started, initial PT/INR goals while on argatroban may require modification.

Additional Information Platelet counts recovered by day 3 in 53% of patients with heparin-induced thrombocytopenia and in 58% of patients with heparin-induced thrombocytopenia with thrombosis syndrome.

Dosage Forms Excipient information presented when available (limited, particularly for generics); consult specific product labeling.

Injection, solution: 100 mg/mL (2.5 mL) [contains dehydrated alcohol 1000 mg/mL]

Arginine (AR ji neen)

U.S. Brand Names R-Gene®

Index Terms Arginine Hydrochloride

Pharmacologic Category Diagnostic Agent

Use Pituitary function test (growth hormone)

Unlabeled/Investigational Use Management of severe, uncompensated, metabolic alkalosis (pH ≥7.55) **after optimizing therapy with sodium and potassium** supplements

Pregnancy Risk Factor B

Dosage I.V.: Pituitary function test:

Children: 500 mg/kg/dose administered over 30 minutes

Adults: 30 g (300 mL) administered over 30 minutes

Additional Information Complete prescribing information for this medication should be consulted for additional detail.

Dosage Forms Excipient information presented when available (limited, particularly for generics); consult specific product labeling.

Injection, solution, as hydrochloride:

R-Gene®: 10% (300 mL) [100 mg/mL = 950 mOsm/L; contains chloride 0.475 mEq/mL]

◆ **Arginine Hydrochloride** *see* Arginine *on page* 133

◆ **8-Arginine Vasopressin** *see* Vasopressin *on page* 1552

◆ **Aricept®** *see* Donepezil *on page* 478

◆ **Aricept® ODT** *see* Donepezil *on page* 478

◆ **Aricept® RDT (Can)** *see* Donepezil *on page* 478

◆ **Arimidex®** *see* Anastrozole *on page* 116

Aripiprazole (ay ri PIP ray zole)

U.S. Brand Names Abilify®; Abilify® Discmelt™

Index Terms BMS 337039; OPC-14597

Pharmacologic Category Antipsychotic Agent, Atypical

Additional Appendix Information

Antipsychotic Agents *on page* 1644

Use

Oral: Acute and maintenance treatment of schizophrenia; stabilization, maintenance, and adjunctive therapy (to lithium or valproate) of bipolar disorder (with acute manic or mixed episodes); adjunctive treatment of major depressive disorder

Injection: Agitation associated with schizophrenia or bipolar mania

Unlabeled/Investigational Use Depression with psychotic features; aggression (children); conduct disorder (children); Tourette syndrome (children); psychosis/agitation related to Alzheimer's dementia

Restrictions An FDA-approved medication guide concerning the use of antidepressants in children, adolescents, and young adults must be distributed when dispensing an outpatient prescription (new or refill) where this medication is to be used without direct supervision of a healthcare provider. Medication guides are available at http://www.fda.gov/cder/Offices/ODS/medication_guides.htm. Dispense to parents or guardians of children and adolescents receiving this medication.

Pregnancy Risk Factor C

Pregnancy Considerations Aripiprazole demonstrated developmental toxicity and teratogenic effects in animal models. There are no adequate and well-controlled trials in pregnant women. Should be used in pregnancy only when potential benefit to mother outweighs possible risk to the fetus. Healthcare providers are encouraged to enroll women 18-45 years of age exposed to aripiprazole during pregnancy in the Atypical Antipsychotics Pregnancy Registry (1-866-961-2388).

Lactation Excretion in breast milk unknown/not recommended

Medication Safety Issues

Sound-alike/look-alike issues:

Aripiprazole may be confused with proton pump inhibitors (eg, rabeprazole)

Contraindications Hypersensitivity to aripiprazole or any component of the formulation

Warnings/Precautions **[U.S. Boxed Warning]: Elderly patients with dementia-related psychosis treated with atypical antipsychotics are at an increased risk of death compared to placebo.** An increased incidence of cerebrovascular adverse events (including fatalities) has been reported in elderly patients with dementia-related psychosis. Aripiprazole is not approved for this indication.

[U.S. Boxed Warning]: Antidepressants increase the risk of suicidal thinking and behavior in children, adolescents, and young adults (18-24 years of age) with major depressive disorder (MDD) and other psychiatric disorders; consider risk prior to prescribing. The possibility of a suicide attempt is inherent in major depression and may persist until remission occurs. Patients treated with antidepressants should be observed for clinical worsening and suicidality, especially during the initial few months of a course of drug therapy, or at times of dose changes, either increases or decreases. Prescriptions should be written for the smallest quantity consistent with good patient care. The patient's family or caregiver should be alerted to monitor patients for the emergence of suicidality and associated behaviors; patients should be instructed to notify their healthcare provider if any of these symptoms or worsening depression or psychosis occur.

A medication guide concerning the use of antidepressants should be dispensed with each prescription. **Aripiprazole is not FDA approved for adjunctive treatment of depression in children.**

May cause extrapyramidal symptoms (EPS), including pseudoparkinsonism, acute dystonic reactions, akathisia, and tardive dyskinesia (risk of these reactions is very low relative to typical/conventional antipsychotics, frequencies reported are similar to placebo). Risk of dystonia (and probably other EPS) may be greater with increased doses, use of conventional antipsychotics, males, and younger patients. May be associated with neuroleptic malignant syndrome (NMS).

May be sedating, use with caution in disorders where CNS depression is a feature. May cause orthostatic hypotension (although reported rates are similar to placebo); use caution in patients at risk of this effect or those who would not tolerate transient hypotensive episodes (cerebrovascular disease, cardiovascular disease, or other medications which may predispose).

Use caution in patients with Parkinson's disease; predisposition to seizures; and severe cardiac disease. May alter cardiac conduction; life-threatening arrhythmias have occurred with therapeutic doses of antipsychotics. Esophageal dysmotility and aspiration have been associated with antipsychotic use; use caution in patients at risk of pneumonia (eg, Alzheimer's disease). May alter temperature regulation. Significant weight gain has been observed with antipsychotic therapy; incidence varies with product. Monitor waist circumference and BMI.

Atypical antipsychotics have been associated with development of hyperglycemia; in some cases, may be extreme and associated with ketoacidosis, hyperosmolar coma, or death. Reports of hyperglycemia with aripiprazole therapy have been few and specific risk associated with this agent is not known. Use caution in patients with diabetes or other disorders of glucose regulation; monitor for worsening of glucose control.

Abilify® Discmelt™: Use caution in phenylketonuria; contains phenylalanine. Safety and efficacy in patients <10 years of age have not been established.

Adverse Reactions Unless otherwise noted, frequency of adverse reactions is shown as reported for adult patients receiving oral administration. Spectrum and incidence of adverse effects similar in children; exceptions noted when incidence much higher in children.

>10%:

Central nervous system: Headache (27%; children 16%; injection 12%), agitation (19%), insomnia (18%), anxiety (17%), akathisia (10% to 13%; injection 2%), lightheadedness (11%)

Gastrointestinal: Weight gain (8% to 30%; highest frequency in patients with BMI <23; children 3%), nausea (15%; injection 9%), dyspepsia (9% to 15%; injection 1%), constipation (11% to 13%), vomiting (11%; injection 3%)

1% to 10%:

Cardiovascular: Orthostatic hypotension (1% to 5%), tachycardia (injection 2%), chest pain, hypertension, peripheral edema

Central nervous system: Dizziness (10%; children 5%; injection 8%), sedation (dose-related 5% to 8%; children 20% to 23%; injection: 7%), EPS (5% to 6%; children 19% to 20%), restlessness (5% to 6%), fatigue (6%; children 7% to 11%), pain (3%), dystonia (children 2%), irritability, suicidal ideation

Dermatologic: Rash

Gastrointestinal: Salivation increased (children 4% to 8%), xerostomia (5%; children 2%; injection 1%), toothache (4%), abdominal discomfort (3%), diarrhea (children 3%), weight loss

Neuromuscular & skeletal: Tremor (5% to 9%), weakness (8%), arthralgia (5%; children 2%), extremity pain (4%), stiffness (4%), myalgia (2% to 4%), spasm (2%)

Ocular: Blurred vision (3%; children 5% to 8%)

Respiratory: Pharyngolaryngeal pain (3%), cough (3%), nasal congestion

<1% (Limited to important or life-threatening): Aggression, agitation, agranulocytosis, alopecia, akinesia, amenorrhea, anaphylactic reaction, anger, angina pectoris, angioedema, anorexia, anorgasmia, asphyxia, aspiration pneumonia, atrial fibrillation, atrial flutter, atrioventricular block, bilirubin increased, bradycardia, bradykinesia, breast pain, bundle branch block, cardiopulmonary failure, cardiorespiratory arrest, catatonia, cerebrovascular accident, cholelithiasis, choreoathetosis, cogwheel rigidity, complete atrioventricular block, creatine phosphokinase increased, creatinine increased, deep vein thrombosis, delirium, diplopia, diabetes mellitus, DKA, dysphagia, dyspnea, edema (facial), erectile dysfunction, esophagitis, extrasystoles, galactorrhea, gastrointestinal hemorrhage, GGT increased, glycosylated hemoglobin increased, gynecomastia, heat stroke, hepatic enzyme increased, hepatitis, homicidal ideation, hostility, hyper-/hypoglycemia, hyperlipidemia, hypersensitivity, hyper-/hypotonia, hypotension, hypokalemia, hypokinesia, hyponatremia, hypothermia cholecystitis, idiopathic thrombocytopenic purpura, intentional self injury, jaundice, lactate dehydrogenase increased, leukopenia, libido changes, memory impairment, menstrual irregularities, MI, muscle rigidity, muscle spasms, myocardial ischemia, myoclonus, neutropenia, nocturia, oropharyngeal spasm, palpitation, pancreatitis, parkinsonism, phlebitis, photophobia, polydypsia, polyuria, priapism, prolactin increased, pruritus, psychomotor agitation, pulmonary embolism, QT_c prolonged, respiratory distress, rhabdomyolysis, seizure (grand mal), shock, speech disorder, suicide, suicide attempt, supraventricular tachycardia, swollen tongue, tardive dyskinesia, thrombocytopenia, thrombophlebitis, tic, ulcer, urea increased, urinary retention, urticaria, ventricular tachycardia

Drug Interactions

Metabolism/Transport Effects Substrate (major) of CYP2D6, 3A4

Avoid Concomitant Use There are no known interactions where it is recommended to avoid concomitant use.

Increased Effect/Toxicity

Aripiprazole may increase the levels/effects of: Alcohol (Ethyl); CNS Depressants

The levels/effects of Aripiprazole may be increased by: Acetylcholinesterase Inhibitors (Central); CYP2D6 Inhibitors (Moderate); CYP2D6 Inhibitors (Strong); CYP3A4 Inhibitors (Moderate); CYP3A4 Inhibitors (Strong); Darunavir; Dasatinib; Lithium formulations; Tetrabenazine

Decreased Effect

Aripiprazole may decrease the levels/effects of: Amphetamines; Anti-Parkinson's Agents (Dopamine Agonist)

The levels/effects of Aripiprazole may be decreased by: CarBAMazepine; CYP3A4 Inducers (Strong); Deferasirox; Herbs (CYP3A4 Inducers); Lithium formulations

Ethanol/Nutrition/Herb Interactions

Ethanol: Avoid ethanol (may increase CNS depression).

Food: Ingestion with a high-fat meal delays time to peak plasma level.

Herb/Nutraceutical: St John's wort may decrease aripiprazole levels. Avoid kava kava, gotu kola, valerian, St John's wort (may increase CNS depression).

Stability

Injection solution: Store at controlled room temperature of 25°C (77°F); excursions permitted to 15°C to 30°C (59°F to 86°F). Protect from light.

Oral solution: Store at controlled room temperature of 25°C (77°F); excursions permitted to 15°C to 30°C (59°F to 86°F). Use within 6 months after opening.

Tablet: Store at controlled room temperature of 25°C (77°F); excursions permitted to 15°C to 30°C (59°F to 86°F).

Mechanism of Action Aripiprazole is a quinolinone antipsychotic which exhibits high affinity for D_2, D_3, 5-HT_{1A}, and 5-HT_{2A} receptors; moderate affinity for D_4, 5-HT_{2C}, 5-HT_7, $alpha_1$ adrenergic, and H_1 receptors. It also possesses moderate affinity for the serotonin reuptake transporter; has no affinity for muscarinic (cholinergic) receptors. Aripiprazole functions as a partial agonist at the D_2 and 5-HT_{1A} receptors, and as an antagonist at the 5-HT_{2A} receptor.

Pharmacodynamics/Kinetics

Onset of action: Initial: 1-3 weeks

Absorption: Well absorbed

Distribution: V_d: 4.9 L/kg

Protein binding: ≥99%, primarily to albumin

Metabolism: Hepatic, via CYP2D6, CYP3A4 (dehydro-aripiprazole metabolite has affinity for D_2 receptors similar to the parent drug and represents 40% of the parent drug exposure in plasma)

Bioavailability: I.M.: 100%; Tablet: 87%

Half-life elimination: Aripiprazole: 75 hours; dehydro-aripiprazole: 94 hours

CYP2D6 poor metabolizers: Aripiprazole: 146 hours

Time to peak, plasma: I.M.: 1-3 hours; Tablet: 3-5 hours

With high-fat meal: Aripiprazole: Delayed by 3 hours; dehydro-aripiprazole: Delayed by 12 hours

Excretion: Feces (55%, ~18% unchanged drug); urine (25%, <1% unchanged drug)

Dosage Note: Oral solution may be substituted for the oral tablet on a mg-per-mg basis, up to 25 mg. Patients receiving 30 mg tablets should be given 25 mg oral solution. Orally disintegrating tablets (Abilify® Discmelt™) are bioequivalent to the immediate release tablets (Abilify®).

Children: Oral: Aggression, conduct disorder, Tourette syndrome (unlabeled uses): 5-20 mg/day

Children ≥10 years: Oral: Bipolar I disorder (acute manic or mixed episodes): Initial: 2 mg daily for 2 days, followed by 5 mg daily for 2 days with a further increase to target dose of 10 mg daily as monotherapy or adjunctive therapy; subsequent dose increases may be made in 5 mg increments, up to a maximum of 30 mg/day

Adolescents ≥13 years: Oral: Schizophrenia: Initial: 2 mg daily for 2 days, followed by 5 mg daily for 2 days with a further increase to target dose of 10 mg daily; subsequent dose increases may be made in 5 mg increments up to a maximum of 30 mg/day (30 mg/day not shown to be more efficacious than 10 mg/day)

Adults:

Acute agitation (schizophrenia/bipolar mania): I.M.: 9.75 mg as a single dose (range: 5.25-15 mg); repeated doses may be given at ≥2-hour intervals to a maximum of 30 mg/day. **Note:** If ongoing therapy with aripiprazole is necessary, transition to oral therapy as soon as possible.

Bipolar disorder (acute manic or mixed episodes): Oral:

Stabilization: Initial: 15 mg once daily as monotherapy or adjunctive to lithium or valproic acid. May increase to 30 mg once daily if clinically indicated; safety of doses >30 mg/day has not been evaluated.

Maintenance: Continue stabilization dose for up to 6 weeks; efficacy of continued treatment >6 weeks has not been established

Depression (adjunctive with antidepressants): Oral: Initial: 2-5 mg/day (range: 2-15 mg/day); dose adjustments of up to 5 mg/day may be made in intervals of ≥1 week. **Note:** Dosing based on patients already receiving antidepressant therapy.

Schizophrenia: Oral: 10-15 mg once daily; may be increased to a maximum of 30 mg once daily (efficacy at dosages above 10-15 mg has not been shown to be increased). Dosage titration should not be more frequent than every 2 weeks.

Dosage adjustment with concurrent CYP450 inducer or inhibitor therapy: Oral:

CYP3A4 inducers (eg, carbamazepine): Aripiprazole dose should be doubled (20-30 mg/day); dose should be subsequently reduced (10-15 mg/day) if concurrent inducer agent discontinued.

CYP3A4 inhibitors (eg, ketoconazole): Aripiprazole dose should be reduced to 1/2 of the usual dose, and proportionally increased upon discontinuation of the inhibitor agent.

CYP2D6 inhibitors (eg, fluoxetine, paroxetine): Aripiprazole dose should be reduced to 1/2 of the usual dose, and proportionally increased upon discontinuation of the inhibitor agent.

Dosage adjustment in renal impairment: No dosage adjustment required

Dosage adjustment in hepatic impairment: No dosage adjustment required

Dietary Considerations May be taken with or without food. Oral solution contains sucrose 400 mg/mL and fructose 200 mg/mL. Orally-disintegrating tablet contains phenylalanine; avoid use in phenylketonuria.

Administration

Injection: For I.M. use only; do not administer SubQ or I.V.; inject slowly into deep muscle mass

Oral: May be administered with or without food. Tablet and oral solution may be interchanged on a mg-per-mg basis, up to 25 mg. Doses using 30 mg tablets should be exchanged for 25 mg oral solution. Orally disintegrating tablets (Abilify® Discmelt™) are bioequivalent to the immediate release tablets (Abilify®).

Orally-disintegrating tablet: Remove from foil blister by peeling back (do not push tablet through the foil). Place tablet in mouth immediately upon removal. Tablet dissolves rapidly in saliva and may be swallowed without liquid. If needed, can be taken with liquid. Do not split tablet.

Monitoring Parameters Vital signs; fasting lipid profile and fasting blood glucose/Hb A_{1c} (prior to treatment, at 3 months, then annually); BMI, personal/family history of diabetes, waist circumference, blood pressure, mental status, abnormal involuntary movement scale (AIMS), extrapyramidal symptoms (EPS). Weight should be assessed prior to treatment, at 4 weeks, 8 weeks, 12 weeks, and then at quarterly intervals. Consider titrating to a different antipsychotic agent for a weight gain ≥5% of the initial weight.

Dosage Forms Excipient information presented when available (limited, particularly for generics); consult specific product labeling.

Injection, solution:

Abilify®: 7.5 mg/mL (1.3 mL)

Solution, oral:

Abilify®: 1 mg/mL (150 mL) [contains propylene glycol, sucrose 400 mg/mL, and fructose 200 mg/mL; orange cream flavor]

Tablet:

Abilify®: 2 mg, 5 mg, 10 mg, 15 mg, 20 mg, 30 mg

Tablet, orally disintegrating:

Abilify® Discmelt™: 10 mg [contains phenylalanine 1.12 mg; creme de vanilla flavor]; 15 mg [contains phenylalanine 1.68 mg; creme de vanilla flavor]

◆ **Aristospan®** *see* Triamcinolone *on page 1510*

◆ **Arixtra®** *see* Fondaparinux *on page 660*

Armodafinil (ar moe DAF i nil)

U.S. Brand Names Nuvigil™

Index Terms R-modafinil

Pharmacologic Category Stimulant

Use Improve wakefulness in patients with excessive daytime sleepiness associated with narcolepsy and shift work sleep disorder (SWSD); adjunctive therapy for obstructive sleep apnea/hypopnea syndrome (OSAHS)

Restrictions C-IV

Pregnancy Risk Factor C

Pregnancy Considerations There are no well-controlled studies of armodafinil in pregnant women. There have been reports of intrauterine growth retardation and spontaneous abortions in women using the both armodafinil and modafinil, but relationship to the drug is unknown. Adverse events have been observed in animal studies. Armodafinil and modafinil have been studied in both rats and rabbits. Developmental toxicity (including visceral and skeletal abnormalities and decreased fetal weight) in rats (armodafinil and modafinil) and rabbits (modafinil) has been observed at doses correlating to those used clinically. Efficacy of steroidal contraceptives may be decreased; alternate means of contraception should be considered during therapy and for 1 month after modafinil is discontinued.

Lactation Excretion in breast milk unknown/use caution

Contraindications Hypersensitivity to armodafinil, modafinil, or any component of the formulation

Warnings/Precautions For use following complete evaluation of sleepiness and in conjunction with other standard treatments (eg, CPAP). The degree of sleepiness should be reassessed frequently; some patients may not return to a normal level of wakefulness. Use is not recommended with a history of angina, cardiac ischemia, recent history of myocardial infarction, left ventricular hypertrophy, or patients with mitral valve prolapse who have developed mitral valve prolapse syndrome with previous CNS stimulant use. Blood pressure monitoring may be required in patients on armodafinil. New or additional antihypertensive therapy may be needed.

Serious and life-threatening rashes including Stevens-Johnson syndrome, toxic epidermal necrolysis, and drug rash with eosinophilia and systemic symptoms have been reported with modafinil, the racemate of armodafinil. In clinical trials of modafinil, these rashes were more likely to occur in children; however, in the postmarketing period, serious reactions have occurred in both adults and children. Most cases have been reported within the first 5 weeks of initiating therapy; however, rare cases have occurred after prolonged therapy.

Caution should be exercised when modafinil is given to patients with a history of psychosis; may impair the ability to engage in potentially hazardous activities. Stimulants may unmask tics in individuals with coexisting Tourette's syndrome. Use caution with renal or hepatic impairment (dosage adjustment in hepatic dysfunction is recommended). Use reduced doses in elderly patients. Safety and efficacy in children <17 years of age have not been established.

Adverse Reactions

>10%: Central nervous system: Headache (14% to 23%; dose-related)

1% to 10%:

Cardiovascular: Palpitation (2%), increased heart rate (1%)

Central nervous system: Dizziness (5%), insomnia (4% to 6%; dose related), anxiety (4%), depression (1% to 3%; dose related), fatigue (2%), agitation (1%), attention disturbance (1%), depressed mood (1%), migraine (1%), nervousness (1%), pain (1%), pyrexia (1%), tremor (1%)

Dermatologic: Rash (1% to 4%; dose related), contact dermatitis (1%), hyperhidrosis (1%)

Gastrointestinal: Nausea (6% to 9%; dose related), xerostomia (2% to 7%; dose related), diarrhea (4%), abdominal pain (2%), dyspepsia (2%), anorexia (1%), appetite decreased (1%), constipation (1%), loose stools (1%), vomiting (1%)

Genitourinary: Polyuria (1%)

Hepatic: GGT increased (1%)

Neuromuscular & skeletal: Paresthesia (1%)

Respiratory: Dyspnea (1%)

Miscellaneous: Flu-like syndrome (1%), thirst (1%)

Postmarketing and/or case reports: Anaphylactoid reaction, angioedema, hypersensitivity, liver enzymes increased, pancytopenia, systolic blood pressure increased

Drug Interactions

Metabolism/Transport Effects

Substrate of CYP3A4 (major); **Inhibits** CYP2C19 (moderate); **Induces** CYP1A2 (weak), 3A4 (moderate)

Avoid Concomitant Use

Avoid concomitant use of Armodafinil with any of the following: Iobenguane I 123

Increased Effect/Toxicity

Armodafinil may increase the levels/effects of: CYP2C19 Substrates; Sympathomimetics

The levels/effects of Armodafinil may be increased by: Cannabinoids; CYP3A4 Inhibitors (Moderate); CYP3A4 Inhibitors (Strong); Dasatinib

Decreased Effect

Armodafinil may decrease the levels/effects of: Iobenguane I 123; Maraviroc; Oral Contraceptive (Estrogens)

The levels/effects of Armodafinil may be decreased by: CYP3A4 Inducers (Strong); Deferasirox; Herbs (CYP3A4 Inducers)

Ethanol/Nutrition/Herb Interactions

Ethanol: Avoid or limit ethanol.

Food: Delays absorption, but minimal effects on bioavailability. Food may affect the onset and time course of armodafinil.

Stability Store at 20°C to 25°C (68°F to 77°F).

Mechanism of Action The exact mechanism of action of armodafinil is unknown. It is the R-enantiomer of modafinil. Armodafinil binds to the dopamine transporter and inhibits dopamine reuptake, which may result in increased extracellular dopamine levels in the brain. However, it does not appear to be a dopamine receptor agonist and also does not appear to bind to or inhibit the most common receptors or enzymes that are relevant for sleep/wake regulation.

Pharmacodynamics/Kinetics

Absorption: Readily absorbed

Distribution: V_d: 42 L

Protein binding: ~60% (based on modafinil; primarily albumin)

Metabolism: Hepatic, multiple pathways, including CYP3A4/5; metabolites include R-modafinil acid and modafinil sulfone

Clearance: 33 mL/minute, mainly via hepatic metabolism

Half-life elimination: 15 hours; Steady state: ~7 days

Time to peak, plasma: 2 hours (fasted)

Excretion: Urine (80% predominantly as metabolites; <10% as unchanged drug)

Dosage Oral:

Adults:

Narcolepsy: 150-250 mg once daily in the morning

Obstructive sleep apnea/hypopnea syndrome (OSAHS): 150-250 mg once daily in the morning; 250 mg was not shown to have any increased benefit over 150 mg

Shift work sleep disorder (SWSD): 150 mg given once daily ~1 hour prior to work shift

Elderly: Consider lower initial dosage. Concentrations were almost doubled in clinical trials (based on modafinil)

Dosage adjustment in renal impairment: Inadequate data to determine safety and efficacy in severe renal impairment.

Dosage adjustment in hepatic impairment: Severe hepatic impairment (Child-Pugh classes B and C): Based on modafinil, dose should be reduced by half

Dietary Considerations Take with or without meals.

Administration May be administered without regard to food.

Monitoring Parameters Signs of hypersensitivity, rash, psychiatric symptoms, levels of sleepiness, blood pressure, and drug abuse

Dosage Forms Excipient information presented when available (limited, particularly for generics); consult specific product labeling.

Tablet:

Nuvigil™: 50 mg, 150 mg, 250 mg

◆ **Armour® Thyroid** *see* Thyroid, Desiccated *on page 1464*

◆ **Aromasin®** *see* Exemestane *on page 595*

◆ **Arranon®** *see* Nelarabine *on page 1047*

Arsenic Trioxide (AR se nik tri OKS id)

U.S. Brand Names Trisenox®

Index Terms As_2O_3; NSC-706363

Pharmacologic Category Antineoplastic Agent, Miscellaneous

Use Induction of remission and consolidation in patients with relapsed or refractory acute promyelocytic leukemia (APL) which is specifically characterized by t(15;17) translocation or PML/RAR-alpha gene expression

Unlabeled/Investigational Use Treatment of myelodysplastic syndrome (MDS), multiple myeloma

Pregnancy Risk Factor D

Pregnancy Considerations Increased resorptions, neural-tube defects, and ophthalmic abnormalities have been observed in animal studies. Arsenic crosses the human placenta. In studies of women exposed to high levels of arsenic from drinking water, cord blood levels were similar to maternal serum levels. Dimethylarsinic acid (DMA) was the form of arsenic found in the fetus. An increased risk of low birth weight and still births were observed in women who ingested high levels of dietary arsenic. There are no studies of arsenic trioxide therapy in pregnant women. Women of childbearing potential should avoid pregnancy.

Lactation Enters breast milk/not recommended

Medication Safety Issues

High alert medication: The Institute for Safe Medication Practices (ISMP) includes this medication among its list of drugs which have a heightened risk of causing significant patient harm when used in error.

Contraindications Hypersensitivity to arsenic or any component of the formulation

Warnings/Precautions Hazardous agent - use appropriate precautions for handling and disposal. **[U.S. Boxed Warnings]: May prolong the QT interval. May lead to torsade de pointes or complete AV block.** Risk factors for torsade de pointes include HF, a history of torsade de pointes, pre-existing QT interval prolongation, patients taking potassium-wasting diuretics, and conditions which cause hypokalemia or hypomagnesemia. If possible, discontinue all medications known to prolong the QT interval. **[U.S. Boxed Warning]: A baseline 12-lead ECG, serum electrolytes (potassium, calcium, magnesium), and creatinine should be obtained prior to treatment.** Correct electrolyte abnormalities prior to treatment and monitor potassium and magnesium levels during therapy (potassium should stay >4 mEq/dL and magnesium >1.8 mg/dL). Correct QT_c >500 msec prior to treatment. Discontinue therapy and hospitalize patient if QT_c >500 msec, syncope, or irregular heartbeats develop during therapy; do not reinitiate until QT_c <460 msec.

[U.S. Boxed Warning]: May cause retinoic-acid-acute promyelocytic leukemia (RA-APL) syndrome or APL differentiation syndrome (dyspnea, fever, weight gain, pulmonary infiltrates, and pleural or pericardial effusions) in patients with APL. High-dose steroids have been used for treatment. May lead to the development of hyperleukocytosis (leukocytes ≥10,000/mm^3). Use with caution in renal impairment; arsenic is eliminated renally. **[U.S. Boxed Warning]: Should be administered under the supervision of an experienced cancer chemotherapy physician.** Safety and efficacy in children <5 years of age have not been established (limited experience with children 5-16 years of age).

Adverse Reactions

>10%:

Cardiovascular: Tachycardia (55%), edema (40%), QT interval >500 msec (40%), chest pain (25%; grades 3/4: 5%), hypotension (25%; grades 3/4: 5%)

Central nervous system: Fatigue (63%), fever (63%), headache (60%), insomnia (43%), anxiety (30%), dizziness (23%), depression (20%), pain (15%)

Dermatologic: Dermatitis (43%), pruritus (33%), bruising (20%), dry skin (13%)

Endocrine & metabolic: Hypokalemia (50%; grades 3/4: 13%), hyperglycemia (45%; grades 3/4: 13%), hypomagnesemia (45%; grades 3/4: 13%), hyperkalemia (18%; grades 3/4: 5%)

Gastrointestinal: Nausea (75%), abdominal pain (58%), vomiting (58%), diarrhea (53%), sore throat (35% to 40%), constipation (28%), anorexia (23%), appetite decreased (15%), weight gain (13%)

Genitourinary: Vaginal hemorrhage (13%)

Hematologic: Leukocytosis (50%; grades 3/4: 3%), APL differentiation syndrome (23%), anemia (20%; grades 3/4: 5%), thrombocytopenia (18%; grades 3/4: 13%), febrile neutropenia (13%; grades 3/4: 8%)

Hepatic: ALT increased (20%; grades 3/4: 5%), AST increased (13%; grades 3/4: 3%)

Local: Injection site: Pain (20%), erythema (13%)

Neuromuscular & skeletal: Neuropathy (43%), rigors (38%), arthralgia (33%), paresthesia (33%), myalgia (25%), bone pain (23%), back pain (18%), limb pain (13%), neck pain (13%), tremor (13%)

Respiratory: Cough (65%), dyspnea (38% to 53%; grades 3/4: 10%), epistaxis (25%), hypoxia (23%), pleural effusion (20%), sinusitis (20%), postnasal drip (13%), upper respiratory tract infection (13%), wheezing (13%)

Miscellaneous: Herpes simplex (13%)

1% to 10%:

Cardiovascular: Hypertension (10%), flushing (10%), pallor (10%), palpitation (10%), facial edema (8%), abnormal ECG (not QT prolongation) (7%)

Central nervous system: Convulsion (8%; grades 3/4: 5%), somnolence (8%), agitation (5%), coma (5%), confusion (5%)

Dermatologic: Erythema (10%), hyperpigmentation (8%), petechia (8%), skin lesions (8%), urticaria (8%), local exfoliation (5%)

Endocrine & metabolic: Hypocalcemia (10%), hypoglycemia (8%), acidosis (5%)

Gastrointestinal: Dyspepsia (10%), loose stools (10%), abdominal distension (8%), abdominal tenderness (8%), xerostomia (8%), fecal incontinence (8%), gastrointestinal hemorrhage (8%), hemorrhagic diarrhea (8%), oral blistering (8%), weight loss (8%), oral candidiasis (5%)

Genitourinary: Intermenstrual bleeding (8%), incontinence (5%)

Hematologic: Neutropenia (10%; grades 3/4: 10%), DIC (8%), hemorrhage (8%), lymphadenopathy (8%)

Local: Injection site edema (10%)

Neuromuscular & skeletal: Weakness (10%)

Ocular: Blurred vision (10%), eye irritation (10%), dry eye (8%), eyelid edema (5%), painful eye (5%)

Otic: Earache (8%), tinnitus (5%)

Renal: Renal failure (8%; grades 3/4: 3%), renal impairment (8%), oliguria (5%)

Respiratory: Crepitations (10%), breath sounds decreased (10%), rales (10%), hemoptysis (8%), rhonchi (8%), tachypnea (8%), nasopharyngitis (5%)

Miscellaneous: Diaphoresis increased (10%), APL differentiation syndrome (8%), bacterial infection (8%), herpes zoster (8%), night sweats (8%), hypersensitivity (5%), sepsis (5%; grades 3/4: 5%)

Postmarketing and/or case reports: Atrial dysrhythmia, AV block, torsade de pointes

Drug Interactions

Avoid Concomitant Use

Avoid concomitant use of Arsenic Trioxide with any of the following: Nilotinib; Tetrabenazine; Thioridazine; Ziprasidone

Increased Effect/Toxicity

Arsenic Trioxide may increase the levels/effects of: QTc-Prolonging Agents; Tetrabenazine; Thioridazine; Ziprasidone

The levels/effects of Arsenic Trioxide may be increased by: Alfuzosin; Ciprofloxacin; Gadobutrol; Herbs (Hypoglycemic Properties); Nilotinib

Decreased Effect There are no known significant interactions involving a decrease in effect.

Ethanol/Nutrition/Herb Interactions Herb/Nutraceutical: Avoid homeopathic products (arsenic is present in some homeopathic medications). Avoid hypoglycemic herbs, including alfalfa, aloe, bilberry, bitter melon, burdock, celery, damiana, fenugreek, garcinia, garlic, ginger, ginseng, gymnema, marshmallow, and stinging nettle (may enhance the hypoglycemic effect of arsenic trioxide).

Stability Store at room temperature of 15°C to 30°C (59°F to 86°F); do not freeze. Following dilution, stable for 24 hours at room temperature or 48 hours when refrigerated. Dilute in 100-250 mL D_5W or 0.9% NaCl. Discard unused portion.

Mechanism of Action Not fully understood; causes *in vitro* morphological changes and DNA fragmentation to NB4 human promyelocytic leukemia cells; also damages or degrades the fusion protein PML-RAR alpha

Pharmacodynamics/Kinetics

Distribution: V_d: ~4 L

Metabolism: Hepatic; pentavalent arsenic is reduced to trivalent arsenic (active) by arsenate reductase; trivalent arsenic is methylated to monomethylarsinic acid, which is then converted to dimethylarsinic acid via methyltransferases

Half-life elimination: Initial: 0.6-1.2 hours; Elimination: 9-15 hours

Excretion: Urine (as methylated metabolite)

Dosage I.V.:

APL: Children ≥5 years and Adults:

Induction: 0.15 mg/kg/day; administer daily until bone marrow remission; maximum induction: 60 doses

Consolidation: 0.15 mg/kg/day starting 3-6 weeks after completion of induction therapy; maximum consolidation: 25 doses over 5 weeks

MDS, multiple myeloma (unlabeled uses): Adults: 0.25 mg/kg/day 5 consecutive days/week for 2 weeks, followed by a 2-week rest period

Elderly: Safety and efficacy have not been established; clinical trials included patients ≤72 years of age; use with caution due to the increased risk of renal impairment in the elderly

Dosage adjustment in renal impairment: Safety and efficacy have not been established; use with caution due to renal elimination

Dosage adjustment in hepatic impairment: Safety and efficacy have not been established

Administration Administer as I.V. infusion over 1-2 hours. If acute vasomotor reactions occur, infuse over a maximum of 4 hours. Does not require administration via a central venous catheter.

Monitoring Parameters Baseline then weekly 12-lead ECG, baseline then twice weekly serum electrolytes, hematologic and coagulation profiles at least twice weekly during induction and at least weekly during consolidation; more frequent monitoring may be necessary in unstable patients

Additional Information Arsenic is stored in liver, kidney, heart, lung, hair, and nails. Arsenic trioxide is a human carcinogen.

Oncology Comment: Arsenic trioxide is listed within National Comprehensive Cancer Network (NCCN) guidelines for the treatment of acute myeloid leukemia as the recommended salvage therapy for relapsed or persistent APL. For patients with APL in their second complete response, who are not candidates for stem cell transplant, in the absence of an appropriate clinical trial, maintenance therapy with arsenic trioxide is an option.

Dosage Forms Excipient information presented when available (limited, particularly for generics); consult specific product labeling.

Injection, solution [preservative free]:

Trisenox®: 1 mg/mL (10 mL)

◆ **Artane** *see* Trihexyphenidyl *on page* *1518*

◆ **Arthrotec®** *see* Diclofenac and Misoprostol *on page* *440*

◆ **As_2O_3** *see* Arsenic Trioxide *on page* *137*

◆ **ASA** *see* Aspirin *on page* *142*

◆ **5-ASA** *see* Mesalamine *on page* *949*

◆ **ASA and Diphenhydramine** *see* Aspirin and Diphenhydramine *on page* *145*

◆ **Asacol®** *see* Mesalamine *on page* *949*

◆ **Asacol® 800 (Can)** *see* Mesalamine *on page* *949*

◆ **Asaphen (Can)** *see* Aspirin *on page* *142*

◆ **Asaphen E.C. (Can)** *see* Aspirin *on page* *142*

◆ **Asco-Caps [OTC]** *see* Ascorbic Acid *on page* *139*

◆ **Ascocid® [OTC]** *see* Ascorbic Acid *on page* *139*

◆ **Ascor L 500®** *see* Ascorbic Acid *on page* *139*

◆ **Ascor L NC®** *see* Ascorbic Acid *on page* *139*

Ascorbic Acid (a SKOR bik AS id)

U.S. Brand Names Acerola [OTC]; Asco-Caps [OTC]; Asco-Tabs [OTC]; Ascocid® [OTC]; Ascor L 500®; Ascor L NC®; C-Gel [OTC]; C-Gram [OTC]; C-Time [OTC]; Cecon® [OTC]; Cemill [OTC]; Cenolate®; Chew-C [OTC]; Dull-C® [OTC]; Mild-C® [OTC]; One Gram C [OTC]; Time-C [OTC]; Time-C-Bio [OTC]; Vicks® Vitamin C [OTC]; Vita-C® [OTC]

Canadian Brand Names Proflavanol C™; Revitalose C-1000®

Index Terms Vitamin C

Pharmacologic Category Vitamin, Water Soluble

Use Prevention and treatment of scurvy; acidify the urine

Unlabeled/Investigational Use Investigational: In large doses, to decrease the severity of "colds"; dietary supplementation; a 20-year study was recently completed involving 730 individuals which indicates a possible decreased risk of death by stroke when ascorbic acid at doses ≥45 mg/day was administered

Pregnancy Risk Factor A/C (dose exceeding RDA recommendation)

Medication Safety Issues

International issues:

Rubex® [Ireland] may be confused with Revex® which is a brand name for nalmefene in the U.S.

Rubex® [Ireland]: Brand name for doxurbicin in the U.S.

Dosage Oral, I.M., I.V., SubQ:

Recommended daily allowance (RDA):

<6 months: 30 mg

6 months to 1 year: 35 mg

1-3 years: 15 mg; upper limit of intake should not exceed 400 mg/day

4-8 years: 25 mg; upper limit of intake should not exceed 650 mg/day

9-13 years: 45 mg; upper limit of intake should not exceed 1200 mg/day

14-18 years: Upper limit of intake should not exceed 1800 mg/day

Male: 75 mg

Female: 65 mg

Adults: Upper limit of intake should not exceed 2000 mg/day

Male: 90 mg

Female: 75 mg

Pregnant female:

≤18 years: 80 mg; upper limit of intake should not exceed 1800 mg/day

19-50 years: 85 mg; upper limit of intake should not exceed 2000 mg/day

Lactating female:

≤18 years: 15 mg; upper limit of intake should not exceed 1800 mg/day

19-50 years: 20 mg; upper limit of intake should not exceed 2000 mg/day

Adult smoker: Add an additional 35 mg/day

Children:

Scurvy: 100-300 mg/day in divided doses for at least 2 weeks

Urinary acidification: 500 mg every 6-8 hours

Dietary supplement: 35-100 mg/day

Adults:

Scurvy: 100-250 mg 1-2 times/day for at least 2 weeks

Urinary acidification: 4-12 g/day in 3-4 divided doses

Prevention and treatment of colds: 1-3 g/day

Dietary supplement: 50-200 mg/day

Additional Information Complete prescribing information for this medication should be consulted for additional detail.

Dosage Forms Excipient information presented when available (limited, particularly for generics); consult specific product labeling.

Caplet: 1000 mg
Caplet, timed release: 500 mg, 1000 mg
Capsule:
  Mild-C®: 500 mg
Capsule, softgel:
  C-Gel: 1000 mg
Capsule, sustained release:
  C-Time: 500 mg
Capsule, timed release: 500 mg
  Asco-Caps: 500 mg, 1000 mg [sugar free]
  Time-C®: 500 mg
Crystals for solution, oral: 4 g/teaspoonful (170 g, 1000 g)
  Mild-C®: 3600 mg/teaspoonful [contains calcium 400 mg/teaspoonful]
  Vita-C®: 4 g/teaspoonful (100 g, 454 g)
Injection, solution: 500 mg/mL (50 mL)
  Cenolate®: 500 mg/mL (1 mL, 2 mL) [contains aluminum, sodium hydrosulfite]
Injection, solution [preservative free]:
  Ascor L 500®: 500 mg/mL (50 mL) [contains edetate disodium]
  Ascor L NC®: 500 mg/mL (50 mL) [contains edetate disodium]
Liquid, oral: 500 mg/5 mL
Lozenge:
  Vicks® Vitamin C: 25 mg [contains sodium 5 mg; orange flavor]
Powder, for solution, oral:
  Ascocid®: 4000 mg/5 mL (227 g); 4300 mg/5 mL (227 g, 454 g); 5000 mg/5 mL (227 g, 454 g)
  Dull-C®: 4 g/teaspoonful
Solution, oral:
  Cecon®: 90 mg/mL
Tablet: 100 mg, 250 mg, 500 mg, 1000 mg
  Asco-Tabs: 1000 mg [sugar free]
  Ascocid®: 500 mg [sugar free]
  C-Gram, One Gram C: 1000 mg
Tablet, chewable: 250 mg, 500 mg
  Acerola: 500 mg [cherry flavor]
  Chew-C: 500 mg [orange flavor]
  Mild-C®: 250 mg
Tablet, timed release: 500 mg, 1000 mg
  Cemill: 500 mg, 1000 mg
  Mild-C®: 1000 mg
  Time-C-Bio: 500 mg

- ◆ **Ascorbic Acid and Ferrous Sulfate** *see* Ferrous Sulfate and Ascorbic Acid *on page 617*
- ◆ **Asco-Tabs [OTC]** *see* Ascorbic Acid *on page 139*
- ◆ **Ascriptin® [OTC]** *see* Aspirin *on page 142*
- ◆ **Ascriptin® Maximum Strength [OTC]** *see* Aspirin *on page 142*
- ◆ **Asendin [DSC]** *see* Amoxapine *on page 97*
- ◆ **Asmanex® Twisthaler®** *see* Mometasone *on page 1012*

Asparaginase (a SPEAR a ji nase)

U.S. Brand Names Elspar®

Canadian Brand Names Kidrolase®

Index Terms *E. coli* Asparaginase; *Erwinia* Asparaginase; L-asparaginase; NSC-106977 (*Erwinia*); NSC-109229 (*E. coli*)

Pharmacologic Category Antineoplastic Agent, Miscellaneous

Use Treatment of acute lymphocytic leukemia (ALL)

Unlabeled/Investigational Use Treatment of lymphoma

Pregnancy Risk Factor C

Pregnancy Considerations Decreased weight gain, resorptions, gross abnormalities, and skeletal abnormalities were observed in animal studies. There are no adequate and well-controlled studies in pregnant women. Use during pregnancy only if clearly needed.

Lactation Excretion in breast milk unknown/not recommended

Medication Safety Issues

Sound-alike/look-alike issues:
  Asparaginase may be confused with pegaspargase
  Elspar® may be confused with Elaprase™

High alert medication: The Institute for Safe Medication Practices (ISMP) includes this medication among its list of classes of drugs which have a heightened risk of causing significant patient harm when used in error.

Contraindications History of serious allergic reaction to asparaginase or any *E. coli*-derived asparaginase; history of serious thrombosis with prior asparaginase treatment; history of pancreatitis with prior asparaginase treatment; serious hemorrhagic events with prior asparaginase treatment

Warnings/Precautions Hazardous agent - use appropriate precautions for handling and disposal. Monitor for severe allergic reactions; immediate treatment for hypersensitivity reactions should be available during administration. May alter hepatic function; use caution with preexisting liver impairment. Serious thrombosis, including sagittal sinus thrombosis may occur; discontinue with serious thrombotic events. Increased prothrombin time, partial thromboplastin time and hypofibrinogenemia may occur; cerebrovascular hemorrhage has been reported; monitor coagulation parameters; use cautiously in patients with an underlying coagulopathy. Monitor blood glucose; may cause hyperglycemia/glucose intolerance (possibly irreversible). May cause serious and possibly fatal pancreatitis; promptly evaluate patients with abdominal pain; discontinue permanently if pancreatitis develops. Appropriate measures must be taken to prevent tumor lysis syndrome and subsequent hyperuricemia and uric acid nephropathy; monitor, consider allopurinol, hydration and urinary alkalization.

Severe allergic reactions may occur; monitor; immediate treatment for hypersensitivity reactions should be available during administration. Risk factors for allergic reactions include: I.V. administration, doses >6000-12,000 units/m^2, patients who have received previous cycles of asparaginase, and intervals of even a few days between doses. Up to 33% of patients who have an allergic reaction to *E. coli* asparaginase will also react to the *Erwinia* form or pegaspargase. A test dose may be administered prior to the first dose of asparaginase, or prior to restarting therapy after a hiatus of several days. **False-negative rates of up to 80% to test doses of 2-50 units are reported.** Desensitization may be performed in patients found to be hypersensitive by the intradermal test dose or who have received previous courses of therapy with the drug.

Adverse Reactions Note: Immediate effects: Fever, chills, nausea, and vomiting occur in 50% to 60% of patients.

>10%:
  Central nervous system: Fatigue, fever, chills, depression, agitation, seizure (10% to 60%), somnolence, stupor, confusion, coma (25%)
  Endocrine & metabolic: Hyperglycemia/glucose intolerance (10%)
  Gastrointestinal: Nausea, vomiting (50% to 60%), anorexia, abdominal cramps (70%), acute pancreatitis (15%, may be severe in some patients)

Hematologic: Hypofibrinogenemia and depression of clotting factors V and VIII, variable decrease in factors VII and IX, severe protein C deficiency and decrease in antithrombin III (may be dose limiting or fatal)
Hepatic: Transaminases, bilirubin, and alkaline phosphatase increased (transient)
Hypersensitivity: Acute allergic reactions (fever, rash, urticaria, arthralgia, hypotension, angioedema, bronchospasm, anaphylaxis (15% to 35%); may be dose limiting in some patients, may be fatal)
Renal: Azotemia (66%)

1% to 10%:
Endocrine & metabolic: Hyperuricemia
Gastrointestinal: Stomatitis
Miscellaneous: Allergic reaction (including anaphylaxis), antibody formation/immunogenicity (~25%)

<1% (Limited to important or life-threatening) and/or frequency not defined: Acute renal failure, albumin decreased, cerebrovascular hemorrhage, cerebrovascular thrombosis, cough, disorientation, drowsiness, fatty liver, fibrinogen decreased, glucosuria, hallucinations, headache, hemorrhagic pancreatitis, hyper-/hypolipidemia, hyperthermia, hypocholesterolemia, hypotension, insulin-dependent diabetes, intracranial hemorrhage, irritability, ketoacidosis, laryngospasm, malabsorption syndrome, pancreatic pseudocyst, Parkinsonian symptoms (including tremor and increased muscle tone), partial thromboplastin time increased, peripheral edema, polyuria, proteinuria, prothrombin time increased, pruritus, rash, renal insufficiency, serum ammonia increased, serum cholesterol decreased, sagittal sinus thrombosis, thrombosis, urticaria, venous thrombosis, weight loss; mild-to-moderate myelosuppression, leukopenia, anemia, thrombocytopenia (onset: 7 days, nadir: 14 days, recovery: 21 days)

Drug Interactions

Avoid Concomitant Use

Avoid concomitant use of Asparaginase with any of the following: Natalizumab; Vaccines (Live)

Increased Effect/Toxicity

Asparaginase may increase the levels/effects of: Natalizumab; Vaccines (Live)

The levels/effects of Asparaginase may be increased by: Trastuzumab

Decreased Effect

Asparaginase may decrease the levels/effects of: Vaccines (Inactivated)

The levels/effects of Asparaginase may be decreased by: Echinacea

Stability Intact vials of powder should be refrigerated at 2°C to 8°C (36°F to 48°F). Lyophilized powder should be reconstituted with 1-5 mL sterile water for injection or NS for I.V. administration; NS for I.M. use. Shake well, but not too vigorously. A 5 micron filter may be used to remove fiber-like particles in the solution (do not use a 0.2 micron filter; has been associated with loss of potency). Reconstituted solutions are stable 1 week refrigerated at 8°C (Stecher, 1999), although the manufacturer recommends use within 8 hours.

Standard I.M. dilution: 2000, 5000, or 10,000 int. units/mL
Standard I.V. dilution: Dilute in 50-250 mL NS or D_5W; solutions for I.V. infusion are stable for 8 hours at room temperature or under refrigeration

Test dose preparation: Reconstitute a 10,000 unit vial with 5 mL NS or SWFI (concentration = 2000 units/mL); withdraw 0.1 mL and add to 9.9 mL NS (concentration = 20 units/mL); test dose is 0.1 mL (2 units)

Mechanism of Action Asparaginase inhibits protein synthesis by hydrolyzing asparagine to aspartic acid and ammonia. Leukemia cells, especially lymphoblasts, require exogenous asparagine; normal cells can synthesize asparagine. Asparaginase is cycle-specific for the G_1 phase.

Pharmacodynamics/Kinetics

Absorption: I.M.: Produces peak blood levels 50% lower than those from I.V. administration
Distribution: V_d: 4-5 L/kg; 70% to 80% of plasma volume; <1% CSF penetration
Metabolism: Systemically degraded
Half-life elimination: I.M.: 39-49 hours; I.V.: 8-30 hours
Time to peak, plasma: I.M.: 14-24 hours

Dosage Refer to individual protocols. **Note:** Dose, frequency, number of doses, and start date may vary by protocol and treatment phase.

Children:

I.V.:
6000 units/m^2/dose 3 times/week for ~6-9 doses **or** 1000 units/kg/day for 10 days **or**
High-dose therapy (unlabeled dose): 10,000 units/m^2/dose every ~3 days for ~4-8 doses

I.M.:
6000 units/m^2/dose 3 times/week **or** 6000 units/m^2/dose every ~3 days for ~6-9 doses
High-dose therapy (unlabeled dose): 10,000 units/m^2/dose every ~3 days for ~4-8 doses **or** 25,000 units/m^2/dose weekly for ~9 doses (generally used in high-risk continuation therapy)

Adults:

I.V.:
6000 units/m^2/dose 3 times/week for ~6-9 doses **or** 1000 units/kg/day for 10 days **or**
High-dose therapy (unlabeled dose): 10,000 units/m^2/day for ~3-12 doses
Single agent therapy (rare): 200 units/kg/day for 28 days

I.M.:
6000 units/m^2/dose 3 times/week for ~6-9 doses **or** 6000 units/m^2/dose every ~3 days for ~6-9 doses
High-dose therapy (unlabeled dose): 10,000 units/m^2/day for ~3-12 doses

Asparaginase Desensitization

Injection No.	Elspar Dose (int. units)	Accumulated Total Dose
1	1	1
2	2	3
3	4	7
4	8	15
5	16	31
6	32	63
7	64	127
8	128	255
9	256	511
10	512	1023
11	1024	2047
12	2048	4095
13	4096	8191
14	8192	16,383
15	16,384	32,767
16	32,768	65,535
17	65,536	131,071
18	131,072	262,143

Test dose: A test dose is often recommended prior to the first dose of asparaginase, or prior to restarting therapy after a hiatus of several days. Most commonly, 0.1 mL of a 20 units/mL (2 units) asparaginase dilution is injected intradermally, and the patient observed for at least 1 hour.

False-negative rates of up to 80% to test doses of 2-50 units are reported.

Some practitioners recommend an asparaginase desensitization regimen for patients who react to a test dose, or are being retreated following a break in therapy. Doses are doubled and given every 10 minutes until the total daily dose for that day has been administered. One schedule begins with a total of 1 unit given I.V. and doubles the dose every 10 minutes until the total amount given is the planned dose for that day. For example, if a patient was to receive a total dose of 4000 units, he/she would receive injections 1 through 12 during the desensitization. See table on previous page.

Administration May be administered I.M., I.V., or intradermal (skin test only); has been administered SubQ in specific protocols

I.M.: Doses should be given as a deep intramuscular injection into a large muscle; volumes >2 mL should be divided and administered in 2 separate sites

Note: I.V. administration greatly increases the risk of allergic reactions and should be avoided if possible.

I.V.: I.V. infusion in 50-250 mL of D_5W or NS over at least 30-60 minutes. The manufacturer recommends a test dose (0.1 mL of a dilute 20 unit/mL solution) prior to initial administration and when given after an interval of 7 days or more. Institutional policies vary. The skin test site should be observed for at least 1 hour for a wheal or erythema. Note that a negative skin test does not preclude the possibility of an allergic reaction. Desensitization may be performed in patients who have been found to be hypersensitive by the intradermal skin test or who have received previous courses of therapy with the drug. Have epinephrine, diphenhydramine, and hydrocortisone at the bedside. Have a running I.V. in place. A physician should be readily accessible.

Gelatinous fiber-like particles may develop on standing. Filtration through a 5-micron filter during administration will remove the particles with no loss of potency.

Monitoring Parameters Vital signs during administration; CBC with differential, urinalysis, amylase, liver enzymes, coagulation parameters (baseline and periodic), renal function tests, urine dipstick for glucose, blood glucose, uric acid. Monitor for allergic reaction, be prepared to treat anaphylaxis at each administration; monitor for onset of abdominal pain and mental status changes.

Test Interactions Decreased thyroxine and thyroxine-binding globulin

Additional Information Some institutions recommended the following precautions for asparaginase administration: Parenteral epinephrine, diphenhydramine, and hydrocortisone available at bedside; freely running I.V. in place; physician readily accessible; monitor the patient closely for 30-60 minutes; avoid administering at night.

The *E. coli* and the *Erwinia* strains of asparaginase differ slightly in their gene sequencing, and have slight differences in their enzyme characteristics. Both are highly specific for asparagine and have <10% activity for the D-isomer. The *E. coli* form is more commonly used. The *Erwinia* variety is no longer commercially available in the U.S., although may be obtained through clinical trials or on a compassionate use basis.

Dosage Forms Excipient information presented when available (limited, particularly for generics); consult specific product labeling.

Injection, powder for reconstitution:

Elspar®: 10,000 units

◆ **Aspart Insulin** *see* Insulin Aspart *on page* 792

◆ **Aspercin [OTC]** *see* Aspirin *on page* 142

◆ ***Aspergillus niger*** *see* Alpha-Galactosidase *on page* 68

◆ **Aspergum® [OTC]** *see* Aspirin *on page* 142

Aspirin (AS pir in)

U.S. Brand Names Ascriptin® Maximum Strength [OTC]; Ascriptin® [OTC]; Aspercin [OTC]; Aspergum® [OTC]; Aspirtab [OTC]; Bayer® Aspirin Extra Strength [OTC]; Bayer® Aspirin Regimen Adult Low Dose [OTC]; Bayer® Aspirin Regimen Children's [OTC]; Bayer® Aspirin Regimen Regular Strength [OTC]; Bayer® Genuine Aspirin [OTC]; Bayer® Plus Extra Strength [OTC]; Bayer® with Heart Advantage [OTC]; Bayer® Women's Aspirin Plus Calcium [OTC]; Buffasal [OTC]; Bufferin® Extra Strength [OTC]; Bufferin® [OTC]; Buffinol [OTC]; Easprin®; Ecotrin® Low Strength [OTC]; Ecotrin® Maximum Strength [OTC]; Ecotrin® [OTC]; Genacote™ [OTC]; Halfprin® [OTC]; St. Joseph® Adult Aspirin [OTC]; ZORprin®

Canadian Brand Names Asaphen; Asaphen E.C.; Entrophen®; Novasen

Index Terms Acetylsalicylic Acid; ASA

Pharmacologic Category Salicylate

Use Treatment of mild-to-moderate pain, inflammation, and fever; may be used as prophylaxis of myocardial infarction; prophylaxis of stroke and/or transient ischemic episodes; management of rheumatoid arthritis, rheumatic fever, osteoarthritis, and gout (high dose); adjunctive therapy in revascularization procedures (coronary artery bypass graft [CABG], percutaneous transluminal coronary angioplasty [PTCA], carotid endarterectomy), stent implantation

Unlabeled/Investigational Use Low doses have been used in the prevention of pre-eclampsia, complications associated with autoimmune disorders such as lupus or antiphospholipid syndrome

Pregnancy Risk Factor C/D (full-dose aspirin in 3rd trimester - expert analysis)

Pregnancy Considerations Salicylates have been noted to cross the placenta and enter fetal circulation. Adverse effects reported in the fetus include mortality, intrauterine growth retardation, salicylate intoxication, bleeding abnormalities, and neonatal acidosis. Use of aspirin close to delivery may cause premature closure of the ductus arteriosus. Adverse effects reported in the mother include anemia, hemorrhage, prolonged gestation, and prolonged labor. Aspirin has been used for the prevention of pre-eclampsia; however, the ACOG currently recommends that it not be used in low-risk women. Low-dose aspirin is used to treat complications resulting from antiphospholipid syndrome in pregnancy (either primary or secondary to SLE). In general, low doses during pregnancy needed for the treatment of certain medical conditions have not been shown to cause fetal harm, however, discontinuing therapy prior to delivery is recommended. Use of safer agents for routine management of pain or headache should be considered.

Lactation Enters breast milk/use caution

Medication Safety Issues

Sound-alike/look-alike issues:

Aspirin may be confused with Afrin®, Asendin®

Ascriptin® may be confused with Aricept®

Ecotrin® may be confused with Akineton®, Edecrin®, Epogen®

Halfprin® may be confused with Halfan®, Haltran®

ZORprin® may be confused with Zyloprim®

International issues:

Cartia® [multiple international markets] may be confused with Cartia XT™ which is a brand name for diltiazem in the U.S.

Contraindications Hypersensitivity to salicylates, other NSAIDs, or any component of the formulation; asthma; rhinitis; nasal polyps; inherited or acquired bleeding disorders (including factor VII and factor IX deficiency); do not use in children (<16 years of age) for viral infections (chickenpox or flu symptoms), with or without fever, due to a potential association with Reye's syndrome; pregnancy (3rd trimester especially)

Warnings/Precautions Use with caution in patients with platelet and bleeding disorders, renal dysfunction, dehydration, erosive gastritis, or peptic ulcer disease. Heavy ethanol use (>3 drinks/day) can increase bleeding risks. Avoid use in severe renal failure or in severe hepatic failure. Discontinue use if tinnitus or impaired hearing occurs. Caution in mild-to-moderate renal failure (only at high dosages). Patients with sensitivity to tartrazine dyes, nasal polyps, and asthma may have an increased risk of salicylate sensitivity. In the treatment of acute ischemic stroke, avoid aspirin for 24 hours following administration of alteplase; administration within 24 hours increases the risk of hemorrhagic transformation. Surgical patients should avoid ASA if possible, for 1-2 weeks prior to surgery, to reduce the risk of excessive bleeding (except in patients with cardiac stents that have not completed their full course of dual antiplatelet therapy [aspirin, clopidogrel]; patient-specific situations need to be discussed with cardiologist; AHA/ACC/SCAI/ACS/ADA Science Advisory provides recommendations).

When used for self-medication (OTC labeling): Children and teenagers who have or are recovering from chickenpox or flu-like symptoms should not use this product. Changes in behavior (along with nausea and vomiting) may be an early sign of Reye's syndrome; patients should be instructed to contact their healthcare provider if these occur.

Adverse Reactions As with all drugs which may affect hemostasis, bleeding is associated with aspirin. Hemorrhage may occur at virtually any site. Risk is dependent on multiple variables including dosage, concurrent use of multiple agents which alter hemostasis, and patient susceptibility. Many adverse effects of aspirin are dose related, and are extremely rare at low dosages. Other serious reactions are idiosyncratic, related to allergy or individual sensitivity. Accurate estimation of frequencies is not possible.

Cardiovascular: Hypotension, tachycardia, dysrhythmias, edema

Central nervous system: Fatigue, insomnia, nervousness, agitation, confusion, dizziness, headache, lethargy, cerebral edema, hyperthermia, coma

Dermatologic: Rash, angioedema, urticaria

Endocrine & metabolic: Acidosis, hyperkalemia, dehydration, hypoglycemia (children), hyperglycemia, hypernatremia (buffered forms)

Gastrointestinal: Nausea, vomiting, dyspepsia, epigastric discomfort, heartburn, stomach pain, gastrointestinal ulceration (6% to 31%), gastric erosions, gastric erythema, duodenal ulcers

Hematologic: Anemia, disseminated intravascular coagulation (DIC), prothrombin times prolonged, coagulopathy, thrombocytopenia, hemolytic anemia, bleeding, iron-deficiency anemia

Hepatic: Hepatotoxicity, transaminases increased, hepatitis (reversible)

Neuromuscular & skeletal: Rhabdomyolysis, weakness, acetabular bone destruction (OA)

Otic: Hearing loss, tinnitus

Renal: Interstitial nephritis, papillary necrosis, proteinuria, renal failure (including cases caused by rhabdomyolysis), BUN increased, serum creatinine increased

Respiratory: Asthma, bronchospasm, dyspnea, laryngeal edema, hyperpnea, tachypnea, respiratory alkalosis, noncardiogenic pulmonary edema

Miscellaneous: Anaphylaxis, prolonged pregnancy and labor, stillbirths, low birth weight, peripartum bleeding, Reye's syndrome

Postmarketing and/or case reports: Colonic ulceration, esophageal stricture, esophagitis with esophageal ulcer, esophageal hematoma, oral mucosal ulcers (aspirin-containing chewing gum), coronary artery spasm, conduction defect and atrial fibrillation (toxicity), delirium, ischemic brain infarction, colitis, rectal stenosis (suppository), cholestatic jaundice, periorbital edema, rhinosinusitis

Drug Interactions

Metabolism/Transport Effects **Substrate** of CYP2C9 (minor)

Avoid Concomitant Use

Avoid concomitant use of Aspirin with any of the following: Ketorolac

Increased Effect/Toxicity

Aspirin may increase the levels/effects of: Alendronate; Anticoagulants; Carbonic Anhydrase Inhibitors; Corticosteroids (Systemic); Drotrecogin Alfa; Heparin; Ibritumomab; Methotrexate; Salicylates; Sulfonylureas; Thrombolytic Agents; Tositumomab and Iodine I 131 Tositumomab; Valproic Acid; Varicella Virus-Containing Vaccines; Vitamin K Antagonists

The levels/effects of Aspirin may be increased by: Antidepressants (Tricyclic, Tertiary Amine); Antiplatelet Agents; Calcium Channel Blockers (Nondihydropyridine); Dasatinib; Ginkgo Biloba; Herbs (Anticoagulant/Antiplatelet Properties); Ketorolac; Nonsteroidal Anti-Inflammatory Agents; NSAID (Nonselective); Omega-3-Acid Ethyl Esters; Pentosan Polysulfate Sodium; Prostacyclin Analogues; Selective Serotonin Reuptake Inhibitors; Serotonin/Norepinephrine Reuptake Inhibitors; Treprostinil

Decreased Effect

Aspirin may decrease the levels/effects of: ACE Inhibitors; NSAID (Nonselective); Tiludronate; Uricosuric Agents

The levels/effects of Aspirin may be decreased by: Corticosteroids (Systemic); Nonsteroidal Anti-Inflammatory Agents; NSAID (Nonselective)

Ethanol/Nutrition/Herb Interactions

Ethanol: Avoid ethanol (may enhance gastric mucosal damage).

Food: Food may decrease the rate but not the extent of oral absorption.

Folic acid: Hyperexcretion of folate; folic acid deficiency may result, leading to macrocytic anemia.

Iron: With chronic aspirin use and at doses of 3-4 g/day, iron-deficiency anemia may result.

Sodium: Hypernatremia resulting from buffered aspirin solutions or sodium salicylate containing high sodium content. Avoid or use with caution in CHF or any condition where hypernatremia would be detrimental.

Benedictine liqueur, prunes, raisins, tea, and gherkins: Potential salicylate accumulation.

Fresh fruits containing vitamin C: Displace drug from binding sites, resulting in increased urinary excretion of aspirin.

Herb/Nutraceutical: Avoid cat's claw, dong quai, evening primrose, feverfew, garlic, ginger, ginkgo, red clover, horse chestnut, green tea, ginseng (all have additional antiplatelet activity). Limit curry powder, paprika, licorice; may cause salicylate accumulation. These foods contain 6 mg salicylate/100 g. An ordinarily American diet contains 10-200 mg/day of salicylate.

Stability Keep suppositories in refrigerator; do not freeze. Hydrolysis of aspirin occurs upon exposure to water or moist air, resulting in salicylate and acetate, which possess a vinegar-like odor. Do not use if a strong odor is present.

Mechanism of Action Irreversibly inhibits cyclooxygenase-1 and 2 (COX-1 and 2) enzymes, which result in decreased formation of prostaglandin precursors; has antiplatelet, antipyretic, analgesic, and anti-inflammatory properties

Pharmacodynamics/Kinetics

Duration: 4-6 hours

Absorption: Rapid

Distribution: V_d: 10 L; readily into most body fluids and tissues

Metabolism: Hydrolyzed to salicylate (active) by esterases in GI mucosa, red blood cells, synovial fluid, and blood; metabolism of salicylate occurs primarily by hepatic conjugation; metabolic pathways are saturable

Bioavailability: 50% to 75% reaches systemic circulation

Half-life elimination: Parent drug: 15-20 minutes; Salicylates (dose dependent): 3 hours at lower doses (300-600 mg), 5-6 hours (after 1 g), 10 hours with higher doses

Time to peak, serum: ~1-2 hours

Excretion: Urine (75% as salicyluric acid, 10% as salicylic acid)

Dosage

Children:

Analgesic and antipyretic: Oral, rectal: 10-15 mg/kg/dose every 4-6 hours, up to a total of 4 g/day

Anti-inflammatory: Oral: Initial: 60-90 mg/kg/day in divided doses; usual maintenance: 80-100 mg/kg/day divided every 6-8 hours; monitor serum concentrations

Antiplatelet effects: Adequate pediatric studies have not been performed; pediatric dosage is derived from adult studies and clinical experience and is not well established; suggested doses have ranged from 3-5 mg/kg/day to 5-10 mg/kg/day given as a single daily dose. Doses are rounded to a convenient amount (eg, 1/2 of 81 mg tablet).

Mechanical prosthetic heart valves: 6-20 mg/kg/day given as a single daily dose (used in combination with an oral anticoagulant in children who have systemic embolism despite adequate oral anticoagulation therapy (INR 2.5-3.5) and used in combination with low-dose anticoagulation (INR 2-3) and dipyridamole when full-dose oral anticoagulation is contraindicated)

Blalock-Taussig shunts: 3-5 mg/kg/day given as a single daily dose

Kawasaki disease: Oral: 80-100 mg/kg/day divided every 6 hours; monitor serum concentrations; after fever resolves: 3-5 mg/kg/day once daily; in patients without coronary artery abnormalities, give lower dose for at least 6-8 weeks or until ESR and platelet count are normal; in patients with coronary artery abnormalities, low-dose aspirin should be continued indefinitely

Antirheumatic: Oral: 60-100 mg/kg/day in divided doses every 4 hours

Adults:

Acute ischemic stroke: Oral: 150-325 mg once daily, initiated within 48 hours (in patients who are not candidates for alteplase and not receiving systemic anticoagulation)

Analgesic and antipyretic:

Oral: 325-650 mg every 4-6 hours up to 4 g/day

Rectal: 300-600 mg every 4-6 hours up to 4 g/day

Anti-inflammatory: Oral: Initial: 2.4-3.6 g/day in divided doses; usual maintenance: 3.6-5.4 g/day; monitor serum concentrations

Atrial fibrillation (in patients not candidates for warfarin or at low risk of ischemic stroke): Oral: 75-325 mg once daily

Bioprosthetic aortic valve: Oral: 50-100 mg once daily; usual dose: 81 mg once daily

Bioprosthetic mitral valve (following 3 months of anticoagulation): Oral: 50-100 mg once daily; usual dose: 81 mg once daily

CABG: Oral: 75-100 mg once daily (usual dose: 81 mg) initiated 6 hours following surgery; if bleeding prevents administration at 6 hours after CABG, initiate as soon as possible

CABG (internal mammary bypass graft): Oral: 75-162 mg once daily

Carotid artery stenting: Oral: 81-325 mg once daily beginning at least 24 hours (preferably 4 days) prior to procedure with concomitant clopidogrel

Carotid endarterectomy: Oral: 50-100 mg once daily preoperatively and daily thereafter; usual dose: 81 mg once daily

Infrainguinal arterial reconstruction/bypass: Oral: 75-100 mg once daily (begin preoperatively); usual dose: 81 mg once daily

Mechanical heart valve (with additional risk factors for thromboembolism): Oral: 50-100 mg once daily (in addition to warfarin); usual dose: 81 mg once daily

Mitral annular calcification (with documented stroke, TIA, or systemic embolism): Oral: 50-100 mg once daily; usual dose: 81 mg once daily

Mitral valve prolapse (with documented stroke or TIA): Oral: 50-100 mg once daily; usual dose: 81 mg once daily

Myocardial infarction (primary prevention): Oral: 75-162 mg once daily (Antman, 2004) **or** 75-100 mg (usual dose: 81 mg) once daily (Hirsh, 2008)

Non-ST-segment elevation myocardial infarction (NSTEMI): Oral: Initial: 162-325 mg; Maintenance: 75-100 mg once daily indefinitely; usual maintenance dose: 81 mg once daily

PCI: Oral: Initial: 75-325 mg (300-325 mg in aspirin naive patients) starting at least 2 hours (preferably 24 hours) before procedure; post procedure: 162-325 mg once daily (dose and duration varies with type of stent implanted); **Note:** Dose may be reduced to 75-162 mg once daily after appropriate duration based on stent-type is complete

Pericarditis associated with myocardial infarction: Oral: 162-325 mg once daily; doses as high as 650 mg every 4-6 hours may be required

Peripheral arterial disease: Oral: 75-100 mg once daily; usual dose: 81 mg once daily

Pre-eclampsia prevention (unlabeled use): Oral: 60-81 mg once daily (usual dose: 81 mg) during gestational weeks 13-26 (patient selection criteria not established)

Prosthetic valve thromboprophylaxis in pregnancy: Oral:75-100 mg once daily; usual dose: 81 mg once daily

ST-segment elevation myocardial infarction (STEMI): Oral: Initial: 162-325 mg given on presentation (patient should chew nonenteric-coated aspirin especially if not taking before presentation); for patients unable to take oral, may use rectal suppository (300 mg). Maintenance (secondary prevention): 75-162 mg once daily indefinitely

Stroke (cardioembolic, anticoagulation contraindicated): Oral: 75-325 mg once daily

Stroke/TIA (noncardioembolic, secondary prevention): Oral: 50-325 mg once daily (Adams, 2008) **or** 50-100 mg once daily; usual dose: 81 mg once daily (Hirsh, 2008)

Dosing adjustment in renal impairment: Cl_{cr} <10 mL/minute: Avoid use.

Hemodialysis: Dialyzable (50% to 100%)

Dosing adjustment in hepatic disease: Avoid use in severe liver disease.

Dietary Considerations Take with food or large volume of water or milk to minimize GI upset.

Administration Do not crush sustained release or enteric coated tablet. Administer with food or a full glass of water to minimize GI distress. For acute myocardial infarction, have patient chew tablet.

Reference Range Timing of serum samples: Peak levels usually occur 2 hours after ingestion. Salicylate serum concentrations correlate with the pharmacological actions and adverse effects observed. The serum salicylate concentration (mcg/mL) and the corresponding clinical correlations are as follows: See table.

Serum Salicylate: Clinical Correlations

Serum Salicylate Concentration (mcg/mL)	Desired Effects	Adverse Effects / Intoxication
~100	Antiplatelet Antipyresis Analgesia	GI intolerance and bleeding, hypersensitivity, hemostatic defects
150-300	Anti-inflammatory	Mild salicylism
250-400	Treatment of rheumatic fever	Nausea/vomiting, hyperventilation, salicylism, flushing, sweating, thirst, headache, diarrhea, and tachycardia
>400-500		Respiratory alkalosis, hemorrhage, excitement, confusion, asterixis, pulmonary edema, convulsions, tetany, metabolic acidosis, fever, coma, cardiovascular collapse, renal and respiratory failure

Test Interactions False-negative results for glucose oxidase urinary glucose tests (Clinistix®); false-positives using the cupric sulfate method (Clinitest®); also, interferes with Gerhardt test, VMA determination; 5-HIAA, xylose tolerance test and T_3 and T_4

Dosage Forms Excipient information presented when available (limited, particularly for generics); consult specific product labeling. [DSC] = Discontinued product

Caplet:
- Bayer® Aspirin Extra Strength: 500 mg
- Bayer® Aspirin Regimen Regular Strength: 325 mg
- Bayer® Genuine Aspirin: 325 mg
- Bayer® Plus Extra Strength: 500 mg [contains calcium carbonate]
- Bayer® with Heart Advantage: 81 mg [contains phytosterols, tartrazine]
- Bayer® Women's Aspirin Plus Calcium: 81 mg [contains elemental calcium 300 mg]

Caplet, buffered:
- Ascriptin® Maximum Strength: 500 mg [contains aluminum hydroxide, calcium carbonate, and magnesium hydroxide]

Gum:
- Aspergum®: 227 mg [cherry or orange flavor]

Suppository, rectal: 300 mg, 600 mg

Tablet: 325 mg
- Aspercin, Aspirtab: 325 mg
- Bayer® Genuine Aspirin: 325 mg

Tablet, buffered: 325 mg
- Ascriptin®: 325 mg [contains aluminum hydroxide, calcium carbonate, and magnesium hydroxide]
- Buffasal: 325 mg [contains magnesium oxide]
- Bufferin®: 325 mg [contains calcium carbonate, magnesium oxide, and magnesium carbonate; contains calcium 65 mg/tablet, magnesium 50 mg/tablet]
- Bufferin® Extra Strength: 500 mg [contains calcium carbonate, magnesium oxide, and magnesium carbonate; contains calcium 90 mg/tablet, magnesium 70 mg/tablet]
- Buffinol: 325 mg [contains magnesium oxide]

Tablet, chewable: 81 mg
- Bayer® Aspirin Regimen Children's: 81 mg [cherry or orange flavor]
- St. Joseph® Adult Aspirin: 81 mg [orange flavor]

Tablet, controlled release:
- ZORprin®: 800 mg

Tablet, delayed release, enteric coated:
- Easprin®: 975 mg

Tablet, enteric coated: 81 mg, 325 mg, 500 mg, 650 mg, 975 mg [DSC]
- Bayer® Aspirin Regimen Adult Low Dose, Ecotrin® Low Strength, St. Joseph Adult Aspirin: 81 mg
- Ecotrin®, Genacote™: 325 mg
- Ecotrin® Maximum Strength: 500 mg
- Halfprin®: 81 mg, 162 mg

◆ **Aspirin, Acetaminophen, and Caffeine** *see* Acetaminophen, Aspirin, and Caffeine *on page 31*

◆ **Aspirin and Carisoprodol** *see* Carisoprodol and Aspirin *on page 261*

Aspirin and Diphenhydramine

(AS pir in & dye fen HYE dra meen)

U.S. Brand Names Alka-Seltzer® P.M. [OTC]; Bayer® PM [OTC]

Index Terms ASA and Diphenhydramine; Aspirin and Diphenhydramine Citrate; Diphenhydramine and ASA; Diphenhydramine and Aspirin; Diphenhydramine Citrate and Aspirin

Pharmacologic Category Analgesic, Miscellaneous

Use Aid in the relief of insomnia accompanied by minor pain or headache

Dosage

Oral: Children ≥12 years and Adults: Pain-associated insomnia: Two tablets (650 mg aspirin/76 mg diphenhydramine citrate) **or** 2 caplets (1000 mg aspirin/76 mg diphenhydramine citrate) at bedtime or as directed by physician; do not exceed recommended dosage; not for use in children <12 years of age

Additional Information Complete prescribing information for this medication should be consulted for additional detail.

Dosage Forms Excipient information presented when available (limited, particularly for generics); consult specific product labeling.

Caplet:
- Bayer® PM: Aspirin 500 mg and diphenhydramine citrate 38.3 mg

Tablet, effervescent:
- Alka-Seltzer® PM: Aspirin 325 mg and diphenhydramine citrate 38 mg [contains phenylalanine 4 mg/tablet and sodium 504 mg/tablet]

◆ **Aspirin and Diphenhydramine Citrate** *see* Aspirin and Diphenhydramine *on page 145*

Aspirin and Dipyridamole

(AS pir in & dye peer ID a mole)

U.S. Brand Names Aggrenox®

Canadian Brand Names Aggrenox®

Index Terms Aspirin and Extended-Release Dipyridamole; Dipyridamole and Aspirin

Pharmacologic Category Antiplatelet Agent

Use Reduction in the risk of stroke in patients who have had transient ischemia of the brain or completed ischemic stroke due to thrombosis

Pregnancy Risk Factor D

Medication Safety Issues

Sound-alike/look-alike issues:
- Aggrenox® may be confused with Aggrastat®

Dosage Adults: Oral: 1 capsule (dipyridamole 200 mg, aspirin 25 mg) twice daily

Alternative regimen for patients with intolerable headache: 1 capsule at bedtime and low-dose aspirin in the morning. Return to usual dose (1 capsule twice daily) as soon as tolerance to headache develops (usually within a week).

Dosage adjustment in renal impairment: Avoid use in patients with severe renal dysfunction (Cl_{cr} <10 mL/minute). Studies have not been done in patients with renal impairment.

Dosage adjustment in hepatic impairment: Avoid use in patients with severe hepatic impairment. Studies have not been done in patients with varying degrees of hepatic impairment.

Elderly: Plasma concentrations were 40% higher, but specific dosage adjustments have not been recommended.

Additional Information Complete prescribing information for this medication should be consulted for additional detail.

Dosage Forms Excipient information presented when available (limited, particularly for generics); consult specific product labeling.

Capsule, variable release:

Aggrenox®: Aspirin 25 mg (immediate release) and dipyridamole 200 mg (extended release)

◆ **Aspirin and Extended-Release Dipyridamole** *see* Aspirin and Dipyridamole *on page 145*

◆ **Aspirin and Meprobamate** *see* Meprobamate and Aspirin *on page 946*

◆ **Aspirin and Oxycodone** *see* Oxycodone and Aspirin *on page 1123*

Aspirin and Pravastatin (AS pir in & PRA va stat in)

U.S. Brand Names Pravigard™ PAC [DSC]

Canadian Brand Names PravASA

Index Terms Buffered Aspirin and Pravastatin Sodium; Pravastatin and Aspirin

Pharmacologic Category Antilipemic Agent, HMG-CoA Reductase Inhibitor; Salicylate

Use Combination therapy in patients who need treatment with aspirin and pravastatin to reduce the incidence of cardiovascular events, including myocardial infarction, stroke, and death

Pregnancy Risk Factor X

Dosage Oral: Adults:

Initial: Pravastatin 40 mg with aspirin (either 81 mg or 325 mg); both medications taken once daily. If pravastatin 40 mg does not achieve the desired cholesterol result, dosage may be increased to 80 mg once daily with aspirin (either 81 mg or 325 mg) once daily. Some patients may achieve/maintain goal cholesterol levels at a pravastatin dosage of 20 mg.

See Pravastatin for dosing in renal or hepatic impairment, as well as, dosing with concurrent cyclosporine therapy.

Additional Information Complete prescribing information for this medication should be consulted for additional detail.

Dosage Forms Excipient information presented when available (limited, particularly for generics); consult specific product labeling. [DSC] = Discontinued product

Combination package (Pravigard™ PAC) [each administration card contains] [DSC]:

81/20:

Tablet: Aspirin, buffered 81 mg (5/card) [contains calcium carbonate, and magnesium oxide, and magnesium carbonate]

Tablet (Pravachol®): Pravastatin sodium 20 mg (5/card) [contains lactose]

81/40:

Tablet: Aspirin, buffered 81 mg (5/card) [contains calcium carbonate, and magnesium oxide, and magnesium carbonate]

Tablet (Pravachol®): Pravastatin sodium 40 mg (5/card) [contains lactose]

81/80:

Tablet: Aspirin, buffered 81 mg (5/card) [contains calcium carbonate, and magnesium oxide, and magnesium carbonate]

Tablet (Pravachol®): Pravastatin sodium 80 mg (5/card) [contains lactose]

325/20:

Tablet: Aspirin, buffered 325 mg (5/card) [contains calcium carbonate, and magnesium oxide, and magnesium carbonate]

Tablet (Pravachol®): Pravastatin sodium 20 mg (5/card) [contains lactose]

325/40:

Tablet: Aspirin, buffered 325 mg (5/card) [contains calcium carbonate, and magnesium oxide, and magnesium carbonate]

Tablet (Pravachol®): Pravastatin sodium 40 mg (5/card) [contains lactose]

325/80:

Tablet: Aspirin, buffered 325 mg (5/card) [contains calcium carbonate, and magnesium oxide, and magnesium carbonate]

Tablet (Pravachol®): Pravastatin sodium 80 mg (5/card) [contains lactose]

◆ **Aspirin, Caffeine and Acetaminophen** *see* Acetaminophen, Aspirin, and Caffeine *on page 31*

◆ **Aspirin, Caffeine, and Butalbital** *see* Butalbital, Aspirin, and Caffeine *on page 230*

◆ **Aspirin, Caffeine, and Propoxyphene** *see* Propoxyphene, Aspirin, and Caffeine *on page 1258*

◆ **Aspirin, Carisoprodol, and Codeine** *see* Carisoprodol, Aspirin, and Codeine *on page 262*

◆ **Aspirin Free Anacin® Maximum Strength [OTC]** *see* Acetaminophen *on page 25*

◆ **Aspirin, Orphenadrine, and Caffeine** *see* Orphenadrine, Aspirin, and Caffeine *on page 1108*

◆ **Aspirtab [OTC]** *see* Aspirin *on page 142*

◆ **Astelin®** *see* Azelastine *on page 165*

◆ **Astepro™** *see* Azelastine *on page 165*

◆ **Astramorph/PF™** *see* Morphine Sulfate *on page 1016*

◆ **AT-III** *see* Antithrombin III *on page 124*

◆ **Atacand®** *see* Candesartan *on page 244*

◆ **Atacand HCT®** *see* Candesartan and Hydrochlorothiazide *on page 245*

◆ **Atacand® Plus (Can)** *see* Candesartan and Hydrochlorothiazide *on page 245*

◆ **Atarax® (Can)** *see* HydrOXYzine *on page 754*

◆ **Atasol® (Can)** *see* Acetaminophen *on page 25*

Atazanavir (at a za NA veer)

U.S. Brand Names Reyataz®

Canadian Brand Names Reyataz®

Index Terms Atazanavir Sulfate; BMS-232632

Pharmacologic Category Antiretroviral Agent, Protease Inhibitor

Additional Appendix Information

Antiretroviral Therapy for HIV Infection: Adults and Adolescents *on page 1758*

Management of Healthcare Worker Exposures to HBV, HCV, and HIV *on page 1719*

Perinatal HIV Guidelines *on page 1730*

Use Treatment of HIV-1 infections in combination with at least two other antiretroviral agents

Note: In patients with prior virologic failure, coadministration with ritonavir is recommended.

Pregnancy Risk Factor B

Pregnancy Considerations Teratogenic effects not observed in animal studies. Pregnancy and protease inhibitors are both associated with an increased risk of hyperglycemia. Glucose levels should be closely monitored. Atazanavir crosses the human placenta in low/variable amounts; it is not known if atazanavir will exacerbate hyperbilirubinemia in neonates. Based on limited studies, normal dosing achieves adequate serum concentrations in pregnant women. Atazanavir is currently not recommended for use during pregnancy. Health professionals are encouraged to contact the antiretroviral pregnancy registry to monitor outcomes of pregnant women exposed to antiretroviral medications (1-800-258-4263 or www.APRegistry.com).

Lactation Excretion in breast milk unknown/contraindicated

Contraindications Hypersensitivity (eg, Stevens-Johnson syndrome, erythema multiforme, or toxic skin eruptions) to atazanavir or any component of the formulation; concurrent therapy with cisapride, ergot derivatives (dihydroergotamine, ergonovine, ergotamine, methylergonovine), indinavir, irinotecan, lovastatin, midazolam (oral), pimozide, rifampin, simvastatin, St John's wort, or triazolam

Warnings/Precautions Use with caution in patients taking strong CYP3A4 inhibitors, moderate or strong CYP3A4 inducers, and major CYP2C8 substrates; consider alternative agents that avoid or lessen the potential for CYP- or glucuronidation-mediated interactions. Contraindicated with drugs that are major CYP3A4 or UGT1A1 substrates (see Drug Interactions).

Atazanavir may prolong PR interval, use with caution in patients with pre-existing conduction abnormalities or with medications which prolong AV conduction (dosage adjustment required with some agents); rare cases of second-degree AV block have been reported. May exacerbate pre-existing hepatic dysfunction; use caution in patients with hepatitis B or C or in patients with elevated transaminases. Asymptomatic elevations in bilirubin (unconjugated) occur commonly during therapy with atazanavir; consider alternative therapy if bilirubin is >5 times ULN. Evaluate alternative etiologies if transaminase elevations also occur.

Cases of nephrolithiasis have been reported in postmarketing surveillance; temporary or permanent discontinuation of therapy should be considered if symptoms develop.

Protease inhibitors have been associated with a variety of hypersensitivity events (some severe), including rash, anaphylaxis (rare), angioedema, bronchospasm, erythema multiforme, and/or Stevens-Johnson syndrome (rare). It is generally recommended to discontinue treatment if severe rash or moderate symptoms accompanied by other systemic symptoms occur.

Use with caution in patients with hemophilia A or B; increased bleeding during protease inhibitor therapy has been reported. Changes in glucose tolerance, hyperglycemia, exacerbation of diabetes, DKA, and new-onset diabetes mellitus have been reported in patients receiving protease inhibitors. May be associated with fat redistribution (buffalo hump, increased abdominal girth, breast engorgement, facial atrophy). Immune reconstitution syndrome may develop resulting in the occurrence of an inflammatory response to an indolent or residual opportunistic infection; further evaluation and treatment may be required. Optimal dosing in pediatric patients <6 years of age has not been established; do not use in children <3 months of age due to potential for kernicterus.

Adverse Reactions Includes data from both treatment-naive and treatment-experienced patients. Percentages listed for adults unless otherwise specified.

>10%:

- Dermatologic: Rash (5% to 21%; median onset 8 weeks)
- Endocrine & metabolic: Cholesterol increased (≥240 mg/dL: 6% to 25%)
- Gastrointestinal: Nausea (3% to 14%), amylase increased (14%)
- Hepatic: Bilirubin increased (≥2.6 times ULN: 34% to 49%)
- Neuromuscular & skeletal: CPK increased (5% to 11%)
- Respiratory: Cough (children 21%)

2% to 10%:

- Cardiovascular: AV block (first degree: 6%; second degree [children] 2%)
- Central nervous system: Headache (1% to 6%; children 7%), peripheral neuropathy (<1% to 4%), insomnia (<1% to 3%), depression (2%), fever (2%; children 19%), dizziness (<1% to 2%)
- Endocrine & metabolic: Triglycerides increased (<1% to 8%), hyperglycemia (≥251 mg/dL: 5%)
- Gastrointestinal: Lipase increased (<1% to 5%), abdominal pain (4%), vomiting (3% to 4%; children 8%), diarrhea (1% to 3%; children 8%)
- Hematologic: Neutropenia (3% to 7%), hemoglobin decreased (<1% to 5%), thrombocytopenia (up to 2%)
- Hepatic: ALT increased (>5 times ULN: 4% to 9%; 15% to 25% in patients seropositive for hepatitis B and/or C), AST increased (>5 times ULN: 2% to 7%; 9% to 10% in patients seropositive for hepatitis B and/or C), jaundice (4% to 9%; children 13%)
- Neuromuscular & skeletal: Myalgia (4%)
- Respiratory: Rhinorrhea (children 6%)

<2%, postmarketing and/or case reports: Alopecia, arthralgia, AV block (second- and third-degree, rare), cholecystitis, cholelithiasis, cholestasis, diabetes mellitus, edema, erythema multiforme, immune reconstitution syndrome, left bundle branch block, macropapular rash, nephrolithiasis, pancreatitis, pruritus, QT_c prolongation, Stevens-Johnson syndrome

Drug Interactions

Metabolism/Transport Effects **Substrate** of CYP3A4 (major); **Inhibits** CYP1A2 (weak), 2C8 (strong), 2C9 (weak), 3A4 (strong), UGT1A1 (strong)

Avoid Concomitant Use

Avoid concomitant use of Atazanavir with any of the following: Alfuzosin; Amiodarone; Cisapride; Eplerenone; Ergot Derivatives; Etravirine; Irinotecan; Nilotinib; Nisoldipine; Pimozide; QuiNIDine; Ranolazine; Rifampin; Rivaroxaban; Salmeterol; Silodosin; St Johns Wort

Increased Effect/Toxicity

Atazanavir may increase the levels/effects of: Alfuzosin; Alosetron; Amiodarone; Antifungal Agents (Azole Derivatives, Systemic); Benzodiazepines (metabolized by oxidation); Buprenorphine; Calcium Channel Blockers (Dihydropyridine); Calcium Channel Blockers (Nondihydropyridine); CarBAMazepine; Ciclesonide; Cisapride; Clarithromycin; Corticosteroids (Orally Inhaled); CycloSPORINE; CYP2C8 Substrates (High risk); CYP3A4 Substrates; Digoxin; Enfuvirtide; Eplerenone; Ergot Derivatives; Etravirine; FentaNYL; Fesoterodine; Fusidic Acid; HMG-CoA Reductase Inhibitors; Irinotecan; Ixabepilone; Maraviroc; Meperidine; Nefazodone; Nilotinib; Nisoldipine; Phosphodiesterase 5 Inhibitors; Pimecrolimus; Pimozide; Protease Inhibitors; QuiNIDine; Ranolazine; Rifamycin Derivatives; Rivaroxaban; Salmeterol; Silodosin; Sirolimus; Sorafenib; Tacrolimus; Temsirolimus; Tenofovir; TraZODone; Tricyclic Antidepressants; Warfarin

The levels/effects of Atazanavir may be increased by: Antifungal Agents (Azole Derivatives, Systemic); Clarithromycin; CycloSPORINE; CYP3A4 Inhibitors (Moderate); CYP3A4 Inhibitors (Strong); Dasatinib; Delavirdine; Enfuvirtide; Fusidic Acid

Decreased Effect

Atazanavir may decrease the levels/effects of: Abacavir; Clarithromycin; Delavirdine; Didanosine; Meperidine; Oral Contraceptive (Estrogens); Theophylline Derivatives; Valproic Acid; Zidovudine

The levels/effects of Atazanavir may be decreased by: Antacids; CarBAMazepine; CYP3A4 Inducers (Strong); Deferasirox; Didanosine; Efavirenz; Etravirine; Garlic; H2-Antagonists; Nevirapine; Oral Contraceptive (Estrogens); Proton Pump Inhibitors; Rifampin; Rifamycin Derivatives; St Johns Wort; Tenofovir

Ethanol/Nutrition/Herb Interactions

Food: Bioavailability of atazanavir increased when taken with food.

Herb/Nutraceutical: St John's wort (*Hypericum perforatum*) decreases serum concentrations of protease inhibitors and may lead to treatment failures; concurrent use is contraindicated.

Stability Store at controlled room temperature of 25°C (77°F).

Mechanism of Action Inhibits the HIV-1 protease; inhibition of the viral protease prevents cleavage of the gag-pol polyprotein resulting in the production of immature, noninfectious virus

Pharmacodynamics/Kinetics

Absorption: Rapid; enhanced with food

Protein binding: 86%

Metabolism: Hepatic, via multiple pathways including CYP3A4; forms two metabolites (inactive)

Half-life elimination: Unboosted therapy: 7-8 hours; Boosted therapy (with ritonavir): 9-18 hours

Time to peak, plasma: 2-3 hours

Excretion: Feces (79%, 20% as unchanged drug); urine (13%, 7% as unchanged drug)

Dosage Oral:

Children ≥6 years and Adolescents:

Antiretroviral-naive patients:

15-24 kg: Atazanavir 150 mg once daily **plus** ritonavir 80 mg once daily

25-31 kg: Atazanavir 200 mg once daily **plus** ritonavir 100 mg once daily

32-38 kg: Atazanavir 250 mg once daily **plus** ritonavir 100 mg once daily

≥39 kg: Atazanavir 300 mg once daily **plus** 100 mg ritonavir once daily. **Note:** Treatment-naive patients ≥39 kg and ≥13 years of age who are unable to tolerate ritonavir, refer to adult dosing.

or

15-19 kg: Atazanavir 8.5 mg/kg/dose once daily (rounded to available capsule strengths) **plus** ritonavir 4 mg/kg once daily

≥20 kg: Atazanavir 7 mg/kg/dose once daily (round to available capsule strengths) (maximum 300 mg) **plus** ritonavir 4 mg/kg once daily

Antiretroviral-experienced patients: **Note:** Atazanavir without ritonavir is not recommended in antiretroviral-experienced patients with prior virologic failure:

25-31 kg: Atazanavir 200 mg once daily **plus** ritonavir 100 mg once daily

32-38 kg: Atazanavir 250 mg once daily **plus** ritonavir 100 mg once daily

≥39 kg: Atazanavir 300 mg once daily **plus** 100 mg ritonavir once daily

Adults:

Antiretroviral-naive patients: Atazanavir 300 mg once daily **plus** ritonavir 100 mg once daily **or** 400 mg once daily in patients unable to tolerate ritonavir.

Antiretroviral-experienced patients: Atazanavir 300 mg once daily **plus** ritonavir 100 mg once daily. **Note:** Atazanavir without ritonavir is not recommended in antiretroviral-experienced patients with prior virologic failure.

Dosage adjustments for concomitant therapy: Adolescents >13 years and Adults:

Coadministration with efavirenz:

Antiretroviral-naive patients: Atazanavir 400 mg plus ritonavir 100 mg given with efavirenz 600 mg (all as a single daily dose)

Antiretroviral-experienced patients: Concurrent use not recommended due to decreased atazanavir exposure.

Coadministration with didanosine buffered or enteric-coated formulations: Administer atazanavir 2 hours before or 1 hour after didanosine buffered formulations

Coadministration with H_2 antagonists:

Antiretroviral-naive patients: Atazanavir 300 mg plus ritonavir 100 mg given simultaneously with, or at least 10 hours after an H_2 antagonist equivalent dose of ≤80 mg famotidine/day

Patients unable to tolerate ritonavir: Atazanavir 400 mg once daily given at least 2 hours before or at least 10 hours after an H_2 antagonist equivalent daily dose of ≤40 mg famotidine (single dose ≤20 mg)

Antiretroviral-experienced patients: Atazanavir 300 mg plus ritonavir 100 mg given simultaneously with, or at least 10 hours after an H_2 antagonist equivalent dose of ≤40 mg famotidine/day

With tenofovir: Increase atazanavir to 400 mg (plus ritonavir 100 mg) once daily

Coadministration with proton pump inhibitors:

Antiretroviral-naive patients: Atazanavir 300 mg plus ritonavir 100 mg given 12 hours after a proton pump inhibitor equivalent dose of ≤20 mg omeprazole/day

Antiretroviral-experienced patients: Concurrent use not recommended.

Coadministration with tenofovir: Atazanavir 300 mg plus ritonavir 100 mg given with tenofovir 300 mg (all as a single daily dose); if H_2 antagonist coadministered, increase atazanavir to 400 mg (plus ritonavir 100 mg) once daily

Dosage adjustment in renal impairment:

Not on hemodialysis: No adjustment necessary

Hemodialysis:

Antiretroviral-naive patients: Use boosted therapy of atazanavir 300 mg with ritonavir 100 mg once daily

Antiretroviral-experienced patients: Not recommended

Dosage adjustment in hepatic impairment:

Mild-to-moderate hepatic insufficiency: Use with caution; if moderate insufficiency (Child-Pugh class B) and no prior virologic failure, reduce dose to 300 mg once daily.

Severe hepatic insufficiency (Child-Pugh class C): Not recommended

Note: Patients with underlying hepatitis B or C may be at increased risk of hepatic decompensation. Combination therapy (with ritonavir) in patients with hepatic impairment not recommended.

Dietary Considerations Should be taken with food to enhance absorption.

Administration Administer with food.

Monitoring Parameters Viral load, CD4, serum glucose; liver function tests, bilirubin, drug levels (with certain concomitant medications), ECG monitoring in patients with prolonged PR interval or with concurrent AV nodal blocking drugs

Additional Information A listing of medications that should not be used concurrently is available with each bottle and patients should be provided with this information.

Dosage Forms Excipient information presented when available (limited, particularly for generics); consult specific product labeling.

Capsule, as sulfate:

Reyataz®: 100 mg, 150 mg, 200 mg, 300 mg

◆ **Atazanavir Sulfate** *see* Atazanavir *on page 146*

Atenolol (a TEN oh lole)

U.S. Brand Names Tenormin®

Canadian Brand Names Apo-Atenol®; Gen-Atenolol; Novo-Atenol; Nu-Atenol; PMS-Atenolol; RAN™-Atenolol; Rhoxal-atenolol; Riva-Atenolol; Sandoz-Atenolol; Tenolin; Tenormin®

Pharmacologic Category Beta Blocker, $Beta_1$ Selective

Additional Appendix Information

Beta-Blockers *on page 1648*

Use Treatment of hypertension, alone or in combination with other agents; management of angina pectoris, postmyocardial infarction patients

Unlabeled/Investigational Use Acute ethanol withdrawal, supraventricular and ventricular arrhythmias, and migraine headache prophylaxis

Pregnancy Risk Factor D

Pregnancy Considerations Atenolol crosses the placenta; beta-blockers have been associated with persistent bradycardia, hypotension, and IUGR; IUGR is probably related to maternal hypertension. Available evidence suggests beta-blockers are generally safe during pregnancy (JNC 7). Cases of neonatal hypoglycemia have been reported following maternal use of beta-blockers at parturition or during breast-feeding. Monitor breast-fed infant for symptoms of beta-blockade.

Lactation Enters breast milk/use caution

Medication Safety Issues

Sound-alike/look-alike issues:

Atenolol may be confused with albuterol, Altenol®, timolol, Tylenol®

Tenormin® may be confused with Imuran®, Norpramin®, thiamine, Trovan®

International issues:

Betanol® [Bangladesh] may be confused with Patanol® which is a brand name for olopatadine in the U.S.

Contraindications Hypersensitivity to atenolol or any component of the formulation; sinus bradycardia; sinus node dysfunction; heart block greater than first-degree (except in patients with a functioning artificial pacemaker); cardiogenic shock; uncompensated cardiac failure; pulmonary edema; pregnancy

Warnings/Precautions Consider pre-existing conditions such as sick sinus syndrome before initiating. Administer cautiously in compensated heart failure and monitor for a worsening of the condition (efficacy of atenolol in heart failure has not been established). **[U.S. Boxed Warning]: Beta-blocker therapy should not be withdrawn abruptly (particularly in patients with CAD), but gradually tapered to avoid acute tachycardia, hypertension, and/or ischemia.** Use caution with concurrent use of beta-blockers and either verapamil or diltiazem; bradycardia or heart block can occur. Avoid concurrent I.V. use of both agents. Beta-blockers should be avoided in patients with bronchospastic disease (asthma). Atenolol, with B_1 selectivity, has been used cautiously in bronchospastic disease with close monitoring. Use cautiously in peripheral arterial disease, especially if severe disease is present. Use cautiously in patients with diabetes - may mask hypoglycemic symptoms. Use cautiously in the renally impaired (dosage adjustment required). Use care with anesthetic agents which decrease myocardial function. Caution in myasthenia gravis or psychiatric disease (may cause CNS depression). Adequate alpha-blockade is required prior to use of any beta-blocker for patients with untreated pheochromocytoma. Use caution with history of severe anaphylaxis to allergens; patients taking beta-blockers may become more sensitive to repeated challenges. Treatment of anaphylaxis (eg, epinephrine) in patients taking beta-blockers may be ineffective or promote undesirable effects. Safety and efficacy have not been established in children.

Adverse Reactions

1% to 10%:

Cardiovascular: Persistent bradycardia, hypotension, chest pain, edema, heart failure, second- or third-degree AV block, Raynaud's phenomenon

Central nervous system: Dizziness, fatigue, insomnia, lethargy, confusion, mental impairment, depression, headache, nightmares

Gastrointestinal: Constipation, diarrhea, nausea

Genitourinary: Impotence

Miscellaneous: Cold extremities

<1% (Limited to important or life-threatening): Alopecia, dyspnea (especially with large doses), hallucinations, impotence, liver enzymes increased, lupus syndrome, Peyronie's disease, positive ANA, psoriasiform rash, psychosis, thrombocytopenia, wheezing

Drug Interactions

Avoid Concomitant Use

Avoid concomitant use of Atenolol with any of the following: Methacholine

Increased Effect/Toxicity

Atenolol may increase the levels/effects of: Alpha-/Beta-Agonists (Direct-Acting); Alpha1-Blockers; Alpha2-Agonists; Amifostine; Cardiac Glycosides; Insulin; Lidocaine; Methacholine; Midodrine; RiTUXimab

The levels/effects of Atenolol may be increased by: Acetylcholinesterase Inhibitors; Amiodarone; Anilidopiperidine Opioids; Calcium Channel Blockers (Nondihydropyridine); Diazoxide; Dipyridamole; Disopyramide; Herbs (Hypotensive Properties); Prostacyclin Analogues; Reserpine

Decreased Effect

Atenolol may decrease the levels/effects of: Beta2-Agonists; Theophylline Derivatives

The levels/effects of Atenolol may be decreased by: Ampicillin; Herbs (Hypertensive Properties); Methylphenidate; Nonsteroidal Anti-Inflammatory Agents; Yohimbine

Ethanol/Nutrition/Herb Interactions

Food: Atenolol serum concentrations may be decreased if taken with food.

Herb/Nutraceutical: Avoid dong quai if using for hypertension (has estrogenic activity). Avoid ephedra, yohimbe, ginseng (may worsen hypertension). Avoid garlic (may have increased antihypertensive effect).

Stability Protect from light.

Mechanism of Action Competitively blocks response to beta-adrenergic stimulation, selectively blocks $beta_1$-receptors with little or no effect on $beta_2$-receptors except at high doses

Pharmacodynamics/Kinetics

Onset of action: Peak effect: Oral: 2-4 hours

Duration: Normal renal function: 12-24 hours

Absorption: Incomplete

Distribution: Low lipophilicity; does not cross blood-brain barrier

Protein binding: 3% to 15%

Metabolism: Limited hepatic

Half-life elimination: Beta:

Neonates: ≤35 hours; Mean: 16 hours

Children: 4.6 hours; children >10 years may have longer half-life (>5 hours) compared to children 5-10 years (<5 hours)

Adults: Normal renal function: 6-9 hours, prolonged with renal impairment; End-stage renal disease: 15-35 hours

Excretion: Feces (50%); urine (40% as unchanged drug)

Dosage

Oral:

Children: Hypertension: 0.5-1 mg/kg/dose given daily; range of 0.5-1.5 mg/kg/day; maximum dose: 2 mg/kg/day up to 100 mg/day

Adults:

Hypertension: 25-50 mg once daily, may increase to 100 mg/day. Doses >100 mg are unlikely to produce any further benefit.

Angina pectoris: 50 mg once daily, may increase to 100 mg/day. Some patients may require 200 mg/day.

Postmyocardial infarction: Follow I.V. dose with 100 mg/day or 50 mg twice daily for 6-9 days postmyocardial infarction.

I.V.:

Hypertension: Dosages of 1.25-5 mg every 6-12 hours have been used in short-term management of patients unable to take oral enteral beta-blockers

Postmyocardial infarction: Early treatment: 5 mg slow I.V. over 5 minutes; may repeat in 10 minutes. If both doses are tolerated, may start oral atenolol 50 mg every 12 hours or 100 mg/day for 6-9 days postmyocardial infarction.

Dosing interval for oral atenolol in renal impairment:

Cl_{cr} 15-35 mL/minute: Administer 50 mg/day maximum.

Cl_{cr} <15 mL/minute: Administer 50 mg every other day maximum.

Hemodialysis: Moderately dialyzable (20% to 50%) via hemodialysis; administer dose postdialysis or administer 25-50 mg supplemental dose.

Peritoneal dialysis: Elimination is not enhanced; supplemental dose is not necessary.

Dietary Considerations May be taken without regard to meals.

Administration When administered acutely for cardiac treatment, monitor ECG and blood pressure. The injection can be administered undiluted or diluted with a compatible I.V. solution. May administer by rapid infusion (I.V. push) at a rate of 1 mg/minute or by slow infusion over ~30 minutes. Necessary monitoring for surgical patients who are unable to take oral beta-blockers (prolonged ileus) has not been defined. Some institutions require monitoring of baseline and postinfusion heart rate and blood pressure when a patient's response to beta-blockade has not been characterized (ie, the patient's initial dose or following a change in dose). Consult individual institutional policies and procedures.

Monitoring Parameters Acute cardiac treatment: Monitor ECG and blood pressure with I.V. administration; heart rate and blood pressure with oral administration

Test Interactions Increased glucose; decreased HDL

Dosage Forms Excipient information presented when available (limited, particularly for generics); consult specific product labeling. [DSC] = Discontinued product

Injection, solution:

Tenormin®: 0.5 mg/mL (10 mL) [DSC]

Tablet: 25 mg, 50 mg, 100 mg

Tenormin®: 25 mg, 50 mg, 100 mg

Extemporaneous Preparations A 2 mg/mL atenolol oral liquid compounded from tablets and a commercially available oral diluent was found to be stable for up to 40 days when stored at 5°C or 25°C.

Garner SS, Wiest DB, and Reynolds ER, "Stability of Atenolol in an Extemporaneously Compounded Oral Liquid," *Am J Hosp Pharm*, 1994, 51(4):508-11.

Atenolol and Chlorthalidone

(a TEN oh lole & klor THAL i done)

U.S. Brand Names Tenoretic®

Canadian Brand Names Apo-Atenidone®; Novo-Atenolthalidone; Tenoretic®

Index Terms Chlorthalidone and Atenolol

Pharmacologic Category Beta Blocker, $Beta_1$ Selective; Diuretic, Thiazide

Use Treatment of hypertension with a cardioselective beta-blocker and a diuretic

Pregnancy Risk Factor D

Dosage Adults: Oral: Initial (based on atenolol component): 50 mg once daily, then individualize dose until optimal dose is achieved

Dosage adjustment in renal impairment:

Cl_{cr} 15-35 mL/minute: Administer 50 mg/day.

Cl_{cr} <15 mL/minute: Administer 50 mg every other day.

Additional Information Complete prescribing information for this medication should be consulted for additional detail.

Dosage Forms Excipient information presented when available (limited, particularly for generics); consult specific product labeling.

Tablet:

50: Atenolol 50 mg and chlorthalidone 25 mg

100: Atenolol 100 mg and chlorthalidone 25 mg

Tenoretic®:

50: Atenolol 50 mg and chlorthalidone 25 mg

100: Atenolol 100 mg and chlorthalidone 25 mg

◆ **ATG** *see* Antithymocyte Globulin (Equine) *on page 124*

◆ **Atgam®** *see* Antithymocyte Globulin (Equine) *on page 124*

◆ **Ativan®** *see* LORazepam *on page 905*

◆ **ATNAA** *see* Atropine and Pralidoxime *on page 159*

Atomoxetine (AT oh mox e teen)

U.S. Brand Names Strattera®

Canadian Brand Names Strattera®

Index Terms Atomoxetine Hydrochloride; LY139603; Methylphenoxy-Benzene Propanamine; Tomoxetine

Pharmacologic Category Norepinephrine Reuptake Inhibitor, Selective

Use Treatment of attention deficit/hyperactivity disorder (ADHD)

Restrictions An FDA-approved medication guide must be distributed when dispensing an outpatient prescription (new or refill) for this medication. Medication guides are available at http://www.fda.gov/cder/Offices/ODS/medication_guides.htm. Dispense to all patients or parents or guardians of children and teenagers receiving this medication.

Pregnancy Risk Factor C

Pregnancy Considerations Decreased pup weight and survival were observed in animal studies. There are no adequate and well-controlled studies in pregnant women. Use only if potential benefit to the mother outweighs possible risk to fetus.

Lactation Excretion in breast milk unknown/use caution

Contraindications Hypersensitivity to atomoxetine or any component of the formulation; use with or within 14 days of MAO inhibitors; narrow-angle glaucoma

Warnings/Precautions [U.S. Boxed Warning]: Use caution in pediatric patients; may be an increased risk of suicidal ideation. Closely monitor for clinical worsening, suicidality, or unusual changes in behavior; especially during the initial few months of a course of drug therapy, or at times of dose changes, either increases or decreases. The child's family or caregiver should be instructed to closely observe the patient and communicate condition with healthcare provider. New or worsening symptoms of hostility or aggressive behaviors have been associated with atomoxetine, particularly with the initiation of therapy. Use caution in patients with a history of psychotic illness or bipolar disorder; therapy may induce mixed/manic disorder or psychotic symptoms. Atomoxetine is not approved for major depressive disorder. Patients presenting with depressive symptoms should be screened for bipolar disorder. Recommended to be used as part of a comprehensive treatment program for attention deficit disorders. Atomoxetine does not worsen anxiety in patients with existing anxiety disorders or tics related to Tourette's disorder.

Use caution with hepatic (dosage adjustments necessary in hepatic impairment). Use may be associated with rare but severe hepatotoxicity; discontinue and do not restart if signs or symptoms of hepatotoxic reaction (eg, jaundice, pruritus, flu-like symptoms) are noted. Use caution in patients who are poor metabolizers of CYP2D6 metabolized drugs ("poor metabolizers"), bioavailability increases.

CNS stimulant use has been associated with serious cardiovascular events including sudden death in patients with pre-existing structural cardiac abnormalities or other serious heart problems (sudden death in children and adolescents; sudden death, stroke, and MI in adults). These products should be avoided in patients with known serious structural cardiac abnormalities, cardiomyopathy, serious heart rhythm abnormalities, or other serious cardiac problems that could increase the risk of sudden death that these conditions alone carry. Patients should be carefully evaluated for cardiac disease prior to initiation of therapy. May cause increased heart rate or blood pressure; use caution with hypertension or other cardiovascular disease. Use caution with renal impairment. May cause urinary retention/hesitancy; use caution in patients with history of urinary retention or bladder outlet obstruction. Priapism has been associated with use (rarely). Allergic reactions (including angioneurotic edema, urticaria, and rash) may occur (rare).

Growth should be monitored during treatment. Height and weight gain may be reduced during the first 9-12 months of treatment, but should recover by 3 years of therapy. Safety and efficacy have not been evaluated in pediatric patients <6 years of age.

Adverse Reactions Percentages as reported in children and adults; some adverse reactions may be increased in "poor metabolizers" (CYP2D6).

>10%:
- Central nervous system: Headache (2% to 19%), insomnia (2% to 15%), somnolence (4% to 11%)
- Gastrointestinal: Xerostomia (21%), nausea (7% to 21%), abdominal pain (7% to 18%), appetite decreased (11% to 16%), vomiting (3% to 11%)

1% to 10%:
- Cardiovascular: Systolic blood pressure increased (4% to 5%), diastolic pressure increased (≤4%), palpitation (3%), flushing (≥2%), tachycardia (≤2%), orthostatic hypotension (<2%)
- Central nervous system: Fatigue/lethargy (6% to 9%), dizziness (5% to 6%), irritability (≤6%), chills (3%), sleep disturbance (3%), mood swings (1% to 2%)
- Dermatologic: Hyperhidrosis (4%), rash (2%)
- Endocrine & metabolic: Hot flashes (8%), dysmenorrhea (6%), libido decreased (4%), menstruation disturbance (2%), orgasm abnormal (2%)
- Gastrointestinal: Constipation (1% to 9%), dyspepsia (4%), anorexia (<3%), weight loss (2% to 3%)
- Genitourinary: Erectile disturbance (9%), urinary hesitation/retention (7%), dysuria (3%), ejaculatory disturbance (3%), prostatitis (2%)
- Neuromuscular & skeletal: Tremor (2%)
- Ocular: Mydriasis (≥2%)
- Respiratory: Sinus headache (3%)
- Miscellaneous: Jittery feeling (2%)

Postmarketing and/or case reports: Allergic reactions, aggressiveness, agitation, akathisia, allergy, angioedema, anxiety, delusional thinking, growth suppression (children), hallucinations, hepatotoxicity, hostility, hypomania, impulsiveness, jaundice, mania, MI, panic attacks, pelvic pain, peripheral vascular instability, priapism, pruritus, QT prolongation, Raynaud's phenomenon, seizure (including patients with no prior history or known risk factors for seizure), stroke, suicidal ideation, syncope, urticaria

Drug Interactions

Metabolism/Transport Effects **Substrate** of CYP2C19 (minor), 2D6 (major)

Avoid Concomitant Use

Avoid concomitant use of Atomoxetine with any of the following: Iobenguane I 123; MAO Inhibitors

Increased Effect/Toxicity

Atomoxetine may increase the levels/effects of: Alcohol (Ethyl); Beta2-Agonists; CNS Depressants

The levels/effects of Atomoxetine may be increased by: CYP2D6 Inhibitors (Moderate); CYP2D6 Inhibitors (Strong); Darunavir; MAO Inhibitors; PARoxetine

Decreased Effect

Atomoxetine may decrease the levels/effects of: Iobenguane I 123

Ethanol/Nutrition/Herb Interactions Ethanol: Avoid ethanol (may increase CNS depression).

Stability Store at room temperature of 25°C (77°F).

Mechanism of Action Selectively inhibits the reuptake of norepinephrine (Ki 4.5nM) with little to no activity at the other neuronal reuptake pumps or receptor sites.

Pharmacodynamics/Kinetics
- Absorption: Rapid
- Distribution: V_d: I.V.: 0.85 L/kg
- Protein binding: 98%, primarily albumin
- Metabolism: Hepatic, via CYP2D6 and CYP2C19; forms metabolites (4-hydroxyatomoxetine, active, equipotent to atomoxetine; N-desmethylatomoxetine in poor metabolizers, limited activity)
- Bioavailability: 63% in extensive metabolizers; 94% in poor metabolizers
- Half-life elimination: Atomoxetine: 5 hours (up to 24 hours in poor metabolizers); Active metabolites: 4-hydroxyatomoxetine: 6-8 hours; N-desmethylatomoxetine: 6-8 hours (34-40 hours in poor metabolizers)
- Time to peak, plasma: 1-2 hours
- Excretion: Urine (80%, as conjugated 4-hydroxy metabolite); feces (17%)

Dosage Oral: **Note:** Atomoxetine may be discontinued without the need for tapering dose.

Children ≥6 years and ≤70 kg: ADHD: Initial: 0.5 mg/kg/day, increase after minimum of 3 days to ~1.2 mg/kg/day; may administer as either a single daily dose or 2 evenly divided doses in morning and late afternoon/early evening. Maximum daily dose: 1.4 mg/kg or 100 mg, whichever is less.

Dosage adjustment in patients receiving strong CYP2D6 inhibitors (eg, paroxetine, fluoxetine, quinidine) or patients known to be CYP2D6 poor metabolizers: Do not exceed 1.2 mg/kg/day; dose adjustments should occur only after 4 weeks.

Children ≥6 years and >70 kg and Adults: ADHD: Initial: 40 mg/day, increased after minimum of 3 days to ~80 mg/day; may administer as either a single daily dose or two evenly divided doses in morning and late afternoon/early evening. May increase to 100 mg/day in 2-4 additional weeks to achieve optimal response.

Dosage adjustment in patients receiving strong CYP2D6 inhibitors (eg, paroxetine, fluoxetine, quinidine) or patients known to be CYP2D6 poor metabolizers: Do not exceed 80 mg/day; dose adjustments should occur only after 4 weeks.

Elderly: Use has not been evaluated in the elderly

Dosage adjustment in renal impairment: No adjustment needed

Dosage adjustment in hepatic impairment:

Moderate hepatic insufficiency (Child-Pugh class B): All doses should be reduced to 50% of normal

Severe hepatic insufficiency (Child-Pugh class C): All doses should be reduced to 25% of normal

Dietary Considerations May be taken with or without food.

Administration May be administered with or without food. Swallow capsules whole; do not open capsules. Powder in capsules is an ocular irritant.

Monitoring Parameters Patient growth (weight/height gain in children); attention, hyperactivity, anxiety, worsening of aggressive behavior or hostility; blood pressure and pulse (baseline and following dose increases and periodically during treatment)

Family members and caregivers need to monitor patient daily for emergence of irritability, agitation, unusual changes in behavior, and suicidal ideation. Pediatric patients should be monitored closely for suicidality, clinical worsening, or unusual changes in behavior, especially during the initial for months of therapy or at times of dose changes. Appearance of symptoms needs to be immediately reported to healthcare provider. Weekly office visits from patient or caregiver are necessary for the first 4 weeks, then every other week for the next 4 weeks, then at 12 weeks, and as clinically indicated beyond 12 weeks. Additional contact may be required between office visits.

When used for the treatment of ADHD, thoroughly evaluate for cardiovascular risk. Monitor heart rate, blood pressure, and consider obtaining ECG prior to initiation (Vetter, 2008)

Dosage Forms Excipient information presented when available (limited, particularly for generics); consult specific product labeling.

Capsule:

Strattera®: 10 mg, 18 mg, 25 mg, 40 mg, 60 mg, 80 mg, 100 mg

◆ **Atomoxetine Hydrochloride** *see* Atomoxetine *on page 150*

Atorvastatin (a TORE va sta tin)

U.S. Brand Names Lipitor®

Canadian Brand Names Lipitor®

Pharmacologic Category Antilipemic Agent, HMG-CoA Reductase Inhibitor

Additional Appendix Information

Hyperlipidemia Management *on page 1815*

Lipid-Lowering Agents *on page 1661*

Use Treatment of dyslipidemias or primary prevention of cardiovascular disease (atherosclerotic) as detailed below:

Primary prevention of cardiovascular disease (high-risk for CVD): To reduce the risk of MI or stroke in patients without evidence of heart disease who have multiple CVD risk factors or type 2 diabetes. Treatment reduces the risk for angina or revascularization procedures in patients with multiple risk factors.

Secondary prevention of cardiovascular disease: To reduce the risk of MI, stroke, revascularization procedures, and angina in patients with evidence of heart disease. To reduce the risk of hospitalization for heart failure.

Treatment of dyslipidemias: To reduce elevations in total cholesterol, LDL-C, apolipoprotein B, and triglycerides in patients with elevations of one or more components, and/or to increase HDL-C as present in Fredrickson type IIa, IIb, III, and IV hyperlipidemias; treatment of primary dysbetalipoproteinemia, homozygous familial hypercholesterolemia

Treatment of heterozygous familial hypercholesterolemia (HeFH) in adolescent patients (10-17 years of age, females >1 year postmenarche) having LDL-C ≥190 mg/dL or LDL-C ≥160 mg/dL with positive family history of premature cardiovascular disease (CVD) or with two or more CVD risk factors.

Pregnancy Risk Factor X

Pregnancy Considerations Cholesterol biosynthesis may be important in fetal development. Contraindicated in pregnancy. Administer to women of childbearing potential only when conception is highly unlikely and patients have been informed of potential hazards.

Lactation Enters breast milk/contraindicated

Medication Safety Issues

Sound-alike/look-alike issues:

Lipitor® may be confused with Levatol®

Contraindications Hypersensitivity to atorvastatin or any component of the formulation; active liver disease; unexplained persistent elevations of serum transaminases; pregnancy

Warnings/Precautions Secondary causes of hyperlipidemia should be ruled out prior to therapy. Liver function must be monitored by periodic laboratory assessment. May cause hepatic dysfunction. Use with caution in patients who consume large amounts of ethanol or have a history of liver disease. Monitoring is recommended. Patients with a history of hemorrhagic stroke may be at increased risk for another with use.

Rhabdomyolysis with acute renal failure has occurred. Risk is dose related and is increased with concurrent use of lipid-lowering agents which may cause rhabdomyolysis (fibric acid derivatives or niacin at doses ≥1 g/day) or during concurrent use with potent CYP3A4 inhibitors (including amiodarone, clarithromycin, cyclosporine, erythromycin, itraconazole, ketoconazole, nefazodone, grapefruit juice in large quantities, verapamil, or protease inhibitors such as indinavir, nelfinavir, or ritonavir). Ensure patient is on the lowest effective atorvastatin dose. If concurrent use of clarithromycin or combination protease inhibitors (eg, lopinavir/ritonavir or ritonavir/saquinavir) is warranted consider dose adjustment of atorvastatin. Monitor closely if used with other drugs associated with myopathy. Weigh the risk versus benefit when combining any of these drugs with atorvastatin. Discontinue in any patient experiencing an acute or serious condition predisposing to renal failure secondary to rhabdomyolysis. Based upon current evidence, HMG-CoA reductase inhibitor therapy should be continued in the perioperative period unless risk outweighs cardioprotective benefit. Use with caution in patients with advanced age, these patients are predisposed to myopathy. Safety and efficacy have not been established in patients <10 years of age or in premenarcheal girls.

Adverse Reactions

>10%: Central nervous system: Headache (3% to 17%)

2% to 10%:

Cardiovascular: Chest pain, peripheral edema

Central nervous system: Insomnia, dizziness

Dermatologic: Rash (1% to 4%)

Gastrointestinal: Abdominal pain (up to 4%), constipation (up to 3%), diarrhea (up to 4%), dyspepsia (1% to 3%), flatulence (1% to 3%), nausea

Genitourinary: Urinary tract infection

Hepatic: Transaminases increased (2% to 3% with 80 mg/day dosing)

Neuromuscular & skeletal: Arthralgia (up to 5%), arthritis, back pain (up to 4%), myalgia (up to 6%), weakness (up to 4%)

Respiratory: Sinusitis (up to 6%), pharyngitis (up to 3%), bronchitis, rhinitis

Miscellaneous: Infection (3% to 10%), flu-like syndrome (up to 3%), allergic reaction (up to 3%)

<2% (Limited to important or life-threatening): Alopecia, anaphylaxis, angina, angioneurotic edema, arrhythmia, bullous rash, cholestatic jaundice, deafness, dyspnea, erythema multiforme, esophagitis, facial paralysis, fatigue, glaucoma, gout, hepatitis, hyperkinesias, impotence, migraine, myasthenia, myopathy, myositis, nephritis, pancreatitis, paresthesia, peripheral neuropathy, petechiae, photosensitivity, postural hypotension, pruritus, rectal hemorrhage, rhabdomyolysis, somnolence, Stevens-Johnson syndrome, syncope, tendinous contracture, tendon rupture, thrombocytopenia, tinnitus, torticollis, toxic epidermal necrolysis, urticaria, vaginal hemorrhage, vomiting

Drug Interactions

Metabolism/Transport Effects Substrate of CYP3A4 (major); **Inhibits** CYP3A4 (weak)

Avoid Concomitant Use

Avoid concomitant use of Atorvastatin with any of the following: Rivaroxaban; Silodosin; Topotecan

Increased Effect/Toxicity

Atorvastatin may increase the levels/effects of: Aliskiren; DAPTOmycin; Digoxin; Midazolam; P-Glycoprotein Substrates; Rivaroxaban; Silodosin; Topotecan

The levels/effects of Atorvastatin may be increased by: Amiodarone; Antifungal Agents (Azole Derivatives, Systemic); Calcium Channel Blockers (Nondihydropyridine); Colchicine; CycloSPORINE; CYP3A4 Inhibitors (Moderate); CYP3A4 Inhibitors (Strong); Danazol; Dasatinib; Eltrombopag; Fenofibrate; Fenofibric Acid; Fluconazole; Gemfibrozil; Grapefruit Juice; Macrolide Antibiotics; Nefazodone; Niacin; Niacinamide; P-Glycoprotein Inhibitors; Protease Inhibitors; Sildenafil

Decreased Effect

Atorvastatin may decrease the levels/effects of: Dabigatran Etexilate

The levels/effects of Atorvastatin may be decreased by: Bosentan; CYP3A4 Inducers (Strong); Deferasirox; Etravirine; P-Glycoprotein Inducers; Phenytoin; Rifamycin Derivatives; St Johns Wort

Ethanol/Nutrition/Herb Interactions

Ethanol: Avoid excessive ethanol consumption (due to potential hepatic effects).

Food: Atorvastatin serum concentrations may be increased by grapefruit juice; avoid concurrent intake of large quantities (>1 quart/day). Red yeast rice contains an estimated 2.4 mg lovastatin per 600 mg rice.

Herb/Nutraceutical: St John's wort may decrease atorvastatin levels.

Mechanism of Action Inhibitor of 3-hydroxy-3-methylglutaryl coenzyme A (HMG-CoA) reductase, the rate-limiting enzyme in cholesterol synthesis (reduces the production of mevalonic acid from HMG-CoA); this then results in a compensatory increase in the expression of LDL receptors on hepatocyte membranes and a stimulation of LDL catabolism

Pharmacodynamics/Kinetics

Onset of action: Initial changes: 3-5 days; Maximal reduction in plasma cholesterol and triglycerides: 2 weeks

Absorption: Rapid

Distribution: V_d: 318 L

Protein binding: ≥98%

Metabolism: Hepatic; forms active ortho- and parahydroxylated derivates and an inactive beta-oxidation product

Bioavailability: ~14% (parent drug); ~30% (parent drug and equipotent metabolites)

Half-life elimination: Parent drug: 14 hours; Equipotent metabolites: 20-30 hours

Time to peak, serum: 1-2 hours

Excretion: Bile; urine (2% as unchanged drug)

Dosage Oral: **Note:** Doses should be individualized according to the baseline LDL-cholesterol levels, the recommended goal of therapy, and patient response; adjustments should be made at intervals of 2-4 weeks

Children 10-17 years (females >1 year postmenarche): Heterozygous familial hypercholesterolemia (HeFH): 10 mg once daily (maximum: 20 mg/day)

Adults:

Hypercholesterolemia (heterozygous familial and nonfamilial) and mixed hyperlipidemia (Fredrickson types IIa and IIb): Initial: 10-20 mg once daily; patients requiring >45% reduction in LDL-C may be started at 40 mg once daily; range: 10-80 mg once daily

Homozygous familial hypercholesterolemia: 10-80 mg once daily

Dosing adjustment in renal impairment: No dosage adjustment is necessary.

Dosing adjustment in hepatic impairment: Do not use in active liver disease.

Dietary Considerations May take with food if desired; may take without regard to time of day. Before initiation of therapy, patients should be placed on a standard cholesterol-lowering diet for 3-6 months and the diet should be continued during drug therapy. Red yeast rice contains an estimated 2.4 mg lovastatin per 600 mg rice.

Administration May be administered with food if desired; may take without regard to time of day.

Monitoring Parameters Lipid levels after 2-4 weeks; LFTs, CPK

It is recommended that liver function tests (LFTs) be performed prior to and at 12 weeks following both the initiation of therapy and any elevation in dose, and periodically (eg, semiannually) thereafter.

Dosage Forms Excipient information presented when available (limited, particularly for generics); consult specific product labeling.

Tablet:

Lipitor®: 10 mg, 20 mg, 40 mg, 80 mg

◆ **Atorvastatin Calcium and Amlodipine Besylate** *see* Amlodipine and Atorvastatin *on page 94*

Atovaquone (a TOE va kwone)

U.S. Brand Names Mepron®

Canadian Brand Names Mepron®

Pharmacologic Category Antiprotozoal

Additional Appendix Information

Guidelines for the Prevention of Opportunistic Infections in HIV Infected Persons *on page 1740*

Malaria Treatment *on page 1770*

Use Acute oral treatment of mild-to-moderate *Pneumocystis jirovecii* pneumonia (PCP) in patients who are intolerant to co-trimoxazole; prophylaxis of PCP in patients who are intolerant to co-trimoxazole

Unlabeled/Investigational Use Treatment of babesiosis; treatment/suppression of *Toxoplasma gondii* encephalitis; primary prophylaxis of HIV-infected persons at high risk for developing *Toxoplasma gondii* encephalitis

Pregnancy Risk Factor C

Pregnancy Considerations There are no adequate and well-controlled studies of atovaquone in pregnant women. Use in pregnant women only if the potential benefit outweighs the possible risk to the fetus.

Lactation Excretion in breast milk unknown/use caution

Contraindications Life-threatening allergic reaction to atovaquone or any component of the formulation

Warnings/Precautions When used for treatment, has only been indicated in mild-to-moderate *Pneumocystis jirovecii* pneumonia (PCP); not studied for use in severe PCP. Use with caution in elderly patients due to potentially impaired renal, hepatic, and cardiac function. Absorption may be decreased in patients who have diarrhea or vomiting; monitor closely and consider use of an antiemetic. If severe, consider use of an alternative antimalarial. Use with caution in patients with severe hepatic impairment; rare cases of hepatitis, elevated liver function tests, and liver failure have been reported.

Adverse Reactions Note: Adverse reaction statistics have been compiled from studies including patients with advanced HIV disease. Consequently, it is difficult to distinguish reactions attributed to atovaquone from those caused by the underlying disease or a combination thereof.

>10%:
- Central nervous system: Fever (14% to 40%), headache (16% to 31%), insomnia (10% to 19%), depression, pain
- Dermatologic: Rash (22% to 46%), pruritus (5% to ≥10%)
- Gastrointestinal: Diarrhea (19% to 42%), nausea (21% to 32%), vomiting (14% to 22%), abdominal pain (4% to 21%)
- Neuromuscular & skeletal: Weakness (8% to 31%), myalgia
- Respiratory: Cough (14% to 25%), rhinitis (5% to 24%), dyspnea (15% to 21%), sinusitis (7% to ≥10%)
- Miscellaneous: Infection (18% to 22%), diaphoresis, flu-like syndrome

1% to 10%:
- Cardiovascular: Hypotension (≤1%)
- Central nervous system: Dizziness (3% to 8%), anxiety (≤7%)
- Endocrine & metabolic: Hyponatremia (7% to 10%), hyperglycemia (≤9%), hypoglycemia (≤1%)
- Gastrointestinal: Amylase increased (7% to 8%), anorexia (≤7%), dyspepsia (≤5%), constipation (≤3%), taste perversion (≤3%)
- Hematologic: Anemia (4% to 6%), neutropenia (3% to 5%)
- Hepatic: Liver enzymes increased (4% to 8%)
- Renal: BUN increased (≤1%), creatinine increased (≤1%)
- Respiratory: Bronchospasm (2% to 4%)
- Miscellaneous: Oral moniliasis (5% to 10%)

Postmarketing and/or case reports: Acute renal failure, allergic reaction, angioedema, erythema multiforme, hepatitis (rare), hypersensitivity reactions, liver failure (rare), methemoglobinemia, pancreatitis, skin desquamation, Stevens-Johnson syndrome, throat tightness, thrombocytopenia, urticaria, vortex keratopathy

Drug Interactions

Avoid Concomitant Use There are no known interactions where it is recommended to avoid concomitant use.

Increased Effect/Toxicity

The levels/effects of Atovaquone may be increased by: Herbs (Hypoglycemic Properties)

Decreased Effect

Atovaquone may decrease the levels/effects of: Indinavir

The levels/effects of Atovaquone may be decreased by: Rifamycin Derivatives; Ritonavir; Tetracycline

Ethanol/Nutrition/Herb Interactions

Food: Ingestion with a fatty meal increases absorption.

Herb/Nutraceutical: Herbs with hypoglycemic properties may enhance the hypoglycemic effect of atovaquone. This includes alfalfa, aloe, bilberry, bitter melon, burdock, celery, damiana, fenugreek, garcinia, garlic, ginger, ginseng (American), gymnema, marshmallow, stinging nettle.

Stability Store at 15°C to 25°C (59°F to 77°F). Do not freeze.

Mechanism of Action Inhibits electron transport in mitochondria resulting in the inhibition of key metabolic enzymes responsible for the synthesis of nucleic acids and ATP

Pharmacodynamics/Kinetics

Absorption: Significantly increased with a high-fat meal

Distribution: V_{dss}: 0.6 ± 17 L/kg

Protein binding: >99%

Metabolism: Undergoes enterohepatic recirculation

Bioavailability: 32% to 62%

Half-life elimination: 1.5-4 days

Excretion: Feces (>94% as unchanged drug); urine (<1%)

Dosage Oral:

Children <13 years (unlabeled uses, AIDSinfo guidelines):
- Prevention of PCP:
  - 1-3 months: 30 mg/kg once daily with food
  - 4-24 months: 45 mg/kg once daily with food
  - >24 months: 30 mg/kg once daily with food
- Treatment of mild-to-moderate PCP:
  - Birth to 3 months: 30-40 mg/kg/day in 2 divided doses with food (maximum: 1500 mg/day)
  - 3-24 months: 45 mg/kg/day in 2 divided doses with food
  - ≥24 months: 30-40 mg/kg/day in 2 divided doses with food (maximum: 1500 mg/day)
- *Toxoplasma gondii* prophylaxis:
  - 1-3 months: 30 mg/kg once daily with food
  - 4-24 months: 45 mg/kg once daily with food
  - >24 months: 30 mg/kg once daily with food
- Babesiosis: 20 mg/kg/day in 2 divided doses with food for 7-10 days

Adolescents 13-16 years and Adults:
- Prevention of PCP: 1500 mg once daily with food
- Treatment of mild-to-moderate PCP: 750 mg twice daily with food for 21 days
- *Toxoplasma gondii* encephalitis (unlabeled use; AIDSinfo guidelines):
  - Prophylaxis: 1500 mg once daily with food
  - Treatment: 750 mg 4 times daily or 1500 mg twice daily with food for at least 6 weeks after resolution of signs and symptoms
  - Suppression after treatment: 750 mg 2-4 times/day with food
- Babesiosis (unlabeled use): 750 mg twice daily with azithromycin for 7-10 days

Dietary Considerations Must be taken with meals.

Administration Must be administered with meals. Shake suspension gently before use. Once opened, the foil pouch can be emptied on a dosing spoon, in a cup, or directly into the mouth.

Dosage Forms Excipient information presented when available (limited, particularly for generics); consult specific product labeling.

Suspension, oral:

Mepron®: 750 mg/5 mL (5 mL, 210 mL) [contains benzyl alcohol; citrus flavor]

Atovaquone and Proguanil

(a TOE va kwone & pro GWA nil)

U.S. Brand Names Malarone®

Canadian Brand Names Malarone®; Malarone® Pediatric

Index Terms Atovaquone and Proguanil Hydrochloride; Proguanil and Atovaquone; Proguanil Hydrochloride and Atovaquone

Pharmacologic Category Antimalarial Agent

Additional Appendix Information

Malaria Treatment *on page 1770*

Use Prevention or treatment of acute, uncomplicated *P. falciparum* malaria

Pregnancy Risk Factor C

Pregnancy Considerations Use in pregnant women only if the potential benefit outweighs the possible risk to the fetus. There are no adequate and well-controlled studies of atovaquone and/or proguanil in pregnant women. Because *P. falciparum* malaria can cause maternal death and fetal loss, pregnant women traveling to malaria-endemic areas must use personal protection against mosquito bites.

Lactation

Atovaquone: Excretion in breast milk unknown/use caution

Proguanil: Enters breast milk (small amounts)/use caution

Contraindications Hypersensitivity to atovaquone, proguanil, or any component of the formulation; prophylactic use in severe renal impairment (Cl_{cr} <30 mL/minute)

Warnings/Precautions Not indicated for severe or complicated malaria. Absorption of atovaquone may be decreased in patients who have diarrhea or vomiting; monitor closely and consider use of an antiemetic. If severe, consider use of an alternative antimalarial. Increased transaminase levels and hepatitis (rare) have been reported with prophylactic use; single case report of hepatic failure requiring transplantation documented. Monitor closely and use caution in patients with existing hepatic impairment. Data from clinical trials indicates that elevations in AST/ALT may persist for up to 4 weeks following treatment. Administer with caution to patients with pre-existing renal disease. May use for 3-day treatment in patients with severe renal impairment if benefit outweighs risk. Contraindicated for prophylactic use in severe renal impairment (Cl_{cr} <30 mL/minute). Not for use in patients <5 kg (treatment) or <11 kg (prophylaxis). Delayed cases of *P. falciparum* malaria may occur after stopping prophylaxis. Recrudescent infections or infections following prophylaxis with this agent should be treated with an alternative agent(s).

Adverse Reactions The following adverse reactions were reported in patients being treated for malaria. When used for prophylaxis, reactions are similar to those seen with placebo.

>10%:

- Gastrointestinal: Abdominal pain (17%), nausea (12%), vomiting (children 10% to 13%, adults 12%)
- Hepatic: Transaminase increases (ALT 27%, AST 17%; increased LFT values typically normalized after ~4 weeks)

1% to 10%:

- Central nervous system: Headache (10%), dizziness (5%)
- Dermatologic: Pruritus (children 6%)
- Gastrointestinal: Diarrhea (children 6%, adults 8%), anorexia (5%)
- Neuromuscular & skeletal: Weakness (8%)

Postmarketing and/or case reports: Anaphylaxis, anemia (rare), angioedema, erythema multiforme, hallucinations, hepatitis, hepatic failure (case report), neutropenia, pancytopenia (with severe renal impairment), photosensitivity, psychotic episodes, rash, seizure, Stevens-Johnson syndrome, urticaria

Drug Interactions

Metabolism/Transport Effects Proguanil: **Substrate** (minor) of 1A2, 2C19, 3A4

Avoid Concomitant Use There are no known interactions where it is recommended to avoid concomitant use.

Increased Effect/Toxicity

Atovaquone and Proguanil may increase the levels/effects of: Antipsychotic Agents (Phenothiazines)

The levels/effects of Atovaquone and Proguanil may be increased by: Herbs (Hypoglycemic Properties)

Decreased Effect

Atovaquone and Proguanil may decrease the levels/effects of: Indinavir

The levels/effects of Atovaquone and Proguanil may be decreased by: Rifamycin Derivatives; Ritonavir; Tetracycline

Ethanol/Nutrition/Herb Interactions

Food: Atovaquone taken with dietary fat increases the rate and extent of absorption.

Herb/Nutraceutical: Herbs with hypoglycemic properties may enhance the hypoglycemic effect of atovaquone. This includes alfalfa, aloe, bilberry, bitter melon, burdock, celery, damiana, fenugreek, garcinia, garlic, ginger, ginseng (American), gymnema, marshmallow, stinging nettle.

Stability Store tablets at controlled room temperature of 25°C (77°F).

Mechanism of Action

Atovaquone: Selectively inhibits parasite mitochondrial electron transport.

Proguanil: The metabolite cycloguanil inhibits dihydrofolate reductase, disrupting deoxythymidylate synthesis. Together, atovaquone/cycloguanil affect the erythrocytic and exoerythrocytic stages of development.

Pharmacodynamics/Kinetics

Atovaquone: See Atovaquone.

Proguanil:

- Absorption: Extensive
- Distribution: 42 L/kg
- Protein binding: 75%
- Metabolism: Hepatic to active metabolites, cycloguanil (via CYP2C19) and 4-chlorophenylbiguanide
- Half-life elimination: 12-21 hours
- Excretion: Urine (40% to 60%)

Dosage Oral:

Children (dosage based on body weight):

Prevention of malaria: Start 1-2 days prior to entering a malaria-endemic area, continue throughout the stay and for 7 days after returning. Take as a single dose, once daily.

- 11-20 kg: Atovaquone/proguanil 62.5 mg/25 mg
- 21-30 kg: Atovaquone/proguanil 125 mg/50 mg
- 31-40 kg: Atovaquone/proguanil 187.5 mg/75 mg
- >40 kg: Atovaquone/proguanil 250 mg/100 mg

Treatment of acute malaria: Take as a single dose, once daily for 3 consecutive days.

- 5-8 kg: Atovaquone/proguanil 125 mg/50 mg
- 9-10 kg: Atovaquone/proguanil 187.5 mg/75 mg
- 11-20 kg: Atovaquone/proguanil 250 mg/100 mg
- 21-30 kg: Atovaquone/proguanil 500 mg/200 mg
- 31-40 kg: Atovaquone/proguanil 750 mg/300 mg
- >40 kg: Atovaquone/proguanil 1 g/400 mg

Adults:

Prevention of malaria: Atovaquone/proguanil 250 mg/100 mg once daily; start 1-2 days prior to entering a malaria-endemic area, continue throughout the stay and for 7 days after returning

Treatment of acute malaria: Atovaquone/proguanil 1 g/400 mg as a single dose, once daily for 3 consecutive days

Elderly: Use with caution due to possible decrease in renal and hepatic function, as well as possible decreases in cardiac function, concomitant diseases, or other drug therapy.

Dosage adjustment in renal impairment: No dosage adjustment required in mild-to-moderate renal impairment. Contraindicated as prophylaxis in severe renal impairment (Cl_{cr} <30 mL/minute). May use for 3-day treatment in patients with severe renal impairment if benefit outweighs risk.

Dosage adjustment in hepatic impairment: No dosage adjustment required in mild-to-moderate hepatic impairment. No data available for use in severe hepatic impairment.

Dietary Considerations Must be taken with food or a milky drink.

Administration Administer with food or milk-based drink at the same time each day. If vomiting occurs within 1 hour of administration, repeat the dose. For children who have difficulty swallowing tablets, tablets may be crushed and mixed with condensed milk just prior to administration.

Dosage Forms Excipient information presented when available (limited, particularly for generics); consult specific product labeling.

Tablet, oral:

Malarone®: Atovaquone 250 mg and proguanil hydrochloride 100 mg

Tablet, oral [pediatric]:

Malarone®: Atovaquone 62.5 mg and proguanil hydrochloride 25 mg

♦ **Atovaquone and Proguanil Hydrochloride** *see* Atovaquone and Proguanil *on page 154*

♦ **ATRA** *see* Tretinoin (Oral) *on page 1508*

Atracurium (a tra KYOO ree um)

Canadian Brand Names Atracurium Besylate Injection

Index Terms Atracurium Besylate

Pharmacologic Category Neuromuscular Blocker Agent, Nondepolarizing

Additional Appendix Information

Neuromuscular-Blocking Agents *on page 1665*

Use Adjunct to general anesthesia to facilitate endotracheal intubation and to relax skeletal muscles during surgery; to facilitate mechanical ventilation in ICU patients; does not relieve pain or produce sedation

Pregnancy Risk Factor C

Lactation Excretion in breast milk unknown/use caution

Medication Safety Issues

High alert medication: The Institute for Safe Medication Practices (ISMP) includes this medication among its list of drugs which have a heightened risk of causing significant patient harm when used in error.

Contraindications Hypersensitivity to atracurium besylate or any component of the formulation

Warnings/Precautions Reduce initial dosage and inject slowly (over 1-2 minutes) in patients in whom substantial histamine release would be potentially hazardous (eg, patients with clinically-important cardiovascular disease). Maintenance of an adequate airway and respiratory support is critical. Certain clinical conditions may result in potentiation or antagonism of neuromuscular blockade:

Potentiation: Electrolyte abnormalities, severe hyponatremia, severe hypocalcemia, severe hypokalemia, hypermagnesemia, neuromuscular diseases, acidosis, acute intermittent porphyria, renal failure, hepatic failure

Antagonism: Alkalosis, hypercalcemia, demyelinating lesions, peripheral neuropathies, diabetes mellitus

Increased sensitivity in patients with myasthenia gravis, Eaton-Lambert syndrome; resistance in burn patients (>30% of body) for period of 5-70 days postinjury; resistance in patients with muscle trauma, denervation, immobilization, infection, chronic treatment with atracurium. Cross-sensitivity with other neuromuscular-blocking agents may occur; use extreme caution in patients with previous anaphylactic reactions. Use caution in the elderly. Bradycardia may be more common with atracurium than with other neuromuscular-blocking agents since it has no clinically-significant effects on heart rate to counteract the bradycardia produced by anesthetics. Should be administered by adequately trained individuals familiar with its use.

Adverse Reactions Mild, rare, and generally suggestive of histamine release

1% to 10%: Cardiovascular: Flushing

<1%: Bronchial secretions, erythema, hives, itching, wheezing

Postmarketing and/or case reports: Allergic reaction, bradycardia, bronchospasm, dyspnea, hypotension, injection site reaction, seizure, acute quadriplegic myopathy syndrome (prolonged use), laryngospasm, myositis ossificans (prolonged use), tachycardia, urticaria

Causes of prolonged neuromuscular blockade: Excessive drug administration; cumulative drug effect, metabolism/excretion decreased (hepatic and/or renal impairment); accumulation of active metabolites; electrolyte imbalance (hypokalemia, hypocalcemia, hypermagnesemia, hypernatremia); hypothermia

Drug Interactions

Avoid Concomitant Use There are no known interactions where it is recommended to avoid concomitant use.

Increased Effect/Toxicity

Atracurium may increase the levels/effects of: Botulinum Toxin Type A; Botulinum Toxin Type B; Cardiac Glycosides; Corticosteroids (Systemic)

The levels/effects of Atracurium may be increased by: Aminoglycosides; Calcium Channel Blockers; Capreomycin; Colistimethate; Inhalational Anesthetics; Ketorolac; Lincosamide Antibiotics; Lithium; Loop Diuretics; Magnesium Salts; Polymyxin B; Procainamide; QuiNIDine; Tetracycline Derivatives; Vancomycin

Decreased Effect

The levels/effects of Atracurium may be decreased by: Acetylcholinesterase Inhibitors; Loop Diuretics

Stability Refrigerate intact vials at 2°C to 8°C (36°F to 46°F). Protect from freezing. Use vials within 14 days upon removal from the refrigerator to room temperature of 25°C (77°F). Dilutions of 0.2 mg/mL or 0.5 mg/mL in 0.9% sodium chloride, dextrose 5% in water, or 5% dextrose in sodium chloride 0.9% are stable for up to 24 hours at room temperature or under refrigeration. Atracurium should not be mixed with alkaline solutions.

Mechanism of Action Blocks neural transmission at the myoneural junction by binding with cholinergic receptor sites

Pharmacodynamics/Kinetics

Onset of action (dose dependent): 2-3 minutes

Duration: Recovery begins in 20-35 minutes following initial dose of 0.4-0.5 mg/kg under balanced anesthesia; recovery to 95% of control takes 60-70 minutes

Metabolism: Undergoes ester hydrolysis and Hofmann elimination (nonbiologic process independent of renal, hepatic, or enzymatic function); metabolites have no neuromuscular blocking properties; laudanosine, a product of Hofmann elimination, is a CNS stimulant and can accumulate with prolonged use. Laudanosine is hepatically metabolized.

Half-life elimination: Biphasic: Adults: Initial (distribution): 2 minutes; Terminal: 20 minutes

Excretion: Urine (<5%)

Dosage I.V. (not to be used I.M.): Dose to effect; doses must be individualized due to interpatient variability; use ideal body weight for obese patients

Children 1 month to 2 years: Initial: 0.3-0.4 mg/kg followed by maintenance doses as needed to maintain neuromuscular blockade

Children >2 years to Adults: 0.4-0.5 mg/kg, then 0.08-0.1 mg/kg 20-45 minutes after initial dose to maintain neuromuscular block, followed by repeat doses of 0.08-0.1 mg/kg at 15- to 25-minute intervals

Initial dose after succinylcholine for intubation (balanced anesthesia): Adults: 0.2-0.4 mg/kg

Pretreatment/priming: 10% of intubating dose given 3-5 minutes before initial dose

Continuous infusion:

Surgery: Initial: 9-10 mcg/kg/minute at initial signs of recovery from bolus dose; block usually maintained by a rate of 5-9 mcg/kg/minute under balanced anesthesia

ICU: Block usually maintained by rate of 11-13 mcg/kg/minute (rates for pediatric patients may be higher)

See table on next page.

Atracurium Besylate Infusion Chart

Drug Delivery Rate (mcg/kg/min)	Infusion Rate (mL/kg/min) 0.2 mg/mL (20 mg/100 mL)	Infusion Rate (mL/kg/min) 0.5 mg/mL (50 mg/100 mL)
5	0.025	0.01
6	0.03	0.012
7	0.035	0.014
8	0.04	0.016
9	0.045	0.018
10	0.05	0.02

Dosage adjustment for hepatic or renal impairment is not necessary

Administration May be given undiluted as a bolus injection; not for I.M. injection due to tissue irritation; administration via infusion requires the use of an infusion pump; use infusion solutions within 24 hours of preparation

Monitoring Parameters Vital signs (heart rate, blood pressure, respiratory rate); degree of muscle relaxation (via peripheral nerve stimulator and presence of spontaneous movement); renal function (serum creatinine, BUN) and liver function when in ICU

In the ICU setting, prolonged paralysis and generalized myopathy, following discontinuation of agent, may be minimized by appropriately monitoring degree of blockade.

Additional Information Atracurium is classified as an intermediate-duration neuromuscular-blocking agent. It does not appear to have a cumulative effect on the duration of blockade. It does not relieve pain or produce sedation.

Dosage Forms Excipient information presented when available (limited, particularly for generics); consult specific product labeling.

Injection, as besylate: 10 mg/mL (10 mL) [contains benzyl alcohol]

Injection, as besylate [preservative free]: 10 mg/mL (5 mL)

- ◆ **Atracurium Besylate** *see* Atracurium *on page 156*
- ◆ **Atracurium Besylate Injection (Can)** *see* Atracurium *on page 156*
- ◆ **Atralin™** *see* Tretinoin (Topical) *on page 1509*
- ◆ **Atriance™ (Can)** *see* Nelarabine *on page 1047*
- ◆ **Atripla®** *see* Efavirenz, Emtricitabine, and Tenofovir *on page 509*
- ◆ **AtroPen®** *see* Atropine *on page 157*

Atropine (A troe peen)

U.S. Brand Names AtroPen®; Atropine-Care®; Isopto® Atropine; Sal-Tropine™

Canadian Brand Names Dioptic's Atropine Solution; Isopto® Atropine

Index Terms Atropine Sulfate

Pharmacologic Category Anticholinergic Agent; Anticholinergic Agent, Ophthalmic; Antidote; Antispasmodic Agent, Gastrointestinal; Ophthalmic Agent, Mydriatic

Additional Appendix Information

Cycloplegic Mydriatics *on page 1655*

Use

Injection: Preoperative medication to inhibit salivation and secretions; treatment of symptomatic sinus bradycardia; AV block (nodal level); ventricular asystole; antidote for anticholinesterase inhibitor poisoning (carbamate insecticides, nerve agents, organophosphate insecticides)

Ophthalmic: Produce mydriasis and cycloplegia for examination of the retina and optic disc and accurate measurement of refractive errors; uveitis

Oral: Inhibit salivation and secretions

Unlabeled/Investigational Use Pulseless electric activity, asystole, neuromuscular blockade reversal

Restrictions The AtroPen® formulation is available for use primarily by the Department of Defense.

Pregnancy Risk Factor C

Pregnancy Considerations Animal reproduction studies have not been conducted. Atropine has been found to cross the human placenta.

Lactation Enters breast milk (trace amounts)/use caution (AAP rates "compatible")

Medication Safety Issues

International issues:

Genatropine® [France] may be confused with Genotropin®

Contraindications Hypersensitivity to atropine or any component of the formulation; narrow-angle glaucoma; adhesions between the iris and lens; tachycardia; obstructive GI disease; paralytic ileus; intestinal atony of the elderly or debilitated patient; severe ulcerative colitis; toxic megacolon complicating ulcerative colitis; hepatic disease; obstructive uropathy; renal disease; myasthenia gravis (unless used to treat side effects of acetylcholinesterase inhibitor); asthma; thyrotoxicosis; Mobitz type II block

Warnings/Precautions Use with caution in children with spastic paralysis; use with caution in elderly patients. Low doses cause a paradoxical decrease in heart rates. Some commercial products contain sodium metabisulfite, which can cause allergic-type reactions. May accumulate with multiple inhalational administration, particularly in the elderly. Heat prostration may occur in hot weather. Use with caution in patients with autonomic neuropathy, prostatic hyperplasia, hyperthyroidism, HF, cardiac arrhythmias, chronic lung disease, biliary tract disease; anticholinergic agents are generally not well tolerated in the elderly and their use should be avoided when possible. Atropine is rarely used except as a preoperative agent or in the acute treatment of bradyarrhythmias.

AtroPen®: There are no absolute contraindications for the use of atropine in severe organophosphate poisonings, however in mild poisonings, use caution in those patients where the use of atropine would be otherwise contraindicated. Formulation for use by trained personnel only.

Adverse Reactions Severity and frequency of adverse reactions are dose related and vary greatly; listed reactions are limited to significant and/or life-threatening.

Cardiovascular: Arrhythmia, flushing, hypotension, palpitation, tachycardia

Central nervous system: Ataxia, coma, delirium, disorientation, dizziness, drowsiness, excitement, fever, hallucinations, headache, insomnia, nervousness

Dermatologic: Anhidrosis, urticaria, rash, scarlatiniform rash

Gastrointestinal: Bloating, constipation, delayed gastric emptying, loss of taste, nausea, paralytic ileus, vomiting, xerostomia, dry throat, nasal dryness

Genitourinary: Urinary hesitancy, urinary retention

Neuromuscular & skeletal: Weakness

Ocular: Angle-closure glaucoma, blurred vision, cycloplegia, dry eyes, mydriasis, ocular tension increased

Respiratory: Dyspnea, laryngospasm, pulmonary edema

Miscellaneous: Anaphylaxis

Drug Interactions

Avoid Concomitant Use There are no known interactions where it is recommended to avoid concomitant use.

Increased Effect/Toxicity

Atropine may increase the levels/effects of: Anticholinergics; Cannabinoids; Potassium Chloride

The levels/effects of Atropine may be increased by: Pramlintide

Decreased Effect

Atropine may decrease the levels/effects of: Acetylcholinesterase Inhibitors (Central); Secretin

The levels/effects of Atropine may be decreased by: Acetylcholinesterase Inhibitors (Central)

Stability Store injection at controlled room temperature of 15°C to 30°C (59°F to 86°F); avoid freezing. In addition, AtroPen® should be protected from light.

Mechanism of Action Blocks the action of acetylcholine at parasympathetic sites in smooth muscle, secretory glands, and the CNS; increases cardiac output, dries secretions. Atropine reverses the muscarinic effects of cholinergic poisoning. The primary goal in cholinergic poisonings is reversal of bronchorrhea and bronchoconstriction. Atropine has no effect on the nicotinic receptors responsible for muscle weakness, fasciculations, and paralysis.

Pharmacodynamics/Kinetics

Onset of action: I.V.: Rapid

Absorption: Complete

Distribution: Widely throughout the body; crosses placenta; trace amounts enter breast milk; crosses blood-brain barrier

Metabolism: Hepatic

Half-life elimination: 2-3 hours

Excretion: Urine (30% to 50% as unchanged drug and metabolites)

Dosage

Neonates, Infants, and Children: Doses <0.1 mg have been associated with paradoxical bradycardia.

Inhibit salivation and secretions (preanesthesia): Oral, I.M., I.V., SubQ:

<5 kg: 0.02 mg/kg/dose 30-60 minutes preop then every 4-6 hours as needed. Use of a minimum dosage of 0.1 mg in neonates <5 kg will result in dosages >0.02 mg/kg. There is no documented minimum dosage in this age group.

>5 kg: 0.01-0.02 mg/kg/dose to a maximum 0.4 mg/dose 30-60 minutes preop; minimum dose: 0.1 mg

Alternate dosing:

3-7 kg (7-16 lb): 0.1 mg

8-11 kg (17-24 lb): 0.15 mg

11-18 kg (24-40 lb): 0.2 mg

18-29 kg (40-65 lb): 0.3 mg

>30 kg (>65 lb): 0.4 mg

Bradycardia: I.V., intratracheal: 0.02 mg/kg, minimum dose 0.1 mg, maximum single dose: 0.5 mg in children and 1 mg in adolescents; may repeat in 5-minute intervals to a maximum total dose of 1 mg in children or 2 mg in adolescents. (**Note:** For intratracheal administration, the dosage must be diluted with normal saline to a total volume of 1-5 mL). When treating bradycardia in neonates, reserve use for those patients unresponsive to improved oxygenation and epinephrine.

Infants and Children: Nerve agent toxicity management: See **Note** under adult dosing.

Prehospital ("in the field"): I.M.:

Birth to <2 years: Mild-to-moderate symptoms: 0.05 mg/kg; severe symptoms: 0.1 mg/kg

2-10 years: Mild-to-moderate symptoms: 1 mg; severe symptoms: 2 mg

>10 years: Mild-to-moderate symptoms: 2 mg; severe symptoms: 4 mg

Hospital/emergency department: I.M.:

Birth to <2 years: Mild-to-moderate symptoms: 0.05 mg/kg I.M. **or** 0.02 mg/kg I.V.; severe symptoms: 0.1 mg/kg I.M. **or** 0.02 mg/kg I.V.

2-10 years: Mild-to-moderate symptoms: 1 mg; severe symptoms: 2 mg

>10 years: Mild-to-moderate symptoms: 2 mg; severe symptoms: 4 mg

Note: Pralidoxime is a component of the management of nerve agent toxicity; consult Pralidoxime for specific route and dose. For prehospital ("in the field") management, repeat atropine I.M. (children: 0.05-0.1 mg/kg) at 5-10 minute intervals until secretions have diminished and breathing is comfortable or airway resistance has returned to near normal. For hospital management, repeat atropine I.M. (infants 1 mg; all others: 2 mg) at 5-10 minute intervals until secretions have diminished and breathing is comfortable or airway resistance has returned to near normal.

Children: Organophosphate or carbamate poisoning:

I.V.: 0.03-0.05 mg/kg every 10-20 minutes until atropine effect, then every 1-4 hours for at least 24 hours

I.M. (AtroPen®): Mild symptoms: Administer dose listed below as soon as exposure is known or suspected. If severe symptoms develop after first dose, 2 additional doses should be repeated in 10 minutes; do not administer more than 3 doses. Severe symptoms: Immediately administer 3 doses as follows:

<6.8 kg (15 lb): Use of **AtroPen® formulation not recommended;** administer atropine 0.05 mg/kg

6.8-18 kg (15-40 lb): 0.5 mg/dose

18-41 kg (40-90 lb): 1 mg/dose

>41 kg (>90 lb): 2 mg/dose

Adults (doses <0.5 mg have been associated with paradoxical bradycardia):

Asystole or pulseless electrical activity:

I.V.: 1 mg; repeat in 3-5 minutes if asystole persists; total dose of 0.04 mg/kg.

Intratracheal: Administer 2-2.5 times the recommended I.V. dose; dilute in 10 mL NS or distilled water. **Note:** Absorption is greater with distilled water, but causes more adverse effects on PaO_2.

Inhibit salivation and secretions (preanesthesia):

I.M., I.V., SubQ: 0.4-0.6 mg 30-60 minutes preop and repeat every 4-6 hours as needed

Oral: 0.4 mg; may repeat in 4 hours if necessary; 0.4 mg initial dose may be exceeded in certain cases and may repeat in 4 hours if necessary

Bradycardia: I.V.: 0.5-1 mg every 5 minutes, not to exceed a total of 3 mg or 0.04 mg/kg; may give intratracheally in 10 mL NS (intratracheal dose should be 2-2.5 times the I.V. dose)

Neuromuscular blockade reversal: I.V.: 25-30 mcg/kg 30-60 seconds before neostigmine or 7-10 mcg/kg 30-60 seconds before edrophonium

Organophosphate or carbamate poisoning: **Note:** The dose of atropine required varies considerably with the severity of poisoning. Total amount of atropine used in carbamate poisoning is usually less. Severely poisoned patients may exhibit significant tolerance to atropine; ≥2 times the suggested doses may be needed. Titrate to pulmonary status (decreased bronchial secretions). Once patient is stable for a period of time, the dose/dosing frequency may be decreased. If atropinization occurs after 1-2 mg of atropine then re-evaluate working diagnosis.

I.V.: Initial: 1-5 mg; doses should be doubled every 5 minutes until signs of muscarinic excess abate (clearing of bronchial secretions, bronchospasm, and adequate oxygenation). Overly aggressive dosing may cause anticholinergic toxicity (eg, delirium, hyperthermia, and muscle twitching).

I.V. Infusion: 0.5-1 mg/hour or 10% to 20% of loading dose/hour

I.M. (AtroPen®): Mild symptoms: Administer 2 mg as soon as exposure is known or suspected. If severe symptoms develop after first dose, 2 additional doses should be repeated in 10 minutes; do not administer more than 3 doses. Severe symptoms: Immediately administer three 2 mg doses.

Nerve agent toxicity management: I.M.: See **Note**. Prehospital ("in the field") or hospital/emergency department: Mild-to-moderate symptoms: 2-4 mg; severe symptoms: 6 mg

Note: Pralidoxime is a component of the management of nerve agent toxicity; consult Pralidoxime for specific route and dose. For prehospital ("in the field") management, repeat atropine I.M. (2 mg) at 5-10 minute intervals until secretions have diminished and breathing is comfortable or airway resistance has returned to near normal. For hospital management, repeat atropine I.M. (2 mg) at 5-10 minute intervals until secretions have diminished and breathing is comfortable or airway resistance has returned to near normal.

Mydriasis, cycloplegia (preprocedure): Ophthalmic (1% solution): Instill 1-2 drops 1 hour before procedure.

Uveitis: Ophthalmic:

1% solution: Instill 1-2 drops 4 times/day

Ointment: Apply a small amount in the conjunctival sac up to 3 times/day; compress the lacrimal sac by digital pressure for 1-3 minutes after instillation

Elderly, frail patients: Nerve agent toxicity management (unlabeled use): I.M.: See **Note** under adult dosing.

Prehospital ("in the field"): Mild-to-moderate symptoms: 1 mg; severe symptoms: 2-4 mg

Hospital/emergency department: Mild-to-moderate symptoms: 1 mg; severe symptoms: 2 mg

Administration

I.M.: AtroPen®: Administer to outer thigh. May be given through clothing as long as pockets at the injection site are empty. Hold autoinjector in place for 10 seconds following injection; massage the injection site.

I.V.: Administer undiluted by rapid I.V. injection; slow injection may result in paradoxical bradycardia.

Intratracheal: Dilute in NS or distilled water. Absorption is greater with distilled water, but causes more adverse effects on PaO_2. Pass catheter beyond tip of tracheal tube, stop compressions, spray drug quickly down tube. Follow immediately with several quick insufflations and continue chest compressions.

Monitoring Parameters Heart rate, blood pressure, pulse, mental status; intravenous administration requires a cardiac monitor

Dosage Forms Excipient information presented when available (limited, particularly for generics); consult specific product labeling.

Injection, solution, as sulfate: 0.05 mg/mL (5 mL); 0.1 mg/mL (5 mL, 10 mL); 0.4 mg/0.5 mL (0.5 mL); 0.4 mg/mL (0.5 mL, 1 mL, 20 mL); 1 mg/mL (1 mL)

AtroPen®: 0.25 mg/0.3 mL (0.3 mL); 0.5 mg/0.7 mL (0.7 mL); 1 mg/0.7 mL (0.7 mL); 2 mg/0.7 mL (0.7 mL) [prefilled autoinjector]

Ointment, ophthalmic, as sulfate: 1% (3.5 g)

Solution, ophthalmic, as sulfate: 1% (2 mL, 5 mL, 15 mL)

Atropine-Care®: 1% (2 mL) [contains benzalkonium chloride]

Isopto® Atropine: 1% (5 mL, 15 mL) [contains benzalkonium chloride]

Tablet, as sulfate:

Sal-Tropine™: 0.4 mg

◆ **Atropine and Difenoxin** *see* Difenoxin and Atropine *on page 443*

◆ **Atropine and Diphenoxylate** *see* Diphenoxylate and Atropine *on page 459*

Atropine and Pralidoxime

(A troe peen & pra li DOKS eem)

U.S. Brand Names ATNAA; Duodote™

Index Terms Atropine and Pralidoxime Chloride; Mark 1™; NAAK; Nerve Agent Antidote Kit; Pralidoxime and Atropine

Pharmacologic Category Anticholinergic Agent; Antidote

Use

ATNAA: Treatment of poisoning by susceptible organophosphorous nerve agents having anticholinesterase activity for self or buddy-administration by military personnel

Duodote™: Treatment of poisoning by organophosphorous nerve agents (eg, tabun, sarin, soman) or organophosphorous insecticide for use by trained emergency medical services personnel

Restrictions

ATNAA (**A**ntidote **T**reatment-**N**erve **A**gent **A**uto-Injector) is only available for use by U.S. Armed Forces military personnel. Information on distribution is available at Defense Services Supply Center-Philadelphia at https://dmmonline.dscp.dla.mil/pharm/nerve.asp.

Duodote™ is only available for use by trained emergency medical services personnel to treat civilians. Distribution is limited to directly from manufacturer (Meridian Medical Technologies, Inc.) to emergency medical service organizations or their suppliers.

Pregnancy Risk Factor C

Dosage I.M.: Adults: Organophosphorous poisoning: **Note:** If suspected, antidotal therapy should be given immediately as soon as symptoms appear (critical to administer immediately in case of soman exposure). Definitive medical care should be sought after any injection given. One injection only may be given as self-aid. If repeat injections needed, administration must be done by another trained individual. Emergency medical personnel who have self-administered a dose must determine capacity to continue to provide care.

ATNAA:

Mild symptoms (some or all mild symptoms): Self-Aid or Buddy-Aid: 1 injection (wait 10-15 minutes for effect); if patient is able to ambulate, and knows who and where they are, then no more injections are needed. If symptoms still present: Buddy-Aid: May repeat 1-2 more injections

Severe symptoms (if most or all): Buddy-Aid: If no self-aid given, 3 injections in rapid succession; if 1 self-aid injection given, 2 injections in rapid succession

Maximum cumulative dose: 3 injections

Symptoms provided by manufacturer in ATNAA product labeling to guide therapy:

Mild symptoms: Breathing difficulties, chest tightness, coughing, difficulty in seeing, drooling, headache, localized sweating and muscular twitching, miosis, nausea (with or without vomiting), runny nose, stomach cramps, tachycardia (followed by bradycardia), wheezing

Severe symptoms: Bradycardia, confused/strange behavior, convulsions, increased wheezing and breathing difficulties, involuntary urination/defecation, miosis (severe), muscular twitching/generalized weakness (severe), red/teary eyes, respiratory failure, unconsciousness, vomiting

Duodote™:

Mild symptoms (≥2 mild symptoms): 1 injection (wait 10-15 minutes for effect); if after 10-15 minutes no severe symptoms emerge, no further injections are indicated; if any severe symptoms emerge at any point following initial injection, repeat dose by giving 2 additional injections in rapid succession. Transport to medical care facility.

Severe symptoms (≥1 severe symptom): 3 injections in rapid succession. Transport to medical care facility.

Maximum cumulative dose: 3 injections unless medical care support (eg, hospital, respiratory support) is available

Symptoms provided by manufacturer in Duodote™ product labeling to guide therapy:

Mild symptoms: Airway secretions increased, blurred vision, bradycardia, breathing difficulties, chest tightness, drooling miosis, nausea, vomiting, runny nose, salivation, stomach cramps (acute onset), tachycardia, teary eyes, tremors/muscular twitching, wheezing/coughing

Severe symptoms: Breathing difficulties (severe), confused/strange behavior, convulsions, copious secretions from lung or airway, involuntary urination/defecation, muscular twitching/generalized weakness (severe)

Dosage adjustment in renal impairment: Use caution in renal impairment; pralidoxime is renally eliminated

Additional Information Complete prescribing information for this medication should be consulted for additional detail.

Dosage Forms Excipient information presented when available (limited, particularly for generics); consult specific product labeling.

Injection, solution:

ATNAA, Duodote™: Atropine 2.1 mg/0.7 mL and pralidoxime chloride 600 mg/2 mL [contains benzyl alcohol; prefilled autoinjector]

- ◆ **Atropine and Pralidoxime Chloride** *see* Atropine and Pralidoxime *on page 159*
- ◆ **Atropine-Care®** *see* Atropine *on page 157*
- ◆ **Atropine, Hyoscyamine, Scopolamine, and Phenobarbital** *see* Hyoscyamine, Atropine, Scopolamine, and Phenobarbital *on page 756*
- ◆ **Atropine Sulfate** *see* Atropine *on page 157*
- ◆ **Atropine Sulfate and Edrophonium Chloride** *see* Edrophonium and Atropine *on page 506*
- ◆ **Atrovent®** *see* Ipratropium *on page 811*
- ◆ **Atrovent® HFA** *see* Ipratropium *on page 811*
- ◆ **Attenuvax®** *see* Measles Virus Vaccine (Live) *on page 924*
- ◆ **Atuss® HX [DSC]** *see* Hydrocodone and Guaifenesin *on page 741*
- ◆ **Augmentin®** *see* Amoxicillin and Clavulanate Potassium *on page 100*
- ◆ **Augmentin ES-600®** *see* Amoxicillin and Clavulanate Potassium *on page 100*
- ◆ **Augmentin XR®** *see* Amoxicillin and Clavulanate Potassium *on page 100*
- ◆ **Auralgan® (Can)** *see* Antipyrine and Benzocaine *on page 124*

Auranofin (au RANE oh fin)

U.S. Brand Names Ridaura®

Canadian Brand Names Ridaura®

Pharmacologic Category Gold Compound

Use Management of active stage of classic or definite rheumatoid arthritis in patients who do not respond to or tolerate other agents; psoriatic arthritis; adjunctive or alternative therapy for pemphigus

Pregnancy Risk Factor C

Medication Safety Issues

Sound-alike/look-alike issues:

Ridaura® may be confused with Cardura®

Dosage Oral:

Children: Initial: 0.1 mg/kg/day divided daily; usual maintenance: 0.15 mg/kg/day in 1-2 divided doses; maximum: 0.2 mg/kg/day in 1-2 divided doses

Adults: 6 mg/day in 1-2 divided doses; after 3 months may be increased to 9 mg/day in 3 divided doses; if still no response after 3 months at 9 mg/day, discontinue drug

Dosing adjustment in renal impairment:

Cl_{cr} 50-80 mL/minute: Reduce dose to 50%.

Cl_{cr} <50 mL/minute: Avoid use

Additional Information Complete prescribing information for this medication should be consulted for additional detail.

Dosage Forms Excipient information presented when available (limited, particularly for generics); consult specific product labeling.

Capsule:

Ridaura®: 3 mg [29% gold]

- ◆ **Auraphene® B [OTC]** *see* Carbamide Peroxide *on page 254*
- ◆ **Auro® [OTC]** *see* Carbamide Peroxide *on page 254*
- ◆ **Aurodex** *see* Antipyrine and Benzocaine *on page 124*
- ◆ **Autoplex® T [DSC]** *see* Anti-inhibitor Coagulant Complex *on page 123*
- ◆ **AVA** *see* Anthrax Vaccine Adsorbed *on page 118*
- ◆ **Avagard™ [OTC]** *see* Chlorhexidine Gluconate *on page 305*
- ◆ **Avage™** *see* Tazarotene *on page 1427*
- ◆ **Avalide®** *see* Irbesartan and Hydrochlorothiazide *on page 814*
- ◆ **Avamys™ (Can)** *see* Fluticasone *on page 644*
- ◆ **Avandamet®** *see* Rosiglitazone and Metformin *on page 1343*
- ◆ **Avandaryl®** *see* Rosiglitazone and Glimepiride *on page 1342*
- ◆ **Avandia®** *see* Rosiglitazone *on page 1340*
- ◆ **Avapro®** *see* Irbesartan *on page 813*
- ◆ **Avapro® HCT** *see* Irbesartan and Hydrochlorothiazide *on page 814*
- ◆ **AVAR™ [DSC]** *see* Sulfur and Sulfacetamide *on page 1411*
- ◆ **AVAR™-e** *see* Sulfur and Sulfacetamide *on page 1411*
- ◆ **AVAR™-e Green [DSC]** *see* Sulfur and Sulfacetamide *on page 1411*
- ◆ **Avastin®** *see* Bevacizumab *on page 193*
- ◆ **Avaxim® (Can)** *see* Hepatitis A Vaccine *on page 726*
- ◆ **Avaxim®-Pediatric (Can)** *see* Hepatitis A Vaccine *on page 726*
- ◆ **Avelox®** *see* Moxifloxacin *on page 1021*
- ◆ **Avelox® I.V.** *see* Moxifloxacin *on page 1021*
- ◆ **Aventyl® (Can)** *see* Nortriptyline *on page 1081*
- ◆ **Aviane™** *see* Ethinyl Estradiol and Levonorgestrel *on page 577*
- ◆ **Aviane® (Can)** *see* Ethinyl Estradiol and Levonorgestrel *on page 577*
- ◆ **Avian Influenza Virus Vaccine** *see* Influenza Virus Vaccine (H5N1) *on page 791*
- ◆ **Avinza®** *see* Morphine Sulfate *on page 1016*
- ◆ **Avita®** *see* Tretinoin (Topical) *on page 1509*
- ◆ **Avitene®** *see* Collagen Hemostat *on page 367*
- ◆ **Avitene® Flour** *see* Collagen Hemostat *on page 367*
- ◆ **Avitene® Ultrafoam** *see* Collagen Hemostat *on page 367*
- ◆ **Avitene® UltraWrap™** *see* Collagen Hemostat *on page 367*
- ◆ **Avodart®** *see* Dutasteride *on page 500*
- ◆ **Avonex®** *see* Interferon Beta-1a *on page 806*

◆ **Axert™** *see* Almotriptan *on page 67*
◆ **Axid®** *see* Nizatidine *on page 1076*
◆ **Axid® AR [OTC]** *see* Nizatidine *on page 1076*
◆ **AY-25650** *see* Triptorelin *on page 1523*
◆ **Aygestin®** *see* Norethindrone *on page 1078*
◆ **Ayr® Allergy Sinus [OTC]** *see* Sodium Chloride *on page 1381*
◆ **Ayr® Baby Saline [OTC]** *see* Sodium Chloride *on page 1381*
◆ **Ayr® Saline [OTC]** *see* Sodium Chloride *on page 1381*
◆ **Ayr® Saline No-Drip [OTC]** *see* Sodium Chloride *on page 1381*
◆ **5-Aza-2'-deoxycytidine** *see* Decitabine *on page 409*
◆ **5-AzaC** *see* Decitabine *on page 409*

AzaCITIDine (ay za SYE ti deen)

U.S. Brand Names Vidaza®

Index Terms 5-Azacytidine; 5-AZC; AZA-CR; Azacytidine; Ladakamycin; NSC-102816

Pharmacologic Category Antineoplastic Agent, DNA Methylation Inhibitor

Use Treatment of myelodysplastic syndrome (MDS)

Unlabeled/Investigational Use Treatment of acute myelogenous leukemia (AML)

Pregnancy Risk Factor D

Pregnancy Considerations Embryotoxicity, fetal death, and fetal abnormalities were observed in animal studies. There are no adequate and well-controlled studies in pregnant women. Women of childbearing potential should be advised to avoid pregnancy during treatment. In addition, males should be advised to avoid fathering a child while on azacitidine therapy.

Lactation Excretion in breast milk unknown/not recommended

Medication Safety Issues

Sound-alike/look-alike issues:

AzaCITIDine may be confused with azaTHIOprine

High alert medication: The Institute for Safe Medication Practices (ISMP) includes this medication among its list of drug classes which have a heightened risk of causing significant patient harm when used in error.

Contraindications Hypersensitivity to azacitidine, mannitol, or any component of the formulation; advanced malignant hepatic tumors

Warnings/Precautions Hazardous agent - use appropriate precautions for handling and disposal. Azacitidine may be hepatotoxic, use caution with hepatic impairment; use is contraindicated in patients with advanced malignant hepatic tumors. Progressive hepatic coma leading to death has been reported (rare) in patients with extensive tumor burden, especially those with a baseline albumin <30 g/L. Use caution with renal impairment; dose adjustment may be required. Serum creatinine elevations, renal tubular acidosis, and renal failure have been reported with combination chemotherapy; decrease or withhold dose for unexplained elevations in BUN or serum creatinine or reductions in serum bicarbonate to <20 mEq/L. Patients with renal and hepatic impairment were excluded from clinical studies. Neutropenia, thrombocytopenia, and anemia are common; may cause therapy delays and/or dosage reductions. Not FDA approved for use in children.

Adverse Reactions

>10%:

Cardiovascular: Peripheral edema (7% to 19%), chest pain (16%), pallor (16%), pitting edema (15%)

Central nervous system: Fever (30% to 52%), fatigue (13% to 36%), headache (22%), dizziness (19%), anxiety (5% to 13%), depression (12%), insomnia (9% to 11%), malaise (11%), pain (11%)

Dermatologic: Bruising (19% to 31%), petechiae (11% to 24%), erythema (7% to 17%), skin lesion (15%), rash (10% to 14%), pruritus (12%)

Endocrine & metabolic: Hypokalemia (6% to 13%)

Gastrointestinal: Nausea (48% to 71%), vomiting (27% to 54%), diarrhea (36%), constipation (34% to 50%), anorexia (13% to 21%), weight loss (16%), abdominal pain (11% to 16%), abdominal tenderness (12%)

Hematologic: Thrombocytopenia (66% to 70%; grades 3/4: 58%), anemia (51% to 70%; grades 3/4: 14%), neutropenia (32% to 66%; grades 3/4: 61%), leukopenia (18% to 48%; grades 3/4: 15%), febrile neutropenia (14% to 16%; grades 3/4: 13%), myelosuppression (nadir: days 10-17; recovery: days 28-31)

Local: Injection site reactions (14% to 29%): Erythema (35% to 43%; more common with I.V. administration), pain (19% to 23%; more common with I.V. administration), bruising (5% to 14%)

Neuromuscular & skeletal: Weakness (29%), rigors (26%), arthralgia (22%), limb pain (20%), back pain (19%), myalgia (16%)

Respiratory: Cough (11% to 30%), dyspnea (5% to 29%), pharyngitis (20%), epistaxis (16%), nasopharyngitis (15%), upper respiratory tract infection (9% to 13%), pneumonia (11%), crackles (11%)

Miscellaneous: Diaphoresis (11%)

5% to 10%:

Cardiovascular: Cardiac murmur (10%), hypertension (≤9%), tachycardia (9%), hypotension (7%), syncope (6%), chest wall pain (5%)

Central nervous system: Lethargy (7% to 8%), hypoesthesia (5%), postprocedural pain (5%)

Dermatologic: Cellulitis (8%), urticaria (6%), dry skin (5%), skin nodule (5%)

Gastrointestinal: Gingival bleeding (10%), oral mucosal petechiae (8%), stomatitis (8%), weight loss (≤8%), dyspepsia (6% to 7%), hemorrhoids (7%), abdominal distension (6%), loose stools (6%), dysphagia (5%), oral hemorrhage (5%), tongue ulceration (5%)

Genitourinary: Dysuria (8%), urinary tract infection (8% to 9%)

Hematologic: Hematoma (9%), postprocedural hemorrhage (6%)

Local: Injection site reactions: Pruritus (7%), hematoma (6%), rash (6%), granuloma (5%), induration (5%), pigmentation change (5%), swelling (5%)

Neuromuscular & skeletal: Muscle cramps (6%)

Renal: Hematuria (≤6%)

Respiratory: Rhinorrhea (10%), rales (9%), wheezing (9%), breath sounds decreased (8%), pharyngolaryngeal pain (6%), pleural effusion (6%), postnasal drip (6%), rhinitis (6%), rhonchi (6%), nasal congestion (6%), atelectasis (5%), sinusitis (5%)

Miscellaneous: Lymphadenopathy (10%), herpes simplex (9%), night sweats (9%), transfusion reaction (7%), mouth hemorrhage (5%)

<5% (Limited to important or life-threatening): Abscess (limb), agranulocytosis, anaphylactic shock, atrial fibrillation, azotemia, blastomycosis, bone marrow depression/failure, bone pain aggravated, cardiac failure, cardiorespiratory arrest, catheter site hemorrhage, cellulitis, cerebral hemorrhage, CHF, cholecystectomy, cholecystitis, congestive cardiomyopathy, dehydration, diverticulitis, eye hemorrhage, fibrosis (interstitial and alveolar), gastrointestinal hemorrhage, glycosuria, hemoptysis, hepatic coma, hypersensitivity reaction, hypophosphatemia, infection (bacterial), injection site infection, intracranial hemorrhage, leukemia cutis, lung infiltration, melena, neutropenic sepsis, orthostatic hypotension, pancytopenia, pneumonitis, polyuria, pyoderma gangrenosum, renal failure, renal tubular acidosis, seizure, respiratory distress, sepsis, septic shock, serum bicarbonate levels decreased, serum creatinine increased, splenomegaly,

systemic inflammatory response syndrome, toxoplasmosis

Drug Interactions

Avoid Concomitant Use

Avoid concomitant use of AzaCITIDine with any of the following: Natalizumab; Vaccines (Live)

Increased Effect/Toxicity

AzaCITIDine may increase the levels/effects of: Natalizumab; Vaccines (Live)

The levels/effects of AzaCITIDine may be increased by: Trastuzumab

Decreased Effect

AzaCITIDine may decrease the levels/effects of: Vaccines (Inactivated)

The levels/effects of AzaCITIDine may be decreased by: Echinacea

Stability Prior to reconstitution, store powder at room temperature of 25°C (77°F); excursions permitted to 15°C to 30°C (59°F to 86°F). Use appropriate precautions for handling and disposal.

SubQ: To prepare a 25 mg/mL suspension, slowly add 4 mL SWFI to each vial. Vigorously shake or roll vial until a suspension is formed (suspension will be cloudy). Following reconstitution, suspension may be stored at room temperature for up to 1 hour, or immediately refrigerated at 2°C to 8°C (36°F to 46°F) and stored for up to 8 hours.

I.V.: **Solutions for I.V. administration have very limited stability and must be prepared immediately prior to each dose.** Reconstitute vial with 10 mL SWFI to form a 10 mg/mL solution; vigorously shake until solution is dissolved and clear. Mix in 50-100 mL of NS or lactated Ringer's injection for infusion. Administration must be completed within 1 hour of (vial) reconstitution.

Mechanism of Action Antineoplastic effects may be a result of azacitidine's ability to promote hypomethylation of DNA leading to direct toxicity of abnormal hematopoietic cells in the bone marrow.

Pharmacodynamics/Kinetics

Absorption: SubQ: Rapid and complete

Distribution: V_d: I.V.: 76 ± 26 L; does not cross blood-brain barrier

Metabolism: Hepatic; hydrolysis to several metabolites

Bioavailability: SubQ: ~89%

Half-life elimination: I.V., SubQ: ~4 hours

Time to peak, plasma: SubQ: 30 minutes

Excretion: Urine (50% to 85%); feces (minor)

Dosage

Children: I.V.:

Pediatric AML and ANLL (unlabeled uses): 250 mg/m^2 days 4 and 5 every 4 weeks

Pediatric AML induction (unlabeled use): 300 mg/m^2 days 5 and 6

Adults:

MDS: I.V., SubQ: 75 mg/m^2/day for 7 days repeated every 4 weeks. Dose may be increased to 100 mg/m^2/day if no benefit is observed after 2 cycles and no toxicity other than nausea and vomiting have occurred. Treatment is recommended for at least 4 cycles; treatment may be continued as long as patient continues to benefit.

AML (unlabeled use): SubQ: 75 mg/m^2/day for 7 days repeated every 4 weeks (Sudan, 2006)

Elderly: Refer to adult dosing; due to the potential for decreased renal function in the elderly, select dose carefully and closely monitor renal function

Dosage adjustment based on hematology: Adults: MDS: I.V., SubQ:

For baseline WBC ≥3.0 x 10^9/L, ANC ≥1.5 x 10^9/L, and platelets ≥75 x 10^9/L:

Nadir count: ANC <0.5 x 10^9/L or platelets <25 x 10^9/L: Administer 50% of dose during next treatment course

Nadir count: ANC 0.5-1.5 x 10^9/L or platelets 25-50 x 10^9/L: Administer 67% of dose during next treatment course

Nadir count: ANC >1.5 x 10^9/L or platelets >50 x 10^9/L: Administer 100% of dose during next treatment course

For baseline WBC <3 x 10^9/L, ANC <1.5 x 10^9/L, or platelets <75 x 10^9/L: Adjust dose as follows based on nadir counts and bone marrow biopsy cellularity at the time of nadir, unless clear improvement in differentiation at the time of the next cycle:

WBC or platelet nadir decreased 50% to 75% from baseline and bone marrow biopsy cellularity at time of nadir 30% to 60%: Administer 100% of dose during next treatment course

WBC or platelet nadir decreased 50% to 75% from baseline and bone marrow biopsy cellularity at time of nadir 15% to 30%: Administer 50% of dose during next treatment course

WBC or platelet nadir decreased 50% to 75% from baseline and bone marrow biopsy cellularity at time of nadir <15%: Administer 33% of dose during next treatment course

WBC or platelet nadir decreased >75% from baseline and bone marrow biopsy cellularity at time of nadir 30% to 60%: Administer 75% of dose during next treatment course

WBC or platelet nadir decreased >75% from baseline and bone marrow biopsy cellularity at time of nadir 15% to 30%: Administer 50% of dose during next treatment course

WBC or platelet nadir decreased >75% from baseline and bone marrow biopsy cellularity at time of nadir <15%: Administer 33% of dose during next treatment course

Note: If a nadir defined above occurs, administer the next treatment course 28 days after the start of the preceding course as long as WBC and platelet counts are >25% above the nadir and rising. If a >25% increase above the nadir is not seen by day 28, reassess counts every 7 days. If a 25% increase is not seen by day 42, administer 50% of the scheduled dose.

Dosage adjustment based on serum electrolytes: The manufacturer recommends that if serum bicarbonate falls to <20 mEq/L (unexplained decrease): Reduce dose by 50% for next treatment course

Dosage adjustment based on renal toxicity: If increases in BUN or serum creatinine (unexplained) occur, delay next cycle until values reach baseline or normal, then reduce dose by 50% for next treatment course.

Dosage adjustment in renal impairment: Not studied in patients with renal impairment; select dose carefully (excretion is primarily renal; consider dose reduction); monitor closely for toxicity

Dosage adjustment in hepatic impairment: Not studied in patients with hepatic impairment; use caution. Contraindicated in patients with advanced malignant hepatic tumors.

Administration

SubQ: Premedication for nausea and vomiting is recommended. The manufacturer recommends equally dividing volumes >4 mL into 2 syringes and injecting into 2 separate sites; however, policies for maximum SubQ administration volume may vary by institution; interpatient variations may also apply. Administer subsequent injections at least 1 inch from previous injection sites. Allow refrigerated suspensions to come to room temperature (up to 30 minutes) prior to administration.

Resuspend by inverting the syringe 2-3 times and then rolling the syringe between the palms for 30 seconds. If azacitidine suspension comes in contact with the skin, immediately wash with soap and water.

I.V.: Premedication for nausea and vomiting is recommended. Infuse over 10-40 minutes; infusion must be completed within 1 hour of (vial) reconstitution.

Monitoring Parameters Liver function tests, electrolytes, CBC with differential and platelets, renal function tests (BUN and serum creatinine) should be obtained prior to initiation of therapy. Electrolytes, renal function (BUN and creatinine), CBC should be monitored prior to each cycle and periodically as needed to monitor response and toxicity.

Dosage Forms Excipient information presented when available (limited, particularly for generics); consult specific product labeling.

Injection, powder for suspension [preservative free]:
 Vidaza®: 100 mg [contains mannitol 100 mg]

◆ **AZA-CR** *see* AzaCITIDine *on page 161*
◆ **Azactam®** *see* Aztreonam *on page 169*
◆ **Azacytidine** *see* AzaCITIDine *on page 161*
◆ **5-Azacytidine** *see* AzaCITIDine *on page 161*
◆ **Azasan®** *see* AzaTHIOprine *on page 163*
◆ **AzaSite™** *see* Azithromycin *on page 166*

AzaTHIOprine (ay za THYE oh preen)

U.S. Brand Names Azasan®; Imuran®

Canadian Brand Names Alti-Azathioprine; Apo-Azathioprine®; Gen-Azathioprine; Imuran®; Novo-Azathioprine

Index Terms Azathioprine Sodium

Pharmacologic Category Immunosuppressant Agent

Use Adjunctive therapy in prevention of rejection of kidney transplants; management of active rheumatoid arthritis (RA)

Unlabeled/Investigational Use Adjunct in prevention of rejection of solid organ (nonrenal) transplants; steroid-sparing agent for corticosteroid-dependent Crohn's disease (CD) and ulcerative colitis (UC); maintenance of remission in CD; fistulizing Crohn's disease

Pregnancy Risk Factor D

Pregnancy Considerations Azathioprine was found to be teratogenic in animal studies; temporary depression in spermatogenesis and reduction in sperm viability and sperm count were also reported in mice. Azathioprine crosses the placenta in humans; congenital anomalies, immunosuppression, hematologic toxicities (lymphopenia, pancytopenia), and intrauterine growth retardation have been reported. There are no adequate and well-controlled studies in pregnant women. Azathioprine should not be used to treat arthritis during pregnancy. The potential benefit to the mother versus possible risk to the fetus should be considered when treating other disease states.

The National Transplantation Pregnancy Registry (NTPR, Temple University) is a registry for pregnant women taking immunosuppressants following any solid organ transplant. The NTPR encourages reporting of all immunosuppressant exposures during pregnancy in transplant recipients at 877-955-6877.

Lactation Enters breast milk/not recommended

Medication Safety Issues

Sound-alike/look-alike issues:

AzaTHIOprine may be confused with azaCITIDine, azatadine, azidothymidine, azithromycin, Azulfidine®

Imuran® may be confused with Elmiron®, Enduron®, Imdur®, Inderal®, Tenormin®

Azathioprine is metabolized to mercaptopurine; concurrent use of these commercially-available products has resulted in profound myelosuppression.

Contraindications Hypersensitivity to azathioprine or any component of the formulation; pregnancy (in patients with rheumatoid arthritis); patients with rheumatoid arthritis and a history of treatment with alkylating agents (eg, cyclophosphamide, chlorambucil, melphalan) may have a prohibitive risk of neoplasia with azathioprine treatment

Warnings/Precautions [U.S. Boxed Warning]: Chronic immunosuppression increases the risk of neoplasia and serious infections. Azathioprine has mutagenic potential to both men and women. Dose-related, delayed hematologic toxicities (leukopenia, thrombocytopenia, macrocytic anemia, pancytopenia) may occur; may be more severe with renal transplants undergoing rejection; dosage modification for hematologic toxicity may be necessary. Use with caution in patients with liver disease or renal impairment; monitor hematologic function closely. Azathioprine is metabolized to mercaptopurine; concomitant use may result in profound myelosuppression and should be avoided. Patients with genetic deficiency of thiopurine methyltransferase (TPMT) or concurrent therapy with drugs which may inhibit TPMT may be sensitive to myelosuppressive effects. Patients with intermediate TPMT activity may be at risk for increased myelosuppression; those with low or absent TPMT activity are at risk for developing severe myelotoxicity. TPMT genotyping or phenotyping may assist in identifying patients at risk for developing toxicity. TPMT testing does not substitute for CBC monitoring. Xanthine oxidase inhibitors may increase risk for hematologic toxicity; reduce azathioprine dose when used concurrently with allopurinol; patients with low or absent TPMT activity may require further dose reductions or discontinuation.

Hepatotoxicity (transaminase, bilirubin, and alkaline phosphatase elevations) may occur, usually in renal transplant patients and generally within 6 months of transplant; normally reversible with discontinuation; monitor liver function periodically. Rarely, hepatic veno-occlusive disease (VOD) has been reported; discontinue if hepatic VOD is suspected. Gastrointestinal toxicity may occur within the first several weeks of therapy and is reversible. Symptoms may include severe nausea, vomiting, diarrhea, rash, fever, malaise, myalgia, hypotension, and liver enzyme abnormalities. **[U.S. Boxed Warning]: Should be prescribed by physicians familiar with the risks, including hematologic toxicities and mutagenic potential.** Immune response to vaccines may be diminished. Hazardous agent - use appropriate precautions for handling and disposal.

Adverse Reactions Frequency not always defined; dependent upon dose, duration, indication, and concomitant therapy.

Central nervous system: Fever, malaise

Gastrointestinal: Nausea/vomiting (RA: 12%), diarrhea

Hematologic: Leukopenia (renal transplant: >50%; RA: 28%), thrombocytopenia

Hepatic: Alkaline phosphatase increased, bilirubin increased, hepatotoxicity, transaminases increased

Neuromuscular & skeletal: Myalgia

Miscellaneous: Infection (renal transplant: 20%; RA: <1%; includes bacterial, fungal, protozoal, viral); neoplasia (other than lymphoma: 3%)

<1%, postmarketing, and/or case reports: Abdominal pain, alopecia, arthralgia, bleeding, bone marrow suppression, fever, hepatic veno-occlusive disease, hepatosplenic T-cell lymphoma, hypersensitivity, hypotension, interstitial pneumonitis, lymphoma, macrocytic anemia, negative nitrogen balance, pancreatitis, pancytopenia, rash, steatorrhea

Drug Interactions

Avoid Concomitant Use

Avoid concomitant use of AzaTHIOprine with any of the following: Natalizumab; Vaccines (Live)

Increased Effect/Toxicity

AzaTHIOprine may increase the levels/effects of: Mercaptopurine; Natalizumab; Vaccines (Live)

The levels/effects of AzaTHIOprine may be increased by: 5-ASA Derivatives; ACE Inhibitors; Allopurinol; Sulfamethoxazole; Trastuzumab; Trimethoprim

Decreased Effect

AzaTHIOprine may decrease the levels/effects of: Vaccines (Inactivated); Vitamin K Antagonists

The levels/effects of AzaTHIOprine may be decreased by: Echinacea

Ethanol/Nutrition/Herb Interactions Herb/Nutraceutical: Avoid cat's claw, echinacea (have immunostimulant properties).

Stability

Tablet: Store at room temperature of 15°C to 25°C (59°F to 77°F); protect from light.

Powder for injection: Store intact vials at room temperature of 15°C to 25°C (59°F to 77°F). Protect from light. Reconstitute each vial with 10 mL sterile water for injection; may further dilute for infusion (in D_5W, 1/2NS, or NS). Reconstituted solution is stable for up to 2 weeks at room temperature or up to 4 days refrigerated; solutions diluted in D_5W, 1/2NS, or NS for infusion are stable at room temperature or refrigerated for up to 16 days; however, the manufacturer recommends use within 24 hours of reconstitution. Use appropriate precautions for handling and disposal.

Mechanism of Action Azathioprine is an imidazolyl derivative of mercaptopurine; antagonizes purine metabolism and may inhibit synthesis of DNA, RNA, and proteins; may also interfere with cellular metabolism and inhibit mitosis. The 6-thioguanine nucleotides appear to mediate the majority of azathioprine's immunosuppressive and toxic effects.

Pharmacodynamics/Kinetics

Absorption: Oral: Well absorbed

Distribution: Crosses placenta

Protein binding: ~30%

Metabolism: Hepatic, to 6-mercaptopurine (6-MP), possibly by glutathione S-transferase (GST). Further metabolism of 6-MP (in the liver and GI tract), via three major pathways: Hypoxanthine guanine phosphoribosyltransferase (to 6-thioguanine-nucleotides, or 6-TGN), xanthine oxidase (to 6-thiouric acid), and thiopurine methyltransferase (TPMT), which forms 6-methylmercapotpurine (6-MMP).

Half-life elimination: Parent drug: 12 minutes; mercaptopurine: 0.7-3 hours; End-stage renal disease: Slightly prolonged

Time to peak, plasma: 1-2 hours (including metabolites)

Excretion: Urine (primarily as metabolites)

Dosage Note: Patients with intermediate TPMT activity may be at risk for increased myelosuppression; those with low or absent TPMT activity receiving conventional azathioprine doses are at risk for developing severe, life-threatening myelotoxicity. Dosage reductions are recommended for patients with reduced TPMT activity.

I.V. dose is equivalent to oral dose (dosing should be transitioned from I.V. to oral as soon as tolerated):

Children (unlabeled) and Adults:

Renal transplantation (treatment usually started the day of transplant, however, has been initiated [rarely] 1-3 days prior to transplant): Oral, I.V.: Initial: 3-5 mg/kg/day usually given as a single daily dose, then 1-3 mg/kg/day maintenance

Rheumatoid arthritis: Oral:

Initial: 1 mg/kg/day given once daily or divided twice daily for 6-8 weeks; increase by 0.5 mg/kg every 4 weeks until response or up to 2.5 mg/kg/day; an adequate trial should be a minimum of 12 weeks

Maintenance dose: Reduce dose by 0.5 mg/kg every 4 weeks until lowest effective dose is reached; optimum duration of therapy not specified; may be discontinued abruptly

Adults: Oral:

Adjunctive management of severe recurrent aphthous stomatitis (unlabeled use): 50 mg once daily in conjunction with prednisone

Reduction of steroid use in CD or UC, maintenance of remission in CD or fistulizing disease (unlabeled uses): Initial: 50 mg once daily; may increase by 25 mg/day every 1-2 weeks as tolerated to target dose of 2-3 mg/kg/day

Dosage adjustment for concomitant use with allopurinol: Reduce azathioprine dose to one-third or one-fourth the usual dose when used concurrently with allopurinol. Patients with low or absent TPMT activity may require further dose reductions or discontinuation.

Dosage adjustment for toxicity:

Rapid WBC count decrease, persistently low WBC count, or serious infection: Reduce dose or temporarily withhold treatment

Severe toxicity in renal transplantation: May require discontinuation

Hepatic veno-occlusive disease: Permanently discontinue

Dosing adjustment in renal impairment: Although dosage reductions are recommended, specific guidelines are not available in the FDA-approved labeling; the following guidelines have been used by some clinicians (Aronoff, 2007):

Cl_{cr} >50 mL/minute: No adjustment recommended

Cl_{cr} 10-50 mL/minute: Administer 75% of normal dose

Cl_{cr} <10 mL/minute: Administer 50% of normal dose

Hemodialysis (dialyzable; ~45% removed in 8 hours): Children: Administer 50% of normal dose; Adults: Supplement: 0.25 mg/kg

CAPD: Children: Administer 50% of normal dose; Adults: Unknown

CRRT: Children and Adults: Administer 75% of normal dose

Dietary Considerations May be taken with food.

Administration

I.V.: Azathioprine can be administered IVP over 5 minutes at a concentration not to exceed 10 mg/mL **or** azathioprine can be further diluted with normal saline or D_5W and administered by intermittent infusion usually over 30-60 minutes; may be extended up to 8 hours.

Oral: Administering tablets after meals or in divided doses may decrease adverse GI events.

Monitoring Parameters CBC with differential and platelets (weekly during first month, twice monthly for months 2 and 3, then monthly; monitor more frequently with dosage modifications), total bilirubin, liver function tests, TPMT genotyping or phenotyping

For use as immunomodulatory therapy in CD or UC, monitor CBC with differential weekly for 1 month, then biweekly for 1 month, followed by monitoring every 1-2 months throughout the course of therapy. LFTs should be assessed every 3 months.

Test Interactions TPMT phenotyping results will not be accurate following recent blood transfusions.

Dosage Forms Excipient information presented when available (limited, particularly for generics); consult specific product labeling.

Injection, powder for reconstitution: 100 mg

Tablet [scored]: 50 mg

Azasan®: 75 mg, 100 mg

Imuran®: 50 mg

Extemporaneous Preparations A 50 mg/mL oral suspension can be prepared by crushing one hundred twenty (120) 50 mg tablets in a mortar (reducing to a fine powder), and then mixing in a small amount of vehicle (a 1:1 combination of Ora-Sweet® or Ora-Sweet® SF and Ora-Plus®) to create a uniform paste. Continue to add vehicle in geometric amounts (while mixing) until near-final volume is achieved. Transfer to a graduate and add sufficient quantity to make 120 mL. Label "shake well" and "refrigerate." Refrigerated stability is 60 days.

Allen LV Jr and Erickson MA III, "Stability of Acetazolamide, Allopurinol, Azathioprine, Clonazepam, and Flucytosine in Extemporaneously Compounded Oral Liquids," *Am J Health Syst Pharm*, 1996, 53 (16):1944-9.

Nahata MC, Morosco RS, and Hipple TF, 4th ed, *Pediatric Drug Formulations*, Cincinnati, OH: Harvey Whitney Books Co, 2000.

◆ **Azathioprine Sodium** *see* AzaTHIOprine *on page 163*

◆ **5-AZC** *see* AzaCITIDine *on page 161*

Azelaic Acid (a zeh LAY ik AS id)

U.S. Brand Names Azelex®; Finacea®

Canadian Brand Names Finacea®

Pharmacologic Category Topical Skin Product, Acne

Use Topical treatment of inflammatory papules and pustules of mild-to-moderate rosacea; mild-to-moderate inflammatory acne vulgaris

Finacea®: Not FDA-approved for the treatment of acne

Pregnancy Risk Factor B

Dosage Topical:

Adolescents ≥12 years and Adults: Acne vulgaris: Cream 20%: After skin is thoroughly washed and patted dry, gently but thoroughly massage a thin film of azelaic acid cream into the affected areas twice daily, in the morning and evening. The duration of use can vary and depends on the severity of the acne. In the majority of patients with inflammatory lesions, improvement of the condition occurs within 4 weeks.

Adults: Rosacea: Gel 15%: Massage gently into affected areas of the face twice daily; use beyond 12 weeks has not been studied

Additional Information Complete prescribing information for this medication should be consulted for additional detail.

Dosage Forms Excipient information presented when available (limited, particularly for generics); consult specific product labeling.

Cream:

Azelex®: 20% (30 g, 50 g) [contains benzoic acid and propylene glycol]

Gel:

Finacea®: 15% (50 g) [contains benzoic acid and propylene glycol]

Azelastine (a ZEL as teen)

U.S. Brand Names Astelin®; Astepro™; Optivar®

Canadian Brand Names Astelin®

Index Terms Azelastine Hydrochloride

Pharmacologic Category Histamine H_1 Antagonist; Histamine H_1 Antagonist, Second Generation

Use

Nasal spray: Treatment of the symptoms of seasonal allergic rhinitis such as rhinorrhea, sneezing, and nasal pruritus in children ≥5 years of age and adults; treatment of the symptoms of vasomotor rhinitis in children ≥12 years of age and adults

Ophthalmic: Treatment of itching of the eye associated with seasonal allergic conjunctivitis in children ≥3 years of age and adults

Pregnancy Risk Factor C

Pregnancy Considerations There are no adequate and well-controlled studies in pregnant women. Animal reproduction studies have shown toxic effects to the fetus at maternally toxic doses. Use during pregnancy only if the potential benefit to the mother outweighs the possible risk to the fetus.

Lactation Excretion in breast milk unknown/use caution

Medication Safety Issues

Sound-alike/look-alike issues:

Optivar® may be confused with Optiray®, Optive™

International issues:

Optivar® may be confused with Opthavir® which is a brand name for acyclovir in Mexico

Contraindications Hypersensitivity to azelastine or any component of the formulation

Warnings/Precautions

Nasal spray: May cause drowsiness in some patients; instruct patient to use caution when driving or operating machinery. Effects may be additive with CNS depressants and/or ethanol. Safety and efficacy in children <5 years of age have not been established.

Ophthalmic: Solution contains benzalkonium chloride; wait at least 10 minutes after instilling solution before inserting soft contact lenses. Do not use contact lenses if eyes are red. Safety and efficacy have not been established in children <3 years of age.

Adverse Reactions

Nasal spray:

>10%:

Central nervous system: Headache (8% to 15%), somnolence (<1% to 12%)

Gastrointestinal: Bitter taste (8% to 20%)

Respiratory: Cold symptoms/rhinitis (2% to 17%), cough (11%)

2% to 10%:

Central nervous system: Dysesthesia (8%), dizziness (2%), fatigue (2%)

Gastrointestinal: Nausea (3%), weight gain (2%), xerostomia (3%)

Neuromuscular & skeletal: Myalgia (≤2%)

Ocular: Conjunctivitis (<2% to 5%)

Respiratory: Asthma (5%), nasal burning (4%), pharyngitis (4%), paroxysmal sneezing (3%), sinusitis (3%), epistaxis (2% to 3%)

<2%:

Cardiovascular: Flushing, hypertension, tachycardia

Central nervous system: Abnormal thinking, anxiety, depersonalization, depression, drowsiness, fever, hypoesthesia, malaise, nervousness, sleep disorder, vertigo

Dermatologic: Contact dermatitis, eczema, furunculosis, hair and follicle infection, skin laceration

Endocrine & metabolic: Amenorrhea, breast pain

Gastrointestinal: Abdominal pain, aphthous stomatitis, appetite increased, constipation, diarrhea, gastroenteritis, glossitis, loss of taste, ulcerative stomatitis, toothache, vomiting

Genitourinary: Albuminuria, hematuria, polyuria

Hepatic: ALT increased

Neuromuscular & skeletal: Back pain, extremity pain, hyperkinesia, rheumatoid arthritis, temporomandibular dislocation

Ocular: Eye pain, watery eyes

Respiratory: Bronchitis, bronchospasm, laryngitis, nasal congestion, nocturnal dyspnea, postnasal drip, sinus hypersecretion, throat burning

Miscellaneous: Allergic reactions, viral infection

<1% (Limited to important or life-threatening): Anaphylactoid reaction, atrial fibrillation, chest pain, confusion, dyspnea, facial edema, involuntary muscle contractions, loss of smell, palpitation, paresthesia, parosmia, pruritus, rash, skin irritation, tolerance, transaminases increased, urinary retention, visual abnormalities, xerophthalmia

Ophthalmic:

>10%:

Central nervous system: Headache (15%)

Ocular: Transient burning/stinging (30%)

1% to 10%:

Central nervous system: Fatigue

Dermatologic: Pruritus

Gastrointestinal: Bitter taste (10%)

Ocular: Conjunctivitis, eye pain, blurred vision (temporary)

Respiratory: Asthma, dyspnea, pharyngitis, rhinitis

Miscellaneous: Flu-like syndrome

Drug Interactions

Metabolism/Transport Effects Substrate (minor) of CYP1A2, 2C19, 2D6, 3A4; **Inhibits** CYP2B6 (weak), 2C9 (weak), 2C19 (weak), 2D6 (weak), 3A4 (weak)

Avoid Concomitant Use There are no known interactions where it is recommended to avoid concomitant use.

Increased Effect/Toxicity

Azelastine may increase the levels/effects of: Alcohol (Ethyl); Anticholinergics; CNS Depressants

The levels/effects of Azelastine may be increased by: Pramlintide

Decreased Effect

Azelastine may decrease the levels/effects of: Acetylcholinesterase Inhibitors (Central); Betahistine

The levels/effects of Azelastine may be decreased by: Acetylcholinesterase Inhibitors (Central); Amphetamines

Ethanol/Nutrition/Herb Interactions Ethanol: Avoid ethanol (may cause increased somnolence or fatigue).

Stability

Nasal spray: Store upright at controlled room temperature of 20°C to 25°C (68°F to 77°F). Protect from freezing.

Ophthalmic solution: Store upright at controlled room temperature of 2°C to 25°C (36°F to 77°F).

Mechanism of Action Competes with histamine for H_1-receptor sites on effector cells and inhibits the release of histamine and other mediators involved in the allergic response; when used intranasally, reduces hyper-reactivity of the airways; increases the motility of bronchial epithelial cilia, improving mucociliary transport

Pharmacodynamics/Kinetics

Onset of action: Peak effect: Nasal spray: 3 hours; Ophthalmic solution: 3 minutes

Duration: Nasal spray: 12 hours; Ophthalmic solution: 8 hours

Distribution: V_d: 14.5 L/kg

Protein binding: Azelastine: 88%; Desmethylazelastine: 97%

Metabolism: Hepatic via CYP; active metabolite, desmethylazelastine

Bioavailability: Intranasal: 40%

Half-life elimination: 22 hours

Time to peak, serum: 2-3 hours

Excretion: Feces (75 %, <10% as unchanged drug)

Dosage

Children 5-11 years: Seasonal allergic rhinitis: Intranasal: 1 spray each nostril twice daily

Children ≥3 years and Adults: Itching eyes due to seasonal allergic conjunctivitis: Ophthalmic: Instill 1 drop into affected eye(s) twice daily

Children ≥12 years and Adults:

Seasonal allergic rhinitis: Intranasal: 1-2 sprays each nostril twice daily

Vasomotor rhinitis: Intranasal: 2 sprays each nostril twice daily.

Administration Intranasal: Before initial use of the nasal spray, the delivery system should be primed with 4 sprays or until a fine mist appears. If 3 or more days have elapsed since last use, the delivery system should be reprimed with 2 sprays or until a fine mist appears. Blow nose to clear nostrils. Keep head tilted downward when spraying. Insert applicator into nostril, keeping bottle upright, and close off the other nostril. Breathe in through nose. While inhaling, press pump to release spray. Alternate sprays between nostrils. After each use, wipe the spray tip with a clean tissue or cloth.

Dosage Forms Excipient information presented when available (limited, particularly for generics); consult specific product labeling.

Solution, intranasal, as hydrochloride [spray]:

Astelin®, Astepro™: 1 mg/mL (30 mL) [contains benzalkonium chloride; 137 mcg/spray; 200 metered sprays]

Solution, ophthalmic, as hydrochloride:

Optivar®: 0.05% (6 mL) [contains benzalkonium chloride]

◆ **Azelastine Hydrochloride** *see* Azelastine *on page* 165

◆ **Azelex®** *see* Azelaic Acid *on page* 165

◆ **Azidothymidine** *see* Zidovudine *on page* 1581

◆ **Azidothymidine, Abacavir, and Lamivudine** *see* Abacavir, Lamivudine, and Zidovudine *on page* 19

◆ **Azilect®** *see* Rasagiline *on page* 1298

Azithromycin (az ith roe MYE sin)

U.S. Brand Names AzaSite™; Zithromax®; Zmax®

Canadian Brand Names Apo-Azithromycin®; CO Azithromycin; Dom-Azithromycin; GMD-Azithromycin; Novo-Azithromycin; PHL-Azithromycin; PMS-Azithromycin; ratio-Azithromycin; Sandoz-Azithromycin; Zithromax®

Index Terms Azithromycin Dihydrate; Azithromycin Hydrogencitrate; Azithromycin Monohydrate; Zithromax® TRI-PAK™; Zithromax® Z-PAK®

Pharmacologic Category Antibiotic, Macrolide; Antibiotic, Ophthalmic

Additional Appendix Information

Antimicrobial Drugs of Choice *on page* 1752

Community-Acquired Pneumonia in Adults *on page* 1766

Guidelines for the Prevention of Opportunistic Infections in HIV Infected Persons *on page* 1740

Prevention of Infective Endocarditis *on page* 1736

Treatment of Sexually Transmitted Infections *on page* 1773

Use

Oral, I.V.: Treatment of acute otitis media due to *H. influenzae*, *M. catarrhalis*, or *S. pneumoniae*; pharyngitis/tonsillitis due to *S. pyogenes*; treatment of mild-to-moderate upper and lower respiratory tract infections, infections of the skin and skin structure, community-acquired pneumonia, pelvic inflammatory disease (PID), sexually-transmitted diseases (urethritis/cervicitis), pharyngitis/tonsillitis (alternative to first-line therapy), and genital ulcer disease (chancroid) due to susceptible strains of *Chlamydophila pneumoniae, C. trachomatis, M. catarrhalis, H. influenzae, S. aureus, S. pneumoniae, Mycoplasma pneumoniae*, and *C. psittaci*; acute bacterial exacerbations of chronic obstructive pulmonary disease (COPD) due to *H. influenzae, M. catarrhalis,* or *S. pneumoniae*; acute bacterial sinusitis

Ophthalmic: Bacterial conjunctivitis

Unlabeled/Investigational Use Prevention of (or to delay onset of) or treatment of MAC in patients with advanced HIV infection; prophylaxis of infective endocarditis in patients who are allergic to penicillin and undergoing surgical or dental procedures; pertussis

Pregnancy Risk Factor B

Pregnancy Considerations Adverse events were not observed in animal studies; therefore, azithromycin is classified as pregnancy category B. Low levels of azithromycin have been shown to cross the placenta. Azithromycin may be used for the treatment of some infections during pregnancy. The CDC and IDSA provide recommendations for the treatment of chlamydial infections and MAC in pregnant patients. Since serum concentrations determine fetal exposure and azithromycin has much higher concentrations in tissue than serum, treatment results in the mother may be obtained with lower exposure to the fetus. Although no adverse reports in human or animal fetuses have been documented, information in pregnant women is limited.

Lactation Enters breast milk/use caution

Medication Safety Issues

Sound-alike/look-alike issues:

Azithromycin may be confused with azathioprine, erythromycin

Zithromax® may be confused with Zinacef®, Zovirax®

Contraindications Hypersensitivity to azithromycin, other macrolide (eg, azalide or ketolide) antibiotics, or any component of the formulation

Warnings/Precautions Use with caution in patients with pre-existing liver disease; hepatic impairment, including hepatocellular and/or cholestatic hepatitis, with or without jaundice, has been observed. Discontinue if symptoms of malaise, nausea, vomiting, abdominal colic, and fever. Allergic reactions have been reported (rare); reappearance of allergic reaction may occur without further azithromycin exposure. May mask or delay symptoms of incubating gonorrhea or syphilis, so appropriate culture and susceptibility tests should be performed prior to initiating azithromycin. Prolonged use may result in fungal or bacterial superinfection, including *C. difficile*-associated diarrhea (CDAD) and pseudomembranous colitis; CDAD has been observed >2 months postantibiotic treatment. Use caution with renal dysfunction. Prolongation of the QT_c interval has been reported with macrolide antibiotics; use caution in patients at risk of prolonged cardiac repolarization. Use with caution in patients with myasthenia gravis. Safety and efficacy of systemically-administered azithromycin (oral, intravenous) have not been established in children <6 months of age with acute otitis media, acute bacterial sinusitis, or community-acquired pneumonia, or in children <2 years of age with pharyngitis/tonsillitis.

Ophthalmic solution should not be injected subconjunctivally or introduced directly into the anterior chamber of the eye. Ophthalmic solution contains benzalkonium chloride which may be absorbed by contact lenses; contact lens should not be worn during treatment of ophthalmic infections. Safety and efficacy for ophthalmic use have not been established in children <1 year of age.

Oral suspensions (immediate release and extended release) are not interchangeable.

Adverse Reactions

>10%: Gastrointestinal: Diarrhea (4% to 9%; high single-dose regimens 12% to 14%), nausea (≤7%; high single-dose regimens 18%)

2% to 10%:

Dermatologic: Pruritus, rash

Gastrointestinal: Abdominal pain, anorexia, cramping, vomiting (especially with high single-dose regimens)

Genitourinary: Vaginitis

Local: (with I.V. administration): Injection site pain, inflammation

Ocular (with ophthalmic solution use): Eye irritation (1% to 2%)

≤1% (Limited to important or life-threatening): Systemic therapy: Agitation, allergic reaction, anemia, angioedema, bronchospasm, candidiasis, chest pain, cholestatic jaundice, conjunctivitis, constipation, cough increased, dermatitis (fungal), diaphoresis, dizziness, dyspepsia, eczema, enteritis, facial edema, fatigue, fever, flatulence, fungal infection, gastritis, headache, hyperkinesia, insomnia, jaundice, leukopenia, malaise, melena, mucositis, nephritis, nervousness, oral moniliasis, pain, palpitation, pharyngitis, photosensitivity, pleural effusion, rhinitis, somnolence, taste perversion, urticaria, vertigo, vesiculobullous rash, weakness

1%: Ophthalmic solution: Contact dermatitis, corneal erosion, dysgeusia, nasal congestion, ocular discharge, ocular dryness; ocular stinging, burning, and irritation upon instillation; punctate keratitis, sinusitis

Postmarketing and/or case reports (all formulations): Acute renal failure, aggressive behavior, anaphylaxis, anxiety, arrhythmia (including ventricular tachycardia), arthralgia, deafness, dehydration, edema, erythema multiforme (rare), hearing disturbance, hearing loss, hepatic failure (rare), hepatic necrosis (rare), hepatitis, hyperactivity, hypertrophic pyloric stenosis, hypotension, interstitial nephritis, loss of smell, loss of taste, LFTs increased, neutropenia (mild), oral candidiasis, pancreatitis, paresthesia, pseudomembranous colitis, QT_c prolongation (rare), seizure, smell perversion, somnolence, Stevens-Johnson syndrome (rare), syncope, thrombocytopenia, tinnitus, tongue discoloration (rare), torsade de pointes (rare), toxic epidermal necrolysis (rare)

Drug Interactions

Metabolism/Transport Effects **Substrate** of CYP3A4 (minor); **Inhibits** CYP3A4 (weak)

Avoid Concomitant Use There are no known interactions where it is recommended to avoid concomitant use.

Increased Effect/Toxicity

Azithromycin may increase the levels/effects of: Amiodarone; Cardiac Glycosides; CycloSPORINE; Tacrolimus; Vitamin K Antagonists

The levels/effects of Azithromycin may be increased by: Nelfinavir

Decreased Effect

Azithromycin may decrease the levels/effects of: Typhoid Vaccine

Ethanol/Nutrition/Herb Interactions Food: Rate and extent of GI absorption may be altered depending upon the formulation. Azithromycin suspension, not tablet form, has significantly increased absorption (46%) with food.

Stability

Injection (Zithromax®): Store intact vials of injection at room temperature. Reconstitute the 500 mg vial with 4.8 mL of sterile water for injection and shake until all of the drug is dissolved. Each mL contains 100 mg azithromycin. Reconstituted solution is stable for 24 hours when stored below 30°C (86°F). Use of a standard syringe is recommended due to the vacuum in the vial (which may draw additional solution through an automated syringe).

The initial solution should be further diluted to a concentration of 1 mg/mL (500 mL) to 2 mg/mL (250 mL) in 0.9% sodium chloride, 5% dextrose in water, or lactated Ringer's. The diluted solution is stable for 24 hours at or below room temperature (30°C or 86°F) and for 7 days if stored under refrigeration (5°C or 41°F).

Ophthalmic solution: Prior to use, store unopened under refrigeration at 2°C to 8°C (36°F to 46°F). After opening, store at 2°C to 25°C (36°F to 77°F) for ≤14 days; discard any remaining solution after 14 days.

Suspension, immediate release (Zithromax®): Store dry powder below 30°C (86°F). Following reconstitution, store at 5°C to 30°C (41°F to 86°F).

Suspension, extended release (Zmax®): Store dry powder ≤30°C (86°F). Following reconstitution, store at 25°C (77°F); excursions permitted to 15°C to 30°C (59°F to 86°F); do not refrigerate freeze. Should be consumed within 12 hours following reconstitution.

Tablet (Zithromax®): Store between 15°C to 30°C (59°F to 86°F).

Mechanism of Action Inhibits RNA-dependent protein synthesis at the chain elongation step; binds to the 50S ribosomal subunit resulting in blockage of transpeptidation

Pharmacodynamics/Kinetics

Absorption: Oral: Rapid; Ophthalmic: Negligible

Distribution: Extensive tissue; distributes well into skin, lungs, sputum, tonsils, and cervix; penetration into CSF is poor; I.V.: 33.3 L/kg; Oral: 31.1 L/kg

Protein binding (concentration dependent): Oral, I.V.: 7% to 51%

Metabolism: Hepatic

Bioavailability: Oral: 38%, decreased by 17% with extended release suspension; variable effect with food (increased with immediate or delayed release oral suspension, unchanged with tablet)

Half-life elimination: Oral, I.V.: Terminal: Immediate release: 68-72 hours; Extended release: 59 hours

Time to peak, serum: Oral: Immediate release: 2-3 hours; Extended release: 5 hours

Excretion: Oral, I.V.: Biliary (major route); urine (6%)

Dosage Note: Extended release suspension (Zmax®) is not interchangeable with immediate release formulations. Use should be limited to approved indications. All doses are expressed as immediate release azithromycin unless otherwise specified.

Usual dosage range:

Children ≥6 months: Oral: 5-12 mg/kg given once daily (maximum: 500 mg/day) **or** 30 mg/kg as a single dose (maximum: 1500 mg)

Extended release suspension (Zmax®): 60 mg/kg as a single dose; **Note:** Extended release suspension (Zmax®): Dose in mL is equal to the weight in lbs for patients <75 lbs (34 kg). Pediatric patients ≥75 lbs should receive the adult dose.

Children ≥1 year and Adults: Ophthalmic: Instill 1 drop into affected eye(s) twice daily (8-12 hours apart) for 2 days, then 1 drop once daily for 5 days

Adolescents ≥16 years and Adults:

Oral: 250-600 mg once daily **or** 1-2 g as a single dose

Extended release suspension (Zmax®): 2 g as a single dose

I.V.: 250-500 mg once daily

Indication-specific dosing:

Children: Oral:

Bacterial sinusitis: 10 mg/kg once daily for 3 days (maximum: 500 mg/day)

Cat scratch disease (unlabeled use): <45.5 kg: 10 mg/kg as a single dose, then 5 mg/kg once daily for 4 days

Community-acquired pneumonia: 10 mg/kg on day 1 (maximum: 500 mg/day) followed by 5 mg/kg/day once daily on days 2-5 (maximum: 250 mg/day)

Extended release suspension (Zmax®):

<75 lbs (34 kg): 60 mg/kg as a single dose; dose in mL is equal to the weight in lbs for patients <75 lbs (34 kg)

≥75 lbs (34 kg): Refer to adult dose

Disseminated *M. avium* (unlabeled use):

HIV-infected patients: 5 mg/kg/day once daily (maximum: 250 mg/day) or 20 mg/kg (maximum: 1200 mg) once weekly given alone or in combination with rifabutin

Treatment and secondary prevention in HIV-negative patients: 5 mg/kg/day once daily (maximum: 250 mg/day) in combination with ethambutol, with or without rifabutin

Prophylaxis against infective endocarditis (unlabeled use): 15 mg/kg 30-60 minutes before procedure (maximum: 500 mg). **Note:** American Heart Association (AHA) guidelines now recommend prophylaxis only in patients undergoing invasive procedures and in whom underlying cardiac conditions may predispose to a higher risk of adverse outcomes should infection occur. As of April 2007, routine prophylaxis for GI/GU procedures is no longer recommended by the AHA.

Otitis media:

1-day regimen: 30 mg/kg as a single dose (maximum: 1500 mg)

3-day regimen: 10 mg/kg once daily for 3 days (maximum: 500 mg/day)

5-day regimen: 10 mg/kg on day 1 (maximum: 500 mg/day) followed by 5 mg/kg/day once daily on days 2-5 (maximum: 250 mg/day)

Pharyngitis, tonsillitis: Children ≥2 years: 12 mg/kg/day once daily for 5 days (maximum: 500 mg/day)

Pertussis (CDC guidelines):

Children <6 months: 10 mg/kg/day for 5 days

Children ≥6 months: 10 mg/kg on day 1 (maximum: 500 mg/day) followed by 5 mg/kg/day once daily on days 2-5 (maximum: 250 mg/day)

Uncomplicated chlamydial urethritis or cervicitis (unlabeled use): Children ≥45 kg: 1 g as a single dose

Children ≥1 year and Adults: Ophthalmic:

Bacterial conjunctivitis: Instill 1 drop into affected eye(s) twice daily (8-12 hours apart) for 2 days, then 1 drop once daily for 5 days

Adolescents ≥16 years and Adults:

Bacterial sinusitis: Oral: 500 mg/day for a total of 3 days

Extended release suspension (Zmax®): 2 g as a single dose

Cat scratch disease (unlabeled use): Oral: >45.5 kg: 500 mg as a single dose, then 250 mg once daily for 4 days

Chancroid due to *H. ducreyi*: Oral: 1 g as a single dose

Community-acquired pneumonia:

Oral: Extended release suspension (Zmax®): 2 g as a single dose

I.V.: 500 mg as a single dose for at least 2 days, follow I.V. therapy by the oral route with a single daily dose of 500 mg to complete a 7- to 10-day course of therapy.

Disseminated *M. avium* complex disease in patients with advanced HIV infection (unlabeled use): Oral:

Prophylaxis: 1200 mg once weekly (may be combined with rifabutin)

Treatment: 600 mg daily (in combination with ethambutol 15 mg/kg)

Prophylaxis against infective endocarditis (unlabeled use): Oral: 500 mg 30-60 minutes prior to the procedure. **Note:** American Heart Association (AHA) guidelines now recommend prophylaxis only in patients undergoing invasive procedures and in whom underlying cardiac conditions may predispose to a higher risk of adverse outcomes should infection occur. As of April 2007, routine prophylaxis for GI/GU procedures is no longer recommended by the AHA.

Mild-to-moderate respiratory tract, skin, and soft tissue infections: Oral: 500 mg in a single loading dose on day 1 followed by 250 mg/day as a single dose on days 2-5

Alternative regimen: Bacterial exacerbation of COPD: 500 mg/day for a total of 3 days

Pelvic inflammatory disease (PID): I.V.: 500 mg as a single dose for 1-2 days, follow I.V. therapy by the oral route with a single daily dose of 250 mg to complete a 7-day course of therapy

Pertussis (CDC guidelines): Oral: 500 mg on day 1 followed by 250 mg/day on days 2-5 (maximum: 500 mg/day)

Urethritis/cervicitis: Oral:
Due to C. trachomatis: 1 g as a single dose
Due to N. gonorrhoeae: 2 g as a single dose

Dosage adjustment in renal impairment: Use caution in patients with GFR <10 mL/minute

Dosage adjustment in hepatic impairment: Use with caution due to potential for hepatotoxicity (rare). Specific guidelines for dosing in hepatic impairment have not been established.

Dietary Considerations
Oral suspension, immediate release, may be administered with or without food.
Oral suspension, extended release, should be taken on an empty stomach (at least 1 hour before or 2 hours following a meal).
Tablet may be administered with food to decrease GI effects.
Sodium content:
Injection: 114 mg (4.96 mEq) per vial
Oral suspension, immediate release: 3.7 mg per 100 mg/5 mL of constituted suspension; 7.4 mg per 200 mg/5 mL of constituted suspension; 37 mg per 1 g single-dose packet
Oral suspension, extended release: 148 mg per 2 g constituted suspension
Tablet: 0.9 mg/250 mg tablet; 1.8 mg/500 mg tablet; 2.1 mg/600 mg tablet

Administration
I.V.: Infusate concentration and rate of infusion for azithromycin for injection should be either 1 mg/mL over 3 hours or 2 mg/mL over 1 hour. Other medications should not be infused simultaneously through the same I.V. line.
Ophthalmic: Shake bottle once prior to each administration. Wash hands before and after instillation.
Oral: Immediate release suspension and tablet may be taken without regard to food; extended release suspension should be taken on an empty stomach (at least 1 hour before or 2 hours following a meal), within 12 hours of reconstitution.

Monitoring Parameters Liver function tests, CBC with differential

Additional Information Zithromax® tablets and immediate release suspension may be interchanged (eg, two Zithromax® 250 mg tablets may be substituted for one Zithromax® 500 mg tablet or the tablets may be substituted with the immediate release suspension); however, the extended release suspension (Zmax®) is not bioequivalent with Zithromax® and therefore should not be interchanged.

Dosage Forms Excipient information presented when available (limited, particularly for generics); consult specific product labeling.
Note: Strength expressed as base
Injection, powder for reconstitution, as dihydrate: 500 mg
Zithromax®: 500 mg [contains sodium 114 mg (4.96 mEq) per vial]
Injection, powder for reconstitution, as hydrogencitrate: 500 mg
Injection, powder for reconstitution, as monohydrate: 500 mg
Microspheres for oral suspension, extended release, as dihydrate:
Zmax®: 2 g [60 mL single-dose bottle; contains sodium 148 mg per bottle; cherry/banana flavor]
Powder for oral suspension, as monohydrate: 100 mg/5 mL (15 mL); 200 mg/5 mL (15 mL, 22.5 mL, 30 mL)
Powder for oral suspension, immediate release, as dihydrate:
Zithromax®: 100 mg/5 mL (15 mL) [contains sodium 3.7 mg/ 5 mL; cherry creme de vanilla and banana flavor]; 200 mg/5 mL (15 mL, 22.5 mL, 30 mL) [contains sodium 7.4 mg/5 mL; cherry creme de vanilla and banana flavor]; 1 g/packet (3s, 10s) [single-dose packet; contains sodium 37 mg per packet; cherry creme de vanilla and banana flavor]
Solution, ophthalmic:
AzaSite™: 1% (2.5 mL) [contains benzalkonium chloride]
Tablet, as dihydrate:
Zithromax®: 250 mg [contains sodium 0.9 mg per tablet]; 500 mg [contains sodium 1.8 mg per tablet]; 600 mg [contains sodium 2.1 mg per tablet]
Zithromax® TRI-PAK™ [unit-dose pack]: 500 mg (3s) [contains sodium 1.8 mg per tablet]
Zithromax® Z-PAK® [unit-dose pack]: 250 mg (6s) [contains sodium 0.9 mg per tablet]
Tablet, as monohydrate: 250 mg, 500 mg, 600 mg

- **Azithromycin Dihydrate** *see* Azithromycin *on page 166*
- **Azithromycin Hydrogencitrate** *see* Azithromycin *on page 166*
- **Azithromycin Monohydrate** *see* Azithromycin *on page 166*
- **Azmacort®** *see* Triamcinolone *on page 1510*
- **AZO-Gesic® [OTC]** *see* Phenazopyridine *on page 1177*
- **Azopt®** *see* Brinzolamide *on page 213*
- **Azor™** *see* Amlodipine and Olmesartan *on page 95*
- **AZO-Standard® [OTC]** *see* Phenazopyridine *on page 1177*
- **AZO-Standard® Maximum Strength [OTC]** *see* Phenazopyridine *on page 1177*
- **AZT™ (Can)** *see* Zidovudine *on page 1581*
- **AZT + 3TC (error-prone abbreviation)** *see* Zidovudine and Lamivudine *on page 1583*
- **AZT, Abacavir, and Lamivudine** *see* Abacavir, Lamivudine, and Zidovudine *on page 19*
- **AZT (error-prone abbreviation)** *see* Zidovudine *on page 1581*
- **Azthreonam** *see* Aztreonam *on page 169*

Aztreonam (AZ tree oh nam)

U.S. Brand Names Azactam®
Canadian Brand Names Azactam®
Index Terms Azthreonam
Pharmacologic Category Antibiotic, Miscellaneous
Additional Appendix Information
Antimicrobial Drugs of Choice *on page 1752*
Community-Acquired Pneumonia in Adults *on page 1766*

Use Treatment of patients with urinary tract infections, lower respiratory tract infections, septicemia, skin/skin structure infections, intra-abdominal infections, and gynecological infections caused by susceptible gram-negative bacilli

Pregnancy Risk Factor B

Pregnancy Considerations Adverse events have not been observed in animal reproduction studies; therefore, the manufacturer classifies aztreonam as pregnancy category B. Aztreonam crosses the placenta and enters cord blood during middle and late pregnancy. Distribution to the fetus is minimal in early pregnancy. Aztreonam is used therapeutically in newborns.

Lactation Enters breast milk/not recommended (AAP rates "compatible")

Medication Safety Issues
Sound-alike/look-alike issues:
Aztreonam may be confused with azidothymidine

Contraindications Hypersensitivity to aztreonam or any component of the formulation

Warnings/Precautions Rare cross-allergenicity to penicillins and cephalosporins has been reported. Use caution in renal impairment; dosing adjustment required.

Prolonged use may result in fungal or bacterial superinfection, including *C. difficile*-associated diarrhea (CDAD) and pseudomembranous colitis; CDAD has been observed >2 months postantibiotic treatment.

Adverse Reactions As reported in adults:

1% to 10%:

Dermatologic: Rash

Gastrointestinal: Diarrhea, nausea, vomiting

Local: Thrombophlebitis, pain at injection site

<1% (Limited to important or life-threatening): Abdominal cramps, abnormal taste, anaphylaxis, anemia, angioedema, aphthous ulcer, breast tenderness, bronchospasm, *C. difficile*-associated diarrhea, chest pain, confusion, diaphoresis, diplopia, dizziness, dyspnea, eosinophilia, erythema multiforme, exfoliative dermatitis, fever, flushing, halitosis, headache, hepatitis, hypotension, insomnia, jaundice, leukopenia, liver enzymes increased, muscular aches myalgia, neutropenia, numb tongue, pancytopenia, paresthesia, petechiae, pruritus, pseudomembranous colitis, purpura, seizure, sneezing, thrombocytopenia, tinnitus, toxic epidermal necrolysis, urticaria, vaginitis, vertigo, weakness, wheezing

Drug Interactions

Avoid Concomitant Use There are no known interactions where it is recommended to avoid concomitant use.

Increased Effect/Toxicity There are no known significant interactions involving an increase in effect.

Decreased Effect

Aztreonam may decrease the levels/effects of: Typhoid Vaccine

Stability Prior to reconstitution, store at room temperature; avoid excessive heat. Reconstituted solutions are colorless to light yellow straw and may turn pink upon standing without affecting potency. Use reconstituted solutions and I.V. solutions (in NS and D_5W) within 48 hours if kept at room temperature (25°C) or 7 days under refrigeration (4°C).

I.M.: Reconstitute with at least 3 mL SWFI, sterile bacteriostatic water for injection, NS, or bacteriostatic sodium chloride.

I.V.:

Bolus injection: Reconstitute with 6-10 mL SWFI.

Infusion: Reconstitute to a final concentration ≤2%; the final concentration should not exceed 20 mg/mL. Solution for infusion may be frozen at less than -2°C (less than -4°F) for up to 3 months. Thawed solution should be used within 24 hours if thawed at room temperature or within 72 hours if thawed under refrigeration. **Do not refreeze.**

Mechanism of Action Inhibits bacterial cell wall synthesis by binding to one or more of the penicillin binding proteins (PBPs) which in turn inhibits the final transpeptidation step of peptidoglycan synthesis in bacterial cell walls, thus inhibiting cell wall biosynthesis. Bacteria eventually lyse due to ongoing activity of cell wall autolytic enzymes (autolysins and murein hydrolases) while cell wall assembly is arrested. Monobactam structure makes cross-allergenicity with beta-lactams unlikely.

Pharmacodynamics/Kinetics

Absorption: I.M.: Well absorbed; I.M. and I.V. doses produce comparable serum concentrations; Oral: <1%

Distribution: Widely to most body fluids and tissues

V_d: Children: 0.2-0.29 L/kg; Adults: 0.2 L/kg

Relative diffusion of antimicrobial agents from blood into CSF: Good only with inflammation (exceeds usual MICs)

CSF:blood level ratio: Meninges: Inflamed: 8% to 40%; Normal: ~1%

Protein binding: 56%

Metabolism: Hepatic (minor %)

Half-life elimination:

Children 2 months to 12 years: 1.7 hours

Adults: Normal renal function: 1.7-2.9 hours

End-stage renal disease: 6-8 hours

Time to peak: I.M., I.V. push: Within 60 minutes; I.V. infusion: 1.5 hours

Excretion: Urine (60% to 70% as unchanged drug); feces (~13% to 15%)

Dosage

Children >1 month: I.M., I.V.:

Mild-to-moderate infections: I.M., I.V.: 30 mg/kg every 8 hours

Moderate-to-severe infections: I.M., I.V.: 30 mg/kg every 6-8 hours; maximum: 120 mg/kg/day (8 g/day)

Cystic fibrosis: I.V.: 50 mg/kg/dose every 6-8 hours (ie, up to 200 mg/kg/day); maximum: 8 g/day

Adults:

Urinary tract infection: I.M., I.V.: 500 mg to 1 g every 8-12 hours

Moderately-severe systemic infections: 1 g I.V. or I.M. or 2 g I.V. every 8-12 hours

Severe systemic or life-threatening infections (especially caused by *Pseudomonas aeruginosa*): I.V.: 2 g every 6-8 hours; maximum: 8 g/day

Meningitis (gram-negative): I.V.: 2 g every 6-8 hours

Dosing adjustment in renal impairment: Adults: Following initial dose, maintenance doses should be given as follows:

Cl_{cr} 10-30 mL/minute: 50% of usual dose at the usual interval

Cl_{cr} <10 mL/minute: 25% of usual dosage at the usual interval

Hemodialysis: Moderately dialyzable (20% to 50%); Loading dose of 500 mg, 1 g, or 2 g, followed by 25% of initial dose at usual interval; for serious/life-threatening infections, administer 1/8 of initial dose after each hemodialysis session (given in addition to the maintenance doses)

Continuous ambulatory peritoneal dialysis (CAPD): Administer as for Cl_{cr} <10 mL/minute

Continuous renal replacement therapy (CRRT): Drug clearance is highly dependent on the method of renal replacement, filter type, and flow rate. Appropriate dosing requires close monitoring of pharmacologic response, signs of adverse reactions due to drug accumulation, as well as drug levels in relation to target trough (if appropriate). The following are general recommendations only (based on dialysate flow/ultrafiltration rates of 1 L/hour) and should not supersede clinical judgment:

CVVH: 1-2 g every 12 hours

CVVHD/CVVHDF: 2 g every 12 hours

Administration Doses >1 g should be administered I.V.

I.M.: Administer by deep injection into large muscle mass, such as upper outer quadrant of gluteus maximus or the lateral part of the thigh

I.V.: Administer by slow I.V. push over 3-5 minutes or by intermittent infusion over 20-60 minutes.

Monitoring Parameters Periodic liver function test; monitor for signs of anaphylaxis during first dose

Test Interactions May interfere with urine glucose tests containing cupric sulfate (Benedict's solution, Clinitest®); positive Coombs' test

Additional Information Although marketed as an agent similar to aminoglycosides, aztreonam is a monobactam antimicrobial with almost pure gram-negative aerobic activity. It cannot be used for gram-positive infections. Aminoglycosides are often used for synergy in gram-positive infections.

Dosage Forms Excipient information presented when available (limited, particularly for generics); consult specific product labeling. [DSC] = Discontinued product

Infusion premixed iso-osmotic solution:

Azactam®: 1 g (50 mL); 2 g (50 mL)

Injection, powder for reconstitution:

Azactam®: 500 mg [DSC], 1 g, 2 g

Bacitracin (bas i TRAY sin)

U.S. Brand Names Baci-Rx; Baciguent® [OTC]; BaciiM®

Canadian Brand Names Baciguent®; Baciject®

Pharmacologic Category Antibiotic, Miscellaneous; Antibiotic, Ophthalmic; Antibiotic, Topical

Use Treatment of susceptible bacterial infections mainly; has activity against gram-positive bacilli; due to toxicity risks, systemic and irrigant uses of bacitracin should be limited to situations where less toxic alternatives would not be effective

Unlabeled/Investigational Use Oral administration: Successful in antibiotic-associated colitis; has been used for enteric eradication of vancomycin-resistant enterococci (VRE)

Medication Safety Issues

Sound-alike/look-alike issues:

Bacitracin may be confused with Bactrim®, Bactroban®

Dosage Do not administer I.V.:

Infants: I.M.:

≤2.5 kg: 900 units/kg/day in 2-3 divided doses

>2.5 kg: 1000 units/kg/day in 2-3 divided doses

Children: I.M.: 800-1200 units/kg/day divided every 8 hours

Adults: Oral:

Antibiotic-associated colitis: 25,000 units 4 times/day for 7-10 days

VRE eradication (unlabeled use): 25,000 units 4 times/day for 7-10 days

Children and Adults:

Topical: Apply 1-5 times/day

Ophthalmic, ointment: Instill 1/4" to 1/2" ribbon every 3-4 hours into conjunctival sac for acute infections, or 2-3 times/day for mild-to-moderate infections for 7-10 days

Irrigation, solution: 50-100 units/mL in normal saline, lactated Ringer's, or sterile water for irrigation; soak sponges in solution for topical compresses 1-5 times/day or as needed during surgical procedures

Additional Information Complete prescribing information for this medication should be consulted for additional detail.

Dosage Forms Excipient information presented when available (limited, particularly for generics); consult specific product labeling.

Injection, powder for reconstitution: 50,000 units

BaciiM®: 50,000 units

Ointment, ophthalmic: 500 units/g (3.5 g)

Ointment, topical: 500 units/g (0.9 g, 15 g, 30 g, 120 g, 454 g)

Baciguent®: 500 units/g (15 g, 30 g)

Powder, for prescription compounding [micronized]:

Baci-Rx: 5 million units

Bacitracin and Polymyxin B

(bas i TRAY sin & pol i MIKS in bee)

U.S. Brand Names AK-Poly-Bac™; Betadine® First Aid Antibiotics + Moisturizer [OTC] [DSC]; Polysporin® [OTC]

Canadian Brand Names LID-Pack®; Optimyxin®

Index Terms Polymyxin B and Bacitracin

Pharmacologic Category Antibiotic, Ophthalmic; Antibiotic, Topical

Use Treatment of superficial infections caused by susceptible organisms

Pregnancy Risk Factor C

Medication Safety Issues

Sound-alike/look-alike issues:

Betadine® may be confused with Betagan®, betaine

Dosage Children and Adults:

Ophthalmic ointment: Instill 1/2" ribbon in the affected eye(s) every 3-4 hours for acute infections or 2-3 times/day for mild-to-moderate infections for 7-10 days

Topical ointment/powder: Apply to affected area 1-4 times/day; may cover with sterile bandage if needed

Additional Information Complete prescribing information for this medication should be consulted for additional detail.

Dosage Forms Excipient information presented when available (limited, particularly for generics); consult specific product labeling. [DSC] = Discontinued product

Ointment, ophthalmic: Bacitracin 500 units and polymyxin B 10,000 units per g (3.5 g)

AK-Poly-Bac™: Bacitracin 500 units and polymyxin 10,000 units per g (3.5 g)

Ointment, topical: Bacitracin 500 units and polymyxin B 10,000 units per g in white petrolatum (15 g, 30 g)

Betadine® First Aid Antibiotics + Moisturizer: Bacitracin 500 units and polymyxin B 10,000 units per g (14 g) [DSC]

Polysporin®: Bacitracin 500 units and polymyxin B 10,000 units per g (0.9 g, 15 g, 30 g)

Powder, topical:

Polysporin®: Bacitracin 500 units and polymyxin B 10,000 units per g (10 g)

Bacitracin, Neomycin, and Polymyxin B

(bas i TRAY sin, nee oh MYE sin, & pol i MIKS in bee)

U.S. Brand Names Neosporin® Neo To Go® [OTC]; Neosporin® Ophthalmic Ointment [DSC]; Neosporin® Topical [OTC]

Canadian Brand Names Neosporin® Ophthalmic Ointment

Index Terms Neomycin, Bacitracin, and Polymyxin B; Polymyxin B, Bacitracin, and Neomycin; Triple Antibiotic

Pharmacologic Category Antibiotic, Ophthalmic; Antibiotic, Topical

Use Helps prevent infection in minor cuts, scrapes, and burns; short-term treatment of superficial external ocular infections caused by susceptible organisms

Pregnancy Risk Factor C

Dosage Children and Adults:

Ophthalmic: Ointment: Instill 1/2" into the conjunctival sac every 3-4 hours for 7-10 days for acute infections

Topical: Apply 1-3 times/day to infected area; may cover with sterile bandage as needed

Additional Information Complete prescribing information for this medication should be consulted for additional detail.

Dosage Forms Excipient information presented when available (limited, particularly for generics); consult specific product labeling. [DSC] = Discontinued product

Ointment, ophthalmic (Neosporin® [DSC]): Bacitracin 400 units, neomycin 3.5 mg, and polymyxin B 10,000 units per g (3.5 g)

Ointment, topical: Bacitracin 400 units, neomycin 3.5 mg, and polymyxin B 5000 units per g (0.9 g, 15 g, 30 g, 454 g)

Neosporin®: Bacitracin 400 units, neomycin 3.5 mg, and polymyxin B 5000 units per g (15 g, 30 g)

Neosporin® Neo To Go®: Bacitracin 400 units, neomycin 3.5 mg, and polymyxin B 5000 units per g (0.9 g)

Bacitracin, Neomycin, Polymyxin B, and Hydrocortisone

(bas i TRAY sin, nee oh MYE sin, pol i MIKS in bee, & hye droe KOR ti sone)

U.S. Brand Names Cortisporin® Ointment

Canadian Brand Names Cortisporin® Topical Ointment

Index Terms Hydrocortisone, Bacitracin, Neomycin, and Polymyxin B; Neomycin, Bacitracin, Polymyxin B, and Hydrocortisone; Polymyxin B, Bacitracin, Neomycin, and Hydrocortisone

Pharmacologic Category Antibiotic, Ophthalmic; Antibiotic, Topical; Corticosteroid, Ophthalmic; Corticosteroid, Topical

Use Prevention and treatment of susceptible inflammatory conditions where bacterial infection (or risk of infection) is present

Pregnancy Risk Factor C

Dosage Children and Adults:

Ophthalmic: Ointment: Instill 1/2 inch ribbon to inside of lower lid every 3-4 hours until improvement occurs

Topical: Apply sparingly 2-4 times/day. Therapy should be discontinued when control is achieved; if no improvement is seen, reassessment of diagnosis may be necessary.

Additional Information Complete prescribing information for this medication should be consulted for additional detail.

Dosage Forms Excipient information presented when available (limited, particularly for generics); consult specific product labeling.

Ointment, ophthalmic: Bacitracin 400 units, neomycin 3.5 mg, polymyxin B 10,000 units, and hydrocortisone 10 mg per g (3.5 g)

Ointment, topical:

Cortisporin®: Bacitracin 400 units, neomycin 3.5 mg, polymyxin B 5000 units, and hydrocortisone 10 mg per g (15 g)

Baclofen (BAK loe fen)

U.S. Brand Names Lioresal®

Canadian Brand Names Apo-Baclofen®; Gen-Baclofen; Lioresal®; Liotec; Nu-Baclo; PMS-Baclofen

Pharmacologic Category Skeletal Muscle Relaxant

Use Treatment of reversible spasticity associated with multiple sclerosis or spinal cord lesions

Orphan drug: Intrathecal: Treatment of intractable spasticity caused by spinal cord injury, multiple sclerosis, and other spinal disease (spinal ischemia or tumor, transverse myelitis, cervical spondylosis, degenerative myelopathy)

Unlabeled/Investigational Use Intractable hiccups, intractable pain relief, bladder spasticity, trigeminal neuralgia, cerebral palsy, Huntington's chorea

Pregnancy Risk Factor C

Lactation Enters breast milk (small amounts)/compatible

Medication Safety Issues

Sound-alike/look-alike issues:

Baclofen may be confused with Bactroban®

Lioresal® may be confused with lisinopril, Lotensin®

High alert medication: The Institute for Safe Medication Practices (ISMP) includes this medication (intrathecal administration) among its list of drugs which have a heightened risk of causing significant patient harm when used in error.

Contraindications Hypersensitivity to baclofen or any component of the formulation

Warnings/Precautions Use with caution in patients with seizure disorder or impaired renal function. **[U.S. Boxed Warning]: Avoid abrupt withdrawal of the drug; abrupt withdrawal of intrathecal baclofen has resulted in severe sequelae (hyperpyrexia, obtundation, rebound/exaggerated spasticity, muscle rigidity, and rhabdomyolysis), leading to organ failure and some fatalities.** Risk may be higher in patients with injuries at T-6 or above, history of baclofen withdrawal, or limited ability to communicate. May cause CNS depression, which may impair physical or mental abilities; patients must be cautioned about performing tasks which require mental alertness (eg, operating machinery or driving). Elderly are more sensitive to the effects of baclofen and are more likely to experience adverse CNS effects at higher doses.

Adverse Reactions

>10%:

Central nervous system: Drowsiness, vertigo, dizziness, psychiatric disturbances, insomnia, slurred speech, ataxia, hypotonia

Neuromuscular & skeletal: Weakness

1% to 10%:

Cardiovascular: Hypotension

Central nervous system: Fatigue, confusion, headache

Dermatologic: Rash

Gastrointestinal: Nausea, constipation

Genitourinary: Polyuria

<1% (Limited to important or life-threatening): Chest pain, dyspnea, dysuria, enuresis, hematuria, impotence, inability to ejaculate, nocturia, palpitation, syncope, urinary retention; withdrawal reactions have occurred with abrupt discontinuation (particularly severe with intrathecal use).

Drug Interactions

Avoid Concomitant Use There are no known interactions where it is recommended to avoid concomitant use.

Increased Effect/Toxicity

Baclofen may increase the levels/effects of: Alcohol (Ethyl); CNS Depressants

Decreased Effect There are no known significant interactions involving a decrease in effect.

Ethanol/Nutrition/Herb Interactions

Ethanol: Avoid ethanol (may increase CNS depression).

Herb/Nutraceutical: Avoid valerian, St John's wort, kava kava, gotu kola.

Mechanism of Action Inhibits the transmission of both monosynaptic and polysynaptic reflexes at the spinal cord level, possibly by hyperpolarization of primary afferent fiber terminals, with resultant relief of muscle spasticity

Pharmacodynamics/Kinetics

Onset of action: 3-4 days

Peak effect: 5-10 days

Absorption (dose dependent): Oral: Rapid

Protein binding: 30%

Metabolism: Hepatic (15% of dose)

Half-life elimination: 3.5 hours

Time to peak, serum: Oral: Within 2-3 hours

Excretion: Urine and feces (85% as unchanged drug)

Dosage

Oral (avoid abrupt withdrawal of drug):

Children (unlabeled use): Caution: Pediatric dosing expressed as a daily amount, and **NOT** in mg/kg. Limited published data in children; the following is a compilation of small prospective studies (Albright, 1996; Milla, 1977; Scheinberg, 2006) and one large retrospective study (Lubsch, 2006):

<2 years: 10-20 mg daily divided every 8 hours; titrate dose every 3 days in increments of 5-15mg/day to a maximum of 40 mg daily

2-7 years: Initial: 20-30 mg daily divided every 8 hours; titrate dose every 3 days in increments of 5-15 mg/day to a maximum of 60 mg daily

≥8 years: 30-40 mg daily divided every 8 hours; titrate dose every 3 days in increments of 5-15 mg/day to a maximum of 120 mg daily

Note: Baclofen dose may need to be increased over time. One retrospective analysis (Lubsch, 2006) suggested that increased doses were needed as the time increased from spasticity onset, as age increased, and as the number of concomitant antispasticity medications increased. A small number of patients required daily doses exceeding 200 mg.

Adults: 5 mg 3 times/day, may increase 5 mg/dose every 3 days to a maximum of 80 mg/day

Hiccups (unlabeled use): Usual effective dose: 10-20 mg 2-3 times/day

Intrathecal: Children and Adults:

Test dose: 50-100 mcg, doses >50 mcg should be given in 25 mcg increments, separated by 24 hours. A screening dose of 25 mcg may be considered in very small patients. Patients not responding to screening dose of 100 mcg should not be considered for chronic infusion/implanted pump.

Maintenance: After positive response to test dose, a maintenance intrathecal infusion can be administered via an implanted intrathecal pump. Initial dose via pump: Infusion at a 24-hour rate dosed at twice the test dose. Avoid abrupt discontinuation.

Elderly: Oral (the lowest effective dose is recommended): Initial: 5 mg 2-3 times/day, increasing gradually as needed; if benefits are not seen, withdraw the drug slowly.

Dosing adjustment in renal impairment: May be necessary to reduce dosage in renal impairment, but there are no specific guidelines available

Hemodialysis: Poor water solubility allows for accumulation during chronic hemodialysis. Low-dose therapy is recommended. There have been several case reports of accumulation of baclofen resulting in toxicity symptoms (organic brain syndrome, myoclonia, deceleration and steep potentials in EEG) in patients with renal failure who have received normal doses of baclofen.

Administration Intrathecal: For screening dosages, dilute with preservative-free sodium chloride to a final concentration of 50 mcg/mL for bolus injection into the subarachnoid space. For maintenance infusions, concentrations of 500-2000 mcg/mL may be used.

Test Interactions Increased alkaline phosphatase, AST, glucose, ammonia (B); decreased bilirubin (S)

Dosage Forms Excipient information presented when available (limited, particularly for generics); consult specific product labeling.

Injection, solution, intrathecal [preservative free]:

Lioresal®: 50 mcg/mL (1 mL); 500 mcg/mL (20 mL); 2000 mcg/mL (5 mL, 20 mL)

Tablet: 10 mg, 20 mg

Extemporaneous Preparations Make a 5 mg/mL suspension by crushing fifteen 20 mg tablets; wet with glycerin, gradually add 45 mL simple syrup in 3 x 5 mL aliquots to make a total volume of 60 mL; refrigerate; stable 35 days

Johnson CE and Hart SM, "Stability of an Extemporaneously Compounded Baclofen Oral Liquid," *Am J Hosp Pharm*, 1993, 50:2353-5.

- ◆ **BactoShield® CHG [OTC]** *see* Chlorhexidine Gluconate *on page 305*
- ◆ **Bactrim™** *see* Sulfamethoxazole and Trimethoprim *on page 1407*
- ◆ **Bactrim™ DS** *see* Sulfamethoxazole and Trimethoprim *on page 1407*
- ◆ **Bactroban®** *see* Mupirocin *on page 1024*
- ◆ **Bactroban® Nasal** *see* Mupirocin *on page 1024*
- ◆ **Baking Soda** *see* Sodium Bicarbonate *on page 1380*
- ◆ **BAL** *see* Dimercaprol *on page 453*
- ◆ **Balacet 325™** *see* Propoxyphene and Acetaminophen *on page 1258*
- ◆ **BAL in Oil®** *see* Dimercaprol *on page 453*
- ◆ **Balmex® [OTC]** *see* Zinc Oxide *on page 1584*
- ◆ **Balminil Decongestant (Can)** *see* Pseudoephedrine *on page 1265*
- ◆ **Balminil DM D (Can)** *see* Pseudoephedrine and Dextromethorphan *on page 1266*
- ◆ **Balminil DM + Decongestant + Expectorant (Can)** *see* Guaifenesin, Pseudoephedrine, and Dextromethorphan *on page 715*
- ◆ **Balminil DM E (Can)** *see* Guaifenesin and Dextromethorphan *on page 710*
- ◆ **Balminil Expectorant (Can)** *see* GuaiFENesin *on page 709*

Balsalazide (bal SAL a zide)

U.S. Brand Names Colazal®

Index Terms Balsalazide Disodium

Pharmacologic Category 5-Aminosalicylic Acid Derivative; Anti-inflammatory Agent

Use Treatment of mild-to-moderate active ulcerative colitis

Pregnancy Risk Factor B

Pregnancy Considerations Teratogenic effects were not observed in animal studies. There are no adequate and well-controlled studies have been done in pregnant women. Balsalazide should be used in pregnant women only if clearly needed.

Lactation Excretion in breast milk unknown/use caution

Medication Safety Issues

Sound-alike/look-alike issues:

Colazal® may be confused with Clozaril®

Contraindications Hypersensitivity to balsalazide, metabolites to balsalazide, salicylates, or any component of the formulation

Warnings/Precautions Pyloric stenosis may prolong gastric retention of balsalazide capsules. Renal toxicity has been observed with other mesalamine (5-aminosalicylic acid) products; use with caution in patients with known renal disease. May exacerbate symptoms of ulcerative colitis. Safety and efficacy of use beyond 12 weeks in adults or 8 weeks in children has not been established. Safety and efficacy have not been established in children <5 years of age.

Adverse Reactions

>10%:

Central nervous system: Headache (children 15%; adults 8%)

Gastrointestinal: Abdominal pain (children 12% to 13%; adults 6%)

1% to 10%:

Central nervous system: Insomnia (adults 2%), fatigue (children 4%; adults 2%), fever (children 6%; adults 2%)

Endocrine & metabolic: Dysmenorrhea (children 3%)

Gastrointestinal: Diarrhea (children 9%; adults 5%), ulcerative colitis exacerbation (children 6%; adults 1%), nausea (children 4%; adults 5%), vomiting (children 10%; adults 4%), hematochezia (children 4%), stomatitis (children 3%), anorexia (adults 2%), dyspepsia (adults 2%), flatulence (adults 2%), cramps (adults 1%), constipation (adults 1%), xerostomia (adults 1%)

Genitourinary: Urinary tract infection (adults 1%)

Neuromuscular & skeletal: Arthralgia (adults 4%), back pain (adults 2%), myalgia (adults 1%)

Respiratory: Respiratory infection (adults 4%), cough (children 3%; adults 2%), pharyngitis (children 6%; adults 2%), pharyngolaryngeal pain (children 3%), rhinitis (adults 2%)

Miscellaneous: Flu-like syndrome (children 4%; adults 1%)

<1% (Limited to important or life-threatening): Alopecia, cholestatic jaundice, cirrhosis, hepatocellular damage, hepatotoxicity, jaundice, hypersensitivity pericarditis, Kawasaki-like syndrome, liver failure, liver necrosis, liver function tests increased, myocarditis

Drug Interactions

Avoid Concomitant Use There are no known interactions where it is recommended to avoid concomitant use.

Increased Effect/Toxicity

Balsalazide may increase the levels/effects of: Thiopurine Analogs; Varicella Virus-Containing Vaccines

Decreased Effect

Balsalazide may decrease the levels/effects of: Cardiac Glycosides

Stability Store at controlled room temperature of 20°C to 25°C (68°F to 77°F).

Mechanism of Action Balsalazide is a prodrug, converted by bacterial azoreduction to 5-aminosalicylic acid (mesalamine, active), 4-aminobenzoyl-β-alanine (inert), and their metabolites. 5-aminosalicylic acid may decrease inflammation by blocking the production of arachidonic acid metabolites topically in the colon mucosa.

Pharmacodynamics/Kinetics

Onset of action: Delayed; may require several days to weeks

Absorption: Very low and variable

Protein binding: Balsalazide: ≥99%

Metabolism: Azoreduced in the colon to 5-aminosalicylic acid (active), 4-aminobenzoyl-β-alanine (inert), and N-acetylated metabolites

Half-life elimination: Primary effect is topical (colonic mucosa); systemic half-life not determined

Time to peak: Balsalazide: 1-2 hours

Excretion: Feces (65% as 5-aminosalicylic acid, 4-aminobenzoyl-β-alanine, and N-acetylated metabolites); urine (25% as N-acetylated metabolites); Parent drug: Urine or feces (<1%)

Dosage Oral:

Children 5-17 years: 750 mg 3 times/day for up to 8 weeks **or** 2.25 g (three 750 mg capsules) 3 times/day for 8 weeks

Adults: 2.25 g (three 750 mg capsules) 3 times/day for 8-12 weeks

Elderly: No specific dosage adjustment available

Dosage adjustment in renal impairment: No information available with balsalazide; renal toxicity has been observed with other 5-aminosalicylic acid products, use with caution

Dosage adjustment in hepatic impairment: No specific dosage adjustment available

Dietary Considerations Colazal® 750 mg capsule contains sodium ~86 mg.

Administration Capsules should be swallowed whole or may be opened and sprinkled on applesauce. Applesauce mixture may be chewed; swallow immediately, do not store mixture for later use. When sprinkled on food, may cause staining of teeth or tongue.

Monitoring Parameters Improvement or worsening of symptoms

Additional Information Balsalazide 750 mg is equivalent to mesalamine 267 mg

Dosage Forms Excipient information presented when available (limited, particularly for generics); consult specific product labeling.

Capsule, as disodium: 750 mg

Colazal®: 750 mg [contains sodium ~86 mg/capsule]

◆ **Balsalazide Disodium** *see* Balsalazide *on page 173*

◆ **Balsam Peru, Trypsin, and Castor Oil** *see* Trypsin, Balsam Peru, and Castor Oil *on page 1526*

◆ **Baltussin** *see* Dihydrocodeine, Chlorpheniramine, and Phenylephrine *on page 448*

◆ **Balziva™** *see* Ethinyl Estradiol and Norethindrone *on page 581*

◆ **Band-Aid® Hurt-Free™ Antiseptic Wash [OTC]** *see* Lidocaine *on page 884*

◆ **Banophen® [OTC]** *see* DiphenhydrAMINE *on page 456*

◆ **Banophen® Anti-Itch [OTC]** *see* DiphenhydrAMINE *on page 456*

◆ **Banzel™** *see* Rufinamide *on page 1349*

◆ **Baraclude®** *see* Entecavir *on page 523*

◆ **Baridium® [OTC]** *see* Phenazopyridine *on page 1177*

◆ **Basaljel® (Can)** *see* Aluminum Hydroxide *on page 75*

◆ **Base Ointment** *see* Zinc Oxide *on page 1584*

Basiliximab (ba si LIK si mab)

U.S. Brand Names Simulect®

Canadian Brand Names Simulect®

Pharmacologic Category Monoclonal Antibody

Use Prophylaxis of acute organ rejection in renal transplantation

Pregnancy Risk Factor B (manufacturer)

Pregnancy Considerations Teratogenic effects were not observed in animal studies. IL-2 receptors play an important role in the development of the immune system. Use in pregnant women only when benefit exceeds potential risk to the fetus. Women of childbearing potential should use effective contraceptive measures before beginning treatment and for 4 months after completion of therapy with this agent.

Lactation Excretion in breast milk unknown/not recommended

Contraindications Hypersensitivity to basiliximab, murine proteins, or any component of the formulation

Warnings/Precautions To be used as a component of immunosuppressive regimen which includes cyclosporine and corticosteroids. The incidence of lymphoproliferative disorders and/or opportunistic infections may be increased by immunosuppressive therapy. Severe hypersensitivity reactions, occurring within 24 hours, have been reported. Reactions, including anaphylaxis, have occurred both with the initial exposure and/or following re-exposure after several months. Use caution during re-exposure to a subsequent course of therapy in a patient who has previously received basiliximab. Discontinue the drug permanently if a reaction occurs. Medications for the treatment of hypersensitivity reactions should be available for immediate use. Treatment may result in the development of human antimurine antibodies (HAMA); however, limited evidence suggesting the use of muromonab-CD3 or other murine products is not precluded. **[U.S. Boxed Warning]: Should be administered under the supervision of a physician experienced in immunosuppression therapy.**

Adverse Reactions Administration of basiliximab did not appear to increase the incidence or severity of adverse effects in clinical trials. Adverse events were reported in 96% of both the placebo and basiliximab groups.

>10%:
- Cardiovascular: Hypertension, peripheral edema
- Central nervous system: Fever, headache, insomnia, pain
- Dermatologic: Acne, wound complications
- Endocrine & metabolic: Hypercholesterolemia, hyperglycemia, hyper-/hypokalemia, hyperuricemia, hypophosphatemia
- Gastrointestinal: Abdominal pain, constipation, diarrhea, dyspepsia, nausea, vomiting
- Genitourinary: Urinary tract infection
- Hematologic: Anemia
- Neuromuscular & skeletal: Tremor
- Respiratory: Dyspnea, infection (upper respiratory)
- Miscellaneous: Viral infection

3% to 10%:
- Cardiovascular: Abnormal heart sounds, angina pectoris, arrhythmia, atrial fibrillation, cardiac failure, chest pain, generalized edema, hypotension, tachycardia
- Central nervous system: Agitation, anxiety, depression, dizziness, fatigue, hypoesthesia, malaise, neuropathy, rigors
- Dermatologic: Cyst, hypertrichosis, pruritus, rash, skin disorder, skin ulceration
- Endocrine & metabolic: Acidosis, dehydration, diabetes mellitus, fluid overload, hyper-/hypocalcemia, hyperlipidemia, hypertriglyceridemia, hypoglycemia, hypomagnesemia, hyponatremia
- Gastrointestinal: Abdomen enlarged, esophagitis, flatulence, gastroenteritis, GI hemorrhage, gingival hyperplasia, melena, moniliasis, stomatitis (including ulcerative), weight gain
- Genitourinary: Albuminuria, bladder disorder, dysuria, genital edema, hematuria, impotence, oliguria, renal function abnormal, renal tubular necrosis, ureteral disorder, urinary frequency, urinary retention
- Hematologic: Hematoma, hemorrhage, leukopenia, polycythemia, purpura, thrombocytopenia, thrombosis
- Neuromuscular & skeletal: Arthralgia, arthropathy, back pain, cramps, fracture, hernia, leg pain, myalgia, paresthesia, weakness
- Ocular: Abnormal vision, cataract, conjunctivitis
- Respiratory: Bronchitis, bronchospasm, cough, pharyngitis, pneumonia, pulmonary edema, sinusitis, rhinitis
- Miscellaneous: Accidental trauma, facial edema, glucocorticoids increased, herpes infection, sepsis

Postmarketing and/or case reports: Capillary leak syndrome, cytokine release syndrome; severe hypersensitivity reactions, including anaphylaxis, have been reported (symptoms may include hypotension, tachycardia, cardiac failure, dyspnea, bronchospasm, pulmonary edema, urticaria, rash, pruritus, sneezing, and respiratory failure)

Drug Interactions

Avoid Concomitant Use

Avoid concomitant use of Basiliximab with any of the following: Natalizumab; Vaccines (Live)

Increased Effect/Toxicity

Basiliximab may increase the levels/effects of: Natalizumab; Vaccines (Live)

The levels/effects of Basiliximab may be increased by: Abciximab; Herbs (Hypoglycemic Properties); Trastuzumab

Decreased Effect

Basiliximab may decrease the levels/effects of: Vaccines (Inactivated)

The levels/effects of Basiliximab may be decreased by: Echinacea

Ethanol/Nutrition/Herb Interactions Herb/Nutraceutical: Echinacea may diminish the therapeutic effect of basiliximab. Avoid hypoglycemic herbs, including alfalfa, bilberry, bitter melon, burdock, celery, damiana, fenugreek, garcinia, garlic, ginger, ginseng, gymnema, marshmallow, and stinging nettle (may enhance the hypoglycemic effect of basiliximab).

Stability Store intact vials under refrigeration 2°C to 8°C (36°F to 46°F). Reconstitute vials with sterile water for injection, USP. Shake the vial gently to dissolve. It is recommended that after reconstitution, the solution should be used immediately. If not used immediately, it can be stored at 2°C to 8°C for up to 24 hours or at room temperature for up to 4 hours. Discard the reconstituted solution within 24 hours. Further dilute reconstituted solution with 25-50 mL 0.9% sodium chloride or dextrose 5% in water. When mixing the solution, gently invert the bag to avoid foaming. Do not shake.

Mechanism of Action Chimeric (murine/human) monoclonal antibody which blocks the alpha-chain of the interleukin-2 (IL-2) receptor complex; this receptor is expressed on activated T lymphocytes and is a critical pathway for activating cell-mediated allograft rejection

Pharmacodynamics/Kinetics
- Duration: Mean: 36 days (determined by IL-2R alpha saturation)
- Distribution: Mean: V_d: Children 1-11 years: 4.8 ± 2.1 L; Adolescents 12-16 years: 7.8 ± 5.1 L; Adults: 8.6 ± 4.1 L
- Half-life elimination: Children 1-11 years: 9.5 days; Adolescents 12-16 years: 9.1 days; Adults: Mean: 7.2 days
- Excretion: Clearance: Children 1-11 years: 17 mL/hour; Adolescents 12-16 years: 31 mL/hour; Adults: Mean: 41 mL/hour

Dosage Note: Patients previously administered basiliximab should only be re-exposed to a subsequent course of therapy with extreme caution.

I.V.:
- Children <35 kg: Renal transplantation: 10 mg within 2 hours prior to transplant surgery, followed by a second 10 mg dose 4 days after transplantation; the second dose should be withheld if complications occur (including severe hypersensitivity reactions or graft loss)
- Children ≥35 kg and Adults: Renal transplantation: 20 mg within 2 hours prior to transplant surgery, followed by a second 20 mg dose 4 days after transplantation; the second dose should be withheld if complications occur (including severe hypersensitivity reactions or graft loss)

Dosing adjustment/comments in renal or hepatic impairment: No specific dosing adjustment recommended

Administration For intravenous administration only. Infuse as a bolus or I.V. infusion over 20-30 minutes. (Bolus dosing is associated with nausea, vomiting, and local pain at the injection site.)

Monitoring Parameters Signs and symptoms of acute rejection

Dosage Forms Excipient information presented when available (limited, particularly for generics); consult specific product labeling.

Injection, powder for reconstitution [preservative free]:
Simulect®: 10 mg, 20 mg

- ◆ **BAY 43-9006** *see* Sorafenib *on page 1392*
- ◆ **Bayer® Aspirin Extra Strength [OTC]** *see* Aspirin *on page 142*
- ◆ **Bayer® Aspirin Regimen Adult Low Dose [OTC]** *see* Aspirin *on page 142*
- ◆ **Bayer® Aspirin Regimen Children's [OTC]** *see* Aspirin *on page 142*

◆ **Bayer® Aspirin Regimen Regular Strength [OTC]** *see* Aspirin *on page* *142*

◆ **Bayer® Genuine Aspirin [OTC]** *see* Aspirin *on page* *142*

◆ **Bayer® Plus Extra Strength [OTC]** *see* Aspirin *on page* *142*

◆ **Bayer® PM [OTC]** *see* Aspirin and Diphenhydramine *on page* *145*

◆ **Bayer® with Heart Advantage [OTC]** *see* Aspirin *on page* *142*

◆ **Bayer® Women's Aspirin Plus Calcium [OTC]** *see* Aspirin *on page* *142*

◆ **BayGam® (Can)** *see* Immune Globulin (Intramuscular) *on page* *776*

◆ **Baza® Antifungal [OTC]** *see* Miconazole *on page* *989*

◆ **Baza® Clear [OTC]** *see* Vitamin A and Vitamin D *on page* *1565*

◆ **B-Caro-T™** *see* Beta-Carotene *on page* *188*

◆ **BCG, Live** *see* BCG Vaccine *on page* *176*

BCG Vaccine (bee see jee vak SEEN)

U.S. Brand Names TheraCys®; TICE® BCG

Canadian Brand Names ImmuCyst®; Oncotice™; Pacis™

Index Terms Bacillus Calmette-Guérin (BCG) Live; BCG Vaccine U.S.P. *(percutaneous use product)*; BCG, Live

Pharmacologic Category Biological Response Modulator; Vaccine

Use Immunization against tuberculosis and immunotherapy for cancer; treatment and prophylaxis of carcinoma *in situ* of the bladder; prophylaxis of primary or recurrent superficial papillary tumors following transurethral resection

Pregnancy Risk Factor C

Medication Safety Issues

High alert medication: The Institute for Safe Medication Practices (ISMP) includes this medication among its list of drugs which have a heightened risk of causing significant patient harm when used in error.

Dosage

Immunization against tuberculosis: Percutaneous: **Note:** Initial lesion usually appears after 10-14 days consisting of small, red papule at injection site and reaches maximum diameter of 3 mm in 4-6 weeks.

Children <1 month: 0.2-0.3 mL (half-strength dilution). Administer tuberculin test (5 TU) after 2-3 months; repeat vaccination after 1 year of age for negative tuberculin test if indications persist.

Children >1 month and Adults: 0.2-0.3 mL (full strength dilution); conduct postvaccinal tuberculin test (5 TU of PPD) in 2-3 months; if test is negative, repeat vaccination.

Immunotherapy for bladder cancer: Intravesicular: Adults:

TheraCys®: One dose instilled into bladder (for 2 hours) once weekly for 6 weeks followed by one treatment at 3, 6, 12, 18, and 24 months after initial treatment

TICE® BCG: One dose instilled into the bladder (for 2 hours) once weekly for 6 weeks followed by once monthly for 6-12 months

Additional Information Complete prescribing information for this medication should be consulted for additional detail.

Dosage Forms Excipient information presented when available (limited, particularly for generics); consult specific product labeling.

Injection, powder for reconstitution, intravesical [preservative free]:

TheraCys®: 81 mg [contains natural rubber/natural latex in packaging, polysorbate 80 (in diluent)]

TICE® BCG: 50 mg

Injection, powder for reconstitution, percutaneous [preservative free]:

BCG Vaccine: 50 mg

◆ **BCG Vaccine U.S.P. *(percutaneous use product)*** *see* BCG Vaccine *on page* *176*

◆ **BCI-Ranitidine (Can)** *see* Ranitidine *on page* *1295*

◆ **BCNU** *see* Carmustine *on page* *262*

◆ **beano® [OTC]** *see* Alpha-Galactosidase *on page* *68*

◆ **Bebulin® VH** *see* Factor IX Complex (Human) *on page* *601*

Becaplermin (be KAP ler min)

U.S. Brand Names Regranex®

Canadian Brand Names Regranex®

Index Terms Recombinant Human Platelet-Derived Growth Factor B; rPDGF-BB

Pharmacologic Category Growth Factor, Platelet-Derived; Topical Skin Product

Use Adjunctive treatment of diabetic neuropathic ulcers occurring on the lower limbs and feet that extend into subcutaneous tissue (or beyond) and have adequate blood supply

Pregnancy Risk Factor C

Medication Safety Issues

Sound-alike/look-alike issues:

Regranex® may be confused with Granulex®, Repronex®

Dosage Topical: Adults: Diabetic ulcers: Apply appropriate amount of gel once daily with a cotton swab or similar tool, as a coating over the ulcer. The amount of becaplermin to be applied will vary depending on the size of the ulcer area.

Note: If the ulcer does not decrease in size by ~30% after 10 weeks of treatment or complete healing has not occurred in 20 weeks, continued treatment with becaplermin gel should be reassessed.

To calculate the length of gel applied to the ulcer, measure the greatest length of the ulcer by the greatest width of the ulcer. Tube size and unit of measure will determine the formula used in the calculation. Recalculate amount of gel needed every 1-2 weeks, depending on the rate of change in ulcer area.

Centimeters:

15 g tube: [ulcer length (cm) x width (cm)] divided by 4 = length of gel (cm)

2 g tube: [ulcer length (cm) x width (cm)] divided by 2 = length of gel (cm)

Inches:

15 g tube: [length (in) x width (in)] x 0.6 = length of gel (in)

2 g tube: [length (in) x width (in)] x 1.3 = length of gel (in)

Additional Information Complete prescribing information for this medication should be consulted for additional detail.

Dosage Forms Excipient information presented when available (limited, particularly for generics); consult specific product labeling.

Gel, topical:

Regranex®: 0.01% (2 g, 15 g)

Beclomethasone (be kloe METH a sone)

U.S. Brand Names Beconase® AQ; QVAR®

Canadian Brand Names Apo-Beclomethasone®; Gen-Beclo; Nu-Beclomethasone; Propaderm®; QVAR®; Rivanase AQ; Vanceril® AEM

Index Terms Beclomethasone Dipropionate

Pharmacologic Category Corticosteroid, Inhalant (Oral); Corticosteroid, Nasal

Additional Appendix Information

Asthma *on page 1793*

Use

Oral inhalation: Maintenance and prophylactic treatment of asthma; includes those who require corticosteroids and those who may benefit from a dose reduction/elimination of systemically-administered corticosteroids. Not for relief of acute bronchospasm.

Nasal aerosol: Symptomatic treatment of seasonal or perennial rhinitis; prevent recurrence of nasal polyps following surgery.

Pregnancy Risk Factor C

Pregnancy Considerations Teratogenic effects were observed in animal studies. No human data on beclomethasone crossing the placenta or effects on the fetus. A decrease in fetal growth has not been observed with inhaled corticosteroid use during pregnancy. Inhaled corticosteroids are recommended for the treatment of asthma (most information available using budesonide) and allergic rhinitis during pregnancy.

Lactation Excretion in breast milk unknown/use caution

Medication Safety Issues

Sound-alike/look-alike issues:

Vanceril® may be confused with Vancenase®

Contraindications Hypersensitivity to beclomethasone or any component of the formulation; status asthmaticus

Warnings/Precautions May cause hypercorticism or suppression of hypothalamic-pituitary-adrenal (HPA) axis, particularly in younger children or in patients receiving high doses for prolonged periods. HPA axis suppression may lead to adrenal crisis. Withdrawal and discontinuation of a corticosteroid should be done slowly and carefully. Particular care is required when patients are transferred from systemic corticosteroids to inhaled products due to possible adrenal insufficiency or withdrawal from steroids, including an increase in allergic symptoms. Patients receiving >20 mg per day of prednisone (or equivalent) may be most susceptible. Fatalities have occurred due to adrenal insufficiency in asthmatic patients during and after transfer from systemic corticosteroids to aerosol steroids; aerosol steroids do not provide the systemic steroid needed to treat patients having trauma, surgery, or infections.

Bronchospasm may occur with wheezing after inhalation; if this occurs, stop steroid and treat with a fast-acting bronchodilator. Supplemental steroids (oral or parenteral) may be needed during stress or severe asthma attacks. Not to be used in status asthmaticus or for the relief of acute bronchospasm. Corticosteroid use may cause psychiatric disturbances, including depression, euphoria, insomnia, mood swings, and personality changes. Pre-existing psychiatric conditions may be exacerbated by corticosteroid use. Prolonged use of corticosteroids may also increase the incidence of secondary infection, mask acute infection (including fungal infections), prolong or exacerbate viral infections, or limit response to vaccines. Exposure to chickenpox should be avoided; corticosteroids should not be used to treat ocular herpes simplex. Corticosteroids should not be used for cerebral malaria. Close observation is required in patients with latent tuberculosis and/or TB reactivity; restrict use in active TB (only in conjunction with antituberculosis treatment). Prolonged treatment with corticosteroids has been associated with the development of Kaposi's sarcoma (case reports); if noted, discontinuation of therapy should be considered.

Use with caution in patients with thyroid disease, hepatic impairment, renal impairment, cardiovascular disease, diabetes, glaucoma, cataracts, myasthenia gravis, patients at risk for osteoporosis, patients at risk for seizures, or GI diseases (diverticulitis, peptic ulcer, ulcerative colitis) due to perforation risk. Use caution following acute MI (corticosteroids have been associated with myocardial rupture). Because of the risk of adverse effects, systemic corticosteroids should be used cautiously in the elderly in the smallest possible effective dose for the shortest duration. Avoid nasal corticosteroid use in patients with recent nasal septal ulcers, nasal surgery or nasal trauma until healing has occurred.

Orally-inhaled and intranasal corticosteroids may cause a reduction in growth velocity in pediatric patients (~1 centimeter per year [range: 0.3-1.8 cm per year] and related to dose and duration of exposure). To minimize the systemic effects of orally-inhaled and intranasal corticosteroids, each patient should be titrated to the lowest effective dose. Growth should be routinely monitored in pediatric patients. Safety and efficacy have not been established in children <5 years of age. There have been reports of systemic corticosteroid withdrawal symptoms (eg, joint/muscle pain, lassitude, depression) when withdrawing oral inhalation therapy.

Adverse Reactions Frequency not defined.

Central nervous system: Agitation, depression, dizziness, dysphonia, headache, lightheadedness, mental disturbances

Dermatologic: Acneiform lesions, angioedema, atrophy, bruising, pruritus, purpura, striae, rash, urticaria

Endocrine & metabolic: Cushingoid features, growth velocity reduction in children and adolescents, HPA function suppression

Gastrointestinal: Dry/irritated nose, throat and mouth, hoarseness, localized *Candida* or *Aspergillus* infection, loss of smell, loss of taste, nausea, unpleasant smell, unpleasant taste, vomiting, weight gain

Local: Nasal spray: Burning, epistaxis, localized *Candida* infection, nasal septum perforation (rare), nasal stuffiness, nosebleeds, rhinorrhea, sneezing, transient irritation, ulceration of nasal mucosa (rare)

Ocular: Cataracts, glaucoma, intraocular pressure increased

Respiratory: Cough, paradoxical bronchospasm, pharyngitis, sinusitis, wheezing

Miscellaneous: Anaphylactic/anaphylactoid reactions, death (due to adrenal insufficiency, reported during and after transfer from systemic corticosteroids to aerosol in asthmatic patients), immediate and delayed hypersensitivity reactions

Drug Interactions

Avoid Concomitant Use There are no known interactions where it is recommended to avoid concomitant use.

Increased Effect/Toxicity

Beclomethasone may increase the levels/effects of: Amphotericin B; Loop Diuretics; Thiazide Diuretics

Decreased Effect

Beclomethasone may decrease the levels/effects of: Antidiabetic Agents; Corticorelin

Stability Do not store near heat or open flame. Do not puncture canisters. Store at 25°C (77°F); excursions permitted between 15°C to 30°C (59°F to 86°F). Rest QVAR® on concave end of canister with actuator on top.

Mechanism of Action Controls the rate of protein synthesis; depresses the migration of polymorphonuclear leukocytes, fibroblasts; reverses capillary permeability and lysosomal stabilization at the cellular level to prevent or control inflammation

Pharmacodynamics/Kinetics

Onset of action: Oral inhalation: Therapeutic effect: 1-4 weeks

Absorption: Readily; quickly hydrolyzed by pulmonary esterases to active metabolite (beclomethasone-17-monoproprionate [17-BMP]) prior to absorption

Distribution: Beclomethasone dipropionate (BDP): 20 L; 17-BMP: 424 L

Protein binding: 17-BMP: 94% to 96%
Metabolism: Pro-drug; undergoes rapid conversion to 17-BMP during absorption; followed by additional metabolism via CYP3A4 to other, less active metabolites (beclomethasone-21-monopropionate [21-BMP] and beclomethasone [BOH])
Bioavailability: Nasal inhalation: 17-BMP: 44% (43% from swallowed portion)
Half-life elimination: BDP: 0.5 hours; 17-BMP: 3 hours
Time to peak, plasma: Oral inhalation: BDP: 0.5 hours; 17-BMP: 0.7 hours
Excretion: Feces (60%); urine (<10% to 12%)

Dosage Nasal inhalation and oral inhalation dosage forms are not to be used interchangeably
Inhalation, nasal: Rhinitis, nasal polyps (Beconase® AQ): Children ≥6 years and Adults: 1-2 inhalations each nostril twice daily; total dose 168-336 mcg/day
Inhalation, oral: Asthma (doses should be titrated to the lowest effective dose once asthma is controlled) (QVAR®):
Children 5-11 years: Initial: 40 mcg twice daily; maximum dose: 80 mcg twice daily
Children ≥12 years and Adults:
Patients previously on bronchodilators only: Initial dose 40-80 mcg twice daily; maximum dose: 320 mcg twice day
Patients previously on inhaled corticosteroids: Initial dose 40-160 mcg twice daily; maximum dose: 320 mcg twice daily
NIH Asthma Guidelines (NIH, 2007): HFA formulation (eg, QVAR®): Administer in divided doses:
Children 5-11 years:
"Low" dose: 80-160 mcg/day
"Medium" dose: >160-320 mcg/day
"High" dose: >320 mcg/day
Children ≥12 years and Adults:
"Low" dose: 80-240 mcg/day
"Medium" dose: >240-480 mcg/day
"High" dose: >480 mcg/day

Administration
Beconase AQ®: Shake well before use. Nasal applicator and dust cap may be washed in warm water and dry thoroughly.
QVAR®: Rinse mouth and throat after use to prevent *Candida* infection. Do not wash or put inhaler in water; mouth piece may be cleaned with a dry tissue or cloth. Prime canister before using.

Additional Information Effects of inhaled/intranasal steroids on growth have been observed in the absence of laboratory evidence of HPA axis suppression, suggesting that growth velocity is a more sensitive indicator of systemic corticosteroid exposure in pediatric patients than some commonly used tests of HPA axis function. The long-term effects of this reduction in growth velocity associated with orally-inhaled and intranasal corticosteroids, including the impact on final adult height, are unknown. The potential for "catch up" growth following discontinuation of treatment with inhaled corticosteroids has not been adequately studied.

Dosage Forms Excipient information presented when available (limited, particularly for generics); consult specific product labeling.
Aerosol for oral inhalation, as dipropionate:
QVAR®: 40 mcg/inhalation [100 metered actuations] (7.3 g); 80 mcg/inhalation [100 metered actuations] (7.3 g)
Suspension, intranasal, as dipropionate [aqueous spray]:
Beconase® AQ: 42 mcg/inhalation [180 metered sprays (25 g)

◆ **Beclomethasone Dipropionate** *see* Beclomethasone *on page 176*

◆ **Beconase® AQ** *see* Beclomethasone *on page 176*

◆ **BeFlex** *see* Acetaminophen and Phenyltoloxamine *on page 29*

◆ **Behenyl Alcohol** *see* Docosanol *on page 473*

◆ **Belladonna Alkaloids With Phenobarbital** *see* Hyoscyamine, Atropine, Scopolamine, and Phenobarbital *on page 756*

Belladonna and Opium (bel a DON a & OH pee um)

U.S. Brand Names B&O Supprettes® [DSC]
Index Terms Opium and Belladonna
Pharmacologic Category Analgesic Combination (Opioid); Antispasmodic Agent, Urinary
Use Relief of moderate-to-severe pain associated with ureteral spasms not responsive to nonopioid analgesics and to space intervals between injections of opiates
Restrictions C-II
Pregnancy Risk Factor C
Dosage Rectal: Children >12 years and Adults: 1 suppository 1-2 times/day, up to 4 doses/day
Additional Information Complete prescribing information for this medication should be consulted for additional detail.
Dosage Forms Excipient information presented when available (limited, particularly for generics); consult specific product labeling. [DSC] = Discontinued product
Suppository: Belladonna extract 16.2 mg and opium 30 mg; belladonna extract 16.2 mg and opium 60 mg
B&O Supprettes® #15 A: Belladonna extract 16.2 mg and opium 30 mg [DSC]
B&O Supprettes® #16 A: Belladonna extract 16.2 mg and opium 60 mg [DSC]

Belladonna, Phenobarbital, and Ergotamine
(bel a DON a, fee noe BAR bi tal, & er GOT a meen)

U.S. Brand Names Bellamine S [DSC]; Eperbel-S [DSC]; Spastrin® [DSC]
Canadian Brand Names Bellergal® Spacetabs®
Index Terms Ergotamine Tartrate, Belladonna, and Phenobarbital; Phenobarbital, Belladonna, and Ergotamine Tartrate
Pharmacologic Category Ergot Derivative
Use Management and treatment of menopausal disorders, GI disorders, and recurrent throbbing headache
Pregnancy Risk Factor X
Dosage Oral: Adults: 1 tablet each morning and evening
Additional Information Complete prescribing information for this medication should be consulted for additional detail.
Dosage Forms Excipient information presented when available (limited, particularly for generics); consult specific product labeling. [DSC] = Discontinued product
Tablet:
Bellamie S [DSC], Eperbel-S [DSC], Spastrin® [DSC]: Belladonna alkaloids 0.2 mg, phenobarbital 40 mg, and ergotamine 0.6 mg

◆ **Bellamine S [DSC]** *see* Belladonna, Phenobarbital, and Ergotamine *on page 178*

◆ **Bellergal® Spacetabs® (Can)** *see* Belladonna, Phenobarbital, and Ergotamine *on page 178*

◆ **Benadryl® (Can)** *see* DiphenhydrAMINE *on page 456*

◆ **Benadryl-D™ Allergy and Sinus Fastmelt™ [OTC]** *see* Diphenhydramine and Pseudoephedrine *on page 459*

◆ **Benadryl-D™ Children's Allergy and Sinus [OTC]** *see* Diphenhydramine and Pseudoephedrine *on page 459*

◆ **Benadryl® Allergy [OTC]** *see* DiphenhydrAMINE *on page 456*

◆ **Benadryl® Allergy and Cold [OTC]** *see* Acetaminophen, Diphenhydramine, and Phenylephrine *on page 33*

◆ **Benadryl® Allergy and Sinus Headache [OTC]** *see* Acetaminophen, Diphenhydramine, and Phenylephrine *on page 33*

◆ **Benadryl® Children's Allergy [OTC]** *see* DiphenhydrAMINE *on page 456*

◆ **Benadryl® Children's Allergy and Cold Fastmelt™ [OTC]** *see* Diphenhydramine and Pseudoephedrine *on page 459*

◆ **Benadryl® Children's Allergy Fastmelt® [OTC]** *see* DiphenhydrAMINE *on page 456*

◆ **Benadryl® Children's Dye-Free Allergy [OTC]** *see* DiphenhydrAMINE *on page 456*

◆ **Benadryl® Itch Stopping [OTC]** *see* DiphenhydrAMINE *on page 456*

◆ **Benadryl® Itch Stopping Extra Strength [OTC]** *see* DiphenhydrAMINE *on page 456*

Benazepril (ben AY ze pril)

U.S. Brand Names Lotensin®

Canadian Brand Names Apo-Benazepril®; Lotensin®

Index Terms Benazepril Hydrochloride

Pharmacologic Category Angiotensin-Converting Enzyme (ACE) Inhibitor

Additional Appendix Information

Angiotensin Agents *on page 1632*

Use Treatment of hypertension, either alone or in combination with other antihypertensive agents

Pregnancy Risk Factor D

Pregnancy Considerations Due to adverse events observed in humans, benazepril is considered pregnancy category D. Benazepril crosses the placenta. First trimester exposure to ACE inhibitors may cause major congenital malformations. An increased risk of cardiovascular and/or central nervous system malformations was observed in one study; however, an increased risk of teratogenic events was not observed in other studies. Second and third trimester use of an ACE inhibitor is associated with oligohydramnios. Oligohydramnios due to decreased fetal renal function may lead to fetal limb contractures, craniofacial deformation, and hypoplastic lung development. The use of ACE inhibitors during the second and third trimesters is also associated with anuria, hypotension, renal failure (reversible or irreversible), skull hypoplasia, and death in the fetus/neonate. Chronic maternal hypertension itself is also associated with adverse events in the fetus/infant. ACE inhibitors are not recommended during pregnancy to treat maternal hypertension or heart failure. Those who are planning a pregnancy should be considered for other medication options if an ACE inhibitor is currently prescribed or the ACE inhibitor should be discontinued as soon as possible once pregnancy is detected. The exposed fetus should be monitored for fetal growth, amniotic fluid volume, and organ formation. Infants exposed to an ACE inhibitor *in utero*, especially during the second and third trimester, should be monitored for hyperkalemia, hypotension, and oliguria.

[U.S. Boxed Warning]: Based on human data, ACE inhibitors can cause injury and death to the developing fetus. ACE inhibitors should be discontinued as soon as possible once pregnancy is detected.

Lactation Enters breast milk

Medication Safety Issues

Sound-alike/look-alike issues:

Benazepril may be confused with Benadryl®

Lotensin® may be confused with Lioresal®, lovastatin

International issues:

Lotensin® may be confused with Latensin® which is a brand name for bacillus cereus in Germany

Contraindications Hypersensitivity to benazepril or any component of the formulation; angioedema or serious hypersensitivity related to previous treatment with an ACE inhibitor

Warnings/Precautions Anaphylactic reactions may occur rarely with ACE inhibitors. At any time during treatment (especially following first dose) angioedema may occur rarely with ACE inhibitors. It may involve the head and neck (potentially compromising airway) or the intestine (presenting with abdominal pain). African-Americans and patients with idiopathic or hereditary angioedema may be at an increased risk. Prolonged frequent monitoring may be required especially if tongue, glottis, or larynx are involved as they are associated with airway obstruction. Patients with a history of airway surgery may have a higher risk of airway obstruction. Aggressive early and appropriate management is critical. Use in patients with previous angioedema associated with ACE inhibitor therapy is contraindicated. Hypersensitivity reactions may be seen during hemodialysis (eg, CVVHD) with high-flux dialysis membranes (eg, AN69), and rarely, during low density lipoprotein apheresis with dextran sulfate cellulose. Rare cases of anaphylactoid reactions have been reported in patients undergoing sensitization treatment with hymenoptera (bee, wasp) venom while receiving ACE inhibitors.

Symptomatic hypotension with or without syncope can occur with ACE inhibitors (usually with the first several doses); effects are most often observed in volume depleted patients; close monitoring of patient is required especially with initial dosing and dosing increases; blood pressure must be lowered at a rate appropriate for the patient's clinical condition. Initiation of therapy in patients with ischemic heart disease or cerebrovascular disease warrants close observation due to the potential consequences posed by falling blood pressure (eg, MI, stroke). **[U.S. Boxed Warning]: Based on human data, ACEIs can cause injury and death to the developing fetus when used in the second and third trimesters. ACEIs should be discontinued as soon as possible once pregnancy is detected.** Use with caution in hypertrophic cardiomyopathy with outflow tract obstruction, severe aortic stenosis, or before, during, or immediately after major surgery.

Hyperkalemia may occur with ACE inhibitors; risk factors include renal dysfunction, diabetes mellitus, concomitant use of potassium-sparing diuretics, potassium supplements and/or potassium containing salts. Use cautiously, if at all, with these agents and monitor potassium closely. Cough may occur with ACE inhibitors. Other causes of cough should be considered (eg, pulmonary congestion in patients with heart failure) and excluded prior to discontinuation. Use with caution in patients with diabetes receiving insulin or oral anti-diabetic agents; may be at increased risk for episodes of hypoglycemia.

May be associated with deterioration of renal function and/or increases in serum creatinine, particularly in patients with low renal blood flow (eg, renal artery stenosis, heart failure) whose glomerular filtration rate (GFR) is dependent on efferent arteriolar vasoconstriction by angiotensin II; deterioration may result in oliguria, acute renal failure, and progressive azotemia. Small increases in serum creatinine may occur following initiation; consider discontinuation only in patients with progressive and/or significant deterioration in renal function. Use with caution in patients with unstented unilateral/bilateral renal artery stenosis. When unstented bilateral renal artery stenosis is present, use is generally avoided due to the elevated risk of deterioration in renal function unless possible benefits outweigh risks.

Rare toxicities associated with ACE inhibitors include cholestatic jaundice (which may progress to fulminant hepatic necrosis), agranulocytosis, neutropenia, or leukopenia with myeloid hypoplasia. Patients with collagen vascular diseases (especially with concomitant renal impairment) or renal impairment alone may be at increased risk for hematologic toxicity; periodically monitor CBC with differential in these patients. Safety and efficacy have not been established in children <6 years of age.

Adverse Reactions

1% to 10%:

Cardiovascular: Postural dizziness (2%)

Central nervous system: Headache (6%), dizziness (4%), fatigue (2%), somnolence (2%)

Gastrointestinal: Nausea (1%)

Renal: Serum creatinine increased (2%), worsening of renal function may occur in patients with bilateral renal artery stenosis or hypovolemia

Respiratory: Cough (1% to 10%)

<1% (Limited to important or life-threatening): Agranulocytosis, alopecia, anaphylactoid reaction, angina, angioedema (includes head, neck and intestinal angioedema), arthralgia, arthritis, asthma, BUN increased (transient), dermatitis, dyspnea, ECG changes, eosinophilia, flushing, gastritis, hemolytic anemia, hyperbilirubinemia, hyperglycemia, hyperkalemia, hypersensitivity, hypertonia, hyponatremia, hypotension, impotence, insomnia, leukopenia, myalgia, neutropenia, palpitations, pancreatitis, paresthesia, pemphigus, peripheral edema, photosensitivity, postural hypotension, proteinuria, pruritis, rash, shock, Stevens-Johnson syndrome, syncope, thrombocytopenia, transaminases increased, uric acid increased, vomiting

Eosinophilic pneumonitis, anaphylaxis, renal insufficiency, and renal failure have been reported with other ACE inhibitors. In addition, a syndrome including fever, myalgia, arthralgia, interstitial nephritis, vasculitis, rash, eosinophilia, and elevated ESR has been reported to be associated with ACE inhibitors.

Drug Interactions

Avoid Concomitant Use There are no known interactions where it is recommended to avoid concomitant use.

Increased Effect/Toxicity

Benazepril may increase the levels/effects of: Allopurinol; Amifostine; AzaTHIOprine; CycloSPORINE; Ferric Gluconate; Gold Sodium Thiomalate; Lithium; RiTUXimab

The levels/effects of Benazepril may be increased by: Angiotensin II Receptor Blockers; Diazoxide; Eplerenone; Herbs (Hypotensive Properties); Loop Diuretics; Potassium Salts; Potassium-Sparing Diuretics; Prostacyclin Analogues; Sirolimus; Temsirolimus; Thiazide Diuretics; Trimethoprim

Decreased Effect

The levels/effects of Benazepril may be decreased by: Antacids; Aprotinin; Herbs (Hypertensive Properties); Methylphenidate; Nonsteroidal Anti-Inflammatory Agents; Salicylates; Yohimbine

Ethanol/Nutrition/Herb Interactions Herb/Nutraceutical: Avoid bayberry, blue cohosh, cayenne, ephedra, ginger, ginseng (American), kola, licorice (may worsen hypertension). Avoid black cohosh, California poppy, coleus, golden seal, hawthorn, mistletoe, periwinkle, quinine, shepherd's purse (may have increased antihypertensive effect).

Mechanism of Action Competitive inhibition of angiotensin I being converted to angiotensin II, a potent vasoconstrictor, through the angiotensin I-converting enzyme (ACE) activity, with resultant lower levels of angiotensin II which causes an increase in plasma renin activity and a reduction in aldosterone secretion

Pharmacodynamics/Kinetics

Reduction in plasma angiotensin-converting enzyme (ACE) activity:

Onset of action: Peak effect: 1-2 hours after 2-20 mg dose

Duration: >90% inhibition for 24 hours after 5-20 mg dose

Reduction in blood pressure:

Peak effect: Single dose: 2-4 hours; Continuous therapy: 2 weeks

Absorption: Rapid (37%); food does not alter significantly; metabolite (benazeprilat) itself unsuitable for oral administration due to poor absorption

Distribution: V_d: ~8.7 L

Protein binding:

Benazepril: ~97%

Benazeprilat: ~95%

Metabolism: Rapidly and extensively hepatic to its active metabolite, benazeprilat, via enzymatic hydrolysis; extensive first-pass effect

Half-life elimination: Benazeprilat: Effective: 10-11 hours; Terminal: Children: 5 hours, Adults: 22 hours

Time to peak: Parent drug: 0.5-1 hour

Excretion:

Urine (trace amounts as benazepril; 20% as benazeprilat; 12% as other metabolites)

Clearance: Nonrenal clearance (ie, biliary, metabolic) appears to contribute to the elimination of benazeprilat (11% to 12%), particularly patients with severe renal impairment; hepatic clearance is the main elimination route of unchanged benazepril

Dialysis: ~6% of metabolite removed within 4 hours of dialysis following 10 mg of benazepril administered 2 hours prior to procedure; parent compound not found in dialysate

Dosage Oral: Hypertension:

Children ≥6 years: Initial: 0.2 mg/kg/day (up to 10 mg/day) as monotherapy; dosing range: 0.1-0.6 mg/kg/day (maximum dose: 40 mg/day)

Adults: Initial: 10 mg/day in patients not receiving a diuretic; 20-80 mg/day as a single dose or 2 divided doses; the need for twice-daily dosing should be assessed by monitoring peak (2-6 hours after dosing) and trough responses.

Note: Patients taking diuretics should have them discontinued 2-3 days prior to starting benazepril. If they cannot be discontinued, then initial dose should be 5 mg; restart after blood pressure is stabilized if needed.

Elderly: Oral: Initial: 5-10 mg/day in single or divided doses; usual range: 20-40 mg/day; adjust for renal function; also see **Note** in adult dosing.

Dosing interval in renal impairment: Cl_{cr} <30 mL/minute:

Children: Use is not recommended.

Adults: Administer 5 mg/day initially; maximum daily dose: 40 mg.

Hemodialysis: Moderately dialyzable (20% to 50%); administer dose postdialysis or administer 25% to 35% supplemental dose.

Peritoneal dialysis: Supplemental dose is not necessary.

Monitoring Parameters Blood pressure; serum creatinine and potassium; if patient has collagen vascular disease and/or renal impairment, periodically monitor CBC with differential

Dosage Forms Excipient information presented when available (limited, particularly for generics); consult specific product labeling.

Tablet, as hydrochloride: 5 mg, 10 mg, 20 mg, 40 mg

Lotensin®: 5 mg, 10 mg, 20 mg, 40 mg

Extemporaneous Preparations To prepare a 2 mg/mL suspension, mix 15 benazepril 20 mg tablets in a bottle with Ora-Plus® 75 mL. Shake for 2 minutes, allow suspension to stand for ≥1 hour, then shake again for at least 1 additional minute. Add Ora-Sweet® 75 mL to suspension and shake to disperse. Will make 150 mL of a 2 mg/mL suspension. Store under refrigeration at 2°C to 8°C (36°F to 46°F) for up to 30 days. Shake prior to each use.

Benazepril and Hydrochlorothiazide
(ben AY ze pril & hye droe klor oh THYE a zide)

U.S. Brand Names Lotensin® HCT

Index Terms Hydrochlorothiazide and Benazepril

Pharmacologic Category Angiotensin-Converting Enzyme (ACE) Inhibitor; Diuretic, Thiazide

Use Treatment of hypertension

Pregnancy Risk Factor C/D (2nd and 3rd trimesters)

Dosage Oral: Dose is individualized (range: benazepril: 5-20 mg; hydrochlorothiazide: 6.25-25 mg/day)

Cl_{cr} <30 mL/minute: Not recommended; loop diuretics are preferred.

Additional Information Complete prescribing information for this medication should be consulted for additional detail.

Dosage Forms Excipient information presented when available (limited, particularly for generics); consult specific product labeling.

Tablet: 5/6.25: Benazepril hydrochloride 5 mg and hydrochlorothiazide 6.25 mg; 10/12.5: Benazepril hydrochloride 10 mg and hydrochlorothiazide 12.5 mg; 20/12.5: Benazepril hydrochloride 20 mg and hydrochlorothiazide 12.5 mg; 20/25: Benazepril hydrochloride 20 mg and hydrochlorothiazide 25 mg

Lotensin® HCT 5/6.25: Benazepril hydrochloride 5 mg and hydrochlorothiazide 6.25 mg

Lotensin® HCT 10/12.5: Benazepril hydrochloride 10 mg and hydrochlorothiazide 12.5 mg

Lotensin® HCT 20/12.5: Benazepril hydrochloride 20 mg and hydrochlorothiazide 12.5 mg

Lotensin® HCT 20/25: Benazepril hydrochloride 20 mg and hydrochlorothiazide 25 mg

◆ **Benazepril Hydrochloride** *see* Benazepril *on page 179*

◆ **Benazepril Hydrochloride and Amlodipine Besylate** *see* Amlodipine and Benazepril *on page 95*

Bendamustine (ben da MUS teen)

U.S. Brand Names Treanda®

Index Terms Bendamustine Hydrochloride; Cytostasan; SDX-105

Pharmacologic Category Antineoplastic Agent, Alkylating Agent

Use Treatment of chronic lymphocytic leukemia (CLL); treatment of progressed indolent B-cell non-Hodgkin's lymphoma (NHL)

Unlabeled/Investigational Use Treatment of mantle cell lymphoma; salvage therapy for relapsed multiple myeloma

Pregnancy Risk Factor D

Pregnancy Considerations Teratogenic and nonteratogenic events were observed in animal studies following intraperitoneal dosing. There are no adequate and well-controlled studies in pregnant women. May cause fetal harm if administered during pregnancy. Effective contraception is recommended during and for 3 months after treatment for women and men of reproductive potential.

Lactation Excretion in breast milk unknown/not recommended

Medication Safety Issues

Sound-alike/look-alike issues:

Bendamustine may be confused with carmustine

High alert medication: The Institute for Safe Medication Practices (ISMP) includes this medication among its list of drug classes which have a heightened risk of causing significant patient harm when used in error.

Contraindications Hypersensitivity to bendamustine, mannitol, or any component of the formulation

Warnings/Precautions Hazardous agent - use appropriate precautions for handling and disposal. Myelosuppression (neutropenia, thrombocytopenia and anemia) is a common toxicity; may require therapy delay and/or dose reduction; monitor. Complications due to febrile neutropenia and severe thrombocytopenia have been reported. ANC should recover to ≥1000/mm^3 and platelets to ≥75,000/mm^3 prior to therapy/cycle initiation. Infections, including pneumonia and sepsis have been reported with use; may require hospitalization; septic shock and fatalities have occurred. Patients with myelosuppression are more susceptible to infection; monitor closely.

Infusion reactions, including chills, fever, pruritus, and rash are common; rarely, anaphylactic and anaphylactoid reactions have occurred, particularly with the second or subsequent cycle(s). In general, patients who experienced grade 3 or 4 allergic reactions were not rechallenged in CLL clinical trials. Consider premedication with antihistamines, antipyretics and/or corticosteroids for patients with a history of grade 1 or 2 infusion reaction. Discontinue for severe allergic reaction; consider discontinuation with grade 3 or 4 infusion reaction. Rash, toxic skin reactions and bullous exanthema have been reported with monotherapy and in combination with other antineoplastics; may be progressive or worsen with continued treatment; discontinue bendamustine treatment for severe or progressive skin reaction. Toxic epidermal necrolysis has been reported when used in combination with rituximab.

Tumor lysis syndrome may occur as a consequence of leukemia treatment, including treatment with bendamustine, usually occurring in the first treatment cycle. May lead to life threatening acute renal failure; adequate hydration and prophylactic allopurinol should be instituted prior to treatment in high risk patients; monitor closely.

Use is not recommended in patients with moderate (AST or ALT 2.5-10 times ULN and total bilirubin 1.5-3 times ULN) or severe (total bilirubin >3 times ULN) hepatic impairment; use with caution in patients with mild hepatic impairment. Use is not recommended in patient with Cl_{cr} <40 mL/minute; use with caution in patients with mild-to-moderate renal impairment. Malignancies (including myelodysplastic syndrome, myeloproliferative disorders, acute myeloid leukemia and bronchial cancer) have been reported in patients who have received bendamustine. Safety and efficacy have not been established in children.

Adverse Reactions

>10%:

Cardiovascular: Peripheral edema (≤13%)

Central nervous system: Fatigue (9% to 57%), fever (24% to 34%), headache (≤21%), chills (6% to 14%), dizziness (≤14%), insomnia (≤13%)

Dermatologic: Rash (8% to 16%; grades 3/4: ≤3%)

Endocrine & metabolic: Dehydration (≤14%)

Gastrointestinal: Nausea (20% to 75%), vomiting (16% to 40%), diarrhea (9% to 37%), constipation (≤29%), anorexia (≤23%), weight loss (7% to 18%), stomatitis (≤15%), abdominal pain (5% to 13%), appetite loss (≤13%), dyspepsia (≤11%)

Hematologic: Myelosuppression (nadir: in week 3), lymphopenia (68% to 99%; grades 3/4: 47% to 94%), leukopenia (61% to 94%; grades 3/4: 28% to 56%), anemia (88% to 89%; grades 3/4: 11% to 13%), thrombocytopenia (77% to 86%; grades 3/4: 11% to 25%), neutropenia (75% to 86%; grades 3/4: 43% to 60%)

Hepatic: Bilirubin increased (≤34%; grades 3/4: 3%)

Neuromuscular & skeletal: Back pain (≤14%), weakness (8% to 11%)

Respiratory: Cough (4% to 22%), dyspnea (≤16%)

1% to 10%:

Cardiovascular: Tachycardia (≤7%), hypotension (≤6%), chest pain (≤6%), hypertension aggravated (≤3%)

Central nervous system: Anxiety (≤8%), depression (≤6%), pain (≤6%)

Dermatologic: Pruritus (5% to 6%), dry skin (≤5%)

Endocrine & metabolic: Hypokalemia (≤9%), hyperuricemia (≤7%; grades 3/4: 2%), hyperglycemia (grades 3/4: ≤3%), hypocalcemia (grades 3/4: ≤2%), hyponatremia (grades 3/4: ≤2%)

Gastrointestinal: Gastroesophageal reflux disease (≤10%), xerostomia (9%), taste alteration (≤7%), oral candidiasis (≤6%), abdominal distention (≤5%)

Genitourinary: Urinary tract infection (≤10%)

Hematologic: Febrile neutropenia (3% to 6%)

Hepatic: ALT increased (grades 3/4: ≤3%), AST increased (grades 3/4: ≤1%)

Local: Infusion site pain (≤6%), catheter site pain (≤5%)

Neuromuscular & skeletal: Arthralgia (≤6%), bone pain (≤5%), limb pain (≤5%)

Renal: Creatinine increased (grades 3/4: ≤2%)

Respiratory: Upper respiratory infection (10%), sinusitis (≤9%), pharnygolaryngeal pain (≤8%), pneumonia (≤8%), nasopharyngitis (6% to 7%), wheezing (≤5%), nasal congestion (≤5%)

Miscellaneous: Herpes infection (3% to 10%), infection (≤6%; grades 3/4: 2%), hypersensitivity (≤5%; grades 3/4: 1%), diaphoresis (≤5%), night sweats (≤5%)

<1% (Limited to important or life-threatening): Acute renal failure, alopecia, anaphylaxis, bullous exanthema, cardiac failure, dermatitis, erythema, hemolysis, infusion reaction, injection/infusion site reaction (irritation, pruritus, swelling), malaise, mucosal inflammation, myelodysplastic syndrome, pulmonary fibrosis, sepsis, septic shock, skin necrosis, somnolence, toxic epidermal necrolysis, toxic skin reactions, tumor lysis syndrome

Drug Interactions

Metabolism/Transport Effects Substrate of CYP1A2; P-glycoprotein (ABCB1); BCRP (ABCG2)

Avoid Concomitant Use There are no known interactions where it is recommended to avoid concomitant use.

Increased Effect/Toxicity

The levels/effects of Bendamustine may be increased by: CYP1A2 Inhibitors (Strong)

Decreased Effect

The levels/effects of Bendamustine may be decreased by: CYP1A2 Inducers (Strong)

Stability Prior to reconstitution, store intact vials at 25°C (77°F); excursions permitted up to 30°C (86°F). Protect from light. Use appropriate precautions for handling and disposal. Reconstitute 100 mg vial with 20 mL of sterile water for injection to a concentration of 5 mg/mL; powder usually dissolves within 5 minutes. Prior to administration, dilute appropriate dose in 500 mL NS (or $D_{2.5}$½NS) to a final concentration of 0.2-0.6 mg/mL; mix thoroughly. The solution in the vial (reconstituted with SWFI) is stable for 30 minutes (transfer to 500 mL infusion bag within that 30 minutes). The solution diluted in 500 mL for infusion is stable for 24 hours refrigerated or 3 hours at room temperature and room light. Infusion must be completed within these time frames.

Mechanism of Action Bendamustine is an alkylating agent (nitrogen mustard derivative) with a benzimidazole ring (purine analog) which demonstrates only partial cross-resistance (in vitro) with other alkylating agents. It leads to cell death via single and double strand DNA cross-linking. Bendamustine is active against quiescent and dividing cells. The primary cytotoxic activity is due to bendamustine (as compared to metabolites).

Pharmacodynamics/Kinetics

Distribution: V_{ss}: ~25 L

Protein binding: 94% to 96%

Metabolism: Hepatic, via CYP1A2 to active (minor) metabolites gamma-hydroxy bendamustine (M3) and N-desmethyl-bendamustine (M4)

Half-life elimination: Bendamustine: ~40 minutes; M3: ~3 hours; M4: ~30 minutes

Time to peak, serum: At end of infusion

Excretion: Feces (~90%); urine (1% to 10%)

Dosage I.V.: Adults:

CLL: 100 mg/m^2 on days 1 and 2 of a 28-day treatment cycle (for up to 6 cycles)

NHL: 120 mg/m^2 on days 1 and 2 of a 21-day treatment cycle for up to 8 cycles

Mantle cell lymphoma (unlabeled use): 90 mg/m^2 days 2 and 3 of a 28-day treatment cycle for up to 4 cycles (Rummel, 2005)

Multiple myeloma (unlabeled use): 90-100 mg/m^2 on days 1 and 2 of a 28-day treatment cycle for at least 2 cycles (Knop, 2005)

Dosage adjustment for toxicity:

Treatment delay:

Hematologic toxicity ≥grade 4: Delay treatment until resolves (ANC ≥1000/mm^3, platelets ≥75,000/mm^3)

Nonhematologic toxicity ≥grade 2 (clinically significant): Delay treatment until resolves to ≤grade 1

Dose modification in CLL:

Hematologic toxicity ≥grade 3: Reduce dose to 50 mg/m^2 on days 1 and 2 of each treatment cycle. For recurrent hematologic toxicity (≥grade 3), further reduce dose to 25 mg/m^2 on days 1 and 2 of the treatment cycle. May cautiously re-escalate dose in subsequent cycles.

Nonhematologic toxicity ≥grade 3 (clinically significant): Reduce dose to 50 mg/m^2 on days 1 and 2 of the treatment cycle with discretion. May cautiously re-escalate dose in subsequent cycles.

Dose modification in NHL:

Hematologic toxicity grade 4: Reduce dose to 90 mg/m^2 on days 1 and 2 of each treatment cycle. For recurrent hematologic toxicity (grade 4), further reduce dose to 60 mg/m^2 on days 1 and 2 of each treatment cycle.

Nonhematologic toxicity ≥grade 3: Reduce dose to 90 mg/m^2 on days 1 and 2 of the treatment cycle with discretion. For recurrent toxicity ≥grade 3, further reduce dose to 60 mg/m^2 on days 1 and 2 of each treatment cycle.

Dosage adjustment in renal impairment:

Mild-to-moderate renal impairment: Use with caution

Cl_{cr} <40 mL/minute: Use is not recommended

Dosage adjustment in hepatic impairment:

Mild hepatic impairment: Use with caution

Moderate hepatic impairment (AST or ALT 2.5-10 times ULN and total bilirubin 1.5-3 times ULN): Use is not recommended

Severe hepatic impairment (total bilirubin >3 times ULN): Use is not recommended

Dietary Considerations Patients should maintain adequate hydration.

Administration Infuse over 30 minutes for the treatment of CLL and over 60 minutes for NHL. Prophylactic treatment with allopurinol may be needed in patients at risk for tumor lysis syndrome. Consider premedication with antihistamines, antipyretics, and/or corticosteroids for patients with a previous grade 1 or 2 infusion reaction to bendamustine.

Monitoring Parameters CBC with differential (in clinical trials, WBC with differential and hemoglobin were monitored weekly; platelets were monitored with each cycle); serum creatinine (pretreatment); ALT, AST, and total bilirubin (pretreatment); monitor potassium and uric acid levels in patients at risk for tumor lysis syndrome

Dosage Forms Excipient information presented when available (limited, particularly for generics); consult specific product labeling.

Injection, powder for reconstitution:
Treanda®: 100 mg [contains mannitol 170 mg]

◆ **Bendamustine Hydrochloride** *see* Bendamustine *on page 181*

◆ **BeneFix®** *see* Factor IX *on page 599*

◆ **Benemid [DSC]** *see* Probenecid *on page 1239*

◆ **Benicar®** *see* Olmesartan *on page 1096*

◆ **Benicar HCT®** *see* Olmesartan and Hydrochlorothiazide *on page 1097*

◆ **Benoxinate Hydrochloride and Fluorescein Sodium** *see* Fluorescein and Benoxinate *on page 634*

◆ **Ben-Tann** *see* DiphenhydrAMINE *on page 456*

Bentoquatam (BEN toe kwa tam)

U.S. Brand Names IvyBlock® [OTC]

Index Terms Quaternium-18 Bentonite

Pharmacologic Category Topical Skin Product

Use Skin protectant for the prevention of allergic contact dermatitis to poison oak, ivy, and sumac

Dosage Children >6 years and Adults: Topical: Apply to skin 15 minutes prior to potential exposure to poison ivy, poison oak, or poison sumac, and reapply every 4 hours

Additional Information Complete prescribing information for this medication should be consulted for additional detail.

Dosage Forms Excipient information presented when available (limited, particularly for generics); consult specific product labeling.

Lotion:
IvyBlock®: 5% (120 mL) [contains alcohol 25% and benzyl alcohol]

◆ **Bentyl®** *see* Dicyclomine *on page 441*

◆ **Bentylol® (Can)** *see* Dicyclomine *on page 441*

◆ **Benuryl™ (Can)** *see* Probenecid *on page 1239*

◆ **Benylin® 3.3 mg-D-E (Can)** *see* Guaifenesin, Pseudoephedrine, and Codeine *on page 715*

◆ **Benylin® D for Infants (Can)** *see* Pseudoephedrine *on page 1265*

◆ **Benylin® DM-D (Can)** *see* Pseudoephedrine and Dextromethorphan *on page 1266*

◆ **Benylin® DM-D-E (Can)** *see* Guaifenesin, Pseudoephedrine, and Dextromethorphan *on page 715*

◆ **Benylin® DM-E (Can)** *see* Guaifenesin and Dextromethorphan *on page 710*

◆ **Benylin® E Extra Strength (Can)** *see* GuaiFENesin *on page 709*

◆ **Benzamycin®** *see* Erythromycin and Benzoyl Peroxide *on page 547*

◆ **Benzamycin® Pak** *see* Erythromycin and Benzoyl Peroxide *on page 547*

◆ **Benzathine Benzylpenicillin** *see* Penicillin G Benzathine *on page 1163*

◆ **Benzathine Penicillin G** *see* Penicillin G Benzathine *on page 1163*

◆ **Benzazoline Hydrochloride** *see* Tolazoline *on page 1485*

◆ **Benzene Hexachloride** *see* Lindane *on page 889*

◆ **Benzhexol Hydrochloride** *see* Trihexyphenidyl *on page 1518*

◆ **Benzmethyzin** *see* Procarbazine *on page 1242*

Benzocaine (BEN zoe kane)

U.S. Brand Names Americaine® Hemorrhoidal [OTC]; Anbesol® Baby [OTC]; Anbesol® Cold Sore Therapy [OTC]; Anbesol® Jr. [OTC]; Anbesol® Maximum Strength [OTC]; Anbesol® [OTC]; Benzodent® [OTC]; Bi-Zets; Boil-Ease® Pain Relieving; Cepacol® Sore Throat [OTC]; Chiggerex® Plus; Chiggerex® [OTC]; Chiggertox® [OTC]; Cylex® [OTC]; Dent's Extra Strength Toothache [OTC]; Dentapaine [OTC]; Dermoplast® Antibacterial [OTC]; Dermoplast® Pain Relieving [OTC]; Detane® [OTC]; Foille® [OTC]; HDA® Toothache [OTC]; Hurricaine® [OTC]; Ivy-Rid® [OTC]; Kank-A® Soft Brush™ [OTC]; Lanacane® Maximum Strength [OTC]; Lanacane® [OTC]; Little Teethers® [OTC]; Mycinettes® [OTC]; Orabase® with Benzocaine [OTC]; Orajel PM® Maximum Strength [OTC]; Orajel® Baby Daytime and Nighttime [OTC]; Orajel® Baby Teething Nighttime [OTC]; Orajel® Baby Teething [OTC]; Orajel® Denture Plus [OTC]; Orajel® Maximum Strength [OTC]; Orajel® Medicated Toothache [OTC]; Orajel® Mouth Sore [OTC]; Orajel® Multi-Action Cold Sore [OTC]; Orajel® Ultra Mouth Sore [OTC]; Outgro® [OTC]; Red Cross™ Canker Sore [OTC]; Rid-A-Pain Dental [OTC]; Sepasoothe®; Skeeter Stik [OTC]; Sting-Kill [OTC]; Tanac® [OTC]; Thorets [OTC]; Trocaine® [OTC]; Zilactin Toothache and Gum Pain® [OTC]; Zilactin®-B [OTC]

Canadian Brand Names Anbesol® Baby; Zilactin Baby®; Zilactin-B®

Index Terms Ethyl Aminobenzoate

Pharmacologic Category Local Anesthetic

Use Temporary relief of pain associated with pruritic dermatosis, pruritus, minor burns, acute congestive, bee stings, and insect bites; mouth and gum irritations (toothache, minor sore throat pain, canker sores, dentures, orthodontia, teething, mucositis, stomatitis); sunburn; hemorrhoids; anesthetic lubricant for passage of catheters and endoscopic tubes

Pregnancy Risk Factor C

Pregnancy Considerations Reproduction studies have not been conducted.

Lactation Excretion in breast milk unknown/use caution

Medication Safety Issues

Sound-alike/look-alike issues:
Orabase®-B may be confused with Orinase®

Contraindications Hypersensitivity to benzocaine, other ester-type local anesthetics, or any component of the formulation; secondary bacterial infection of area; ophthalmic use

Warnings/Precautions Methemoglobinemia has been reported following topical use (rare), particularly with higher concentration (14% to 20%) spray formulations applied to the mouth or mucous membranes. When applied as a spray to the mouth or throat, multiple sprays (or sprays of longer than indicated duration) are not recommended. Use caution with breathing problems (asthma, bronchitis, emphysema, in smokers), inflamed/damaged mucosa, heart disease, children <6 months of age, and hemoglobin or enzyme abnormalities (glucose-6-phosphate dehydrogenase deficiency, hemoglobin-M disease, NADH-methemoglobin reductase deficiency, pyruvate-kinase deficiency). Alternatives to benzocaine sprays, such as topical lidocaine preparations, should be considered for patients at higher risk of this reaction.

The classical clinical finding of methemoglobinemia is chocolate brown-colored arterial blood. However, suspected cases should be confirmed by co-oximetry, which yields a direct and accurate measure of methemoglobin levels. Standard pulse oximetry readings or arterial blood gas values are not reliable. Clinically significant methemoglobinemia requires immediate treatment.

When used for self-medication (OTC), notify healthcare provider if condition worsens or does not improve within 7 days, or if swelling, rash, or fever develops. Do not use on open wounds. Avoid contact with the eyes.

Adverse Reactions Frequency not defined.

Hematologic: Methemoglobinemia

Local: Burning, contact dermatitis, edema, erythema, pruritus, rash, stinging, tenderness, urticaria

Miscellaneous: Hypersensitivity

Drug Interactions

Avoid Concomitant Use There are no known interactions where it is recommended to avoid concomitant use.

Increased Effect/Toxicity There are no known significant interactions involving an increase in effect.

Decreased Effect There are no known significant interactions involving a decrease in effect.

Mechanism of Action Ester local anesthetic blocks both the initiation and conduction of nerve impulses by decreasing the neuronal membrane's permeability to sodium ions, which results in inhibition of depolarization with resultant blockade of conduction

Pharmacodynamics/Kinetics

Absorption: Topical: Poor to intact skin; well absorbed from mucous membranes and traumatized skin

Metabolism: Hepatic (to a lesser extent) and plasma via hydrolysis by cholinesterase

Excretion: Urine (as metabolites)

Dosage Note: These are general dosing guidelines; refer to specific product labeling for dosing instructions.

Children ≥4 months: Topical (oral): Teething pain: 7.5% to 10%: Apply to affected gum area up to 4 times daily

Children ≥2 years and Adults:

Topical:

Bee stings, insect bites, minor burns, sunburn: 5% to 20%: Apply to affected area 3-4 times a day as needed. In cases of bee stings, remove stinger before treatment.

Lubricant for passage of catheters and instruments: 20%: Apply evenly to exterior of instrument prior to use.

Topical (oral): Mouth and gum irritation: 10% to 20%: Apply thin layer to affected area up to 4 times daily

Children ≥5 years and Adults: Oral: Sore throat: Allow 1 lozenge (10-15 mg) to dissolve slowly in mouth; may repeat every 2 hours as needed

Children ≥12 years and Adults: Rectal: Hemorrhoids: 5% to 20%: Apply externally to affected area up to 6 times daily

Monitoring Parameters Monitor patients for signs and symptoms of methemoglobinemia such as pallor, cyanosis, nausea, muscle weakness, dizziness, confusion, agitation, dyspnea and tachycardia. The classical clinical finding of methemoglobinemia is chocolate brown-colored arterial blood. However, suspected cases should be confirmed by co-oximetry, which yields a direct and accurate measure of methemoglobin levels. Standard pulse oximetry readings or arterial blood gas values are not reliable. Clinically significant methemoglobinemia requires immediate treatment.

Dosage Forms Excipient information presented when available (limited, particularly for generics); consult specific product labeling. [DSC] = Discontinued product

Aerosol, oral spray:

Hurricaine®: 20% (60 mL) [dye free; cherry flavor]

Aerosol, topical spray:

Dermoplast® Antibacterial: 20% (83 mL) [contains aloe vera, benzethonium chloride, menthol]

Dermoplast® Pain Relieving: 20% (60 mL, 83 mL) [contains menthol]

Foille®: 5% (92 g) [contains chloroxylenol 0.63% and corn oil]

Ivy-Rid®: 2% (83 mL)

Lanacane® Maximum Strength: 20% (120 mL) [contains ethanol 36%]

Combination package (Orajel® Baby Daytime and Nighttime):

Gel, oral [Daytime Regular Formula]: 7.5% (5.3 g)

Gel, oral [Nighttime Formula]: 10% (5.3 g)

Cream, oral:

Benzodent®: 20% (7.5 g, 30 g)

Orajel PM® Maximum Strength: 20% (5.3 g, 7 g) [contains menthol]

Cream, topical:

Lanacane®: 6% (30 g, 60 g)

Lanacane® Maximum Strength: 20% (30 g)

Gel, oral:

Anbesol®: 10% (7.5 g) [contains benzyl alcohol; cool mint flavor]

Anbesol® Baby: 7.5% (7.5 g) [contains benzoic acid; grape flavor]

Anbesol® Jr.: 10% (7 g) [contains benzyl alcohol; bubble gum flavor]

Anbesol® Maximum Strength: 20% (7.5 g, 10 g) [contains benzyl alcohol]

Dentapaine: 20% (11 g) [contains clove oil]

HDA® Toothache: 6.5% (15 mL) [contains benzyl alcohol]

Hurricaine®: 20% (5 g) [dye free; wild cherry flavor]; (30 g) [dye free; mint, pina colada, watermelon, and wild cherry flavors]

Kank-A® Soft Brush™: 20% (2 mL) [packaged in applicator with brush tip]

Little Teethers®: 7.5% (9.4 g) [cherry flavor]

Orabase® with Benzocaine®: 20% (7 g) [contains ethanol 48%; mild mint flavor]

Orajel®: 10% (5.3 g, 7 g, 9.4 g)

Orajel® Baby Teething: 7.5% (9.4 g, 11.9 g) [cherry flavor]

Orajel® Baby Teething Nighttime: 10% (5.3 g)

Orajel® Denture Plus: 15% (9 g) [contains menthol 2%, ethanol 66.7%]

Orajel® Maximum Strength: 20% (5.3 g, 7 g, 9.4 g, 11.9 g)

Orajel® Mouth Sore: 20% (5.3 g, 9.4 g, 11.9 g) [contains allantoin, benzalkonium chloride 0.02%, zinc chloride 0.1%]

Orajel® Multi-Action Cold Sore: 20% (9.4 g) [contains allantoin 0.5%, camphor 3%, dimethicone 2%]

Orajel® Ultra Mouth Sore: 15% (9.4 g) [contains ethanol 66.7%, menthol 2%]

Zilactin®-B: 10% (7.5 g)

Gel, topical:

Detane®: 7.5% (15 g)

Liquid, oral:

Anbesol®: 10% (9 mL) [cool mint flavor; contains benzyl alcohol]

Anbesol® Maximum Strength: 20% (9 mL) [contains benzyl alcohol]

Hurricaine®: 20% (30 mL) [pina colada and wild cherry flavors; dye free]

Orajel® Baby Teething: 7.5% (13 mL) [very berry flavor]

Orajel® Maximum Strength: 20% (13 mL) [contains ethanol 44%, tartrazine]

Tanac®: 10% (13 mL) [contains benzalkonium chloride]

Liquid, oral [drops]:

Rid-A-Pain Dental: 6.3% (30 mL) [contains ethanol 70%]

Liquid, topical:

Chiggertox®: 2% (30 mL)

Outgro®: 20% (9 mL)

Skeeter Stik: 5% (14 mL) [contains menthol]

Lozenge: 6 mg (18s) [contains menthol]; 15 mg (10s)

Bi-Zets: 15 mg (10s)

Cepacol® Sore Throat: 15 mg (18s) [contains cetylpyridinium, menthol; cherry, citrus, and honey lemon flavors]

Cepacol® Sore Throat: 15 mg (16s) [sugar free; contains cetylpyridinium, menthol; cherry and menthol flavors]
Cylex®: 15 mg (12s) [sugar free; contains cetylpyridinium chloride 5 mg; cherry flavor]
Mycinettes®: 15 mg (12s) [sugar free; contains sodium 9 mg; cherry or regular flavor]
Sepasoothe®: 10 mg (6s, 24s, 100s, 250s, 500s) [sugar free; contains cetylpyridium 0.5 mg/lozenge; wild cherry flavor]
Thorets: 18 mg (300s) [sugar free]
Trocaine®: 10 mg (50s, 300s)
Ointment, oral:
Anbesol® Cold Sore Therapy: 20% (7.1 g) [contains benzyl alcohol, allantoin, aloe, camphor, menthol, vitamin E]
Red Cross™ Canker Sore: 20% (7.5 g) [contains coconut oil]
Ointment, rectal:
Americaine® Hemorrhoidal: 20% (30 g)
Ointment, topical:
Boil-Ease® Pain Relieving: 20% (30 g)
Chiggerex®: 2% (50 g) [contains aloe vera] [DSC]
Chiggerex® Plus: 6% (50 g) [contains aloe]
Foille®: 5% (3.5 g, 14 g, 28 g) [contains chloroxylenol 0.1%, benzyl alcohol; corn oil base]
Pads, topical:
Sting-Kill: 20% (8s) [contains menthol and tartrazine]
Paste, oral:
Orabase® with Benzocaine: 20% (6 g)
Swabs, oral:
Hurricaine®: 20% (6s, 100s) [dye free; wild cherry flavor]
Orajel® Baby Teething: 7.5% (12s) [berry flavor]
Orajel® Medicated Mouth Sore, Orajel® Medicated Toothache: 20% (8s, 12s) [contains tartrazine]
Zilactin® Toothache and Gum Pain: 20% (8s) [grape flavor]
Swabs, topical:
Boil-Ease® Pain Relieving: 20% (12s) [contains tartrazine]
Sting-Kill: 20% (5s) [contains menthol and tartrazine]
Wax, oral:
Dent's Extra Strength Toothache Gum: 20% (1 g)

- **Benzocaine and Antipyrine** *see* Antipyrine and Benzocaine *on page 124*

Benzocaine, Butamben, and Tetracaine
(BEN zoe kane, byoo TAM ben, & TET ra kane)

U.S. Brand Names Cetacaine®; Exactacain™
Index Terms Benzocaine, Butamben, and Tetracaine Hydrochloride; Benzocaine, Butyl Aminobenzoate, and Tetracaine; Butamben, Tetracaine, and Benzocaine; Tetracaine, Benzocaine, and Butamben
Pharmacologic Category Local Anesthetic
Use Topical anesthetic to control pain in surgical or endoscopic procedures; anesthetic for accessible mucous membranes except for the eyes
Dosage Topical anesthetic: **Note:** Decrease dose in the acutely-ill patient.
Children: Dose has not been established; dose reduction is suggested
Adults:
Cetacaine®:
Aerosol: Apply for ≤1 second; use of sprays >2 seconds is contraindicated
Gel: Apply ~1/2 inch (13 mm) x 3/16 inch (5 mm); application of >1 inch (26 cm) x 3/16 inch (5 mm) is contraindicated
Liquid: Apply 6-7 drops (0.2 mL); application of >12-14 drops (0.4 mL) is contraindicated
Exactacain™: 3 metered sprays (use of >6 metered sprays is contraindicated)
Elderly: Dose reduction is suggested
Additional Information Complete prescribing information for this medication should be consulted for additional detail.
Dosage Forms Excipient information presented when available (limited, particularly for generics); consult specific product labeling.
Aerosol, topical [spray]:
Cetacaine®: Benzocaine 14%, butamben 2%, and tetracaine hydrochloride 2% (56 g) [delivers benzocaine 28 mg, butamben 4 mg, and tetracaine hydrochloride 4 mg per second; contains benzalkonium chloride and CFCs; packaged with cannula]
Exactacain™: Benzocaine 14%, butamben 2%, and tetracaine hydrochloride 2% (60 g) [delivers benzocaine 9.3 mg, butamben 1.3 mg, and tetracaine 1.3 mg per metered spray; contains benzalkonium chloride; cherry flavor; packaged with 100 disposable applicators]
Gel, topical:
Cetacaine®: Benzocaine 14%, butamben 2%, and tetracaine hydrochloride 2% (29 g) [provides benzocaine 28 mg, butamben 4 mg and tetracaine hydrochloride 4 mg per 0.5 inch (13 mm) x 3/16 inch (5 mm) application; contains benzalkonium chloride]
Liquid, topical:
Cetacaine®: Benzocaine 14%, butamben 2%, and tetracaine hydrochloride 2% (56 g) [provides benzocaine 28 mg, butamben 4 mg, and tetracaine hydrochloride 4 mg per 6-7 drops (0.2 mL); contains benzalkonium chloride]

- **Benzocaine, Butamben, and Tetracaine Hydrochloride** *see* Benzocaine, Butamben, and Tetracaine *on page 185*
- **Benzocaine, Butyl Aminobenzoate, and Tetracaine** *see* Benzocaine, Butamben, and Tetracaine *on page 185*
- **Benzodent® [OTC]** *see* Benzocaine *on page 183*
- **Benzoic Acid, Methenamine, Methylene Blue, Phenyl Salicylate, and Hyoscyamine** *see* Methenamine, Phenyl Salicylate, Methylene Blue, Benzoic Acid, and Hyoscyamine *on page 962*

Benzonatate (ben ZOE na tate)

U.S. Brand Names Tessalon®
Canadian Brand Names Tessalon®
Pharmacologic Category Antitussive
Use Symptomatic relief of nonproductive cough
Pregnancy Risk Factor C
Dosage Children >10 years and Adults: Oral: 100 mg 3 times/day or every 4 hours up to 600 mg/day
Additional Information Complete prescribing information for this medication should be consulted for additional detail.
Dosage Forms Excipient information presented when available (limited, particularly for generics); consult specific product labeling.
Capsule, softgel: 100 mg, 200 mg
Tessalon®: 100 mg, 200 mg

- **Benzoyl Peroxide and Erythromycin** *see* Erythromycin and Benzoyl Peroxide *on page 547*

Benzoyl Peroxide and Hydrocortisone
(BEN zoe il peer OKS ide & hye droe KOR ti sone)

U.S. Brand Names Vanoxide-HC®
Canadian Brand Names Vanoxide-HC®
Index Terms Hydrocortisone and Benzoyl Peroxide
Pharmacologic Category Acne Products; Topical Skin Product; Topical Skin Product, Acne

Use Treatment of acne vulgaris and oily skin

Pregnancy Risk Factor C

Dosage Adolescents and Adults: Topical: Shake well; apply thin film 1-3 times/day; gently massage into skin

Additional Information Complete prescribing information for this medication should be consulted for additional detail.

Dosage Forms Excipient information presented when available (limited, particularly for generics); consult specific product labeling.

Lotion: Benzoyl peroxide 5% and hydrocortisone acetate 0.5% (25 mL)

Benztropine (BENZ troe peen)

U.S. Brand Names Cogentin®

Canadian Brand Names Apo-Benztropine®

Index Terms Benztropine Mesylate

Pharmacologic Category Anti-Parkinson's Agent, Anticholinergic; Anticholinergic Agent

Additional Appendix Information

Antiparkinsonian Agents *on page 1643*

Use Adjunctive treatment of Parkinson's disease; treatment of drug-induced extrapyramidal symptoms (except tardive dyskinesia)

Pregnancy Risk Factor C

Lactation Excretion in breast milk unknown/use caution

Medication Safety Issues

Sound-alike/look-alike issues:

Benztropine may be confused with bromocriptine

Contraindications Hypersensitivity to benztropine or any component of the formulation; pyloric or duodenal obstruction, stenosing peptic ulcers; bladder neck obstructions; achalasia; myasthenia gravis; children <3 years of age

Warnings/Precautions Use with caution in older children (dose has not been established). Use with caution in hot weather or during exercise. May cause anhydrosis and hyperthermia, which may be severe. The risk is increased in hot environments, particularly in the elderly, alcoholics, patients with CNS disease, and those with prolonged outdoor exposure.

Elderly patients frequently develop increased sensitivity and require strict dosage regulation - side effects may be more severe in elderly patients with atherosclerotic changes. Use with caution in patients with tachycardia, cardiac arrhythmias, hypertension, hypotension, glaucoma, prostatic hyperplasia (especially in the elderly), any tendency toward urinary retention, liver or kidney disorders, and obstructive disease of the GI or GU tract. When given in large doses or to susceptible patients, may cause weakness and inability to move particular muscle groups.

May be associated with confusion or hallucinations (generally at higher dosages). Intensification of symptoms or toxic psychosis may occur in patients with mental disorders. May cause CNS depression, which may impair physical or mental abilities; patients must be cautioned about performing tasks which require mental alertness (eg, operating machinery or driving). Benztropine does not relieve symptoms of tardive dyskinesia.

Adverse Reactions Frequency not defined.

Cardiovascular: Tachycardia

Central nervous system: Confusion, disorientation, memory impairment, toxic psychosis, visual hallucinations

Dermatologic: Rash

Endocrine & metabolic: Heat stroke, hyperthermia

Gastrointestinal: Constipation, dry throat, ileus, nasal dryness, nausea, vomiting, xerostomia

Genitourinary: Urinary retention, dysuria

Ocular: Blurred vision, mydriasis

Miscellaneous: Fever

Drug Interactions

Metabolism/Transport Effects Substrate of CYP2D6 (minor)

Avoid Concomitant Use There are no known interactions where it is recommended to avoid concomitant use.

Increased Effect/Toxicity

Benztropine may increase the levels/effects of: Anticholinergics; Cannabinoids; Potassium Chloride

The levels/effects of Benztropine may be increased by: Pramlintide

Decreased Effect

Benztropine may decrease the levels/effects of: Acetylcholinesterase Inhibitors (Central); Secretin

The levels/effects of Benztropine may be decreased by: Acetylcholinesterase Inhibitors (Central)

Ethanol/Nutrition/Herb Interactions Ethanol: Avoid ethanol (may increase CNS depression).

Mechanism of Action Possesses both anticholinergic and antihistaminic effects. *In vitro* anticholinergic activity approximates that of atropine; *in vivo* it is only about half as active as atropine. Animal data suggest its antihistaminic activity and duration of action approach that of pyrilamine maleate. May also inhibit the reuptake and storage of dopamine, thereby prolonging the action of dopamine.

Pharmacodynamics/Kinetics

Onset of action: Oral: Within 1 hour; Parenteral: Within 15 minutes

Duration: 6-48 hours

Metabolism: Hepatic (N-oxidation, N-dealkylation, and ring hydroxylation)

Bioavailability: 29%

Dosage Use in children ≤3 years of age should be reserved for life-threatening emergencies

Drug-induced extrapyramidal symptom: Oral, I.M., I.V.:

Children >3 years: 0.02-0.05 mg/kg/dose 1-2 times/day

Adults: 1-4 mg/dose 1-2 times/day

Acute dystonia: Adults: I.M., I.V.: 1-2 mg

Parkinsonism: Oral:

Adults: 0.5-6 mg/day in 1-2 divided doses; if one dose is greater, administer at bedtime; titrate dose in 0.5 mg increments at 5- to 6-day intervals

Elderly: Initial: 0.5 mg once or twice daily; increase by 0.5 mg as needed at 5-6 days; maximum: 4 mg/day

Monitoring Parameters Symptoms of EPS or Parkinson's, pulse, anticholinergic effects

Additional Information No significant difference in onset of I.M. or I.V. injection; therefore, there is usually no need to use the I.V. route. Improvement is sometimes noticeable a few minutes after injection.

Dosage Forms Excipient information presented when available (limited, particularly for generics); consult specific product labeling.

Injection, solution, as mesylate (Cogentin®): 1 mg/mL (2 mL)

Tablet, as mesylate: 0.5 mg, 1 mg, 2 mg

◆ **Benztropine Mesylate** *see* Benztropine *on page 186*

◆ **Benzylpenicillin Benzathine** *see* Penicillin G Benzathine *on page 1163*

◆ **Benzylpenicillin Potassium** *see* Penicillin G (Parenteral/Aqueous) *on page 1164*

◆ **Benzylpenicillin Sodium** *see* Penicillin G (Parenteral/Aqueous) *on page 1164*

Benzylpenicilloyl-polylysine
(BEN zil pen i SIL oyl pol i LIE seen)

U.S. Brand Names Pre-Pen® [DSC]

Index Terms Penicilloyl-polylysine; PPL

Pharmacologic Category Diagnostic Agent

Use Adjunct in assessing the risk of administering penicillin (penicillin or benzylpenicillin) in adults with a history of clinical penicillin hypersensitivity

Pregnancy Risk Factor C

Dosage PPL is administered by a scratch technique or by intradermal injection. For initial testing, PPL should always be applied via the scratch technique. **Do not administer intradermally to patients who have positive reactions to a scratch test.** PPL test alone does not identify those patients who react to a minor antigenic determinant and does not appear to predict reliably the occurrence of late reactions.

Scratch test: Use scratch technique with a 20-gauge needle to make 3-5 mm nonbleeding scratch on epidermis, apply a small drop of solution to scratch, rub in gently with applicator or toothpick. A positive reaction consists of a pale wheal surrounding the scratch site which develops within 10 minutes and ranges from 5-15 mm or more in diameter.

Intradermal test: Use intradermal test with a tuberculin syringe with a 26- to 30-gauge short bevel needle; a dose of 0.01-0.02 mL is injected intradermally. A control of 0.9% sodium chloride should be injected at least 1.5" from the PPL test site. Most skin responses to the intradermal test will develop within 5-15 minutes.

Interpretation:

(-) Negative: No reaction

(±) Ambiguous: Wheal only slightly larger than original bleb with or without erythematous flare and larger than control site

(+) Positive: Itching and marked increase in size of original bleb

Control site should be reactionless

Additional Information Complete prescribing information for this medication should be consulted for additional detail.

Dosage Forms Excipient information presented when available (limited, particularly for generics); consult specific product labeling. [DSC] = Discontinued product

Injection, solution: 6 x 10^{-5} M (0.25 mL) [DSC]

Beractant (ber AKT ant)

U.S. Brand Names Survanta®

Canadian Brand Names Survanta®

Index Terms Bovine Lung Surfactant; Natural Lung Surfactant

Pharmacologic Category Lung Surfactant

Use Prevention and treatment of respiratory distress syndrome (RDS) in premature infants

Prophylactic therapy: Body weight <1250 g in infants at risk for developing, or with evidence of, surfactant deficiency (administer within 15 minutes of birth)

Rescue therapy: Treatment of infants with RDS confirmed by x-ray and requiring mechanical ventilation (administer as soon as possible - within 8 hours of age)

Medication Safety Issues

Sound-alike/look-alike issues:

Survanta® may be confused with Sufenta®

Warnings/Precautions For intratracheal administration only. Rapidly affects oxygenation and lung compliance; restrict use to a highly-supervised clinical setting with immediate availability of clinicians experienced in intubation and ventilatory management of premature infants. Transient episodes of bradycardia and decreased oxygen saturation occur. Discontinue dosing procedure and initiate measures to alleviate the condition; may reinstitute after the patient is stable. Produces rapid improvements in lung oxygenation and compliance that may require frequent adjustments to oxygen delivery and ventilator settings.

Adverse Reactions During the dosing procedure:

>10%: Cardiovascular: Transient bradycardia

1% to 10%: Respiratory: Oxygen desaturation

<1% (Limited to important or life-threatening): Apnea, endotracheal tube blockage, hypercarbia, hyper-/hypotension, post-treatment nosocomial sepsis probability increased, pulmonary air leaks, pulmonary interstitial emphysema, vasoconstriction

Drug Interactions

Avoid Concomitant Use There are no known interactions where it is recommended to avoid concomitant use.

Increased Effect/Toxicity There are no known significant interactions involving an increase in effect.

Decreased Effect There are no known significant interactions involving a decrease in effect.

Stability Refrigerate; protect from light. Prior to administration, warm by standing at room temperature for 20 minutes or held in hand for 8 minutes. **Artificial warming methods should not be used.** Unused, unopened vials warmed to room temperature may be returned to the refrigerator within 8 hours of warming only once.

Mechanism of Action Replaces deficient or ineffective endogenous lung surfactant in neonates with respiratory distress syndrome (RDS) or in neonates at risk of developing RDS. Surfactant prevents the alveoli from collapsing during expiration by lowering surface tension between air and alveolar surfaces.

Pharmacodynamics/Kinetics Excretion: Clearance: Alveolar clearance is rapid

Dosage

Prophylactic treatment: Administer 100 mg phospholipids (4 mL/kg) intratracheal as soon as possible; as many as 4 doses may be administered during the first 48 hours of life, no more frequently than 6 hours apart. The need for additional doses is determined by evidence of continuing respiratory distress; if the infant is still intubated and requiring at least 30% inspired oxygen to maintain a PaO_2 ≤80 torr.

Rescue treatment: Administer 100 mg phospholipids (4 mL/kg) as soon as the diagnosis of RDS is made; may repeat if needed, no more frequently than every 6 hours to a maximum of 4 doses

Administration

For intratracheal administration only

Suction infant prior to administration. Inspect solution to verify complete mixing of the suspension.

Administer intratracheally by instillation through a 5-French end-hole catheter inserted into the infant's endotracheal tube.

Administer the dose in four 1 mL/kg aliquots. Each quarter-dose is instilled over 2-3 seconds; each quarter-dose is administered with the infant in a different position. Slightly downward inclination with head turned to the right, then repeat with head turned to the left; then slightly upward inclination with head turned to the right, then repeat with head turned to the left.

Monitoring Parameters Continuous ECG and transcutaneous O_2 saturation should be monitored during administration; frequent arterial blood gases are necessary to prevent postdosing hyperoxia and hypocarbia

Additional Information Each mL contains 25 mg phospholipids suspended in 0.9% sodium chloride solution. Contents of 1 mL: 0.5-1.75 mg triglycerides, 1.4-3.5 mg free fatty acids, and <1 mg protein.

Dosage Forms Excipient information presented when available (limited, particularly for generics); consult specific product labeling.

Suspension, intratracheal [preservative free; bovine derived]:

Survanta®: 25 mg/mL (4 mL, 8 mL)

◆ **9-Beta-D-Ribofuranosyladenine** *see* Adenosine *on page 46*

◆ **Betacaine® (Can)** *see* Lidocaine *on page 884*

Beta-Carotene (BAY ta KARE oh teen)

U.S. Brand Names A-Caro-25; B-Caro-T™; Lumitene™

Pharmacologic Category Vitamin, Fat Soluble

Unlabeled/Investigational Use Prophylaxis and treatment of polymorphous light eruption; prophylaxis against photosensitivity reactions in erythropoietic protoporphyria

Pregnancy Risk Factor C

Dosage Oral:

Children <14 years: 30-150 mg/day

Adults: 30-300 mg/day

Additional Information Complete prescribing information for this medication should be consulted for additional detail.

Dosage Forms Excipient information presented when available (limited, particularly for generics); consult specific product labeling.

Capsule, softgel: 10,000 int. units (6 mg); 25,000 int. units (15 mg)

A-Caro-25: 25,000 int. units (15 mg) [contains soy]

B-Caro-T™: 25,000 int. units (15 mg) [contains soybean lecithin and soybean oil]

Capsule:

Lumitene™: 50,000 int. units (30 mg)

Tablet: 10,000 int. units

◆ **Betaderm (Can)** *see* Betamethasone *on page 188*

◆ **Betadine®** *see* Povidone-Iodine *on page 1222*

◆ **Betadine® First Aid Antibiotics + Moisturizer [OTC] [DSC]** *see* Bacitracin and Polymyxin B *on page 171*

◆ **Betagan®** *see* Levobunolol *on page 873*

◆ **Beta-HC®** *see* Hydrocortisone *on page 743*

Betaine (BAY ta een)

U.S. Brand Names Cystadane®

Canadian Brand Names Cystadane®

Index Terms Betaine Anhydrous

Pharmacologic Category Homocystinuria, Treatment Agent

Use Treatment of homocystinuria (eg, deficiencies or defects in cystathionine beta-synthase [CBS], 5,10-methylene tetrahydrofolate reductase [MTHFR], and cobalamin cofactor metabolism [CBL])

Pregnancy Risk Factor C

Medication Safety Issues

Sound-alike/look-alike issues:

Betaine may be confused with Betadine®

Cystadane® may be confused with cysteamine, cysteine

Dosage Oral:

Children <3 years: Initial dose: 100 mg/kg/day given once daily or in 2 divided doses; increase weekly by 50 mg/kg increments, as needed

Children ≥3 years and Adults: Usual dose: 6 g/day administered in divided doses of 3 g twice daily; dosages of up to 20 g/day have been necessary to control homocysteine levels in some patients

Note: Dosage in all patients can be gradually increased until plasma total homocysteine is undetectable or present only in small amounts. One study in six patients with CBS deficiency, ranging from 6-17 years of age, showed minimal benefit from exceeding a twice daily dosing schedule and a 150 mg/kg/day dosage.

Additional Information Complete prescribing information for this medication should be consulted for additional detail.

Dosage Forms Excipient information presented when available (limited, particularly for generics); consult specific product labeling.

Powder for oral solution, anhydrous:

Cystadane®: 1 g/scoop (180 g) [1 scoop = 1.7 mL]

◆ **Betaine Anhydrous** *see* Betaine *on page 188*

◆ **Betaject™ (Can)** *see* Betamethasone *on page 188*

◆ **Betaloc® (Can)** *see* Metoprolol *on page 982*

◆ **Betaloc® Durules® (Can)** *see* Metoprolol *on page 982*

Betamethasone (bay ta METH a sone)

U.S. Brand Names Beta-Val®; Celestone®; Celestone® Soluspan®; Diprolene®; Diprolene® AF; Luxiq®

Canadian Brand Names Betaderm; Betaject™; Betnesol®; Betnovate®; Celestone® Soluspan®; Diprolene® Glycol; Diprosone®; Ectosone; Prevex® B; Taro-Sone®; Topilene®; Topisone®; Valisone® Scalp Lotion

Index Terms Betamethasone Dipropionate; Betamethasone Dipropionate, Augmented; Betamethasone Sodium Phosphate; Betamethasone Valerate; Flubenisolone

Pharmacologic Category Corticosteroid, Systemic; Corticosteroid, Topical

Additional Appendix Information

Corticosteroids *on page 1652*

Use Inflammatory dermatoses such as seborrheic or atopic dermatitis, neurodermatitis, anogenital pruritus, psoriasis, inflammatory phase of xerosis

Unlabeled/Investigational Use Accelerate fetal lung maturation in patients with preterm labor

Pregnancy Risk Factor C

Pregnancy Considerations Adverse events have been observed with corticosteroids in animal reproduction studies. Betamethasone crosses the placenta; approximately 25% is metabolized by placental enzymes to an inactive metabolite. Due to its positive effect on stimulating fetal lung maturation, the injection is often used in patients with premature labor (24-34 weeks gestation). Topical products are not recommended for extensive use, in large quantities, or for long periods of time in pregnant women. Some studies have shown an association between first trimester systemic corticosteroid use and oral clefts; adverse events in the fetus/neonate have been noted in case reports following large doses of systemic corticosteroids during pregnancy. Women exposed to betamethasone during pregnancy for the treatment of an autoimmune disease may contact the OTIS Autoimmune Diseases Study at 877-311-8972.

Lactation Excretion in breast milk unknown/use caution

Medication Safety Issues

Sound-alike/look-alike issues:

Luxiq® may be confused with Lasix®

International issues:

Beta-Val® may be confused with Betanol® which is a brand name for metipranolol in Monaco

Contraindications Hypersensitivity to betamethasone, other corticosteroids, or any component of the formulation; systemic fungal infections; I.M. administration contraindicated in idiopathic thrombocytopenia purpura

Warnings/Precautions Very high potency topical products are not for treatment of rosacea, perioral dermatitis; not for use on face, groin, or axillae; not for use in a diapered area. Avoid concurrent use of other corticosteroids.

May cause hypercorticism or suppression of hypothalamic-pituitary-adrenal (HPA) axis, particularly in younger children or in patients receiving high doses for prolonged periods. HPA axis suppression may lead to adrenal crisis. Withdrawal and discontinuation of a corticosteroid should be done slowly and carefully. Particular care is required when patients are transferred from systemic corticosteroids to inhaled products due to possible adrenal insufficiency or withdrawal from steroids, including an increase in allergic symptoms. Patients receiving >20 mg per day of prednisone (or equivalent) may be most susceptible. Fatalities have occurred due to adrenal insufficiency in asthmatic patients during and after transfer from systemic corticosteroids to aerosol steroids; aerosol steroids do not provide the systemic steroid needed to treat patients having trauma, surgery, or infections. In stressful situations, HPA axis-suppressed patients should receive adequate supplementation with natural glucocorticoids (hydrocortisone or cortisone) rather than betamethasone (due to lack of mineralocorticoid activity).

Acute myopathy has been reported with high dose corticosteroids, usually in patients with neuromuscular transmission disorders; may involve ocular and/or respiratory muscles; monitor creatine kinase; recovery may be delayed. Corticosteroid use may cause psychiatric disturbances, including depression, euphoria, insomnia, mood swings, and personality changes. Pre-existing psychiatric conditions may be exacerbated by corticosteroid use. Prolonged use of corticosteroids may also increase the incidence of secondary infection, mask acute infection (including fungal infections), prolong or exacerbate viral infections, or limit response to vaccines. Exposure to chickenpox should be avoided; corticosteroids should not be used to treat ocular herpes simplex. Corticosteroids should not be used for cerebral malaria or viral hepatitis. Close observation is required in patients with latent tuberculosis and/or TB reactivity; restrict use in active TB (only in conjunction with antituberculosis treatment). Prolonged treatment with corticosteroids has been associated with the development of Kaposi's sarcoma (case reports); if noted, discontinuation of therapy should be considered. High-dose corticosteroids should not be used to manage acute head injury.

Use with caution in patients with thyroid disease, hepatic impairment, renal impairment, cardiovascular disease, diabetes, glaucoma, cataracts, myasthenia gravis, patients at risk for osteoporosis, patients at risk for seizures, or GI diseases (diverticulitis, peptic ulcer, ulcerative colitis) due to perforation risk. Use caution following acute MI (corticosteroids have been associated with myocardial rupture). Because of the risk of adverse effects, systemic corticosteroids should be used cautiously in the elderly in the smallest possible effective dose for the shortest duration. Do not use occlusive dressings on weeping or exudative lesions and general caution with occlusive dressings should be observed; adverse effects may be increased. Discontinue if skin irritation or contact dermatitis should occur; do not use in patients with decreased skin circulation. Withdraw therapy with gradual tapering of dose. May affect growth velocity; growth should be routinely monitored in pediatric patients. Topical use in patients ≤12 years of age is not recommended.

Adverse Reactions

Systemic:

Cardiovascular: Congestive heart failure, edema, hyper-/hypotension

Central nervous system: Dizziness, headache, insomnia, intracranial pressure increased, lightheadedness, nervousness, pseudotumor cerebri, seizure, vertigo

Dermatologic: Ecchymoses, facial erythema, fragile skin, hirsutism, hyper-/hypopigmentation, perioral dermatitis (oral), petechiae, striae, wound healing impaired

Endocrine & metabolic: Amenorrhea, Cushing's syndrome, diabetes mellitus, growth suppression, hyperglycemia, hypokalemia, menstrual irregularities, pituitary-adrenal axis suppression, protein catabolism, sodium retention, water retention

Gastrointestinal: Abdominal distention, appetite increased, hiccups, indigestion, peptic ulcer, pancreatitis, ulcerative esophagitis

Local: Injection site reactions (intra-articular use), sterile abscess

Neuromuscular & skeletal: Arthralgia, muscle atrophy, fractures, muscle weakness, myopathy, osteoporosis, necrosis (femoral and humeral heads)

Ocular: Cataracts, glaucoma, intraocular pressure increased

Miscellaneous: Anaphylactoid reaction, diaphoresis, hypersensitivity, secondary infection

Topical:

Dermatologic: Acneiform eruptions, allergic dermatitis, burning, dry skin, erythema, folliculitis, hypertrichosis, irritation, miliaria, pruritus, skin atrophy, striae, vesiculation

Endocrine and metabolic effects have occasionally been reported with topical use.

Drug Interactions

Metabolism/Transport Effects **Inhibits** CYP3A4 (weak)

Avoid Concomitant Use

Avoid concomitant use of Betamethasone with any of the following: Natalizumab; Vaccines (Live)

Increased Effect/Toxicity

Betamethasone may increase the levels/effects of: Acetylcholinesterase Inhibitors; Amphotericin B; CycloSPORINE; Loop Diuretics; Natalizumab; NSAID (COX-2 Inhibitor); NSAID (Nonselective); Thiazide Diuretics; Vaccines (Live); Warfarin

The levels/effects of Betamethasone may be increased by: Antifungal Agents (Azole Derivatives, Systemic); Aprepitant; Calcium Channel Blockers (Nondihydropyridine); CycloSPORINE; Estrogen Derivatives; Fluconazole; Fosaprepitant; Macrolide Antibiotics; Neuromuscular-Blocking Agents (Nondepolarizing); Quinolone Antibiotics; Salicylates; Trastuzumab

Decreased Effect

Betamethasone may decrease the levels/effects of: Antidiabetic Agents; Calcitriol; Corticorelin; Isoniazid; Salicylates; Vaccines (Inactivated)

The levels/effects of Betamethasone may be decreased by: Aminoglutethimide; Antacids; Barbiturates; Bile Acid Sequestrants; Echinacea; Primidone; Rifamycin Derivatives

Ethanol/Nutrition/Herb Interactions

Ethanol: Avoid ethanol (may enhance gastric mucosal irritation).

Food: Betamethasone interferes with calcium absorption.

Herb/Nutraceutical: Avoid cat's claw, echinacea (have immunostimulant properties).

Mechanism of Action Controls the rate of protein synthesis; depresses the migration of polymorphonuclear leukocytes, fibroblasts; reverses capillary permeability and lysosomal stabilization at the cellular level to prevent or control inflammation

Pharmacodynamics/Kinetics

Protein binding: 64%

Metabolism: Hepatic

Half-life elimination: 6.5 hours

Time to peak, serum: I.V.: 10-36 minutes

Excretion: Urine (<5% as unchanged drug)

Dosage Base dosage on severity of disease and patient response

Children: Use lowest dose listed as initial dose for adrenocortical insufficiency (physiologic replacement)

I.M.: 0.0175-0.125 mg base/kg/day divided every 6-12 hours **or** 0.5-7.5 mg base/m^2/day divided every 6-12 hours

Oral: 0.0175-0.25 mg/kg/day divided every 6-8 hours **or** 0.5-7.5 mg/m^2/day divided every 6-8 hours

Topical:

≤12 years: Use is not recommended.

≥13 years: Use minimal amount for shortest period of time to avoid HPA axis suppression
Gel, augmented formulation: Apply once or twice daily; rub in gently. **Note:** Do not exceed 2 weeks of treatment or 50 g/week.
Lotion: Apply a few drops twice daily
Augmented formulation: Apply a few drops once or twice daily; rub in gently. **Note:** Do not exceed 2 weeks of treatment or 50 mL/week.
Cream/ointment: Apply once or twice daily.
Augmented formulation: Apply once or twice daily. **Note:** Do not exceed 2 weeks of treatment or 45 g/week.

Adolescents and Adults:
Oral: 2.4-4.8 mg/day in 2-4 doses; range: 0.6-7.2 mg/day
I.M.: Betamethasone sodium phosphate and betamethasone acetate: 0.6-9 mg/day (generally, 1/3 to 1/2 of oral dose) divided every 12-24 hours

Adults:
Intrabursal, intra-articular, intradermal: 0.25-2 mL
Intralesional: Rheumatoid arthritis/osteoarthritis:
Very large joints: 1-2 mL
Large joints: 1 mL
Medium joints: 0.5-1 mL
Small joints: 0.25-0.5 mL
Topical:
Foam: Apply to the scalp twice daily, once in the morning and once at night
Gel, augmented formulation: Apply once or twice daily; rub in gently. **Note:** Do not exceed 2 weeks of treatment or 50 g/week.
Lotion: Apply a few drops twice daily
Augmented formulation: Apply a few drops once or twice daily; rub in gently. **Note:** Do not exceed 2 weeks of treatment or 50 mL/week.
Cream/ointment: Apply once or twice daily
Augmented formulation: Apply once or twice daily. **Note:** Do not exceed 2 weeks of treatment or 45 g/week.

Dosing adjustment in hepatic impairment: Adjustments may be necessary in patients with liver failure because betamethasone is extensively metabolized in the liver

Dietary Considerations May be taken with food to decrease GI distress.

Administration
Oral: Not for alternate day therapy; once daily doses should be given in the morning.
I.M.: Do **not** give injectable sodium phosphate/acetate suspension I.V.
Topical: Apply topical sparingly to areas. Not for use on broken skin or in areas of infection. Do not apply to wet skin unless directed; do not cover with occlusive dressing. Do not apply very high potency agents to face, groin, axillae, or diaper area.
Foam: Invert can and dispense a small amount onto a saucer or other cool surface. Do not dispense directly into hands. Pick up small amounts of foam and gently massage into affected areas until foam disappears. Repeat until entire affected scalp area is treated.

Additional Information
Very high potency: Augmented betamethasone dipropionate ointment, lotion
High potency: Augmented betamethasone dipropionate cream, betamethasone dipropionate cream and ointment
Intermediate potency: Betamethasone dipropionate lotion, betamethasone valerate cream

Dosage Forms Excipient information presented when available (limited, particularly for generics); consult specific product labeling.
Note: Potency expressed as betamethasone base.
Aerosol, topical, as valerate [foam]:
Luxiq®: 0.12% (50 g, 100 g, 150 g) [strength expressed as salt; contains ethanol 60.4%]
Cream, topical, as dipropionate: 0.05% (15 g, 45 g)
Cream, topical, as dipropionate augmented: 0.05% (15 g, 50 g)
Diprolene® AF: 0.05% (15 g, 50 g)
Cream, topical, as valerate (Beta-Val®): 0.1% (15 g, 45 g)
Beta-Val®: 0.1% (15 g, 45 g)
Gel, topical, as dipropionate augmented: 0.05% (15 g, 50 g)
Injection, suspension:
Celestone® Soluspan®: Betamethasone sodium phosphate 3 mg and betamethasone acetate 3 mg per 1 mL (5 mL) [6 mg/mL]
Lotion, topical, as dipropionate: 0.05% (60 mL)
Lotion, topical, as dipropionate augmented:
Diprolene®: 0.05% (30 mL, 60 mL)
Lotion, topical, as valerate: 0.1% (60 mL)
Beta-Val®: 0.1% (60 mL)
Ointment, topical, as dipropionate: 0.05% (15 g, 45 g)
Ointment, topical, as dipropionate augmented: 0.05% (15 g, 50 g)
Diprolene®: 0.05% (15 g, 50 g)
Ointment, topical, as valerate: 0.1% (15 g, 45 g)
Solution, as base:
Celestone®: 0.6 mg/5 mL (118 mL) [contains alcohol and sodium benzoate; cherry-orange flavor]

Betamethasone and Clotrimazole
(bay ta METH a sone & kloe TRIM a zole)

U.S. Brand Names Lotrisone®
Canadian Brand Names Lotriderm®
Index Terms Clotrimazole and Betamethasone
Pharmacologic Category Antifungal Agent, Topical; Corticosteroid, Topical
Use Topical treatment of various dermal fungal infections (including tinea pedis, cruris, and corpora in patients ≥17 years of age)
Pregnancy Risk Factor C
Medication Safety Issues
Sound-alike/look-alike issues:
Clotrimazole may be confused with co-trimoxazole
Lotrisone® may be confused with Lotrimin®

Dosage
Children <17 years: Do not use
Children ≥17 years and Adults:
Allergic or inflammatory diseases: Topical: Apply to affected area twice daily, morning and evening
Tinea corporis, tinea cruris: Topical: Massage into affected area twice daily, morning and evening; do not use for longer than 2 weeks; re-evaluate after 1 week if no clinical improvement; do not exceed 45 g cream/week or 45 mL lotion/week
Tinea pedis: Topical: Massage into affected area twice daily, morning and evening; do not use for longer than 4 weeks; re-evaluate after 2 weeks if no clinical improvement; do not exceed 45 g cream/week or 45 mL lotion/week
Elderly: Use with caution; skin atrophy and skin ulceration (rare) have been reported in patients with thinning skin; do not use for diaper dermatitis or under occlusive dressings

Additional Information Complete prescribing information for this medication should be consulted for additional detail.

Dosage Forms Excipient information presented when available (limited, particularly for generics); consult specific product labeling.
Cream: Betamethasone dipropionate 0.05% (base) and clotrimazole 1% (15 g, 45 g) [contains benzyl alcohol]
Lotrisone®: Betamethasone dipropionate 0.05% (base) and clotrimazole 1% (15 g, 45 g) [contains benzyl alcohol]

Lotion: Betamethasone dipropionate 0.05% (base) and clotrimazole 1% (30 mL) [contains benzyl alcohol]
Lotrisone®: Betamethasone dipropionate 0.05% (base) and clotrimazole 1% (30 mL) [contains benzyl alcohol]

- ◆ **Betamethasone Dipropionate** *see* Betamethasone *on page 188*
- ◆ **Betamethasone Dipropionate and Calcipotriene Hydrate** *see* Calcipotriene and Betamethasone *on page 234*
- ◆ **Betamethasone Dipropionate, Augmented** *see* Betamethasone *on page 188*
- ◆ **Betamethasone Sodium Phosphate** *see* Betamethasone *on page 188*
- ◆ **Betamethasone Valerate** *see* Betamethasone *on page 188*
- ◆ **Betapace®** *see* Sotalol *on page 1394*
- ◆ **Betapace AF®** *see* Sotalol *on page 1394*
- ◆ **Betasept® [OTC]** *see* Chlorhexidine Gluconate *on page 305*
- ◆ **Betaseron®** *see* Interferon Beta-1b *on page 807*
- ◆ **Beta-Val®** *see* Betamethasone *on page 188*
- ◆ **Betaxin® (Can)** *see* Thiamine *on page 1458*

Betaxolol (be TAKS oh lol)

U.S. Brand Names Betoptic® S; Kerlone®

Canadian Brand Names Betoptic® S; Sandoz-Betaxolol

Index Terms Betaxolol Hydrochloride

Pharmacologic Category Beta Blocker, Beta$_1$ Selective; Ophthalmic Agent, Antiglaucoma

Additional Appendix Information

Beta-Blockers *on page 1648*
Glaucoma Drug Therapy *on page 1808*

Use

Ophthalmic: Treatment of chronic open-angle glaucoma or ocular hypertension
Oral: Management of hypertension

Pregnancy Risk Factor C

Pregnancy Considerations Teratogenic effects were not observed in animal studies; however, there was drug-related postimplantation loss in rats and rabbits. There are no adequate and well-controlled studies in pregnant women.

Lactation Oral: Enters breast milk/use caution

Medication Safety Issues

Sound-alike/look-alike issues:
Betaxolol may be confused with bethanechol, labetalol
Betoptic® S may be confused with Betagan®, Timoptic®

Contraindications Hypersensitivity to betaxolol or any component of the formulation; sinus bradycardia; heart block greater than first-degree (except in patients with a functioning artificial pacemaker); cardiogenic shock; uncompensated cardiac failure

Warnings/Precautions Consider pre-existing conditions (such as sick sinus syndrome) before initiating. Administer cautiously in compensated heart failure and monitor for a worsening of the condition. Beta-blocker therapy should not be withdrawn abruptly (particularly in patients with CAD), but gradually tapered to avoid acute tachycardia, hypertension, and/or ischemia. Use caution with concurrent use of beta-blockers, either verapamil or diltiazem, or digoxin; bradycardia or heart block can occur. Bradycardia may be observed more frequently in elderly patients (>65 years of age); dosage reductions may be necessary.

May precipitate or aggravate symptoms of arterial insufficiency in patients with peripheral vascular disease (PVD) and Raynaud's disease; use with caution; monitor for progression of arterial obstruction. In general, beta-blockers should be avoided in patients with bronchospastic disease. Betaxolol, with beta$_1$ selectivity, may be used cautiously in bronchospastic disease with the lowest possible dose (eg, 5-10 mg/day), availability of a bronchodilator, and close monitoring; if dosage increase is indicated, administer in divided doses. Use cautiously in patients with diabetes because it may potentiate and/or mask prominent hypoglycemic symptoms. May mask signs of hyperthyroidism (eg, tachycardia); use caution if hyperthyroidism is suspected, abrupt withdrawal may precipitate thyroid storm. Use with caution in patients with cerebrovascular insufficiency; hypotension and decreased heart rate may reduce cerebral blood flow. Dosage adjustment required in severe renal impairment and in patients on dialysis. Use care with anesthetic agents which decrease myocardial function. Use with caution in patients with myasthenia gravis (may potentiate myasthenia-related muscle weakness, including diplopia and ptosis) or psychiatric disease (may cause CNS depression). Adequate alpha-blockade is required prior to use of any beta-blocker for patients with untreated pheochromocytoma. Use caution with history of severe anaphylaxis to allergens; patients taking beta-blockers may become more sensitive to repeated challenges. Treatment of anaphylaxis (eg, epinephrine) in patients taking beta-blockers may be ineffective or promote undesirable effects. Safety and efficacy of the oral formulation have not been established in children.

Discontinue ophthalmic preparations with signs of cardiac failure. Should not be used alone in angle-closure glaucoma (has no effect on pupillary constriction). Ophthalmic suspension contains benzalkonium chloride which may be absorbed by contact lenses; remove contact lens prior to administration and wait 15 minutes before reinserting. Inadvertent contamination of multiple-dose ophthalmic solutions has caused bacterial keratitis. Choroidal detachment has been reported with aqueous suppressant therapy after filtration procedures.

Adverse Reactions

Ophthalmic:

>10%: Ocular: Short-term discomfort (≤25%)

<1%: Alopecia, asthma, bradycardia, bronchial secretions thickened, bronchospasm, depression, dizziness, dyspnea, glossitis, heart block, heart failure, headache, hives, insomnia, lethargy, myasthenia gravis exacerbation, respiratory failure, smell/taste perversion, toxic epidermal necrolysis, vertigo

Frequency not defined: Ocular: Allergic reaction, anisocoria, blurred vision, choroidal detachment, corneal punctate keratitis, corneal punctate staining (with or without dendritic formations), corneal sensitivity decreased, corneal staining, crusty lashes, discharge, dry eyes, edema, erythema, foreign body sensation, inflammation, keratitis, ocular pain, photophobia, sensation of itching, tearing, visual acuity decreased

Systemic:

2% to 10%:

Cardiovascular: Bradycardia (6% to 8%; symptomatic bradycardia: <1% to 2%; dose-dependent), chest pain (2% to 7%), palpitation (2%), edema (≤2%; similar to placebo)

Central nervous system: Fatigue (3% to 10%), insomnia (1% to 5%), lethargy (3%)

Gastrointestinal: Nausea (2% to 6%), dyspepsia (4% to 5%), diarrhea (2%)

Neuromuscular & Skeletal: Arthralgia (3% to 5%), paresthesia (2%)

Respiratory: Dyspnea (2%), pharyngitis (2%)

Miscellaneous: Antinuclear antibody positive (5%), cold extremities (2%)

<2% (Limited to important or life-threatening): Acidosis, allergy, alopecia, ALT increased, AST increased, anemia, angina, anorexia, arrhythmia, arthropathy, ataxia, atrioventricular block, blepharitis, breast fibroadenosis, bronchitis, bronchospasm, cataract, cerebrovascular disorder, conjunctivitis, constipation, cough, cystitis, deafness, depression (<1%), diabetes, diaphoresis, dreams abnormal (1%), dysphagia, dysuria, epistaxis, erythematous rash, fever, flu, flushing, hallucinations, heart failure, hyper-/hypotension, hypercholesterolemia, hyperglycemia, hypo/hyperkalemia, hyperlipemia, hypertrichosis, hyperuricemia, impotence (1%), intermittent claudication, iritis, labyrinth disorder, LDH increased, leukocytosis, libido decreased, lymphadenopathy, malaise, menstrual disorder, MI, muscle cramps, nervousness (1%), neuralgia, neuropathy, numbness, ocular hemorrhage, oliguria, peripheral ischemia, Peyronie's disease, pneumonia, prostatitis, proteinuria, pruritus, purpura, rash (1%), renal function abnormal, rhinitis (1%), rigors, scotoma, stupor, syncope, tendonitis, thrombophlebitis, thrombosis, tinnitus, tremor, thrombocytopenia, vision abnormal, vomiting, weight gain/loss, xerostomia

Drug Interactions

Metabolism/Transport Effects Substrate (major) of CYP1A2, 2D6; **Inhibits** CYP2D6 (weak)

Avoid Concomitant Use

Avoid concomitant use of Betaxolol with any of the following: Methacholine

Increased Effect/Toxicity

Betaxolol may increase the levels/effects of: Alpha-/Beta-Agonists (Direct-Acting); Alpha1-Blockers; Alpha2-Agonists; Amifostine; Antipsychotic Agents (Phenothiazines); Cardiac Glycosides; Insulin; Lidocaine; Methacholine; Midodrine; RiTUXimab

The levels/effects of Betaxolol may be increased by: Acetylcholinesterase Inhibitors; Aminoquinolines (Antimalarial); Amiodarone; Anilidopiperidine Opioids; Antipsychotic Agents (Phenothiazines); Calcium Channel Blockers (Nondihydropyridine); CYP1A2 Inhibitors (Moderate); CYP1A2 Inhibitors (Strong); Diazoxide; Dipyridamole; Disopyramide; Herbs (Hypotensive Properties); Propafenone; Propoxyphene; Prostacyclin Analogues; QuiNIDine; Reserpine; Selective Serotonin Reuptake Inhibitors

Decreased Effect

Betaxolol may decrease the levels/effects of: Beta2-Agonists; Theophylline Derivatives

The levels/effects of Betaxolol may be decreased by: Barbiturates; CYP1A2 Inducers (Strong); Herbs (Hypertensive Properties); Methylphenidate; Nonsteroidal Anti-Inflammatory Agents; Rifamycin Derivatives; Yohimbine

Ethanol/Nutrition/Herb Interactions Herb/Nutraceutical: Avoid bayberry; blue cohosh, cayenne, ephedra, ginger, ginseng (American), gotu kola, and licorice (may worsen hypertension). Avoid black cohosh, California poppy, coleus, golden seal, hawthorn, mistletoe, periwinkle, quinine, shepherd's purse (may have increased antihypertensive effects).

Stability Avoid freezing. Store tablets at room temperature of 15°C to 25°C (59°F to 77°F). Store ophthalmic suspension upright at 2°C to 25°C (36°F to 77°F). Store ophthalmic solution at room temperature.

Mechanism of Action Competitively blocks beta$_1$-receptors, with little or no effect on beta$_2$-receptors; with ophthalmic use, reduces intraocular pressure by reducing the production of aqueous humor

Pharmacodynamics/Kinetics

Onset of action: Ophthalmic: 30 minutes; Oral: 1-1.5 hours

Duration: Ophthalmic: ≥12 hours

Absorption: Ophthalmic: Some systemic; Oral: ~100%

Metabolism: Hepatic to multiple metabolites

Protein binding: Oral: ~50%

Bioavailability: Oral: 89%

Half-life elimination: Oral: 14-22 hours; prolonged in hepatic disease and/or chronic renal failure

Time to peak: Ophthalmic: ~2 hours; Oral: 1.5-6 hours

Excretion: Urine (>80%; as unchanged drug [15%] and inactive metabolites)

Dosage

Children and Adults: Ophthalmic suspension (Betoptic® S): Instill 1 drop into affected eye(s) twice daily.

Adults:

Ophthalmic solution: Instill 1-2 drops into affected eye(s) twice daily.

Oral: 5-10 mg/day; may increase dose to 20 mg/day after 7-14 days if desired response is not achieved.

Elderly:

Ophthalmic: Refer to adult dosing.

Oral: Refer to adult dosing; initial dose: 5 mg/day

Dosage adjustment in renal impairment: Severe impairment: Initial dose: 5 mg/day; may increase every 2 weeks up to a maximum of 20 mg/day

Hemodialysis: Initial dose: 5 mg/day; may increase every 2 weeks up to a maximum of 20 mg/day. Supplemental dose not required.

Administration

Ophthalmic: Shake suspension well before using. Tilt head back and instill in eye. Keep eye open and do not blink for 30 seconds. Apply gentle pressure to lacrimal sac for 1 minute. Wipe away excess from skin. Do not touch applicator to eye and do not contaminate tip of applicator.

Oral: Absorption is not affected by food.

Monitoring Parameters Ophthalmic: Intraocular pressure. Systemic: Blood pressure, pulse; baseline renal function

Test Interactions Oral betaxolol may interfere with glaucoma screening tests.

Dosage Forms Excipient information presented when available (limited, particularly for generics); consult specific product labeling. [DSC] = Discontinued product

Solution, ophthalmic: 0.5% (5 mL, 10 mL, 15 mL) [contains benzalkonium chloride]

Suspension, ophthalmic:

Betoptic® S: 0.25% (5 mL [DSC], 10 mL, 15 mL) [contains benzalkonium chloride]

Tablet, as hydrochloride: 10 mg, 20 mg

Kerlone®: 10 mg, 20 mg

◆ **Betaxolol Hydrochloride** *see* Betaxolol *on page 191*

Bethanechol (be THAN e kole)

U.S. Brand Names Urecholine®

Canadian Brand Names Duvoid®; PMS-Bethanechol

Index Terms Bethanechol Chloride

Pharmacologic Category Cholinergic Agonist

Use Treatment of acute postoperative and postpartum nonobstructive (functional) urinary retention; treatment of neurogenic atony of the urinary bladder with retention

Unlabeled/Investigational Use Gastroesophageal reflux

Pregnancy Risk Factor C

Pregnancy Considerations Reproduction studies have not been conducted.

Lactation Excretion in breast milk unknown/not recommended

Medication Safety Issues

Sound-alike/look-alike issues:

Bethanechol may be confused with betaxolol

Contraindications Hypersensitivity to bethanechol or any component of the formulation; mechanical obstruction of the GI or GU tract or when the strength or integrity of the GI or bladder wall is in question; hyperthyroidism, peptic ulcer disease, epilepsy, asthma, bradycardia, vasomotor instability, coronary artery disease, hypotension, or parkinsonism

Warnings/Precautions Potential for reflux infection if the sphincter fails to relax as bethanechol contracts the bladder. Safety and efficacy in children have not been established.

Adverse Reactions Frequency not defined.

Cardiovascular: Hypotension, tachycardia, flushed skin

Central nervous system: Headache, malaise, seizure

Gastrointestinal: Abdominal cramps, belching, borborygmi, colicky pain, diarrhea, nausea, vomiting, salivation

Genitourinary: Urinary urgency

Ocular: Lacrimation, miosis

Respiratory: Asthmatic attacks, bronchial constriction

Miscellaneous: Diaphoresis

Drug Interactions

Avoid Concomitant Use There are no known interactions where it is recommended to avoid concomitant use.

Increased Effect/Toxicity

The levels/effects of Bethanechol may be increased by: Acetylcholinesterase Inhibitors

Decreased Effect There are no known significant interactions involving a decrease in effect.

Stability Store at room temperature of 15°C to 30°C (59°F to 86°F).

Mechanism of Action Due to stimulation of the parasympathetic nervous system, bethanechol increases bladder muscle tone causing contractions which initiate urination. Bethanechol also stimulates gastric motility, increases gastric tone and may restore peristalsis.

Pharmacodynamics/Kinetics

Onset of action: 30-90 minutes

Duration: Up to 6 hours

Absorption: Variable

Dosage Oral:

Children:

Urinary retention (unlabeled use): 0.3-0.6 mg/kg/day in 3-4 divided doses

Gastroesophageal reflux (unlabeled use): 0.3-0.6 mg/kg/day in 3-4 divided doses

Adults:

Urinary retention, neurogenic bladder: Initial: 10-50 mg 3-4 times/day (some patients may require dosages of 50-100 mg 4 times/day). To determine effective dose, may initiate at a dose of 5-10 mg, with additional doses of 5-10 mg hourly until an effective cumulative dose is reached. Cholinergic effects at higher oral dosages may be cumulative.

Gastroesophageal reflux (unlabeled): 25 mg 4 times/day

Elderly: Use the lowest effective dose

Dietary Considerations Should be taken 1 hour before meals or 2 hours after meals.

Monitoring Parameters Observe closely for side effects.

Test Interactions Increased lipase, amylase (S), bilirubin, aminotransferase [ALT/AST] (S)

Dosage Forms Excipient information presented when available (limited, particularly for generics); consult specific product labeling. [CAN] = Canadian brand name

Tablet, as chloride: 5 mg, 10 mg, 25 mg, 50 mg

Duvoid® [CAN]: 10 mg, 25 mg, 50 mg [not available in U.S.]

Urecholine®: 5 mg, 10 mg, 25 mg, 50 mg

◆ **Bethanechol Chloride** *see* Bethanechol *on page 192*

◆ **Betimol®** *see* Timolol *on page 1472*

◆ **Betnesol® (Can)** *see* Betamethasone *on page 188*

◆ **Betnovate® (Can)** *see* Betamethasone *on page 188*

◆ **Betoptic® S** *see* Betaxolol *on page 191*

Bevacizumab (be vuh SIZ uh mab)

U.S. Brand Names Avastin®

Canadian Brand Names Avastin®

Index Terms Anti-VEGF Monoclonal Antibody; NSC-704865; rhuMAb-VEGF

Pharmacologic Category Antineoplastic Agent, Monoclonal Antibody; Vascular Endothelial Growth Factor (VEGF) Inhibitor

Use Treatment of metastatic colorectal cancer; treatment of nonsquamous, nonsmall cell lung cancer; treatment of breast cancer (metastatic, HER-2 negative)

Unlabeled/Investigational Use Treatment of ovarian cancer (early stage), renal cell cancer, age-related macular degeneration (AMD)

Pregnancy Risk Factor C

Pregnancy Considerations There are no adequate or well-controlled studies in pregnant women, however, bevacizumab is teratogenic in animal models. Angiogenesis is of critical importance to fetal development, and bevacizumab is likely to have adverse consequences in terms of fetal development. Adequate contraception during therapy is recommended. The risk and benefit of treatment should be evaluated in pregnant women. Patients should also be counseled regarding prolonged exposure following discontinuation of therapy due to the long half-life of bevacizumab.

Based on animal studies, bevacizumab may disrupt normal menstrual cycles and impair fertility by several effects, including reduced endometrial proliferation and follicular developmental arrest. Some parameters do not recover completely, or recover very slowly following discontinuation.

Lactation Excretion in breast milk unknown/not recommended

Medication Safety Issues

Sound-alike/look-alike issues:

Bevacizumab may be confused with cetuximab

High alert medication: The Institute for Safe Medication Practices (ISMP) includes this medication among its list of drug classes which have a heightened risk of causing significant patient harm when used in error.

Contraindications There are no contraindications listed in the manufacturer's labeling.

Warnings/Precautions [U.S. Boxed Warning]: Gastrointestinal perforation, fistula (including gastrointestinal, enterocutaneous, esophageal, duodenal, and rectal fistulas), intra-abdominal abscess, and wound dehiscence/wound healing complications have been reported in patients receiving bevacizumab (not related to treatment duration); monitor patients for signs/symptoms (eg, abdominal pain with constipation and/or vomiting). Permanently discontinue in patients who develop these complications. Nongastrointestinal fistula formation (including tracheoesophageal, bronchopleural, biliary, vaginal, and bladder fistulas) has been observed, most commonly within the first 6 months of treatment; permanently discontinue in patients who develop internal organ fistulas. The appropriate intervals between administration of bevacizumab and surgical procedures to avoid impairment in wound healing has not been established. Therapy should not be initiated within 28 days of major surgery and only following complete healing of the incision. Bevacizumab should be discontinued prior to elective surgery and the estimated half-life (20 days) should be considered.

Use with caution in patients with cardiovascular disease; patients with significant recent cardiovascular disease were excluded from clinical trials. An increased risk for arterial thromboembolic events (eg, stroke, MI, TIA, angina) is associated with bevacizumab use in combination with chemotherapy. History of arterial thromboembolism or ≥65 years of age may present an even greater risk; permanently discontinue if serious arterial thromboembolic events occur. Although patients with cancer are at risk for venous thromboembolism, a meta-analysis of 15 controlled trials has demonstrated an increased risk for venous thromboembolism in patients who received bevacizumab (Nalluri, 2008).

The risk for heart failure, including left ventricular dysfunction, is higher in patients receiving bevacizumab plus chemotherapy when compared to chemotherapy alone. May potentiate the cardiotoxic effects of anthracyclines. Heart failure is more common with prior anthracycline exposure and/or left chest wall irradiation. The safety of therapy resumption or continuation in patients with cardiac dysfunction has not been studied. Bevacizumab may cause and/or worsen hypertension significantly; use caution in patients with pre-existing hypertension and monitor BP closely in all patients. Permanent discontinuation is recommended in patients who experience a hypertensive crisis or encephalopathy. Temporarily discontinue in patients who develop uncontrolled hypertension. Cases of reversible posterior leukoencephalopathy syndrome (RPLS) have been reported. Symptoms (which include headache, seizure, confusion, lethargy, blindness and/or other vision, or neurologic disturbances) may occur from 16 hours to 1 year after treatment initiation. RPLS may be associated with hypertension; discontinue bevacizumab and begin management of hypertension, if present.

[U.S. Boxed Warning]: Avoid use in patients with recent hemoptysis (>2.5 mL blood); significant pulmonary bleeding has been reported in patients receiving bevacizumab (primarily in patients with nonsmall cell lung cancer with squamous cell histology [not an FDA-approved indication]). Avoid use in patients with CNS metastases; patients with CNS metastases were excluded from clinical trials due to concerns for bleeding. Other serious bleeding events may occur, but with a lower frequency; discontinuation of treatment is recommended in all patients with serious hemorrhage.

Infusion reactions (eg, hypertension, hypertensive crisis, wheezing, hypersensitivity, chest pain, headache, diaphoresis) may occur with the first infusion (uncommon); interrupt therapy in patients experiencing severe infusion reactions; there are no data to address reinstitution of therapy in patients who experience severe infusion reactions. Proteinuria and/or nephrotic syndrome has been associated with bevacizumab; discontinue in patients with nephrotic syndrome. Elderly patients (≥65 years of age) are at higher risk for adverse events, including thromboembolic events and proteinuria. Microangiopathic hemolytic anemia (MAHA) has been reported when bevacizumab has been used in combination with sunitinib. When used in combination with myelosuppressive chemotherapy, increased rates of severe or febrile neutropenia and neutropenic infection were reported. Safety and efficacy in children have not been established.

Adverse Reactions Percentages reported as monotherapy and as part of combination chemotherapy regimens. Some studies only reported hematologic toxicities grades ≥4 and nonhematologic toxicities grades ≥3.

>10%:

Cardiovascular: Hypertension (23% to 67%; grades 3/4: 8% to 18%), thromboembolic event (grades 3/4: 15%), hypotension (7% to 15%)

Central nervous system: Pain (61% to 62%), headache (26%; grades 3/4: 2% to 4%), dizziness (19% to 26%), fatigue (grades 3/4: 5% to 19%), sensory neuropathy (grades 3/4: 1% to 17%; in combination with paclitaxel: 24%)

Dermatologic: Alopecia (6% to 32%), dry skin (7% to 20%), exfoliative dermatitis (3% to 19%), skin discoloration (2% to 16%)

Endocrine & metabolic: Hypokalemia (12% to 16%)

Gastrointestinal: Abdominal pain (50% to 61%; grades 3/4: 8%), vomiting (47% to 52%; grades 3/4: 6% to 11%), anorexia (35% to 43%), constipation (29% to 40%), diarrhea (grades 3/4: 2% to 34%), stomatitis (30% to 32%), gastrointestinal hemorrhage (19% to 24%), dyspepsia (17% to 24%), taste disorder (14% to 21%), flatulence (11% to 19%), weight loss (15% to 16%), nausea (grades 3/4: 4% to 12%)

Hematologic: Leukopenia (grades 3/4: 37%), neutropenia (grade 4: 6% to 27%)

Neuromuscular & skeletal: Weakness (73% to 74%), myalgia (8% to 15%)

Ocular: Tearing increased (6% to 18%)

Renal: Proteinuria (36%; grades 3/4: 3%)

Respiratory: Upper respiratory infection (40% to 47%), epistaxis (32% to 35%), dyspnea (25% to 26%)

Miscellaneous: Infection (serious: 9% to 14%; pneumonia, catheter, or wound infections)

1% to 10%:

Cardiovascular: DVT (6% to 9%; grades 3/4: 9%), venous thrombus/embolus (grades 3/4: 5%), arterial thrombosis (3% to 4%), syncope (grades 3/4: 3%), intra-abdominal venous thrombosis (grades 3/4: 3%), cardio-/cerebrovascular arterial thrombotic event (2% to 4%), CHF (2%)

Central nervous system: Confusion (1% to 6%), abnormal gait (1% to 5%)

Dermatologic: Nail disorder (2% to 8%), rash desquamation (grades 3/4: 3%), wound dehiscence (1%)

Endocrine & metabolic: Dehydration (grades 3/4: 3% to 10%), hyponatremia (grades 3/4: 4%)

Gastrointestinal: Xerostomia (4% to 7%), colitis (1% to 6%), ileus (grades 3/4: 4% to 5%), gingival bleeding (2%), fistula (1%), gastrointestinal perforation (≤4%), intra-abdominal abscess (1%)

Genitourinary: Polyuria/urgency (3% to 6%), vaginal hemorrhage (4%)

Hematologic: Neutropenic fever/infection (5%; grades 3 and/or 4: 4% to 5%), thrombocytopenia (5%), hemorrhage (grades 3/4: 4% to 5%)

Hepatic: Bilirubinemia (1% to 6%)

Neuromuscular & skeletal: Bone pain (grades 3/4: 4%)

Respiratory: Voice alteration (6% to 9%), pneumonitis/pulmonary infiltrates (grades 3/4: 5%), hemoptysis (nonsquamous histology 2%)

Miscellaneous: Infusion reactions (<3%)

<1% (Limited to important or life-threatening): Anastomotic ulceration, angina, cerebral infarction; fistula (biliary, bladder, bronchopleural, duodenal, endophthalmitis, enterocutaneous, esophageal, eye inflammation, gastrointestinal, rectal, tracheoesophageal [TE] and vaginal); hemorrhagic stroke, hypertensive crises, hypertensive encephalopathy, intestinal necrosis, intestinal obstruction, mesenteric venous occlusion, microangiopathic hemolytic anemia (when used in combination with sunitinib), MI, nasal septum perforation, nephrotic syndrome, pancytopenia, polyserositis, pulmonary embolism, pulmonary hemorrhage, pulmonary hypertension, reversible posterior leukoencephalopathy syndrome (RPLS), subarachnoid hemorrhage, toxic anterior segment syndrome (TASS), transient ischemic attack, ureteral stricture, vision blurred, wound healing complications

Drug Interactions

Avoid Concomitant Use

Avoid concomitant use of Bevacizumab with any of the following: Sunitinib

Increased Effect/Toxicity

Bevacizumab may increase the levels/effects of: Antineoplastic Agents (Anthracycline); Irinotecan

The levels/effects of Bevacizumab may be increased by: Sunitinib

Decreased Effect There are no known significant interactions involving a decrease in effect.

Stability Store vials at 2°C to 8°C (36°F to 46°F). Protect from light; do not freeze or shake. Prior to infusion, dilute prescribed dose of bevacizumab in 100 mL NS. Do not mix with dextrose-containing solutions. Diluted solutions are stable for up to 8 hours under refrigeration.

Mechanism of Action Bevacizumab is a recombinant, humanized monoclonal antibody which binds to, and neutralizes, vascular endothelial growth factor (VEGF), preventing its association with endothelial receptors, Flt-1 and KDR. VEGF binding initiates angiogenesis (endothelial proliferation and the formation of new blood vessels). The inhibition of microvascular growth is believed to retard the growth of all tissues (including metastatic tissue).

Pharmacodynamics/Kinetics

Distribution: V_d: 46 mL/kg

Half-life elimination: ~20 days (range: 11-50 days)

Excretion: Clearance: 2.75-5 mL/kg/day

Dosage Adults: Details concerning dosing in combination regimens should also be consulted.

I.V.:

Breast cancer: 10 mg/kg every 2 weeks (in combination with paclitaxel)

Colorectal cancer: 5 or 10 mg/kg every 2 weeks (in combination with fluorouracil-based chemotherapy)

Lung cancer, nonsquamous cell nonsmall cell: 15 mg/kg every 3 weeks (in combination with carboplatin and paclitaxel)

Renal cell cancer (unlabeled use): 10 mg/kg every 2 weeks

Intravitreal: AMD (unlabeled use): 1.25 mg (0.05 mL) monthly until improvement/resolution, usually ~1-3 injections (Avery, 2006) or 2.5 mg (0.1 mL) every 4 weeks for 3 doses (Bashshur, 2006)

Dosage adjustment for toxicity: I.V. administration (systemic): Temporary suspension is recommended in moderate-to-severe proteinuria (in most studies, treatment was withheld for ≥2 g proteinuria/24 hours) or in patients with severe hypertension which is not controlled with medical management. Permanent discontinuation is recommended (by the manufacturer) in patients who develop wound dehiscence requiring intervention, fistula (gastrointestinal and nongastrointestinal), gastrointestinal perforation, hypertensive crisis, hypertensive encephalopathy, intra-abdominal abscess, serious bleeding, severe arterial thrombotic event, nephrotic syndrome, or RPLS.

Administration

I.V. infusion, usually after the other antineoplastic agents. Infuse the initial dose over 90 minutes. Infusion may be shortened to 60 minutes if the initial infusion is well tolerated. The third and subsequent infusions may be shortened to 30 minutes if the 60-minute infusion is well tolerated. Monitor closely during the infusion for signs/symptoms of an infusion reaction. Some institutions use a 10-minute infusion (0.5 mg/kg/minute) for bevacizumab dosed at 5 mg/kg (Reidy, 2007).

Intravitreal injection (unlabeled use): Adequate anesthesia and a broad-spectrum antimicrobial agent should be administered prior to the procedure; administer topical antibiotics for 3 days after procedure.

Monitoring Parameters Monitor closely during the infusion for signs/symptoms of an infusion reaction. Monitor CBC with differential; signs/symptoms of gastrointestinal perforation, fistula, or abscess (including abdominal pain, constipation, vomiting, and fever); signs/symptoms of bleeding, including hemoptysis, gastrointestinal, and/or CNS bleeding, and/or epistaxis. Monitor blood pressure every 2-3 weeks; more frequently if hypertension develops during therapy. Continue to monitor blood pressure after discontinuing due to bevacizumab-induced hypertension. Monitor for proteinuria/nephrotic syndrome.

AMD: Monitor intraocular pressure and retinal artery perfusion

Dosage Forms Excipient information presented when available (limited, particularly for generics); consult specific product labeling.

Injection, solution [preservative free]:

Avastin®: 25 mg/mL (4 mL, 16 mL)

Bexarotene (beks AIR oh teen)

U.S. Brand Names Targretin®

Canadian Brand Names Targretin®

Pharmacologic Category Antineoplastic Agent, Miscellaneous

Use

Oral: Treatment of cutaneous manifestations of cutaneous T-cell lymphoma in patients who are refractory to at least one prior systemic therapy

Topical: Treatment of cutaneous lesions in patients with refractory cutaneous T-cell lymphoma (stage 1A and 1B) or who have not tolerated other therapies

Pregnancy Risk Factor X

Pregnancy Considerations **[U.S. Boxed Warning]: Bexarotene is a retinoid, a drug class associated with birth defects in humans; do not administer during pregnancy.** Bexarotene caused birth defects when administered orally to pregnant rats. It must not be given to a pregnant woman or a woman who intends to become pregnant. If a woman becomes pregnant while taking the drug, it must be stopped immediately and appropriate counseling be given. Women of childbearing potential should use two forms of reliable contraception, one should be nonhormonal.

Lactation Excretion in breast milk unknown/contraindicated

Medication Safety Issues

High alert medication: The Institute for Safe Medication Practices (ISMP) includes this medication among its list of drugs which have a heightened risk of causing significant patient harm when used in error.

Contraindications Hypersensitivity to bexarotene or any component of the formulation; pregnancy

Warnings/Precautions Hazardous agent - use appropriate precautions for handling and disposal. **[U.S. Boxed Warning]: Bexarotene is a retinoid, a drug class associated with birth defects in humans; do not administer during pregnancy.** Pregnancy test needed 1 week before initiation and every month thereafter. Effective contraception must be in place 1 month before initiation, during therapy, and for at least 1 month after discontinuation. Male patients with sexual partners who are pregnant, possibly pregnant, or who could become pregnant, must use condoms during sexual intercourse during treatment and for 1 month after last dose. Induces significant lipid abnormalities in a majority of patients (triglyceride, total cholesterol, and HDL); reversible on discontinuation. Use extreme caution in patients with underlying hypertriglyceridemia. Pancreatitis secondary to hypertriglyceridemia has been reported. Patients with risk factors for pancreatitis (eg, prior pancreatitis, uncontrolled hyperlipidemia, excess ethanol consumption, uncontrolled diabetes, biliary tract disease) should generally not receive bexarotene (oral). Monitor for liver function test abnormalities and discontinue drug if tests are three times the upper limit of normal values for AST, ALT, or bilirubin. Hypothyroidism occurs in about a third of patients. Monitor for signs and symptoms of infection about 4-8 weeks after initiation (leukopenia may occur). Any new visual abnormalities experienced by the patient should be evaluated by an ophthalmologist (cataracts can form, or worsen, especially in the geriatric population). May cause photosensitization. Safety and efficacy are not established in the pediatric population. Use only with extreme caution in patients with hepatic impairment. Limit additional vitamin A intake to <15,000 int. units/day. Use caution with diabetic patients.

Adverse Reactions First percentage is at a dose of 300 mg/m^2/day; the second percentage is at a dose >300 mg/m^2/day.

Oral:

>10%:

Cardiovascular: Peripheral edema (13% to 11%)

Central nervous system: Headache (30% to 42%), chills (10% to 13%)

Dermatologic: Rash (17% to 23%), exfoliative dermatitis (10% to 28%)

Endocrine & metabolic: Hyperlipidemia (about 79% in both dosing ranges), hypercholesteremia (32% to 62%), hypothyroidism (29% to 53%)

Hematologic: Leukopenia (17% to 47%)

Neuromuscular & skeletal: Weakness (20% to 45%)

Miscellaneous: Infection (13% to 23%)

<10% (Limited to important or life-threatening):

Cardiovascular: Hemorrhage, hypertension, angina pectoris, right heart failure, tachycardia, cerebrovascular accident, syncope

Central nervous system: Fever (5% to 17%), insomnia (5% to 11%), subdural hematoma, depression, agitation, ataxia

Dermatologic: Dry skin (about 10% for both dosing ranges), alopecia (4% to 11%), skin ulceration, maculopapular rash, vesicular bullous rash, cheilitis

Endocrine & metabolic: Hypoproteinemia, hyperglycemia

Gastrointestinal: Abdominal pain (11% to 4%), nausea (16% to 8%), diarrhea (7% to 42%), vomiting (4% to 13%), anorexia (2% to 23%), colitis, gastroenteritis, gingivitis, melena, pancreatitis

Genitourinary: Albuminuria, hematuria, dysuria

Hematologic: Hypochromic anemia (4% to 13%), anemia (6% to 25%), eosinophilia, thrombocythemia, coagulation time increased, lymphocytosis, thrombocytopenia

Hepatic: LDH increased (7% to 13%), hepatic failure

Neuromuscular & skeletal: Back pain (2% to 11%), arthralgia, myalgia, myasthenia, neuropathy

Ocular: Conjunctivitis, blepharitis, corneal lesion, visual field defects, keratitis

Otic: Ear pain, otitis externa

Renal: Renal dysfunction

Respiratory: Pharyngitis, rhinitis, dyspnea, pleural effusion, bronchitis, cough increased, lung edema, hemoptysis, hypoxia

Miscellaneous: Flu-like syndrome (4% to 13%), infection (1% to 13%)

Topical:

Cardiovascular: Edema (10%)

Central nervous system: Headache (14%), weakness (6%), pain (30%)

Dermatologic: Rash (14% to 72%), pruritus (6% to 40%), contact dermatitis (14%), exfoliative dermatitis (6%)

Hematologic: Leukopenia (6%), lymphadenopathy (6%)

Neuromuscular & skeletal: Paresthesia (6%)

Respiratory: Cough (6%), pharyngitis (6%)

Miscellaneous: Diaphoresis (6%), infection (18%)

Drug Interactions

Metabolism/Transport Effects **Substrate** of CYP3A4 (minor); **Induces** CYP3A4 (weak)

Avoid Concomitant Use

Avoid concomitant use of Bexarotene with any of the following: Tetracycline Derivatives

Increased Effect/Toxicity

The levels/effects of Bexarotene may be increased by: Tetracycline Derivatives

Decreased Effect

Bexarotene may decrease the levels/effects of: Maraviroc; Oral Contraceptive (Estrogens); Oral Contraceptive (Progestins)

Ethanol/Nutrition/Herb Interactions

Food: Take with a fat-containing meal. Bexarotene serum levels may be increased by grapefruit juice; avoid concurrent use.

Herb/Nutraceutical: Avoid dong quai, St John's wort (may also cause photosensitization). St John's wort may decrease bexarotene levels. Additional vitamin A supplements may lead to vitamin A toxicity (dry skin, irritation, arthralgias, myalgias, abdominal pain, hepatic changes).

Stability Store at 2°C to 25°C (36°F to 77°F); protect from light.

Mechanism of Action The exact mechanism is unknown. Binds and activates retinoid X receptor subtypes. Once activated, these receptors function as transcription factors that regulate the expression of genes which control cellular differentiation and proliferation. Bexarotene inhibits the growth *in vitro* of some tumor cell lines of hematopoietic and squamous cell origin.

Pharmacodynamics/Kinetics

Absorption: Significantly improved by a fat-containing meal

Protein binding: >99%

Metabolism: Hepatic via CYP3A4 isoenzyme; four metabolites identified; further metabolized by glucuronidation

Half-life elimination: 7 hours

Time to peak: 2 hours

Excretion: Primarily feces; urine (<1% as unchanged drug and metabolites)

Dosage Adults:

Oral: 300-400 mg/m^2/day taken as a single daily dose.

Topical: Apply once every other day for first week, then increase on a weekly basis to once daily, 2 times/day, 3 times/day, and finally 4 times/day, according to tolerance

Dosing adjustment in renal impairment: No studies have been conducted; however, renal insufficiency may result in significant protein binding changes and alter pharmacokinetics of bexarotene

Dosing adjustment in hepatic impairment: No studies have been conducted; however, hepatic impairment would be expected to result in decreased clearance of bexarotene due to the extensive hepatic contribution to elimination

Dietary Considerations It is preferable to take the oral capsule following a fat-containing meal.

Administration

Oral: Administer capsule following a fat-containing meal.

Topical: Allow gel to dry before covering with clothing. Avoid application to normal skin. Use of occlusive dressings is not recommended.

Monitoring Parameters If female, pregnancy test 1 week before initiation then monthly while on bexarotene; lipid panel before initiation, then weekly until lipid response established and then at 8-week intervals thereafter; baseline LFTs, repeat at 1, 2, and 4 weeks after initiation then at 8-week intervals thereafter if stable; baseline and periodic thyroid function tests; baseline CBC with periodic monitoring

Dosage Forms Excipient information presented when available (limited, particularly for generics); consult specific product labeling.

Capsule:

Targretin®: 75 mg

Gel: 1% (60 g)

Targretin®: 1% (60 g) [contains dehydrated alcohol]

◆ **Bexxar®** *see* Tositumomab and Iodine I 131 Tositumomab *on page* 1495

◆ **BG 9273** *see* Alefacept *on page* 55

◆ **Biaxin®** *see* Clarithromycin *on page* 341

◆ **Biaxin® XL** *see* Clarithromycin *on page* 341

Bicalutamide (bye ka LOO ta mide)

U.S. Brand Names Casodex®

Canadian Brand Names Casodex®; CO Bicalutamide; Gen-Bicalutamide; Novo-Bicalutamide; PHL-Bicalutamide; PMS-Bicalutamide; Pro-Bicalutamide; ratio-Bicalutamide; Sandoz-Bicalutamide

Index Terms CDX; ICI-176334; NC-722665

Pharmacologic Category Antineoplastic Agent, Antiandrogen

Use In combination therapy with LHRH agonist analogues in treatment of metastatic prostate cancer

Unlabeled/Investigational Use Monotherapy for locally-advanced prostate cancer

Pregnancy Risk Factor X

Pregnancy Considerations Animal studies have demonstrated teratogenicity. Bicalutamide is not indicated for women.

Lactation Excretion in breast milk unknown/ contraindicated

Contraindications Hypersensitivity to bicalutamide or any component of the formulation; female patients; pregnancy

Warnings/Precautions Hazardous agent - use appropriate precautions for handling and disposal. Rare cases of death or hospitalization due to hepatitis have been reported postmarketing. Use with caution in moderate-to-severe hepatic dysfunction. Hepatotoxicity generally occurs within the first 3-4 months of use; patients should be monitored for signs and symptoms of liver dysfunction. Bicalutamide should be discontinued if patients have jaundice or ALT is >2 times the upper limit of normal. May cause gynecomastia, breast pain, or lead to spermatogenesis inhibition.

Adverse Reactions Adverse reaction percentages reported as part of combination regimen with an LHRH analogue.

>10%:

Cardiovascular: Peripheral edema (13%)

Central nervous system: Pain (35%)

Endocrine & metabolic: Hot flashes (53%)

Gastrointestinal: Constipation (22%), nausea (15%), diarrhea (12%), abdominal pain (11%)

Genitourinary: Pelvic pain (21%), nocturia (12%), hematuria (12%)

Hematologic: Anemia (11%)

Neuromuscular & skeletal: Back pain (25%), weakness (22%)

Respiratory: Dyspnea (13%)

Miscellaneous: Infection (18%)

≥2% to 10%:

Cardiovascular: Chest pain (8%), hypertension (8%), angina pectoris (2% to <5%), CHF (2% to <5%), edema (2% to <5%), MI (2% to <5%), coronary artery disorder (2% to <5%), syncope (2% to <5%)

Central nervous system: Dizziness (10%), headache (7%), insomnia (7%), anxiety (5%), depression (4%), chills (2% to <5%), confusion (2% to <5%), fever (2% to <5%), nervousness (2% to <5%), somnolence (2% to <5%)

Dermatologic: Rash (9%), alopecia (2% to <5%), dry skin (2% to <5%), pruritus (2% to <5%), skin carcinoma (2% to <5%)

Endocrine & metabolic: Gynecomastia (9%), breast pain (6%; up to 39% as monotherapy), hyperglycemia (6%), dehydration (2% to <5%), gout (2% to <5%), hypercholesterolemia (2% to <5%), libido decreased (2% to <5%)

Gastrointestinal: Dyspepsia (7%), weight loss (7%), anorexia (6%), flatulence (6%), vomiting (6%), weight gain (5%), dysphagia (2% to <5%), gastrointestinal carcinoma (2% to <5%), melena (2% to <5%), periodontal abscess (2% to <5%), rectal hemorrhage (2% to <5%), xerostomia (2% to <5%)

Genitourinary: Urinary tract infection (9%), impotence (7%), polyuria (6%), urinary retention (5%), urinary impairment (5%), urinary incontinence (4%), dysuria (2% to <5%), urinary urgency (2% to <5%)

Hepatic: LFTs increased (7%), alkaline phosphatase increased (5%)

Neuromuscular & skeletal: Bone pain (9%), paresthesia (8%), myasthenia (7%), arthritis (5%), pathological fracture (4%), hypertonia (2% to <5%), leg cramps (2% to <5%), myalgia (2% to <5%), neck pain (2% to <5%), neuropathy (2% to <5%)

Ocular: Cataract (2% to <5%)

Renal: BUN increased, creatinine increased, hydronephrosis

Respiratory: Cough (8%), pharyngitis (8%), bronchitis (6%), pneumonia (4%), rhinitis (4%), asthma (2% to <5%), epistaxis (2% to <5%), sinusitis (2% to <5%)

Miscellaneous: Flu syndrome (7%), diaphoresis (6%), cyst (2% to <5%), hernia (2% to <5%), herpes zoster (2% to <5%), sepsis (2% to <5%)

Postmarketing and/or case reports: Bilirubin increased, hemoglobin decreased, hepatitis, hypersensitivity reactions (including angioneurotic edema and urticaria), interstitial pneumonitis, pulmonary fibrosis, WBC decreased

Drug Interactions

Avoid Concomitant Use There are no known interactions where it is recommended to avoid concomitant use.

Increased Effect/Toxicity There are no known significant interactions involving an increase in effect.

Decreased Effect There are no known significant interactions involving a decrease in effect.

Stability Store at room temperature of 20°C to 25°C (68°F to 77°F).

Mechanism of Action Pure nonsteroidal antiandrogen that binds to androgen receptors; specifically a competitive inhibitor for the binding of dihydrotestosterone and testosterone; prevents testosterone stimulation of cell growth in prostate cancer

Pharmacodynamics/Kinetics

Absorption: Rapid and complete

Protein binding: 96%

Metabolism: Extensively hepatic; glucuronidation and oxidation of the R (active) enantiomer to inactive metabolites

Half-life elimination: Active enantiomer ~6 days, ~10 days in severe liver disease

Time to peak, plasma: 31 hours

Excretion: Urine (36%, as inactive metabolites); feces (42%, as unchanged drug and inactive metabolites)

Dosage Adults: Oral:

Metastatic prostate cancer: 50 mg once daily (in combination with an LHRH analogue)

Locally-advanced prostate cancer (unlabeled use): Oral: 150 mg once daily (as monotherapy)

Dosage adjustment in renal impairment: No adjustment required

Dosage adjustment in hepatic impairment: No adjustment required for mild, moderate, or severe hepatic impairment; use caution with moderate-to-severe impairment. Discontinue if ALT >2 times ULN or patient develops jaundice.

Dietary Considerations May be taken with or without food.

Administration Dose should be taken at the same time each day with or without food. Treatment should be started concomitantly with an LHRH analogue.

Monitoring Parameters Periodically monitor CBC, ECG, echocardiograms, serum testosterone, luteinizing hormone, and prostate specific antigen. Liver function tests should be obtained at baseline and repeated regularly during the first 4 months of treatment, and periodically thereafter; monitor for signs and symptoms of liver dysfunction (discontinue if jaundice is noted or ALT is >2 times the upper limit of normal).

Dosage Forms Excipient information presented when available (limited, particularly for generics); consult specific product labeling.

Tablet: 50 mg

- **Bicillin® L-A** *see* Penicillin G Benzathine *on page 1163*
- **Bicillin® C-R** *see* Penicillin G Benzathine and Penicillin G Procaine *on page 1164*
- **Bicillin® C-R 900/300** *see* Penicillin G Benzathine and Penicillin G Procaine *on page 1164*
- **Bicitra®** *see* Sodium Citrate and Citric Acid *on page 1383*
- **BiCNU®** *see* Carmustine *on page 262*
- **Bidhist** *see* Brompheniramine *on page 214*
- **BiDil®** *see* Isosorbide Dinitrate and Hydralazine *on page 824*
- **BIG-IV** *see* Botulism Immune Globulin (Intravenous-Human) *on page 211*
- **Biltricide®** *see* Praziquantel *on page 1229*

Bimatoprost (bi MAT oh prost)

U.S. Brand Names Latisse™; Lumigan®

Canadian Brand Names Lumigan®

Pharmacologic Category Ophthalmic Agent, Antiglaucoma; Ophthalmic Agent, Miscellaneous; Prostaglandin, Ophthalmic

Additional Appendix Information

Glaucoma Drug Therapy *on page 1808*

Use Reduction of intraocular pressure (IOP) in patients with open-angle glaucoma or ocular hypertension; hypotrichosis treatment of the eyelashes

Pregnancy Risk Factor C

Dosage Adults:

Ophthalmic: Open-angle glaucoma or ocular hypertension: Instill 1 drop into affected eye(s) once daily in the evening; do not exceed once-daily dosing (may decrease IOP-lowering effect). If used with other topical ophthalmic agents, separate administration by at least 5 minutes.

Ophthalmic, topical: Hypotrichosis of the eyelashes: Place one drop on applicator and apply evenly along the skin of the upper eyelid at base of eyelashes once daily at bedtime; repeat procedure for second eye (use a clean applicator)

Additional Information Complete prescribing information for this medication should be consulted for additional detail.

Product Availability Latisse™: FDA approved: December 2008; availability anticipated during first quarter of 2009

Dosage Forms Excipient information presented when available (limited, particularly for generics); consult specific product labeling.

Solution, ophthalmic:

Latisse™: 0.03% (3 mL) [contains benzalkonium chloride]

Lumigan®: 0.03% (2.5 mL, 5 mL, 7.5 mL) [contains benzalkonium chloride]

- **Bio-Carbamazepine (Can)** *see* CarBAMazepine *on page 252*
- **Biolon™ [DSC]** *see* Hyaluronate and Derivatives *on page 734*
- **Bionect®** *see* Hyaluronate and Derivatives *on page 734*
- **Bioniche Promethazine (Can)** *see* Promethazine *on page 1249*
- **Bio-Oxazepam (Can)** *see* Oxazepam *on page 1116*
- **BioQuin® Durules™ (Can)** *see* QuiNIDine *on page 1280*
- **Bio-Statin®** *see* Nystatin *on page 1087*
- **BioThrax®** *see* Anthrax Vaccine Adsorbed *on page 118*
- **Biphentin® (Can)** *see* Methylphenidate *on page 973*
- **Bird Flu Vaccine** *see* Influenza Virus Vaccine (H5N1) *on page 791*
- **Bisac-Evac™ [OTC]** *see* Bisacodyl *on page 198*

Bisacodyl (bis a KOE dil)

U.S. Brand Names Alophen® [OTC]; Bisac-Evac™ [OTC]; Bisacodyl Uniserts® [OTC] [DSC]; Biscolax™ [OTC]; Correctol® Tablets [OTC]; Dacodyl™ [OTC]; Doxidan® [OTC]; Dulcolax® [OTC]; ex-lax® Ultra [OTC]; Fematrol [OTC]; Femilax™ [OTC]; Fleet® Bisacodyl [OTC]; Fleet® Stimulant Laxative [OTC]; Veracolate [OTC]

Canadian Brand Names Apo-Bisacodyl®; Carter's Little Pills®; Dulcolax®; Gentlax®

Pharmacologic Category Laxative, Stimulant

Additional Appendix Information

Laxatives, Classification and Properties *on page 1660*

Use Treatment of constipation; colonic evacuation prior to procedures or examination

Pregnancy Risk Factor C

Medication Safety Issues

Sound-alike/look-alike issues:

Doxidan® may be confused with doxepin

Modane® may be confused with Matulane®, Moban®

Dosage

Children:

Oral: >6 years: 5-10 mg (0.3 mg/kg) at bedtime or before breakfast

Rectal suppository:

<2 years: 5 mg as a single dose

>2 years: 10 mg

Adults:

Oral: 5-15 mg as single dose (up to 30 mg when complete evacuation of bowel is required)

Rectal suppository: 10 mg as single dose

Additional Information Complete prescribing information for this medication should be consulted for additional detail.

Dosage Forms Excipient information presented when available (limited, particularly for generics); consult specific product labeling. [DSC] = Discontinued product

Solution, rectal [enema]:

Fleet® Bisacodyl: 10 mg/30 mL (37 mL)

Suppository, rectal: 10 mg

Bisac-Evac™, Bisacodyl Uniserts® [DSC], Biscolax™, Dulcolax®: 10 mg

Tablet [enteric coated]: 5 mg

Alophen®, Bisac-Evac™, Correctol®, Dacodyl™, Dulcolax®, ex-lax® Ultra, Fematrol, Femilax™, Veracolate: 5 mg

Tablet, delayed release: 5 mg

Doxidan®, Fleet® Stimulant Laxative: 5 mg

- **Bisacodyl Uniserts® [OTC] [DSC]** *see* Bisacodyl *on page 198*
- **bis-chloronitrosourea** *see* Carmustine *on page 262*
- **Biscolax™ [OTC]** *see* Bisacodyl *on page 198*
- **Bismatrol** *see* Bismuth *on page 199*
- **Bismatrol [OTC]** *see* Bismuth *on page 199*
- **Bismatrol Maximum Strength [OTC]** *see* Bismuth *on page 199*

Bismuth (BIZ muth)

U.S. Brand Names Bismatrol Maximum Strength [OTC]; Bismatrol [OTC]; Diotame® [OTC]; Kao-Tin [OTC]; Kaopectate® Extra Strength [OTC]; Kaopectate® [OTC]; Kapectolin [OTC]; Maalox® Total Stomach Relief® [OTC]; Peptic Relief [OTC]; Pepto Relief [OTC]; Pepto-Bismol® Maximum Strength [OTC]; Pepto-Bismol® [OTC]

Index Terms Bismatrol; Bismuth Subsalicylate; Pink Bismuth

Pharmacologic Category Antidiarrheal

Use Subsalicylate formulation: Symptomatic treatment of mild, nonspecific diarrhea; control of traveler's diarrhea (enterotoxigenic *Escherichia coli*); as part of a multidrug regimen for *H. pylori* eradication to reduce the risk of duodenal ulcer recurrence

Pregnancy Risk Factor C/D (3rd trimester)

Medication Safety Issues

Sound-alike/look-alike issues:

Kaopectate® may be confused with Kayexalate®

Maalox® Total Stomach Relief® is a different formulation than Maalox®

Note: Canadian formulation of Kaopectate® does not contain bismuth; the active ingredient in the Canadian formulation is attapulgite.

Dosage Oral:

Treatment of nonspecific diarrhea, control/relieve traveler's diarrhea: Subsalicylate (doses based on 262 mg/15 mL liquid or 262 mg tablets):

Children: Up to 8 doses/24 hours:

3-6 years: 1/3 tablet or 5 mL every 30 minutes to 1 hour as needed

6-9 years: 2/3 tablet or 10 mL every 30 minutes to 1 hour as needed

9-12 years: 1 tablet or 15 mL every 30 minutes to 1 hour as needed

Children >12 years and Adults: 2 tablets or 30 mL every 30 minutes to 1 hour as needed up to 8 doses/24 hours

Helicobacter pylori eradication: Subsalicylate: Adults: 524 mg 4 times/day with meals and at bedtime; requires combination therapy

Dosing adjustment in renal impairment: Should probably be avoided in patients with renal failure

Additional Information Complete prescribing information for this medication should be consulted for additional detail.

Dosage Forms Excipient information presented when available (limited, particularly for generics); consult specific product labeling.

Caplet, as subsalicylate:

Kaopectate®: 262 mg

Pepto-Bismol®: 262 mg [sugar free; contains sodium 2 mg/caplet]

Liquid, as subsalicylate: 262 mg/15 mL (240 mL)

Bismatrol: 262 mg/15 mL (240 mL)

Bismatrol Maximum Strength: 525 mg/15 mL (240 mL)

Diotame®: 262 mg/15 mL (30 mL) [sugar free]

Kaopectate®: 262 mg/15 mL (240 mL, 360 mL) [contains potassium 5 mg/15 mL, sodium 10 mg/15 mL; regular and peppermint flavors]

Kaopectate®: 262 mg/15 mL (180 mL) [contains sodium 10 mg/15 mL; cherry flavor]

Kaopectate® Extra Strength: 525 mg/15 mL (240 mL) [contains potassium 5 mg/15 mL, sodium 10 mg/15 mL; peppermint flavor]

Kao-Tin: 262 mg/15 mL (240 mL, 480 mL) [contains sodium benzoate]

Maalox® Total Stomach Relief®: 525 mg/15 mL (360 mL) [contains sodium 3.3 mg/15mL; strawberry and peppermint flavor]

Peptic Relief: 262 mg/15 mL (240 mL) [sugar free; mint flavor]

Pepto-Bismol®: 262 mg/15 mL (120 mL, 240 mL, 360 mL, 480 mL) [sugar free; contains sodium 6 mg/15 mL and benzoic acid; cherry and wintergreen flavors]

Pepto-Bismol® Maximum Strength: 525 mg/15 mL (120 mL, 240 mL, 360 mL) [sugar free; contains sodium 6 mg/15 mL and benzoic acid; wintergreen flavor]

Suspension, as subsalicylate:

Kapectolin: 262 mg/15 mL (480 mL) [mint flavor]

Tablet, chewable, as subsalicylate: 262 mg

Bismatrol: 262 mg

Diotame®: 262 mg [sugar free]

Peptic Relief, Pepto Relief: 262 mg

Pepto-Bismol®: 262 mg [sugar free; contains sodium <1 mg; cherry and wintergreen flavors]

Bismuth, Metronidazole, and Tetracycline

(BIZ muth, me troe NI da zole, & tet ra SYE kleen)

U.S. Brand Names Helidac®; Pylera™

Index Terms Bismuth Subcitrate Potassium, Tetracycline, and Metronidazole; Bismuth Subsalicylate, Tetracycline, and Metronidazole; Metronidazole, Bismuth Subcitrate Potassium, and Tetracycline; Metronidazole, Bismuth Subsalicylate, and Tetracycline; Tetracycline, Metronidazole, and Bismuth Subcitrate Potassium; Tetracycline, Metronidazole, and Bismuth Subsalicylate

Pharmacologic Category Antibiotic, Miscellaneous; Antibiotic, Tetracycline Derivative; Antidiarrheal

Use As part of a multidrug regimen for *H. pylori* eradication to reduce the risk of duodenal ulcer recurrence in combination with an H_2 agonist (Helidac®) or omeprazole (Pylera™)

Pregnancy Risk Factor D

Dosage Oral: Adults:

Helidac®: Two bismuth subsalicylate 262.4 mg tablets, 1 metronidazole 250 mg tablet, and 1 tetracycline 500 mg capsule 4 times/day at meals and bedtime, plus an H_2 antagonist (at the appropriate dose) for 14 days; follow with 8 oz of water; the H_2 antagonist should be continued for a total of 28 days

Pylera™: Three capsules 4 times/day after meals and at bedtime, plus omeprazole 20 mg twice daily for 10 days; follow each dose with 8 oz of water (each capsule contains bismuth subcitrate potassium 140 mg, metronidazole 125 mg, and tetracycline 125 mg)

Additional Information Complete prescribing information for this medication should be consulted for additional detail.

Dosage Forms Excipient information presented when available (limited, particularly for generics); consult specific product labeling.

Capsule:

Pylera™: Bismuth subcitrate potassium 140 mg, metronidazole 125 mg, and tetracycline hydrochloride 125 mg

Combination package:

Helidac® [each package contains 14 blister cards (2-week supply); each card contains the following]:

Capsule: Tetracycline hydrochloride: 500 mg (4)

Tablet, chewable: Bismuth subsalicylate: 262.4 mg (8)

Tablet: Metronidazole: 250 mg (4)

◆ **Bismuth Subcitrate Potassium, Tetracycline, and Metronidazole** *see* Bismuth, Metronidazole, and Tetracycline *on page 199*

◆ **Bismuth Subsalicylate** *see* Bismuth *on page 199*

◆ **Bismuth Subsalicylate, Tetracycline, and Metronidazole** *see* Bismuth, Metronidazole, and Tetracycline *on page 199*

Bisoprolol (bis OH proe lol)

U.S. Brand Names Zebeta®

Canadian Brand Names Apo-Bisoprolol®; Monocor®; Novo-Bisoprolol; PMS-Bisoprolol; PRO-Bisoprolol; Sandoz-Bisoprolol; Zebeta®

Index Terms Bisoprolol Fumarate

Pharmacologic Category Beta Blocker, $Beta_1$ Selective

Additional Appendix Information

Beta-Blockers *on page 1648*

Heart Failure (Systolic) *on page 1809*

Use Treatment of hypertension, alone or in combination with other agents

Unlabeled/Investigational Use Chronic stable angina, supraventricular arrhythmias, PVCs, heart failure (HF)

Pregnancy Risk Factor C (manufacturer); D (2nd and 3rd trimesters - expert analysis)

Pregnancy Considerations No data available on whether bisoprolol crosses the placenta. Beta-blockers have been associated with persistent bradycardia, hypotension, and IUGR; IUGR is probably related to maternal hypertension. Available evidence suggests beta-blockers are generally safe during pregnancy (JNC 7). Cases of neonatal hypoglycemia have been reported following maternal use of beta-blockers at parturition or during breast-feeding. Monitor breast-fed infant for symptoms of beta-blockade.

Lactation Enters breast milk/use caution

Medication Safety Issues

Sound-alike/look-alike issues:

Zebeta® may be confused with DiaBeta®, Zetia®

Contraindications Cardiogenic shock; overt cardiac failure; marked sinus bradycardia; heart block greater than first-degree (except in patients with a functioning artificial pacemaker)

Warnings/Precautions Consider pre-existing conditions such as sick sinus syndrome before initiating. Use caution in patients with heart failure; use gradual and careful titration; monitor for symptoms of congestive heart failure. Use with caution in patients with myasthenia gravis, psychiatric disease (may cause CNS depression), bronchospastic disease, undergoing anesthesia; and in those with impaired hepatic function. Beta-blocker therapy should not be withdrawn abruptly (particularly in patients with CAD), but gradually tapered to avoid acute tachycardia, hypertension, and/or ischemia. Use caution in patients with PVD (can aggravate arterial insufficiency). Use caution with concurrent use of verapamil or diltiazem; bradycardia or heart block may occur. Bisoprolol, with $beta_1$-selectivity, may be used cautiously in bronchospastic disease with close monitoring. Use cautiously in patients with diabetes because it can mask prominent hypoglycemic symptoms. Use caution in hyperthyroidism since beta-blockade may mask signs of thyrotoxicosis. Dosage adjustment is required in patients with significant hepatic or renal dysfunction. Use care with anesthetic agents which decrease myocardial function. Adequate alpha-blockade is required prior to use of any beta-blocker for patients with untreated pheochromocytoma. Use caution with history of severe anaphylaxis to allergens; patients taking beta-blockers may become more sensitive to repeated challenges. Treatment of anaphylaxis (eg, epinephrine) in patients taking beta-blockers may be ineffective or promote undesirable effects. Safety and efficacy have not been established in children.

Adverse Reactions

1% to 10%:

Cardiovascular: Chest pain (1% to 2%)

Central nervous system: Fatigue (dose related; 6% to 8%), insomnia (2% to 3%), hypoesthesia (1% to 2%)

Gastrointestinal: Diarrhea (dose related; 3% to 4%), nausea (2%), vomiting (1% to 2%)

Neuromuscular & skeletal: Arthralgia, asthenia (dose related; ≤2%)

Respiratory: Upper respiratory infection (5%), rhinitis (3% to 4%), sinusitis (dose related; 2%), dyspnea (1% to 2%)

<1% (Limited to important or life-threatening): Abdominal pain, acne, alopecia, angioedema, anxiety, arrhythmia, asthma, back/neck pain, bradycardia (dose related), bronchitis, bronchospasm, BUN/creatinine increased, claudication, cold extremities, confusion (especially in the elderly), congestive heart failure, constipation, coughing, cutaneous vasculitis, cystitis, depression, dermatitis, dizziness, dyspepsia, dyspnea on exertion, eczema, edema, flushing, gastritis, gout, hallucinations, headache, hearing decreased, hyper-/hypoesthesia, hyperglycemia, hyperkalemia, hyperphosphatemia, hypertriglyceridemia, hypotension, impotence, lacrimation (abnormal), leukopenia, libido decreased, malaise, memory loss, muscle cramps, muscle/joint pain, nervousness, ocular pain/pressure, orthostatic hypotension, palpitations, paresthesia, peptic ulcer, Peyronie's disease, pharyngitis, polyuria, positive ANA titers, pruritus, psoriasis, psoriasiform eruption, purpura, rash, renal colic, restlessness, rhythm disturbances, sleep disturbances, somnolence, syncope, taste abnormality, thrombocytopenia, tinnitus, transaminases increased, tremor, twitching, uric acid increased, vasculitis, vertigo, visual disturbances, weight gain, xerostomia

Drug Interactions

Metabolism/Transport Effects Substrate of CYP2D6 (minor), 3A4 (major)

Avoid Concomitant Use

Avoid concomitant use of Bisoprolol with any of the following: Methacholine

Increased Effect/Toxicity

Bisoprolol may increase the levels/effects of: Alpha-/Beta-Agonists (Direct-Acting); Alpha1-Blockers; Alpha2-Agonists; Amifostine; Antipsychotic Agents (Phenothiazines); Cardiac Glycosides; Insulin; Lidocaine; Methacholine; Midodrine; RiTUXimab

The levels/effects of Bisoprolol may be increased by: Acetylcholinesterase Inhibitors; Aminoquinolines (Antimalarial); Amiodarone; Anilidopiperidine Opioids; Antipsychotic Agents (Phenothiazines); Calcium Channel Blockers (Nondihydropyridine); CYP3A4 Inhibitors (Moderate); CYP3A4 Inhibitors (Strong); Dasatinib; Diazoxide; Dipyridamole; Disopyramide; Herbs (Hypotensive Properties); Propafenone; Propoxyphene; Prostacyclin Analogues; QuiNIDine; Reserpine; Selective Serotonin Reuptake Inhibitors

Decreased Effect

Bisoprolol may decrease the levels/effects of: Beta2-Agonists; Theophylline Derivatives

The levels/effects of Bisoprolol may be decreased by: Barbiturates; CYP3A4 Inducers (Strong); Deferasirox; Herbs (CYP3A4 Inducers); Herbs (Hypertensive Properties); Methylphenidate; Nonsteroidal Anti-Inflammatory Agents; Rifamycin Derivatives; Yohimbine

Ethanol/Nutrition/Herb Interactions Herb/Nutraceutical: Avoid dong quai if using for hypertension (has estrogenic activity). Avoid ephedra, yohimbe, ginseng (may worsen hypertension). Avoid garlic (may have increased antihypertensive effect).

Mechanism of Action Selective inhibitor of $beta_1$-adrenergic receptors; competitively blocks $beta_1$-receptors, with little or no effect on $beta_2$-receptors at doses ≤20 mg

Pharmacodynamics/Kinetics

Onset of action: 1-2 hours

Absorption: Rapid and almost complete

Distribution: Widely; highest concentrations in heart, liver, lungs, and saliva; crosses blood-brain barrier; enters breast milk
Protein binding: ~30%
Metabolism: Extensively hepatic; significant first-pass effect (~20%)
Bioavailability: ~80%
Half-life elimination: Normal renal function: 9-12 hours; Cl_{cr} <40 mL/minute: 27-36 hours; Hepatic cirrhosis: 8-22 hours
Time to peak: 2-4 hours
Excretion: Urine (50% as unchanged drug, remainder as inactive metabolites); feces (<2%)

Dosage Oral:
Adults: 2.5-5 mg once daily; may be increased to 10 mg and then up to 20 mg once daily, if necessary
Hypertension (JNC 7): 2.5-10 mg once daily
HF (unlabeled use): Initial: 1.25 mg once daily; maximum recommended dose: 10 mg once daily. **Note:** Increase dose gradually and monitor for signs and symptoms of CHF.
Elderly: Initial dose: 2.5 mg/day; may be increased by 2.5-5 mg/day; maximum recommended dose: 20 mg/day
Dosing adjustment in renal/hepatic impairment: Cl_{cr} <40 mL/minute: Initial: 2.5 mg/day; increase cautiously.
Hemodialysis: Not dialyzable

Dietary Considerations May be taken without regard to meals.

Monitoring Parameters Blood pressure, ECG, neurologic status

Dosage Forms Excipient information presented when available (limited, particularly for generics); consult specific product labeling.
Tablet, as fumarate: 5 mg, 10 mg

Bisoprolol and Hydrochlorothiazide
(bis OH proe lol & hye droe klor oh THYE a zide)

U.S. Brand Names Ziac®
Canadian Brand Names Ziac®
Index Terms Hydrochlorothiazide and Bisoprolol
Pharmacologic Category Beta Blocker, $Beta_1$ Selective; Diuretic, Thiazide
Use Treatment of hypertension
Unlabeled/Investigational Use Pediatric hypertension
Pregnancy Risk Factor C/D (2nd and 3rd trimesters)
Medication Safety Issues
Sound-alike/look-alike issues:
Ziac® may be confused with Tiazac®, Zerit®

Dosage Oral: Hypertension:
Children (unlabeled use): Initial: Bisoprolol 2.5 mg/hydrochlorothiazide 6.25 mg once daily; up to a maximum of bisoprolol 10 mg/hydrochlorothiazide 6.25 mg daily
Adults: Dose is individualized, given once daily
Dosage adjustment in hepatic impairment: Caution should be used in dosing/titrating patients.

Additional Information Complete prescribing information for this medication should be consulted for additional detail.

Dosage Forms Excipient information presented when available (limited, particularly for generics); consult specific product labeling.
Tablet:
2.5/6.25: Bisoprolol fumarate 2.5 mg and hydrochlorothiazide 6.25 mg
5/6.25: Bisoprolol fumarate 5 mg and hydrochlorothiazide 6.25 mg
10/6.25: Bisoprolol fumarate 10 mg and hydrochlorothiazide 6.25 mg

◆ **Bisoprolol Fumarate** *see* Bisoprolol *on page* 200
◆ **Bis-POM PMEA** *see* Adefovir *on page* 45
◆ **Bistropamide** *see* Tropicamide *on page* 1525

Bivalirudin (bye VAL i roo din)

U.S. Brand Names Angiomax®
Canadian Brand Names Angiomax®
Index Terms Hirulog
Pharmacologic Category Anticoagulant, Thrombin Inhibitor
Use Anticoagulant used in conjunction with aspirin for patients with unstable angina undergoing percutaneous transluminal coronary angioplasty (PTCA) or percutaneous coronary intervention (PCI) with provisional glycoprotein IIb/IIIa inhibitor; anticoagulant used in patients undergoing PCI with (or at risk of) heparin-induced thrombocytopenia (HIT) / thrombosis syndrome (HITTS)
Unlabeled/Investigational Use Heparin-induced thrombocytopenia (HIT)
Pregnancy Risk Factor B
Pregnancy Considerations Although animal studies have not shown harm to the fetus, safety and efficacy for use in pregnant women have not been established. Bivalirudin is used in conjunction with aspirin, which may lead to maternal or fetal adverse effects, especially during the third trimester. Use during pregnancy only if clearly needed.
Lactation Excretion in breast milk unknown/use caution
Medication Safety Issues
High alert medication: The Institute for Safe Medication Practices (ISMP) includes this medication among its list of drugs which have a heightened risk of causing significant patient harm when used in error.

Contraindications Hypersensitivity to bivalirudin or any component of the formulation; active major bleeding

Warnings/Precautions Not for intramuscular use. Safety and efficacy have not been established in patients with unstable angina or acute coronary syndromes who are not undergoing PTCA or PCI. Increased risk of thrombus formation (some fatal) has been reported with bivalirudin use in gamma brachytherapy. As with all anticoagulants, bleeding may occur at any site and should be considered following an unexplained fall in blood pressure or hematocrit, or any unexplained symptom. Use with caution in patients with disease states associated with increased risk of bleeding. Use with caution in patients with renal impairment; dosage reduction required. Safety and efficacy in pediatric patients have not been established.

Adverse Reactions As with all anticoagulants, bleeding is the major adverse effect of bivalirudin. Hemorrhage may occur at virtually any site. Risk is dependent on multiple variables, including the intensity of anticoagulation and patient susceptibility. Additional adverse effects are often related to idiosyncratic reactions, and the frequency is difficult to estimate. Adverse reactions reported were generally less than those seen with heparin.

>10%:
Cardiovascular: Hypotension (3% to 12%)
Central nervous system: Pain (15%), headache (3% to 12%)
Gastrointestinal: Nausea (3% to 15%)
Neuromuscular & skeletal: Back pain (9% to 42%)

1% to 10%:
Cardiovascular: Hypertension (6%), bradycardia (5%), angina (up to 5%)
Central nervous system: Insomnia (7%), anxiety (6%), fever (5%), nervousness (5%)
Gastrointestinal: Vomiting (6%), dyspepsia (5%), abdominal pain (5%)
Genitourinary: Urinary retention (4%)
Hematologic: Major hemorrhage (2% to 4%, compared to 4% to 9% with heparin); transfusion required (1% to 2%,

compared to 2% to 6% with heparin), thrombocytopenia (<1% to 4%)

Local: Injection site pain (3% to 8%)

Neuromuscular & skeletal: Pelvic pain (6%)

<1% (Limited to important or life-threatening): Allergic reaction (including anaphylaxis), cerebral ischemia, confusion, facial paralysis, fatal bleeding, intracranial bleeding, kidney failure, pulmonary edema, retroperitoneal bleeding, syncope, thrombus formation (during PCI, including intracoronary brachytherapy), ventricular fibrillation

Drug Interactions

Avoid Concomitant Use There are no known interactions where it is recommended to avoid concomitant use.

Increased Effect/Toxicity

Bivalirudin may increase the levels/effects of: Anticoagulants; Ibritumomab; Tositumomab and Iodine I 131 Tositumomab

The levels/effects of Bivalirudin may be increased by: Antiplatelet Agents; Dasatinib; Herbs (Anticoagulant/Antiplatelet Properties); Nonsteroidal Anti-Inflammatory Agents; Pentosan Polysulfate Sodium; Prostacyclin Analogues; Salicylates; Thrombolytic Agents

Decreased Effect There are no known significant interactions involving a decrease in effect.

Stability Store unopened vials at 15°C to 30°C. Reconstitute each 250 mg with 5 mL SWFI. Gently swirl to dissolve. Further dilution in D_5W or NS (50 mL to make 5 mg/mL solution **or** 500 mL to make 0.5 mg/mL solution) is required prior to infusion. Do not administer in same line with other medications. Following reconstitution, vials should be stored at 2°C to 8°C. Do not freeze. Final dilutions of 0.5 mg/mL or 5 mg/mL are stable at room temperature for up to 24 hours.

Mechanism of Action Bivalirudin acts as a specific and reversible direct thrombin inhibitor; it binds to the catalytic and anionic exosite of both circulating and clot-bound thrombin. Catalytic binding site occupation functionally inhibits coagulant effects by preventing thrombin-mediated cleavage of fibrinogen to fibrin monomers, and activation of factors V, VIII, and XIII. Shows linear dose- and concentration-dependent prolongation of ACT, aPTT, PT, and TT.

Pharmacodynamics/Kinetics

Onset of action: Immediate

Duration: Coagulation times return to baseline ~1 hour following discontinuation of infusion

Distribution: 0.2 L/kg

Protein binding, plasma: Does not bind other than thrombin

Metabolism: Blood proteases

Half-life elimination: Normal renal function: 25 minutes; Cl_{cr} 10-29 mL/minute: 57 minutes; Dialysis-dependent patients (off dialysis): 3.5 hours

Excretion: Urine (20%), proteolytic cleavage

Dosage I.V.: Adults:

Acute coronary syndromes (moderate-high risk) undergoing invasive strategy (unlabeled dose): Initial dose: 0.1 mg/kg bolus, followed by 0.25 mg/kg/hour. Prior to PCI, give an additional bolus of 0.5 mg/kg and increase infusion rate to 1.75 mg/kg/hour.

Anticoagulant in patients undergoing PTCA/PCI or PCI with HITS/HITTS (treatment should be started just prior to procedure): Initial: Bolus: 0.75 mg/kg, followed by continuous infusion: 1.75 mg/kg/hour for the duration of procedure and up to 4 hours postprocedure if needed; determine ACT 5 minutes after bolus dose; may administer additional bolus of 0.3 mg/kg if necessary.

A glycoprotein IIb/IIIa inhibitor may be administered concomitantly during the procedure.

If needed, infusion may be continued beyond initial 4 hours at 0.2 mg/kg/hour for up to 20 hours.

Cardiac surgery (unlabeled; Warkentin, 2008):

Off-pump: Initial bolus: 0.75 mg/kg, followed by continuous infusion 1.75 mg/kg/hour to maintain ACT >300 seconds

On-pump: Initial bolus: 1 mg/kg, followed by continuous infusion 2.5 mg/kg/hour; 50 mg bolus added to priming solution of cardiopulmonary bypass (CPB) circuit

Additional boluses of 0.1-0.5 mg may be given to maintain ACT >2.5 times baseline ACT. **Note:** Special maneuvers needed to prevent stasis and consequent clotting within CPB circuit during or after surgery.

HIT (unlabeled use; Warkentin, 2008): Normal renal function: Initial dose: ~0.15 mg/kg/hour; adjust to aPTT 1.5-2.5 times baseline value

Dosage adjustment in renal impairment: Infusion dose should be reduced based on degree of renal impairment; initial bolus dose remains unchanged; monitor activated coagulation time (ACT) or aPTT depending on indication.

For use in PCI:

Cl_{cr} ≥30 mL/minute: No adjustment required

Cl_{cr} 10-29 mL/minute: Decrease infusion rate to 1 mg/kg/hour

Dialysis-dependent patients (off dialysis): Decrease infusion rate to 0.25 mg/kg/hour

Clearance of bivalirudin remains 1.8-fold greater than the glomerular filtration rate, regardless of the degree in renal impairment.

Hemodialysis: Approximately 25% removed during hemodialysis

Dosage adjustment in hepatic impairment: No dosage adjustment is needed

Elderly: No dosage adjustment is needed in elderly patients with normal renal function. Puncture site hemorrhage and catheterization site hemorrhage were seen in more patients ≥65 years of age than in patients <65 years of age

Administration For I.V. administration only.

Monitoring Parameters Depends upon indication for use of bivalirudin: ACT or aPTT

Test Interactions PT/INR levels may become elevated in the absence of warfarin. If warfarin is initiated, initial PT/INR goals while on bivalirudin may require modification.

Dosage Forms Excipient information presented when available (limited, particularly for generics); consult specific product labeling.

Injection, powder for reconstitution: 250 mg

◆ **Bi-Zets** *see* Benzocaine *on page 183*

◆ **BL4162A** *see* Anagrelide *on page 115*

◆ **Blenoxane® [DSC]** *see* Bleomycin *on page 202*

◆ **Blenoxane® (Can)** *see* Bleomycin *on page 202*

◆ **Bleo** *see* Bleomycin *on page 202*

Bleomycin (blee oh MYE sin)

U.S. Brand Names Blenoxane® [DSC]

Canadian Brand Names Blenoxane®; Bleomycin Injection, USP

Index Terms Bleo; Bleomycin Sulfate; BLM; NSC-125066

Pharmacologic Category Antineoplastic Agent, Antibiotic

Use Treatment of squamous cell carcinomas, melanomas, sarcomas, testicular carcinoma, Hodgkin's lymphoma, and non-Hodgkin's lymphoma; sclerosing agent for malignant pleural effusion

Pregnancy Risk Factor D

Pregnancy Considerations Animal studies have demonstrated teratogenic and abortifacient effects. There are no adequate and well-controlled studies in pregnant women.

Women of childbearing potential should avoid becoming pregnant during treatment.

Lactation Excretion in breast milk unknown/not recommended

Medication Safety Issues

Sound-alike/look-alike issues:

Bleomycin may be confused with Cleocin®

High alert medication: The Institute for Safe Medication Practices (ISMP) includes this medication among its list of drugs which have a heightened risk of causing significant patient harm when used in error.

Contraindications Hypersensitivity to bleomycin or any component of the formulation; severe pulmonary disease; pregnancy

Warnings/Precautions Hazardous agent - use appropriate precautions for handling and disposal. **[U.S. Boxed Warnings]: Occurrence of pulmonary fibrosis (commonly presenting as pneumonitis) is higher in elderly patients, patients receiving >400 units total lifetime dose or single doses >30 units, smokers, and patients with prior radiation therapy or receiving concurrent oxygen. A severe idiosyncratic reaction consisting of hypotension, mental confusion, fever, chills, and wheezing (similar to anaphylaxis) has been reported in 1% of lymphoma patients treated with bleomycin.** Since these reactions usually occur after the first or second dose, careful monitoring is essential after these doses. Use caution when administering O_2 during surgery to patients who have received bleomycin. Use caution with renal impairment, may require dose adjustment. May cause renal or hepatic toxicity. **[U.S. Boxed Warning]: Should be administered under the supervision of an experienced cancer chemotherapy physician.**

Adverse Reactions

>10%:

Dermatologic: Pain at the tumor site, phlebitis. About 50% of patients develop erythema, rash, striae, induration, hyperkeratosis, vesiculation, and peeling of the skin, particularly on the palmar and plantar surfaces of the hands and feet. Hyperpigmentation (50%), alopecia, nailbed changes may also occur. These effects appear dose related and reversible with discontinuation.

Gastrointestinal: Stomatitis and mucositis (30%), anorexia, weight loss

Respiratory: Tachypnea, rales, acute or chronic interstitial pneumonitis, and pulmonary fibrosis (5% to 10%); hypoxia and death (1%). Symptoms include cough, dyspnea, and bilateral pulmonary infiltrates. The pathogenesis is not certain, but may be due to damage of pulmonary, vascular, or connective tissue. Response to steroid therapy is variable and somewhat controversial.

Miscellaneous: Acute febrile reactions (25% to 50%)

1% to 10%:

Dermatologic: Skin thickening, diffuse scleroderma, onycholysis, pruritus

Miscellaneous: Anaphylactoid-like reactions (characterized by hypotension, confusion, fever, chills, and wheezing; onset may be immediate or delayed for several hours); idiosyncratic reactions (1% in lymphoma patients)

<1% (Limited to important or life-threatening): Angioedema, cerebrovascular accident, cerebral arteritis, hepatotoxicity, malaise, MI, nausea, Raynaud's phenomenon, renal toxicity, scleroderma-like skin changes, thrombotic microangiopathy, vomiting; Myelosuppression (rare); Onset: 7 days, Nadir: 14 days, Recovery: 21 days

Drug Interactions

Avoid Concomitant Use

Avoid concomitant use of Bleomycin with any of the following: Natalizumab; Vaccines (Live)

Increased Effect/Toxicity

Bleomycin may increase the levels/effects of: Natalizumab; Vaccines (Live)

The levels/effects of Bleomycin may be increased by: Gemcitabine; Trastuzumab

Decreased Effect

Bleomycin may decrease the levels/effects of: Cardiac Glycosides; Vaccines (Inactivated)

The levels/effects of Bleomycin may be decreased by: Echinacea

Stability

Refrigerate intact vials of powder. Intact vials are stable for up to 1 month at 45°C. Solutions for infusion are stable for 96 hours at room temperature and 14 days under refrigeration.

Reconstitute powder with 1-5 mL BWFI or BNS which is stable at room temperature or under refrigeration for 28 days.

Standard I.V. dilution: Dose/50-1000 mL NS.

Mechanism of Action Inhibits synthesis of DNA; binds to DNA leading to single- and double-strand breaks

Pharmacodynamics/Kinetics

Absorption: I.M. and intrapleural administration: 30% to 50% of I.V. serum concentrations; intraperitoneal and SubQ routes produce serum concentrations equal to those of I.V.

Distribution: V_d: 22 L/m^2; highest concentrations in skin, kidney, lung, heart tissues; lowest in testes and GI tract; does not cross blood-brain barrier

Protein binding: 1%

Metabolism: Via several tissues including hepatic, GI tract, skin, pulmonary, renal, and serum

Half-life elimination: Biphasic (renal function dependent):

Normal renal function: Initial: 1.3 hours; Terminal: 9 hours

End-stage renal disease: Initial: 2 hours; Terminal: 30 hours

Time to peak, serum: I.M.: Within 30 minutes

Excretion: Urine (50% to 70% as active drug)

Dosage Maximum cumulative lifetime dose: 400 units; refer to individual protocols; 1 unit = 1 mg

May be administered I.M., I.V., SubQ, or intracavitary

Children and Adults:

Test dose for lymphoma patients: I.M., I.V., SubQ: Because of the possibility of an anaphylactoid reaction, administer 1-2 units of bleomycin before the first 1-2 doses; monitor vital signs every 15 minutes; wait a minimum of 1 hour before administering remainder of dose; if no acute reaction occurs, then the regular dosage schedule may be followed. **Note:** Test doses may produce false-negative results.

Single-agent therapy:

I.M./I.V./SubQ: Squamous cell carcinoma, lymphoma, testicular carcinoma: 0.25-0.5 units/kg (10-20 units/m^2) 1-2 times/week

CIV: 15 units/m^2 over 24 hours daily for 4 days

Pleural sclerosing: Intrapleural: 60 units as a single instillation (some recommend limiting the dose in the elderly to 40 units/m^2; usual maximum: 60 units). Dose may be repeated at intervals of several days if fluid continues to accumulate (mix in 50-100 mL of NS); may add lidocaine 100-200 mg to reduce local discomfort.

Dosing adjustment in renal impairment:

The FDA-approved labeling recommends the following adjustments:

Cl_{cr} 40-50 mL/minute: Administer 70% of normal dose

Cl_{cr} 30-40 mL/minute: Administer 60% of normal dose

Cl_{cr} 20-30 mL/minute: Administer 55% of normal dose

Cl_{cr} 10-20 mL/minute: Administer 45% of normal dose

Cl_{cr} 5-10 mL/minute: Administer 40% of normal dose

The following guidelines have been used by some clinicians:

Aronoff, 2007: Adults: Continuous renal replacement therapy (CRRT): Administer 75% of dose

Kintzel, 1995:

Cl_{cr} 46-60 mL/minute: Administer 70% of dose

Cl_{cr} 31-45 mL/minute: Administer 60% of dose

Cl_{cr} <30 mL/minute: Consider use of alternative drug

Dosing adjustment in hepatic impairment: Not studied in patients with hepatic impairment; adjustment for hepatic impairment may be needed.

Administration

I.V. doses should be administered slowly (over 10-60 minutes).

I.M. or SubQ: May cause pain at injection site

Intrapleural: 60 units in 50-100 mL NS; use of topical anesthetics or narcotic analgesia is usually not necessary

Monitoring Parameters Pulmonary function tests (total lung volume, forced vital capacity, carbon monoxide diffusion), renal function, liver function, chest x-ray, temperature initially; check body weight at regular intervals

Dosage Forms Excipient information presented when available (limited, particularly for generics); consult specific product labeling. [DSC] = Discontinued product

Injection, powder for reconstitution, as sulfate: 15 units, 30 units

Blenoxane®: 15 units [DSC], 30 units [DSC]

- ◆ **Bleomycin Injection, USP (Can)** *see* Bleomycin *on page 202*
- ◆ **Bleomycin Sulfate** *see* Bleomycin *on page 202*
- ◆ **Bleph®-10** *see* Sulfacetamide *on page 1405*
- ◆ **Blephamide®** *see* Sulfacetamide and Prednisolone *on page 1405*
- ◆ **Blis-To-Sol® [OTC]** *see* Tolnaftate *on page 1487*
- ◆ **BLM** *see* Bleomycin *on page 202*
- ◆ **BMS-232632** *see* Atazanavir *on page 146*
- ◆ **BMS-247550** *see* Ixabepilone *on page 832*
- ◆ **BMS 337039** *see* Aripiprazole *on page 134*
- ◆ **BMS-354825** *see* Dasatinib *on page 404*
- ◆ **Boil-Ease® Pain Relieving** *see* Benzocaine *on page 183*
- ◆ **Bonamine™ (Can)** *see* Meclizine *on page 928*
- ◆ **Bondronat® (Can)** *see* Ibandronate *on page 757*
- ◆ **Bonine® [OTC]** *see* Meclizine *on page 928*
- ◆ **Bonine® (Can)** *see* Meclizine *on page 928*
- ◆ **Boniva®** *see* Ibandronate *on page 757*
- ◆ **Boostrix®** *see* Diphtheria and Tetanus Toxoids, and Acellular Pertussis Vaccine *on page 463*

Bortezomib (bore TEZ oh mib)

U.S. Brand Names Velcade®

Canadian Brand Names Velcade®

Index Terms LDP-341; MLN341; NSC-681239; PS-341

Pharmacologic Category Antineoplastic Agent; Proteasome Inhibitor

Use Treatment of multiple myeloma; treatment of relapsed or refractory mantle cell lymphoma

Unlabeled/Investigational Use Treatment of non-Hodgkin's lymphomas (other than mantle cell lymphoma)

Pregnancy Risk Factor D

Pregnancy Considerations Adverse effects (fetal loss and decreased fetal weight) were observed in animal studies. There are no adequate and well-controlled studies in pregnant women. Effective contraception is recommended for women of childbearing potential.

Lactation Excretion in breast milk unknown/not recommended

Medication Safety Issues

High alert medication: The Institute for Safe Medication Practices (ISMP) includes this medication among its list of drug classes which have a heightened risk of causing significant patient harm when used in error.

Contraindications Hypersensitivity to bortezomib, boron, mannitol, or any component of the formulation

Warnings/Precautions Hazardous agent - use appropriate precautions for handling and disposal. May cause peripheral neuropathy (usually sensory but may be mixed sensorimotor); risk may be increased with previous use of neurotoxic agents or pre-existing peripheral neuropathy; adjustment of dose and schedule may be required. May cause hypotension (including postural and orthostatic); use caution with dehydration, history of syncope, or medications associated with hypotension. Has been associated with the development or exacerbation of congestive heart failure and decreased left ventricular ejection fraction; use caution in patients with risk factors or existing heart disease. Has also been associated with QT_c prolongation.

Pulmonary disorders including pneumonitis, interstitial pneumonia, lung infiltrates, and acute respiratory distress syndrome (ARDS) have been reported. Pulmonary hypertension (without left heart failure or significant pulmonary disease has been reported rarely). May cause tumor lysis syndrome; risk is increased in patients with high tumor burden prior to treatment. Reversible posterior leukoencephalopathy syndrome (RPLS) has been reported (rarely). Symptoms of RPLS include confusion, headache, hypertension, lethargy, seizure, blindness and/or other vision, or neurologic disturbances; discontinue if RPLS occurs. The safety of reinitiating bortezomib in patients previously experiencing RPLS is unknown. Herpes (zoster and simplex) reactivation has been reported with bortezomib; consider antiviral prophylaxis during therapy. Hematologic toxicity, including neutropenia and severe thrombocytopenia, may occur; risk is increased in patients with pretreatment platelet counts <75,000/µL; frequent monitoring is required throughout treatment; may require dosage adjustments; withhold treatment for platelets <25,000/µL. Hemorrhage (gastrointestinal and intracerebral) due to low platelet count has been observed. Acute liver failure has been reported (rarely) in patients receiving multiple concomitant medications; hepatitis, transaminase increases, and hyperbilirubinemia have also been reported. Use caution in patients with hepatic dysfunction; toxicities may be increased. Hyper- and hypoglycemia may occur in diabetic patients receiving oral hypoglycemics; may require adjustment of diabetes medications. Safety and efficacy have not been established in pediatric patients.

Adverse Reactions

>10%:

Cardiovascular: Edema (11% to 28%), hypotension (12% to 15%; grades 3/4: 3%)

Central nervous system: Fever (19% to 37%), psychiatric disturbance (35%), headache (17% to 26%), dysesthesia (9% to 27%), insomnia (18% to 21%), dizziness (14% to 23%; excludes vertigo), anxiety (5% to 11%)

Dermatologic: Rash (17% to 28%), pruritus (11%)

Endocrine & metabolic: Dehydration (7% to 11%)

Gastrointestinal: Diarrhea (47% to 57%), nausea (44% to 57%), constipation (40% to 50%), anorexia (34% to 39%), vomiting (27% to 35%), abdominal pain (14% to 16%), abnormal taste (13%), dyspepsia (13%)

Hematologic: Thrombocytopenia (21% to 38%; grade 4: 4% to 5%; nadir: day 11; recovery: by day 21), anemia (17% to 30%; grade 4: <1%), neutropenia (6% to 19%; grade 4: 2% to 3%; nadir: day 11; recovery: by day 21)

Neuromuscular & skeletal: Weakness (61% to 72%; grades 3/4: 12% to 19%), peripheral neuropathy (36% to 55%; grade 3: 7% to 11%; grade 4: <1%), paresthesia (9% to 27%), arthralgia (13% to 18%), limb pain (5% to 17%), bone pain (2% to 16%), back pain (<1 % to 15%), myalgia (10% to 12%), muscle cramps (5% to 12%), rigors (11%)

Ocular: Blurred vision (11%)

Respiratory: Dyspnea (20% to 23%), cough (19% to 21%), lower respiratory infection (15%), upper respiratory tract infection (11% to 15%), nasopharyngitis (8% to 14%), pneumonia (9% to 12%)

Miscellaneous: Herpesvirus infections (7% to 13%)

1% to 10%:

Cardiovascular: Syncope (2%)

Endocrine & metabolic: Hypercalcemia (grade 4: 2%)

Frequency not defined (limited to important or life-threatening): Acute diffuse infiltrative pulmonary disease, acute respiratory distress syndrome, alkaline phosphatase increased, allergic reaction, amyloidosis, anaphylaxis, angina, angioedema, ascites, aspergillosis, atelectasis, atrial fibrillation, atrial flutter, AV block, bacteremia, bradycardia, cardiac amyloidosis, cardiac arrest, cardiac tamponade, cardiogenic shock, cardiopulmonary arrest, cerebral hemorrhage, cerebrovascular accident, CHF, cholestasis, coma, complete heart block, confusion, cranial palsy, deafness, deep venous thrombosis, diplopia, disseminated intravascular coagulation (DIC), duodenitis (hemorrhagic), dysautonomia, dysphagia, edema (facial), encephalopathy, embolism, epistaxis, fecal impaction, fracture, gastritis (hemorrhagic), gastroenteritis, GGT increased, glomerular nephritis, hematemesis, hematuria, hemoptysis, hemorrhagic cystitis, hepatic failure, hepatic hemorrhage, hepatitis, hepatocellular damage, herpes meningoencephalitis, hyperbilirubinemia, hyper-/hypoglycemia, hyper-/hypokalemia, hyper-/hyponatremia, hypersensitivity, hyperuricemia, hypocalcemia, hypoxia, immune complex hypersensitivity, injection site reaction, intestinal obstruction, intestinal perforation, intracerebral hemorrhage, ischemic colitis, ischemic stroke, laryngeal edema, leukocytoclastic vasculitis, leukopenia, listeriosis, lymphopenia, melena, mental status change, MI, myocardial ischemia, neuralgia, neutropenic fever, ophthalmic herpes, oral candidiasis, pancreatitis, paralytic ileus, paraplegia, pericardial effusion, pericarditis, peritonitis, pleural effusion, pneumonia, pneumonitis, portal vein thrombosis, proliferative glomerular nephritis, psychosis, pulmonary alveolar hemorrhage, pulmonary edema, pulmonary embolism, pulmonary hypertension, psychosis, QT_c prolongation, renal calculus, renal failure, respiratory failure, respiratory insufficiency, reversible posterior leukoencephalopathy syndrome (RPLS), seizure, septic shock, sepsis, sinus arrest, spinal cord compression, stomatitis, stroke (hemorrhagic), stroke, subarachnoid hemorrhage, subdural hematoma, suicidal ideation, tachycardia, torsade de pointes, toxic epidermal necrolysis, toxoplasmosis, transaminases increased, transient ischemic attack, tumor lysis syndrome, urinary incontinence, urinary retention, urinary tract infection, urticaria, ventricular tachycardia

Drug Interactions

Metabolism/Transport Effects **Substrate** of CYP1A2 (minor), 2C9 (minor), 2C19 (major), 2D6 (minor), 3A4 (major); **Inhibits** CYP1A2 (weak), 2C9 (weak), 2C19 (moderate), 2D6 (weak), 3A4 (weak)

Avoid Concomitant Use There are no known interactions where it is recommended to avoid concomitant use.

Increased Effect/Toxicity

Bortezomib may increase the levels/effects of: CYP2C19 Substrates

The levels/effects of Bortezomib may be increased by: CYP2C19 Inhibitors (Moderate); CYP2C19 Inhibitors (Strong); CYP3A4 Inhibitors (Moderate); CYP3A4 Inhibitors (Strong); Dasatinib

Decreased Effect

The levels/effects of Bortezomib may be decreased by: CYP2C19 Inducers (Strong); CYP3A4 Inducers (Strong); Deferasirox; Herbs (CYP3A4 Inducers)

Ethanol/Nutrition/Herb Interactions Herb/Nutraceutical: Avoid St John's wort (may decrease bortezomib levels).

Stability Prior to reconstitution, store at room temperature of 25°C (77°F); excursions permitted between 15°C to 30°C (59°F to 86°F). Protect from light. Dilute each 3.5 mg vial with 3.5 mL NS to a final concentration of 1 mg/mL. Once reconstituted, although the manufacturer recommends use within 8 hours, solution may be stored at room temperature for up to 3 days, or under refrigeration for up to 5 days, in vial or syringe (Andre, 2005). Protect from light. Use appropriate precautions for handling and disposal.

Mechanism of Action Bortezomib inhibits proteasomes, enzyme complexes which regulate protein homeostasis within the cell. Specifically, it reversibly inhibits chymotrypsin-like activity at the 26S proteasome, leading to activation of signaling cascades, cell-cycle arrest, and apoptosis.

Pharmacodynamics/Kinetics

Distribution: 498-1884 L/m^2

Protein binding: ~83%

Metabolism: Hepatic primarily via CYP2C19 and 3A4 and to a lesser extent CYP1A2; forms metabolites (inactive) via deboronization followed by hydroxylation

Half-life elimination: Single dose: 9-15 hours; multiple dosing: 1 mg/m^2: 40-193 hours; 1.3 mg/m^2: 76-108 hours

Dosage Details concerning dosing in combination regimens should also be consulted. I.V.: Adults:

Multiple myeloma (first-line therapy; in combination with melphalan and prednisone): 1.3 mg/m^2 days 1, 4, 8, 11, 22, 25, 29, and 32 of a 42-day treatment cycle for 4 cycles, followed by 1.3 mg/m^2 days 1, 8, 22, and 29 of a 42-day treatment cycle for 5 cycles.

Relapsed multiple myeloma and mantle cell lymphoma: 1.3 mg/m^2 twice weekly for 2 weeks on days 1, 4, 8, and 11 of a 21-day treatment cycle. Consecutive doses should be separated by at least 72 hours. Therapy extending beyond 8 cycles may be given once weekly for 4 weeks (days 1, 8, 15, and 22), followed by a 13-day rest (days 23 through 35).

Non-Hodgkin's lymphoma, other than mantle cell (unlabeled use): 1.3-1.5 mg/m^2 twice weekly for 2 weeks on days 1, 4, 8, and 11 of a 21-day treatment cycle.

Dosage adjustment in renal impairment: Dosage adjustment not necessary. **Note:** Dialysis may reduce bortezomib concentrations; administer postdialysis.

Dosage adjustment in hepatic impairment: Specific guidelines are not available; clearance may be decreased; monitor closely for toxicity

Dosage adjustment for toxicity:

Myeloma (first-line therapy):

Platelets should be ≥70,000/mm^3, ANC should be ≥1000/mm^3, and nonhematologic toxicities should resolve to grade 1 or baseline prior to therapy initiation.

Platelets ≤30,000/mm^3 or ANC <750/mm^3 on bortezomib day(s): Withhold bortezomib; if several consecutive bortezomib doses are withheld, reduce dose 1 level (1.3 mg/m^2/dose reduced to 1 mg/m^2/dose; 1 mg/m^2/dose reduced to 0.7 mg/m^2/dose)

Grade ≥3 nonhematological toxicity (other than neuropathy): Withhold bortezomib until toxicity resolves to grade 1 or baseline. May reinitiate bortezomib at 1 dose level reduction (1.3 mg/m^2/dose reduced to 1 mg/m^2/dose; 1 mg/m^2/dose reduced to 0.7 mg/m^2/dose).

Neuropathic pain and/or peripheral sensory neuropathy: See "Neuropathic pain and/or peripheral sensory neuropathy" toxicity adjustment guidelines below.

Relapsed multiple myeloma and mantle cell lymphoma:

Grade 3 nonhematological (excluding neuropathy) or Grade 4 hematological toxicity: Withhold until toxicity resolved; may reinitiate with a 25% dose reduction (1.3 mg/m^2/dose reduced to 1 mg/m^2/dose; 1 mg/m^2/dose reduced to 0.7 mg/m^2/dose)

Neuropathic pain and/or peripheral sensory neuropathy:

Grade 1 without pain or loss of function: No action needed

Grade 1 with pain or Grade 2 interfering with function but not activities of daily living: Reduce dose to 1 mg/m^2

Grade 2 with pain or Grade 3 interfering with activities of daily living: Withhold until toxicity resolved, may reinitiate at 0.7 mg/m^2 once weekly

Grade 4: Discontinue therapy

Administration Administer via rapid I.V. push (3-5 seconds)

Monitoring Parameters Signs/symptoms of peripheral neuropathy, dehydration, or hypotension; CBC with differential and platelets (monitor frequently throughout therapy); renal function, pulmonary function (with new or worsening pulmonary symptoms), liver function tests (in patients with existing hepatic impairment)

Dosage Forms Excipient information presented when available (limited, particularly for generics); consult specific product labeling.

Injection, powder for reconstitution [preservative free]:

Velcade®: 3.5 mg [contains mannitol 35 mg]

Bosentan (boe SEN tan)

U.S. Brand Names Tracleer®

Canadian Brand Names Tracleer®

Pharmacologic Category Endothelin Antagonist; Vasodilator

Use Treatment of pulmonary artery hypertension (PAH) (WHO Group I) in patients with World Health Organization (WHO) Class III or IV symptoms to improve exercise capacity and decrease the rate of clinical deterioration

Restrictions Bosentan (Tracleer®) is available only through a limited distribution program directly from the manufacturer (Actelion Pharmaceuticals 1-866-228-3546). It will not be available through wholesalers or individual pharmacies. An FDA-approved medication guide must be distributed when dispensing an outpatient prescription (new or refill) where this medication is to be used without direct supervision of a healthcare provider. Medication guides are available at http://www.fda.gov/cder/Offices/ODS/medication_guides.htm.

Pregnancy Risk Factor X

Pregnancy Considerations [U.S. Boxed Warning]: Use in pregnancy is contraindicated. Based on animal studies, bosentan is likely to produce major birth defects if used by pregnant women. Pregnancy must be excluded prior to initiation of therapy and follow-up pregnancy tests should be obtained monthly. Effective contraception must be maintained throughout treatment. Hormonal contraception is not recommended as the sole contraceptive therapy due to a potential lack of efficacy in patients receiving bosentan. Women of childbearing potential should avoid exposure to dust generated from broken or split tablets, especially if repeated exposure is expected (tablet splitting is currently outside of product labeling). Irreversible testicular atrophy and decreased fertility in males was observed in animal studies with long-term exposure.

Lactation Excretion in breast milk unknown/not recommended

Medication Safety Issues

Sound-alike/look-alike issues:

Tracleer® may be confused with TriCor®

Contraindications Hypersensitivity to bosentan or any component of the formulation; concurrent use of cyclosporine or glyburide; pregnancy

Warnings/Precautions Hazardous agent - use appropriate precautions for handling and disposal. **[U.S. Boxed Warning]: Avoid use in moderate-to-severe hepatic impairment.** Has been associated with a high incidence (12%) of significant transaminase elevations, and rare cases of unexplained hepatic cirrhosis have occurred, including after long-term therapy. Transaminase elevations are dose dependent, generally asymptomatic, occur both early and late in therapy, progress slowly, and are usually reversible after treatment interruption or discontinuation. Avoid use in patients with elevated serum transaminases (>3 times upper limit of normal) at baseline. Monitor hepatic function closely (at least monthly) for the duration of treatment. Treatment should be stopped in patients who develop elevated transaminases (ALT or AST) in combination with symptoms of hepatic injury (unusual fatigue, jaundice, nausea, vomiting, abdominal pain, and/or fever) or elevated serum bilirubin ≥2 times upper limit of normal. Safety of reintroduction is unknown.

[U.S. Boxed Warning]: Use in pregnancy is contraindicated; exclude pregnancy prior to initiation of therapy and shipment of each monthly refill. Efficacy of hormonal contraceptive may be decreased, and should not be the sole contraceptive method in patients receiving bosentan. A missed menses should be reported to healthcare provider and prompt immediate pregnancy testing. Women of childbearing potential should avoid excessive handling of broken tablets.

Use caution in patients with low hemoglobin levels or ischemic cardiovascular disease. May cause dose-related decreases in hemoglobin and hematocrit (monitoring of hemoglobin is recommended).

May cause fluid retention evidenced by signs and symptoms of CHF, weight gain, and leg edema. Bosentan should be discontinued in any patient with pulmonary edema suggestive of pulmonary veno-occlusive disease (PVOD). Safety and efficacy in pediatric patients ≤12 years of age have not been established.

Adverse Reactions

>10%:

Central nervous system: Headache (16% to 22%)

Hematologic: Hemoglobin decreased (≥1 g/dL in up to 57%; <11 g/dL: 3% to 6%; typically in first 6 weeks of therapy)

Hepatic: Transaminases increased (>3 times upper limit of normal; up to 12%; dose-related)

Respiratory: Nasopharyngitis (11%)

1% to 10%:

Cardiovascular: Flushing (7% to 9%), edema (lower limb, 5% to 8%; generalized 4%), hypotension (7%), palpitation (5%)

Central nervous system: Fatigue (4%)

Dermatologic: Pruritus (4%)

Gastrointestinal: Dyspepsia (4%)

Hematologic: Anemia (3%)

Hepatic: Abnormal hepatic function (6% to 8%)

<1% (Limited to important or life-threatening): Angioneurotic edema, heart failure (exacerbation), cirrhosis (prolonged therapy), hyperbilirubinemia, hypersensitivity, leukocytoclastic vasculitis, liver failure (rare), peripheral edema, rash, thrombocytopenia, weight gain

Drug Interactions

Metabolism/Transport Effects Substrate (major) of CYP2C9, 3A4; **Induces** CYP2C9 (strong), 3A4 (strong)

Avoid Concomitant Use

Avoid concomitant use of Bosentan with any of the following: CycloSPORINE; GlyBURIDE; Nilotinib; Nisoldipine; Ranolazine

Increased Effect/Toxicity

The levels/effects of Bosentan may be increased by: Antifungal Agents (Azole Derivatives, Systemic); CycloSPORINE; CYP2C9 Inhibitors (Moderate); CYP2C9 Inhibitors (Strong); CYP3A4 Inhibitors (Moderate); CYP3A4 Inhibitors (Strong); Dasatinib; Eltrombopag; GlyBURIDE; Sildenafil

Decreased Effect

Bosentan may decrease the levels/effects of: CycloSPORINE; CYP2C9 Substrates (High risk); CYP3A4 Substrates; GlyBURIDE; HMG-CoA Reductase Inhibitors; Maraviroc; Nilotinib; Nisoldipine; Ranolazine; Sildenafil; Sorafenib; Vitamin K Antagonists

The levels/effects of Bosentan may be decreased by: CYP2C9 Inducers (Highly Effective); CYP3A4 Inducers (Strong); Deferasirox; GlyBURIDE; Herbs (CYP3A4 Inducers)

Ethanol/Nutrition/Herb Interactions

Food: Bioavailability of bosentan is not affected by food.

Herb/Nutraceutical: Avoid St John's wort (may decrease serum concentrations of bosentan).

Stability Store at 15°C to 30°C (59°F to 86°F).

Mechanism of Action Blocks endothelin receptors on vascular endothelium and smooth muscle. Stimulation of these receptors is associated with vasoconstriction. Although bosentan blocks both ET_A and ET_B receptors, the affinity is higher for the A subtype. Improvement in symptoms of pulmonary artery hypertension and a decrease in the rate of clinical deterioration have been demonstrated in clinical trials.

Pharmacodynamics/Kinetics

Distribution: V_d: 18 L

Protein binding, plasma: >98% primarily to albumin

Metabolism: Hepatic via CYP2C9 and 3A4 to three primary metabolites (one contributing ~10% to 20% pharmacologic activity)

Bioavailability: 50%

Half-life elimination: 5 hours; prolonged with heart failure, possibly in PAH

Time to peak, plasma: 3-5 hours

Excretion: Feces (as metabolites); urine (<3% as unchanged drug)

Dosage Oral:

Children ≤12 years (unlabeled use):

10-20 kg: Initial: 31.25 mg once daily for 4 weeks; increase to maintenance dose of 31.25 mg twice daily

>20-40 kg: Initial: 31.25 mg twice daily for 4 weeks; increase to maintenance dose of 62.5 mg twice daily

>40 kg: Initial: 62.5 mg twice daily for 4 weeks; increase to maintenance dose of 125 mg twice daily

Adolescents >12 years and ≥40 kg and Adults: Initial: 62.5 mg twice daily for 4 weeks; increase to maintenance dose of 125 mg twice daily; patients <40 kg should be maintained at 62.5 mg twice daily. Doses >125 mg twice daily do not appear to confer additional clinical benefit but may increase risk of liver toxicity.

Note: When discontinuing treatment, consider a reduction in dosage to 62.5 mg twice daily for 3-7 days (to avoid clinical deterioration).

Dosage adjustment in renal impairment: No dosage adjustment required.

Dosage adjustment in hepatic impairment: Avoid use in patients with **pretreatment** moderate to severe hepatic insufficiency.

Modification based on transaminase elevation:

If any elevation, regardless of degree, is accompanied by clinical symptoms of hepatic injury (unusual fatigue, nausea, vomiting, abdominal pain, fever, or jaundice) or a serum bilirubin ≥2 times the upper limit of normal, treatment should be stopped.

AST/ALT >3 times but ≤5 times upper limit of normal: Confirm with additional test; if confirmed, reduce dose or interrupt treatment. Monitor transaminase levels at least every 2 weeks. May continue or reintroduce treatment, as appropriate, following return to pretreatment values. Begin with initial dose (above) and recheck transaminases within 3 days

AST/ALT >5 times but ≤8 times upper limit of normal: Confirm with additional test; if confirmed, stop treatment. Monitor transaminase levels at least every 2 weeks. May reintroduce treatment, as appropriate, at starting dose, following return to pretreatment values. Recheck within 3 days and thereafter following reinitiation.

AST/ALT >8 times upper limit of normal: Stop treatment and do not reintroduce.

Dietary Considerations May be taken with or without food. Avoid grapefruit and grapefruit juice.

Administration May be administered with or without food, once in the morning and once in the evening. Women of childbearing potential should avoid excessive handling broken tablets.

Monitoring Parameters Serum transaminase (AST and ALT) and bilirubin should be determined prior to the initiation of therapy and at monthly intervals thereafter. Monitor for clinical signs and symptoms of liver injury (eg, abdominal pain, fatigue, fever, jaundice, nausea, vomiting).

A woman of childbearing potential must have a negative pregnancy test prior to the initiation of therapy and monthly thereafter (prior to shipment of monthly refill). Hemoglobin and hematocrit should be measured at baseline, at 1 month and 3 months of treatment, and every 3 months thereafter (generally stabilizes after 4-12 weeks of treatment).

Monitor for clinical signs and symptoms of liver injury.

Dosage Forms Excipient information presented when available (limited, particularly for generics); consult specific product labeling.

Tablet:

Tracleer®: 62.5 mg, 125 mg

Extemporaneous Preparations Use a commercial pill cutter to prepare a 31.25 mg dose from the 62.5 mg tablet. Half-cut 62.5 mg tablets are stable for up to 4 weeks, when stored at room temperature in the high-density polyethylene plastic bottle provided by the manufacturer of the drug.

Women of childbearing potential should avoid exposure to dust generated from broken or split tablets, especially if repeated exposure is expected.

Suspension preparation: Dissolve the 62.5 mg tablet in 10-20 mL water. Tablets will disintegrate rapidly without crushing (within ~5 minutes); stirring will accelerate disintegration. Bosentan should not be mixed or dissolved in liquids with an acidic pH (eg, fruit juices) due to poor solubility; the drug is most soluble in solutions with a pH >8.5. Bosentan is soluble in water, and sediment will form quickly when left to rest. Homogeneity of suspension cannot be assured; therefore, the manufacturer emphasizes that division of the dose by volume of suspension may not be particularly accurate.

◆ **B&O Supprettes® [DSC]** *see* Belladonna and Opium *on page 178*

◆ **Botox®** *see* Botulinum Toxin Type A *on page 208*

◆ **Botox® Cosmetic** *see* Botulinum Toxin Type A *on page 208*

Botulinum Pentavalent (ABCDE) Toxoid

(BOT yoo lin num pen ta VAY lent [aye, bee, cee, dee, ee] TOKS oyd)

Index Terms Botulinum Toxoid, Pentavalent Vaccine (Against Types A / B / C / D / E Strains of *C. botulinum*)

Pharmacologic Category Toxoid

Unlabeled/Investigational Use Investigational: Prophylaxis for *C. botulinum* exposure (high-risk research laboratory personnel actively working with, or expect to work with, known cultures and purified botulinum toxin)

Dosage Do not inject intracutaneously or into superficial structures.

Initial vaccination series: 0.5 mL deep SubQ at 0-, 2-, and 12 weeks

First booster: 0.5 mL deep SubQ 12 months after first injection of the initial series

Subsequent boosters: 0.5 mL deep SubQ at 2-year intervals based on antitoxin titers as checked by CDC

Additional Information Complete prescribing information for this medication should be consulted for additional detail.

Dosage Forms Excipient information presented when available (limited, particularly for generics); consult specific product labeling.

Botulinum Toxin Type A

(BOT yoo lin num TOKS in type aye)

U.S. Brand Names Botox®; Botox® Cosmetic

Canadian Brand Names Botox®; Botox® Cosmetic

Index Terms BTX-A

Pharmacologic Category Neuromuscular Blocker Agent, Toxin; Ophthalmic Agent, Toxin

Use Treatment of strabismus and blepharospasm associated with dystonia (including benign essential blepharospasm or VII nerve disorders) in patients ≥12 years of age; cervical dystonia (spasmodic torticollis) in patients ≥16 years of age; temporary improvement in the appearance of lines/wrinkles of the face (moderate to severe glabellar lines associated with corrugator and/or procerus muscle activity) in adult patients ≤65 years of age; treatment of severe primary axillary hyperhidrosis in adults not adequately controlled with topical treatments

Canadian labeling: Additional use (not in U.S. labeling): Focal spasticity, including treatment of stroke related upper limb spasticity; dynamic equines foot deformity in pediatric cerebral palsy patients

Unlabeled/Investigational Use Treatment of oromandibular dystonia, spasmodic dysphonia (laryngeal dystonia) and other dystonias (ie, writer's cramp, focal task-specific dystonias); migraine treatment and prophylaxis; treatment of dynamic muscle contracture in pediatric cerebral palsy patients

Pregnancy Risk Factor C

Pregnancy Considerations Decreased fetal body weight, delayed ossification, maternal toxicity, abortions, and fetal malformations were observed in animal studies. Human reproduction studies have not been conducted. Avoid use in pregnancy. Based on limited case reports, adverse fetal effects have not been observed with inadvertent administration during pregnancy. It is currently recommended to ensure adequate contraception in women of childbearing potential.

Lactation Excretion in breast milk unknown/use caution

Contraindications Hypersensitivity to albumin, botulinum toxin, or any component of the formulation; infection at the proposed injection site(s)

Canadian labeling: Additional contraindications (not in U.S. labeling): Myasthenia gravis or Eaton-Lambert syndrome

Warnings/Precautions Higher doses or more frequent administration may result in neutralizing antibody formation and loss of efficacy. Product contains albumin and may carry a remote risk of virus transmission. Use caution if there is excessive weakness or atrophy at the proposed injection site(s); use is contraindicated if infection is present at injection site. Have appropriate support in case of anaphylactic reaction. Use with caution in patients with neuromuscular diseases (such as myasthenia gravis), neuropathic disorders (such as amyotrophic lateral sclerosis), patients taking aminoglycosides, neuromuscular-blocking agents, or other drugs that interfere with neuromuscular transmission and patients with preexisting cardiovascular disease (rare reports of arrhythmia and MI). Long-term effects of chronic therapy unknown.

Cervical dystonia: Dysphagia is common. It may be severe requiring alternative feeding methods and may persist anywhere from 2 weeks up to 5 months after administration. Risk of upper respiratory infection may be increased. Risk factors include smaller neck muscle mass, bilateral injections into the sternocleidomastoid muscle, or injections into the levator scapulae.

Ocular disease: Blepharospasm: Reduced blinking from injection of the orbicularis muscle can lead to corneal exposure and ulceration. Strabismus: Retrobulbar hemorrhages may occur from needle penetration into orbit. Spatial disorientation, double vision, or past pointing may occur if one or more extraocular muscles are paralyzed. Covering the affected eye may help. Careful testing of corneal sensation, avoidance of lower lid injections, and treatment of epithelial defects are necessary. Use with caution in angle closure glaucoma.

Primary axillary hyperhidrosis: Evaluate for secondary causes prior to treatment (eg, hyperthyroidism). Safety and efficacy for treatment of hyperhidrosis in other areas of the body have not been established.

Temporary reduction in glabellar lines: Do not use more frequently than every 3 months. Patients with marked facial asymmetry, ptosis, excessive dermatochalasis, deep dermal scarring, thick sebaceous skin, or the inability to substantially lessen glabellar lines by physically spreading them apart were excluded from clinical trials. Reduced blinking from injection of the orbicularis muscle can lead to corneal exposure and ulceration. Spatial disorientation, double vision, or past pointing may occur if one or more extraocular muscles are paralyzed.

Adverse Reactions Adverse effects usually occur in 1 week and may last up to several months

>10%:

Cervical dystonia:

Central nervous system: Pain (32%), headache (up to 11%)

Gastrointestinal: Dysphagia (19%)

Neuromuscular & skeletal: Focal weakness (17%), neck pain (11%)

Respiratory: Upper respiratory infection (12%)

Other indications (blepharospasm, primary axillary hyperhidrosis, strabismus):

Neuromuscular & skeletal: Primary axillary hyperhidrosis (3% to 10%)

Ocular: Ptosis (blepharospasm 21%; strabismus 1% to 38%), vertical deviation (strabismus 17%)

2% to 10%:

Cervical dystonia:

Central nervous system: Dizziness, drowsiness, fever, malaise, speech disorder

Gastrointestinal: Nausea, xerostomia

Local: Injection site reaction: Soreness

Neuromuscular & skeletal: Back pain, hypertonia, weakness, stiffness

Respiratory: Cough, rhinitis

Miscellaneous: Flu-like syndrome

Cerebral palsy spasticity:
Central nervous system: Pain (1% to 2%), fever (1%), lethargy (1%)
Neuromuscular & skeletal: Falling, weakness
Focal spasticity:
Central nervous system: Arm pain (1% to 3%)
Dermatologic: Bruising (1% to 3%)
Local: Injection site reactions: burning, pain (1% to 3%)
Neuromuscular & skeletal: Hypertonia (1% to 3%), weakness (1% to 3%)
Other indications (blepharospasm, primary axillary hyperhidrosis, reduction of glabellar lines, strabismus):
Central nervous system: Anxiety, dizziness
Dermatologic: Pruritus
Gastrointestinal: Nausea
Local: Injection site reaction: Soreness
Neuromuscular & skeletal: Back pain, facial pain, weakness
Ocular: Irritation/tearing (includes dry eye, lagophthalmos, photophobia); ptosis, superficial punctate keratitis
Respiratory: Pharyngitis
Miscellaneous: Flu-like syndrome, infection, nonaxillary sweating

<2% (Limited to important or life-threatening): *Any indication:* Abdominal pain, acute angle closure glaucoma, allergic reactions, anaphylaxis, ankle pain, anterior segment eye ischemia, appetite decreased, arrhythmia, arthralgia, aspiration pneumonia, blurred vision, brachial plexopathy, bruising, ciliary ganglion damage, corneal perforation, dermatitis, diaphoresis, diarrhea, diplopia, dyspepsia, dysphonia, dyspnea, ectropion, entropion, erythema multiforme, eyelid edema, facial weakness, focal facial paralysis, glaucoma, hearing loss, hypoesthesia, hypertension, knee pain, leg cramps, lethargy, malaise, MI, myalgia, myasthenia gravis exacerbation, neutralizing antibody formation, numbness, pneumonia, pruritus, psoriasiform eruption, ptosis, rash, reduced blinking leading to corneal ulceration, retinal vein occlusion, retrobulbar hemorrhage, seizure, skin tightness, syncope, tooth disorder, urticaria, vertigo with nystagmus, vitreous hemorrhage, vomiting

Drug Interactions

Avoid Concomitant Use There are no known interactions where it is recommended to avoid concomitant use.

Increased Effect/Toxicity

Botulinum Toxin Type A may increase the levels/effects of: Botulinum Toxin Type B

The levels/effects of Botulinum Toxin Type A may be increased by: Aminoglycosides; Neuromuscular-Blocking Agents

Decreased Effect There are no known significant interactions involving a decrease in effect.

Stability Store undiluted vials under refrigeration at 2°C to 8°C for up to 24 months (Botox® Cosmetic) or up to 36 months (Botox®). Reconstitute with sterile, preservative free 0.9% sodium chloride. Mix gently. After reconstitution, store in refrigerator (2°C to 8°C) and use within 4 hours (does not contain preservative).

Botox®: Reconstitute vials with 1 mL of diluent to obtain concentration of 10 units per 0.1 mL; 2 mL of diluent to obtain concentration of 5 units per 0.1 mL; 4 mL of diluent to obtain concentration of 2.5 units per 0.1 mL; 8 mL of diluent to obtain concentration of 1.25 units per 0.1 mL.
Botox® Cosmetic: Reconstitute vials with 2.5 mL of diluent to obtain concentration of 4 units per 0.1 mL (20 units per 0.5 mL).

Mechanism of Action Botulinum A toxin is a neurotoxin produced by *Clostridium botulinum*, spore-forming anaerobic bacillus, which appears to affect only the presynaptic membrane of the neuromuscular junction in humans, where it prevents calcium-dependent release of acetylcholine and produces a state of denervation. Muscle inactivation persists until new fibrils grow from the nerve and form junction plates on new areas of the muscle-cell walls. Intradermal injection results in temporary sweat gland denervation, reducing local sweating.

Pharmacodynamics/Kinetics

Onset of action (improvement):
Blepharospasm: ~3 days
Cervical dystonia: ~2 weeks
Reduction of glabellar lines (Botox® Cosmetic): 1-2 days, increasing in intensity during first week
Spasticity (focal and cerebral palsy related): <2 weeks
Strabismus: ~1-2 days

Duration:
Blepharospasm: ~3 months
Cervical dystonia: <3 months
Primary axillary hyperhidrosis: 201 days (mean)
Reduction of glabellar lines (Botox® Cosmetic): ~3-4 months
Spasticity (cerebral palsy related): ~3-3.5 months
Strabismus: ~2-6 weeks

Absorption: Not expected to be present in peripheral blood at recommended doses following intramuscular (I.M.) injection

Time to peak:
Blepharospasm: 1-2 weeks
Cervical dystonia: ~6 weeks
Spasticity (focal): 4-6 weeks
Strabismus: Within first week

Dosage

Cervical dystonia: Children ≥16 years and Adults: I.M.: For dosing guidance, the mean dose is 236 units (25th to 75th percentile range 198-300 units) divided among the affected muscles in patients previously treated with botulinum toxin. Initial dose in previously untreated patients should be lower. Sequential dosing should be based on the patient's head and neck position, localization of pain, muscle hypertrophy, patient response, and previous adverse reactions. The total dose injected into the sternocleidomastoid muscles should be ≤100 units to decrease the occurrence of dysphagia.
Canadian labeling (not in U.S. labeling): Effective range of 200-360 units has been used in clinical practice; maximum dose: 6 units/kg every 2 months

Blepharospasm: Children ≥12 years and Adults: I.M.: Initial dose: 1.25-2.5 units injected into the medial and lateral pretarsal orbicularis oculi of the upper lid and lateral pretarsal orbicularis oculi of lower lid; dose may be increased up to twice the previous dose if the response from the initial dose lasted ≤2 months; maximum dose per site: 5 units. Tolerance may occur if treatments are given more often than every 3 months, but the effect is not usually permanent. Cumulative dose:
U.S. labeling: ≤200 units in 30-day period
Canadian labeling (not in U.S. labeling): ≤200 units in 60-day period

Strabismus: Children ≥12 years and Adults: I.M.: **Note:** Several minutes prior to injection, administration of local anesthetic and ocular decongestant drops are recommended.
Initial dose:
Vertical muscles and for horizontal strabismus <20 prism diopters: 1.25-2.5 units in any one muscle
Horizontal strabismus of 20-50 prism diopters: 2.5-5 units in any one muscle
Persistent VI nerve palsy ≥1 month: 1.25-2.5 units in the medial rectus muscle
Re-examine patients 7-14 days after each injection to assess the effect of that dose. Subsequent doses for patients experiencing incomplete paralysis of the target may be increased up to twice the previous administered dose. The maximum recommended dose as a single injection for any one muscle is 25 units. Do not

administer subsequent injections until the effects of the previous dose are gone.

Primary axillary hyperhidrosis: Adults ≥18 years: Intradermal: 50 units/axilla. Injection area should be defined by standard staining techniques. Injections should be evenly distributed into multiple sites (10-15), administered in 0.1-0.2 mL aliquots, ~1-2 cm apart. May repeat when clinical effect diminishes.

Reduction of glabellar lines: Adults ≤65 years: I.M.: An effective dose is determined by gross observation of the patient's ability to activate the superficial muscles injected. The location, size and use of muscles may vary markedly among individuals. Inject 0.1 mL (4 units) dose into each of five sites, two in each corrugator muscle and one in the procerus muscle for a total dose 0.5 mL (20 units) administered no more frequently than every 3-4 months.

Spasticity (cerebral palsy related; Canadian labeling [not approved in U.S. labeling]): Children ≥2 years: I.M.: 4 units/kg (total dose) divided into two injections into medial and lateral heads of the gastrocnemius of affected limb; if clinically indicated, may repeat every 2 months (maximum dose: 200 units)

Spasticity (focal; Canadian labeling [not approved in U.S. labeling]): Adults ≥18 years: I.M.: Individualize dose based on patient size, extent, and location of muscle involvement, degree of spasticity, local muscle weakness, and response to prior treatment. In clinical trials total doses up to 360 units were administered as separate injections typically divided among flexor muscles of the elbow, wrist, and fingers; may repeat therapy at 3-4 months with appropriate dosage based upon the clinical condition of patient at time of retreatment.

Suggested guidelines for the treatment of stroke-related upper limb spasticity: **Note:** Dose listed is total dose administered as individual or separate intramuscular injection(s):

Biceps brachii: 100-200 units (up to 4 sites)
Flexor digitorum profundus: 15-50 units (1-2 sites)
Flexor digitorum sublimes: 15-50 units (1-2 sites)
Flexor carpi radialis: 15-60 units (1-2 sites)
Flexor carpi ulnaris: 10-50 units (1-2 sites)
Adductor pollicis: 20 units (1-2 sites)
Flexor pollicis longus: 20 units (1-2 sites)

Elderly: No specific adjustment recommended

Dosage adjustment in renal impairment: No specific adjustment recommended

Dosage adjustment in hepatic impairment: No specific adjustment recommended

Administration

Cervical dystonia: Use 25-, 27-, or 30-gauge needle for superficial muscles and a longer 22-gauge needle for deeper musculature; electromyography may help localize the involved muscles.

Blepharospasm: Use a 27- or 30-gauge needle without electromyography guidance. Avoid injecting near the levator palpebrae superioris (may decrease ptosis); avoid medial lower lid injections (may decrease diplopia). Apply pressure at the injection site to prevent ecchymosis in the soft eyelid tissues.

Spasticity (cerebral palsy related; Canadian labeling [not in U.S. labeling]): Use a 23- to 26-gauge needle for administration into the medial and lateral heads of the gastrocnemius muscle of the affected limb.

Spasticity (focal; Canadian labeling [not in U.S. labeling]): Use a 25-, 27-, or 30-gauge needle for superficial muscles and a longer 22-gauge needle for deeper musculature; electromyography or nerve stimulation may help localize the involved muscles.

Strabismus injections: Must use surgical exposure or electromyographic guidance; use the electrical activity recorded from the tip of the injections needle as a guide to placement within the target muscle. Local anesthetic and ocular decongestant should be given before injection. The volume of injection should be 0.05-0.15 mL per muscle. Many patients will require additional doses because of inadequate response to initial dose.

Primary axillary hyperhidrosis: Inject each dose intradermally to a depth of ~2 mm and at a 45° angle. Do not inject directly into areas marked in ink (to avoid permanent tattoo effect). Prior to administration, injection area should be defined by standard staining techniques such as Minor's Iodine-Starch Test.

Instructions for Minor's Iodine-Starch Test: Patient should shave underarms and refrain from using deodorants or antiperspirants for 24 hours prior to test. At 30 minutes prior to test, patient should be at rest, no exercise, and not consume hot beverages. Underarm area should be dried and immediately painted with iodine solution. After area dries, lightly sprinkle with starch powder. Gently blow off excess powder. A deep blue-black color will develop over the hyperhidrotic area in ~10 minutes.

Reduction of glabellar lines (Botox® Cosmetic): Use a 30-gauge needle. Ensure injected volume/dose is accurate and where feasible keep to a minimum. Avoid injection near the levator palpebrae superioris. Medial corrugator injections should be at least 1 cm above the bony supraorbital ridge. Do not inject toxin closer than 1 cm above the central eyebrow.

Additional Information Units of biological activity of Botox® cannot be compared with units of any other botulinum toxin.

Dosage Forms Excipient information presented when available (limited, particularly for generics); consult specific product labeling.

Injection, powder for reconstitution [preservative free]: *Clostridium botulinum* toxin type A 100 units [contains human albumin]

Botulinum Toxin Type B

(BOT yoo lin num TOKS in type bee)

U.S. Brand Names Myobloc®

Pharmacologic Category Neuromuscular Blocker Agent, Toxin

Use Treatment of cervical dystonia (spasmodic torticollis)

Unlabeled/Investigational Use Treatment of cervical dystonia in patients who have developed resistance to botulinum toxin type A

Pregnancy Risk Factor C (manufacturer)

Pregnancy Considerations Reproduction studies have not been conducted. Based on limited case reports using botulinum toxin A, adverse fetal effects have not been observed with inadvertent administration during pregnancy. It is currently recommended to ensure adequate contraception in women of childbearing years.

Lactation Excretion in breast milk unknown/use caution

Contraindications Hypersensitivity to albumin, botulinum toxin, or any component of the formulation; infection at the injection site(s). Relative contraindications include diseases of neuromuscular transmission; coagulopathy, including therapeutic anticoagulation; inability of patient to cooperate.

Warnings/Precautions Higher doses or more frequent administration may result in neutralizing antibody formation and loss of efficacy. Product contains albumin and may carry a remote risk of virus transmission. Use caution if there is inflammation, excessive weakness, or atrophy at the proposed injection site(s). Concurrent use of botulinum toxin type A or within <4 months of type B is not recommended. Have appropriate support in case of anaphylactic reaction. Use with caution in patients taking aminoglycosides or other drugs that interfere with neuromuscular transmission. Long-term effects of chronic therapy unknown. Increased risk of dysphagia and respiratory complications. Safety and efficacy in children have not been established.

Adverse Reactions

>10%:

Central nervous system: Headache (10% to 16%), pain (6% to 13%; placebo 10%)

Gastrointestinal: Dysphagia (10% to 25%), xerostomia (3% to 34%)

Local: Injection site pain (12% to 16%)

Neuromuscular & skeletal: Neck pain (up to 17%; placebo: 16%)

Miscellaneous: Infection (13% to 19%; placebo: 15%)

1% to 10%:

Cardiovascular: Chest pain, vasodilation, peripheral edema

Central nervous system: Dizziness (3% to 6%), fever, malaise, migraine, anxiety, tremor, hyperesthesia, somnolence, confusion, vertigo

Dermatologic: Pruritus, bruising

Gastrointestinal: Nausea (3% to 10%; placebo: 5%), dyspepsia (up to 10%; placebo: 5%), vomiting, stomatitis, taste perversion

Genitourinary: Urinary tract infection, cystitis, vaginal moniliasis

Hematologic: Serum neutralizing activity

Neuromuscular & skeletal: Torticollis (up to 8%; placebo: 7%), arthralgia (up to 7%; placebo: 5%), back pain (3% to 7%; placebo: 3%), myasthenia (3% to 6%; placebo: 3%), weakness (up to 6%; placebo: 4%), arthritis

Ocular: Amblyopia, abnormal vision

Otic: Otitis media, tinnitus

Respiratory: Cough (3% to 7%; placebo: 3%), rhinitis (1% to 5%; placebo: 6%), dyspnea, pneumonia

Miscellaneous: Flu-syndrome (6% to 9%), allergic reaction, viral infection, abscess, cyst

Drug Interactions

Avoid Concomitant Use There are no known interactions where it is recommended to avoid concomitant use.

Increased Effect/Toxicity

The levels/effects of Botulinum Toxin Type B may be increased by: Aminoglycosides; Botulinum Toxin Type A; Neuromuscular-Blocking Agents

Decreased Effect There are no known significant interactions involving a decrease in effect.

Stability Store vials under refrigeration at 2°C to 8°C (36°F to 46°F) for up to 21 months. May be diluted with normal saline; once diluted, use within 4 hours. Does not contain preservative. Single-use vial. Do not shake; do not freeze.

Mechanism of Action Botulinum B toxin is a neurotoxin produced by *Clostridium botulinum*, spore-forming anaerobic bacillus. It cleaves synaptic Vesicle Association Membrane Protein (VAMP; synaptobrevin) which is a component of the protein complex responsible for docking and fusion of the synaptic vesicle to the presynaptic membrane. By blocking neurotransmitter release, botulinum B toxin paralyzes the muscle.

Pharmacodynamics/Kinetics

Duration: 12-16 weeks

Absorption: Not expected to be present in peripheral blood at recommended doses

Dosage

Children: Not established in pediatric patients

Adults: Cervical dystonia: I.M.: Initial: 2500-5000 units divided among the affected muscles in patients **previously treated** with botulinum toxin; initial dose in **previously untreated** patients should be lower. Subsequent dosing should be optimized according to patient's response.

Elderly: No dosage adjustments required, but limited experience in patients ≥75 years old

Dosage adjustment in renal impairment: No specific adjustment recommended

Dosage adjustment in hepatic impairment: No specific adjustment recommended

Additional Information Units of biological activity of Myobloc® cannot be compared with units of any other botulinum toxin.

Dosage Forms Excipient information presented when available (limited, particularly for generics); consult specific product labeling.

Injection, solution [preservative free]:

Myobloc®: 5000 units/mL (0.5 mL, 1 mL, 2 mL) [contains albumin 0.05%]

◆ **Botulinum Toxoid, Pentavalent Vaccine (Against Types A / B / C / D / E Strains of *C. botulinum*)** *see* Botulinum Pentavalent (ABCDE) Toxoid *on page 208*

Botulism Immune Globulin (Intravenous-Human)

(BOT yoo lism i MYUN GLOB you lin, in tra VEE nus, YU man)

U.S. Brand Names BabyBIG®

Index Terms BIG-IV

Pharmacologic Category Immune Globulin

Use Treatment of infant botulism caused by toxin type A or B

Restrictions Available from the California Department of Health

Pregnancy Considerations Reproduction studies have not been conducted.

Medication Safety Issues

Sound-alike/look-alike issues:

BabyBIG® may be confused with HBIG

Contraindications Hypersensitivity to human immune globulin preparations or any component of the formulation; selective immunoglobulin A deficiency

Warnings/Precautions Hypersensitivity and anaphylactic reactions can occur; immediate treatment (including epinephrine 1:1000) should be available. Aseptic meningitis syndrome (AMS) has been reported with intravenous immune globulin administration (rare); may occur with high doses (≥2 g/kg). Acute renal dysfunction (increased serum creatinine, oliguria, acute renal failure) can rarely occur; usually within 7 days of use (more likely with products stabilized with sucrose). Use with caution in the elderly, patients with renal disease, diabetes mellitus, volume depletion, sepsis, paraproteinemia, and nephrotoxic medications due to risk of renal dysfunction. In patients at risk of renal dysfunction, the rate of infusion and concentration of solution should be minimized. discontinue if renal function deteriorates. Patients should not be volume depleted prior to therapy. Product of human plasma; may potentially contain infectious agents which could transmit disease. Screening of donors, as well as testing and/or inactivation or removal of certain viruses, reduces the risk. Infections thought to be transmitted by this product should be reported to the manufacturer. For I.V. infusion only; do not exceed recommended rate of administration. Not indicated for use in adults. Safety and efficacy established for infants <1 year of age; not indicated for children ≥1 year of age.

Adverse Reactions Percentages reported in open-label study except where otherwise noted; may reflect pathophysiology of infant botulism.

>10%:

Cardiovascular: Blood pressure increased (transient, 75%), pallor (28%), edema (18%); blood pressure decreased (transient, 16%), cardiac murmur (15%)

Central nervous system: Irritability (41%), pyrexia (17%), body temperature decreased (16%)

Dermatologic: Contact dermatitis (24%), erythematous rash (22%, reported as 14% vs 8% in placebo-controlled study)

Gastrointestinal: Dysphagia (65%), loose stools (25%), vomiting (20%), abdominal distension (11%)
Otic: Otitis media (11%, reported in placebo-controlled study)
Respiratory: Atelectasis (39%), rhonchi (34%), nasal congestion (18%), oxygen saturation decreased (17%), cough (13%), rales (13%)
1% to 10%:
Cardiovascular: Tachycardia (7%), peripheral coldness (7%)
Central nervous system: Agitation (10%)
Endocrine & metabolic: Dehydration (10%), hyponatremia (6%), metabolic acidosis (5%)
Hematologic: Hemoglobin decreased (9%), anemia (5%)
Local: Injection site reaction (7%), injection site erythema (5%)
Renal: Neurogenic bladder
Respiratory: Breath sounds decreased (10%), stridor (9%), lower respiratory tract infection (8%), dyspnea (6%), tachypnea (5%)
Miscellaneous: Oral candidiasis (8%), intubation (5%), infusion rate reactions (<5%, includes chills, back pain, fever, muscle cramps, nausea, vomiting, wheezing)

Drug Interactions

Avoid Concomitant Use There are no known interactions where it is recommended to avoid concomitant use.

Increased Effect/Toxicity There are no known significant interactions involving an increase in effect.

Decreased Effect
Botulism Immune Globulin (Intravenous-Human) may decrease the levels/effects of: Vaccines (Live)

Stability Prior to reconstitution, store between 2°C to 8°C (35.6°F to 46.4°F). Infusion should begin within 2 hours of reconstitution and be completed within 4 hours of reconstitution. Reconstitute with SWFI 2 mL. Swirl gently to wet powder; do not shake. Powder should dissolve in ~30 minutes.

Mechanism of Action BIG-IV is purified immunoglobulin derived from the plasma of adults immunized with botulinum toxoid types A and B. BIG-IV provides antibodies to neutralize circulating toxins.

Pharmacodynamics/Kinetics
Duration: Protective neutralizing antibody levels: 6 months
Half-life elimination: 28 days

Dosage I.V.: Children <1 year: Infant botulism: 1 mL/kg (50 mg/kg) as a single dose; infuse at 0.5 mL/kg/hour (25 mg/kg/hour) for the first 15 minutes; if well tolerated, may increase to 1 mL/kg/hour (50 mg/kg/hour)

Administration For I.V. infusion only. Do not administer if solution is turbid. Epinephrine should be available for the treatment of acute allergic reaction. Administer using low volume tubing and infusion pump with an in-line or syringe tip 18 µm filter. Infuse at 0.5 mL/kg/hour (25 mg/kg/hour) for the first 15 minutes; if well tolerated, may increase to 1 mL/kg/hour (50 mg/kg/hour). Infusion should take ~67.5 minutes. Infusion should be slowed or temporarily interrupted for minor side effects; discontinue in case of hypotension or anaphylaxis.

Monitoring Parameters Renal function (BUN, serum creatinine, urinary output); vital signs (continuously during infusion); aseptic meningitis syndrome (may occur hours to days following IGIV therapy); signs of relapse (may occur up to 1 month following recovery)

Dosage Forms Excipient information presented when available (limited, particularly for generics); consult specific product labeling.
Injection, powder for reconstitution [preservative free]:
BabyBIG®: ~100 mg [contains albumin and sucrose; packaged with SWFI]

◆ **Boudreaux's® Butt Paste [OTC]** *see* Zinc Oxide *on page* 1584
◆ **Bovine Lung Surfactant** *see* Beractant *on page* 187
◆ **Bravelle®** *see* Urofollitropin *on page* 1531
◆ **Breathe Free® [OTC]** *see* Sodium Chloride *on page* 1381
◆ **Brethaire [DSC]** *see* Terbutaline *on page* 1442
◆ **Brevibloc®** *see* Esmolol *on page* 550
◆ **Brevicon®** *see* Ethinyl Estradiol and Norethindrone *on page* 581
◆ **Brevicon® 0.5/35 (Can)** *see* Ethinyl Estradiol and Norethindrone *on page* 581
◆ **Brevicon® 1/35 (Can)** *see* Ethinyl Estradiol and Norethindrone *on page* 581
◆ **Brevital® (Can)** *see* Methohexital *on page* 965
◆ **Brevital® Sodium** *see* Methohexital *on page* 965
◆ **Bricanyl [DSC]** *see* Terbutaline *on page* 1442
◆ **Bricanyl® (Can)** *see* Terbutaline *on page* 1442

Brimonidine (bri MOE ni deen)

U.S. Brand Names Alphagan® P

Canadian Brand Names Alphagan®; Apo-Brimonidine P; Apo-Brimonidine®; PMS-Brimonidine Tartrate; ratio-Brimonidine; Sandoz-Brimonidine

Index Terms Brimonidine Tartrate

Pharmacologic Category Alpha$_2$ Agonist, Ophthalmic; Ophthalmic Agent, Antiglaucoma

Additional Appendix Information
Glaucoma Drug Therapy *on page* 1808

Use Lowering of intraocular pressure (IOP) in patients with open-angle glaucoma or ocular hypertension

Pregnancy Risk Factor B

Medication Safety Issues
Sound-alike/look-alike issues:
Brimonidine may be confused with bromocriptine

Dosage Ophthalmic: Children ≥2 years of age and Adults: Glaucoma: Instill 1 drop in affected eye(s) 3 times/day (approximately every 8 hours)

Additional Information Complete prescribing information for this medication should be consulted for additional detail.

Dosage Forms Excipient information presented when available (limited, particularly for generics); consult specific product labeling.
Solution, ophthalmic, as tartrate: 0.2% (5 mL, 10 mL, 15 mL) [may contain benzalkonium chloride]
Alphagan® P: 0.1% (5 mL, 10 mL, 15 mL) [contains Purite® as preservative]; 0.15% (5 mL, 10 mL, 15 mL) [contains Purite® as preservative]

Brimonidine and Timolol
(bri MOE ni deen & TIM oh lol)

U.S. Brand Names Combigan™

Canadian Brand Names Combigan®

Index Terms Brimonidine Tartrate and Timolol Maleate; Timolol and Brimonidine

Pharmacologic Category Alpha$_2$ Agonist, Ophthalmic; Beta Blocker, Nonselective; Ophthalmic Agent, Antiglaucoma

Use Reduction of intraocular pressure (IOP) in patients with glaucoma or ocular hypertension

Pregnancy Risk Factor C

Medication Safety Issues
International issues:
Combigan® may be confused with Combivent® which is a brand name for ipratropium/albuterol in the U.S.; may be confused with Comtan® which is a brand name for entacapone in the U.S.

Dosage Ophthalmic: Children ≥2 years and Adults: Instill 1 drop into affected eye(s) twice daily

Note: In the Canadian labeling, use in children (at any age) is not recommended

Additional Information Complete prescribing information for this medication should be consulted for additional detail.

Dosage Forms Excipient information presented when available (limited, particularly for generics); consult specific product labeling. [CAN] = Canadian availability

Solution, ophthalmic [drops]:

Combigan™: Brimonidine tartrate 0.2% and timolol maleate 0.5% (5 mL,10 mL) [contains benzalkonium chloride]

Combigan® [CAN]: Brimonidine tartrate 0.2% and timolol maleate 0.5% (2.5 mL, 5 mL,10 mL) [contains benzalkonium chloride]

◆ **Brimonidine Tartrate** *see* Brimonidine *on page 212*

◆ **Brimonidine Tartrate and Timolol Maleate** *see* Brimonidine and Timolol *on page 212*

Brinzolamide (brin ZOH la mide)

U.S. Brand Names Azopt®

Canadian Brand Names Azopt®

Pharmacologic Category Carbonic Anhydrase Inhibitor; Ophthalmic Agent, Antiglaucoma

Additional Appendix Information

Glaucoma Drug Therapy *on page 1808*

Use Lowers intraocular pressure in patients with ocular hypertension or open-angle glaucoma

Pregnancy Risk Factor C

Dosage Ophthalmic: Adults: Instill 1 drop in affected eye(s) 3 times/day

Additional Information Complete prescribing information for this medication should be consulted for additional detail.

Dosage Forms Excipient information presented when available (limited, particularly for generics); consult specific product labeling. [DSC] = Discontinued product

Suspension, ophthalmic:

Azopt®: 1% (5 mL [DSC], 10 mL, 15 mL) [contains benzalkonium chloride]

◆ **Brioschi® [OTC]** *see* Sodium Bicarbonate *on page 1380*

◆ **British Anti-Lewisite** *see* Dimercaprol *on page 453*

◆ **BRL 43694** *see* Granisetron *on page 706*

◆ **Bromaline® [OTC]** *see* Brompheniramine and Pseudoephedrine *on page 214*

Bromfenac (BROME fen ak)

U.S. Brand Names Xibrom™

Index Terms Bromfenac Sodium

Pharmacologic Category Nonsteroidal Anti-inflammatory Drug (NSAID), Ophthalmic

Use Treatment of postoperative inflammation and reduction in ocular pain following cataract removal

Pregnancy Risk Factor C/D (3rd trimester)

Dosage Ophthalmic: Adults: Instill 1 drop into affected eye(s) twice daily beginning 24 hours after surgery and continuing for 2 weeks postoperatively

Dosage adjustment in renal impairment: No adjustment required

Additional Information Complete prescribing information for this medication should be consulted for additional detail.

Dosage Forms Excipient information presented when available (limited, particularly for generics); consult specific product labeling.

Solution, ophthalmic:

Xibrom™: 0.09% (2.5 mL, 5 mL) [contains benzalkonium chloride and sodium sulfite]

◆ **Bromfenac Sodium** *see* Bromfenac *on page 213*

◆ **Bromfenex® [DSC]** *see* Brompheniramine and Pseudoephedrine *on page 214*

◆ **Bromfenex® PD [DSC]** *see* Brompheniramine and Pseudoephedrine *on page 214*

◆ **Bromhist-NR** *see* Brompheniramine and Pseudoephedrine *on page 214*

◆ **Bromhist Pediatric** *see* Brompheniramine and Pseudoephedrine *on page 214*

Bromocriptine (broe moe KRIP teen)

U.S. Brand Names Parlodel®; Parlodel® SnapTabs®

Canadian Brand Names Apo-Bromocriptine®; Parlodel®; PMS-Bromocriptine

Index Terms Bromocriptine Mesylate

Pharmacologic Category Anti-Parkinson's Agent, Dopamine Agonist; Ergot Derivative

Additional Appendix Information

Antiparkinsonian Agents *on page 1643*

Use Treatment of hyperprolactinemia associated with amenorrhea with or without galactorrhea, infertility, or hypogonadism; treatment of prolactin-secreting adenomas; treatment of acromegaly; treatment of Parkinson's disease

Unlabeled/Investigational Use Neuroleptic malignant syndrome

Pregnancy Risk Factor B

Medication Safety Issues

Sound-alike/look-alike issues:

Bromocriptine may be confused with benztropine, brimonidine

Parlodel® may be confused with pindolol, Provera®

Dosage Oral:

Children: Hyperprolactinemia:

11-15 years (based on limited information): Initial: 1.25-2.5 mg daily; dosage may be increased as tolerated to achieve a therapeutic response (range: 2.5-10 mg daily).

≥16 years: Refer to adult dosing

Adults:

Parkinsonism: 1.25 mg twice daily, increased by 2.5 mg/day in 2- to 4-week intervals (usual dose range is 30-90 mg/day in 3 divided doses; maximum: 100 mg/day), though elderly patients can usually be managed on lower doses

Neuroleptic malignant syndrome (unlabeled use): 2.5-10 mg every 6-8 hours; continue therapy until NMS is controlled, then taper slowly

Acromegaly: Initial: 1.25-2.5 mg daily increasing by 1.25-2.5 mg daily as necessary every 3-7 days; usual dose: 20-30 mg/day (maximum: 100 mg/day)

Hyperprolactinemia: Initial: 1.25-2.5 mg/day; may be increased by 2.5 mg/day as tolerated every 2-7 days until optimal response (range: 2.5-15 mg/day)

Dosing adjustment in hepatic impairment: No guidelines are available, however, may be necessary

Additional Information Complete prescribing information for this medication should be consulted for additional detail.

Dosage Forms Excipient information presented when available (limited, particularly for generics); consult specific product labeling.

Capsule, as mesylate: 5 mg

Parlodel®: 5 mg

Tablet, as mesylate: 2.5 mg

Parlodel® SnapTabs®: 2.5 mg

◆ **Bromocriptine Mesylate** *see* Bromocriptine *on page 213*

Brompheniramine (brome fen IR a meen)

U.S. Brand Names B-Vex; Bidhist; BroveX™; BroveX™ CT; Lodrane® 12 Hour; Lodrane® 24; Lodrane® XR; LoHist-12; TanaCof-XR

Index Terms Brompheniramine Maleate; Brompheniramine Tannate

Pharmacologic Category Histamine H_1 Antagonist; Histamine H_1 Antagonist, First Generation

Use Symptomatic relief of perennial and seasonal allergic rhinitis, vasomotor rhinitis, and other respiratory allergies

Pregnancy Risk Factor C

Dosage Allergic rhinitis, allergic symptoms, vasomotor rhinitis: Oral:

Children:
- 1-2 years (B-Vex, BroveX™): 1.25 mL every 12 hours (maximum: 2.5 mL/day)
- 2-6 years:
  - B-Vex, BroveX™: 2.5 mL every 12 hours (maximum: 5 mL/day)
  - BroveX™ CT: 1/2 tablet every 12 hours (maximum: 1 tablet/day)
  - Lodrane® XR, TanaCof-XR: 1.25 mL every 12 hours (maximum: 2.5 mL/day)
- 6-12 years:
  - B-Vex, BroveX™: 5 mL every 12 hours (maximum: 10 mL/day)
  - BroveX™ CT: 1/2 to 1 tablet every 12 hours (maximum: 2 tablets/day)
  - Lodrane® 12 Hour, LoHist-12: One tablet every 12 hours (maximum: 2 tablets/day)
  - Lodrane® 24: One capsule once daily
  - Lodrane® XR, TanaCof-XR: 2.5 mL every 12 hours (maximum: 5 mL/day)
- >12 years (B-Vex, BroveX™, BroveX™ CT, Lodrane® 12 Hour, Lodrane® 24, Lodrane® XR, LoHist-12, TanaCof-XR): Refer to adult dosing

Adults:
- B-Vex, BroveX™: 5-10 mL every 12 hours (maximum: 20 mL/day)
- BroveX™ CT: 1-2 tablets every 12 hours (maximum: 4 tablets/day)
- Lodrane® 12 Hour, LoHist: 1-2 tablets every 12 hours (maximum: 4 tablets/day)
- Lodrane® 24: 1-2 capsules once daily
- Lodrane® XR, TanaCof-XR: 5 mL every 12 hours (maximum: 10 mL/day)

Elderly (also refer to adult dosing): Initial:
- B-Vex, BroveX™: 5 mL every 12 hours
- BroveX™ CT, Lodrane® 12 Hour, LoHist: 1 tablet every 12 hours
- Lodrane® 24: 1 capsule/24 hours
- Lodrane® XR, TanaCof-XR: 2.5 mL every 12 hours

Additional Information Complete prescribing information for this medication should be consulted for additional detail.

Dosage Forms Excipient information presented when available (limited, particularly for generics); consult specific product labeling.

Capsule, extended release:
- Lodrane® 24: 12 mg [dye free]

Suspension, as tannate:
- B-Vex, BroveX™: 12 mg/5 mL (120 mL) [contains sodium benzoate and tartrazine; banana flavor]
- Lodrane® XR: 8 mg/5 mL (480 mL) [alcohol free, sugar free; strawberry flavor]
- TanaCof-XR: 8 mg/5 mL (480 mL) [alcohol free, sugar free; contains phenylalanine; strawberry creme flavor]

Tablet, chewable, as tannate: 12 mg
- BroveX™ CT: 12 mg [banana flavor]

Tablet, extended release, as maleate:
- Bidhist: 6 mg

Tablet, extended release, as maleate [scored]:
- Lodrane® 12 Hour, LoHist-12: 6 mg [dye free]

Tablet, timed release, as maleate: 6 mg

Brompheniramine and Pseudoephedrine
(brome fen IR a meen & soo doe e FED rin)

U.S. Brand Names AccuHist®; Andehist NR Syrup; Bromaline® [OTC]; Bromfenex® PD [DSC]; Bromfenex® [DSC]; Bromhist Pediatric; Bromhist-NR; Brotapp; Brovex SR; Dimaphen [OTC]; Histex® SR; Lodrane® 12D; Lodrane® 24D; Lodrane® D; Lodrane® [DSC]; LoHist 12D; LoHist LQ; LoHist PD; Respahist®; Sildec Syrup; Touro® Allergy

Index Terms Brompheniramine Maleate and Pseudoephedrine Hydrochloride; Brompheniramine Maleate and Pseudoephedrine Sulfate; Pseudoephedrine and Brompheniramine

Pharmacologic Category Alpha/Beta Agonist; Histamine H_1 Antagonist; Histamine H_1 Antagonist, First Generation

Use Temporary relief of symptoms of seasonal and perennial allergic rhinitis, and vasomotor rhinitis, including nasal obstruction

Pregnancy Risk Factor C

Medication Safety Issues

Sound-alike/look-alike issues:
- Bromfed® may be confused with Bromphen®

Dosage Oral:

Capsule, long acting:
- Based on 60 mg pseudoephedrine:
  - Children 6-12 years: 1 capsule every 12 hours
  - Children ≥12 years and Adults: 1-2 capsules every 12 hours
- Based on 120 mg pseudoephedrine: Children ≥12 years and Adults: 1 capsule every 12 hours

Liquid:
- Based on brompheniramine 1 mg/pseudoephedrine 15 mg per 1 mL: Children:
  - 1-3 months: 0.25 mL 4 times/day
  - 3-6 months: 0.5 mL 4 times/day
  - 6-12 months: 0.75 mL 4 times/day
  - 12-24 months: 1 mL 4 times/day
- Based on brompheniramine 1 mg/pseudoephedrine 15 mg per 5 mL: Children:
  - 6-11 months (6-8 kg): 2.5 mL every 6-8 hours (maximum: 4 doses/24 hours)
  - 12-23 months (8-10 kg): 3.75 mL every 6-8 hours (maximum: 4 doses/24 hours)
  - 2-6 years: 5 mL every 6-8 hours (maximum: 4 doses/24 hours)
  - 6-12 years: 10 mL every 6-8 hours (maximum: 4 doses/24 hours)
  - >12 years and Adults: 20 mL every 4 hours (maximum: 4 doses/24 hours)
- Based on brompheniramine 4 mg/pseudoephedrine 30 mg:
  - Children 2-6 years: 2.5 mL 3 times/day
  - Children >6 years and Adults: 5 mL 3 times/day
- Brompheniramine 4 mg/pseudoephedrine 45 mg per 5 mL:
  - Children 2-6 years: 2.5 mL 4 times/day
  - Children >6 years and Adults: 5 mL 4 times/day

Tablet, extended release: Based on pseudoephedrine 45 mg:
- Children 6-12 years: 1 tablet every 12 hours
- Children ≥12 years and Adults: 1-2 tablets every 12 hours

Additional Information Complete prescribing information for this medication should be consulted for additional detail.

Dosage Forms Excipient information presented when available (limited, particularly for generics); consult specific product labeling. [DSC] = Discontinued product

Caplet, extended release:

Histex® SR: Brompheniramine maleate 10 mg and pseudoephedrine hydrochloride 120 mg

Capsule, extended release:

Bromfenex®: Brompheniramine maleate 12 mg and pseudoephedrine hydrochloride 120 mg [DSC]

Bromfenex® PD: Brompheniramine maleate 6 mg and pseudoephedrine hydrochloride 60 mg [DSC]

Lodrane® 24D: Brompheniramine maleate 12 mg and pseudoephedrine hydrochloride 90 mg

Capsule, sustained release:

Brovex SR: Brompheniramine maleate 9 mg and pseudoephedrine hydrochloride 90 mg

Respahist®: Brompheniramine maleate 6 mg and pseudoephedrine hydrochloride 60 mg

Touro® Allergy: Brompheniramine maleate 5.75 mg and pseudoephedrine hydrochloride 60 mg [DSC]

Elixir:

Dimaphen: Brompheniramine maleate 1 mg and pseudoephedrine hydrochloride 15 mg per 5 mL (120 mL, 480 mL)

Liquid: Brompheniramine maleate 4 mg and pseudoephedrine hydrochloride 60 mg per 5 mL (480 mL)

Brotapp: Brompheniramine maleate 1 mg and pseudoephedrine hydrochloride 15 mg per 5 mL (120 mL, 240 mL, 480 mL) [grape flavor]

Lodrane®: Brompheniramine maleate 4 mg and pseudoephedrine hydrochloride 60 mg per 5 mL (480 mL) [alcohol free, dye free, sugar free; cherry flavor] [DSC]

LoHist LQ: Brompheniramine maleate 4 mg and pseudoephedrine hydrochloride 60 mg per 5 mL (480 mL) [cherry flavor]

Liquid, oral [drops]:

AccuHist®: Brompheniramine maleate 1 mg and pseudoephedrine hydrochloride 12.5 mg per 1 mL (30 mL) [sugar free; cherry flavor]

Bromhist NR: Brompheniramine maleate 1 mg and pseudoephedrine hydrochloride 12.5 mg per 1 mL (30 mL) [cherry flavor]

Bromhist Pediatric: Brompheniramine maleate 1 mg and pseudoephedrine hydrochloride 15 mg per 1 mL (30 mL) [cherry flavor]

LoHist PD: Brompheniramine maleate 1 mg and pseudoephedrine hydrochloride 12.5 mg per 1 mL (30 mL) [cherry flavor]

Solution:

Bromaline®: Brompheniramine maleate 1 mg and pseudoephedrine hydrochloride 15 mg per 5 mL (120 mL, 480 mL) [alcohol free; contains sodium benzoate; grape flavor]

Suspension:

Lodrane® D: Brompheniramine tannate 8 mg and pseudoephedrine tannate 90 mg per 5 mL (480 mL) [alcohol free, sugar free; strawberry flavor]

Syrup:

Andehist NR: Brompheniramine maleate 4 mg and pseudoephedrine sulfate 45 mg per 5 mL (473 mL) [raspberry flavor]

Sildec: Brompheniramine maleate 4 mg and pseudoephedrine hydrochloride 45 mg per 5 mL (480 mL) [raspberry flavor]

Tablet, extended release:

Lodrane® 12D: Brompheniramine maleate 6 mg and pseudoephedrine hydrochloride 45 mg [dye free]

LoHist 12D: Brompheniramine maleate 6 mg and pseudoephedrine hydrochloride 45 mg

Tablet, prolonged release:

Touro® Allergy: Brompheniramine maleate 6 mg and pseudoephedrine hydrochloride 45 mg

Tablet, sustained release: Brompheniramine maleate 6 mg and pseudoephedrine hydrochloride 45 mg

- **Brompheniramine Maleate** *see* Brompheniramine *on page 214*
- **Brompheniramine Maleate and Pseudoephedrine Hydrochloride** *see* Brompheniramine and Pseudoephedrine *on page 214*
- **Brompheniramine Maleate and Pseudoephedrine Sulfate** *see* Brompheniramine and Pseudoephedrine *on page 214*
- **Brompheniramine Tannate** *see* Brompheniramine *on page 214*
- **Brontex®** *see* Guaifenesin and Codeine *on page 710*
- **Brotapp** *see* Brompheniramine and Pseudoephedrine *on page 214*
- **Brovana®** *see* Arformoterol *on page 131*
- **BroveX™** *see* Brompheniramine *on page 214*
- **BroveX™ CT** *see* Brompheniramine *on page 214*
- **Brovex SR** *see* Brompheniramine and Pseudoephedrine *on page 214*
- **BSF208075** *see* Ambrisentan *on page 80*
- **BTX-A** *see* Botulinum Toxin Type A *on page 208*
- **B-type Natriuretic Peptide (Human)** *see* Nesiritide *on page 1054*
- **Budeprion XL®** *see* BuPROPion *on page 223*
- **Budeprion SR®** *see* BuPROPion *on page 223*

Budesonide (byoo DES oh nide)

U.S. Brand Names Entocort® EC; Pulmicort Flexhaler™; Pulmicort Respules®; Rhinocort® Aqua®

Canadian Brand Names Entocort®; Gen-Budesonide AQ; Pulmicort®; Rhinocort® Aqua™; Rhinocort® Turbuhaler®

Pharmacologic Category Corticosteroid, Inhalant (Oral); Corticosteroid, Nasal; Corticosteroid, Systemic

Additional Appendix Information

Asthma *on page 1793*

Use

Intranasal: Management of symptoms of seasonal or perennial rhinitis

Canadian labeling: Additional use (not in U.S. labeling): Prevention and treatment of nasal polyps

Nebulization: Maintenance and prophylactic treatment of asthma

Oral capsule: Treatment of active Crohn's disease (mild-to-moderate) involving the ileum and/or ascending colon; maintenance of remission (for up to 3 months) of Crohn's disease (mild-to-moderate) involving the ileum and/or ascending colon

Oral inhalation: Maintenance and prophylactic treatment of asthma; includes patients who require oral corticosteroids and those who may benefit from systemic dose reduction/elimination

Pregnancy Risk Factor C (capsule)/B (inhalation)

Pregnancy Considerations Adverse events have been observed with corticosteroids in animal reproduction studies. Studies of pregnant women using inhaled budesonide have not demonstrated an increased risk of abnormalities. Some studies have shown an association between first trimester systemic corticosteroid use and oral clefts; adverse events in the fetus/neonate have been noted in case reports following large doses of systemic corticosteroids during pregnancy. Budesonide is the preferred inhaled corticosteroid for the treatment of asthma in pregnant women.

Lactation Enters breast milk/use caution

Contraindications Hypersensitivity to budesonide or any component of the formulation

Inhalation: Contraindicated in primary treatment of status asthmaticus, acute episodes of asthma; not for relief of acute bronchospasm

Canadian labeling: Additional contraindications (not in U.S. labeling): Moderate-to-severe bronchiectasis, pulmonary tuberculosis (active or quiescent), untreated respiratory infection (bacterial, fungal, or viral); use of Rhinocort® Aqua™ and Rhinocort® Turbuhaler® in patients <6 years of age

Warnings/Precautions May cause hypercorticism or suppression of hypothalamic-pituitary-adrenal (HPA) axis, particularly in younger children or in patients receiving high doses for prolonged periods. HPA axis suppression may lead to adrenal crisis. Withdrawal and discontinuation of a corticosteroid should be done slowly and carefully. Particular care is required when patients are transferred from systemic corticosteroids to inhaled products due to possible adrenal insufficiency or withdrawal from steroids, including an increase in allergic symptoms. Patients receiving >20 mg per day of prednisone (or equivalent) may be most susceptible. Fatalities have occurred due to adrenal insufficiency in asthmatic patients during and after transfer from systemic corticosteroids to aerosol steroids; aerosol steroids do not provide the systemic steroid needed to treat patients having trauma, surgery, or infections. Do not use this product to transfer patients directly from oral corticosteroid therapy.

Bronchospasm may occur with wheezing after inhalation; if this occurs stop steroid and treat with a fast-acting bronchodilator (eg, albuterol). Supplemental steroids (oral or parenteral) may be needed during stress or severe asthma attacks. Not to be used in status asthmaticus or for the relief of acute bronchospasm. Acute myopathy has been reported with high-dose corticosteroids, usually in patients with neuromuscular transmission disorders; may involve ocular and/or respiratory muscles; monitor creatine kinase; recovery may be delayed. Corticosteroid use may cause psychiatric disturbances, including depression, euphoria, insomnia, mood swings, and personality changes. Pre-existing psychiatric conditions may be exacerbated by corticosteroid use. Prolonged use of corticosteroids may also increase the incidence of secondary infection, mask acute infection (including fungal infections), prolong or exacerbate viral infections, or limit response to vaccines. Exposure to chickenpox should be avoided; corticosteroids should not be used to treat ocular herpes simplex. Corticosteroids should not be used for cerebral malaria or viral hepatitis. Close observation is required in patients with latent tuberculosis and/or TB reactivity; restrict use in active TB (only in conjunction with antituberculosis treatment). *Candida albicans* infections may occur in the mouth and pharynx; rinsing (and spitting) with water after inhaler use may decrease risk. Prolonged treatment with corticosteroids has been associated with the development of Kaposi's sarcoma (case reports); if noted, discontinuation of therapy should be considered.

Use with caution in patients with thyroid disease, hepatic impairment, renal impairment, cardiovascular disease, diabetes, glaucoma, cataracts, myasthenia gravis, patients at risk for osteoporosis, patients at risk for seizures, or GI diseases (diverticulitis, peptic ulcer, ulcerative colitis) due to perforation risk. Use caution following acute MI (corticosteroids have been associated with myocardial rupture). Because of the risk of adverse effects, systemic corticosteroids should be used cautiously in the elderly in the smallest possible effective dose for the shortest duration. Avoid nasal corticosteroid use in patients with recent nasal septal ulcers, nasal surgery or nasal trauma until healing has occurred.

Orally-inhaled and intranasal corticosteroids may cause a reduction in growth velocity in pediatric patients (~1 centimeter per year [range 0.3-1.8 cm per year] and related to dose and duration of exposure). To minimize the systemic effects of orally-inhaled and intranasal corticosteroids, each patient should be titrated to the lowest effective dose. Growth should be routinely monitored in pediatric patients. Withdraw systemic therapy with gradual tapering of dose. There have been reports of systemic corticosteroid withdrawal symptoms (eg, joint/muscle pain, lassitude, depression) when withdrawing oral inhalation therapy. Pulmicort Flexhaler™ contains lactose; very rare anaphylactic reactions have been reported in patients with severe milk protein allergy.

Adverse Reactions Reaction severity varies by dose and duration; not all adverse reactions have been reported with each dosage form.

>10%:

Central nervous system: Headache (≤21%)

Gastrointestinal: Nausea (≤11%)

Respiratory: Respiratory infection, rhinitis

Miscellaneous: Symptoms of HPA axis suppression and/or hypercorticism may occur in >10% of patients following administration of dosage forms which result in higher systemic exposure (ie, oral capsule), but may be less frequent than rates observed with comparator drugs (prednisolone). These symptoms may be rare (<1%) following administration via methods which result in lower exposures (topical).

1% to 10%:

Cardiovascular: Chest pain, edema, flushing, hypertension, palpitation, syncope, tachycardia

Central nervous system: Dizziness, dysphonia, emotional lability, fatigue, fever, insomnia, migraine, nervousness, pain, vertigo

Dermatologic: Acne, alopecia, bruising, contact dermatitis, eczema, hirsutism, pruritus, pustular rash, rash, striae

Endocrine & metabolic: Adrenal insufficiency, hypokalemia, menstrual disorder

Gastrointestinal: Abdominal pain, anorexia, diarrhea, dyspepsia, flatulence, gastroenteritis (including viral), oral candidiasis, taste perversion, vomiting, weight gain, xerostomia

Genitourinary: Dysuria, hematuria, nocturia, pyuria

Hematologic: Cervical lymphadenopathy, leukocytosis, purpura

Hepatic: Alkaline phosphatase increased

Neuromuscular & skeletal: Arthralgia, back pain, fracture, hyperkinesis, hypertonia, myalgia, neck pain, paresthesia, weakness

Ocular: Conjunctivitis, eye infection

Otic: Earache, ear infection, external ear infection

Respiratory: Bronchitis, bronchospasm, cough, epistaxis, hoarseness, nasal congestion, nasal irritation, pharyngitis, sinusitis, stridor, throat irritation

Miscellaneous: Abscess, allergic reaction, C-reactive protein increased, erythrocyte sedimentation rate increased, fat distribution (moon face, buffalo hump); flu-like syndrome, herpes simplex, infection, moniliasis, viral infection, voice alteration

<1% (Limited to important or life-threatening): Aggressive reactions, alopecia, angioedema, anxiety, avascular necrosis of the femoral head, benign intracranial hypertension, bone mineral density decreased, cataracts, depression, dyspnea, glaucoma, growth suppression, hypersensitivity reactions (immediate and delayed [includes rash, contact dermatitis, angioedema, bronchospasm]), hypocorticism, intermenstrual bleeding, irritability, nasal septum perforation, osteoporosis, psychosis, somnolence, urticaria, wheezing (patients with severe milk allergy)

Drug Interactions

Metabolism/Transport Effects Substrate of CYP3A4 (major)

Avoid Concomitant Use There are no known interactions where it is recommended to avoid concomitant use.

Increased Effect/Toxicity

Budesonide may increase the levels/effects of: Amphotericin B; Loop Diuretics; Thiazide Diuretics

The levels/effects of Budesonide may be increased by: Antifungal Agents (Azole Derivatives, Systemic); CYP3A4 Inhibitors (Moderate); CYP3A4 Inhibitors (Strong); Dasatinib; Protease Inhibitors

Decreased Effect

Budesonide may decrease the levels/effects of: Antidiabetic Agents; Corticorelin

The levels/effects of Budesonide may be decreased by: Antacids; Bile Acid Sequestrants

Ethanol/Nutrition/Herb Interactions Food: Grapefruit juice may double systemic exposure of orally-administered budesonide. Administration of capsules with a high-fat meal delays peak concentration, but does not alter the extent of absorption.

Stability

Suspension for nebulization: Store upright at 20°C to 25°C (68°F to 77°F). Protect from light. Do not refrigerate or freeze. Once aluminum package is opened, solution should be used within 2 weeks. Continue to protect from light.

Nasal inhaler: Store with valve up at 15°C to 30°C (59°F to 86°F). Protect from high humidity.

Nasal spray: Store with valve up at 20°C to 25°C (68°F to 77°F); do not freeze. Protect from light.

Oral inhaler (Pulmicort Flexhaler™): Store at controlled room temperature of 20°C to 25°C (68°F to 77°F). Protect from moisture.

Mechanism of Action Controls the rate of protein synthesis; depresses the migration of polymorphonuclear leukocytes, fibroblasts; reverses capillary permeability and lysosomal stabilization at the cellular level to prevent or control inflammation. Has potent glucocorticoid activity and weak mineralocorticoid activity.

Pharmacodynamics/Kinetics

Onset of action: Pulmicort Respules®: 2-8 days; Rhinocort® Aqua®: ~10 hours; Inhalation: 24 hours

Peak effect: Pulmicort Respules®: 4-6 weeks; Rhinocort® Aqua®: ~2 weeks; Inhalation: 1-2 weeks

Distribution: 2.2-3.9 L/kg

Protein binding: 85% to 90%

Metabolism: Hepatic via CYP3A4 to two metabolites: 16 alpha-hydroxyprednisolone and 6 beta-hydroxybudesonide; minor activity

Bioavailability: Limited by high first-pass effect; Capsule: 9% to 21%; Pulmicort Respules®: 6%; Inhalation: 6% to 13%; Nasal: 34%

Half-life elimination: 2-3.6 hours

Time to peak: Capsule: 0.5-10 hours (variable in Crohn's disease); Pulmicort Respules®: 10-30 minutes; Inhalation: 1-2 hours; Nasal: 1 hour

Excretion: Urine (60%) and feces as metabolites

Dosage

Nasal inhalation:

U.S. labeling (Rhinocort® Aqua®): Rhinitis: Children ≥6 years and Adults: 64 mcg/day as a single 32 mcg spray in each nostril. Some patients who do not achieve adequate control may benefit from increased dosage. A reduced dosage may be effective after initial control is achieved.

Maximum dose: Children <12 years: 128 mcg/day; Adults: 256 mcg/day

Canadian labeling:

Rhinocort® Aqua®: Children ≥6 years and Adults:

Nasal polyps: 256 mcg/day administered as a single 64 mcg spray in each nostril twice daily

Rhinitis: Initial: 256 mcg/day administered as two 64 mcg sprays in each nostril once daily or a single 64 mcg spray in each nostril twice daily; Maintenance: Individualize, lowest effective dose

Maximum dose: 256 mcg/day

Rhinocort® Turbuhaler®: Children ≥6 years and Adults:

Nasal polyps: 100 mcg into each nostril twice daily (maximum: 400 mcg/day)

Rhinitis: Initial: 200 mcg into each nostril once daily; Maintenance: Individualize, lowest effective dose (maximum: 400 mcg/day)

Nebulization: Children 12 months to 8 years: Asthma: Pulmicort Respules®: Titrate to lowest effective dose once patient is stable; start at 0.25 mg/day or use as follows:

Previous therapy of bronchodilators alone: 0.5 mg/day administered as a single dose or divided twice daily (maximum daily dose: 0.5 mg)

Previous therapy of inhaled corticosteroids: 0.5 mg/day administered as a single dose or divided twice daily (maximum daily dose: 1 mg)

Previous therapy of oral corticosteroids: 1 mg/day administered as a single dose or divided twice daily (maximum daily dose: 1 mg)

NIH Asthma Guidelines (NIH, 2007):

Children 0-4 years:

"Low" dose: 0.25-0.5 mg/day

"Medium" dose: >0.5-1 mg/day

"High" dose: >1 mg/day

Children 5-11 years:

"Low" dose: 0.5 mg/day

"Medium" dose: 1 mg/day

"High" dose: 2 mg/day

Oral inhalation: Asthma:

Children ≥6 years:

Pulmicort Flexhaler™: Initial: 180 mcg twice daily (some patients may be initiated at 360 mcg twice daily); maximum 360 mcg twice daily

NIH Asthma Guidelines (NIH, 2007) (administer in divided doses twice daily):

Children 5-11 years:

"Low" dose: 180-400 mcg/day

"Medium" dose: >400-800 mcg/day

"High" dose: >800 mcg/day

Children ≥12 years: Refer to adult dosing.

Pulmicort® Turbuhaler®: [CAN, not available in the U.S.]: Initial (during periods of severe asthma or when switching from oral corticosteroid therapy): 200-400 mcg daily in 2 divided doses; Maintenance: Individualized, lowest effective dose.

Adults:

Pulmicort Flexhaler™: Initial: 360 mcg twice daily (selected patients may be initiated at 180 mcg twice daily); maximum 720 mcg twice daily

NIH Asthma Guidelines (NIH, 2007) (administer in divided doses twice daily):

"Low" dose: 180-600 mcg/day

"Medium" dose: >600-1200 mcg/day

"High" dose: >1200 mcg/day

Pulmicort® Turbuhaler® [CAN, not available in the U.S.]: Initial (during periods of severe asthma or when switching from oral corticosteroid therapy): 400-2400 mcg daily in 2-4 divided doses; Maintenance: 200-400 mcg twice daily (higher doses may be needed for short periods of time). **Note:** Patients taking 400 mcg/day may take as a single daily dose

Oral: Crohn's disease (active): Adults: 9 mg once daily in the morning for up to 8 weeks; recurring episodes may be treated with a repeat 8-week course of treatment

Note: Patients receiving CYP3A4 inhibitors should be monitored closely for signs and symptoms of hypercorticism; dosage reduction may be required. If switching from oral prednisolone, prednisolone dosage should be tapered while budesonide (Entocort™ EC) treatment is initiated.

Maintenance of remission: Following treatment of active disease (control of symptoms with CDAI <150), treatment may be continued at a dosage of 6 mg once daily for up to 3 months. If symptom control is maintained for 3 months, tapering of the dosage to complete cessation is recommended. Continued dosing beyond 3 months has not been demonstrated to result in substantial benefit.

Dosage adjustment in hepatic impairment: Monitor closely for signs and symptoms of hypercorticism; dosage reduction may be required.

Dietary Considerations Avoid grapefruit juice when using oral capsules.

Administration

Oral capsule: Capsule should be swallowed whole; do not crush or chew.

Powder for inhalation:

Pulmicort Flexhaler™: Hold inhaler in upright position (mouthpiece up) to load dose. Do not shake prior to use. Unit should be primed prior to first use only. It will not need primed again, even if not used for a long time. Place mouthpiece between lips and inhale forcefully and deeply. Do not exhale through inhaler; do not use a spacer. Dose indicator does not move with every dose, usually only after 5 doses. Discard when dose indicator reads "0". Rinse mouth with water after each use to reduce incidence of candidiasis.

Pulmicort Turbuhaler® [CAN, not available in the U.S.]: Hold inhaler in upright position (mouthpiece up) to load dose. Do not shake inhaler after dose is loaded. Unit should be primed prior to first use. Place mouthpiece between lips and inhale forcefully and deeply; mouthpiece should face up. Do not exhale through inhaler; do not use a spacer. When a red mark appears in the dose indicator window, 20 doses are left. When the red mark reaches the bottom of the window, the inhaler should be discarded. Rinse mouth with water after use to reduce incidence of candidiasis.

Rhinocort® Turbuhaler® [CAN, not available in the U.S.]: Hold inhaler in upright position and turn grey grip as far as it will go in one direction and then back to original position. Clicking sound means inhaler is loaded with dose and ready for use. Place nasal adapter into nostril and ensure firm fit. Cover opposite nostril with finger and inhale (sniff) quickly and forcefully. Do not exhale through inhaler. When a red mark appears in the dose indicator window, 20 doses are left. When the red mark reaches the bottom of the window, the inhaler should be discarded

Suspension for nebulization: Shake well before using. Use Pulmicort Respules® with jet nebulizer connected to an air compressor; administer with mouthpiece or facemask. Do not use ultrasonic nebulizer. Do not mix with other medications in nebulizer. Rinse mouth following treatments to decrease risk of oral candidiasis (wash face if using face mask).

Suspension for nasal inhalation: Shake gently before use. Prime before first use; discard after 120 sprays.

Monitoring Parameters Monitor growth in pediatric patients; blood pressure, serum glucose, weight with high-dose or long-term oral use

Asthma: FEV_1, peak flow, and/or other pulmonary function tests

Additional Information Effects of inhaled/intranasal steroids on growth have been observed in the absence of laboratory evidence of HPA axis suppression, suggesting that growth velocity is a more sensitive indicator of systemic corticosteroid exposure in pediatric patients than some commonly used tests of HPA axis function. The long-term effects of this reduction in growth velocity associated with orally-inhaled and intranasal corticosteroids, including the impact on final adult height, are unknown. The potential for "catch up" growth following discontinuation of treatment with inhaled corticosteroids has not been adequately studied.

Dosage Forms Excipient information presented when available (limited, particularly for generics); consult specific product labeling. [CAN] = Canadian brand name; [DSC] = Discontinued product

Capsule, enteric coated:

Entocort® EC: 3 mg

Powder for nasal inhalation:

Rhinocort® Turbuhaler® [CAN]: 100 mcg/inhalation [delivers 200 metered actuations] [not available in the U.S.]

Powder for oral inhalation:

Pulmicort Flexhaler™: 90 mcg/inhalation (165 mg) [contains lactose; delivers ~80 mcg/inhalation; 60 actuations]

Pulmicort Flexhaler™: 180 mcg/inhalation (225 mg) [contains lactose; delivers ~160 mcg/inhalation; 120 actuations]

Pulmicort Turbuhaler® [CAN]: 100 mcg/inhalation [delivers 200 metered actuations]; 200 mcg/inhalation [delivers 200 metered actuations]; 400 mcg/inhalation [delivers 200 metered actuations] [not available in the U.S.]

Suspension, intranasal [spray]:

Rhinocort® Aqua®: 32 mcg/inhalation (8.6 g) [120 metered actuations]

Rhinocort® Aqua® [CAN]: 64 mcg/inhalation [120 metered actuations] [not available in the U.S.]

Suspension for nebulization:

Pulmicort Respules®: 0.25 mg/2 mL (2 mL); 0.5 mg/2 mL (2 mL); 1 mg/2 mL (2 mL)

◆ **Budesonide and Eformoterol** *see* Budesonide and Formoterol *on page* 218

Budesonide and Formoterol

(byoo DES oh nide & for MOH te rol)

U.S. Brand Names Symbicort®

Canadian Brand Names Symbicort®

Index Terms Budesonide and Eformoterol; Eformoterol and Budesonide; Formoterol Fumarate Dihydrate and Budesonide

Pharmacologic Category Beta2-Adrenergic Agonist, Long-Acting; $Beta_2$-Adrenergic Agonist; Corticosteroid, Inhalant (Oral)

Use Treatment of asthma in patients ≥12 years of age where combination therapy is indicated

Unlabeled/Investigational Use Treatment of asthma in children 5-11 years of age where combination therapy is indicated

Restrictions An FDA-approved medication guide must be distributed when dispensing an outpatient prescription (new or refill) where this medication is to be used without direct supervision of a healthcare provider. Medication guides are available at http://www.fda.gov/cder/Offices/ODS/medication_guides.htm.

Pregnancy Risk Factor C

Dosage Oral inhalation:

Children 5-11 years (NIH Guidelines): Symbicort® 80/4.5: 2 inhalations twice daily. Do not exceed 4 inhalations per day.

Children ≥12 years and Adults:

U.S. labeling: Symbicort® 80/4.5, Symbicort® 160/4.5: 2 inhalations twice daily. Patients currently receiving a low-to-medium dose inhaled corticosteroid may be started on the lower strength combination; those receiving a medium-to-high dose inhaled corticosteroid may be started on the higher strength combination. Consider the higher dose combination for patients not adequately controlled on the lower combination following 1-2 weeks of therapy. Do not use more than 2 inhalations twice daily of either strength.

Canadian labeling:

Symbicort® 100 Turbuhaler® [CAN; not available in U.S.], Symbicort® 200 Turbuhaler® [CAN; not available in U.S.]:

Initial: 1-2 inhalations twice daily until symptom control, then titrate to lowest effective dosage to maintain control

Maintenance: 1-2 inhalations once or twice daily (maximum: 8 inhalations/day as temporary treatment in periods of worsening asthma)

Symbicort® Maintenance and Reliever Therapy (Symbicort® SMART): **Note:** Not approved in the U.S.:

Maintenance: Symbicort® 100 Turbuhaler® [CAN] **or** Symbicort® 200 Turbuhaler® [CAN]: 1-2 inhalations twice daily **or** 2 inhalations once daily

Reliever therapy: Symbicort® 100 Turbuhaler [CAN] **or** Symbicort® 200 Turbuhaler® [CAN.]: 1 additional inhalation as needed, may repeat if no relief for up to 6 inhalations total (maximum: 8 inhalations/day)

Additional Information Complete prescribing information for this medication should be consulted for additional detail.

Dosage Forms Excipient information presented when available (limited, particularly for generics); consult specific product labeling. [CAN] = Canadian product

Aerosol for oral inhalation:

Symbicort® 80/4.5: Budesonide 80 mcg and formoterol fumarate dihydrate 4.5 mcg per actuation (6.9 g) [60 metered inhalations]; budesonide 80 mcg and formoterol fumarate dihydrate 4.5 mcg per actuation (10.2 g) [120 metered inhalations]

Symbicort® 160/4.5: Budesonide 160 mcg and formoterol fumarate dihydrate 4.5 mcg per actuation (6 g) [60 metered inhalations]; budesonide 160 mcg and formoterol fumarate dihydrate 4.5 mcg per actuation (10.2 g) [120 metered inhalations]

Powder for oral inhalation:

Symbicort® 100 Turbuhaler® [CAN]: Budesonide 100 mcg and formoterol dihydrate 6 mcg per inhalation (available in 60 or 120 metered doses) [delivers ~80 mcg budesonide and 4.5 mcg formoterol per inhalation; contains lactose] [not available in the U.S]

Symbicort® 200 Turbuhaler® [CAN]: Budesonide 200 mcg and formoterol dihydrate 6 mcg per inhalation (available in 60 or 120 metered doses) [delivers ~160 mcg budesonide and 4.5 mcg formoterol per inhalation; contains lactose] [not available in the U.S]

◆ **Buffasal [OTC]** *see* Aspirin *on page 142*

◆ **Buffered Aspirin and Pravastatin Sodium** *see* Aspirin and Pravastatin *on page 146*

◆ **Bufferin® [OTC]** *see* Aspirin *on page 142*

◆ **Bufferin® Extra Strength [OTC]** *see* Aspirin *on page 142*

◆ **Buffinol [OTC]** *see* Aspirin *on page 142*

◆ **Bulk-K [OTC]** *see* Psyllium *on page 1268*

Bumetanide (byoo MET a nide)

U.S. Brand Names Bumex®

Canadian Brand Names Bumex®; Burinex®

Pharmacologic Category Diuretic, Loop

Additional Appendix Information

Heart Failure (Systolic) *on page 1809*

Sulfonamide Derivatives *on page 1671*

Use Management of edema secondary to congestive heart failure or hepatic or renal disease including nephrotic syndrome; may be used alone or in combination with antihypertensives in the treatment of hypertension; can be used in furosemide-allergic patients

Pregnancy Risk Factor C (manufacturer); D (expert analysis)

Lactation Excretion in breast milk unknown/use caution

Medication Safety Issues

Sound-alike/look-alike issues:

Bumetanide may be confused with Buminate®

Bumex® may be confused with Brevibloc®, Buprenex®, Permax®

Contraindications Hypersensitivity to bumetanide, any component of the formulation, or sulfonylureas; anuria; patients with hepatic coma or in states of severe electrolyte depletion until the condition improves or is corrected; pregnancy (based on expert analysis)

Warnings/Precautions [U.S. Boxed Warning]: Excessive amounts can lead to profound diuresis with fluid and electrolyte loss; close medical supervision and dose evaluation are required. In cirrhosis, avoid electrolyte and acid/base imbalances that might lead to hepatic encephalopathy. *In vitro* studies using pooled sera from critically-ill neonates have shown bumetanide to be a potent displacer of bilirubin; avoid use in neonates at risk for kernicterus. Coadministration of antihypertensives may increase the risk of hypotension.

Monitor fluid status and renal function in an attempt to prevent oliguria, azotemia, and reversible increases in BUN and creatinine; close medical supervision of aggressive diuresis required. Rapid I.V. administration, renal impairment, excessive doses, and concurrent use of other ototoxins is associated with ototoxicity. Asymptomatic hyperuricemia has been reported with use.

Chemical similarities are present among sulfonamides, sulfonylureas, carbonic anhydrase inhibitors, thiazides, and loop diuretics (except ethacrynic acid). Use in patients with sulfonylurea allergy is specifically contraindicated in product labeling, however, a risk of cross-reaction exists in patients with allergy to any of these compounds; avoid use when previous reaction has been severe. Discontinue if signs of hypersensitivity are noted.

Adverse Reactions

>10%:

Endocrine & metabolic: Hyperuricemia (18%), hypochloremia (15%), hypokalemia (15%)

Renal: Azotemia (11%)

1% to 10%:

Central nervous system: Dizziness (1%)

Endocrine & metabolic: Hyponatremia (9%); hyperglycemia (7%); variations in phosphorus (5%), CO_2 content (4%), bicarbonate (3%), and calcium (2%)

Neuromuscular & skeletal: Muscle cramps (1%)

Otic: Ototoxicity (1%)

Renal: Serum creatinine increased (7%)

<1% (Limited to important or life-threatening): Asterixis, dehydration, encephalopathy, hearing impaired, hypernatremia, hypotension, orthostatic hypotension, pruritus, rash, renal failure, vertigo, vomiting

Drug Interactions

Avoid Concomitant Use There are no known interactions where it is recommended to avoid concomitant use.

Increased Effect/Toxicity

Bumetanide may increase the levels/effects of: ACE Inhibitors; Allopurinol; Amifostine; Aminoglycosides; Dofetilide; Neuromuscular-Blocking Agents; RiTUXimab

The levels/effects of Bumetanide may be increased by: Corticosteroids (Orally Inhaled); Corticosteroids (Systemic); Diazoxide; Herbs (Hypotensive Properties); Prostacyclin Analogues

Decreased Effect

Bumetanide may decrease the levels/effects of: Neuromuscular-Blocking Agents

The levels/effects of Bumetanide may be decreased by: Bile Acid Sequestrants; Herbs (Hypertensive Properties); Methylphenidate; Nonsteroidal Anti-Inflammatory Agents; Phenytoin; Yohimbine

Ethanol/Nutrition/Herb Interactions Herb/Nutraceutical: Avoid ephedra, yohimbe, ginseng (may worsen hypertension). Avoid dong quai if using for hypertension (has estrogenic activity). Avoid garlic (may have increased antihypertensive effect).

Stability

I.V.: Store vials at 15°C to 30°C (59°F to 86°F). Infusion solutions should be used within 24 hours after preparation. Light sensitive; discoloration may occur when exposed to light.

Tablet: Store at 15°C to 30°C (59°F to 86°F).

Mechanism of Action Inhibits reabsorption of sodium and chloride in the ascending loop of Henle and proximal renal tubule, interfering with the chloride-binding cotransport system, thus causing increased excretion of water, sodium, chloride, magnesium, phosphate, and calcium; it does not appear to act on the distal tubule

Pharmacodynamics/Kinetics

Onset of action: Oral, I.M.: 0.5-1 hour; I.V.: 2-3 minutes

Duration: 4-6 hours

Distribution: V_d: 13-25 L/kg

Protein binding: 95%

Metabolism: Partially hepatic

Half-life elimination: Neonates: ~6 hours; Infants (1 month): ~2.4 hours; Adults: 1-1.5 hours

Excretion: Primarily urine (as unchanged drug and metabolites)

Dosage

Oral, I.M., I.V.:

Neonates (see Warnings/Precautions): 0.01-0.05 mg/kg/dose every 24-48 hours

Infants and Children: 0.015-0.1 mg/kg/dose every 6-24 hours (maximum dose: 10 mg/day)

Adults:

Edema:

Oral: 0.5-2 mg/dose (maximum dose: 10 mg/day) 1-2 times/day

I.M., I.V.: 0.5-1 mg/dose; may repeat in 2-3 hours for up to 2 doses if needed (maximum dose: 10 mg/day)

Continuous I.V. infusion: Initial: 1 mg I.V. load then 0.5-2 mg/hour (ACC/AHA 2005 practice guidelines for chronic heart failure)

Hypertension: Oral: 0.5 mg daily (maximum dose: 5 mg/day); usual dosage range (JNC 7): 0.5-2 mg/day in 2 divided doses

Dietary Considerations May require increased intake of potassium-rich foods.

Administration Administer I.V. slowly, over 1-2 minutes. An alternate-day schedule or a 3-4 daily dosing regimen with rest periods of 1-2 days in between may be the most tolerable and effective regimen for the continued control of edema. Reserve I.V. administration for those unable to take oral medications.

Monitoring Parameters Blood pressure, serum electrolytes, renal function

Dosage Forms Excipient information presented when available (limited, particularly for generics); consult specific product labeling. [DSC] = Discontinued product

Injection, solution: 0.25 mg/mL (2 mL, 4 mL, 10 mL)

Tablet: 0.5 mg, 1 mg, 2 mg

Bumex®: 0.5 mg [DSC]; 1 mg; 2 mg [DSC]

◆ **Bumex®** *see* Bumetanide *on page* 219

◆ **Buminate®** *see* Albumin *on page* 49

◆ **Bupap** *see* Butalbital and Acetaminophen *on page* 230

◆ **Buphenyl®** *see* Sodium Phenylbutyrate *on page* 1385

Bupivacaine (byoo PIV a kane)

U.S. Brand Names Marcaine®; Marcaine® Spinal; Sensorcaine®; Sensorcaine®-MPF; Sensorcaine®-MPF Spinal

Canadian Brand Names Marcaine®; Sensorcaine®

Index Terms Bupivacaine Hydrochloride

Pharmacologic Category Local Anesthetic

Use Local anesthetic (injectable) for peripheral nerve block, infiltration, sympathetic block, caudal or epidural block, retrobulbar block

Pregnancy Risk Factor C

Pregnancy Considerations Decreased pup survival and embryocidal effects were observed in animal studies. Bupivacaine is approved for use at term in obstetrical anesthesia or analgesia. **[U.S. Boxed Warning]: The 0.75% is not recommended for obstetrical anesthesia.** Bupivacaine 0.75% solutions have been associated with cardiac arrest following epidural anesthesia in obstetrical patients and use of this concentration is not recommended for this purpose. Use in obstetrical paracervical block anesthesia is contraindicated.

Lactation Enters breast milk/not recommended

Medication Safety Issues

Sound-alike/look-alike issues:

Bupivacaine may be confused with mepivacaine, ropivacaine

Marcaine® may be confused with Narcan®

High alert medication: The Institute for Safe Medication Practices (ISMP) includes this medication (epidural administration) among its list of drug classes which have a heightened risk of causing significant patient harm when used in error.

Contraindications Hypersensitivity to bupivacaine hydrochloride, amide-type local anesthetics, or any component of the formulation; obstetrical paracervical block anesthesia

Warnings/Precautions Use with caution in patients with hepatic impairment. Not recommended for use in children <12 years of age. The solution for spinal anesthesia should not be used in children <18 years of age. **Do not use solutions containing preservatives for caudal or epidural block.** Local anesthetics have been associated with rare occurrences of sudden respiratory arrest; convulsions due to systemic toxicity leading to cardiac arrest have also been reported, presumably following unintentional intravascular injection. **[U.S. Boxed Warning]: The 0.75% is not recommended for obstetrical anesthesia.** A test dose is recommended prior to epidural administration (prior to initial dose) and all reinforcing doses with continuous catheter technique. Use caution with cardiovascular dysfunction. Use caution in debilitated, elderly, or acutely ill patients; dose reduction may be required. Resuscitative equipment, oxygen, and other resuscitative drugs should be available for immediate use.

Adverse Reactions Note: Incidence of adverse reactions is difficult to define. Most effects are dose related, and are often due to accelerated absorption from the injection site, unintentional intravascular injection, or slow metabolic degradation. The development of any central nervous system symptoms may be an early indication of more significant toxicity (seizure).

Cardiovascular: Hypotension, bradycardia, palpitation, heart block, ventricular arrhythmia, cardiac arrest

Central nervous system: Restlessness, anxiety, dizziness, seizure (0.1%); rare symptoms (usually associated with unintentional subarachnoid injection during high spinal anesthesia) include persistent anesthesia, paresthesia, paralysis, headache, septic meningitis, and cranial nerve palsies

Gastrointestinal: Nausea, vomiting; rare symptoms (usually associated with unintentional subarachnoid injection during high spinal anesthesia) include fecal incontinence and loss of sphincter control

Genitourinary: Rare symptoms (usually associated with unintentional subarachnoid injection during high spinal anesthesia) include urinary incontinence, loss of perineal sensation, and loss of sexual function

Neuromuscular & skeletal: Weakness

Ocular: Blurred vision, pupillary constriction

Otic: Tinnitus

Respiratory: Apnea, hypoventilation (usually associated with unintentional subarachnoid injection during high spinal anesthesia)

Miscellaneous: Allergic reactions (urticaria, pruritus, angioedema), anaphylactoid reactions

Drug Interactions

Metabolism/Transport Effects **Substrate** (minor) of CYP1A2, 2C19, 2D6, 3A4

Avoid Concomitant Use There are no known interactions where it is recommended to avoid concomitant use.

Increased Effect/Toxicity There are no known significant interactions involving an increase in effect.

Decreased Effect There are no known significant interactions involving a decrease in effect.

Stability Store at controlled room temperature of 15°C to 30°C (59°F to 86°F).

Mechanism of Action Blocks both the initiation and conduction of nerve impulses by decreasing the neuronal membrane's permeability to sodium ions, which results in inhibition of depolarization with resultant blockade of conduction

Pharmacodynamics/Kinetics

Onset of action: Anesthesia (route and dose dependent): 1-17 minutes

Duration (route and dose dependent): 2-9 hours

Protein binding: ~95%

Metabolism: Hepatic; forms metabolite (PPX)

Half-life elimination (age dependent): Neonates: 8.1 hours; Adults: 1.5-5.5 hours

Excretion: Urine (~6% unchanged)

Dosage Dose varies with procedure, depth of anesthesia, vascularity of tissues, duration of anesthesia, and condition of patient. Do not use solutions containing preservatives for caudal or epidural block.

Children >12 years and Adults:

Local anesthesia: Infiltration: 0.25% infiltrated locally; maximum: 175 mg

Caudal block (preservative free): 15-30 mL of 0.25% or 0.5%

Epidural block (other than caudal block; preservative free): Administer in 3-5 mL increments, allowing sufficient time to detect toxic manifestations of inadvertent I.V. or I.T. administration: 10-20 mL of 0.25% or 0.5%

Surgical procedures requiring a high degree of muscle relaxation and prolonged effects **only**: 10-20 mL of 0.75% (**Note:** Not to be used in obstetrical cases)

Peripheral nerve block: 5 mL of 0.25 or 0.5%; maximum: 400 mg/day

Sympathetic nerve block: 20-50 mL of 0.25%

Retrobulbar anesthesia: 2-4 mL of 0.75%

Adults: Spinal anesthesia: Preservative free solution of 0.75% bupivacaine in 8.25% dextrose:

Lower extremity and perineal procedures: 1 mL

Lower abdominal procedures: 1.6 mL

Normal vaginal delivery: 0.8 mL (higher doses may be required in some patients)

Cesarean section: 1-1.4 mL

Administration Solutions containing preservatives should not be used for epidural or caudal blocks.

Monitoring Parameters Vital signs, state of consciousness; signs of CNS toxicity; fetal heart rate during paracervical anesthesia

Dosage Forms Excipient information presented when available (limited, particularly for generics); consult specific product labeling.

Injection, solution, as hydrochloride [preservative free]: 0.25% (10 mL, 20 mL, 30 mL, 50 mL); 0.5% (10 mL, 20 mL, 30 mL); 0.75% (10 mL, 20 mL, 30 mL)

Marcaine®: 0.25% (10 mL, 30 mL); 0.5% (10 mL, 30 mL); 0.75% (10 mL, 30 mL)

Sensorcaine®-MPF: 0.25% (10 mL, 30 mL); 0.5% (10 mL, 30 mL); 0.75% (10 mL, 30 mL)

Injection, solution, as hydrochloride [preservative free]: 0.75% (2 mL) [in dextrose 8.25%]

Marcaine® Spinal: 0.75% (2 mL) [in dextrose 8.25%]

Sensorcaine®-MPF Spinal: 0.75% (2 mL) [in dextrose 8.25%]

Injection, solution, as hydrochloride:

Marcaine®, Sensorcaine®: 0.25% (50 mL); 0.5% (50 mL) [contains methylparaben]

◆ **Bupivacaine and Lidocaine** *see* Lidocaine and Bupivacaine *on page 886*

◆ **Bupivacaine Hydrochloride** *see* Bupivacaine *on page 220*

◆ **Buprenex®** *see* Buprenorphine *on page 221*

Buprenorphine (byoo pre NOR feen)

U.S. Brand Names Buprenex®; Subutex®

Canadian Brand Names Buprenex®; Subutex®

Index Terms Buprenorphine Hydrochloride

Pharmacologic Category Analgesic, Opioid

Additional Appendix Information

Narcotic / Opioid Analgesics *on page 1663*

Use

Injection: Management of moderate to severe pain

Tablet: Treatment of opioid dependence

Unlabeled/Investigational Use Injection: Heroin and opioid withdrawal

Restrictions Injection: C-V/C-III; Tablet: C-III

Prescribing of tablets for opioid dependence is limited to physicians who have met the qualification criteria and have received a DEA number specific to prescribing this product. Tablets will be available through pharmacies and wholesalers which normally provide controlled substances.

Pregnancy Risk Factor C

Pregnancy Considerations Withdrawal has been reported in infants of women receiving buprenorphine during pregnancy. Onset of symptoms ranged from day 1 to day 8 of life, most occurring on day 1.

Lactation Enters breast milk/not recommended

Medication Safety Issues

Sound-alike/look-alike issues:

Buprenex® may be confused with Brevibloc®, Bumex®

High alert medication: The Institute for Safe Medication Practices (ISMP) includes this medication among its list of drug classes which have a heightened risk of causing significant patient harm when used in error.

Contraindications Hypersensitivity to buprenorphine or any component of the formulation

Warnings/Precautions An opioid-containing analgesic regimen should be tailored to each patient's needs and based upon the type of pain being treated (acute versus chronic), the route of administration, degree of tolerance for opioids (naive versus chronic user), age, weight, and medical condition. The optimal analgesic dose varies widely among patients. Doses should be titrated to pain relief/prevention.

May cause CNS depression, which may impair physical or mental abilities. Effects with other sedative drugs or ethanol may be potentiated. Elderly may be more sensitive to CNS depressant and constipating effects. May cause respiratory depression - use caution in patients with respiratory disease or pre-existing respiratory depression. Potential for drug dependency exists, abrupt cessation may precipitate withdrawal. Use caution in elderly, debilitated, pediatric patients, depression or suicidal tendencies. Tolerance, psychological and physical dependence may occur with prolonged use. Partial antagonist activity may precipitate acute narcotic withdrawal in opioid-dependent individuals.

Use with caution in patients with hepatic, pulmonary, or renal function impairment. Also use caution in patients with head injury or increased ICP, biliary tract dysfunction, patients with history of hyperthyroidism, morbid obesity, adrenal insufficiency, prostatic hyperplasia, urinary stricture, CNS depression, toxic psychosis, pancreatitis, alcoholism, delirium tremens, or kyphoscoliosis. May cause hypotension; use with caution in patients with hypovolemia, cardiovascular disease (including acute MI), or drugs which may exaggerate hypotensive effects (including phenothiazines or general anesthetics). May obscure diagnosis or clinical course of patients with acute abdominal conditions.

Tablets, which are used for induction treatment of opioid dependence, should not be started until effects of withdrawal are evident. Safety and efficacy of the tablet formulation have not been established in children <16 years of age; safety and efficacy of the injection formulation have not been established in children <2 years of age.

Adverse Reactions

Injection:

>10%: Central nervous system: Sedation

1% to 10%:

- Cardiovascular: Hypotension
- Central nervous system: Respiratory depression, dizziness, headache
- Gastrointestinal: Vomiting, nausea
- Ocular: Miosis
- Otic: Vertigo
- Miscellaneous: Diaphoresis

<1% (Limited to important or life-threatening): Agitation, allergic reaction, apnea, appetite decreased, blurred vision, bradycardia, confusion, constipation, convulsion, coma, cyanosis, depersonalization, depression, diplopia, dyspnea, dysphoria, euphoria, fatigue, flatulence, flushing, hallucinations, hypertension, injection site reaction, malaise, nervousness, pallor, paresthesia, pruritus, psychosis, rash, slurred speech, tachycardia, tinnitus, tremor, urinary retention, urticaria, weakness, Wenckebach block, xerostomia

Tablet:

>10%:

- Central nervous system: Headache (30%), pain (24%), insomnia (21% to 25%), anxiety (12%), depression (11%)
- Gastrointestinal: Nausea (10% to 14%), abdominal pain (12%), constipation (8% to 11%)
- Neuromuscular & skeletal: Back pain (14%), weakness (14%)
- Respiratory: Rhinitis (11%)
- Miscellaneous: Withdrawal syndrome (19%; placebo 37%), infection (12% to 20%), diaphoresis (12% to 13%)

1% to 10%:

- Central nervous system: Chills (6%), nervousness (6%), somnolence (5%), dizziness (4%), fever (3%)
- Gastrointestinal: Vomiting (5% to 8%), diarrhea (5%), dyspepsia (3%)
- Ocular: Lacrimation (5%)
- Respiratory: Cough (4%), pharyngitis (4%)
- Miscellaneous: Flu-like syndrome (6%)

Drug Interactions

Metabolism/Transport Effects Substrate of CYP3A4 (major); **Inhibits** CYP1A2 (weak), 2A6 (weak), 2C19 (weak), 2D6 (weak)

Avoid Concomitant Use There are no known interactions where it is recommended to avoid concomitant use.

Increased Effect/Toxicity

Buprenorphine may increase the levels/effects of: Alcohol (Ethyl); Alvimopan; CNS Depressants; Desmopressin; Selective Serotonin Reuptake Inhibitors

The levels/effects of Buprenorphine may be increased by: Amphetamines; Antipsychotic Agents (Phenothiazines); Atazanavir; CYP3A4 Inhibitors (Moderate); CYP3A4 Inhibitors (Strong); Dasatinib; Succinylcholine

Decreased Effect

Buprenorphine may decrease the levels/effects of: Pegvisomant

The levels/effects of Buprenorphine may be decreased by: Ammonium Chloride; CYP3A4 Inducers (Strong); Deferasirox; Herbs (CYP3A4 Inducers)

Ethanol/Nutrition/Herb Interactions

Ethanol: Avoid ethanol (may increase CNS depression).

Herb/Nutraceutical: Avoid valerian, St John's wort, kava kava, gotu kola (may increase CNS depression).

Stability

Injection: Protect from excessive heat >40°C (>104°F) and light.

Tablet: Store at room temperature of 25°C (77°F).

Mechanism of Action Buprenorphine exerts its analgesic effect via high affinity binding to μ opiate receptors in the CNS; displays both agonist and antagonist activity

Pharmacodynamics/Kinetics

Onset of action: Analgesic: 10-30 minutes

Duration: 6-8 hours

Absorption: I.M., SubQ: 30% to 40%

Distribution: V_d: 97-187 L/kg

Protein binding: High

Metabolism: Primarily hepatic; extensive first-pass effect

Half-life elimination: 2.2-3 hours

Excretion: Feces (70%); urine (20% as unchanged drug)

Dosage Long-term use is not recommended

Note: These are guidelines and do not represent the maximum doses that may be required in all patients. Doses should be titrated to pain relief/prevention. In high-risk patients (eg, elderly, debilitated, presence of respiratory disease) and/or concurrent CNS depressant use, reduce dose by one-half. Buprenorphine has an analgesic ceiling.

Acute pain (moderate to severe):

- Children 2-12 years: I.M., slow I.V.: 2-6 mcg/kg every 4-6 hours
- Children ≥13 years and Adults:
  - I.M.: Initial: Opiate-naive: 0.3 mg every 6-8 hours as needed; initial dose (up to 0.3 mg) may be repeated once in 30-60 minutes after the initial dose if needed; usual dosage range: 0.15-0.6 mg every 4-8 hours as needed
  - Slow I.V.: Initial: Opiate-naive: 0.3 mg every 6-8 hours as needed; initial dose (up to 0.3 mg) may be repeated once in 30-60 minutes after the initial dose if needed
- Elderly: I.M., slow I.V.: 0.15 mg every 6 hours; elderly patients are more likely to suffer from confusion and drowsiness compared to younger patients

Heroin or opiate withdrawal (unlabeled use): Children ≥13 years and Adults: I.M., slow I.V.: Variable; 0.1-0.4 mg every 6 hours

Sublingual: Children ≥16 years and Adults: Opioid dependence:

Induction: Range: 12-16 mg/day (doses during an induction study used 8 mg on day 1, followed by 16 mg on day 2; induction continued over 3-4 days). Treatment should begin at least 4 hours after last use of heroin or short-acting opioid, preferably when first signs of withdrawal appear. Titrating dose to clinical effectiveness should be done as rapidly as possible to prevent undue withdrawal symptoms and patient drop-out during the induction period.

Maintenance: Target dose: 16 mg/day; range: 4-24 mg/day; patients should be switched to the buprenorphine/naloxone combination product for maintenance and unsupervised therapy

Administration

I.V.: Administer slowly, over at least 2 minutes.

Sublingual: Tablet should be placed under the tongue until dissolved; should not be swallowed. If two or more tablets are needed per dose, all may be placed under the tongue at once, or two at a time. To ensure consistent bioavailability, subsequent doses should always be taken the same way.

Monitoring Parameters Pain relief, respiratory and mental status, CNS depression, blood pressure; LFTs

Additional Information Subutex® (buprenorphine) should be limited to supervised use whenever possible; patients should be switched to Suboxone® (buprenorphine/naloxone) for maintenance and unsupervised therapy

Dosage Forms Excipient information presented when available (limited, particularly for generics); consult specific product labeling.

Injection, solution: 0.3 mg/mL (1 mL) [C-III]

Buprenex®: 0.3 mg/mL (1 mL) [C-V]

Tablet, sublingual:

Subutex®: 2 mg, 8 mg

Buprenorphine and Naloxone

(byoo pre NOR feen & nal OKS one)

U.S. Brand Names Suboxone®

Index Terms Buprenorphine Hydrochloride and Naloxone Hydrochloride Dihydrate; Naloxone and Buprenorphine; Naloxone Hydrochloride Dihydrate and Buprenorphine Hydrochloride

Pharmacologic Category Analgesic, Opioid

Use Treatment of opioid dependence

Restrictions C-III; Prescribing of tablets for opioid dependence is limited to physicians who have met the qualification criteria and have received a DEA number specific to prescribing this product. Tablets will be available through pharmacies and wholesalers which normally provide controlled substances.

Pregnancy Risk Factor C

Medication Safety Issues

High alert medication: The Institute for Safe Medication Practices (ISMP) includes this medication among its list of drug classes which have a heightened risk of causing significant patient harm when used in error.

Dosage Sublingual: Children ≥16 years and Adults: Opioid dependence: **Note:** This combination product is not recommended for use during the induction period; initial treatment should begin using buprenorphine oral tablets. Patients should be switched to the combination product for maintenance and unsupervised therapy.

Maintenance: Target dose (based on buprenorphine content): 16 mg/day; range: 4-24 mg/day

Additional Information Complete prescribing information for this medication should be consulted for additional detail.

Dosage Forms Excipient information presented when available (limited, particularly for generics); consult specific product labeling.

Tablet, sublingual: Buprenorphine 2 mg and naloxone 0.5 mg; buprenorphine 8 mg and naloxone 2 mg [lemon-lime flavor]

◆ **Buprenorphine Hydrochloride** *see* Buprenorphine *on page 221*

◆ **Buprenorphine Hydrochloride and Naloxone Hydrochloride Dihydrate** *see* Buprenorphine and Naloxone *on page 223*

◆ **Buproban™** *see* BuPROPion *on page 223*

BuPROPion (byoo PROE pee on)

U.S. Brand Names Budeprion SR®; Budeprion XL®; Buproban™; Wellbutrin SR®; Wellbutrin XL®; Wellbutrin®; Zyban®

Canadian Brand Names Novo-Bupropion SR; PMS-Bupropion SR; RATIO-Bupropion SR; SANDOZ-Bupropion SR; Wellbutrin XL®; Wellbutrin®; Zyban®

Pharmacologic Category Antidepressant, Dopamine-Reuptake Inhibitor; Smoking Cessation Aid

Additional Appendix Information

Antidepressant Agents *on page 1638*

Use Treatment of major depressive disorder, including seasonal affective disorder (SAD); adjunct in smoking cessation

Unlabeled/Investigational Use Attention-deficit/hyperactivity disorder (ADHD); depression associated with bipolar disorder

Restrictions An FDA-approved medication guide concerning the use of antidepressants in children, adolescents, and young adults must be distributed when dispensing an outpatient prescription (new or refill) where this medication is to be used without direct supervision of a healthcare provider. Medication guides are available at http://www.fda.gov/cder/Offices/ODS/medication_guides.htm. Dispense to parents or guardians of children and adolescents receiving this medication.

Pregnancy Risk Factor C

Pregnancy Considerations Due to adverse events observed in some animal studies, bupropion is classified as pregnancy category C. A significant increase in major teratogenic effects has not been observed following exposure to bupropion during pregnancy; however, the risk of spontaneous abortions may be increased (additional studies are needed to confirm). The long-term effects on development and behavior have not been studied.

Pregnancy itself does not provide protection against depression. The ACOG recommends that therapy with antidepressants during pregnancy be individualized and should incorporate the clinical expertise of the mental health clinician, obstetrician, primary care provider, and pediatrician. If treatment is needed, consider gradually stopping antidepressants 10-14 days before the expected date of delivery to prevent potential withdrawal symptoms in the infant. If this is done and the woman is considered to be at risk of relapse from her major depressive disorder, the medication can be restarted following delivery, although the dose should be readjusted to that required before pregnancy. Bupropion has also been evaluated for smoking cessation during pregnancy; current recommendations suggest that pharmacologic treatments be considered only after other therapies have failed. A registry has been established for women exposed to bupropion during pregnancy (800-336-2176).

Lactation Enters breast milk/not recommended (AAP rates "of concern")

Medication Safety Issues

Sound-alike/look-alike issues:

BuPROPion may be confused with busPIRone

Wellbutrin SR® may be confused with Wellbutrin XL®

Wellbutrin XL® may be confused with Wellbutrin SR®

Zyban® may be confused with Zagam®, Diovan®

Contraindications Hypersensitivity to bupropion or any component of the formulation; seizure disorder; anorexia/bulimia; use of MAO inhibitors within 14 days; patients undergoing abrupt discontinuation of ethanol or sedatives (including benzodiazepines); patients receiving other dosage forms of bupropion

Warnings/Precautions [U.S. Boxed Warning]: Antidepressants increase the risk of suicidal thinking and behavior in children, adolescents, and young adults (18-24 years of age) with major depressive disorder (MDD) and other psychiatric disorders; consider risk prior to prescribing. Short-term studies did not show an increased risk in patients >24 years of age and showed a decreased risk in patients ≥65 years. All patients must be closely monitored for clinical worsening, suicidality, or unusual changes in behavior, especially during the initiation of therapy (generally first 1-2 months) or following an increase or decrease in dosage. The patient's family or caregiver should be instructed to closely observe the patient and communicate condition with healthcare provider. A medication guide should be dispensed with each prescription. **Bupropion is not FDA approved for use in children.**

The possibility of a suicide attempt is inherent in major depression and may persist until remission occurs. Use caution in high-risk patients. Worsening depression and severe abrupt suicidality that are not part of the presenting symptoms may require discontinuation or modification of drug therapy. The patient's family or caregiver should be alerted to monitor patients for the emergence of suicidality and associated behaviors (such as agitation, irritability, hostility, impulsivity, and hypomania) and notify the healthcare provider.

May worsen psychosis in some patients or precipitate a shift to mania or hypomania in patients with bipolar disorder. Patients presenting with depressive symptoms should be screened for bipolar disorder. Monotherapy in patients with bipolar disorder should be avoided. **Bupropion is not FDA approved for bipolar depression.**

The risk of seizures is dose-dependent and increased in patients with a history of seizures, anorexia/bulimia, head trauma, CNS tumor, severe hepatic cirrhosis, abrupt discontinuation of sedative-hypnotics or ethanol, medications which lower seizure threshold (antipsychotics, antidepressants, theophyllines, systemic steroids), stimulants, or hypoglycemic agents. Discontinue and do not restart in patients experiencing a seizure. May cause CNS stimulation (restlessness, anxiety, insomnia) or anorexia. May increase the risks associated with electroconvulsive therapy. Consider discontinuing, when possible, prior to elective surgery. May cause weight loss; use caution in patients where weight loss is not desirable. The incidence of sexual dysfunction with bupropion is generally lower than with SSRIs.

Use caution in patients with cardiovascular disease, history of hypertension, or coronary artery disease; treatment-emergent hypertension (including some severe cases) has been reported, both with bupropion alone and in combination with nicotine transdermal systems. Use with caution in patients with hepatic or renal dysfunction and in elderly patients; reduced dose recommended. Elderly patients may be at greater risk of accumulation during chronic dosing. May cause motor or cognitive impairment in some patients; use with caution if tasks requiring alertness such as operating machinery or driving are undertaken. Arthralgia, myalgia, and fever with rash and other symptoms suggestive of delayed hypersensitivity resembling serum sickness have been reported.

Extended release tablet: Insoluble tablet shell may remain intact and be visible in the stool.

Adverse Reactions Frequencies, when reported, reflect highest incidence reported with sustained release product.

>10%:

Cardiovascular: Tachycardia (11%)

Central nervous system: Headache (25% to 34%), insomnia (11% to 20%), dizziness (6% to 11%)

Gastrointestinal: Xerostomia (17% to 26%), weight loss (14% to 23%), nausea (1% to 18%)

Respiratory: Pharyngitis (3% to 13%)

1% to 10%:

Cardiovascular: Palpitation (2% to 6%), arrhythmias (5%), chest pain (3% to 4%), hypertension (2% to 4%; may be severe), flushing (1% to 4%), hypotension (3%)

Central nervous system: Agitation (2% to 9%), confusion (8%), anxiety (5% to 7%), hostility (6%), nervousness (3% to 5%), sleep disturbance (4%), sensory disturbance (4%), migraine (1% to 4%), abnormal dreams (3%), irritability (2% to 3%), somnolence (2% to 3%), pain (2% to 3%), memory decreased (up to 3%), fever (1% to 2%), CNS stimulation (1% to 2%), depression

Dermatologic: Rash (1% to 5%), pruritus (2% to 4%), urticaria (1% to 2%)

Endocrine & metabolic: Menstrual complaints (2% to 5%), hot flashes (1% to 3%), libido decreased (3%)

Gastrointestinal: Constipation (5% to 10%), abdominal pain (2% to 9%), diarrhea (5% to 7%), flatulence (6%), anorexia (3% to 5%), appetite increased (4%), taste perversion (2% to 4%), vomiting (2% to 4%), dyspepsia (3%), dysphagia (up to 2%)

Genitourinary: Urinary frequency (2% to 5%), urinary urgency (up to 2%), vaginal hemorrhage (up to 2%), UTI (up to 1%)

Neuromuscular & skeletal: Tremor (3% to 6%), myalgia (2% to 6%), weakness (2% to 4%), arthralgia (1% to 4%), arthritis (2%), akathisia (2%), paresthesia (1% to 2%), twitching (1% to 2%), neck pain

Ocular: Amblyopia (2%), blurred vision (2% to 3%)

Otic: Tinnitus (3% to 6%), auditory disturbance (5%)

Respiratory: Upper respiratory infection (9%), cough increased (1% to 4%), sinusitis (1% to 5%)

Miscellaneous: Infection (8% to 9%), diaphoresis increased (5% to 6%), allergic reaction (including anaphylaxis, pruritus, urticaria)

Postmarketing and/or case reports: Accommodation abnormality, aggression, akinesia, alopecia, amnesia, anemia, angioedema, aphasia, ataxia, atrioventricular block, bronchospasm, bruxism, chills, colitis, coma, coordination abnormal, cystitis, deafness, delirium, delusions, depersonalization, derealization, diplopia, dry eye, dysarthria, dyskinesia, dyspareunia, dysphoria, dystonia, ecchymosis, EEG abnormality, ejaculation abnormality, emotional lability, esophagitis, euphoria, exfoliative dermatitis, extrapyramidal syndrome, extrasystoles, facial edema, fever with rash (and other symptoms suggestive of delayed hypersensitivity resembling serum sickness), gastric reflux, gastrointestinal hemorrhage, gingivitis, glossitis, glycosuria, gum hemorrhage, gynecomastia, hallucinations, hepatic damage, hepatitis, hirsutism, hostility, hyper-/hypokinesia, hypertonia, hypoesthesia, hyper-/hypoglycemia, hypomania, impotence, intestinal perforation, intraocular pressure increased, jaundice, leg cramps, leukocytosis, leukopenia, libido increased, liver function abnormal, lymphadenopathy, maculopapular rash, malaise, manic reaction, menopause, MI, mouth ulcers, muscle rigidity, muscle weakness, musculoskeletal chest pain, mydriasis, myoclonus, neuralgia, neuropathy, painful erection, pancreatitis, pancytopenia, paranoia, paranoid reaction, phlebitis, pneumonia, photosensitivity, postural hypotension, prostate disorder, pulmonary embolism, restlessness, rhabdomyolysis, salivation increased, salpingitis, sciatica, seizure, SIADH, stomach ulcer, stomatitis, stroke, suicidal ideation, syncope, tardive dyskinesia, thirst, thrombocytopenia, tongue edema, urinary incontinence, urinary retention, vaginitis, vasodilation, vertigo

Drug Interactions

Metabolism/Transport Effects Substrate of CYP1A2 (minor), 2A6 (minor), 2B6 (major), 2C9 (minor), 2D6 (minor), 2E1 (minor), 3A4 (minor); **Inhibits** CYP2D6 (weak)

Avoid Concomitant Use

Avoid concomitant use of BuPROPion with any of the following: MAO Inhibitors

Increased Effect/Toxicity

BuPROPion may increase the levels/effects of: Alcohol (Ethyl); CNS Depressants; Tricyclic Antidepressants

The levels/effects of BuPROPion may be increased by: CYP2B6 Inhibitors (Moderate); CYP2B6 Inhibitors (Strong); MAO Inhibitors

Decreased Effect

The levels/effects of BuPROPion may be decreased by: CYP2B6 Inducers (Strong); Lopinavir; Ritonavir

Ethanol/Nutrition/Herb Interactions

Ethanol: Avoid ethanol (may increase CNS depression).

Herb/Nutraceutical: Avoid valerian, St John's wort, SAMe, gotu kola, kava kava (may increase CNS depression).

Stability

Store at controlled room temperature of 20°C to 25°C (68°F to 77°F).

Wellbutrin XL®: Store at 15°C to 30°C (59°F to 86°F).

Mechanism of Action Aminoketone antidepressant structurally different from all other marketed antidepressants; like other antidepressants the mechanism of bupropion's activity is not fully understood. Bupropion is a relatively weak inhibitor of the neuronal uptake of norepinephrine and dopamine, and does not inhibit monoamine oxidase or the reuptake of serotonin. Metabolite inhibits the reuptake of norepinephrine. The primary mechanism of action is thought to be dopaminergic and/or noradrenergic.

Pharmacodynamics/Kinetics

Absorption: Rapid

Distribution: V_d: 19-21 L/kg

Protein binding: 82% to 88%

Metabolism: Extensively hepatic via CYP2B6 to hydroxybupropion; non-CYP-mediated metabolism to erythrohydrobupropion and threohydrobupropion. Metabolite activity ranges from 20% to 50% potency of bupropion.

Bioavailability: 5% to 20% in animals

Half-life:

Distribution: 3-4 hours

Elimination: 21 ± 9 hours; Metabolites: Hydroxybupropion: 20 ± 5 hours; Erythrohydrobupropion: 33 ± 10 hours; Threohydrobupropion: 37 ± 13 hours (metabolite accumulation has been noted in ESRD).

Time to peak, serum: Bupropion: ~3 hours; bupropion extended release: ~5 hours

Metabolites: Hydroxybupropion, erythrohydrobupropion, threohydrobupropion: 6 hours

Excretion: Urine (87%); feces (10%)

Dosage Oral:

Children and Adolescents: ADHD (unlabeled use): 1.4-6 mg/kg/day

Adults:

Depression:

Immediate release: 100 mg 3 times/day; begin at 100 mg twice daily; may increase to a maximum dose of 450 mg/day

Sustained release: Initial: 150 mg/day in the morning; may increase to 150 mg twice daily by day 4 if tolerated; target dose: 300 mg/day given as 150 mg twice daily; maximum dose: 400 mg/day given as 200 mg twice daily

Extended release: Initial: 150 mg/day in the morning; may increase as early as day 4 of dosing to 300 mg/day; maximum dose: 450 mg/day

SAD (Wellbutrin XL®): Initial: 150 mg/day in the morning; if tolerated, may increase after 1 week to 300 mg/day

Note: Prophylactic treatment should be reserved for those patients with frequent depressive episodes and/or significant impairment. Initiate treatment in the Autumn prior to symptom onset, and discontinue in early Spring with dose tapering to 150 mg/day for 2 weeks

Smoking cessation (Zyban®): Initiate with 150 mg once daily for 3 days; increase to 150 mg twice daily; treatment should continue for 7-12 weeks

Elderly: Depression: 50-100 mg/day, increase by 50-100 mg every 3-4 days as tolerated; there is evidence that the elderly respond at 150 mg/day in divided doses, but some may require a higher dose. **Note:** Patients with Alzheimer's dementia-related depression may require a lower starting dosage of 37.5 mg once or twice daily (100 mg/day sustained release), increased as needed up to 300 mg/day in divided doses (300 mg/day for sustained release)

Dosing conversion between immediate, sustained, and extended release products: Convert using same total daily dose (up to the maximum recommended dose for a given dosage form), but adjust frequency as indicated for sustained (twice daily) or extended (once daily) release products.

Dosing adjustment/comments in renal impairment: Per the manufacturer, the elimination of hydroxybupropion and threohydrobupropion are reduced in patients with end-stage renal failure. Other research has noted a reduction in bupropion clearance (Turpeinen, 2007). Consider a reduction in frequency and/or dosage in this patient population.

Dosing adjustment in hepatic impairment:

Note: The mean AUC increased by ~1.5-fold for hydroxybupropion and ~2.5-fold for erythro/threohydrobupropion; median T_{max} was observed 19 hours later for hydroxybupropion, 31 hours later for erythro/threohydrobupropion; mean half-life for hydroxybupropion increased fivefold, and increased twofold for erythro/threohydrobupropion in patients with severe hepatic cirrhosis compared to healthy volunteers.

Mild-to-moderate hepatic impairment: Use with caution and/or reduced dose/frequency

Severe hepatic cirrhosis: Use with extreme caution; maximum dose:

Wellbutrin®: 75 mg/day

Wellbutrin SR®: 100 mg/day or 150 mg every other day

Wellbutrin XL®: 150 mg every other day

Zyban®: 150 mg every other day

Administration May be taken without regard to meals. Zyban® and extended release tablets should be swallowed whole; do not crush, chew, or divide. The insoluble shell of the extended-release tablet may remain intact during GI transit and is eliminated in the feces. Data from the manufacturer states that dividing Wellbutrin SR® tablets resulted in an increased rate of release at 15 minutes: "However, the divided tablet retained its sustained-release characteristics with similar increases of released bupropion at each sampling point beyond

15 minutes when compared to the intact Wellbutrin SR® tablet..." Bupropion is hydroscopic and therefore should be stored in a dry place. Splitting of large quantities in advance of administration is not advised since loss of potency may result. If necessary, splitting should be done cleanly without crushing.

Monitoring Parameters Body weight; mental status for depression, suicidal ideation (especially at the beginning of therapy or when doses are increased or decreased), anxiety, social functioning, mania, panic attacks

When used for the treatment of ADHD, thoroughly evaluate for cardiovascular risk. Monitor heart rate, blood pressure, and consider obtaining ECG prior to initiation (Vetter, 2008).

Reference Range Therapeutic levels (trough, 12 hours after last dose): 50-100 ng/mL

Additional Information Risk of seizures: When using immediate release tablets, seizure risk is increased at total daily dosage >450 mg, individual dosages >150 mg, or by sudden, large increments in dose. Data for the immediate-release formulation of bupropion revealed a seizure incidence of 0.4% in patients treated at doses in the 300-450 mg/day range. The estimated seizure incidence increases almost 10-fold between 450 mg and 600 mg per day. Data for the sustained release dosage form revealed a seizure incidence of 0.1% in patients treated at a dosage range of 100-300 mg/day, and increases to ~0.4% at the maximum recommended dose of 400 mg/day.

Dosage Forms Excipient information presented when available (limited, particularly for generics); consult specific product labeling.

Tablet, as hydrochloride: 75 mg [generic for Wellbutrin®], 100 mg [generic for Wellbutrin®]
- Wellbutrin®: 75 mg, 100 mg

Tablet, extended release, as hydrochloride: 100 mg [generic for Wellbutrin SR®], 150 mg [generic for Wellbutrin SR®], 150 mg [generic for Zyban®], 200 mg [generic for Wellbutrin SR®], 300 mg [generic for Wellbutrin XL®]
- Budeprion SR®: 100 mg [generic for Wellbutrin SR®; contains tartrazine], 150 mg [generic for Wellbutrin SR®]
- Budeprion XL®: 150 mg [generic for Wellbutrin XL®], 300 mg [contains tartrazine; generic for Wellbutrin XL®]
- Buproban™: 150 mg [generic for Zyban®]
- Wellbutrin XL®: 150 mg, 300 mg

Tablet, sustained release, as hydrochloride: 100 mg [generic for Wellbutrin SR®], 150 mg [generic for Wellbutrin SR®], 150 mg [generic for Zyban®], 200 mg [generic for Wellbutrin SR®]
- Wellbutrin SR®: 100 mg, 150 mg, 200 mg
- Zyban®: 150 mg

- ◆ **Burinex® (Can)** *see* Bumetanide *on page* 219
- ◆ **Burnamycin [OTC]** *see* Lidocaine *on page* 884
- ◆ **Burn Jel® [OTC]** *see* Lidocaine *on page* 884
- ◆ **Burn-O-Jel [OTC]** *see* Lidocaine *on page* 884
- ◆ **Buscopan® (Can)** *see* Scopolamine Derivatives *on page* 1356
- ◆ **BuSpar®** *see* BusPIRone *on page* 226
- ◆ **Buspirex (Can)** *see* BusPIRone *on page* 226

BusPIRone (byoo SPYE rone)

U.S. Brand Names BuSpar®

Canadian Brand Names Apo-Buspirone®; BuSpar®; Buspirex; Bustab®; CO Buspirone; Dom-Buspirone; Gen-Buspirone; Lin-Buspirone; Novo-Buspirone; Nu-Buspirone; PMS-Buspirone; ratio-Buspirone; Riva-Buspirone

Index Terms Buspirone Hydrochloride

Pharmacologic Category Antianxiety Agent, Miscellaneous

Use Management of generalized anxiety disorder (GAD)

Unlabeled/Investigational Use Management of aggression in mental retardation and secondary mental disorders; major depression; potential augmenting agent for antidepressants; premenstrual syndrome

Pregnancy Risk Factor B

Pregnancy Considerations No impairment of fertility or fetotoxic effects were noted in animal studies with doses 30 times maximum recommended human dose. There are no adequate and well-controlled studies in pregnant women.

Lactation Excretion in breast milk unknown/not recommended

Medication Safety Issues

Sound-alike/look-alike issues:
- BusPIRone may be confused with buPROPion

Contraindications Hypersensitivity to buspirone or any component of the formulation

Warnings/Precautions Use in severe hepatic or renal impairment is not recommended; does not prevent or treat withdrawal from benzodiazepines. Low potential for cognitive or motor impairment. Use with MAO inhibitors may result in hypertensive reactions. Restlessness syndrome has been reported in small number of patients; monitor for signs of any dopamine-related movement disorders. Buspirone does not exhibit cross-tolerance with benzodiazepines or other sedative/hypnotic agents. If substituting buspirone for any of these agents, gradually withdraw the drug(s) prior to initiating buspirone. Safety and efficacy of buspirone have not been established in children <6 years of age; no long-term safety/efficacy data available in children.

Adverse Reactions

>10%: Central nervous system: Dizziness (12%)

1% to 10%:
- Cardiovascular: Chest pain (≥1%)
- Central nervous system: Drowsiness (10%), headache (6%), nervousness (5%), lightheadedness (3%), anger/hostility (2%), confusion (2%), excitement (2%), dream disturbance (≥1%)
- Dermatologic: Rash (1%)
- Gastrointestinal: Nausea (8%), diarrhea (2%)
- Neuromuscular & skeletal: Numbness (2%), weakness (2%), musculoskeletal pain (1%), paresthesia (1%), incoordination (1%), tremor (1%)
- Ocular: Blurred vision (2%)
- Otic: Tinnitus (≥1%)
- Respiratory: Nasal congestion (≥1%), sore throat (≥1%)
- Miscellaneous: Diaphoresis (1%)

<1% (Limited to important or life-threatening): Akathisia, allergic reaction, angioedema, anorexia, bradycardia, bruising, cardiomyopathy, cogwheel rigidity, conjunctivitis, CVA, dyskinesia, dyspnea, dystonia, edema, enuresis, eosinophilia, epistaxis, EPS, galactorrhea, hallucination, heart failure, hyper-/hypotension, hyperventilation, irritable colon, leukopenia, menstrual irregularity, MI, muscle spasms, parkinsonism, personality disorders, PID, psychosis, rectal bleeding, restless leg syndrome, seizure, serotonin syndrome, suicidal ideation, syncope, thrombocytopenia, thyroid abnormality, transaminase increases, visual disturbances (tunnel vision)

Drug Interactions

Metabolism/Transport Effects **Substrate** of CYP2D6 (minor), 3A4 (major)

Avoid Concomitant Use

Avoid concomitant use of BusPIRone with any of the following: MAO Inhibitors; Sibutramine

Increased Effect/Toxicity

BusPIRone may increase the levels/effects of: Antidepressants (Serotonin Reuptake Inhibitor/Antagonist);

MAO Inhibitors; Selective Serotonin Reuptake Inhibitors; Serotonin Modulators

The levels/effects of BusPIRone may be increased by: Antifungal Agents (Azole Derivatives, Systemic); Calcium Channel Blockers (Nondihydropyridine); CYP3A4 Inhibitors (Moderate); CYP3A4 Inhibitors (Strong); Dasatinib; Grapefruit Juice; Macrolide Antibiotics; Selective Serotonin Reuptake Inhibitors; Sibutramine

Decreased Effect

The levels/effects of BusPIRone may be decreased by: CYP3A4 Inducers (Strong); Deferasirox; Herbs (CYP3A4 Inducers); Rifamycin Derivatives; Yohimbine

Ethanol/Nutrition/Herb Interactions

Ethanol: Ethanol (may increase CNS depression).

Food: Food may decrease the absorption of buspirone, but it may also decrease the first-pass metabolism, thereby increasing the bioavailability of buspirone. Grapefruit juice may cause increased buspirone concentrations; avoid intake of large quantities of grapefruit juice.

Herb/Nutraceutical: St John's wort may decrease buspirone levels or increase CNS depression. Avoid valerian, gotu kola, kava kava (may increase CNS depression).

Stability Store at USP controlled room temperature of 25°C (77°F). Protect from light.

Mechanism of Action The mechanism of action of buspirone is unknown. Buspirone has a high affinity for serotonin 5-HT_{1A} and 5-HT_2 receptors, without affecting benzodiazepine-GABA receptors. Buspirone has moderate affinity for dopamine D_2 receptors.

Pharmacodynamics/Kinetics

Absorption: Rapid

Distribution: V_d: 5.3 L/kg

Protein binding: 86% to 95%

Metabolism: Hepatic oxidation, primarily via CYP3A4; extensive first-pass effect

Bioavailability: ~4%

Half-life elimination: 2-3 hours

Time to peak, serum: 40-90 minutes

Excretion: Urine: 29% to 63% (<0.1% dose excreted unchanged); feces: 18% to 38%

Dosage Oral:

Generalized anxiety disorder:

Children ≥6 years and Adolescents: Initial: 5 mg daily; increase in increments of 5 mg/day at weekly intervals as needed, to a maximum dose of 60 mg/day divided into 2-3 doses

Adults: 15 mg/day (7.5 mg twice daily); may increase in increments of 5 mg/day every 2-3 days to a maximum of 60 mg/day; target dose for most people is 20-30 mg/day (10-15 mg twice daily)

Elderly: Initial: 5 mg twice daily, increase by 5 mg/day every 2-3 days as needed up to 20-30 mg/day; maximum daily dose: 60 mg/day.

Dosing adjustment in renal impairment: Patients with impaired renal function demonstrated increased plasma levels and a prolonged half-life of buspirone. Use in patients with severe renal impairment not recommended.

Dosing adjustment in hepatic impairment: Patients with impaired hepatic function demonstrated increased plasma levels and a prolonged half-life of buspirone. Use in patients with severe hepatic impairment not recommended.

Monitoring Parameters Mental status, symptoms of anxiety

Additional Information Has shown little potential for abuse; needs continuous use. Because of slow onset, not appropriate for "as needed" (prn) use or for brief, situational anxiety. Ineffective for treatment of benzodiazepine or ethanol withdrawal.

Dosage Forms Excipient information presented when available (limited, particularly for generics); consult specific product labeling.

Tablet, as hydrochloride: 5 mg, 7.5 mg, 10 mg, 15 mg, 30 mg

BuSpar®: 5 mg, 10 mg, 15 mg, 30 mg

- **Buspirone Hydrochloride** *see* BusPIRone *on page 226*
- **Bustab® (Can)** *see* BusPIRone *on page 226*

Busulfan (byoo SUL fan)

U.S. Brand Names Busulfex®; Myleran®

Canadian Brand Names Busulfex®; Myleran®

Index Terms NSC-750

Pharmacologic Category Antineoplastic Agent, Alkylating Agent

Use

Oral: Chronic myelogenous leukemia (CML); conditioning regimens for bone marrow transplantation

I.V.: Combination therapy with cyclophosphamide as a conditioning regimen prior to allogeneic hematopoietic progenitor cell transplantation for chronic myelogenous leukemia

Unlabeled/Investigational Use Oral: Bone marrow disorders, such as polycythemia vera and myeloid metaplasia; thrombocytosis

Pregnancy Risk Factor D

Pregnancy Considerations Animal studies have demonstrated teratogenic effects. May cause fetal harm if administered during pregnancy. The solvent in I.V. busulfan, DMA, is associated with teratogenic effects and may impair fertility. There are no adequate and well-controlled studies in pregnant women. Women of childbearing potential should avoid pregnancy while receiving treatment.

Lactation Excretion in breast milk unknown/not recommended

Medication Safety Issues

Sound-alike/look-alike issues:

Busulfan may be confused with Butalan®

Myleran® may be confused with Alkeran®, Leukeran®, melphalan, Mylicon®

High alert medication: The Institute for Safe Medication Practices (ISMP) includes this medication among its list of drugs which have a heightened risk of causing significant patient harm when used in error.

Contraindications Hypersensitivity to busulfan or any component of the formulation; oral busulfan is contraindicated in patients without a definitive diagnosis of CML

Warnings/Precautions Hazardous agent - use appropriate precautions for handling and disposal. **[U.S. Boxed Warning]: May induce severe bone marrow suppression.** May result in severe neutropenia, thrombocytopenia and/or anemia. Seizures have been reported with use; use caution in patients predisposed to seizures; initiate prophylactic anticonvulsant therapy (eg, phenytoin) prior to treatment; use caution with history of seizures or head trauma. May cause delayed pulmonary toxicity (known as "busulfan lung" - bronchopulmonary dysplasia with pulmonary fibrosis); the average onset is 4 years (range: 4 months to 10 years). Cardiac tamponade as been reported in children with thalassemia treated with high-dose oral busulfan in combination with cyclophosphamide. Busulfan has been causally related to the development of secondary malignancies (tumors and acute leukemias). Busulfan has been associated with ovarian failure (including failure to achieve puberty).

High busulfan area under the concentration versus time curve (AUC) values (>1500 μM/minute) are associated with increased risk of hepatic veno-occlusive disease during conditioning for allogenic BMT; patients with of history of radiation therapy, prior chemotherapy (≥3 cycles) and prior stem cell transplantation are at increased risk.

Oral busulfan doses above 16 mg/kg (based on IBW) and concurrent use with alkylating agents may also increase the risk for hepatic VOD. The solvent in I.V. busulfan, DMA, may impair fertility. DMA may also be associated with hepatotoxicity, hallucinations, somnolence, lethargy, and confusion. **[U.S. Boxed Warning]: Should be administered under the supervision of an experienced cancer chemotherapy physician.**

Adverse Reactions

I.V.:

>10%:

Cardiovascular: Tachycardia (44%), hypertension (36%; grades 3/4: 7%), edema (28% to 79%), thrombosis (33%), chest pain (26%), vasodilation (25%), hypotension (11%; grades 3/4: 3%)

Central nervous system: Insomnia (84%), fever (80%), anxiety (72% to 75%), headache (69%), chills (46%), pain (44%), dizziness (30%), depression (23%), confusion (11%)

Dermatologic: Rash (57%), pruritus (28%), alopecia (2% to 15%)

Endocrine & metabolic: Hypomagnesemia (77%), hyperglycemia (66%; grades 3/4: 15%), hypokalemia (64%), hypocalcemia (49%), hypophosphatemia (17%)

Gastrointestinal: Nausea (98%), mucositis/stomatitis (97%; grades 3/4: 26%), vomiting (43% to 95%), anorexia (85%), diarrhea (84%; grades 3/4: 5%), abdominal pain (72%), dyspepsia (44%), constipation (38%), xerostomia (26%), rectal disorder (25%), abdominal fullness (23%)

Hematologic: Myelosuppression (≤100%), neutropenia (100%; median recovery: 13 days), thrombocytopenia (98%; median onset: 5-6 days), lymphopenia (children: 79%), anemia (69%)

Hepatic: Hyperbilirubinemia (49%; grades 3/4: 30%), ALT increased (31%; grades 3/4: 7%), veno-occlusive disease (adults: 8% to 12%; children: 21%), jaundice (12%)

Local: Injection site inflammation (25%), injection site pain (15%)

Neuromuscular & skeletal: Weakness (51%), back pain (23%), myalgia (16%), arthralgia (13%)

Renal: Creatinine increased (21%), oliguria (15%)

Respiratory: Rhinitis (44%), lung disorder (34%), cough (28%), epistaxis (25%), dyspnea (25%), pneumonia (children: 21%), hiccup (18%), pharyngitis (18%)

Miscellaneous: Infection (51%), allergic reaction (26%)

1% to 10%:

Cardiovascular: Arrhythmia (5%), cardiomegaly (5%), atrial fibrillation (2%), ECG abnormal (2%), heart block (2%), heart failure (grade 3/4: 2%), pericardial effusion (2%), tamponade (children with thalassemia: 2%), ventricular extrasystoles (2%), hypervolemia

Central nervous system: Lethargy (7%), hallucination (5%), agitation (2%), delirium (2%), encephalopathy (2%), seizure (2%), somnolence (2%), cerebral hemorrhage (1%)

Dermatologic: Vesicular rash (10%), vesiculobullous rash (10%), skin discoloration (8%), maculopapular rash (8%), acne (7%), exfoliative dermatitis (5%), erythema nodosum (2%)

Endocrine & metabolic: Hyponatremia (2%)

Gastrointestinal: Ileus (8%), weight gain (8%), hematemesis (2%), pancreatitis (2%)

Hematologic: Prothrombin time increased (2%)

Hepatic: Hepatomegaly (6%)

Renal: Hematuria (8%), dysuria (7%), hemorrhagic cystitis (grade 3/4: 7%), BUN increased (3%)

Respiratory: Asthma (8%), alveolar hemorrhage (5%), hyperventilation (5%), hemoptysis (3%), pleural effusion (3%), sinusitis (3%), atelectasis (2%), hypoxia (2%)

Oral: Frequency not defined:

Central nervous system: Seizure

Dermatologic: Hyperpigmentation of skin (busulfan tan 5% to 10%), alopecia, rash, urticaria

Endocrine & metabolic: Amenorrhea, ovarian suppression

Hematologic: Myelosuppression (anemia, leukopenia, thrombocytopenia), pancytopenia

I.V. and/or Oral: Infrequent, postmarketing, and/or case reports: Acute leukemias, adrenal suppression, alopecia (permanent), aplastic anemia (may be irreversible), azoospermia, blurred vision, cataracts, cheilosis, cholestatic jaundice, corneal thinning, dry skin, endocardial fibrosis, erythema multiforme, erythema nodosum, esophageal varices, gynecomastia, hemorrhagic cystitis, hepatic dysfunction, hepatocellular atrophy, hyperuricemia, hyperuricosuria, interstitial pulmonary fibrosis (busulfan lung; manifested by a diffuse interstitial pulmonary fibrosis and persistent cough, fever, rales, and dyspnea; may be relieved by corticosteroids); malignant tumors, myasthenia gravis, ocular (lens) changes, ovarian failure, porphyria cutanea tarda, radiation myelopathy, radiation recall (skin rash), sepsis, sterility, testicular atrophy

Drug Interactions

Metabolism/Transport Effects Substrate of CYP3A4 (major)

Avoid Concomitant Use

Avoid concomitant use of Busulfan with any of the following: Natalizumab; Vaccines (Live)

Increased Effect/Toxicity

Busulfan may increase the levels/effects of: Natalizumab; Vaccines (Live); Vitamin K Antagonists

The levels/effects of Busulfan may be increased by: Antifungal Agents (Azole Derivatives, Systemic); CYP3A4 Inhibitors (Moderate); CYP3A4 Inhibitors (Strong); Dasatinib; MetroNIDAZOLE; Trastuzumab

Decreased Effect

Busulfan may decrease the levels/effects of: Vaccines (Inactivated); Vitamin K Antagonists

The levels/effects of Busulfan may be decreased by: CYP3A4 Inducers (Strong); Deferasirox; Echinacea; Herbs (CYP3A4 Inducers)

Ethanol/Nutrition/Herb Interactions

Ethanol: Avoid ethanol due to GI irritation.

Food: No clear or firm data on the effect of food on busulfan bioavailability.

Herb/Nutraceutical: Avoid St John's wort (may decrease busulfan levels).

Stability

Injection: Store unopened ampuls and vials under refrigeration at 2°C to 8°C (36°F to 46°F). Dilute (using manufacturer provided 5-micron filters for ampuls) in 0.9% sodium chloride injection or dextrose 5% in water. The dilution volume should be ten times the volume of busulfan injection, ensuring that the final concentration of busulfan is 0.5 mg/mL. This solution is stable for up to 8 hours at room temperature (25°C); the infusion must also be completed within that 8-hour timeframe. Dilution of busulfan injection in 0.9% sodium chloride is stable for up to 12 hours at refrigeration (2°C to 8°C); the infusion must be completed within that 12-hour timeframe.

Tablet: Store at room temperature at 15°C to 30°C (59°F to 86°F).

Mechanism of Action Busulfan is an alkylating agent which reacts with the N-7 position of guanosine and interferes with DNA replication and transcription of RNA. Busulfan has a more marked effect on myeloid cells than on lymphoid cells and is also very toxic to hematopoietic stem cells. Busulfan exhibits little immunosuppressive activity. Interferes with the normal function of DNA by alkylation and cross-linking the strands of DNA.

Pharmacodynamics/Kinetics
Duration: 28 days
Absorption: Rapid and complete
Distribution: V_d: ~1 L/kg; into CSF and saliva with levels similar to plasma
Protein binding: 32% to plasma proteins and 47% to red blood cells
Metabolism: Extensively hepatic (may increase with multiple doses); glutathione conjugation followed by oxidation
Half-life elimination: After first dose: 3.4 hours; After last dose: 2.3 hours
Time to peak, serum: Oral: Within 4 hours; I.V.: Within 5 minutes
Excretion: Urine (10% to 50% as metabolites) within 24 hours (<2% as unchanged drug)

Dosage Note: Premedicate with prophylactic anticonvulsant therapy (eg, phenytoin) prior to high-dose busulfan treatment.
Children:
CML, remission induction: Oral: 0.06-0.12 mg/kg/day **or** 1.8-4.6 mg/m^2/day; titrate dosage to maintain leukocyte count above 40,000/mm^3; reduce dosage by 50% if the leukocyte count reaches 30,000-40,000/mm^3; discontinue drug if counts fall to ≤20,000/mm^3
BMT marrow-ablative conditioning regimen:
Oral: 1 mg/kg/dose (ideal body weight) every 6 hours for 16 doses
I.V.:
≤12 kg: 1.1 mg/kg/dose (ideal body weight) every 6 hours for 16 doses
>12 kg: 0.8 mg/kg/dose (ideal body weight) every 6 hours for 16 doses
Adjust dose to desired AUC [1125 µmol(min)] using the following formula:
Adjusted dose (mg) = Actual dose (mg) x [target AUC µmol(min) / actual AUC µmol(min)]
Adults:
CML, remission induction: Oral: 60 mcg/kg/day or 1.8 mg/m^2/day; usual range: 4-8 mg/day (may be as high as 12 mg/day); Maintenance doses: 1-4 mg/day to 2 mg/week to maintain WBC 10,000-20,000 cells/mm^3
BMT marrow-ablative conditioning regimen:
Oral: 1 mg/kg/dose (ideal body weight) every 6 hours for 16 doses
I.V.: 0.8 mg/kg (ideal body weight or actual body weight, whichever is lower); for obese or severely-obese patients adjusted ideal body weight is recommended) every 6 hours for 4 days (a total of 16 doses)
Polycythemia vera (unlabeled use): Oral: 2-6 mg/day
Thrombocytosis (unlabeled use): Oral: 4-6 mg/day

Dosing adjustment in renal impairment: I.V.: Has not been studied in patients with renal impairment per the FDA-approved labeling. Some clinicians suggest adjustment is not necessary (Aronoff, 2007).

Dosing adjustment in hepatic impairment: I.V.: Has not been administered in clinical studies in patients with hepatic impairment per the FDA-approved labeling. Busulfan has extensive hepatic metabolism and risk of hepatic veno-occlusive disease with high doses; dosage adjustment may be needed.

Administration Intravenous busulfan should be administered as a 2-hour via central line.

BMT only: To facilitate ingestion of high oral doses, insert multiple tablets into gelatin capsules.

Monitoring Parameters CBC with differential and platelet count, liver function tests (evaluate transaminases, alkaline phosphatase, and bilirubin daily for at least 28 days post transplant)

Additional Information Oncology Comment: Low-dose monotherapy with oral busulfan for the palliative treatment of CML is no longer common. Treatment with imatinib or hematopoietic stem cell transplant (HSCT) are considered the primary treatments for CML (NCCN v1.2008).

Dosage Forms Excipient information presented when available (limited, particularly for generics); consult specific product labeling.
Injection, solution:
Busulfex®: 6 mg/mL (10 mL) [contains N,N-dimethylacetamide (DMA)]
Tablet:
Myleran®: 2 mg

◆ **Busulfex®** *see* Busulfan *on page* 227

Butabarbital (byoo ta BAR bi tal)

U.S. Brand Names Butisol Sodium®
Pharmacologic Category Barbiturate
Use Sedative; hypnotic
Restrictions C-III
Pregnancy Risk Factor D
Medication Safety Issues
Sound-alike/look-alike issues:
Butabarbital may be confused with butalbital
Dosage Oral:
Children: Preoperative sedation: 2-6 mg/kg/dose (maximum: 100 mg)
Adults:
Sedative: 15-30 mg 3-4 times/day
Hypnotic: 50-100 mg at bedtime. When used for insomnia, treatment should be limited since barbiturates lose effectiveness for sleep induction and maintenance after 2 weeks.
Preop: 50-100 mg 1-1½ hours before surgery
Elderly: Use with caution; reduce dose if use is needed

Dosage adjustment in renal impairment: Reduce dose if use is needed

Dosage adjustment in hepatic impairment: Reduce dose if use is needed

Additional Information Complete prescribing information for this medication should be consulted for additional detail.

Dosage Forms Excipient information presented when available (limited, particularly for generics); consult specific product labeling.
Elixir, as sodium:
Butisol Sodium®: 30 mg/5 mL (480 mL) [contains alcohol 7%, propylene glycol, sodium benzoate, and tartrazine]
Tablet, as sodium:
Butisol Sodium®: 30 mg [contains tartrazine], 50 mg [contains tartrazine]

Butalbital, Acetaminophen, and Caffeine
(byoo TAL bi tal, a seet a MIN oh fen, & KAF een)

U.S. Brand Names Anolor 300; Dolgic® LQ; Dolgic® Plus; Esgic-Plus™; Esgic®; Fioricet®; Medigesic®; Repan®; Zebutal™
Index Terms Acetaminophen, Butalbital, and Caffeine
Pharmacologic Category Barbiturate
Use Relief of the symptomatic complex of tension or muscle contraction headache
Pregnancy Risk Factor C
Medication Safety Issues
Sound-alike/look-alike issues:
Fioricet® may be confused with Fiorinal®, Lorcet®
Repan® may be confused with Riopan®

Duplicate therapy issues: This product contains acetaminophen, which may be a component of other combination products. Do not exceed the maximum recommended daily dose of acetaminophen.

Dosage
Adults: Oral: 1-2 tablets or capsules (or 15-30 mL solution) every 4 hours; not to exceed 6 tablets or capsules (or 180 mL solution) daily
Elderly: Not recommended for use in the elderly
Dosing interval in renal or hepatic impairment: Should be reduced

Additional Information Complete prescribing information for this medication should be consulted for additional detail.

Dosage Forms Excipient information presented when available (limited, particularly for generics); consult specific product labeling.
Capsule:
Anolor 300, Esgic®, Medigesic®: Butalbital 50 mg, acetaminophen 325 mg, and caffeine 40 mg
Dolgic® Plus: Butalbital 50 mg, acetaminophen 750 mg, and caffeine 40 mg
Esgic-Plus™, Zebutal™: Butalbital 50 mg, acetaminophen 500 mg, and caffeine 40 mg
Solution:
Dolgic® LQ: Butalbital 50 mg, acetaminophen 325 mg, and caffeine 40 mg per 15 mL (480 mL) [contains alcohol 7%; tropical fruit punch flavor]
Tablet: Butalbital 50 mg, acetaminophen 325 mg, and caffeine 40 mg; butalbital 50 mg, acetaminophen 500 mg, and caffeine 40 mg
Esgic®, Fioricet®, Repan®: Butalbital 50 mg, acetaminophen 325 mg, and caffeine 40 mg
Esgic-Plus™: Butalbital 50 mg, acetaminophen 500 mg, and caffeine 40 mg

Butalbital and Acetaminophen
(byoo TAL bi tal & a seet a MIN oh fen)

U.S. Brand Names Bupap; Cephadyn; Phrenilin®; Phrenilin® Forte; Promacet; Sedapap®

Index Terms Acetaminophen and Butalbital

Pharmacologic Category Analgesic, Miscellaneous; Barbiturate

Use Relief of the symptomatic complex of tension or muscle contraction headache

Pregnancy Risk Factor C

Medication Safety Issues
Duplicate therapy issues: This product contains acetaminophen, which may be a component of other combination products. Do not exceed the maximum recommended daily dose of acetaminophen.

Dosage Oral: Adults: One tablet/capsule every 4 hours as needed (maximum dose: 6 tablets/day)
Phrenilin®: 1-2 tablets every 4 hours as needed (maximum: 6 tablets in 24 hours)
Elderly: Use with caution; see adult dosing
Dosage adjustment in renal impairment: Mild-to-moderate: Should decrease dose; in severe impairment, use with caution
Dosage adjustment in hepatic impairment: Mild-to-moderate: Should decrease dose; in severe impairment, use with caution

Additional Information Complete prescribing information for this medication should be consulted for additional detail.

Dosage Forms Excipient information presented when available (limited, particularly for generics); consult specific product labeling.
Tablet:
Phrenilin®: Butalbital 50 mg and acetaminophen 325 mg
Bupap, Cephadyn, Promacet, Sedapap®: Butalbital 50 mg and acetaminophen 650 mg
Capsule:
Phrenilin® Forte: Butalbital 50 mg and acetaminophen 650 mg [may contain benzyl alcohol]

Butalbital, Aspirin, and Caffeine
(byoo TAL bi tal, AS pir in, & KAF een)

U.S. Brand Names Fiorinal®

Canadian Brand Names Fiorinal®

Index Terms Aspirin, Caffeine, and Butalbital; Butalbital Compound

Pharmacologic Category Barbiturate

Use Relief of the symptomatic complex of tension or muscle contraction headache

Restrictions C-III

Pregnancy Risk Factor C/D (prolonged use or high doses at term)

Medication Safety Issues
Sound-alike/look-alike issues:
Fiorinal® may be confused with Fioricet®, Florical®, Florinef®

Dosage
Oral: Adults: 1-2 tablets or capsules every 4 hours; not to exceed 6/day
Elderly: Not recommended for use in the elderly
Dosing interval in renal or hepatic impairment: Should be reduced

Additional Information Complete prescribing information for this medication should be consulted for additional detail.

Dosage Forms Excipient information presented when available (limited, particularly for generics); consult specific product labeling.
Capsule: Butalbital 50 mg, aspirin 325 mg, and caffeine 40 mg
Fiorinal®: Butalbital 50 mg, aspirin 325 mg, and caffeine 40 mg
Tablet: Butalbital 50 mg, aspirin 325 mg, and caffeine 40 mg

◆ **Butalbital Compound** *see* Butalbital, Aspirin, and Caffeine *on page 230*

◆ **Butamben, Tetracaine, and Benzocaine** *see* Benzocaine, Butamben, and Tetracaine *on page 185*

Butenafine (byoo TEN a feen)

U.S. Brand Names Lotrimin® Ultra™ [OTC]; Mentax®

Index Terms Butenafine Hydrochloride

Pharmacologic Category Antifungal Agent, Topical

Use Topical treatment of tinea pedis (athlete's foot), tinea cruris (jock itch), tinea corporis (ringworm), and tinea versicolor

Pregnancy Risk Factor C

Medication Safety Issues
Sound-alike/look-alike issues:
Lotrimin may be confused with Lotrisone®, Otrivin®

Dosage Children >12 years and Adults: Topical:
Tinea corporis, tinea cruris (Lotrimin® Ultra™): Apply once daily for 2 weeks to affected area and surrounding skin
Tinea versicolor (Mentax®): Apply once daily for 2 weeks to affected area and surrounding skin
Tinea pedis (Lotrimin® Ultra™): Apply to affected skin between and around the toes, twice daily for 1 week, or once daily for 4 weeks

Additional Information Complete prescribing information for this medication should be consulted for additional detail.

Dosage Forms Excipient information presented when available (limited, particularly for generics); consult specific product labeling.
Cream, as hydrochloride:
Lotrimin® Ultra™: 1% (12 g, 24 g) [contains benzyl alcohol and sodium benzoate]

Mentax®: 1% (15 g, 30 g) [contains benzyl alcohol and sodium benzoate]

◆ **Butenafine Hydrochloride** *see* Butenafine *on page 230*
◆ **Butisol Sodium®** *see* Butabarbital *on page 229*

Butoconazole (byoo toe KOE na zole)

U.S. Brand Names Gynazole-1®
Canadian Brand Names Femstat® One; Gynazole-1®
Index Terms Butoconazole Nitrate
Pharmacologic Category Antifungal Agent, Vaginal
Additional Appendix Information
Treatment of Sexually Transmitted Infections *on page 1773*
Use Local treatment of vulvovaginal candidiasis
Pregnancy Risk Factor C (use only in 2nd or 3rd trimester)
Dosage Adults: Female: Gynazole-1®: Insert 1 applicatorful (~5 g) intravaginally as a single dose; treatment may need to be extended for up to 6 days in pregnant women (use in pregnancy during 2nd or 3rd trimester only)
Additional Information Complete prescribing information for this medication should be consulted for additional detail.
Dosage Forms Excipient information presented when available (limited, particularly for generics); consult specific product labeling.
Cream, vaginal, as nitrate:
Gynazole-1®: 2% (5 g) [prefilled applicator]

◆ **Butoconazole Nitrate** *see* Butoconazole *on page 231*

Butorphanol (byoo TOR fa nole)

U.S. Brand Names Stadol® [DSC]
Canadian Brand Names Apo-Butorphanol®; PMS-Butorphanol
Index Terms Butorphanol Tartrate
Pharmacologic Category Analgesic, Opioid
Additional Appendix Information
Narcotic / Opioid Analgesics *on page 1663*
Use
Parenteral: Management of moderate-to-severe pain; preoperative medication; supplement to balanced anesthesia; management of pain during labor
Nasal spray: Management of moderate-to-severe pain, including migraine headache pain
Restrictions C-IV
Pregnancy Risk Factor C/D (prolonged use or high doses at term)
Medication Safety Issues
Sound-alike/look-alike issues:
Stadol® may be confused with Haldol®, sotalol

High alert medication: The Institute for Safe Medication Practices (ISMP) includes this medication among its list of drug classes which have a heightened risk of causing significant patient harm when used in error.
Dosage Note: These are guidelines and do not represent the maximum doses that may be required in all patients. Doses should be titrated to pain relief/prevention. Butorphanol has an analgesic ceiling.
Adults:
Parenteral:
Acute pain (moderate to severe):
I.M.: Initial: 2 mg, may repeat every 3-4 hours as needed; usual range: 1-4 mg every 3-4 hours as needed
I.V.: Initial: 1 mg, may repeat every 3-4 hours as needed; usual range: 0.5-2 mg every 3-4 hours as needed
Preoperative medication: I.M.: 2 mg 60-90 minutes before surgery
Supplement to balanced anesthesia: I.V.: 2 mg shortly before induction and/or an incremental dose of 0.5-1 mg (up to 0.06 mg/kg), depending on previously administered sedative, analgesic, and hypnotic medications
Pain during labor (fetus >37 weeks gestation and no signs of fetal distress):
I.M., I.V.: 1-2 mg; may repeat in 4 hours
Note: Alternative analgesia should be used for pain associated with delivery or if delivery is anticipated within 4 hours

Nasal spray:
Moderate to severe pain (including migraine headache pain): Initial: 1 spray (~1 mg per spray) in 1 nostril; if adequate pain relief is not achieved within 60-90 minutes, an additional 1 spray in 1 nostril may be given; may repeat initial dose sequence in 3-4 hours after the last dose as needed
Alternatively, an initial dose of 2 mg (1 spray in each nostril) may be used in patients who will be able to remain recumbent (in the event drowsiness or dizziness occurs); additional 2 mg doses should not be given for 3-4 hours
Note: In some clinical trials, an initial dose of 2 mg (as 2 doses 1 hour apart or 2 mg initially - 1 spray in each nostril) has been used, followed by 1 mg in 1 hour; side effects were greater at these dosages

Elderly:
I.M., I.V.: Initial dosage should generally be 1/2 of the recommended dose; repeated dosing must be based on initial response rather than fixed intervals, but generally should be at least 6 hours apart
Nasal spray: Initial dose should not exceed 1 mg; a second dose may be given after 90-120 minutes

Dosage adjustment in renal impairment:
I.M., I.V.: Initial dosage should generally be 1/2 of the recommended dose; repeated dosing must be based on initial response rather than fixed intervals, but generally should be at least 6 hours apart
Nasal spray: Initial dose should not exceed 1 mg; a second dose may be given after 90-120 minutes
Dosage adjustment in hepatic impairment:
I.M., I.V.: Initial dosage should generally be 1/2 of the recommended dose; repeated dosing must be based on initial response rather than fixed intervals, but generally should be at least 6 hours apart
Nasal spray: Initial dose should not exceed 1 mg; a second dose may be given after 90-120 minutes
Additional Information Complete prescribing information for this medication should be consulted for additional detail.
Dosage Forms Excipient information presented when available (limited, particularly for generics); consult specific product labeling.
Injection, solution, as tartrate [preservative free]: 1 mg/mL (1 mL); 2 mg/mL (1 mL, 2 mL)
Injection, solution, as tartrate [with preservative]: 2 mg/mL (10 mL)
Solution, intranasal, as tartrate [spray]: 10 mg/mL (2.5 mL) [14-15 doses]

◆ **Butorphanol Tartrate** *see* Butorphanol *on page 231*
◆ **B-Vex** *see* Brompheniramine *on page 214*
◆ **BW-430C** *see* LamoTRIgine *on page 850*
◆ **BW524W91** *see* Emtricitabine *on page 513*
◆ **Byetta®** *see* Exenatide *on page 595*
◆ **Bystolic™** *see* Nebivolol *on page 1046*

C1 Inhibitor (Human) (cee won in HIB i ter HYU man)

U.S. Brand Names Cinryze™

Index Terms C1 Esterase Inhibitor; C1-INH; C1-Inhibitor; C1INHRP; Human C1 Inhibitor

Pharmacologic Category Blood Product Derivative

Use Routine prophylaxis against angioedema attacks in patients with hereditary angioedema (HAE) or inherited C1 inhibitor deficiency

Unlabeled/Investigational Use Treatment of acute or severe angioedema attacks (eg, laryngeal swelling) in patients with HAE

Pregnancy Risk Factor C

Dosage I.V.: Adolescents and Adults: Routine prophylaxis against HAE attacks: 1000 units every 3-4 days

Additional Information Complete prescribing information for this medication should be consulted for additional detail.

Dosage Forms

Injection, powder for reconstitution:

Cinryze™: 500 units [contains sucrose 21 mg/mL]

Cabergoline (ca BER goe leen)

U.S. Brand Names Dostinex® [DSC]

Canadian Brand Names CO Cabergoline; Dostinex®

Pharmacologic Category Ergot Derivative

Additional Appendix Information

Antiparkinsonian Agents *on page 1643*

Use Treatment of hyperprolactinemic disorders, either idiopathic or due to pituitary adenomas

Pregnancy Risk Factor B

Dosage Initial dose: Oral: 0.25 mg twice weekly; the dose may be increased by 0.25 mg twice weekly up to a maximum of 1 mg twice weekly according to the patient's serum prolactin level. Dosage increases should not occur more rapidly than every 4 weeks. Once a normal serum prolactin level is maintained for 6 months, the dose may be discontinued and prolactin levels monitored to determine if cabergoline is still required. The durability of efficacy beyond 24 months of therapy has not been established.

Elderly: No dosage recommendations suggested, but start at the low end of the dosage range

Dosage adjustment in renal dysfunction: No adjustment required.

Dosage adjustment in hepatic dysfunction:

Mild-to-moderate dysfunction (Child-Pugh Class B): No adjustment required

Severe dysfunction (Child-Pugh Class C): Use caution; significant increase in AUC

Additional Information Complete prescribing information for this medication should be consulted for additional detail.

Dosage Forms Excipient information presented when available (limited, particularly for generics); consult specific product labeling. [DSC] = Discontinued product

Tablet: 0.5 mg

Dostinex®: 0.5 mg [DSC]

Caffeine (KAF een)

U.S. Brand Names Cafcit®; Enerjets [OTC]; No Doz® Maximum Strength [OTC]; Vivarin® [OTC]

Index Terms Caffeine and Sodium Benzoate; Caffeine Citrate; Sodium Benzoate and Caffeine

Pharmacologic Category Stimulant

Use

Caffeine citrate: Treatment of idiopathic apnea of prematurity

Caffeine and sodium benzoate: Treatment of acute respiratory depression (not a preferred agent)

Caffeine [OTC labeling]: Restore mental alertness or wakefulness when experiencing fatigue

Unlabeled/Investigational Use Caffeine and sodium benzoate: Treatment of spinal puncture headache; CNS stimulant; diuretic; augmentation of seizure induction during electroconvulsive therapy (ECT)

Pregnancy Risk Factor C

Pregnancy Considerations Caffeine crosses the placenta; serum levels in the fetus are similar to those in the mother. When large bolus doses are administered to animals, teratogenic effects have been reported. Similar doses are not probable following normal caffeine consumption and moderate consumption is not associated with congenital malformations, spontaneous abortions, preterm birth or low birth weight. According to one source, pregnant women who do not smoke or drink alcohol could consume ≤5 mg/kg of caffeine over the course of a day without reproductive risk. Another source recommends limiting caffeine intake to <150 mg/day. The half-life of caffeine is prolonged during the second and third trimesters of pregnancy.

Lactation Enters breast milk/use caution (AAP rates "compatible")

Contraindications Hypersensitivity to caffeine or any component of the formulation; sodium benzoate is not for use in neonates

Warnings/Precautions Use with caution in patients with a history of peptic ulcer, gastroesophageal reflux, impaired renal or hepatic function, seizure disorders, or cardiovascular disease. Avoid use in patients with symptomatic cardiac arrhythmias, agitation, anxiety, or tremor. Over-the-counter [OTC] products contain an amount of caffeine similar to one cup of coffee; limit the use of other caffeine-containing beverages or foods.

Caffeine citrate should not be interchanged with caffeine and sodium benzoate. Avoid use of products containing sodium benzoate in neonates; has been associated with a potentially fatal toxicity ("gasping syndrome"). Neonates receiving caffeine citrate should be closely monitored for the development of necrotizing enterocolitis. Caffeine serum levels should be closely monitored to optimize therapy and prevent serious toxicity.

Adverse Reactions Frequency not specified; primarily serum-concentration related.

Cardiovascular: Angina, arrhythmia (ventricular), chest pain, flushing, palpitation, sinus tachycardia, tachycardia (supraventricular), vasodilation

Central nervous system: Agitation, delirium, dizziness, hallucinations, headache, insomnia, irritability, psychosis, restlessness

Dermatologic: Urticaria

Gastrointestinal: Esophageal sphincter tone decreased, gastritis

Neuromuscular & skeletal: Fasciculations

Ocular: Intraocular pressure increased (>180 mg caffeine), miosis

Renal: Diuresis

Drug Interactions

Metabolism/Transport Effects Substrate of CYP1A2 (major), 2C9 (minor), 2D6 (minor), 2E1 (minor), 3A4 (minor); **Inhibits** CYP1A2 (weak), 3A4 (moderate)

Avoid Concomitant Use

Avoid concomitant use of Caffeine with any of the following: Iobenguane I 123

Increased Effect/Toxicity

Caffeine may increase the levels/effects of: CYP3A4 Substrates; Eplerenone; FentaNYL; Maraviroc; Pimecrolimus; Ranolazine; Salmeterol; Sympathomimetics

The levels/effects of Caffeine may be increased by: Cannabinoids; CYP1A2 Inhibitors (Moderate); CYP1A2 Inhibitors (Strong); Quinolone Antibiotics

Decreased Effect

Caffeine may decrease the levels/effects of: Iobenguane I 123; Regadenoson

Stability Store at 20°C to 25°C (68°F to 77°F).

Caffeine citrate: Injection and oral solution contain no preservatives; injection is chemically stable for at least 24 hours at room temperature when diluted to 10 mg/mL (as caffeine citrate) with D_5W, $D_{50}W$, Intralipid® 20%, and Aminosyn® 8.5%; also compatible with dopamine (600 mcg/mL), calcium gluconate 10%, heparin (1 unit/mL), and fentanyl (10 mcg/mL) at room temperature for 24 hours.

Mechanism of Action Increases levels of 3'5' cyclic AMP by inhibiting phosphodiesterase; CNS stimulant which increases medullary respiratory center sensitivity to carbon dioxide, stimulates central inspiratory drive, and improves skeletal muscle contraction (diaphragmatic contractility); prevention of apnea may occur by competitive inhibition of adenosine

Pharmacodynamics/Kinetics

Distribution: V_d:

Neonates: 0.8-0.9 L/kg

Children >9 months to Adults: 0.6 L/kg

Protein binding: 17% (children) to 36% (adults)

Metabolism: Hepatic, via demethylation by CYP1A2. **Note:** In neonates, interconversion between caffeine and theophylline has been reported (caffeine levels are ~25% of measured theophylline after theophylline administration and ~3% to 8% of caffeine would be expected to be converted to theophylline)

Half-life elimination:

Neonates: 72-96 hours (range: 40-230 hours)

Children >9 months and Adults: 5 hours

Time to peak, serum: Oral: Within 30 minutes to 2 hours

Excretion:

Neonates ≤1 month: 86% excreted unchanged in urine

Infants >1 month and Adults: In urine, as metabolites

Dosage

Note: Caffeine citrate should not be interchanged with the caffeine sodium benzoate formulation.

Caffeine citrate: Neonates: Apnea of prematurity: Oral, I.V.:

Loading dose: 10-20 mg/kg as caffeine citrate (5-10 mg/kg as caffeine base). If theophylline has been administered to the patient within the previous 3 days, a full or modified loading dose (50% to 75% of a loading dose) may be given.

Maintenance dose: 5 mg/kg/day as caffeine citrate (2.5 mg/kg/day as caffeine base) once daily starting 24 hours after the loading dose. Maintenance dose is adjusted based on patient's response and serum caffeine concentrations.

Caffeine and sodium benzoate:

Children: Stimulant: I.M., I.V., SubQ: 8 mg/kg every 4 hours as needed

Children ≥12 years and Adults: OTC labeling (stimulant): Oral: 100-200 mg every 3-4 hours as needed

Adults:

Electroconvulsive therapy: I.V.: 300-2000 mg

Respiratory depression: I.M., I.V.: 250 mg as a single dose; may repeat as needed. Maximum single dose should be limited to 500 mg; maximum amount in any 24-hour period should generally be limited to 2500 mg.

Spinal puncture headache (unlabeled use):

I.V.: 500 mg in 1000 mL NS infused over 1 hour, followed by 1000 mL NS infused over 1 hour; a second course of caffeine can be given for unrelieved headache pain in 4 hours.

Oral: 300 mg as a single dose

Stimulant/diuretic (unlabeled use): I.M., I.V.: 500 mg, maximum single dose: 1 g

Dosage adjustment in renal impairment: No dosage adjustment required.

Administration

Oral: May be administered without regard to feedings or meals. May administer injectable formulation (caffeine citrate) orally.

Parenteral:

Caffeine citrate: Infuse loading dose over at least 30 minutes; maintenance dose may be infused over at least 10 minutes. May administer without dilution or diluted with D_5W to 10 mg caffeine citrate/mL.

Caffeine and sodium benzoate: I.V. as slow direct injection. For spinal headaches, dilute in 1000 mL NS and infuse over 1 hour. Follow with 1000 mL NS; infuse over 1 hour. May administer I.M. undiluted.

Reference Range

Therapeutic: Apnea of prematurity: 8-20 mcg/mL

Potentially toxic: >20 mcg/mL

Toxic: >50 mcg/mL

Dosage Forms Excipient information presented when available (limited, particularly for generics); consult specific product labeling. [DSC] = Discontinued product

Caplet:

NoDoz® Maximum Strength, Vivarin®: 200 mg

Injection, solution, as citrate [preservative free]: 20 mg/mL (3 mL) [equivalent to 10 mg/mL caffeine base]

Cafcit®: 20 mg/mL (3 mL) [equivalent to 10 mg/mL caffeine base]

Injection, solution [with sodium benzoate]: Caffeine 125 mg/mL and sodium benzoate 125 mg/mL (2 mL); caffeine 121 mg/mL and sodium benzoate 129 mg/mL (2 mL) [DSC]

Lozenge:

Enerjets®: 75 mg [classic coffee, hazelnut cream, or mochamint flavor]

Solution, oral, as citrate [preservative free]: 20 mg/mL (3 mL) [equivalent to 10 mg/mL caffeine base]

Cafcit®: 20 mg/mL (3 mL) [equivalent to 10 mg/mL caffeine base]

Tablet: 200 mg

Vivarin®: 200 mg

◆ **Caffeine, Acetaminophen, and Aspirin** *see* Acetaminophen, Aspirin, and Caffeine *on page* 31

◆ **Caffeine and Sodium Benzoate** *see* Caffeine *on page* 232

◆ **Caffeine, Aspirin, and Acetaminophen** *see* Acetaminophen, Aspirin, and Caffeine *on page* 31

◆ **Caffeine Citrate** *see* Caffeine *on page* 232

◆ **Caffeine, Orphenadrine, and Aspirin** *see* Orphenadrine, Aspirin, and Caffeine *on page 1108*

◆ **Caffeine, Propoxyphene, and Aspirin** *see* Propoxyphene, Aspirin, and Caffeine *on page 1258*

◆ **Cal-C-Caps [OTC]** *see* Calcium Citrate *on page 241*

◆ **Calan®** *see* Verapamil *on page 1557*

◆ **Calan® SR** *see* Verapamil *on page 1557*

◆ **Calcarb 600 [OTC]** *see* Calcium Carbonate *on page 238*

◆ **Cal-Cee [OTC]** *see* Calcium Citrate *on page 241*

◆ **Calci-Chew® [OTC]** *see* Calcium Carbonate *on page 238*

◆ **Calcijex®** *see* Calcitriol *on page 235*

◆ **Calcimar® (Can)** *see* Calcitonin *on page 234*

◆ **Calci-Mix® [OTC]** *see* Calcium Carbonate *on page 238*

◆ **Calcionate [OTC]** *see* Calcium Glubionate *on page 241*

Calcipotriene (kal si POE try een)

U.S. Brand Names Dovonex®

Canadian Brand Names Dovonex®

Pharmacologic Category Topical Skin Product; Vitamin D Analog

Use Treatment of plaque psoriasis; chronic, moderate-to-severe psoriasis of the scalp

Unlabeled/Investigational Use Vitiligo

Pregnancy Risk Factor C

Dosage Topical: Adults:

Cream: Apply a thin film to the affected skin twice daily and rub in gently and completely, for up to 8 weeks

Solution: Apply to the affected scalp twice daily and rub in gently and completely, for up to 8 weeks

Additional Information Complete prescribing information for this medication should be consulted for additional detail.

Dosage Forms Excipient information presented when available (limited, particularly for generics); consult specific product labeling. [DSC] = Discontinued product

Cream:

Dovonex®: 0.005% (60 g, 120 g)

Ointment:

Dovonex®: 0.005% (60 g, 120 g) [DSC]

Solution, topical: 0.005% (60 mL)

Dovonex®: 0.005% (60 mL)

Calcipotriene and Betamethasone

(kal si POE try een & bay ta METH a sone)

U.S. Brand Names Taclonex Scalp®; Taclonex®

Canadian Brand Names Dovobet®

Index Terms Betamethasone Dipropionate and Calcipotriene Hydrate; Calcipotriol and Betamethasone Dipropionate

Pharmacologic Category Corticosteroid, Topical; Vitamin D Analog

Use Treatment of psoriasis vulgaris

Unlabeled/Investigational Use Treatment of corticosteroid-responsive dermatoses

Pregnancy Risk Factor C

Dosage Topical: Adults: Psoriasis vulgaris:

Cream/ointment: Apply to affected area once daily for up to 4 weeks (maximum recommended dose: 100 g/week). Application to >30% of body surface area is not recommended.

Suspension: Apply to affected area of the scalp once daily for 2 weeks or until clear; may continue for up to 8 weeks (maximum recommended dose: 100 g/week)

Dosing adjustment in renal impairment: Safety and efficacy have not been established with severe renal impairment.

Dosing adjustment in hepatic impairment: Safety and efficacy have not been established with severe hepatic impairment.

Additional Information Complete prescribing information for this medication should be consulted for additional detail.

Dosage Forms Excipient information presented when available (limited, particularly for generics); consult specific product labeling. [CAN] = Canadian brand name

Cream, topical:

Dovobet® [CAN]: Calcipotriol 50 mcg and betamethasone 0.5 mg per gram (3 g, 30 g, 60 g, 100 g, 120 g) [not available in the U.S.]

Ointment, topical:

Taclonex®: Calcipotriene 0.005% and betamethasone dipropionate 0.064% (60 g, 100 g)

Suspension, topical:

Taclonex Scalp®: Calcipotriene 0.005% and betamethasone dipropionate 0.064% (15 g, 30 g, 60 g, 2 x 60 g)

◆ **Calcipotriol and Betamethasone Dipropionate** *see* Calcipotriene and Betamethasone *on page 234*

◆ **Calcite-500 (Can)** *see* Calcium Carbonate *on page 238*

Calcitonin (kal si TOE nin)

U.S. Brand Names Fortical®; Miacalcin®

Canadian Brand Names Apo-Calcitonin®; Calcimar®; Caltine®; Miacalcin® NS; Pro-Calcitonin

Index Terms Calcitonin (Salmon)

Pharmacologic Category Antidote; Hormone

Use Calcitonin (salmon): Treatment of Paget's disease of bone (osteitis deformans); adjunctive therapy for hypercalcemia; treatment of osteoporosis in women >5 years postmenopause

Pregnancy Risk Factor C

Pregnancy Considerations Decreased birth weight was observed in animal studies. Calcitonin does not cross the placental barrier. There are no adequate and well-controlled studies in pregnant women.

Lactation Excretion in breast milk unknown/not recommended

Medication Safety Issues

Sound-alike/look-alike issues:

Calcitonin may be confused with calcitriol

Miacalcin® may be confused with Micatin®

Calcitonin nasal spray is administered as a single spray into **one** nostril daily, using alternate nostrils each day.

Contraindications Hypersensitivity to calcitonin salmon or any component of the formulation

Warnings/Precautions A skin test should be performed prior to initiating therapy of calcitonin salmon in patients with suspected sensitivity; have epinephrine immediately available for a possible hypersensitivity reaction. A detailed skin testing protocol is available from the manufacturers. Temporarily withdraw use of nasal spray if ulceration of nasal mucosa occurs. Patients >65 years of age may experience a higher incidence of nasal adverse events with calcitonin nasal spray. Safety and efficacy have not been established in pediatric patients.

Adverse Reactions Unless otherwise noted, frequencies reported are with nasal spray.

>10%: Respiratory: Rhinitis (12%)

1% to 10%:

Cardiovascular: Flushing (nasal spray: <1%; injection: 2% to 5%), angina (1% to 3%), hypertension (1% to 3%)

Central nervous system: Depression (1% to 3%), dizziness (1% to 3%), fatigue (1% to 3%)

Dermatologic: Erythematous rash (1% to 3%)

Gastrointestinal: Abdominal pain (1% to 3%), constipation (1% to 3%), diarrhea (1% to 3%), dyspepsia (1% to 3%), nausea (injection: 10%; nasal spray: 1% to 3%)

Genitourinary: Cystitis (1% to 3%)
Local: Injection site reactions (injection: 10%)
Neuromuscular & skeletal: Back pain (5%), arthrosis (1% to 3%), myalgia (1% to 3%), paresthesia (1% to 3%)
Ocular: Conjunctivitis (1% to 3%), lacrimation abnormality (1% to 3%)
Respiratory: Bronchospasm (1% to 3%), sinusitis (1% to 3%), upper respiratory tract infection (1% to 3%)
Miscellaneous: Flu-like syndrome (1% to 3%), infection (1% to 3%), lymphadenopathy (1% to 3%)

<1% (Limited to important or life-threatening): Agitation, allergic reactions, alopecia, anaphylaxis, anemia, anorexia, anxiety, appetite increased, arthritis, blurred vision, bronchitis, bundle branch block, cerebrovascular accident, cholelithiasis, cough, diaphoresis, dyspnea, earache, eczema, fever, flatulence, gastritis, goiter, hearing loss, hematuria, hepatitis, hyperthyroidism, insomnia, migraine, myocardial infarction, neuralgia, nocturia, palpitation, parosmia, periorbital edema, pharyngitis, pneumonia, polymyalgia rheumatica, pruritus, pyelonephritis, rash, renal calculus, skin ulceration, stiffness, tachycardia, taste perversion, thirst, thrombophlebitis, tinnitus, vertigo, vitreous floater, vomiting, weight gain, xerostomia

Drug Interactions

Avoid Concomitant Use There are no known interactions where it is recommended to avoid concomitant use.

Increased Effect/Toxicity There are no known significant interactions involving an increase in effect.

Decreased Effect There are no known significant interactions involving a decrease in effect.

Ethanol/Nutrition/Herb Interactions Ethanol: Avoid ethanol (may increase risk of osteoporosis).

Stability

Injection: Store under refrigeration at 2°C to 8°C (36°F to 46°F); protect from freezing. NS has been recommended for the dilution to prepare a skin test in patients with suspected sensitivity.

Nasal: Store unopened bottle under refrigeration at 2°C to 8°C (36°F to 46°F); do not freeze.
Fortical®: After opening, store for up to 30 days at 20°C to 25°C (68°F to 77°F); excursions permitted to 15°C to 30°C (59°F to 86°F). Store in upright position.
Miacalcin®: After opening, store for up to 35 days at room temperature of 15°C to 30°C (59°F to 86°F). Store in upright position.

Mechanism of Action Peptide sequence similar to human calcitonin; functionally antagonizes the effects of parathyroid hormone. Directly inhibits osteoclastic bone resorption; promotes the renal excretion of calcium, phosphate, sodium, magnesium, and potassium by decreasing tubular reabsorption; increases the jejunal secretion of water, sodium, potassium, and chloride

Pharmacodynamics/Kinetics

Hypercalcemia: I.M. or SubQ:
Onset of action: ~2 hours
Duration: 6-8 hours
Absorption: Nasal: ~3% of I.M. level (range: 0.3% to 31%)
Distribution: Does not cross placenta
Half-life elimination: SubQ: 1.2 hours; Nasal: 43 minutes
Time to peak: Nasal: ~30-40 minutes
Excretion: Urine (as inactive metabolites)

Dosage

Children: Dosage not established
Adults:
Paget's disease (Miacalcin®): I.M., SubQ: Initial: 100 units/day; maintenance: 50 units/day or 50-100 units every 1-3 days
Hypercalcemia (Miacalcin®): Initial: I.M., SubQ: 4 units/kg every 12 hours; may increase up to 8 units/kg every 12 hours to a maximum of every 6 hours
Postmenopausal osteoporosis:
I.M., SubQ: Miacalcin®: 100 units/every other day
Intranasal: Fortical®, Miacalcin®: 200 units (1 spray) in one nostril daily

Dietary Considerations Adequate vitamin D and calcium intake is essential for preventing/treating osteoporosis. Patients with Paget's disease and hypercalcemia should follow a low calcium diet as prescribed.

Administration

Injection solution: Administer I.M. or SubQ; intramuscular route is recommended over the subcutaneous route when the volume of calcitonin to be injected exceeds 2 mL.

Nasal spray: Before first use, allow bottle to reach room temperature, then prime pump by releasing at least 5 sprays until full spray is produced. To administer, place nozzle into nostril with head in upright position. Alternate nostrils daily. Do not prime pump before each daily use. Discard after 30 doses.

Monitoring Parameters Serum electrolytes and calcium; alkaline phosphatase and 24-hour urine collection for hydroxyproline excretion (Paget's disease), urinalysis (urine sediment); bone mineral density

Nasal formulation: Visualization of nasal mucosa, turbinate, septum, and mucosal blood vessels)

Reference Range Therapeutic: <19 pg/mL (SI: 19 ng/L) basal, depending on the assay

Dosage Forms Excipient information presented when available (limited, particularly for generics); consult specific product labeling.

Injection, solution [calcitonin-salmon]:
Miacalcin®: 200 int. units/mL (2 mL)
Solution, intranasal [spray, calcitonin-salmon]:
Fortical®: 200 int. units/0.09 mL (3.7 mL) [rDNA origin; contains benzyl alcohol; delivers 30 doses, 200 units/actuation]
Miacalcin®: 200 int. units/0.09 mL (3.7 mL) [contains benzalkonium chloride; delivers 30 doses, 200 units/actuation]

◆ **Calcitonin (Salmon)** *see* Calcitonin *on page 234*

◆ **Cal-Citrate-225** *see* Calcium Citrate *on page 241*

◆ **Cal-Citrate® 250 [OTC] [DSC]** *see* Calcium Citrate *on page 241*

Calcitriol (kal si TRYE ole)

U.S. Brand Names Calcijex®; Rocaltrol®

Canadian Brand Names Calcijex®; Rocaltrol®

Index Terms 1,25 Dihydroxycholecalciferol

Pharmacologic Category Vitamin D Analog

Use Management of hypocalcemia in patients on chronic renal dialysis; management of secondary hyperparathyroidism in patients with chronic kidney disease (CKD); management of hypocalcemia in hypoparathyroidism and pseudohypoparathyroidism

Unlabeled/Investigational Use Decrease severity of psoriatic lesions in psoriatic vulgaris; vitamin D-dependent rickets

Pregnancy Risk Factor C (manufacturer); A/D (dose exceeding RDA recommendation) (expert analysis)

Pregnancy Considerations Teratogenic effects have been observed in animal studies. Mild hypercalcemia has been reported in a newborn following maternal use of calcitriol during pregnancy. If calcitriol is used for the management of hypoparathyroidism in pregnancy, dose adjustments may be needed as pregnancy progresses and again following delivery. Vitamin D and calcium levels should be monitored closely and kept in the lower normal range.

Lactation Enters breast milk/not recommended

Medication Safety Issues

Sound-alike/look-alike issues:

Calcitriol may be confused with calcifediol, Calciferol®, calcitonin

Dosage is expressed in mcg (micrograms), **not** mg (milligrams); rare cases of acute overdose have been reported

Contraindications Hypersensitivity to calcitriol or any component of the formulation; hypercalcemia, vitamin D toxicity

Warnings/Precautions Adequate dietary (supplemental) calcium is necessary for clinical response to vitamin D. Excessive vitamin D may cause severe hypercalcemia, hypercalciuria, and hyperphosphatemia; calcium-phosphate product (serum calcium times phosphorus) must not exceed 70 mg^2/dL^2. Other forms of vitamin D should be withheld during therapy. Immobilization may increase risk of hypercalcemia and/or hypercalciuria. Maintain adequate hydration. Use caution in patients with malabsorption syndromes (efficacy may be limited and/or response may be unpredictable). Use of calcitriol for the treatment of secondary hyperparathyroidism associated with CKD is not recommended in patients with rapidly worsening kidney function or in noncompliant patients. Increased serum phosphate levels in patients with renal failure may lead to calcification; the use of an aluminum-containing phosphate binder is recommended along with a low phosphate diet in these patients. Use with caution in patients taking cardiac glycosides; digitalis toxicity is potentiated by hypocalcemia. Products may contain coconut (capsule) or palm seed oil (oral solution). Some products may contain tartrazine.

Adverse Reactions Frequency not defined.

Cardiovascular: Cardiac arrhythmia, hypertension

Central nervous system: Apathy, headache, hypothermia, psychosis, sensory disturbances, somnolence

Dermatologic: Erythema multiforme, pruritus

Endocrine & metabolic: Dehydration, growth suppression, hypercalcemia, hypercholesterolemia, hypermagnesemia, hyperphosphatemia, libido decreased, polydipsia

Gastrointestinal: Abdominal pain, anorexia, constipation, metallic taste, nausea, pancreatitis, stomach ache, vomiting, weight loss, xerostomia

Genitourinary: Nocturia, urinary tract infection

Hepatic: ALT increased, AST increased

Local: Injection site pain (mild)

Neuromuscular & skeletal: Bone pain, myalgia, dystrophy, soft tissue calcification, weakness

Ocular: Conjunctivitis, photophobia

Renal: Albuminuria, BUN increased, creatinine increased, hypercalciurianephrocalcinosis, polyuria

Respiratory: Rhinorrhea

Miscellaneous: Allergic reaction

Drug Interactions

Metabolism/Transport Effects **Induces** CYP3A4 (weak)

Avoid Concomitant Use There are no known interactions where it is recommended to avoid concomitant use.

Increased Effect/Toxicity

Calcitriol may increase the levels/effects of: Cardiac Glycosides; Magnesium Salts

The levels/effects of Calcitriol may be increased by: CYP3A4 Inhibitors (Moderate); CYP3A4 Inhibitors (Strong); Dasatinib; Thiazide Diuretics

Decreased Effect

Calcitriol may decrease the levels/effects of: Maraviroc

The levels/effects of Calcitriol may be decreased by: Bile Acid Sequestrants; Corticosteroids (Systemic); CYP3A4 Inducers (Strong); Deferasirox; Herbs (CYP3A4 Inducers)

Stability Store at room temperature of 15°C to 30°C (59°F to 86°F). Protect from light.

Mechanism of Action Calcitriol is a potent active metabolite of vitamin D. Vitamin D promotes absorption of calcium in the intestines and retention at the kidneys thereby increasing calcium levels in the serum; decreases excessive serum phosphatase levels, parathyroid hormone levels, and decreases bone resorption; increases renal tubule phosphate resorption

Pharmacodynamics/Kinetics

Onset of action: ~2-6 hours

Duration: 3-5 days

Absorption: Oral: Rapid

Protein binding: 99.9%

Metabolism: Primarily to 1,24,25-trihydroxycholecalciferol and 1,24,25-trihydroxy ergocalciferol

Half-life elimination: Children ~27 hours; Normal adults: 5-8 hours; Hemodialysis: 16-22 hours

Time to peak, serum: Oral: 3-6 hours; Hemodialysis: 8-12 hours

Excretion: Primarily feces; urine

Dosage

Hypocalcemia in patients on chronic renal dialysis (manufacturer labeling): *Adults:*

Oral: 0.25 mcg/day or every other day (may require 0.5-1 mcg/day); increases should be made at 4- to 8-week intervals

I.V.: Initial: 1-2 mcg 3 times/week (0.02 mcg/kg) approximately every other day. Adjust dose at 2-4 week intervals; dosing range: 0.5-4 mcg 3 times/week

Hypocalcemia in hypoparathyroidism/pseudohypoparathyroidism (manufacturers labeling): Oral (evaluate dosage at 2- to 4-week intervals):

Children <1 year (unlabeled use): 0.04-0.08 mcg/kg once daily

Children 1-5 years: 0.25-0.75 mcg once daily

Children ≥6 years and Adults: Initial: 0.25 mcg/day, range: 0.5-2 mcg once daily

Secondary hyperparathyroidism associated with moderate-to-severe CKD in patients not on dialysis (manufacturer labeling): Oral:

Children <3 years: Initial dose: 0.01-0.015 mcg/kg/day

Children ≥3 years and Adults: 0.25 mcg/day; may increase to 0.5 mcg/day

K/DOQI guidelines for vitamin D therapy in CKD:

Children:

CKD stage 2, 3: Oral:

<10 kg: 0.05 mcg every other day

10-20 kg: 0.1-0.15 mcg/day

>20 kg: 0.25 mcg/day

Note: Treatment should only be started with serum 25 (OH) D >30 ng/mL, serum iPTH >70 pg/mL, serum calcium <10 mg/dL and serum phosphorus less than or equal to the age appropriate level.

CKD stage 4: Oral:

<10 kg: 0.05 mcg every other day

10-20 kg: 0.1-0.15 mcg/day

>20 kg: 0.25 mcg/day

Note: Treatment should only be started with serum 25 (OH) D >30 ng/mL, serum iPTH >110 pg/mL, serum calcium <10 mg/dL and serum phosphorus less than or equal to the age appropriate level.

CKD stage 5: Oral, I.V.: **Note:** The following initial doses are based on plasma PTH and serum calcium levels for patients with serum phosphorus <5.5 mg/dL in adolescents or <6.5 in infants and children, and Ca-P product <55 in adolescents or <65 in infants and children <12 years. Adjust dose based on serum phosphate, calcium and PTH levels. Administer dose with each dialysis session (3 times/week). Intermittent I.V./oral administration is more effective than daily oral dosing.

Plasma PTH 300-500 pg/mL and serum Ca <10 mg/dL: 0.0075 mcg/kg (maximum: 0.25 mcg/day)

Plasma PTH >500-1000 pg/mL and serum Ca <10 mg/dL: 0.015 mcg/kg (maximum: 0.5 mcg/day)

Plasma PTH >1000 pg/mL and serum Ca <10.5 mg/dL: 0.025 mcg/kg (maximum: 1 mcg/day)

Adults:

CKD stage 3: Oral: 0.25 mcg/day. Treatment should only be started with serum 25(OH) D >30 ng/mL, serum iPTH >70 pg/mL, serum calcium <9.5 mg/dL and serum phosphorus <4.6 mg/dL

CKD stage 4: Oral: 0.25 mcg/day. Treatment should only be started with serum 25(OH) D >30 ng/mL, serum iPTH >110 pg/mL, serum calcium <9.5 mg/dL and serum phosphorus <4.6 mg/dL

CKD stage 5:

Peritoneal dialysis: Oral: Initial: 0.5-1 mcg 2-3 times/week or 0.25 mcg/day

Hemodialysis: **Note:** The following initial doses are based on plasma PTH and serum calcium levels for patients with serum phosphorus <5.5 mg/dL and Ca-P product <55. Adjust dose based on serum phosphate, calcium, and PTH levels. Intermittent I.V. administration may be more effective than daily oral dosing.

Plasma PTH 300-600 pg/mL and serum Ca <9.5 mg/dL: Oral, I.V.: 0.5-1.5 mcg

Plasma PTH 600-1000 pg/mL and serum Ca <9.5 mg/dL:

Oral: 1-4 mcg

I.V.: 1-3 mcg

Plasma PTH >1000 pg/mL and serum Ca <10 mg/dL:

Oral: 3-7 mcg

I.V.: 3-5 mcg

Vitamin D-dependent rickets (unlabeled use): Children and Adults: Oral: 1 mcg once daily

Elderly: No dosage recommendations, but start at the lower end of the dosage range

Dosage adjustment for toxicity: K/DOQI guidelines: Children and Adults: CKD stage 3 and 4:

iPTH below target: Hold calcitriol until levels rise then resume treatment at half the previous dose. If the lowest dose was being used, switch to alternate day therapy.

Corrected total calcium >9.5 mg/dL (adults) or 10.2 mg/dL (children): Hold calcitriol until serum calcium returns to <9.5 mg/dL (adults) or <9.8 mg/dL (children) then resume treatment at half the previous dose. If the lowest dose was being used, switch to alternate day therapy.

Serum phosphorus >4.6 mg/dL (adults) or greater than the age appropriate limits in children: Hold calcitriol (or add/increase dose of phosphate binder) until levels of phosphorous decrease, then resume at half the prior dose.

Dietary Considerations May be taken without regard to food. Give with meals to reduce GI problems. Adequate calcium intake should be maintained during therapy; dietary phosphorous may need to be restricted. Rocaltrol® capsules contain coconut oil; Rocaltrol® solution contains palm seed oil.

Administration May be administered without regard to food. Give with meals to reduce GI problems. May be administered as a bolus dose I.V. through the catheter at the end of hemodialysis.

Monitoring Parameters Signs and symptoms of vitamin D intoxication; alkaline phosphatase, serum creatinine

Serum calcium and phosphorus:

CKD stage 2-4: Every month for the first 3 months, then every 3 months

CKD stage 5: Every 2 weeks for 1 month, then monthly

Serum or plasma intact PTH (iPTH):

CKD stage 3 and 4: Every 3 months for 6 months, then every 3 months

CKD stage 5: Monthly for 3 months, then every 3 months

Reference Range

CKD K/DOQI guidelines definition of stages; chronic disease is kidney damage or GFR <60 mL/minute/1.73 m^2 for ≥3 months:

Stage 2: GFR 60-89 mL/minute/1.73 m^2 (kidney damage with mild decrease GFR)

Stage 3: GFR 30-59 mL/minute/1.73 m^2 (moderate decrease GFR)

Stage 4: GFR 15-29 mL/minute/1.73 m^2 (severe decrease GFR)

Stage 5: GFR <15 mL/minute/1.73 m^2 or dialysis (kidney failure)

Target range for iPTH:

Stage 2 CKD: 35-70 pg/mL (children)

Stage 3 CKD: 35-70 pg/mL (children and adults)

Stage 4 CKD: 70-110 pg/mL (children and adults)

Stage 5 CKD: 150-300 pg/mL (adults); 200-300 pg/mL (children)

Serum phosphorus:

Stage 3 and 4 CKD: ≥2.7 to <4.6 mg/dL (adults); within age appropriate limits (children)

Stage 5 CKD: 3.5-5.5 mg/dL (children >12 years and adults); 4-6 mg/dL (children 1-12 years)

Serum calcium-phosphorus product:

Stage 3-5 CKD: <55 mg^2/dL^2 (children >12 years and adults); <65 mg^2/dL^2 (children ≤12 years)

Dosage Forms Excipient information presented when available (limited, particularly for generics); consult specific product labeling.

Capsule, softgel: 0.25 mcg, 0.5 mcg

Rocaltrol®: 0.25 mcg [contains coconut oil]; 0.5 mcg [contains coconut oil]

Injection, solution: 1 mcg/mL (1 mL)

Calcijex®: 1 mcg/mL (1 mL) [contains aluminum]

Solution, oral: 1 mcg/mL (15 mL)

Rocaltrol®: 1 mcg/mL (15 mL) [contains palm seed oil]

Calcium Acetate (KAL see um AS e tate)

U.S. Brand Names PhosLo®

Canadian Brand Names PhosLo®

Pharmacologic Category Antidote; Calcium Salt; Phosphate Binder

Use Control of hyperphosphatemia in end-stage renal failure; does not promote aluminum absorption

Pregnancy Risk Factor C

Medication Safety Issues

Sound-alike/look-alike issues:

PhosLo® may be confused with Phos-Flur®, ProSom™

Dosage

Dietary Reference Intake:

0-6 months: 210 mg/day

7-12 months: 270 mg/day

1-3 years: 500 mg/day

4-8 years: 800 mg/day

Adults, Male/Female:

9-18 years: 1300 mg/day

19-50 years: 1000 mg/day

≥51 years: 1200 mg/day

Female: Pregnancy/Lactating: Same as for Adults, Male/Female

Oral: Adults, on dialysis: Initial: 1334 mg with each meal, can be increased gradually to bring the serum phosphate value to <6 mg/dL as long as hypercalcemia does not develop (usual dose: 2001-2868 mg calcium acetate with each meal); do not give additional calcium supplements

Additional Information Complete prescribing information for this medication should be consulted for additional detail.

Dosage Forms Excipient information presented when available (limited, particularly for generics); consult specific product labeling.

Gelcap: 667 mg

PhosLo®: 667 mg [equivalent to elemental calcium 169 mg (8.45 mEq)]

- **Calcium Acetate and Aluminum Sulfate** *see* Aluminum Sulfate and Calcium Acetate *on page 77*
- **Calcium Acetylhomotaurinate** *see* Acamprosate *on page 23*
- **Calcium and Risedronate** *see* Risedronate and Calcium *on page 1323*

Calcium and Vitamin D

(KAL see um & VYE ta min dee)

U.S. Brand Names Cal-CYUM [OTC]; Caltrate® 600+ Soy™ [OTC]; Caltrate® 600+D [OTC]; Caltrate® Colon-Health™ [OTC]; Chew-Cal [OTC]; Liqua-Cal [OTC]; Os-Cal® 500+D [OTC]; Oysco 500+D [OTC]; Oysco D [OTC]; Oyst-Cal-D 500 [OTC]; Oyst-Cal-D [OTC]

Index Terms Vitamin D and Calcium Carbonate

Pharmacologic Category Calcium Salt; Electrolyte Supplement, Oral; Vitamin, Fat Soluble

Use Dietary supplement, antacid

Dosage Oral: Adults: Refer to individual monographs for dietary reference intake.

Dosage adjustment in renal impairment: Use caution in severe renal impairment

Additional Information Complete prescribing information for this medication should be consulted for additional detail.

Dosage Forms Excipient information presented when available (limited, particularly for generics); consult specific product labeling.

Capsule, softgel: Calcium 500 mg and vitamin D 500 int. units; calcium 600 mg and vitamin D 100 int. units; calcium 600 mg and vitamin D 200 int. units

Liqua-Cal: Calcium 600 mg and vitamin D 200 int. units [contains beeswax, lecithin, and soybean oil]

Tablet: Calcium 250 mg and vitamin D 125 int. units; calcium 500 mg and vitamin D 125 int. units; calcium 500 mg and vitamin D 200 int. units; calcium 600 mg and vitamin D 125 int. units; calcium 600 mg and vitamin D 200 int. units

Caltrate® 600+D: Calcium 600 mg and vitamin D 200 int. units [contains soybean oil]

Caltrate® 600+ Soy™: Calcium 600 mg and vitamin D 200 int. units [contains soy isoflavones 25 mg]

Caltrate® ColonHealth™: Calcium 600 mg and vitamin D 200 int. units [contains soybean oil]

Oysco D: Calcium 250 mg and vitamin D 125 int. units

Oysco 500+D: Calcium 500 mg and vitamin D 200 int. units [contains tartrazine]

Oyst-Cal-D: Calcium 250 mg and vitamin D 125 int. units [sodium free, sugar free; contains tartrazine]

Oyst-Cal-D 500: Calcium 500 mg and vitamin D 200 int. units [sodium free, sugar free; contains tartrazine]

Tablet, chewable: Calcium 500 mg and vitamin D 100 int. units; Calcium 600 mg and vitamin D 400 int. units

Os-Cal® 500+D: Calcium 500 mg and vitamin D 400 int. units [sugar free; contains phenylalanine; light lemon flavor]

Wafer, chewable:

Cal-CYUM: Calcium 519 mg and vitamin D 150 int. units (50s) [dye free; vanilla flavor]

Chew-Cal: Calcium 333 mg and vitamin D 40 int. units (100s, 250s)

Calcium Carbonate (KAL see um KAR bun ate)

U.S. Brand Names Alcalak [OTC]; Alka-Mints® [OTC]; Cal-Gest [OTC]; Cal-Mint [OTC]; Calcarb 600 [OTC]; Calci-Chew® [OTC]; Calci-Mix® [OTC]; Caltrate® 600 [OTC]; Children's Pepto [OTC]; Chooz® [OTC]; Florical® [OTC]; Maalox® Regular Chewable [OTC]; Mylanta® Children's [OTC]; Nephro-Calci® [OTC]; Nutralox® [OTC]; Os-Cal® 500 [OTC] [DSC]; Oysco 500 [OTC]; Oyst-Cal 500 [OTC]; Rolaids® Softchews [OTC]; Titralac™ [OTC]; Tums® E-X [OTC]; Tums® Extra Strength Sugar Free [OTC]; Tums® Smoothies™ [OTC]; Tums® Ultra [OTC]; Tums® [OTC]

Canadian Brand Names Apo-Cal®; Calcite-500; Caltrate®; Caltrate® Select; Os-Cal®

Pharmacologic Category Antacid; Antidote; Calcium Salt; Electrolyte Supplement, Oral

Use As an antacid; treatment and prevention of calcium deficiency or hyperphosphatemia (eg, osteoporosis, osteomalacia, mild/moderate renal insufficiency, hypoparathyroidism, postmenopausal osteoporosis, rickets); has been used to bind phosphate

Medication Safety Issues

Sound-alike/look-alike issues:

Florical® may be confused with Fiorinal®

Mylanta® may be confused with Mynatal®

Nephro-Calci® may be confused with Nephrocaps®

Os-Cal® may be confused with Asacol®

International issues:

Remegel® [Great Britain, Ireland, Italy] may be confused with Renagel® which is a brand name for sevelamer in the U.S.

Dosage Oral (dosage is in terms of elemental calcium):

Dietary Reference Intake:

0-6 months: 210 mg/day

7-12 months: 270 mg/day

1-3 years: 500 mg/day

4-8 years: 800 mg/day

Adults, Male/Female:

9-18 years: 1300 mg/day

19-50 years: 1000 mg/day

≥51 years: 1200 mg/day

Female: Pregnancy/Lactating: Same as for Adults, Male/Female

Hypocalcemia (dose depends on clinical condition and serum calcium level): Dose expressed in mg of **elemental calcium**

Neonates: 50-150 mg/kg/day in 4-6 divided doses; not to exceed 1 g/day

Children: 45-65 mg/kg/day in 4 divided doses

Adults: 1-2 g or more/day in 3-4 divided doses

Antacid:

Children 2-5 years (24-47 lb): Elemental calcium 161 mg as needed; maximum 483 mg per 24 hours

Children 6-11 years (48-95 lb): Elemental calcium 322 mg as needed; maximum: 966 mg per 24 hours

Adults: Dosage based on acid-neutralizing capacity of specific product; generally, 1-2 tablets or 5-10 mL every 2 hours; maximum: 7000 mg calcium carbonate per 24 hours; specific product labeling should be consulted

Dietary supplementation: Adults: 500 mg to 2 g divided 2-4 times/day

Osteoporosis: Adults >51 years: 1200 mg/day

Dosing adjustment in renal impairment: Cl_{cr} <25 mL/minute: Dosage adjustments may be necessary depending on the serum calcium levels

Additional Information Complete prescribing information for this medication should be consulted for additional detail.

Dosage Forms Excipient information presented when available (limited, particularly for generics); consult specific product labeling. [DSC] = Discontinued product

Capsule:

Calci-Mix®: 1250 mg [equivalent to elemental calcium 500 mg]

Florical®: 364 mg [equivalent to elemental calcium 145.6 mg; contains sodium fluoride 3.75 mg]

Gum, chewing: 250 mg (30s)

Chooz®: 500 mg [equivalent to elemental calcium 200 mg; mint flavor]
Powder: 4000 mg/teaspoonful (480 g) [equivalent to 1600 mg elemental calcium/teaspoonful]
Suspension, oral: 1250 mg/5 mL (5 mL, 500 mL) [equivalent to elemental calcium 500 mg/5 mL; mint flavor]
Tablet: 1250 mg [equivalent to elemental calcium 500 mg]; 1500 mg [equivalent to elemental calcium 600 mg]
Calcarb 600, Caltrate® 600, Nephro-Calci®: 1500 mg [equivalent to elemental calcium 600 mg]
Florical®: 364 mg [equivalent to elemental calcium 145.6 mg; contains sodium fluoride 8.3 mg]
Os-Cal® 500: 1250 mg [equivalent to elemental calcium 500 mg; contains tartrazine] [DSC]
Oysco 500, Oyst-Cal 500: 1250 mg [equivalent to elemental calcium 500 mg]
Tablet, chewable: 500 mg [equivalent to elemental calcium 200 mg]; 650 mg [equivalent to elemental calcium 260 mg]; 750 mg [equivalent to elemental calcium 300 mg]
Alcalak: 420 mg [equivalent to elemental calcium 168 mg; mint flavor]
Alka-Mints®: 850 mg [equivalent to elemental calcium 340 mg; spearmint flavor]
Cal-Gest: 500 mg [equivalent to elemental calcium 200 mg; assorted flavors]
Calci-Chew®: 1250 mg [equivalent to elemental calcium 500 mg; cherry, lemon, and orange flavors]
Cal-Mint: 650 mg [equivalent to elemental calcium 260 mg; mint flavor]
Children's Pepto: 400 mg [equivalent to elemental calcium 161 mg; bubble gum or watermelon flavors]
Maalox® Regular: 600 mg [equivalent to elemental calcium 222 mg; contains phenylalanine 0.5 mg/tablet; lemon flavor]
Mylanta® Children's: 400 mg [equivalent to elemental calcium 160 mg; bubble gum flavor]
Nutralox®: 420 mg [equivalent to elemental calcium 168 mg; sugar free; mint flavor]
Os-Cal® 500: 1250 mg [equivalent to elemental calcium 500 mg; Bavarian cream flavor] [DSC]
Titralac™: 420 mg [equivalent to elemental calcium 168 mg; sugar free; contains sodium 1.1 mg/tablet; spearmint flavor]
Tums®: 500 mg [equivalent to elemental calcium 200 mg; contains tartrazine; assorted fruit and peppermint flavors]
Tums® E-X: 750 mg [equivalent to elemental calcium 300 mg; contains tartrazine; assorted fruit, cool relief mint, fresh blend, tropical assorted fruit, wintergreen, and assorted berry flavors]
Tums® Extra Strength Sugar Free: 750 mg [equivalent to elemental calcium 300 mg; sugar free; contains phenylalanine <1 mg/tablet; orange cream flavor]
Tums® Smoothies™: 750 mg [equivalent to elemental calcium 300 mg; contains tartrazine; assorted fruit, assorted tropical fruit, peppermint flavors]
Tums® Ultra®: 1000 mg [equivalent to elemental calcium 400 mg; contains tartrazine; assorted berry, assorted fruit, assorted tropical fruit, peppermint, and spearmint flavors]
Tablet, softchew:
Rolaids®: 1177 mg [equivalent to elemental calcium 471 mg; contains coconut oil and soy lecithin; vanilla creme and wild cherry flavors]

Calcium Carbonate and Magnesium Hydroxide

(KAL see um KAR bun ate & mag NEE zhum hye DROKS ide)

U.S. Brand Names Mi-Acid™ Double Strength [OTC]; Mylanta® Gelcaps® [OTC]; Mylanta® Supreme [OTC]; Mylanta® Ultra [OTC]; Rolaids® Extra Strength [OTC]; Rolaids® [OTC]

Index Terms Magnesium Hydroxide and Calcium Carbonate

Pharmacologic Category Antacid

Use Hyperacidity

Medication Safety Issues
Sound-alike/look-alike issues:
Mylanta® may be confused with Mynatal®

Dosage Adults: Oral: 2-4 tablets between meals, at bedtime, or as directed by healthcare provider

Additional Information Complete prescribing information for this medication should be consulted for additional detail.

Dosage Forms Excipient information presented when available (limited, particularly for generics); consult specific product labeling.
Gelcap (Mylanta® Gelcaps®): Calcium carbonate 550 mg and magnesium hydroxide 125 mg
Liquid (Mylanta® Supreme): Calcium carbonate 400 mg and magnesium hydroxide 135 mg per 5 mL (360 mL, 720 mL) [cherry flavor]
Tablet, chewable:
Mi-Acid™ Double Strength: Calcium carbonate 700 mg and magnesium hydroxide 300 mg
Mylanta® Ultra: Calcium carbonate 700 mg and magnesium hydroxide 300 mg [cherry créme and cool mint flavors]
Rolaids®: Calcium carbonate 550 mg and magnesium hydroxide 110 mg [sodium free; contains elemental calcium 220 mg and elemental magnesium 45 mg; original (peppermint), cherry, and spearmint flavors]
Rolaids® Extra Strength: Calcium carbonate 675 mg and magnesium hydroxide 135 mg [sodium free; contains elemental calcium 271 mg and elemental magnesium 56 mg, fruit flavor contains tartrazine; cool strawberry, fresh mint, fruit, and tropical fruit punch flavors]

◆ **Calcium Carbonate, Magnesium Hydroxide, and Famotidine** *see* Famotidine, Calcium Carbonate, and Magnesium Hydroxide *on page 604*

Calcium Chloride (KAL see um KLOR ide)

Pharmacologic Category Calcium Salt; Electrolyte Supplement, Parenteral

Use Treatment of acute symptomatic hypocalcemia; cardiac disturbances of hyperkalemia or hypocalcemia; emergent treatment of hypocalcemic tetany; treatment of severe hypermagnesemia

Unlabeled/Investigational Use Calcium channel blocker overdose; severe hyperkalemia ($K+$ >7 mEq/L with toxic ECG changes) [ACLS guidelines]; malignant arrhythmias associated with hypermagnesemia [ACLS guidelines]

Pregnancy Risk Factor C

Medication Safety Issues
Dosing issues:
Calcium chloride may be confused with calcium gluconate
Confusion with the different intravenous salt forms of calcium has occurred. There is a threefold difference in the primary cation concentration between calcium chloride (in which 1g = 13.6 mEq [270 mg] of elemental Ca^{++}) and calcium gluconate (in which 1g = 4.65 mEq [90 mg] of elemental Ca^{++}).
Prescribers should specify which salt form is desired. Dosages should be expressed either as mEq, mg, or grams of the salt form.

Contraindications Hypercalcemia, known or suspected digoxin toxicity; not recommended as routine treatment in cardiac arrest (includes asystole, ventricular fibrillation, pulseless ventricular tachycardia, or pulseless electrical activity)

Warnings/Precautions For I.V. use only; do not inject SubQ or I.M.; avoid rapid I.V. administration (<100 mg/minute) unless being given emergently. Avoid extravasation. Use with caution in patients with hyperphosphatemia, respiratory acidosis, renal impairment, or respiratory failure; acidifying effect of calcium chloride may potentiate acidosis. Use with caution in patients with chronic renal failure to avoid hypercalcemia; frequent monitoring of serum calcium and phosphorus is necessary. Use with caution in hypokalemic or digitalized patients since acute rises in serum calcium levels may precipitate cardiac arrhythmias. Solutions may contain aluminum; toxic levels may occur following prolonged administration in premature neonates or patients with renal impairment. Avoid metabolic acidosis (ie, administer only 2-3 days then change to another calcium salt).

Adverse Reactions Frequency not defined. I.V.:

Cardiovascular: Arrhythmia, bradycardia, cardiac arrest, hypotension, syncope, vasodilation

Endocrine & metabolic: Hypercalcemia

Gastrointestinal: Irritation, chalky taste

Hepatic: Elevated serum amylase

Neuromuscular & skeletal: Tingling sensation

Renal: Renal calculi

Miscellaneous: Hot flashes

Postmarketing and/or case reports: Calcinosis cutis

Drug Interactions

Avoid Concomitant Use

Avoid concomitant use of Calcium Chloride with any of the following: CefTRIAXone

Increased Effect/Toxicity

Calcium Chloride may increase the levels/effects of: CefTRIAXone

The levels/effects of Calcium Chloride may be increased by: Thiazide Diuretics

Decreased Effect

Calcium Chloride may decrease the levels/effects of: Bisphosphonate Derivatives; Calcium Channel Blockers; DOBUTamine; Eltrombopag; Phosphate Supplements; Trientine

The levels/effects of Calcium Chloride may be decreased by: Trientine

Stability Do not refrigerate solutions; IVPB solutions/I.V. infusion solutions are stable for 24 hours at room temperature.

Although calcium chloride is not routinely used in the preparation of parenteral nutrition, it is important to note that phosphate salts may precipitate when mixed with calcium salts. Solubility is improved in amino acid parenteral nutrition solutions. Check with a pharmacist to determine compatibility.

Mechanism of Action Moderates nerve and muscle performance via action potential excitation threshold regulation

Pharmacodynamics/Kinetics

Distribution: Crosses placenta; enters breast milk

Excretion: Primarily feces (80% as insoluble calcium); urine (20%)

Dosage Note: One gram of calcium chloride is equal to 270 mg of elemental calcium.

Dosages are expressed in terms of the calcium chloride salt based on a solution concentration of 100 mg/mL (10%) containing 1.4 mEq (27.3 mg)/mL elemental calcium.

Acute, symptomatic ionized hypocalcemia, hyperkalemia, or magnesium toxicity: **Note:** Routine use in cardiac arrest is not recommended due to the lack of improved survival [PALS, ACLS 2005 Guidelines]: I.V.:

Neonates: 20 mg/kg; may repeat as necessary

Infants and Children: 20 mg/kg; may repeat as necessary [PALS 2005 Guidelines]

Adults: 500-1000 mg, may repeat as necessary [ACLS 2005 Guidelines]

Calcium channel blocker overdose (unlabeled use):

Neonates, Infants, and Children [PALS 2005 Guidelines]:

I.V., I.O.: 20 mg/kg (maximum: 1000 mg/dose) over 5-10 minutes; if favorable response obtained, consider I.V. infusion

I.V. infusion: 20-50 mg/kg/hour

Adults:

I.V.: 1000 mg every 10-20 minutes (total of 4 doses) **or** 1000 mg every 2-3 minutes until clinical effect is achieved; if favorable response obtained, consider I.V. infusion

I.V. infusion: 20-50 mg/kg/hour

Hypocalcemia secondary to citrated blood transfusion: I.V.:

Note: Routine administration of calcium, in the absence of signs/symptoms of hypocalcemia, is generally not recommended. A number of recommendations have been published seeking to address potential hypocalcemia during massive transfusion of citrated blood; however, many practitioners recommend replacement only as guided by clinical evidence of hypocalcemia and/or serial monitoring of ionized calcium. In adults, clinically-significant hypocalcemia usually dose not occur until >5 units of packed red blood cells have been administered.

Neonates, Infants, and Children: Give 32 mg (0.45 mEq elemental calcium) for each 100 mL citrated blood infused

Adults: 200-500 mg per 500 mL of citrated blood (infused into another vein)

Hypocalcemic tetany: I.V.:

Neonates: 40-60 mg/kg/dose repeated every 6-8 hours

Infants and Children: 10 mg/kg over 5-10 minutes; may repeat after 6-8 hours or follow with an infusion with a maximum dose of 200 mg/kg/day; alternatively, higher doses of 35-50 mg/kg/dose repeated every 6-8 hours have been used

Adults: 1000 mg over 10-30 minutes; may repeat after 6 hours

Dosing adjustment in renal impairment: Cl_{cr} <25 mL/minute: Dosage adjustments may be necessary depending on the serum calcium levels

Administration For I.V. administration only; avoid extravasation. Avoid rapid administration (do not exceed 100 mg/minute). May be given over 2-5 minutes if rapid increase in serum calcium concentration is required. For I.V. infusion, dilute to a maximum concentration of 20 mg/mL and infuse over 1 hour or no greater than 45-90 mg/kg/hour (0.6-1.2 mEq/kg/hour); administration via a central or deep vein is preferred; do not use scalp, small hand or foot veins for I.V. administration since severe necrosis and sloughing may occur. Monitor ECG if calcium is infused faster than 2.5 mEq/minute; **stop the infusion if the patient complains of pain or discomfort.** Warm to body temperature. **Do not infuse calcium chloride in the same I.V. line as phosphate-containing solutions.**

Monitoring Parameters Monitor infusion site, ECG when appropriate; serum calcium and ionized calcium (normal: 8.5-10.2 mg/dL [total]; 4.5-5.0 mg/dL [ionized]), albumin, serum phosphate

Reference Range

Serum calcium: 8.4-10.2 mg/dL

Due to a poor correlation between the serum ionized calcium (free) and total serum calcium, particularly in states of low albumin or acid/base imbalances, direct measurement of ionized calcium is recommended.

In low albumin states, the corrected **total** serum calcium may be estimated by the following equation (assuming a normal albumin of 4 g/dL).

Corrected total calcium = total serum calcium + 0.8 (4.0 - measured serum albumin)

or

Corrected calcium = measured calcium - measured albumin + 4.0

Serum/plasma chloride: 95-108 mEq/L

Test Interactions Increased calcium

Additional Information 14 mEq calcium/g (10 mL); 270 mg elemental calcium/g calcium chloride (27% elemental calcium)

Dosage Forms Excipient information presented when available (limited, particularly for generics); consult specific product labeling.

Injection, solution [preservative free]: 10% (10 mL) [present as calcium chloride 100 mg (1.36 mEq)/mL; provides elemental calcium 27.2 mg/mL (1.36 mEq)/mL]

Injection, solution: 10% (10 mL) [present as calcium chloride 100 mg (1.36 mEq)/mL; provides elemental calcium 27.2 mg (1.36 mEq)/mL]

Calcium Citrate (KAL see um SIT rate)

U.S. Brand Names Cal-C-Caps [OTC]; Cal-Cee [OTC]; Cal-Citrate-225; Cal-Citrate® 250 [OTC] [DSC]; Citracal® Kosher [OTC]

Canadian Brand Names Osteocit®

Pharmacologic Category Calcium Salt

Use Antacid; treatment and prevention of calcium deficiency or hyperphosphatemia (eg, osteoporosis, osteomalacia, mild/moderate renal insufficiency, hypoparathyroidism, postmenopausal osteoporosis, rickets)

Pregnancy Risk Factor C

Medication Safety Issues

Sound-alike/look-alike issues:

Citracal® may be confused with Citrucel®

Dosage Oral: Dosage is in terms of elemental calcium

Dietary Reference Intake:

0-6 months: 210 mg/day

7-12 months: 270 mg/day

1-3 years: 500 mg/day

4-8 years: 800 mg/day

Adults, Male/Female:

9-18 years: 1300 mg/day

19-50 years: 1000 mg/day

≥51 years: 1200 mg/day

Female: Pregnancy/Lactating: Same as for Adults, Male/Female

Dietary supplement: Usual dose: 500 mg to 2 g 2-4 times/day

Additional Information Complete prescribing information for this medication should be consulted for additional detail.

Dosage Forms Excipient information presented when available (limited, particularly for generics); consult specific product labeling. [DSC] = Discontinued product

Capsule:

Cal-C-Caps: Elemental calcium 180 mg

Cal-Citrate-225: Elemental calcium 225 mg

Granules: Elemental calcium 760 mg/teaspoonful (480 g)

Tablet: Elemental calcium 200 mg, 250 mg

Cal-Citrate®: Elemental calcium 250 mg [DSC]

Cal-Cee: Elemental calcium 250 mg

Citracal® Kosher: Elemental calcium 200 mg

◆ **Calcium Disodium Edetate** *see* Edetate CALCIUM Disodium *on page* 503

◆ **Calcium Disodium Versenate®** *see* Edetate CALCIUM Disodium *on page* 503

Calcium Glubionate (KAL see um gloo BYE oh nate)

U.S. Brand Names Calcionate [OTC]

Pharmacologic Category Calcium Salt

Use Dietary supplement

Medication Safety Issues

Sound-alike/look-alike issues:

Calcium glubionate may be confused with calcium gluconate

Dosage Dosage is in terms of **elemental** calcium

Dietary Reference Intake:

0-6 months: 210 mg/day

7-12 months: 270 mg/day

1-3 years: 500 mg/day

4-8 years: 800 mg/day

Adults, Male/Female:

9-18 years: 1300 mg/day

19-50 years: 1000 mg/day

≥51 years: 1200 mg/day

Female: Pregnancy/Lactating: Same as for Adults, Male/Female

Dietary supplement: Oral:

Infants <12 months: 1 teaspoonful 5 times a day; may mix with juice or formula

Children <4 years: 2 teaspoonsful 3 times a day

Children ≥4 years and Adults: 1 tablespoonful 3 times a day

Pregnant or lactating women: 1 tablespoonful 4 times a day

Dosing adjustment in renal impairment: Cl_{cr} <25 mL/minute: Dosage adjustments may be necessary depending on the serum calcium levels

Additional Information Complete prescribing information for this medication should be consulted for additional detail.

Dosage Forms Excipient information presented when available (limited, particularly for generics); consult specific product labeling.

Syrup:

Calcionate: 1.8 g/5 mL (480 mL) [equivalent to elemental calcium 115 mg/5 mL; contains benzoic acid; caramel and orange flavor]

Calcium Gluconate (KAL see um GLOO koe nate)

U.S. Brand Names Cal-G [OTC]; Cal-GLU™

Pharmacologic Category Calcium Salt; Electrolyte Supplement, Oral; Electrolyte Supplement, Parenteral

Use Treatment and prevention of hypocalcemia; treatment of tetany, cardiac disturbances of hyperkalemia, cardiac resuscitation when epinephrine fails to improve myocardial contractions, hypocalcemia; calcium supplementation; hydrofluoric acid (HF) burns

Unlabeled/Investigational Use Calcium channel blocker overdose

Pregnancy Risk Factor C

Pregnancy Considerations Reproduction studies have not been completed.

Lactation Enters breast milk

Medication Safety Issues

Sound-alike/look-alike issues:

Calcium gluconate may be confused with calcium glubionate

Contraindications Hypersensitivity to calcium gluconate or any component of the formulation; ventricular fibrillation during cardiac resuscitation; digitalis toxicity or suspected digoxin toxicity; hypercalcemia

Warnings/Precautions Injection solution is for I.V. use only; do not inject SubQ or I.M. Avoid too rapid I.V. administration and avoid extravasation. Use with caution in digitalized patients, severe hyperphosphatemia, respiratory failure, or acidosis. May produce cardiac arrest. Hypercalcemia may occur in patients with renal failure; frequent determination of serum calcium is necessary. Use caution with renal disease. Use caution when administering calcium supplements to patients with a history of kidney stones. Solutions may contain aluminum; toxic levels may occur following prolonged administration in premature neonates or patients with renal dysfunction. Oral: Constipation, bloating, and gas are common with oral calcium supplements (especially carbonate salt). Taking calcium (≤500 mg) with food improves absorption. Calcium administration interferes with absorption of some minerals and drugs; use with caution. It is recommended to concomitantly administer vitamin D for optimal calcium absorption.

Adverse Reactions Frequency not defined.

I.V.:
- Cardiovascular: Arrhythmia, bradycardia, cardiac arrest, hypotension, vasodilation, and syncope may occur following rapid I.V. injection
- Central nervous system: Sense of oppression
- Gastrointestinal: Chalky taste
- Local: Abscess and necrosis following I.M. administration
- Neuromuscular & skeletal: Tingling sensation
- Miscellaneous: Heat waves
- Postmarketing and/or case reports: Calcinosis cutis

Oral: Gastrointestinal: Constipation

Drug Interactions

Avoid Concomitant Use

Avoid concomitant use of Calcium Gluconate with any of the following: CefTRIAXone

Increased Effect/Toxicity

Calcium Gluconate may increase the levels/effects of: CefTRIAXone

The levels/effects of Calcium Gluconate may be increased by: Thiazide Diuretics

Decreased Effect

Calcium Gluconate may decrease the levels/effects of: Bisphosphonate Derivatives; Calcium Channel Blockers; DOBUTamine; Eltrombopag; Estramustine; Phosphate Supplements; Quinolone Antibiotics; Trientine

The levels/effects of Calcium Gluconate may be decreased by: Trientine

Stability

Do not refrigerate solutions. IVPB solutions/I.V. infusion solutions are stable for 24 hours at room temperature.

Standard diluent: 1 g/100 mL D_5W or NS; 2 g/100 mL D_5W or NS.

Maximum concentration in parenteral nutrition solutions is variable depending upon concentration and solubility (consult detailed reference).

Mechanism of Action As dietary supplement, used to prevent or treat negative calcium balance; in osteoporosis, it helps to prevent or decrease the rate of bone loss. The calcium in calcium salts moderates nerve and muscle performance and allows normal cardiac function.

Pharmacodynamics/Kinetics

Absorption: Requires vitamin D; calcium is absorbed in soluble, ionized form; solubility of calcium is increased in an acid environment

Distribution: Primarily in bones and teeth; crosses placenta; enters breast milk

Protein binding: Primarily albumin

Excretion: Primarily feces (as unabsorbed calcium); urine (20%)

Dosage

Adequate Intake (as elemental calcium):
- 0-6 months: 210 mg/day
- 7-12 months: 270 mg/day
- 1-3 years: 500 mg/day
- 4-8 years: 800 mg/day
- 9-18 years: 1300 mg/day

Adults, Male/Female:
- 19-50 years: 1000 mg/day
- ≥51 years: 1200 mg/day

Female: Pregnancy/Lactating: Same as for Adults, Male/Female

Dosage note: Calcium chloride has 3 times more elemental calcium than calcium gluconate. Calcium chloride is 27% elemental calcium; calcium gluconate is 9% elemental calcium. One gram of calcium chloride is equal to 270 mg of elemental calcium; 1 gram of calcium gluconate is equal to 90 mg of elemental calcium. The following dosages are expressed in terms of the calcium gluconate salt based on a solution concentration of 100 mg/mL (10%) containing 0.465 mEq (9.3 mg)/mL elemental calcium:

Hypocalcemia: I.V.:
- Neonates: 200-800 mg/kg/day as a continuous infusion or in 4 divided doses (maximum: 1 g/dose)
- Infants and Children: 200-500 mg/kg/day as a continuous infusion or in 4 divided doses (maximum: 2-3 g/dose)
- Adults: 2-15 g/24 hours as a continuous infusion or in divided doses

Hypocalcemia: Oral:
- Children: 200-500 mg/kg/day divided every 6 hours
- Adults: 500 mg to 2 g 2-4 times/day

Hypocalcemia secondary to citrated blood infusion: I.V.:

Note: Routine administration of calcium, in the absence of signs/symptoms of hypocalcemia, is generally not recommended. A number of recommendations have been published seeking to address potential hypocalcemia during massive transfusion of citrated blood; however, many practitioners recommend replacement only as guided by clinical evidence of hypocalcemia and/or serial monitoring of ionized calcium.
- Neonates, Infants, and Children: Give 98 mg (0.45 mEq **elemental** calcium) for each 100 mL citrated blood infused
- Adults: 500 mg to 1 g per 500 mL of citrated blood (infused into another vein). Single doses up to 2 g have also been recommended.

Hypocalcemic tetany: I.V.:
- Neonates, Infants, and Children: 100-200 mg/kg/dose over 5-10 minutes; may repeat every 6-8 hours **or** follow with an infusion of 500 mg/kg/day
- Adults: 1-3 g may be administered until therapeutic response occurs

Magnesium intoxication, cardiac arrest in the presence of hyperkalemia or hypocalcemia: I.V.:
- Infants and Children: 60-100 mg/kg/dose (maximum: 3 g/dose)
- Adults: 500-800 mg/dose (maximum: 3 g/dose)

Maintenance electrolyte requirements for total parenteral nutrition: I.V.: Daily requirements: Adults: 1.7-3.4 g/1000 kcal/24 hours

Calcium channel blocker overdose (unlabeled use): Adults: I.V. infusion: 10% solution: 0.6-1.2 mL/kg/hour or I.V. 0.2-0.5 ml/kg every 15-20 minutes for 4 doses (maximum: 2-3 g/dose). In life-threatening situations, 1 g has been given every 1-10 minutes until clinical effect is achieved (case reports of resistant hypotension reported use of 12-18 g total).

Dosing adjustment in renal impairment: Cl_{cr} <25 mL/minute: Dosage adjustments may be necessary depending on the serum calcium levels

Administration Not for I.M. or SubQ administration. For I.V. administration only; administer slowly (~1.5 mL calcium gluconate 10% per minute) through a small needle into a large vein in order to avoid too rapid increased in serum calcium and extravasation.

Extravasation treatment example: Hyaluronidase: Add 1 mL NS to 150 unit vial to make 150 units/mL of concentration; mix 0.1 mL of above with 0.9 mL NS in 1 mL syringe to make final concentration = 15 units/mL

Reference Range

Serum calcium: 8.4-10.2 mg/dL: Monitor plasma calcium levels if using calcium salts as electrolyte supplements for deficiency

Due to a poor correlation between the serum ionized calcium (free) and total serum calcium, particularly in states of low albumin or acid/base imbalances, direct measurement of ionized calcium is recommended

In low albumin states, the corrected **total** serum calcium may be estimated by: Corrected total calcium = total serum calcium + 0.8 (4.0 - measured serum albumin)

Test Interactions Increased calcium (S); decreased magnesium

Additional Information A topical 2.5% to 5% calcium gel for the treatment of hydrofluoric acid (HF) burns can be prepared by adding calcium gluconate to a surgical lubricant (water soluble such as K-Y® Jelly). Calcium chloride should not be used for this purpose. Use of injectable calcium gluconate (I.V., SubQ) has also been reported in the literature for the treatment of HF burns not amenable to topical treatment.

Dosage Forms Excipient information presented when available (limited, particularly for generics); consult specific product labeling.

Capsule, oral:

Cal-G: 700 mg [gluten free, wheat free; equivalent to elemental calcium 65 mg]

Capsule, oral [preservative free]:

Cal-GLU™: 515 mg [dye free, sugar free; equivalent to elemental calcium 50 mg]

Injection, solution [preservative free]: 10% (10 mL, 50 mL, 100 mL, 200 mL) [100 mg/mL; equivalent to elemental calcium 9 mg/mL; calcium 0.46 mEq/mL]

Powder: 347 mg/tablespoonful (480 g)

Tablet: 500 mg [equivalent to elemental calcium 45 mg]; 650 mg [equivalent to elemental calcium 58.5 mg]; 975 mg [equivalent to elemental calcium 87.75 mg]

Extemporaneous Preparations To make calcium gluconate gel, 3.5 g of calcium gluconate can be added to 5 oz tube of a surgical lubricant (water soluble such as K-Y® Jelly).

◆ **Calcium Leucovorin** *see* Leucovorin Calcium *on page 866*

◆ **Calcium Levoleucovorin** *see* LEVOleucovorin *on page 878*

◆ **Cal-CYUM [OTC]** *see* Calcium and Vitamin D *on page 238*

◆ **Caldecort® [OTC]** *see* Hydrocortisone *on page 743*

Calfactant (kaf AKT ant)

U.S. Brand Names Infasurf®

Pharmacologic Category Lung Surfactant

Use Prevention of respiratory distress syndrome (RDS) in premature infants at high risk for RDS and for the treatment ("rescue") of premature infants who develop RDS

Prophylaxis: Therapy at birth with calfactant is indicated for premature infants <29 weeks of gestational age at significant risk for RDS. Should be administered as soon as possible, preferably within 30 minutes after birth.

Treatment: For infants ≤72 hours of age with RDS (confirmed by clinical and radiologic findings) and requiring endotracheal intubation.

Warnings/Precautions For intratracheal administration only. Rapidly affects oxygenation and lung compliance; restrict use to a highly-supervised clinical setting with immediate availability of clinicians experienced in intubation and ventilatory management of premature infants. Transient episodes of bradycardia, decreased oxygen saturation, endotracheal tube blockage or reflux of calfactant into endotracheal tube may occur. Discontinue dosing procedure and initiate measures to alleviate the condition; may reinstitute after the patient is stable. Produces rapid improvements in lung oxygenation and compliance that may require frequent adjustments to oxygen delivery and ventilator settings.

Adverse Reactions

Cardiovascular: Bradycardia (34%), cyanosis (65%)

Respiratory: Airway obstruction (39%), reflux (21%), requirement for manual ventilation (16%), reintubation (1% to 10%)

Drug Interactions

Avoid Concomitant Use There are no known interactions where it is recommended to avoid concomitant use.

Increased Effect/Toxicity There are no known significant interactions involving an increase in effect.

Decreased Effect There are no known significant interactions involving a decrease in effect.

Stability Gentle swirling or agitation of the vial of suspension is often necessary for redispersion. **Do not shake**. Visible flecks of the suspension and foaming under the surface are normal. Calfactant should be stored at refrigeration (2°C to 8°C/36°F to 46°F). Warming before administration is not necessary. Unopened and unused vials of calfactant that have been warmed to room temperature can be returned to the refrigeration storage within 24 hours for future use. Repeated warming to room temperature should be avoided. Each single-use vial should be entered only once and the vial with any unused material should be discarded after the initial entry.

Mechanism of Action Endogenous lung surfactant is essential for effective ventilation because it modifies alveolar surface tension, thereby stabilizing the alveoli. Lung surfactant deficiency is the cause of respiratory distress syndrome (RDS) in premature infants and lung surfactant restores surface activity to the lungs of these infants.

Pharmacodynamics/Kinetics No human studies of absorption, biotransformation, or excretion have been performed

Dosage Intratracheal administration **only**: Each dose is 3 mL/kg body weight at birth; should be administered every 12 hours for a total of up to 3 doses

Administration Gentle swirling or agitation of the vial is often necessary for redispersion as suspension settles during storage; do **not** shake; visible flecks in the suspension and foaming at the surface are normal; does not require reconstitution; do not dilute or sonicate.

Should be administered intratracheally through an endotracheal tube. Dose is drawn into a syringe from the single-use vial using a 20-gauge or larger needle with care taken to avoid excessive foaming. Should be administered in two aliquots of 1.5 mL/kg each. After each aliquot is instilled, the infant should be positioned with either the right or the left side dependent. Administration is made while ventilation is continued over 20-30 breaths for each aliquot, with small bursts timed only during the inspiratory cycles. A pause followed by evaluation of the respiratory status and repositioning should separate the two aliquots.

Monitoring Parameters Following administration, patients should be carefully monitored so that oxygen therapy and ventilatory support can be modified in response to changes in respiratory status.

Additional Information Each mL = 35 mg total phospholipids (including 26 mg phosphatidylcholine, of which 16 mg is desaturated phosphatidylcholine) and 0.65 protein (including 0.26 mg SP-B)

Dosage Forms Excipient information presented when available (limited, particularly for generics); consult specific product labeling.

Suspension, intratracheal [preservative free; calf lung derived]:
Infasurf®: 35 mg/mL (3 mL, 6 mL)

- **Cal-G [OTC]** *see* Calcium Gluconate *on page* 241
- **Cal-Gest [OTC]** *see* Calcium Carbonate *on page* 238
- **Cal-GLU™** *see* Calcium Gluconate *on page* 241
- **Cal-Mint [OTC]** *see* Calcium Carbonate *on page* 238
- **Calmylin with Codeine (Can)** *see* Guaifenesin, Pseudoephedrine, and Codeine *on page* 715
- **CaloMist™** *see* Cyanocobalamin *on page* 374
- **Caltine® (Can)** *see* Calcitonin *on page* 234
- **Caltrate® (Can)** *see* Calcium Carbonate *on page* 238
- **Caltrate® 600 [OTC]** *see* Calcium Carbonate *on page* 238
- **Caltrate® 600+D [OTC]** *see* Calcium and Vitamin D *on page* 238
- **Caltrate® 600+ Soy™ [OTC]** *see* Calcium and Vitamin D *on page* 238
- **Caltrate® ColonHealth™ [OTC]** *see* Calcium and Vitamin D *on page* 238
- **Caltrate® Select (Can)** *see* Calcium Carbonate *on page* 238
- **Camila™** *see* Norethindrone *on page* 1078
- **Campath®** *see* Alemtuzumab *on page* 56
- **Campath-1H** *see* Alemtuzumab *on page* 56
- **Camphorated Tincture of Opium (error-prone synonym)** *see* Paregoric *on page* 1144
- **Campral®** *see* Acamprosate *on page* 23
- **Camptosar®** *see* Irinotecan *on page* 814
- **Camptothecin-11** *see* Irinotecan *on page* 814
- **Canasa®** *see* Mesalamine *on page* 949
- **Cancidas®** *see* Caspofungin *on page* 266

Candesartan (kan de SAR tan)

U.S. Brand Names Atacand®

Canadian Brand Names Atacand®

Index Terms Candesartan Cilexetil

Pharmacologic Category Angiotensin II Receptor Blocker

Additional Appendix Information

Angiotensin Agents *on page* 1632
Heart Failure (Systolic) *on page* 1809

Use Alone or in combination with other antihypertensive agents in treating essential hypertension; treatment of heart failure (NYHA class II-IV)

Pregnancy Risk Factor C (1st trimester); D (2nd and 3rd trimesters)

Pregnancy Considerations Medications which act on the renin-angiotensin system are reported to have the following fetal/neonatal effects: Hypotension, neonatal skull hypoplasia, anuria, renal failure, and death; oligohydramnios is also reported. These effects are reported to occur with exposure during the second and third trimesters. There are no adequate and well-controlled studies in pregnant women. **[U.S. Boxed Warning]: Based on human data, drugs that act on the angiotensin system can cause injury and death to the developing fetus when used in the second and third trimesters. Angiotensin receptor blockers should be discontinued as soon as possible once pregnancy is detected.**

Lactation Enters breast milk/contraindicated

Contraindications Hypersensitivity to candesartan or any component of the formulation; severe hepatic impairment and/or cholestasis; pregnancy; breast-feeding

Warnings/Precautions [U.S. Boxed Warning]: Based on human data, drugs that act on the angiotensin system can cause injury and death to the developing fetus when used in the second and third trimesters. Angiotensin receptor blockers should be discontinued as soon as possible once pregnancy is detected. May cause hyperkalemia; avoid potassium supplementation unless specifically required by healthcare provider. Avoid use or use a smaller dose in patients who are volume depleted; correct depletion first. May be associated with deterioration of renal function and/or increases in serum creatinine, particularly in patients with low renal blood flow (eg, renal artery stenosis, heart failure) whose glomerular filtration rate (GFR) is dependent on efferent arteriolar vasoconstriction by angiotensin II. Use with caution in unstented unilateral/bilateral renal artery stenosis, pre-existing renal insufficiency, or significant aortic/mitral stenosis. Use with caution in patients with moderate hepatic impairment. Contraindicated with severe hepatic impairment and/or cholestasis. Use caution when initiating in heart failure; may need to adjust dose, and/or concurrent diuretic therapy, because of candesartan-induced hypotension. Hypotension may occur during major surgery and anesthesia; use cautiously before, during, and immediately after such interventions. Although some properties may be shared between these agents, concurrent therapy with ACE inhibitor may be rational in selected patients. Safety and efficacy have not been established in children.

Adverse Reactions

Cardiovascular: Angina, hypotension (CHF 19%), MI, palpitation, tachycardia

Central nervous system: Dizziness, lightheadedness, drowsiness, headache, vertigo, anxiety, depression, somnolence, fever

Dermatologic: Angioedema, rash

Endocrine & metabolic: Hyperglycemia, hyperkalemia (CHF <1% to 6%), hypertriglyceridemia, hyperuricemia

Gastrointestinal: Dyspepsia, gastroenteritis

Genitourinary: Hematuria

Neuromuscular & skeletal: Back pain, CPK increased, myalgia, paresthesia, weakness

Renal: Serum creatinine increased (up to 13% in patients with CHF with drug discontinuation required in 6%)

Respiratory: Dyspnea, epistaxis, pharyngitis, rhinitis, upper respiratory tract infection

Miscellaneous: Diaphoresis increased

<1%, postmarketing, and/or case reports: Abnormal hepatic function, agranulocytosis, anemia, hepatitis, hyponatremia, leukopenia, neutropenia, pruritus, renal failure, renal impairment, rhinitis, sinusitis, thrombocytopenia, urticaria; rhabdomyolysis has been reported (rarely) with angiotensin-receptor antagonists

Drug Interactions

Metabolism/Transport Effects Substrate of CYP2C9 (minor); **Inhibits** CYP2C8 (weak), 2C9 (weak)

Avoid Concomitant Use There are no known interactions where it is recommended to avoid concomitant use.

Increased Effect/Toxicity

Candesartan may increase the levels/effects of: ACE Inhibitors; Amifostine; Lithium; Potassium-Sparing Diuretics; RiTUXimab

The levels/effects of Candesartan may be increased by: Diazoxide; Eplerenone; Herbs (Hypotensive Properties); Potassium Salts; Prostacyclin Analogues; Trimethoprim

Decreased Effect

The levels/effects of Candesartan may be decreased by: Herbs (Hypertensive Properties); Methylphenidate; Nonsteroidal Anti-Inflammatory Agents; Yohimbine

Ethanol/Nutrition/Herb Interactions

Food: Food reduces the time to maximal concentration and increases the C_{max}.

Herb/Nutraceutical: Avoid dong quai if using for hypertension (has estrogenic activity). Avoid ephedra, yohimbe, ginseng (may worsen hypertension). Avoid garlic (may have increased antihypertensive effect).

Mechanism of Action Candesartan is an angiotensin receptor antagonist. Angiotensin II acts as a vasoconstrictor. In addition to causing direct vasoconstriction, angiotensin II also stimulates the release of aldosterone. Once aldosterone is released, sodium as well as water are reabsorbed. The end result is an elevation in blood pressure. Candesartan binds to the AT1 angiotensin II receptor. This binding prevents angiotensin II from binding to the receptor thereby blocking the vasoconstriction and the aldosterone secreting effects of angiotensin II.

Pharmacodynamics/Kinetics

Onset of action: 2-3 hours

Peak effect: 6-8 hours

Duration: >24 hours

Distribution: V_d: 0.13 L/kg

Protein binding: 99%

Metabolism: To candesartan by the intestinal wall cells

Bioavailability: 15%

Half-life elimination (dose dependent): 5-9 hours

Time to peak: 3-4 hours

Excretion: Urine (26%)

Clearance: Total body: 0.37 mL/kg/minute; Renal: 0.19 mL/kg/minute

Dosage Adults: Oral:

Hypertension: Usual dose is 4-32 mg once daily; dosage must be individualized. Blood pressure response is dose related over the range of 2-32 mg. The usual recommended starting dose of 16 mg once daily when it is used as monotherapy in patients who are not volume depleted. It can be administered once or twice daily with total daily doses ranging from 8-32 mg. Larger doses do not appear to have a greater effect and there is relatively little experience with such doses.

Congestive heart failure: Initial: 4 mg once daily; double the dose at 2-week intervals, as tolerated; target dose: 32 mg

Note: In selected cases, concurrent therapy with an ACE inhibitor may provide additional benefit.

Elderly: No initial dosage adjustment is necessary for elderly patients (although higher concentrations (C_{max}) and AUC were observed in these populations), for patients with mildly impaired renal function, or for patients with mildly impaired hepatic function.

Dosage adjustment in hepatic impairment:

Mild hepatic impairment: No initial dosage adjustment required

Moderate hepatic impairment: Consider initiation at lower dosages (AUC increased by 145%).

Severe hepatic impairment and/or cholestasis: Contraindicated

Monitoring Parameters Supine blood pressure, electrolytes, serum creatinine, BUN, urinalysis, symptomatic hypotension, and tachycardia; in CHF, serum potassium during dose escalation and periodically thereafter

Additional Information May have an advantage over losartan due to minimal metabolism requirements and consequent use in mild-to-moderate hepatic impairment

Dosage Forms Excipient information presented when available (limited, particularly for generics); consult specific product labeling.

Tablet, as cilexetil:

Atacand®: 4 mg, 8 mg, 16 mg, 32 mg

Candesartan and Hydrochlorothiazide

(kan de SAR tan & hye droe klor oh THYE a zide)

U.S. Brand Names Atacand HCT®

Canadian Brand Names Atacand® Plus

Index Terms Candesartan Cilexetil and Hydrochlorothiazide

Pharmacologic Category Angiotensin II Receptor Blocker; Diuretic, Thiazide

Use Treatment of hypertension; combination product should not be used for initial therapy

Pregnancy Risk Factor C/D (2nd and 3rd trimesters)

Dosage Oral: Adults: Replacement therapy: Combination product can be substituted for individual agents; maximum therapeutic effect would be expected within 4 weeks

Usual dosage range:

Candesartan: 16-32 mg/day, given once daily or twice daily in divided doses

Hydrochlorothiazide: 12.5-25 mg once daily

Elderly: No initial dosage adjustment is recommended in patients with normal renal and hepatic function; some patients may have increased sensitivity.

Dosage adjustment in renal impairment: Serum levels of candesartan are increased and the half-life of hydrochlorothiazide is prolonged in patients with renal impairment.

Cl_{cr} <30 mL/minute: Contraindicated

Dosage adjustment in hepatic impairment: Use with caution with moderate hepatic impairment.

Severe hepatic impairment and/or cholestasis: Use is contraindicated.

Additional Information Complete prescribing information for this medication should be consulted for additional detail.

Dosage Forms Excipient information presented when available (limited, particularly for generics); consult specific product labeling.

Tablet:

Atacand HCT®:

16/12.5: Candesartan cilexetil 16 mg and hydrochlorothiazide 12.5 mg

32/12.5: Candesartan cilexetil 32 mg and hydrochlorothiazide 12.5 mg

32/25: Candesartan cilexetil 32 mg and hydrochlorothiazide 25 mg

- **Candesartan Cilexetil** *see* Candesartan *on page 244*
- **Candesartan Cilexetil and Hydrochlorothiazide** *see* Candesartan and Hydrochlorothiazide *on page 245*
- **Candistatin® (Can)** *see* Nystatin *on page 1087*
- **Canesten® Topical (Can)** *see* Clotrimazole *on page 359*
- **Canesten® Vaginal (Can)** *see* Clotrimazole *on page 359*
- **Cankaid® [OTC]** *see* Carbamide Peroxide *on page 254*
- **Capastat® Sulfate** *see* Capreomycin *on page 247*

Capecitabine (ka pe SITE a been)

U.S. Brand Names Xeloda®

Canadian Brand Names Xeloda®

Index Terms NSC-712807

Pharmacologic Category Antineoplastic Agent, Antimetabolite; Antineoplastic Agent, Antimetabolite (Pyrimidine Analog)

Use Treatment of metastatic colorectal cancer; adjuvant therapy of Dukes' C colon cancer; treatment of metastatic breast cancer

Unlabeled/Investigational Use Treatment of gastric cancer, pancreatic cancer, esophageal cancer, ovarian cancer, metastatic renal cell cancer, neuroendocrine tumors, metastatic CNS lesions

Pregnancy Risk Factor D

Pregnancy Considerations Animal studies have demonstrated teratogenicity and fetal loss. There are no adequate and well-controlled studies in pregnant women;

however, fetal harm may occur. Women of childbearing potential should avoid pregnancy.

Lactation Excretion in breast milk unknown/not recommended

Medication Safety Issues

Sound-alike/look-alike issues:

Xeloda® may be confused with Xenical®

High alert medication: The Institute for Safe Medication Practices (ISMP) includes this medication among its list of drug classes which have a heightened risk of causing significant patient harm when used in error.

Contraindications Hypersensitivity to capecitabine, fluorouracil, or any component of the formulation; known deficiency of dihydropyrimidine dehydrogenase (DPD); severe renal impairment (Cl_{cr} <30 mL/minute)

Warnings/Precautions Hazardous agent - use appropriate precautions for handling and disposal. Use with caution in patients with bone marrow suppression, ≥80 years of age, or renal or hepatic dysfunction. Patients with baseline moderate renal impairment require dose reduction. Patients with mild-to-moderate renal impairment require careful monitoring and subsequent dose reduction with any grade 2 or higher adverse event. Use with caution in patients who have received extensive pelvic radiation or alkylating therapy. Use cautiously with warfarin. Rare and unexpected severe toxicity may be attributed to dihydropyrimidine dehydrogenase (DPD) deficiency. Necrotizing enterocolitis (typhlitis) has been reported.

Capecitabine can cause severe diarrhea; median time to first occurrence is 34 days. Subsequent doses should be reduced after grade 3 or 4 diarrhea or recurrence of grade 2 diarrhea.

Hand-and-foot syndrome is characterized by numbness, dysesthesia/paresthesia, tingling, painless or painful swelling, erythema, desquamation, blistering, and severe pain. If grade 2 or 3 hand-and-foot syndrome occurs, interrupt administration of capecitabine until decreases to grade 1. Following grade 3 hand-and-foot syndrome, decrease subsequent doses of capecitabine. In patients with colorectal cancer, treatment with capecitabine immediately following 6 weeks of fluorouracil/leucovorin (FU/LV) therapy has been associated with an increased incidence of grade ≥3 toxicity, when compared to patients receiving the reverse sequence, capecitabine (two 3-week courses) followed by FU/LV (Hennig, 2008).

There has been cardiotoxicity associated with fluorinated pyrimidine therapy. May be more common in patients with a history of coronary artery disease. **[U.S. Boxed Warning]: Capecitabine may increase the anticoagulant effects of warfarin; monitor closely.**

Safety and efficacy in children <18 years of age have not been established.

Adverse Reactions Frequency listed derived from monotherapy trials.

>10%:

Cardiovascular: Edema (9% to 15%)

Central nervous system: Fatigue (16% to 42%), fever (7% to 18%), pain (12%)

Dermatologic: Palmar-plantar erythrodysesthesia (hand-and-foot syndrome) (54% to 60%; grade 3: 11% to 17%; may be dose limiting), dermatitis (27% to 37%)

Gastrointestinal: Diarrhea (47% to 57%; may be dose limiting; grade 3: 12% to 13%; grade 4: 2% to 3%), nausea (34% to 53%), vomiting (15% to 37%), abdominal pain (7% to 35%), stomatitis (22% to 25%), appetite decreased (26%), anorexia (9% to 23%), constipation (9% to 15%)

Hematologic: Lymphopenia (94%; grade 4: 14%), anemia (72% to 80%; grade 4: <1% to 1%), neutropenia (2% to 26%; grade 4: 2%), thrombocytopenia (24%; grade 4: 1%)

Hepatic: Bilirubin increased (22% to 48%; grades 3/4: 11% to 23%)

Neuromuscular & skeletal: Paresthesia (21%)

Ocular: Eye irritation (13% to 15%)

Respiratory: Dyspnea (14%)

5% to 10%:

Cardiovascular: Venous thrombosis (8%), chest pain (6%)

Central nervous system: Headache (5% to 10%), lethargy (10%), dizziness (6% to 8%), insomnia (7% to 8%), mood alteration (5%), depression (5%)

Dermatologic: Nail disorder (7%), rash (7%), skin discoloration (7%), alopecia (6%), erythema (6%)

Endocrine & metabolic: Dehydration (7%)

Gastrointestinal: Motility disorder (10%), oral discomfort (10%), dyspepsia (6% to 8%), upper GI inflammatory disorders (colorectal cancer: 8%), hemorrhage (6%), ileus (6%), taste perversion (colorectal cancer: 6%)

Neuromuscular & skeletal: Back pain (10%), weakness (10%), neuropathy (10%), myalgia (9%), arthralgia (8%), limb pain (6%)

Ocular: Abnormal vision (colorectal cancer: 5%), conjunctivitis (5%)

Respiratory: Cough (7%)

Miscellaneous: Viral infection (colorectal cancer: 5%)

<5% (Limited to important or life-threatening): Angina, ascites, asthma, atrial fibrillation, bradycardia, bronchitis, bronchopneumonia, bronchospasm, cachexia, cardiac arrest, cardiac failure, cardiomyopathy, cerebral vascular accident, cholestasis, coagulation disorder, colitis, deep vein thrombosis, diaphoresis, duodenitis, dysphagia, dysrhythmia, ECG changes, encephalopathy, epistaxis, fungal infection, gastric ulcer, gastroenteritis, hematemesis, hemoptysis, hepatic failure, hepatic fibrosis, hepatitis, hypokalemia, hypomagnesemia, hyper-/hypotension, hypersensitivity, hypertriglyceridemia, idiopathic thrombocytopenia purpura, ileus, infection, intestinal obstruction (~1%), keratoconjunctivitis, lacrimal duct stenosis, leukopenia, loss of consciousness, lymphedema, MI, multifocal leukoencephalopathy, myocardial ischemia, myocarditis, necrotizing enterocolitis (typhlitis), oral candidiasis, pericardial effusion, thrombocytopenic purpura, pancytopenia, photosensitivity reaction, pneumonia, pruritus, pulmonary embolism, radiation recall syndrome, renal impairment, respiratory distress, sedation, sepsis, skin ulceration, tachycardia, thrombophlebitis, toxic megacolon, tremor, ventricular extrasystoles

Drug Interactions

Avoid Concomitant Use

Avoid concomitant use of Capecitabine with any of the following: Natalizumab; Vaccines (Live)

Increased Effect/Toxicity

Capecitabine may increase the levels/effects of: CYP2C9 Substrates (High risk); Natalizumab; Phenytoin; Vaccines (Live); Vitamin K Antagonists

The levels/effects of Capecitabine may be increased by: Leucovorin-Levoleucovorin; Trastuzumab

Decreased Effect

Capecitabine may decrease the levels/effects of: Vaccines (Inactivated)

The levels/effects of Capecitabine may be decreased by: Echinacea

Ethanol/Nutrition/Herb Interactions Food: Food reduced the rate and extent of absorption of capecitabine.

Stability Store at room temperature of 25°C (77°F); excursions between 15°C and 30°C (59°F and 86°F) permitted.

Mechanism of Action Capecitabine is a prodrug of fluorouracil. It undergoes hydrolysis in the liver and tissues to form fluorouracil which is the active moiety. Fluorouracil is a fluorinated pyrimidine antimetabolite that inhibits thymidylate synthetase, blocking the methylation of deoxyuridylic acid to thymidylic acid, interfering with DNA, and to a lesser degree, RNA synthesis. Fluorouracil appears to be phase specific for the G_1 and S phases of the cell cycle.

Pharmacodynamics/Kinetics

Absorption: Rapid and extensive

Protein binding: <60%; ~35% to albumin

Metabolism:

Hepatic: Inactive metabolites: 5′-deoxy-5-fluorocytidine, 5′-deoxy-5-fluorouridine

Tissue: Active metabolite: Fluorouracil

Half-life elimination: 0.5-1 hour

Time to peak: 1.5 hours; Fluorouracil: 2 hours

Excretion: Urine (96%, 57% as α-fluoro-β-alanine); feces (<3%)

Dosage Oral:

Adults: **Note:** Details concerning dosing in combination regimens should also be consulted. Capecitabine toxicities, particularly hand-foot syndrome, may be higher in North American populations (for the treatment of colorectal cancer); therapy initiation at doses of 1000 mg/m^2 twice daily (for 2 weeks every 21 days) may be considered (Haller, 2006; NCCN Colon Cancer Guidelines)

Metastatic breast cancer, metastatic colorectal cancer: 1250 mg/m^2 twice daily (morning and evening) for 2 weeks, every 21 days

Adjuvant therapy of Dukes' C colon cancer: Recommended for a total of 24 weeks (8 cycles of 2 weeks of drug administration and 1 week rest period.

Pancreatic cancer (unlabeled use): 1000-1250 mg/m^2 twice daily (morning and evening) for 2 weeks, every 21 days

Elderly: The elderly may be more sensitive to the toxic effects of fluorouracil. Insufficient data are available to provide dosage modifications.

Dosing adjustment in renal impairment:

Cl_{cr} 51-80 mL/minute: No adjustment of initial dose

Cl_{cr} 30-50 mL/minute: Administer 75% of normal dose

Cl_{cr} <30 mL/minute: Use is contraindicated

Dosing adjustment in hepatic impairment:

Mild-to-moderate impairment: No starting dose adjustment is necessary; however, carefully monitor patients

Severe hepatic impairment: Patients have not been studied

Dosage modification guidelines: See table.

Refer to package labeling for modifications when administered in combination with docetaxel.

Dosage adjustments for hematologic toxicity in combination therapy with ixabepilone:

Neutrophils <500/mm^3 for ≥7 days or neutropenic fever: Hold for concurrent diarrhea or stomatitis until neutrophils recover to >1000/mm3, then continue at same dose

Platelets <25,000/mm^3 (or <50,000/mm^3 with bleeding): Hold for concurrent diarrhea or stomatitis until platelets recover to >50,000/mm^3, then continue at same dose

Dietary Considerations Because current safety and efficacy data are based upon administration with food, it is recommended that capecitabine be administered with food. In all clinical trials, patients were instructed to take with water within 30 minutes after a meal.

Administration Usually administered in 2 divided doses taken 12 hours apart. Doses should be taken with water within 30 minutes after a meal.

Recommended Dose Modifications

Toxicity NCI Grades	During a Course of Therapy (Monotherapy)	Dose Adjustment for Next Cycle (% of starting dose)
Grade 1	Maintain dose level	Maintain dose level
Grade 2		
1st appearance	Interrupt until resolved to grade 0-1	100%
2nd appearance	Interrupt until resolved to grade 0-1	75%
3rd appearance	Interrupt until resolved to grade 0-1	50%
4th appearance	Discontinue treatment permanently	
Grade 3		
1st appearance	Interrupt until resolved to grade 0-1	75%
2nd appearance	Interrupt until resolved to grade 0-1	50%
3rd appearance	Discontinue treatment permanently	
Grade 4		
1st appearance	Discontinue permanently **or** If physician deems it to be in the patient's best interest to continue, interrupt until resolved to grade 0-1	50%

Monitoring Parameters Renal function should be estimated at baseline to determine initial dose. During therapy, CBC with differential, hepatic function, and renal function should be monitored.

Dosage Forms Excipient information presented when available (limited, particularly for generics); consult specific product labeling.

Tablet:

Xeloda®: 150 mg, 500 mg

Extemporaneous Preparations Capecitabine oral solution: A solution of capecitabine in water may be prepared by adding 2000 mg capecitabine (powder) to 200 mL water. Capecitabine tablets are water soluble (data on file from Roche). Administer immediately after preparation, 30 minutes after a meal. Use appropriate precautions for handling and disposal.

Judson IR, Beale PJ, Trigo JM, et al, "A Human Capecitabine Excretion Balance and Pharmacokinetic Study After Administration of a Single Oral Dose of ^{14}C-Labelled Drug," *Invest New Drugs*, 1999, 17(1):49-56.

◆ **Capex®** *see* Fluocinolone *on page 633*

◆ **Capital® and Codeine** *see* Acetaminophen and Codeine *on page 27*

◆ **Capoten®** *see* Captopril *on page 249*

◆ **Capoten™ (Can)** *see* Captopril *on page 249*

◆ **Capozide®** *see* Captopril and Hydrochlorothiazide *on page 251*

Capreomycin (kap ree oh MYE sin)

U.S. Brand Names Capastat® Sulfate

Index Terms Capreomycin Sulfate

Pharmacologic Category Antibiotic, Miscellaneous; Antitubercular Agent

Additional Appendix Information

Tuberculosis *on page 1776*

Use Treatment of tuberculosis in conjunction with at least one other antituberculosis agent

Pregnancy Risk Factor C

Pregnancy Considerations Capreomycin has been shown to be teratogenic in animal studies. **[U.S. Boxed Warning]: Safety has not been established in pregnant women**; use during pregnancy only if the potential benefit to the mother outweighs the possible risk to the fetus.

Lactation Excretion in breast milk unknown/use caution

Medication Safety Issues

Sound-alike/look-alike issues:

Capastat® may be confused with Cepastat®

Contraindications Hypersensitivity to capreomycin or any component of the formulation

Warnings/Precautions [U.S. Boxed Warnings]: Use in patients with renal insufficiency or pre-existing auditory impairment must be undertaken with great caution, and the risk of additional eighth nerve impairment or renal injury should be weighed against the benefits to be derived from therapy. Since other parenteral antituberculous agents (eg, streptomycin) also have similar and sometimes irreversible toxic effects, particularly on eighth cranial nerve and renal function, simultaneous administration of these agents with capreomycin is not recommended. Use with nonantituberculous drugs (ie, aminoglycoside antibiotics) having ototoxic or nephrotoxic potential should be undertaken only with great caution. Use caution with renal dysfunction and in the elderly; dosage reductions are recommended for known or suspected renal impairment. Electrolyte imbalances (hypocalcemia, hypokalemia, and hypomagnesemia) have been reported with use. Prolonged use may result in fungal or bacterial superinfection, including *C. difficile*-associated diarrhea (CDAD) and pseudomembranous colitis; CDAD has been observed >2 months postantibiotic treatment. **[U.S. Boxed Warning]: Safety in pregnant women or pediatric patients not established.**

Adverse Reactions

>10%:

Otic: Ototoxicity (subclinical hearing loss: 11%; clinical loss: 3%)

Renal: Nephrotoxicity (36%, increased BUN)

1% to 10%: Hematologic: Eosinophilia (dose related, mild)

<1% (Limited to important or life-threatening): Acute tubular necrosis, Bartter's syndrome, creatinine increased, hypersensitivity (maculopapular rash, urticaria and/or fever), hypocalcemia, hypokalemia, hypomagnesemia, injection site reactions (abscess, bleeding, induration and pain), leukocytosis, leukopenia, liver function decreased (BSP excretion decreased), renal injury, thrombocytopenia (rare), tinnitus, toxic nephritis, urinary sediment abnormal, vertigo

Drug Interactions

Avoid Concomitant Use There are no known interactions where it is recommended to avoid concomitant use.

Increased Effect/Toxicity

Capreomycin may increase the levels/effects of: Aminoglycosides; Colistimethate; Neuromuscular-Blocking Agents; Polymyxin B

Decreased Effect There are no known significant interactions involving a decrease in effect.

Stability Powder for injection should be stored at room temperature of 15°C to 30°C (59°F to 86°F). Dissolve powder with 2 mL of NS or SWFI; allow 2-3 minutes for dissolution.

For I.V. administration: Further dilute in NS 100 mL.

For I.M. administration:

1 g dose: Administer contents of reconstituted vial

<1 g dose: See table:

Capreomycin Dilution for Doses <1 g (I.M. Administration)

Diluent Volume (mL)	Capreomycin Solution Volume (mL)	Final Concentration (approximate)
2.15	2.85	370 mg/mL
2.63	3.33	315 mg/mL
3.3	4	260 mg/mL
4.3	5	210 mg/mL

Following reconstitution, may store under refrigeration for up to 24 hours.

Mechanism of Action Capreomycin is a cyclic polypeptide antimicrobial. It is administered as a mixture of capreomycin IA and capreomycin IB. The mechanism of action of capreomycin is not well understood. Mycobacterial species that have become resistant to other agents are usually still sensitive to the action of capreomycin. However, significant cross-resistance with viomycin, kanamycin, and neomycin occurs.

Pharmacodynamics/Kinetics

Half-life elimination: Normal renal function: 4-6 hours; Cl_{cr} 100-110 mL/minute: 5-6 hours; Cl_{cr} 50-80 mL/minute: 7-10 hours; Cl_{cr} 20-40 mL/minute: 12-20 hours; Cl_{cr} 10 mL/minute: 29 hours; Cl_{cr} 0 mL/minute: 55 hours

Time to peak, serum: I.M.: 1-2 hours

Excretion: Urine (52% within 12 hours)

Dosage I.M., I.V.:

Infants and Children <15 years and ≤40 kg (unlabeled use): 15-30 mg/kg/day (maximum: 1 g/day) for 2-4 months, followed by 15-30 mg/kg (maximum: 1 g/day) twice weekly (*MMWR*, 2003)

Children ≥15 years or >40 kg (unlabeled use): 15 mg/kg/day (maximum: 1 g/dose) for 2-4 months followed by 15 mg/kg (maximum: 1 g/dose) 2-3 times/week (*MMWR*, 2003)

Adults: 1 g/day (maximum: 20 mg/kg/day) for 60-120 days, followed by 1 g 2-3 times/week **or** 15 mg/kg/day (maximum: 1 g/dose) for 2-4 months, followed by 15 mg/kg (maximum: 1 g/dose) 2-3 times/week (*MMWR*, 2003)

Elderly: Use with caution due to the increased potential for pre-existing renal dysfunction or impaired hearing. The manufacturer recommends initiating at lower end of dosing range. Adults >59 years of age: 10 mg/kg (maximum: 750 mg/dose) for 5-7 days per week for 2-4 months, followed by 10 mg/kg (maximum: 750 mg/dose) 2-3 times/week (*MMWR*, 2003).

Dosing interval in renal impairment: Adults:

The FDA-approved labeling contains the following renal dosing adjustment guidelines (maximum: 1 g/dose):

Cl_{cr} 110 mL/minute: Administer 13.9 mg/kg every 24 hours

Cl_{cr} 100 mL/minute: Administer 12.7 mg/kg every 24 hours

Cl_{cr} 80 mL/minute: Administer 10.4 mg/kg every 24 hours

Cl_{cr} 60 mL/minute: Administer 8.2 mg/kg every 24 hours

Cl_{cr} 50 mL/minute: Administer 7 mg/kg every 24 hours **or** 14 mg/kg every 48 hours

Cl_{cr} 40 mL/minute: Administer 5.9 mg/kg every 24 hours **or** 11.7 mg/kg every 48 hours

Cl_{cr} 30 mL/minute: Administer 4.7 mg/kg every 24 hours **or** 9.5 mg/kg every 48 hours **or** 14.2 mg/kg every 72 hours

Cl_{cr} 20 mL/minute: Administer 3.6 mg/kg every 24 hours **or** 7.2 mg/kg every 48 hours **or** 10.7 mg/kg every 72 hours

Cl_{cr} 10 mL/minute: Administer 2.4 mg/kg every 24 hours **or** 4.9 mg/kg every 48 hours **or** 7.3 mg/kg every 72 hours

Cl_{cr} 0 mL/minute: Administer 1.3 mg/kg every 24 hours **or** 2.6 mg/kg every 48 hours **or** 3.9 mg/kg every 72 hours

The following (unlabeled) guidelines may also be used:
MMWR, 2003:
Cl_{cr} ≥30 mL/minute: No adjustment required
Cl_{cr} <30 mL/minute and hemodialysis: 12-15 mg/kg (maximum: 1 g/dose) 2-3 days per week (**NOT** daily)
Aronoff, 2007:
Cl_{cr} ≥10 mL/minute: 1 g every 24 hours
Cl_{cr} <10 mL/minute: 1 g every 48 hours
Hemodialysis: Administer dose after hemodialysis only
Continuous renal replacement therapy (CRRT): 5 mg/kg every 24 hours

Administration
I.M.: Administer by deep I.M. injection into a large muscle mass.
I.V.: Administer over 60 minutes.

Monitoring Parameters Audiometric measurements and vestibular function at baseline and during therapy; renal function at baseline and weekly during therapy; frequent assessment of serum electrolytes (including calcium, magnesium, and potassium), liver function tests

Reference Range Recommended concentration for susceptibility testing: 10 mcg/mL

Dosage Forms Excipient information presented when available (limited, particularly for generics); consult specific product labeling.
Injection, powder for reconstitution, as sulfate:
Capastat® Sulfate: 1 g

◆ **Capreomycin Sulfate** *see* Capreomycin *on page 247*

Captopril (KAP toe pril)

U.S. Brand Names Capoten®

Canadian Brand Names Alti-Captopril; Apo-Capto®; Capoten™; Gen-Captopril; Novo-Captopril; Nu-Capto; PMS-Captopril

Index Terms ACE

Pharmacologic Category Angiotensin-Converting Enzyme (ACE) Inhibitor

Additional Appendix Information
Angiotensin Agents *on page 1632*
Heart Failure (Systolic) *on page 1809*
Hypertension *on page 1820*

Use Management of hypertension; treatment of heart failure, left ventricular dysfunction after myocardial infarction, diabetic nephropathy

Unlabeled/Investigational Use To delay the progression of nephropathy and reduce risks of cardiovascular events in hypertensive patients with type 1 or 2 diabetes mellitus; treatment of hypertensive crisis, rheumatoid arthritis; diagnosis of anatomic renal artery stenosis, hypertension secondary to scleroderma renal crisis; diagnosis of aldosteronism, idiopathic edema, Bartter's syndrome, postmyocardial infarction for prevention of ventricular failure; increase circulation in Raynaud's phenomenon, hypertension secondary to Takayasu's disease

Pregnancy Risk Factor C (1st trimester); D (2nd and 3rd trimesters)

Pregnancy Considerations Due to adverse events observed in some animal studies, captopril is considered pregnancy category C during the first trimester. Based on human data, captopril is considered pregnancy category D if used during the second and third trimesters (per the manufacturer; however, one study suggests that fetal injury may occur at anytime during pregnancy). Captopril crosses the placenta and may affect ACE activity in the fetus. First trimester exposure to ACE inhibitors may cause major congenital malformations. An increased risk of cardiovascular and/or central nervous system malformations was observed in one study; however, an increased risk of teratogenic events was not observed in other studies. Second and third trimester use of an ACE inhibitor is associated with oligohydramnios. Oligohydramnios due to decreased fetal renal function may lead to fetal limb contractures, craniofacial deformation, and hypoplastic lung development. The use of ACE inhibitors during the second and third trimesters is also associated with anuria, hypotension, renal failure (reversible or irreversible), skull hypoplasia, and death in the fetus/neonate. Chronic maternal hypertension itself is also associated with adverse events in the fetus/infant. ACE inhibitors are not recommended during pregnancy to treat maternal hypertension or heart failure. Those who are planning a pregnancy should be considered for other medication options if an ACE inhibitor is currently prescribed or the ACE inhibitor should be discontinued as soon as possible once pregnancy is detected. The exposed fetus should be monitored for fetal growth, amniotic fluid volume, and organ formation. Infants exposed to an ACE inhibitor *in utero*, especially during the second and third trimester, should be monitored for hyperkalemia, hypotension, and oliguria.

[U.S. Boxed Warning]: Based on human data, ACE inhibitors can cause injury and death to the developing fetus when used in the second and third trimesters. ACE inhibitors should be discontinued as soon as possible once pregnancy is detected.

Lactation Enters breast milk/not recommended (AAP rates "compatible")

Medication Safety Issues
Sound-alike/look-alike issues:
Captopril may be confused with Capitrol®, carvedilol

International issues:
Acepril® [Great Britain] may be confused with Accupril® which is a brand name for quinapril in the U.S.
Acepril®: Brand name for enalapril in Hungary and Switzerland; brand name for lisinopril in Denmark

Contraindications Hypersensitivity to captopril, any other ACE inhibitor, or any component of the formulation; angioedema related to previous treatment with an ACE inhibitor

Warnings/Precautions Anaphylactic reactions may occur rarely with ACE inhibitors. At any time during treatment (especially following first dose) angioedema may occur rarely with ACE inhibitors; may involve the head and neck (potentially compromising airway) or the intestine (presenting with abdominal pain). African-Americans and patients with idiopathic or hereditary angioedema may be at an increased risk. Prolonged frequent monitoring may be required especially if tongue, glottis, or larynx are involved as they are associated with airway obstruction. Patients with a history of airway surgery may have a higher risk of airway obstruction. Aggressive early and appropriate management is critical. Use in patients with previous angioedema associated with ACE inhibitor therapy is contraindicated. Severe anaphylactoid reactions may be seen during hemodialysis (eg, CVVHD) with high-flux dialysis membranes (eg, AN69), and rarely, during low density lipoprotein apheresis with dextran sulfate cellulose. Rare cases of anaphylactoid reactions have been reported in patients undergoing sensitization treatment with hymenoptera (bee, wasp) venom while receiving ACE inhibitors.

Symptomatic hypotension with or without syncope can occur with ACE inhibitors (usually with the first several doses); effects are most often observed in volume depleted patients; close monitoring of patient is required especially with initial dosing and dosing increases; blood pressure must be lowered at a rate appropriate for the patient's clinical condition. Initiation of therapy in patients with ischemic heart disease or cerebrovascular disease ▶

warrants close observation due to the potential consequences posed by falling blood pressure (eg, MI, stroke). Use with caution in hypertrophic cardiomyopathy with outflow tract obstruction, severe aortic stenosis, or before, during, or immediately after major surgery. **[U.S. Boxed Warning]: Based on human data, ACEIs can cause injury and death to the developing fetus when used in the second and third trimesters. ACEIs should be discontinued as soon as possible once pregnancy is detected.**

Hyperkalemia may occur with ACE inhibitors; risk factors include renal dysfunction, diabetes mellitus, concomitant use of potassium-sparing diuretics, potassium supplements and/or potassium containing salts. Use cautiously, if at all, with these agents and monitor potassium closely. Cough may occur with ACE inhibitors. Other causes of cough should be considered (eg, pulmonary congestion in patients with heart failure) and excluded prior to discontinuation.

May be associated with deterioration of renal function and/or increases in serum creatinine, particularly in patients with low renal blood flow (eg, renal artery stenosis, heart failure) whose glomerular filtration rate (GFR) is dependent on efferent arteriolar vasoconstriction by angiotensin II; deterioration may result in oliguria, acute renal failure, and progressive azotemia. Small increases in serum creatinine may occur following initiation; consider discontinuation only in patients with progressive and/or significant deterioration in renal function. Use with caution in patients with unstented unilateral/bilateral renal artery stenosis. When unstented bilateral renal artery stenosis is present, use is generally avoided due to the elevated risk of deterioration in renal function unless possible benefits outweigh risks.

Rare toxicities associated with ACE inhibitors include cholestatic jaundice (which may progress to fulminant hepatic necrosis), agranulocytosis, neutropenia, or leukopenia with myeloid hypoplasia. Patients with collagen vascular diseases (especially with concomitant renal impairment) or renal impairment alone may be at increased risk for hematologic toxicity; closely monitor CBC with differential for the first 3 months of therapy and periodically thereafter in these patients.

Adverse Reactions

1% to 10%:

- Cardiovascular: Hypotension (1% to 2.5%), tachycardia (1%), chest pain (1%), palpitation (1%)
- Dermatologic: Rash (maculopapular or urticarial) (4% to 7%), pruritus (2%); in patients with rash, a positive ANA and/or eosinophilia has been noted in 7% to 10%.
- Endocrine & metabolic: Hyperkalemia (1% to 11%)
- Hematologic: Neutropenia may occur in up to 3.7% of patients with renal insufficiency or collagen-vascular disease.
- Renal: Proteinuria (1%), serum creatinine increased, worsening of renal function (may occur in patients with bilateral renal artery stenosis or hypovolemia)
- Respiratory: Cough (0.5% to 2%)
- Miscellaneous: Hypersensitivity reactions (rash, pruritus, fever, arthralgia, and eosinophilia) have occurred in 4% to 7% of patients (depending on dose and renal function); dysgeusia - loss of taste or diminished perception (2% to 4%)

Frequency not defined:

- Cardiovascular: Angioedema, cardiac arrest, cerebrovascular insufficiency, rhythm disturbances, orthostatic hypotension, syncope, flushing, pallor, angina, MI, Raynaud's syndrome, CHF
- Central nervous system: Ataxia, confusion, depression, nervousness, somnolence
- Dermatologic: Bullous pemphigus, erythema multiforme, Stevens-Johnson syndrome, exfoliative dermatitis
- Endocrine & metabolic: Alkaline phosphatase increased, bilirubin increased, gynecomastia
- Gastrointestinal: Pancreatitis, glossitis, dyspepsia
- Genitourinary: Urinary frequency, impotence
- Hematologic: Anemia, thrombocytopenia, pancytopenia, agranulocytosis
- Hepatic: Jaundice, hepatitis, hepatic necrosis (rare), cholestasis, hyponatremia (symptomatic), transaminases increased
- Neuromuscular & skeletal: Asthenia, myalgia, myasthenia
- Ocular: Blurred vision
- Renal: Renal insufficiency, renal failure, nephrotic syndrome, polyuria, oliguria
- Respiratory: Bronchospasm, eosinophilic pneumonitis, rhinitis
- Miscellaneous: Anaphylactoid reactions

Postmarketing and/or case reports: Alopecia, aplastic anemia, exacerbations of Huntington's disease, Guillain-Barré syndrome, hemolytic anemia, Kaposi's sarcoma, pericarditis, seizure (in premature infants), systemic lupus erythematosus. A syndrome which may include fever, myalgia, arthralgia, interstitial nephritis, vasculitis, rash, eosinophilia, and elevated ESR has been reported for captopril and other ACE inhibitors.

Drug Interactions

Metabolism/Transport Effects Substrate of CYP2D6 (major)

Avoid Concomitant Use There are no known interactions where it is recommended to avoid concomitant use.

Increased Effect/Toxicity

Captopril may increase the levels/effects of: Allopurinol; Amifostine; AzaTHIOprine; CycloSPORINE; Ferric Gluconate; Gold Sodium Thiomalate; Lithium; RiTUXimab

The levels/effects of Captopril may be increased by: Angiotensin II Receptor Blockers; CYP2D6 Inhibitors (Moderate); CYP2D6 Inhibitors (Strong); Darunavir; Diazoxide; Eplerenone; Herbs (Hypotensive Properties); Loop Diuretics; Potassium Salts; Potassium-Sparing Diuretics; Prostacyclin Analogues; Sirolimus; Temsirolimus; Thiazide Diuretics; Trimethoprim

Decreased Effect

The levels/effects of Captopril may be decreased by: Antacids; Aprotinin; Herbs (Hypertensive Properties); Methylphenidate; Nonsteroidal Anti-Inflammatory Agents; Salicylates; Yohimbine

Ethanol/Nutrition/Herb Interactions

- Food: Captopril serum concentrations may be decreased if taken with food. Long-term use of captopril may result in a zinc deficiency which can result in a decrease in taste perception.
- Herb/Nutraceutical: Avoid bayberry, blue cohosh, cayenne, ephedra, ginger, ginseng (American), kola, licorice (may worsen hypertension). Avoid black cohosh, california poppy, coleus, golden seal, hawthorn, mistletoe, periwinkle, quinine, shepherd's purse (may have increased antihypertensive effect).

Mechanism of Action Competitive inhibitor of angiotensin-converting enzyme (ACE); prevents conversion of angiotensin I to angiotensin II, a potent vasoconstrictor; results in lower levels of angiotensin II which causes an increase in plasma renin activity and a reduction in aldosterone secretion

Pharmacodynamics/Kinetics

- Onset of action: Peak effect: Blood pressure reduction: 1-1.5 hours after dose
- Duration: Dose related, may require several weeks of therapy before full hypotensive effect
- Absorption: 60% to 75%; reduced 30% to 40% by food
- Protein binding: 25% to 30%
- Metabolism: 50%

Half-life elimination (renal and cardiac function dependent):

Adults, healthy volunteers: 1.9 hours; Heart failure: 2.06 hours; Anuria: 20-40 hours

Time to peak: 1 hour

Excretion: Urine (>95%) within 24 hours (40% to 50% as unchanged drug)

Dosage Note: Titrate dose according to patient's response; use lowest effective dose. Oral:

Infants: Initial: 0.15-0.3 mg/kg/dose; titrate dose upward to maximum of 6 mg/kg/day in 1-4 divided doses; usual required dose: 2.5-6 mg/kg/day

Children: Initial: 0.5 mg/kg/dose; titrate upward to maximum of 6 mg/kg/day in 2-4 divided doses

Older Children: Initial: 6.25-12.5 mg/dose every 12-24 hours; titrate upward to maximum of 6 mg/kg/day

Adolescents: Initial: 12.5-25 mg/dose given every 8-12 hours; increase by 25 mg/dose to maximum of 450 mg/day

Adults:

Acute hypertension (urgency/emergency): 12.5-25 mg, may repeat as needed (may be given sublingually, but no therapeutic advantage demonstrated)

Hypertension:

Initial dose: 12.5-25 mg 2-3 times/day; may increase by 12.5-25 mg/dose at 1- to 2-week intervals up to 50 mg 3 times/day; maximum dose: 150 mg 3 times/day; add diuretic before further dosage increases

Usual dose range (JNC 7): 25-100 mg/day in 2 divided doses

Congestive heart failure:

Initial dose: 6.25-12.5 mg 3 times/day in conjunction with cardiac glycoside and diuretic therapy; initial dose depends upon patient's fluid/electrolyte status

Target dose: 50 mg 3 times/day

LVD after MI: Initial dose: 6.25 mg followed by 12.5 mg 3 times/day; then increase to 25 mg 3 times/day during next several days and then over next several weeks to target dose of 50 mg 3 times/day

Diabetic nephropathy: 25 mg 3 times/day; other antihypertensives often given concurrently

Dosing adjustment in renal impairment:

Cl_{cr} 10-50 mL/minute: Administer at 75% of normal dose.

Cl_{cr} <10 mL/minute: Administer at 50% of normal dose.

Note: Smaller dosages given every 8-12 hours are indicated in patients with renal dysfunction; renal function and leukocyte count should be carefully monitored during therapy.

Hemodialysis: Moderately dialyzable (20% to 50%); administer dose postdialysis or administer 25% to 35% supplemental dose.

Peritoneal dialysis: Supplemental dose is not necessary.

Dietary Considerations Should be taken at least 1 hour before or 2 hours after eating.

Administration Unstable in aqueous solutions; to prepare solution for oral administration, mix prior to administration and use within 10 minutes.

Monitoring Parameters BUN, electrolytes, serum creatinine; blood pressure. In patients with renal impairment and/or collagen vascular disease, closely monitor CBC with differential for the first 3 months of therapy and periodically thereafter.

Test Interactions Positive Coombs' [direct]; may cause false-positive results in urine acetone determinations using sodium nitroprusside reagent

Dosage Forms Excipient information presented when available (limited, particularly for generics); consult specific product labeling.

Tablet: 12.5 mg, 25 mg, 50 mg, 100 mg

Extemporaneous Preparations Captopril has limited stability in aqueous preparations. The addition of an antioxidant (sodium ascorbate) has been shown to increase the stability of captopril in solution; captopril (1 mg/mL) in syrup with methylcellulose is stable for 7 days stored either at 4°C or 22°C; captopril (1 mg/mL) in distilled water (no additives) is stable for 14 days if stored at 4°C and 7 days if stored at 22°C; captopril (1 mg/mL) with sodium ascorbate (5 mg/mL) in distilled water is stable for 56 days at 4°C and 14 days at 22°C.

Captopril (0.75 mg/mL) in cherry syrup is stable for only 2 days in amber clear plastic containers stored at room temperature or under refrigeration; captopril (0.75 mg/mL) in either a 1:1 mixture of Ora-Sweet® and Ora-Plus® or a 1:1 mixture of Ora-Sweet® SF and Ora-Plus® is stable for 10 days or less depending on the storage temperature (see Allen, 1996).

Powder papers can also be made; powder papers are stable for 12 weeks when stored at room temperature

Allen LV and Erickson III MA, "Stability of Baclofen, Captopril, Diltiazem Hydrochloride, Dipyridamole, and Flecainide Acetate in Extemporaneously Compounded Oral Liquids," *Am J Health Syst Pharm*, 1996, 53:2179-84.

Nahata MC, Morosco RS, and Hipple TF, "Stability of Captopril in Three Liquid Dosage Forms," *Am J Hosp Pharm*, 1994, 51(1):95-6.

Taketomo CK, Chu SA, Cheng MH, et al, "Stability of Captopril in Powder Papers Under Three Storage Conditions," *Am J Hosp Pharm*, 1990, 47(8):1799-1801.

Captopril and Hydrochlorothiazide

(KAP toe pril & hye droe klor oh THYE a zide)

U.S. Brand Names Capozide®

Canadian Brand Names Capozide®

Index Terms Hydrochlorothiazide and Captopril

Pharmacologic Category Angiotensin-Converting Enzyme (ACE) Inhibitor; Diuretic, Thiazide

Use Management of hypertension

Pregnancy Risk Factor C/D (2nd and 3rd trimesters)

Dosage Oral: Adults: Hypertension, CHF: May be substituted for previously titrated dosages of the individual components; alternatively, may initiate as follows:

Initial: Single tablet (captopril 25 mg/hydrochlorothiazide 15 mg) taken once daily; daily dose of captopril should not exceed 150 mg; daily dose of hydrochlorothiazide should not exceed 50 mg

Additional Information Complete prescribing information for this medication should be consulted for additional detail.

Dosage Forms Excipient information presented when available (limited, particularly for generics); consult specific product labeling.

Tablet:

25/15: Captopril 25 mg and hydrochlorothiazide 15 mg

25/25: Captopril 25 mg and hydrochlorothiazide 25 mg

50/15: Captopril 50 mg and hydrochlorothiazide 15 mg

50/25: Captopril 50 mg and hydrochlorothiazide 25 mg

◆ **Carac®** *see* Fluorouracil *on page 636*

◆ **Carafate®** *see* Sucralfate *on page 1404*

◆ **Carapres® (Can)** *see* CloNIDine *on page 354*

Carbachol (KAR ba kole)

U.S. Brand Names Isopto® Carbachol; Miostat®

Canadian Brand Names Isopto® Carbachol; Miostat®

Index Terms Carbacholine; Carbamylcholine Chloride

Pharmacologic Category Cholinergic Agonist; Ophthalmic Agent, Antiglaucoma; Ophthalmic Agent, Miotic

Additional Appendix Information

Glaucoma Drug Therapy *on page 1808*

Use Lowers intraocular pressure in the treatment of glaucoma; cause miosis during surgery

Pregnancy Risk Factor C

Medication Safety Issues

Sound-alike/look-alike issues:

Isopto® Carbachol may be confused with Isopto® Carpine

Dosage Adults:

Ophthalmic: Instill 1-2 drops up to 3 times/day

Intraocular: 0.5 mL instilled into anterior chamber before or after securing sutures

Additional Information Complete prescribing information for this medication should be consulted for additional detail.

Dosage Forms Excipient information presented when available (limited, particularly for generics); consult specific product labeling.

Solution, intraocular:

Miostat®): 0.01% (1.5 mL)

Solution, ophthalmic:

Isopto® Carbachol: 1.5% (15 mL); 3% (15 mL) [contains benzalkonium chloride]

◆ **Carbacholine** *see* Carbachol *on page* 251

CarBAMazepine (kar ba MAZ e peen)

U.S. Brand Names Carbatrol®; Epitol®; Equetro®; Tegretol®; Tegretol®-XR

Canadian Brand Names Apo-Carbamazepine®; Bio-Carbamazepine; Carbamazepine; Dom-Carbamazepine; Gen-Carbamazepine CR; Mapezine®; Novo-Carbamaz; Nu-Carbamazepine; PHL-Carbamazepine; PMS-Carbamazepine; Sandoz-Carbamazepine; Taro-Carbamazepine Chewable; Tegretol®

Index Terms CBZ; SPD417

Pharmacologic Category Anticonvulsant, Miscellaneous

Additional Appendix Information

Anticonvulsant Drugs of Choice *on page* 1637

Use

Carbatrol®, Tegretol®, Tegretol®-XR: Partial seizures with complex symptomatology (psychomotor, temporal lobe), generalized tonic-clonic seizures (grand mal), mixed seizure patterns, trigeminal neuralgia

Equetro®: Acute manic and mixed episodes associated with bipolar 1 disorder

Unlabeled/Investigational Use Treatment of resistant schizophrenia, ethanol withdrawal, restless leg syndrome, post-traumatic stress disorders

Pregnancy Risk Factor D

Pregnancy Considerations Crosses the placenta. Dysmorphic facial features, cranial defects, cardiac defects, spina bifida, IUGR, and multiple other malformations reported. Epilepsy itself, number of medications, genetic factors, or a combination of these probably influences the teratogenicity of anticonvulsant therapy. Benefit:risk ratio usually favors continued use during pregnancy and breast-feeding. Contraceptives may be rendered less effective by the coadministration of carbamazepine; alternative methods of contraception should be considered.

Lactation Enters breast milk/not recommended (AAP rates "compatible")

Medication Safety Issues

Sound-alike/look-alike issues:

CarBAMazepine may be confused with OXcarbazepine

Carbatrol® may be confused with Cartrol®

Epitol® may be confused with Epinal®

Tegretol®, Tegretol®-XR may be confused with Mebaral®, Tegrin®, Toprol-XL®, Toradol®, Trental®

Contraindications Hypersensitivity to carbamazepine, tricyclic antidepressants, or any component of the formulation; bone marrow depression; with or within 14 days of MAO inhibitor use; concurrent use of nefazodone

Warnings/Precautions **[U.S. Boxed Warning]: Potentially fatal blood cell abnormalities have been reported.** Patients with a previous history of adverse hematologic reaction to any drug may be at increased risk. Administer carbamazepine with caution to patients with history of cardiac damage, ECG abnormalities (or at risk for ECG abnormalities), hepatic or renal disease. When used to treat bipolar disorder, the smallest effective dose is suggested to reduce the risk for overdose/suicide; high-risk patients should be monitored for suicidal ideations. Prescription should be written for the smallest quantity consistent with good patient care. May activate latent psychosis and/or cause confusion or agitation; elderly patients may be at an increased risk for psychiatric effects. Potentially serious, sometimes fatal multiorgan hypersensitivity reactions have been reported with some antiepileptic drugs; monitor for signs and symptoms of possible disparate manifestations associated with lymphatic, hepatic, renal, and/or hematologic organ systems; gradual discontinuation and conversion to alternate therapy may be required.

Carbamazepine is not effective in absence, myoclonic, or akinetic seizures; exacerbation of certain seizure types have been seen after initiation of carbamazepine therapy in children with mixed seizure disorders. Abrupt discontinuation is not recommended in patients being treated for seizures. Dizziness or drowsiness may occur; caution should be used when performing tasks which require alertness until the effects are known. Effects with other sedative drugs or ethanol may be potentiated. Carbamazepine has a high potential for drug interactions; use caution in patients taking strong CYP3A4 inducers or inhibitors or medications significantly metabolized via CYP1A2, 2B6, 2C9, 2C19, and 3A4. Coadministration of carbamazepine and nefazodone may lead to insufficient plasma levels of nefazodone; combination is contraindicated. Carbamazepine has mild anticholinergic activity; use with caution in patients with increased intraocular pressure, or sensitivity to anticholinergic effects. Severe dermatologic reactions, including toxic epidermal necrolysis and Stevens-Johnson syndrome, although rarely reported, have resulted in fatalities. **[U.S. Boxed Warning]: Use caution and screen for the genetic susceptibility genotype (*HLA-B*1502* allele) in Asian patients. Patients with a positive result should not be started on carbamazepine.** Discontinue if there are any signs of hypersensitivity. Elderly patients may have an increased risk of SIADH-like syndrome.

Administration of the suspension will yield higher peak and lower trough serum levels than an equal dose of the tablet form; consider a lower starting dose given more frequently (same total daily dose) when using the suspension.

Adverse Reactions Frequency not defined, unless otherwise specified.

Cardiovascular: Arrhythmias, AV block, bradycardia, chest pain (bipolar use), CHF, edema, hyper-/hypotension, lymphadenopathy, syncope, thromboembolism, thrombophlebitis

Central nervous system: Amnesia (bipolar use), anxiety (bipolar use), aseptic meningitis (case report), ataxia (bipolar use 15%), confusion, depression (bipolar use), dizziness (bipolar use 44%), fatigue, headache (bipolar use 22%), sedation, slurred speech, somnolence (bipolar use 32%)

Dermatologic: Alopecia, alterations in skin pigmentation, erythema multiforme, exfoliative dermatitis, photosensitivity reaction, pruritus (bipolar use 8%), purpura, rash, Stevens-Johnson syndrome, toxic epidermal necrolysis, urticaria

Endocrine & metabolic: Chills, fever, hyponatremia, syndrome of inappropriate ADH secretion (SIADH)

Gastrointestinal: Abdominal pain, anorexia, constipation, diarrhea, dyspepsia (bipolar use), gastric distress, nausea (bipolar use 29%), pancreatitis, vomiting (bipolar use 18%), xerostomia (bipolar use)

Genitourinary: Azotemia, impotence, renal failure, urinary frequency, urinary retention

Hematologic: Acute intermittent porphyria, agranulocytosis, aplastic anemia, bone marrow suppression, eosinophilia, leukocytosis, leukopenia, pancytopenia, thrombocytopenia

Hepatic: Abnormal liver function tests, hepatic failure, hepatitis, jaundice

Neuromuscular & skeletal: Back pain, pain (bipolar use 12%), peripheral neuritis, weakness

Ocular: Blurred vision, conjunctivitis, lens opacities, nystagmus

Otic: Hyperacusis, tinnitus

Miscellaneous: Diaphoresis, hypersensitivity (including multiorgan reactions, may include disorders mimicking lymphoma, eosinophilia, hepatosplenomegaly, vasculitis); infection (bipolar use 12%)

Postmarketing and/or case reports: Suicidal ideation

Drug Interactions

Metabolism/Transport Effects Substrate of CYP2C8 (minor), 3A4 (major); **Induces** CYP1A2 (strong), 2B6 (strong), 2C8 (strong), 2C9 (strong), 2C19 (strong), 3A4 (strong)

Avoid Concomitant Use

Avoid concomitant use of CarBAMazepine with any of the following: Darunavir; Etravirine; Nilotinib; Ranolazine; Voriconazole

Increased Effect/Toxicity

CarBAMazepine may increase the levels/effects of: Alcohol (Ethyl); ClomiPRAMINE; CNS Depressants; Desmopressin; Lithium; Phenytoin

The levels/effects of CarBAMazepine may be increased by: Allopurinol; Antifungal Agents (Azole Derivatives, Systemic); Calcium Channel Blockers (Nondihydropyridine); Carbonic Anhydrase Inhibitors; Cimetidine; CYP3A4 Inhibitors (Moderate); CYP3A4 Inhibitors (Strong); Danazol; Dasatinib; Fluconazole; Grapefruit Juice; Isoniazid; LamoTRIgine; Macrolide Antibiotics; Propoxyphene; Protease Inhibitors; Selective Serotonin Reuptake Inhibitors

Decreased Effect

CarBAMazepine may decrease the levels/effects of: Acetaminophen; Aminocamptothecin; Aripiprazole; Bendamustine; Benzodiazepines (metabolized by oxidation); Calcium Channel Blockers (Dihydropyridine); Calcium Channel Blockers (Nondihydropyridine); Caspofungin; Clozapine; Contraceptive (Progestins); CycloSPORINE; CYP1A2 Substrates; CYP2B6 Substrates; CYP2C19 Substrates; CYP2C8 Substrates (High risk); CYP2C9 Substrates (High risk); CYP3A4 Substrates; Dabigatran Etexilate; Darunavir; Doxycycline; Etravirine; Flunarizine; Haloperidol; Lacosamide; LamoTRIgine; Maraviroc; Mebendazole; Methadone; Nilotinib; Oral Contraceptive (Estrogens); Paliperidone; P-Glycoprotein Substrates; Phenytoin; Protease Inhibitors; Ranolazine; Risperidone; Rufinamide; Selective Serotonin Reuptake Inhibitors; Sorafenib; Temsirolimus; Theophylline Derivatives; Thyroid Products; Topiramate; Tricyclic Antidepressants; Valproic Acid; Vecuronium; Vitamin K Antagonists; Voriconazole; Ziprasidone

The levels/effects of CarBAMazepine may be decreased by: CYP3A4 Inducers (Strong); Deferasirox; Herbs (CYP3A4 Inducers); Ketorolac; Mefloquine; Methylfolate; Phenytoin; Rufinamide; Valproic Acid

Ethanol/Nutrition/Herb Interactions

Ethanol: Avoid ethanol (may increase CNS depression).

Food: Carbamazepine serum levels may be increased if taken with food. Carbamazepine serum concentration may be increased if taken with grapefruit juice; avoid concurrent use.

Herb/Nutraceutical: Avoid evening primrose (seizure threshold decreased). Avoid valerian, St John's wort, kava kava, gotu kola (may increase CNS depression).

Mechanism of Action In addition to anticonvulsant effects, carbamazepine has anticholinergic, antineuralgic, antidiuretic, muscle relaxant, antimanic, antidepressive, and antiarrhythmic properties; may depress activity in the nucleus ventralis of the thalamus or decrease synaptic transmission or decrease summation of temporal stimulation leading to neural discharge by limiting influx of sodium ions across cell membrane or other unknown mechanisms; stimulates the release of ADH and potentiates its action in promoting reabsorption of water; chemically related to tricyclic antidepressants

Pharmacodynamics/Kinetics

Absorption: Slow

Distribution: V_d: Neonates: 1.5 L/kg; Children: 1.9 L/kg; Adults: 0.59-2 L/kg

Protein binding: Carbamazepine: 75% to 90%, may be decreased in newborns; Epoxide metabolite: 50%

Metabolism: Hepatic via CYP3A4 to active epoxide metabolite; induces hepatic enzymes to increase metabolism

Bioavailability: 85%

Half-life elimination: **Note:** Half-life is variable because of autoinduction which is usually complete 3-5 weeks after initiation of a fixed carbamazepine regimen.

Carbamazepine: Initial: 25-65 hours; Extended release: 35-40 hours; Multiple doses: Children: 8-14 hours; Adults: 12-17 hours

Epoxide metabolite: Initial: 25-43 hours

Time to peak, serum: Unpredictable:

Immediate release: Suspension: 1.5 hour; tablet: 4-5 hours

Extended release: Carbatrol®, Equetro®: 12-26 hours (single dose), 4-8 hours (multiple doses); Tegretol®-XR: 3-12 hours

Excretion: Urine 72% (1% to 3% as unchanged drug); feces (28%)

Dosage Dosage must be adjusted according to patient's response and serum concentrations. Administer tablets (chewable or conventional) in 2-3 divided doses daily and suspension in 4 divided doses daily. Oral:

Epilepsy:

Children:

<6 years: Initial: 10-20 mg/kg/day divided twice or 3 times daily as tablets or 4 times/day as suspension; increase dose every week until optimal response and therapeutic levels are achieved

Maintenance dose: Divide into 3-4 doses daily (tablets or suspension); maximum recommended dose: 35 mg/kg/day

6-12 years: Initial: 200 mg/day in 2 divided doses (tablets or extended release tablets) or 4 divided doses (oral suspension); increase by up to 100 mg/day at weekly intervals using a twice daily regimen of extended release tablets or 3-4 times daily regimen of other formulations until optimal response and therapeutic levels are achieved

Maintenance: Usual: 400-800 mg/day; maximum recommended dose: 1000 mg/day

Note: Children <12 years who receive ≥400 mg/day of carbamazepine may be converted to extended release capsules (Carbatrol®) using the same total daily dosage divided twice daily

Children >12 years and Adults: Initial: 400 mg/day in 2 divided doses (tablets or extended release tablets) or 4 divided doses (oral suspension); increase by up to 200 mg/day at weekly intervals using a twice daily regimen of extended release tablets or capsules, or a 3-4 times/day regimen of other formulations until optimal response and therapeutic levels are achieved; usual dose: 800-1200 mg/day

Maximum recommended doses:

Children 12-15 years: 1000 mg/day

Children >15 years: 1200 mg/day

Adults: 1600 mg/day; however, some patients have required up to 1.6-2.4 g/day

Trigeminal or glossopharyngeal neuralgia: Adults: Initial: 200 mg/day in 2 divided doses (tablets, extended release tablets, or extended release capsules) or 4 divided doses (oral suspension) with food, gradually increasing in increments of 200 mg/day as needed

Maintenance: Usual: 400-800 mg daily in 2 divided doses (tablets, extended release tablets, or extended release capsules) or 4 divided doses (oral suspension); maximum dose: 1200 mg/day

Bipolar disorder: Adults: Initial: 400 mg/day in 2 divided doses (tablets, extended release tablets, or extended release capsules) or 4 divided doses (oral suspension), may adjust by 200 mg/day increments; maximum dose: 1600 mg/day.

Note: Equetro® is the only formulation specifically approved by the FDA for the management of bipolar disorder.

Dietary Considerations Drug may cause GI upset, take with large amount of water or food to decrease GI upset. May need to split doses to avoid GI upset.

Administration

Suspension: Must be given on a 3-4 times/day schedule versus tablets which can be given 2-4 times/day. Since a given dose of suspension will produce higher peak and lower trough levels than the same dose given as the tablet form, patients given the suspension should be started on lower doses given more frequently (same total daily dose) and increased slowly to avoid unwanted side effects. When carbamazepine suspension has been combined with chlorpromazine or thioridazine solutions, a precipitate forms which may result in loss of effect. Therefore, it is recommended that the carbamazepine suspension dosage form not be administered at the same time with other liquid medicinal agents or diluents. Should be administered with meals.

Extended release capsule (Carbatrol®, Equetro®): Consists of three different types of beads: Immediate release, extended-release, and enteric release. The bead types are combined in a ratio to allow twice daily dosing. May be opened and contents sprinkled over food such as a teaspoon of applesauce; may be administered with or without food; do not crush or chew.

Extended release tablet: Should be inspected for damage. Damaged extended release tablets (without release portal) should not be administered. Should be administered with meals; swallow whole, do not crush or chew.

Monitoring Parameters CBC with platelet count, reticulocytes, serum iron, lipid panel, liver function tests, urinalysis, BUN, serum carbamazepine levels, thyroid function tests, serum sodium; pregnancy test; ophthalmic exams (pupillary reflexes); observe patient for excessive sedation, especially when instituting or increasing therapy; signs of rash; *HLA-B*1502* genotype screening prior to therapy initiation in patients of Asian descent.

Reference Range

Timing of serum samples: Absorption is slow, peak levels occur 6-8 hours after ingestion of the first dose; the half-life ranges from 8-60 hours, therefore, steady-state is achieved in 2-5 days

Therapeutic levels: 4-12 mcg/mL (SI: 17-51 μmol/L)

Toxic concentration: >15 mcg/mL; patients who require higher levels of 8-12 mcg/mL (SI: 34-51 μmol/L) should be watched closely. Side effects including CNS effects occur commonly at higher dosage levels. If other anticonvulsants are given therapeutic range is 4-8 mcg/mL.

Test Interactions May interact with some pregnancy tests; increased BUN, AST, ALT, bilirubin, alkaline phosphatase (S); decreased calcium, T_3, T_4, sodium (S)

Dosage Forms Excipient information presented when available (limited, particularly for generics); consult specific product labeling.

Capsule, extended release:

Carbatrol®, Equetro®: 100 mg, 200 mg, 300 mg

Suspension, oral: 100 mg/5 mL (5 mL, 10 mL, 450 mL)

Tegretol®: 100 mg/5 mL (450 mL) [contains propylene glycol; citrus vanilla flavor]

Tablet: 200 mg

Epitol®, Tegretol®: 200 mg

Tablet, chewable: 100 mg

Tegretol®: 100 mg

Tablet, extended release:

Tegretol®-XR: 100 mg, 200 mg, 400 mg

◆ **Carbamazepine (Can)** *see* CarBAMazepine *on page 252*

◆ **Carbamide** *see* Urea *on page 1530*

Carbamide Peroxide (KAR ba mide per OKS ide)

U.S. Brand Names Auraphene® B [OTC]; Auro® [OTC]; Cankaid® [OTC]; Debrox® [OTC]; Dent's Ear Wax [OTC] [DSC]; E•R•O [OTC]; Gly-Oxide® [OTC]; Murine® Ear Wax Removal System [OTC]; Orajel® Perioseptic® Spot Treatment [OTC]; Otix® [OTC]

Index Terms Urea Peroxide

Pharmacologic Category Anti-inflammatory, Locally Applied; Otic Agent, Cerumenolytic

Use Relief of minor inflammation of gums, oral mucosal surfaces, and lips including canker sores and dental irritation; emulsify and disperse ear wax

Pregnancy Risk Factor C

Dosage Children and Adults:

Oral: Inflammation/dental irritation: Solution (should not be used for >7 days): Oral preparation should not be used in children <2 years of age; apply several drops undiluted on affected area 4 times/day after meals and at bedtime; expectorate after 2-3 minutes **or** place 10 drops onto tongue, mix with saliva, swish for several minutes, expectorate

Otic:

Children <12 years: Tilt head sideways and individualize the dose according to patient size; 3 drops (range: 1-5 drops) twice daily for up to 4 days, tip of applicator should not enter ear canal; keep drops in ear for several minutes by keeping head tilted and placing cotton in ear

Children ≥12 years and Adults: Tilt head sideways and instill 5-10 drops twice daily up to 4 days, tip of applicator should not enter ear canal; keep drops in ear for several minutes by keeping head tilted and placing cotton in ear

Additional Information Complete prescribing information for this medication should be consulted for additional detail.

Dosage Forms Excipient information presented when available (limited, particularly for generics); consult specific product labeling. [DSC] = Discontinued product

Liquid, oral: 10% (60 mL)

Cankaid®: 10% (22 mL)

Gly-Oxide®: 10% (15 mL, 60 mL)

Solution, otic [drops]: 6.5% (15 mL)

Auraphene® B, Otix®: 6.5% (15 mL)

Auro®: 6.5% (22.2 mL)

Debrox®: 6.5% (15 mL, 30 mL)

Dent's Ear Wax: 6.5% (3.7 mL) [DSC]

E•R•O: 6.5% (15 mL) [alcohol free]

Murine® Ear Wax Removal System: 6.5% (15 mL) [contains alcohol 6.3%]

◆ **Carbamylcholine Chloride** *see* Carbachol *on page 251*

◆ **Carbatrol®** *see* CarBAMazepine *on page 252*

◆ **Carbaxefed RF [DSC]** *see* Carbinoxamine and Pseudoephedrine *on page 258*

Carbetapentane and Phenylephrine

(kar bay ta PEN tane & fen il EF rin)

U.S. Brand Names L-All 12

Index Terms Phenylephrine Tannate and Carbetapentane Tannate

Pharmacologic Category Antitussive; Antitussive/Decongestant; Sympathomimetic

Use Symptomatic relief of upper respiratory tract conditions such as the common cold, bronchial asthma, and bronchitis (acute and chronic)

Pregnancy Risk Factor C

Dosage Oral:

Children:

2-6 years: 2.5 mL every 12 hours, not to exceed 5 mL/24 hours

6-12 years: 5 mL every 12 hours, not to exceed 10 mL/24 hours

Children >12 years and Adults: 5-10 mL every 12 hours, not to exceed 20 mL/24 hours

Additional Information Complete prescribing information for this medication should be consulted for additional detail.

Dosage Forms Excipient information presented when available (limited, particularly for generics); consult specific product labeling.

Suspension:

L-All 12: Carbetapentane tannate 30 mg and phenylephrine tannate 30 mg per 5 mL (120 mL) [contains sodium benzoate and phenylalanine; strawberry flavor]

Carbetapentane and Pseudoephedrine

(kar bay ta PEN tane & soo doe e FED rin)

U.S. Brand Names Pseudacarb™; Respi-Tann™

Index Terms Carbetapentane Tannate and Pseudoephedrine Tannate; Pseudoephedrine and Carbetapentane

Pharmacologic Category Antitussive/Decongestant

Use Relief of cough and congestion due to the common cold, influenza, sinusitis, or bronchitis

Pregnancy Risk Factor C

Dosage Relief of cough and congestion: Oral:

Children:

2-6 years: 1/2 tablet or 2.5 mL suspension every 12 hours (maximum: 4 doses/24 hours)

6-12 years: 1 tablet or 5 mL suspension every 12 hours (maximum: 4 doses/24 hours)

Children >12 years and Adults: 2 tablets or 10 mL suspension every 12 hours (maximum: 4 doses/24 hours)

Additional Information Complete prescribing information for this medication should be consulted for additional detail.

Dosage Forms Excipient information presented when available (limited, particularly for generics); consult specific product labeling.

Suspension: Carbetapentane tannate 25 mg and pseudoephedrine tannate 75 mg per 5 mL (480 mL)

Respi-Tann™: Carbetapentane tannate 25 mg and pseudoephedrine tannate 75 mg per 5 mL (480 mL) [dye free; contains sodium benzoate; cherry flavor]

Tablet, chewable:

Respi-Tann™: Carbetapentane tannate 25 mg and pseudoephedrine tannate 75 mg [dye free; cherry flavor]

Pseudacarb™: Carbetapentane tannate 25 mg and pseudoephedrine tannate 75 mg [dye free; grape flavor]

◆ **Carbetapentane, Ephedrine, Phenylephrine, and Chlorpheniramine** *see* Chlorpheniramine, Ephedrine, Phenylephrine, and Carbetapentane *on page 311*

Carbetapentane, Guaifenesin, and Phenylephrine

(kar bay ta PEN tane, gwye FEN e sin, & fen il EF rin)

U.S. Brand Names Carbetaplex; Extendryl® GCP; Gentex LQ; Levall™; Phencarb GG

Index Terms Guaifenesin, Carbetapentane Citrate, and Phenylephrine Hydrochloride; Phenylephrine Hydrochloride, Carbetapentane Citrate, and Guaifenesin

Pharmacologic Category Antitussive; Expectorant; Expectorant/Decongestant/Antitussive; Sympathomimetic

Use Relief of nonproductive cough accompanying respiratory tract congestion associated with the common cold, influenza, sinusitis, and bronchitis

Pregnancy Risk Factor C

Dosage Oral:

Children <2 years: Dosage not established

Children 2-6 years:

Gentex LQ: 2.5 mL every 4-6 hours

Levall™: 1.25 mL every 4-6 hours; maximum dose of phenylephrine: 15 mg/24 hours

Children 6-12 years:

Gentex LQ: 5 mL every 4-6 hours

Levall™: 2.5 mL every 4-6 hours; maximum dose of phenylephrine: 30 mg/24 hours

Children ≥12 years and Adults:

Gentex LQ: 5-10 mL every 4-6 hours

Levall™: 5 mL every 4-6 hours; maximum dose of phenylephrine: 60 mg/24 hours

Additional Information Complete prescribing information for this medication should be consulted for additional detail.

Dosage Forms Excipient information presented when available (limited, particularly for generics); consult specific product labeling.

Liquid:

Carbetaplex: Carbetapentane citrate 20 mg, guaifenesin 100 mg, and phenylephrine hydrochloride 15 mg per 5 mL (480 mL) [alcohol free, sugar free, dye free; strawberry flavor]

Gentex LQ: Carbetapentane citrate 20 mg, guaifenesin 100 mg, and phenylephrine hydrochloride 10 mg per 5 mL [contains edetate disodium and benzoic acid; spearmint flavor]

Levall™: Carbetapentane citrate 15 mg, guaifenesin 100 mg, and phenylephrine hydrochloride 5 mg per 5 mL (480 mL) [alcohol free; strawberry flavor]

Phencarb GG: Carbetapentane citrate 20 mg, guaifenesin 100 mg, and phenylephrine hydrochloride 10 mg per 5 mL (480 mL) [spearmint flavor]

Solution, oral:

Extendryl® GCP: Carbetapentane citrate 15 mg, guaifenesin 100 mg, and phenylephrine hydrochloride 5 mg per 5 mL (473 mL) [alcohol free; contains propylene glycol; strawberry flavor]

◆ **Carbetapentane Tannate and Pseudoephedrine Tannate** *see* Carbetapentane and Pseudoephedrine *on page 255*

◆ **Carbetaplex** *see* Carbetapentane, Guaifenesin, and Phenylephrine *on page 255*

Carbidopa (kar bi DOE pa)

U.S. Brand Names Lodosyn®

Pharmacologic Category Anti-Parkinson's Agent, Dopamine Agonist

Use Given with levodopa in the treatment of parkinsonism to enable a lower dosage of levodopa to be used and a more rapid response to be obtained and to decrease side effects; for details of administration and dosage, see Levodopa; has no effect without levodopa

Pregnancy Risk Factor C

Medication Safety Issues

International issues:

Lodosyn® may be confused with Lidosen® which is a brand name for lidocaine in Italy

Dosage Oral: Adults: 70-100 mg/day; maximum daily dose: 200 mg

Additional Information Complete prescribing information for this medication should be consulted for additional detail.

Dosage Forms Excipient information presented when available (limited, particularly for generics); consult specific product labeling.

Tablet: 25 mg

Carbidopa and Levodopa
(kar bi DOE pa & lee voe DOE pa)

U.S. Brand Names Parcopa™; Sinemet®; Sinemet® CR

Canadian Brand Names Apo-Levocarb®; Apo-Levocarb® CR; Endo®-Levodopa/Carbidopa; Novo-Levocarbidopa; Nu-Levocarb; Pro-Levocarb; Sinemet®; Sinemet® CR

Index Terms Levodopa and Carbidopa

Pharmacologic Category Anti-Parkinson's Agent, Dopamine Agonist

Additional Appendix Information

Antiparkinsonian Agents *on page 1643*

Use Idiopathic Parkinson's disease; postencephalitic parkinsonism; symptomatic parkinsonism

Unlabeled/Investigational Use Restless leg syndrome

Pregnancy Risk Factor C

Pregnancy Considerations Teratogenic effects were observed with levodopa and carbidopa in animal studies. There are case reports of levodopa crossing the placenta in humans.

Lactation Excretion in breast milk unknown/use caution

Medication Safety Issues

Sound-alike/look-alike issues:

Sinemet® may be confused with Serevent®

Contraindications Hypersensitivity to levodopa, carbidopa, or any component of the formulation; narrow-angle glaucoma; use of MAO inhibitors within prior 14 days (however, may be administered concomitantly with the manufacturer's recommended dose of an MAO inhibitor with selectivity for MAO type B); history of melanoma or undiagnosed skin lesions

Warnings/Precautions Use with caution in patients with history of cardiovascular disease (including myocardial infarction and arrhythmias), pulmonary dieases such as asthma, psychosis, wide-angle glaucoma, peptic ulcer disease, as well as in severe renal and hepatic dysfunction. Use with caution when interpreting plasma/urine catecholamine levels; falsely diagnosed pheochromocytoma has been rarely reported. Severe cases or rhabdomyolysis have been reported. Sudden discontinuation of levodopa may cause a worsening of Parkinson's disease. Elderly may be more sensitive to CNS effects of levodopa. May cause or exacerbate dyskinesias. Patients have reported falling asleep while engaging in activities of daily living; this has been reported to occur without significant warning signs. May cause orthostatic hypotension; Parkinson's disease patients appear to have an impaired capacity to respond to a postural challenge; use with caution in patients at risk of hypotension (such as those receiving antihypertensive drugs) or where transient hypotensive episodes would be poorly tolerated (cardiovascular disease or cerebrovascular disease). Observe patients closely for development of depression with concomitant suicidal tendencies.

Dopamine agonists have been associated with compulsive behaviors and/or loss of impulse control, which has manifested as pathological gambling, libido increases (hypersexuality), and/or binge eating. Causality has not been established, and controversy exists as to whether this phenomenon is related to the underlying disease, prior behaviors/addictions and/or drug therapy. Dose reduction or discontinuation of therapy has been reported to reverse these behaviors in some, but not all cases. Dopaminergic agents have been associated with a syndrome resembling neuroleptic malignant syndrome on abrupt withdrawal or significant dosage reduction after long-term use. Protein in the diet should be distributed throughout the day to avoid fluctuations in levodopa absorption. Safety and efficacy have not been established in children.

Adverse Reactions Frequency not defined.

Cardiovascular: Orthostatic hypotension, arrhythmia, chest pain, hypertension, syncope, palpitation, phlebitis

Central nervous system: Dizziness, anxiety, confusion, nightmares, headache, hallucinations, on-off phenomenon, decreased mental acuity, memory impairment, disorientation, delusions, euphoria, agitation, somnolence, insomnia, gait abnormalities, nervousness, ataxia, EPS, falling, psychosis, peripheral neuropathy, seizure (causal relationship not established)

Dermatologic: Rash, alopecia, malignant melanoma, hypersensitivity (angioedema, urticaria, pruritus, bullous lesions, Henoch-Schönlein purpura)

Endocrine & metabolic: Increased libido

Gastrointestinal: Anorexia, nausea, vomiting, constipation, GI bleeding, duodenal ulcer, diarrhea, dyspepsia, taste alterations, sialorrhea, heartburn

Genitourinary: Discoloration of urine, urinary frequency

Hematologic: Hemolytic anemia, agranulocytosis, thrombocytopenia, leukopenia; decreased hemoglobin and hematocrit; abnormalities in AST and ALT, LDH, bilirubin, BUN, Coombs' test

Neuromuscular & skeletal: Choreiform and involuntary movements, paresthesia, bone pain, shoulder pain, muscle cramps, weakness

Ocular: Blepharospasm, oculogyric crises (may be associated with acute dystonic reactions)

Renal: Difficult urination

Respiratory: Dyspnea, cough

Miscellaneous: Hiccups, discoloration of sweat, diaphoresis (increased)

Reported with dopamine agonists: Impulsive/compulsive behaviors (eg, pathological gambling, hypersexuality, binge eating)

Drug Interactions

Avoid Concomitant Use There are no known interactions where it is recommended to avoid concomitant use.

Increased Effect/Toxicity

Carbidopa and Levodopa may increase the levels/effects of: MAO Inhibitors

The levels/effects of Carbidopa and Levodopa may be increased by: Sapropterin

Decreased Effect

The levels/effects of Carbidopa and Levodopa may be decreased by: Antipsychotics (Atypical); Antipsychotics (Typical); Iron Salts; Methionine; Metoclopramide; Phenytoin; Pyridoxine

Ethanol/Nutrition/Herb Interactions

Ethanol: Avoid ethanol (due to CNS depression).

Food: Avoid high protein diets and high intakes of vitamin B_6.

Herb/Nutraceutical: Avoid kava kava (may decrease effects). Pyridoxine in doses >10-25 mg (for levodopa alone) or higher doses >200 mg/day (for levodopa/carbidopa) may decrease efficacy.

Stability Store at 20°C to 25°C (68°F to 77°F); excursions permitted between 15°C to 30°C (59°F to 86°F). Protect from light and moisture.

Mechanism of Action Parkinson's symptoms are due to a lack of striatal dopamine; levodopa circulates in the plasma to the blood-brain-barrier (BBB), where it crosses, to be converted by striatal enzymes to dopamine; carbidopa inhibits the peripheral plasma breakdown of levodopa by inhibiting its decarboxylation, and thereby increases available levodopa at the BBB

Pharmacodynamics/Kinetics

Duration: Variable, 6-12 hours; longer with sustained release forms

See individual agents.

Dosage Oral: Adults:

Parkinson's disease:

Immediate release tablet:

Initial: Carbidopa 25 mg/levodopa 100 mg 3 times/day

Dosage adjustment: Alternate tablet strengths may be substituted according to individual carbidopa/levodopa requirements. Increase by 1 tablet every other day as necessary, except when using the carbidopa 25 mg/levodopa 250 mg tablets where increases should be made using 1/2-1 tablet every 1-2 days. Use of more than 1 dosage strength or dosing 4 times/day may be required (maximum: 8 tablets of any strength/day or 200 mg of carbidopa and 2000 mg of levodopa)

Sustained release tablet:

Initial: Carbidopa 50 mg/levodopa 200 mg 2 times/day, at intervals not <6 hours

Dosage adjustment: May adjust every 3 days; intervals should be between 4-8 hours during the waking day (maximum: 8 tablets/day)

Restless leg syndrome (unlabeled use): Carbidopa 25 mg/levodopa 100 mg given 30-60 minutes before bedtime; may repeat dose once

Elderly: Initial: Carbidopa 25 mg/levodopa 100 mg twice daily, increase as necessary

Dietary Considerations Levodopa peak serum concentrations may be decreased if taken with food. High protein diets (>2 g/kg) may decrease the efficacy of levodopa via competition with amino acids in crossing the blood-brain barrier.

Parcopa™: Contains phenylalanine 3.4 mg per 10/100 mg and 25/100 mg strengths; phenylalanine 8.4 mg in 25/250 mg strength

Administration Space doses evenly over the waking hours. Give with meals to decrease GI upset. Sustained release product should not be crushed. Orally-disintegrating tablets do not require water; the tablet should disintegrate on the tongue's surface before swallowing.

Monitoring Parameters Blood pressure, standing and sitting/supine; symptoms of parkinsonism, dyskinesias, mental status

Test Interactions False-positive reaction for urinary glucose with Clinitest®; false-negative reaction using Clinistix®; false-positive urine ketones with Acetest®, Ketostix®, Labstix®

Additional Information 50-100 mg/day of carbidopa is needed to block the peripheral conversion of levodopa to dopamine. "On-off" (a clinical syndrome characterized by sudden periods of drug activity/inactivity), can be managed by giving smaller, more frequent doses of Sinemet® or adding a dopamine agonist or selegiline; when adding a new agent, doses of Sinemet® can usually be decreased. Protein in the diet should be distributed throughout the day to avoid fluctuations in levodopa absorption. Levodopa is the drug of choice when rigidity is the predominant presenting symptom.

Conversion from levodopa to carbidopa/levodopa: **Note:** Levodopa must be discontinued at least 12 hours prior to initiation of levodopa/carbidopa:

Initial dose: Levodopa portion of carbidopa/levodopa should be at least 25% of previous levodopa therapy.

Levodopa <1500 mg/day: Sinemet® or Parcopa™ (levodopa 25 mg/carbidopa 100 mg) 3-4 times/day

Levodopa ≥1500 mg/day: Sinemet® or Parcopa™ (levodopa 25 mg/carbidopa 250 mg) 3-4 times/day

Conversion from immediate release carbidopa/levodopa (Sinemet® or Parcopa™) to Sinemet® CR (50/200):

Sinemet® or Parcopa™ [total daily dose of levodopa]/Sinemet® CR:

Sinemet® or Parcopa™ (levodopa 300-400 mg/day): Sinemet® CR (50/200) 1 tablet twice daily

Sinemet® or Parcopa™ (levodopa 500-600 mg/day): Sinemet® CR (50/200) 1 1/2 tablets twice daily or 1 tablet 3 times/day

Sinemet® or Parcopa™ (levodopa 700-800 mg/day): Sinemet® CR (50/200) 4 tablets in 3 or more divided doses

Sinemet® or Parcopa™ (levodopa 900-1000 mg/day): Sinemet® CR (50/200) 5 tablets in 3 or more divided doses

Intervals between doses of Sinemet® CR should be 4-8 hours while awake; when divided doses are not equal, smaller doses should be given toward the end of the day.

Dosage Forms Excipient information presented when available (limited, particularly for generics); consult specific product labeling.

Tablet: 10/100: Carbidopa 10 mg and levodopa 100 mg; 25/100: Carbidopa 25 mg and levodopa 100 mg; 25/250: Carbidopa 25 mg and levodopa 250 mg

Sinemet®:

10/100: Carbidopa 10 mg and levodopa 100 mg

25/100: Carbidopa 25 mg and levodopa 100 mg

25/250: Carbidopa 25 mg and levodopa 250 mg

Tablet, extended release: 25/100: Carbidopa 25 mg and levodopa 100 mg; 50/200: Carbidopa 50 mg and levodopa 200 mg

Tablet, orally disintegrating: 10/100: Carbidopa 10 mg and levodopa 100 mg; 25/100: Carbidopa 25 mg and levodopa 100 mg; 25/250: Carbidopa 25 mg and levodopa 250 mg

Parcopa™:

10/100: Carbidopa 10 mg and levodopa 100 mg [contains phenylalanine 3.4 mg/tablet; mint flavor]

25/100: Carbidopa 25 mg and levodopa 100 mg [contains phenylalanine 3.4 mg/tablet; mint flavor]

25/250: Carbidopa 25 mg and levodopa 250 mg [contains phenylalanine 8.4 mg/tablet; mint flavor]

Tablet, sustained release: 25/100: Carbidopa 25 mg and levodopa 100 mg; 50/200: Carbidopa 50 mg and levodopa 200 mg

Sinemet® CR:

25/100: Carbidopa 25 mg and levodopa 100 mg

50/200: Carbidopa 50 mg and levodopa 200 mg

◆ **Carbidopa, Levodopa, and Entacapone** *see* Levodopa, Carbidopa, and Entacapone *on page 875*

Carbinoxamine (kar bi NOKS a meen)

U.S. Brand Names Palgic®

Index Terms Carbinoxamine Maleate

Pharmacologic Category Histamine H_1 Antagonist; Histamine H_1 Antagonist, First Generation

Use Seasonal and perennial allergic rhinitis; vasomotor rhinitis; urticaria; decrease severity of other allergic reactions

Pregnancy Risk Factor C

Dosage Oral (Palgic®):
Children:
>3-6 years: 2-5 mg 3-4 times/day
>6 years: 4-6 mg 3-4 times/day
Adults: 4-8 mg 3-4 times/day

Additional Information Complete prescribing information for this medication should be consulted for additional detail.

Dosage Forms Excipient information presented when available (limited, particularly for generics); consult specific product labeling.
Solution, as maleate:
Palgic®: 4 mg/5 mL (480 mL) [bubble gum flavor]
Tablet, as maleate [scored]:
Palgic®: 4 mg

Carbinoxamine and Pseudoephedrine
(kar bi NOKS a meen & soo doe e FED rin)

U.S. Brand Names Andehist NR Drops [DSC]; Carbaxefed RF [DSC]; Carboxine-PSE [DSC]; Cordron-D NR [DSC]; Hydro-Tussin™-CBX [DSC]; Palgic®-D [DSC]; Palgic®-DS [DSC]; Pediatex™-D [DSC]; Sildec [DSC]

Index Terms Pseudoephedrine and Carbinoxamine

Pharmacologic Category Alpha/Beta Agonist; Histamine H_1 Antagonist; Histamine H_1 Antagonist, First Generation

Use Seasonal and perennial allergic rhinitis; vasomotor rhinitis

Pregnancy Risk Factor C

Dosage Oral:
Children:
Drops (Andehist NR, Carbaxefed RF, Sildec):
1-3 months: 0.25 mL 4 times/day
3-6 months: 0.5 mL 4 times/day
6-12 months: 0.75 mL 4 times/day
12-24 months: 1 mL 4 times/day
Liquid (Pediatex™-D):
1-3 months: 1.25 mL up to 4 times/day
3-6 months: 2.5 mL up to 4 times/day
6-9 months: 3.75 mL up to 4 times/day
9-18 months: 3.75-5 mL up to 4 times/day
18 months to 6 years: 5 mL 3-4 times/day
>6 years: Refer to adult dosing
Syrup (Hydro-Tussin™-CBX, Palgic®-DS):
1-3 months: 1.25 mL up to 4 times/day
3-6 months: 2.5 mL up to 4 times/day
6-9 months: 3.75 mL up to 4 times/day
9-18 months: 3.75-5 mL up to 4 times/day
18 months to 6 years: 5 mL 3-4 times/day
>6 years: Refer to adult dosing
Tablet, timed release:
6-12 years (Palgic®-D): One-half tablet every 12 hours
≥12 years (Palgic®-D): Refer to adult dosing
Adults:
Liquid (Pediatex™-D): 10 mL 4 times/day
Syrup (Hydro-Tussin™-CBX, Palgic®-DS): 10 mL 4 times/day
Tablet, timed release (Palgic®-D): 1 tablet every 12 hours

Additional Information Complete prescribing information for this medication should be consulted for additional detail.

Dosage Forms Excipient information presented when available (limited, particularly for generics); consult specific product labeling. [DSC] = Discontinued product
Liquid:
Cordron-D NR: Carbinoxamine maleate 2 mg and pseudoephedrine hydrochloride 12.5 mg per 5 mL (480 mL) [cotton candy flavor] [DSC]
Pediatex™-D: Carbinoxamine maleate 2 mg and pseudoephedrine hydrochloride 20 mg per 5 mL (480 mL) [alcohol free, dye free, sugar free; cotton candy flavor] [DSC]
Solution: Carbinoxamine maleate 2 mg and pseudoephedrine hydrochloride 25 mg per 5 mL (480 mL) [DSC]
Carboxine-PSE: Carbinoxamine maleate 2 mg and pseudoephedrine hydrochloride 20 mg per 5 mL (480 mL) [peach flavor] [DSC]
Solution, oral drops:
Andehist NR: Carbinoxamine maleate 1 mg and pseudoephedrine hydrochloride 15 mg per mL (30 mL) [alcohol and sugar free; raspberry flavor] [DSC]
Carbaxefed RF: Carbinoxamine maleate 1 mg and pseudoephedrine hydrochloride 15 mg per mL (30 mL) [alcohol free; contains sodium benzoate; cherry flavor] [DSC]
Sildec: Carbinoxamine maleate 1 mg and pseudoephedrine hydrochloride 15 mg per mL (30 mL) [raspberry flavor] [DSC]
Syrup: Carbinoxamine maleate 2 mg and pseudoephedrine hydrochloride 25 mg per 5 mL (480 mL)
Hydro-Tussin™-CBX [DSC], Palgic®-DS [DSC]: Carbinoxamine maleate 2 mg and pseudoephedrine hydrochloride 25 mg per 5 mL (480 mL) [alcohol, dye, and sugar free; strawberry/pineapple flavor]
Tablet, timed release:
Palgic®-D: Carbinoxamine maleate 8 mg and pseudoephedrine hydrochloride 80 mg [dye free] [DSC]

◆ **Carbinoxamine Maleate** *see* Carbinoxamine *on page 257*

◆ **Carbinoxamine, Pseudoephedrine, and Hydrocodone** *see* Hydrocodone, Carbinoxamine, and Pseudoephedrine *on page 743*

◆ **Carbocaine®** *see* Mepivacaine *on page 945*

◆ **Carbolith™ (Can)** *see* Lithium *on page 897*

CARBOplatin (KAR boe pla tin)

Canadian Brand Names Paraplatin-AQ

Index Terms CBDCA; NSC-241240

Pharmacologic Category Antineoplastic Agent, Alkylating Agent; Antineoplastic Agent, Platinum Analog

Use Treatment of ovarian cancer

Unlabeled/Investigational Use Lung cancer, head and neck cancer, endometrial cancer, esophageal cancer, bladder cancer, breast cancer, cervical cancer, CNS tumors, germ cell tumors, osteogenic sarcoma, and high-dose therapy with stem cell/bone marrow support

Pregnancy Risk Factor D

Lactation Excretion in breast milk unknown/contraindicated

Medication Safety Issues
Sound-alike/look-alike issues:
CARBOplatin may be confused with CISplatin, oxaliplatin
Paraplatin® may be confused with Platinol®

High alert medication: The Institute for Safe Medication Practices (ISMP) includes this medication among its list of drugs which have a heightened risk of causing significant patient harm when used in error.

Contraindications History of severe allergic reaction to cisplatin, carboplatin, other platinum-containing formulations, or any component of the formulation; pregnancy; breast-feeding

Warnings/Precautions Hazardous agent - use appropriate precautions for handling and disposal. High doses have resulted in severe abnormalities of liver function tests. **[U.S. Boxed Warning]: Bone marrow suppression, which may be severe, and vomiting are dose related;** reduce dosage in patients with bone marrow suppression and impaired renal function. Anemia is cumulative. Clinically significant hearing loss has been reported to occur in pediatric patients when carboplatin was administered at higher than recommended doses in combination with other ototoxic agents.

[U.S. Boxed Warning]: Increased risk of allergic reactions in patients previously exposed to platinum therapy. When administered as sequential infusions, taxane derivatives (docetaxel, paclitaxel) should be administered before the platinum derivatives (carboplatin, cisplatin) to limit myelosuppression and to enhance efficacy. Loss of vision (reversible) has been reported with higher than recommended doses. The elderly (≥65 years) and patients who have previously received cisplatin have an increased incidence of peripheral neuropathy. **[U.S. Boxed Warning]: Should be administered under the supervision of an experienced cancer chemotherapy physician.**

Adverse Reactions Percentages reported with single-agent therapy.

>10%:

- Central nervous system: Pain (23%)
- Endocrine & metabolic: Hyponatremia (29% to 47%), hypomagnesemia (29% to 43%), hypocalcemia (22% to 31%), hypokalemia (20% to 28%)
- Gastrointestinal: Vomiting (65% to 81%), abdominal pain (17%), nausea (10% to 15%)
- Hematologic: Myelosuppression (dose related and dose limiting; nadir at ~21 days; recovery by ~28 days), leukopenia (85%; grades 3/4: 15% to 26%), anemia (71% to 90%; grades 3/4: 21%), neutropenia (67%; grades 3/4: 16% to 21%), thrombocytopenia (62%; grades 3/4: 25% to 35%)
- Hepatic: Alkaline phosphatase increased (24% to 37%), AST increased (15% to 19%)
- Neuromuscular & skeletal: Weakness (11%)
- Renal: Creatinine clearance decreased (27%), BUN increased (14% to 22%)

1% to 10%:

- Central nervous system: Neurotoxicity (5%)
- Dermatologic: Alopecia (2% to 3%)
- Gastrointestinal: Constipation (5%), diarrhea (6%), stomatitis/mucositis (1%), taste dysgeusia (1%)
- Hematologic: Hemorrhagic complications (5%)
- Hepatic: Bilirubin increased (5%)
- Local: Pain at injection site
- Neuromuscular & skeletal: Peripheral neuropathy (4% to 6%; up to 10% in older and/or previously-treated patients)
- Ocular: Visual disturbance (1%)
- Otic: Ototoxicity (1%)
- Renal: Creatinine increased (6% to 10%)
- Miscellaneous: Infection (5%), hypersensitivity (2%)

<1% (Limited to important or life-threatening): Anaphylaxis, anorexia, bronchospasm, cardiac failure, cerebrovascular accident, embolism, erythema, fever, hemolytic uremic syndrome (HUS), hyper-/hypotension, malaise, necrosis (associated with extravasation), nephrotoxicity, neurotoxicity, pruritus, rash, secondary malignancies, urticaria, vision loss

Drug Interactions

Avoid Concomitant Use

Avoid concomitant use of CARBOplatin with any of the following: Natalizumab; Vaccines (Live)

Increased Effect/Toxicity

CARBOplatin may increase the levels/effects of: Natalizumab; Taxane Derivatives; Topotecan; Vaccines (Live)

The levels/effects of CARBOplatin may be increased by: Aminoglycosides; Trastuzumab

Decreased Effect

CARBOplatin may decrease the levels/effects of: Vaccines (Inactivated)

The levels/effects of CARBOplatin may be decreased by: Echinacea

Ethanol/Nutrition/Herb Interactions Herb/Nutraceutical: Avoid black cohosh, dong quai in estrogen-dependent tumors.

Stability Store intact vials at room temperature of 15°C to 30°C (59°F to 86°F); protect from light. Further dilution to a concentration as low as 0.5 mg/mL is stable at room temperature (25°C) for 8 hours in NS; stable at room temperature or under refrigeration for at least 9 days in D_5W, although the manufacturer states to use within 8 hours due to lack of preservative.

Powder for reconstitution: Reconstitute powder to yield a final concentration of 10 mg/mL which is stable for 5 days at room temperature (25°C). Reconstituted carboplatin 10 mg/mL should be further diluted to a final concentration of 0.5-2 mg/mL with D_5W or NS for administration.

Solution for injection: Multidose vials are stable for up to 14 days after opening when stored at room temperature.

Mechanism of Action Carboplatin is an alkylating agent which covalently binds to DNA; possible cross-linking and interference with the function of DNA

Pharmacodynamics/Kinetics

- Distribution: V_d: 16 L/kg; into liver, kidney, skin, and tumor tissue
- Protein binding: 0%; platinum is 30% irreversibly bound
- Metabolism: Minimally hepatic to aquated and hydroxylated compounds
- Half-life elimination: Terminal: 22-40 hours; Cl_{cr} >60 mL/minute: 2.5-5.9 hours
- Excretion: Urine (~60% to 90%) within 24 hours

Dosage Refer to individual protocols: **Note:** Doses for adults are usually determined by the AUC using the Calvert formula.

IVPB, I.V. infusion:

Children:

- Solid tumor (unlabeled use): 300-600 mg/m^2 once every 4 weeks
- Brain tumor (unlabeled use): 175 mg/m^2 weekly for 4 weeks every 6 weeks, with a 2-week recovery period between courses

Adults:

- Ovarian cancer: 300-360 mg/m^2 every 4 weeks
- Autologous BMT (unlabeled use): 1600 mg/m^2 (total dose) divided over 4 days
- In adults, dosing is commonly calculated using the Calvert formula:
  - Total dose (mg) = Target AUC x (GFR+ 25)
  - Usual target AUCs:
    - Previously untreated patients: 6-8
    - Previously treated patients: 4-6

Elderly: The Calvert formula should be used to calculate dosing for elderly patients.

Intraperitoneal (unlabeled use): Adults: 200-650 mg/m^2 in 2 L of dialysis fluid have been administered into the peritoneum of ovarian cancer patients **or** target AUC: 5-7

Dosage adjustment for toxicity: Platelets <50,000 cells/mm^3 or ANC <500 cells/mm^3: Administer 75% of dose

Dosing adjustment in renal impairment: Note: Dose determination with Calvert formula uses GFR and, therefore, inherently adjusts for renal dysfunction.

The FDA-approved labeling recommends the following dosage adjustment guidelines:

- Baseline Cl_{cr} 41-59 mL/minute: Initiate at 250 mg/m^2 and adjust subsequent doses based on bone marrow toxicity
- Baseline Cl_{cr} 16-40 mL/minute: Initiate at 200 mg/m^2 and adjust subsequent doses based on bone marrow toxicity

Baseline Cl_{cr} ≤15 mL/minute: No guidelines are available.

The following dosage adjustments have been used by some clinicians (Aronoff, 2007): Adults (for dosing based on mg/m^2):

Hemodialysis: Administer 50% of dose

Continuous ambulatory peritoneal dialysis (CAPD): Administer 25% of dose

Continuous renal replacement therapy (CRRT): 200 mg/m^2

Dosing adjustment in hepatic impairment: Minimal hepatic metabolism; dosage adjustment may not be needed. No specific dosage adjustment guidelines are available.

Administration Infuse over 15 minutes to 24 hours. May also be administered intraperitoneally. When administered as sequential infusions, taxane derivatives (docetaxel, paclitaxel) should be administered before platinum derivatives to limit myelosuppression and to enhance efficacy.

Monitoring Parameters CBC (with differential and platelet count), serum electrolytes, creatinine clearance, liver function tests, BUN, creatinine

Dosage Forms Excipient information presented when available (limited, particularly for generics); consult specific product labeling. [DSC] = Discontinued product

Injection, powder for reconstitution: 50 mg, 150 mg, 450 mg

Injection, solution: 10 mg/mL (5 mL, 15 mL, 45 mL, 60 mL)

Injection, solution [preservative free]: 10 mg/mL (5 mL, 15 mL, 45 mL)

◆ **Carboprost** *see* Carboprost Tromethamine *on page 260*

Carboprost Tromethamine

(KAR boe prost tro METH a meen)

U.S. Brand Names Hemabate®

Canadian Brand Names Hemabate®

Index Terms Carboprost; Prostaglandin F_2

Pharmacologic Category Abortifacient; Prostaglandin

Use Termination of pregnancy; treatment of refractory postpartum uterine bleeding

Unlabeled/Investigational Use Investigational: Hemorrhagic cystitis

Pregnancy Risk Factor C

Pregnancy Considerations Teratogenic effects were not observed in animal studies. Carboprost tromethamine is not considered feticidal, but is used to terminate pregnancy due to its ability to stimulate uterine contractions. Use is not indicated if the fetus has reached a stage of viability *in utero*. Complete abortion may not be induced in ~20% of cases.

Lactation Excretion in breast milk unknown

Contraindications Hypersensitivity to carboprost tromethamine or any component of the formulation; acute pelvic inflammatory disease; active cardiac, pulmonary, renal, or hepatic dysfunction

Warnings/Precautions [U.S. Boxed Warning] Potent oxytocic agent; use with strict adherence to recommended dosing. Immediate intensive care and acute surgical facilities must be available. Transient pyrexia and increased blood pressure may be observed with treatment. Use caution with history of asthma; hypotension or hypertension; cardiovascular, adrenal, renal, or hepatic disease; anemia; jaundice; diabetes; epilepsy; or compromised uteri. Concomitant use of antiemetic and antidiarrheal agents is recommended to decrease incidence of GI side effects. Safety and efficacy have not been established in pediatric patients.

Adverse Reactions Frequency not defined. Effects due to increased smooth muscle contractility are most common.

Cardiovascular: Chest pain, flushing, hypertension, syncope, palpitation, tachycardia, tightness of chest

Central nervous system: Anxiety, chills/shivering, dizziness, drowsiness, dystonia, faintness, headache, lethargy, lightheadedness, nervousness, sleep disturbance, temperature elevation (may be drug induced or due to postabortion endometritis), vasovagal syndrome, vertigo

Dermatologic: Rash

Endocrine & metabolic: Breast tenderness, dysmenorrhea-like pain, endometritis, hot flashes, thyroid storm

Gastrointestinal: Choking sensation, diarrhea (~2/3 patients), dry throat, epigastric pain, gagging/retching, hematemesis, nausea (~1/3 patients), taste alteration, thirst, throat fullness, vomiting (~2/3 patients), xerostomia

Genitourinary: Perforated uterus, posterior cervical perforation, urinary tract infection, uterine bleeding (excessive), uterine rupture, uterine sacculation

Local: Injection site pain

Neuromuscular & skeletal: Backache, leg cramps, muscular pain, paresthesia, torticollis, weakness

Ocular: Blurred vision, eye pain, eyelid twitching

Otic: Tinnitus

Respiratory: Asthma, cough, bronchospasm, dyspnea, epistaxis, hyperventilation, pulmonary edema, respiratory distress, upper respiratory tract infection, wheezing

Miscellaneous: Diaphoresis, hiccups, retained placental fragment, septic shock

Drug Interactions

Avoid Concomitant Use There are no known interactions where it is recommended to avoid concomitant use.

Increased Effect/Toxicity There are no known significant interactions involving an increase in effect.

Decreased Effect There are no known significant interactions involving a decrease in effect.

Stability Store under refrigeration at 2°C to 8°C (36°F to 46°F).

Bladder irrigation: Dilute immediately prior to administration in NS; stability unknown.

Mechanism of Action Carboprost tromethamine is a prostaglandin similar to prostaglandin F_2 alpha (dinoprost) except for the addition of a methyl group at the C-15 position. This substitution produces longer duration of activity than dinoprost; carboprost stimulates uterine contractility which usually results in expulsion of the products of conception and is used to induce abortion between 13-20 weeks of pregnancy. Hemostasis at the placentation site is achieved through the myometrial contractions produced by carboprost.

Pharmacodynamics/Kinetics Excretion: Urine

Dosage I.M.: Adults:

Abortion: Initial: 250 mcg, then 250 mcg at 1.5- to 3.5-hour intervals, depending on uterine response; a 500 mcg dose may be given if uterine response is not adequate after several 250 mcg doses; do not exceed 12 mg total dose or continuous administration for >2 days

Refractory postpartum uterine bleeding: Initial: 250 mcg; if needed, may repeat at 15- to 90-minute intervals; maximum total dose: 2 mg (8 doses)

Bladder irrigation for hemorrhagic cystitis (unlabeled use): [0.1-1.0 mg/dL as solution] 50 mL instilled into bladder 4 times/day for 1 hour

Administration Do not inject I.V.; may result in bronchospasm, hypertension, vomiting, or anaphylaxis. Administer deep I.M.; rotate site if repeat injections are required.

Dosage Forms Excipient information presented when available (limited, particularly for generics); consult specific product labeling.

Injection, solution:

Hemabate®: Carboprost 250 mcg and tromethamine 83 mcg per mL (1 mL) [contains benzyl alcohol]

Carisoprodol (kar eye soe PROE dole)

U.S. Brand Names Soma®

Canadian Brand Names Soma®

Index Terms Carisoprodate; Isobamate

Pharmacologic Category Skeletal Muscle Relaxant

Use Short-term (2-3 weeks) relief of skeletal muscle pain

Pregnancy Risk Factor C

Pregnancy Considerations Animal data suggests that carisoprodol crosses placenta and adverse events have been observed in animal studies. Limited postmarketing data with meprobamate (the active metabolite) demonstrate a possible risk for congenital malformations. Use only if benefit outweighs the risk.

Lactation Enters breast milk/use caution

Contraindications Hypersensitivity to carisoprodol, meprobamate, or any component of the formulation; acute intermittent porphyria

Warnings/Precautions May cause CNS depression, which may impair physical or mental abilities. Effects with other sedative drugs or ethanol may be potentiated. Use with caution in patients with hepatic/renal dysfunction. Tolerance or drug dependence may result from extended use. Limit to 2-3 weeks; use caution in patients who may be prone to addiction. Idiosyncratic reactions and/or severe allergic reactions may occur. Idiosyncratic reactions occur following the initial dose and may include severe weakness, transient quadriplegia, euphoria, or vision loss (temporary). Has been associated (rarely) with seizures in patients with and without seizure history. Carisoprodol should be used with caution in patients who are poor metabolizers of CYP2C19; poor metabolizers have been shown to have a fourfold increase in exposure to carisoprodol and a 50% reduced exposure to the metabolite meprobamate compared to normal metabolizers. Safety and efficacy in children <16 years of age have not been established.

Adverse Reactions

>10%: Central nervous system: Drowsiness (13% to 17%)

1% to 10%: Central nervous system: Dizziness (7% to 8%), headache (3% to 5%)

Postmarketing and/or case reports: Agitation, anaphylaxis, angioedema, asthma exacerbation, ataxia, burning eyes, depression, dermatitis (allergic), dyspnea, epigastric pain, eosinophilia, erythema multiforme, fixed drug eruption, flushing of face, headache, hiccups, hypersensitivity reactions, hypotension (postural), idiosyncratic reaction (symptoms may include agitation, ataxia, confusion, diplopia, disorientation, dysarthria, euphoria, extreme weakness, mydriasis, temporary vision loss, and/or transient quadriplegia); insomnia, irritability, leukopenia, nausea, pancytopenia, paradoxical CNS stimulation, pruritus, rash, seizure, syncope, tachycardia, tremor, urticaria, vertigo, vomiting, weakness, withdrawal syndrome (abdominal cramps, headache, insomnia, nausea, seizure)

Drug Interactions

Metabolism/Transport Effects **Substrate** of CYP2C19 (major)

Avoid Concomitant Use There are no known interactions where it is recommended to avoid concomitant use.

Increased Effect/Toxicity

Carisoprodol may increase the levels/effects of: Alcohol (Ethyl); CNS Depressants

The levels/effects of Carisoprodol may be increased by: CYP2C19 Inhibitors (Moderate); CYP2C19 Inhibitors (Strong)

Decreased Effect There are no known significant interactions involving a decrease in effect.

Ethanol/Nutrition/Herb Interactions Ethanol: Avoid ethanol (may increase CNS depression).

Stability Store at controlled room temperature of 20°C to 25°C (68°F to 77°F).

Mechanism of Action Precise mechanism is not yet clear, but many effects have been ascribed to its central depressant actions. In animals, carisoprodol blocks interneuronal activity and depresses polysynaptic neuron transmission in the spinal cord and reticular formation of the brain. It is also metabolized to meprobamate, which has anxiolytic and sedative effects.

Pharmacodynamics/Kinetics

Onset of action: ~30 minutes

Duration: 4-6 hours

Metabolism: Hepatic, via CYP2C19 to active metabolite (meprobamate)

Half-life elimination: 2.4 hours; Meprobamate: 10 hours

Time to peak, plasma: 1.5-2 hours

Excretion: Urine, as metabolite

Dosage Note: Carisoprodol should only be used for short periods (2-3 weeks) due to lack of evidence of effectiveness with prolonged use.

Oral: Children ≥16 years and Adults: 250-350 mg 3 times/day and at bedtime

Dietary Considerations May give with or without food.

Administration Administer with or without food.

Monitoring Parameters Look for relief of pain and/or muscle spasm and avoid excessive drowsiness; signs of drug abuse in addiction-prone individuals

Dosage Forms Excipient information presented when available (limited, particularly for generics); consult specific product labeling.

Tablet: 350 mg

Soma®: 250 mg, 350 mg

Carisoprodol and Aspirin
(kar eye soe PROE dole & AS pir in)

U.S. Brand Names Soma® Compound

Index Terms Aspirin and Carisoprodol

Pharmacologic Category Skeletal Muscle Relaxant

Use Skeletal muscle relaxant

Pregnancy Risk Factor C/D (full-dose aspirin in 3rd trimester)

Dosage Oral: Adults: 1-2 tablets 4 times/day

Additional Information Complete prescribing information for this medication should be consulted for additional detail.

Dosage Forms Excipient information presented when available (limited, particularly for generics); consult specific product labeling.

Tablet: Carisoprodol 200 mg and aspirin 325 mg

Carisoprodol, Aspirin, and Codeine

(kar eye soe PROE dole, AS pir in, and KOE deen)

U.S. Brand Names Soma® Compound w/Codeine [DSC]

Index Terms Aspirin, Carisoprodol, and Codeine; Codeine, Aspirin, and Carisoprodol

Pharmacologic Category Skeletal Muscle Relaxant

Use Skeletal muscle relaxant

Restrictions C-III

Pregnancy Risk Factor D

Dosage Oral:

Adults: 1 or 2 tablets 4 times/day (maximum: 8 tablets/day); treatment should be temporary (2-3 weeks)

Elderly: Avoid or use with caution in the elderly (>65 years of age); adverse effects (eg, orthostatic hypotension and CNS depression) may be potentiated.

Additional Information Complete prescribing information for this medication should be consulted for additional detail.

Dosage Forms Excipient information presented when available (limited, particularly for generics); consult specific product labeling. [DSC] = Discontinued product

Tablet: Carisoprodol 200 mg, aspirin 325 mg, and codeine phosphate 16 mg

Soma® Compound w/Codeine: Carisoprodol 200 mg, aspirin 325 mg, and codeine phosphate 16 mg [DSC]

◆ **Carmol® 10 [OTC]** *see* Urea *on page* 1530

◆ **Carmol® 20 [OTC]** *see* Urea *on page* 1530

◆ **Carmol® 40** *see* Urea *on page* 1530

◆ **Carmol® Deep Cleaning** *see* Urea *on page* 1530

◆ **Carmol-HC®** *see* Urea and Hydrocortisone *on page* 1531

◆ **Carmol® Scalp Treatment** *see* Sulfacetamide *on page* 1405

Carmustine (kar MUS teen)

U.S. Brand Names BiCNU®; Gliadel®

Canadian Brand Names BiCNU®; Gliadel Wafer®

Index Terms BCNU; bis-chloronitrosourea; Carmustinum; NSC-409962; WR-139021

Pharmacologic Category Antineoplastic Agent; Antineoplastic Agent, Alkylating Agent (Nitrosourea); Antineoplastic Agent, DNA Adduct-Forming Agent; Antineoplastic Agent, DNA Binding Agent

Use

Injection: Treatment of brain tumors (glioblastoma, brainstem glioma, medulloblastoma, astrocytoma, ependymoma, and metastatic brain tumors), multiple myeloma, Hodgkin's disease (relapsed or refractory), non-Hodgkin's lymphomas (relapsed or refractory)

Wafer (implant): Adjunct to surgery in patients with recurrent glioblastoma multiforme; adjunct to surgery and radiation in patients with high-grade malignant glioma

Unlabeled/Investigational Use Melanoma

Pregnancy Risk Factor D

Pregnancy Considerations Teratogenicity and embryotoxicity have been demonstrated in animal studies. Carmustine can cause fetal harm if administered to a pregnant woman. There are no adequate and well-controlled studies in pregnant women. Women of child-bearing potential should avoid becoming pregnant while on treatment.

Lactation Excretion in breast milk unknown/not recommended

Medication Safety Issues

Sound-alike/look-alike issues:

Carmustine may be confused with bendamustine, lomustine

High alert medication: The Institute for Safe Medication Practices (ISMP) includes this medication among its list of drugs which have a heightened risk of causing significant patient harm when used in error.

Contraindications Hypersensitivity to carmustine or any component of the formulation

Warnings/Precautions Hazardous agent - use appropriate precautions for handling and disposal. **[U.S. Boxed Warning]: Bone marrow suppression (thrombocytopenia, leukopenia) is the major toxicity and may be delayed; monitor blood counts weekly for at least 6 weeks after administration. Myelosuppression is cumulative; consider nadir blood counts from prior dose for dosage adjustment. May cause bleeding (due to thrombocytopenia) or infections (due to neutropenia); monitor closely.** Administer with caution to patients with depressed platelet, leukocyte, or erythrocyte counts; renal or hepatic impairment. Diluent contains significant amounts of ethanol; use caution with aldehyde dehydrogenase-2 deficiency or history of "alcohol-flushing syndrome."

[U.S. Boxed Warning]: Dose-related pulmonary toxicity may occur; patients receiving cumulative doses >1400 mg/m^2 are at higher risk. Baseline pulmonary function tests are recommended. **[U.S. Boxed Warning]: Delayed onset of pulmonary fibrosis has occurred up to 17 years after treatment** in children (1-16 years) who received carmustine in cumulative doses ranging from 770-1800 mg/m^2 combined with cranial radiotherapy for intracranial tumors. **[U.S. Boxed Warning]: Should be administered under the supervision of an experienced cancer chemotherapy physician.** Long-term use may be associated with the development of secondary malignancies. Safety and efficacy in children have not been established.

Adverse Reactions

>10%:

Cardiovascular: Hypotension (with high-dose I.V. therapy, due to the alcohol content of the diluent)

Central nervous system: Ataxia, dizziness

Postoperatively: Seizure (wafer 5% to 54%), brain edema (wafer 4% to 23%)

Dermatologic: Burning (with skin contact), hyperpigmentation of skin (with skin contact)

Gastrointestinal: Severe nausea and vomiting, usually begins within 2-4 hours of drug administration and lasts for 4-6 hours; dose related. Patients should receive a prophylactic antiemetic regimen.

Hematologic: Myelosuppression (cumulative, dose related, delayed, and dose limiting), thrombocytopenia (onset: 28 days; recovery: 35-42 days), leukopenia (onset: 35-42 days; recovery: 42-56 days)

Hepatic: Reversible increases in bilirubin, alkaline phosphatase, and AST occur in 20% to 25% of patients

Local: Pain and burning at injection site, phlebitis

Neuromuscular & skeletal: Weakness (wafer 22%)

Ocular: Ocular toxicities (transient conjunctival flushing and blurred vision), retinal hemorrhages

Respiratory: Interstitial fibrosis occurs in up to 50% of patients receiving a cumulative dose >1400 mg/m^2, or bone marrow transplantation doses; may be delayed up to 3 years; rare in patients receiving lower doses. A history of lung disease or concomitant bleomycin therapy may increase the risk of this reaction. Patients with forced vital capacity (FVC) or carbon monoxide diffusing capacity of the lungs (DLCO) <70% of predicted are at higher risk.

Miscellaneous: Disease progression/performance deterioration (wafer 82%)

1% to 10%:

Cardiovascular: Chest pain, deep thrombophlebitis (wafer), facial edema (wafer), peripheral edema (wafer)

Central nervous system: Wafer: Amnesia, anxiety, aphasia, ataxia, brain abscess, confusion, convulsion, CSF leaks, depression, diplopia, dizziness, facial paralysis, headache, hemiplegia, hydrocephalus, hypoesthesia, insomnia, intracranial hypertension, meningitis, somnolence, speech disorder, stupor

Dermatologic: Facial flushing, probably due to the alcohol diluent; alopecia, rash (wafer), wound healing abnormal (wafer)

Gastrointestinal: Abdominal pain, anorexia, constipation, diarrhea, stomatitis

Hematologic: Anemia, hemorrhage (wafer)

Local: Abscess (wafer)

Neuromuscular & skeletal: Back pain

<1% (Limited to important or life-threatening): Allergic reaction, azotemia (progressive), cerebral hemorrhage infarction (wafer), cyst formation (wafer), dermatitis, hepatic coma, hyperpigmentation, hypotension, kidney size decreased, neuroretinitis, painless jaundice, renal failure, subacute hepatitis, tachycardia, thrombosis

Drug Interactions

Avoid Concomitant Use

Avoid concomitant use of Carmustine with any of the following: Natalizumab; Vaccines (Live)

Increased Effect/Toxicity

Carmustine may increase the levels/effects of: Natalizumab; Vaccines (Live)

The levels/effects of Carmustine may be increased by: Cimetidine; Trastuzumab

Decreased Effect

Carmustine may decrease the levels/effects of: Cardiac Glycosides; Vaccines (Inactivated)

The levels/effects of Carmustine may be decreased by: Echinacea

Ethanol/Nutrition/Herb Interactions Ethanol: Diluent for infusion contains ethanol; avoid concurrent use of medications that inhibit aldehyde dehydrogenase-2 or cause disulfiram-like reactions.

Stability

Injection: Store intact vials under refrigeration at 2°C to 8°C (36°F to 46°F); vials are stable for 36 days at room temperature. Initially, dilute with 3 mL of absolute alcohol. Further dilute with SWFI (27 mL) to a concentration of 3.3 mg/mL; protect from light; may further dilute with D_5W or NS, using a non-PVC container. Solutions are stable for 8 hours at room temperature (25°C) and 24 hours under refrigeration (2°C to 8°C) and protected from light. Further dilution in D_5W or NS is stable for 8 hours at room temperature (25°C) and 48 hours under refrigeration (4°C) in glass or polyolefin containers and protected from light.

Wafer: Store at or below -20°C (-4°F). Unopened foil pouches may be kept at room temperature for up to 6 hours.

Mechanism of Action Interferes with the normal function of DNA and RNA by alkylation and cross-linking the strands of DNA and RNA, and by possible protein modification; may also inhibit enzyme processes by carbamylation of amino acids in protein

Pharmacodynamics/Kinetics

Distribution: 3.3 L/kg; readily crosses blood-brain barrier producing CSF levels equal to >50% of blood plasma levels; highly lipid soluble

Metabolism: Rapidly hepatic; forms active metabolites

Half-life elimination: Biphasic: Initial: 1.4 minutes; Secondary: 20 minutes (active metabolites: plasma half-life of 67 hours)

Excretion: Urine (~60% to 70%) within 96 hours; lungs (6% to 10% as CO_2)

Dosage

I.V. (refer to individual protocols):

Children (unlabeled use): 200-250 mg/m^2 every 4-6 weeks as a single dose

Adults: Usual dosage (per manufacturer labeling): 150-200 mg/m^2 every 6 weeks **or** 75-100 mg/m^2/day for 2 days every 6 weeks

Alternative regimens (unlabeled):

75-120 mg/m^2 days 1 and 2 every 6-8 weeks **or**

50-80 mg/m^2 days 1,2,3 every 6-8 weeks

Primary brain cancer:

150-200 mg/m^2 every 6-8 weeks as a single dose **or**

75-120 mg/m^2 days 1 and 2 every 6-8 weeks **or**

20-65 mg/m^2 every 4-6 weeks **or**

0.5-1 mg/kg every 4-6 weeks **or**

40-80 mg/m^2/day for 3 days every 6-8 weeks

Autologous BMT: ALL OF THE FOLLOWING DOSES ARE FATAL WITHOUT BMT

Combination therapy: Up to 300-900 mg/m^2

Single-agent therapy: Up to 1200 mg/m^2 (fatal necrosis is associated with doses >2 g/m^2)

Implantation (wafer): Adults: Recurrent glioblastoma multiforme, malignant glioma: Up to 8 wafers may be placed in the resection cavity (total dose 62.6 mg); should the size and shape not accommodate 8 wafers, the maximum number of wafers allowed should be placed

Dosing adjustment in renal impairment: I.V.: The FDA-approved labeling does not contain renal dosing adjustment guidelines. The following dosage adjustments have been used by some clinicians (Kintzel, 1995):

Cl_{cr} 46-60 mL/minute: Administer 80% of dose

Cl_{cr} 31-45 mL/minute: Administer 75% of dose

Cl_{cr} ≤30 mL/minute: Consider use of alternative drug

Dosing adjustment in hepatic impairment: Dosage adjustment may be necessary; however, no specific guidelines are available.

Administration

Injection: Significant absorption to PVC containers - should be administered in either glass or polyolefin containers. I.V. infusion over 1-2 hours is recommended; infusion through a free-flowing saline or dextrose infusion, or administration through a central catheter can alleviate venous pain/irritation.

High-dose carmustine: Maximum rate of infusion of ≤3 mg/m^2/minute to avoid excessive flushing, agitation, and hypotension; infusions should run over at least 2 hours; some investigational protocols dictate shorter infusions. **(High-dose carmustine is fatal if not followed by bone marrow or peripheral stem cell infusions.)**

Extravasation management: Elevate extremity. Inject long-acting dexamethasone (Decadron® LA) or by hyaluronidase throughout tissue with a 25- to 37-gauge needle. Apply warm, moist compresses.

Implant: Use appropriate precautions for handling and disposal; double glove before handling; outer gloves should be discarded as chemotherapy waste after handling wafers. Any wafer or remnant that is removed upon repeat surgery should be discarded as chemotherapy waste. The outer surface of the external foil pouch is not sterile. Open pouch gently; avoid pressure on the wafers to prevent breakage. Wafer that are broken in half may be used, however, wafers broken into more than 2 pieces should be discarded. Oxidized regenerated cellulose (Surgicel®) may be placed over the wafer to secure; irrigate cavity prior to closure.

Monitoring Parameters CBC with differential and platelet count, pulmonary function, liver function, and renal function tests; monitor blood pressure during administration

Wafer: Complications of craniotomy (seizures, intracranial infection, brain edema)

Additional Information Accidental skin contact may cause transient burning and brown discoloration of the skin. Delayed onset pulmonary fibrosis occurring up to 17 years after treatment has been reported in patients who received cumulative doses >1400 mg/m^2.

Dosage Forms Excipient information presented when available (limited, particularly for generics); consult specific product labeling.

Implant:

Gliadel®: 7.7 mg (8s)

Injection, powder for reconstitution:

BiCNU®: 100 mg [packaged with 3 mL of absolute alcohol as diluent]

- ◆ **Carmustinum** *see* Carmustine *on page* 262
- ◆ **Carrington Antifungal [OTC]** *see* Miconazole *on page* 989
- ◆ **Carter's Little Pills® (Can)** *see* Bisacodyl *on page* 198
- ◆ **Cartia XT™** *see* Diltiazem *on page* 450

Carvedilol (KAR ve dil ole)

U.S. Brand Names Coreg CR®; Coreg®

Canadian Brand Names Apo-Carvedilol®; Coreg®; DOM-Carvedilol; Novo-Carvedilol; PHL-Carvedilol; PMS-Carvedilol; RAN™-Carvedilol; ratio-Carvedilol

Pharmacologic Category Beta Blocker With Alpha-Blocking Activity

Additional Appendix Information

Beta-Blockers *on page* 1648

Heart Failure (Systolic) *on page* 1809

Use Mild-to-severe heart failure of ischemic or cardiomyopathic origin (usually in addition to standard therapy); left ventricular dysfunction following myocardial infarction (MI) (clinically stable with LVEF ≤40%); management of hypertension

Unlabeled/Investigational Use Angina pectoris

Pregnancy Risk Factor C (manufacturer); D (2nd and 3rd trimesters - expert analysis)

Pregnancy Considerations Postimplantation losses were observed in animal studies. No data available on whether carvedilol crosses the placenta. Beta-blockers have been associated with persistent bradycardia, hypotension, and IUGR; IUGR probably related to maternal hypertension. Cases of neonatal hypoglycemia have been reported following maternal use of beta-blockers at parturition or during breast-feeding.

Lactation Excretion in breast milk unknown/not recommended

Medication Safety Issues

Sound-alike/look-alike issues:

Carvedilol may be confused with atenolol, captopril, carbidopa, carteolol

Coreg® may be confused with Corgard®, Cortef®, Cozaar®

International issues:

Talliton® [Hungary] may be confused with Talacen® which is a brand name for pentazocine/acetaminophen combination in the U.S.

Contraindications Serious hypersensitivity to carvedilol or any component of the formulation; decompensated cardiac failure requiring intravenous inotropic therapy; bronchial asthma or related bronchospastic conditions; second- or third-degree AV block, sick sinus syndrome, and severe bradycardia (except in patients with a functioning artificial pacemaker); cardiogenic shock; severe hepatic impairment

Warnings/Precautions Consider pre-existing conditions such as sick sinus syndrome before initiating. Heart failure patients may experience a worsening of renal function (rare); risk factors include ischemic heart disease, diffuse vascular disease, underlying renal dysfunction, and systolic BP <100 mm Hg. Initiate cautiously and monitor for possible deterioration in patient status (eg, symptoms of HF). Worsening heart failure or fluid retention may occur during upward titration; dose reduction or temporary discontinuation may be necessary. Adjustment of other medications (ACE inhibitors and/or diuretics) may also be required.

Symptomatic hypotension with or without syncope may occur with carvedilol (usually within the first 30 days of therapy); close monitoring of patient is required especially with initial dosing and dosing increases; blood pressure must be lowered at a rate appropriate for the patient's clinical condition. Initiation with a low dose, gradual up-titration, and administration with food may help to decrease the occurrence of hypotension or syncope. Patients should be advised to avoid driving or other hazardous tasks during initiation of therapy due to the risk of syncope. Beta-blocker therapy should not be withdrawn abruptly (particularly in patients with CAD), but gradually tapered to avoid acute tachycardia, hypertension, and/or ischemia.

In general, patients with bronchospastic disease should not receive beta-blockers; if used at all, should be used cautiously with close monitoring. May precipitate or aggravate symptoms of arterial insufficiency in patients with PVD and Raynaud's disease; use with caution and monitor for progression of arterial obstruction. Use caution with concurrent use of verapamil or diltiazem; bradycardia or heart block can occur. Use cautiously in patients with diabetes because it can mask prominent hypoglycemic symptoms. May mask signs of hyperthyroidism (eg, tachycardia); if hyperthyroidism is suspected, carefully manage and monitor; abrupt withdrawal may exacerbate symptoms of hyperthyroidism or precipitate thyroid storm. Use with caution in patients with myasthenia gravis or psychiatric disease (may cause CNS depression). Use with caution in patients with mild-to-moderate hepatic impairment; use is contraindicated in patients with severe impairment. Manufacturer recommends discontinuation of therapy if liver injury occurs (confirmed by laboratory testing). Adequate alpha-blockade is required prior to use of any beta-blocker for patients with untreated pheochromocytoma. Use caution with history of severe anaphylaxis to allergens; patients taking beta-blockers may become more sensitive to repeated challenges. Treatment of anaphylaxis (eg, epinephrine) in patients taking beta-blockers may be ineffective or promote undesirable effects. Use care with anesthetic agents that decrease myocardial function. Safety and efficacy in children <18 years of age have not been established.

Adverse Reactions Note: Frequency ranges include data from hypertension and heart failure trials. Higher rates of adverse reactions have generally been noted in patients with heart failure. However, the frequency of adverse effects associated with placebo is also increased in this population.

>10%:

Cardiovascular: Hypotension (9% to 20%)

Central nervous system: Dizziness (2% to 32%), fatigue (4% to 24%)

Endocrine & metabolic: Hyperglycemia (5% to 12%)

Gastrointestinal: Diarrhea (1% to 12%), weight gain (10% to 12%)

Neuromuscular & skeletal: Weakness (7% to 11%)

1% to 10%:

Cardiovascular: Bradycardia (2% to 10%), syncope (3% to 8%), peripheral edema (1% to 7%), generalized edema (5% to 6%), angina (1% to 6%), dependent edema (≤4%), AV block, cerebrovascular accident, hypertension, hyper-/hypovolemia, postural hypotension, palpitation

Central nervous system: Headache (5% to 8%), depression, fever, hypoesthesia, hypotonia, insomnia, malaise, somnolence, vertigo

Endocrine & metabolic: Hypercholesterolemia (1% to 4%), hypertriglyceridemia (1%), diabetes mellitus, gout, hyperkalemia, hyperuricemia, hypoglycemia, hyponatremia

Gastrointestinal: Nausea (2% to 9%), vomiting (1% to 6%), abdominal pain, melena, periodontitis, weight loss

Genitourinary: Impotence

Hematologic: Anemia, prothrombin decreased, purpura, thrombocytopenia

Hepatic: Alkaline phosphatase increased (1% to 3%), GGT increased, transaminases increased

Neuromuscular & skeletal: Back pain (2% to 7%), arthralgia (1% to 6%), arthritis, muscle cramps, paresthesia

Ocular: Blurred vision (1% to 5%)

Renal: BUN increased (≤6%), nonprotein nitrogen increased (6%), albuminuria, creatinine increased, glycosuria, hematuria, renal insufficiency

Respiratory: Cough (5% to 8%), nasopharyngitis (4%), rales (4%), dyspnea (>3%), pulmonary edema (>3%), rhinitis (2%), nasal congestion (1%), sinus congestion (1%)

Miscellaneous: Injury (3% to 6%), allergy, flu-like syndrome, sudden death

<1% (Limited to important or life-threatening): Anaphylactoid reaction, alopecia, aplastic anemia (rare, all events occurred in patients receiving other medications capable of causing this effect), amnesia, asthma, bronchospasm, bundle branch block, cholestatic jaundice, concentration decreased, diaphoresis, erythema multiforme, exfoliative dermatitis, GI hemorrhage, HDL decreased, hearing decreased, hyperbilirubinemia, hypokalemia, hypokinesia, interstitial pneumonitis, leukopenia, libido decreased, migraine, myocardial ischemia, nervousness, neuralgia, nightmares, pancytopenia, paresis, peripheral ischemia, photosensitivity, pruritus, rash (erythematous, maculopapular, and psoriaform), respiratory alkalosis, seizure, Stevens-Johnson syndrome, tachycardia, tinnitus, toxic epidermal necrolysis, urinary incontinence, xerostomia

Drug Interactions

Metabolism/Transport Effects Substrate of CYP1A2 (minor), 2C9 (major), 2D6 (major), 2E1 (minor), 3A4 (minor)

Avoid Concomitant Use

Avoid concomitant use of Carvedilol with any of the following: Dabigatran Etexilate; Methacholine; Rivaroxaban; Topotecan

Increased Effect/Toxicity

Carvedilol may increase the levels/effects of: Alpha-/Beta-Agonists (Direct-Acting); Alpha1-Blockers; Alpha2-Agonists; Amifostine; Antipsychotic Agents (Phenothiazines); Cardiac Glycosides; CycloSPORINE; Dabigatran Etexilate; Digoxin; Insulin; Lidocaine; Methacholine; Midodrine; P-Glycoprotein Substrates; RiTUXimab; Rivaroxaban; Topotecan

The levels/effects of Carvedilol may be increased by: Acetylcholinesterase Inhibitors; Aminoquinolines (Antimalarial); Amiodarone; Anilidopiperidine Opioids; Antipsychotic Agents (Phenothiazines); Calcium Channel Blockers (Nondihydropyridine); Cimetidine; CYP2D6 Inhibitors (Moderate); CYP2D6 Inhibitors (Strong); Darunavir; Diazoxide; Dipyridamole; Disopyramide; Herbs (Hypotensive Properties); P-Glycoprotein Inhibitors; Propafenone; Propoxyphene; Prostacyclin Analogues; QuiNIDine; Reserpine; Selective Serotonin Reuptake Inhibitors

Decreased Effect

Carvedilol may decrease the levels/effects of: Beta2-Agonists; Theophylline Derivatives

The levels/effects of Carvedilol may be decreased by: Barbiturates; Herbs (Hypertensive Properties); Methylphenidate; Nonsteroidal Anti-Inflammatory Agents; P-Glycoprotein Inducers; Rifamycin Derivatives; Yohimbine

Ethanol/Nutrition/Herb Interactions

Food: Food decreases rate but not extent of absorption. Administration with food minimizes risks of orthostatic hypotension.

Herb/Nutraceutical: Avoid herbs with hypertensive properties (bayberry, blue cohosh, cayenne, ephedra, ginger, ginseng [American], kola, licorice); may diminish the antihypertensive effect of carvedilol. Avoid herbs with hypotensive properties (black cohosh, California poppy, coleus, golden seal, hawthorn, mistletoe, periwinkle, quinine, shepherd's purse); may enhance the hypotensive effect of carvedilol.

Stability

Coreg®: Store at <30°C (<86°F). Protect from moisture.

Coreg CR®: Store at 25°C (77°F); excursions permitted to 15°C to 30°C (59°F to 86°F).

Mechanism of Action As a racemic mixture, carvedilol has nonselective beta-adrenoreceptor and alpha-adrenergic blocking activity. No intrinsic sympathomimetic activity has been documented. Associated effects in hypertensive patients include reduction of cardiac output, exercise- or beta-agonist-induced tachycardia, reduction of reflex orthostatic tachycardia, vasodilation, decreased peripheral vascular resistance (especially in standing position), decreased renal vascular resistance, reduced plasma renin activity, and increased levels of atrial natriuretic peptide. In CHF, associated effects include decreased pulmonary capillary wedge pressure, decreased pulmonary artery pressure, decreased heart rate, decreased systemic vascular resistance, increased stroke volume index, and decreased right arterial pressure (RAP).

Pharmacodynamics/Kinetics

Onset of action: 1-2 hours

Peak antihypertensive effect: ~1-2 hours

Absorption: Rapid and extensive

Distribution: V_d: 115 L

Protein binding: >98%, primarily to albumin

Metabolism: Extensively hepatic, via CYP2C9, 2D6, 3A4, and 2C19 (2% excreted unchanged); three active metabolites (4-hydroxyphenyl metabolite is 13 times more potent than parent drug for beta-blockade); first-pass effect; plasma concentrations in the elderly and those with cirrhotic liver disease are 50% and 4-7 times higher, respectively

Bioavailability: Immediate release: 25% to 35% (due to significant first-pass metabolism); Extended release: 85% of immediate release

Half-life elimination: 7-10 hours

Time to peak, plasma: Extended release: 5 hours

Excretion: Primarily feces

Dosage Oral: Adults: Reduce dosage if heart rate drops to <55 beats/minute.

Hypertension:

Immediate release: 6.25 mg twice daily; if tolerated, dose should be maintained for 1-2 weeks, then increased to 12.5 mg twice daily. If necessary, dosage may be increased to a maximum of 25 mg twice daily after 1-2 weeks.

Extended release: Initial: 20 mg once daily, if tolerated, dose should be maintained for 1-2 weeks then increased to 40 mg once daily if necessary; maximum dose: 80 mg once daily

Heart failure:

Immediate release: 3.125 mg twice daily for 2 weeks; if this dose is tolerated, may increase to 6.25 mg twice daily. Double the dose every 2 weeks to the highest dose tolerated by patient. (Prior to initiating therapy, other heart failure medications should be stabilized and fluid retention minimized.)

Maximum recommended dose:

Mild-to-moderate heart failure:

<85 kg: 25 mg twice daily

>85 kg: 50 mg twice daily

Severe heart failure: 25 mg twice daily

Extended release: Initial: 10 mg once daily for 2 weeks; if the dose is tolerated, increase dose to 20 mg, 40 mg, and 80 mg over successive intervals of at least 2 weeks. Maintain on lower dose if higher dose is not tolerated.

Left ventricular dysfunction following MI: **Note**: Should be initiated only after patient is hemodynamically stable and fluid retention has been minimized.

Immediate release: Initial 3.125-6.25 mg twice daily; increase dosage incrementally (ie, from 6.25-12.5 mg twice daily) at intervals of 3-10 days, based on tolerance, to a target dose of 25 mg twice daily.

Extended release: Initial: 10-20 mg once daily; increase dosage incrementally at intervals of 3-10 days, based on tolerance, to a target dose of 80 mg once daily.

Angina pectoris (unlabeled use): Immediate release: 25-50 mg twice daily

Conversion from immediate release to extended release (Coreg CR®):

Current dose immediate release tablets 3.125 mg twice daily: Convert to extended release capsules 10 mg once daily

Current dose immediate release tablets 6.25 mg twice daily: Convert to extended release capsules 20 mg once daily

Current dose immediate release tablets 12.5 mg twice daily: Convert to extended release capsules 40 mg once daily

Current dose immediate release tablets 25 mg twice daily: Convert to extended release capsules 80 mg once daily

Dosing adjustment in renal impairment: None necessary

Dosing adjustment in hepatic impairment: Use is contraindicated in severe liver dysfunction.

Dietary Considerations Should be taken with food to minimize the risk of orthostatic hypotension.

Administration Administer with food. Extended release capsules should not be crushed or chewed. Capsules may be opened and sprinkled on applesauce for immediate use.

Monitoring Parameters Heart rate, blood pressure (base need for dosage increase on trough blood pressure measurements and for tolerance on standing systolic pressure 1 hour after dosing); renal studies, BUN, liver function; in patient with increase risk for developing renal dysfunction, monitor during dosage titration.

Additional Information Fluid retention during therapy should be treated with an increase in diuretic dosage.

Dosage Forms Excipient information presented when available (limited, particularly for generics); consult specific product labeling.

Capsule, extended release; as phosphate:

Coreg CR®: 10 mg, 20 mg, 40 mg, 80 mg

Tablet: 3.125 mg, 6.25 mg, 12.5 mg, 25 mg

Coreg®: 3.125 mg, 6.25 mg, 12.5 mg, 25 mg

◆ **Casodex®** *see* Bicalutamide *on page 197*

Caspofungin (kas poe FUN jin)

U.S. Brand Names Cancidas®

Canadian Brand Names Cancidas®

Index Terms Caspofungin Acetate

Pharmacologic Category Antifungal Agent, Parenteral; Echinocandin

Additional Appendix Information

Antifungal Agents *on page 1640*

Use Treatment of invasive *Aspergillus* infections in patients who are refractory or intolerant of other therapy; treatment of candidemia and other *Candida* infections (intra-abdominal abscesses, esophageal, peritonitis, pleural space); empirical treatment for presumed fungal infections in febrile neutropenic patient

Pregnancy Risk Factor C

Pregnancy Considerations Adverse events have been observed in animal studies. There are no adequate and well-controlled studies in pregnant women. Should be used during pregnancy only if potential benefit justifies the potential risk to the fetus.

Lactation Excretion in breast milk unknown/use caution

Contraindications Hypersensitivity to caspofungin or any component of the formulation

Warnings/Precautions Concurrent use of cyclosporine should be limited to patients for whom benefit outweighs risk, due to a high frequency of hepatic transaminase elevations observed during concurrent use. Limited data are available concerning treatment durations longer than 4 weeks, however, treatment appears to be well tolerated. Use caution in hepatic impairment; dosage reduction required with moderate impairment. Safety and efficacy have not been established in children <3 months of age.

Adverse Reactions

>10%:

Cardiovascular: Hypotension (6% to 20%), peripheral edema (6% to 11%), tachycardia (4% to 11%)

Central nervous system: Fever (13% to 30%), chills (8% to 23%), headache (5% to 15%)

Dermatologic: Rash (4% to 23%)

Endocrine & metabolic: Hypokalemia (5% to 23%)

Gastrointestinal: Diarrhea (7% to 27%), vomiting (7% to 17%), nausea (4% to 15%)

Hematologic: Hemoglobin decreased (5% to 21%), hematocrit decreased (13% to 18%), WBC decreased (12%), anemia (2% to 11%)

Hepatic: Serum alkaline phosphatase increased (13% to 22%), transaminases increased (2% to 18%), bilirubin increased (5% to 13%)

Local: Phlebitis/thrombophlebitis (18%)

Renal: Serum creatinine increased (3% to 11%), urinary RBCs increased (10%)

Respiratory: Respiratory failure (11% to 20%), cough (6% to 11%), pneumonia (4% to 11%)

Miscellaneous: Infusion reactions (20% to 35%), septic shock (11%)

1% to 10%:

Cardiovascular: Hypertension (children 9% to 10%), edema (3% to 4%)

Dermatologic: Erythema (4% to 9%), pruritus (5% to 7%)

Endocrine & metabolic: Hypomagnesemia (7%), hyperglycemia (6%), hyperkalemia (3%)

Gastrointestinal: Mucosal inflammation (4% to 10%), abdominal pain (4% to 9%)

Hepatic: Albumin decreased (7%)

Local: Infection (1% to 9%, central line)

Neuromuscular & skeletal: Back pain (children up to 4%)

Renal: Nephrotoxicity (13%), blood urea nitrogen increased (4% to 9%)

Note: Nephrotoxicity defined as serum creatinine ≥2x baseline value or ≥1 mg/dL in patients with serum creatinine above ULN range (patients with Cl_{cr} <30 mL/minute were excluded)

Respiratory: Dyspnea (9%), pleural effusion (9%), respiratory distress (children up to 8%), rales (7%), tachypnea (1%)

<1% (Limited to important or life-threatening): Abdominal distention, anaphylaxis, anorexia, anxiety, appetite decrease, arrhythmia, arthralgia, atrial fibrillation, bradycardia, coagulopathy, confusion, constipation, depression, dizziness, dyspepsia, dystonia, epistaxis, erythema multiforme, fatigue, febrile neutropenia, fluid overload, flushing, hematuria, hepatic necrosis, hepatomegaly, hepatotoxicity, hypercalcemia, hypoxia, infusion site reactions (pain/pruritus/swelling), insomnia, jaundice, liver failure, MI, pain (extremities), pancreatitis, petechiae, pulmonary edema, renal failure/insufficiency, seizure, skin exfoliation, skin lesion, somnolence, stridor, Stevens-Johnson syndrome, tachypnea, thrombocytopenia, tremor, urinary tract infection, urticaria, weakness; histamine-mediated reactions (including facial swelling, bronchospasm, sensation of warmth) have been reported

Drug Interactions

Avoid Concomitant Use There are no known interactions where it is recommended to avoid concomitant use.

Increased Effect/Toxicity

The levels/effects of Caspofungin may be increased by: CycloSPORINE

Decreased Effect

Caspofungin may decrease the levels/effects of: Saccharomyces boulardii; Tacrolimus

The levels/effects of Caspofungin may be decreased by: Inducers of Drug Clearance; Rifampin

Stability Store vials at 2°C to 8°C (36°F to 46°F). Reconstituted solution may be stored at ≤25°C (≤77°F) for 1 hour prior to preparation of infusion solution. Infusion solutions may be stored at ≤25°C (≤77°F) and should be used within 24 hours; up to 48 hours if stored at 2°C to 8°C (36°F to 46°F).

Bring refrigerated vial to room temperature. Reconstitute vials using 0.9% sodium chloride for injection, SWFI, or bacteriostatic water for injection. Mix gently until clear solution is formed; do not use if cloudy or contains particles. Solution should be further diluted with 0.9%, 0.45%, or 0.225% sodium chloride or LR (do not exceed final concentration of 0.5 mg/mL).

Mechanism of Action Inhibits synthesis of β(1,3)-D-glucan, an essential component of the cell wall of susceptible fungi. Highest activity in regions of active cell growth. Mammalian cells do not require β(1,3)-D-glucan, limiting potential toxicity.

Pharmacodynamics/Kinetics

Protein binding: ~97% to albumin

Metabolism: Slowly, via hydrolysis and *N*-acetylation as well as by spontaneous degradation, with subsequent metabolism to component amino acids. Overall metabolism is extensive.

Half-life elimination: Beta (distribution): 9-11 hours; Terminal: 40-50 hours

Excretion: Urine (41% as metabolites, 1% to 9% unchanged) and feces (35% as metabolites)

Dosage I.V.:

Children: 3 months to 17 years: Initial dose: 70 mg/m^2 on day 1, subsequent dosing: 50 mg/m^2 once daily, if clinical response inadequate, may increase to 70 mg/m^2 once daily if tolerated, but increased efficacy not demonstrated (maximum dose: 70 mg/day)

Adults: **Note:** Duration of caspofungin treatment should be determined by patient status and clinical response. Empiric therapy should be given until neutropenia resolves. In patients with positive cultures, treatment should continue until 14 days after last positive culture. In neutropenic patients, treatment should be given at least 7 days after both signs and symptoms of infection **and** neutropenia resolve.

Aspergillosis, invasive: Initial dose: 70 mg on day 1; subsequent dosing: 50 mg/day. If clinical response inadequate, may increase up to 70 mg/day if tolerated, but increased efficacy not demonstrated. **Note:** Duration of therapy should be a minimum of 6-12 weeks or throughout period of immunosuppression.

Candidiasis: Initial dose: 70 mg on day 1; subsequent dosing: 50 mg/day

Esophageal: 50 mg/day; **Note:** The majority of patients studied for this indication also had oropharyngeal involvement.

Empiric therapy: Initial dose: 70 mg on day 1; subsequent dosing: 50 mg/day; if clinical response inadequate, may increase up to 70 mg/day if tolerated, but increased efficacy not demonstrated

Concomitant use of an enzyme inducer:

Children: Patients receiving carbamazepine, dexamethasone, efavirenz, nevirapine, phenytoin, or rifampin (and possibly other enzyme inducers): Consider 70 mg/m^2 once daily (maximum: 70 mg/day)

Adults:

Patients receiving rifampin: 70 mg caspofungin daily

Patients receiving carbamazepine, dexamethasone, efavirenz, nevirapine, **or** phenytoin (and possibly other enzyme inducers) may require an increased daily dose of caspofungin (70 mg/day).

Elderly: The number of patients >65 years of age in clinical studies was not sufficient to establish whether a difference in response may be anticipated.

Dosage adjustment in renal impairment: No specific dosage adjustment is required; supplemental dose is not required following dialysis

Dosage adjustment in hepatic impairment:

Children: Mild-to-severe hepatic insufficiency: No clinical experience

Adults:

Mild hepatic insufficiency (Child-Pugh score 5-6): No adjustment necessary

Moderate hepatic insufficiency (Child-Pugh score 7-9): 35 mg/day; initial 70 mg loading dose should still be administered in treatment of invasive infections

Severe hepatic insufficiency (Child-Pugh score >9): No clinical experience

Administration Infuse slowly, over 1 hour; monitor during infusion. Isolated cases of possible histamine-related reactions have occurred during clinical trials (rash, flushing, pruritus, facial edema).

Monitoring Parameters Liver function

Dosage Forms Excipient information presented when available (limited, particularly for generics); consult specific product labeling.

Injection, powder for reconstitution, as acetate:

Cancidas®: 50 mg [contains sucrose 39 mg], 70 mg [contains sucrose 54 mg]

- ◆ **Caspofungin Acetate** *see* Caspofungin *on page* 266
- ◆ **Castor Oil, Trypsin, and Balsam Peru** *see* Trypsin, Balsam Peru, and Castor Oil *on page* 1526
- ◆ **Cataflam®** *see* Diclofenac *on page* 437
- ◆ **Catapres®** *see* CloNIDine *on page* 354
- ◆ **Catapres-TTS®** *see* CloNIDine *on page* 354
- ◆ **Cathflo® Activase®** *see* Alteplase *on page* 72
- ◆ **Caverject®** *see* Alprostadil *on page* 70
- ◆ **Caverject Impulse®** *see* Alprostadil *on page* 70
- ◆ **CaviRinse™** *see* Fluoride *on page* 635
- ◆ **CB-1348** *see* Chlorambucil *on page* 301
- ◆ **CBDCA** *see* CARBOplatin *on page* 258
- ◆ **CBZ** *see* CarBAMazepine *on page* 252
- ◆ **CC-5013** *see* Lenalidomide *on page* 861
- ◆ **CCI-779** *see* Temsirolimus *on page* 1434
- ◆ **CCNU** *see* Lomustine *on page* 899
- ◆ **2-CdA** *see* Cladribine *on page* 339

- **CDDP** *see* CISplatin *on page* 335
- **CDP870** *see* Certolizumab Pegol *on page* 293
- **CDX** *see* Bicalutamide *on page* 197
- **CE** *see* Estrogens (Conjugated/Equine) *on page* 563
- **Ceclor® (Can)** *see* Cefaclor *on page* 268
- **Cecon® [OTC]** *see* Ascorbic Acid *on page* 139
- **Cedax®** *see* Ceftibuten *on page* 283
- **Cedocard®-SR (Can)** *see* Isosorbide Dinitrate *on page* 823
- **CEE** *see* Estrogens (Conjugated/Equine) *on page* 563
- **CeeNU®** *see* Lomustine *on page* 899

Cefaclor (SEF a klor)

U.S. Brand Names Raniclor™

Canadian Brand Names Apo-Cefaclor®; Ceclor®; Novo-Cefaclor; Nu-Cefaclor; PMS-Cefaclor

Pharmacologic Category Antibiotic, Cephalosporin (Second Generation)

Additional Appendix Information

Antimicrobial Drugs of Choice *on page* 1752

Use Treatment of susceptible bacterial infections including otitis media, lower respiratory tract infections, acute exacerbations of chronic bronchitis, pharyngitis and tonsillitis, urinary tract infections, skin and skin structure infections

Pregnancy Risk Factor B

Pregnancy Considerations Adverse events were not observed in animal reproduction studies; therefore, cefaclor is classified as pregnancy category B. It is not known if cefaclor crosses the placenta; other cephalosporins cross the placenta and are considered safe for use during pregnancy. An increased risk of teratogenic effects has not been observed following maternal use of cefaclor.

Lactation Enters breast milk/use caution

Medication Safety Issues

Sound-alike/look-alike issues:

Cefaclor may be confused with cephalexin

Contraindications Hypersensitivity to cefaclor, any component of the formulation, or other cephalosporins

Warnings/Precautions Modify dosage in patients with severe renal impairment. Prolonged use may result in fungal or bacterial superinfection, including *C. difficile*-associated diarrhea (CDAD) and pseudomembranous colitis; CDAD has been observed >2 months postantibiotic treatment. Use with caution in patients with a history of penicillin allergy, especially IgE-mediated reactions (eg, anaphylaxis, urticaria). Beta-lactamase-negative, ampicillin-resistant (BLNAR) strains of *H. influenzae* should be considered resistant to cefaclor. Extended release tablets are not approved for use in children <16 years of age. Some products may contain phenylalanine.

Adverse Reactions

1% to 10%:

Dermatologic: Rash (maculopapular, erythematous, or morbilliform) (1% to 2%)

Gastrointestinal: Diarrhea (3%)

Genitourinary: Vaginitis (2%)

Hematologic: Eosinophilia (2%)

Hepatic: Transaminases increased (3%)

Miscellaneous: Moniliasis (2%)

<1% (Limited to important or life-threatening): Agitation, agranulocytosis, anaphylaxis, angioedema, aplastic anemia, arthralgia, cholestatic jaundice, CNS irritability, confusion, dizziness, hallucinations, hemolytic anemia, hepatitis, hyperactivity, insomnia, interstitial nephritis, nausea, nervousness, neutropenia, paresthesia, PT prolonged, pruritus, pseudomembranous colitis, seizure, serum-sickness, somnolence, Stevens-Johnson syndrome, thrombocytopenia, toxic epidermal necrolysis, urticaria, vomiting

Reactions reported with other cephalosporins: Abdominal pain, cholestasis, fever, hemorrhage, renal dysfunction, superinfection, toxic nephropathy

Drug Interactions

Avoid Concomitant Use There are no known interactions where it is recommended to avoid concomitant use.

Increased Effect/Toxicity

The levels/effects of Cefaclor may be increased by: Uricosuric Agents

Decreased Effect

Cefaclor may decrease the levels/effects of: Typhoid Vaccine

Ethanol/Nutrition/Herb Interactions

Food: Cefaclor serum levels may be decreased slightly if taken with food. The bioavailability of cefaclor extended release tablets is decreased 23% and the maximum concentration is decreased 67% when taken on an empty stomach.

Stability Store at controlled room temperature. Refrigerate suspension after reconstitution. Discard after 14 days. Do not freeze.

Mechanism of Action Inhibits bacterial cell wall synthesis by binding to one or more of the penicillin-binding proteins (PBPs) which in turn inhibits the final transpeptidation step of peptidoglycan synthesis in bacterial cell walls, thus inhibiting cell wall biosynthesis. Bacteria eventually lyse due to ongoing activity of cell wall autolytic enzymes (autolysins and murein hydrolases) while cell wall assembly is arrested.

Pharmacodynamics/Kinetics

Absorption: Well absorbed, acid stable

Distribution: Widely throughout the body and reaches therapeutic concentration in most tissues and body fluids, including synovial, pericardial, pleural, peritoneal fluids; bile, sputum, and urine; bone, myocardium, gallbladder, skin and soft tissue

Protein binding: 25%

Metabolism: Partially hepatic

Half-life elimination: 0.5-1 hour; prolonged with renal impairment

Time to peak: Capsule: 60 minutes; Suspension: 45 minutes

Excretion: Urine (80% as unchanged drug)

Dosage

Usual dosage range:

Children >1 month: Oral: 20-40 mg/kg/day divided every 8-12 hours (maximum dose: 1 g/day)

Adults: Oral: 250-500 mg every 8 hours

Indication-specific dosing:

Children: Oral:

Otitis media: 40 mg/kg/day divided every 12 hours

Pharyngitis: 20 mg/kg/day divided every 12 hours

Dosing adjustment in renal impairment:

Cl_{cr} 10-50 mL/minute: Administer 50% to 100% of dose

Cl_{cr} <10 mL/minute: Administer 50% of dose

Hemodialysis: Moderately dialyzable (20% to 50%)

Dietary Considerations Capsule, chewable tablet, and suspension may be taken with or without food. Raniclor™ contains phenylalanine 2.8 mg/cefaclor 125 mg.

Administration Administer around-the-clock to promote less variation in peak and trough serum levels.

Chewable tablet: Should be chewed before swallowing; should not be swallowed whole.

Oral suspension: Shake well before using.

Monitoring Parameters Assess patient at beginning and throughout therapy for infection; monitor for signs of anaphylaxis during first dose

Test Interactions Positive direct Coombs', false-positive urinary glucose test using cupric sulfate (Benedict's solution, Clinitest®, Fehling's solution), false-positive serum or urine creatinine with Jaffé reaction

Dosage Forms Excipient information presented when available (limited, particularly for generics); consult specific product labeling.

Capsule: 250 mg, 500 mg

Powder for oral suspension: 125 mg/5 mL (75 mL, 150 mL); 250 mg/5 mL (75 mL, 150 mL); 375 mg/5 mL (50 mL, 100 mL)

Tablet, chewable:

Raniclor™: 250 mg [contains phenylalanine 5.6 mg/tablet and tartrazine; fruity flavor]; 375 mg [contains phenylalanine 8.4 mg/tablet and tartrazine; fruity flavor]

Tablet, extended release: 500 mg

Cefadroxil (sef a DROKS il)

U.S. Brand Names Duricef® [DSC]

Canadian Brand Names Apo-Cefadroxil®; Duricef®; Novo-Cefadroxil; Pro-Cefadroxil

Index Terms Cefadroxil Monohydrate

Pharmacologic Category Antibiotic, Cephalosporin (First Generation)

Use Treatment of susceptible bacterial infections, including those caused by group A beta-hemolytic *Streptococcus*

Pregnancy Risk Factor B

Pregnancy Considerations Adverse events were not observed in animal reproduction studies; therefore, cefadroxil is classified as pregnancy category B. Cefadroxil crosses the placenta. Limited data is available concerning the use of cefadroxil in pregnancy; however, adverse fetal effects were not noted in a small clinical trial. Adequate and well-controlled studies have been not completed in pregnant women.

Lactation Enters breast milk (small amounts)/use caution (AAP rates "compatible")

Contraindications Hypersensitivity to cefadroxil, any component of the formulation, or other cephalosporins

Warnings/Precautions Modify dosage in patients with severe renal impairment. Use with caution in patients with a history of penicillin allergy, especially IgE-mediated reactions (eg, anaphylaxis, angioedema, urticaria). Prolonged use may result in fungal or bacterial superinfection, including *C. difficile*-associated diarrhea (CDAD) and pseudomembranous colitis; CDAD has been observed >2 months postantibiotic treatment.

Adverse Reactions

1% to 10%: Gastrointestinal: Diarrhea

<1% (Limited to important or life-threatening): Abdominal pain, agranulocytosis, anaphylaxis, angioedema, arthralgia, cholestasis, dyspepsia, erythema multiforme, fever, nausea, neutropenia, pruritus, pseudomembranous colitis, rash (maculopapular and erythematous), serum sickness, Stevens-Johnson syndrome, thrombocytopenia, transaminases increased, urticaria, vaginitis, vomiting

Reactions reported with other cephalosporins: Abdominal pain, aplastic anemia, BUN increased, creatinine increased, eosinophilia, hemolytic anemia, hemorrhage, pancytopenia, prothrombin time prolonged, renal dysfunction, seizure, superinfection, toxic epidermal necrolysis, toxic nephropathy

Drug Interactions

Avoid Concomitant Use There are no known interactions where it is recommended to avoid concomitant use.

Increased Effect/Toxicity

The levels/effects of Cefadroxil may be increased by: Uricosuric Agents

Decreased Effect

Cefadroxil may decrease the levels/effects of: Typhoid Vaccine

Ethanol/Nutrition/Herb Interactions Food: Concomitant administration with food, infant formula, or cow's milk does **not** significantly affect absorption.

Stability Refrigerate suspension after reconstitution; discard after 14 days.

Mechanism of Action Inhibits bacterial cell wall synthesis by binding to one or more of the penicillin-binding proteins (PBPs) which in turn inhibits the final transpeptidation step of peptidoglycan synthesis in bacterial cell walls, thus inhibiting cell wall biosynthesis. Bacteria eventually lyse due to ongoing activity of cell wall autolytic enzymes (autolysins and murein hydrolases) while cell wall assembly is arrested.

Pharmacodynamics/Kinetics

Absorption: Rapid and well absorbed

Distribution: Widely throughout the body and reaches therapeutic concentrations in most tissues and body fluids, including synovial, pericardial, pleural, and peritoneal fluids; bile, sputum, and urine; bone, myocardium, gallbladder, skin, and soft tissue

Protein binding: 20%

Half-life elimination: 1-2 hours; Renal failure: 20-24 hours

Time to peak, serum: 70-90 minutes

Excretion: Urine (>90% as unchanged drug)

Dosage

Usual dosage range: Oral:

Children: 30 mg/kg/day divided twice daily up to a maximum of 2 g/day

Adults: 1-2 g/day in 2 divided doses

Indication-specific dosing: Orofacial infections: Adults: 250-500 mg every 8 hours

Dosing interval in renal impairment:

Cl_{cr} 10-25 mL/minute: Administer every 24 hours

Cl_{cr} <10 mL/minute: Administer every 36 hours

Administration Administer around-the-clock to promote less variation in peak and trough serum levels.

Monitoring Parameters Observe for signs and symptoms of anaphylaxis during first dose.

Test Interactions Positive direct Coombs', false-positive urinary glucose test using cupric sulfate (Benedict's solution, Clinitest®, Fehling's solution), false-positive serum or urine creatinine with Jaffé reaction

Dosage Forms Excipient information presented when available (limited, particularly for generics); consult specific product labeling. [DSC] = Discontinued product

Note: Strength is expressed as base

Capsule, as hemihydrate: 500 mg

Capsule, as monohydrate: 500 mg

Powder for oral suspension, as monohydrate: 250 mg/5 mL (100 mL); 500 mg/5 mL (75 mL, 100 mL)

Duricef®: 250 mg/5 mL (50 mL, 100 mL) [DSC]; 500 mg/5 mL (75 mL, 100 mL) [contains sodium benzoate; orange-pineapple flavor] [DSC]

Tablet, as hemihydrate: 1 g

Tablet, as monohydrate: 1 g

◆ **Cefadroxil Monohydrate** *see* Cefadroxil *on page 269*

CeFAZolin (sef A zoe lin)

Index Terms Ancef; Cefazolin Sodium

Pharmacologic Category Antibiotic, Cephalosporin (First Generation)

Additional Appendix Information

Animal and Human Bites *on page 1747*

Antibiotic Treatment of Adults With Infective Endocarditis *on page 1748*

Prevention of Infective Endocarditis *on page 1736*

Prevention of Wound Infection and Sepsis in Surgical Patients *on page 1738*

Use Treatment of respiratory tract, skin and skin structure, genital, urinary tract, biliary tract, bone and joint infections, and septicemia due to susceptible gram-positive cocci (except enterococcus); some gram-negative bacilli including *E. coli*, *Proteus*, and *Klebsiella* may be susceptible; perioperative prophylaxis

Unlabeled/Investigational Use Prophylaxis against infective endocarditis

Pregnancy Risk Factor B

Pregnancy Considerations Adverse effects were not observed in animal reproduction studies; therefore, cefazolin is classified as pregnancy category B. Cefazolin crosses the placenta. Adverse events have not been reported in the fetus following administration of cefazolin prior to caesarean section. Cefazolin is recommended for group B streptococcus prophylaxis in pregnant patients with a nonanaphylactic penicillin allergy.

Due to pregnancy-induced physiologic changes, the pharmacokinetics of cefazolin are altered. The half-life is shorter and the AUC is smaller. The volume of distribution is unchanged.

Lactation Enters breast milk (small amounts)/use caution (AAP rates "compatible")

Medication Safety Issues

Sound-alike/look-alike issues:

CeFAZolin may be confused with cefprozil, cefTRIAXone, cephalexin, cephalothin

Kefzol® may be confused with Cefzil®

Contraindications Hypersensitivity to cefazolin sodium, any component of the formulation, or other cephalosporins

Warnings/Precautions Modify dosage in patients with severe renal impairment. Use with caution in patients with a history of penicillin allergy, especially IgE-mediated reactions (eg, anaphylaxis, angioedema, urticaria). Prolonged use may result in fungal or bacterial superinfection, including *C. difficile*-associated diarrhea (CDAD) and pseudomembranous colitis; CDAD has been observed >2 months postantibiotic treatment. May be associated with increased INR, especially in nutritionally-deficient patients, prolonged treatment, hepatic or renal disease. Use with caution in patients with a history of seizure disorder; high levels, particularly in the presence of renal impairment, may increase risk of seizures.

Adverse Reactions Frequency not defined.

Central nervous system: Fever, seizure

Dermatologic: Rash, pruritus, Stevens-Johnson syndrome

Gastrointestinal: Diarrhea, nausea, vomiting, abdominal cramps, anorexia, pseudomembranous colitis, oral candidiasis

Genitourinary: Vaginitis

Hepatic: Transaminases increased, hepatitis

Hematologic: Eosinophilia, neutropenia, leukopenia, thrombocytopenia, thrombocytosis

Local: Pain at injection site, phlebitis

Renal: BUN increased, serum creatinine increased, renal failure

Miscellaneous: Anaphylaxis

Reactions reported with other cephalosporins: Toxic epidermal necrolysis, abdominal pain, cholestasis, superinfection, toxic nephropathy, aplastic anemia, hemolytic anemia, hemorrhage, prothrombin time prolonged, pancytopenia

Drug Interactions

Avoid Concomitant Use There are no known interactions where it is recommended to avoid concomitant use.

Increased Effect/Toxicity

CeFAZolin may increase the levels/effects of: Vitamin K Antagonists

The levels/effects of CeFAZolin may be increased by: Uricosuric Agents

Decreased Effect

CeFAZolin may decrease the levels/effects of: Typhoid Vaccine

Stability Store intact vials at room temperature and protect from temperatures exceeding 40°C. Dilute large vial with 2.5 mL SWFI; 10 g vial may be diluted with 45 mL to yield 1 g/5 mL or 96 mL to yield 1 g/10 mL. May be injected or further dilution for I.V. administration in 50-100 mL compatible solution. Standard diluent is 1 g/50 mL D_5W or 2 g/50 mL D_5W.

Reconstituted solutions of cefazolin are light yellow to yellow. Protection from light is recommended for the powder and for the reconstituted solutions. Reconstituted solutions are stable for 24 hours at room temperature and for 10 days under refrigeration. Stability of parenteral admixture at room temperature (25°C) is 48 hours. Stability of parenteral admixture at refrigeration temperature (4°C) is 14 days.

DUPLEX™: Store at 20°C to 25°C (68°F to 77°F); excursions permitted to 15°C to 30°C (59°F to 86°F) prior to activation. Following activation, stable for 24 hours at room temperature and for 7 days under refrigeration.

Mechanism of Action Inhibits bacterial cell wall synthesis by binding to one or more of the penicillin-binding proteins (PBPs) which in turn inhibits the final transpeptidation step of peptidoglycan synthesis in bacterial cell walls, thus inhibiting cell wall biosynthesis. Bacteria eventually lyse due to ongoing activity of cell wall autolytic enzymes (autolysins and murein hydrolases) while cell wall assembly is arrested.

Pharmacodynamics/Kinetics

Distribution: Widely into most body tissues and fluids including gallbladder, liver, kidneys, bone, sputum, bile, pleural, and synovial; CSF penetration is poor

Protein binding: 74% to 86%

Metabolism: Minimally hepatic

Half-life elimination: 90-150 minutes; prolonged with renal impairment

Time to peak, serum: I.M.: 0.5-2 hours

Excretion: Urine (80% to 100% as unchanged drug)

Dosage

Usual dosage range: I.M., I.V.:

Children >1 month: 25-100 mg/kg/day divided every 6-8 hours; maximum: 6 g/day

Adults: 250 mg to 2 g every 6-12 (usually 8) hours, depending on severity of infection; maximum dose: 12 g/day

Indication-specific dosing:

Infants and Children: I.M., I.V.:

Prophylaxis against infective endocarditis (unlabeled use): 50 mg/kg 30-60 minutes before procedure; maximum dose: 1 g. Intramuscular injections should be avoided in patients who are receiving anticoagulant therapy. In these circumstances, orally administered regimens should be given whenever possible. Intravenously administered antibiotics should be used for patients who are unable to tolerate or absorb oral medications.

Note: American Heart Association (AHA) guidelines now recommend prophylaxis only in patients undergoing invasive procedures and in whom underlying cardiac conditions may predispose to a higher risk of adverse outcomes should infection occur. As of April 2007, routine prophylaxis for GI/GU procedures is no longer recommended by the AHA.

Adults: I.M., I.V.:

Prophylaxis against infective endocarditis (unlabeled use): 1 g 30-60 minutes before procedure. Intramuscular injections should be avoided in patients who are receiving anticoagulant therapy. In these circumstances, orally administered regimens should be given whenever possible. Intravenously administered antibiotics should be used for patients who are unable to tolerate or absorb oral medications.

Note: American Heart Association (AHA) guidelines now recommend prophylaxis only in patients undergoing invasive procedures and in whom underlying cardiac conditions may predispose to a higher risk of adverse outcomes should infection occur. As of April

2007, routine prophylaxis for GI/GU procedures is no longer recommended by the AHA.

Prophylaxis in total joint replacement patient: 1 g 1 hour prior to the procedure

Mild-to-moderate infections: 500 mg to 1 g every 6-8 hours

Mild infection with gram-positive cocci: 250-500 mg every 8 hours

Perioperative prophylaxis: 1 g given 30 minutes prior to surgery (repeat with 500 mg to 1 g during prolonged surgery); followed by 500 mg to 1 g every 6-9 hours for 24 hours postop

Pneumococcal pneumonia: 500 mg every 12 hours

Severe infection: 1-2 g every 6 hours

UTI (uncomplicated): 1 g every 12 hours

Dosing adjustment in renal impairment:

Cl_{cr} 35-54 mL/minute: Administer full dose in intervals of ≥8 hours

Cl_{cr} 11-34 mL/minute: Administer 1/2 usual dose every 12 hours

Cl_{cr} ≤10 mL/minute: Administer 1/2 usual dose every 18-24 hours

Hemodialysis: Moderately dialyzable (20% to 50%); administer dose postdialysis or administer supplemental dose of 0.5-1 g after dialysis

Continuous ambulatory peritoneal dialysis (CAPD): Administer 0.5 g every 12 hours

Continuous renal replacement therapy (CRRT): Drug clearance is highly dependent on the method of renal replacement, filter type, and flow rate. Appropriate dosing requires close monitoring of pharmacologic response, signs of adverse reactions due to drug accumulation, as well as drug levels in relation to target trough (if appropriate). The following are general recommendations only (based on dialysate flow/ultrafiltration rates of 1 L/hour) and should not supersede clinical judgment:

CVVH: 1-2 g every 12 hours

CVVHD/CVVHDF: 2 g every 12 hours

Dietary Considerations Sodium content of 1 g: 48 mg (2 mEq)

Administration

I.M.: Inject deep I.M. into large muscle mass.

I.V.: Inject direct I.V. over 5 minutes. Infuse intermittent infusion over 30-60 minutes.

Some penicillins (eg, carbenicillin, ticarcillin and piperacillin) have been shown to inactivate aminoglycosides *in vitro*. This has been observed to a greater extent with tobramycin and gentamicin, while amikacin has shown greater stability against inactivation. Concurrent use of these agents may pose a risk of reduced antibacterial efficacy *in vivo*, particularly in the setting of profound renal impairment. However, definitive clinical evidence is lacking. If combination penicillin/aminoglycoside therapy is desired in a patient with renal dysfunction, separation of doses (if feasible), and routine monitoring of aminoglycoside levels, CBC, and clinical response should be considered.

Monitoring Parameters Renal function periodically when used in combination with other nephrotoxic drugs, hepatic function tests, CBC; monitor for signs of anaphylaxis during first dose

Test Interactions Positive direct Coombs', false-positive urinary glucose test using cupric sulfate (Benedict's solution, Clinitest®, Fehling's solution), false-positive serum or urine creatinine with Jaffé reaction.

Some penicillin derivatives may accelerate the degradation of aminoglycosides *in vitro*, leading to a potential underestimation of aminoglycoside serum concentration.

Dosage Forms Excipient information presented when available (limited, particularly for generics); consult specific product labeling.

Infusion [iso-osmotic dextrose solution]: 1 g (50 mL)

Injection, powder for reconstitution: 500 mg, 1 g, 10 g, 20 g

◆ **Cefazolin Sodium** *see* CeFAZolin *on page 269*

Cefdinir (SEF di ner)

U.S. Brand Names Omnicef®

Canadian Brand Names Omnicef®

Index Terms CFDN

Pharmacologic Category Antibiotic, Cephalosporin (Third Generation)

Use Treatment of community-acquired pneumonia, acute exacerbations of chronic bronchitis, acute bacterial otitis media, acute maxillary sinusitis, pharyngitis/tonsillitis, and uncomplicated skin and skin structure infections.

Pregnancy Risk Factor B

Pregnancy Considerations Teratogenic events have not been observed in animal studies; therefore, cefdinir is classified as pregnancy category B. It is not known if cefdinir crosses the human placenta.

Lactation Excretion in breast milk unknown

Contraindications Hypersensitivity to cefdinir, any component of the formulation, other cephalosporins, or related antibiotics

Warnings/Precautions Administer cautiously to penicillin-sensitive patients, especially IgE-mediated reactions (eg, anaphylaxis, urticaria). Prolonged use may result in fungal or bacterial superinfection, including *C. difficile*-associated diarrhea (CDAD) and pseudomembranous colitis; CDAD has been observed >2 months postantibiotic treatment. Use caution with renal dysfunction; dose adjustment may be required. Safety and efficacy in infants <6 months of age have not been established.

Adverse Reactions

>10%: Gastrointestinal: Diarrhea (8% to 15%)

1% to 10%:

Central nervous system: Headache (2%)

Dermatologic: Rash (≤3%)

Gastrointestinal: Nausea (≤3%), abdominal pain (≤1%), vomiting (≤1%)

Genitourinary: Vaginal moniliasis (≤4%), urine leukocytes increased (2%), urine protein increased (1% to 2%), vaginitis (≤1%)

Hematologic: Eosinophils increased (1%)

Hepatic: Alkaline phosphatase increased (≤1%), platelets increased (1%)

Renal: Microhematuria (1%)

Miscellaneous: Lymphocytes increased (≤2%), GGT increased (1%), lactate dehydrogenase increased (≤1%), bicarbonate decreased (≤1%), lymphocytes decreased (≤1%), PMN changes (≤1%)

<1% (Limited to important or life-threatening): Allergic vasculitis, anaphylaxis, anorexia, bloody diarrhea, cardiac failure, chest pain, cholestasis, coagulation disorder, constipation, cutaneous moniliasis, disseminated intravascular coagulation (DIC), enterocolitis (acute), eosinophilic pneumonia, erythema multiforme, erythema nodosum, exfoliative dermatitis, facial edema, fulminant hepatitis, granulocytopenia, hemolytic anemia, hemorrhagic colitis, hepatic failure, hepatitis (acute), hyperkinesia, hypertension, idiopathic thrombocytopenia purpura, ileus, interstitial pneumonia (idiopathic), involuntary movement, jaundice, laryngeal edema, leukopenia, loss of consciousness, maculopapular rash, melena, MI, nephropathy, pancytopenia, pruritus, pseudomembranous colitis, renal failure (acute), respiratory failure (acute), rhabdomyolysis, serum sickness, shock, Stevens-Johnson syndrome, thrombocytopenia, toxic epidermal necrolysis, upper GI bleed, weakness, xerostomia

Reactions reported with other cephalosporins: Dizziness, fever, encephalopathy, asterixis, neuromuscular excitability, seizure, aplastic anemia, interstitial nephritis, toxic nephropathy, angioedema, hemorrhage, PT prolonged, and superinfection

Drug Interactions

Avoid Concomitant Use There are no known interactions where it is recommended to avoid concomitant use.

Increased Effect/Toxicity

The levels/effects of Cefdinir may be increased by: Uricosuric Agents

Decreased Effect

Cefdinir may decrease the levels/effects of: Typhoid Vaccine

The levels/effects of Cefdinir may be decreased by: Iron Salts

Stability Capsules and unmixed powder should be stored at room temperature of 15°C to 30°C (59°F to 86°F). Oral suspension should be mixed with 38 mL water for the 60 mL bottle and 63 mL of water for the 100 mL bottle. After mixing, the suspension can be stored at room temperature of 25°C (77°F) for 10 days.

Mechanism of Action Inhibits bacterial cell wall synthesis by binding to one or more of the penicillin-binding proteins (PBPs) which in turn inhibits the final transpeptidation step of peptidoglycan synthesis in bacterial cell walls, thus inhibiting cell wall biosynthesis. Bacteria eventually lyse due to ongoing activity of cell wall autolytic enzymes (autolysins and murein hydrolases) while cell wall assembly is arrested.

Pharmacodynamics/Kinetics

Distribution: V_d:

Children 6 months to 12 years: 0.29-1.05 L/kg

Adults: 0.06-0.64 L/kg

Protein binding: 60% to 70%

Metabolism: Minimally hepatic

Bioavailability: Capsule: 16% to 21%; suspension 25%

Half-life elimination: 100 minutes

Time to peak, plasma: 3 hours

Excretion: Primarily urine

Dosage

Usual dosage range:

Children 6 months to 12 years: Oral: 7 mg/kg/dose twice daily or 14 mg/kg/dose once daily (maximum: 600 mg/day)

Adolescents and Adults: Oral: 300 mg twice daily or 600 mg once daily

Indication-specific dosing:

Children 6 months to 12 years: Oral:

Acute bacterial otitis media, pharyngitis/tonsillitis: 7 mg/kg/dose twice daily for 5-10 days **or** 14 mg/kg/dose once daily for 10 days (maximum: 600 mg/day)

Acute maxillary sinusitis: 7 mg/kg/dose twice daily **or** 14 mg/kg/dose once daily for 10 days (maximum: 600 mg/day)

Uncomplicated skin and skin structure infections: 7 mg/kg/dose twice daily for 10 days (maximum: 600 mg/day)

Adolescents and Adults:

Acute exacerbations of chronic bronchitis, pharyngitis/tonsillitis: 300 mg twice daily for 5-10 days **or** 600 mg once daily for 10 days

Acute maxillary sinusitis: 300 mg twice daily **or** 600 mg once daily for 10 days

Community-acquired pneumonia, uncomplicated skin and skin structure infections: 300 mg twice daily for 10 days

Dosing adjustment in renal impairment: Cl_{cr} <30 mL/minute:

Children: 7 mg/kg once daily (maximum: 300 mg/day)

Adults: 300 mg once daily

Hemodialysis removes cefdinir; recommended initial dose: 300 mg (or 7 mg/kg/dose) every other day. At the conclusion of each hemodialysis session, 300 mg (or 7 mg/kg/dose) should be given. Subsequent doses (300 mg or 7 mg/kg/dose) should be administered every other day.

Dosing adjustment in hepatic impairment: No adjustment necessary.

Dietary Considerations Suspension contains sucrose 2.86 g/5 mL

Administration Twice daily doses should be given every 12 hours. May be taken with or without food. Manufacturer recommends administering at least 2 hours before or after antacids or iron supplements. Shake suspension well before use.

Monitoring Parameters Observe for signs and symptoms of anaphylaxis during first dose.

Test Interactions False-positive reaction for urinary ketones may occur with nitroprusside- but not nitroferricyanide-based tests. False-positive urine glucose results may occur when using Clinitest®, Benedict's solution, or Fehling's solution; glucose-oxidase-based reaction systems (eg, Clinistix®, Tes-Tape®) are recommended. May cause positive direct Coombs' test.

Dosage Forms Excipient information presented when available (limited, particularly for generics); consult specific product labeling.

Capsule: 300 mg

Omnicef®: 300 mg

Powder for oral suspension: 125 mg/5 mL (60 mL, 100 mL); 250 mg/5 mL (60 mL, 100 mL)

Omnicef®: 125 mg/5 mL (60 mL, 100 mL) [contains sodium benzoate and sucrose 2.86 g/5 mL; strawberry flavor]; 250 mg/5 mL (60 mL, 100 mL) [contains sodium benzoate and sucrose 2.86 g/5 mL; strawberry flavor]

Cefditoren (sef de TOR en)

U.S. Brand Names Spectracef®

Index Terms Cefditoren Pivoxil

Pharmacologic Category Antibiotic, Cephalosporin (Third Generation)

Use Treatment of acute bacterial exacerbation of chronic bronchitis or community-acquired pneumonia (due to susceptible organisms including *Haemophilus influenzae*, *Haemophilus parainfluenzae*, *Streptococcus pneumoniae*-penicillin susceptible only, *Moraxella catarrhalis*); pharyngitis or tonsillitis (*Streptococcus pyogenes*); and uncomplicated skin and skin-structure infections (*Staphylococcus aureus* - not MRSA, *Streptococcus pyogenes*)

Pregnancy Risk Factor B

Pregnancy Considerations Adverse events have not been observed in animal reproduction studies; therefore, the manufacturer classifies cefditoren as pregnancy category B. Other cephalosporins cross the placenta and are considered safe in pregnancy.

Lactation Excretion in breast milk unknown/use caution

Medication Safety Issues

International issues:

Spectracef® may be confused with Spectrocef® which is a brand name for cefotaxime in Italy

Contraindications Hypersensitivity to cefditoren, any component of the formulation, other cephalosporins, or milk protein; carnitine deficiency

Warnings/Precautions Use with caution in patients with a history of penicillin allergy, especially IgE-mediated reactions (eg, anaphylaxis, urticaria). Prolonged use may result in fungal or bacterial superinfection, including *C. difficile*-associated diarrhea (CDAD) and pseudomembranous colitis; CDAD has been observed >2 months postantibiotic treatment. Caution in individuals with seizure disorders; high levels, particularly in the presence of renal impairment, may increase risk of seizures. Use caution in patients with renal or hepatic impairment; modify dosage in patients with severe renal impairment. Cefditoren causes renal excretion of carnitine; do not use in patients with carnitine deficiency; not for long-term therapy due to the possible development of carnitine deficiency over time. May prolong prothrombin time; use with caution in patients with a history of bleeding disorder. Cefditoren tablets contain sodium caseinate, which may cause hypersensitivity reactions in patients with milk protein hypersensitivity; this does not affect patients with lactose intolerance. Safety and efficacy have not been established in children <12 years of age.

Adverse Reactions

>10%: Gastrointestinal: Diarrhea (11% to 15%)

1% to 10%:

Central nervous system: Headache (2% to 3%)

Endocrine & metabolic: Glucose increased (1% to 2%)

Gastrointestinal: Nausea (4% to 6%), abdominal pain (2%), dyspepsia (1% to 2%), vomiting (1%)

Genitourinary: Vaginal moniliasis (3% to 6%)

Hematologic: Hematocrit decreased (2%)

Renal: Hematuria (3%), urinary white blood cells increased (2%)

<1% (Limited to important or life-threatening): Acute renal failure, albumin decreased, allergic reaction, arthralgia, asthma, BUN increased, calcium decreased, eosinophilic pneumonia, coagulation time increased, erythema multiforme, fungal infection, hyperglycemia, interstitial pneumonia, leukopenia, leukorrhea, positive direct Coombs' test, potassium increased, pseudomembranous colitis, rash, sodium decreased, Stevens-Johnson syndrome, thrombocythemia, thrombocytopenia, toxic epidermal necrolysis, white blood cells increased/decreased

Reactions reported with other cephalosporins: Anaphylaxis, aplastic anemia, cholestasis, hemorrhage, hemolytic anemia, renal dysfunction, reversible hyperactivity, serum sickness-like reaction, toxic nephropathy

Drug Interactions

Avoid Concomitant Use There are no known interactions where it is recommended to avoid concomitant use.

Increased Effect/Toxicity

Cefditoren may increase the levels/effects of: Vitamin K Antagonists

The levels/effects of Cefditoren may be increased by: Uricosuric Agents

Decreased Effect There are no known significant interactions involving a decrease in effect.

Ethanol/Nutrition/Herb Interactions Food: Moderate- to high-fat meals increase bioavailability and maximum plasma concentration.

Stability Store at controlled room temperature of 15°C to 30°C (59°F to 86°F). Protect from light and moisture.

Mechanism of Action Inhibits bacterial cell wall synthesis by binding to one or more of the penicillin binding proteins (PBPs) which in turn inhibits the final transpeptidation step of peptidoglycan synthesis in bacterial cell walls, thus inhibiting cell wall biosynthesis. Bacteria eventually lyse due to ongoing activity of cell wall autolytic enzymes (autolysins and murein hydrolases) while cell wall assembly is arrested.

Pharmacodynamics/Kinetics

Distribution: 9.3 ± 1.6 L

Protein binding: 88% (*in vitro*), primarily to albumin

Metabolism: Cefditoren pivoxil is hydrolyzed to cefditoren (active) and pivalate

Bioavailability: ~14% to 16%, increased by moderate to high-fat meal

Half-life elimination: 1.6 ± 0.4 hours

Time to peak: 1.5-3 hours

Excretion: Urine (as cefditoren and pivaloylcarnitine)

Dosage

Usual dosage range:

Children ≥12 years and Adults: Oral: 200-400 mg twice daily

Indication-specific dosing:

Children ≥12 years and Adults: Oral:

Acute bacterial exacerbation of chronic bronchitis: 400 mg twice daily for 10 days

Dental infections (unlabeled use): 400 mg twice daily for 10 days

Community-acquired pneumonia: 400 mg twice daily for 14 days

Pharyngitis, tonsillitis, uncomplicated skin and skin structure infections: 200 mg twice daily for 10 days

Dosage adjustment in renal impairment:

Cl_{cr} 30-49 mL/minute/1.73 m^2: Maximum dose: 200 mg twice daily

Cl_{cr} <30 mL/minute/1.73 m^2: Maximum dose: 200 mg once daily

End-stage renal disease: Appropriate dosing not established

Dosage adjustment in hepatic impairment:

Mild-to-moderate impairment: Adjustment not required

Severe impairment (Child-Pugh Class C): Specific guidelines not available

Dietary Considerations Cefditoren should be taken with meals. Plasma carnitine levels are decreased during therapy (39% with 200 mg dosing, 63% with 400 mg dosing); normal concentrations return within 7-10 days after treatment is discontinued.

Administration Should be administered with meals.

Monitoring Parameters Assess patient at beginning and throughout therapy for infection; monitor for signs of anaphylaxis during first dose.

Test Interactions May induce a positive direct Coomb's test. May cause a false-negative ferricyanide test. Glucose oxidase or hexokinase methods recommended for blood/plasma glucose determinations. False-positive urine glucose test when using copper reduction based assays (eg, Clinitest®).

Dosage Forms Excipient information presented when available (limited, particularly for generics); consult specific product labeling.

Tablet:

Spectracef®: 200 mg, 400 mg [contains sodium caseinate]

◆ **Cefditoren Pivoxil** *see* Cefditoren *on page 272*

Cefepime (SEF e pim)

U.S. Brand Names Maxipime®

Canadian Brand Names Maxipime®

Index Terms Cefepime Hydrochloride

Pharmacologic Category Antibiotic, Cephalosporin (Fourth Generation)

Additional Appendix Information

Antimicrobial Drugs of Choice *on page 1752*

Community-Acquired Pneumonia in Adults *on page 1766*

Use Treatment of uncomplicated and complicated urinary tract infections, including pyelonephritis caused by typical urinary tract pathogens; monotherapy for febrile neutropenia; uncomplicated skin and skin structure infections caused by *Streptococcus pyogenes*; moderate-to-severe pneumonia caused by pneumococcus, *Pseudomonas aeruginosa*, and other gram-negative organisms; complicated intra-abdominal infections (in combination with metronidazole). Also active against methicillin-susceptible staphylococci, *Enterobacter* sp, and many other gram-negative bacilli.

Children 2 months to 16 years: Empiric therapy of febrile neutropenia patients, uncomplicated skin/soft tissue infections, pneumonia, and uncomplicated/complicated urinary tract infections.

Pregnancy Risk Factor B

Pregnancy Considerations Teratogenic effects were not observed in animal studies; therefore, cefepime is classified as pregnancy category B. It is not known if cefepime crosses the human placenta.

Lactation Enters breast milk/use caution

Contraindications Hypersensitivity to cefepime, any component of the formulation, or other cephalosporins

Warnings/Precautions Modify dosage in patients with severe renal impairment; use with caution in patients with a history of penicillin or cephalosporin allergy, especially IgE-mediated reactions (eg, anaphylaxis, urticaria). Prolonged use may result in fungal or bacterial superinfection, including *C. difficile*-associated diarrhea (CDAD) and pseudomembranous colitis; CDAD has been observed >2 months postantibiotic treatment. May be associated with increased INR, especially in nutritionally-deficient patients, prolonged treatment, hepatic or renal disease. Use with caution in patients with a history of seizure disorder; high levels, particularly in the presence of renal impairment, may increase risk of seizures.

Adverse Reactions

>10%: Hematologic: Positive Coombs' test without hemolysis

1% to 10%:

Central nervous system: Fever (1%), headache (1%)

Dermatologic: Rash, pruritus

Gastrointestinal: Diarrhea, nausea, vomiting

Local: Pain, erythema at injection site

<1% (Limited to important or life-threatening): Agranulocytosis, anaphylactic shock, anaphylaxis, coma, encephalopathy, hallucinations, leukopenia, myoclonus, neuromuscular excitability, neutropenia, seizure, status epilepticus (nonconvulsive), thrombocytopenia

Reactions reported with other cephalosporins: Aplastic anemia, erythema multiforme, hemolytic anemia, hemorrhage, pancytopenia, PT prolonged, renal dysfunction, Stevens-Johnson syndrome, superinfection, toxic epidermal necrolysis, toxic nephropathy, vaginitis

Drug Interactions

Avoid Concomitant Use There are no known interactions where it is recommended to avoid concomitant use.

Increased Effect/Toxicity

The levels/effects of Cefepime may be increased by: Uricosuric Agents

Decreased Effect

Cefepime may decrease the levels/effects of: Typhoid Vaccine

Stability Stable with normal saline, D_5W, and a variety of other solutions for 24 hours at room temperature and 7 days refrigerated.

Mechanism of Action Inhibits bacterial cell wall synthesis by binding to one or more of the penicillin-binding proteins (PBPs) which in turn inhibits the final transpeptidation step of peptidoglycan synthesis in bacterial cell walls, thus inhibiting cell wall biosynthesis. Bacteria eventually lyse due to ongoing activity of cell wall autolytic enzymes (autolysis and murein hydrolases) while cell wall assembly is arrested.

Pharmacodynamics/Kinetics

Absorption: I.M.: Rapid and complete

Distribution: V_d: Adults: 14-20 L; penetrates into inflammatory fluid at concentrations ~80% of serum levels and into bronchial mucosa at levels ~60% of those reached in the plasma; crosses blood-brain barrier

Protein binding, plasma: 16% to 19%

Metabolism: Minimally hepatic

Half-life elimination: 2 hours

Time to peak: 0.5-1.5 hours

Excretion: Urine (85% as unchanged drug)

Dosage

Usual dosage range:

Children: I.M., I.V.: 50 mg/kg every 8-12 hours (maximum not to exceed adult dosing)

Adults: I.V.: 1-2 g every 8-12 hours; I.M.: 500-1000 mg every 12 hours

Indication-specific dosing:

Children ≥2 months to 16 years (<40 kg):

Febrile neutropenia: I.V.: 50 mg/kg every 8 hours for 7 days or until neutropenia resolves

Skin and skin structure infections (uncomplicated) and pneumonia: I.V.: 50 mg/kg every 12 hours for 10 days

Urinary tract infections, complicated and uncomplicated: I.M., I.V.: 50 mg/kg every 12 hours for 7-10 days; **Note:** I.M. may be considered for mild-to-moderate infection only

Adults:

Brain abscess, postneurosurgical prevention (unlabeled use): I.V.: 2 g every 8 hours with vancomycin

Febrile neutropenia, monotherapy: I.V: 2 g every 8 hours for 7 days or until the neutropenia resolves

Intra-abdominal infections, complicated: I.V.: 2 g every 12 hours for 7-10 days with metronidazole

Otitis externa, malignant (unlabeled use): I.V.: 2 g every 12 hours

Pneumonia: I.V.:

Nosocomial (HAP/VAP): 1-2 g every 8-12 hours; **Note:** Duration of therapy may vary considerably (7-21 days); usually longer courses are required if *Pseudomonas*. In absence of *Pseudomonas*, and if appropriate empiric treatment used and patient responsive, it may be clinically appropriate to reduce duration of therapy to 7-10 days (American Thoracic Society Guidelines, 2005).

Community-acquired (including pseudomonal): 1-2 g every 12 hours for 10 days

Septic lateral/cavernous sinus thrombosis (unlabeled use): I.V.: 2 g every 8-12 hours; with metronidazole for lateral

Skin and skin structure, uncomplicated: I.V.: 2 g every 12 hours for 10 days

Urinary tract infections, complicated and uncomplicated:

Mild-to-moderate: I.M., I.V.: 500-1000 mg every 12 hours for 7-10 days

Severe: I.V.: 2 g every 12 hours for 10 days

Dosing adjustment in renal impairment: Adults: Recommended maintenance schedule based on creatinine clearance (mL/minute), compared to normal dosing schedule: See table.

Cefepime Hydrochloride

Creatinine Clearance (mL/minute)	Recommended Maintenance Schedule			
>60 (normal recommended dosing schedule)	500 mg every 12 hours	1 g every 12 hours	2 g every 12 hours	2 g every 8 hours
30-60	500 mg every 24 hours	1 g every 24 hours	2 g every 24 hours	2 g every 12 hours
11-29	500 mg every 24 hours	500 mg every 24 hours	1 g every 24 hours	2 g every 24 hours
<11	250 mg every 24 hours	250 mg every 24 hours	500 mg every 24 hours	1 g every 24 hours

Hemodialysis: Initial: 1 g (single dose) on day 1. Maintenance: 500 mg once daily (1 g once daily in febrile neutropenic patients). Dosage should be administered after dialysis on dialysis days.

Continuous ambulatory peritoneal dialysis (CAPD): Removed to a lesser extent than hemodialysis; administer normal recommended dose every 48 hours

Continuous renal replacement therapy (CRRT) (Trotman, 2005): Drug clearance is highly dependent on the method of renal replacement, filter type, and flow rate. Appropriate dosing requires close monitoring of pharmacologic response, signs of adverse reactions due to drug accumulation, as well as drug levels in relation to target trough (if appropriate). The following are general recommendations only (based on dialysate flow/ultrafiltration rates of 1 L/hour) and should not supersede clinical judgment:

CVVH: 1-2 g every 12 hours

CVVHDF: 2 g every 12 hours

Note: Consider higher dosage of 4 g/day if treating *Pseudomonas* or life-threatening infections in order to maximize time above MIC.

Administration May be administered either I.M. or I.V.

Inject deep I.M. into large muscle mass. Inject direct I.V. over 5 minutes. Infuse intermittent infusion over 30 minutes.

Monitoring Parameters Obtain specimen for culture and sensitivity prior to the first dose. Monitor for signs of anaphylaxis during first dose.

Test Interactions Positive direct Coombs', false-positive urinary glucose test using cupric sulfate (Benedict's solution, Clinitest®, Fehling's solution), false-positive serum or urine creatinine with Jaffé reaction, false-positive urinary proteins and steroids

Dosage Forms Excipient information presented when available (limited, particularly for generics); consult specific product labeling.

Injection, powder for reconstitution, as hydrochloride: 500 mg, 1 g, 2 g

Maxipime®: 500 mg, 1 g, 2 g

◆ **Cefepime Hydrochloride** *see* Cefepime *on page 273*

Cefixime (sef IKS eem)

U.S. Brand Names Suprax®

Canadian Brand Names Suprax®

Index Terms Cefixime Trihydrate

Pharmacologic Category Antibiotic, Cephalosporin (Third Generation)

Additional Appendix Information

Antimicrobial Drugs of Choice *on page 1752*

Treatment of Sexually Transmitted Infections *on page 1773*

Use Treatment of urinary tract infections, otitis media, respiratory infections due to susceptible organisms including *S. pneumoniae* and *S. pyogenes*, *H. influenzae*, and many Enterobacteriaceae; uncomplicated cervical/urethral gonorrhea due to *N. gonorrhoeae*

Pregnancy Risk Factor B

Pregnancy Considerations Teratogenic effects were not observed in animal studies; therefore cefixime is classified as pregnancy category B. It is not known if cefixime crosses the human placenta; other cephalosporins cross the placenta and are considered safe in pregnancy. Congenital anomalies have not been associated with cefixime use during pregnancy (limited data). Cefixime is recommended for use in pregnant women for the treatment of gonococcal infections.

Lactation Excretion in breast milk unknown

Medication Safety Issues

Sound-alike/look-alike issues:

Suprax® may be confused with Sporanox®, Surbex®

International issues:

Cefiton® [Portugal] may be confused with Cefotan® which is a brand name for cefotetan in the U.S.

Cefiton® [Portugal] may be confused with Ceftim® which is a brand name for ceftazidime in Italy

Cefiton® [Portugal] may be confused with Ceftin® which is a brand name for cefuroxime in the U.S.

Cefiton® [Portugal] may be confused with Lexotan® which is a brand name for bromazepam in multiple international markets

Contraindications Hypersensitivity to cefixime, any component of the formulation, or other cephalosporins

Warnings/Precautions Prolonged use may result in fungal or bacterial superinfection, including *C. difficile*-associated diarrhea (CDAD) and pseudomembranous colitis; CDAD has been observed >2 months postantibiotic treatment. Modify dosage in patients with renal impairment. Use with caution in patients with a history of penicillin allergy, especially IgE-mediated reactions (eg, anaphylaxis, urticaria).

Adverse Reactions

>10%: Gastrointestinal: Diarrhea (16%)

2% to 10%: Gastrointestinal: Abdominal pain, nausea, dyspepsia, flatulence, loose stools

<2% (Limited to important or life-threatening): Acute renal failure, anaphylactic/anaphylactoid reactions, angioedema, BUN increased, candidiasis, creatinine increased, dizziness, drug fever, eosinophilia, erythema multiforme, facial edema, fever, headache, hepatitis, hyperbilirubinemia, jaundice, leukopenia, neutropenia, pruritus, pseudomembranous colitis, PT prolonged, rash, seizure, serum sickness-like reaction, Stevens-Johnson syndrome, thrombocytopenia, toxic epidermal necrolysis, transaminases increased, urticaria, vaginitis, vomiting

Reactions reported with other cephalosporins: Agranulocytosis, aplastic anemia, colitis, hemolytic anemia, hemorrhage, interstitial nephritis, pancytopenia, superinfection

Drug Interactions

Avoid Concomitant Use There are no known interactions where it is recommended to avoid concomitant use.

Increased Effect/Toxicity

The levels/effects of Cefixime may be increased by: Uricosuric Agents

Decreased Effect

Cefixime may decrease the levels/effects of: Typhoid Vaccine

Ethanol/Nutrition/Herb Interactions Food: Delays cefixime absorption.

Stability After reconstitution, suspension may be stored for 14 days at room temperature or under refrigeration.

Mechanism of Action Inhibits bacterial cell wall synthesis by binding to one or more of the penicillin binding proteins (PBPs); which in turn inhibits the final transpeptidation step of peptidoglycan synthesis in bacterial cell walls, thus inhibiting cell wall biosynthesis. Bacteria eventually lyse due to ongoing activity of cell wall autolytic enzymes (autolysins and murein hydrolases) while cell wall assembly is arrested.

Pharmacodynamics/Kinetics

Absorption: 40% to 50%

Distribution: Widely throughout the body and reaches therapeutic concentration in most tissues and body fluids, including synovial, pericardial, pleural, peritoneal; bile, sputum, and urine; bone, myocardium, gallbladder, and skin and soft tissue

Protein binding: 65%

Half-life elimination: Normal renal function: 3-4 hours; Renal failure: Up to 11.5 hours

Time to peak, serum: 2-6 hours; delayed with food

Excretion: Urine (50% of absorbed dose as active drug); feces (10%)

Dosage

Usual dosage range:

Children ≥6 months: Oral: 8-20 mg/kg/day divided every 12-24 hours (maximum: 400 mg/day)

Children >50 kg or >12 years and Adults: Oral: 400 mg/day divided every 12-24 hours

Indication-specific dosing:

Children: Oral:

***S. pyogenes* infections:** Treat for 10 days

Typhoid fever: 20 mg/kg/day for 10-14 days; maximum 400 mg

Adults: Oral:

***S. pyogenes* infections:** Treat for 10 days

Typhoid fever: 20-30 mg/kg/day in 2 divided doses for 7-14 days after I.V. therapy

Uncomplicated cervical/urethral gonorrhea due to *N. gonorrhoeae:* 400 mg as a single dose

Dosing adjustment in renal impairment:

Cl_{cr} 21-60 mL/minute or with renal hemodialysis: Administer 75% of the standard dose

Cl_{cr} <20 mL/minute or with CAPD: Administer 50% of the standard dose

Moderately dialyzable (10%)

Dietary Considerations May be taken with food.

Administration May be administered with or without food; administer with food to decrease GI distress. Shake oral suspension well before use.

Monitoring Parameters With prolonged therapy, monitor renal and hepatic function periodically. Observe for signs and symptoms of anaphylaxis during first dose.

Test Interactions Positive direct Coombs', false-positive urinary glucose test using cupric sulfate (Benedict's solution, Clinitest®, Fehling's solution), false-positive serum or urine creatinine with Jaffé reaction

Dosage Forms Excipient information presented when available (limited, particularly for generics); consult specific product labeling. [DSC] = Discontinued product

Powder for oral suspension, as trihydrate:

Suprax®: 100 mg/5 mL (50 mL, 75 mL [DSC], 100 mL) [contains sodium benzoate; strawberry flavor]; 200 mg/5 mL (50 mL, 75 mL) [contains sodium benzoate; strawberry flavor]

Tablet, oral, as trihydrate:

Suprax®: 400 mg

◆ **Cefixime Trihydrate** *see* Cefixime *on page 275*

◆ **Cefizox®** *see* Ceftizoxime *on page 284*

Cefotaxime (sef oh TAKS eem)

U.S. Brand Names Claforan®

Canadian Brand Names Claforan®

Index Terms Cefotaxime Sodium

Pharmacologic Category Antibiotic, Cephalosporin (Third Generation)

Additional Appendix Information

Antibiotic Treatment of Adults With Infective Endocarditis *on page 1748*

Antimicrobial Drugs of Choice *on page 1752*

Community-Acquired Pneumonia in Adults *on page 1766*

Treatment of Sexually Transmitted Infections *on page 1773*

Use Treatment of susceptible infection in respiratory tract, skin and skin structure, bone and joint, urinary tract, gynecologic as well as septicemia, and documented or suspected meningitis. Active against most gram-negative bacilli (not *Pseudomonas*) and gram-positive cocci (not enterococcus). Active against many penicillin-resistant pneumococci.

Pregnancy Risk Factor B

Pregnancy Considerations Teratogenic effects were not observed in animal studies; therefore, cefotaxime is classified as pregnancy category B. Cefotaxime crosses the placenta and can be found in fetal tissue. An increased risk of teratogenic effects has not been observed following maternal use. During pregnancy, peak cefotaxime serum concentrations are decreased and the serum half-life is shorter.

Lactation Enters breast milk/use caution (AAP rates "compatible")

Medication Safety Issues

Sound-alike/look-alike issues:

Cefotaxime may be confused with cefoxitin, ceftizoxime, cefuroxime

International issues:

Spectrocef® [Italy] may be confused with Spectracef® which is a brand name for cefditoren in the U.S.

Contraindications Hypersensitivity to cefotaxime, any component of the formulation, or other cephalosporins

Warnings/Precautions Modify dosage in patients with severe renal impairment. Prolonged use may result in superinfection. A potentially life-threatening arrhythmia has been reported in patients who received a rapid bolus injection via central line. Granulocytopenia and more rarely agranulocytosis may develop during prolonged treatment (>10 days). Minimize tissue inflammation by changing infusion sites when needed. Use with caution in patients with a history of penicillin allergy, especially IgE-mediated reactions (eg, anaphylaxis, urticaria). Prolonged use may result in fungal or bacterial superinfection, including *C. difficile*-associated diarrhea (CDAD) and pseudomembranous colitis; CDAD has been observed >2 months postantibiotic treatment.

Adverse Reactions

1% to 10%:

Dermatologic: Rash, pruritus

Gastrointestinal: Diarrhea, nausea, vomiting, colitis

Local: Pain at injection site

<1% (Limited to important or life-threatening): Anaphylaxis, arrhythmia (after rapid I.V. injection via central catheter), BUN increased, candidiasis, creatinine increased, eosinophilia, erythema multiforme, fever, headache, interstitial nephritis, neutropenia, phlebitis, pseudomembranous colitis, Stevens-Johnson syndrome, thrombocytopenia, transaminases increased, toxic epidermal necrolysis, urticaria, vaginitis

Reactions reported with other cephalosporins: Agranulocytosis, aplastic anemia, cholestasis, hemolytic anemia, hemorrhage, pancytopenia, renal dysfunction, seizure, superinfection, toxic nephropathy.

Drug Interactions

Avoid Concomitant Use There are no known interactions where it is recommended to avoid concomitant use.

Increased Effect/Toxicity

The levels/effects of Cefotaxime may be increased by: Uricosuric Agents

Decreased Effect

Cefotaxime may decrease the levels/effects of: Typhoid Vaccine

Stability Reconstituted solution is stable for 12-24 hours at room temperature and 7-10 days when refrigerated and for 13 weeks when frozen. For I.V. infusion in NS or D_5W solution is stable for 24 hours at room temperature, 5 days when refrigerated, or 13 weeks when frozen in Viaflex® plastic containers. Thawed solutions previously of frozen premixed bags are stable for 24 hours at room temperature or 10 days when refrigerated.

Mechanism of Action Inhibits bacterial cell wall synthesis by binding to one or more of the penicillin-binding proteins (PBPs) which in turn inhibits the final transpeptidation step of peptidoglycan synthesis in bacterial cell walls, thus inhibiting cell wall biosynthesis. Bacteria eventually lyse due to ongoing activity of cell wall autolytic enzymes (autolysins and murein hydrolases) while cell wall assembly is arrested.

Pharmacodynamics/Kinetics

Distribution: Widely to body tissues and fluids including aqueous humor, ascitic and prostatic fluids, bone; penetrates CSF best when meninges are inflamed

Metabolism: Partially hepatic to active metabolite, desacetylcefotaxime

Half-life elimination:

Cefotaxime: Premature neonates <1 week: 5-6 hours; Full-term neonates <1 week: 2-3.4 hours; Adults: 1-1.5 hours; prolonged with renal and/or hepatic impairment

Desacetylcefotaxime: 1.5-1.9 hours; prolonged with renal impairment

Time to peak, serum: I.M.: Within 30 minutes

Excretion: Urine (as unchanged drug and metabolites)

Dosage

Usual dosage range:

Infants and Children 1 month to 12 years <50 kg: I.M., I.V.: 50-200 mg/kg/day in divided doses every 6-8 hours

Children >12 years and Adults: I.M., I.V.: 1-2 g every 4-12 hours

Indication-specific dosing:

Infants and Children 1 month to 12 years:

Epiglottitis: I.M., I.V.: 150-200 mg/kg/day in 4 divided doses with clindamycin for 7-10 days

Meningitis: I.M., I.V.: 200 mg/kg/day in divided doses every 6 hours

Pneumonia: I.V.: 200 mg/kg/day divided every 8 hours

Sepsis: I.V.: 150 mg/kg/day divided every 8 hours

Typhoid fever: I.M., I.V.: 150-200 mg/kg/day in 3-4 divided doses (maximum: 12 g/day); fluoroquinolone resistant: 80 mg/kg/day in 3-4 divided doses (maximum: 12 g/day)

Children >12 years and Adults:

Arthritis (septic): I.V.: 1 g every 8 hours

Brain abscess, meningitis: I.V.: 2 g every 4-6 hours

Caesarean section: I.M., I.V.: 1 g as soon as the umbilical cord is clamped, then 1 g at 6- and 12-hour intervals

Epiglottitis: I.V.: 2 g every 4-8 hours

Gonorrhea: I.M.: 1 g as a single dose

Disseminated: I.V.: 1 g every 8 hours

Life-threatening infections: I.V.: 2 g every 4 hours

Liver abscess: I.V.: 1-2 g every 6 hours

Lyme disease:

Cardiac manifestations: I.V.: 2 g every 4 hours

CNS manifestations: I.V.: 2 g every 8 hours for 14-28 days

Moderate-to-severe infections: I.M., I.V.: 1-2 g every 8 hours

Orbital cellulitis: I.V.: 2 g every 4 hours

Peritonitis (spontaneous): I.V.: 2 g every 8 hours, unless life-threatening then 2 g every 4 hours

Septicemia: I.V.: 2 g every 6-8 hours

Skin and soft tissue:

Mixed, necrotizing: I.V.: 2 g every 6 hours, with metronidazole or clindamycin

Bite wounds (animal): I.V.: 2 g every 6 hours

Surgical prophylaxis: I.M., I.V.: 1 g 30-90 minutes before surgery

Uncomplicated infections: I.M., I.V.: 1 g every 12 hours

Dosing interval in renal impairment:

Cl_{cr} 10-50 mL/minute: Administer every 8-12 hours

Cl_{cr} <10 mL/minute: Administer every 24 hours

Hemodialysis: Moderately dialyzable

Continuous ambulatory peritoneal dialysis (CAPD): Administer 0.5-1 g every 24 hours

Continuous renal replacement therapy (CRRT): Drug clearance is highly dependent on the method of renal replacement, filter type, and flow rate. Appropriate dosing requires close monitoring of pharmacologic response, signs of adverse reactions due to drug accumulation, as well as drug levels in relation to target trough (if appropriate). The following are general recommendations only (based on dialysate flow/ultrafiltration rates of 1 L/hour) and should not supersede clinical judgment:

CVVH: 1-2 g every 12 hours

CVVHD/CVVHDF: 2 g every 12 hours

Dosing adjustment in hepatic impairment: Moderate dosage reduction is recommended in severe liver disease

Continuous arteriovenous or venovenous hemodiafiltration effects: Administer 1 g every 12 hour

Dietary Considerations Sodium content of 1 g: 50.5 mg (2.2 mEq)

Administration Can be administered IVP over 3-5 minutes or I.V. intermittent infusion over 15-30 minutes.

Monitoring Parameters Observe for signs and symptoms of anaphylaxis during first dose; CBC with differential (especially with long courses)

Test Interactions Positive direct Coombs', false-positive urinary glucose test using cupric sulfate (Benedict's solution, Clinitest®, Fehling's solution), false-positive serum or urine creatinine with Jaffé reaction

Dosage Forms Excipient information presented when available (limited, particularly for generics); consult specific product labeling.

Infusion [premixed iso-osmotic solution]:

Claforan®: 1 g (50 mL); 2 g (50 mL) [contains sodium 50.5 mg (2.2 mEq) per cefotaxime 1 g]

Injection, powder for reconstitution: 500 mg, 1 g, 2 g, 10 g, 20 g

Claforan®: 500 mg, 1 g, 2 g, 10 g [contains sodium 50.5 mg (2.2 mEq) per cefotaxime 1 g]

◆ **Cefotaxime Sodium** *see* Cefotaxime *on page 276*

Cefotetan (SEF oh tee tan)

Index Terms Cefotetan Disodium

Pharmacologic Category Antibiotic, Cephalosporin (Second Generation)

Additional Appendix Information

Animal and Human Bites *on page 1747*

Antimicrobial Drugs of Choice *on page 1752*

Use Surgical prophylaxis; intra-abdominal infections and other mixed infections; respiratory tract, skin and skin structure, bone and joint, urinary tract and gynecologic as well as septicemia; active against gram-negative enteric bacilli including *E. coli*, *Klebsiella*, and *Proteus*; less active against staphylococci and streptococci than first generation cephalosporins, but active against anaerobes including *Bacteroides fragilis*

Pregnancy Risk Factor B

Pregnancy Considerations Adverse events have not been observed in animal reproduction studies; therefore, the manufacturer classifies cefotetan as pregnancy category B. Cefotetan crosses the placenta and produces therapeutic concentrations in the amniotic fluid and cord serum.

Lactation Enters breast milk (small amounts)/use caution

Medication Safety Issues

Sound-alike/look-alike issues:

Cefotetan may be confused with cefoxitin, Ceftin®

Cefotan® may be confused with Ceftin®

International issues:

Cefotan® may be confused with Lexotan® which is a brand name for bromazepam in multiple international markets

Cefotan® may be confused with Cefiton® which is a brand name for cefixime in Portugal

Contraindications Hypersensitivity to cefotetan, any component of the formulation, or other cephalosporins; previous cephalosporin-associated hemolytic anemia

Warnings/Precautions Modify dosage in patients with severe renal impairment. Although cefotetan contains the methyltetrazolethiol side chain, bleeding has not been a significant problem. Use with caution in patients with a history of penicillin allergy, especially IgE-mediated reactions (eg, anaphylaxis, urticaria). Cefotetan has been associated with a higher risk of hemolytic anemia relative to other cephalosporins (approximately threefold); monitor carefully during use and consider cephalosporin-associated immune anemia in patients who have received cefotetan within 2-3 weeks (either as treatment or prophylaxis). Prolonged use may result in fungal or bacterial superinfection, including *C. difficile*-associated diarrhea (CDAD) and pseudomembranous colitis; CDAD has been observed >2 months postantibiotic treatment. May be associated with increased INR, especially in nutritionally-deficient patients, prolonged treatment, hepatic or renal disease.

Adverse Reactions

1% to 10%:

Gastrointestinal: Diarrhea (1%)

Hepatic: Transaminases increased (1%)

Miscellaneous: Hypersensitivity reactions (1%)

<1%: Anaphylaxis, urticaria, rash, pruritus, pseudomembranous colitis, nausea, vomiting, eosinophilia, thrombocytosis, agranulocytosis, hemolytic anemia, leukopenia, thrombocytopenia, prolonged PT, bleeding, BUN increased, creatinine increased, nephrotoxicity, phlebitis, fever

Reactions reported with other cephalosporins: Seizure, Stevens-Johnson syndrome, toxic epidermal necrolysis, renal dysfunction, toxic nephropathy, cholestasis, aplastic anemia, hemolytic anemia, hemorrhage, pancytopenia, agranulocytosis, colitis, superinfection

Drug Interactions

Avoid Concomitant Use There are no known interactions where it is recommended to avoid concomitant use.

Increased Effect/Toxicity

Cefotetan may increase the levels/effects of: Alcohol (Ethyl); Vitamin K Antagonists

The levels/effects of Cefotetan may be increased by: Uricosuric Agents

Decreased Effect

Cefotetan may decrease the levels/effects of: Typhoid Vaccine

Ethanol/Nutrition/Herb Interactions Ethanol: Avoid ethanol (may cause a disulfiram-like reaction).

Stability Reconstituted solution is stable for 24 hours at room temperature and 96 hours when refrigerated. For I.V. infusion in NS or D_5W solution and after freezing, thawed solution is stable for 24 hours at room temperature or 96 hours when refrigerated. Frozen solution is stable for 12 weeks.

Mechanism of Action Inhibits bacterial cell wall synthesis by binding to one or more of the penicillin-binding proteins (PBPs) which in turn inhibits the final transpeptidation step of peptidoglycan synthesis in bacterial cell walls, thus inhibiting cell wall biosynthesis. Bacteria eventually lyse due to ongoing activity of cell wall autolytic enzymes (autolysins and murein hydrolases) while cell wall assembly is arrested.

Pharmacodynamics/Kinetics

Distribution: Widely to body tissues and fluids including bile, sputum, prostatic, peritoneal; low concentrations enter CSF

Protein binding: 76% to 90%

Half-life elimination: 3-5 hours

Time to peak, serum: I.M.: 1.5-3 hours

Excretion: Primarily urine (as unchanged drug); feces (20%)

Dosage

Usual dosage range:

Children (unlabeled use): I.M., I.V.: 20-40 mg/kg/dose every 12 hours (maximum: 6 g/day)

Adults: I.M., I.V.: 1-6 g/day in divided doses every 12 hours

Indication-specific dosing:

Children (unlabeled use):

Preoperative prophylaxis: I.M., I.V.: 40 mg/kg 30-60 minutes prior to surgery

Adolescents and Adults:

Pelvic inflammatory disease: I.V.: 2 g every 12 hours; used in combination with doxycycline

Adults:

Orbital cellulitis, odontogenic infections: I.V.: 2 g every 12 hours

Preoperative prophylaxis: I.M., I.V.: 1-2 g 30-60 minutes prior to surgery; when used for cesarean section, dose should be given as soon as umbilical cord is clamped

Urinary tract infection: I.M., I.V.: 1-2 g may be given every 24 hours

Dosing interval in renal impairment:

Cl_{cr} 10-30 mL/minute: Administer every 24 hours

Cl_{cr} <10 mL/minute: Administer every 48 hours

Hemodialysis: Dialyzable (5% to 20%); administer 1/4 the usual dose every 24 hours on days between dialysis; administer 1/2 the usual dose on the day of dialysis.

Continuous arteriovenous or venovenous hemodiafiltration effects: Administer 750 mg every 12 hours

Dietary Considerations Contains sodium of 80 mg (3.5 mEq) per cefotetan 1 g

Administration

I.M.: Inject deep I.M. into large muscle mass.

I.V.: Inject direct I.V. over 3-5 minutes. Infuse intermittent infusion over 30 minutes.

Monitoring Parameters Observe for signs and symptoms of anaphylaxis during first dose; monitor for signs and symptoms of hemolytic anemia, including hematologic parameters where appropriate.

Test Interactions Positive direct Coombs', false-positive urinary glucose test using cupric sulfate (Benedict's solution, Clinitest®, Fehling's solution), false-positive serum or urine creatinine with Jaffé reaction

Dosage Forms Excipient information presented when available (limited, particularly for generics); consult specific product labeling.

Injection, powder for reconstitution: 1 g, 2 g [contains sodium 80 mg/g (3.5 mEq/g)]

◆ **Cefotetan Disodium** *see* Cefotetan *on page* 277

Cefoxitin (se FOKS i tin)

Canadian Brand Names Apo-Cefoxitin®

Index Terms Cefoxitin Sodium

Pharmacologic Category Antibiotic, Cephalosporin (Second Generation)

Use Less active against staphylococci and streptococci than first generation cephalosporins, but active against anaerobes including *Bacteroides fragilis*; active against gram-negative enteric bacilli including *E. coli*, *Klebsiella*, and *Proteus*; used predominantly for respiratory tract, skin and skin structure, bone and joint, urinary tract and gynecologic as well as septicemia; surgical prophylaxis; intra-abdominal infections and other mixed infections; indicated for bacterial *Eikenella corrodens* infections

Pregnancy Risk Factor B

Pregnancy Considerations

Adverse events have not been observed in animal reproduction studies; therefore, cefoxitin is classified as pregnancy category B. Cefoxitin crosses the placenta and reaches the cord serum and amniotic fluid. Adequate well-controlled studies are not available in pregnant women.

Peak serum concentrations of cefoxitin during pregnancy may be similar to or decreased compared to nonpregnant values. Maternal half-life may be shorter at term. Pregnancy-induced hypertension increases trough concentrations in the immediate postpartum period.

Lactation Enters breast milk (small amounts)/use caution (AAP rates "compatible")

Medication Safety Issues

Sound-alike/look-alike issues:

Cefoxitin may be confused with cefotaxime, cefotetan, Cytoxan®

Mefoxin® may be confused with Lanoxin®

Contraindications Hypersensitivity to cefoxitin, any component of the formulation, or other cephalosporins

Warnings/Precautions Modify dosage in patients with severe renal impairment. Prolonged use may result in superinfection. Use with caution in patients with a history of penicillin allergy, especially IgE-mediated reactions (eg, anaphylaxis, urticaria). Prolonged use may result in fungal or bacterial superinfection, including *C. difficile*-associated diarrhea (CDAD) and pseudomembranous colitis; CDAD has been observed >2 months postantibiotic treatment.

Adverse Reactions

1% to 10%: Gastrointestinal: Diarrhea

<1% (Limited to important or life-threatening): Anaphylaxis, angioedema, bone marrow suppression, BUN increased, creatinine increased, dyspnea, eosinophilia, exacerbation of myasthenia gravis, exfoliative dermatitis, fever, hemolytic anemia, hypotension, interstitial nephritis, jaundice, leukopenia, nausea, nephrotoxicity (with aminoglycosides), phlebitis, prolonged PT, pruritus, pseudomembranous colitis, rash, thrombocytopenia, thrombophlebitis, toxic epidermal necrolysis, transaminases increased, urticaria, vomiting

Reactions reported with other cephalosporins: Agranulocytosis, aplastic anemia, cholestasis, colitis, erythema multiforme, hemolytic anemia, hemorrhage, pancytopenia, renal dysfunction, seizure, serum-sickness reactions, Stevens-Johnson syndrome, superinfection, toxic nephropathy, vaginitis

Drug Interactions

Avoid Concomitant Use There are no known interactions where it is recommended to avoid concomitant use.

Increased Effect/Toxicity

Cefoxitin may increase the levels/effects of: Vitamin K Antagonists

The levels/effects of Cefoxitin may be increased by: Uricosuric Agents

Decreased Effect

Cefoxitin may decrease the levels/effects of: Typhoid Vaccine

Stability Reconstitute vials with SWFI, bacteriostatic water for injection, NS, or D_5W. For I.V. infusion, solutions may be further diluted in NS, $D_5{}^1/_4NS$, $D_5{}^1/_2NS$, D_5NS, D_5W, $D_{10}W$, LR, D_5LR, mannitol 10%, or sodium bicarbonate 5%. Reconstituted solution is stable for 6 hours at room temperature or 7 days when refrigerated; I.V. infusion in NS or D_5W solution is stable for 18 hours at room temperature or 48 hours when refrigerated. Premixed frozen solution, when thawed, is stable for 24 hours at room temperature or 21 days when refrigerated.

Mechanism of Action Inhibits bacterial cell wall synthesis by binding to one or more of the penicillin-binding proteins (PBPs) which in turn inhibits the final transpeptidation step of peptidoglycan synthesis in bacterial cell walls, thus inhibiting cell wall biosynthesis. Bacteria eventually lyse due to ongoing activity of cell wall autolytic enzymes (autolysins and murein hydrolases) while cell wall assembly is arrested.

Pharmacodynamics/Kinetics

Distribution: Widely to body tissues and fluids including pleural, synovial, ascitic, bile; poorly penetrates into CSF even with inflammation of the meninges

Protein binding: 65% to 79%

Half-life elimination: 45-60 minutes; significantly prolonged with renal impairment

Time to peak, serum: I.M.: 20-30 minutes

Excretion: Urine (85% as unchanged drug)

Dosage

Usual dosage range:

Infants >3 months and Children: I.M., I.V.: 80-160 mg/kg/day in divided doses every 4-6 hours (maximum dose: 12 g/day)

Adults: I.M., I.V.: 1-2 g every 6-8 hours (maximum dose: 12 g/day)

Note: I.M. injection is painful

Indication-specific dosing:

Infants >3 months and Children:

Mild-to-moderate infection: I.M., I.V.: 80-100 mg/kg/day in divided doses every 4-6 hours

Perioperative prophylaxis: I.V.: 30-40 mg/kg 30-60 minutes prior to surgery followed by 30-40 mg/kg/dose every 6 hours for no more than 24 hours after surgery depending on the procedure

Severe infection: I.M., I.V.: 100-160 mg/kg/day in divided doses every 4-6 hours

Adolescents and Adults:

Perioperative prophylaxis: I.M., I.V.: 1-2 g 30-60 minutes prior to surgery followed by 1-2 g every 6-8 hours for no more than 24 hours after surgery depending on the procedure

Adults:

Amnionitis, endomyometritis: I.M., I.V.: 2 g every 6-8 hours

Aspiration pneumonia, empyema, orbital cellulitis, parapharyngeal space, human bites: I.M., I.V.: 2 g every 8 hours

Liver abscess: I.V.: 1 g every 4 hours

Mycobacterium species, not MTB or MAI: I.V.: 12 g/day with amikacin

Pelvic inflammatory disease:

Inpatients: I.V.: 2 g every 6 hours **plus** doxycycline 100 mg I.V. or 100 mg orally every 12 hours until improved, followed by doxycycline 100 mg orally twice daily to complete 14 days

Outpatients: I.M.: 2 g **plus** probenecid 1 g orally as a single dose, followed by doxycycline 100 mg orally twice daily for 14 days

Dosing interval in renal impairment:

Cl_{cr} 30-50 mL/minute: Administer 1-2 g every 8-12 hours

Cl_{cr} 10-29 mL/minute: Administer 1-2 g every 12-24 hours

Cl_{cr} 5-9 mL/minute: Administer 0.5-1 g every 12-24 hours

Cl_{cr} <5 mL/minute: Administer 0.5-1 g every 24-48 hours

Hemodialysis: Moderately dialyzable (20% to 50%); administer a loading dose of 1-2 g after each hemodialysis; maintenance dose as noted above based on Cl_{cr}

Continuous arteriovenous or venovenous hemodiafiltration effects: Dose as for Cl_{cr} 10-50 mL/minute

Dietary Considerations Sodium content of 1 g: 53 mg (2.3 mEq)

Administration

I.M.: Inject deep I.M. into large muscle mass.

I.V.: Can be administered IVP over 3-5 minutes at a maximum concentration of 100 mg/mL or I.V. intermittent infusion over 10-60 minutes at a final concentration for I.V. administration not to exceed 40 mg/mL

Monitoring Parameters Monitor renal function periodically when used in combination with other nephrotoxic drugs; observe for signs and symptoms of anaphylaxis during first dose

Test Interactions Positive direct Coombs', false-positive urinary glucose test using cupric sulfate (Benedict's solution, Clinitest®, Fehling's solution), false-positive serum or urine creatinine with Jaffé reaction

Dosage Forms Excipient information presented when available (limited, particularly for generics); consult specific product labeling.

Injection, powder for reconstitution: 1 g, 2 g, 10 g [contains sodium 53.8 mg/g (2.3 mEq/g)]

Powder for prescription compounding: 100 g

◆ **Cefoxitin Sodium** *see* Cefoxitin *on page 278*

Cefpodoxime (sef pode OKS eem)

U.S. Brand Names Vantin®

Canadian Brand Names Vantin®

Index Terms Cefpodoxime Proxetil

Pharmacologic Category Antibiotic, Cephalosporin (Third Generation)

Additional Appendix Information

Antimicrobial Drugs of Choice *on page 1752*
Community-Acquired Pneumonia in Adults *on page 1766*
Treatment of Sexually Transmitted Infections *on page 1773*

Use Treatment of susceptible acute, community-acquired pneumonia caused by *S. pneumoniae* or nonbeta-lactamase producing *H. influenzae*; acute uncomplicated gonorrhea caused by *N. gonorrhoeae*; uncomplicated skin and skin structure infections caused by *S. aureus* or *S. pyogenes*; acute otitis media caused by *S. pneumoniae*, *H. influenzae*, or *M. catarrhalis*; pharyngitis or tonsillitis; and uncomplicated urinary tract infections caused by *E. coli*, *Klebsiella*, and *Proteus*

Pregnancy Risk Factor B

Pregnancy Considerations Teratogenic events were not observed in animal studies; therefore, cefpodoxime is classified as pregnancy category B. It is not known if cefpodoxime crosses the human placenta. Other cephalosporins cross the placenta and are considered safe in pregnancy.

Lactation Enters breast milk (small amounts)/not recommended

Medication Safety Issues

Sound-alike/look-alike issues:

Vantin® may be confused with Ventolin®

Contraindications Hypersensitivity to cefpodoxime, any component of the formulation, or other cephalosporins

Warnings/Precautions Modify dosage in patients with severe renal impairment. Prolonged use may result in fungal or bacterial superinfection, including *C. difficile*-associated diarrhea (CDAD) and pseudomembranous colitis; CDAD has been observed >2 months postantibiotic treatment. Use with caution in patients with a history of penicillin allergy, especially IgE-mediated reactions (eg, anaphylaxis, urticaria).

Adverse Reactions

>10%:

Dermatologic: Diaper rash (12.1%)

Gastrointestinal: Diarrhea in infants and toddlers (15.4%)

1% to 10%:

Central nervous system: Headache (1.1%)

Dermatologic: Rash (1.4%)

Gastrointestinal: Diarrhea (7.2%), nausea (3.8%), abdominal pain (1.6%), vomiting (1.1% to 2.1%)

Genitourinary: Vaginal infection (3.1%)

<1% (Limited to important or life-threatening): Anaphylaxis, anxiety, appetite decreased, chest pain, cough, dizziness, epistaxis, eye itching, fatigue, fever, flatulence, flushing, fungal skin infection, hypotension, insomnia, malaise, nightmares, pruritus, pseudomembranous colitis, purpuric nephritis, salivation decreased, taste alteration, tinnitus, vaginal candidiasis, weakness

Reactions reported with other cephalosporins: Agranulocytosis, aplastic anemia, cholestasis, colitis, erythema multiforme, hemolytic anemia, hemorrhage, interstitial nephritis, toxic nephropathy, pancytopenia, renal dysfunction, seizure, serum-sickness reactions, Stevens-Johnson syndrome, superinfection, toxic epidermal necrolysis, urticaria, vaginitis

Drug Interactions

Avoid Concomitant Use There are no known interactions where it is recommended to avoid concomitant use.

Increased Effect/Toxicity

The levels/effects of Cefpodoxime may be increased by: Uricosuric Agents

Decreased Effect

Cefpodoxime may decrease the levels/effects of: Typhoid Vaccine

The levels/effects of Cefpodoxime may be decreased by: Antacids; H2-Antagonists

Ethanol/Nutrition/Herb Interactions Food: Food delays absorption; cefpodoxime serum levels may be increased if taken with food.

Stability Shake well before using. After mixing, keep suspension in refrigerator. Discard unused portion after 14 days.

Mechanism of Action Inhibits bacterial cell wall synthesis by binding to one or more of the penicillin-binding proteins (PBPs) which in turn inhibits the final transpeptidation step of peptidoglycan synthesis in bacterial cell walls, thus inhibiting cell wall biosynthesis. Bacteria eventually lyse due to ongoing activity of cell wall autolytic enzymes (autolysins and murein hydrolases) while cell wall assembly is arrested.

Pharmacodynamics/Kinetics

Absorption: Rapid and well absorbed (50%), acid stable; enhanced in the presence of food or low gastric pH

Distribution: Good tissue penetration, including lung and tonsils; penetrates into pleural fluid

Protein binding: 18% to 23%

Metabolism: De-esterified in GI tract to active metabolite, cefpodoxime

Half-life elimination: 2.2 hours; prolonged with renal impairment

Time to peak: Within 1 hour

Excretion: Urine (80% as unchanged drug) in 24 hours

Dosage

Usual dosage range:

Children 2 months to 12 years: Oral: 10 mg/kg/day divided every 12 hours (maximum dose: 400 mg/day)

Children ≥12 years and Adults: Oral: 100-400 mg every 12 hours

Indication-specific dosing:

Children 2 months to 12 years: Oral:

Acute maxillary sinusitis: 10 mg/kg/day divided every 12 hours for 10 days (maximum: 200 mg/dose)

Acute otitis media: 10 mg/kg/day divided every 12 hours (400 mg/day) for 5 days (maximum: 200 mg/dose)

Pharyngitis/tonsillitis: 10 mg/kg/day in 2 divided doses for 5-10 days (maximum: 100 mg/dose)

Children ≥12 years and Adults: Oral:

Acute community-acquired pneumonia and bacterial exacerbations of chronic bronchitis: 200 mg every 12 hours for 14 days and 10 days, respectively

Acute maxillary sinusitis: 200 mg every 12 hours for 10 days

Pharyngitis/tonsillitis: 100 mg every 12 hours for 5-10 days

Skin and skin structure: 400 mg every 12 hours for 7-14 days

Uncomplicated gonorrhea (male and female) and rectal gonococcal infections (female): 200 mg as a single dose

Uncomplicated urinary tract infection: 100 mg every 12 hours for 7 days

Dosing adjustment in renal impairment: Cl_{cr} <30 mL/minute: Administer every 24 hours

Hemodialysis: Administer dose 3 times/week following hemodialysis

Dietary Considerations May be taken with food.

Administration Administer around-the-clock to promote less variation in peak and trough serum levels.

Monitoring Parameters Observe for signs and symptoms of anaphylaxis during first dose

Test Interactions Positive direct Coombs', false-positive urinary glucose test using cupric sulfate (Benedict's solution, Clinitest®, Fehling's solution), false-positive serum or urine creatinine with Jaffé reaction

Dosage Forms Excipient information presented when available (limited, particularly for generics); consult specific product labeling. [DSC] = Discontinued product

Granules for oral suspension: 50 mg/5 mL (50 mL, 75 mL, 100 mL); 100 mg/5 mL (50 mL, 75 mL, 100 mL)

Vantin®: 50 mg/5 mL (100 mL) [contains sodium benzoate; lemon creme flavor] [DSC]; 100 mg/5 mL (100 mL) [contains sodium benzoate; lemon creme flavor] [DSC]

Tablet: 100 mg, 200 mg

Vantin®: 100 mg, 200 mg

◆ **Cefpodoxime Proxetil** *see* Cefpodoxime *on page 280*

Cefprozil (sef PROE zil)

Canadian Brand Names Apo-Cefprozil®; Cefzil®; Ran-Cefprozil; Sandoz-Cefprozil

Pharmacologic Category Antibiotic, Cephalosporin (Second Generation)

Additional Appendix Information

Community-Acquired Pneumonia in Adults *on page 1766*

Use Treatment of otitis media and infections involving the respiratory tract and skin and skin structure; active against methicillin-sensitive staphylococci, many streptococci, and various gram-negative bacilli including *E. coli*, some *Klebsiella*, *P. mirabilis*, *H. influenzae*, and *Moraxella*.

Pregnancy Risk Factor B

Pregnancy Considerations Adverse events were not observed in animal reproduction studies; therefore, cefprozil is classified as pregnancy category B. It is not known if cefprozil crosses the human placenta. Other cephalosporins cross the placenta and are considered safe for use during pregnancy.

Lactation Enters breast milk/use caution (AAP rates "compatible")

Medication Safety Issues

Sound-alike/look-alike issues:

Cefprozil may be confused with ceFAZolin, cefuroxime

Cefzil® may be confused with Cefol®, Ceftin®, Kefzol®

Contraindications Hypersensitivity to cefprozil, any component of the formulation, or other cephalosporins

Warnings/Precautions Modify dosage in patients with severe renal impairment. Use with caution in patients with a history of penicillin allergy, especially IgE-mediated reactions (eg, anaphylaxis, urticaria). Prolonged use may result in fungal or bacterial superinfection, including *C. difficile*-associated diarrhea (CDAD) and pseudomembranous colitis; CDAD has been observed >2 months postantibiotic treatment. Some products may contain phenylalanine.

Adverse Reactions

1% to 10%:

Central nervous system: Dizziness (1%)

Dermatologic: Diaper rash (1.5%)

Gastrointestinal: Diarrhea (2.9%), nausea (3.5%), vomiting (1%), abdominal pain (1%)

Genitourinary: Vaginitis, genital pruritus (1.6%)

Hepatic: Transaminases increased (2%)

Miscellaneous: Superinfection

<1% (Limited to important or life-threatening): Anaphylaxis, angioedema, arthralgia, BUN increased, cholestatic jaundice, confusion, creatinine increased, eosinophilia, erythema multiforme, fever, headache, hyperactivity, insomnia, leukopenia, pseudomembranous colitis, rash, serum sickness, somnolence, Stevens-Johnson syndrome, thrombocytopenia, urticaria

Reactions reported with other cephalosporins: Agranulocytosis, aplastic anemia, colitis, hemolytic anemia, hemorrhage, interstitial nephritis, pancytopenia, renal dysfunction, seizure, superinfection, toxic epidermal necrolysis, toxic nephropathy, vaginitis

Drug Interactions

Avoid Concomitant Use There are no known interactions where it is recommended to avoid concomitant use.

Increased Effect/Toxicity

The levels/effects of Cefprozil may be increased by: Uricosuric Agents

Decreased Effect

Cefprozil may decrease the levels/effects of: Typhoid Vaccine

Ethanol/Nutrition/Herb Interactions Food: Food delays cefprozil absorption.

Mechanism of Action Inhibits bacterial cell wall synthesis by binding to one or more of the penicillin-binding proteins (PBPs) which in turn inhibits the final transpeptidation step of peptidoglycan synthesis in bacterial cell walls, thus inhibiting cell wall biosynthesis. Bacteria eventually lyse due to ongoing activity of cell wall autolytic enzymes (autolysins and murein hydrolases) while cell wall assembly is arrested.

Pharmacodynamics/Kinetics

Absorption: Well absorbed (94%)

Protein binding: 35% to 45%

Half-life elimination: Normal renal function: 1.3 hours

Time to peak, serum: Fasting: 1.5 hours

Excretion: Urine (61% as unchanged drug)

Dosage

Usual dosage range:

Infants and Children >6 months to 12 years: Oral: 7.5-15 mg/kg/day divided every 12 hours

Children >12 years and Adults: Oral: 250-500 mg every 12 hours or 500 mg every 24 hours

Indication-specific dosing:

Infants and Children >6 months to 12 years: Oral:

Otitis media: 15 mg/kg every 12 hours for 10 days

Children 2-12 years: Oral:

Pharyngitis/tonsillitis: 7.5-15 mg/kg/day divided every 12 hours for 10 days (administer for >10 days if due to *S. pyogenes*); maximum: 1 g/day

Uncomplicated skin and skin structure infections: 20 mg/kg every 24 hours for 10 days; maximum: 1 g/day

Children >12 years and Adults: Oral:

Pharyngitis/tonsillitis: 500 mg every 24 hours for 10 days

Secondary bacterial infection of acute bronchitis or acute bacterial exacerbation of chronic bronchitis: 500 mg every 12 hours for 10 days

Uncomplicated skin and skin structure infections: 250 mg every 12 hours or 500 mg every 12-24 hours for 10 days

Dosing adjustment in renal impairment: Cl_{cr} <30 mL/minute: Reduce dose by 50%

Hemodialysis: Reduced by hemodialysis; administer dose after the completion of hemodialysis

Dietary Considerations May be taken with food. Oral suspension contains phenylalanine 28 mg/5 mL.

Administration Administer around-the-clock to promote less variation in peak and trough serum levels. Chilling the reconstituted oral suspension improves flavor (do not freeze).

Monitoring Parameters Assess patient at beginning and throughout therapy for infection; monitor for signs of anaphylaxis during first dose

Test Interactions Positive direct Coombs', false-positive urinary glucose test using cupric sulfate (Benedict's solution, Clinitest®, Fehling's solution), false-positive serum or urine creatinine with Jaffé reaction

Dosage Forms Excipient information presented when available (limited, particularly for generics); consult specific product labeling.

Powder for oral suspension, as anhydrous: 125 mg/5 mL (50 mL, 75 mL, 100 mL); 250 mg/5 mL (50 mL, 75 mL, 100 mL)

Tablet, as anhydrous: 250 mg, 500 mg

Ceftazidime (SEF tay zi deem)

U.S. Brand Names Fortaz®; Tazicef®

Canadian Brand Names Fortaz®

Pharmacologic Category Antibiotic, Cephalosporin (Third Generation)

Additional Appendix Information

Antimicrobial Drugs of Choice *on page 1752*

Use Treatment of documented susceptible *Pseudomonas aeruginosa* infection and infections due to other susceptible aerobic gram-negative organisms; empiric therapy of a febrile, granulocytopenic patient

Unlabeled/Investigational Use Bacterial endophthalmitis

Pregnancy Risk Factor B

Pregnancy Considerations Teratogenic effects were not observed in animal studies; therefore, ceftazidime is classified as pregnancy category B. Ceftazidime crosses the placenta and reaches the cord serum and amniotic fluid. Maternal peak serum concentration is unchanged in the first trimester. After the first trimester, serum concentrations decrease by approximately 50% of those in nonpregnant patients. Renal clearance is increased during pregnancy.

Lactation Enters breast milk (small amounts)/use caution (AAP rates "compatible")

Medication Safety Issues

Sound-alike/look-alike issues:

Ceftazidime may be confused with ceftizoxime
Ceptaz® may be confused with Septra®
Tazicef® may be confused with Tazidime®
Tazidime® may be confused with Tazicef®

International issues:

Ceftim® [Italy] may be confused with Ceftin® which is a brand name for cefuroxime in the U.S.
Ceftim® [Italy] may be confused with Cefiton® which is a brand name for cefixime in Portugal
Ceftim® [Italy] may be confused with Ceftina® which is a brand name for cefalotin in Mexico

Contraindications Hypersensitivity to ceftazidime, any component of the formulation, or other cephalosporins

Warnings/Precautions Modify dosage in patients with severe renal impairment. Use with caution in patients with a history of penicillin allergy, especially IgE-mediated reactions (eg, anaphylaxis, urticaria). Prolonged use may result in fungal or bacterial superinfection, including *C. difficile*-associated diarrhea (CDAD) and pseudomembranous colitis; CDAD has been observed >2 months postantibiotic treatment. May be associated with increased INR, especially in nutritionally-deficient patients, prolonged treatment, hepatic or renal disease. Use with caution in patients with a history of seizure disorder; high levels, particularly in the presence of renal impairment, may increase risk of seizures.

Adverse Reactions

1% to 10%:

Gastrointestinal: Diarrhea (1%)
Local: Pain at injection site (1%)
Miscellaneous: Hypersensitivity reactions (2%)

<1% (Limited to important or life-threatening): Anaphylaxis, angioedema, asterixis, BUN increased, candidiasis, creatinine increased, dizziness, encephalopathy, eosinophilia, erythema multiforme, fever, headache, hemolytic anemia, hyperbilirubinemia, jaundice, leukopenia, myoclonus, nausea, neuromuscular excitability, paresthesia, phlebitis, pruritus, pseudomembranous colitis, rash, Stevens-Johnson syndrome, thrombocytosis, toxic epidermal necrolysis, transaminases increased, vaginitis, vomiting

Reactions reported with other cephalosporins: Agranulocytosis, aplastic anemia, cholestasis, colitis, hemolytic anemia, hemorrhage, interstitial nephritis, pancytopenia, prolonged PT, renal dysfunction, seizure, serum-sickness reactions, superinfection, toxic nephropathy, urticaria

Drug Interactions

Avoid Concomitant Use There are no known interactions where it is recommended to avoid concomitant use.

Increased Effect/Toxicity

The levels/effects of Ceftazidime may be increased by: Uricosuric Agents

Decreased Effect

Ceftazidime may decrease the levels/effects of: Typhoid Vaccine

Stability

Vials: Reconstituted solution and solution further diluted for I.V. infusion are stable for 12 hours at room temperature, for 3 days when refrigerated, or for 12 weeks when frozen at -20°C (-4°F). After freezing, thawed solution in SWFI for I.M. administration is stable for 3 hours at room temperature or for 3 days when refrigerated, thawed solution in NS in a Viaflex® small volume container for I.V. administration is stable for 12 hours at room temperature or for 3 days when refrigerated, and thawed solution in SWFI in the original container is stable for 8 hours at room temperature or for 3 days when refrigerated.

Premixed frozen solution: Store frozen at -20°C (-4°F). Thawed solution is stable for 8 hours at room temperature or for 3 days under refrigeration; do not refreeze.

Mechanism of Action Inhibits bacterial cell wall synthesis by binding to one or more of the penicillin-binding proteins (PBPs) which in turn inhibits the final transpeptidation step of peptidoglycan synthesis in bacterial cell walls, thus inhibiting cell wall biosynthesis. Bacteria eventually lyse due to ongoing activity of cell wall autolytic enzymes (autolysins and murein hydrolases) while cell wall assembly is arrested.

Pharmacodynamics/Kinetics

Distribution: Widely throughout the body including bone bile, skin, CSF (higher concentrations achieved when meninges are inflamed), endometrium, heart, pleural and lymphatic fluids

Protein binding: 17%

Half-life elimination: 1-2 hours, prolonged with renal impairment; Neonates <23 days: 2.2-4.7 hours

Time to peak, serum: I.M.: ~1 hour

Excretion: Urine (80% to 90% as unchanged drug)

Dosage

Usual dosage range:

Infants and Children 1 month to 12 years: I.V.: 30-50 mg/kg/dose every 8 hours (maximum dose: 6 g/day)

Adults: I.M., I.V.: 500 mg to 2 g every 8-12 hours

Indication-specific dosing:

Bacterial arthritis (gram-negative bacilli): I.V.: 1-2 g every 8 hours

Cystic fibrosis: I.V.: 30-50 mg/kg every 8 hours (maximum: 6 g/day)

Endophthalmitis, bacterial (unlabeled use): Intravitreal: 2.25 mg/0.1 mL NS in combination with vancomycin

Melioidosis: I.V.: 40 mg/kg every 8 hours for 10 days, followed by oral therapy with doxycycline or TMP/SMX

Otitis externa: I.V.: 2 g every 8 hours

Peritonitis (CAPD):

Anuric, intermittent: 1000-1500 mg/day

Anuric, continuous (per liter exchange): Loading dose: 250 mg; maintenance dose: 125 mg

Severe infections, including meningitis, complicated pneumonia, endophthalmitis, CNS infection, osteomyelitis, intra-abdominal and gynecological, skin and soft tissue: I.V.: 2 g every 8 hours

Dosing interval in renal impairment:

Cl_{cr} 30-50 mL/minute: Administer every 12 hours

Cl_{cr} 10-30 mL/minute: Administer every 24 hours

Cl_{cr} <10 mL/minute: Administer every 48-72 hours

Hemodialysis: Dialyzable (50% to 100%)

Continuous renal replacement therapy (CRRT): Drug clearance is highly dependent on the method of renal replacement, filter type, and flow rate. Appropriate dosing requires close monitoring of pharmacologic response, signs of adverse reactions due to drug accumulation, as well as drug levels in relation to target trough (if appropriate). The following are general recommendations only (based on dialysate flow/ultrafiltration rates of 1 L/hour) and should not supersede clinical judgment:

CVVH: 1-2 g every 12 hours

CVVHD/CVVHDF: 2 g every 12 hours

Dietary Considerations Sodium content of 1 g: 2.3 mEq

Administration Any carbon dioxide bubbles that may be present in the withdrawn solution should be expelled prior to injection. Administer around-the-clock to promote less variation in peak and trough serum levels. Ceftazidime can be administered deep I.M. into large mass muscle, IVP over 3-5 minutes, or I.V. intermittent infusion over 15-30 minutes. Do not admix with aminoglycosides in same bottle/bag. Final concentration for I.V. administration should not exceed 100 mg/mL.

Monitoring Parameters Observe for signs and symptoms of anaphylaxis during first dose

Test Interactions Positive direct Coombs', false-positive urinary glucose test using cupric sulfate (Benedict's solution, Clinitest®, Fehling's solution), false-positive serum or urine creatinine with Jaffé reaction

Additional Information With some organisms, resistance may develop during treatment (including *Enterobacter* spp and *Serratia* spp). Consider combination therapy or periodic susceptibility testing for organisms with inducible resistance.

Dosage Forms Excipient information presented when available (limited, particularly for generics); consult specific product labeling.

Infusion [premixed iso-osmotic solution, frozen]:

Fortaz®: 1 g (50 mL) [contains sodium carbonate, sodium ~54 mg (2.3 mEq)/g]; 2 g (50 mL) [contains sodium ~54 mg (2.3 mEq)/g]

Injection, powder for reconstitution: 1 g, 2 g, 6 g

Fortaz®: 500 mg, 1 g, 2 g, 6 g [contains sodium ~54 mg (2.3 mEq)/g]

Tazicef®: 1 g, 2 g, 6 g [contains sodium ~54 mg (2.3 mEq)/g]

Ceftibuten (sef TYE byoo ten)

U.S. Brand Names Cedax®

Pharmacologic Category Antibiotic, Cephalosporin (Third Generation)

Use Oral cephalosporin for treatment of bronchitis, otitis media, and pharyngitis/tonsillitis due to *H. influenzae* and *M. catarrhalis*, both beta-lactamase-producing and non-producing strains, as well as *S. pneumoniae* (weak) and *S. pyogenes*

Pregnancy Risk Factor B

Pregnancy Considerations Teratogenic effects were not observed in animal studies; therefore, ceftibuten is classified as pregnancy category B. It is not know if ceftibuten crosses the placenta; other cephalosporins cross the placenta and are considered safe for use during pregnancy. Adequate and well-controlled studies have been completed in pregnant women.

Lactation Excretion in breast milk unknown/use caution

Medication Safety Issues

International issues:

Cedax® may be confused with Codex which is a brand name for *Saccharomyces boulardii* in Italy

Contraindications Hypersensitivity to ceftibuten, any component of the formulation, or other cephalosporins

Warnings/Precautions Modify dosage in patients with severe renal impairment. Prolonged use may result in fungal or bacterial superinfection, including *C. difficile*-associated diarrhea (CDAD) and pseudomembranous colitis; CDAD has been observed >2 months postantibiotic treatment. Use with caution in patients with a history of penicillin allergy, especially IgE-mediated reactions (eg, anaphylaxis, urticaria).

Adverse Reactions

1% to 10%:

Central nervous system: Headache (3%), dizziness (1%)

Gastrointestinal: Nausea (4%), diarrhea (3%), dyspepsia (2%), vomiting (1%), abdominal pain (1%)

Hematologic: Eosinophils increased (3%), hemoglobin decreased (2%), thrombocytosis

Hepatic: ALT increased (1%), bilirubin increased (1%)

Renal: BUN increased (4%)

<1% (Limited to important or life-threatening): Agitation, anorexia, candidiasis, constipation, creatinine increased, diaper rash, dry mouth, dyspnea, dysuria, fatigue, insomnia, irritability, leukopenia, nasal congestion, paresthesia, rash, rigors, transaminases increased, urticaria

Reactions reported with other cephalosporins: Agranulocytosis, anaphylaxis, angioedema, aplastic anemia, asterixis, candidiasis, cholestasis, colitis, encephalopathy, erythema multiforme, fever, hemolytic anemia, hemorrhage, interstitial nephritis, neuromuscular excitability, pancytopenia, paresthesia, prolonged PT, pruritus, pseudomembranous colitis, renal dysfunction, seizure, serum-sickness reactions, Stevens-Johnson syndrome, superinfection, toxic epidermal necrolysis, toxic nephropathy, vaginitis

Drug Interactions

Avoid Concomitant Use There are no known interactions where it is recommended to avoid concomitant use.

Increased Effect/Toxicity

The levels/effects of Ceftibuten may be increased by: Uricosuric Agents

Decreased Effect

Ceftibuten may decrease the levels/effects of: Typhoid Vaccine

Stability Reconstituted suspension is stable for 14 days when refrigerated.

Mechanism of Action Inhibits bacterial cell wall synthesis by binding to one or more of the penicillin-binding proteins (PBPs) which in turn inhibits the final transpeptidation step of peptidoglycan synthesis in bacterial cell walls, thus inhibiting cell wall biosynthesis. Bacteria eventually lyse due to ongoing activity of cell wall autolytic enzymes (autolysins and murein hydrolases) while cell wall assembly is arrested.

Pharmacodynamics/Kinetics

Absorption: Rapid; food decreases peak concentrations, delays T_{max}, and lowers AUC

Distribution: V_d: Children: 0.5 L/kg; Adults: 0.21 L/kg

Protein binding: 65%

Half-life elimination: 2 hours

Time to peak: 2-3 hours

Excretion: Urine (52%); feces (39%)

Dosage

Usual dosage range:

Children <12 years: Oral: 9 mg/kg/day for 10 days (maximum dose: 400 mg/day)

Children ≥12 years and Adults: Oral: 400 mg once daily for 10 days (maximum dose: 400 mg/day)

Dosage adjustment in renal impairment:

Cl_{cr} 30-49 mL//minute: Administer 4.5 mg/kg or 200 mg every 24 hours

Cl_{cr} 5-29 mL/minute: Administer 2.25 mg/kg or 100 mg every 24 hours.

Hemodialysis: Administer 400 mg or 9 mg/kg (maximum: 400 mg) after hemodialysis

Dietary Considerations

Capsule: Take without regard to food.

Suspension: Take 2 hours before or 1 hour after meals; contains 1 g of sucrose per 5 mL

Administration Shake suspension well before use.

Monitoring Parameters Observe for signs and symptoms of anaphylaxis during first dose; with prolonged therapy, monitor renal, hepatic, and hematologic function periodically

Test Interactions Positive direct Coombs', false-positive urinary glucose test using cupric sulfate (Benedict's solution, Clinitest®, Fehling's solution), false-positive serum or urine creatinine with Jaffé reaction

Dosage Forms Excipient information presented when available (limited, particularly for generics); consult specific product labeling.

Capsule:

Cedax®: 400 mg

Powder for oral suspension:

Cedax®: 90 mg/5 mL (30 mL, 60 mL, 90 mL, 120 mL) [contains sucrose 1g/5 mL and sodium benzoate; cherry flavor]

◆ **Ceftin®** *see* Cefuroxime *on page* 288

Ceftizoxime (sef ti ZOKS eem)

U.S. Brand Names Cefizox®

Canadian Brand Names Cefizox®

Index Terms Ceftizoxime Sodium

Pharmacologic Category Antibiotic, Cephalosporin (Third Generation)

Additional Appendix Information

Antimicrobial Drugs of Choice *on page* 1752

Treatment of Sexually Transmitted Infections *on page* 1773

Use Treatment of susceptible bacterial infections, mainly respiratory tract, skin and skin structure, bone and joint, urinary tract and gynecologic, as well as septicemia; active against many gram-negative bacilli (not *Pseudomonas*), some gram-positive cocci (not *Enterococcus*), and some anaerobes

Pregnancy Risk Factor B

Pregnancy Considerations Teratogenic effects have not been observed in animal studies; therefore, ceftizoxime is classified as pregnancy category B. Ceftizoxime crosses the placenta and is found in the cord blood and amniotic fluid in amounts that are higher than the maternal serum. The maternal peak concentrations at term are similar to those in nonpregnant volunteers.

Lactation Enters breast milk (small amounts)/use caution

Medication Safety Issues

Sound-alike/look-alike issues:

Ceftizoxime may be confused with cefotaxime, ceftazidime, cefuroxime

Contraindications Hypersensitivity to ceftizoxime, any component of the formulation, or other cephalosporins

Warnings/Precautions Modify dosage in patients with severe renal impairment. Prolonged use may result in fungal or bacterial superinfection, including *C. difficile*-associated diarrhea (CDAD) and pseudomembranous colitis; CDAD has been observed >2 months postantibiotic treatment. Use with caution in patients with a history of penicillin allergy, especially IgE-mediated reactions (eg, anaphylaxis, urticaria).

Adverse Reactions

1% to 10%:

Central nervous system: Fever

Dermatologic: Rash, pruritus

Hematologic: Eosinophilia, thrombocytosis

Hepatic: Alkaline phosphatase increased, transaminases increased

Local: Pain, burning at injection site

<1% (Limited to important or life-threatening): Anaphylaxis, anemia, bilirubin increased, BUN increased, creatinine increased, diarrhea, injection site reactions, leukopenia, nausea, neutropenia, numbness, paresthesia, phlebitis, thrombocytopenia, vaginitis, vomiting

Reactions reported with other cephalosporins: Agranulocytosis, angioedema, aplastic anemia, asterixis, candidiasis, cholestasis, colitis, encephalopathy, erythema multiforme, hemolytic anemia, hemorrhage, interstitial nephritis, neuromuscular excitability, pancytopenia, prolonged PT, pseudomembranous colitis, renal dysfunction, seizure, serum-sickness reactions, Stevens-Johnson syndrome, superinfection, toxic epidermal necrolysis, toxic nephropathy

Drug Interactions

Avoid Concomitant Use There are no known interactions where it is recommended to avoid concomitant use.

Increased Effect/Toxicity

The levels/effects of Ceftizoxime may be increased by: Uricosuric Agents

Decreased Effect

Ceftizoxime may decrease the levels/effects of: Typhoid Vaccine

Stability Reconstituted solution is stable for 24 hours at room temperature and 96 hours when refrigerated. For I.V. infusion in NS or D_5W solution is stable for 24 hours at room temperature, 96 hours when refrigerated, or 12 weeks when frozen. After freezing, thawed solution is stable for 24 hours at room temperature or 10 days when refrigerated.

Mechanism of Action Inhibits bacterial cell wall synthesis by binding to one or more of the penicillin-binding proteins (PBPs) which in turn inhibits the final transpeptidation step of peptidoglycan synthesis in bacterial cell walls, thus inhibiting cell wall biosynthesis. Bacteria eventually lyse due to ongoing activity of cell wall autolytic enzymes (autolysins and murein hydrolases) while cell wall assembly is arrested.

Pharmacodynamics/Kinetics

Distribution: V_d: 0.35-0.5 L/kg; widely into most body tissues and fluids including gallbladder, liver, kidneys, bone, sputum, bile, pleural and synovial fluids; has good CSF penetration

Protein binding: 30%

Half-life elimination: 1.6 hours; Cl_{cr} <10 mL/minute: 25 hours

Time to peak, serum: I.M.: 0.5-1 hour

Excretion: Urine (as unchanged drug)

Dosage

Usual dosage range:

Children ≥6 months: I.M., I.V.: 150-200 mg/kg/day divided every 6-8 hours (maximum: 12 g/24 hours)

Adults: I.M., I.V.: 1-4 g every 8-12 hours

Indication-specific dosing:

Adults:

Gonococcal:

Disseminated infection: I.M., I.V.: 1 g every 8 hours

Uncomplicated: I.M.: 1 g as single dose

Life-threatening infections: I.V.: 2 g every 4 hours or 4 g every 8 hours

Dosing adjustment in renal impairment: Adults:

Cl_{cr} 50-79 mL/minute: Administer 500-1500 mg every 8 hours.

Cl_{cr} 5-49 mL/minute: Administer 250-1000 mg every 12 hours.

Cl_{cr} 0-4 mL/minute: Administer 500-1000 mg every 48 hours or 250-500 mg every 24 hours.

Moderately dialyzable (20% to 50%)

Continuous arteriovenous hemofiltration: Dose as for Cl_{cr} 10-50 mL/minute.

Dietary Considerations Sodium content of 1 g: 60 mg (2.6 mEq)

Administration

I.M.: Inject deep I.M. into large muscle mass.

I.V.: Inject direct I.V. over 3-5 minutes. Infuse intermittent infusion over 30 minutes.

Monitoring Parameters Observe for signs and symptoms of anaphylaxis during first dose

Test Interactions Positive direct Coombs', false-positive urinary glucose test using cupric sulfate (Benedict's solution, Clinitest®, Fehling's solution), false-positive serum or urine creatinine with Jaffé reaction

Dosage Forms Excipient information presented when available (limited, particularly for generics); consult specific product labeling.

Infusion [premixed iso-osmotic solution]:

Cefizox®: 1 g (50 mL); 2 g (50 mL)

Injection, powder for reconstitution:

Cefizox®: 1 g, 2 g, 10 g [DSC]

◆ **Ceftizoxime Sodium** *see* Ceftizoxime *on page 284*

CefTRIAXone (sef trye AKS one)

U.S. Brand Names Rocephin®

Canadian Brand Names Rocephin®

Index Terms Ceftriaxone Sodium

Pharmacologic Category Antibiotic, Cephalosporin (Third Generation)

Use Treatment of lower respiratory tract infections, acute bacterial otitis media, skin and skin structure infections, bone and joint infections, intra-abdominal and urinary tract infections, pelvic inflammatory disease (PID), uncomplicated gonorrhea, bacterial septicemia, and meningitis; used in surgical prophylaxis

Unlabeled/Investigational Use Treatment of chancroid, epididymitis, complicated gonococcal infections; sexually-transmitted diseases (STD); periorbital or buccal cellulitis; salmonellosis or shigellosis; atypical community-acquired pneumonia; epiglottitis, Lyme disease; used in chemoprophylaxis for high-risk contacts and persons with invasive meningococcal disease; sexual assault; typhoid fever, Whipple's disease

Pregnancy Risk Factor B

Pregnancy Considerations Teratogenic effects have not been observed in animal studies; therefore, ceftriaxone is classified as pregnancy category B. The pharmacokinetics of ceftriaxone in the third trimester are similar to those of nonpregnant patients, with the possible exception of lower peak concentrations during labor. Ceftriaxone crosses the placenta and distributes to amniotic fluid. Ceftriaxone is recommended for use in pregnant women for the treatment of gonococcal infections.

Lactation Enters breast milk/use caution (AAP rates "compatible")

Medication Safety Issues

Sound-alike/look-alike issues:

Rocephin® may be confused with Roferon®

Contraindications Hypersensitivity to ceftriaxone sodium, any component of the formulation, or other cephalosporins; **do not use in hyperbilirubinemic neonates**, particularly those who are premature since ceftriaxone is reported to displace bilirubin from albumin binding sites; concomitant use with intravenous calcium-containing solutions/products in neonates (≤28 days)

Warnings/Precautions Use with caution in patients with a history of penicillin allergy, especially IgE-mediated reactions (eg, anaphylaxis, urticaria). Abnormal gallbladder sonograms have been reported, possibly due to cetriaxone-calcium precipitates; discontinue in patients with signs and symptoms of gallbladder disease. Secondary to biliary obstruction, pancreatitis has been reported rarely. Use with caution in patients with a history of GI disease, especially colitis. Prolonged use may result in fungal or bacterial superinfection, including *C. difficile*-associated diarrhea (CDAD) and pseudomembranous colitis; CDAD has been observed >2 months postantibiotic treatment. May be associated with increased INR (rarely), especially in nutritionally-deficient patients, prolonged treatment, hepatic or renal disease. No adjustment is generally necessary in patients with renal impairment; if severe renal impairment, particularly with concurrent hepatic dysfunction, do not exceed 2 g/day without serum concentration monitoring. Ceftriaxone may complex with calcium causing precipitation. Fatal lung and kidney damage associated with calcium-ceftriaxone precipitates has been observed in premature and term neonates. Do not reconstitute, admix, or coadminister with calcium-containing solutions, even via separate infusion lines/sites or at different times in any patient, regardless of age, due to concerns of potential precipitation reactions (contraindicated in neonates). Further recommendations include avoiding intravenous calcium-containing solutions within 48 hours of the last ceftriaxone dose in all patients. However, extending these recommendations to all patients is based solely on theoretical data, as there have been no reports of precipitant-induced adverse effects in non-neonatal patients.

Adverse Reactions

>10%: Local: Induration (I.M. 5% to 17%), warmth (I.M.), tightness (I.M.)

1% to 10%:

Dermatologic: Rash (2%)

Gastrointestinal: Diarrhea (3%)

Hematologic: Eosinophilia (6%), thrombocytosis (5%), leukopenia (2%)

Hepatic: Transaminases increased (3%)

Local: Tenderness at injection site (I.V. 1%), pain

Renal: BUN increased (1%)

<1% (Limited to important or life-threatening): Abdominal pain, agranulocytosis, alkaline phosphatase increased, allergic dermatitis, allergic pneumonitis, anaphylaxis, anemia, basophilia, biliary lithiasis, bilirubin increased, bronchospasm, chills, colitis, creatinine increased, diaphoresis, dizziness, dysgeusia, dyspepsia, edema, epistaxis, erythema multiforme, exanthema, fever, flatulence, flushing, gallbladder sludge, gallstones, glossitis, glycosuria, headache, hematuria, hemolytic anemia, jaundice, leukocytosis, Lyell's syndrome, lymphocytosis, lymphopenia, moniliasis, monocytosis, nausea, nephrolithiasis, neutropenia, oliguria, palpitation, pancreatitis, phlebitis, prolonged or decreased PT, pruritus, pseudomembranous colitis, renal and pulmonary ceftriaxone-calcium precipitations (neonates including some

fatalities), seizure, serum sickness Stevens-Johnson syndrome, stomatitis, thrombocytopenia , toxic epidermal necrolysis, urinary casts, urticaria, vaginitis, vomiting

Reactions reported with other cephalosporins: Angioedema, allergic reaction, aplastic anemia, asterixis, cholestasis, encephalopathy, hemorrhage, hepatic dysfunction, hyperactivity (reversible), hypertonia, interstitial nephritis, LDH increased, neuromuscular excitability, pancytopenia, paresthesia, renal dysfunction, superinfection, toxic nephropathy

Drug Interactions

Avoid Concomitant Use

Avoid concomitant use of CefTRIAXone with any of the following: Calcium Salts (Intravenous); Ringer's Injection (Lactated)

Increased Effect/Toxicity

CefTRIAXone may increase the levels/effects of: Vitamin K Antagonists

The levels/effects of CefTRIAXone may be increased by: Calcium Salts (Intravenous); Ringer's Injection (Lactated); Uricosuric Agents

Decreased Effect

CefTRIAXone may decrease the levels/effects of: Typhoid Vaccine

Stability

Powder for injection: Prior to reconstitution, store at room temperature ≤25°C (≤77°F). Protect from light.

Premixed solution (manufacturer premixed): Store at -20°C. Once thawed, solutions are stable for 3 days at room temperature of 25°C (77°F) or for 21 days refrigerated at 5°C (41°F). Do not refreeze.

Stability of reconstituted solutions:

10-40 mg/mL: Reconstituted in D_5W, $D_{10}W$, NS, or SWFI: Stable for 2 days at room temperature of 25°C (77°F) or for 10 days when refrigerated at 4°C (39°F). Stable for 26 weeks when frozen at -20°C when reconstituted with D_5W or NS. Once thawed (at room temperature), solutions are stable for 2 days at room temperature of 25°C (77°F) or for 10 days when refrigerated at 4°C (39°F); does not apply to manufacturer's premixed bags. Do not refreeze.

100 mg/mL:

Reconstituted in D_5W, SWFI, or NS: Stable for 2 days at room temperature of 25°C (77°F) or for 10 days when refrigerated at 4°C (39°F).

Reconstituted in lidocaine 1% solution or bacteriostatic water: Stable for 24 hours at room temperature of 25°C (77°F) or for 10 days when refrigerated at 4°C (39°F).

250-350 mg/mL: Reconstituted in D_5W, NS, lidocaine 1% solution, bacteriostatic water, or SWFI: Stable for 24 hours at room temperature of 25°C (77°F) or for 3 days when refrigerated at 4°C (39°F).

Reconstitution:

I.M. injection: Vials should be reconstituted with appropriate volume of diluent (including D_5W, NS, SWFI, bacteriostatic water, or 1% lidocaine) to make a final concentration of 250 mg/mL or 350 mg/mL.

Volume to add to create a **250 mg/mL** solution:

250 mg vial: 0.9 mL
500 mg vial: 1.8 mL
1 g vial: 3.6 mL
2 g vial: 7.2 mL

Volume to add to create a **350 mg/mL** solution:

500 mg vial: 1.0 mL
1 g vial: 2.1 mL
2 g vial: 4.2 mL

I.V. infusion: Infusion is prepared in two stages: Initial reconstitution of powder, followed by dilution to final infusion solution.

Vials: Reconstitute powder with appropriate I.V. diluent (including SWFI, D_5W, $D_{10}W$, NS) to create an initial solution of ~100 mg/mL. Recommended volume to add:

250 mg vial: 2.4 mL
500 mg vial: 4.8 mL
1 g vial: 9.6 mL
2 g vial: 19.2 mL

Note: After reconstitution of powder, further dilution into a volume of compatible solution (eg, 50-100 mL of D_5W or NS) is recommended.

Piggyback bottle: Reconstitute powder with appropriate I.V. diluent (D_5W or NS) to create a resulting solution of ~100 mg/mL. Recommended initial volume to add:

1 g bottle:10 mL
2 g bottle: 20 mL

Note: After reconstitution, to prepare the final infusion solution, further dilution to 50 mL or 100 mL volumes with the appropriate I.V. diluent (including D_5W or NS) is recommended.

Mechanism of Action Inhibits bacterial cell wall synthesis by binding to one or more of the penicillin-binding proteins (PBPs) which in turn inhibits the final transpeptidation step of peptidoglycan synthesis in bacterial cell walls, thus inhibiting cell wall biosynthesis. Bacteria eventually lyse due to ongoing activity of cell wall autolytic enzymes (autolysins and murein hydrolases) while cell wall assembly is arrested.

Pharmacodynamics/Kinetics

Absorption: I.M.: Well absorbed

Distribution: V_d: 6-14 L; widely throughout the body including gallbladder, lungs, bone, bile, CSF (higher concentrations achieved when meninges are inflamed)

Protein binding: 85% to 95%

Half-life elimination: Normal renal and hepatic function: 5-9 hours; Renal impairment (mild-to-severe): 12-16 hours

Time to peak, serum: I.M.: 2-3 hours

Excretion: Urine (33% to 67% as unchanged drug); feces (as inactive drug)

Dosage

Usual dosage range:

Infants and Children: I.M., I.V.: 50-100 mg/kg/day in 1-2 divided doses (maximum: 4 g/day [meningitis]; 2 g/day [nonmeningeal infections])

Adults: I.M., I.V.: 1-2 g every 12-24 hours

Indication-specific dosing:

Infants and Children:

Epiglottitis (unlabeled use): I.M., I.V.: 50-100 mg/kg once daily; reported duration of treatment ranged from 2-14 days

Gonococcal infections:

Conjunctivitis, complicated (unlabeled use): I.M.:
<45 kg: 50 mg/kg in a single dose (maximum: 1 g)
≥45 kg: 1 g in a single dose

Disseminated (unlabeled use): I.M., I.V.:
<45 kg: 25-50 mg/kg once daily (maximum: 1 g)
≥45 kg: 1 g once daily for 7 days

Endocarditis (unlabeled use):
<45 kg: I.M., I.V.: 50 mg/kg/day every 12 hours (maximum: 2 g/day) for at least 28 days
≥45 kg: I.V.: 1-2 g every 12 hours, for at least 28 days

Prophylaxis (due to maternal gonococcal infection): I.M., I.V.: 25-50 mg/kg as a single dose (maximum 125 mg)

Uncomplicated: I.M.: 125 mg in a single dose

Infective endocarditis: I.M., I.V.:

Native valve: 100 mg/kg once daily for 2-4 weeks
Note: If using 2-week regimen, concurrent gentamicin is recommended

Prosthetic valve: 100 mg/kg once daily for 6 weeks (with or without 2 weeks of gentamicin [dependent on penicillin MIC]); **Note:** For HACEK organisms duration of therapy is 4 weeks

Enterococcus faecalis (resistant to penicillin, aminoglycoside, and vancomycin), native or prosthetic valve: 100 mg/kg once daily for ≥8 weeks administered concurrently with ampicillin

Prophylaxis: 50 mg/kg 30-60 minutes before procedure; maximum dose: 1 g. Intramuscular injections should be avoided in patients who are receiving anticoagulant therapy. In these circumstances, orally administered regimens should be given whenever possible. Intravenously administered antibiotics should be used for patients who are unable to tolerate or absorb oral medications.

Note: American Heart Association (AHA) guidelines now recommend prophylaxis only in patients undergoing invasive procedures and in whom underlying cardiac conditions may predispose to a higher risk of adverse outcomes should infection occur. As of April 2007, routine prophylaxis for GI/GU procedures is no longer recommended by the AHA.

Lyme disease, persistent arthritis (unlabeled use): I.M., I.V.: 75-100 mg/kg (maximum: 2 g) for 2-4 weeks

Mild-to-moderate infections: I.M., I.V.: 50-75 mg/kg/day in 1-2 divided doses every 12-24 hours (maximum: 2 g/day); continue until at least 2 days after signs and symptoms of infection have resolved

Meningitis:

Gonococcal, complicated:

<45 kg: I.V.: 50 mg/kg/day given every 12 hours (maximum: 2 g/day); usual duration of treatment is 10-14 days

>45 kg: I.V.: 1-2 g every 12 hours; usual duration of treatment is 10-14 days

Uncomplicated: I.M., I.V.: Loading dose of 100 mg/kg (maximum: 4 g), followed by 100 mg/kg/day divided every 12-24 hours (maximum: 4 g/day); usual duration of treatment is 7-14 days

Otitis media:

Acute: I.M.: 50 mg/kg in a single dose (maximum: 1 g)

Persistent or relapsing (unlabeled use): I.M., I.V.: 50 mg/kg once daily for 3 days

Pneumonia: I.V.: 50-75 mg/kg once daily

Serious infections: I.V.: 80-100 mg/kg/day in 1-2 divided doses (maximum: 4 g/day)

Skin/skin structure infections: I.M., I.V.: 50-75 mg/kg/day in 1-2 divided doses (maximum: 2 g/day)

STD, sexual assault (unlabeled use): I.M.: 125 mg in a single dose

Typhoid fever (unlabeled use): I.V.: 75-80 mg/kg once daily for 5-14 days

Children >8 years (≥45 kg) and Adolescents:

Epididymitis, acute (unlabeled use): I.M.: 125 mg in a single dose

Children ≤15 years:

Chemoprophylaxis for high-risk contacts and persons with invasive meningococcal disease (unlabeled use): I.M.: 125 mg in a single dose. Children >15 years: Refer to adult dosing.

Adults:

Arthritis, septic (unlabeled use): I.V.: 1-2 g once daily

Brain abscess (unlabeled use): I.V.: 2 g every 12 hours with metronidazole

Cavernous sinus thrombosis (unlabeled use): I.V.: 2 g once daily with vancomycin or linezolid

Chancroid (unlabeled use): I.M.: 250 mg as single dose

Chemoprophylaxis for high-risk contacts and persons with invasive meningococcal disease (unlabeled use): I.M.: 250 mg in a single dose

Gonococcal infections:

Conjunctivitis, complicated (unlabeled use): I.M.: 1 g in a single dose

Disseminated (unlabeled use): I.M., I.V.: 1 g once daily for 7 days

Endocarditis (unlabeled use): I.M., I.V.: 1-2 g every 12 hours for at least 28 days

Epididymitis, acute (unlabeled use): I.M.: 250 mg in a single dose with doxycycline

Prostatitis (unlabeled use): I.M.: 125-250 mg in a single dose with doxycycline

Uncomplicated: I.M.: 125-250 mg in a single dose

Infective endocarditis: I.M., I.V.:

Native valve: 2 g once daily for 2-4 weeks; **Note:** If using 2-week regimen, concurrent gentamicin is recommended

Prosthetic valve: I.M., I.V.: 2 g once daily for 6 weeks (with or without 2 weeks of gentamicin [dependent on penicillin MIC]); **Note:** For HACEK organisms, duration of therapy is 4 weeks

Enterococcus faecalis (resistant to penicillin, aminoglycoside, and vancomycin), native or prosthetic valve: 2 g twice daily for ≥8 weeks administered concurrently with ampicillin

Prophylaxis: I.M., I.V.: 1 g 30-60 minutes before procedure. Intramuscular injections should be avoided in patients who are receiving anticoagulant therapy. In these circumstances, orally administered regimens should be given whenever possible. Intravenously administered antibiotics should be used for patients who are unable to tolerate or absorb oral medications.

Note: American Heart Association (AHA) guidelines now recommend prophylaxis only in patients undergoing invasive procedures and in whom underlying cardiac conditions may predispose to a higher risk of adverse outcomes should infection occur. As of April 2007, routine prophylaxis for GI/GU procedures is no longer recommended by the AHA.

Lyme disease (unlabeled use): I.V.: 2 g once daily for 14-28 days

Mastoiditis (hospitalized; unlabeled use): I.V.: 2 g once daily; >60 years old: 1 g once daily

Meningitis: I.V.: 2 g every 12 hours for 7-14 days (longer courses may be necessary for selected organisms)

Orbital cellulitis (unlabeled use) and endophthalmitis: I.V.: 2 g once daily

Pelvic inflammatory disease: I.M.: 250 mg in a single dose

Pneumonia, community-acquired: I.V.: 1 g once daily, usually in combination with a macrolide; consider 2 g/day for patients at risk for more severe infection and/or resistant organisms (ICU status, age >65 years, disseminated infection)

Septic/toxic shock/necrotizing fasciitis (unlabeled use): I.V.: 2 g once daily; with clindamycin for toxic shock

STD prophylaxis in sexual assault victims: I.M.: 125 mg as a single dose

Surgical prophylaxis: I.V.: 1 g 30 minutes to 2 hours before surgery

Syphilis (unlabeled use): I.M., I.V.: 1 g once daily for 8-10 days

Typhoid fever (unlabeled use): I.V.: 2 g once daily for 14 days

Whipple's disease (unlabeled use): Initial: 2 g once daily for 10-14 days, then oral therapy for ~ 1 year.

Dosage adjustment in renal impairment: No adjustment is generally necessary; if severe impairment, particularly with concurrent hepatic dysfunction, do not exceed 2 g/day without serum concentration monitoring.

Hemodialysis: Not dialyzable (0% to 5%); administer dose postdialysis

Continuous ambulatory peritoneal dialysis (CAPD): Administer 1 g every 12 hours

Continuous renal replacement therapy (CRRT): Drug clearance is highly dependent on the method of renal replacement, filter type, and flow rate. Appropriate dosing requires close monitoring of pharmacologic response, signs of adverse reactions due to drug accumulation, as well as drug levels in relation to target trough (if appropriate). The following are general recommendations only (based on dialysate flow/ultrafiltration rates of 1 L/hour) and should not supersede clinical judgment:

CVVH or CVVHD/CVVHDF: 2 g every 12-24 hours

Dosage adjustment in hepatic impairment: No adjustment necessary

Dietary Considerations Sodium contents: ~83 mg (3.6 mEq) per ceftriaxone 1 g

Administration Do not admix with aminoglycosides in same bottle/bag. Do not reconstitute, admix, or coadminister with calcium-containing solutions. Infuse intermittent infusion over 30 minutes.

I.M.: Inject deep I.M. into large muscle mass; a concentration of 250 mg/mL or 350 mg/mL is recommended for all vial sizes except the 250 mg size (250 mg/mL is suggested); can be diluted with 1:1 water and 1% lidocaine for I.M. administration.

I.V.: Infuse intermittent infusion over 30 minutes.

Monitoring Parameters Observe for signs and symptoms of anaphylaxis

Test Interactions Positive direct Coombs', false-positive urinary glucose test using cupric sulfate (Benedict's solution, Clinitest®, Fehling's solution), false-positive serum or urine creatinine with Jaffé reaction

Dosage Forms Excipient information presented when available (limited, particularly for generics); consult specific product labeling. [DSC] = Discontinued product

Infusion [premixed in dextrose]: 1 g (50 mL); 2 g (50 mL)

Injection, powder for reconstitution: 250 mg, 500 mg, 1 g, 2 g, 10 g

Rocephin®: 250 mg [DSC], 500 mg, 1 g, 2 g [DSC], 10 g [contains sodium ~83 mg (3.6 mEq) per ceftriaxone 1 g] [DSC]

◆ **Ceftriaxone Sodium** *see* CefTRIAXone *on page* 285

Cefuroxime (se fyoor OKS eem)

U.S. Brand Names Ceftin®; Zinacef®

Canadian Brand Names Apo-Cefuroxime®; Ceftin®; Cefuroxime For Injection; Pro-Cefuroxime; Ratio-Cefuroxime; Zinacef®

Index Terms Cefuroxime Axetil; Cefuroxime Sodium

Pharmacologic Category Antibiotic, Cephalosporin (Second Generation)

Additional Appendix Information

Antimicrobial Drugs of Choice *on page* 1752

Community-Acquired Pneumonia in Adults *on page* 1766

Prevention of Wound Infection and Sepsis in Surgical Patients *on page* 1738

Use Treatment of infections caused by staphylococci, group B streptococci, *H. influenzae* (type A and B), *E. coli, Enterobacter, Salmonella*, and *Klebsiella*; treatment of susceptible infections of the upper and lower respiratory tract, otitis media, urinary tract, uncomplicated skin and soft tissue, bone and joint, sepsis, uncomplicated gonorrhea, and early Lyme disease; preoperative prophylaxis of susceptible infections

Pregnancy Risk Factor B

Pregnancy Considerations Adverse events were not observed in animal studies; therefore, cefuroxime is classified as pregnancy category B. Cefuroxime crosses the placenta and reaches the cord serum and amniotic fluid. Placental transfer is decreased in the presence of oligohydraminios. Several studies have failed to identify a teratogenic risk to the fetus from maternal cefuroxime use. During pregnancy, mean plasma concentrations of cefuroxime are 50% lower, the AUC is 25% lower, and the plasma half-life is shorter than nonpregnant values. At term, plasma half-life is similar to nonpregnant values and peak maternal concentrations after I.M. administration are slightly decreased. Pregnancy does not alter the volume of distribution.

Lactation Enters breast milk/use caution

Medication Safety Issues

Sound-alike/look-alike issues:

Cefuroxime may be confused with cefotaxime, cefprozil, ceftizoxime, deferoxamine

Ceftin® may be confused with Cefzil®, Cipro®

Zinacef® may be confused with Zithromax®

International issues:

Ceftin® may be confused with Cefiton® which is a brand name for cefixime in Portugal

Ceftin® may be confused with Ceftina® which is a brand name for cefalotin in Mexico

Ceftin® may be confused with Ceftim® which is a brand name for ceftazidime in Italy

Contraindications Hypersensitivity to cefuroxime, any component of the formulation, or other cephalosporins

Warnings/Precautions Modify dosage in patients with severe renal impairment. Use with caution in patients with a history of penicillin allergy, especially IgE-mediated reactions (eg, anaphylaxis, urticaria). Prolonged use may result in fungal or bacterial superinfection, including *C. difficile*-associated diarrhea (CDAD) and pseudomembranous colitis; CDAD has been observed >2 months postantibiotic treatment. May be associated with increased INR, especially in nutritionally-deficient patients, prolonged treatment, hepatic or renal disease. Tablets and oral suspension are not bioequivalent (do not substitute on a mg-per-mg basis). Some products may contain phenylalanine.

Adverse Reactions

>10%: Gastrointestinal: Diarrhea (4% to 11%, duration-dependent)

1% to 10%:

Dermatologic: Diaper rash (3%)

Endocrine & metabolic: Alkaline phosphatase increased (2%), lactate dehydrogenase increased (1%)

Gastrointestinal: Nausea/vomiting (3% to 7%)

Genitourinary: Vaginitis (≤5%)

Hematologic: Eosinophilia (7%), hemoglobin and hematocrit decreased (10%)

Hepatic: Transaminases increased (2% to 4%)

Local: Thrombophlebitis (2%)

<1% (Limited to important or life-threatening): Anaphylaxis, angioedema, BUN increased, chest pain, cholestasis, colitis, creatinine increased, dyspnea, erythema multiforme, fever, GI bleeding, hemolytic anemia, hepatitis, hives, hyperbilirubinemia, hypersensitivity, interstitial nephritis, jaundice, leukopenia, neutropenia, pain at injection site, pancytopenia, positive Coombs test, prolonged PT/INR, pseudomembranous colitis, rash, renal dysfunction, seizure, Stevens-Johnson syndrome, stomach cramps, tachycardia, thrombocytopenia (rare), tongue swelling, toxic epidermal necrolysis, urticaria

Reactions reported with other cephalosporins: Agranulocytosis, aplastic anemia, asterixis, colitis, encephalopathy, hemorrhage, neuromuscular excitability, serum-sickness reactions, superinfection, toxic nephropathy

Drug Interactions

Avoid Concomitant Use There are no known interactions where it is recommended to avoid concomitant use.

Increased Effect/Toxicity

The levels/effects of Cefuroxime may be increased by: Uricosuric Agents

Decreased Effect

Cefuroxime may decrease the levels/effects of: Typhoid Vaccine

The levels/effects of Cefuroxime may be decreased by: Antacids; H2-Antagonists

Ethanol/Nutrition/Herb Interactions Food: Bioavailability is increased with food; cefuroxime serum levels may be increased if taken with food or dairy products.

Stability

Injection: Reconstituted solution is stable for 24 hours at room temperature and 48 hours when refrigerated. I.V. infusion in NS or D_5W solution is stable for 24 hours at room temperature, 7 days when refrigerated, or 26 weeks when frozen. After freezing, thawed solution is stable for 24 hours at room temperature or 21 days when refrigerated.

Oral suspension: Prior to reconstitution, store at 2°C to 30°C (36°F to 86°F). Reconstituted suspension is stable for 10 days at 2°C to 8°C (36°F to 46°F).

Tablet: Store at 15°C to 30°C (59°F to 86°F).

Mechanism of Action Inhibits bacterial cell wall synthesis by binding to one or more of the penicillin-binding proteins (PBPs) which in turn inhibits the final transpeptidation step of peptidoglycan synthesis in bacterial cell walls, thus inhibiting cell wall biosynthesis. Bacteria eventually lyse due to ongoing activity of cell wall autolytic enzymes (autolysins and murein hydrolases) while cell wall assembly is arrested.

Pharmacodynamics/Kinetics

Absorption: Oral (cefuroxime axetil): Increases with food

Distribution: Widely to body tissues and fluids; crosses blood-brain barrier; therapeutic concentrations achieved in CSF even when meninges are not inflamed

Protein binding: 33% to 50%

Bioavailability: Tablet: Fasting: 37%; Following food: 52%

Half-life elimination: Children 1-2 hours; Adults: 1-2 hours; prolonged with renal impairment

Time to peak, serum: I.M.: ~15-60 minutes; I.V.: 2-3 minutes; Oral: Children: 3-4 hours; Adults: 2-3 hours

Excretion: Urine (66% to 100% as unchanged drug)

Dosage Note: Cefuroxime axetil film-coated tablets and oral suspension are not bioequivalent and are not substitutable on a mg/mg basis

Usual dosage range:

Children 3 months to 12 years:

Oral: 20-30 mg/kg/day in 2 divided doses

I.M., I.V.: 75-150 mg/kg/day divided every 8 hours (maximum dose: 6 g/day)

Children ≥13 years and Adults:

Oral: 250-500 mg twice daily

I.M., I.V.: 750 mg to 1.5 g every 6-8 hours or 100-150 mg/kg/day in divided doses every 6-8 hours (maximum: 6 g/day)

Indication-specific dosing:

Children ≥3 months to 12 years:

Acute bacterial maxillary sinusitis, acute otitis media, and impetigo:

Oral: Suspension: 30 mg/kg/day in 2 divided doses for 10 days (maximum dose: 1 g/day); tablet: 250 mg twice daily for 10 days

I.M., I.V.: 75-150 mg/kg/day divided every 8 hours (maximum dose: 6 g/day)

Epiglottitis: Oral: 150 mg/kg/day in 3 divided doses for 7-10 days

Pharyngitis/tonsillitis:

Oral: Suspension: 20 mg/kg/day (maximum: 500 mg/day) in 2 divided doses for 10 days; tablet: 125 mg every 12 hours for 10 days

I.M., I.V.: 75-150 mg/kg day divided every 8 hours (maximum: 6 g/day)

Children ≥13 years and Adults (all oral doses listed are for tablet formulation):

Bronchitis (acute and exacerbations of chronic bronchitis):

Oral: 250-500 mg every 12 hours for 10 days

I.V.: 500-750 mg every 8 hours (complete therapy with oral dosing)

Cellulitis, orbital: I.V.: 1.5 g every 8 hours

Gonorrhea:

Disseminated: I.M., I.V.: 750 mg every 8 hours

Uncomplicated:

Oral: 1 g as a single dose

I.M.: 1.5 g as single dose (administer in 2 different sites with probenecid)

Lyme disease (early): Oral: 500 mg twice daily for 20 days

Pharyngitis/tonsillitis and sinusitis: Oral: 250 mg twice daily for 10 days

Pneumonia (uncomplicated): I.V.: 750 mg every 8 hours

Severe or complicated infections: I.M., I.V.: 1.5 g every 8 hours (up to 1.5 g every 6 hours in life-threatening infections)

Skin/skin structure infection (uncomplicated):

Oral: 250-500 mg every 12 hours for 10 days

I.M., I.V.: 750 mg every 8 hours

Surgical prophylaxis:

I.V.: 1.5 g 30 minutes to 1 hour prior to procedure (if procedure is prolonged can give 750 mg every 8 hours I.M.)

Open heart: I.V.: 1.5 g every 12 hours to a total of 6 g

Urinary tract infection (uncomplicated):

Oral: 125-250 mg every 12 hours for 7-10 days

I.M., I.V.: 750 mg every 8 hours

Dosing adjustment in renal impairment:

Cl_{cr} 10-20 mL/minute: Administer every 12 hours

Cl_{cr} <10 mL/minute: Administer every 24 hours

Hemodialysis: Dialyzable (25%)

Peritoneal dialysis: Dose every 24 hours

Continuous renal replacement therapy (CRRT): 1 g every 12 hours

Dietary Considerations May be taken with food.

Zinacef®: Sodium content: 1.8 mEq (41 mg) per 750 mg

Ceftin®: Powder for oral suspension 125 mg/5 mL contains phenylalanine 11.8 mg/5 mL; 250 mg/5 mL contains phenylalanine 25.2 mg/5 mL.

Administration

Oral: Administer around-the-clock to promote less variation in peak and trough serum levels.

Oral suspension: Administer with food. Shake well before use.

I.M.: Inject deep I.M. into large muscle mass.

I.V.: Inject direct I.V. over 3-5 minutes. Infuse intermittent infusion over 15-30 minutes.

Monitoring Parameters Observe for signs and symptoms of anaphylaxis during first dose; with prolonged therapy, monitor renal, hepatic, and hematologic function periodically; monitor prothrombin time in patients at risk of prolongation during cephalosporin therapy (nutritionally-deficient, prolonged treatment, renal or hepatic disease)

Test Interactions Positive direct Coombs', false-positive urinary glucose test using cupric sulfate (Benedict's solution, Clinitest®, Fehling's solution); false-negative may occur with ferricyanide test. Glucose oxidase or hexokinase-based methods should be used.

Dosage Forms Excipient information presented when available (limited, particularly for generics); consult specific product labeling.

Note: Strength expressed as base

Infusion, as sodium [premixed]: 750 mg (50 mL); 1.5 g (50 mL)

Zinacef®: 750 mg (50 mL); 1.5 g (50 mL) [contains sodium 4.8 mEq (111 mg) per 750 mg]

Injection, powder for reconstitution, as sodium: 750 mg, 1.5 g, 7.5 g, 75 g, 225 g
  Zinacef®: 750 mg, 1.5 g, 7.5 g [contains sodium 1.8 mEq (41 mg) per 750 mg]
Powder for suspension, oral, as axetil: 125 mg/5 mL (100 mL); 250 mg/5 mL (50 mL, 100 mL)
  Ceftin®: 125 mg/5 mL (100 mL) [contains phenylalanine 11.8 mg/5 mL; tutti-frutti flavor]; 250 mg/5 mL (50 mL, 100 mL) [contains phenylalanine 25.2 mg/5 mL; tutti-frutti flavor]
Tablet, as axetil: 250 mg, 500 mg
  Ceftin®: 250 mg, 500 mg

◆ **Cefuroxime Axetil** *see* Cefuroxime *on page 288*
◆ **Cefuroxime For Injection (Can)** *see* Cefuroxime *on page 288*
◆ **Cefuroxime Sodium** *see* Cefuroxime *on page 288*
◆ **Cefzil® (Can)** *see* Cefprozil *on page 281*
◆ **Celebrex®** *see* Celecoxib *on page 290*

Celecoxib (se le KOKS ib)

U.S. Brand Names Celebrex®
Canadian Brand Names Celebrex®; GD-Celecoxib
Pharmacologic Category Nonsteroidal Anti-inflammatory Drug (NSAID), COX-2 Selective
Additional Appendix Information
Nonsteroidal Anti-inflammatory Agents *on page 1669*
Sulfonamide Derivatives *on page 1671*

Use Relief of the signs and symptoms of osteoarthritis, ankylosing spondylitis, juvenile rheumatoid arthritis (JRA), and rheumatoid arthritis; management of acute pain; treatment of primary dysmenorrhea; to reduce the number of intestinal polyps in familial adenomatous polyposis (FAP)

Canadian note: Celecoxib is only indicated for relief of symptoms of rheumatoid arthritis, osteoarthritis, and relief of acute pain in adults

Restrictions An FDA-approved medication guide must be distributed when dispensing an oral outpatient prescription (new or refill) where this medication is to be used without direct supervision of a healthcare provider. Medication guides are available at http://www.fda.gov/cder/Offices/ODS/medication_guides.htm.

Pregnancy Risk Factor C/D (3rd trimester)

Pregnancy Considerations Teratogenic effects were observed in animal studies. Avoid use in the 3rd trimester of pregnancy, this drug may cause premature closure of the ductus arteriosus.

Lactation Enters breast milk/not recommended

Medication Safety Issues
Sound-alike/look-alike issues:
Celebrex® may be confused with Celexa®, cerebra, Cerebyx®

Contraindications Hypersensitivity to celecoxib, sulfonamides, aspirin, other NSAIDs, or any component of the formulation; perioperative pain in the setting of coronary artery bypass surgery (CABG); pregnancy (3rd trimester)

Canadian labeling: Additional contraindications (not in U.S. labeling): Pregnancy (3rd trimester); women who are breast-feeding; severe, uncontrolled heart failure; active gastrointestinal ulcer (gastric, duodenal, peptic) or bleeding; inflammatory bowel disease; cerebrovascular bleeding; severe liver impairment or active hepatic disease; severe renal impairment (Cl_{cr} <30 mL/minute) or deteriorating renal disease; known hyperkalemia; use in children

Warnings/Precautions [U.S. Boxed Warning]: NSAIDs are associated with an increased risk of adverse cardiovascular thrombotic events, including MI, and new onset or worsening of pre-existing hypertension. Risk may be increased with duration of use or pre-existing cardiovascular risk factors or disease. Carefully evaluate individual cardiovascular risk profiles prior to prescribing. May cause sodium and fluid retention; use with caution in patients with CHF, edema, cerebrovascular disease, ischemic heart disease, or hypertension. Long-term cardiovascular risk in children has not been evaluated.

[U.S. Boxed Warning]: Celecoxib is contraindicated for treatment of perioperative pain in the setting of coronary artery bypass surgery (CABG). Risk of MI and stroke may be increased with use following CABG surgery.

[U.S. Boxed Warning]: NSAIDs may increase risk of gastrointestinal irritation, ulceration, bleeding, and perforation. These events may occur at any time during therapy and without warning. Use caution with a history of GI disease (bleeding or ulcers), concurrent therapy with aspirin, anticoagulants and/or corticosteroids, smoking, use of alcohol, the elderly or debilitated patients.

Use the lowest effective dose for the shortest duration of time, consistent with individual patient goals, to reduce risk of cardiovascular or GI adverse events. Alternate therapies should be considered for patients at high risk.

NSAIDs may cause serious skin adverse events including exfoliative dermatitis, Stevens-Johnson syndrome (SJS), and toxic epidermal necrolysis (TEN). Anaphylactoid reactions may occur, even without prior exposure; patients with "aspirin triad" (bronchial asthma, aspirin intolerance, rhinitis) may be at increased risk. Do not use in patients who experience bronchospasm, asthma, rhinitis, or urticaria with NSAID or aspirin therapy. Use caution in other forms of asthma.

Use with caution in patients with decreased hepatic (dosage adjustments are recommended for moderate hepatic impairment; not recommended for patients with severe hepatic impairment) or renal function. Closely monitor patients with any abnormal LFT. Severe hepatic reactions (eg, fulminant hepatitis, liver failure) have occurred with NSAID use, rarely; discontinue if signs or symptoms of liver disease develop, or if systemic manifestations occur. NSAID use may compromise existing renal function; dose-dependent decreases in prostaglandin synthesis may result from NSAID use, causing a reduction in renal blood flow which may cause renal decompensation. Patients with impaired renal function, dehydration, heart failure, liver dysfunction, those taking diuretics and ACEI, and the elderly are at greater risk for renal toxicity. Rehydrate patient before starting therapy; monitor renal function closely. Not recommended for use in patients with advanced renal disease. Long-term NSAID use may result in renal papillary necrosis.

Anaphylactoid reactions may occur, even with no prior exposure to celecoxib. Use with caution in patients with known or suspected deficiency of cytochrome P450 isoenzyme 2C9; poor metabolizers may have higher plasma levels due to reduced metabolism.

When used for the treatment of FAP, routine monitoring and care should be continued. When used for JRA, celecoxib is not FDA-approved in children <2 years of age or in children <10 kg. Use caution with systemic onset JRA (may be at risk for disseminated intravascular coagulation). Safety and efficacy have not been established for use in children for indications other than JRA.

Adverse Reactions
>10%:
Cardiovascular: Hypertension (≤13%)
Central nervous system: Headache (10% to 16%)
Gastrointestinal: Diarrhea (4% to 11%)

2% to 10%:

Cardiovascular: Peripheral edema (2%)

Central nervous system: Fever (≤9%), insomnia (2%), dizziness (1% to 2%)

Dermatologic: Skin rash (2%)

Gastrointestinal: Dyspepsia (9%), nausea (4% to 7%), gastroesophageal reflux (≤5%), abdominal pain (4% to 8%), vomiting (≤6%), flatulence (2%)

Neuromuscular & skeletal: Arthralgia (≤7%), back pain (3%)

Respiratory: Upper respiratory tract infection (8%), cough (≤7%), nasopharyngitis (≤6%), sinusitis (5%), dyspnea (≤3%), pharyngitis (2%), rhinitis (2%)

Miscellaneous: Accidental injury (3%)

0.1% to 2%:

Cardiovascular: Angina, aortic valve incompetence, chest pain, coronary artery disorder, DVT, edema, facial edema, hypertension (aggravated), MI, palpitation, sinus bradycardia, tachycardia, ventricular hypertrophy

Central nervous system: Anxiety, cerebral infarction, depression, fatigue, hypoesthesia, migraine, nervousness, pain, somnolence, vertigo

Dermatologic: Alopecia, bruising, cellulitis, dermatitis, dry skin, nail disorder, photosensitivity, pruritus, rash (erythematous), rash (maculopapular), urticaria

Endocrine & metabolic: Breast fibroadenosis, breast neoplasm, breast pain, diabetes mellitus, dysmenorrhea, hot flashes, hypercholesterolemia, hyperglycemia, hyper-/hypokalemia, hypernatremia, menstrual disturbances, ovarian cyst, testosterone decreased

Gastrointestinal: Anorexia, appetite increased, constipation, diverticulitis, dysphagia, eructation, esophagitis, gastritis, gastroenteritis, gastrointestinal ulcer, hemorrhoids, hiatal hernia, melena, stomatitis, taste disturbance, tenesmus, tooth disorder, weight gain, xerostomia

Genitourinary: Cystitis, dysuria, incontinence, monilial vaginitis, prostate disorder, urinary frequency, urinary tract infection, vaginal bleeding, vaginitis

Hematologic: Anemia, thrombocytopenia

Hepatic: Alkaline phosphatase increased, transaminases increased

Neuromuscular & skeletal: Arthrosis, bone disorder, CPK increased, fracture, leg cramps, myalgia, neck stiffness, neuralgia, neuropathy, paresthesia, hypertonia, synovitis, tendon rupture, tendonitis, weakness

Ocular: Blurred vision, cataract, conjunctival hemorrhage, conjunctivitis, eye pain, glaucoma, vitreous floaters

Otic: Deafness, earache, labyrinthitis, otitis media, tinnitus

Renal: Albuminuria, BUN increased, creatinine increased, hematuria, nonprotein nitrogen increased, renal calculi

Respiratory: Bronchitis, bronchospasm, epistaxis, laryngitis, pneumonia

Miscellaneous: Allergic reactions, allergy aggravated, diaphoresis, flu-like syndrome, herpes infection, infection (bacterial, fungal, viral), moniliasis

<0.1% (Limited to important or life-threatening): Acute renal failure, agranulocytosis, anaphylactoid reactions, angioedema, aplastic anemia, aseptic meningitis, ataxia, cerebrovascular accident, CHF, cholelithiasis, colitis, erythema multiforme, esophageal perforation, exfoliative dermatitis, gangrene, gastrointestinal bleeding, hepatic failure, hepatic necrosis, hepatitis (including fulminant), hypoglycemia, hyponatremia, ileus, interstitial nephritis, intestinal obstruction, intestinal perforation, intracranial hemorrhage, jaundice, leukopenia, pancreatitis, pancytopenia, pulmonary embolism, renal papillary necrosis, sepsis, Stevens-Johnson syndrome, sudden death, suicide, syncope, thrombophlebitis, toxic epidermal necrolysis, vasculitis, ventricular fibrillation

Drug Interactions

Metabolism/Transport Effects Substrate of CYP2C9 (major), 3A4 (minor); **Inhibits** CYP2C8 (moderate), 2D6 (weak)

Avoid Concomitant Use

Avoid concomitant use of Celecoxib with any of the following: Ketorolac

Increased Effect/Toxicity

Celecoxib may increase the levels/effects of: Aminoglycosides; Anticoagulants; Antiplatelet Agents; Bisphosphonate Derivatives; CycloSPORINE; CYP2C8 Substrates (High risk); Desmopressin; Lithium; Methotrexate; Nonsteroidal Anti-Inflammatory Agents; Quinolone Antibiotics; Thrombolytic Agents; Vancomycin; Vitamin K Antagonists

The levels/effects of Celecoxib may be increased by: Antidepressants (Tricyclic, Tertiary Amine); Corticosteroids (Systemic); CYP2C9 Inhibitors (Moderate); CYP2C9 Inhibitors (Strong); Herbs (Anticoagulant/Antiplatelet Properties); Ketorolac; Probenecid; Selective Serotonin Reuptake Inhibitors; Treprostinil

Decreased Effect

Celecoxib may decrease the levels/effects of: ACE Inhibitors; Angiotensin II Receptor Blockers; Antiplatelet Agents; Beta-Blockers; Eplerenone; HydrALAZINE; Loop Diuretics; Thiazide Diuretics

The levels/effects of Celecoxib may be decreased by: Bile Acid Sequestrants; CYP2C9 Inducers (Highly Effective)

Ethanol/Nutrition/Herb Interactions

Ethanol: Avoid ethanol (increased GI irritation).

Food: Peak concentrations are delayed and AUC is increased by 10% to 20% when taken with a high-fat meal.

Herb/Nutraceutical: Avoid concomitant use with herbs possessing anticoagulation/antiplatelet properties, including alfalfa, anise, bilberry, bladderwrack, bromelain, cat's claw, celery, chamomile, coleus, cordyceps, dong quai, evening primrose, fenugreek, feverfew, garlic, ginger, ginkgo biloba, ginseng (American, Panax, Siberian), grapeseed, green tea, guggul, horse chestnuts, horseradish, licorice, prickly ash, red clover, reishi, SAMe (S-adenosylmethionine), sweet clover, turmeric, white willow.

Stability Store at controlled room temperature of 25°C (77°F); excursions permitted to 15°C to 30°C (59°F to 86°F).

Mechanism of Action Inhibits prostaglandin synthesis by decreasing the activity of the enzyme, cyclooxygenase-2 (COX-2), which results in decreased formation of prostaglandin precursors; has antipyretic, analgesic, and anti-inflammatory properties

Pharmacodynamics/Kinetics

Distribution: V_d (apparent): ~400 L

Protein binding: ~97% primarily to albumin

Metabolism: Hepatic via CYP2C9; forms inactive metabolites

Bioavailability: Absolute: Unknown

Half-life elimination: ~11 hours (fasted)

Time to peak: ~3 hours

Excretion: Feces (57% as metabolites, <3% as unchanged drug); urine (27% as metabolites, <3% as unchanged drug)

Dosage Note: Use the lowest effective dose for the shortest duration of time, consistent with individual patient goals. Oral:

Children ≥2 years: JRA

≥10 kg to ≤25 kg: 50 mg twice daily

>25 kg: 100 mg twice daily

Adults:

Acute pain or primary dysmenorrhea: Initial dose: 400 mg, followed by an additional 200 mg if needed on day 1; maintenance dose: 200 mg twice daily as needed

Ankylosing spondylitis: 200 mg/day as a single dose or in divided doses twice daily; if no effect after 6 weeks, may increase to 400 mg/day. If no response following 6 weeks of treatment with 400 mg/day, consider discontinuation and alternative treatment.

Familial adenomatous polyposis: 400 mg twice daily

Osteoarthritis: 200 mg/day as a single dose or in divided dose twice daily

Rheumatoid arthritis: 100-200 mg twice daily

Elderly: No specific adjustment based on age is recommended. However, the AUC in elderly patients may be increased by 50% as compared to younger subjects. Initiate at the lowest recommended dose in patients weighing <50 kg.

Dosing adjustment in renal impairment: No specific dosage adjustment is recommended; not recommended in patients with severe renal dysfunction

Dosing adjustment in hepatic impairment: Reduced dosage is recommended (AUC may be increased by 40% to 180%); decrease dose by 50% in patients with moderate hepatic impairment (Child-Pugh class B). Not recommended for use with severe impairment.

Dietary Considerations Lower doses (200 mg twice daily) may be taken without regard to meals. Larger doses should be taken with food to improve absorption.

Administration Lower doses (200 mg twice daily) may be taken without regard to meals. Larger doses should be taken with food to improve absorption. Capsules may be swallowed whole or the entire contents emptied onto a teaspoon of cool or room temperature applesauce. The contents of the capsules sprinkled onto applesauce may be stored under refrigeration for up to 6 hours.

Monitoring Parameters CBC; blood chemistry profile; occult blood loss and periodic liver function tests; monitor renal function (urine output, serum BUN and creatinine; monitor response (pain, range of motion, grip strength, mobility, ADL function), inflammation; observe for weight gain, edema; observe for bleeding, bruising; evaluate gastrointestinal effects (abdominal pain, bleeding, dyspepsia); blood pressure

FAP: Continue routine endoscopic exams

JRA: Monitor for development of abnormal coagulation tests with systemic onset JRA

Additional Information Celecoxib does not inhibit cyclooxygenase-1 (COX-1) at therapeutic concentrations. Celecoxib does not affect platelet aggregation.

Dosage Forms Excipient information presented when available (limited, particularly for generics); consult specific product labeling.

Capsule:

Celebrex®: 50 mg, 100 mg, 200 mg, 400 mg

◆ **Celestone®** *see* Betamethasone *on page 188*

◆ **Celestone® Soluspan®** *see* Betamethasone *on page 188*

◆ **Celexa®** *see* Citalopram *on page 337*

◆ **CellCept®** *see* Mycophenolate *on page 1026*

◆ **Celontin®** *see* Methsuximide *on page 970*

◆ **Celsentri™ (Can)** *see* Maraviroc *on page 921*

◆ **Cemill [OTC]** *see* Ascorbic Acid *on page 139*

◆ **Cenestin®** *see* Estrogens (Conjugated A/Synthetic) *on page 560*

◆ **Cenestin (Can)** *see* Estrogens (Conjugated A/Synthetic) *on page 560*

◆ **Cenolate®** *see* Ascorbic Acid *on page 139*

◆ **Centany™ [DSC]** *see* Mupirocin *on page 1024*

◆ **Cepacol® Sore Throat [OTC]** *see* Benzocaine *on page 183*

◆ **Cephadyn** *see* Butalbital and Acetaminophen *on page 230*

Cephalexin (sef a LEKS in)

U.S. Brand Names Keflex®

Canadian Brand Names Apo-Cephalex®; Keftab®; Novo-Lexin; Nu-Cephalex

Index Terms Cephalexin Monohydrate

Pharmacologic Category Antibiotic, Cephalosporin (First Generation)

Additional Appendix Information

Animal and Human Bites *on page 1747*

Prevention of Infective Endocarditis *on page 1736*

Use Treatment of susceptible bacterial infections including respiratory tract infections, otitis media, skin and skin structure infections, bone infections, and genitourinary tract infections, including acute prostatitis; alternative therapy for acute infective endocarditis prophylaxis

Pregnancy Risk Factor B

Pregnancy Considerations Adverse events were not observed in animal reproduction studies; therefore, cephalexin is classified as pregnancy category B. Cephalexin crosses the placenta and produces therapeutic concentrations in the fetal circulation and amniotic fluid. An increased risk of teratogenic effects has not been observed following maternal use of cephalexin; however, adequate and well-controlled studies have not been completed in pregnant women. Peak concentrations in pregnant patients are similar to those in nonpregnant patients. Prolonged labor may decrease oral absorption.

Lactation Enters breast milk (small amounts)/use caution

Medication Safety Issues

Sound-alike/look-alike issues:

Cephalexin may be confused with cefaclor, ceFAZolin, cephalothin, ciprofloxacin

Contraindications Hypersensitivity to cephalexin, any component of the formulation, or other cephalosporins

Warnings/Precautions Modify dosage in patients with severe renal impairment. Use with caution in patients with a history of penicillin allergy, especially IgE-mediated reactions (eg, anaphylaxis, urticaria). Prolonged use may result in fungal or bacterial superinfection, including *C. difficile*-associated diarrhea (CDAD) and pseudomembranous colitis; CDAD has been observed >2 months postantibiotic treatment. May be associated with increased INR, especially in nutritionally-deficient patients, prolonged treatment, hepatic or renal disease.

Adverse Reactions Frequency not defined.

Central nervous system: Agitation, confusion, dizziness, fatigue, hallucinations, headache

Dermatologic: Angioedema, erythema multiforme (rare), rash, Stevens-Johnson syndrome (rare), toxic epidermal necrolysis (rare), urticaria

Gastrointestinal: Abdominal pain, diarrhea, dyspepsia, gastritis, nausea (rare), pseudomembranous colitis, vomiting (rare)

Genitourinary: Genital pruritus, genital moniliasis, vaginitis, vaginal discharge

Hematologic: Eosinophilia, hemolytic anemia, neutropenia, thrombocytopenia

Hepatic: ALT increased, AST increased, cholestatic jaundice (rare), transient hepatitis (rare)

Neuromuscular & skeletal: Arthralgia, arthritis, joint disorder

Renal: Interstitial nephritis (rare)

Miscellaneous: Allergic reactions, anaphylaxis

Drug Interactions

Avoid Concomitant Use There are no known interactions where it is recommended to avoid concomitant use.

Increased Effect/Toxicity

Cephalexin may increase the levels/effects of: MetFORMIN

The levels/effects of Cephalexin may be increased by: Uricosuric Agents

Decreased Effect

Cephalexin may decrease the levels/effects of: Typhoid Vaccine

Ethanol/Nutrition/Herb Interactions Food: Peak antibiotic serum concentration is lowered and delayed, but total drug absorbed is not affected. Cephalexin serum levels may be decreased if taken with food.

Stability

Capsule: Store at 15°C to 30°C (59°F to 86°F).

Powder for oral suspension: Refrigerate suspension after reconstitution; discard after 14 days.

Mechanism of Action Inhibits bacterial cell wall synthesis by binding to one or more of the penicillin-binding proteins (PBPs) which in turn inhibits the final transpeptidation step of peptidoglycan synthesis in bacterial cell walls, thus inhibiting cell wall biosynthesis. Bacteria eventually lyse due to ongoing activity of cell wall autolytic enzymes (autolysins and murein hydrolases) while cell wall assembly is arrested.

Pharmacodynamics/Kinetics

Absorption: Delayed in young children

Distribution: Widely into most body tissues and fluids, including gallbladder, liver, kidneys, bone, sputum, bile, and pleural and synovial fluids; CSF penetration is poor

Protein binding: 6% to 15%

Half-life elimination: Adults: 0.5-1.2 hours; prolonged with renal impairment

Time to peak, serum: ~1 hour

Excretion: Urine (80% to 100% as unchanged drug) within 8 hours

Dosage

Usual dosage range:

Children >1 year: Oral: 25-100 mg/kg/day every 6-8 hours (maximum: 4 g/day)

Adults: Oral: 250-1000 mg every 6 hours; maximum: 4 g/day

Indication-specific dosing:

Children >1 year: Oral:

Furunculosis: 25-50 mg/kg/day in 4 divided doses

Impetigo: 25 mg/kg/day in 4 divided doses

Otitis media: 75-100 mg/kg/day in 4 divided doses

Prophylaxis against infective endocarditis (dental, oral, or respiratory tract procedures): 50 mg/kg 30-60 minutes prior to procedure (maximum: 2 g). **Note:** American Heart Association (AHA) guidelines now recommend prophylaxis only in patients undergoing invasive procedures and in whom underlying cardiac conditions may predispose to a higher risk of adverse outcomes should infection occur.

Severe infections: 50-100 mg/kg/day in divided doses every 6-8 hours

Skin abscess: 50 mg/kg/day in 4 divided doses (maximum: 4 g)

Streptococcal pharyngitis, skin and skin structure infections: 25-50 mg/kg/day divided every 12 hours

Children >15 years and Adults: Oral:

Cellulitis and mastitis: 500 mg every 6 hours

Furunculosis/skin abscess: 250 mg 4 times/day

Prophylaxis against infective endocarditis (dental, oral, or respiratory tract procedures): 2 g 30-60 minutes prior to procedure. **Note:** American Heart Association (AHA) guidelines now recommend prophylaxis only in patients undergoing invasive procedures and in whom underlying cardiac conditions may predispose to a higher risk of adverse outcomes should infection occur.

Prophylaxis in total joint replacement patients undergoing dental procedures which produce bacteremia: 2 g 1 hour prior to procedure

Streptococcal pharyngitis, skin and skin structure infections: 500 mg every 12 hours

Uncomplicated cystitis: 500 mg every 12 hours for 7-14 days

Dosing adjustment in renal impairment: Adults:

Cl_{cr} 10-50 mL/minute: 500 mg every 8-12 hours

Cl_{cr} <10: 250-500 mg every 12-24 hours

Hemodialysis: 250 mg every 12-24 hours; moderately dialyzable (20% to 50%); give dose after dialysis session

Dietary Considerations Take without regard to food. If GI distress, take with food. Panixine DisperDose™ contains phenylalanine 2.8 mg/cephalexin 125 mg.

Administration Take without regard to food. If GI distress, take with food. Give around-the-clock to promote less variation in peak and trough serum levels.

Monitoring Parameters With prolonged therapy monitor renal, hepatic, and hematologic function periodically; monitor for signs of anaphylaxis during first dose

Test Interactions Positive direct Coombs', false-positive urinary glucose test using cupric sulfate (Benedict's solution, Clinitest®, Fehling's solution), false-positive serum or urine creatinine with Jaffé reaction, false-positive urinary proteins and steroids

Dosage Forms Excipient information presented when available (limited, particularly for generics); consult specific product labeling.

Capsule: 250 mg, 500 mg

Keflex®: 250 mg, 500 mg, 750 mg

Powder for oral suspension: 125 mg/5 mL (100 mL, 200 mL); 250 mg/5 mL (100 mL, 200 mL)

Keflex®: 125 mg/5 mL (100 mL, 200 mL); 250 mg/5 mL (100 mL, 200 mL)

Tablet: 250 mg, 500 mg

- ◆ **Cephalexin Monohydrate** *see* Cephalexin *on page* 292
- ◆ **Ceprotin** *see* Protein C Concentrate (Human) *on page* 1264
- ◆ **Cerebyx®** *see* Fosphenytoin *on page* 671
- ◆ **Ceredase®** *see* Alglucerase *on page* 62
- ◆ **Cerezyme®** *see* Imiglucerase *on page* 771
- ◆ **Ceron** *see* Chlorpheniramine and Phenylephrine *on page* 309
- ◆ **Ceron-DM** *see* Chlorpheniramine, Phenylephrine, and Dextromethorphan *on page* 311
- ◆ **Cerovel™** *see* Urea *on page* 1530

Certolizumab Pegol (cer to LIZ u mab PEG ol)

U.S. Brand Names Cimzia®

Index Terms CDP870

Pharmacologic Category Gastrointestinal Agent, Miscellaneous; Tumor Necrosis Factor (TNF) Blocking Agent

Use Treatment of moderately- to severely-active Crohn's disease in patients who have inadequate response to conventional therapy

Restrictions An FDA-approved medication guide is available, distribute to each patient to whom this medication is dispensed.

Pregnancy Risk Factor B

Pregnancy Considerations Adverse effects were not observed in animal studies. There are no adequate and well-controlled studies in pregnant women.

Lactation Excretion in breast milk unknown/not recommended

Contraindications There are no contraindications listed within the manufacturer's labeling.

Warnings/Precautions [U.S. Boxed Warning]: Serious infections (including tuberculosis, invasive fungal and

other opportunistic infections), some with fatalities, have been reported in patients receiving TNF-blocking agents, including certolizumab. Cases of unrecognized invasive fungal infections (eg, histoplasmosis, blastomycosis, coccidioidomycosis) have also been reported with anti-TNF agent use. Many of the serious infections have occurred in patients on concomitant immunosuppressive therapy. Caution should be exercised when considering the use in patients with a history of chronic or recurrent infection, concomitant immunosuppressive therapy, predisposition to infection (eg, diabetes or residence/travel from areas of endemic mycoses). Do not give to patients with an active chronic or localized infection. Patients who develop a new infection while undergoing treatment should be monitored closely. If a patient develops a serious infection, therapy should be discontinued. Use of TNF blockers may affect defenses against malignancies; impact on the development and course of malignancies is not fully defined. Chronic immunosuppressant therapy use may be a predisposing factor for malignancy development.

Tuberculosis has been reported with certolizumab treatment. **[U.S. Boxed Warnings]: Patients should be evaluated for tuberculosis risk factors and for latent tuberculosis infection (with a tuberculin skin test) prior to therapy. Treatment of latent tuberculosis should be initiated before use. Patients with initial negative tuberculin skin tests should receive continued monitoring for tuberculosis throughout treatment;** active tuberculosis has developed in this population during treatment. Use with caution in patients who have resided in regions where tuberculosis is endemic. If appropriate, antituberculosis therapy should be considered (prior to certolizumab treatment) in patients with several or with highly significant risk factors for tuberculosis development.

Rare and sometimes fatal reactivation of hepatitis B virus (HBV) has occurred in chronic virus carriers; evaluate prior to initiation, during, and for several months after treatment. Evaluate patients at risk for HBV infection prior to therapy to determine HBV status. Use with extreme caution in patients identified as HBV carriers, use has not been evaluated in this population.

Hypersensitivity reactions, including angioedema, dyspnea, rash, serum sickness and urticaria have been reported (rarely) with treatment; discontinue further therapy if hypersensitivity occurs. Use with caution in patients who have experienced hypersensitivity with other TNF blockers. Use with caution in heart failure patients; worsening heart failure and new onset heart failure have been reported with TNF blockers; monitor closely. Rare cases of pancytopenia and other significant cytopenias, including aplastic anemia and have been reported with TNF-blocking agents. Leukopenia and thrombocytopenia have occurred with certolizumab; use with caution in patients with underlying hematologic disorders; consider discontinuing therapy with significant hematologic abnormalities. Autoantibody formation may develop; rarely resulting in autoimmune disorder, including lupus-like syndrome; monitor and discontinue if symptoms develop. A small number of patients (8%) develop antibodies to certolizumab during therapy. Antibody-positive patients may have an increased inicidence of adverse events (including injection site pain/erythema, abdominal pain and erythema nodosom). Use with caution in patients with pre-existing or recent-onset CNS demyelinating disorders; rare cases of optic neuritis, seizure, peripheral neuropathy, and demyelinating disease (new onset or exacerbation) have been reported.

The manufacturer does not recommend concurrent use with anakinra due to the risk of serious infections. Patients should be brought up to date with all immunizations before initiating therapy; live vaccines should not be given concurrently. There is no data available concerning the effects of therapy on vaccination or secondary transmission of live vaccines in patients receiving therapy. Use with caution in the elderly, may be at higher risk for infections. Safety and efficacy have not been established in children.

Adverse Reactions

>10%:

- Central nervous system: Headache (7% to 18%)
- Gastrointestinal: Nausea (≤11%)
- Respiratory: Upper respiratory infection (20%), nasopharyngitis (4% to 13%)
- Miscellaneous: Infection (14% to 38%; serious: 3%)

1% to 10%:

- Central nervous system: Dizziness (≤6%), fever (≤5%)
- Gastrointestinal: Abdominal pain (≤6%), vomiting (5%)
- Genitourinary: Urinary tract infection (≤8%)
- Local: Injection site reactions (includes bleeding, burning, erythema, inflammation, pain, rash: ≤7%; incidence higher with placebo)
- Neuromuscular & skeletal: Arthralgia (6% to 7%)
- Respiratory: Cough (≤6%)
- Miscellaneous: Antibody formation (8%), positive ANA (4%)

<1% (Limited to important or life-threatening): Abdominal mass, abscess, alopecia, anemia, angina, anxiety, aphthous stomatitis, aplastic anemia, arrhythmia, bipolar disorder, blurred vision, cytopenia, demyelinating disorder exacerbation, dermatitis, diarrhea, erythema nodosum, gastroenteritis, heart failure, hepatitis, hepatitis B reactivation; hypersensitivity reaction (eg, allergic dermatitis, angioedema, dizziness [postural], dyspnea, hot flush, hypotension, malaise, serum sickness, syncope); hypertension, leukopenia, lupus-like syndrome, lymphadenopathy, malignancy, menstrual disorder, MI, myocardial ischemia, nephrotic syndrome, optic neuritis, pancytopenia, paralytic ileus, pericardial effusion, pericarditis, peripheral neuropathy, pneumonia, pyelonephritis, rash, rectal hemorrhage, renal failure, retinal hemorrhage, seizure, suicide attempt, thrombocytopenia, thrombophilia, transaminases increased, tuberculosis (pulmonary and disseminated), urticaria, uveitis, vasculitis, visual acuity decreased

Drug Interactions

Avoid Concomitant Use

Avoid concomitant use of Certolizumab Pegol with any of the following: Anakinra; Natalizumab; Rilonacept; Vaccines (Live)

Increased Effect/Toxicity

Certolizumab Pegol may increase the levels/effects of: Abatacept; Anakinra; Natalizumab; Rilonacept; Vaccines (Live)

The levels/effects of Certolizumab Pegol may be increased by: Trastuzumab

Decreased Effect

Certolizumab Pegol may decrease the levels/effects of: Vaccines (Inactivated)

The levels/effects of Certolizumab Pegol may be decreased by: Echinacea

Ethanol/Nutrition/Herb Interactions Herb/Nutraceutical: Echinacea may decrease the therapeutic effects of certolizumab; avoid concurrent use.

Stability Prior to reconstitution, store intact vials under refrigeration at 2°C to 8°C (36°F to 46°F). Allow to reach room temperature prior to reconstitution. Using aseptic technique, reconstitute each vial with 1 mL sterile water for injection (provided) to a concentration of ~200 mg/mL; the manufacturer recommends using a 20-gauge needle (provided). Gently swirl to facilitate wetting of powder; do not shake. Allow vials to set undisturbed (may take up to 30 minutes) until fully reconstituted. Reconstituted solutions should not contain visible particles or gels in the solution. Reconstituted vials may be retained at room temperature for ≤2 hours or refrigerated for ≤24 hours prior to administration. Do not freeze. Bring to room temperature prior to administration.

Mechanism of Action Certolizumab pegol is a pegylated humanized antibody Fab' fragment of tumor necrosis factor alpha (TNF-alpha) monoclonal antibody. Certolizumab pegol binds to and selectively neutralizes human TNF-alpha activity. (Elevated levels of TNF-alpha have a role in the inflammatory process associated with Crohn's disease.) Since it is not a complete antibody (lacks Fc region), it does not induce complement activation, antibody-dependent cell-mediated cytotoxicity, or apoptosis. Pegylation of certolizumab allows for delayed elimination and therefore an extended half-life.

Pharmacodynamics/Kinetics

Distribution: V_{ss}: 6.4 L

Bioavailability: SubQ: ~80% (range: 76% to 88%)

Half-life elimination: ~14 days

Time to peak, plasma: 54-171 hours

Dosage Note: Each 400 mg dose should be administered as 2 injections of 200 mg each

SubQ: Adults: Crohn's disease: Initial: 400 mg, repeat dose 2 and 4 weeks after initial dose; Maintenance: 400 mg every 4 weeks

Administration SubQ: Bring to room temperature prior to administration. Total dose requires 2 vials; after reconstitution, draw each vial into separate syringes, administer each syringe subcutaneously (using provided 23-gauge needle) to separate sites on abdomen or thigh.

Monitoring Parameters Signs and symptoms of infection, signs and symptoms of hypersensitivity reaction, symptoms of lupus-like syndrome; hepatitis B virus and TB screening prior to therapy initiation

Dosage Forms Excipient information presented when available (limited, particularly for generics); consult specific product labeling.

Injection, powder for reconstitution:

Cimzia®: 200 mg [contains sterile water for reconstitution, syringes, and needles]

- ◆ **Cerubidine®** *see* DAUNOrubicin Hydrochloride *on page 407*
- ◆ **Cerumenex® [DSC]** *see* Triethanolamine Polypeptide Oleate-Condensate *on page 1516*
- ◆ **Cerumenex® (Can)** *see* Triethanolamine Polypeptide Oleate-Condensate *on page 1516*
- ◆ **Cervidil®** *see* Dinoprostone *on page 454*
- ◆ **C.E.S.** *see* Estrogens (Conjugated/Equine) *on page 563*
- ◆ **C.E.S.® (Can)** *see* Estrogens (Conjugated/Equine) *on page 563*
- ◆ **Cesia™** *see* Ethinyl Estradiol and Desogestrel *on page 575*
- ◆ **Cetacaine®** *see* Benzocaine, Butamben, and Tetracaine *on page 185*
- ◆ **Cetacort® [DSC]** *see* Hydrocortisone *on page 743*
- ◆ **Cetafen® [OTC]** *see* Acetaminophen *on page 25*
- ◆ **Cetafen Extra® [OTC]** *see* Acetaminophen *on page 25*
- ◆ **Cetamide™ (Can)** *see* Sulfacetamide *on page 1405*

Cetirizine (se TI ra zeen)

U.S. Brand Names Zyrtec® Allergy [OTC]; Zyrtec® [OTC]; Zyrtec®, Children's Allergy [OTC]; Zyrtec®, Children's Hives Relief [OTC]

Canadian Brand Names Apo-Cetirizine®; PMS-Cetirizine; Reactine™

Index Terms Cetirizine Hydrochloride; P-071; UCB-P071

Pharmacologic Category Histamine H_1 Antagonist; Histamine H_1 Antagonist, Second Generation

Use Perennial and seasonal allergic rhinitis and other allergic symptoms including urticaria; chronic idiopathic urticaria

Pregnancy Risk Factor B

Pregnancy Considerations Cetirizine was not shown to be teratogenic in animal studies; however, adequate studies have not been conducted in pregnant women. Use during pregnancy only if clearly needed.

Lactation Enters breast milk/not recommended

Medication Safety Issues

Sound-alike/look-alike issues:

Zyrtec® may be confused with Serax®, Xanax®, Zantac®, Zyprexa®

Contraindications Hypersensitivity to cetirizine, hydroxyzine, or any component of the formulation

Warnings/Precautions Cetirizine should be used cautiously in patients with hepatic or renal dysfunction; dosage adjustment recommended. Use with caution in the elderly; may be more sensitive to adverse effects. May cause drowsiness; use caution performing tasks which require alertness (eg, operating machinery or driving). Effects may be potentiated when used with other sedative drugs or ethanol. Safety and efficacy in pediatric patients <6 months of age have not been established.

Adverse Reactions

>10%: Central nervous system: Headache (children 11% to 14%, placebo 12%), somnolence (adults 14%, children 2% to 4%)

2% to 10%:

Central nervous system: Insomnia (children 9%, adults <2%), fatigue (adults 6%), malaise (4%), dizziness (adults 2%)

Gastrointestinal: Abdominal pain (children 4% to 6%), dry mouth (adults 5%), diarrhea (children 2% to 3%), nausea (children 2% to 3%, placebo 2%), vomiting (children 2% to 3%)

Respiratory: Epistaxis (children 2% to 4%, placebo 3%), pharyngitis (children 3% to 6%, placebo 3%), bronchospasm (children 2% to 3%, placebo 2%)

<2% (Limited to important or life-threatening; as reported in adults and/or children): Aggressive reaction, anaphylaxis, angioedema, ataxia, chest pain, confusion, convulsions, depersonalization, depression, edema, fussiness, hallucinations, hemolytic anemia, hepatitis, hypertension, hypotension (severe), irritability, liver function abnormal, nervousness, ototoxicity, palpitation, paralysis, paresthesia, photosensitivity, rash, suicidal ideation, suicide, taste perversion, tongue discoloration, tongue edema, tremor, visual field defect, weakness

Drug Interactions

Metabolism/Transport Effects **Substrate** of CYP3A4 (minor)

Avoid Concomitant Use There are no known interactions where it is recommended to avoid concomitant use.

Increased Effect/Toxicity

Cetirizine may increase the levels/effects of: Alcohol (Ethyl); Anticholinergics; CNS Depressants

The levels/effects of Cetirizine may be increased by: P-Glycoprotein Inhibitors; Pramlintide

Decreased Effect

Cetirizine may decrease the levels/effects of: Acetylcholinesterase Inhibitors (Central); Betahistine

The levels/effects of Cetirizine may be decreased by: Acetylcholinesterase Inhibitors (Central); Amphetamines; P-Glycoprotein Inducers

Ethanol/Nutrition/Herb Interactions Ethanol: Avoid ethanol (may increase CNS depression).

Stability

Syrup: Store at room temperature of 15°C to 30°C (59°F to 86°F), or under refrigeration at 2°C to 8°C (36°F to 46°F).

Tablet: Store at room temperature of 15°C to 30°C (59°F to 86°F).

Mechanism of Action Competes with histamine for H_1-receptor sites on effector cells in the gastrointestinal tract, blood vessels, and respiratory tract

Pharmacodynamics/Kinetics

Onset of action: 15-30 minutes

Absorption: Rapid

Protein binding, plasma: Mean: 93%

Metabolism: Limited hepatic

Half-life elimination: 8 hours

Time to peak, serum: 1 hour

Excretion: Urine (70%); feces (10%)

Dosage Oral:

Children:

6-12 months: Chronic urticaria, perennial allergic rhinitis: 2.5 mg once daily

12 months to <2 years: Chronic urticaria, perennial allergic rhinitis: 2.5 mg once daily; may increase to 2.5 mg every 12 hours if needed

2-5 years: Chronic urticaria, perennial or seasonal allergic rhinitis: Initial: 2.5 mg once daily; may be increased to 2.5 mg every 12 hours **or** 5 mg once daily

Children ≥6 years and Adults: Chronic urticaria, perennial or seasonal allergic rhinitis: 5-10 mg once daily, depending upon symptom severity

Elderly: Initial: 5 mg once daily; may increase to 10 mg/day. **Note:** Manufacturer recommends 5 mg/day in patients ≥77 years of age.

Dosage adjustment in renal/hepatic impairment:

Children <6 years: Cetirizine use not recommended

Children 6-11 years: <2.5 mg once daily

Children ≥12 and Adults:

Cl_{cr} 11-31 mL/minute, hemodialysis, or hepatic impairment: Administer 5 mg once daily

Cl_{cr} <11 mL/minute, not on dialysis: Cetirizine use not recommended

Dietary Considerations May be taken with or without food.

Administration May be administered with or without food.

Monitoring Parameters Relief of symptoms, sedation and anticholinergic effects

Dosage Forms Excipient information presented when available (limited, particularly for generics); consult specific product labeling. [DSC] = Discontinued product

Syrup, as hydrochloride: 5 mg/5 mL (120 mL, 473 mL)

Zyrtec®: 5 mg/5 mL (120 mL, 480 mL) [contains propylene glycol; banana-grape flavor]

Zyrtec®, Children's Allergy, Zyrtec®, Children's Hives Relief: 5 mg/5 mL (120 mL) [contains propylene glycol; grape flavor]

Tablet, as hydrochloride: 5 mg, 10 mg

Zyrtec®: 5 mg, 10 mg [DSC]

Zyrtec® Allergy: 10 mg

Tablet, chewable, as hydrochloride:

Zyrtec®: 5 mg, 10 mg [grape flavor] [DSC]

Zyrtec®, Children's Allergy: 5 mg, 10 mg [grape flavor]

◆ **Cetirizine Hydrochloride** *see* Cetirizine *on page 295*

Cetrorelix (set roe REL iks)

U.S. Brand Names Cetrotide®

Canadian Brand Names Cetrotide®

Index Terms Cetrorelix Acetate

Pharmacologic Category Gonadotropin Releasing Hormone Antagonist

Use Inhibits premature luteinizing hormone (LH) surges in women undergoing controlled ovarian stimulation

Pregnancy Risk Factor X

Pregnancy Considerations Animal studies have shown fetal resorption and implantation losses following administration. Resorption resulting in fetal loss would be expected if used in a pregnant woman.

Lactation Excretion in breast milk unknown/contraindicated

Contraindications Hypersensitivity to cetrorelix or any component of the formulation; extrinsic peptide hormones, mannitol, gonadotropin releasing hormone (GnRH) or GnRH analogs; severe renal impairment; pregnancy; breast-feeding

Warnings/Precautions Should only be prescribed by fertility specialists. Monitor carefully after first injection for possible hypersensitivity reactions. Use caution in women with active allergic conditions or a history of allergies; use in women with severe allergic conditions is not recommended. Pregnancy should be excluded before treatment is begun.

Adverse Reactions

1% to 10%:

Central nervous system: Headache (1%)

Endocrine & metabolic: Ovarian hyperstimulation syndrome, WHO grade II or III (4%)

Gastrointestinal: Nausea (1%)

Hepatic: ALT, AST, GGT, and alkaline phosphatase increased (1% to 2%)

Postmarketing and/or case reports: Severe anaphylactic reaction (cough, rash, hypotension) occurred in one patient following several months of treatment in a study not related to fertility. Congenital abnormalities and stillbirths have been reported, however, the relationship to cetrorelix treatment has not been established. Local injection site reactions (bruising, erythema, itching, pruritus, redness, swelling) have also been reported.

Drug Interactions

Avoid Concomitant Use There are no known interactions where it is recommended to avoid concomitant use.

Increased Effect/Toxicity There are no known significant interactions involving an increase in effect.

Decreased Effect There are no known significant interactions involving a decrease in effect.

Stability Store in outer carton. Once mixed, solution should be used immediately.

0.25 mg vials: Store under refrigeration at 2°C to 8°C (36°F to 46°F).

3 mg vials: Store at controlled room temperature at 25°C (77°F).

Mechanism of Action Competes with naturally-occurring GnRH for binding on receptors of the pituitary. This delays luteinizing hormone surge, preventing ovulation until the follicles are of adequate size.

Pharmacodynamics/Kinetics

Onset of action: 0.25 mg dose: 2 hours; 3 mg dose: 1 hour

Duration: 3 mg dose (single dose): 4 days

Absorption: Rapid

Distribution: V_d: ~1 L/kg

Protein binding: 86%

Metabolism: Transformed by peptidases; cetrorelix and peptides (1-9), (1-7), (1-6), and (1-4) are found in the bile; peptide (1-4) is the predominant metabolite

Bioavailability: 85%

Half-life elimination: 0.25 mg dose: 5 hours; 0.25 mg multiple doses: 20.6 hours; 3 mg dose: 62.8 hours

Time to peak: 0.25 mg dose: 1 hour; 3 mg dose: 1.5 hours

Excretion: Feces (5% to 10% as unchanged drug and metabolites); urine (2% to 4% as unchanged drug); within 24 hours

Dosage Adults: Females: SubQ: Used in conjunction with controlled ovarian stimulation therapy using gonadotropins (FSH, HMG):

Single-dose regimen: 3 mg given when serum estradiol levels show appropriate stimulation response, usually stimulation day 7 (range days 5-9). If hCG is not administered within 4 days, continue cetrorelix at 0.25 mg/day until hCG is administered.

Multiple-dose regimen: 0.25 mg morning or evening of stimulation day 5, or morning of stimulation day 6; continue until hCG is administered.

Dosing adjustment in renal impairment:

Severe impairment: Use is contraindicated

Mild-to-moderate impairment: No specific guidelines are available

Dosing adjustment in hepatic impairment: No specific guidelines are available

Elderly: Not intended for use in women ≥65 years of age (Phase 2 and Phase 3 studies included women 19-40 years of age)

Administration Cetrorelix is administered by SubQ injection following proper aseptic technique procedures. Injections should be to the lower abdomen, preferably around the navel (but staying at least 1 inch from the navel). The injection site should be rotated daily. The needle should be inserted completely into the skin at a 45-degree angle.

Monitoring Parameters Ultrasound to assess follicle size

Dosage Forms Excipient information presented when available (limited, particularly for generics); consult specific product labeling.

Injection, powder for reconstitution:

Cetrotide®: 0.25 mg, 3 mg [contains mannitol]

◆ **Cetrorelix Acetate** *see* Cetrorelix *on page 296*

◆ **Cetrotide®** *see* Cetrorelix *on page 296*

Cetuximab (se TUK see mab)

U.S. Brand Names Erbitux®

Canadian Brand Names Erbitux®

Index Terms C225; IMC-C225; NSC-714692

Pharmacologic Category Antineoplastic Agent, Monoclonal Antibody; Epidermal Growth Factor Receptor (EGFR) Inhibitor

Use Treatment of metastatic colorectal cancer; treatment of squamous cell cancer of the head and neck

Unlabeled/Investigational Use Treatment of EGFR-expressing advanced nonsmall cell lung cancer (NSCLC)

Pregnancy Risk Factor C

Pregnancy Considerations In pregnant cynomolgus monkeys, cetuximab was detected in the amniotic fluid and in the serum of embryos. Although teratogenic effects were not observed in animal studies, increases in embryolethality and fetal loss were noted. There are no adequate and well-controlled studies in pregnant women. It is not known whether cetuximab can cause fetal harm or affect reproductive capacity. Because cetuximab inhibits epidermal growth factor (EGF), a component of fetal development, adverse effects on pregnancy would be expected. Cetuximab should only be given to a pregnant woman if the potential benefit justifies the potential risk to the fetus.

Lactation Excretion in breast milk is unknown/not recommended

Medication Safety Issues

Sound-alike/look-alike issues:

Cetuximab may be confused with bevacizumab

Contraindications There are no contraindications listed in the manufacturer's labeling

Warnings/Precautions [U.S. Boxed Warning]: Severe infusion reactions (bronchospasm, stridor, hoarseness, urticaria, hypotension, loss of consciousness, shock, MI, cardiac arrest) have been reported in ~3% of patients; fatal outcome has been reported rarely. Approximately 90% of reactions occur with the first infusion despite the use of prophylactic antihistamines. **Note:** Although a 20 mg test dose was used in some studies, it did not reliably predict the risk of an infusion reaction, and is not recommended. In case of severe reaction, treatment should be stopped and permanently discontinued. Immediate treatment for anaphylactic/anaphylactoid reactions should be available during administration. The manufacturer recommends monitoring patients for at least 1 hour following completion of infusion, or longer if a reaction occurs. Mild-to-moderate infusion reactions are managed by slowing the infusion rate (by 50%) and administering antihistamines. Patients with pre-existing IgE antibody against cetuximab (specific for galactose-α-1,3-galactose) are reported to have a higher incidence of severe hypersensitivity reaction. Severe hypersensitivity reaction has been reported more frequently in patients living in the middle south area of the United States, including North Carolina and Tennessee (O'Neil, 2007; Chung, 2008).

[U.S. Boxed Warning]: Cardiopulmonary arrest has been reported in patients receiving radiation therapy in combination with cetuximab; closely monitor serum electrolytes during and after (for at least 8 weeks) cetuximab therapy; use caution with history of coronary artery disease, HF, and arrhythmias. Interstitial lung disease (ILD) has been reported; use caution with pre-existing lung disease; permanently discontinue with confirmed ILD. Acneiform rash has been reported in 76% to 88% of patients (severe in 1% to 17%), usually developing within the first 2 weeks of therapy; may require dose modification. Acneiform rash should be treated with topical and/or oral antibiotics; topical corticosteroids are not recommended. Other dermatologic toxicities, including dry skin, fissures, hypertrichosis, paronychial inflammation, and skin infections have been reported; related ocular toxicities (blepharitis, conjunctivitis, keratitis) may also occur. Sunlight may exacerbate skin reactions. Hypomagnesemia is common; the onset of electrolyte disturbance may occur within days to months after initiation of treatment. Non-neutralizing anticetuximab antibodies were detected in 5% of evaluable patients. Safety and efficacy have not been established when used in combination with radiation therapy and cisplatin. Safety and efficacy in children have not been established.

Adverse Reactions Except where noted, percentages reported for cetuximab monotherapy.

>10%:

Central nervous system: Fatigue (89%), pain (17% to 51%), headache (26% to 33%), insomnia (10% to 30%), fever (27% to 30%), confusion (15%), anxiety (14%), chills/rigors (13%), depression (7% to 13%)

Dermatologic: Acneiform rash (76% to 90%; grades 3/4: 1% to 17%; onset: ≤14 days), rash (89%), dry skin (49%), pruritus (11% to 40%), nail changes/disorder (16% to 21%)

Endocrine & metabolic: Hypomagnesemia (55%; grades 3/4: 6% to 17%)

Gastrointestinal: Abdominal pain (26% to 59%), constipation (26% to 46%), diarrhea (25% to 39%), vomiting (25% to 37%), nausea (mild-to-moderate 29%), weight loss (7% to 27%), anorexia (23%), stomatitis (10% to 25%), xerostomia (11%)

Neuromuscular & skeletal: Weakness (45% to 48%), bone pain (15%)

Respiratory: Dyspnea (17% to 48%), cough (11% to 29%)

Miscellaneous: Infection (13% to 35%), infusion reaction (15% to 21%; grades 3/4: 2% to 5%; 90% of severe reactions occurred with first infusion)

1% to 10%:

Cardiovascular: Peripheral edema (10%), cardiopulmonary arrest (2%; with radiation therapy)

Dermatologic: Alopecia (4%), skin disorder (4%)

Endocrine & metabolic: Dehydration (2% to 10%)

Gastrointestinal: Dyspepsia (6%)

Hematologic: Anemia (9%)

Hepatic: Alkaline phosphatase increased (5% to 10%), transaminases increased (5% to 10%)

Neuromuscular & skeletal: Back pain (10%)
Ocular: Conjunctivitis (7%)
Renal: Renal failure (1%)
Respiratory: Pulmonary embolus (1%)
Miscellaneous: Sepsis (1% to 4%)

<1% (Limited to important or life-threatening): Abscess formation, arrhythmia, blepharitis, bronchospasm, cardiac arrest, cellulitis, cheilitis, hoarseness, hypertrichosis, hypotension, interstitial lung disease (occurred between the fourth and eleventh doses), keratitis, leukopenia, loss of consciousness, MI, paronychial inflammation, sepsis, shock, skin fissure, skin infection, stridor

Drug Interactions

Avoid Concomitant Use There are no known interactions where it is recommended to avoid concomitant use.

Increased Effect/Toxicity There are no known significant interactions involving an increase in effect.

Decreased Effect There are no known significant interactions involving a decrease in effect.

Stability Store unopened vials under refrigeration at 2°C to 8°C (36°F to 46°F). Do not freeze. Reconstitution is not required. Appropriate dose should be added to empty sterile container; do not shake or dilute. Preparations in infusion containers are stable for up to 12 hours under refrigeration at 2°C to 8°C (36°F to 46°F) and up to 8 hours at room temperature of 20°C to 25°C (68°F to 77°F).

Mechanism of Action Recombinant human/mouse chimeric monoclonal antibody which binds specifically to the epidermal growth factor receptor (EGFR, HER1, c-ErbB-1) and competitively inhibits the binding of epidermal growth factor (EGF) and other ligands. Binding to the EGFR blocks phosphorylation and activation of receptor-associated kinases, resulting in inhibition of cell growth, induction of apoptosis, and decreased matrix metalloproteinase and vascular endothelial growth factor production.

Pharmacodynamics/Kinetics

Distribution: V_d: ~2-3 L/m^2

Half-life elimination: ~112 hours (range: 63-230 hours)

Dosage I.V.: Adults: **Note:** Premedicate with an H_1 antagonist (eg, diphenhydramine) I.V. 30-60 minutes prior to the first dose; premedication for subsequent doses is based on clinical judgement.

Colorectal cancer:
- Initial loading dose: 400 mg/m^2 infused over 120 minutes
- Maintenance dose: 250 mg/m^2 infused over 60 minutes weekly
- Biweekly administration (unlabeled dosing): 500 mg/m^2 every 2 weeks (initial dose infused over 120 minutes, subsequent doses infused over 60 minutes) (Pfeiffer, 2007)

Head and neck cancer:
- Initial loading dose: 400 mg/m^2 infused over 120 minutes
- Maintenance dose: 250 mg/m^2 infused over 60 minutes weekly
- **Note:** If given in combination with radiation therapy, administer loading dose 1 week prior to initiation of radiation course. Weekly maintenance dose should be completed 1 hour prior to radiation for the duration of radiation therapy (6-7 weeks).

NSCLC (unlabeled use): Initial loading dose: 400 mg/m^2, followed by maintenance dose: 250 mg/m^2 weekly (Pirker, 2008)

Dosage adjustment for toxicity:

Infusion reactions, grade 1 or 2 and nonserious grades 3 or 4: Reduce the infusion rate by 50% and continue to use prophylactic antihistamines

Infusion reactions, severe: Immediately and permanently discontinue treatment

Pulmonary toxicity:
- Acute onset or worsening pulmonary symptoms: Hold treatment
- Interstitial lung disease: Permanently discontinue

Skin toxicity, mild to moderate: No dosage modification required

Acneiform rash, severe (grade 3 or 4):
- First occurrence: Delay cetuximab infusion 1-2 weeks
  - If improvement, continue at 250 mg/m^2
  - If no improvement, discontinue therapy
- Second occurrence: Delay cetuximab infusion 1-2 weeks
  - If improvement, continue at reduced dose of 200 mg/m^2
  - If no improvement, discontinue therapy
- Third occurrence: Delay cetuximab infusion 1-2 weeks
  - If improvement, continue at reduced dose of 150 mg/m^2
  - If no improvement, discontinue therapy
- Fourth occurrence: Discontinue therapy
  - **Note:** Dose adjustments are not recommended for severe **radiation** dermatitis.

Dosage adjustment for renal/hepatic impairment: No adjustment required.

Administration Administer via I.V. infusion; loading dose over 2 hours, weekly maintenance dose over 1 hour. Do not administer as I.V. push or bolus. Do not shake or dilute. Administer via infusion pump or syringe pump. Following the infusion, an observation period (1 hour) is recommended; longer observation time (following an infusion reaction) may be required. Premedication with an H_1 antagonist prior to the initial dose is recommended. The maximum infusion rate is 10 mg/minute. Administer through a low protein-binding 0.22 micrometer in-line filter. Use 0.9% NaCl to flush line at the end of infusion.

For biweekly administration (unlabeled frequency and dose), the initial dose was infused over 120 minutes and subsequent doses infused over 60 minutes (Pfeiffer, 2007).

Monitoring Parameters Vital signs during infusion and observe for at least 1 hour postinfusion. Patients developing dermatologic toxicities should be monitored for the development of complications. Periodic monitoring of serum magnesium, calcium, and potassium are recommended to continue over an interval consistent with the half-life (8 weeks); monitor closely (during and after treatment) for cetuximab plus radiation therapy. KRAS genotyping of tumor tissue in patients with colorectal cancer.

Additional Information Oncology Comment: EGFR expression is detected in nearly all patients with head and neck cancer; laboratory evidence of EGFR expression is not necessary for head and neck cancers.

The National Comprehensive Cancer Network® (NCCN) guidelines for colon cancer (v.3.2008) recommend genotyping tumor tissue for KRAS mutation in all patients with metastatic colorectal cancer (genotyping may be done on archived specimens). Patients with known codon 12 or 13 KRAS gene mutations are unlikely to respond to EGFR inhibitors and should not receive cetuximab. Favorable progression-free survival and overall survival has been demonstrated with cetuximab in patients with KRAS wild-type (Karapetis, 2008; Van Cutsem, 2008). Because EGFR testing in colorectal tumors does not correlate with response, the NCCN guidelines do not recommend routine EGFR testing in colorectal cancer. Dermatologic toxicity with cetuximab is predictive for response; the presence of acneiform rash correlates with treatment response and prolonged survival (Cunningham, 2004).

The NCCN Non-Small Cell Lung cancer guidelines (v.2.2009) recommend cetuximab in combination with cisplatin and vinorelbine as a first-line therapy option in patients with advanced (stage IIIB or IV disease), with EGFR expression and a performance status of 0-2.

Dosage Forms Excipient information presented when available (limited, particularly for generics); consult specific product labeling.

Injection, solution [preservative free]:

Erbitux®: 2 mg/mL (50 mL, 100 mL)

Cevimeline (se vi ME leen)

U.S. Brand Names Evoxac®

Canadian Brand Names Evoxac®

Index Terms Cevimeline Hydrochloride

Pharmacologic Category Cholinergic Agonist

Use Treatment of symptoms of dry mouth in patients with Sjögren's syndrome

Pregnancy Risk Factor C

Medication Safety Issues

Sound-alike/look-alike issues:

Cevimeline may be confused with Savella™

Evoxac® may be confused with Eurax®

Dosage Adults: Oral: 30 mg 3 times/day

Dosage adjustment in renal/hepatic impairment: Not studied; no specific dosage adjustment is recommended

Elderly: No specific dosage adjustment is recommended; however, use caution when initiating due to potential for increased sensitivity

Additional Information Complete prescribing information for this medication should be consulted for additional detail.

Dosage Forms Excipient information presented when available (limited, particularly for generics); consult specific product labeling.

Capsule, as hydrochloride: 30 mg

- **Cevimeline Hydrochloride** *see* Cevimeline *on page 299*
- **CFDN** *see* Cefdinir *on page 271*
- **CG** *see* Chorionic Gonadotropin (Human) *on page 320*
- **C-Gel [OTC]** *see* Ascorbic Acid *on page 139*
- **CGP 33101** *see* Rufinamide *on page 1349*
- **CGP-42446** *see* Zoledronic Acid *on page 1587*
- **CGP-57148B** *see* Imatinib *on page 768*
- **C-Gram [OTC]** *see* Ascorbic Acid *on page 139*
- **CGS-20267** *see* Letrozole *on page 865*
- **Champix® (Can)** *see* Varenicline *on page 1548*
- **Chantix®** *see* Varenicline *on page 1548*
- **Charcadole® (Can)** *see* Charcoal *on page 299*
- **Charcadole®, Aqueous (Can)** *see* Charcoal *on page 299*
- **Charcadole® TFS (Can)** *see* Charcoal *on page 299*
- **Char-Caps [OTC]** *see* Charcoal *on page 299*
- **CharcoAid® G [OTC]** *see* Charcoal *on page 299*

Charcoal (CHAR kole)

U.S. Brand Names Actidose-Aqua® [OTC]; Actidose® with Sorbitol [OTC]; Char-Caps [OTC]; CharcoAid® G [OTC]; Charcoal Plus® DS [OTC]; CharcoCaps® [OTC]; EZ-Char™ [OTC]; Kerr Insta-Char® [OTC]; Requa® Activated Charcoal [OTC]

Canadian Brand Names Charcadole®; Charcadole® TFS; Charcadole®, Aqueous

Index Terms Activated Carbon; Activated Charcoal; Adsorbent Charcoal; Liquid Antidote; Medicinal Carbon; Medicinal Charcoal

Pharmacologic Category Antidote

Use Emergency treatment in poisoning by drugs and chemicals; aids the elimination of certain drugs and improves decontamination of excessive ingestions of sustained-release products or in the presence of bezoars; repetitive doses have proven useful to enhance the elimination of certain drugs (eg, carbamazepine, dapsone, phenobarbital, quinine, or theophylline); repetitive doses for gastric dialysis in uremia to adsorb various waste products; dietary supplement (digestive aid)

Pregnancy Risk Factor C

Lactation Does not enter breast milk/compatible

Medication Safety Issues

Sound-alike/look-alike issues:

Actidose® may be confused with Actos®

Contraindications Hypersensitivity to charcoal or any component of the formulation; intestinal obstruction; GI tract not anatomically intact; patients at risk of hemorrhage or GI perforation; patients with an unprotected airway (eg, CNS depression without intubation); if use would increase risk and severity of aspiration

Warnings/Precautions When using ipecac with charcoal, ensure ipecac-induced vomiting has ceased prior to administering charcoal. Charcoal may cause vomiting; avoid in hydrocarbon and caustic ingestions. Use caution with decreased peristalsis. Coadministration of a cathartic (eg, sorbitol, mannitol, magnesium sulfate) is not recommended secondary to lack of compelling evidence and the increased morbidity associated with their use. If charcoal is administered with a cathartic, avoid excessive fluid and electrolyte losses, especially in children <1 year of age. Charcoal with sorbitol not recommended in children <1 year of age.

Not effective for cyanide, mineral acids, caustic alkalis, organic solvents, iron, ethanol, methanol, or lithium poisoning. Most effective when administered within 30-60 minutes of ingestion. Commercial charcoal products may contain propylene glycol.

Adverse Reactions Frequency not defined.

Endocrine & metabolic: Hypernatremia, hypokalemia, and hypermagnesemia may occur with coadministration of cathartics

Gastrointestinal: Vomiting (incidence may increase with sorbitol), diarrhea (with sorbitol), constipation, swelling of abdomen, bowel obstruction, appendicitis

Respiratory: Aspiration (both gastric contents and charcoal)

Miscellaneous: Fecal discoloration (black)

Drug Interactions

Avoid Concomitant Use There are no known interactions where it is recommended to avoid concomitant use.

Increased Effect/Toxicity There are no known significant interactions involving an increase in effect.

Decreased Effect There are no known significant interactions involving a decrease in effect.

Ethanol/Nutrition/Herb Interactions Food: Do not mix with milk, ice cream, sherbet, or marmalade (may reduce charcoal's effectiveness).

Stability Adsorbs gases from air, store in closed container. Dilute powder with at least 8 mL of water per 1 g of charcoal, or mix in a charcoal to water ratio of 1:4 to 1:8. Mix to form a slurry.

Mechanism of Action Adsorbs toxic substances or irritants, thus inhibiting GI absorption; adsorbs intestinal gas; the addition of sorbitol results in hyperosmotic laxative action causing catharsis

Pharmacodynamics/Kinetics Excretion: Feces (as charcoal)

Dosage Oral:

Acute poisoning: **Note:** ~10 g of activated charcoal for each 1 g of toxin is considered adequate; this may require multiple doses. If sorbitol is also used, sorbitol dose should not exceed 1.5 g/kg. When using multiple doses of charcoal, sorbitol should be given with every other dose (not to exceed 2 doses/day).

Children:
<1 year: 0.5-1 g/kg (10-25 g) as a single dose; if multiple doses are needed, give as 0.25 g/kg/hour or equivalent (eg, 0.5 g/kg every 2 hours)
1-12 years: 0.5-1 g/kg (25-50 g) as a single dose; if multiple doses are needed, give as 0.25 g/kg/hour or equivalent (eg, 0.5 g/kg every 2 hours)
Children >12 years and Adults: 25-100 g as a single dose; if multiple doses are needed, additional doses may be given as 12.5 g/hour or equivalent (eg, 25 g every 2 hours)
Dietary supplement: Adult: 500-520 mg after meals; may repeat in 2 hours if needed (maximum: 10 g/day)

Administration Flavoring agents (eg, chocolate, concentrated fruit juice) or thickening agents (eg, bentonite, carboxymethylcellulose) can enhance charcoal's palatability. If treatment includes ipecac syrup, induce vomiting prior to administration of charcoal. Often given with a laxative or cathartic; check for presence of bowel sounds before administration. I.V. antiemetics may be required to reduce the risk of vomiting during multiple-dose therapy with charcoal.

Dosage Forms Excipient information presented when available (limited, particularly for generics); consult specific product labeling.
Capsule:
Char-Caps, CharcoCaps®: 260 mg
Pellets, for suspension:
EZ-Char™: 25 g
Powder for suspension: 30 g, 240 g
CharcoAid® G: 15 g
Suspension:
Actidose-Aqua®: 15 g (72 mL); 25 g (120 mL); 50 g (240 mL)
Kerr Insta-Char®: 25 g (120 mL) [contains sodium benzoate; packaged with cherry flavor (cherry flavor contains propylene glycol and sodium benzoate)]; 50 g (240 mL) [contains sodium benzoate; unflavored or packaged with cherry flavor (cherry flavor contains propylene glycol and sodium benzoate)]
Suspension [with sorbitol]:
Actidose® with Sorbitol: 25 g (120 mL); 50 g (240 mL)
Kerr Insta-Char®: 25 g (120 mL) [contains sodium benzoate; packaged with cherry flavor (cherry flavor contains propylene glycol and sodium benzoate)]; 50 g (240 mL) [contains sodium benzoate; packaged with cherry flavor (cherry flavor contains propylene glycol and sodium benzoate)]
Tablet:
Requa® Activated Charcoal: 250 mg
Tablet, enteric coated:
Charcoal Plus® DS: 250 mg

- **Charcoal Plus® DS [OTC]** *see* Charcoal *on page 299*
- **CharcoCaps® [OTC]** *see* Charcoal *on page 299*
- **Chemet®** *see* Succimer *on page 1401*
- **Cheracol®** *see* Guaifenesin and Codeine *on page 710*
- **Cheracol® D [OTC]** *see* Guaifenesin and Dextromethorphan *on page 710*
- **Cheracol® Plus [OTC]** *see* Guaifenesin and Dextromethorphan *on page 710*
- **Chew-C [OTC]** *see* Ascorbic Acid *on page 139*
- **Chew-Cal [OTC]** *see* Calcium and Vitamin D *on page 238*
- **CHG** *see* Chlorhexidine Gluconate *on page 305*
- **Chickenpox Vaccine** *see* Varicella Virus Vaccine *on page 1549*
- **Chiggerex® [OTC]** *see* Benzocaine *on page 183*
- **Chiggerex® Plus** *see* Benzocaine *on page 183*
- **Chiggertox® [OTC]** *see* Benzocaine *on page 183*
- **Children's Advil® Cold (Can)** *see* Pseudoephedrine and Ibuprofen *on page 1267*
- **Children's Pepto [OTC]** *see* Calcium Carbonate *on page 238*
- **Children's Motion Sickness Liquid (Can)** *see* DimenhyDRINATE *on page 453*
- **Children's Tylenol® Plus Cold and Allergy [OTC]** *see* Acetaminophen, Diphenhydramine, and Phenylephrine *on page 33*
- **Chirocaine® [DSC]** *see* Levobupivacaine *on page 874*
- **Chirocaine® (Can)** *see* Levobupivacaine *on page 874*
- **Chloral** *see* Chloral Hydrate *on page 300*

Chloral Hydrate (KLOR al HYE drate)

U.S. Brand Names Aquachloral® Supprettes® [DSC]; Somnote®
Canadian Brand Names PMS-Chloral Hydrate
Index Terms Chloral; Hydrated Chloral; Trichloroacetaldehyde Monohydrate
Pharmacologic Category Hypnotic, Nonbenzodiazepine
Use Short-term sedative and hypnotic (<2 weeks); sedative/hypnotic for diagnostic procedures; sedative prior to EEG evaluations
Restrictions C-IV
Pregnancy Risk Factor C
Medication Safety Issues
High alert medication: The Institute for Safe Medication Practices (ISMP) includes this medication among its list of drugs which have a heightened risk of causing significant patient harm when used in error.

Dosage
Children:
Sedation or anxiety: Oral, rectal: 5-15 mg/kg/dose every 8 hours (maximum: 500 mg/dose)
Prior to EEG: Oral, rectal: 20-25 mg/kg/dose, 30-60 minutes prior to EEG; may repeat in 30 minutes to maximum of 100 mg/kg or 2 g total
Hypnotic: Oral, rectal: 20-40 mg/kg/dose up to a maximum of 50 mg/kg/24 hours or 1 g/dose or 2 g/24 hours
Conscious sedation: Oral: 50-75 mg/kg/dose 30-60 minutes prior to procedure; may repeat 30 minutes after initial dose if needed, to a total maximum dose of 120 mg/kg or 1 g total
Adults: Oral, rectal:
Sedation, anxiety: 250 mg 3 times/day
Hypnotic: 500-1000 mg at bedtime or 30 minutes prior to procedure, not to exceed 2 g/24 hours
Discontinuation: Withdraw gradually over 2 weeks if patient has been maintained on high doses for prolonged period of time. Do not stop drug abruptly; sudden withdrawal may result in delirium.
Dosing adjustment/comments in renal impairment: Cl_{cr} <50 mL/minute: Avoid use
Hemodialysis: Dialyzable (50% to 100%); supplemental dose is not necessary
Dosing adjustment/comments in hepatic impairment: Avoid use in patients with severe hepatic impairment

Additional Information Complete prescribing information for this medication should be consulted for additional detail.

Dosage Forms Excipient information presented when available (limited, particularly for generics); consult specific product labeling. [DSC] = Discontinued product
Capsule:
Somnote®: 500 mg
Suppository, rectal: 500 mg
Aquachloral® Supprettes®: 325 mg [contains tartrazine] [DSC]
Syrup: 500 mg/5 mL (5 mL, 480 mL)

Chlorambucil (klor AM byoo sil)

U.S. Brand Names Leukeran®

Canadian Brand Names Leukeran®

Index Terms CB-1348; Chlorambucilum; Chloraminophene; Chlorbutinum; NSC-3088; WR-139013

Pharmacologic Category Antineoplastic Agent, Alkylating Agent

Use Management of chronic lymphocytic leukemia (CLL), Hodgkin's lymphoma, non-Hodgkin's lymphoma (NHL)

Unlabeled/Investigational Use Nephrotic syndrome, Waldenström's macroglobulinemia

Pregnancy Risk Factor D

Pregnancy Considerations Animal studies have demonstrated teratogenicity. Chlorambucil crosses the human placenta. Following exposure during the first trimester, case reports have noted adverse renal effects (unilateral agenesis). There are no adequate and well-controlled studies in pregnant women. Women of childbearing potential should avoid becoming pregnant while receiving treatment. **[U.S. Boxed Warning]: Affects human fertility; probably mutagenic and teratogenic as well**; chromosomal damage has been documented. Fertility effects (reversible and irreversible sterility) include azoospermia (when administered to prepubertal and pubertal males) and amenorrhea.

Lactation Excretion in breast milk unknown/not recommended

Medication Safety Issues

Sound-alike/look-alike issues:

Chlorambucil may be confused with Chloromycetin®

Leukeran® may be confused with Alkeran®, leucovorin, Leukine®, Myleran®

High alert medication: The Institute for Safe Medication Practices (ISMP) includes this medication among its list of drugs which have a heightened risk of causing significant patient harm when used in error.

Contraindications Hypersensitivity to chlorambucil or any component of the formulation; hypersensitivity to other alkylating agents (may have cross-hypersensitivity); pregnancy

Warnings/Precautions Hazardous agent - use appropriate precautions for handling and disposal. Seizures have been observed; use with caution in patients with seizure disorder or head trauma; history of nephrotic syndrome and high pulse doses are at higher risk of seizures. **[U.S. Boxed Warning]: May cause bone marrow suppression;** reduce initial dosage if patient has received myelosuppressive or radiation therapy, or has a depressed baseline leukocyte or platelet count within the previous 4 weeks. Lymphopenia may occur. Avoid administration of live vaccines to immunocompromised patients. Rare instances of severe skin reactions (eg, erythema multiforme, Stevens-Johnson syndrome) have been reported; discontinue if a reaction occurs.

[U.S. Boxed Warning]: Affects human fertility; carcinogenic in humans and probably mutagenic and teratogenic as well; chromosomal damage has been documented. Fertility effects (reversible and irreversible sterility) include azoospermia (when administered to prepubertal and pubertal males) and amenorrhea. Secondary malignancies and acute myelocytic leukemia may be associated with chronic therapy. Safety and efficacy in pediatric patients have not been established.

Adverse Reactions Frequency not always defined.

Central nervous system: Agitation (rare), ataxia (rare), confusion (rare), drug fever, focal/generalized seizure (rare), hallucinations (rare)

Dermatologic: Angioneurotic edema, erythema multiforme (rare), rash, skin hypersensitivity, Stevens-Johnson syndrome (rare), toxic epidermal necrolysis (rare), urticaria

Endocrine & metabolic: Amenorrhea, infertility, SIADH (rare)

Gastrointestinal: Diarrhea (infrequent), nausea (infrequent), oral ulceration (infrequent), vomiting (infrequent)

Genitourinary: Azoospermia, cystitis (sterile)

Hematologic: Neutropenia (25%; dose- and duration-related; onset: 3 weeks; recovery: 10 days after last dose), bone marrow failure (irreversible), bone marrow suppression, anemia, leukemia (secondary), leukopenia, lymphopenia, pancytopenia, thrombocytopenia

Hepatic: Hepatotoxicity, jaundice

Neuromuscular & skeletal: Flaccid paresis (rare), muscular twitching (rare), myoclonia (rare), peripheral neuropathy, tremor (rare)

Respiratory: Interstitial pneumonia, pulmonary fibrosis

Miscellaneous: Allergic reactions, malignancies (secondary)

Drug Interactions

Avoid Concomitant Use

Avoid concomitant use of Chlorambucil with any of the following: Natalizumab; Vaccines (Live)

Increased Effect/Toxicity

Chlorambucil may increase the levels/effects of: Natalizumab; Vaccines (Live)

The levels/effects of Chlorambucil may be increased by: Trastuzumab

Decreased Effect

Chlorambucil may decrease the levels/effects of: Vaccines (Inactivated)

The levels/effects of Chlorambucil may be decreased by: Echinacea

Stability Store in refrigerator at 2°C to 8°C (36°F to 46°F); protect from light.

Mechanism of Action Interferes with DNA replication and RNA transcription by alkylation and cross-linking the strands of DNA

Pharmacodynamics/Kinetics

Absorption: Rapid and complete

Distribution: V_d: 0.14-0.24 L/kg

Protein binding: ~99%

Metabolism: Hepatic; forms a major active metabolite (phenylacetic acid mustard) and inactive metabolites

Bioavailability: Reduced 10% to 20% with food

Half-life elimination: ~1.5 hours; Phenylacetic acid mustard: ~1.8 hours

Time to peak, plasma: Within 1 hour; Phenylacetic acid mustard: 1.2-2.6 hours

Excretion: Urine (15% to 60% primarily as inactive metabolites, <1% as unchanged drug or phenylacetic acid mustard)

Dosage Oral (refer to individual protocols):

Children (unlabeled uses):

General short courses: 0.1-0.2 mg/kg/day for 3-6 weeks **or** maintenance therapy: 0.03-0.1 mg/kg/day

Nephrotic syndrome: 0.1-0.2 mg/kg/day every day for ~8-12 weeks with low-dose prednisone

Chronic lymphocytic leukemia (CLL):

Biweekly regimen: Initial: 0.4 mg/kg/dose every 2 weeks; increase dose by 0.1 mg/kg every 2 weeks until a response occurs and/or myelosuppression occurs

Monthly regimen: Initial: 0.4 mg/kg, increase dose by 0.1 mg/kg every 4 weeks until a response occurs and/ or myelosuppression occurs

Malignant lymphomas:

Non-Hodgkin's lymphoma: 0.1 mg/kg/day

Hodgkin's lymphoma: 0.2 mg/kg/day

Adults:

CLL, NHL: 0.1 mg/kg/day for 3-6 weeks **or** 0.4 mg/kg (increased by 0.1mg/kg/dose until response/toxicity observed) biweekly **or** 0.4 mg/kg (increased by 0.1mg/kg/dose until response/toxicity observed) monthly **or** 0.03-0.1 mg/kg/day continuously

Hodgkin's lymphoma: 0.2 mg/kg/day for 3-6 weeks **or** 0.4 mg/kg (increased by 0.1mg/kg/dose until response/toxicity observed) biweekly **or** 0.4 mg/kg (increased by 0.1mg/kg/dose until response/toxicity observed) monthly **or** 0.03-0.1 mg/kg/day continuously

Waldenström's macroglobulinemia (unlabeled use): 0.1 mg/kg/day (continuously) for at least 6 months **or** 0.3 mg/kg/day for 7 days every 6 weeks for at least 6 months

Elderly: Refer to adult dosing; begin at the lower end of dosing range(s)

Dosage adjustment for toxicity:

Skin reactions: Discontinue treatment

Hematologic: Persistent neutropenia, thrombocytopenia, and/or lymphocytosis: Do not exceed 0.1 mg/kg/day

Concurrent or within 4 weeks of chemotherapy/radiotherapy: Initiate treatment cautiously; reduce dose; monitor closely. (May use the usual dose if radiation therapy is small doses of palliative radiation over isolated foci remote from bone marrow.)

Dosing adjustment in renal impairment: The FDA-appproved labeling does not contain renal dosing adjustment guidelines. The following guidelines have been used by some clinicians (Aronoff, 2007): Adults:

Cl_{cr} 10-50 mL/minute: Administer 75% of dose

Cl_{cr} <10 mL/minute: Administer 50% of dose

Continuous ambulatory peritoneal dialysis (CAPD): Administer 50% of dose

Dosing adjustment in hepatic impairment: The FDA-approved labeling does not contain hepatic dosing adjustment guidelines. Chlorambucil is hepatically metabolized into active and inactive metabolites; dosage adjustment may be needed in patients with hepatic impairment.

Administration Usually administered as a single dose; preferably on an empty stomach.

Monitoring Parameters Liver function tests, CBC with differential and platelets (weekly, with WBC monitored twice weekly during the first 3-6 weeks of treatment), serum uric acid

Dosage Forms Excipient information presented when available (limited, particularly for generics); consult specific product labeling.

Tablet:

Leukeran®: 2 mg

Extemporaneous Preparations A 2 mg/mL oral suspension can be prepared by crushing sixty 2 mg tablets in a mortar and then mixing in small amounts of methylcellulose (mix in a total of 30 mL of methylcellulose). Next, add a sufficient quantity of syrup to make 60 mL of final product. Transfer to amber container. Label "shake well," "refrigerate," and "protect from light." Refrigerated stability is 7 days.

Nahata MC and Hipple TF, *Pediatric Drug Formulations*, 4th ed, Cincinnati, OH: Harvey Whitney Books Co, 2000.

Dressman JB and Poust RI, "Stability of Allopurinol and of Five Antineoplastics in Suspension," *Am J Hosp Pharm*, 1983, 40(4):616-8.

◆ **Chlorambucilum** *see* Chlorambucil *on page 301*

◆ **Chloraminophene** *see* Chlorambucil *on page 301*

Chloramphenicol (klor am FEN i kole)

Canadian Brand Names Chloromycetin®; Chloromycetin® Succinate; Diochloram®; Pentamycetin®

Pharmacologic Category Antibiotic, Miscellaneous

Use Treatment of serious infections due to organisms resistant to other less toxic antibiotics or when its penetrability into the site of infection is clinically superior to other antibiotics to which the organism is sensitive; useful in infections caused by *Bacteroides*, *H. influenzae*, *Neisseria meningitidis*, *Salmonella*, and *Rickettsia*; active against many vancomycin-resistant enterococci

Pregnancy Considerations Chloramphenicol crosses the placenta producing cord concentrations approaching maternal serum concentrations. An increased risk of teratogenic effects has not been identified for chloramphenicol and there have been no reports of fetal harm related to use of chloramphenicol in pregnancy. "Gray Syndrome" has occurred in premature infants and newborns receiving chloramphenicol. In most cases, chloramphenicol was started during the first 48 hours of life, but it has also occurred in older patients after high doses. Symptoms began after 3-4 days of therapy, starting with abdominal distention and continuing to progressive pallid cyanosis, vasomotor collapse, irregular respiration, and death within a few hours of symptom onset. Stopping therapy can reverse the process and allow complete recovery. There is one case report of an infant with gray baby syndrome after *in utero* exposure to a single maternal dose during labor, followed by a 10-fold overdose of chloramphenicol in the first day of life. The extent of the contribution of the single dose given during labor is unknown. The manufacturer recommends caution if used in a pregnant patient near term or during labor.

Lactation Enters breast milk/use with caution (AAP rates "of concern")

Medication Safety Issues

Sound-alike/look-alike issues:

Chloromycetin® may be confused with chlorambucil, Chlor-Trimeton®

Contraindications Hypersensitivity to chloramphenicol or any component of the formulation; treatment of trivial or viral infections; bacterial prophylaxis

Warnings/Precautions Gray syndrome characterized by circulatory collapse, cyanosis, acidosis, abdominal distention, myocardial depression, coma, and death has occurred. Use with caution in patients with impaired renal or hepatic function and in neonates. Reduce dose with impaired liver function. Use with care in patients with glucose 6-phosphate dehydrogenase deficiency. **[U.S. Boxed Warning]: Serious and fatal blood dyscrasias (aplastic anemia, hypoplastic anemia, thrombocytopenia, and granulocytopenia) have occurred after both short-term and prolonged therapy. Monitor CBC frequently in all patients;** discontinue if evidence of myelosuppression. Irreversible bone marrow suppression may occur weeks or months after therapy. Avoid repeated courses of treatment. Should not be used for minor infections or when less potentially toxic agents are effective. Prolonged use may result in fungal or bacterial superinfection, including *C. difficile*-associated diarrhea (CDAD) and pseudomembranous colitis; CDAD has been observed >2 months postantibiotic treatment.

Adverse Reactions Frequency not defined.

Central nervous system: Confusion, delirium, depression, fever, headache

Dermatologic: Angioedema, rash, urticaria

Gastrointestinal: Diarrhea, enterocolitis, glossitis, nausea, stomatitis, vomiting

Hematologic: Aplastic anemia, bone marrow suppression, granulocytopenia, hypoplastic anemia, pancytopenia, thrombocytopenia

Ocular: Optic neuritis

Miscellaneous: Anaphylaxis, hypersensitivity reactions, Gray syndrome

Drug Interactions

Metabolism/Transport Effects Inhibits CYP2C9 (weak), 3A4 (weak)

Avoid Concomitant Use There are no known interactions where it is recommended to avoid concomitant use.

Increased Effect/Toxicity

Chloramphenicol may increase the levels/effects of: Anticonvulsants (Hydantoin); Barbiturates; Sulfonylureas

Decreased Effect

Chloramphenicol may decrease the levels/effects of: Cyanocobalamin; Typhoid Vaccine

The levels/effects of Chloramphenicol may be decreased by: Anticonvulsants (Hydantoin); Barbiturates; Rifampin

Ethanol/Nutrition/Herb Interactions Food: May decrease intestinal absorption of vitamin B_{12} may have increased dietary need for riboflavin, pyridoxine, and vitamin B_{12}.

Stability Store at room temperature prior to reconstitution. Reconstituted solutions remain stable for 30 days. Use only clear solutions. Frozen solutions remain stable for 6 months.

Mechanism of Action Reversibly binds to 50S ribosomal subunits of susceptible organisms preventing amino acids from being transferred to growing peptide chains thus inhibiting protein synthesis

Pharmacodynamics/Kinetics

Distribution: To most tissues and body fluids
- Chloramphenicol: V_d: 0.5-1 L/kg
- Chloramphenicol succinate: V_d: 0.2-3.1 L/kg; decreased with hepatic or renal dysfunction

Protein binding: Chloramphenicol: ~60%; decreased with hepatic or renal dysfunction and in newborn infants

Metabolism:
- Chloramphenicol: Hepatic to metabolites (inactive)
- Chloramphenicol succinate: Hydrolyzed in the liver, kidney and lungs to chloramphenicol (active)

Bioavailability:
- Chloramphenicol: Oral: ~80%
- Chloramphenicol succinate: I.V.: ~70%; highly variable, dependant upon rate and extent of metabolism to chloramphenicol

Half-life elimination:
- Normal renal function:
  - Chloramphenicol: Adults: ~4 hours; Children 4-6 hours; Infants: Significantly prolonged
  - Chloramphenicol succinate: Adults: ~3 hours
- End-stage renal disease: Chloramphenicol: 3-7 hours
- Hepatic disease: Prolonged

Excretion: Urine (~30% as unchanged chloramphenicol succinate in adults, 6% to 80% in children; 5% to 15% as chloramphenicol)

Dosage

Neonates: Initial loading dose: I.V. (I.M. administration is not recommended): 20 mg/kg (the first maintenance dose should be given 12 hours after the loading dose)
- Maintenance dose: Postnatal age:
  - ≤7 days: 25 mg/kg/day once every 24 hours
  - >7 days, ≤2000 g: 25 mg/kg/day once every 24 hours
  - >7 days, >2000 g: 50 mg/kg/day divided every 12 hours

Children: Usual dosing range: I.V.: 50-100 mg/kg/day in divided doses every 6 hours; maximum daily dose: 4 g/day
- Meningitis: I.V.: Infants >30 days and Children: 75-100 mg/kg/day divided every 6 hours

Adults: 50-100 mg/kg/day in divided doses every 6 hours; maximum daily dose: 4 g/day

Dosing adjustment in renal impairment: Use with caution; monitor serum concentrations

Dosing adjustment/comments in hepatic impairment: Use with caution; monitor serum concentrations

Dietary Considerations May have increased dietary need for riboflavin, pyridoxine, and vitamin B_{12}. Sodium content of 1 g injection: ~52 mg (2.25 mEq).

Administration Do not administer I.M.; can be administered IVP over at least 1 minute at a concentration of 100 mg/mL, or I.V. intermittent infusion over 15-30 minutes at a final concentration for administration of ≤20 mg/mL.

Monitoring Parameters CBC with differential (baseline and every 2 days during therapy), periodic liver and renal function tests, serum drug concentration

Reference Range

Therapeutic levels:
- Meningitis:
  - Peak: 15-25 mcg/mL; toxic concentration: >40 mcg/mL
  - Trough: 5-15 mcg/mL
- Other infections:
  - Peak: 10-20 mcg/mL
  - Trough: 5-10 mcg/mL

Timing of serum samples: Draw levels 0.5-1.5 hours after completion of I.V. dose

Test Interactions May cause false-positive results in urine glucose tests when using cupric sulfate (Benedict's solution, Clinitest®).

Dosage Forms Excipient information presented when available (limited, particularly for generics); consult specific product labeling.

Injection, powder for reconstitution: 1 g [contains sodium ~52 mg/g (2.25 mEq/g)]

- ◆ **ChloraPrep® [OTC]** *see* Chlorhexidine Gluconate *on page 305*
- ◆ **ChloraPrep® Frepp® [OTC]** *see* Chlorhexidine Gluconate *on page 305*
- ◆ **ChloraPrep® Sepp® [OTC]** *see* Chlorhexidine Gluconate *on page 305*
- ◆ **Chlorascrub™ [OTC]** *see* Chlorhexidine Gluconate *on page 305*
- ◆ **Chlorascrub™ Maxi [OTC]** *see* Chlorhexidine Gluconate *on page 305*
- ◆ **Chlorbutinum** *see* Chlorambucil *on page 301*
- ◆ **Chlordex GP** *see* Dextromethorphan, Chlorpheniramine, Phenylephrine, and Guaifenesin *on page 434*

ChlordiazePOXIDE (klor dye az e POKS ide)

U.S. Brand Names Librium®

Canadian Brand Names Apo-Chlordiazepoxide®

Index Terms Methaminodiazepoxide Hydrochloride

Pharmacologic Category Benzodiazepine

Additional Appendix Information

Benzodiazepines *on page 1646*

Use Management of anxiety disorder or for the short-term relief of symptoms of anxiety; withdrawal symptoms of acute alcoholism; preoperative apprehension and anxiety

Restrictions C-IV

Pregnancy Risk Factor D

Lactation Enters breast milk/not recommended

Medication Safety Issues

Sound-alike/look-alike issues:
- ChlordiazePOXIDE may be confused with chlorproMAZINE
- Librium® may be confused with Librax®

Contraindications Hypersensitivity to chlordiazepoxide or any component of the formulation (cross-sensitivity with other benzodiazepines may also exist); narrow-angle glaucoma; pregnancy

Warnings/Precautions Active metabolites with extended half-lives may lead to delayed accumulation and adverse effects. Use with caution in elderly or debilitated patients, pediatric patients, patients with hepatic disease (including alcoholics) or renal impairment, patients with respiratory disease or impaired gag reflex, patients with porphyria.

Parenteral administration should be avoided in comatose patients or shock. Adequate resuscitative equipment/personnel should be available, and appropriate monitoring should be conducted at the time of injection and for several hours following administration. The parenteral formulation should be diluted for I.M. administration with the supplied diluent only. This diluent should not be used when preparing the drug for intravenous administration.

Causes CNS depression (dose related) resulting in sedation, dizziness, confusion, or ataxia which may impair physical and mental capabilities. Patients must be cautioned about performing tasks which require mental alertness (eg, operating machinery or driving). Use with caution in patients receiving other CNS depressants or psychoactive agents (lithium, phenothiazines). Effects with other sedative drugs or ethanol may be potentiated. Benzodiazepines have been associated with falls and traumatic injury and should be used with extreme caution in patients who are at risk of these events (especially the elderly).

Use caution in patients with depression, particularly if suicidal risk may be present. Use with caution in patients with a history of drug dependence. Benzodiazepines have been associated with dependence and acute withdrawal symptoms on discontinuation or reduction in dose. Acute withdrawal, including seizures, may be precipitated in patients after administration of flumazenil to patients receiving long-term benzodiazepine therapy.

Benzodiazepines have been associated with anterograde amnesia. Paradoxical reactions, including hyperactive or aggressive behavior have been reported with benzodiazepines, particularly in adolescent/pediatric or psychiatric patients. Does not have analgesic, antidepressant, or antipsychotic properties.

Adverse Reactions

>10%:

Central nervous system: Drowsiness, fatigue, ataxia, lightheadedness, memory impairment, dysarthria, irritability

Dermatologic: Rash

Endocrine & metabolic: Libido decreased, menstrual disorders

Gastrointestinal: Xerostomia, salivation decreased, appetite increased or decreased, weight gain/loss

Genitourinary: Micturition difficulties

1% to 10%:

Cardiovascular: Hypotension

Central nervous system: Confusion, dizziness, disinhibition, akathisia

Dermatologic: Dermatitis

Endocrine & metabolic: Libido increased

Gastrointestinal: Salivation increased

Genitourinary: Sexual dysfunction, incontinence

Neuromuscular & skeletal: Rigidity, tremor, muscle cramps

Otic: Tinnitus

Respiratory: Nasal congestion

<1% (Limited to important or life-threatening): Photosensitivity

Drug Interactions

Metabolism/Transport Effects Substrate of CYP3A4 (major)

Avoid Concomitant Use There are no known interactions where it is recommended to avoid concomitant use.

Increased Effect/Toxicity

ChlordiazePOXIDE may increase the levels/effects of: Alcohol (Ethyl); Clozapine; CNS Depressants; Phenytoin

The levels/effects of ChlordiazePOXIDE may be increased by: Antifungal Agents (Azole Derivatives, Systemic); Aprepitant; Calcium Channel Blockers (Nondihydropyridine); Cimetidine; CYP3A4 Inhibitors (Moderate); CYP3A4 Inhibitors (Strong); Dasatinib; Disulfiram; Fluconazole; Fosaprepitant; Grapefruit Juice; Isoniazid; Macrolide Antibiotics; Nefazodone; Oral Contraceptive (Estrogens); Oral Contraceptive (Progestins); Protease Inhibitors; Proton Pump Inhibitors; Selective Serotonin Reuptake Inhibitors

Decreased Effect

The levels/effects of ChlordiazePOXIDE may be decreased by: CarBAMazepine; CYP3A4 Inducers (Strong); Deferasirox; Rifamycin Derivatives; St Johns Wort; Theophylline Derivatives; Yohimbine

Ethanol/Nutrition/Herb Interactions

Ethanol: Avoid ethanol (may increase CNS depression).

Food: Serum concentrations/effects may be increased with grapefruit juice, but unlikely because of high oral bioavailability of chlordiazepoxide.

Herb/Nutraceutical: Avoid valerian, St John's wort, kava kava, gotu kola (may increase CNS depression).

Stability Injection: Prior to reconstitution, store under refrigeration and protect from light. Solution should be used immediately following reconstitution.

I.M. use: Reconstitute by adding 2 mL of provided diluent; agitate gently until dissolved. Provided diluent is **not** for I.V. use.

I.V. use: Reconstitute by adding 5 mL NS or SWFI; agitate gently until dissolved; **do not administer this dilution I.M.**

Mechanism of Action Binds to stereospecific benzodiazepine receptors on the postsynaptic GABA neuron at several sites within the central nervous system, including the limbic system, reticular formation. Enhancement of the inhibitory effect of GABA on neuronal excitability results by increased neuronal membrane permeability to chloride ions. This shift in chloride ions results in hyperpolarization (a less excitable state) and stabilization.

Pharmacodynamics/Kinetics

Distribution: V_d: 3.3 L/kg; crosses placenta; enters breast milk

Protein binding: 90% to 98%

Metabolism: Extensively hepatic to desmethyldiazepam (active and long-acting)

Half-life elimination: 6.6-25 hours; End-stage renal disease: 5-30 hours; Cirrhosis: 30-63 hours

Time to peak, serum: Oral: Within 2 hours; I.M.: Results in lower peak plasma levels than oral

Excretion: Urine (minimal as unchanged drug)

Dosage

Children:

<6 years: Not recommended

>6 years: Anxiety: Oral, I.M.: 0.5 mg/kg/24 hours divided every 6-8 hours

Adults:

Anxiety:

Oral: 15-100 mg divided 3-4 times/day

I.M., I.V.: Initial: 50-100 mg followed by 25-50 mg 3-4 times/day as needed

Preoperative anxiety: I.M.: 50-100 mg prior to surgery

Ethanol withdrawal symptoms: Oral, I.V.: 50-100 mg to start, dose may be repeated in 2-4 hours as necessary to a maximum of 300 mg/24 hours

Note: Up to 300 mg may be given I.M. or I.V. during a 6-hour period, but not more than this in any 24-hour period.

Dosing adjustment in renal impairment: Cl_{cr} <10 mL/minute: Administer 50% of dose

Hemodialysis: Not dialyzable (0% to 5%)

Dosing adjustment/comments in hepatic impairment: Avoid use

Administration

I.M.: Administer by deep I.M. injection slowly into the upper outer quadrant of the gluteus muscle. Use only the diluent provided for I.M. use. Solutions made with SWFI or NS cause pain with I.M. administration.

I.V.: Administer slowly over at least 1 minute. Do not use the diluent provided for I.M. use. Air bubbles form during reconstitution.

Monitoring Parameters Respiratory and cardiovascular status, mental status, check for orthostasis

Reference Range Therapeutic: 0.1-3 mcg/mL (SI: 0-10 µmol/L); Toxic: >23 mcg/mL (SI: >77 µmol/L)

Additional Information Abrupt discontinuation after sustained use (generally >10 days) may cause withdrawal symptoms.

Dosage Forms Excipient information presented when available (limited, particularly for generics); consult specific product labeling.

Capsule, as hydrochloride: 5 mg, 10 mg, 25 mg

Injection, powder for reconstitution, as hydrochloride: 100 mg [diluent contains benzyl alcohol, polysorbate 80, and propylene glycol]

◆ **Chlordiazepoxide and Amitriptyline Hydrochloride** *see* Amitriptyline and Chlordiazepoxide *on page 92*

◆ **Chlordiazepoxide and Clidinium** *see* Clidinium and Chlordiazepoxide *on page 344*

Chlordiazepoxide and Methscopolamine

(klor dye az e POKS ide & meth skoe POL a meen)

U.S. Brand Names Librax® *[reformulation]* [DSC]

Index Terms Methscopolamine Nitrate and Chlordiazepoxide Hydrochloride

Pharmacologic Category Anticholinergic Agent; Benzodiazepine

Use Adjunctive treatment of peptic ulcer; treatment of irritable bowel syndrome, acute enterocolitis

Restrictions C-IV

Pregnancy Risk Factor C

Medication Safety Issues

Librax® formulation may be cause for confusion:

In November 2004, Valeant Pharmaceuticals licensed the Librax® trademark to Victory Pharmaceuticals. Subsequently, the product was reformulated to contain chlordiazepoxide and methscopolamine. In January 2006, Valeant Pharmaceuticals began redistributing the original formulation of Librax®, containing clidinium and chlordiazepoxide. Victory Pharmaceuticals has discontinued their product. **Note:** The formulation of Librax® distributed in Canada (Valeant Canada Ltd) always contained clidinium and chlordiazepoxide.

Dosage Oral: Peptic ulcer, irritable bowel syndrome, acute enterocolitis:

Adults: 1-2 capsules 3-4 times/day; adjust dose based on individual response

Elderly: Initial dose should not exceed 2 capsules/day; adjust dose as tolerated

Additional Information Complete prescribing information for this medication should be consulted for additional detail.

Dosage Forms Excipient information presented when available (limited, particularly for generics); consult specific product labeling.

Capsule: Chlordiazepoxide hydrochloride 5 mg and methscopolamine nitrate 2.5 mg [DSC]

◆ **Chlorethazine** *see* Mechlorethamine *on page 927*

◆ **Chlorethazine Mustard** *see* Mechlorethamine *on page 927*

◆ **Chlorex-A** *see* Chlorpheniramine, Phenylephrine, and Phenyltoloxamine *on page 314*

◆ **Chlorex-A 12 [DSC]** *see* Chlorpheniramine, Pyrilamine, and Phenylephrine *on page 315*

Chlorhexidine Gluconate

(klor HEKS i deen GLOO koe nate)

U.S. Brand Names Avagard™ [OTC]; BactoShield® CHG [OTC]; Betasept® [OTC]; ChloraPrep® Frepp® [OTC]; ChloraPrep® Sepp® [OTC]; ChloraPrep® [OTC]; Chlorascrub™ Maxi [OTC]; Chlorascrub™ [OTC]; Dyna-Hex® [OTC]; Hibiclens® [OTC]; Hibistat® [OTC]; Operand® Chlorhexidine Gluconate [OTC]; Peridex®; PerioChip®; PerioGard®

Canadian Brand Names Hibidil® 1:2000; ORO-Clense; Peridex® Oral Rinse

Index Terms 3M™ Avagard™ [OTC]; CHG

Pharmacologic Category Antibiotic, Oral Rinse; Antibiotic, Topical

Use Skin cleanser for surgical scrub, cleanser for skin wounds, preoperative skin preparation, germicidal hand rinse, and as antibacterial dental rinse. Chlorhexidine is active against gram-positive and gram-negative organisms, facultative anaerobes, aerobes, and yeast.

Orphan drug: Peridex®: Oral mucositis with cytoreductive therapy when used for patients undergoing bone marrow transplant

Pregnancy Risk Factor B

Medication Safety Issues

Sound-alike/look-alike issues:

Peridex® may be confused with Precedex™

Dosage Adults:

Oral rinse (Peridex®, PerioGard®):

Floss and brush teeth, completely rinse toothpaste from mouth and swish 15 mL (one capful) undiluted oral rinse around in mouth for 30 seconds, then expectorate. Caution patient not to swallow the medicine and instruct not to eat for 2-3 hours after treatment. (Cap on bottle measures 15 mL.)

Treatment of gingivitis: Oral prophylaxis: Swish for 30 seconds with 15 mL chlorhexidine, then expectorate; repeat twice daily (morning and evening). Patient should have a re-evaluation followed by a dental prophylaxis every 6 months.

Periodontal chip: One chip is inserted into a periodontal pocket with a probing pocket depth ≥5 mm. Up to 8 chips may be inserted in a single visit. Treatment is recommended every 3 months in pockets with a remaining depth ≥5 mm. If dislodgment occurs 7 days or more after placement, the subject is considered to have had the full course of treatment. If dislodgment occurs within 48 hours, a new chip should be inserted. The chip biodegrades completely and does not need to be removed. Patients should avoid dental floss at the site of PerioChip® insertion for 10 days after placement because flossing might dislodge the chip.

Insertion of periodontal chip: Pocket should be isolated and surrounding area dried prior to chip insertion. The chip should be grasped using forceps with the rounded edges away from the forceps. The chip should be inserted into the periodontal pocket to its maximum depth. It may be maneuvered into position using the tips of the forceps or a flat instrument.

Cleanser:

Surgical scrub: Scrub 3 minutes and rinse thoroughly, wash for an additional 3 minutes

Hand sanitizer (Avagard™): Dispense 1 pumpful in palm of one hand; dip fingertips of opposite hand into solution and work it under nails. Spread remainder evenly over hand and just above elbow, covering all surfaces. Repeat on other hand. Dispense another pumpful in each hand and reapply to each hand up to the wrist. Allow to dry before gloving.

Hand wash: Wash for 15 seconds and rinse

Hand rinse: Rub 15 seconds and rinse

Additional Information Complete prescribing information for this medication should be consulted for additional detail.

Dosage Forms Excipient information presented when available (limited, particularly for generics); consult specific product labeling.

Chip, for periodontal pocket insertion:
PerioChip®: 2.5 mg

Liquid, topical [surgical scrub]:
BactoShield® CHG: 2% (120 mL, 480 mL, 750 mL, 960 mL, 3840 mL); 4% (120 mL, 480 mL, 960 mL, 3840 mL) [contains isopropyl alcohol]
Betasept®: 4% (120 mL, 240 mL, 480 mL, 960 mL, 3840 mL) [contains isopropyl alcohol]
ChloraPrep®: 2% (0.67 mL, 1.5 mL, 3 mL, 10.5 mL, 26 mL) [contains isopropyl alcohol 70%; prefilled applicator]
Dyna-Hex®: 2% (120 mL, 480 mL, 960 mL, 3840 mL) [contains isopropyl alcohol]; 4% (120 mL, 480 mL, 960 mL, 3840 mL) [contains isopropyl alcohol]
Hibiclens®: 4% (15 mL, 120 mL, 240 mL, 480 mL, 960 mL, 3840 mL) [contains isopropyl alcohol]
Operand® Chlorhexidine Gluconate: 2% (120 mL); 4% (120 mL, 240 mL, 480 mL, 960 mL, 3840 mL) [contains isopropyl alcohol]

Liquid, oral [rinse]: 0.12% (480 mL)
Peridex®: 0.12% (120 mL, 480 mL, 1920 mL) [contains alcohol 11.6%; mint flavor]
PerioGard®: 0.12% (480 mL) [contains alcohol 11.6%; mint flavor]

Lotion, topical [surgical scrub]:
Avagard™: 1% (500 mL) [contains ethyl alcohol and moisturizers]

Sponge/Brush, topical:
BactoShield® CHG): 4% [contains isopropyl alcohol]

Sponge, topical [surgical scrub]:
ChloraPrep® 3 mL: 2% (25s) [contains isopropyl alcohol; available in clear or Hi-Lite Orange™]
ChloraPrep® 10.5 mL: 2% (25s) [contains isopropyl alcohol; available in clear, Hi-Lite Orange™, and Scrub Teal™]
ChloraPrep® 26 mL: 2% (25s) [contains isopropyl alcohol; available in clear, Hi-Lite Orange™, and Scrub Teal™]
ChloraPrep® Frepp® 1.5 mL: 2% (20s) [contains isopropyl alcohol]
ChloraPrep® Sepp® 0.67 mL: 2% (200s) [contains isopropyl alcohol]

Swab, topical [prep pad]:
Chlorascrub™: 3.15% (100s) [contains isopropyl alcohol]

Swabstick, topical [surgical scrub]:
ChloraPrep® 1.75 mL: 2% (48s) [contains isopropyl alcohol]
ChloraPrep® 5.25 mL: 2% (40s) [contains isopropyl alcohol]
Chlorascrub™ 1.6 mL: 3.15% (50s) [contains isopropyl alcohol]
Chlorascrub™ Maxi 5.1 mL: 3.15% (30s) [contains isopropyl alcohol]

Wipe, topical [towlette]:
Hibistat®: 0.5% (50s) [contains isopropyl alcohol]

- **Chlormeprazine** *see* Prochlorperazine *on page 1244*
- **Chlor-Mes** *see* Chlorpheniramine, Phenylephrine, and Methscopolamine *on page 313*
- **Chlor-Mes-D** *see* Chlorpheniramine, Phenylephrine, and Methscopolamine *on page 313*
- **2-Chlorodeoxyadenosine** *see* Cladribine *on page 339*
- **Chloromag®** *see* Magnesium Chloride *on page 914*
- **Chloromycetin® (Can)** *see* Chloramphenicol *on page 302*
- **Chloromycetin® Succinate (Can)** *see* Chloramphenicol *on page 302*
- **Chlorophyllin Copper Complex Sodium, Papain, and Urea** *see* Chlorophyllin, Papain, and Urea *on page 306*

Chlorophyllin, Papain, and Urea

(KLOR oh fil in, pa PAY in, & yoor EE a)

U.S. Brand Names Allanfil 405; Allanfil Spray; Panafil®; Panafil® SE; Papfyll™; Ziox 405™; Ziox™

Index Terms Chlorophyllin Copper Complex Sodium, Papain, and Urea; Papain, Urea, and Chlorophyllin; Urea, Chlorophyllin, and Papain

Pharmacologic Category Enzyme, Topical Debridement

Use Treatment of acute and chronic lesions, such as venous, diabetic, and decubitus ulcers, burns, post-operative wounds, pilonidal cyst wounds, carbuncles, and miscellaneous traumatic or infected wounds

Medication Safety Issues
Sound-alike/look-alike issues:
Ziox™ may be confused with Zyvox®

Dosage Topical: Adults: Apply with each dressing change; daily or twice daily dressing changes are preferred, but some products may be applied every 2-3 days. Cover with dressing following application.
Foam: Apply a single even layer
Ointment: Apply 1/8" thickness over the wound with clean applicator.
Spray: Completely cover the wound site so that the wound is not visible.

Additional Information Complete prescribing information for this medication should be consulted for additional detail.

Dosage Forms Excipient information presented when available (limited, particularly for generics); consult specific product labeling. [DSC] = Discontinued product

Aerosol, topical [foam]:
Papfyll™: Chlorophyllin copper complex sodium 0.5%, papain ≥520,000 USP units/g, and urea 10% (45 g)

Emulsion [spray]:
Panafil® SE: Chlorophyllin copper complex sodium 0.5%, papain ≥521,700 USP units/g, and urea 10% (34 mL)

Ointment:
Allanfil 405, Panafil®: Chlorophyllin copper complex sodium 0.5%, papain ≥521,700 USP units/g, and urea 10% (6 g, 30 g)
Ziox™: Chlorophyllin copper complex sodium 0.5%, papain ≥521,700 units/g, and urea 10% (30 g)
Ziox 405™: Chlorophyllin copper complex sodium 0.5%, papain ≥521,700 USP units/g, and urea 10% (30 g)

Solution [spray]:
Allanfil, Panafil® [DSC]: Chlorophyllin copper complex sodium 0.5%, papain ≥521,700 USP units/g, and urea 10% (33 mL)

Chloroprocaine (klor oh PROE kane)

U.S. Brand Names Nesacaine®; Nesacaine®-MPF

Canadian Brand Names Nesacaine®-CE

Index Terms Chloroprocaine Hydrochloride

Pharmacologic Category Local Anesthetic

Use Infiltration anesthesia and peripheral and epidural anesthesia

Pregnancy Risk Factor C

Medication Safety Issues
Sound-alike/look-alike issues:
Nesacaine® may be confused with Neptazane®

High alert medication: The Institute for Safe Medication Practices (ISMP) includes this medication (epidural administration) among its list of drug classes which have a heightened risk of causing significant patient harm when used in error.

Dosage Dosage varies with anesthetic procedure, the area to be anesthetized, the vascularity of the tissues, depth of anesthesia required, degree of muscle relaxation required, and duration of anesthesia; range.

Children >3 years (normally developed): Maximum dose (without epinephrine): 11 mg/kg; for infiltration, concentrations of 0.5% to 1% are recommended; for nerve block, concentrations of 1% to 1.5% are recommended

Adults:

Maximum single dose (without epinephrine): 11 mg/kg; maximum dose: 800 mg

Maximum single dose (with epinephrine): 14 mg/kg; maximum dose: 1000 mg

Infiltration and peripheral nerve block:

Mandibular: 2%: 2-3 mL; total dose 40-60 mg

Infraorbital: 2%: 0.5-1 mL; total dose 10-20 mg

Brachial plexus: 2%; 30-40 mL; total dose 600-800 mg

Digital (without epinephrine): 1%; 3-4 mL; total dose: 30-40 mg

Pudendal: 2%; 10 mL each side; total dose: 400 mg

Paracervical: 1%; 3 mL per each of four sites

Caudal block: Preservative-free: 2% or 3%: 15-25 mL; may repeat at 40-60 minute intervals

Lumbar epidural block: Preservative-free: 2% or 3%: 2-2.5 mL per segment; usual total volume: 15-25 mL; may repeat with doses that are 2-6 mL less than initial dose every 40-50 minutes.

Additional Information Complete prescribing information for this medication should be consulted for additional detail.

Dosage Forms Excipient information presented when available (limited, particularly for generics); consult specific product labeling.

Injection, solution, as hydrochloride:

Nesacaine®: 1% (30 mL); 2% (30 mL) [contains disodium EDTA and methylparaben]

Injection, solution, as hydrochloride [preservative free]: 2% (20 mL); 3% (20 mL)

Nesacaine®-MPF: 2% (20 mL); 3% (20 mL)

◆ **Chloroprocaine Hydrochloride** *see* Chloroprocaine *on page 306*

Chloroquine (KLOR oh kwin)

U.S. Brand Names Aralen®

Canadian Brand Names Aralen®; Novo-Chloroquine

Index Terms Chloroquine Phosphate

Pharmacologic Category Aminoquinoline (Antimalarial)

Additional Appendix Information

Malaria Treatment *on page 1770*

Use Suppression or chemoprophylaxis of malaria; treatment of uncomplicated or mild-to-moderate malaria; extraintestinal amebiasis

Unlabeled/Investigational Use Rheumatoid arthritis; discoid lupus erythematosus

Pregnancy Risk Factor C

Pregnancy Considerations There are no adequate and well-controlled studies using chloroquine during pregnancy. However, based on clinical experience and because malaria infection in pregnant women may be more severe than in nonpregnant women, chloroquine prophylaxis may be considered in areas of chloroquine-sensitive *P. falciparum* malaria. Pregnant women should be advised not to travel to areas of *P. falciparum* resistance to chloroquine.

Lactation Enters breast milk/not recommended (AAP considers "compatible")

Medication Safety Issues

International issues:

Aralen® may be confused with Oralon® which is a brand name for povidone-iodine in Japan

Aralen® may be confused with Paralen® which is a brand name for acetaminophen in the Czech Republic

Contraindications Hypersensitivity to chloroquine or any component of the formulation; retinal or visual field changes

Warnings/Precautions Use with caution in patients with liver disease, alcoholism or in conjunction with hepatotoxic drugs. May exacerbate psoriasis or porphyria. Use caution in patients with seizure disorders. Use caution in G6PD deficiency; 4-aminoquinolines such as chloroquine has been associated with hemolysis and renal impairment. Use with caution in patients with pre-existing auditory damage; discontinue immediately if hearing defects are noted. Retinopathy (irreversible) and neuropathy/myopathy have occurred with long or high-dose therapy; discontinue drug if any abnormality in the visual field or if muscular weakness develops during treatment. Chloroquine has been associated with ECG changes, AV block, and cardiomyopathy. Aminoquinolones have been associated with rare hematologic reactions including agranulocytosis, aplastic anemia, and thrombocytopenia; monitoring (CBC) is recommended in prolonged therapy.

Adverse Reactions Frequency not defined.

Cardiovascular: Hypotension (rare), ECG changes (rare; including T-wave inversion), cardiomyopathy

Central nervous system: Fatigue, personality changes, headache, psychosis, seizure, delirium, depression

Dermatologic: Pruritus, hair bleaching, pleomorphic skin eruptions, lichen planus eruptions, alopecia, mucosal pigmentary changes (blue-black), photosensitivity

Gastrointestinal: Nausea, diarrhea, vomiting, anorexia, stomatitis, abdominal cramps

Hematologic: Aplastic anemia, agranulocytosis (reversible), neutropenia, thrombocytopenia

Neuromuscular & skeletal: Rare cases of myopathy, neuromyopathy, proximal muscle atrophy, and depression of deep tendon reflexes have been reported

Ocular: Retinopathy (including irreversible changes in some patients long-term or high-dose therapy), blurred vision

Otic: Nerve deafness, tinnitus, hearing reduced (risk increased in patients with pre-existing auditory damage)

Drug Interactions

Metabolism/Transport Effects Substrate (major) of CYP2D6, 3A4; **Inhibits** CYP2D6 (moderate)

Avoid Concomitant Use

Avoid concomitant use of Chloroquine with any of the following: Mefloquine

Increased Effect/Toxicity

Chloroquine may increase the levels/effects of: Antipsychotic Agents (Phenothiazines); Beta-Blockers; Cardiac Glycosides; CYP2D6 Substrates; Fesoterodine; Mefloquine; Tamoxifen

The levels/effects of Chloroquine may be increased by: CYP2D6 Inhibitors (Moderate); CYP2D6 Inhibitors (Strong); CYP3A4 Inhibitors (Moderate); CYP3A4 Inhibitors (Strong); Darunavir; Dasatinib; Mefloquine

Decreased Effect

Chloroquine may decrease the levels/effects of: Anthelmintics; Codeine; TraMADol

The levels/effects of Chloroquine may be decreased by: CYP3A4 Inducers (Strong); Deferasirox; Herbs (CYP3A4 Inducers)

Ethanol/Nutrition/Herb Interactions Ethanol: Avoid ethanol (may increase GI irritation).

Stability Store tablets at 25°C (77°F); excursions permitted to 15°C to 30°C (59°F to 86°F).

Mechanism of Action Binds to and inhibits DNA and RNA polymerase; interferes with metabolism and hemoglobin utilization by parasites; inhibits prostaglandin effects; chloroquine concentrates within parasite acid vesicles and raises internal pH resulting in inhibition of parasite growth; may involve aggregates of ferriprotoporphyrin IX acting as chloroquine receptors causing membrane damage; may also interfere with nucleoprotein synthesis

Pharmacodynamics/Kinetics

Duration: Small amounts may be present in urine months following discontinuation of therapy

Absorption: Oral: Rapid (~89%)

Distribution: Widely in body tissues (eg, eyes, heart, kidneys, liver, lungs) where retention prolonged; crosses placenta; enters breast milk

Metabolism: Partially hepatic

Half-life elimination: 3-5 days

Time to peak, serum: 1-2 hours

Excretion: Urine (~70% as unchanged drug); acidification of urine increases elimination

Dosage Oral:

Suppression or prophylaxis of malaria:

Children: Administer 5 mg base/kg/week on the same day each week (not to exceed 300 mg base/dose); begin 1-2 weeks prior to exposure; continue for 4-6 weeks after leaving endemic area; if suppressive therapy is not begun prior to exposure, double the initial loading dose to 10 mg base/kg and administer in 2 divided doses 6 hours apart, followed by the usual dosage regimen

Adults: 500 mg/week (300 mg base) on the same day each week; begin 1-2 weeks prior to exposure; continue for 4-6 weeks after leaving endemic area; if suppressive therapy is not begun prior to exposure, double the initial loading dose to 1 g (600 mg base) and administer in 2 divided doses 6 hours apart, followed by the usual dosage regimen

Acute attack:

Children: 10 mg/kg (base) on day 1, followed by 5 mg/kg (base) 6 hours later and 5 mg/kg (base) on days 2 and 3

Adults: 1 g (600 mg base) on day 1, followed by 500 mg (300 mg base) 6 hours later, followed by 500 mg (300 mg base) on days 2 and 3

Extraintestinal amebiasis:

Children: 10 mg/kg (base) once daily for 2-3 weeks (up to 300 mg base/day)

Adults: 1 g/day (600 mg base) for 2 days followed by 500 mg/day (300 mg base) for at least 2-3 weeks

Rheumatoid arthritis, lupus erythematosus (unlabeled uses): Adults: 250 mg (150 mg base) once daily; reduce dosage following maximal response (taper to discontinue after response in lupus); generally requires 3-6 weeks

Note: Not considered first-line agent.

Dosing adjustment in renal impairment: Cl_{cr} <10 mL/minute: Administer 50% of dose

Hemodialysis: Minimally removed by hemodialysis

Dietary Considerations May be taken with meals to decrease GI upset.

Administration Chloroquine phosphate tablets have also been mixed with chocolate syrup or enclosed in gelatin capsules to mask the bitter taste.

Monitoring Parameters Ophthalmic exams at baseline and every 3 months during prolonged therapy. Visual acuity, slit-lamp, fundoscopic and visual field examination are recommended. Evaluate neuormuscular function during prolonged therapy. Periodic CBC in patients receiving prolonged therapy

Dosage Forms Excipient information presented when available (limited, particularly for generics); consult specific product labeling.

Tablet, as phosphate: 250 mg [equivalent to 150 mg base]; 500 mg [equivalent to 300 mg base]

Aralen®: 500 mg [equivalent to 300 mg base]

Extemporaneous Preparations A 10 mg chloroquine base/mL suspension is made by pulverizing two Aralen® 500 mg phosphate = 300 mg base/tablet, levigating with sterile water, and adding by geometric proportion, a significant amount of the cherry syrup and levigating until a uniform mixture is obtained; qs ad to 60 mL with cherry syrup, stable for up to 4 weeks when stored in the refrigerator or at a temperature of 29°C

Mirochnick M, Barnett E, Clarke DF, et al, "Stability of Chloroquine in an Extemporaneously Prepared Suspension Stored at Three Temperatures," *Pediatr Infect Dis J*, 1994, 13(9):827-8.

◆ **Chloroquine Phosphate** *see* Chloroquine *on page 307*

Chlorothiazide (klor oh THYE a zide)

U.S. Brand Names Diuril®; Sodium Diuril®

Canadian Brand Names Diuril®

Pharmacologic Category Diuretic, Thiazide

Additional Appendix Information

Sulfonamide Derivatives *on page 1671*

Use Management of mild-to-moderate hypertension; adjunctive treatment of edema

Pregnancy Risk Factor C (manufacturer); D (expert analysis)

Medication Safety Issues

International issues:

Diuril® may be confused with Duorol® which is a brand name for acetaminophen in Spain

Dosage Note: The manufacturer states that I.V. and oral dosing are equivalent. Some clinicians may use lower I.V. doses; however, because of chlorothiazide's poor oral absorption. I.V. dosing in infants and children has not been well established.

Infants <6 months:

Oral: 10-30 mg/kg/day in 2 divided doses (maximum dose: 375 mg/day); anecdotal reports have used up to 40 mg/kg/day (unlabeled).

I.V. (unlabeled): 2-8 mg/kg/day in 2 divided doses; anecdotal reports have used up to 20 mg/kg/day

Infants >6 months and Children:

Oral: 10-20 mg/kg/day in 1-2 divided doses (maximum dose: 375 mg/day in children <2 years or 1 g/day in children 2-12 years)

I.V. (unlabeled route): 4 mg/kg/day in 1-2 divided doses; anecdotal reports have used up to 20 mg/kg/day

Adults:

Hypertension: Oral: 500-2000 mg/day divided in 1-2 doses (manufacturer labeling); doses of 125-500 mg/day have also been recommended (JNC 7)

Edema: Oral, I.V.: 500-1000 mg once or twice daily; intermittent treatment (eg, therapy on alternative days) may be appropriate for some patients

ACC/AHA 2005 Heart Failure guidelines:

Oral: 250-500 mg once or twice daily (maximum daily dose: 1000 mg)

I.V.: 500-1000 mg once daily plus a loop diuretic

Dosage adjustment in renal impairment: Cl_{cr} <10 mL/minute: Avoid use. Ineffective with Cl_{cr} <30 mL/minute unless in combination with a loop diuretic (Aronoff, 2007)

Note: ACC/AHA 2005 Heart Failure guidelines suggest that thiazides lose their efficacy when Cl_{cr} <40 mL/minute

Additional Information Complete prescribing information for this medication should be consulted for additional detail.

Dosage Forms Excipient information presented when available (limited, particularly for generics); consult specific product labeling.

Injection, powder for reconstitution, as sodium:
Sodium Diuril®: 500 mg
Suspension, oral:
Diuril®: 250 mg/5 mL (237 mL) [contains alcohol 0.5% and benzoic acid]
Tablet: 250 mg, 500 mg

◆ **Chlorpheniramine, Acetaminophen, and Pseudoephedrine** *see* Acetaminophen, Chlorpheniramine, and Pseudoephedrine *on page 31*

Chlorpheniramine and Acetaminophen

(klor fen IR a meen & a seet a MIN oh fen)

U.S. Brand Names Coricidin HBP® Cold and Flu [OTC]

Index Terms Acetaminophen and Chlorpheniramine

Pharmacologic Category Analgesic, Miscellaneous; Histamine H_1 Antagonist; Histamine H_1 Antagonist, First Generation

Use Symptomatic relief of congestion, headache, aches and pains of colds and flu

Medication Safety Issues

Duplicate therapy issues: This product contains acetaminophen, which may be a component of other combination products. Do not exceed the maximum recommended daily dose of acetaminophen.

Dosage Adults: Oral: 2 tablets every 4 hours

Additional Information Complete prescribing information for this medication should be consulted for additional detail.

Dosage Forms Excipient information presented when available (limited, particularly for generics); consult specific product labeling.

Tablet: Chlorpheniramine maleate 2 mg and acetaminophen 325 mg

◆ **Chlorpheniramine and Dextromethorphan** *see* Dextromethorphan and Chlorpheniramine *on page 433*

Chlorpheniramine and Phenylephrine

(klor fen IR a meen & fen il EF rin)

U.S. Brand Names Actifed® Cold & Allergy [OTC] *[reformulation]*; AllanTan Pediatric [DSC]; AlleRx™ Suspension; C-Phen; Ceron; Dallergy Drops; Dallergy®-JR; Dec-Chlorphen; Ed A-Hist™; Ed ChlorPed D; NoHist; P-Tann D; PD-Hist-D; PediaTan™ D; Phenabid®; R-Tanna; R-Tanna Pediatric; Rescon-Jr®; Rinate™ Pediatric; Rondec® ; Rynatan®; Rynatan® Pediatric; Sildec PE [DSC]; Sudafed PE® Sinus & Allergy [OTC]; Tannate Pediatric; Triaminic® Cold and Allergy [OTC]

Index Terms Chlorpheniramine Maleate and Phenylephrine Hydrochloride; Chlorpheniramine Tannate and Phenylephrine Tannate; Phenylephrine and Chlorpheniramine

Pharmacologic Category Alpha/Beta Agonist; Histamine H_1 Antagonist; Histamine H_1 Antagonist, First Generation

Use Temporary relief of upper respiratory conditions such as nasal congestion, runny nose, and sneezing due to the common cold, hay fever, or allergic or vasomotor rhinitis

Pregnancy Risk Factor C

Medication Safety Issues

Sound-alike/look-alike issues:
Rynatan® may be confused with Rynatuss®

Dosage Antihistamine/decongestant: Oral:

Children:
6-12 months: Rondec® drops: 0.75 mL 4 times/day
1-2 years: Rondec® drops: 1 mL 4 times/day
2-6 years:
AlleRx™: 1.25 -2.5 mL every 12 hours
Dallergy®-JR suspension: 2.5 mL every 12 hours
Rondec® syrup: 1.25 mL every 4-6 hours; maximum 7.5 mL/24 hours
Rynatan® suspension: 2.5 -5 mL every 12 hours
6-12 years:
AlleRx™: 2.5- 5 mL every 12 hours
Dallergy®-JR: One capsule every 12 hours; maximum 2 capsules/24 hours
Dallergy®-JR suspension: 5 mL every 12 hours
Ed A-Hist™: One-half caplet every 12 hours
Rondec® syrup: 2.5 mL every 4-6 hours; maximum 15 mL/24 hours
Rynatan® suspension: 5-10 mL every 12 hours
≥12 years: Refer to adult dosing.

Adults:
AlleRx™: 15 mL every 12 hours
Dallergy®-JR: Two capsules every 12 hours; maximum 4 capsules/24 hours
Dallergy®-JR suspension: 10 mL every 12 hours
Ed A-Hist™: One caplet every 12 hours
R-Tanna: 1-2 tablets every 12 hours
Rondec® syrup: 5 mL every 4-6 hours; maximum 30 mL/24 hours
Rynatan® tablet: 1-2 tablets every 12 hours

Additional Information Complete prescribing information for this medication should be consulted for additional detail.

Dosage Forms Excipient information presented when available (limited, particularly for generics); consult specific product labeling. [DSC] = Discontinued product

Caplet, prolonged release:
Ed A-Hist™, NoHist: Chlorpheniramine maleate 8 mg and phenylephrine hydrochloride 20 mg

Capsule, extended release:
Dallergy®-JR: Chlorpheniramine maleate 4 mg and phenylephrine hydrochloride 20 mg

Liquid:
Ed A-Hist™: Chlorpheniramine maleate 4 mg and phenylephrine hydrochloride 10 mg per 5 mL (480 mL) [sugar free; contains alcohol 5%; grape flavor]
Triaminic® Cold and Allergy: Chlorpheniramine maleate 1 mg and phenylephrine hydrochloride 2.5 mg per 5 mL (120 mL) [contains sodium 5 mg/5 mL and benzoic acid; orange flavor]

Liquid, oral [drops]:
Dallergy: Chlorpheniramine maleate 1 mg and phenylephrine hydrochloride 2 mg per 1 mL (30 mL) [alcohol free, sugar free; contains propylene glycol; peach flavor]

Solution, oral [drops]:
C-Phen, PD-Hist-D: Chlorpheniramine maleate 1 mg and phenylephrine hydrochloride 3.5 mg per mL (30 mL) [alcohol free, sugar free; bubblegum flavor]
Ceron: Chlorpheniramine maleate 1 mg and phenylephrine hydrochloride 3.5 mg per mL (30 mL) [raspberry flavor]
Dec-Chlorphen: Chlorpheniramine maleate 1 mg and phenylephrine hydrochloride 3.5 mg per mL (30 mL) [alcohol free, dye free, sugar free; grape flavor]
Rondec®: Chlorpheniramine maleate 1 mg and phenylephrine hydrochloride 3.5 mg per mL (30 mL) [alcohol free, sugar free; contains propylene glycol; bubble gum flavor] [DSC]
Sildec PE: Chlorpheniramine maleate 1 mg and phenylephrine hydrochloride 3.5 mg per 1 mL (30 mL) [alcohol free, sugar free; raspberry flavor] [DSC]

Suspension, oral: Chlorpheniramine tannate 4 mg and phenylephrine tannate 20 mg per 5 mL (473 mL)
AllanTan Pediatric: Chlorpheniramine tannate 4.5 mg and phenylephrine tannate 5 mg per 5 mL (473 mL) [contains sodium benzoate; strawberry flavor] [DSC]
AlleRx™: Chlorpheniramine tannate 3 mg and phenylephrine tannate 7.5 per 5 mL (480 mL) [contains benzoic acid; raspberry flavor]
Dallergy®-JR: Chlorpheniramine tannate 4 mg and phenylephrine tannate 20 mg per 5 mL (480 mL) [contains sodium benzoate; peaches and cream flavor]

P-Tann D, PediaTan™ D: Chlorpheniramine tannate 8 mg and phenylephrine tannate 10 mg per 5 mL (480 mL) [sugar free; contains sodium benzoate; bubblegum flavor]

R-Tanna Pediatric: Chlorpheniramine tannate 4.5 mg and phenylephrine tannate 5 mg per 5 mL (480 mL) [contains benzoic acid and tartrazine]

Rinate™ Pediatric: Chlorpheniramine tannate 4.5 mg and phenylephrine tannate 5 mg per 5 mL (120 mL, 480 mL) [contains sodium benzoate; blueberry flavor]

Rynatan® Pediatric: Chlorpheniramine tannate 4.5 mg and phenylephrine tannate 5 mg per 5 mL (480 mL) [contains benzoic acid and tartrazine; strawberry-currant flavor]

Tannate Pediatric: Chlorpheniramine tannate 4.5 mg and phenylephrine tannate 5 mg per 5 mL (480 mL) [contains sodium benzoate; raspberry flavor]

Suspension, oral [drops]:

Ed ChlorPed D: Chlorpheniramine tannate 2 mg and phenylephrine tannate 6 mg per 1 mL (60 mL) [apple sauce flavor]

Syrup:

C-Phen: Chlorpheniramine maleate 4 mg and phenylephrine hydrochloride 12. 5 mg per 5 mL (120 mL, 480 mL) [alcohol free, sugar free; contains sodium benzoate; bubble gum flavor]

Ceron, Sildec PE: Chlorpheniramine maleate 4 mg and phenylephrine hydrochloride 12. 5 mg per 5 mL (480 mL) [raspberry flavor]

PD-Hist-D: Chlorpheniramine maleate 4 mg and phenylephrine hydrochloride 12. 5 mg per 5 mL (480 mL) [alcohol free, sugar free; bubblegum flavor]

Rondec®: Chlorpheniramine maleate 4 mg and phenylephrine hydrochloride 12.5 mg per 5 mL (120 mL, 480 mL) [alcohol free, sugar free; contains propylene glycol; bubble gum flavor]

Tablet:

Actifed® Cold & Allergy, Sudafed PE® Sinus & Allergy: Chlorpheniramine maleate 4 mg and phenylephrine hydrochloride 10 mg

R-Tanna, Rynatan®: Chlorpheniramine tannate 9 mg and phenylephrine tannate 25 mg

Tablet, chewable:

Rynatan®: Chlorpheniramine tannate 4.5 mg and phenylephrine tannate 5 mg [grape flavor]

Tablet, sustained release:

Rescon-Jr®: Chlorpheniramine maleate 4 mg and phenylephrine hydrochloride 20 mg

Tablet, timed release:

Phenabid®: Chlorpheniramine maleate 8 mg and phenylephrine hydrochloride 20 mg [dye free, sugar free]

Chlorpheniramine and Pseudoephedrine

(klor fen IR a meen & soo doe e FED rin)

U.S. Brand Names Allerest® Maximum Strength Allergy and Hay Fever [OTC]; Deconamine® SR; Dicel™; Duratuss® DA; Dynahist-ER Pediatric® [DSC]; Histade™ [DSC]; Histex™; LoHist-D; QDALL® [DSC]; Suclor™; Sudafed® Sinus & Allergy [OTC]; SudaHist®; Sudal® 12

Canadian Brand Names Triaminic® Cold & Allergy

Index Terms Chlorpheniramine Maleate and Pseudoephedrine Hydrochloride; Chlorpheniramine Tannate and Pseudoephedrine Tannate; Pseudoephedrine and Chlorpheniramine

Pharmacologic Category Alpha/Beta Agonist; Histamine H_1 Antagonist; Histamine H_1 Antagonist, First Generation

Use Relief of nasal congestion associated with the common cold, hay fever, and other allergies, sinusitis, eustachian tube blockage, and vasomotor and allergic rhinitis

Pregnancy Risk Factor C

Medication Safety Issues

Sound-alike/look-alike issues:

Allerest® may be confused with Sinarest®

Chlor-Trimeton® may be confused with Chloromycetin®

Sudafed® may be confused with Sufenta®

Dosage General dosing guidelines; consult specific product labeling. Rhinitis/decongestant: Oral:

Children:

2-6 years:

Chlorpheniramine maleate 1 mg and pseudoephedrine hydrochloride 15 mg every 4-6 hours

Chlorpheniramine tannate 4.5 mg and pseudoephedrine tannate 75 mg: 2.5-5 mL every 12 hours (maximum: 10 mL/24 hours)

6-12 years: Chlorpheniramine maleate 2 mg and pseudoephedrine hydrochloride 30 mg every 4-6 hours (immediate release products)

Children ≥12 years and Adults:

Chlorpheniramine maleate 4 mg and pseudoephedrine hydrochloride 60 mg every 4-6 hours (immediate release products)

Chlorpheniramine tannate 4.5 mg and pseudoephedrine tannate 75 mg: 10-20 mL every 12 hours (maximum: 40 mL/24 hours)

Deconamine® SR: Chlorpheniramine maleate 8 mg and pseudoephedrine hydrochloride 120 mg every 12 hours

Additional Information Complete prescribing information for this medication should be consulted for additional detail.

Dosage Forms Excipient information presented when available (limited, particularly for generics); consult specific product labeling. [DSC] = Discontinued product

Capsule, extended release: Chlorpheniramine maleate 8 mg and pseudoephedrine hydrochloride 120 mg; chlorpheniramine maleate 12 mg and pseudoephedrine hydrochloride 100 mg

Duratuss® DA: Chlorpheniramine maleate 12 mg and pseudoephedrine hydrochloride 100 mg

Dynahist-ER Pediatric®: Chlorpheniramine maleate 4 mg and pseudoephedrine hydrochloride 60 mg [DSC]

Histade™: Chlorpheniramine maleate 12 mg and pseudoephedrine hydrochloride 120 mg [DSC]

QDALL®: Chlorpheniramine maleate 12 mg and pseudoephedrine hydrochloride 100 mg [DSC]

Suclor™: Chlorpheniramine maleate 8 mg and pseudoephedrine hydrochloride 120 mg

Capsule, sustained release: Chlorpheniramine maleate 8 mg and pseudoephedrine hydrochloride 120 mg

Deconamine® SR: Chlorpheniramine maleate 8 mg and pseudoephedrine hydrochloride 120 mg

Liquid:

Histex™: Chlorpheniramine maleate 2 mg and pseudoephedrine sulfate 30 mg per 5 mL (480 mL) [peach flavor]

LoHist-D: Chlorpheniramine maleate 2 mg and pseudoephedrine hydrochloride 30 mg per 5 mL (480 mL) [alcohol free, dye free; peach flavor]

Suspension:

Dicel™: Chlorpheniramine tannate 5 mg and pseudoephedrine tannate 75 mg per 5 mL (480 mL) [contains sodium benzoate; strawberry banana flavor]

Syrup: Chlorpheniramine maleate 2 mg and pseudoephedrine hydrochloride 30 mg per 5 mL (480 mL)

Tablet: Chlorpheniramine maleate 4 mg and pseudoephedrine hydrochloride 60 mg

Allerest® Maximum Strength Allergy and Hay Fever: Chlorpheniramine maleate 2 mg and pseudoephedrine hydrochloride 30 mg

Sudafed® Sinus & Allergy: Chlorpheniramine maleate 4 mg and pseudoephedrine hydrochloride 60 mg

Tablet, chewable:

Sudal® 12: Chlorpheniramine maleate 4 mg and pseudoephedrine hydrochloride 30 mg [contains phenylalanine 25 mg/tablet; grape flavor]

Tablet, sustained release:

SudaHist: Chlorpheniramine maleate 12 mg and pseudoephedrine hydrochloride 120 mg

- **Chlorpheniramine, Dextromethorphan, Phenylephrine, and Guaifenesin** *see* Dextromethorphan, Chlorpheniramine, Phenylephrine, and Guaifenesin *on page 434*

Chlorpheniramine, Ephedrine, Phenylephrine, and Carbetapentane

(klor fen IR a meen, e FED rin, fen il EF rin, & kar bay ta PEN tane)

U.S. Brand Names Quad Tann®; Quad Tann® Pediatric; Rynatuss®; Tetra Tannate Pediatric

Index Terms Carbetapentane, Ephedrine, Phenylephrine, and Chlorpheniramine; Ephedrine, Chlorpheniramine, Phenylephrine, and Carbetapentane; Phenylephrine, Ephedrine, Chlorpheniramine, and Carbetapentane

Pharmacologic Category Alpha/Beta Agonist; Antitussive; Histamine H_1 Antagonist; Histamine H_1 Antagonist, First Generation

Use Symptomatic relief of cough with a decongestant and an antihistamine

Pregnancy Risk Factor C

Medication Safety Issues

Sound-alike/look-alike issues:

Rynatuss® may be confused with Rynatan®

Dosage Oral:

Children:

<2 years: Titrate dose individually

2-6 years: 2.5-5 mL every 12 hours

>6 years: 5-10 mL every 12 hours

Adults: 1-2 tablets every 12 hours

Additional Information Complete prescribing information for this medication should be consulted for additional detail.

Dosage Forms Excipient information presented when available (limited, particularly for generics); consult specific product labeling.

Suspension:

Quad Tann® Pediatric: Chlorpheniramine tannate 4 mg, ephedrine tannate 5 mg, phenylephrine tannate 5 mg, and carbetapentane tannate 30 mg per 5 mL (480 mL) [contains sodium benzoate; grape flavor]

Tetra Tannate Pediatric: Chlorpheniramine tannate 4 mg, ephedrine tannate 5 mg, phenylephrine tannate 5 mg, and carbetapentane tannate 30 mg per 5 mL (240 mL, 480 mL) [alcohol free; strawberry flavor]

Tablet:

Rynatuss®: Chlorpheniramine tannage 5 mg, ephedrine tannate 10 mg, phenylephrine tannate 10 mg, and carbetapentane tannate 60 mg

Tablet, long acting:

Quad Tann®: Chlorpheniramine tannage 5 mg, ephedrine tannate 10 mg, phenylephrine tannate 10 mg, and carbetapentane tannate 60 mg

- **Chlorpheniramine Maleate and Dextromethorphan Hydrobromide** *see* Dextromethorphan and Chlorpheniramine *on page 433*
- **Chlorpheniramine Maleate and Hydrocodone Bitartrate** *see* Hydrocodone and Chlorpheniramine *on page 741*
- **Chlorpheniramine Maleate and Phenylephrine Hydrochloride** *see* Chlorpheniramine and Phenylephrine *on page 309*
- **Chlorpheniramine Maleate and Pseudoephedrine Hydrochloride** *see* Chlorpheniramine and Pseudoephedrine *on page 310*
- **Chlorpheniramine Maleate, Dihydrocodeine Bitartrate, and Phenylephrine Hydrochloride** *see* Dihydrocodeine, Chlorpheniramine, and Phenylephrine *on page 448*
- **Chlorpheniramine Maleate, Phenylephrine Hydrochloride, and Guaifenesin** *see* Chlorpheniramine, Phenylephrine, and Guaifenesin *on page 312*
- **Chlorpheniramine Maleate, Pseudoephedrine Hydrochloride, and Dextromethorphan Hydrobromide** *see* Chlorpheniramine, Pseudoephedrine, and Dextromethorphan *on page 315*

Chlorpheniramine, Phenylephrine, and Dextromethorphan

(klor fen IR a meen, fen il EF rin, & deks troe meth OR fan)

U.S. Brand Names C-Phen DM; Ceron-DM; Corfen DM; De-Chlor DM; De-Chlor DR; Dec-Chlorphen DM [DSC]; Dex PC; Donatussin DM [DSC]; Ed A-Hist DM; Father John's® Plus [OTC]; Mintuss DR; Neo DM; Norel DM™; PD-Cof; PE-Hist DM; Phenabid DM®; Poly Tussin DM; Robitussin® Cough and Allergy [OTC] [DSC]; Robitussin® Cough and Cold Nighttime [OTC]; Robitussin® Pediatric Cough and Cold Nighttime [OTC]; Rondec®-DM; Sildec PE-DM [DSC]; Statuss™ DM; Tri-Vent™ DPC [DSC]; Trital DM; Tussplex™ DM

Index Terms Dextromethorphan, Chlorpheniramine, and Phenylephrine; Phenylephrine, Chlorpheniramine, and Dextromethorphan

Pharmacologic Category Alpha/Beta Agonist; Antitussive; Histamine H_1 Antagonist; Histamine H_1 Antagonist, First Generation

Use Temporary relief of cough and upper respiratory symptoms associated with allergies or the common cold

Pregnancy Risk Factor C

Dosage Oral: Relief of cough and cold symptoms:

Children:

6-12 months (Rondec®-DM drops): 0.75 mL 4 times/day

1-2 years (Rondec®-DM drops): 1 mL 4 times/day

2-6 years:

Rondec®-DM syrup: 1.25 mL every 4-6 hours (maximum: 7.5 mL/24 hours)

Tri-Vent™ DPC: 2.5 mL every 6 hours (maximum: 10 mL/24 hours)

6-12 years:

Rondec®-DM syrup: 2.5 mL every 4-6 hours (maximum: 15 mL/24 hours)

Tri-Vent™ DPC: 5 mL every 6 hours (maximum: 20 mL/24 hours)

Children ≥12 years and Adults:

Rondec®-DM syrup: 5 mL every 4-6 hours (maximum: 30 mL/24 hours)

Tri-Vent™ DPC: 10 mL every 6 hours (maximum: 40 mL/24 hours)

Additional Information Complete prescribing information for this medication should be consulted for additional detail.

Dosage Forms Excipient information presented when available (limited, particularly for generics); consult specific product labeling. [DSC] = Discontinued product

Liquid:

Corfen DM: Chlorpheniramine maleate 4 mg, phenylephrine hydrochloride 10 mg, and dextromethorphan hydrobromide 15 mg per 5 mL (480 mL) [grape flavor]

De-Chlor DM: Chlorpheniramine maleate 2 mg, phenylephrine hydrochloride 10 mg, and dextromethorphan hydrobromide 15 mg per 5 mL (480 mL) [strawberry flavor]

De-Chlor DR: Chlorpheniramine maleate 2 mg, phenylephrine hydrochloride 6 mg, and dextromethorphan hydrobromide 15 mg per 5 mL (480 mL) [strawberry flavor]

Father John's® Plus: Chlorpheniramine maleate 2 mg, phenylephrine hydrochloride 5 mg, and dextromethorphan hydrobromide 5 mg per 15 mL (118 mL) [alcohol free]

Norel DM™: Chlorpheniramine maleate 4 mg, phenylephrine hydrochloride 10 mg, and dextromethorphan hydrobromide 15 mg per 5 mL (480 mL) [alcohol free, dye free, sugar free; contains propylene glycol; grape flavor]

Trital DM: Chlorpheniramine maleate 4 mg, phenylephrine hydrochloride 10 mg, and dextromethorphan hydrobromide 15 mg per 5 mL (480 mL) [alcohol free, dye free, sugar free; contains sodium benzoate; grape flavor]

Liquid, oral [drops]:

Ceron DM: Chorpheniramine maleate 1 mg, phenylephrine hydrochloride 3.5 mg, and dextromethorphan hydrobromide 3 mg per 1 mL (30 mL) [alcohol free, sugar free; contains sodium benzoate; grape flavor] [DSC]

C-Phen DM: Chlorpheniramine maleate 1 mg, phenylephrine hydrochloride 3.5 mg, and dextromethorphan hydrobromide 3 mg per 1 mL (30 mL) [grape flavor]

Donatussin DM: Chlorpheniramine maleate 1 mg, phenylephrine hydrochloride 1.5 mg, and dextromethorphan hydrobromide 3 mg per 1 mL (30 mL) [alcohol free, sugar free; contains propylene glycol; bubblegum flavor] [DSC]

Neo DM: Chlorpheniramine maleate 0.75 mg, phenylephrine hydrochloride 1.75 mg, and dextromethorphan hydrobromide 2.75 mg per 1 mL (30 mL) [alcohol free, sugar free; contains propylene glycol; black cherry flavor]

PD-Cof: Chlorpheniramine maleate 1 mg, phenylephrine hydrochloride 3.5 mg, and dextromethorphan hydrobromide 3 mg per 1 mL (30 mL) [alcohol free, sugar free; grape flavor]

Rondec® DM, Sildec PE-DM [DSC]: Chlorpheniramine maleate 1 mg, phenylephrine hydrochloride 3.5 mg, and dextromethorphan hydrobromide 3 mg per 1 mL (30 mL) [alcohol free, sugar free; grape flavor]

Suspension:

Donatussin DM: Dexchlorpheniramine tannate 2 mg, phenylephrine tannate 20 mg, and dextromethorphan tannate 30 mg per 5 mL (480 mL) [alcohol free, sugar free; contains phenylalanine 7 mg/5 mL, propylene glycol; cotton candy strawberry flavor] [DSC]

Syrup:

Ceron-DM: Chlorpheniramine maleate 4 mg, phenylephrine hydrochloride 12.5 mg, and dextromethorphan hydrobromide 15 mg per 5 mL (480 mL) [alcohol free, sugar free; contains sodium benzoate; grape flavor]

C-Phen DM: Chlorpheniramine maleate 4 mg, phenylephrine hydrochloride 12.5 mg, and dextromethorphan hydrobromide 15 mg per 5 mL (120 mL, 480 mL) [grape flavor]

Dec-Chlorphen DM: Chlorpheniramine maleate 4 mg, phenylephrine hydrochloride 12.5 mg, and dextromethorphan hydrobromide 15 mg per 5 mL (120 mL, 480 mL) [alcohol free, dye free, sugar free; grape flavor] [DSC]

Dex PC: Chlorpheniramine maleate 2 mg, phenylephrine hydrochloride 6 mg, and dextromethorphan hydrobromide 15 mg per 5 mL (480 mL) [strawberry flavor]

Ed A-Hist DM: Chlorpheniramine maleate 4 mg, phenylephrine hydrochloride 10 mg, and dextromethorphan hydrobromide 15 mg per 5 mL (480 mL) [alcohol free, sugar free; contains propylene glycol; banana flavor]

Mintuss DR: Chlorpheniramine maleate 2 mg, phenylephrine hydrochloride 6 mg, and dextromethorphan hydrobromide 15 mg per 5 mL (480 mL) [alcohol free; strawberry flavor]

PD-Cof: Chlorpheniramine maleate 4 mg, phenylephrine hydrochloride 12.5 mg, and dextromethorphan hydrobromide 15 mg per 5 mL (480 mL) [alcohol free, sugar free; grape flavor]

PE-Hist DM: Chlorpheniramine maleate 2 mg, phenylephrine hydrochloride 5 mg, and dextromethorphan hydrobromide 15 mg per 5 mL (480 mL) [strawberry flavor]

Poly Tussin DM: Chlorpheniramine maleate 2 mg, phenylephrine hydrochloride 5 mg, and dextromethorphan hydrobromide 15 mg per 5 mL (480 mL) [alcohol free, sugar free]

Robitussion® Cough and Allergy: Chlorpheniramine maleate 2 mg, phenylephrine hydrochloride 5 mg, and dextromethorphan hydrobromide 10 mg per 5 mL (120 mL) [alcohol free; contains sodium 3 mg/5 mL, sodium benzoate, and propylene glycol] [DSC]

Robitussin® Cough and Cold Nighttime: Chlorpheniramine maleate 1 mg, phenylephrine hydrochloride 2.5 mg, and dextromethorphan hydrobromide 5 mg per 5 mL (120 mL) [alcohol free; contains sodium 3 mg/5 mL, sodium benzoate, and propylene glycol]

Robitussin® Pediatric Cough and Cold Nighttime: Chlorpheniramine maleate 1 mg, phenylephrine hydrochloride 2.5 mg, and dextromethorphan hydrobromide 5 mg per 5 mL (120 mL) [alcohol free; contains sodium 3 mg/5 mL, sodium benzoate, and propylene glycol; fruit punch flavor]

Rondec®-DM: Chlorpheniramine maleate 4 mg, phenylephrine hydrochloride 12.5 mg, and dextromethorphan hydrobromide 15 mg per 5 mL (120 mL, 480 mL) [alcohol free, sugar free; contains propylene glycol; grape flavor]

Sildec PE-DM: Chlorpheniramine maleate 4 mg, phenylephrine hydrochloride 12.5 mg, and dextromethorphan hydrobromide 15 mg per 5 mL (480 mL) [grape flavor]

Statuss™: DM: Chlorpheniramine maleate 2 mg, phenylephrine hydrochloride 10 mg, and dextromethorphan hydrobromide 15 mg per 5 mL (480 mL) [alcohol free, sugar free; raspberry flavor]

Tri-Vent™ DPC: Chlorpheniramine maleate 2 mg, phenylephrine hydrochloride 6 mg, and dextromethorphan hydrobromide 15 mg per 5 mL (480 mL) [alcohol free; contains sodium benzoate, propylene glycol; strawberry flavor] [DSC]

Tussplex™ DM: Chlorpheniramine maleate 2 mg, phenylephrine hydrochloride 5 mg, and dextromethorphan hydrobromide 15 mg per 5 mL (480 mL) [alcohol free, sugar free; contains sodium benzoate; strawberry flavor]

Tablet, timed release:

Phenabid DM®: Chlorpheniramine maleate 8 mg, phenylephrine hydrochloride 20 mg, and dextromethorphan hydrobromide 30 mg [scored; dye free, sugar free]

Chlorpheniramine, Phenylephrine, and Guaifenesin

(klor fen IR a meen, fen il EF rin, & gwye FEN e sin)

U.S. Brand Names P Chlor GG

Index Terms Chlorpheniramine Maleate, Phenylephrine Hydrochloride, and Guaifenesin; Chlorpheniramine Tannate, Phenylephrine Tannate, and Guaifenesin; Guaifenesin, Phenylephrine, and Chlorpheniramine; Phenylephrine, Chlorpheniramine, and Guaifenesin

Pharmacologic Category Alpha/Beta Agonist; Expectorant; Histamine H_1 Antagonist; Histamine H_1 Antagonist, First Generation

Use Symptomatic relief of upper respiratory symptoms associated with infections such as the common cold or allergies

Pregnancy Risk Factor C

Dosage General dosing guidelines; consult specific product labeling.

Antihistamine/decongestant/expectorant: Oral:

Children <3 months: 2-3 drops per month of age every 4-6 hours as needed; not to exceed 4 doses/24 hours

Children 3-6 months: 0.3-0.6 mL every 4-6 hours as needed; not to exceed 4 doses/24 hours

Children 6 months to 1 year: 0.6-1 mL every 4-6 hours as needed; not to exceed 4 doses/24 hours

Children 1-2 years: 1-2 mL every 4-6 hours as needed; not to exceed 4 doses/24 hours

Additional Information Complete prescribing information for this medication should be consulted for additional detail.

Dosage Forms Excipient information presented when available (limited, particularly for generics); consult specific product labeling.

Liquid:

P Chlor GG [drops]: Chlorpheniramine maleate 1 mg, phenylephrine hydrochloride 2 mg, and guaifenesin 20 mg per 1 mL (30 mL) [peach flavor]

Chlorpheniramine, Phenylephrine, and Methscopolamine

(klor fen IR a meen, fen il EF rin, & meth skoe POL a meen)

U.S. Brand Names aerohist plus™; aeroKid™; AH-Chew®; AH-Chew™ Ultra; Chlor-Mes; Chlor-Mes-D; Dallergy®; Dehistine; Duradryl®; Durahist™ PE; Extendryl®; Extendryl® JR; Extendryl® SR; Hista-Vent® DA [DSC]; Histatab PH; OMNIhist® II L.A.; PCM; PCM Allergy [DSC]; Phenylephrine CM; Ralix; Rescon®; Rescon® MX; Triall™

Index Terms Methscopolamine Nitrate, Chlorpheniramine Maleate, and Phenylephrine Hydrochloride; Phenylephrine Tannate, Chlorpheniramine Tannate, and Methscopolamine Nitrate

Pharmacologic Category Alpha/Beta Agonist; Anticholinergic Agent; Histamine H_1 Antagonist; Histamine H_1 Antagonist, First Generation

Use Treatment of upper respiratory symptoms such as respiratory congestion, allergic rhinitis, vasomotor rhinitis, sinusitis, and allergic skin reactions of urticaria and angioedema

Pregnancy Risk Factor C

Dosage

Children 6-11 years: Relief of respiratory symptoms: Oral:

aeroKid™: 2.5-5 mL every 4 hours

Ah-Chew® suspension: 2.5-5 mL every 12 hours

Dallergy®, Durahist™ PE, OMNIhist® II L.A., Rescon® MX: One-half caplet/tablet every 12 hours

Duradryl® syrup, Extendryl® syrup: 2.5-5 mL, may repeat up to every 4 hours depending on age and body weight

Extendryl® chewable tablet: One tablet every 4 hours; do not exceed 4 doses in 24 hours

Extendryl® JR: One tablet every 12 hours

Children ≥12 years and Adults: Relief of respiratory symptoms: Oral: **Note:** If disturbances in urination occur in patients without renal impairment, medication should be discontinued for 1-2 days and should then be restarted at a lower dose

aeroKid™: 5-10 mL every 3-4 hours

Ah-Chew® suspension: 5-10 mL every 12 hours

Dallergy®, Durahist™ PE, Extendryl® SR, OMNIhist® II L.A., Rescon® MX: One capsule/tablet every 12 hours

Duradryl® syrup, Extendryl® syrup: 5-10 mL every 3-4 hours (4 times/day)

Extendryl®: 1-2 chewable tablets every 4 hours

Elderly: Use with caution, may have increased adverse reactions

Dosage adjustment in renal impairment: Use is not recommended

Additional Information Complete prescribing information for this medication should be consulted for additional detail.

Dosage Forms Excipient information presented when available (limited, particularly for generics); consult specific product labeling. [DSC] = Discontinued product

Caplet, extended release:

aerohist plus™: Chlorpheniramine maleate 8 mg, phenylephrine hydrochloride 20 mg, and methscopolamine nitrate 2.5 mg

Chlor-Mes: Chlorpheniramine maleate 12 mg, phenylephrine hydrochloride 20 mg, and methscopolamine nitrate 2.5 mg [dye free, sugar free]

Dallergy®: Chlorpheniramine maleate 12 mg, phenylephrine hydrochloride 20 mg, and methscopolamine nitrate 2.5 mg [scored]

Liquid:

Chlor-Mes-D: Chlorpheniramine maleate 2 mg, phenylephrine hydrochloride 10 mg, and methscopolamine nitrate 0.625 mg per 5 mL (480 mL) [grape flavor]

Suspension:

AH-Chew®: Chlorpheniramine tannate [equivalent to chlorpheniramine maleate 2 mg], phenylephrine tannate [equivalent to phenylephrine hydrochloride 10 mg], and methscopalamine nitrate 1.5 mg per 5 mL (120 mL) [grape flavor]

Syrup:

aeroKid™: Chlorpheniramine maleate 4 mg, phenylephrine hydrochloride 10 mg, and methscopolamine nitrate 1.25 mg per 5 mL (120 mL, 480 mL) [contains propylene glycol; blue raspberry flavor]

Dallergy: Chlorpheniramine maleate 2 mg, phenylephrine hydrochloride 8 mg, and methscopolamine nitrate 0.75 mg per 5 mL (480 mL) [contains propylene glycol; grape flavor]

Dehistine: Chlorpheniramine maleate 2 mg, phenylephrine hydrochloride 10 mg, and methscopolamine nitrate 1.25 mg per 5 mL (480 mL) [root beer flavor]

Duradryl®: Chlorpheniramine maleate 2 mg, phenylephrine hydrochloride 10 mg, and methscopolamine nitrate 1.25 mg per 5 mL (480 mL) [contains sodium benzoate; cherry flavor]

Extendryl®: Dexchlorpheniramine maleate 1 mg, phenylephrine hydrochloride 10 mg, and methscopolamine nitrate 1.25 mg per 5 mL (480 mL) [root beer flavor]

Triall™: Chlorpheniramine maleate 2 mg, phenylephrine hydrochloride 8 mg, and methscopolamine nitrate 0.75 mg per 5 mL (473 mL) [contains sodium benzoate; alcohol free; grape flavor]

Tablet [scored]:

Dallergy®: Chlorpheniramine maleate 4 mg, phenylephrine hydrochloride 10 mg, and methscopolamine nitrate 1.25 mg

Tablet, chewable:

AH-Chew™ Ultra: Chlorpheniramine tannate [equivalent to chlorpheniramine maleate 2 mg], phenylephrine tanneate [equivalent to phenylephrine hydrochloride 10 mg], and methscopolamine nitrate 1.5 mg [scored; grape flavor]

Extendryl: Chlorpheniramine maleate 2 mg, phenylephrine hydrochloride 10 mg, and methscopolamine nitrate 1.25 mg [root beer flavor]

PCM: Chlorpheniramine maleate 2 mg, phenylephrine hydrochloride 10 mg, and methscopolamine nitrate 1.25 mg [grape flavor]

Tablet, extended release: Chlorpheniramine maleate 8 mg, phenylephrine hydrochloride 20 mg, and methscopolamine nitrate 1.25 mg

Durahist™ PE: Chlorpheniramine maleate 8 mg, phenylephrine hydrochloride 20 mg, and methscopolamine nitrate 1.25 mg [scored]

Extendryl SR: Chlorpheniramine maleate 8 mg, phenylephrine hydrochloride 20 mg, and methscopolamine nitrate 2.5 mg [scored]
Extendryl® JR: Chlorpheniramine maleate 4 mg, phenylephrine hydrochloride 10 mg, and methscopolamine nitrate 1.25 mg [scored]
Hista-Vent® DA: Chlorpheniramine maleate 8 mg, phenylephrine hydrochloride 20 mg, and methscopolamine nitrate 2.5 mg [scored] [DSC]
PCM Allergy: Chlorpheniramine maleate 12 mg, phenylephrine hydrochloride 20 mg, and methscopolamine nitrate 2.5 mg [DSC]

Tablet, long acting [scored]:
OMNIhist® II L.A.: Chlorpheniramine maleate 8 mg, phenylephrine hydrochloride 25 mg, and methscopolamine nitrate 2.5 mg
Rescon® MX: Chlorpheniramine maleate 8 mg, phenylephrine hydrochloride 40 mg, and methscopolamine nitrate 2.5 mg

Tablet, sustained release:
Histatab PH: Chlorpheniramine maleate 8 mg, phenylephrine hydrochloride 20 mg, and methscopolamine nitrate 1.25 mg
Ralix: Chlorpheniramine maleate 8 mg, phenylephrine hydrochloride 40 mg, and methscopolamine nitrate 2 mg

Tablet, timed release:
Phenylephrine CM: Chlorpheniramine maleate 8 mg, phenylephrine hydrochloride 40 mg, and methscopolamine nitrate 2.5 mg

Tablet, variable release:
Rescon®: Chlorpheniramine maleate 12 mg and phenylephrine hydrochloride 40 mg [sustained release] and methscopolamine nitrate 2 mg [immediate release] [MaxRelent release]

Chlorpheniramine, Phenylephrine, and Phenyltoloxamine

(klor fen IR a meen, fen il EF rin, & fen il tole LOKS a meen)

U.S. Brand Names Chlorex-A; Comhist® [DSC]; Nalex®-A; NoHist-A; Rhinacon A

Index Terms Phenylephrine, Chlorpheniramine, and Phenyltoloxamine; Phenyltoloxamine, Chlorpheniramine, and Phenylephrine

Pharmacologic Category Alpha/Beta Agonist; Histamine H_1 Antagonist; Histamine H_1 Antagonist, First Generation

Use Symptomatic relief of rhinitis and nasal congestion due to colds or allergy

Pregnancy Risk Factor C

Dosage Oral:

Children:
2-6 years: Nalex®-A liquid: 1.25-2.5 mL every 4-6 hours
6-12 years:
Nalex®-A liquid: 5 mL every 4-6 hours
Nalex®-A tablet: 1/2 tablet 2-3 times/day

Children >12 years and Adults:
Nalex®-A liquid: 10 mL every 4-6 hours
Nalex®-A tablet: 1 tablet 2-3 times/day

Additional Information Complete prescribing information for this medication should be consulted for additional detail.

Dosage Forms Excipient information presented when available (limited, particularly for generics); consult specific product labeling. [DSC] = Discontinued product

Liquid: Chlorpheniramine maleate 2.5 mg, phenylephrine hydrochloride 5 mg, and phenyltoloxamine citrate 7.5 mg per 5 mL (480 mL)
Nalex®-A, NoHist-A, Rhinacon A: Chlorpheniramine maleate 2.5 mg, phenylephrine hydrochloride 5 mg, and phenyltoloxamine citrate 7.5 mg per 5 mL (480 mL) [alcohol free, sugar free; cotton candy flavor]

Tablet:
Comhist®: Chlorpheniramine maleate 2 mg, phenylephrine hydrochloride 10 mg, and phenyltoloxamine citrate 25 mg [DSC]

Tablet, extended release:
Rhinacon A: Chlorpheniramine maleate 4 mg, phenylephrine hydrochloride 20 mg, and phenyltoloxamine citrate 40 mg

Tablet, prolonged release:
Nalex®-A: Chlorpheniramine maleate 4 mg, phenylephrine hydrochloride 20 mg, and phenyltoloxamine citrate 40 mg

Tablet, sustained release:
Chlorex-A: Chlorpheniramine maleate 4 mg, phenylephrine hydrochloride 20 mg, and phenyltoloxamine citrate 40 mg

Chlorpheniramine, Phenylephrine, Codeine, and Potassium Iodide

(klor fen IR a meen, fen il EF rin, KOE deen, & poe TASS ee um EYE oh dide)

U.S. Brand Names Pediacof® [DSC]

Index Terms Codeine, Chlorpheniramine, Phenylephrine, and Potassium Iodide; Phenylephrine, Chlorpheniramine, Codeine, and Potassium Iodide; Potassium Iodide, Chlorpheniramine, Phenylephrine, and Codeine

Pharmacologic Category Alpha/Beta Agonist; Analgesic, Opioid; Antitussive; Expectorant; Histamine H_1 Antagonist; Histamine H_1 Antagonist, First Generation

Use Symptomatic relief of rhinitis, nasal congestion and cough due to colds or allergy

Restrictions C-V

Dosage Children 6 months to 12 years: 1.25-10 mL every 4-6 hours

Additional Information Complete prescribing information for this medication should be consulted for additional detail.

Dosage Forms Excipient information presented when available (limited, particularly for generics); consult specific product labeling.

Syrup: Chlorpheniramine maleate 0.75 mg, phenylephrine hydrochloride 2.5 mg, codeine phosphate 5 mg, and potassium iodide 75 mg per 5 mL (480 mL) [contains alcohol 5% and sodium benzoate; raspberry flavor] [DSC]

◆ **Chlorpheniramine, Pseudoephedrine, and Acetaminophen** *see* Acetaminophen, Chlorpheniramine, and Pseudoephedrine *on page 31*

Chlorpheniramine, Pseudoephedrine, and Codeine

(klor fen IR a meen, soo doe e FED rin, & KOE deen)

U.S. Brand Names Dihistine® DH [DSC]

Index Terms Codeine, Chlorpheniramine, and Pseudoephedrine; Pseudoephedrine, Chlorpheniramine, and Codeine

Pharmacologic Category Alpha/Beta Agonist; Analgesic, Opioid; Antitussive; Histamine H_1 Antagonist; Histamine H_1 Antagonist, First Generation

Use Temporary relief of cough associated with minor throat or bronchial irritation or nasal congestion due to common cold, allergic rhinitis, or sinusitis

Restrictions C-V

Pregnancy Risk Factor C

Dosage Oral:

Children:
25-50 lb: 1.25-2.5 mL every 4-6 hours, up to 4 doses in 24-hour period

50-90 lb: 2.5-5 mL every 4-6 hours, up to 4 doses in 24-hour period

Adults: 10 mL every 4-6 hours, up to 4 doses in 24-hour period

Additional Information Complete prescribing information for this medication should be consulted for additional detail.

Dosage Forms Excipient information presented when available (limited, particularly for generics); consult specific product labeling. [DSC] = Discontinued product

Elixir:

Dihistine® DH: Chlorpheniramine maleate 2 mg, pseudoephedrine hydrochloride 30 mg, and codeine phosphate 10 mg per 5 mL (120 mL, 480 mL) [contains alcohol; grape flavor] [DSC]

Chlorpheniramine, Pseudoephedrine, and Dextromethorphan

(klor fen IR a meen, soo doe e FED rin, & deks troe meth OR fan)

U.S. Brand Names Dicel™ DM; DuraTan™ Forte; Kidkare Children's Cough and Cold [OTC]; Pedia Relief™ [OTC]; Rescon DM [OTC]; Tanafed DMX™; Tannate PD-DM

Index Terms Chlorpheniramine Maleate, Pseudoephedrine Hydrochloride, and Dextromethorphan Hydrobromide; Chlorpheniramine Tannate, Pseudoephedrine Tannate, and Dextromethorphan Tannate; Dexchlorpheniramine Tannate, Pseudoephedrine Tannate, and Dextromethorphan Tannate; Dextromethorphan, Chlorpheniramine, and Pseudoephedrine; Pseudoephedrine, Chlorpheniramine, and Dextromethorphan

Pharmacologic Category Alpha/Beta Agonist; Antitussive; Histamine H_1 Antagonist; Histamine H_1 Antagonist, First Generation

Use Temporarily relieves nasal congestion, runny nose, cough, and sneezing due to the common cold, hay fever, or allergic rhinitis

Pregnancy Risk Factor C

Dosage General dosing guidelines; consult specific product labeling. Relief of cold symptoms: Oral:

Children:

2-6 years:

Dexchlorpheniramine tannate 2.5 mg, pseudoephedrine tannate 75 mg, and dextromethorphan tannate 25 mg (Tanafed DMX™): 2.5-5 mL every 12 hours (maximum: 10 mL/24 hours)

Dexchlorpheniramine tannate 3.5 mg, pseudoephedrine tannate 45 mg, and dextromethorphan tannate 30 mg (DuraTan™ Forte): 1.25-2.5 mL every 12 hours (maximum: 5 mL/24 hours)

6-12 years:

Chlorpheniramine maleate 1 mg, pseudoephedrine 15 mg, and dextromethorphan hydrobromide 7.5 mg per 5 mL: 10 mL every 6 hours

Chlorpheniramine maleate 1 mg, pseudoephedrine 15 mg, and dextromethorphan hydrobromide 5 mg per tablet or 5 mL: 2 tablets or 10 mL every 4-6 hours (maximum: 4 doses/24 hours)

Chlorpheniramine maleate 2 mg, pseudoephedrine 30 mg, and dextromethorphan hydrobromide 10 mg per tablet or 5 mL (Rescon DM): 5 mL every 4-6 hours (maximum: 4 doses/24 hours)

Dexchlorpheniramine tannate 2.5 mg, pseudoephedrine tannate 75 mg, and dextromethorphan tannate 25 mg (Tanafed DMX™): 5-10 mL every 12 hours (maximum: 20 mL/24 hours)

Dexchlorpheniramine tannate 3.5 mg, pseudoephedrine tannate 45 mg, and dextromethorphan tannate 30 mg (DuraTan™ Forte): 2.5-5 mL every 12 hours (maximum: 10 mL/24 hours)

>12 years: Refer to adult dosing

Adults:

Chlorpheniramine maleate 1 mg, pseudoephedrine 15 mg, and dextromethorphan hydrobromide 7.5 mg per 5 mL: 20 mL every 6 hours

Chlorpheniramine maleate 2 mg, pseudoephedrine 30 mg, and dextromethorphan hydrobromide 10 mg per tablet or 5 mL (Rescon DM): 10 mL every 4-6 hours (maximum: 4 doses/24 hours)

Dexchlorpheniramine tannate 2.5 mg, pseudoephedrine tannate 75 mg, and dextromethorphan tannate 25 mg (Tanafed DMX™): 10-20 mL every 12 hours (maximum: 40 mL/24 hours)

Dexchlorpheniramine tannate 3.5 mg, pseudoephedrine tannate 45 mg, and dextromethorphan tannate 30 mg (DuraTan™ Forte): 5-15 mL every 12 hours (maximum: 30 mL/24 hours)

Additional Information Complete prescribing information for this medication should be consulted for additional detail.

Dosage Forms Excipient information presented when available (limited, particularly for generics); consult specific product labeling. [DSC] = Discontinued product

Liquid: Chlorpheniramine maleate 1 mg, pseudoephedrine hydrochloride 15 mg, and dextromethorphan hydrobromide 5 mg per 5 mL (120 mL)

Kidkare Children's Cough and Cold: Chlorpheniramine maleate 1 mg, pseudoephedrine hydrochloride 15 mg, and dextromethorphan hydrobromide 5 mg per 5 mL (120 mL) [alcohol free; contains propylene glycol and sodium benzoate; cherry flavor]

Pedia Relief™: Chlorpheniramine maleate 1 mg, pseudoephedrine hydrochloride 15 mg, and dextromethorphan hydrobromide 5 mg per 5 mL (120 mL) [alcohol free; contains propylene glycol and sodium benzoate; cherry flavor]

Rescon DM: Chlorpheniramine maleate 2 mg, pseudoephedrine hydrochloride 30 mg, and dextromethorphan hydrobromide 10 mg per 5 mL (120 mL, 480 mL) [dye free; contains propylene glycol; cherry flavor]

Suspension:

Dicel™ DM: Chlorpheniramine tannate 5 mg, pseudoephedrine tannate 75 mg, and dextromethorphan tannate 25 mg per 5 mL (480 mL) [contains sodium benzoate; cotton candy flavor]

DuraTan™ Forte: Dexchlorpheniramine tannate 3.5 mg, pseudoephedrine tannate 45 mg, and dextromethorphan tannate 30 mg per 5 mL (480 mL) [contains sodium benzoate; grape flavor]

Tanafed DMX™: Dexchlorpheniramine tannate 2.5 mg, pseudoephedrine tannate 75 mg, and dextromethorphan tannate 25 mg (120 mL, 480 mL) [contains sodium benzoate; cotton candy flavor]

Tannate PD-DM: Dexchlorpheniramine tannate 3 mg, pseudoephedrine tannate 50 mg, and dextromethorphan tannate 27.5 mg per 5 mL (473 mL) [contains sodium benzoate; grape flavor]

Chlorpheniramine, Pyrilamine, and Phenylephrine

(klor fen IR a meen, pye RIL a meen, & fen il EF rin)

U.S. Brand Names AllerTan™; Chlor-Tan A 12 [DSC]; Chlorex-A 12 [DSC]; Conal; MyHist-PD; Nalex A 12; Poly Hist Forte®; Poly Hist PD; Ru-Hist Forte; Tri-Hist; Triplex™ AD

Pharmacologic Category Alpha/Beta Agonist; Histamine H_1 Antagonist; Histamine H_1 Antagonist, First Generation

Use Symptomatic relief of rhinitis and nasal congestion due to colds or allergy

Pregnancy Risk Factor C

Dosage Oral:

Tablet (Ru-Hist Forte, Poly Hist Forte®):

Children <6 years: Dosage not established.

Children 6-12 years: 1/2 tablet 2-3 times/day
Children >12 years and Adults: 1 tablet 2-3 times/day
Liquid (MyHist-PD, Poly Hist PD):
Children 2-6 years: 2.5 mL every 4-6 hours (maximum: 10 mL/day)
Children 6-12 years: 5 mL every 4-6 hours (maximum: 20 mL/day)
Children >12 years and Adults: 5-10 mL every 4-6 hours (maximum: 40 mL/day)
Liquid (Triplex™ AD):
Children <6 years: Dosage not established
Children 6-12 years: 5 mL every 4-6 hours (maximum: 20 mL/day)
Children >12 and Adults: 5-10 mL every 4-6 hours (maximum: 40 mL/day)
Suspension (AllerTan™, Conal):
Children 2-6 years: 2.5 mL every 12 hours (maximum: 5 mL/day)
Children 6-12 years: 5 mL every 12 hours (maximum: 10 mL/day)
Children >12 years and Adults: 5-10 mL every 12 hours (maximum: 20 mL/day)

Additional Information Complete prescribing information for this medication should be consulted for additional detail.

Dosage Forms Excipient information presented when available (limited, particularly for generics); consult specific product labeling.
Liquid, oral:
MyHist-PD: Chlorpheniramine maleate 2 mg, pyrilamine maleate 12.5 mg, and phenylephrine hydrochloride 7.5 mg per 5 mL (473 mL) [dye free, ethanol free, sugar free; bubblegum flavor]
Poly Hist PD: Chlorpheniramine maleate 2 mg, pyrilamine maleate 12.5 mg, and phenylephrine hydrochloride 7.5 mg per 5 mL (480 mL) [dye free, ethanol free, sugar free; contains propylene glycol; bubblegum flavor]
Triplex™ AD: Chlorpheniramine maleate 2 mg, pyrilamine maleate 12.5 mg, and phenylephrine hydrochloride 7.5 mg per 5 mL (473 mL) [dye free, ethanol free, sugar free; contains sodium benzoate; bubblegum flavor]
Suspension, oral:
AllerTan™: Chlorpheniramine maleate 8 mg, pyrilamine maleate 12.5 mg, and phenylephrine hydrochloride 15 mg per 5 mL (473 mL) [contains sodium benzoate; grape flavor]
Chlor-Tan A 12: Chlorpheniramine maleate 2 mg, pyrilamine maleate 12.5 mg, and phenylephrine hydrochloride 5 mg per 5 mL (118 mL) [ethanol free, sugar free; raspberry flavor] [DSC]
Chlorex-A 12: Chlorpheniramine maleate 2 mg, pyrilamine maleate 12.5 mg, and phenylephrine hydrochloride 5 mg per 5 mL (120 mL) [raspberry flavor] [DSC]
Conal: Chlorpheniramine maleate 8 mg, pyrilamine maleate 12.5 mg, and phenylephrine hydrochloride 15 mg per 5 mL (473 mL) [contains phenylalanine 7 mg/5 mL, propylene glycol; raspberry flavor]
Nalex A 12: Chlorpheniramine tannate 2 mg, pyrilamine tannate 12.5 mg, and phenylephrine tannate 5 mg per 5 mL (120 mL) [contains benzoic acid; raspberry flavor]
Tri-Hist: Chlorpheniramine maleate 2 mg, pyrilamine maleate 12.5 mg, and phenylephrine hydrochloride 5 mg per 5 mL (120 mL)
Tablet, sustained release, oral:
Poly Hist Forte®: Chlorpheniramine maleate 4 mg, pyrilamine maleate 25 mg, and phenylephrine hydrochloride 10 mg
Tablet, time-released, oral: Chlorpheniramine maleate 4 mg, pyrilamine maleate 25 mg, and phenylephrine hydrochloride 10 mg
Ru-Hist Forte: Chlorpheniramine maleate 4 mg, pyrilamine maleate 25 mg, and phenylephrine hydrochloride 10 mg

◆ **Chlorpheniramine Tannate and Phenylephrine Tannate** *see* Chlorpheniramine and Phenylephrine *on page 309*

◆ **Chlorpheniramine Tannate and Pseudoephedrine Tannate** *see* Chlorpheniramine and Pseudoephedrine *on page 310*

◆ **Chlorpheniramine Tannate, Phenylephrine Tannate, and Guaifenesin** *see* Chlorpheniramine, Phenylephrine, and Guaifenesin *on page 312*

◆ **Chlorpheniramine Tannate, Pseudoephedrine Tannate, and Dextromethorphan Tannate** *see* Chlorpheniramine, Pseudoephedrine, and Dextromethorphan *on page 315*

ChlorproMAZINE (klor PROE ma zeen)

Canadian Brand Names Largactil®; Novo-Chlorpromazine

Index Terms Chlorpromazine Hydrochloride; CPZ

Pharmacologic Category Antimanic Agent; Antipsychotic Agent, Typical, Phenothiazine

Additional Appendix Information
Antipsychotic Agents *on page 1644*

Use Control of mania; treatment of schizophrenia; control of nausea and vomiting; relief of restlessness and apprehension before surgery; acute intermittent porphyria; adjunct in the treatment of tetanus; intractable hiccups; combativeness and/or explosive hyperexcitable behavior in children 1-12 years of age and in short-term treatment of hyperactive children

Unlabeled/Investigational Use Management of psychotic disorders; behavioral symptoms associated with dementia (elderly); psychosis/agitation related to Alzheimer's dementia

Pregnancy Risk Factor C

Lactation Enters breast milk/not recommended (AAP rates "of concern")

Medication Safety Issues
Sound-alike/look-alike issues:
ChlorproMAZINE may be confused with chlordiazePOXIDE, chlorproPAMIDE, clomiPRAMINE, prochlorperazine, promethazine
Thorazine® may be confused with thiamine, thioridazine

Contraindications Hypersensitivity to chlorpromazine or any component of the formulation (cross-reactivity between phenothiazines may occur); severe CNS depression; coma

Warnings/Precautions Highly sedating, use with caution in disorders where CNS depression is a feature and in patients with Parkinson's disease. Use with caution in patients with hemodynamic instability, bone marrow suppression, predisposition to seizures, subcortical brain damage, severe cardiac, hepatic, renal, or respiratory disease. Esophageal dysmotility and aspiration have been associated with antipsychotic use; use with caution in patients at risk of aspiration pneumonia (ie, Alzheimer's disease). Caution in breast cancer or other prolactin-dependent tumors (may elevate prolactin levels). May alter temperature regulation or mask toxicity of other drugs due to antiemetic effects. May alter cardiac conduction; life-threatening arrhythmias have occurred with therapeutic doses of neuroleptics.

Elderly patients with dementia-related psychosis treated with antipsychotics are at an increased risk of death compared to placebo. An increased incidence of cerebrovascular adverse events (including fatalities) has been reported in elderly patients with dementia-related psychosis. Chlorpromazine is not approved for this indication. Use with caution in patients at risk of hypotension (orthostasis is common) or those who would tolerate transient hypotensive episodes (cerebrovascular disease, cardiovascular disease, or other medications which may predispose). Significant hypotension may occur, particularly with parenteral administration. Injection contains sulfites.

Use with caution in patients with decreased gastrointestinal motility, urinary retention, BPH, xerostomia, or visual problems (ie, narrow-angle glaucoma - screening is recommended) and myasthenia gravis. Relative to other neuroleptics, chlorpromazine has a moderate potency of cholinergic blockade.

May cause extrapyramidal symptoms (EPS), including pseudoparkinsonism, acute dystonic reactions, akathisia, and tardive dyskinesia (risk of these reactions is low-moderate relative to other neuroleptics). Risk of dystonia (and possibly other EPS) may be greater with increased doses, use of conventional antipsychotics, males, and younger patients. May cause neuroleptic malignant syndrome (NMS) or pigmentary retinopathy.

Adverse Reactions Frequency not defined.

Cardiovascular: Postural hypotension, tachycardia, dizziness, nonspecific QT changes

Central nervous system: Drowsiness, dystonias, akathisia, pseudoparkinsonism, tardive dyskinesia, neuroleptic malignant syndrome, seizure

Dermatologic: Photosensitivity, dermatitis, skin pigmentation (slate gray)

Endocrine & metabolic: Lactation, breast engorgement, false-positive pregnancy test, amenorrhea, gynecomastia, hyper- or hypoglycemia

Gastrointestinal: Xerostomia, constipation, nausea

Genitourinary: Urinary retention, ejaculatory disorder, impotence

Hematologic: Agranulocytosis, eosinophilia, leukopenia, hemolytic anemia, aplastic anemia, thrombocytopenic purpura

Hepatic: Jaundice

Ocular: Blurred vision, corneal and lenticular changes, epithelial keratopathy, pigmentary retinopathy

Drug Interactions

Metabolism/Transport Effects **Substrate** of CYP1A2 (minor), 2D6 (major), 3A4 (minor); **Inhibits** CYP2D6 (strong), 2E1 (weak)

Avoid Concomitant Use

Avoid concomitant use of ChlorproMAZINE with any of the following: Nilotinib; Tamoxifen; Thioridazine; Ziprasidone

Increased Effect/Toxicity

ChlorproMAZINE may increase the levels/effects of: Alcohol (Ethyl); Analgesics (Opioid); Anticholinergics; Beta-Blockers; CNS Depressants; CYP2D6 Substrates; Desmopressin; Fesoterodine; Haloperidol; QTc-Prolonging Agents; Tamoxifen; Thioridazine; Valproic Acid; Ziprasidone

The levels/effects of ChlorproMAZINE may be increased by: Acetylcholinesterase Inhibitors (Central); Alfuzosin; Antimalarial Agents; Beta-Blockers; Ciprofloxacin; CYP2D6 Inhibitors (Moderate); CYP2D6 Inhibitors (Strong); Darunavir; Gadobutrol; Haloperidol; Lithium formulations; Nilotinib; Pramlintide; Tetrabenazine

Decreased Effect

ChlorproMAZINE may decrease the levels/effects of: Amphetamines; Anti-Parkinson's Agents (Dopamine Agonist); TraMADol

The levels/effects of ChlorproMAZINE may be decreased by: Antacids; Lithium formulations

Ethanol/Nutrition/Herb Interactions

Ethanol: Avoid ethanol (may increase CNS depression).

Herb/Nutraceutical: Avoid St John's wort (may decrease chlorpromazine levels, increase photosensitization, or enhance sedative effect). Avoid dong quai (may enhance photosensitization). Avoid kava kava, gotu kola, valerian (may increase CNS depression).

Stability Injection: Protect from light. A slightly yellowed solution does not indicate potency loss, but a markedly discolored solution should be discarded. Diluted injection (1 mg/mL) with NS and stored in 5 mL vials remains stable for 30 days.

Mechanism of Action Chlorpromazine is an aliphatic phenothiazine antipsychotic which blocks postsynaptic mesolimbic dopaminergic receptors in the brain; exhibits a strong alpha-adrenergic blocking effect and depresses the release of hypothalamic and hypophyseal hormones; believed to depress the reticular activating system, thus affecting basal metabolism, body temperature, wakefulness, vasomotor tone, and emesis

Pharmacodynamics/Kinetics

Onset of action: I.M.: 15 minutes; Oral: 30-60 minutes

Absorption: Rapid

Distribution: V_d: 20 L/kg; crosses the placenta; enters breast milk

Protein binding: 92% to 97%

Metabolism: Extensively hepatic to active and inactive metabolites

Bioavailability: 20%

Half-life, biphasic: Initial: 2 hours; Terminal: 30 hours

Excretion: Urine (<1% as unchanged drug) within 24 hours

Dosage

Children ≥6 months:

Schizophrenia/psychoses:

Oral: 0.5-1 mg/kg/dose every 4-6 hours; older children may require 200 mg/day or higher

I.M., I.V.: 0.5-1 mg/kg/dose every 6-8 hours

<5 years (22.7 kg): Maximum: 40 mg/day

5-12 years (22.7-45.5 kg): Maximum: 75 mg/day

Nausea and vomiting:

Oral: 0.5-1 mg/kg/dose every 4-6 hours as needed

I.M., I.V.: 0.5-1 mg/kg/dose every 6-8 hours

<5 years (22.7 kg): Maximum: 40 mg/day

5-12 years (22.7-45.5 kg): Maximum: 75 mg/day

Adults:

Schizophrenia/psychoses:

Oral: Range: 30-2000 mg/day in 1-4 divided doses, initiate at lower doses and titrate as needed; usual dose: 400-600 mg/day; some patients may require 1-2 g/day

I.M., I.V.: Initial: 25 mg, may repeat (25-50 mg) in 1-4 hours, gradually increase to a maximum of 400 mg/dose every 4-6 hours until patient is controlled; usual dose: 300-800 mg/day

Intractable hiccups: Oral, I.M.: 25-50 mg 3-4 times/day

Nausea and vomiting:

Oral: 10-25 mg every 4-6 hours

I.M., I.V.: 25-50 mg every 4-6 hours

Elderly: Behavioral symptoms associated with dementia (unlabeled use): Initial: 10-25 mg 1-2 times/day; increase at 4- to 7-day intervals by 10-25 mg/day. Increase dose intervals (bid, tid, etc) as necessary to control behavior response or side effects; maximum daily dose: 800 mg; gradual increases (titration) may prevent some side effects or decrease their severity.

Dosing comments in renal impairment: Hemodialysis: Not dialyzable (0% to 5%)

Dosing adjustment/comments in hepatic impairment: Avoid use in severe hepatic dysfunction

Administration Note: Avoid skin contact with oral solution or injection solution; may cause contact dermatitis.

I.V.: Direct or intermittent infusion: Infuse 1 mg or portion thereof over 1 minute.

Monitoring Parameters Vital signs; lipid profile, fasting blood glucose/Hgb A_{1c}; BMI; mental status; abnormal involuntary movement scale (AIMS); extrapyramidal symptoms (EPS)

Reference Range

Therapeutic: 50-300 ng/mL (SI: 157-942 nmol/L)

Toxic: >750 ng/mL (SI: >2355 nmol/L); serum concentrations poorly correlate with expected response

Test Interactions False-positives for phenylketonuria, amylase, uroporphyrins, urobilinogen. May cause false-positive pregnancy test.

Dosage Forms Excipient information presented when available (limited, particularly for generics); consult specific product labeling.

Injection, solution, as hydrochloride: 25 mg/mL (1 mL, 2 mL)

Tablet, as hydrochloride: 10 mg, 25 mg, 50 mg, 100 mg, 200 mg

◆ **Chlorpromazine Hydrochloride** *see* ChlorproMAZINE *on page 316*

ChlorproPAMIDE (klor PROE pa mide)

U.S. Brand Names Diabinese® [DSC]

Canadian Brand Names Apo-Chlorpropamide®; Novo-Propamide

Pharmacologic Category Antidiabetic Agent, Sulfonylurea

Additional Appendix Information

Diabetes Mellitus Management, Adults *on page 1801*

Sulfonamide Derivatives *on page 1671*

Use Management of blood sugar in type 2 diabetes mellitus (noninsulin dependent, NIDDM)

Unlabeled/Investigational Use Neurogenic diabetes insipidus

Pregnancy Risk Factor C

Medication Safety Issues

Sound-alike/look-alike issues:

ChlorproPAMIDE may be confused with chlorproMAZINE

Diabinese® may be confused with DiaBeta®, Dialume®, Diamox®

High alert medication: The Institute for Safe Medication Practices (ISMP) includes this medication among its list of drugs which have a heightened risk of causing significant patient harm when used in error.

Dosage Oral: The dosage of chlorpropamide is variable and should be individualized based upon the patient's response

Initial dose:

Adults: 250 mg/day in mild-to-moderate diabetes in middle-aged, stable diabetic

Elderly: 100-125 mg/day in older patients

Subsequent dosages may be increased or decreased by 50-125 mg/day at 3- to 5-day intervals

Maintenance dose: 100-250 mg/day; severe diabetics may require 500 mg/day; avoid doses >750 mg/day

Dosing adjustment/comments in renal impairment: Cl_{cr} <50 mL/minute: Avoid use

Hemodialysis: Removed with hemoperfusion

Peritoneal dialysis: Supplemental dose is not necessary

Dosing adjustment in hepatic impairment: Dosage reduction is recommended. Conservative initial and maintenance doses are recommended in patients with liver impairment because chlorpropamide undergoes extensive hepatic metabolism.

Additional Information Complete prescribing information for this medication should be consulted for additional detail.

Dosage Forms Excipient information presented when available (limited, particularly for generics); consult specific product labeling. [DSC] = Discontinued product

Tablet: 100 mg, 250 mg

Diabinese®: 100 mg, 250 mg [DSC]

◆ **Chlor-Tan A 12 [DSC]** *see* Chlorpheniramine, Pyrilamine, and Phenylephrine *on page 315*

Chlorthalidone (klor THAL i done)

U.S. Brand Names Thalitone®

Canadian Brand Names Apo-Chlorthalidone®

Index Terms Hygroton

Pharmacologic Category Diuretic, Thiazide

Additional Appendix Information

Sulfonamide Derivatives *on page 1671*

Use Management of mild-to-moderate hypertension when used alone or in combination with other agents; treatment of edema associated with congestive heart failure or nephrotic syndrome. Recent studies have found chlorthalidone effective in the treatment of isolated systolic hypertension in the elderly.

Unlabeled/Investigational Use Pediatric hypertension

Pregnancy Risk Factor B (manufacturer); D (expert analysis)

Dosage Oral:

Children (nonapproved): 2 mg/kg/dose 3 times/week or 1-2 mg/kg/day

Hypertension (unlabeled use): Initial: 0.3 mg/kg once daily, up to 2 mg/kg/day; maximum: 50 mg/day

Adults:

Hypertension: 25-100 mg/day or 100 mg 3 times/week; usual dosage range (JNC 7): 12.5-25 mg/day

Edema: Initial: 50-100 mg/day or 100 mg on alternate days; maximum dose: 200 mg/day

Heart failure-associated edema: 12.5-25 mg once daily; maximum daily dose: 100 mg (ACC/AHA 2005 Heart Failure Guidelines)

Elderly: Initial: 12.5-25 mg/day or every other day; there is little advantage to using doses >25 mg/day

Dosage adjustment in renal impairment: Cl_{cr} <10 mL/minute: Avoid use. Ineffective with low GFR (Aronoff G, 2002)

Note: ACC/AHA 2005 Heart Failure Guidelines suggest that thiazides lose their efficacy when Cl_{cr} <40 mL/minute

Additional Information Complete prescribing information for this medication should be consulted for additional detail.

Dosage Forms Excipient information presented when available (limited, particularly for generics); consult specific product labeling.

Tablet: 25 mg, 50 mg, 100 mg

Thalitone®: 15 mg

◆ **Chlorthalidone and Atenolol** *see* Atenolol and Chlorthalidone *on page 150*

◆ **Chlorthalidone and Clonidine** *see* Clonidine and Chlorthalidone *on page 356*

◆ **Chlor-Tripolon ND® (Can)** *see* Loratadine and Pseudoephedrine *on page 905*

Chlorzoxazone (klor ZOKS a zone)

U.S. Brand Names Parafon Forte® DSC

Canadian Brand Names Parafon Forte®; Strifon Forte®

Pharmacologic Category Skeletal Muscle Relaxant

Use Symptomatic treatment of muscle spasm and pain associated with acute musculoskeletal conditions

Pregnancy Risk Factor C

Medication Safety Issues

Sound-alike/look-alike issues:

Parafon Forte® may be confused with Fam-Pren Forte

Dosage Oral:

Children: 20 mg/kg/day or 600 mg/m²/day in 3-4 divided doses

Adults: 250-500 mg 3-4 times/day up to 750 mg 3-4 times/day

Additional Information Complete prescribing information for this medication should be consulted for additional detail.

Dosage Forms Excipient information presented when available (limited, particularly for generics); consult specific product labeling.

Caplet (Parafon Forte® DSC): 500 mg

Tablet: 250 mg, 500 mg

◆ **Cholecalciferol and Alendronate** *see* Alendronate and Cholecalciferol *on page 60*

Cholestyramine Resin (koe LES teer a meen REZ in)

U.S. Brand Names Prevalite®; Questran®; Questran® Light

Canadian Brand Names Novo-Cholamine; Novo-Cholamine Light; PMS-Cholestyramine; Questran®; Questran® Light Sugar Free

Pharmacologic Category Antilipemic Agent, Bile Acid Sequestrant

Additional Appendix Information

Hyperlipidemia Management *on page 1815*

Lipid-Lowering Agents *on page 1661*

Use Adjunct in the management of primary hypercholesterolemia; pruritus associated with elevated levels of bile acids; diarrhea associated with excess fecal bile acids; binding toxicologic agents; pseudomembraneous colitis

Pregnancy Risk Factor C

Dosage Oral (dosages are expressed in terms of anhydrous resin):

Children: 240 mg/kg/day in 3 divided doses; need to titrate dose depending on indication

Adults: 4 g 1-2 times/day to a maximum of 24 g/day and 6 doses/day

Dialysis: Not removed by hemo- or peritoneal dialysis; supplemental doses not necessary with dialysis or continuous arteriovenous or venovenous hemofiltration

Additional Information Complete prescribing information for this medication should be consulted for additional detail.

Dosage Forms Excipient information presented when available (limited, particularly for generics); consult specific product labeling.

Powder for oral suspension: Cholestyramine resin 4 g/5 g packet (60s); cholestyramine resin 4 g/5 g of powder (210 g); cholestyramine resin 4 g/5.7 g packet (60s); cholestyramine resin 4 g/5.7 g of powder (240 g can); cholestyramine resin 4 g/9 g packet (60s); cholestyramine resin 4 g of resin/9 g of powder (378 g)

Prevalite®: Cholestyramine resin 4 g/5.5 g packet (42s, 60s) [contains phenylalanine 14.1 mg/5.5 g; orange flavor]; cholestyramine resin 4 g/5.5 g of powder (231 g) [contains phenylalanine 14.1 mg/5.5 g; orange flavor]

Questran®: Cholestyramine resin 4 g/9 g packet (60s); cholestyramine resin 4 g/9 g of powder (378 g)

Questran® Light: Cholestyramine resin 4 g/5 g packet (60s) [contains phenylalanine 14 mg/5 g]; cholestyramine resin 4 g/5 g of powder (210 g) [contains phenylalanine 14 mg/5 g]

◆ **Choline Fenofibrate** *see* Fenofibric Acid *on page 609*

Choline Magnesium Trisalicylate

(KOE leen mag NEE zhum trye sa LIS i late)

Index Terms Tricosal

Pharmacologic Category Salicylate

Use Management of osteoarthritis, rheumatoid arthritis, and other arthritis; acute painful shoulder

Pregnancy Risk Factor C/D (3rd trimester)

Pregnancy Considerations Animal reproduction studies have not been conducted. Due to the known effects of other salicylates (closure of ductus arteriosus), use during late pregnancy should be avoided.

Lactation Enters breast milk/use caution

Contraindications Hypersensitivity to salicylates, other nonacetylated salicylates, other NSAIDs, or any component of the formulation; bleeding disorders; pregnancy (3rd trimester)

Warnings/Precautions Salicylate salts may not inhibit platelet aggregation and, therefore, should not be substituted for aspirin in the prophylaxis of thrombosis. Use with caution in patients with impaired hepatic or renal function, dehydration, erosive gastritis, asthma, or peptic ulcer. Children and teenagers who have or are recovering from chickenpox or flu-like symptoms should not use this product. Changes in behavior (along with nausea and vomiting) may be an early sign of Reye's syndrome; patients should be instructed to contact their healthcare provider if these occur.

Elderly are a high-risk population for adverse effects from NSAIDs. As many as 60% of elderly can develop peptic ulceration and/or hemorrhage asymptomatically. Use lowest effective dose for shortest period possible. Tinnitus or impaired hearing may indicate toxicity. Tinnitus may be a difficult and unreliable indication of toxicity due to age-related hearing loss or eighth cranial nerve damage. CNS adverse effects may be observed in the elderly at lower doses than younger adults.

Adverse Reactions

<20%:

Gastrointestinal: Nausea, vomiting, diarrhea, heartburn, dyspepsia, epigastric pain, constipation

Otic: Tinnitus

<2%:

Central nervous system: Headache, lightheadedness, dizziness, drowsiness, lethargy

Otic: Hearing impairment

<1%: Anorexia, asthma, BUN and creatinine increased, bruising, confusion, duodenal ulceration, dysgeusia, edema, epistaxis, erythema multiforme, esophagitis, hallucinations, hearing loss (irreversible), hepatic enzymes increased, gastric ulceration, occult bleeding, pruritus, rash, weight gain

Drug Interactions

Avoid Concomitant Use There are no known interactions where it is recommended to avoid concomitant use.

Increased Effect/Toxicity

Choline Magnesium Trisalicylate may increase the levels/effects of: Anticoagulants; Carbonic Anhydrase Inhibitors; Corticosteroids (Systemic); Drotrecogin Alfa; Methotrexate; Salicylates; Sulfonylureas; Thrombolytic Agents; Valproic Acid; Varicella Virus-Containing Vaccines; Vitamin K Antagonists

The levels/effects of Choline Magnesium Trisalicylate may be increased by: Antiplatelet Agents; Calcium Channel Blockers (Nondihydropyridine); Ginkgo Biloba; Herbs (Anticoagulant/Antiplatelet Properties); Treprostinil

Decreased Effect

Choline Magnesium Trisalicylate may decrease the levels/effects of: ACE Inhibitors; Uricosuric Agents

The levels/effects of Choline Magnesium Trisalicylate may be decreased by: Corticosteroids (Systemic)

Ethanol/Nutrition/Herb Interactions

Ethanol: Avoid ethanol (may enhance gastric mucosal irritation).

Food: May decrease the rate but not the extent of oral absorption.

Herb/Nutraceutical: Avoid cat's claw, dong quai, evening primrose, feverfew, garlic, ginger, ginkgo, red clover, horse chestnut, green tea, ginseng (all have additional antiplatelet activity). Limit curry powder, paprika, licorice, Benedictine liqueur, prunes, raisins, tea, and gherkins; may cause salicylate accumulation. These foods contain 6 mg salicylate/100 g.

Stability Store at controlled room temperature of 15°C to 30°C (59°F to 86°F).

Mechanism of Action Weakly inhibits cyclooxygenase enzymes, which result in decreased formation of prostaglandin precursors; antipyretic, analgesic, and anti-inflammatory properties.

Pharmacodynamics/Kinetics

Onset of action: Peak effect: ~2 hours

Absorption: Stomach and small intestines

Distribution: Readily into most body fluids and tissues; crosses placenta; enters breast milk

Half-life elimination (dose dependent): Low dose: 2-3 hours; High dose: 30 hours

Time to peak, serum: ~2 hours

Dosage Oral (based on total salicylate content):

Children <37 kg: 50 mg/kg/day given in 2 divided doses; 2250 mg/day for heavier children

Adults: 500 mg to 1.5 g 2-3 times/day **or** 3 g at bedtime; usual maintenance dose: 1-4.5 g/day

Elderly: 750 mg 3 times/day

Dosing adjustment/comments in renal impairment: Avoid use in severe renal impairment

Dietary Considerations Take with food or large volume of water or milk to minimize GI upset. Liquid may be mixed with fruit juice just before drinking. Hypermagnesemia resulting from magnesium salicylate; avoid or use with caution in renal insufficiency.

Administration Liquid may be mixed with fruit juice just before drinking. Do not administer with antacids. Take with a full glass of water and remain in an upright position for 15-30 minutes after administration.

Monitoring Parameters Serum magnesium with high dose therapy or in patients with impaired renal function; serum salicylate levels, renal function, hearing changes or tinnitus, abnormal bruising, weight gain and response (ie, pain)

Reference Range Salicylate blood levels for anti-inflammatory effect: 150-300 mcg/mL; analgesia and antipyretic effect: 30-50 mcg/mL

Test Interactions False-negative results for glucose oxidase urinary glucose tests (Clinistix®); false-positives using the cupric sulfate method (Clinitest®); also, interferes with Gerhardt test (urinary ketone analysis), VMA determination; 5-HIAA, xylose tolerance test, and T_3 and T_4; increased PBI

Dosage Forms Excipient information presented when available (limited, particularly for generics); consult specific product labeling.

Liquid: 500 mg/5 mL (240 mL) [choline salicylate 293 mg and magnesium salicylate 362 mg per 5 mL; cherry cordial flavor]

Tablet: 500 mg [choline salicylate 293 mg and magnesium salicylate 362 mg]; 750 mg [choline salicylate 440 mg and magnesium salicylate 544 mg]; 1000 mg [choline salicylate 587 mg and magnesium salicylate 725 mg]

◆ **Chondroitin Sulfate and Sodium Hyaluronate** *see* Sodium Chondroitin Sulfate and Sodium Hyaluronate *on page 1383*

◆ **Chooz® [OTC]** *see* Calcium Carbonate *on page 238*

◆ **Choriogonadotropin Alfa** *see* Chorionic Gonadotropin (Recombinant) *on page 321*

Chorionic Gonadotropin (Human)

(kor ee ON ik goe NAD oh troe pin, HYU man)

U.S. Brand Names Novarel®; Pregnyl®

Canadian Brand Names Humegon®; Pregnyl®; Profasi® HP

Index Terms CG; hCG

Pharmacologic Category Gonadotropin; Ovulation Stimulator

Use Induces ovulation and pregnancy in anovulatory, infertile females; treatment of hypogonadotropic hypogonadism, prepubertal cryptorchidism; spermatogenesis induction with follitropin alfa

Pregnancy Risk Factor X

Pregnancy Considerations Teratogenic effects (forelimb, CNS) have been noted in animal studies at doses intended to induce superovulation (used in combination with gonadotropin). Testicular tumors in otherwise healthy men have been reported when treating secondary infertility.

Lactation Excretion in breast milk unknown/use caution

Contraindications Hypersensitivity to chorionic gonadotropin or any component of the formulation; precocious puberty; prostatic carcinoma or similar neoplasms; pregnancy

Warnings/Precautions Use with caution in asthma, seizure disorders, migraine, cardiac or renal disease. **Not** effective in the treatment of obesity. Safety and efficacy in children <4 years of age have not been established.

Cryptorchidism: May induce precocious puberty in children being treated for cryptorchidism; discontinue if signs of precocious puberty occur.

Ovulation induction: These medications should only be used by physicians who are thoroughly familiar with infertility problems and their management. May cause ovarian hyperstimulation syndrome (OHSS); characterized by severe ovarian enlargement, abdominal pain/distention, nausea, vomiting, diarrhea, dyspnea, and oliguria, and may be accompanied by ascites, pleural effusion, hypovolemia, electrolyte imbalance, hemoperitoneum, and thromboembolic events. If severe hyperstimulation occurs, stop treatment and hospitalize patient. This syndrome develops rapidly with 24 hours to several days and generally occurs during the 7-10 days immediately following treatment. Ovarian enlargement ay be accompanied by abdominal distention or abdominal pain and generally regresses without treatment within 2-3 weeks. If ovaries are abnormally enlarged on the last day of treatment, withhold hCG to reduce the risk of OHSS. In association with and separate from OHSS, thromboembolic events have been reported. May result from the use of these medications; advise patients of the potential risk of multiple births before starting the treatment.

Adverse Reactions Frequency not defined.

Cardiovascular: Edema

Central nervous system: Depression, fatigue, headache, irritability, restlessness

Endocrine & metabolic: Gynecomastia, precocious puberty

Local: Injection site reaction

Miscellaneous: Hypersensitivity reaction (local or systemic)

Drug Interactions

Avoid Concomitant Use There are no known interactions where it is recommended to avoid concomitant use.

Increased Effect/Toxicity There are no known significant interactions involving an increase in effect.

Decreased Effect There are no known significant interactions involving a decrease in effect.

Stability Following reconstitution with the provided diluent, solutions are stable for 30-60 days, depending on the specific preparation, when stored at 2°C to 15°C.

Mechanism of Action Luteinizing hormone obtained from the urine of pregnant women. Stimulates production of gonadal steroid hormones by causing production of androgen by the testes; as a substitute for luteinizing hormone (LH) to stimulate ovulation

Pharmacodynamics/Kinetics
Half-life elimination: Biphasic: Initial: 11 hours; Terminal: 23 hours
Excretion: Urine

Dosage I.M.:
Children: Various regimens:
Prepubertal cryptorchidism:
4000 units 3 times/week for 3 weeks **or**
5000 units every second day for 4 injections **or**
500 units 3 times/week for 4-6 weeks **or**
15 injections of 500-1000 units given over 6 weeks

Hypogonadotropic hypogonadism: Males:
500-1000 units 3 times/week for 3 weeks, followed by the same dose twice weekly for 3 weeks **or**
4000 units 3 times/week for 6-9 months, then reduce dosage to 2000 units 3 times/week for additional 3 months

Adults:
Induction of ovulation: Females: 5000-10,000 units one day following last dose of menotropins
Spermatogenesis induction associated with hypogonadotropic hypogonadism: Males: Treatment regimens vary (range: 1000-2000 units 2-3 times a week). Administer hCG until serum testosterone levels are normal (may require 2-3 months of therapy), then may add follitropin alfa or menopausal gonadotropin if needed to induce spermatogenesis; continue hCG at the dose required to maintain testosterone levels.

Administration I.M. administration only

Monitoring Parameters
Male: Serum testosterone levels, semen analysis
Female: Ultrasound and/or estradiol levels to assess follicle development; ultrasound to assess number and size of follicles; ovulation (basal body temperature, serum progestin level, menstruation, sonography)

Reference Range Depends on application and methodology; <3 mIU/mL (SI: <3 units/L) usually normal (nonpregnant)

Dosage Forms Excipient information presented when available (limited, particularly for generics); consult specific product labeling.
Injection, powder for reconstitution: 10,000 units [packaged with diluent; diluent contains benzyl alcohol and mannitol]
Novarel®: 10,000 units [packaged with diluent; diluent contains benzyl alcohol and mannitol]
Pregnyl®: 10,000 units [packaged with diluent; diluent contains benzyl alcohol]

Chorionic Gonadotropin (Recombinant)
(kor ee ON ik goe NAD oh troe pin ree KOM be nant)

U.S. Brand Names Ovidrel®
Canadian Brand Names Ovidrel®
Index Terms Choriogonadotropin Alfa; r-hCG
Pharmacologic Category Gonadotropin; Ovulation Stimulator
Use As part of an assisted reproductive technology (ART) program, induces ovulation in infertile females who have been pretreated with follicle stimulating hormones (FSH); induces ovulation and pregnancy in infertile females when the cause of infertility is functional
Pregnancy Risk Factor X
Pregnancy Considerations Intrauterine death and impaired birth were observed in animal studies. Ectopic pregnancy, premature labor, postpartum fever, and spontaneous abortion have been reported in clinical trials. Congenital abnormalities have also been observed, however, the incidence is similar during natural conception.

Lactation Excretion in breast milk unknown/use caution

Contraindications Hypersensitivity to hCG preparations or any component of the formulation; primary ovarian failure; uncontrolled thyroid or adrenal dysfunction; uncontrolled organic intracranial lesion (ie, pituitary tumor); abnormal uterine bleeding, ovarian cyst or enlargement of undetermined origin; sex hormone dependent tumors; pregnancy

Warnings/Precautions Ovarian enlargement may occur; may be accompanied by abdominal distention or abdominal pain and generally regresses without treatment within 2-3 weeks. If ovaries are abnormally enlarged on the last day of treatment, withhold hCG to reduce the risk of ovarian hyperstimulation syndrome (OHSS). OHSS is characterized by severe ovarian enlargement, abdominal pain/distention, nausea, vomiting, diarrhea, dyspnea, and oliguria, and may be accompanied by ascites, pleural effusion, hypovolemia, electrolyte imbalance, hemoperitoneum, and thromboembolic events. If severe hyperstimulation occurs, stop treatment and hospitalize patient. This syndrome develops rapidly with 24 hours to several days and generally occurs during the 7-10 days immediately following treatment.

Arterial thromboembolic events have been reported in association with and separate from OHSS. These medications should only be used by healthcare providers who are thoroughly familiar with infertility problems and their management. Multiple births may result from the use of these medications; advise patients of the potential risk of multiple births before starting the treatment. Safety and efficacy have not been established in the elderly or in children.

Adverse Reactions
2% to 10%:
Endocrine & metabolic: Ovarian cyst (3%), ovarian hyperstimulation (<2% to 3%)
Gastrointestinal: Abdominal pain (3% to 4%), nausea (3%), vomiting (3%)
Local: Injection site: Pain (8%), bruising (3% to 5%), reaction (<2% to 3%), inflammation (<2% to 2%)
Miscellaneous: Postoperative pain (5%)
<2% (Limited to important or life-threatening): Abdominal enlargement, albuminuria, allergic reaction, back pain, breast pain, cardiac arrhythmia, cervical carcinoma, cervical lesion, cough, diarrhea, dizziness, dysuria, ectopic pregnancy, emotional lability, fever, flatulence, genital herpes, genital moniliasis, headache, heart murmur, hiccups, hot flashes, hyperglycemia, insomnia, intermenstrual bleeding, leukocytosis, leukorrhea, malaise, paresthesia, pharyngitis, pruritus, rash, upper respiratory tract infection, urinary incontinence, urinary tract infection, vaginal discomfort, vaginal hemorrhage, vaginitis
In addition, the following have been reported with menotropin therapy: Adnexal torsion, hemoperitoneum, mild-to-moderate ovarian enlargement, pulmonary and vascular complications. Ovarian neoplasms have also been reported (rare) with multiple drug regimens used for ovarian induction (relationship not established).

Drug Interactions
Avoid Concomitant Use There are no known interactions where it is recommended to avoid concomitant use.
Increased Effect/Toxicity There are no known significant interactions involving an increase in effect.
Decreased Effect There are no known significant interactions involving a decrease in effect.

Stability Prefilled syringe: Prior to dispensing, store at 2°C to 8°C (36°F to 46°F). Patient may store at 25°C (77°F) for up to 30 days. Protect from light.

Mechanism of Action Luteinizing hormone analogue produced by recombinant DNA techniques; stimulates late follicular maturation and intitates rupture of the ovarian follicle once follicular development has occurred

Pharmacodynamics/Kinetics

Distribution: V_d: 21.4L

Bioavailability: 40%

Half-life elimination: Initial: 4 hours; Terminal: 29 hours

Time to peak: 12-24 hours

Excretion: Urine (10% of dose)

Dosage SubQ:

Adults: Female:

Assisted reproductive technologies (ART) and ovulation induction: 250 mcg given 1 day following the last dose of follicle stimulating agent. Use only after adequate follicular development has been determined. Hold treatment when there is an excessive ovarian response.

Elderly: Safety and efficacy have not been established

Dosage adjustment in renal impairment: Safety and efficacy have not been established

Dosage adjustment in hepatic impairment: Safety and efficacy have not been established

Administration For SubQ use only; inject into stomach area.

Monitoring Parameters Ultrasound and/or estradiol levels to assess follicle development; ultrasound to assess number and size of follicles; ovulation (basal body temperature, serum progestin level, menstruation, sonography)

Test Interactions May interfere with interpretation of pregnancy tests; may cross-react with radioimmunoassay of luteinizing hormone and other gonadotropins

Additional Information Clinical studies have shown r-hCG to be clinically and statistically equivalent to urinary-derived hCG products.

Dosage Forms Excipient information presented when available (limited, particularly for generics); consult specific product labeling.

Injection, solution:

Ovidrel®: 257.5 mcg/0.515 mL (0.515 mL) [prefilled syringe; delivers 250 mcg r-hCG/0.5 mL]

◆ **Chronovera® (Can)** *see* Verapamil *on page 1557*

◆ **CI-1008** *see* Pregabalin *on page 1234*

◆ **Cialis®** *see* Tadalafil *on page 1422*

Ciclesonide (sye KLES oh nide)

U.S. Brand Names Alvesco®; Omnaris™

Canadian Brand Names Alvesco®; Omnaris™

Pharmacologic Category Corticosteroid, Inhalant (Oral); Corticosteroid, Nasal

Use

Intranasal: Management of seasonal and perennial allergic rhinitis

Oral inhalation: Prophylactic management of bronchial asthma

Pregnancy Risk Factor C

Pregnancy Considerations Teratogenic effects were reported in some, but not all animal studies. There are no adequate and well-controlled studies in pregnant women. The extent of intranasal absorption of ciclesonide systemically is low but variable; use during pregnancy with caution. Hypoadrenalism may occur in infants born to mothers receiving corticosteroids during pregnancy.

Lactation Excretion in breast milk unknown/use caution

Contraindications Hypersensitivity to ciclesonide or any component of the formulation

Oral inhalation (Alvesco®): Primary treatment of acute asthma or status asthmaticus; moderate-to-severe bronchiectasis

Canadian labeling (Alvesco®): Additional contraindications (not in U.S. labeling): Untreated fungal, bacterial, or tuberculosis infections of the respiratory tract; moderate-to-severe bronchiectasis

Warnings/Precautions May cause hypercorticism or suppression of hypothalamic-pituitary-adrenal (HPA) axis, particularly in younger children or in patients receiving high doses for prolonged periods. HPA axis suppression may lead to adrenal crisis. Withdrawal and discontinuation of a corticosteroid should be done slowly and carefully. Particular care is required when patients are transferred from systemic corticosteroids to inhaled products due to possible adrenal insufficiency or withdrawal from steroids, including an increase in allergic symptoms. Patients receiving >20 mg per day of prednisone (or equivalent) may be most susceptible. Fatalities have occurred due to adrenal insufficiency in asthmatic patients during and after transfer from systemic corticosteroids to aerosol steroids; aerosol steroids do **not** provide the systemic steroid needed to treat patients having trauma, surgery, or infections.

Bronchospasm may occur with wheezing after inhalation; if this occurs stop steroid and treat with a fast-acting bronchodilator. Supplemental steroids (oral or parenteral) may be needed during stress or severe asthma attacks. Not to be used in status asthmaticus or for the relief of acute bronchospasm. Oropharyngeal thrush due to candida albicans infection may occur with use. Prolonged use of corticosteroids may also increase the incidence of secondary infection, mask acute infection (including fungal infections), prolong or exacerbate viral infections, or limit response to vaccines. Exposure to chickenpox and measles should be avoided; corticosteroids should not be used to treat ocular herpes simplex. Close observation is required in patients with latent tuberculosis and/or TB reactivity; restrict use in active TB (only in conjunction with antituberculosis treatment). Use in patients with TB is contraindicated in the Canadian labeling. Prolonged treatment with corticosteroids has been associated with the development of Kaposi's sarcoma (case reports); if noted, discontinuation of therapy should be considered.

Use with caution in patients with thyroid disease, severe hepatic impairment, glaucoma, cataracts, patients at risk for osteoporosis, and patients at risk for seizures. Avoid nasal corticosteroid use in patients with recent nasal septal ulcers, nasal surgery or nasal trauma until healing has occurred.

Orally-inhaled and intranasal corticosteroids may cause a reduction in growth velocity in pediatric patients (~1 cm per year [range 0.3-1.8 cm per year] and related to dose and duration of exposure). To minimize the systemic effects of orally-inhaled and intranasal corticosteroids, each patient should be titrated to the lowest effective dose. Growth should be routinely monitored in pediatric patients. Safety and efficacy of intranasal use have not been established in children <6 years of age and of oral inhalation use in patients <12 years.

Adverse Reactions

>10%:

Central nervous system: Headache (≤11%)

Respiratory: Nasopharyngitis (≤11%)

1% to 10%:

Cardiovascular: Facial edema (≥3%)

Central nervous system: Dizziness (≥3%), fatigue (≥3%)

Dermatologic: Urticaria (≥3%)

Gastrointestinal: Gastroenteritis (≥3%), oral candidiasis (≥3%)

Neuromuscular & skeletal: Arthralgia (≤4%), musculoskeletal chest pain (≥3%), back pain (≥3%), extremity pain (≥3%)

Ocular: Conjunctivitis (≥3%)

Otic: Ear pain (2%)

Respiratory: Upper respiratory infection (≤9%), epistaxis (≤8%), nasal congestion (≤6%), sinusitis (≤6%), pharyngolaryngeal pain (≤ 5%), hoarseness (≥3%), pneumonia (≥3%), paradoxical bronchospasm (2%), dysphonia (1%)

Miscellaneous: Influenza (≥3%)

<1% (Limited to important or life-threatening): ALT increased, angioedema (with swelling of lip/pharynx/tongue), bruising, candidiasis (nasal/pharyngeal/systemic), cataract, chest discomfort, cough, dry throat, dysgeusia, dyspepsia, GGT increased, intraocular pressure increased, nausea, nasal septum disorder, palpitation, pharyngitis, rash, rhinorrhea, throat irritation, WBC increased, weight gain, xerostomia

Drug Interactions

Metabolism/Transport Effects Substrate of CYP3A4 (major), 2D6 (minor)

Avoid Concomitant Use There are no known interactions where it is recommended to avoid concomitant use.

Increased Effect/Toxicity

The levels/effects of Ciclesonide may be increased by: CYP3A4 Inhibitors (Moderate); CYP3A4 Inhibitors (Strong); Dasatinib

Decreased Effect

Ciclesonide may decrease the levels/effects of: Corticorelin

Stability Store at 15°C to 30°C (59°F to 86°F); do not freeze. Nasal spray: Use within 4 months after opening aluminum pouch.

Mechanism of Action Ciclesonide is a nonhalogenated, glucocorticoid prodrug that is hydrolyzed to the pharmacologically active metabolite des-ciclesonide following administration. Des-ciclesonide has a high affinity for the glucocorticoid receptor and exhibits anti-inflammatory activity. The mechanism of action for corticosteroids is believed to be a combination of three important properties - anti-inflammatory activity, immunosuppressive properties, and antiproliferative actions.

Pharmacodynamics/Kinetics

Onset of action: Intranasal: 24-48 hours; further improvement observed over 1-2 weeks in seasonal allergic rhinitis or 5 weeks in perennial allergic rhinitis

Absorption: Intranasal: Minimal systemic absorption; Oral inhalation: 52% (lung deposition)

Distribution: I.V.: V_d: Ciclesonide 2.9 L/kg; Des-ciclesonide 12.1 L/kg

Protein binding: ≥99%

Metabolism: Ciclesonide hydrolyzed to active metabolite, des-ciclesonide via esterases in nasal mucosa and lungs; further metabolism via hepatic CYP3A4 and 2D6

Bioavailability: Intranasal <1%; oral inhalation: >50% (active metabolite)

Half-life elimination: Oral inhalation: ~5-7 hours

Time to peak: Oral inhalation: ~1 hour (active metabolite)

Excretion:

Intranasal: Feces (~66%); urine (≤20%)

Oral inhalation: Feces (78%)

Dosage

Intranasal (Omnaris™):

Seasonal allergic rhinitis:

U.S. labeling: Children ≥6 years and Adults: 2 sprays (50 mcg/spray) per nostril once daily; maximum: 200 mcg/day

Canadian labeling: Children ≥12 years and Adults: 2 sprays (50 mcg/spray) per nostril once daily; maximum: 200 mcg/day

Perennial allergic rhinitis: Children ≥12 years and Adults: 2 sprays (50 mcg/spray) per nostril once daily; maximum: 200 mcg/day

Oral inhalation (Alvesco®):

Asthma: **Note:** Titrate to the lowest effective dose once asthma stability is achieved:

U.S. labeling: Children ≥12 years and Adults:

Prior therapy with bronchodilators alone: Initial: 80 mcg twice daily (maximum dose: 320 mcg/day)

Prior therapy with inhaled corticosteroids: Initial: 80 mcg twice daily (maximum dose: 640 mcg/day)

Prior therapy with oral corticosteroids: Initial: 320 mcg twice daily (maximum dose: 640 mcg/day)

Canadian labeling: Children ≥12 years and Adults: Initial: 400 mcg once daily; maintenance: 100-800 mcg/day (1-2 puffs once or twice daily)

Conversion from oral to inhaled steroid: Initiation of oral inhalation therapy should begin in patients who have previously been stabilized on oral corticosteroids (OCS). A gradual dose reduction of OCS should begin ~7-10 days after starting inhaled therapy. U.S. labeling recommends reducing prednisone dose no more rapidly than ≤2.5 mg/day on a weekly basis. The Canadian labeling recommends decreasing the daily dose of prednisone by 1 mg (or equivalent of other OCS) every 7 days in closely monitored patients, and every 10 days in patients whom close monitoring is not possible. In the presence of withdrawal symptoms, resume previous OCS dose for 1 week before attempting further dose reductions.

Administration

Intranasal: Shake bottle gently before using. Prime pump prior to first use (press 8 times until fine mist appears) or if spray has not been used in 4 consecutive days (press 1 time or until a fine mist appears). Blow nose to clear nostrils. Insert applicator into nostril, keeping bottle upright, and close off the other nostril. Breathe in through nose. While inhaling, press pump to release spray. Avoid spraying directly onto the nasal septum. Nasal applicator may be removed and rinsed with warm water to clean. Discard after the "discard by" date or after labeled number of doses has been used, even if bottle is not completely empty.

Oral inhalation: Remove mouthpiece cover, place inhaler in mouth, close lips around mouthpiece, and inhale slowly and deeply. Press down on top of inhaler after slow inhalation has begun. Remove inhaler while holding breath for approximately 10 seconds. Breathe out slowly and replace mouthpiece on inhaler. Do not wash or place inhaler in water. Clean mouthpiece using a dry cloth or tissue once weekly. Discard after the "discard by" date or after labeled number of doses has been used, even if container is not completely empty.

Shaking is not necessary since drug is formulated as a solution aerosol. Prime inhaler prior to initial use or if not in use for ≥1 week by releasing 3 puffs into the air.

Monitoring Parameters Growth (adolescents) and signs/symptoms of HPA axis suppression/adrenal insufficiency; ocular effects (eg, cataracts, increased intraocular pressure, glaucoma)

Additional Information The incidence of oral candidiasis, as well as other localized oropharyngeal effects, observed with ciclesonide use has been reported to be approximately one-half of that seen with other commonly inhaled corticosteroids such as budesonide and fluticasone. Small particle size, minimal activation, and deposition in the oropharynx may explain this decreased incidence.

Dosage Forms Excipient information presented when available (limited, particularly for generics); consult specific product labeling. [CAN] = Canadian brand name

Aerosol for oral inhalation:

Alvesco® [U.S.]: 80 mcg/inhalation (6.1 g) [60 metered actuations]; 160 mcg/inhalation (6.1 g) [60 metered actuations]

Alvesco® [CAN]: 50 mcg/inhalation [30-, 60-, and 120 metered actuations] [not available in the U.S.]; 100 mcg/inhalation [30-, 60-, and 120 metered actuations] [not available in the U.S.]; 200 mcg/inhalation [30-, 60-, and 120 metered actuations] [not available in the U.S.]

Suspension, intranasal [spray]:

Omnaris™: 50 mcg/inhalation (12.5 g) [120 metered actuations]

Ciclopirox (sye kloe PEER oks)

U.S. Brand Names Loprox®; Penlac®
Canadian Brand Names Loprox®; Penlac®; Stieprox®
Index Terms Ciclopirox Olamine
Pharmacologic Category Antifungal Agent, Topical
Use
Cream/suspension: Treatment of tinea pedis (athlete's foot), tinea cruris (jock itch), tinea corporis (ringworm), cutaneous candidiasis, and tinea versicolor (pityriasis)
Gel: Treatment of tinea pedis (athlete's foot), tinea corporis (ringworm); seborrheic dermatitis of the scalp
Lacquer (solution): Topical treatment of mild-to-moderate onychomycosis of the fingernails and toenails due to *Trichophyton rubrum* (not involving the lunula) and the immediately-adjacent skin
Shampoo: Treatment of seborrheic dermatitis of the scalp
Pregnancy Risk Factor B
Medication Safety Issues
Sound-alike/look-alike issues:
Loprox® may be confused with Lonox®
Dosage Topical:
Children >10 years and Adults: Tinea pedis, tinea cruris, tinea corporis, cutaneous candidiasis, and tinea versicolor: Cream/suspension: Apply twice daily, gently massage into affected areas; if no improvement after 4 weeks of treatment, re-evaluate the diagnosis.
Children ≥12 years and Adults: Onychomycosis of the fingernails and toenails: Lacquer (solution): Apply to adjacent skin and affected nails daily (as a part of a comprehensive management program for onychomycosis). Remove with alcohol every 7 days.
Children >16 years and Adults:
Tinea pedis, tinea corporis: Gel: Apply twice daily, gently massage into affected areas and surrounding skin; if no improvement after 4 weeks of treatment, re-evaluate diagnosis
Seborrheic dermatitis of the scalp:
Gel: Apply twice daily, gently massage into affected areas and surrounding skin; if no improvement after 4 weeks of treatment, re-evaluate diagnosis.
Shampoo: Apply ~5 mL (1 teaspoonful) to wet hair; lather, and leave in place ~3 minutes; rinse. May use up to 10 mL for longer hair. Repeat twice weekly for 4 weeks; allow a minimum of 3 days between applications.
Additional Information Complete prescribing information for this medication should be consulted for additional detail.
Dosage Forms Excipient information presented when available (limited, particularly for generics); consult specific product labeling. [DSC] = Discontinued product
Cream, topical, as olamine: 0.77% (15 g, 30 g, 90 g)
Loprox®: 0.77% (15 g, 30 g, 90 g) [contains benzyl alcohol] [DSC]
Gel, topical: 0.77% (30 g, 45 g, 100 g)
Loprox®: 0.77% (30 g, 45 g, 100 g) [contains isopropyl alcohol]
Shampoo, topical:
Loprox®: 1% (120 mL)
Solution, topical [nail lacquer]: 8% (6.6 mL)
Penlac®: 8% (6.6 mL) [contains isopropyl alcohol]
Suspension, topical, as olamine: 0.77% (30 mL, 60 mL)
Loprox®: 0.77% (30 mL, 60 mL) [contains benzyl alcohol] [DSC]

◆ **Ciclopirox Olamine** *see* Ciclopirox *on page 324*
◆ **Cidecin** *see* DAPTOmycin *on page 397*

Cidofovir (si DOF o veer)

U.S. Brand Names Vistide®
Pharmacologic Category Antiviral Agent
Additional Appendix Information
Guidelines for the Prevention of Opportunistic Infections in HIV Infected Persons *on page 1740*
Use Treatment of cytomegalovirus (CMV) retinitis in patients with acquired immunodeficiency syndrome (AIDS). **Note:** Should be administered with probenecid.
Pregnancy Risk Factor C
Pregnancy Considerations [U.S. Boxed Warning]: Possibly carcinogenic and teratogenic based on animal data. May cause hypospermia. Cidofovir was shown to be teratogenic and embryotoxic in animal studies, some at doses which also produced maternal toxicity. Reduced testes weight and hypospermia were also noted in animal studies. There are no adequate and well-controlled studies in pregnant women; use during pregnancy only if the potential benefit to the mother outweighs the possible risk to the fetus. Women of childbearing potential should use effective contraception during therapy and for 1 month following treatment. Males should use a barrier contraceptive during therapy and for 3 months following treatment.
Lactation Excretion in breast milk unknown/contraindicated
Contraindications Hypersensitivity to cidofovir; history of clinically-severe hypersensitivity to probenecid or other sulfa-containing medications; serum creatinine >1.5 mg/dL; Cl_{cr} <55 mL/minute; urine protein ≥100 mg/dL (≥2+ proteinuria); use with or within 7 days of nephrotoxic agents; direct intraocular injection
Warnings/Precautions Hazardous agent - use appropriate precautions for handling and disposal. **[U.S. Boxed Warning]: Dose-dependent nephrotoxicity requires dose adjustment or discontinuation if changes in renal function occur during therapy (eg, proteinuria, glycosuria, decreased serum phosphate, uric acid or bicarbonate, and elevated creatinine). Neutropenia has been reported;** monitor counts during therapy. Cases of ocular hypotony have also occurred; monitor intraocular pressure. Monitor for signs of metabolic acidosis. Safety and efficacy have not been established in children or the elderly. Administration must be accompanied by oral probenecid and intravenous saline prehydration. **[U.S. Boxed Warning]: Indicated only for CMV retinitis treatment in HIV patients; possibly carcinogenic and teratogenic based on animal data. May cause hypospermia.**
Adverse Reactions
>10%:
Central nervous system: Chills, fever, headache, pain
Dermatologic: Alopecia, rash
Gastrointestinal: Nausea, vomiting, diarrhea, anorexia
Hematologic: Anemia, neutropenia
Neuromuscular & skeletal: Weakness
Ocular: Intraocular pressure decreased, iritis, ocular hypotony, uveitis
Renal: Creatinine increased, proteinuria, renal toxicity
Respiratory: Cough, dyspnea
Miscellaneous: Infection, oral moniliasis, serum bicarbonate decreased
1% to 10%:
Renal: Fanconi syndrome
Respiratory: Pneumonia
<1%: Hepatic failure, metabolic acidosis, pancreatitis
Frequency not defined (limited to important or life-threatening reactions):
Cardiovascular: Cardiomyopathy, cardiovascular disorder, CHF, edema, postural hypotension, shock, syncope, tachycardia
Central nervous system: Agitation, amnesia, anxiety, confusion, convulsion, dizziness, hallucinations, insomnia, malaise, vertigo

Dermatologic: Photosensitivity reaction, skin discoloration, urticaria
Endocrine & metabolic: Adrenal cortex insufficiency
Gastrointestinal: Abdominal pain, aphthous stomatitis, colitis, constipation, dysphagia, fecal incontinence, gastritis, GI hemorrhage, gingivitis, melena, proctitis, splenomegaly, stomatitis, tongue discoloration
Genitourinary: Urinary incontinence
Hematologic: Hypochromic anemia, leukocytosis, leukopenia, lymphadenopathy, lymphoma-like reaction, pancytopenia, thrombocytopenia, thrombocytopenic purpura
Hepatic: Hepatomegaly, hepatosplenomegaly, jaundice, liver function tests abnormal, liver damage, liver necrosis
Local: Injection site reaction
Neuromuscular & skeletal: Tremor
Ocular: Amblyopia, blindness, cataract, conjunctivitis, corneal lesion, diplopia, vision abnormal
Otic: Hearing loss
Miscellaneous: Allergic reaction, sepsis

Drug Interactions

Avoid Concomitant Use There are no known interactions where it is recommended to avoid concomitant use.

Increased Effect/Toxicity There are no known significant interactions involving an increase in effect.

Decreased Effect There are no known significant interactions involving a decrease in effect.

Stability Store at controlled room temperature 20°C to 25°C (68°F to 77°F). Dilute dose in NS 100 mL prior to infusion. Store admixtures under refrigeration for ≤24 hours. Cidofovir infusion admixture should be administered within 24 hours of preparation at room temperature or refrigerated. Admixtures should be allowed to equilibrate to room temperature prior to use.

Mechanism of Action Cidofovir is converted to cidofovir diphosphate which is the active intracellular metabolite; cidofovir diphosphate suppresses CMV replication by selective inhibition of viral DNA synthesis. Incorporation of cidofovir into growing viral DNA chain results in reductions in the rate of viral DNA synthesis.

Pharmacodynamics/Kinetics The following pharmacokinetic data is based on a combination of cidofovir administered with probenecid:
Distribution: V_d: 0.54 L/kg; does not cross significantly into CSF
Protein binding: <6%
Metabolism: Minimal; phosphorylation occurs intracellularly
Half-life elimination, plasma: ~2.6 hours
Excretion: Urine

Dosage Adults:
Induction: 5 mg/kg I.V. over 1 hour once weekly for 2 consecutive weeks
Maintenance: 5 mg/kg over 1 hour once every other week
Note: Administer with probenecid 2 g orally 3 hours prior to each cidofovir dose and 1 g at 2 hours and 8 hours after completion of the infusion (total: 4 g)
Hydrate with 1 L of 0.9% NS I.V. prior to cidofovir infusion; a second liter may be administered over a 1- to 3-hour period immediately following infusion, if tolerated

Dosing adjustment in renal impairment:
Changes in renal function during therapy: If the creatinine increases by 0.3-0.4 mg/dL, reduce the cidofovir dose to 3 mg/kg; discontinue therapy for increases ≥0.5 mg/dL or development of ≥3+ proteinuria
Pre-existing renal impairment: Use is contraindicated with serum creatinine >1.5 mg/dL, Cl_{cr} <55 mL/minute, or urine protein ≥100 mg/dL (≥2+ proteinuria)

Administration For I.V. infusion only. Infuse over 1 hour. Hydrate with 1 L of 0.9% NS I.V. prior to cidofovir infusion. A second liter may be administered over a 1- to 3-hour period immediately following infusion, if tolerated.

Monitoring Parameters Renal function (Cr, BUN, UAs) within 48 hours of each dose, LFTs, WBCs; intraocular pressure and visual acuity, signs and symptoms of uveitis/iritis

Dosage Forms Excipient information presented when available (limited, particularly for generics); consult specific product labeling.
Injection, solution [preservative free]: 75 mg/mL (5 mL)

Cilazapril and Hydrochlorothiazide
(sye LAY za pril & hye droe klor oh THYE a zide)

Canadian Brand Names Apo-Cilazapril/Hctz; Inhibace® Plus

Index Terms Cilazapril Monohydrate and Hydrochlorothiazide; Hydrochlorothiazide and Cilazapril

Pharmacologic Category Angiotensin-Converting Enzyme (ACE) Inhibitor; Diuretic, Thiazide

Use Treatment of mild-to-moderate hypertension in patients who have been stabilized on the individual agents given in the same proportions; not indicated for initial treatment of hypertension

Restrictions Not available in U.S.

Dosage Note: Initiate therapy with combination product only after successful titration of individual agents to adequate blood pressure response.
Oral: Adults: One tablet administered once daily; dose is individualized (range: Cilazapril: 2.5-10 mg; hydrochlorothiazide: 6.25-25 mg/day)

Dosage adjustment in renal impairment:
Mild-to-moderate renal impairment: Use with caution; reduced dosage may be appropriate
Cl_{cr} <30 mL/minute: Not recommended

Additional Information Complete prescribing information for this medication should be consulted for additional detail.

Dosage Forms Excipient information presented when available (limited, particularly for generics); consult specific product labeling. [CAN] = Canadian brand name
Tablet: 5/12.5: Cilazapril monohydrate 5 mg and hydrochlorothiazide 12.5 mg [not available in the U.S.]
Inhibace® Plus 5/12.5 [CAN]: Cilazapril monohydrate 5 mg and hydrochlorothiazide 12.5 mg [not available in the U.S.; contains lactose]

◆ **Cilazapril Monohydrate and Hydrochlorothiazide** *see* Cilazapril and Hydrochlorothiazide *on page* 325

Cilostazol (sil OH sta zol)

U.S. Brand Names Pletal®

Canadian Brand Names Pletal®

Index Terms OPC-13013

Pharmacologic Category Antiplatelet Agent; Phosphodiesterase Enzyme Inhibitor

Use Symptomatic management of peripheral vascular disease, primarily intermittent claudication

Unlabeled/Investigational Use Adjunct with aspirin and clopidogrel for prevention of stent thrombosis and restenosis after coronary stent placement

Pregnancy Risk Factor C

Pregnancy Considerations In animal studies, abnormalities of the skeletal, renal and cardiovascular system were increased. In addition, the incidence of stillbirth and decreased birth weights were increased.

Lactation Excretion in breast milk unknown/not recommended

Medication Safety Issues
Sound-alike/look-alike issues:
Pletal® may be confused with Plendil®

Contraindications Hypersensitivity to cilostazol or any component of the formulation; heart failure (HF) of any severity; hemostatic disorders or active bleeding

Warnings/Precautions Use with caution in patients receiving other platelet aggregation inhibitors or in patients with thrombocytopenia. Discontinue therapy if thrombocytopenia or leukopenia occur; progression to agranulocytosis (reversible) has been reported when cilostazol was not immediately stopped. When cilostazol and clopidogrel are used concurrently, manufacturer recommends checking bleeding times. Withhold for at least 4-6 half-lives prior to elective surgical procedures. Use with caution in patients receiving CYP3A4 inhibitors (eg, ketoconazole or erythromycin) or CYP2C19 inhibitors (eg, omeprazole). If concurrent use is warranted, consider dosage adjustment of cilostazol. Use with caution in severe underlying heart disease. Use caution in moderate-to-severe hepatic impairment. Use cautiously in severe renal impairment (Cl_{cr} <25 mL/minute). Safety and efficacy in pediatric patients have not been established.

Adverse Reactions

>10%:

Central nervous system: Headache (27% to 34%)

Gastrointestinal: Abnormal stools (12% to 15%), diarrhea (12% to 19%)

Respiratory: Rhinitis (7% to 12%)

Miscellaneous: Infection (10% to 14%)

2% to 10%:

Cardiovascular: Peripheral edema (7% to 9%), palpitation (5% to 10%), tachycardia (4%)

Central nervous system: Dizziness (9% to 10%), vertigo (up to 3%)

Gastrointestinal: Dyspepsia (6%), nausea (6% to 7%), abdominal pain (4% to 5%), flatulence (2% to 3%)

Neuromuscular & skeletal: Back pain (6% to 7%), myalgia (2% to 3%)

Respiratory: Pharyngitis (7% to 10%), cough (3% to 4%)

<2% (Limited to important or life-threatening): Agranulocytosis, anemia, aplastic anemia, asthma, atrial fibrillation, atrial flutter, blindness, blood pressure increased, bursitis, cardiac arrest, cerebral infarction/ischemia, cerebrovascular accident, chest pain, CHF, cholelithiasis, colitis, coronary stent thrombosis, cystitis, diabetes mellitus, duodenal ulcer, duodenitis, esophageal hemorrhage, esophagitis, extradural hematoma, gastrointestinal hemorrhage, gout, granulocytopenia, hemorrhage, hepatic dysfunction, hot flashes, hyperglycemia, hypotension, interstitial pneumonia, intracranial hemorrhage, jaundice, leukopenia, myocardial infarction/ischemia, neuralgia, nodal arrhythmia, pain, periodontal abscess, peptic ulcer, pneumonia, polycythemia, postural hypotension, pulmonary hemorrhage, pruritus, QT_c prolongation, rectal hemorrhage, retinal hemorrhage, retroperitoneal hemorrhage, Stevens-Johnson syndrome, subcutaneous hemorrhage, subdural hematoma, supraventricular tachycardia, syncope, thrombocytopenia, thrombosis, torsade de pointes, uric acid increased, ventricular tachycardia

Drug Interactions

Metabolism/Transport Effects **Substrate** of CYP1A2 (minor), 2C19 (minor), 2D6 (minor), 3A4 (major)

Avoid Concomitant Use There are no known interactions where it is recommended to avoid concomitant use.

Increased Effect/Toxicity

Cilostazol may increase the levels/effects of: Anticoagulants; Antiplatelet Agents; Drotrecogin Alfa; Ibritumomab; Salicylates; Thrombolytic Agents; Tositumomab and Iodine I 131 Tositumomab

The levels/effects of Cilostazol may be increased by: Antifungal Agents (Azole Derivatives, Systemic); CYP2C19 Inhibitors (Moderate); CYP2C19 Inhibitors (Strong); CYP3A4 Inhibitors (Moderate); CYP3A4 Inhibitors (Strong); Dasatinib; Herbs (Anticoagulant/Antiplatelet Properties); Macrolide Antibiotics; Nonsteroidal Anti-Inflammatory Agents; Omega-3-Acid Ethyl Esters; Omeprazole; Pentosan Polysulfate Sodium; Prostacyclin Analogues

Decreased Effect

The levels/effects of Cilostazol may be decreased by: CYP3A4 Inducers (Strong); Deferasirox; Herbs (CYP3A4 Inducers); Nonsteroidal Anti-Inflammatory Agents

Ethanol/Nutrition/Herb Interactions

Food: Taking cilostazol with a high-fat meal may increase peak concentration by 90%. Avoid concurrent ingestion of grapefruit juice due to the potential to inhibit CYP3A4.

Herb/Nutraceutical: St John's wort may decrease the levels/effects of cilostazol. Avoid alfalfa, anise, bilberry, bladderwrack, bromelain, cat's claw, chamomile, coleus, cordyceps, dong quai, evening primrose oil, fenugreek, feverfew, garlic, ginger, ginkgo biloba, ginseng (American), ginseng (Panax), ginseng (Siberian), grape seed, green tea, guggul, horse chestnut seed, horseradish, licorice, prickly ash, red clover, reishi, SAMe (S-adenosylmethionine), sweet clover, turmeric, white willow (all have additional antiplatelet activity).

Stability Store at 25°C (77°F); excursions permitted to 15°C to 30°C (59°F to 86°F).

Mechanism of Action Cilostazol and its metabolites are inhibitors of phosphodiesterase III. As a result, cyclic AMP is increased leading to reversible inhibition of platelet aggregation, vasodilation, and inhibition of vascular smooth muscle cell proliferation.

Pharmacodynamics/Kinetics

Onset of action: 2-4 weeks; may require up to 12 weeks

Protein binding: Cilostazol 95% to 98%; active metabolites 66% to 97%

Metabolism: Hepatic via CYP3A4 (primarily), 1A2, 2C19, and 2D6; at least one metabolite has significant activity

Half-life elimination: 11-13 hours

Excretion: Urine (74%) and feces (20%) as metabolites

Dosage Adults: Oral: 100 mg twice daily

Dosage adjustment for cilostazol with concomitant medications:

CYP2C19 inhibitors (see Drug Interactions): Dosage of cilostazol should be reduced to 50 mg twice daily

CYP3A4 inhibitors (see Drug Interactions): Dosage of cilostazol should be reduced to 50 mg twice daily

Dietary Considerations It is best to take cilostazol 30 minutes before or 2 hours after meals.

Administration Administer cilostazol 30 minutes before or 2 hours after meals.

Dosage Forms Excipient information presented when available (limited, particularly for generics); consult specific product labeling.

Tablet: 50 mg, 100 mg

Pletal®: 50 mg, 100 mg

◆ **Ciloxan®** *see* Ciprofloxacin *on page* 329

Cimetidine (sye MET i deen)

U.S. Brand Names Tagamet® HB 200 [OTC]

Canadian Brand Names Apo-Cimetidine®; Gen-Cimetidine; Novo-Cimetidine; Nu-Cimet; PMS-Cimetidine; Tagamet® HB

Pharmacologic Category Histamine H_2 Antagonist

Use Short-term treatment of active duodenal ulcers and benign gastric ulcers; long-term prophylaxis of duodenal ulcer; gastric hypersecretory states; gastroesophageal reflux; prevention of upper GI bleeding in critically-ill patients; labeled for OTC use for prevention or relief of heartburn, acid indigestion, or sour stomach

Unlabeled/Investigational Use Part of a multidrug regimen for *H. pylori* eradication to reduce the risk of duodenal ulcer recurrence

Pregnancy Risk Factor B

Pregnancy Considerations Teratogenic events were not observed in animal studies.

Lactation Enters breast milk/not recommended

Medication Safety Issues

Sound-alike/look-alike issues:

Cimetidine may be confused with simethicone

Contraindications Hypersensitivity to cimetidine, any component of the formulation, or other H_2 antagonists

Warnings/Precautions Reversible confusional states, usually clearing within 3-4 days after discontinuation, have been linked to use. Increased age (>50 years) and renal or hepatic impairment are thought to be associated. Dosage should be adjusted in renal/hepatic impairment or in patients receiving drugs metabolized through the P450 system. Rapid intravenous administration has been associated with rare cases of arrhythmia and/or hypotension.

Over the counter (OTC) cimetidine should not be taken by individuals experiencing painful swallowing, vomiting with blood, or bloody or black stools; medical attention should be sought. A physician should be consulted prior to use when pain in the stomach, shoulder, arms or neck is present; if heartburn has occurred for >3 months; or if unexplained weight loss, or nausea and vomiting occur. Frequent wheezing, shortness of breath, lightheadedness, or sweating, especially with chest pain or heartburn, should also be reported. Consultation of a healthcare provider should occur by patients if also taking theophylline, phenytoin, or warfarin; if heartburn or stomach pain continues or worsens; or if use is required for >14 days. Symptoms of GI distress may be associated with a variety of conditions; symptomatic response to H_2 antagonists does not rule out the potential for significant pathology (eg, malignancy). OTC cimetidine is not approved for use in patients <12 years of age.

Adverse Reactions

1% to 10%:

Central nervous system: Headache (2% to 4%), dizziness (1%), somnolence (1%), agitation

Endocrine & metabolic: Gynecomastia (<1% to 4%)

Gastrointestinal: Diarrhea (1%)

Frequency not defined:

Cardiovascular: AV block, bradycardia, hypotension, tachycardia, vasculitis

Central nervous system: Confusion, fever

Dermatologic: Alopecia, erythema multiforme, exfoliative dermatitis, Stevens-Johnson syndrome, toxic epidermal necrolysis, rash

Endocrine & metabolic: Edema of the breasts, sexual ability decreased

Gastrointestinal: Nausea, pancreatitis, vomiting

Hematologic: Agranulocytosis, aplastic anemia, hemolytic anemia (immune-based), neutropenia, pancytopenia, thrombocytopenia

Hepatic: ALT increased, AST increased, hepatic fibrosis (case report)

Neuromuscular & skeletal: Arthralgia, myalgia, polymyositis

Renal: Creatinine increased, interstitial nephritis

Miscellaneous: Anaphylaxis, pneumonia (causal relationship not established)

Drug Interactions

Metabolism/Transport Effects Inhibits CYP1A2 (moderate), 2C9 (weak), 2C19 (moderate), 2D6 (moderate), 2E1 (weak), 3A4 (moderate)

Avoid Concomitant Use

Avoid concomitant use of Cimetidine with any of the following: Erlotinib; Mesalamine; Thioridazine

Increased Effect/Toxicity

Cimetidine may increase the levels/effects of: Alfentanil; Amiodarone; Anticonvulsants (Hydantoin); Benzodiazepines (metabolized by oxidation); Calcium Channel Blockers; CarBAMazepine; Carmustine; Carvedilol; Cisapride; Clozapine; CYP1A2 Substrates; CYP2C19 Substrates; CYP2D6 Substrates; CYP3A4 Substrates; Dofetilide; Eplerenone; FentaNYL; Fesoterodine; Maraviroc; MetFORMIN; Moclobemide; Moricizine; Nebivolol; Nicotine; Pimecrolimus; Praziquantel; Procainamide; Propafenone; QuiNIDine; Ranolazine; Salmeterol; Saquinavir; Selective Serotonin Reuptake Inhibitors; Sulfonylureas; Tamoxifen; Theophylline Derivatives; Thioridazine; Tricyclic Antidepressants; Vitamin K Antagonists; Zaleplon; Zolmitriptan

The levels/effects of Cimetidine may be increased by: P-Glycoprotein Inhibitors

Decreased Effect

Cimetidine may decrease the levels/effects of: Antifungal Agents (Azole Derivatives, Systemic); Atazanavir; Cefpodoxime; Cefuroxime; Codeine; Dasatinib; Erlotinib; Fosamprenavir; Indinavir; Iron Salts; Mesalamine; Nelfinavir; TraMADol

The levels/effects of Cimetidine may be decreased by: P-Glycoprotein Inducers

Ethanol/Nutrition/Herb Interactions

Ethanol: Avoid ethanol (may enhance gastric mucosal irritation).

Food: Cimetidine may increase serum caffeine levels if taken with caffeine. Cimetidine peak serum levels may be decreased if taken with food.

Herb/Nutraceutical: St John's wort may decrease cimetidine levels.

Stability

Tablet: Store between 15°C and 30°C (59°F to 86°F); protect from light.

Solution for injection/infusion: Intact vials should be stored at room temperature, between 15°C and 30°C (59°F to 86°F); protect from light. May precipitate from solution upon exposure to cold, but can be redissolved by warming without degradation.

Stability at room temperature:

Prepared bags: 7 days

Premixed bags: Manufacturer expiration dating and out of overwrap stability: 15 days

Stable in parenteral nutrition solutions for up to 7 days when protected from light.

Mechanism of Action Competitive inhibition of histamine at H_2 receptors of the gastric parietal cells resulting in reduced gastric acid secretion, gastric volume and hydrogen ion concentration reduced

Pharmacodynamics/Kinetics

Onset of action: 1 hour

Duration: 4-8 hours

Absorption: Rapid

Distribution: Crosses placenta; enters breast milk

Protein binding: 20%

Metabolism: Partially hepatic, forms metabolites

Bioavailability: 60% to 70%

Half-life elimination: Neonates: 3.6 hours; Children: 1.4 hours; Adults: Normal renal function: 2 hours

Time to peak, serum: Oral: 1-2 hours

Excretion: Primarily urine (48% as unchanged drug); feces (some)

Dosage

Children: Oral, I.M., I.V.: 20-40 mg/kg/day in divided doses every 6 hours

Children ≥12 years and Adults: Oral: Heartburn, acid indigestion, sour stomach (OTC labeling): 200 mg up to twice daily; may take 30 minutes prior to eating foods or beverages expected to cause heartburn or indigestion

Adults:

Short-term treatment of active ulcers:

Oral: 300 mg 4 times/day or 800 mg at bedtime or 400 mg twice daily for up to 8 weeks

Note: Higher doses of 1600 mg at bedtime for 4 weeks may be beneficial for a subpopulation of patients with larger duodenal ulcers (>1 cm defined endoscopically) who are also heavy smokers (≥1 pack/day).

I.M., I.V.: 300 mg every 6 hours or 37.5 mg/hour by continuous infusion; I.V. dosage should be adjusted to maintain an intragastric pH ≥5

Prevention of upper GI bleed in critically-ill patients: 50 mg/hour by continuous infusion; I.V. dosage should be adjusted to maintain an intragastric pH ≥5

Note: Reduce dose by 50% if Cl_{cr} <30 mL/minute; treatment >7 days has not been evaluated.

Duodenal ulcer prophylaxis: Oral: 400 mg at bedtime

Gastric hypersecretory conditions: Oral, I.M., I.V.: 300-600 mg every 6 hours; dosage not to exceed 2.4 g/day

Gastroesophageal reflux disease: Oral: 400 mg 4 times/day or 800 mg twice daily for 12 weeks

Helicobacter pylori eradication (unlabeled use): 400 mg twice daily; requires combination therapy with antibiotics

Dosing adjustment/interval in renal impairment: Children and Adults:

Cl_{cr} 10-50 mL/minute: Administer 50% of normal dose

Cl_{cr} <10 mL/minute: Administer 25% of normal dose

Hemodialysis: Slightly dialyzable (5% to 20%); administer after dialysis

Dosing adjustment/comments in hepatic impairment: Usual dose is safe in mild liver disease but use with caution and in reduced dosage in severe liver disease; increased risk of CNS toxicity in cirrhosis suggested by enhanced penetration of CNS

Administration

Oral: Administer with meals so that the drug's peak effect occurs at the proper time (peak inhibition of gastric acid secretion occurs at 1 and 3 hours after dosing in fasting subjects and approximately 2 hours in nonfasting subjects; this correlates well with the time food is no longer in the stomach offering a buffering effect)

Injection: May be administered as a slow I.V. push or preferably as an I.V. intermittent or I.V. continuous infusion. Administer each 300 mg (or fraction thereof) over a minimum of 5 minutes when giving I.V. push. Rapid intravenous administration has been associated with rare cases of arrhythmia and/or hypotension. Give intermittent infusion over 15-30 minutes for each 300 mg dose. Intermittent infusions are administered over 15-30 minutes at a final concentration not to exceed 6 mg/mL; for patients with an active bleed, preferred method of administration is continuous infusion.

Monitoring Parameters CBC, gastric pH, occult blood with GI bleeding; monitor renal function to correct dose.

Dosage Forms Excipient information presented when available (limited, particularly for generics); consult specific product labeling.

Note: Strength is expressed as base

Infusion [premixed in NS]: 300 mg (50 mL)

Injection, solution: 150 mg/mL (2 mL, 8 mL)

Solution, oral: 300 mg/5 mL (240 mL, 480 mL)

Tablet: 200 mg [OTC], 300 mg, 400 mg, 800 mg

Tagamet® HB 200: 200 mg

◆ **Cimzia®** *see* Certolizumab Pegol *on page* 293

Cinacalcet (sin a KAL cet)

U.S. Brand Names Sensipar®

Canadian Brand Names Sensipar®

Index Terms AMG 073; Cinacalcet Hydrochloride

Pharmacologic Category Calcimimetic

Use Treatment of secondary hyperparathyroidism in patients with chronic kidney disease (CKD) on dialysis; treatment of hypercalcemia in patients with parathyroid carcinoma

Note: In Canada, cinacalcet is approved only for the treatment of secondary hyperparathyroidism in patients with chronic kidney disease (CKD) on dialysis

Unlabeled/Investigational Use Primary hyperparathyroidism

Pregnancy Risk Factor C

Pregnancy Considerations In animal studies, there were no teratogenic effects seen. There are no adequate or well-controlled studies in pregnant women.

Lactation Excretion in breast milk unknown/not recommended

Contraindications Hypersensitivity to cinacalcet or any component of the formulation

Warnings/Precautions If hypocalcemia develops or symptoms of hypocalcemia (eg, cramps, myalgia, paresthesia, seizure, tetany) occur during treatment, consider initiating supplemental calcium, calcium-based phosphate binder, or vitamin D or temporarily withholding cinacalcet (dosage reductions may be necessary upon reinitiation of cinacalcet). Serum calcium levels should be ≥8.4 mg/dL prior to initiating treatment. Use caution in patients with a seizure disorder; monitor calcium levels closely. Adynamic bone disease may develop if iPTH levels are suppressed (<100 pg/mL). Use caution in patients with moderate-to-severe hepatic impairment (Child-Pugh classes B & C). In the U.S., the long-term safety and efficacy of cinacalcet has not been evaluated in chronic kidney disease (CKD) patients with hyperparathyroidism not requiring dialysis. Not indicated for CKD patients not receiving dialysis. Although possibly related to lower baseline calcium levels, clinical studies have shown an increased incidence of hypocalcemia (<8.4 mg/dL) in patients not requiring dialysis. May cause a decrease in testosterone levels (free and total); although below normal testosterone levels may occur in patients with end-stage renal disease, the clinical significance has not been determined. Use with caution in patients with cardiovascular disease; idiosyncratic hypotension and/or worsening of heart failure have been reported in patients with impaired cardiovascular function. Safety and efficacy have not been established in pediatric patients.

Adverse Reactions

>10%:

Endocrine & metabolic: Hypocalcemia

Gastrointestinal: Nausea (31%), vomiting (27%), diarrhea (21%)

Neuromuscular & skeletal: Myalgia (15%)

1% to 10%:

Cardiovascular: Hypertension (7%)

Central nervous system: Dizziness (10%), seizure (1%)

Endocrine & metabolic: Testosterone decreased

Gastrointestinal: Anorexia (6%)

Neuromuscular & skeletal: Weakness (7%), chest pain (noncardiac; 6%)

Postmarketing and/or case reports: Adynamic bone disease, heart failure (worsening; in patients with cardiac dysfunction), hypersensitivity reactions, hypotension (idiosyncratic; in patients with cardiac dysfunction), rash

Drug Interactions

Metabolism/Transport Effects Substrate of CYP1A2, 2D6, 3A4; **Inhibits** CYP2D6 (major)

Avoid Concomitant Use

Avoid concomitant use of Cinacalcet with any of the following: Tamoxifen; Thioridazine

Increased Effect/Toxicity

Cinacalcet may increase the levels/effects of: CYP2D6 Substrates; Fesoterodine; Nebivolol; Tamoxifen; Tetrabenazine; Thioridazine; Tricyclic Antidepressants

The levels/effects of Cinacalcet may be increased by: Antifungal Agents (Azole Derivatives, Systemic);

CYP3A4 Inhibitors (Moderate); CYP3A4 Inhibitors (Strong); Dasatinib

Decreased Effect

Cinacalcet may decrease the levels/effects of: Codeine; Tacrolimus; TraMADol

Ethanol/Nutrition/Herb Interactions Food: Food increases bioavailability.

Stability Store at 25°C (77°F); excursions permitted to 15°C to 30°C (59°F to 86°F).

Mechanism of Action Increases the sensitivity of the calcium-sensing receptor on the parathyroid gland thereby, concomitantly lowering PTH and serum calcium levels.

Pharmacodynamics/Kinetics

Distribution: V_d: ~1000 L

Protein binding: ~93% to 97%

Metabolism: Hepatic (extensive) via CYP3A4, 2D6, 1A2; forms inactive metabolites

Half-life elimination: Terminal: 30-40 hours; moderate hepatic impairment: prolonged 33%; severe hepatic impairment: prolonged 70%

Time to peak, plasma: Nadir in iPTH levels: 2-6 hours postdose

Excretion: Urine 80% (as metabolites); feces 15%

Dosage Oral: Adults: **Do not titrate dose more frequently than every 2-4 weeks.**

Secondary hyperparathyroidism: Initial: 30 mg once daily (maximum daily dose: 180 mg); increase dose incrementally (60 mg, 90 mg, 120 mg, 180 mg once daily) as necessary to maintain iPTH level between 150-300 pg/mL.

Parathyroid carcinoma: Initial: 30 mg twice daily (maximum daily dose: 360 mg daily as 90 mg 4 times/day); increase dose incrementally (60 mg twice daily, 90 mg twice daily, 90 mg 3-4 times/day) as necessary to normalize serum calcium levels.

Elderly: No adjustment required; refer to adult dosing

Dosage adjustment for hypocalcemia:

If serum calcium >7.5 mg/dL but <8.4 mg/dL **or** if hypocalcemia symptoms occur: Use calcium-containing phosphate binders and/or vitamin D to raise calcium levels.

If serum calcium <7.5 mg/dL **or** if hypocalcemia symptoms persist and the dose of vitamin D cannot be increased: Withhold cinacalcet until serum calcium ≥8 mg/dL and/or symptoms of hypocalcemia resolve. Reinitiate cinacalcet at the next lowest dose.

If iPTH <150-300 pg/mL: Reduce dose or discontinue cinacalcet and/or vitamin D.

Dosage adjustment in renal impairment: No adjustment required.

Dosage adjustment in hepatic impairment: Patients with moderate-to-severe dysfunction (Child-Pugh classes B and C) have an increased exposure to cinacalcet and increased half-life.

Dietary Considerations Take with food or shortly after a meal. May be taken with vitamin D and/or phosphate binders.

Administration Administer with food or shortly after a meal. Do not break tablet; should be taken whole.

Monitoring Parameters

Hyperparathyroidism: Serum calcium and phosphorus levels prior to initiation and within a week of initiation or dosage adjustment; iPTH should be measured 1-4 weeks after initiation or dosage adjustment. After the maintenance dose is established, monthly calcium and phosphorus levels and iPTH every 1-3 months are required. Wait at least 12 hours after dose before drawing PTH levels.

Parathyroid carcinoma: Serum calcium levels prior to initiation and within a week of initiation or dosage adjustment; once maintenance dose is established, obtain serum calcium level every 2 months.

Reference Range

CKD K/DOQI guidelines definition of stages; chronic disease is kidney damage or GFR <60 mL/minute/1.73 m^2 for ≥3 months:

Stage 2: GFR 60-89 mL/minute/1.73 m^2 (kidney damage with mild decrease GFR)

Stage 3: GFR 30-59 mL/minute/1.73 m^2 (moderate decrease GFR)

Stage 4: GFR 15-29 mL/minute/1.73 m^2 (severe decrease GFR)

Stage 5: GFR <15 mL/minute/1.73 m^2 or dialysis (kidney failure)

Target range for iPTH: Adults:

Stage 3 CKD: 35-70 pg/mL

Stage 4 CKD: 70-110 pg/mL

Stage 5 CKD: 150-300 pg/mL

Serum phosphorus: Adults:

Stage 3 and 4 CKD: ≥2.7 to <4.6 mg/dL

Stage 5 CKD: 3.5-5.5 mg/dL

Serum calcium-phosphorus product: Adults: Stage 3-5 CKD: <55 mg^2/dL^2

Dosage Forms Excipient information presented when available (limited, particularly for generics); consult specific product labeling.

Tablet:

Sensipar®: 30 mg, 60 mg, 90 mg

- **Cinacalcet Hydrochloride** *see* Cinacalcet *on page* *328*
- **Cinryze™** *see* C1 Inhibitor (Human) *on page* *232*
- **Cipralex® (Can)** *see* Escitalopram *on page* *547*
- **Cipro®** *see* Ciprofloxacin *on page* *329*
- **Cipro® XL (Can)** *see* Ciprofloxacin *on page* *329*
- **Ciprodex®** *see* Ciprofloxacin and Dexamethasone *on page* *333*

Ciprofloxacin (sip roe FLOKS a sin)

U.S. Brand Names Ciloxan®; Cipro®; Cipro® XR; Proquin® XR

Canadian Brand Names Apo-Ciproflox®; Ciloxan®; Cipro®; Cipro® XL; CO Ciprofloxacin; Dom-Ciprofloxacin; Gen-Ciprofloxacin; Novo-Ciprofloxacin; PHL-Ciprofloxacin; PMS-Ciprofloxacin; RAN™-Ciprofloxacin; ratio-Ciprofloxacin; Riva-Ciprofloxacin; Sandoz-Ciprofloxacin; Taro-Ciprofloxacin

Index Terms Ciprofloxacin Hydrochloride

Pharmacologic Category Antibiotic, Ophthalmic; Antibiotic, Quinolone

Additional Appendix Information

Antibiotic Treatment of Adults With Infective Endocarditis *on page* *1748*

Antimicrobial Drugs of Choice *on page* *1752*

Community-Acquired Pneumonia in Adults *on page* *1766*

Desensitization Protocols *on page* *1691*

Guidelines for the Prevention of Opportunistic Infections in HIV Infected Persons *on page* *1740*

Prevention of Wound Infection and Sepsis in Surgical Patients *on page* *1738*

Treatment of Sexually Transmitted Infections *on page* *1773*

Tuberculosis *on page* *1776*

Use

Children: Complicated urinary tract infections and pyelonephritis due to *E. coli.* **Note:** Although effective, ciprofloxacin is not the drug of first choice in children.

Children and Adults: To reduce incidence or progression of disease following exposure to aerolized *Bacillus anthracis.* Ophthalmologically, for superficial ocular infections (corneal ulcers, conjunctivitis) due to susceptible strains

Adults: Treatment of the following infections when caused by susceptible bacteria: Urinary tract infections; acute uncomplicated cystitis in females; chronic bacterial prostatitis; lower respiratory tract infections (including acute exacerbations of chronic bronchitis); acute sinusitis; skin and skin structure infections; bone and joint infections; complicated intra-abdominal infections (in combination with metronidazole); infectious diarrhea; typhoid fever due to *Salmonella typhi* (eradication of chronic typhoid carrier state has not been proven); uncomplicated cervical and urethra gonorrhea (due to *N. gonorrhoeae*); nosocomial pneumonia; empirical therapy for febrile neutropenic patients (in combination with piperacillin)

Note: As of April 2007, the CDC no longer recommends the use of fluoroquinolones for the treatment of gonococcal disease.

Unlabeled/Investigational Use Acute pulmonary exacerbations in cystic fibrosis (children); cutaneous/gastrointestinal/oropharyngeal anthrax (treatment, children and adults); disseminated gonococcal infection (adults); chancroid (adults); prophylaxis to *Neisseria meningitidis* following close contact with an infected person; empirical therapy (oral) for febrile neutropenia in low-risk cancer patients; HACEK group endocarditis; infectious diarrhea (children)

Restrictions An FDA-approved patient medication guide is available and must be distributed when dispensing an outpatient prescription (new or refill) where this medication is to be used without direct supervision of a healthcare provider. Medication guides are available at http://www.fda.gov/cder/Offices/ODS/medication_guides.htm.

Pregnancy Risk Factor C

Pregnancy Considerations Adverse events have been observed in some animal studies; therefore, the manufacturer classifies ciprofloxacin as pregnancy category C. Ciprofloxacin crosses the placenta and produces measurable concentrations in the amniotic fluid and cord serum. An increased risk of teratogenic effects has not been observed in animals or humans following ciprofloxacin use during pregnancy; however, because of concerns of cartilage damage in immature animals, ciprofloxacin should only be used during pregnancy if a safer option is not available. Ciprofloxacin is recommended for prophylaxis and treatment of pregnant women exposed to anthrax. Serum concentrations of ciprofloxacin may be lower during pregnancy than in nonpregnant patients.

Lactation Enters breast milk/not recommended (AAP rates "compatible")

Medication Safety Issues

Sound-alike/look-alike issues:

Ciprofloxacin may be confused with cephalexin

Ciloxan® may be confused with cinoxacin, Cytoxan®

Cipro® may be confused with Ceftin®

Contraindications Hypersensitivity to ciprofloxacin, any component of the formulation, or other quinolones; concurrent administration of tizanidine

Warnings/Precautions [U.S. Boxed Warning]: There have been reports of tendon inflammation and/or rupture with quinolone antibiotics; risk may be increased with concurrent corticosteroids, organ transplant recipients, and in patients >60 years of age. Rupture of the Achilles tendon sometimes requiring surgical repair has been reported most frequently; but other tendon sites (eg, rotator cuff, biceps) have also been reported. Strenuous physical activity, rheumatoid arthritis, and renal impairment may be an independent risk factor for tendonitis. Discontinue at first sign of tendon inflammation or pain. May occur even after discontinuation of therapy. Use with caution in patients with rheumatoid arthritis; may increase risk of tendon rupture. CNS stimulation may occur (tremor, restlessness, confusion, and very rarely hallucinations or seizures). Use with caution in patients with known or suspected CNS disorder. Potential for seizures, although very rare, may be increased with concomitant NSAID therapy. Use with caution in individuals at risk of seizures. Fluoroquinolones may prolong QT_c interval; avoid use in patients with a history of QT_c prolongation, uncorrected hypokalemia, hypomagnesemia, or concurrent administration of other medications known to prolong the QT interval (including Class Ia and Class III antiarrhythmics, cisapride, erythromycin, antipsychotics, and tricyclic antidepressants). Prolonged use may result in fungal or bacterial superinfection, including *C. difficile*-associated diarrhea (CDAD) and pseudomembranous colitis; CDAD has been observed >2 months postantibiotic treatment. Rarely crystalluria has occurred; urine alkalinity may increase the risk. Ensure adequate hydration during therapy. Adverse effects, including those related to joints and/or surrounding tissues, are increased in pediatric patients and therefore, ciprofloxacin should not be considered as drug of choice in children (exception is anthrax treatment). Rare cases of peripheral neuropathy may occur.

Fluoroquinolones have been associated with the development of serious, and sometimes fatal, hypoglycemia, most often in elderly diabetics but also in patients without diabetes. This occurred most frequently with gatifloxicain (no longer available systemically), but may occur at a lower frequency with other quinolones.

Severe hypersensitivity reactions, including anaphylaxis, have occurred with quinolone therapy. Reactions may present as typical allergic symptoms after a single dose, or may manifest as severe idiosyncratic dermatologic, vascular, pulmonary, renal, hepatic, and/or hematologic events, usually after multiple doses. Prompt discontinuation of drug should occur if skin rash or other symptoms arise. Quinolones may exacerbate myasthenia gravis, use with caution (rare, potentially life-threatening weakness of respiratory muscles may occur). Use caution in renal impairment. Avoid excessive sunlight and take precautions to limit exposure (eg, loose fitting clothing, sunscreen); may cause moderate-to-severe phototoxicity reactions. Discontinue use if photosensitivity occurs. Since ciprofloxacin is ineffective in the treatment of syphilis and may mask symptoms, all patients should be tested for syphilis at the time of gonorrheal diagnosis and 3 months later. Hemolytic reactions may (rarely) occur with quinolone use in patients with latent or actual G6PD deficiency.

Ciprofloxacin is a potent inhibitor of CYP1A2. Coadministration of drugs which depend on this pathway may lead to substantial increases in serum concentrations and adverse effects.

Adverse Reactions

1% to 10%:

Central nervous system: Neurologic events (children 2%, includes dizziness, insomnia, nervousness, somnolence); fever (children 2%); headache (I.V. administration); restlessness (I.V. administration)

Dermatologic: Rash (children 2%, adults 1%)

Gastrointestinal: Nausea (children/adults 3%); diarrhea (children 5%, adults 2%); vomiting (children 5%, adults 1%); abdominal pain (children 3%, adults <1%); dyspepsia (children 3%)

Hepatic: ALT increased, AST increased (adults 1%)

Local: Injection site reactions (I.V. administration)

Respiratory: Rhinitis (children 3%)

<1% (Limited to important or life-threatening): Abnormal gait, acute renal failure, agitation, agranulocytosis, albuminuria, allergic reactions, anaphylactic shock, anaphylaxis, anemia, angina pectoris, angioedema, anorexia, anosmia, arthralgia, ataxia, atrial flutter, bone marrow depression (life-threatening), breast pain, bronchospasm, candidiasis, candiduria, cardiopulmonary arrest, cerebral thrombosis, chills, cholestatic jaundice, chromatopsia, confusion, constipation, crystalluria (particularly in alkaline urine), cylindruria, delirium, depersonalization, depression, dizziness, drowsiness, dyspepsia

(adults), dysphagia, dyspnea, edema, eosinophilia, erythema multiforme, erythema nodosum, exfoliative dermatitis, fever (adults), fixed eruption, flatulence, gastrointestinal bleeding, hallucinations, headache (oral), hematuria, hemolytic anemia, hepatic failure (some fatal), hepatic necrosis, hyperesthesia, hyperglycemia, hyperpigmentation, hyper-/hypotension, hypertonia, insomnia, interstitial nephritis, intestinal perforation, irritability, jaundice, joint pain, laryngeal edema, lightheadedness, lymphadenopathy, malaise, manic reaction, methemoglobinemia, MI, migraine, moniliasis, myalgia, myasthenia gravis, myoclonus, nephritis, nightmares, nystagmus, orthostatic hypotension, palpitation, pancreatitis, pancytopenia (life-threatening or fatal), paranoia, paresthesia, peripheral neuropathy, petechia, photosensitivity, pneumonitis, prolongation of PT/INR, pseudomembranous colitis, psychosis, pulmonary edema, renal calculi, seizure; serum cholesterol, glucose, triglycerides increased; serum sickness-like reactions, Stevens-Johnson syndrome, syncope, tachycardia, taste loss, tendon rupture, tendonitis, thrombophlebitis, tinnitus, torsade de pointes, toxic epidermal necrolysis (Lyell's syndrome), tremor, twitching, urethral bleeding, vaginal candidiasis, vaginitis, vasculitis, ventricular ectopy, visual disturbance, weakness

Drug Interactions

Metabolism/Transport Effects **Inhibits** CYP1A2 (strong), 3A4 (weak)

Avoid Concomitant Use

Avoid concomitant use of Ciprofloxacin with any of the following: TiZANidine

Increased Effect/Toxicity

Ciprofloxacin may increase the levels/effects of: Bendamustine; Caffeine; Corticosteroids (Systemic); CYP1A2 Substrates; Methotrexate; Pentoxifylline; QTc-Prolonging Agents; Ropinirole; Ropivacaine; Sulfonylureas; Theophylline Derivatives; TiZANidine; Vitamin K Antagonists

The levels/effects of Ciprofloxacin may be increased by: Insulin; Nonsteroidal Anti-Inflammatory Agents; P-Glycoprotein Inhibitors; Probenecid

Decreased Effect

Ciprofloxacin may decrease the levels/effects of: Mycophenolate; Phenytoin; Sulfonylureas; Typhoid Vaccine

The levels/effects of Ciprofloxacin may be decreased by: Antacids; Calcium Salts; Didanosine; Iron Salts; Magnesium Salts; P-Glycoprotein Inducers; Quinapril; Sevelamer; Sucralfate; Zinc Salts

Ethanol/Nutrition/Herb Interactions

Food: Food decreases rate, but not extent, of absorption. Ciprofloxacin serum levels may be decreased if taken with dairy products or calcium-fortified juices. Ciprofloxacin may increase serum caffeine levels if taken with caffeine.

Enteral feedings may decrease plasma concentrations of ciprofloxacin probably by >30% inhibition of absorption. Ciprofloxacin should not be administered with enteral feedings. The feeding would need to be discontinued for 1-2 hours prior to and after ciprofloxacin administration. Nasogastric administration produces a greater loss of ciprofloxacin bioavailability than does nasoduodenal administration.

Herb/Nutraceutical: Avoid dong quai, St John's wort (may also cause photosensitization).

Stability

Injection:

Premixed infusion: Store between 5°C to 25°C (41°F to 77°F); avoid freezing. Protect from light.

Vial: Store between 5°C to 30°C (41°F to 86°F); avoid freezing. Protect from light. May be diluted with NS, D_5W, SWFI, $D_{10}W$, $D_5{}^1/_4NS$, $D_5{}^1/_2NS$, LR. Diluted solutions of 0.5-2 mg/mL are stable for up to 14 days refrigerated or at room temperature.

Ophthalmic solution/ointment: Store at 36°F to 77°F (2°C to 25°C); protect from light.

Microcapsules for oral suspension: Prior to reconstitution, store below 25°C (77°F); protect from freezing. Following reconstitution, store below 30°C (86°F) for up to 14 days; protect from freezing.

Tablet:

Immediate release: Store below 30°C (86°F).

Extended release: Store at room temperature of 15°C to 30°C (59°F to 86°F).

Mechanism of Action Inhibits DNA-gyrase in susceptible organisms; inhibits relaxation of supercoiled DNA and promotes breakage of double-stranded DNA

Pharmacodynamics/Kinetics

Absorption: Oral: Immediate release tablet: Rapid (~50% to 85%)

Distribution: V_d: 2.1-2.7 L/kg; tissue concentrations often exceed serum concentrations especially in kidneys, gallbladder, liver, lungs, gynecological tissue, and prostatic tissue; CSF concentrations: 10% of serum concentrations (noninflamed meninges), 14% to 37% (inflamed meninges)

Protein binding: 20% to 40%

Metabolism: Partially hepatic; forms 4 metabolites (limited activity)

Half-life elimination: Children: 2.5 hours; Adults: Normal renal function: 3-5 hours

Time to peak: Oral:

Immediate release tablet: 0.5-2 hours

Extended release tablet: Cipro® XR: 1-2.5 hours, Proquin® XR: 3.5-8.7 hours

Excretion: Urine (30% to 50% as unchanged drug); feces (15% to 43%)

Dosage Note: Extended release tablets and immediate release formulations are not interchangeable. Unless otherwise specified, oral dosing reflects the use of immediate release formulations.

Usual dosage ranges:

Children (see Warnings/Precautions):

Oral: 20-30 mg/kg/day in 2 divided doses; maximum dose: 1.5 g/day

I.V.: 20-30 mg/kg/day divided every 12 hours; maximum dose: 800 mg/day

Adults:

Oral: 250-750 mg every 12 hours

I.V.: 200-400 mg every 12 hours

Indication-specific dosing:

Children:

Anthrax:

Inhalational (postexposure prophylaxis):

Oral: 15 mg/kg/dose every 12 hours for 60 days; maximum: 500 mg/dose

I.V.: 10 mg/kg/dose every 12 hours for 60 days; do **not** exceed 400 mg/dose (800 mg/day)

Cutaneous (treatment, CDC guidelines): Oral: 10-15 mg/kg every 12 hours for 60 days (maximum: 1 g/day); amoxicillin 80 mg/kg/day divided every 8 hours is an option for completion of treatment after clinical improvement. **Note:** In the presence of systemic involvement, extensive edema, lesions on head/neck, refer to I.V. dosing for treatment of inhalational/gastrointestinal/oropharyngeal anthrax.

Inhalational/gastrointestinal/oropharyngeal (treatment, CDC guidelines): I.V.: Initial: 10-15 mg/kg every 12 hours for 60 days (maximum: 500 mg/dose); switch to oral therapy when clinically appropriate; refer to adult dosing for notes on combined therapy and duration

Bacterial conjunctivitis: See adult dosing

Corneal ulcer: See adult dosing

Cystic fibrosis (unlabeled use):

Oral: 40 mg/kg/day divided every 12 hours administered following 1 week of I.V. therapy has been reported in a clinical trial; total duration of therapy: 10-21 days

I.V.: 30 mg/kg/day divided every 8 hours for 1 week, followed by oral therapy, has been reported in a clinical trial

Urinary tract infection (complicated) or pyelonephritis:

Oral: 20-30 mg/kg/day in 2 divided doses (every 12 hours) for 10-21 days; maximum: 1.5 g/day

I.V.: 6-10 mg/kg every 8 hours for 10-21 days (maximum: 400 mg/dose)

Adults:

Anthrax:

Inhalational (postexposure prophylaxis):

Oral: 500 mg every 12 hours for 60 days

I.V.: 400 mg every 12 hours for 60 days

Cutaneous (treatment, CDC guidelines): Oral: Immediate release formulation: 500 mg every 12 hours for 60 days. **Note:** In the presence of systemic involvement, extensive edema, lesions on head/neck, refer to I.V. dosing for treatment of inhalational/gastrointestinal/oropharyngeal anthrax

Inhalational/gastrointestinal/oropharyngeal (treatment, CDC guidelines): I.V.: 400 mg every 12 hours. **Note:** Initial treatment should include two or more agents predicted to be effective (per CDC recommendations). Continue combined therapy for 60 days.

Bacterial conjunctivitis:

Ophthalmic solution: Instill 1-2 drops in eye(s) every 2 hours while awake for 2 days and 1-2 drops every 4 hours while awake for the next 5 days

Ophthalmic ointment: Apply a 1/2" ribbon into the conjunctival sac 3 times/day for the first 2 days, followed by a 1/2" ribbon applied twice daily for the next 5 days

Bone/joint infections:

Oral: 500-750 mg twice daily for 4-6 weeks

I.V.: Mild to moderate: 400 mg every 12 hours for 4-6 weeks; Severe/complicated: 400 mg every 8 hours for 4-6 weeks

Chancroid (CDC guidelines): Oral: 500 mg twice daily for 3 days

Corneal ulcer: Ophthalmic solution: Instill 2 drops into affected eye every 15 minutes for the first 6 hours, then 2 drops into the affected eye every 30 minutes for the remainder of the first day. On day 2, instill 2 drops into the affected eye hourly. On days 3-14, instill 2 drops into affected eye every 4 hours. Treatment may continue after day 14 if re-epithelialization has not occurred.

Endocarditis due to HACEK organisms (AHA guidelines, unlabeled use): Note: Not first-line option; use only if intolerant of beta-lactam therapy:

Oral: 500 mg every 12 hours for 4 weeks

I.V.: 400 mg every 12 hours for 4 weeks

Febrile neutropenia*: I.V.: 400 mg every 8 hours for 7-14 days

Gonococcal infections:

Urethral/cervical gonococcal infections: Oral: 250-500 mg as a single dose (CDC recommends concomitant doxycycline or azithromycin due to possible coinfection with *Chlamydia*; **Note:** As of April 2007, the CDC no longer recommends the use of fluoroquinolones for the treatment of uncomplicated gonococcal disease.

Disseminated gonococcal infection (CDC guidelines): Oral: 500 mg twice daily to complete 7 days of therapy (initial treatment with ceftriaxone 1 g I.M./I.V. daily for 24-48 hours after improvement begins); **Note:** As of April 2007, the CDC no longer recommends the use of fluoroquinolones for the treatment of more serious gonococcal disease, unless no other options exist and susceptibility can be confirmed via culture.

Infectious diarrhea: Oral:

Salmonella: 500 mg twice daily for 5-7 days

Shigella: 500 mg twice daily for 3 days

Traveler's diarrhea: Mild: 750 mg for one dose; Severe: 500 mg twice daily for 3 days

Vibrio cholerae: 1 g for one dose

Intra-abdominal*:

Oral: 500 mg every 12 hours for 7-14 days

I.V.: 400 mg every 12 hours for 7-14 days

Lower respiratory tract, skin/skin structure infections:

Oral: 500-750 mg twice daily for 7-14 days

I.V.: Mild to moderate: 400 mg every 12 hours for 7-14 days; Severe/complicated: 400 mg every 8 hours for 7-14 days

Nosocomial pneumonia: I.V.: 400 mg every 8 hours for 10-14 days

Prostatitis (chronic, bacterial): Oral: 500 mg every 12 hours for 28 days

Sinusitis (acute): Oral: 500 mg every 12 hours for 10 days

Typhoid fever: Oral: 500 mg every 12 hours for 10 days

Urinary tract infection:

Acute uncomplicated, cystitis:

Oral:

Immediate release formulation: 250 mg every 12 hours for 3 days

Extended release formulation (Cipro® XR, Proquin® XR): 500 mg every 24 hours for 3 days

I.V.: 200 mg every 12 hours for 7-14 days

Complicated (including pyelonephritis):

Oral:

Immediate release formulation: 500 mg every 12 hours for 7-14 days

Extended release formulation (Cipro® XR): 1000 mg every 24 hours for 7-14 days

I.V.: 400 mg every 12 hours for 7-14 days

*Combination therapy generally recommended.

Elderly: No adjustment needed in patients with normal renal function

Dosing adjustment in renal impairment: Adults:

Cl_{cr} 30-50 mL/minute: Oral: 250-500 mg every 12 hours

Cl_{cr} <30 mL/minute: Acute uncomplicated pyelonephritis or complicated UTI: Oral: Extended release formulation: 500 mg every 24 hours

Cl_{cr} 5-29 mL/minute:

Oral: 250-500 mg every 18 hours

I.V.: 200-400 mg every 18-24 hours

Dialysis: Only small amounts of ciprofloxacin are removed by hemo- or peritoneal dialysis (<10%); usual dose: Oral: 250-500 mg every 24 hours following dialysis

Continuous renal replacement therapy (CRRT): I.V.:

CVVH: 200 mg every 12 hours

CVVHD or CVVHDF: 200-400 mg every 12 hours

Dietary Considerations

Food: Drug may cause GI upset; take without regard to meals (manufacturer prefers that immediate release tablet is taken 2 hours after meals). Extended release tablet may be taken with meals that contain dairy products (calcium content <800 mg), but not with dairy products alone.

Dairy products, calcium-fortified juices, oral multivitamins, and mineral supplements: Absorption of ciprofloxacin is decreased by divalent and trivalent cations. The manufacturer states that the usual dietary intake of calcium (including meals which include dairy products) has not been shown to interfere with ciprofloxacin absorption. Immediate release ciprofloxacin and Cipro® XR may be taken 2 hours before or 6 hours after, and

Proquin® XR may be taken 4 hours before or 6 hours after, any of these products.

Caffeine: Patients consuming regular large quantities of caffeinated beverages may need to restrict caffeine intake if excessive cardiac or CNS stimulation occurs.

Administration

Oral: May administer with food to minimize GI upset; avoid antacid use; maintain proper hydration and urine output. Administer immediate release ciprofloxacin and Cipro® XR at least 2 hours before or 6 hours after, and Proquin® XR at least 4 hours before or 6 hours after antacids or other products containing calcium, iron, or zinc (including dairy products or calcium-fortified juices). Separate oral administration from drugs which may impair absorption (see Drug Interactions).

Oral suspension: Should not be administered through feeding tubes (suspension is oil-based and adheres to the feeding tube). Patients should avoid chewing on the microcapsules.

Nasogastric/orogastric tube: Crush immediate-release tablet and mix with water. Flush feeding tube before and after administration. Hold tube feedings at least 1 hour before and 2 hours after administration.

Tablet, extended release: Do not crush, split, or chew. May be administered with meals containing dairy products (calcium content <800 mg), but not with dairy products alone. Proquin® XR should be administered with a main meal of the day; evening meal is preferred.

Parenteral: Administer by slow I.V. infusion over 60 minutes to reduce the risk of venous irritation (burning, pain, erythema, and swelling); final concentration for administration should not exceed 2 mg/mL.

Monitoring Parameters Patients receiving concurrent ciprofloxacin, theophylline, or cyclosporine should have serum levels monitored; CBC, renal and hepatic function during prolonged therapy

Reference Range Therapeutic: 2.6-3 mcg/mL; Toxic: >5 mcg/mL

Test Interactions Some quinolones may produce a false-positive urine screening result for opiates using commercially-available immunoassay kits. This has been demonstrated most consistently for levofloxacin and ofloxacin, but other quinolones have shown cross-reactivity in certain assay kits. Confirmation of positive opiate screens by more specific methods should be considered.

Additional Information Although the systemic use of ciprofloxacin is only FDA approved in children for the treatment of complicated UTI and postexposure treatment of inhalation anthrax, use of the fluoroquinolones in pediatric patients is increasing. Current recommendations by the American Academy of Pediatrics note that the systemic use of these agents in children should be restricted to infections caused by multidrug resistant pathogens with no safe or effective alternative, and when parenteral therapy is not feasible or other oral agents are not available.

Dosage Forms Excipient information presented when available (limited, particularly for generics); consult specific product labeling.

Infusion [premixed in D_5W]: 200 mg (100 mL); 400 mg (200 mL)

Cipro®: 200 mg (100 mL); 400 mg (200 mL)

Injection, solution [concentrate]: 10 mg/mL (20 mL, 40 mL, 120 mL)

Cipro®: 10 mg/mL (20 mL, 40 mL)

Microcapsules for suspension, oral:

Cipro®: 250 mg/5 mL (100 mL); 500 mg/5 mL (100 mL) [strawberry flavor]

Ointment, ophthalmic, as hydrochloride:

Ciloxan®: 3.33 mg/g (3.5 g) [0.3% base]

Solution, ophthalmic, as hydrochloride: 3.5 mg/mL (2.5 mL, 5mL, 10 mL) [0.3% base]

Ciloxan®: 3.5 mg/mL (5 mL) [0.3% base; contains benzalkonium chloride]

Tablet, as hydrochloride: 100 mg [strength expressed as base], 250 mg [strength expressed as base], 500 mg [strength expressed as base], 750 mg [strength expressed as base]

Cipro®: 250 mg [strength expressed as base], 500 mg [strength expressed as base], 750 mg [strength expressed as base]

Tablet, extended release, as base and hydrochloride: 500 mg [strength expressed as base], 1000 mg [strength expressed as base]

Cipro® XR: 500 mg [strength expressed as base], 1000 mg [strength expressed as base]

Tablet, extended release, as hydrochloride:

Proquin® XR: 500 mg [strength expressed as base]

Tablet, extended release, as hydrochloride [dose pack]:

Proquin® XR: 500 mg (3s)

Ciprofloxacin and Dexamethasone

(sip roe FLOKS a sin & deks a METH a sone)

U.S. Brand Names Ciprodex®

Canadian Brand Names Ciprodex®

Index Terms Ciprofloxacin Hydrochloride and Dexamethasone; Dexamethasone and Ciprofloxacin

Pharmacologic Category Antibiotic/Corticosteroid, Otic

Use Treatment of acute otitis media in pediatric patients with tympanostomy tubes or acute otitis externa in children and adults

Pregnancy Risk Factor C

Dosage Otic:

Children: Acute otitis media in patients with tympanostomy tubes or acute otitis externa: Instill 4 drops into affected ear(s) twice daily for 7 days

Adults: Acute otitis externa: Instill 4 drops into affected ear (s) twice daily for 7 days

Additional Information Complete prescribing information for this medication should be consulted for additional detail.

Dosage Forms Excipient information presented when available (limited, particularly for generics); consult specific product labeling.

Suspension, otic: Ciprofloxacin 0.3% and dexamethasone 0.1% (7.5 mL) [contains benzalkonium chloride]

Ciprofloxacin and Hydrocortisone

(sip roe FLOKS a sin & hye droe KOR ti sone)

U.S. Brand Names Cipro® HC

Canadian Brand Names Cipro® HC

Index Terms Ciprofloxacin Hydrochloride and Hydrocortisone; Hydrocortisone and Ciprofloxacin

Pharmacologic Category Antibiotic/Corticosteroid, Otic

Use Treatment of acute otitis externa, sometimes known as "swimmer's ear"

Dosage Children >1 year of age and Adults: Otic: The recommended dosage for all patients is three drops of the suspension in the affected ear twice daily for 7 days; twice-daily dosing schedule is more convenient for patients than that of existing treatments with hydrocortisone, which are typically administered three or four times a day; a twice-daily dosage schedule may be especially helpful for parents and caregivers of young children

Additional Information Complete prescribing information for this medication should be consulted for additional detail.

Dosage Forms Excipient information presented when available (limited, particularly for generics); consult specific product labeling.

Suspension, otic: Ciprofloxacin hydrochloride 0.2% and hydrocortisone 1% (10 mL) [contains benzyl alcohol]

◆ **Ciprofloxacin Hydrochloride** *see* Ciprofloxacin *on page 329*

◆ **Ciprofloxacin Hydrochloride and Dexamethasone** *see* Ciprofloxacin and Dexamethasone *on page 333*

◆ **Ciprofloxacin Hydrochloride and Hydrocortisone** *see* Ciprofloxacin and Hydrocortisone *on page 333*

◆ **Cipro® HC** *see* Ciprofloxacin and Hydrocortisone *on page 333*

◆ **Cipro® XR** *see* Ciprofloxacin *on page 329*

Cisapride (SIS a pride)

U.S. Brand Names Propulsid®

Pharmacologic Category Gastrointestinal Agent, Prokinetic

Use Treatment of nocturnal symptoms of gastroesophageal reflux disease (GERD); has demonstrated effectiveness for gastroparesis, refractory constipation, and nonulcer dyspepsia

Restrictions In U.S., available via limited-access protocol only (1-800-JANSSEN).

Pregnancy Risk Factor C

Medication Safety Issues

Sound-alike/look-alike issues:

Propulsid® may be confused with propranolol

Dosage Oral:

Children: 0.15-0.3 mg/kg/dose 3-4 times/day; maximum: 10 mg/dose

Adults: Initial: 10 mg 4 times/day at least 15 minutes before meals and at bedtime; in some patients the dosage will need to be increased to 20 mg to obtain a satisfactory result

Additional Information Complete prescribing information for this medication should be consulted for additional detail.

Cisatracurium (sis a tra KYOO ree um)

U.S. Brand Names Nimbex®

Canadian Brand Names Nimbex®

Index Terms Cisatracurium Besylate

Pharmacologic Category Neuromuscular Blocker Agent, Nondepolarizing

Additional Appendix Information

Neuromuscular-Blocking Agents *on page 1665*

Use Adjunct to general anesthesia to facilitate endotracheal intubation and to relax skeletal muscles during surgery; to facilitate mechanical ventilation in ICU patients; does not relieve pain or produce sedation

Pregnancy Risk Factor B

Lactation Excretion in breast milk unknown/use caution

Medication Safety Issues

Sound-alike/look-alike issues:

Nimbex® may be confused with Revex®

High alert medication: The Institute for Safe Medication Practices (ISMP) includes this medication among its list of drugs which have a heightened risk of causing significant patient harm when used in error.

Contraindications Hypersensitivity to cisatracurium besylate or any component of the formulation

Warnings/Precautions Maintenance of an adequate airway and respiratory support is critical; certain clinical conditions may result in potentiation or antagonism of neuromuscular blockade:

Potentiation: Electrolyte abnormalities, severe hyponatremia, severe hypocalcemia, severe hypokalemia, hypermagnesemia, neuromuscular diseases, acidosis, acute intermittent porphyria, renal failure, hepatic failure

Antagonism: Alkalosis, hypercalcemia, demyelinating lesions, peripheral neuropathies, diabetes mellitus

Increased sensitivity in patients with myasthenia gravis, Eaton-Lambert syndrome; resistance in burn patients (>30% of body) for period of 5-70 days postinjury; resistance in patients with muscle trauma, denervation, immobilization, infection. Cross-sensitivity with other neuromuscular-blocking agents may occur; use extreme caution in patients with previous anaphylactic reactions. Bradycardia may be more common with cisatracurium than with other neuromuscular blocking agents since it has no clinically significant effects on heart rate to counteract the bradycardia produced by anesthetics. Use caution in the elderly. Should be administered by adequately trained individuals familiar with its use.

Adverse Reactions <1%: Effects are minimal and transient, bradycardia and hypotension, flushing, pruritus, rash, bronchospasm, acute quadriplegic myopathy syndrome (prolonged use), myositis ossificans (prolonged use)

Drug Interactions

Avoid Concomitant Use There are no known interactions where it is recommended to avoid concomitant use.

Increased Effect/Toxicity

Cisatracurium may increase the levels/effects of: Botulinum Toxin Type A; Botulinum Toxin Type B; Cardiac Glycosides; Corticosteroids (Systemic)

The levels/effects of Cisatracurium may be increased by: Aminoglycosides; Calcium Channel Blockers; Capreomycin; Colistimethate; Inhalational Anesthetics; Ketorolac; Lincosamide Antibiotics; Lithium; Loop Diuretics; Magnesium Salts; Polymyxin B; Procainamide; QuiNIDine; Tetracycline Derivatives; Vancomycin

Decreased Effect

The levels/effects of Cisatracurium may be decreased by: Acetylcholinesterase Inhibitors; Loop Diuretics

Stability Refrigerate intact vials at 2°C to 8°C/36°F to 46°F; use vials within 21 days upon removal from the refrigerator to room temperature (25°C to 77°F). Dilutions of 0.1-0.2 mg/mL in 0.9% sodium chloride or dextrose 5% in water are stable for up to 24 hours at room temperature.

Mechanism of Action Blocks neural transmission at the myoneural junction by binding with cholinergic receptor sites

Pharmacodynamics/Kinetics

Onset of action: I.V.: 2-3 minutes

Peak effect: 3-5 minutes

Duration: Recovery begins in 20-35 minutes when anesthesia is balanced; recovery is attained in 90% of patients in 25-93 minutes

Metabolism: Undergoes rapid nonenzymatic degradation in the bloodstream (Hofmann elimination), additional metabolism occurs via ester hydrolysis; some active metabolites

Half-life elimination: 22-29 minutes

Dosage I.V. (not to be used I.M.):

Operating room administration:

Infants 1-23 months: 0.15 mg/kg over 5-10 seconds during either halothane or opioid anesthesia

Children 2-12 years: Intubating doses: 0.1-0.15 mg/kg over 5-15 seconds during either halothane or opioid anesthesia. (**Note:** When given during stable opioid/nitrous oxide/oxygen anesthesia, 0.1 mg/kg produces maximum neuromuscular block in an average of 2.8 minutes and clinically effective block for 28 minutes.)

Adults: Intubating doses: 0.15-0.2 mg/kg as component of propofol/nitrous oxide/oxygen induction-intubation technique. (**Note:** May produce generally good or excellent conditions for tracheal intubation in 1.5-2 minutes with clinically effective duration of action during propofol anesthesia of 55-61 minutes.); initial dose after succinylcholine for intubation: 0.1 mg/kg; maintenance dose: 0.03 mg/kg 40-60 minutes after initial dose, then at ~20-minute intervals based on clinical criteria

Children ≥2 years and Adults: Continuous infusion: After an initial bolus, a diluted solution can be given by continuous infusion for maintenance of neuromuscular blockade during extended surgery; adjust the rate of administration according to the patient's response as determined by peripheral nerve stimulation. An initial infusion rate of 3 mcg/kg/minute may be required to rapidly counteract the spontaneous recovery of neuromuscular function; thereafter, a rate of 1-2 mcg/kg/minute should be adequate to maintain continuous neuromuscular block in the 89% to 99% range in most pediatric and adult patients. Consider reduction of the infusion rate by 30% to 40% when administering during stable isoflurane, enflurane, sevoflurane, or desflurane anesthesia. Spontaneous recovery from neuromuscular blockade following discontinuation of infusion of cisatracurium may be expected to proceed at a rate comparable to that following single bolus administration.

Intensive care unit administration: Follow the principles for infusion in the operating room. At initial signs of recovery from bolus dose, begin the infusion at a dose of 3 mcg/kg/minute and adjust rates accordingly; dosage ranges of 0.5-10 mcg/kg/minute have been reported. If patient is allowed to recover from neuromuscular blockade, readministration of a bolus dose may be necessary to quickly re-establish neuromuscular block prior to reinstituting the infusion. See table.

Cisatracurium Besylate Infusion Chart

Drug Delivery Rate (mcg/kg/min)	Infusion Rate (mL/kg/min) 0.1 mg/mL (10 mg/100 mL)	Infusion Rate (mL/kg/min) 0.4 mg/mL (40 mg/100 mL)
1	0.01	0.0025
1.5	0.015	0.00375
2	0.02	0.005
3	0.03	0.0075
5	0.05	0.0125

Dosing adjustment in renal impairment: Because slower times to onset of complete neuromuscular block were observed in renal dysfunction patients, extending the interval between the administration of cisatracurium and intubation attempt may be required to achieve adequate intubation conditions.

Administration Administer I.V. only; the use of a peripheral nerve stimulator will permit the most advantageous use of cisatracurium, minimize the possibility of overdosage or underdosage and assist in the evaluation of recovery

Give undiluted as a bolus injection; not for I.M. injection, too much tissue irritation; continuous administration requires the use of an infusion pump

Monitoring Parameters Vital signs (heart rate, blood pressure, respiratory rate)

Additional Information Cisatracurium is classified as an intermediate-duration neuromuscular-blocking agent. It does not appear to have a cumulative effect on the duration of blockade. Neuromuscular-blocking potency is 3 times that of atracurium; maximum block is up to 2 minutes longer than for equipotent doses of atracurium.

Dosage Forms Excipient information presented when available (limited, particularly for generics); consult specific product labeling.

Injection, solution: 2 mg/mL (5 mL); 10 mg/mL (20 mL)

Injection, solution: 2 mg/mL (10 mL) [contains benzyl alcohol]

◆ **Cisatracurium Besylate** *see* Cisatracurium *on page* 334

CISplatin (SIS pla tin)

Index Terms CDDP

Pharmacologic Category Antineoplastic Agent, Alkylating Agent; Antineoplastic Agent, Platinum Analog

Use Treatment of bladder, testicular, and ovarian cancer

Unlabeled/Investigational Use Treatment of head and neck, breast, gastric, lung, esophageal, cervical, prostate and small cell lung cancer; Hodgkin's and non-Hodgkin's lymphoma; neuroblastoma; sarcomas, myeloma, melanoma, mesothelioma, and osteosarcoma

Pregnancy Risk Factor D

Pregnancy Considerations Animal studies have demonstrated teratogenicity and embryotoxicity. There are no adequate and well-controlled studies in pregnant women. Women of childbearing potential should be advised to avoid pregnancy. If used in pregnancy, or if patient becomes pregnant during treatment, the patient should be apprised of potential hazard to the fetus.

Lactation Enters breast milk/contraindicated

Medication Safety Issues

Sound-alike/look-alike issues:

CISplatin may be confused with CARBOplatin

High alert medication: The Institute for Safe Medication Practices (ISMP) includes this medication among its list of drugs which have a heightened risk of causing significant patient harm when used in error.

Doses >100 mg/m^2 once every 3-4 weeks are rarely used and should be verified with the prescriber.

Contraindications Hypersensitivity to cisplatin, other platinum-containing compounds, or any component of the formulation (anaphylactic-like reactions have been reported); pre-existing renal insufficiency; myelosuppression; hearing impairment; pregnancy

Warnings/Precautions Hazardous agent - use appropriate precautions for handling and disposal. **[U.S. Boxed Warning]: Doses >100 mg/m^2 once every 3-4 weeks are rarely used and should be verified with the prescriber.** Patients should receive adequate hydration, with or without diuretics, prior to and for 24 hours after cisplatin administration. Reduce dosage in renal impairment. **[U.S. Boxed Warning]: Cumulative renal toxicity may be severe.** Elderly patients may be more susceptible to nephrotoxicity and peripheral neuropathy; select dose cautiously and monitor closely. **[U.S. Boxed Warnings]: Dose-related toxicities include myelosuppression, nausea, and vomiting. Ototoxicity, especially pronounced in children, is manifested by tinnitus or loss of high frequency hearing and occasionally, deafness.** Severe and possibly irreversible neuropathies may occur with higher than recommended doses or more frequent regimen. Serum electrolytes, particularly magnesium and potassium, should be monitored and replaced as needed during and after cisplatin therapy. When administered as sequential infusions, taxane derivatives (docetaxel, paclitaxel) should be administered before platinum derivatives (carboplatin, cisplatin). **[U.S. Boxed Warnings]: Anaphylactic-like reactions have been reported; may be managed with epinephrine, corticosteroids, and/or antihistamines. Should be administered under the supervision of an experienced cancer chemotherapy physician.**

Adverse Reactions

>10%:

Central nervous system: Neurotoxicity: Peripheral neuropathy is dose- and duration-dependent.

Dermatologic: Mild alopecia

Gastrointestinal: Nausea and vomiting (76% to 100%)

Hematologic: Myelosuppression (25% to 30%; mild with moderate doses, mild to moderate with high-dose therapy)

WBC: Mild
Platelets: Mild
Onset: 10 days
Nadir: 14-23 days
Recovery: 21-39 days
Hepatic: Liver enzymes increased
Renal: Nephrotoxicity (acute renal failure and chronic renal insufficiency)
Otic: Ototoxicity (10% to 30%; manifested as high frequency hearing loss; ototoxicity is especially pronounced in children)

1% to 10%:
Gastrointestinal: Diarrhea
Local: Tissue irritation

<1% (Limited to important or life-threatening): Anaphylactic reaction, arrhythmias, blurred vision, bradycardia, cerebral blindness, hemolytic anemia, liver enzymes increased, mild alopecia, mouth sores, optic neuritis, papilledema

BMT:
Central nervous system: Peripheral and autonomic neuropathy, ototoxicity
Endocrine & metabolic: Hypokalemia, hypomagnesemia
Gastrointestinal: Highly emetogenic
Hematologic: Myelosuppression
Renal: Acute renal failure, increased serum creatinine, azotemia
Miscellaneous: Transient pain at tumor, transient autoimmune disorders

Drug Interactions

Avoid Concomitant Use

Avoid concomitant use of CISplatin with any of the following: Natalizumab; Vaccines (Live)

Increased Effect/Toxicity

CISplatin may increase the levels/effects of: Aminoglycosides; Natalizumab; Taxane Derivatives; Topotecan; Vaccines (Live); Vinorelbine

The levels/effects of CISplatin may be increased by: Trastuzumab

Decreased Effect

CISplatin may decrease the levels/effects of: Vaccines (Inactivated)

The levels/effects of CISplatin may be decreased by: Echinacea

Ethanol/Nutrition/Herb Interactions Herb/Nutraceutical: Avoid black cohosh, dong quai in estrogen-dependent tumors.

Stability

Store intact vials at room temperature of 15°C to 25°C (59°F to 77°F); protect from light. Do not refrigerate solution, a precipitate may form. Further dilution **stability is dependent on the chloride ion concentration** and should be mixed in solutions of NS (at least 0.3% NaCl). Further dilutions in NS, D_5/0.45% NaCl or D_5/NS to a concentration of 0.05-2 mg/mL are stable for 72 hours at 4°C to 25°C. The infusion solution should have a final sodium chloride concentration ≥0.2%.

After initial entry into the vial, solution is stable for 28 days protected from light or for at least 7 days under fluorescent room light at room temperature.

Standard I.V. dilution: Dose/250-1000 mL NS, D_5/NS, or D_5/0.45% NaCl

Mechanism of Action Inhibits DNA synthesis by the formation of DNA cross-links; denatures the double helix; covalently binds to DNA bases and disrupts DNA function; may also bind to proteins; the *cis*-isomer is 14 times more cytotoxic than the *trans*-isomer; both forms cross-link DNA but cis-platinum is less easily recognized by cell enzymes and, therefore, not repaired. Cisplatin can also bind two adjacent guanines on the same strand of DNA producing intrastrand cross-linking and breakage.

Pharmacodynamics/Kinetics

Distribution: I.V.: Rapidly into tissue; high concentrations in kidneys, liver, ovaries, uterus, and lungs
Protein binding: >90%
Metabolism: Nonenzymatic; inactivated (in both cell and bloodstream) by sulfhydryl groups; covalently binds to glutathione and thiosulfate
Half-life elimination: Initial: 20-30 minutes; Beta: 60 minutes; Terminal: ~24 hours; Secondary half-life: 44-73 hours
Excretion: Urine (>90%); feces (10%)

Dosage Refer to individual protocols. **VERIFY ANY CISPLATIN DOSE EXCEEDING 100 mg/m^2 PER COURSE.**

Children (unlabeled uses):
Intermittent dosing schedule: 37-75 mg/m^2 once every 2-3 weeks or 50-100 mg/m^2 over 4-6 hours, once every 21-28 days
Daily dosing schedule: 15-20 mg/m^2/day for 5 days every 3-4 weeks
Osteogenic sarcoma or neuroblastoma: 60-100 mg/m^2 on day 1 every 3-4 weeks
Recurrent brain tumors: 60 mg/m^2 once daily for 2 consecutive days every 3-4 weeks
Bone marrow/blood cell transfusion: Continuous Infusion: High dose: 55 mg/m^2/day for 72 hours; total dose = 165 mg/m^2

Adults:
Advanced bladder cancer: 50-70 mg/m^2 every 3-4 weeks
Head and neck cancer (unlabeled use): 100-120 mg/m^2 every 3-4 weeks
Malignant pleural mesothelioma in combination with pemetrexed: 75 mg/m^2 on day 1 of each 21-day cycle; see Pemetrexed monograph for additional details
Metastatic ovarian cancer: 75-100 mg/m^2 every 3-4 weeks
Intraperitoneal: Cisplatin has been administered intraperitoneal with systemic sodium thiosulfate for ovarian cancer; doses up to 90-270 mg/m^2 have been administered and retained for 4 hours before draining
Testicular cancer: 10-20 mg/m^2/day for 5 days repeated every 3-4 weeks

Dosing adjustment in renal impairment: Note: The manufacturer(s) recommend that repeat courses of cisplatin should not be given until serum creatinine is <1.5 mg/dL and/or BUN is <25 mg/dL. The FDA-approved labeling does not contain renal dosing adjustment guidelines. The following guidelines have been used by some clinicians:

Aronoff, 2007:
Cl_{cr} 10-50 mL/minute: Administer 75% of dose
Cl_{cr} <10 mL/minute: Administer 50% of dose
Hemodialysis: Partially cleared by hemodialysis
Administer 50% of dose posthemodialysis
Continuous ambulatory peritoneal dialysis (CAPD): Administer 50% of dose
Continuous renal replacement therapy (CRRT): Administer 75% of dose

Kintzel, 1995:
Cl_{cr} 46-60 mL/minute: Administer 75% of dose
Cl_{cr} 31-45 mL/minute: Administer 50% of dose
Cl_{cr} <30 mL/minute: Consider use of alternative drug

Dietary Considerations Sodium content: 9 mg/mL (equivalent to 0.9% sodium chloride solution)

Administration Pretreatment hydration with 1-2 L of fluid is recommended prior to cisplatin administration; adequate hydration and urinary output (>100 mL/hour) should be maintained for 24 hours after administration.

I.V.: Rate of administration has varied from a 15- to 120-minute infusion, 1 mg/minute infusion, 6- to 8-hour infusion, 24-hour infusion, or per protocol; maximum rate of infusion of 1 mg/minute in patients with CHF.

Monitoring Parameters Renal function (serum creatinine, BUN, Cl_{cr}); electrolytes (particularly magnesium, calcium, potassium) before and within 48 hours after cisplatin therapy; audiography (baseline and prior to each subsequent dose), neurologic exam (with high dose); liver function tests periodically, CBC with differential and platelet count; urine output, urinalysis

Dosage Forms Excipient information presented when available (limited, particularly for generics); consult specific product labeling.

Injection, solution [preservative free]: 1 mg/mL (50 mL, 100 mL, 200 mL)

◆ **13-*cis*-Retinoic Acid** *see* Isotretinoin *on page 825*

Citalopram (sye TAL oh pram)

U.S. Brand Names Celexa®

Canadian Brand Names Apo-Citalopram®; Celexa®; Citalopram-ODAN; CO Citalopram; CTP 30; Dom-Citalopram; Gen-Citalopram; IPG-Citalopram; JAMP-Citalopram; Mint-Citalopram; Novo-Citalopram; PHL-Citalopram; PMS-Citalopram; RAN™-Citalopram; ratio-Citalopram; Riva-Citalopram; Sandoz-Citalopram

Index Terms Citalopram Hydrobromide; Nitalapram

Pharmacologic Category Antidepressant, Selective Serotonin Reuptake Inhibitor

Additional Appendix Information

Antidepressant Agents *on page 1638*

Selective Serotonin Reuptake Inhibitors (SSRIs) Pharmacokinetics *on page 1670*

Use Treatment of depression

Unlabeled/Investigational Use Treatment of mild dementia-associated agitation in nonpsychotic patients; smoking cessation; ethanol abuse; obsessive-compulsive disorder (OCD) in children; diabetic neuropathy

Restrictions An FDA-approved medication guide concerning the use of antidepressants in children, adolescents, and young adults must be distributed when dispensing an outpatient prescription (new or refill) where this medication is to be used without direct supervision of a healthcare provider. Medication guides are available at http://www.fda.gov/cder/Offices/ODS/medication_guides.htm. Dispense to parents or guardians of children and adolescents receiving this medication.

Pregnancy Risk Factor C

Pregnancy Considerations Due to adverse effects observed in animal studies, citalopram is classified as pregnancy category C. Citalopram and its metabolites cross the human placenta. Nonteratogenic effects in the newborn following SSRI exposure late in the third trimester include respiratory distress, cyanosis, apnea, seizures, temperature instability, feeding difficulty, vomiting, hypoglycemia, hypo- or hypertonia, hyper-reflexia, jitteriness, irritability, constant crying, and tremor. An increased risk of low birth weight and lower APGAR scores have also been reported. Exposure to SSRIs after the twentieth week of gestation has been associated with persistent pulmonary hypertension of the newborn (PPHN). Adverse effects may be due to toxic effects of the SSRI or drug withdrawal without a taper. The long term effects of *in utero* SSRI exposure on infant development and behavior are not known.

Due to pregnancy-induced physiologic changes, women who are pregnant may require increased doses of citalopram to achieve euthymia. Women treated for major depression and who are euthymic prior to pregnancy are more likely to experience a relapse when medication is discontinued as compared to pregnant women who continue taking antidepressant medications. The ACOG recommends that therapy with SSRIs or SNRIs during pregnancy be individualized; treatment of depression during pregnancy should incorporate the clinical expertise of the mental health clinician, obstetrician, primary healthcare provider, and pediatrician (ACOG, 2007). If treatment during pregnancy is required, consider tapering therapy during the third trimester in order to prevent withdrawal symptoms in the infant. If this is done and the woman is considered to be at risk from her major depressive disorder, the medication can be restarted following delivery, although the dose should be readjusted to that required before pregnancy.

Lactation Enters breast milk/consider risk:benefit

Medication Safety Issues

Sound-alike/look-alike issues:

Celexa® may be confused with Celebrex®, Cerebra®, Cerebyx®, Ranexa™, Zyprexa®

Contraindications Hypersensitivity to citalopram or any component of the formulation; concomitant use with MAO inhibitors or within 2 weeks of discontinuing MAO inhibitors; concomitant use with pimozide

Warnings/Precautions **[U.S. Boxed Warning]: Antidepressants increase the risk of suicidal thinking and behavior in children, adolescents, and young adults (18-24 years of age) with major depressive disorder (MDD) and other psychiatric disorders;** consider risk prior to prescribing. Short-term studies did not show an increased risk in patients >24 years of age and showed a decreased risk in patients ≥65 years. Closely monitor patients for clinical worsening, suicidality, or unusual changes in behavior, particularly during the initial 1-2 months of therapy or during periods of dosage adjustments (increases or decreases); the patient's family or caregiver should be instructed to closely observe the patient and communicate condition with healthcare provider. A medication guide concerning the use of antidepressants should be dispensed with each prescription. **Citalopram is not FDA approved for use in children.**

The possibility of a suicide attempt is inherent in major depression and may persist until remission occurs. Use caution in high-risk patients. Worsening depression and severe abrupt suicidality that are not part of the presenting symptoms may require discontinuation or modification of drug therapy. The patient's family or caregiver should be alerted to monitor patients for the emergence of suicidality and associated behaviors (such as agitation, irritability, hostility, impulsivity, and hypomania) and call healthcare provider.

May worsen psychosis in some patients or precipitate a shift to mania or hypomania in patients with bipolar disorder. Patients presenting with depressive symptoms should be screened for bipolar disorder. Monotherapy in patients with bipolar disorder should be avoided. **Citalopram is not FDA approved for the treatment of bipolar depression.**

The potential for severe reaction exists when used with MAO inhibitors, SSRIs/SNRIs or triptans; serotonin syndrome (hyperthermia, muscular rigidity, mental status changes/agitation, and autonomic instability) may occur. Concurrent use with MAO inhibitors is contraindicated. May increase the risks associated with electroconvulsive therapy. Has a low potential to impair cognitive or motor performance; caution operating hazardous machinery or driving.

Use with caution in patients with hepatic or renal dysfunction, in elderly patients, concomitant CNS depressants, and pregnancy (high doses of citalopram have been associated with teratogenicity in animals). Use caution with concomitant use of aspirin, NSAIDs, warfarin, or other drugs that affect coagulation; the risk of bleeding may be potentiated. May cause hyponatremia/SIADH (elderly at increased risk); volume depletion and diuretics may increase risk. May cause or exacerbate sexual dysfunction. Upon discontinuation of citalopram therapy, gradually taper dose. If intolerable symptoms occur following a decrease in dosage or upon discontinuation of therapy, then resuming the previous dose with a more gradual taper should be considered.

Adverse Reactions

>10%:

Central nervous system: Somnolence (18%; dose related), insomnia (15%; dose related)

Gastrointestinal: Nausea (21%), xerostomia (20%)

Miscellaneous: Diaphoresis (11%; dose related)

1% to 10%:

Cardiovascular: Heart rate decreased, postural hypotension, tachycardia

Central nervous system: Fatigue (5%; dose related), anorexia (4%), anxiety (4%), agitation (3%), fever (2%), yawning (2%; dose related), amnesia, apathy, concentration impaired, confusion, depression, migraine, suicide attempt

Dermatologic: Rash, pruritus

Endocrine & metabolic: Libido decreased (1% to 4%), dysmenorrhea (3%), amenorrhea, sexual dysfunction

Gastrointestinal: Diarrhea (8%), dyspepsia (5%), vomiting (4%), abdominal pain (3%), flatulence, salivation increased, taste perversion, weight gain/loss

Genitourinary: Ejaculation disorder (6%), impotence (3%; dose related), polyuria

Neuromuscular & skeletal: Tremor (8%), arthralgia (2%), myalgia (2%), paresthesia

Ocular: Abnormal accommodation

Respiratory: Rhinitis (5%), upper respiratory tract infection (5%), sinusitis (3%), cough

<1% (Limited to important or life threatening): Acute renal failure, aggressiveness, akathisia, alkaline phosphatase increased, allergic reaction, alopecia, anaphylaxis, anemia, angina pectoris, angioedema, ataxia, cardiac failure, cerebral vascular accident, chest pain, choreoathetosis, delirium, dyskinesia, dyspnea, dystonia, ecchymosis, eczema, edema (extremities), epidermal necrolysis, epistaxis, erythema multiforme, extrapyramidal symptoms, extrasystoles, gastrointestinal hemorrhage, glaucoma, grand mal seizure, hallucinations, hemolytic anemia, hepatic necrosis, hypertension, hyponatremia, leukocytosis, leukopenia, liver enzymes increased, lymphadenopathy, muscle weakness, myocardial infarction, myoclonus, neuralgia, neuroleptic malignant syndrome, nystagmus, pancreatitis, photosensitivity, priapism, prolactinemia, prothrombin decreased, purpura, QT prolonged, rhabdomyolysis, rigors, serotonin syndrome, SIADH, spontaneous abortion, thrombocytopenia, thrombosis, tinnitus, torsade de pointes, urinary incontinence, urinary retention, urticaria, ventricular arrhythmia, withdrawal syndrome

Drug Interactions

Metabolism/Transport Effects Substrate of CYP2C19 (major), 2D6 (minor), 3A4 (major); **Inhibits** CYP1A2 (weak), 2B6 (weak), 2C19 (weak), 2D6 (weak)

Avoid Concomitant Use

Avoid concomitant use of Citalopram with any of the following: Iobenguane I 123; MAO Inhibitors; Pimozide; Sibutramine

Increased Effect/Toxicity

Citalopram may increase the levels/effects of: Alcohol (Ethyl); Alpha-/Beta-Blockers; Anticoagulants; Antidepressants (Serotonin Reuptake Inhibitor/Antagonist); Antiplatelet Agents; Aspirin; Beta-Blockers; BusPIRone; CarBAMazepine; Clozapine; CNS Depressants; Desmopressin; Dextromethorphan; Drotrecogin Alfa; Haloperidol; Ibritumomab; Lithium; Methadone; Mexiletine; NSAID (COX-2 Inhibitor); NSAID (Nonselective); Phenytoin; Pimozide; Propafenone; Risperidone; Salicylates; Serotonin Modulators; Thrombolytic Agents; Tositumomab and Iodine I 131 Tositumomab; TraMADol; Tricyclic Antidepressants; Vitamin K Antagonists

The levels/effects of Citalopram may be increased by: Analgesics (Opioid); BusPIRone; Cimetidine; CYP2C19 Inhibitors (Moderate); CYP2C19 Inhibitors (Strong); CYP3A4 Inhibitors (Moderate); CYP3A4 Inhibitors (Strong); Dasatinib; Herbs (Anticoagulant/Antiplatelet Properties); Macrolide Antibiotics; MAO Inhibitors; Omega-3-Acid Ethyl Esters; Pentosan Polysulfate Sodium; Prostacyclin Analogues; Sibutramine; TraMADol; Tryptophan

Decreased Effect

Citalopram may decrease the levels/effects of: Iobenguane I 123

The levels/effects of Citalopram may be decreased by: CarBAMazepine; CYP2C19 Inducers (Strong); CYP3A4 Inducers (Strong); Cyproheptadine; Deferasirox; Herbs (CYP3A4 Inducers)

Ethanol/Nutrition/Herb Interactions

Ethanol: Avoid ethanol (may increase CNS depression).

Herb/Nutraceutical: Avoid valerian, St John's wort, SAMe, kava kava, and gotu kola (may increase CNS depression).

Stability Store at 25°C (77°F); excursions permitted to 15°C to 30°C (59°F to 86°F).

Mechanism of Action A racemic bicyclic phthalane derivative, citalopram selectively inhibits serotonin reuptake in the presynaptic neurons and has minimal effects on norepinephrine or dopamine. Uptake inhibition of serotonin is primarily due to the *S*-enantiomer of citalopram. Displays little to no affinity for serotonin, dopamine, adrenergic, histamine, GABA, or muscarinic receptor subtypes.

Pharmacodynamics/Kinetics

Onset of action: Depression: The onset of action is within a week, however, individual response varies greatly and full response may not be seen until 8-12 weeks after initiation of treatment.

Distribution: V_d: 12 L/kg

Protein binding, plasma: ~80%

Metabolism: Extensively hepatic, via CYP3A4 and 2C19 (major pathways), and 2D6 (minor pathway); forms metabolites, N-demethylcitalopram (DCT) and didemethylcitalopram (DDCT) which are at least eight times less potent than citalopram

Bioavailability: 80%

Half-life elimination: 24-48 hours (average: 35 hours); doubled with hepatic impairment

Time to peak, serum: 1-6 hours, average within 4 hours

Excretion: Urine (Citalopram 10% and DCT 5%)

Note: Clearance was decreased, while AUC and half-life were significantly increased in elderly patients and in patients with hepatic impairment. Mild-to-moderate renal impairment may reduce clearance (17%) and prolong half-life of citalopram. No pharmacokinetic information is available concerning patients with severe renal impairment.

Dosage Oral:

Children and Adolescents: Obsessive-compulsive disorder (unlabeled use): 10-40 mg/day

Adults: Depression: Initial: 20 mg/day, generally with an increase to 40 mg/day; doses of more than 40 mg are not usually necessary. Should a dose increase be necessary, it should occur in 20 mg increments at intervals of no less than 1 week. Maximum dose: 60 mg/day; reduce dosage in elderly or those with hepatic impairment.

Elderly:

Depression: Initial: 20 mg once daily; increase dose to 40 mg/day in nonresponsive patients

Alzheimer's dementia-related depression (unlabeled use): Initial: 5-10 mg/day; may increase at multi-week intervals to maximum of 40 mg/day

Dosage adjustment in renal impairment:
Mild-to-moderate impairment: No dosage adjustment needed
Severe impairment: Cl_{cr} <20 mL/minute: Use with caution
Dosage adjustment in hepatic impairment: 20 mg once daily; increase dose to 40 mg/day in nonresponsive patients
Dietary Considerations May be taken without regard to food.
Monitoring Parameters Monitor patient periodically for symptom resolution; mental status for depression, suicidal ideation (especially at the beginning of therapy or when doses are increased or decreased), anxiety, social functioning, mania, panic attacks; akathisia
Dosage Forms Excipient information presented when available (limited, particularly for generics); consult specific product labeling.
Solution, oral: 10 mg/5 mL (240 mL)
Celexa®: 10 mg/5 mL (240 mL) [alcohol free, sugar free; contains propylene glycol; peppermint flavor]
Tablet: 10 mg, 20 mg, 40 mg
Celexa®: 10 mg, 20 mg, 40 mg

- ◆ **Citalopram Hydrobromide** *see* Citalopram *on page 337*
- ◆ **Citalopram-ODAN (Can)** *see* Citalopram *on page 337*
- ◆ **Citracal® Kosher [OTC]** *see* Calcium Citrate *on page 241*
- ◆ **Citrate of Magnesia** *see* Magnesium Citrate *on page 914*
- ◆ **Citric Acid and Potassium Citrate** *see* Potassium Citrate and Citric Acid *on page 1218*

Citric Acid, Sodium Citrate, and Potassium Citrate
(SIT rik AS id, SOW dee um SIT rate, & poe TASS ee um SIT rate)

U.S. Brand Names Cytra-3; Polycitra®; Polycitra®-LC; Tricitrates
Index Terms Potassium Citrate, Citric Acid, and Sodium Citrate; Sodium Citrate, Citric Acid, and Potassium Citrate
Pharmacologic Category Alkalinizing Agent, Oral
Use Conditions where long-term maintenance of an alkaline urine is desirable as in control and dissolution of uric acid and cystine calculi of the urinary tract
Pregnancy Risk Factor Not established
Dosage Oral:
Children: 5-15 mL diluted in water after meals and at bedtime
Adults: 15-30 mL diluted in water after meals and at bedtime
Additional Information Complete prescribing information for this medication should be consulted for additional detail.
Dosage Forms Excipient information presented when available (limited, particularly for generics); consult specific product labeling.
Solution, oral:
Cytra-3: Citric acid 334 mg, sodium citrate 500 mg, and potassium citrate 550 mg per 5 mL (480 mL) [equivalent to potassium 1 mEq, sodium 1 mEq, and bicarbonate 2 mEq per 1 mL; alcohol free, sugar free; contains sodium benzoate and propylene glycol; raspberry flavor]
Polycitra®-LC: Citric acid 334 mg, sodium citrate 500 mg, and potassium citrate 550 mg per 5 mL (480 mL) [equivalent to potassium 1 mEq, sodium 1 mEq, and bicaronate 2 mEq per 1 mL; alcohol free, sugar free]
Tricitrates: Citric acid 334 mg, sodium citrate 500 mg, and potassium citrate 550 mg per 5 mL (480 mL) [equivalent to potassium 1 mEq, sodium 1 mEq, and bicaronate 2 mEq per 1 mL; alcohol free; contains sodium benzoate; raspberry flavor]
Tricitrates: Citric acid 334 mg, sodium citrate 500 mg, and potassium citrate 550 mg per 5 mL (15 mL, 30 mL, 480 mL) [equivalent to potassium 1 mEq, sodium 1 mEq, and bicaronate 2 mEq per 1 mL; alcohol free, sugar free; contains sodiuim benzoate and propylene glycol; raspberry flavor]
Syrup, oral:
Polycitra®: Citric acid 334 mg, sodium citrate 500 mg, and potassium citrate 550 mg per 5 mL (480 mL) [equivalent to potassium 1 mEq, sodium 1 mEq and bicarbonate 2 mEq per 1 mL; alcohol free]

- ◆ **Citroma® [OTC]** *see* Magnesium Citrate *on page 914*
- ◆ **Citro-Mag® (Can)** *see* Magnesium Citrate *on page 914*
- ◆ **Citrovorum Factor** *see* Leucovorin Calcium *on page 866*
- ◆ **CL-118,532** *see* Triptorelin *on page 1523*
- ◆ **Cl-719** *see* Gemfibrozil *on page 687*
- ◆ **CL-184116** *see* Porfimer *on page 1212*
- ◆ **CL-232315** *see* Mitoxantrone *on page 1007*

Cladribine (KLA dri been)

U.S. Brand Names Leustatin®
Canadian Brand Names Leustatin®
Index Terms 2-CdA; 2-Chlorodeoxyadenosine; NSC-105014
Pharmacologic Category Antineoplastic Agent, Antimetabolite; Antineoplastic Agent, Antimetabolite (Purine Antagonist)
Use Treatment of hairy cell leukemia
Unlabeled/Investigational Use Treatment of chronic lymphocytic leukemia (CLL), chronic myelogenous leukemia (CML), non-Hodgkin's lymphomas, progressive multiple sclerosis
Pregnancy Risk Factor D
Pregnancy Considerations Teratogenic effects and fetal mortality were observed in animal studies. There are no adequate and well-controlled studies in pregnant women. Women of childbearing potential should avoid becoming pregnant.
Lactation Excretion in breast milk unknown/not recommended
Medication Safety Issues
Sound-alike/look-alike issues:
Cladribine may be confused with cleVIDipine, clofarabine, fludarabine
Leustatin® may be confused with lovastatin

High alert medication: The Institute for Safe Medication Practices (ISMP) includes this medication among its list of drugs which have a heightened risk of causing significant patient harm when used in error.
Contraindications Hypersensitivity to cladribine or any component of the formulation
Warnings/Precautions Hazardous agent - use appropriate precautions for handling and disposal. **[U.S. Boxed Warnings]: Dose-dependent, reversible myelosuppression will occur; use with caution in patients with pre-existing hematologic or immunologic abnormalities. Neurologic toxicity has been reported, usually with higher doses, but may occur at normal doses. Acute renal toxicity has been reported with high doses; use caution when administering with other nephrotoxic agents.** Use caution with renal or hepatic impairment. Fever may occur, with or without neutropenia. Use caution in patients with high tumor burden; tumor lysis syndrome may occur. **[U.S. Boxed Warning]: Should be administered under the supervision of an experienced cancer chemotherapy physician.** Safety and efficacy in children have not been established.

Adverse Reactions

>10%:

Central nervous system: Fever (69%; ≥104°F: 11%), fatigue (11% to 45%), headache (7% to 22%)

Dermatologic: Rash (10% to 27%)

Gastrointestinal: Nausea (28%), appetite decreased (17%), vomiting (13%)

Hematologic: Myelosuppression, common, dose limiting (nadir: 5-10 days, recovery: 4-8 weeks); neutropenia (70%); anemia (37%); thrombocytopenia (12%)

Local: Injection site reactions (9% to 19%)

Respiratory: Abnormal breath sounds (11%)

Miscellaneous: Infection (28%)

1% to 10%:

Cardiovascular: Edema (6%), tachycardia (6%), thrombosis (2%)

Central nervous system: Dizziness (9%), chills (9%), insomnia (7%), malaise (5% to 7%), pain (6%)

Dermatologic: Purpura (10%), petechiae (8%), pruritus (6%), erythema (6%)

Gastrointestinal: Diarrhea (10%), constipation (9%), abdominal pain (6%)

Local: Phlebitis (2%)

Neuromuscular & skeletal: Weakness (9%), myalgia (7%), arthralgia (5%)

Respiratory: Cough (7% to 10%), abnormal chest sounds (9%), dyspnea (7%), epistaxis (5%)

Miscellaneous: Diaphoresis (9%)

<1% (Limited to important or life-threatening): Aplastic anemia, bilirubin increased, hemolytic anemia, hypereosinophilia, myelodysplastic syndrome, neurologic toxicity, opportunistic infections, pancytopenia, paraparesis, pneumonia, polyneuropathy (with high doses), pulmonary interstitial infiltrates, quadriplegia (reported at high doses); renal dysfunction (with high doses), Stevens-Johnson syndrome, toxic epidermal necrolysis, transaminases increased, tumor lysis syndrome, urticaria

Drug Interactions

Avoid Concomitant Use

Avoid concomitant use of Cladribine with any of the following: Natalizumab; Vaccines (Live)

Increased Effect/Toxicity

Cladribine may increase the levels/effects of: Natalizumab; Vaccines (Live)

The levels/effects of Cladribine may be increased by: Trastuzumab

Decreased Effect

Cladribine may decrease the levels/effects of: Vaccines (Inactivated)

The levels/effects of Cladribine may be decreased by: Echinacea

Ethanol/Nutrition/Herb Interactions Ethanol: Avoid ethanol (due to GI irritation).

Stability Store intact vials under refrigeration 2°C to 8°C (36°F to 46°F); protect from light. Dilutions in 500 mL NS are stable for 72 hours. Stable in PVC containers for 24 hours at room temperature of 15°C to 30°C (59°F to 86°F) and 7 days in Pharmacia Deltec® cassettes. Dilute in 500 mL; dilute to a total volume of 100 mL for 7-day infusion. Solutions for 7-day infusion should be prepared in bacteriostatic NS. The manufacturer recommends filtering with a 0.22 micron filter when preparing 7-day infusions.

Mechanism of Action A purine nucleoside analogue; prodrug which is activated via phosphorylation by deoxycytidine kinase to a 5'-triphosphate derivative. This active form incorporates into DNA to result in the breakage of DNA strand and shutdown of DNA synthesis. This also results in a depletion of nicotinamide adenine dinucleotide and adenosine triphosphate (ATP). Cladribine is cell-cycle nonspecific.

Pharmacodynamics/Kinetics

Absorption: Oral: 55%; SubQ: 100%; Rectal: 20%

Distribution: V_d: 4.52 ± 2.82 L/kg

Protein binding: 20%

Metabolism: Hepatic; 5'-triphosphate moiety-active

Half-life elimination: Biphasic: Alpha: 25 minutes; Beta: 6.7 hours; Terminal, mean: Normal renal function: 5.4 hours

Excretion: Urine (18% to 44%)

Clearance: Estimated systemic: 640 mL/hour/kg

Dosage I.V.: Refer to individual protocols.

Children (unlabeled use): Acute leukemias: 6.2-7.5 mg/m^2/day continuous infusion for days 1-5; maximum tolerated dose was 8.9 mg/m^2/day.

Adults:

Hairy cell leukemia: Continuous infusion:

0.09 mg/kg/day days 1-7; may be repeated every 28-35 days **or**

3.4 mg/m^2/day SubQ days 1-7 (unlabeled dose)

Chronic lymphocytic leukemia (unlabeled use): Continuous infusion:

0.1 mg/kg/day days 1-7 **or**

0.028-0.14 mg/kg/day as a 2-hour infusion days 1-5

Chronic myelogenous leukemia (unlabeled use): 15 mg/m^2/day as a 1-hour infusion days 1-5; if no response, increase dose to 20 mg/m^2/day in the second course.

Dosing adjustment in renal impairment: The FDA-approved labeling recommends that caution should be used in patients with renal impairment; however, no specific dosage adjustment guidelines are available due to lack of data. The following guidelines have been used by some clinicians (Aronoff, 2007):

Children:

Cl_{cr} 10-50 mL/minute: Administer 50% of dose

Cl_{cr} <10 mL/minute: Administer 30% of dose

Hemodialysis: Administer 30% of dose

Continuous renal replacement therapy (CRRT): Administer 50% of dose

Adults:

Cl_{cr} 10-50 mL/minute: Administer 75% of dose

Cl_{cr} <10 mL/minute: Administer 50% of dose

Continuous ambulatory peritoneal dialysis (CAPD): Administer 50% of dose

Dosing adjustment in hepatic impairment: The FDA-approved labeling recommends that caution should be used in patients with hepatic impairment; however, no specific dosage adjustment guidelines are available due to lack of data.

Administration I.V.: Administer as a 1- to 2-hour infusion or by continuous infusion

Monitoring Parameters CBC with differential, renal and hepatic function; monitor for fever

Periodic assessment of peripheral blood counts, particularly during the first 4-8 weeks post-treatment, is recommended to detect the development of anemia, neutropenia, and thrombocytopenia and for early detection of any potential sequelae (eg, infection or bleeding)

Dosage Forms Excipient information presented when available (limited, particularly for generics); consult specific product labeling.

Injection, solution [preservative free]: 1 mg/mL (10 mL)

◆ **Claforan®** *see* Cefotaxime *on page* 276

◆ **Claravis™** *see* Isotretinoin *on page* 825

◆ **Clarifoam™ EF** *see* Sulfur and Sulfacetamide *on page* 1411

◆ **Clarinex®** *see* Desloratadine *on page* 420

◆ **Clarinex-D® 12 Hour** *see* Desloratadine and Pseudoephedrine *on page* 421

◆ **Clarinex-D® 24 Hour** *see* Desloratadine and Pseudoephedrine *on page* 421

◆ **Claripel™ [DSC]** *see* Hydroquinone *on page* 749

Clarithromycin (kla RITH roe mye sin)

U.S. Brand Names Biaxin®; Biaxin® XL

Canadian Brand Names Apo-Clarithromycin; Biaxin®; Biaxin® XL; Gen-Clarithromycin; PMS-Clarithromycin; ratio-Clarithromycin; Sandoz-Clarithromycin

Pharmacologic Category Antibiotic, Macrolide

Additional Appendix Information

Antimicrobial Drugs of Choice *on page 1752*
Community-Acquired Pneumonia in Adults *on page 1766*
Guidelines for the Prevention of Opportunistic Infections in HIV Infected Persons *on page 1740*
Helicobacter pylori Treatment *on page 1813*
Prevention of Infective Endocarditis *on page 1736*

Use

Children:

- Acute otitis media (*H. influenzae, M. catarrhalis*, or *S. pneumoniae*)
- Community-acquired pneumonia due to susceptible *Mycoplasma pneumoniae, S. pneumoniae*, or *Chlamydia pneumoniae* (TWAR)
- Pharyngitis/tonsillitis due to susceptible *S. pyogenes*, acute maxillary sinusitis due to susceptible *H. influenzae, S. pneumoniae*, or *Moraxella catarrhalis*, uncomplicated skin/skin structure infections due to susceptible *S. aureus, S. pyogenes*, and mycobacterial infections
- Prevention of disseminated mycobacterial infections due to MAC disease in patients with advanced HIV infection

Adults:

- Pharyngitis/tonsillitis due to susceptible *S. pyogenes*
- Acute maxillary sinusitis and acute exacerbation of chronic bronchitis due to susceptible *H. influenzae, H. parainfluenzae, M. catarrhalis*, or *S. pneumoniae*
- Community-acquired pneumonia due to susceptible *H. influenzae, H. parainfluenzae, Mycoplasma pneumoniae, S. pneumoniae*, or *Chlamydia pneumoniae* (TWAR), *Moraxella catarrhalis*
- Uncomplicated skin/skin structure infections due to susceptible *S. aureus, S. pyogenes*
- Disseminated mycobacterial infections due to *M. avium* or *M. intracellulare*
- Prevention of disseminated mycobacterial infections due to *M. avium* complex (MAC) disease (eg, patients with advanced HIV infection)
- Duodenal ulcer disease due to *H. pylori* in regimens with other drugs including amoxicillin and lansoprazole or omeprazole, ranitidine bismuth citrate, bismuth subsalicylate, tetracycline, and/or an H_2 antagonist

Unlabeled/Investigational Use Pertussis (CDC guidelines); alternate antibiotic for prophylaxis of infective endocarditis in patients who are allergic to penicillin and undergoing surgical or dental procedures (ACC/AHA guidelines)

Pregnancy Risk Factor C

Pregnancy Considerations Clarithromycin crosses the placenta. Although no teratogenic effects have been reported in humans, adverse fetal effects have been documented in animal studies; therefore, clarithromycin is classified as pregnancy category C. The manufacturer recommends that clarithromycin not be used in a pregnant woman unless there are no alternative therapies. No adequate and well-controlled studies have been completed in pregnant women.

Lactation Excretion in breast milk unknown/use caution

Medication Safety Issues

Sound-alike/look-alike issues:

Clarithromycin may be confused with Claritin®, clindamycin, erythromycin

Contraindications Hypersensitivity to clarithromycin, erythromycin, or any macrolide antibiotic; use with ergot derivatives, pimozide, cisapride

Warnings/Precautions Dosage adjustment required with severe renal impairment; decreased dosage or prolonged dosing interval may be appropriate. Use with caution in patients with myasthenia gravis. Colchicine toxicity (including fatalities) has been reported with concomitant use. Prolonged use may result in fungal or bacterial superinfection, including *C. difficile*-associated diarrhea (CDAD) and pseudomembranous colitis; CDAD has been observed >2 months postantibiotic treatment. Macrolides (including clarithromycin) have been associated with rare QT prolongation and ventricular arrhythmias, including torsade de pointes. Use caution in patients with coronary artery disease. Avoid use of extended release tablets (Biaxin® XL) in patients with known stricture/narrowing of the GI tract. Safety and efficacy in children <6 months of age have not been established.

Adverse Reactions

1% to 10%:

- Central nervous system: Headache (adults and children 2%)
- Dermatologic: Rash (children 3%)
- Gastrointestinal: Abnormal taste (adults 3% to 7%), diarrhea (adults 3% to 6%; children 6%), vomiting (children 6%), nausea (adults 3%), abdominal pain (adults 2%; children 3%), dyspepsia (adults 2%)
- Hepatic: Prothrombin time increased (1%)
- Renal: BUN increased (4%)

<1% (Limited to important or life-threatening): *Clostridium difficile* colitis, alkaline phosphatase increased, anaphylaxis, anorexia, anxiety, behavioral changes, bilirubin increased, confusion, disorientation, GGT increased, glossitis, hallucinations, hearing loss (reversible), hepatic dysfunction, hepatic failure, hepatitis, hypoglycemia, insomnia, interstitial nephritis, jaundice, leukopenia, manic behavior, neutropenia, oral moniliasis, pancreatitis, psychosis, QT prolongation, seizure, serum creatinine increased, Stevens-Johnson syndrome, stomatitis, thrombocytopenia, tinnitus, tongue discoloration, tooth discoloration (reversible), torsade de pointes, toxic epidermal necrolysis, transaminases increased, tremor, urticaria, ventricular tachycardia, ventricular arrhythmia, vertigo

Drug Interactions

Metabolism/Transport Effects Substrate of CYP3A4 (major); **Inhibits** CYP1A2 (weak), 3A4 (strong)

Avoid Concomitant Use

Avoid concomitant use of Clarithromycin with any of the following: Alfuzosin; Cisapride; Dabigatran Etexilate; Disopyramide; Nilotinib; Pimozide; Ranolazine; Rivaroxaban; Salmeterol; Silodosin; Tetrabenazine; Thioridazine; Topotecan; Ziprasidone

Increased Effect/Toxicity

Clarithromycin may increase the levels/effects of: Alfentanil; Alfuzosin; Alosetron; Antifungal Agents (Azole Derivatives, Systemic); Benzodiazepines (metabolized by oxidation); BusPIRone; Calcium Channel Blockers; CarBAMazepine; Cardiac Glycosides; Ciclesonide; Cilostazol; Cisapride; Clozapine; Colchicine; Corticosteroids (Systemic); CycloSPORINE; CYP3A4 Substrates; Dabigatran Etexilate; Disopyramide; Eletriptan; Eplerenone; Ergot Derivatives; FentaNYL; Fesoterodine; HMG-CoA Reductase Inhibitors; Ixabepilone; Maraviroc; Nilotinib; P-Glycoprotein Substrates; Phosphodiesterase 5 Inhibitors; Pimecrolimus; Pimozide; Protease Inhibitors; QTc-Prolonging Agents; QuiNIDine; Ranolazine; Repaglinide; Rifamycin Derivatives; Rivaroxaban; Salmeterol; Selective Serotonin Reuptake Inhibitors; Silodosin; Sirolimus; Sorafenib; Tacrolimus; Temsirolimus; Tetrabenazine; Theophylline Derivatives; Thioridazine; Topotecan; Vitamin K Antagonists; Ziprasidone; Zopiclone

The levels/effects of Clarithromycin may be increased by: Alfuzosin; Antifungal Agents (Azole Derivatives, Systemic); Ciprofloxacin; CYP3A4 Inhibitors (Moderate);

CYP3A4 Inhibitors (Strong); Dasatinib; Gadobutrol; Nilotinib; Protease Inhibitors

Decreased Effect

Clarithromycin may decrease the levels/effects of: Clopidogrel; Typhoid Vaccine

The levels/effects of Clarithromycin may be decreased by: CYP3A4 Inducers (Strong); Deferasirox; Etravirine; Herbs (CYP3A4 Inducers); Protease Inhibitors

Ethanol/Nutrition/Herb Interactions

Food: Immediate release: Food delays rate, but not extent of absorption; Extended release: Food increases clarithromycin AUC by ~30% relative to fasting conditions.

Herb/Nutraceutical: St John's wort may decrease clarithromycin levels.

Stability Store tablets and granules for oral suspension at controlled room temperature. Reconstituted oral suspension should not be refrigerated because it might gel; microencapsulated particles of clarithromycin in suspension is stable for 14 days when stored at room temperature

Mechanism of Action Exerts its antibacterial action by binding to 50S ribosomal subunit resulting in inhibition of protein synthesis. The 14-OH metabolite of clarithromycin is twice as active as the parent compound against certain organisms.

Pharmacodynamics/Kinetics

Absorption: Immediate release: Rapid; food delays rate, but not extent of absorption

Distribution: Widely into most body tissues except CNS

Protein binding: 42% to 50%

Metabolism: Partially hepatic via CYP3A4; converted to 14-OH clarithromycin (active metabolite)

Bioavailability: ~50%

Half-life elimination: Immediate release: Clarithromycin: 3-7 hours; 14-OH-clarithromycin: 5-9 hours

Time to peak: Immediate release: 2-3 hours

Excretion: Primarily urine (20% to 40% as unchanged drug; additional 10% to 15% as metabolite)

Clearance: Approximates normal GFR

Dosage

Usual dosage range:

Children ≥6 months: Oral: 7.5 mg/kg every 12 hours (maximum: 500 mg/dose)

Adults: Oral: 250-500 mg every 12 hours **or** 1000 mg (two 500 mg extended release tablets) once daily for 7-14 days

Indication-specific dosing:

Children: Oral:

Community-acquired pneumonia, sinusitis, bronchitis, skin infections: 15 mg/kg/day divided every 12 hours for 10 days

Mycobacterial infection (prevention and treatment): 7.5 mg/kg (up to 500 mg) twice daily. **Note:** Safety of clarithromycin for MAC not studied in children <20 months.

Pertussis (unlabeled use; CDC guidelines):

Children 1-5 months: 15 mg/kg/day divided every 12 hours for 7 days

Children ≥6 months: 15 mg/kg/day divided every 12 hours for 7 days (maximum: 1 g/day)

Prophylaxis against infective endocarditis (unlabeled use): 15 mg/kg 30-60 minutes before procedure. **Note:** American Heart Association (AHA) guidelines now recommend prophylaxis only in patients undergoing invasive procedures and in whom underlying cardiac conditions may predispose to a higher risk of adverse outcomes should infection occur. As of April 2007, routine prophylaxis for GI/GU procedures is no longer recommended by the AHA.

Adults: Oral:

Acute exacerbation of chronic bronchitis:

M. catarrhalis and *S. pneumoniae*: 250 mg every 12 hours for 7-14 days **or** 1000 mg (two 500 mg extended release tablets) once daily for 7 days

H. influenzae: 500 mg every 12 hours for 7-14 days or 1000 mg (two 500 mg extended release tablets) once daily for 7 days

H. parainfluenzae: 500 mg every 12 hours for 7 days or 1000 mg (two 500 mg extended release tablets) once daily for 7 days

Acute maxillary sinusitis: 500 mg every 12 hours **or** 1000 mg (two 500 mg extended release tablets) once daily for 14 days

Mycobacterial infection (prevention and treatment): 500 mg twice daily (use with other antimycobacterial drugs, eg, ethambutol or rifampin)

Peptic ulcer disease: Eradication of *Helicobacter pylori*: Dual or triple combination regimens with bismuth subsalicylate, amoxicillin, an H_2-receptor antagonist, or proton-pump inhibitor: 500 mg every 8-12 hours for 10-14 days

Pertussis (unlabeled use; CDC guidelines): 500 mg twice daily for 7 days

Pharyngitis, tonsillitis: 250 mg every 12 hours for 10 days

Pneumonia:

C. pneumoniae, *M. pneumoniae*, and *S. pneumoniae*: 250 mg every 12 hours for 7-14 days **or** 1000 mg (two 500 mg extended release tablets) once daily for 7 days

H. influenzae: 250 mg every 12 hours for 7 days **or** 1000 mg (two 500 mg extended release tablets) once daily for 7 days

H. parainfluenzae and *M. catarrhalis*: 1000 mg (two 500 mg extended release tablets) once daily for 7 days

Prophylaxis against infective endocarditis (unlabeled use): 500 mg 30-60 minutes prior to procedure. **Note:** American Heart Association (AHA) guidelines now recommend prophylaxis only in patients undergoing invasive procedures and in whom underlying cardiac conditions may predispose to a higher risk of adverse outcomes should infection occur. As of April 2007, routine prophylaxis for GI/GU procedures is no longer recommended by the AHA.

Skin and skin structure infection, uncomplicated: 250 mg every 12 hours for 7-14 days

Elderly: Pharmacokinetics are similar to those in younger adults; may have age-related reductions in renal function; monitor and adjust dose if necessary

Dosing adjustment in renal impairment:

Cl_{cr} <30 mL/minute: Half the normal dose or double the dosing interval

In combination with ritonavir:

Cl_{cr} 30-60 mL/minute: Decrease clarithromycin dose by 50%

Cl_{cr} <30 mL/minute: Decrease clarithromycin dose by 75%

Dosing adjustment in hepatic impairment: No dosing adjustment is needed as long as renal function is normal

Dietary Considerations Clarithromycin immediate release tablets and oral solution may be given with or without meals. May be taken with milk. Biaxin® XL should be taken with food.

Administration Clarithromycin immediate release tablets and oral solution may be given with or without meals. Give every 12 hours rather than twice daily to avoid peak and trough variation.

Biaxin® XL: Should be given with food. Do not crush or chew extended release tablet.

Monitoring Parameters CBC with differential, BUN, creatinine; perform culture and sensitivity studies prior to initiating drug therapy

Dosage Forms Excipient information presented when available (limited, particularly for generics); consult specific product labeling.

Granules for oral suspension: 125 mg/5 mL (50 mL, 100 mL); 250 mg/5 mL (50 mL, 100 mL)

Biaxin®: 125 mg/5 mL (50 mL, 100 mL); 250 mg/5 mL (50 mL, 100 mL) [fruit punch flavor]

Tablet: 250 mg, 500 mg

Biaxin®: 250 mg, 500 mg

Tablet, extended release: 500 mg

Biaxin® XL: 500 mg

◆ **Clarithromycin, Lansoprazole, and Amoxicillin** *see* Lansoprazole, Amoxicillin, and Clarithromycin *on page 855*

◆ **Claritin® (Can)** *see* Loratadine *on page 904*

◆ **Claritin® 24 Hour Allergy [OTC]** *see* Loratadine *on page 904*

◆ **Claritin-D® 12 Hour Allergy & Congestion [OTC]** *see* Loratadine and Pseudoephedrine *on page 905*

◆ **Claritin-D® 24 Hour Allergy & Congestion [OTC]** *see* Loratadine and Pseudoephedrine *on page 905*

◆ **Claritin® Children's [OTC]** *see* Loratadine *on page 904*

◆ **Claritin® Children's Allergy [OTC]** *see* Loratadine *on page 904*

◆ **Claritin® Extra (Can)** *see* Loratadine and Pseudoephedrine *on page 905*

◆ **Claritin® Hives Relief [OTC]** *see* Loratadine *on page 904*

◆ **Claritin® Kids (Can)** *see* Loratadine *on page 904*

◆ **Claritin® Liberator (Can)** *see* Loratadine and Pseudoephedrine *on page 905*

◆ **Clarus™ (Can)** *see* Isotretinoin *on page 825*

◆ **Clavulanic Acid and Amoxicillin** *see* Amoxicillin and Clavulanate Potassium *on page 100*

◆ **Clavulin® (Can)** *see* Amoxicillin and Clavulanate Potassium *on page 100*

◆ **Clear eyes® for Dry Eyes and ACR Relief [OTC]** *see* Naphazoline *on page 1040*

◆ **Clear eyes® for Dry Eyes and Redness Relief [OTC]** *see* Naphazoline *on page 1040*

◆ **Clear eyes® Redness Relief [OTC]** *see* Naphazoline *on page 1040*

◆ **Clear eyes® Seasonal Relief [OTC]** *see* Naphazoline *on page 1040*

Clemastine (KLEM as teen)

U.S. Brand Names Dayhist® Allergy [OTC]; Tavist® Allergy [OTC]

Index Terms Clemastine Fumarate

Pharmacologic Category Histamine H_1 Antagonist; Histamine H_1 Antagonist, First Generation

Use Perennial and seasonal allergic rhinitis and other allergic symptoms including urticaria

Pregnancy Risk Factor B

Lactation Enters breast milk/not recommended

Contraindications Hypersensitivity to clemastine or any component of the formulation; narrow-angle glaucoma

Warnings/Precautions Use caution with bladder neck obstruction, symptomatic prostate hypertrophy, asthmatic attacks, stenosing peptic ulcer, increased intraocular pressure, hyperthyroidism, cardiovascular disease, hypertension, and in the elderly. May cause drowsiness; use caution in performing tasks which require alertness. Effects may be potentiated when used with other sedative drugs or ethanol. Safety and efficacy have not been established in children <6 years of age.

Adverse Reactions Frequency not defined.

Cardiovascular: Palpitation, hypotension, tachycardia

Central nervous system: Dyscoordination, sedation, somnolence slight to moderate, sleepiness, confusion, restlessness, nervousness, insomnia, irritability, fatigue, headache, dizziness increased

Dermatologic: Rash, photosensitivity

Gastrointestinal: Diarrhea, nausea, xerostomia, epigastric distress, vomiting, constipation

Genitourinary: Urinary frequency, difficult urination, urinary retention

Hematologic: Hemolytic anemia, thrombocytopenia, agranulocytosis

Ocular: Blurred vision

Otic: Tinnitus

Respiratory: Thickening of bronchial secretions

Miscellaneous: Anaphylaxis

Drug Interactions

Metabolism/Transport Effects **Inhibits** CYP2D6 (weak), 3A4 (weak)

Avoid Concomitant Use There are no known interactions where it is recommended to avoid concomitant use.

Increased Effect/Toxicity

Clemastine may increase the levels/effects of: Alcohol (Ethyl); Anticholinergics; CNS Depressants

The levels/effects of Clemastine may be increased by: Pramlintide

Decreased Effect

Clemastine may decrease the levels/effects of: Acetylcholinesterase Inhibitors (Central); Betahistine

The levels/effects of Clemastine may be decreased by: Acetylcholinesterase Inhibitors (Central); Amphetamines

Ethanol/Nutrition/Herb Interactions Ethanol: Avoid ethanol (may increase CNS depression).

Mechanism of Action Competes with histamine for H_1-receptor sites on effector cells in the gastrointestinal tract, blood vessels, and respiratory tract

Pharmacodynamics/Kinetics

Onset of action: Peak effect: Therapeutic: 5-7 hours

Duration: 8-16 hours

Absorption: Almost complete

Metabolism: Hepatic

Excretion: Urine

Dosage Oral:

Infants and Children <6 years: 0.05 mg/kg/day as **clemastine base** or 0.335-0.67 mg/day clemastine fumarate (0.25-0.5 mg base/day) divided into 2 or 3 doses; maximum daily dosage: 1.34 mg (1 mg base)

Children 6-12 years: 0.67-1.34 mg clemastine fumarate (0.5-1 mg base) twice daily; do not exceed 4.02 mg/day (3 mg/day base)

Children ≥12 years and Adults:

1.34 mg clemastine fumarate (1 mg base) twice daily to 2.68 mg (2 mg base) 3 times/day; do not exceed 8.04 mg/day (6 mg base)

OTC labeling: 1.34 mg clemastine fumarate (1 mg base) twice daily; do not exceed 2 mg base/24 hours

Elderly: Lower doses should be considered in patients >60 years

Monitoring Parameters Look for a reduction of rhinitis, urticaria, eczema, pruritus, or other allergic symptoms

Dosage Forms Excipient information presented when available (limited, particularly for generics); consult specific product labeling.

Syrup, as fumarate: 0.67 mg/5 mL (120 mL, 480 mL) [prescription formulation; 0.5 mg base/5 mL]

Tablet, as fumarate: 1.34 mg [1 mg base; OTC], 2.68 mg [2 mg base; prescription formulation]

Dayhist® Allergy, Tavist® Allergy: 1.34 mg [1 mg base]

◆ **Clemastine Fumarate** *see* Clemastine *on page* *343*

◆ **Clenia™** *see* Sulfur and Sulfacetamide *on page* *1411*

◆ **Cleocin®** *see* Clindamycin *on page* *344*

◆ **Cleocin HCl®** *see* Clindamycin *on page* *344*

◆ **Cleocin Pediatric®** *see* Clindamycin *on page* *344*

◆ **Cleocin Phosphate®** *see* Clindamycin *on page* *344*

◆ **Cleocin T®** *see* Clindamycin *on page* *344*

◆ **Cleocin® Vaginal Ovule** *see* Clindamycin *on page* *344*

Clevidipine (klev ID i peen)

U.S. Brand Names Cleviprex™

Index Terms Clevidipine Butyrate

Pharmacologic Category Calcium Channel Blocker

Additional Appendix Information

Calcium Channel Blockers *on page* *1651*

Hypertension *on page* *1820*

Use Management of hypertension when oral treatment is not feasible or not desirable

Pregnancy Risk Factor C

Medication Safety Issues

Sound-alike/look-alike issues:

Clevidipine may be confused with cladribine, clofarabine, clomiPRAMINE

Cleviprex™ may be confused with Claravis™

Dosage I.V.:

Adults: Initial: 1-2 mg/hour

Titration: Initial: dose may be doubled at 90-second intervals toward blood pressure goal. As blood pressure approaches goal, dose may be increased by less than double every 5-10 minutes. **Note:** For every 1-2 mg/hour increase in dose, an approximate reduction of 2-4 mm Hg in systolic blood pressure may occur.

Usual maintenance: 4-6 mg/hour; maximum: 21 mg/hour (1000 mL within a 24-hour period). There is limited short-term experience with doses up to 32 mg/hour. Data is limited beyond 72 hours.

Elderly: Initiate at the low end of the dosage range. Specific guidelines for adjustment of clevidipine are not available, but careful monitoring is warranted.

Dosing adjustment in renal impairment: No adjustment required with initial infusion rate

Dosing adjustment in hepatic impairment: No adjustment required with initial infusion rate

Additional Information Complete prescribing information for this medication should be consulted for additional detail.

Dosage Forms Excipient information presented when available (limited, particularly for generics); consult specific product labeling.

Injection, emulsion:

Cleviprex™: 0.5 mg/mL (50 mL, 100 mL) [contains eggs, soy products]

◆ **Clevidipine Butyrate** *see* Clevidipine *on page* *344*

◆ **Cleviprex™** *see* Clevidipine *on page* *344*

Clidinium and Chlordiazepoxide

(kli DI nee um & klor dye az e POKS ide)

U.S. Brand Names Librax® *[original formulation]*

Canadian Brand Names Apo-Chlorax®; Librax®

Index Terms Chlordiazepoxide and Clidinium

Pharmacologic Category Antispasmodic Agent, Gastrointestinal; Benzodiazepine

Use Adjunct treatment of peptic ulcer; treatment of irritable bowel syndrome

Pregnancy Risk Factor D

Medication Safety Issues

Sound-alike/look-alike issues:

Librax® may be confused with Librium®

Librax® formulation may be cause for confusion:

In November 2004, Valeant Pharmaceuticals licensed the Librax® trademark to Victory Pharmaceuticals. Subsequently, the product was reformulated to contain chlordiazepoxide and methscopolamine. In January 2006, Valeant Pharmaceuticals began redistributing the original formulation of Librax®, containing clidinium and chlordiazepoxide. Victory Pharmaceuticals has discontinued their product. **Note:** The formulation of Librax® distributed in Canada (Valeant Canada Ltd) always contained clidinium and chlordiazepoxide.

Dosage Oral: 1-2 capsules 3-4 times/day, before meals or food and at bedtime

Additional Information Complete prescribing information for this medication should be consulted for additional detail.

Dosage Forms Excipient information presented when available (limited, particularly for generics); consult specific product labeling.

Capsule: Clidinium bromide 2.5 mg and chlordiazepoxide hydrochloride 5 mg

Librax® [original formulation]: Clidinium bromide 2.5 mg and chlordiazepoxide hydrochloride 5 mg

◆ **Climara®** *see* Estradiol *on page* *554*

◆ **ClimaraPro®** *see* Estradiol and Levonorgestrel *on page* *558*

◆ **Clindagel®** *see* Clindamycin *on page* *344*

◆ **ClindaMax®** *see* Clindamycin *on page* *344*

Clindamycin (klin da MYE sin)

U.S. Brand Names Cleocin HCl®; Cleocin Pediatric®; Cleocin Phosphate®; Cleocin T®; Cleocin®; Cleocin® Vaginal Ovule; Clindagel®; ClindaMax®; ClindaReach™; Clindesse™; Evoclin®

Canadian Brand Names Alti-Clindamycin; Apo-Clindamycin®; Clindamycin Injection, USP; Clindoxyl®; Dalacin® C; Dalacin® T; Dalacin® Vaginal; Gen-Clindamycin; Novo-Clindamycin; PMS-Clindamycin; ratio-Clindamycin; Riva-Clindamycin; Taro-Clindamycin

Index Terms Clindamycin Hydrochloride; Clindamycin Palmitate; Clindamycin Phosphate

Pharmacologic Category Antibiotic, Lincosamide; Topical Skin Product, Acne

Additional Appendix Information

Animal and Human Bites *on page* *1747*

Antimicrobial Drugs of Choice *on page* *1752*

Community-Acquired Pneumonia in Adults *on page* *1766*

Guidelines for the Prevention of Opportunistic Infections in HIV Infected Persons *on page* *1740*

Malaria Treatment *on page* *1770*

Prevention of Infective Endocarditis *on page* *1736*

Prevention of Wound Infection and Sepsis in Surgical Patients *on page* *1738*

Treatment of Sexually Transmitted Infections *on page* *1773*

Use Treatment of susceptible bacterial infections, mainly those caused by anaerobes, streptococci, pneumococci, and staphylococci; bacterial vaginosis (vaginal cream, vaginal suppository); pelvic inflammatory disease (I.V.); topically in treatment of severe acne; vaginally for *Gardnerella vaginalis*

Unlabeled/Investigational Use May be useful in PCP; alternate treatment for toxoplasmosis

Pregnancy Risk Factor B

Pregnancy Considerations Teratogenic effects were not observed in animal studies. There are no adequate and well-controlled studies in pregnant women.

Lactation Enters breast milk/not recommended

Medication Safety Issues

Sound-alike/look-alike issues:

Cleocin® may be confused with bleomycin, Clinoril®, Cubicin®, Lincocin®

Clindamycin may be confused with clarithromycin, Claritin®, vancomycin

Contraindications Hypersensitivity to clindamycin, lincomycin, or any component of the formulation

Topical and vaginal products: Additional contraindications: Previous pseudomembranous colitis, regional enteritis, ulcerative colitis

Warnings/Precautions Dosage adjustment may be necessary in patients with severe hepatic dysfunction. **[U.S. Boxed Warning]: Can cause severe and possibly fatal colitis.** Prolonged use may result in fungal or bacterial superinfection, including *C. difficile*-associated diarrhea (CDAD) and pseudomembranous colitis; CDAD has been observed >2 months postantibiotic treatment. Use with caution in patients with a history of gastrointestinal disease. Discontinue drug if significant diarrhea, abdominal cramps, or passage of blood and mucus occurs. Vaginal products may weaken condoms, or contraceptive diaphragms. Barrier contraceptives are not recommended concurrently or for 3-5 days (depending on the product) following treatment. Some dosage forms contain benzyl alcohol or tartrazine. Use caution in atopic patients.

Adverse Reactions

Systemic: Frequency not defined:

Cardiovascular: Cardiac arrest (rare; I.V. administration), hypotension (rare; I.V. administration)

Dermatologic: Erythema multiforme (rare), exfoliative dermatitis (rare), pruritus, rash, Stevens-Johnson syndrome (rare), urticaria

Gastrointestinal: Abdominal pain, diarrhea, esophagitis, nausea, pseudomembranous colitis, vomiting

Genitourinary: Vaginitis

Hematologic: Agranulocytosis, eosinophilia (transient), neutropenia (transient), thrombocytopenia

Hepatic: Jaundice, liver function test abnormal

Local: Induration/pain/sterile abscess (I.M.), thrombophlebitis (I.V.)

Neuromuscular & skeletal: Polyarthritis (rare)

Renal: Renal dysfunction (rare)

Miscellaneous: Anaphylactoid reactions (rare)

Topical:

>10%: Dermatologic: Dryness, burning, itching, scaliness, erythema, or peeling of skin (lotion, solution); oiliness (gel, lotion)

<1% (Limited to important or life-threatening): Pseudomembranous colitis, nausea, vomiting, diarrhea (severe), abdominal pain, folliculitis, hypersensitivity reactions

Vaginal:

>10%: Genitourinary: Vaginal candidiasis (≤13%), vulvovaginal pruritus (from *Candida albicans*)

1% to 10%:

Dermatologic: Pruritus (≤1%)

Genitourinary: Vulvovaginal disorder (3% to 7%), vulvovaginitis (4% to 6%), vaginal pain (≤2%), trichomonal vaginitis (1%)

Miscellaneous: Fungal infection (1% to 2%)

<1% (Limited to important or life-threatening): Abdominal cramps, allergic reaction, atrophic vaginitis, bacterial infection, diarrhea, dizziness, dysuria, endometriosis, epistaxis, erythema, fever, hypersensitivity, hyperthyroidism, local edema, menstrual disorder, metrorrhagia, nausea, pain, pruritus, pyelonephritis, rash, urinary tract infection, urticaria, vaginal burning, vertigo, vomiting

Drug Interactions

Avoid Concomitant Use

Avoid concomitant use of Clindamycin with any of the following: Erythromycin

Increased Effect/Toxicity

Clindamycin may increase the levels/effects of: Neuromuscular-Blocking Agents

Decreased Effect

Clindamycin may decrease the levels/effects of: Erythromycin; Typhoid Vaccine

The levels/effects of Clindamycin may be decreased by: Kaolin

Ethanol/Nutrition/Herb Interactions

Food: Peak concentrations may be delayed with food.

Herb/Nutraceutical: St John's wort may decrease clindamycin levels.

Stability

Capsule: Store at room temperature of 20°C to 25°C (68°F to 77°F).

Cream: Store at room temperature.

Foam: Store at room temperature of 20°C to 25°C (68°F to 77°F); avoid fire, flame, or smoking during or following application.

Gel: Store at room temperature.

Clindagel®: Do not store in direct sunlight.

I.V.: Infusion solution in NS or D_5W solution is stable for 16 days at room temperature, 32 days refrigerated, or 8 weeks frozen. Prior to use, store vials and premixed bags at controlled room temperature 20°C to 25°C (68°F to 77°F). After initial use, discard any unused portion of vial after 24 hours.

Lotion: Store at room temperature of 20°C to 25°C (68°F to 77°F).

Oral solution: Do not refrigerate reconstituted oral solution (it will thicken); following reconstitution, oral solution is stable for 2 weeks at room temperature of 20°C to 25°C (68°F to 77°F).

Ovule: Store at room temperature of 15°C to 30°C (68°F to 77°F).

Pledget: Store at room temperature.

Topical solution: Store at room temperature of 20°C to 25°C (68°F to 77°F).

Mechanism of Action Reversibly binds to 50S ribosomal subunits preventing peptide bond formation thus inhibiting bacterial protein synthesis; bacteriostatic or bactericidal depending on drug concentration, infection site, and organism

Pharmacodynamics/Kinetics

Absorption: Topical: ~10%; Oral: Rapid (90%)

Distribution: High concentrations in bone and urine; no significant levels in CSF, even with inflamed meninges; crosses placenta; enters breast milk

Metabolism: Hepatic

Bioavailability: Topical: <1%

Half-life elimination: Neonates: Premature: 8.7 hours; Full-term: 3.6 hours; Adults: 1.6-5.3 hours (average: 2-3 hours)

Time to peak, serum: Oral: Within 60 minutes; I.M.: 1-3 hours

Excretion: Urine (10%) and feces (~4%) as active drug and metabolites

Dosage

Usual dosage ranges:

Infants and Children:

Oral: 8-20 mg/kg/day as hydrochloride; 8-25 mg/kg/day as palmitate in 3-4 divided doses (minimum dose of palmitate: 37.5 mg 3 times/day)

I.M., I.V.:

<1 month: 15-20 mg/kg/day in 3-4 divided doses

>1 month: 20-40 mg/kg/day in 3-4 divided doses

Adults:

Oral: 150-450 mg/dose every 6-8 hours; maximum dose: 1.8 g/day

I.M., I.V.: 1.2-2.7 g/day in 2-4 divided doses; maximum dose: 4.8 g/day

Indication-specific dosing:

Children:

Anthrax: I.V.: 7.5 mg/kg every 6 hours

Babesiosis (unlabeled use): Oral: 20-40 mg/kg/day divided every 8 hours for 7 days plus quinine

Orofacial infections:

Oral: 10-20 mg/kg in 3-4 equally divided doses

I.V.: 15-25 mg/kg in 3-4 equally divided doses

Prophylaxis against infective endocarditis (unlabeled use):

Oral: 20 mg/kg 30-60 minutes before procedure

I.M., I.V.: 20 mg/kg 30-60 minutes before procedure. Intramuscular injections should be avoided in patients who are receiving anticoagulant therapy. In these circumstances, orally administered regimens should be given whenever possible. Intravenously administered antibiotics should be used for patients who are unable to tolerate or absorb oral medications.

Note: American Heart Association (AHA) guidelines now recommend prophylaxis only in patients undergoing invasive procedures and in whom underlying cardiac conditions may predispose to a higher risk of adverse outcomes should infection occur. As of April 2007, routine prophylaxis for GI/GU procedures is no longer recommended by the AHA.

Children ≥12 years and Adults:

Acne vulgaris: Topical:

Gel, pledget, lotion, solution: Apply a thin film twice daily

Foam (Evoclin®): Apply once daily

Adults:

Amnionitis: I.V.: 450-900 mg every 8 hours

Anthrax: I.V.: 900 mg every 8 hours with ciprofloxacin or doxycycline

Babesiosis (unlabeled use):

Oral: 600 mg 3 times/day for 7 days with quinine

I.V.: 1.2 g twice daily for 7 days with quinine

Bacterial vaginosis: Intravaginal:

Suppositories: Insert one ovule (100 mg clindamycin) daily into vagina at bedtime for 3 days

Cream:

Cleocin®: One full applicator inserted intravaginally once daily before bedtime for 3 or 7 consecutive days in nonpregnant patients or for 7 consecutive days in pregnant patients

Clindesse™: One full applicator inserted intravaginally as a single dose at anytime during the day in nonpregnant patients

Bite wounds (canine): Oral: 300 mg 4 times/day with a fluoroquinolone

Gangrenous pyomyositis: I.V.: 900 mg every 8 hours with penicillin G

Group B streptococcus (neonatal prophylaxis): I.V.: 900 mg every 8 hours until delivery

Orofacial/parapharyngeal space infections:

Oral: 150-450 mg every 6 hours for 7 days, maximum 1.8 g/day

I.V.: 600-900 mg every 8 hours

Pelvic inflammatory disease: I.V.: 900 mg every 8 hours with gentamicin 2 mg/kg, then 1.5 mg/kg every 8 hours; continue after discharge with doxycycline 100 mg twice daily to complete 14 days of total therapy

***Pneumocystis jiroveci* pneumonia (unlabeled use):** I.V.: 600 mg every 8 hours with primaquine or pentamidine for 21 days

Prophylaxis against infective endocarditis (unlabeled use):

Oral: 600 mg 30-60 minutes before procedure

I.M., I.V.: 600 mg 30-60 minutes before procedure. Intramuscular injections should be avoided in patients who are receiving anticoagulant therapy. In these circumstances, orally administered regimens should be given whenever possible. Intravenously administered antibiotics should be used for patients who are unable to tolerate or absorb oral medications.

Note: American Heart Association (AHA) guidelines now recommend prophylaxis only in patients undergoing invasive procedures and in whom underlying cardiac conditions may predispose to a higher risk of adverse outcomes should infection occur. As of April 2007, routine prophylaxis for GI/GU procedures is no longer recommended by the AHA.

Prophylaxis in total joint replacement patients undergoing dental procedures which produce bacteremia:

Oral: 600 mg 1 hour prior to procedure

I.V.: 600 mg 1 hour prior to procedure (for patients unable to take oral medication)

Toxic shock syndrome: I.V.: 900 mg every 8 hours with penicillin G or ceftriaxone

Toxoplasmosis (unlabeled use): Oral, I.V.: 600 mg every 6 hours with pyrimethamine and folinic acid

Dosing adjustment in renal impairment: No adjustment required.

Dosing adjustment in hepatic impairment: Adjustment recommended in patients with severe hepatic disease

Dietary Considerations May be taken with food.

Administration

I.M.: Deep I.M. sites, rotate sites; do not exceed 600 mg in a single injection.

Intravaginal:

Cream: Insertion should be as far as possible into the vagina without causing discomfort.

Ovule: The foil should be removed; if the applicator is used for insertion, it should be washed for additional use.

I.V.: **Never administer as bolus**; administer by I.V. intermittent infusion over at least 10-60 minutes, at a rate **not** to exceed 30 mg/minute (do not exceed 1200 mg/hour); final concentration for administration should not exceed 18 mg/mL.

Oral: Administer with a full glass of water to minimize esophageal ulceration; give around-the-clock to promote less variation in peak and trough serum levels.

Topical foam: Dispense directly into cap or onto a cool surface; do not dispense directly into hands.

Monitoring Parameters Observe for changes in bowel frequency. Monitor for colitis and resolution of symptoms. During prolonged therapy monitor CBC, liver and renal function tests periodically.

Dosage Forms Excipient information presented when available (limited, particularly for generics); consult specific product labeling.

Note: Strength is expressed as base

Capsule, as hydrochloride: 75 mg, 150 mg, 300 mg

Cleocin HCl®: 75 mg [contains tartrazine], 150 mg [contains tartrazine], 300 mg

Cream, vaginal, as phosphate:

Cleocin®: 2% (40 g) [contains benzyl alcohol and mineral oil; packaged with 7 disposable applicators]

ClindaMax®: 2% (40 g) [contains benzyl alcohol and mineral oil; packaged with 7 disposable applicators]

Clindesse™: 2% (5 g) [contains mineral oil; prefilled single disposable applicator]

Foam, topical, as phosphate:

Evoclin®: 1% (50 g, 100 g) [contains ethanol 58%]

Gel, topical, as phosphate: 1% (30 g, 60 g)

Cleocin T®: 1% (30 g, 60 g)
Clindagel®: 1% (40 mL, 75 mL)
ClindaMax®: 1% (30 g, 60 g)
Granules for oral solution, as palmitate:
Cleocin Pediatric®: 75 mg/5 mL (100 mL) [cherry flavor]
Infusion, as phosphate [premixed in D_5W]:
Cleocin Phosphate®: 300 mg (50 mL); 600 mg (50 mL); 900 mg (50 mL) [contains benzyl alcohol and edetate disodium 0.5 mg/mL]
Injection, solution, as phosphate: 150 mg/mL (2 mL, 4 mL, 6 mL, 60 mL)
Cleocin Phosphate®: 150 mg/mL (2 mL, 4 mL, 6 mL, 60 mL) [contains benzyl alcohol and edetate disodium 0.5 mg/mL]
Lotion, as phosphate: 1% (60 mL)
Cleocin T®, ClindaMax®: 1% (60 mL)
Pledgets, topical: 1% (60s, 69s)
Cleocin T®: 1% (60s) [contains isopropyl alcohol 50%]
ClindaReach™: 1% (120s) [contains isopropyl alcohol 50%; packaged as a kit containing 1 collapsible applicator, 64 appliques, and 64 unmedicated pads]
Solution, topical, as phosphate: 1% (30 mL, 60 mL)
Cleocin T®: 1% (30 mL, 60 mL) [contains isopropyl alcohol 50%]
Suppository, vaginal, as phosphate:
Cleocin® Vaginal Ovule: 100 mg (3s) [contains oleaginous base; single reusable applicator]

Clindamycin and Tretinoin

(klin da MYE sin & TRET i noyn)

U.S. Brand Names Ziana™

Index Terms Clindamycin Phosphate and Tretinoin; Tretinoin and Clindamycin

Pharmacologic Category Acne Products; Retinoic Acid Derivative; Topical Skin Product; Topical Skin Product, Acne

Use Treatment of acne vulgaris

Pregnancy Risk Factor C

Dosage Topical: Children ≥12 years and Adults: Apply pea-size amount to entire face once daily at bedtime

Additional Information Complete prescribing information for this medication should be consulted for additional detail.

Dosage Forms Excipient information presented when available (limited, particularly for generics); consult specific product labeling.
Gel, topical:
Ziana™: Clindamycin phosphate 1.2% and tretinoin 0.025% (30 g, 60 g)

◆ **Clindamycin Hydrochloride** *see* Clindamycin *on page 344*
◆ **Clindamycin Injection, USP (Can)** *see* Clindamycin *on page 344*
◆ **Clindamycin Palmitate** *see* Clindamycin *on page 344*
◆ **Clindamycin Phosphate** *see* Clindamycin *on page 344*
◆ **Clindamycin Phosphate and Tretinoin** *see* Clindamycin and Tretinoin *on page 347*
◆ **ClindaReach™** *see* Clindamycin *on page 344*
◆ **Clindesse™** *see* Clindamycin *on page 344*
◆ **Clindoxyl® (Can)** *see* Clindamycin *on page 344*
◆ **Clinoril®** *see* Sulindac *on page 1412*

Clobetasol (kloe BAY ta sol)

U.S. Brand Names Clobevate® [DSC]; Clobex®; Cormax®; Olux-E™; Olux®; Temovate E®; Temovate®

Canadian Brand Names Clobex®; Dermovate®; Gen-Clobetasol; Novo-Clobetasol; PMS-Clobetasol; RATIO-Clobetasol; Taro-Clobetasol

Index Terms Clobetasol Propionate

Pharmacologic Category Corticosteroid, Topical

Additional Appendix Information
Corticosteroids *on page 1652*

Use Short-term relief of inflammation of moderate-to-severe corticosteroid-responsive dermatoses (very high potency topical corticosteroid)

Pregnancy Risk Factor C

Medication Safety Issues
International issues:
Clobex® may be confused with Codex® which is a brand name for *Saccharomyces boulardii* in Italy

Dosage Topical: Discontinue when control achieved; if improvement not seen within 2 weeks, reassessment of diagnosis may be necessary.

Children <12 years: Use is not recommended
Children ≥12 years and Adults:
Oral mucosal inflammation, dental (unlabeled use): Cream: Apply twice daily for up to 2 weeks (maximum dose: 50 g/week); discontinue application when control is achieved; if no improvement is seen, reassessment of diagnosis may be necessary
Steroid-responsive dermatoses:
Cream, emollient cream, gel, ointment: Apply twice daily for up to 2 weeks (maximum dose: 50 g/week)
Foam (Olux-E™): Apply to affected area twice daily for up to 2 weeks (maximum dose: 50 g/week); do not apply to face or intertriginous areas
Steroid-responsive dermatoses: Foam (Olux®), solution: Apply to affected scalp twice daily for up to 2 weeks (maximum dose: 50 g/week or 50 mL/week)
Mild-to-moderate plaque-type psoriasis of nonscalp areas: Foam (Olux®): Apply to affected area twice daily for up to 2 weeks (maximum dose: 50 g/week); do not apply to face or intertriginous areas
Children ≥16 years and Adults: Moderate-to-severe plaque-type psoriasis: Emollient cream, lotion: Apply twice daily for up to 2 weeks, has been used for up to 4 weeks when application is <10% of body surface area; use with caution (maximum dose: 50 g/week)
Children ≥18 years and Adults:
Moderate-to-severe plaque-type psoriasis: Spray: Apply by spraying directly onto affected area twice daily; should be gently rubbed into skin. Should be used for not longer than 4 weeks; treatment beyond 2 weeks should be limited to localized lesions which have not improved sufficiently. Total dose should not exceed 50 g/week or 59 mL/week.
Scalp psoriasis: Shampoo: Apply thin film to dry scalp once daily; leave in place for 15 minutes, then add water, lather; rinse thoroughly
Steroid-responsive dermatoses: Lotion: Apply twice daily for up to 2 weeks (maximum dose: 50 g/week)

Additional Information Complete prescribing information for this medication should be consulted for additional detail.

Dosage Forms Excipient information presented when available (limited, particularly for generics); consult specific product labeling. [DSC] = Discontinued product
Aerosol, topical, as propionate [foam]: 0.05% (50 g, 100 g)
Olux®: 0.05% (50 g, 100 g) [contains ethanol 60%]
Olux-E™: 0.05% (50 g, 100 g)
Cream, as propionate: 0.05% (15 g, 30 g, 45 g, 60 g)
Cormax®: 0.05% (15 g, 30 g, 45 g)
Temovate®: 0.05% (30 g, 60 g)
Cream, as propionate [in emollient base]: 0.05% (15 g, 30 g, 60 g)
Temovate E®: 0.05% (60 g)
Gel, as propionate: 0.05% (15 g, 30 g, 60 g)
Clobevate®: 0.05% (45 g) [DSC]
Temovate®: 0.05% (60 g)

Lotion, as propionate:
Clobex®: 0.05% (30 mL, 59 mL, 118 mL)
Ointment, as propionate: 0.05% (15 g, 30 g, 45 g, 60 g)
Cormax®: 0.05% (15 g, 45 g)
Temovate®: 0.05% (15 g, 30 g)
Shampoo, as propionate:
Clobex®: 0.05% (120 mL) [contains alcohol]
Solution, topical, as propionate [for scalp application]: 0.05% (25 mL, 50 mL)
Cormax®: 0.05% (25 mL, 50 mL) [contains isopropyl alcohol 40%]
Temovate®: 0.05% (50 mL) [contains isopropyl alcohol 40%]
Solution, topical, as propionate [spray]:
Clobex®: 0.05% (60 mL, 125 mL) [contains alcohol]

◆ **Clobetasol Propionate** *see* Clobetasol *on page 347*

◆ **Clobevate® [DSC]** *see* Clobetasol *on page 347*

◆ **Clobex®** *see* Clobetasol *on page 347*

Clocortolone (kloe KOR toe lone)

U.S. Brand Names Cloderm®
Canadian Brand Names Cloderm®
Index Terms Clocortolone Pivalate
Pharmacologic Category Corticosteroid, Topical
Additional Appendix Information
Corticosteroids *on page 1652*
Use Inflammation of corticosteroid-responsive dermatoses (intermediate-potency topical corticosteroid)
Pregnancy Risk Factor C
Medication Safety Issues
Sound-alike/look-alike issues:
Cloderm® may be confused with Clocort®

International issues:
Cloderm®: Brand name for clotrimazole in Germany
Dosage Adults: Apply sparingly and gently; rub into affected area from 1-4 times/day. Therapy should be discontinued when control is achieved; if no improvement is seen, reassessment of diagnosis may be necessary.
Additional Information Complete prescribing information for this medication should be consulted for additional detail.
Dosage Forms Excipient information presented when available (limited, particularly for generics); consult specific product labeling.
Cream, as pivalate:
Cloderm®: 0.1% (30 g, 45 g, 90 g)

◆ **Clocortolone Pivalate** *see* Clocortolone *on page 348*

◆ **Cloderm®** *see* Clocortolone *on page 348*

Clofarabine (klo FARE a been)

U.S. Brand Names Clolar®
Index Terms CAFdA; Clofarex; NSC606869
Pharmacologic Category Antineoplastic Agent, Antimetabolite (Purine Antagonist)
Use Treatment of relapsed or refractory acute lymphoblastic leukemia (ALL)
Unlabeled/Investigational Use Relapsed and refractory acute myeloid leukemia (AML) and myelodysplastic syndrome (MDS)
Pregnancy Risk Factor D
Pregnancy Considerations Teratogenic effects were observed in animal studies. There are no adequate or well-controlled studies in pregnant women. Women of childbearing potential should be advised to use effective contraception and avoid becoming pregnant during therapy.
Lactation Excretion in breast milk unknown/not recommended
Medication Safety Issues
Sound-alike/look-alike issues:
Clofarabine may be confused with cladribine, cleVIDipine

High alert medication: The Institute for Safe Medication Practices (ISMP) includes this medication among its list of drug classes which have a heightened risk of causing significant patient harm when used in error.
Contraindications There are no contraindications listed within the manufacturer's labeling.
Warnings/Precautions Hazardous agent - use appropriate precautions for handling and disposal. Tumor lysis syndrome may occur. Cytokine release may develop into systemic inflammatory response syndrome (SIRS)/capillary leak syndrome, and organ dysfunction; discontinuation of clofarabine should be considered with the presentation of SIRS or capillary leak syndrome. Myelosuppression (dose-dependent) is common. Safety and efficacy have not been established with renal or hepatic dysfunction; use with caution. Safety and efficacy in pediatric patients <1 year of age or adults >21 years have not been established.
Adverse Reactions
>10%:
Cardiovascular: Tachycardia (35%), hypotension (29%), flushing (19%), hypertension (13%), edema (12%)
Central nervous system: Headache (43%), fever (39%), chills (34%), fatigue (34%), anxiety (21%), pain (15%)
Dermatologic: Pruritus (43%), rash (38%), petechiae (26%), palmar-plantar erythrodysesthesia syndrome (16%), erythema (11%)
Gastrointestinal: Vomiting (78%; grades 3/4: 9%), nausea (73%; grades 3/4: 15%), diarrhea (56%), abdominal pain (8% to 35%), anorexia (30%), mucosal inflammation (16%), gingival bleeding (14%), oral candidiasis (11%)
Genitourinary: Hematuria (13%)
Hematologic: Leukopenia (grades 3/4: 88%), anemia (83%; grades 3/4: 75%), lymphopenia (grades 3/4: 82%), thrombocytopenia (81%; grades 3/4: 80%), neutropenia (grades 3/4: 10% to 64%), febrile neutropenia (55%; grade 4: 3%)
Hepatic: ALT increased (81%; grades 3/4: 43% to 44%), AST increased (74%; grades 3/4: 36%), bilirubin increased (45%; grades 3/4: 13%)
Neuromuscular & skeletal: Limb pain (30%), myalgia (14%)
Renal: Creatinine increased (50%; grades 3/4: 8%)
Respiratory: Epistaxis (27%), dyspnea (13%), pleural effusion (12%)
Miscellaneous: Infection (83%; includes bacterial, fungal, and viral), catheter-related infection (12%)
1% to 10%:
Cardiovascular: Pericardial effusion (8%)
Central nervous system: Irritability (10%), lethargy (10%), somnolence (10%), agitation (5%), mental status change
Dermatologic: Cellulitis (8%), pruritic rash (8%)
Gastrointestinal: Proctalgia (8%), clostridium colitis (7%), stomatitis (7%), mouth hemorrhage (5%), oral mucosal petechiae (5%), cecitis (1% to 4%), pancreatitis (1% to 4%)
Hepatic: Jaundice (8%)
Neuromuscular & skeletal: Back pain (10%), bone pain (10%), weakness (10%), arthralgia (9%)
Respiratory: Pneumonia (10%), respiratory distress (10%), tachypnea (9%), upper respiratory tract infection (5%), pulmonary edema (1% to 4%)
Miscellaneous: Herpes simplex (10%), sepsis (10%), bacteremia (9%), candidiasis (7%), herpes zoster (7%), septic shock (7%), staphylococcus bacteremia (6%), tumor lysis syndrome (grade 3: 6%), capillary leak syndrome (4%), hypersensitivity (1% to 4%), SIRS (2%)

<1% (Limited to important or life-threatening): Bone marrow failure, dermatitis, hallucination, hepatic veno-occlusive disease, hepatomegaly, hypokalemia, hypophosphatemia, left ventricular systolic function decreased, right ventricular pressure increased, Stevens-Johnson syndrome, toxic epidermal necrolysis

Drug Interactions

Avoid Concomitant Use

Avoid concomitant use of Clofarabine with any of the following: Natalizumab; Vaccines (Live)

Increased Effect/Toxicity

Clofarabine may increase the levels/effects of: Natalizumab; Vaccines (Live); Vitamin K Antagonists

The levels/effects of Clofarabine may be increased by: Trastuzumab

Decreased Effect

Clofarabine may decrease the levels/effects of: Cardiac Glycosides; Vaccines (Inactivated); Vitamin K Antagonists

The levels/effects of Clofarabine may be decreased by: Echinacea

Stability Store undiluted and diluted solutions at room temperature of 25°C (77°F); excursions permitted to 15°C to 30°C (59°F to 86°F). Clofarabine should be diluted with 100-500 mL NS or D_5W to a final concentration of 0.15-0.4 mg/mL. The manufacturer recommends the product be filtered through a 0.2 micrometer filter before dilution. Solutions diluted in 100-500 mL of D_5W or NS are stable for 24 hours at room temperature. Use appropriate precautions for handling and disposal.

Mechanism of Action Clofarabine, a purine (deoxyadenosine) nucleoside analog, is metabolized to clofarabine 5'-triphosphate. Clofarabine 5'-triphosphate decreases cell replication and repair as well as causing cell death. To decrease cell replication and repair, clofarabine 5'-triphosphate competes with deoxyadenosine triphosphate for the enzymes ribonucleotide reductase and DNA polymerase. Cell replication is decreased when clofarabine 5'-triphosphate inhibits ribonucleotide reductase from reacting with deoxyadenosine triphosphate to produce deoxynucleotide triphosphate which is needed for DNA synthesis. Cell replication is also decreased when clofarabine 5'-triphosphate competes with DNA polymerase for incorporation into the DNA chain; when done during the repair process, cell repair is affected. To cause cell death, clofarabine 5'-triphosphate alters the mitochondrial membrane by releasing proteins, an inducing factor and cytochrome C.

Pharmacodynamics/Kinetics

Distribution: V_d: 172 L/m^2

Protein binding: 47%, primarily to albumin

Metabolism: Intracellulary by deoxycytidine kinase and mono- and diphosphokinases to active metabolite clofarabine 5'-triphosphate; limited hepatic metabolism (0.2%)

Half-life elimination: ~5.2 hours

Excretion: Urine (49% to 60%, as unchanged drug)

Dosage Consider prophylactic corticosteroids (hydrocortisone 100 mg/m^2 on days 1-3; to prevent signs/symptoms of capillary leak syndrome or SIRS), hydration and allopurinol (to reduce the risk of tumor lysis syndrome/hyperuricemia), and prophylactic antiemetics.

I.V.: Children ≥1 year and Adults ≤21 years: ALL: 52 mg/m^2/day days 1 through 5; repeat every 2-6 weeks; subsequent cycles should begin no sooner than 14 days from day 1 of the previous cycle (subsequent cycles may be administered when ANC ≥750/mm^3)

Dosage adjustment for toxicity:

Hematologic toxicity: ANC <500/mm^3 lasting ≥4 weeks: Reduce clofarabine dose by 25% for next cycle

Nonhematologic toxicity:

Clinically significant infection: Withhold treatment until infection is under control, then restart clofarabine at full dose

Grade 3 toxicity excluding infection, nausea and vomiting, and transient elevations in transaminases and bilirubin: Withhold treatment; may reinitiate clofarabine with a 25% dose-reduction with resolution or return to baseline

Grade ≥3 increase in creatinine or bilirubin: Discontinue clofarabine; may reinitiate with 25% dosage reduction when creatinine or bilirubin return to baseline and patient is stable; administer allopurinol for hyperuricemia

Grade 4 toxicity (noninfectious): Discontinue clofarabine treatment

Capillary leak or systemic inflammatory response syndrome (SIRS) signs/symptoms (eg, hypotension, tachycardia, tachypnea, pulmonary edema): Discontinue clofarabine; institute supportive measures

Dosage adjustment in renal/hepatic impairment: Safety not established; use with caution

Administration I.V. infusion: Over 2 hours. Continuous I.V. fluids are encouraged to decrease adverse events and tumor lysis effects. Hypotension may be a sign of capillary leak syndrome or systemic inflammatory response syndrome (SIRS). Discontinue if the patient becomes hypotensive during administration. Retreatment should only be considered if the hypotension is not related to capillary leak syndrome or SIRS.

Monitoring Parameters Blood pressure, cardiac function, and respiratory status during infusion; periodic CBC with platelet count (increase frequency in patients who develop cytopenias); liver and kidney function during 5 days of clofarabine administration; signs and symptoms of tumor lysis syndrome and cytokine release syndrome (tachypnea, tachycardia, hypotension, pulmonary edema); hydration status

Dosage Forms Excipient information presented when available (limited, particularly for generics); consult specific product labeling.

Injection, solution [preservative free]:

Clolar®: 1 mg/mL (20 mL)

◆ **Clofarex** *see* Clofarabine *on page 348*

◆ **Clolar®** *see* Clofarabine *on page 348*

◆ **Clomid®** *see* ClomiPHENE *on page 349*

ClomiPHENE (KLOE mi feen)

U.S. Brand Names Clomid®; Serophene®

Canadian Brand Names Clomid®; Milophene®; Serophene®

Index Terms Clomiphene Citrate

Pharmacologic Category Ovulation Stimulator; Selective Estrogen Receptor Modulator (SERM)

Use Treatment of ovulatory failure in patients desiring pregnancy

Pregnancy Risk Factor X

Pregnancy Considerations Embryotoxic effects were observed in animal studies. The incidence of adverse fetal effects following maternal use of clomiphene for ovulation induction is similar to those seen in the general population. Clomiphene is not indicated for use in women who are already pregnant.

Lactation Excretion in breast milk unknown/use caution

Medication Safety Issues

Sound-alike/look-alike issues:

ClomiPHENE may be confused with clomiPRAMINE, clonidine

Clomid® may be confused with clonidine

Serophene® may be confused with Sarafem™

Contraindications Hypersensitivity to clomiphene citrate or any of its components; liver disease; abnormal uterine bleeding; enlargement or development of ovarian cyst (not due to polycystic ovarian syndrome); uncontrolled thyroid or adrenal dysfunction; presence of an organic intracranial lesion such as pituitary tumor; pregnancy

Warnings/Precautions Ovarian enlargement may occur with use; may be accompanied by abdominal distention or abdominal pain and generally regresses without treatment within 2-3 weeks. Do not continue dosing until ovaries are of normal size. Ovarian hyperstimulation syndrome (OHSS) is characterized by severe ovarian enlargement, abdominal pain/distention, nausea, vomiting, diarrhea, dyspnea, and oliguria, and may be accompanied by ascites, pleural effusion, hypovolemia, electrolyte imbalance, hemoperitoneum, and thromboembolic events. If severe hyperstimulation occurs, stop treatment and hospitalize patient. This syndrome develops rapidly within 24 hours to several days and generally occurs during the 7-10 days immediately following treatment. Use with caution in patients unusually sensitive to pituitary gonadotropins (eg, PCOS). To minimize risks, use only at the lowest effective dose. Blurring or other visual symptoms can occur; patients with visual disturbances should discontinue therapy and have an eye exam. Multiple births may result from the use of these medications; advise patient of the potential risk of multiple births before starting the treatment.

Adverse Reactions

>10%: Endocrine & metabolic: Ovarian enlargement (14%)

1% to 10%:

Central nervous system: Headache (1%)

Endocrine & metabolic: Hot flashes (10%), breast discomfort (2%), abnormal uterine bleeding (1%)

Gastrointestinal: Distention/bloating/discomfort (6%), nausea (2%), vomiting (2%)

Ocular: Visual symptoms (2%, includes blurring of vision, diplopia, floaters, lights, phosphenes, photophobia, scotomata, waves)

<1% (Limited to important or life-threatening): Abnormal accommodation, acne, acute abdomen, allergic reaction, appetite increased, arrhythmia, chest pain, constipation, depression, dermatitis, diarrhea, dizziness, dry hair, edema, endometriosis, erythema multiforme, erythema nodosum, eye pain, fatigue, fever, hypertension, hypertrichosis, insomnia, lightheadedness, macular edema, migraine, mood changes, neoplasms, nervousness, optic neuritis, ovarian cyst, ovarian hemorrhage, palpitation, PE, pruritus, rash, retinal hemorrhage, retinal thrombosis, seizure, stroke, syncope, tachycardia, temporary loss of vision, thrombophlebitis, thyroid disorder, tinnitus, transaminase increased, tubal pregnancy, urinary frequency/volume increased, uterine hemorrhage, vaginal dryness, vertigo, weight gain/loss

Drug Interactions

Avoid Concomitant Use There are no known interactions where it is recommended to avoid concomitant use.

Increased Effect/Toxicity There are no known significant interactions involving an increase in effect.

Decreased Effect There are no known significant interactions involving a decrease in effect.

Stability Store at room temperature of 15°C to 30°C (59°F to 86°F). Protect from light, heat, and excessive humidity.

Mechanism of Action Clomiphene is a racemic mixture consisting of zuclomiphene (~38%) and enclomiphene (~62%), each with distinct pharmacologic properties. Enclomiphene is much less potent in inducing ovulation; however, it is more rapidly absorbed and metabolized, allowing the more potent activity of zuclomiphene to predominate. Zuclomiphene acts at the level of the hypothalamus, occupying cell surface and intracellular estrogen receptors (ERs) for longer durations than estrogen. This interferes with receptor recycling, effectively depleting hypothalamic ERs and inhibiting normal estrogenic negative feedback. Impairment of the feedback signal results in increased pulsatile GnRH secretion from the hypothalamus and subsequent pituitary gonadotropin (FSH, LH) release, causing growth of the ovarian follicle, followed by follicular rupture.

Pharmacodynamics/Kinetics

Onset of action: Ovulation: 5-10 days following course of treatment

Duration: Effects are cumulative; ovulation may occur in the cycle following the last treatment

Metabolism: Hepatic; undergoes enterohepatic recirculation

Half-life elimination: 5-7 days

Time to peak, plasma: ~6 hours

Excretion: Primarily feces; urine (small amounts)

Dosage Oral: Adults: Ovulation induction: Females:

Initial course: 50 mg once daily for 5 days. Begin on or about the fifth day of cycle if progestin-induced bleeding is scheduled or spontaneous uterine bleeding occurs prior to therapy.

Dose adjustment: Subsequent doses may be increased to 100 mg once daily for 5 days only if ovulation does not occur at the initial dose. A low dose or duration of course is recommended in patients where unusual sensitivity to pituitary gonadotropin is suspected (eg, PCOS).

Repeat courses: If needed, the 5-day cycle may be repeated as early as 30 days after the previous one. Exclude the presence of pregnancy.

Maximum dose: 100 mg once daily for 5 days for 6 cycles. Discontinue if ovulation does not occur after 3 courses of treatment; or if 3 ovulatory responses occur but pregnancy is not achieved. Re-evaluate if menses does not occur following ovulatory response. Doses larger than 150 mg have been reported, however, pregnancy rates are low.

Administration The total daily dose should be taken at one time to maximize effectiveness.

Monitoring Parameters Basal body temperature, serum progesterone, urinary luteinizing hormone; follicular growth and endometrial thickness may be useful in some cases; pregnancy test prior to repeat courses

Reference Range Serum progesterone: Ovulation generally occurs with levels ≥3 ng/mL; best results with levels >10 ng/mL

Test Interactions Clomiphene may increase levels of serum thyroxine and thyroxine-binding globulin (TBG)

Dosage Forms Excipient information presented when available (limited, particularly for generics); consult specific product labeling.

Tablet, as citrate [scored]: 50 mg

Clomid®, Serophene®: 50 mg

◆ **Clomiphene Citrate** *see* ClomiPHENE *on page 349*

ClomiPRAMINE (kloe MI pra meen)

U.S. Brand Names Anafranil®

Canadian Brand Names Anafranil®; Apo-Clomipramine®; CO Clomipramine; Gen-Clomipramine

Index Terms Clomipramine Hydrochloride

Pharmacologic Category Antidepressant, Tricyclic (Tertiary Amine)

Additional Appendix Information

Antidepressant Agents *on page 1638*

Use Treatment of obsessive-compulsive disorder (OCD)

Unlabeled/Investigational Use Depression, panic attacks, chronic pain

Restrictions An FDA-approved medication guide concerning the use of antidepressants in children, adolescents, and young adults must be distributed when dispensing an outpatient prescription (new or refill) where this medication is to be used without direct supervision of a healthcare provider. Medication guides are available at http://www.fda.gov/cder/Offices/ODS/medication_guides.htm. Dispense to parents or guardians of children and adolescents receiving this medication.

Pregnancy Risk Factor C

Pregnancy Considerations There are no adequate and well-controlled studies in pregnant women. Withdrawal symptoms (including dizziness, nausea, vomiting, headache, malaise, sleep disturbance, hyperthermia, and/or irritability) have been observed in neonates whose mothers took clomipramine up to delivery. Use in pregnancy only if the benefits to the mother outweigh the potential risks to the fetus.

Lactation Enters breast milk/not recommended (AAP rates "of concern")

Medication Safety Issues

Sound-alike/look-alike issues:

ClomiPRAMINE may be confused with chlorproMAZINE, cleVIDipine, clomiPHENE, desipramine, Norpramin®

Anafranil® may be confused with alfentanil, enalapril, nafarelin

Contraindications Hypersensitivity to clomipramine, other tricyclic agents, or any component of the formulation; use of MAO inhibitors within 14 days; use in a patient during the acute recovery phase of MI

Warnings/Precautions **[U.S. Boxed Warning]: Antidepressants increase the risk of suicidal thinking and behavior in children, adolescents, and young adults (18-24 years of age) with major depressive disorder (MDD) and other psychiatric disorders;** consider risk prior to prescribing. Short-term studies did not show an increased risk in patients >24 years of age and showed a decreased risk in patients ≥65 years. Closely monitor for clinical worsening, suicidality, or unusual changes in behavior; the patient's family or caregiver should be instructed to closely observe the patient and communicate condition with healthcare provider. A medication guide should be dispensed with each prescription. **Clomipramine is FDA approved for the treatment of OCD in children ≥10 years of age.**

The possibility of a suicide attempt is inherent in major depression and may persist until remission occurs. Monitor for worsening of depression or suicidality, especially during initiation of therapy (generally first 1-2 months) or with dose increases or decreases. Use caution in high-risk patients. Worsening depression and severe abrupt suicidality that are not part of the presenting symptoms may require discontinuation or modification of drug therapy. The patient's family or caregiver should be alerted to monitor patients for the emergence of suicidality and associated behaviors (such as agitation, irritability, hostility, impulsivity, and hypomania) and notify the healthcare provider.

May worsen psychosis in some patients or precipitate a shift to mania or hypomania in patients with bipolar disorder. Patients presenting with depressive symptoms should be screened for bipolar disorder. Monotherapy in patients with bipolar disorder should be avoided. **Clomipramine is not FDA approved for bipolar depression.**

TCAs may rarely cause bone marrow suppression; monitor for any signs of infection and obtain CBC if symptoms (eg, fever, sore throat) evident. May cause seizures (relationship to dose and/or duration of therapy) - do not exceed maximum doses. Use caution in patients with a previous seizure disorder or condition predisposing to seizures such as brain damage, alcoholism, or concurrent therapy with other drugs which lower the seizure threshold. May increase the risks associated with electroconvulsive therapy. Has been associated with a high incidence of sexual dysfunction. Weight gain may occur. Hyperpyrexia has been observed with TCAs in combination with anticholinergics and/or neuroleptics, particularly during hot weather.

The degree of sedation, anticholinergic effects, and conduction abnormalities are high relative to other antidepressants. Clomipramine often causes drowsiness/sedation, resulting in impaired performance of tasks requiring alertness (eg, operating machinery or driving). Sedative effects may be additive with other CNS depressants and/or ethanol. The risk of orthostasis is moderate to high relative to other antidepressants. Use with caution in patients with a history of cardiovascular disease (including previous MI, stroke, tachycardia, or conduction abnormalities). Use with caution in patients with urinary retention, benign prostatic hyperplasia, narrow-angle glaucoma, xerostomia, visual problems, constipation, or a history of bowel obstruction.

Consider discontinuing, when possible, prior to elective surgery. Therapy should not be abruptly discontinued in patients receiving high doses for prolonged periods. Use with caution in hyperthyroid patients or those receiving thyroid supplementation. Use with caution in patients with hepatic or renal dysfunction and in elderly patients.

Adverse Reactions Data shown for children reflects both children and adolescents studied in clinical trials.

>10%:

Central nervous system: Dizziness (54%), somnolence (54%), drowsiness, headache (52%; children 28%), fatigue (39%), insomnia (25%; children 11%), malaise, nervousness (18%; children 4%)

Endocrine & metabolic: Libido changes (21%), hot flushes (5%)

Gastrointestinal: Xerostomia (84%, children 63%) constipation (47%; children 22%), nausea (33%; children 9%), dyspepsia (22%; children 13%), weight gain (18%; children 2%), diarrhea (13%; children 7%), anorexia (12%; children 22%), abdominal pain (11%), appetite increased (11%)

Genitourinary: Ejaculation failure (42%), impotence (20%), micturition disorder (14%; children 4%)

Neuromuscular & skeletal: Tremor (54%), myoclonus (13%; children 2%), myalgia (13%)

Ocular: Abnormal vision (18%; children 7%)

Respiratory: Pharyngitis (14%), rhinitis (12%)

Miscellaneous: Diaphoresis increased (29%; children 9%)

1% to 10%:

Cardiovascular: Flushing (8%), postural hypotension (6%), palpitation (4%), tachycardia (4%; children 2%), chest pain (4%), edema (2%)

Central nervous system: Anxiety (9%), memory impairment (9%), twitching (7%), depression (5%), concentration impaired (5%), fever (4%), hypertonia (4%), abnormal dreaming (3%), agitation (3%), confusion (3%), migraine (3%), pain (3%), psychosomatic disorder (3%), speech disorder (3%), yawning (3%), aggressiveness (children 2%), chills (2%), depersonalization (2%), emotional lability (2%), irritability (2%), panic reaction (1%)

Dermatologic: Rash (8%), pruritus (6%), purpura (3%), dermatitis (2%), acne (2%), dry skin (2%), urticaria (1%)

Endocrine & metabolic: Amenorrhea (1%), breast enlargement (2%), breast pain (1%), hot flashes (5%), lactation (nonpuerperal) (4%)

Gastrointestinal: Taste disturbance (8%), vomiting (7%), flatulence (6%), tooth disorder (5%), dysphagia (2%), esophagitis (1%)

Genitourinary: UTI (2% to 6%), micturition frequency (5%), dysuria (2%), leucorrhea (2%), vaginitis (2%), urinary retention (2%)

Neuromuscular & skeletal: Paresthesia (9%), back pain (6%), arthralgia (3%), paresis (children 2%), weakness (1%)

Ocular: Lacrimation abnormal (3%), mydriasis (2%), conjunctivitis (1%)

Otic: Tinnitus (6%)

Respiratory: Sinusitis (6%), coughing (6%), bronchospasm (2%; children 7%), epistaxis (2%)

<1% (Limited to important or life-threatening): Accommodation abnormal, albuminuria, aneurysm, anticholinergic syndrome, aphasia, apraxia, arrhythmia, ataxia, atrial flutter, blepharitis, blood in stool, bradycardia, breast fibroadenosis, bronchitis, bundle branch block, cardiac arrest, cardiac failure, catalepsy, cellulitis, cerebral hemorrhage, cervical dysplasia, cheilitis, cholinergic syndrome, choreoathetosis, chromatopsia, chronic enteritis, coma, conjunctival hemorrhage, cyanosis, deafness, dehydration, delirium, delusion, diabetes mellitus, diplopia, dyskinesia, dysphonia, dystonia, EEG abnormal, encephalopathy, endometrial hyperplasia, endometriosis, epididymitis, erythematous rash, exophthalmos, extrapyramidal disorder, extrasystoles, gastric ulcer, generalized spasm, glaucoma, glycosuria, goiter, gynecomastia, hallucinations, heart block, hematuria, hemiparesis, hemoptysis, hepatitis, hostility, hyperacusis, hypercholesterolemia, hyper-/hypoesthesia, hyperglycemia, hyper-/hypokinesia, hyperreflexia, hyper-/hypothyroidism, hyperuricemia, hyper-/hypoventilation, hypnagogic hallucination, hypokalemia, ideation, intestinal obstruction, irritable bowel syndrome, keratitis, laryngismus, leukemoid reaction, lupus erythematosus rash, lymphadenopathy, lymphoma-like disorder, maculopapular rash, manic reaction, marrow depression, myocardial infarction, myocardial ischemia, myopathy, myositis, neuralgia, neuropathy, oculogyric crisis, oculomotor nerve paralysis, oral/pharyngeal edema, ovarian cyst, paralytic ileus, paranoia, parosmia, peptic ulcer, peripheral ischemia, phobic disorder, photophobia, photosensitivity reaction, pneumonia, polyarteritis nodosa, premature ejaculation, psychosis, pyelonephritis, pyuria, rectal hemorrhage, renal calculus, renal cyst, schizophrenic reaction, scleritis, seizure, sensory disturbance, skin ulceration, strabismus, stupor, suicidal ideation, suicide, suicide attempt, thrombophlebitis, tongue ulceration, tooth caries, torticollis, urinary incontinence, uterine hemorrhage, uterine inflammation, vaginal hemorrhage, vasospasm, ventricular tachycardia, visual field defect, withdrawal syndrome

Drug Interactions

Metabolism/Transport Effects Substrate of CYP1A2 (major), 2C19 (major), 2D6 (major), 3A4 (minor); **Inhibits** CYP2D6 (moderate)

Avoid Concomitant Use

Avoid concomitant use of ClomiPRAMINE with any of the following: Iobenguane I 123; MAO Inhibitors; Nilotinib; Sibutramine; Tetrabenazine; Thioridazine; Ziprasidone

Increased Effect/Toxicity

ClomiPRAMINE may increase the levels/effects of: Alcohol (Ethyl); Alpha-/Beta-Agonists (Direct-Acting); Alpha1-Agonists; Amphetamines; Anticholinergics; Aspirin; Beta2-Agonists; CNS Depressants; CYP2D6 Substrates; Desmopressin; Fesoterodine; Milnacipran; Nebivolol; NSAID (COX-2 Inhibitor); NSAID (Nonselective); QTc-Prolonging Agents; QuiNIDine; Serotonin Modulators; Sulfonylureas; Tamoxifen; Tetrabenazine; Thioridazine; TraMADol; Vitamin K Antagonists; Yohimbine; Ziprasidone

The levels/effects of ClomiPRAMINE may be increased by: Alfuzosin; Altretamine; BuPROPion; CarBAMazepine; Cimetidine; Cinacalcet; Ciprofloxacin; CYP1A2 Inhibitors (Moderate); CYP1A2 Inhibitors (Strong); CYP2C19 Inhibitors (Moderate); CYP2C19 Inhibitors (Strong); CYP2D6 Inhibitors (Moderate); CYP2D6 Inhibitors (Strong); Darunavir; Dexmethylphenidate; DULoxetine; Gadobutrol; Lithium; MAO Inhibitors; Methylphenidate; Nilotinib; Pramlintide; Propoxyphene; Protease Inhibitors; QuiNIDine; Selective Serotonin Reuptake Inhibitors; Sibutramine; Terbinafine; Valproic Acid

Decreased Effect

ClomiPRAMINE may decrease the levels/effects of: Acetylcholinesterase Inhibitors (Central); Alpha2-Agonists; Codeine; Iobenguane I 123

The levels/effects of ClomiPRAMINE may be decreased by: Acetylcholinesterase Inhibitors (Central); Barbiturates; CYP1A2 Inducers (Strong); CYP2C19 Inducers (Strong); St Johns Wort

Ethanol/Nutrition/Herb Interactions

Ethanol: Avoid ethanol (may increase CNS depression).

Food: Serum concentrations/toxicity may be increased by grapefruit juice.

Herb/Nutraceutical: Avoid valerian, St John's wort, SAMe, kava kava.

Mechanism of Action Clomipramine appears to affect serotonin uptake while its active metabolite, desmethylclomipramine, affects norepinephrine uptake

Pharmacodynamics/Kinetics

Absorption: Rapid

Protein binding: 97%, primarily to albumin

Metabolism: Hepatic to desmethylclomipramine (DMI; active); extensive first-pass effect

Half-life elimination: Clomipramine: mean 32 hours (19-37 hours); DMI: mean 69 hours (range 54-77 hours)

Time to peak, plasma: 2-6 hours

Excretion: Urine and feces

Dosage Oral:

Children:

<10 years: Safety and efficacy have not been established.

≥10 years: OCD:

Initial: 25 mg/day; may gradually increase as tolerated over the first 2 weeks to 3 mg/kg/day or 100 mg/day (whichever is less) in divided doses

Maintenance: May further increase to recommended maximum of 3 mg/kg/day or 200 mg/day (whichever is less); may give as a single daily dose at bedtime once tolerated

Adults: OCD:

Initial: 25 mg/day; may gradually increase as tolerated over the first 2 weeks to 100 mg/day in divided doses

Maintenance: May further increase to recommended maximum of 250 mg/day; may give as a single daily dose at bedtime once tolerated

Administration During titration, may divide doses and administer with meals to decrease gastrointestinal side effects. After titration, may administer total daily dose at bedtime to decrease daytime sedation.

Monitoring Parameters Pulse rate and blood pressure prior to and during therapy; ECG/cardiac status in older adults and patients with cardiac disease; suicidal ideation (especially at the beginning of therapy or when doses are increased or decreased)

Test Interactions Increased glucose

Dosage Forms Excipient information presented when available (limited, particularly for generics); consult specific product labeling.

Capsule, as hydrochloride: 25 mg, 50 mg, 75 mg

Anafranil®: 25 mg, 50 mg, 75 mg

◆ **Clomipramine Hydrochloride** *see* ClomiPRAMINE *on page 350*

◆ **Clonapam (Can)** *see* ClonazePAM *on page 352*

ClonazePAM (kloe NA ze pam)

U.S. Brand Names Klonopin®; Klonopin® Wafers

Canadian Brand Names Alti-Clonazepam; Apo-Clonazepam®; Clonapam; CO Clonazepam; Gen-Clonazepam;

Klonopin®; Novo-Clonazepam; Nu-Clonazepam; PMS-Clonazepam; Pro-Clonazepam; Rho®-Clonazepam; Rivotril®; Sandoz-Clonazepam

Pharmacologic Category Benzodiazepine

Additional Appendix Information

Anticonvulsant Drugs of Choice *on page 1637*
Benzodiazepines *on page 1646*

Use Alone or as an adjunct in the treatment of petit mal variant (Lennox-Gastaut), akinetic, and myoclonic seizures; petit mal (absence) seizures unresponsive to succimides; panic disorder with or without agoraphobia

Unlabeled/Investigational Use Restless legs syndrome; neuralgia; multifocal tic disorder; parkinsonian dysarthria; bipolar disorder; adjunct therapy for schizophrenia

Restrictions C-IV

Pregnancy Risk Factor D

Pregnancy Considerations Clonazepam was shown to be teratogenic in some animal studies. Clonazepam crosses the placenta. Benzodiazepine use during pregnancy is associated with increased risk of congenital malformations. Nonteratogenic effects (including neonatal flaccidity, respiratory and feeding problems, and withdrawal symptoms) during the postnatal period have also been reported with benzodiazepine use. Epilepsy itself, number of medications, genetic factors, or a combination of these probably influence the teratogenicity of anticonvulsant therapy.

Lactation Enters breast milk/not recommended

Medication Safety Issues

Sound-alike/look-alike issues:

ClonazePAM may be confused with clofazimine, cloNIDine, clorazepate, clozapine, LORazepam

Klonopin® may be confused with clofazimine, clonNIDine, clorazepate, clozapine, LORazepam

Contraindications Hypersensitivity to clonazepam or any component of the formulation (cross-sensitivity with other benzodiazepines may exist); significant liver disease; narrow-angle glaucoma; pregnancy

Warnings/Precautions Use with caution in elderly or debilitated patients, patients with hepatic disease (including alcoholics), or renal impairment. Use with caution in patients with respiratory disease or impaired gag reflex or ability to protect the airway from secretions (salivation may be increased). Worsening of seizures may occur when added to patients with multiple seizure types. Concurrent use with valproic acid may result in absence status. Monitoring of CBC and liver function tests has been recommended during prolonged therapy.

Causes CNS depression (dose related) resulting in sedation, dizziness, confusion, or ataxia which may impair physical and mental capabilities. Patients must be cautioned about performing tasks which require mental alertness (eg, operating machinery or driving). Use with caution in patients receiving other CNS depressants or psychoactive agents. Effects with other sedative drugs or ethanol may be potentiated. Benzodiazepines have been associated with falls and traumatic injury and should be used with extreme caution in patients who are at risk of these events (especially the elderly).

Use caution in patients with depression, particularly if suicidal risk may be present. Use with caution in patients with a history of drug dependence. Benzodiazepines have been associated with dependence and acute withdrawal symptoms, including seizures, on discontinuation or reduction in dose. Acute withdrawal, including seizures, may be precipitated in patients after administration of flumazenil to patients receiving long-term benzodiazepine therapy.

Benzodiazepines have been associated with anterograde amnesia. Paradoxical reactions, including hyperactive or aggressive behavior, have been reported with benzodiazepines, particularly in adolescent/pediatric or psychiatric patients. Does not have analgesic, antidepressant, or antipsychotic properties.

Adverse Reactions Reactions reported in patients with seizure and/or panic disorder. Frequency not defined.

Cardiovascular: Edema (ankle or facial), palpitation

Central nervous system: Amnesia, ataxia (seizure disorder ~30%; panic disorder 5%), behavior problems (seizure disorder ~25%), coma, confusion, depression, dizziness, drowsiness (seizure disorder ~50%), emotional lability, fatigue, fever, hallucinations, headache, hypotonia, hysteria, insomnia, intellectual ability reduced, memory disturbance, nervousness; paradoxical reactions (including aggressive behavior, agitation, anxiety, excitability, hostility, irritability, nervousness, nightmares, sleep disturbance, vivid dreams); psychosis, slurred speech, somnolence (panic disorder 37%), suicidal attempt, vertigo

Dermatologic: Hair loss, hirsutism, skin rash

Endocrine & metabolic: Dysmenorrhea, libido increased/decreased

Gastrointestinal: Abdominal pain, anorexia, appetite increased/decreased, coated tongue, constipation, dehydration, diarrhea, gastritis, gum soreness, nausea, weight changes (loss/gain), xerostomia

Genitourinary: Colpitis, dysuria, ejaculation delayed, enuresis, impotence, micturition frequency, nocturia, urinary retention, urinary tract infection

Hematologic: Anemia, eosinophilia, leukopenia, thrombocytopenia

Hepatic: Alkaline phosphatase increased (transient), hepatomegaly, transaminases increased (transient)

Neuromuscular & skeletal: Choreiform movements, coordination abnormal, dysarthria, muscle pain, muscle weakness, myalgia, tremor

Ocular: Blurred vision, eye movements abnormal, diplopia, nystagmus

Respiratory: Chest congestion, cough, bronchitis, hypersecretions, pharyngitis, respiratory depression, respiratory tract infection, rhinitis, rhinorrhea, shortness of breath, sinusitis

Miscellaneous: Allergic reaction, aphonia, dysdiadochokinesis, encopresis, "glassy-eyed" appearance, hemiparesis, lymphadenopathy

Drug Interactions

Metabolism/Transport Effects Substrate of CYP3A4 (major)

Avoid Concomitant Use There are no known interactions where it is recommended to avoid concomitant use.

Increased Effect/Toxicity

ClonazePAM may increase the levels/effects of: Alcohol (Ethyl); Clozapine; CNS Depressants; Phenytoin

The levels/effects of ClonazePAM may be increased by: Antifungal Agents (Azole Derivatives, Systemic); Aprepitant; Calcium Channel Blockers (Nondihydropyridine); Cimetidine; CYP3A4 Inhibitors (Moderate); CYP3A4 Inhibitors (Strong); Dasatinib; Disulfiram; Fluconazole; Fosaprepitant; Grapefruit Juice; Isoniazid; Macrolide Antibiotics; Nefazodone; Oral Contraceptive (Estrogens); Oral Contraceptive (Progestins); Protease Inhibitors; Proton Pump Inhibitors; Selective Serotonin Reuptake Inhibitors

Decreased Effect

The levels/effects of ClonazePAM may be decreased by: CarBAMazepine; CYP3A4 Inducers (Strong); Deferasirox; Rifamycin Derivatives; St Johns Wort; Theophylline Derivatives; Yohimbine

Ethanol/Nutrition/Herb Interactions

Ethanol: Avoid ethanol (may increase CNS depression).

Food: Clonazepam serum concentration is unlikely to be increased by grapefruit juice because of clonazepam's high oral bioavailability.

Herb/Nutraceutical: St John's wort may decrease clonazepam levels. Avoid valerian, St John's wort, kava kava, gotu kola (may increase CNS depression).

Mechanism of Action The exact mechanism is unknown, but believed to be related to its ability to enhance the activity of GABA; suppresses the spike-and-wave discharge in absence seizures by depressing nerve transmission in the motor cortex

Pharmacodynamics/Kinetics

Onset of action: 20-60 minutes

Duration: Infants and young children: 6-8 hours; Adults: ≤12 hours

Absorption: Well absorbed

Distribution: Adults: V_d: 1.5-4.4 L/kg

Protein binding: 85%

Metabolism: Extensively hepatic via glucuronide and sulfate conjugation

Half-life elimination: Children: 22-33 hours; Adults: 19-50 hours

Time to peak, serum: 1-3 hours; Steady-state: 5-7 days

Excretion: Urine (<2% as unchanged drug); metabolites excreted as glucuronide or sulfate conjugates

Dosage Oral:

Children <10 years or 30 kg: Seizure disorders:

Initial daily dose: 0.01-0.03 mg/kg/day (maximum: 0.05 mg/kg/day) given in 2-3 divided doses; increase by no more than 0.5 mg every third day until seizures are controlled or adverse effects seen

Usual maintenance dose: 0.1-0.2 mg/kg/day divided 3 times/day, not to exceed 0.2 mg/kg/day

Adults:

Burning mouth syndrome (dental use): 0.25-3 mg/day in 2 divided doses, in morning and evening

Seizure disorders:

Initial daily dose not to exceed 1.5 mg given in 3 divided doses; may increase by 0.5-1 mg every third day until seizures are controlled or adverse effects seen (maximum: 20 mg/day)

Usual maintenance dose: 0.05-0.2 mg/kg; do not exceed 20 mg/day

Panic disorder: 0.25 mg twice daily; increase in increments of 0.125-0.25 mg twice daily every 3 days; target dose: 1 mg/day (maximum: 4 mg/day)

Discontinuation of treatment: To discontinue, treatment should be withdrawn gradually. Decrease dose by 0.125 mg twice daily every 3 days until medication is completely withdrawn.

Elderly: Initiate with low doses and observe closely

Hemodialysis: Supplemental dose is not necessary

Administration Orally-disintegrating tablet: Open pouch and peel back foil on the blister; do not push tablet through foil. Use dry hands to remove tablet and place in mouth. May be swallowed with or without water. Use immediately after removing from package.

Monitoring Parameters CBC, liver function tests; observe patient for excess sedation, respiratory depression

Reference Range Relationship between serum concentration and seizure control is not well established

Timing of serum samples: Peak serum levels occur 1-3 hours after oral ingestion; the half-life is 20-40 hours; therefore, steady-state occurs in 5-7 days

Therapeutic levels: 20-80 ng/mL; Toxic concentration: >80 ng/mL

Additional Information Ethosuximide or valproic acid may be preferred for treatment of absence (petit mal) seizures. Clonazepam-induced behavioral disturbances may be more frequent in mentally handicapped patients. Abrupt discontinuation after sustained use (generally >10 days) may cause withdrawal symptoms. Flumazenil, a competitive benzodiazepine antagonist at the CNS receptor site, reverses benzodiazepine-induced CNS depression.

Dosage Forms Excipient information presented when available (limited, particularly for generics); consult specific product labeling.

Tablet: 0.5 mg, 1 mg, 2 mg

Klonopin®: 0.5 mg, 1 mg, 2 mg

Tablet, orally disintegrating: 0.125 mg, 0.25 mg, 0.5 mg, 1 mg, 2 mg

Klonopin® Wafers: 0.125 mg, 0.25 mg, 0.5 mg, 1 mg, 2 mg

Extemporaneous Preparations A 0.1 mg/mL oral suspension has been made using five 2 mg tablets, purified water USP (10 mL), and methylcellulose 1% (qs ad 100 mL). The expected stability of this preparation is 2 weeks if stored under refrigeration; shake well before use.

Nahata MC and Hipple TF, *Pediatric Drug Formulations*, 2nd ed, Cincinnati, OH: Harvey Whitney Books Co, 1992.

CloNIDine (KLON i deen)

U.S. Brand Names Catapres-TTS®; Catapres®; Duraclon®

Canadian Brand Names Apo-Clonidine®; Carapres®; Dixarit®; DOM-Clonidine; Novo-Clonidine; Nu-Clonidine

Index Terms Clonidine Hydrochloride

Pharmacologic Category Alpha$_2$-Adrenergic Agonist

Additional Appendix Information

Hypertension *on page 1820*

Use Management of mild-to-moderate hypertension; either used alone or in combination with other antihypertensives

Orphan drug: Duraclon®: For continuous epidural administration as adjunctive therapy with intraspinal opiates for treatment of cancer pain in patients tolerant to or unresponsive to intraspinal opiates

Unlabeled/Investigational Use Heroin or nicotine withdrawal; severe pain; dysmenorrhea; vasomotor symptoms associated with menopause; ethanol dependence; prophylaxis of migraines; glaucoma; diabetes-associated diarrhea; impulse control disorder, attention-deficit/hyperactivity disorder (ADHD), clozapine-induced sialorrhea

Pregnancy Risk Factor C

Pregnancy Considerations Clonidine crosses the placenta. Caution should be used with this drug due to the potential of rebound hypertension with abrupt discontinuation.

Lactation Enters breast milk/not recommended

Medication Safety Issues

Sound-alike/look-alike issues:

CloNIDine may be confused with Clomid®, clomiPHENE, clonazePAM, clozapine, Klonopin®, quiNIDine

Catapres® may be confused with Cataflam®, Cetapred®, Combipres®

High alert medication: The Institute for Safe Medication Practices (ISMP) includes this medication (epidural administration) among its list of drug classes which have a heightened risk of causing significant patient harm when used in error.

Transdermal patch may contain conducting metal (eg, aluminum); remove patch prior to MRI.

Contraindications Hypersensitivity to clonidine hydrochloride or any component of the formulation

Warnings/Precautions Gradual withdrawal is needed (over 1 week for oral, 2-4 days with epidural) if drug needs to be stopped. Patients should be instructed about abrupt discontinuation (causes rapid increase in BP and symptoms of sympathetic overactivity). In patients on both a beta-blocker and clonidine where withdrawal of clonidine is necessary, withdraw the beta-blocker first and several days before clonidine. Then slowly decrease clonidine.

Use with caution in patients with severe coronary insufficiency; conduction disturbances; recent MI, CVA, or chronic renal insufficiency. Caution in sinus node dysfunction. Discontinue within 4 hours of surgery then restart as soon as possible after. Clonidine injection should be administered via a continuous epidural infusion device. **[U.S. Boxed Warning]: Epidural clonidine is not recommended for perioperative, obstetrical, or postpartum pain.** It is not recommended for use in patients with severe cardiovascular disease or hemodynamic instability. In all cases, the epidural may lead to cardiovascular instability (hypotension, bradycardia). Transdermal patch may contain conducting metal (eg, aluminum); remove patch prior to MRI. Due to the potential for altered electrical conductivity, remove transdermal patch before cardioversion or defibrillation. Clonidine cause significant CNS depression and xerostomia. Caution in patients with pre-existing CNS disease or depression. Elderly may be at greater risk for CNS depressive effects, favoring other agents in this population.

Adverse Reactions Incidence of adverse events is not always reported.

>10%:

- Central nervous system: Drowsiness (35% oral, 12% transdermal), dizziness (16% oral, 2% transdermal)
- Dermatologic: Transient localized skin reactions characterized by pruritus, and erythema (15% to 50% transdermal)
- Gastrointestinal: Dry mouth (40% oral, 25% transdermal)
- Neuromuscular & skeletal: Weakness (10% transdermal)

1% to 10%:

- Cardiovascular: Orthostatic hypotension (3% oral)
- Central nervous system: Headache (1% oral, 5% transdermal), sedation (3% transdermal), fatigue (6% transdermal), lethargy (3% transdermal), insomnia (2% transdermal), nervousness (3% oral, 1% transdermal), mental depression (1% oral)
- Dermatologic: Rash (1% oral), allergic contact sensitivity (5% transdermal), localized vesiculation (7%), hyperpigmentation (5% at application site), edema (3%), excoriation (3%), burning (3%), throbbing, blanching (1%), papules (1%), and generalized macular rash (1%) has occurred in patients receiving transdermal clonidine.
- Endocrine & metabolic: Sodium and water retention, sexual dysfunction (3% oral, 2% transdermal), impotence (3% oral, 2% transdermal), weakness (10% transdermal)
- Gastrointestinal: Nausea (5% oral, 1% transdermal), vomiting (5% oral), anorexia and malaise (1% oral), constipation (10% oral, 1% transdermal), dry throat (2% transdermal), taste disturbance (1% transdermal), weight gain (1% oral)
- Genitourinary: Nocturia (1% oral)
- Hepatic: Liver function test (mild abnormalities, 1% oral)
- Miscellaneous: Withdrawal syndrome (1% oral)

<1% (Limited to important or life-threatening): Abdominal pain, agitation, alopecia, angioedema, AV block, behavioral changes, blurred vision, bradycardia, chest pain, CHF, contact dermatitis (transdermal), CVA, delirium, depression, dryness of eyes, ECG abnormalities, ethanol sensitivity increased, gynecomastia, hallucinations, hepatitis, localized hypo- or hyperpigmentation (transdermal), nightmares, orthostatic symptoms, pseudo-obstruction, rash, Raynaud's phenomenon, syncope, tachycardia, thrombocytopenia, urinary retention, urticaria, vomiting, withdrawal syndrome

Drug Interactions

Avoid Concomitant Use

Avoid concomitant use of CloNIDine with any of the following: Iobenguane I 123

Increased Effect/Toxicity

CloNIDine may increase the levels/effects of: Amifostine; RiTUXimab

The levels/effects of CloNIDine may be increased by: Beta-Blockers; Diazoxide; Herbs (Hypotensive Properties); Methylphenidate; Prostacyclin Analogues

Decreased Effect

CloNIDine may decrease the levels/effects of: Iobenguane I 123

The levels/effects of CloNIDine may be decreased by: Antidepressants (Alpha2-Antagonist); Herbs (Hypertensive Properties); Serotonin/Norepinephrine Reuptake Inhibitors; Tricyclic Antidepressants; Yohimbine

Ethanol/Nutrition/Herb Interactions

Ethanol: Avoid ethanol (may increase CNS depression).

Herb/Nutraceutical: Avoid dong quai if using for hypertension (has estrogenic activity). Avoid ephedra, yohimbe, ginseng (may worsen hypertension). Avoid valerian, St John's wort, kava kava, gotu kola (may increase CNS depression).

Mechanism of Action Stimulates alpha$_2$-adrenoceptors in the brain stem, thus activating an inhibitory neuron, resulting in reduced sympathetic outflow from the CNS, producing a decrease in peripheral resistance, renal vascular resistance, heart rate, and blood pressure; epidural clonidine may produce pain relief at spinal presynaptic and postjunctional alpha$_2$-adrenoceptors by preventing pain signal transmission; pain relief occurs only for the body regions innervated by the spinal segments where analgesic concentrations of clonidine exist

Pharmacodynamics/Kinetics

Onset of action: Oral: 0.5-1 hour; Transdermal: Initial application: 2-3 days

Duration: 6-10 hours

Distribution: V_d: Adults: 2.1 L/kg; highly lipid soluble; distributes readily into extravascular sites

Protein binding: 20% to 40%

Metabolism: Extensively hepatic to inactive metabolites; undergoes enterohepatic recirculation

Bioavailability: 75% to 95%

Half-life elimination: Adults: Normal renal function: 6-20 hours; Renal impairment: 18-41 hours

Time to peak: 2-4 hours

Excretion: Urine (65%, 32% as unchanged drug); feces (22%)

Dosage

Children:

Oral:

Hypertension: Children ≥12 years: Initial: 0.2 mg/day in 2 divided doses; increase gradually at 5- to 7-day intervals; maximum: 2.4 mg/day

Clonidine tolerance test (test of growth hormone release from pituitary): 0.15 mg/m^2 or 4 mcg/kg as single dose

ADHD (unlabeled use): Initial: 0.05 mg/day; increase every 3-7 days by 0.05 mg/day to 3-5 mcg/kg/day given in divided doses 3-4 times/day (maximum dose: 0.3-0.4 mg/day)

Epidural infusion: Pain management: Reserved for patients with severe intractable pain, unresponsive to other analgesics or epidural or spinal opiates: Initial: 0.5 mcg/kg/hour; adjust with caution, based on clinical effect

Adults:

Oral:

Acute hypertension (urgency): Initial 0.1-0.2 mg; may be followed by additional doses of 0.1 mg every hour, if necessary, to a maximum total dose of 0.6 mg.

Unlabeled route of administration: Sublingual clonidine 0.1-0.2 mg twice daily may be effective in patients unable to take oral medication

Hypertension: Initial dose: 0.1 mg twice daily (maximum recommended dose: 2.4 mg/day); usual dose range (JNC 7): 0.1-0.8 mg/day in 2 divided doses

Nicotine withdrawal symptoms: 0.1 mg twice daily to maximum of 0.4 mg/day for 3-4 weeks

Transdermal: Hypertension: Apply once every 7 days; for initial therapy start with 0.1 mg and increase by 0.1 mg at 1- to 2-week intervals (dosages >0.6 mg do not improve efficacy); usual dose range (JNC 7): 0.1-0.3 mg once weekly

Note: If transitioning from oral to transdermal therapy, overlap oral regimen for 1-2 days; transdermal route takes 2-3 days to achieve therapeutic effects.

Conversion from oral to transdermal:

Day 1: Place Catapres-TTS® 1; administer 100% of oral dose.

Day 2: Administer 50% of oral dose.

Day 3: Administer 25% of oral dose.

Day 4: Patch remains, no further oral supplement necessary.

Epidural infusion: Pain management: Starting dose: 30 mcg/hour; titrate as required for relief of pain or presence of side effects; minimal experience with doses >40 mcg/hour; should be considered an adjunct to intraspinal opiate therapy

Elderly: Initial: 0.1 mg once daily at bedtime, increase gradually as needed

Dosing adjustment in renal impairment: Cl_{cr} <10 mL/minute: Administer 50% to 75% of normal dose initially

Dialysis: Not dialyzable (0% to 5%) via hemo- or peritoneal dialysis; supplemental dose not necessary

Dietary Considerations Hypertensive patients may need to decrease sodium and calories in diet.

Administration

Oral: Do not discontinue clonidine abruptly. If needed, gradually reduce dose over 2-4 days to avoid rebound hypertension

Transdermal patch: Patches should be applied weekly at bedtime to a clean, hairless area of the upper outer arm or chest. Rotate patch sites weekly. Redness under patch may be reduced if a topical corticosteroid spray is applied to the area before placement of the patch.

Monitoring Parameters Blood pressure, standing and sitting/supine, mental status, heart rate

When used for the treatment of ADHD, thoroughly evaluate for cardiovascular risk. Monitor heart rate, blood pressure (when started and weaned), and consider obtaining ECG prior to initiation (Vetter, 2008).

Reference Range Therapeutic: 1-2 ng/mL (SI: 4.4-8.7 nmol/L)

Additional Information Transdermal clonidine should only be used in patients unable to take oral medication. The transdermal product is much more expensive than oral clonidine and produces no better therapeutic effects.

Dosage Forms Excipient information presented when available (limited, particularly for generics); consult specific product labeling.

Injection, solution, as hydrochloride [epidural; preservative free]:

Duraclon®: 100 mcg/mL (10 mL); 500 mcg/mL (10 mL)

Tablet, as hydrochloride: 0.1 mg, 0.2 mg, 0.3 mg

Catapres®: 0.1 mg, 0.2 mg, 0.3 mg

Transdermal system, topical [once-weekly patch]:

Catapres-TTS®-1: 0.1 mg/24 hours (4s)

Catapres-TTS®-2: 0.2 mg/24 hours (4s)

Catapres-TTS®-3: 0.3 mg/24 hours (4s)

Clonidine and Chlorthalidone

(KLON i deen & klor THAL i done)

U.S. Brand Names Clorpres®; Combipres® [DSC]

Index Terms Chlorthalidone and Clonidine

Pharmacologic Category $Alpha_2$-Adrenergic Agonist; Diuretic, Thiazide

Use Management of mild-to-moderate hypertension

Pregnancy Risk Factor C

Medication Safety Issues

Sound-alike/look-alike issues:

Combipres® may be confused with Catapres®

Dosage Oral: 1 tablet 1-2 times/day; maximum: 0.6 mg clonidine and 30 mg chlorthalidone

Additional Information Complete prescribing information for this medication should be consulted for additional detail.

Dosage Forms Excipient information presented when available (limited, particularly for generics); consult specific product labeling.

Tablet:

0.1: Clonidine hydrochloride 0.1 mg and chlorthalidone 15 mg

0.2: Clonidine hydrochloride 0.2 mg and chlorthalidone 15 mg

0.3: Clonidine hydrochloride 0.3 mg and chlorthalidone 15 mg

◆ **Clonidine Hydrochloride** *see* CloNIDine *on page* 354

Clopidogrel (kloh PID oh grel)

U.S. Brand Names Plavix®

Canadian Brand Names Plavix®

Index Terms Clopidogrel Bisulfate

Pharmacologic Category Antiplatelet Agent

Use Reduces rate of atherothrombotic events (myocardial infarction, stroke, vascular deaths) in patients with recent MI or stroke, or established peripheral arterial disease; reduces rate of atherothrombotic events in patients with unstable angina or non-ST-segment elevation acute coronary syndromes (unstable angina and non-ST-segment elevation MI) managed medically or through percutaneous coronary intervention (PCI) (with or without stent) or CABG; reduces rate of death and atherothrombotic events in patients with ST-segment elevation MI (STEMI) managed medically

Unlabeled/Investigational Use In aspirin-allergic patients, initial treatment of acute coronary syndromes (ACS) or prevention of coronary artery bypass graft closure (saphenous vein)

Pregnancy Risk Factor B

Pregnancy Considerations Teratogenic effects were not observed in animal studies. Use during pregnancy only if clearly needed.

Lactation Excretion in breast milk unknown/not recommended

Medication Safety Issues

Sound-alike/look-alike issues:

Plavix® may be confused with Elavil®, Paxil®

Contraindications Hypersensitivity to clopidogrel or any component of the formulation; active pathological bleeding such as peptic ulcer disease (PUD) or intracranial hemorrhage; coagulation disorders

Warnings/Precautions Use with caution in patients who may be at risk of increased bleeding, including patients with PUD, trauma, or surgery. Consider discontinuing 5 days before elective surgery (except in patients with cardiac stents that have not completed their full course of dual antiplatelet therapy; patient-specific situations need to be discussed with cardiologist; AHA/ACC/SCAI/ACS/ADA Science Advisory provides recommendations). Use caution in concurrent treatment with anticoagulants (eg, heparin, warfarin) or other antiplatelet drugs; bleeding risk is increased. Use with caution in patients with severe liver or renal disease (experience is limited). Cases of thrombotic thrombocytopenic purpura (usually occurring within the first 2 weeks of therapy), resulting in some fatalities, have been reported; urgent plasmapheresis is required. Safety and efficacy have not been established in pediatric patients.

Adverse Reactions As with all drugs which may affect hemostasis, bleeding is associated with clopidogrel. Hemorrhage may occur at virtually any site. Risk is dependent on multiple variables, including the concurrent use of multiple agents which alter hemostasis and patient susceptibility.

>10%: Gastrointestinal: The overall incidence of gastrointestinal events (including abdominal pain, vomiting, dyspepsia, gastritis, and constipation) has been documented to be 27% compared to 30% in patients receiving aspirin.

3% to 10%:

Cardiovascular: Chest pain (8%), edema (4%), hypertension (4%)

Central nervous system: Headache (3% to 8%), dizziness (2% to 6%), depression (4%), fatigue (3%), general pain (6%)

Dermatologic: Rash (4%), pruritus (3%)

Endocrine & metabolic: Hypercholesterolemia (4%)

Gastrointestinal: Abdominal pain (2% to 6%), dyspepsia (2% to 5%), diarrhea (2% to 5%), nausea (3%)

Genitourinary: Urinary tract infection (3%)

Hematologic: Bleeding (major 4%; minor 5%), purpura (5%), epistaxis (3%)

Hepatic: Liver function test abnormalities (<3%; discontinued in 0.11%)

Neuromuscular & skeletal: Arthralgia (6%), back pain (6%)

Respiratory: Dyspnea (5%), rhinitis (4%), bronchitis (4%), cough (3%), upper respiratory infection (9%)

Miscellaneous: Flu-like syndrome (8%)

1% to 3%:

Cardiovascular: Atrial fibrillation, cardiac failure, palpitation, syncope

Central nervous system: Fever, insomnia, vertigo, anxiety

Dermatologic: Eczema

Endocrine & metabolic: Gout, hyperuricemia

Gastrointestinal: Constipation, GI hemorrhage, vomiting

Genitourinary: Cystitis

Hematologic: Hematoma, anemia

Neuromuscular & skeletal: Arthritis, leg cramps, neuralgia, paresthesia, weakness

Ocular: Cataract, conjunctivitis

<1% (Limited to important or life-threatening): Acute liver failure, agranulocytosis, allergic reaction, anaphylactoid reaction, angioedema, aplastic anemia, bilirubinemia, bronchospasm, bullous eruption, confusion, erythema multiforme, fatty liver, fever, granulocytopenia, hallucination, hematuria, hemoptysis, hemothorax, hepatitis, hypersensitivity, hypochromic anemia, interstitial pneumonitis, intracranial hemorrhage (0.4%), ischemic necrosis, leukopenia, lichen planus, maculopapular rash, menorrhagia, neutropenia (0.05%), ocular hemorrhage, pancreatitis, pancytopenia, pulmonary hemorrhage, purpura, retroperitoneal bleeding, serum sickness, Stevens-Johnson syndrome, stomatitis, taste disorder, thrombocytopenia, thrombotic thrombocytopenic purpura (TTP), toxic epidermal necrolysis, urticaria, vasculitis

Drug Interactions

Metabolism/Transport Effects **Substrate** of CYP2C19, CYP3A4; CYP1A2 (minor) **Inhibits** CYP2C9 (weak)

Avoid Concomitant Use There are no known interactions where it is recommended to avoid concomitant use.

Increased Effect/Toxicity

Clopidogrel may increase the levels/effects of: Anticoagulants; Antiplatelet Agents; Drotrecogin Alfa; Ibritumomab; Salicylates; Thrombolytic Agents; Tositumomab and Iodine I 131 Tositumomab; Warfarin

The levels/effects of Clopidogrel may be increased by: Dasatinib; Herbs (Anticoagulant/Antiplatelet Properties); Nonsteroidal Anti-Inflammatory Agents; Omega-3-Acid Ethyl Esters; Pentosan Polysulfate Sodium; Prostacyclin Analogues; Rifamycin Derivatives

Decreased Effect

The levels/effects of Clopidogrel may be decreased by: Calcium Channel Blockers; Macrolide Antibiotics; Nonsteroidal Anti-Inflammatory Agents; Proton Pump Inhibitors

Ethanol/Nutrition/Herb Interactions Herb/Nutraceutical: Avoid alfalfa, anise, bilberry, bladderwrack, bromelain, cat's claw, chamomile, coleus, cordyceps, dong quai, evening primrose oil, fenugreek, feverfew, garlic, ginger, ginkgo biloba, ginseng (American), ginseng (Panax), ginseng (Siberian), grape seed, green tea, guggul, horse chestnut seed, horseradish, licorice, prickly ash, red clover, reishi, SAMe (S-adenosylmethionine), sweet clover, turmeric, white willow (all have additional antiplatelet activity).

Stability Store at 25°C (77°F); excursions permitted to 15°C to 30°C (59°F to 86°F).

Mechanism of Action Clopidogrel requires *in vivo* biotransformation to an unidentified active metabolite. This active metabolite irreversibly blocks the $P2Y_{12}$ component of ADP receptors on the platelet surface, which prevents activation of the GPIIb/IIIa receptor complex, thereby reducing platelet aggregation. Platelets blocked by clopidogrel are affected for the remainder of their lifespan.

Pharmacodynamics/Kinetics

Onset of action: Inhibition of platelet aggregation detected: 2 hours after 300 mg administered; after second day of treatment with 50-100 mg/day. At steady-state with 75 mg/day, the average inhibition level observed was 40% to 60%.

Peak effect: 50-100 mg/day: Bleeding time: 5-6 days; Platelet function: 3-7 days

Absorption: Well absorbed

Protein binding: Parent drug: 98%; metabolite: 94%

Metabolism: Extensively hepatic via hydrolysis; biotransformation primarily to carboxyl acid derivative (inactive). The active metabolite that inhibits platelet aggregation has not been isolated.

Half-life elimination: ~8 hours

Time to peak, serum: ~1 hour

Excretion: Urine (50%); feces (46%)

Dosage Oral: Adults:

Recent MI, recent stroke, or established arterial disease: 75 mg once daily

Acute coronary syndrome (ACS):

Unstable angina, non-ST-segment elevation myocardial infarction (UA/NSTEMI): Initial: 300 mg loading dose, followed by 75 mg once daily (in combination with aspirin 75-325 mg once daily). **Note:** A loading dose of 600 mg given at least 2 hours (or 24 hours in patients unable to take aspirin) prior to PCI followed by 75 mg once daily is recommended (*Chest* guidelines, 2008)

ST-segment elevation myocardial infarction (STEMI): 75 mg once daily (in combination with aspirin 75-162 mg/day). CLARITY used a 300 mg loading dose of clopidogrel (with thrombolysis). The duration of therapy was <28 days (usually until hospital discharge) (Sabatine, 2005).

The American College of Chest Physicians (Goodman, 2008) recommends:

Patients ≤75 years: Initial: 300 mg loading dose, followed by 75 mg once daily for up to 28 days (in combination with aspirin)

Patients >75 years: 75 mg once daily for up to 28 days (with or without thrombolysis)

Note: *Coronary artery stents:* Duration of clopidogrel (in combination with aspirin): According to the ACC/AHA/SCAI guidelines, ideally 12 months following drug-eluting stent (DES) placement in patients not at high risk for bleeding; at a minimum, 1, 3, and 6 months for bare metal (BMS), sirolimus eluting, and paclitaxel eluting stents, respectively, for uninterrupted therapy (Smith, 2005). The 2008 *Chest* guidelines recommend for patients who undergo PCI and receive a BMS (with ongoing ACS) or a DES (with or without ongoing ACS) that clopidogrel be continued for at least 12 months. In patients receiving a BMS without ongoing ACS, clopidogrel may be continued for at least 1 month. In patients receiving a DES, therapy with clopidogrel beyond 12 months may be considered in patients without bleeding or tolerability issues (Becker, 2008). Premature interruption of therapy may result in stent thrombosis with subsequent fatal and nonfatal myocardial infarction.

Prevention of coronary artery bypass graft closure (saphenous vein) [*Chest* guidelines, 2008]: Aspirin-allergic patients (unlabeled use): Loading dose: 300 mg 6 hours following procedure; maintenance: 75 mg/day

Dosing adjustment in renal impairment and elderly: None necessary

Dosing adjustment in hepatic impairment: No specific guidelines for patients with hepatic impairment; use with caution

Dietary Considerations May be taken without regard to meals.

Monitoring Parameters Signs of bleeding; hemoglobin and hematocrit periodically

Dosage Forms Excipient information presented when available (limited, particularly for generics); consult specific product labeling.

Tablet:

Plavix®: 75 mg, 300 mg

◆ **Clopidogrel Bisulfate** *see* Clopidogrel *on page 356*

Clorazepate (klor AZ e pate)

U.S. Brand Names Tranxene® SD™; Tranxene® SD™-Half Strength; Tranxene® T-Tab®

Canadian Brand Names Apo-Clorazepate®; Novo-Clopate

Index Terms Clorazepate Dipotassium; Tranxene T-Tab®

Pharmacologic Category Benzodiazepine

Additional Appendix Information

Benzodiazepines *on page 1646*

Use Treatment of generalized anxiety disorder; management of ethanol withdrawal; adjunct anticonvulsant in management of partial seizures

Restrictions C-IV

Pregnancy Risk Factor D

Lactation Excretion in breast milk unknown/not recommended

Medication Safety Issues

Sound-alike/look-alike issues:

Clorazepate may be confused with clofibrate, clonazepam

Contraindications Hypersensitivity to clorazepate or any component of the formulation (cross-sensitivity with other benzodiazepines may exist); narrow-angle glaucoma; pregnancy

Warnings/Precautions Not recommended for use in patients <9 years of age or patients with depressive or psychotic disorders. Use with caution in elderly or debilitated patients, patients with hepatic disease (including alcoholics), or renal impairment. Active metabolites with extended half-lives may lead to delayed accumulation and adverse effects. Use with caution in patients with respiratory disease or impaired gag reflex. Avoid use in patients with sleep apnea.

Causes CNS depression (dose related) resulting in sedation, dizziness, confusion, or ataxia which may impair physical and mental capabilities. Patients must be cautioned about performing tasks which require mental alertness (eg, operating machinery or driving). Use with caution in patients receiving other CNS depressants or psychoactive agents. Effects with other sedative drugs or ethanol may be potentiated. Benzodiazepines have been associated with falls and traumatic injury and should be used with extreme caution in patients who are at risk of these events (especially the elderly).

Use caution in patients with depression, particularly if suicidal risk may be present. Use with caution in patients with a history of drug dependence. Benzodiazepines have been associated with dependence and acute withdrawal symptoms on discontinuation or reduction in dose. Acute withdrawal, including seizures, may be precipitated in patients after administration of flumazenil to patients receiving long-term benzodiazepine therapy.

Benzodiazepines have been associated with anterograde amnesia. Paradoxical reactions, including hyperactive or aggressive behavior, have been reported with benzodiazepines, particularly in adolescent/pediatric or psychiatric patients. Does not have analgesic, antidepressant, or antipsychotic properties.

Adverse Reactions Frequency not defined.

Cardiovascular: Hypotension

Central nervous system: Drowsiness, fatigue, ataxia, lightheadedness, memory impairment, insomnia, anxiety, headache, depression, slurred speech, confusion, nervousness, dizziness, irritability

Dermatologic: Rash

Endocrine & metabolic: Libido decreased

Gastrointestinal: Xerostomia, constipation, diarrhea, salivation decreased, nausea, vomiting, appetite increased or decreased

Neuromuscular & skeletal: Dysarthria, tremor

Ocular: Blurred vision, diplopia

Drug Interactions

Metabolism/Transport Effects Substrate of CYP3A4 (major)

Avoid Concomitant Use There are no known interactions where it is recommended to avoid concomitant use.

Increased Effect/Toxicity

Clorazepate may increase the levels/effects of: Alcohol (Ethyl); Clozapine; CNS Depressants; Phenytoin

The levels/effects of Clorazepate may be increased by: Antifungal Agents (Azole Derivatives, Systemic); Aprepitant; Calcium Channel Blockers (Nondihydropyridine); Cimetidine; CYP3A4 Inhibitors (Moderate); CYP3A4 Inhibitors (Strong); Dasatinib; Disulfiram; Fluconazole; Fosaprepitant; Grapefruit Juice; Isoniazid; Macrolide Antibiotics; Nefazodone; Oral Contraceptive (Estrogens); Oral Contraceptive (Progestins); Protease Inhibitors; Proton Pump Inhibitors; Selective Serotonin Reuptake Inhibitors

Decreased Effect

The levels/effects of Clorazepate may be decreased by: CarBAMazepine; CYP3A4 Inducers (Strong); Deferasirox; Rifamycin Derivatives; St Johns Wort; Theophylline Derivatives; Yohimbine

Ethanol/Nutrition/Herb Interactions

Ethanol: Avoid ethanol (may increase CNS depression).

Food: Serum concentrations/toxicity may be increased by grapefruit juice.

Herb/Nutraceutical: Avoid valerian, St John's wort, kava kava, gotu kola (may increase CNS depression).

Mechanism of Action Binds to stereospecific benzodiazepine receptors on the postsynaptic GABA neuron at several sites within the central nervous system, including the limbic system, reticular formation. Enhancement of the inhibitory effect of GABA on neuronal excitability results by increased neuronal membrane permeability to chloride ions. This shift in chloride ions results in hyperpolarization (a less excitable state) and stabilization.

Pharmacodynamics/Kinetics

Onset of action: 1-2 hours

Duration: Variable, 8-24 hours

Distribution: Crosses placenta; appears in urine

Metabolism: Rapidly decarboxylated to desmethyldiazepam (active) in acidic stomach prior to absorption; hepatically to oxazepam (active)

Half-life elimination: Adults: Desmethyldiazepam: 48-96 hours; Oxazepam: 6-8 hours

Time to peak, serum: ~1 hour

Excretion: Primarily urine

Dosage Oral:

Children 9-12 years: Anticonvulsant: Initial: 3.75-7.5 mg/dose twice daily; increase dose by 3.75 mg at weekly intervals, not to exceed 60 mg/day in 2-3 divided doses

Children >12 years and Adults: Anticonvulsant: Initial: Up to 7.5 mg/dose 2-3 times/day; increase dose by 7.5 mg at weekly intervals, not to exceed 90 mg/day

Adults:

Anxiety:

Regular release tablets (Tranxene® T-Tab®): 7.5-15 mg 2-4 times/day

Sustained release (Tranxene® SD™): 11.25 or 22.5 mg once daily at bedtime

Ethanol withdrawal: Initial: 30 mg, then 15 mg 2-4 times/day on first day; maximum daily dose: 90 mg; gradually decrease dose over subsequent days

Monitoring Parameters Respiratory and cardiovascular status, excess CNS depression

Reference Range Therapeutic: 0.12-1 mcg/mL (SI: 0.36-3.01 µmol/L)

Test Interactions Decreased hematocrit; abnormal liver and renal function tests

Additional Information Abrupt discontinuation after sustained use (generally >10 days) may cause withdrawal symptoms.

Dosage Forms Excipient information presented when available (limited, particularly for generics); consult specific product labeling.

Tablet, as dipotassium: 3.75 mg, 7.5 mg, 15 mg

Tranxene® SD™: 22.5 mg [once daily]

Tranxene® SD™-Half Strength: 11.25 mg [once daily]

Tranxene® T-Tab®: 3.75 mg, 7.5 mg, 15 mg

◆ **Clorazepate Dipotassium** *see* Clorazepate *on page* 358

◆ **Clorpres®** *see* Clonidine and Chlorthalidone *on page* 356

◆ **Clotrimaderm (Can)** *see* Clotrimazole *on page* 359

Clotrimazole (kloe TRIM a zole)

U.S. Brand Names Cruex® Cream [OTC]; Gyne-Lotrimin® 3 [OTC]; Gyne-Lotrimin® 7 [OTC]; Lotrimin® AF Athlete's Foot Cream [OTC]; Lotrimin® AF for Her [OTC]; Lotrimin® AF Jock Itch Cream [OTC]; Mycelex®

Canadian Brand Names Canesten® Topical; Canesten® Vaginal; Clotrimaderm; Trivagizole-3®

Pharmacologic Category Antifungal Agent, Oral Nonabsorbed; Antifungal Agent, Topical; Antifungal Agent, Vaginal

Additional Appendix Information

Guidelines for the Prevention of Opportunistic Infections in HIV Infected Persons *on page* 1740

Treatment of Sexually Transmitted Infections *on page* 1773

Use Treatment of susceptible fungal infections, including oropharyngeal candidiasis, dermatophytoses, superficial mycoses, and cutaneous candidiasis, as well as vulvovaginal candidiasis; limited data suggest that clotrimazole troches may be effective for prophylaxis against oropharyngeal candidiasis in neutropenic patients

Pregnancy Risk Factor B (topical); C (troches)

Medication Safety Issues

Sound-alike/look-alike issues:

Clotrimazole may be confused with co-trimoxazole

Lotrimin® may be confused with Lotrisone®, Otrivin®

Mycelex® may be confused with Myoflex®

International issues:

Cloderm®: Brand name for clocortolone in the United States

Canesten® [multiple international markets] may be confused with Cenestin® which is a brand name for estrogens (conjugated a/synthetic) in the U.S.

Canesten® [multiple international markets]: Brand name for fluconazole in Great Britain

Mycelex® may be confused with Mucolex® which is a brand name for carbocysteine in Ireland, Portugal, and Thailand; a brand name for guaifenesin in Hong Kong

Dosage

Children >3 years and Adults:

Oral:

Prophylaxis: 10 mg troche dissolved 3 times/day for the duration of chemotherapy or until steroids are reduced to maintenance levels

Treatment: 10 mg troche dissolved slowly 5 times/day for 14 consecutive days

Topical (cream, solution): Apply twice daily; if no improvement occurs after 4 weeks of therapy, reevaluate diagnosis

Children >12 years and Adults:

Vaginal:

Cream:

1%: Insert 1 applicatorful vaginal cream daily (preferably at bedtime) for 7 consecutive days

2%: Insert 1 applicatorful vaginal cream daily (preferably at bedtime) for 3 consecutive days

Tablet: Insert 100 mg/day for 7 days or 500 mg single dose

Topical (cream, solution): Apply to affected area twice daily (morning and evening) for 7 consecutive days

Additional Information Complete prescribing information for this medication should be consulted for additional detail.

Dosage Forms Excipient information presented when available (limited, particularly for generics); consult specific product labeling. [DSC] = Discontinued product

Cream, topical: 1% (15 g, 30 g, 45 g)

Cruex®: 1% (15 g) [contains benzyl alcohol]

Lotrimin® AF Athlete's Foot: 1% (12 g) [contains benzyl alcohol]

Lotrimin® AF Jock Itch: 1% (12 g) [contains benzyl alcohol]

Lotrimin® AF for Her: 1% (24 g) [contains benzyl alcohol]

Cream, topical/vaginal: 1% (45 g)

Gyne-Lotrimin® 7: 1% (45 g) [contains benzyl alcohol; packaged with refillable applicator]

Cream, vaginal: 2% (21 g)

Gyne-Lotrimin® 3: 2% (21 g) [contains benzyl alcohol; packaged with 3 disposable applicators]

Solution, topical: 1% (10 mL, 30 mL)

Tablet, vaginal:

Gyne-Lotrimin® 3: 200 mg (3s) [DSC]

Troche, oral: 10 mg

Mycelex®: 10 mg

◆ **Clotrimazole and Betamethasone** *see* Betamethasone and Clotrimazole *on page* 190

Clozapine (KLOE za peen)

U.S. Brand Names Clozaril®; FazaClo®

Canadian Brand Names Apo-Clozapine®; Clozaril®; Gen-Clozapine; PMS-Clozapine

Pharmacologic Category Antipsychotic Agent, Atypical

Use Treatment-refractory schizophrenia; to reduce risk of recurrent suicidal behavior in schizophrenia or schizoaffective disorder

Unlabeled/Investigational Use Schizoaffective disorder, bipolar disorder, childhood psychosis, severe obsessive-compulsive disorder; psychosis/agitation related to Alzheimer's dementia

Restrictions Patient-specific registration is required to dispense clozapine. Monitoring systems for individual clozapine manufacturers are independent. If a patient is switched from one brand/manufacturer of clozapine to another, the patient must be entered into a new registry (must be completed by the prescriber and delivered to the dispensing pharmacy). Healthcare providers, including pharmacists dispensing clozapine, should verify the patient's hematological status and qualification to receive clozapine with all existing registries. The manufacturer of Clozaril® requests that healthcare providers submit all WBC/ANC values following discontinuation of therapy to the Clozaril National Registry for all nonrechallengable patients until WBC is ≥3500/mm^3 and ANC is ≥2000/mm^3.

Pregnancy Risk Factor B

Pregnancy Considerations Teratogenic effects were not seen in animal studies; however, there are no adequate and well-controlled studies in pregnant women. Use during pregnancy only if clearly needed. Healthcare providers are encouraged to enroll women 18-45 years of age exposed to clozapine during pregnancy in the Atypical Antipsychotics Pregnancy Registry (1-866-961-2388).

Lactation Enters breast milk/not recommended (AAP rates "of concern")

Medication Safety Issues

Sound-alike/look-alike issues:

Clozapine may be confused with clofazimine, clonidine, Klonopin®

Clozaril® may be confused with Clinoril®, Colazal®

Contraindications Hypersensitivity to clozapine or any component of the formulation; history of agranulocytosis or granulocytopenia with clozapine; uncontrolled epilepsy, severe central nervous system depression or comatose state; paralytic ileus; myeloproliferative disorders or use with other agents which have a well-known risk of agranulocytosis or bone marrow suppression

Warnings/Precautions **[U.S. Boxed Warning]: Elderly patients with dementia-related psychosis treated with atypical antipsychotics are at an increased risk of death compared to placebo.** An increased incidence of cerebrovascular adverse events (including fatalities) has been reported in elderly patients with dementia-related psychosis. Clozapine is not approved for this indication.

[U.S. Boxed Warning]: Significant risk of agranulocytosis, potentially life-threatening. Therapy should not be initiated in patients with WBC <3500 cells/mm^3 or ANC <2000 cells/mm^3 or history of myeloproliferative disorder. WBC testing should occur periodically on an on-going basis (see prescribing information for monitoring details) to ensure that acceptable WBC/ANC counts are maintained. Initial episodes of moderate leukopenia or granulopoietic suppression confer up to a 12-fold increased risk for subsequent episodes of agranulocytosis. WBCs must be monitored weekly for at least 4 weeks after therapy discontinuation or until WBC is ≥3500/mm^3 and ANC is ≥2000/mm^3. Use with caution in patients receiving other marrow suppressive agents. Eosinophilia has been reported to occur with clozapine and may require temporary or permanent interruption of therapy. Due to the significant risk of agranulocytosis, it is strongly recommended that a patient must fail at least two trials of other primary medications for the treatment of schizophrenia (of adequate dose and duration) before initiating therapy with clozapine.

Cognitive and/or motor impairment (sedation) is common with clozapine, resulting in impaired performance of tasks requiring alertness (eg, operating machinery or driving); use caution in patients receiving general anesthesia. **[U.S. Boxed Warning]: Seizures have been associated with clozapine use in a dose-dependent manner;** use with caution in patients at risk of seizures, including those with a history of seizures, head trauma, brain damage, alcoholism, or concurrent therapy with medications which may lower seizure threshold. Has been associated with benign, self-limiting fever (<100.4°F, usually within first 3 weeks). However, clozapine may also be associated with severe febrile reactions, including neuroleptic malignant syndrome (NMS). Clozapine's potential for extrapyramidal symptoms (including tardive dyskinesia) appears to be extremely low. Risk of dystonia (and probably other EPS) may be greater with increased doses, use of conventional antipsychotics, males, and younger patients.

Deep vein thrombosis, myocarditis, pericarditis, pericardial effusion, cardiomyopathy, and HF have also been associated with clozapine. **[U.S. Boxed Warning]: Fatalities due to myocarditis have been reported; highest risk in the first month of therapy, however, later cases also reported.** Myocarditis or cardiomyopathy should be considered in patients who present with signs/symptoms of heart failure (dyspnea, fatigue, orthopnea, paroxysmal nocturnal dyspnea, peripheral edema), chest pain, palpitations, new electrocardiographic abnormalities (arrhythmias, ST-T wave abnormalities), or unexplained fever. Patients with tachycardia during the first month of therapy should be closely monitored for other signs of myocarditis. Discontinue clozapine if myocarditis is suspected; do not rechallenge in patients with clozapine-related myocarditis. The reported rate of myocarditis in clozapine-treated patients appears to be 17-322 times greater than in the general population. Clozapine should be discontinued in patients with confirmed cardiomyopathy unless benefit clearly outweighs risk. Rare cases of thromboembolism, including pulmonary embolism and stroke resulting in fatalities, have been associated with clozapine.

May cause anticholinergic effects; use with caution in patients with urinary retention, benign prostatic hyperplasia, narrow-angle glaucoma, xerostomia, visual problems, constipation, or history of bowel obstruction. May cause hyperglycemia; in some cases may be extreme and associated with ketoacidosis, hyperosmolar coma, or death. Use with caution in patients with diabetes or other disorders of glucose regulation; monitor for worsening of glucose control. Use with caution in patients with hepatic disease or impairment; hepatitis has been reported as a consequence of therapy.

Use caution with cardiovascular or renal disease. **[U.S. Boxed Warning]: May cause orthostatic hypotension (with or without syncope)** and tachycardia; use with caution in patients at risk of hypotension or in patients where transient hypotensive episodes would be poorly tolerated (cardiovascular disease or cerebrovascular disease). Concurrent use with benzodiazepines may increase the risk of severe cardiopulmonary reactions.

The possibility of a suicide attempt is inherent in psychotic illness or bipolar disorder; use caution in high-risk patients during initiation of therapy. Prescriptions should be written for the smallest quantity consistent with good patient care.

Medication should not be stopped abruptly; taper off over 1-2 weeks. If conditions warrant abrupt discontinuation (leukopenia, myocarditis, cardiomyopathy), monitor patient for psychosis and cholinergic rebound (headache, nausea, vomiting, diarrhea). Significant weight gain has been observed with antipsychotic therapy; incidence varies with product. Monitor waist circumference and BMI. Elderly patients are more susceptible to adverse effects (including agranulocytosis, cardiovascular, anticholinergic, and tardive dyskinesia). Safety and efficacy have not been established in children.

Adverse Reactions

>10%:

Cardiovascular: Tachycardia (25%)

Central nervous system: Drowsiness (39% to 46%), dizziness (19% to 27%), insomnia (2% to 20%)

Gastrointestinal: Constipation (14% to 25%), weight gain (4% to 31%), sialorrhea (31% to 48%), nausea/vomiting (3% to 17%)

1% to 10%:

Cardiovascular: Angina (1%), ECG changes (1%), hypertension (4%), hypotension (9%), syncope (6%)

Central nervous system: Akathisia (3%), seizure (3%), headache (7%), nightmares (4%), akinesia (4%), confusion (3%), myoclonic jerks (1%), restlessness (4%), agitation (4%), lethargy (1%), ataxia (1%), slurred speech (1%), depression (1%), anxiety (1%)

Dermatologic: Rash (2%)

Gastrointestinal: Abdominal discomfort/heartburn (4% to 14%), anorexia (1%), diarrhea (2%), xerostomia (6%), throat discomfort (1%)

Genitourinary: Urinary abnormalities (eg, abnormal ejaculation, retention, urgency, incontinence; 1% to 2%)

Hematologic: Eosinophilia (1%), leukopenia, leukocytosis, agranulocytosis (1%)

Hepatic: Liver function tests abnormal (1%)

Neuromuscular & skeletal: Tremor (6%), hypokinesia (4%), rigidity (3%), hyperkinesia (1%), weakness (1%), pain (1%), spasm (1%)

Ocular: Visual disturbances (5%)

Respiratory: Dyspnea (1%), nasal congestion (1%)

Miscellaneous: Diaphoresis increased, fever, tongue numbness (1%)

<1%, postmarketing, and/or case reports (limited to important or life-threatening): Amentia, amnesia, anemia, arrhythmia (atrial or ventricular), aspiration, blurred vision, bradycardia, bronchitis, cardiomyopathy (usually dilated), cataplexy, CHF, cholestasis, cyanosis, delusions, diabetes mellitus, difficult urination, edema, erythema multiforme, ESR increased, fecal impaction, gastroenteritis, granulocytopenia, hallucinations, hematemesis, hepatitis, hypercholesterolemia (rare), hyperglycemia, hypertriglyceridemia (rare), hyponatremia, hypothermia, impotence, interstitial nephritis (acute), intestinal obstruction, jaundice, loss of speech, MI, myasthenia syndrome, myocarditis, narrow-angle glaucoma, neuroleptic malignant syndrome, palpitations, pancreatitis (acute), paralytic ileus, Parkinsonism, pericardial effusion, pericarditis, phlebitis, pleural effusion, pneumonia, priapism, pulmonary embolism, rhabdomyolysis, rectal bleeding, salivary gland swelling, sepsis, status epilepticus, stroke, Stevens-Johnson syndrome, tardive dyskinesia, thrombocytopenia, thrombocytosis, thromboembolism, thrombophlebitis, vasculitis, wheezing

Drug Interactions

Metabolism/Transport Effects Substrate of CYP1A2 (major), 2A6 (minor), 2C9 (minor), 2C19 (minor), 2D6 (minor), 3A4 (minor); **Inhibits** CYP1A2 (weak), 2C9 (weak), 2C19 (weak), 2D6 (moderate), 2E1 (weak), 3A4 (weak)

Avoid Concomitant Use

Avoid concomitant use of Clozapine with any of the following: Thioridazine

Increased Effect/Toxicity

Clozapine may increase the levels/effects of: Alcohol (Ethyl); Anticholinergics; CNS Depressants; CYP2D6 Substrates; Fesoterodine; Nebivolol; Tamoxifen; Thioridazine

The levels/effects of Clozapine may be increased by: Acetylcholinesterase Inhibitors (Central); Benzodiazepines; Cimetidine; CYP1A2 Inhibitors (Moderate); CYP1A2 Inhibitors (Strong); Lithium formulations; Macrolide Antibiotics; Nefazodone; Omeprazole; Pramlintide; Selective Serotonin Reuptake Inhibitors; Tetrabenazine

Decreased Effect

Clozapine may decrease the levels/effects of: Amphetamines; Anti-Parkinson's Agents (Dopamine Agonist); Codeine; TraMADol

The levels/effects of Clozapine may be decreased by: CarBAMazepine; CYP1A2 Inducers (Strong); Lithium formulations; Omeprazole; Phenytoin

Ethanol/Nutrition/Herb Interactions

Ethanol: Avoid ethanol (may increase CNS depression).

Herb/Nutraceutical: St John's wort may decrease clozapine levels. Avoid kava kava, gotu kola, valerian, St John's wort (may increase CNS depression).

Stability Dispensed in "clozapine patient system" packaging. Store at controlled room temperature. FazaClo™: Protect from moisture; do not remove from package until ready to use.

Mechanism of Action Clozapine (dibenzodiazepine antipsychotic) exhibits weak antagonism of D_1, D_2, D_3, and D_5 dopamine receptor subtypes, but shows high affinity for D_4; in addition, it blocks the serotonin ($5HT_2$), alpha-adrenergic, histamine H_1, and cholinergic receptors

Pharmacodynamics/Kinetics

Protein binding: 97% to serum proteins

Metabolism: Extensively hepatic; forms metabolites with limited or no activity

Bioavailability: 12% to 81% (not affected by food)

Half-life elimination: Steady state: 12 hours (range: 4-66 hours)

Time to peak: 2.5 hours (range: 1-6 hours)

Excretion: Urine (~50%) and feces (30%) with trace amounts of unchanged drug

Dosage Oral:

Children and Adolescents: Childhood psychosis (unlabeled use): Initial: 25 mg/day; increase to a target dose of 25-400 mg/day

Adults:

Schizophrenia: Initial: 12.5 mg once or twice daily; increased, as tolerated, in increments of 25-50 mg/day to a target dose of 300-450 mg/day after 2-4 weeks; may require doses as high as 600-900 mg/day

Reduce risk of suicidal behavior: Initial: 12.5 mg once or twice daily; increased, as tolerated, in increments of 25-50 mg/day to a target dose of 300-450 mg/day after 2-4 weeks; median dose is ~300 mg/day (range: 12.5-900 mg)

Elderly:

Schizophrenia: Dose selection and titration should be cautious

Psychosis/agitation related to Alzheimer's dementia (unlabeled use): Initial: 12.5 mg/day; if necessary, gradually increase as tolerated not to exceed 75-100 mg/day

Termination of therapy: If dosing is interrupted for ≥48 hours, therapy must be reinitiated at 12.5-25 mg/day; may be increased more rapidly than with initial titration, unless cardiopulmonary arrest occurred during initial titration.

In the event of planned termination of clozapine, gradual reduction in dose over a 1- to 2-week period is recommended. If conditions warrant abrupt discontinuation (leukopenia), monitor patient for psychosis and cholinergic rebound (headache, nausea, vomiting, diarrhea).

Patients discontinued on clozapine therapy due to WBC $<2000/mm^3$ or ANC $<1000/mm^3$ should not be restarted on clozapine.

Dosage adjustment for toxicity:

Moderate leukopenia or granulocytopenia (WBC <3000/ mm^3 and/or ANC <1500/mm^3): Discontinue therapy; may rechallenge patient when WBC is >3500/mm^3 and ANC is >2000/mm^3. **Note:** Patient is at greater risk for developing agranulocytosis.

Severe leukopenia or granulocytopenia (WBC <2000/ mm^3 and/or ANC <1000/mm^3): Discontinue therapy and do not rechallenge patient.

Dietary Considerations May be taken without regard to food. Fazaclo™ contains phenylalanine 0.87 mg per 12.5 mg tablet, phenylalanine 1.74 mg per 25 mg tablet, and phenylalanine 6.96 mg per 100 mg tablet.

Administration Orally-disintegrating tablet: Should be removed from foil blister by peeling apart (do not push tablet through the foil). Remove immediately prior to use. Place tablet in mouth and allow to dissolve; swallow with saliva. If dosing requires splitting tablet, throw unused portion away.

Monitoring Parameters Mental status, ECG, WBC (see below), vital signs, fasting lipid profile and fasting blood glucose/Hgb A_{1c} (prior to treatment, at 3 months, then annually; BMI, personal/family history of obesity; waist circumference (weight should be assessed prior to treatment, at 4 weeks, 8 weeks, 12 weeks, and then at quarterly intervals. Consider titrating to a different antipsychotic agent for a weight gain ≥5% of the initial weight); blood pressure; abnormal involuntary movement scale (AIMS).

WBC and ANC should be obtained at baseline and at least weekly for the first 6 months of continuous treatment. If counts remain acceptable (WBC ≥3500/mm^3, ANC ≥2000/ mm^3) during this time period, then they may be monitored every other week for the next 6 months. If WBC/ANC continue to remain within these acceptable limits after the second 6 months of therapy, monitoring can be decreased to every 4 weeks. (**Note**: The decrease in monitoring to every 4 weeks is applicable in the United States. Blood monitoring requirements related to the use of clozapine have not changed in Canada). If clozapine is discontinued, a weekly WBC should be conducted for an additional 4 weeks or until WBC is ≥3500/mm^3 and ANC is ≥2000/mm^3. If clozapine therapy is interrupted due to moderate leukopenia, weekly WBC/ANC monitoring is required for 12 months in patients restarted on clozapine treatment. If therapy is interrupted for reasons other than leukopenia/ granulocytopenia, the 6-month time period for initiation of biweekly WBCs may need to be reset. This determination depends upon the treatment duration, the length of the break in therapy, and whether or not an abnormal blood event occurred.

Consult full prescribing information for determination of appropriate WBC/ANC monitoring interval (http://www.-clozaril.com/index.jsp).

Dosage Forms Excipient information presented when available (limited, particularly for generics); consult specific product labeling.

Tablet: 25 mg, 50 mg, 100 mg, 200 mg

Clozaril®: 25 mg [scored], 100 mg [scored]

Tablet, orally disintegrating:

FazaClo®: 12.5 mg [contains phenylalanine 0.87 mg/ tablet; mint flavor], 25 mg [contains phenylalanine 1.74 mg/tablet; mint flavor], 100 mg [contains phenylalanine 6.96 mg/tablet; mint flavor]

- **Clozaril®** *see* Clozapine *on page 359*
- **CMA-676** *see* Gemtuzumab Ozogamicin *on page 689*
- **CMV-IGIV** *see* Cytomegalovirus Immune Globulin (Intravenous-Human) *on page 387*
- **CNJ-016™** *see* Vaccinia Immune Globulin (Intravenous) *on page 1534*
- **CoActifed® (Can)** *see* Triprolidine, Pseudoephedrine, and Codeine *on page 1523*
- **Coagulant Complex Inhibitor** *see* Anti-inhibitor Coagulant Complex *on page 123*
- **Coagulation Factor I** *see* Fibrinogen Concentrate (Human) *on page 619*
- **Coagulation Factor VIIa** *see* Factor VIIa (Recombinant) *on page 598*
- **CO Alendronate (Can)** *see* Alendronate *on page 58*
- **CO Azithromycin (Can)** *see* Azithromycin *on page 166*
- **CO Bicalutamide (Can)** *see* Bicalutamide *on page 197*
- **CO Buspirone (Can)** *see* BusPIRone *on page 226*
- **CO Cabergoline (Can)** *see* Cabergoline *on page 232*

Cocaine (koe KANE)

Index Terms Cocaine Hydrochloride

Pharmacologic Category Local Anesthetic

Use Topical anesthesia for mucous membranes

Restrictions C-II

Pregnancy Risk Factor C/X (nonmedicinal use)

Dosage Topical application (ear, nose, throat, bronchoscopy): Dosage depends on the area to be anesthetized, tissue vascularity, technique of anesthesia, and individual patient tolerance; the lowest dose necessary to produce adequate anesthesia should be used; concentrations of 1% to 10% are used (not to exceed 1 mg/kg). Use reduced dosages for children, elderly, or debilitated patients.

Additional Information Complete prescribing information for this medication should be consulted for additional detail.

Dosage Forms Excipient information presented when available (limited, particularly for generics); consult specific product labeling. [DSC] = Discontinued product

Powder, for prescription compounding, as hydrochloride: 1 g, 5 g, 25 g

Solution, topical, as hydrochloride: 4% (4 mL, 10 mL); 10% (4 mL, 10 mL) [DSC]

- **Cocaine Hydrochloride** *see* Cocaine *on page 362*
- **CO Ciprofloxacin (Can)** *see* Ciprofloxacin *on page 329*
- **CO Citalopram (Can)** *see* Citalopram *on page 337*
- **CO Clomipramine (Can)** *see* ClomiPRAMINE *on page 350*
- **CO Clonazepam (Can)** *see* ClonazePAM *on page 352*

Codeine (KOE deen)

Canadian Brand Names Codeine Contin®

Index Terms Codeine Phosphate; Codeine Sulfate; Methylmorphine

Pharmacologic Category Analgesic, Opioid; Antitussive

Additional Appendix Information

Narcotic / Opioid Analgesics *on page 1663*

Use Treatment of mild-to-moderate pain; antitussive in lower doses; dextromethorphan has equivalent antitussive activity but has much lower toxicity in accidental overdose

Restrictions C-II

Pregnancy Risk Factor C/D (prolonged use or high doses at term)

Pregnancy Considerations Animal reproduction studies have not been conducted. Neonatal abstinence syndrome (NAS) has been observed in the newborn following maternal use of codeine during pregnancy. Symptoms of opiate withdrawal may include excessive crying, diarrhea, fever, hyperreflexia, irritability, tremors, or vomiting. Perinatal stroke has also been reported.

Lactation Enters breast milk/use caution (AAP rates "compatible")

Medication Safety Issues

Sound-alike/look-alike issues:

Codeine may be confused with Cardene®, Cophene®, Cordran®, iodine, Lodine®

High alert medication: The Institute for Safe Medication Practices (ISMP) includes this medication among its list of drug classes which have a heightened risk of causing significant patient harm when used in error.

Contraindications Hypersensitivity to codeine or any component of the formulation; pregnancy (prolonged use or high doses at term)

Warnings/Precautions Use with caution in patients with hypersensitivity reactions to other phenanthrene-derivative opioid agonists (morphine, hydrocodone, hydromorphone, levorphanol, oxycodone, oxymorphone); respiratory diseases including asthma, emphysema, COPD, adrenal insufficiency, biliary tract impairment, CNS depression/coma, head trauma, morbid obesity, prostatic hyperplasia, urinary stricture, thyroid dysfunction, or severe liver or renal insufficiency; some preparations contain sulfites which may cause allergic reactions; tolerance or drug dependence may result from extended use. May obscure diagnosis or clinical course of patients with acute abdominal conditions. May cause CNS depression, which may impair physical or mental abilities; patients must be cautioned about performing tasks which require mental alertness (eg, operating machinery or driving). May cause hypotension; use with caution in patients with hypovolemia, cardiovascular disease (including acute MI), or drugs which may exaggerate hypotensive effects (including phenothiazines or general anesthetics). Use caution in patients with two or more copies of the variant CYP2D6*2 allele; may have extensive conversion to morphine and thus increased opioid-mediated effects.

Not recommended for use for cough control in patients with a productive cough; not recommended as an antitussive for children <2 years of age; the elderly and debilitated patients may be particularly susceptible to adverse effects of narcotics

Not approved for I.V. administration (although this route has been used clinically). If given intravenously, must be given slowly and the patient should be lying down. Rapid intravenous administration of narcotics may increase the incidence of serious adverse effects, in part due to limited opportunity to assess response prior to administration of the full dose. Access to respiratory support should be immediately available.

Concurrent use of agonist/antagonist analgesics may precipitate withdrawal symptoms and/or reduced analgesic efficacy in patients following prolonged therapy with mu opioid agonists. Abrupt discontinuation following prolonged use may also lead to withdrawal symptoms.

Adverse Reactions

Frequency not defined: ALT increased, AST increased

>10%:

- Central nervous system: Drowsiness
- Gastrointestinal: Constipation

1% to 10%:

- Cardiovascular: Hypotension, tachycardia or bradycardia
- Central nervous system: Confusion, dizziness, false feeling of well being, headache, lightheadedness, malaise, paradoxical CNS stimulation, restlessness
- Dermatologic: Rash, urticaria
- Gastrointestinal: Anorexia, nausea, vomiting, xerostomia
- Genitourinary: Ureteral spasm, u rination decreased
- Hepatic: LFTs increased
- Local: Burning at injection site
- Neuromuscular & skeletal: Weakness
- Ocular: Blurred vision
- Respiratory: Dyspnea
- Miscellaneous: Histamine release

<1% (Limited to important or life-threatening): Biliary spasm, convulsions, hallucinations, insomnia, mental depression, muscle rigidity, nightmares, paralytic ileus, stomach cramps

Drug Interactions

Metabolism/Transport Effects Substrate of CYP2D6 (major), 3A4 (minor); **Inhibits** CYP2D6 (weak)

Avoid Concomitant Use There are no known interactions where it is recommended to avoid concomitant use.

Increased Effect/Toxicity

Codeine may increase the levels/effects of: Alcohol (Ethyl); Alvimopan; CNS Depressants; Desmopressin; Selective Serotonin Reuptake Inhibitors

The levels/effects of Codeine may be increased by: Amphetamines; Antipsychotic Agents (Phenothiazines); Somatostatin Analogs; Succinylcholine

Decreased Effect

Codeine may decrease the levels/effects of: Pegvisomant

The levels/effects of Codeine may be decreased by: Ammonium Chloride; CYP2D6 Inhibitors (Moderate); CYP2D6 Inhibitors (Strong)

Ethanol/Nutrition/Herb Interactions

Ethanol: Avoid or limit ethanol (may increase CNS depression).

Herb/Nutraceutical: St John's wort may decrease codeine levels. Avoid valerian, St John's wort, kava kava, gotu kola (may increase CNS depression).

Stability Store injection between 15°C to 30°C; avoid freezing. Do not use if injection is discolored or contains a precipitate. Protect injection from light.

Mechanism of Action Binds to opiate receptors in the CNS, causing inhibition of ascending pain pathways, altering the perception of and response to pain; causes cough supression by direct central action in the medulla; produces generalized CNS depression

Pharmacodynamics/Kinetics

Onset of action: Oral: 0.5-1 hour; I.M.: 10-30 minutes

Peak effect: Oral: 1-1.5 hours; I.M.: 0.5-1 hour

Duration: 4-6 hours

Absorption: Oral: Adequate

Distribution: Crosses placenta; enters breast milk

Protein binding: 7%

Metabolism: Hepatic to morphine (active)

Half-life elimination: 2.5-3.5 hours

Excretion: Urine (3% to 16% as unchanged drug, norcodeine, and free and conjugated morphine)

Dosage Note: These are guidelines and do not represent the maximum doses that may be required in all patients. Doses should be titrated to pain relief/prevention. Doses >1.5 mg/kg body weight are not recommended.

Analgesic:

Children: Oral, I.M., SubQ: 0.5-1 mg/kg/dose every 4-6 hours as needed; maximum: 60 mg/dose

Adults:

Oral: 30 mg every 4-6 hours as needed; patients with prior opiate exposure may require higher initial doses. Usual range: 15-120 mg every 4-6 hours as needed

Oral, controlled release formulation (Codeine Contin®, not available in U.S.): 50-300 mg every 12 hours. **Note:** A patient's codeine requirement should be established using prompt release formulations; conversion to long acting products may be considered when chronic, continuous treatment is required. Higher dosages should be reserved for use only in opioid-tolerant patients.

I.M., SubQ: 30 mg every 4-6 hours as needed; patients with prior opiate exposure may require higher initial doses. Usual range: 15-120 mg every 4-6 hours as needed; more frequent dosing may be needed

Antitussive: Oral (for nonproductive cough):
- Children: 1-1.5 mg/kg/day in divided doses every 4-6 hours as needed: Alternative dose according to age:
  - 2-6 years: 2.5-5 mg every 4-6 hours as needed; maximum: 30 mg/day
  - 6-12 years: 5-10 mg every 4-6 hours as needed; maximum: 60 mg/day
- Adults: 10-20 mg/dose every 4-6 hours as needed; maximum: 120 mg/day

Dosing adjustment in renal impairment:
- Cl_{cr} 10-50 mL/minute: Administer 75% of dose
- Cl_{cr} <10 mL/minute: Administer 50% of dose

Dosing adjustment in hepatic impairment: Probably necessary in hepatic insufficiency

Administration Not approved for I.V. administration (although this route has been used clinically). If given intravenously, must be given slowly and the patient should be lying down. Rapid intravenous administration of narcotics may increase the incidence of serious adverse effects, in part due to limited opportunity to assess response prior to administration of the full dose. Access to respiratory support should be immediately available.

Monitoring Parameters Pain relief, respiratory and mental status, blood pressure, heart rate

Reference Range Therapeutic: Not established; Toxic: >1.1 mcg/mL

Test Interactions Some quinolones may produce a false-positive urine screening result for opiates using commercially-available immunoassay kits. This has been demonstrated most consistently for levofloxacin and ofloxacin, but other quinolones have shown cross-reactivity in certain assay kits. Confirmation of positive opiate screens by more specific methods should be considered.

Dosage Forms Excipient information presented when available (limited, particularly for generics); consult specific product labeling. [CAN] = Canadian brand name
- Injection, as phosphate: 15 mg/mL (2 mL); 30 mg/mL (2 mL) [contains sodium metabisulfite]
- Powder, for prescription compounding: 10 g, 25 g
- Tablet, as phosphate: 30 mg, 60 mg
- Tablet, as sulfate: 15 mg, 30 mg, 60 mg
- Tablet, controlled release (Codeine Contin®) [CAN]: 50 mg, 100 mg, 150 mg, 200 mg [not available in U.S.]

◆ **Codeine and Acetaminophen** *see* Acetaminophen and Codeine *on page* 27

◆ **Codeine and Guaifenesin** *see* Guaifenesin and Codeine *on page* 710

◆ **Codeine and Promethazine** *see* Promethazine and Codeine *on page* 1251

◆ **Codeine and Pseudoephedrine** *see* Pseudoephedrine and Codeine *on page* 1266

◆ **Codeine, Aspirin, and Carisoprodol** *see* Carisoprodol, Aspirin, and Codeine *on page* 262

◆ **Codeine, Chlorpheniramine, and Pseudoephedrine** *see* Chlorpheniramine, Pseudoephedrine, and Codeine *on page* 314

◆ **Codeine, Chlorpheniramine, Phenylephrine, and Potassium Iodide** *see* Chlorpheniramine, Phenylephrine, Codeine, and Potassium Iodide *on page* 314

◆ **Codeine Contin® (Can)** *see* Codeine *on page* 362

◆ **Codeine, Guaifenesin, and Pseudoephedrine** *see* Guaifenesin, Pseudoephedrine, and Codeine *on page* 715

◆ **Codeine Phosphate** *see* Codeine *on page* 362

◆ **Codeine Phosphate and Pseudoephedrine Hydrochloride** *see* Pseudoephedrine and Codeine *on page* 1266

◆ **Codeine, Promethazine, and Phenylephrine** *see* Promethazine, Phenylephrine, and Codeine *on page* 1251

◆ **Codeine, Pseudoephedrine, and Triprolidine** *see* Triprolidine, Pseudoephedrine, and Codeine *on page* 1523

◆ **Codeine Sulfate** *see* Codeine *on page* 362

◆ **Codeine, Triprolidine, and Pseudoephedrine** *see* Triprolidine, Pseudoephedrine, and Codeine *on page* 1523

◆ **Codiclear® DH [DSC]** *see* Hydrocodone and Guaifenesin *on page* 741

◆ **Cod Liver Oil** *see* Vitamin A and Vitamin D *on page* 1565

◆ **CO Enalapril (Can)** *see* Enalapril *on page* 515

◆ **Co-Famciclovir (Can)** *see* Famciclovir *on page* 602

◆ **Co-Fluconazole (Can)** *see* Fluconazole *on page* 625

◆ **CO Fluoxetine (Can)** *see* FLUoxetine *on page* 638

◆ **CO-Gabapentin (Can)** *see* Gabapentin *on page* 678

◆ **Cogentin®** *see* Benztropine *on page* 186

◆ **Co-Gesic® [DSC]** *see* Hydrocodone and Acetaminophen *on page* 740

◆ **CO Glimepiride (Can)** *see* Glimepiride *on page* 696

◆ **Cognex®** *see* Tacrine *on page* 1418

◆ **CO Ipra-Sal (Can)** *see* Ipratropium and Albuterol *on page* 812

◆ **Colace® [OTC]** *see* Docusate *on page* 473

◆ **Colace® (Can)** *see* Docusate *on page* 473

◆ **Colax-C® (Can)** *see* Docusate *on page* 473

◆ **Colazal®** *see* Balsalazide *on page* 173

◆ **ColBenemid** *see* Colchicine and Probenecid *on page* 365

Colchicine (KOL chi seen)

Pharmacologic Category Colchicine

Use Treatment of acute gouty arthritis attacks and prevention of recurrences of such attacks

Unlabeled/Investigational Use Primary biliary cirrhosis; management of familial Mediterranean fever; pericarditis

Pregnancy Risk Factor C (oral); D (parenteral)

Lactation Enters breast milk/use caution (AAP rates "compatible")

Medication Safety Issues

Sound-alike/look-alike issues:

Colchicine may be confused with Cortrosyn®

High alert medication: The Institute for Safe Medication Practices (ISMP) includes this medication (I.V. formulation) among its list of drugs which have a heightened risk of causing significant patient harm when used in error.

Contraindications Hypersensitivity to colchicine or any component of the formulation; severe renal, gastrointestinal, hepatic, or cardiac disorders; blood dyscrasias; pregnancy (parenteral)

Warnings/Precautions Use with caution in debilitated patients or elderly patients; use caution in patients with mild-to-moderate cardiac, GI, renal, or liver disease. Severe local irritation can occur following SubQ or I.M. administration. Dosage reduction is recommended in patients who develop weakness or gastrointestinal symptoms (anorexia, diarrhea, nausea, vomiting) related to drug therapy.

Intravenous: Use only with extreme caution; potential for serious, life-threatening complications. Should not be administered to patients with renal insufficiency, hepatobiliary obstruction, patients >70 years of age, or recent oral colchicine use. Should be reserved for hospitalized patients who are under the care of a physician experienced in the use of intravenous colchicine.

Adverse Reactions

>10%: Gastrointestinal: Nausea, vomiting, diarrhea, abdominal pain

1% to 10%:

Dermatologic: Alopecia

Gastrointestinal: Anorexia

<1% (Limited to important or life-threatening): Agranulocytosis, aplastic anemia, arrhythmia (with intravenous administration), azoospermia, bone marrow suppression, dermatosis, hepatotoxicity, hypersensitivity reaction, myopathy, peripheral neuritis, purpura, rash

Drug Interactions

Metabolism/Transport Effects **Substrate** of CYP3A4 (major); **Induces** CYP2C8 (weak), 2C9 (weak), 2E1 (weak), 3A4 (weak)

Avoid Concomitant Use There are no known interactions where it is recommended to avoid concomitant use.

Increased Effect/Toxicity

Colchicine may increase the levels/effects of: CycloSPORINE; HMG-CoA Reductase Inhibitors; Verapamil

The levels/effects of Colchicine may be increased by: CycloSPORINE; CYP3A4 Inhibitors (Moderate); CYP3A4 Inhibitors (Strong); Dasatinib; Macrolide Antibiotics; P-Glycoprotein Inhibitors; Verapamil

Decreased Effect

Colchicine may decrease the levels/effects of: Maraviroc

The levels/effects of Colchicine may be decreased by: P-Glycoprotein Inducers

Ethanol/Nutrition/Herb Interactions

Ethanol: Avoid ethanol.

Food: Cyanocobalamin (vitamin B_{12}): Malabsorption of the substrate. May result in macrocytic anemia or neurologic dysfunction.

Herb/Nutraceutical: Vitamin B_{12} absorption may be decreased by colchicine.

Stability Protect tablets from light.

Mechanism of Action Decreases leukocyte motility, decreases phagocytosis in joints and lactic acid production, thereby reducing the deposition of urate crystals that perpetuates the inflammatory response

Pharmacodynamics/Kinetics

Onset of action: Oral: Pain relief: ~12 hours if adequately dosed

Distribution: Concentrates in leukocytes, kidney, spleen, and liver; does not distribute in heart, skeletal muscle, and brain

Protein binding: 10% to 31%

Metabolism: Partially hepatic via deacetylation

Half-life elimination: 12-30 minutes; End-stage renal disease: 45 minutes

Time to peak, serum: Oral: 0.5-2 hours, declining for the next 2 hours before increasing again due to enterohepatic recycling

Excretion: Primarily feces; urine (10% to 20%)

Dosage

Familial Mediterranean fever (unlabeled use): Prophylaxis: Oral:

Children:

≤5 years: 0.5 mg/day

>5 years: 1-1.5 mg/day in 2-3 divided doses

Adults: 1-2 mg daily in divided doses (occasionally reduced to 0.6 mg/day in patients with GI intolerance)

Gouty arthritis: Adults:

Prophylaxis of acute attacks: Oral: 0.6 mg twice daily; initial and/or subsequent dosage may be decreased (ie, 0.6 mg once daily) in patients at risk of toxicity or in those who are intolerant (including weakness, loose stools, or diarrhea); range: 0.6 mg every other day to 0.6 mg 3 times/day

Acute attacks:

Oral: Initial: 0.6-1.2 mg, followed by 0.6 every 1-2 hours; some clinicians recommend a maximum of 3 doses; more aggressive approaches have recommended a maximum dose of up to 6 mg. Wait at least 3 days before initiating another course of therapy

I.V.: Initial: 1-2 mg, then 0.5 mg every 6 hours until response, not to exceed total dose of 4 mg. If pain recurs, it may be necessary to administer additional daily doses. The amount of colchicine administered intravenously in an acute treatment period (generally ~1 week) should not exceed a total dose of 4 mg. Do not administer more colchicine by any route for at least 7 days after a full course of I.V. therapy.

Note: Many experts would avoid use because of potential for serious, life-threatening complications. Should not be administered to patients with renal insufficiency, hepatobiliary obstruction, patients >70 years of age, or recent oral colchicine use. Should be reserved for hospitalized patients who are under the care of a physician experienced in the use of intravenous colchicine.

Surgery: Gouty arthritis, prophylaxis of recurrent attacks: Adults: Oral: 0.6 mg/day or every other day; patients who are to undergo surgical procedures may receive 0.6 mg 3 times/day for 3 days before and 3 days after surgery

Primary biliary cirrhosis (unlabeled use): Adults: Oral: 0.6 mg twice daily

Pericarditis (unlabeled use): Adults: Oral: 0.6 mg twice daily

Elderly: Reduce maintenance/prophylactic dose by 50% in individuals >70 years

Dosing adjustment in renal impairment: Gouty arthritis, acute attacks: Oral: Specific dosing recommendations not available from the manufacturer:

Prophylaxis:

Cl_{cr} 35-49 mL/minute: 0.6 mg once daily

Cl_{cr} 10-34 mL/minute: 0.6 mg every 2-3 days

Cl_{cr} <10 mL/minute: Avoid chronic use of colchicine. Use in serious renal impairment is contraindicated by the manufacturer.

Treatment: Cl_{cr} <10 mL/minute: Use in serious renal impairment is contraindicated by the manufacturer. If a decision is made to use colchicine, decrease dose by 75%.

Peritoneal dialysis: Supplemental dose is not necessary

Dosage adjustment in hepatic impairment: Avoid in hepatobiliary dysfunction and in patients with hepatic disease.

Dietary Considerations May need to supplement with vitamin B_{12}.

Administration

I.V.: Injection should be made over 2-5 minutes into tubing of free-flowing I.V. with compatible fluid. Do not administer I.M. or SubQ; severe local irritation can occur following SubQ or I.M. administration. Extravasation can cause tissue irritation.

Tablet: Administer orally with water and maintain adequate fluid intake.

Monitoring Parameters CBC and renal function test

Test Interactions May cause false-positive results in urine tests for erythrocytes or hemoglobin

Dosage Forms Excipient information presented when available (limited, particularly for generics); consult specific product labeling.

Injection, solution: 0.5 mg/mL (2 mL)

Tablet: 0.6 mg

Colchicine and Probenecid

(KOL chi seen & proe BEN e sid)

Index Terms ColBenemid; Probenecid and Colchicine

Pharmacologic Category Anti-inflammatory Agent; Antigout Agent; Uricosuric Agent

Use Treatment of chronic gouty arthritis when complicated by frequent, recurrent acute attacks of gout

Pregnancy Risk Factor C

Dosage Adults: Oral: 1 tablet daily for 1 week, then 1 tablet twice daily thereafter

Additional Information Complete prescribing information for this medication should be consulted for additional detail.

Dosage Forms Excipient information presented when available (limited, particularly for generics); consult specific product labeling.

Tablet: Colchicine 0.5 mg and probenecid 0.5 g

◆ **Coldcough PD** *see* Dihydrocodeine, Chlorpheniramine, and Phenylephrine *on page 448*

◆ **Coldmist DM [DSC]** *see* Guaifenesin, Pseudoephedrine, and Dextromethorphan *on page 715*

Colesevelam (koh le SEV a lam)

U.S. Brand Names WelChol®

Canadian Brand Names WelChol®

Pharmacologic Category Antilipemic Agent, Bile Acid Sequestrant

Additional Appendix Information

Diabetes Mellitus Management, Adults *on page 1801*

Hyperlipidemia Management *on page 1815*

Lipid-Lowering Agents *on page 1661*

Use Management of elevated LDL in primary hypercholesterolemia (Fredrickson type IIa) when used alone or in combination with an HMG-CoA reductase inhibitor; improve control of type 2 diabetes mellitus (noninsulin dependent, NIDDM) in conjunction with insulin or oral antidiabetic agents

Pregnancy Risk Factor B

Dosage Oral: Adults: 3 tablets twice daily with meals or 6 tablets once daily with a meal

Dosage adjustment in renal impairment: No recommendations made

Dosage adjustment in hepatic impairment: No recommendations made

Elderly: No recommendations made

Additional Information Complete prescribing information for this medication should be consulted for additional detail.

Dosage Forms Excipient information presented when available (limited, particularly for generics); consult specific product labeling.

Tablet, as hydrochloride:

WelChol®: 625 mg

◆ **Colestid®** *see* Colestipol *on page 366*

Colestipol (koe LES ti pole)

U.S. Brand Names Colestid®

Canadian Brand Names Colestid®

Index Terms Colestipol Hydrochloride

Pharmacologic Category Antilipemic Agent, Bile Acid Sequestrant

Additional Appendix Information

Hyperlipidemia Management *on page 1815*

Lipid-Lowering Agents *on page 1661*

Use Adjunct in management of primary hypercholesterolemia; regression of arteriolosclerosis; relief of pruritus associated with elevated levels of bile acids; possibly used to decrease plasma half-life of digoxin in toxicity

Pregnancy Risk Factor C

Dosage Adults: Oral:

Granules: 5-30 g/day given once or in divided doses 2-4 times/day; initial dose: 5 g 1-2 times/day; increase by 5 g at 1- to 2-month intervals

Tablets: 2-16 g/day; initial dose: 2 g 1-2 times/day; increase by 2 g at 1- to 2-month intervals

Additional Information Complete prescribing information for this medication should be consulted for additional detail.

Dosage Forms Excipient information presented when available (limited, particularly for generics); consult specific product labeling.

Granules for suspension, as hydrochloride, oral: 5 g/packet (30s, 90s); 5 g/scoopful (500 g)

Colestid®: 5 g/packet (30s, 90s); 5 g/teaspoon (300 g, 500 g) [unflavored]

Colestid®, flavored: 5 g/packet (60s) [contains phenylalanine (18.2 mg/packet); orange flavor]

Colestid®, flavored: 5 g/scoopful (450 g) [contains phenylalanine (18.2 mg/scoopful); orange flavor]

Tablet, as hydrochloride: 1 g

Tablet, as hydrochloride, oral [micronized]:

Colestid®: 1 g

◆ **Colestipol Hydrochloride** *see* Colestipol *on page 366*

◆ **CO Levetiracetam (Can)** *see* Levetiracetam *on page 872*

◆ **CO Lisinopril (Can)** *see* Lisinopril *on page 894*

Colistimethate (koe lis ti METH ate)

U.S. Brand Names Coly-Mycin® M

Canadian Brand Names Coly-Mycin® M

Index Terms Colistimethate Sodium; Colistin Methanesulfonate; Colistin Sulfomethate; Pentasodium Colistin Methanesulfonate

Pharmacologic Category Antibiotic, Miscellaneous

Use Treatment of infections due to sensitive strains of certain gram-negative bacilli which are resistant to other antibacterials or in patients allergic to other antibacterials

Unlabeled/Investigational Use Used as nebulized inhalation in the prevention of *Pseudomonas aeruginosa* respiratory tract infections in immunocompromised patients, and used as nebulized inhalation adjunct agent for the treatment of *P. aeruginosa* infections in patients with cystic fibrosis and other seriously ill or chronically ill patients

Pregnancy Risk Factor C

Pregnancy Considerations Adverse events have been observed in animal reproduction studies; therefore, the manufacturer classifies colistimethate as pregnancy category C. Colistimethate crosses the placenta in humans. There are no adequate and well-controlled studies in pregnant women.

Lactation Excretion in breast milk unknown/use caution

Contraindications Hypersensitivity to colistimethate, colistin, or any component of the formulation

Warnings/Precautions Nephrotoxicity has been reported; use with caution in patients with pre-existing renal disease; dosage adjustments may be required. Respiratory arrest has been reported with use; impaired renal function may increase the risk for neuromuscular blockade and apnea. Transient, reversible neurological disturbances (eg, dizziness, numbness, paresthesia, tingling, vertigo) may occur. Prolonged use may result in fungal or bacterial superinfection, including *C. difficile*-associated diarrhea (CDAD) and pseudomembranous colitis; CDAD has been observed >2 months postantibiotic treatment.

Adverse Reactions Frequency not defined.

Central nervous system: Dizziness, fever, headache, slurred speech, vertigo

Dermatologic: Pruritus, rash, urticaria

Gastrintestinal: GI upset

Neuromuscular & skeletal: Paresthesia (extremities, oral); weakness (lower limb)

Renal: BUN increased, creatinine increased, nephrotoxicity, proteinuria, urine output decreased

Respiratory: Apnea, respiratory arrest

Postmarketing, and/or case reports: Lung toxicity (bronchoconstriction, bronchospasm, chest tightness, respiratory distress, acute respiratory failure following inhalation)

Drug Interactions

Avoid Concomitant Use There are no known interactions where it is recommended to avoid concomitant use.

Increased Effect/Toxicity

Colistimethate may increase the levels/effects of: Neuromuscular-Blocking Agents

The levels/effects of Colistimethate may be increased by: Aminoglycosides; Amphotericin B; Capreomycin; Polymyxin B; Vancomycin

Decreased Effect

Colistimethate may decrease the levels/effects of: Typhoid Vaccine

Stability Store intact vials (prior to reconstitution) at 20°C to 25°C (68°F to 77°F); reconstituted vials may be refrigerated at 2°C to 8°C (36°F to 46°F) or stored at 20°C to 25°C (68°F to 77°F) for up to 24 hours. Solutions for infusion should be freshly prepared; do not use beyond 24 hours. For I.V. use, reconstitute each vial with 2 mL of SWFI; swirl gently to avoid foaming. May further dilute in D_5W or NS for I.V. infusion. For nebulized inhalation (unlabeled use), reconstitute with NS; should be used promptly after preparation; do not use after 24 hours.

Mechanism of Action Hydrolyzed to colistin, which acts as a cationic detergent which damages the bacterial cytoplasmic membrane causing leaking of intracellular substances and cell death

Pharmacodynamics/Kinetics

Distribution: Widely, except for CNS, synovial, pleural, and pericardial fluids

Metabolism: Colistimethate is hydrolyzed to colistin

Half-life elimination: I.M., I.V.: 2-3 hours; Anuria: ≤2-3 days

Time to peak: I.V.: 10 minutes

Excretion: Primarily urine (as unchanged drug)

Dosage Note: Doses should be based on ideal body weight in obese patients; dosage expressed in terms of colistin.

Children and Adults:

Susceptible infections:

I.M., I.V.: 2.5-5 mg/kg/day in 2-4 divided doses

Inhalation (unlabeled use): 50-75 mg in NS (3-4 mL total) via nebulizer 2-3 times/day

Cystic fibrosis (unlabeled use): I.V.:

Children: 3-8 mg/kg/day in 3 divided doses (maximum dose: 70 mg)

Adults: 3-8 mg/kg/day in 3 divided doses **or** 60-70 mg every 8 hours, if tolerated, may increase to 80-100 mg every 8 hours

Dosing interval in renal impairment: Adults:

S_{cr} 1.3-1.5 mg/dL: 75-115 mg twice daily (approximately 2.5-3.8 mg/kg/day)

S_{cr} 1.6-2.5 mg/dL: 66-150 mg once or twice daily (approximately 2.5 mg/kg/day)

S_{cr} 2.6-4 mg/dL: 100-150 mg every 36 hours (approximately 1.5 mg/kg/day)

Continuous renal replacement therapy (CRRT): Drug clearance is highly dependent on the method of renal replacement, filter type, and flow rate. Appropriate dosing requires close monitoring of pharmacologic response, signs of adverse reactions due to drug accumulation, as well as drug levels in relation to target trough (if appropriate). The following are general recommendations only (based on dialysate flow/ultrafiltration rates of 1 L/hour) and should not supersede clinical judgment:

CVVH or CVVHD/CVVHDF: 2.5 mg/kg every 48 hours

Note: A single case report has demonstrated that the use of 2.5 mg/kg every 48 hours with a dialysate flow rate of 1 L/hour may be inadequate and that dosing every 24 hours was well-tolerated. Based on pharmacokinetic analysis, the authors recommend dosing as frequent as every 12 hours in patients receiving CRRT (Li, 2005).

Administration

Parenteral: Reconstitute vial with 2 mL SWFI resulting in a concentration of 75 mg colistin/mL; swirl gently to avoid frothing. Administer by I.M., direct I.V. injection over 3-10 minutes, intermittent infusion over 30 minutes, or by continuous I.V. infusion. For continuous I.V. infusion, one-half of the total daily dose is administered by direct I.V. injection over 3-10 minutes followed 1-2 hours later by the remaining one-half of the total daily dose diluted in a compatible I.V. solution infused over 22-23 hours. The final concentration for administration should be based on the patient's fluid needs.

Inhalation (unlabeled): Further dilute dose to a total volume of 3-4 mL in NS and administer via nebulizer. If patient is on a ventilator, place medicine in a T-piece at the midinspiratory circuit of the ventilator. Administer solution promptly following preparation to decrease possibility of high concentrations of colistin from forming which may lead to potentially life-threatening lung toxicity.

Monitoring Parameters Serum creatinine, BUN; urine output; signs of neurotoxicity

Dosage Forms Excipient information presented when available (limited, particularly for generics); consult specific product labeling.

Injection, powder for reconstitution, as colistin base: 150 mg

Coly-Mycin® M: 150 mg

◆ **Colistimethate Sodium** *see* Colistimethate *on page 366*

◆ **Colistin Methanesulfonate** *see* Colistimethate *on page 366*

◆ **Colistin, Neomycin, Hydrocortisone, and Thonzonium** *see* Neomycin, Colistin, Hydrocortisone, and Thonzonium *on page 1051*

◆ **Colistin Sulfomethate** *see* Colistimethate *on page 366*

◆ **Collagen** *see* Collagen Hemostat *on page 367*

◆ **Collagen Absorbable Hemostat** *see* Collagen Hemostat *on page 367*

Collagenase (KOL la je nase)

U.S. Brand Names Santyl®

Pharmacologic Category Enzyme, Topical Debridement

Use Promotes debridement of necrotic tissue in dermal ulcers and severe burns

Orphan drug: Injection: Treatment of Peyronie's disease; treatment of Dupytren's disease

Pregnancy Risk Factor C

Dosage Topical: Apply once daily (or more frequently if the dressing becomes soiled)

Additional Information Complete prescribing information for this medication should be consulted for additional detail.

Dosage Forms Excipient information presented when available (limited, particularly for generics); consult specific product labeling.

Ointment:

Santyl®: 250 units/g (15 g, 30 g)

Collagen Hemostat (KOL la jen HEE moe stat)

U.S. Brand Names Avitene®; Avitene® Flour; Avitene® Ultrafoam; Avitene® UltraWrap™; EndoAvitene®; Helistat®; Helitene®; Instat™; Instat™ MCH; SyringeAvitene™

Index Terms Collagen; Collagen Absorbable Hemostat; MCH; Microfibrillar Collagen Hemostat

Pharmacologic Category Hemostatic Agent

Use Adjunct to hemostasis when control of bleeding by ligature is ineffective or impractical

Medication Safety Issues

Sound-alike/look-alike issues:

Avitene® may be confused with Ativan®

Over 100 reports of paralysis or other neural deficits have been received by the FDA, attributable to collagen hemostat-associated neuronal impingement

Dosage Apply dry directly to source of bleeding; remove excess material after ~10-15 minutes

Additional Information Complete prescribing information for this medication should be consulted for additional detail.

Dosage Forms Excipient information presented when available (limited, particularly for generics); consult specific product labeling.

Pad (Instat™) [bovine derived]: 1 inch x 2 inch (24s); 3 inch x 4 inch (24s)

Powder:

Avitene® Flour [microfibrillar product, bovine derived]: 0.5 g, 1 g, 5 g

Helitene® [bovine derived]: 0.5 g, 1 g

Instat™ MCH [microfibrillar product, bovine derived]: 0.5 g, 1 g

SyringeAvitene™ [microfibrillar product, bovine derived, prefilled syringe]: 1 g

Sheet:

Avitene® [microfibrillar product, bovine derived, nonwoven web]: 35 mm x 35 mm (1s); 70 mm x 35 mm (6s, 12s); 70 mm x 70 mm (6s, 12s)

EndoAvitene® [microfibrillar product, bovine derived, preloaded applicator]: 5 mm diameter (6s); 10 mm diameter (6s)

Sponge:

Avitene® Ultrafoam [microfibrillar product, bovine derived]: 2 cm x 6.25 cm x 7 mm (12s); 8 cm x 6.25 cm x 1 cm (6s); 8 cm x 12.5 cm x 1 cm (6s); 8 cm x 12.5 cm x 3 mm (6s)

Avitene® UltraWrap™ [microfibrillar product, bovine derived]: 8 cm x 12.5 cm (6s)

Helistat® [bovine derived]: 0.5 inch x 1 inch x 7 mm (18s) [packaged as 3 strips of 6 sponges]; 3 inch x 4 inch x 5 inch (10s)

◆ **Colocort®** *see* Hydrocortisone *on page* 743

◆ **CO Lovastatin (Can)** *see* Lovastatin *on page* 910

◆ **Coly-Mycin® M** *see* Colistimethate *on page* 366

◆ **Coly-Mycin® S** *see* Neomycin, Colistin, Hydrocortisone, and Thonzonium *on page* 1051

◆ **Colyte®** *see* Polyethylene Glycol-Electrolyte Solution *on page* 1209

◆ **Colyte™ (Can)** *see* Polyethylene Glycol-Electrolyte Solution *on page* 1209

◆ **Combantrin™ (Can)** *see* Pyrantel Pamoate *on page* 1270

◆ **ComBgen™** *see* Folic Acid, Cyanocobalamin, and Pyridoxine *on page* 655

◆ **Combigan™** *see* Brimonidine and Timolol *on page* 212

◆ **Combigan® (Can)** *see* Brimonidine and Timolol *on page* 212

◆ **CombiPatch®** *see* Estradiol and Norethindrone *on page* 558

◆ **Combipres® [DSC]** *see* Clonidine and Chlorthalidone *on page* 356

◆ **Combivent®** *see* Ipratropium and Albuterol *on page* 812

◆ **Combivir®** *see* Zidovudine and Lamivudine *on page* 1583

◆ **Combunox™** *see* Oxycodone and Ibuprofen *on page* 1123

◆ **CO Meloxicam (Can)** *see* Meloxicam *on page* 935

◆ **CO-Metformin (Can)** *see* MetFORMIN *on page* 954

◆ **Comhist® [DSC]** *see* Chlorpheniramine, Phenylephrine, and Phenyltoloxamine *on page* 314

◆ **CO Mirtazapine (Can)** *see* Mirtazapine *on page* 1002

◆ **Commit® [OTC]** *see* Nicotine *on page* 1062

◆ **Compazine** *see* Prochlorperazine *on page* 1244

◆ **Compound E** *see* Cortisone *on page* 370

◆ **Compound F** *see* Hydrocortisone *on page* 743

◆ **Compound S** *see* Zidovudine *on page* 1581

◆ **Compound S, Abacavir, and Lamivudine** *see* Abacavir, Lamivudine, and Zidovudine *on page* 19

◆ **Compoz® Nighttime Sleep Aid [OTC]** *see* DiphenhydrAMINE *on page* 456

◆ **Compro™** *see* Prochlorperazine *on page* 1244

◆ **Comtan®** *see* Entacapone *on page* 522

◆ **Comtrex® Flu Therapy Nighttime [OTC]** *see* Acetaminophen, Chlorpheniramine, and Pseudoephedrine *on page* 31

◆ **Comtrex® Sore Throat Maximum Strength [OTC]** *see* Acetaminophen *on page* 25

◆ **Comvax®** *see Haemophilus* b Conjugate and Hepatitis B Vaccine *on page* 717

◆ **Conal** *see* Chlorpheniramine, Pyrilamine, and Phenylephrine *on page* 315

◆ **Conceptrol® [OTC]** *see* Nonoxynol 9 *on page* 1077

◆ **Concerta®** *see* Methylphenidate *on page* 973

◆ **Congestac® [OTC]** *see* Guaifenesin and Pseudoephedrine *on page* 713

Conivaptan (koe NYE vap tan)

U.S. Brand Names Vaprisol®

Index Terms Conivaptan Hydrochloride; YM087

Pharmacologic Category Vasopressin Antagonist

Use Treatment of euvolemic and hypervolemic hyponatremia in hospitalized patients

Pregnancy Risk Factor C

Pregnancy Considerations Animal studies indicate that conivaptan accumulates in the placenta (2.2-fold relative to maternal plasma); systemic exposure to fetus is likely. No teratogenic effects have been observed in animal studies; however, these studies have shown decreased neonatal viability and delayed growth and development at doses lower than those required for therapeutic efficacy. There are no adequate and well-controlled studies in pregnant women. Use only if benefit outweighs risk.

Lactation Excretion in breast milk unknown/use caution

Contraindications Hypersensitivity to conivaptan or any component of the formulation; use in hypovolemic hyponatremia; concurrent use with strong CYP3A4 inhibitors (eg, ketoconazole, itraconazole, ritonavir, indinavir, and clarithromycin)

Warnings/Precautions Monitor closely for rate of serum sodium increase and neurological status; overly rapid serum sodium correction (>12 mEq/L/24 hours) can lead to permanent neurological damage. Discontinue use if rate of serum sodium increase is undesirable; may reinitiate infusion (at reduced dose) if hyponatremia persists in the absence of neurological symptoms typically associated with rapid sodium rise. Discontinue if hypovolemia or hypotension occurs. Safety and efficacy in heart failure patients have not been established. Use in small numbers of hypervolemic, hyponatremic heart failure patients led to increased adverse events. In other heart failure studies, conivaptan did not show significant improvements in outcomes over placebo. Use with caution in patients with hepatic and renal impairment. May cause injection-site reactions. Safety and efficacy in pediatric patients have not been established.

Adverse Reactions

>10%:

Cardiovascular: Orthostatic hypotension (6% to 14%)

Central nervous system: Fever (5% to 11%)

Endocrine & metabolic: Hypokalemia (10% to 22%)

Local: Injection site reactions including pain, erythema, phlebitis, swelling (63% to 73%)

1% to 10%:

Cardiovascular: Hypertension (6% to 8%), hypotension (5% to 8%), edema (3% to 8%), phlebitis (5%), atrial fibrillation (2% to 5%), ECG abnormality (up to 5%)

Central nervous system: Headache (8% to 10%), insomnia (4% to 5%), confusion (up to 5%), pain (2%)

Dermatologic: Pruritus (1% to 5%), erythema (3%)

Endocrine & metabolic: Hyponatremia (3% to 8%), hypomagnesemia (2% to 5%), hyper-/hypoglycemia (3%)

Gastrointestinal: Constipation (6% to 8%), vomiting (5% to 7%), diarrhea (up to 7%), nausea (5%), dry mouth (4%), dehydration (2%), oral candidiasis (2%)

Genitourinary: Urinary tract infection (4% to 5%)

Hematologic: Anemia (4%)

Renal: Polyuria (5% to 6%), hematuria (2%)

Respiratory: Pneumonia (2% to 5%)

Miscellaneous: Thirst (3% to 6%)

<1%, postmarketing, and/or case reports (limited to important or life-threatening): Atrial arrhythmias, sepsis

Drug Interactions

Metabolism/Transport Effects Substrate of CYP3A4 (major); **Inhibits** CYP3A4 (strong)

Avoid Concomitant Use

Avoid concomitant use of Conivaptan with any of the following: Alfuzosin; Antifungal Agents (Azole Derivatives, Systemic); Eplerenone; Nilotinib; Nisoldipine; Ranolazine; Rivaroxaban; Salmeterol; Silodosin

Increased Effect/Toxicity

Conivaptan may increase the levels/effects of: Alfuzosin; Alosetron; Ciclesonide; CYP3A4 Substrates; Digoxin; Eplerenone; FentaNYL; Fesoterodine; Ixabepilone; Maraviroc; Nilotinib; Nisoldipine; Pimecrolimus; Ranolazine; Rivaroxaban; Salmeterol; Silodosin; Sorafenib

The levels/effects of Conivaptan may be increased by: Antifungal Agents (Azole Derivatives, Systemic); CYP3A4 Inhibitors (Moderate); CYP3A4 Inhibitors (Strong); Dasatinib

Decreased Effect

The levels/effects of Conivaptan may be decreased by: CYP3A4 Inducers (Strong); Deferasirox; Herbs (CYP3A4 Inducers)

Ethanol/Nutrition/Herb Interactions Herb/Nutraceutical: St John's wort may decrease the levels/effects of conivaptan.

Stability Store ampuls in original cardboard container at 15°C to 30°C (59°F to 86°F); protect from light. Dilute loading dose of 20 mg in 100 mL D_5W and continuous infusion dose of 20-40 mg in 250 mL D_5W. After dilution, infusion bag (final concentration of 0.08-0.2 mg/mL) is stable at room temperature for 24 hours.

Mechanism of Action Conivaptan is an arginine vasopressin (AVP) receptor antagonist with affinity for AVP receptor subtypes V_{1A} and V_2. The antidiuretic action of AVP is mediated through activation of the V_2 receptor, which functions to regulate water and electrolyte balance at the level of the collecting ducts in the kidney. Serum levels of AVP are commonly elevated in euvolemic or hypervolemic hyponatremia, which results in the dilution of serum sodium and the relative hyponatremic state. Antagonism of the V_2 receptor by conivaptan promotes the excretion of free water (without loss of serum electrolytes) resulting in net fluid loss, increased urine output, decreased urine osmolality, and subsequent restoration of normal serum sodium levels.

Pharmacodynamics/Kinetics

Protein binding: 99%

Metabolism: Hepatic via CYP3A4 to four minimally-active metabolites

Half-life elimination: 6.7-8.6 hours

Excretion: Feces (83%); urine (12%, primarily as metabolites)

Dosage I.V.: Adults:

Loading dose: 20 mg infused over 30 minutes, followed by continuous infusion of 20 mg over 24 hours

Maintenance: 20 mg/day as continuous infusion over 24 hours; may titrate to maximum of 40 mg/day if serum sodium not rising sufficiently; total duration of therapy not to exceed 4 days

Administration For intravenous use only; do not administer undiluted; infuse into large veins and change infusion site every 24 hours to minimize vascular irritation

Monitoring Parameters Rate of serum sodium increase, blood pressure, volume status, urine output

Dosage Forms Excipient information presented when available (limited, particularly for generics); consult specific product labeling.

Injection, solution:

Vaprisol®: 5 mg/mL (4 mL) [single-use ampul; contains propylene glycol and ethanol]

- **Conivaptan Hydrochloride** *see* Conivaptan *on page 368*
- **Conjugated Estrogen** *see* Estrogens (Conjugated/Equine) *on page 563*
- **Conjugated Estrogen and Methyltestosterone** *see* Estrogens (Esterified) and Methyltestosterone *on page 568*
- **CO Norfloxacin (Can)** *see* Norfloxacin *on page 1080*
- **Constulose** *see* Lactulose *on page 847*
- **Contac® Cold 12 Hour Relief Non Drowsy (Can)** *see* Pseudoephedrine *on page 1265*
- **Contac® Cold and Sore Throat, Non Drowsy, Extra Strength (Can)** *see* Acetaminophen and Pseudoephedrine *on page 30*
- **Contac® Cold-Chest Congestion, Non Drowsy, Regular Strength (Can)** *see* Guaifenesin and Pseudoephedrine *on page 713*
- **Contac® Cold + Flu Maximum Strength Non-Drowsy [OTC]** *see* Acetaminophen and Phenylephrine *on page 29*
- **Contac® Complete (Can)** *see* Acetaminophen, Dextromethorphan, and Pseudoephedrine *on page 33*
- **Contac® Cough, Cold and Flu Day & Night™ (Can)** *see* Acetaminophen, Dextromethorphan, and Pseudoephedrine *on page 33*
- **Continuous Renal Replacement Therapy** *see* Electrolyte Solution, Renal Replacement *on page 510*
- **ControlRx®** *see* Fluoride *on page 635*
- **Co-Pantoprazole (Can)** *see* Pantoprazole *on page 1140*
- **CO Paroxetine (Can)** *see* PARoxetine *on page 1146*
- **Copaxone®** *see* Glatiramer Acetate *on page 695*
- **COPD** *see* Dyphylline and Guaifenesin *on page 501*
- **Copegus®** *see* Ribavirin *on page 1310*
- **CO Pioglitazone (Can)** *see* Pioglitazone *on page 1195*
- **Copolymer-1** *see* Glatiramer Acetate *on page 695*
- **CO Pravastatin (Can)** *see* Pravastatin *on page 1227*
- **CO-Quetiapine (Can)** *see* QUEtiapine *on page 1275*
- **CO Ramipril (Can)** *see* Ramipril *on page 1292*

- **CO Ranitidine (Can)** *see* Ranitidine *on page 1295*
- **Cordarone®** *see* Amiodarone *on page 87*
- **Cordran®** *see* Flurandrenolide *on page 642*
- **Cordran® SP** *see* Flurandrenolide *on page 642*
- **Cordron-D NR [DSC]** *see* Carbinoxamine and Pseudoephedrine *on page 258*
- **Coreg®** *see* Carvedilol *on page 264*
- **Coreg CR®** *see* Carvedilol *on page 264*
- **Corfen DM** *see* Chlorpheniramine, Phenylephrine, and Dextromethorphan *on page 311*
- **Corgard®** *see* Nadolol *on page 1031*
- **Coricidin HBP® Chest Congestion and Cough [OTC]** *see* Guaifenesin and Dextromethorphan *on page 710*
- **Coricidin HBP® Cold and Flu [OTC]** *see* Chlorpheniramine and Acetaminophen *on page 309*
- **Coricidin® HBP Cough & Cold [OTC]** *see* Dextromethorphan and Chlorpheniramine *on page 433*
- **CO Risperidone (Can)** *see* Risperidone *on page 1323*
- **Corlopam®** *see* Fenoldopam *on page 609*
- **Cormax®** *see* Clobetasol *on page 347*
- **Coronex® (Can)** *see* Isosorbide Dinitrate *on page 823*
- **Correctol® [OTC]** *see* Docusate *on page 473*
- **Correctol® Tablets [OTC]** *see* Bisacodyl *on page 198*
- **Cortaid® Intensive Therapy [OTC]** *see* Hydrocortisone *on page 743*
- **Cortaid® Maximum Strength [OTC]** *see* Hydrocortisone *on page 743*
- **Cortaid® Sensitive Skin [OTC]** *see* Hydrocortisone *on page 743*
- **Cortamed® (Can)** *see* Hydrocortisone *on page 743*
- **Cortef®** *see* Hydrocortisone *on page 743*
- **Cortenema®** *see* Hydrocortisone *on page 743*
- **Corticool® [OTC]** *see* Hydrocortisone *on page 743*

Corticorelin (kor ti koe REL in)

U.S. Brand Names Acthrel®

Index Terms Corticorelin Ovine Triflutate; Human Corticotrophin-Releasing Hormone, Analogue; Ovine Corticotrophin-Releasing Hormone

Pharmacologic Category Diagnostic Agent, ACTH-Dependent Hypercortisolism

Use Diagnostic test used in adrenocorticotropic hormone (ACTH)-dependent Cushing's syndrome to differentiate between pituitary and ectopic production of ACTH

Pregnancy Risk Factor C

Medication Safety Issues

Sound-alike/look-alike issues:

Acthrel® may be confused with Acthar®

Corticorelin may be confused with corticotropin

Dosage I.V.: Adults: Testing pituitary corticotrophin function: 1 mcg/kg; dosages >100 mcg have been associated with an increase in adverse effects

Note: Venous blood samples should be drawn 15 minutes before and immediately prior to corticorelin administration to determine baseline ACTH and cortisol. At 15-, 30-, and 60 minutes after administration, venous blood samples should be drawn again to determine response. **Basal and peak responses differ depending on AM or PM administration; therefore, any repeat evaluations are recommended to be done at the same time of day as initial testing.**

Additional Information Complete prescribing information for this medication should be consulted for additional detail.

Dosage Forms Excipient information presented when available (limited, particularly for generics); consult specific product labeling.

Injection, powder for reconstitution, as trifluoroacetate:

Acthrel®: 100 mcg [ovine derived; contains lactose 10 mg]

- **Corticorelin Ovine Triflutate** *see* Corticorelin *on page 370*
- **Cortifoam®** *see* Hydrocortisone *on page 743*
- **Cortifoam™ (Can)** *see* Hydrocortisone *on page 743*
- **Cortimyxin® (Can)** *see* Neomycin, Polymyxin B, and Hydrocortisone *on page 1052*
- **Cortisol** *see* Hydrocortisone *on page 743*

Cortisone (KOR ti sone)

Index Terms Compound E; Cortisone Acetate

Pharmacologic Category Corticosteroid, Systemic

Additional Appendix Information

Corticosteroids *on page 1652*

Use Management of adrenocortical insufficiency

Pregnancy Considerations Adverse events have been observed with corticosteroids in animal reproduction studies. Cortisone is found in cord blood; endogenous maternal cortisol (active) is metabolized by placental enzymes to cortisone (inactive), regulating the amount of maternal glucocorticoids reaching the fetus. Some studies have shown an association between first trimester systemic corticosteroid use and oral clefts; adverse events in the fetus/neonate have been noted in case reports following large doses of systemic corticosteroids during pregnancy. Women exposed to cortisone during pregnancy for the treatment of an autoimmune disease may contact the OTIS Autoimmune Diseases Study at 877-311-8972.

Lactation Excretion in breast milk unknown/use caution

Medication Safety Issues

Sound-alike/look-alike issues:

Cortisone may be confused with Cortizone®

Contraindications Hypersensitivity to cortisone acetate or any component of the formulation; serious infections, except septic shock or tuberculous meningitis; administration of live virus vaccines

Warnings/Precautions Use with caution in patients with thyroid disease, hepatic impairment, renal impairment, cardiovascular disease, diabetes, glaucoma, cataracts, myasthenia gravis, patients at risk for osteoporosis, patients at risk for seizures, or GI diseases (diverticulitis, peptic ulcer, ulcerative colitis) due to perforation risk. Use caution following acute MI (corticosteroids have been associated with myocardial rupture). Because of the risk of adverse effects, systemic corticosteroids should be used cautiously in the elderly in the smallest possible effective dose for the shortest duration. May affect growth velocity; growth should be routinely monitored in pediatric patients. Withdraw therapy with gradual tapering of dose.

May cause hypercorticism or suppression of hypothalamic-pituitary-adrenal (HPA) axis, particularly in younger children or in patients receiving high doses for prolonged periods. HPA axis suppression may lead to adrenal crisis. Withdrawal and discontinuation of a corticosteroid should be done slowly and carefully. Particular care is required when patients are transferred from systemic corticosteroids to inhaled products due to possible adrenal insufficiency or withdrawal from steroids, including an increase in allergic symptoms. Patients receiving >20 mg per day of prednisone (or equivalent) may be most susceptible. Fatalities have occurred due to adrenal insufficiency in asthmatic patients during and after transfer from systemic corticosteroids to aerosol steroids; aerosol steroids do not provide the systemic steroid needed to treat patients having trauma, surgery, or infections.

Acute myopathy has been reported with high dose corticosteroids, usually in patients with neuromuscular transmission disorders; may involve ocular and/or respiratory muscles; monitor creatine kinase; recovery may be delayed. Corticosteroid use may cause psychiatric disturbances, including depression, euphoria, insomnia, mood swings, and personality changes. Pre-existing psychiatric conditions may be exacerbated by corticosteroid use. Prolonged use of corticosteroids may also increase the incidence of secondary infection, mask acute infection (including fungal infections), prolong or exacerbate viral infections, or limit response to vaccines. Exposure to chickenpox should be avoided; corticosteroids should not be used to treat ocular herpes simplex. Corticosteroids should not be used for cerebral malaria or viral hepatitis. Close observation is required in patients with latent tuberculosis and/or TB reactivity; restrict use in active TB (only in conjunction with antituberculosis treatment). Prolonged treatment with corticosteroids has been associated with the development of Kaposi's sarcoma (case reports); if noted, discontinuation of therapy should be considered.

Adverse Reactions

>10%:

Central nervous system: Insomnia, nervousness
Gastrointestinal: Increased appetite, indigestion

1% to 10%:

Dermatologic: Hirsutism
Endocrine & metabolic: Diabetes mellitus
Neuromuscular & skeletal: Arthralgia
Ocular: Cataracts, glaucoma
Respiratory: Epistaxis

<1% (Limited to important or life-threatening): Alkalosis, Cushing's syndrome, delirium, edema, euphoria, fractures, hallucinations, hypersensitivity reactions, hypertension, hypokalemia, muscle wasting, myalgia, osteoporosis, pancreatitis, peptic ulcer, pituitary-adrenal axis suppression, pseudotumor cerebri, psychoses, seizure, skin atrophy, ulcerative esophagitis

Drug Interactions

Avoid Concomitant Use

Avoid concomitant use of Cortisone with any of the following: Natalizumab; Vaccines (Live)

Increased Effect/Toxicity

Cortisone may increase the levels/effects of: Acetylcholinesterase Inhibitors; Amphotericin B; CycloSPORINE; Loop Diuretics; Natalizumab; NSAID (COX-2 Inhibitor); NSAID (Nonselective); Thiazide Diuretics; Vaccines (Live); Warfarin

The levels/effects of Cortisone may be increased by: Antifungal Agents (Azole Derivatives, Systemic); Aprepitant; Calcium Channel Blockers (Nondihydropyridine); CycloSPORINE; Estrogen Derivatives; Fluconazole; Fosaprepitant; Macrolide Antibiotics; Neuromuscular-Blocking Agents (Nondepolarizing); Quinolone Antibiotics; Salicylates; Trastuzumab

Decreased Effect

Cortisone may decrease the levels/effects of: Antidiabetic Agents; Calcitriol; Corticorelin; Isoniazid; Salicylates; Vaccines (Inactivated)

The levels/effects of Cortisone may be decreased by: Aminoglutethimide; Antacids; Barbiturates; Bile Acid Sequestrants; Echinacea; Primidone; Rifamycin Derivatives; Somatropin

Ethanol/Nutrition/Herb Interactions Food: Limit caffeine intake.

Mechanism of Action Decreases inflammation by suppression of migration of polymorphonuclear leukocytes and reversal of increased capillary permeability

Pharmacodynamics/Kinetics

Onset of action: Peak effect: Oral: ~2 hours; I.M.: 20-48 hours
Duration: 30-36 hours
Absorption: Slow
Distribution: Muscles, liver, skin, intestines, and kidneys; crosses placenta; enters breast milk
Metabolism: Hepatic to inactive metabolites
Half-life elimination: 0.5-2 hours; End-stage renal disease: 3.5 hours
Excretion: Urine and feces

Dosage If possible, administer glucocorticoids before 9 AM to minimize adrenocortical suppression; dosing depends upon the condition being treated and the response of the patient. **Note:** Supplemental doses may be warranted during times of stress in the course of withdrawing therapy.

Children:

Anti-inflammatory or immunosuppressive: Oral: 2.5-10 mg/kg/day **or** 20-300 mg/m^2/day in divided doses every 6-8 hours
Physiologic replacement: Oral: 0.5-0.75 mg/kg/day **or** 20-25 mg/m^2/day in divided doses every 8 hours

Adults:

Anti-inflammatory or immunosuppressive: Oral: 25-300 mg/day in divided doses every 12-24 hours
Physiologic replacement: Oral: 25-35 mg/day

Hemodialysis: Supplemental dose is not necessary
Peritoneal dialysis: Supplemental dose is not necessary

Dietary Considerations May need diet with increased potassium, pyridoxine, vitamin C, vitamin D, folate, calcium, and phosphorus and decreased sodium; may be taken with food to decrease GI distress.

Administration Insoluble in water.

Dosage Forms Excipient information presented when available (limited, particularly for generics); consult specific product labeling.

Tablet, as acetate: 25 mg

- ◆ **Cortisone Acetate** *see* Cortisone *on page 370*
- ◆ **Cortisporin® Cream** *see* Neomycin, Polymyxin B, and Hydrocortisone *on page 1052*
- ◆ **Cortisporin® Ointment** *see* Bacitracin, Neomycin, Polymyxin B, and Hydrocortisone *on page 172*
- ◆ **Cortisporin® Ophthalmic [DSC]** *see* Neomycin, Polymyxin B, and Hydrocortisone *on page 1052*
- ◆ **Cortisporin® Otic** *see* Neomycin, Polymyxin B, and Hydrocortisone *on page 1052*
- ◆ **Cortisporin®-TC** *see* Neomycin, Colistin, Hydrocortisone, and Thonzonium *on page 1051*
- ◆ **Cortisporin® Topical Ointment (Can)** *see* Bacitracin, Neomycin, Polymyxin B, and Hydrocortisone *on page 172*
- ◆ **Cortizone®-10 Maximum Strength [OTC]** *see* Hydrocortisone *on page 743*
- ◆ **Cortizone®-10 Plus Maximum Strength [OTC]** *see* Hydrocortisone *on page 743*
- ◆ **Cortizone®-10 Quick Shot [OTC]** *see* Hydrocortisone *on page 743*
- ◆ **Cortrosyn®** *see* Cosyntropin *on page 372*
- ◆ **Corvert®** *see* Ibutilide *on page 763*
- ◆ **CO Sertraline (Can)** *see* Sertraline *on page 1362*
- ◆ **CO Simvastatin (Can)** *see* Simvastatin *on page 1370*
- ◆ **Cosmegen®** *see* DACTINomycin *on page 390*
- ◆ **Cosopt®** *see* Dorzolamide and Timolol *on page 482*
- ◆ **CO Sotalol (Can)** *see* Sotalol *on page 1394*
- ◆ **CO Sumatriptan (Can)** *see* SUMAtriptan *on page 1414*

Cosyntropin (koe sin TROE pin)

U.S. Brand Names Cortrosyn®
Canadian Brand Names Cortrosyn®
Index Terms Synacthen; Tetracosactide
Pharmacologic Category Diagnostic Agent
Use Diagnostic test to differentiate primary adrenal from secondary (pituitary) adrenocortical insufficiency
Pregnancy Risk Factor C
Lactation Excretion in breast milk unknown/use caution
Medication Safety Issues
Sound-alike/look-alike issues:
Cortrosyn® may be confused with colchicine, Cotazym®
Contraindications Hypersensitivity to cosyntropin or any component of the formulation
Warnings/Precautions Use with caution in patients with pre-existing allergic disease or a history of allergic reactions to corticotropin.
Adverse Reactions Frequency not defined.
Cardiovascular: Bradycardia, hypertension, peripheral edema, tachycardia
Dermatologic: Rash
Local: Whealing with redness at the injection site
Miscellaneous: Anaphylaxis, hypersensitivity reaction
Drug Interactions
Avoid Concomitant Use There are no known interactions where it is recommended to avoid concomitant use.
Increased Effect/Toxicity There are no known significant interactions involving an increase in effect.
Decreased Effect There are no known significant interactions involving a decrease in effect.
Stability Powder for injection: Store at controlled room temperature of 15°C to 30°C (59°F to 86°F).
I.M.: Reconstitute cosyntropin 0.25 mg with NS 1 mL.
I.V. push: Reconstitute cosyntropin 0.25 mg with NS 2-5 mL.
I.V. infusion: Mix in NS or D_5W. Stable for 12 hours at room temperature; stable for 21 days under refrigeration.
Mechanism of Action Stimulates the adrenal cortex to secrete adrenal steroids (including hydrocortisone, cortisone), androgenic substances, and a small amount of aldosterone
Pharmacodynamics/Kinetics Time to peak, serum: I.M., IVP: ~1 hour; plasma cortisol levels rise in healthy individuals within 5 minutes
Dosage
Adrenocortical insufficiency: I.M., I.V. (over 2 minutes): Peak plasma cortisol concentrations usually occur 45-60 minutes after cosyntropin administration
Children <2 years: 0.125 mg
Children >2 years and Adults: 0.25-0.75 mg
When greater cortisol stimulation is needed, an I.V. infusion may be used:
Children >2 years and Adults: 0.25 mg administered at 0.04 mg/hour over 6 hours
Administration Administer I.V. doses over 2 minutes
Reference Range Normal baseline cortisol; increase in serum cortisol after cosyntropin injection of >7 mcg/dL or peak response >18 mcg/dL; plasma cortisol concentrations should be measured immediately before and exactly 30 minutes after a dose
Test Interactions Decreased effect: Spironolactone, hydrocortisone, cortisone, etomidate
Additional Information Each 0.25 mg of cosyntropin is equivalent to 25 units of corticotropin.
Patient should not receive corticosteroids or spironolactone the day prior and the day of the test.
Dosage Forms Excipient information presented when available (limited, particularly for generics); consult specific product labeling.
Injection, powder for reconstitution: 0.25 mg

- ◆ **Cotazym® (Can)** *see* Pancrelipase *on page 1136*
- ◆ **CO Temazepam (Can)** *see* Temazepam *on page 1432*
- ◆ **CO Terbinafine (Can)** *see* Terbinafine *on page 1441*
- ◆ **Co-Topiramate (Can)** *see* Topiramate *on page 1489*
- ◆ **Co-Trimoxazole** *see* Sulfamethoxazole and Trimethoprim *on page 1407*
- ◆ **Coughcold HCM [DSC]** *see* Hydrocodone and Pseudoephedrine *on page 742*
- ◆ **Coumadin®** *see* Warfarin *on page 1570*
- ◆ **Covan® (Can)** *see* Triprolidine, Pseudoephedrine, and Codeine *on page 1523*
- ◆ **Covaryx™** *see* Estrogens (Esterified) and Methyltestosterone *on page 568*
- ◆ **Covaryx™ HS** *see* Estrogens (Esterified) and Methyltestosterone *on page 568*
- ◆ **Co-Venlafaxine XR (Can)** *see* Venlafaxine *on page 1554*
- ◆ **Covera® (Can)** *see* Verapamil *on page 1557*
- ◆ **Covera-HS®** *see* Verapamil *on page 1557*
- ◆ **Coversyl® (Can)** *see* Perindopril Erbumine *on page 1174*
- ◆ **Co-Vidarabine** *see* Pentostatin *on page 1171*
- ◆ **Coviracil** *see* Emtricitabine *on page 513*
- ◆ **Cozaar®** *see* Losartan *on page 907*
- ◆ **CP358774** *see* Erlotinib *on page 541*
- ◆ **C-Phen** *see* Chlorpheniramine and Phenylephrine *on page 309*
- ◆ **C-Phen DM** *see* Chlorpheniramine, Phenylephrine, and Dextromethorphan *on page 311*
- ◆ **CPM** *see* Cyclophosphamide *on page 376*
- ◆ **CPT-11** *see* Irinotecan *on page 814*
- ◆ **CPZ** *see* ChlorproMAZINE *on page 316*
- ◆ **Cramp Tabs [OTC]** *see* Acetaminophen and Pamabrom *on page 28*
- ◆ **Crantex LA** *see* Guaifenesin and Phenylephrine *on page 712*
- ◆ **Creon®** *see* Pancrelipase *on page 1136*
- ◆ **Crestor®** *see* Rosuvastatin *on page 1343*
- ◆ **Crinone®** *see* Progesterone *on page 1247*
- ◆ **Critic-Aid® Clear AF [OTC]** *see* Miconazole *on page 989*
- ◆ **Critic-Aid Skin Care® [OTC]** *see* Zinc Oxide *on page 1584*
- ◆ **Crixivan®** *see* Indinavir *on page 782*
- ◆ **Crolom®** *see* Cromolyn *on page 372*
- ◆ **Cromoglycic Acid** *see* Cromolyn *on page 372*

Cromolyn (KROE moe lin)

U.S. Brand Names Crolom®; Gastrocrom®; Intal®; NasalCrom® [OTC]
Canadian Brand Names Apo-Cromolyn®; Intal®; Nalcrom®; Nu-Cromolyn; Opticrom®; Rhinaris-CS Anti-Allergic Nasal Mist
Index Terms Cromoglycic Acid; Cromolyn Sodium; Disodium Cromoglycate; DSCG
Pharmacologic Category Mast Cell Stabilizer
Use
Inhalation: May be used as an adjunct in the prophylaxis of allergic disorders, including asthma; prevention of exercise-induced bronchospasm
Nasal: Prevention and treatment of seasonal and perennial allergic rhinitis

Oral: Systemic mastocytosis
Ophthalmic: Treatment of vernal keratoconjunctivitis, vernal conjunctivitis, and vernal keratitis

Unlabeled/Investigational Use Oral: Food allergy, treatment of inflammatory bowel disease

Pregnancy Risk Factor B

Pregnancy Considerations No data available on whether cromolyn crosses the placenta or clinical effects on the fetus. Available evidence suggests safe use during pregnancy.

Lactation Excretion in breast milk unknown/use caution

Medication Safety Issues

Sound-alike/look-alike issues:
Intal® may be confused with Endal®
NasalCrom® may be confused with Nasacort®, Nasalide®

Contraindications Hypersensitivity to cromolyn or any component of the formulation; acute asthma attacks

Warnings/Precautions Severe anaphylactic reactions may occur rarely; cromolyn is a prophylactic drug with no benefit for acute situations; caution should be used when withdrawing the drug or tapering the dose as symptoms may reoccur; use with caution in patients with a history of cardiac arrhythmias. Transient burning or stinging may occur with ophthalmic use. Dosage of oral product should be decreased with hepatic or renal dysfunction.

Adverse Reactions

Inhalation: >10%: Gastrointestinal: Unpleasant taste in mouth

Nasal:

>10%: Respiratory: Increase in sneezing, burning, stinging, or irritation inside of nose

1% to 10%:
Central nervous system: Headache
Gastrointestinal: Unpleasant taste
Respiratory: Hoarseness, cough, postnasal drip

<1% (Limited to important or life-threatening): Anaphylactic reactions, epistaxis

Ophthalmic: Frequency not defined:

Ocular: Conjunctival injection, dryness around the eye, edema, eye irritation, immediate hypersensitivity reactions, itchy eyes, puffy eyes, styes, rash, watery eyes
Respiratory: Dyspnea

Systemic: Frequency not defined:

Cardiovascular: Angioedema, chest pain, edema, flushing, palpitation, premature ventricular contractions, tachycardia
Central nervous system: Anxiety, behavior changes, convulsions, depression, dizziness, fatigue, hallucinations, headache, irritability, insomnia, lethargy, migraine, nervousness, hypoesthesia, postprandial lightheadedness, psychosis
Dermatologic: Erythema, photosensitivity, pruritus, purpura, rash, urticaria
Gastrointestinal: Abdominal pain, constipation, diarrhea, dyspepsia, dysphagia, esophagospasm, flatulence, glossitis, nausea, stomatitis, unpleasant taste, vomiting
Genitourinary: Dysuria, urinary frequency
Hematologic: Neutropenia, pancytopenia, polycythemia
Hepatic: Liver function test abnormal
Local: Burning
Neuromuscular & skeletal: Arthralgia, leg stiffness, leg weakness, myalgia, paresthesia
Otic: Tinnitus
Respiratory: Dyspnea, pharyngitis
Miscellaneous: Lupus erythematosus

Drug Interactions

Avoid Concomitant Use There are no known interactions where it is recommended to avoid concomitant use.

Increased Effect/Toxicity There are no known significant interactions involving an increase in effect.

Decreased Effect There are no known significant interactions involving a decrease in effect.

Stability Store at room temperature of 15°C to 30°C (59°F to 86°F); protect from light. Do not use oral solution if solution becomes discolored or forms a precipitate.

Mechanism of Action Prevents the mast cell release of histamine, leukotrienes, and slow-reacting substance of anaphylaxis by inhibiting degranulation after contact with antigens

Pharmacodynamics/Kinetics

Onset: Response to treatment:
Nasal spray: May occur at 1-2 weeks
Ophthalmic: May be seen within a few days; treatment for up to 6 weeks is often required
Oral: May occur within 2-6 weeks

Absorption:
Inhalation: ~8% reaches lungs upon inhalation; well absorbed
Oral: <1% of dose absorbed

Half-life elimination: 80-90 minutes
Time to peak, serum: Inhalation: ~15 minutes
Excretion: Urine and feces (equal amounts as unchanged drug); exhaled gases (small amounts)

Dosage

Oral:

Systemic mastocytosis:
Children 2-12 years: 100 mg 4 times/day; not to exceed 40 mg/kg/day; given 1/2 hour prior to meals and at bedtime
Children >12 years and Adults: 200 mg 4 times/day; given 1/2 hour prior to meals and at bedtime; if control of symptoms is not seen within 2-3 weeks, dose may be increased to a maximum 40 mg/kg/day

Food allergy and inflammatory bowel disease (unlabeled use):
Children <2 years: Not recommended
Children 2-12 years: Initial dose: 100 mg 4 times/day; may double the dose if effect is not satisfactory within 2-3 weeks; not to exceed 40 mg/kg/day
Children >12 years and Adults: Initial dose: 200 mg 4 times/day; may double the dose if effect is not satisfactory within 2-3 weeks; up to 400 mg 4 times/day
Note: Once desired effect is achieved, dose may be tapered to lowest effective dose

Inhalation:

For chronic control of asthma, taper frequency to the lowest effective dose (ie, 4 times/day to 3 times/day to twice daily): **Note:** Not effective for immediate relief of symptoms in acute asthmatic attacks; must be used at regular intervals for 2-4 weeks to be effective.
Nebulization solution: Children >2 years and Adults: Initial: 20 mg 4 times/day; usual dose: 20 mg 3-4 times/day
Metered spray:
Children 5-12 years: Initial: 2 inhalations 4 times/day; usual dose: 1-2 inhalations 3-4 times/day
Children ≥12 years and Adults: Initial: 2 inhalations 4 times/day; usual dose: 2-4 inhalations 3-4 times/day

Prevention of allergen- or exercise-induced bronchospasm: Administer 10-15 minutes prior to exercise or allergen exposure but no longer than 1 hour before:
Nebulization solution: Children >2 years and Adults: Single dose of 20 mg
Metered spray: Children >5 years and Adults: Single dose of 2 inhalations

Ophthalmic: Children >4 years and Adults: 1-2 drops in each eye 4-6 times/day

Nasal: Allergic rhinitis (treatment and prophylaxis): Children ≥2 years and Adults: 1 spray into each nostril 3-4 times/day; may be increased to 6 times/day (symptomatic relief may require 2-4 weeks)

Dosage adjustment in renal/hepatic impairment: Specific guidelines not available; consider lower dose of oral product.

Dietary Considerations Oral: Should be taken at least 30 minutes before meals.

Administration

Oral solution: Open ampul and squeeze contents into glass of water; stir well; administer at least 30 minutes before meals and at bedtime

Oral inhalation: Shake canister gently before use; do not immerse canister in water.

Nasal inhalation: Clear nasal passages by blowing nose prior to use.

Monitoring Parameters Periodic pulmonary function tests

Dosage Forms Excipient information presented when available (limited, particularly for generics); consult specific product labeling.

Aerosol, for oral inhalation, as sodium:

Intal®: 800 mcg/inhalation (8.1 g) [112 metered inhalations; 56 doses], (14.2 g) [200 metered inhalations; 100 doses]

Solution for nebulization, as sodium: 20 mg/2 mL (60s, 120s)

Intal®: 20 mg/2 mL (60s, 120s)

Solution, intranasal, as sodium [spray]:

NasalCrom®: 40 mg/mL (13 mL, 26 mL) [5.2 mg/inhalation; contains benzalkonium chloride]

Solution, ophthalmic, as sodium: 4% (10 mL)

Crolom®: 4% (10 mL) [contains benzalkonium chloride]

Solution, oral, as sodium [concentrate]:

Gastrocrom®: 100 mg/5 mL (96s)

◆ **Cromolyn Sodium** *see* Cromolyn *on page* 372

Crotamiton (kroe TAM i tonn)

U.S. Brand Names Eurax®

Pharmacologic Category Scabicidal Agent

Use Treatment of scabies (*Sarcoptes scabiei*) and symptomatic treatment of pruritus

Pregnancy Risk Factor C

Medication Safety Issues

Sound-alike/look-alike issues:

Eurax® may be confused with Efudex®, Eulexin®, Evoxac™, Serax®, Urex®

International issues:

Eurax® may be confused with Urex® which is a brand name for furosemide in Australia

Dosage Topical:

Scabicide: Children and Adults: Wash thoroughly and scrub away loose scales, then towel dry; apply a thin layer and massage drug onto skin of the entire body from the neck to the toes (with special attention to skin folds, creases, and interdigital spaces). Repeat application in 24 hours. Take a cleansing bath 48 hours after the final application. Treatment may be repeated after 7-10 days if live mites are still present.

Pruritus: Massage into affected areas until medication is completely absorbed; repeat as necessary

Additional Information Complete prescribing information for this medication should be consulted for additional detail.

Dosage Forms Excipient information presented when available (limited, particularly for generics); consult specific product labeling.

Cream: 10% (60 g)

Lotion: 10% (60 mL, 480 mL)

◆ **CRRT** *see* Electrolyte Solution, Renal Replacement *on page* 510

◆ **Cruex® Cream [OTC]** *see* Clotrimazole *on page* 359

◆ **Cryselle™** *see* Ethinyl Estradiol and Norgestrel *on page* 585

◆ **Crystalline Penicillin** *see* Penicillin G (Parenteral/Aqueous) *on page* 1164

◆ **Crystal Violet** *see* Gentian Violet *on page* 695

◆ **Crystapen® (Can)** *see* Penicillin G (Parenteral/Aqueous) *on page* 1164

◆ **CsA** *see* CycloSPORINE *on page* 379

◆ **C-Time [OTC]** *see* Ascorbic Acid *on page* 139

◆ **CTLA-4Ig** *see* Abatacept *on page* 20

◆ **CTP 30 (Can)** *see* Citalopram *on page* 337

◆ **CTX** *see* Cyclophosphamide *on page* 376

◆ **Cubicin®** *see* DAPTOmycin *on page* 397

◆ **Cuprimine®** *see* Penicillamine *on page* 1161

◆ **Cutivate®** *see* Fluticasone *on page* 644

◆ **Cutivate™ (Can)** *see* Fluticasone *on page* 644

◆ **CyA** *see* CycloSPORINE *on page* 379

Cyanocobalamin (sye an oh koe BAL a min)

U.S. Brand Names CaloMist™; Nascobal®; Twelve Resin-K

Index Terms Vitamin B_{12}

Pharmacologic Category Vitamin, Water Soluble

Use Treatment of pernicious anemia; vitamin B_{12} deficiency due to dietary deficiencies or malabsorption diseases, inadequate secretion of intrinsic factor, and inadequate utilization of B_{12} (eg, during neoplastic treatment); increased B_{12} requirements due to pregnancy, thyrotoxicosis, hemorrhage, malignancy, liver or kidney disease

CaloMist™: Maintenance of vitamin B_{12} concentrations after initial correction in patients with B_{12} deficiency without CNS involvement

Pregnancy Risk Factor A/C (dose exceeding RDA recommendation); C (intranasal)

Dosage

Adequate intake:

Children:

0-6 months: 0.4 mcg/day

7-12 months: 0.5 mcg/day

Recommended intake:

Children:

1-3 years: 0.9 mcg/day

4-8 years: 1.2 mcg/day

9-13 years: 1.8 mcg/day

Children >14 years and Adults: 2.4 mcg/day

Pregnancy: 2.6 mcg/day

Lactation: 2.8 mcg/day

Vitamin B_{12} deficiency:

I.M., deep SubQ:

Children (dosage not well established): 0.2 mcg/kg for 2 days, followed by 1000 mcg/day for 2-7 days, followed by 100 mcg/week for one month; for malabsorptive causes of B_{12} deficiency, monthly maintenance doses of 100 mcg have been recommended **or** as an alternative 100 mcg/day for 10-15 days, then once or twice weekly for several months

Adults: Initial: 30 mcg/day for 5-10 days; maintenance: 100-200 mcg/month

Intranasal: Adults:

Nascobal®: 500 mcg in one nostril once weekly

CaloMist™: Maintenance therapy (following correction of vitamin B_{12} deficiency): 25 mcg in each nostril daily (50 mcg/day). If inadequate response, 25 mcg in each nostril twice daily (100 mcg/day).

Oral: Adults: 250 mcg/day

Pernicious anemia: I.M., deep SubQ (administer concomitantly with folic acid if needed, 1 mg/day for 1 month):

Children: 30-50 mcg/day for 2 or more weeks (to a total dose of 1000-5000 mcg), then follow with 100 mcg/month as maintenance dosage

Adults: 100 mcg/day for 6-7 days; if improvement, administer same dose on alternate days for 7 doses, then every 3-4 days for 2-3 weeks; once hematologic values have returned to normal, maintenance dosage: 100 mcg/month. **Note:** Alternative dosing of 1000 mcg/day for 5 days (followed by 500-1000 mcg/month) has been used.

Hematologic remission (without evidence of nervous system involvement): Adults:

Intranasal (Nascobal®): 500 mcg in one nostril once weekly

Oral: 1000-2000 mcg/day

I.M., SubQ: 100-1000 mcg/month

Schilling test: Adults: I.M.: 1000 mcg

Additional Information Complete prescribing information for this medication should be consulted for additional detail.

Dosage Forms Excipient information presented when available (limited, particularly for generics); consult specific product labeling.

Injection, solution: 1000 mcg/mL (1 mL, 10 mL, 30 mL) [may contain benzyl alcohol]

Lozenge: 50 mcg, 100 mcg, 250 mcg, 500 mcg

Lozenge, sublingual: 500 mcg

Solution, intranasal [spray]:

CaloMist™: 25 mcg/0.1 mL actuation (18 mL) [contains benzyl alcohol, benzalkonium chloride; 60 metered sprays]

Nascobal®: 500 mcg/0.1 mL actuation (2.3 mL) [contains benzalkonium chloride; delivers 8 sprays]

Tablet: 50 mcg, 100 mcg, 250 mcg, 500 mcg, 1000 mcg

Twelve Resin-K: 1000 mcg [may be used as oral, sublingual, or buccal]

Tablet, timed release: 1000 mcg, 1500 mcg

Tablet, sublingual: 1000 mcg, 2500 mcg, 5000 mcg

- **Cyanocobalamin, Folic Acid, and Pyridoxine** *see* Folic Acid, Cyanocobalamin, and Pyridoxine *on page 655*
- **Cyanokit®** *see* Hydroxocobalamin *on page 750*
- **Cyclen® (Can)** *see* Ethinyl Estradiol and Norgestimate *on page 584*
- **Cyclessa®** *see* Ethinyl Estradiol and Desogestrel *on page 575*

Cyclobenzaprine (sye kloe BEN za preen)

U.S. Brand Names Amrix®; Fexmid™; Flexeril®

Canadian Brand Names Apo-Cyclobenzaprine®; Flexeril®; Flexitec; Gen-Cyclobenzaprine; Novo-Cycloprine; Nu-Cyclobenzaprine

Index Terms Cyclobenzaprine Hydrochloride

Pharmacologic Category Skeletal Muscle Relaxant

Use Treatment of muscle spasm associated with acute painful musculoskeletal conditions

Pregnancy Risk Factor B

Pregnancy Considerations Teratogenic effects were not observed in animal studies. There are no adequate and well-controlled studies in pregnant women. Use during pregnancy only if clearly needed.

Lactation Excretion in breast milk unknown/use caution

Medication Safety Issues

Sound-alike/look-alike issues:

Cyclobenzaprine may be confused with cycloSERINE, cyproheptadine

Flexeril® may be confused with Floxin®

Contraindications Hypersensitivity to cyclobenzaprine or any component of the formulation; do not use concomitantly or within 14 days of MAO inhibitors; hyperthyroidism; congestive heart failure, arrhythmias, heart block; acute recovery phase of MI

Warnings/Precautions May cause CNS depression, which may impair physical or mental abilities; patients must be cautioned about performing tasks which require mental alertness (eg, operating machinery or driving). Cyclobenzaprine shares the toxic potentials of the tricyclic antidepressants (including arrhythmias, tachycardia, and conduction time prolongation) and the usual precautions of tricyclic antidepressant therapy should be observed; use with caution in patients with urinary hesitancy or retention, angle-closure glaucoma or increased intraocular pressure, hepatic impairment, or in the elderly. Do not use concomitantly or within 14 days after MAO inhibitors; combination may cause hypertensive crisis, severe convulsions. Effects may be potentiated when used with other CNS depressants or ethanol. Safety and efficacy have not been established in patients <15 years of age.

Adverse Reactions

>10%:

Central nervous system: Drowsiness (29% to 39%), dizziness (1% to 11%)

Gastrointestinal: Xerostomia (21% to 32%)

1% to 10%:

Central nervous system: Fatigue (1% to 6%), confusion (1% to 3%), headache (1% to 3%), irritability (1% to 3%), mental acuity decreased (1% to 3%), nervousness (1% to 3%), somnolence (1% to 2%)

Gastrointestinal: Abdominal pain (1% to 3%), constipation (1% to 3%), diarrhea (1% to 3%), dyspepsia (≤4%), nausea (1% to 3%), unpleasant taste (1% to 3%)

Neuromuscular & skeletal: Weakness (1% to 3%)

Ocular: Blurred vision (1% to 3%)

Respiratory: Pharyngitis (1% to 3%), upper respiratory infection (1% to 3%)

<1% (Limited to important or life-threatening): Ageusia, agitation, anaphylaxis, angioedema, anorexia, anxiety, arrhythmia, ataxia, cholestasis, depression, diaphoresis, diplopia, disorientation, dysarthria, facial edema, flatulence, gastritis, hallucinations, hepatitis (rare), hypertonia, hypotension, insomnia, jaundice, liver function tests abnormal, malaise, muscle twitching, palpitation, paresthesia, pruritus, psychosis, rash, seizure, syncope, tachycardia, thirst, tinnitus, tongue edema, tremor, urinary retention, urticaria, vasodilation, vertigo, vomiting

Drug Interactions

Metabolism/Transport Effects **Substrate** of CYP1A2 (major), 2D6 (minor), 3A4 (minor)

Avoid Concomitant Use

Avoid concomitant use of Cyclobenzaprine with any of the following: MAO Inhibitors

Increased Effect/Toxicity

Cyclobenzaprine may increase the levels/effects of: Alcohol (Ethyl); Anticholinergics; CNS Depressants; MAO Inhibitors

The levels/effects of Cyclobenzaprine may be increased by: CYP1A2 Inhibitors (Moderate); CYP1A2 Inhibitors (Strong); Pramlintide

Decreased Effect

Cyclobenzaprine may decrease the levels/effects of: Acetylcholinesterase Inhibitors (Central)

The levels/effects of Cyclobenzaprine may be decreased by: Acetylcholinesterase Inhibitors (Central)

Ethanol/Nutrition/Herb Interactions

Food: Food increases bioavailability (peak plasma concentrations increased by 35% and area under the curve by 20%) of the extended release capsule.

Ethanol: Avoid ethanol (may increase CNS depression).

Herb/Nutraceutical: Avoid valerian, kava kava, gotu kola (may increase CNS depression).

Stability

Amrix®, Flexeril®: Store at room temperature of 15°C to 30°C (59°F to 86°F).

Fexmid™: Store at room temperature of 20°C to 25°C (68°F to 77°F).

Mechanism of Action Centrally-acting skeletal muscle relaxant pharmacologically related to tricyclic antidepressants; reduces tonic somatic motor activity influencing both alpha and gamma motor neurons

Pharmacodynamics/Kinetics

Onset of action: Immediate release tablet: ~1 hour

Duration: Immediate release tablet: 12-24 hours

Absorption: Complete

Metabolism: Hepatic via CYP3A4, 1A2, and 2D6; may undergo enterohepatic recirculation

Bioavailability: 33% to 55%

Half-life elimination: Range: 8-37 hours; Immediate release tablet: 18 hours; Extended release capsule: 32 hours

Time to peak, serum: Immediate release tablet: 3-8 hours; Extended release capsule: 7-8 hours

Excretion: Urine (as inactive metabolites); feces (as unchanged drug)

Dosage Oral: **Note:** Do not use longer than 2-3 weeks

Capsule, extended release:

Adults: Usual: 15 mg once daily; some patients may require up to 30 mg once daily

Elderly: Use not recommended

Tablet, immediate release:

Children ≥15 years and Adults: Initial: 5 mg 3 times/day; may increase to 7.5-10 mg 3 times/day if needed

Elderly: Initial: 5 mg; titrate dose slowly and consider less frequent dosing

Dosage adjustment in hepatic impairment:

Capsule, extended release: Mild-to-severe impairment: Use not recommended.

Tablet, immediate release:

Mild impairment: Initial: 5 mg; use with caution; titrate slowly and consider less frequent dosing

Moderate-to-severe impairment: Use not recommended

Administration Oral: Extended release capsules: Administer at the same time each day. Do not crush or chew.

Dosage Forms Excipient information presented when available (limited, particularly for generics); consult specific product labeling.

Capsule, extended release, as hydrochloride:

Amrix®: 15 mg, 30 mg

Tablet, as hydrochloride: 5 mg, 10 mg

Fexmid™: 7.5 mg

Flexeril®: 5 mg, 10 mg

◆ **Cyclobenzaprine Hydrochloride** *see* Cyclobenzaprine *on page 375*

◆ **Cyclocort® (Can)** *see* Amcinonide *on page 81*

◆ **Cyclogyl®** *see* Cyclopentolate *on page 376*

◆ **Cyclomen® (Can)** *see* Danazol *on page 394*

◆ **Cyclomydril®** *see* Cyclopentolate and Phenylephrine *on page 376*

Cyclopentolate (sye kloe PEN toe late)

U.S. Brand Names AK-Pentolate™; Cyclogyl®; Cylate™

Canadian Brand Names Cyclogyl®; Diopentolate®

Index Terms Cyclopentolate Hydrochloride

Pharmacologic Category Anticholinergic Agent, Ophthalmic

Additional Appendix Information

Cycloplegic Mydriatics *on page 1655*

Use Diagnostic procedures requiring mydriasis and cycloplegia

Pregnancy Risk Factor C

Dosage Ophthalmic:

Neonates and Infants: **Note:** Cyclopentolate and phenylephrine combination formulation is the preferred agent for use in neonates and infants due to lower cyclopentolate concentration and reduced risk for systemic reactions

Children: Instill 1 drop of 0.5%, 1%, or 2% in eye followed by 1 drop of 0.5% or 1% in 5 minutes, if necessary

Adults: Instill 1 drop of 1% followed by another drop in 5 minutes; 2% solution in heavily pigmented iris

Additional Information Complete prescribing information for this medication should be consulted for additional detail.

Dosage Forms Excipient information presented when available (limited, particularly for generics); consult specific product labeling.

Solution, ophthalmic, as hydrochloride: 1% (2 mL, 15 mL)

AK-Pentolate™, Cylate™: 1% (2 mL, 15 mL) [contains benzalkonium chloride]

Cyclogyl®: 0.5% (15 mL); 1% (2 mL, 5 mL, 15 mL); 2% (2 mL, 5 mL, 15 mL) [contains benzalkonium chloride]

Cyclopentolate and Phenylephrine
(sye kloe PEN toe late & fen il EF rin)

U.S. Brand Names Cyclomydril®

Index Terms Phenylephrine and Cyclopentolate

Pharmacologic Category Ophthalmic Agent, Antiglaucoma

Use Induce mydriasis greater than that produced with cyclopentolate HCl alone

Pregnancy Risk Factor C

Dosage Ophthalmic: Neonates, Infants, Children, and Adults: Instill 1 drop into the eye every 5-10 minutes, for up to 3 doses, approximately 40-50 minutes before the examination

Additional Information Complete prescribing information for this medication should be consulted for additional detail.

Dosage Forms Excipient information presented when available (limited, particularly for generics); consult specific product labeling.

Solution, ophthalmic: Cyclopentolate hydrochloride 0.2% and phenylephrine hydrochloride 1% (2 mL, 5 mL) [contains benzalkonium chloride]

◆ **Cyclopentolate Hydrochloride** *see* Cyclopentolate *on page 376*

Cyclophosphamide (sye kloe FOS fa mide)

U.S. Brand Names Cytoxan® [DSC]

Canadian Brand Names Cytoxan®; Procytox®

Index Terms CPM; CTX; CYT; Neosar; NSC-26271

Pharmacologic Category Antineoplastic Agent, Alkylating Agent

Use

Oncologic: Treatment of Hodgkin's and non-Hodgkin's lymphoma, Burkitt's lymphoma, chronic lymphocytic leukemia (CLL), chronic myelocytic leukemia (CML), acute myelocytic leukemia (AML), acute lymphocytic leukemia (ALL), mycosis fungoides, multiple myeloma, neuroblastoma, retinoblastoma, rhabdomyosarcoma, Ewing's sarcoma; breast, testicular, endometrial, ovarian, and lung cancers, and in conditioning regimens for bone marrow transplantation

Nononcologic: Prophylaxis of rejection for kidney, heart, liver, and bone marrow transplants, severe rheumatoid disorders, nephrotic syndrome, Wegener's granulomatosis, idiopathic pulmonary hemosideroses, myasthenia gravis, multiple sclerosis, systemic lupus erythematosus, lupus nephritis, autoimmune hemolytic anemia, idiopathic thrombocytic purpura (ITP), macroglobulinemia, and antibody-induced pure red cell aplasia

Pregnancy Risk Factor D

Lactation Enters breast milk/contraindicated

Medication Safety Issues

Sound-alike/look-alike issues:

Cyclophosphamide may be confused with cycloSPORINE, ifosfamide

Cytoxan® may be confused with cefoxitin, Centoxin®, Ciloxan®, cytarabine, CytoGam®, Cytosar®, Cytosar-U®, Cytotec®

High alert medication: The Institute for Safe Medication Practices (ISMP) includes this medication among its list of drugs which have a heightened risk of causing significant patient harm when used in error.

Contraindications Hypersensitivity to cyclophosphamide or any component of the formulation; pregnancy

Warnings/Precautions Hazardous agent - use appropriate precautions for handling and disposal. Dosage adjustment may be needed for renal or hepatic failure. Hemorrhagic cystitis may occur; increased hydration and frequent voiding is recommended. Immunosuppression may occur; monitor for infections. May cause cardiotoxicity (HF, usually with higher doses); may potentiate the cardiotoxicity of anthracyclines. May impair fertility; interferes with oogenesis and spermatogenesis. Secondary malignancies (usually delayed) have been reported

Adverse Reactions

>10%:

Dermatologic: Alopecia (40% to 60%) but hair will usually regrow although it may be a different color and/or texture. Hair loss usually begins 3-6 weeks after the start of therapy.

Endocrine & metabolic: Fertility: May cause sterility; interferes with oogenesis and spermatogenesis; may be irreversible in some patients; gonadal suppression (amenorrhea)

Gastrointestinal: Nausea and vomiting, usually beginning 6-10 hours after administration; anorexia, diarrhea, mucositis, and stomatitis are also seen

Genitourinary: Severe, potentially fatal acute hemorrhagic cystitis (7% to 40%)

Hematologic: Thrombocytopenia and anemia are less common than leukopenia

Onset: 7 days

Nadir: 10-14 days

Recovery: 21 days

1% to 10%:

Cardiovascular: Facial flushing

Central nervous system: Headache

Dermatologic: Skin rash

Renal: SIADH may occur, usually with doses >50 mg/kg (or 1 g/m^2); renal tubular necrosis, which usually resolves with discontinuation of the drug, is also reported

Respiratory: Nasal congestion occurs when I.V. doses are administered too rapidly; patients experience runny eyes, rhinorrhea, sinus congestion, and sneezing during or immediately after the infusion.

<1% (Limited to important or life-threatening): High-dose therapy may cause cardiac dysfunction manifested as CHF; cardiac necrosis or hemorrhagic myocarditis has occurred rarely, but may be fatal. Interstitial pneumonitis and pulmonary fibrosis are occasionally seen with high doses. Cyclophosphamide may also potentiate the cardiac toxicity of anthracyclines. Other adverse reactions include anaphylactic reactions, darkening of skin/fingernails, dizziness, hemorrhagic colitis, hemorrhagic ureteritis, hepatotoxicity, hyperuricemia, hypokalemia, jaundice, malaise, neutrophilic eccrine hidradenitis, radiation recall, renal tubular necrosis, secondary malignancy (eg, bladder carcinoma), SAIDH, Stevens-Johnson syndrome, toxic epidermal necrolysis, weakness.

BMT:

Cardiovascular: Heart failure, cardiac necrosis, pericardial tamponade

Endocrine & metabolic: Hyponatremia

Hematologic: Methemoglobinemia

Gastrointestinal: Severe nausea and vomiting

Miscellaneous: Hemorrhagic cystitis, secondary malignancy

Drug Interactions

Metabolism/Transport Effects **Substrate** of CYP2A6 (minor), 2B6 (major), 2C9 (minor), 2C19 (minor), 3A4 (major); **Inhibits** CYP3A4 (weak); **Induces** CYP2B6 (weak), 2C8 (weak), 2C9 (weak)

Avoid Concomitant Use

Avoid concomitant use of Cyclophosphamide with any of the following: Natalizumab; Vaccines (Live)

Increased Effect/Toxicity

Cyclophosphamide may increase the levels/effects of: Mivacurium [Off Market]; Natalizumab; Succinylcholine; Vaccines (Live); Vitamin K Antagonists

The levels/effects of Cyclophosphamide may be increased by: Allopurinol; CYP2B6 Inhibitors (Moderate); CYP2B6 Inhibitors (Strong); Etanercept; Pentostatin; Trastuzumab

Decreased Effect

Cyclophosphamide may decrease the levels/effects of: Cardiac Glycosides; Vaccines (Inactivated); Vitamin K Antagonists

The levels/effects of Cyclophosphamide may be decreased by: CYP2B6 Inducers (Strong); Echinacea

Ethanol/Nutrition/Herb Interactions Herb/Nutraceutical: Avoid black cohosh, dong quai in estrogen-dependent tumors.

Stability Store intact vials of powder at room temperature of 15°C to 30°C (59°F to 86°F). Reconstitute vials with sterile water, normal saline, or 5% dextrose to a concentration of 20 mg/mL. Reconstituted solutions are stable for 24 hours at room temperature and 6 days under refrigeration at 2°C to 8°C (36°F to 46°F). Further dilutions in D_5W or NS are stable for 24 hours at room temperature and 6 days at refrigeration.

Mechanism of Action Cyclophosphamide is an alkylating agent that prevents cell division by cross-linking DNA strands and decreasing DNA synthesis. It is a cell cycle phase nonspecific agent. Cyclophosphamide also possesses potent immunosuppressive activity. Cyclophosphamide is a prodrug that must be metabolized to active metabolites in the liver.

Pharmacodynamics/Kinetics

Absorption: Oral: Well absorbed

Distribution: V_d: 0.48-0.71 L/kg; crosses placenta; crosses into CSF (not in high enough concentrations to treat meningeal leukemia)

Protein binding: 10% to 60%

Metabolism: Hepatic to active metabolites acrolein, 4-aldophosphamide, 4-hydroperoxycyclophosphamide, and nor-nitrogen mustard

Bioavailability: >75%

Half-life elimination: 3-12 hours

Time to peak, serum: Oral: ~1 hour

Excretion: Urine (<30% as unchanged drug, 85% to 90% as metabolites)

Dosage Refer to individual protocols

Children:

SLE: I.V.: 500-750 mg/m^2 every month; maximum dose: 1 g/m^2

JRA/vasculitis: I.V.: 10 mg/kg every 2 weeks

Children and Adults:

Oral: 50-100 mg/m^2/day as continuous therapy or 400-1000 mg/m^2 in divided doses over 4-5 days as intermittent therapy

I.V.:

Single doses: 400-1800 mg/m^2 (30-50 mg/kg) per treatment course (1-5 days) which can be repeated at 2-4 week intervals

Continuous daily doses: 60-120 mg/m^2 (1-2.5 mg/kg) per day

Autologous BMT: IVPB: 50 mg/kg/dose x 4 days or 60 mg/kg/dose for 2 days; total dose is usually divided over 2-4 days

Nephrotic syndrome: Oral: 2-3 mg/kg/day every day for up to 12 weeks when corticosteroids are unsuccessful

Dosing adjustment in renal impairment: The FDA-approved labeling states there is insufficiant evidence to recommend dosage adjustment and therefore, does not contain renal dosing adjustment guidelines. The following guidelines have been used by some clinicians (Aronoff, 2007): Children and Adults:

Cl_{cr} <10 mL/minute: Administer 75% of normal dose

Hemodialysis effects: Moderately dialyzable (20% to 50%)

Administer 50% of dose posthemodialysis

Continuous ambulatory peritoneal dialysis (CAPD): Administer 75% of normal dose

Continuous renal replacement therapy (CRRT): Administer 100% of normal dose

Dosing adjustment in hepatic impairment: The pharmacokinetics of cyclophosphamide are not significantly altered in the presence of hepatic insufficiency. The FDA-approved labeling does not contain hepatic dosing adjustment guidelines. The following guidelines have been used by some clinicians (Floyd, 2006):

Serum bilirubin 3.1-5 mg/dL or transaminases >3 times ULN: Administer 75% of dose

Serum bilirubin >5 mg/mL: Avoid use

Dietary Considerations Tablets should be administered during or after meals.

Administration Administer I.P., intrapleurally, IVPB, or continuous I.V. infusion; may also be administered slow IVP in doses ≤1 g.

I.V. infusions may be administered over 1-24 hours

Doses >500 mg to approximately 2 g may be administered over 20-30 minutes

To minimize bladder toxicity, increase normal fluid intake during and for 1-2 days after cyclophosphamide dose. Most adult patients will require a fluid intake of at least 2 L/day. High-dose regimens should be accompanied by vigorous hydration with or without mesna therapy.

Oral: Tablets are not scored and should not be cut or crushed. To minimize the risk of bladder irritation, do not administer tablets at bedtime.

Monitoring Parameters CBC with differential and platelet count, BUN, UA, serum electrolytes, serum creatinine

Additional Information In patients with CYP2B6 G516T variant allele, cyclophosphamide metabolism is markedly increased; metabolism is not influenced by CYP2C9 and CYP2C19 isotypes.

Dosage Forms Excipient information presented when available (limited, particularly for generics); consult specific product labeling. [DSC] = Discontinued product

Injection, powder for reconstitution: 500 mg, 1 g, 2 g

Cytoxan®: 500 mg, 1 g, 2 g [DSC]

Tablet: 25 mg, 50 mg

Cytoxan®: 25 mg, 50 mg [DSC]

Extemporaneous Preparations A 2 mg/mL oral elixir was stable for 14 days when refrigerated when made as follows: Reconstitute a 200 mg vial with aromatic elixir, withdraw the solution, and add sufficient aromatic elixir to make a final volume of 100 mL (store in amber glass container).

Brook D, Davis RE, and Bequette RJ, "Chemical Stability of Cyclophosphamide in Aromatic Elixir U.S.P.," *Am J Health Syst Pharm*, 1973, 30:618-20.

CycloSERINE (sye kloe SER een)

U.S. Brand Names Seromycin®

Pharmacologic Category Antibiotic, Miscellaneous; Antitubercular Agent

Additional Appendix Information

Antimicrobial Drugs of Choice *on page* 1752

Tuberculosis *on page* 1776

Use Adjunctive treatment in pulmonary or extrapulmonary tuberculosis

Unlabeled/Investigational Use Treatment of Gaucher's disease

Pregnancy Risk Factor C

Lactation Enters breast milk/compatible

Medication Safety Issues

Sound-alike/look-alike issues:

CycloSERINE may be confused with cyclobenzaprine, cycloSPORINE

Contraindications Hypersensitivity to cycloserine or any component of the formulation

Warnings/Precautions Has been associated with CNS toxicity, including seizures, psychosis, depression, and confusion; decrease dosage or discontinue use if occurs. Use with caution in patients with epilepsy, depression, severe anxiety, psychosis, severe renal insufficiency, chronic alcoholism and patients with potential folate deficiency (malnourished, chronic anticonvulsant therapy, or elderly). Prolonged use may result in fungal or bacterial superinfection, including *C. difficile*-associated diarrhea (CDAD) and pseudomembranous colitis; CDAD has been observed >2 months postantibiotic treatment.

Adverse Reactions Frequency not defined.

Cardiovascular: Cardiac arrhythmia

Central nervous system: Drowsiness, headache, dizziness, vertigo, seizure, confusion, psychosis, paresis, coma

Dermatologic: Rash

Endocrine & metabolic: Vitamin B_{12} deficiency

Hematologic: Folate deficiency

Hepatic: Liver enzymes increased

Neuromuscular & skeletal: Tremor

Drug Interactions

Avoid Concomitant Use There are no known interactions where it is recommended to avoid concomitant use.

Increased Effect/Toxicity

CycloSERINE may increase the levels/effects of: Isoniazid

Decreased Effect

CycloSERINE may decrease the levels/effects of: Typhoid Vaccine

Ethanol/Nutrition/Herb Interactions

Ethanol: Avoid ethanol (may increase CNS depression).

Food: May increase vitamin B_{12} and folic acid dietary requirements.

Mechanism of Action Inhibits bacterial cell wall synthesis by competing with amino acid (D-alanine) for incorporation into the bacterial cell wall; bacteriostatic or bactericidal

Pharmacodynamics/Kinetics

Absorption: ~70% to 90%

Distribution: Widely to most body fluids and tissues including CSF, breast milk, bile, sputum, lymph tissue, lungs, and ascitic, pleural, and synovial fluids; crosses placenta

Half-life elimination: Normal renal function: 10 hours

Metabolism: Hepatic

Time to peak, serum: 3-4 hours

Excretion: Urine (60% to 70% as unchanged drug) within 72 hours; feces (small amounts); remainder metabolized

Dosage Some neurotoxic effects may be relieved or prevented by concomitant administration of pyridoxine

Tuberculosis: Oral:

Children: 10-20 mg/kg/day in 2 divided doses up to 1000 mg/day for 18-24 months

Adults: Initial: 250 mg every 12 hours for 14 days, then administer 500 mg to 1 g/day in 2 divided doses for 18-24 months (maximum daily dose: 1 g)

Dosing interval in renal impairment:

Cl_{cr} 10-50 mL/minute: Administer every 24 hours

Cl_{cr} <10 mL/minute: Administer every 36-48 hours

Dietary Considerations May be taken with food; may increase vitamin B_{12} and folic acid dietary requirements.

Monitoring Parameters Periodic renal, hepatic, hematological tests, and plasma cycloserine concentrations

Reference Range Toxicity is greatly increased at levels >30 mcg/mL

Dosage Forms Excipient information presented when available (limited, particularly for generics); consult specific product labeling.

Capsule: 250 mg

◆ **Cyclosporin A** *see* CycloSPORINE *on page 379*

CycloSPORINE (SYE kloe spor een)

U.S. Brand Names Gengraf®; Neoral®; Restasis®; Sandimmune®

Canadian Brand Names Neoral®; Rhoxal-cyclosporine; Sandimmune® I.V.; Sandoz-Cyclosporine

Index Terms CsA; CyA; Cyclosporin A

Pharmacologic Category Immunosuppressant Agent

Use Prophylaxis of organ rejection in kidney, liver, and heart transplants, has been used with azathioprine and/or corticosteroids; severe, active rheumatoid arthritis (RA) not responsive to methotrexate alone; severe, recalcitrant plaque psoriasis in nonimmunocompromised adults unresponsive to or unable to tolerate other systemic therapy

Ophthalmic emulsion (Restasis®): Increase tear production when suppressed tear production is presumed to be due to keratoconjunctivitis sicca-associated ocular inflammation (in patients not already using topical anti-inflammatory drugs or punctal plugs)

Unlabeled/Investigational Use Short-term, high-dose cyclosporine as a modulator of multidrug resistance in cancer treatment; allogenic bone marrow transplants for prevention and treatment of graft-versus-host disease; also used in some cases of severe autoimmune disease (eg, SLE, myasthenia gravis, inflammatory bowel disease) that are resistant to corticosteroids and other therapy; focal segmental glomerulosclerosis

Pregnancy Risk Factor C

Pregnancy Considerations Reproductive toxicity has been observed in animal studies; mutagenic and teratogenic effects were not observed in the standard test systems following oral administration. In humans, cyclosporine crosses the placenta. Based on clinical use, premature births and low birth weight were consistently observed. Use only if the benefit to the mother outweighs the possible risks to the fetus.

A pregnancy registry has been established for pregnant women taking immunosuppressants following any solid organ transplant (National Transplantation Pregnancy Registry, Temple University, 877-955-6877).

Lactation Enters breast milk/not recommended

Medication Safety Issues

Sound-alike/look-alike issues:

CycloSPORINE may be confused with cyclophosphamide, Cyklokapron®, cycloSERINE

CycloSPORINE modified (Neoral®, Gengraf®) may be confused with cycloSPORINE non-modified (Sandimmne®)

Gengraf® may be confused with Prograf®

Neoral® may be confused with Neurontin®, Nizoral®

Sandimmune® may be confused with Sandostatin®

Contraindications Hypersensitivity to cyclosporine or any component of the formulation. Rheumatoid arthritis and psoriasis: Abnormal renal function, uncontrolled hypertension, malignancies. Concomitant treatment with PUVA or UVB therapy, methotrexate, other immunosuppressive agents, coal tar, or radiation therapy are also contraindications for use in patients with psoriasis. Ophthalmic emulsion is contraindicated in patients with active ocular infections.

Warnings/Precautions **[U.S. Boxed Warning]: Renal impairment, including structural kidney damage has occurred (when used at high doses); monitor renal function closely.** Use caution with other potentially nephrotoxic drugs (eg, acyclovir, aminoglycoside antibiotics, amphotericin B, ciprofloxacin). **[U.S. Boxed Warning]: Increased risk of lymphomas and other malignancies, particularly those of the skin;** risk is related to intensity/duration of therapy and the use of >1 immunosuppressive agent; all patients should avoid excessive sun/UV light exposure. **[U.S. Boxed Warning]: Increased risk of infection; fatal infections have been reported. [U.S. Boxed Warning]: May cause hypertension.** Use caution when changing dosage forms. **[U.S. Boxed Warning]: Cyclosporine (modified) has increased bioavailability as compared to cyclosporine (non-modified) and cannot be used interchangeably without close monitoring.** Monitor cyclosporine concentrations closely following the addition, modification, or deletion of other medications; live, attenuated vaccines may be less effective; use should be avoided. Increased hepatic enzymes and bilirubin have occurred (when used at high doses); improvement usually seen with dosage reduction.

Transplant patients: To be used initially with corticosteroids. May cause significant hyperkalemia and hyperuricemia, seizures (particularly if used with high dose corticosteroids), and encephalopathy. Make dose adjustments based on cyclosporine blood concentrations. **[U.S. Boxed Warning]: Adjustment of dose should only be made under the direct supervision of an experienced physician.** Anaphylaxis has been reported with I.V. use; reserve for patients who cannot take oral form. **[U.S. Boxed Warning]: Risk of skin cancer may be increased in transplant patients.**

Psoriasis: Patients should avoid excessive sun exposure; safety and efficacy in children <18 years of age have not been established. **[U.S. Boxed Warning]: Risk of skin cancer may be increased with a history of PUVA and possibly methotrexate or other immunosuppressants, UVB, coal tar, or radiation.**

Rheumatoid arthritis: Safety and efficacy for use in juvenile rheumatoid arthritis have not been established. If receiving other immunosuppressive agents, radiation or UV therapy, concurrent use of cyclosporine is not recommended.

Ophthalmic emulsion: Safety and efficacy have not been established in patients <16 years of age.

Products may contain corn oil, ethanol, or propylene glycol; injection also contains Cremophor® EL (polyoxyethylated castor oil), which has been associated with rare anaphylactic reactions.

Adverse Reactions Adverse reactions reported with systemic use, including rheumatoid arthritis, psoriasis, and transplantation (kidney, liver, and heart). Percentages noted include the highest frequency regardless of indication/dosage. Frequencies may vary for specific conditions or formulation.

>10%:
- Cardiovascular: Hypertension (8% to 53%), edema (5% to 14%)
- Central nervous system: Headache (2% to 25%)
- Dermatologic: Hirsutism (21% to 45%), hypertrichosis (5% to 19%)
- Endocrine & metabolic: Triglycerides increased (15%), female reproductive disorder (9% to 11%)
- Gastrointestinal: Nausea (23%), diarrhea (3% to 13%), gum hyperplasia (2% to 16%), abdominal discomfort (<1% to 15%), dyspepsia (2% to 12%)
- Neuromuscular & skeletal: Tremor (7% to 55%), paresthesia (1% to 11%), leg cramps/muscle contractions (2% to 12%)
- Renal: Renal dysfunction/nephropathy (10% to 38%), creatinine increased (16% to ≥50%)
- Respiratory: Upper respiratory infection (1% to 14%)
- Miscellaneous: Infection (3% to 25%)

1% to 10%:
- Cardiovascular: Chest pain (4% to 6%), arrhythmia (2% to 5%), abnormal heart sounds, cardiac failure, flushes (<1% to 5%), MI, peripheral ischemia
- Central nervous system: Dizziness (8%), pain (6%), convulsions (1% to 5%), insomnia (4%), psychiatric events (4% to 5%), pain (3% to 4%), depression (1% to 6%), migraine (2% to 3%), anxiety, confusion, fever, hypoesthesia, emotional lability, impaired concentration, lethargy, malaise, nervousness, paranoia, somnolence, vertigo
- Dermatologic: Purpura (3% to 4%), acne (1% to 6%), brittle fingernails, hair breaking, abnormal pigmentation, angioedema, cellulitis, dermatitis, dry skin, eczema, folliculitis, keratosis, pruritus, rash, skin disorder, skin malignancies, urticaria
- Endocrine & metabolic: Gynecomastia (<1% to 4%), menstrual disorder (1% to 3%), breast fibroadenosis, breast pain, hyper-/hypoglycemia, diabetes mellitus, goiter, hot flashes, hyperkalemia, hyperuricemia, libido increased/decreased
- Gastrointestinal: Vomiting (2% to 10%), flatulence (5%), gingivitis (up to 4%), cramps (up to 4%), anorexia, constipation, dry mouth, dysphagia, enanthema, eructation, esophagitis, gastric ulcer, gastritis, gastroenteritis, gastrointestinal bleeding (upper), gingival bleeding, glossitis, mouth sores, peptic ulcer, pancreatitis, swallowing difficulty, salivary gland enlargement, taste perversion, tongue disorder, tooth disorder, weight loss/gain
- Genitourinary: Leukorrhea (1%), abnormal urine, micturition increased, micturition urgency, nocturia, polyuria, pyelonephritis, urinary incontinence, uterine hemorrhage
- Hematologic: Leukopenia (<1% to 6%), anemia, bleeding disorder, clotting disorder, platelet disorder, red blood cell disorder, thrombocytopenia
- Hepatic: Hepatotoxicity (<1% to 7%), hyperbilirubinemia
- Neuromuscular & skeletal: Arthralgia (1% to 6%), bone fracture, joint dislocation, joint pain, muscle pain, myalgia, neuropathy, stiffness, synovial cyst, tendon disorder, tingling, weakness
- Ocular: Abnormal vision, cataract, conjunctivitis, eye pain, visual disturbance
- Otic: Deafness, hearing loss, tinnitus, vestibular disorder
- Renal: BUN increased, hematuria, renal abscess
- Respiratory: Sinusitis (<1% to 7%), bronchospasm (up to 5%), cough (3% to 5%), pharyngitis (3% to 5%), dyspnea (1% to 5%), rhinitis (up to 5%), abnormal chest sounds, epistaxis, respiratory infection, pneumonia (up to 1%)
- Miscellaneous: Flu-like syndrome (8% to 10%), lymphoma (<1% to 6% reported in transplant), abscess, allergic reactions, bacterial infection, carcinoma, diaphoresis increased, fungal infection, herpes simplex, herpes zoster, hiccups, lymphadenopathy, moniliasis, night sweats, tonsillitis, viral infection

Postmarketing and/or case reports (any indication): Anaphylaxis/anaphylactoid reaction (possibly associated with Cremophor® EL vehicle in injection formulation), benign intracranial hypertension, cholesterol increased, death (due to renal deterioration), encephalopathy, gout, hyperbilirubinemia, hyperkalemia, hypomagnesemia (mild), impaired consciousness, neurotoxicity, papilloedema, pulmonary edema (noncardiogenic), uric acid increased

Ophthalmic emulsion (Restasis®):

>10%: Ocular: Burning (17%)

1% to 10%: Ocular: Hyperemia (conjunctival 5%), eye pain, pruritus, stinging

Drug Interactions

Metabolism/Transport Effects Substrate of CYP3A4 (major); **Inhibits** CYP2C9 (weak), 3A4 (moderate)

Avoid Concomitant Use

Avoid concomitant use of CycloSPORINE with any of the following: Aliskiren; Bosentan; Dabigatran Etexilate; Natalizumab; Rivaroxaban; Silodosin; Sitaxsentan; Topotecan; Vaccines (Live)

Increased Effect/Toxicity

CycloSPORINE may increase the levels/effects of: Aliskiren; Ambrisentan; Bosentan; Calcium Channel Blockers (Dihydropyridine); Calcium Channel Blockers (Nondihydropyridine); Cardiac Glycosides; Caspofungin; Colchicine; Corticosteroids (Systemic); CYP3A4 Substrates; Dabigatran Etexilate; DOXOrubicin; Eplerenone; Etoposide; Etoposide Phosphate; Ezetimibe; Fenofibric Acid; FentaNYL; HMG-CoA Reductase Inhibitors; Maraviroc; Methotrexate; Minoxidil; Natalizumab; P-Glycoprotein Substrates; Pimecrolimus; Protease Inhibitors; Ranolazine; Repaglinide; Rivaroxaban; Salmeterol; Silodosin; Sirolimus; Sitaxsentan; Topotecan; Vaccines (Live)

The levels/effects of CycloSPORINE may be increased by: ACE Inhibitors; Aminoglycosides; Amiodarone; Amphotericin B; Androgens; Antifungal Agents (Azole Derivatives, Systemic); Bromocriptine; Calcium Channel Blockers (Nondihydropyridine); Carvedilol; Colchicine; Corticosteroids (Systemic); CYP3A4 Inhibitors (Moderate); CYP3A4 Inhibitors (Strong); Dasatinib; Ezetimibe; Fenofibric Acid; Fluconazole; Grapefruit Juice; Imatinib; Macrolide Antibiotics; Melphalan; Methotrexate; Metoclopramide; MetroNIDAZOLE; Nonsteroidal Anti-Inflammatory Agents; Norfloxacin; P-Glycoprotein Inhibitors; Protease Inhibitors; Quinupristin; Sirolimus; Sulfonamide Derivatives; Sulfonylureas; Temsirolimus; Trastuzumab

Decreased Effect

CycloSPORINE may decrease the levels/effects of: Mycophenolate; Vaccines (Inactivated)

The levels/effects of CycloSPORINE may be decreased by: Antacids; Barbiturates; Bosentan; CarBAMazepine; CYP3A4 Inducers (Strong); Deferasirox; Echinacea; Griseofulvin; Nafcillin; P-Glycoprotein Inducers; Phenytoin; Probucol; Pyrazinamide; Rifamycin Derivatives; Somatostatin Analogs; St Johns Wort; Sulfinpyrazone [Off Market]; Sulfonamide Derivatives; Terbinafine

Ethanol/Nutrition/Herb Interactions

Food: Grapefruit juice increases cyclosporine absorption

Herb/Nutraceutical: Avoid St John's wort; as an enzyme inducer, it may increase the metabolism of and decrease plasma levels of cyclosporine; organ rejection and graft loss have been reported. Avoid cat's claw, echinacea (have immunostimulant properties).

Stability

Capsule: Store at controlled room temperature.

Injection: Store at controlled room temperature; do not refrigerate. Ampuls should be protected from light.

Stability of injection of parenteral admixture at room temperature (25°C) is 6 hours in PVC; 24 hours in Excel®, PAB® containers, or glass.

Sandimmune® injection: Injection should be further diluted [1 mL (50 mg) of concentrate in 20-100 mL of D_5W or NS] for administration by intravenous infusion.

Ophthalmic emulsion: Store at 15°C to 25°C (59°F to 77°F). Vials are single-use; discard immediately following administration.

Oral solution: Store at controlled room temperature; do not refrigerate. Use within 2 months after opening; should be mixed in glass containers.

Neoral® oral solution: Orange juice, apple juice; avoid changing diluents frequently; mix thoroughly and drink at once.

Sandimmune® oral solution: Milk, chocolate milk, orange juice; avoid changing diluents frequently; mix thoroughly and drink at once.

Mechanism of Action Inhibition of production and release of interleukin II and inhibits interleukin II-induced activation of resting T-lymphocytes.

Pharmacodynamics/Kinetics

Absorption:

Ophthalmic emulsion: Serum concentrations not detectable.

Oral:

Cyclosporine (non-modified): Erratic and incomplete; dependent on presence of food, bile acids, and GI motility; larger oral doses are needed in pediatrics due to shorter bowel length and limited intestinal absorption

Cyclosporine (modified): Erratic and incomplete; increased absorption, up to 30% when compared to cyclosporine (non-modified); less dependent on food, bile acids, or GI motility when compared to cyclosporine (non-modified)

Distribution: Widely in tissues and body fluids including the liver, pancreas, and lungs; crosses placenta; enters breast milk

V_{dss}: 4-6 L/kg in renal, liver, and marrow transplant recipients (slightly lower values in cardiac transplant patients; children <10 years have higher values)

Protein binding: 90% to 98% to lipoproteins

Metabolism: Extensively hepatic via CYP3A4; forms at least 25 metabolites; extensive first-pass effect following oral administration

Bioavailability: Oral:

Cyclosporine (non-modified): Dependent on patient population and transplant type (<10% in adult liver transplant patients and as high as 89% in renal transplant patients); bioavailability of Sandimmune® capsules and oral solution are equivalent; bioavailability of oral solution is ~30% of the I.V. solution

Children: 28% (range: 17% to 42%); gut dysfunction common in BMT patients and oral bioavailability is further reduced

Cyclosporine (modified): Bioavailability of Neoral® capsules and oral solution are equivalent:

Children: 43% (range: 30% to 68%)

Adults: 23% greater than with cyclosporine (non-modified) in renal transplant patients; 50% greater in liver transplant patients

Half-life elimination: Oral: May be prolonged in patients with hepatic impairment and shorter in pediatric patients due to the higher metabolism rate

Cyclosporine (non-modified): Biphasic: Alpha: 1.4 hours; Terminal: 19 hours (range: 10-27 hours)

Cyclosporine (modified): Biphasic: Terminal: 8.4 hours (range: 5-18 hours)

Time to peak, serum: Oral:

Cyclosporine (non-modified): 2-6 hours; some patients have a second peak at 5-6 hours

Cyclosporine (modified): Renal transplant: 1.5-2 hours

Excretion: Primarily feces; urine (6%, 0.1% as unchanged drug and metabolites)

Dosage Neoral®/Genraf® and Sandimmune® are not bioequivalent and cannot be used interchangeably.

Children: Transplant: Refer to adult dosing; children may require, and are able to tolerate, larger doses than adults.

Adults:

Newly-transplanted patients: Adjunct therapy with corticosteroids is recommended. Initial dose should be given 4-12 hours prior to transplant or may be given postoperatively; adjust initial dose to achieve desired plasma concentration

Oral: Dose is dependent upon type of transplant and formulation:

Cyclosporine (modified):

Renal: 9 ± 3 mg/kg/day, divided twice daily

Liver: 8 ± 4 mg/kg/day, divided twice daily

Heart: 7 ± 3 mg/kg/day, divided twice daily

Cyclosporine (non-modified): Initial dose: 15 mg/kg/day as a single dose (range 14-18 mg/kg); lower doses of 10-14 mg/kg/day have been used for renal transplants. Continue initial dose daily for 1-2 weeks; taper by 5% per week to a maintenance dose of 5-10 mg/kg/day; some renal transplant patients may be dosed as low as 3 mg/kg/day

Note: When using the non-modified formulation, cyclosporine levels may increase in liver transplant patients when the T-tube is closed; dose may need decreased

I.V.: Cyclosporine (non-modified): Manufacturer's labeling: Initial dose: 5-6 mg/kg/day as a single dose (1/3 the oral dose), infused over 2-6 hours; use should be limited to patients unable to take capsules or oral solution; patients should be switched to an oral dosage form as soon as possible

Note: Many transplant centers administer cyclosporine as "divided dose" infusions (in 2-3 doses/day) or as a continuous (24-hour) infusion; dosages range from 3-7.5 mg/kg/day. Specific institutional protocols should be consulted.

Conversion to cyclosporine (modified) from cyclosporine (non-modified): Start with daily dose previously used and adjust to obtain preconversion cyclosporine trough concentration. Plasma concentrations should be monitored every 4-7 days and dose adjusted as necessary, until desired trough level is obtained. When transferring patients with previously poor absorption of cyclosporine (non-modified), monitor trough levels at least twice weekly (especially if initial dose exceeds 10 mg/kg/day); high plasma levels are likely to occur.

Rheumatoid arthritis: Oral: Cyclosporine (modified): Initial dose: 2.5 mg/kg/day, divided twice daily; salicylates, NSAIDs, and oral glucocorticoids may be continued (refer to Drug Interactions); dose may be increased by 0.5-0.75 mg/kg/day if insufficient response is seen after 8 weeks of treatment; additional dosage increases may be made again at 12 weeks (maximum dose: 4 mg/kg/day). Discontinue if no benefit is seen by 16 weeks of therapy.

Note: Increase the frequency of blood pressure monitoring after each alteration in dosage of cyclosporine. Cyclosporine dosage should be decreased by 25% to 50% in patients with no history of hypertension who develop sustained hypertension during therapy and, if hypertension persists, treatment with cyclosporine should be discontinued.

Psoriasis: Oral: Cyclosporine (modified): Initial dose: 2.5 mg/kg/day, divided twice daily; dose may be increased by 0.5 mg/kg/day if insufficient response is seen after 4 weeks of treatment. Additional dosage increases may be made every 2 weeks if needed (maximum dose: 4 mg/kg/day). Discontinue if no benefit is seen by 6 weeks of therapy. Once patients are adequately controlled, the dose should be decreased to the lowest effective dose. Doses lower than 2.5 mg/kg/day may be effective. Treatment longer than 1 year is not recommended.

Note: Increase the frequency of blood pressure monitoring after each alteration in dosage of cyclosporine. Cyclosporine dosage should be decreased by 25% to 50% in patients with no history of hypertension who develop sustained hypertension during therapy and, if hypertension persists, treatment with cyclosporine should be discontinued.

Focal segmental glomerulosclerosis (unlabeled use): Initial: 3 mg/kg/day divided every 12 hours

Autoimmune diseases (unlabeled use): 1-3 mg/kg/day

Keratoconjunctivitis sicca: Ophthalmic (Restasis®): Children ≥16 years and Adults: Instill 1 drop in each eye every 12 hours

Dosage adjustment in renal impairment: For severe psoriasis:

Serum creatinine levels ≥25% above pretreatment levels: Take another sample within 2 weeks; if the level remains ≥25% above pretreatment levels, decrease dosage of cyclosporine (modified) by 25% to 50%. If two dosage adjustments do not reverse the increase in serum creatinine levels, treatment should be discontinued.

Serum creatinine levels ≥50% above pretreatment levels: Decrease cyclosporine dosage by 25% to 50%. If two dosage adjustments do not reverse the increase in serum creatinine levels, treatment should be discontinued.

Hemodialysis: Supplemental dose is not necessary.

Peritoneal dialysis: Supplemental dose is not necessary.

Dosage adjustment in hepatic impairment: Probably necessary; monitor levels closely

Dietary Considerations Administer this medication consistently with relation to time of day and meals. Avoid grapefruit juice.

Administration

Oral solution: Do not administer liquid from plastic or styrofoam cup. May dilute Neoral® oral solution with orange juice or apple juice. May dilute Sandimmune® oral solution with milk, chocolate milk, or orange juice. Avoid changing diluents frequently. Mix thoroughly and drink at once. Use syringe provided to measure dose. Mix in a glass container and rinse container with more diluent to ensure total dose is taken. Do not rinse syringe before or after use (may cause dose variation).

I.V.: The manufacturer recommends that following dilution, intravenous admixture be administered over 2-6 hours. However, many transplant centers administer as divided doses (2-3 doses/day) or as a 24-hour continuous infusion. Discard solution after 24 hours. Anaphylaxis has been reported with I.V. use; reserve for patients who cannot take oral form. Patients should be under continuous observation for at least the first 30 minutes of the infusion, and should be monitored frequently thereafter. Maintain patent airway; other supportive measures and agents for treating anaphylaxis should be present when I.V. drug is given.

Ophthalmic emulsion: Prior to use, invert vial several times to obtain a uniform emulsion. Remove contact lenses prior to instillation of drops; may be reinserted 15 minutes after administration. May be used with artificial tears; allow 15 minute interval between products.

Monitoring Parameters Monitor blood pressure and serum creatinine after any cyclosporine dosage changes or addition, modification, or deletion of other medications. Monitor plasma concentrations periodically.

Transplant patients: Cyclosporine trough levels, serum electrolytes, renal function, hepatic function, blood pressure, lipid profile

Psoriasis therapy: Baseline blood pressure, serum creatinine (2 levels each), BUN, CBC, serum magnesium, potassium, uric acid, lipid profile. Biweekly monitoring of blood pressure, complete blood count, and levels of BUN, uric acid, potassium, lipids, and magnesium during the first 3 months of treatment for psoriasis. Monthly monitoring is recommended after this initial period. Also evaluate any atypical skin lesions prior to therapy. Increase the frequency of blood pressure monitoring after each alteration in dosage of cyclosporine. Cyclosporine dosage should be decreased by 25% to 50% in patients with no history of hypertension who develop sustained hypertension during therapy and, if hypertension persists, treatment with cyclosporine should be discontinued.

Rheumatoid arthritis: Baseline blood pressure, and serum creatinine (2 levels each); serum creatinine every 2 weeks for first 3 months, then monthly if patient is stable. Increase the frequency of blood pressure monitoring after each alteration in dosage of cyclosporine. Cyclosporine dosage should be decreased by 25% to 50% in patients with no history of hypertension who develop sustained hypertension during therapy and, if hypertension persists, treatment with cyclosporine should be discontinued.

Reference Range Reference ranges are method dependent and specimen dependent; use the same analytical method consistently

Method-dependent and specimen-dependent: Trough levels should be obtained:

Oral: 12-18 hours after dose (chronic usage)

I.V.: 12 hours after dose **or** immediately prior to next dose

Therapeutic range: Not absolutely defined, dependent on organ transplanted, time after transplant, organ function and CsA toxicity:

General range of 100-400 ng/mL

Toxic level: Not well defined, nephrotoxicity may occur at any level

Test Interactions Specific whole blood, HPLC assay for cyclosporine may be falsely elevated if sample is drawn from the same line through which dose was administered (even if flush has been administered and/or dose was given hours before).

Additional Information Cyclosporine (modified): Refers to the capsule dosage formulation of cyclosporine in an aqueous dispersion (previously referred to as "microemulsion"). Cyclosporine (modified) has increased bioavailability as compared to cyclosporine (non-modified) and cannot be used interchangeably without close monitoring.

Dosage Forms Excipient information presented when available (limited, particularly for generics); consult specific product labeling.

Capsule [modified]:
- Gengraf®: 25 mg [contains alcohol 12.8%]; 100 mg [contains alcohol 12.8%]

Capsule [non-modified]: 25 mg, 100 mg

Capsule, soft gel [modified]: 25 mg, 50 mg, 100 mg
- Neoral®: 25 mg [contains alcohol 11.9% and corn oil]; 100 mg [contains alcohol 11.9% and corn oil]

Capsule, soft gel [non-modified]:
- Sandimmune®: 25 mg [contains alcohol 12.7% and corn oil]; 100 mg [contains alcohol 12.7% and corn oil]

Emulsion, ophthalmic [preservative free]:
- Restasis®: 0.05% (0.4 mL) [contains 30 single-use vials/box]

Injection, solution [non-modified]: 50 mg/mL (5 mL)
- Sandimmune®: 50 mg/mL (5 mL) [contains Cremophor® EL (polyoxyethylated castor oil) and alcohol 32.9%]

Solution, oral [modified]: 100 mg/mL (50 mL)
- Gengraf®: 100 mg/mL (50 mL) [contains propylene glycol]
- Neoral®: 100 mg/mL (50 mL) [contains alcohol 11.9%, corn oil, and propylene glycol]

Solution, oral [non-modified]: 100 mg/mL (50 mL)

Sandimmune®: 100 mg/mL (50 mL) [contains alcohol 12.5%]

- ◆ **Cyklokapron®** *see* Tranexamic Acid *on page 1501*
- ◆ **Cylate™** *see* Cyclopentolate *on page 376*
- ◆ **Cylex® [OTC]** *see* Benzocaine *on page 183*
- ◆ **Cymbalta®** *see* DULoxetine *on page 498*

Cyproheptadine (si proe HEP ta deen)

Index Terms Cyproheptadine Hydrochloride; Periactin

Pharmacologic Category Histamine H_1 Antagonist; Histamine H_1 Antagonist, First Generation

Use Perennial and seasonal allergic rhinitis and other allergic symptoms including urticaria

Unlabeled/Investigational Use Appetite stimulation, blepharospasm, cluster headaches, migraine headaches, Nelson's syndrome, pruritus, schizophrenia, spinal cord damage associated spasticity, and tardive dyskinesia

Pregnancy Risk Factor B

Lactation Excretion in breast milk unknown/contra-indicated

Medication Safety Issues

Sound-alike/look-alike issues:

Cyproheptadine may be confused with cyclobenzaprine

Periactin may be confused with Perative®, Percodan®, Persantine®

Contraindications Hypersensitivity to cyproheptadine or any component of the formulation; narrow-angle glaucoma; bladder neck obstruction; symptomatic prostatic hyperplasia; acute asthmatic attack; stenosing peptic ulcer; GI tract obstruction; concurrent use of MAO inhibitors; avoid use in premature and term newborns due to potential association with SIDS

Warnings/Precautions May cause CNS depression, which may impair physical or mental abilities; patients must be cautioned about performing tasks which require mental alertness (eg, operating machinery or driving). Effects may be potentiated when used with other sedative drugs or ethanol. Use with caution in patients with cardiovascular disease; increased intraocular pressure; respiratory disease; or thyroid dysfunction. Use with caution in the elderly; may be more sensitive to adverse effects. In case reports, cyproheptadine has promoted weight gain in anorexic adults, though it has not been specifically studied in the elderly. All cases of weight loss or decreased appetite should be adequately assessed. Antihistamines may cause excitation in young children. Safety and efficacy have not been established in children <2 years of age.

Adverse Reactions

>10%:

Central nervous system: Slight to moderate drowsiness

Respiratory: Thickening of bronchial secretions

1% to 10%:

Central nervous system: Dizziness, fatigue, headache, nervousness

Gastrointestinal: Abdominal pain, appetitie stimulation, diarrhea, nausea, xerostomia

Neuromuscular & skeletal: Arthralgia

Respiratory: Pharyngitis

<1% (Limited to important or life-threatening): Bronchospasm, CNS stimulation, depression, epistaxis, hemolytic anemia, hepatitis, leukopenia, sedation, seizure, thrombocytopenia

Drug Interactions

Avoid Concomitant Use There are no known interactions where it is recommended to avoid concomitant use.

Increased Effect/Toxicity

Cyproheptadine may increase the levels/effects of: Alcohol (Ethyl); Anticholinergics; CNS Depressants

The levels/effects of Cyproheptadine may be increased by: Pramlintide

Decreased Effect

Cyproheptadine may decrease the levels/effects of: Acetylcholinesterase Inhibitors (Central); Betahistine; Selective Serotonin Reuptake Inhibitors

The levels/effects of Cyproheptadine may be decreased by: Acetylcholinesterase Inhibitors (Central); Amphetamines

Ethanol/Nutrition/Herb Interactions Ethanol: Avoid ethanol (may increase CNS sedation).

Mechanism of Action A potent antihistamine and serotonin antagonist, competes with histamine for H_1-receptor sites on effector cells in the gastrointestinal tract, blood vessels, and respiratory tract

Pharmacodynamics/Kinetics

Absorption: Completely

Metabolism: Almost completely hepatic

Excretion: Urine (>50% primarily as metabolites); feces (~25%)

Dosage Oral:

Children:

Allergic conditions: 0.25 mg/kg/day or 8 mg/m^2/day in 2-3 divided doses **or**

2-6 years: 2 mg every 8-12 hours (not to exceed 12 mg/day)

7-14 years: 4 mg every 8-12 hours (not to exceed 16 mg/day)

Migraine headaches: 4 mg 2-3 times/day

Children ≥12 years and Adults: Spasticity associated with spinal cord damage: 4 mg at bedtime; increase by a 4 mg dose every 3-4 days; average daily dose: 16 mg in divided doses; not to exceed 36 mg/day

Children >13 years and Adults: Appetite stimulation (anorexia nervosa): 2 mg 4 times/day; may be increased gradually over a 3-week period to 8 mg 4 times/day

Adults:

Allergic conditions: 4-20 mg/day divided every 8 hours (not to exceed 0.5 mg/kg/day)

Cluster headaches: 4 mg 4 times/day

Migraine headaches: 4-8 mg 3 times/day

Dosage adjustment in hepatic impairment: Reduce dosage in patients with significant hepatic dysfunction

Test Interactions Diagnostic antigen skin test results may be suppressed; false positive serum TCA screen

Additional Information May stimulate appetite. In case reports, cyproheptadine has promoted weight gain in anorexic adults.

Dosage Forms Excipient information presented when available (limited, particularly for generics); consult specific product labeling.

Syrup, as hydrochloride: 2 mg/5 mL (473 mL) [contains alcohol 5%; mint flavor]

Tablet, as hydrochloride: 4 mg

- ◆ **Cyproheptadine Hydrochloride** *see* Cyproheptadine *on page 383*
- ◆ **Cystadane®** *see* Betaine *on page 188*
- ◆ **Cystagon®** *see* Cysteamine *on page 383*

Cysteamine (sis TEE a meen)

U.S. Brand Names Cystagon®

Index Terms Cysteamine Bitartrate

Pharmacologic Category Anticystine Agent; Urinary Tract Product

Use Treatment of nephropathic cystinosis

Pregnancy Risk Factor C

Dosage Oral: Initiate therapy with 1/4 to 1/6 of maintenance dose; titrate slowly upward over 4-6 weeks. **Note:** Dosage may be increased if cystine levels are <1 nmol/½ cystine/mg protein, although intolerance and incidence of adverse events may be increased.

Children <12 years: Maintenance: 1.3 g/m²/day or 60 mg/kg/day divided into 4 doses (maximum dose: 1.95 g/m²/day or 90 mg/kg/day)

Children >12 years and Adults (>110 lb): 2 g/day in 4 divided doses; maximum dose: 1.95 g/m²/day or 90 mg/kg/day

Additional Information Complete prescribing information for this medication should be consulted for additional detail.

Dosage Forms Excipient information presented when available (limited, particularly for generics); consult specific product labeling.

Capsule:

Cystagon®: 50 mg, 150 mg

- **Cysteamine Bitartrate** *see* Cysteamine *on page* 383
- **Cystistat® (Can)** *see* Hyaluronate and Derivatives *on page* 734
- **Cystospaz®** *see* Hyoscyamine *on page* 756
- **CYT** *see* Cyclophosphamide *on page* 376
- **Cytadren®** *see* Aminoglutethimide *on page* 86

Cytarabine (sye TARE a been)

Canadian Brand Names Cytosar®

Index Terms Ara-C; Arabinosylcytosine; Cytarabine (Conventional); Cytarabine Hydrochloride; Cytosar-U; Cytosine Arabinosine Hydrochloride; NSC-63878

Pharmacologic Category Antineoplastic Agent, Antimetabolite; Antineoplastic Agent, Antimetabolite (Pyrimidine Analog)

Use Treatment of acute myeloid leukemia (AML), acute lymphocytic leukemia (ALL), chronic myelocytic leukemia (CML; blast phase), and lymphomas; prophylaxis and treatment of meningeal leukemia

Pregnancy Risk Factor D

Pregnancy Considerations Cytarabine is teratogenic in animal studies. Limb and ear defects have been noted in case reports when cytarabine has been used during pregnancy. The following have also been noted in the neonate: Pancytopenia, WBC depression, electrolyte abnormalities, prematurity, low birth weight, decreased hematocrit or platelets. Risk to the fetus is decreased if therapy is avoided during the 1st trimester; however, women of childbearing potential should be advised of the potential risks.

Lactation Excretion in breast milk unknown/not recommended

Medication Safety Issues

Sound-alike/look-alike issues:

Cytarabine may be confused with Cytadren®, Cytosar®, Cytoxan®, vidarabine

Cytarabine (conventional) may be confused with cytarabine liposomal

Cytosar-U may be confused with cytarabine, Cytovene®, Cytoxan®, Neosar®

High alert medication: The Institute for Safe Medication Practices (ISMP) includes this medication among its list of drugs which have a heightened risk of causing significant patient harm when used in error.

Contraindications Hypersensitivity to cytarabine or any component of the formulation

Warnings/Precautions Hazardous agent - use appropriate precautions for handling and disposal. **[U.S. Boxed Warning]: Potent myelosuppressive agent;** use with caution in patients with prior bone marrow suppression; monitor for signs of febrile neutropenia. High-dose regimens are associated with CNS, gastrointestinal, ocular (prophylaxis with ophthalmic corticosteroid drops is recommended), pulmonary toxicities and cardiomyopathy. Neurotoxicity associated with high dose treatment may present as acute cerebellar toxicity, or may be severe with seizure and/or coma; may be delayed, occurring up to 3 to 8 days after treatment has begun. Risk factors for neurotoxicity include cumulative cytarabine dose, prior CNS disease and renal impairment. Tumor lysis syndrome and subsequent hyperuricemia may occur with high dose cytarabine; monitor, consider allopurinol and hydrate accordingly. There have been case reports of fatal cardiomyopathy when high dose cytarabine was used in combination with cyclophosphamide as a preparation regimen for transplantation.

Use with caution in patients with impaired renal and hepatic function; may be at higher risk for CNS toxicities; dosage adjustments may be necessary. Cytarabine syndrome is characterized by fever, myalgia, bone pain, chest pain, maculopapular rash, conjunctivitis, and malaise, and may occur 6-12 hours following administration; may be managed with corticosteroids. There have been reports of acute pancreatitis in patients receiving continuous infusion and in patients previously treated with L-asparaginase. **[U.S. Boxed Warning]: Should be administered under the supervision of an experienced cancer chemotherapy physician.** Some products may contain benzyl alcohol; do not use products containing benzyl alcohol or products reconstituted with bacteriostatic diluent intrathecally or for high-dose cytarabine regimens.

Adverse Reactions Note: Frequency not defined.

Frequent:

Central nervous system: Fever

Dermatologic: Rash

Gastrointestinal: Anal inflammation, anal ulceration, anorexia, diarrhea, mucositis, nausea, vomiting

Hematologic: Myelosuppression, neutropenia (onset: 1-7 days; nadir [biphasic]: 7-9 days and at 15-24 days; recovery [biphasic]: 9-12 and at 24-34 days), thrombocytopenia (onset: 5 days; nadir: 12-15 days; recovery 15-25 days), anemia, bleeding, leukopenia, megaloblastosis, reticulocytes decreased

Hepatic: Hepatic dysfunction, transaminases increased (acute)

Local: Thrombophlebitis

Less frequent:

Cardiovascular: Chest pain, pericarditis

Central nervous system: Dizziness, headache, neural toxicity, neuritis

Dermatologic: Alopecia, pruritus, skin freckling, skin ulceration, urticaria

Gastrointestinal: Abdominal pain, bowel necrosis, esophageal ulceration, esophagitis, pancreatitis, sore throat

Genitourinary: Urinary retention

Hepatic: Jaundice

Local: Injection site cellulitis

Ocular: Conjunctivitis

Renal: Renal dysfunction

Respiratory: Dyspnea

Miscellaneous: Allergic edema, anaphylaxis, sepsis

Infrequent and/or case reports: Amylase increased, aseptic meningitis, cardiopulmonary arrest (acute), cerebral dysfunction, cytarabine syndrome (bone pain, chest pain, conjunctivitis, fever, maculopapular rash, malaise, myalgia); exanthematous pustulosis, hyperuricemia, injection site inflammation (SubQ injection), injection site pain (SubQ injection), interstitial pneumonitis, lipase increased, paralysis (intrathecal and I.V. combination therapy), rhabdomyolysis, veno-occlusive liver disease

Adverse events associated with high-dose cytarabine (CNS, gastrointestinal, ocular, and pulmonary toxicities are more common with high-dose regimens):

Cardiovascular: Cardiomegaly, cardiomyopathy (in combination with cyclophosphamide)

Central nervous system: Coma, neurotoxicity (dose-related, cerebellar toxicity may occur in patients receiving high-dose cytarabine [>36-48 g/m^2/cycle]; incidence may up to 55% in patients with renal impairment), personality change, somnolence

Dermatologic: Alopecia (complete), desquamation, rash (severe)

Gastrointestinal: Gastrointestinal ulcer, peritonitis, pneumatosis cystoides intestinalis

Hepatic: Hyperbilirubinemia, liver abscess, liver damage, necrotizing colitis

Neuromuscular & skeletal: Peripheral neuropathy (motor and sensory)

Ocular: Corneal toxicity, hemorrhagic conjunctivitis

Respiratory: Pulmonary edema, syndrome of sudden respiratory distress

Miscellaneous: Sepsis

Adverse events associated with intrathecal cytarabine administration:

Central nervous system: Accessory nerve paralysis, fever, necrotizing leukoencephalopathy (with concurrent cranial irradiation, I.T. methotrexate, and I.T. hydrocortisone), neurotoxicity, paraplegia

Gastrointestinal: Dysphagia, nausea, vomiting

Ocular: Blindness (with concurrent systemic chemotherapy and cranial irradiation), diplopia

Respiratory: Cough, hoarseness

Miscellaneous: Aphonia

Drug Interactions

Avoid Concomitant Use

Avoid concomitant use of Cytarabine with any of the following: Natalizumab; Vaccines (Live)

Increased Effect/Toxicity

Cytarabine may increase the levels/effects of: Natalizumab; Vaccines (Live)

The levels/effects of Cytarabine may be increased by: Trastuzumab

Decreased Effect

Cytarabine may decrease the levels/effects of: Cardiac Glycosides; Flucytosine; Vaccines (Inactivated)

The levels/effects of Cytarabine may be decreased by: Echinacea

Stability

Powder for reconstitution: Store intact vials of powder at room temperature 15°C to 30°C (59°F to 86°F). Reconstitute with bacteriostatic water for injection. Reconstituted solutions are stable for up to 8 days at room temperature, although the manufacturer recommends use within 48 hours.

Solution: Prior to dilution, store at room temperature, 15°C to 30°C (59°F to 86°F); protect from light. Do not refrigerate solution; precipitate may form.

Further dilution in D_5W or NS is stable for 8 days at room temperature (25°C). Intrathecal solutions in 3-20 mL lactated Ringer's are stable for 7 days at room temperature (30°C); however, should be used within 24 hours due to sterility concerns.

Reconstitute powder with bacteriostatic water for injection, bacteriostatic 0.9% NaCl.

For I.T. use: Reconstitute with preservative free diluent.

For I.V. infusion: Dilute in 250-1000 mL 0.9% NaCl or D_5W.

Note: Solutions containing bacteriostatic agents should not be used for the preparation of either high doses or intrathecal doses of cytarabine; may be used for I.M., SubQ, and low-dose (100-200 mg/m^2) I.V. solution.

Mechanism of Action Inhibits DNA synthesis. Cytosine gains entry into cells by a carrier process, and then must be converted to its active compound, aracytidine triphosphate. Cytosine is a pyrimidine analog and is incorporated into DNA; however, the primary action is inhibition of DNA polymerase resulting in decreased DNA synthesis and repair. The degree of cytotoxicity correlates linearly with incorporation into DNA; therefore, incorporation into the DNA is responsible for drug activity and toxicity. Cytarabine is specific for the S phase of the cell cycle (blocks progression from the G_1 to the S phase).

Pharmacodynamics/Kinetics

Distribution: V_d: Total body water; widely and rapidly since it enters the cells readily; crosses blood-brain barrier with CSF levels of 40% to 50% of plasma level

Metabolism: Primarily hepatic; metabolized by deoxycytidine kinase and other nucleotide kinases to aracytidine triphosphate (active); about 86% to 96% of dose is metabolized to inactive uracil arabinoside (ARA-U); intrathecal administration results in little conversion to ARA-U due to the low levels of deaminase in the cerebral spinal fluid

Half-life elimination: I.V.: Initial: 7-20 minutes; Terminal: 1-3 hours

Time to peak, plasma: I.M., SubQ: 20-60 minutes

Excretion: Urine (~80%; 90% as metabolite ARA-U) within 24 hours

Dosage Refer to individual protocols. Children and Adults:

Remission induction:

I.V.: 75-200 mg/m^2/day for 5-10 days; a second course, beginning 2-4 weeks after the initial therapy, may be required in some patients.

or 100 mg/m^2 for 7 days

or 100 mg/m^2/dose every 12 hours for 7 days

I.T.: Usual dose 30 mg/m^2 every 4 days; range: 5-75 mg/m^2 every 2-7 days until CNS findings normalize; or age-based dosing (frequency of administration usually defined by protocol):

<1 year of age: 15-20 mg per dose

1-2 years of age: 16-30 mg per dose

2-3 years of age: 20-50 mg per dose

>3 years of age: 24-75 mg per dose

Remission maintenance:

I.V.: 70-200 mg/m^2/day for 2-5 days at monthly intervals

I.M., SubQ: 1-1.5 mg/kg single dose for maintenance at 1- to 4-week intervals

High-dose therapies (unlabeled use):

Doses as high as 1-3 g/m^2 have been used for refractory or secondary leukemias or refractory non-Hodgkin's lymphoma.

Doses of 1-3 g/m^2 every 12 hours for up to 12 doses have been used for leukemia

Bone marrow transplant (unlabeled use): 1.5 g/m^2 continuous infusion over 48 hours

Dosage adjustment in renal impairment: The FDA-approved labeling does not contain renal dosing adjustment guidelines; the following guidelines have been used by some clinicians:

Aronoff, 2007 (Cytarabine 100-200 mg/m^2): Children and Adults: No adjustment necessary

Kintzel, 1995 (High-dose cytarabine 1-3 g/m^2):

Cl_{cr} 46-60 mL/minute: Administer 60% of dose

Cl_{cr} 31-45 mL/minute: Administer 50% of dose

Cl_{cr} <30 mL/minute: Consider use of alternative drug

Smith, 1997 (High-dose cytarabine ≥2 g/m^2/dose):

Serum creatinine 1.5-1.9 mg/dL or increase (from baseline) of 0.5-1.2 mg/dL: Reduce dose to 1 g/m^2/dose

Serum creatinine ≥2 mg/dL or increase (from baseline) of >1.2 mg/dL: Reduce dose to 0.1 g/m^2/day as a continuous infusion

Dosage adjustment in hepatic impairment: Dose may need to be adjusted in patients with liver failure since cytarabine is partially detoxified in the liver. The FDA-approved labeling does not contain hepatic dosing adjustment guidelines; the following guideline has been used by some clinicians:

Floyd, 2006: Transaminases (any elevation): Administer 50% of dose; may increase subsequent doses in the absence of toxicities

Koren, 1992 (dose level not specified): Bilirubin >2 mg/dL: Administer 50% of dose; may increase subsequent doses in the absence of toxicities

Administration May be administered I.M., I.T., or SubQ at a concentration not to exceed 100 mg/mL. When administered via I.V. infusion, infuse over 1-3 hours or as a continuous infusion. GI effects may be more pronounced with divided I.V. bolus doses than with continuous infusion.

Monitoring Parameters Liver function tests, CBC with differential and platelet count, serum creatinine, BUN, serum uric acid

Additional Information I.V. doses ≥1.5 g/m^2 may produce conjunctivitis which can be ameliorated with prophylactic use of corticosteroid (0.1% dexamethasone) eye drops. Dexamethasone eye drops should be administered at 1-2 drops every 6 hours during and for 2-7 days after cytarabine is done.

Dosage Forms Excipient information presented when available (limited, particularly for generics); consult specific product labeling.

Injection, powder for reconstitution: 100 mg, 500 mg, 1 g, 2 g

Injection, solution: 20 mg/mL (5 mL, 25 mL, 50 mL); 100 mg/mL (20 mL)

◆ **Cytarabine (Conventional)** *see* Cytarabine *on page 384*

◆ **Cytarabine Hydrochloride** *see* Cytarabine *on page 384*

Cytarabine (Liposomal)

(sye TARE a been lip po SOE mal)

U.S. Brand Names DepoCyt®

Canadian Brand Names DepoCyt®

Pharmacologic Category Antineoplastic Agent, Antimetabolite (Pyrimidine Antagonist)

Use Treatment of lymphomatous meningitis

Pregnancy Risk Factor D

Pregnancy Considerations Reproductive studies have not been conducted with cytarabine liposomal. Cytarabine, the active component, has been associated with fetal malformations when given as a component of combination chemotherapy during the first trimester. Systemic exposure following intrathecal administration of cytarabine liposomal is negligible. There are no adequate and well-controlled studies in pregnant women. Women of childbearing potential should avoid becoming pregnant during treatment.

Lactation Excretion in breast milk unknown/not recommended

Medication Safety Issues

Sound-alike/look-alike issues:

Cytarabine may be confused with Cytadren®, Cytosar®, Cytoxan®, vidarabine

Cytarabine liposomal may be confused with conventional cytarabine

DepoCyt® may be confused with Depoject®

High alert medication: The Institute for Safe Medication Practices (ISMP) includes this medication among its list of drugs which have a heightened risk of causing significant patient harm when used in error.

Contraindications Hypersensitivity to cytarabine or any component of the formulation; active meningeal infection

Warnings/Precautions Hazardous agent - use appropriate precautions for handling and disposal. **[U.S. Boxed Warning]: Chemical arachnoiditis (nausea, vomiting, headache, fever) occurs commonly; may be fatal if untreated. The incidence and severity of chemical arachnoiditis is reduced by coadministration with dexamethasone.** Hydrocephalus has been reported and may be precipitated by chemical arachnoiditis. May cause neurotoxicity (including myelopathy), which may lead to permanent neurologic deficit. Blockage to CSF flow may increase the risk of neurotoxicity. Peripheral neurotoxicity has also been reported. Monitor for neurotoxicity; reduce subsequent doses; discontinue with persistent neurotoxicity. The risk of adverse events, including neurotoxicity, is increased with concurrent radiation therapy or systemic chemotherapy. Infectious meningitis may be associated with intrathecal administration. **[U.S. Boxed Warning]: Should be administered under the supervision of an experienced cancer chemotherapy physician.** For intrathecal use only. Safety and efficacy in pediatric patients have not been established.

Adverse Reactions

>10%:

Cardiovascular: Peripheral edema (11%)

Central nervous system: Chemical arachnoiditis (without dexamethasone premedication: 100%; with dexamethasone premedication: 33% to 42%; grade 4: 19% to 30%; onset: ≤5 days); headache (56%), confusion (33%), fever (32%), fatigue (25%), seizure (20% to 22%), dizziness (18%), lethargy (16%), insomnia (14%), memory impairment (14%), pain (14%)

Endocrine & metabolic: Dehydration (13%)

Gastrointestinal: Nausea (46%), vomiting (44%), constipation (25%), diarrhea (12%), appetite decreased (11%)

Genitourinary: Urinary tract infection (14%)

Hematologic: Anemia (12%), thrombocytopenia (3% to 11%)

Neuromuscular & skeletal: Weakness (40%), back pain (24%), abnormal gait (23%), limb pain (15%), neck pain (14%), arthralgia (11%), neck stiffness (11%)

Ocular: Blurred vision (11%)

1% to 10%:

Cardiovascular: Tachycardia (9%), hypotension (8%), hypertension (6%), syncope (3%), edema (2%)

Central nervous system: Agitation (10%), hypoesthesia (10%), depression (8%), anxiety (7%), sensory neuropathy (3%)

Dermatologic: Pruritus (2%)

Endocrine & metabolic: Hypokalemia (7%), hyponatremia (7%), hyperglycemia (6%)

Gastrointestinal: Abdominal pain (9%), dysphagia (8%), anorexia (5%), hemorrhoids (3%), mucosal inflammation (3%)

Genitourinary: Incontinence (7%), urinary retention (5%)

Hematologic: Neutropenia (10%), contusion (2%)

Neuromuscular & skeletal: Muscle weakness (10%), tremor (9%), peripheral neuropathy (4%), abnormal reflexes (3%)

Otic: Hypoacusis (6%)

Respiratory: Dyspnea (10%), cough (7%), pneumonia (6%)

Miscellaneous: Diaphoresis (2%)

1% (Limited to important or life-threatening): Anaphylaxis, bladder control impaired, blindness, bowel control impaired, cauda equine syndrome, cranial nerve palsies, CSF protein increased, CSF WBC increased, deafness, encephalopathy, hemiplegia, hydrocephalus, infectious meningitis, intracranial pressure increased, myelopathy, neurologic deficit, numbness, papilledema, somnolence, visual disturbance

Drug Interactions

Avoid Concomitant Use

Avoid concomitant use of Cytarabine (Liposomal) with any of the following: Natalizumab; Vaccines (Live)

Increased Effect/Toxicity

Cytarabine (Liposomal) may increase the levels/effects of: Natalizumab; Vaccines (Live)

The levels/effects of Cytarabine (Liposomal) may be increased by: Trastuzumab

Decreased Effect

Cytarabine (Liposomal) may decrease the levels/effects of: Vaccines (Inactivated)

The levels/effects of Cytarabine (Liposomal) may be decreased by: Echinacea

Stability Store under refrigeration at 2°C to 8°C (36°F to 46°F). Protect from freezing and avoid aggressive agitation. Solutions should be used within 4 hours of withdrawal from the vial. Allow vial to warm to room temperature prior to withdrawal from vial. Particles may settle in diluent over time, and may be resuspended by gentle agitation or inversion of the vial.

Mechanism of Action Cytarabine liposomal is a sustained-release formulation of the active ingredient cytarabine, an antimetabolite which acts through inhibition of DNA synthesis and is cell cycle-specific for the S phase of cell division. Cytarabine is converted intracellularly to its active metabolite cytarabine-5'-triphosphate (ara-CTP). Ara-CTP also appears to be incorporated into DNA and RNA; however, the primary action is inhibition of DNA polymerase, resulting in decreased DNA synthesis and repair. The liposomal formulation allows for gradual release, resulting in prolonged exposure.

Pharmacodynamics/Kinetics

Absorption: Systemic exposure following intrathecal administration is negligible since transfer rate from CSF to plasma is slow

Half-life elimination, CSF: 6-82 hours

Time to peak, CSF: Intrathecal: <1 hour

Dosage Note: Patients should be started on dexamethasone 4 mg twice daily (oral or I.V.) for 5 days, beginning on the day of cytarabine liposomal injection.

Intrathecal: Adults:
- Induction: 50 mg every 14 days for a total of 2 doses (weeks 1 and 3)
- Consolidation: 50 mg every 14 days for 3 doses (weeks 5, 7, and 9), followed by an additional dose at week 13
- Maintenance: 50 mg every 28 days for 4 doses (weeks 17, 21, 25, and 29)

Dosage reduction for toxicity: If drug-related neurotoxicity develops, reduce dose to 25 mg. If toxicity persists, discontinue treatment.

Administration For intrathecal use only. Dose should be removed from vial immediately before administration (must be administered within 4 hours of removal). An in-line filter should **not** be used. Administer directly into the CSF via an intraventricular reservoir or by direct injection into the lumbar sac. Injection should be made slowly (over 1-5 minutes). Patients should lie flat for 1 hour after lumbar puncture.

Monitoring Parameters Monitor closely for signs of an immediate reaction; neurotoxicity

Test Interactions Since cytarabine liposomes are similar in appearance to WBCs, care must be taken in interpreting CSF examinations in patients receiving cytarabine liposomal.

Dosage Forms Excipient information presented when available (limited, particularly for generics); consult specific product labeling.

Injection, suspension, intrathecal [preservative free]:
- Depocyt®: 10 mg/mL (5 mL)

◆ **CytoGam®** *see* Cytomegalovirus Immune Globulin (Intravenous-Human) *on page 387*

Cytomegalovirus Immune Globulin (Intravenous-Human)

(sye toe meg a low VYE rus i MYUN GLOB yoo lin in tra VEE nus HYU man)

U.S. Brand Names CytoGam®

Canadian Brand Names CytoGam®

Index Terms CMV-IGIV

Pharmacologic Category Immune Globulin

Use Prophylaxis of cytomegalovirus (CMV) disease associated with kidney, lung, liver, pancreas, and heart transplants; concomitant use with ganciclovir should be considered in organ transplants (other than kidney) from CMV seropositive donors to CMV seronegative recipients

Unlabeled/Investigational Use Adjunct therapy in the treatment of CMV disease in immunocompromised patients

Pregnancy Risk Factor C

Pregnancy Considerations Reproduction studies have not been conducted.

Lactation Excretion in breast milk unknown

Medication Safety Issues

Sound-alike/look-alike issues:
- CytoGam® may be confused with Cytoxan®, Gamimune® N

Contraindications Hypersensitivity to CMV-IGIV, other immunoglobulins, or any component of the formulation; immunoglobulin A deficiency

Warnings/Precautions Hypersensitivity and anaphylactic reactions can occur; immediate treatment (including epinephrine 1:1000) should be available. Aseptic meningitis syndrome (AMS) has been reported with intravenous immune globulin administration (rare); may occur with high doses (≥2 g/kg). Intravenous immune globulin has been associated with antiglobulin hemolysis; monitor for signs of hemolytic anemia. Monitor for transfusion-related acute lung injury (TRALI); noncardiogenic pulmonary edema has been reported with intravenous immune globulin use. Acute renal dysfunction (increased serum creatinine, oliguria, acute renal failure) can rarely occur; usually within 7 days of use (more likely with products stabilized with sucrose). Use with caution in the elderly, patients with renal disease, diabetes mellitus, volume depletion, sepsis, paraproteinemia, and nephrotoxic medications due to risk of renal dysfunction. In patients at risk of renal dysfunction, the rate of infusion and concentration of solution should be minimized. discontinue if renal function deteriorates. Patients should not be volume depleted prior to therapy. Thrombotic events have been reported with administration of intravenous immune globulin; use with caution in patients with cardiovascular risk factors. Use with caution in patients >65 years of age. Product is stabilized with albumin. Product of human plasma; may potentially contain infectious agents which could transmit disease. Screening of donors, as well as testing and/or inactivation or removal of certain viruses, reduces the risk. Infections thought to be transmitted by this product should be reported to the manufacturer. Product is stabilized with sucrose.

Adverse Reactions

<6%:
- Cardiovascular: Flushing
- Central nervous system: Chills, fever
- Gastrointestinal: Nausea, vomiting
- Neuromuscular & skeletal: Arthralgia, back pain, muscle cramps
- Respiratory: Wheezing

<1% (Limited to important or life-threatening): Acute renal failure, acute tubular necrosis, AMS, anaphylactic shock,

angioneurotic edema, anuria, blood presure decreased, BUN increase, oliguria, osmotic nephrosis, proximal tubular nephropathy, serum creatinine increased

Drug Interactions

Avoid Concomitant Use There are no known interactions where it is recommended to avoid concomitant use.

Increased Effect/Toxicity There are no known significant interactions involving an increase in effect.

Decreased Effect

Cytomegalovirus Immune Globulin (Intravenous-Human) may decrease the levels/effects of: Vaccines (Live)

Stability Store between 2°C and 8°C (35.6°F and 46.4°F). Use reconstituted product within 6 hours; do not admix with other medications; do not use if turbid. Do not shake vials. Dilution is not recommended. Infusion with other products is not recommended.

Mechanism of Action CMV-IGIV is a preparation of immunoglobulin G derived from pooled healthy blood donors with a high titer of CMV antibodies; administration provides a passive source of antibodies against cytomegalovirus

Dosage I.V.: Adults:

Kidney transplant:

Initial dose (within 72 hours of transplant): 150 mg/kg/dose

2-, 4-, 6-, and 8 weeks after transplant: 100 mg/kg/dose

12 and 16 weeks after transplant: 50 mg/kg/dose

Liver, lung, pancreas, or heart transplant:

Initial dose (within 72 hours of transplant): 150 mg/kg/dose

2-, 4-, 6-, and 8 weeks after transplant: 150 mg/kg/dose

12 and 16 weeks after transplant: 100 mg/kg/dose

Severe CMV pneumonia (unlabeled): Various regimens have been used, including 400 mg/kg CMV-IGIV in combination with ganciclovir on days 1, 2, 7, or 8, followed by 200 mg/kg CMV-IGIV on days 14 and 21

Elderly: Use with caution in patients >65 years of age, may be at increased risk of renal insufficiency

Dosage adjustment in renal impairment: Use with caution; specific dosing adjustments are not available. Infusion rate should be the minimum practical; do not exceed 180 mg/kg/hour

Dietary Considerations

CytoGam® solution for injection 50 mg (± 10 mg/mL) contains sodium 20-30 mEq/L

Administration Administer through an I.V. line containing an in-line filter (pore size 15 micron) using an infusion pump. Do not mix with other infusions; do not use if turbid. Begin infusion within 6 hours of entering vial, complete infusion within 12 hours.

Infuse at 15 mg/kg/hour. If no adverse reactions occur within 30 minutes, may increase rate to 30 mg/kg/hour. If no adverse reactions occur within the second 30 minutes, may increase rate to 60 mg/kg/hour; maximum rate of infusion: 75 mL/hour. When infusing subsequent doses, may decrease titration interval from 30 minutes to 15 minutes. If patient develops nausea, back pain, or flushing during infusion, slow the rate or temporarily stop the infusion. Discontinue if blood pressure drops or in case of anaphylactic reaction.

Monitoring Parameters Vital signs (throughout infusion), flushing, chills, muscle cramps, back pain, fever, nausea, vomiting, wheezing, decreased blood pressure, or anaphylaxis; renal function and urine output

Dosage Forms Excipient information presented when available (limited, particularly for generics); consult specific product labeling.

Injection, solution [preservative free]:

CytoGam®: 50 mg ± 10 mg/mL (50 mL) [contains sodium 20-30 mEq/L, human albumin, and sucrose]

◆ **Cytomel®** *see* Liothyronine *on page 892*

◆ **Cytosar® (Can)** *see* Cytarabine *on page 384*

◆ **Cytosar-U** *see* Cytarabine *on page 384*

◆ **Cytosine Arabinosine Hydrochloride** *see* Cytarabine *on page 384*

◆ **Cytostasan** *see* Bendamustine *on page 181*

◆ **Cytotec®** *see* Misoprostol *on page 1004*

◆ **Cytovene®** *see* Ganciclovir *on page 681*

◆ **Cytoxan® [DSC]** *see* Cyclophosphamide *on page 376*

◆ **Cytoxan® (Can)** *see* Cyclophosphamide *on page 376*

◆ **Cytra-2** *see* Sodium Citrate and Citric Acid *on page 1383*

◆ **Cytra-3** *see* Citric Acid, Sodium Citrate, and Potassium Citrate *on page 339*

◆ **Cytra-K** *see* Potassium Citrate and Citric Acid *on page 1218*

◆ **Cēpacol® Dual Action Maximum Strength [OTC]** *see* Dyclonine *on page 501*

◆ **D2E7** *see* Adalimumab *on page 43*

◆ **D-3-Mercaptovaline** *see* Penicillamine *on page 1161*

◆ **d4T** *see* Stavudine *on page 1398*

◆ **$DAB_{389}IL-2$** *see* Denileukin Diftitox *on page 417*

◆ **DAB389 Interleukin-2** *see* Denileukin Diftitox *on page 417*

Dacarbazine (da KAR ba zeen)

Canadian Brand Names DTIC®

Index Terms DIC; Dimethyl Triazeno Imidazole Carboxamide; DTIC; Imidazole Carboxamide; Imidazole Carboxamide Dimethyltriazene; WR-139007

Pharmacologic Category Antineoplastic Agent, Alkylating Agent (Triazene)

Use Treatment of malignant melanoma, Hodgkin's disease, soft-tissue sarcomas, fibrosarcomas, rhabdomyosarcoma, islet cell carcinoma, medullary carcinoma of the thyroid, and neuroblastoma

Pregnancy Risk Factor C

Pregnancy Considerations [U.S. Boxed Warning]: This agent is carcinogenic and/or teratogenic when used in animals.

Lactation Excretion in breast milk unknown/not recommended

Medication Safety Issues

Sound-alike/look-alike issues:

Dacarbazine may be confused with Dicarbosil®, procarbazine

High alert medication: The Institute for Safe Medication Practices (ISMP) includes this medication among its list of drugs which have a heightened risk of causing significant patient harm when used in error.

Contraindications Hypersensitivity to dacarbazine or any component of the formulation

Warnings/Precautions Hazardous agent - use appropriate precautions for handling and disposal. **[U.S. Boxed Warnings]: Bone marrow suppression is a common toxicity; monitor closely. Hepatotoxicity with hepatocellular necrosis and hepatic vein thrombosis has been reported,** usually with combination chemotherapy, but may occur with dacarbazine alone. The half-life is increased in patients with renal and/or hepatic impairment; use caution, monitor for toxicity and consider dosage reduction. Anaphylaxis may occur. Extravasation may result in tissue damage and pain. **[U.S. Boxed Warnings]: May be carcinogenic and/or teratogenic. Should be administered under the supervision of an experienced cancer chemotherapy physician.**

Adverse Reactions

>10%:

Gastrointestinal: Nausea and vomiting (>90%), can be severe and dose limiting; nausea and vomiting decrease on successive days when dacarbazine is given daily for 5 days; diarrhea

Hematologic: Myelosuppression, leukopenia, thrombocytopenia - dose limiting

Onset: 5-7 days

Nadir: 7-10 days

Recovery: 21-28 days

Local: Pain on infusion, may be minimized by administration through a central line, or by administration as a short infusion (eg, 1-2 hours as opposed to bolus injection)

1% to 10%:

Dermatologic: Alopecia, rash, photosensitivity

Gastrointestinal: Anorexia, metallic taste

Miscellaneous: Flu-like syndrome (fever, myalgia, malaise)

<1% (Limited to important or life-threatening): Anaphylactic reactions, diarrhea (following high-dose bolus injection), eosinophilia, headache, hepatic necrosis, hepatic vein occlusion, liver enzymes increased (transient), paresthesia

Drug Interactions

Metabolism/Transport Effects Substrate (major) of CYP1A2, 2E1

Avoid Concomitant Use

Avoid concomitant use of Dacarbazine with any of the following: Natalizumab; Vaccines (Live)

Increased Effect/Toxicity

Dacarbazine may increase the levels/effects of: Natalizumab; Vaccines (Live)

The levels/effects of Dacarbazine may be increased by: CYP1A2 Inhibitors (Moderate); CYP1A2 Inhibitors (Strong); CYP2E1 Inhibitors (Moderate); CYP2E1 Inhibitors (Strong); Trastuzumab

Decreased Effect

Dacarbazine may decrease the levels/effects of: Vaccines (Inactivated)

The levels/effects of Dacarbazine may be decreased by: CYP1A2 Inducers (Strong); Echinacea; Sorafenib

Ethanol/Nutrition/Herb Interactions

Ethanol: Avoid ethanol (due to GI irritation).

Herb/Nutraceutical: Avoid dong quai, St John's wort (may also cause photosensitization).

Stability Store intact vials under refrigeration (2°C to 8°C) and protect from light; vials are stable for 4 weeks at room temperature. Reconstituted solution is stable for 24 hours at room temperature (20°C) and 96 hours under refrigeration (4°C). Solutions for infusion (in D_5W or NS) are stable for 24 hours at room temperature and protected from light. Decomposed drug turns pink.

The manufacturer recommends reconstituting 100 mg and 200 mg vials with 9.9 mL and 19.7 mL SWFI, respectively, to a concentration of 10 mg/mL; some institutions use different standard dilutions (eg, 20 mg/mL).

Standard I.V. dilution: Dilute in 250-1000 mL D_5W or NS.

Mechanism of Action Alkylating agent which appears to form methylcarbonium ions that attack nucleophilic groups in DNA; cross-links strands of DNA resulting in the inhibition of DNA, RNA, and protein synthesis, the exact mechanism of action is still unclear.

Pharmacodynamics/Kinetics

Onset of action: I.V.: 18-24 days

Distribution: V_d: 0.6 L/kg, exceeding total body water; suggesting binding to some tissue (probably liver)

Protein binding: 5%

Metabolism: Extensively hepatic; hepatobiliary excretion is probably of some importance; metabolites may also have an antineoplastic effect

Half-life elimination: Biphasic: Initial: 20-40 minutes; Terminal: 5 hours

Excretion: Urine (~30% to 50% as unchanged drug)

Dosage Refer to individual protocols. Some dosage regimens include:

Intra-arterial: 50-400 mg/m^2 for 5-10 days

I.V.:

Hodgkin's disease, ABVD: 375 mg/m^2 days 1 and 15 every 4 weeks **or** 100 mg/m^2/day for 5 days

Metastatic melanoma (alone or in combination with other agents): 150-250 mg/m^2 days 1-5 every 3-4 weeks

Metastatic melanoma: 850 mg/m^2 every 3 weeks

High dose: Bone marrow/blood cell transplantation: I.V.: 1-3 g/m^2; maximum dose as a single agent: 3.38 g/m^2; generally combined with other high-dose chemotherapeutic drugs

Dosage adjustment in renal impairment: The FDA-approved labeling does not contain dosage adjustment guidelines. The following guidelines have been used by some clinicians (Kintzel, 1995):

Cl_{cr} 46-60 mL/minute: Administer 80% of dose

Cl_{cr} 31-45 mL/minute: Administer 75% of dose

Cl_{cr} <30 mL/minute: Administer 70% of dose

Dosage adjustment in hepatic impairment: The FDA-approved labeling does not contain adjustment guidelines. May cause hepatotoxicity; monitor closely for signs of toxicity.

Administration Infuse over 30-60 minutes; rapid infusion may cause severe venous irritation.

Extravasation management: Local pain, burning sensation, and irritation at the injection site may be relieved by local application of hot packs. If extravasation occurs, apply cold packs. Protect exposed tissue from light following extravasation.

Monitoring Parameters CBC with differential, liver function

Dosage Forms Excipient information presented when available (limited, particularly for generics); consult specific product labeling.

Injection, powder for reconstitution: 100 mg, 200 mg

Daclizumab (dac KLYE zue mab)

U.S. Brand Names Zenapax®

Canadian Brand Names Zenapax®

Pharmacologic Category Immunosuppressant Agent

Use Part of an immunosuppressive regimen (including cyclosporine and corticosteroids) for the prophylaxis of acute organ rejection in patients receiving renal transplant

Unlabeled/Investigational Use Graft-versus-host disease; prevention of organ rejection after heart transplant

Pregnancy Risk Factor C

Pregnancy Considerations Animal reproduction studies have not been conducted. Generally, IgG molecules cross the placenta. Do not use during pregnancy unless the potential benefit to the mother outweighs the possible risk to the fetus. Women of childbearing potential should use effective contraception before, during, and for 4 months following treatment.

Lactation Excretion in breast milk unknown/use caution

Contraindications Hypersensitivity to daclizumab or any component of the formulation

Warnings/Precautions Patients on immunosuppressive therapy are at increased risk for infectious complications and secondary malignancies. Long-term effects of daclizumab on immune function are unknown. Severe hypersensitivity reactions have been rarely reported; anaphylaxis has been observed on initial exposure and following re-exposure; medications for the management of severe allergic reaction should be available for immediate use. Anti-idiotype antibodies have been measured in patients who have received daclizumab (adults 14%; children 34%); detection of antibodies may be influenced by multiple factors and may therefore be misleading.

In cardiac transplant patients, the combined use of daclizumab, cyclosporine, mycophenolate mofetil, and corticosteroids has been associated with an increased mortality. Higher mortality may be associated with the use of antilymphocyte globulin and a higher incidence of severe infections. **[U.S. Boxed Warning]: Should be administered under the supervision of a physician experienced in immunosuppressive therapy.**

Adverse Reactions Although reported adverse events are frequent, when daclizumab is compared with placebo the incidence of adverse effects is similar between the two groups. Many of the adverse effects reported during clinical trial use of daclizumab may be related to the patient population, transplant procedure, and concurrent transplant medications. Diarrhea, fever, postoperative pain, pruritus, respiratory tract infection, urinary tract infection, and vomiting occurred more often in children than adults.

≥5%:
- Cardiovascular: Chest pain, edema, hyper-/hypotension, tachycardia, thrombosis
- Central nervous system: Dizziness, fatigue, fever, headache, insomnia, pain, post-traumatic pain, tremor
- Dermatologic: Acne, cellulitis, wound healing impaired
- Gastrointestinal: Abdominal distention, abdominal pain, constipation, diarrhea, dyspepsia, epigastric pain, nausea, pyrosis, vomiting
- Genitourinary: Dysuria
- Hematologic: Bleeding
- Neuromuscular & skeletal: Back pain, musculoskeletal pain
- Renal: Oliguria, renal tubular necrosis
- Respiratory: Cough, dyspnea, pulmonary edema
- Miscellaneous: Lymphocele, wound infection

≥2% to <5%:
- Central nervous system: Anxiety, depression, shivering
- Dermatologic: Hirsutism, pruritus, rash
- Endocrine & metabolic: Dehydration, diabetes mellitus, fluid overload
- Gastrointestinal: Flatulence, gastritis, hemorrhoids
- Genitourinary: Urinary retention, urinary tract bleeding
- Local: Application site reaction
- Neuromuscular & skeletal: Arthralgia, leg cramps, myalgia, weakness
- Ocular: Vision blurred
- Renal: Hydronephrosis, renal damage, renal insufficiency
- Respiratory: Atelectasis, congestion, hypoxia, pharyngitis, pleural effusion, rales, rhinitis
- Miscellaneous: Night sweats, prickly sensation, diaphoresis

<1% (Limited to important or life-threatening): Severe hypersensitivity reactions (rare): Anaphylaxis, bronchospasm, cardiac arrest, cytokine release syndrome, hypotension, laryngeal edema, pulmonary edema, pruritus, urticaria

Drug Interactions

Avoid Concomitant Use

Avoid concomitant use of Daclizumab with any of the following: Natalizumab; Vaccines (Live)

Increased Effect/Toxicity

Daclizumab may increase the levels/effects of: Natalizumab; Vaccines (Live)

The levels/effects of Daclizumab may be increased by: Trastuzumab

Decreased Effect

Daclizumab may decrease the levels/effects of: Vaccines (Inactivated)

The levels/effects of Daclizumab may be decreased by: Echinacea

Stability Refrigerate vials at 2°C to 8°C (36°F to 46°F). Do not shake or freeze; protect undiluted solution against direct sunlight. Dose should be further diluted in 50 mL 0.9% sodium chloride solution. When mixing, gently invert bag to avoid foaming; do not shake. Do not use if solution is discolored. Diluted solution is stable for 24 hours at 4°C or for 4 hours at room temperature. Do not mix with other medications or infuse other medications through same I.V. line.

Mechanism of Action Daclizumab is a chimeric (90% human, 10% murine) monoclonal IgG antibody produced by recombinant DNA technology. Daclizumab inhibits immune reactions by binding and blocking the alpha-chain of the interleukin-2 receptor (CD25) located on the surface of activated lymphocytes.

Pharmacodynamics/Kinetics

Distribution: V_d:
- Adults: Central compartment: 0.031 L/kg; Peripheral compartment: 0.043 L/kg
- Children: Central compartment: 0.067 L/kg; Peripheral compartment: 0.047 L/kg

Half-life elimination (estimated): Adults: Terminal: 20 days; Children: 13 days

Dosage Daclizumab is used adjunctively with other immunosuppressants (eg, cyclosporine, corticosteroids, mycophenolate mofetil, and azathioprine): I.V.:

Children: Use same weight-based dose as adults

Adults:
- Immunoprophylaxis against acute renal allograft rejection: 1 mg/kg infused over 15 minutes within 24 hours before transplantation (day 0), then every 14 days for 4 additional doses
- Treatment of graft-versus-host disease (unlabeled use, limited data): 0.5-1.5 mg/kg, repeat same dosage for transient response. Repeat doses have been administered 11-48 days following the initial dose.
- Prevention of organ rejection after heart transplant (unlabeled use): 1 mg/kg up to a maximum of 100 mg; administer within 12 hours after heart transplant and on days 8, 22, 36, and 50 post-transplant

Dosage adjustment in renal impairment: No adjustment needed.

Dosage adjustment in hepatic impairment: No data available for patients with severe impairment.

Administration For I.V. administration following dilution. Daclizumab solution should be administered within 4 hours of preparation if stored at room temperature; infuse over a 15-minute period via a peripheral or central vein.

Dosage Forms Excipient information presented when available (limited, particularly for generics); consult specific product labeling.

Injection, solution [concentrate; preservative free]:
- Zenapax®: 5 mg/mL (5 mL) [contains polysorbate 80]

◆ **Dacodyl™ [OTC]** *see* Bisacodyl *on page 198*
◆ **Dacogen™** *see* Decitabine *on page 409*
◆ **DACT** *see* DACTINomycin *on page 390*

DACTINomycin (dak ti noe MYE sin)

U.S. Brand Names Cosmegen®

Canadian Brand Names Cosmegen®

Index Terms ACT; Act-D; Actinomycin; Actinomycin Cl; Actinomycin D; DACT; NSC-3053

Pharmacologic Category Antineoplastic Agent, Antibiotic

Use Treatment of testicular tumors, melanoma, gestational trophoblastic neoplasm, Wilms' tumor, neuroblastoma, retinoblastoma, rhabdomyosarcoma, uterine sarcomas, Ewing's sarcoma, Kaposi's sarcoma, sarcoma botryoides, and soft tissue sarcoma

Pregnancy Risk Factor D

Pregnancy Considerations Animal studies have demonstrated teratogenic effects and fetal loss There are no adequate and well-controlled studies in pregnant women. Women of childbearing potential are advised not to become pregnant. Use only when potential benefit justifies potential risk to the fetus. **[U.S. Boxed Warning]: Avoid exposure during pregnancy.**

Lactation Excretion in breast milk unknown/not recommended

Medication Safety Issues

Sound-alike/look-alike issues:

DACTINomycin may be confused with DAPTOmycin, DAUNOrubicin

Actinomycin may be confused with achromycin

High alert medication: The Institute for Safe Medication Practices (ISMP) includes this medication among its list of drugs which have a heightened risk of causing significant patient harm when used in error.

Contraindications Hypersensitivity to dactinomycin or any component of the formulation; patients with concurrent or recent chickenpox or herpes zoster; avoid in infants <6 months of age

Warnings/Precautions **[U.S. Boxed Warnings]: Hazardous agent - use appropriate precautions for handling and disposal. Dactinomycin is extremely irritating to tissues and must be administered I.V.; if extravasation occurs during I.V. use, severe damage to soft tissues will occur. Avoid inhalation of vapors or contact with skin, mucous membrane, or eyes; avoid exposure during pregnancy.** Dosage is usually expressed in **MICRO**grams, **NOT** milligrams, and must be calculated on the basis of body surface area (BSA) in obese or edematous adult patients. Dactinomycin potentiates the effects of radiation therapy; use with caution in patients who have received radiation therapy; reduce dosages in patients who are receiving dactinomycin and radiation therapy simultaneously; combination with radiation therapy may result in increased GI toxicity and myelosuppression. Avoid dactinomycin use within 2 months of radiation treatment for right-sided Wilms' tumor, may increase the risk of hepatotoxicity. Toxic effects may be delayed in onset (2-4 days following a course of treatment) and may require 1-2 weeks to reach maximum severity. Avoid administration of live vaccines. Use caution in hepatobiliary dysfunction; may cause veno-occlusive liver disease, increased risk in children <4 years of age. Long-term observation of cancer survivors is recommended due to the potential for secondary primary tumors following treatment with radiation and antineoplastic agents. **[U.S. Boxed Warning]: Should be administered under the supervision of an experienced cancer chemotherapy physician.**

Adverse Reactions Frequency not defined.

Central nervous system: Fatigue, fever, lethargy, malaise

Dermatologic: Acne, alopecia (reversible), cheilitis; increased pigmentation, sloughing, or erythema of previously irradiated skin; skin eruptions

Endocrine & metabolic: Growth retardation, hypocalcemia

Gastrointestinal: Abdominal pain, anorexia, diarrhea, dysphagia, esophagitis, GI ulceration, mucositis, nausea, pharyngitis, proctitis, stomatitis, vomiting

Hematologic: Agranulocytosis, anemia, aplastic anemia, leukopenia, pancytopenia, reticulocytopenia, thrombocytopenia, myelosuppression (onset: 7 days, nadir: 14-21 days, recovery: 21-28 days)

Hepatic: Ascites, hepatic failure, hepatitis, hepatomegaly, hepatotoxicity, liver function test abnormality, veno-occlusive disease

Local: Erythema, edema, epidermolysis, pain, tissue necrosis, and ulceration (following extravasation)

Neuromuscular & skeletal: Myalgia

Renal: Renal function abnormality

Respiratory: Pneumonitis

Miscellaneous: Anaphylactoid reaction, infection

Drug Interactions

Avoid Concomitant Use

Avoid concomitant use of DACTINomycin with any of the following: Natalizumab; Vaccines (Live)

Increased Effect/Toxicity

DACTINomycin may increase the levels/effects of: Natalizumab; Vaccines (Live)

The levels/effects of DACTINomycin may be increased by: Trastuzumab

Decreased Effect

DACTINomycin may decrease the levels/effects of: Vaccines (Inactivated)

The levels/effects of DACTINomycin may be decreased by: Echinacea

Stability Store at controlled room temperature of 15°C to 30°C (59°F to 86°F); protect from light and humidity. Dilute with 1.1 mL of preservative-free SWI to yield a final concentration of 500 mcg/mL. Solutions in 50 mL D_5W or NS are stable for 24 hours at room temperature. Do not use preservative diluent as precipitation may occur. Cellulose ester membrane filters should not be used during preparation.

Mechanism of Action Binds to the guanine portion of DNA intercalating between guanine and cytosine base pairs inhibiting DNA and RNA synthesis and protein synthesis

Pharmacodynamics/Kinetics

Distribution: High concentrations found in bone marrow and tumor cells, submaxillary gland, liver, and kidney; crosses placenta; poor CSF penetration

Metabolism: Hepatic, minimal

Half-life elimination: ~36 hours

Time to peak, serum: I.V.: 2-5 minutes

Excretion: Bile (50%); feces (14%); urine (~10% as unchanged drug)

Dosage Refer to individual protocols:

Note: Medication orders for dactinomycin are commonly written in MICROgrams (eg, 150 mcg) although many regimens list the dose in MILLIgrams (eg, mg/kg or mg/m^2). One-time doses for >1000 mcg, or multiple-day doses for >500 mcg/day are not common. The dose intensity per 2-week cycle for adults and children should not exceed 15 mcg/kg/day for 5 days or 400-600 mcg/m^2/day for 5 days. Some practitioners recommend calculation of the dosage for obese or edematous adult patients on the basis of body surface area in an effort to relate dosage to lean body mass.

Children >6 months: I.V.: Usual dose: 15 mcg/kg/day **or** 400-600 mcg/m^2/day for 5 days every 3-6 weeks

Wilms' tumor, rhabdomyosarcoma, Ewing's sarcoma: 15 mcg/kg/day for 5 days (in various combination regimens and schedules)

Adults: I.V.:

Usual doses:

2.5 mg/m^2 in divided doses over 1 week, repeated every 2 weeks **or**

0.75-2 mg/m^2 every 1-4 weeks **or**

400-600 mcg/m^2/day for 5 days, repeated every 3-6 weeks

Testicular cancer: 1000 mcg/m^2 on day 1 (as part of a combination chemotherapy regimen)

Gestational trophoblastic neoplasm: 12 mcg/kg/day for 5 days **or** 500 mcg days 1 and 2 (as part of a combination chemotherapy regimen)

Wilms' tumor, Ewing's sarcoma: 15 mcg/kg/day for 5 days (in various combination regimens and schedules)

Elderly: Elderly patients are at increased risk of myelosuppression; dosing should begin at the low end of the dosing range.

Dosage adjustment in renal impairment: No adjustment required

Administration Do not administer I.M. or SubQ. Administer by slow I.V. push or infuse over 10-15 minutes. Avoid extravasation. Do not filter with cellulose ester membrane filters.

Monitoring Parameters CBC with differential and platelet count, liver function tests, and renal function tests

Test Interactions May interfere with bioassays of antibacterial drug levels

Dosage Forms Excipient information presented when available (limited, particularly for generics); consult specific product labeling.

Injection, powder for reconstitution:

Cosmegen®: 0.5 mg [contains mannitol 20 mg]

- **Dakin's Solution** *see* Sodium Hypochlorite Solution *on page 1384*
- **Dalacin® C (Can)** *see* Clindamycin *on page 344*
- **Dalacin® T (Can)** *see* Clindamycin *on page 344*
- **Dalacin® Vaginal (Can)** *see* Clindamycin *on page 344*
- **Dallergy®** *see* Chlorpheniramine, Phenylephrine, and Methscopolamine *on page 313*
- **Dallergy Drops** *see* Chlorpheniramine and Phenylephrine *on page 309*
- **Dallergy®-JR** *see* Chlorpheniramine and Phenylephrine *on page 309*
- **Dalmane®** *see* Flurazepam *on page 643*
- **d-Alpha-Gems™ [OTC]** *see* Vitamin E *on page 1566*
- ***d*-Alpha Tocopherol** *see* Vitamin E *on page 1566*

Dalteparin (dal TE pa rin)

U.S. Brand Names Fragmin®

Canadian Brand Names Fragmin®

Index Terms Dalteparin Sodium; NSC-714371

Pharmacologic Category Low Molecular Weight Heparin

Use Prevention of deep vein thrombosis which may lead to pulmonary embolism, in patients requiring abdominal surgery who are at risk for thromboembolism complications (eg, patients >40 years of age, obesity, patients with malignancy, history of deep vein thrombosis or pulmonary embolism, and surgical procedures requiring general anesthesia and lasting >30 minutes); prevention of DVT in patients undergoing hip-replacement surgery; patients immobile during an acute illness; acute treatment of unstable angina or non-Q-wave myocardial infarction; prevention of ischemic complications in patients on concurrent aspirin therapy; in patients with cancer, extended treatment (6 months) of acute symptomatic venous thromboembolism (DVT and/or PE) to reduce the recurrence of venous thromboembolism

Unlabeled/Investigational Use Active treatment of deep vein thrombosis (noncancer patients)

Pregnancy Risk Factor B

Pregnancy Considerations Multiple-dose vials contain benzyl alcohol (avoid in pregnant women due to association with gasping syndrome in premature infants). Adverse effects were not observed in animal studies. There are no adequate and well-controlled studies in pregnant women. Use during pregnancy only if clearly needed.

Lactation Enters breast milk/use caution

Medication Safety Issues

High alert medication: The Institute for Safe Medication Practices (ISMP) includes this medication among its list of drugs which have a heightened risk of causing significant patient harm when used in error.

2009 National Patient Safety Goals: The Joint Commission on Accreditation of Healthcare Organizations requires healthcare organizations that provide anticoagulant therapy to have a process in place to reduce the risk of anticoagulant-associated patient harm. Patients receiving anticoagulants should receive individualized care through a defined process that includes standardized ordering, dispensing, administration, monitoring and education. This does not apply to routine short-term use of anticoagulants for prevention of venous thromboembolism when the expectation is that the patient's laboratory values will remain within or close to normal values (NPSG.03.05.01).

Contraindications Hypersensitivity to dalteparin or any component of the formulation; thrombocytopenia associated with a positive *in vitro* test for antiplatelet antibodies in the presence of dalteparin; hypersensitivity to heparin or pork products; patients with active major bleeding; patients with unstable angina, non-Q-wave MI, or acute venous thromboembolism undergoing regional anesthesia; not for I.M. or I.V. use

Warnings/Precautions [U.S. Boxed Warning]: Patients with recent or anticipated neuraxial anesthesia (epidural or spinal anesthesia) are at risk of spinal or epidural hematoma and subsequent paralysis. Consider risk versus benefit prior to neuraxial anesthesia. Risk is increased by concomitant agents which may alter hemostasis, as well as traumatic or repeated epidural or spinal puncture. Patient should be observed closely for bleeding if dalteparin is administered during or immediately following diagnostic lumbar puncture, epidural anesthesia, or spinal anesthesia.

Use with caution in patients with pre-existing thrombocytopenia, recent childbirth, subacute bacterial endocarditis, peptic ulcer disease, pericarditis or pericardial effusion, liver or renal function impairment, recent lumbar puncture, vasculitis, concurrent use of aspirin (increased bleeding risk), previous hypersensitivity to heparin, heparin-associated thrombocytopenia. Monitor platelet count closely. Rare thrombocytopenia may occur. Consider discontinuation of dalteparin in any patient developing significant thrombocytopenia related to initiation of dalteparin. Rare cases of thrombocytopenia with thrombosis have occurred. Use caution in patients with congenital or drug-induced thrombocytopenia or platelet defects. Cancer patients with thrombocytopenia may require dose adjustments for treatment of acute venous thromboembolism.

Use with caution in patients with known hypersensitivity to methylparaben or propylparaben. Monitor patient closely for signs or symptoms of bleeding. Certain patients are at increased risk of bleeding. Risk factors include bacterial endocarditis; congenital or acquired bleeding disorders; active ulcerative or angiodysplastic GI diseases; severe uncontrolled hypertension; hemorrhagic stroke; or use shortly after brain, spinal, or ophthalmology surgery; in patient treated concomitantly with platelet inhibitors; recent GI bleeding; thrombocytopenia or platelet defects; severe liver disease; hypertensive or diabetic retinopathy; or in patients undergoing invasive procedures.

Use with caution in patients with severe renal failure (has not been studied). Safety and efficacy in pediatric patients have not been established. Rare cases of thrombocytopenia with thrombosis have occurred. Multidose vials contain benzyl alcohol and should not be used in pregnant women. In neonates, large amounts of benzyl alcohol

(>100 mg/kg/day) have been associated with fatal toxicity (gasping syndrome). Heparin can cause hyperkalemia by affecting aldosterone. Similar reactions could occur with dalteparin. Monitor for hyperkalemia. Do **not** administer intramuscularly. Not to be used interchangeably (unit for unit) with heparin or any other low molecular weight heparins.

Adverse Reactions

Note: As with all anticoagulants, bleeding is the major adverse effect of dalteparin. Hemorrhage may occur at virtually any site. Risk is dependent on multiple variables.

>10%:

Hematologic: Bleeding (3% to 14%)

1% to 10%:

Hematologic: Wound hematoma (up to 3%)

Hepatic: AST >3 times upper limit of normal (5% to 9%), ALT >3 times upper limit of normal (4% to 10%)

Local: Pain at injection site (up to 12%), injection site hematoma (up to 7%)

<1% (Limited to important or life-threatening): Thrombocytopenia (including heparin-induced thrombocytopenia), allergic reaction (fever, pruritus, rash, injections site reaction, bullous eruption), alopecia, anaphylactoid reaction, operative site bleeding, gastrointestinal bleeding, hemoptysis, skin necrosis, subdural hematoma, thrombosis (associated with heparin-induced thrombocytopenia). Spinal or epidural hematomas can occur following neuraxial anesthesia or spinal puncture, resulting in paralysis.

Drug Interactions

Avoid Concomitant Use There are no known interactions where it is recommended to avoid concomitant use.

Increased Effect/Toxicity

Dalteparin may increase the levels/effects of: Anticoagulants; Drotrecogin Alfa; Ibritumomab; Tositumomab and Iodine I 131 Tositumomab

The levels/effects of Dalteparin may be increased by: Antiplatelet Agents; Dasatinib; Herbs (Anticoagulant/Antiplatelet Properties); Nonsteroidal Anti-Inflammatory Agents; Pentosan Polysulfate Sodium; Prostacyclin Analogues; Salicylates; Thrombolytic Agents

Decreased Effect There are no known significant interactions involving a decrease in effect.

Ethanol/Nutrition/Herb Interactions Herb/Nutraceutical: Alfalfa, anise, bilberry, bladderwrack, bromelain, cat's claw, celery, chamomile, coleus, cordyceps, dong quai, evening primrose oil, fenugreek, feverfew, garlic, ginger, ginkgo biloba, Ginseng (american), Ginseng (panax), Ginseng (siberian), grapeseed, green tea, guggul, horse chestnut seed, horseradish, licorice, prickly ash, red clover, reishi, SAMe (s-adenosylmethionine), sweet clover, turmeric, white willow (all have additional antiplatelet/anticoagulant activity)

Stability Store at temperatures of 20°C to 25°C (68°F to 77°F). Multidose vials may be stored for up to 2 weeks at room temperature after entering.

Mechanism of Action Low molecular weight heparin analog with a molecular weight of 4000-6000 daltons; the commercial product contains 3% to 15% heparin with a molecular weight <3000 daltons, 65% to 78% with a molecular weight of 3000-8000 daltons and 14% to 26% with a molecular weight >8000 daltons; while dalteparin has been shown to inhibit both factor Xa and factor IIa (thrombin), the antithrombotic effect of dalteparin is characterized by a higher ratio of antifactor Xa to antifactor IIa activity (ratio = 4)

Pharmacodynamics/Kinetics

Onset of action: 1-2 hours

Duration: >12 hours

Distribution: V_d: 40-60 mL/kg

Bioavailability: SubQ: 81% to 93%

Half-life elimination (route dependent): 2-5 hours

Time to peak, serum: 4 hours

Dosage Adults: SubQ:

Abdominal surgery:

Low-to-moderate DVT risk: 2500 int. units 1-2 hours prior to surgery, then once daily for 5-10 days postoperatively

High DVT risk: 5000 int. units the evening prior to surgery and then once daily for 5-10 days postoperatively. Alternatively in patients with malignancy: 2500 int. units 1-2 hours prior to surgery, 2500 int. units 12 hours later, then 5000 int. units once daily for 5-10 days postoperatively.

Patients undergoing total hip surgery: **Note:** Three treatment options are currently available. Dose is given for 5-10 days, although up to 14 days of treatment have been tolerated in clinical trials:

Postoperative start:

Initial: 2500 int. units 4-8 hours* after surgery

Maintenance: 5000 int. units once daily; start at least 6 hours after postsurgical dose

Preoperative (starting day of surgery):

Initial: 2500 int. units within 2 hours before surgery

Adjustment: 2500 int. units 4-8 hours* after surgery

Maintenance: 5000 int. units once daily; start at least 6 hours after postsurgical dose

Preoperative (starting evening prior to surgery):

Initial: 5000 int. units 10-14 hours before surgery

Adjustment: 5000 int. units 4-8 hours* after surgery

Maintenance: 5000 int. units once daily, allowing 24 hours between doses.

***Dose may be delayed if hemostasis is not yet achieved.**

Unstable angina or non-Q-wave myocardial infarction: 120 int. units/kg body weight (maximum dose: 10,000 int. units) every 12 hours for 5-8 days with concurrent aspirin therapy. Discontinue dalteparin once patient is clinically stable.

Venous thromboembolism: Cancer patients:

Initial (month 1): 200 int. units/kg (maximum dose: 18,000 int. units) once daily for 30 days

Maintenance (months 2-6): ~150 int. units/kg (maximum dose: 18,000 int. units) once daily. If platelet count between 50,000-100,000/mm^3, reduce dose by 2,500 int. units until platelet count recovers to ≥100,000/mm^3. If platelet count <50,000/mm^3, discontinue dalteparin until platelet count recover to >50,000/mm^3.

Immobility during acute illness: 5000 int. units once daily

Dosing adjustment in renal impairment: Half-life is increased in patients with chronic renal failure, use with caution, accumulation can be expected; specific dosage adjustments have not been recommended. In cancer patients, receiving treatment for venous thromboembolism, if Cl_{cr} <30 mL/minute, manufacturer recommends monitoring anti-Xa levels to determine appropriate dose.

Dosing adjustment in hepatic impairment: Use with caution in patients with hepatic insufficiency; specific dosage adjustments have not been recommended

Administration For deep SubQ injection only. May be injected in a U-shape to the area surrounding the navel, the upper outer side of the thigh, or the upper outer quadrangle of the buttock. Apply pressure to injection site; do not massage. Use thumb and forefinger to lift a fold of skin when injecting dalteparin to the navel area or thigh. Insert needle at a 45- to 90-degree angle. The entire length of needle should be inserted. Do not expel air bubble from fixed-dose syringe prior to injection. Air bubble (and extra solution, if applicable) may be expelled from graduated syringes.

Administration once daily beginning prior to surgery and continuing 5-10 days after surgery prevents deep vein thrombosis in patients at risk for thromboembolic complications. For unstable angina or non-Q-wave myocardial infarction, dalteparin is administered every 12 hours until the patient is stable (5-8 days).

Monitoring Parameters Periodic CBC including platelet count; stool occult blood tests; monitoring of PT and PTT is not necessary. Once patient has received 3-4 doses, anti-Xa levels, drawn 4-6 hours after dalteparin administration, may be used to monitor effect in patients with severe renal dysfunction or if abnormal coagulation parameters or bleeding should occur.

Reference Range Treatment: Venous thromboembolism: Target anti-Xa range: 0.5-1.5 int. units/mL

Additional Information Multidose vial contains 14 mg/mL benzyl alcohol.

Dosage Forms Excipient information presented when available (limited, particularly for generics); consult specific product labeling.

Injection, solution:

Fragmin®: Antifactor Xa 10,000 int. units per 1 mL (9.5 mL) [contains benzyl alcohol]; antifactor Xa 25,000 units per 1 mL (3.8 mL) [contains benzyl alcohol]

Injection, solution [preservative free]:

Fragmin®: Antifactor Xa 2500 int. units per 0.2 mL (0.2 mL); antifactor Xa 5000 int. units per 0.2 mL (0.2 mL); antifactor Xa 7500 int. units per 0.3 mL (0.3 mL); antifactor Xa 10,000 int. units per 1 mL (1 mL); antifactor Xa 12,500 int. units per 0.5 mL (0.5 mL); antifactor Xa 15,000 int. units per 0.6 mL (0.6 mL); antifactor Xa 18,000 int. units per 0.72 mL (0.72 mL)

◆ **Dalteparin Sodium** *see* Dalteparin *on page* 392

Danazol (DA na zole)

U.S. Brand Names Danocrine® [DSC]

Canadian Brand Names Cyclomen®; Danocrine®

Pharmacologic Category Androgen

Use Treatment of endometriosis, fibrocystic breast disease, and hereditary angioedema

Pregnancy Risk Factor X

Pregnancy Considerations **[U.S. Boxed Warning]: Pregnancy should be ruled out prior to treatment** using a sensitive test (beta subunit test, if available). Nonhormonal contraception should be used during therapy. May cause androgenic effects to the female fetus; clitoral hypertrophy, labial fusion, urogenital sinus defect, vaginal atresia, and ambiguous genitalia have been reported.

Lactation Enters breast milk/contraindicated

Medication Safety Issues

Sound-alike/look-alike issues:

Danazol may be confused with Dantrium®

Danocrine® may be confused with Dacriose®

Contraindications Hypersensitivity to danazol or any component of the formulation; undiagnosed genital bleeding; pregnancy; breast-feeding; porphyria; markedly impaired hepatic, renal, or cardiac function

Warnings/Precautions Use with caution in patients with seizure disorders, migraine, or conditions influenced by edema. **[U.S. Boxed Warning]: Thromboembolism, thrombotic, and thrombophlebitic events have been reported (including life-threatening or fatal strokes). [U.S. Boxed Warning]: Peliosis hepatis and benign hepatic adenoma have been reported with long-term use. [U.S. Boxed Warning]: May cause benign intracranial hypertension.** Breast cancer should be ruled out prior to treatment for fibrocystic breast disease. May increase risk of atherosclerosis and coronary artery disease. May cause nonreversible androgenic effects. Use with caution in patients with conditions influenced by edema (eg, cardiovascular disease, migraine, seizure disorder, renal impairment), porphyria, hepatic impairment and diabetes. **[U.S. Boxed Warning]: Pregnancy must be ruled out prior to treatment.** Safety and efficacy in pediatric patients have not been established.

Adverse Reactions Frequency not defined.

Cardiovascular: Benign intracranial hypertension (rare), edema, flushing, hypertension

Central nervous system: Anxiety (rare), chills (rare), convulsions (rare), depression, dizziness, emotional lability, fainting, fever (rare), Guillain-Barré syndrome, headache, nervousness, sleep disorders, tremor

Dermatologic: Acne, hair loss, mild hirsutism, maculopapular rash, papular rash, petechial rash, pruritus, purpuric rash, seborrhea, Stevens-Johnson syndrome (rare), photosensitivity (rare), urticaria, vesicular rash

Endocrine & metabolic: Amenorrhea (which may continue post therapy), breast size reduction, clitoris hypertrophy, glucose intolerance, HDL decreased, LDL increased, libido changes, nipple discharge, menstrual disturbances (spotting, altered timing of cycle), semen abnormalities (changes in volume, viscosity, sperm count/motility), spermatogenesis reduction

Gastrointestinal: Appetite changes (rare), bleeding gums (rare), constipation, gastroenteritis, nausea, pancreatitis (rare), vomiting, weight gain

Genitourinary: Vaginal dryness, vaginal irritation, pelvic pain

Hematologic: Eosinophilia, erythrocytosis (reversible), leukocytosis, leukopenia, platelet count increased, polycythemia, RBC increased, thrombocytopenia

Hepatic: Cholestatic jaundice, hepatic adenoma, jaundice, liver enzymes (elevated), malignant tumors (after prolonged use), peliosis hepatis

Neuromuscular & skeletal: Back pain, carpal tunnel syndrome (rare), CPK abnormalities, extremity pain, joint lockup, joint pain, joint swelling, muscle cramps, neck pain, paresthesia, spasms, weakness

Ocular: Cataracts (rare), visual disturbances

Renal: Hematuria

Respiratory: Nasal congestion (rare)

Miscellaneous: Voice change (hoarseness, sore throat, instability, deepening of pitch), diaphoresis

Drug Interactions

Metabolism/Transport Effects **Inhibits** CYP3A4 (weak)

Avoid Concomitant Use There are no known interactions where it is recommended to avoid concomitant use.

Increased Effect/Toxicity

Danazol may increase the levels/effects of: CarBAMazepine; CycloSPORINE; HMG-CoA Reductase Inhibitors; Vitamin K Antagonists

Decreased Effect There are no known significant interactions involving a decrease in effect.

Ethanol/Nutrition/Herb Interactions Food: Delays time to peak; high-fat meal increases plasma concentration

Stability Store at controlled room temperature of 15°C to 30°C (59°F to 86°F).

Mechanism of Action Suppresses pituitary output of follicle-stimulating hormone and luteinizing hormone that causes regression and atrophy of normal and ectopic endometrial tissue; decreases rate of growth of abnormal breast tissue; reduces attacks associated with hereditary angioedema by increasing levels of C4 component of complement

Pharmacodynamics/Kinetics

Onset of action: Therapeutic: ~4 weeks

Metabolism: Extensively hepatic, primarily to 2-hydroxymethylethisterone

Half-life elimination: 4.5 hours (variable)

Time to peak, serum: Within 2 hours

Excretion: Urine

Dosage Adults: Oral:

Females: Endometriosis: Initial: 200-400 mg/day in 2 divided doses for mild disease; individualize dosage. Usual maintenance dose: 800 mg/day in 2 divided doses to achieve amenorrhea and rapid response to painful symptoms. Continue therapy uninterrupted for 3-6 months (up to 9 months).

Females: Fibrocystic breast disease: Range: 100-400 mg/day in 2 divided doses

Males/Females: Hereditary angioedema: Initial: 200 mg 2-3 times/day; after favorable response, decrease the dosage by 50% or less at intervals of 1-3 months or longer if the frequency of attacks dictates. If an attack occurs, increase the dosage by up to 200 mg/day.

Monitoring Parameters Signs and symptoms of intracranial hypertension (papilledema, headache, nausea, vomiting), lipoproteins, androgenic changes, hepatic function

Test Interactions Testosterone, androstenedione, dehydroepiandrosterone

Dosage Forms Excipient information presented when available (limited, particularly for generics); consult specific product labeling. [DSC] = Discontinued product

Capsule: 50 mg, 100 mg, 200 mg

Danocrine®: 50 mg, 100 mg, 200 mg [DSC]

- ◆ **Dandrex [OTC]** *see* Selenium Sulfide *on page 1361*
- ◆ **Danocrine® [DSC]** *see* Danazol *on page 394*
- ◆ **Danocrine® (Can)** *see* Danazol *on page 394*
- ◆ **Dantrium®** *see* Dantrolene *on page 395*

Dantrolene (DAN troe leen)

U.S. Brand Names Dantrium®

Canadian Brand Names Dantrium®

Index Terms Dantrolene Sodium

Pharmacologic Category Skeletal Muscle Relaxant

Use Treatment of spasticity associated with upper motor neuron disorders (eg, spinal cord injury, stroke, cerebral palsy, or multiple sclerosis); management of malignant hyperthermia; prevention of malignant hyperthermia in susceptible individuals (preoperative/postoperative administration)

Unlabeled/Investigational Use Neuroleptic malignant syndrome (NMS)

Pregnancy Risk Factor C

Lactation Enters breast milk/not recommended

Medication Safety Issues

Sound-alike/look-alike issues:

Dantrium® may be confused with danazol, Daraprim®

Contraindications

I.V.: There are no contraindications listed within the manufacturers labeling.

Oral: Active hepatic disease; should not be used when spasticity is used to maintain posture/balance during locomotion or to obtain/maintain increased function

Warnings/Precautions [U.S. Boxed Warning]: Has potential for hepatotoxicity. Overt hepatitis has been most frequently observed between the third and twelfth month of therapy. Hepatic injury appears to be greater in females and in patients >35 years of age. Idiosyncratic and hypersensitivity reactions (sometimes fatal) of the liver have also occurred.

Use with caution in patients with impaired cardiac, hepatic, or pulmonary function. May cause photosensitivity. Patients should be cautioned about performing tasks which require mental alertness (eg, operating machinery or driving). The combination of I.V. dantrolene and calcium channel blockers is not recommended. Injection contains 3 g mannitol/vial; caution if additional mannitol required. Alkaline solution may cause tissue necrosis if extravasated. In addition to I.V. dantrolene, supportive measures must also be utilized for management of malignant hyperthermia. Long-term use in patients <5 years of age has not been established.

Adverse Reactions Frequency not defined.

Cardiovascular: Blood pressure (altered), heart failure, tachycardia

Central nervous system: Chills, confusion, dizziness, drowsiness, fatigue, fever, headache, insomnia, lightheadedness, malaise, mental depression, nervousness, seizure, speech disturbance

Dermatologic: Eczematoid eruption, hair growth (abnormal), pruritus, rash, urticaria

Gastrointestinal: Abdominal cramps, anorexia, constipation, diarrhea, dysphagia, gastric irritation, gastrointestinal hemorrhage, nausea, taste change, vomiting

Genitourinary: Crystalluria, difficult erection, difficult urination, nocturia, polyuria, urinary frequency, urinary incontinence, urinary retention

Hematologic: Anemia (aplastic), leukopenia, thrombocytopenia

Hepatic: Hepatitis

Local: Injection site reaction, thrombophlebitis, tissue necrosis

Neuromuscular & skeletal: Back pain, muscle weakness, myalgia

Ocular: Blurred vision, diplopia, tearing (excessive)

Renal: Hematuria

Respiratory: Feeling of suffocation, pleural effusion (associated with pericarditis), pulmonary edema, respiratory depression

Miscellaneous: Anaphylaxis, diaphoresis, lymphocytic lymphoma, sialorrhea

Drug Interactions

Metabolism/Transport Effects Substrate of CYP3A4 (major)

Avoid Concomitant Use There are no known interactions where it is recommended to avoid concomitant use.

Increased Effect/Toxicity

Dantrolene may increase the levels/effects of: Alcohol (Ethyl); CNS Depressants

The levels/effects of Dantrolene may be increased by: CYP3A4 Inhibitors (Moderate); CYP3A4 Inhibitors (Strong); Dasatinib

Decreased Effect

The levels/effects of Dantrolene may be decreased by: CYP3A4 Inducers (Strong); Deferasirox; Herbs (CYP3A4 Inducers)

Ethanol/Nutrition/Herb Interactions

Ethanol: Avoid ethanol (may increase CNS depression).

Herb/Nutraceutical: Avoid valerian, St John's wort, kava kava, gotu kola (may increase CNS depression).

Stability Reconstitute vial by adding 60 mL of sterile water for injection USP (**not bacteriostatic water for injection**). Protect from light. Use within 6 hours; avoid glass bottles for I.V. infusion.

Mechanism of Action Acts directly on skeletal muscle by interfering with release of calcium ion from the sarcoplasmic reticulum; prevents or reduces the increase in myoplasmic calcium ion concentration that activates the acute catabolic processes associated with malignant hyperthermia

Pharmacodynamics/Kinetics

Absorption: Oral: Slow and incomplete

Metabolism: Hepatic

Half-life elimination: 8.7 hours

Excretion: Feces (45% to 50%); urine (25% as unchanged drug and metabolites)

Dosage

Spasticity: Oral:

Children: Initial: 0.5 mg/kg/dose twice daily, increase frequency to 3-4 times/day at 4- to 7-day intervals, then increase dose by 0.5 mg/kg to a maximum of 3 mg/kg/dose 2-4 times/day up to 400 mg/day

Adults: 25 mg/day to start, increase frequency to 2-4 times/day, then increase dose by 25 mg every 4-7 days to a maximum of 100 mg 2-4 times/day or 400 mg/day

Malignant hyperthermia: Children and Adults:

Preoperative prophylaxis:

Oral: 4-8 mg/kg/day in 4 divided doses, begin 1-2 days prior to surgery with last dose 3-4 hours prior to surgery

I.V.: 2.5 mg/kg ~1¼ hours prior to anesthesia and infused over 1 hour with additional doses as needed and individualized

Crisis: I.V.: 2.5 mg/kg; may repeat dose up to cumulative dose of 10 mg/kg; if physiologic and metabolic abnormalities reappear, repeat regimen

Postcrisis follow-up: Oral: 4-8 mg/kg/day in 4 divided doses for 1-3 days; I.V. dantrolene may be used when oral therapy is not practical; individualize dosage beginning with 1 mg/kg or more as the clinical situation dictates

Neuroleptic malignant syndrome (unlabeled use): I.V.: 1 mg/kg; may repeat dose up to maximum cumulative dose of 10 mg/kg, then switch to oral dosage

Administration I.V.: Therapeutic or emergency dose can be administered with rapid continuous I.V. push. Follow-up doses should be administered over 2-3 minutes.

Monitoring Parameters Motor performance should be monitored for therapeutic outcomes; nausea, vomiting, and liver function tests should be monitored for potential hepatotoxicity; intravenous administration requires cardiac monitor and blood pressure monitor

Dosage Forms Excipient information presented when available (limited, particularly for generics); consult specific product labeling.

Capsule, as sodium: 25 mg, 50 mg, 100 mg

Dantrium®: 25 mg, 50 mg, 100 mg

Injection, powder for reconstitution, as sodium:

Dantrium®: 20 mg [contains mannitol 3 g]

Extemporaneous Preparations A 5 mg/mL suspension may be made by adding five 100 mg capsules to a citric acid solution (150 mg citric acid powder in 10 mL water) and then adding syrup to a total volume of 100 mL; stable 2 days in refrigerator

Nahata MC and Hipple TF, *Pediatric Drug Formulations*, 1st ed, Cincinnati, OH: Harvey Whitney Books Co, 1990.

◆ **Dantrolene Sodium** *see* Dantrolene *on page* 395

◆ **Dapcin** *see* DAPTOmycin *on page* 397

Dapsone (DAP sone)

U.S. Brand Names Aczone®

Index Terms Diaminodiphenylsulfone

Pharmacologic Category Antibiotic, Miscellaneous; Topical Skin Product, Acne

Additional Appendix Information

Antimicrobial Drugs of Choice *on page* 1752

Guidelines for the Prevention of Opportunistic Infections in HIV Infected Persons *on page* 1740

Sulfonamide Derivatives *on page* 1671

Use Treatment of leprosy and dermatitis herpetiformis (infections caused by *Mycobacterium leprae*); topical treatment of acne vulgaris

Unlabeled/Investigational Use Prophylaxis of toxoplasmosis in severely-immunocompromised patients; alternative agent for *Pneumocystis carinii* pneumonia prophylaxis (monotherapy) and treatment (in combination with trimethoprim)

Pregnancy Risk Factor C

Pregnancy Considerations There are no adequate and well-controlled studies in pregnant women. Use during pregnancy when the benefit to the mother outweighs the potential risk to the fetus.

Lactation Enters breast milk/not recommended (AAP rates "compatible")

Medication Safety Issues

Sound-alike/look-alike issues:

Dapsone may be confused with Diprosone®

Contraindications Hypersensitivity to dapsone or any component of the formulation

Warnings/Precautions Use with caution in patients with severe anemia, G6PD, methemoglobin reductase deficiency or hemoglobin M deficiency; hypersensitivity to other sulfonamides; aplastic anemia, agranulocytosis and other severe blood dyscrasias have resulted in death; monitor carefully; serious dermatologic reactions (including toxic epidermal necrolysis) are rare but potential occurrences; sulfone reactions may also occur as potentially fatal hypersensitivity reactions; these, but not leprosy reactional states, require drug discontinuation. Motor loss and muscle weakness have been reported with use. Prolonged use may result in fungal or bacterial superinfection, including *C. difficile*-associated diarrhea and pseudomembranous colitis. Safety and efficacy of topical dapsone has not been established in children <12 years of age.

Adverse Reactions Adverse reactions reported for oral formulation unless otherwise noted.

>10%: Hematologic: Hemolysis (dose related; seen in patients with and without G6PD deficiency), hemoglobin decrease (1-2 g/dL; almost all patients), reticulocyte increase (2% to 12%), methemoglobinemia, red cell life span shortened

Frequency not always defined.

Cardiovascular: Facial edema (topical), tachycardia

Central nervous system: Depression (topical), fever, headache, insomnia, psychosis (oral/topical), suicide attempt (topical), tonic clonic movement (topical), vertigo

Dermatologic: Bullous and exfoliative dermatitis, erythema nodosum, exfoliative dermatitis, morbilliform and scarlatiniform reactions, phototoxicity, Stevens-Johnson syndrome, toxic epidural necrolysis, urticaria

Endocrine & metabolic: Hypoalbuminemia (without proteinuria), male infertility

Gastrointestinal: Abdominal pain (oral/topical), nausea, pancreatitis (oral/topical), vomiting (oral/topical)

Hematologic: Agranulocytosis, anemia, leukopenia, pure red cell aplasia (case report)

Hepatic: Cholestatic jaundice, hepatitis

Neuromuscular & skeletal: Drug-induced lupus erythematosus, lower motor neuron toxicity (prolonged therapy), peripheral neuropathy (rare, nonleprosy patients)

Ocular: Blurred vision

Otic: Tinnitus

Renal: Albuminuria, nephrotic syndrome, renal papillary necrosis

Respiratory: Interstitial pneumonitis, pulmonary eosinophilia, sinusitis (topical 2%)

Miscellaneous: Infectious mononucleosis-like syndrome (rash, fever, lymphadenopathy, hepatic dysfunction)

Drug Interactions

Metabolism/Transport Effects Substrate of CYP2C8 (minor), 2C9 (major), 2C19 (minor), 2E1 (minor), 3A4 (major)

Avoid Concomitant Use There are no known interactions where it is recommended to avoid concomitant use.

Increased Effect/Toxicity

Dapsone may increase the levels/effects of: Trimethoprim

The levels/effects of Dapsone may be increased by: CYP2C9 Inhibitors (Moderate); CYP2C9 Inhibitors

(Strong); CYP3A4 Inhibitors (Moderate); CYP3A4 Inhibitors (Strong); Dasatinib; Trimethoprim; Uricosuric Agents

Decreased Effect

Dapsone may decrease the levels/effects of: Typhoid Vaccine

The levels/effects of Dapsone may be decreased by: CYP2C9 Inducers (Highly Effective); CYP3A4 Inducers (Strong); Deferasirox; Didanosine; Herbs (CYP3A4 Inducers); Rifamycin Derivatives

Ethanol/Nutrition/Herb Interactions Herb/Nutraceutical: St John's wort may decrease dapsone levels.

Stability Store at 20°C to 25°C (68°F to 76°F). Protect tablets from light. Do not freeze gel.

Mechanism of Action Competitive antagonist of para-aminobenzoic acid (PABA) and prevents normal bacterial utilization of PABA for the synthesis of folic acid

Pharmacodynamics/Kinetics

Absorption:

Oral: Well absorbed

Topical: ~1% of the absorption of 100 mg tablet

Distribution: V_d: 1.5 L/kg; throughout total body water and present in all tissues, especially liver and kidney

Metabolism: Hepatic; forms metabolite

Half-life elimination: 30 hours (range: 10-50 hours)

Excretion: Urine (~85%)

Dosage Oral:

Leprosy:

Children: 1-2 mg/kg/24 hours, up to a maximum of 100 mg/day

Adults: 50-100 mg/day for 3-10 years

Dermatitis herpetiformis: Adults: Start at 50 mg/day, increase to 300 mg/day, or higher to achieve full control, reduce dosage to minimum level as soon as possible

Pneumocystis carinii pneumonia (unlabeled use):

Prophylaxis:

Children >1 month: 2 mg/kg/day once daily (maximum dose: 100 mg/day) or 4 mg/kg/dose once weekly (maximum dose: 200 mg)

Adults: 100 mg/day

Treatment: Adults: 100 mg/day in combination with trimethoprim (15-20 mg/kg/day) for 21 days

Topical: Acne: Children ≥12 years and Adults: Apply pea-sized amount (approximately) in a thin layer to affected areas twice daily; reevaluate patient if no improvement after 12 weeks of therapy

Dosing in renal impairment: No specific guidelines are available

Dietary Considerations Oral: Do not give with antacids, alkaline foods, or drugs.

Administration

Oral: May administer with meals if GI upset occurs.

Topical: Skin should be clean and dry before applying. Rub in gently and completely. Wash hands after applying. Gel may be gritty. For external use only; avoid applying to inside nose, mouth, eyes, and mucous membranes.

Monitoring Parameters

Oral: Check G6PD levels prior to initiation. Monitor patients for signs of jaundice and hemolysis; CBC weekly for first month, monthly for 6 months and semiannually thereafter.

Topical: For patients at risk of anemia, monitor with CBC, reticulocyte counts at baseline and routinely thereafter.

Dosage Forms Excipient information presented when available (limited, particularly for generics); consult specific product labeling.

Gel, topical:

Aczone®: 5% (30 g)

Tablet: 25 mg, 100 mg

Extemporaneous Preparations One report indicated that dapsone may not be well absorbed when administered to children as suspensions made from pulverized tablets

Mirochnick M, Clarke D, Brenn A, et al, "Low Serum Dapsone Concentrations in Children Receiving an Extemporaneously Prepared Oral Formulation," [Abstract Th B 365], APS-SPR, Baltimore, MD: 1992.

Jacobus Pharmaceutical Company (609) 921-7447 makes a 2 mg/mL proprietary liquid formulation available under an IND for the prophylaxis of *Pneumocystis carinii* pneumonia

◆ **Daptacel®** *see* Diphtheria and Tetanus Toxoids, and Acellular Pertussis Vaccine *on page 463*

DAPTOmycin (DAP toe mye sin)

U.S. Brand Names Cubicin®

Canadian Brand Names Cubicin®

Index Terms Cidecin; Dapcin; LY146032

Pharmacologic Category Antibiotic, Cyclic Lipopeptide

Additional Appendix Information

Antimicrobial Drugs of Choice *on page 1752*

Use Treatment of complicated skin and skin structure infections caused by susceptible aerobic gram-positive organisms; *Staphylococcus aureus* bacteremia, including right-sided infective endocarditis caused by MSSA or MRSA

Unlabeled/Investigational Use Treatment of severe infections caused by MRSA or VRE

Pregnancy Risk Factor B

Pregnancy Considerations Because adverse events were not observed in animal reproduction studies, daptomycin is classified as pregnancy category B. There are no adequate and well-controlled studies in pregnant women

Lactation Excretion in breast milk unknown/use caution

Medication Safety Issues

Sound-alike/look-alike issues:

Cubicin® may be confused with Cleocin®

DAPTOmycin may be confused with DACTINomycin

Contraindications Hypersensitivity to daptomycin or any component of the formulation

Warnings/Precautions May be associated with an increased incidence of myopathy; discontinue in patients with signs and symptoms of myopathy in conjunction with an increase in CPK (>5 times ULN or 1000 units/L) or in asymptomatic patients with a CPK ≥10 times ULN. Myopathy may occur more frequently at dose and/or frequency in excess of recommended dosages. Use caution in patients receiving other drugs associated with myopathy (eg, HMG-CoA reductase inhibitors). Not indicated for the treatment of pneumonia (poor lung penetration). Use caution in renal impairment (dosage adjustment required). Symptoms suggestive of peripheral neuropathy have been observed with treatment; monitor for new-onset or worsening neuropathy. Prolonged use may result in fungal or bacterial superinfection, including *C. difficile*-associated diarrhea and pseudomembranous colitis. Safety and efficacy in patients <18 years of age have not been established.

Adverse Reactions

>10%:

Gastrointestinal: Diarrhea (5% to 12%), vomiting (3% to 12%), constipation (6% to 11%)

Hematologic: Anemia (2% to 13%)

1% to 10%:

Cardiovascular: Peripheral edema (7%), chest pain (7%), hypertension (1% to 6%), hypotension (2% to 5%)

Central nervous system: Insomnia (5% to 9%), headache (5% to7%), fever (2% to 7%), dizziness (2% to 6%), anxiety (5%)

Dermatologic: Rash (4% to 7%), pruritus (3% to 6%), erythema (5%)

Endocrine & metabolic: Hypokalemia (9%), hyperkalemia (5%), hyperphosphatemia (3%)

Gastrointestinal: Nausea (6% to 10%), abdominal pain (6%), dyspepsia (1% to 4%), loose stool (4%), GI hemorrhage (2%)
Genitourinary: Urinary tract infection (2% to 7%)
Hematologic: INR increased (2%), eosinophilia (2%)
Hepatic: Transaminases increased (2% to 3%), alkaline phosphatase increased (2%)
Local: Injection site reaction (3% to 6%)
Neuromuscular & skeletal: CPK increased (3% to 9%), limb pain (2% to 9%), back pain (7%), weakness (5%), arthralgia (1% to 3%)
Renal: Renal failure (2% to 3%)
Respiratory: Pharyngolaryngeal pain (8%), pleural effusion (6%), cough (3%), pneumonia (3%), dyspnea (2% to 3%)
Miscellaneous: Osteomyelitis (6%), bacteremia (5%), diaphoresis (5%), sepsis (5%), infection (fungal, 2% to 3%)

<1% (Limited to important or life-threatening): Anaphylaxis, appetite decreased, arthralgia, atrial fibrillation, atrial flutter, cardiac arrest, dyskinesia, dysphagia, eczema, electrolyte disturbance, eosinophilia, erythema (truncal), eye irritation, fatigue, flatulence, flushing, GI discomfort, gingival pain, hallucination, hives, hypomagnesemia, hypersensitivity, hypoesthesia, jaundice, jitteriness, LDH increased, leukocytosis, lymphadenopathy, mental status change, muscle cramps, muscle weakness, myalgia, osteomyelitis, paresthesia, proteinuria, prothrombin time prolonged, rhabdomyolysis, rigors, serum bicarbonate increased, stomatitis, supraventricular arrhythmia, taste disturbance, thrombocytopenia, thrombocythemia, tinnitus, vertigo, vision blurred, xerostomia

Drug Interactions

Avoid Concomitant Use There are no known interactions where it is recommended to avoid concomitant use.

Increased Effect/Toxicity

The levels/effects of DAPTOmycin may be increased by: HMG-CoA Reductase Inhibitors

Decreased Effect There are no known significant interactions involving a decrease in effect.

Stability Store under refrigeration at 2°C to 8°C (36°F to 46°F). Reconstitute vial with 10 mL NS. Add NS to vial and rotate gently to wet powder. Allow to stand for 10 minutes, then gently swirl to obtain completely reconstituted solution. Do not shake or agitate vial vigorously. Should be further diluted following reconstitution in an appropriate volume of NS. Reconstituted solution (either in vial or in infusion bag) is stable for a cumulative time of 12 hours at room temperature and 48 hours if refrigerated (2°C to 8°C).

Mechanism of Action Daptomycin binds to components of the cell membrane of susceptible organisms and causes rapid depolarization, inhibiting intracellular synthesis of DNA, RNA, and protein. Daptomycin is bactericidal in a concentration-dependent manner.

Pharmacodynamics/Kinetics

Distribution: 0.1 L/kg
Protein binding: 90% to 93%; 84% to 88% in patients with Cl_{cr}<30 mL/minute
Half-life elimination: 8-9 hours (up to 28 hours in renal impairment)
Excretion: Urine (78%; primarily as unchanged drug); feces (6%)

Dosage I.V.: Adults:

Skin and soft tissue: 4 mg/kg once daily for 7-14 days
Bacteremia, right-sided endocarditis caused by MSSA or MRSA: 6 mg/kg once daily for 2-6 weeks

Dosage adjustment in renal impairment: Cl_{cr} <30 mL/minute:
Skin and soft tissue infections: 4 mg/kg every 48 hours
Staphylococcal bacteremia: 6 mg/kg every 48 hours

Hemodialysis (administer after hemodialysis) and/or CAPD: Dose as in Cl_{cr} <30 mL/minute
Continuous renal replacement therapy (CRRT): Dose as in Cl_{cr} <30 mL/minute

Dosage adjustment in hepatic impairment: No adjustment required for mild-to-moderate impairment (Child-Pugh Class A or B); not evaluated in severe hepatic impairment

Administration Infuse over 30 minutes.

Monitoring Parameters Monitor signs and symptoms of infection. CPK should be monitored at least weekly during therapy; more frequent monitoring if current or prior statin therapy, unexplained CPK increases, and/or renal impairment. Monitor for muscle pain or weakness, especially if noted in distal extremities.

Reference Range

Trough concentrations at steady-state:
4 mg/kg once daily: 5.9 ± 1.6 mcg/mL
6 mg/kg once daily: 6.7 ± 1.6 mcg/mL

Note: Trough concentrations are not predictive of efficacy/toxicity. Drug exhibits concentration-dependent bactericidal activity, so C_{max}:MIC ratios may be a more useful parameter.

Test Interactions Daptomycin may cause false prolongation of the PT and increase of INR with certain reagents. This appears to be a dose-dependent phenomenon. Therefore, it is recommended to obtain blood samples immediately prior to next daptomycin dose (eg, trough). If PT/INR elevated, clinicians should repeat PT/INR and evaluate for other causes of hypocoagulation.

Dosage Forms Excipient information presented when available (limited, particularly for generics); consult specific product labeling.

Injection, powder for reconstitution:
Cubicin®: 500 mg

◆ **Daraprim®** *see* Pyrimethamine *on page* 1274

Darbepoetin Alfa (dar be POE e tin AL fa)

U.S. Brand Names Aranesp®

Canadian Brand Names Aranesp®

Index Terms Erythropoiesis-Stimulating Agent (ESA); Erythropoiesis-Stimulating Protein; NSC-729969

Pharmacologic Category Colony Stimulating Factor; Growth Factor; Recombinant Human Erythropoietin

Use Treatment of anemia (elevate/maintain red blood cell level and decrease the need for transfusions) associated with chronic renal failure (including patients on dialysis and not on dialysis); treatment of anemia due to concurrent chemotherapy in patients with metastatic cancer (non-myeloid malignancies)

Note: Darbepoetin is **not** indicated for use in cancer patients under the following conditions:

- receiving hormonal therapy, therapeutic biologic products, or radiation therapy unless also receiving concurrent myelosuppressive chemotherapy
- receiving myelosuppressive therapy when the expected outcome is curative

Unlabeled/Investigational Use Treatment of symptomatic anemia in myelodysplastic syndrome (MDS)

Restrictions An FDA-approved medication guide is available; distribute to each patient to whom this medication is dispensed.

Pregnancy Risk Factor C

Pregnancy Considerations There are no adequate and well-controlled studies in pregnant women. Darbepoetin alfa should be used in a pregnant woman only if potential benefit justifies the potential risk to the fetus.

Lactation Excretion in breast milk unknown/use caution

Medication Safety Issues

Sound-alike/look-alike issues:
Aranesp® may be confused with Aralast, Aricept®

Darbepoetin alfa may be confused with dalteparin, epoetin alfa, epoetin beta

Contraindications Hypersensitivity to darbepoetin or any component of the formulation; uncontrolled hypertension

Warnings/Precautions [U.S. Boxed Warning]: ESAs increased the risk of serious cardiovascular events, thromboembolic events, mortality, and/or tumor progression in clinical studies; a rapid rise in hemoglobin (>1 g/dL over 2 weeks) or maintaining higher hemoglobin levels may contribute to these risks. **[U.S. Boxed Warning]: A shortened overall survival and/or increased risk of tumor progression or recurrence has been reported in studies with breast,cervical, head and neck, lymphoid, and non small cell lung cancer patients.** It is of note that in these studies, patients received ESAs to a target hemoglobin of ≥12 g/dL; although risk has not been excluded when dosed to achieve a target hemoglobin of <12 g/dL. **[U.S. Boxed Warnings]: To decrease these risks, and risk of cardio- and thrombovascular events, use ESAs in cancer patients only for the treatment of anemia related to concurrent chemotherapy and use the lowest dose needed to avoid red blood cell transfusions. Discontinue ESA following completion of the chemotherapy course. ESAs are not indicated for patients receiving myelosuppressive therapy when the anticipated outcome is curative. [U.S. Boxed Warning]: An increased risk of death and serious cardiovascular events was reported in chronic renal failure patients administered ESAs to target higher versus lower hemoglobin levels (13.5 vs 11.3 g/dL; 14 vs 10 g/dL) in two clinical studies; dosing should be individualized to achieve and maintain hemoglobin levels within 10-12 g/dL range.** Hemoglobin rising >1 g/dL in a 2-week period may contribute to the risk. Chronic renal failure patients who exhibit an inadequate hemoglobin response to ESA therapy may be at a higher risk for cardiovascular events and mortality compared to other patients. ESA therapy may reduce dialysis efficacy (due to increase in red blood cells and decrease in plasma volume); adjustments in dialysis parameters may be needed. An increased risk of DVT has been observed in patients treated with epoetin undergoing surgical orthopedic procedures. Darbepoetin is **not** approved for reduction in red blood cell transfusions in patients scheduled for surgical procedures. During therapy in any patient, hemoglobin levels should not exceed a target range of 10-12 g/dL and should not rise >1 g/dL per 2-week time period.

Use with caution in patients with hypertension or with a history of seizures; hypertensive encephalopathy and seizures have been reported. If hypertension is difficult to control, reduce or hold darbepoetin alfa. **Not** recommended for acute correction of severe anemia or as a substitute for transfusion. Consider discontinuing in patients who receive a renal transplant.

Prior to treatment, correct or exclude deficiencies of iron, vitamin B_{12}, and/or folate, as well as other factors which may impair erythropoiesis (aluminum toxicity, inflammatory conditions, infections). Prior to and during therapy, iron stores must be evaluated. Supplemental iron is recommended if serum ferritin <100 mcg/L or serum transferrin saturation <20%. Poor response should prompt evaluation of these potential factors, as well as possible malignant processes, occult blood loss, hemolysis, and/or bone marrow fibrosis. Severe anemia and pure red cell aplasia (PRCA) with associated neutralizing antibodies to erythropoietin has been reported, predominantly in patients with CRF receiving SubQ darbepoetin (the I.V. route is preferred for hemodialysis patients). Patients with loss of response to darbepoetin should be evaluated; discontinue treatment in patients with PRCA secondary to neutralizing antibodies to erythropoietin. Antibodies may cross-react; do not switch to another ESA in patients who develop antibody-mediated anemia.

Due to the delayed onset of erythropoiesis, darbepoetin is of no value in the acute treatment of anemia. Safety and efficacy in patients with underlying hematologic diseases have not been established, including porphyria, thalassemia, hemolytic anemia, and sickle cell disease. Potentially serious allergic reactions have been reported. Some products may contain albumin and the packaging of some formulations may contain latex. Safety and efficacy in children with cancer have not been established; children >1 year of age with CRF have been converted from epoetin alfa to darbepoetin.

Adverse Reactions

>10%:

Cardiovascular: Edema (21%), hypertension (4% to 20%), hypotension (20%)

Central nervous system: Fatigue (9% to 33%), fever (4% to 19%), headache (12% to 16%), dizziness (7% to 14%)

Gastrointestinal: Diarrhea (14% to 22%), constipation (5% to 18%), vomiting (2% to 14%), nausea (11%)

Neuromuscular & skeletal: Muscle spasm (17%), arthralgia (9% to 13%)

Respiratory: Upper respiratory infection (15%)

Miscellaneous: Infection (24%)

1% to 10%:

Cardiovascular: Peripheral edema (10%), arrhythmia/arrest (8%), angina/chest pain (7% to 8%), fluid overload (6%), thrombosis (6%), CHF (5%), MI (2%)

Central nervous system: Stroke (2%), seizure (≤1%), TIA (≤1%)

Dermatologic: Rash (7%), pruritus (6%)

Endocrine & metabolic: Dehydration (3% to 5%)

Gastrointestinal: Abdominal pain (10%)

Local: Vascular access hemorrhage (7%), injection site pain (6%), vascular access infection (6%), vascular access thrombosis (6%)

Neuromuscular & skeletal: Limb pain (8%), myalgia (8%), back pain (7%), weakness (5%)

Respiratory: Dyspnea (2% to 10%), cough (9%), bronchitis (5%), pneumonia (3%), pulmonary embolism (1%)

Miscellaneous: Death (7% to 10 %; similar to placebo), flu-like syndrome (6%)

<1% (Limited to important or life-threatening): Abscess, allergic reaction, bacteremia, deep vein thrombosis, GI hemorrhage, hypertensive encephalopathy, peritonitis, pure red cell aplasia (PRCA), sepsis, severe anemia (with or without other cytopenias), thromboembolism, thrombophlebitis, thrombosis, tumor progression (cancer patients)

Drug Interactions

Avoid Concomitant Use There are no known interactions where it is recommended to avoid concomitant use.

Increased Effect/Toxicity There are no known significant interactions involving an increase in effect.

Decreased Effect There are no known significant interactions involving a decrease in effect.

Ethanol/Nutrition/Herb Interactions Ethanol: Should be avoided due to adverse effects on erythropoiesis.

Stability Store at 2°C to 8°C (36°F to 46°F). Do not freeze or shake. Protect from light. Do not dilute or administer with other solutions.

Mechanism of Action Induces erythropoiesis by stimulating the division and differentiation of committed erythroid progenitor cells; induces the release of reticulocytes from the bone marrow into the bloodstream, where they mature to erythrocytes. There is a dose response relationship with this effect. This results in an increase in reticulocyte counts followed by a rise in hematocrit and hemoglobin levels.

When administered SubQ or I.V., darbepoetin's half-life is ~3 times that of epoetin alfa concentrations.

Pharmacodynamics/Kinetics

Onset of action: Increased hemoglobin levels not generally observed until 2-6 weeks after initiating treatment

Absorption: SubQ: Slow

Distribution: V_d: 0.06 L/kg

Bioavailability: CRF: SubQ: Adults: ~37% (range: 30% to 50%); Children: 54% (range: 32% to 70%)

Half-life elimination:

CRF: Adults:

I.V.: 21 hours

SubQ: Nondialysis patients: 70 hours (range: 35-139 hours); Dialysis patients: 46 hours (range: 12-89 hours)

Cancer: Adults: SubQ: 74 hours (range: 24-144 hours); Children: 49 hours

Note: Darbepoetin half-life is approximately threefold longer than epoetin alfa following I.V. administration

Time to peak: SubQ:

CRF: Adults: 48 hours (range: 12-72 hours; independent of dialysis); Children: 36 hours (range: 10-58 hours)

Cancer: Adults: 71-90 hours (range: 28-123 hours); Children: 71 hours (range: 21-143 hours)

Dosage Note: Hemoglobin levels should not exceed 12 g/dL and should not rise >1 g/dL per 2-week time period during therapy in any patient.

Anemia associated with CRF: Individualize dosing to achieve and maintain hemoglobin levels at a target range of 10-12 g/dL. Hemoglobin levels should not exceed 12 g/dL. **Note:** I.V. route is preferred in hemodialysis patients.

Children ≥1 year: Conversion from epoetin alfa: I.V., SubQ: Initial dose: Epoetin alfa doses of 1500 to ≥90,000 units per week may be converted to doses ranging from 6.25-200 mcg darbepoetin alfa per week (see pediatric column in conversion table below).

Children 11-18 years: Initial treatment (unlabeled use): I.V., SubQ: Initial dose: 0.45 mcg/kg once weekly; titrate to hemoglobin response

Adults: I.V., SubQ: Initial: 0.45 mcg/kg once weekly; alternative dose for nondialysis patients: 0.75 mcg/kg once every 2 weeks; Maintenance: titrate to maintain hemoglobin levels between 10-12 g/dL as described below (may be administered once weekly or every 2 weeks; nondialysis patients may require lower maintenance doses)

Dosage adjustment:

Decrease dose by ~25%: If hemoglobin approaches 12 g/dL **or** hemoglobin increases >1 g/dL in any 2-week period. If hemoglobin continues to increase, temporarily discontinue therapy until hemoglobin begins to decrease, then resume therapy with a ~25% reduction from previous dose.

Increase dose by ~25%: If hemoglobin does not increase by 1 g/dL after 4 weeks of therapy (with adequate iron stores). Do not increase dose more frequently than at 4-week intervals.

Inadequate or lack of response: If patient does not attain target hemoglobin range of 10-12 g/dL after appropriate dose titrations over 12 weeks:

Do not continue to increase dose and use the minimum effective dose that will maintain a hemoglobin level sufficient to avoid red blood cell transfusions **and** evaluate patient for other causes of anemia.

Monitor hemoglobin closely thereafter, and if responsiveness improves, may resume making dosage adjustments as recommended above. If responsiveness does not improve and recurrent red blood cell transfusions continue to be needed, discontinue therapy.

Maintenance dose: Individualize to target hemoglobin range of 10-12 g/dL; limit additional dosage increase to every 4 weeks or longer. Patients generally require lower maintenance doses than initial doses to maintain target range.

Conversion from epoetin alfa: I.V., SubQ: Initial dose: Epoetin alfa doses may be converted to doses ranging from 6.25-200 mcg darbepoetin alfa per week (see conversion table below).

Anemia associated with chemotherapy: Titrate dosage to use the minimum effective dose that will maintain a hemoglobin level sufficient to avoid red blood cell transfusions. Do not initiate therapy if hemoglobin ≥10 g/dL. Discontinue darbepoetin following completion of chemotherapy.

Children (unlabeled use): SubQ: 2.25 mcg/kg once weekly

Adults: SubQ: Initial: 2.25 mcg/kg once weekly **or** 500 mcg once every 3 weeks

Dosage adjustment:

Increase dose: If hemoglobin does not increase by 1 g/dL after 6 weeks of therapy (for patients receiving weekly therapy), the dose should be increased up to 4.5 mcg/kg once weekly.

Decrease dose by 40%: If hemoglobin increases >1g/dL in any 2-week period **or** hemoglobin reaches a level sufficient to avoid red blood cell transfusion.

Withhold dose: If hemoglobin exceeds a level needed to avoid red blood cell transfusion. Resume treatment with a dose 40% below the previous dose when hemoglobin approaches a level where transfusions may be required.

Discontinue: On completion of chemotherapy or if after 8 weeks of therapy there is no hemoglobin response or transfusions still required

Anemia associated with MDS (unlabeled use): Adults: SubQ: 150-300 mcg once weekly

Conversion from epoetin alfa to darbepoetin alfa: See table.

Conversion From Epoetin Alfa to Darbepoetin Alfa (Initial Dose)

Previous Dosage of Epoetin Alfa (units/week)	Children Darbepoetin Alfa Dosage (mcg/week)	Adults Darbepoetin Alfa Dosage (mcg/week)
<1500	Not established	6.25
1500-2499	6.25	6.25
2500-4999	10	12.5
5000-10,999	20	25
11,000-17,999	40	40
18,000-33,999	60	60
34,000-89,999	100	100
≥90,000	200	200

Note: In patients receiving epoetin alfa 2-3 times per week, darbepoetin alfa is administered once weekly. In patients receiving epoetin alfa once weekly, darbepoetin alfa is administered once every 2 weeks. The darbepoetin dose to be administered every 2 weeks is derived by adding together 2 weekly epoetin alfa doses and then converting to the appropriate darbepoetin dose. Titrate dose to hemoglobin response thereafter (see dosage adjustment in renal impairment).

Dosage adjustment in renal impairment: Dosage requirements for patients with chronic renal failure who do not require dialysis may be lower than in dialysis patients. Monitor patients closely during the time period in which a dialysis regimen is initiated, dosage requirement may increase. The National Kidney Foundation Clinical Practice Guidelines for Anemia in Chronic Kidney

Disease: 2007 Update of Hemoglobin Target (September, 2007) recommend hemoglobin levels in the range of 11-12 g/dL for dialysis and nondialysis patients receiving ESAs; hemoglobin levels should not be maintained >13 g/dL.

Hemodialysis: I.V. route is preferred in hemodialysis patients.

Dietary Considerations Supplemental iron intake may be required in patients with low iron stores.

Administration May be administered by SubQ or I.V. injection. The I.V. route is recommended in hemodialysis patients. Do not shake; vigorous shaking may denature darbepoetin alfa, rendering it biologically inactive. Do not dilute or administer in conjunction with other drug solutions. Discard any unused portion of the vial; do not pool unused portions.

Monitoring Parameters Hemoglobin (at least once per week until maintenance dose established and after dosage changes; monitor at regular intervals at least once per month once hemoglobin is stabilized); iron stores (transferrin saturation and ferritin) prior to and during therapy; serum chemistry (CRF patients); blood pressure

Additional Information Oncology Comment: The American Society of Hematology (ASH) and American Society of Clinical Oncology (ASCO) 2007 updates to the clinical practice guidelines for the use of erythropoiesis-stimulating agents (ESAs) indicate that ESAs are most appropriate when used according to the dosage parameters within the Food and Drug Administration (FDA) approved labeling for epoetin and darbepoetin (Rizzo, 2008). While the previous guidelines addressed only the use of epoetin, the 2007 guidelines also address the use of darbepoetin, which is assessed as being equivalent to epoetin with respect to safety and efficacy. When used as an option for the treatment of chemotherapy-associated anemia (to increase hemoglobin and decrease red blood cell transfusions), therapy with ESAs should begin as the hemoglobin level approaches or falls below 10 g/dL. The ASH/ASCO guidelines recommend following the FDA approved dosing (and dosing adjustment) guidelines and target hemoglobin ranges as alternate dosing and schedules have not demonstrated consistent differences in effectiveness with regard to hemoglobin response. In patients who do not have a response within 6-8 weeks (hemoglobin rise <1-2 g/dL or no reduction in transfusions) ESA therapy should be discontinued.

The guidelines note that patients with an increased risk of thromboembolism (generally includes previous history of thrombosis, surgery, and/or prolonged periods of immobilization) and patients receiving concomitant medications that may increase thromboembolic risk, should begin ESA therapy only after careful consideration. With the exception of low-risk myelodysplasia-associated anemia (which has evidence supporting the use of ESAs without concurrent chemotherapy), the guidelines do not support the use of ESAs in the absence of concurrent chemotherapy.

Dosage Forms Excipient information presented when available (limited, particularly for generics); consult specific product labeling.

Injection, solution [preservative free]:

Aranesp®: 25 mcg/0.42 mL (0.42 mL); 40 mcg/ 0.4 mL (0.4 mL); 60 mcg/0.3 mL (0.3 mL); 100 mcg/0.5 mL (0.5 mL); 150 mcg/0.3 mL (0.3 mL); 200 mcg/0.4 mL (0.4 mL); 300 mcg/0.6 mL (0.6 mL); 500 mcg/mL (1 mL) [contains polysorbate 80; prefilled syringe; needle cover contains latex]

Aranesp®: 25 mcg/mL (1 mL); 40 mcg/mL (1 mL); 60 mcg/mL (1 mL); 100 mcg/mL (1 mL); 150 mcg/0.75 mL (0.75 mL); 200 mcg/mL (1 mL); 300 mcg/mL (1 mL) [contains polysorbate 80; single-dose vial]

Darifenacin (dar i FEN a sin)

U.S. Brand Names Enablex®

Canadian Brand Names Enablex®

Index Terms Darifenacin Hydrobromide; UK-88,525

Pharmacologic Category Anticholinergic Agent

Use Management of symptoms of bladder overactivity (urge incontinence, urgency, and frequency)

Pregnancy Risk Factor C

Pregnancy Considerations Teratogenic effects and developmental delay were observed in some animal studies. There are no adequate and well-controlled studies in pregnant women; should be used only if potential benefit outweighs possible risk to the fetus.

Lactation Excretion in breast milk unknown/use caution

Contraindications Hypersensitivity to darifenacin or any component of the formulation; uncontrolled narrow-angle glaucoma; urinary retention, paralytic ileus, GI or GU obstruction

Warnings/Precautions May cause drowsiness and/or blurred vision, which may impair physical or mental abilities; patients must be cautioned about performing tasks which require mental alertness (eg, operating machinery or driving). May occur in the presence of increased environmental temperature; use caution in hot weather and/or exercise. Use with caution with hepatic impairment; dosage limitation is required in moderate hepatic impairment (Child-Pugh class B). Not recommended for use in severe hepatic impairment (Child-Pugh class C). Use with caution in patients with clinically-significant bladder outlet obstruction or prostatic hyperplasia (nonobstructive).Use caution in patients with decreased GI motility, constipation, hiatal hernia, reflux esophagitis, and ulcerative colitis. Use caution in patients with myasthenia gravis. In patients with controlled narrow-angle glaucoma, darifenacin should be used with extreme caution and only when the potential benefit outweighs risks of treatment. Use with caution in patients taking strong CYP3A4 inhibitors (see Drug Interactions); dosage limitation of darifenacin is required. Safety and efficacy have not been established in pediatric patients.

Adverse Reactions

>10%: Gastrointestinal: Xerostomia (19% to 35%), constipation (15% to 21%)

1% to 10%:

- Cardiovascular: Hypertension (≥1%), peripheral edema (≥1%)
- Central nervous system: Headache (7%), dizziness (<2%), pain (≥1%)
- Dermatological: Dry skin (≥1%), pruritus (≥1%), rash (≥1%)
- Gastrointestinal: Dyspepsia (3% to 8%), abdominal pain (2% to 4%), nausea (2% to 4%), vomiting (≥1%), weight gain (≥1%)
- Genitourinary: Urinary tract infection (4% to 5%), vaginitis (≥1%), urinary retention (acute)
- Neuromuscular & skeletal: Weakness (<3%), arthralgia (≥1%), back pain (≥1%)
- Ocular: Dry eyes (2%), abnormal vision (≥1%)
- Respiratory: Bronchitis (≥1%), pharyngitis (≥1%), rhinitis (≥1%), sinusitis (≥1%)
- Miscellaneous: Flu-like syndrome (1% to 3%)

Postmarketing and/or case reports: Angioedema, confusion, hallucinations, hypersensitivity reactions, palpitation

Drug Interactions

Metabolism/Transport Effects Substrate of CYP2D6 (minor), CYP3A4 (major); **Inhibits** CYP2D6 (moderate), 3A4 (weak)

Avoid Concomitant Use

Avoid concomitant use of Darifenacin with any of the following: Thioridazine

Increased Effect/Toxicity

Darifenacin may increase the levels/effects of: Anticholinergics; Cannabinoids; CYP2D6 Substrates; Fesoterodine; Nebivolol; Potassium Chloride; Tamoxifen; Thioridazine

The levels/effects of Darifenacin may be increased by: CYP3A4 Inhibitors (Moderate); CYP3A4 Inhibitors (Strong); Dasatinib; Pramlintide

Decreased Effect

Darifenacin may decrease the levels/effects of: Acetylcholinesterase Inhibitors (Central); Codeine; Secretin; TraMADol

The levels/effects of Darifenacin may be decreased by: Acetylcholinesterase Inhibitors (Central); CYP3A4 Inducers (Strong); Deferasirox; Herbs (CYP3A4 Inducers)

Ethanol/Nutrition/Herb Interactions Herb/Nutraceutical: Darifenacin serum concentration may be decreased by St John's wort (avoid concurrent use.)

Stability Store at 25°C (77°F); excursions permitted to 15°C to 30°C (59°F to 86°F). Protect from light.

Mechanism of Action Selective antagonist of the M3 muscarinic (cholinergic) receptor subtype. Blockade of the receptor limits bladder contractions, reducing the symptoms of bladder irritability/overactivity (urge incontinence, urgency and frequency).

Pharmacodynamics/Kinetics

Distribution: V_{dss}: ~163 L

Protein binding: ~98% (primarily alpha$_1$-acid glycoprotein)

Metabolism: Hepatic, via CYP3A4 (major) and CYP2D6 (minor)

Bioavailability: 15% to 19%

Half-life elimination: ~13-19 hours

Time to peak, plasma: ~7 hours

Excretion: As metabolites (inactive); urine (60%), feces (40%)

Dosage Oral: Adults: Initial: 7.5 mg once daily. If response is not adequate after a minimum of 2 weeks, dosage may be increased to 15 mg once daily.

Dosage adjustment with concomitant potent CYP3A4 inhibitors (eg, azole antifungals, erythromycin, isoniazid, protease inhibitors): Daily dosage should not exceed 7.5 mg/day

Dosage adjustment in renal impairment: No adjustment required.

Dosage adjustment in hepatic impairment:

Moderate impairment (Child-Pugh class B): Daily dosage should not exceed 7.5 mg/day

Severe impairment (Child-Pugh class C): Has not been evaluated; use is not recommended

Dietary Considerations May be taken without regard to meals, with or without food.

Administration Tablet should be taken with liquid and swallowed whole; do not chew, crush or split tablet. May be taken without regard to food.

Dosage Forms Excipient information presented when available (limited, particularly for generics); consult specific product labeling.

Tablet, extended release: 7.5 mg, 15 mg

◆ **Darifenacin Hydrobromide** *see* Darifenacin *on page 401*

Darunavir (dar OO na veer)

U.S. Brand Names Prezista®

Index Terms Darunavir Ethanolate; TMC-114

Pharmacologic Category Antiretroviral Agent, Protease Inhibitor

Additional Appendix Information

Antiretroviral Therapy for HIV Infection: Adults and Adolescents *on page 1758*

Perinatal HIV Guidelines *on page 1730*

Use Treatment of HIV-1 infections in combination with ritonavir and other antiretroviral agents

Pregnancy Risk Factor C

Pregnancy Considerations It is not known if darunavir crosses the human placenta. No teratogenicity has been demonstrated in animal studies. However, there are no adequate and well-controlled studies in pregnant women. Pregnancy and protease inhibitors are both associated with an increased risk of hyperglycemia. Glucose levels should be closely monitored. Women receiving estrogen (as hormonal contraception or replacement therapy) have an increased incidence of rash. Alternative forms of contraception may be needed. Health professionals are encouraged to contact the antiretroviral pregnancy registry to monitor outcomes of pregnant women exposed to antiretroviral medications (1-800-258-4263 or www.APRegistry.com).

Lactation Excretion in breast milk unknown/not recommended

Contraindications Coadministration with medications highly dependent upon CYP3A4 for clearance and for which increased levels are associated with serious and/or life-threatening events (includes cisapride, ergot alkaloids (eg, dihydroergotamine, ergonovine, ergotamine, methylergonovine), lovastatin, midazolam (oral), pimozide, rifampin, simvastatin, St John's wort, triazolam)

Warnings/Precautions Coadministration with ritonavir is required. Use with caution in patients taking strong CYP3A4 inhibitors, moderate or strong CYP3A4 inducers and major CYP3A4 substrates (see Drug Interactions); consider alternative agents that avoid or lessen the potential for CYP-mediated interactions. Use with caution in patients with hepatic impairment, including active chronic hepatitis; consider interruption or discontinuation with worsening hepatic function. Not recommended in severe hepatic impairment. Infrequent cases of drug-induced hepatitis (including acute and cytolytic) have been reported. Liver injury has been reported with use (including some fatalities), though generally in patients on multiple medications, with advanced HIV disease, hepatitis B/C coinfection, and/or immune reconstitution syndrome. Monitor patients closely; consider interrupting or discontinuing therapy if signs/symptoms of liver impairment occur.

May cause fat redistribution (buffalo hump, increased abdominal girth, breast engorgement, facial atrophy). Immune reconstitution syndrome, including inflammatory responses to indolent infections, has been associated with antiretroviral therapy; additional evaluation and treatment may be required. May increase cholesterol and/or triglycerides. Protease inhibitors have been associated with glucose dysregulation; use caution in diabetic patients. Use with caution in patients with sulfonamide allergy (contains sulfa moiety) or hemophilia. Protease inhibitors have been associated with a variety of hypersensitivity events (some severe), including rash, anaphylaxis (rare), angioedema, bronchospasm, erythema multiforme, and/or Stevens-Johnson syndrome (rare). It is generally recommended to discontinue treatment if severe rash or moderate symptoms accompanied by other systemic symptoms occur. Treatment history and resistance data should guide use of darunavir with ritonavir. Safety and efficacy have not been established in children.

Adverse Reactions As a class, protease inhibitors potentially cause dyslipidemias which includes elevated cholesterol and triglycerides and a redistribution of body fat centrally to cause increased abdominal girth, buffalo hump, facial atrophy, and breast enlargement. These agents also cause hyperglycemia. Frequency of adverse events is reported for darunavir/ritonavir. See also Ritonavir monograph.

>10%:
Endocrine & metabolic: Hypercholesterolemia (grade 2: 12% to 24%; grade 3: 1% to 8%), LDL increased (grade 2: 11% to 13%; grade 3: 2% to 7%), triglycerides increased (grade 2: 2% to 11%; grade 3: 1% to 7%; grade 4: ≤2%)
Gastrointestinal: Diarrhea (6% to 12%)
Hematologic: Neutropenia (7% to 12%)
Respiratory: Nasopharyngitis (14%)

2% to 10%:
Central nervous system: Headache (2% to 5%)
Dermatologic: Rash (2% to 10%)
Endocrine & metabolic: Hyperglycemia (grade 2: 6% to 8%; grade 3: ≤1%; grade 4: <1%), hypoglycemia (2% to 4%), hypocalcemia (up to 4%), hyponatremia (1% to 3%), hypernatremia (up to 2%)
Gastrointestinal: Nausea (3% to 7%), amylase increased (grade 2: 4% to 6%; grade 3: 3% to 6%), abdominal pain (4% to 5%), vomiting (2% to 4%), abdominal distention (≤2%), dyspepsia (≤2%), lipase increased (grade 2: 2%; grade 3: ≤2%; grade 4: <1%)
Hematologic: Thromboplastin time increased (4% to 8%), hypoalbuminemia (3% to 4%), prothrombin time increased (1% to 4%), thrombocytopenia (3%)
Hepatic: ALT increased (grade 2: 5% to 6%, grade 3: 2% to 3%; grade 4: ≤1%), AST increased (grade 2: 4% to 6%; grade 3: 2% to 3%; grade 4: <1%)
Neuromuscular & skeletal: Weakness (≤3%)

<2% (Limited to important or life-threatening): Acute renal failure, alkaline phosphatase increased, allergic dermatitis, alopecia, anorexia, anxiety, appetite decreased, arthralgia, confusion, cough, dermatitis medicamentosa, diabetes mellitus, disorientation, dreams abnormal, dyspnea, erythema multiforme, extremity pain; fat redistribution (eg, buffalo hump, increased abdominal girth, breast engorgement, facial atrophy); fatigue, fever, flatulence, folliculitis, hepatitis (acute and cytolytic), gynecomastia, hiccups, hyperbilirubinemia, hyperhidrosis, hyperlipidemia, hypersensitivity reactions (including facial edema), hypertension, hyperthermia, hypoesthesia, immune reconstitution syndrome, irritability, lipoatrophy, maculopapular rash, memory impairment, MI, mood changes, myalgia, nephrolithiasis, night sweats, nightmare, obesity, osteopenia, osteoporosis, pancreatitis, paresthesia, peripheral edema, peripheral neuropathy, polydipsia, polyuria, pruritus, renal insufficiency, rhabdomyolysis (coadministration with HMG-CoA reductase inhibitors), rigors, skin inflammation, somnolence, Stevens-Johnson syndrome, tachycardia, toxic skin eruption, transient ischemic attack, vertigo, xerostomia

Drug Interactions

Metabolism/Transport Effects **Substrate** of CYP3A4 (major); **Inhibits** P-glycoprotein

Avoid Concomitant Use

Avoid concomitant use of Darunavir with any of the following: Alfuzosin; Amiodarone; CarBAMazepine; Cisapride; Dabigatran Etexilate; Eplerenone; Ergot Derivatives; Lopinavir; Nilotinib; Nisoldipine; PHENobarbital; Phenytoin; Pimozide; QuiNIDine; Ranolazine; Rivaroxaban; Salmeterol; Saquinavir; Silodosin; St Johns Wort; Topotecan; Voriconazole

Increased Effect/Toxicity

Darunavir may increase the levels/effects of: Alfuzosin; Alosetron; Amiodarone; Antifungal Agents (Azole Derivatives, Systemic); Benzodiazepines (metabolized by oxidation); Calcium Channel Blockers (Dihydropyridine); Calcium Channel Blockers (Nondihydropyridine); Ciclesonide; Cisapride; Clarithromycin; Corticosteroids (Orally Inhaled); CycloSPORINE; CYP2D6 Substrates; CYP3A4 Substrates; Dabigatran Etexilate; Digoxin; Efavirenz; Enfuvirtide; Eplerenone; Ergot Derivatives; Etravirine; FentaNYL; Fesoterodine; Fusidic Acid; HMG-CoA Reductase Inhibitors; Ixabepilone; Lidocaine; Maraviroc; Meperidine; Methadone; Nefazodone; Nilotinib; Nisoldipine; P-Glycoprotein Substrates; Phosphodiesterase 5 Inhibitors; Pimecrolimus; Pimozide; Protease Inhibitors; QuiNIDine; Ranolazine; Rifamycin Derivatives; Rivaroxaban; Salmeterol; Silodosin; Sirolimus; Sorafenib; Tacrolimus; Temsirolimus; Tenofovir; Topotecan; TraZODone; Tricyclic Antidepressants

The levels/effects of Darunavir may be increased by: Antifungal Agents (Azole Derivatives, Systemic); Clarithromycin; CycloSPORINE; CYP3A4 Inhibitors (Moderate); CYP3A4 Inhibitors (Strong); Dasatinib; Delavirdine; Enfuvirtide; Etravirine; Fusidic Acid

Decreased Effect

Darunavir may decrease the levels/effects of: Abacavir; Clarithromycin; Delavirdine; Didanosine; Etravirine; Meperidine; Norethindrone; Oral Contraceptive (Estrogens); PARoxetine; Sertraline; Theophylline Derivatives; Valproic Acid; Voriconazole; Warfarin; Zidovudine

The levels/effects of Darunavir may be decreased by: CarBAMazepine; CYP3A4 Inducers (Strong); Deferasirox; Efavirenz; Garlic; Lopinavir; Nevirapine; Oral Contraceptive (Estrogens); PHENobarbital; Phenytoin; Rifamycin Derivatives; Saquinavir; St Johns Wort; Tenofovir

Ethanol/Nutrition/Herb Interactions

Food: Bioavailability is increased with a high-fat meal.
Herb/nutraceutical: St John's wort may decrease the plasma levels of darunavir (concomitant use not recommended).

Stability Store at 25°C (77°F); excursions permitted to 15°C to 30°C (59°F to 86°F).

Mechanism of Action Darunavir binds to the HIV-1 protease activity site and inhibits the activity of the enzyme. HIV protease is required for the cleavage of viral Gag-Pol polyprotein precursors into individual functional proteins found in infectious HIV. Inhibition prevents cleavage of these polyproteins, resulting in the formation of immature, noninfectious viral particles.

Pharmacodynamics/Kinetics All kinetic parameters derived in the presence of ritonavir coadministration.
Absorption: Increased 30% with food
Protein binding: ~95%
Metabolism: Hepatic, via CYP3A4 to minimally-active metabolites
Bioavailability: 82% (with ritonavir)
Half-life elimination: ~15 hours (with ritonavir)
Time to peak, plasma: 2.5-4 hours
Excretion: Feces (~80%, 41% as unchanged drug); urine (~14%, 8% as unchanged drug)

Dosage Oral: Adults:
Therapy-naive: 800 mg once daily with food; coadministration with ritonavir 100 mg once daily is required
Therapy-experienced: 600 mg twice daily with food; coadministration with ritonavir 100 mg twice daily is required
Dosage adjustment for toxicity:
Severe rash: Discontinue treatment
New or worsening liver dysfunction: Consider interrupting or discontinuing treatment

Dosage adjustment in renal impairment: No adjustment required for mild-to-moderate impairment. No data available for use in severe renal failure failure or end-stage renal disease.

Dosage adjustment in hepatic impairment: No adjustment for mild-to-moderate impairment. Not recommended for patients with severe impairment.

Dietary Considerations Absorption increased with food. Take with meals.

Administration Administer with food (bioavailability is increased). Coadministration with ritonavir is required.

Monitoring Parameters Viral load, CD4, serum glucose; transaminase levels prior to and during therapy (increase monitoring in patients at risk for liver impairment), cholesterol, triglycerides

Dosage Forms Excipient information presented when available (limited, particularly for generics); consult specific product labeling.

Tablet:

Prezista®: 300 mg, 400 mg, 600 mg

- **Darunavir Ethanolate** *see* Darunavir *on page 402*
- **Darvocet A500®** *see* Propoxyphene and Acetaminophen *on page 1258*
- **Darvocet-N® 50** *see* Propoxyphene and Acetaminophen *on page 1258*
- **Darvocet-N® 100** *see* Propoxyphene and Acetaminophen *on page 1258*
- **Darvon®** *see* Propoxyphene *on page 1256*
- **Darvon® Compound [DSC]** *see* Propoxyphene, Aspirin, and Caffeine *on page 1258*
- **Darvon-N®** *see* Propoxyphene *on page 1256*

Dasatinib (da SA ti nib)

U.S. Brand Names Sprycel®

Canadian Brand Names Sprycel®

Index Terms BMS-354825; NSC-732517

Pharmacologic Category Antineoplastic Agent, Tyrosine Kinase Inhibitor

Use Treatment of chronic myelogenous leukemia (CML) in chronic, accelerated or blast (myeloid or lymphoid) phase resistant or intolerant to prior therapy (including imatinib); treatment of Philadelphia chromosome-positive (Ph+) acute lymphoblastic leukemia (ALL) resistant or intolerant to prior therapy

Pregnancy Risk Factor D

Pregnancy Considerations Animal studies have demonstrated fetal abnormalities (skeletal malformations, reduced ossification, edema, microhepatia) and fetal death. There are no adequate and well-controlled studies in pregnant women. May cause fetal harm if administered to a pregnant woman. Not recommended for use during pregnancy or if contemplating pregnancy. Effective contraception is recommended for men and women of childbearing potential. Pregnant women are advised to avoid contact with crushed or broken tablets.

Lactation Excretion in breast milk unknown/not recommended

Medication Safety Issues

High alert medication: The Institute for Safe Medication Practices (ISMP) includes this medication among its list of drug classes which have a heightened risk of causing significant patient harm when used in error.

Contraindications There are no contraindications listed within the FDA-approved manufacturer's labeling.

Canadian labeling: Hypersensitivity to dasatinib or any other component of the formulation

Warnings/Precautions Hazardous agent - use appropriate precautions for handling and disposal. Severe dose-related bone marrow suppression (thrombocytopenia, neutropenia, anemia) is associated with treatment; dosage adjustment or temporary interruption may be required for severe myelosuppression; the incidence of myelosuppression is higher in patients with advanced CML and Ph+ ALL. Fatal intracranial hemorrhage has been reported in association with dasatinib use. Severe hemorrhage (including CNS, GI) may occur due to thrombocytopenia; in addition to thrombocytopenia, dasatinib may also cause platelet dysfunction. Use caution with patients taking anticoagulants or medications interfering with platelet function; not studied in clinical trials. Use with caution in patients receiving concurrent therapy which alters CYP3A4 activity; avoid concomitant use or consider dasatinib dosage adjustments. Fluid retention, including pleural and pericardial effusions, severe ascites, severe pulmonary edema, and generalized edema were reported; may be dose-related. Use caution in patients where fluid accumulation may be poorly tolerated, such as in cardiovascular disease (HF or hypertension) and pulmonary disease. Elderly may be more likely to experience fluid retention.

May prolong QT interval; use caution in patients at risk for QT prolongation, including patients with long QT syndrome; patients taking antiarrhythmic medications or other medications that lead to QT prolongation or potassium-wasting diuretics; patients with cumulative high-dose anthracycline therapy, and conditions which cause hypokalemia or hypomagnesemia. Correct hypokalemia and hypomagnesemia prior to initiation of therapy. Use caution with hepatic impairment due to extensive hepatic metabolism; patients with ALT or AST >2.5 times the upper limit of normal (ULN) or total bilirubin >2 times the ULN were excluded from clinical trials. Safety and efficacy in children <18 years of age have not been established.

Adverse Reactions

≥10%:

Cardiovascular: Fluid retention (37%; grades 3/4: 8%), superficial edema (20%)

Central nervous system: Headache (24%), fatigue (21%), fever (13%)

Dermatologic: Rash (22%; includes erythema, erythema multiforme, erythematous rash, exfoliative rash, follicular rash, heat rash, maculopapular rash, milia, papular rash, pruritic rash, pustular rash, skin exfoliation, skin irritation, systemic lupus erythematosus rash, urticaria vesiculosa, vesicular rash)

Endocrine & metabolic: Hypophosphatemia (grades 3/4: 6% to 20%), hypocalcemia (grades 3/4: 1% to 16%)

Gastrointestinal: Diarrhea (31%; grades 3/4: 3%), nausea (22%), vomiting (13%)

Hematologic: Neutropenia (grades 3/4: 34% to 80%), thrombocytopenia (grades 3/4: 22% to 81%), anemia (grades 3/4: 10% to 75%), hemorrhage (21%; grades 3/4: 6%)

Neuromuscular & skeletal: Musculoskeletal pain (14%)

Respiratory: Pleural effusion (22%; grades 3/4: 5%), dyspnea (20%; grades 3/4: 4%)

1% to <10%:

Cardiovascular: Generalized edema (3%), pericardial effusion (3%; grades 3/4: 1%), CHF/cardiac dysfunction (2%; grades 3/4: 1%; includes cardiac failure, cardiomyopathy, diastolic dysfunction, ejection fraction decreased, left ventricular dysfunction, ventricular failure); arrhythmia, chest pain, flushing, hypertension, palpitation

Central nervous system: CNS bleeding (1%), chills, depression, dizziness, insomnia, pain, somnolence

Dermatologic: Acne, alopecia, dermatitis, dry skin, eczema, hyperhydrosis, pruritus, urticaria

Gastrointestinal: Abdominal pain (10%), gastrointestinal bleeding (7%; grades 3/4: 4%), abdominal distention, colitis, constipation, dysgeusia, dyspepsia, enterocolitis, gastritis, mucositis/stomatitis, oral soft tissue disorder, weight loss/gain

Hematologic: Contusion, neutropenic fever, pancytopenia

Hepatic: ALT increased (grades 3/4: ≤7%), AST increased (grades 3/4: ≤5%), bilirubin increased (grades 3/4: ≤5%)

Neuromuscular & skeletal: Arthralgia, muscle inflammation, muscle weakness, myalgia, neuropathy, peripheral neuropathy, weakness

Ocular: Visual disorder, xerophthalmia

Renal: Serum creatinine increased (grades 3/4: ≤3%)

Respiratory: Pulmonary edema (2%; grades 3/4: 1%), pulmonary hypertension (1%), cough, lung infiltration, pneumonia, pneumonitis, upper respiratory tract infection/inflammation

Miscellaneous: Infection (bacterial, fungal, viral), herpes virus infection

<1% (Limited to important or life-threatening): Acute coronary syndrome, acute febrile neutrophilic dermatosis, acute respiratory distress syndrome, affect lability, amnesia, anal fissure, angina, ascites, asthma, bronchospasm, bullous conditions, cardiomegaly, cerebrovascular accident, cholecystitis, cholestasis, coagulopathy, confusion, conjunctivitis, creatine phosphokinase increased, dysphagia, erythema nodosum, esophagitis, gynecomastia, hand-foot syndrome, hepatitis, hypersensitivity, hyperuricemia, hypoalbuminemia, hypotension, ileus, libido decreased, livedo reticularis, menstrual irregularities, MI, musculoskeletal stiffness, myocarditis, neutropenic colitis, pancreatitis, panniculitis, pericarditis, periorbital edema, photosensitivity, platelet aggregation abnormal, polyuria, proteinuria, pure red cell aplasia, QT_c prolongation, renal failure, reversible posterior leukoencephalopathy syndrome, rhabdomyolysis, seizure, sepsis, skin ulcer, syncope, tendonitis, thrombophlebitis, TIA, tinnitus, tremor, troponin increased, tumor lysis syndrome, upper gastrointestinal ulcer, ventricular arrhythmia, ventricular tachycardia, vertigo

Drug Interactions

Metabolism/Transport Effects Substrate of CYP3A4 (major); **Inhibits** CYP3A4 (weak)

Avoid Concomitant Use

Avoid concomitant use of Dasatinib with any of the following: Nilotinib; Tetrabenazine; Thioridazine; Ziprasidone

Increased Effect/Toxicity

Dasatinib may increase the levels/effects of: Anticoagulants; Antiplatelet Agents; CYP3A4 Substrates; QTc-Prolonging Agents; Tetrabenazine; Thioridazine; Ziprasidone

The levels/effects of Dasatinib may be increased by: Alfuzosin; Ciprofloxacin; CYP3A4 Inhibitors (Moderate); CYP3A4 Inhibitors (Strong); Gadobutrol; Nilotinib

Decreased Effect

The levels/effects of Dasatinib may be decreased by: Antacids; CYP3A4 Inducers (Strong); Deferasirox; H2-Antagonists; Herbs (CYP3A4 Inducers); Proton Pump Inhibitors

Ethanol/Nutrition/Herb Interactions Herb/Nutraceutical: Avoid St John's wort (may increase metabolism and decrease dasatinib plasma concentration).

Stability Store at 25°C (77°F); excursions permitted to 15°C to 30°C (59°F to 86°F).

Mechanism of Action BCR-ABL tyrosine kinase inhibitor; targets most imatinib-resistant BCR-ABL mutations (except the T315I and F317V mutants) by distinctly binding to ABL-kinase. Kinase inhibition halts proliferation of leukemia cells. Also inhibits SRC family (including SRC, LKC, YES, FYN); c-KIT, EPHA2 and platelet derived growth factor receptor (PDGFRβ)

Pharmacodynamics/Kinetics

Distribution: 2505 L

Protein binding: Dasatinib: 96%; metabolite (active): 93%

Metabolism: Hepatic (extensive); metabolized by CYP3A4 (primarily), flavin-containing mono-oxygenase-3 (FOM-3) and uridine diphosphate-glucuronosyltransferase (UGT) to an active metabolite and other inactive metabolites (the active metabolite plays only a minor role in the pharmacology of dasatinib)

Half-life elimination: Terminal: 3-5 hours

Time to peak, plasma: 0.5-6 hours

Excretion: Feces (85%, 19% as unchanged drug); urine (4%, 0.1% as unchanged drug)

Dosage Oral: Adults:

CML:

Chronic phase: 100 mg once daily. In clinical studies, a dose escalation to 140 mg once daily was allowed in patients not achieving cytogenetic response at recommended initial dosage.

Accelerated or blast phase: 70 mg twice daily. In clinical studies, a dose escalation to 100 mg twice daily was allowed in patients not achieving cytogenetic response at recommended initial dosage.

Ph+ ALL: 70 mg twice daily. In clinical studies, a dose escalation to 100 mg twice daily was allowed in patients not achieving cytogenetic response at recommended initial dosage.

Dosage adjustment for concomitant CYP3A4 inhibitors/inducers: Dose reductions are likely to be needed when dasatinib is administered concomitantly with a strong CYP3A4 inhibitor (an alternate medication for CYP3A4 enzyme inhibitors should be investigated first). In the event that dasatinib must be administered concomitantly with a potent enzyme inhibitor, consider reducing dasatinib to 20 mg daily with careful monitoring. (Canadian labeling recommend reducing dose to 20-40 mg daily). If reduced dose is not tolerated, the strong CYP3A4 inhibitor must be discontinued or dasatinib therapy temporarily held until concomitant inhibitor use has ceased. When a strong CYP3A4 inhibitor is discontinued, allow a washout period (~1 week) prior to adjusting dasatinib dose upward.

Concomitant administration with CYP3A4 inducers may require increased dasatinib doses, with careful monitoring; alternatives to the enzyme-inducing agent should be utilized first.

Dosage adjustment for toxicity:

Hematologic toxicity:

Chronic phase CML (100 mg daily starting dose): For ANC <0.5 x 10^9/L or platelets <50 x 10^9/L, withhold treatment until ANC ≥1 x 10^9/L and platelets ≥50 x 10^9/L; then resume treatment at the original starting dose if recovery occurs in ≤7 days. If platelets <25 x 10^9/L or recurrence of ANC <0.5 x 10^9/L for >7 days, withhold treatment until ANC ≥1 x 10^9/L and platelets ≥50 x 10^9/L; then resume treatment at 80 mg once daily (2nd episode) or discontinue (3rd episode)

Accelerated or blast phase CML and Ph+ ALL (70 mg twice daily starting dose): For ANC <0.5 x 10^9/L or platelets <10 x 10^9/L, if cytopenia unrelated to leukemia, withhold treatment until ANC ≥1 x 10^9/L and platelets ≥20 x 10^9/L; then resume treatment at the original starting dose. If cytopenia recurs, withhold treatment until ANC ≥1 x 10^9/L and platelets ≥20 x 10^9/L; then resume treatment at 50 mg twice daily (2nd episode) or 40 mg twice daily (3rd episode). For cytopenias related to leukemia (confirm with marrow aspirate or biopsy), consider dose escalation to 100 mg twice daily with careful monitoring.

Nonhematologic toxicity: Withhold treatment until toxicity improvement or resolution; if appropriate, resume treatment at a reduced dose based on the event severity.

Dietary Considerations May be taken without regard to food. Avoid grapefruit juice.

Administration Administer once daily (morning or evening) or twice daily (morning and evening). May be taken without regard to food. Do not break, crush, or chew tablets.

Monitoring Parameters CBC with differential (weekly for 2 months, then monthly); bone marrow biopsy; liver function tests, electrolytes including calcium, phosphorus, magnesium; monitor for fluid retention; ECG monitoring if at risk for QT_c prolongation; chest x-ray is recommended for symptoms suggestive of pleural effusion (eg, cough, dyspnea)

Additional Information Oncology Comment: In a dose finding study in chronic-phase CML, dasatininb 100 mg once daily provided comparable efficacy to the original FDA-approved dose of 70 mg twice daily. The 100 mg once daily dose was better tolerated (lower rates of pleural effusion and grades 3/4 thrombocytopenia), required fewer dose reductions, and fewer dosing interruptions or discontinuations (Shah, 2008).

Dosage Forms Excipient information presented when available (limited, particularly for generics); consult specific product labeling.

Tablet, oral:

Sprycel®: 20 mg, 50 mg, 70 mg, 100 mg

◆ **Daunomycin** *see* DAUNOrubicin Hydrochloride *on page 407*

DAUNOrubicin Citrate (Liposomal)

(daw noe ROO bi sin SI trate lip po SOE mal)

U.S. Brand Names DaunoXome®

Index Terms DAUNOrubicin Liposomal; Liposomal DAUNOrubicin; NSC-697732

Pharmacologic Category Antineoplastic Agent, Anthracycline

Use First-line treatment of advanced HIV-associated Kaposi's sarcoma (KS)

Pregnancy Risk Factor D

Pregnancy Considerations Teratogenic effects and embryotoxicity were noted in animal studies. There are no adequate and well-controlled studies in pregnant women. Women of childbearing potential should avoid becoming pregnant while receiving treatment.

Lactation Excretion in breast milk unknown/not recommended

Medication Safety Issues

Sound-alike/look-alike issues:

DAUNOrubicin liposomal may be confused with DACTINomycin, DOXOrubicin, DOXOrubicin liposomal, epirubicin, IDArubicin

Liposomal formulation (DaunoXome®) may be confused with the conventional formulation (Cerubidine®, Rubex®)

High alert medication: The Institute for Safe Medication Practices (ISMP) includes this medication among its list of drug classes which have a heightened risk of causing significant patient harm when used in error.

Contraindications Hypersensitivity to daunorubicin citrate (liposomal), daunorubicin, or any component of the formulation

Warnings/Precautions Hazardous agent - use appropriate precautions for handling and disposal. **[U.S. Boxed Warning]: Monitor cardiac function regularly; especially in patients with previous therapy with high cumulative doses of anthracyclines, cyclophosphamide, or thoracic radiation, or who have pre-existing cardiac disease.** Although the risk increases with cumulative dose, irreversible cardiotoxicity may occur with anthracycline treatment at any dose level. Patients with pre-existing heart disease, hypertension, concurrent administration of other antineoplastic agents, prior or concurrent chest irradiation, and advanced age are at increased risk. Evaluate left ventricular ejection fraction (LVEF) prior to treatment and periodically during treatment.

[U.S. Boxed Warning]: May cause bone marrow suppression, particularly neutropenia; monitor closely for infections. **[U.S. Boxed Warning]: Use caution with hepatic impairment;** dosage reduction is recommended. Use caution with renal impairment; may require dose adjustment. **[U.S. Boxed Warning]: The lipid component is associated with infusion-related reactions (back pain, flushing, chest tightness) usually within the first 5 minutes of infusion;** monitor, interrupt infusion, and resume at reduced infusion rate. Safety and efficacy in children and the elderly have not been established. **[U.S. Boxed Warning]: Should be administered under the supervision of an experienced cancer chemotherapy physician.**

Adverse Reactions

>10%:

Cardiovascular: Edema (11%)

Central nervous system: Fatigue (49%), fever (47%), headache (25%), neutropenic fever (17%)

Gastrointestinal: Nausea (54%), diarrhea (38%), abdominal pain (23%), anorexia (23%), vomiting (23%)

Hematologic: Myelosuppression (onset: 7 days; nadir: 14 days; recovery 21 days), neutropenia (up to 55%; grade 4: 15%), anemia (up to 55%; grade 4: 2%), thrombocytopenia (up to 12%; grade 4: 1%)

Neuromuscular & skeletal: Rigors (19%), back pain (16%), neuropathy (13%)

Respiratory: Cough (28%), dyspnea (26%), rhinitis (12%)

Miscellaneous: Opportunistic infections (40%), allergic reactions (24%), diaphoresis (14%), infusion-related reactions (14%; includes back pain, flushing, chest tightness)

1% to 10%:

Cardiovascular: Chest pain (10%), hypertension (≤5%), palpitation (≤5%), syncope (≤5%), tachycardia (≤5%), LVEF decreased (3%), CHF/cardiomyopathy

Central nervous system: Depression (10%), malaise (10%), dizziness (8%), insomnia (6%), abnormal thinking (≤5%), amnesia (≤5%), anxiety (≤5%), ataxia (≤5%), confusion (≤5%), emotional lability (≤5%), hallucination (≤5%), meningitis (≤5%), seizure (≤5%), somnolence (≤5%)

Dermatologic: Alopecia (8%), pruritus (7%), dry skin (≤5%), folliculitis (≤5%), seborrhea (≤5%)

Endocrine & metabolic: Dehydration (≤5%), hot flashes (≤5%)

Gastrointestinal: Stomatitis (10%), constipation (7%), tenesmus (5%), appetite increased (≤5%), dental caries (≤5%), dysphagia (≤5%), gastrointestinal hemorrhage (≤5%), gastritis (≤5%), gingival bleeding (≤5%), hemorrhoids (≤5%), melena (≤5%), splenomegaly (≤5%), taste perversion (≤5%), xerostomia (≤5%)

Genitourinary: Dysuria (≤5%), nocturia (≤5%), polyuria (≤5%)

Hepatic: Hepatomegaly (≤5%)

Local: Injection site inflammation (≤5%)

Neuromuscular & skeletal: Arthralgia (7%), myalgia (7%), gait abnormal (≤5%), hyperkinesia (≤5%), hypertonia (≤5%), tremor (≤5%)

Ocular: Abnormal vision (5%) conjunctivitis (≤5%), eye pain (≤5%)

Otic: Deafness (≤5%), earache (≤5%), tinnitus (≤5%)

Respiratory: Sinusitis (8%), hemoptysis (≤5%), pulmonary infiltrate (≤5%), sputum increased (≤5%)

Miscellaneous: Flu-like syndrome (5%), hiccups (≤5%), lymphadenopathy (≤5%), thirst (≤5%)

Postmarketing and/or case reports: Angina, atrial fibrillation, cardiac arrest, MI, pericardial effusion, pericardial tamponade, pulmonary hypertension, supraventricular tachycardia, ventricular extrasystoles

Drug Interactions

Avoid Concomitant Use

Avoid concomitant use of DAUNOrubicin Citrate (Liposomal) with any of the following: Natalizumab; Vaccines (Live)

Increased Effect/Toxicity

DAUNOrubicin Citrate (Liposomal) may increase the levels/effects of: Natalizumab; Vaccines (Live)

The levels/effects of DAUNOrubicin Citrate (Liposomal) may be increased by: Bevacizumab; P-Glycoprotein Inhibitors; Taxane Derivatives; Trastuzumab

Decreased Effect

DAUNOrubicin Citrate (Liposomal) may decrease the levels/effects of: Cardiac Glycosides; Vaccines (Inactivated)

The levels/effects of DAUNOrubicin Citrate (Liposomal) may be decreased by: Cardiac Glycosides; Echinacea; P-Glycoprotein Inducers

Stability Store intact vials of solution under refrigeration at 2°C to 8°C (36°F to 46°F); do not freeze. Protect from light. Only fluid which may be mixed with DaunoXome® is D_5W. Dilute to a 1:1 solution (1 mg daunorubicin liposomal/mL D_5W). Must **not** be mixed with saline, bacteriostatic agents (such as benzyl alcohol), or any other solution. Diluted daunorubicin liposomal for infusion may be refrigerated at 2°C to 8°C (36°F to 46°F) for a maximum of 6 hours. Do not use with in-line filters.

Mechanism of Action Liposomes have been shown to penetrate solid tumors more effectively, possibly because of their small size and longer circulation time. Once in tissues, daunorubicin is released. Daunorubicin inhibits DNA and RNA synthesis by intercalation between DNA base pairs and by steric obstruction; and intercalates at points of local uncoiling of the double helix. Although the exact mechanism is unclear, it appears that direct binding to DNA (intercalation) and inhibition of DNA repair (topoisomerase II inhibition) result in blockade of DNA and RNA synthesis and fragmentation of DNA.

Pharmacodynamics/Kinetics

Distribution: V_d: 5-8 L

Metabolism: Similar to daunorubicin, but metabolite plasma levels are low

Half-life elimination: Distribution: 4.4 hours; Terminal: 3-5 hours

Excretion: Primarily feces; some urine

Clearance, plasma: 17.3 mL/minute

Dosage Refer to individual protocols. I.V.:

Adults: HIV-associated KS: 40 mg/m^2 every 2 weeks

Elderly: Use with caution.

Dosage adjustment for toxicity: Withhold treatment for ANC <750/mm^3

Elderly: Use with caution.

Dosing adjustment in renal impairment: Serum creatinine >3 mg/dL: Administer 50% of normal dose

Dosing adjustment in hepatic impairment:

Bilirubin 1.2-3 mg/dL: Administer 75% of normal dose

Bilirubin >3 mg/dL: Administer 50% of normal dose

Administration Infuse over 1 hour; do not mix with other drugs. Avoid extravasation.

Monitoring Parameters CBC with differential and platelets (prior to each dose), liver function tests, renal function tests; evaluate cardiac function (baseline left ventricular ejection fraction [LVEF] prior to treatment initiation; repeat LVEF at total cumulative doses of 320 mg/m^2, and every 160 mg/m^2 thereafter; patients with pre-existing cardiac disease, history of prior chest irradiation, or history of prior anthracycline treatment should have baseline LVEF and every 160 mg/m^2 thereafter); signs and symptoms of infection or disease progression; monitor closely for infusion reactions

Dosage Forms Excipient information presented when available (limited, particularly for generics); consult specific product labeling.

Injection, solution [preservative free]:

DaunoXome®: 2 mg/mL (25 mL) [contains sucrose 2125 mg/25 mL]

DAUNOrubicin Hydrochloride

(daw noe ROO bi sin hye droe KLOR ide)

U.S. Brand Names Cerubidine®

Canadian Brand Names Cerubidine®

Index Terms Daunomycin; NSC-82151; Rubidomycin Hydrochloride

Pharmacologic Category Antineoplastic Agent, Anthracycline

Use Treatment of acute lymphocytic (ALL) and nonlymphocytic (ANLL) leukemias

Pregnancy Risk Factor D

Pregnancy Considerations May cause fetal harm when administered to a pregnant woman. Animal studies have shown an increased incidence of fetal abnormalities.

Lactation Excretion in breast milk unknown/not recommended

Medication Safety Issues

Sound-alike/look-alike issues:

DAUNOrubicin may be confused with DACTINomycin, DOXOrubicin, DOXOrubicin liposomal, epirubicin, IDArubicin

Conventional formulation (Cerubidine®, DAUNOrubicin hydrochloride) may be confused with the liposomal formulation (DaunoXome®)

High alert medication: The Institute for Safe Medication Practices (ISMP) includes this medication among its list of drug classes which have a heightened risk of causing significant patient harm when used in error.

Contraindications Hypersensitivity to daunorubicin or any component of the formulation

Warnings/Precautions Hazardous agent - use appropriate precautions for handling and disposal. Use with caution in patients who have received radiation therapy; reduce dosage in patients who are receiving radiation therapy simultaneously. **[U.S. Boxed Warnings]: Use caution with renal impairment or in the presence of hepatic dysfunction; dosage reduction is recommended. Potent vesicant; if extravasation occurs, severe local tissue damage leading to ulceration and necrosis, and pain may occur. For I.V. administration only. Severe bone marrow suppression may occur.**

[U.S. Boxed Warning]: May cause cumulative, dose-related myocardial toxicity (concurrent or delayed). Total cumulative dose should take into account previous or concomitant treatment with cardiotoxic agents or irradiation of chest. The incidence of irreversible myocardial toxicity increases as the total cumulative (lifetime) dosages approach:

550 mg/m^2 in adults

400 mg/m^2 in adults receiving chest radiation

300 mg/m^2 in children >2 years of age

10 mg/kg in children <2 years of age

Although the risk increases with cumulative dose, irreversible cardiotoxicity may occur at any dose level. Patients with pre-existing heart disease, hypertension, concurrent administration of other antineoplastic agents, prior or concurrent chest irradiation, advanced age; and infants and children are at increased risk. Monitor left ventricular (LV) function (baseline and periodic) with ECHO or MUGA scan; monitor ECG.

Secondary leukemias may occur when used with combination chemotherapy or radiation therapy. **[U.S. Boxed Warning]: Should be administered under the supervision of an experienced cancer chemotherapy physician].**

Adverse Reactions

>10%:

Cardiovascular: Transient ECG abnormalities (supraventricular tachycardia, S-T wave changes, atrial or ventricular extrasystoles); generally asymptomatic and self-limiting. CHF, dose related, may be delayed for 7-8 years after treatment.

Dermatologic: Alopecia (reversible), radiation recall

Gastrointestinal: Mild nausea or vomiting, stomatitis

Genitourinary: Discoloration of urine (red)

Hematologic: Myelosuppression (onset: 7 days; nadir: 10-14 days; recovery: 21-28 days), primarily leukopenia; thrombocytopenia and anemia

1% to 10%:

Dermatologic: Skin "flare" at injection site; discoloration of saliva, sweat, or tears

Endocrine & metabolic: Hyperuricemia

Gastrointestinal: Abdominal pain, GI ulceration, diarrhea

<1% (Limited to important or life-threatening): Anaphylactoid reaction, bilirubin increased, hepatitis, infertility; local (cellulitis, pain, thrombophlebitis at injection site); MI, myocarditis, nail banding, onycholysis, pericarditis, pigmentation of nailbeds, secondary leukemia, skin rash, sterility, systemic hypersensitivity (including urticaria, pruritus, angioedema, dysphagia, dyspnea); transaminases increased

Drug Interactions

Avoid Concomitant Use

Avoid concomitant use of DAUNOrubicin Hydrochloride with any of the following: Natalizumab; Vaccines (Live)

Increased Effect/Toxicity

DAUNOrubicin Hydrochloride may increase the levels/effects of: Natalizumab; Vaccines (Live)

The levels/effects of DAUNOrubicin Hydrochloride may be increased by: Bevacizumab; P-Glycoprotein Inhibitors; Taxane Derivatives; Trastuzumab

Decreased Effect

DAUNOrubicin Hydrochloride may decrease the levels/effects of: Cardiac Glycosides; Vaccines (Inactivated)

The levels/effects of DAUNOrubicin Hydrochloride may be decreased by: Cardiac Glycosides; Echinacea; P-Glycoprotein Inducers

Ethanol/Nutrition/Herb Interactions Ethanol: Avoid ethanol (due to GI irritation).

Stability Store intact vials of powder for injection at room temperature of 15°C to 30°C (59°F to 86°F); intact vials of solution for injection should be refrigerated at 2°C to 8°C (36°F to 46°F). Protect from light. Dilute vials of powder for injection with 4 mL SWFI for a final concentration of 5 mg/mL. May further dilute in 100 mL D_5W or NS. Reconstituted solution is stable for 4 days at 15°C to 25°C. Further dilution in D_5W, LR, or NS is stable at room temperature (25°C) for up to 4 weeks if protected from light.

Mechanism of Action Inhibition of DNA and RNA synthesis by intercalation between DNA base pairs and by steric obstruction. Daunomycin intercalates at points of local uncoiling of the double helix. Although the exact mechanism is unclear, it appears that direct binding to DNA (intercalation) and inhibition of DNA repair (topoisomerase II inhibition) result in blockade of DNA and RNA synthesis and fragmentation of DNA.

Pharmacodynamics/Kinetics

Distribution: Many body tissues, particularly the liver, kidneys, lung, spleen, and heart; not into CNS; crosses placenta; V_d: 40 L/kg

Metabolism: Primarily hepatic to daunorubicinol (active), then to inactive aglycones, conjugated sulfates, and glucuronides

Half-life elimination: Distribution: 2 minutes; Elimination: 14-20 hours; Terminal: 18.5 hours; Daunorubicinol plasma half-life: 24-48 hours

Excretion: Feces (40%); urine (~25% as unchanged drug and metabolites)

Dosage I.V. (refer to individual protocols):

Children: **Note:** Cumulative dose should not exceed 300 mg/m^2 in children >2 years or 10 mg/kg in children <2 years of age; maximum cumulative doses for younger children are unknown.

Children <2 years or BSA <0.5 m^2: ALL combination therapy: 1 mg/kg/dose per protocol, with frequency dependent on regimen employed

Children ≥2 years and BSA ≥0.5 m^2:

ALL combination therapy: Remission induction: 25 mg/m^2 on day 1 every week for up to 4-6 cycles

AML combination therapy: Induction: I.V. continuous infusion: 30-60 mg/m^2/day on days 1-3 of cycle

Adults: **Note:** Cumulative dose should not exceed 550 mg/m^2 in adults without risk factors for cardiotoxicity and should not exceed 400 mg/m^2 in adults receiving chest irradiation.

Range: 30-60 mg/m^2/day for 3 days, repeat dose in 3-4 weeks

ALL combination therapy: 45 mg/m^2/day for 3 days

AML combination therapy:

Adults <60 years: Induction: 45 mg/m^2/day for 3 days of the first course of induction therapy; subsequent courses: 45 mg/m^2/day for 2 days

Adults ≥60 years: Induction: 30 mg/m^2/day for 3 days of the first course of induction therapy; subsequent courses: 30 mg/m^2/day for 2 days

Dosing adjustment in renal impairment:

The FDA-approved labeling recommends the following adjustment: S_{cr} >3 mg/dL: Administer 50% of normal dose

The following guidelines have been used by some clinicians (Aronoff, 2007):

Children:

Cl_{cr} <30 mL/minute: Administer 50% of dose

Hemodialysis/continuous ambulatory peritoneal dialysis (CAPD): Administer 50% of dose

Adults: No adjustment recommended

Dosing adjustment in hepatic impairment:

The FDA-approved labeling recommends the following adjustments:

Serum bilirubin 1.2-3 mg/dL: Administer 75% of dose

Serum bilirubin >3 mg/dL: Administer 50% of dose

The following guidelines have been used by some clinicians (Floyd, 2006):

Serum bilirubin 1.2-3 mg/dL: Administer 75% of dose

Serum bilirubin 3.1-5 mg/dL: Administer 50% of dose

Serum bilirubin >5 mg/dL: Avoid use

Administration Not for I.M. or SubQ administration. Administer as slow I.V. push over 1-5 minutes into the tubing of a rapidly infusing I.V. solution of D_5W or NS or dilute in 100 mL of D_5W or NS and infuse over 15-30 minutes.

Monitoring Parameters CBC with differential and platelet count, liver function test, ECG, left ventricular ejection function (echocardiography [ECHO] or multigated radionuclide angiography [MUGA] scan), renal function test

Dosage Forms Excipient information presented when available (limited, particularly for generics); consult specific product labeling. **Note: Strength expressed as base**

Injection, powder for reconstitution: 20 mg

Cerubidine®: 20 mg [contains mannitol 100 mg]

Injection, solution: 5 mg/mL (4 mL, 10 mL)

◆ **DAUNOrubicin Liposomal** *see* DAUNOrubicin Citrate (Liposomal) *on page 406*

◆ **DaunoXome®** *see* DAUNOrubicin Citrate (Liposomal) *on page 406*

◆ **1-Day™ [OTC]** *see* Tioconazole *on page 1475*

◆ **Dayhist® Allergy [OTC]** *see* Clemastine *on page 343*

◆ **Daypro®** *see* Oxaprozin *on page 1114*

◆ **Daytrana™** *see* Methylphenidate *on page 973*

◆ **dCF** *see* Pentostatin *on page 1171*

◆ **DDAVP®** *see* Desmopressin *on page 421*

- **DDAVP® Melt (Can)** *see* Desmopressin *on page 421*
- **ddI** *see* Didanosine *on page 441*
- **1-Deamino-8-D-Arginine Vasopressin** *see* Desmopressin *on page 421*
- **Debrox® [OTC]** *see* Carbamide Peroxide *on page 254*
- **Deca-Durabolin® (Can)** *see* Nandrolone *on page 1040*
- **Decavac®** *see* Diphtheria and Tetanus Toxoid *on page 460*
- **Dec-Chlorphen** *see* Chlorpheniramine and Phenylephrine *on page 309*
- **Dec-Chlorphen DM [DSC]** *see* Chlorpheniramine, Phenylephrine, and Dextromethorphan *on page 311*
- **De-Chlor DM** *see* Chlorpheniramine, Phenylephrine, and Dextromethorphan *on page 311*
- **De-Chlor DR** *see* Chlorpheniramine, Phenylephrine, and Dextromethorphan *on page 311*

Decitabine (de SYE ta been)

U.S. Brand Names Dacogen™

Index Terms 5-Aza-2'-deoxycytidine; 5-AzaC; NSC-127716

Pharmacologic Category Antineoplastic Agent, DNA Methylation Inhibitor

Use Treatment of myelodysplastic syndrome (MDS)

Unlabeled/Investigational Use Treatment of acute myelogenous leukemia (AML), chronic myelogenous leukemia (CML), sickle cell anemia

Pregnancy Risk Factor D

Pregnancy Considerations Teratogenic effects, decreased fetal weight, and increased fetal deaths were observed in animal studies. There are no adequate and well-controlled studies in pregnant women. Women of childbearing potential should be advised to avoid pregnancy during treatment. In addition, males should be advised to avoid fathering a child while on decitabine therapy and for 2 months after treatment.

Lactation Excretion in breast milk unknown/not recommended

Medication Safety Issues

High alert medication: The Institute for Safe Medication Practices (ISMP) includes this medication among its list of drug classes which have a heightened risk of causing significant patient harm when used in error.

Contraindications Hypersensitivity to decitabine or any component of the formulation

Warnings/Precautions Hazardous agent - use appropriate precautions for handling and disposal. The dose-limiting toxicity is bone marrow suppression; worsening neutropenia is common in first two treatment cycles and may not correlate with progression of underlying MDS; may require growth factor support. Not studied in hepatic and renal disease; use caution. Safety and efficacy in children have not been established.

Adverse Reactions

>10%:

Cardiovascular: Peripheral edema (25%), pallor (23%), edema (18%), cardiac murmur (16%)

Central nervous system: Pyrexia (6% to 53%), headache (28%), insomnia (28%), dizziness (18%), pain (13%), confusion (12%), lethargy (12%), anxiety (11%), hypoesthesia (11%)

Dermatologic: Petechiae (39%), bruising (22%), rash (19%), erythema (14%), cellulitis (12%), lesions (11%), pruritus (11%)

Endocrine & metabolic: Hyperglycemia (33%), hypoalbuminemia (7% to 24%), hypomagnesemia (24%), hypokalemia (22%), hyperkalemia (13%), hyponatremia (13%)

Gastrointestinal: Nausea (42%), constipation (35%), diarrhea (34%), vomiting (25%), anorexia (16%), appetite decreased (16%), abdominal pain (5% to 14%), oral mucosal petechiae (13%), stomatitis (12%), dyspepsia (12%)

Hematologic: Neutropenia (90%; recovery 28-50 days), thrombocytopenia (89%), anemia (82%), febrile neutropenia (29%), leukopenia (28%), lymphadenopathy (12%)

Hepatic: Hyperbilirubinemia (14%), alkaline phosphatase increased (11%)

Local: Tenderness (11%)

Neuromuscular & skeletal: Rigors (22%), arthralgia (20%), limb pain (19%), back pain (17%)

Respiratory: Cough (40%), pneumonia (22%), pharyngitis (16%), lung crackles (14%)

5% to 10%:

Cardiovascular: Chest discomfort (7%), facial swelling (6%), hypotension (6%)

Central nervous system: Malaise (5%)

Dermatologic: Alopecia (8%), urticaria (6%)

Endocrine & metabolic: Hyperuricemia (10%), LDH increased (8%), bicarbonate increased (6%), dehydration (6%), hypochloremia (6%), bicarbonate decreased (5%), hypoproteinemia (5%)

Gastrointestinal: Gingival bleeding (8%), hemorrhoids (8%), loose stools (7%), tongue ulceration (7%), dysphagia (6%), oral candidiasis (6%), lip ulceration (5%), abdominal distension (5%), gastroesophageal reflux (5%), glossodynia (5%)

Genitourinary: Urinary tract infection (7%), dysuria (6%), polyuria (5%)

Hematologic: Hematoma (5%), thrombocythemia (5%), bacteremia (5%)

Hepatic: Ascites (10%), AST increased (10%), hypobilirubinemia (5%)

Local: Catheter infection (8%), catheter site erythema (5%), catheter site pain (5%), injection site swelling (5%)

Neuromuscular & skeletal: Falling (8%), chest wall pain (7%), musculoskeletal discomfort (6%), crepitation (5%), myalgia (5%)

Ocular: Blurred vision (6%)

Respiratory: Breath sounds diminished (10%), hypoxia (10%), rales (8%), pulmonary edema (6%), postnasal drip (5%), sinusitis (5%)

Miscellaneous: Candidal infection (10%), staphylococcal infection (7%), transfusion reaction (7%)

<5% (Limited to important or life-threatening): Anaphylactic reaction, atrial fibrillation, bronchopulmonary aspergillosis, cardiomyopathy, cardiorespiratory failure, catheter site hemorrhage, chest pain, CHF, cholecystitis, dyspnea, fungal infection, gastrointestinal hemorrhage, hemoptysis, hypersensitivity, intracranial hemorrhage, MI, peridiverticular abscess, pseudomonal lung infection, pulmonary embolism, pulmonary infiltrates, pulmonary mass, renal failure, respiratory arrest, respiratory tract infection, sepsis, splenomegaly, supraventricular tachycardia, urethral hemorrhage, weakness

Drug Interactions

Avoid Concomitant Use There are no known interactions where it is recommended to avoid concomitant use.

Increased Effect/Toxicity There are no known significant interactions involving an increase in effect.

Decreased Effect There are no known significant interactions involving a decrease in effect.

Stability Store vials at 15°C to 30°C (59°F to 86°F). Vials should be reconstituted with 10 mL SWFI to a concentration of 5 mg/mL. Further dilute with 50-250 mL NS, D_5W, or lactated Ringer's to a final concentration of 0.1-1 mg/mL. Solutions not administered within 15 minutes of preparation should be prepared with cold (2°C to 8°C [36°F to 46°F]) infusion solutions. Solutions diluted for infusion may be stored for up to 7 hours under refrigeration at 2°C to 8°C (36°F to 46°F) if prepared with cold infusion fluids.

Mechanism of Action After phosphorylation, decitabine is incorporated into DNA and inhibits DNA methyltransferase causing hypomethylation and subsequent cell death.

Pharmacodynamics/Kinetics

Distribution: 63-89 L/m^2

Protein binding: <1%

Metabolism: Extrahepatic; possibly via deamination by cytidine deaminase

Half-life elimination: ~30-35 minutes

Time to peak: At end of infusion

Dosage Adults:

MDS: I.V.: 15 mg/m^2 over 3 hours every 8 hours (45 mg/m^2/day) for 3 days (135 mg/m^2/cycle) every 6 weeks (treatment is recommended for at least 4 cycles and may continue until the patient no longer continues to benefit)

or

Low-dose schedule (unlabeled): 20 mg/m^2 over 1 hour daily for 5 days every 28 days

AML (investigational use): I.V.:

5-15 mg/m^2 over 1 hour daily, 5 days/week for 2 weeks (5 days on, 2 days off, 5 days on; 10 doses total) every 6 weeks

or

15 mg/m^2 over 1 hour daily for 10 days every 6 weeks

CML (investigational use): I.V.:

20 mg/m^{2}over 1 hour daily for 5 days every 28 days

or

10-15 mg/m^2 over 1 hour daily, 5 days/week for 2 weeks (5 days on, 2 days off, 5 days on; 10 doses total) every 6 weeks

or

50-75 mg/m^2 over 6 hours every 12 hours for 5 days every 4-8 weeks

Sickle cell anemia (investigational use): I.V., SubQ: 0.15-0.3 mg/kg/day over 2 minutes 5 days/week for 2 weeks (5 days on, 2 days off, 5 days on; 10 doses total) every 6 weeks

Dosage adjustment for toxicity:

For delayed hematologic recovery (ANC ≥1000/mm^3 and platelets ≥50,000/mm^3):

Greater than 6 weeks but less than 8 weeks: Delay dose for up to 2 weeks and temporarily reduce dose to 11 mg/m^2 every 8 hours (33 mg/m^2/day) for 3 days

Greater than 8 weeks but less than 10 weeks: Assess for disease progression; if no disease progression, delay dose for up to 2 weeks and reduce dose to 11 mg/m^2 every 8 hours (33 mg/m^2/day) for 3 days; maintain or increase dose with subsequent cycles if clinically indicated

Temporarily hold treatment until resolution for any of the following nonhematologic toxicities:

Serum creatinine ≥2 mg/dL

ALT, bilirubin ≥2 times ULN

Active or uncontrolled infection

Administration Infuse over 1-6 hours. Premedication with antiemetics is recommended.

Monitoring Parameters CBC and platelets with each cycle, more frequently if needed; liver enzymes; serum creatinine

Dosage Forms Excipient information presented when available (limited, particularly for generics); consult specific product labeling.

Injection, powder for reconstitution:

Dacogen™: 50 mg

◆ **Declomycin®** *see* Demeclocycline *on page 416*

◆ **Deconamine® SR** *see* Chlorpheniramine and Pseudoephedrine *on page 310*

◆ **Deconsal® II** *see* Guaifenesin and Phenylephrine *on page 712*

◆ **Deep Sea [OTC]** *see* Sodium Chloride *on page 1381*

Deferasirox (de FER a sir ox)

U.S. Brand Names Exjade®

Canadian Brand Names Exjade®

Index Terms ICL670

Pharmacologic Category Antidote; Chelating Agent

Use Treatment of chronic iron overload due to blood transfusions (transfusional hemosiderosis)

Pregnancy Risk Factor B

Pregnancy Considerations Teratogenic effects were not observed in animal studies. There are no adequate and well-controlled studies in pregnant women. Use during pregnancy only if clearly needed.

Lactation Excretion in breast milk unknown/use caution

Medication Safety Issues

Sound-alike/look-alike issues:

Deferasirox may be confused with deferoxamine

Contraindications Hypersensitivity to deferasirox or any component of the formulation

Canadian labeling: Additional contraindications (not in U.S. labeling): Cl_{cr} <60 mL/minute

Warnings/Precautions Cases of acute renal failure (some fatal) and dose-related elevations in serum creatinine have been reported. Monitor serum creatinine in patients at risk for renal complications (eg, pre-existing renal conditions, elderly, comorbid conditions, and/or with concurrent medications that may affect renal function); consider dose reduction, interruption, or discontinuation for serum creatinine elevations. Has not been studied in patients with renal impairment; patients with baseline serum creatinine above the upper limit of normal (ULN) were excluded from clinical trials. May cause proteinuria; closely monitor.

Severe hepatic dysfunction or failure (including fatalities) have occurred (postmarketing reports), mostly in patients >55 years of age with underlying comorbidities (including hepatic cirrhosis and multiorgan failure). Hepatitis and elevated transaminases have also been reported; monitor transaminases and consider dose modification or interruption of therapy with severe or persistent hepatic function test abnormalities. Has not been studied in patients with hepatic impairment, although has been used in patients with baseline transaminases ≤5 times ULN (deferasirox pharmacokinetics were not altered with these transaminase levels); use with caution. Gastrointestinal (GI) irritation, as well as upper GI ulceration and hemorrhage have been reported. Use caution with concurrent medications that may increase risk of adverse GI effects (eg, NSAIDs, corticosteroids, anticoagulants). Monitor patients closely for signs/symptoms of GI ulceration/bleeding.

May cause skin rash (dose-related); mild-to-moderate rashes may resolve without treatment interruption; for severe rash, interrupt and consider restarting at a lower dose with dose escalation and oral steroids. Hypersensitivity reactions, including severe reactions (anaphylaxis and angioedema) have been reported, usually within the first month of treatment. Discontinuation of therapy may be necessary. Auditory (decreased hearing and high frequency hearing loss) or ocular disturbances (lens opacities, cataracts, intraocular pressure elevation, and retinal disorders) have been reported; monitor and consider dose reduction or treatment interruption. Cytopenias (including agranulocytosis, neutropenia, and thrombocytopenia) have been reported, predominately in patients with preexisting hematologic disorders; monitor closely; interrupt treatment for unexplained cytopenias. Do not combine with other iron chelation therapies; safety of combinations has not been established. Safety and efficacy in children <2 years of age have not been established.

Adverse Reactions

>10%:

Central nervous system: Fever (19%), headache (16%)

Dermatologic: Rash (8% to 11%)

Gastrointestinal: Abdominal pain (21% to 28%), diarrhea (12% to 20%), nausea (11% to 23%), vomiting (10% to 21%)

Renal: Serum creatinine increased (dose related; 7% to 38%), proteinuria (19%)

Respiratory: Cough (14%), nasopharyngitis (13%), pharyngolaryngeal pain (11%)

Miscellaneous: Influenza (11%)

1% to 10%:

Central nervous system: Fatigue (6%)

Dermatologic: Urticaria (4%)

Hepatic: ALT increased (2% to 8%), transaminitis (4%)

Neuromuscular & skeletal: Arthralgia (7%), back pain (6%)

Otic: Ear infection (5%)

Respiratory: Respiratory tract infection (10%), bronchitis (9%), pharyngitis (8%), acute tonsillitis (6%), rhinitis (6%)

<1% (Limited to important or life-threatening): Acute renal failure, agranulocytosis, anaphylaxis, angioedema, anxiety, ascites, bilirubin increased, cataract, cholecystitis, cholelithiasis, constipation, cytopenias, dizziness, drug fever, duodenal ulcer, edema, erythema multiforme, esophagitis, gastric ulcer, gastritis, gastrointestinal bleeding, glomerulonephritis, glucosuria, hearing loss (including high frequency), hematuria, Henoch-Schönlein purpura, hepatic dysfunction, hepatic encephalopathy, hepatic failure (including fatalities), hepatic transaminases increased, hepatitis, hyperactivity, hypersensitivity reaction, insomnia, interstitial nephritis, intraocular pressure increased, jaundice, lens opacities, leukocytoclastic vasculitis, maculopathy, neutropenia, optic neuritis, pigment disorder, purpura, renal tubular necrosis, renal tubulopathy, retinal disorder, sleep disorder, thrombocytopenia, visual disturbance

Drug Interactions

Avoid Concomitant Use There are no known interactions where it is recommended to avoid concomitant use.

Increased Effect/Toxicity There are no known significant interactions involving an increase in effect.

Decreased Effect

Deferasirox may decrease the levels/effects of: CYP3A4 Substrates

The levels/effects of Deferasirox may be decreased by: Aluminum Hydroxide

Stability Store at room temperature of 25°C (77°F); excursions between 15°C and 30°C (59°F and 86°F) permitted. Protect from moisture.

Mechanism of Action Selectively binds iron, forming a complex which is excreted primarily through the feces.

Pharmacodynamics/Kinetics

Distribution: Adults: 11.7-17.1 L

Protein binding: ~99% to serum albumin

Metabolism: Hepatic via glucuronidation by UGT1A1 (primarily) and UGT1A3; minor oxidation by CYP450; undergoes enterohepatic recirculation

Bioavailability: 70%

Half-life elimination: 8-16 hours

Time to peak, plasma: ~1.5 hours

Excretion: Feces (84%), urine (8%)

Dosage Oral: Children ≥2 years and Adults:

Initial: 20 mg/kg daily (calculate dose to nearest whole tablet)

Maintenance: Adjust dose every 3-6 months based on serum ferritin levels; increase by 5-10 mg/kg/day (calculate dose to nearest whole tablet); titrate. Maximum dose: 30 mg/kg/day; consider interrupting therapy for serum ferritin <500 mcg/L. In clinical trials, doses were individualized based on iron burden determined by liver iron concentrations (LIC); transfusional iron intake should be considered when individualizing maintenance dose. **Note:** Consider dose reduction or interruption for hearing loss or visual disturbances.

Dosage adjustment in renal impairment: Interrupt treatment for progressive increase in serum creatinine above the age-appropriate ULN; once serum creatinine recovers to within the normal range, reinitiate treatment at a reduced dose; gradually escalate the dose if the clinical benefit outweighs potential risk.

Children: For increase in serum creatinine >33% on 2 consecutive measures and above the age-appropriate ULN for 2 consecutive levels, reduce daily dose by 10 mg/kg

Adults: For increase in serum creatinine >33% above the average pretreatment level at 2 consecutive levels (and cannot be attributed to other causes), reduce daily dose by 10 mg/kg

Dosage adjustment in hepatic impairment: Consider dose adjustment or discontinuation for severe or persistent elevations in liver function tests.

Dietary Considerations Bioavailability increased variably when taken with food; take on empty stomach 30 minutes before a meal.

Administration Do not chew or swallow whole tablets. Take at same time each day on an empty stomach, 30 minutes before food. Disperse tablets in water, orange juice, or apple juice (use 3.5 ounces for total doses <1 g; 7 ounces for doses ≥1 g); stir to form suspension and drink entire contents. Rinse remaining residue with more fluid; drink. Do not take simultaneously with aluminum-containing antacids.

Monitoring Parameters

CBC with differential, serum creatinine (twice prior to initiation, then monthly thereafter; monitor patients with renal risk factors or with changes in therapy weekly for the first month and then monthly thereafter, urine protein (monthly), liver function tests (monthly), and serum ferritin (monthly); baseline and annual auditory and ophthalmic function (including slit lamp exam and dilated fundoscopy)

Additional Information Deferasirox has a low affinity for binding with zinc and copper, may cause variable decreases in the serum concentration of these trace minerals.

Oncology Comment: The National Comprehensive Cancer Network (NCCN) guidelines for myelodysplastic syndromes (MDS) recommend iron chelation therapy in relatively low-risk MDS patients to reverse adverse effects (on cardiac, hepatic and endocrine function) from chronic iron overload due to multiple transfusions. Treatment is generally recommended in MDS patients who have received ≥20 units of RBC transfusions and for those with serum ferritin levels >2500 mcg/L. Although clinical trials in MDS are ongoing, deferasirox may be useful in the management of iron overload of these patients.

Dosage Forms Excipient information presented when available (limited, particularly for generics); consult specific product labeling.

Tablet, for oral suspension:

Exjade®: 125 mg, 250 mg, 500 mg

Deferoxamine (de fer OKS a meen)

U.S. Brand Names Desferal®

Canadian Brand Names Desferal®; PMS-Deferoxamine

Index Terms Deferoxamine Mesylate; Desferrioxamine; NSC-644468

Pharmacologic Category Antidote; Chelating Agent

Use Acute iron intoxication or when clinical signs of significant iron toxicity exist; chronic iron overload secondary to multiple transfusions

Unlabeled/Investigational Use Removal of corneal rust rings following surgical removal of foreign bodies; diagnosis or treatment of aluminum induced toxicity associated with chronic kidney disease (CKD)

Pregnancy Risk Factor C

Pregnancy Considerations Skeletal anomalies and delayed ossification were observed in some but not all animal studies. Toxic amounts of iron or deferoxamine have not been noted to cross the placenta. In case of acute toxicity, treatment during pregnancy should not be withheld.

Lactation Excretion in breast milk unknown/use caution

Medication Safety Issues

Sound-alike/look-alike issues:

Deferoxamine may be confused with cefuroxime, deferasirox

Desferal® may be confused with desflurane, Dexferrum®, Disophrol®

International issues:

Desferal® may be confused with Deseril® which is a brand name for methysergide in multiple international markets

Contraindications Hypersensitivity to deferoxamine or any component of the formulation; patients with severe renal disease or anuria, primary hemochromatosis

Warnings/Precautions Patients with iron overload are at increased susceptibility to infection with *Yersinia enterocolitica* and *Yersinia pseudotuberculosis;* treatment with deferoxamine may enhance this risk; if infection develops, discontinue deferoxamine until resolved. Rare and serious cases of mucormycosis have been reported with use; withhold treatment with signs and symptoms of mucormycosis. Combination treatment with ascorbic acid may impair cardiac function (rare). If combination treatment is warranted, therapy may need adjusted; monitor cardiac function. Do not administer deferoxamine in combination with ascorbic acid in patients with pre-existing cardiac failure.

High doses may exacerbate neurological symptoms, including seizure in patients with aluminum-related encephalopathy. Deferoxamine treatment in patients with aluminum toxicity may cause hypocalcemia and aggravate hyperparathyroidism. Deferoxamine is associated with dialysis dementia onset. Ocular and auditory disturbances have been reported following prolonged administration at high doses, or in patients with low ferritin levels; elderly patients are at increased risk for ocular and auditory disorders. Has been associated with adult respiratory distress syndrome (ARDS) following excessively high-dose treatment of acute intoxication or thalassemia; has also been reported in children. Flushing, hypotension, urticaria and shock are associated with rapid infusions. Patients should be informed that urine may have a reddish color. High deferoxamine doses and low ferritin levels are also associated with growth retardation. Safety and efficacy have not been established in children <3 years of age.

Adverse Reactions Frequency not defined.

Cardiovascular: Flushing, hypotension, tachycardia, shock, edema

Central nervous system: Fever, dizziness, neuropathy, seizure, exacerbation of aluminum-related encephalopathy (dialysis), headache

Dermatologic: Angioedema, rash, urticaria

Endocrine & metabolic: Growth retardation (children), hypocalcemia

Gastrointestinal: Abdominal discomfort, abdominal pain, diarrhea, nausea, vomiting

Genitourinary: Dysuria

Hematologic: Thrombocytopenia, leukopenia

Local: Injection site: Burning, crust, edema, erythema, eschar, induration, infiltration, irritation, pain, pruritus, swelling, vesicles, wheal formation

Neuromuscular & skeletal: Arthralgia, leg cramps, metaphyseal dysplasia (dose related), myalgia, paresthesia

Ocular: Acuity decreased, blurred vision, dichromatopsia, maculopathy, night vision impaired, peripheral vision impaired, visual loss, scotoma, visual field defects, optic neuritis, cataracts, retinal pigmentary abnormalities, night blindness

Otic: Hearing loss, tinnitus

Renal: Renal impairment, urine discoloration (vin-rose color)

Respiratory: Acute/adult respiratory distress syndrome, asthma

Miscellaneous: Anaphylaxis, hypersensitivity reaction, infections (*Yersinia*, mucormycosis)

Drug Interactions

Avoid Concomitant Use There are no known interactions where it is recommended to avoid concomitant use.

Increased Effect/Toxicity

The levels/effects of Deferoxamine may be increased by: Ascorbic Acid

Decreased Effect There are no known significant interactions involving a decrease in effect.

Stability Prior to reconstitution, do not store above 25°C (77°F). Following reconstitution, may be stored at room temperature for 7 days; protect from light. Do not refrigerate reconstituted solution.

Reconstitution:

I.M.: Reconstitute with sterile water for injection (500 mg vial with 2 mL to a final concentration of 210 mg/mL; 2000 mg vial with 8 mL to a final concentration of 213 mg/mL)

I.V.: Reconstitute with sterile water for injection to a final solution of 100 mg/mL

SubQ: Reconstitute with sterile water for injection (500 mg vial with 5 mL; 2000 mg vial with 20 mL) to a final concentration of 95 mg/mL

Mechanism of Action Complexes with trivalent ions (ferric ions) to form ferrioxamine, which are removed by the kidneys

Pharmacodynamics/Kinetics

Absorption: I.M.: Erratic

Metabolism: Plasma enzymes; binds with iron to form ferrioxamine

Half-life elimination: Parent drug: 6.1 hours; Ferrioxamine: 5.8 hours

Excretion: Primarily urine (as unchanged drug and ferrioxamine); feces (via bile)

Dosage

Acute iron toxicity: **Note:** I.V. route is used when severe toxicity is evidenced by systemic symptoms (coma, shock, metabolic acidosis, or severe gastrointestinal bleeding) or potentially severe intoxications (serum iron level >500 mcg/dL). When severe symptoms are not present, the I.M. route may be preferred (per manufacturer); however, the use of deferoxamine in situations where the serum iron concentration is <500 mcg/dL or when severe toxicity is not evident is a subject of some clinical debate.

Children ≥3 years:

I.M.: 90 mg/kg/dose every 8 hours (maximum: 6 g/24 hours)

I.V.: 15 mg/kg/hour (maximum: 6 g/24 hours)

Adults: I.M., I.V.: Initial: 1000 mg, may be followed by 500 mg every 4 hours for up to 2 doses; subsequent doses of 500 mg have been administered every 4-12 hours

Maximum recommended dose: 6 g/day (per manufacturer, however, higher doses have been administered)

Chronic iron overload:
Children ≥3 years:
I.V.: 15 mg/kg/hour (maximum: 12 g/24 hours)
SubQ: 20-40 mg/kg/day over 8-12 hours (maximum: 1000-2000 mg/day)
Adults:
I.M., I.V.: 500-1000 mg/day I.M.; in addition, 2000 mg should be given I.V. with each unit of blood transfused (administer separately from blood); maximum: 1 g/day in absence of transfusions; 6 g/day if patient received transfusions
SubQ: 1-2 g every day or 20-40 mg/kg/day over 8-24 hours
Diagnosis of aluminum induced toxicity with CKD (unlabeled use): Children and Adults: I.V.: Test dose: 5 mg/kg during the last hour of dialysis if serum aluminum levels are 60-200 mcg/L and there are clinical signs/symptoms of toxicity. Do not use if aluminum serum levels are >200 mcg/L
Treatment of aluminum toxicity with CKD (unlabeled use): Children and Adults: I.V.: 5-10 mg/kg 4-6 hours before dialysis. Administer every 7-10 days with 3-4 dialysis procedures between doses. Do not use if aluminum serum levels are >200 mcg/L.

Dosing adjustment in renal impairment: Cl_{cr} <10 mL/minute: Administer 50% of dose

Dietary Considerations Vitamin C supplements may need to be limited. The manufacturer recommends a maximum of 200 mg/day in adults (given in divided doses) and avoiding use in patients with heart failure.

Administration
I.V.: Urticaria, hypotension, and shock have occurred following rapid I.V. administration; limiting infusion rate to 15mg/kg/hour may help avoid infusion-related adverse effects.
Acute iron toxicity: The manufacturer states that the I.M. route is preferred; however, the I.V. route is generally preferred in patients with severe toxicity (ie, patients in shock). For the first 1000 mg, infuse at 15 mg/kg/hour (although rates up to 40-50 mg/kg/hour have been given in patients with massive iron intoxication). Subsequent doses may be given over 4-12 hours at a rate not to exceed 125 mg/hour.
Diagnosis or treatment of aluminum induced toxicity with CKD: Administer dose over 1 hour
SubQ: When administered for chronic iron overload, daily dose should be given over 8-24 hours using portable pump.

Monitoring Parameters Serum iron; ophthalmologic exam (fundoscopy, slit-lamp exam) and audiometry with chronic therapy; growth and body weight in children (every 3 months)

Dialysis patients: Serum aluminum (yearly; every 3 months in patients on aluminum-containing medications)
Aluminum-induced bone disease: Serum aluminum 2 days following test dose; test is considered positive if serum aluminum increases ≥50 mcg/L

Reference Range
Iron, serum: Normal: 50-150 mcg/dL; levels >500 mcg/dL associated with toxicity. Consider treatment with symptomatic patients with levels ≥350 mcg/dL; toxicity cannot be excluded with serum iron levels <350 mcg/dL
Aluminum, serum: <20 mcg/L recommended baseline level in dialysis patients

Test Interactions TIBC may be falsely elevated with high serum iron concentrations or deferoxamine therapy. Imaging results may be distorted due to rapid urinary excretion of deferoxamine-bound gallium-67; discontinue deferoxamine 48 hours prior to scintigraphy.

Dosage Forms Excipient information presented when available (limited, particularly for generics); consult specific product labeling.

Injection, powder for reconstitution, as mesylate: 500 mg, 2 g
Desferal®: 500 mg, 2 g

◆ **Deferoxamine Mesylate** *see* Deferoxamine *on page 411*

Degarelix (deg a REL ix)

Index Terms Degarelix Acetate; FE200486

Pharmacologic Category Antineoplastic Agent, Gonadotropin-Releasing Hormone Antagonist; Gonadotropin Releasing Hormone Antagonist

Use Treatment of advanced prostate cancer

Pregnancy Risk Factor X

Pregnancy Considerations Animal studies have demonstrated embryo and fetal loss. Use is contraindicated in women who are or may become pregnant.

Lactation Excretion in breast milk unknown/not recommended

Medication Safety Issues
Sound-alike/look-alike issues:
Degarelix may be confused with cetrorelix, ganirelix

Contraindications Hypersensitivity to degarelix or any component of the formulation; pregnancy (or potential to become pregnant)

Warnings/Precautions Hazardous agent - use appropriate precautions for handling and disposal. Androgen deprivation therapy may prolong the QT interval; use with caution in patients with a known history of QT prolongation or other risk factors for QT prolongation (eg, concomitant use of medications known to prolong QT interval, heart failure, and/or electrolyte abnormalities). Androgen deprivation therapy may increase the risk for cardiovascular disease and decreased bone mineral density. Androgen deprivation therapy may cause obesity and insulin resistance; the risk for diabetes is increased.

Degarelix exposure is decreased in patients with hepatic impairment, dosage adjustment is not recommended in patients with mild-to-moderate hepatic impairment, although testosterone levels should be monitored. Has not been studied in patients with severe hepatic impairment; use with caution. Data for use in patients with moderate-to-severe renal impairment (Cl_{cr} <50 mL/minute) is limited; use with caution. Safety and efficacy have not been established in children.

Adverse Reactions
>10%:
Endocrine & metabolic: Hot flashes (26%)
Local: Injections site reactions (35%, grade 3: ≤2%; pain 28%, erythema 17%, swelling 6%, induration 4%, nodule 3%)
1% to 10%:
Cardiovascular: Hypertension (6%)
Central nervous system: Chills (5%), dizziness (1% to 5%), fever (1% to 5%), headache (1% to 5%), insomnia (1% to 5%), fatigue (3%)
Dermatologic: Hyperhydrosis
Endocrine & metabolic: Hypercholesterolemia (3%), gynecomastia, testicular atrophy
Gastrointestinal: Weight gain (9%), constipation (5%), nausea (1% to 5%), diarrhea
Genitourinary: Urinary tract infection (5%), erectile dysfunction
Hepatic: ALT increased (10%; grade 3: <1%), AST increased (5%; grade 3: <1%), GGT increased
Neuromuscular & skeletal: Back pain (6%), arthralgia (5%), weakness (1% to 5%)
Miscellaneous: Antidegarelix antibody formation (10%), night sweats (1% to 5%)
<1% (Limited to important or life-threatening): Bone metastases worsening, cerebral stroke, depression, injection site pruritus, injection site soreness, lymphoma

(malignant), mental status changes, MI, osteoarthritis, QT interval prolongation, squamous cell cancer, unstable angina

Drug Interactions

Avoid Concomitant Use

Avoid concomitant use of Degarelix with any of the following: Nilotinib; Tetrabenazine; Thioridazine; Ziprasidone

Increased Effect/Toxicity

Degarelix may increase the levels/effects of: QTc-Prolonging Agents; Tetrabenazine; Thioridazine; Ziprasidone

The levels/effects of Degarelix may be increased by: Alfuzosin; Ciprofloxacin; Gadobutrol; Nilotinib

Decreased Effect There are no known significant interactions involving a decrease in effect.

Stability Store at 25°C (77°F); excursions permitted to 15°C to 30°C (59°F to 86°F). Use appropriate precautions (wear gloves for preparation and administration) for handling and disposal. Reconstitute with preservative free sterile water for injection (reconstitute each 120 mg vial with 3 mL; reconstitute the 80 mg vial with 4.2 mL). Swirl gently; do not shake (to prevent foaming). Dissolution may take up to 15 minutes. Keep vial upright at all times. Tilt vial slightly, keeping needle in lowest section of vial to withdraw for administration. Administer within 1 hour of reconstitution.

Mechanism of Action Gonadotropin-releasing hormone (GnRH) antagonist which reversibly binds to GnRH receptors in the anterior pituitary gland, blocking the receptor and decreasing secretion of luteinizing hormone (LH) and follicle stimulation hormone (FSH), resulting in rapid androgen deprivation by decreasing testosterone production, thereby decreasing testosterone levels. Testosterone levels do not exhibit an initial surge, or flare, as is typical with GnRH agonists.

Pharmacodynamics/Kinetics

Onset of action: Rapid; ~96% of patients had testosterone levels ≤50 ng/dL within 3 days (Klotz, 2008)

Distribution: V_d: >1000 L

Protein binding: ~90%

Metabolism: Hepatobiliary, via peptide hydrolysis

Bioavailability: Biphasic release: Rapid release initially, then slow release from depot formed after subcutaneous injection administration (Tornoe, 2007)

Half-life elimination: Loading dose: SubQ: ~53 days

Time to peak, plasma: Loading dose: SubQ: Within 2 days

Excretion: Feces (~70% to 80%, primarily as peptide fragments); urine (~20% to 30%)

Dosage SubQ: Adults: Prostate cancer:

Loading dose: 240 mg administered as two 120 mg (3 mL) injections

Maintenance dose: 80 mg every 28 days (beginning 28 days after initial loading dose)

Dosage adjustment in renal impairment: Cl_{cr} <50 mL/minute: Use with caution

Dosage adjustment in hepatic impairment:

Mild-to-moderate hepatic impairment: No adjustment required; monitor serum testosterone levels

Severe hepatic impairment: Has not been studied; use with caution

Dietary Considerations Supplementation with 500 mg calcium and 400 int. units of vitamin D is recommended (due to the increased risk for osteoporosis with androgen deprivation therapy).

Administration Not for I.V. use. Administer SubQ in the abdominal area by grasping skin and elevating SubQ tissue; inject at an angle ≤45 degrees. Avoid pressure exposed areas (eg, waistband, near ribs); rotate injection site. Inject loading dose as two 3 mL injections (40 mg/mL); maintenance dose should be administered as one 4mL injection (20 mg/mL); begin maintenance dose 28 days after initial loading dose.

Monitoring Parameters Prostate-specific antigen (PSA) periodically, serum testosterone levels (if PSA increases; in patients with hepatic impairment: monitor testosterone levels monthly until achieve castration levels, then consider monitoring every other month), liver function tests (at baseline), serum electrolytes (calcium, magnesium, potassium, sodium); bone mineral density

Screen for diabetes and cardiovascular risk prior to initiating treatment.

Test Interactions Suppression of pituitary-gonadal function may affect diagnostic tests of pituitary gonadotropic and gonadal functions.

Product Availability Degarelix (brand name pending): FDA approved December 2008; availability anticipated towards the end of 2009

Dosage Forms Excipient information presented when available (limited, particularly for generics); consult specific product labeling.

Injection, powder for reconstitution, as acetate: 80 mg, 120 mg

- **Degarelix Acetate** *see* Degarelix *on page 413*
- **Dehistine** *see* Chlorpheniramine, Phenylephrine, and Methscopolamine *on page 313*
- **Dehydral® (Can)** *see* Methenamine *on page 961*
- **Dehydrobenzperidol** *see* Droperidol *on page 495*
- **Delatestryl®** *see* Testosterone *on page 1445*

Delavirdine (de la VIR deen)

U.S. Brand Names Rescriptor®

Canadian Brand Names Rescriptor®

Index Terms U-90152S

Pharmacologic Category Antiretroviral Agent, Reverse Transcriptase Inhibitor (Non-nucleoside)

Additional Appendix Information

Management of Healthcare Worker Exposures to HBV, HCV, and HIV *on page 1719*

Perinatal HIV Guidelines *on page 1730*

Use Treatment of HIV-1 infection in combination with at least two additional antiretroviral agents

Pregnancy Risk Factor C

Pregnancy Considerations It is not known if delavirdine crosses the human placenta. Delavirdine was shown to be teratogenic in some animal studies. There are no adequate and well-controlled studies in pregnant women and use during pregnancy is not recommended unless other alternatives are not available. Health professionals are encouraged to contact the antiretroviral pregnancy registry to monitor outcomes of pregnant women exposed to antiretroviral medications (1-800-258-4263 or www.APRegistry.com).

Lactation Excretion in breast milk unknown/contraindicated

Contraindications Hypersensitivity to delavirdine or any component of the formulation; concurrent use of alprazolam, cisapride, ergot alkaloids, midazolam, pimozide, rifampin, or triazolam

Warnings/Precautions Use with caution in patients with hepatic or renal dysfunction; due to rapid emergence of resistance, delavirdine should not be used as monotherapy; cross-resistance may be conferred to other non-nucleoside reverse transcriptase inhibitors, although potential for cross-resistance with protease inhibitors is low. Long-term effects of delavirdine are not known. May cause redistribution of fat (eg, buffalo hump, peripheral wasting with increased abdominal girth, cushingoid appearance). Immune reconstitution syndrome may develop resulting in the occurrence of an inflammatory response to an indolent or residual opportunistic infection; further evaluation and treatment may be required. Safety and efficacy have not been established in children. Rash, which occurs frequently, may require discontinuation of therapy; usually occurs within 1-3 weeks and lasts <2 weeks. Most patients may resume therapy following a treatment interruption. Use with caution in patients taking strong CYP3A4 inhibitors, moderate or strong CYP3A4 inducers and major CYP3A4 substrates (see Drug Interactions); consider alternative agents that avoid or lessen the potential for CYP-mediated interactions.

Adverse Reactions

Frequency of adverse reactions reported from occurrence in clinical trials with delavirdine when used as part of combination antiretroviral therapy.

>10%:

Central nervous system: Headache (19% to 20%), depressive symptoms (10% to 15%), fever (4% to 12%)

Dermatologic: Rash (16% to 32%)

Gastrointestinal: Nausea (20% to 25%), vomiting (3% to 11%)

1% to 10%:

Central nervous system: Anxiety (6% to 8%)

Endocrine & metabolic: Transaminases increased (2% to 5%), amylase increased (3%), bilirubin increased (2%)

Gastrointestinal: Diarrhea, vomiting, abdominal pain (4% to 6%)

Hematologic: Prothrombin time increased (2%), hemoglobin decreased (1% to 3%)

Respiratory: Bronchitis (6% to 8%)

Frequency not defined (limited to important or life threatening): Abscess, adenopathy, alkaline phosphatase increased, allergic reaction, angioedema, anorexia, arrhythmia, bloody stool, bone pain, bruising, cardiac insufficiency, cardiac rate abnormal, cardiomyopathy, chest congestion, cognitive impairment, colitis, confusion, conjunctivitis, dermal leukocytoclastic vasculitis, desquamation, diverticulitis, dyspnea, emotional lability, eosinophilia, erythema multiforme, fecal incontinence, fungal dermatitis, gamma glutamyl transpeptidase increased, gastroenteritis, gastrointestinal bleeding, granulocytosis, gum hemorrhage, hallucination, hematuria, hepatomegaly, hyperglycemia, hyperkalemia, hypertension, hypertriglyceridemia, hyperuricemia, hypocalcemia, hyponatremia, hypophosphatemia, infection, jaundice, kidney pain, leukopenia, lipase increased, menstrual irregularities, moniliasis (oral/vaginal), pancreatitis, pancytopenia, paralysis, peripheral vascular disorder, pneumonia, postural hypotension, purpura, redistribution of body fat, renal calculi, serum creatinine increased, spleen disorder, Stevens-Johnson syndrome, tetany, thrombocytopenia, urinary tract infection, vertigo

Postmarketing and/or case reports: Acute renal failure, hemolytic anemia, hepatic failure, immune reconstitution syndrome, rhabdomyolysis

Drug Interactions

Metabolism/Transport Effects **Substrate** of CYP2D6 (minor), 3A4 (major); **Inhibits** CYP1A2 (weak), 2C9 (strong), 2C19 (strong), 2D6 (strong), 3A4 (strong)

Avoid Concomitant Use

Avoid concomitant use of Delavirdine with any of the following: Alfuzosin; Amprenavir; Eplerenone; Etravirine; Fosamprenavir; Nilotinib; Nisoldipine; Ranolazine; Rivaroxaban; Salmeterol; Silodosin; Tamoxifen; Thioridazine

Increased Effect/Toxicity

Delavirdine may increase the levels/effects of: Alfuzosin; Alosetron; Amprenavir; Ciclesonide; CYP2C19 Substrates; CYP2C9 Substrates (High risk); CYP2D6 Substrates; CYP3A4 Substrates; Eplerenone; Etravirine; FentaNYL; Fesoterodine; Fosamprenavir; Ixabepilone; Maraviroc; Nebivolol; Nilotinib; Nisoldipine; Pimecrolimus; Protease Inhibitors; Ranolazine; Rifamycin Derivatives; Rivaroxaban; Salmeterol; Silodosin; Sorafenib; Tamoxifen; Tetrabenazine; Thioridazine

Decreased Effect

Delavirdine may decrease the levels/effects of: Codeine; Etravirine; TraMADol

The levels/effects of Delavirdine may be decreased by: Amprenavir; Antacids; CYP3A4 Inducers (Strong); Deferasirox; Fosamprenavir; Herbs (CYP3A4 Inducers); Protease Inhibitors; Rifamycin Derivatives

Ethanol/Nutrition/Herb Interactions Herb/Nutraceutical: Delavirdine serum concentration may be decreased by St John's wort; avoid concurrent use.

Stability Store at 20°C to 25°C (68°F to 77°F); protect from humidity.

Mechanism of Action Delavirdine binds directly to reverse transcriptase, blocking RNA-dependent and DNA-dependent DNA polymerase activities

Pharmacodynamics/Kinetics

Absorption: Rapid

Distribution: Low concentration in saliva and semen; CSF 0.4% concurrent plasma concentration

Protein binding: ~98%, primarily albumin

Metabolism: Hepatic via CYP3A4 and 2D6 (**Note:** May reduce CYP3A activity and inhibit its own metabolism.)

Bioavailability: Tablet: 85% as tablet; ~100% as oral slurry

Half-life elimination: 5.8 hours (range: 2-11 hours)

Time to peak, plasma: 1 hour

Excretion: Urine (51%, <5% as unchanged drug); feces (44%); nonlinear kinetics exhibited

Dosage Adolescents ≥16 years and Adults: Oral: 400 mg 3 times/day

Dietary Considerations May be taken without regard to food.

Administration Patients with achlorhydria should take the drug with an acidic beverage; antacids and delavirdine should be separated by 1 hour. A dispersion of delavirdine may be prepared by adding four 100 mg tablets to at least 3 oz of water. Allow to stand for a few minutes and stir until uniform dispersion. Drink immediately. Rinse glass and mouth, then swallow the rinse to ensure total dose administered. The 200 mg tablets should be taken intact.

Monitoring Parameters Liver function tests if administered with saquinavir

Additional Information Potential compliance problems, frequency of administration, and adverse effects should be discussed with patients before initiating therapy to help prevent the emergence of resistance.

Dosage Forms Excipient information presented when available (limited, particularly for generics); consult specific product labeling.

Tablet, as mesylate: 100 mg, 200 mg

Extemporaneous Preparations A dispersion of delavirdine may be prepared by adding four 100 mg tablets to at least 3 oz of water; allow to stand for a few minutes and stir until uniform dispersion; drink immediately; rinse glass and mouth following ingestion to ensure total dose administered

- **Delestrogen®** *see* Estradiol *on page 554*
- **Delfen® [OTC]** *see* Nonoxynol 9 *on page 1077*
- **Delta-9-tetrahydro-cannabinol** *see* Dronabinol *on page 494*
- **Delta-9 THC** *see* Dronabinol *on page 494*
- **Deltacortisone** *see* PredniSONE *on page 1232*
- **Deltadehydrocortisone** *see* PredniSONE *on page 1232*
- **Deltahydrocortisone** *see* PrednisoLONE *on page 1230*
- **Demadex®** *see* Torsemide *on page 1494*

Demeclocycline (dem e kloe SYE kleen)

U.S. Brand Names Declomycin®

Canadian Brand Names Declomycin®

Index Terms Demeclocycline Hydrochloride; Demethylchlortetracycline

Pharmacologic Category Antibiotic, Tetracycline Derivative

Use Treatment of susceptible bacterial infections (acne, gonorrhea, pertussis, and urinary tract infections) caused by both gram-negative and gram-positive organisms

Unlabeled/Investigational Use Treatment of chronic syndrome of inappropriate secretion of antidiuretic hormone (SIADH)

Pregnancy Risk Factor D

Pregnancy Considerations Demeclocycline has been shown to cross the placenta in rats and other tetracyclines cross the placenta in humans causing permanent discoloration of teeth if used during the second or third trimester. Because use during pregnancy may cause fetal harm, demeclocyline is classified as pregnancy category D.

Lactation Enters breast milk/not recommended

Contraindications Hypersensitivity to demeclocycline, tetracyclines, or any component of the formulation; children <8 years of age; concomitant use with methoxyflurane; pregnancy

Warnings/Precautions Photosensitivity reactions occur frequently with this drug; avoid prolonged exposure to sunlight and do not use tanning equipment. Use caution in patients with renal or hepatic impairment (eg, elderly); dosage modification required in patients with renal impairment. May act as an antianabolic agent and increase BUN. Pseudotumor cerebri has been reported with tetracycline use (usually resolves with discontinuation). Outdated drug can cause nephropathy. Prolonged use may result in fungal or bacterial superinfection, including *C. difficile*-associated diarrhea (CDAD) and pseudomembranous colitis; CDAD has been observed >2 months postantibiotic treatment. May cause tissue hyperpigmentation, enamel hypoplasia, or permanent tooth discoloration; use of tetracyclines should be avoided during tooth development (children ≤8 years of age) unless other drugs are not likely to be effective or are contraindicated. However, recommended in treatment of anthrax exposure. Do not use during pregnancy. In addition to affecting tooth development, tetracycline use has been associated with retardation of skeletal development and reduced bone growth.

Adverse Reactions Frequency not defined.

Cardiovascular: Pericarditis

Central nervous system: Bulging fontanels (infants), dizziness, headache, pseudotumor cerebri (adults)

Dermatologic: Angioneurotic edema, erythema multiforme, erythematous rash, maculopapular rash, photosensitivity, pigmentation of skin, Stevens-Johnson syndrome (rare), urticaria

Endocrine & metabolic: Discoloration of thyroid gland (brown/black), nephrogenic diabetes insipidus

Gastrointestinal: Anorexia, diarrhea, dysphagia, enterocolitis, esophageal ulcerations, glossitis, nausea, pancreatitis, vomiting

Genitourinary: Balanitis

Hematologic: Eosinophilia, neutropenia, hemolytic anemia, thrombocytopenia

Hepatic: Hepatitis (rare), hepatotoxicity (rare), liver enzymes increased, liver failure (rare)

Neuromuscular & skeletal: Myasthenic syndrome, polyarthralgia, tooth discoloration (children <8 years, rarely in adults)

Ocular: Visual disturbances

Otic: Tinnitus

Renal: Acute renal failure

Respiratory: Pulmonary infiltrates

Miscellaneous: Anaphylaxis, anaphylactoid purpura, lupus-like syndrome, systemic lupus erythematosus exacerbation

Drug Interactions

Avoid Concomitant Use

Avoid concomitant use of Demeclocycline with any of the following: Retinoic Acid Derivatives

Increased Effect/Toxicity

Demeclocycline may increase the levels/effects of: Neuromuscular-Blocking Agents; Retinoic Acid Derivatives; Vitamin K Antagonists

Decreased Effect

Demeclocycline may decrease the levels/effects of: Desmopressin; Penicillins; Typhoid Vaccine

The levels/effects of Demeclocycline may be decreased by: Antacids; Bile Acid Sequestrants; Bismuth; Bismuth Subsalicylate; Iron Salts; Magnesium Salts; Quinapril; Zinc Salts

Ethanol/Nutrition/Herb Interactions

Food: Demeclocycline serum levels may be decreased if taken with food.

Herb/Nutraceutical: Avoid dong quai, St John's wort (may also cause photosensitization).

Stability Tetracyclines form toxic products when outdated or when exposed to light, heat, or humidity (Fanconi-like syndrome).

Mechanism of Action Inhibits protein synthesis by binding with the 30S and possibly the 50S ribosomal subunit(s) of susceptible bacteria; may also cause alterations in the cytoplasmic membrane; inhibits the action of ADH in patients with chronic SIADH

Pharmacodynamics/Kinetics

Onset of action: SIADH: Several days

Absorption: ~50% to 80%; reduced by food and dairy products

Protein binding: 41% to 50%

Metabolism: Hepatic (small amounts) to inactive metabolites; undergoes enterohepatic recirculation

Half-life elimination: 10-17 hours

Time to peak, serum: 3-6 hours

Excretion: Urine (42% to 50% as unchanged drug)

Dosage Oral:

Children ≥8 years: 8-12 mg/kg/day divided every 6-12 hours

Adults: 150 mg 4 times/day or 300 mg twice daily

SIADH (unlabeled use): 900-1200 mg/day or 13-15 mg/kg/day divided every 6-8 hours initially, then decrease to 600-900 mg/day

Dosing adjustment/comments in renal/hepatic impairment: Should be avoided in patients with renal/hepatic dysfunction

Dietary Considerations Should be taken 1 hour before or 2 hours after food or milk with plenty of fluid.

Administration Administer 1 hour before or 2 hours after food or milk with plenty of fluid.

Monitoring Parameters CBC, renal and hepatic function

Test Interactions May interfere with tests for urinary glucose (false-negative urine glucose using Clinistix®, Tes-Tape®)

Dosage Forms Excipient information presented when available (limited, particularly for generics); consult specific product labeling.

Tablet, as hydrochloride: 150 mg, 300 mg

Declomycin®: 150 mg, 300 mg

◆ **Demeclocycline Hydrochloride** *see* Demeclocycline *on page 416*

◆ **Demerol®** *see* Meperidine *on page 943*

◆ **4-Demethoxydaunorubicin** *see* IDArubicin *on page 765*

◆ **Demethylchlortetracycline** *see* Demeclocycline *on page 416*

◆ **Demser®** *see* Metyrosine *on page 986*

◆ **Demulen® 30 (Can)** *see* Ethinyl Estradiol and Ethynodiol Diacetate *on page 576*

◆ **Denavir®** *see* Penciclovir *on page 1161*

Denileukin Diftitox (de ni LOO kin DIF ti toks)

U.S. Brand Names ONTAK®

Index Terms DAB389 Interleukin-2; DAB_{389}IL-2; NSC-714744

Pharmacologic Category Antineoplastic Agent, Miscellaneous

Use Treatment of persistent or recurrent cutaneous (peripheral) T-cell lymphoma (CTCL) whose malignant cells express the CD25 component of the IL-2 receptor

Unlabeled/Investigational Use Treatment of CTCL types mycosis fungoides (MF) and Sézary syndrome (SS)

Pregnancy Considerations Animal reproduction studies have not been conducted. There are no adequate and well-controlled studies in pregnant women. Should be given to a pregnant woman only if clearly needed

Lactation Excretion in breast milk unknown/not recommended

Medication Safety Issues

High alert medication: The Institute for Safe Medication Practices (ISMP) includes this medication among its list of drug classes which have a heightened risk of causing significant patient harm when used in error.

Contraindications There are no contraindications listed within the manufacturer's labeling.

Warnings/Precautions Hazardous agent - use appropriate precautions for handling and disposal. **[U.S. Boxed Warning]: Has been associated with a potentially severe, including life-threatening, capillary leak syndrome; monitor weight, edema, blood pressure, and serum albumin prior to and during treatment.** Symptoms of capillary leak syndrome (hypotension, edema, hypoalbuminemia) may be delayed, occurring up to 2 weeks post infusion; symptoms may persist or worsen after cessation of denileukin diftitox. Withhold treatment if serum albumin <3 g/dL; pre-existing low serum albumin levels may correlate with capillary leak syndrome. **[U.S. Boxed Warning]: Serious and fatal infusion reactions have occurred. Administer in a facility appropriate for cardiopulmonary resuscitation. Discontinue immediately and permanently with serious infusion reaction.** Infusion reaction symptoms usually occur within 24 hours of infusion and resolve within 48 hours of last infusion of cycle. Incidence of infusion reaction has been reported to be lower in cycles 3 and 4 (compared to cycles 1 and 2). **[U.S. Boxed Warning]: Loss of visual acuity, usually associated with loss of color vision (with or without retinal pigment mottling) has been reported;** most patients have persistent visual impairment.

Confirm CD25 expression on malignant cells prior to treatment. May develop immunogenicity; patients with antibodies have a two- to threefold increase in clearance; the presence of antibodies does not correlate with risk for hypersensitivity/infusion related reactions. Monitor closely for infection; may impair immune function. Use with caution in patients >65 years of age; adverse events (anemia, anorexia, confusion, hypotension, rash, nausea/vomiting) may occur more frequently. Safety and efficacy in children have not been established. Should be administered under the supervision of an experienced cancer chemotherapy physician.

Adverse Reactions

>10%:

Cardiovascular: Capillary leak syndrome (33%; serious: 11%), peripheral edema (20% to 26%), vasodilation (22%), hypotension (7% to 16%), chest pain (4% to 13%), tachycardia (12%), thrombosis-related events (7% to 11%)

Central nervous system: Fever (49% to 64%), fatigue (44% to 47%), headache (26% to 29%), dizziness (11% to 13%), pain (11% to 13%)

Dermatologic: Rash (20% to 24%), pruritus (16% to 18%)

Endocrine & metabolic: Hypoalbuminemia (14% to 17%)

Gastrointestinal: Nausea (47% to 60%), vomiting (13% to 35%), diarrhea (22%), anorexia (9% to 20%), taste disturbance (11% to 13%)

Hematologic: Lymphopenia (70%; 24% had lymphopenia at baseline)

Hepatic: ALT increased (84%), AST increased (84%)

Neuromuscular & skeletal: Rigors (42% to 47%), myalgia (18% to 20%), weakness (18%), back pain (16% to 18%), arthralgia (13% to 16%)

Respiratory: Cough (18% to 20%), upper respiratory infection (13%), dyspnea (11% to 13%)

Miscellaneous: Antibody formation (76% to 100%) neutralizing antibodies (45% to 97%), flu-like syndrome (≤85%), infusion reaction (71%; serious: 8%), infection (48%)

1% to 10%:

Cardiovascular: Arrhythmia (6%), hypertension (6%)

Hematologic: Leukopenia (grades 3/4: 3% to 6%), neutropenia (grades 3/4: 3%), thrombocytopenia (grades 3/4: 3%)

Local: Injection site reaction (8%)

Ocular: Visual changes (serious: 4%; includes loss of visual acuity)

Renal: Serum creatinine increased (3% to 10%), proteinuria/casts/hematuria (6%)

Postmarketing and/or case reports: Acute renal insufficiency, hyper-/hypothyroidism, oral ulcer, pancreatitis, thyroiditis, thyrotoxicosis, toxic epidermal necrolysis

Drug Interactions

Avoid Concomitant Use

Avoid concomitant use of Denileukin Diftitox with any of the following: Natalizumab; Vaccines (Live)

Increased Effect/Toxicity

Denileukin Diftitox may increase the levels/effects of: Natalizumab; Vaccines (Live)

The levels/effects of Denileukin Diftitox may be increased by: Trastuzumab

Decreased Effect

Denileukin Diftitox may decrease the levels/effects of: Vaccines (Inactivated)

The levels/effects of Denileukin Diftitox may be decreased by: Echinacea

Stability Store intact vials frozen at or below -10°C (14°F). Must be brought to room temperature (25°C or 77°F) before preparing the dose. Do not refreeze after thawing. Do **not** heat vials. Thaw in refrigerator for not >24 hours or at room temperature for 1-2 hours. Solution may be mixed by gentle swirling; avoid vigorous agitation. Dilute with NS to a concentration of ≥15 mcg/mL; the concentration must be ≥15 mcg/mL during all steps of preparation. This solution should be used within 6 hours. Add drug to the empty sterile I.V. bag first, then add NS. Do not prepare with glass syringes or in glass containers.

Mechanism of Action Denileukin diftitox is a fusion protein (a combination of amino acid sequences from diphtheria toxin and interleukin-2) which selectively delivers the cytotoxic activity of diphtheria toxin to targeted cells. It interacts with the high-affinity IL-2 receptor on the surface of malignant cells to inhibit intracellular protein synthesis, rapidly leading to cell death.

Pharmacodynamics/Kinetics

Distribution: V_d: 0.06-0.09 L/kg

Metabolism: Hepatic via proteolytic degradation (animal studies)

Half-life elimination: Distribution: 2-5 minutes; Terminal: 70-80 minutes

Dosage Note: Premedicate with an antihistamine and acetaminophen prior to each infusion; withhold treatment if serum albumin <3 g/dL

I.V.: Adults: CTCL: 9 or 18 mcg/kg/day days 1 through 5 every 21 days for 8 cycles

Dosage adjustment for toxicity:

Serum albumin <3 g/dL: Withhold treatment

Severe infusion reaction: Permanently discontinue treatment

Administration For I.V. use only. Infuse over 30-60 minutes. Should **not** be given as a rapid I.V. bolus. Discontinue or reduce infusion rate for infusion related reactions; discontinue for severe infusion reaction. Do not administer through an in-line filter. Premedicate with an antihistamine and acetaminophen.

Monitoring Parameters Baseline CD25 expression (on malignant cells); serum albumin level (prior to each treatment), CBC, blood chemistry panel, renal and hepatic function tests (prior to initiation of therapy and weekly during therapy). During the infusion, the patient should be monitored for symptoms of an infusion reaction. After infusion, the patient should be monitored for the development of a delayed capillary leak syndrome (usually in the first 2 weeks), including careful monitoring of weight, blood pressure, and serum albumin.

Information on assay for malignant cell CD25 expression is available at 1-877-873-4724.

Additional Information Oncology Comment: The National Comprehensive Cancer Network (NCCN) Non-Hodgkin's Lymphoma Guidelines (v.3.2008) list denileukin diftitox as a second-line treatment option for systemic therapy of peripheral (cutaneous) T-cell lymphoma in patients who are not candidates for high dose therapy or autologous stem cell rescue. In mycosis fungoides (MF) and Sézary syndrome (SS), denileukin diftitox is a therapy option, either as monotherapy or in combination with bexarotene; participation in a clinical trial is encouraged for this patient population.

Dosage Forms Excipient information presented when available (limited, particularly for generics); consult specific product labeling.

Injection, solution [frozen]:

ONTAK®: 150 mcg/mL (2 mL) [contains EDTA]

- ◆ **Denta 5000 Plus** *see* Fluoride *on page 635*
- ◆ **DentaGel** *see* Fluoride *on page 635*
- ◆ **Dentapaine [OTC]** *see* Benzocaine *on page 183*
- ◆ **Dent's Ear Wax [OTC] [DSC]** *see* Carbamide Peroxide *on page 254*
- ◆ **Dent's Extra Strength Toothache [OTC]** *see* Benzocaine *on page 183*
- ◆ **Deoxycoformycin** *see* Pentostatin *on page 1171*
- ◆ **2'-Deoxycoformycin** *see* Pentostatin *on page 1171*
- ◆ **Depacon®** *see* Valproic Acid and Derivatives *on page 1538*
- ◆ **Depade®** *see* Naltrexone *on page 1039*
- ◆ **Depakene®** *see* Valproic Acid and Derivatives *on page 1538*
- ◆ **Depakote®** *see* Valproic Acid and Derivatives *on page 1538*
- ◆ **Depakote® ER** *see* Valproic Acid and Derivatives *on page 1538*
- ◆ **Depakote® Sprinkle** *see* Valproic Acid and Derivatives *on page 1538*
- ◆ **Depen®** *see* Penicillamine *on page 1161*
- ◆ **DepoCyt®** *see* Cytarabine (Liposomal) *on page 386*
- ◆ **DepoDur®** *see* Morphine Sulfate *on page 1016*
- ◆ **Depo®-Estradiol** *see* Estradiol *on page 554*
- ◆ **Depo-Medrol®** *see* MethylPREDNISolone *on page 976*
- ◆ **Depo-Prevera® (Can)** *see* MedroxyPROGESTERone *on page 930*
- ◆ **Depo-Provera®** *see* MedroxyPROGESTERone *on page 930*
- ◆ **Depo-Provera® Contraceptive** *see* MedroxyPROGESTERone *on page 930*
- ◆ **depo-subQ provera 104™** *see* MedroxyPROGESTERone *on page 930*
- ◆ **Depotest® 100 (Can)** *see* Testosterone *on page 1445*
- ◆ **Depo®-Testosterone** *see* Testosterone *on page 1445*
- ◆ **Deprenyl** *see* Selegiline *on page 1359*
- ◆ **DermaFungal [OTC]** *see* Miconazole *on page 989*
- ◆ **Dermagran® [OTC]** *see* Aluminum Hydroxide *on page 75*
- ◆ **Dermagran® AF [OTC]** *see* Miconazole *on page 989*
- ◆ **Dermamycin® [OTC]** *see* DiphenhydrAMINE *on page 456*
- ◆ **Dermarest Dricort® [OTC]** *see* Hydrocortisone *on page 743*
- ◆ **Dermarest® Skin Correction Cream Plus [OTC]** *see* Hydroquinone *on page 749*
- ◆ **Derma-Smoothe/FS®** *see* Fluocinolone *on page 633*
- ◆ **Dermatop®** *see* Prednicarbate *on page 1229*
- ◆ **Dermazene®** *see* Iodoquinol and Hydrocortisone *on page 810*
- ◆ **Dermazole (Can)** *see* Miconazole *on page 989*
- ◆ **Dermoplast® Antibacterial [OTC]** *see* Benzocaine *on page 183*
- ◆ **Dermoplast® Pain Relieving [OTC]** *see* Benzocaine *on page 183*
- ◆ **DermOtic®** *see* Fluocinolone *on page 633*
- ◆ **Dermovate® (Can)** *see* Clobetasol *on page 347*
- ◆ **Dermtex® HC [OTC]** *see* Hydrocortisone *on page 743*
- ◆ **Desferal®** *see* Deferoxamine *on page 411*
- ◆ **Desferrioxamine** *see* Deferoxamine *on page 411*
- ◆ **Desiccated Thyroid** *see* Thyroid, Desiccated *on page 1464*

Desipramine (des IP ra meen)

U.S. Brand Names Norpramin®

Canadian Brand Names Alti-Desipramine; Apo-Desipramine®; Norpramin®; Nu-Desipramine; PMS-Desipramine

Index Terms Desipramine Hydrochloride; Desmethylimipramine Hydrochloride

Pharmacologic Category Antidepressant, Tricyclic (Secondary Amine)

Additional Appendix Information

Antidepressant Agents *on page 1638*

Use Treatment of depression

Unlabeled/Investigational Use Analgesic adjunct in chronic pain; peripheral neuropathies; substance-related disorders (eg, cocaine withdrawal); attention-deficit/hyperactivity disorder (ADHD); depression in children ≤12 years of age

Restrictions An FDA-approved medication guide concerning the use of antidepressants in children, adolescents, and young adults must be distributed when dispensing an outpatient prescription (new or refill) where this medication is to be used without direct supervision of a healthcare provider. Medication guides are available at http://www.fda.gov/cder/Offices/ODS/medication_guides.htm. Dispense to parents or guardians of children and adolescents receiving this medication.

Pregnancy Risk Factor C

Lactation Enters breast milk/not recommended (AAP rates "of concern")

Medication Safety Issues

Sound-alike/look-alike issues:

Desipramine may be confused with clomiPRAMINE, deserpidine, diphenhydrAMINE, disopyramide, imipramine, nortriptyline

Norpramin® may be confused with clomiPRAMINE, imipramine, Norpace®, nortriptyline, Tenormin®

International issues:

Norpramin®: Brand name for omeprazole in Spain

Contraindications Hypersensitivity to desipramine, drugs of similar chemical class, or any component of the formulation; use of MAO inhibitors within 14 days; use in a patient during the acute recovery phase of MI; concurrent use of thioridazine

Warnings/Precautions [U.S. Boxed Warning]: Antidepressants increase the risk of suicidal thinking and behavior in children, adolescents, and young adults (18-24 years of age) with major depressive disorder (MDD) and other psychiatric disorders; consider risk prior to prescribing. Short-term studies did not show an increased risk in patients >24 years of age and showed a decreased risk in patients ≥65 years. Closely monitor for clinical worsening, suicidality, or unusual changes in behavior; the patient's family or caregiver should be instructed to closely observe the patient and communicate condition with healthcare provider. A medication guide should be dispensed with each prescription. **Desipramine is FDA approved for the treatment of depression in adolescents.**

The possibility of a suicide attempt is inherent in major depression and may persist until remission occurs. Monitor for worsening of depression or suicidality, especially during initiation of therapy (generally first 1-2 months) or with dose increases or decreases. Use caution in high-risk patients. Worsening depression and severe abrupt suicidality that are not part of the presenting symptoms may require discontinuation or modification of drug therapy. The patient's family or caregiver should be alerted to monitor patients for the emergence of suicidality and associated behaviors (such as agitation, irritability, hostility, impulsivity, and hypomania) and notify healthcare provider.

May worsen psychosis in some patients or precipitate a shift to mania or hypomania in patients with bipolar disorder. Patients presenting with depressive symptoms should be screened for bipolar disorder. Monotherapy in patients with bipolar disorder should be avoided. **Desipramine is not FDA approved for the treatment of bipolar depression.**

TCAs may rarely cause bone marrow suppression; monitor for any signs of infection and obtain CBC if symptoms (eg, fever, sore throat) evident. The degree of anticholinergic blockade produced by this agent is low relative to other cyclic antidepressants - however, caution should be used in patients with urinary retention, benign prostatic hyperplasia, narrow-angle glaucoma, xerostomia, visual problems, constipation, or a history of bowel obstruction. The degree of sedation and conduction disturbances with desipramine are low relative to other antidepressants. However, desipramine may cause drowsiness/sedation, resulting in impaired performance of tasks requiring alertness (eg, operating machinery or driving). Sedative effects may be additive with other CNS depressants and/or ethanol. The risk of orthostasis is moderate relative to other antidepressants. Use with caution in patients with a history of cardiovascular disease (including previous MI, stroke, tachycardia, or conduction abnormalities). Use with caution in patients with diabetes mellitus; may alter glucose regulation.

Consider discontinuing, when possible, prior to elective surgery. Therapy should not be abruptly discontinued in patients receiving high doses for prolonged periods. May lower seizure threshold - use caution in patients with a previous seizure disorder or condition predisposing to seizures such as brain damage, alcoholism, or concurrent therapy with other drugs which lower the seizure threshold. May increase the risks associated with electroconvulsive therapy. Use with caution in hyperthyroid patients or those receiving thyroid supplementation. Use with caution in patients with hepatic or renal dysfunction and in elderly patients. Safety and efficacy have not been established in children.

Adverse Reactions Frequency not defined.

Cardiovascular: Arrhythmias, edema, flushing, heart block, hyper-/hypotension, MI, palpitation, stroke, tachycardia

Central nervous system: Agitation, anxiety, ataxia, confusion, delirium, disorientation, dizziness, drowsiness, drug fever, exacerbation of psychosis, extrapyramidal symptoms, fatigue, hallucinations, headache, hypomania, incoordination, insomnia, nervousness, parkinsonian syndrome, restlessness, seizure

Dermatologic: Alopecia, itching, petechiae, photosensitivity, skin rash, urticaria

Endocrine & metabolic: Breast enlargement, galactorrhea, hyper-/hypoglycemia, impotence, libido changes, SIADH

Gastrointestinal: Abdominal cramps, anorexia, black tongue, constipation, decreased lower esophageal sphincter tone may cause GE reflux, diarrhea, heartburn, nausea, paralytic ileus, stomatitis, unpleasant taste, vomiting, weight gain/loss, xerostomia

Genitourinary: Difficult urination, polyuria, sexual dysfunction, testicular edema, urinary retention

Hematologic: Agranulocytosis, eosinophilia, purpura, thrombocytopenia

Hepatic: Cholestatic jaundice, hepatitis, liver enzymes increased

Neuromuscular & skeletal: Fine muscle tremor, numbness, paresthesia of extremities, peripheral neuropathy, tingling, weakness

Ocular: Blurred vision, disturbances of accommodation, intraocular pressure increased, mydriasis

Otic: Tinnitus

Miscellaneous: Allergic reaction, diaphoresis (excessive)

Drug Interactions

Metabolism/Transport Effects Substrate of CYP1A2 (minor), 2D6 (major); **Inhibits** CYP2A6 (moderate), 2B6 (moderate), 2D6 (moderate), 2E1 (weak), 3A4 (moderate)

Avoid Concomitant Use

Avoid concomitant use of Desipramine with any of the following: Iobenguane I 123; MAO Inhibitors; Nilotinib; Sibutramine; Tetrabenazine; Thioridazine; Ziprasidone

Increased Effect/Toxicity

Desipramine may increase the levels/effects of: Alcohol (Ethyl); Alpha-/Beta-Agonists (Direct-Acting); Alpha1-Agonists; Amphetamines; Anticholinergics; Beta2-Agonists; CNS Depressants; CYP2A6 Substrates; CYP2B6 Substrates; CYP2D6 Substrates; CYP3A4 Substrates; Desmopressin; Eplerenone; FentaNYL; Fesoterodine; Maraviroc; Nebivolol; Pimecrolimus; QTc-Prolonging Agents; QuiNIDine; Ranolazine; Serotonin Modulators; Sulfonylureas; Tamoxifen; Tetrabenazine; Thioridazine; TraMADol; Vitamin K Antagonists; Yohimbine; Ziprasidone

The levels/effects of Desipramine may be increased by: Alfuzosin; Altretamine; BuPROPion; Cimetidine; Cinacalcet; Ciprofloxacin; CYP2D6 Inhibitors (Moderate);

CYP2D6 Inhibitors (Strong); Darunavir; Dexmethylphenidate; DULoxetine; Gadobutrol; Lithium; MAO Inhibitors; Methylphenidate; Nilotinib; Pramlintide; Propoxyphene; Protease Inhibitors; QuiNIDine; Selective Serotonin Reuptake Inhibitors; Sibutramine; Terbinafine; Valproic Acid

Decreased Effect

Desipramine may decrease the levels/effects of: Acetylcholinesterase Inhibitors (Central); Alpha2-Agonists; Codeine; Iobenguane I 123

The levels/effects of Desipramine may be decreased by: Acetylcholinesterase Inhibitors (Central); Barbiturates; CarBAMazepine; St Johns Wort

Ethanol/Nutrition/Herb Interactions

Ethanol: Avoid ethanol (may increase CNS depression).

Food: Grapefruit juice may inhibit the metabolism of some TCAs and clinical toxicity may result.

Herb/Nutraceutical: Avoid valerian, St John's wort, SAMe, kava kava (may increase risk of serotonin syndrome and/or excessive sedation).

Mechanism of Action Traditionally believed to increase the synaptic concentration of norepinephrine (and to a lesser extent, serotonin) in the central nervous system by inhibition of its reuptake by the presynaptic neuronal membrane. However, additional receptor effects have been found including desensitization of adenyl cyclase, down regulation of beta-adrenergic receptors, and down regulation of serotonin receptors.

Pharmacodynamics/Kinetics

Onset of action: 1-3 weeks; Maximum antidepressant effect: >2 weeks

Absorption: Well absorbed

Metabolism: Hepatic

Half-life elimination: Adults: 7-60 hours

Time to peak, plasma: 4-6 hours

Excretion: Urine (70%)

Dosage Oral (dose is generally administered at bedtime):

Children 6-12 years: Depression (unlabeled use): 10-30 mg/day or 1-3 mg/kg/day in divided doses; do not exceed 5 mg/kg/day

Adolescents: Depression: Initial: 25-50 mg/day; gradually increase to 100 mg/day in single or divided doses (maximum: 150 mg/day)

Adults:

Depression: Initial: 75 mg/day in divided doses; increase gradually to 150-200 mg/day in divided or single dose (maximum: 300 mg/day)

Cocaine withdrawal (unlabeled use): 50-200 mg/day in divided or single dose

Elderly: Depression: Initial dose: 10-25 mg/day; increase by 10-25 mg every 3 days for inpatients and every week for outpatients if tolerated; usual maintenance dose: 75-100 mg/day, but doses up to 150 mg/day may be necessary

Hemodialysis/peritoneal dialysis: Supplemental dose is not necessary

Monitoring Parameters Monitor blood pressure and pulse rate prior to and during initial therapy; evaluate mental status, suicidal ideation (especially at the beginning of therapy or when doses are increased or decreased); monitor weight; ECG in older adults and those patients with cardiac disease; blood levels are useful for therapeutic monitoring

When used for the treatment of ADHD, thoroughly evaluate for cardiovascular risk. Monitor heart rate, blood pressure, and consider obtaining ECG prior to initiation (Vetter, 2008); ensure PR interval ≤200 ms, QRS duration ≤120 ms, and QT_c ≤460 ms.

Reference Range

Plasma levels do not always correlate with clinical effectiveness

Timing of serum samples: Draw trough just before next dose

Therapeutic: 50-300 ng/mL

In elderly patients the response rate is greatest with steady-state plasma concentrations >115 ng/mL

Possible toxicity: >300 ng/mL

Toxic: >1000 ng/mL

Additional Information Less sedation and anticholinergic effects than with amitriptyline or imipramine

Dosage Forms Excipient information presented when available (limited, particularly for generics); consult specific product labeling.

Tablet, as hydrochloride: 10 mg, 25 mg, 50 mg, 75 mg, 100 mg, 150 mg

Norpramin®: 10 mg, 25 mg, 50 mg, 75 mg, 100 mg, 150 mg [contains soy oil]

- **Desipramine Hydrochloride** *see* Desipramine *on page 418*
- **Desitin® [OTC]** *see* Zinc Oxide *on page 1584*
- **Desitin® Creamy [OTC]** *see* Zinc Oxide *on page 1584*

Desloratadine (des lor AT a deen)

U.S. Brand Names Clarinex®

Canadian Brand Names Aerius®

Pharmacologic Category Histamine H_1 Antagonist; Histamine H_1 Antagonist, Second Generation

Use Relief of nasal and non-nasal symptoms of seasonal allergic rhinitis (SAR) and perennial allergic rhinitis (PAR); treatment of chronic idiopathic urticaria (CIU)

Pregnancy Risk Factor C

Pregnancy Considerations There are no adequate and well-controlled studies in pregnant women. Use during pregnancy only if clearly needed.

Lactation Enters breast milk/not recommended

Contraindications Hypersensitivity to desloratadine, loratadine, or any component of the formulation

Warnings/Precautions Dose should be adjusted in patients with liver or renal impairment. Use with caution in patients known to be slow metabolizers of desloratadine (incidence of side effects may be increased). Some products may contain phenylalanine. Safety and efficacy have not been established for children <6 months of age.

Adverse Reactions

>10%: Central nervous system: Headache (14%)

1% to 10%:

Central nervous system: Fatigue (2% to 5%), somnolence (2%), dizziness (4%)

Endocrine & metabolic: Dysmenorrhea (2%)

Gastrointestinal: Xerostomia (3%), nausea (5%), dyspepsia (3%)

Neuromuscular & skeletal: Myalgia (2% to 3%)

Respiratory: Pharyngitis (3% to 4%)

Postmarketing and/or case reports: Anaphylaxis, bilirubin increased, dyspnea, edema, hepatitis, hypersensitivity reactions, palpitation, pruritus, psychomotor hyperactivity, rash, seizure, tachycardia, transaminases increased, urticaria

Drug Interactions

Avoid Concomitant Use There are no known interactions where it is recommended to avoid concomitant use.

Increased Effect/Toxicity

Desloratadine may increase the levels/effects of: Alcohol (Ethyl); Anticholinergics; CNS Depressants

The levels/effects of Desloratadine may be increased by: P-Glycoprotein Inhibitors; Pramlintide

Decreased Effect

Desloratadine may decrease the levels/effects of: Acetylcholinesterase Inhibitors (Central); Betahistine

The levels/effects of Desloratadine may be decreased by: Acetylcholinesterase Inhibitors (Central); Amphetamines; P-Glycoprotein Inducers

Ethanol/Nutrition/Herb Interactions

Ethanol: Avoid ethanol (may increase risk of sedation).

Food: Does not affect bioavailability.

Stability Syrup, tablet, orally-disintegrating tablet: Store at 25°C (77°F); excursions permitted between 15°C to 30°C (59°F to 86°F). Protect from moisture and excessive heat (85°F). Use orally-disintegrating tablet immediately after opening blister package. Syrup should be protected from light.

Mechanism of Action Desloratadine, a major metabolite of loratadine, is a long-acting tricyclic antihistamine with selective peripheral histamine H_1 receptor antagonistic activity and additional anti-inflammatory properties.

Pharmacodynamics/Kinetics

Protein binding: Desloratadine: 82% to 87%; 3-hydroxydesloratadine: 85% to 89%

Metabolism: Hepatic to active metabolite, 3-hydroxydesloratadine (specific enzymes not identified); undergoes glucuronidation. Decreased in slow metabolizers of desloratadine. Not expected to affect or be affected by medications metabolized by CYP with normal doses.

Half-life elimination: 27 hours

Time to peak: 3 hours

Excretion: Urine and feces (as metabolites)

Dosage Oral:

Children:

6-11 months: 1 mg once daily

12 months to 5 years: 1.25 mg once daily

6-11 years: 2.5 mg once daily

Children ≥12 years and Adults: 5 mg once daily

Dosage adjustment in renal/hepatic impairment:

Children: Not established

Adults: 5 mg every other day

Dietary Considerations May be taken with or without food. Orally-disintegrating tablets contain phenylalanine.

Administration May be taken with or without food.

RediTabs® should be placed on the tongue; tablet will disintegrate immediately. May be taken with or without water.

Syrup: A commercially-available measuring dropper or syringe calibrated to deliver 2 mL or 2.5 mL should be used to administer age-appropriate doses in children.

Dosage Forms Excipient information presented when available (limited, particularly for generics); consult specific product labeling.

Syrup:

Clarinex®: 0.5 mg/mL (480 mL) [contains propylene glycol, sodium benzoate; bubble gum flavor]

Tablet:

Clarinex®: 5 mg

Tablet, orally disintegrating:

Clarinex® RediTabs®: 2.5 mg [contains phenylalanine 1.4 mg/tablet; tutti-frutti flavor]; 5 mg [contains phenylalanine 2.9 mg/tablet; tutti-frutti flavor]

Desloratadine and Pseudoephedrine

(des lor AT a deen & soo doe e FED rin)

U.S. Brand Names Clarinex-D® 12 Hour; Clarinex-D® 24 Hour

Index Terms Pseudoephedrine and Desloratadine

Pharmacologic Category Alpha/Beta Agonist; Histamine H_1 Antagonist; Histamine H_1 Antagonist, Second Generation

Use Relief of symptoms of seasonal allergic rhinitis, in children ≥12 years of age and adults

Pregnancy Risk Factor C

Dosage Oral: Children ≥12 years and Adults:

Clarinex-D® 12 Hour: One tablet twice daily

Clarinex-D® 24 Hour: One tablet daily

Dosage adjustment in renal impairment:

Clarinex-D® 12 Hour: Not recommended

Clarinex-D® 24 Hour: One tablet every other day

Dosage adjustment in hepatic impairment: Not recommended

Additional Information Complete prescribing information for this medication should be consulted for additional detail.

Dosage Forms Excipient information presented when available (limited, particularly for generics); consult specific product labeling.

Tablet, variable release:

Clarinex-D® 12 Hour: Desloratadine 2.5 mg [immediate release] and pseudoephedrine 120 mg [extended release]

Clarinex-D® 24 Hour: Desloratadine 5 mg [immediate release] and pseudoephedrine 240 mg [extended release]

◆ **Desmethylimipramine Hydrochloride** *see* Desipramine *on page 418*

Desmopressin (des moe PRES in)

U.S. Brand Names DDAVP®; Stimate®

Canadian Brand Names Apo-Desmopressin®; DDAVP®; DDAVP® Melt; Minirin®; Novo-Desmopressin; Octostim®; PMS-Desmopressin

Index Terms 1-Deamino-8-D-Arginine Vasopressin; Desmopressin Acetate

Pharmacologic Category Antihemophilic Agent; Hemostatic Agent; Vasopressin Analog, Synthetic

Use

Injection: Treatment of diabetes insipidus; maintenance of hemostasis and control of bleeding in hemophilia A with factor VIII coagulant activity levels >5% and mild-to-moderate classic von Willebrand's disease (type 1) with factor VIII coagulant activity levels >5%

Nasal solutions (DDAVP® Nasal Spray and DDAVP® Rhinal Tube): Treatment of central diabetes insipidus

Nasal spray (Stimate®): Maintenance of hemostasis and control of bleeding in hemophilia A with factor VIII coagulant activity levels >5% and mild to moderate classic von Willebrand's disease (type 1) with factor VIII coagulant activity levels >5%

Tablet: Treatment of central diabetes insipidus, temporary polyuria and polydipsia following pituitary surgery or head trauma, primary nocturnal enuresis

Unlabeled/Investigational Use Uremic bleeding associated with acute or chronic renal failure; prevention of surgical bleeding in patients with uremia

Pregnancy Risk Factor B

Pregnancy Considerations Adverse events were not observed in animal reproductive studies. There are no adequate and well-controlled studies in pregnant women. Anecdotal reports suggest congenital anomalies and low birth weight. However, causal relationship has not been established. Desmopressin has been used safely during pregnancy.

Lactation Excretion in breast milk unknown/use caution

Contraindications Hypersensitivity to desmopressin or any component of the formulation; hyponatremia or a history of hyponatremia; moderate-to-severe renal impairment (Cl_{cr}<50 mL/minute)

Canadian labeling: Additional contraindications (not in U.S. labeling): Type 2B or platelet-type (pseudo) von Willebrand's disease (injection, intranasal, oral, sublingual); known hyponatremia, habitual or psychogenic polydipsia, cardiac insufficiency or other conditions requiring diuretic therapy (intranasal, sublingual); nephrosis, severe hepatic dysfunction (sublingual); primary nocturnal enuresis (intranasal)

Warnings/Precautions Allergic reactions and anaphylaxis have been reported rarely with both the I.V. and intranasal formulations. Fluid intake should be adjusted downward in the elderly and very young patients to decrease the possibility of water intoxication and hyponatremia. Use may rarely lead to extreme decreases in plasma osmolality, resulting in seizures, coma, and death. Use caution with cystic fibrosis, heart failure, renal dysfunction, polydipsia (habitual or psychogenic [contraindicated in Canadian labeling]), or other conditions associated with fluid and electrolyte imbalance due to potential hyponatremia. Use caution with coronary artery insufficiency or hypertensive cardiovascular disease; may increase or decrease blood pressure leading to changes in heart rate. Consider switching from nasal to intravenous solution if changes in the nasal mucosa (scarring, edema) occur leading to unreliable absorption. Use caution in patients predisposed to thrombus formation; thrombotic events (acute cerebrovascular thrombosis, acute myocardial infarction) have occurred (rare).

Desmopressin (intranasal and I.V.), when used for hemostasis in hemophilia, is not for use in hemophilia B, type 2B von Willebrand disease, severe classic von Willebrand disease (type 1), or in patients with factor VIII antibodies. In general, desmopressin is also not recommended for use in patients with ≤5% factor VIII activity level, although it may be considered in selected patients with activity levels between 2% and 5%.

Consider switching from nasal to intravenous administration if changes in the nasal mucosa (scarring, edema) occur leading to unreliable absorption. Consider alternative rout of administration (I.V. or intranasal) with inadequate therapeutic response at maximum recommended oral doses. Therapy should be interrupted if patient experiences an acute illness (eg, fever, recurrent vomiting or diarrhea), vigorous exercise, or any condition associated with an increase in water consumption. Some patients may demonstrate a change in response after long-term therapy (>6 months) characterized as decreased response or a shorter duration of response.

Adverse Reactions Frequency may not be defined (may be dose or route related).

Cardiovascular: Blood pressure increased/decreased (I.V.), facial flushing

Central nervous system: Headache (2% to 5%), dizziness (intranasal; ≤3%), chills (intranasal; 2%)

Dermatologic: Rash

Endocrine & metabolic: Hyponatremia, water intoxication

Gastrointestinal: Abdominal pain (intranasal; 2%), gastrointestinal disorder (intranasal; ≤2%), nausea (intranasal; ≤2%), abdominal cramps, sore throat

Hepatic: Transient increases in liver transaminases (associated primarily with tablets)

Local: Injection: Burning pain, erythema, and swelling at the injection site

Neuromuscular & Skeletal: Weakness (intranasal; ≤2%)

Ocular: Conjunctivitis (intranasal; ≤2%), eye edema (intranasal; ≤2%), lacrimation disorder (intranasal; ≤2%)

Respiratory: Rhinitis (intranasal; 3% to 8%), epistaxis (intranasal; ≤3%), nostril pain (intranasal; ≤2%), cough, nasal congestion, upper respiratory infection

<1% (Limited to important or life-threatening): Acute cerebrovascular thrombosis (I.V.), acute MI (I.V.), agitation, allergic reactions (rare), anaphylaxis (rare), balanitis, chest pain, coma, diarrhea, dyspepsia, edema, insomnia, itching eyes, light-sensitive eyes, pain, palpitation, seizure, somnolence, tachycardia, thinking abnormal, vomiting, vulval pain, warmth

Drug Interactions

Avoid Concomitant Use There are no known interactions where it is recommended to avoid concomitant use.

Increased Effect/Toxicity

Desmopressin may increase the levels/effects of: Lithium

The levels/effects of Desmopressin may be increased by: Analgesics (Opioid); CarBAMazepine; ChlorproMAZINE; LamoTRIgine; Nonsteroidal Anti-Inflammatory Agents; Selective Serotonin Reuptake Inhibitors; Tricyclic Antidepressants

Decreased Effect

The levels/effects of Desmopressin may be decreased by: Demeclocycline; Lithium

Ethanol/Nutrition/Herb Interactions Ethanol: Avoid ethanol (may decrease antidiuretic effect).

Stability

DDAVP®:

Nasal spray: Store at controlled room temperature of 20°C to 25°C (68°F to 77°F). Keep nasal spray in upright position.

Rhinal Tube solution: Store refrigerated at 2°C to 8°C (36°F to 46°F). May store at controlled room temperature of 20°C to 25°C (68°F to 77°F) for up to 3 weeks.

Solution for injection: Store refrigerated at 2°C to 8°C (36°F to 46°F). Dilute solution for injection in 10-50 mL NS for I.V. infusion (10 mL for children ≤10 kg: 50 mL for adults and children >10 kg).

Tablet: Store at controlled room temperature of 20°C to 25°C (68°F to 77°F).

DDAVP® Melt (CAN; not available in U.S.): Store at 15°C to 25°C (59°F to 77°F) in original container. Protect from moisture.

Stimate® nasal spray: Store at controlled room temperature of 20°C to 25°C (68°F to 77°F). Keep nasal spray in upright position. Discard 6 months after opening.

Mechanism of Action In a dose dependent manner, desmopressin increases cyclic adenosine monophosphate (cAMP) in renal tubular cells which increases water permeability resulting in decreased urine volume and increased urine osmolality; increases plasma levels of von Willebrand factor, factor VIII, and t-PA contributing to a shortened activated partial thromboplastin time (aPTT) and bleeding time.

Pharmacodynamics/Kinetics

Onset of action:

Intranasal: Antidiuretic: 15-30 minutes; Increased factor VIII and von Willebrand factor (vWF) activity (dose related): 30 minutes

Peak effect: Antidiuretic: 1 hour; Increased factor VIII and vWF activity: 1.5 hours

I.V. infusion: Increased factor VIII and vWF activity: 30 minutes (dose related)

Peak effect: 1.5-2 hours

Oral tablet: Antidiuretic: ~1 hour

Peak effect: 4-7 hours

Duration: Intranasal, I.V. infusion, Oral tablet: ~6-14 hours

Absorption: Sublingual: Rapid

Bioavailability: Intranasal: ~3.5%; Oral tablet: 5% compared to intranasal, 0.16% compared to I.V.

Half-life elimination: Intranasal: ~3.5 hours; I.V. infusion: 3 hours; Oral tablet: 2-3 hours

Renal impairment: ≤9 hours

Excretion: Urine

Dosage

Children:

Diabetes insipidus:

I.M., I.V., SubQ: Canadian labeling (not in U.S. labeling): ≥3 months: 0.4 mcg (0.1 mL) once daily or 1/10 of the maintenance intranasal dose. Fluid restriction should be observed.

I.V., SubQ: Children <12 years: No definitive dosing available. Adult dosing should **not** be used in this age group; adverse events such as hyponatremia-induced seizures may occur. Dose should be reduced. Some have suggested an initial dosage range of 0.1-1 mcg in 1 or 2 divided doses (Cheetham, 2002). Initiate at low dose and increase as necessary. Closely monitor serum sodium levels and urine output; fluid restriction is recommended.

Intranasal (using 100 mcg/mL nasal solution): 3 months to 12 years: Initial: 5 mcg/day (0.05 mL/day) divided 1-2 times/day; range: 5-30 mcg/day (0.05-0.3 mL/day) divided 1-2 times/day; adjust morning and evening doses separately for an adequate diurnal rhythm of water turnover. **Note:** The nasal spray pump can only deliver doses of 10 mcg (0.1 mL) or multiples of 10 mcg (0.1 mL); if doses other than this are needed, the rhinal tube delivery system is preferred. Fluid restriction should be observed.

Oral:

U.S. labeling: ≥4 years: Initial: 0.05 mg twice daily; total daily dose should be increased or decreased as needed to obtain adequate antidiuresis (range: 0.1-1.2 mg divided 2-3 times/day). Fluid restriction should be observed.

Canadian labeling (not in U.S. labeling): ≥5 years: Initial: 0.1 mg 3 times/day; total daily dose should be increased or decreased as needed to obtain adequate antidiuresis (range: 0.3-1.2 mg divided 3 times/day). Divide daily doses so that the evening dose is 2 times higher than the morning or afternoon dose to ensure adequate antidiuresis during the night. Fluid restriction should be observed.

Sublingual formulation: Canadian labeling (not in U.S. labeling): ≥3 months: Initial: 60 mcg 3 times/day; total daily dose should be increased or decreased as needed to obtain adequate antidiuresis. Usual maintenance: 60-120 mcg 3 times/day (range: 120-720 mcg divided 2-3 times/day); divide daily doses so that the evening dose is 2 times higher than the morning or afternoon dose to ensure adequate antidiuresis during the night. Fluid restriction should be observed.

Hemophilia A and von Willebrand disease (type 1):

I.V.: ≥3 months: 0.3 mcg/kg by slow infusion; may repeat dose if needed; if used preoperatively, administer 30 minutes before procedure

Canadian labeling (not in U.S. labeling): Maximum I.V. dose: 20 mcg

Note: Adverse events such as hyponatremia-induced seizures have been reported especially in young children using this dosing regimen (Das, 2005; Molnar, 2005; Smith, 1989; Thumfart, 2005; Weinstein, 1989). Fluid restriction and careful monitoring of serum sodium levels and urine output are necessary.

Intranasal (using high concentration spray [1.5 mg/mL]): ≥11 months: Refer to adult dosing.

Nocturnal enuresis:

Oral: ≥6 years: 0.2 mg at bedtime; dose may be titrated up to 0.6 mg to achieve desired response. Fluid intake should be limited 1 hour prior to dose until the next morning, or at least 8 hours after administration. **Note:** In the Canadian labeling, use is approved for patients ≥5 years.

Sublingual formulation: Canadian labeling (not in U.S. labeling): ≥5 years: Initial: 120 mcg at bedtime; dose may be titrated up to 360 mcg to achieve desired response. Fluid intake should be limited 1 hour prior to dose until the next morning, or at least 8 hours after administration.

Children ≥12 years and Adults:

Diabetes insipidus:

I.V., SubQ: 2-4 mcg/day (0.5-1 mL) in 2 divided doses or 1/10 of the maintenance intranasal dose. Fluid restriction should be observed.

Intranasal (using 100 mcg/mL nasal solution): 10-40 mcg/day (0.1-0.4 mL) divided 1-3 times/day; adjust morning and evening doses separately for an adequate diurnal rhythm of water turnover. **Note:** The nasal spray pump can only deliver doses of 10 mcg (0.1 mL) or multiples of 10 mcg (0.1 mL); if doses other than this are needed, the rhinal tube delivery system is preferred. Fluid restriction should be observed.

Oral:

U.S. labeling: Initial: 0.05 mg twice daily; total daily dose should be increased or decreased as needed to obtain adequate antidiuresis (range: 0.1-1.2 mg divided 2-3 times/day). Fluid restriction should be observed.

Canadian labeling (not in U.S. labeling): Initial: 0.1 mg 3 times/day; total daily dose should be increased or decreased as needed to obtain adequate antidiuresis (range: 0.3-1.2 mg divided 3 times/day). Fluid restriction should be observed.

Sublingual formulation: Canadian labeling (not in U.S. labeling): Initial: 60 mcg 3 times/day; total daily dose should be increased or decreased as needed to obtain adequate antidiuresis. Usual maintenance: 60-120 mcg 3 times/day (range: 120-720 mcg divided 2-3 times/day). Fluid restriction should be observed.

Hemophilia A and mild-to-moderate von Willebrand disease (type 1):

I.V.: 0.3 mcg/kg by slow infusion; if used preoperatively, administer 30 minutes before procedure

Canadian labeling (not in U.S. labeling): Maximum I.V. dose: 20 mcg

Intranasal (using high concentration spray [1.5 mg/mL]): <50 kg: 150 mcg (1 spray); >50 kg: 300 mcg (1 spray each nostril); repeat use is determined by the patient's clinical condition and laboratory work; if using preoperatively, administer 2 hours before surgery

Adults:

Diabetes insipidus: I.M., I.V., SubQ: Canadian label (not in U.S. labeling): 1-4 mcg (0.25-1 mL) once daily or 1/10 of the maintenance intranasal dose. Fluid restriction should be observed.

Uremic bleeding associated with acute or chronic renal failure (unlabeled use; Watson, 1984): I.V.: 0.4 mcg/kg over 10 minutes

Prevention of surgical bleeding in patients with uremia (unlabeled use; Mannucci, 1983): I.V.: 0.3 mcg/kg over 30 minutes

Dosage adjustment in renal impairment: Cl_{cr} <50 mL/minute: Use is contraindicated according to the manufacturer; however, has been used in acute and chronic renal failure patients experiencing uremic bleeding or for prevention of surgical bleeding (unlabeled uses; Mannuccio, 1983; Watson, 1984)

Administration

I.M., I.V. push, SubQ injection: Central diabetes insipidus: Withdraw dose from ampul into appropriate syringe size (eg, insulin syringe). Further dilution is not required. Administer as direct injection.

I.V. infusion:

Hemophilia A, von Willebrand disease (type 1), and prevention of surgical bleeding in patients with uremia (unlabeled; Mannucci, 1983): Infuse over 15-30 minutes

Acute uremic bleeding (unlabeled; Watson, 1984): May infuse over 10 minutes

Intranasal:

DDAVP®: Nasal pump spray: Delivers 0.1 mL (10 mcg); for doses <10 mcg or for other doses which are not multiples, use rhinal tube. DDAVP® Nasal spray delivers fifty 10 mcg doses. For 10 mcg dose, administer in one nostril. Any solution remaining after 50 doses should be discarded. Pump must be primed prior to first use.

DDAVP® Rhinal tube: Insert top of dropper into tube (arrow marked end) in downward position. Squeeze dropper until solution reaches desired calibration mark. Disconnect dropper. Grasp the tube 3/4 inch from the end and insert tube into nostril until the fingertips reach the nostril. Place opposite end of tube into the mouth (holding breath). Tilt head back and blow with a strong, short puff into the nostril (for very young patients, an adult should blow solution into the child's nose). Reseal dropper after use.

Monitoring Parameters Blood pressure and pulse should be monitored during I.V. infusion

Note: For all indications, fluid intake, urine volume, and signs and symptoms of hyponatremia should be closely monitored especially in high-risk patient subgroups (eg, young children, elderly, patients with heart failure).

Diabetes insipidus: Urine specific gravity, plasma and urine osmolality, serum electrolytes

Hemophilia A: Factor VIII coagulant activity, factor VIII ristocetin cofactor activity, and factor VIII antigen levels, aPTT

von Willebrand disease: Factor VIII coagulant activity, factor VIII ristocetin cofactor activity, and factor VIII von Willebrand antigen levels, bleeding time

Nocturnal enuresis: Serum electrolytes if used for >7 days

Additional Information 10 mcg of desmopressin acetate is equivalent to 40 int. units

Dosage Forms Excipient information presented when available (limited, particularly for generics); consult specific product labeling. [CAN] = Canadian product

Injection, solution, as acetate: 4 mcg/mL (1 mL, 10 mL)
DDAVP®: 5 mcg/mL (1 mL, 10 mL)
Solution, intranasal, as acetate: 100 mcg/mL (2.5 mL)
DDAVP®: 100 mcg/mL (2.5 mL) [contains benzalkonium chloride; with rhinal tube]
Solution, as acetate, intranasal [spray]: 100 mcg/mL (5 mL)
DDAVP®: 100 mcg/mL (5 mL) [contains benzalkonium chloride; delivers 10 mcg/spray]
Stimate®: 1.5 mg/mL (2.5 mL) [delivers 150 mcg/spray]
Tablet, as acetate, oral: 0.1 mg, 0.2 mg
DDAVP®: 0.1 mg, 0.2 mg [scored]
Tablet, as acetate, sublingual:
DDAVP® Melt (CAN) [not available in U.S.]: 60 mcg, 120 mcg, 240 mcg

- ◆ **Desmopressin Acetate** *see* Desmopressin *on page 421*
- ◆ **Desocort® (Can)** *see* Desonide *on page 424*
- ◆ **Desogen®** *see* Ethinyl Estradiol and Desogestrel *on page 575*
- ◆ **Desogestrel and Ethinyl Estradiol** *see* Ethinyl Estradiol and Desogestrel *on page 575*
- ◆ **Desonate™** *see* Desonide *on page 424*

Desonide (DES oh nide)

U.S. Brand Names Desonate™; DesOwen®; LoKara™; Verdeso™

Canadian Brand Names Desocort®; PMS-Desonide

Pharmacologic Category Corticosteroid, Topical

Additional Appendix Information
Corticosteroids *on page 1652*

Use Adjunctive therapy for inflammation in acute and chronic corticosteroid responsive dermatosis (low potency corticosteroid); mild-to-moderate atopic dermatitis

Pregnancy Risk Factor C

Dosage Topical:

Corticosteroid responsive dermatoses: Children and Adults: Therapy should be discontinued when control is achieved. If no improvement is seen within 2 weeks, reassessment of diagnosis may be necessary.
Cream, ointment: Apply 2-4 times/day sparingly
Lotion: Apply 2-3 times/day sparingly

Atopic dermatitis: Children ≥3 months and Adults: Aerosol, gel: Apply 2 times/day sparingly. Therapy should be discontinued when control is achieved. If no improvement is seen within 4 weeks, reassessment of diagnosis may be necessary.

Additional Information Complete prescribing information for this medication should be consulted for additional detail.

Dosage Forms Excipient information presented when available (limited, particularly for generics); consult specific product labeling. [DSC] = Discontinued product

Aerosol, topical [foam]:
Verdeso®: 0.05% (50 g, 100 g)
Cream, topical: 0.05% (15 g, 60 g)
DesOwen®: 0.05% (60 g)
Gel, topical [aqueous]:
Desonate™: 0.05% (15 g [DSC], 30 g [DSC], 60 g)
Lotion, topical: 0.05% (60 mL, 120 mL)
DesOwen® [DSC], LoKara™: 0.05% (60 mL, 120 mL)
Ointment, topical: 0.05% (15 g, 60 g)
DesOwen®: 0.05% (60 g)

- ◆ **DesOwen®** *see* Desonide *on page 424*

Desoximetasone (des oks i MET a sone)

U.S. Brand Names Topicort®; Topicort®-LP

Canadian Brand Names Taro-Desoximetasone; Topicort®

Pharmacologic Category Corticosteroid, Topical

Additional Appendix Information
Corticosteroids *on page 1652*

Use Relieves inflammation and pruritic symptoms of corticosteroid-responsive dermatosis (intermediate- to high-potency topical corticosteroid)

Pregnancy Risk Factor C

Medication Safety Issues
Sound-alike/look-alike issues:
Desoximetasone may be confused with dexamethasone
Topicort® may be confused with Topic®

Dosage Desoximetasone is a potent fluorinated topical corticosteroid. Therapy should be discontinued when control is achieved; if no improvement is seen, reassessment of diagnosis may be necessary.

Cream, gel: Children and Adults: Apply a thin film to affected area twice daily
Ointment: Children ≥10 years and Adults: Apply a thin film to affected area twice daily

Additional Information Complete prescribing information for this medication should be consulted for additional detail.

Dosage Forms Excipient information presented when available (limited, particularly for generics); consult specific product labeling.

Cream, topical: 0.25% (15 g, 60 g); 0.05% (15 g, 60 g)
Topicort®: 0.25% (15 g, 60 g)
Topicort®-LP: 0.05% (15 g, 60 g)
Gel, topical: 0.05% (15 g, 60 g)
Topicort®: 0.05% (15 g, 60 g) [contains alcohol]
Ointment, topical: 0.25% (15 g, 60 g)
Topicort®: 0.25% (15 g, 60 g) [contains coconut oil]

- ◆ **Desoxyephedrine Hydrochloride** *see* Methamphetamine *on page 960*
- ◆ **Desoxyn®** *see* Methamphetamine *on page 960*
- ◆ **Desoxyphenobarbital** *see* Primidone *on page 1238*

Desvenlafaxine (des ven la FAX een)

U.S. Brand Names Pristiq™

Index Terms O-desmethylvenlafaxine; ODV

Pharmacologic Category Antidepressant, Serotonin/Norepinephrine Reuptake Inhibitor

Additional Appendix Information

Antidepressant Agents *on page 1638*

Use Treatment of major depressive disorder

Restrictions An FDA-approved medication guide concerning the use of antidepressants in children, adolescents, and young adults must be distributed when dispensing an outpatient prescription (new or refill) where this medication is to be used without direct supervision of a healthcare provider. Medication guides are available at http://www.wyeth.com/content/showlabeling.asp?id=498.

Pregnancy Risk Factor C

Dosage Oral: Adults: Depression: 50 mg once daily; up to 400 mg once daily have been studied; however, the manufacturer states there is no evidence that higher doses confer any additional benefit. A flat dose response curve for efficacy between 50-400 mg/day has been noted as well as an increase in adverse events.

Note: Gradually taper dose (by increasing dosing interval) if discontinuing.

Dosing adjustment in renal impairment:

Cl_{cr} ≥30 mL/minute: No dosage adjustment required

Cl_{cr} <30 mL/minute: 50 mg every other day (maximum).

Hemodialysis: 50 mg every other day (maximum). Supplemental doses not required after HD.

Dosing adjustment in hepatic impairment: Usual adult dose recommended; maximum dose: 100 mg/day

Additional Information Complete prescribing information for this medication should be consulted for additional detail.

Dosage Forms Excipient information presented when available (limited, particularly for generics); consult specific product labeling.

Tablet, extended release:

Pristiq™: 50 mg, 100 mg

- ◆ **Desyrel® (Can)** *see* TraZODone *on page 1505*
- ◆ **Detane® [OTC]** *see* Benzocaine *on page 183*
- ◆ **Detemir Insulin** *see* Insulin Detemir *on page 793*
- ◆ **Detrol®** *see* Tolterodine *on page 1488*
- ◆ **Detrol® LA** *see* Tolterodine *on page 1488*

Dexamethasone (deks a METH a sone)

U.S. Brand Names Dexamethasone Intensol™; DexPak® 10 Day TaperPak®; DexPak® TaperPak®; Maxidex®

Canadian Brand Names Apo-Dexamethasone®; Dexasone®; Diodex®; Maxidex®; PMS-Dexamethasone

Index Terms Dexamethasone Sodium Phosphate

Pharmacologic Category Anti-inflammatory Agent; Anti-inflammatory Agent, Ophthalmic; Antiemetic; Corticosteroid, Ophthalmic; Corticosteroid, Otic; Corticosteroid, Systemic

Additional Appendix Information

Corticosteroids *on page 1652*

Use Systemic: Primarily as an anti-inflammatory or immunosuppressant agent in the treatment of a variety of diseases including those of allergic, dermatologic, endocrine, hematologic, inflammatory, neoplastic, nervous system, renal, respiratory, rheumatic, and autoimmune origin; may be used in management of cerebral edema, chronic swelling, as a diagnostic agent, diagnosis of Cushing's syndrome, antiemetic

Unlabeled/Investigational Use

Dexamethasone suppression test: General indicator consistent with depression and/or suicide

Accelerate fetal lung maturation in patients with preterm labor

Pregnancy Risk Factor C

Pregnancy Considerations Adverse events have been observed with corticosteroids in animal reproduction studies. Dexamethasone crosses the placenta; and is partially metabolized to an inactive metabolite by placental enzymes. Due to its positive effect on stimulating fetal lung maturation, the injection is often used in patients with premature labor (24-34 weeks gestation). Some studies have shown an association between first trimester systemic corticosteroid use and oral clefts; adverse events in the fetus/neonate have been noted in case reports following large doses of systemic corticosteroids during pregnancy. Women exposed to dexamethasone during pregnancy for the treatment of an autoimmune disease may contact the OTIS Autoimmune Diseases Study at 877-311-8972.

Lactation Excretion in breast milk unknown/use caution

Medication Safety Issues

Sound-alike/look-alike issues:

Dexamethasone may be confused with desoximetasone, dextroamphetamine

Decadron® may be confused with Percodan®

Maxidex® may be confused with Maxzide®

Contraindications Hypersensitivity to dexamethasone or any component of the formulation; systemic fungal infections, cerebral malaria; ophthalmic use in viral (active ocular herpes simplex), fungal, or tuberculosis diseases of the eye

Warnings/Precautions Use with caution in patients with thyroid disease, hepatic impairment, renal impairment, cardiovascular disease, diabetes, glaucoma, cataracts, myasthenia gravis, patients at risk for osteoporosis, patients at risk for seizures, or GI diseases (diverticulitis, peptic ulcer, ulcerative colitis) due to perforation risk. Use caution following acute MI (corticosteroids have been associated with myocardial rupture). Because of the risk of adverse effects, systemic corticosteroids should be used cautiously in the elderly in the smallest possible effective dose for the shortest duration. May affect growth velocity; growth should be routinely monitored in pediatric patients. Withdraw therapy with gradual tapering of dose.

May cause hypercorticism or suppression of hypothalamic-pituitary-adrenal (HPA) axis, particularly in younger children or in patients receiving high doses for prolonged periods. HPA axis suppression may lead to adrenal crisis. Withdrawal and discontinuation of a corticosteroid should be done slowly and carefully. Particular care is required when patients are transferred from systemic corticosteroids to inhaled products due to possible adrenal insufficiency or withdrawal from steroids, including an increase in allergic symptoms. Patients receiving >20 mg per day of prednisone (or equivalent) may be most susceptible. Fatalities have occurred due to adrenal insufficiency in asthmatic patients during and after transfer from systemic corticosteroids to aerosol steroids; aerosol steroids do not provide the systemic steroid needed to treat patients having trauma, surgery, or infections. Dexamethasone does not provide adequate mineralocorticoid activity in adrenal insufficiency (may be employed as a single dose while cortisol assays are performed). The lowest possible dose should be used during treatment; discontinuation and/or dose reductions should be gradual.

Acute myopathy has been reported with high dose corticosteroids, usually in patients with neuromuscular transmission disorders; may involve ocular and/or respiratory muscles; monitor creatine kinase; recovery may be delayed. Corticosteroid use may cause psychiatric disturbances, including depression, euphoria, insomnia, mood swings, and personality changes. Pre-existing psychiatric conditions may be exacerbated by corticosteroid use. Prolonged use of corticosteroids may also increase the incidence of secondary infection, mask acute infection (including fungal infections), prolong or exacerbate viral infections, or limit response to vaccines. Exposure to chickenpox should be avoided; corticosteroids should not be used to treat ocular herpes simplex. Corticosteroids should not be used for cerebral malaria or viral hepatitis. Close observation is required in patients with latent tuberculosis and/or TB reactivity; restrict use in active TB (only in conjunction with antituberculosis treatment). Prolonged treatment with corticosteroids has been associated with the development of Kaposi's sarcoma (case reports); if noted, discontinuation of therapy should be considered. High-dose corticosteroids should not be used to manage acute head injury.

Adverse Reactions Frequency not defined.

Cardiovascular: Arrhythmia, bradycardia, cardiac arrest, cardiomyopathy, CHF, circulatory collapse, edema, hypertension, myocardial rupture (post-MI), syncope, thromboembolism, vasculitis

Central nervous system: Depression, emotional instability, euphoria, headache, intracranial pressure increased, insomnia, malaise, mood swings, neuritis, personality changes, pseudotumor cerebri (usually following discontinuation), psychic disorders, seizure, vertigo

Dermatologic: Acne, allergic dermatitis, alopecia, angioedema, bruising, dry skin, erythema, fragile skin, hirsutism, hyper-/hypopigmentation, hypertrichosis, perianal pruritus (following I.V. injection), petechiae, rash, skin atrophy, skin test reaction impaired, striae, urticaria, wound healing impaired

Endocrine & metabolic: Adrenal suppression, carbohydrate tolerance decreased, Cushing's syndrome, diabetes mellitus, glucose intolerance decreased, growth suppression (children), hyperglycemia, hypokalemic alkalosis, menstrual irregularities, negative nitrogen balance, pituitary-adrenal axis suppression, protein catabolism, sodium retention

Gastrointestinal: Abdominal distention, appetite increased, gastrointestinal hemorrhage, gastrointestinal perforation, nausea, pancreatitis, peptic ulcer, ulcerative esophagitis, weight gain

Genitourinary: Altered (increased or decreased) spermatogenesis

Hepatic: Hepatomegaly, transaminases increased

Local: Postinjection flare (intra-articular use), thrombophlebitis

Neuromuscular & skeletal: Arthropathy, aseptic necrosis (femoral and humoral heads), fractures, muscle mass loss, myopathy (particularly in conjunction with neuromuscular disease or neuromuscular-blocking agents), neuropathy, osteoporosis, parasthesia, tendon rupture, vertebral compression fractures, weakness

Ocular: Cataracts, exophthalmos, glaucoma, intraocular pressure increased

Renal: Glucosuria

Respiratory: Pulmonary edema

Miscellaneous: Abnormal fat deposition, anaphylactoid reaction, anaphylaxis, avascular necrosis, diaphoresis, hiccups, hypersensitivity, impaired wound healing, infections, Kaposi's sarcoma, moon face, secondary malignancy

Drug Interactions

Metabolism/Transport Effects **Substrate** of CYP3A4 (major); **Induces** CYP2A6 (weak), 2B6 (weak), 2C8 (weak), 2C9 (weak), 3A4 (strong)

Avoid Concomitant Use

Avoid concomitant use of Dexamethasone with any of the following: Natalizumab; Nilotinib; Nisoldipine; Ranolazine; Vaccines (Live)

Increased Effect/Toxicity

Dexamethasone may increase the levels/effects of: Acetylcholinesterase Inhibitors; Amphotericin B; CycloSPORINE; Lenalidomide; Loop Diuretics; Natalizumab; NSAID (COX-2 Inhibitor); NSAID (Nonselective); Thalidomide; Thiazide Diuretics; Vaccines (Live); Warfarin

The levels/effects of Dexamethasone may be increased by: Antifungal Agents (Azole Derivatives, Systemic); Aprepitant; Calcium Channel Blockers (Nondihydropyridine); CycloSPORINE; CYP3A4 Inhibitors (Moderate); CYP3A4 Inhibitors (Strong); Dasatinib; Estrogen Derivatives; Fluconazole; Fosaprepitant; Macrolide Antibiotics; Neuromuscular-Blocking Agents (Nondepolarizing); P-Glycoprotein Inhibitors; Quinolone Antibiotics; Salicylates; Trastuzumab

Decreased Effect

Dexamethasone may decrease the levels/effects of: Antidiabetic Agents; Calcitriol; Caspofungin; Corticorelin; CYP3A4 Substrates; Dabigatran Etexilate; Isoniazid; Maraviroc; Nilotinib; Nisoldipine; P-Glycoprotein Substrates; Ranolazine; Salicylates; Sorafenib; Vaccines (Inactivated)

The levels/effects of Dexamethasone may be decreased by: Aminoglutethimide; Antacids; Barbiturates; Bile Acid Sequestrants; CYP3A4 Inducers (Strong); Deferasirox; Echinacea; Herbs (CYP3A4 Inducers); P-Glycoprotein Inducers; Primidone; Rifamycin Derivatives

Ethanol/Nutrition/Herb Interactions

Ethanol: Avoid ethanol (may enhance gastric mucosal irritation).

Food: Dexamethasone interferes with calcium absorption. Limit caffeine.

Herb/Nutraceutical: Avoid cat's claw, echinacea (have immunostimulant properties).

Stability

Injection solution: Store at room temperature; protect from light and freezing.

Stability of injection of parenteral admixture at room temperature (25°C): 24 hours

Stability of injection of parenteral admixture at refrigeration temperature (4°C): 2 days; protect from light and freezing.

Injection should be diluted in 50-100 mL NS or D_5W.

Mechanism of Action Decreases inflammation by suppression of neutrophil migration, decreased production of inflammatory mediators, and reversal of increased capillary permeability; suppresses normal immune response. Dexamethasone's mechanism of antiemetic activity is unknown.

Pharmacodynamics/Kinetics

Onset of action: Acetate: Prompt

Duration of metabolic effect: 72 hours; acetate is a long-acting repository preparation

Metabolism: Hepatic

Half-life elimination: Normal renal function: 1.8-3.5 hours; Biological half-life: 36-54 hours

Time to peak, serum: Oral: 1-2 hours; I.M.: ~8 hours

Excretion: Urine and feces

Dosage Refer to individual protocols.

Children:

Antiemetic (prior to chemotherapy): I.V.: 10 mg/m^2 (initial dose) followed by 5 mg/m^2 every 6 hours as needed **or** 5-20 mg given 15-30 minutes before treatment

Anti-inflammatory immunosuppressant: Oral, I.M., I.V.: 0.08-0.3 mg/kg/day **or** 2.5-10 mg/m^2/day in divided doses every 6-12 hours

Extubation or airway edema: Oral, I.M., I.V.: 0.5-2 mg/kg/day in divided doses every 6 hours beginning 24 hours prior to extubation and continuing for 4-6 doses afterwards

Cerebral edema: I.V.: Loading dose: 1-2 mg/kg/dose as a single dose; maintenance: 1-1.5 mg/kg/day (maximum: 16 mg/day) in divided doses every 4-6 hours, taper off over 1-6 weeks

Bacterial meningitis in infants and children >2 months: I.V.: 0.6 mg/kg/day in 4 divided doses every 6 hours for the first 4 days of antibiotic treatment; start dexamethasone at the time of the first dose of antibiotic

Physiologic replacement: Oral, I.M., I.V.: 0.03-0.15 mg/kg/day **or** 0.6-0.75 mg/m^2/day in divided doses every 6-12 hours

Adults:

Antiemetic:

Prophylaxis: Oral, I.V.: 10-20 mg 15-30 minutes before treatment on each treatment day

Continuous infusion regimen: Oral or I.V.: 10 mg every 12 hours on each treatment day

Mildly emetogenic therapy: Oral, I.M., I.V.: 4 mg every 4-6 hours

Delayed nausea/vomiting: Oral: 4-10 mg 1-2 times/day for 2-4 days **or**

8 mg every 12 hours for 2 days; then

4 mg every 12 hours for 2 days **or**

20 mg 1 hour before chemotherapy; then

10 mg 12 hours after chemotherapy; then

8 mg every 12 hours for 4 doses; then

4 mg every 12 hours for 4 doses

Anti-inflammatory:

Oral, I.M., I.V. (injections should be given as sodium phosphate): 0.75-9 mg/day in divided doses every 6-12 hours

Intra-articular, intralesional, or soft tissue (as sodium phosphate): 0.4-6 mg/day

Ophthalmic:

Solution: Instill 1-2 drops into conjunctival sac every hour during the day and every other hour during the night; gradually reduce dose to every 3-4 hours, then to 3-4 times/day

Suspension: Instill 1-2 drops into conjunctival sac up to 4-6 times per day; may use hourly in severe disease; taper prior to discontinuation

Otic: Instill 3-4 drops 2-3 times a day; reduce dose gradually prior to discontinuation

Multiple myeloma: Oral, I.V.: 40 mg/day, days 1 to 4, 9 to 12, and 17 to 20, repeated every 4 weeks (alone or as part of a regimen)

Cerebral edema: I.V. 10 mg stat, 4 mg I.M./I.V. every 6 hours until response is maximized, then switch to oral regimen, then taper off if appropriate; dosage may be reduced after 24 days and gradually discontinued over 5-7 days

Extubation or airway edema: Oral, I.M., I.V. (injections should be given as sodium phosphate): 0.5-2 mg/kg/day in divided doses every 6 hours beginning 24 hours prior to extubation and continuing for 4-6 doses afterwards

Dexamethasone suppression test (depression/suicide indicator) (unlabeled use): Oral: 1 mg at 11 PM, draw blood at 8 AM the following day for plasma cortisol determination

Cushing's syndrome, diagnostic: Oral: 1 mg at 11 PM, draw blood at 8 AM; greater accuracy for Cushing's syndrome may be achieved by the following:

Dexamethasone 0.5 mg by mouth every 6 hours for 48 hours (with 24-hour urine collection for 17-hydroxycorticosteroid excretion)

Differentiation of Cushing's syndrome due to ACTH excess from Cushing's due to other causes: Oral: Dexamethasone 2 mg every 6 hours for 48 hours (with 24-hour urine collection for 17-hydroxycorticosteroid excretion)

Multiple sclerosis (acute exacerbation): 30 mg/day for 1 week, followed by 4-12 mg/day for 1 month

Physiological replacement: Oral, I.M., I.V. (should be given as sodium phosphate): 0.03-0.15 mg/kg/day **or** 0.6-0.75 mg/m^2/day in divided doses every 6-12 hours

Treatment of shock:

Addisonian crisis/shock (ie, adrenal insufficiency/responsive to steroid therapy): I.V. (given as sodium phosphate): 4-10 mg as a single dose, which may be repeated if necessary

Unresponsive shock (ie, unresponsive to steroid therapy): I.V. (given as sodium phosphate): 1-6 mg/kg as a single I.V. dose or up to 40 mg initially followed by repeat doses every 2-6 hours while shock persists

Hemodialysis: Supplemental dose is not necessary

Peritoneal dialysis: Supplemental dose is not necessary

Dietary Considerations May be taken with meals to decrease GI upset. May need diet with increased potassium, pyridoxine, vitamin C, vitamin D, folate, calcium, and phosphorus.

Administration

Oral: Administer with meals to decrease GI upset.

I.V.: Administer as a 5-10 minute bolus; rapid injection is associated with a high incidence of perineal discomfort.

Ophthalmic: Remove soft contact lenses prior to using solutions containing benzalkonium chloride. Do not touch tip of container to eye.

Otic: Use ophthalmic solution for otic administration. Instill directly into aural canal or may pack canal with gauze saturated with solution. Keep wick moist and remove after 12-24 hours.

Monitoring Parameters Hemoglobin, occult blood loss, serum potassium, and glucose; intraocular pressure (with use >6 weeks)

Reference Range Dexamethasone suppression test, overnight: 8 AM cortisol <6 mcg/100 mL (dexamethasone 1 mg); plasma cortisol determination should be made on the day after giving dose

Additional Information Effects of inhaled/intranasal steroids on growth have been observed in the absence of laboratory evidence of HPA axis suppression, suggesting that growth velocity is a more sensitive indicator of systemic corticosteroid exposure in pediatric patients than some commonly used tests of HPA axis function. The long-term effects of this reduction in growth velocity associated with orally-inhaled and intranasal corticosteroids, including the impact on final adult height, are unknown. The potential for "catch up" growth following discontinuation of treatment with inhaled corticosteroids has not been adequately studied.

Withdrawal/tapering of therapy: Corticosteroid tapering following short-term use is limited primarily by the need to control the underlying disease state; tapering may be accomplished over a period of days. Following longer-term use, tapering over weeks to months may be necessary to avoid signs and symptoms of adrenal insufficiency and to allow recovery of the HPA axis. Testing of HPA axis responsiveness may be of value in selected patients. Subtle deficits in HPA response may persist for months after discontinuation of therapy, and may require supplemental dosing during periods of acute illness or surgical stress.

Dosage Forms Excipient information presented when available (limited, particularly for generics); consult specific product labeling.

Elixir, as base: 0.5 mg/5 mL (240 mL)

Injection, solution, as sodium phosphate: 4 mg/mL (1 mL, 5 mL, 30 mL); 10 mg/mL (10 mL)

Injection, solution, as sodium phosphate [preservative free]: 10 mg/mL (1 mL)

Solution, ophthalmic, as sodium phosphate [drops]: 0.1% (5 mL)

Solution, oral: 0.5 mg/5 mL (500 mL)

Solution, oral [concentrate]:

Dexamethasone Intensol™: 1 mg/mL (30 mL) [dye free, sugar free; contains alcohol 30% and propylene glycol]

Suspension, ophthalmic [drops]:

Maxidex®: 0.1% (5 mL) [contains benzalkonium chloride]

Tablet [scored]: 0.5 mg, 0.75 mg, 1 mg, 1.5 mg, 2 mg, 4 mg, 6 mg

DexPak® 10 Day TaperPak®: 1.5 mg [35 tablets on taper dose card]

DexPak® TaperPak®: 1.5 mg [51 tablets on taper dose card]

- **Dexamethasone and Ciprofloxacin** *see* Ciprofloxacin and Dexamethasone *on page 333*
- **Dexamethasone and Tobramycin** *see* Tobramycin and Dexamethasone *on page 1484*
- **Dexamethasone Intensol™** *see* Dexamethasone *on page 425*
- **Dexamethasone, Neomycin, and Polymyxin B** *see* Neomycin, Polymyxin B, and Dexamethasone *on page 1052*
- **Dexamethasone Sodium Phosphate** *see* Dexamethasone *on page 425*
- **Dexasone® (Can)** *see* Dexamethasone *on page 425*

Dexbrompheniramine and Pseudoephedrine

(deks brom fen EER a meen & soo doe e FED rin)

U.S. Brand Names Drixoral® Cold & Allergy [OTC]

Canadian Brand Names Drixoral®

Index Terms Pseudoephedrine and Dexbrompheniramine

Pharmacologic Category Alpha/Beta Agonist; Histamine H_1 Antagonist; Histamine H_1 Antagonist, First Generation

Use Relief of symptoms of upper respiratory mucosal congestion in seasonal and perennial nasal allergies, acute rhinitis, rhinosinusitis, and eustachian tube blockage

Pregnancy Risk Factor B

Dosage Children >12 years and Adults: Oral: 1 timed release tablet every 12 hours, may require 1 tablet every 8 hours

Additional Information Complete prescribing information for this medication should be consulted for additional detail.

Dosage Forms Excipient information presented when available (limited, particularly for generics); consult specific product labeling.

Tablet, sustained action: Dexbrompheniramine maleate 6 mg and pseudoephedrine sulfate 120 mg

Dexchlorpheniramine (deks klor fen EER a meen)

Index Terms Dexchlorpheniramine Maleate

Pharmacologic Category Histamine H_1 Antagonist; Histamine H_1 Antagonist, First Generation

Use Perennial and seasonal allergic rhinitis and other allergic symptoms including urticaria

Pregnancy Risk Factor B

Dosage Oral:

Children:

2-5 years: 0.5 mg every 4-6 hours (do not use timed release)

6-11 years: 1 mg every 4-6 hours or 4 mg timed release at bedtime

Adults: 2 mg every 4-6 hours or 4-6 mg timed release at bedtime or every 8-10 hours

Additional Information Complete prescribing information for this medication should be consulted for additional detail.

Dosage Forms Excipient information presented when available (limited, particularly for generics); consult specific product labeling. [DSC] = Discontinued product

Syrup, as maleate: 2 mg/5 mL (480 mL) [contains alcohol 6%; orange flavor]

Tablet, sustained action, as maleate: 4 mg [DSC]

Dexchlorpheniramine and Pseudoephedrine

(deks klor fen EER a meen & soo doe e FED rin)

U.S. Brand Names AllerDur™; Duotan PD [DSC]; SuTan

Index Terms Pseudoephedrine Tannate and Dexchlorpheniramine Tannate

Pharmacologic Category Alpha/Beta Agonist; Histamine H_1 Antagonist; Histamine H_1 Antagonist, First Generation

Use Relief of nasal congestion associated with the common cold, hay fever, and other allergies, sinusitis, and vasomotor and allergic rhinitis

Pregnancy Risk Factor C

Dosage Oral: Rhinitis/decongestant:

Children:

2-6 years:

AllerDur™: 2.5-5 mL every 12 hours (maximum: 10 mL/24 hours)

DuoTan PD: 2.5-5 mL every 12 hours (maximum: 10 mL/24 hours)

6-12 years:

AllerDur™: 5-7.5 mL every 12 hours (maximum: 15 mL/24 hours)

DuoTan PD: 5-10 mL every 12 hours (maximum: 20 mL/24 hours)

Children ≥12 years and Adults:

AllerDur™: 15 mL every 12 hours (maximum: 30 mL/24 hours)

DuoTan PD: 10-20 mL every 12 hours (maximum: 40 mL/24 hours)

Additional Information Complete prescribing information for this medication should be consulted for additional detail.

Dosage Forms Excipient information presented when available (limited, particularly for generics); consult specific product labeling. [DSC] = Discontinued product

Suspension:

AllerDur™: Dexchlorpheniramine tannate 3 mg and pseudoephedrine tannate 50 mg per 5 mL (480 mL) [sugar free; contains sodium benzoate; candy-apple flavor]

Duotan PD: Dexchlorpheniramine tannate 2.5 mg and pseudoephedrine tannate 75 mg per 5 mL (120 mL, 480 mL) [contains sodium benzoate; strawberry-banana flavor] [DSC]

SuTan: Dexchlorpheniramine tannate 3 mg and pseudoephedrine tannate 50 mg per 5 mL (480 mL) [candy-apple flavor]

- **Dexchlorpheniramine Maleate** *see* Dexchlorpheniramine *on page 428*
- **Dexchlorpheniramine Tannate, Pseudoephedrine Tannate, and Dextromethorphan Tannate** *see* Chlorpheniramine, Pseudoephedrine, and Dextromethorphan *on page 315*
- **Dexedrine®** *see* Dextroamphetamine *on page 431*
- **Dexferrum®** *see* Iron Dextran Complex *on page 817*
- **Dexiron™ (Can)** *see* Iron Dextran Complex *on page 817*

Dexmedetomidine (deks MED e toe mi deen)

U.S. Brand Names Precedex®

Canadian Brand Names Precedex®

Index Terms Dexmedetomidine Hydrochloride

Pharmacologic Category $Alpha_2$-Adrenergic Agonist; Sedative

Use Sedation of initially intubated and mechanically ventilated patients during treatment in an intensive care setting; sedation prior to and/or during surgical or other procedures of nonintubated patients; duration of infusion should not exceed 24 hours

Unlabeled/Investigational Use Unlabeled uses include premedication prior to anesthesia induction with thiopental; relief of pain and reduction of opioid dose following laparoscopic tubal ligation; as an adjunct anesthetic in ophthalmic surgery; treatment of shivering; premedication to attenuate the cardiostimulatory and postanesthetic delirium of ketamine; use in children

Pregnancy Risk Factor C

Pregnancy Considerations Teratogenic effects were not observed in animal studies. There are no adequate and well-controlled studies in pregnant women.

Lactation Excretion in breast milk unknown/use caution

Medication Safety Issues

Sound-alike/look-alike issues:

Precedex® may be confused with Peridex®

Contraindications There are no contraindications listed in the manufacturer's labeling.

Warnings/Precautions Should be administered only by persons skilled in management of patients in intensive care setting or operating room. Patients should be continuously monitored. Episodes of bradycardia, hypotension, and sinus arrest have been associated with dexmedetomidine. Use caution in patients with heart block, severe ventricular dysfunction, hypovolemia, diabetes, chronic hypertension, and elderly. Use with caution in patients with hepatic impairment; dosage reductions recommended. Use with caution in patients receiving vasodilators or drugs which decrease heart rate. If medical intervention is required, treatment may include stopping or decreasing the infusion; increasing the rate of I.V. fluid administration, use of pressor agents, and elevation of the lower extremities. Transient hypertension has been primarily observed during the loading dose administration and is associated with the initial peripheral vasoconstrictive effects of dexmedetomidine. Treatment of this is generally unnecessary; however, reduction of infusion rate may be required. Patients may be arousable and alert when stimulated. This alone should not be considered as lack of efficacy in the absence of other clinical signs/symptoms. When withdrawn abruptly in patients who have received >24 hours, withdrawal symptoms similar to clonidine withdrawal may result (eg, hypertension, nervousness, agitation, headaches). Use for >24 hours is not recommended.

Adverse Reactions

>10%:

Cardiovascular: Hypotension (24% to 54%), bradycardia (5% to 14%)

Respiratory: Respiratory depression (37%)

1% to 10%:

Cardiovascular: Atrial fibrillation (4% to 5%), hypovolemia (3%)

Endocrine & metabolic: Hypocalcemia (1%)

Gastrointestinal: Nausea (3% to 9%), xerostomia (3% to 4%)

Renal: Urine output decreased (1%)

Respiratory: Pleural effusion (32%), wheezing (≤1%)

Postmarketing and/or case reports: Abdominal pain, abnormal vision, acidosis, agitation, alkaline phosphatase increased, ALT increased, anemia, apnea, arrhythmia, AST increased, atrioventricular block, BUN increased, bronchospasm, cardiac arrest, confusion, delirium, diaphoresis, diarrhea, dizziness, dyspnea, extrasystoles, fever, GGT increased, hallucination, headache, heart block, hemorrhage, hepatic impairment, hyperbilirubinemia, hypercapnia, hyperkalemia, hypertension, hypoglycemia, hypoventilation, hypoxia, illusion, MI, neuralgia, neuritis, oliguria, pain, photopsia, pulmonary congestion, respiratory acidosis, rigors, seizure, speech disorder, supraventricular tachycardia, tachycardia, thirst, T-wave inversion, ventricular arrhythmia, ventricular tachycardia, vomiting

Drug Interactions

Metabolism/Transport Effects **Substrate** of CYP2A6 (major); **Inhibits** CYP1A2 (weak), 2C9 (weak), 2D6 (strong), 3A4 (weak)

Avoid Concomitant Use

Avoid concomitant use of Dexmedetomidine with any of the following: Iobenguane I 123

Increased Effect/Toxicity

Dexmedetomidine may increase the levels/effects of: Amifostine; RiTUXimab

The levels/effects of Dexmedetomidine may be increased by: Beta-Blockers; CYP2A6 Inhibitors (Moderate); CYP2A6 Inhibitors (Strong); Diazoxide; Herbs (Hypotensive Properties); Prostacyclin Analogues

Decreased Effect

Dexmedetomidine may decrease the levels/effects of: Iobenguane I 123

The levels/effects of Dexmedetomidine may be decreased by: Antidepressants (Alpha2-Antagonist); Herbs (Hypertensive Properties); Methylphenidate; Serotonin/Norepinephrine Reuptake Inhibitors; Tricyclic Antidepressants; Yohimbine

Stability Store at controlled room temperature of 25°C (77°F); excursions permitted to 15°C to 30°C (59°F to 86°F). Add 2 mL (200 mcg) of dexmedetomidine to 48 mL of 0.9% sodium chloride for a total volume of 50 mL (4 mcg/mL). Shake gently to mix.

Mechanism of Action Selective alpha$_2$-adrenoceptor agonist with anesthetic and sedative properties thought to be due to activation of G-proteins by apha$_{2a}$-adrenoceptors in the brainstem resulting in inhibition of norepinephrine release; peripheral alpha$_{2b}$-adrenoceptors are activated at high doses or with rapid I.V. administration resulting in vasoconstriction.

Pharmacodynamics/Kinetics

Onset of action: Rapid

Distribution: V_{ss}: ~118 L; rapid

Protein binding: ~94%

Metabolism: Hepatic via N-glucuronidation, N-methylation, and CYP2A6

Half-life elimination: ~6 minutes; Terminal: ~2 hours

Excretion: Urine (95%); feces (4%)

Dosage Individualized and titrated to desired clinical effect; duration of infusion should not exceed 24 hours.

ICU sedation:

Adults: I.V.: Initial: Loading infusion of 1 mcg/kg over 10 minutes, followed by a maintenance infusion of 0.2-0.7 mcg/kg/hour; adjust rate to desired level of sedation

Elderly (>65 years of age): Dosage reduction may need to be considered. No specific guidelines available. Dose selections should be cautious, at the low end of dosage range; titration should be slower, allowing adequate time to evaluate response.

Procedural sedation:

Adults: I.V.: Initial: Loading infusion of 1 mcg/kg (or 0.5 mcg/kg for less invasive procedures [eg, ophthalmic]) over 10 minutes, followed by a maintenance infusion of 0.6 mcg/kg/hour, titrate to desired effect; usual range: 0.2-1 mcg/kg/hour

Elderly (>65 years of age): Initial: Loading infusion of 0.5 mcg/kg over 10 minutes; Maintenance infusion: Dosage reduction should be considered

Fiberoptic intubation (awake): I.V. Initial: Loading infusion of 1 mcg/kg over 10 minutes, followed by a maintenance infusion of 0.7 mcg/kg/hour until endotracheal tube is secured.

Dosage adjustment in renal impairment: Dosage reduction may need to be considered. No specific guidelines available.

Dosage adjustment in hepatic impairment: Dosage reduction may need to be considered. No specific guidelines available.

Administration Administer using a controlled infusion device. Must be diluted in 0.9% sodium chloride solution to achieve the required concentration (4 mcg/mL) prior to administration. Advisable to use administration components made with synthetic or coated natural rubber gaskets. Parenteral products should be inspected visually for particulate matter and discoloration prior to administration. If loading dose used, administer over 10 minutes; may extend to 20 minutes to further reduce vasoconstrictive effects.

Monitoring Parameters Level of sedation; heart rate, respiration, rhythm, blood pressure; pain control

Dosage Forms Excipient information presented when available (limited, particularly for generics); consult specific product labeling.

Injection, solution [preservative free]:
Precedex®: 100 mcg/mL (2 mL)

◆ **Dexmedetomidine Hydrochloride** *see* Dexmedetomidine *on page 428*

Dexmethylphenidate (dex meth il FEN i date)

U.S. Brand Names Focalin®; Focalin® XR

Index Terms Dexmethylphenidate Hydrochloride

Pharmacologic Category Central Nervous System Stimulant

Use Treatment of attention-deficit/hyperactivity disorder (ADHD)

Restrictions C-II

An FDA-approved medication guide must be distributed when dispensing an outpatient prescription (new or refill) where this medication is to be used without direct supervision of a healthcare provider. Medication guides are available at http://www.fda.gov/cder/Offices/ODS/medication_guides.htm.

Pregnancy Risk Factor C

Medication Safety Issues

Sound-alike/look-alike issues:
Dexmethylphenidate may be confused with methadone

Dosage Treatment of ADHD: Oral:

Children ≥6 years: Patients not currently taking methylphenidate:

Tablet: Initial: 2.5 mg twice daily; dosage may be adjusted in increments of 2.5-5 mg at weekly intervals (maximum dose: 20 mg/day); doses should be taken at least 4 hours apart

Capsule: Initial: 5 mg/day; dosage may be adjusted in increments of 5 mg/day at weekly intervals (maximum dose: 20 mg/day)

Adults: Patients not currently taking methylphenidate:

Tablet: Initial: 2.5 mg twice daily; dosage may be adjusted in increments of 2.5-5 mg at weekly intervals (maximum dose: 20 mg/day); doses should be taken at least 4 hours apart

Capsule: Initial: 10 mg/day; dosage may be adjusted in increments of 10 mg/day at weekly intervals (maximum dose: 20 mg/day)

Conversion to dexmethylphenidate from methylphenidate: Tablet, capsule: Initial: Half the total daily dose of racemic methylphenidate (maximum dexmethylphenidate dose: 20 mg/day)

Conversion from dexmethylphenidate immediate release to dexmethylphenidate extended release: When changing from Focalin® tablets to Focalin® XR capsules, patients may be switched to the same daily dose using Focalin® XR (maximum dose: 20 mg/day)

Dose reductions and discontinuation: Reduce dose or discontinue in patients with paradoxical aggravation of symptoms. Discontinue if no improvement is seen after one month of treatment.

Dosage adjustment in renal impairment: No data available. However, considering extensive metabolism to inactive compounds, renal insufficiency expected to have minimal effect on kinetics of dexmethylphenidate.

Dosage adjustment in hepatic impairment: No data available.

Additional Information Complete prescribing information for this medication should be consulted for additional detail.

Dosage Forms Excipient information presented when available (limited, particularly for generics); consult specific product labeling.

Capsule, extended release:
Focalin® XR: 5 mg, 10 mg, 15 mg, 20 mg [bimodal release]

Tablet, as hydrochloride: 2.5 mg, 5 mg, 10 mg
Focalin®: 2.5 mg, 5 mg; 10 mg [dye free]

◆ **Dexmethylphenidate Hydrochloride** *see* Dexmethylphenidate *on page 430*

◆ **DexPak® 10 Day TaperPak®** *see* Dexamethasone *on page 425*

◆ **DexPak® TaperPak®** *see* Dexamethasone *on page 425*

Dexpanthenol (deks PAN the nole)

Index Terms Pantothenyl Alcohol

Pharmacologic Category Gastrointestinal Agent, Stimulant; Topical Skin Product

Use Prophylactic use to minimize paralytic ileus; treatment of postoperative distention; topical to relieve itching and to aid healing of minor dermatoses

Pregnancy Risk Factor C

Dosage I.M.: Adults:

Prevention of postoperative ileus: 250-500 mg stat, repeat in 2 hours, followed by doses every 6 hours until danger passes

Paralytic ileus: 500 mg stat, repeat in 2 hours, followed by doses every 6 hours, if needed

Additional Information Complete prescribing information for this medication should be consulted for additional detail.

Dosage Forms Excipient information presented when available (limited, particularly for generics); consult specific product labeling.

Injection, solution [preservative free]: 250 mg/mL (2 mL)

◆ **Dex PC** *see* Chlorpheniramine, Phenylephrine, and Dextromethorphan *on page 311*

Dexrazoxane (deks ray ZOKS ane)

U.S. Brand Names Totect™; Zinecard®

Canadian Brand Names Zinecard®

Index Terms ICRF-187; NSC-169780

Pharmacologic Category Antidote; Cardioprotectant

Use

Zinecard®: Reduction of the incidence and severity of cardiomyopathy associated with doxorubicin administration in women with metastatic breast cancer who have received a cumulative doxorubicin dose of 300 mg/m^2 and who would benefit from continuing therapy with doxorubicin. (Not recommended for use with initial doxorubicin therapy.)

Totect™: Treatment of anthracycline-induced extravasation.

Unlabeled/Investigational Use Reduction of the incidence and severity of cardiomyopathy associated with doxorubicin administration (cumulative doses >300 mg/m^2) in patients with malignancies other than metastatic breast cancer who would benefit from continuing therapy with doxorubicin; reduction of the incidence and severity of cardiomyopathy associated with continued epirubicin administration for advanced breast cancer

Pregnancy Risk Factor C (Zinecard®) / D (Totect™)

Medication Safety Issues

Sound-alike/look-alike issues:

Zinecard® may be confused with Gemzar®

Dosage Adults: I.V.:

Prevention of doxorubicin cardiomyopathy: A 10:1 ratio of dexrazoxane:doxorubicin (500 mg/m^2 dexrazoxane: 50 mg/m^2 doxorubicin). **Note:** Cardiac monitoring should continue during dexrazoxane therapy; doxorubicin/dexrazoxane should be discontinued in patients who develop a decline in LVEF or clinical CHF.

Treatment of anthracycline extravasation: 1000 mg/m^2 on days 1 and 2 (maximum dose: 2000 mg), followed by 500 mg/m^2 on day 3 (maximum dose: 1000 mg); begin treatment as soon as possible, within 6 hours of extravasation

Dosage adjustment in renal impairment: Moderate-to-severe (Cl_{cr}<40 mL/minute):

Prevention of cardiomyopathy: Reduce dose by 50%, using a 5:1 ratio (250 mg/m^2 dexrazoxane: 50 mg/m^2 doxorubicin)

Anthracycline-induced extravasation: Reduce dose by 50%

Dosage adjustment in hepatic impairment: Since doxorubicin dosage is reduced in hyperbilirubinemia, a proportional reduction in dexrazoxane dosage is recommended (maintain ratio of 10:1).

Additional Information Complete prescribing information for this medication should be consulted for additional detail.

Dosage Forms Excipient information presented when available (limited, particularly for generics); consult specific product labeling.

Injection, powder for reconstitution: 250 mg, 500 mg

Totect™: 500 mg [provided with 0.167 Molar sodium lactate injection, USP]

Zinecard®: 250 mg, 500 mg [provided with 0.167 Molar sodium lactate injection, USP]

Dextran (DEKS tran)

U.S. Brand Names Gentran®; LMD®

Canadian Brand Names Gentran®

Index Terms Dextran 40; Dextran 70; Dextran, High Molecular Weight; Dextran, Low Molecular Weight

Pharmacologic Category Plasma Volume Expander

Use Blood volume expander used in treatment of shock or impending shock when blood or blood products are not available; dextran 40 is also used as a priming fluid in cardiopulmonary bypass and for prophylaxis of venous thrombosis and pulmonary embolism in surgical procedures associated with a high risk of thromboembolic complications

Pregnancy Risk Factor C

Medication Safety Issues

Sound-alike/look-alike issues:

Dextran may be confused with Dexatrim®, Dexedrine®

Dosage I.V. (requires an infusion pump): Dose and infusion rate are dependent upon the patient's fluid status and must be individualized:

Volume expansion/shock:

Children (Dextran 40 or 70): Total dose should not exceed 20 mL/kg during first 24 hours

Adults:

Dextran 40: 500-1000 mL at a rate of 20-40 mL/minute (maximum: 20 mL/kg/day for first 24 hours); 10 mL/kg/day thereafter; therapy should not be continued beyond 5 days

Dextran 70: 500-1000 mL at a rate of 20-40 mL/minute (maximum: 20 mL/kg/day for first 24 hours)

Pump prime (Dextran 40): Varies with the volume of the pump oxygenator; generally, the 10% solution is added in a dose of 1-2 g/kg

Prophylaxis of venous thrombosis/pulmonary embolism (Dextran 40): Begin during surgical procedure and give 50-100 g on the day of surgery; an additional 50 g (500 mL) should be administered every 2-3 days during the period of risk (up to 2 weeks postoperatively); usual maximum infusion rate for nonemergency use: 4 mL/minute

Dosing in renal and/or hepatic impairment: Use with extreme caution

Additional Information Complete prescribing information for this medication should be consulted for additional detail.

Dosage Forms Excipient information presented when available (limited, particularly for generics); consult specific product labeling.

Infusion [premixed in D_5W; low molecular weight]:

LMD®: 10% Dextran 40 (500 mL)

Infusion [premixed in NS; high molecular weight]:

Gentran®: 6% Dextran 70 (500 mL)

Infusion [premixed in NS; low molecular weight]:

LMD®: 10% Dextran (500 mL)

◆ **Dextran 40** *see* Dextran *on page 431*

◆ **Dextran 70** *see* Dextran *on page 431*

Dextran 1 (DEKS tran won)

U.S. Brand Names Promit® [DSC]

Pharmacologic Category Plasma Volume Expander

Use Prophylaxis of serious anaphylactic reactions to I.V. infusion of dextran

Pregnancy Risk Factor C

Medication Safety Issues

Sound-alike/look-alike issues:

Dextran may be confused with Dexatrim®, Dexedrine®

Dosage I.V. (time between dextran 1 and dextran solution should not exceed 15 minutes):

Children: 0.3 mL/kg 1-2 minutes before I.V. infusion of dextran

Adults: 20 mL 1-2 minutes before I.V. infusion of dextran

Additional Information Complete prescribing information for this medication should be consulted for additional detail.

Dosage Forms Excipient information presented when available (limited, particularly for generics); consult specific product labeling. [DSC] = Discontinued product

Injection, solution:

Promit®: 150 mg/mL (20 mL) [DSC]

◆ **Dextran, High Molecular Weight** *see* Dextran *on page 431*

◆ **Dextran, Low Molecular Weight** *see* Dextran *on page 431*

Dextroamphetamine (deks troe am FET a meen)

U.S. Brand Names Dexedrine®; DextroStat®; Liquadd™

Canadian Brand Names Dexedrine®

Index Terms Dextroamphetamine Sulfate

Pharmacologic Category Stimulant

Use Narcolepsy; attention-deficit/hyperactivity disorder (ADHD)

Unlabeled/Investigational Use Exogenous obesity; depression; abnormal behavioral syndrome in children (minimal brain dysfunction)

Restrictions C-II

An FDA-approved medication guide must be distributed when dispensing an outpatient prescription (new or refill) where this medication is to be used without direct supervision of a healthcare provider. Medication guides are available at http://www.fda.gov/cder/Offices/ODS/medication_guides.htm.

Pregnancy Risk Factor C

Medication Safety Issues

Sound-alike/look-alike issues:

Dexedrine® may be confused with dextran, Excedrin®

Dextroamphetamine may be confused with dexamethasone

Dosage Oral:

Children:

Narcolepsy: 6-12 years: Initial: 5 mg/day; may increase at 5 mg increments in weekly intervals until side effects appear (maximum dose: 60 mg/day)

ADHD:

3-5 years: Initial: 2.5 mg/day given every morning; increase by 2.5 mg/day in weekly intervals until optimal response is obtained; usual range: 0.1-0.5 mg/kg/dose every morning with maximum of 40 mg/day

≥6 years: 5 mg once or twice daily; increase in increments of 5 mg/day at weekly intervals until optimal response is obtained; usual range: 0.1-0.5 mg/kg/dose every morning (5-20 mg/day) with maximum of 40 mg/day

Children >12 years and Adults:

Narcolepsy: Initial: 10 mg/day, may increase at 10 mg increments in weekly intervals until side effects appear; maximum: 60 mg/day

Exogenous obesity (unlabeled use): 5-30 mg/day in divided doses of 5-10 mg 30-60 minutes before meals

Additional Information Complete prescribing information for this medication should be consulted for additional detail.

Dosage Forms Excipient information presented when available (limited, particularly for generics); consult specific product labeling.

Capsule, extended release, as sulfate: 5 mg, 10 mg, 15 mg

Capsule, sustained release, as sulfate:

Dexedrine® Spansule®: 5 mg, 10 mg, 15 mg

Tablet, as sulfate: 5 mg, 10 mg

DextroStat®: 5 mg, 10 mg [contains tartrazine]

Solution, oral, as sulfate:

Liquadd™: 5 mg/5 mL (480 mL) [contains benzoic acid; bubblegum flavor]

Dextroamphetamine and Amphetamine

(deks troe am FET a meen & am FET a meen)

U.S. Brand Names Adderall XR®; Adderall®

Canadian Brand Names Adderall XR®

Index Terms Amphetamine and Dextroamphetamine

Pharmacologic Category Stimulant

Use Attention-deficit/hyperactivity disorder (ADHD); narcolepsy

Restrictions C-II

An FDA-approved medication guide must be distributed when dispensing an outpatient prescription (new or refill) where this medication is to be used without direct supervision of a healthcare provider. Medication guides are available at http://www.fda.gov/cder/Offices/ODS/medication_guides.htm.

Pregnancy Risk Factor C

Medication Safety Issues

Sound-alike/look-alike issues:

Adderall® may be confused with Inderal®

Dosage Oral: **Note:** Use lowest effective individualized dose; administer first dose as soon as awake

ADHD:

Children: <3 years: Not recommended

Children: 3-5 years (Adderall®): Initial 2.5 mg/day given every morning; increase daily dose in 2.5 mg increments at weekly intervals until optimal response is obtained (maximum dose: 40 mg/day given in 1-3 divided doses); use intervals of 4-6 hours between additional doses

Children: ≥6 years:

Adderall®: Initial: 5 mg 1-2 times/day; increase daily dose in 5 mg increments at weekly intervals until optimal response is obtained (usual maximum dose: 40 mg/day given in 1-3 divided doses); use intervals of 4-6 hours between additional doses

Adderall XR®: 5-10 mg once daily in the morning; if needed, may increase daily dose in 5-10 mg increments at weekly intervals (maximum dose: 30 mg/day)

Adolescents 13-17 years (Adderall XR®): 10 mg once daily in the morning; maybe increased to 20 mg/day after 1 week if symptoms are not controlled; higher doses (up to 60 mg/day) have been evaluated; however, there is not adequate evidence that higher doses afford additional benefit.

Adults (Adderall XR®): Initial: 20 mg once daily in the morning; higher doses (up to 60 mg once daily) have been evaluated; however, there is not adequate evidence that higher doses afforded additional benefit

Narcolepsy (Adderall®):

Children: 6-12 years: Initial: 5 mg/day; increase daily dose in 5 mg at weekly intervals until optimal response is obtained (maximum dose: 60 mg/day given in 1-3 divided doses with intervals of 4-6 hours between doses)

Children >12 years and Adults: Initial: 10 mg/day; increase daily dose in 10 mg increments at weekly intervals until optimal response is obtained (maximum dose: 60 mg/day given in 1-3 divided doses with intervals of 4-6 hours between doses)

Additional Information Complete prescribing information for this medication should be consulted for additional detail.

Dosage Forms Excipient information presented when available (limited, particularly for generics); consult specific product labeling.

Capsule, extended release:

Adderall XR®:

5 mg [dextroamphetamine sulfate 1.25 mg, dextroamphetamine saccharate 1.25 mg, amphetamine aspartate monohydrate 1.25 mg, amphetamine sulfate 1.25 mg (equivalent to amphetamine base 3.1 mg)]

10 mg [dextroamphetamine sulfate 2.5 mg, dextroamphetamine saccharate 2.5 mg, amphetamine aspartate monohydrate 2.5 mg, amphetamine sulfate 2.5 mg (equivalent to amphetamine base 6.3 mg)]

15 mg [dextroamphetamine sulfate 3.75 mg, dextroamphetamine saccharate 3.75 mg, amphetamine aspartate monohydrate 3.75 mg, amphetamine sulfate 3.75 mg (equivalent to amphetamine base 9.4 mg)]

20 mg [dextroamphetamine sulfate 5 mg, dextroamphetamine saccharate 5 mg, amphetamine aspartate monohydrate 5 mg, amphetamine sulfate 5 mg (equivalent to amphetamine base 12.5 mg)]

25 mg [dextroamphetamine sulfate 6.25 mg, dextroamphetamine saccharate 6.25 mg, amphetamine aspartate monohydrate 6.25 mg, amphetamine sulfate 6.25 mg (equivalent to amphetamine base 15.6 mg)]

30 mg [dextroamphetamine sulfate 7.5 mg, dextroamphetamine saccharate 7.5 mg, amphetamine aspartate monohydrate 7.5 mg, amphetamine sulfate 7.5 mg (equivalent to amphetamine base 18.8 mg)]

Tablet:

5 mg [dextroamphetamine sulfate 1.25 mg, dextroamphetamine saccharate 1.25 mg, amphetamine aspartate monohydrate 1.25 mg, amphetamine sulfate 1.25 mg (equivalent to amphetamine base 3.13 mg)]

7.5 mg [dextroamphetamine 1.875 mg, dextroamphetamine saccharate 1.875 mg, amphetamine aspartate monohydrate 1.875 mg, amphetamine sulfate 1.875 mg (equivalent to amphetamine base 4.7 mg)]

10 mg [dextroamphetamine sulfate 2.5 mg, dextroamphetamine saccharate 2.5 mg, amphetamine aspartate monohydrate 2.5 mg, amphetamine sulfate 2.5 mg (equivalent to amphetamine base 6.3 mg)]

12.5 mg [dextroamphetamine sulfate 3.125 mg, dextroamphetamine saccharate 3.125 mg, amphetamine aspartate monohydrate 3.125 mg, amphetamine sulfate 3.125 mg (equivalent to amphetamine base 7.8 mg)]

15 mg [dextroamphetamine sulfate 3.75 mg, dextroamphetamine saccharate 3.75 mg, amphetamine aspartate monohydrate 3.75 mg, amphetamine sulfate 3.75 mg (equivalent to amphetamine base 9.4 mg)]

20 mg [dextroamphetamine sulfate 5 mg, dextroamphetamine saccharate 5 mg, amphetamine aspartate monohydrate 5 mg, amphetamine sulfate 5 mg (equivalent to amphetamine base 12.6 mg)]

30 mg [dextroamphetamine sulfate 7.5 mg, dextroamphetamine saccharate 7.5 mg, amphetamine aspartate monohydrate 7.5 mg, amphetamine sulfate 7.5 mg (equivalent to amphetamine base 18.8 mg)]

Adderall®:

5 mg [dextroamphetamine sulfate 1.25 mg, dextroamphetamine saccharate 1.25 mg, amphetamine aspartate monohydrate 1.25 mg, amphetamine sulfate 1.25 mg (equivalent to amphetamine base 3.13 mg)]

7.5 mg [dextroamphetamine 1.875 mg, dextroamphetamine saccharate 1.875 mg, amphetamine aspartate monohydrate 1.875 mg, amphetamine sulfate 1.875 mg (equivalent to amphetamine base 4.7 mg)]

10 mg [dextroamphetamine sulfate 2.5 mg, dextroamphetamine saccharate 2.5 mg, amphetamine aspartate monohydrate 2.5 mg, amphetamine sulfate 2.5 mg (equivalent to amphetamine base 6.3 mg)]

12.5 mg [dextroamphetamine sulfate 3.125 mg, dextroamphetamine saccharate 3.125 mg, amphetamine aspartate monohydrate 3.125 mg, amphetamine sulfate 3.125 mg (equivalent to amphetamine base 7.8 mg)]

15 mg [dextroamphetamine sulfate 3.75 mg, dextroamphetamine saccharate 3.75 mg, amphetamine aspartate monohydrate 3.75 mg, amphetamine sulfate 3.75 mg (equivalent to amphetamine base 9.4 mg)]

20 mg [dextroamphetamine sulfate 5 mg, dextroamphetamine saccharate 5 mg, amphetamine aspartate monohydrate 5 mg, amphetamine sulfate 5 mg (equivalent to amphetamine base 12.6 mg)]

30 mg [dextroamphetamine sulfate 7.5 mg, dextroamphetamine saccharate 7.5 mg, amphetamine aspartate monohydrate 7.5 mg, amphetamine sulfate 7.5 mg (equivalent to amphetamine base 18.8 mg)]

◆ **Dextroamphetamine Sulfate** *see* Dextroamphetamine *on page 431*

◆ **Dextromethorphan, Acetaminophen, and Pseudoephedrine** *see* Acetaminophen, Dextromethorphan, and Pseudoephedrine *on page 33*

Dextromethorphan and Chlorpheniramine

(deks troe meth OR fan & klor fen IR a meen)

U.S. Brand Names Coricidin® HBP Cough & Cold [OTC]; Dimetapp® Children's Long Acting Cough Plus Cold [OTC]; Robitussin® Children's Cough & Cold Long-Acting [OTC]; Robitussin® Cough & Cold Long-Acting [OTC]; Scot-Tussin® DM Maximum Strength [OTC]

Index Terms Chlorpheniramine and Dextromethorphan; Chlorpheniramine Maleate and Dextromethorphan Hydrobromide; Dextromethorphan Hydrobromide and Chlorpheniramine Maleate

Pharmacologic Category Antitussive; Histamine H_1 Antagonist; Histamine H_1 Antagonist, First Generation

Use Symptomatic relief of runny nose, sneezing, itchy/watery eyes, cough, and other upper respiratory symptoms associated with hay fever, common cold, or upper respiratory allergies

Dosage General dosing guidelines; consult specific product labeling.

Antitussive/antihistamine: Oral:

Children: 6-11 years: Dextromethorphan 15 mg and chlorpheniramine 2 mg every 6 hours as needed (maximum: 60 mg dextromethorphan and 8 mg chlorpheniramine/24 hours)

Children ≥12 years and Adults: Dextromethorphan 30 mg and chlorpheniramine 4 mg every 6 hours as needed (maximum: 120 mg dextromethorphan and 16 mg chlorpheniramine/24 hours)

Additional Information Complete prescribing information for this medication should be consulted for additional detail.

Dosage Forms Excipient information presented when available (limited, particularly for generics); consult specific product labeling. [DSC] = Discontinued product

Syrup:

Dimetapp® Children's Long Acting Cough Plus Cold: Dextromethorphan hydrobromide 7.5 mg and chlorpheniramine maleate 1 mg per 5 mL (118 mL) [alcohol free, sugar free; contains sodium benzoate, propylene glycol; grape flavor]

Robitussin® Children's Cough and Cold Long-Acting: Dextromethorphan hydrobromide 15 mg and chlorpheniramine maleate 2 mg per 5 mL (118 mL) [alcohol free, sugar free; contains sodium benzoate, propylene glycol, fruit punch flavor]

Robitussin® Cough and Cold Long-Acting: Dextromethorphan hydrobromide 7.5 mg and chlorpheniramine maleate 1 mg per 5 mL (118 mL) [alcohol free, sugar free; contains sodium benzoate, propylene glycol]

Scot-Tussin® DM Maximum Strength: Dextromethorphan hydrobromide 15 mg and chlorpheniramine maleate 2 mg per 5 mL (118 mL) [alcohol free, sugar free, cherry-strawberry flavor]

Tablet:

Coricidin® HBP Cough and Cold: Dextromethorphan hydrobromide 30 mg and chlorpheniramine maleate 4 mg

◆ **Dextromethorphan and Guaifenesin** *see* Guaifenesin and Dextromethorphan *on page 710*

◆ **Dextromethorphan and Promethazine** *see* Promethazine and Dextromethorphan *on page 1251*

◆ **Dextromethorphan and Pseudoephedrine** *see* Pseudoephedrine and Dextromethorphan *on page 1266*

◆ **Dextromethorphan, Chlorpheniramine, and Phenylephrine** *see* Chlorpheniramine, Phenylephrine, and Dextromethorphan *on page 311*

◆ **Dextromethorphan, Chlorpheniramine, and Pseudoephedrine** *see* Chlorpheniramine, Pseudoephedrine, and Dextromethorphan *on page 315*

Dextromethorphan, Chlorpheniramine, Phenylephrine, and Guaifenesin

(deks troe meth OR fan, klor fen IR a meen, fen il EF rin, & gwye FEN e sin)

U.S. Brand Names Chlordex GP; Donatussin; Quartuss™

Index Terms Chlorpheniramine, Dextromethorphan, Phenylephrine, and Guaifenesin; Guaifenesin, Chlorpheniramine, Phenylephrine, and Dextromethorphan; Phenylephrine Hydrochloride, Chlorpheniramine maleate, Dextromethorphan Hydrobromide, and Guaifenesin

Pharmacologic Category Alpha/Beta Agonist; Antitussive; Expectorant; Histamine H_1 Antagonist; Histamine H_1 Antagonist, First Generation

Use Symptomatic relief of dry, nonproductive cough and upper respiratory symptoms associated with infections such as the common cold, bronchitis, or sinusitis

Pregnancy Risk Factor C

Dosage General dosing guidelines; consult specific product labeling.

Antitussive/antihistamine/decongestant/expectorant: Oral (Donatussin):

Children:

2-6 years: 2.5 mL every 6 hours as needed (maximum: 10 mL/24 hours)

6-12 years: 5 mL every 6 hours as needed (maximum: 20 mL/24 hours)

Children ≥12 years and Adults: 10 mL every 6 hours as needed (maximum: 40 mL/24 hours)

Additional Information Complete prescribing information for this medication should be consulted for additional detail.

Dosage Forms Excipient information presented when available (limited, particularly for generics); consult specific product labeling.

Syrup:

Chlordex GP®: Dextromethorphan hydrobromide 7.5 mg, chlorpheniramine maleate 2 mg, phenylephrine hydrochloride 10 mg, and guaifenesin 100 mg per 5 mL (480 mL) [grape flavor]

Donatussin: Dextromethorphan hydrobromide 15 mg, chlorpheniramine maleate 2 mg, phenylephrine hydrochloride 10 mg, and guaifenesin 100 mg per 5 mL (480 mL) [alcohol free; contains propylene glycol; cherry flavor]

Quartuss™: Dextromethorphan hydrobromide 15 mg, chlorpheniramine maleate 2 mg, phenylephrine hydrochloride 10 mg, and guaifenesin 100 mg per 5 mL (480 mL) [alcohol free, sugar free; contains sodium benzoate, propylene glycol; cherry flavor]

◆ **Dextromethorphan, Guaifenesin, and Pseudoephedrine** *see* Guaifenesin, Pseudoephedrine, and Dextromethorphan *on page 715*

◆ **Dextromethorphan Hydrobromide, Acetaminophen, and Phenylephrine Hydrochloride** *see* Acetaminophen, Dextromethorphan, and Phenylephrine *on page 32*

◆ **Dextromethorphan Hydrobromide and Chlorpheniramine Maleate** *see* Dextromethorphan and Chlorpheniramine *on page 433*

◆ **Dextropropoxyphene** *see* Propoxyphene *on page 1256*

◆ **DextroStat®** *see* Dextroamphetamine *on page 431*

◆ **DFMO** *see* Eflornithine *on page 510*

◆ **DHAD** *see* Mitoxantrone *on page 1007*

◆ **DHAQ** *see* Mitoxantrone *on page 1007*

◆ **DHE** *see* Dihydroergotamine *on page 449*

◆ **D.H.E. 45®** *see* Dihydroergotamine *on page 449*

◆ **DHPG Sodium** *see* Ganciclovir *on page 681*

◆ **DHT™ [DSC]** *see* Dihydrotachysterol *on page 450*

◆ **DHT™ Intensol™ [DSC]** *see* Dihydrotachysterol *on page 450*

◆ **Diabeta** *see* GlyBURIDE *on page 701*

◆ **DiabetAid™ Antifungal Foot Bath [OTC]** *see* Miconazole *on page 989*

◆ **Diabetic Tussin C®** *see* Guaifenesin and Codeine *on page 710*

◆ **Diabetic Tussin® DM [OTC]** *see* Guaifenesin and Dextromethorphan *on page 710*

◆ **Diabetic Tussin® DM Maximum Strength [OTC]** *see* Guaifenesin and Dextromethorphan *on page 710*

◆ **Diabetic Tussin® EX [OTC]** *see* GuaiFENesin *on page 709*

◆ **Diabinese® [DSC]** *see* ChlorproPAMIDE *on page 318*

◆ **Diaβeta®** *see* GlyBURIDE *on page 701*

◆ **Diaminocyclohexane Oxalatoplatinum** *see* Oxaliplatin *on page 1112*

◆ **Diaminodiphenylsulfone** *see* Dapsone *on page 396*

◆ **Diamode [OTC]** *see* Loperamide *on page 900*

◆ **Diamox® (Can)** *see* AcetaZOLAMIDE *on page 34*

◆ **Diamox® Sequels®** *see* AcetaZOLAMIDE *on page 34*

◆ **Diarr-Eze (Can)** *see* Loperamide *on page 900*

◆ **Diastat®** *see* Diazepam *on page 434*

◆ **Diastat® AcuDial™** *see* Diazepam *on page 434*

◆ **Diastat® Rectal Delivery System (Can)** *see* Diazepam *on page 434*

◆ **Diazemuls® (Can)** *see* Diazepam *on page 434*

Diazepam (dye AZ e pam)

U.S. Brand Names Diastat®; Diastat® AcuDial™; Diazepam Intensol™; Valium®

Canadian Brand Names Apo-Diazepam®; Diastat®; Diastat® Rectal Delivery System; Diazemuls®; Novo-Dipam; Valium®

Pharmacologic Category Benzodiazepine

Additional Appendix Information

Benzodiazepines *on page 1646*

Use Management of anxiety disorders, ethanol withdrawal symptoms; skeletal muscle relaxant; status epilepticus; muscle spasm associated with tetanus

Rectal gel: Management of selected, refractory epilepsy patients on stable regimens of antiepileptic drugs (AEDs) requiring intermittent use of diazepam to control episodes of increased seizure activity

Unlabeled/Investigational Use Panic disorders; preoperative sedation, light anesthesia, amnesia

Restrictions C-IV

Pregnancy Risk Factor D

Pregnancy Considerations Teratogenic effects have been reported in animal studies. In humans, diazepam crosses the placenta. An increased risk of congenital malformations and other developmental abnormalities have been associated with diazepam; epilepsy itself may also increase the risk. Hypotonia, hypothermia, withdrawal symptoms, respiratory and feeding difficulties have been reported in the infant following maternal use of benzodiazepines near time of delivery.

Lactation Enters breast milk/contraindicated (AAP rates "of concern")

Medication Safety Issues

Sound-alike/look-alike issues:

Diazepam may be confused with diazoxide, Ditropan®, LORazepam

Valium® may be confused with Valcyte™

Contraindications Hypersensitivity to diazepam or any component of the formulation (cross-sensitivity with other benzodiazepines may exist); myasthenia gravis; severe respiratory insufficiency; severe hepatic insufficiency; sleep apnea syndrome; acute narrow-angle glaucoma; not for use in children <6 months of age (oral)

Warnings/Precautions Withdrawal has also been associated with an increase in the seizure frequency. Use with caution with drugs which may decrease diazepam metabolism. Use with caution in elderly or debilitated patients, obese patients, patients with hepatic disease (including alcoholics), or renal impairment. Active metabolites with extended half-lives may lead to delayed accumulation and adverse effects. Use with caution in patients with respiratory disease or impaired gag reflex.

Acute hypotension, muscle weakness, apnea, and cardiac arrest have occurred with parenteral administration. Acute effects may be more prevalent in patients receiving concurrent barbiturates, narcotics, or ethanol. Appropriate resuscitative equipment and qualified personnel should be available during administration and monitoring. Avoid use of the injection in patients with shock, coma, or acute ethanol intoxication. Intra-arterial injection or extravasation of the parenteral formulation should be avoided. Parenteral formulation contains propylene glycol, which has been associated with toxicity when administered in high dosages. Administration of rectal gel should only be performed by individuals trained to recognize characteristic seizure activity and monitor response.

Causes CNS depression (dose-related) resulting in sedation, dizziness, confusion, or ataxia which may impair physical and mental capabilities. Patients must be cautioned about performing tasks which require mental alertness (eg, operating machinery or driving). Use with caution in patients receiving other CNS depressants or psychoactive agents. Effects with other sedative drugs or ethanol may be potentiated. The dosage of narcotics should be reduced by approximately 1/3 when diazepam is added. Benzodiazepines have been associated with falls and traumatic injury and should be used with extreme caution in patients who are at risk of these events (especially the elderly). Use with caution in patients taking strong CYP3A4 inhibitors, moderate or strong CYP3A4 and CYP2C19 inducers and major CYP3A4 substrates.

Use caution in patients with depression or anxiety associated with depression, particularly if suicidal risk may be present. Use with caution in patients with a history of drug dependence. Benzodiazepines have been associated with dependence and acute withdrawal symptoms on discontinuation or reduction in dose. Acute withdrawal, including seizures, may be precipitated in patients after administration of flumazenil to patients receiving long-term benzodiazepine therapy.

Diazepam has been associated with anterograde amnesia. Psychiatric and paradoxical reactions, including hyperactive or aggressive behavior, have been reported with benzodiazepines, particularly in adolescent/pediatric or elderly patients. Does not have analgesic, antidepressant, or antipsychotic properties.

Rectal gel: Safety and efficacy have not been established in children <2 years of age.

Oral: Safety and efficacy have not been established in children <6 months of age.

Injection: Safety and efficacy have not been established in children <30 days of age. Solution for injection may contain sodium benzoate, benzyl alcohol, or benzoic acid. Large amounts have been associated with "gasping syndrome" in neonates.

Adverse Reactions Frequency not defined. Adverse reactions may vary by route of administration.

Cardiovascular: Hypotension, vasodilatation

Central nervous system: Amnesia, ataxia, confusion, depression, drowsiness, fatigue, headache, slurred speech, paradoxical reactions (eg, aggressiveness, agitation, anxiety, delusions, hallucinations, inappropriate behavior, increased muscle spasms, insomnia, irritability, psychoses, rage, restlessness, sleep disturbances, stimulation), vertigo

Dermatologic: Rash

Endocrine & metabolic: Libido changes

Gastrointestinal: Constipation, diarrhea, nausea, salivation changes (dry mouth or hypersalivation)

Genitourinary: Incontinence, urinary retention

Hepatic: Jaundice

Local: Phlebitis, pain with injection

Neuromuscular & skeletal: Dysarthria, tremor, weakness

Ocular: Blurred vision, diplopia

Respiratory: Apnea, asthma, respiratory rate decreased

Drug Interactions

Metabolism/Transport Effects **Substrate** of CYP1A2 (minor), 2B6 (minor), 2C9 (minor), 2C19 (major), 3A4 (major); **Inhibits** CYP2C19 (weak), 3A4 (weak)

Avoid Concomitant Use There are no known interactions where it is recommended to avoid concomitant use.

Increased Effect/Toxicity

Diazepam may increase the levels/effects of: Alcohol (Ethyl); Clozapine; CNS Depressants; Phenytoin

The levels/effects of Diazepam may be increased by: Antifungal Agents (Azole Derivatives, Systemic); Aprepitant; Calcium Channel Blockers (Nondihydropyridine); Cimetidine; CYP2C19 Inhibitors (Moderate); CYP2C19 Inhibitors (Strong); CYP3A4 Inhibitors (Moderate); CYP3A4 Inhibitors (Strong); Dasatinib; Disulfiram; Fluconazole; Fosaprepitant; Grapefruit Juice; Isoniazid; Macrolide Antibiotics; Nefazodone; Oral Contraceptive (Estrogens); Oral Contraceptive (Progestins); Protease Inhibitors; Proton Pump Inhibitors; Selective Serotonin Reuptake Inhibitors

Decreased Effect

The levels/effects of Diazepam may be decreased by: CarBAMazepine; CYP2C19 Inducers (Strong); CYP3A4 Inducers (Strong); Deferasirox; Rifamycin Derivatives; St Johns Wort; Theophylline Derivatives; Yohimbine

Ethanol/Nutrition/Herb Interactions

Ethanol: Avoid ethanol (may increase CNS depression).

Food: Diazepam serum levels may be increased if taken with food. Diazepam effect/toxicity may be increased by grapefruit juice; avoid concurrent use.

Herb/Nutraceutical: St John's wort may decrease diazepam levels. Avoid valerian, St John's wort, kava kava, gotu kola (may increase CNS depression).

Stability

Injection: Store at 20° to 25°C (68° to 77°F); excursions permitted to 15°C to 30°C (59°F to 86°F). Protect from light. Potency is retained for up to 3 months when kept at room temperature. Most stable at pH 4-8; hydrolysis occurs at pH <3. Per manufacturer, do not mix I.V. product with other medications.

Rectal gel: Store at 25°C (77°F); excursion permitted to 15°C to 30°C (59°F to 86°F).

Tablet: Store at 15°C to 30°C (59°F to 86°F).

Mechanism of Action Binds to stereospecific benzodiazepine receptors on the postsynaptic GABA neuron at several sites within the central nervous system, including the limbic system, reticular formation. Enhancement of the inhibitory effect of GABA on neuronal excitability results by increased neuronal membrane permeability to chloride ions. This shift in chloride ions results in hyperpolarization (a less excitable state) and stabilization.

Pharmacodynamics/Kinetics

I.V.: Status epilepticus:

Onset of action: Almost immediate

Duration: 20-30 minutes

Absorption: Oral: 85% to 100%, more reliable than I.M.

Protein binding: 98%

Metabolism: Hepatic

Half-life elimination: Parent drug: Adults: 20-50 hours; increased half-life in neonates, elderly, and those with severe hepatic disorders; Active major metabolite (desmethyldiazepam): 50-100 hours; may be prolonged in neonates

Dosage Oral absorption is more reliable than I.M.

Children:

Conscious sedation for procedures: Oral: 0.2-0.3 mg/kg (maximum: 10 mg) 45-60 minutes prior to procedure

Muscle spasm associated with tetanus: I.V., I.M.:

Infants >30 days: 1-2 mg/dose every 3-4 hours as needed

Children ≥5 years: 5-10 mg/dose every 3-4 hours as needed

Sedation/muscle relaxant/anxiety:

Oral: 0.12-0.8 mg/kg/day in divided doses every 6-8 hours

I.M., I.V.: 0.04-0.3 mg/kg/dose every 2-4 hours to a maximum of 0.6 mg/kg within an 8-hour period if needed

Status epilepticus:

I.V.: Infants >30 days and Children: 0.1-0.3 mg/kg given over ≤5 mg/minute; may repeat dose after 5-10 minutes; maximum: 10 mg/dose (Hegenbarth, 2008)

Rectal gel: 0.5 mg/kg, then 0.25 mg/kg in 10 minutes if needed

Anticonvulsant (acute treatment): Rectal gel:

Children <2 years: Safety and efficacy have not been studied

Children 2-5 years: 0.5 mg/kg

Children 6-11 years: 0.3 mg/kg

Children ≥12 years: 0.2 mg/kg

Note: Dosage should be rounded upward to the next available dose, 2.5, 5, 7.5, 10, 12.5, 15, 17.5, and 20 mg/dose; dose may be repeated in 4-12 hours if needed; do not use for more than 5 episodes per month or more than one episode every 5 days

Adolescents: Conscious sedation for procedures:

Oral: 10 mg

I.V.: 5 mg, may repeat with 1/2 dose if needed

Adults:

Acute ethanol withdrawal: Oral: 10 mg 3-4 times during first 24 hours, then decrease to 5 mg 3-4 times/day as needed

Anticonvulsant (acute treatment): Rectal gel: 0.2 mg/kg

Note: Dosage should be rounded upward to the next available dose, 2.5, 5, 7.5, 10, 12.5, 15, 17.5, and 20 mg/dose; dose may be repeated in 4-12 hours if needed; do not use for more than 5 episodes per month or more than one episode every 5 days.

Anxiety (symptoms/disorders):

Oral: 2-10 mg 2-4 times/day

I.M., I.V.: 2-10 mg, may repeat in 3-4 hours if needed

Muscle spasm: I.V., I.M.: Initial: 5-10 mg; then 5-10 mg in 3-4 hours, if necessary. Larger doses may be required if associated with tetanus.

Sedation in the ICU patient: I.V.: 0.03-0.1 mg/kg every 30 minutes to 6 hours

Skeletal muscle relaxant (adjunct therapy): Oral: 2-10 mg 3-4 times/day

Status epilepticus:

I.V.: 5-10 mg every 5-10 minutes given over ≤5 mg/minute; maximum dose: 30 mg

Rectal gel: Premonitory/out-of-hospital treatment: 10 mg once; may repeat once if necessary

Rapid tranquilization of agitated patient (administer every 30-60 minutes): Oral: 5-10 mg; average total dose for tranquilization: 20-60 mg

Elderly/debilitated patients:

Oral: 2-2.5 mg 1-2 times/day initially; increase gradually as needed and tolerated

Rectal gel: Due to the increased half-life in elderly and debilitated patients, consider reducing dose.

Dosing adjustment in renal impairment: No dose adjustment recommended; decrease dose if administered for prolonged periods.

I.V.: Risk of propylene glycol toxicity; monitor closely if using for prolonged periods or at high doses

Hemodialysis: Not dialyzable (0% to 5%); supplemental dose is not necessary

Dosing adjustment in hepatic impairment: Use with caution

Administration Intensol™ should be diluted before use.

In children, do not exceed 1-2 mg/minute IVP; adults 5 mg/minute.

Rectal gel: Prior to administration, confirm that prescribed dose is visible and correct, and that the green "ready" band is visible. Patient should be positioned on side (facing person responsible for monitoring), with top leg bent forward. Insert rectal tip (lubricated) into rectum and push in plunger gently over 3 seconds. Remove tip of rectal syringe after 3 additional seconds. Buttocks should be held together for 3 seconds after removal. Dispose of syringe appropriately.

Monitoring Parameters Respiratory, cardiovascular, and mental status; check for orthostasis

Reference Range Therapeutic: Diazepam: 0.2-1.5 mcg/mL (SI: 0.7-5.3 µmol/L); N-desmethyldiazepam (nordiazepam): 0.1-0.5 mcg/mL (SI: 0.35-1.8 µmol/L)

Test Interactions False-negative urinary glucose determinations when using Clinistix® or Diastix®

Additional Information Diazepam does not have any analgesic effects.

Diastat® AcuDial™: When dispensing, consult package information for directions on setting patient's dose; confirm green "ready" band is visible prior to dispensing product.

Dosage Forms Excipient information presented when available (limited, particularly for generics); consult specific product labeling.

Gel, rectal [adult rectal tip (6 cm)]:

Diastat® AcuDial™: 20 mg (4 mL) [contains benzoic acid, bentyl alcohol, ethanol 10%, propylene glycol, and sodium benzoate; delivers set doses of 10 mg, 12.5 mg, 15 mg, 17.5 mg, and 20 mg]

Gel, rectal [pediatric rectal tip (4.4 cm)]:

Diastat®: 5 mg/mL (0.5 mg) [contains benzoic acid, benzyl alcohol, ethanol 10%, propylene glycol, and sodium benzoate]

Injection, solution: 5 mg/mL (2 mL, 10 mL)

Solution, oral: 5 mg/5 mL (5 mL, 500 mL)

Solution, oral [concentrate]:

Diazepam Intensol™: 5 mg/mL (30 mL) [contains ethanol 19%, propylene glycol]

Tablet: 2 mg, 5 mg, 10 mg

Valium®: 2 mg, 5 mg, 10 mg

◆ **Diazepam Intensol™** *see* Diazepam *on page 434*

Diazoxide (dye az OKS ide)

U.S. Brand Names Proglycem®

Canadian Brand Names Proglycem®

Pharmacologic Category Antihypoglycemic Agent; Vasodilator, Direct-Acting

Additional Appendix Information

Hypertension *on page 1820*

Use Hypoglycemia related to islet cell adenoma, carcinoma, hyperplasia, or adenomatosis; nesidioblastosis; leucine sensitivity; extrapancreatic malignancy

Pregnancy Risk Factor C

Medication Safety Issues

Sound-alike/look-alike issues:

Diazoxide may be confused with diazepam, Dyazide®

Dosage Oral: Hyperinsulinemic hypoglycemia:

Newborns and Infants: Initial dose: 10 mg/kg/day; dosing range: 8-15 mg/kg/day in divided doses every 8-12 hours

Children and Adults: Initial dose: 3 mg/kg/day; dosing range: 3-8 mg/kg/day in divided doses every 8-12 hours. **Note:** In certain instances, patients with refractory hypoglycemia may require higher doses.

Dosing adjustment in renal impairment: Half-life may be prolonged with renal impairment; a reduced dose should be considered.

Additional Information Complete prescribing information for this medication should be consulted for additional detail.

Dosage Forms Excipient information presented when available (limited, particularly for generics); consult specific product labeling.

Capsule, oral:

Proglycem®: 50 mg [not available in the U.S.]

Suspension, oral:

Proglycem®: 50 mg/mL (30 mL) [contains ethanol 7.25%, sodium benzoate, propylene glycol; chocolate-mint flavor]

- **Dibenzyline®** *see* Phenoxybenzamine *on page 1181*
- **DIC** *see* Dacarbazine *on page 388*
- **Dicel™** *see* Chlorpheniramine and Pseudoephedrine *on page 310*
- **Dicel™ DM** *see* Chlorpheniramine, Pseudoephedrine, and Dextromethorphan *on page 315*
- **Dichloralphenazone, Acetaminophen, and Isometheptene** *see* Acetaminophen, Isometheptene, and Dichloralphenazone *on page 34*
- **Dichloralphenazone, Isometheptene, and Acetaminophen** *see* Acetaminophen, Isometheptene, and Dichloralphenazone *on page 34*

Dichlorodifluoromethane and Trichloromonofluoromethane

(dye klor oh dye flor oh METH ane & tri klor oh mon oh flor oh METH ane)

U.S. Brand Names Fluori-Methane®

Index Terms Trichloromonofluoromethane and Dichlorodifluoromethane

Pharmacologic Category Analgesic, Topical

Use Management of pain associated with injections

Dosage Invert bottle over treatment area approximately 12" away from site of application; open dispenseal spring valve completely, allowing liquid to flow in a stream from the bottle. The rate of spraying is approximately 10 cm/second and should be continued until entire muscle has been covered.

Additional Information Complete prescribing information for this medication should be consulted for additional detail.

Dosage Forms Excipient information presented when available (limited, particularly for generics); consult specific product labeling.

Aerosol, topical: Dichlorodifluoromethane 15% and trichloromonofluoromethane 85% (103 mL) [contains chlorofluorocarbons]

- **Dichysterol** *see* Dihydrotachysterol *on page 450*

Diclofenac (dye KLOE fen ak)

U.S. Brand Names Cataflam®; Flector®; Solaraze®; Voltaren Ophthalmic®; Voltaren®; Voltaren® Gel; Voltaren®-XR

Canadian Brand Names Apo-Diclo Rapide®; Apo-Diclo SR®; Apo-Diclo®; Cataflam®; Dom-Diclofenac; Dom-Diclofenac SR; Novo-Difenac; Novo-Difenac K; Novo-Difenac-SR; Nu-Diclo; Nu-Diclo-SR; Pennsaid®; PMS-Diclofenac; PMS-Diclofenac SR; Pro-Diclo-Rapide; Riva-Diclofenac; Riva-Diclofenac-K; Sab-Diclofenac; Sandoz-Diclofenac; Voltaren Ophtha®; Voltaren Rapide®; Voltaren®

Index Terms Diclofenac Epolamine; Diclofenac Potassium; Diclofenac Sodium

Pharmacologic Category Nonsteroidal Anti-inflammatory Drug (NSAID); Nonsteroidal Anti-inflammatory Drug (NSAID), Ophthalmic; Nonsteroidal Anti-inflammatory Drug (NSAID), Oral; Nonsteroidal Anti-inflammatory Drug (NSAID), Topical

Additional Appendix Information

Nonsteroidal Anti-inflammatory Agents *on page 1669*

Use

Immediate release tablet: Ankylosing spondylitis; primary dysmenorrhea; acute and chronic treatment of rheumatoid arthritis, osteoarthritis

Delayed-release tablet: Acute and chronic treatment of rheumatoid arthritis, osteoarthritis, ankylosing spondylitis

Extended-release tablet: Chronic treatment of osteoarthritis, rheumatoid arthritis

Ophthalmic solution: Postoperative inflammation following cataract extraction; temporary relief of pain and photophobia in patients undergoing corneal refractive surgery

Topical gel 1%: Relief of osteoarthritis pain in joints amenable to topical therapy (eg, ankle, elbow, foot, hand, knee, wrist)

Topical gel 3%: Actinic keratosis (AK) in conjunction with sun avoidance

Topical patch: Acute pain due to minor strains, sprains, and contusions

Unlabeled/Investigational Use Juvenile rheumatoid arthritis

Restrictions An FDA-approved medication guide must be distributed when dispensing an oral outpatient prescription (new or refill) where this medication is to be used without direct supervision of a healthcare provider. Medication guides are available at http://www.fda.gov/cder/Offices/ODS/medication_guides.htm.

Pregnancy Risk Factor B (topical gel 3%); C (oral, topical gel 1%, topical patch); D (3rd trimester)

Pregnancy Considerations Safety and efficacy in pregnant women have not been established. Exposure late in pregnancy may lead to premature closure of the ductus arteriosus and may inhibit uterine contractions. Avoid use of diclofenac (all forms) in late pregnancy.

Lactation Excretion in breast milk unknown/not recommended

Medication Safety Issues

Sound-alike/look-alike issues:

Diclofenac may be confused with Diflucan®, Duphalac®

Cataflam® may be confused with Catapres®

Voltaren® may be confused with traMADol, Ultram®, Verelan®

Contraindications Hypersensitivity to diclofenac, aspirin, other NSAIDs, or any component of the formulation; perioperative pain in the setting of coronary artery bypass graft (CABG) surgery

Topical patch: Do not apply to nonintact or damaged skin (eg, exudative dermatitis, eczema, infected lesions, burns or wounds)

Warnings/Precautions [U.S. Boxed Warning]: NSAIDs are associated with an increased risk of adverse

cardiovascular thrombotic events, including MI, stroke, and new onset or worsening of pre-existing hypertension. Risk may be increased with duration of use or pre-existing cardiovascular risk factors or disease. Carefully evaluate individual cardiovascular risk profiles prior to prescribing. Use caution with fluid retention, HF, or hypertension. Concurrent administration of ibuprofen, and potentially other nonselective NSAIDs, may interfere with aspirin's cardioprotective effect. **[U.S. Boxed Warning]: Use is contraindicated for treatment of perioperative pain in the setting of coronary artery bypass graft (CABG) surgery.** Risk of MI and stroke may be increased with use following CABG surgery.

NSAID use may compromise existing renal function; dose-dependent decreases in prostaglandin synthesis may result from NSAID use, reducing renal blood flow which may cause renal decompensation. Patients with impaired renal function, dehydration, heart failure, liver dysfunction, those taking diuretics and ACEI, and the elderly are at greater risk of renal toxicity.. Rehydrate patient before starting therapy; monitor renal function closely. Not recommended for use in patients with advanced renal disease. Long-term NSAID use may result in renal papillary necrosis.

[U.S. Boxed Warning]: NSAIDs may increase risk of gastrointestinal irritation, inflammation, ulceration, bleeding, and perforation. These events may occur at any time during therapy and without warning. Use caution with a history of GI disease (bleeding or ulcers), concurrent therapy with aspirin, anticoagulants and/or corticosteroids, smoking, use of alcohol, the elderly or debilitated patients.

Use the lowest effective dose for the shortest duration of time, consistent with individual patient goals, to reduce risk of cardiovascular or GI adverse events. Alternate therapies should be considered for patients at high risk.

NSAIDs may cause serious skin adverse events including exfoliative dermatitis, Stevens-Johnson syndrome (SJS), and toxic epidermal necrolysis (TEN); discontinue use at first sign of skin rash or hypersensitivity. Anaphylactoid reactions may occur, even without prior exposure; patients with "aspirin triad" (bronchial asthma, aspirin intolerance, rhinitis) may be at increased risk. Do not use in patients who experience bronchospasm, asthma, rhinitis, or urticaria with NSAID or aspirin therapy. Use caution in other forms of asthma. Platelet adhesion and aggregation may be decreased; may prolong bleeding time; patients with coagulation disorders or who are receiving anticoagulants should be monitored closely. Anemia may occur; patients on long-term NSAID therapy should be monitored for anemia.

Use with caution in patients with decreased hepatic function. Closely monitor patients with any abnormal LFT. Rarely, severe hepatic reactions (eg, fulminant hepatitis, liver failure) have occurred with oral NSAID; rarely; discontinue all formulations if signs or symptoms of liver disease develop, or if systemic manifestations occur.

The elderly are at increased risk for adverse effects (especially peptic ulceration, CNS effects, and renal toxicity) from NSAIDs even at low doses.

Withhold for at least 4-6 half-lives prior to surgical or dental procedures. Safety and efficacy have not been established in children.

Topical gel: Should not be applied to the eyes, open wounds, infected areas, or to exfoliative dermatitis. Avoid use of occlusive dressings. Should not be used concomitantly with sunscreens, cosmetics, lotions, moisturizers, insect repellents, or other topical medication on the same skin sites. Minimize or avoid sun exposure on treated areas; may increase risk of UV light-induced skin tumors.

Topical patch: Do not apply topical patch to the eyes, mucous membranes, open wounds, infected areas, or to exudative dermatitis. Patch should not be worn during bathing or showering.

Ophthalmic drops: Monitor patients for 1 year following application of ophthalmic drops for corneal refractive procedures. Patients using ophthalmic drops should not wear soft contact lenses. Ophthalmic drops may slow/delay healing or prolong bleeding time following surgery.

Adverse Reactions

Ophthalmic solution (drops):

>10%: Ocular: Lacrimation (30%), keratitis (28%), intraocular pressure increased (15%), transient burning/stinging (15%)

1% to 10%:

- Cardiovascular: Facial edema (≤3%)
- Central nervous system: ≤3%: Dizziness, fever, headache, insomnia, pain
- Gastrointestinal: ≤3%: Abdominal pain, nausea, vomiting
- Neuromuscular & skeletal: ≤3%: Pain, weakness
- Ocular: 5%: Abnormal vision, blurred vision, conjunctivitis, corneal deposits, corneal edema, corneal lesions, corneal opacity, discharge, eyelid swelling, injection, iritis, irritation, itching, lacrimation disorder, ocular allergy
- Respiratory: Rhinitis (≤3%)
- Miscellaneous: Viral infection (≤3%)

<1% (Limited to important or life-threatening): Corneal erosion, corneal infiltrates, corneal perforation, corneal thinning, corneal ulceration, epithelial breakdown, superficial punctuate keratitis

Oral:

1% to 10%:

- Cardiovascular: Edema
- Central nervous system: Dizziness, headache
- Dermatologic: Pruritus, rash
- Endocrine & metabolic: Fluid retention
- Gastrointestinal: Abdominal distension, abdominal pain, constipation, diarrhea, dyspepsia, flatulence, GI perforation, heartburn, nausea, peptic ulcer/GI bleed, vomiting
- Hematologic: Anemia, bleeding time increased
- Hepatic: Liver enzyme abnormalities
- Otic: Tinnitus
- Renal: Renal function abnormal

<1% (Limited to important or life-threatening): Abnormal coordination, agranulocytosis, alopecia, amblyopia, anaphylactoid reactions, anaphylaxis, anxiety, angioedema, aphthous stomatitis, aplastic anemia, appetite changes, arrhythmia, aseptic meningitis, asthma, azotemia, blurred vision, bruising, chest pain, cirrhosis, CHF, colitis, confusion, coma, cystitis, depression, dermatitis, diaphoresis, diplopia, disorientation, drowsiness, dyspnea, epistaxis, eructation, erythema multiforme, esophageal lesions, exfoliative dermatitis, dysuria, flushing, hallucination, hearing impairment, hearing loss, hematuria, hemoglobin decreased, hemolytic anemia, hepatitis, hepatic failure, hepatic necrosis, hyper-/hypotension, hyper-/hypoglycemia, hyperventilation, impotence, infection, interstitial nephritis, intestinal perforation, jaundice, laryngeal edema, leukopenia, lymphadenopathy, malaise, melena, memory disturbance, meningitis, MI, nervousness, night blindness, nocturia, oliguria, palpitation, pancreatitis, pancytopenia, paresthesia, pharynx edema, photosensitivity, pneumonia, polyuria, purpura, psychotic reactions, PVCs, rectal bleeding, renal failure, respiratory depression, scotoma, seizure, sepsis, somnolence, Stevens-Johnson syndrome, swelling of lips and tongue, stomatitis, syncope, tachycardia, taste disorder, thrombocytopenia, tic, toxic epidermal

necrolysis, tremor, urinary frequency, urticaria, vaginal bleeding, vertigo, vitreous floaters, weight change, weakness, vasculitis, xerostomia

Topical gel:

>10%: Local: Application site reactions (incidence increased with 3% gel): Pruritus (≤52%), rash (35% to 46%), contact dermatitis (4% to 33%), dry skin (≤27%), pain (15% to 26%), exfoliation (3% gel; 6% to 24%), paresthesia (≤20%)

1% to 10% (reported for 3% gel):

Cardiovascular: Chest pain, hypertension

Central nervous system: Headache, pain

Dermatologic: Pruritus, rash, skin ulcer

Endocrine & metabolic: Hypercholesterolemia, hyperglycemia

Gastrointestinal: Abdominal pain, diarrhea, dyspepsia

Genitourinary: Hematuria

Hepatic: Liver enzymes increased

Local: Alopecia, edema, photosensitivity

Neuromuscular and skeletal: Arthralgia, arthrosis, back pain, CPK increased, hypokinesia, myalgia, neck pain, weakness

Ocular: Conjunctivitis

Respiratory: Asthma, dyspnea, pneumonia, sinusitis

Miscellaneous: Flu-like syndrome

Topical patch:

1% to 10%:

Central nervous system: Dizziness, hypaesthesia

Dermatologic: Dermatitis (2%), dermal allergic reaction

Gastrointestinal: Nausea (3%), dysgeusia (2%), abdominal pain, constipation, diarrhea, gastritis, vomiting, xerostomia

Local: Application site dryness, irritation, erythema, atrophy, discoloration, hyperhidrosis, and vesicles, edema, itching

Neuromuscular & skeletal: Hyperkinesia

Drug Interactions

Metabolism/Transport Effects **Substrate** (minor) of CYP1A2, 2B6, 2C8, 2C9, 2C19, 2D6, 3A4; **Inhibits** CYP1A2 (moderate), 2C9 (weak), 2E1 (weak), 3A4 (weak)

Avoid Concomitant Use

Avoid concomitant use of Diclofenac with any of the following: Ketorolac

Increased Effect/Toxicity

Diclofenac may increase the levels/effects of: Aminoglycosides; Anticoagulants; Antiplatelet Agents; Bisphosphonate Derivatives; CycloSPORINE; CYP1A2 Substrates; Desmopressin; Lithium; Methotrexate; Nonsteroidal Anti-Inflammatory Agents; Pemetrexed; Quinolone Antibiotics; Thrombolytic Agents; Vancomycin; Vitamin K Antagonists

The levels/effects of Diclofenac may be increased by: Antidepressants (Tricyclic, Tertiary Amine); Corticosteroids (Systemic); Herbs (Anticoagulant/Antiplatelet Properties); Ketorolac; Probenecid; Selective Serotonin Reuptake Inhibitors; Serotonin/Norepinephrine Reuptake Inhibitors; Treprostinil; Voriconazole

Decreased Effect

Diclofenac may decrease the levels/effects of: ACE Inhibitors; Angiotensin II Receptor Blockers; Antiplatelet Agents; Beta-Blockers; Eplerenone; HydrALAZINE; Latanoprost; Loop Diuretics; Thiazide Diuretics

The levels/effects of Diclofenac may be decreased by: Bile Acid Sequestrants

Ethanol/Nutrition/Herb Interactions

Ethanol: Avoid ethanol (may enhance gastric mucosal irritation).

Herb/Nutraceutical: Avoid alfalfa, anise, bilberry, bladderwrack, bromelain, cat's claw, celery, chamomile, coleus, cordyceps, dong quai, evening primrose, fenugreek, feverfew, garlic, ginger, ginkgo biloba, grapeseed, green tea, ginseng (Siberian), guggul, horse chestnut, horseradish, licorice, prickly ash, red clover, reishi, SAMe (s-adenosylmethionine), sweet clover, turmeric, white willow (all have additional antiplatelet activity).

Stability

Ophthalmic solution: Store at 15°C to 25°C (59°F to 77°F).

Tablet: Store below 30°C (86°F). Protect from moisture; store in tight container.

Topical gel: Store at controlled room temperature of 20°C to 25°C (68°F to 77°F); do not freeze.

Topical patch: Store at controlled room temperature 25°C (77°F); excursions permitted to 15°C to 30°C (59°F to 86°F). Keep envelope sealed when not being used.

Mechanism of Action Reversibly inhibits cyclooxygenase-1 and 2 (COX-1 and 2) enzymes, which result in decreased formation of prostaglandin precursors; has antipyretic, analgesic, and anti-inflammatory properties

Pharmacodynamics/Kinetics

Onset of action: Cataflam® is more rapid than sodium salt (Voltaren®) because it dissolves in the stomach instead of the duodenum

Absorption: Topical gel: 6% to 10%

Protein binding: 99% to albumin

Metabolism: Hepatic to several metabolites

Half-life elimination: 2 hours; Patch: ~12 hours

Time to peak, serum: Cataflam®: ~1 hour; Flector®: 10-20 hours; Solaraze® Gel: ~5 hours; Voltaren®: ~2 hours; Voltaren® Gel: 10-14 hours

Excretion: Urine (65%); feces (35%)

Dosage Adults:

Oral:

Analgesia/primary dysmenorrhea: Starting dose: 50 mg 3 times/day; maximum dose: 150 mg/day

Rheumatoid arthritis: 150-200 mg/day in 2-4 divided doses (100-200 mg/day of sustained release product)

Osteoarthritis: 100-150 mg/day in 2-3 divided doses (100-200 mg/day of sustained release product)

Ankylosing spondylitis: 100-125 mg/day in 4-5 divided doses

Ophthalmic:

Cataract surgery: Instill 1 drop into affected eye 4 times/day beginning 24 hours after cataract surgery and continuing for 2 weeks

Corneal refractive surgery: Instill 1-2 drops into affected eye within the hour prior to surgery, within 15 minutes following surgery, and then continue for 4 times/day, up to 3 days

Topical gel:

Actinic keratoses (Solaraze® Gel): Apply 3% gel to lesion area twice daily for 60-90 days

Osteoarthritis (Voltaren® Gel): **Note:** Maximum total body dose of 1% gel should not exceed 32 g per day

Lower extremities: Apply 4 g of 1% gel to affected area 4 times daily (maximum: 16 g per joint per day)

Upper extremities: Apply 2 g of 1% gel to affected area 4 times daily (maximum: 8 g per joint per day)

Topical patch: Acute pain (strains, sprains, contusions): Apply 1 patch twice daily to most painful area of skin

Dosage adjustment in renal impairment: Not recommended in patients with advanced renal disease or significant renal impairment

Dosage adjustment in hepatic impairment: No specific dosing recommendations

Elderly: No specific dosing recommendations; elderly may demonstrate adverse effects at lower doses than younger adults, and >60% may develop asymptomatic peptic ulceration with or without hemorrhage; monitor renal function

Dietary Considerations Oral formulations may be taken with food to decrease GI distress.

Diclofenac potassium = Cataflam®; potassium content: 5.8 mg (0.15 mEq) per 50 mg tablet

Administration

Oral: Do not crush tablets. Administer with food or milk to avoid gastric distress. Take with full glass of water to enhance absorption.

Ophthalmic: Wait at least 5 minutes before administering other types of eye drops.

Topical gel:

1% formulation: Apply gel to affected joint and rub into skin gently, making sure to apply to entire joint. Do not cover area with occlusive dressings or apply sunscreens, cosmetics, or other medications to affected area. Do not wash area for one hour following application. Wash hands immediately after application (unless hands are treated joint).

3% formulation: Apply to lesion with gel and smooth into skin gently. Do not cover lesion with occlusive dressings or apply sunscreens, cosmetics, or other medications to affected area.

Topical patch: Apply to intact, nondamaged skin. Remove transparent liner prior to applying to skin. Wash hands after applying as well as after removal of patch. May tape down edges of patch, if peeling occurs. Should not be worn while bathing or showering. Fold used patches so the adhesive side sticks to itself; dispose of used patches out of reach of children and pets.

Monitoring Parameters Monitor CBC, liver enzymes; monitor urine output and BUN/serum creatinine; occult blood loss, hemoglobin, hematocrit

Dosage Forms Excipient information presented when available (limited, particularly for generics); consult specific product labeling. [DSC] = Discontinued product

Gel, as sodium:

Solaraze®: 3% (50 g, 100 g)

Voltaren® Gel: 1% (100 g)

Solution, ophthalmic, as sodium [drops]: 0.1% (2.5 mL, 5 mL)

Voltaren Ophthalmic®: 0.1% (2.5 mL, 5 mL)

Tablet, as potassium: 50 mg

Cataflam®: 50 mg

Tablet, delayed release, enteric coated, as sodium: 50 mg, 75 mg

Voltaren®: 25 mg [DSC], 50 mg [DSC], 75 mg

Tablet, extended release, as sodium: 100 mg

Voltaren®-XR: 100 mg

Transdermal system, topical, as epolamine:

Flector®: 1.3% (30s) [180 mg]

Diclofenac and Misoprostol

(dye KLOE fen ak & mye soe PROST ole)

U.S. Brand Names Arthrotec®

Canadian Brand Names Arthrotec®

Index Terms Misoprostol and Diclofenac

Pharmacologic Category Nonsteroidal Anti-inflammatory Drug (NSAID), Oral; Prostaglandin

Use The diclofenac component is indicated for the treatment of osteoarthritis and rheumatoid arthritis; the misoprostol component is indicated for the prophylaxis of NSAID-induced gastric and duodenal ulceration

Restrictions An FDA-approved medication guide must be distributed when dispensing an oral outpatient prescription (new or refill) where this medication is to be used without direct supervision of a healthcare provider. Medication guides are available at http://www.fda.gov/cder/Offices/ODS/medication_guides.htm.

Pregnancy Risk Factor X

Dosage Oral:

Adults:

Arthrotec® 50:

Osteoarthritis: 1 tablet 2-3 times/day

Rheumatoid arthritis: 1 tablet 3-4 times/day

For both regimens, if not tolerated by patient, the dose may be reduced to 1 tablet twice daily

Arthrotec® 75:

Patients who cannot tolerate full daily Arthrotec® 50 regimens: 1 tablet twice daily

Note: The use of these tablets may not be as effective at preventing GI ulceration

Elderly: No specific dosage adjustment is recommended; may require reduced dosage due to lower body weight; monitor renal function

Dosage adjustment in renal impairment: Not recommended in patients with advanced renal disease. In renal insufficiency, diclofenac should be used with caution due to potential detrimental effects on renal function, and misoprostol dosage reduction may be required if adverse effects occur (misoprostol is renally eliminated).

Additional Information Complete prescribing information for this medication should be consulted for additional detail.

Dosage Forms Excipient information presented when available (limited, particularly for generics); consult specific product labeling.

Tablet: Diclofenac sodium 50 mg and misoprostol 200 mcg; diclofenac sodium 75 mg and misoprostol 200 mcg

◆ **Diclofenac Epolamine** *see* Diclofenac *on page* 437

◆ **Diclofenac Potassium** *see* Diclofenac *on page* 437

◆ **Diclofenac Sodium** *see* Diclofenac *on page* 437

Dicloxacillin (dye kloks a SIL in)

Canadian Brand Names Dycill®; Pathocil®

Index Terms Dicloxacillin Sodium

Pharmacologic Category Antibiotic, Penicillin

Use Treatment of systemic infections such as pneumonia, skin and soft tissue infections, and osteomyelitis caused by penicillinase-producing staphylococci

Pregnancy Risk Factor B

Dosage

Usual dosage range:

Newborns: Use not recommended

Children <40 kg: Oral: 12.5-100 mg/kg/day divided every 6 hours

Children >40 kg: Oral: 125-250 mg every 6 hours

Adults: Oral: 125-1000 mg every 6 hours

Indication-specific dosing:

Children: Oral:

Furunculosis: 25-50 mg/kg/day divided every 6 hours

Osteomyelitis: 50-100 mg/kg/day in divided doses every 6 hours

Adults: Oral:

Erysipelas, furunculosis, mastitis, otitis externa, septic bursitis, skin abscess: 500 mg every 6 hours

Impetigo: 250 mg every 6 hours

Prosthetic joint (long-term suppression therapy): 250 mg twice daily

***Staphylococcus aureus*, methicillin susceptible infection if no I.V. access:** 500-1000 mg every 6-8 hours

Dosage adjustment in renal impairment: Not necessary

Hemodialysis: Not dialyzable (0% to 5%); supplemental dosage not necessary

Peritoneal dialysis: Supplemental dosage not necessary

Continuous arteriovenous or venovenous hemofiltration: Supplemental dosage not necessary

Additional Information Complete prescribing information for this medication should be consulted for additional detail.

Dosage Forms Excipient information presented when available (limited, particularly for generics); consult specific product labeling.

Capsule: 250 mg, 500 mg

◆ **Dicloxacillin Sodium** *see* Dicloxacillin *on page* 440

Dicyclomine (dye SYE kloe meen)

U.S. Brand Names Bentyl®

Canadian Brand Names Bentylol®; Formulex®; Lomine; Riva-Dicyclomine

Index Terms Dicyclomine Hydrochloride; Dicycloverine Hydrochloride

Pharmacologic Category Anticholinergic Agent

Use Treatment of functional bowel/irritable bowel syndrome

Unlabeled/Investigational Use Urinary incontinence

Pregnancy Risk Factor B

Medication Safety Issues

Sound-alike/look-alike issues:

Dicyclomine may be confused with diphenhydrAMINE, doxycycline, dyclonine

Bentyl® may be confused with Aventyl®, Benadryl®, Bontril®, Cantil®, Proventil®, Trental®

Dosage Adults:

Oral: Initiate with 80 mg/day in 4 equally divided doses, then increase up to 160 mg/day. Duration: Safety data not available for duration >2 weeks.

I.M. **(should not be used I.V.)**: 80 mg/day in 4 divided doses (20 mg/dose)

Additional Information Complete prescribing information for this medication should be consulted for additional detail.

Dosage Forms Excipient information presented when available (limited, particularly for generics); consult specific product labeling.

Capsule, as hydrochloride: 10 mg

Bentyl®: 10 mg

Injection, solution, as hydrochloride: 10 mg/mL (2 mL)

Bentyl®: 10 mg/mL (2 mL)

Syrup, as hydrochloride:

Bentyl®: 10 mg/5 mL (480 mL)

Tablet, as hydrochloride: 20 mg

Bentyl®: 20 mg

◆ **Dicyclomine Hydrochloride** *see* Dicyclomine *on page 441*

◆ **Dicycloverine Hydrochloride** *see* Dicyclomine *on page 441*

◆ **Di-Dak-Sol** *see* Sodium Hypochlorite Solution *on page 1384*

Didanosine (dye DAN oh seen)

U.S. Brand Names Videx®; Videx® EC

Canadian Brand Names Videx®; Videx® EC

Index Terms ddI; Dideoxyinosine

Pharmacologic Category Antiretroviral Agent, Reverse Transcriptase Inhibitor (Nucleoside)

Additional Appendix Information

Antiretroviral Therapy for HIV Infection: Adults and Adolescents *on page 1758*

Management of Healthcare Worker Exposures to HBV, HCV, and HIV *on page 1719*

Perinatal HIV Guidelines *on page 1730*

Use Treatment of HIV infection; always to be used in combination with at least two other antiretroviral agents

Pregnancy Risk Factor B

Pregnancy Considerations Cases of fatal and nonfatal lactic acidosis, with or without pancreatitis, have been reported in pregnant women. It is not known if pregnancy itself potentiates this known side effect; however, pregnant women may be at increased risk of lactic acidosis and liver damage. Hepatic enzymes and electrolytes should be monitored frequently during the 3rd trimester of pregnancy. Use during pregnancy only if the potential benefit to the mother outweighs the potential risk of this complication. Didanosine has been shown to cross the placenta. Preliminary information from the antiretroviral pregnancy registry note an increased risk of birth defects with 1st trimester exposure compared to exposure later in pregnancy; no pattern of defects have been noted. Pharmacokinetics are not significantly altered during pregnancy; dose adjustments are not needed. The Perinatal HIV Guidelines Working Group considers didanosine to be an alternative NRTI in dual nucleoside combination regimens; use with stavudine only if no other alternatives are available. Health professionals are encouraged to contact the antiretroviral pregnancy registry to monitor outcomes of pregnant women exposed to antiretroviral medications (1-800-258-4263 or www.APRegistry.com).

Lactation Excretion in breast milk unknown/contraindicated

Medication Safety Issues

Sound-alike/look-alike issues:

Videx® may be confused with Lidex®

Contraindications There are no contraindications listed in manufacturer's labeling.

Warnings/Precautions **[U.S. Boxed Warning]: Pancreatitis (sometimes fatal) has been reported;** incidence is dose related. Risk factors for developing pancreatitis may include a previous history of the condition, concurrent cytomegalovirus or *Mycobacterium avium-intracellulare* infection, renal impairment, advanced age, and concomitant use of stavudine, pentamidine, or hydroxyurea. Discontinue didanosine if clinical signs of pancreatitis occur. **[U.S. Boxed Warning]: Lactic acidosis, symptomatic hyperlactatemia, and severe hepatomegaly with steatosis (sometimes fatal) have occurred with antiretroviral nucleoside analogues, including didanosine.** Hepatotoxicity may occur even in the absence of marked transaminase elevations; suspend therapy in any patient developing clinical/laboratory findings which suggest hepatotoxicity. Hepatotoxicity and hepatic failure (including fatal cases) have been reported in HIV patients receiving combination drug therapy with hydroxyurea, didanosine, and stavudine; avoid combination. Pregnant women may be at increased risk of lactic acidosis and liver damage. Use with caution in patients with hepatic impairment; safety and efficacy have not been established in patients with significant hepatic disease. Patients on combination antiretroviral therapy with hepatic impairment may be at increased risk of potentially severe and fatal hepatic toxicity; consider interruption or discontinuation of therapy if hepatic impairment worsens.

Peripheral neuropathy occurs in ~20% of patients receiving the drug. If symptomatic, discontinue therapy; after resolution of symptoms, reinitiation of therapy at a reduced dose may be tolerated. Permanently discontinue if neuropathy recurs. Retinal changes (including retinal depigmentation) and optic neuritis have been reported in adults and children using didanosine. Patients should undergo retinal examination every 6-12 months. Hepatotoxicity and hepatic failure (including fatal cases) have been reported in HIV patients receiving combination drug therapy with hydroxyurea, didanosine, and stavudine; avoid combination. Use with caution in patients on sodium-restricted diets or with edema, HF, or hyperuricemia. Use caution in renal impairment; dose reduction recommended for Cl_{cr} <60 mL/minute. May cause redistribution of fat (eg, buffalo hump, peripheral wasting with increased abdominal girth, cushingoid appearance). Patients may develop immune reconstitution syndrome resulting in the occurrence of an inflammatory response to an indolent or residual opportunistic infection; further evaluation and treatment may be required. Didanosine delayed release capsules are indicated for once-daily use.

Adverse Reactions As reported in monotherapy studies; risk of toxicity may increase when combined with other agents.

>10%:

Gastrointestinal: Diarrhea (19% to 28%), amylase increased (15% to 17%), abdominal pain (7% to 13%)

Neuromuscular & skeletal: Peripheral neuropathy (17% to 20%)

1% to 10%:

Dermatologic: Rash/pruritus (7% to 9%)

Endocrine & metabolic: Uric acid increased (2% to 3%)

Gastrointestinal: Pancreatitis (1% to 7% dose dependent); patients >65 years of age had a higher frequency of pancreatitis than younger patients

Hepatic: Alkaline phosphatase increased (1% to 4%), ALT increased (6% to 9%), AST increased (6% to 9%)

Postmarketing and/or case reports: Acute renal impairment, alopecia, anaphylactoid reaction, anemia, anorexia, arthralgia, chills/fever, diabetes mellitus, dry eyes, dyspepsia, flatulence, granulocytopenia, hepatic steatosis, hepatitis, hyper-/hypoglycemia, hyperlactatemia (symptomatic), hypersensitivity, immune reconstitution syndrome, lactic acidosis/hepatomegaly, leukopenia, lipodystrophy, liver failure, MI, myalgia, myopathy, optic neuritis, pain, parotid gland enlargement, retinal depigmentation, rhabdomyolysis, seizure, sialoadenitis, thrombocytopenia, weakness, xerostomia

Drug Interactions

Avoid Concomitant Use There are no known interactions where it is recommended to avoid concomitant use.

Increased Effect/Toxicity

Didanosine may increase the levels/effects of: Hydroxyurea

The levels/effects of Didanosine may be increased by: Allopurinol; Ganciclovir-Valganciclovir; Ribavirin; Stavudine; Tenofovir

Decreased Effect

Didanosine may decrease the levels/effects of: Antifungal Agents (Azole Derivatives, Systemic); Atazanavir; Dapsone; Indinavir; Quinolone Antibiotics

The levels/effects of Didanosine may be decreased by: Atazanavir; Darunavir; Lopinavir; Methadone; Tenofovir; Tipranavir

Ethanol/Nutrition/Herb Interactions

Ethanol: Avoid ethanol (increases risk of pancreatitis).

Food: Decreases AUC and C_{max}. Didanosine serum levels may be decreased by 55% if taken with food.

Stability Delayed release capsules should be stored in tightly closed bottles at controlled room temperature of 25°C (77°F). Unreconstituted powder should be stored at 15°C to 30°C (59°F to 86°F). Reconstituted pediatric solution is stable for 30 days if refrigerated.

Videx® pediatric powder: Add 100 mL or 200 mL purified water, USP to the 2 g or 4 g container, respectively, to achieve a 20 mg/mL solution. Immediately mix the resulting solution with an equal volume of Mylanta® Maximum Strength (or equivalent) to achieve a final concentration of 10 mg/mL.

Mechanism of Action Didanosine, a purine nucleoside (adenosine) analog and the deamination product of dideoxyadenosine (ddA), inhibits HIV replication *in vitro* in both T cells and monocytes. Didanosine is converted within the cell to the mono-, di-, and triphosphates of ddA. These ddA triphosphates act as substrate and inhibitor of HIV reverse transcriptase substrate and inhibitor of HIV reverse transcriptase thereby blocking viral DNA synthesis and suppressing HIV replication.

Pharmacodynamics/Kinetics

Absorption: Subject to degradation by acidic pH of stomach; some formulations are buffered to resist acidic pH; ≤50% reduction in peak plasma concentration is observed in presence of food. Delayed release capsules contain enteric-coated beadlets which dissolve in the small intestine.

Distribution: V_d: Children: 28 L/m^2; Adults: 1.08 L/kg

Protein binding: <5%

Metabolism: Has not been evaluated in humans; studies conducted in dogs show extensive metabolism with allantoin, hypoxanthine, xanthine, and uric acid being the major metabolites found in urine

Bioavailability: Children: 25%; Adults: 42%

Half-life elimination:

Children and Adolescents: 0.8 hour

Adults: Normal renal function: 1.5 hours; active metabolite, ddATP, has an intracellular half-life >12 hours *in vitro*; Renal impairment: 2.5-5 hours

Time to peak: Delayed release capsules: 2 hours; Powder for suspension: 0.25-1.5 hours

Excretion: Urine (~55% as unchanged drug)

Clearance: Total body: Averages 800 mL/minute

Dosage Treatment of HIV infection: Oral (administer on an empty stomach):

Pediatric powder for oral solution (Videx®):

Infants: 2 weeks to 8 months: 100 mg/m^2 twice daily is recommended by the manufacturer; 50 mg/m^2 may be considered in infants 2 weeks to 4 months (AIDSinfo guidelines)

Infants and Children >8 months: 120 mg/m^2 twice daily is recommended by the manufacturer. **Note:** AIDSinfo guidelines suggest a range of 90-150 mg/m^2 twice daily

Children 3-21 years (AIDSinfo guidelines): Treatment-naive: 240 mg/m^2/dose once daily (maximum: 400 mg/dose)

Adolescents and Adults: Dosing based on patient weight:

<60 kg: 125 mg twice daily (preferred) or 250 mg once daily

≥60 kg: 200 mg twice daily (preferred) or 400 mg once daily

Delayed release capsule (Videx® EC): Children and Adults:

20 kg to <25 kg: 200 mg once daily

25 kg to <60 kg: 250 mg once daily

≥60 kg: 400 mg once daily

Elderly patients have a higher frequency of pancreatitis (10% versus 5% in younger patients); monitor renal function and dose accordingly

When taken with tenofovir: Adults:

<60 kg and Cl_{cr} ≥60 mL/minute: 200 mg once daily

≥60 kg and Cl_{cr} ≥60 mL/minute: 250 mg once daily

Dosage adjustment in renal impairment: Children: No specific guidelines available; consider dosage reduction. Adults: Dosing based on patient weight, creatinine clearance, and dosage form: See table.

Recommended Dose (mg) of Didanosine by Body Weight – Adults

Creatinine Clearance (mL/min)	≥60 kg		<60 kg	
	Powder for Oral Solution	Delayed Release Capsule	Powder for Oral Solution	Delayed Release Capsule
≥60	400 mg daily or 200 mg twice daily	400 mg daily	250 mg daily or 125 mg twice daily	250 mg daily
30-59	200 mg daily or 100 mg twice daily	200 mg daily	150 mg daily or 75 mg twice daily	125 mg daily
10-29	150 mg daily	125 mg daily	100 mg daily	125 mg daily
<10	100 mg daily	125 mg daily	75 mg daily	See Note.

Note: Per manufacturer, not suitable for use in patients <60 kg with Cl_{cr} <10 mL/minute; use alternate formulation.

Patients requiring hemodialysis or CAPD: Dose per Cl_{cr} <10 mL/minute. No didanosine removed via CAPD.

Hemodialysis: Minimal amount of dose (≤7%) removed by hemodialysis; no supplemental dosing necessary

Dosing adjustment in hepatic impairment: Should be considered; monitor for toxicity

Dietary Considerations Videx® EC: Take on an empty stomach; administer at least 1 hour before or 2 hours after eating

Administration Pediatric powder for oral solution: Prior to dispensing, the powder should be mixed with purified water USP to an initial concentration of 20 mg/mL and then further diluted with an appropriate antacid suspension to a final mixture of 10 mg/mL. Shake well prior to use. Videx® EC: Administer on an empty stomach at least 1 hour before or 2 hours after eating; swallow capsule whole.

Monitoring Parameters Serum potassium, uric acid, creatinine; hemoglobin, CBC with neutrophil and platelet count, CD4 cells; viral load; liver function tests, amylase; weight gain; perform dilated retinal exam every 6 months

Additional Information A high rate of early virologic nonresponse was observed when didanosine, lamivudine, and tenofovir were used as the initial regimen in treatment-naive patients. Use of this combination is not recommended; patients currently on this regimen should be closely monitored for modification of therapy. Early virologic failure was also observed with tenofovir and didanosine delayed release capsules, plus either efavirenz or nevirapine; use caution in treatment-naive patients with high baseline viral loads.

Dosage Forms Excipient information presented when available (limited, particularly for generics); consult specific product labeling.

Capsule, delayed release, enteric coated pellets: 200 mg, 250 mg, 400 mg

Capsule, delayed release, enteric coated beadlets:

Videx® EC: 125 mg, 200 mg, 250 mg, 400 mg

Powder for oral solution, pediatric:

Videx®: 2 g, 4 g [makes 10 mg/mL solution after final mixing]

◆ **Dideoxyinosine** *see* Didanosine *on page 441*

◆ **Didronel®** *see* Etidronate Disodium *on page 586*

Diethylpropion (dye eth il PROE pee on)

Canadian Brand Names Tenuate®; Tenuate® Dospan®

Index Terms Amfepramone; Diethylpropion Hydrochloride

Pharmacologic Category Anorexiant; Sympathomimetic

Use Short-term (few weeks) adjunct in the management of exogenous obesity

Restrictions C-IV

Pharmacotherapy for weight loss is recommended only for obese patients with a body mass index ≥30 kg/m^2, or ≥27 kg/m^2 in the presence of other risk factors such as hypertension, diabetes, and/or dyslipidemia or a high waist circumference; therapy should be used in conjunction with a comprehensive weight management program. Rule out organic causes of obesity (eg, untreated hypothyroidism) prior to use.

Note: Diethylpropion is not approved for long-term use. The limited usefulness of medications in this class should be weighed against possible risks associated with their use. Consult weight loss guidelines for current pharmacotherapy recommendations.

Pregnancy Risk Factor B

Dosage Children >16 years and Adults: Oral:

Tablet: 25 mg 3 times/day before meals or food

Tablet, controlled release: 75 mg at midmorning

Additional Information Complete prescribing information for this medication should be consulted for additional detail.

Dosage Forms Excipient information presented when available (limited, particularly for generics); consult specific product labeling.

Tablet, as hydrochloride: 25 mg

Tablet, controlled release, as hydrochloride: 75 mg

◆ **Diethylpropion Hydrochloride** *see* Diethylpropion *on page 443*

Difenoxin and Atropine
(dye fen OKS in & A troe peen)

U.S. Brand Names Motofen® [DSC]

Index Terms Atropine and Difenoxin

Pharmacologic Category Antidiarrheal

Use Treatment of diarrhea

Restrictions C-IV

Pregnancy Risk Factor C

Dosage Adults: Oral: Initial: 2 tablets (each tablet contains difenoxin hydrochloride 1 mg and atropine sulfate 0.025 mg), then 1 tablet after each loose stool; 1 tablet every 3-4 hours, up to 8 tablets in a 24-hour period; if no improvement after 48 hours, continued administration is not indicated

Additional Information Complete prescribing information for this medication should be consulted for additional detail.

Dosage Forms Excipient information presented when available (limited, particularly for generics); consult specific product labeling. [DSC] = Discontinued product

Tablet, oral:

Motofen®: Difenoxin hydrochloride 1 mg and atropine sulfate 0.025 mg [DSC]

◆ **Differin®** *see* Adapalene *on page 44*

◆ **Differin® XP (Can)** *see* Adapalene *on page 44*

◆ **Difil-G** *see* Dyphylline and Guaifenesin *on page 501*

◆ **Difil®-G Forte** *see* Dyphylline and Guaifenesin *on page 501*

Diflorasone (dye FLOR a sone)

U.S. Brand Names ApexiCon™; ApexiCon™ E

Index Terms Diflorasone Diacetate

Pharmacologic Category Corticosteroid, Topical

Additional Appendix Information

Corticosteroids *on page 1652*

Use Relieves inflammation and pruritic symptoms of corticosteroid-responsive dermatosis (high to very high potency topical corticosteroid)

Pregnancy Risk Factor C

Medication Safety Issues

Sound-alike/look-alike issues:

International issues:

Florone® may be confused with Fluoron® which is a brand name for fluorine in Canada

Florone® may be confused with Flogene® which is a brand name for fentiazac in Italy and a brand name for piroxicam in Brazil

Dosage Topical: Apply ointment sparingly 1-3 times/day; apply cream sparingly 2-4 times/day. Therapy should be discontinued when control is achieved; if no improvement is seen, reassessment of diagnosis may be necessary.

Additional Information Complete prescribing information for this medication should be consulted for additional detail.

Dosage Forms Excipient information presented when available (limited, particularly for generics); consult specific product labeling.

Cream, as diacetate: 0.05% (15 g, 30 g, 60 g)

ApexiCon™ E: 0.05% (30 g, 60 g)

Ointment, as diacetate: 0.05% (15 g, 30 g, 60 g)

ApexiCon™: 0.05% (30 g, 60 g)

- **Diflorasone Diacetate** *see* Diflorasone *on page 443*
- **Diflucan®** *see* Fluconazole *on page 625*

Difluprednate (dye floo PRED nate)

U.S. Brand Names Durezol™

Pharmacologic Category Corticosteroid, Ophthalmic

Use Treatment of inflammation and pain following ocular surgery

Pregnancy Risk Factor C

Dosage Ophthalmic: Adults: Instill 1 drop in conjunctival sac of the affected eye(s) 4 times/day beginning 24 hours after surgery, continue for 2 weeks, then decrease to 2 times/day for 1 week, then taper based on response

Additional Information Complete prescribing information for this medication should be consulted for additional detail.

Dosage Forms Excipient information presented when available (limited, particularly for generics); consult specific product labeling.

Emulsion, ophthalmic:

Durezol™: 0.05% (5 mL) [contains sorbic acid]

- **Digibind®** *see* Digoxin Immune Fab *on page 446*
- **DigiFab™** *see* Digoxin Immune Fab *on page 446*
- **Digitek®** *see* Digoxin *on page 444*

Digoxin (di JOKS in)

U.S. Brand Names Digitek®; Lanoxicaps® [DSC]; Lanoxin®

Canadian Brand Names Apo-Digoxin®; Digoxin CSD; Lanoxicaps®; Lanoxin®; Novo-Digoxin; Pediatric Digoxin CSD

Pharmacologic Category Antiarrhythmic Agent, Class IV; Cardiac Glycoside

Additional Appendix Information

Heart Failure (Systolic) *on page 1809*

Use Treatment of congestive heart failure and to slow the ventricular rate in tachyarrhythmias such as atrial fibrillation, atrial flutter, and supraventricular tachycardia (paroxysmal atrial tachycardia); cardiogenic shock

Pregnancy Risk Factor C

Lactation Enters breast milk (small amounts)/compatible

Medication Safety Issues

Sound-alike/look-alike issues:

Digoxin may be confused with Desoxyn®, doxepin

Lanoxin® may be confused with Lasix®, Levoxyl®, Levsinex®, Lomotil®, Lonox®, Mefoxin®, Xanax®

High alert medication: The Institute for Safe Medication Practices (ISMP) includes this medication among its list of drugs which have a heightened risk of causing significant patient harm when used in error.

International issues:

Dilacor®: Brand name for diltiazem in the U.S.; brand name for verapamil in Brazil; brand name for barnidipine in Argentina

Lanoxin® may be confused with Lemoxin® which is a brand bane for cefuroxime in Mexico

Lanoxin® may be confused with Limoxin® which is a brand name for amoxicillin in Mexico

Contraindications Hypersensitivity to digoxin or any component of the formulation; hypersensitivity to cardiac glycosides (another may be tried); history of toxicity; ventricular tachycardia or fibrillation; idiopathic hypertrophic subaortic stenosis; constrictive pericarditis; amyloid disease; second- or third-degree heart block (except in patients with a functioning artificial pacemaker); Wolff-Parkinson-White syndrome and atrial fibrillation concurrently

Warnings/Precautions Watch for proarrhythmic effects (especially with digoxin toxicity). Withdrawal in HF patients may lead to recurrence of HF symptoms. Use with caution in patients with hypoxia, myxedema, hypothyroidism, acute myocarditis; patients with incomplete AV block (Stokes-Adams attack) may progress to complete block with digitalis drug administration; use with caution in patients with acute myocardial infarction, severe pulmonary disease, advanced heart failure, idiopathic hypertrophic subaortic stenosis, Wolff-Parkinson-White syndrome, sick-sinus syndrome (bradyarrhythmias), amyloid heart disease, and constrictive cardiomyopathies; adjust dose with renal impairment and when verapamil, quinidine or amiodarone are added to a patient on digoxin; elderly and neonates may develop exaggerated serum/tissue concentrations due to age-related alterations in clearance and pharmacodynamic differences; exercise will reduce serum concentrations of digoxin due to increased skeletal muscle uptake; recent studies indicate photopsia, chromatopsia and decreased visual acuity may occur even with therapeutic serum drug levels; reduce or hold dose 1-2 days before elective electrical cardioversion. In the Cardiac Arrhythmia Suppression Trial (CAST), recent (>6 days but <2 years ago) myocardial infarction patients with asymptomatic, non-life-threatening ventricular arrhythmias did not benefit and may have been harmed by attempts to suppress the arrhythmia with flecainide or encainide. An increased mortality or nonfatal cardiac arrest rate (7.7%) was seen in the active treatment group compared with patients in the placebo group (3%). The applicability of the CAST results to other populations is unknown. Antiarrhythmic agents should be reserved for patients with life-threatening ventricular arrhythmias.

Adverse Reactions Incidence not always reported.

Cardiovascular: Heart block; first-, second- (Wenckebach), or third-degree heart block; asystole; atrial tachycardia with block; AV dissociation; accelerated junctional rhythm; ventricular tachycardia or ventricular fibrillation; PR prolongation; ST segment depression

Central nervous system: Visual disturbances (blurred or yellow vision), headache (3.2%), dizziness (4.9%), apathy, confusion, mental disturbances (4.1%), anxiety, depression, delirium, hallucinations, fever

Dermatologic: Maculopapular rash (1.6%); erythematous, scarlatiniform, papular, vesicular, or bullous rash; urticaria; pruritus; facial, angioneurotic, or laryngeal edema; shedding of fingernails or toenails; alopecia

Gastrointestinal: Nausea (3.2%), vomiting (1.6%), diarrhea (3.2%), abdominal pain

Neuromuscular & skeletal: Weakness

<1% (Limited to important or life-threatening): Abdominal pain, anorexia, eosinophilia, gynecomastia, hemorrhagic necrosis of the intestines, increased plasma estrogen and decreased serum luteinizing hormone in men and postmenopausal women and decreased plasma testosterone in men, intestinal ischemia, palpitation, sexual dysfunction, thrombocytopenia, unifocal or multiform ventricular premature contractions (especially bigeminy or trigeminy), vaginal cornification

Any arrhythmia seen in a child on digoxin should be considered as digoxin toxicity. The gastrointestinal and central nervous system symptoms are not frequently seen in children.

Drug Interactions

Metabolism/Transport Effects Substrate of CYP3A4 (minor)

Avoid Concomitant Use There are no known interactions where it is recommended to avoid concomitant use.

Increased Effect/Toxicity

Digoxin may increase the levels/effects of: Midodrine

The levels/effects of Digoxin may be increased by: Aminoquinolines (Antimalarial); Amiodarone; Antifungal

Agents (Azole Derivatives, Systemic); Atorvastatin; Beta-Blockers; Calcitriol; Calcium Channel Blockers (Nondihydropyridine); Carvedilol; Conivaptan; CycloSPORINE; Macrolide Antibiotics; Milnacipran; Nefazodone; Neuromuscular-Blocking Agents; P-Glycoprotein Inhibitors; Propafenone; Protease Inhibitors; QuiNIDine; QuiNINE; Ranolazine; Telmisartan

Decreased Effect

Digoxin may decrease the levels/effects of: Antineoplastic Agents (Anthracycline)

The levels/effects of Digoxin may be decreased by: 5-ASA Derivatives; Acarbose; Aminoglycosides; Antineoplastic Agents; Antineoplastic Agents (Anthracycline); Bile Acid Sequestrants; Kaolin; Penicillamine; P-Glycoprotein Inducers; Potassium-Sparing Diuretics; St Johns Wort

Ethanol/Nutrition/Herb Interactions

Food: Digoxin peak serum levels may be decreased if taken with food. Meals containing increased fiber (bran) or foods high in pectin may decrease oral absorption of digoxin.

Herb/Nutraceutical: Avoid ephedra (risk of cardiac stimulation). Avoid natural licorice (causes sodium and water retention and increases potassium loss).

Stability Protect elixir and injection from light.

Mechanism of Action

Congestive heart failure: Inhibition of the sodium/potassium ATPase pump which acts to increase the intracellular sodium-calcium exchange to increase intracellular calcium leading to increased contractility

Supraventricular arrhythmias: Direct suppression of the AV node conduction to increase effective refractory period and decrease conduction velocity - positive inotropic effect, enhanced vagal tone, and decreased ventricular rate to fast atrial arrhythmias. Atrial fibrillation may decrease sensitivity and increase tolerance to higher serum digoxin concentrations.

Pharmacodynamics/Kinetics

Onset of action: Oral: 1-2 hours; I.V.: 5-30 minutes

Peak effect: Oral: 2-8 hours; I.V.: 1-4 hours

Duration: Adults: 3-4 days both forms

Absorption: By passive nonsaturable diffusion in the upper small intestine; food may delay, but does not affect extent of absorption

Distribution:

Normal renal function: 6-7 L/kg

V_d: Extensive to peripheral tissues, with a distinct distribution phase which lasts 6-8 hours; concentrates in heart, liver, kidney, skeletal muscle, and intestines. Heart/serum concentration is 70:1. Pharmacologic effects are delayed and do not correlate well with serum concentrations during distribution phase.

Hyperthyroidism: Increased V_d

Hyperkalemia, hyponatremia: Decreased digoxin distribution to heart and muscle

Hypokalemia: Increased digoxin distribution to heart and muscles

Concomitant quinidine therapy: Decreased V_d

Chronic renal failure: 4-6 L/kg

Decreased sodium/potassium ATPase activity - decreased tissue binding

Neonates, full-term: 7.5-10 L/kg

Children: 16 L/kg

Adults: 7 L/kg, decreased with renal disease

Protein binding: 30%; in uremic patients, digoxin is displaced from plasma protein binding sites

Metabolism: Via sequential sugar hydrolysis in the stomach or by reduction of lactone ring by intestinal bacteria (in ~10% of population, gut bacteria may metabolize up to 40% of digoxin dose); metabolites may contribute to therapeutic and toxic effects of digoxin; metabolism is reduced with CHF

Bioavailability: Oral (formulation dependent): Elixir: 75% to 85%; Tablet: 70% to 80%

Half-life elimination (age, renal and cardiac function dependent):

Neonates: Premature: 61-170 hours; Full-term: 35-45 hours

Infants: 18-25 hours

Children: 35 hours

Adults: 38-48 hours

Adults, anephric: 4-6 days

Half-life elimination: Parent drug: 38 hours; Metabolites: Digoxigenin: 4 hours; Monodigitoxoside: 3-12 hours

Time to peak, serum: Oral: ~1 hour

Excretion: Urine (50% to 70% as unchanged drug)

Dosage When changing from oral (tablets or liquid) or I.M. to I.V. therapy, dosage should be reduced by 20% to 25%. Refer to the following: See table.

Dosage Recommendations for Digoxin

Age	Total Digitalizing Dose[2] (mcg/kg[1])		Daily Maintenance Dose[3] (mcg/kg[1])	
	P.O.	I.V. or I.M.	P.O.	I.V. or I.M.
Preterm infant[1]	20-30	15-25	5-7.5	4-6
Full-term infant[1]	25-35	20-30	6-10	5-8
1 mo - 2 y[1]	35-60	30-50	10-15	7.5-12
2-5 y[1]	30-40	25-35	7.5-10	6-9
5-10 y[1]	20-35	15-30	5-10	4-8
>10 y[1]	10-15	8-12	2.5-5	2-3
Adults	0.75-1.5 mg	0.5-1 mg	0.125-0.5 mg	0.1-0.4 mg

[1]Based on lean body weight and normal renal function for age. Decrease dose in patients with ↓ renal function; digitalizing dose often not recommended in infants and children.

[2]Give one-half of the total digitalizing dose (TDD) in the initial dose, then give one-quarter of the TDD in each of two subsequent doses at 6- to 8-hour intervals. Obtain ECG 6 hours after each dose to assess potential toxicity.

[3]Divided every 12 hours in infants and children <10 years of age. Given once daily to children >10 years of age and adults.

Dosing adjustment/interval in renal impairment:

Cl_{cr} 10-50 mL/minute: Administer 25% to 75% of dose or every 36 hours

Cl_{cr} <10 mL/minute: Administer 10% to 25% of dose or every 48 hours

Reduce loading dose by 50% in ESRD

Hemodialysis: Not dialyzable (0% to 5%)

Dietary Considerations Maintain adequate amounts of potassium in diet to decrease risk of hypokalemia (hypokalemia may increase risk of digoxin toxicity).

Administration

I.M.: Inject no more than 2 mL per injection site. May cause intense pain.

I.V.: May be administered undiluted or diluted fourfold in D_5W, NS, or SWFI for direct injection. Less than fourfold dilution may lead to drug precipitation. Inject slowly over ≥5 minutes.

Monitoring Parameters

When to draw serum digoxin concentrations: Digoxin serum concentrations are monitored because digoxin possesses a narrow therapeutic serum range; the therapeutic endpoint is difficult to quantify and digoxin toxicity may be life-threatening. Digoxin serum levels should be drawn **at least 4 hours after an intravenous dose** and **at least 6 hours after an oral dose (optimally 12-24 hours after a dose).**

Initiation of therapy:

If a loading dose is given: Digoxin serum concentration may be drawn within 12-24 hours after the initial loading dose administration. Levels drawn this early may confirm the relationship of digoxin plasma levels and response but are of little value in determining maintenance doses.

If a loading dose is not given: Digoxin serum concentration should be obtained after 3-5 days of therapy.

Maintenance therapy:

Trough concentrations should be followed just prior to the next dose or at a minimum of 4 hours after an I.V. dose and at least 6 hours after an oral dose.

Digoxin serum concentrations should be obtained within 5-7 days (approximate time to steady-state) after any dosage changes. Continue to obtain digoxin serum concentrations 7-14 days after any change in maintenance dose. **Note:** In patients with end-stage renal disease, it may take 15-20 days to reach steady-state.

Additionally, patients who are receiving potassium-depleting medications such as diuretics, should be monitored for potassium, magnesium, and calcium levels.

Digoxin serum concentrations should be obtained whenever any of the following conditions occur:

Questionable patient compliance or to evaluate clinical deterioration following an initial good response

Changing renal function

Suspected digoxin toxicity

Initiation or discontinuation of therapy with drugs (amiodarone, quinidine, verapamil) which potentially interact with digoxin; if quinidine therapy is started, the digoxin dose should be reduced by 25% to 50% and digoxin levels should be monitored closely. Any disease changes (hypothyroidism)

Any disease changes (hypothyroidism)

Heart rate and rhythm should be monitored along with periodic ECGs to assess both desired effects and signs of toxicity

Follow closely (especially in patients receiving diuretics or amphotericin) for decreased serum potassium and magnesium or increased calcium, all of which predispose to digoxin toxicity

Assess renal function

Be aware of drug interactions

Observe patients for noncardiac signs of toxicity, confusion, and depression

Reference Range

Digoxin therapeutic serum concentrations:

Congestive heart failure: 0.5-0.8 ng/mL

Arrhythmias: 0.8-2 ng/mL

Adults: <0.5 ng/mL; probably indicates underdigitalization unless there are special circumstances

Toxic: >2.5 ng/mL

Digoxin-like immunoreactive substance (DLIS) may cross-react with digoxin immunoassay. DLIS has been found in patients with renal and liver disease, congestive heart failure, neonates, and pregnant women (3rd trimester).

Dosage Forms Excipient information presented when available (limited, particularly for generics); consult specific product labeling. [CAN] = Canadian brand name; [DSC] = Discontinued product

Capsule:

Lanoxicaps®: 100 mcg [contains ethanol; DSC]; 200 mcg [contains ethanol; DSC]

Injection, solution: 250 mcg/mL (1 mL, 2 mL)

Lanoxin®: 250 mcg/mL (2 mL) [contains ethanol 10% and propylene glycol 40%]

Injection, solution [pediatric]: 100 mcg/mL (1 mL)

Solution, oral: 50 mcg/mL (2.5 mL, 5 mL, 60 mL)

Tablet: 125 mcg, 250 mcg

Digitek®, Lanoxin®: 125 mcg, 250 mcg

Apo-Digoxin® [CAN]: 62.5 mcg, 125 mcg, 250 mcg

◆ **Digoxin CSD (Can)** *see* Digoxin *on page 444*

Digoxin Immune Fab (di JOKS in i MYUN fab)

U.S. Brand Names Digibind®; DigiFab™

Canadian Brand Names Digibind®

Index Terms Antidigoxin Fab Fragments, Ovine

Pharmacologic Category Antidote

Use Treatment of life-threatening or potentially life-threatening digoxin intoxication, including:

- acute digoxin ingestion (ie, >10 mg in adults or >4 mg in children)
- chronic ingestions leading to steady-state digoxin concentrations >6 ng/mL in adults or >4 ng/mL in children
- manifestations of digoxin toxicity due to overdose (life-threatening ventricular arrhythmias, progressive bradycardia, second- or third-degree heart block not responsive to atropine, serum potassium >5 mEq/L in adults or >6 mEq in children)

Pregnancy Risk Factor C

Pregnancy Considerations Animal reproduction studies have not been conducted. Safety and efficacy in pregnant women have not been established. Use during pregnancy only if clearly needed.

Lactation Excretion in breast milk unknown/use caution

Contraindications Hypersensitivity to digoxin immune Fab, sheep products, or any component of the formulation

Warnings/Precautions Suicidal attempts often involve multiple drugs; consider other drug toxicities as well. Hypersensitivity reactions can occur. Epinephrine should be immediately available. Serum potassium levels should be monitored, especially during the first few hours after administration. Total serum digoxin concentrations will rise precipitously following administration of this drug (has no clinical meaning; avoid monitoring serum concentrations). If digoxin was being used to treat heart failure, may see exacerbation of symptoms as digoxin level is reduced. Use with caution in renal failure (experience limited); the complex will be removed from the body more slowly. Monitor for reoccurrence of digoxin toxicity. Failure of response to adequate treatment may call diagnosis of digitalis toxicity into question. Digoxin immune Fab is processed with papain and may cause hypersensitivity reactions in patients allergic to papaya, other papaya extracts, papain, chymopapain, or the pineapple enzyme bromelain. There may also be cross allergy with dust mite and latex allergens.

Adverse Reactions Frequency not defined.

Cardiovascular: Effects (due to withdrawal of digitalis) include exacerbation of heart failure, rapid ventricular response in patients with atrial fibrillation; postural hypotension

Endocrine & metabolic: Hypokalemia

Local: Phlebitis

Miscellaneous: Allergic reactions, serum sickness

Drug Interactions

Avoid Concomitant Use There are no known interactions where it is recommended to avoid concomitant use.

Increased Effect/Toxicity There are no known significant interactions involving an increase in effect.

Decreased Effect There are no known significant interactions involving a decrease in effect.

Stability Should be refrigerated (2°C to 8°C).

Digibind®: Reconstitute by adding 4 mL sterile water, resulting in 9.5 mg/mL for I.V. infusion. Reconstituted solutions should be used within 4 hours if refrigerated. For very small doses, reconstituted vial can be further diluted by adding an additional 34 mL of sterile isotonic saline to achieve a final concentration of 1 mg/mL.

DigiFab™: Reconstitute by adding 4 mL sterile water, resulting in 10 mg/mL for I.V. infusion. Reconstituted solutions should be used within 4 hours if refrigerated. For very small doses, reconstituted vial can be further diluted by adding an additional 36 mL of sterile isotonic saline to achieve a final concentration of 1 mg/mL.

Mechanism of Action Digoxin immune antigen-binding fragments (Fab) are specific antibodies for the treatment of digitalis intoxication in carefully selected patients; binds with molecules of digoxin or digitoxin and then is excreted by the kidneys and removed from the body

Pharmacodynamics/Kinetics

Onset of action: I.V.: Improvement in 2-30 minutes for toxicity

Half-life elimination: 15-20 hours; prolonged with renal impairment

Excretion: Urine; undetectable amounts within 5-7 days

Dosage Each vial of Digibind® 38 mg or DigiFab™ 40 mg will bind ~0.5 mg of digoxin or digitoxin.

Note: Estimation of the dose is based on the body burden of digitalis. This may be calculated if the amount ingested is known or the postdistribution serum drug level is known (round dose to the nearest whole vial). If the amount of ingestion is unknown, general dosing guidelines should be used.

Acute ingestion of *unknown* amount: I.V.: Children and Adults: 20 vials is adequate to treat most life-threatening ingestions. May give as a single dose or give 10 vials, observe response, and give a second 10-vial dose if indicated.

Acute ingestion of *known* amount: I.V.:

Based on number of tablets/capsules ingested: Children and Adults:

Step 1:

Total body load (mg) = Amount (mg) digoxin capsules/ digitoxin ingested

Step 2:

Dose (vials) = Total body load (mg) / (0.5 mg digitalis bound/vial)

Alternatively, the following table gives an estimation of the number of vials needed based on the number of digoxin tablets or capsules ingested.

Number of Digoxin Tablets or Capsules Ingested[1]	Dose of Digoxin Immune Fab (# of Vials)
25	10
50	20
75	30
100	40
150	60
200	80

[1]250 mcg tablets with 80% bioavailability or 200 mcg Lanoxicaps® capsules with 100% bioavailability.

Based on steady-state serum digoxin concentration:

Infants and Children ≤20 kg: May require smaller doses; calculate dose in milligrams, reconstitute with NS, and administer dose via tuberculin syringe

Step 1:

Dose (mg) = [(serum digoxin concentration [ng/mL] x weight [kg]) / 10] x (mg/vial)[1]

[1]Digibind® 38 mg/vial or DigiFab™ 40 mg/vial

Alternatively, the following table gives an estimation of the amount of **Digibind®** needed based on the steady-state serum digoxin concentration.

Infants and Small Children Dose Estimates of Digibind® (in mg) From Steady-State Serum Digoxin Concentration

Patient Weight (kg)	Serum Digoxin Concentration (ng/mL)						
	1	2	4	8	12	16	20
1	0.4 mg[1]	1 mg[1]	1.5 mg[1]	3 mg[1]	5 mg	6 mg	8 mg
3	1 mg[1]	2 mg[1]	5 mg	9 mg	14 mg	18 mg	23 mg
5	2 mg[1]	4 mg	8 mg	15 mg	23 mg	30 mg	38 mg
10	4 mg	8 mg	15 mg	30 mg	46 mg	61 mg	76 mg
20	8 mg	15 mg	30 mg	61 mg	91 mg	122 mg	152 mg

[1]Dilution of reconstituted vial to 1 mg/mL may be desirable.

Alternatively, the following table gives an estimation of the amount of **DigiFab™** needed based on the steady-state serum digoxin concentration.

Infants and Small Children Dose Estimates of DigiFab™ (in mg) From Steady-State Serum Digoxin Concentration

Patient Weight (kg)	Serum Digoxin Concentration (ng/mL)						
	1	2	4	8	12	16	20
1	0.4 mg[1]	1 mg[1]	1.5 mg[1]	3 mg[1]	5 mg	6.5 mg	8 mg
3	1 mg[1]	2.5 mg[1]	5 mg	10 mg	14 mg	19 mg	24 mg
5	2 mg[1]	4 mg	8 mg	16 mg	24 mg	32 mg	40 mg
10	4 mg	8 mg	16 mg	32 mg	48 mg	64 mg	80 mg
20	8 mg	16 mg	32 mg	64 mg	96 mg	128 mg	160 mg

[1]Dilution of reconstituted vial to 1 mg/mL may be desirable.

Adults:

Step 1:

Dose (vials) = [(serum digoxin concentration [ng/mL] x weight [kg]) / 100

Alternatively, the following table gives an estimation of the number of vials needed based on the steady-state serum digoxin concentration.

Adult Dose Estimates of Digibind® (in # of Vials) From Steady-State Serum Digoxin Concentration

Patient Weight (kg)	Serum Digoxin Concentration (ng/mL)						
	1	2	4	8	12	16	20
40	0.5 v	1 v	2 v	3 v	5 v	7 v	8 v
60	0.5 v	1 v	3 v	5 v	7 v	10 v	12 v
70	1 v	2 v	3 v	6 v	9 v	11 v	14 v
80	1 v	2 v	3 v	7 v	10 v	13 v	16 v
100	1 v	2 v	4 v	8 v	12 v	16 v	20 v

v = vials.

Based on steady-state serum digitoxin concentration: Children and Adults: If the calculated dose based on the **digitoxin** concentration is different than that for the digoxin concentration, use the higher dose.

Step 1:

Dose (vials) = [serum **digitoxin** concentration (ng/mL) x weight (kg)] / 1000

Chronic toxicity (serum digoxin concentration unavailable): I.V.:

Infants and Children ≤20 kg: 1 vial is adequate to reverse most cases of toxicity

Adults: 6 vials is adequate to reverse most cases of toxicity

Administration Continuous I.V. infusion over ≥30 minutes is preferred. May give by bolus injection if cardiac arrest is imminent. Small doses (infants/small children) may be administered using tuberculin syringe. Stopping the infusion and restarting at a slower rate may help if infusion-related reactions occur.

Monitoring Parameters Serum potassium, serum digoxin concentration prior to first dose of digoxin immune Fab; **digoxin levels will greatly increase with digoxin immune Fab use and are not an accurate determination of body stores** (has no clinical meaning; avoid monitoring serum concentrations); standard digoxin concentration measurements may be misleading until Fab fragments are eliminated from the body.

Patients with renal failure should be monitored for a prolonged period for reintoxication with digoxin following the rerelease of bound digoxin into the blood.

Test Interactions Digibind® will interfere with digitalis immunoassay measurements - this will result in clinically misleading serum digoxin concentrations fragment is eliminated from the body (several days to >1 week after Digibind® administration).

Dosage Forms Excipient information presented when available (limited, particularly for generics); consult specific product labeling.

Injection, powder for reconstitution [ovine derived]:

Digibind®: 38 mg [derived from or manufactured using papain]

DigiFab™: 40 mg [derived from or manufactured using papain]

- **Dihematoporphyrin Ether** *see* Porfimer *on page* *1212*
- **Dihistine® DH [DSC]** *see* Chlorpheniramine, Pseudoephedrine, and Codeine *on page* *314*

Dihydrocodeine, Aspirin, and Caffeine

(dye hye droe KOE deen, AS pir in, & KAF een)

U.S. Brand Names Synalgos®-DC

Index Terms Dihydrocodeine Compound

Pharmacologic Category Analgesic, Opioid

Use Management of mild to moderate pain that requires relaxation

Restrictions C-III

Pregnancy Risk Factor B/D (prolonged use or high doses at term)

Medication Safety Issues

Sound-alike/look-alike issues:

Synalgos®-DC may be confused with Synagis®

High alert medication: The Institute for Safe Medication Practices (ISMP) includes this medication among its list of drug classes which have a heightened risk of causing significant patient harm when used in error.

Dosage

Adults: Oral: 1-2 capsules every 4-6 hours as needed for pain

Elderly: Initial dosing should be cautious (low end of adult dosing range)

Additional Information Complete prescribing information for this medication should be consulted for additional detail.

Dosage Forms Excipient information presented when available (limited, particularly for generics); consult specific product labeling.

Capsule: Dihydrocodeine bitartrate 16 mg, aspirin 356.4 mg, and caffeine 30 mg

Dihydrocodeine, Chlorpheniramine, and Phenylephrine

(dye hye droe KOE deen, klor fen IR a meen, & fen il EF rin)

U.S. Brand Names Baltussin; Coldcough PD; Novahistine DH

Index Terms Chlorpheniramine Maleate, Dihydrocodeine Bitartrate, and Phenylephrine Hydrochloride; Phenylephrine, Chlorpheniramine, and Dihydrocodeine

Pharmacologic Category Alpha/Beta Agonist; Analgesic, Opioid; Antitussive; Histamine H_1 Antagonist; Histamine H_1 Antagonist, First Generation

Use Symptomatic relief of cough and congestion associated with the upper respiratory tract

Restrictions C-III/C-V

Pregnancy Risk Factor C

Dosage Cough and congestion: Oral:

Children 2-6 years (Novahistine DH): 1.25-2.5 mL every 4-6 hours as needed (maximum: 10 mL/24 hours)

Children 6-12 years:

Baltussin: 2.5 mL every 4-6 hours as needed

Novahistine DH: 2.5-5 mL every 4-6 hours as needed (maximum: 20 mL/24 hours)

Children ≥12 years and adults:

Baltussin: 5 mL every 4-6 hours as needed

Novahistine DH: 5-10 mL every 4-6 hours as needed (maximum: 40 mL/24 hours)

Additional Information Complete prescribing information for this medication should be consulted for additional detail.

Dosage Forms Excipient information presented when available (limited, particularly for generics); consult specific product labeling.

Liquid:

Novahistine DH: Dihydrocodeine bitartrate 7.5 mg, chlorpheniramine maleate 2 mg and phenylephrine hydrochloride 5 mg per 5 mL (480 mL) [alcohol free, sugar free; contains propylene glycol; strawberry flavor; C-III]

Syrup:

Baltussin: Dihydrocodeine bitartrate 3 mg, chlorpheniramine maleate 5 mg, and phenylephrine hydrochloride 20 mg per 5 mL (480 mL) [alcohol free, sugar free; contains propylene glycol; fruit flavor; C-III]

Coldcough PD: Dihydrocodeine bitartrate 3 mg, chlorpheniramine maleate 2 mg, and phenylephrine hydrochloride 7.5 mg per 5 mL (120 mL) [alcohol free, sugar free; grape flavor; C-V]

- **Dihydrocodeine Compound** *see* Dihydrocodeine, Aspirin, and Caffeine *on page* *448*

Dihydrocodeine, Pseudoephedrine, and Guaifenesin

(dye hye droe KOE deen, soo doe e FED rin, & gwye FEN e sin)

U.S. Brand Names DiHydro-GP; Hydro-Tussin™ EXP [DSC]; Pancof®-EXP

Index Terms Guaifenesin, Dihydrocodeine, and Pseudoephedrine; Pseudoephedrine Hydrochloride, Guaifenesin, and Dihydrocodeine Bitartrate

Pharmacologic Category Antitussive/Decongestant/Expectorant

Use Temporary relief of cough and congestion associated with upper respiratory tract infections and allergies

Pregnancy Risk Factor C

Dosage Oral: Cough/congestion (Hydro-Tussin™ EXP, Pancof®-EXP):

Children:

2-6 years: 1.25-2.5 mL every 4-6 hours as needed

6-12 years: 2.5-5 mL every 4-6 hours as needed

Children ≥12 years and Adults: 5-10 mL every 4-6 hours as needed

Additional Information Complete prescribing information for this medication should be consulted for additional detail.

Dosage Forms Excipient information presented when available (limited, particularly for generics); consult specific product labeling. [DSC] = Discontinued product

Syrup:

DiHydro-GP: Dihydrocodeine bitartrate 7.5 mg, pseudoephedrine hydrochloride 15 mg, and guaifenesin 100 mg per 5 mL (480 mL) [vanilla flavor]

Hydro-Tussin™ EXP [DSC], Pancof®-EXP: Dihydrocodeine bitartrate 7.5 mg, pseudoephedrine hydrochloride 15 mg, and guaifenesin 100 mg per 5 mL (480 mL) [alcohol free, dye free, sugar free]

Dihydroergotamine (dye hye droe er GOT a meen)

U.S. Brand Names D.H.E. 45®; Migranal®

Canadian Brand Names Migranal®

Index Terms DHE; Dihydroergotamine Mesylate

Pharmacologic Category Antimigraine Agent; Ergot Derivative

Use Treatment of migraine headache with or without aura; injection also indicated for treatment of cluster headaches

Unlabeled/Investigational Use Adjunct for DVT prophylaxis for hip surgery, for orthostatic hypotension, xerostomia secondary to antidepressant use, and pelvic congestion with pain

Pregnancy Risk Factor X

Pregnancy Considerations Dihydroergotamine is oxytocic and should not be used during pregnancy.

Lactation May be excreted in breast milk/contraindicated

Contraindications Hypersensitivity to dihydroergotamine or any component of the formulation; high-dose aspirin therapy; uncontrolled hypertension, ischemic heart disease, angina pectoris, history of MI, silent ischemia, or coronary artery vasospasm including Prinzmetal's angina; hemiplegic or basilar migraine; peripheral vascular disease; sepsis; severe hepatic or renal dysfunction; following vascular surgery; avoid use within 24 hours of sumatriptan, zolmitriptan, other serotonin agonists, or ergot-like agents; avoid during or within 2 weeks of discontinuing MAO inhibitors; ergot alkaloids are contraindicated with potent inhibitors of CYP3A4 (includes protease inhibitors, azole antifungals, and some macrolide antibiotics); pregnancy

Warnings/Precautions **[U.S. Boxed Warning]: Ergot alkaloids are contraindicated with potent inhibitors of CYP3A4 (includes protease inhibitors, azole antifungals, and some macrolide antibiotics); concomitant use associated with acute ergot toxicity (ergotism).** Do not give to patients with risk factors for CAD until a cardiovascular evaluation has been performed; if evaluation is satisfactory, the healthcare provider should administer the first dose and cardiovascular status should be periodically evaluated. May cause vasospastic reactions; persistent vasospasm may lead to gangrene or death in patients with compromised circulation. Discontinue if signs of vasoconstriction develop. Rare reports of increased blood pressure in patients without history of hypertension. Rare reports of adverse cardiac events (acute MI, life-threatening arrhythmias, death) have been reported following use of the injection. Cerebral hemorrhage, subarachnoid hemorrhage, and stroke have also occurred following use of the injection. Not for prolonged use. Pleural and peritoneal fibrosis have been reported with prolonged daily use. Cardiac valvular fibrosis has also been associated with ergot alkaloids. Use with caution in the elderly. Safety and efficacy in pediatric patients have not been established.

Migranal® Nasal Spray: Local irritation to nose and throat (usually transient and mild-moderate in severity) can occur; long-term consequences on nasal or respiratory mucosa have not been extensively evaluated.

Adverse Reactions

>10%: Nasal spray: Respiratory: Rhinitis (26%)

1% to 10%: Nasal spray:

- Central nervous system: Dizziness (4%), somnolence (3%)
- Endocrine & metabolic: Hot flashes (1%)
- Gastrointestinal: Nausea (10%), taste disturbance (8%), vomiting (4%), diarrhea (2%)
- Local: Application site reaction (6%)
- Neuromuscular & skeletal: Weakness (1%), stiffness (1%)
- Respiratory: Pharyngitis (3%)

<1% (Limited to important or life-threatening): Injection and nasal spray: Cerebral hemorrhage, coronary artery vasospasm, hypertension, MI, paresthesia, peripheral cyanosis, peripheral ischemia, rash, stroke, subarachnoid hemorrhage, ventricular fibrillation, ventricular tachycardia. Pleural and retroperitoneal fibrosis have been reported following prolonged use of the injection; cardiac valvular fibrosis has been associated with ergot alkaloids.

Drug Interactions

Metabolism/Transport Effects **Substrate** of CYP3A4 (major); **Inhibits** CYP3A4 (weak)

Avoid Concomitant Use

Avoid concomitant use of Dihydroergotamine with any of the following: Efavirenz; Posaconazole; Protease Inhibitors; Serotonin 5-HT1D Receptor Agonists; Sibutramine; Voriconazole

Increased Effect/Toxicity

Dihydroergotamine may increase the levels/effects of: Serotonin 5-HT1D Receptor Agonists; Serotonin Modulators

The levels/effects of Dihydroergotamine may be increased by: CYP3A4 Inhibitors (Moderate); CYP3A4 Inhibitors (Strong); Dasatinib; Efavirenz; Macrolide Antibiotics; Posaconazole; Protease Inhibitors; Serotonin 5-HT1D Receptor Agonists; Sibutramine; Voriconazole

Decreased Effect There are no known significant interactions involving a decrease in effect.

Stability

Injection: Store below 25°C (77°F); do not refrigerate or freeze. Protect from heat and light.

Nasal spray: Prior to use, store below 25°C (77°F); do not refrigerate or freeze. Once spray applicator has been prepared, use within 8 hours; discard any unused solution.

Mechanism of Action Ergot alkaloid alpha-adrenergic blocker directly stimulates vascular smooth muscle to vasoconstrict peripheral and cerebral vessels; also has effects on serotonin receptors

Pharmacodynamics/Kinetics

Onset of action: 15-30 minutes

Duration: 3-4 hours

Distribution: V_d: 14.5 L/kg

Protein binding: 93%

Metabolism: Extensively hepatic

Half-life elimination: 1.3-3.9 hours

Time to peak, serum: I.M.: 15-30 minutes

Excretion: Primarily feces; urine (10% mostly as metabolites)

Dosage Adults:

I.M., SubQ: 1 mg at first sign of headache; repeat hourly to a maximum dose of 3 mg total; maximum dose: 6 mg/week

I.V.: 1 mg at first sign of headache; repeat hourly up to a maximum dose of 2 mg total; maximum dose: 6 mg/week

Intranasal: 1 spray (0.5 mg) of nasal spray should be administered into each nostril; if needed, repeat after 15 minutes, up to a total of 4 sprays. **Note:** Do not exceed 3 mg (6 sprays) in a 24-hour period and no more than 8 sprays in a week.

Elderly: Patients >65 years of age were not included in controlled clinical studies

Dosing adjustment in renal impairment: Contraindicated in severe renal impairment

Dosing adjustment in hepatic impairment: Dosage reductions are probably necessary but specific guidelines are not available; contraindicated in severe hepatic dysfunction

Administration Prior to administration of nasal spray, the nasal spray applicator must be primed (pumped 4 times); in order to let the drug be absorbed through the skin in the nose, patients should not inhale deeply through the nose while spraying or immediately after spraying; for best results, treatment should be initiated at the first symptom or sign of an attack; however, nasal spray can be used at any stage of a migraine attack

Reference Range Minimum concentration for vasoconstriction is reportedly 0.06 ng/mL

Dosage Forms Excipient information presented when available (limited, particularly for generics); consult specific product labeling.

Injection, solution, as mesylate: 1 mg/mL (1 mL) [contains ethanol 6.2%]

D.H.E. 45®: 1 mg/mL (1 mL) [contains ethanol 6.2%]

Solution, intranasal spray, as mesylate (Migranal®): 4 mg/mL [0.5 mg/spray] (1 mL) [contains caffeine 10 mg/mL]

- **Dihydroergotamine Mesylate** *see* Dihydroergotamine *on page 449*
- **Dihydroergotoxine** *see* Ergoloid Mesylates *on page 539*
- **Dihydrogenated Ergot Alkaloids** *see* Ergoloid Mesylates *on page 539*
- **DiHydro-GP** *see* Dihydrocodeine, Pseudoephedrine, and Guaifenesin *on page 448*
- **Dihydrohydroxycodeinone** *see* OxyCODONE *on page 1120*
- **Dihydromorphinone** *see* HYDROmorphone *on page 747*

Dihydrotachysterol (dye hye droe tak ISS ter ole)

U.S. Brand Names DHT™ Intensol™ [DSC]; DHT™ [DSC]; Hytakerol® [DSC]

Canadian Brand Names Hytakerol®

Index Terms Dichysterol

Pharmacologic Category Vitamin D Analog

Use Treatment of hypocalcemia associated with hypoparathyroidism; prophylaxis of hypocalcemic tetany following thyroid surgery

Pregnancy Risk Factor A/D (dose exceeding RDA recommendation)

Dosage Oral:

Hypoparathyroidism:

Infants and young Children: Initial: 1-5 mg/day for 4 days, then 0.1-0.5 mg/day

Older Children and Adults: Initial: 0.8-2.4 mg/day for several days followed by maintenance doses of 0.2-1 mg/day

Nutritional rickets: 0.5 mg as a single dose or 13-50 mcg/day until healing occurs

Renal osteodystrophy: Maintenance: 0.25-0.6 mg/24 hours adjusted as necessary to achieve normal serum calcium levels and promote bone healing

Additional Information Complete prescribing information for this medication should be consulted for additional detail.

Dosage Forms Excipient information presented when available (limited, particularly for generics); consult specific product labeling. [DSC] = Discontinued product

Capsule (Hytakerol®): 0.125 mg [contains sesame oil] [DSC]

Solution, oral concentrate (DHT™ Intensol™): 0.2 mg/mL (30 mL) [contains alcohol 20%] [DSC]

Tablet (DHT™): 0.125 mg, 0.2 mg, 0.4 mg [DSC]

- **Dihydroxyanthracenedione Dihydrochloride** *see* Mitoxantrone *on page 1007*
- **1,25 Dihydroxycholecalciferol** *see* Calcitriol *on page 235*
- **Dihydroxydeoxynorvinkaleukoblastine** *see* Vinorelbine *on page 1563*
- **Diiodohydroxyquin** *see* Iodoquinol *on page 810*
- **Dilacor® XR** *see* Diltiazem *on page 450*
- **Dilantin®** *see* Phenytoin *on page 1186*
- **Dilatrate®-SR** *see* Isosorbide Dinitrate *on page 823*
- **Dilaudid®** *see* HYDROmorphone *on page 747*
- **Dilaudid-HP®** *see* HYDROmorphone *on page 747*
- **Dilaudid-HP-Plus® (Can)** *see* HYDROmorphone *on page 747*
- **Dilaudid® Sterile Powder (Can)** *see* HYDROmorphone *on page 747*
- **Dilaudid-XP® (Can)** *see* HYDROmorphone *on page 747*
- **Dilex-G** *see* Dyphylline and Guaifenesin *on page 501*
- **Dilor-G®** *see* Dyphylline and Guaifenesin *on page 501*
- **Dilt-CD** *see* Diltiazem *on page 450*

Diltiazem (dil TYE a zem)

U.S. Brand Names Cardizem®; Cardizem® CD; Cardizem® LA; Cartia XT™; Dilacor® XR; Dilt-CD; Dilt-XR; Taztia XT™; Tiazac®

Canadian Brand Names Alti-Diltiazem CD; Apo-Diltiaz CD®; Apo-Diltiaz SR®; Apo-Diltiaz TZ®; Apo-Diltiaz®; Apo-Diltiaz® Injectable; Cardizem®; Cardizem® CD; Cardizem® SR; Diltiazem HCl ER®; Diltiazem Hydrochloride Injection; Gen-Diltiazem; Gen-Diltiazem CD; Med-Diltiazem; Novo-Diltazem; Novo-Diltazem-CD; Novo-Diltiazem HCl ER; Nu-Diltiaz; Nu-Diltiaz-CD; ratio-Diltiazem CD; Rhoxal-diltiazem CD; Rhoxal-diltiazem SR; Rhoxal-diltiazem T; Sandoz-Diltiazem CD; Sandoz-Diltiazem T; Syn-Diltiazem®; Tiazac® ; Tiazac® XC

Index Terms Diltiazem Hydrochloride

Pharmacologic Category Calcium Channel Blocker

Additional Appendix Information

Calcium Channel Blockers *on page 1651*

Hypertension *on page 1820*

Use

Oral: Essential hypertension; chronic stable angina or angina from coronary artery spasm

Injection: Atrial fibrillation or atrial flutter; paroxysmal supraventricular tachycardia (PSVT)

Unlabeled/Investigational Use Investigational: Therapy of Duchenne muscular dystrophy

Pregnancy Risk Factor C

Pregnancy Considerations Teratogenic and embryotoxic effects have been demonstrated in small animals. There are no adequate and well-controlled studies in pregnant women.

Lactation Enters breast milk/not recommended (AAP considers "compatible")

Medication Safety Issues

Sound-alike/look-alike issues:

Cardizem® may be confused with Cardene®, Cardene SR®, Cardizem CD®, Cardizem SR®, cardiem

Cartia XT™ may be confused with Procardia XL®

Diltiazem may be confused with Dilantin®

Tiazac® may be confused with Tigan®, Tiazac® XC [CAN], Ziac®

High alert medication: The Institute for Safe Medication Practices (ISMP) includes this medication (I.V. formulation) among its list of drug classes which have a heightened risk of causing significant patient harm when used in error.

Significant differences exist between oral and I.V. dosing. Use caution when converting from one route of administration to another.

International issues:

Cardizem® may be confused with Cardem® which is a brand name for celiprolol in Spain

Cartia XT™ may be confused with Cartia® which is a brand name for aspirin in multiple international markets

Dilacor®: Brand name for digoxin in Serbia, a brand name for verapamil in Brazil, and a brand name for barnidipine in Argentina

Tiazac® may be confused with Tazac® which is a brand name for nizatidine in Australia

Tiazac® may be confused with Tiazac® XC which is a brand name for diltiazem available in Canada (not available in U.S.)

Contraindications

Oral: Hypersensitivity to diltiazem or any component of the formulation; sick sinus syndrome; second- or third-degree AV block (except in patients with a functioning artificial pacemaker); severe hypotension (systolic <90 mm Hg); acute MI and pulmonary congestion

Intravenous (I.V.): Hypersensitivity to diltiazem or any component of the formulation; sick sinus syndrome; second- or third-degree AV block (except in patients with a functioning artificial pacemaker); severe hypotension (systolic <90 mm Hg); acute MI and pulmonary congestion; administration concomitantly or within a few hours of the administration of I.V. beta-blockers; atrial fibrillation or flutter associated with accessory bypass tract (eg, Wolff-Parkinson-White syndrome); ventricular tachycardia (with wide-complex tachycardia, must determine whether origin is supraventricular or ventricular)

Canadian labeling: Additional contraindications (not in U.S. labeling): I.V. and oral: Pregnancy; use in women of childbearing potential

Warnings/Precautions Can cause first-, second-, and third-degree AV block or sinus bradycardia and risk increases with agents known to slow cardiac conduction. The most common side effect is peripheral edema; occurs within 2-3 weeks of starting therapy. Symptomatic hypotension with or without syncope can rarely occur; blood pressure must be lowered at a rate appropriate for the patient's clinical condition. Concomitant use with beta-blockers or digoxin can result in conduction disturbances. I.V. administration concomitantly or within a few hours of I.V. beta-blockers is contraindicated. Use caution in left ventricular dysfunction (may exacerbate condition). Use with caution with hypertrophic obstructive cardiomyopathy. Use with caution in hepatic or renal dysfunction.

Adverse Reactions Note: Frequencies represent ranges for various dosage forms. Patients with impaired ventricular function and/or conduction abnormalities may have higher incidence of adverse reactions.

>10%:

Cardiovascular: Edema (2% to 15%)

Central nervous system: Headache (5% to 12%)

2% to 10%:

Cardiovascular: AV block (first degree 2% to 8%), edema (lower limb, 2% to 8%), pain (6%), bradycardia (2% to 6%), hypotension (<2% to 4%), vasodilation (2% to 3%), extrasystoles (2%), flushing (1% to 2%), palpitation (1% to 2%)

Central nervous system: Dizziness (3% to 10%), nervousness (2%)

Dermatologic: Rash (1% to 4%)

Endocrine & metabolic: Gout (1% to 2%)

Gastrointestinal: Dyspepsia (1% to 6%), constipation (<2% to 4%), vomiting (2%), diarrhea (1% to 2%)

Local: Injection site reactions: Burning, itching (4%)

Neuromuscular & skeletal: Weakness (1% to 4%), myalgia (2%)

Respiratory: Rhinitis (<2% to 10%), pharyngitis (2% to 6%), dyspnea (1% to 6%), bronchitis (1% to 4%), sinus congestion (1% to 2%)

<2% (Limited to important or life-threatening): Alkaline phosphatase increased, allergic reaction, ALT increased, AST increased, amblyopia, amnesia, arrhythmia, AV block (second or third degree), bundle branch block, CHF, depression, dysgeusia, extrapyramidal symptoms, gingival hyperplasia, hemolytic anemia, petechiae, photosensitivity, Stevens-Johnson syndrome, syncope, tachycardia, thrombocytopenia, tremor, toxic epidermal necrolysis

Drug Interactions

Metabolism/Transport Effects Substrate of CYP2C9 (minor), 2D6 (minor), 3A4 (major); **Inhibits** CYP2C9 (weak), 2D6 (weak), 3A4 (moderate)

Avoid Concomitant Use

Avoid concomitant use of Diltiazem with any of the following: Ranolazine

Increased Effect/Toxicity

Diltiazem may increase the levels/effects of: Alfentanil; Amifostine; Amiodarone; Aprepitant; Benzodiazepines (metabolized by oxidation); Beta-Blockers; BusPIRone; Calcium Channel Blockers (Dihydropyridine); CarBAMazepine; Cardiac Glycosides; Corticosteroids (Systemic); CycloSPORINE; CYP3A4 Substrates; Eletriptan; Eplerenone; Fosaprepitant; HMG-CoA Reductase Inhibitors; Lithium; Magnesium Salts; Maraviroc; Midodrine; Neuromuscular-Blocking Agents (Nondepolarizing); Nitroprusside; Phenytoin; Pimecrolimus; QuiNIDine; Ranolazine; RiTUXimab; Salicylates; Salmeterol; Tacrolimus

The levels/effects of Diltiazem may be increased by: Alpha1-Blockers; Anilidopiperidine Opioids; Antifungal Agents (Azole Derivatives, Systemic); Aprepitant; Cimetidine; CycloSPORINE; CYP3A4 Inhibitors (Moderate); CYP3A4 Inhibitors (Strong); Dasatinib; Diazoxide; Fluconazole; Fosaprepitant; Grapefruit Juice; Herbs (Hypotensive Properties); Macrolide Antibiotics; Magnesium Salts; P-Glycoprotein Inhibitors; Prostacyclin Analogues; Protease Inhibitors; Quinupristin

Decreased Effect

Diltiazem may decrease the levels/effects of: Clopidogrel

The levels/effects of Diltiazem may be decreased by: Barbiturates; Calcium Salts; CarBAMazepine; Colestipol; CYP3A4 Inducers (Strong); Deferasirox; Herbs (CYP3A4 Inducers); Herbs (Hypertensive Properties); Methylphenidate; Nafcillin; P-Glycoprotein Inducers; Rifamycin Derivatives; Yohimbine

Ethanol/Nutrition/Herb Interactions

Ethanol: Avoid ethanol (may increase risk of hypotension or vasodilation).

Food: Diltiazem serum levels may be elevated if taken with food. Serum concentrations were not altered by grapefruit juice in small clinical trials.

Herb/Nutraceutical: St John's wort may decrease diltiazem levels. Avoid bayberry, blue cohosh, cayenne, ephedra, ginger, ginseng (American), kola, licorice, yohimbe (may worsen hypertension). Avoid black cohosh, California poppy, coleus, garlic, golden seal, hawthorn, mistletoe, periwinkle, quinine, shepherd's purse (may have increased antihypertensive effect).

Stability

Capsule, tablet: Store at 15°C to 30°C (59°F to 86°F). Protect from light.

Solution for injection: Store in refrigerator at 2°C to 8°C (36°F to 46°F). May be stored at room temperature for up to 1 month; do not freeze. Following dilution with $D_5$1/2NS, D_5W, or NS, solution is stable for 24 hours at room temperature or under refrigeration.

Mechanism of Action Inhibits calcium ion from entering the "slow channels" or select voltage-sensitive areas of vascular smooth muscle and myocardium during depolarization, producing a relaxation of coronary vascular smooth muscle and coronary vasodilation; increases myocardial oxygen delivery in patients with vasospastic angina

Pharmacodynamics/Kinetics

Onset of action: Oral: Immediate release tablet: 30-60 minutes

Absorption: Immediate release tablet: >90%; Extended release capsule: ~93%

Distribution: V_d: 3-13 L/kg

Protein binding: 70% to 80%

Metabolism: Hepatic; extensive first-pass effect; following single I.V. injection, plasma concentrations of N-monodesmethyldiltiazem and desacetyldiltiazem are typically undetectable; however, these metabolites accumulate to detectable concentrations following 24-hour constant rate infusion. N-monodesmethyldiltiazem appears to have 20% of the potency of diltiazem; desacetyldiltiazem is about 25% to 50% as potent as the parent compound.

Bioavailability: Oral: ~40% (undergoes extensive first-pass metabolism)

Half-life elimination: Immediate release tablet: 3-4.5 hours, may be prolonged with renal impairment; Extended release tablet: 6-9 hours; Extended release capsules: 5-10 hours

Time to peak, serum: Immediate release tablet: 2-4 hours; Extended release tablet: 11-18 hours; Extended release capsule: 10-14 hours

Excretion: Urine (2% to 4% as unchanged drug; 6% to 7% as metabolites); feces

Dosage

Children (unlabeled use): Oral: Hypertension: Immediate release tablets: Initial: 1.5-2 mg/kg/day 3 times daily (maximum dose 6 mg/kg/day up to 360 mg/day)

Note: Doses up to 8 mg/kg/day given in 4 divided doses have been used for investigational therapy of Duchenne muscular dystrophy

Adults:

Oral:

Angina:

Capsule, extended release (Cardizem® CD, Cartia XT™, Dilacor® XR, Tiazac®): Initial: 120-180 mg once daily (maximum dose: 480 mg/day)

Tablet, extended release (Cardizem® LA), Tiazac® XC [CAN; not available in U.S.]): 180 mg once daily; may increase at 7- to 14-day intervals (maximum recommended dose: 360 mg/day)

Tablet, immediate release (Cardizem®): Usual starting dose: 30 mg 4 times/day; usual range: 180-360 mg/day

Hypertension:

Capsule, extended release (Cardizem® CD, Cartia XT™, Dilacor® XR, Tiazac®): Initial: 180-240 mg once daily; dose adjustment may be made after 14 days; usual dose range (JNC 7): 180-420 mg/day; Tiazac®: usual dose range: 120-540 mg/day

Capsule, sustained release: Initial: 60-120 mg twice daily; dose adjustment may be made after 14 days; usual range: 240-360 mg/day

Tablet, extended release (Cardizem® LA, Tiazac® XC [CAN; not available in U.S.]): Initial: 180-240 mg once daily; dose adjustment may be made after 14 days; usual dose range (JNC 7): 120-540 mg/day

Note: Elderly: Patients ≥60 years may respond to a lower initial dose (ie, 120 mg once daily using extended release capsule)

I.V.: Atrial fibrillation, atrial flutter, PSVT:

Initial bolus dose: 0.25 mg/kg actual body weight over 2 minutes (average adult dose: 20 mg)

Repeat bolus dose (may be administered after 15 minutes if the response is inadequate.): 0.35 mg/kg actual body weight over 2 minutes (average adult dose: 25 mg)

Continuous infusion (requires an infusion pump; infusions >24 hours or infusion rates >15 mg/hour are not recommended.): Initial infusion rate of 10 mg/hour; rate may be increased in 5 mg/hour increments up to 15 mg/hour as needed; some patients may respond to an initial rate of 5 mg/hour.

If diltiazem injection is administered by continuous infusion for >24 hours, the possibility of decreased diltiazem clearance, prolonged elimination half-life, and increased diltiazem and/or diltiazem metabolite plasma concentrations should be considered.

Conversion from I.V. diltiazem to oral diltiazem:

Oral dose (mg/day) is approximately equal to [rate (mg/hour) x 3 + 3] x 10.

3 mg/hour = 120 mg/day

5 mg/hour = 180 mg/day

7 mg/hour = 240 mg/day

11 mg/hour = 360 mg/day

Dosing comments in renal/hepatic impairment: Use with caution as extensively metabolized by the liver and excreted in the kidneys and bile.

Dialysis: Not removed by hemo- or peritoneal dialysis; supplemental dose is not necessary.

Administration

Oral: Do not crush long acting dosage forms.

Taztia XT™, Tiazac®: Capsules may be opened and sprinkled on a spoonful of applesauce. Applesauce should be swallowed without chewing, followed by drinking a glass of water.

Tiazac® XC [CAN; not available in U.S.]: Administer at bedtime

I.V.: Bolus doses given over 2 minutes with continuous ECG and blood pressure monitoring. Continuous infusion should be via infusion pump.

Monitoring Parameters Liver function tests, blood pressure, ECG

Dosage Forms Excipient information presented when available (limited, particularly for generics); consult specific product labeling. [CAN] = Canadian brand name

Capsule, extended release, as hydrochloride [once-daily dosing]: 120 mg, 180 mg, 240 mg, 300 mg, 360 mg, 420 mg

Cardizem® CD: 120 mg, 180 mg, 240 mg, 300 mg, 360 mg

Cartia XT™: 120 mg, 180 mg, 240 mg, 300 mg

Dilacor® XR, Dilt-XR: 120 mg, 180 mg, 240 mg

Dilt-CD: 120 mg, 180 mg, 240 mg, 300 mg

Taztia XT™: 120 mg, 180 mg, 240 mg, 300 mg, 360 mg

Tiazac®: 120 mg, 180 mg, 240 mg, 300 mg, 360 mg, 420 mg

Capsule, extended release, as hydrochloride [twice-daily dosing]: 60 mg, 90 mg, 120 mg

Injection, solution, as hydrochloride: 5 mg/mL (5 mL, 10 mL, 25 mL)

Injection, powder for reconstitution, as hydrochloride: 100 mg

Tablet, as hydrochloride: 30 mg, 60 mg, 90 mg, 120 mg

Cardizem®: 30 mg, 60 mg, 90 mg, 120 mg

Tablet, extended release, as hydrochloride:

Cardizem® LA: 120 mg, 180 mg, 240 mg, 300 mg, 360 mg, 420 mg

Tiazac® XC [CAN; not available in U.S.]: 120 mg, 180 mg, 240 mg, 300 mg, 360 mg

Extemporaneous Preparations A 12 mg/mL oral liquid preparation made from tablets (regular, not sustained release) and 3 different vehicles (cherry syrup, a 1:1 mixture of Ora-Sweet® and Ora-Plus®, or a 1:1 mixture of Ora-Sweet® SF and Ora-Plus®) was stable for 60 days when stored in amber plastic prescription bottles in the dark at room temperature (25°C) or under refrigeration (5°C); grind sixteen 90 mg tablets in a mortar into a fine powder; add 10 mL of the vehicle and mix well to form a uniform paste; mix while adding the vehicle in geometric proportions to **almost** 120 mL; transfer to a calibrated bottle and qs ad with vehicle to 120 mL; label "shake well" and "protect from light."

Allen LV and Erickson MA, "Stability of Baclofen, Captopril, Diltiazem Hydrochloride, Dipyridamole, and Flecainide Acetate in Extemporaneously Compounded Oral Liquids," *Am J Health Syst Pharm*, 1996, 53 (18):2179-84.

- **Diltiazem HCl ER® (Can)** *see* Diltiazem *on page 450*
- **Diltiazem Hydrochloride** *see* Diltiazem *on page 450*
- **Diltiazem Hydrochloride Injection (Can)** *see* Diltiazem *on page 450*
- **Dilt-XR** *see* Diltiazem *on page 450*
- **Dimaphen [OTC]** *see* Brompheniramine and Pseudoephedrine *on page 214*

DimenhyDRINATE (dye men HYE dri nate)

U.S. Brand Names Dramamine® [OTC]; Driminate® [OTC]; TripTone® [OTC]

Canadian Brand Names Apo-Dimenhydrinate®; Children's Motion Sickness Liquid; Dinate®; Gravol®; Jamp® Travel Tablet; Nauseatol; Novo-Dimenate; SAB-Dimenhydrinate

Pharmacologic Category Histamine H_1 Antagonist; Histamine H_1 Antagonist, First Generation

Use Treatment and prevention of nausea, vertigo, and vomiting associated with motion sickness

Dosage forms available in Canada (not available in the U.S.), including parenteral formulations and suppositories, are also approved for the treatment of postoperative nausea and vomiting and treatment of radiation sickness.

Unlabeled/Investigational Use Treatment of Meniere's disease

Pregnancy Risk Factor B

Medication Safety Issues

Sound-alike/look-alike issues:

DimenhyDRINATE may be confused with diphenhydrAMINE

Dosage Oral:

Children:

2-5 years: 12.5-25 mg every 6-8 hours, maximum: 75 mg/day

6-12 years: 25-50 mg every 6-8 hours, maximum: 150 mg/day

Adults: 50-100 mg every 4-6 hours, not to exceed 400 mg/ day

Gravol® L/A (not available in the U.S.): 75-150 mg every 8-12 hours, up to a maximum of five 75 mg caplets or three 100 mg caplets in 24 hours

Additional formulations/uses (approved in Canada) for parenteral/suppository formulations (not available in U.S.):

I.M., I.V., rectal: Adults:

Postoperative nausea and vomiting: 50-100 mg administered 30-60 minutes prior to radiation therapy; may be repeated as needed up to a maximum of 400 mg in 24 hours

Radiation sickness: 50-100 mg administered 30-60 minutes prior to radiation therapy. May be repeated as needed up to a maximum of 400 mg in 24 hours

Additional Information Complete prescribing information for this medication should be consulted for additional detail.

Dosage Forms Excipient information presented when available (limited, particularly for generics); consult specific product labeling. [CAN] = Canadian brand name

Capsule, softgel (Gravol®) [CAN]: 50 mg [not available in the U.S.]

Capsule, long-acting (Gravol® L/A) [CAN]: 75 mg, 100 mg [not available in the U.S.]

Injection, solution: 50 mg/mL (1 mL)

Gravol® I.M. [CAN]: 50 mg/mL (1 mL, 5 mL) [not available in the U.S.]

Gravol® I.V. [CAN]: 10 mg/mL (5 mL) [not available in the U.S.]

Solution, oral (Gravol® [CAN], Children's Motion Sickness [CAN]): 3 mg/mL (75 mL) [not available in the U.S.]

Suppository, rectal (Gravol® [CAN], Sab-Dimenhydrinate [CAN]): 75 mg, 100 mg [not available in the U.S.]

Tablet:

Dinate® [CAN], Jamp® Travel Tablet [CAN], Nauseatol® [CAN]: 50 mg

Dramamine®: 50 mg

Driminate®: 50 mg [scored]

Gravol® Filmkote Jr [CAN]: 25 mg [not available in the U.S.]

Gravol® Filmkote [CAN]: 50 mg [not available in the U.S.]

TripTone®: 50 mg

Tablet, chewable:

Dramamine®: 50 mg [contains phenylalanine 1.5 mg/ tablet and tartrazine; orange flavor]

Gravol® Chewable for Children [CAN]: 25 mg [not available in the U.S.]

Gravol® Chewable for Adults [CAN]: 50 mg [not available in the U.S.]

Dimercaprol (dye mer KAP role)

U.S. Brand Names BAL in Oil®

Index Terms BAL; British Anti-Lewisite; Dithioglycerol

Pharmacologic Category Antidote

Use Antidote to gold, arsenic (except arsine), or acute mercury poisoning (except nonalkyl mercury); adjunct to edetate CALCIUM disodium in lead poisoning

Pregnancy Risk Factor C

Pregnancy Considerations Animal reproduction studies have not been conducted. There are no adequate and well-controlled studies in pregnant women.

Lead poisoning: Following maternal occupational exposure, lead was found to cross the placenta in amounts related to maternal plasma levels. Possible outcomes of maternal lead exposure >10 mcg/dL include spontaneous abortion, postnatal developmental delay, and reduced birth weight. Chelation therapy during pregnancy is for maternal benefit only and should be limited to the treatment of severe, symptomatic lead poisoning.

Lactation Excretion in breast milk unknown/use caution

Contraindications Hepatic insufficiency (unless due to arsenic poisoning); iron, cadmium, or selenium poisoning

Warnings/Precautions Potentially a nephrotoxic drug, use with caution in patients with oliguria; keep urine alkaline to protect kidneys (prevents dimercaprol-metal complex breakdown). Discontinue or use with extreme caution if renal insufficiency develops during treatment. Hemodialysis may be used to remove dimercaprol-metal chelate in patients with renal dysfunction. Use with caution in patients with glucose 6-phosphate dehydrogenase deficiency; may increase risk of hemolytic anemia. Administer all injections deep I.M. at different sites. Fevers may occur in ~30% of children and may persistent for the duration of therapy. Product contains peanut oil; use caution in patients with peanut allergy; medication for the treatment of hypersensitivity reactions should be available for immediate use. When used in the treatment of lead poisoning, investigate, identify, and remove sources of lead exposure prior to treatment. Primary care providers should consult experts in chemotherapy of heavy metal toxicity before using chelation drug therapy.

Adverse Reactions

Frequency not always defined.

Cardiovascular: Chest pain, hypertension (dose related), tachycardia (dose related)

Central nervous system: Anxiety, fever (children ~30%), headache, nervousness

Dermatologic: Abscess

Gastrointestinal: Abdominal pain, burning sensation (lips, mouth, throat), nausea, salivation, throat irritation/pain, vomiting

Genitourinary: Burning sensation (penis)

Hematologic: Leukopenia (polymorphonuclear)

Local: Injection site pain

Neuromuscular & skeletal: Paresthesias (hand), weakness

Ocular: Blepharospasm, conjunctivitis, lacrimation

Renal: Acute renal insufficiency

Respiratory: Rhinorrhea, throat constriction

Miscellaneous: Diaphoresis

Drug Interactions

Avoid Concomitant Use

Avoid concomitant use of Dimercaprol with any of the following: Iron Salts

Increased Effect/Toxicity

Dimercaprol may increase the levels/effects of: Iron Salts

Decreased Effect There are no known significant interactions involving a decrease in effect.

Stability Store at 20°C to 25°C (68°F to 77°F).

Mechanism of Action Sulfhydryl group combines with ions of various heavy metals to form relatively stable, nontoxic, soluble chelates which are excreted in urine

Pharmacodynamics/Kinetics

Absorption: I.M.: Rapid; Oral: Not absorbed

Distribution: To all tissues including the brain

Metabolism: Rapidly hepatic to inactive metabolites

Time to peak, serum: 0.5-1 hour

Excretion: Urine

Dosage Note: Premedication with a histamine H_1 antagonist (eg, diphenhydramine) is recommended.

Children and Adults: Deep I.M.:

Mild arsenic or gold poisoning: 2.5 mg/kg every 6 hours for 2 days, then every 12 hours for 1 day, followed by once daily for 10 days

Severe arsenic or gold poisoning: 3 mg/kg every 4 hours for 2 days, then every 6 hours for 1 day, followed every 12 hours for 10 days

Mercury poisoning: 5 mg/kg initially, followed by 2.5 mg/kg 1-2 times/day for 10 days

Lead poisoning: **Note:** For the treatment of high blood lead levels in children, the CDC recommends chelation treatment when blood lead levels are >45 mcg/dL (CDC, 2002). Combination parenteral therapy is indicated when blood lead levels are ≥70 mcg/dL, or patients are symptomatic (AAP, 2005). In adults, available guidelines recommend chelation therapy with blood lead levels >50 mcg/dL and significant symptoms; chelation therapy may also be indicated with blood lead levels ≥100 mcg/dL and/or symptoms. (Kosnett, 2007).

Lead encephalopathy (in conjunction with edetate CALCIUM disodium): Dimercaprol 4 mg/kg (75 mg/m^2) loading dose, followed by dimercaprol 4 mg/kg (75 mg/m^2) every 4 hours for 2-7 days (edetate CALCIUM disodium is **not** administered with the loading dose; begin edetate CALCIUM disodium with the second dose)

Symptomatic lead poisoning or blood lead levels ≥70 mcg/dL (in conjunction with edetate CALCIUM disodium): Dimercaprol 4 mg/kg (75 mg/m^2) loading dose, followed by dimercaprol 3 mg/kg/dose (50 mg/m^2) every 4 hours for 2-7 days (edetate CALCIUM disodium is **not** administered with the loading dose; begin edetate CALCIUM disodium with the second dose)

Administration Administer all injections deep I.M. at different sites. Keep urine alkaline to protect renal function. When used in the treatment of lead poisoning, administer in a separate site from edetate CALCIUM disodium.

Monitoring Parameters Renal function, urine pH, infusion-related reactions

For lead poisoning: Blood lead levels (baseline and 7-21 days after completing chelation therapy); hemoglobin or hematocrit, iron status, free erythrocyte protoporphyrin or zinc protoporphyrin; neurodevelopmental changes

Test Interactions Iodine ^{131}I thyroidal uptake values may be decreased

Dosage Forms Excipient information presented when available (limited, particularly for generics); consult specific product labeling.

Injection, oil:

BAL in Oil®: 100 mg/mL (3 mL) [contains benzyl benzoate and peanut oil]

◆ **Dimetapp® Children's Long Acting Cough Plus Cold [OTC]** *see* Dextromethorphan and Chlorpheniramine *on page 433*

◆ **Dimetapp® Children's Nighttime Cold & Congestion [OTC]** *see* Diphenhydramine and Phenylephrine *on page 458*

◆ **Dimetapp® ND Children's [OTC]** *see* Loratadine *on page 904*

◆ **Dimetapp® Toddler's [OTC]** *see* Phenylephrine *on page 1183*

◆ **β,β-Dimethylcysteine** *see* Penicillamine *on page 1161*

◆ **Dimethyl Triazeno Imidazole Carboxamide** *see* Dacarbazine *on page 388*

◆ **Dinate® (Can)** *see* DimenhyDRINATE *on page 453*

Dinoprostone (dye noe PROST one)

U.S. Brand Names Cervidil®; Prepidil®; Prostin E_2®

Canadian Brand Names Cervidil®; Prepidil®; Prostin E_2®

Index Terms PGE_2; Prostaglandin E_2

Pharmacologic Category Abortifacient; Prostaglandin

Use

Gel: Promote cervical ripening in patients at or near term in whom there is a medical or obstetrical indication for the induction of labor

Suppositories: Terminate pregnancy from 12th through 20th week of gestation; evacuate uterus in cases of missed abortion or intrauterine fetal death up to 28 weeks of gestation; manage benign hydatidiform mole (nonmetastatic gestational trophoblastic disease)

Vaginal insert: Initiation and/or continuation of cervical ripening in patients at or near term in whom there is a medical or obstetrical indication for the induction of labor

Pregnancy Risk Factor C

Pregnancy Considerations Skeletal anomalies and embryotoxicity have been observed in animal studies. Although these effects would not be expected in humans when administered after the period of organogenesis, a sustained increase in uterine tone may have increased risks of adverse events to the fetus.

Fetal distress without corresponding maternal uterine hyperstimulation was observed in 3% to 4% of infants exposed to Cervidil® *in utero*. No adverse effects on physical or psychomotor function were observed in a 3 year follow-up study of exposed infants. Abnormal fetal heart rates were observed in 17% of infants exposed to Prepidil® gel *in utero*. Deceleration, intrauterine fetal sepsis, fetal depression and fetal acidosis have also been reported with administration of the gel.

When used for termination of pregnancy, dinoprostone is not considered feticidal, but is used to terminate pregnancy due to its ability to stimulate uterine contractions; do not use if fetus has reached the stage of viability.

Lactation Excretion in breast milk unknown

Medication Safety Issues

Sound-alike/look-alike issues:

Prepidil® may be confused with Bepridil®

International issues:

Cervidil®: Brand name for gemeprost in Italy

Contraindications

Gel, vaginal insert: Hypersensitivity to prostaglandins or any component of the formulation; fetal distress (suspicion or clinical evidence unless delivery is imminent); unexplained vaginal bleeding during this pregnancy; strong suspicion of marked cephalopelvic disproportion; patients in whom oxytocic drugs are contraindicated or when prolonged contraction of the uterus may be detrimental to fetal safety or uterine integrity (including previous cesarean section or major uterine surgery); >6 previous term pregnancies; patients already receiving oxytocic drugs; hyperactive or hypotonic uterine patterns; when vaginal delivery is not indicated (vasa previa, active herpes genitalia); obstetrical emergencies when surgical intervention would be favorable

Suppository: Hypersensitivity to dinoprostone or any component of the formulation; acute pelvic inflammatory disease; active cardiac, pulmonary, renal or hepatic disease

Warnings/Precautions [U.S. Boxed Warning]: Dinoprostone should be used only by medically-trained personnel in a hospital.

Gel, vaginal insert: Use caution with ruptured membranes; nonvertex or nonsingleton pregnancy; previous uterine hypertony; glaucoma; history of asthma. Vaginal insert must be removed prior to administration of oxytocin; in case of hyperstimulation or if labor begins; fetal or maternal distress; and prior to amniotomy.

Suppository: Transient pyrexia and decreased blood pressure may be observed with treatment. Use caution with history of asthma; hypotension or hypertension; cardiovascular, renal, or hepatic disease; anemia; jaundice; diabetes; epilepsy; compromised uteri; cervicitis, endocervical infections or acute vaginitis. Measures should be taken to ensure complete abortion. Commercially available suppositories should not be used for extemporaneous preparation of any other dosage form of drug. Do not use for cervical ripening or other indications in patients with term pregnancy.

Adverse Reactions

Gel:

1% to 10%:

Central nervous system: Fever (1%)

Gastrointestinal: GI upset (6%)

Genitourinary: Abnormal uterine contractions (7%), warm feeling in vagina (2%)

Neuromuscular & skeletal: Back pain (3%)

Postmarketing and/or case reports: Amnionitis, premature rupture of membranes, uterine rupture (with intracervical administration)

Suppository:

Frequency not defined:

Cardiovascular: Arrhythmia, chest pain, chest tightness, hypotension, syncope

Central nervous system: Chills, dizziness, fever, headache, shivering, tension

Dermatologic: Rash, skin discoloration

Endocrine & metabolic: Breast tenderness, endometritis, hot flashes

Gastrointestinal: Dehydration, diarrhea, nausea, vomiting

Genitourinary: uterine rupture, urinary retention, vaginal pain, vaginismus, vaginitis, vulvitis

Neuromuscular & skeletal: Arthralgia, backache, joint inflammation/pain (new or exacerbated), leg cramps (nocturnal), muscle cramp/pain, myalgia, paresthesia, stiff neck, tremor, weakness

Ocular: Blurred vision, eye pain

Otic: Hearing impairment

Respiratory: Cough, dyspnea, laryngitis, pharyngitis, wheezing

Miscellaneous: Diaphoresis

Postmarketing and/or case reports: MI

Vaginal insert:

1% to 10%: Genitourinary: Uterine hyperstimulation *without* fetal distress (2% to 5%), uterine hyperstimulation *with* fetal distress (3%)

<1% (Limited to important or life-threatening): Abdominal pain, diarrhea, fever, nausea, uterine rupture, vomiting

Drug Interactions

Avoid Concomitant Use There are no known interactions where it is recommended to avoid concomitant use.

Increased Effect/Toxicity

Dinoprostone may increase the levels/effects of: Oxytocin

Decreased Effect There are no known significant interactions involving a decrease in effect.

Stability

Cervical gel should be stored under refrigeration 2°C to 8°C (36°F to 46°F).

Suppositories must be kept frozen; store in freezer not above -20°C (-4°F).

Vaginal insert should be stored in freezer between -20°C and -10°C (-4°F and 14°F).

Mechanism of Action A synthetic prostaglandin E_2 abortifacient that stimulates uterine contractions similar to those seen during natural labor. Prostaglandin E_2 plays a role in cervical ripening, which allows the fetus to pass through the birth canal.

Pharmacodynamics/Kinetics

Onset of action (uterine contractions): Vaginal suppository: Within 10 minutes

Duration: Vaginal insert: 0.3 mg/hour over 12 hours; Vaginal suppository: Up to 2-3 hours

Absorption: Vaginal suppository: Slow

Metabolism: In many tissues including lungs, liver, and kidney

Half-life elimination: 2.5-5 minutes

Time to peak, plasma: Gel: 30-45 minutes

Excretion: Primarily urine; feces (small amounts)

Dosage Females of reproductive age:

Abortifacient: Vaginal suppository: Insert 20 mg (1 suppository) high in vagina, repeat at 3- to 5-hour intervals until abortion occurs; continued administration for longer than 2 days is not advisable

Cervical ripening:

Endocervical gel: Using catheter supplied with gel, insert 0.5 mg into the cervical canal. May repeat every 6 hours if needed. Maximum cumulative dose: 1.5 mg/24 hours

Vaginal insert: Insert 10 mg transversely into the posterior fornix of the vagina (to be removed at the onset of active labor or after 12 hours)

Administration

Endocervical gel: Bring to room temperature just prior to use. Do not force the warming process (eg, water bath, microwave). Avoid contact with skin while handling; wash hands thoroughly with soap and water after administration. For cervical ripening, patient should be supine in the dorsal position. The appropriate catheter length should be based on degree of effacement; 20 mm for no effacement; 10 mm if 50% effaced. Patient should remain supine for 15-30 minutes following administration.

Vaginal insert: One vaginal insert is placed transversely in the posterior fornix of the vagina immediately after removal from its foil package. Patients should remain in the recumbent position for 2 hours after insertion, but thereafter may be ambulatory. Do not use without retrieval system. Product does not need warmed prior to use. A water miscible lubricant may be used to facilitate insertion (avoid excessive use of lubricant). Ensure complete removal of system at completion of therapy.

Vaginal suppository: Bring to room temperature just prior to use. Patient should remain supine for 10 minutes following insertion.

Monitoring Parameters

Gel, insert: Fetal heart rate and uterine activity

Suppository: Confirmation of fetal death

Dosage Forms Excipient information presented when available (limited, particularly for generics); consult specific product labeling.

Gel, endocervical (Prepidil®): 0.5 mg/3 g syringe [each package contains a 10 mm and 20 mm shielded catheter]

Insert, vaginal (Cervidil®): 10 mg [releases 0.3 mg/hour]

Suppository, vaginal (Prostin E_2®): 20 mg

- **Diocaine® (Can)** *see* Proparacaine *on page 1253*
- **Diocarpine (Can)** *see* Pilocarpine *on page 1192*
- **Diochloram® (Can)** *see* Chloramphenicol *on page 302*
- **Diocto® [OTC]** *see* Docusate *on page 473*
- **Dioctyl Calcium Sulfosuccinate** *see* Docusate *on page 473*
- **Dioctyl Sodium Sulfosuccinate** *see* Docusate *on page 473*
- **Diodex® (Can)** *see* Dexamethasone *on page 425*
- **Diodoquin® (Can)** *see* Iodoquinol *on page 810*
- **Diogent® (Can)** *see* Gentamicin *on page 692*
- **Diomycin® (Can)** *see* Erythromycin *on page 544*
- **Dionephrine® (Can)** *see* Phenylephrine *on page 1183*
- **Diopentolate® (Can)** *see* Cyclopentolate *on page 376*
- **Diopred® (Can)** *see* PrednisoLONE *on page 1230*
- **Dioptic's Atropine Solution (Can)** *see* Atropine *on page 157*
- **Dioptimyd® (Can)** *see* Sulfacetamide and Prednisolone *on page 1405*
- **Dioptrol® (Can)** *see* Neomycin, Polymyxin B, and Dexamethasone *on page 1052*
- **Diosulf™ (Can)** *see* Sulfacetamide *on page 1405*
- **Diotame® [OTC]** *see* Bismuth *on page 199*
- **Diotrope® (Can)** *see* Tropicamide *on page 1525*
- **Diovan®** *see* Valsartan *on page 1542*
- **Diovan HCT®** *see* Valsartan and Hydrochlorothiazide *on page 1544*
- **Diovol® (Can)** *see* Aluminum Hydroxide and Magnesium Hydroxide *on page 76*
- **Diovol® Ex (Can)** *see* Aluminum Hydroxide and Magnesium Hydroxide *on page 76*
- **Diovol Plus® (Can)** *see* Aluminum Hydroxide, Magnesium Hydroxide, and Simethicone *on page 76*
- **Dipentum®** *see* Olsalazine *on page 1098*
- **Diphen® [OTC]** *see* DiphenhydrAMINE *on page 456*
- **Diphen® AF [OTC]** *see* DiphenhydrAMINE *on page 456*
- **Diphenhist [OTC]** *see* DiphenhydrAMINE *on page 456*

DiphenhydrAMINE (dye fen HYE dra meen)

U.S. Brand Names Aler-Cap [OTC]; Aler-Dryl [OTC]; Aler-Tab [OTC]; AllerMax® [OTC]; Altaryl [OTC]; Banophen® Anti-Itch [OTC]; Banophen® [OTC]; Ben-Tann; Benadryl® Allergy [OTC]; Benadryl® Children's Allergy Fastmelt® [OTC]; Benadryl® Children's Allergy [OTC]; Benadryl® Children's Dye-Free Allergy [OTC]; Benadryl® Itch Stopping Extra Strength [OTC]; Benadryl® Itch Stopping [OTC]; Compoz® Nighttime Sleep Aid [OTC]; Dermamycin® [OTC]; Diphenhist [OTC]; Diphen® AF [OTC]; Diphen® [OTC]; Dytan™; Genahist® [OTC]; Hydramine® [OTC]; Nytol® Quick Caps [OTC]; Nytol® Quick Gels [OTC]; Siladryl® Allergy [OTC]; Silphen® [OTC]; Simply Sleep® [OTC]; Sleep-ettes D [OTC]; Sleepinal® [OTC]; Sominex® Maximum Strength [OTC]; Sominex® [OTC]; Triaminic® Thin Strips™ Cough and Runny Nose [OTC]; Twilite® [OTC]; Unisom® Maximum Strength SleepGels® [OTC]

Canadian Brand Names Allerdryl®; Allernix; Benadryl®; Nytol®; Nytol® Extra Strength; PMS-Diphenhydramine; Simply Sleep®

Index Terms Diphenhydramine Citrate; Diphenhydramine Hydrochloride; Diphenhydramine Tannate

Pharmacologic Category Histamine H_1 Antagonist; Histamine H_1 Antagonist, First Generation

Additional Appendix Information

Antiparkinsonian Agents *on page 1643*

Contrast Media Reactions, Premedication for Prophylaxis *on page 1799*

Use Symptomatic relief of allergic symptoms caused by histamine release including nasal allergies and allergic dermatosis; adjunct to epinephrine in the treatment of anaphylaxis; nighttime sleep aid; prevention or treatment of motion sickness; antitussive; management of Parkinsonian syndrome including drug-induced extrapyramidal symptoms; topically for relief of pain and itching associated with insect bites, minor cuts and burns, or rashes due to poison ivy, poison oak, and poison sumac

Pregnancy Risk Factor B

Pregnancy Considerations Teratogenic effects were not observed in animal studies. Diphenhydramine crosses the human placenta. One retrospective study showed an increased risk of cleft palate formation following maternal use of diphenhydramine during the 1st trimester of pregnancy; however, later studies have not confirmed this finding. Signs of toxicity and symptoms of withdrawal have been reported in infants following high doses or chronic maternal use close to term. Diphenhydramine has been evaluated for the treatment of hyperemesis gravidarum. It is generally not considered the antihistamine of choice for treating allergic rhinitis or nausea and vomiting during pregnancy.

Lactation Enters breast milk/contraindicated

Medication Safety Issues

ISMP has reported cases of patients mistakenly *swallowing* Benadryl® Itch Stopping [OTC] gel intended for topical application. Unclear labeling and similar packaging of the topical gel in containers resembling an oral liquid are factors believed to be contributing to the administration errors. The topical gel contains camphor which can be toxic if swallowed. ISMP has requested the manufacturer to make the necessary changes to prevent further confusion.

Sound-alike/look-alike issues:

DiphenhydrAMINE may be confused with desipramine, dicyclomine, dimenhyDRINATE

Benadryl® may be confused with benazepril, Bentyl®, Benylin®, Caladryl®

Contraindications Hypersensitivity to diphenhydramine or any component of the formulation; acute asthma; neonates or premature infants; breast-feeding; use as a local anesthetic (injection)

Warnings/Precautions Causes sedation, caution must be used in performing tasks which require alertness (eg, operating machinery or driving). Sedative effects of CNS depressants or ethanol are potentiated. Use with caution in the elderly; may be more sensitive to adverse effects. Antihistamines may cause excitation in young children. Use with caution in patients with angle-closure glaucoma, pyloroduodenal obstruction (including stenotic peptic ulcer), urinary tract obstruction (including bladder neck obstruction and symptomatic prostatic hyperplasia), asthma, hyperthyroidism, increased intraocular pressure, and cardiovascular disease (including hypertension and tachycardia). Some preparations contain soy protein; avoid use in patients with soy protein or peanut allergies. Some products may contain phenylalanine.

Self-medication (OTC use): Do not use with other products containing diphenhydramine, even ones used on the skin. Oral products are not for OTC use in children <6 years of age. Topical products should not be used on large areas of the body, or on chicken pox or measles. Healthcare provider should be contacted if topical use is needed for >7 days. Topical products are not for OTC use in children <2 years of age.

Adverse Reactions Frequency not defined.

Cardiovascular: Chest tightness, extrasystoles, hypotension, palpitation, tachycardia

Central nervous system: Chills, confusion, convulsion, disturbed coordination, dizziness, euphoria, excitation, fatigue, headache, insomnia, irritability, nervousness, paradoxical excitement, restlessness, sedation, sleepiness, vertigo

Dermatologic: Photosensitivity, rash, urticaria

Endocrine & metabolic: Menstrual irregularities (early menses)

Gastrointestinal: Anorexia, constipation, diarrhea, dry mucous membranes, epigastric distress, nausea, throat tightness, vomiting, xerostomia

Genitourinary: Difficult urination, urinary frequency, urinary retention

Hematologic: Agranulocytosis, hemolytic anemia, thrombocytopenia

Neuromuscular & skeletal: Neuritis, paresthesia, tremor

Ocular: Blurred vision, diplopia

Otic: Labyrinthitis (acute), tinnitus

Respiratory: Nasal stuffiness, thickening of bronchial secretions, wheezing

Miscellaneous: Anaphylactic shock, diaphoresis

Drug Interactions

Metabolism/Transport Effects **Inhibits** CYP2D6 (moderate)

Avoid Concomitant Use There are no known interactions where it is recommended to avoid concomitant use.

Increased Effect/Toxicity

DiphenhydrAMINE may increase the levels/effects of: Alcohol (Ethyl); Anticholinergics; CNS Depressants; CYP2D6 Substrates; Fesoterodine; Nebivolol; Tamoxifen

The levels/effects of DiphenhydrAMINE may be increased by: Pramlintide

Decreased Effect

DiphenhydrAMINE may decrease the levels/effects of: Acetylcholinesterase Inhibitors (Central); Betahistine; Codeine; TraMADol

The levels/effects of DiphenhydrAMINE may be decreased by: Acetylcholinesterase Inhibitors (Central); Amphetamines

Ethanol/Nutrition/Herb Interactions

Ethanol: Avoid ethanol (may increase CNS depression).

Herb/Nutraceutical: Avoid valerian, St John's wort, kava kava, gotu kola (may increase CNS depression).

Stability Injection: Store at room temperature of 15°C to 30°C (59°F to 86°F). Protect from light and freezing

Mechanism of Action Competes with histamine for H_1-receptor sites on effector cells in the gastrointestinal tract, blood vessels, and respiratory tract; anticholinergic and sedative effects are also seen

Pharmacodynamics/Kinetics

Onset of action: Maximum sedative effect: 1-3 hours

Duration: 4-7 hours

Distribution: V_d: 3-22 L/kg

Protein binding: 78%

Metabolism: Extensively hepatic n-demethylation via CYP2D6; minor demethylation via CYP1A2, 2C9 and 2C19; smaller degrees in pulmonary and renal systems; significant first-pass effect

Bioavailability: Oral: ~40% to 70%

Half-life elimination: 2-10 hours; Elderly: 13.5 hours

Time to peak, serum: 2-4 hours

Excretion: Urine (as unchanged drug)

Dosage Note: Dosages are expressed as the hydrochloride salt.

Children:

- Allergic reactions or motion sickness: Oral, I.M., I.V.: 5 mg/kg/day or 150 mg/m²/day in divided doses every 6-8 hours, not to exceed 300 mg/day
  - Alternate dosing by age: Oral:
    - 2 to <6 years: 6.25 mg every 4-6 hours; maximum: 37.5 mg/day
    - 6 to <12 years: 12.5-25 mg every 4-6 hours; maximum: 150 mg/day
    - ≥12 years: 25-50 mg every 4-6 hours; maximum: 300 mg/day
- Night-time sleep aid: Oral: Children ≥12 years: 50 mg at bedtime
- Antitussive: Oral:
  - 2 to <6 years: 6.25 mg every 4 hours; maximum 37.5 mg/day
  - 6 to <12 years: 12.5 mg every 4 hours; maximum 75 mg/day
  - ≥12 years: 25 mg every 4 hours; maximum 150 mg/day
- Treatment of dystonic reactions: I.M., I.V.: 0.5-1 mg/kg/dose
- Relief of pain and itching: Topical: Children ≥2 years: Apply 1% or 2% to affected area up to 3-4 times/day

Adults:

- Allergic reactions or motion sickness: Oral: 25-50 mg every 6-8 hours
- Antitussive: Oral: 25 mg every 4 hours; maximum 150 mg/24 hours
- Nighttime sleep aid: Oral: 50 mg at bedtime
- Allergic reactions or motion sickness: I.M., I.V.: 10-50 mg per dose; single doses up to 100 mg may be used if needed; not to exceed 400 mg/day
- Dystonic reaction: I.M., I.V.: 50 mg in a single dose; may repeat in 20-30 minutes if necessary
- Relief of pain and itching: Topical: Apply 1% or 2% to affected area up to 3-4 times/day

Elderly: Initial: 25 mg 2-3 times/day increasing as needed

Dietary Considerations

Benadryl® Allergy strips contain sodium 4 mg per 25 mg strip.

Benadryl® Children's Allergy chewable tablets contain phenylalanine 4.2 mg, magnesium 15 mg, and sodium 2 mg per 12.5 mg tablet.

Benadryl® Children's Allergy Fastmelt® contains phenylalanine 4.5 mg/tablet and soy protein isolate (contraindicated in patients with soy protein allergies; use caution in peanut allergic individuals, ~10% are estimated to also have soy protein allergies).

Dytan™ chewable tablets contain phenylalanine.

Administration When used to prevent motion sickness, first dose should be given 30 minutes prior to exposure. Injection solution is for I.V. or I.M. administration only; local necrosis may result with SubQ or intradermal use. For I.V. administration, inject at a rate ≤25 mg/minute.

Monitoring Parameters Relief of symptoms, mental alertness

Reference Range

Antihistamine effects at levels >25 ng/mL

Drowsiness at levels 30-40 ng/mL

Mental impairment at levels >60 ng/mL

Therapeutic: Not established

Toxic: >0.1 mcg/mL

Test Interactions May suppress the wheal and flare reactions to skin test antigens

Additional Information Diphenhydramine citrate 19 mg is equivalent to diphenhydramine hydrochloride 12.5 mg

Dosage Forms Excipient information presented when available (limited, particularly for generics); consult specific product labeling. [DSC] = Discontinued product

Caplet, as hydrochloride: 25 mg, 50 mg

Aler-Dryl, AllerMax®, Compoz® Nighttime Sleep Aid, Sleep-ettes D, Sominex® Maximum Strength, Twilite®: 50 mg

Nytol® Quick Caps, Simply Sleep®: 25 mg

Capsule, as hydrochloride: 25 mg, 50 mg

Aler-Cap, Banophen®, Benadryl® Allergy, Diphen®, Diphenhist, Genahist®: 25 mg

Sleepinal®: 50 mg

Capsule, softgel, as hydrochloride: 50 mg

Benadryl® Dye-Free Allergy: 25 mg [dye-free]

Compoz® Nighttime Sleep Aid, Nytol® Quick Gels, Sleepinal®, Unisom® Maximum Strength SleepGels®: 50 mg

Captab, as hydrochloride:

Diphenhist®: 25 mg

Cream, as hydrochloride: 2% (30 g)

Banophen® Anti-Itch: 2% (30 g) [contains zinc acetate 0.1%]

Benadryl® Itch Stopping: 1% (30 g) [contains zinc acetate 0.1%]

Benadryl® Itch Stopping Extra Strength: 2% (30 g) [contains zinc acetate 0.1%]

Diphenhist®: 2% (30 g) [contains zinc acetate 0.1%]

Elixir, as hydrochloride:

Altaryl: 12.5 mg/5 mL (120 mL, 480 mL, 3840 mL) [cherry flavor]

Banophen®: 12.5 mg/5 mL (120 mL)

Diphen AF: 12.5 mg/5 mL (240 mL, 480 mL) [alcohol free; cherry flavor]

Gel, topical, as hydrochloride:

Benadryl® Itch Stopping Extra Strength: 2% (120 mL)

Injection, solution, as hydrochloride: 50 mg/mL (1 mL, 10 mL)

Liquid, as hydrochloride:

AllerMax®: 12.5 mg/5 mL (120 mL)

Benadryl® Allergy: 12.5 mg/5 mL (120 mL, 240 mL) [alcohol free; contains sodium benzoate; cherry flavor]

Benadryl® Children's Dye-Free Allergy: 12.5 mg/5 mL (120 mL) [alcohol free, dye free, sugar free; contains sodium benzoate; bubble gum flavor]

Genahist®: 12.5 mg/5 mL (120 mL) [alcohol free, sugar free; contains sodium benzoate; cherry flavor]

Hydramine®: 12.5 mg/5 mL (120 mL, 480 mL) [alcohol free]

Siladryl® Allergy: 12.5 mg/5 mL (120 mL, 240 mL, 480 mL) [alcohol free, sugar free; black cherry flavor]

Liquid, topical, as hydrochloride [stick]:

Benadryl® Itch Stopping Extra Strength: 2% (14 mL) [contains zinc acetate 0.1% and alcohol]

Solution, oral, as hydrochloride:

Diphenhist: 12.5 mg/5 mL (120 mL, 480 mL) [alcohol free; contains sodium benzoate]

Solution, topical, as hydrochloride [spray]:

Benadryl® Itch Stopping Extra Strength: 2% (60 mL) [contains zinc acetate 0.1% and alcohol]

Dermamycin®: 2% (60 mL) [contains menthol 1%]

Strips, oral, as hydrochloride:

Benadryl® Allergy: 25 mg (10s) [contains sodium 4 mg/strip; vanilla mint flavor]

Benadryl® Children's Allergy: 12.5 mg (10s) [vanilla mint flavor]

Triaminic® Thin Strips™ Cough and Runny Nose: 12.5 mg (16s) [grape flavor]

Suspension, as tannate:

Ben-Tann: 25 mg/5 mL (120 ml) [contains sodium benzoate; strawberry flavor]

Dytan™: 25 mg/5 mL (120 mL) [strawberry flavor] [DSC]

Syrup, as hydrochloride:

Silphen® Cough: 12.5 mg/5 mL (120 mL, 240 mL, 480 mL) [contains alcohol; 5%; strawberry flavor]

Tablet, as hydrochloride: 25 mg, 50 mg

Aler-Tab, Benadryl® Allergy, Genahist®, Sominex®: 25 mg

Tablet, chewable, as hydrochloride:

Benadryl® Children's Allergy: 12.5 mg [contains phenylalanine 4.2 mg, magnesium 15 mg, and sodium 2 mg per tablet; grape flavor]

Tablet, chewable, as tannate:

Dytan™: 25 mg [contains phenylalanine; strawberry flavor]

Tablet, orally disintegrating, as citrate:

Benadryl® Children's Allergy Fastmelt®: 19 mg [equivalent to diphenhydramine hydrochloride 12.5 mg; contains phenylalanine 4.5 mg/tablet and soy protein isolate; cherry flavor]

◆ **Diphenhydramine and Acetaminophen** *see* Acetaminophen and Diphenhydramine *on page 28*

◆ **Diphenhydramine and ASA** *see* Aspirin and Diphenhydramine *on page 145*

◆ **Diphenhydramine and Aspirin** *see* Aspirin and Diphenhydramine *on page 145*

Diphenhydramine and Phenylephrine

(dye fen HYE dra meen & fen il EF rin)

U.S. Brand Names Aldex® CT; D-Tann; Dimetapp® Children's Nighttime Cold & Congestion [OTC]; Robitussin® Night Time Cough & Cold [OTC]

Index Terms Diphenhydramine Hydrochloride and Phenylephrine Hydrochloride; Diphenhydramine Tannate and Phenylephrine Tannate; Phenylephrine and Diphenhydramine; Phenylephrine Hydrochloride and Diphenhydramine Hydrochloride; Phenylephrine Tannate and Diphenhydramine Tannate

Pharmacologic Category Alpha/Beta Agonist; Histamine H_1 Antagonist; Histamine H_1 Antagonist, First Generation

Use Temporary relief of symptoms of allergic rhinitis, sinusitis, and other upper respiratory conditions, including sinus/nasal congestion, sneezing, stuffy/runny nose, itchy/watery eyes, and cough

Pregnancy Risk Factor C

Dosage Oral:

Aldex® CT:

Children 6-11 years: One-half to 1 tablet every 6 hours

Children ≥12 years and Adults: 1-2 tablets every 6 hours

D-Tann:

Children 2-5 years: 1.25-2.5 mL every 12 hours

Children 6-11 years: 2.5-5 mL **or** 1/2 to 1 tablet every 12 hours

Children ≥12 years and Adults: 5-10 mL **or** 1-2 tablets every 12 hours

OTC labeling:

Children <6 years: Use not recommended

Children 6-11 years (Dimetapp® Children's Nighttime Cold and Congestion): 10 mL every 4 hours as needed, maximum 6 doses/24 hours

Children ≥12 years and Adults: 20 mL every 4 hours as needed, maximum 6 doses/24 hours

Additional Information Complete prescribing information for this medication should be consulted for additional detail.

Dosage Forms Excipient information presented when available (limited, particularly for generics); consult specific product labeling.

Suspension:

D-Tann: Diphenhydramine tannate 25 mg and phenylephrine tannate 7.5 mg per 5 mL [118 mL] [contains sodium benzoate, bubblegum flavor]

Syrup:

Dimetapp® Children's Nighttime Cold and Congestion: Diphenhydramine hydrochloride 6.25 mg and phenylephrine hydrochloride 2.5 mg per 5 mL [120 mL] [alcohol free, sugar free; grape flavor]

Robitussin® Night Time Cough and Cold: Diphenhydramine hydrochloride 6.25 mg and phenylephrine hydrochloride 2.5 mg per 5 mL [120 mL] [alcohol free, contains sodium benzoate]

Tablet, chewable:

Aldex® CT: Diphenhydramine hydrochloride 12.5 mg and phenylephrine hydrochloride 5 mg [strawberry flavor]

D-Tann: Diphenhydramine tannate 25 mg and phenylephrine tannate 10 mg [contains phenylalanine 5.7 mg/tablet, berry flavor]

Diphenhydramine and Pseudoephedrine

(dye fen HYE dra meen & soo doe e FED rin)

U.S. Brand Names Benadryl-D™ Allergy and Sinus Fastmelt™ [OTC]; Benadryl-D™ Children's Allergy and Sinus [OTC]; Benadryl® Children's Allergy and Cold Fastmelt™ [OTC]

Index Terms Pseudoephedrine and Diphenhydramine

Pharmacologic Category Alpha/Beta Agonist; Histamine H_1 Antagonist; Histamine H_1 Antagonist, First Generation

Use Relief of symptoms of upper respiratory mucosal congestion in seasonal and perennial nasal allergies, acute rhinitis, rhinosinusitis, and eustachian tube blockage

Medication Safety Issues

Sound-alike/look-alike issues:

Benadryl® may be confused with benazepril, Bentyl®, Benylin®, Caladryl®

Dosage Based on **pseudoephedrine** component:

Adults: Oral: 60 mg every 4-6 hours, maximum: 240 mg/day

Additional Information Complete prescribing information for this medication should be consulted for additional detail.

Dosage Forms Excipient information presented when available (limited, particularly for generics); consult specific product labeling.

Liquid:

Benadryl-D™ Children's Allergy and Sinus: Diphenhydramine hydrochloride 12.5 mg and pseudoephedrine hydrochloride 30 mg per 5 mL [alcohol free, sugar free; contains sodium 10 mg/5 mL and sodium benzoate; grape flavor]

Tablet, quick dissolving:

Benadryl® Children's Allergy and Cold Fastmelt™, Benadryl-D™ Allergy and Sinus Fastmelt™: Diphenhydramine citrate 19 mg [equivalent to diphenhydramine hydrochloride 12.5 mg] and pseudoephedrine 30 mg [contains phenylalanine 4.6 mg/tablet; cherry flavor]

◆ **Diphenhydramine Citrate** *see* DiphenhydrAMINE *on page 456*

◆ **Diphenhydramine Citrate and Aspirin** *see* Aspirin and Diphenhydramine *on page 145*

◆ **Diphenhydramine Hydrochloride** *see* DiphenhydrAMINE *on page 456*

◆ **Diphenhydramine Hydrochloride and Phenylephrine Hydrochloride** *see* Diphenhydramine and Phenylephrine *on page 458*

◆ **Diphenhydramine, Phenylephrine Hydrochloride, and Acetaminophen** *see* Acetaminophen, Diphenhydramine, and Phenylephrine *on page 33*

◆ **Diphenhydramine Tannate** *see* DiphenhydrAMINE *on page 456*

◆ **Diphenhydramine Tannate and Phenylephrine Tannate** *see* Diphenhydramine and Phenylephrine *on page 458*

Diphenoxylate and Atropine

(dye fen OKS i late & A troe peen)

U.S. Brand Names Lomotil®; Lonox®

Canadian Brand Names Lomotil®

Index Terms Atropine and Diphenoxylate

Pharmacologic Category Antidiarrheal

Use Treatment of diarrhea

Restrictions C-V

Pregnancy Risk Factor C

Pregnancy Considerations Teratogenic effects were not noted in animal studies; decreased maternal weight, fertility and litter sizes were observed. There are no adequate and well-controlled studies in pregnant women.

Lactation Enters breast milk/use caution

Medication Safety Issues

Sound-alike/look-alike issues:

Lomotil® may be confused with Lamictal®, Lamisil®, lamotrigine, Lanoxin®, Lasix®, ludiomil

Lonox® may be confused with Lanoxin®, Loprox®

International issues:

Lomotil® may be confused with Lemesil® which is a brand name for nimesulide in Greece

Lonox® may be confused with Flomox® which is a brand of cefcapene in Japan

Contraindications Hypersensitivity to diphenoxylate, atropine, or any component of the formulation; obstructive jaundice; diarrhea associated with pseudomembranous enterocolitis or enterotoxin-producing bacteria; not for use in children <2 years of age

Warnings/Precautions Use in conjunction with fluid and electrolyte therapy when appropriate. In case of severe dehydration or electrolyte imbalance, withhold diphenoxylate/atropine treatment until corrective therapy has been initiated. Inhibiting peristalsis may lead to fluid retention in the intestine aggravating dehydration and electrolyte imbalance. Reduction of intestinal motility may be deleterious in diarrhea resulting from *Shigella, Salmonella,* toxigenic strains of *E. coli*, and pseudomembranous enterocolitis associated with broad-spectrum antibiotics; use is not recommended.

Use with caution in children. Younger children may be predisposed to toxicity; signs of atropinism may occur even at recommended doses, especially in patients with Down syndrome. Overdose in children may result in severe respiratory depression, coma, and possibly permanent brain damage.

Use caution with acute ulcerative colitis, hepatic or renal dysfunction. If there is no response with 48 hours, this medication is unlikely to be effective and should be discontinued; if chronic diarrhea is not improved symptomatically within 10 days at maximum dosage, control is unlikely with further use. Physical and psychological dependence have been reported with higher than recommended dosing.

Adverse Reactions Frequency not defined.

Cardiovascular: Tachycardia

Central nervous system: Confusion, depression, dizziness, drowsiness, euphoria, flushing, headache, hyperthermia, lethargy, malaise, restlessness, sedation
Dermatologic: Angioneurotic edema, dry skin, pruritus, urticaria
Gastrointestinal: Abdominal discomfort, anorexia, gum swelling, nausea, pancreatitis, paralytic ileus, toxic megacolon, vomiting, xerostomia
Genitourinary: Urinary retention
Neuromuscular & skeletal: Numbness
Miscellaneous: Anaphylaxis

Drug Interactions

Avoid Concomitant Use There are no known interactions where it is recommended to avoid concomitant use.

Increased Effect/Toxicity

Diphenoxylate and Atropine may increase the levels/effects of: Anticholinergics; Cannabinoids; Potassium Chloride

The levels/effects of Diphenoxylate and Atropine may be increased by: Pramlintide

Decreased Effect

Diphenoxylate and Atropine may decrease the levels/effects of: Acetylcholinesterase Inhibitors (Central); Secretin

The levels/effects of Diphenoxylate and Atropine may be decreased by: Acetylcholinesterase Inhibitors (Central)

Ethanol/Nutrition/Herb Interactions Ethanol: Avoid ethanol (may increase CNS depression).

Mechanism of Action Diphenoxylate inhibits excessive GI motility and GI propulsion; commercial preparations contain a subtherapeutic amount of atropine to discourage abuse

Pharmacodynamics/Kinetics

Atropine: See Atropine monograph.

Diphenoxylate:

Onset of action: Antidiarrheal: 45-60 minutes
Duration: Antidiarrheal: 3-4 hours
Absorption: Well absorbed
Metabolism: Extensively hepatic via ester hydrolysis to diphenoxylic acid (active)
Half-life elimination: Diphenoxylate: 2.5 hours; Diphenoxylic acid: 12-14 hours
Time to peak, serum: 2 hours
Excretion: Primarily feces (49% as unchanged drug and metabolites); urine (~14%, <1% as unchanged drug)

Dosage Oral:

Children 2-12 years (use with caution in young children due to variable responses): Liquid: Diphenoxylate 0.3-0.4 mg/kg/day in 4 divided doses until control achieved (maximum: 10 mg/day), then reduce dose as needed; some patients may be controlled on doses as low as 25% of the initial daily dose

Adults: Diphenoxylate 5 mg 4 times/day until control achieved (maximum: 20 mg/day), then reduce dose as needed; some patients may be controlled on doses of 5 mg/day

Administration If there is no response within 48 hours of continuous therapy, this medication is unlikely to be effective and should be discontinued; if chronic diarrhea is not improved symptomatically within 10 days at maximum dosage, control is unlikely with further use. Use of the liquid preparation is recommended in children <13 years of age; use plastic dropper provided when measuring liquid.

Monitoring Parameters Watch for signs of atropinism (dryness of skin and mucous membranes, tachycardia, thirst, flushing); monitor number and consistency of stools; observe for signs of toxicity, fluid and electrolyte loss, hypotension, and respiratory depression

Dosage Forms Excipient information presented when available (limited, particularly for generics); consult specific product labeling.

Solution, oral: Diphenoxylate hydrochloride 2.5 mg and atropine sulfate 0.025 mg per 5 mL (5 mL, 10 mL, 60 mL)
Lomotil®: Diphenoxylate hydrochloride 2.5 mg and atropine sulfate 0.025 mg per 5 mL (60 mL) [contains alcohol 15%; cherry flavor]

Tablet: Diphenoxylate hydrochloride 2.5 mg and atropine sulfate 0.025 mg
Lomotil®, Lonox®: Diphenoxylate hydrochloride 2.5 mg and atropine sulfate 0.025 mg

◆ **Diphenylhydantoin** *see* Phenytoin *on page 1186*

Diphtheria and Tetanus Toxoid

(dif THEER ee a & TET a nus TOKS oyds)

U.S. Brand Names Decavac®

Canadian Brand Names Td Adsorbed

Index Terms DT; Td; Tetanus and Diphtheria Toxoid

Pharmacologic Category Vaccine, Inactivated (Bacterial)

Additional Appendix Information

Immunization Recommendations *on page 1708*

Use

Diphtheria and tetanus toxoids adsorbed for pediatric use (DT): Infants and children through 6 years of age: Active immunization against diphtheria and tetanus when pertussis vaccine is contraindicated

Tetanus and diphtheria toxoids adsorbed for adult use (Td) (Decavac™): Children ≥7 years of age and Adults: Active immunization against diphtheria and tetanus; tetanus prophylaxis in wound management

The Advisory Committee on Immunization Practices (ACIP) recommends routine vaccination for the following:

- Adults and children ≥7 years should receive a booster dose of Td every 10 years; persons <65 years of age may substitute a single Td booster dose with Tdap
- Children 7-10 years, adults, and the elderly (≥65 years) who are wounded in bombings or similar mass casualty events who have penetrating injuries or nonintact skin exposure and who cannot confirm receipt of a tetanus booster within the previous 5 years, may also receive a single dose of Td; children ≥11 years may also received Td if Tdap is unavailable

Pregnancy Risk Factor C

Pregnancy Considerations Reproduction studies have not been conducted. DT is not recommended for use in persons ≥7 years of age. The Advisory Committee on Immunization Practices (ACIP) recommends booster injections for previously vaccinated pregnant women who have not had Td vaccination within the past 10 years. Pregnant women who are not immunized or are only partially immunized should complete the primary series. Vaccination may be deferred until the postpartum period in women who are likely to have sufficient diphtheria and tetanus protection until delivery; Tdap may be substituted for Td after delivery to add extra protection against pertussis. Td should be administered during pregnancy to women who do not have sufficient tetanus immunity to protect against maternal and neonatal tetanus, and if booster protection for diphtheria is required (eg, travel to where diphtheria is endemic). Tetanus immune globulin and a tetanus toxoid containing vaccine are recommended by the ACIP as part of the standard wound management to prevent tetanus in pregnant women; the use of Td during pregnancy is recommended for wound management if ≥5 years have passed since the last Td vaccination.

Lactation Excretion in breast milk unknown/use caution

Contraindications Hypersensitivity to diphtheria, tetanus toxoid, or any component of the formulation

Warnings/Precautions Do not confuse pediatric diphtheria and tetanus (DT) with adult tetanus and diphtheria (Td). Immediate treatment for anaphylactic/anaphylactoid reaction should be available during administration. Patients with a history of severe local reaction

(Arthus-type) or temperature of >39.4°C (103°F) following a previous dose should not be given further routine or emergency doses of Td more frequently than every 10 years. Continue use with caution if Guillain-Barré syndrome occurs within 6 weeks of prior tetanus toxoid. For I.M. administration; use caution with history of bleeding disorders or anticoagulant therapy. Defer administration during moderate or severe illness (with or without fever) or during outbreaks of poliomyelitis. Immune response may be decreased in immunocompromised patients. Safety and efficacy of DT have not been established in children <6 weeks of age; Td should be administered to children ≥7 years of age and adults. Some products may contain natural latex/natural rubber or thimerosal. In order to maximize vaccination rates, the ACIP recommends simultaneous administration of all age-appropriate vaccines (live or inactivated) for which a person is eligible at a single clinic visit, unless contraindications exist.

Adverse Reactions All serious adverse reactions must be reported to the U.S. Department of Health and Human Services (DHHS) Vaccine Adverse Event Reporting System (VAERS) 1-800-822-7967.

>10%: Local: Injection site (19%; including erythema, induration, tenderness)

<10%: Central nervous system: Headache (2%), malaise (2%), temperature increased (2%)

Postmarketing and/or case reports: Allergic reactions (facial edema, pruritus, rash, urticaria); anaphylactoid reactions, arthralgia, chills, convulsions, dizziness, fatigue, fever; injection site reactions (cellulitis, nodules, redness, swelling, warmth); lymphadenopathy, musculoskeletal stiffness, myalgia, nausea, pain, paresthesia, peripheral edema, syncope, vomiting, weakness. Guillain-Barré syndrome and brachial neuritis may also occur with tetanus toxoid-containing vaccines.

Drug Interactions

Avoid Concomitant Use There are no known interactions where it is recommended to avoid concomitant use.

Increased Effect/Toxicity There are no known significant interactions involving an increase in effect.

Decreased Effect

The levels/effects of Diphtheria and Tetanus Toxoids may be decreased by: Immunosuppressants

Stability Store at 2°C to 8°C (35°F to 46°F); do not freeze. Discard if product has been frozen.

Dosage I.M.:

Infants and Children ≤6 years (DT): Primary immunization:

6 weeks to 1 year: Three 0.5 mL doses at least 4 weeks apart; administer a reinforcing dose 6-12 months after the third injection

1-6 years: Two 0.5 mL doses at least 4-8 weeks apart; reinforcing dose 6-12 months after second injection; if final dose is given after seventh birthday, use adult preparation

4-6 years (booster immunization): 0.5 mL; not necessary if the fourth dose was given after fourth birthday; routinely administer booster doses at 10-year intervals with the adult preparation

Children ≥7 years and Adults (Td):

Primary immunization: Patients previously not immunized should receive 2 primary doses of 0.5 mL each, given at an interval of 4-8 weeks; third (reinforcing) dose of 0.5 mL 6-12 months later

Booster immunization: 0.5 mL every 10 years; to be given to children 11-12 years of age if at least 5 years have elapsed since last dose of toxoid containing vaccine. Subsequent routine doses are not recommended more often than every 10 years. The ACIP prefers Tdap for use in adolescents 11-18 years; refer to Diphtheria and Tetanus Toxoids and Acellular Pertussis Vaccine monograph for additional information.

Tetanus prophylaxis in wound management; use of tetanus toxoid (Td) and/or tetanus immune globulin (TIG) depends upon the number of prior tetanus toxoid doses and type of wound: See table.

Tetanus Prophylaxis in Wound Management

Number of Prior Tetanus Toxoid Doses	Clean, Minor Wounds		All Other Wounds	
	Td[1]	TIG[2]	Td[1]	TIG[2]
Unknown or <3	Yes	No	Yes	Yes
≥3[3]	No[4]	No	No[5]	No

[1]Adult tetanus and diphtheria toxoids; use pediatric preparations (DT or DTP) if the patient is <7 years old.

[2]Tetanus immune globulin.

[3]If only three doses of fluid tetanus toxoid have been received, a fourth dose of toxoid, preferably an adsorbed toxoid, should be given.

[4]Yes, if >10 years since last dose.

[5]Yes, if >5 years since last dose.

Adapted from Centers for Disease Control, "Diphtheria, Tetanus, and Pertussis: Recommendations for Vaccine Use and Other Preventive Measures: Recommendations of the Immunization Practices Advisory Committee (ACIP)," *MMWR* 1991:40(RR-10).

Administration For I.M. administration; prior to use, shake suspension well

Td: Administer in the deltoid muscle; do not inject in the gluteal area

DT: Administer in the anterolateral aspect of the thigh or the deltoid muscle; do not inject in the gluteal area

For patients at risk of hemorrhage following intramuscular injection, the ACIP recommends "it should be administered intramuscularly if, in the opinion of the physician familiar with the patients bleeding risk, the vaccine can be administered with reasonable safety by this route. If the patient receives antihemophilia or other similar therapy, intramuscular vaccination can be scheduled shortly after such therapy is administered. A fine needle (23 gauge or smaller) can be used for the vaccination and firm pressure applied to the site (without rubbing) for at least 2 minutes. The patient should be instructed concerning the risk of hematoma from the injection."

Administration with other vaccines:

Diphtheria and Tetanus Toxoids vaccine with other inactivated vaccines: May be given simultaneously or at any interval between doses.

Diphtheria and Tetanus Toxoids vaccine with live vaccines: May be given simultaneously or at any interval between doses.

Vaccine administration with antibody-containing products: Diphtheria and tetanus toxoids vaccine may be given simultaneously at different sites or at any interval between doses. Examples of antibody containing products include I.M. and I.V. immune globulin, hepatitis B immune globulin, tetanus immune globulin, varicella zoster immune globulin, rabies immune globulin, whole blood, packed red cells, plasma, and platelet products.

Monitoring Parameters Monitor for syncope for ≥15 minutes following vaccination

Additional Information Pediatric dosage form should only be used in patients ≤6 years of age. Federal law requires that the date of administration, the vaccine manufacturer, lot number of vaccine, and the administering person's name, title, and address be entered into the patient's permanent medical record.

Since protective tetanus and diphtheria antibodies decline with age, only 28% of persons >70 years of age in the U.S. are believed to be immune to tetanus, and most of the tetanus-induced deaths occur in people >60 years of age, it is advisable to offer Td especially to the elderly concurrent with their influenza and other immunization programs if history of vaccination is unclear; boosters should be given at 10-year intervals; earlier for wounds

DT contains higher proportions of diphtheria toxoid than Td.

Dosage Forms Excipient information presented when available (limited, particularly for generics); consult specific product labeling.

Injection, suspension [Td, adult]: Diphtheria 2 Lf units and tetanus 2 Lf units per 0.5 mL (5 mL, 7.5 mL); Diphtheria 2 Lf units and tetanus 5 Lf units per 0.5 mL (5 mL, 7.5 mL)

Injection, suspension [Td, adult; preservative free]: Diphtheria 2 Lf units and tetanus 2 Lf units per 0.5 mL (0.5 mL); diphtheria 2 Lf units and tetanus 5 Lf units per 0.5 mL (0.5 mL)

Decavac®: Diphtheria 2 Lf units and tetanus 5 Lf units per 0.5 mL (0.5 mL) [contains aluminum, thimerosal (may have trace amounts)]

Injection, suspension [DT, pediatric; preservative free]: Diphtheria 6.7 Lf units and tetanus 5 Lf units per 0.5 mL (0.5 mL)

Diphtheria and Tetanus Toxoids, Acellular Pertussis, and *Haemophilus influenzae* b Conjugate Vaccine

(dif THEER ee a & TET a nus TOKS oyds, ay CEL yoo lar per TUS sis & hem OF fi lus in floo EN za bee KON joo gate vak SEEN)

U.S. Brand Names TriHIBit®

Index Terms *Haemophilus influenzae* b Conjugate Vaccine and Diphtheria, Tetanus Toxoids, and Acellular Pertussis Vaccine; DTaP/Hib

Pharmacologic Category Vaccine, Inactivated (Bacterial)

Use Active immunization of children 15-18 months of age for prevention of diphtheria, tetanus, pertussis, and invasive disease caused by *H. influenzae* type b

The Advisory Committee on Immunization Practices (ACIP) recommends the use of TriHIBit® for the fourth dose of the diphtheria, tetanus, pertussis, and *Haemophilus* vaccine series. Whenever feasible, the same manufacturer should be used to provide the pertussis component; however, vaccination should not be deferred if a specific brand is not known or is not available.

Dosage Children 15-18 months: I.M.: 0.5 mL: **Note:** For use as the fourth dose of the DTaP and Hib series (see individual vaccines). May be used as a booster in children 12-20 months of age as long as 6 months have elapsed since the third dose.

Additional Information Complete prescribing information for this medication should be consulted for additional detail.

Dosage Forms Excipient information presented when available (limited, particularly for generics); consult specific product labeling.

Injection, suspension [preservative free]:

TriHIBit®: Diphtheria 6.7 Lf units, tetanus 5 Lf units, acellular pertussis antigens [inactivated pertussis toxin 23.4 mcg, filamentous hemagglutinin 23.4 mcg], and *Haemophilus* b capsular polysaccharide 10 mcg [bound to tetanus toxoid 24 mcg] per 0.5 mL (0.5 mL) [contains aluminum, natural rubber/natural latex in packaging, polysorbate 80, sucrose, and trace amounts of thimerosal; Tripedia® vaccine used to reconstitute ActHIB® forms TriHIBit®]

Diphtheria and Tetanus Toxoids, Acellular Pertussis, and Poliovirus Vaccine

(dif THEER ee a & TET a nus TOKS oyds, ay CEL yoo lar per TUS sis & POE lee oh VYE rus vak SEEN)

U.S. Brand Names Kinrix™

Index Terms Diphtheria and Tetanus Toxoids and Acellular Pertussis Adsorbed, and Inactivated Poliovirus Vaccine Combined; Diphtheria, Tetanus Toxoids, Acellular Pertussis (DTaP); DTaP-IPV; Poliovirus, inactivated (IPV)

Pharmacologic Category Vaccine, Inactivated (Bacterial); Vaccine, Inactivated (Viral)

Additional Appendix Information

Immunization Recommendations *on page 1708*

Use Active immunization against diphtheria, tetanus, pertussis, and poliomyelitis, used as the 5th dose in the DTaP series and the 4th dose in the IPV series

The Advisory Committee on Immunization Practices (ACIP) recommends routine vaccination for use as the fifth dose in the DTaP series and the fourth dose in the IPV series in children who received DTaP (Infanrix®) and/or DTaP-Hepatitis B-IPV (Pediarix®) as the first 3 doses and DTaP (Infanrix®) as the fourth dose. Whenever feasible, the same manufacturer should be used to provide the pertussis component; however, vaccination should not be deferred if a specific brand is not known or is not available.

Pregnancy Risk Factor C

Dosage I.M.: Children 4-6 years: Immunization: 0.5 mL; **Note:** For use as the 5th dose in the DTaP series and the 4th dose in the IPV series

Additional Information Complete prescribing information for this medication should be consulted for additional detail.

Dosage Forms Excipient information presented when available (limited, particularly for generics); consult specific product labeling.

Injection, suspension [preservative free]:

Kinrix™: Diphtheria toxoid 25 Lf, tetanus toxoid 10 Lf, PT 25 mcg, FHA 25 mcg, pertactin 8 mcg, poliovirus type 1 40 DU, poliovirus type 2 8 DU, and poliovirus type 3 32 DU per 0.5 mL (0.5 mL) [contains aluminum, neomycin sulfate, polymyxin B, polysorbate 80, natural rubber/natural latex in packaging]

Diphtheria and Tetanus Toxoids, Acellular Pertussis, Poliovirus and *Haemophilus* b Conjugate Vaccine

(dif THEER ee a & TET a nus TOKS oyds ay CEL yoo lar per TUS sis POE lee oh VYE rus & hem OF fi lus in floo EN za bee KON joo gate vak SEEN)

U.S. Brand Names Pentacel®

Index Terms *Haemophilus* B Conjugate (Hib); *Haemophilus* B Polysaccharide; Diphtheria Toxoid; Diphtheria, Tetanus Toxoids, Acellular Pertussis (DTaP); DTaP-IPV/Hib; Pertussis, Acellular (Adsorbed); Poliovirus, Inactivated (IPV); Tetanus Toxoid

Pharmacologic Category Vaccine, Inactivated (Bacterial); Vaccine, Inactivated (Viral)

Additional Appendix Information

Immunization Recommendations *on page 1708*

Use Active immunization against diphtheria, tetanus, pertussis, poliomyelitis, and invasive disease caused by *H. influenzae* type b in children 6 weeks through 4 years of age

Advisory Committee on Immunization Practices (ACIP) recommends that Pentacel® (DTaP-IPV/Hib) may be used to provide the recommended DTaP, IPV, and Hib immunization in children <5 years of age. Whenever feasible, the same manufacturer should be used to provide the pertussis component; however, vaccination should not be deferred if a specific brand is not known or is not available. The Hib component in Pentacel® contains a tetanus toxoid conjugate. A Hib vaccine containing the PRP-OMP conjugate (PedvaxHIB®) may provide a more rapid seroconversion following the first dose and may be preferable to use in certain populations (eg, American Indian or Alaska Native children).

Pregnancy Risk Factor C

Dosage I.M.: Children:

Primary immunization: Children 6 weeks to ≤4 years: 0.5 mL per dose administered at 2, 4, 6 and 15-18 months of age (total of 4 doses). The first dose may be administered as early as 6 weeks of age. Following completion of the 4-dose series, children should receive a dose of DTaP vaccine at 4-6 years of age (Daptacel® recommended due to same pertussis antigen used in both products).

Children previously vaccinated with ≥1 dose of Daptacel® or IPV vaccines: Pentacel® may be used to complete the first 4 doses of the DTaP or IPV series in children scheduled to receive the other components in the vaccine.

Children previously vaccinated with ≥1 dose of *Haemophilus* b conjugate vaccine: Pentacel® may be used to complete the series in children scheduled to receive the other components in the vaccine; however, if different brands of *Haemophilus* b conjugate vaccine are administered to complete the series, 3 primary immunizing doses are needed, followed by a booster dose.

Note: Completion of 3 doses of Pentacel® provides primary immunization against diphtheria, tetanus, *H. influenzae* type B, and poliomyelitis. Completion of the 4-dose series with Pentacel® provides primary immunization against pertussis. It also provides a booster vaccination against diphtheria, tetanus, *H. influenzae* type B, and poliomyelitis.

Additional Information Federal law requires that the date of administration, the vaccine manufacturer, lot number of vaccine, and the administering person's name, title, and address be entered into the patient's permanent medical record. Lot numbers are different for each component of the DTaP-IPV/Hib vaccine; numbers should be recorded separately for the DTaP-IPV and Hib components. The vaccine components should not be administered separately.

Dosage Forms Excipient information presented when available (limited, particularly for generics); consult specific product labeling.

Injection, suspension:

Pentacel®: Diphtheria toxoid 15 Lf, tetanus toxoid 5 Lf, acellular pertussis antigens (pertussis toxin detoxified 20 mcg, filamentous hemagglutinin 20 mcg, pertactin 3 mcg, fimbriae [types 2 and 3] 5 mcg), poliovirus (type 1: 40 D-antigen units; type 2: 8 D antigen units; type 3: 32 D antigen units), and *Haemophilus* b capsular polysaccharide 10 mcg (bound to tetanus toxoid 24 mcg) per 0.5 mL (0.5 mL) [contains albumin, aluminum, neomycin, polymyxin B sulfate, and polysorbate 80; supplied in two vials, one containing DTaP-IPV liquid and one containing Hib powder]

◆ **Diphtheria and Tetanus Toxoids and Acellular Pertussis Adsorbed, and Inactivated Poliovirus Vaccine Combined** *see* Diphtheria and Tetanus Toxoids, Acellular Pertussis, and Poliovirus Vaccine *on page 462*

◆ **Diphtheria and Tetanus Toxoids and Acellular Pertussis Adsorbed, Hepatitis B (Recombinant) and Inactivated Poliovirus Vaccine Combined** *see* Diphtheria, Tetanus Toxoids, Acellular Pertussis, Hepatitis B (Recombinant), and Poliovirus Vaccine *on page 466*

Diphtheria and Tetanus Toxoids, and Acellular Pertussis Vaccine

(dif THEER ee a & TET a nus TOKS oyds & ay CEL yoo lar per TUS sis vak SEEN)

U.S. Brand Names Adacel®; Boostrix®; Daptacel®; Infanrix®; Tripedia®

Canadian Brand Names Adacel®

Index Terms DTaP; dTpa; Tdap; Tetanus Toxoid, Reduced Diphtheria Toxoid, and Acellular Pertussis, Adsorbed

Pharmacologic Category Vaccine, Inactivated (Bacterial)

Additional Appendix Information

Immunization Recommendations *on page 1708*

Use

Daptacel®, Infanrix®, Tripedia® (DTaP): Active immunization against diphtheria, tetanus, and pertussis from age 6 weeks through 6 years of age (prior to seventh birthday)

Adacel®, Boostrix® (Tdap): Active booster immunization against diphtheria, tetanus, and pertussis

The Advisory Committee on Immunization Practices (ACIP) recommends routine vaccination for the following:

Children 6 weeks to <7 years (DTaP): For primary immunization against diphtheria, tetanus and pertussis

Adolescents 11-18 years [Adacel® (Tdap)]; Adolescents and Adults 10-64 years of age [Boostrix® (Tdap)]:

- A single dose of Tdap as a booster dose in adolescents who have completed the recommended childhood DTaP vaccination series (preferred age of administration is 11-12 years)
- A single dose of Tdap should be given to replace a single dose of Td if the last dose of Td was ≥5 years earlier; lesser intervals may be used if the benefit outweighs the risk (not for multiple administrations; recommendations are for the replacement of a single dose of Td only)
- Persons wounded in bombings or similar mass casualty events and who cannot confirm receipt of a tetanus booster within the previous 5 years and who have penetrating injuries or nonintact skin exposure should receive a single dose of Tdap

Adults aged 19-64 (Adacel®): A single dose of Tdap should be given to replace a single dose of Td if the last dose of Td was ≥10 years earlier (not for multiple administrations; recommendations are for the replacement of a single dose of Td only). A shorter interval (<10 years but at least 2 years since last dose of Td) may be considered in the following situations:

- To protect against pertussis
- To protect against pertussis transmission to infants in adults who anticipate close contact with children <12 months of age; Tdap should be administered at least 2 weeks prior to beginning close contact
- Healthcare providers with direct patient contact
- Persons wounded in bombings or similar mass casualty events and who cannot confirm receipt of a tetanus booster within the previous 5 years and who have penetrating injuries or nonintact skin exposure, should receive a single dose of Tdap

Pregnancy Risk Factor C

Pregnancy Considerations Animal reproduction studies have not been conducted. It is not known whether the vaccine can cause fetal harm when administered to a pregnant woman or can affect reproductive capacity. Daptacel®, Infanrix®, and Tripedia® are not recommended for use in a pregnant woman or any patient ≥7 years of age. Although pregnancy itself is generally not considered a contraindication to Tdap (Adacel®, Boostrix®) vaccination, Td is preferred to Tdap when vaccination cannot be delayed during pregnancy. In order to help prevent pertussis exposure among infants, the use of Tdap, is recommended in women of childbearing potential prior to pregnancy. Due to lack of information with Tdap, a pregnancy registry has been established for women who may become exposed to Boostrix® (888-825-5249) or Adacel® (800-822-2463) while pregnant.

Lactation Excretion in breast milk unknown/use caution

Medication Safety Issues

Carefully review product labeling to prevent inadvertent administration of Tdap when DTaP is indicated. Tdap contains lower amounts of diphtheria toxoid and some pertussis antigens than DTaP.

Tdap is not indicated for use in children <10 years of age

DTaP is not indicated for use in persons ≥7 years of age

Guidelines are available in case of inadvertent administration of these products; refer to ACIP recommendations, February 2006 available at http://www.cdc.gov/mmwr/preview/mmwrhtml/rr55e223a1.htm

Note:

DTaP: Diphtheria and tetanus toxoids and acellular pertussis vaccine

DTP: Diphtheria and tetanus toxoids and pertussis vaccine (unspecified pertussis antigens)

DTwP: Diphtheria and tetanus toxoids and whole-cell pertussis vaccine (no longer available on U.S. market)

Tdap: Tetanus toxoid, reduced diphtheria toxoid, and acellular pertussis vaccine

Contraindications Hypersensitivity to diphtheria, tetanus toxoids, pertussis, or any component of the formulation; history of any of the following effects from previous administration of pertussis-containing vaccine - progressive neurologic disorder, including infantile spasms, uncontrolled epilepsy or progressive epilepsy (postpone until condition stabilized); encephalopathy occurring within 7 days of administration and not attributable to another cause

Warnings/Precautions Defer administration during moderate or severe illness (with or without fever). Carefully consider use in patients with history of any of the following effects from previous administration of whole-cell DTP or acellular pertussis vaccine: Fever ≥105°F (40.5°C) within 48 hours of unknown cause; seizures with or without fever occurring within 3 days; persistent, inconsolable crying episodes lasting ≥3 hours and occurring within 48 hours; shock or collapse within 48 hours. Carefully consider use in patients with history of Guillain-Barré syndrome occurring within 6 weeks of a vaccine containing tetanus toxoid. Td or Tdap vaccines and emergency doses of Td vaccine should not be given more frequently than every 10 years in patients who have experienced a serious Arthus-type hypersensitivity reaction following a prior use of tetanus toxoid even if the wound is not clean or minor; these patients generally have high serum antitoxin levels.

Use caution in patients with coagulation disorders (including thrombocytopenia) where intramuscular injections should not be used. Patients who are immunocompromised may have reduced response; may be used in patients with HIV infection. Defer immunization during outbreaks of poliomyelitis. Use caution in patients with history of seizure disorder, progressive neurologic disease, or conditions predisposing to seizures; ACIP and APP guidelines recommend deferring immunization until health status can be assessed and condition stabilized. Products may contain thimerosal; packaging may contain natural latex rubber. Immediate treatment for anaphylactic/anaphylactoid reaction should be available during vaccine use. In order to maximize vaccination rates, the ACIP recommends simultaneous administration of all age-appropriate vaccines (live or inactivated) for which a person is eligible at a single clinic visit, unless contraindications exist.

Adacel® is formulated with the same antigens found in Daptacel®, but with reduced quantities of tetanus and pertussis. Safety and efficacy have not been established in children <11 years or adults ≥65 years of age.

Boostrix® is formulated with the same antigens found in Infanrix®, but in reduced quantities. Safety and efficacy have not been established in patients <10 years or ≥65 years of age. Use of Adacel® or Boostrix® in the primary immunization series or to complete the primary series has not been evaluated.

Daptacel®, Infanrix®, Tripedia®: Safety and efficacy in children <6 weeks of age or ≥7 years of age have not been established.

Adverse Reactions All serious adverse reactions must be reported to the U.S. Department of Health and Human Services (DHHS) Vaccine Adverse Event Reporting System (VAERS) 1-800-822-7967.

Daptacel®, Infanrix®, Tripedia® (incidence of erythema, swelling, and fever increases with successive doses):

Frequency not defined:

Central nervous system: Drowsiness, fever, fussiness, irritability, lethargy

Gastrointestinal: Appetite decreased, vomiting

Local: Pain, redness, swelling, tenderness

Miscellaneous: Prolonged or persistent crying, refusal to play

Postmarketing and/or case reports: Allergic reaction, anaphylactic reactions, cellulitis, cyanosis, diarrhea, ear pain, encephalopathy, erythema, hypersensitivity, hypotonia, hypotonic-hyporesponsive episode, idiopathic thrombocytopenic purpura, infantile spasm, injection site reaction (abscess, cellulitis, mass, nodule, rash), intussusception, irritability, limb swelling, lymphadenopathy, nausea, pruritus, rash, respiratory tract infection, seizure, screaming, somnolence, sudden infant death syndrome, thrombocytopenia, urticaria

Adacel®, Boostrix®: Note: Ranges presented, actual percent varies by product and age group

>10%:

Central nervous system: Fatigue, tiredness (24% to 37%; grade 3/severe: 1% to 4%), headache (34% to 44%; grade 3/severe: 2% to 4%), chills (8% to 15%; severe: <1%)

Gastrointestinal: Gastrointestinal symptoms, includes abdominal pain, diarrhea, nausea and/or vomiting (3% to 26%; grade 3/severe: ≤3%)

Local: Injection site pain (66% to 78%; grade 3/severe: 1% to 5%), arm circumference increased (28%; >40 mm: 0.5%), redness (21% to 25%; ≥50 mm: 2% to 4%), swelling (21%; ≥50 mm: 3%)

Neuromuscular & skeletal: Body aches/muscle weakness (22% to 30%; severe: 1%), soreness/swollen joints (9% to 11%; severe: <1%)

1% to 10%:

Central nervous system: Fever ≥38°C (≥100.4°F: 1% to 5%)

Dermatologic: Rash (2% to 3%)

Miscellaneous: Lymph node swelling (7%; severe: <1%)

Postmarketing and/or case reports: Arthralgia, back pain, bruising, diabetes mellitus, encephalitis, exanthema, facial palsy, Henoch-Schönlein purpura, injection site reaction (induration, inflammation, mass, nodule, warmth), limb swelling (extensive), lymphadenitis, lymphadenopathy, myalgia, myocarditis, nerve compression, paresthesia, pruritus, seizure, sterile abscess, urticaria

Additional adverse reactions associated with diphtheria, tetanus, and/or pertussis antigens: Arthus hypersensitivity, brachial neuritis, GBS, peripheral/central mononeuropathies

Drug Interactions

Avoid Concomitant Use There are no known interactions where it is recommended to avoid concomitant use.

Increased Effect/Toxicity There are no known significant interactions involving an increase in effect.

Decreased Effect

The levels/effects of Diphtheria and Tetanus Toxoids, and Acellular Pertussis Vaccine may be decreased by: Immunosuppressants

Stability Refrigerate at 2°C to 8°C (35°F to 46°F); do not freeze.

Mechanism of Action Promotes active immunity to diphtheria, tetanus, and pertussis by inducing production of specific antibodies.

Dosage

Primary immunization: Children 6 weeks to <7 years: I.M.: **Note:** Whenever possible, the same product should be used for all doses. Interruption of recommended schedule does not require starting the series over; a delay between doses should not interfere with final immunity.

Daptacel®, Infanrix®, Tripedia®: 0.5 mL per dose, total of 5 doses administered as follows:

Three doses, usually given at 2-, 4-, and 6 months of age; may be given as early as 6 weeks of age and repeated every 6-8 weeks

Fourth dose: Given at ~15-20 months of age, but at least 6 months after third dose

Fifth dose: Given at 4-6 years of age, prior to starting school or kindergarten; if the fourth dose is given at ≥4 years of age, the fifth dose may be omitted

Booster immunization:

ACIP recommendations:

Adolescents 11-18 years: I.M.: 0.5 mL. A single dose of Tdap should be given instead of Td in adolescents who have completed the recommended childhood DTP/DTaP series and have not received Td or Tdap; preferred age of vaccination with Tdap is 11-12 years. Adolescents who received Td but not Tdap and who have completed the recommended childhood DTP/DTaP series are encouraged to receive Tdap; an interval of at least 5 years between Td and Tdap is recommended, but lesser intervals may be used if the benefit outweighs the risk.

Adults 19-64 years (Adacel®): I.M.: 0.5 mL. A single dose should be given instead of Td in adults if they received their last dose of Td ≥10 years previous. Shorter intervals (as short as 2 years) may used among healthcare providers, adults in contact with infants, or others in settings with increased risk for pertussis, including during pertussis outbreaks. Adacel® should only be used to replace a single booster dose of Td.

Manufacturer's labeling:

Children ≥10 and Adults ≤64 years (Boostrix®): I.M.: 0.5 mL as a single dose, administered 5 years after last dose of DTwP or DTaP vaccine.

Children ≥11 years and Adults ≤64 years (Adacel®): I.M.: 0.5 mL as a single dose, administered 5 years after last dose of DTwP or DTaP vaccine.

Wound management: Adacel® (in patients 11-64 years of age) or Boostrix® (in patients 10-64 years of age) may be used as an alternative to Td vaccine when a tetanus toxoid-containing vaccine is needed for wound management, and in whom the pertussis component is also indicated.

Administration Shake suspension well.

Adacel®, Boostrix®: Administer only I.M. in deltoid muscle of upper arm.

Daptacel®, Infanrix®, Tripedia®: Administer only I.M. in anterolateral aspect of thigh or deltoid muscle of upper arm.

For patients at risk of hemorrhage following intramuscular injection, the ACIP recommends "it should be administered intramuscularly if, in the opinion of the physician familiar with the patients bleeding risk, the vaccine can be administered with reasonable safety by this route. If the patient receives antihemophilia or other similar therapy, intramuscular vaccination can be scheduled shortly after such therapy is administered. A fine needle (23 gauge or smaller) can be used for the vaccination and firm pressure applied to the site (without rubbing) for at least 2 minutes. The patient should be instructed concerning the risk of hematoma from the injection."

Administration with other vaccines:

Diphtheria and Tetanus Toxoids, and Acellular Pertussis vaccine with other inactivated vaccines: May be given simultaneously or at any interval between doses.

Diphtheria and Tetanus Toxoids, and Acellular Pertussis vaccine with live vaccines: May be given simultaneously or at any interval between doses.

Vaccine administration with antibody-containing products: Diphtheria and Tetanus Toxoids, and Acellular Pertussis vaccine may be given simultaneously at different sites or at any interval between doses. Examples of antibody containing products include I.M. and I.V. immune globulin, hepatitis B immune globulin, tetanus immune globulin, varicella zoster immune globulin, rabies immune globulin, whole blood, packed red cells, plasma, and platelet products.

Monitoring Parameters Monitor for syncope for ≥15 minutes following vaccination

Additional Information DTaP may be given for the fourth and fifth doses in children who started immunization with DTP vaccine. In patients who cannot be given pertussis vaccine, DT for pediatric use should be given to complete the series.

TriHIBit® is Tripedia® vaccine used to reconstitute ActHIB® (*Haemophilus* b conjugate) vaccine. The combination can be used for the DTaP dose given at 15-18 months when Tripedia® was used for the initial doses and a primary series of HIB vaccine has been given.

Adacel® is formulated with the same antigens found in Daptacel® but with reduced quantities of pertussis and tetanus. It is intended for use as a booster dose in children and adults, 11-64 years of age, and **not** for primary immunization.

Boostrix® is formulated with the same antigens found in Infanrix® but in reduced quantities. It is intended for use as a booster dose in children and adults, 10-64 years of age, and is **not** for primary immunization.

The ACIP considers Adacel® and Boostrix® to be interchangeable when administered to adolescents for childhood vaccination according to the Child and Adolescent Immunization Schedule.

Acetaminophen or ibuprofen may reduce or prevent fever; the child's medical record should document that the small risk of postvaccination seizure and the benefits of the pertussis vaccination were discussed with the patient; parents or guardians should be questioned prior to administration of vaccine as to any adverse reactions from previous dose. Provide Vaccine Information Materials, as required by National Childhood Vaccine Injury Act of 1986, prior to immunization.

Federal law requires that the date of administration, the vaccine manufacturer, lot number of vaccine, and the administering person's name, title and address be entered into the patient's permanent medical record.

Dosage Forms Excipient information presented when available (limited, particularly for generics); consult specific product labeling.

Injection, suspension [Tdap, booster formulation]:

Adacel®: Diphtheria 2 Lf units, tetanus 5 Lf units, and acellular pertussis antigens (detoxified pertussis toxin

2.5 mcg, filamentous hemagglutinin 5 mcg, pertactin 3 mcg, fimbriae [types 2 and 3] 5 mcg) per 0.5 mL (0.5 mL) [contains aluminum]

Boostrix®: Diphtheria 2.5 Lf units, tetanus 5 Lf units, and acellular pertussis antigens (inactivated pertussis toxin 8 mcg, filamentous hemagglutinin 8 mcg, pertactin 2.5 mcg) per 0.5 mL (0.5 mL) [preservative free; contains aluminum and polysorbate 80; prefilled syringes contain natural rubber/natural latex]

Injection, suspension [DTaP, active immunization formulation]:

Daptacel®: Diphtheria 15 Lf units, tetanus 5 Lf units, and acellular pertussis antigens (detoxified pertussis toxin 10 mcg, filamentous hemagglutinin 5 mcg, pertactin 3 mcg, fimbriae [types 2 and 3] 5 mcg) per 0.5 mL (0.5 mL) [contains aluminum; contains natural rubber/natural latex in packaging]

Infanrix®: Diphtheria 25 Lf units, tetanus 10 Lf units, and acellular pertussis antigens (inactivated pertussis toxin 25 mcg, filamentous hemagglutinin 25 mcg, pertactin 8 mcg) per 0.5 mL (0.5 mL) [contains aluminum and polysorbate 80; prefilled syringes contain natural rubber/natural latex]

Tripedia®: Diphtheria 6.7 Lf units, tetanus 5 Lf units, and acellular pertussis antigens (inactivated pertussis toxin 23.4 mcg, filamentous hemagglutinin 23.4 mcg) per 0.5 mL (0.5 mL) [contains aluminum, natural rubber/natural latex in packaging, polysorbate 80, and thimerosal (trace amounts)]

Note: Tripedia® vaccine is also used to reconstitute ActHIB® to prepare TriHIBit® vaccine (diphtheria, tetanus toxoids, and acellular pertussis and *Haemophilus influenzae* b conjugate vaccine combination)

◆ **Diphtheria CRM_{197} Protein** *see* Pneumococcal Conjugate Vaccine (7-Valent) *on page 1204*

◆ **Diphtheria, Tetanus Toxoids, Acellular Pertussis (DTaP)** *see* Diphtheria and Tetanus Toxoids, Acellular Pertussis, and Poliovirus Vaccine *on page 462*

◆ **Diphtheria, Tetanus Toxoids, Acellular Pertussis (DTaP)** *see* Diphtheria and Tetanus Toxoids, Acellular Pertussis, Poliovirus and *Haemophilus* b Conjugate Vaccine *on page 462*

Diphtheria, Tetanus Toxoids, Acellular Pertussis, Hepatitis B (Recombinant), and Poliovirus Vaccine

(dif THEER ee a, TET a nus TOKS oyds, ay CEL yoo lar per TUS sis, hep a TYE tis bee ree KOM be nant, & POE lee oh VYE rus vak SEEN)

U.S. Brand Names Pediarix®

Canadian Brand Names Pediarix®

Index Terms Diphtheria and Tetanus Toxoids and Acellular Pertussis Adsorbed, Hepatitis B (Recombinant) and Inactivated Poliovirus Vaccine Combined; DTaP/IPV/HepB

Pharmacologic Category Vaccine, Inactivated (Bacterial); Vaccine, Inactivated (Viral)

Use Combination vaccine for the active immunization against diphtheria, tetanus, pertussis, hepatitis B virus (all known subtypes), and poliomyelitis (caused by poliovirus types 1, 2, and 3)

The Advisory Committee on Immunization Practices (ACIP) recommends Pediarix® for the following:

- Primary vaccination for DTaP, Hep B, and IPV in children at 2-, 4-, and 6 months of age.
- To complete the primary vaccination series in children who have received DTaP (Infanrix®) and who are scheduled to received the other components of the vaccine. Whenever feasible, the same manufacturer should be used to provide the pertussis component; however, vaccination should not be deferred if a specific brand is not known or is not available. HepB and IPV from different manufacturers are interchangeable.

Pregnancy Risk Factor C

Dosage I.M.: Children 6 weeks to <7 years:

Primary immunization: 0.5 mL; repeat in 6-8 week intervals (preferably 8-week intervals) for a total of 3 doses. Vaccination usually begins at 2 months, but may be started as early as 6 weeks of age.

Use in children previously vaccinated with one or more component, and who are also scheduled to receive all vaccine components:

Hepatitis B vaccine: Infants born of HBsAg-negative mothers who received 1 dose of hepatitis B vaccine at birth may be given Pediarix® (safety data limited); use in infants who received more than 1 dose of hepatitis B vaccine has not been studied. Infants who received 1 or more doses of hepatitis B vaccine (recombinant) may be given Pediarix® to complete the hepatitis B series (safety and efficacy not established).

Diphtheria and tetanus toxoids, and acellular pertussis vaccine (DTaP): Infants previously vaccinated with 1 or 2 doses of Infanrix® may use Pediarix® to complete the first 3 doses of the series (safety and efficacy not established); use of Pediarix® to complete DTaP vaccination started with products other than Infanrix® is not recommended.

Inactivated polio vaccine (IPV): Infants previously vaccinated with 1 or 2 doses of IPV may use Pediarix® to complete the first 3 doses of the series (safety and efficacy not established).

Additional Information Complete prescribing information for this medication should be consulted for additional detail.

Dosage Forms Excipient information presented when available (limited, particularly for generics); consult specific product labeling.

Injection, suspension [preservative free]:

Pediarix®: Diphtheria toxoid 25 Lf, tetanus toxoid 10 Lf, acellular pertussis antigens [inactivated pertussis toxin 25 mcg, filamentous hemagglutin 25 mcg, pertactin 8 mcg, HBsAg 10 mcg, type 1 poliovirus 40 D antigen units, type 2 poliovirus 8 D antigen units and type 3 poliovirus 32 D antigen units] per 0.5 mL (0.5 mL) [contains aluminum, neomycin sulfate (trace amounts), polymyxin B (trace amounts), polysorbate 80, and yeast protein ≤5%; prefilled syringes contain natural rubber/natural latex]

◆ **Diphtheria Toxoid** *see* Diphtheria and Tetanus Toxoids, Acellular Pertussis, Poliovirus and *Haemophilus* b Conjugate Vaccine *on page 462*

◆ **Diphtheria Toxoid Conjugate** *see Haemophilus* b Conjugate Vaccine *on page 718*

◆ **Dipivalyl Epinephrine** *see* Dipivefrin *on page 466*

Dipivefrin (dye PI ve frin)

U.S. Brand Names Propine®

Canadian Brand Names Ophtho-Dipivefrin™; PMS-Dipivefrin; Propine®

Index Terms Dipivalyl Epinephrine; Dipivefrin Hydrochloride; DPE

Pharmacologic Category Alpha/Beta Agonist; Ophthalmic Agent, Antiglaucoma; Ophthalmic Agent, Vasoconstrictor

Additional Appendix Information

Glaucoma Drug Therapy *on page 1808*

Use Reduces elevated intraocular pressure in chronic open-angle glaucoma; also used to treat ocular hypertension, low tension, and secondary glaucomas

Pregnancy Risk Factor B

Dosage Adults: Ophthalmic: Instill 1 drop every 12 hours into the eyes

Additional Information Complete prescribing information for this medication should be consulted for additional detail.

Dosage Forms Excipient information presented when available (limited, particularly for generics); consult specific product labeling.

Solution, ophthalmic, as hydrochloride: 0.1% (5 mL, 10 mL, 15 mL) [contains benzalkonium chloride]

Propine®: 0.1% (5 mL [DSC], 10 mL, 15 mL) [contains benzalkonium chloride]

◆ **Dipivefrin Hydrochloride** *see* Dipivefrin *on page 466*

◆ **Diprivan®** *see* Propofol *on page 1254*

◆ **Diprolene®** *see* Betamethasone *on page 188*

◆ **Diprolene® AF** *see* Betamethasone *on page 188*

◆ **Diprolene® Glycol (Can)** *see* Betamethasone *on page 188*

◆ **Dipropylacetic Acid** *see* Valproic Acid and Derivatives *on page 1538*

◆ **Diprosone® (Can)** *see* Betamethasone *on page 188*

Dipyridamole (dye peer ID a mole)

U.S. Brand Names Persantine®

Canadian Brand Names Apo-Dipyridamole FC®; Dipyridamole For Injection; Persantine®

Pharmacologic Category Antiplatelet Agent; Vasodilator

Use

Oral: Used with warfarin to decrease thrombosis in patients after artificial heart valve replacement

I.V.: Diagnostic agent in CAD

Pregnancy Risk Factor B

Pregnancy Considerations Teratogenic effects were not observed in animal studies.

Lactation Enters breast milk/use caution

Medication Safety Issues

Sound-alike/look-alike issues:

Dipyridamole may be confused with disopyramide

Persantine® may be confused with Periactin®, Permitil®

Contraindications Hypersensitivity to dipyridamole or any component of the formulation

Warnings/Precautions Use with in patients with hypotension, unstable angina, and/or recent MI. Use with caution in hepatic impairment. Use caution in patients on other antiplatelet agents or anticoagulation. Severe adverse reactions have occurred with I.V. administration (rarely); use the I.V. form with caution in patients with bronchospastic disease or unstable angina. Aminophylline should be available in case of urgency or emergency with I.V. use. Safety and efficacy in children <12 years of age have not been established.

Adverse Reactions

Oral:

>10%: Dizziness (14%)

1% to 10%:

Central nervous system: Headache (2%)

Dermatologic: Rash (2%)

Gastrointestinal: Abdominal distress (6%)

Frequency not defined: Diarrhea, vomiting, flushing, pruritus, angina pectoris, liver dysfunction

Postmarketing and/or case reports: Alopecia, arthritis, cholelithiasis, dyspepsia, fatigue, hepatitis, hypersensitivity reaction, hypotension, larynx edema, malaise, myalgia, nausea, palpitation, paresthesia, tachycardia, thrombocytopenia

I.V.:

>10%:

Cardiovascular: Exacerbation of angina pectoris (20%)

Central nervous system: Dizziness (12%), headache (12%)

1% to 10%:

Cardiovascular: Hypotension (5%), hypertension (2%), blood pressure lability (2%), ECG abnormalities (ST-T changes, extrasystoles; 5% to 8%), pain (3%), tachycardia (3%)

Central nervous system: Flushing (3%), fatigue (1%)

Gastrointestinal: Nausea (5%)

Neuromuscular & skeletal: Paresthesia (1%)

Respiratory: Dyspnea (3%)

<1% (Limited to important or life-threatening): Abdominal pain, abnormal coordination, allergic reaction (pruritus, rash, urticaria), appetite increased, arrhythmia (ventricular tachycardia, bradycardia, AV block, SVT, atrial fibrillation, asystole), arthralgia, asthenia, back pain, breast pain, bronchospasm, cardiomyopathy, cough, depersonalization, diaphoresis, dry mouth, dysgeusia, dyspepsia, dysphagia, earache, ECG abnormalities (unspecified), edema, eructation, flatulence, hypertonia, hyperventilation, injection site reaction, intermittent claudication leg cramping, malaise, MI, myalgia, orthostatic hypotension, palpitation, perineal pain, pharyngitis, pleural pain, renal pain, rhinitis, rigor, syncope, tenesmus, thirst, tinnitus, tremor, vertigo, vision abnormalities, vomiting

Drug Interactions

Avoid Concomitant Use

Avoid concomitant use of Dipyridamole with any of the following: Dabigatran Etexilate; Rivaroxaban; Silodosin

Increased Effect/Toxicity

Dipyridamole may increase the levels/effects of: Adenosine; Amifostine; Anticoagulants; Antiplatelet Agents; Beta-Blockers; Dabigatran Etexilate; Drotrecogin Alfa; Ibritumomab; P-Glycoprotein Substrates; Regadenoson; RiTUXimab; Rivaroxaban; Salicylates; Silodosin; Thrombolytic Agents; Topotecan; Tositumomab and Iodine I 131 Tositumomab

The levels/effects of Dipyridamole may be increased by: Dasatinib; Diazoxide; Herbs (Anticoagulant/Antiplatelet Properties); Herbs (Hypotensive Properties); Nonsteroidal Anti-Inflammatory Agents; Omega-3-Acid Ethyl Esters; Pentosan Polysulfate Sodium; Prostacyclin Analogues

Decreased Effect

The levels/effects of Dipyridamole may be decreased by: Herbs (Hypertensive Properties); Methylphenidate; Nonsteroidal Anti-Inflammatory Agents; Yohimbine

Ethanol/Nutrition/Herb Interactions Herb/Nutraceutical: Avoid cat's claw, dong quai, evening primrose, feverfew, garlic, ginger, ginkgo, red clover, horse chestnut, green tea, ginseng (all have additional antiplatelet activity).

Stability I.V.: Store between 15°C to 25°C (59°F to 77°F). Do not freeze, protect from light. Prior to administration, dilute to a ≥1:2 ratio in NS, 1/2NS, or D_5W. Total volume should be ~20-50 mL.

Mechanism of Action Inhibits the activity of adenosine deaminase and phosphodiesterase, which causes an accumulation of adenosine, adenine nucleotides, and cyclic AMP; these mediators then inhibit platelet aggregation and may cause vasodilation; may also stimulate release of prostacyclin or PGD_2; causes coronary vasodilation

Pharmacodynamics/Kinetics

Absorption: Readily, but variable

Distribution: Adults: V_d: 2-3 L/kg

Protein binding: 91% to 99%

Metabolism: Hepatic

Half-life elimination: Terminal: 10-12 hours

Time to peak, serum: 2-2.5 hours

Excretion: Feces (as glucuronide conjugates and unchanged drug)

Dosage

Oral: Children ≥12 years and Adults: Adjunctive therapy for prophylaxis of thromboembolism with cardiac valve replacement: 75-100 mg 4 times/day

I.V.: Adults: Evaluation of coronary artery disease: 0.14 mg/kg/minute for 4 minutes; maximum dose: 60 mg

Dietary Considerations Should be taken with water 1 hour before meals.

Administration

I.V.: Infuse diluted solution over 4 minutes; following dipyridamole infusion, inject thallium-201 within 5 minutes. **Note:** Aminophylline should be available for urgent/emergent use; dosing of 50-100 mg (range: 50-250 mg) IVP over 30-60 seconds.

Tablet: Administer with water 1 hour before meals.

Monitoring Parameters Blood pressure, heart rate, ECG (stress test)

Dosage Forms Excipient information presented when available (limited, particularly for generics); consult specific product labeling.

Injection, solution: 5 mg/mL (2 mL, 10 mL)

Tablet: 25 mg, 50 mg, 75 mg

Persantine®: 25 mg, 50 mg, 75 mg

Extemporaneous Preparations A 10 mg/mL oral suspension has been made using four 25 mg tablets and purified water USP qs ad to 10 mL; expected stability is 3 days. Dipyridamole 10 mg/mL was stable for up to 60 days at 5°C and 25°C in 1:1 mixtures of Ora-Sweet® and Ora-Plus®, Ora-Sweet® SF and Ora-Plus® and in cherry syrup

Allen LV and Erickson III MA, "Stability of Baclofen, Captopril, Diltiazem, Hydrochloride, Dipyridamole, and Flecainide Acetate in Extemporaneously Compounded Oral Liquids," *Am J Health Syst Pharm*, 1996, 53:2179-84.

Nahata MC and Hipple TF, *Pediatric Drug Formulations*, 2nd ed, Cincinnati, OH: Harvey Whitney Books Co, 1992.

- **Dipyridamole and Aspirin** *see* Aspirin and Dipyridamole *on page 145*
- **Dipyridamole For Injection (Can)** *see* Dipyridamole *on page 467*
- **Disalicylic Acid** *see* Salsalate *on page 1352*
- **DisCoVisc®** *see* Sodium Chondroitin Sulfate and Sodium Hyaluronate *on page 1383*
- **Disodium Cromoglycate** *see* Cromolyn *on page 372*
- **Disodium Thiosulfate Pentahydrate** *see* Sodium Thiosulfate *on page 1386*
- ***d*-Isoephedrine Hydrochloride** *see* Pseudoephedrine *on page 1265*

Disopyramide (dye soe PEER a mide)

U.S. Brand Names Norpace®; Norpace® CR

Canadian Brand Names Norpace®; Rythmodan®; Rythmodan®-LA

Index Terms Disopyramide Phosphate

Pharmacologic Category Antiarrhythmic Agent, Class Ia

Use Suppression and prevention of unifocal and multifocal atrial and premature, ventricular premature complexes, coupled ventricular tachycardia; effective in the conversion of atrial fibrillation, atrial flutter, and paroxysmal atrial tachycardia to normal sinus rhythm and prevention of the recurrence of these arrhythmias after conversion by other methods

Unlabeled/Investigational Use Hypertrophic obstructive cardiomyopathy (HOCM)

Pregnancy Risk Factor C

Lactation Enters breast milk/compatible

Medication Safety Issues

Sound-alike/look-alike issues:

Disopyramide may be confused with desipramine, dipyridamole

Norpace® may be confused with Norpramin®

Contraindications Hypersensitivity to disopyramide or any component of the formulation; cardiogenic shock; pre-existing second- or third-degree heart block (except in patients with a functioning artificial pacemaker); congenital QT syndrome; sick sinus syndrome

Warnings/Precautions Monitor and adjust dose to prevent QT_c prolongation. Avoid concurrent use with other medications that prolong QT interval or decrease myocardial contractility. Correct hypokalemia before initiating therapy; may worsen toxicity. Watch for proarrhythmic effects. **[U.S. Boxed Warning]: In the Cardiac Arrhythmia Suppression Trial (CAST), recent (>6 days but <2 years ago) myocardial infarction patients with asymptomatic, non-life-threatening ventricular arrhythmias did not benefit and may have been harmed by attempts to suppress the arrhythmia with flecainide or encainide. An increased mortality or nonfatal cardiac arrest rate (7.7%) was seen in the active treatment group compared with patients in the placebo group (3%). The applicability of the CAST results to other populations is unknown. Antiarrhythmic agents should be reserved for patients with life-threatening ventricular arrhythmias.** May precipitate or exacerbate HF. Due to significant anticholinergic effects, do not use in patients with urinary retention, BPH, glaucoma, or myasthenia gravis. Reduce dosage in renal or hepatic impairment. The extended release form is not recommended for Cl_{cr} <40 mL/minute. In patients with atrial fibrillation or flutter, block the AV node before initiating. Use caution in Wolff-Parkinson-White syndrome or bundle branch block. Monitor closely for hypotension during the initiation of therapy.

Adverse Reactions The most common adverse effects are related to cholinergic blockade. The most serious adverse effects of disopyramide are hypotension and CHF.

>10%:

Gastrointestinal: Xerostomia (32%), constipation (11%)

Genitourinary: Urinary hesitancy (14% to 23%)

1% to 10%:

Cardiovascular: CHF, hypotension, cardiac conduction disturbance, edema, syncope, chest pain

Central nervous system: Fatigue, headache, malaise, dizziness, nervousness

Dermatologic: Rash, generalized dermatoses, pruritus

Endocrine & metabolic: Hypokalemia, elevated cholesterol, elevated triglycerides

Gastrointestinal: Dry throat, nausea, abdominal distension, flatulence, abdominal bloating, anorexia, diarrhea, vomiting, weight gain

Genitourinary: Urinary retention, urinary frequency, urinary urgency, impotence (1% to 3%)

Neuromuscular & skeletal: Muscle weakness, muscular pain

Ocular: Blurred vision, dry eyes

Respiratory: Dyspnea

<1% (Limited to important or life-threatening): Agranulocytosis, AV block, cholestatic jaundice, depression, dysuria, creatinine increased, gynecomastia, hepatotoxicity, hypoglycemia, BUN increased, insomnia, new or worsened arrhythmia (proarrhythmic effect), paresthesia, psychotic reaction, respiratory distress, thrombocytopenia, transaminases increased. Rare cases of lupus have been reported (generally in patients previously receiving procainamide), peripheral neuropathy, psychosis, toxic cutaneous blisters.

Drug Interactions

Metabolism/Transport Effects **Substrate** of CYP3A4 (major)

Avoid Concomitant Use

Avoid concomitant use of Disopyramide with any of the following: Macrolide Antibiotics; Nilotinib; Tetrabenazine; Thioridazine; Ziprasidone

Increased Effect/Toxicity

Disopyramide may increase the levels/effects of: Amiodarone; Anticholinergics; Beta-Blockers; Cannabinoids; Lidocaine; Potassium Chloride; QTc-Prolonging Agents; Tetrabenazine; Thioridazine; Ziprasidone

The levels/effects of Disopyramide may be increased by: Alfuzosin; Ciprofloxacin; CYP3A4 Inhibitors (Moderate); CYP3A4 Inhibitors (Strong); Dasatinib; Gadobutrol; Macrolide Antibiotics; Nilotinib; Pramlintide

Decreased Effect

Disopyramide may decrease the levels/effects of: Acetylcholinesterase Inhibitors (Central); Secretin

The levels/effects of Disopyramide may be decreased by: Acetylcholinesterase Inhibitors (Central); Amiodarone; Barbiturates; CYP3A4 Inducers (Strong); Deferasirox; Herbs (CYP3A4 Inducers); Phenytoin; Rifamycin Derivatives

Ethanol/Nutrition/Herb Interactions

Ethanol: Avoid ethanol (may increase CNS depression).

Herb/Nutraceutical: St John's wort may decrease disopyramide levels. Avoid ephedra (may worsen arrhythmia).

Stability Extemporaneously prepared suspension is stable for 4 weeks refrigerated.

Mechanism of Action Class Ia antiarrhythmic: Decreases myocardial excitability and conduction velocity; reduces disparity in refractory between normal and infarcted myocardium; possesses anticholinergic, peripheral vasoconstrictive, and negative inotropic effects

Pharmacodynamics/Kinetics

Onset of action: 0.5-3.5 hours

Duration: 1.5-8.5 hours

Absorption: 60% to 83%

Protein binding (concentration dependent): 20% to 60%

Metabolism: Hepatic to inactive metabolites

Half-life elimination: Adults: 4-10 hours; prolonged with hepatic or renal impairment

Excretion: Urine (40% to 60% as unchanged drug); feces (10% to 15%)

Dosage Oral:

Children:

<1 year: 10-30 mg/kg/24 hours in 4 divided doses

1-4 years: 10-20 mg/kg/24 hours in 4 divided doses

4-12 years: 10-15 mg/kg/24 hours in 4 divided doses

12-18 years: 6-15 mg/kg/24 hours in 4 divided doses

Adults:

<50 kg: 100 mg every 6 hours or 200 mg every 12 hours (controlled release)

>50 kg: 150 mg every 6 hours or 300 mg every 12 hours (controlled release); if no response, increase to 200 mg every 6 hours. Maximum dose required for patients with severe refractory ventricular tachycardia is 400 mg every 6 hours.

Hypertrophic obstructive cardiomyopathy (unlabeled use): Initial: Controlled release: 200 mg twice daily. If symptoms do not improve, increase by 100 mg/day at 2-week intervals to a maximum daily dose of 600 mg.

Elderly: Dose with caution, starting at the lower end of dosing range

Dosing adjustment in renal impairment: 100 mg (nonsustained release) given at the following intervals, based on creatinine clearance (mL/minute):

Cl_{cr} 30-40 mL/minute: Administer every 8 hours

Cl_{cr} 15-30 mL/minute: Administer every 12 hours

Cl_{cr} <15 mL/minute: Administer every 24 hours

or alter the dose as follows:

Cl_{cr} 30-<40 mL/minute: Reduce dose 50%

Cl_{cr} 15-30 mL/minute: Reduce dose 75%

Dialysis: Not dialyzable (0% to 5%) by hemo- or peritoneal methods; supplemental dose is not necessary.

Dosing interval in hepatic impairment: 100 mg every 6 hours or 200 mg every 12 hours (controlled release)

Dietary Considerations Should be taken on an empty stomach.

Administration Do not break or chew controlled release capsules. Administer around-the-clock to Administer around-the-clock rather than 4 times/day (ie, 12-6-12-6, not 9-1-5-9) to promote less variation in peak and trough serum levels

Monitoring Parameters ECG, blood pressure, urinary retention, CNS anticholinergic effects (confusion, agitation, hallucinations, etc)

Reference Range

Therapeutic concentration:

Atrial arrhythmias: 2.8-3.2 mcg/mL

Ventricular arrhythmias 3.3-7.5 mcg/mL

Toxic concentration: >7 mcg/mL

Dosage Forms Excipient information presented when available (limited, particularly for generics); consult specific product labeling.

Capsule (Norpace®): 100 mg, 150 mg

Capsule, controlled release (Norpace® CR): 100 mg, 150 mg

Extemporaneous Preparations Extemporaneous suspensions in cherry syrup (1 mg/mL and 10 mg/mL) are stable for 4 weeks in amber glass bottles stored at 5°C, 30°C, or at room temperature; shake well before use; do not use extended release capsules for this suspension

Mathur LK, Lai PK, and Shively CD, "Stability of Disopyramide Phosphate in Cherry Syrup," *Am J Hosp Pharm*, 1982, 39(2):309-10.

◆ **Disopyramide Phosphate** *see* Disopyramide *on page 468*

Disulfiram (dye SUL fi ram)

U.S. Brand Names Antabuse®

Pharmacologic Category Aldehyde Dehydrogenase Inhibitor

Use Management of chronic alcoholism

Pregnancy Risk Factor C

Medication Safety Issues

Sound-alike/look-alike issues:

Disulfiram may be confused with Diflucan®

Antabuse® may be confused with Anturane®

Dosage Adults: Oral: Do not administer until the patient has abstained from ethanol for at least 12 hours

Initial: 500 mg/day as a single dose for 1-2 weeks; maximum daily dose is 500 mg

Average maintenance dose: 250 mg/day; range: 125-500 mg; duration of therapy is to continue until the patient is fully recovered socially and a basis for permanent self control has been established; maintenance therapy may be required for months or even years

Additional Information Complete prescribing information for this medication should be consulted for additional detail.

Dosage Forms Excipient information presented when available (limited, particularly for generics); consult specific product labeling.

Tablet:

Antabuse®: 250 mg, 500 mg

◆ **Dithioglycerol** *see* Dimercaprol *on page 453*

◆ **Dithranol** *see* Anthralin *on page 118*

- ◆ **Ditropan®** *see* Oxybutynin *on page 1119*
- ◆ **Ditropan® XL** *see* Oxybutynin *on page 1119*
- ◆ **Diuril®** *see* Chlorothiazide *on page 308*
- ◆ **Divalproex Sodium** *see* Valproic Acid and Derivatives *on page 1538*
- ◆ **Divigel®** *see* Estradiol *on page 554*
- ◆ **Dixarit® (Can)** *see* CloNIDine *on page 354*
- ◆ **5071-1DL(6)** *see* Megestrol *on page 934*
- ◆ ***dl*-Alpha Tocopherol** *see* Vitamin E *on page 1566*
- ◆ ***D*-Mannitol** *see* Mannitol *on page 919*
- ◆ **4-DMDR** *see* IDArubicin *on page 765*
- ◆ **DMSA** *see* Succimer *on page 1401*
- ◆ **Doan's® Extra Strength [OTC]** *see* Magnesium Salicylate *on page 917*

DOBUTamine (doe BYOO ta meen)

Canadian Brand Names Dobutamine Injection, USP; Dobutrex®

Index Terms Dobutamine Hydrochloride

Pharmacologic Category Adrenergic Agonist Agent

Additional Appendix Information

Hemodynamic Support, Intravenous *on page 1657*

Use Short-term management of patients with cardiac decompensation

Unlabeled/Investigational Use Positive inotropic agent for use in myocardial dysfunction related to sepsis; stress echocardiography

Pregnancy Risk Factor B

Lactation Excretion in breast milk unknown

Medication Safety Issues

Sound-alike/look-alike issues:

DOBUTamine may be confused with DOPamine

High alert medication: The Institute for Safe Medication Practices (ISMP) includes this medication among its list of drugs which have a heightened risk of causing significant patient harm when used in error.

Contraindications Hypersensitivity to dobutamine or sulfites (some contain sodium metabisulfate), or any component of the formulation; idiopathic hypertrophic subaortic stenosis (IHSS)

Warnings/Precautions May increase heart rate. Patients with atrial fibrillation may experience an increase in ventricular response. An increase in blood pressure is more common, but occasionally a patient may become hypotensive. May exacerbate ventricular ectopy. If needed, correct hypovolemia first to optimize hemodynamics. Ineffective therapeutically in the presence of mechanical obstruction such as severe aortic stenosis. Use caution post-MI (can increase myocardial oxygen demand). Use cautiously in the elderly starting at lower end of the dosage range. Use with extreme caution in patients taking MAO inhibitors. Dobutamine in combination with stress echo may be used diagnostically. Product may contain sodium sulfite.

Adverse Reactions Incidence of adverse events is not always reported.

Cardiovascular: Increased heart rate, increased blood pressure, increased ventricular ectopic activity, hypotension, premature ventricular beats (5%, dose related), anginal pain (1% to 3%), nonspecific chest pain (1% to 3%), palpitation (1% to 3%)

Central nervous system: Fever (1% to 3%), headache (1% to 3%), paresthesia

Endocrine & metabolic: Slight decrease in serum potassium

Gastrointestinal: Nausea (1% to 3%)

Hematologic: Thrombocytopenia (isolated cases)

Local: Phlebitis, local inflammatory changes and pain from infiltration, cutaneous necrosis (isolated cases)

Neuromuscular & skeletal: Mild leg cramps

Respiratory: Dyspnea (1% to 3%)

Drug Interactions

Avoid Concomitant Use

Avoid concomitant use of DOBUTamine with any of the following: Iobenguane I 123

Increased Effect/Toxicity

DOBUTamine may increase the levels/effects of: Sympathomimetics

The levels/effects of DOBUTamine may be increased by: Cannabinoids; COMT Inhibitors

Decreased Effect

DOBUTamine may decrease the levels/effects of: Iobenguane I 123

The levels/effects of DOBUTamine may be decreased by: Calcium Salts

Stability Remix solution every 24 hours. Store reconstituted solution under refrigeration for 48 hours or 6 hours at room temperature. Pink discoloration of solution indicates slight oxidation but **no** significant loss of potency.

Stability of parenteral admixture at room temperature (25°C): 48 hours; at refrigeration (4°C): 7 days.

Standard adult diluent: 250 mg/500 mL D_5W; 500 mg/500 mL D_5W.

Mechanism of Action Stimulates $beta_1$-adrenergic receptors, causing increased contractility and heart rate, with little effect on $beta_2$- or alpha-receptors

Pharmacodynamics/Kinetics

Onset of action: I.V.: 1-10 minutes

Peak effect: 10-20 minutes

Metabolism: In tissues and hepatically to inactive metabolites

Half-life elimination: 2 minutes

Excretion: Urine (as metabolites)

Dosage Administration requires the use of an infusion pump; I.V. infusion:

Neonates: 2-15 mcg/kg/minute, titrate to desired response

Children and Adults: 2.5-20 mcg/kg/minute; maximum: 40 mcg/kg/minute, titrate to desired response. See table.

Infusion Rates of Various Dilutions of Dobutamine

Desired Delivery Rate (mcg/kg/min)	Infusion Rate (mL/kg/min)	
	500 mcg/mL[1]	1000 mcg/mL[2]
2.5	0.005	0.0025
5	0.01	0.005
7.5	0.015	0.0075
10	0.02	0.01

[1]500 mg per liter or 250 mg per 500 mL of diluent.

[2]1000 mg per liter or 250 mg per 250 mL of diluent.

To prepare for infusion:

$$\frac{6 \text{ x weight (kg) x desired dose (mcg/kg/min)}}{\text{I.V. infusion rate (mL/h)}} = \text{mg of drug to be added to 100 mL of I.V. fluid}$$

Administration Use infusion device to control rate of flow; administer into large vein. Do not administer through same I.V. line as heparin, hydrocortisone sodium succinate, cefazolin, or penicillin.

Monitoring Parameters Blood pressure, ECG, heart rate, CVP, RAP, MAP, urine output; if pulmonary artery catheter is in place, monitor CI, PCWP, and SVR; also monitor serum potassium

Additional Information Dobutamine lowers central venous pressure and wedge pressure but has little effect on pulmonary vascular resistance.

Dobutamine therapy should be avoided in patients with stable heart failure due to an increase in mortality. In patients with intractable heart failure, dobutamine may be used as a short-term infusion to provide symptomatic benefit. It is not known whether short-term dobutamine therapy in end-stage heart failure has any outcome benefit.

Dobutamine infusion during echocardiography is used as a cardiovascular stress. Wall motion abnormalities developing with increasing doses of dobutamine may help to identify ischemic and/or hibernating myocardium.

Dosage Forms Excipient information presented when available (limited, particularly for generics); consult specific product labeling.

Infusion, as hydrochloride [premixed in dextrose]: 1 mg/mL (250 mL, 500 mL); 2 mg/mL (250 mL); 4 mg/mL (250 mL)

Injection, solution, as hydrochloride: 12.5 mg/mL (20 mL, 40 mL, 100 mL) [contains sodium bisulfite]

- **Dobutamine Hydrochloride** *see* DOBUTamine *on page 470*
- **Dobutamine Injection, USP (Can)** *see* DOBUTamine *on page 470*
- **Dobutrex® (Can)** *see* DOBUTamine *on page 470*

Docetaxel (doe se TAKS el)

U.S. Brand Names Taxotere®

Canadian Brand Names Taxotere®

Index Terms NSC-628503; RP-6976

Pharmacologic Category Antineoplastic Agent, Antimicrotubular; Antineoplastic Agent, Natural Source (Plant) Derivative; Antineoplastic Agent, Taxane Derivative

Use Treatment of breast cancer; locally-advanced or metastatic nonsmall cell lung cancer (NSCLC); hormone refractory, metastatic prostate cancer; advanced gastric adenocarcinoma; locally-advanced squamous cell head and neck cancer

Unlabeled/Investigational Use Treatment of bladder cancer, ovarian cancer, small cell lung cancer, and soft tissue sarcoma

Pregnancy Risk Factor D

Pregnancy Considerations Animal studies have demonstrated embryotoxicity, fetal toxicity, and maternal toxicity. There are no adequate and well-controlled studies in pregnant women; however, fetal harm may occur. Women of childbearing potential should avoid becoming pregnant. A pregnancy registry is available for all cancers diagnosed during pregnancy at Cooper Health (856-757-7876).

Lactation Excretion in breast milk unknown/not recommended

Medication Safety Issues

Sound-alike/look-alike issues:

Taxotere® may be confused with Taxol®

High alert medication: The Institute for Safe Medication Practices (ISMP) includes this medication among its list of drug classes which have a heightened risk of causing significant patient harm when used in error.

Contraindications Hypersensitivity to docetaxel or any component of the formulation; prior hypersensitivity to medications containing polysorbate 80; pre-existing bone marrow suppression (neutrophils <1500 cells/mm^3)

Warnings/Precautions Hazardous agent - use appropriate precautions for handling and disposal. **[U.S. Boxed Warnings]: Use caution in hepatic disease; avoid use in patients with bilirubin exceeding upper limit of normal (ULN) or AST and/or ALT >1.5 times ULN in conjunction with alkaline phosphatase >2.5 times ULN; patients with abnormal liver function are at increased risk of treatment-related adverse events. Severe hypersensitivity reactions characterized by rash/erythema, hypotension, bronchospasms, or anaphylaxis may occur; minor reactions including flushing or localized skin reactions may also occur. Fluid retention syndrome characterized by pleural effusions, ascites, edema, and weight gain (2-15 kg) has also been reported.** The incidence and severity of the syndrome increase sharply at cumulative doses ≥400 mg/m^2. Patients should be premedicated with a corticosteroid to prevent hypersensitivity reactions and fluid retention; severity is reduced with dexamethasone premedication starting one day prior to docetaxel administration.

[U.S. Boxed Warning]: Patients with abnormal liver function, those receiving higher doses, and patients with nonsmall cell lung cancer and a history of prior treatment with platinum derivatives who receive docetaxel doses higher than 100 mg/m^2 are at higher risk for treatment-related mortality.

Neutropenia is the dose-limiting toxicity; however, this rarely results in treatment delays and prophylactic colony stimulating factors have not been routinely used. Patients with increased liver function tests experienced more episodes of neutropenia with a greater number of severe infections. **[U.S. Boxed Warning]: Patients with an absolute neutrophil count <1500 cells/mm^3 should not receive docetaxel.** When administered as sequential infusions, taxane derivatives (docetaxel, paclitaxel) should be administered before platinum derivatives (carboplatin, cisplatin) to limit myelosuppression and to enhance efficacy.

Cutaneous reactions including erythema and desquamation have been reported; may require dose reduction. Dosage adjustment is recommended with severe neurosensory symptoms (paresthesia, dysesthesia, pain). Safety and efficacy in children have not been established.

Adverse Reactions Percentages reported for docetaxel monotherapy; frequency may vary depending on diagnosis, dose, liver function, prior treatment, and premedication. The incidence of adverse events was usually higher in patients with elevated liver function tests.

>10%:

- Cardiovascular: Fluid retention (13% to 60%; dose dependent)
- Central nervous system: Neurosensory events (20% to 58%; including neuropathy), fever (31% to 35%), neuromotor events (16%)
- Dermatologic: Alopecia (56% to 76%), cutaneous events (20% to 48%), nail disorder (11% to 41%)
- Gastrointestinal: Stomatitis (19% to 53%; severe 1% to 8%), diarrhea (23% to 43%; severe: 5% to 6%), nausea (34% to 42%), vomiting (22% to 23%)
- Hematologic: Neutropenia (84% to 99%; grade 4: 75% to 86%; onset: 4-7 days, nadir: 5-9 days, recovery: 21 days; dose dependent), leukopenia (84% to 99%; grade 4: 32% to 44%), anemia (65% to 94%; dose dependent; grades 3/4: 8% to 9%), thrombocytopenia (8% to 14%; grade 4: 1%; dose dependent), febrile neutropenia (6% to 12%; dose dependent)
- Hepatic: Transaminases increased (4% to 19%)
- Neuromuscular & skeletal: Weakness (53% to 66%; severe 13% to 18%), myalgia (3% to 23%)
- Respiratory: Pulmonary events (41%)
- Miscellaneous: Infection (1% to 34%; dose dependent), hypersensitivity (1% to 21%; with premedication 15%)

1% to 10%:

- Cardiovascular: Left ventricular ejection fraction decreased (prostate cancer: 10%; metastatic breast cancer: 8%), hypotension (3%)

Dermatologic: Rash/erythema (2%)
Gastrointestinal: Taste perversion (6%)
Hepatic: Bilirubin increased (9%), alkaline phosphatase increased (4% to 7%)
Local: Infusion-site reactions (4%, including hyperpigmentation, inflammation, redness, dryness, phlebitis, extravasation, swelling of the vein)
Neuromuscular and skeletal: Arthralgia (3% to 9%)
Ocular: Epiphora associated with canalicular stenosis (≤77% with weekly administration; ≤1% with every-3-week administration)

<1% (Limited to important or life-threatening): Acute myeloid leukemia (AML), acute respiratory distress syndrome (ARDS), anaphylactic shock, angina, ascites, atrial fibrillation, atrial flutter, bleeding episodes, bronchospasm, cardiac tamponade, chest pain, chest tightness, colitis, conjunctivitis, constipation, cutaneous lupus erythematosus, deep vein thrombosis, dehydration, disseminated intravascular coagulation (DIC), drug fever, duodenal ulcer, dyspnea, dysrhythmia, ECG abnormalities, erythema multiforme, esophagitis, gastrointestinal hemorrhage, gastrointestinal obstruction, gastrointestinal perforation, hand and foot syndrome, hearing loss, heart failure, hepatitis, hypertension, ileus, interstitial pneumonia, ischemic colitis, lacrimal duct obstruction, loss of consciousness (transient), MI, multiorgan failure, myelodysplastic syndrome, neutropenic enterocolitis, ototoxicity, pleural effusion, pruritus, pulmonary edema, pulmonary embolism, pulmonary fibrosis, radiation pneumonitis, radiation recall, renal insufficiency, seizure, sepsis, sinus tachycardia, Stevens-Johnson syndrome, syncope, toxic epidermal necrolysis, tachycardia, thrombophlebitis, unstable angina, visual disturbances (transient)

Drug Interactions

Metabolism/Transport Effects **Substrate** of CYP3A4 (major); **Inhibits** CYP3A4 (weak)

Avoid Concomitant Use

Avoid concomitant use of Docetaxel with any of the following: Natalizumab; Vaccines (Live)

Increased Effect/Toxicity

Docetaxel may increase the levels/effects of: Antineoplastic Agents (Anthracycline); Natalizumab; Vaccines (Live)

The levels/effects of Docetaxel may be increased by: Antifungal Agents (Azole Derivatives, Systemic); CYP3A4 Inhibitors (Moderate); CYP3A4 Inhibitors (Strong); Dasatinib; P-Glycoprotein Inhibitors; Platinum Derivatives; Trastuzumab

Decreased Effect

Docetaxel may decrease the levels/effects of: Vaccines (Inactivated)

The levels/effects of Docetaxel may be decreased by: CYP3A4 Inducers (Strong); Deferasirox; Echinacea; Herbs (CYP3A4 Inducers); P-Glycoprotein Inducers

Ethanol/Nutrition/Herb Interactions

Ethanol: Avoid ethanol (due to GI irritation).
Herb/Nutraceutical: Avoid St John's wort (may decrease docetaxel levels).

Stability Intact vials should be stored at 2°C to 25°C (36°F to 77°F) and protected from light. Freezing does not adversely affect the product. If refrigerated, vials should be stored at room temperature for approximately 5 minutes before using. Vials should be diluted with 13% (w/w) ethanol/water (provided with the drug) to a final concentration of 10 mg/mL. Do not shake. The solution should be further diluted in 250-1000 mL of NS or D_5W to a final concentration of 0.3-0.9 mg/mL (although the manufacturer recommends a final concentration of 0.3-0.74) and dispensed in a non-DEHP container (eg, glass, polypropylene, polyolefin). Diluted solutions in the vial are stable for 8 hours at room temperature or under refrigeration. Solutions diluted for infusion in D_5W or NS are stable for up to 4 weeks at room temperature of 15°C to 25°C (59°F to 77°F) in polyolefin containers; however, the manufacturer recommends use within 4 hours.

Mechanism of Action Docetaxel promotes the assembly of microtubules from tubulin dimers, and inhibits the depolymerization of tubulin which stabilizes microtubules in the cell. This results in inhibition of DNA, RNA, and protein synthesis. Most activity occurs during the M phase of the cell cycle.

Pharmacodynamics/Kinetics Exhibits linear pharmacokinetics at the recommended dosage range
Distribution: Extensive extravascular distribution and/or tissue binding; V_d: 80-90 L/m^2, V_{dss}: 113 L (mean steady state)
Protein binding: ~94% to 97%, primarily to alpha$_1$-acid glycoprotein, albumin, and lipoproteins
Metabolism: Hepatic; oxidation via CYP3A4 to metabolites
Half-life elimination: Terminal: 11 hours
Excretion: Feces (75%, <8% as unchanged drug); urine (6%); ~80% within 48 hours
Clearance: Total body: Mean: 21 L/hour/m^2

Dosage Adults: I.V. infusion: Refer to individual protocols: **Note:** Premedicate with corticosteroids, beginning the day before docetaxel administration, (administer for 1-5 days) to reduce the severity of hypersensitivity reactions and pulmonary/peripheral edema

Breast cancer:
Locally-advanced or metastatic: 60-100 mg/m^2 every 3 weeks; patients initially started at 60 mg/m^2 who do not develop toxicity may tolerate higher doses
Operable, node-positive (adjuvant treatment): 75 mg/m^2 every 3 weeks for 6 courses (in combination with doxorubicin and cyclophosphamide)
Nonsmall cell lung cancer: 75 mg/m^2 every 3 weeks (as monotherapy or in combination with cisplatin)
Prostate cancer: 75 mg/m^2 every 3 weeks (in combination with prednisone)
Gastric adenocarcinoma: 75 mg/m^2 every 3 weeks (in combination with cisplatin and fluorouracil)
Head and neck cancer: 75 mg/m^2 every 3 weeks (in combination with cisplatin and fluorouracil) for 3 or 4 cycles, followed by radiation therapy

Dosing adjustment for toxicity:

Note: Toxicity includes febrile neutropenia, neutrophils ≤500/mm^3 for >1 week, severe or cumulative cutaneous reactions; in nonsmall cell lung cancer, this may also include platelets <25,000/mm^3 and other grade 3/4 nonhematologic toxicities.

Breast cancer: Patients dosed initially at 100 mg/m^2; reduce dose to 75 mg/m^2; **Note:** If the patient continues to experience these adverse reactions, the dosage should be reduced to 55 mg/m^2 or therapy should be discontinued; discontinue for peripheral neuropathy ≥ grade 3

Breast cancer, adjuvant treatment: TAC regimen should be administered when neutrophils are ≥1500 cells/mm^3. Patients experiencing febrile neutropenia should receive G-CSF in all subsequent cycles. Patients with persistent febrile neutropenia (while on G-CSF) or patients experiencing severe/cumulative cutaneous reactions or moderate neurosensory effects (signs/symptoms) should receive a reduced dose (60 mg/m^2) of docetaxel. Patients who experience grade 3 or 4 stomatitis should also receive a reduced dose (60 mg/m^2) of docetaxel. Discontinue therapy with persistent toxicities after dosage reduction.

Nonsmall cell lung cancer:
Monotherapy: Patients dosed initially at 75 mg/m^2 should have dose held until toxicity is resolved, then

resume at 55 mg/m^2; discontinue for peripheral neuropathy ≥ grade 3.

Combination therapy (with cisplatin): Patients dosed initially at 75 mg/m^2 should have the docetaxel dosage reduced to 65 mg/m^2 in subsequent cycles; if further adjustment is required, dosage may be reduced to 50 mg/m^2

Prostate cancer: Reduce dose to 60 mg/m^2; discontinue therapy if toxicities persist at lower dose.

Gastric cancer, head and neck cancer: **Note:** Cisplatin may require dose reductions/therapy delays for peripheral neuropathy, ototoxicity, and/or nephrotoxicity. Patients experiencing febrile neutropenia, documented infection with neutropenia or neutropenia >7 days should receive G-CSF in all subsequent cycles. For neutropenic complications despite G-CSF use, further reduce dose to 60 mg/m^2. Neutropenic complications in subsequent cycles should be further dose reduced to 45 mg/m^2. Patients who experience grade 4 thrombocytopenia should receive a dose reduction from 75 mg/m^2 to 60 mg/m^2. Discontinue therapy for persistent toxicities.

Gastrointestinal toxicity for docetaxel in combination with cisplatin and fluorouracil for treatment of gastric cancer or head and neck cancer:

Diarrhea, grade 3:
- First episode: Reduce fluorouracil dose by 20%
- Second episode: Reduce docetaxel dose by 20%

Diarrhea, grade 4:
- First episode: Reduce fluorouracil and docetaxel doses by 20%
- Second episode: Discontinue treatment

Stomatitis, grade 3:
- First episode: Reduce fluorouracil dose by 20%
- Second episode: Discontinue fluorouracil for all subsequent cycles
- Third episode: Reduce docetaxel dose by 20%

Stomatitis, grade 4:
- First episode: Discontinue fluorouracil for all subsequent cycles
- Second episode: Reduce docetaxel dose by 20%

Dosing adjustment in renal impairment: Docetaxel has minimal renal excretion; dosage adjustments for renal dysfunction may not be needed.

Dosing adjustment in hepatic impairment:

The FDA-approved labeling recommends the following adjustments:

Total bilirubin greater than the ULN, or AST and/or ALT >1.5 times ULN concomitant with alkaline phosphatase >2.5 times ULN: Docetaxel **generally should not be administered**.

Hepatic impairment dosing adjustment specific for gastric adenocarcinoma:
- AST/ALT >2.5 to ≤5 times ULN and alkaline phosphatase ≤2.5 times ULN: Administer 80% of dose
- AST/ALT >1.5 to ≤5 times ULN and alkaline phosphatase >2.5 to ≤5 times ULN: Administer 80% of dose
- AST/ALT >5 times ULN and /or alkaline phosphatase >5 times ULN: Discontinue docetaxel

The following guidelines have been used by some clinicians (Floyd, 2006):
- Transaminases 1.6-6 times ULN: Administer 75% of dose
- Transaminases >6 times ULN: Use clinical judgment

Administration Administer I.V. infusion over 1-hour through nonsorbing polyethylene lined (non-DEHP) tubing; in-line filter is not necessary (the use of a filter during administration is not recommended by the manufacturer). **Note:** Premedication with corticosteroids for 1-5 days, beginning the day before docetaxel administration, is recommended to prevent hypersensitivity reactions and pulmonary/peripheral edema (see Additional Information).

Monitoring Parameters CBC with differential, liver function tests, bilirubin, alkaline phosphatase, renal function; monitor for hypersensitivity reactions, fluid retention, epiphora, and canalicular stenosis

Additional Information Premedication with oral corticosteroids is recommended to decrease the incidence and severity of fluid retention and severity of hypersensitivity reactions. Dexamethasone 8-10 mg orally twice daily for 3-5 days, starting the day before docetaxel administration, is usually recommended. When prednisone is part of the antineoplastic regimen (eg, prostate cancer), the prednisone is sometimes withheld on the days dexamethasone is administered.

Dosage Forms Excipient information presented when available (limited, particularly for generics); consult specific product labeling.

Injection, solution [concentrate]:

Taxotere®: 20 mg/0.5 mL (0.5 mL, 2 mL) [contains Polysorbate 80®; diluent contains ethanol 13%]

Docosanol (doe KOE san ole)

U.S. Brand Names Abreva® [OTC]

Index Terms *n*-Docosanol; Behenyl Alcohol

Pharmacologic Category Antiviral Agent, Topical

Use Treatment of herpes simplex of the face or lips

Dosage Children ≥12 years and Adults: Topical: Apply 5 times/day to affected area of face or lips. Start at first sign of cold sore or fever blister and continue until healed.

Additional Information Complete prescribing information for this medication should be consulted for additional detail.

Dosage Forms Excipient information presented when available (limited, particularly for generics); consult specific product labeling.

Cream, topical:

Abreva®: 10% (2 g) [contains benzyl alcohol]

Docusate (DOK yoo sate)

U.S. Brand Names Colace® [OTC]; Correctol® [OTC]; D-S-S® [OTC]; Diocto® [OTC]; Docu-Soft [OTC]; Docusoft-S™ [OTC]; DOK™ [OTC]; DOS® [OTC]; Dulcolax® Stool Softener [OTC]; Enemeez® Plus [OTC]; Enemeez® [OTC]; Fleet® Sof-Lax® [OTC]; Genasoft® [OTC]; Phillips'® Stool Softener Laxative [OTC]; Silace [OTC]; Surfak® [OTC]

Canadian Brand Names Apo-Docusate-Sodium®; Colace®; Colax-C®; Novo-Docusate Calcium; Novo-Docusate Sodium; PMS-Docusate Calcium; PMS-Docusate Sodium; Regulex®; Selax®; Soflax™

Index Terms Dioctyl Calcium Sulfosuccinate; Dioctyl Sodium Sulfosuccinate; Docusate Calcium; Docusate Potassium; Docusate Sodium; DOSS; DSS

Pharmacologic Category Stool Softener

Additional Appendix Information

Laxatives, Classification and Properties *on page 1660*

Use Stool softener in patients who should avoid straining during defecation and constipation associated with hard, dry stools; prophylaxis for straining (Valsalva) following myocardial infarction. A safe agent to be used in elderly; some evidence that doses <200 mg are ineffective; stool softeners are unnecessary if stool is well hydrated or "mushy" and soft; shown to be ineffective used long-term.

Unlabeled/Investigational Use Ceruminolytic

Pregnancy Risk Factor C

Medication Safety Issues

Sound-alike/look-alike issues:
- Colace® may be confused with Calan®, Cozaar®
- Docusate may be confused with Doxinate®
- Surfak® may be confused with Surbex®

Dosage Docusate salts are interchangeable; the amount of sodium or calcium per dosage unit is clinically insignificant

Infants and Children <3 years: Oral: 10-40 mg/day in 1-4 divided doses
Children: Oral:
3-6 years: 20-60 mg/day in 1-4 divided doses
6-12 years: 40-150 mg/day in 1-4 divided doses
Adolescents and Adults: Oral: 50-500 mg/day in 1-4 divided doses
Older Children and Adults: Rectal: Add 50-100 mg of docusate liquid to enema fluid (saline or water); administer as retention or flushing enema

Ceruminolytic (unlabeled use): Intra-aural: Administer 1 mL of docusate sodium in 2 mL syringes; if no clearance in 15 minutes, irrigate with 50-100 mL normal saline (this method is 80% effective)

Additional Information Complete prescribing information for this medication should be consulted for additional detail.

Dosage Forms Excipient information presented when available (limited, particularly for generics); consult specific product labeling. [DSC] = Discontinued product
Capsule, oral, as calcium: 240 mg
Capsule, oral, as sodium: 100 mg, 250 mg [DSC]
Colace®: 50 mg [contains sodium 3 mg/capsule]; 100 mg [contains sodium 5 mg/capsule]
Capsule, liquid, oral, as calcium:
Surfak®: 240 mg
Capsule, liquid, oral, as sodium:
Docusoft-S™: 100 mg [contains sodium 5 mg/capsule]
Capsule, softgel, oral, as calcium: 240 mg
Capsule, softgel, oral, as sodium: 100 mg, 250 mg
Correctol®: 100 mg
Docu-Soft: 100 mg
DOK™: 100 mg, 250 mg
Dulcolax® Stool Softener: 100 mg [contains sodium 5 mg/softgel]
Fleet® Sof-Lax®: 100 mg [contains sodium 5 mg/softgel]
DOS®, D-S-S®: 100 mg, 250 mg
Genasoft®: 100 mg
Phillips'® Stool Softener Laxative: 100 mg [contains sodium 5.2 mg/softgel]
Liquid, oral, as sodium: 150 mg/15 mL (480 mL)
Colace®: 150 mg/15 mL (30 mL) [contains propylene glycol, sodium 1 mg/mL]
Diocto®: 150 mg/15 mL (480 mL)
Silace: 150 mg/15 mL (480 mL) [lemon-vanilla flavor]
Solution, rectal, as sodium [enema]:
Enemeez®: 283 mg/5 mL
Enemeez® Plus: 283 mg/5 mL [contains benzocaine]
Syrup, oral, as sodium: 60 mg/15 mL (480 mL)
Colace®: 60 mg/15 mL (480 mL) [alcohol free, sugar free; contains sodium 36 mg/5 mL]
Diocto®: 60 mg/15 mL (480 mL)
Silace: 20 mg/5 mL (480 mL) [peppermint flavor]

Docusate and Senna (DOK yoo sate & SEN na)

U.S. Brand Names Peri-Colace® [OTC]; Senokot-S® [OTC]; SenoSol™-SS [OTC]

Index Terms Senna and Docusate; Senna-S

Pharmacologic Category Laxative, Stimulant; Stool Softener

Additional Appendix Information
Laxatives, Classification and Properties *on page 1660*

Use Short-term treatment of constipation

Unlabeled/Investigational Use Evacuate the colon for bowel or rectal examinations; management/prevention of opiate-induced constipation

Medication Safety Issues
Sound-alike/look-alike issues:
Senokot® may be confused with Depakote®

Dosage Oral: Constipation: OTC ranges:
Children:
2-6 years: Initial: 4.3 mg sennosides plus 25 mg docusate (1/2 tablet) once daily (maximum: 1 tablet twice daily)
6-12 years: Initial: 8.6 sennosides plus 50 mg docusate (1 tablet) once daily (maximum: 2 tablets twice daily)
Children ≥12 years and Adults: Initial: 2 tablets (17.2 mg sennosides plus 100 mg docusate) once daily (maximum: 4 tablets twice daily)
Elderly: Consider half the initial dose in older, debilitated patients

Additional Information Complete prescribing information for this medication should be consulted for additional detail.

Dosage Forms Excipient information presented when available (limited, particularly for generics); consult specific product labeling.
Tablet: Docusate sodium 50 mg and sennosides 8.6 mg
Peri-Colace®: Docusate sodium 50 mg and sennosides 8.6 mg
Senokot-S®: Docusate sodium 50 mg and sennosides 8.6 mg [sugar free; contains sodium 4 mg/tablet]
SenoSol™-SS: Docusate sodium 50 mg and sennosides 8.6 mg [contains sodium 3 mg/tablet]

◆ **Docusate Calcium** *see* Docusate *on page 473*
◆ **Docusate Potassium** *see* Docusate *on page 473*
◆ **Docusate Sodium** *see* Docusate *on page 473*
◆ **Docu-Soft [OTC]** *see* Docusate *on page 473*
◆ **Docusoft-S™ [OTC]** *see* Docusate *on page 473*

Dofetilide (doe FET il ide)

U.S. Brand Names Tikosyn®

Canadian Brand Names Tikosyn®

Pharmacologic Category Antiarrhythmic Agent, Class III

Use Maintenance of normal sinus rhythm in patients with chronic atrial fibrillation/atrial flutter of longer than 1-week duration who have been converted to normal sinus rhythm; conversion of atrial fibrillation and atrial flutter to normal sinus rhythm

Restrictions Tikosyn® is only available to prescribers and hospitals that have confirmed their participation in a designated Tikosyn® Education Program. The program provides comprehensive education about the importance of in-hospital treatment initiation and individualized dosing.

T.I.P.S. is the Tikosyn® In Pharmacy System designated to allow retail pharmacies to stock and dispense Tikosyn® once they have been enrolled. A participating pharmacy must confirm receipt of the T.I.P.S. program materials and educate its pharmacy staff about the procedures required to fill an outpatient prescription for Tikosyn®. The T.I.P.S. enrollment form is available at www.tikosyn.com. Tikosyn® is only available from a special mail order pharmacy, and enrolled retail pharmacies. Pharmacists must verify that the hospital/prescriber is a confirmed participant before Tikosyn® is provided. For participant verification, the pharmacist may call 1-800-788-7353 or use the web site located at www.tikosynlist.com. Further details and directions on the program are provided at www.tikosyn.com.

Dofetilide therapy must be initiated/adjusted in a hospital setting with proper monitoring under the guidance of experienced personnel.

Pregnancy Risk Factor C

Pregnancy Considerations Dofetilide has been shown to adversely affect *in utero* growth, organogenesis, and survival of rats and mice. There are no adequate and well-controlled studies in pregnant women. Dofetilide should be used with extreme caution in pregnant women and in women of childbearing age only when the benefit to the patient unequivocally justifies the potential risk to the fetus.

Lactation Excretion in breast milk unknown/not recommended

Contraindications Hypersensitivity to dofetilide or any component of the formulation; patients with congenital or acquired long QT syndromes, do not use if a baseline QT interval or QT_c is >440 msec (500 msec in patients with ventricular conduction abnormalities); severe renal impairment (estimated Cl_{cr} <20 mL/minute); concurrent use with verapamil, cimetidine, hydrochlorothiazide (alone or in combinations), trimethoprim (alone or in combination with sulfamethoxazole), itraconazole, ketoconazole, prochlorperazine, or megestrol; baseline heart rate <50 beats/minute; other drugs that prolong QT intervals (phenothiazines, cisapride, bepridil, tricyclic antidepressants, moxifloxacin; hypokalemia or hypomagnesemia; concurrent amiodarone, clarithromycin, or erythromycin

Warnings/Precautions [U.S. Boxed Warning]: Must be initiated (or reinitiated) in a setting with continuous monitoring and staff familiar with the recognition and treatment of life-threatening arrhythmias. Patients must be monitored with continuous ECG for a minimum of 3 days, or for a minimum of 12 hours after electrical or pharmacological cardioversion to normal sinus rhythm, whichever is greater. Patients should be readmitted for continuous monitoring if dosage is later increased.

Reserve for patients who are highly symptomatic with atrial fibrillation/atrial flutter; torsade de pointes significantly increases with doses >500 mcg twice daily; hold Class Ia or Class II antiarrhythmics for at least three half-lives prior to starting dofetilide; use in patients on amiodarone therapy only if serum amiodarone level is <0.3 mg/L or if amiodarone was stopped for >3 months previously; correct hypokalemia or hypomagnesemia before initiating dofetilide and maintain within normal limits during treatment. Risk of hypokalemia and/or hypomagnesemia may be increased by potassium-depleting diuretics, increasing the risk of torsade de pointes. Concurrent use with other drugs known to prolong QT_c interval is not recommended.

Patients with sick sinus syndrome or with second or third-degree heart block should not receive dofetilide unless a functional pacemaker is in place. Defibrillation threshold is reduced in patients with ventricular tachycardia or ventricular fibrillation undergoing implantation of a cardioverter-defibrillator device. Safety and efficacy in children (<18 years of age) have not been established. Use with caution in renal impairment; not recommended in patients receiving drugs which may compete for renal secretion via cationic transport. Use with caution in patients with severe hepatic impairment.

In the Cardiac Arrhythmia Suppression Trial (CAST), recent (>6 days but <2 years ago) myocardial infarction patients with asymptomatic, non-life-threatening ventricular arrhythmias did not benefit and may have been harmed by attempts to suppress the arrhythmia with flecainide or encainide. An increased mortality or nonfatal cardiac arrest rate (7.7%) was seen in the active treatment group compared with patients in the placebo group (3%). The applicability of the CAST results to other populations is unknown. Antiarrhythmic agents should be reserved for patients with life-threatening ventricular arrhythmias.

Adverse Reactions

Supraventricular arrhythmia patients (incidence > placebo)

>10%: Central nervous system: Headache (11%)

2% to 10%:

Central nervous system: Dizziness (8%), insomnia (4%)

Cardiovascular: Ventricular tachycardia (2.6% to 3.7%), chest pain (10%), torsade de pointes (3.3% in CHF patients and 0.9% in patients with a recent MI; up to 10.5% in patients receiving doses in excess of those recommended). Torsade de pointes occurs most frequently within the first 3 days of therapy.

Dermatologic: Rash (3%)

Gastrointestinal: Nausea (5%), diarrhea (3%), abdominal pain (3%)

Neuromuscular & skeletal: Back pain (3%)

Respiratory: Dyspnea (6%), respiratory tract infection (7%)

Miscellaneous: Flu syndrome (4%)

<2% (Limited to important or life-threatening): Angioedema, AV block (0.4% to 1.5%), bundle branch block, cardiac arrest, facial paralysis, flaccid paralysis, heart block, hepatotoxicity, MI, paralysis, paresthesia, stroke, syncope, ventricular fibrillation (0% to 0.4%)

Drug Interactions

Metabolism/Transport Effects Substrate of CYP3A4 (minor)

Avoid Concomitant Use

Avoid concomitant use of Dofetilide with any of the following: Antifungal Agents (Azole Derivatives, Systemic); Nilotinib; Tetrabenazine; Thioridazine; Trimethoprim; Verapamil; Ziprasidone

Increased Effect/Toxicity

Dofetilide may increase the levels/effects of: QTc-Prolonging Agents; Tetrabenazine; Thioridazine; Ziprasidone

The levels/effects of Dofetilide may be increased by: Alfuzosin; Antifungal Agents (Azole Derivatives, Systemic); Cimetidine; Ciprofloxacin; Gadobutrol; Loop Diuretics; Nilotinib; Thiazide Diuretics; Trimethoprim; Verapamil

Decreased Effect There are no known significant interactions involving a decrease in effect.

Ethanol/Nutrition/Herb Interactions Herb/Nutraceutical: St John's wort may decrease dofetilide levels. Avoid ephedra (may worsen arrhythmia).

Mechanism of Action Vaughan Williams Class III antiarrhythmic activity. Blockade of the cardiac ion channel carrying the rapid component of the delayed rectifier potassium current. Dofetilide has no effect on sodium channels, adrenergic alpha-receptors, or adrenergic beta-receptors. It increases the monophasic action potential duration due to delayed repolarization. The increase in the QT interval is a function of prolongation of both effective and functional refractory periods in the His-Purkinje system and the ventricles. Changes in cardiac conduction velocity and sinus node function have not been observed in patients with or without structural heart disease. PR and QRS width remain the same in patients with pre-existing heart block and or sick sinus syndrome.

Pharmacodynamics/Kinetics

Absorption: >90%

Distribution: V_d: 3 L/kg

Protein binding: 60% to 70%

Metabolism: Hepatic via CYP3A4, but low affinity for it; metabolites formed by N-dealkylation and N-oxidation

Bioavailability: >90%

Half-life elimination: 10 hours

Time to peak: Fasting: 2-3 hours

Excretion: Urine (80%, 80% as unchanged drug, 20% as inactive or minimally active metabolites); renal elimination consists of glomerular filtration and active tubular secretion via cationic transport system

Dosage Adults: Oral:

Note: QT or QT_c must be determined prior to first dose. If QT_c >440 msec (>500 msec in patients with ventricular conduction abnormalities), dofetilide is contraindicated (see Contraindications and Warnings/Precautions).

Initial: 500 mcg orally twice daily. Initial dosage must be adjusted in patients with estimated Cl_{cr} <60 mL/minute (see Dosage Adjustment in Renal Impairment). Dofetilide may be initiated at lower doses than recommended based on physician discretion.

Modification of dosage in response to initial dose: QT_c interval should be measured 2-3 hours after the initial dose. If the QT_c >15% of baseline, or if the QT_c is >500 msec (550 msec in patients with ventricular conduction abnormalities) dofetilide should be adjusted. If the starting dose is 500 mcg twice daily, then adjust to 250 mcg twice daily. If the starting dose was 250 mcg twice daily, then adjust to 125 mcg twice daily. If the starting dose was 125 mcg twice daily then adjust to 125 mcg every day.

Continued monitoring for doses 2-5: QT_c interval must be determined 2-3 hours after each subsequent dose of dofetilide for in-hospital doses 2-5. If the measured QT_c is >500 msec (550 msec in patients with ventricular conduction abnormalities) at any time, dofetilide should be discontinued.

Chronic therapy (following the 5th dose):

QT or QT_c and creatinine clearance should be evaluated every 3 months. If QT_c >500 msec (>550 msec in patients with ventricular conduction abnormalities), dofetilide should be discontinued.

Dosage adjustment in renal impairment:

Cl_{cr} >60 mL/minute: Administer 500 mcg twice daily.

Cl_{cr} 40-60 mL/minute: Administer 250 mcg twice daily.

Cl_{cr} 20-39 mL/minute: Administer 125 mcg twice daily.

Cl_{cr} <20 mL/minute: Contraindicated in this group.

Dosage adjustment in hepatic impairment: No dosage adjustments required in Child-Pugh Class A and B. Patients with severe hepatic impairment were not studied.

Elderly: No specific dosage adjustments are recommended based on age, however, careful assessment of renal function is particularly important in this population.

Administration Do not open capsules.

Monitoring Parameters ECG monitoring with attention to QT_c and occurrence of ventricular arrhythmias, baseline serum creatinine and changes in serum creatinine. Check serum potassium and magnesium levels if on medications where these electrolyte disturbances can occur, or if patient has a history of hypokalemia or hypomagnesemia. QT or QT_c must be monitored at specific times prior to the first dose and during the first 3 days of therapy. Thereafter, QT or QT_c and creatinine clearance must be evaluated at 3-month intervals.

Dosage Forms Excipient information presented when available (limited, particularly for generics); consult specific product labeling.

Capsule: 125 mcg, 250 mcg, 500 mcg

◆ **DOK™ [OTC]** *see* Docusate *on page* 473

Dolasetron (dol A se tron)

U.S. Brand Names Anzemet®

Canadian Brand Names Anzemet®

Index Terms Dolasetron Mesylate; MDL 73,147EF

Pharmacologic Category Antiemetic; Selective 5-HT_3 Receptor Antagonist

Use Prevention of nausea and vomiting associated with emetogenic cancer chemotherapy; prevention of postoperative nausea and vomiting; treatment of postoperative nausea and vomiting (injectable form only).

Note: In Canada, the use of dolasetron is contraindicated for all uses in children <18 years of age or in the treatment of postoperative nausea and vomiting in adults. These are not labeled contraindications in the U.S.

Pregnancy Risk Factor B

Pregnancy Considerations

Teratogenic effects were not observed in animal studies. There are no adequate and well-controlled studies in pregnant women.

Lactation Excretion in breast milk unknown/use caution

Medication Safety Issues

Sound-alike/look-alike issues:

Anzemet® may be confused with Aldomet® and Avandamet®

Dolasetron may be confused with granisetron, ondansetron, palonosetron

Contraindications Hypersensitivity to dolasetron or any component of the formulation

Note: In Canada, the use of dolasetron is contraindicated for all uses in children <18 years of age or in the treatment of postoperative nausea and vomiting in adults. These are not labeled contraindications in the U.S.

Warnings/Precautions Dolasetron should be administered with caution in patients with congenital long QT syndrome or other risk factors for QT prolongation (eg, medications known to prolong QT interval, electrolyte abnormalities, and cumulative high-dose anthracycline therapy). Dolasetron has been associated with a number of dose-dependent increases in ECG intervals (eg, PR, QRS duration, QT/QT_c, JT), usually occurring 1-2 hours after I.V. administration and usually lasting 6-8 hours; however, may last ≥24 hours and rarely lead to heart block or arrhythmia. Clinically relevant QT interval prolongation may occur resulting in torsade de pointes, when used in conjunction with other agents that prolong the QT interval (eg, Class I and III antiarrhythmics). Use with caution in patients at risk of QT prolongation and/or ventricular arrhythmia. Reduction in heart rate may also occur with the 5-HT_3 antagonists. I.V. formulations of 5-HT_3 antagonists have more association with ECG interval changes, compared to oral formulations. Use with caution in children and adolescents who have or may develop QT_c prolongation; rare cases of supraventricular and ventricular arrhythmias, cardiac arrest, and MI have been reported in this population.

Use with caution in patients allergic to other 5-HT_3 receptor antagonists; cross-reactivity has been reported. **For chemotherapy, should be used on a scheduled basis, not on an "as needed" (PRN) basis,** since data support the use of this drug only in the prevention of nausea and vomiting (due to antineoplastic therapy) and not in the rescue of nausea and vomiting. Not intended for treatment of nausea and vomiting or for chronic continuous therapy. Safety and efficacy in children <2 years of age have not been established.

Adverse Reactions Adverse events may vary according to indication

>10%:

Central nervous system: Headache (7% to 24%)

Gastrointestinal: Diarrhea (2% to 12%)

1% to 10%:

Cardiovascular: Bradycardia (4% to 5%), hypotension (5%), hypertension (2% to 3%), tachycardia (2% to 3%)

Central nervous system: Dizziness (1% to 6%), fatigue (3% to 6%), fever (4% to 5%), pain (≤3%), chills/shivering (1% to 2%), sedation (2%)

Dermatological: Pruritus (3% to 4%)

Gastrointestinal: Dyspepsia (2% to 3%), abdominal pain (≤3%)

Hepatic: Abnormal hepatic function (4%)

Neuromuscular & skeletal: Pain (3%)

Renal: Oliguria (1% to 3%)

<1% (Limited to important or life-threatening): Abnormal vision, abnormal dreaming, acute renal failure, alkaline phosphatase increased, ALT increased, anaphylactic reaction, anemia, anorexia, anxiety, arrhythmia

(supraventricular and ventricular), AST increased, ataxia, AV block, bronchospasm, cardiac arrest, cardiac conduction abnormalities, chest pain, confusion, constipation, diaphoresis, dyspnea, dysuria, edema, epistaxis, facial edema, flushing, GGT increased, heart block, hematuria, hyperbilirubinemia, ischemia (peripheral), local injection site reaction, MI, myocardial ischemia, orthostatic hypotension, palpitation, pancreatitis, paresthesia, peripheral edema, photophobia, polyuria; prolonged PR, QRS, JT, and QT_c intervals; prothrombin time increased, PTT increased, purpura/hematoma, rash, sleep disorder, syncope, taste perversion, thrombocytopenia, thrombophlebitis/phlebitis, tinnitus, tremor, twitching, urticaria, vertigo

Drug Interactions

Metabolism/Transport Effects Substrate (minor) of CYP2C9, 3A4; **Inhibits** CYP2D6 (weak)

Avoid Concomitant Use

Avoid concomitant use of Dolasetron with any of the following: Apomorphine; Nilotinib; Tetrabenazine; Thioridazine; Ziprasidone

Increased Effect/Toxicity

Dolasetron may increase the levels/effects of: Apomorphine; QTc-Prolonging Agents; Tetrabenazine; Thioridazine; Ziprasidone

The levels/effects of Dolasetron may be increased by: Alfuzosin; Ciprofloxacin; Gadobutrol; Nilotinib

Decreased Effect There are no known significant interactions involving a decrease in effect.

Stability Store intact vials and tablets at room temperature; protect from light. A 20 mg/mL solution in syringes is stable for 8 months at room temperature. Dilute in 50-100 mL of a compatible solution (ie, 0.9% NS, D_5W, $D_5{}^1/_2NS$, D_5LR, LR, and 10% mannitol injection). Solutions diluted for infusion are stable at room temperature for 24 hours or under refrigeration for 48 hours.

Mechanism of Action Selective serotonin receptor ($5\text{-}HT_3$) antagonist, blocking serotonin both peripherally (primary site of action) and centrally at the chemoreceptor trigger zone

Pharmacodynamics/Kinetics

Absorption: Rapid and complete

Distribution: Hydrodolasetron: 5.8 L/kg

Protein binding: Hydrodolasetron: 69% to 77% (50% bound to $alpha_1$-acid glycoprotein)

Metabolism: Hepatic; reduction by carbonyl reductase to hydrodolasetron (active metabolite); further metabolized by CYP2D6, CYP3A, and flavin monooxygenase

Bioavailability: 75%

Half-life elimination: Dolasetron: 10 minutes; hydrodolasetron: Adults: 6-8 hours; Children: 4-6 hours

Time to peak, plasma: Hydrodolasetron: I.V.: 0.6 hours; Oral: 1 hour

Excretion: Urine ~67% (53% to 61% as active metabolite hydrodolasetron); feces ~33%

Dosage Note: In Canada, the use of dolasetron is contraindicated in children <18 years of age or in the treatment of postoperative nausea and vomiting in adults. These are not labeled contraindications in the U.S.

Prevention of chemotherapy-associated nausea and vomiting (including initial and repeat courses):

Children 2-16 years:

Oral: 1.8 mg/kg within 1 hour before chemotherapy; maximum: 100 mg/dose

I.V.: 1.8 mg/kg ~30 minutes before chemotherapy; maximum: 100 mg/dose

Adults:

Oral:100 mg single dose 1 hour prior to chemotherapy

I.V.: 1.8 mg/kg or 100 mg 30 minutes prior to chemotherapy

Prevention of postoperative nausea and vomiting:

Children 2-16 years:

Oral: 1.2 mg/kg within 2 hours before surgery; maximum: 100 mg/dose

I.V.: 0.35 mg/kg (maximum: 12.5 mg) ~15 minutes before stopping anesthesia

Adults:

Oral: 100 mg within 2 hours before surgery

I.V.: 12.5 mg ~15 minutes before stopping anesthesia

Treatment of postoperative nausea and vomiting: I.V. (only):

Children: 0.35 mg/kg (maximum: 12.5 mg) as soon as needed

Adults: 12.5 mg as soon as needed

Dosing adjustment for elderly, renal/hepatic impairment: No dosage adjustment is recommended

Administration I.V. injection may be given either undiluted IVP over 30 seconds or diluted in 50 mL of compatible fluid and infused over 15 minutes. Line should be flushed, prior to and after, dolasetron administration. Dolasetron injection may be diluted in apple or apple-grape juice and taken orally; this dilution is stable for 2 hours at room temperature.

Monitoring Parameters Liver function tests, blood pressure and pulse, and ECG in patients with cardiovascular disease

Additional Information Efficacy of dolasetron, for chemotherapy treatment, is enhanced with concomitant administration of dexamethasone 20 mg (increases complete response by 10% to 20%). Oral administration of the intravenous solution is equivalent to tablets. A single I.V. dose of dolasetron mesylate (1.8 or 2.4 mg/kg) has comparable safety and efficacy to a single 32 mg I.V. dose of ondansetron in patients receiving cisplatin chemotherapy.

Dosage Forms Excipient information presented when available (limited, particularly for generics); consult specific product labeling.

Injection, solution, as mesylate:

Anzemet®: 20 mg/mL (0.625 mL) [single-use Carpuject® or vial; contains mannitol 38.2 mg/mL]; 20 mg/mL (5 mL) [single-use vial; contains mannitol 38.2 mg/mL]; 20 mg/mL (25 mL) [multidose vial; contains mannitol 29 mg/mL]

Tablet, as mesylate:

Anzemet®: 50 mg, 100 mg

Extemporaneous Preparations Dolasetron injection may be diluted in apple or apple-grape juice and taken orally; this dilution is stable for 2 hours at room temperature.

- **Dolasetron Mesylate** *see* Dolasetron *on page 476*
- **Dolgic® LQ** *see* Butalbital, Acetaminophen, and Caffeine *on page 229*
- **Dolgic® Plus** *see* Butalbital, Acetaminophen, and Caffeine *on page 229*
- **Dologesic®** *see* Acetaminophen and Phenyltoloxamine *on page 29*
- **Dolophine®** *see* Methadone *on page 957*
- **Doloral (Can)** *see* Morphine Sulfate *on page 1016*
- **Dom-Alendronate (Can)** *see* Alendronate *on page 58*
- **Dom-Amiodarone (Can)** *see* Amiodarone *on page 87*
- **Dom-Anagrelide (Can)** *see* Anagrelide *on page 115*
- **Dom-Azithromycin (Can)** *see* Azithromycin *on page 166*
- **Dom-Buspirone (Can)** *see* BusPIRone *on page 226*
- **Dom-Carbamazepine (Can)** *see* CarBAMazepine *on page 252*
- **DOM-Carvedilol (Can)** *see* Carvedilol *on page 264*
- **Dom-Ciprofloxacin (Can)** *see* Ciprofloxacin *on page 329*

◆ **Dom-Citalopram (Can)** *see* Citalopram *on page 337*

◆ **DOM-Clonidine (Can)** *see* CloNIDine *on page 354*

◆ **Dom-Diclofenac (Can)** *see* Diclofenac *on page 437*

◆ **Dom-Diclofenac SR (Can)** *see* Diclofenac *on page 437*

◆ **Dom-Divalproex (Can)** *see* Valproic Acid and Derivatives *on page 1538*

◆ **Domeboro® [OTC]** *see* Aluminum Sulfate and Calcium Acetate *on page 77*

◆ **Dome Paste Bandage** *see* Zinc Gelatin *on page 1584*

◆ **Dom-Fenofibrate Supra (Can)** *see* Fenofibrate *on page 607*

◆ **Dom-Fluconazole (Can)** *see* Fluconazole *on page 625*

◆ **Dom-Fluoxetine (Can)** *see* FLUoxetine *on page 638*

◆ **Dom-Furosemide (Can)** *see* Furosemide *on page 676*

◆ **DOM-Gabapentin (Can)** *see* Gabapentin *on page 678*

◆ **Dom-Indapamide (Can)** *see* Indapamide *on page 781*

◆ **DOM-Leflunomide (Can)** *see* Leflunomide *on page 859*

◆ **DOM-Levetiracetam (Can)** *see* Levetiracetam *on page 872*

◆ **Dom-Loperamide (Can)** *see* Loperamide *on page 900*

◆ **DOM-Lovastatin (Can)** *see* Lovastatin *on page 910*

◆ **Dom-Mefenamic Acid (Can)** *see* Mefenamic Acid *on page 932*

◆ **DOM-Metformin (Can)** *see* MetFORMIN *on page 954*

◆ **Dom-Methimazole (Can)** *see* Methimazole *on page 963*

◆ **Dom-Metoprolol (Can)** *see* Metoprolol *on page 982*

◆ **DOM-Mirtazapine (Can)** *see* Mirtazapine *on page 1002*

◆ **DOM-Ondansetron (Can)** *see* Ondansetron *on page 1102*

◆ **DOM-Pravastatin (Can)** *see* Pravastatin *on page 1227*

◆ **Dom-Propranolol (Can)** *see* Propranolol *on page 1259*

◆ **Dom-Ranitidine (Can)** *see* Ranitidine *on page 1295*

◆ **Dom-Risperidone (Can)** *see* Risperidone *on page 1323*

◆ **Dom-Sertraline (Can)** *see* Sertraline *on page 1362*

◆ **Dom-Simvastatin (Can)** *see* Simvastatin *on page 1370*

◆ **DOM-Sotalol (Can)** *see* Sotalol *on page 1394*

◆ **Dom-Sumatriptan (Can)** *see* SUMAtriptan *on page 1414*

◆ **Dom-Temazepam (Can)** *see* Temazepam *on page 1432*

◆ **Dom-Topiramate (Can)** *see* Topiramate *on page 1489*

◆ **DOM-Ursodiol C (Can)** *see* Ursodiol *on page 1534*

◆ **Dom-Verapamil SR (Can)** *see* Verapamil *on page 1557*

◆ **Donatussin** *see* Dextromethorphan, Chlorpheniramine, Phenylephrine, and Guaifenesin *on page 434*

◆ **Donatussin DM [DSC]** *see* Chlorpheniramine, Phenylephrine, and Dextromethorphan *on page 311*

◆ **Donatussin Drops** *see* Guaifenesin and Phenylephrine *on page 712*

Donepezil (doh NEP e zil)

U.S. Brand Names Aricept®; Aricept® ODT

Canadian Brand Names Aricept®; Aricept® RDT

Index Terms E2020

Pharmacologic Category Acetylcholinesterase Inhibitor (Central)

Use Treatment of mild, moderate, or severe dementia of the Alzheimer's type

Unlabeled/Investigational Use Attention-deficit/hyperactivity disorder (ADHD); behavioral syndromes in dementia; mild-to-moderate dementia associated with Parkinson's disease; Lewy body dementia

Pregnancy Risk Factor C

Pregnancy Considerations Teratogenic effects were not observed in animal studies. There are no adequate and well-controlled studies in pregnant women.

Lactation Excretion in breast milk unknown/not recommended

Medication Safety Issues

Sound-alike/look-alike issues:

Aricept® may be confused with AcipHex®, Ascriptin®, and Azilect®

Contraindications Hypersensitivity to donepezil, piperidine derivatives, or any component of the formulation

Warnings/Precautions Cholinesterase inhibitors may have vagotonic effects which may cause bradycardia and/or heart block with or without a history of cardiac disease; syncopal episodes have been associated with donepezil. Alzheimer's treatment guidelines consider bradycardia to be a relative contraindication for use of centrally-active cholinesterase inhibitors. Use with caution with sick sinus syndrome or other supraventricular cardiac conduction abnormalities, with seizures, COPD, or asthma. Use with caution in patients at risk of ulcer disease (eg, previous history or NSAID use), or in patients with bladder outlet obstruction. May cause diarrhea, nausea, and/or vomiting, which may be dose-related. May exaggerate neuromuscular blockade effects of depolarizing neuromuscular-blocking agents like succinylcholine. Safety and efficacy in children have not been established.

Adverse Reactions

>10%:

Central nervous system: Insomnia (5% to 14%)

Gastrointestinal: Nausea (5% to 19%), diarrhea (8% to 15%)

Miscellaneous: Accident (7% to 13%), infection (11%)

1% to 10%:

Cardiovascular: Hypertension (3%), chest pain (2%), hemorrhage (2%), syncope (2%), hypotension, atrial fibrillation, bradycardia, ECG abnormal, edema, heart failure, hot flashes, peripheral edema, vasodilation

Central nervous system: Headache (4% to 10%), pain (3% to 9%), fatigue (3% to 8%), dizziness (2% to 8%), abnormal dreams (3%), depression (2% to 3%), hostility (3%), nervousness (3%), hallucinations (3%), confusion (2%), emotional lability (2%), personality disorder (2%), fever (2%), somnolence (2%), abnormal crying, aggression, agitation, anxiety, aphasia, delusions, irritability, restlessness, seizure

Dermatologic: Bruising (4% to 5%), eczema (3%), pruritus, rash, skin ulcer, urticaria

Endocrine & metabolic: Dehydration (2%), hyperlipemia (2%), libido increased

Gastrointestinal: Anorexia (3% to 8%), vomiting (3% to 8%), weight loss (3%), abdominal pain, constipation, dyspepsia, fecal incontinence, gastroenteritis, GI bleeding, bloating, epigastric pain, toothache

Genitourinary: Urinary frequency (2%), urinary incontinence (2%), hematuria, glycosuria, nocturia, UTI

Hematologic: Anemia

Hepatic: Alkaline phosphatase increased

Neuromuscular & skeletal: Muscle cramps (3% to 8%), back pain (3%), CPK increased (3%), arthritis (2%), ataxia, bone fracture, gait abnormal, lactate dehydrogenase increased, paresthesia, tremor, weakness

Ocular: Blurred vision, cataract, eye irritation

Respiratory: Cough increased, dyspnea, bronchitis, pharyngitis, pneumonia, sore throat

Miscellaneous: Diaphoresis, fungal infection, flu symptoms, wandering

<1%, postmarketing, and/or case reports (limited to important or life-threatening): Abscess, breast fibroadenosis, cellulitis, cerebrovascular accident, CHF, cholecystitis, conjunctival hemorrhage, conjunctivitis, deep

vein thrombosis, diabetes mellitus, diverticulitis, ear pain, eosinophilia, fibrocystic breast, gastrointestinal ulcer, glaucoma, goiter, heart block, hemolytic anemia, hepatitis, hostility, hyperglycemia, hypertonia, hypokalemia, hypokinesia, hyponatremia, hypoxia, intracranial hemorrhage, jaundice, LFTs increased, MI, neuroleptic malignant syndrome, pancreatitis, pleurisy, pulmonary collapse, pulmonary congestion, pyelonephritis, renal failure, retinal hemorrhage, SVT, thrombocythemia, thrombocytopenia, tongue edema, transient ischemic attack, vision abnormal

Drug Interactions

Metabolism/Transport Effects Substrate (minor) of CYP2D6, 3A4

Avoid Concomitant Use There are no known interactions where it is recommended to avoid concomitant use.

Increased Effect/Toxicity

Donepezil may increase the levels/effects of: Antipsychotics; Beta-Blockers; Cholinergic Agonists; Succinylcholine

The levels/effects of Donepezil may be increased by: Corticosteroids (Systemic); Ginkgo Biloba

Decreased Effect

Donepezil may decrease the levels/effects of: Anticholinergics; Neuromuscular-Blocking Agents (Nondepolarizing)

The levels/effects of Donepezil may be decreased by: Anticholinergics

Ethanol/Nutrition/Herb Interactions Herb/Nutraceutical: St John's wort may decrease donepezil levels. Gingko biloba may increase adverse effects/toxicity of acetylcholinesterase inhibitors.

Stability Store at 15°C to 30°C (59°F to 86°F).

Mechanism of Action Alzheimer's disease is characterized by cholinergic deficiency in the cortex and basal forebrain, which contributes to cognitive deficits. Donepezil reversibly and noncompetitively inhibits centrally-active acetylcholinesterase, the enzyme responsible for hydrolysis of acetylcholine. This appears to result in increased concentrations of acetylcholine available for synaptic transmission in the central nervous system.

Pharmacodynamics/Kinetics

Absorption: Well absorbed

Protein binding: 96%, primarily to albumin (75%) and α_1-acid glycoprotein (21%)

Metabolism: Extensively to four major metabolites (two are active) via CYP2D6 and 3A4; undergoes glucuronidation

Bioavailability: 100%

Half-life elimination: 70 hours; time to steady-state: 15 days

Time to peak, plasma: 3-4 hours

Excretion: Urine 57% (17% as unchanged drug); feces 15%

Dosage Oral:

Children: ADHD (unlabeled use): 5 mg/day

Adults: Dementia of Alzheimer's type: Initial: 5 mg/day at bedtime; may increase to 10 mg/day at bedtime after 4-6 weeks

Dietary Considerations May take with or without food.

Administration Administer at bedtime without regard to food.

Aricept® ODT: Allow tablet to dissolve completely on tongue and follow with water.

Monitoring Parameters Behavior, mood, bowel function, cognitive function, general function (eg, activities of daily living)

Dosage Forms Excipient information presented when available (limited, particularly for generics); consult specific product labeling.

Tablet, as hydrochloride:

Aricept®: 5 mg, 10 mg

Tablet, orally disintegrating, as hydrochloride:

Aricept® ODT: 5 mg, 10 mg

- **Donnatal®** *see* Hyoscyamine, Atropine, Scopolamine, and Phenobarbital *on page 756*
- **Donnatal Extentabs®** *see* Hyoscyamine, Atropine, Scopolamine, and Phenobarbital *on page 756*

DOPamine (DOE pa meen)

Index Terms Dopamine Hydrochloride; Intropin

Pharmacologic Category Adrenergic Agonist Agent

Additional Appendix Information

Hemodynamic Support, Intravenous *on page 1657*

Use Adjunct in the treatment of shock (eg, MI, open heart surgery, renal failure, cardiac decompensation) which persists after adequate fluid volume replacement

Unlabeled/Investigational Use Symptomatic bradycardia or heart block unresponsive to atropine or pacing

Pregnancy Risk Factor C

Lactation Excretion in breast milk unknown

Medication Safety Issues

Sound-alike/look-alike issues:

DOPamine may be confused with DOBUTamine, Dopram®

High alert medication: The Institute for Safe Medication Practices (ISMP) includes this medication among its list of drugs which have a heightened risk of causing significant patient harm when used in error.

Contraindications Hypersensitivity to sulfites (commercial preparation contains sodium bisulfite); pheochromocytoma; ventricular fibrillation

Warnings/Precautions Use with caution in patients with cardiovascular disease or cardiac arrhythmias or patients with occlusive vascular disease. Correct hypovolemia and electrolytes when used in hemodynamic support. May cause increases in HR and arrhythmia. Use with caution in post-MI patients. Use with extreme caution in patients taking MAO inhibitors. Avoid extravasation; infuse into a large vein if possible. Avoid infusion into leg veins. Watch I.V. site closely. **[U.S. Boxed Warning]: If extravasation occurs, infiltrate the area with diluted phentolamine (5-10 mg in 10-15 mL of saline) with a fine hypodermic needle. Phentolamine should be administered as soon as possible after extravasation is noted.** Product may contain sodium metabisulfite.

Adverse Reactions Frequency not defined.

Most frequent:

Cardiovascular: Ectopic beats, tachycardia, anginal pain, palpitation, hypotension, vasoconstriction

Central nervous system: Headache

Gastrointestinal: Nausea and vomiting

Respiratory: Dyspnea

Infrequent:

Cardiovascular: Aberrant conduction, bradycardia, widened QRS complex, ventricular arrhythmia (high dose), gangrene (high dose), hypertension

Central nervous system: Anxiety

Endocrine & metabolic: Piloerection, serum glucose increased (usually not above normal limits)

Local: Extravasation of dopamine can cause tissue necrosis and sloughing of surrounding tissues

Ocular: Intraocular pressure increased, dilated pupils

Renal: Azotemia, polyuria

Drug Interactions

Avoid Concomitant Use

Avoid concomitant use of DOPamine with any of the following: Iobenguane I 123

Increased Effect/Toxicity

DOPamine may increase the levels/effects of: Sympathomimetics

The levels/effects of DOPamine may be increased by: Cannabinoids; COMT Inhibitors

Decreased Effect

DOPamine may decrease the levels/effects of: Iobenguane I 123

Stability Protect from light; solutions that are darker than slightly yellow should not be used.

Mechanism of Action Stimulates both adrenergic and dopaminergic receptors, lower doses are mainly dopaminergic stimulating and produce renal and mesenteric vasodilation, higher doses also are both dopaminergic and $beta_1$-adrenergic stimulating and produce cardiac stimulation and renal vasodilation; large doses stimulate alpha-adrenergic receptors

Pharmacodynamics/Kinetics

Children: Dopamine has exhibited nonlinear kinetics in children; with medication changes, may not achieve steady-state for ~1 hour rather than 20 minutes

Onset of action: Adults: 5 minutes

Duration: Adults: <10 minutes

Metabolism: Renal, hepatic, plasma; 75% to inactive metabolites by monoamine oxidase and 25% to norepinephrine

Half-life elimination: 2 minutes

Excretion: Urine (as metabolites)

Clearance: Neonates: Varies and appears to be age related; clearance is more prolonged with combined hepatic and renal dysfunction

Dosage I.V. infusion (administration requires the use of an infusion pump):

Neonates: 1-20 mcg/kg/minute continuous infusion, titrate to desired response.

Children: 1-20 mcg/kg/minute, maximum: 50 mcg/kg/minute continuous infusion, titrate to desired response.

Adults: 1-5 mcg/kg/minute up to 20 mcg/kg/minute, titrate to desired response (maximum: 50 mcg/kg/minute). Infusion may be increased by 1-4 mcg/kg/minute at 10- to 30-minute intervals until optimal response is obtained.

If dosages >20-30 mcg/kg/minute are needed, a more direct-acting pressor may be more beneficial (ie, epinephrine, norepinephrine).

The hemodynamic effects of dopamine are dose dependent:

Low-dose: 1-3 mcg/kg/minute, increased renal blood flow and urine output

Intermediate-dose: 3-10 mcg/kg/minute, increased renal blood flow, heart rate, cardiac contractility, and cardiac output

High-dose: >10 mcg/kg/minute, alpha-adrenergic effects begin to predominate, vasoconstriction, increased blood pressure

Administration Administer into large vein to prevent the possibility of extravasation (central line administration); monitor continuously for free flow; use infusion device to control rate of flow; administration into an umbilical arterial catheter is not recommended; when discontinuing the infusion, gradually decrease the dose of dopamine (sudden discontinuation may cause hypotension).

To prepare for infusion:

$$\frac{6 \times \text{weight (kg)} \times \text{desired dose (mcg/kg/min)}}{\text{I.V. infusion rate (mL/h)}} = \frac{\text{mg of drug to be added to}}{\text{100 mL of I.V. fluid}}$$

Extravasation management: Due to short half-life, withdrawal of drug is often only necessary treatment. Use phentolamine as antidote. Mix 5 mg with 9 mL of NS; inject a small amount of this dilution into extravasated area. Blanching should reverse immediately. Monitor site. If blanching should recur, additional injections of phentolamine may be needed.

Monitoring Parameters Blood pressure, ECG, heart rate, CVP, RAP, MAP, urine output; if pulmonary artery catheter is in place, monitor CI, PCWP, SVR, and PVR

Additional Information Dopamine is most frequently used for treatment of hypotension because of its peripheral vasoconstrictor action. In this regard, dopamine is often used together with dobutamine and minimizes hypotension secondary to dobutamine-induced vasodilation. Thus, pressure is maintained by increased cardiac output (from dobutamine) and vasoconstriction (by dopamine). It is critical neither dopamine nor dobutamine be used in patients in the absence of correcting any hypovolemia as a cause of hypotension.

Low-dose dopamine is often used in the intensive care setting for presumed beneficial effects on renal function. However, there is no clear evidence that low-dose dopamine confers any renal or other benefit. Indeed, dopamine may act on dopamine receptors in the carotid bodies causing chemoreflex suppression. In patients with heart failure, dopamine may inhibit breathing and cause pulmonary shunting. Both these mechanisms would act to decrease minute ventilation and oxygen saturation. This could potentially be deleterious in patients with respiratory compromise and patients being weaned from ventilators.

Dosage Forms Excipient information presented when available (limited, particularly for generics); consult specific product labeling.

Infusion, as hydrochloride [premixed in D_5W]: 0.8 mg/mL (250 mL, 500 mL); 1.6 mg/mL (250 mL, 500 mL); 3.2 mg/mL (250 mL)

Injection, solution, as hydrochloride: 40 mg/mL (5 mL, 10 mL); 80 mg/mL (5 mL); 160 mg/mL (5 mL) [contains sodium metabisulfite]

◆ **Dopamine Hydrochloride** *see* DOPamine *on page 479*

◆ **Dopram®** *see* Doxapram *on page 482*

◆ **Doral®** *see* Quazepam *on page 1275*

◆ **Doribax™** *see* Doripenem *on page 480*

Doripenem (dore i PEN em)

U.S. Brand Names Doribax™

Index Terms S-4661

Pharmacologic Category Antibiotic, Carbapenem

Use Treatment of complicated intra-abdominal infections and complicated urinary tract infections (including pyelonephritis) due to susceptible gram-positive, gram-negative (including *Pseudomonas aeruginosa*), and anaerobic bacteria

Unlabeled/Investigational Use Treatment of nosocomial pneumonia

Pregnancy Risk Factor B

Pregnancy Considerations Adverse events have not been observed in animal studies; therefore, the manufacturer classifies doripenem as pregnancy category B. There are no adequate and well-controlled studies completed in pregnant women.

Lactation Excretion in breast milk unknown/use caution

Contraindications Known serious hypersensitivity to doripenem or other carbapenems (eg, imipenem, ertapenem, meropenem); anaphylactic reactions to beta-lactam antibiotics

Warnings/Precautions Serious hypersensitivity reactions, including anaphylaxis, and skin reactions have been reported in patients receiving beta-lactams. Prolonged use may result in fungal or bacterial superinfection, including *C. difficile*-associated diarrhea (CDAD) and pseudomembranous colitis; CDAD has been observed >2 months postantibiotic treatment. Use with caution in patients with renal impairment; dosage adjustment required in patients with moderate-to-severe renal dysfunction. Levels of valproic acid may be decreased during concomitant use to subtherapeutic levels, increasing potential for breakthrough seizures. Administer via intravenous infusion only. Per manufacturer's labeling, investigational experience of doripenem via inhalation resulted in pneumonitis. Safety and efficacy have not been established in children <18 years of age.

Adverse Reactions

>10%:

Central nervous system: Headache (4% to 16%)

Gastrointestinal: Nausea (4% to 12%), diarrhea (6% to 11%)

1% to 10%:

Dermatologic: Rash (1% to 5%; includes allergic/bullous dermatitis, erythema, macular/papular eruptions, urticaria, and erythema multiforme), pruritus (≤3%)

Gastrointestinal: Oral candidiasis (1%)

Hematologic: Anemia (2% to 10%)

Hepatic: Transaminases increased (1% to 2%)

Local: Phlebitis (4% to 8%)

Renal: Renal impairment/failure (≤1%)

Miscellaneous: Vulvomycotic infection (1% to 2%)

Postmarketing and/or case reports: Anaphylaxis, interstitial pneumonia, Stevens-Johnson syndrome, seizure, toxic epidermal necrolysis

Drug Interactions

Avoid Concomitant Use There are no known interactions where it is recommended to avoid concomitant use.

Increased Effect/Toxicity

The levels/effects of Doripenem may be increased by: Probenecid; Uricosuric Agents

Decreased Effect

Doripenem may decrease the levels/effects of: Typhoid Vaccine; Valproic Acid

Stability Store dry powder vials at 15°C to 30°C (59°F to 86°F). Reconstitute 500 mg vial with 10 mL of SWFI or NS. Shake gently until clear. Further dilute for infusion with 100 mL of NS or D_5W. Reconstituted vial may be stored for up to 1 hour prior to preparation of infusion solution. Stability of solution (concentration: 4.5 mg/mL) when diluted in NS is 8 hours at room temperature or 24 hours under refrigeration; stability in D_5W is 4 hours at room temperature and 24 hours under refrigeration.

Renal impairment: For preparation of a 250 mg dose in renal impairment, reconstitute 500 mg vial with 10 mL of SWFI or NS and further dilute with 100 mL of compatible solution as above, but remove and discard 55 mL from the infusion bag to leave the remaining solution containing the 250 mg dose (concentration: 4.5 mg/mL).

Mechanism of Action Inhibits bacterial cell wall synthesis by binding to several of the penicillin-binding proteins, which in turn inhibits the final transpeptidation step of peptidoglycan synthesis in bacterial cell walls, thus inhibiting cell wall biosynthesis; bacteria eventually lyse due to ongoing activity of cell wall autolytic enzymes (autolysins and murein hydrolases) while cell wall assembly is arrested.

Pharmacodynamics/Kinetics

Distribution: V_d: 16.8 L

Protein binding: 8% to 9%

Metabolism: Non-CYP-mediated metabolism via dehydropeptidase-I to doripenem-M1 (inactive metabolite)

Half-life elimination: ~1 hour

Excretion: Urine (70% as unchanged drug; 15% as doripenem-M1 metabolite); feces (<1%)

Dosage

Usual dosage: Adults: I.V.: 500 mg every 8 hours

Indication-specific dosing: Adults: I.V.:

Intra-abdominal infection (complicated): 500 mg every 8 hours for 5-14 days

Urinary tract infection (complicated) or pyelonephritis: 500 mg every 8 hours for 10-14 days

Dosing adjustment in renal impairment:

Cl_{cr} 30-50 mL/minute: 250 mg every 8 hours

Cl_{cr} 11-29 mL/minute: 250 mg every 12 hours

Hemodialysis: Dialyzable (~52% of dose removed during 4-hour session in ESRD patients)

Administration Administer I.V. infusion over 1 hour

Monitoring Parameters Monitor for signs of anaphylaxis during first dose; periodic renal assessment; consider hematologic monitoring during prolonged therapy

Dosage Forms Excipient information presented when available (limited, particularly for generics); consult specific product labeling.

Injection, powder for reconstitution:

Doribax™: 500 mg

Dornase Alfa (DOOR nase AL fa)

U.S. Brand Names Pulmozyme®

Canadian Brand Names Pulmozyme®

Index Terms Recombinant Human Deoxyribonuclease; rhDNase

Pharmacologic Category Enzyme

Use Management of cystic fibrosis patients to reduce the frequency of respiratory infections that require parenteral antibiotics in patients with FVC ≥40% of predicted; in conjunction with standard therapies, to improve pulmonary function in patients with cystic fibrosis

Pregnancy Risk Factor B

Pregnancy Considerations Teratogenic effects were not observed in animal studies. There are no adequate and well-controlled studies in pregnant women.

Lactation Excretion in breast milk unknown/use caution

Contraindications Hypersensitivity to dornase alfa, Chinese hamster ovary cell products, or any component of the formulation

Warnings/Precautions Safety and efficacy have not been established for daily administration >12 months. In patients with pulmonary function <40% of normal, dornase alfa does not significantly reduce the risk of respiratory infections that require parenteral antibiotics. Safety studies included children ≥3 months, however experience is limited in children <5 years of age

Adverse Reactions Adverse events were similar in children using the PARI BABY™ nebulizer (facemask as opposed to mouthpiece) with the addition of cough (45% in children 3 months to <5 years; 30% in children 5 to ≤10 years).

>10%:

Cardiovascular: Chest pain (18% to 25%)

Central nervous system: Fever (32% in patients with FVC <40%)

Dermatologic: Rash (3% to 12%)

Respiratory: Pharyngitis (32% to 40%), rhinitis (30% in patients with FVC <40%); FVC decrease ≥10% of predicted (22% in patients with FVC <40%), dyspnea (17% in patients with FVC <40%)

Miscellaneous: Voice alteration (12% to 18%)

1% to 10%:

Gastrointestinal: Dyspepsia (≤3%)

Ocular: Conjunctivitis (1% to 5%)

Respiratory: Laryngitis (3% to 4%)

Miscellaneous: Dornase alfa serum antibodies (2% to 4%)

Postmarketing and/or case reports: Headache, urticaria

Drug Interactions

Avoid Concomitant Use There are no known interactions where it is recommended to avoid concomitant use.

Increased Effect/Toxicity There are no known significant interactions involving an increase in effect.

Decreased Effect There are no known significant interactions involving a decrease in effect.

Stability Must be stored in the refrigerator at 2°C to 8°C (36°F to 46°F) and protected from strong light.

Mechanism of Action The hallmark of cystic fibrosis lung disease is the presence of abundant, purulent airway secretions composed primarily of highly polymerized DNA. The principal source of this DNA is the nuclei of degenerating neutrophils, which is present in large concentrations in infected lung secretions. The presence of this DNA produces a viscous mucous that may contribute to the decreased mucociliary transport and persistent infections that are commonly seen in this population. Dornase alfa is a deoxyribonuclease (DNA) enzyme produced by recombinant gene technology. Dornase selectively cleaves DNA, thus reducing mucous viscosity and as a result, airflow in the lung is improved and the risk of bacterial infection may be decreased.

Pharmacodynamics/Kinetics

Onset of action: Nebulization: Enzyme levels are measured in sputum in ~15 minutes

Duration: Rapidly declines

Dosage Inhalation:

Children ≥3 months to Adults: 2.5 mg once daily through selected nebulizers; experience in children <5 years is limited

Patients unable to inhale or exhale orally throughout the entire treatment period may use Pari-Baby™ nebulizer. Some patients may benefit from twice daily administration.

Administration Nebulization: Should not be diluted or mixed with any other drugs in the nebulizer, this may inactivate the drug

Dosage Forms Excipient information presented when available (limited, particularly for generics); consult specific product labeling.

Solution for nebulization [preservative free]:

Pulmozyme®: 1 mg/mL (2.5 mL) [derived from Chinese hamster cells]

◆ **Doryx®** *see* Doxycycline *on page 491*

Dorzolamide (dor ZOLE a mide)

U.S. Brand Names Trusopt®

Canadian Brand Names Trusopt®

Index Terms Dorzolamide Hydrochloride

Pharmacologic Category Carbonic Anhydrase Inhibitor; Ophthalmic Agent, Antiglaucoma

Additional Appendix Information

Glaucoma Drug Therapy *on page 1808*

Use Treatment of elevated intraocular pressure in patients with ocular hypertension or open-angle glaucoma

Pregnancy Risk Factor C

Dosage Children and Adults: Reduction of intraocular pressure: Instill 1 drop in the affected eye(s) 3 times/day

Additional Information Complete prescribing information for this medication should be consulted for additional detail.

Dosage Forms Excipient information presented when available (limited, particularly for generics); consult specific product labeling.

Solution, ophthalmic: 2% (10 mL)

Trusopt®: 2% (10 mL) [contains benzalkonium chloride]

Dorzolamide and Timolol
(dor ZOLE a mide & TYE moe lole)

U.S. Brand Names Cosopt®

Canadian Brand Names Cosopt®; Preservative-Free Cosopt®

Index Terms Timolol and Dorzolamide

Pharmacologic Category Beta-Adrenergic Blocker, Nonselective; Carbonic Anhydrase Inhibitor; Ophthalmic Agent, Antiglaucoma

Use Treatment of elevated intraocular pressure in patients with ocular hypertension or open-angle glaucoma

Pregnancy Risk Factor C

Dosage Ophthalmic: Children ≥2 years and Adults: Instill 1 drop in affected eye(s) twice daily

Additional Information Complete prescribing information for this medication should be consulted for additional detail.

Dosage Forms Excipient information presented when available (limited, particularly for generics); consult specific product labeling. [DSC] = Discontinued product

Solution, ophthalmic: Dorzolamide hydrochloride 2% (as base) and timolol maleate 0.5% (as base) (10 mL)

Cosopt®: Dorzolamide hydrochloride 2% (as base) and timolol maleate 0.5% (as base) (5 mL [DSC]; 10 mL) [contains benzalkonium chloride]

◆ **Dorzolamide Hydrochloride** *see* Dorzolamide *on page 482*

◆ **DOS® [OTC]** *see* Docusate *on page 473*

◆ **DOSS** *see* Docusate *on page 473*

◆ **Dostinex® [DSC]** *see* Cabergoline *on page 232*

◆ **Dostinex® (Can)** *see* Cabergoline *on page 232*

◆ **Double Tussin DM [OTC]** *see* Guaifenesin and Dextromethorphan *on page 710*

◆ **Dovobet® (Can)** *see* Calcipotriene and Betamethasone *on page 234*

◆ **Dovonex®** *see* Calcipotriene *on page 234*

Doxapram (DOKS a pram)

U.S. Brand Names Dopram®

Index Terms Doxapram Hydrochloride

Pharmacologic Category Respiratory Stimulant; Stimulant

Use Respiratory and CNS stimulant for respiratory depression secondary to anesthesia, drug-induced CNS depression; acute hypercapnia secondary to COPD

Pregnancy Risk Factor B

Medication Safety Issues

Sound-alike/look-alike issues:

Doxapram may be confused with doxacurium, doxazosin, doxepin, Doxinate®, DOXOrubicin

Dopram® may be confused with DOPamine

Dosage

Respiratory depression following anesthesia:

Intermittent injection: Initial: 0.5-1 mg/kg; may repeat at 5-minute intervals (only in patients who demonstrate initial response); maximum total dose: 2 mg/kg

I.V. infusion: Initial: 5 mg/minute until adequate response or adverse effects seen; decrease to 1-3 mg/minute; maximum total dose: 4 mg/kg

Drug-induced CNS depression:

Intermittent injection: Initial: Priming dose of 1-2 mg/kg, repeat after 5 minutes; may repeat at 1-2 hour intervals (until sustained consciousness); maximum: 3 g/day. May repeat in 24 hours if necessary.

I.V. infusion: Initial: Priming dose of 1-2 mg/kg, repeat after 5 minutes. If no response, wait 1-2 hours and repeat. If some stimulation is noted, initiate infusion at 1-3 mg/minute (depending on size of patient/depth of CNS depression); suspend infusion if patient begins to awaken. Infusion should not be continued for >2 hours. May reinstitute infusion as described above, including bolus, after rest interval of 30 minutes to 2 hours; maximum: 3 g/day

Acute hypercapnia secondary to COPD: I.V. infusion Initial: Initiate infusion at 1-2 mg/minute (depending on size of patient/depth of CNS depression); may increase to maximum rate of 3 mg/minute; infusion should not be continued for >2 hours. Monitor arterial blood gases prior to initiation of infusion and at 30-minute intervals during the infusion (to identify possible development of acidosis/ CO_2 retention). Additional infusions are not recommended (per manufacturer).

Additional Information Complete prescribing information for this medication should be consulted for additional detail.

Dosage Forms Excipient information presented when available (limited, particularly for generics); consult specific product labeling.

Injection, solution, as hydrochloride: 20 mg/mL (20 mL) [contains benzyl alcohol]

◆ **Doxapram Hydrochloride** *see* Doxapram *on page 482*

Doxazosin (doks AY zoe sin)

U.S. Brand Names Cardura®; Cardura® XL

Canadian Brand Names Alti-Doxazosin; Apo-Doxazosin®; Cardura-1™; Cardura-2™; Cardura-4™; Gen-Doxazosin; Novo-Doxazosin

Index Terms Doxazosin Mesylate

Pharmacologic Category Alpha$_1$ Blocker

Use Treatment of hypertension alone or in conjunction with diuretics, ACE inhibitors, beta-blockers, or calcium antagonists; treatment of urinary outflow obstruction and/or obstructive and irritative symptoms associated with benign prostatic hyperplasia (BPH), particularly useful in patients with troublesome symptoms who are unable or unwilling to undergo invasive procedures, but who require rapid symptomatic relief; can be used in combination with finasteride

Unlabeled/Investigational Use Pediatric hypertension

Pregnancy Risk Factor C

Pregnancy Considerations Some studies demonstrated embryolethality resulting from doxazosin exposure during organogenesis. Delayed postnatal development was also noted. There are no adequate and well-controlled studies in pregnant women. Use only if benefit outweighs risk.

Lactation Excretion in breast milk unknown/not recommended

Medication Safety Issues

Sound-alike/look-alike issues:

Doxazosin may be confused with doxapram, doxepin, DOXOrubicin

Cardura® may be confused with Cardene®, Cordarone®, Cordran®, Coumadin®, K-Dur®, Ridaura®

Contraindications Hypersensitivity to quinazolines (prazosin, terazosin), doxazosin, or any component of the formulation

Warnings/Precautions Can cause significant orthostatic hypotension and syncope, especially with first dose; anticipate a similar effect if therapy is interrupted for a few days, if dosage is rapidly increased, or if another antihypertensive drug (particularly vasodilators) or a PDE-5 inhibitor is introduced. Discontinue if symptoms of angina occur or worsen. Patients should be cautioned about performing hazardous tasks when starting new therapy or adjusting dosage upward. Prostate cancer should be ruled out before starting for BPH. Use with caution in mild to moderate hepatic impairment; not recommended in severe dysfunction. Intraoperative floppy iris syndrome has been observed in cataract surgery patients who were on or were previously treated with alpha$_1$-blockers. Causality has not been established and there appears to be no benefit in discontinuing alpha-blocker therapy prior to surgery. Safety and efficacy in children have not been established.

The extended release formulation consists of drug within a nondeformable matrix; following drug release/absorption, the matrix/shell is expelled in the stool. The use of nondeformable products in patients with known stricture/narrowing of the GI tract has been associated with symptoms of obstruction. Use caution in patients with increased GI retention (eg, chronic constipation) as doxazosin exposure may be increased. Extended release formulation is not approved for the treatment of hypertension.

Adverse Reactions Note: Type and frequency of adverse reactions reflect combined data from trials with immediate release and extended release products.

>10%: Central nervous system: Dizziness (5% to 19%), headache (5% to 14%)

1% to 10%:

Cardiovascular: Orthostatic hypotension (dose related; 0.3% up to 2%), edema (3% to 4%), hypotension (2%), palpitation (1% to 2%), chest pain (1% to 2%), arrhythmia (1%), syncope (2%), flushing (1%)

Central nervous system: Fatigue (8% to 12%), somnolence (1% to 5%), nervousness (2%), pain (2%), vertigo (2% to 4%), insomnia (1%), anxiety (1%), paresthesia (1%), movement disorder (1%), ataxia (1%), hypertonia (1%), depression (1%)

Dermatologic: Rash (1%), pruritus (1%)

Endocrine & metabolic: Sexual dysfunction (2%)

Gastrointestinal: Abdominal pain (2%), diarrhea (2%), dyspepsia (1% to 2%), nausea (1% to 3%), xerostomia (1% to 2%), constipation (1%), flatulence (1%)

Genitourinary: Urinary tract infection (1%), impotence (1%), polyuria (2%), incontinence (1%)

Neuromuscular & skeletal: Back pain (2% to 3%), weakness (1% to 7%), arthritis (1%), muscle weakness (1%), myalgia (≤1%), muscle cramps (1%)

Ocular: Abnormal vision (1% to 2%), conjunctivitis (1%)

Otic: Tinnitus (1%)

Respiratory: Respiratory tract infection (5%), rhinitis (3%), dyspnea (1% to 3%), respiratory disorder (1%), epistaxis (1%)

Miscellaneous: Diaphoresis increased (1%), flu-like syndrome (1%)

<1% (Limited to important or life-threatening): Abnormal thinking, agitation, allergic reaction, amnesia, angina, anorexia, bradycardia, breast pain, bronchospasm, cataplexy, cerebrovascular accident, cholestasis, confusion, depersonalization, emotional lability, enuresis, fecal incontinence, fever, gastroenteritis, gout, hematuria, hepatitis, hypoesthesia, hypokalemia, infection, intraoperative floppy iris syndrome (cataract surgery), jaundice, leukopenia, liver function tests increased, lymphadenopathy, MI, micturition abnormality, migraine, neutropenia, nocturia, pallor, paranoia, paresis, paresthesia, parosmia, peripheral ischemia, priapism, purpura, renal calculus, rigors stroke, syncope, systemic lupus erythematosus, tachycardia, thrombocytopenia, vomiting

Drug Interactions

Avoid Concomitant Use

Avoid concomitant use of Doxazosin with any of the following: Alfuzosin; Silodosin; Tamsulosin

Increased Effect/Toxicity

Doxazosin may increase the levels/effects of: Alfuzosin; Amifostine; Calcium Channel Blockers; RiTUXimab; Silodosin; Tamsulosin

The levels/effects of Doxazosin may be increased by: Alfuzosin; Beta-Blockers; Diazoxide; Herbs (Hypotensive Properties); Phosphodiesterase 5 Inhibitors; Prostacyclin Analogues; Silodosin; Tamsulosin

Decreased Effect

The levels/effects of Doxazosin may be decreased by: Herbs (Hypertensive Properties); Methylphenidate; Yohimbine

Ethanol/Nutrition/Herb Interactions Herb/Nutraceutical: Avoid dong quai if using for hypertension (has estrogenic activity). Avoid ephedra, yohimbe, ginseng (may worsen hypertension). Avoid saw palmetto when used for BPH (due to limited experience with this combination). Avoid garlic (may have increased antihypertensive effect).

Mechanism of Action
Hypertension: Competitively inhibits postsynaptic alpha$_1$-adrenergic receptors which results in vasodilation of veins and arterioles and a decrease in total peripheral resistance and blood pressure; ~50% as potent on a weight by weight basis as prazosin.

BPH: Competitively inhibits postsynaptic alpha$_1$-adrenergic receptors in prostatic stromal and bladder neck tissues. This reduces the sympathetic tone-induced urethral stricture causing BPH symptoms.

Pharmacodynamics/Kinetics Not significantly affected by increased age
Duration: >24 hours
Protein binding: Extended release: 98%
Metabolism: Extensively hepatic to active metabolites; primarily via CYP3A4; secondary pathways involve CYP2D6 and 2C19
Bioavailability: Extended release relative to immediate release: 54% to 59%
Half-life elimination: 15-22 hours
Time to peak, serum: Immediate release: 2-3 hours; extended release: 8-9 hours
Excretion: Feces (63% primarily as metabolites); urine (9%)

Dosage Oral:
Children (unlabeled use): Hypertension: Immediate release: Initial: 1 mg once daily; maximum: 4 mg/day
Adults:
Immediate release: 1 mg once daily in morning or evening; may be increased to 2 mg once daily. Thereafter titrate upwards, if needed, over several weeks, balancing therapeutic benefit with doxazosin-induced postural hypotension. In the elderly, initiate at 0.5 mg once daily
Hypertension: Maximum dose: 16 mg/day
BPH: Goal: 4-8 mg/day; maximum dose: 8 mg/day
Extended release: BPH: 4 mg once daily with breakfast; titrate based on response and tolerability every 3-4 weeks to maximum recommended dose of 8 mg/day
Reinitiation of therapy: If therapy is discontinued for several days, restart at 4 mg dose and titrate as before.
Conversion to extended release from immediate release: Initiate with 4 mg once daily; omit final evening dose of immediate release prior to starting morning dosing with extended release product.

Dosing adjustment in hepatic impairment: Use with caution in mild-to-moderate hepatic dysfunction. Do not use with severe impairment.

Dietary Considerations Cardura® XL: Take with morning meal.

Administration Cardura® XL: Tablets should be swallowed whole; do not crush, chew, or divide.

Monitoring Parameters Blood pressure, standing and sitting/supine; syncope may occur usually within 90 minutes of the initial dose

Additional Information First-dose hypotension occurs less frequently with doxazosin as compared to prazosin; this may be due to its slower onset of action.

Dosage Forms Excipient information presented when available (limited, particularly for generics); consult specific product labeling.
Tablet: 1 mg, 2 mg, 4 mg, 8 mg
Cardura®: 1 mg, 2 mg, 4 mg, 8 mg
Tablet, extended release:
Cardura® XL: 4 mg, 8 mg

◆ **Doxazosin Mesylate** *see* Doxazosin *on page* 483

Doxepin (DOKS e pin)

U.S. Brand Names Prudoxin™; Sinequan® [DSC]; Zonalon®

Canadian Brand Names Apo-Doxepin®; Novo-Doxepin; Sinequan®; Zonalon®

Index Terms Doxepin Hydrochloride

Pharmacologic Category Antidepressant, Tricyclic (Tertiary Amine); Topical Skin Product

Additional Appendix Information
Antidepressant Agents *on page* 1638

Use
Oral: Depression
Topical: Short-term (<8 days) management of moderate pruritus in adults with atopic dermatitis or lichen simplex chronicus

Unlabeled/Investigational Use Analgesic for certain chronic and neuropathic pain; anxiety

Restrictions An FDA-approved medication guide concerning the use of antidepressants in children, adolescents and young adults must be distributed when dispensing an outpatient prescription (new or refill) where this medication is to be used without direct supervision of a healthcare provider. Medication guides are available at http://www.fda.gov/cder/Offices/ODS/medication_guides.htm. Dispense to parents or guardians of children and adolescents receiving this medication.

Pregnancy Risk Factor B (cream); C (all other forms)

Pregnancy Considerations Teratogenic effects were not observed in animal studies; however, there are no adequate and well-controlled studies in pregnant women. Use during pregnancy only if clearly needed.

Lactation Enters breast milk/not recommended (AAP rates "of concern")

Medication Safety Issues
Sound-alike/look-alike issues:
Doxepin may be confused with digoxin, doxapram, doxazosin, Doxidan®, doxycycline
Sinequan® may be confused with saquinavir, Serentil®, Seroquel®, Singulair®
Zonalon® may be confused with Zone-A Forte®

International issues:
Doxal® [Finland] may be confused with Doxil® which is a brand name for doxorubicin in the U.S.
Doxal® [Finland]: Brand name for doxycycline in Austria; brand name for pyridoxine/thiamine in Brazil

Contraindications Hypersensitivity to doxepin, drugs from similar chemical class, or any component of the formulation; narrow-angle glaucoma; urinary retention; use of MAO inhibitors within 14 days; use in a patient during acute recovery phase of MI

Warnings/Precautions [U.S. Boxed Warning]: Antidepressants increase the risk of suicidal thinking and behavior in children, adolescents, and young adults (18-24 years of age) with major depressive disorder (MDD) and other psychiatric disorders; consider risk prior to prescribing. Short-term studies did not show an increased risk in patients >24 years of age and showed a decreased risk in patients ≥65 years. Closely monitor for clinical worsening, suicidality, or unusual changes in behavior; the patient's family or caregiver should be instructed to closely observe the patient and communicate condition with healthcare provider. A medication guide should be dispensed with each prescription. **Doxepin is approved for treatment of depression in adolescents.**

The possibility of a suicide attempt is inherent in major depression and may persist until remission occurs. Monitor for worsening of depression or suicidality, especially during initiation of therapy (generally first 1-2 months) or with dose increases or decreases. Use caution in high-risk patients. Worsening depression and severe abrupt suicidality that are not part of the presenting symptoms may require discontinuation or modification of drug therapy. The patient's family or caregiver should be alerted to monitor patients for the emergence of suicidality and associated behaviors (such as agitation, irritability, hostility, impulsivity, and hypomania) and call healthcare provider.

May worsen psychosis in some patients or precipitate a shift to mania or hypomania in patients with bipolar disorder. Patients presenting with depressive symptoms should be screened for bipolar disorder. Monotherapy in patients with bipolar disorder should be avoided. **Doxepin is not FDA approved for the treatment of bipolar depression.**

The risks of sedative and anticholinergic effects are high relative to other antidepressant agents. Doxepin frequently causes sedation, which may result in impaired performance of tasks requiring alertness (eg, operating machinery or driving). Sedative effects may be additive with other CNS depressants and/or ethanol. Also use caution in patients with benign prostatic hyperplasia, xerostomia, visual problems, constipation, or history of bowel obstruction.

May cause orthostatic hypotension or conduction disturbances (risks are moderate relative to other antidepressants). Use with caution in patients with a history of cardiovascular disease (including previous MI, stroke, tachycardia, or conduction abnormalities). Consider discontinuation, when possible, prior to elective surgery. Therapy should not be abruptly discontinued in patients receiving high doses for prolonged periods.

Use caution in patients with a previous seizure disorder or condition predisposing to seizures such as brain damage, alcoholism, or concurrent therapy with other drugs which lower the seizure threshold. Use with caution in hyperthyroid patients or those receiving thyroid supplementation. Use with caution in patients with hepatic or renal dysfunction and in elderly patients.

Cream formulation is for external use only (not for ophthalmic, vaginal, or oral use). Do not use occlusive dressings. Use for >8 days may increase risk of contact sensitization. Doxepin is significantly absorbed following topical administration; plasma levels may be similar to those achieved with oral administration.

Adverse Reactions

Oral: Frequency not defined.

Cardiovascular: Hyper-/hypotension, tachycardia

Central nervous system: Drowsiness, dizziness, headache, disorientation, ataxia, confusion, seizure

Dermatologic: Alopecia, photosensitivity, rash, pruritus

Endocrine & metabolic: Breast enlargement, galactorrhea, SIADH, blood sugar increased/decreased, libido increased/decreased

Gastrointestinal: Xerostomia, constipation, vomiting, indigestion, anorexia, aphthous stomatitis, nausea, unpleasant taste, weight gain, diarrhea, trouble with gums, lower esophageal sphincter tone decrease may cause GE reflux

Genitourinary: Urinary retention, testicular edema

Hematologic: Agranulocytosis, leukopenia, eosinophilia, thrombocytopenia, purpura

Neuromuscular & skeletal: Weakness, tremor, numbness, paresthesia, extrapyramidal symptoms, tardive dyskinesia

Ocular: Blurred vision

Otic: Tinnitus

Miscellaneous: Diaphoresis (excessive), allergic reactions

Topical:

>10%:

Central nervous system: Drowsiness (22%)

Dermatologic: Stinging/burning (23%)

1% to 10%:

Cardiovascular: Edema: (1%)

Central nervous system: Dizziness (2%), emotional changes (2%)

Gastrointestinal: Xerostomia (10%), taste alteration (2%)

<1% (Limited to important or life-threatening): Contact dermatitis, tongue numbness, anxiety

Drug Interactions

Metabolism/Transport Effects Substrate (major) of CYP1A2, 2D6, 3A4

Avoid Concomitant Use

Avoid concomitant use of Doxepin with any of the following: Iobenguane I 123; MAO Inhibitors; Nilotinib; Sibutramine; Tetrabenazine; Thioridazine; Ziprasidone

Increased Effect/Toxicity

Doxepin may increase the levels/effects of: Alcohol (Ethyl); Alpha-/Beta-Agonists (Direct-Acting); Alpha1-Agonists; Amphetamines; Anticholinergics; Aspirin; Beta2-Agonists; CNS Depressants; Desmopressin; NSAID (COX-2 Inhibitor); NSAID (Nonselective); QTc-Prolonging Agents; QuiNIDine; Serotonin Modulators; Sulfonylureas; Tetrabenazine; Thioridazine; TraMADol; Vitamin K Antagonists; Yohimbine; Ziprasidone

The levels/effects of Doxepin may be increased by: Alfuzosin; Altretamine; BuPROPion; Cimetidine; Cinacalcet; Ciprofloxacin; CYP1A2 Inhibitors (Moderate); CYP1A2 Inhibitors (Strong); CYP2D6 Inhibitors (Moderate); CYP2D6 Inhibitors (Strong); CYP3A4 Inhibitors (Moderate); CYP3A4 Inhibitors (Strong); Darunavir; Dasatinib; Dexmethylphenidate; DULoxetine; Gadobutrol; Lithium; MAO Inhibitors; Methylphenidate; Nilotinib; Pramlintide; Propoxyphene; Protease Inhibitors; QuiNIDine; Selective Serotonin Reuptake Inhibitors; Sibutramine; Terbinafine; Valproic Acid

Decreased Effect

Doxepin may decrease the levels/effects of: Acetylcholinesterase Inhibitors (Central); Alpha2-Agonists; Iobenguane I 123

The levels/effects of Doxepin may be decreased by: Acetylcholinesterase Inhibitors (Central); Barbiturates; CarBAMazepine; CYP1A2 Inducers (Strong); CYP3A4 Inducers (Strong); Deferasirox; St Johns Wort

Ethanol/Nutrition/Herb Interactions

Ethanol: Avoid ethanol (may increase CNS depression).

Food: Grapefruit juice may inhibit the metabolism of some TCAs and clinical toxicity may result.

Herb/Nutraceutical: Avoid valerian, St John's wort, SAMe, kava kava (may increase risk of serotonin syndrome and/or excessive sedation).

Stability Protect from light.

Mechanism of Action Increases the synaptic concentration of serotonin and norepinephrine in the central nervous system by inhibition of their reuptake by the presynaptic neuronal membrane

Pharmacodynamics/Kinetics

Onset of action: Peak effect: Antidepressant: Usually >2 weeks; Anxiolytic: may occur sooner

Absorption: Following topical application, plasma levels may be similar to those achieved with oral administration

Distribution: Crosses placenta; enters breast milk

Protein binding: 80% to 85%

Metabolism: Hepatic; metabolites include desmethyldoxepin (active)

Half-life elimination: Adults: 6-8 hours

Excretion: Urine

Dosage

Oral: Topical: Burning mouth syndrome (dental use): Cream: Apply 3-4 times daily

Oral (entire daily dose may be given at bedtime):

Depression or anxiety:

Children (unlabeled use): 1-3 mg/kg/day in single or divided doses

Adolescents: Initial: 25-50 mg/day in single or divided doses; gradually increase to 100 mg/day

Adults: Initial: 25-150 mg/day at bedtime or in 2-3 divided doses; may gradually increase up to 300 mg/day; single dose should not exceed 150 mg; select patients may respond to 25-50 mg/day

Elderly: Use a lower dose and adjust gradually

Chronic urticaria, angioedema, nocturnal pruritus: Adults and Elderly: 10-30 mg/day

Dosing adjustment in hepatic impairment: Use a lower dose and adjust gradually

Topical: Pruritus: Adults and Elderly: Apply a thin film 4 times/day with at least 3- to 4-hour interval between applications; not recommended for use >8 days. **Note:** Low-dose (25-50 mg) oral administration has also been used to treat pruritus, but systemic effects are increased.

Administration

Oral: Do not mix oral concentrate with carbonated beverages (physically incompatible).

Topical: Apply thin film to affected area; use of occlusive dressings is not recommended.

Monitoring Parameters Monitor blood pressure and pulse rate prior to and during initial therapy; monitor mental status, suicidal ideation (especially at the beginning of therapy or when doses are increased or decreased); weight; ECG in older adults; adverse effects may be increased if topical formulation is applied to >10% of body surface area

Reference Range Proposed therapeutic concentration (doxepin plus desmethyldoxepin): 110-250 ng/mL. Toxic concentration (doxepin plus desmethyldoxepin): >500 ng/mL. Utility of serum level monitoring is controversial.

Test Interactions Increased glucose

Dosage Forms Excipient information presented when available (limited, particularly for generics); consult specific product labeling. [DSC] = Discontinued product

Capsule, as hydrochloride: 10 mg, 25 mg, 50 mg, 75 mg, 100 mg, 150 mg

Sinequan®: 10 mg, 25 mg, 50 mg, 75 mg, 100 mg, 150 mg [DSC]

Cream, as hydrochloride:

Prudoxin™: 5% (45 g) [contains benzyl alcohol]

Zonalon®: 5% (30 g, 45 g) [contains benzyl alcohol]

Solution, oral concentrate, as hydrochloride: 10 mg/mL (120 mL)

Sinequan®: 10 mg/mL (120 mL) [DSC]

◆ **Doxepin Hydrochloride** *see* Doxepin *on page* 484

Doxercalciferol (doks er kal si fe FEER ole)

U.S. Brand Names Hectorol®

Canadian Brand Names Hectorol®

Index Terms 1α-Hydroxyergocalciferol

Pharmacologic Category Vitamin D Analog

Use Treatment of secondary hyperparathyroidism in patients with chronic kidney disease

Pregnancy Risk Factor B

Dosage

Oral:

Dialysis patients: Dose should be titrated to lower iPTH to 150-300 pg/mL; dose is adjusted at 8-week intervals (maximum dose: 20 mcg 3 times/week)

Initial dose: iPTH >400 pg/mL: 10 mcg 3 times/week at dialysis

Dose titration:

iPTH level decreased by 50% and >300 pg/mL: Dose can be increased to 12.5 mcg 3 times/week for 8 more weeks; this titration process can continue at 8-week intervals; each increase should be by 2.5 mcg/dose

iPTH level 150-300 pg/mL: Maintain current dose

iPTH level <100 pg/mL: Suspend doxercalciferol for 1 week; resume at a reduced dose; decrease each dose (not weekly dose) by at least 2.5 mcg

Predialysis patients: Dose should be titrated to lower iPTH to 35-70 pg/mL with stage 3 disease or to 70-110 pg/mL with stage 4 disease: Dose may be adjusted at 2-week intervals (maximum dose: 3.5 mcg/day)

Initial dose: 1 mcg/day

Dose titration:

iPTH level >70 pg/mL with stage 3 disease or >110 pg/mL with stage 4 disease: Increase dose by 0.5 mcg every 2 weeks as necessary

iPTH level 35-70 pg/mL with stage 3 disease or 70-110 pg/mL with stage 4 disease: Maintain current dose

iPTH level is <35 pg/mL with stage 3 disease or <70 pg/mL with stage 4 disease: Suspend doxercalciferol for 1 week, then resume at a reduced dose (at least 0.5 mcg lower)

I.V.:

Dialysis patients: Dose should be titrated to lower iPTH to 150-300 pg/mL; dose is adjusted at 8-week intervals (maximum dose: 18 mcg/week)

Initial dose: iPTH level >400 pg/mL: 4 mcg 3 times/week after dialysis, administered as a bolus dose

Dose titration:

iPTH level decreased by <50% and >300 pg/mL: Dose can be increased by 1-2 mcg at 8-week intervals, as necessary

iPTH level decreased by >50% and >300 pg/mL: Maintain current dose

iPTH level 150-300 pg/mL: Maintain the current dose

iPTH level <100 pg/mL: Suspend doxercalciferol for 1 week; resume at a reduced dose (at least 1 mcg lower)

Additional Information Complete prescribing information for this medication should be consulted for additional detail.

Dosage Forms Excipient information presented when available (limited, particularly for generics); consult specific product labeling.

Capsule, softgel:

Hectorol®: 0.5 mcg, 2.5 mcg [contains coconut oil]

Injection, solution:

Hectorol®: 2 mcg/mL (2 mL) [contains disodium edetate]

◆ **Doxidan® [OTC]** *see* Bisacodyl *on page* 198

◆ **Doxil®** *see* DOXOrubicin (Liposomal) *on page* 488

DOXOrubicin (doks oh ROO bi sin)

U.S. Brand Names Adriamycin®; Rubex® [DSC]

Canadian Brand Names Adriamycin®

Index Terms ADR (error-prone abbreviation); Adria; Doxorubicin Hydrochloride; Hydroxydaunomycin Hydrochloride; Hydroxyldaunorubicin Hydrochloride; NSC-123127

Pharmacologic Category Antineoplastic Agent, Anthracycline

Use Treatment of leukemias, lymphomas, multiple myeloma, osseous and nonosseous sarcomas, mesotheliomas, germ cell tumors of the ovary or testis, and carcinomas of the head and neck, thyroid, lung, breast, stomach, pancreas, liver, ovary, bladder, prostate, uterus, neuroblastoma, and Wilms' tumor.

Pregnancy Risk Factor D

Pregnancy Considerations Teratogenicity and embryotoxicity were observed in animal studies. There are no adequate and well-controlled studies in pregnant women. Advise patients to avoid becoming pregnant (females) and to avoid causing pregnancy (males) during treatment. According to the National Comprehensive Cancer Network (NCCN) breast cancer guidelines, doxorubicin, if indicated, may be administered to pregnant women with breast cancer as part of a combination chemotherapy regimen, although chemotherapy should not be administered during the first trimester or after 35 weeks gestation.

Lactation Enters breast milk/not recommended

Medication Safety Issues

Sound-alike/look-alike issues:

DOXOrubicin may be confused with DACTINomycin, DAUNOrubicin, DAUNOrubicin liposomal, doxacurium, doxapram, doxazosin, DOXOrubicin liposomal, epirubicin, IDArubicin

Adriamycin PFS® may be confused with achromycin, Aredia®, Idamycin®

Conventional formulation (Adriamycin PFS®, Adriamycin RDF®) may be confused with the liposomal formulation (Doxil®)

Use caution when selecting product for preparation and dispensing; indications, dosages and adverse event profiles differ between conventional DOXOrubicin hydrochloride solution and DOXOrubicin liposomal. Both formulations are the same concentration. As a result, serious errors have occurred.

High alert medication: The Institute for Safe Medication Practices (ISMP) includes this medication among its list of drug classes which have a heightened risk of causing significant patient harm when used in error.

ADR is an error-prone abbreviation

International issues:

Doxil® may be confused with Doxal® which is a brand name for doxepin in Finland, a brand name for doxycycline in Austria, and a brand name for pyridoxine/thiamine combination in Brazil

Rubex®: Brand name for ascorbic acid in Ireland

Contraindications Hypersensitivity to doxorubicin, any component of the formulation, or to other anthracyclines or anthracenediones; recent MI, severe myocardial insufficiency, severe arrhythmia; previous therapy with high cumulative doses of doxorubicin, daunorubicin, idarubicin, or other anthracycline and anthracenediones; baseline neutrophil count <1500/mm^3; severe hepatic impairment

Warnings/Precautions Hazardous agent - use appropriate precautions for handling and disposal. **[U.S. Boxed Warning]: May cause cumulative, dose-related, myocardial toxicity (early or delayed).** Cardiotoxicity is dose-limiting. Total cumulative dose should take into account previous or concomitant treatment with cardiotoxic agents or irradiation of chest. The incidence of irreversible myocardial toxicity increases as the total cumulative (lifetime) dosages approach 450-500 mg/m^2. Although the risk increases with cumulative dose, irreversible cardiotoxicity may occur at any dose level. Patients with pre-existing heart disease, hypertension, concurrent administration of other antineoplastic agents, prior or concurrent chest irradiation, advanced age; and infants and children are at increased risk. Alternative administration schedules (weekly or continuous infusions) have are associated with less cardiotoxicity Baseline and periodic monitoring of ECG and LVEF (with either ECHO or MUGA scan) is recommended. **[U.S. Boxed Warnings]: Reduce dose in patients with impaired hepatic function; dose-limiting severe myelosuppression (primarily leukopenia and neutropenia) may occur. Secondary acute myelogenous leukemia and myelodysplastic syndrome have been reported following treatment.** May cause tumor lysis syndrome and hyperuricemia (in patients with rapidly growing tumors).

Children are at increased risk for developing delayed cardiotoxicity; follow-up cardiac function monitoring is recommended. Doxorubicin may contribute to prepubertal growth failure in children; may also contribute to gonadal impairment (usually temporary). Radiation recall pneumonitis has been reported in children receiving concomitant dactinomycin and doxorubicin. **[U.S. Boxed Warnings]: For I.V. administration only. Potent vesicant; if extravasation occurs, severe local tissue damage leading to ulceration, necrosis, and pain may occur. Should be administered under the supervision of an experienced cancer chemotherapy physician.**

Adverse Reactions Frequency not defined.

Cardiovascular:

Acute cardiotoxicity: Atrioventricular block, bradycardia, bundle branch block, ECG abnormalities, extrasystoles (atrial or ventricular), sinus tachycardia, ST-T wave changes, supraventricular tachycardia, tachyarrhythmia, ventricular tachycardia

Delayed cardiotoxicity: LVEF decreased, CHF (manifestations include ascites, cardiomegaly, dyspnea, edema, gallop rhythm, hepatomegaly, oliguria, pleural effusion, pulmonary edema, tachycardia); myocarditis, pericarditis

Central nervous system: Malaise

Dermatologic: Alopecia, itching, photosensitivity, radiation recall, rash; discoloration of saliva, sweat, or tears

Endocrine & metabolic: Amenorrhea, dehydration, infertility (may be temporary), hyperuricemia

Gastrointestinal: Abdominal pain, anorexia, colon necrosis, diarrhea, GI ulceration, mucositis, nausea, vomiting

Genitourinary: Discoloration of urine

Hematologic: Leukopenia/neutropenia (75%; nadir: 10-14 days; recovery: by day 21); thrombocytopenia and anemia

Local: Skin "flare" at injection site, urticaria

Neuromuscular & skeletal: Weakness

Postmarketing and/or case reports: Anaphylaxis, azoospermia, bilirubin increased, chills, coma (when in combination with cisplatin or vincristine), conjunctivitis, fever, gonadal impairment (children), growth failure (prepubertal), hepatitis, hyperpigmentation (nail, skin & oral mucosa), infection, keratitis, lacrimation, myelodysplastic syndrome, neutropenic fever, oligospermia, onycholysis, peripheral neurotoxicity (with intra-arterial doxorubicin), phlebosclerosis, radiation recall pneumonitis (children), secondary acute myelogenous leukemia, seizure (when in combination with cisplatin or vincristine), sepsis, shock, systemic hypersensitivity (including urticaria, pruritus, angioedema, dysphagia, and dyspnea), transaminases increased, urticaria

Drug Interactions

Metabolism/Transport Effects Substrate (major) of CYP2D6, 3A4; **Inhibits** CYP2B6 (moderate), 2D6 (weak), 3A4 (weak)

Avoid Concomitant Use

Avoid concomitant use of DOXOrubicin with any of the following: Natalizumab; Vaccines (Live)

Increased Effect/Toxicity

DOXOrubicin may increase the levels/effects of: CYP2B6 Substrates; Natalizumab; Vaccines (Live); Vitamin K Antagonists; Zidovudine

The levels/effects of DOXOrubicin may be increased by: Bevacizumab; CycloSPORINE; CYP2D6 Inhibitors (Moderate); CYP2D6 Inhibitors (Strong); CYP3A4 Inhibitors (Moderate); CYP3A4 Inhibitors (Strong); Darunavir; Dasatinib; P-Glycoprotein Inhibitors; Sorafenib; Taxane Derivatives; Trastuzumab

Decreased Effect

DOXOrubicin may decrease the levels/effects of: Cardiac Glycosides; Dabigatran Etexilate; P-Glycoprotein Substrates; Stavudine; Vaccines (Inactivated); Vitamin K Antagonists; Zidovudine

The levels/effects of DOXOrubicin may be decreased by: Cardiac Glycosides; CYP3A4 Inducers (Strong);

Deferasirox; Echinacea; Herbs (CYP3A4 Inducers); P-Glycoprotein Inducers

Ethanol/Nutrition/Herb Interactions Herb/Nutraceutical: Avoid St John's wort (may decrease doxorubicin levels). Avoid black cohosh, dong quai in estrogen-dependent tumors.

Stability Store intact vials of solution under refrigeration (2°C to 8°C) and protect from light; store intact vials of lyophilized powder at room temperature (15°C to 30°C). Reconstitute lyophilized powder with NS to a final concentration of 2 mg/mL. Reconstituted vials are stable for 7 days at room temperature (25°C) and 15 days under refrigeration (5°C) when protected from light. Infusions are stable for 48 hours at room temperature (25°C) when protected from light. Solutions diluted in 50-1000 mL D_5W or NS are stable for 48 hours at room temperature (25°C) when protected from light.

Unstable in solutions with a pH <3 or >7.

Mechanism of Action Inhibition of DNA and RNA synthesis by intercalation between DNA base pairs by inhibition of topoisomerase II and by steric obstruction. Doxorubicin intercalates at points of local uncoiling of the double helix. Although the exact mechanism is unclear, it appears that direct binding to DNA (intercalation) and inhibition of DNA repair (topoisomerase II inhibition) result in blockade of DNA and RNA synthesis and fragmentation of DNA. Doxorubicin is also a powerful iron chelator; the iron-doxorubicin complex can bind DNA and cell membranes and produce free radicals that immediately cleave the DNA and cell membranes.

Pharmacodynamics/Kinetics

Absorption: Oral: Poor (<50%)

Distribution: V_d: 809-1214 L/m^2; to many body tissues, particularly liver, spleen, kidney, lung, heart; does not distribute into the CNS; crosses placenta

Protein binding, plasma: 70% to 76%

Metabolism: Primarily hepatic to doxorubicinol (active), then to inactive aglycones, conjugated sulfates, and glucuronides

Half-life elimination:

Distribution: 5-10 minutes

Elimination: Doxorubicin: 1-3 hours; Metabolites: 3-3.5 hours

Terminal: 17-48 hours

Male: 54 hours; Female: 35 hours

Excretion: Feces (~40% to 50% as unchanged drug); urine (~5% to 12% as unchanged drug and metabolites)

Clearance: Male: 113 L/hour; Female: 44 L/hour

Dosage I.V.: Refer to individual protocols. **Note:** Lower dosage should be considered for patients with inadequate marrow reserve (due to old age, prior treatment or neoplastic marrow infiltration)

Children:

35-75 mg/m^2/dose every 21 days **or**

20-30 mg/m^2/dose once weekly **or**

60-90 mg/m^2/dose given as a continuous infusion over 96 hours every 3-4 weeks

Adults: Usual or typical dose: 60-75 mg/m^2/dose every 21 days **or**

60 mg/m^2/dose every 2 weeks (dose dense) **or**

40-60 mg/m^2/dose every 3-4 weeks **or**

20-30 mg/m^2/day for 2-3 days every 4 weeks **or**

20 mg/m^2/dose once weekly

Dosing adjustment in toxicity: The following delays and/or dose reductions have been used:

Neutropenic fever/infection: Consider reducing to 75% of dose in subsequent cycles

ANC <1000/mm^3: Delay treatment until ANC recovers to ≥1000/mm^3

Platelets <100,000/mm^3: Delay treatment until platelets recover to ≥100,000/mm^3

Dosing adjustment in renal impairment: Adjustments are not required.

Hemodialysis: Supplemental dose is not necessary.

Dosing adjustment in hepatic impairment:

The FDA-approved labeling recommends the following adjustments:

Serum bilirubin 1.2-3 mg/dL: Administer 50% of dose

Serum bilirubin 3.1-5 mg/dL: Administer 25% of dose

Severe hepatic impairment: Use is contraindicated

The following guidelines have been used by some clinicians: Floyd, 2006:

Transaminases 2-3 times ULN: Administer 75% of dose

Transaminases >3 times ULN or serum bilirubin 1.2-3 mg/dL: Administer 50% of dose

Serum bilirubin 3.1-5 mg/dL: Administer 25% of dose

Serum bilirubin >5 mg/dL: Do not administer

Administration Administer I.V. push over at least 3-5 minutes, IVPB over 15-60 minutes, or continuous infusion.

Monitoring Parameters CBC with differential and platelet count; liver function tests (bilirubin, ALT/AST, alkaline phosphatase); serum uric acid, calcium, potassium, phosphate and creatinine; cardiac function (baseline, periodic, and followup): ECG, left ventricular ejection fraction (echocardiography [ECHO] or multigated radionuclide angiography [MUGA])

Dosage Forms Excipient information presented when available (limited, particularly for generics); consult specific product labeling.

Injection, powder for reconstitution, as hydrochloride: 10 mg, 50 mg

Adriamycin®: 10 mg, 20 mg, 50 mg, [contains lactose]

Rubex®: 50 mg, 100 mg [contains lactose] [DSC]

Injection, solution, as hydrochloride: 2 mg/mL (5 mL, 10 mL, 25 mL, 100 mL)

Adriamycin®: 2 mg/mL (5 mL, 10 mL, 25 mL, 100 mL)

◆ **Doxorubicin Hydrochloride** *see* DOXOrubicin *on page 486*

◆ **DOXOrubicin Hydrochloride (Liposomal)** *see* DOXOrubicin (Liposomal) *on page 488*

◆ **DOXOrubicin Hydrochloride Liposome** *see* DOXOrubicin (Liposomal) *on page 488*

DOXOrubicin (Liposomal)

(doks oh ROO bi sin lip pah SOW mal)

U.S. Brand Names Doxil®

Canadian Brand Names Caelyx®

Index Terms DOXOrubicin Hydrochloride (Liposomal); DOXOrubicin Hydrochloride Liposome; Liposomal DOXOrubicin; Pegylated DOXOrubicin Liposomal; Pegylated Liposomal DOXOrubicin

Pharmacologic Category Antineoplastic Agent, Anthracycline

Use Treatment of ovarian cancer, multiple myeloma, and AIDS-related Kaposi's sarcoma

Unlabeled/Investigational Use Treatment of metastatic breast cancer, Hodgkin's lymphoma, cutaneous T-cell lymphomas (mycosis fungoides and Sézary syndrome), advanced soft tissue sarcomas

Pregnancy Risk Factor D

Pregnancy Considerations May cause fetal harm if administered during pregnancy. There are no adequate and well-controlled studies in pregnant women. Women of childbearing potential should avoid becoming pregnant during treatment.

Lactation Excretion in breast milk unknown/contraindicated

Medication Safety Issues

Sound-alike/look-alike issues:

DOXOrubicin liposomal may be confused with DACTINomycin, DAUNOrubicin, DAUNOrubicin liposomal, doxacurium, doxapram, doxazosin, DOXOrubicin, epirubicin, IDArubicin

DOXOrubicin liposomal may be confused with DAUNOrubicin liposomal

Doxil® may be confused with Doxy®, Paxil®

Liposomal formulation (Doxil®) may be confused with the conventional formulation (Adriamycin PFS®, Adriamycin RDF®)

High alert medication: The Institute for Safe Medication Practices (ISMP) includes this medication among its list of drug classes which have a heightened risk of causing significant patient harm when used in error.

Use caution when selecting product for preparation and dispensing; indications, dosages and adverse event profiles differ between conventional DOXOrubicin hydrochloride solution and DOXOrubicin liposomal. Both formulations are the same concentration. As a result, serious errors have occurred. Liposomal formulation of doxorubicin should NOT be substituted for doxorubicin hydrochloride on a mg-per-mg basis.

Contraindications Hypersensitivity to doxorubicin liposomal, conventional doxorubicin, or any component of the formulation; breast-feeding

Warnings/Precautions Hazardous agent - use appropriate precautions for handling and disposal.

[U.S. Boxed Warning]: Doxorubicin may cause cumulative, dose-related myocardial toxicity (concurrent or delayed). Doxorubicin liposomal should be used with caution in patients with high cumulative doses of any anthracycline. Total cumulative dose should also account for previous or concomitant treatment with other cardiotoxic agents or irradiation of chest. The incidence of irreversible myocardial toxicity increases as the total cumulative (lifetime) dosages approach 450-550 mg/m^2; or 400 mg/m^2 in patients who have received prior mediastinal radiation therapy or concurrent therapy with other cardiotoxic agents (eg, cyclophosphamide). Although the risk increases with cumulative dose, irreversible cardiotoxicity may occur with anthracycline treatment at any dose level. Patients with pre-existing heart disease, hypertension, concurrent administration of other antineoplastic agents, prior or concurrent chest irradiation, and advanced age are at increased risk. Evaluate left ventricular ejection fraction (LVEF) prior to treatment and periodically during treatment. The onset of symptoms of anthracycline-induced HF and/or cardiomyopathy may be delayed.

[U.S. Boxed Warning]: Acute infusion reactions may occur, some may be serious/life-threatening, including fatal allergic/anaphylactoid-like reactions. Infusion reactions typically occur with the first infusion and may include flushing, dyspnea, facial swelling, headache, chills, back pain, hypotension, and/or tightness of chest/throat. Reactions usually resolve with termination of infusion, or in some cases, slowing the infusion rate. Medication for the treatment of reactions should be readily available in the event of severe reactions. Infuse doxorubicin liposomal at 1 mg/minute initially to minimize risk of infusion reaction.

[U.S. Boxed Warning]: Use with caution in patients with hepatic impairment; dosage reduction is recommended. Use in patients with hepatic impairment has not been adequately studied; dosing adjustment recommendations in multiple myeloma patients with hepatic impairment is not available. **[U.S. Boxed Warning]: Severe myelosuppression may occur.** Palmar-plantar erythrodysesthesia (hand-foot syndrome) has been reported in up to 51% of patients with ovarian cancer, 19% of patients with multiple myeloma, and ~3% in patients with Kaposi's sarcoma. May occur early in treatment, but is usually seen after 2-3 treatment cycles. Dosage modification may be required. In severe cases, treatment discontinuation may be required. **[U.S. Boxed Warning]: Liposomal formulations of doxorubicin should NOT be substituted for conventional doxorubicin hydrochloride on a mg-per-mg basis.**

Doxorubicin may potentiate the toxicity of cyclophosphamide (hemorrhagic cystitis) and mercaptopurine (hepatotoxicity). Radiation recall reaction has been reported with doxorubicin liposomal treatment after radiation therapy. Radiation-induced toxicity (to the myocardium, mucosa, skin, and liver) may be increased by doxorubicin. Safety and efficacy in children have not been established.

Adverse Reactions

>10%:

Cardiovascular: Peripheral edema (≤11%)

Central nervous system: Fever (8% to 21%), headache (≤11%), pain (≤21%)

Dermatologic: Palmar-plantar erythrodysesthesia/hand-foot syndrome (≤51% in ovarian cancer [grades 3/4: 24%]; 3% in Kaposi's sarcoma), rash (≤29% in ovarian cancer, ≤5% in Kaposi's sarcoma), alopecia (9% to 19%)

Gastrointestinal: Nausea (17% to 46%), stomatitis (5% to 41%), vomiting (8% to 33%), constipation (≤30%), diarrhea (5% to 21%), anorexia (≤20%), mucositis (≤14%), dyspepsia (≤12%), intestinal obstruction (≤11%)

Hematologic: Myelosuppression (onset: 7 days; nadir: 10-14 days; recovery: 21-28 days), thrombocytopenia (13% to 65%; grades 3/4: 1%), neutropenia (12% to 62%; grade 4: 4%), leukopenia (36%), anemia (6% to 74%; grade 4: <1%)

Neuromuscular & skeletal: Weakness (7% to 40%), back pain (≤12%)

Respiratory: Pharyngitis (≤16%), dyspnea (≤15%)

Miscellaneous: Infection (≤12%)

1% to 10%:

Cardiovascular: Cardiac arrest, chest pain, deep thrombophlebitis, edema, hypotension, pallor, tachycardia, vasodilation

Central nervous system: Agitation, anxiety, chills, confusion, depression, dizziness, emotional lability, insomnia, somnolence, vertigo

Dermatologic: Acne, bruising, dry skin (6%), exfoliative dermatitis, fungal dermatitis, furunculosis, maculopapular rash, pruritus, skin discoloration, vesiculobullous rash

Endocrine & metabolic: Dehydration, hypercalcemia, hyperglycemia, hypokalemia, hyponatremia

Gastrointestinal: Abdomen enlarged, anorexia, ascites, cachexia, dyspepsia, dysphagia, esophagitis, flatulence, gingivitis, glossitis, ileus, mouth ulceration, oral moniliasis, rectal bleeding, taste perversion, weight loss, xerostomia

Genitourinary: Cystitis, dysuria, leukorrhea, pelvic pain, polyuria, urinary incontinence, urinary tract infection, urinary urgency, vaginal bleeding, vaginal moniliasis

Hematologic: Hemolysis, prothrombin time increased

Hepatic: ALT increased, alkaline phosphatase increased, hyperbilirubinemia

Local: Thrombophlebitis

Neuromuscular & skeletal: Arthralgia, hypertonia, myalgia, neuralgia, neuritis (peripheral), neuropathy, paresthesia (≤10%), pathological fracture

Ocular: Conjunctivitis, dry eyes, retinitis

Otic: Ear pain

Renal: Albuminuria, hematuria

Respiratory: Apnea, cough (≤10%), epistaxis, pleural effusion, pneumonia, rhinitis, sinusitis

Miscellaneous: Allergic reaction; infusion-related reactions (7%; includes bronchospasm, chest tightness, chills, dyspnea, facial edema, flushing, headache, herpes simplex/zoster, hypotension, pruritus); moniliasis, diaphoresis

<1% (Limited to important or life-threatening): Abscess, acute brain syndrome, abnormal vision, acute myeloid leukemia (secondary), alkaline phosphatase increased, anaphylactic or anaphylactoid reaction, asthma, balanitis, blindness, bone pain, bronchitis, BUN increased, bundle branch block, cardiomegaly, cardiomyopathy, cellulitis, CHF, colitis, creatinine increased, cryptococcosis, diabetes mellitus, erythema multiforme, erythema nodosum, eosinophilia, fecal impaction, flu-like syndrome, gastritis, glucosuria, hemiplegia, hemorrhage, hepatic failure, hepatitis, hepatosplenomegaly, hyperkalemia, hypernatremia, hyperuricemia, hyperventilation, hypoglycemia, hypolipidemia, hypomagnesemia, hypophosphatemia, hypoproteinemia, hypothermia, injection site hemorrhage, injection site pain, jaundice, ketosis, lactic dehydrogenase increased, kidney failure, lymphadenopathy, lymphangitis, migraine, myositis, optic neuritis, palpitation, pancreatitis, pericardial effusion, petechia, pneumothorax, pulmonary embolism, radiation injury, sclerosing cholangitis, seizure, sepsis, skin necrosis, skin ulcer, syncope, Stevens-Johnson syndrome, tenesmus, thromboplastin decreased, thrombosis, tinnitus, toxic epidermal necrolysis, urticaria, visual field defect, ventricular arrhythmia

Drug Interactions

Metabolism/Transport Effects Substrate (major) of CYP2D6, 3A4; **Inhibits** CYP2B6 (moderate), 2D6 (weak), 3A4 (weak)

Avoid Concomitant Use

Avoid concomitant use of DOXOrubicin (Liposomal) with any of the following: Natalizumab; Vaccines (Live)

Increased Effect/Toxicity

DOXOrubicin (Liposomal) may increase the levels/effects of: CYP2B6 Substrates; Natalizumab; Vaccines (Live); Zidovudine

The levels/effects of DOXOrubicin (Liposomal) may be increased by: Bevacizumab; CYP2D6 Inhibitors (Moderate); CYP2D6 Inhibitors (Strong); CYP3A4 Inhibitors (Moderate); CYP3A4 Inhibitors (Strong); Darunavir; Dasatinib; Taxane Derivatives; Trastuzumab

Decreased Effect

DOXOrubicin (Liposomal) may decrease the levels/effects of: Cardiac Glycosides; Stavudine; Vaccines (Inactivated); Zidovudine

The levels/effects of DOXOrubicin (Liposomal) may be decreased by: Cardiac Glycosides; CYP3A4 Inducers (Strong); Deferasirox; Echinacea; Herbs (CYP3A4 Inducers)

Ethanol/Nutrition/Herb Interactions

Ethanol: Avoid ethanol (due to GI irritation).

Herb/Nutraceutical: St John's wort may decrease doxorubicin levels.

Stability Store intact vials of solution under refrigeration at 2°C to 8°C (36°F to 46°F); avoid freezing. Prolonged freezing may adversely affect liposomal drug products, however, short-term freezing (<1 month) does not appear to have a deleterious effect.

Doses of doxorubicin liposomal ≤90 mg must be diluted in 250 mL of D_5W prior to administration. Doses >90 mg should be diluted in 500 mL D_5W. Solution is not a clear, but has a red, translucent appearance due to the liposomal dispersion. Use appropriate precautions for handling and disposal. Diluted doxorubicin hydrochloride liposome injection may be refrigerated at 2°C to 8°C (36°F to 46°F); administer within 24 hours. **Do not infuse with in-line filters.**

Mechanism of Action Doxorubicin inhibits DNA and RNA synthesis by intercalating between DNA base pairs causing steric obstruction and inhibits topoisomerase-II at the point of DNA cleavage. Doxorubicin is also a powerful iron chelator. The iron-doxorubicin complex can bind DNA and cell membranes, producing free hydroxyl (OH) radicals that cleave DNA and cell membranes. Active throughout entire cell cycle. Doxorubicin liposomal is a pegylated formulation which protects the liposomes, and thereby increases blood circulation time.

Pharmacodynamics/Kinetics

Distribution: V_{dss}: 2.7-2.8 L/m^2

Protein binding, plasma: Unknown; nonliposomal (conventional) doxorubicin: 70%

Half-life elimination: Terminal: Distribution: 4.7-5.2 hours, Elimination: 44-55 hours

Metabolism: Hepatic and in plasma to doxorubicinol and the sulfate and glucuronide conjugates of 4-demethyl,7-deoxyaglycones

Excretion: Urine (5% as doxorubicin or doxorubicinol)

Dosage Details concerning dosing in combination regimens should also be consulted. **Liposomal formulations of doxorubicin should NOT be substituted for conventional doxorubicin hydrochloride on a mg-per-mg basis.**

AIDS-related Kaposi's sarcoma: I.V.: 20 mg/m^2/dose once every 3 weeks

Multiple myeloma: I.V.: 30 mg/m^2/dose every 3 weeks (in combination with bortezomib) **or**

Unlabeled dosing: I .V.: 40 mg/m^2/dose every 4 weeks (in combination with vincristine and dexamethasone) (Rifkin, 2006)

Ovarian cancer: I.V.: 50 mg/m^2/dose every 4 weeks (minimum of 4 cycles is recommended)

Breast cancer (unlabeled use): I.V.: 50 mg/m^2/dose every 4 weeks (Keller, 2004)

Dosing adjustment in hepatic impairment: Note: Dosage adjustment information is not available in patients with multiple myeloma.

Bilirubin 1.2-3 mg/dL: Administer 50% of dose

Bilirubin >3 mg/dL: Administer 25% of dose

Dosing Adjustment for Toxicity in Treatment with Bortezomib (for Multiple Myeloma) (see Bortezomib monograph for bortezomib dosage reduction with toxicity guidelines):

Fever ≥38°C and ANC <1000/mm^3: If prior to doxorubicin liposomal treatment (day 4), do not administer; if after doxorubicin liposomal administered, reduce dose by 25% in next cycle.

ANC <500/mm^3, platelets <25,000/mm^3, hemoglobin <8 g/dL: If prior to doxorubicin liposomal treatment (day 4); do not administer; if after doxorubicin liposomal administered, reduce dose by 25% in next cycle if bortezomib dose reduction occurred for hematologic toxicity.

Grade 3 or 4 nonhematologic toxicity: Delay dose until resolved to grade <2; reduce dose by 25% for all subsequent doses.

Neuropathic pain or peripheral neuropathy: No dose reductions needed for doxorubicin liposomal, refer to Bortezomib monograph for bortezomib dosing adjustment.

Dosing adjustment for toxicity:

Recommended Dose Modification Guidelines

Toxicity Grade	Dose Adjustment
HAND FOOT SYNDROME (HFS)	
1 (Mild erythema, swelling, or desquamation not interfering with daily activities)	Redose unless patient has experienced previous Grade 3 or 4 HFS toxicity. If so, delay up to 2 weeks and decrease dose by 25%; return to original dosing interval.
2 (Erythema, desquamation, or swelling interfering with, but not precluding, normal physical activities; small blisters or ulcerations <2 cm in diameter)	Delay dosing up to 2 weeks or until resolved to Grade 0-1. If after 2 weeks there is no resolution, discontinue liposomal doxorubicin. Otherwise, if no prior Grade 3-4 HFS, continue treatment at previous dose and dosage interval. If a prior Grade 3-4 HFS has occurred, continue prior dosage interval, but decrease dose by 25%.
3 (Blistering, ulceration, or swelling interfering with walking or normal daily activities; cannot wear regular clothing)	Delay dosing up to 2 weeks or until resolved to Grade 0-1. Decrease dose by 25% and return to original dosing interval; if after 2 weeks there is no resolution, discontinue liposomal doxorubicin.
4 (Diffuse or local process causing infectious complications, or a bedridden state or hospitalization)	Delay dosing up to 2 weeks or until resolved to Grade 0-1. Decrease dose by 25% and return to original dosing interval. If after 2 weeks there is no resolution, discontinue liposomal doxorubicin.
STOMATITIS	
1 (Painless ulcers, erythema, or mild soreness)	Redose unless patient has experienced previous Grade 3 or 4 toxicity. If so, delay up to 2 weeks and decrease by 25%. Return to original dosing interval.
2 (Painful erythema, edema, or ulcers, but can eat)	Delay dosing up to 2 weeks or until resolved to Grade 0-1. If after 2 weeks there is no resolution, discontinue liposomal doxorubicin. Otherwise, if not prior Grade 3-4 stomatitis, continue treatment at previous dose and dosage interval. If prior Grade 3-4 toxicity, continue treatment with previous dosage interval, but decrease dose by 25%.
3 (Painful erythema, edema, or ulcers, and cannot eat)	Delay dosing up to 2 weeks or until resolved to Grade 0-1. Decrease dose by 25% and return to original dosing interval. If after 2 weeks there is no resolution, discontinue liposomal doxorubicin.
4 (Requires parenteral or enteral support)	Delay dosing up to 2 weeks or until resolved to Grade 0-1. Decrease dose by 25% and return to original dosing interval. If after 2 weeks there is no resolution, discontinue liposomal doxorubicin.

See table: "Hematological Toxicity"

Hematological Toxicity (see below for multiple myeloma)

Grade	ANC	Platelets	Modification
1	1500-1900	75,000-150,000	Resume treatment with no dose reduction.
2	1000-<1500	50,000-<75,000	Wait until ANC ≥1500 and platelets ≥75,000; redose with no dose reduction.
3	500-999	25,000-<50,000	Wait until ANC ≥1500 and platelets ≥75,000; redose with no dose reduction.
4	<500	<25,000	Wait until ANC ≥1500 and platelets ≥75,000; redose at 25% dose reduction or continue full dose with cytokine support.

Administration Administer IVPB over 60 minutes; manufacturer recommends administering at initial rate of 1 mg/minute to minimize risk of infusion reactions until the absence of a reaction has been established, then increase the infusion rate for completion over 1 hour. **Do not administer I.M. or SubQ. Do not infuse with in-line filters.** Avoid extravasation (irritant), monitor site; extravasation may occur without stinging or burning. Flush with 5-10 mL of D_5W solution before and after drug administration (do not rapidly flush through the I.V. line), incompatible with heparin flushes. Monitor for local erythematous streaking along vein and/or facial flushing (may indicate rapid infusion rate).

Monitoring Parameters CBC with differential and platelet count, liver function tests (ALT/AST, bilirubin, alkaline phosphatase); monitor for infusion reactions

Cardiac function (left ventricular ejection fraction [LVEF]), should be carefully monitored; echocardiography, or MUGA scan may be used. Endomyocardial biopsy is the most definitive test for anthracycline myocardial injury.

Additional Information Oncology Comment: Pegylated liposomal doxorubicin is listed within National Comprehensive Cancer Network® (NCCN) guidelines for the treatment of the following types of malignancies:

Breast cancer: As a preferred single-agent therapy for recurrent or metastatic breast cancer

Hodgkin's lymphoma: As second-line chemotherapy (in combination with gemcitabine and vinorelbine)

Non-Hodgkin's lymphomas: As a first-line systemic treatment for cutaneous T-cell lymphomas, mycosis fungoides, and Sezary syndrome, in patients with generalized tumor disease or tumor disease with blood involvement

Ovarian cancer: As a preferred agent for recurrent ovarian cancer

Multiple myeloma: As primary induction therapy for both transplant candidates and nontransplant candidates (in combination with vincristine and dexamethasone), and as salvage therapy (in combination with bortezomib)

Soft tissue sarcoma: As a systemic single-agent treatment for metastatic disease for extremity, retroperitoneal, or intra-abdominal (other than GIST) soft tissue sarcomas

Dosage Forms Excipient information presented when available (limited, particularly for generics); consult specific product labeling.

Injection, solution, as hydrochloride:

Doxil®: 2 mg/mL (10 mL, 25 mL)

◆ **Doxy-100®** *see* Doxycycline *on page 491*

◆ **Doxycin (Can)** *see* Doxycycline *on page 491*

Doxycycline (doks i SYE kleen)

U.S. Brand Names Adoxa®; Doryx®; Doxy-100®; Monodox®; Oracea™; Periostat®; Vibra-Tabs®; Vibramycin®

Canadian Brand Names Apo-Doxy Tabs®; Apo-Doxy®; Doxycin; Doxytec; Novo-Doxylin; Nu-Doxycycline; Periostat®; Vibra-Tabs®

Index Terms Doxycycline Calcium; Doxycycline Hyclate; Doxycycline Monohydrate

Pharmacologic Category Antibiotic, Tetracycline Derivative

Additional Appendix Information

Animal and Human Bites *on page 1747*

Antimicrobial Drugs of Choice *on page 1752*

Community-Acquired Pneumonia in Adults *on page 1766*

Malaria Treatment *on page 1770*

Prevention of Wound Infection and Sepsis in Surgical Patients *on page 1738*

Treatment of Sexually Transmitted Infections *on page 1773*

Use Principally in the treatment of infections caused by susceptible *Rickettsia*, *Chlamydia*, and *Mycoplasma*; alternative to mefloquine for malaria prophylaxis; treatment for syphilis, uncomplicated *Neisseria gonorrhoeae*, *Listeria*, *Actinomyces israelii*, and *Clostridium* infections in penicillin-allergic patients; used for community-acquired pneumonia and other common infections due to susceptible organisms; anthrax due to *Bacillus anthracis,* including inhalational anthrax (postexposure); treatment of infections caused by uncommon susceptible gram-negative and gram-positive organisms including *Borrelia recurrentis*, *Ureaplasma urealyticum*, *Haemophilus ducreyi*, *Yersinia pestis*, *Francisella tularensis*, *Vibrio cholerae*, *Campylobacter fetus*, *Brucella* spp, *Bartonella bacilliformis*, and *Calymmatobacterium granulomatis,* Q fever, Lyme disease; treatment of inflammatory lesions associated with rosacea; intestinal amebiasis; severe acne

Unlabeled/Investigational Use Sclerosing agent for pleural effusion injection; vancomycin-resistant enterococci (VRE)

Pregnancy Risk Factor D

Pregnancy Considerations Because use during pregnancy may cause fetal harm, doxycycline is classified as pregnancy category D. Exposure to tetracyclines during the second or third trimester may cause permanent discoloration of the teeth. Most reports do not show an increase risk for teratogenicity with the exception of a potential small increased risk for cleft palate or esophageal atresia/stenosis. When considering treatment for life-threatening infection and/or prolonged duration of therapy (such as in anthrax), the potential risk to the fetus must be balanced against the severity of the potential illness.

Lactation Enters breast milk/not recommended

Medication Safety Issues

Sound-alike/look-alike issues:

- Doxycycline may be confused with dicyclomine, doxepin, doxylamine
- Doxy-100® may be confused with Doxil®
- Monodox® may be confused with Maalox®
- Oracea™ may be confused with Orencia®
- Vibramycin® may be confused with vancomycin

Contraindications Hypersensitivity to doxycycline, tetracycline or any component of the formulation; children ≤8 years of age, except in treatment of anthrax (including inhalational anthrax postexposure prophylaxis)

Warnings/Precautions Photosensitivity reaction may occur with this drug; avoid prolonged exposure to sunlight or tanning equipment. Antianabolic effects of tetracyclines can increase BUN (dose-related). Autoimmune syndromes have been reported. Hepatotoxicity rarely occurs: if symptomatic, conduct LFT and discontinue drug. Pseudotumor cerebri has been (rarely) reported with tetracycline use; usually resolves with discontinuation. Prolonged use may result in fungal or bacterial superinfection, including *C. difficile*-associated diarrhea (CDAD) and pseudomembranous colitis; CDAD has been observed >2 months postantibiotic treatment. May cause tissue hyperpigmentation, enamel hypoplasia, or permanent tooth discoloration; use of tetracyclines should be avoided during tooth development (children ≤8 years of age) unless other drugs are not likely to be effective or are contraindicated. However, recommended in treatment of anthrax exposure. Do not use during pregnancy. In addition to affecting tooth development, tetracycline use has been associated with retardation of skeletal development and reduced bone growth.

Additional specific warnings: Periostat®: Effectiveness has not been established in patients with coexistent oral candidiasis; use with caution in patients with a history or predisposition to oral candidiasis. Oracea™: Should not be used for the treatment or prophylaxis of bacterial infections, since the lower dose of drug per capsule may be subefficacious and promote resistance. Syrup contains sodium metabisulfite.

Adverse Reactions Frequency not defined.

Cardiovascular: Intracranial hypertension, pericarditis

Dermatologic: Angioneurotic edema, exfoliative dermatitis (rare), photosensitivity, rash, skin hyperpigmentation, urticaria

Endocrine & metabolic: Brown/black discoloration of thyroid gland (no dysfunction reported), hypoglycemia

Gastrointestinal: Anorexia, diarrhea, dysphagia, enterocolitis, esophagitis (rare), esophageal ulcerations (rare), glossitis, inflammatory lesions in anogenital region, nausea, oral (mucosal) pigmentation, pseudomembranous colitis, tooth discoloration (children), vomiting

Hematologic: Eosinophilia, hemolytic anemia, neutropenia, thrombocytopenia

Hepatic: Hepatotoxicity (rare)

Renal: BUN increased (dose related)

Miscellaneous: Anaphylactoid purpura, anaphylaxis, bulging fontanels (infants), serum sickness, SLE exacerbation

Note: Adverse effects in clinical trials with Periostat® occurring at a frequency more than 1% greater than placebo included nausea, dyspepsia, joint pain, diarrhea, menstrual cramp, and pain.

Drug Interactions

Metabolism/Transport Effects Inhibits CYP3A4 (moderate)

Avoid Concomitant Use

Avoid concomitant use of Doxycycline with any of the following: Retinoic Acid Derivatives

Increased Effect/Toxicity

Doxycycline may increase the levels/effects of: CYP3A4 Substrates; Eplerenone; FentaNYL; Maraviroc; Neuromuscular-Blocking Agents; Pimecrolimus; Ranolazine; Retinoic Acid Derivatives; Salmeterol; Vitamin K Antagonists

Decreased Effect

Doxycycline may decrease the levels/effects of: Penicillins; Typhoid Vaccine

The levels/effects of Doxycycline may be decreased by: Antacids; Barbiturates; Bile Acid Sequestrants; Bismuth; Bismuth Subsalicylate; CarBAMazepine; Iron Salts; Magnesium Salts; Phenytoin; Quinapril

Ethanol/Nutrition/Herb Interactions

Ethanol: Chronic ethanol ingestion may reduce the serum concentration of doxycycline.

Food: Doxycycline serum levels may be slightly decreased if taken with food or milk. Administration with iron or calcium may decrease doxycycline absorption. May decrease absorption of calcium, iron, magnesium, zinc, and amino acids.

Herb/Nutraceutical: St John's wort may decrease doxycycline levels. Avoid dong quai, St John's wort (may also cause photosensitization).

Stability

Capsule, tablet: Store at controlled room temperature of 25°C (77°F); excursions permitted to 15°C to 30°C (59°F to 86°F). Protect from light.

I.V. infusion: Following reconstitution with sterile water for injection, dilute to a final concentration of 0.1-1 mg/mL using a compatible solution. Solutions for I.V. infusion may be prepared using 0.9% sodium chloride, D_5W, Ringer's injection, lactated Ringer's, D_5LR. Protect from light. Stability varies based on solution.

Mechanism of Action Inhibits protein synthesis by binding with the 30S and possibly the 50S ribosomal subunit(s) of susceptible bacteria; may also cause alterations in the cytoplasmic membrane

Periostat® capsules (proposed mechanism): Has been shown to inhibit collagenase activity *in vitro*. Also has been noted to reduce elevated collagenase activity in the gingival crevicular fluid of patients with periodontal disease. Systemic levels do not reach inhibitory concentrations against bacteria.

Pharmacodynamics/Kinetics

Absorption: Oral: Almost complete

Distribution: Widely into body tissues and fluids including synovial, pleural, prostatic, seminal fluids, and bronchial secretions; saliva, aqueous humor, and CSF penetration is poor

Protein binding: 90%

Metabolism: Not hepatic; partially inactivated in GI tract by chelate formation

Half-life elimination: 12-15 hours (usually increases to 22-24 hours with multiple doses); End-stage renal disease: 18-25 hours

Time to peak, serum: 1.5-4 hours

Excretion: Feces (30%); urine (23%)

Dosage

Usual dosage range:

Children >8 years (<45 kg): Oral, I.V.: 2-5 mg/kg/day in 1-2 divided doses, not to exceed 200 mg/day

Children >8 years (>45 kg) and Adults: Oral, I.V.: 100-200 mg/day in 1-2 divided doses

Indication-specific dosing:

Children:

Anthrax: Doxycycline should be used in children if antibiotic susceptibility testing, exhaustion of drug supplies, or allergic reaction preclude use of penicillin or ciprofloxacin. For treatment, the consensus recommendation does not include a loading dose for doxycycline.

Inhalational (postexposure prophylaxis) (*MMWR*, 2001, 50:889-893): Oral, I.V. (use oral route when possible):

≤8 years: 2.2 mg/kg every 12 hours for 60 days

>8 years and ≤45 kg: 2.2 mg/kg every 12 hours for 60 days

>8 years and >45 kg: 100 mg every 12 hours for 60 days

Cutaneous (treatment): Oral: See dosing for "Inhalational (postexposure prophylaxis)"

Note: In the presence of systemic involvement, extensive edema, and/or lesions on head/neck, doxycycline should initially be administered I.V.

Inhalational/gastrointestinal/oropharyngeal (treatment): I.V.: Refer to dosing for inhalational anthrax (postexposure prophylaxis); switch to oral therapy when clinically appropriate

Note: Initial treatment should include two or more agents predicted to be effective (per CDC recommendations). Agents suggested for use in conjunction with doxycycline or ciprofloxacin include rifampin, vancomycin, imipenem, penicillin, ampicillin, chloramphenicol, clindamycin, and clarithromycin. May switch to oral antimicrobial therapy when clinically appropriate. Continue combined therapy for 60 days

Children ≥8 years:

Malaria prophylaxis: Oral: 2 mg/kg/day (maximum 100 mg/day). Start 1-2 days prior to travel to endemic area; continue daily during travel and for 4 weeks after leaving endemic area

Children ≥8 years (and >45 kg) and Adults:

Chlamydial infections, uncomplicated: Oral: 100 mg twice daily for ≥7 days

Lyme disease, Q fever, or tularemia: Oral: 100 mg twice daily for 14-21 days

Rickettsial disease or ehrlichiosis: Oral, I.V.: 100 mg twice daily for 7-14 days

Adults:

Anthrax:

Inhalational (postexposure prophylaxis): Oral, I.V. (use oral route when possible): 100 mg every 12 hours for 60 days (*MMWR*, 2001, 50:889-93)

Cutaneous (treatment): Oral: 100 mg every 12 hours for 60 days. **Note:** In the presence of systemic involvement, extensive edema, lesions on head/neck, refer to I.V. dosing for treatment of inhalational/gastrointestinal/oropharyngeal anthrax

Inhalational/gastrointestinal/oropharyngeal (treatment): I.V.: Initial: 100 mg every 12 hours; switch to oral therapy when clinically appropriate; some recommend initial loading dose of 200 mg, followed by 100 mg every 8-12 hours (*JAMA*, 1997, 278:399-411). **Note:** Initial treatment should include two or more agents predicted to be effective (per CDC recommendations). Agents suggested for use in conjunction with doxycycline or ciprofloxacin include rifampin, vancomycin, imipenem, penicillin, ampicillin, chloramphenicol, clindamycin, and clarithromycin. May switch to oral antimicrobial therapy when clinically appropriate. Continue combined therapy for 60 days

Brucellosis: Oral: 100 mg twice daily for 6 weeks with rifampin or streptomycin

Community-acquired pneumonia, bronchitis: Oral, I.V.: 100 mg twice daily

Endometritis, salpingitis, parametritis, or peritonitis: I.V.: 100 mg twice daily with cefoxitin 2 g every 6 hours for 4 days and for ≥48 hours after patient improves; then continue with oral therapy 100 mg twice daily to complete a 10- to 14-day course of therapy

Gonococcal infection, acute (PID) in combination with another antibiotic: I.V.: 100 mg every 12 hours until improved, followed by 100 mg orally twice daily to complete 14 days

Malaria prophylaxis: 100 mg/day. Start 1-2 days prior to travel to endemic area; continue daily during travel and for 4 weeks after leaving endemic area

Nongonococcal urethritis: Oral: 100 mg twice daily for 7 days

Periodontitis: Oral (Periostat®): 20 mg twice daily as an adjunct following scaling and root planing; may be administered for up to 9 months. Safety beyond 12 months of treatment and efficacy beyond 9 months of treatment have not been established.

Rosacea: (Oracea™): Oral: 40 mg once daily in the morning

Sclerosing agent for pleural effusion injection (unlabeled use): Irrigation: 500 mg as a single dose in 30-50 mL of NS or SWI

Syphilis:

Early syphilis: Oral, I.V.: 200 mg/day in divided doses for 14 days

Late syphilis: Oral, I.V.: 200 mg/day in divided doses for 28 days

***Yersinia pestis* (plague):** Oral: 100 mg twice daily for 7 days

Vibrio cholerae: Oral: 300 mg as a single dose

Dosing adjustment in renal impairment: No adjustment necessary

Dialysis: Not dialyzable; 0% to 5% by hemo- and peritoneal methods or by continuous arteriovenous or venovenous hemofiltration: No supplemental dosage necessary

Dietary Considerations

Tetracyclines (in general): Take with food if gastric irritation occurs. While administration with food may decrease GI absorption of doxycycline by up to 20%, administration on an empty stomach is not recommended due to GI intolerance. Of currently available tetracyclines, doxycycline has the least affinity for calcium.

Oracea™: Take on an empty stomach 1 hour before or 2 hours after meals.

Doryx®: 75 mg, 100 mg, and 150 mg tablets contain sodium 4.5 mg, 6 mg, and 9 mg respectively.

Administration
Oral: May give with meals to decrease GI upset. Capsule and tablet: Administer with at least 8 ounces of water and have patient sit up for at least 30 minutes after taking to reduce the risk of esophageal irritation and ulceration.
Oracea™: Take on an empty stomach 1 hour before or 2 hours after meals.
Doryx®: May be administered by carefully breaking up the tablet and sprinkling tablet contents on a spoonful of cold applesauce. The delayed release pellets must not be crushed or damaged when breaking up tablet. Should be administered immediately after preparation and without chewing.
I.V.: Infuse I.V. doxycycline over 1-4 hours; avoid extravasation

Monitoring Parameters Perform culture and sensitivity testing prior to initiating therapy. CBC, renal and liver function tests periodically with prolonged therapy.

Test Interactions False elevations of urine catecholamine levels; false-negative urine glucose using Clinistix®, Tes-Tape®

Dosage Forms Excipient information presented when available (limited, particularly for generics); consult specific product labeling. [DSC] = Discontinued product
Note: Strength expressed as base.
Capsule, as hyclate: 50 mg, 100 mg
Vibramycin®: 100 mg
Capsule, as monohydrate: 50 mg, 100 mg
Monodox®: 50 mg, 75 mg, 100 mg
Capsule, variable release:
Oracea™: 40 mg [30 mg (immediate-release) and 10 mg (delayed-release)]
Injection, powder for reconstitution, as hyclate: 100 mg
Doxy-100®: 100 mg
Powder for oral suspension, as monohydrate: 25 mg/5 mL (60 mL)
Vibramycin®: 25 mg/5 mL (60 mL) [raspberry flavor]
Syrup, as calcium:
Vibramycin®: 50 mg/5 mL (480 mL) [contains sodium metabisulfite; raspberry-apple flavor]
Tablet, as hyclate: 20 mg, 100 mg
Periostat®: 20 mg
Vibra-Tabs®: 100 mg
Tablet, as monohydrate: 50 mg, 75 mg, 100 mg, 150 mg
Adoxa®: 50 mg, 75 mg, 100 mg
Adoxa® Pak™ 1/75 [unit-dose pack]: 75 mg (31s)
Adoxa® Pak™ 1/100 [unit-dose pack]: 100 mg (31s)
Adoxa® Pak™ 1/150 [unit-dose pack]: 150 mg (30s)
Adoxa® Pak™ 2/100 [unit-dose pack]: 100 mg (60s)
Tablet, delayed-release coated pellets, as hyclate:
Doryx®: 75 mg [contains sodium 4.5 mg (0.196 mEq); 100 mg [contains sodium 6 mg (0.261 mEq)]; 150 mg [contains sodium 9 mg (0.392 mEq)]

Extemporaneous Preparations If liquid doxycycline is unavailable for the treatment of anthrax, emergency doses may be prepared for children using the tablets.

Crush one 100 mg tablet and grind into a fine powder. Mix with 4 teaspoons of food or drink (lowfat milk, chocolate milk, chocolate pudding, or apple juice). Appropriate dose may be taken from this mixture. Mixture may be stored for up to 24 hours. Dairy mixtures should be refrigerated; apple juice may be stored at room temperature.

U.S. Food and Drug Administration, Center for Drug Evaluation and Research, "How to Prepare Emergency Dosages of Doxycycline at Home for Infants and Children," April 25, 2003, viewable at http://www.fda.gov/cder/drug/infopage/penG_doxy/doxycyclinePeds.htm, last accessed May 8, 2003.

- **Doxycycline Calcium** *see* Doxycycline *on page 491*
- **Doxycycline Hyclate** *see* Doxycycline *on page 491*
- **Doxycycline Monohydrate** *see* Doxycycline *on page 491*
- **Doxytec (Can)** *see* Doxycycline *on page 491*
- **DPA** *see* Valproic Acid and Derivatives *on page 1538*
- **DPE** *see* Dipivefrin *on page 466*
- **D-Penicillamine** *see* Penicillamine *on page 1161*
- **DPH** *see* Phenytoin *on page 1186*
- **D-Phen 1000** *see* Guaifenesin and Phenylephrine *on page 712*
- **DPM™ [OTC]** *see* Urea *on page 1530*
- **Dramamine® [OTC]** *see* DimenhyDRINATE *on page 453*
- **Dramamine® Less Drowsy Formula [OTC]** *see* Meclizine *on page 928*
- **Dried Smallpox Vaccine** *see* Smallpox Vaccine *on page 1377*
- **Driminate® [OTC]** *see* DimenhyDRINATE *on page 453*
- **Drinex [OTC]** *see* Acetaminophen, Chlorpheniramine, and Pseudoephedrine *on page 31*
- **Drisdol®** *see* Ergocalciferol *on page 538*
- **Dristan® N.D. (Can)** *see* Acetaminophen and Pseudoephedrine *on page 30*
- **Dristan® N.D., Extra Strength (Can)** *see* Acetaminophen and Pseudoephedrine *on page 30*
- **Dritho-Scalp®** *see* Anthralin *on page 118*
- **Drixoral® (Can)** *see* Dexbrompheniramine and Pseudoephedrine *on page 428*
- **Drixoral® Cold & Allergy [OTC]** *see* Dexbrompheniramine and Pseudoephedrine *on page 428*
- **Drixoral® ND (Can)** *see* Pseudoephedrine *on page 1265*

Dronabinol (droe NAB i nol)

U.S. Brand Names Marinol®
Canadian Brand Names Marinol®
Index Terms Delta-9 THC; Delta-9-tetrahydro-cannabinol; Tetrahydrocannabinol; THC
Pharmacologic Category Antiemetic; Appetite Stimulant
Use Chemotherapy-associated nausea and vomiting refractory to other antiemetic(s); AIDS-related anorexia
Unlabeled/Investigational Use Cancer-related anorexia
Restrictions C-III
Pregnancy Risk Factor C
Lactation Enters breast milk/contraindicated
Medication Safety Issues
Sound-alike/look-alike issues:
Dronabinol may be confused with droperidol
Contraindications Hypersensitivity to dronabinol, cannabinoids, sesame oil, or any component of the formulation, or marijuana; should be avoided in patients with a history of schizophrenia
Warnings/Precautions Use with caution in patients with hepatic disease or seizure disorders. Reduce dosage in patients with severe hepatic impairment. May cause additive CNS effects with sedatives, hypnotics or other psychoactive agents; patients must be cautioned about performing tasks which require mental alertness (eg, operating machinery or driving).

May have potential for abuse; drug is psychoactive substance in marijuana; use caution in patients with a history of substance abuse or potential. May cause withdrawal symptoms upon abrupt discontinuation. Use with caution in patients with mania, depression, or schizophrenia; careful psychiatric monitoring is recommended. Use caution in elderly; they are more sensitive to adverse effects. Safety and efficacy have not been established in children.

Adverse Reactions Frequency not always specified.

>1%:

Cardiovascular: Palpitations, tachycardia, vasodilation/facial flushing

Central nervous system: Euphoria (8% to 24%, dose related), abnormal thinking (3% to 10%), dizziness (3% to 10%), paranoia (3% to 10%), somnolence (3% to 10%), amnesia, anxiety, ataxia, confusion, depersonalization, hallucination

Gastrointestinal: Abdominal pain (3% to 10%), nausea (3% to 10%), vomiting (3% to 10%)

Neuromuscular & skeletal: Weakness

<1% (Limited to important or life-threatening): Conjunctivitis, depression, diarrhea, fatigue, fecal incontinence, flushing, hypotension, myalgia, nightmares, seizure, speech difficulties, tinnitus, vision difficulties

Drug Interactions

Avoid Concomitant Use There are no known interactions where it is recommended to avoid concomitant use.

Increased Effect/Toxicity

Dronabinol may increase the levels/effects of: Alcohol (Ethyl); CNS Depressants; Sympathomimetics

The levels/effects of Dronabinol may be increased by: Anticholinergic Agents; Cocaine; Ritonavir

Decreased Effect There are no known significant interactions involving a decrease in effect.

Ethanol/Nutrition/Herb Interactions

Ethanol: Avoid ethanol (may increase CNS depression).

Food: Administration with high-lipid meals may increase absorption.

Herb/Nutraceutical: St John's wort may decrease dronabinol levels.

Stability Store under refrigeration (or in a cool environment) between 8°C and 15°C (46°F and 59°F). Protect from freezing.

Mechanism of Action Unknown, may inhibit endorphins in the brain's emetic center, suppress prostaglandin synthesis, and/or inhibit medullary activity through an unspecified cortical action. Some pharmacologic effects appear to involve sympathimometic activity; tachyphylaxis to some effect (eg, tachycardia) may occur, but appetite-stimulating effects do not appear to wane over time. Antiemetic activity may be due to effect on cannabinoid receptors (CB1) within the central nervous system.

Pharmacodynamics/Kinetics

Onset of action: Within 1 hour

Peak effect: 2-4 hours

Duration: 24 hours (appetite stimulation)

Absorption: Oral: 90% to 95%; 10% to 20% of dose gets into systemic circulation

Distribution: V_d: 10 L/kg; dronabinol is highly lipophilic and distributes to adipose tissue

Protein binding: 97% to 99%

Metabolism: Hepatic to at least 50 metabolites, some of which are active; 11-hydroxy-delta-9-tetrahydrocannabinol (11-OH-THC) is the major metabolite; extensive first-pass effect

Half-life elimination: Dronabinol: 25-36 hours (terminal); Dronabinol metabolites: 44-59 hours

Time to peak, serum: 0.5-4 hours

Excretion: Feces (50% as unconjugated metabolites, 5% as unchanged drug); urine (10% to 15% as acid metabolites and conjugates)

Dosage Refer to individual protocols. Oral:

Antiemetic: Children and Adults: 5 mg/m^2 1-3 hours before chemotherapy, then 5 mg/m^2/dose every 2-4 hours after chemotherapy for a total of 4-6 doses/day; increase doses in increments of 2.5 mg/m^2 to a maximum of 15 mg/m^2/dose.

Appetite stimulant: Adults: Initial: 2.5 mg twice daily (before lunch and dinner); titrate up to a maximum of 20 mg/day.

Dietary Considerations Capsules contain sesame oil.

Monitoring Parameters CNS effects, heart rate, blood pressure, behavioral profile

Reference Range Antinauseant effects: 5-10 ng/mL

Test Interactions Decreased FSH, LH, growth hormone, and testosterone

Dosage Forms Excipient information presented when available (limited, particularly for generics); consult specific product labeling.

Capsule, soft gelatin: 2.5 mg, 5 mg, 10 mg

Marinol®: 2.5 mg, 5 mg, 10 mg [contains sesame oil]

Droperidol (droe PER i dole)

U.S. Brand Names Inapsine®

Canadian Brand Names Droperidol Injection, USP

Index Terms Dehydrobenzperidol

Pharmacologic Category Antiemetic; Antipsychotic Agent, Typical

Use Antiemetic in surgical and diagnostic procedures; preoperative medication in patients when other treatments are ineffective or inappropriate

Pregnancy Risk Factor C

Pregnancy Considerations Crosses the placenta

Lactation Excretion in breast milk unknown

Medication Safety Issues

Sound-alike/look-alike issues:

Droperidol may be confused with dronabinol

Inapsine® may be confused with Nebcin®

Contraindications Hypersensitivity to droperidol or any component of the formulation; known or suspected QT prolongation, including congenital long QT syndrome (prolonged QT_c is defined as >440 msec in males or >450 msec in females)

Warnings/Precautions May alter cardiac conduction. **[U.S. Boxed Warning]: Cases of QT prolongation and torsade de pointes, including some fatal cases, have been reported.** Use extreme caution in patients with bradycardia (<50 bpm), cardiac disease, concurrent MAO inhibitor therapy, Class I and Class III antiarrhythmics or other drugs known to prolong QT interval, and electrolyte disturbances (hypokalemia or hypomagnesemia), including concomitant drugs which may alter electrolytes (diuretics).

Use with caution in patients with seizures or severe liver disease. May be sedating, use with caution in disorders where CNS depression is a feature. Caution in patients with hemodynamic instability, predisposition to seizures, subcortical brain damage, pheochromocytoma or renal disease. Esophageal dysmotility and aspiration have been associated with antipsychotic use - use with caution in patients at risk of pneumonia (ie, Alzheimer's disease). Caution in breast cancer or other prolactin-dependent tumors (may elevate prolactin levels). May alter temperature regulation or mask toxicity of other drugs due to antiemetic effects. May cause orthostatic hypotension - use with caution in patients at risk of this effect or those who would tolerate transient hypotensive episodes (cerebrovascular disease, cardiovascular disease, or other medications which may predispose). Significant hypotension may occur; injection contains benzyl alcohol; injection also contains sulfites which may cause allergic reaction.

May cause anticholinergic effects (confusion, agitation, constipation, xerostomia, blurred vision, urinary retention). Therefore, they should be used with caution in patients with decreased gastrointestinal motility, urinary retention, BPH, xerostomia, or visual problems. Conditions which also may be exacerbated by cholinergic blockade include narrow-angle glaucoma (screening is recommended) and worsening of myasthenia gravis. Relative to other neuroleptics, droperidol has a low potency of cholinergic blockade.

May cause extrapyramidal symptoms (EPS), including pseudoparkinsonism, acute dystonic reactions, akathisia, and tardive dyskinesia (risk of these reactions is high relative to other neuroleptics). Risk of dystonia (and possibly other EPS) may be greater with increased doses, use of conventional antipsychotics, males, and younger patients. May be associated with neuroleptic malignant syndrome (NMS) or pigmentary retinopathy. May mask toxicity of other drugs or conditions (eg, intestinal obstruction, Reye's syndrome, brain tumor) due to antiemetic effects. Use with caution in the elderly; reduce initial dose. Safety in children <2 years of age has not been established.

Adverse Reactions

>10%:

Cardiovascular: QT_c prolongation (dose dependent)

Central nervous system: Restlessness, anxiety, extrapyramidal symptoms, dystonic reactions, pseudoparkinsonian signs and symptoms, tardive dyskinesia, seizure, altered central temperature regulation, sedation, drowsiness

Endocrine & metabolic: Swelling of breasts

Gastrointestinal: Weight gain, constipation

1% to 10%:

Cardiovascular: Hypotension (especially orthostatic), tachycardia, abnormal T waves with prolonged ventricular repolarization, hypertension

Central nervous system: Hallucinations, persistent tardive dyskinesia, akathisia

Gastrointestinal: Nausea, vomiting

Genitourinary: Dysuria

<1% (Limited to important or life-threatening): Adynamic ileus, agranulocytosis, alopecia, arrhythmia, cholestatic jaundice, heat stroke, hyperpigmentation, laryngospasm, leukopenia, neuroleptic malignant syndrome (NMS), obstructive jaundice, photosensitivity (rare), priapism, rash, respiratory depression, retinal pigmentation, tardive dystonia, torsade de pointes, urinary retention, ventricular tachycardia, visual acuity decreased (may be irreversible)

Drug Interactions

Avoid Concomitant Use

Avoid concomitant use of Droperidol with any of the following: Nilotinib; Thioridazine; Ziprasidone

Increased Effect/Toxicity

Droperidol may increase the levels/effects of: Alcohol (Ethyl); Anticholinergics; CNS Depressants; QTc-Prolonging Agents; Thioridazine; Ziprasidone

The levels/effects of Droperidol may be increased by: Acetylcholinesterase Inhibitors (Central); Alfuzosin; Ciprofloxacin; Gadobutrol; Lithium formulations; Nilotinib; Pramlintide; Tetrabenazine

Decreased Effect

Droperidol may decrease the levels/effects of: Amphetamines; Anti-Parkinson's Agents (Dopamine Agonist)

The levels/effects of Droperidol may be decreased by: Lithium formulations

Stability Droperidol ampuls/vials should be stored at room temperature and protected from light. Solutions diluted in NS or D_5W are stable at room temperature for up to 7 days.

Mechanism of Action Droperidol is a butyrophenone antipsychotic; antiemetic effect is a result of blockade of dopamine stimulation of the chemoreceptor trigger zone. Other effects include alpha-adrenergic blockade, peripheral vascular dilation, and reduction of the pressor effect of epinephrine resulting in hypotension and decreased peripheral vascular resistance; may also reduce pulmonary artery pressure

Pharmacodynamics/Kinetics

Onset of action: Peak effect: Parenteral: ~30 minutes

Duration: Parenteral: 2-4 hours, may extend to 12 hours

Absorption: I.M.: Rapid

Distribution: Crosses blood-brain barrier and placenta

V_d: Children: ~0.25-0.9 L/kg; Adults: ~2 L/kg

Protein binding: Extensive

Metabolism: Hepatic, to *p*-fluorophenylacetic acid, benzimidazolone, *p*-hydroxypiperidine

Half-life elimination: Adults: 2.3 hours

Excretion: Urine (75%, <1% as unchanged drug); feces (22%, 11% to 50% as unchanged drug)

Dosage Titrate carefully to desired effect

Children 2-12 years: Nausea and vomiting: I.M., I.V.: 0.05-0.06 mg/kg (maximum initial dose: 0.1 mg/kg); additional doses may be repeated to achieve effect; administer additional doses with caution

Adults: Prevention of postoperative nausea and vomiting (PONV): I.M., I.V.: Initial: 0.625-2.5 mg; additional doses of 1.25 mg may be administered to achieve desired effect; administer additional doses with caution. Consensus guidelines recommend 0.625-1.25 mg I.V. administered after surgery (Gan, 2003).

Administration Administer I.M. or I.V.; according to the manufacturer, I.V. push administration should be slow (generally regarded as 2-5 minutes); however, many clinicians administer I.V. doses rapidly (over 30-60 seconds) in an effort to reduce the incidence of EPS. The effect, if any, of rapid administration on QT prolongation is unclear. For I.V. infusion, dilute in 50-100 mL NS or D_5W; ECG monitoring for 2-3 hours after administration is recommended regardless of rate of infusion.

Monitoring Parameters To identify QT prolongation, a 12-lead ECG prior to use is recommended; continued ECG monitoring for 2-3 hours following administration is recommended. Vital signs; lipid profile, fasting blood glucose/Hgb A_{1c}, serum magnesium and potassium; BMI; mental status, abnormal involuntary movement scale (AIMS); observe for dystonias, extrapyramidal side effects, and temperature changes

Additional Information Does not possess analgesic effects; has little or no amnesic properties.

Dosage Forms Excipient information presented when available (limited, particularly for generics); consult specific product labeling.

Injection, solution [preservative free]: 2.5 mg/mL (1 mL, 2 mL)

Inapsine®: 2.5 mg/mL (1 mL, 2 mL)

◆ **Droperidol Injection, USP (Can)** *see* Droperidol *on page 495*

◆ **Drospirenone and Ethinyl Estradiol** *see* Ethinyl Estradiol and Drospirenone *on page 576*

Drotrecogin Alfa (dro TRE coe jin AL fa)

U.S. Brand Names Xigris®

Canadian Brand Names Xigris®

Index Terms Activated Protein C, Human, Recombinant; Drotrecogin Alfa, Activated; Protein C (Activated), Human, Recombinant

Pharmacologic Category Protein C (Activated)

Use Reduction of mortality from severe sepsis (associated with organ dysfunction) in adults at high risk of death (eg, APACHE II score ≥25)

Unlabeled/Investigational Use Purpura fulminans

Pregnancy Risk Factor C

Lactation Excretion in breast milk unknown/not recommended

Contraindications Hypersensitivity to drotrecogin alfa or any component of the formulation; active internal bleeding;

recent hemorrhagic stroke (within 3 months); severe head trauma (within 2 months); recent intracranial or intraspinal surgery (within 2 months); intracranial neoplasm or mass lesion; evidence of cerebral herniation; presence of an epidural catheter; trauma with an increased risk of life-threatening bleeding

Warnings/Precautions Increases risk of bleeding; careful evaluation of risks and benefit is required prior to initiation. Bleeding risk is increased in patients receiving concurrent therapeutic heparin, oral anticoagulants, glycoprotein IIb/IIIa antagonists, platelet aggregation inhibitors, or aspirin at a dosage of >650 mg/day (within 7 days). In addition, an increased bleeding risk is associated with prolonged INR (>3), gastrointestinal bleeding (within 6 weeks), decreased platelet count (<30,000/mm^3), thrombolytic therapy (within 3 days), recent ischemic stroke (within 3 months), intracranial AV malformation or aneurysm, known bleeding diathesis, severe hepatic disease (chronic), or other condition where bleeding is a significant hazard or difficult to manage due to its location. Discontinue if significant bleeding occurs (may consider continued use after stabilization). Treatment interruption required for invasive procedures. During treatment, aPTT cannot be used to assess coagulopathy (PT/INR not affected).

Efficacy not established in adult patients at a low risk of death. Patients with pre-existing nonsepsis-related medical conditions with a poor prognosis (anticipated survival <28 days), patients with acute pancreatitis (no established source of infection), HIV-infected patients with a CD4 count ≤50 cells/mm^3, chronic dialysis patients, pre-existing hypercoagulable conditions, and patients who had received bone marrow, liver, lung, pancreas, or small bowel transplants were excluded from the clinical trial which established benefit. In addition, patients weighing >135 kg were not evaluated. Safety and efficacy have not been established in pediatric patients.

Adverse Reactions As with all drugs which may affect hemostasis, bleeding is the major adverse effect associated with drotrecogin alfa. Hemorrhage may occur at virtually any site. Risk is dependent on multiple variables, including the dosage administered, concurrent use of multiple agents which alter hemostasis, and patient predisposition.

>10%:

Dermatologic: Bruising

Gastrointestinal: Gastrointestinal bleeding

1% to 10%: Hematologic: Bleeding (serious 2.4% during infusion vs 3.5% during 28-day study period; individual events listed as <1%)

<1% (Limited to important or life-threatening): Gastrointestinal hemorrhage, genitourinary bleeding, immune reaction (antibody production), intracranial hemorrhage (0.2%; frequencies up to 2% noted in a previous trial without placebo control), intrathoracic hemorrhage, retroperitoneal bleeding, skin/soft tissue bleeding

Drug Interactions

Avoid Concomitant Use There are no known interactions where it is recommended to avoid concomitant use.

Increased Effect/Toxicity

Drotrecogin Alfa may increase the levels/effects of: Anticoagulants; Fondaparinux; Ibritumomab; Tositumomab and Iodine I 131 Tositumomab

The levels/effects of Drotrecogin Alfa may be increased by: Antiplatelet Agents; Antithrombin III; Danaparoid; Dasatinib; Heparin; Heparin (Low Molecular Weight); Herbs (Anticoagulant/Antiplatelet Properties); Nonsteroidal Anti-Inflammatory Agents; Pentosan Polysulfate Sodium; Prostacyclin Analogues; Salicylates; Thrombolytic Agents; Vitamin K Antagonists

Decreased Effect There are no known significant interactions involving a decrease in effect.

Ethanol/Nutrition/Herb Interactions Herb/Nutraceutical: Recent use/intake of herbs with anticoagulant or antiplatelet activity (including cat's claw, feverfew, garlic, ginkgo, ginseng, and horse chestnut seed) may increase the risk of bleeding.

Stability Store vials under refrigeration at 2°C to 8°C (36°F to 46°F). Protect from light. Do not freeze. Reconstitute 5 mg vials with 2.5 mL and 20 mg vials with 10 mL sterile water for injection (resultant solution ~2 mg/mL). Must be further diluted (within 3 hours of reconstitution) in 0.9% sodium chloride, typically to a concentration between 100 mcg/mL and 200 mcg/mL when using infusion pump and between 100 mcg/mL and 1000 mcg/mL when infused via syringe pump. Although product information states administration must be completed within 12 hours of preparation, additional studies (data on file, Lilly Research Laboratories) show that the final solution is stable for 14 hours at 15°C to 30°C (59°F to 86°F). If not used immediately, a prepared solution may be stored in the refrigerator for up to 12 hours. The total expiration time (refrigeration and administration) should be ≤24 hours from time of preparation.

Mechanism of Action Inhibits factors Va and VIIIa, limiting thrombotic effects. Additional *in vitro* data suggest inhibition of plasminogen activator inhibitor-1 (PAF-1) resulting in profibrinolytic activity, inhibition of macrophage production of tumor necrosis factor, blocking of leukocyte adhesion, and limitation of thrombin-induced inflammatory responses. Relative contribution of effects on the reduction of mortality from sepsis is not completely understood.

Pharmacodynamics/Kinetics

Duration: Plasma nondetectable within 2 hours of discontinuation

Metabolism: Inactivated by endogenous plasma protease inhibitors; mean clearance: 40 L/hour; increased with severe sepsis (~50%)

Half-life elimination: 1.6 hours

Dosage I.V.:

Children and Adults: Purpura fulminans (unlabeled use): 24 mcg/kg/hour

Adults: Sepsis: 24 mcg/kg/hour for a total of 96 hours; stop infusion **immediately** if clinically-important bleeding is identified. **Note:** Use actual body weight for dosing.

Dosage adjustment in renal impairment: No specific adjustment recommended.

Administration Infuse separately from all other medications. Only dextrose, normal saline, dextrose/saline combinations, and lactated Ringer's solution may be infused through the same line. May administer via infusion pump. Administration of prepared solution must be completed within 12 hours of preparation. Suspend administration for 2 hours prior to invasive procedures or other procedure with significant bleeding risk; may continue treatment immediately following uncomplicated, minimally-invasive procedures, but delay for 12 hours after major invasive procedures/surgery.

Monitoring Parameters Monitor for signs and symptoms of bleeding, hemoglobin/hematocrit, PT/INR, platelet count

Test Interactions May interfere with one-stage coagulation assays based on the aPTT (such as factor VIII, IX, and XI assays).

Additional Information Prepared by recombinant DNA technology in human cell line

Dosage Forms Excipient information presented when available (limited, particularly for generics); consult specific product labeling.

Injection, powder for reconstitution [preservative free]: 5 mg [contains sucrose 31.8 mg], 20 mg [contains sucrose 124.9 mg]

◆ **Drotrecogin Alfa, Activated** *see* Drotrecogin Alfa *on page 496*

◆ **Droxia®** *see* Hydroxyurea *on page 753*

DULoxetine (doo LOX e teen)

U.S. Brand Names Cymbalta®

Canadian Brand Names Cymbalta®

Index Terms (+)-(*S*)-*N*-Methyl-γ-(1-naphthyloxy)-2-thiophenepropylamine Hydrochloride; Duloxetine Hydrochloride; LY248686

Pharmacologic Category Antidepressant, Serotonin/Norepinephrine Reuptake Inhibitor

Additional Appendix Information

Antidepressant Agents *on page 1638*

Use Acute and maintenance treatment of major depressive disorder (MDD); treatment of generalized anxiety disorder (GAD); management of pain associated with diabetic neuropathy; management of fibromyalgia

Unlabeled/Investigational Use Treatment of stress incontinence; management of chronic pain syndromes

Restrictions An FDA-approved medication guide concerning the use of antidepressants in children, adolescents, and young adults must be distributed when dispensing an outpatient prescription (new or refill) where this medication is to be used without direct supervision of a healthcare provider. Medication guides are available at http://www.fda.gov/cder/Offices/ODS/medication_guides.htm. Dispense to parents or guardians of children and adolescents receiving this medication.

Pregnancy Risk Factor C

Pregnancy Considerations Duloxetine is classified as pregnancy category C due to adverse effects observed in animal studies. Nonteratogenic effects in the newborn following SSRI/SNRI exposure late in the third trimester include respiratory distress, cyanosis, apnea, seizures, temperature instability, feeding difficulty, vomiting, hypoglycemia, hyper- or hypotonia, hyper-reflexia, jitteriness, irritability, constant crying, and tremor. The long-term effects on neurobehavior have not been studied.

Women treated for major depression and who are euthymic prior to pregnancy are more likely to experience a relapse when medication is discontinued as compared to pregnant women who continue taking antidepressant medications. The ACOG recommends that therapy with SSRIs or SNRIs during pregnancy be individualized; treatment of depression during pregnancy should incorporate the clinical expertise of the mental health clinician, obstetrician, primary healthcare provider, and pediatrician. If treatment during pregnancy is required, consider tapering therapy during the third trimester in order to prevent withdrawal symptoms in the infant. If this is done and the woman is considered to be at risk of relapse from her major depressive disorder, the medication can be restarted following delivery, although the dose should be readjusted to that required before pregnancy.

Lactation Enters breast milk/not recommended

Medication Safety Issues

Sound-alike/look-alike issues:

DULoxetine may be confused with FLUoxetine

Contraindications Concomitant use or within 2 weeks of MAO inhibitors; uncontrolled narrow-angle glaucoma

Canadian labeling: Additional contraindications (not in U.S. labeling): Hypersensitivity to duloxetine or any component of the formulation; hepatic impairment; severe renal impairment (eg, Cl_{cr} <30 mL/minute) or end-stage renal disease (ESRD); concomitant use with thioridazine or with CYP1A2 inhibitors

Warnings/Precautions [U.S. Boxed Warning]: Antidepressants increase the risk of suicidal thinking and behavior in children, adolescents, and young adults (18-24 years of age) with major depressive disorder (MDD) and other psychiatric disorders; consider risk prior to prescribing. Short-term studies did not show an increased risk in patients >24 years of age and showed a decreased risk in patients ≥65 years. Closely monitor for clinical worsening, suicidality, or unusual changes in behavior; the patient's family or caregiver should be instructed to closely observe the patient and communicate condition with healthcare provider. A medication guide concerning the use of antidepressants in children and teenagers should be dispensed with each prescription. **Duloxetine is not FDA approved for use in children.**

The possibility of a suicide attempt is inherent in major depression and may persist until remission occurs. Patients treated with antidepressants should be observed for clinical worsening and suicidality, especially during the initial (generally first 1-2 months) few months of a course of drug therapy, or at times of dose changes, either increases or decreases. Use caution in high-risk patients. Worsening depression and severe abrupt suicidality that are not part of the presenting symptoms may require discontinuation or modification of drug therapy. The patient's family or caregiver should be alerted to monitor patients for the emergence of suicidality and associated behaviors (such as agitation, irritability, hostility, impulsivity, and hypomania) and call healthcare provider.

May worsen psychosis in some patients or precipitate a shift to mania or hypomania in patients with bipolar disorder. Patients presenting with depressive symptoms should be screened for bipolar disorder. Monotherapy in patients with bipolar disorder should be avoided. **Duloxetine is not FDA approved for the treatment of bipolar depression.**

May cause orthostatic hypotension/syncope at therapeutic doses especially within the first week of therapy and after dose increases. Monitor blood pressure with initiation of therapy, dose increases (especially in patients receiving >60 mg/day), or with concomitant use of vasodilators or CYP1A2 inhibitors. Use caution in patients with hypertension. May increase blood pressure. Rare cases of hypertensive crisis have been reported in patients with pre-existing hypertension; evaluate blood pressure prior to initiating therapy and periodically thereafter; consider dose reduction or gradual discontinuation of therapy in individuals with sustained hypertension during therapy.

Modest increases in serum glucose and hemoglobin A_{1c} (Hb A_{1c}) levels have been observed in some diabetic patients receiving duloxetine therapy for diabetic peripheral neuropathy (DPN). Duloxetine may cause increased urinary resistance; advise patient to report symptoms of urinary hesitation/difficulty. Has a low potential to impair cognitive or motor performance. Use caution with a previous seizure disorder or condition predisposing to seizures such as brain damage or alcoholism. Avoid use in patients with substantial ethanol intake, evidence of chronic liver disease, or hepatic impairment (contraindicated in Canadian labeling). Rare cases of hepatic failure (including fatalities) have been reported with use. Hepatitis with abdominal pain, hepatomegaly, elevated transaminase levels >20 times the upper limit of normal (ULN) with and without jaundice have all been observed. Discontinue therapy with the presentation of jaundice or other signs of hepatic dysfunction and do not reinitiate therapy unless another source or cause is identified.

May cause hyponatremia/SIADH (elderly at increased risk); volume depletion (diuretics may increase risk). Use with caution in patients with controlled narrow angle glaucoma. May cause or exacerbate sexual dysfunction. Use caution with renal impairment (contraindicated in Canadian labeling for severe renal impairment or ESRD). Use caution with concomitant CNS depressants. May impair platelet aggregation; use caution with concomitant use of NSAIDs, ASA, or other drugs that affect coagulation; the risk of bleeding may be potentiated.

A potential exists for severe reactions when used with MAO inhibitors, SSRIs/SNRIs or triptans; serotonin syndrome (hyperthermia, muscular rigidity, mental status changes/agitation, autonomic instability) may occur. Use caution during concurrent therapy with other drugs which lower the seizure threshold. To discontinue therapy with duloxetine, gradually taper dose. If intolerable symptoms occur following a decrease in dosage or upon discontinuation of therapy, then resuming the previous dose with a more gradual taper should be considered. May increase the risks associated with electroconvulsive therapy. Consider discontinuing, when possible, prior to elective surgery. Formulation contains sucrose; patients with fructose intolerance, glucose-galactose malabsorption, or sucrose-isomaltase deficiency should avoid use. Safety and efficacy have not been established in patients <18 years of age.

Adverse Reactions

>10%:

Central nervous system: Fatigue (2% to 15%), somnolence (7% to 21%), dizziness (6% to 17%), headache (13% to 20%), insomnia (8% to 16%)

Gastrointestinal: Nausea (14% to 30%), xerostomia (5% to 18%), diarrhea (7% to 13%), constipation (5% to 15%), appetite decreased (3% to 11%)

1% to 10%:

Cardiovascular: Palpitation (1% to 2%)

Central nervous system: Agitation (5% to 6%), anxiety (3%), sleep disorder (3%), dreams abnormal (2% to 3%), fever (1% to 3%), yawning (1% to 2%), hypoesthesia (1%), lethargy (1%), nightmares (1%), vertigo (1%)

Dermatologic: Hyperhydrosis (6% to 8%), rash (4%), pruritus (3%)

Endocrine & metabolic: Libido decreased (2% to 4%), orgasm abnormality (3%), hot flushes (2% to 3%), anorgasmia (1%)

Gastrointestinal: Vomiting (5% to 6%), dyspepsia (4% to 5%), anorexia (3% to 5%), loose stools (2% to 3%), taste abnormal (1% to 3%), weight gain/loss (2%), flatulence (1%)

Genitourinary: Erectile dysfunction (1% to 5%), pollakiuria (1% to 5%), ejaculatory dysfunction (2% to 4%), ejaculation delayed (3%), penis disorder (2%)

Hepatic: ALT >3x ULN (1%)

Neuromuscular & skeletal: Weakness (2% to 8%), musculoskeletal pain (1% to 5%), muscle cramp (4% to 5%), muscle spasms (4%), tremor (3% to 4%), myalgia (1% to 4%), paresthesia (1%), rigors (1%)

Ocular: Blurred vision (1% to 3%)

Respiratory: Nasopharyngitis (7% to 9%), upper respiratory infection (7%), cough (3% to 6%), pharyngolaryngeal pain (1% to 6%)

Miscellaneous: Diaphoresis increased (6%), seasonal allergies (3%)

<1% (Limited to important or life-threatening): Abdominal pain, acne, agitation, aggression, alkaline phosphatase increased, alopecia, anaphylactic reaction, anger, anemia, angioneurotic edema, aphthous stomatitis, ataxia, atrial fibrillation, bloody stools, bundle branch block, CHF, colitis, CPK increased, dehydration, diastolic blood pressure increased, diplopia, disorientation, diverticulitis, dysarthria, dyskinesia, dyslipidemia, dysphagia, dysuria, ecchymosis, eczema, edema (peripheral), erythema, erythema multiforme, esophageal stenosis, EPS, facial edema, flu-like syndrome, flushing, gastric emptying impaired, gastric ulcer, gastritis, gastroenteritis, GI bleeding, gingivitis, glaucoma, hallucinations, Hb A_{1c} increased, hematochezia, hepatic failure, hepatic steatosis, hepatitis, hepatomegaly, hyperbilirubinemia, hypercholesterolemia, hyperglycemia, hyperlipidemia, hypersensitivity, hypertensive crisis, hyponatremia, hypothyroidism, irritability, irritable bowel syndrome, jaundice, keroconjunctivitis sicca, laryngitis, leukopenia, lymphadenopathy, macular degeneration, maculopathy, malaise, mania, melena, MI, micturition urgency, mood swings, muscle spasm, muscle tightness, muscle twitching, nephropathy, night sweats, nocturia, oropharyngeal edema, orthostatic hypotension, peripheral coldness, phlebitis, photosensitivity, polyuria, retinal detachment, seizure, serotonin syndrome, sexual dysfunction, SIADH, Stevens-Johnson syndrome, stomatitis, suicide, supraventricular arrhythmia, syncope, systolic blood pressure increased, tachycardia, thirst, throat tightness, thrombocytopenia, tinnitus, transaminases increased, trismus, urinary retention, urticaria, visual disturbance; withdrawal syndrome (including headache, dizziness, nightmares, irritability, paresthesia, and/or vomiting)

Drug Interactions

Metabolism/Transport Effects Substrate (major) of CYP1A2, 2D6; **inhibits** CYP2D6 (moderate)

Avoid Concomitant Use

Avoid concomitant use of DULoxetine with any of the following: Iobenguane I 123; MAO Inhibitors; Sibutramine; Thioridazine

Increased Effect/Toxicity

DULoxetine may increase the levels/effects of: Alcohol (Ethyl); Alpha-/Beta-Agonists; Aspirin; CNS Depressants; CYP2D6 Substrates; Fesoterodine; Nebivolol; NSAID (Nonselective); Serotonin Modulators; Tamoxifen; Thioridazine; Tricyclic Antidepressants

The levels/effects of DULoxetine may be increased by: CYP1A2 Inhibitors (Moderate); CYP1A2 Inhibitors (Strong); CYP2D6 Inhibitors (Moderate); CYP2D6 Inhibitors (Strong); Darunavir; Fluvoxamine; MAO Inhibitors; PARoxetine; Sibutramine

Decreased Effect

DULoxetine may decrease the levels/effects of: Alpha2-Agonists; Codeine; Iobenguane I 123; TraMADol

The levels/effects of DULoxetine may be decreased by: CYP1A2 Inducers (Strong)

Ethanol/Nutrition/Herb Interactions

Ethanol: Avoid ethanol (may increase CNS depression and/or hepatotoxic potential of duloxetine).

Herb/Nutraceutical: Avoid valerian, St John's wort, SAMe, kava kava, and gotu kola (may increase CNS depression).

Stability Store at 25°C (77°F); excursions permitted to 15°C to 30°C (59°F to 86°F)

Mechanism of Action Duloxetine is a potent inhibitor of neuronal serotonin and norepinephrine reuptake and a weak inhibitor of dopamine reuptake. Duloxetine has no significant activity for muscarinic cholinergic, H_1-histaminergic, or $alpha_2$-adrenergic receptors. Duloxetine does not possess MAO-inhibitory activity.

Pharmacodynamics/Kinetics

Absorption: Well absorbed, 2-hour delay in absorption after ingestion; food decreases extent of absorption ~10% (no effect on C_{max})

Distribution: 1640 L (range: 701-3800 L)

Protein binding: >90%; primarily to albumin and α_1-acid glycoprotein

Metabolism: Hepatic, via CYP1A2 and CYP2D6; forms multiple metabolites (inactive)

Half-life elimination: 12 hours (range 8-17 hours)

Time to peak: 6 hours; 10 hours when ingested with food

Excretion: As metabolites; urine (72%), feces (19%)

Dosage Oral:

Adults:

Major depressive disorder: Initial: 40-60 mg/day; dose may be divided (ie, 20 or 30 mg twice daily) or given as a single daily dose of 60 mg; maintenance: 60 mg once daily; for doses >60 mg/day, titrate dose in increments of 30 mg/day over 1 week as tolerated to a maximum dose: 120 mg/day. **Note:** Doses >60 mg/day have not been demonstrated to be more effective.

Diabetic neuropathy: 60 mg once daily; lower initial doses may be considered in patients where tolerability is a concern and/or renal impairment is present. **Note:** Doses up to 120 mg/day administered in clinical trials offered no additional benefit and were less well tolerated than dose of 60 mg/day.

Fibromyalgia: Initial: 30 mg/day for 1 week, then increase to 60 mg/day as tolerated. **Note:** Doses up to 120 mg/day administered in clinical trials offered no additional benefit and were less well tolerated than dose of 60 mg/day.

Generalized anxiety disorder: Initial: 30-60 mg/day as a single daily dose; patients initiated at 30 mg/day should be titrated to 60 mg/day after 1 week; maximum dose: 120 mg/day. **Note:** Doses >60 mg/day have not been demonstrated to be more effective than 60 mg/day.

Chronic pain syndromes (unlabeled use): 60 mg once daily

Stress incontinence (unlabeled use): 40 mg twice daily

Elderly:

Major depressive disorder: Manufacturer does not recommend specific dosage adjustment. Conservatively, may initiate at a dose of 20 mg 1-2 times/day; increase to 40-60 mg/day as a single daily dose or in divided doses **or** initiate therapy at 30 mg/day for 1 week then increase to 60 mg/day as tolerated.

Other indications: Refer to adult dosing

Dosage adjustment in renal impairment: Not recommended for use in Cl_{cr} <30 mL/minute or ESRD (contraindicated in Canadian labeling); in mild-moderate impairment, lower initial doses may be considered with titration guided by response and tolerability

Dosage adjustment in hepatic impairment: Not recommended for use in hepatic impairment (contraindicated in Canadian labeling)

Dietary Considerations May be taken without regard to meals.

Administration Capsule should be swallowed whole; do not break open or crush.

Monitoring Parameters Blood pressure should be checked prior to initiating therapy and then regularly monitored, especially in patients with a high baseline blood pressure; mental status for depression, suicidal ideation (especially at the beginning of therapy or when doses are increased or decreased), anxiety, social functioning, mania, panic attacks; glucose levels and Hb A_{1c} levels in diabetic patients, creatinine, BUN, transaminases

Dosage Forms Excipient information presented when available (limited, particularly for generics); consult specific product labeling.

Capsule, delayed release, enteric coated pellets:

Cymbalta®: 20 mg, 30 mg, 60 mg

- **Duloxetine Hydrochloride** *see* DULoxetine *on page 498*
- **Duocaine™** *see* Lidocaine and Bupivacaine *on page 886*
- **Duodote™** *see* Atropine and Pralidoxime *on page 159*
- **Duomax** *see* Guaifenesin and Phenylephrine *on page 712*
- **DuoNeb®** *see* Ipratropium and Albuterol *on page 812*
- **Duotan PD [DSC]** *see* Dexchlorpheniramine and Pseudoephedrine *on page 428*
- **DuP 753** *see* Losartan *on page 907*
- **Durabolin® (Can)** *see* Nandrolone *on page 1040*
- **Duraclon®** *see* CloNIDine *on page 354*
- **Duradrin® [DSC]** *see* Acetaminophen, Isometheptene, and Dichloralphenazone *on page 34*
- **Duradryl®** *see* Chlorpheniramine, Phenylephrine, and Methscopolamine *on page 313*
- **Duragesic®** *see* FentaNYL *on page 610*
- **Durahist™ PE** *see* Chlorpheniramine, Phenylephrine, and Methscopolamine *on page 313*
- **Duralith® (Can)** *see* Lithium *on page 897*
- **Duramorph®** *see* Morphine Sulfate *on page 1016*
- **DuraTan™ Forte** *see* Chlorpheniramine, Pseudoephedrine, and Dextromethorphan *on page 315*
- **Duratuss®** *see* Guaifenesin and Phenylephrine *on page 712*
- **Duratuss® DA** *see* Chlorpheniramine and Pseudoephedrine *on page 310*
- **Duratuss® DM** *see* Guaifenesin and Dextromethorphan *on page 710*
- **Duratuss GP®** *see* Guaifenesin and Phenylephrine *on page 712*
- **Durezol™** *see* Difluprednate *on page 444*
- **Duricef® [DSC]** *see* Cefadroxil *on page 269*
- **Duricef® (Can)** *see* Cefadroxil *on page 269*
- **Durolane® (Can)** *see* Hyaluronate and Derivatives *on page 734*

Dutasteride (doo TAS teer ide)

U.S. Brand Names Avodart®

Canadian Brand Names Avodart®

Pharmacologic Category 5 Alpha-Reductase Inhibitor

Use Treatment of symptomatic benign prostatic hyperplasia (BPH) as monotherapy or combination therapy with tamsulosin

Unlabeled/Investigational Use Treatment of male patterned baldness

Pregnancy Risk Factor X

Dosage Oral: Adults: Males: 0.5 mg once daily alone or in combination with tamsulosin

Dosage adjustment in renal impairment: No adjustment required

Dosage adjustment in hepatic impairment: Use caution; no specific adjustments recommended

Additional Information Complete prescribing information for this medication should be consulted for additional detail.

Dosage Forms Excipient information presented when available (limited, particularly for generics); consult specific product labeling.

Capsule, softgel:

Avodart®: 0.5 mg

- ◆ **Duvoid® (Can)** *see* Bethanechol *on page 192*
- ◆ **DW286** *see* Gemifloxacin *on page 688*
- ◆ **Dyazide®** *see* Hydrochlorothiazide and Triamterene *on page 739*
- ◆ **Dycill® (Can)** *see* Dicloxacillin *on page 440*

Dyclonine (DYE kloe neen)

U.S. Brand Names Cēpacol® Dual Action Maximum Strength [OTC]; Sucrets® [OTC]

Index Terms Dyclonine Hydrochloride

Pharmacologic Category Local Anesthetic, Oral

Use Temporary relief of pain associated with oral mucosa

Medication Safety Issues

Sound-alike/look-alike issues:

Dyclonine may be confused with dicyclomine

Dosage Oral:

Lozenge: Children ≥2 years and Adults: One lozenge every 2 hours as needed (maximum: 10 lozenges/day)

Spray:

Children ≥3-12 years: 1-3 sprays, up to 4 times a day

Children ≥12 years and Adults: 1-4 sprays, up to 4 times a day

Additional Information Complete prescribing information for this medication should be consulted for additional detail.

Dosage Forms Excipient information presented when available (limited, particularly for generics); consult specific product labeling.

Lozenge, as hydrochloride (Sucrets®): 1.2 mg [children's cherry flavor]; 2 mg [wild cherry and assorted flavors]; 3 mg [vapor black cherry and wintergreen flavors]

Spray, oral, as hydrochloride (Cēpacol® Dual Action Maximum Strength): 0.1% (120 mL) [contains glycerin 33%; cherry, honey lemon and cool menthol flavors]

- ◆ **Dyclonine Hydrochloride** *see* Dyclonine *on page 501*
- ◆ **Dynacin®** *see* Minocycline *on page 999*
- ◆ **DynaCirc® (Can)** *see* Isradipine *on page 827*
- ◆ **DynaCirc® CR** *see* Isradipine *on page 827*
- ◆ **Dyna-Hex® [OTC]** *see* Chlorhexidine Gluconate *on page 305*
- ◆ **Dynahist-ER Pediatric® [DSC]** *see* Chlorpheniramine and Pseudoephedrine *on page 310*
- ◆ **Dynex [DSC]** *see* Guaifenesin and Pseudoephedrine *on page 713*

Dyphylline and Guaifenesin
(DYE fi lin & gwye FEN e sin)

U.S. Brand Names COPD; Difil-G; Difil®-G Forte; Dilex-G; Dilor-G®; Lufyllin®-GG

Index Terms Guaifenesin and Dyphylline

Pharmacologic Category Expectorant; Theophylline Derivative

Use Treatment of bronchial asthma and reversible bronchospasm associated with chronic bronchitis and emphysema

Pregnancy Risk Factor C

Dosage Oral:

Children 6-12 years:

Elixir: Lufyllin®-GG: 15-30 mL 3 or 4 times/day

Syrup: Dilex-G:

18-27 kg: 1.25-1.6 mL 4 times/day

27-36 kg: 2.5-3.3 mL 4 times/day

36.5-45 kg: 3.3-3.7 mL 4 times/day

Tablet: Lufyllin®-GG: 1/2 -1 tablet 3 or 4 times/day

Children >12 years and Adults:

Elixir: Lufyllin®-GG: 30 mL 4 times/day

Syrup:

Dilex-G: 5-10 mL 4 times/day

Difil®-G Forte: 5-10 mL 3 or 4 times/day; may double or triple (in severe cases) according to patient response

Tablet: Difil®-G, Dilex-G, Lufyllin®-GG: One tablet 3 or 4 times/day

Dosage adjustment in renal impairment: Dosage reduction should be considered in severe renal impairment. Half-life of dyphylline is significantly prolonged in anuria.

Additional Information Complete prescribing information for this medication should be consulted for additional detail.

Dosage Forms Excipient information presented when available (limited, particularly for generics); consult specific product labeling.

Elixir: Dyphylline 100 mg and guaifenesin 100 mg per 15 mL (480 mL)

Lufyllin®-GG: Dyphylline 100 mg and guaifenesin 100 mg per 15 mL (480 mL) [contains alcohol 17%; wine-like flavor]

Liquid: Dyphylline 100 mg and guaifenesin 100 mg per 5 mL (480 mL)

Difil®-G Forte: Dyphylline 100 mg and guaifenesin 100 mg per 5 mL (240 mL) [menthol flavor]

Syrup:

Dilex-G: Dyphylline 100 mg and guaifenesin 200 mg per 5 mL (480 mL) [alcohol free, dye free, and sugar free]

Tablet: Dyphylline 200 mg and guaifenesin 200 mg

COPD, Lufyllin®-GG: Dyphylline 200 mg and guaifenesin 200 mg

Difil®-G: Dyphylline 200 mg and guaifenesin 300 mg

Dilex-G: Dyphylline 200 mg and guaifenesin 400 mg

- ◆ **Dyrenium®** *see* Triamterene *on page 1514*
- ◆ **Dytan™** *see* DiphenhydrAMINE *on page 456*
- ◆ **7E3** *see* Abciximab *on page 21*
- ◆ **E2020** *see* Donepezil *on page 478*
- ◆ **E 2080** *see* Rufinamide *on page 1349*
- ◆ **EACA** *see* Aminocaproic Acid *on page 85*
- ◆ **EarSol® HC** *see* Hydrocortisone *on page 743*
- ◆ **Easprin®** *see* Aspirin *on page 142*
- ◆ **Ebixa® (Can)** *see* Memantine *on page 938*

Echothiophate Iodide
(ek oh THYE oh fate EYE oh dide)

U.S. Brand Names Phospholine Iodide®

Index Terms Ecostigmine Iodide

Pharmacologic Category Acetylcholinesterase Inhibitor; Ophthalmic Agent, Antiglaucoma; Ophthalmic Agent, Miotic

Additional Appendix Information
Glaucoma Drug Therapy *on page 1808*

Use Used as miotic in treatment of chronic, open-angle glaucoma; may be useful in specific cases of angle-closure glaucoma (postiridectomy or where surgery refused/contraindicated); postcataract surgery-related glaucoma; accommodative esotropia

Pregnancy Risk Factor C

Dosage Ophthalmic:
Children: Accommodative esotropia:
Diagnosis: Instill 1 drop (0.125%) once daily into both eyes at bedtime for 2-3 weeks
Treatment: Usual dose: Instill 1 drop of 0.06% once daily or 0.125% every other day (maximum: 0.125% daily). **Note:** Use lowest concentration and frequency which gives satisfactory response; if necessary, doses >0.125% daily may be used for short periods of time.
Adults: Open-angle or secondary glaucoma:
Initial: Instill 1 drop (0.03%) twice daily into eyes with 1 dose just prior to bedtime
Maintenance: Some patients have been treated with 1 dose daily or every other day
Conversion from other ophthalmic agents: If IOP control was unsatisfactory, patients may be expected to require higher doses of echothiophate (eg, ≥0.06%); however, patients should be initially started on the 0.03% strength for a short period to better tolerance.

Additional Information Complete prescribing information for this medication should be consulted for additional detail.

Dosage Forms Excipient information presented when available (limited, particularly for generics); consult specific product labeling.
Powder for reconstitution, ophthalmic:
Phospholine Iodide®: 6.25 mg (5 mL) [0.125%; packaged with sterile diluent containing mannitol]

◆ **EC-Naprosyn®** *see* Naproxen *on page 1041*

◆ ***E. coli* Asparaginase** *see* Asparaginase *on page 140*

Econazole (e KONE a zole)

U.S. Brand Names Spectazole® [DSC]

Index Terms Econazole Nitrate

Pharmacologic Category Antifungal Agent, Topical

Use Topical treatment of tinea pedis (athlete's foot), tinea cruris (jock itch), tinea corporis (ringworm), tinea versicolor, and cutaneous candidiasis

Pregnancy Risk Factor C

Dosage Children and Adults: Topical:
Tinea pedis: Apply sufficient amount to cover affected areas once daily for 1 month
Tinea cruris, tinea corporis, tinea versicolor: Apply sufficient amount to cover affected areas once daily for 2 weeks
Cutaneous candidiasis: Apply sufficient quantity twice daily (morning and evening) for 2 weeks

Additional Information Complete prescribing information for this medication should be consulted for additional detail.

Dosage Forms Excipient information presented when available (limited, particularly for generics); consult specific product labeling.
Cream, topical, as nitrate: 1% (15 g, 30 g, 85 g)
Spectazole®: 1% (15 g, 30 g, 85 g) [DSC]

◆ **Econazole Nitrate** *see* Econazole *on page 502*

◆ **Econopred® Plus [DSC]** *see* PrednisoLONE *on page 1230*

◆ **Ecostigmine Iodide** *see* Echothiophate Iodide *on page 501*

◆ **Ecotrin® [OTC]** *see* Aspirin *on page 142*

◆ **Ecotrin® Low Strength [OTC]** *see* Aspirin *on page 142*

◆ **Ecotrin® Maximum Strength [OTC]** *see* Aspirin *on page 142*

◆ **Ectosone (Can)** *see* Betamethasone *on page 188*

Eculizumab (e kue LIZ oo mab)

U.S. Brand Names Soliris™

Pharmacologic Category Monoclonal Antibody; Monoclonal Antibody, Complement Inhibitor

Use Treatment of paroxysmal nocturnal hemoglobinuria (PNH) to reduce hemolysis

Restrictions Patients and providers must enroll with Soliris™ OneSource™ (1-888-765-4747) prior to treatment initiation.

An FDA-approved medication guide is available at http://www.fda.gov/cder/Offices/ODS/medication_guides.htm; distribute to each patient to whom this medication is dispensed.

Pregnancy Risk Factor C

Pregnancy Considerations Animal studies have demonstrated fetal abnormalities. Human IgG is known to cross the placenta; therefore, eculizumab (a recombinant IgG molecule) may also. There are no adequate and well-controlled studies in pregnant women. Pregnant women with PNH and their fetuses have high rates of morbidity and mortality during pregnancy and the postpartum period. Use during pregnancy only if clearly needed.

Lactation Excretion in breast milk unknown/use caution

Medication Safety Issues
Sound-alike/look-alike issues:
Eculizumab may be confused with efalizumab

Contraindications Hypersensitivity to eculizumab or any component of the formulation; unresolved serious *Neisseria meningitidis* infection; use in patients who have not received *Neisseria meningitidis* vaccination at least 2 weeks prior to first treatment

Warnings/Precautions [U.S. Boxed Warning]: The risk for meningococcal *(Neisseria meningitides)* infections (septicemia and/or meningitis) is increased with PNH and may be further increased in patients receiving eculizumab; vaccinate with meningococcal vaccine at least 2 weeks prior to initiation of treatment; revaccinate according to current guidelines. Quadravalent, conjugated meningococcal vaccines are recommended. Meningococcal infections developed in some patients despite vaccination. Monitor for early signs of meningococcal infections; evaluate and treat promptly. Consider withholding eculizumab during the treatment of serious meningococcal infections. In addition to meningitis, the risk of other infections, especially with encapsulated bacteria (eg, *Streptococcus pneumoniae, H. influenzae*) is increased with eculizumab treatment. Use caution in patients with concurrent systemic infection. Patients should be brought up to date with all immunizations before initiating therapy.

Infusion reactions, including anaphylaxis or hypersensitivity, may occur; interrupt infusion for severe reaction. Continue monitoring for 1 hour after completion of infusion. Patients with PNH who discontinue treatment may be at increased risk for serious hemolysis; monitor closely for at least 8 weeks after treatment discontinuation. In clinical trials, anticoagulant therapy was continued in patients who were receiving these agents prior to initiation of eculizumab. The effect of anticoagulant therapy withdrawal is unknown. Safety and efficacy have not been established in children.

Adverse Reactions
>10%:
Central nervous system: Headache (2% to 44%), fatigue (12%)

Gastrointestinal: Nausea (16%)
Neuromuscular & skeletal: Back pain (19%)
Respiratory: Nasopharyngitis (23%), cough (12%)

1% to 10%:
Central nervous system: Fever (2%)
Gastrointestinal: Constipation (7%)
Hematologic: Anemia (2%)
Neuromuscular & skeletal: Limb pain (7%), myalgia (7%)
Respiratory: Respiratory tract infection (7%), sinusitis (7%)
Miscellaneous: Herpes infections (7%), flu-like syndrome (5%), viral infection (2%), meningococcal infection (1%)

<1% (Limited to important or life-threatening): Chills, dizziness, infusion reaction, vomiting

Drug Interactions

Avoid Concomitant Use There are no known interactions where it is recommended to avoid concomitant use.

Increased Effect/Toxicity There are no known significant interactions involving an increase in effect.

Decreased Effect There are no known significant interactions involving a decrease in effect.

Stability Prior to dilution, store vials at 2°C to 8°C (36°F to 46°F). Protect from light; do not freeze; do not shake. Dilute with an equal volume of D_5W, sodium chloride 0.9% sodium chloride 0.45%, or Ringer's injection to a final concentration of 5 mg/mL. (eg, 600 mg in a total volume of 120 mL or 900 mg in a total volume of 180 mL). Gently invert bag to mix. Following dilution, store at room temperature or refrigerate; protect from light; use within 24 hours.

Mechanism of Action Eculizumab is a humanized monoclonal IgG antibody that binds to complement protein C5, preventing cleavage into C5a and C5b. Blocking the formation of C5b inhibits the subsequent formation of terminal complex C5b-9 or membrane attack complex (MAC). Terminal complement-mediated intravascular hemolysis is a key clinical feature of paroxysmal nocturnal hemoglobinuria. Blocking the formation of MAC results in stabilization of hemoglobin and a reduction in the need for RBC transfusions.

Pharmacodynamics/Kinetics
Onset of action: PNH: Reduced hemolysis: ≤1 week
Distribution: 7.7 L
Half-life elimination: ~11 days (range: ~8-15 days)

Dosage Note: Patients must receive meningococcal vaccine at least 2 weeks prior to treatment initiation; revaccinate according to current guidelines.

I.V.: Adults: PNH: 600 mg once weekly (±2 days) for 4 weeks, followed by 900 mg 1 week (±2 days) later; then maintenance: 900 mg every 2 weeks (±2 days) thereafter

Treatment should be administered at the recommended time interval, however, the administration day may be varied by ±2 days if serum LDH levels suggest increased hemolysis before the end of the dosing interval.

Dosage adjustment in renal impairment: Not studied in renal dysfunction

Dosage adjustment in hepatic impairment: Not studied in hepatic dysfunction

Administration I.V.: Allow to warm to room temperature prior to administration. Infuse over 35 minutes. Decrease infusion rate or discontinue for infusion reactions; do not exceed a maximum 2-hour duration of infusion. Monitor for at least 1 hour following completion of infusion.

Monitoring Parameters Signs and symptoms of infusion reaction (during infusion and for 1 hour after infusion complete); CBC with differential, lactic dehydrogenase (LDH), AST, urinalysis

After discontinuation: Signs and symptoms of intravascular hemolysis, serum LDH (monitor for at least 8 weeks after discontinuation)

Dosage Forms Excipient information presented when available (limited, particularly for generics); consult specific product labeling.

Injection, solution [preservative free]:
Soliris™: 10 mg/mL (30 mL) [contains polysorbate 80]

- **Ed A-Hist™** *see* Chlorpheniramine and Phenylephrine *on page 309*
- **Ed A-Hist DM** *see* Chlorpheniramine, Phenylephrine, and Dextromethorphan *on page 311*
- **Edathamil Disodium** *see* Edetate Disodium *on page 505*
- **Ed ChlorPed D** *see* Chlorpheniramine and Phenylephrine *on page 309*
- **Edecrin®** *see* Ethacrynic Acid *on page 573*

Edetate CALCIUM Disodium

(ED e tate KAL see um dye SOW dee um)

U.S. Brand Names Calcium Disodium Versenate®

Index Terms CaEDTA ; Calcium Disodium Edetate; Edetate Disodium CALCIUM; EDTA (CALCIUM Disodium) (error-prone abbreviation)

Pharmacologic Category Chelating Agent

Use Treatment of symptomatic acute and chronic lead poisoning or for symptomatic patients with high blood lead levels

Unlabeled/Investigational Use Possibly useful in poisoning by zinc, manganese, and certain heavy radioisotopes

Pregnancy Risk Factor B

Pregnancy Considerations Adverse events were observed in some animal reproduction studies; there are no well controlled studies of edetate CALCIUM disodium in pregnant women. Following maternal occupational exposure, lead was found to cross the placenta in amounts related to maternal plasma levels. Possible outcomes of maternal lead exposure >10 mcg/dL includes spontaneous abortion, postnatal developmental delay, and reduced birth weight. Chelation therapy during pregnancy is for maternal benefit only and should be limited to the treatment of severe, symptomatic lead poisoning.

Lactation Excretion in breast milk unknown/use caution

Medication Safety Issues

Sound-alike look-alike issues:

To avoid potentially serious errors, the abbreviation "EDTA" should **never** be used.

Edetate CALCIUM disodium (CaEDTA) may be confused with edetate disodium (Na_2EDTA). CDC recommends that edetate disodium should **never** be used for chelation therapy in children. Fatal hypocalcemia may result if edetate disodium is used for chelation therapy instead of edetate calcium disodium. ISMP recommends confirming the diagnosis to help distinguish between the two drugs prior to dispensing and/or administering either drug.

Edetate CALCIUM disodium may be confused with etomidate

Contraindications
Active renal disease or anuria; hepatitis

Warnings/Precautions [U.S. Boxed Warning]: Use with extreme caution in patients with lead encephalopathy and cerebral edema. In these patients, I.V. infusion has been associated with lethal increase in intracranial pressure; I.M. injection is preferred.

Edetate CALCIUM disodium is potentially nephrotoxic; renal tubular acidosis and fatal nephrosis may occur, especially with high doses; ECG changes may occur during therapy; do not exceed recommended daily dose. If anuria, increasing proteinuria, or hematuria occurs during therapy, discontinue edetate CALCIUM disodium. ▶

Minimize nephrotoxicity by adequate hydration, establishment of good urine output, avoidance of excessive doses, and limitation of continuous administration to ≤5 days.

Exercise caution in the ordering, dispensing, and administration of this drug. Edetate CALCIUM disodium (CaEDTA) may be confused with edetate disodium (Na_2EDTA). The CDC and FDA recommend that edetate disodium should never be used for chelation therapy (especially in children). Death has occurred following the use of edetate disodium for chelation therapy in pediatric patients with autism. Fatal hypocalcemia may result if edetate disodium is used for the treatment of lead poisoning instead of edetate CALCIUM disodium. Investigate, identify, and remove sources of lead exposure prior to treatment. Primary care providers should consult experts in chemotherapy of lead toxicity before using chelation drug therapy.

Adverse Reactions Frequency not defined.

Cardiovascular: Arrhythmia, ECG changes, hypotension

Central nervous system: Chills, fatigue, fever, headache, malaise

Dermatologic: Cheilosis, dermatitis, rash

Endocrine & metabolic: Hypercalcemia

Gastrointestinal: Anorexia, GI upset, nausea, thirst (excessive), vomiting

Hematologic: Anemia, bone marrow suppression (transient)

Hepatic: Liver function test increased (mild)

Local: Thrombophlebitis following I.V. infusion (when concentration >5 mg/mL), pain at injection site following I.M. injection

Neuromuscular & skeletal: Arthralgia, myalgia, numbness, tremor

Ocular: Lacrimation

Renal: Glucosuria, nephrotoxicity, renal tubular necrosis, microscopic hematuria, proteinuria, urinary frequency/urgency

Respiratory: Nasal congestion, sneezing

Miscellaneous: Iron, magnesium, and/or zinc deficiency (with chronic therapy)

Drug Interactions

Avoid Concomitant Use There are no known interactions where it is recommended to avoid concomitant use.

Increased Effect/Toxicity

Edetate CALCIUM Disodium may increase the levels/effects of: Insulin

Decreased Effect There are no known significant interactions involving a decrease in effect.

Stability Store at controlled room temperature of 15°C to 30°C (59°F to 86°F). For I.V. infusion, dilute total daily dose into 250-500 mL of 0.9% sodium chloride or D_5W. Concentrations >0.5% (5 mg/mL) should be avoided. Procaine or lidocaine may be added to solutions given by I.M. injection.

Mechanism of Action Calcium is displaced by divalent and trivalent heavy metals, forming a nonionizing soluble complex that is excreted in urine

Pharmacodynamics/Kinetics

Onset of action: Chelation of lead: I.V.: 1 hour

Absorption: I.M., SubQ: Well absorbed; Oral: <5%

Distribution: Into extracellular fluid; minimal CSF penetration (~5%)

Half-life elimination, plasma: 20-60 minutes

Excretion: Urine (as metal chelates or unchanged drug); decreased GFR decreases elimination

Dosage

Treatment of lead poisoning: Children and Adults: **Note:** For the treatment of high blood lead levels in children, the CDC recommends chelation treatment when blood lead levels are >45 mcg/dL (CDC, 2002). In adults, available guidelines recommend chelation therapy with blood lead levels >50 mcg/dL and significant symptoms; chelation therapy may also be indicated with blood lead levels ≥100 mcg/dL and/or symptoms (Kosnett, 2007). Depending upon the blood lead level, additional courses may be necessary; repeat at least 2-4 days and preferably 2-4 weeks apart:

Asymptomatic lead poisoning with blood lead level >20 mcg/dL and <70 mcg/dL (manufacturer labeling): I.M., I.V.: 1000 mg/m²/day (25-50 mg/kg/day) for 5 days. **Note:** The AAP recommends succimer as the drug used for initial management in asymptomatic children when blood lead levels are >45 mcg/dL and <70 mcg/dL. Edetate CALCIUM disodium can be used in children allergic to to succimer (AAP, 2005).

Symptomatic lead poisoning or blood lead levels ≥70 mcg/dL: I.M., I.V.: 1000 mg/m²/day (25-50 mg/kg/day) for 5 days. Edetate CALCIUM disodium should be administered 4 hours after the initial dimercaprol dose. Edetate CALCIUM disodium should be used in conjunction with dimercaprol when blood lead levels are >70 mcg/dL or when symptoms of lead poisoning are present.

Lead encephalopathy: I.M., I.V.: 1500 mg/m²/day (50-75 mg/kg/day). Edetate CALCIUM disodium should be administered 4 hours after the initial dimercaprol dose. Edetate CALCIUM disodium should be used in conjunction with dimercaprol when blood lead levels are >70 mcg/dL or when symptoms of lead poisoning are present.

Lead nephropathy: Adults: An alternative dosing regimen reflecting the reduction in renal clearance is based upon the serum creatinine. Dose of edetate CALCIUM disodium based on serum creatinine (Morgan, 1975): **Note:** Repeat regimen monthly until lead levels are reduced to an acceptable level:

S_{cr} >2-3 mg/dL / Cl_{cr} 30-50 mL/minute: Reduce recommended dose by 50% and administer daily

S_{cr} >3-4 mg/dL / Cl_{cr} 20-30 mL/minute: Reduce recommended dose by 50% and administer every 48 hours

S_{cr} >4 mg/dL / Cl_{cr} <20 mL/minute: Reduce recommended dose by 50% and administer once weekly

Dosage adjustment in renal impairment: Dose should be reduced with pre-existing mild renal disease. Limiting daily dose to 1 g in children and 2 g in adults may decrease risk of nephrotoxicity, although larger doses may be needed in the treatment of lead encephalopathy.

Administration For I.M. or I.V. use; I.V. is generally preferred, however, I.M. route is preferred when cerebral edema is present.

I.V. infusion: Administer daily dose in diluted solution over 8-12 hours or continuously over 24 hours

For I.M. injection: Daily dose should be divided into 2-3 equal doses spaced 8-12 hours apart. Procaine hydrochloride or lidocaine may be added to edetate CALCIUM disodium to minimize pain at injection site. Administer by deep I.M. injection. When used in conjunction with dimercaprol, inject in a separate site.

Monitoring Parameters Urinary output; ECG changes (with I.V. therapy); blood lead levels (baseline and 7-21 days after completing chelation therapy); hemoglobin or hematocrit, iron status, free erythrocyte protoporphyrin or zinc protoporphyrin; neurodevelopmental changes

Test Interactions If edetate CALCIUM disodium is given as a continuous I.V. infusion, stop the infusion for at least

1 hour before blood is drawn for lead concentration to avoid a falsely elevated value

Dosage Forms Excipient information presented when available (limited, particularly for generics); consult specific product labeling.

Injection, solution: 200 mg/mL (5 mL)

Edetate Disodium (ED e tate dye SOW dee um)

U.S. Brand Names Endrate® [DSC]

Index Terms Edathamil Disodium; EDTA (Disodium) (error-prone abbreviation); Na_2EDTA; Sodium Edetate

Pharmacologic Category Chelating Agent

Use Emergency treatment of hypercalcemia in adults

Unlabeled/Investigational Use Emergency treatment of hypercalcemia in children

Pregnancy Risk Factor C

Medication Safety Issues

Sound-alike look-alike issues:

To avoid potentially serious errors, the abbreviation "EDTA" should **never** be used.

Edetate disodium (Na_2EDTA) may be confused with edetate calcium disodium (CaEDTA). CDC recommends that edetate disodium should **never** be used for chelation therapy in children. Fatal hypocalcemia may result if edetate disodium is used for chelation therapy instead of edetate calcium disodium. ISMP recommends confirming the diagnosis to help distinguish between the two drugs prior to dispensing and/or administering either drug.

Edetate disodium may be confused with etomidate

Contraindications Hypersensitivity to edetate disodium or any component of the formulation; severe renal disease or anuria

Warnings/Precautions **[U.S. Boxed Warning]: Use of this drug is recommended only when the severity of the clinical condition justifies the aggressive measures associated with this type of therapy;** use with caution in patients with renal dysfunction, diabetes, hypokalemia, intracranial lesions, seizure disorders, vascular disease

Not recommended for the treatment of atherosclerotic cardiovascular disease; no evidence of a beneficial effect with chelation therapy.

Exercise caution in the ordering, dispensing, and administration of this drug. Edetate disodium (Na_2EDTA) may be confused with edetate CALCIUM disodium (CaEDTA). The CDC and FDA recommend that edetate disodium should never be used for chelation therapy (especially in children). Death has occurred following the use of edetate disodium for chelation therapy in pediatric patients with autism. Fatal hypocalcemia may result if edetate disodium is used for the treatment of lead poisoning instead of edetate CALCIUM disodium. Rapid I.V. administration or excessive doses may cause a sudden drop in serum calcium concentration which may lead to hypocalcemic tetany, seizure, arrhythmia, and death from respiratory arrest. Do not exceed recommended dosage and rate of administration. Safety and efficacy have not been established in pediatric patients.

Adverse Reactions Frequency not always defined.

Gastrointestinal: Nausea, vomiting, abdominal cramps, diarrhea

<1% (Limited to important or life-threatening): Arrhythmias, transient hypotension, acute tubular necrosis, seizure, fever, headache, tetany, chills, eruptions, dermatologic lesions, hypomagnesemia, hypokalemia, anemia, thrombophlebitis, pain at the site of injection, paresthesia, back pain, muscle cramps, nephrotoxicity, death from respiratory arrest

Drug Interactions

Avoid Concomitant Use There are no known interactions where it is recommended to avoid concomitant use.

Increased Effect/Toxicity

Edetate Disodium may increase the levels/effects of: Insulin

Decreased Effect There are no known significant interactions involving a decrease in effect.

Mechanism of Action Chelates with divalent or trivalent metals to form a soluble complex that is then eliminated in urine

Pharmacodynamics/Kinetics

Metabolism: None

Half-life elimination: 20-60 minutes

Time to peak: I.V.: 24-48 hours

Excretion: Following chelation: Urine (95%); chelates within 24-48 hours

Dosage Note: Confirm the diagnosis prior to dispensing.

Hypercalcemia: I.V.:

Children (unlabeled use): 40-70 mg/kg/day slow infusion over 3-4 hours or more to a maximum of 3 g/24 hours; administer for 5 days and allow 5 days between courses of therapy

Adults: 50 mg/kg/day over 3 or more hours to a maximum of 3 g/24 hours; a suggested regimen of 5 days followed by 2 days without drug and repeated courses up to 15 total doses

Dietary Considerations Sodium content of 1 g: 5.4 mEq

Administration Parenteral: I.V.: Must be diluted before I.V. use in D_5W or NS to a maximum concentration of 30 mg/mL (3%) and infused over at least 3 hours; avoid extravasation; not for I.M. use

Monitoring Parameters ECG monitoring; blood pressure during infusion; renal function should be assessed before and during therapy; monitor calcium, magnesium, and potassium levels

Dosage Forms Excipient information presented when available (limited, particularly for generics); consult specific product labeling. [DSC] = Discontinued product

Injection, solution: 150 mg/mL (20 mL)

Endrate®: 150 mg/mL (20 mL) [DSC]

◆ **Edetate Disodium CALCIUM** *see* Edetate CALCIUM Disodium *on page 503*

◆ **Edex®** *see* Alprostadil *on page 70*

Edrophonium (ed roe FOE nee um)

U.S. Brand Names Enlon® [DSC]

Canadian Brand Names Enlon®; Tensilon®

Index Terms Edrophonium Chloride

Pharmacologic Category Antidote; Cholinergic Agonist; Diagnostic Agent

Use Diagnosis of myasthenia gravis; differentiation of cholinergic crises from myasthenia crises; reversal of nondepolarizing neuromuscular blockers; adjunct treatment of respiratory depression caused by curare overdose

Pregnancy Risk Factor C

Lactation Excretion in breast milk unknown

Contraindications Hypersensitivity to edrophonium, sulfites, or any component of the formulation; GI or GU obstruction

Warnings/Precautions Use with caution in patients with bronchial asthma and those receiving a cardiac glycoside; atropine sulfate should always be readily available as an antagonist. Overdosage can cause cholinergic crisis which may be fatal. I.V. atropine should be readily available for treatment of cholinergic reactions. Use with caution in patients with cardiac arrhythmias (eg, bradyarrhythmias). Avoid use in myasthenia gravis; may exacerbate muscular weakness. Products may contain sodium sulfite.

▶

Adverse Reactions Frequency not defined.

Cardiovascular: Arrhythmias (especially bradycardia), AV block, cardiac arrest, decreased carbon monoxide, flushing, hypotension, nodal rhythm, nonspecific ECG changes, syncope, tachycardia

Central nervous system: Convulsions, dizziness, drowsiness, dysarthria, dysphonia, headache, loss of consciousness

Dermatologic: Skin rash, thrombophlebitis (I.V.), urticaria

Gastrointestinal: Diarrhea, dysphagia, flatulence, hyperperistalsis, nausea, salivation, stomach cramps, vomiting

Genitourinary: Urinary urgency

Neuromuscular & skeletal: Arthralgias, fasciculations, muscle cramps, spasms, weakness

Ocular: Lacrimation, small pupils

Respiratory: Bronchiolar constriction, bronchospasm, dyspnea, bronchial secretions increased, laryngospasm, respiratory arrest, respiratory depression, respiratory muscle paralysis

Miscellaneous: Allergic reactions, anaphylaxis, diaphoresis increased

Drug Interactions

Avoid Concomitant Use There are no known interactions where it is recommended to avoid concomitant use.

Increased Effect/Toxicity

The levels/effects of Edrophonium may be increased by: Acetylcholinesterase Inhibitors

Decreased Effect There are no known significant interactions involving a decrease in effect.

Mechanism of Action Inhibits destruction of acetylcholine by acetylcholinesterase. This facilitates transmission of impulses across myoneural junction and results in increased cholinergic responses such as miosis, increased tonus of intestinal and skeletal muscles, bronchial and ureteral constriction, bradycardia, and increased salivary and sweat gland secretions.

Pharmacodynamics/Kinetics

Onset of action: I.M.: 2-10 minutes; I.V.: 30-60 seconds

Duration: I.M.: 5-30 minutes: I.V.: 10 minutes

Distribution: V_d: Adults: 1.1 L/kg

Half-life elimination: Adults: 1.2-2.4 hours; Anephric patients: 2.4-4.4 hours

Excretion: Adults: Primarily urine (67%)

Dosage Usually administered I.V., however, if not possible, I.M. or SubQ may be used:

Infants:

I.M.: 0.5-1 mg

I.V.: Initial: 0.1 mg, followed by 0.4 mg if no response; total dose = 0.5 mg

Children:

Diagnosis: Initial: 0.04 mg/kg over 1 minute followed by 0.16 mg/kg if no response, to a maximum total dose of 5 mg for children <34 kg, or 10 mg for children >34 kg

or

Alternative dosing (manufacturer's recommendation):

≤34 kg: 1 mg; if no response after 45 seconds, repeat dosage in 1 mg increments every 30-45 seconds, up to a total of 5 mg

>34 kg: 2 mg; if no response after 45 seconds, repeat dosage in 1 mg increments every 30-45 seconds, up to a total of 10 mg

I.M.:

<34 kg: 1 mg

>34 kg: 5 mg

Titration of oral anticholinesterase therapy: 0.04 mg/kg once given 1 hour after oral intake of the drug being used in treatment; if strength improves, an increase in neostigmine or pyridostigmine dose is indicated

Adults:

Diagnosis:

I.V.: 2 mg test dose administered over 15-30 seconds; 8 mg given 45 seconds later if no response is seen; test dose may be repeated after 30 minutes

I.M.: Initial: 10 mg; if no cholinergic reaction occurs, administer 2 mg 30 minutes later to rule out false-negative reaction

Titration of oral anticholinesterase therapy: 1-2 mg given 1 hour after oral dose of anticholinesterase; if strength improves, an increase in neostigmine or pyridostigmine dose is indicated

Reversal of nondepolarizing neuromuscular blocking agents (neostigmine with atropine usually preferred): I.V.: 10 mg over 30-45 seconds; may repeat every 5-10 minutes up to 40 mg

Termination of paroxysmal atrial tachycardia: I.V. rapid injection: 5-10 mg

Differentiation of cholinergic from myasthenic crisis: I.V.: 1 mg; may repeat after 1 minute. **Note:** Intubation and controlled ventilation may be required if patient has cholinergic crisis

Dosing adjustment in renal impairment: Dose may need to be reduced in patients with chronic renal failure

Administration Edrophonium is administered by direct I.V. injection; see Dosage

Monitoring Parameters Pre- and postinjection strength (cranial musculature is most useful); heart rate, respiratory rate, blood pressure

Test Interactions Increased aminotransferase [ALT/AST] (S), amylase (S)

Additional Information Atropine should be administered along with edrophonium when reversing the effects of nondepolarizing agents to antagonize the cholinergic effects at the muscarinic receptors, especially bradycardia. It is important to recognize the difference in dose for diagnosis of myasthenia gravis versus reversal of muscle relaxant, a much larger dose is needed for desired effect of reversal of muscle paralysis.

Dosage Forms Excipient information presented when available (limited, particularly for generics); consult specific product labeling.

Injection, solution, as chloride:

Enlon®: 10 mg/mL (15 mL) [contains sodium sulfite]

Edrophonium and Atropine

(ed roe FOE nee um & A troe peen)

U.S. Brand Names Enlon-Plus™ [DSC]

Index Terms Atropine Sulfate and Edrophonium Chloride; Edrophonium Chloride and Atropine Sulfate

Pharmacologic Category Anticholinergic Agent; Antidote; Cholinergic Agonist

Use Reversal of nondepolarizing neuromuscular blockers; adjunct treatment of respiratory depression caused by curare overdose

Pregnancy Risk Factor C

Dosage I.V.: Adults: Reversal of neuromuscular blockade: 0.05 mL/kg given over 45-60 seconds. The dose delivered is 0.5-1 mg/kg of edrophonium and 0.007-0.015 mg/kg of atropine. An edrophonium dose of 1 mg/kg should rarely be exceeded. **Note:** Monitor closely for bradyarrhythmias. Have atropine on hand in case needed.

Dosage adjustment in renal impairment: Adjustment not required.

Dosage adjustment in hepatic impairment: Adjustment not required.

Additional Information Complete prescribing information for this medication should be consulted for additional detail.

Dosage Forms Excipient information presented when available (limited, particularly for generics); consult specific product labeling. [DSC] = Discontinued product

Injection, solution:

Enlon-Plus™: Edrophonium chloride 10 mg/mL and atropine sulfate 0.14 mg/mL (5 mL, 15 mL) [contains sodium sulfite] [DSC]

◆ **Edrophonium Chloride** *see* Edrophonium *on page 505*

◆ **Edrophonium Chloride and Atropine Sulfate** *see* Edrophonium and Atropine *on page 506*

◆ **EDTA (CALCIUM Disodium) (error-prone abbreviation)** *see* Edetate CALCIUM Disodium *on page 503*

◆ **EDTA (Disodium) (error-prone abbreviation)** *see* Edetate Disodium *on page 505*

◆ **E.E.M.T. D.S.** *see* Estrogens (Esterified) and Methyltestosterone *on page 568*

◆ **E.E.M.T. H.S.** *see* Estrogens (Esterified) and Methyltestosterone *on page 568*

◆ **E.E.S.®** *see* Erythromycin *on page 544*

◆ **EES® (Can)** *see* Erythromycin *on page 544*

Efalizumab (e fa li ZOO mab)

U.S. Brand Names Raptiva®

Index Terms Anti-CD11a; hu1124

Pharmacologic Category Immunosuppressant Agent; Monoclonal Antibody

Use Treatment of chronic moderate-to-severe plaque psoriasis in patients who are candidates for systemic therapy or phototherapy

Pregnancy Risk Factor C

Pregnancy Considerations Reproduction studies have not been conducted. A decreased ability to mount an antibody response was observed in the offspring of female mice who received efalizumab during toxicity studies. There are no adequate and well-controlled studies in pregnant women. Healthcare providers are encouraged to enroll patients who may become pregnant during therapy or within 6 weeks of discontinuing treatment in the Raptiva® registry (877-727-8482).

Lactation Excretion in breast milk unknown/not recommended

Medication Safety Issues

Sound-alike/look-alike issues:

Efalizumab may be confused with eculizumab

Raptiva® maybe confused with Rapaflo®

Contraindications Hypersensitivity to efalizumab or any component of the formulation

Warnings/Precautions **[U.S. Boxed Warning]: Infections (bacterial, viral, fungal and other opportunistic infections), some serious and even fatal, have been reported with efalizumab use.** May result in increased susceptibility to infections or reactivation of latent infection; use caution with chronic infections, history of recurrent infection, or the elderly. Avoid administration to patients with clinically important infection. Discontinue therapy if serious infection develops. Neurologic events, including chronic inflammatory demyelinating polyneuropathy, facial palsy, Guillain-Barré syndrome, and transverse myelitis, have been observed; discontinue therapy if signs of a neurologic event occurs. **[U.S. Boxed Warning]: Progressive multifocal leukoencephalopathy (PML), a demyelinating central nervous system disease due to latent JC virus infection, has been reported with efalizumab use.** Evaluate any neurological change promptly; if clinically indicated, consider neurology consultation, brain MRI, and lumbar puncture for suspected PML. Discontinue efalizumab in patients who develop PML. Thrombocytopenia has been reported (rare) and may require treatment; discontinue if thrombocytopenia develops. Hemolytic anemia, which may occur after 4-6 months of treatment, has been reported; discontinue if signs and symptoms of hemolytic anemia occur. Use caution in patients at high risk for malignancy or history of malignancy; effects of efalizumab on the development of malignancies is unknown. Psoriasis and/or arthritis may worsen with efalizumab treatment or following discontinuation (rare). First-dose reactions have been reported; a lower, conditioning dose is recommended to reduce the incidence and severity of reactions. Concomitant use with other immunosuppressant agents is not recommended. Patients should be brought up to date with all immunizations before initiating therapy. Live vaccines should not be given concurrently; there is no data available concerning secondary transmission of live vaccines in patients receiving therapy. Inactivated immunizations may not elicit adequate response to prevent disease. Produced in a Chinese hamster cell medium. Safety and efficacy in pediatric patients or patients with renal or hepatic impairment have not been established.

Adverse Reactions

>10%:

Central nervous system: Headache (32%), chills (13%)

Gastrointestinal: Nausea (11%)

Hematologic: Lymphocytosis (40%), leukocytosis (26%)

Miscellaneous: First-dose reaction (29%, described as chills, fever, headache, myalgia, and nausea occurring within 2 days of the first injection; percent reported in patients receiving a 1 mg/kg dose; severity decreased with 0.7 mg/kg dose); infection (29%, serious infection <1%)

1% to 10%:

Cardiovascular: Peripheral edema (1% to 2%)

Central nervous system: Pain (10%), fever (7%)

Dermatologic: Acne (4%), psoriasis (1% to 2%), urticaria (1%)

Hepatic: Alkaline phosphatase elevated (4%)

Neuromuscular & skeletal: Myalgia (8%), back pain (4%), arthralgia (1% to 2%), weakness (1% to 2%)

Miscellaneous: Antibodies to efalizumab (6%); hypersensitivity reaction, including asthma, dyspnea, angioedema, urticaria, or maculopapular rash (8%); flu-like syndrome (7%)

<1% (Limited to important or life-threatening): Arthritis, aseptic meningitis, asthma, bacterial sepsis (with seeding of distant sites), bronchiolitis obliterans, chronic inflammatory demyelinating polyneuropathy, drug eruption (allergic), erythema multiforme, facial palsy, fungal infection, Guillain-Barré syndrome, hemolytic anemia (immune mediated), inflammatory arthritis, idiopathic hepatitis, interstitial pneumonitis, laryngospasm, lymphoma, malignancies, necrotizing fasciitis, opportunistic infection, photoallergic dermatitis, photosensitivity, pneumonia (severe with neutropenia), progressive multifocal leukoencephalopathy (PML), serious psoriasis events (include erythrodermic, guttate, and pustular subtypes); psoriatic arthritis, serum sickness-like reaction, sialadenitis, sensorineural hearing loss, thrombocytopenia (immune mediated), toxic epidermal necrolysis, transverse myelitis, tuberculous pneumonia, viral infection

Drug Interactions

Avoid Concomitant Use

Avoid concomitant use of Efalizumab with any of the following: Natalizumab; Vaccines (Live)

Increased Effect/Toxicity

Efalizumab may increase the levels/effects of: Natalizumab; Vaccines (Live)

The levels/effects of Efalizumab may be increased by: Trastuzumab

Decreased Effect

Efalizumab may decrease the levels/effects of: Vaccines (Inactivated)

The levels/effects of Efalizumab may be decreased by: Echinacea

Stability Powder should be stored under refrigeration at 2°C to 8°C (36°F to 46°F) and protected from light. Slowly inject 1.3 mL of the provided diluent into vial. Gently swirl to mix; do not shake. Following reconstitution, solution should be stored at room temperature and used within 8 hours. Discard unused solution.

Mechanism of Action Efalizumab is a recombinant monoclonal antibody which binds to CD11a, a subunit of leukocyte function antigen-1 (LFA-1) found on leukocytes. By binding to CD11a, efalizumab blocks multiple T-cell mediated responses involved in the pathogenesis of psoriatic plaques.

Pharmacodynamics/Kinetics

Onset of action: Reduction of CD11a expression and free CD11a-binding sites seen 1-2 days after the first dose; time to steady state serum concentration: 4 weeks

Response to therapy (75% reduction from baseline of PASI score): Observed after 12 weeks

Duration: CD11a expression was ~74% of baseline at 5-13 weeks after discontinuing dose; free CD11a binding sites were at ~86% of baseline at 8-13 weeks following discontinuation; response to therapy (75% reduction from baseline PASI score) continued 1-2 months after discontinuation

Bioavailability: SubQ: 50%

Excretion: Time to eliminate (at steady state): 25 days (range: 13-35 days)

Dosage SubQ: Adults: Psoriasis: Initial: 0.7 mg/kg, followed by weekly dose of 1 mg/kg (maximum: 200 mg/dose)

Administration For SubQ injection in the abdomen, buttocks, thigh, or upper arm. Rotate injection sites.

Monitoring Parameters Platelet counts (at least monthly at the start of treatment, every 3 months as therapy continues); signs of infection; worsening of psoriasis; any neurologic impairment

Signs or symptoms of progressive multifocal leukoencephalopathy (focal neurologic deficits, which may present as hemiparesis, visual field deficits, cognitive impairment, aphasia, ataxia, and/or cranial nerve deficits); if PML is suspected, obtain brain MRI scan and lumbar puncture

Test Interactions Increased lymphocytes (related to mechanism of action)

Dosage Forms Excipient information presented when available (limited, particularly for generics); consult specific product labeling.

Injection, powder for reconstitution:

Raptiva®: 150 mg [contains sucrose 123.2 mg/vial; delivers 125 mg/1.25 mL; packaged with prefilled syringe containing sterile water for injection]

Efavirenz (e FAV e renz)

U.S. Brand Names Sustiva®

Canadian Brand Names Sustiva®

Pharmacologic Category Antiretroviral Agent, Reverse Transcriptase Inhibitor (Non-nucleoside)

Additional Appendix Information

Antiretroviral Therapy for HIV Infection: Adults and Adolescents *on page 1758*

Management of Healthcare Worker Exposures to HBV, HCV, and HIV *on page 1719*

Perinatal HIV Guidelines *on page 1730*

Use Treatment of HIV-1 infections in combination with at least two other antiretroviral agents

Pregnancy Risk Factor D

Pregnancy Considerations Teratogenic effects have been observed in Primates receiving efavirenz. Severe CNS defects have been reported in infants following efavirenz exposure in the first trimester. Pregnancy should be avoided and alternate therapy should be considered in women of childbearing potential. Women of childbearing potential should undergo pregnancy testing prior to initiation of efavirenz. Barrier contraception should be used in combination with other (hormonal) methods of contraception and for 12 weeks after efavirenz is discontinued. If therapy with efavirenz is administered during pregnancy, avoid use during the first trimester. Health professionals are encouraged to contact the antiretroviral pregnancy registry to monitor outcomes of pregnant women exposed to antiretroviral medications (1-800-258-4263 or www.APRegistry.com).

Lactation Excretion is breast milk unknown/contraindicated

Contraindications Hypersensitivity to efavirenz or any component of the formulation; concurrent use of cisapride, midazolam, pimozide, triazolam, voriconazole (with standard [eg, unadjusted] voriconazole and efavirenz doses), or ergot alkaloids (includes dihydroergotamine, ergotamine, ergonovine, methylergonovine)

Warnings/Precautions Do not use as single-agent therapy; avoid pregnancy; women of childbearing potential should undergo pregnancy testing prior to initiation of therapy; use caution with other agents metabolized by cytochrome P450 isoenzyme 3A4 (see Contraindications); use caution with history of mental illness/drug abuse (predisposition to psychological reactions); may cause CNS and psychiatric symptoms, which include impaired concentration, dizziness or drowsiness (avoid potentially hazardous tasks such as driving or operating machinery if these effects are noted); CNS effects may be potentiated when used with other sedative drugs or ethanol. Serious psychiatric side effects have been associated with efavirenz, including severe depression, suicide, paranoia, and mania. Discontinue if severe rash (involving blistering, desquamation, mucosal involvement or fever) develops. Children are more susceptible

Caution in patients with known or suspected hepatitis B or C infection (monitoring of liver function is recommended); hepatic impairment. Persistent elevations of serum transaminases >5 times the upper limit of normal should prompt evaluation - benefit of continued therapy should be weighed against possible risk of hepatotoxicity. Increases in total cholesterol and triglycerides have been reported; screening should be done prior to therapy and periodically throughout treatment. May cause redistribution of fat (eg, buffalo hump, peripheral wasting with increased abdominal girth, cushingoid appearance). Patients may develop immune reconstitution syndrome resulting in the occurrence of an inflammatory response to an indolent or residual opportunistic infection; further evaluation and treatment may be required. Use with caution in patients with a history of seizure disorder; seizures have been associated with use.

Adverse Reactions

Unless otherwise noted, frequency of adverse events is as reported in adults receiving combination antiretroviral therapy.

>10%:

Central nervous system: Dizziness (2% to 28%; children 16%), fever (children 21%), depression (up to 19%; severe: 1% to 2%), insomnia (up to 16%), anxiety (2% to 13%), pain (1% to 13%; children 14%), headache (2% to 8%; children 11%)

Dermatologic: Rash (5% to 26%, grade 3/4: <1%; children up to 46%, grade 3/4: 2% to 4%)

Endocrine & metabolic: HDL increased (25% to 35%), total cholesterol increased (20% to 40%), triglycerides increased (≥751 mg/dL: 6% to 11%)

Gastrointestinal: Diarrhea (3% to 14%; children: up to 39%), nausea (2% to 12%; children 12%), vomiting (3% to 6%; children 12%)

Respiratory: Cough (children 16%)

1% to 10%:

Central nervous system: Impaired concentration (up to 8%), somnolence (up to 7%), fatigue (up to 8%), abnormal dreams (1% to 6%), nervousness (2% to 7%), hallucinations (1%)

Dermatologic: Pruritus (up to 9%)

Endocrine & metabolic: Hyperglycemia (>250 mg/dL: 2% to 5%)

Gastrointestinal: Dyspepsia (up to 4%), abdominal pain (2% to 3%), anorexia (up to 2%), amylase increased (grade 3/4: up to 6%)

Hematologic: Neutropenia (grade 3/4: 2% to 10%)

Hepatic: Transaminases increased (grade 3/4: 2% to 8%, incidence higher with hepatitis B and/or C coinfection)

Miscellaneous: Diaphoresis increased (1% to 2%)

<1% (Limited to important or life-threatening): Allergic reaction, aggressive reaction, agitation, arthralgia, ataxia, balance disturbances, body fat accumulation/redistribution, cerebellar coordination disturbances, constipation, coordination abnormal, delusions, dermatitis (photoallergic), dyspnea, emotional lability, erythema multiforme, flushing, gynecomastia, hepatic failure, hepatitis, hypoesthesia, immune reconstitution syndrome, malabsorption, mania, myalgia, myopathy, nail disorder, neuropathy, neurosis, palpitation, paranoia, paresthesia, psychosis, seizure, skin discoloration, Stevens-Johnson syndrome, suicide attempts, suicidal ideation, tinnitus, tremor, visual abnormality, weakness

Drug Interactions

Metabolism/Transport Effects Substrate (major) of CYP2B6, 3A4; **Inhibits** CYP2C9 (moderate), 2C19 (moderate), 3A4 (moderate); **Induces** CYP2B6 (weak), 3A4 (strong)

Avoid Concomitant Use

Avoid concomitant use of Efavirenz with any of the following: Cisapride; Ergot Derivatives; Etravirine; Midazolam; Nilotinib; Nisoldipine; Pimozide; Posaconazole; Ranolazine; St Johns Wort; Triazolam

Increased Effect/Toxicity

Efavirenz may increase the levels/effects of: Cisapride; CYP2C19 Substrates; CYP2C9 Substrates (High risk); CYP3A4 Substrates; Eplerenone; Ergot Derivatives; Etravirine; FentaNYL; Maraviroc; Midazolam; Phenytoin; Pimecrolimus; Pimozide; Protease Inhibitors; Ranolazine; Salmeterol; Triazolam; Vitamin K Antagonists

The levels/effects of Efavirenz may be increased by: Darunavir; Voriconazole

Decreased Effect

Efavirenz may decrease the levels/effects of: Atazanavir; Caspofungin; CYP3A4 Substrates; Darunavir; Etravirine; Itraconazole; Lopinavir; Maraviroc; Methadone; Nilotinib; Nisoldipine; Posaconazole; Protease Inhibitors; Raltegravir; Ranolazine; Rifabutin; Sertraline; Sorafenib; Voriconazole

The levels/effects of Efavirenz may be decreased by: CYP2B6 Inducers (Strong); CYP3A4 Inducers (Strong); Deferasirox; Phenytoin; Rifabutin; Rifampin; St Johns Wort

Ethanol/Nutrition/Herb Interactions

Ethanol: Avoid ethanol (hepatic and CNS adverse effects).

Food: Avoid high-fat meals (increase the absorption of efavirenz).

Herb/Nutraceutical: St John's wort may decrease efavirenz serum levels. Avoid concurrent use.

Stability Store at controlled room temperature of 25°C (77°F), excursion permitted to 15°C to 30°C (59°F to 86°F).

Mechanism of Action As a non-nucleoside reverse transcriptase inhibitor, efavirenz has activity against HIV-1 by binding to reverse transcriptase. It consequently blocks the RNA-dependent and DNA-dependent DNA polymerase activities including HIV-1 replication. It does not require intracellular phosphorylation for antiviral activity.

Pharmacodynamics/Kinetics

Absorption: Increased by fatty meals

Distribution: CSF concentrations exceed free fraction in serum

Protein binding: >99%, primarily to albumin

Metabolism: Hepatic via CYP3A4 and 2B6 to inactive hydroxylated metabolites; may induce its own metabolism

Half-life elimination: Single dose: 52-76 hours; Multiple doses: 40-55 hours

Time to peak: 3-5 hours

Excretion: Feces (16% to 61% primarily as unchanged drug); urine (14% to 34% as metabolites)

Dosage Oral:

Children ≥3 years: Dosage is based on body weight:
- 10 kg to <15 kg: 200 mg once daily
- 15 kg to <20 kg: 250 mg once daily
- 20 kg to <25 kg: 300 mg once daily
- 25 kg to <32.5 kg: 350 mg once daily
- 32.5 kg to <40 kg: 400 mg once daily
- ≥40 kg: 600 mg once daily

Adults: 600 mg once daily

Dosage adjustment for concomitant voriconazole: Reduce efavirenz dose to 300 mg once daily and increase voriconazole to 400 mg every 12 hours

Dosing adjustment in renal impairment: None recommended

Dosing comments in hepatic impairment: Limited clinical experience, use with caution

Dietary Considerations Should be taken on an empty stomach.

Administration Administer on an empty stomach. Dosing at bedtime is recommended to limit central nervous system effects. Tablets should not be broken. Capsules may be opened and added to liquid or food.

Monitoring Parameters Serum transaminases (discontinuation of treatment should be considered for persistent elevations greater than five times the upper limit of normal), cholesterol, triglycerides, signs and symptoms of infection

Test Interactions False-positive test for cannabinoids have been reported when the CEDIA DAU Multilevel THC assay is used. False-positive results with other assays for cannabinoids have not been observed.

Additional Information Efavirenz oral solution is available only through an expanded access (compassionate use) program. Enrollment information may be obtained by calling 1-877-372-7097.

Early virologic failure was observed with tenofovir and didanosine delayed release capsules, plus either efavirenz or nevirapine; use caution in treatment-naive patients with high baseline viral loads.

Dosage Forms Excipient information presented when available (limited, particularly for generics); consult specific product labeling. [DSC] = Discontinued product

Capsule:
Sustiva®: 50 mg; 100 mg [DSC]; 200 mg

Tablet:
Sustiva®: 600 mg

Efavirenz, Emtricitabine, and Tenofovir

(e FAV e renz, em trye SYE ta been, & te NOE fo veer)

U.S. Brand Names Atripla®

Canadian Brand Names Atripla®

Index Terms Emtricitabine, Efavirenz, and Tenofovir; FTC, TDF, and EFV; Tenofovir Disoproxil Fumarate, Efavirenz, and Emtricitabine

Pharmacologic Category Antiretroviral Agent, Reverse Transcriptase Inhibitor (Non-nucleoside); Antiretroviral Agent, Reverse Transcriptase Inhibitor (Nucleoside); Antiretroviral Agent, Reverse Transcriptase Inhibitor (Nucleotide)

Additional Appendix Information

Antiretroviral Therapy for HIV Infection: Adults and Adolescents *on page 1758*

Management of Healthcare Worker Exposures to HBV, HCV, and HIV *on page 1719*

Use Treatment of HIV infection

Pregnancy Risk Factor D

Dosage Oral: Adults: One tablet once daily

Dosage adjustment in renal impairment: Moderate-to-severe renal impairment (Cl_{cr} <50 mL/minute): Use not recommended

Additional Information Complete prescribing information for this medication should be consulted for additional detail.

Dosage Forms Excipient information presented when available (limited, particularly for generics); consult specific product labeling.

Tablet:

Atripla™: Efavirenz 600 mg, emtricitabine 200 mg, and tenofovir disoproxil fumarate 300 mg

- ◆ **Effer-K™** *see* Potassium Bicarbonate and Potassium Citrate *on page 1216*
- ◆ **Effexor®** *see* Venlafaxine *on page 1554*
- ◆ **Effexor XR®** *see* Venlafaxine *on page 1554*
- ◆ **Effexor® XR (Can)** *see* Venlafaxine *on page 1554*

Eflornithine (ee FLOR ni theen)

U.S. Brand Names Vaniqa™

Canadian Brand Names Vaniqa™

Index Terms DFMO; Eflornithine Hydrochloride

Pharmacologic Category Antiprotozoal; Topical Skin Product

Use Cream: Females ≥12 years: Reduce unwanted hair from face and adjacent areas under the chin

Orphan status: Injection: Treatment of meningoencephalitic stage of *Trypanosoma brucei gambiense* infection (sleeping sickness)

Pregnancy Risk Factor C

Medication Safety Issues

Sound-alike/look-alike issues:

Vaniqa™ may be confused with Viagra®

Dosage

Children ≥12 years and Adults: Females: Topical: Apply thin layer of cream to affected areas of face and adjacent chin twice daily, at least 8 hours apart

Adults: I.V. infusion: 100 mg/kg/dose given every 6 hours (over at least 45 minutes) for 14 days

Dosing adjustment in renal impairment: Injection: Dose should be adjusted although no specific guidelines are available

Additional Information Complete prescribing information for this medication should be consulted for additional detail.

Dosage Forms Excipient information presented when available (limited, particularly for generics); consult specific product labeling.

Cream, topical, as hydrochloride: 13.9% (30 g)

Injection, solution, as hydrochloride: 200 mg/mL (100 mL) [orphan drug status]

- ◆ **Eflornithine Hydrochloride** *see* Eflornithine *on page 510*
- ◆ **Eformoterol and Budesonide** *see* Budesonide and Formoterol *on page 218*
- ◆ **Efudex®** *see* Fluorouracil *on page 636*
- ◆ **E-Gems® [OTC]** *see* Vitamin E *on page 1566*
- ◆ **E-Gems Elite® [OTC]** *see* Vitamin E *on page 1566*
- ◆ **E-Gems Plus® [OTC]** *see* Vitamin E *on page 1566*
- ◆ **EHDP** *see* Etidronate Disodium *on page 586*
- ◆ **Elaprase™** *see* Idursulfase *on page 766*
- ◆ **Elavil** *see* Amitriptyline *on page 90*
- ◆ **Eldepryl®** *see* Selegiline *on page 1359*
- ◆ **Eldopaque® [OTC]** *see* Hydroquinone *on page 749*
- ◆ **Eldopaque® (Can)** *see* Hydroquinone *on page 749*
- ◆ **Eldopaque Forte®** *see* Hydroquinone *on page 749*
- ◆ **Eldoquin® [OTC]** *see* Hydroquinone *on page 749*
- ◆ **Eldoquin® (Can)** *see* Hydroquinone *on page 749*
- ◆ **Eldoquin Forte®** *see* Hydroquinone *on page 749*
- ◆ **Electrolyte Lavage Solution** *see* Polyethylene Glycol-Electrolyte Solution *on page 1209*

Electrolyte Solution, Renal Replacement
(ee LEK trow lite soe LOO shun REE nil ree PLASE ment)

U.S. Brand Names Normocarb HF™; PrismaSol

Index Terms Continuous Renal Replacement Therapy; CRRT; Renal Replacement Solution

Pharmacologic Category Alkalinizing Agent; Electrolyte Supplement

Use Used as a replacement solution to replenish water, correct electrolytes, and adjust acid-base balance depleted by hemofiltration or hemodiafiltration (continuous renal replacement therapy [CRRT])

Medication Safety Issues

High alert medication: The Institute for Safe Medication Practices (ISMP) includes this medication among its list of drug classes which have a heightened risk of causing significant patient harm when used in error.

Dosage Note: If using PrismaSol™, ensure that compartment A and B are mixed.

Continuous renal replacement circuit: Children and Adults:

Pre- or post-filter: Volume of solution administered depends upon the patient's fluid balance, target fluid balance, body weight, and amount of fluid removed during hemofiltration process.

Post-filter replacement: Volume infused/hour should not be greater than 1/3 of blood flow rate (eg, blood flow rate 100 mL/minute [6000 mL/hour], post-filter replacement rate ≤2000 mL/hour)

Dosage adjustment in hepatic impairment: Ability to convert lactate to bicarbonate may be impaired; use solutions containing lactate cautiously.

Additional Information Complete prescribing information for this medication should be consulted for additional detail.

Dosage Forms Excipient information presented when available (limited, particularly for generics); consult specific product labeling.

Injection, solution [concentrate; preservative free]:

Normocarb HF™ 25: Bicarbonate 25 mEq/L, chloride 116.5 mEq/L, magnesium 1.5 mEq/L, sodium 140 mEq/L (240 mL) [strength represents final solution after mixing; when diluted as directed, makes 3240 mL of infusate]

Normocarb HF™ 35: Bicarbonate 35 mEq/L, chloride 106.5 mEq/L, magnesium 1.5 mEq/L, sodium 140 mEq/L (240 mL) [strength represents final solution after mixing; when diluted as directed, makes 3240 mL of infusate]

Injection, solution [preservative free]:

PrismaSol BGK 0/2.5: Bicarbonate 32 mEq/L, calcium 2.5 mEq/L, chloride 109 mEq/L, dextrose 100 mg/dL, lactate 3 mEq/L, magnesium 1.5 mEq/L, sodium 140 mEq/L (5000 mL) [strength represents final solution after mixing]

PrismaSol BGK 2/0: Bicarbonate 32 mEq/L, chloride 108 mEq/L, dextrose 100 mg/dL, lactate 3 mEq/L, magnesium 1 mEq/L, potassium 2 mEq/L, sodium 140 mEq/L (5000 mL) [strength represents final solution after mixing]

PrismaSol BGK 2/3.5: Bicarbonate 32 mEq/L, calcium 3.5 mEq/L, chloride 111.5 mEq/L, dextrose 100 mg/dL, lactate 3 mEq/L, magnesium 1 mEq/L, potassium 2 mEq/L, sodium 140 mEq/L (5000 mL) [strength represents final solution after mixing]

PrismaSol BGK 4/2.5: Bicarbonate 32 mEq/L, calcium 2.5 mEq/L, chloride 113 mEq/L, dextrose 100 mg/dL, lactate 3 mEq/L, magnesium 1.5 mEq/L, potassium 4 mEq/L, sodium 140 mEq/L (5000 mL) [strength represents final solution after mixing]

PrismaSol BK 0/3.5: Bicarbonate 32 mEq/L, calcium 3.5 mEq/L, chloride 109.5 mEq/L, lactate 3 mEq/L, magnesium 1 mEq/L, sodium 140 mEq/L (5000 mL) [strength represents final solution after mixing]

◆ **Elestat™** *see* Epinastine *on page 525*

◆ **Elestrin™** *see* Estradiol *on page 554*

Eletriptan (el e TRIP tan)

U.S. Brand Names Relpax®

Canadian Brand Names Relpax®

Index Terms Eletriptan Hydrobromide

Pharmacologic Category Antimigraine Agent; Serotonin 5-$HT_{1B,\ 1D}$ Receptor Agonist

Use Acute treatment of migraine, with or without aura

Pregnancy Risk Factor C

Pregnancy Considerations There are no adequate and well-controlled studies in pregnant women; use during pregnancy only if the potential benefit to the mother outweighs the possible risk to the fetus. Teratogenic effects were observed in animal studies.

Lactation Enters breast milk/use caution

Contraindications Hypersensitivity to eletriptan or any component of the formulation; ischemic heart disease or signs or symptoms of ischemic heart disease (including Prinzmetal's angina, angina pectoris, MI, silent myocardial ischemia); cerebrovascular syndromes (including strokes, transient ischemic attacks); peripheral vascular syndromes (including ischemic bowel disease); uncontrolled hypertension; use within 24 hours of ergotamine derivatives; use within 24 hours of another 5-HT_1 agonist; use within 72 hours of potent CYP3A4 inhibitors; management of hemiplegic or basilar migraine; prophylactic treatment of migraine; severe hepatic impairment

Warnings/Precautions Eletriptan is indicated only in patients ≥18 years of age with a clear diagnosis of migraine headache. If a patient does not respond to the first dose, the diagnosis of migraine should be reconsidered. Do not give to patients with risk factors for CAD until a cardiovascular evaluation has been performed; if evaluation is satisfactory, the healthcare provider should administer the first dose and cardiovascular status should be periodically evaluated. Cardiac events (coronary artery vasospasm, transient ischemia, MI, ventricular tachycardia/fibrillation, cardiac arrest, and death), cerebral/subarachnoid hemorrhage, stroke, peripheral vascular ischemia, and colonic ischemia have been reported with 5-HT_1 agonist administration. Significant elevation in blood pressure, including hypertensive crisis, has also been reported on rare occasions in patients with and without a history of hypertension. Use with caution with mild to moderate hepatic impairment. Symptoms of agitation, confusion, hallucinations, hyper-reflexia, myoclonus, shivering, and tachycardia (serotonin syndrome) may occur with concomitant proserotonergic drugs (ie, SSRIs/SNRIs or triptans) or agents which reduce eletriptan's metabolism. Concurrent use of serotonin precursors (eg, tryptophan) is not recommended. Safety and efficacy in pediatric patients have not been established.

Adverse Reactions

1% to 10%:

Cardiovascular: Chest pain/tightness (1% to 4%; placebo 1%), palpitation

Central nervous system: Dizziness (3% to 7%; placebo 3%), somnolence (3% to 7%; placebo 4%), headache (3% to 4%; placebo 3%), chills, pain, vertigo

Gastrointestinal: Nausea (4% to 8%; placebo 5%), xerostomia (2% to 4%, placebo 2%), dysphagia (1% to 2%), abdominal pain/discomfort (1% to 2%; placebo 1%), dyspepsia (1% to 2%; placebo 1%)

Neuromuscular & skeletal: Weakness (4% to 10%), paresthesia (3% to 4%), back pain, hypertonia, hypoesthesia

Respiratory: Pharyngitis

Miscellaneous: Diaphoresis

<1% (Limited to important or life-threatening): Agitation, allergic reaction, angina, arrhythmia, ataxia, confusion, constipation, CPK increased, depersonalization, depression, diarrhea, dreams (abnormal), dyspnea, edema, emotional lability, esophagitis, euphoria, hyperesthesia, hyperkinesia, hypertension, impotence, incoordination, insomnia, lacrimation disorder, liver function tests abnormal, myalgia, myasthenia, nervousness, peripheral vascular disorder, photophobia, polyuria, pruritus, rash, salivation increased, shock, speech disorder, stupor, tachycardia, taste perversion, thrombophlebitis, tinnitus, tongue edema, tremor, urinary frequency, vasospasm, vision abnormal

Drug Interactions

Metabolism/Transport Effects Substrate of CYP3A4 (major)

Avoid Concomitant Use

Avoid concomitant use of Eletriptan with any of the following: Ergot Derivatives; Sibutramine

Increased Effect/Toxicity

Eletriptan may increase the levels/effects of: Ergot Derivatives; Serotonin Modulators

The levels/effects of Eletriptan may be increased by: Antifungal Agents (Azole Derivatives, Systemic); Calcium Channel Blockers (Nondihydropyridine); CYP3A4 Inhibitors (Moderate); CYP3A4 Inhibitors (Strong); Dasatinib; Ergot Derivatives; Fluconazole; Macrolide Antibiotics; Sibutramine

Decreased Effect There are no known significant interactions involving a decrease in effect.

Ethanol/Nutrition/Herb Interactions Food: High-fat meal increases bioavailability.

Stability Store at 25°C (77°F); excursions permitted to 15°C to 30°C (59°F to 86°F).

Mechanism of Action Selective agonist for serotonin (5-HT_{1B}, 5-HT_{1D}, 5-HT_{1F} receptors) in cranial arteries; causes vasoconstriction and reduce sterile inflammation associated with antidromic neuronal transmission correlating with relief of migraine

Pharmacodynamics/Kinetics

Absorption: Well absorbed

Distribution: V_d: 138 L

Protein binding: ~85%

Metabolism: Hepatic via CYP3A4; forms one metabolite (active)

Bioavailability: ~50%, increased with high-fat meal

Half-life elimination: 4 hours (Elderly: 4.4-5.7 hours); Metabolite: ~13 hours

Time to peak, plasma: 1.5-2 hours

Dosage Oral: Adults: Acute migraine: 20-40 mg; if the headache improves but returns, dose may be repeated after 2 hours have elapsed since first dose; maximum 80 mg/day.

Note: If the first dose is ineffective, diagnosis needs to be re-evaluated. Safety of treating >3 headaches/month has not been established.

Dosage adjustment in renal impairment: No dosing adjustment needed; monitor for increased blood pressure

Dosage adjustment in hepatic impairment:

Mild to moderate impairment: No adjustment necessary

Severe impairment: Use is contraindicated

Dosage Forms Excipient information presented when available (limited, particularly for generics); consult specific product labeling.

Tablet, as hydrobromide: 20 mg, 40 mg [as base]

- ◆ **Eletriptan Hydrobromide** *see* Eletriptan *on page 511*
- ◆ **Elidel®** *see* Pimecrolimus *on page 1193*
- ◆ **Eligard®** *see* Leuprolide *on page 868*
- ◆ **Elimite®** *see* Permethrin *on page 1176*
- ◆ **Elipten** *see* Aminoglutethimide *on page 86*
- ◆ **Elitek™** *see* Rasburicase *on page 1300*
- ◆ **Elixophyllin®** *see* Theophylline *on page 1455*
- ◆ **Elixophyllin-GG®** *see* Theophylline and Guaifenesin *on page 1457*
- ◆ **Ellence®** *see* Epirubicin *on page 528*
- ◆ **Elmiron®** *see* Pentosan Polysulfate Sodium *on page 1171*
- ◆ **Elocom® (Can)** *see* Mometasone *on page 1012*
- ◆ **Elocon®** *see* Mometasone *on page 1012*
- ◆ **Eloxatin®** *see* Oxaliplatin *on page 1112*
- ◆ **Elspar®** *see* Asparaginase *on page 140*
- ◆ **Eltor® (Can)** *see* Pseudoephedrine *on page 1265*

Eltrombopag (el TROM boe pag)

U.S. Brand Names Promacta®

Index Terms Eltrombopag Olamine; Revolade®; SB-497115; SB-497115-GR

Pharmacologic Category Colony Stimulating Factor; Thrombopoietic Agent

Use Treatment of thrombocytopenia in patients with chronic immune (idiopathic) thrombocytopenic purpura (ITP) at risk for bleeding who have had insufficient response to corticosteroids, immune globulin, or splenectomy

Restrictions Eltrombopag is approved for marketing under a Food and Drug Administration (FDA) approved, risk management, and restricted distribution program called Promacta® Cares™ (1-877-977-6622). Patients, prescribers, and pharmacies must be enrolled in the program.

An FDA-approved medication guide is available, distribute to each patient to whom this medication is dispensed.

Pregnancy Risk Factor C

Pregnancy Considerations Adverse effects were observed in animal studies. There are no adequate and well-controlled studies in pregnant women. Use during pregnancy only if the potential benefit to the mother outweighs the potential risk to the fetus. A Promacta® pregnancy registry has been established to monitor outcomes of women exposed to eltrombopag during pregnancy (1-888-825-5249).

Lactation Excretion in breast milk unknown/not recommended

Contraindications There are no contraindications listed within the manufacturer's labeling.

Warnings/Precautions **[U.S. Boxed Warning]: May cause hepatotoxicity; obtain ALT/AST and bilirubin prior to treatment initiation, every 2 weeks during adjustment phase, then monthly; obtain fractionation for elevated bilirubin levels. Repeat abnormal liver function tests within 3-5 days; if confirmed abnormal, monitor weekly until resolves, stabilizes, or returns to baseline. Discontinue treatment for ALT levels ≥3 times the upper limit of normal (ULN) and which are progressive, or persistent (≥4 weeks), or accompanied by increased direct bilirubin, or accompanied by clinical signs of liver injury or evidence of hepatic decompensation.** Reinitiation is not recommended; hepatotoxicity usually recurred with retreatment after therapy interruption. Use with caution in patients with pre-existing hepatic impairment (clearance may be reduced); dosage reductions are recommended in patients moderate-to-severe hepatic dysfunction; monitor closely.

[U.S. Boxed Warning]: Eltrombopag is available through a restricted access program called Promacta Cares™; prescribers, pharmacies and patients must be registered with the program. The program maintains a patient registry and requires prescribers to monitor and report baseline and periodic safety information related to hepatotoxicity, thromboembolic events, bone marrow reticulin events, rebound thrombocytopenia (after cessation), and malignancies. May increase the risk for bone marrow reticulin formation or progression; collagen fibrosis (not associated with cytopenias) was observed in clinical trials. Monitor peripheral blood smear for cellular morphologic abnormalities; discontinue treatment with onset of new or worsening abnormalities or cytopenias and consider bone marrow biopsy. Upon discontinuation of therapy, thrombocytopenia may worsen; severity may be greater than pretreatment level. Risk of bleeding is increased during rebound thrombocytopenia, particularly in patients receiving anticoagulants or antiplatelet agents; monitor closely; monitor for at least 4 weeks after treatment discontinuation.

Thromboembolism may occur with excess increases in platelet levels. Use with caution in patients with known risk factors for thromboembolism (eg, Factor V Leiden, AT deficiency, antiphospholipid syndrome). Stimulation of cell surface thrombopoietin (TPO) receptors may increase the risk for hematologic malignancies.

Cataract formation or worsening was observed in clinical trials. Monitor regularly for signs and symptoms of cataracts; obtain ophthalmic exam at baseline and during therapy. Use with caution in patients at risk for cataracts (eg, advanced age, long-term glucocorticoid use). Allow at least 4 hours between dosing of eltrombopag and antacids, minerals (eg, iron, calcium, aluminum, magnesium, selenium, zinc), or foods high in calcium; may reduce eltrombopag levels. Patients of East-Asian ethnicity (eg, Chinese, Japanese, Korean, Taiwanese) may have greater drug exposure (compared to non-east Asians); therapy should be initiated with lower starting doses. Safety and efficacy have not been established in renal impairment or in children.

Indicated only when the degree of thrombocytopenia and clinical conditions increase the risk for bleeding; use the lowest dose necessary to achieve and maintain platelet count ≥50,000/mm^3. Do not use to normalize platelet counts. Discontinue if platelet count does not respond to a level to avoid clinically important bleeding after 4 weeks at the maximum recommended dose.

Adverse Reactions

1% to 10%:

Dermatologic: Rash (≤7%), bruising (2%)

Endocrine & metabolic: Menorrhagia (4%)

Gastrointestinal: Nausea (6%), vomiting (4%), dyspepsia (2%)

Hematologic: Rebound thrombocytopenia (10%), thrombocytopenia (2%)

Hepatic: Liver function tests abnormal (10%), ALT increased (2%), AST increased (2%)

Neuromuscular & skeletal: Limb pain (≤7%), myalgia (3%), paresthesia (3%)

Ocular: Cataract (3%), conjunctival hemorrhage (2%)

<1% (Limited to important or life-threatening): Bone marrow collagen fiber deposits, bone marrow reticulin fiber deposits, cataract worsening, epistaxis, headache, hemorrhage (due to thrombocytopenia or rebound thrombocytopenia), non-Hodgkin's lymphoma, thrombotic/thromboembolic complications

Drug Interactions

Metabolism/Transport Effects

Substrate of CYP1A2, CYP2C8, UGT 1A1, UGT1A3; **Inhibits** OATP1B1, UGT1A1, UGT1A3, UGT1A4, UGT1A6, UGT1A9, UGT2B7, and UGT2B15

Avoid Concomitant Use There are no known interactions where it is recommended to avoid concomitant use.

Increased Effect/Toxicity

Eltrombopag may increase the levels/effects of: CYP2C8 Substrates (High risk); OATP1B1/SLCO1B1 Substrates; Rosuvastatin

Decreased Effect

The levels/effects of Eltrombopag may be decreased by: Aluminum Hydroxide; Calcium Salts; Iron Salts; Magnesium Salts; Sucralfate

Ethanol/Nutrition/Herb Interactions Food: Food, especially dairy products, may decrease the absorption of eltrombopag; allow at least 4 hours between dosing of eltrombopag and polyvalent cation intake (eg, dairy products, calcium-rich foods, multivitamins with minerals).

Stability Store at room temperature of 25°C (77°F); excursions permitted to 15°C to 30°C (59°F to 86°F).

Mechanism of Action Thrombopoietin (TPO) nonpeptide agonist which increases platelet counts by binding to and activating the human TPO receptor. Activates intracellular signal transduction pathways to increase proliferation and differentiation of marrow progenitor cells. Does not induce platelet aggregation or activation.

Pharmacodynamics/Kinetics

Onset of action: Platelet count increase: Within 1-2 weeks

Peak platelet count increase: 14-16 days

Duration: Platelets return to baseline: 1-2 weeks after last dose

Protein binding: >99%

Metabolism: Extensive hepatic metabolism; via CYP 1A2, 2C8 oxidation and UGT 1A1, 1A3 glucuronidation

Bioavailability: ~52%

Half-life elimination: ~21-32 hours in healthy individuals; ~26-35 hours in patients with ITP

Time to peak, plasma: 2-6 hours

Excretion: Feces (~59%, 20% as unchanged drug, 21% glutathione-related conjugates); urine (31%, 20% glucuronide of the phenypyrazole moiety)

Dosage Note: Discontinue if platelet count does not respond to a level that avoids clinically important bleeding after 4 weeks at the maximum daily dose of 75 mg.

Oral: Adults: ITP: Initial: 50 mg once daily; adjust dose to achieve and maintain platelet count ≥50,000/mm^3 to reduce the risk of bleeding; Maximum dose: 75 mg once daily

Dosage adjustment recommendations:

Platelet count <50,000/mm^3 (after at least 2 weeks): Increase daily dose by 25 mg; maximum dose: 75 mg/day

Platelet count >200,000/mm^3 (at any time): Reduce daily dose by 25 mg; reassess in 2 weeks

Platelet count >400,000/mm^3: Withhold dose; assess platelet count twice weekly; when platelet count <150,000/mm^3, resume with the daily dose reduced by 25 mg

Platelet count >400,000/mm^3 after 2 weeks at the lowest dose: Permanently discontinue

Dosage adjustment for patients of East-Asian ethnicity (eg, Chinese, Japanese, Korean, Taiwanese): Initial dose: 25 mg once daily

Dosage adjustment for toxicity:

ALT levels ≥3 times the upper limit of normal (ULN) **and** which are progressive, or persistent (≥4 weeks), or accompanied by increased direct bilirubin, or accompanied by clinical signs of liver injury or evidence of hepatic decompensation: Discontinue treatment

New or worsening cellular abnormalities or cytopenias: Discontinue treatment

Dosage adjustment in renal impairment: Has not been evaluated in patients with renal impairment; monitor closely

Dosage adjustment in hepatic impairment:

Mild impairment: No adjustment required

Moderate-to-severe impairment: Initial dose: 25 mg once daily

Dietary Considerations Take on an empty stomach (1 hour before or 2 hours after a meal). Food, especially dairy products, may decrease the absorption of eltrombopag; allow at least 4 hours between dosing of eltrombopag and polyvalent cation intake (eg, dairy products, calcium-rich foods, multivitamins with minerals).

Administration Administer on an empty stomach, 1 hour before or 2 hours after a meal. Do not administer concurrently with antacids, foods high in calcium, or minerals (eg, iron, calcium, aluminum, magnesium, selenium, zinc); separate by at least 4 hours.

Monitoring Parameters Liver tests, including ALT, AST, and bilirubin (baseline, every 2 weeks during dosage titration, then monthly; monitor weekly if retreating [not recommended] after therapy interruption for hepatotoxicity); bilirubin fractionation (for elevated bilirubin); CBC with differential and platelet count (weekly at initiation and during dosage titration, then monthly when stable; continue monitoring for ≥4 weeks after cessation); peripheral blood smear (baseline and monthly when stable), bone marrow biopsy (if peripheral blood smear reveals abnormality); ophthalmic exam (baseline and during treatment)

Reference Range Target platelet count (with treatment) of 50,000-200,000/mm^3; platelet life span: 8-11 days

Dosage Forms Excipient information presented when available (limited, particularly for generics); consult specific product labeling.

Tablet:

Promacta®: 25 mg, 50 mg

- ◆ **Eltrombopag Olamine** *see* Eltrombopag *on page 512*
- ◆ **Eltroxin® (Can)** *see* Levothyroxine *on page 881*
- ◆ **Emcyt®** *see* Estramustine *on page 558*
- ◆ **Emend®** *see* Aprepitant *on page 129*
- ◆ **Emend® for Injection** *see* Fosaprepitant *on page 666*
- ◆ **EMLA®** *see* Lidocaine and Prilocaine *on page 887*
- ◆ **Emo-Cort® (Can)** *see* Hydrocortisone *on page 743*
- ◆ **Emsam®** *see* Selegiline *on page 1359*

Emtricitabine (em trye SYE ta been)

U.S. Brand Names Emtriva®

Canadian Brand Names Emtriva®

Index Terms BW524W91; Coviracil; FTC

Pharmacologic Category Antiretroviral Agent, Reverse Transcriptase Inhibitor (Nucleoside)

Additional Appendix Information

Antiretroviral Therapy for HIV Infection: Adults and Adolescents *on page 1758*

Management of Healthcare Worker Exposures to HBV, HCV, and HIV *on page 1719*

Perinatal HIV Guidelines *on page 1730*

Use Treatment of HIV infection in combination with at least two other antiretroviral agents

Unlabeled/Investigational Use Hepatitis B (with HIV coinfection)

Pregnancy Risk Factor B

Pregnancy Considerations Adverse events were not observed in animal studies, however, there are no studies of emtricitabine during human pregnancy. Cases of fatal and nonfatal lactic acidosis, with or without pancreatitis, have been reported in pregnant women receiving reverse transcriptase inhibitors. It is not known if pregnancy itself potentiates this known side effect; however, pregnant women may be at increased risk of lactic acidosis and liver damage. Hepatic enzymes and electrolytes should be monitored frequently during the 3rd trimester of pregnancy. The Perinatal HIV Guidelines Working Group considers emtricitabine to be an alternative NRTI in dual nucleoside combination regimens. Health professionals are encouraged to contact the antiretroviral pregnancy registry to monitor outcomes of pregnant women exposed to antiretroviral medications (1-800-258-4263 or www.APRegistry.com).

Lactation Excretion in breast milk unknown/contraindicated

Contraindications Hypersensitivity to emtricitabine or any component of the formulation

Warnings/Precautions [U.S. Boxed Warning]: Lactic acidosis, severe hepatomegaly with steatosis, and hepatic failure have occurred rarely with emtricitabine (similar to other nucleoside analogues). Some cases have been fatal; stop treatment if lactic acidosis or hepatotoxicity occur. Prior liver disease, obesity, extended duration of therapy, and female gender may represent risk factors for severe hepatic reactions. Testing for hepatitis B is recommended prior to the initiation of therapy; **[U.S. Boxed Warnings]: Hepatitis B may be exacerbated following discontinuation of emtricitabine; not indicated for treatment of chronic hepatitis B; safety and efficacy in HIV/HBV coinfected patients not established.** May be associated with fat redistribution (buffalo hump, increased abdominal girth, breast engorgement, facial atrophy, and dyslipidemia). Immune reconstitution syndrome may develop resulting in the occurrence of an inflammatory response to an indolent or residual opportunistic infection; further evaluation and treatment may be required. Use caution in patients with renal impairment (dosage adjustment required).

Adverse Reactions Clinical trials were conducted in patients receiving other antiretroviral agents, and it is not possible to correlate frequency of adverse events with emtricitabine alone. The range of frequencies of adverse events is generally comparable to comparator groups, with the exception of hyperpigmentation, which occurred more frequently in patients receiving emtricitabine. Unless otherwise noted, percentages are as reported in adults.

>10%:

Central nervous system: Dizziness (4% to 25%), headache (6% to 22%), fever (children 18%), insomnia (5% to 16%), abnormal dreams (2% to 11%)

Dermatologic: Hyperpigmentation (children 32%; adults 2% to 4%; primarily of palms and/or soles but may include tongue, arms, lip and nails; generally mild and nonprogressive without associated local reactions such as pruritus or rash); rash (17% to 30%; includes pruritus, maculopapular rash, vesiculobullous rash, pustular rash, and allergic reaction)

Gastrointestinal: Diarrhea (children 20%; adults 9% to 23%), vomiting (children 23%; adults 9%), nausea (13% to 18%), abdominal pain (8% to 14%), gastroenteritis (children 11%)

Neuromuscular & skeletal: Weakness (12% to 16%), CPK increased (grades 3/4: 11% to 12%)

Otic: Otitis media (children 23%)

Respiratory: Cough (children 28%; adults 14%), rhinitis (children 20%; adults 12% to 18%), pneumonia (children 15%)

Miscellaneous: Infection (children 44%)

1% to 10%:

Central nervous system: Depression (6% to 9%), neuropathy/neuritis (4%)

Endocrine & metabolic: Serum triglycerides increased (grades 3/4: 4% to 10%), disordered glucose homeostasis (grades 3/4: 2% to 3%), serum amylase increased (grades 3/4: children 9%; adults 2% to 5%), serum lipase increased (grades 3/4: ≤1%)

Gastrointestinal: Dyspepsia (4% to 8%), serum amylase increased (grades 3/4: 8%)

Genitourinary: Hematuria (grades 3/4: 3%)

Hematologic: Anemia (children: 7%), neutropenia (grades 3/4: children 2%; adults 5%)

Hepatic: Transaminases increased (grades 3/4: 2% to 6%), alkaline phosphatase increased (>550 units/L: 1%), bilirubin increased (grades 3/4: 1%)

Neuromuscular & skeletal: Creatinine kinase increased (grades 3/4: 9%), myalgia (4% to 6%), paresthesia (5% to 6%), arthralgia (3% to 5%)

Respiratory: Upper respiratory tract infection (8%), sinusitis (8%), pharyngitis (5%)

Drug Interactions

Avoid Concomitant Use

Avoid concomitant use of Emtricitabine with any of the following: LamiVUDine

Increased Effect/Toxicity

The levels/effects of Emtricitabine may be increased by: Ganciclovir-Valganciclovir; LamiVUDine; Ribavirin

Decreased Effect There are no known significant interactions involving a decrease in effect.

Ethanol/Nutrition/Herb Interactions Food: Food decreases peak plasma concentrations, but does not alter the extent of absorption or overall systemic exposure.

Stability Store capsules at 15°C to 30°C (59°F to 86°F). Solution should be stored under refrigeration at 2°C to 8°C (36°F to 46°F). Once dispensed, may be stored at 15°C to 30°C (59°F to 86°F) if used within 3 months.

Mechanism of Action Nucleoside reverse transcriptase inhibitor; emtricitabine is a cytosine analogue which is phosphorylated intracellularly to emtricitabine 5'-triphosphate which interferes with HIV viral RNA dependent DNA polymerase resulting in inhibition of viral replication.

Pharmacodynamics/Kinetics

Absorption: Rapid, extensive

Protein binding: <4%

Metabolism: Limited, via oxidation and conjugation (not via CYP isoenzymes)

Bioavailability: Capsule: 93%; solution: 75%

Half-life elimination: Normal renal function: Adults: 10 hours; children: 5-18 hours

Time to peak, plasma: 1-2 hours

Excretion: Urine (86% primarily as unchanged drug, 13% as metabolites); feces (14%)

Dosage Oral:

Children:

0-3 months: Solution: 3 mg/kg/day

3 months to 17 years:

Capsule: Children >33 kg: 200 mg once daily

Solution: 6 mg/kg once daily; maximum: 240 mg/day

Adults:

Capsule: 200 mg once daily

Solution: 240 mg once daily

Dosage adjustment in renal impairment: Adults (consider similar adjustments in children):

Cl_{cr} 30-49 mL/minute: Capsule: 200 mg every 48 hours; solution: 120 mg every 24 hours

Cl_{cr} 15-29 mL/minute: Capsule: 200 mg every 72 hours; solution: 80 mg every 24 hours

Cl_{cr} <15 mL/minute (including hemodialysis patients): Capsule: 200 mg every 96 hours; solution: 60 mg every 24 hours; administer after dialysis on dialysis days

Dosage adjustment in hepatic impairment: No adjustment required.

Dietary Considerations May be taken with or without food.

Administration May be administered with or without food.

Monitoring Parameters Viral load, CD4, liver function tests; hepatitis B testing is recommended prior to initiation of therapy

Dosage Forms Excipient information presented when available (limited, particularly for generics); consult specific product labeling.

Capsule:
Emtriva®: 200 mg

Solution:
Emtriva®: 10 mg/mL (170 mL) [contains propylene glycol; cotton candy flavor]

Emtricitabine and Tenofovir

(em trye SYE ta been & te NOE fo veer)

U.S. Brand Names Truvada®

Canadian Brand Names Truvada®

Index Terms Tenofovir and Emtricitabine

Pharmacologic Category Antiretroviral Agent, Reverse Transcriptase Inhibitor (Nucleoside); Antiretroviral Agent, Reverse Transcriptase Inhibitor (Nucleotide)

Additional Appendix Information

Antiretroviral Therapy for HIV Infection: Adults and Adolescents *on page 1758*

Management of Healthcare Worker Exposures to HBV, HCV, and HIV *on page 1719*

Use Treatment of HIV infection in combination with other antiretroviral agents

Pregnancy Risk Factor B

Dosage Adults: Oral: One tablet (emtricitabine 200 mg and tenofovir 300 mg) once daily

Note: Concurrent use with adefovir, emtricitabine, lamivudine, and/or tenofovir alone or as a combination product should be avoided.

Dosage adjustment in renal impairment:

Cl_{cr} ≥50 mL/minute: No adjustment necessary

Cl_{cr} 30-49 mL/minute: Increase interval to every 48 hours.

Cl_{cr} <30 mL/minute or hemodialysis: Not recommended.

Additional Information Complete prescribing information for this medication should be consulted for additional detail.

Dosage Forms Excipient information presented when available (limited, particularly for generics); consult specific product labeling.

Tablet:
Truvada®: Emtricitabine 200 mg and tenofovir disoproxil fumarate 300 mg [equivalent to 245 mg tenofovir disoproxil]

◆ **Emtricitabine, Efavirenz, and Tenofovir** *see* Efavirenz, Emtricitabine, and Tenofovir *on page 509*

◆ **Emtriva®** *see* Emtricitabine *on page 513*

◆ **ENA 713** *see* Rivastigmine *on page 1331*

◆ **Enablex®** *see* Darifenacin *on page 401*

Enalapril (e NAL a pril)

U.S. Brand Names Vasotec®

Canadian Brand Names Apo-Enalapril®; CO Enalapril; Gen-Enalapril; Novo-Enalapril; PMS-Enalapril; Pro-Enalapril; ratio-Enalapril; Riva-Enalapril; Sandoz-Enalapril; Taro-Enalapril; Vasotec®; Vasotec® I.V.

Index Terms Enalapril Maleate; Enalaprilat

Pharmacologic Category Angiotensin-Converting Enzyme (ACE) Inhibitor

Additional Appendix Information

Angiotensin Agents *on page 1632*

Heart Failure (Systolic) *on page 1809*

Use Treatment of hypertension; treatment of symptomatic heart failure; treatment of asymptomatic left ventricular dysfunction

Unlabeled/Investigational Use

Unlabeled: To delay the progression of nephropathy and reduce risks of cardiovascular events in hypertensive patients with type 1 or 2 diabetes mellitus; hypertensive crisis, diabetic nephropathy, hypertension secondary to scleroderma renal crisis, diagnosis of aldosteronism, idiopathic edema, Bartter's syndrome, postmyocardial infarction for prevention of ventricular failure

Investigational: Severe congestive heart failure in infants, neonatal hypertension, acute cardiogenic pulmonary edema (enalaprilat)

Pregnancy Risk Factor C (1st trimester); D (2nd and 3rd trimesters)

Pregnancy Considerations Due to adverse events observed in some animal studies, enalapril is considered pregnancy category C during the first trimester. Based on human data, enalapril is considered pregnancy category D if used during the second and third trimesters (per the manufacturer; however, one study suggests that fetal injury may occur at anytime during pregnancy). Enalaprilat, the active metabolite of enalapril, crosses the placenta. First trimester exposure to ACE inhibitors may cause major congenital malformations. An increased risk of cardiovascular and/or central nervous system malformations was observed in one study; however, an increased risk of teratogenic events was not observed in other studies. Second and third trimester use of an ACE inhibitor is associated with oligohydramnios. Oligohydramnios due to decreased fetal renal function may lead to fetal limb contractures, craniofacial deformation, and hypoplastic lung development. The use of ACE inhibitors during the second and third trimesters is also associated with anuria, hypotension, renal failure (reversible or irreversible), skull hypoplasia, and death in the fetus/neonate. Chronic maternal hypertension itself is also associated with adverse events in the fetus/infant. ACE inhibitors are not recommended during pregnancy to treat maternal hypertension or heart failure. Those who are planning a pregnancy should be considered for other medication options if an ACE inhibitor is currently prescribed or the ACE inhibitor should be discontinued as soon as possible once pregnancy is detected. The exposed fetus should be monitored for fetal growth, amniotic fluid volume, and organ formation. Infants exposed to an ACE inhibitor *in utero*, especially during the second and third trimester, should be monitored for hyperkalemia, hypotension, and oliguria.

[U.S. Boxed Warning]: Based on human data, ACE inhibitors can cause injury and death to the developing fetus when used in the second and third trimesters. ACE inhibitors should be discontinued as soon as possible once pregnancy is detected.

Lactation Enters breast milk/not recommended (AAP rates "compatible")

Medication Safety Issues

Sound-alike/look-alike issues:

Enalapril may be confused with Anafranil®, Elavil®, Eldepryl®, nafarelin, ramipril

Significant differences exist between oral and I.V. dosing. Use caution when converting from one route of administration to another.

International issues:

Acepril® [Hungary, Switzerland] may be confused with Accupril® which is a brand name for quinapril in the U.S.

Acepril®: Brand name for lisinopril in Denmark; brand name for captopril in Great Britain

Nacor® [Spain] may be confused with Niacor® which is a brand name for niacin in the U.S.

Contraindications Hypersensitivity to enalapril or enalaprilat; angioedema related to previous treatment with an ACE inhibitor; patients with idiopathic or hereditary angioedema

Warnings/Precautions Anaphylactic reactions may occur rarely with ACE inhibitors. At any time during treatment (especially following first dose) angioedema may occur rarely with ACE inhibitors; it may involve the head and neck (potentially compromising airway) or the intestine (presenting with abdominal pain). African-Americans may be at an increased risk. Prolonged frequent monitoring may be required especially if tongue, glottis, or larynx are involved as they are associated with airway obstruction. Patients with a history of airway surgery may have a higher risk of airway obstruction. Aggressive early and appropriate management is critical. Use in patients with idiopathic or hereditary angioedema or previous angioedema associated with ACE inhibitor therapy is contraindicated. Severe anaphylactoid reactions may be seen during hemodialysis (eg, CVVHD) with high-flux dialysis membranes (eg, AN69), and rarely, during low density lipoprotein apheresis with dextran sulfate cellulose. Rare cases of anaphylactoid reactions have been reported in patients undergoing sensitization treatment with hymenoptera (bee, wasp) venom while receiving ACE inhibitors.

Symptomatic hypotension with or without syncope can occur with ACE inhibitors (usually with the first several doses); effects are most often observed in volume depleted patients; correct volume depletion prior to initiation; close monitoring of patient is required especially with initial dosing and dosing increases; blood pressure must be lowered at a rate appropriate for the patient's clinical condition. Initiation of therapy in patients with ischemic heart disease or cerebrovascular disease warrants close observation due to the potential consequences posed by falling blood pressure (eg, MI, stroke). Use with caution in hypertrophic cardiomyopathy with outflow tract obstruction, severe aortic stenosis, or before, during, or immediately after major surgery. **[U.S. Boxed Warning]: Based on human data, ACEIs can cause injury and death to the developing fetus when used in the second and third trimesters. ACEIs should be discontinued as soon as possible once pregnancy is detected.**

Hyperkalemia may occur with ACE inhibitors; risk factors include renal dysfunction, diabetes mellitus, concomitant use of potassium-sparing diuretics, potassium supplements, and/or potassium-containing salts. Use cautiously, if at all, with these agents and monitor potassium closely. Cough may occur with ACE inhibitors. Other causes of cough should be considered (eg, pulmonary congestion in patients with heart failure) and excluded prior to discontinuation.

May be associated with deterioration of renal function and/or increases in serum creatinine, particularly in patients with low renal blood flow (eg, renal artery stenosis, heart failure) whose glomerular filtration rate (GFR) is dependent on efferent arteriolar vasoconstriction by angiotensin II; deterioration may result in oliguria, acute renal failure, and progressive azotemia. Small increases in serum creatinine may occur following initiation; consider discontinuation only in patients with progressive and/or significant deterioration in renal function. Use with caution in patients with unstented unilateral/bilateral renal artery stenosis. When unstented bilateral renal artery stenosis is present, use is generally avoided due to the elevated risk of deterioration in renal function unless possible benefits outweigh risks.

Rare toxicities associated with ACE inhibitors include cholestatic jaundice (which may progress to fulminant hepatic necrosis), agranulocytosis, neutropenia or leukopenia with myeloid hypoplasia. Patients with collagen vascular diseases (especially with concomitant renal impairment) or renal impairment alone may be at increased risk for hematologic toxicity; periodically monitor CBC with differential in these patients.

Adverse Reactions Note: Frequency ranges include data from hypertension and heart failure trials. Higher rates of adverse reactions have generally been noted in patients with CHF. However, the frequency of adverse effects associated with placebo is also increased in this population.

1% to 10%:

Cardiovascular: Hypotension (0.9% to 6.7%), chest pain (2%), syncope (0.5% to 2%), orthostasis (2%), orthostatic hypotension (2%)

Central nervous system: Headache (2% to 5%), dizziness (4% to 8%), fatigue (2% to 3%)

Dermatologic: Rash (1.5%)

Gastrointestinal: Abnormal taste, abdominal pain, vomiting, nausea, diarrhea, anorexia, constipation

Neuromuscular & skeletal: Weakness

Renal: Serum creatinine increased (0.2% to 20%), worsening of renal function (in patients with bilateral renal artery stenosis or hypovolemia)

Respiratory (1% to 2%): Bronchitis, cough, dyspnea

<1% (Limited to important or life-threatening): Agranulocytosis, alopecia, anaphylactoid reaction, angina pectoris, angioedema, ataxia, atrial fibrillation, atrial tachycardia, bone marrow suppression, bradycardia, bronchospasm, cardiac arrest, cerebral vascular accident, cholestatic jaundice, depression, eosinophilic pneumonitis, erythema multiforme, exfoliative dermatitis, flushing, giant cell arteritis, gynecomastia, hallucinations, hemolysis with G6PD, Henoch-Schönlein purpura, hepatitis, ileus, impotence, jaundice, lichen-form reaction, melena, MI, neutropenia, ototoxicity, pancreatitis, paresthesia, pemphigus, pemphigus foliaceus, peripheral neuropathy, photosensitivity, psychosis, pulmonary edema, pulmonary embolism, pulmonary infiltrates, Raynaud's phenomenon, sicca syndrome, somnolence, Stevens-Johnson syndrome, systemic lupus erythematosus, thrombocytopenia, toxic epidermal necrolysis, toxic pustuloderma, vertigo.

A syndrome which may include arthralgia, elevated ESR, eosinophilia and positive ANA, fever, interstitial nephritis, myalgia, rash, and vasculitis has been reported for enalapril and other ACE inhibitors.

Drug Interactions

Metabolism/Transport Effects Substrate of CYP3A4 (minor)

Avoid Concomitant Use There are no known interactions where it is recommended to avoid concomitant use.

Increased Effect/Toxicity

Enalapril may increase the levels/effects of: Allopurinol; Amifostine; AzaTHIOprine; CycloSPORINE; Ferric Gluconate; Gold Sodium Thiomalate; Lithium; RiTUXimab

The levels/effects of Enalapril may be increased by: Angiotensin II Receptor Blockers; Diazoxide; Eplerenone; Herbs (Hypotensive Properties); Loop Diuretics; Potassium Salts; Potassium-Sparing Diuretics; Prostacyclin Analogues; Sirolimus; Temsirolimus; Thiazide Diuretics; Trimethoprim

Decreased Effect

The levels/effects of Enalapril may be decreased by: Antacids; Aprotinin; CYP3A4 Inducers (Strong);

Deferasirox; Herbs (CYP3A4 Inducers); Herbs (Hypertensive Properties); Methylphenidate; Nonsteroidal Anti-Inflammatory Agents; Salicylates; Yohimbine

Ethanol/Nutrition/Herb Interactions Herb/Nutraceutical: Avoid bayberry, blue cohosh, cayenne, ephedra, ginger, ginseng (American), kola, licorice (may worsen hypertension). Avoid black cohosh, california poppy, coleus, golden seal, hawthorn, mistletoe, periwinkle, quinine, shepherd's purse (may have increased antihypertensive effect).

Stability Enalaprilat: Clear, colorless solution which should be stored at <30°C. I.V. is 24 hours at room temperature in D_5W or NS.

Mechanism of Action Competitive inhibitor of angiotensin-converting enzyme (ACE); prevents conversion of angiotensin I to angiotensin II, a potent vasoconstrictor; results in lower levels of angiotensin II which causes an increase in plasma renin activity and a reduction in aldosterone secretion

Pharmacodynamics/Kinetics

Onset of action: Oral: ~1 hour

Duration: Oral: 12-24 hours

Absorption: Oral: 55% to 75%

Protein binding: 50% to 60%

Metabolism: Prodrug, undergoes hepatic biotransformation to enalaprilat

Half-life elimination:

Enalapril: Adults: Healthy: 2 hours; Congestive heart failure: 3.4-5.8 hours

Enalaprilat: Infants 6 weeks to 8 months of age: 6-10 hours; Adults: 35-38 hours

Time to peak, serum: Oral: Enalapril: 0.5-1.5 hours; Enalaprilat (active): 3-4.5 hours

Excretion: Urine (60% to 80%); some feces

Dosage Use lower listed initial dose in patients with hyponatremia, hypovolemia, severe congestive heart failure, decreased renal function, or in those receiving diuretics.

Oral: **Enalapril**: Children 1 month to 17 years: Hypertension: Initial: 0.08 mg/kg/day (up to 5 mg) in 1-2 divided doses; adjust dosage based on patient response; doses >0.58 mg/kg (40 mg) have not been evaluated in pediatric patients

Investigational: Congestive heart failure: Initial oral doses of **enalapril**: 0.1 mg/kg/day increasing as needed over 2 weeks to 0.5 mg/kg/day have been used in infants

Investigational: Neonatal hypertension: I.V. doses of **enalaprilat**: 5-10 mcg/kg/dose administered every 8-24 hours have been used; monitor patients carefully; select patients may require higher doses

Adults:

Oral: **Enalapril:**

Hypertension: 2.5-5 mg/day then increase as required, usually at 1- to 2-week intervals; usual dose range (JNC 7): 2.5-40 mg/day in 1-2 divided doses. **Note:** Initiate with 2.5 mg if patient is taking a diuretic which cannot be discontinued. May add a diuretic if blood pressure cannot be controlled with enalapril alone.

Heart failure: Initial: 2.5 mg once or twice daily (usual range: 5-40 mg/day in 2 divided doses). Titrate slowly at 1- to 2-week intervals. Target dose: 10-20 mg twice daily (ACC/AHA 2005 Heart Failure Guidelines)

Asymptomatic left ventricular dysfunction: 2.5 mg twice daily, titrated as tolerated to 20 mg/day

I.V.: **Enalaprilat:**

Hypertension: 1.25 mg/dose, given over 5 minutes every 6 hours; doses as high as 5 mg/dose every 6 hours have been tolerated for up to 36 hours. **Note:** If patients are concomitantly receiving diuretic therapy, begin with 0.625 mg I.V. over 5 minutes; if the effect is not adequate after 1 hour, repeat the dose and administer 1.25 mg at 6-hour intervals thereafter; if adequate, administer 0.625 mg I.V. every 6 hours.

Heart failure: Avoid I.V. administration in patients with unstable heart failure or those suffering acute myocardial infarction.

Conversion from I.V. to oral therapy if not concurrently on diuretics: 5 mg once daily; subsequent titration as needed; if concurrently receiving diuretics and responding to 0.625 mg I.V. every 6 hours, initiate with 2.5 mg/day.

Dosing adjustment in renal impairment:

Oral: Enalapril:

Cl_{cr} 30-80 mL/minute: Administer 5 mg/day titrated upwards to maximum of 40 mg.

Cl_{cr} <30 mL/minute: Administer 2.5 mg day; titrated upward until blood pressure is controlled.

For heart failure patients with sodium <130 mEq/L or serum creatinine >1.6 mg/dL, initiate dosage with 2.5 mg/day, increasing to twice daily as needed. Increase further in increments of 2.5 mg/dose at >4-day intervals to a maximum daily dose of 40 mg.

I.V.: Enalaprilat:

Cl_{cr} >30 mL/minute: Initiate with 1.25 mg every 6 hours and increase dose based on response.

Cl_{cr} <30 mL/minute: Initiate with 0.625 mg every 6 hours and increase dose based on response.

Hemodialysis: Moderately dialyzable (20% to 50%); administer dose postdialysis (eg, 0.625 mg I.V. every 6 hours) or administer 20% to 25% supplemental dose following dialysis; Clearance: 62 mL/minute.

Peritoneal dialysis: Supplemental dose is not necessary, although some removal of drug occurs.

Dosing adjustment in hepatic impairment: Hydrolysis of enalapril to enalaprilat may be delayed and/or impaired in patients with severe hepatic impairment, but the pharmacodynamic effects of the drug do not appear to be significantly altered; no dosage adjustment.

Dietary Considerations Limit salt substitutes or potassium-rich diet.

Administration Administer direct IVP over at least 5 minutes or dilute up to 50 mL and infuse; discontinue diuretic, if possible, for 2-3 days before beginning enalapril therapy

Monitoring Parameters Blood pressure; serum creatinine and potassium; if patient has collagen vascular disease and/or renal impairment, periodically monitor CBC with differential

Test Interactions Positive Coombs' [direct]; may cause false-positive results in urine acetone determinations using sodium nitroprusside reagent

Dosage Forms Excipient information presented when available (limited, particularly for generics); consult specific product labeling.

Injection, solution, as enalaprilat: 1.25 mg/mL (1 mL, 2 mL) [contains benzyl alcohol]

Tablet, as maleate: 2.5 mg, 5 mg, 10 mg, 20 mg

Vasotec®: 2.5 mg, 5 mg, 10 mg, 20 mg

Extemporaneous Preparations

An enalapril oral suspension (0.2 mg/mL) has been made using one 2.5 mg tablet and 12.5 mL sterile water; stability unknown; suspension should be used immediately and the remaining amount discarded

Young TE and Mangum OB, "Neofax®, '95: A Manual of Drugs Used in Neonatal Care," 8th ed, Columbus, OH: Ross Products Division, Abbott Laboratories, 1995, 85.

An enalapril oral suspension (1 mg/mL) has been made using 20 mg tablets and Bicitra®. Add 50 mL Bicitra® to a polyethylene terephthalate (PET) bottle containing ten 20 mg tablets and shake for at least 2 minutes. Let concentrate stand for 60 minutes. Following the 60-minute hold time, shake the concentration for an additional minute. Add 150 mL Bicitra® to the concentrate and shake the suspension to disperse the ingredients. The suspension should refrigerated at 2°C to 8°C (36°F to 46°F); it can be stored for up to 30 days. Shake suspension well before use.

Package labeling, Merck & Co, Inc, issued October 2000.

Enalapril and Felodipine

(e NAL a pril & fe LOE di peen)

U.S. Brand Names Lexxel® [DSC]

Canadian Brand Names Lexxel®

Index Terms Enalapril Maleate and Felodipine; Felodipine and Enalapril

Pharmacologic Category Angiotensin-Converting Enzyme (ACE) Inhibitor; Calcium Channel Blocker

Use Treatment of hypertension, however, not indicated for initial treatment of hypertension; replacement therapy in patients receiving separate dosage forms (for patient convenience); when monotherapy with one component fails to achieve desired antihypertensive effect, or when dose-limiting adverse effects limit upward titration of monotherapy

Pregnancy Risk Factor C/D (2nd and 3rd trimesters)

Dosage Oral:

Adults: Enalapril 5-20 mg and felodipine 2.5-10 mg once daily

Elderly: Initial dose of felodipine is 2.5 mg daily

Additional Information Complete prescribing information for this medication should be consulted for additional detail.

Dosage Forms Excipient information presented when available (limited, particularly for generics); consult specific product labeling. [DSC] = Discontinued product

Tablet, extended release:

Lexxel® 5/2.5: Enalapril maleate 5 mg and felodipine 2.5 mg [DSC]

Lexxel® 5/5: Enalapril maleate 5 mg and felodipine 5 mg [DSC]

Enalapril and Hydrochlorothiazide

(e NAL a pril & hye droe klor oh THYE a zide)

U.S. Brand Names Vaseretic®

Canadian Brand Names Vaseretic®

Index Terms Enalapril Maleate and Hydrochlorothiazide; Hydrochlorothiazide and Enalapril

Pharmacologic Category Angiotensin-Converting Enzyme (ACE) Inhibitor; Diuretic, Thiazide

Use Treatment of hypertension

Pregnancy Risk Factor C/D (2nd and 3rd trimesters)

Dosage Oral: Adults: Enalapril 5-10 mg and hydrochlorothiazide 12.5-25 mg once daily (maximum: 40 mg/day [enalapril]; 50 mg/day [hydrochlorothiazide])

Additional Information Complete prescribing information for this medication should be consulted for additional detail.

Dosage Forms Excipient information presented when available (limited, particularly for generics); consult specific product labeling.

Tablet:

5/12.5: Enalapril maleate 5 mg and hydrochlorothiazide 12.5 mg

10/25: Enalapril maleate 10 mg and hydrochlorothiazide 25 mg

Vaseretic®:

10/25: Enalapril maleate 10 mg and hydrochlorothiazide 25 mg

- ◆ **Enalaprilat** *see* Enalapril *on page* 515
- ◆ **Enalapril Maleate** *see* Enalapril *on page* 515
- ◆ **Enalapril Maleate and Felodipine** *see* Enalapril and Felodipine *on page* 518
- ◆ **Enalapril Maleate and Hydrochlorothiazide** *see* Enalapril and Hydrochlorothiazide *on page* 518
- ◆ **Enbrel®** *see* Etanercept *on page* 571
- ◆ **Encare® [OTC]** *see* Nonoxynol 9 *on page* 1077
- ◆ **Encort™** *see* Hydrocortisone *on page* 743
- ◆ **EndaCof [DSC]** *see* Hydrocodone and Guaifenesin *on page* 741
- ◆ **EndaCof-XP [DSC]** *see* Hydrocodone and Guaifenesin *on page* 741
- ◆ **Endantadine® (Can)** *see* Amantadine *on page* 78
- ◆ **EndoAvitene®** *see* Collagen Hemostat *on page* 367
- ◆ **Endocet®** *see* Oxycodone and Acetaminophen *on page* 1122
- ◆ **Endodan®** *see* Oxycodone and Aspirin *on page* 1123
- ◆ **Endo®-Levodopa/Carbidopa (Can)** *see* Carbidopa and Levodopa *on page* 256
- ◆ **Endometrin®** *see* Progesterone *on page* 1247
- ◆ **Endrate® [DSC]** *see* Edetate Disodium *on page* 505
- ◆ **Enduron® [DSC]** *see* Methyclothiazide *on page* 970
- ◆ **Enduron® (Can)** *see* Methyclothiazide *on page* 970
- ◆ **Enemeez® [OTC]** *see* Docusate *on page* 473
- ◆ **Enemeez® Plus [OTC]** *see* Docusate *on page* 473
- ◆ **Enerjets [OTC]** *see* Caffeine *on page* 232

Enfuvirtide (en FYOO vir tide)

U.S. Brand Names Fuzeon®

Canadian Brand Names Fuzeon®

Index Terms T-20

Pharmacologic Category Antiretroviral Agent, Fusion Protein Inhibitor

Additional Appendix Information

Antiretroviral Therapy for HIV Infection: Adults and Adolescents *on page* 1758

Management of Healthcare Worker Exposures to HBV, HCV, and HIV *on page* 1719

Perinatal HIV Guidelines *on page* 1730

Use Treatment of HIV-1 infection in combination with other antiretroviral agents in treatment-experienced patients with evidence of HIV-1 replication despite ongoing antiretroviral therapy

Pregnancy Risk Factor B

Pregnancy Considerations Teratogenic effects were not observed in animal studies; however, there are no adequate and well-controlled studies in pregnant women. An antiretroviral registry has been established to monitor maternal and fetal outcomes in women receiving antiretroviral drugs. Physicians are encouraged to register patients at 1-800-258-4263 or www.APRegistry.com.

Lactation Excretion in breast milk unknown/contraindicated

Contraindications Hypersensitivity to enfuvirtide or any component of the formulation

Warnings/Precautions Monitor closely for signs/symptoms of pneumonia; associated with an increased incidence during clinical trials, particularly in patients with a low CD4 cell count, high initial viral load, I.V. drug use, smoking, or a history of lung disease. May cause hypersensitivity reactions (symptoms may include rash, fever, nausea, vomiting, hypotension, and elevated transaminases). In addition, local injection site reactions are common. An inflammatory response to indolent or residual opportunistic infections (immune reconstitution syndrome) has occurred with antiretroviral therapy; further investigation is warranted. Administration using a needle-free device has been associated with nerve pain (including neuralgia and/or paresthesia lasting up to 6 months), bruising, and hematomas when administered at sites where large nerves are close to the skin; only administer medication in recommended sites and use caution in patients with coagulation disorders (eg, hemophilia) or receiving anticoagulants. Safety and efficacy have not been established in children <6 years of age.

Adverse Reactions

>10%:

Central nervous system: Fatigue (20%), insomnia (11%)

Gastrointestinal: Diarrhea (32%), nausea (23%)

Local: Injection site reactions (98%; may include pain, erythema, induration, pruritus, ecchymosis, nodule or cyst formation)

1% to 10%:

Dermatologic: Folliculitis (2%)

Gastrointestinal: Weight loss (7%), abdominal pain (4%), appetite decreased (3%), pancreatitis (3%), anorexia (2%), xerostomia (2%)

Hematologic: Eosinophilia (2% to 9%)

Hepatic: Transaminases increased (4%, grade 4: 1%)

Local: Injection site infection (2%)

Neuromuscular & skeletal: CPK increased (3% to 7%), limb pain (3%), myalgia (3%)

Ocular: Conjunctivitis (2%)

Respiratory: Sinusitis (6%), cough (4%), pneumonia (3%)

Miscellaneous: Infections (4% to 6%), herpes simplex (4%), flu-like syndrome (2%)

<1% (Limited to important or life-threatening): Abacavir hypersensitivity worsening, amylase increased, angina, anxiety, constipation, depression, GGT increased, glomerulonephritis, Guillain-Barré syndrome, hepatic steatosis, hyperglycemia; hypersensitivity reactions (symptoms may include rash, fever, nausea, vomiting, hypotension, and transaminase increases); insomnia, lipase increased, lymphadenopathy, neutropenia, peripheral neuropathy, pneumopathy, renal failure, renal insufficiency, respiratory distress, sepsis, sixth nerve palsy, suicide attempt, taste disturbances, thrombocytopenia, toxic hepatitis, triglycerides increased, tubular necrosis, weakness

Drug Interactions

Avoid Concomitant Use There are no known interactions where it is recommended to avoid concomitant use.

Increased Effect/Toxicity

Enfuvirtide may increase the levels/effects of: Protease Inhibitors

The levels/effects of Enfuvirtide may be increased by: Protease Inhibitors

Decreased Effect There are no known significant interactions involving a decrease in effect.

Stability Store powder at 15°C to 30°C (59°F to 86°F). Reconstitute with 1.1 mL SWFI. Tap vial for 10 seconds and roll gently to ensure contact with diluent. Allow to stand until solution is completed. May require up to 45 minutes to form solution. Reconstituted solutions should be refrigerated and must be used within 24 hours.

Mechanism of Action Binds to the first heptad-repeat (HR1) in the gp41 subunit of the viral envelope glycoprotein. Inhibits the fusion of HIV-1 virus with CD4 cells by blocking the conformational change in gp41 required for membrane fusion and entry into CD4 cells

Pharmacodynamics/Kinetics

Distribution: V_d: 5.5 L

Protein binding: 92%

Metabolism: Proteolytic hydrolysis (CYP isoenzymes do not appear to contribute to metabolism)

Clearance: Adults: 24.8 mL/hour/kg

Bioavailability: 84% ± 16%

Half-life elimination: 3.8 hours

Time to peak: 4-8 hours

Dosage SubQ:

Children 6-16 years: 2 mg/kg twice daily (maximum dose: 90 mg twice daily)

Adolescents ≥16 years and Adults: 90 mg twice daily

Dosage adjustment in renal impairment:

Cl_{cr} >35 mL/minute: Clearance not affected; no dosage adjustment required.

Cl_{cr} ≤35 mL/minute: Limited data showed decreased clearance; however, no dosage adjustment recommended.

End-stage renal disease (on dialysis): Limited data showed decreased clearance; however, no dosage adjustment recommended.

Dosage adjustment in hepatic impairment: No dosage adjustment required

Administration Inject subcutaneously into upper arm, abdomen, or anterior thigh. Do not inject into moles, the navel, over a blood vessel or skin abnormalities such as scar tissue, surgical scars, bruises, or tattoos. In addition, do not inject in or near sites where large nerves are close to the skin including the elbow, knee, groin, or buttocks. Rotate injection site, give injections at a site different from the preceding injection site; do not inject into any site where an injection site reaction is evident. Bioequivalence was found to be similar in a study comparing standard administration using a needle versus a needle-free device.

Dosage Forms Excipient information presented when available (limited, particularly for generics); consult specific product labeling.

Injection, powder for reconstitution [preservative free]:

Fuzeon®: 108 mg [90 mg/mL following reconstitution; available in convenience kit of 60 vials, SWFI, syringes, alcohol wipes, patient instructions]

◆ **ENG** *see* Etonogestrel *on page 589*

◆ **Engerix-B®** *see* Hepatitis B Vaccine (Recombinant) *on page 728*

◆ **Engerix-B® and Havrix®** *see* Hepatitis A and Hepatitis B Recombinant Vaccine *on page 725*

◆ **Enhanced-potency Inactivated Poliovirus Vaccine** *see* Poliovirus Vaccine (Inactivated) *on page 1207*

◆ **Enjuvia™** *see* Estrogens (Conjugated B/Synthetic) *on page 561*

◆ **Enlon® [DSC]** *see* Edrophonium *on page 505*

◆ **Enlon® (Can)** *see* Edrophonium *on page 505*

◆ **Enlon-Plus™ [DSC]** *see* Edrophonium and Atropine *on page 506*

Enoxaparin (ee noks a PA rin)

U.S. Brand Names Lovenox®

Canadian Brand Names Enoxaparin Injection; Lovenox®; Lovenox® HP

Index Terms Enoxaparin Sodium

Pharmacologic Category Low Molecular Weight Heparin

Additional Appendix Information

Anticoagulants, Injectable *on page 1636*

Use

Acute coronary syndromes: Unstable angina (UA), non-ST-elevation (NSTEMI), and ST-elevation myocardial infarction (STEMI)

DVT prophylaxis: Following hip or knee replacement surgery, abdominal surgery, or in medical patients with severely-restricted mobility during acute illness who are at risk for thromboembolic complications

DVT treatment (acute): Inpatient treatment (patients with and without pulmonary embolism) and outpatient treatment (patients without pulmonary embolism)

Note: High-risk patients include those with one or more of the following risk factors: >40 years of age, obesity, general anesthesia lasting >30 minutes, malignancy, history of deep vein thrombosis or pulmonary embolism

Unlabeled/Investigational Use Prophylaxis and treatment of thromboembolism in children; anticoagulant bridge therapy during temporary interruption of vitamin K antagonist therapy in patients at high risk for thromboembolism; DVT prophylaxis following moderate-risk general surgery, major gynecologic surgery and following higher-risk general surgery for cancer; management of venous thromboembolism (VTE) during pregnancy (Hirsh, 2008)

Pregnancy Risk Factor B

Pregnancy Considerations Animal studies have not shown teratogenic or fetotoxic effects. Pregnancy itself increases the risk of thromboembolism. Pregnant women with a history of thromboembolic disease are at increased risk of maternal and fetal complications. Enoxaparin does not cross the placenta. Use may be recommended in pregnant women for the management of VTE. Monitoring antifactor Xa levels is recommended. Risk of adverse events may be increased in pregnant women with mechanical heart valves; use is controversial and has not been adequately studied. Postmarketing reports include congenital abnormalities (cause and effect not established) and also fetal death when used in pregnant women. Multiple-dose vials contain benzyl alcohol; use caution in pregnant women.

Lactation Excretion in breast milk unknown/use caution

Medication Safety Issues

Sound-alike/look-alike issues:

Lovenox® may be confused with Levaquin®, Lotronex®, Protonix®

High alert medication: The Institute for Safe Medication Practices (ISMP) includes this medication among its list of drugs which have a heightened risk of causing significant patient harm when used in error.

International issues:

Lovenox® may be confused with Lotanax® which is a brand name for terfenadine in the Czech Republic

2009 National Patient Safety Goals: The Joint Commission on Accreditation of Healthcare Organizations requires healthcare organizations that provide anticoagulant therapy to have a process in place to reduce the risk of anticoagulant-associated patient harm. Patients receiving anticoagulants should receive individualized care through a defined process that includes standardized ordering, dispensing, administration, monitoring and education. This does not apply to routine short-term use of anticoagulants for prevention of venous thromboembolism when the expectation is that the patient's laboratory values will remain within or close to normal values (NPSG.03.05.01).

Contraindications Hypersensitivity to enoxaparin, heparin, or any component of the formulation; thrombocytopenia associated with a positive *in vitro* test for antiplatelet antibodies in the presence of enoxaparin; hypersensitivity to pork products; active major bleeding; not for I.M. use

Warnings/Precautions [U.S. Boxed Warning]: Patients with recent or anticipated neuraxial anesthesia (epidural or spinal anesthesia) are at risk of spinal or epidural hematoma and subsequent paralysis. Consider risk versus benefit prior to neuraxial anesthesia; risk is increased by concomitant agents which may alter hemostasis or by the use of indwelling epidural catheters for analgesia, as well as traumatic or repeated epidural or spinal puncture. Patient should be observed closely for bleeding if enoxaparin is administered during or immediately following diagnostic lumbar puncture, epidural anesthesia, or spinal anesthesia.

Do not administer intramuscularly. Not recommended for thromboprophylaxis in patients with prosthetic heart valves (especially pregnant women). Not to be used interchangeably (unit for unit) with heparin or any other low molecular weight heparins. Use caution in patients with history of heparin-induced thrombocytopenia. Monitor patient closely for signs or symptoms of bleeding. Certain patients are at increased risk of bleeding. Risk factors include bacterial endocarditis; congenital or acquired bleeding disorders; active ulcerative or angiodysplastic GI diseases; severe uncontrolled hypertension; history of hemorrhagic stroke; use shortly after brain, spinal, or ophthalmic surgery; patients treated concomitantly with platelet inhibitors; recent GI bleeding; thrombocytopenia or platelet defects; severe liver disease; hypertensive or diabetic retinopathy; or in patients undergoing invasive procedures. Monitor platelet count closely. Rare cases of thrombocytopenia have occurred. Discontinue therapy and consider alternative treatment if platelets are <100,000/mm^3 and/or thrombosis develops. Rare cases of thrombocytopenia with thrombosis have occurred. Use caution in patients with congenital or drug-induced thrombocytopenia or platelet defects. Risk of bleeding may be increased in women <45 kg and in men <57 kg. Use caution in patients with renal failure; dosage adjustment needed if Cl_{cr} <30 mL/minute. Use with caution in the elderly (delayed elimination may occur); dosage alteration/adjustment may be required (eg, omission of I.V. bolus in acute STEMI in patients ≥75 years of age). Monitor for hyperkalemia; can cause hyperkalemia by suppressing aldosterone production. Multiple-dose vials contain benzyl alcohol (use caution in pregnant women). In neonates, large amounts of benzyl alcohol (>100 mg/kg/day) have been associated with fatal toxicity (gasping syndrome).

Adverse Reactions As with all anticoagulants, bleeding is the major adverse effect of enoxaparin. Hemorrhage may occur at virtually any site. Risk is dependent on multiple variables. At the recommended doses, single injections of enoxaparin do not significantly influence platelet aggregation or affect global clotting time (ie, PT or aPTT).

1% to 10%:

Central nervous system: Fever (5% to 8%), confusion, pain

Dermatologic: Erythema, bruising

Gastrointestinal: Nausea (3%), diarrhea

Hematologic: Hemorrhage (major, <1% to 4%; includes cases of intracranial, retroperitoneal, or intraocular hemorrhage; incidence varies with indication/population), thrombocytopenia (moderate 1%; severe 0.1% - see note below), anemia (<2%)

Hepatic: ALT increased, AST increased

Local: Injection site hematoma (9%), local reactions (irritation, pain, ecchymosis, erythema)

Renal: Hematuria (<2%)

<1% (Limited to important or life-threatening): Allergic reaction, anaphylactoid reaction, cutaneous vasculitis (hypersensitive), eczematous plaques, hematoma (see note on "Spinal or epidural hematomas" below), hyperkalemia, hyperlipidemia, hypertriglyceridemia, intracranial hemorrhage (up to 0.8%), erythematous pruritic patches, pruritus, purpura, retroperitoneal bleeding, skin necrosis, thrombocytopenia with thrombosis, thrombocytosis, urticaria, vesicobullous rash

Notes:

Spinal or epidural hematomas: Can occur following neuraxial anesthesia or spinal puncture, resulting in paralysis. Risk is increased in patients with indwelling epidural catheters or concomitant use of other drugs affecting hemostasis. Prosthetic valve thrombosis, including fatal cases, has been reported in pregnant women receiving enoxaparin as thromboprophylaxis.

Thrombocytopenia with thrombosis: Cases of heparin-induced thrombocytopenia (some complicated by organ infarction, limb ischemia, or death) have been reported.

Drug Interactions

Avoid Concomitant Use There are no known interactions where it is recommended to avoid concomitant use.

Increased Effect/Toxicity

Enoxaparin may increase the levels/effects of: Anticoagulants; Drotrecogin Alfa; Ibritumomab; Tositumomab and Iodine I 131 Tositumomab

The levels/effects of Enoxaparin may be increased by: Antiplatelet Agents; Dasatinib; Herbs (Anticoagulant/Antiplatelet Properties); Nonsteroidal Anti-Inflammatory Agents; Pentosan Polysulfate Sodium; Prostacyclin Analogues; Salicylates; Thrombolytic Agents

Decreased Effect There are no known significant interactions involving a decrease in effect.

Ethanol/Nutrition/Herb Interactions Herb/Nutraceutical: Avoid cat's claw, dong quai, evening primrose, feverfew, garlic, ginger, ginkgo, red clover, horse chestnut, green tea, ginseng (all have additional antiplatelet activity).

Stability Store at 25°C (77°F); excursions permitted to 15°C to 30°C (59°F to 86°F); do not freeze.

Mechanism of Action Standard heparin consists of components with molecular weights ranging from 4000-30,000 daltons with a mean of 16,000 daltons. Heparin acts as an anticoagulant by enhancing the inhibition rate of clotting proteases by antithrombin III impairing normal hemostasis and inhibition of factor Xa. Low molecular weight heparins have a small effect on the activated partial thromboplastin time and strongly inhibit factor Xa. Enoxaparin is derived from porcine heparin that undergoes benzylation followed by alkaline depolymerization. The average molecular weight of enoxaparin is 4500 daltons which is distributed as (≤20%) 2000 daltons (≥68%) 2000-8000 daltons, and (≤15%) >8000 daltons. Enoxaparin has a higher ratio of antifactor Xa to antifactor IIa activity than unfractionated heparin.

Pharmacodynamics/Kinetics

Onset of action: Peak effect: SubQ: Antifactor Xa and antithrombin (antifactor IIa): 3-5 hours

Duration: 40 mg dose: Antifactor Xa activity: ~12 hours

Distribution: 4.3 L (based on antifactor Xa activity)

Metabolism: Hepatic, to lower molecular weight fragments (little activity)

Protein binding: Does not bind to heparin binding proteins

Half-life elimination, plasma: 2-4 times longer than standard heparin, independent of dose; based on anti-Xa activity: 4.5-7 hours

Excretion: Urine (40% of dose; 10% as active fragments)

Dosage SubQ:

Infants and Children (unlabeled use; Monagle, 2008):

Infants <2 months: Initial:

Prophylaxis: 0.75 mg/kg every 12 hours

Treatment: 1.5 mg/kg every 12 hours

Infants >2 months and Children ≤18 years: Initial:

Prophylaxis: 0.5 mg/kg every 12 hours

Treatment: 1 mg/kg every 12 hours

Maintenance: See **Dosage Titration** table:

Enoxaparin Pediatric Dosage Titration

Antifactor Xa	Dose Titration	Time to Repeat Antifactor Xa Level
<0.35 units/mL	Increase dose by 25%	4 h after next dose
0.35-0.49 units/mL	Increase dose by 10%	4 h after next dose
0.5-1 unit/mL	Keep same dosage	Next day, then 1 wk later, then monthly (4 h after dose)
1.1-1.5 units/mL	Decrease dose by 20%	Before next dose
1.6-2 units/mL	Hold dose for 3 h and decrease dose by 30%	Before next dose, then 4 h after next dose
>2 units/mL	Hold all doses until antifactor Xa is 0.5 units/mL, then decrease dose by 40%	Before next dose and every 12 h until antifactor Xa <0.5 units/mL

Modified from Monagle P, Michelson AD, Bovill E, et al, "Antithrombotic Therapy in Children," *Chest*, 2001, 119:344S-70S.

Adults:

DVT prophylaxis:

Hip replacement surgery:

Twice-daily dosing: 30 mg every 12 hours, with initial dose within 12-24 hours after surgery, and every 12 hours for at least 10 days or until risk of DVT has diminished or the patient is adequately anticoagulated on warfarin.

Once-daily dosing: 40 mg once daily, with initial dose within 9-15 hours before surgery, and daily for at least 10 days (or up to 35 days postoperatively) or until risk of DVT has diminished or the patient is adequately anticoagulated on warfarin.

Knee replacement surgery: 30 mg every 12 hours, with initial dose within 12-24 hours after surgery, and every 12 hours for at least 10 days or until risk of DVT has diminished or the patient is adequately anticoagulated on warfarin.

Abdominal surgery: 40 mg once daily, with initial dose given 2 hours prior to surgery; continue until risk of DVT has diminished (usually 7-10 days).

Medical patients with severely-restricted mobility during acute illness: 40 mg once daily; continue until risk of DVT has diminished (usually 6-11 days).

DVT treatment (acute): **Note:** Start warfarin on the first treatment day and continue enoxaparin until INR is between 2 and 3 (usually 5-7 days).

Inpatient treatment (with or without pulmonary embolism): 1 mg/kg/dose every 12 hours or 1.5 mg/kg once daily.

Outpatient treatment (without pulmonary embolism): 1 mg/kg/dose every 12 hours.

ST-elevation myocardial infarction (STEMI):

Patients <75 years of age: Initial: 30 mg I.V. single bolus plus 1 mg/kg (maximum 100 mg for the first 2 doses only) SubQ every 12 hours. The first SubQ dose should be administered with the I.V. bolus. Maintenance: After first 2 doses, administer 1 mg/kg SubQ every 12 hours.

Patients ≥75 years of age: Initial: SubQ: 0.75 mg/kg every 12 hours (**Note:** No I.V. bolus is administered in this population); a maximum dose of 75 mg is recommended for the first 2 doses. Maintenance: After first 2 doses, administer 0.75 mg/kg SubQ every 12 hours

Additional notes on STEMI treatment: Therapy was continued for 8 days or until hospital discharge; optimal duration not defined. Unless contraindicated, all patients received aspirin (75-325 mg daily) in clinical trials. In patients with STEMI receiving thrombolytics, initiate enoxaparin dosing between 15 minutes before and 30 minutes after fibrinolytic therapy. In patients undergoing PCI, if balloon inflation occurs ≤8 hours after the last SubQ enoxaparin dose, no additional dosing is needed. If balloon inflation occurs 8-12 hours after last SubQ enoxaparin dose, a single I.V. dose of 0.3 mg/kg should be administered.

Unstable angina or non-ST-elevation myocardial infarction (NSTEMI): 1 mg/kg every 12 hours in conjunction with oral aspirin therapy (100-325 mg once daily); continue until clinical stabilization (a minimum of at least 2 days)

Elderly: Refer to adult dosing. Increased incidence of bleeding with doses of 1.5 mg/kg/day or 1 mg/kg every 12 hours; injection-associated bleeding and serious adverse reactions are also increased in the elderly. Careful attention should be paid to elderly patients, particularly those <45 kg. **Note:** Dosage alteration/adjustment may be required.

Dosing adjustment in renal impairment: SubQ:

Cl_{cr} ≥30 mL/minute: No specific adjustment recommended (per manufacturer); monitor closely for bleeding

Cl_{cr} <30 mL/minute:

DVT prophylaxis in abdominal surgery, hip replacement, knee replacement, or in medical patients during acute illness: 30 mg once daily

DVT treatment (inpatient or outpatient treatment in conjunction with warfarin): 1 mg/kg once daily

STEMI:

<75 years: Initial: I.V.: 30 mg as a single dose with the first dose of the SubQ maintenance regimen administered at the same time as the I.V. bolus

≥75 years of age: Omit I.V. bolus; Maintenance: SubQ: 1 mg/kg every 24 hours in all patients

Unstable angina, NSTEMI: SubQ: 1 mg/kg once daily

Dialysis: Enoxaparin has not been FDA approved for use in dialysis patients. It's elimination is primarily via the renal route. Serious bleeding complications have been reported with use in patients who are dialysis dependent or have severe renal failure. LMWH administration at fixed doses without monitoring has greater unpredictable anticoagulant effects in patients with chronic kidney disease. If used, dosages should be reduced and anti-Xa levels frequently monitored, as accumulation may occur with repeated doses. Many clinicians would not use enoxaparin in this population especially without timely anti-Xa levels.

Hemodialysis: Supplemental dose is not necessary.

Peritoneal dialysis: Significant drug removal is unlikely based on physiochemical characteristics.

Administration Do **not** administer I.M.; should be administered by deep SubQ injection to the left or right anterolateral and left or right posterolateral abdominal wall. A single dose may be administered I.V. as part of treatment for ST-elevation myocardial infarction (STEMI) to patients <75 years of age; no I.V. bolus is given to patients ≥75 years of age. To avoid loss of drug from the 30 mg and 40 mg syringes, do not expel the air bubble from the syringe prior to injection. In order to minimize bruising, do not rub injection site. An automatic injector (Lovenox EasyInjector™) is available with the 30 mg and 40 mg syringes to aid the patient with self-injections. **Note:** Enoxaparin is available in 100 mg/mL and 150 mg/mL concentrations.

Monitoring Parameters Platelets, occult blood, anti-Xa levels, serum creatinine; monitoring of PT and/or aPTT is not necessary. Routine monitoring of anti-Xa levels is not required, but has been utilized in patients with obesity and/or renal insufficiency. Monitoring anti-Xa levels is recommended in pregnant women receiving therapeutic doses of enoxaparin (Hirsh, 2008).

Reference Range The following therapeutic ranges for anti-Xa levels have been suggested, but have not been validated in a controlled trial. Anti-Xa level measured 4 hours postdose.

DVT treatment (every-12-hour dosing): 0.6-1 units/mL

DVT treatment (once-daily dosing): 1-2 units/mL

Dosage Forms Excipient information presented when available (limited, particularly for generics); consult specific product labeling.

Injection, solution, as sodium [graduated prefilled syringe; preservative free]:

Lovenox®: 60 mg/0.6 mL (0.6 mL); 80 mg/0.8 mL (0.8 mL); 100 mg/mL (1 mL); 120 mg/0.8 mL (0.8 mL); 150 mg/mL (1 mL)

Injection, solution, as sodium [multidose vial]:

Lovenox®: 100 mg/mL (3 mL) [contains benzyl alcohol]

Injection, solution, as sodium [prefilled syringe; preservative free]:

Lovenox®: 30 mg/0.3 mL (0.3 mL); 40 mg/0.4 mL (0.4 mL)

◆ **Enoxaparin Injection (Can)** *see* Enoxaparin *on page 519*

◆ **Enoxaparin Sodium** *see* Enoxaparin *on page 519*

◆ **Enpresse™** *see* Ethinyl Estradiol and Levonorgestrel *on page 577*

Entacapone (en TA ka pone)

U.S. Brand Names Comtan®

Canadian Brand Names Comtan®

Pharmacologic Category Anti-Parkinson's Agent, COMT Inhibitor

Additional Appendix Information

Antiparkinsonian Agents *on page 1643*

Use Adjunct to levodopa/carbidopa therapy in patients with idiopathic Parkinson's disease who experience "wearing-off" symptoms at the end of a dosing interval

Pregnancy Risk Factor C

Pregnancy Considerations Not recommended

Lactation Excretion in breast milk unknown/use caution

Contraindications Hypersensitivity to entacapone or any of component of the formulation

Warnings/Precautions May cause orthostatic hypotension and syncope; Parkinson's disease patients appear to have an impaired capacity to respond to a postural challenge; use with caution in patients at risk of hypotension (such as those receiving antihypertensive drugs) or where transient hypotensive episodes would be poorly tolerated (cardiovascular disease or cerebrovascular disease). Parkinson's patients being treated with dopaminergic agonists ordinarily require careful monitoring for signs and symptoms of postural hypotension, especially during dose escalation, and should be informed of this risk. May cause hallucinations, which may improve with reduction in levodopa therapy. Use with caution in patients with pre-existing dyskinesias; exacerbation of pre-existing dyskinesia and severe rhabdomyolysis has been reported. Levodopa dosage reduction may be required, particularly in patients with levodopa dosages >600 mg daily or with moderate-to-severe dyskinesia prior to initiation. Entacapone, in conjunction with other drug therapy that alters brain biogenic amine concentrations (eg, MAO inhibitors, SSRIs), has been associated with a syndrome resembling neuroleptic malignant syndrome (hyperpyrexia and confusion - some fatal) on abrupt withdrawal or dosage reduction. Concomitant use of entacapone and nonselective MAO inhibitors should be avoided. Selegiline is a selective MAO type B inhibitor (when given orally at ≤10 mg/day) and can be taken with entacapone. Dopaminergic agents from the ergot class have also been associated with fibrotic complications, such as retroperitoneal fibrosis, pulmonary infiltrates or effusion and pleural thickening. It is unknown whether non-ergot, pro-dopaminergic agents like entacapone confer this risk. Use caution in patients with hepatic impairment or severe renal impairment. Do not withdraw therapy abruptly. Safety and efficacy in pediatric patients have not been established.

Adverse Reactions

>10%:

Gastrointestinal: Nausea (14%)

Neuromuscular & skeletal: Dyskinesia (25%), placebo (15%)

1% to 10%:

Cardiovascular: Orthostatic hypotension (4.3%), syncope (1.2%)

Central nervous system: Dizziness (8%), fatigue (6%), hallucinations (4%), anxiety (2%), somnolence (2%), agitation (1%)

Dermatologic: Purpura (2%)

Gastrointestinal: Diarrhea (10%), abdominal pain (8%), constipation (6%), vomiting (4%), dry mouth (3%),

dyspepsia (2%), flatulence (2%), gastritis (1%), taste perversion (1%)
Genitourinary: Brown-orange urine discoloration (10%)
Neuromuscular & skeletal: Hyperkinesia (10%), hypokinesia (9%), back pain (4%), weakness (2%)
Respiratory: Dyspnea (3%)
Miscellaneous: Diaphoresis increased (2%), bacterial infection (1%)

<1% (Limited to important or life-threatening): Hyperpyrexia and confusion (resembling neuroleptic malignant syndrome), pulmonary fibrosis, retroperitoneal fibrosis, rhabdomyolysis

Drug Interactions

Metabolism/Transport Effects Inhibits CYP1A2 (weak), 2A6 (weak), 2C9 (weak), 2C19 (weak), 2D6 (weak), 2E1 (weak), 3A4 (weak)

Avoid Concomitant Use There are no known interactions where it is recommended to avoid concomitant use.

Increased Effect/Toxicity

Entacapone may increase the levels/effects of: Alcohol (Ethyl); CNS Depressants; COMT Substrates; MAO Inhibitors

Decreased Effect There are no known significant interactions involving a decrease in effect.

Ethanol/Nutrition/Herb Interactions

Ethanol: Avoid ethanol (may increase CNS adverse effects).
Food: Entacapone has been reported to chelate iron and decreasing serum iron levels were noted in clinical trials; however, clinically significant anemia has not been observed.

Mechanism of Action Entacapone is a reversible and selective inhibitor of catechol-O-methyltransferase (COMT). When entacapone is taken with levodopa, the pharmacokinetics are altered, resulting in more sustained levodopa serum levels compared to levodopa taken alone. The resulting levels of levodopa provide for increased concentrations available for absorption across the blood-brain barrier, thereby providing for increased CNS levels of dopamine, the active metabolite of levodopa.

Pharmacodynamics/Kinetics

Onset of action: Rapid
Peak effect: 1 hour
Absorption: Rapid
Distribution: I.V.: V_{dss}: 20 L
Protein binding: 98%, primarily to albumin
Metabolism: Isomerization to the *cis*-isomer, followed by direct glucuronidation of the parent and *cis*-isomer
Bioavailability: 35%
Half-life elimination: B phase: 0.4-0.7 hours; Y phase: 2.4 hours
Time to peak, serum: 1 hour
Excretion: Feces (90%); urine (10%)

Dosage Oral: Adults: 200 mg with each dose of levodopa/carbidopa, up to a maximum of 8 times/day (maximum daily dose: 1600 mg/day). To optimize therapy, the dosage of levodopa may need reduced or the dosing interval may need extended. Patients taking levodopa ≥800 mg/day or who had moderate-to-severe dyskinesias prior to therapy required an average decrease of 25% in the daily levodopa dose.

Dosage adjustment in hepatic impairment: Treat with caution and monitor carefully; AUC and C_{max} can be possibly doubled

Dietary Considerations May be taken with or without food.

Administration Always administer in association with levodopa/carbidopa; can be combined with both the immediate and sustained release formulations of levodopa/carbidopa. Can be taken with or without food. Should not be abruptly withdrawn from patient's therapy due to significant worsening of symptoms.

Monitoring Parameters Signs and symptoms of Parkinson's disease; liver function tests, blood pressure, patient's mental status; serum iron (if signs of anemia)

Dosage Forms Excipient information presented when available (limited, particularly for generics); consult specific product labeling.
Tablet: 200 mg

◆ **Entacapone, Carbidopa, and Levodopa** *see* Levodopa, Carbidopa, and Entacapone *on page 875*

Entecavir (en TE ka veer)

U.S. Brand Names Baraclude®

Canadian Brand Names Baraclude®

Pharmacologic Category Antiretroviral Agent, Reverse Transcriptase Inhibitor (Nucleoside)

Use Treatment of chronic hepatitis B infection in adults with evidence of active viral replication and either evidence of persistent transaminase elevations or histologically-active disease

Pregnancy Risk Factor C

Pregnancy Considerations Teratogenic effects have been observed in animal studies. There are no adequate and well-controlled studies in pregnant women. Use only if benefit outweighs risk. Pregnant women taking entecavir should enroll in the pregnancy registry by calling 1-800-258-4263.

Lactation Excretion in breast milk unknown/not recommended

Contraindications Hypersensitivity to entecavir or any component of the formulation

Warnings/Precautions [U.S. Boxed Warning]: Lactic acidosis and severe hepatomegaly with steatosis have been reported. [U.S. Boxed Warning]: Exacerbation of hepatitis B may occur upon discontinuation. Monitor liver function several months after stopping treatment; reinitiation of antihepatitis B therapy may be required. Use caution in patients with renal impairment or in patients receiving concomitant therapy which may reduce renal function; dose adjustment recommended for Cl_{cr} <50 mL/minute. Cross-resistance may develop in patients failing previous therapy with lamivudine.

HIV: **[U.S. Boxed Warning]: May cause the development of HIV resistance in chronic hepatitis B patients with unrecognized or untreated HIV infection.** Determine HIV status prior to initiating treatment with entecavir. Not recommended for HIV/HBV coinfected patients unless also receiving highly active antiretroviral therapy (HAART). The manufacturer's labeling states that entecavir does not exhibit any clinically-relevant activity against human immunodeficiency virus (HIV type 1). However, a small number of case reports have indicated declines in virus levels during entecavir therapy. Reports of HIV resistance to a common HIV drug has been reported in an HIV/HBV-infected patient receiving entecavir as monotherapy for HBV.

Safety and efficacy in patients <16 years of age and liver transplant patients have not been established.

Adverse Reactions

>10%: Hepatic: ALT increased (>5 x ULN: 11% to 12%; post-treatment flare [lamivudine refractory]: >10 x ULN and >2 x baseline: 12%)

1% to 10%:
Central nervous system: Headache (2% to 4%), fatigue (1% to 3%), dizziness
Endocrine & metabolic: Hyperglycemia (2% to 3%)
Gastrointestinal: Lipase increased (7%), amylase increased (2% to 3%), diarrhea (≤1%), dyspepsia (≤1%), nausea
Hepatic: Bilirubin increased (2% to 3%), ALT increased (>10 x ULN and >2 x baseline: 2%; post-treatment flare

[nucleoside-naive]: >10 x ULN and >2 x baseline: 2% to 8%)

Renal: Hematuria (9%), glycosuria (4%), creatinine increased (1% to 2%)

<1% (Limited to important or life-threatening): Dizziness, hypoalbuminemia, insomnia, nausea, rash, somnolence, thrombocytopenia, vomiting

Drug Interactions

Avoid Concomitant Use There are no known interactions where it is recommended to avoid concomitant use.

Increased Effect/Toxicity

The levels/effects of Entecavir may be increased by: Ganciclovir-Valganciclovir; Ribavirin

Decreased Effect There are no known significant interactions involving a decrease in effect.

Ethanol/Nutrition/Herb Interactions

Food: Food delays absorption and reduces AUC by 18% to 20%.

Stability Store at controlled room temperature of 25°C (77°F); excursions permitted to 15°C to 30°C (59°F to 86°F). Protect oral solution from light.

Mechanism of Action Entecavir is intracellularly phosphorylated to guanosine triphosphate which competes with natural substrates to effectively inhibit hepatitis B viral polymerase; enzyme inhibition blocks reverse transcriptase activity thereby reducing viral DNA synthesis.

Pharmacodynamics/Kinetics

Distribution: Extensive (V_d in excess of body water)

Protein binding: ~13%

Metabolism: Minor hepatic glucuronide/sulfate conjugation

Half-life elimination: Terminal: ~5-6 days; accumulation: ~24 hours

Time to peak, plasma: 0.5-1.5 hours

Excretion: Urine (60% to 73% as unchanged drug)

Dosage Oral: Adolescents ≥16 years and Adults:

Nucleoside treatment naive: 0.5 mg daily

Lamivudine-resistant viremia (or known lamivudine- or telbivudine-resistant mutations): 1 mg daily

Note: Usual treatment duration is at least 1 year and varies with HBeAg status; consult current guidelines and literature.

Dosage adjustment in renal impairment:

Cl_{cr} 30-49 mL/minute: Administer 50% of usual dose daily or administer the normal dose every 48 hours

Cl_{cr} 10-29 mL/minute: Administer 30% of usual dose daily or administer the normal dose every 72 hours

Cl_{cr} <10 mL/minute (including hemodialysis and CAPD): Administer 10% of usual dose daily or administer the normal dose every 7 days; administer after hemodialysis

Dosage adjustment in hepatic impairment: No adjustment necessary.

Dietary Considerations Take on an empty stomach (2 hours before or after a meal).

Administration Administer on an empty stomach. Do not dilute or mix oral solution with water or other beverages; use calibrated oral dosing syringe. Oral solution and tablet are bioequivalent on a mg-to-mg basis.

Monitoring Parameters HIV status (prior to initiation of therapy); liver function tests, renal function; in HBV/HIV-coinfected patients, monitor HIV viral load and CD4 count

Dosage Forms Excipient information presented when available (limited, particularly for generics); consult specific product labeling.

Oral solution:

Baraclude®: 0.05 mg/mL (210 mL) [orange flavor]

Tablet:

Baraclude®: 0.5 mg, 1 mg

◆ **Entereg®** *see* Alvimopan *on page* *77*

◆ **Enterex® Glutapak-10® [OTC]** *see* Glutamine *on page* *700*

◆ **Entex® HC [DSC]** *see* Hydrocodone, Pseudoephedrine, and Guaifenesin *on page* *743*

◆ **Entex® LA (Can)** *see* Guaifenesin and Pseudoephedrine *on page* *713*

◆ **Entex® PSE** *see* Guaifenesin and Pseudoephedrine *on page* *713*

◆ **Entocort® (Can)** *see* Budesonide *on page* *215*

◆ **Entocort® EC** *see* Budesonide *on page* *215*

◆ **Entrophen® (Can)** *see* Aspirin *on page* *142*

◆ **Entsol® [OTC]** *see* Sodium Chloride *on page* *1381*

◆ **Enulose** *see* Lactulose *on page* *847*

◆ **Eperbel-S [DSC]** *see* Belladonna, Phenobarbital, and Ergotamine *on page* *178*

EPHEDrine (e FED rin)

U.S. Brand Names Pretz-D® [OTC]

Index Terms Ephedrine Sulfate

Pharmacologic Category Alpha/Beta Agonist

Additional Appendix Information

Contrast Media Reactions, Premedication for Prophylaxis *on page* *1799*

Use Treatment of bronchial asthma, nasal congestion, acute bronchospasm, idiopathic orthostatic hypotension, hypotension induced by spinal anesthesia

Pregnancy Risk Factor C

Lactation Enters breast milk/not recommended

Medication Safety Issues

Sound-alike/look-alike issues:

EPHEDrine may be confused with Epifrin®, EPINEPHrine

Contraindications Hypersensitivity to ephedrine or any component of the formulation; cardiac arrhythmias; angle-closure glaucoma; concurrent use of other sympathomimetic agents

Warnings/Precautions Blood volume depletion should be corrected before injectable ephedrine therapy is instituted; use caution in patients with unstable vasomotor symptoms, diabetes, hyperthyroidism, prostatic hyperplasia or a history of seizures; also use caution in the elderly and those patients with cardiovascular disorders such as coronary artery disease, arrhythmias, and hypertension. Ephedrine may cause hypertension. Long-term use may cause anxiety and symptoms of paranoid schizophrenia. Avoid as a bronchodilator; generally not used as a bronchodilator since other beta$_2$-agents are less toxic. Use with caution in the elderly, since it crosses the blood-brain barrier and may cause confusion. Use with extreme caution in patients taking MAO inhibitors.

Adverse Reactions Frequency not defined.

Cardiovascular: Arrhythmias, chest pain, elevation or depression of blood pressure, hypertension, palpitation, tachycardia, unusual pallor

Central nervous system: Agitation, anxiety, apprehension, CNS stimulating effects, dizziness, excitation, fear, headache hyperactivity, insomnia, irritability, nervousness, restlessness, tension

Gastrointestinal: Anorexia, GI upset, nausea, vomiting, xerostomia

Genitourinary: Painful urination

Neuromuscular & skeletal: Trembling, tremor (more common in the elderly), weakness

Respiratory: Dyspnea

Miscellaneous: Diaphoresis increased

Drug Interactions

Avoid Concomitant Use

Avoid concomitant use of EPHEDrine with any of the following: Iobenguane I 123; MAO Inhibitors

Increased Effect/Toxicity

EPHEDrine may increase the levels/effects of: Bromocriptine; Sympathomimetics

The levels/effects of EPHEDrine may be increased by: Antacids; Cannabinoids; Carbonic Anhydrase Inhibitors; MAO Inhibitors; Serotonin/Norepinephrine Reuptake Inhibitors

Decreased Effect

EPHEDrine may decrease the levels/effects of: Iobenguane I 123

Ethanol/Nutrition/Herb Interactions Herb/Nutraceutical: Avoid ephedra, yohimbe (may cause CNS stimulation).

Stability Protect all dosage forms from light.

Mechanism of Action Releases tissue stores of epinephrine and thereby produces an alpha- and beta-adrenergic stimulation; longer-acting and less potent than epinephrine

Pharmacodynamics/Kinetics

Onset of action: Oral: Bronchodilation: 0.25-1 hour

Duration: Oral: 3-6 hours

Distribution: Crosses placenta; enters breast milk

Metabolism: Minimally hepatic

Half-life elimination: 2.5-3.6 hours

Excretion: Urine (60% to 77% as unchanged drug) within 24 hours

Dosage

Children:

Oral, SubQ: 3 mg/kg/day or 25-100 mg/m^2/day in 4-6 divided doses every 4-6 hours

I.M., slow I.V. push: 0.2-0.3 mg/kg/dose every 4-6 hours

Adults:

Oral: 25-50 mg every 3-4 hours as needed

I.M., SubQ: 25-50 mg, parenteral adult dose should not exceed 150 mg in 24 hours

I.M.: Hypotension induced by anesthesia: 25 mg

I.V.: 5-25 mg/dose slow I.V. push repeated after 5-10 minutes as needed, then every 3-4 hours not to exceed 150 mg/24 hours

Nasal spray:

Children 6-12 years: 1-2 sprays into each nostril, not more frequently than every 4 hours

Children ≥12 years and Adults: 2-3 sprays into each nostril, not more frequently than every 4 hours

Monitoring Parameters Injection solution: Monitor blood pressure, pulse

Test Interactions Can cause a false-positive amphetamine EMIT assay

Dosage Forms Excipient information presented when available (limited, particularly for generics); consult specific product labeling.

Capsule, as sulfate: 25 mg

Injection, solution, as sulfate: 50 mg/mL (1 mL, 10 mL)

Solution, intranasal spray, as sulfate (Pretz-D®): 0.25% (50 mL)

◆ **Ephedrine, Chlorpheniramine, Phenylephrine, and Carbetapentane** *see* Chlorpheniramine, Ephedrine, Phenylephrine, and Carbetapentane *on page 311*

◆ **Ephedrine Sulfate** *see* EPHEDrine *on page 524*

◆ **Epidermal Thymocyte Activating Factor** *see* Aldesleukin *on page 53*

◆ **Epifoam®** *see* Pramoxine and Hydrocortisone *on page 1227*

Epinastine (ep i NAS teen)

U.S. Brand Names Elestat™

Index Terms Epinastine Hydrochloride

Pharmacologic Category Histamine H_1 Antagonist; Histamine H_1 Antagonist, Second Generation

Use Treatment of allergic conjunctivitis

Pregnancy Risk Factor C

Dosage Ophthalmic: Allergic conjunctivitis: Children ≥3 years and Adults: Instill 1 drop into each eye twice daily; continue throughout period of exposure, even in the absence of symptoms

Additional Information Complete prescribing information for this medication should be consulted for additional detail.

Dosage Forms Excipient information presented when available (limited, particularly for generics); consult specific product labeling.

Solution, ophthalmic, as hydrochloride: 0.05% (5 mL) [contains benzalkonium chloride]

◆ **Epinastine Hydrochloride** *see* Epinastine *on page 525*

EPINEPHrine (ep i NEF rin)

U.S. Brand Names Adrenalin®; EpiPen®; EpiPen® Jr; Primatene® Mist [OTC]; Raphon [OTC]; S2® [OTC]; Twinject®

Canadian Brand Names Adrenalin®; EpiPen®; EpiPen® Jr; Twinject®

Index Terms Adrenaline; Epinephrine Bitartrate; Epinephrine Hydrochloride; Racepinephrine

Pharmacologic Category Alpha/Beta Agonist

Additional Appendix Information

Bronchodilators *on page 1650*

Glaucoma Drug Therapy *on page 1808*

Hemodynamic Support, Intravenous *on page 1657*

Use Treatment of bronchospasms, bronchial asthma, nasal congestion, viral croup, anaphylactic reactions, cardiac arrest; added to local anesthetics to decrease systemic absorption of intraspinal and local anesthetics and increase duration of action; decrease superficial hemorrhage

Unlabeled/Investigational Use ACLS guidelines: Ventricular fibrillation (VF) or pulseless ventricular tachycardia (VT) unresponsive to initial defibrillatory shocks; pulseless electrical activity; asystole; hypotension/shock unresponsive to volume resuscitation; symptomatic bradycardia unresponsive to atropine or pacing; inotropic support

Pregnancy Risk Factor C

Pregnancy Considerations Teratogenic effects have been observed in animal reproduction studies. Epinephrine crosses the placenta and may cause fetal anoxia. Use during pregnancy when the potential benefit to the mother outweighs the possible risk to the fetus.

Lactation Excretion in breast milk unknown

Medication Safety Issues

Sound-alike/look-alike issues:

EPINEPHrine may be confused with ePHEDrine

Epifrin® may be confused with ephedrine, EpiPen®

EpiPen® may be confused with Epifrin®

High alert medication: The Institute for Safe Medication Practices (ISMP) includes this medication among its list of drugs which have a heightened risk of causing significant patient harm when used in error.

Medication errors have occurred due to confusion with epinephrine products expressed as ratio strengths (eg, 1:1000 vs 1:10,000).

Epinephrine 1:1000 = 1 mg/mL and is most commonly used I.M.

Epinephrine 1:10,000 = 0.1 mg/mL and is used I.V.

International issues:

EpiPen® may be confused with Epigen® which is a brand name for glycyrrhizinic acid in Mexico

EpiPen® may be confused with Epopen® which is a brand name for epoetin alfa in Spain

Contraindications There are no absolute contraindications to the use of injectable epinephrine (including EpiPen®, EpiPen® Jr, and Twinject®) in a life-threatening situation.

Injectable solution: Per the manufacturer, contraindicated in narrow-angle glaucoma; shock; during general anesthesia with halogenated hydrocarbons or cyclopropane (currently not available); individuals with organic brain damage; with local anesthesia of the digits; during labor; heart failure; coronary insufficiency

Primatene Mist®, S2®: concurrent use or within 2 weeks of MAO inhibitors

Raphon: Hypersensitivity to epinephrine or any component of the formulation

Warnings/Precautions Use with caution in elderly patients, patients with diabetes mellitus, cardiovascular diseases (eg, coronary artery disease, hypertension), thyroid disease, cerebrovascular disease, Parkinson's disease, or patients taking tricyclic antidepressants. Some products contain sulfites as preservatives; the presence of sulfites in some products (eg, EpiPen® and Twinject®) should not deter administration during a serious allergic or other emergency situation even if the patient is sulfite-sensitive. Use with caution in patients taking MAO inhibitors; the concomitant use with some formulations (eg, Primatene Mist®, S2®) of epinephrine is contraindicated. Accidental injection into digits, hands, or feet may result in local reactions including injection site pallor, coldness and hypoesthesia or injury resulting in bruising, bleeding, discoloration, erythema or skeletal injury; patient should seek immediate medical attention if this occurs. Rapid I.V. administration may cause death from cerebrovascular hemorrhage or cardiac arrhythmias; however, rapid I.V. administration during pulseless arrest is necessary. Avoid topical application where reduced perfusion could lead to ischemic tissue damage (eg, penis, ears, digits).

Adverse Reactions Frequency not defined.

Cardiovascular: Angina, cardiac arrhythmia, chest pain, flushing, hypertension, pallor, palpitation, sudden death, tachycardia (parenteral), vasoconstriction, ventricular ectopy

Central nervous system: Anxiety (transient), apprehensiveness, cerebral hemorrhage, dizziness, headache, insomnia, lightheadedness, nervousness, restlessness

Gastrointestinal: Dry throat, loss of appetite, nausea, vomiting, xerostomia

Genitourinary: Acute urinary retention in patients with bladder outflow obstruction

Neuromuscular & skeletal: Tremor, weakness

Ocular: Allergic lid reaction, burning, eye pain, ocular irritation, precipitation of or exacerbation of narrow-angle glaucoma, transient stinging

Respiratory: Dyspnea, pulmonary edema

Miscellaneous: Diaphoresis

Drug Interactions

Avoid Concomitant Use

Avoid concomitant use of EPINEPHrine with any of the following: Iobenguane I 123

Increased Effect/Toxicity

EPINEPHrine may increase the levels/effects of: Bromocriptine; Sympathomimetics

The levels/effects of EPINEPHrine may be increased by: Antacids; Beta-Blockers; Cannabinoids; Carbonic Anhydrase Inhibitors; COMT Inhibitors; Inhalational Anesthetics; MAO Inhibitors; Serotonin/Norepinephrine Reuptake Inhibitors; Tricyclic Antidepressants

Decreased Effect

EPINEPHrine may decrease the levels/effects of: Iobenguane I 123

Ethanol/Nutrition/Herb Interactions Herb/Nutraceutical: Avoid ephedra, yohimbe (may cause CNS stimulation).

Stability

Epinephrine is sensitive to light and air; protection from light is recommended. Oxidation turns drug pink, then a brown color. **Solutions should not be used if they are discolored or contain a precipitate.**

Adrenalin®: Store between 15°C to 25°C (59°F to 77°F); do not freeze. Protect from light. The 1:1000 solution should be discarded 30 days after initial use.

EpiPen® and EpiPen® Jr: Store at 25°C (77°F); excursions permitted to 15°C to 30°C (59°F to 86°F); do not freeze or refrigerate. Protect from light by storing in carrier tube provided.

Primatene® Mist: Store between 20°C to 25°C (68°F to 77°F).

Raphon: Store between 2°C to 25°C (36°F to 77°F). Refrigerate after opening.

S2®: Store between 2°C to 20°C (36°F to 68°F). Protect from light.

Twinject®: Store between 20°C to 25°C (68°F to 77°F); excursions permitted to 15°C to 30°C (59°F to 86°F); do not freeze or refrigerate. Protect from light.

Stability of injection of parenteral admixture at room temperature (25°C) or refrigeration (4°C) is 24 hours.

Standard I.V. diluent: 1 mg/250 mL NS.

Preparation of adult I.V. infusion: Dilute 1 mg in 250 mL of D_5W or NS (4 mcg/mL).

S2®: Dilution not required when administered via hand-bulb nebulizer; dilute with NS 3-5 mL if using jet nebulizer

Mechanism of Action Stimulates alpha-, $beta_1$-, and $beta_2$-adrenergic receptors resulting in relaxation of smooth muscle of the bronchial tree, cardiac stimulation (increasing myocardial oxygen consumption), and dilation of skeletal muscle vasculature; small doses can cause vasodilation via $beta_2$-vascular receptors; large doses may produce constriction of skeletal and vascular smooth muscle

Pharmacodynamics/Kinetics

Onset of action: Bronchodilation: SubQ: ~5-10 minutes; Inhalation: ~1 minute

Distribution: Crosses placenta

Metabolism: Taken up into the adrenergic neuron and metabolized by monoamine oxidase and catechol-o-methyltransferase; circulating drug hepatically metabolized

Excretion: Urine (as inactive metabolites, metanephrine, and sulfate and hydroxy derivatives of mandelic acid, small amounts as unchanged drug)

Dosage

Neonates: Cardiac arrest:

I.V.: 0.01-0.03 mg/kg (0.1-0.3 mL/kg of **1:10,000** solution) every 3-5 minutes until return of spontaneous circulation

Intratracheal: Although I.V. route is preferred, may consider administration of doses up to 0.1 mg/kg (1 mL/kg of **1:10,000** solution) every 3-5 minutes until I.V. access established or return of spontaneous circulation

Infants and Children:

Asystole/pulseless arrest, pulseless VT/VF (after failed defibrillations):

I.V., I.O.: 0.01 mg/kg (0.1 mL/kg of **1:10,000** solution) (maximum single dose: 1 mg) every 3-5 minutes until return of spontaneous circulation

Intratracheal: 0.1 mg/kg (0.1 mL/kg of **1:1000** solution) (maximum single dose: 10 mg) every 3-5 minutes until I.V./I.O access established or return of spontaneous circulation

Bradycardia (symptomatic; unresponsive to atropine or pacing):

I.V., I.O.: 0.01 mg/kg (0.1 mL/kg of **1:10,000** solution) (maximum single dose: 1 mg) every 3-5 minutes as needed

Intratracheal: 0.1 mg/kg or (0.1 mL/kg of **1:1000** solution) (maximum single dose: 10 mg) every 3-5 minutes as needed until I.V./I.O access established

Continuous I.V. infusion: 0.1-1 mcg/kg/minute; doses <0.3 mcg/kg/minute generally produce beta-adrenergic effects and higher doses generally produce alpha-adrenergic vasoconstriction; titrate dosage to desired effect

Bronchodilator:

SubQ: 0.01 mg/kg (0.01 mL/kg of **1:1000** solution) (maximum single dose: 0.5 mg) every 20 minutes for 3 doses

Nebulization: S2® (racepinephrine, OTC labeling):

Children <4 years: Jet nebulizer: Croup: 0.05 mL/kg (maximum dose: 0.5 mL); dilute in 3 mL of NS. Administer over ~15 minutes; do not administer more frequently than every 2 hours

Children ≥4 years: Refer to adult dosing.

Inhalation: Children ≥4 years: Primatene® Mist: Refer to adult dosing.

Decongestant: Children ≥6 years: Refer to adult dosing

Hypersensitivity reaction: **Note:** SubQ administration results in slower absorption and is less reliable. I.M. administration in the anterolateral aspect of the thigh is preferred in the setting of anaphylaxis (ACLS guidelines, 2005; Kemp, 2008).

I.M., SubQ: 0.01 mg/kg (0.01 mL/kg of **1:1000** solution) (maximum single dose: 0.5 mg) every 5-20 minutes; larger I.M. or SubQ doses, use of I.V. route, or continuous infusion may be needed for severe anaphylactic reactions

Self-administration following severe allergic reactions (eg, insect stings, food): **Note:** World Health Organization (WHO) and Anaphylaxis Canada recommend the availability of 1 dose for every 10-20 minutes of travel time to a medical emergency facility:

EpiPen® Jr: I.M., SubQ: Children 15-29 kg: 0.15 mg; if anaphylactic symptoms persist, dose may be repeated in 5-15 minutes using an additional EpiPen® Jr

EpiPen®: I.M., SubQ: Children ≥30 kg: 0.3 mg; if anaphylactic symptoms persist, dose may be repeated in 5-15 minutes using an additional EpiPen®

Twinject®: I.M. SubQ:

Children 15-29 kg: 0.15 mg; if anaphylactic symptoms persist, dose may be repeated in 5-15 minutes using the same device after partial disassembly

Children ≥30 kg: 0.3 mg; if anaphylactic symptoms persist, dose may be repeated in 5-15 minutes using the same device after partial disassembly

Hypotension/shock, fluid-resistant (unlabeled use): Continuous I.V. infusion: 0.1-1 mcg/kg/minute; doses up to 5 mcg/kg/minute may rarely be necessary (Hegenbarth, 2008)

Adults:

Asystole/pulseless arrest, pulseless VT/VF:

I.V., I.O.: 1 mg every 3-5 minutes until return of spontaneous circulation; if this approach fails, higher doses of epinephrine (up to 0.2 mg/kg) have been used for treatment of specific problems (eg, beta-blocker or calcium channel blocker overdose)

Intratracheal: 2-2.5 mg every 3-5 minutes until I.V./I.O access established or return of spontaneous circulation; dilute in 5-10 mL NS or distilled water. **Note:** Absorption is greater with distilled water, but causes more adverse effects on PaO_2.

Bradycardia (symptomatic; unresponsive to atropine or pacing): I.V. infusion: 1-10 mcg/minute; titrate to desired effect

Bronchodilator:

SubQ: 0.3-0.5 mg (**1:1000** solution) every 20 minutes for 3 doses

Nebulization: S2® (racepinephrine, OTC labeling):

Hand-bulb nebulizer: Add 0.5 mL (~10 drops) to nebulizer; 1-3 inhalations up to every 3 hours if needed

Jet nebulizer: Add 0.5 mL (~10 drops) to nebulizer and dilute with 3 mL of NS; administer over ~15 minutes every 3-4 hours as needed

Inhalation: Primatene® Mist (OTC labeling): One inhalation, wait at least 1 minute; if not relieved, may use once more. Do not use again for at least 3 hours.

Decongestant: Intranasal: Apply **1:1000** solution locally as drops or spray or with sterile swab

Hypersensitivity reaction: **Note:** SubQ administration results in slower absorption and is less reliable. I.M. administration in the anterolateral aspect of the thigh is preferred in the setting of anaphylaxis (ACLS guidelines, 2005; Kemp, 2008).

I.M., SubQ: 0.3-0.5 mg (**1:1000** solution) every 15-20 minutes if condition requires

I.V.: 0.1 mg (**1:10,000** solution) over 5 minutes; may infuse at 1-4 mcg/minute to prevent the need to repeat injections frequently

Self-administration following severe allergic reactions (eg, insect stings, food): **Note:** The World Health Organization (WHO) and Anaphylaxis Canada recommend the availability of one dose for every 10-20 minutes of travel time to a medical emergency facility. More than 2 doses should only be administered under direct medical supervision.

Twinject®: I.M., SubQ: 0.3 mg; if anaphylactic symptoms persist, dose may be repeated in 5-15 minutes using the same device after partial disassembly

EpiPen®: I.M., SubQ: 0.3 mg; if anaphylactic symptoms persist, dose may be repeated in 5-15 minutes using an additional EpiPen®

Hypotension/shock, severe and fluid resistant (unlabeled use): I.V. infusion: Initial: 1 mcg/minute; titrate to desired response; usual range: 2-10 mcg/minute (AHA, 2005)

Administration When administering as a continuous infusion, central line administration is preferred. I.V. infusions require an infusion pump. Epinephrine solutions for injection can be administered I.M., I.O., intratracheally, I.V., or SubQ. **Note:** EpiPen® and EpiPen® Jr Auto-Injectors contain a single, fixed-dose of epinephrine. Twinject® Auto-Injectors contain two doses; the first fixed-dose is available for auto-injection; the second dose is available for manual injection following partial disassembly of device.

Subcutaneous: SubQ administration results in slower absorption and is less reliable.

I.M.: I.M. administration into the buttocks should be avoided. I.M. administration in the anterolateral aspect of the thigh is preferred in the setting of anaphylaxis (ACLS guidelines, 2005; Kemp, 2008). EpiPen®, EpiPen® Jr, and Twinject® Auto-Injectors should only be injected into the anterolateral aspect of the thigh, through clothing if necessary.

Inhalation: S2®: If using jet nebulizer: Administer over ~15 minutes; must be diluted.

Intratracheal: Dilute in NS or distilled water. Absorption is greater with distilled water, but causes more adverse effects on PaO_2. Pass catheter beyond tip of tracheal tube, stop compressions, spray drug quickly down tube. Follow immediately with several quick insufflations and continue chest compressions.

Extravasation management: Use phentolamine as antidote. Mix 5 mg with 9 mL of NS. Inject a small amount of this dilution into extravasated area. Blanching should reverse immediately. Monitor site. If blanching should recur, additional injections of phentolamine may be needed.

Monitoring Parameters Pulmonary function, heart rate, blood pressure, site of infusion for blanching, extravasation; cardiac monitor and blood pressure monitor required during continuous infusion. If using to treat hypotension, assess intravascular volume and support as needed.

Additional Information Twinject® and EpiPen® are not interchangeable due to packaging considerations.

Dosage Forms Excipient information presented when available (limited, particularly for generics); consult specific product labeling. [DSC] = Discontinued product

Aerosol for oral inhalation:

Primatene® Mist: 0.22 mg/inhalation (15 mL, 22.5 mL [DSC]) [contains CFCs]

Injection, solution [prefilled auto injector]:

EpiPen®: 0.3 mg/0.3 mL (2 mL) [1:1000 solution; delivers 0.3 mg per injection; contains sodium metabisulfite; available as single unit or in double-unit pack with training unit]

EpiPen® Jr: 0.15 mg/0.3 mL (2 mL) [1:2000 solution; delivers 0.15 mg per injection; contains sodium metabisulfite; available as single unit or in double-unit pack with training unit]

Twinject®: 0.15 mg/0.15 mL (1.1 mL) [1:1000 solution; delivers 0.15 mg per injection; contains sodium bisulfite; two 0.15 mg doses per injector]; 0.3 mg/0.3 mL (1.1 mL) [1:1000 solution; delivers 0.3 mg per injection; contains sodium bisulfite; two 0.3 mg doses per injector]

Injection, solution, as hydrochloride: 0.1 mg/mL (10 mL) [1:10,000 solution]; 1 mg/mL (1 mL) [1:1000 solution]

Adrenalin®: 1 mg/mL (1 mL) [1:1000 solution; contains sodium bisulfite]

Adrenalin®: 1 mg/mL (30 mL) [1:1000 solution; contains chlorobutanol, sodium bisulfite]

Solution for oral inhalation [racepinephrine; preservative free]:

S2®: 2.25% (0.5 mL) [as d-epinephrine 1.125% and l-epinephrine 1.125%]

Solution, intranasal, as hydrochloride [drops, spray]:

Adrenalin®: 1 mg/mL (30 mL) [1:1000 solution; contains sodium bisulfite]

Solution, topical [racepinephrine]:

Raphon: 2.25% (15 mL) [as d-epinephrine 1.125% and l-epinephrine 1.125%; contains benzoic acid, metabisulfites]

◆ **Epinephrine and Lidocaine** *see* Lidocaine and Epinephrine *on page 887*

◆ **Epinephrine Bitartrate** *see* EPINEPHrine *on page 525*

◆ **Epinephrine Hydrochloride** *see* EPINEPHrine *on page 525*

◆ **EpiPen®** *see* EPINEPHrine *on page 525*

◆ **EpiPen® Jr** *see* EPINEPHrine *on page 525*

◆ **Epipodophyllotoxin** *see* Etoposide *on page 591*

◆ **EpiQuin™ Micro** *see* Hydroquinone *on page 749*

Epirubicin (ep i ROO bi sin)

U.S. Brand Names Ellence®

Canadian Brand Names Ellence®; Pharmorubicin®

Index Terms Epirubicin Hydrochloride; NSC-256942; Pidorubicin; Pidorubicin Hydrochloride

Pharmacologic Category Antineoplastic Agent, Anthracycline

Use Adjuvant therapy for primary breast cancer

Pregnancy Risk Factor D

Pregnancy Considerations Teratogenic effects and embryotoxicity were noted in animal studies. There are no adequate and well-controlled studies in pregnant women. If a pregnant woman is treated with epirubicin, or if a woman becomes pregnant while receiving this drug, she should be informed of the potential hazard to the fetus. Women of childbearing potential should be advised to avoid becoming pregnant. Men undergoing treatment should use effective contraception.

Lactation Excretion in breast milk unknown/contraindicated

Medication Safety Issues

Sound-alike/look-alike issues:

Epirubicin may be confused with DOXOrubicin, DAUNOrubicin, idarubicin

Ellence® may be confused with Elase®

High alert medication: The Institute for Safe Medication Practices (ISMP) includes this medication among its list of drugs which have a heightened risk of causing significant patient harm when used in error.

Contraindications Hypersensitivity to epirubicin or any component of the formulation, other anthracyclines, or anthracenediones; previous anthracycline treatment up to maximum cumulative dose; severe myocardial insufficiency, severe arrhythmias; recent myocardial infarction; severe hepatic dysfunction; baseline neutrophil count 1500 cells/mm^3; pregnancy

Warnings/Precautions Hazardous agent - use appropriate precautions for handling and disposal.

[U.S. Boxed Warning]: Potential cardiotoxicity, particularly in patients who have received prior anthracyclines, prior or concomitant radiotherapy to the mediastinal/pericardial area, or who have pre-existing cardiac disease, may occur. Acute toxicity (primarily arrhythmias) and delayed toxicity (HF) have been described. Delayed toxicity usually develops late in the course of therapy or within 2-3 months after completion, however, events with an onset of several months to years after termination of treatment have been described. The risk of delayed cardiotoxicity increases more steeply with cumulative doses >900 mg/m^2, and this dose should be exceeded only with extreme caution. (The risk of HF is ~0.9% at a cumulative dose of 550 mg/m^2, ~1.6% at a cumulative dose of 700 mg/m^2, and ~3.3% at a cumulative dose of 900 mg/m^2.) Toxicity may be additive with other anthracyclines or anthracenediones, and may be increased in pediatric patients. Regular monitoring of LVEF and discontinuation at the first sign of impairment is recommended especially in patients with cardiac risk factors or impaired cardiac function.

[U.S. Boxed Warning]: May cause severe myelosuppression; neutropenia is the dose-limiting toxicity; severe thrombocytopenia or anemia may occur. Thrombophlebitis and thromboembolic phenomena (including pulmonary embolism) have occurred.

[U.S. Boxed Warning]: Reduce dosage and use with caution in mild-to-moderate hepatic impairment or in severe renal dysfunction (serum creatinine >5 mg/dL). May cause tumor lysis syndrome. Radiation recall has been reported; epirubicin may have radiosensitizing activity. **[U.S. Boxed Warnings]: Treatment with anthracyclines may increase the risk of secondary leukemias. For I.V. administration only, severe local tissue damage and necrosis will result if extravasation occurs.** Women ≥70 years of age should be especially monitored for toxicity; women of childbearing age should be advised to avoid becoming pregnant. **[U.S. Boxed Warning]: Should be administered under the supervision of an experienced cancer chemotherapy**

physician. Safety and efficacy in children have not been established.

Adverse Reactions Percentages reported as part of combination chemotherapy regimens.

>10%:

Central nervous system: Lethargy (1% to 46%)

Dermatologic: Alopecia (69% to 96%)

Endocrine & metabolic: Amenorrhea (69% to 72%), hot flashes (5% to 39%)

Gastrointestinal: Nausea/vomiting (83% to 92%), mucositis (9% to 59%), diarrhea (7% to 25%)

Hematologic: Leukopenia (50% to 80%; grades 3/4: 2% to 59%), neutropenia (54% to 80%; grades 3/4: 11% to 67%; nadir: 10-14 days; recovery: 21 days), anemia (13% to 72%; grades 3/4: 6%), thrombocytopenia (5% to 49%; grades 3/4: 5%)

Local: Injection site reactions (3% to 20%)

Ocular: Conjunctivitis (1% to 15%)

Miscellaneous: Infection (15% to 21%)

1% to 10%:

Cardiovascular: CHF (0.4% to 1.5%), decreased LVEF (asymptomatic) (1% to 2%); recommended maximum cumulative dose: 900 mg/m^2

Central nervous system: Fever (1% to 5%)

Dermatologic: Rash (1% to 9%), skin changes (1% to 5%)

Gastrointestinal: Anorexia (2% to 3%)

Hematologic: Neutropenic fever (grades 3/4: 6%)

<1%, postmarketing, case reports, and/or frequency not defined: Acute lymphoid leukemia; acute myelogenous leukemia (0.3% at 3 years, 0.5% at 5 years, 0.6% at 8 years); anaphylaxis, atrioventricular block, bradycardia, bundle-branch block, cardiomyopathy, ECG abnormalities, hypersensitivity, myelodysplastic syndrome, photosensitivity, premature menopause, premature ventricular contractions, pulmonary embolism, radiation recall, sinus tachycardia, skin and nail hyperpigmentation, ST-T wave changes (nonspecific), tachyarrhythmias, thromboembolism, thrombophlebitis, transaminases increased, urticaria, ventricular tachycardia

Drug Interactions

Avoid Concomitant Use

Avoid concomitant use of Epirubicin with any of the following: Natalizumab; Vaccines (Live)

Increased Effect/Toxicity

Epirubicin may increase the levels/effects of: Natalizumab; Vaccines (Live)

The levels/effects of Epirubicin may be increased by: Bevacizumab; Taxane Derivatives; Trastuzumab

Decreased Effect

Epirubicin may decrease the levels/effects of: Cardiac Glycosides; Vaccines (Inactivated)

The levels/effects of Epirubicin may be decreased by: Cardiac Glycosides; Echinacea

Ethanol/Nutrition/Herb Interactions

Ethanol: Avoid ethanol (due to GI irritation).

Herb/Nutraceutical: Avoid black cohosh, dong quai in estrogen-dependent tumors.

Stability Store intact vials of solution under refrigeration at 2°C to 8°C (36°F to 46°F). Store intact vials of lyophilized powder at room temperature 15°C to 30°C (59°F to 86°F). Protect from light. Reconstitute lyophilized powder with SWFI to a final concentration of 2 mg/mL. May administer undiluted for IVP or dilute in 50-250 mL NS or D_5W for infusion. Reconstituted solutions and solutions for infusion are stable for 24 hours when stored at 2°C to 8°C (36°F to 46°F).

Mechanism of Action Epirubicin is an anthracycline antibiotic; known to inhibit DNA and RNA synthesis by steric obstruction after intercalating between DNA base pairs; active throughout entire cell cycle. Intercalation triggers DNA cleavage by topoisomerase II, resulting in cytocidal activity. Also inhibits DNA helicase, and generates cytotoxic free radicals.

Pharmacodynamics/Kinetics

Distribution: V_{ss}: 21-27 L/kg

Protein binding: 77% to albumin

Metabolism: Extensively via hepatic and extrahepatic (including RBCs) routes

Half-life elimination: Triphasic; Mean terminal: 33 hours

Excretion: Feces (34% to 35%); urine (20% to 27%)

Dosage Adults: I.V.: 100-120 mg/m^2 once every 3-4 weeks **or** 50-60 mg/m^2 days 1 and 8 every 3-4 weeks

Breast cancer:

CEF-120: 60 mg/m^2 on days 1 and 8 every 28 days for 6 cycles

FEC-100: 100 mg/m^2 on day 1 every 21 days for 6 cycles

Note: Patients receiving 120 mg/m^2/cycle as part of combination therapy should also receive prophylactic therapy with sulfamethoxazole/trimethoprim or a fluoroquinolone.

Dosage modifications:

Delay day 1 dose until platelets are ≥100,000/mm^3, ANC ≥1500/mm^3, and nonhematologic toxicities have recovered to ≤grade 1

Reduce day 1 dose in subsequent cycles to 75% of previous day 1 dose if patient experiences nadir platelet counts <50,000/mm^3, ANC <250/mm^3, neutropenic fever, or grade 3/4 nonhematologic toxicity during the previous cycle

For divided doses (day 1 and day 8), reduce day 8 dose to 75% of day 1 dose if platelet counts are 75,000-100,000/mm^3 and ANC is 1000-1499/mm^3; omit day 8 dose if platelets are <75,000/mm^3, ANC <1000/mm^3, or grade 3/4 nonhematologic toxicity

Dosage adjustment in bone marrow dysfunction: Heavily-treated patients, patients with pre-existing bone marrow depression or neoplastic bone marrow infiltration: Lower starting doses (75-90 mg/mm^2) should be considered.

Elderly: Plasma clearance of epirubicin in elderly female patients was noted to be reduced by 35%. Although no initial dosage reduction is specifically recommended, particular care should be exercised in monitoring toxicity and adjusting subsequent dosage in elderly patients (particularly females >70 years of age).

Dosage adjustment in renal impairment: The FDA-approved labeling recommends that in patients with severe renal impairment (serum creatinine >5 mg/dL), lower doses should be considered. Aronoff (2007) recommends no dosage adjustment needed for Cl_{cr} <50 mL/minute.

Dosage adjustment in hepatic impairment: The FDA-approved labeling recommends the following guidelines (based on clinical trial information):

Bilirubin 1.2-3 mg/dL or AST 2-4 times the upper limit of normal: Administer 50% of recommended starting dose

Bilirubin >3 mg/dL or AST >4 times the upper limit of normal: Administer 25% of recommended starting dose

Severe hepatic impairment: Use is contraindicated

Administration I.V.: Infuse over 15-20 minutes or slow I.V. push (for lower doses [due to dose modification or organ dysfunction]) over 3-10 minutes

Monitoring Parameters Monitor injection site during infusion for possible extravasation or local reactions; CBC with differential and platelet count, liver function tests, renal function, ECG, and left ventricular ejection fraction. Monitor during therapy for potential cardiotoxicity with ECHO or with MUGA scans (patients with higher cumulative doses).

Dosage Forms Excipient information presented when available (limited, particularly for generics); consult specific product labeling.

Injection, powder for reconstitution, as hydrochloride, [preservative free]: 50 mg, 200 mg [contains lactose]

Injection, solution, as hydrochloride [preservative free]: 2 mg/mL (5 mL, 25 mL, 75 mL, 100 mL)
Ellence®: 2 mg/mL (25 mL, 100 mL)

- **Epirubicin Hydrochloride** *see* Epirubicin *on page 528*
- **Epitol®** *see* CarBAMazepine *on page 252*
- **Epival® I.V. (Can)** *see* Valproic Acid and Derivatives *on page 1538*
- **Epivir®** *see* LamiVUDine *on page 848*
- **Epivir-HBV®** *see* LamiVUDine *on page 848*

Eplerenone (e PLER en one)

U.S. Brand Names Inspra™

Pharmacologic Category Diuretic, Potassium-Sparing; Selective Aldosterone Blocker

Use Treatment of hypertension (may be used alone or in combination with other antihypertensive agents); treatment of heart failure (HF) following acute MI

Pregnancy Risk Factor B

Pregnancy Considerations No teratogenic effects were seen in animal studies, however, there are no adequate and well-controlled studies in pregnant women. Use during pregnancy only if the potential benefit to the mother outweighs the possible risk to the fetus.

Lactation Excretion in breast milk unknown/not recommended

Medication Safety Issues

Sound-alike/look-alike issues:

Inspra™ may be confused with Spiriva®

Contraindications Serum potassium >5.5 mEq/L at initiation; Cl_{cr} ≤30 mL/minute; concomitant use of strong CYP3A4 inhibitors (see Drug Interactions for details)

The following additional contraindications apply to patients with hypertension: Type 2 diabetes mellitus (noninsulin dependent, NIDDM) with microalbuminuria; serum creatinine >2.0 mg/dL in males or >1.8 mg/dL in females; Cl_{cr} <50 mL/minute; concomitant use with potassium supplements or potassium-sparing diuretics

Warnings/Precautions Dosage adjustment needed for patients on moderate CYP3A4 inhibitors. Monitor closely for hyperkalemia; increases in serum potassium were dose related during clinical trials and rates of hyperkalemia also increased with declining renal function. Safety and efficacy have not been established in patients with severe hepatic impairment. Use with caution in HF patients post-MI with diabetes (especially if patient has proteinuria); risk of hyperkalemia is increased. Risk of hyperkalemia is increased with declining renal function. Use with caution in patients with mild renal impairment; contraindicated with moderate-severe impairment (HTN: Cl_{cr} <50 mL/minute; other indications: Cl_{cr} ≤30 mL/minute).

Adverse Reactions

>10%: Endocrine & metabolic: Hyperkalemia ([HF post-MI: K >5.5 mEq/L: 16%; K ≥6 mEq/L: 6%] [HTN: K >5.5 mEq/L at doses ≤100 mg: ≤1%; doses >100 mg: 9%]), hypertriglyceridemia (1% to 15%, dose related)

1% to 10%:

Central nervous system: Dizziness (3%), fatigue (2%)
Endocrine & metabolic: Hyponatremia (2%, dose related), breast pain (males <1% to 1%), gynecomastia (males <1% to 1%), hypercholesterolemia (<1% to 1%)
Gastrointestinal: Diarrhea (2%), abdominal pain (1%)
Genitourinary: Abnormal vaginal bleeding (<1% to 2%)
Renal: Creatinine increased (HF post-MI: 6%), albuminuria (1%)
Respiratory: Cough (2%)
Miscellaneous: Flu-like syndrome (2%)

<1%, postmarketing, and/or case reports: Angioneurotic edema, BUN increased, liver function tests increased, rash, uric acid increased

Drug Interactions

Metabolism/Transport Effects Substrate of CYP3A4 (major)

Avoid Concomitant Use

Avoid concomitant use of Eplerenone with any of the following: CYP3A4 Inhibitors (Strong)

Increased Effect/Toxicity

Eplerenone may increase the levels/effects of: ACE Inhibitors; Amifostine; Angiotensin II Receptor Blockers; Potassium Salts; Potassium-Sparing Diuretics; RiTUXimab

The levels/effects of Eplerenone may be increased by: Antifungal Agents (Azole Derivatives, Systemic); Calcium Channel Blockers (Nondihydropyridine); CYP3A4 Inhibitors (Moderate); CYP3A4 Inhibitors (Strong); Dasatinib; Diazoxide; Fluconazole; Herbs (Hypotensive Properties); Macrolide Antibiotics; Prostacyclin Analogues; Protease Inhibitors

Decreased Effect

The levels/effects of Eplerenone may be decreased by: CYP3A4 Inducers (Strong); Deferasirox; Herbs (CYP3A4 Inducers); Herbs (Hypertensive Properties); Methylphenidate; Nonsteroidal Anti-Inflammatory Agents; Yohimbine

Ethanol/Nutrition/Herb Interactions

Food: Grapefruit juice increases eplerenone AUC ~25%.

Herb/Nutraceutical: St John's wort may decrease levels of eplerenone. Avoid black cohosh, California poppy, coleus, golden seal, hawthorn, mistletoe, periwinkle, quinine, shepherd's purse(may have increased antihypertensive effect). Avoid bayberry, blue cohosh, cayenne, ephedra, ginger, ginseng (American), kola, licorice (may diminish the antihypertensive effect).

Stability Store at controlled room temperature of 25°C (77°F).

Mechanism of Action Aldosterone, a mineralocorticoid, increases blood pressure primarily by inducing sodium and water retention. Overexpression of aldosterone is thought to contribute to myocardial fibrosis (especially following myocardial infarction) and vascular fibrosis. Mineralocorticoid receptors are located in the kidney, heart, blood vessels, and brain. Eplerenone selectively blocks mineralocorticoid receptors reducing blood pressure in a dose-dependent manner and appears to prevent myocardial and vascular fibrosis.

Pharmacodynamics/Kinetics

Distribution: V_d: 43-90 L

Protein binding: ~50%; primarily to $alpha_1$-acid glycoproteins

Metabolism: Primarily hepatic via CYP3A4; metabolites inactive

Bioavailability: 69%

Half-life elimination: 4-6 hours

Time to peak, plasma: ~1.5 hours; may take up to 4 weeks for full antihypertensive effect

Excretion: Urine (~67%); feces (32%); <5% as unchanged drug in urine and feces

Dosage Oral: Adults:

Hypertension: Initial: 50 mg once daily; may increase to 50 mg twice daily if response is not adequate; may take up to 4 weeks for full therapeutic response. Doses >100 mg/day are associated with increased risk of hyperkalemia and no greater therapeutic effect.

Concurrent use with moderate CYP3A4 inhibitors: Initial: 25 mg once daily

Heart failure (post-MI): Initial: 25 mg once daily; dosage goal: Titrate to 50 mg once daily within 4 weeks, as tolerated

Dosage adjustment per serum potassium concentrations for HF (post-MI):

<5.0 mEq/L:

Increase dose from 25 mg every other day to 25 mg daily **or**

Increase dose from 25 mg daily to 50 mg daily

5.0-5.4 mEq/L: No adjustment needed

5.5-5.9 mEq/L:

Decrease dose from 50 mg daily to 25 mg daily **or**

Decrease dose from 25 mg daily to 25 mg every other day **or**

Decrease dose from 25 mg every other day to withhold medication

≥6.0 mEq/L: Withhold medication until potassium <5.5 mEq/L, then restart at 25 mg every other day

Dosage adjustment in renal impairment:

Hypertension: Cl_{cr} <50 mL/minute or serum creatinine >2.0 mg/dL in males or >1.8 mg/dL in females: Use is contraindicated; risk of hyperkalemia increases with declining renal function

All other indications: Cl_{cr} ≤30 mL/minute: Use is contraindicated.

Dosage adjustment in hepatic impairment: No dosage adjustment needed for mild-to-moderate impairment; safety and efficacy not established for severe impairment

Dietary Considerations May be taken with or without food. Do not use salt substitutes containing potassium.

Administration May be administered with or without food.

Monitoring Parameters Blood pressure; serum potassium (levels monitored prior to therapy, within the first week, and at 1 month after start of treatment or dose adjustment, then periodically [monthly in clinical trials]); renal function

Dosage Forms Excipient information presented when available (limited, particularly for generics); consult specific product labeling.

Tablet: 25 mg, 50 mg

Inspra™: 25 mg, 50 mg

◆ **EPO** *see* Epoetin Alfa *on page* 531

Epoetin Alfa (e POE e tin AL fa)

U.S. Brand Names Epogen®; Procrit®

Canadian Brand Names Eprex®

Index Terms *r*HuEPO-α; EPO; Erythropoiesis-Stimulating Agent (ESA); Erythropoietin; NSC-724223

Pharmacologic Category Colony Stimulating Factor

Use Treatment of anemia (elevate/maintain red blood cell level and decrease the need for transfusions) associated with HIV (zidovudine) therapy, chronic renal failure (including patients on dialysis and not on dialysis); reduction of allogeneic blood transfusion for elective, noncardiac, nonvascular surgery; treatment of anemia due to concurrent chemotherapy in patients with metastatic cancer (nonmyeloid malignancies)

Note: Erythropoietin is **not** indicated for use in cancer patients under the following conditions:

- receiving hormonal therapy, therapeutic biologic products, or radiation therapy unless also receiving concurrent myelosuppressive chemotherapy
- receiving myelosuppressive therapy when the expected outcome is curative
- anemia due to other factors (eg, iron deficiency, folate deficiency, or gastrointestinal bleed)

Unlabeled/Investigational Use Treatment of anemia associated with critical illness; anemia of prematurity; symptomatic anemia in myelodysplastic syndrome (MDS)

Restrictions An FDA-approved medication guide is available; distribute to each patient to whom this medication is dispensed.

Pregnancy Risk Factor C

Pregnancy Considerations Epoetin alfa has been shown to have adverse effects (decreased weight gain, delayed development, delayed ossification) in animal studies. Studies suggest that *r*HuEPO-α does not cross the human placenta. Based on case reports, treatment with *r*HuEPO-α may be an option in pregnant women with ESRD on dialysis. Amenorrheic premenopausal women should be cautioned that menstruation may resume following treatment with *r*HuEPO-α and contraception should be considered if pregnancy is to be avoided.

Lactation Excretion in breast milk unknown/use caution

Medication Safety Issues

Sound-alike/look-alike issues:

Epoetin alfa may be confused with darbepoetin alfa, epoetin beta

Epogen® may be confused with Neupogen®

International issues:

Epopen® [Spain] may be confused with EpiPen® which is a brand name for epinephrine in the U.S.

Contraindications Hypersensitivity to albumin (human) or mammalian cell-derived products; uncontrolled hypertension

Warnings/Precautions [U.S. Boxed Warning]: ESAs increased the risk of serious cardiovascular events, thromboembolic events, mortality, and/or tumor progression in clinical studies; a rapid rise in hemoglobin (>1 g/dL over 2 weeks) or maintaining higher hemoglobin levels may contribute to these risks. **[U.S. Boxed Warning]: A shortened overall survival and/or increased risk of tumor progression or recurrence has been reported in studies with breast, cervical, head and neck, lymphoid, and non small cell lung cancer patients.** It is of note that in these studies, patients received ESAs to a target hemoglobin of ≥12 g/dL; although risk has not been excluded when dosed to achieve a target hemoglobin of <12 g/dL. **[U.S. Boxed Warnings]: To decrease these risks, and risk of cardio- and thrombovascular events, use the lowest dose needed to avoid red blood cell transfusions. Use ESAs in cancer patients only for the treatment of anemia related to concurrent chemotherapy; discontinue ESA following completion of the chemotherapy course. ESAs are not indicated for patients receiving myelosuppressive therapy when the anticipated outcome is curative. [U.S. Boxed Warning]: An increased risk of death and serious cardiovascular events was reported in chronic renal failure patients administered ESAs to target higher versus lower hemoglobin levels (13.5 vs 11.3 g/dL; 14 vs 10 g/dL) in two clinical studies; dosing should be individualized to achieve and maintain hemoglobin levels within 10-12 g/dL range.** Hemoglobin rising >1 g/dL in a 2-week period may contribute to the risk. Chronic renal failure patients who exhibit an inadequate hemoglobin response to ESA therapy may be at a higher risk for cardiovascular events and mortality compared to other patients. ESA therapy may reduce dialysis efficacy (due to increase in red blood cells and decrease in plasma volume); adjustments in dialysis parameters may be needed. Patients treated with epoetin may require increased heparinization during dialysis to prevent clotting of the artificial kidney. **[U.S. Boxed Warning]: Epoetin alfa increased the rate of DVT in perisurgery patients not receiving anticoagulant prophylaxis; consider DVT prophylaxis.** Increased mortality was also observed in patients undergoing coronary artery bypass surgery who received epoetin alfa; these deaths were associated with thrombotic events. Epoetin is not approved for reduction of red blood cell transfusion in patients undergoing cardiac or vascular surgery. During therapy in any patient, hemoglobin levels should not exceed a target range of 10-12 g/dL and should not rise >1 g/dL per 2-week time period.

Use with caution in patients with hypertension or with a history of seizures; hypertensive encephalopathy and seizures have been reported. If hypertension is difficult to control, reduce or hold epoetin alfa. An excessive rate of rise of hemoglobin is associated with hypertension or exacerbation of hypertension; decrease the epoetin dose if the hemoglobin increase exceeds 1 g/dL in any 2-week period. Blood pressure should be controlled prior to start of therapy and monitored closely throughout treatment. **Not** recommended for acute correction of severe anemia or as a substitute for transfusion.

Prior to treatment, correct or exclude deficiencies of iron, vitamin B_{12}, and/or folate, as well as other factors which may impair erythropoiesis (aluminum toxicity, inflammatory conditions, infections). Prior to and periodically during therapy, iron stores must be evaluated. Supplemental iron is recommended if serum ferritin <100 mcg/L or serum transferrin saturation <20%. Poor response should prompt evaluation of these potential factors, as well as possible malignant processes, occult blood loss, hemolysis, and/or bone marrow fibrosis. Severe anemia and pure red cell aplasia (PRCA) with associated neutralizing antibodies to erythropoietin has been reported, predominantly in patients with CRF receiving SubQ epoetin (the I.V. route is preferred for hemodialysis patients). Patients with loss of response to epoetin alfa should be evaluated; discontinue treatment in patients with PRCA secondary to neutralizing antibodies to epoetin. Antibodies may cross-react; do not switch to another ESA in patients who develop antibody-mediated anemia.

Due to the delayed onset of erythropoiesis, epoetin is of no value in the acute treatment of anemia. Safety and efficacy in patients with underlying hematologic diseases have not been established, including hypercoagulation disorders and sickle cell disease. Potentially serious allergic reactions have been reported. Use caution with porphyria, exacerbation of porphyria has been reported (rarely) in patients with chronic renal failure. Some products may contain albumin. Multidose vials contain benzyl alcohol; do not use in premature infants. Safety and efficacy in children <1 month of age have not been established.

Adverse Reactions

>10%:

Cardiovascular: Hypertension (5% to 24%), thrombotic/vascular events (coronary artery bypass graft surgery: 23%), edema (6% to 17%), deep vein thrombosis (3% to 11%)

Central nervous system: Fever (29% to 51%), dizziness (<7% to 21%), insomnia (13% to 21%), headache (10% to 19%)

Dermatologic: Pruritus (14% to 22%), skin pain (4% to 18%), rash (≤16%)

Gastrointestinal: Nausea (11% to 58%), constipation (42% to 53%), vomiting (8% to 29%), diarrhea (9% to 21%), dyspepsia (7% to 11%)

Genitourinary: Urinary tract infection (3% to 12%)

Local: Injection site reaction (<10% to 29%)

Neuromuscular & skeletal: Arthralgia (11%), paresthesia (11%)

Respiratory: Cough (18%), congestion (15%), dyspnea (13% to 14%), upper respiratory infection (11%)

1% to 10%:

Central nervous system: Seizure (1% to 3%)

Local: Clotted vascular access (7%)

<1% (Limited to important or life-threatening): Allergic reaction, anemia (severe; with or without other cytopenias), CVA, flu-like syndrome, hyperkalemia, hypersensitivity reactions, hypertensive encephalopathy, microvascular thrombosis, MI, myalgia, neutralizing antibodies, pulmonary embolism, pure red cell aplasia (PRCA), renal vein thrombosis, retinal artery thrombosis, tachycardia, temporal vein thrombosis, thrombophlebitis, thrombosis, TIA, urticaria

Drug Interactions

Avoid Concomitant Use There are no known interactions where it is recommended to avoid concomitant use.

Increased Effect/Toxicity There are no known significant interactions involving an increase in effect.

Decreased Effect There are no known significant interactions involving a decrease in effect.

Stability

Vials should be stored at 2°C to 8°C (36°F to 46°F); **do not freeze or shake**. Protect from light.

Single-dose 1 mL vial contains no preservative: Use one dose per vial. Do not re-enter vial; discard unused portions.

Single-dose vials (except 40,000 units/mL vial) are stable for 2 weeks at room temperature. Single-dose 40,000 units/mL vial is stable for 1 week at room temperature.

Multidose 1 mL or 2 mL vial contains preservative. Store at 2°C to 8°C after initial entry and between doses. Discard 21 days after initial entry.

Multidose vials (with preservative) are stable for 1 week at room temperature.

Prefilled syringes containing the 20,000 units/mL formulation with preservative are stable for 6 weeks refrigerated (2°C to 8°C).

Dilutions of 1:10 and 1:20 (1 part epoetin:19 parts sodium chloride) are stable for 18 hours at room temperature.

Prior to SubQ administration, preservative free solutions may be mixed with bacteriostatic NS containing benzyl alcohol 0.9% in a 1:1 ratio. Dilutions of 1:10 in $D_{10}W$ with human albumin 0.05% or 0.1% are stable for 24 hours.

Mechanism of Action Induces erythropoiesis by stimulating the division and differentiation of committed erythroid progenitor cells; induces the release of reticulocytes from the bone marrow into the bloodstream, where they mature to erythrocytes. There is a dose response relationship with this effect. This results in an increase in reticulocyte counts followed by a rise in hematocrit and hemoglobin levels.

Pharmacodynamics/Kinetics

Onset of action: Several days

Peak effect: 2-3 weeks

Distribution: V_d: 9 L; rapid in the plasma compartment; concentrated in liver, kidneys, and bone marrow

Metabolism: Some degradation does occur

Bioavailability: SubQ: ~21% to 31%; intraperitoneal epoetin: 3% (a few patients)

Half-life elimination: Cancer: SubQ: 16-67 hours; Chronic renal failure: I.V.: 4-13 hours

Time to peak, serum: Chronic renal failure: SubQ: 5-24 hours

Excretion: Feces (majority); urine (small amounts, 10% unchanged in normal volunteers)

Dosage Note: Hemoglobin levels should not exceed 12 g/dL and should not rise >1 g/dL per 2-week time period during therapy in any patient.

Chronic renal failure patients: Individualize dosing to achieve and maintain hemoglobin levels between 10-12 g/dL. Hemoglobin levels should not exceed 12 g/dL. **Note:** I.V. route is preferred for hemodialysis patients.

Children: I.V., SubQ: Initial dose: 50 units/kg 3 times/week

Adults: I.V., SubQ: Initial dose: 50-100 units/kg 3 times/week

Dosage adjustment in Children and Adults: SubQ, I.V.:

Decrease dose by 25%: If hemoglobin approaches 12 g/dL **or** hemoglobin increases >1 g/dL in any 2-week period. If hemoglobin continues to increase, temporarily discontinue therapy until hemoglobin begins to decrease, then resume therapy with a ~25% reduction from previous dose.

Increase dose by 25%: If hemoglobin <10 g/dL and does not increase by 1 g/dL after 4 weeks of therapy (with adequate iron stores) **or** hemoglobin decreases below 10 g/dL. If transferrin saturation >20%, may increase epoetin dose. Do not increase dose more frequently than at 4-week intervals, unless clinically indicated (hemoglobin response time for dose increases may be 2-6 weeks).

Inadequate or lack of response: If patient does not attain target hemoglobin range of 10-12 g/dL after appropriate dose titrations over 12 weeks:

Do not continue to increase dose and use the minimum effective dose that will maintain a hemoglobin level sufficient to avoid red blood cell transfusions **and** evaluate patient for other causes of anemia.

Monitor hemoglobin closely thereafter, and if responsiveness improves, may resume making dosage adjustments as recommended above. If responsiveness does not improve and recurrent red blood cell transfusions continue to be needed, discontinue therapy.

Maintenance dose: Individualize to target hemoglobin range of 10-12 g/dL; limit additional dosage increases to every 4 weeks (or longer)

Dialysis patients: Median dose:

Children: 167 units/kg/week (hemodialysis) **or** 76 units/kg/week (peritoneal dialysis), in 2-3 divided doses per week

Adults: 75 units/kg 3 times/week

Nondialysis patients:

Children: Dosing range: 50-250 units/kg 1-3 times/week

Adults: Dosing range: 75-150 units/kg/week

Zidovudine-treated, HIV-infected patients (patients with erythropoietin levels >500 mU/mL are **unlikely** to respond): Titrate dosage to use the minimum effective dose that will maintain a hemoglobin level sufficient to avoid red blood cell transfusions. Hemoglobin levels should not exceed 12 g/dL.

Children: SubQ, I.V.: Limited data available; reported dosing range: 50-400 units/kg 2-3 times/week

Adults (with serum erythropoietin levels ≤500 and zidovudine doses ≤4200 mg/week): SubQ, I.V.: 100 units/kg 3 times/week for 8 weeks

Dosage adjustment:

Increase dose by 50-100 units/kg 3 times/week: If response is not satisfactory in terms of reducing transfusion requirements **or** increasing hemoglobin after 8 weeks of therapy. Evaluate response every 4-8 weeks thereafter, and adjust the dose accordingly by 50-100 units/kg increments 3 times/week. If patients has not responded satisfactorily to 300 units/kg/dose 3 times/week, a response to higher doses is unlikely.

Withhold dose: If hemoglobin exceeds 12 g/dL. Resume treatment with a 25% dose reduction when hemoglobin drops below 11 g/dL

Cancer patient on chemotherapy: Treatment of patients with erythropoietin levels >200 mU/mL is **not recommended by the manufacturer.** Titrate dosage to use the minimum effective dose that will maintain a hemoglobin level sufficient to avoid red blood cell transfusions. Do not initiate therapy if hemoglobin ≥10 g/dL. Discontinue erythropoietin following completion of chemotherapy.

Children: I.V.: 600 units/kg once weekly (maximum: 40,000 units)

Dosage adjustment:

Increase dose: If response is not satisfactory after a sufficient period of evaluation (no increase in hemoglobin by ≥1 g/dL after 4 weeks of once-weekly therapy), the dose may be increased every 4 weeks (or longer) to 900 units/kg/week; maximum 60,000 units. If patient does not respond, a response to higher doses is unlikely.

Withhold dose: If hemoglobin exceeds a level needed to avoid red blood cell transfusion. Resume treatment with a 25% dose reduction when hemoglobin approaches a level where transfusions may be required.

Reduce dose by 25%: If hemoglobin increases >1 g/dL in any 2-week period **or** hemoglobin reaches a level sufficient to avoid red blood cell transfusion.

Discontinue: If after 8 weeks of therapy there is no response (ie, increased hemoglobin levels) or transfusions still required.

Adults: SubQ: Initial dose: 150 units/kg 3 times/week or 40,000 units once weekly; commonly used doses range from 10,000 units 3 times/week to 40,000-60,000 units once weekly.

Dosage adjustment:

Increase dose: If response is not satisfactory after a sufficient period of evaluation (no reduction in transfusion requirements or increase in hemoglobin after 8 weeks of 3 times/week therapy) **or** (no increase in hemoglobin by ≥1 g/dL after 4 weeks of once-weekly therapy), the dose may be increased every 4 weeks (or longer) to 300 units/kg 3 times/week, **or** when dosed weekly, increased all at once to 60,000 units weekly. If patient does not respond, a response to higher doses is unlikely.

Withhold dose: If hemoglobin exceeds a level needed to avoid red blood cell transfusion. Resume treatment with a 25% dose reduction when hemoglobin approaches a level where transfusions may be required.

Reduce dose by 25%: If hemoglobin increases >1 g/dL in any 2-week period **or** hemoglobin reaches a level sufficient to avoid red blood cell transfusion.

Discontinue: If after 8 weeks of therapy there is no response (ie, increased hemoglobin levels) or transfusions still required.

Surgery patients: Prior to initiating treatment, obtain a hemoglobin to establish that it is >10 g/dL and ≤13 g/dL:

Adults: SubQ: Initial dose: 300 units/kg/day for 10 days before surgery, on the day of surgery, and for 4 days after surgery

Alternative dose: 600 units/kg in once weekly doses (21, 14, and 7 days before surgery) plus a fourth dose on the day of surgery

Anemia of critical illness (unlabeled use): Adults: SubQ: 40,000 units once weekly

Symptomatic anemia associated with MDS (unlabeled use): Adults: SubQ: 40,000-60,000 units 1-3 times/week

Anemia of prematurity (unlabeled use): Infants: I.V., SubQ: Dosing range: 500-1250 units/kg/week; commonly used dose: 250 units/kg 3 times/week; supplement with oral iron therapy 3-8 mg/kg/day

Dosage adjustment in renal impairment: The National Kidney Foundation Clinical Practice Guideline for Anemia in Chronic Kidney Disease: 2007 Update of Hemoglobin Target (September, 2007) recommend hemoglobin levels in the range of 11-12 g/dL for dialysis and nondialysis patients receiving ESAs; hemoglobin levels should not be >13 g/dL.

Hemodialysis: Supplemental dose is not necessary. I.V. route is preferred for hemodialysis patients.

Peritoneal dialysis: Supplemental dose is not necessary.

Administration SubQ, I.V.:

Patients with CRF on dialysis: I.V. route preferred; may be administered I.V. bolus into the venous line after dialysis.

Patients with CRF not on dialysis: May be administered I.V. or SubQ

Monitoring Parameters Blood pressure; hemoglobin, CBC with differential and platelets, transferrin saturation and ferritin, serum chemistry (CRF patients)

Suggested tests to be monitored and their frequency: See table.

Test	Initial Phase Frequency	Maintenance Phase Frequency
Hemoglobin	1-2 x/week	2-4 x/month
Blood pressure	3 x/week	3 x/week
Serum ferritin	Monthly	Quarterly
Transferrin saturation	Monthly	Quarterly
Serum chemistries including CBC with differential, creatinine, blood urea nitrogen, potassium, phosphorous	Regularly per routine	Regularly per routine

Reference Range

Zidovudine-treated HIV patients: Available evidence indicates patients with endogenous serum erythropoietin levels >500 mU/mL are unlikely to respond

Cancer chemotherapy patients: Measurement of endogenous serum erythropoietin levels in patients with cancer is generally not recommended (NCCN Cancer- and Chemotherapy-Induced Anemia Guidelines, v2.2009). Treatment of patients with endogenous serum erythropoietin levels >200 mU/mL is not recommended according to the manufacturer.

Additional Information

Factors limiting response to epoetin alfa: Delayed onset of erythropoiesis (2-6 weeks to increase hemoglobin), iron deficiency (most patients require iron supplementation); underlying infection, inflammatory or malignant process; blood loss (occult), underlying hematologic disease (thalassemia, refractory anemia, MDS); vitamin deficiency (folic acid or cyanocobalamin), hemolysis, aluminum overload, osteitis fibrosa cystica, and PRCA

Oncology Comment: The American Society of Hematology (ASH) and American Society of Clinical Oncology (ASCO) 2007 updates to the clinical practice guidelines for the use of erythropoiesis-stimulating agents (ESAs) indicate that ESAs are most appropriate when used according to the dosage parameters within the Food and Drug Administration (FDA) approved labeling for epoetin and darbepoetin (Rizzo, 2008). While the previous guidelines addressed only the use of epoetin, the 2007 guidelines also address the use of darbepoetin, which is assessed as being equivalent to epoetin with respect to safety and efficacy. When used as an option for the treatment of chemotherapy-associated anemia (to increase hemoglobin and decrease red blood cell transfusions), therapy with ESAs should begin as the hemoglobin level approaches or falls below 10 g/dL. The ASH/ASCO guidelines recommend following the FDA approved dosing (and dosing adjustment) guidelines and target hemoglobin ranges as alternate dosing and schedules have not demonstrated consistent differences in effectiveness with regard to hemoglobin response. In patients who do not have a response within 6-8 weeks (hemoglobin rise <1-2 g/dL or no reduction in transfusions) ESA therapy should be discontinued.

The guidelines note that patients with an increased risk of thromboembolism (generally includes previous history of thrombosis, surgery, and/or prolonged periods of immobilization) and patients receiving concomitant medications that may increase thromboembolic risk, should begin ESA therapy only after careful consideration. With the exception of low-risk myelodysplasia-associated anemia (which has evidence supporting the use of ESAs without concurrent chemotherapy), the guidelines do not support the use of ESAs in the absence of concurrent chemotherapy.

Dosage Forms Excipient information presented when available (limited, particularly for generics); consult specific product labeling.

Injection, solution [preservative free]:

Epogen®, Procrit®: 2000 units/mL (1 mL); 3000 units/mL (1 mL); 4000 units/mL (1 mL); 10,000 units/mL (1 mL); 40,000 units/mL (1 mL) [contains human albumin]

Injection, solution [with preservative]:

Epogen®, Procrit®: 10,000 units/mL (2 mL); 20,000 units/mL (1 mL) [contains human albumin and benzyl alcohol]

◆ **Epogen®** *see* Epoetin Alfa *on page* 531

Epoprostenol (e poe PROST en ole)

U.S. Brand Names Flolan®

Canadian Brand Names Flolan®

Index Terms Epoprostenol Sodium; PGI_2; PGX; Prostacyclin

Pharmacologic Category Prostacyclin; Prostaglandin; Vasodilator

Use Treatment of idiopathic pulmonary arterial hypertension (IPAH); pulmonary hypertension associated with the scleroderma spectrum of disease (SSD) in NYHA Class III and Class IV patients who do not respond adequately to conventional therapy

Restrictions Orders for epoprostenol are distributed by two sources in the United States. Information on orders or reimbursement assistance may be obtained from either Accredo Health, Inc (1-800-935-6526) or TheraCom, Inc (1-877-356-5264).

Pregnancy Risk Factor B

Pregnancy Considerations Teratogenic effects were not reported in animal studies. There are no adequate and well-controlled studies in pregnant women. Pregnant women with IPAH are encouraged to avoid pregnancy.

Lactation Excretion in breast milk unknown/use caution

Medication Safety Issues

High alert medication: The Institute for Safe Medication Practices (ISMP) includes this medication among its list of drugs which have a heightened risk of causing significant patient harm when used in error.

Contraindications Hypersensitivity to epoprostenol or to structurally-related compounds; chronic use in patients with heart failure due to severe left ventricular systolic dysfunction; patients who develop pulmonary edema during dose initiation

Warnings/Precautions Abrupt interruptions or large sudden reductions in dosage may result in rebound pulmonary hypertension; some patients with primary pulmonary hypertension have developed pulmonary edema during dose ranging, which may be associated with pulmonary veno-occlusive disease; during chronic use, unless contraindicated, anticoagulants should be coadministered to reduce the risk of thromboembolism. Use cautiously in patients who have conditions that increase bleeding risk (inhibits platelet aggregation). Use with caution in patients receiving anticoagulants and antiplatelet agents. Chronic continuous I.V. infusion of epoprostenol via a chronic indwelling central venous catheter has been associated with local infections and serious blood stream infections. Clinical studies of epoprostenol in pulmonary hypertension did not include sufficient numbers of patients ≥65 years of age to substantiate its safety and efficacy in the geriatric population. As a result, in general, dose selection for an elderly patient should be cautious usually starting at the low end of the dosing range.

Adverse Reactions

Note: Adverse events reported during dose initiation and escalation include flushing (58%), headache (49%), nausea/vomiting (32%), hypotension (16%), anxiety/nervousness/agitation (11%), chest pain (11%), dizziness, abdominal pain, bradycardia, musculoskeletal pain, dyspnea, back pain, diaphoresis, dyspepsia, hypoesthesia/paresthesia, and tachycardia are also reported. The following adverse events have been reported during chronic administration for IPAH. Although some may be related to the underlying disease state, anxiety, diarrhea, flu-like syndrome, flushing, headache, jaw pain, nausea, nervousness, and vomiting are clearly contributed to epoprostenol.

>10%:

Cardiovascular: Chest pain (52% to 67%), palpitation (63%), tachycardia (35% to 43%), flushing (23% to 42%), arrhythmia (27%), bradycardia (15%), hypotension (13%)

Central nervous system: Dizziness (83%), headache (46% to 83%), chills/fever/sepsis/flu-like syndrome (13% to 25%), anxiety/nervousness/tremor (7% to 21%), depression/depression psychotic (13%)

Dermatologic: Skin ulcer (39%), eczema/rash/urticaria (25%)

Gastrointestinal: Nausea/vomiting (41% to 67%), anorexia (66%), diarrhea (37% to 50%), weight loss (27%)

Hematologic: Hemorrhage (11% to 19%)

Hepatic: Ascites (23%)

Local: Injection site reactions: Infection (21%), pain (13%)

Neuromuscular & skeletal: Weakness (87% to 100%), pain/neck pain/arthralgia (84%), jaw pain (54% to 75%), arthritis (52%), myalgia (44%), musculoskeletal pain (35%; predominantly involving legs and feet), back pain (13%), hypoesthesia/hyperparesthesia/paresthesia (5% to 12%)

Respiratory: Dyspnea (90%)

Miscellaneous: Diaphoresis (41%)

1% to 10%:

Cardiovascular: Supraventricular tachycardia (8%), cerebrovascular accident (4%), MI (4%)

Central nervous system: Insomnia (9%), seizure (4%), somnolence (4%)

Dermatologic: Rash (10%), pruritus (4%)

Endocrine & metabolic: Hypokalemia (6%), hyperkalemia (4%)

Gastrointestinal: Abdominal pain (14%), constipation (4% to 6%), weight gain (6%), flatulence (5%), abdominal enlargement (4%)

Genitourinary: Urinary tract infection (7%)

Hematologic: Thrombocytopenia (4%)

Ocular: Amblyopia (8%), vision abnormality (4%)

Renal: Hematuria (5%)

Respiratory: Epistaxis (4% to 9%), pleural effusion (4% to 7%), pharyngitis (5%), pneumonia (5%), pneumothorax (4%), pulmonary edema (4%)

<1% (Limited to important or life-threatening): Anemia, hepatic failure, hypersplenism, hyperthyroidism, pancytopenia, pulmonary embolism, splenomegaly

Drug Interactions

Avoid Concomitant Use There are no known interactions where it is recommended to avoid concomitant use.

Increased Effect/Toxicity

Epoprostenol may increase the levels/effects of: Anticoagulants; Antihypertensives; Antiplatelet Agents

Decreased Effect There are no known significant interactions involving a decrease in effect.

Stability Prior to use, store vials at 15°C to 25°C (59°F to 77°F); do not freeze. Protect from light. Reconstitute only with provided sterile diluent. Following reconstitution, solution must be stored under refrigeration at 2°C to 8°C (36°F to 46°F) if not used immediately; do not freeze. Protect from light. Discard if refrigerated for >48 hours. See table. During use, a single reservoir of solution may be used at room temperature for a total duration of 8 hours, or used with a cold pouch for administration up to 24 hours. Cold packs should be changed every 12 hours.

Preparation of Epoprostenol Infusion

Note: Only prepare with sterile diluent provided.

To make 100 mL of solution with concentration:	Directions
3000 ng/mL	Dissolve one 0.5 mg vial with 5 mL supplied diluent, withdraw 3 mL, and add to a sufficient volume of supplied diluent to make a total of 100 mL.
5000 ng/mL	Dissolve one 0.5 mg vial with 5 mL supplied diluent, withdraw entire vial contents, and add to a sufficient volume of supplied diluent to make a total of 100 mL.
10,000 ng/mL	Dissolve two 0.5 mg vials each with 5 mL supplied diluent, withdraw entire vial contents, and add to a sufficient volume of supplied diluent to make a total of 100 mL.
15,000 ng/mL	Dissolve one 1.5 mg vial with 5 mL supplied diluent, withdraw entire vial contents, and add to a sufficient volume of supplied diluent to make a total of 100 mL.

Mechanism of Action Epoprostenol is also known as prostacyclin and PGI_2. It is a strong vasodilator of all vascular beds. In addition, it is a potent endogenous inhibitor of platelet aggregation. The reduction in platelet aggregation results from epoprostenol's activation of intracellular adenylate cyclase and the resultant increase in cyclic adenosine monophosphate concentrations within the platelets. Additionally, it is capable of decreasing thrombogenesis and platelet clumping in the lungs by inhibiting platelet aggregation.

Pharmacodynamics/Kinetics

Metabolism: Rapidly hydrolyzed; subject to some enzymatic degradation; forms one active metabolite and 13 inactive metabolites

Half-life elimination: 6 minutes

Excretion: Urine (84%); feces (4%)

Dosage Children (unlabeled use) and Adults: I.V.: Initial: 1-2 ng/kg/minute, increase dose in increments of 1-2 ng/kg/minute every 15 minutes or longer until dose-limiting side effects are noted or tolerance limit to epoprostenol is observed. Significant patient variability in optimal dose exists. Maximum dose with chronic therapy has not been defined; however, doses as high as 195 ng/kg/minute have been described in children (Rosenzweig, 1999).

Note: The need for increased doses should be expected with chronic use; incremental increases occur more frequently during the first few months after the drug is initiated.

Dose adjustment:

Increase dose in 1-2 ng/kg/minute increments at intervals of at least 15 minutes if symptoms persist or recur following improvement. In clinical trials, dosing increases occurred at intervals of 24-48 hours.

Decrease dose in 2 ng/kg/minute decrements at intervals of at least 15 minutes in case of dose-limiting pharmacologic events. Avoid abrupt withdrawal or sudden large dose reductions.

Lung transplant: In patients receiving lung transplants, epoprostenol may be tapered after the initiation of cardiopulmonary bypass.

Administration The ambulatory infusion pump should be small and lightweight, be able to adjust infusion rates in 2 ng/kg/minute increments, have occlusion, end of infusion, and low battery alarms, have ± 6% accuracy of the programmed rate, and have positive continuous or pulsatile pressure with intervals ≤3 minutes between pulses. The reservoir should be made of polyvinyl chloride, polypropylene, or glass. The infusion pump used in the most recent clinical trial was CADD-1 HFX 5100 (Pharmacia Deltec). Immediate access to back up pump, infusion sets and medication is essential to prevent treatment interruptions. Assess patient's and family's ability to manage a central venous catheter in the home setting. Clinicians should routinely review with patient the importance of infection control practices for the management of a central venous catheter.

Monitoring Parameters Monitor for improvements in pulmonary function, decreased exertional dyspnea, fatigue, syncope and chest pain, pulmonary vascular resistance, pulmonary arterial pressure and quality of life. In addition, the pump device and catheters should be monitored frequently to avoid "system" related failure. Monitor arterial pressure; assess all vital functions. Hypoxia, flushing, and tachycardia may indicate overdose.

Dosage Forms Excipient information presented when available (limited, particularly for generics); consult specific product labeling.

Injection, powder for reconstitution: 0.5 mg, 1.5 mg [provided with 50 mL sterile diluent]

Flolan®: 0.5 mg, 1.5 mg

◆ **Epoprostenol Sodium** *see* Epoprostenol *on page 534*

◆ **Eprex® (Can)** *see* Epoetin Alfa *on page 531*

Eprosartan (ep roe SAR tan)

U.S. Brand Names Teveten®

Canadian Brand Names Teveten®

Pharmacologic Category Angiotensin II Receptor Blocker

Additional Appendix Information

Angiotensin Agents *on page 1632*

Use Treatment of hypertension; may be used alone or in combination with other antihypertensives

Pregnancy Risk Factor C (1st trimester); D (2nd and 3rd trimesters)

Pregnancy Considerations Medications which act on the renin-angiotensin system are reported to have the following fetal/neonatal effects: Hypotension, neonatal skull hypoplasia, anuria, renal failure, and death; oligohydramnios is also reported. These effects are reported to occur with exposure during the second and third trimesters. There are no adequate and well-controlled studies in pregnant women. **[U.S. Boxed Warning]: Based on human data, drugs that act on the angiotensin system can cause injury and death to the developing fetus when used in the second and third trimesters. Angiotensin receptor blockers should be discontinued as soon as possible once pregnancy is detected.**

Lactation Not recommended

Contraindications Hypersensitivity to eprosartan or any component of the formulation

Warnings/Precautions [U.S. Boxed Warning]: Based on human data, drugs that act on the angiotensin system can cause injury and death to the developing fetus when used in the second and third trimesters. Angiotensin receptor blockers should be discontinued as soon as possible once pregnancy is detected. May cause hyperkalemia; avoid potassium supplementation unless specifically required by healthcare provider. Avoid use or use a smaller dose in patients who are volume depleted; correct depletion first. May be associated with deterioration of renal function and/or increases in serum creatinine, particularly in patients with low renal blood flow (eg, renal artery stenosis, heart failure) whose glomerular filtration rate (GFR) is dependent on efferent arteriolar vasoconstriction by angiotensin II. Use with caution in unstented unilateral/bilateral renal artery stenosis. When unstented bilateral renal artery stenosis is present, use is generally avoided due to the elevated risk of deterioration in renal function unless possible benefits outweigh risks. Use with caution with pre-existing renal insufficiency; significant aortic/mitral stenosis. Safety and efficacy not established in pediatric patients.

Adverse Reactions

1% to 10%:

Central nervous system: Fatigue (2%), depression (1%)

Endocrine & metabolic: Hypertriglyceridemia (1%)

Gastrointestinal: Abdominal pain (2%)

Genitourinary: Urinary tract infection (1%)

Respiratory: Upper respiratory tract infection (8%), rhinitis (4%), pharyngitis (4%), cough (4%)

Miscellaneous: Viral infection (2%), injury (2%)

<1% (Limited to important or life-threatening): Abnormal ECG, angina, arthritis, asthma, ataxia, bradycardia, BUN increased, creatinine increased, eczema, edema, esophagitis, ethanol intolerance, gingivitis, gout, hypotension, influenza-like symptoms, leg cramps, leukopenia, maculopapular rash, migraine, neuritis, neutropenia, orthostasis, palpitation, paresthesia, peripheral ischemia, purpura, renal calculus, somnolence, tachycardia, tendonitis, thrombocytopenia, tinnitus, tremor, urinary incontinence, vertigo; rhabdomyolysis has been reported (rarely) with angiotensin-receptor antagonists.

Drug Interactions

Metabolism/Transport Effects Inhibits CYP2C9 (weak)

Avoid Concomitant Use There are no known interactions where it is recommended to avoid concomitant use.

Increased Effect/Toxicity

Eprosartan may increase the levels/effects of: ACE Inhibitors; Amifostine; Lithium; Potassium-Sparing Diuretics; RiTUXimab

The levels/effects of Eprosartan may be increased by: Diazoxide; Eplerenone; Herbs (Hypotensive Properties); Potassium Salts; Prostacyclin Analogues; Trimethoprim

Decreased Effect

The levels/effects of Eprosartan may be decreased by: Herbs (Hypertensive Properties); Methylphenidate; Nonsteroidal Anti-Inflammatory Agents; Yohimbine

Ethanol/Nutrition/Herb Interactions Herb/Nutraceutical: Avoid dong quai if using for hypertension (has estrogenic activity). Avoid ephedra, yohimbe, ginseng (may worsen hypertension). Avoid garlic (may have increased antihypertensive effect).

Mechanism of Action Angiotensin II is formed from angiotensin I in a reaction catalyzed by angiotensin-converting enzyme (ACE, kininase II). Angiotensin II is the principal pressor agent of the renin-angiotensin system, with effects that include vasoconstriction, stimulation of synthesis and release of aldosterone, cardiac stimulation, and renal reabsorption of sodium. Eprosartan blocks the vasoconstrictor and aldosterone-secreting effects of angiotensin II by selectively blocking the binding of angiotensin II to the AT1 receptor in many tissues, such as vascular smooth muscle and the adrenal gland. Its action is therefore independent of the pathways for angiotensin II synthesis. Blockade of the renin-angiotensin system with ACE inhibitors, which inhibit the biosynthesis of angiotensin II from angiotensin I, is widely used in the treatment of hypertension. ACE inhibitors also inhibit the degradation of bradykinin, a reaction also catalyzed by ACE. Because eprosartan does not inhibit ACE (kininase II), it does not affect the response to bradykinin. Whether this difference has clinical relevance is not yet known. Eprosartan does not bind to or block other hormone receptors or ion channels known to be important in cardiovascular regulation.

Pharmacodynamics/Kinetics

Protein binding: 98%

Metabolism: Minimally hepatic

Bioavailability: 300 mg dose: 13%

Half-life elimination: Terminal: 5-9 hours

Time to peak, serum: Fasting: 1-2 hours
Excretion: Feces (90%); urine (7%, mostly as unchanged drug)
Clearance: 7.9 L/hour

Dosage Adults: Oral: Dosage must be individualized; can administer once or twice daily with total daily doses of 400-800 mg. Usual starting dose is 600 mg once daily as monotherapy in patients who are euvolemic. Limited clinical experience with doses >800 mg.

Dosage adjustment in renal impairment: No starting dosage adjustment is necessary; however, carefully monitor the patient

Dosage adjustment in hepatic impairment: No starting dosage adjustment is necessary; however, carefully monitor the patient

Elderly: No starting dosage adjustment is necessary; however, carefully monitor the patient

Dosage Forms Excipient information presented when available (limited, particularly for generics); consult specific product labeling.

Tablet: 400 mg, 600 mg

Eprosartan and Hydrochlorothiazide

(ep roe SAR tan & hye droe klor oh THYE a zide)

U.S. Brand Names Teveten® HCT

Canadian Brand Names Teveten® HCT; Teveten® Plus

Index Terms Eprosartan Mesylate and Hydrochlorothiazide; Hydrochlorothiazide and Eprosartan

Pharmacologic Category Angiotensin II Receptor Blocker; Diuretic, Thiazide

Use Treatment of hypertension (not indicated for initial treatment)

Pregnancy Risk Factor C/D (2nd and 3rd trimesters)

Dosage Oral: Adults: Dose is individualized (combination substituted for individual components)

Usual recommended dose: Eprosartan 600 mg/hydrochlorothiazide 12.5 mg once daily (maximum dose: Eprosartan 600 mg/hydrochlorothiazide 25 mg once daily)

Dosage adjustment in renal impairment: Initial dose adjustments not recommended by manufacturer; carefully monitor patient. Hydrochlorothiazide is ineffective in patients with Cl_{cr} <30 mL/minute.

Dosage adjustment in hepatic impairment: Initial dose adjustments not recommended by manufacturer; carefully monitor patient.

Additional Information Complete prescribing information for this medication should be consulted for additional detail.

Dosage Forms Excipient information presented when available (limited, particularly for generics); consult specific product labeling.

Tablet:

600 mg/12.5 mg: Eprosartan 600 mg and hydrochlorothiazide 12.5 mg

600 mg/25 mg: Eprosartan 600 mg and hydrochlorothiazide 25 mg

◆ **Eprosartan Mesylate and Hydrochlorothiazide** *see* Eprosartan and Hydrochlorothiazide *on page 537*

◆ **Epsilon Aminocaproic Acid** *see* Aminocaproic Acid *on page 85*

◆ **Epsom Salts** *see* Magnesium Sulfate *on page 917*

◆ **EPT** *see* Teniposide *on page 1438*

◆ **Eptacog Alfa (Activated)** *see* Factor VIIa (Recombinant) *on page 598*

Eptifibatide (ep TIF i ba tide)

U.S. Brand Names Integrilin®

Canadian Brand Names Integrilin®

Index Terms Intrifiban

Pharmacologic Category Antiplatelet Agent, Glycoprotein IIb/IIIa Inhibitor

Additional Appendix Information

Glycoprotein Antagonists *on page 1656*

Use Treatment of patients with acute coronary syndrome (unstable angina/non-Q wave myocardial infarction [UA/NQMI]), including patients who are to be managed medically and those undergoing percutaneous coronary intervention (PCI including angioplasty, intracoronary stenting)

Pregnancy Risk Factor B

Pregnancy Considerations Teratogenic effects were not observed in animal studies.

Lactation Excretion in breast milk unknown/use caution

Medication Safety Issues

High alert medication: The Institute for Safe Medication Practices (ISMP) includes this medication among its list of drugs which have a heightened risk of causing significant patient harm when used in error.

Contraindications Hypersensitivity to eptifibatide or any component of the product; active abnormal bleeding or a history of bleeding diathesis within the previous 30 days; history of CVA within 30 days or a history of hemorrhagic stroke; severe hypertension (systolic blood pressure >200 mm Hg or diastolic blood pressure >110 mm Hg) not adequately controlled on antihypertensive therapy; major surgery within the preceding 6 weeks; current or planned administration of another parenteral GP IIb/IIIa inhibitor; thrombocytopenia; dependency on renal dialysis

Warnings/Precautions Bleeding is the most common complication. Most major bleeding occurs at the arterial access site where the cardiac catheterization was done. When bleeding can not be controlled with pressure, discontinue infusion and heparin. Use caution in patients with hemorrhagic retinopathy or with other drugs that affect hemostasis. Concurrent use with thrombolytics has not been established as safe. Minimize other procedures including arterial and venous punctures, I.M. injections, nasogastric tubes, etc. Prior to sheath removal, the aPTT or ACT should be checked (do not remove unless aPTT is <45 seconds or the ACT <150 seconds). Use caution in renal dysfunction (estimated Cl_{cr} <50 mL/minute); dosage adjustment required. Safety and efficacy in pediatric patients have not been determined.

Adverse Reactions Bleeding is the major drug-related adverse effect. Access site is often primary source of bleeding complications. Incidence of bleeding is also related to heparin intensity. Patients weighing <70 kg may have an increased risk of major bleeding.

>10%: Hematologic: Bleeding (major: 1% to 11%; minor: 3% to 14%; transfusion required: 2% to 13%)

1% to 10%:

Cardiovascular: Hypotension (up to 7%)
Hematologic: Thrombocytopenia (1% to 3%)
Local: Injection site reaction

<1% (Limited to important or life-threatening): Acute profound thrombocytopenia, anaphylaxis, fatal bleeding events, GI hemorrhage, intracranial hemorrhage (0.5% to 0.7%), pulmonary hemorrhage, stroke

Drug Interactions

Avoid Concomitant Use There are no known interactions where it is recommended to avoid concomitant use.

Increased Effect/Toxicity

Eptifibatide may increase the levels/effects of: Anticoagulants; Antiplatelet Agents; Drotrecogin Alfa; Ibritumomab; Salicylates; Thrombolytic Agents; Tositumomab and Iodine I 131 Tositumomab

The levels/effects of Eptifibatide may be increased by: Dasatinib; Herbs (Anticoagulant/Antiplatelet Properties); Nonsteroidal Anti-Inflammatory Agents; Omega-3-Acid

Ethyl Esters; Pentosan Polysulfate Sodium; Prostacyclin Analogues

Decreased Effect

The levels/effects of Eptifibatide may be decreased by: Nonsteroidal Anti-Inflammatory Agents

Ethanol/Nutrition/Herb Interactions Herb/Nutraceutical: Avoid alfalfa, anise, bilberry, bladderwrack, bromelain, cat's claw, celery, coleus, cordyceps, dong quai, evening primrose oil, fenugreek, feverfew, garlic, ginger, ginkgo biloba, ginseng (American), ginseng (Panax), ginseng (Siberian), grapeseed, green tea, guggul, horse chestnut seed, horseradish, licorice, prickly ash, red clover, reishi, same (s-adenosylmethionine), sweet clover, turmeric, and white willow (all have additional antiplatelet activity).

Stability Vials should be stored refrigerated at 2°C to 8°C (36°F to 46°F). Vials can be kept at room temperature for 2 months. Protect from light until administration. Do not use beyond the expiration date. Discard any unused portion left in the vial.

Mechanism of Action Eptifibatide is a cyclic heptapeptide which blocks the platelet glycoprotein IIb/IIIa receptor, the binding site for fibrinogen, von Willebrand factor, and other ligands. Inhibition of binding at this final common receptor reversibly blocks platelet aggregation and prevents thrombosis.

Pharmacodynamics/Kinetics

Onset of action: Within 1 hour

Duration: Platelet function restored ~4 hours following discontinuation

Protein binding: ~25%

Half-life elimination: 2.5 hours

Excretion: Primarily urine (as eptifibatide and metabolites); significant renal impairment may alter disposition of this compound

Clearance: Total body: 55-58 mL/kg/hour; Renal: ~50% of total in healthy subjects

Dosage I.V.: Adults:

Acute coronary syndrome: Bolus of 180 mcg/kg (maximum: 22.6 mg) over 1-2 minutes, begun as soon as possible following diagnosis, followed by a continuous infusion of 2 mcg/kg/minute (maximum: 15 mg/hour) until hospital discharge or initiation of CABG surgery, up to 72 hours. Concurrent aspirin and heparin therapy (target aPTT 50-70 seconds) are recommended.

Percutaneous coronary intervention (PCI) with or without stenting: Bolus of 180 mcg/kg (maximum: 22.6 mg) administered immediately before the initiation of PCI, followed by a continuous infusion of 2 mcg/kg/minute (maximum: 15 mg/hour). A second 180 mcg/kg bolus (maximum: 22.6 mg) should be administered 10 minutes after the first bolus. Infusion should be continued until hospital discharge or for up to 18-24 hours, whichever comes first. Concurrent aspirin (160-325 mg 1-24 hours before PCI and daily thereafter) and heparin therapy (ACT 200-300 seconds during PCI) are recommended. Heparin infusion after PCI is discouraged. In patients who undergo coronary artery bypass graft surgery, discontinue infusion prior to surgery.

Elderly: No dosing adjustment for the elderly appears to be necessary; adjust carefully to renal function.

Dosing adjustment in renal impairment: Dialysis is a contraindication to use.

Note: The Cockroft-Gault equation using actual body weight sould be used to estimate renal function.

Acute coronary syndrome: Cl_{cr} <50 mL/minute: Use 180 mcg/kg bolus (maximum: 22.6 mg) and 1 mcg/kg/minute infusion (maximum: 7.5 mg/hour)

Percutaneous coronary intervention (PCI) with or without stenting: Cl_{cr} <50 mL/minute: Use 180 mcg/kg bolus (maximum: 22.6 mg) administered immediately before the initiation of PCI and followed by a continuous infusion of 1 mcg/kg/minute (maximum: 7.5 mg/hour). A second 180 mcg/kg (maximum: 22.6 mg) bolus should be administered 10 minutes after the first bolus.

Administration Do not shake vial. Visually inspect for discoloration or particulate matter prior to administration. The bolus dose should be withdrawn from the 10 mL vial into a syringe and administered by I.V. push over 1-2 minutes. Begin continuous infusion immediately following bolus administration, administered directly from the 100 mL vial. The 100 mL vial should be spiked with a vented infusion set.

Monitoring Parameters Coagulation parameters, signs/symptoms of excessive bleeding. Laboratory tests at baseline and monitoring during therapy: hematocrit and hemoglobin, platelet count, serum creatinine, PT/aPTT (maintain aPTT between 50-70 seconds unless PCI is to be performed), and ACT with PCI (maintain ACT between 200-300 seconds during PCI).

Assess sheath insertion site and distal pulses of affected leg every 15 minutes for the first hour and then every 1 hour for the next 6 hours. Arterial access site care is important to prevent bleeding. Care should be taken when attempting vascular access that only the anterior wall of the femoral artery is punctured, avoiding a Seldinger (through and through) technique for obtaining sheath access. Femoral vein sheath placement should be avoided unless needed. While the vascular sheath is in place, patients should be maintained on complete bedrest with the head of the bed at a 30° angle and the affected limb restrained in a straight position.

Observe patient for mental status changes, hemorrhage, assess nose and mouth mucous membranes, puncture sites for oozing, ecchymosis and hematoma formation, and examine urine, stool and emesis for presence of occult or frank blood; gentle care should be provided when removing dressings.

Dosage Forms Excipient information presented when available (limited, particularly for generics); consult specific product labeling.

Injection, solution: 0.75 mg/mL (100 mL); 2 mg/mL (10 mL, 100 mL)

◆ **Epzicom®** *see* Abacavir and Lamivudine *on page 19*
◆ **Equagesic®** *see* Meprobamate and Aspirin *on page 946*
◆ **Equanil** *see* Meprobamate *on page 946*
◆ **Equetro®** *see* CarBAMazepine *on page 252*
◆ **Eraxis™** *see* Anidulafungin *on page 117*
◆ **Erbitux®** *see* Cetuximab *on page 297*

Ergocalciferol (er goe kal SIF e role)

U.S. Brand Names Drisdol®

Canadian Brand Names Drisdol®; Ostoforte®

Index Terms Activated Ergosterol; Viosterol; Vitamin D_2

Pharmacologic Category Vitamin D Analog

Use Treatment of refractory rickets, hypophosphatemia, hypoparathyroidism; dietary supplement

Unlabeled/Investigational Use Prevention and treatment of vitamin D deficiency in patients with chronic kidney disease (CKD)

Pregnancy Risk Factor C (manufacturer); A/C (dose exceeding RDA recommendation; per expert analysis)

Medication Safety Issues

Sound-alike/look-alike issues:

Calciferol™ may be confused with calcitriol

Drisdol® may be confused with Drysol™

Dosage Oral: **Note:** 1 mcg = 40 int. units

Adequate intake:

Infants and Children: 5 mcg/day (200 int. units/day)

Adults:

18-50 years: 5 mcg/day (200 int. units/day)

51-70 years: 10 mcg/day (400 int. units/day)
Elderly >70 years: 15 mcg/day (600 int. units/day)

Dietary supplementation: Infants, Children, and Adults: 10 mcg/day (400 int. units/day)

Vitamin D deficiency/insufficiency in patients with CKD stages 3-4 (K/DOQI guidelines): **Note:** Dose is based on 25-hydroxyvitamin D serum level [25(OH) D]:

Children (treatment duration should be a total of 3 months):
Serum 25(OH)D <5 ng/mL:
8000 int. units/day for 4 weeks, then 4000 int. units/day for 2 months **or**
50,000 int. units/week for 4 weeks, then 50,000 int. units twice a month for 2 months
Serum 25(OH)D 5-15 ng/mL:
4000 int units/day **or**
50,000 int units every other week
Serum 25(OH)D 16-30 ng/mL:
2000 int. units/day **or**
50,000 int. units every 4 weeks

Adults (treatment duration should be a total of 6 months):
Serum 25(OH)D <5 ng/mL:
50,000 int. units/week for 12 weeks, then 50,000 int. units/month
Serum 25(OH)D 5-15 ng/mL:
50,000 int. units/week for 4 weeks, then 50,000 int. units/month
Serum 25(OH)D 16-30 ng/mL:
50,000 int. units/month

Hypoparathyroidism:
Children: 1.25-5 mg/day (50,000-200,000 int. units) and calcium supplements
Adults: 625 mcg to 5 mg/day (25,000-200,000 int. units) and calcium supplements

Nutritional rickets and osteomalacia:
Children and Adults (with normal absorption): 25-125 mcg/day (1000-5000 int. units)
Children with malabsorption: 250-625 mcg/day (10,000-25,000 int. units)
Adults with malabsorption: 250-7500 mcg (10,000-300,000 int. units)

Vitamin D-*dependent* rickets:
Children: 75-125 mcg/day (3000-5000 int. units); maximum: 1500 mcg/day
Adults: 250 mcg to 1.5 mg/day (10,000-60,000 int. units)

Vitamin D-*resistant* rickets: Children and Adults: 12,000-500,000 int. units/day

Familial hypophosphatemia:
Children: 40,000-80,000 int. units plus phosphate supplements; dose may be reduced once growth is complete
Adults: 10,000-60,000 int. units plus phosphate supplements

Additional Information Complete prescribing information for this medication should be consulted for additional detail.

Dosage Forms Excipient information presented when available (limited, particularly for generics); consult specific product labeling.
Capsule:
Drisdol®: 50,000 int. units [1.25 mg; contains tartrazine and soybean oil]
Liquid, oral [drops]:
Drisdol®: 8000 int. units/mL (60 mL) [200 mcg/mL; OTC]
Tablet: 400 int. units [10 mcg; OTC]

Ergoloid Mesylates (ER goe loid MES i lates)

Canadian Brand Names Hydergine®

Index Terms Dihydroergotoxine; Dihydrogenated Ergot Alkaloids; Hydergine [DSC]

Pharmacologic Category Ergot Derivative

Use Treatment of cerebrovascular insufficiency in primary progressive dementia, Alzheimer's dementia, and senile onset

Pregnancy Risk Factor C

Dosage Adults: Oral: 1 mg 3 times/day up to 4.5-12 mg/day; up to 6 months of therapy may be necessary

Additional Information Complete prescribing information for this medication should be consulted for additional detail.

Dosage Forms Excipient information presented when available (limited, particularly for generics); consult specific product labeling.
Tablet: 1 mg
Tablet, sublingual: 1 mg

◆ **Ergomar®** *see* Ergotamine *on page 540*

◆ **Ergometrine Maleate** *see* Ergonovine *on page 539*

Ergonovine (er goe NOE veen)

U.S. Brand Names Ergotrate®

Index Terms Ergometrine Maleate; Ergonovine Maleate

Pharmacologic Category Ergot Derivative

Use Prevention and treatment of postpartum and postabortion hemorrhage caused by uterine atony or subinvolution

Unlabeled/Investigational Use Diagnostically to identify Prinzmetal's angina

Pregnancy Considerations Administration causes hyperstimulation of the uterus and may cause uterine tetany, decreased uteroplacental blood flow, uterine rupture, cervical and perineal lacerations, amniotic fluid embolism, and possible trauma to the infant. Ergonovine is used in the third stage of labor for the prevention and treatment of postpartum hemorrhage; use is contraindicated during pregnancy.

Contraindications Hypersensitivity to ergonovine or any component of the formulation; ergot alkaloids are contraindicated with potent inhibitors of CYP3A4 (includes protease inhibitors, azole antifungals, and some macrolide antibiotics); induction of labor, threatened spontaneous abortion, pregnancy

Warnings/Precautions Use caution in patients with sepsis, obliterative vascular disease, cardiovascular disease, hepatic or renal involvement, or second stage of labor; administer with extreme caution if using intravenously. Pleural and peritoneal fibrosis have been reported with prolonged daily use. Cardiac valvular fibrosis has also been associated with ergot alkaloids. Ergot alkaloid use may result in ergotism (intense vasoconstriction) resulting in peripheral vascular ischemia and possible gangrene. Concomitant use with potent inhibitors of CYP3A4 (includes protease inhibitors, azole antifungals, and some macrolide antibiotics) and ergot alkaloids has been associated with acute ergot toxicity (ergotism); certain ergot alkaloids (eg, ergotamine and dihydroergotamine) are contraindicated by the manufacturer. Use with caution in the elderly. Restore uterine responsiveness in calcium-deficient patients who do not respond to ergonovine by I.V. calcium administration. Safety and efficacy have not been established in children.

Adverse Reactions Frequency not defined.
Cardiovascular: Hypertension, MI, shock
Gastrointestinal: Nausea, vomiting
Miscellaneous: Allergic reactions, ergotism

Drug Interactions

Metabolism/Transport Effects **Substrate** of CYP3A4 (major)

Avoid Concomitant Use

Avoid concomitant use of Ergonovine with any of the following: Efavirenz; Posaconazole; Protease Inhibitors; Serotonin 5-HT1D Receptor Agonists; Sibutramine; Voriconazole

Increased Effect/Toxicity

Ergonovine may increase the levels/effects of: Serotonin 5-HT1D Receptor Agonists; Serotonin Modulators

The levels/effects of Ergonovine may be increased by: CYP3A4 Inhibitors (Moderate); CYP3A4 Inhibitors (Strong); Dasatinib; Efavirenz; Macrolide Antibiotics; Posaconazole; Protease Inhibitors; Serotonin 5-HT1D Receptor Agonists; Sibutramine; Voriconazole

Decreased Effect There are no known significant interactions involving a decrease in effect.

Stability

Injection: Store at <46°F; protect from light. May store at room temperature for up to 60 days. Do not use if discoloration occurs.

Tablet: Store at controlled room temperature of 15°C to 30°C (59°F to 86°F).

Mechanism of Action Similar smooth muscle actions as seen with ergotamine; however, it affects primarily uterine smooth muscles producing sustained contractions and thereby shortens the third stage of labor.

Pharmacodynamics/Kinetics

Onset of action: I.M.: ~2-5 minutes; Oral: 6-15 minutes

Duration: I.M.: Uterine effect: 3 hours; I.V.: ~45 minutes; Oral: 3 hours

Absorption: Oral: Rapid

Metabolism: Hepatic

Half-life elimination: I.V.: 120 minutes

Excretion: Primarily feces; urine

Dosage Adults:

I.M., I.V. (I.V. should be reserved for emergency use only): 0.2 mg, may repeat dose in 2-4 hours if needed

Oral, SL:

Immediate post-partum: 0.2 mg (usually given I.M. or I.V)

Late post-partum: 0.2-0.4 mg every 6-12 hours until danger of uterine atony has passed (usually ~48 hours)

Administration I.V. doses should be administered over a period of not <1 minute. Dilute in NS to 5 mL for I.V. administration. Oral tablets may also be administered sublingually.

Monitoring Parameters Blood pressure, pulse, uterine response; cramping, if severe, may justify a need for dose reduction (oral)

Dosage Forms Excipient information presented when available (limited, particularly for generics); consult specific product labeling.

Injection, as maleate:

Ergotrate®: 0.2 mg/mL (1 mL)

Tablet, as maleate:

Ergotrate®: 0.2 mg

◆ **Ergonovine Maleate** *see* Ergonovine *on page* 539

Ergotamine (er GOT a meen)

U.S. Brand Names Ergomar®

Index Terms Ergotamine Tartrate

Pharmacologic Category Antimigraine Agent; Ergot Derivative

Use Abort or prevent vascular headaches, such as migraine, migraine variants, or so-called "histaminic cephalalgia"

Pregnancy Risk Factor X

Pregnancy Considerations May cause prolonged constriction of the uterine vessels and/or increased myometrial tone leading to reduced placental blood flow. This has contributed to fetal growth retardation in animals.

Lactation Enters breast milk/not recommended

Contraindications Hypersensitivity to ergotamine or any component of the formulation; peripheral vascular disease; hepatic or renal disease; coronary artery disease; hypertension; sepsis; ergot alkaloids are contraindicated with strong inhibitors of CYP3A4 (includes protease inhibitors, azole antifungals, and some macrolide antibiotics); pregnancy

Warnings/Precautions Ergot alkaloids have been associated with fibrotic valve thickening (eg, aortic, mitral, tricuspid); usually associated with long-term, chronic use; vasospasm or vasoconstriction can occur; ergot alkaloid use may result in ergotism (intense vasoconstriction) resulting in peripheral vascular ischemia and possible gangrene; rare cases of pleural and/or retroperitoneal fibrosis have been reported with prolonged daily use. Discontinuation after extended use may result in withdrawal symptoms (eg, rebound headache). Use with caution in the elderly. Safety and efficacy have not been established in children.

[U.S. Boxed Warning]: Ergot alkaloids are contraindicated with potent inhibitors of CYP3A4 (includes protease inhibitors, azole antifungals, and some macrolide antibiotics); concomitant use associated with acute ergot toxicity (ergotism).

Adverse Reactions Frequency not defined.

Cardiovascular: Absence of pulse, bradycardia, cardiac valvular fibrosis, cyanosis, edema, ECG changes, gangrene, hypertension, ischemia, precordial distress and pain, tachycardia, vasospasm

Central nervous system: Vertigo

Dermatologic: Itching

Gastrointestinal: Nausea, vomiting

Genitourinary: Retroperitoneal fibrosis

Neuromuscular & skeletal: Muscle pain, numbness, paresthesia, weakness

Respiratory: Pleuropulmonary fibrosis

Miscellaneous: Cold extremities

Drug Interactions

Metabolism/Transport Effects Substrate of CYP3A4 (major); Inhibits CYP3A4 (weak)

Avoid Concomitant Use

Avoid concomitant use of Ergotamine with any of the following: Efavirenz; Posaconazole; Protease Inhibitors; Serotonin 5-HT1D Receptor Agonists; Sibutramine; Voriconazole

Increased Effect/Toxicity

Ergotamine may increase the levels/effects of: Serotonin 5-HT1D Receptor Agonists; Serotonin Modulators

The levels/effects of Ergotamine may be increased by: CYP3A4 Inhibitors (Moderate); CYP3A4 Inhibitors (Strong); Dasatinib; Efavirenz; Macrolide Antibiotics; Posaconazole; Protease Inhibitors; Serotonin 5-HT1D Receptor Agonists; Sibutramine; Voriconazole

Decreased Effect There are no known significant interactions involving a decrease in effect.

Ethanol/Nutrition/Herb Interactions Food: Avoid tea, cola, and coffee (caffeine may increase GI absorption of ergotamine). Grapefruit juice may cause increased blood levels of ergotamine, leading to increased toxicity.

Stability Store sublingual tablet at room temperature. Protect from light and heat.

Mechanism of Action Has partial agonist and/or antagonist activity against tryptaminergic, dopaminergic and alpha-adrenergic receptors depending upon their site; is a highly active uterine stimulant; it causes constriction of peripheral and cranial blood vessels and produces depression of central vasomotor centers

Pharmacodynamics/Kinetics

Absorption: Oral: Erratic; enhanced by caffeine coadministration

Metabolism: Extensively hepatic

Time to peak, serum: 0.5-3 hours

Half-life elimination: 2 hours

Excretion: Feces (90% as metabolites)

Dosage Sublingual: One tablet under tongue at first sign, then 1 tablet every 30 minutes if needed; maximum dose: 3 tablets/24 hours, 5 tablets/week

Administration Do not crush sublingual tablets.

Dosage Forms Excipient information presented when available (limited, particularly for generics); consult specific product labeling.

Tablet, sublingual, as tartrate:

Ergomar®: 2 mg [peppermint flavor]

- **Ergotamine Tartrate** *see* Ergotamine *on page 540*
- **Ergotamine Tartrate, Belladonna, and Phenobarbital** *see* Belladonna, Phenobarbital, and Ergotamine *on page 178*
- **Ergotrate®** *see* Ergonovine *on page 539*

Erlotinib (er LOE tye nib)

U.S. Brand Names Tarceva®

Canadian Brand Names Tarceva®

Index Terms CP358774; Erlotinib Hydrochloride; NSC-718781; OSI-774; R 14-15

Pharmacologic Category Antineoplastic Agent, Tyrosine Kinase Inhibitor; Epidermal Growth Factor Receptor (EGFR) Inhibitor

Use Treatment of locally advanced or metastatic nonsmall cell lung cancer (NSCLC) as monotherapy; locally advanced, unresectable or metastatic pancreatic cancer (first-line therapy in combination with gemcitabine)

Pregnancy Risk Factor D

Pregnancy Considerations Animal studies have demonstrated fetal harm and abortion. There are no well-controlled studies in pregnant women. Women of child-bearing potential should be advised to avoid pregnancy; adequate contraception is recommended during treatment and for 2 weeks after treatment has been completed.

Lactation Excretion in breast milk unknown/not recommended

Medication Safety Issues

Sound-alike/look-alike issues:

Erlotinib may be confused with gefitinib

High alert medication: The Institute for Safe Medication Practices (ISMP) includes this medication among its list of drug classes which have a heightened risk of causing significant patient harm when used in error.

Contraindications There are no contraindications listed within the manufacturer's labeling.

Warnings/Precautions Hazardous agent - use appropriate precautions for handling and disposal. Rare, sometimes fatal, pulmonary toxicity (interstitial pneumonia, interstitial lung disease [ILD], obliterative bronchiolitis, pulmonary fibrosis) has occurred; symptoms may begin within 5 days to more than 9 months after treatment initiation. Interrupt therapy for unexplained pulmonary symptoms (dyspnea, cough, and fever); discontinue for confirmed ILD.

Liver enzyme elevations have been reported. Hepatic failure and hepatorenal syndrome have also been reported, particularly in patients with baseline hepatic impairment. Monitor patients with any hepatic impairment (total bilirubin >ULN; Child-Pugh class A, B, or C) closely, including those with hepatic disease due to tumor burden; use with extreme caution in patients with total bilirubin >3 times ULN. Dosage reduction, interruption or discontinuation may be recommended for changes in hepatic function. Acute renal failure and renal insufficiency (with/without hypokalemia) have been reported; use with caution in patients with or at risk for renal impairment. Use caution with cardiovascular disease; MI, CVA, and microangiopathic hemolytic anemia with thrombocytopenia have been noted in patients receiving concomitant erlotinib and gemcitabine. Elevated INR and bleeding events have been reported; use caution with concomitant anticoagulant therapy. Generalized or severe acneiform, erythematous or maculopapular rash may occur; skin rash may correlate with treatment response and prolonged survival (Saif, 2008). Management should include alcohol-free lotions, topical antibiotics or topical corticosteroids, or if necessary, oral antibiotics and systemic corticosteroids; severe skin reactions may require dosage modification; avoid sunlight. Erlotinib levels may be lower in patients who smoke; advise patients to stop smoking. Concurrent use with CYP3A4 inhibitors and moderate or strong CYP3A4 inducers may affect erlotinib levels; consider alternative agents to CYP3A4 inducers to avoid the potential for CYP-mediated interactions; use with caution in patients taking strong CYP3A4 inhibitors. Safety and efficacy have not been established in children.

Adverse Reactions

Adverse reactions reported with monotherapy:

>10%:

Central nervous system: Fatigue (52% to 79%)

Dermatologic: Rash (75% to 76%; grade 3: 8%; grade 4: <1%; median onset: 8 days), pruritus (13%), dry skin (12%)

Gastrointestinal: Diarrhea (54% to 55%; grade 3: 6%; grade 4: <1%; median onset: 12 days), anorexia (52% to 69%), nausea (33% to 40%), vomiting (23% to 25%), stomatitis (17% to 19%), abdominal pain (11%)

Ocular: Conjunctivitis (12%), keratoconjunctivitis sicca (12%)

Respiratory: Dyspnea (41%), cough (33%)

Miscellaneous: Infection (24% to 34%)

1% to 10%:

Hepatic: ALT increased (grade 2: 4%)

Respiratory: Pneumonitis/pulmonary infiltrate (3%), pulmonary fibrosis (3%)

Significant adverse reactions reported with combination (erlotinib plus gemcitabine) therapy:

Cardiovascular: Deep venous thrombosis (4%), cerebrovascular accident (2%; including cerebral hemorrhage), MI/myocardial ischemia (2%), arrhythmia, syncope

Central nervous system: Fever (36%), depression (19%), headache (15%)

Dermatologic: Rash (69%)

Gastrointestinal: Diarrhea (48%), weight loss (39%), stomatitis (22%), ileus, pancreatitis

Hematologic: Hemolytic anemia, microangiopathic hemolytic anemia with thrombocytopenia (1%)

Hepatic: ALT increased (grade 2: 31%, grade 3: 13%, grade 4: <1%), AST increased (grade 2: 24%, grade 3: 10%, grade 4 <1%), hyperbilirubinemia (grade 2: 17%, grade 3: 10%, grade 4: <1%)

Renal: Renal insufficiency

Respiratory: Dyspnea (24%), cough (16%), ILD-like events (3%)

Miscellaneous: Infection (39%)

Mono- or combination therapy: <1% (Limited to important or life-threatening): Acute renal failure, bronchiolitis, corneal ulcerations, episcleritis, epistaxis, gastritis, gastroduodenal ulcers, gastrointestinal bleeding, gastrointestinal hemorrhage, hair/nail disorders (alopecia, brittle/loose nails, eyelash/brow changes, hirsutism, paronychia), hearing loss, hematemesis, hematochezia, hepatic failure, hepatorenal syndrome, hepatotoxicity, interstitial lung disease, melena, peptic ulcer bleeding, pulmonary fibrosis, pulmonary infiltrates, rash (acneiform; sparing prior radiation field), tympanic membrane perforation

Drug Interactions

Metabolism/Transport Effects Substrate of CYP1A2 (minor), 3A4 (major)

Avoid Concomitant Use

Avoid concomitant use of Erlotinib with any of the following: H2-Antagonists; Natalizumab; Proton Pump Inhibitors; Vaccines (Live)

Increased Effect/Toxicity

Erlotinib may increase the levels/effects of: Natalizumab; Vaccines (Live); Vitamin K Antagonists

The levels/effects of Erlotinib may be increased by: Antifungal Agents (Azole Derivatives, Systemic); CYP3A4 Inhibitors (Moderate); CYP3A4 Inhibitors (Strong); Dasatinib; Trastuzumab

Decreased Effect

Erlotinib may decrease the levels/effects of: Cardiac Glycosides; Vaccines (Inactivated); Vitamin K Antagonists

The levels/effects of Erlotinib may be decreased by: Antacids; CYP3A4 Inducers (Strong); Deferasirox; Echinacea; H2-Antagonists; Herbs (CYP3A4 Inducers); Proton Pump Inhibitors; Rifampin

Ethanol/Nutrition/Herb Interactions

Food: Erlotinib bioavailability is increased with food. Avoid grapefruit or grapefruit juice (may decrease the metabolism and increase erlotinib levels). Avoid grapefruit juice.

Herb/Nutraceutical: Avoid St John's wort (may increase metabolism and decrease erlotinib concentrations).

Stability Store at room temperature of 25°C (77°F); excursions permitted to 15°C and 30°C (59°F and 86°F).

Mechanism of Action The mechanism of erlotinib's antitumor action is not fully characterized. The drug is known to inhibit overall epidermal growth factor receptor (HER1/EGFR)- tyrosine kinase. Active competitive inhibition of adenosine triphosphate inhibits downstream signal transduction of ligand dependent HER1/EGFR activation.

Pharmacodynamics/Kinetics

Absorption: Oral: 60% on an empty stomach; almost 100% on a full stomach

Distribution: 94-232 L

Protein binding: 92% to 95% to albumin and α_1-acid glycoprotein

Metabolism: Hepatic, via CYP3A4 (major), CYP1A1 (minor), CYP1A2 (minor), and CYP1C (minor)

Bioavailability: Almost 100% when given with food; 60% without food

Half-life elimination: 24-36 hours

Time to peak, plasma: 1-7 hours

Excretion: Primarily as metabolites: Feces (83%; 1% as unchanged drug); urine (8%)

Dosage Oral: Adults: **Note:** Dose adjustments are likely to be needed when erlotinib is administered concomitantly with strong CYP3A4 inducers or inhibitors.

NSCLC: 150 mg once daily

Pancreatic cancer: 100 mg once daily in combination with gemcitabine

Dosage adjustment for concomitant CYP3A4 inhibitors/inducers:

CYP3A4 inhibitors: Dose reductions are more likely to be needed for severe adverse reactions when erlotinib is administered concomitantly with strong CYP3A4 inhibitors (eg, azole antifungals, clarithromycin, erythromycin, nefazodone, protease inhibitors, telithromycin). Dose reduction (if required) should be done in decrements of 50 mg.

CYP3A4 inducers: Concomitant administration with CYP3A4 inducers (eg, carbamazepine, phenobarbital, phenytoin, rifamycins, and St John's wort) may require increased doses (increase as tolerated at 2-week intervals); doses >150 mg/day should be considered with rifampin; alternatives to the enzyme-inducing agent should be utilized first.

Dosage adjustment for toxicity: Dose reductions should be made in 50 mg decrements

Diarrhea: Manage with loperamide; Severe diarrhea: Reduce dose or temporarily interrupt treatment

Pulmonary symptoms: Acute onset (or worsening) of pulmonary symptoms (eg, dyspnea, cough, fever): Interrupt treatment and evaluate for drug-induced interstitial lung disease; discontinue permanently with development of interstitial lung disease

Severe skin reaction: Reduce dose or temporarily interrupt treatment

Dosage adjustment in renal impairment: Interrupt treatment for renal disease due to dehydration; may resume after euvolemia re-established.

Dosage adjustment in hepatic impairment:

The manufacturer recommends the following guidelines:

Patients with normal hepatic function at baseline: Total bilirubin >3 times ULN and/or transaminases >5 times ULN: Interrupt or discontinue treatment

Patients with baseline hepatic impairment:

Total bilirubin >3 times ULN: Use extreme caution

Worsening liver function (not yet severe): Interrupt treatment and/or reduce dose

Severe changes in liver function (eg, doubling of total bilirubin and/or tripling of transaminases): Interrupt or discontinue treatment

A reduced starting dose (75 mg once daily) has been recommended in patients with hepatic dysfunction (AST ≥3 times ULN or direct bilirubin 1-7 mg/dL), with individualized dosage escalation if tolerated (Miller, 2007).

Dietary Considerations Take this medicine an empty stomach, 1 hour before or 2 hours after a meal. Avoid grapefruit juice.

Administration The manufacturer recommends administration on an empty stomach (at least 1 hour before or 2 hours after the ingestion of food) even though this reduces drug absorption by approximately 40%. Administration after a meal results in nearly 100% absorption.

Monitoring Parameters Periodic liver function tests (transaminases, bilirubin, and alkaline phosphatase); periodic renal function tests and serum electrolytes (in patients at risk for dehydration); hydration status

Additional Information Oncology Comment: According to the National Comprehensive Cancer Network (NCCN) pancreatic adenocarcinoma guidelines, gemcitabine combination therapy (including gemcitabine plus erlotinib) is an option for patients with good performance status in the treatment of locally-advanced or metastatic pancreatic cancer.

The NCCN guidelines for NSCLC recommend erlotinib as single agent treatment for disease progression after failure of first- or second-line treatment in patients with a performance status of 0-2. Erlotinib may be considered for patients with a performance status of 3. Erlotinib is considered a first-line therapy (alone or in combination with chemotherapy) in patients with advanced or metastatic NSCLC who have never smoked and have known active EGFR mutation or gene amplification.

Factors (in patients with NSCLC) which correlate positively with response to EGFR-tyrosine kinase inhibitor (TKI) therapy include skin rash (due to EGFR-TKI therapy), patients who have never smoked, EGFR mutation, and patients of Asian origin. KRAS mutation correlated with poorer outcome with EGFR-TKI therapy in patients with NSCLC. (Cooley, 2008; Jackman, 2008; Masarelli, 2007; Shepherd, 2005)

Dosage Forms Excipient information presented when available (limited, particularly for generics); consult specific product labeling.

Tablet:

Tarceva®: 25 mg, 100 mg, 150 mg

◆ **Erlotinib Hydrochloride** *see* Erlotinib *on page* 541

◆ **Errin™** *see* Norethindrone *on page* 1078

◆ **Ertaczo®** *see* Sertaconazole *on page* 1362

Ertapenem (er ta PEN em)

U.S. Brand Names Invanz®
Canadian Brand Names Invanz®
Index Terms Ertapenem Sodium; L-749,345; MK0826
Pharmacologic Category Antibiotic, Carbapenem
Additional Appendix Information

Antimicrobial Drugs of Choice *on page 1752*
Community-Acquired Pneumonia in Adults *on page 1766*

Use Treatment of the following moderate-severe infections: Complicated intra-abdominal infections, complicated skin and skin structure infections (including diabetic foot infections without osteomyelitis), complicated UTI (including pyelonephritis), acute pelvic infections (including postpartum endomyometritis, septic abortion, post surgical gynecologic infections), and community-acquired pneumonia. Prophylaxis of surgical site infection following elective colorectal surgery. Antibacterial coverage includes aerobic gram-positive organisms, aerobic gram-negative organisms, anaerobic organisms.

Note: Methicillin-resistant *Staphylococcus, Enterococcus* spp, penicillin-resistant strains of *Streptococcus pneumoniae*, beta-lactamase-positive strains of *Haemophilus influenzae* are **resistant** to ertapenem, as are most *Pseudomonas aeruginosa*.

Pregnancy Risk Factor B

Pregnancy Considerations With the exception of slightly decreased fetal weights in mice, teratogenic effects and fetal harm have not been shown in animal studies. Adequate and well-controlled studies have not been conducted in pregnant women and it is not known whether ertapenem can cause fetal harm.

Lactation Enters breast milk/use caution

Medication Safety Issues

Sound-alike/look-alike issues:

Ertapenem may be confused with imipenem, meropenem
Invanz® may be confused with Avinza™

Contraindications Hypersensitivity to ertapenem, other carbapenems, or any component of the formulation; anaphylactic reactions to beta-lactam antibiotics. If using intramuscularly, known hypersensitivity to local anesthetics of the amide type (lidocaine is the diluent).

Warnings/Precautions Use caution with renal impairment. Dosage adjustment required in patients with moderate-to-severe renal dysfunction; elderly patients often require lower doses (based upon renal function). Prolonged use may result in fungal or bacterial superinfection, including *C. difficile*-associated diarrhea (CDAD) and pseudomembranous colitis; CDAD has been observed >2 months postantibiotic treatment. Has been associated with CNS adverse effects, including confusional states and seizures; use caution with CNS disorders (eg, brain lesions, history of seizures, or renal impairment). Serious hypersensitivity reactions, including anaphylaxis, have been reported (some without a history of previous allergic reactions to beta-lactams). Doses for I.M. administration are mixed with lidocaine; consult Lidocaine on page *884* information for associated Warnings/Precautions. Serum concentrations of valproic acid may be reduced to subtherapeutic levels with concomitant use. Safety and efficacy have not been established in children <3 months of age.

Adverse Reactions Note: Percentages reported in adults.

1% to 10%:

Cardiovascular: Swelling/edema (3%), chest pain (1% to 2%), hypertension (1% to 2%), hypotension (1% to 2%), tachycardia (1% to 2%)

Central nervous system: Headache (6% to 7%), altered mental status (eg, agitation, confusion, disorientation, decreased mental acuity, changed mental status, somnolence, stupor) (3% to 5%), fever (2% to 5%), insomnia (3%), dizziness (2%), fatigue (1%), anxiety (1%)

Dermatologic: Rash (2% to 3%), pruritus (1% to 2%), erythema (1% to 2%)

Endocrine & metabolic: Hypokalemia (2%), hyperglycemia (1% to 2%), hyperkalemia (≤1%)

Gastrointestinal: Diarrhea (9% to 10%), nausea (6% to 9%), abdominal pain (4%), vomiting (4%), constipation (3% to 4%), acid regurgitation (1% to 2%), dyspepsia (1%), oral candidiasis (≤1%)

Genitourinary: Urine WBCs increased (2% to 3%), urine RBCs increased (1% to 3%), vaginitis (1% to 3%)

Hematologic: Platelet count increased (3% to 7%), hematocrit/hemoglobin decreased (3% to 5%), eosinophils increased (1% to 2%), leukopenia (1% to 2%), neutrophils decreased (1% to 2%), platelet count decreased (1%), prothrombin time increased (<1%)

Hepatic: Hepatic enzyme increased (5% to 9%), alkaline phosphatase increase (3% to 7%), albumin decreased (1% to 2%), bilirubin (total) increased (1% to 2%)

Local: Infused vein complications (5% to 7%), phlebitis/thrombophlebitis (2%), extravasation (1% to 2%)

Neuromuscular & skeletal: Leg pain (≤1%), weakness (1%)

Renal: Serum creatinine increased (1%)

Respiratory: Dyspnea (1% to 3%), cough (1% to 2%), pharyngitis (1%), rales/rhonchi (1%), respiratory distress (≤1%)

<1% (Limited to important or life-threatening): Abdominal distention, aggressive behavior, anaphylactoid reactions, anaphylaxis, anorexia, arrhythmia, asthma, asystole, atrial fibrillation, bicarbonate (serum) decreased, bilirubin (direct and indirect) increased, bladder dysfunction, bradycardia, bronchoconstriction, BUN increased, *C. difficile*-associated diarrhea, candidiasis, cardiac arrest, chills, cholelithiasis, dehydration, depression, dermatitis, desquamation, diaphoresis, duodenitis, dysphagia, epistaxis, epithelial (urine) cells increased, esophagitis, facial edema, flank pain, flatulence, flushing, gastritis, gastrointestinal hemorrhage, gout, hallucinations, heart failure, heart murmur, hematoma, hematuria, hemoptysis, hemorrhoids, hiccups, hypoesthesia, hypoxemia, ileus, injection site induration, injection site pain, jaundice, malaise, monocytes increased, mouth ulcer, muscle spasm, necrosis, nervousness, oliguria/anuria, pain, pancreatitis, paresthesia, pharyngeal discomfort, pleural effusion, pleuritic pain, pseudomembranous colitis, PTT increased, pyloric stenosis, renal insufficiency, seizure (0.5%), septicemia, septic shock, sodium (serum) increased, spasm, stomatitis, subdural hemorrhage, syncope, taste perversion, tremor, urinary retention, urticaria, vaginal candidiasis, vaginal pruritus, ventricular tachycardia, vertigo, voice disturbance, vulvovaginitis, weight loss

Drug Interactions

Avoid Concomitant Use There are no known interactions where it is recommended to avoid concomitant use.

Increased Effect/Toxicity

The levels/effects of Ertapenem may be increased by: Uricosuric Agents

Decreased Effect

Ertapenem may decrease the levels/effects of: Typhoid Vaccine; Valproic Acid

Stability Before reconstitution store at ≤25°C (77°F).

I.M.: Reconstitute 1 g vial with 3.2 mL of 1% lidocaine HCl injection (without epinephrine). Shake well. Use within 1 hour after preparation.

I.V.: Reconstitute 1 g vial with 10 mL of water for injection, 0.9% sodium chloride injection, or bacteriostatic water for injection. Shake well. For adults, transfer dose to 50 mL of 0.9% sodium chloride injection; for children, dilute dose with NS to a final concentration ≤20 mg/mL. Reconstituted I.V. solution may be stored at room temperature and must be used within 6 hours **or** refrigerated, stored for up to 24 hours and used within 4 hours after removal from refrigerator. Do not freeze.

Mechanism of Action Inhibits bacterial cell wall synthesis by binding to one or more of the penicillin binding proteins; which in turn inhibits the final transpeptidation step of peptidoglycan synthesis in bacterial cell walls, thus inhibiting cell wall biosynthesis. Bacteria eventually lyse due to ongoing activity of cell wall autolytic enzymes (autolysins and murein hydrolases) while cell wall assembly is arrested.

Pharmacodynamics/Kinetics

Absorption: I.M.: Almost complete

Distribution: V_{dss}:

Children 3 months to 12 years: ~0.2 L/kg

Children 13-17 years: ~0.16 L/kg

Adults: ~0.12 L/kg

Protein binding (concentration dependent, primarily to albumin): 85% at 300 mcg/mL, 95% at <100 mcg/mL

Metabolism: Non-CYP-mediated hydrolysis to inactive metabolite

Bioavailability: I.M.: ~90%

Half-life elimination:

Children 3 months to 12 years: ~2.5 hours

Children ≥13 years and Adults: ~4 hours

Time to peak: I.M.: ~2.3 hours

Excretion: Urine (~80% as unchanged drug and metabolite); feces (~10%)

Dosage Note: I.V. therapy may be administered for up to 14 days; I.M. therapy for up to 7 days

Usual dosage ranges:

Children 3 months to 12 years: I.M., I.V.: 15 mg/kg twice daily (maximum: 1 g/day)

Children ≥13 years and Adults: I.M., I.V.: 1 g/day

Indication-specific dosing:

Children 3 months to 12 years: I.M., I.V.:

Community-acquired pneumonia, complicated urinary tract infections (including pyelonephritis): 15 mg/kg twice daily (maximum: 1 g/day); duration of total antibiotic treatment: 10-14 days (**Note:** Duration includes possible switch to appropriate oral therapy after at least 3 days of parenteral treatment, once clinical improvement demonstrated.)

Intra-abdominal infection: 15 mg/kg twice daily (maximum: 1 g/day) for 5-14 days

Pelvic infections (acute): 15 mg/kg twice daily (maximum: 1 g/day) for 3-10 days

Skin and skin structure infections: 15 mg/kg twice daily (maximum: 1 g/day) for 7-14 days

Children ≥13 years and Adults: I.M., I.V.:

Community-acquired pneumonia, complicated urinary tract infections (including pyelonephritis): 1 g/day; duration of total antibiotic treatment: 10-14 days (**Note:** Duration includes possible switch to appropriate oral therapy after at least 3 days of parenteral treatment, once clinical improvement demonstrated.)

Intra-abdominal infection: 1 g/day for 5-14 days

Pelvic infections (acute): 1 g/day for 3-10 days

Skin and skin structure infections (including diabetic foot infections): 1 g/day for 7-14 days

Adults: I.V.: **Prophylaxis of surgical site following colorectal surgery:** 1 g given 1 hour preoperatively

Dosage adjustment in renal impairment:

Children: No data available for pediatric patients with renal insufficiency.

Adults:

Cl_{cr} >30 mL/minute/1.73 m^2: No adjustment required

Cl_{cr} ≤30 mL/minute/1.73 m^2 and ESRD: 500 mg/day

Hemodialysis: Adults: When the daily dose is given within 6 hours prior to hemodialysis, a supplementary dose of 150 mg is required following hemodialysis.

Dosage adjustment in hepatic impairment: Adjustments cannot be recommended (lack of experience and research in this patient population).

Dietary Considerations Sodium content: 137 mg (~6 mEq) per gram of ertapenem

Administration

I.M.: Avoid injection into a blood vessel. Make sure patient does not have an allergy to lidocaine or another anesthetic of the amide type. Administer by deep I.M. injection into a large muscle mass (eg, gluteal muscle or lateral part of the thigh). Do not administer I.M. preparation or drug reconstituted for I.M. administration intravenously.

I.V.: Infuse over 30 minutes

Monitoring Parameters Periodic renal, hepatic, and hematopoietic assessment during prolonged therapy; neurological assessment

Dosage Forms Excipient information presented when available (limited, particularly for generics); consult specific product labeling.

Injection, powder for reconstitution:

Invanz®: 1 g [contains sodium 137 mg/g (~6 mEq/g)]

◆ **Ertapenem Sodium** *see* Ertapenem *on page 543*

◆ ***Erwinia* Asparaginase** *see* Asparaginase *on page 140*

◆ **Erybid™ (Can)** *see* Erythromycin *on page 544*

◆ **Eryc® [DSC]** *see* Erythromycin *on page 544*

◆ **Eryc® (Can)** *see* Erythromycin *on page 544*

◆ **Eryderm® [DSC]** *see* Erythromycin *on page 544*

◆ **Erygel® [DSC]** *see* Erythromycin *on page 544*

◆ **EryPed®** *see* Erythromycin *on page 544*

◆ **Ery-Tab®** *see* Erythromycin *on page 544*

◆ **Erythrocin®** *see* Erythromycin *on page 544*

Erythromycin (er ith roe MYE sin)

U.S. Brand Names Akne-Mycin®; E.E.S.®; Ery-Tab®; Eryc® [DSC]; Eryderm® [DSC]; Erygel® [DSC]; EryPed®; Erythro-RX; Erythrocin®; PCE®; Romycin®

Canadian Brand Names Apo-Erythro Base®; Apo-Erythro E-C®; Apo-Erythro-ES®; Apo-Erythro-S®; Diomycin®; EES®; Erybid™; Eryc®; Novo-Rythro Estolate; Novo-Rythro Ethylsuccinate; Nu-Erythromycin-S; PCE®; PMS-Erythromycin; Sans Acne®

Index Terms Erythromycin Base; Erythromycin Ethylsuccinate; Erythromycin Lactobionate; Erythromycin Stearate

Pharmacologic Category Acne Products; Antibiotic, Macrolide; Antibiotic, Ophthalmic; Antibiotic, Topical; Topical Skin Product; Topical Skin Product, Acne

Use

Systemic: Treatment of susceptible bacterial infections including *S. pyogenes*, some *S. pneumoniae*, some *S. aureus*, *M. pneumoniae*, *Legionella pneumophila*, diphtheria, pertussis, *Chlamydia*, erythrasma, *N. gonorrhoeae*, *E. histolytica*, syphilis and nongonococcal urethritis, and *Campylobacter* gastroenteritis; used in conjunction with neomycin for decontaminating the bowel

Ophthalmic: Treatment of superficial eye infections involving the conjunctiva or cornea; neonatal ophthalmia

Topical: Treatment of acne vulgaris

Unlabeled/Investigational Use Systemic: Treatment of gastroparesis, chancroid; preoperative gut sterilization

Pregnancy Risk Factor B

Pregnancy Considerations Adverse events were not observed in animal studies; therefore, erythromycin is classified as pregnancy category B. Low levels of erythromycin have been shown to cross the placenta and erythromycin is considered the drug of choice for certain illnesses in pregnant women. Most studies do not support a link between prenatal exposure to erythromycin and pyloric stenosis in the neonate. No increased risk for congenital abnormalities has been documented, with the exception of a possible slight increase in risk for cardiovascular anomalies. No adequate and well-controlled studies have been completed in pregnant women. The estolate form of erythromycin should not be used in pregnancy due to a potential increased risk for hepatic toxicity.

Lactation Enters breast milk/use caution (AAP considers "compatible")

Medication Safety Issues

Sound-alike/look-alike issues:

Erythromycin may be confused with azithromycin, clarithromycin, Ethmozine®

Akne-Mycin® may be confused with AK-Mycin®

E.E.S.® may be confused with DES®

Eryc® may be confused with Emcyt®, Ery-Tab®

Ery-Tab® may be confused with Eryc®

Erythrocin® may be confused with Ethmozine®

Contraindications Hypersensitivity to erythromycin or any component of the formulation

Systemic: Concomitant use with pimozide or cisapride

Warnings/Precautions Systemic: Use caution with hepatic impairment with or without jaundice has occurred, it may be accompanied by malaise, nausea, vomiting, abdominal colic, and fever; discontinue use if these occur. Use caution with other medication relying on CYP3A4 metabolism; high potential for drug interactions exists. Prolonged use may result in fungal or bacterial superinfection, including *C. difficile*-associated diarrhea (CDAD) and pseudomembranous colitis; CDAD has been observed >2 months postantibiotic treatment. Use in infants has been associated with infantile hypertrophic pyloric stenosis (IHPS). Macrolides have been associated with rare QT_c prolongation and ventricular arrhythmias, including torsade de pointes. Use caution in elderly patients, as risk of adverse events may be increased. Use caution in myasthenia gravis patients; erythromycin may aggravate muscular weakness.

Adverse Reactions Frequency not defined. Incidence may vary with formulation.

Systemic:

Cardiovascular: QT_c prolongation, torsade de pointes, ventricular arrhythmia, ventricular tachycardia

Central nervous system: Seizure

Dermatitis: Pruritus, rash

Gastrointestinal: Abdominal pain, anorexia, diarrhea, infantile hypertrophic pyloric stenosis, nausea, oral candidiasis, pancreatitis, pseudomembranous colitis, vomiting

Hepatic: Cholestatic jaundice (most common with estolate), hepatitis, liver function tests abnormal

Local: Phlebitis at the injection site, thrombophlebitis

Neuromuscular & skeletal: Weakness

Otic: Hearing loss

Miscellaneous: Allergic reactions, anaphylaxis, hypersensitivity reactions, urticaria

Topical: 1% to 10%: Dermatologic: Erythema, desquamation, dryness, pruritus

Drug Interactions

Metabolism/Transport Effects Substrate of CYP2B6 (minor), 3A4 (major); **Inhibits** CYP1A2 (weak), 3A4 (moderate)

Avoid Concomitant Use

Avoid concomitant use of Erythromycin with any of the following: Cisapride; Dabigatran Etexilate; Disopyramide; Lincosamide Antibiotics; Nilotinib; Pimozide; Silodosin; Tetrabenazine; Thioridazine; Topotecan; Ziprasidone

Increased Effect/Toxicity

Erythromycin may increase the levels/effects of: Alfentanil; Antifungal Agents (Azole Derivatives, Systemic); Benzodiazepines (metabolized by oxidation); BusPIRone; Calcium Channel Blockers; CarBAMazepine; Cardiac Glycosides; Cilostazol; Cisapride; Clozapine; Colchicine; Corticosteroids (Systemic); CycloSPORINE; CYP3A4 Substrates; Dabigatran Etexilate; Disopyramide; Eletriptan; Eplerenone; Ergot Derivatives; FentaNYL; Fexofenadine; HMG-CoA Reductase Inhibitors; Maraviroc; P-Glycoprotein Substrates; Phosphodiesterase 5 Inhibitors; Pimecrolimus; Pimozide; QTc-Prolonging Agents; QuiNIDine; Ranolazine; Repaglinide; Rifamycin Derivatives; Rivaroxaban; Salmeterol; Selective Serotonin Reuptake Inhibitors; Silodosin; Sirolimus; Tacrolimus; Temsirolimus; Tetrabenazine; Theophylline Derivatives; Thioridazine; Topotecan; Vitamin K Antagonists; Ziprasidone; Zopiclone

The levels/effects of Erythromycin may be increased by: Alfuzosin; Antifungal Agents (Azole Derivatives, Systemic); Ciprofloxacin; CYP3A4 Inhibitors (Moderate); CYP3A4 Inhibitors (Strong); Dasatinib; Gadobutrol; Nilotinib; P-Glycoprotein Inhibitors

Decreased Effect

Erythromycin may decrease the levels/effects of: Clopidogrel; Typhoid Vaccine; Zafirlukast

The levels/effects of Erythromycin may be decreased by: CYP3A4 Inducers (Strong); Deferasirox; Etravirine; Herbs (CYP3A4 Inducers); Lincosamide Antibiotics; P-Glycoprotein Inducers

Ethanol/Nutrition/Herb Interactions

Ethanol: Avoid ethanol (may decrease absorption of erythromycin or enhance ethanol effects).

Food: Erythromycin serum levels may be altered if taken with food (formulation-dependent).

Herb/Nutraceutical: St John's wort may decrease erythromycin levels.

Stability

Injection:

Store unreconstituted vials at 15°C to 30°C (59°F to 86°F). Erythromycin lactobionate should be reconstituted with sterile water for injection without preservatives to avoid gel formation. The reconstituted solution is stable for 2 weeks when refrigerated or for 8 hours at room temperature.

Erythromycin I.V. infusion solution is stable at pH 6-8. Stability of lactobionate is pH dependent. I.V. form has the longest stability in 0.9% sodium chloride (NS) and should be prepared in this base solution whenever possible. Do not use D_5W as a diluent unless sodium bicarbonate is added to solution. If I.V. must be prepared in D_5W, 0.5 mL of the 8.4% sodium bicarbonate solution should be added per each 100 mL of D_5W.

Stability of parenteral admixture at room temperature (25°C) and at refrigeration temperature (4°C) is 24 hours.

Standard diluent: 500 mg/250 mL D_5W/NS; 750 mg/250 mL D_5W/NS; 1 g/250 mL D_5W/NS.

Oral suspension:

Granules: Prior to mixing, store at <30°C (<86°F). After mixing, store under refrigeration and use within 10 days.

Powder: Refrigerate to preserve taste. Erythromycin ethylsuccinate may be stored at room temperature if used within 14 days. EryPed® drops should be used within 35 days following reconstitution. May store at room temperature or under refrigeration.

Tablet and capsule formulations: Store at <30°C (<86°F).

Topical and ophthalmic formulations: Store at room temperature.

Mechanism of Action Inhibits RNA-dependent protein synthesis at the chain elongation step; binds to the 50S ribosomal subunit resulting in blockage of transpeptidation

Pharmacodynamics/Kinetics

Absorption: Oral: Variable but better with salt forms than with base form; 18% to 45%; ethylsuccinate may be better absorbed with food

Distribution:
- Relative diffusion from blood into CSF: Minimal even with inflammation
- CSF:blood level ratio: Normal meninges: 2% to 13%; Inflamed meninges: 7% to 25%

Protein binding: Base: 73% to 81%

Metabolism: Demethylation primarily via hepatic CYP3A4

Half-life elimination: Peak: 1.5-2 hours; End-stage renal disease: 5-6 hours

Time to peak, serum: Base: 4 hours; Ethylsuccinate: 0.5-2.5 hours; delayed with food due to differences in absorption

Excretion: Primarily feces; urine (2% to 15% as unchanged drug)

Dosage Note: Due to differences in absorption, 400 mg erythromycin ethylsuccinate produces the same serum levels as 250 mg erythromycin base or stearate.

Usual dosage range:

Neonates: Ophthalmic: Prophylaxis of neonatal gonococcal or chlamydial conjunctivitis: 0.5-1 cm ribbon of ointment should be instilled into each conjunctival sac

Infants and Children:

Oral:
- Base: 30-50 mg/kg/day in 2-4 divided doses; maximum: 2 g/day
- Ethylsuccinate: 30-50 mg/kg/day in 2-4 divided doses; maximum: 3.2 g/day
- Stearate: 30-50 mg/kg/day in 2-4 divided doses; maximum: 2 g/day

I.V.: Lactobionate: 15-50 mg/kg/day divided every 6 hours, not to exceed 4 g/day

Children and Adults:

Ophthalmic: Instill 1/2" (1.25 cm) 2-6 times/day depending on the severity of the infection

Topical: Acne: Apply over the affected area twice daily after the skin has been thoroughly washed and patted dry

Adults:

Oral:
- Base: 250-500 mg every 6-12 hours; maximum 4 g/day
- Ethylsuccinate: 400-800 mg every 6-12 hours; maximum: 4 g/day

I.V.: Lactobionate: 15-20 mg/kg/day divided every 6 hours or 500 mg to 1 g every 6 hours, or given as a continuous infusion over 24 hours; maximum: 4 g/24 hours

Indication-specific dosing:

Children:

***Bartonella sp* infections (bacillary angiomatosis [BA], peliosis hepatis [PH]) (unlabeled use):** Oral: 40 mg/kg/day (ethylsuccinate) in 4 divided doses (maximum: 2 g/day) for 3 months (BA) or 4 months (PH)

Conjunctivitis, neonatal *(C. trachomatis)*: Oral: 50 mg/kg/day (base or ethylsuccinate) in 4 divided doses for 14 days

Mild/moderate infection: Oral: 30-50 mg/kg/day in divided doses every 6-12 hours

Pertussis: Oral: 40-50 mg/kg/day in 4 divided doses for 14 days; maximum 2 g/day (not preferred agent for infants <1 month due to IHPS)

Pharyngitis, tonsillitis (streptococcal): Oral: 20 mg (base)/kg/day or 40 mg (ethylsuccinate)/kg/day in 2 divided doses for 10 days. **Note:** No longer preferred therapy due to increased organism resistance.

Pneumonia *(C. trachomatis)*: Oral: 50 mg/kg/day (base or ethylsuccinate) in 4 divided doses for 14-21 days

Preop bowel preparation: Oral: 20 mg (base)/kg at 1, 2, and 11 PM on the day before surgery combined with mechanical cleansing of the large intestine and oral neomycin

Severe infection: I.V.: 15-50 mg/kg/day; maximum: 4 g/day

Adults:

***Bartonella sp* infections (bacillary angiomatosis [BA], peliosis hepatis [PH]) (unlabeled use):** Oral: 500 mg (base) 4 times/day for 3 months (BA) or 4 months (PH)

Chancroid (unlabeled use): Oral: 500 mg (base) 3 times/day for 7 days; Note: Not a preferred agent; isolates with intermediate resistance have been documented

Gastrointestinal prokinetic (unlabeled use): I.V.: 200 mg initially followed by 250 mg (base) orally 3 times/day 30 minutes before meals. Lower dosages have been used in some trials.

Granuloma inguinale (*K. granulomatis*) (unlabeled use): Oral: 500 mg (base) 4 times/day for 21 days

Legionnaires' disease: Oral: 1.6-4 g (ethylsuccinate)/day or 1-4 g (base)/day in divided doses for 21 days. **Note:** No longer preferred therapy and only used in nonhospitalized patients.

Lymphogranuloma venereum: Oral: 500 mg (base) 4 times/day for 21 days

Nongonococcal urethritis (including coinfection with *C. trachomatis*): Oral: 500 mg (base) 4 times/day for 7 days or 800 mg (ethylsuccinate) 4 times/day for 7 days. **Note:** May use 250 mg (base) or 400 mg (ethylsuccinate) 4 times/day for 14 days if gastrointestinal intolerance.

Pelvic inflammatory disease: I.V.: 500 mg every 6 hours for 3 days, followed by 1000 mg (base)/day orally in 2-4 divided doses for 7 days. **Note:** Not recommended therapy per current treatment guidelines.

Pertussis: Oral: 500 mg (base) every 6 hours for 14 days

Preop bowel preparation (unlabeled use): Oral: 1 g erythromycin base at 1, 2, and 11 PM on the day before surgery combined with mechanical cleansing of the large intestine and oral neomycin

Syphilis, primary: Oral: 48-64 g (ethylsuccinate) or 30-40 g (base) in divided doses over 10-15 days. **Note:** Not recommended therapy per current treatment guidelines.

Dosage adjustment in renal impairment: Dialysis: Slightly dialyzable (5% to 20%); no supplemental dosage necessary in hemo- or peritoneal dialysis or in continuous arteriovenous or venovenous hemofiltration

Dietary Considerations

Systemic: Drug may cause GI upset; may take with food.

E.E.S.® granules for oral suspension contain sodium 25.9 mg (1.1 mEq)/5 mL

EryPed® powder for oral suspension contains sodium 117.5 mg (5.1 mEq)/5 mL; powder for oral suspension (drops) contains sodium 58.8 mg (2.6 mEq)/dropperful dose

Administration

Oral: Do not crush enteric coated drug product. GI upset, including diarrhea, is common. May be administered with food to decrease GI upset. Do not give with milk or acidic beverages.

I.V.: Infuse 1 g over 20-60 minutes. I.V. infusion may be very irritating to the vein. If phlebitis/pain occurs with used dilution, consider diluting further (eg, 1:5) if fluid status of the patient will tolerate, or consider administering in larger available vein. The addition of lidocaine or bicarbonate does not decrease the irritation of erythromycin infusions.

Ophthalmic: Avoid contact of tip of ophthalmic ointment tube with affected eye

Test Interactions False-positive urinary catecholamines

Dosage Forms Excipient information presented when available (limited, particularly for generics); consult specific product labeling. [DSC] = Discontinued product; [CAN] = Canadian brand name

Note: Strength expressed as base

Capsule, delayed release, enteric-coated pellets, as base: 250 mg
Eryc®: 250 mg [DSC]

Gel, topical: 2% (30 g, 60 g)
Erygel®: 2% (30 g, 60 g) [DSC] [contains alcohol 92%]

Granules for oral suspension, as ethylsuccinate:
E.E.S.®: 200 mg/5 mL (100 mL, 200 mL) [contains sodium 25.9 mg (1.1 mEq)/5 mL; cherry flavor]

Injection, powder for reconstitution, as lactobionate:
Erythrocin®: 500 mg, 1 g

Ointment, ophthalmic: 0.5% [5 mg/g] (1 g, 3.5 g)
Romycin®: 0.5% [5 mg/g] (3.5 g)

Ointment, topical:
Akne-Mycin®: 2% (25 g)

Powder for oral suspension, as ethylsuccinate:
EryPed®: 200 mg/5 mL (100 mL, 200 mL [DSC]) [contains sodium 117.5 mg (5.1 mEq)/5 mL; fruit flavor]; 400 mg/5 mL (100 mL, 200 mL [DSC]) [contains sodium 117.5 mg (5.1 mEq)/5 mL; banana flavor]

Powder for oral suspension, as ethylsuccinate [drops]:
EryPed®: 100 mg/2.5 mL (50 mL) [DSC] [contains sodium 58.8 mg (2.6 mEq)/dropperful; fruit flavor]

Powder, for prescription compounding:
Erythro-RX: USP (50 g)

Solution, topical: 2% (60 mL)
Eryderm®: 2% (60 mL) [contain alcohol] [DSC]
Sans acne [CAN]: 2% (60 mL) [contains ethyl alcohol 44%; not available in U.S.]

Suspension, oral, as ethylsuccinate: 200 mg/5 mL (480 mL) [DSC]; 400 mg/5 mL (480 mL) [DSC]
E.E.S.®: 200 mg/5 mL (100 mL, 480 mL) [fruit flavor] [DSC]; 400 mg/5 mL (100 mL, 480 mL) [orange flavor]

Tablet, as base: 250 mg, 500 mg

Tablet, as base [polymer-coated particles]:
PCE®: 333 mg, 500 mg

Tablet, as ethylsuccinate: 400 mg
E.E.S.®: 400 mg [DSC]

Tablet, as stearate: 250 mg, 500 mg
Erythrocin®: 250 mg, 500 mg

Tablet, delayed release, enteric coated, as base:
Ery-Tab®: 250 mg, 333 mg, 500 mg

Erythromycin and Benzoyl Peroxide

(er ith roe MYE sin & BEN zoe il per OKS ide)

U.S. Brand Names Benzamycin®; Benzamycin® Pak

Index Terms Benzoyl Peroxide and Erythromycin

Pharmacologic Category Acne Products; Topical Skin Product, Acne

Use Topical control of acne vulgaris

Pregnancy Risk Factor C

Dosage Adolescents ≥12 years and Adults: Apply twice daily, morning and evening

Additional Information Complete prescribing information for this medication should be consulted for additional detail.

Dosage Forms Excipient information presented when available (limited, particularly for generics); consult specific product labeling.

Gel, topical: Erythromycin 30 mg and benzoyl peroxide 50 mg per g (23 g, 47 g)
Benzamycin®: Erythromycin 30 mg and benzoyl peroxide 50 mg per g (47 g) [contains alcohol 20%]
Benzamycin® Pak: Erythromycin 30 mg and benzoyl peroxide 50 mg per 0.8 g packet (60s) [supplied with diluent containing alcohol]

Erythromycin and Sulfisoxazole

(er ith roe MYE sin & sul fi SOKS a zole)

U.S. Brand Names E.S.P.®

Canadian Brand Names Pediazole®

Index Terms Sulfisoxazole and Erythromycin

Pharmacologic Category Antibiotic, Macrolide; Antibiotic, Macrolide Combination; Antibiotic, Sulfonamide Derivative

Use Treatment of susceptible bacterial infections of the upper and lower respiratory tract, otitis media in children caused by susceptible strains of *Haemophilus influenzae*, and many other infections in patients allergic to penicillin

Pregnancy Risk Factor C

Medication Safety Issues

Sound-alike/look-alike issues:
Pediazole® may be confused with Pediapred®

Dosage Oral (dosage recommendation is based on the product's erythromycin content):

Children ≥2 months: 50 mg/kg/day erythromycin and 150 mg/kg/day sulfisoxazole in divided doses every 6 hours; not to exceed 2 g erythromycin/day or 6 g sulfisoxazole/day for 10 days

Adults >45 kg: 400 mg erythromycin and 1200 mg sulfisoxazole every 6 hours

Dosing adjustment in renal impairment (sulfisoxazole must be adjusted in renal impairment):
Cl_{cr} 10-50 mL/minute: Administer every 8-12 hours
Cl_{cr} <10 mL/minute: Administer every 12-24 hours

Additional Information Complete prescribing information for this medication should be consulted for additional detail.

Dosage Forms Excipient information presented when available (limited, particularly for generics); consult specific product labeling.

Powder for oral suspension: Erythromycin ethylsuccinate 200 mg and sulfisoxazole acetyl 600 mg per 5 mL (100 mL, 150 mL, 200 mL)
E.S.P.®: Erythromycin ethylsuccinate 200 mg and sulfisoxazole acetyl 600 mg per 5 mL (100 mL, 150 mL, 200 mL) [cheri beri flavor]

- ◆ **Erythromycin Base** *see* Erythromycin *on page 544*
- ◆ **Erythromycin Ethylsuccinate** *see* Erythromycin *on page 544*
- ◆ **Erythromycin Lactobionate** *see* Erythromycin *on page 544*
- ◆ **Erythromycin Stearate** *see* Erythromycin *on page 544*
- ◆ **Erythropoiesis-Stimulating Agent (ESA)** *see* Darbepoetin Alfa *on page 398*
- ◆ **Erythropoiesis-Stimulating Agent (ESA)** *see* Epoetin Alfa *on page 531*
- ◆ **Erythropoiesis-Stimulating Protein** *see* Darbepoetin Alfa *on page 398*
- ◆ **Erythropoietin** *see* Epoetin Alfa *on page 531*
- ◆ **Erythro-RX** *see* Erythromycin *on page 544*

Escitalopram (es sye TAL oh pram)

U.S. Brand Names Lexapro®

Canadian Brand Names Cipralex®

Index Terms Escitalopram Oxalate; Lu-26-054; S-Citalopram

Pharmacologic Category Antidepressant, Selective Serotonin Reuptake Inhibitor

Additional Appendix Information

Antidepressant Agents *on page 1638*
Selective Serotonin Reuptake Inhibitors (SSRIs) Pharmacokinetics *on page 1670*

Use Treatment of major depressive disorder; generalized anxiety disorders (GAD)

Unlabeled/Investigational Use

Treatment of mild dementia-associated agitation in nonpsychotic patients

Restrictions An FDA-approved medication guide concerning the use of antidepressants in children, adolescents, and young adults must be distributed when dispensing an outpatient prescription (new or refill) where this medication is to be used without direct supervision of a healthcare provider. Medication guides are available at http://www.fda.gov/cder/Offices/ODS/medication_guides.htm. Dispense to parents or guardians of children and adolescents receiving this medication.

Pregnancy Risk Factor C

Pregnancy Considerations Due to adverse effects observed in animal studies, escitalopram is classified as pregnancy category C. Escitalopram is distributed into the amniotic fluid. Limited data is available concerning the use of escitalopram during pregnancy. Nonteratogenic effects in the newborn following SSRI exposure late in the third trimester include respiratory distress, cyanosis, apnea, seizures, temperature instability, feeding difficulty, vomiting, hypoglycemia, hypo- or hypertonia, hyper-reflexia, jitteriness, irritability, constant crying, and tremor. An increased risk of low birth weight and lower APGAR scores have also been reported. Exposure to SSRIs after the twentieth week of gestation has been associated with persistent pulmonary hypertension of the newborn (PPHN). Adverse effects may be due to toxic effects of the SSRI or drug withdrawal without a taper. The long-term effects of *in utero* SSRI exposure on infant development and behavior are not known. Escitalopram is the S-enantiomer of the racemic derivative citalopram; also refer to the Citalopram monograph.

Women treated for major depression and who are euthymic prior to pregnancy are more likely to experience a relapse when medication is discontinued as compared to pregnant women who continue taking antidepressant medications. The ACOG recommends that therapy with SSRIs or SNRIs during pregnancy be individualized; treatment of depression during pregnancy should incorporate the clinical expertise of the mental health clinician, obstetrician, primary healthcare provider, and pediatrician (ACOG, 2007). If treatment during pregnancy is required, consider tapering therapy during the third trimester in order to prevent withdrawal symptoms in the infant. If this is done and the woman is considered to be at risk from her major depressive disorder, the medication can be restarted following delivery, although the dose should be readjusted to that required before pregnancy.

Lactation Enters breast milk/consider risk:benefit

Medication Safety Issues

Sound-alike/look-alike issues:

Lexapro® may be confused with Loxitane®

Contraindications Hypersensitivity to escitalopram, citalopram, or any component of the formulation; concomitant use with pimozide; concomitant use or within 2 weeks of MAO inhibitors

Warnings/Precautions [U.S. Boxed Warning]: Antidepressants increase the risk of suicidal thinking and behavior in children, adolescents, and young adults (18-24 years of age) with major depressive disorder (MDD) and other psychiatric disorders; consider risk prior to prescribing. Short-term studies did not show an increased risk in patients >24 years of age and showed a decreased risk in patients ≥65 years. Closely monitor patients for clinical worsening, suicidality, or unusual changes in behavior, particularly during the initial 1-2 months of therapy or during periods of dosage adjustments (increases or decreases); the patient's family or caregiver should be instructed to closely observe the patient and communicate condition with healthcare provider. A medication guide concerning the use of antidepressants should be dispensed with each prescription. **Escitalopram is not FDA approved for use in children.**

The possibility of a suicide attempt is inherent in major depression and may persist until remission occurs. Use caution in high-risk patients. Worsening depression and severe abrupt suicidality that are not part of the presenting symptoms may require discontinuation or modification of drug therapy. The patient's family or caregiver should be alerted to monitor patients for the emergence of suicidality and associated behaviors (such as agitation, irritability, hostility, impulsivity, and hypomania) and call healthcare provider.

May worsen psychosis in some patients or precipitate a shift to mania or hypomania in patients with bipolar disorder. Patients presenting with depressive symptoms should be screened for bipolar disorder. Monotherapy in patients with bipolar disorder should be avoided. Escitalopram is not FDA approved for the treatment of bipolar depression. Escitalopram is not FDA approved for the treatment of bipolar depression.

The potential for a severe reaction exists when used with MAO inhibitors, SSRIs/SNRIs or triptans; serotonin syndrome (hyperthermia, muscular rigidity, mental status changes/agitation, autonomic instability) may occur. Concurrent use with MAO inhibitors is contraindicated. May increase the risks associated with electroconvulsive therapy. Has a low potential to impair cognitive or motor performance; caution operating hazardous machinery or driving.

Use caution with a previous seizure disorder or condition predisposing to seizures such as brain damage, alcoholism, or concurrent therapy with other drugs which lower the seizure threshold. May cause hyponatremia/SIADH (elderly at increased risk); volume depletion (diuretics may increase risk) may occur. May cause or exacerbate sexual dysfunction. Use caution with renal or liver impairment; concomitant CNS depressants; pregnancy (high doses of citalopram have been associated with teratogenicity in animals). Use caution with concomitant use of aspirin, NSAIDs, warfarin, or other drugs that affect coagulation; the risk of bleeding may be potentiated.

Upon discontinuation of escitalopram therapy, gradually taper dose. If intolerable symptoms occur following a decrease in dosage or upon discontinuation of therapy, then resuming the previous dose with a more gradual taper should be considered.

Adverse Reactions

>10%:

Central nervous system: Headache (24%), somnolence (6% to 13%), insomnia (9% to 12%)

Gastrointestinal: Nausea (15% to 18%)

Genitourinary: Ejaculation disorder (9% to 14%)

1% to 10%:

Cardiovascular: Chest pain, hypertension, palpitation

Central nervous system: Fatigue (5% to 8%), dizziness (5%), dreaming abnormal (3%), lethargy (1% to 3%), yawning (2%), concentration impaired, fever, irritability, lightheadedness, migraine

Dermatologic: Rash

Endocrine & metabolic: Libido decreased (3% to 7%), anorgasmia (2% to 6%), menstrual disorder (2%), hot flashes, menstrual cramps

Gastrointestinal: Xerostomia (6% to 9%), diarrhea (8%), constipation (3% to 5%), appetite decreased (3%), indigestion (3%), vomiting (3%), abdominal pain (2%), flatulence (2%), toothache (2%), abdominal cramps, appetite increased, gastroenteritis, heartburn, weight gain

Genitourinary: Impotence (2% to 3%), urinary tract infection, urinary frequency
Neuromuscular & skeletal: Neck/shoulder pain (3%), paresthesia (2%), arthralgia, limb pain, muscle cramp, myalgia
Ocular: Blurred vision
Otic: Earache, tinnitus
Respiratory: Rhinitis (5%), sinusitis (3%), bronchitis, cough, nasal or sinus congestion, sinus headache
Miscellaneous: Diaphoresis (4% to 5%), flu-like syndrome (5%), allergy

<1% (Limited to important or life threatening): Abdominal discomfort, acute renal failure, aggression, agitation, akathisia, allergic reaction, amnesia, anaphylaxis, anemia, angioedema, anxiety attack, apathy, arthritis, arthropathy, asthma, atrial fibrillation, auditory hallucination, back discomfort, bilirubin increased, bradycardia, bruxism, carpal tunnel syndrome, chest tightness, chills, choreoathetosis, confusion, conjunctivitis, coordination abnormal, delirium, delusion, depersonalization, depression aggravated, depression, dermatitis, diplopia, disorientation, dyskinesia, dyspepsia, dyspnea, dystonia, dysuria, ecchymosis, ECG abnormal, eczema, edema, emotional lability, erythema multiforme, excitability, eye infection, flushing, folliculitis, furunculosis, gastritis, GERD, glaucoma, gout, grand mal seizure, hallucination, hematoma, hematuria, hemolytic anemia, hepatic necrosis, hepatitis, hypercholesterolemia, hyperglycemia, hyper-reflexia, INR increased, kidney stone, leg pain, lipoma, liver enzymes increased, liver failure, malaise, menorrhagia, muscle contractions (involuntary), muscle stiffness, muscle weakness, muscular tone increased, myocardial infarction, nervousness, neuroleptic malignant syndrome, nosebleed, nystagmus, pancreatitis, panic reaction, pneumonia, priapism, prolactinemia, prothrombin decreased, pruritus, pulmonary embolism, pupils dilated, QT prolonged, restless legs, restlessness aggravated, rhabdomyolysis, serotonin syndrome, shaking, SIADH, spontaneous abortion, spotting between menses, Stevens-Johnson syndrome, suicidal tendency, suicide attempt, syncope, tachycardia, taste alteration, thrombocytopenia, thrombosis, tics, torsade de pointes, toxic epidermal necrolysis, tracheitis, tremor, tremulousness nervous, twitching, urinary urgency, varicose vein, ventricular arrhythmia, vertigo, vision abnormal, visual disturbance, weakness, weight loss, withdrawal syndrome

Drug Interactions

Metabolism/Transport Effects Substrate (major) of CYP2C19, 3A4; **Inhibits** CYP2D6 (weak)

Avoid Concomitant Use

Avoid concomitant use of Escitalopram with any of the following: Iobenguane I 123; MAO Inhibitors; Pimozide; Sibutramine

Increased Effect/Toxicity

Escitalopram may increase the levels/effects of: Alcohol (Ethyl); Alpha-/Beta-Blockers; Anticoagulants; Antidepressants (Serotonin Reuptake Inhibitor/Antagonist); Antiplatelet Agents; Aspirin; Beta-Blockers; BusPIRone; CarBAMazepine; Clozapine; CNS Depressants; Desmopressin; Dextromethorphan; Drotrecogin Alfa; Haloperidol; Ibritumomab; Lithium; Methadone; Mexiletine; NSAID (COX-2 Inhibitor); NSAID (Nonselective); Phenytoin; Pimozide; Propafenone; Risperidone; Salicylates; Serotonin Modulators; Thrombolytic Agents; Tositumomab and Iodine I 131 Tositumomab; TraMADol; Tricyclic Antidepressants; Vitamin K Antagonists

The levels/effects of Escitalopram may be increased by: Analgesics (Opioid); BusPIRone; Cimetidine; CYP2C19 Inhibitors (Moderate); CYP2C19 Inhibitors (Strong); CYP3A4 Inhibitors (Moderate); CYP3A4 Inhibitors (Strong); Dasatinib; Herbs (Anticoagulant/Antiplatelet Properties); Macrolide Antibiotics; MAO Inhibitors; Omega-3-Acid Ethyl Esters; Pentosan Polysulfate Sodium; Prostacyclin Analogues; Sibutramine; TraMADol; Tryptophan

Decreased Effect

Escitalopram may decrease the levels/effects of: Iobenguane I 123

The levels/effects of Escitalopram may be decreased by: CarBAMazepine; CYP2C19 Inducers (Strong); CYP3A4 Inducers (Strong); Cyproheptadine; Deferasirox; Herbs (CYP3A4 Inducers)

Ethanol/Nutrition/Herb Interactions
Ethanol: Avoid ethanol (may increase CNS depression).
Herb/Nutraceutical: Avoid valerian, St John's wort, SAMe, kava kava, and gotu kola (may increase CNS depression).

Stability Store at 25°C (77°F); excursions permitted to 15°C to 30°C (59°F to 86°F).

Mechanism of Action Escitalopram is the S-enantiomer of the racemic derivative citalopram, which selectively inhibits the reuptake of serotonin with little to no effect on norepinephrine or dopamine reuptake. It has no or very low affinity for $5\text{-HT}_{1\text{-}7}$, alpha- and beta-adrenergic, $D_{1\text{-}5}$, $H_{1\text{-}3}$, $M_{1\text{-}5}$, and benzodiazepine receptors. Escitalopram does not bind to or has low affinity for Na^+, K^+, Cl^-, and Ca^{++} ion channels.

Pharmacodynamics/Kinetics
Onset of action: Depression: The onset of action is within a week; however, individual response varies greatly and full response may not be seen until 8-12 weeks after initiation of treatment.
Protein binding: 56% to plasma proteins
Metabolism: Hepatic via CYP2C19 and 3A4 to an active metabolite, S-desmethylcitalopram (S-DCT; 1/7 the activity); S-DCT is metabolized to S-didesmethylcitalopram (S-DDCT; active; 1/27 the activity) via CYP2D6
Half-life elimination: Escitalopram: 27-32 hours; S-desmethylcitalopram: 59 hours
Time to peak: Escitalopram: ~5 hours; S-desmethylcitalopram: 14 hours
Excretion: Urine (Escitalopram: 8%; S-DCT: 10%)
Clearance: Total body: 37-40 L/hour; Renal: Escitalopram: 2.7 L/hour; S-desmethylcitalopram: 6.9 L/hour

Dosage Oral:
Adults: Major depressive disorder, generalized anxiety disorder: Initial: 10 mg/day; dose may be increased to 20 mg/day after at least 1 week
Elderly: 10 mg once daily

Dosage adjustment in renal impairment:
Mild-to-moderate impairment: No dosage adjustment needed
Severe impairment: Cl_{cr} <20 mL/minute: Use with caution

Dosage adjustment in hepatic impairment: 10 mg/day

Dietary Considerations May be taken with or without food.

Administration Administer once daily (morning or evening), with or without food.

Monitoring Parameters Mental status for depression, suicidal ideation (especially at the beginning of therapy or when doses are increased or decreased), anxiety, social functioning, mania, panic attacks; akathisia

Additional Information The tablet and oral solution dosage forms are bioequivalent. Clinically, escitalopram 20 mg is equipotent to citalopram 40 mg. Do not coadminister with citalopram.

Dosage Forms Excipient information presented when available (limited, particularly for generics); consult specific product labeling.
Solution, oral:
Lexapro®: 1 mg/mL (240 mL) [contains propylene glycol; peppermint flavor]

Tablet:

Lexapro®: 5 mg, 10 mg, 20 mg

Note: Cipralex® [CAN] is available only in 10 mg and 20 mg strengths.

- **Escitalopram Oxalate** *see* Escitalopram *on page 547*
- **Eserine® (Can)** *see* Physostigmine *on page 1190*
- **Eserine Salicylate** *see* Physostigmine *on page 1190*
- **Esgic®** *see* Butalbital, Acetaminophen, and Caffeine *on page 229*
- **Esgic-Plus™** *see* Butalbital, Acetaminophen, and Caffeine *on page 229*
- **Eskalith® [DSC]** *see* Lithium *on page 897*
- **Eskalith CR® [DSC]** *see* Lithium *on page 897*

Esmolol (ES moe lol)

U.S. Brand Names Brevibloc®

Canadian Brand Names Brevibloc®

Index Terms Esmolol Hydrochloride

Pharmacologic Category Antiarrhythmic Agent, Class II; Beta Blocker, $Beta_1$ Selective

Additional Appendix Information

Beta-Blockers *on page 1648*

Hypertension *on page 1820*

Use Treatment of supraventricular tachycardia (SVT) and atrial fibrillation/flutter (control ventricular rate); treatment of tachycardia and/or hypertension (especially intraoperative or postoperative); treatment of noncompensatory sinus tachycardia

Unlabeled/Investigational Use In children, for SVT and postoperative hypertension

Pregnancy Risk Factor C (manufacturer); D (2nd and 3rd trimesters - expert analysis)

Pregnancy Considerations Teratogenic effects are not noted in animal studies. Fetal bradycardia can occur when administered in the 3rd trimester of pregnancy or at delivery.

Lactation Excretion in breast milk unknown/use with caution

Medication Safety Issues

Sound-alike/look-alike issues:

Esmolol may be confused with Osmitrol®

Brevibloc® may be confused with bretylium, Brevital®, Bumex®, Buprenex®

High alert medication: The Institute for Safe Medication Practices (ISMP) includes this medication among its list of drugs which have a heightened risk of causing significant patient harm when used in error.

Contraindications Hypersensitivity to esmolol or any component of the formulation; sinus bradycardia; heart block greater than first degree (except in patients with a functioning artificial pacemaker); cardiogenic shock; bronchial asthma (relative); uncompensated cardiac failure; hypotension; pregnancy (2nd and 3rd trimesters)

Warnings/Precautions Consider pre-existing conditions such as sick sinus syndrome before initiating. Hypotension is common; patients need close blood pressure monitoring. Administer cautiously in compensated heart failure and monitor for a worsening of the condition. Use caution in patients with PVD (can aggravate arterial insufficiency). Use caution with concurrent use of beta-blockers and either verapamil or diltiazem; bradycardia or heart block can occur. Avoid concurrent I.V. use of both agents. Use beta-blockers cautiously in patients with bronchospastic disease; monitor pulmonary status closely. Use cautiously in patients with diabetes because it can mask prominent hypoglycemic symptoms. Use with caution in patients with myasthenia gravis and psychiatric disease (may cause CNS depression). Use caution in patients with renal dysfunction (active metabolite retained). Adequate alpha-blockade is required prior to use of any beta-blocker for patients with untreated pheochromocytoma. Use caution with history of severe anaphylaxis to allergens; patients taking beta-blockers may become more sensitive to repeated challenges. Treatment of anaphylaxis (eg, epinephrine) in patients taking beta-blockers may be ineffective or promote undesirable effects. Beta-blocker therapy should not be withdrawn abruptly (particularly in patients with CAD), but gradually tapered to avoid acute tachycardia, hypertension, and/or ischemia. Do not use in the treatment of hypertension associated with vasoconstriction related to hypothermia. Concentrations >10 mg/mL or infusion into small veins or through a butterfly catheter should be avoided (can cause thrombophlebitis). Extravasation can lead to skin necrosis and sloughing. Safety and efficacy have not been established in children.

Adverse Reactions

>10%:

Cardiovascular: Asymptomatic hypotension (dose related: 25% to 38%), symptomatic hypotension (dose related: 12%)

Miscellaneous: Diaphoresis (10%)

1% to 10%:

Cardiovascular: Peripheral ischemia (1%)

Central nervous system: Dizziness (3%), somnolence (3%), confusion (2%), headache (2%), agitation (2%), fatigue (1%)

Gastrointestinal: Nausea (7%), vomiting (1%)

Local: Pain on injection (8%), infusion site reaction

<1% (Limited to important or life-threatening): Alopecia, bronchospasm, chest pain, CHF, depression, dyspnea, edema, exfoliative dermatitis, heart block, infusion site reactions, paresthesia, pruritus, pulmonary edema, rigors, seizure, severe bradycardia/asystole (rare), skin necrosis (from extravasation), syncope, thrombophlebitis, urinary retention

Drug Interactions

Avoid Concomitant Use

Avoid concomitant use of Esmolol with any of the following: Methacholine

Increased Effect/Toxicity

Esmolol may increase the levels/effects of: Alpha-/Beta-Agonists (Direct-Acting); Alpha1-Blockers; Alpha2-Agonists; Amifostine; Antipsychotic Agents (Phenothiazines); Cardiac Glycosides; Insulin; Lidocaine; Methacholine; Midodrine; RiTUXimab

The levels/effects of Esmolol may be increased by: Acetylcholinesterase Inhibitors; Aminoquinolines (Antimalarial); Amiodarone; Anilidopiperidine Opioids; Antipsychotic Agents (Phenothiazines); Calcium Channel Blockers (Nondihydropyridine); Diazoxide; Dipyridamole; Disopyramide; Herbs (Hypotensive Properties); Propafenone; Propoxyphene; Prostacyclin Analogues; QuiNIDine; Reserpine

Decreased Effect

Esmolol may decrease the levels/effects of: Beta2-Agonists; Theophylline Derivatives

The levels/effects of Esmolol may be decreased by: Barbiturates; Herbs (Hypertensive Properties); Methylphenidate; Nonsteroidal Anti-Inflammatory Agents; Rifamycin Derivatives; Yohimbine

Stability Clear, colorless to light yellow solution which should be stored at 25°C (77°F); do not freeze. Protect from excessive heat.

Stability of parenteral admixture at room temperature (25°C) is 24 hours.

Mechanism of Action Class II antiarrhythmic: Competitively blocks response to $beta_1$-adrenergic stimulation with little or no effect of $beta_2$-receptors except at high doses, no intrinsic sympathomimetic activity, no membrane stabilizing activity

Pharmacodynamics/Kinetics
Onset of action: Beta-blockade: I.V.: 2-10 minutes (quickest when loading doses are administered)
Duration of hemodynamic effects: 10-30 minutes; prolonged following higher cumulative doses, extended duration of use
Protein binding: 55%
Metabolism: In blood by red blood cell esterases
Half-life elimination: Adults: 9 minutes; elimination of metabolite decreases with end stage renal disease
Excretion: Urine (~69% as metabolites, 2% unchanged drug)

Dosage I.V. infusion requires an infusion pump (must be adjusted to individual response and tolerance):

Children:
SVT (unlabeled use): A limited amount of information regarding esmolol use in pediatric patients is currently available. Some centers have utilized doses of 100-500 mcg/kg given over 1 minute for control of supraventricular tachycardias.
Postoperative hypertension (unlabeled use): Loading doses of 500 mcg/kg/minute over 1 minute with maximal doses of 50-250 mcg/kg/minute (mean = 173) have been used in addition to nitroprusside to treat postoperative hypertension after coarctation of aorta repair.
Adults:
Intraoperative tachycardia and/or hypertension (immediate control): Initial bolus: 80 mg (~1 mg/kg) over 30 seconds, followed by a 150 mcg/kg/minute infusion, if necessary. Adjust infusion rate as needed to maintain desired heart rate and/or blood pressure, up to 300 mcg/kg/minute.
For control of postoperative hypertension, as many as one-third of patients may require higher doses (250-300 mcg/kg/minute) to control blood pressure; the safety of doses >300 mcg/kg/minute has not been studied.
Supraventricular tachycardia or gradual control of postoperative tachycardia/hypertension: Loading dose: 500 mcg/kg over 1 minute; follow with a 50 mcg/kg/minute infusion for 4 minutes; response to this initial infusion rate may be a rough indication of the responsiveness of the ventricular rate.
Infusion may be continued at 50 mcg/kg/minute or, if the response is inadequate, titrated upward in 50 mcg/kg/minute increments (increased no more frequently than every 4 minutes) to a maximum of 200 mcg/kg/minute.
To achieve more rapid response, following the initial loading dose and 50 mcg/kg/minute infusion, rebolus with a second 500 mcg/kg loading dose over 1 minute, and increase the maintenance infusion to 100 mcg/kg/minute for 4 minutes. If necessary, a third (and final) 500 mcg/kg loading dose may be administered, prior to increasing to an infusion rate of 150 mcg/kg/minute. After 4 minutes of the 150 mcg/kg/minute infusion, the infusion rate may be increased to a maximum rate of 200 mcg/kg/minute (without a bolus dose).
Usual dosage range (SVT): 50-200 mcg/kg/minute with average dose of 100 mcg/kg/minute.

Guidelines for transfer to oral therapy (beta-blocker, calcium channel blocker):
Infusion should be reduced by 50% 30 minutes following the first dose of the alternative agent
Manufacturer suggests following the second dose of the alternative drug, patient's response should be monitored and if control is adequate for the first hours, esmolol may be discontinued.

Dialysis: Not removed by hemo- or peritoneal dialysis; supplemental dose is not necessary.

Administration Infusions must be administered with an infusion pump. Concentrations >10 mg/mL or infusion into small veins or through a butterfly catheter should be avoided (can cause thrombophlebitis). Decrease or discontinue infusion if hypotension or congestive heart failure occur. Medication port of premixed bags should be used to withdraw only the initial bolus, if necessary (not to be used for withdrawal of additional bolus doses).

Monitoring Parameters Blood pressure, heart rate, MAP, ECG, respiratory rate, I.V. site; cardiac monitor and blood pressure monitor required

Test Interactions Increases cholesterol (S), glucose

Dosage Forms Excipient information presented when available (limited, particularly for generics); consult specific product labeling.
Infusion [premixed in sodium chloride; preservative free]:
Brevibloc®: 2000 mg (100 mL) [20 mg/mL; double strength]; 2500 mg (250 mL) [10 mg/mL]
Injection, solution, as hydrochloride: 10 mg/mL (10 mL)
Brevibloc®:
10 mg/mL (10 mL) [alcohol free; premixed in sodium chloride]
20 mg/mL (5 mL, 100 mL) [alcohol free; double strength; premixed in sodium chloride]

◆ **Esmolol Hydrochloride** *see* Esmolol *on page* 550

Esomeprazole (es oh ME pray zol)

U.S. Brand Names Nexium®
Canadian Brand Names Nexium®
Index Terms Esomeprazole Magnesium; Esomeprazole Sodium
Pharmacologic Category Proton Pump Inhibitor; Substituted Benzimidazole
Additional Appendix Information
Helicobacter pylori Treatment *on page* 1813

Use
Oral: Short-term (4-8 weeks) treatment of erosive esophagitis; maintaining symptom resolution and healing of erosive esophagitis; treatment of symptomatic gastroesophageal reflux disease (GERD); as part of a multidrug regimen for *Helicobacter pylori* eradication in patients with duodenal ulcer disease (active or history of within the past 5 years); prevention of gastric ulcers in patients at risk (age ≥60 years and/or history of gastric ulcer) associated with continuous NSAID therapy; long-term treatment of pathological hypersecretory conditions including Zollinger-Ellison syndrome
Canadian labeling: Additional use (not in U.S. labeling):
Oral: Treatment of nonerosive reflux disease (NERD)
I.V.: Short-term (≤10 days) treatment of gastroesophageal reflux disease (GERD) when oral therapy is not possible or appropriate

Pregnancy Risk Factor B

Pregnancy Considerations Teratogenic effects were not observed in animal studies. However, there are no adequate and well-controlled studies in pregnant women. Congenital abnormalities have been reported sporadically following omeprazole use during pregnancy.

Lactation Excretion in breast milk unknown/not recommended

Medication Safety Issues
Sound-alike/look-alike issues:
Nexium® may be confused with Nexavar®

Contraindications Hypersensitivity to esomeprazole, substituted benzimidazoles (ie, lansoprazole, omeprazole, pantoprazole, rabeprazole), or any component of the formulation

Warnings/Precautions Use of proton pump inhibitors may increase the risk of gastrointestinal infections (eg, *Salmonella, Campylobacter*). Relief of symptoms does not preclude the presence of a gastric malignancy. Atrophic gastritis (by biopsy) has been noted with long-term omeprazole therapy; this may also occur with esomeprazole. No reports of enterochromaffin-like (ECL) cell ▶

carcinoids, dysplasia, or neoplasia have occurred. Severe liver dysfunction may require dosage reductions. Safety and efficacy of I.V. therapy >10 days have not been established; transition from I.V. to oral therapy as soon possible.

Adverse Reactions Unless otherwise specified, percentages represent adverse reactions identified in clinical trials evaluating the oral formulation.

>10%: Central nervous system: Headache (I.V. 11%; oral ≤8%)

1% to 10%:

Cardiovascular: Hypertension (≤3%), chest pain (>1%)

Central nervous system: Pain (4%), dizziness (oral >1%; I.V. 3%), anxiety (2%), insomnia (2%), pyrexia (2%), fatigue (>1%)

Dermatologic: Rash (>1%), pruritus (I.V. ≤1%)

Endocrine & metabolic: Hypercholesterolemia (2%)

Gastrointestinal: Flatulence (oral ≤5%; I.V. 10%), diarrhea (oral ≤7%; I.V. 4%), abdominal pain (oral ≤6%; I.V. 6%), nausea (oral 5%; I.V. 6%), dyspepsia (oral > 1%; I.V. 6%), gastritis (≤6%), constipation (oral 2%; I.V. 3%), vomiting (≤3%), benign GI neoplasm (>1%), dyspepsia (>1%), duodenitis (>1%), epigastric pain (>1%), esophageal disorder (>1%), gastroenteritis (>1%), GI mucosal discoloration (>1%), serum gastrin increased (>1%), tooth disorder (>1%), xerostomia (1%)

Genitourinary: Urinary tract infection (4%)

Hematologic: Anemia (>1%)

Hepatic: Transaminases increased (>1%)

Local: Injection site reaction (I.V. 2%)

Neuromuscular & skeletal: Arthralgia (3%), back pain (>1%), fracture (>1%), arthropathy (1%), myalgia (1%)

Respiratory: Respiratory infection (oral ≤9%; I.V. 1%), bronchitis (4%), sinusitis (oral ≤4%; I.V. 2%), coughing (>1%), rhinitis (>1%), dyspnea (1%)

Miscellaneous: Accident/injury (≤8%), viral infection (4%), allergy (2%), ear infection (2%), hernia (>1%), flu-like syndrome (1%)

<1% (Limited to important or life-threatening): Abdominal rigidity, aggression, agitation, agranulocytosis, albuminuria, alkaline phosphatase increased, alopecia, anaphylactic reaction/shock, angioedema, anorexia, arthritis exacerbation, asthma exacerbation, benign polyps/nodules, bilirubinemia, blurred vision, bronchospasm, candidiasis (GI and genital), carcinoid tumor of stomach, cervical lymphadenopathy, conjunctivitis, cramps, creatinine increased, cystitis, dehydration, depression, dermatitis, dysmenorrhea, dysphagia, dysuria, edema (including facial, peripheral and tongue), epigastric pain, epistaxis, erythema multiforme, esophageal varices, fibromyalgia syndrome, flushing, fungal infection, gastric retention, GI dysplasia, glycosuria, goiter, gynecomastia, hallucinations, hematuria, hepatic encephalopathy, hepatic failure, hepatitis, hyperhidrosis, hyperparathyroidism, hypertonia, hyperuricemia, hypoesthesia, hypokalemia, hypomagnesemia, hyponatremia, impotence, interstitial nephritis, jaundice, larynx edema, leukocytosis, leukopenia, malaise, micturition increased, migraine, muscular weakness, nervousness, osteoporosis, otitis media, pancreatitis, pancytopenia, paresthesia, pharyngolaryngeal pain, pharyngitis, photosensitivity, polymyalgia rheumatica, polyuria, proteinuria, pruritus ani, rhinorrhea, rigors, sleep disorder, somnolence, Stevens-Johnson syndrome, stomatitis, tachycardia, taste disturbances, thrombocytopenia, thyroid-stimulating hormone increased, tinnitus, total bilirubin increased, toxic epidermal necrolysis, tremor, urticaria, vaginitis, vertigo, vitamin B_{12} deficiency, weight changes

Drug Interactions

Metabolism/Transport Effects Substrate of CYP2C19 (major), 3A4 (major); **Inhibits** CYP2C19 (moderate)

Avoid Concomitant Use

Avoid concomitant use of Esomeprazole with any of the following: Erlotinib; Mesalamine; Nelfinavir

Increased Effect/Toxicity

Esomeprazole may increase the levels/effects of: Benzodiazepines (metabolized by oxidation); CYP2C19 Substrates; Methotrexate; Saquinavir; Voriconazole

The levels/effects of Esomeprazole may be increased by: Fluconazole; Ketoconazole

Decreased Effect

Esomeprazole may decrease the levels/effects of: Atazanavir; Clopidogrel; Dabigatran Etexilate; Dasatinib; Erlotinib; Indinavir; Iron Salts; Itraconazole; Ketoconazole; Mesalamine; Mycophenolate; Nelfinavir

The levels/effects of Esomeprazole may be decreased by: CYP2C19 Inducers (Strong); Tipranavir

Ethanol/Nutrition/Herb Interactions Food: Absorption is decreased by 43% to 53% when taken with food.

Stability

Capsule, granules: Store at 15°C to 30°C (59°F to 86°F). Keep container tightly closed.

Powder for injection: Store at 15°C to 30°C (59°F to 86°F). Protect from light.

For I.V. injection: Reconstitute powder with 5 mL NS.

For I.V. infusion: Initially reconstitute powder with 5 mL of NS, LR, or D_5W, then further dilute to a final volume of 50 mL.

Following reconstitution, solution for injection prepared in NS, and solution for infusion prepared in NS or LR should be used within 12 hours. Following reconstitution, solution for infusion prepared in D_5W should be used within 6 hours. Refrigeration is not required following reconstitution.

Mechanism of Action Proton pump inhibitor suppresses gastric acid secretion by inhibition of the H^+/K^+-ATPase in the gastric parietal cell

Pharmacodynamics/Kinetics

Distribution: V_{dss}: 16 L

Protein binding: 97%

Metabolism: Hepatic via CYP2C19 and 3A4 enzymes to hydroxy, desmethyl, and sulfone metabolites (all inactive)

Bioavailability: Oral: 90% with repeat dosing

Half-life elimination: ~1-1.5 hours

Time to peak: Oral: 1.5-2 hours

Excretion: Urine (80%, primarily as inactive metabolites; <1% as active drug); feces (20%)

Dosage

Children 1-11 years: Oral: **Note:** Safety and efficacy of doses >1 mg/kg/day and/or therapy beyond 8 weeks have not been established.

Symptomatic GERD: 10 mg once daily for up to 8 weeks

Erosive esophagitis (healing):

<20 kg: 10 mg once daily for 8 weeks

≥20 kg: 10-20 mg once daily for 8 weeks

Nonerosive reflux disease (NERD) (Canadian labeling): 10 mg once daily for up to 8 weeks

Adolescents 12-17 years: Oral:

GERD: 20-40 mg once daily for up to 8 weeks

NERD (Canadian labeling): 20 mg once daily for 2-4 weeks; lack of symptom control after 4 weeks warrants further evaluation

Adults:

Oral:

Erosive esophagitis (healing): Initial: 20-40 mg once daily for 4-8 weeks; if incomplete healing, may continue for an additional 4-8 weeks; maintenance: 20 mg once daily (controlled studies did not extend beyond 6 months)

Symptomatic GERD: 20 mg once daily for 4 weeks; may continue an additional 4 weeks if symptoms persist

NERD (Canadian labeling): Initial: 20 mg once daily for 2-4 weeks; lack of symptom control after 4 weeks warrants further evaluation; maintenance (in patients with successful initial therapy): 20 mg once daily as needed

Helicobacter pylori eradication: 40 mg once daily for 10 days; requires combination therapy **Note:** Various regimens available.

Canadian labeling: 20 mg twice daily for 7 days; requires combination therapy

Prevention of NSAID-induced gastric ulcers: 20-40 mg once daily for up to 6 months

Treatment of NSAID-induced gastric ulcers (Canadian labeling): 20 mg once daily for 4-8 weeks.

Pathological hypersecretory conditions (Zollinger-Ellison syndrome): 40 mg twice daily; adjust regimen to individual patient needs; doses up to 240 mg/day have been administered

I.V.: GERD: 20 mg or 40 mg once daily for ≤10 days; change to oral therapy as soon as appropriate

Elderly: No dosage adjustment needed.

Dosage adjustment in renal impairment: No dosage adjustment needed

Dosage adjustment in hepatic impairment:

Safety and efficacy not established in children with hepatic impairment.

Mild-to-moderate hepatic impairment (Child-Pugh class A or B): No dosage adjustment needed

Severe hepatic impairment (Child-Pugh class C): Dose should not exceed 20 mg/day

Dietary Considerations Take at least 1 hour before meals; best if taken before breakfast. The contents of the capsule may be mixed in applesauce or water; pellets also remain intact when exposed to orange juice, apple juice, and yogurt.

Administration

Oral:

Capsule: Should be swallowed whole and taken at least 1 hour before eating (best if taken before breakfast). Capsule can be opened and contents mixed with 1 tablespoon of applesauce. Swallow immediately; mixture should not be chewed or warmed. For patients with difficulty swallowing, use of granules may be easiest.

Granules: Empty into container with 1 tablespoon of water and stir; leave 2-3 minutes to thicken. Stir and drink within 30 minutes. If any medicine remains after drinking, add more water, stir and drink immediately.

Tablet (Canadian formulation, not available in U.S.): Swallow whole or may be dispersed in a half a glass of noncarbonated water. Stir until tablets disintegrate, leaving a liquid containing pellets. Drink contents within 30 minutes. Do not chew or crush pellets. After drinking, rinse glass with water and drink.

I.V.: May be administered by injection (≥3 minutes) or infusion (10-30 minutes). Flush line prior to and after administration with NS, LR, or D_5W.

Nasogastric tube:

Capsule: Open capsule and place intact granules into a 60 mL syringe; mix with 50 mL of water. Replace plunger and shake vigorously for 15 seconds. Ensure that no granules remain in syringe tip. Do not administer if pellets dissolve or disintegrate. Use immediately after preparation. After administration, flush nasogastric tube with additional water.

Granules: Delayed release oral suspension granules can also be given by nasogastric or gastric tube. Add 15 mL of water to a syringe, add granules from packet. Shake the syringe, leave 2-3 minutes to thicken. Shake the syringe and administer through nasogastric or gastric tube (French size 6 or greater) within 30 minutes. Refill the syringe with 15 mL of water, shake and flush nasogastric/gastric tube.

Tablet (Canadian formulation, not available in U.S.): Disperse tablets in 50 mL of noncarbonated water. Stir until tablets disintegrate leaving a liquid containing pellets. After administration, flush with additional 25-50 mL of water to clear the syringe and tube.

Monitoring Parameters Susceptibility testing recommended in patients who fail *H. pylori* eradication regimen (esomeprazole, clarithromycin, and amoxicillin)

Additional Information Esomeprazole is the S-isomer of omeprazole.

Dosage Forms Excipient information presented when available (limited, particularly for generics); consult specific product labeling. [CAN] = Canadian availability

Note: Strength expressed as base

Capsule, delayed release, as magnesium:

Nexium®: 20 mg, 40 mg

Granules, for oral suspension, delayed release, as magnesium:

Nexium®: 10 mg/packet (30s); 20 mg/packet (30s); 40 mg/packet (30s)

Nexium® [CAN]: 10 mg/packet (28s)

Injection, powder for reconstitution, as sodium:

Nexium®: 20 mg, 40 mg [contains edetate sodium]

Tablet, extended release, as magnesium:

Nexium® [CAN]: 20 mg, 40 mg [not available in U.S.]

◆ **Esomeprazole Magnesium** *see* Esomeprazole *on page 551*

◆ **Esomeprazole Sodium** *see* Esomeprazole *on page 551*

◆ **Esoterica® Regular [OTC]** *see* Hydroquinone *on page 749*

◆ **E.S.P.®** *see* Erythromycin and Sulfisoxazole *on page 547*

◆ **Estalis® (Can)** *see* Estradiol and Norethindrone *on page 558*

◆ **Estalis-Sequi® (Can)** *see* Estradiol and Norethindrone *on page 558*

Estazolam (es TA zoe lam)

U.S. Brand Names ProSom® [DSC]

Pharmacologic Category Benzodiazepine

Additional Appendix Information

Benzodiazepines *on page 1646*

Use Short-term management of insomnia

Restrictions C-IV

Pregnancy Risk Factor X

Medication Safety Issues

Sound-alike/look-alike issues:

ProSom® may be confused with PhosLo®, Proscar®, Pro-Sof® Plus, Prozac®, Psorcon®

Dosage Adults: Oral: 1 mg at bedtime, some patients may require 2 mg; start at doses of 0.5 mg in debilitated or small elderly patients

Dosing adjustment in hepatic impairment: May be necessary

Additional Information Complete prescribing information for this medication should be consulted for additional detail.

Dosage Forms Excipient information presented when available (limited, particularly for generics); consult specific product labeling. [DSC] = Discontinued product

Tablet: 1 mg, 2 mg

ProSom®: 1 mg, 2 mg [DSC]

◆ **Ester-E™ [OTC]** *see* Vitamin E *on page 1566*

◆ **Esterified Estrogen and Methyltestosterone** *see* Estrogens (Esterified) and Methyltestosterone *on page 568*

◆ **Esterified Estrogens** *see* Estrogens (Esterified) *on page 566*

◆ **Estrace®** *see* Estradiol *on page 554*

◆ **Estraderm®** *see* Estradiol *on page 554*

Estradiol (es tra DYE ole)

U.S. Brand Names Alora®; Climara®; Delestrogen®; Depo®-Estradiol; Divigel®; Elestrin™; Estrace®; Estraderm®; Estrasorb™; Estring®; EstroGel®; Evamist™; Femring®; Femtrace®; Gynodiol® [DSC]; Menostar®; Vagifem®; Vivelle-Dot®; Vivelle® [DSC]

Canadian Brand Names Climara®; Depo®-Estradiol; Estrace®; Estraderm®; Estradot®; Estring®; EstroGel®; Menostar®; Oesclim®; Sandoz-Estradiol Derm 100; Sandoz-Estradiol Derm 50; Sandoz-Estradiol Derm 75; Vagifem®

Index Terms Estradiol Acetate; Estradiol Cypionate; Estradiol Hemihydrate; Estradiol Transdermal; Estradiol Valerate

Pharmacologic Category Estrogen Derivative

Use Treatment of moderate-to-severe vasomotor symptoms associated with menopause; treatment of vulvar and vaginal atrophy; hypoestrogenism (due to hypogonadism, castration, or primary ovarian failure); prostatic cancer (palliation), breast cancer (palliation), osteoporosis (prophylaxis); abnormal uterine bleeding due to hormonal imbalance; postmenopausal urogenital symptoms of the lower urinary tract (urinary urgency, dysuria)

Pregnancy Risk Factor X

Pregnancy Considerations Estrogens are not indicated for use during pregnancy or immediately postpartum. Increased risk of fetal reproductive tract disorders and other birth defects have been observed with diethylstilbestrol (DES). In general, the use of estrogen and progestin as in combination hormonal contraceptives have not been associated with teratogenic effects when inadvertently taken early in pregnancy. These products are not intended to be used during pregnancy.

Lactation Enters breast milk/use caution

Medication Safety Issues

Sound-alike/look-alike issues:

Alora® may be confused with Aldara®
Elestrin™ may be confused with alosetron
Estraderm® may be confused with Testoderm®

International issues:

Vivelle®: Brand name for ethinyl estradiol and norgestimate in Austria
Estring® may be confused with Estrena® [Finland]
Estrena® [Finland] may be confused with estrone in the U.S.

Transdermal patch may contain conducting metal (eg, aluminum); remove patch prior to MRI.

Contraindications Hypersensitivity to estradiol or any component of the formulation; undiagnosed abnormal vaginal bleeding; history of or current thrombophlebitis or venous thromboembolic disorders (including DVT, PE); active or recent (within 1 year) arterial thromboembolic disease (eg, stroke, MI); carcinoma of the breast, except in appropriately selected patients being treated for metastatic disease; estrogen-dependent tumor; hepatic dysfunction or disease; porphyria; pregnancy

Warnings/Precautions

Cardiovascular-related considerations: **[U.S. Boxed Warning]: Estrogens with or without progestin should not be used to prevent coronary heart disease.** Use caution with cardiovascular disease or dysfunction. May increase the risks of hypertension, myocardial infarction (MI), stroke, pulmonary emboli (PE), and deep vein thrombosis; incidence of these effects was shown to be significantly increased in postmenopausal women using conjugated equine estrogens (CEE) in combination with medroxyprogesterone acetate (MPA). Nonfatal MI, PE, and thrombophlebitis have also been reported in males taking high doses of CEE (eg, for prostate cancer). Estrogen compounds are generally associated with lipid effects such as increased HDL-cholesterol and decreased LDL-cholesterol. Triglycerides may also be increased; use with caution in patients with familial defects of lipoprotein metabolism. Whenever possible, estrogens should be discontinued at least 4 weeks prior to and for 2 weeks following elective surgery associated with an increased risk of thromboembolism or during periods of prolonged immobilization.

Neurological considerations: **[U.S. Boxed Warning]: The risk of dementia may be increased in postmenopausal women;** increased incidence was observed in women ≥65 years of age taking CEE alone or in combination with MPA.

Cancer-related considerations: **[U.S. Boxed Warning]: Adequate diagnostic measures, including endometrial sampling, if indicated, should be performed to rule out malignancy in all cases of undiagnosed abnormal vaginal bleeding. Unopposed estrogens may increase the risk of endometrial carcinoma in postmenopausal women with an intact uterus.** The use of a progestin should be considered when administering estrogens to postmenopausal women with an intact uterus. Estrogens may exacerbate endometriosis. Malignant transformation of residual endometrial implants has been reported posthysterectomy with estrogen only therapy. Consider adding a progestin in women with residual endometriosis posthysterectomy. Estrogens may increase the risk of breast cancer. An increased risk of invasive breast cancer was observed in postmenopausal women using CEE in combination with MPA; a smaller increase in risk was seen with estrogen therapy alone in observational studies. An increase in abnormal mammograms has also been reported with estrogen and progestin therapy. Estrogen use may lead to severe hypercalcemia in patients with breast cancer and bone metastases; discontinue estrogen if hypercalcemia occurs.

Estrogens may cause retinal vascular thrombosis; discontinue permanently if papilledema or retinal vascular lesions are observed on examination. Use with caution in patients with diseases which may be exacerbated by fluid retention, including asthma, epilepsy, migraine, diabetes or renal dysfunction. Use with caution in patients with a history of severe hypocalcemia, SLE, hepatic hemangiomas, porphyria (use is contraindicated with certain products), endometriosis, and gallbladder disease. Use caution with history of cholestatic jaundice associated with past estrogen use or pregnancy. Safety and efficacy in pediatric patients have not been established. Prior to puberty, estrogens may cause premature closure of the epiphyses, premature breast development in girls or gynecomastia in boys. Vaginal bleeding and vaginal cornification may also be induced in girls.

[U.S. Boxed Warning]: Estrogens with or without progestin should be used for shortest duration possible at the lowest effective dose consistent with treatment goals. Before prescribing estrogen therapy to postmenopausal women, the risks and benefits must be weighed for each patient. Women should be informed of these risks and benefits, as well as possible effects of progestin when added to estrogen therapy. Conduct periodic risk:benefit assessments.

When used solely for prevention of osteoporosis in women at significant risk, nonestrogen treatment options should be considered. When used solely for the treatment of vulvar and vaginal atrophy, topical vaginal products should be considered. Use caution applying topical products to severely atrophic vaginal mucosa. Absorption of the topical emulsion (Estrasorb™) and topical gel (Elestrin™) is increased by application of sunscreen; do not apply sunscreen within close proximity of estradiol. When sunscreen is applied ~1 hour prior to the topical spray (Evamist™), no change in absorption was observed (estradiol absorption was decreased when sunscreen is applied 1 hour after Evamist™). Application of Divigel® or EstroGel® with sunscreen has not been evaluated. Transdermal patch may contain conducting metal (eg, aluminum); remove patch prior to MRI. Use of the vaginal ring may not be appropriate in women with narrow vagina, vaginal stenosis, vaginal infections, cervical prolapse, rectoceles, cystoceles, or other conditions which may increase the risk of vaginal irritation, ulceration, or increase the risk of expulsion. Remove ring if vaginal infection develops; reinsert only after infection has been appropriately treated. Ring should also be removed in case of ulceration, erosion, or adherence to vaginal wall; do not reinsert until healing is complete.

Adverse Reactions Frequency not defined. Some adverse reactions observed with estrogen and/or progestin combination therapy.

Cardiovascular: Chest pain, DVT, edema, hypertension, MI, stroke, syncope, venous thromboembolism

Central nervous system: Anxiety, dementia, dizziness, epilepsy exacerbation, headache, insomnia, irritability, mental depression, migraine, mood disturbances, nervousness

Dermatologic: Angioedema, chloasma, dermatitis, erythema multiforme, erythema nodosum, hemorrhagic eruption, hirsutism, loss of scalp hair, melasma, rash, pruritus, urticaria

Endocrine & metabolic: Breast cancer, breast enlargement, breast pain, breast tenderness, fibrocystic breast changes, HDL-cholesterol increased, galactorrhea, glucose intolerance, hot flashes, hypocalcemia, LDL-cholesterol decreased, libido changes, nipple pain, serum triglycerides/phospholipids increased, thyroid-binding globulin increased, total thyroid hormone (T_4) increased

Gastrointestinal: Abdominal cramps, abdominal distension, abdominal pain, bloating, cholecystitis, cholelithiasis, diarrhea, dyspepsia, flatulence, gallbladder disease, gastritis, nausea, pancreatitis, vomiting, weight gain/loss

Genitourinary: Alterations in frequency and flow of menses, cervical secretion changes, cystitis, dysmenorrhea, dysuria, endometrial cancer, endometrial hyperplasia, genital eruption, metrorrhagia, ovarian cancer, Pap smear suspicious, urinary tract infection, uterine leiomyomata size increased, leukorrhea, uterine pain, urinary incontinence, urogenital eruption/pruritus, vaginal candidiasis, vaginal discharge, vaginal moniliasis, vaginitis

Vaginal: Trauma from applicator insertion may occur in women with severely atrophic vaginal mucosa; skin hypertrophy, vaginal discomfort, vaginal hemorrhage, vaginal pain

Hematologic: Aggravation of porphyria, antithrombin III and antifactor Xa decreased, fibrinogen levels increased, platelet aggregability increased, platelet count increased, prothrombin increased; factors VII, VIII, IX, X increased

Hepatic: Cholestatic jaundice, hepatic hemangioma enlargement

Local: Thrombophlebitis

Gel, spray: Application site reaction

Transdermal patches: Burning, erythema, irritation

Neuromuscular & skeletal: Arthralgia, arthritis, back pain, chorea, leg cramps, muscle cramps, skeletal pain

Ocular: Contact lens intolerance, corneal curvature steepening, retinal vascular thrombosis, vision abnormal

Respiratory: Asthma exacerbation, pulmonary thromboembolism

Miscellaneous: Anaphylactoid/anaphylactic reactions

Postmarketing and/or case reports: Liver function tests increased (rare), leg pain

Vaginal ring: Bowel obstruction, ring adherence to vaginal wall, toxic shock syndrome

Drug Interactions

Metabolism/Transport Effects **Substrate** of CYP1A2 (major), 2A6 (minor), 2B6 (minor), 2C9 (minor), 2C19 (minor), 2D6 (minor), 2E1 (minor), 3A4 (major); **Inhibits** CYP1A2 (weak), 2C8 (weak); **Induces** CYP3A4 (weak)

Avoid Concomitant Use There are no known interactions where it is recommended to avoid concomitant use.

Increased Effect/Toxicity

Estradiol may increase the levels/effects of: Corticosteroids (Systemic); Ropinirole; Tipranavir

The levels/effects of Estradiol may be increased by: Herbs (Estrogenic Properties); P-Glycoprotein Inhibitors

Decreased Effect

Estradiol may decrease the levels/effects of: Maraviroc; Somatropin; Thyroid Products

The levels/effects of Estradiol may be decreased by: CYP1A2 Inducers (Strong); CYP3A4 Inducers (Strong); Deferasirox; Herbs (CYP3A4 Inducers); P-Glycoprotein Inducers; Tipranavir

Ethanol/Nutrition/Herb Interactions

Ethanol: Avoid ethanol (routine use increases estrogen level and risk of breast cancer). Ethanol may also increase the risk of osteoporosis.

Food: Folic acid absorption may be decreased

Herb/Nutraceutical: St John's wort may decrease levels. Herbs with estrogenic properties may enhance the adverse/toxic effect of estrogen derivatives; examples include alfalfa, black cohosh, bloodroot, hops, kudzu, licorice, red clover, saw palmetto, soybean, thyme, wild yam, yucca.

Mechanism of Action Estrogens are responsible for the development and maintenance of the female reproductive system and secondary sexual characteristics. Estradiol is the principle intracellular human estrogen and is more potent than estrone and estriol at the receptor level; it is the primary estrogen secreted prior to menopause. Following menopause, estrone and estrone sulfate are more highly produced. Estrogens modulate the pituitary secretion of gonadotropins, luteinizing hormone, and follicle-stimulating hormone through a negative feedback system; estrogen replacement reduces elevated levels of these hormones in postmenopausal women.

Pharmacodynamics/Kinetics

Absorption: Oral, topical: Well absorbed

Protein binding: 37% to sex hormone-binding globulin; 61% to albumin

Metabolism: Hepatic via oxidation and conjugation in GI tract; hydroxylated via CYP3A4 to metabolites; first-pass effect; enterohepatic recirculation; reversibly converted to estrone and estriol

Excretion: Primarily urine (as metabolites estrone and estriol); feces (small amounts)

Dosage All dosage needs to be adjusted based upon the patient's response

Oral:

Prostate cancer (androgen-dependent, inoperable, progressing): 10 mg 3 times/day for at least 3 months

Breast cancer (inoperable, progressing in appropriately selected patients): 10 mg 3 times/day for at least 3 months

Osteoporosis prophylaxis in postmenopausal females: 0.5 mg/day in a cyclic regimen (3 weeks on and 1 week off)

Female hypoestrogenism (due to hypogonadism, castration, or primary ovarian failure): 1-2 mg/day; titrate as necessary to control symptoms using minimal effective dose for maintenance therapy

Moderate-to-severe vasomotor symptoms associated with menopause: 1-2 mg/day, adjusted as necessary to limit symptoms; administration should be cyclic (3 weeks on, 1 week off). Patients should be re-evaluated at 3- to 6-month intervals to determine if treatment is still necessary.

I.M.:

Prostate cancer: Valerate: ≥30 mg or more every 1-2 weeks

Moderate-to-severe vasomotor symptoms associated with menopause:

Cypionate: 1-5 mg every 3-4 weeks

Valerate: 10-20 mg every 4 weeks

Female hypoestrogenism (due to hypogonadism):

Cypionate: 1.5-2 mg monthly

Valerate: 10-20 mg every 4 weeks

Topical:

Emulsion: Moderate-to-severe vasomotor symptoms associated with menopause: 3.84 g applied once daily in the morning

Gel:

Moderate-to-severe vasomotor symptoms associated with menopause:

Divigel®: 0.25 g/day; adjust dose based on patient response. Dosing range: 0.25-1 g/day

Elestrin™: 0.87g/day applied at the same time each day

EstroGel®: 1.25 g/day applied at the same time each day

Vulvar and vaginal atrophy:

Elestrin™: 0.87g/day applied at the same time each day

EstroGel®: 1.25 g/day applied at the same time each day

Spray: Moderate-to-severe vasomotor symptoms associated with menopause (Evamist™): Initial: One spray (1.53 mg) per day. Adjust dose based on patient response. Dosing range: 1-3 sprays per day.

Transdermal: Indicated dose may be used continuously in patients without an intact uterus. May be given continuously or cyclically (3 weeks on, 1 week off) in patients with an intact uterus **(exception - Menostar®, see specific dosing instructions).** When changing patients from oral to transdermal therapy, start transdermal patch 1 week after discontinuing oral hormone (may begin sooner if symptoms reappear within 1 week):

Once-weekly patch:

Moderate to severe vasomotor symptoms associated with menopause, vulvar and vaginal atrophy associated with menopause, female hypoestrogenism (Climara®): Apply 0.025 mg/day patch once weekly. Adjust dose as necessary to control symptoms. Patients should be re-evaluated at 3- to 6-month intervals to determine if treatment is still necessary.

Osteoporosis prophylaxis in postmenopausal women:

Climara®: Apply patch once weekly; minimum effective dose 0.025 mg/day; adjust response to therapy by biochemical markers and bone mineral density

Menostar®: Apply patch once weekly. In women with a uterus, also administer a progestin for 14 days every 6-12 months

Twice-weekly patch:

Moderate-to-severe vasomotor symptoms associated with menopause, vulvar/vaginal atrophy, female hypogonadism: Titrate to lowest dose possible to control symptoms, adjusting initial dose after the first month of therapy; re-evaluate therapy at 3- to 6-month intervals to taper or discontinue medication:

Alora®, Estraderm®, Vivelle-Dot®: Apply 0.05 mg patch twice weekly

Vivelle®: Apply 0.0375 mg patch twice weekly

Prevention of osteoporosis in postmenopausal women:

Alora®, Vivelle®, Vivelle-Dot®: Apply 0.025 mg patch twice weekly, increase dose as necessary

Estraderm®: Apply 0.05 mg patch twice weekly

Vaginal cream: Vulvar and vaginal atrophy: Insert 2-4 g/day intravaginally for 2 weeks, then gradually reduce to 1/2 the initial dose for 2 weeks, followed by a maintenance dose of 1 g 1-3 times/week

Vaginal ring:

Postmenopausal vaginal atrophy, urogenital symptoms: Estring®: 2 mg intravaginally; following insertion, ring should remain in place for 90 days

Moderate-to-severe vasomotor symptoms associated with menopause; vulvar/vaginal atrophy: Femring®: 0.05 mg intravaginally; following insertion, ring should remain in place for 3 months; dose may be increased to 0.1 mg if needed

Vaginal tablets: Atrophic vaginitis: Vagifem®: Initial: Insert 1 tablet once daily for 2 weeks; maintenance: Insert 1 tablet twice weekly; attempts to discontinue or taper medication should be made at 3- to 6-month intervals

Dosing adjustment in hepatic impairment:

Mild-to-moderate liver impairment: Dosage reduction of estrogens is recommended

Severe liver impairment: **Not recommended**

Dietary Considerations Ensure adequate calcium and vitamin D intake when used for the prevention of osteoporosis.

Administration

Injection formulation: Intramuscular use only

Emulsion: Apply to clean, dry skin while in a sitting position. Contents of two pouches (total 3.48 g) are to be applied individually, once daily in the morning. Apply contents of first pouch to left thigh; massage into skin of left thigh and calf until thoroughly absorbed (~3 minutes). Apply excess from both hands to the buttocks. Apply contents of second pouch to the right thigh; massage into skin of right thigh and calf until thoroughly absorbed (~3 minutes). Apply excess from both hands to buttocks. Wash hands with soap and water. Allow skin to dry before covering legs with clothing. Do not apply to other areas of body. Do not apply to red or irritated skin.

Gel: Apply to clean, dry, unbroken skin at the same time each day. Allow to dry for 5 minutes prior to dressing. Gel is flammable; avoid fire or flame until dry. After application, wash hands with soap and water. Prior to the first use, pump must be primed. Do not apply gel to breast.

Divigel®: Apply entire contents of packet to right or left upper thigh each day (alternate sites). Do not apply to face, breasts, vaginal area or irritated skin. Apply over an area ~5x7 inches. Do not wash application site for 1 hour. Allow gel to dry before dressing

Elestrin™: Apply to upper arm and shoulder area using two fingers to spread gel. Apply after bath or shower; allow at least 2 hours between applying gel and going swimming. Wait at least 25 minutes before applying sunscreen to application area. Do not apply sunscreen to application area for ≥7 days (may increase absorption of gel).

EstroGel®: Apply gel to the arm, from the wrist to the shoulder. Spread gel as thinly as possible over one arm.

Spray: Evamist™: Prior to first use, prime pump by spraying 3 sprays with the cover on. To administer dose, hold container upright and vertical and rest the plastic cone flat against the skin while spraying. Spray to the inner surface of the forearm, starting near the elbow. If more than one spray is needed, apply to adjacent but not overlapping areas. Apply at the same time each day. Allow spray to dry for ~2 minutes. Do not wash application site for 30 minutes. Apply to clean, dry, unbroken skin. Do not apply to skin other than that of the forearm. Solution contained in the spray is flammable; avoid fire, flame, or smoking until spray has dried. If needed, sunscreen should be applied ~1 hour prior to application of Evamist™.

Transdermal patch: Aerosol topical corticosteroids applied under the patch may reduce allergic reactions. Do not apply transdermal system to breasts, but place on trunk of body (preferably abdomen). Rotate application sites allowing a 1-week interval between applications at a particular site. Do not apply to oily, damaged or irritated skin; avoid waistline or other areas where tight clothing may rub the patch off. Apply patch immediately after removing from protective pouch. In general, if patch falls off, the same patch may be reapplied or a new system may be used for the remainder of the dosing interval. Swimming, bathing or showering are not expected to affect use of the patch. Note the following exceptions:

Estraderm®: Do not apply to an area exposed to direct sunlight.

Menostar®: Swimming, bathing, or wearing patch while in a sauna have not been studied; adhesion of patch may be decreased or delivery of estradiol may be affected. Remove patch slowly after use to avoid skin irritation. If any adhesive remains on the skin after removal, first allow skin to dry for 15 minutes, then gently rub area with an oil-based cream or lotion. If patch falls off, a new patch should be applied for the remainder of the dosing interval.

Vaginal ring: Exact positioning is not critical for efficacy; however, patient should not feel anything once inserted. In case of discomfort, ring should be pushed further into vagina. If ring is expelled prior to 90 days, it may be rinsed off and reinserted.

Vaginal tablet: Insert tablet with supplied applicator at the same time each day. Once inserted, depress plunger until a click is heard, then remove applicator and discard. If tablet comes out of applicator prior to insertion, do not replace; use a new tablet filled applicator instead.

Monitoring Parameters Routine physical examination that includes blood pressure and Papanicolaou smear, breast exam, mammogram. Monitor for signs of endometrial cancer in female patients with uterus. Adequate diagnostic measures, including endometrial sampling, if indicated, should be performed to rule out malignancy in all cases of undiagnosed abnormal vaginal bleeding. Monitor for loss of vision, sudden onset of proptosis, diplopia, migraine; signs and symptoms of thromboembolic disorders; glycemic control in patients with diabetes; lipid profiles in patients being treated for hyperlipidemias; thyroid function in patients on thyroid hormone replacement therapy.

When using Menostar® in a woman with a uterus, endometrial sampling is recommended at yearly intervals or when clinically indicated.

Menopausal symptoms: Assess need for therapy at 3- to 6-month intervals

Prevention of osteoporosis: Bone density measurement

Reference Range

Children: <10 pg/mL (SI: <37 pmol/L)

Male: 10-50 pg/mL (SI: 37-184 pmol/L)

Female:

Premenopausal: 30-400 pg/mL (SI: 110-1468 pmol/L)

Postmenopausal: 0-30 pg/mL (SI: 0-110 pmol/L)

Test Interactions Pathologist should be advised of estrogen/progesterone therapy when specimens are submitted. Reduced response to metyrapone test.

Dosage Forms Excipient information presented when available (limited, particularly for generics); consult specific product labeling. [DSC] = Discontinued product

Cream, vaginal:

Estrace®: 0.1 mg/g (42.5 g)

Emulsion, topical, as hemihydrate:

Estrasorb™: 2.5 mg/g (56s) [each pouch contains 4.35 mg estradiol hemihydrate; contents of two pouches delivers estradiol 0.05 mg/day]

Gel, topical:

Divigel®: 0.1% (0.25 g) [delivers estradiol 0.25 mg/packet]; (0.5 g) [delivers 0.5 mg estradiol/packet]; (1 g) [delivers estradiol 1 mg/packet]

Elestrin™: 0.06% (144 g) [delivers estradiol 0.52 mg/0.87 g; 100 actuations]

EstroGel®: 0.06% (50 g) [delivers estradiol 0.75 mg/1.25 g; 32 actuations; contains ethanol]

Injection, oil, as cypionate:

Depo®-Estradiol: 5 mg/mL (5 mL) [contains chlorobutanol, cottonseed oil]

Injection, oil, as valerate: 10 mg/mL (5 mL); 20 mg/mL (5 mL); 40 mg/mL (5 mL)

Delestrogen®:

10 mg/mL (5 mL) [contains chlorobutanol, sesame oil]

20 mg/mL (5 mL) [contains benzyl alcohol, castor oil]

40 mg/mL (5 mL) [contains benzyl alcohol, castor oil]

Ring, vaginal, as base:

Estring®: 2 mg (1s) [total estradiol 2 mg; releases 7.5 mcg/day over 90 days]

Ring, vaginal, as acetate:

Femring®: 0.05 mg/day (1s) [total estradiol 12.4 mg; releases 0.05 mg/day over 3 months]; 0.1 mg/day (1s) [total estradiol 24.8 mg; releases 0.1 mg/day over 3 months]

Solution, topical [spray]:

Evamist™: 1.53 mg/spray (8.1 mL) [contains 56 sprays after priming; contains ethanol]

Tablet, oral, as acetate:

Femtrace®: 0.45 mg, 0.9 mg, 1.8 mg

Tablet, oral, micronized: 0.5 mg, 1 mg, 2 mg

Estrace®: 0.5 mg, 1 mg, 2 mg [2 mg tablets contain tartrazine]

Gynodiol®: 0.5 mg [DSC], 1 mg [DSC], 1.5 mg [DSC], 2 mg [DSC]

Tablet, vaginal, as base:

Vagifem®: 25 mcg

Transdermal system: 0.025 mg/24 hours (4s) [once-weekly patch]; 0.0375 mg/24 hours (4s) [once-weekly patch]; 0.05 mg/24 hours (4s) [once-weekly patch]; 0.06 mg/24 hours (4s) [once-weekly patch]; 0.075 mg/24 hours [once-weekly patch]; 0.1 mg/24 hours (4s) [once-weekly patch]

Alora® [twice-weekly patch]:

0.025 mg/24 hours (8s) [9 cm^2, total estradiol 0.77 mg]

0.05 mg/24 hours (8s, 24s [DSC]) [18 cm^2, total estradiol 1.5 mg]

0.075 mg/24 hours (8s) [27 cm^2, total estradiol 2.3 mg]

0.1 mg/24 hours (8s) [36 cm^2, total estradiol 3.1 mg]

Climara® [once-weekly patch]:

0.025 mg/24 hours (4s) [6.5 cm^2, total estradiol 2.04 mg]

0.0375 mg/24 hours (4s) [9.375 cm^2, total estradiol 2.85 mg]

0.05 mg/24 hours (4s) [12.5 cm^2, total estradiol 3.8 mg]

0.06 mg/24 hours (4s) [15 cm^2, total estradiol 4.55 mg]

0.075 mg/24 hours (4s) [18.75 cm^2, total estradiol 5.7 mg]

0.1 mg/24 hours (4s) [25 cm^2, total estradiol 7.6 mg]

Estraderm® [twice-weekly patch]:

0.05 mg/24 hours (8s) [10 cm^2, total estradiol 4 mg]

0.1 mg/24 hours (8s) [20 cm^2, total estradiol 8 mg]

Menostar® [once-weekly patch]: 0.014 mg/24 hours (4s) [3.25 cm^2, total estradiol 1 mg]

Vivelle® [twice-weekly patch]:

0.05 mg/24 hours (8s) [14.5 cm^2, total estradiol 4.33 mg] [DSC]

0.1 mg/24 hours (8s) [29 cm^2, total estradiol 8.66 mg] [DSC]

Vivelle-Dot® [twice-weekly patch]:

0.025 mg/day (24s) [2.5 cm^2, total estradiol 0.39 mg]

0.0375 mg/day (24s) [3.75 cm^2, total estradiol 0.585 mg]

0.05 mg/day (24s) [5 cm^2, total estradiol 0.78 mg]
0.075 mg/day (24s) [7.5 cm^2, total estradiol 1.17 mg]
0.1 mg/day (24s) [10 cm^2, total estradiol 1.56 mg]

◆ **Estradiol Acetate** *see* Estradiol *on page* 554

Estradiol and Levonorgestrel
(es tra DYE ole & LEE voe nor jes trel)

U.S. Brand Names ClimaraPro®
Index Terms Levonorgestrel and Estradiol
Pharmacologic Category Estrogen and Progestin Combination
Use Women with an intact uterus: Treatment of moderate-to-severe vasomotor symptoms associated with menopause; prevention of postmenopausal osteoporosis
Medication Safety Issues
Transdermal patch may contain conducting metal (eg, aluminum); remove patch prior to MRI.
Dosage Topical: Adult females with an intact uterus: Treatment of moderate-to-severe vasomotor symptoms associated with menopause or prevention of postmenopausal osteoporosis:
Estradiol 0.045 mg/levonorgestrel 0.015 mg: Apply one patch weekly
Additional Information Complete prescribing information for this medication should be consulted for additional detail.
Dosage Forms Excipient information presented when available (limited, particularly for generics); consult specific product labeling.
Transdermal system: Estradiol 0.045 mg/24 hours and levonorgestrel 0.015 mg/24 hours (4s) [once-weekly patch; 22 cm^2; contains estradiol 4.4 mg and levonorgestrel 1.39 mg]

Estradiol and Norethindrone
(es tra DYE ole & nor eth IN drone)

U.S. Brand Names Activella®; CombiPatch®
Canadian Brand Names Estalis-Sequi®; Estalis®
Index Terms Norethindrone and Estradiol
Pharmacologic Category Estrogen and Progestin Combination
Use Women with an intact uterus:
Tablet: Treatment of moderate-to-severe vasomotor symptoms associated with menopause; treatment of vulvar and vaginal atrophy; prophylaxis for postmenopausal osteoporosis
Transdermal patch: Treatment of moderate-to-severe vasomotor symptoms associated with menopause; treatment of vulvar and vaginal atrophy; treatment of hypoestrogenism due to hypogonadism, castration, or primary ovarian failure
Medication Safety Issues
Transdermal patch may contain conducting metal (eg, aluminum); remove patch prior to MRI.
Dosage Note: Patients should be treated with the lowest effective dose and for the shortest duration, consistent with treatment goals. Adults:
Oral (Activella®): One tablet daily
Transdermal patch (CombiPatch®):
Continuous combined regimen: Apply 1 patch twice weekly
Continuous sequential regimen: Apply estradiol-only patch for first 14 days of cycle, followed by one CombiPatch® applied twice weekly for the remaining 14 days of a 28-day cycle
Transdermal patch, combination pack (product-specific dosing for Canadian formulation):
Estalis®: Continuous combined regimen: Apply a new patch twice weekly during a 28-day cycle
Estalis-Sequi®: Continuous sequential regimen: Apply estradiol-only patch (Vivelle®) for first 14 days, followed by one Estalis® patch applied twice weekly during the last 14 days of a 28-day cycle
Note: In women previously receiving oral estrogens, initiate upon reappearance of menopausal symptoms following discontinuation of oral therapy.
Additional Information Complete prescribing information for this medication should be consulted for additional detail.
Dosage Forms Excipient information presented when available (limited, particularly for generics); consult specific product labeling.
Combination pack:
Estalis-Sequi® 140/50 [CAN; not available in U.S.]:
Transdermal system (Vivelle®): Estradiol 50 mcg per day (4s) [14.5 sq cm; total estradiol 4.33 mg]
Transdermal system (Estalis®): Norethindrone acetate 140 mcg and estradiol 50 mcg per day (4s) [9 sq cm; total norethindrone acetate 2.7 mg, total estradiol 0.62 mg; not available in U.S.]
Estalis-Sequi® 250/50 [CAN; not available in U.S.]:
Transdermal system (Vivelle®): Estradiol 50 mcg per day (4s) [14.5 sq cm; total estradiol 4.33 mg]
Transdermal system (Estalis®): Norethindrone acetate 250 mcg and estradiol 50 mcg per day (4s) [16 sq cm; total norethindrone acetate 4.8 mg, total estradiol 0.51 mg; not available in U.S.]
Tablet:
Activella® 0.5/0.1: Estradiol 0.5 mg and norethindrone acetate 0.1mg (28s)
Activella® 1/0.5: Estradiol 1 mg and norethindrone acetate 0.5 mg (28s)
Transdermal system:
CombiPatch®:
0.05/0.14: Estradiol 0.05 mg and norethindrone acetate 0.14 mg per day (8s) [9 sq cm]
0.05/0.25: Estradiol 0.05 mg and norethindrone acetate 0.25 mg per day (8s) [16 sq cm]
Estalis® [CAN]:
140/50: Norethindrone acetate 140 mcg and estradiol 50 mcg per day (8s) [9 sq cm; total norethindrone acetate 2.7 mg, total estradiol 0.62 mg; not available in U.S.]
250/50 Norethindrone acetate 250 mcg and estradiol 50 mcg per day (8s) [16 sq cm; total norethindrone acetate 4.8 mg, total estradiol 0.51 mg; not available in U.S.]

◆ **Estradiol Cypionate** *see* Estradiol *on page* 554
◆ **Estradiol Hemihydrate** *see* Estradiol *on page* 554
◆ **Estradiol Transdermal** *see* Estradiol *on page* 554
◆ **Estradiol Valerate** *see* Estradiol *on page* 554
◆ **Estradot® (Can)** *see* Estradiol *on page* 554

Estramustine (es tra MUS teen)

U.S. Brand Names Emcyt®
Canadian Brand Names Emcyt®
Index Terms Estramustine Phosphate; Estramustine Phosphate Sodium; NSC-89199
Pharmacologic Category Antineoplastic Agent, Alkylating Agent; Antineoplastic Agent, Hormone; Antineoplastic Agent, Hormone (Estrogen/Nitrogen Mustard)
Use Palliative treatment of progressive or metastatic prostate cancer
Pregnancy Considerations Estramustine is not indicated for use in women. Men who were impotent on estrogen therapy have regained potency while taking estramustine; effective contraception should be used for male patients with partners of childbearing potential.

Medication Safety Issues

Sound-alike/look-alike issues:

Emcyt® may be confused with Eryc®

Estramustine may be confused with exemestane.

High alert medication: The Institute for Safe Medication Practices (ISMP) includes this medication among its list of drug classes which have a heightened risk of causing significant patient harm when used in error.

Contraindications Hypersensitivity to estramustine, estradiol, nitrogen mustard, or any component of the formulation; active thrombophlebitis or thromboembolic disorders (except where tumor mass is the cause of thromboembolic disorder and the benefit may outweigh the risk)

Canadian labeling: Additional contraindications (not in the U.S. labeling): Severe hepatic or cardiac disease

Warnings/Precautions Hazardous agent - use appropriate precautions for handling and disposal. Glucose tolerance may be decreased; use with caution in patients with diabetes. Elevated blood pressure, peripheral edema (new-onset or exacerbation), or congestive heart disease may occur; use with caution in patients where fluid accumulation may be poorly tolerated, including cardiovascular disease (HF or hypertension), migraine, seizure disorder or renal dysfunction. Estrogen treatment for prostate cancer is associated with an increased risk of thrombosis and MI; use caution with history of cardiovascular disease (eg, thrombophlebitis, thrombosis, or thromboembolic disease) and cerebrovascular or coronary artery disease. Use with caution in patients with hepatic impairment (may be metabolized poorly) or with metabolic bone diseases. Allergic reactions and angioedema, including airway involvement, have been reported with use. Patients with prostate cancer and osteoblastic metastases should have their calcium monitored regularly. Estrogen use may cause gynecomastia and/or impotence. Avoid vaccination with live vaccines during treatment (risk of infection may be increased due to immunosuppression). Although the response to vaccines may be diminished, inactivated vaccines may be administered during treatment.

Adverse Reactions

>10%:

Cardiovascular: Edema (20%)

Endocrine & metabolic: Gynecomastia (75%), breast tenderness (71%), libido decreased

Gastrointestinal: Nausea (16%), diarrhea (13%), gastrointestinal upset (12%)

Hepatic: LDH increased (2% to 33%), AST increased (2% to 33%)

Respiratory: Dyspnea (12%)

1% to 10%:

Cardiovascular: CHF (3%), MI (3%), cerebrovascular accident (2%), chest pain (1%), flushing (1%)

Central nervous system: Lethargy (4%), insomnia (3%), emotional lability (2%), anxiety (1%), headache (1%)

Dermatologic: Bruising (3%), dry skin (2%), pruritus (2%), hair thinning (1%), rash (1%), skin peeling (1%)

Gastrointestinal: Anorexia (4%), flatulence (2%), burning throat (1%), gastrointestinal bleeding (1%), thirst (1%), vomiting (1%)

Hematologic: Leukopenia (4%), thrombocytopenia (1%)

Hepatic: Bilirubin increased (1% to 2%)

Local: Thrombophlebitis (3%)

Neuromuscular & skeletal: Leg cramps (9%)

Ocular: Tearing (1%)

Respiratory: Pulmonary embolism (2%), upper respiratory discharge (1%), hoarseness (1%)

<1% (Limited to important or life-threatening): Allergic reactions, anemia, angina, angioedema, cerebrovascular ischemia, confusion, coronary ischemia, depression, glucose tolerance decreased, hyper-/hypocalcemia, hypertension, impotence, muscle weakness, venous thrombosis

Drug Interactions

Avoid Concomitant Use

Avoid concomitant use of Estramustine with any of the following: Natalizumab; Vaccines (Live)

Increased Effect/Toxicity

Estramustine may increase the levels/effects of: Natalizumab; Vaccines (Live)

The levels/effects of Estramustine may be increased by: Clodronate; Trastuzumab

Decreased Effect

Estramustine may decrease the levels/effects of: Vaccines (Inactivated)

The levels/effects of Estramustine may be decreased by: Calcium Salts; Echinacea

Ethanol/Nutrition/Herb Interactions Food: Estramustine serum levels may be decreased if taken with milk and other dairy products, calcium supplements, and vitamins containing calcium.

Stability Refrigerate at 2°C to 8°C (36°F to 46°F).

Mechanism of Action Combines the effects of estradiol and nitrogen mustard. It appears to bind to microtubule proteins, preventing normal tubulin function. The antitumor effect may be due solely to an estrogenic effect. Estramustine causes a marked decrease in plasma testosterone and an increase in estrogen levels.

Pharmacodynamics/Kinetics

Absorption: Oral: 75%

Metabolism:

GI tract: Initial dephosphorylation

Hepatic: Oxidation and hydrolysis; metabolites include estramustine, estrone analog, estrone, and estradiol

Half-life elimination: Terminal: 15-24 hours

Time to peak, serum: 2-3 hours

Excretion: Feces (2.9% to 4.8% as unchanged drug)

Dosage Details concerning dosing in combination regimens should also be consulted.

Oral: Adults: Males: Prostate cancer: 14 mg/kg/day (range: 10-16 mg/kg/day) in 3 or 4 divided doses

Combination therapy with docetaxel (unlabeled dose): 280 mg 3 times/day for 5 days (days 1 through 5) of a 21-day treatment cycle for up to 12 cycles (Petrylak, 2004)

Dietary Considerations Should be taken at least 1 hour before or 2 hours after eating. Milk products and calcium-rich foods or supplements may impair the oral absorption of estramustine phosphate sodium.

Administration Administer on an empty stomach, at least 1 hour before or 2 hours after eating.

Monitoring Parameters Serum calcium, liver function tests; blood pressure

Dosage Forms Excipient information presented when available (limited, particularly for generics); consult specific product labeling.

Capsule, as phosphate sodium:

Emcyt®: 140 mg

- **Estramustine Phosphate** *see* Estramustine *on page* *558*
- **Estramustine Phosphate Sodium** *see* Estramustine *on page* *558*
- **Estrasorb™** *see* Estradiol *on page* *554*
- **Estratab® (Can)** *see* Estrogens (Esterified) *on page* *566*
- **Estratest®** *see* Estrogens (Esterified) and Methyltestosterone *on page* *568*
- **Estratest® H.S.** *see* Estrogens (Esterified) and Methyltestosterone *on page* *568*
- **Estring®** *see* Estradiol *on page* *554*
- **EstroGel®** *see* Estradiol *on page* *554*

◆ **Estrogenic Substances, Conjugated** *see* Estrogens (Conjugated/Equine) *on page 563*

Estrogens (Conjugated A/Synthetic)

(ES troe jenz, KON joo gate ed, aye, sin THET ik)

U.S. Brand Names Cenestin®

Canadian Brand Names Cenestin

Pharmacologic Category Estrogen Derivative

Use Treatment of moderate-to-severe vasomotor symptoms of menopause; treatment of vulvar and vaginal atrophy

Pregnancy Considerations Use during pregnancy is contraindicated.

Lactation Enters breast milk/use caution

Medication Safety Issues

Sound-alike/look-alike issues:

Cenestin® may be confused with Senexon®

International issues:

Cenestin® may be confused with Canesten® which is a brand name for clotrimazole in multiple international markets and a brand name for fluconazole in Great Britain

Contraindications Hypersensitivity to estrogens or any component of the formulation; undiagnosed abnormal vaginal bleeding; history of or current thrombophlebitis or venous thromboembolic disorders (including DVT, PE); active or recent (within 1 year) arterial thromboembolic disease (eg, stroke, MI); carcinoma of the breast; estrogen-dependent tumor; hepatic dysfunction or disease; pregnancy

Warnings/Precautions

Cardiovascular-related considerations: **[U.S. Boxed Warning]: Estrogens with or without progestin should not be used to prevent coronary heart disease.** Use caution with cardiovascular disease or dysfunction. May increase the risks of hypertension, myocardial infarction (MI), stroke, pulmonary emboli (PE), and deep vein thrombosis; incidence of these effects was shown to be significantly increased in postmenopausal women using conjugated equine estrogens (CEE) in combination with medroxyprogesterone acetate (MPA). Nonfatal MI, PE, and thrombophlebitis have also been reported in males taking high doses of CEE (eg, for prostate cancer). Estrogen compounds are generally associated with lipid effects such as increased HDL-cholesterol and decreased LDL-cholesterol. Triglycerides may also be increased; use with caution in patients with familial defects of lipoprotein metabolism. Whenever possible, estrogens should be discontinued at least 4 weeks prior to and for 2 weeks following elective surgery associated with an increased risk of thromboembolism or during periods of prolonged immobilization.

Neurological considerations: **[U.S. Boxed Warning]: The risk of dementia may be increased in postmenopausal women;** increased incidence was observed in women ≥65 years of age taking CEE alone or in combination with MPA.

Cancer-related considerations: **[U.S. Boxed Warning]: Unopposed estrogens may increase the risk of endometrial carcinoma in postmenopausal women.** Estrogens may exacerbate endometriosis. Malignant transformation of residual endometrial implants has been reported posthysterectomy with estrogen only therapy. Consider adding a progestin in women with residual endometriosis posthysterectomy. Estrogens may increase the risk of breast cancer. An increased risk of invasive breast cancer was observed in postmenopausal women using CEE in combination with MPA; a smaller increase in risk was seen with estrogen therapy alone in observational studies. An increase in abnormal mammograms has also been reported with estrogen and progestin therapy. Estrogen use may lead to severe hypercalcemia in patients with breast cancer and bone metastases; discontinue estrogen if hypercalcemia occurs.

Estrogens may cause retinal vascular thrombosis; discontinue permanently if papilledema or retinal vascular lesions are observed on examination. Use with caution in patients with diseases which may be exacerbated by fluid retention, including asthma, epilepsy, migraine, diabetes or renal dysfunction. Use with caution in patients with a history of severe hypocalcemia, SLE, hepatic hemangiomas, porphyria, endometriosis, and gallbladder disease. Use caution with history of cholestatic jaundice associated with past estrogen use or pregnancy. Safety and efficacy in pediatric patients have not been established. Prior to puberty, estrogens may cause premature closure of the epiphyses, premature breast development in girls or gynecomastia in boys. Vaginal bleeding and vaginal cornification may also be induced in girls.

Before prescribing estrogen therapy to postmenopausal women, the risks and benefits must be weighed for each patient. Women should be informed of these risks and benefits, as well as possible effects of progestin when added to estrogen therapy. Estrogens with or without progestin should be used for shortest duration possible consistent with treatment goals. Conduct periodic risk: benefit assessments.

When used solely for prevention of osteoporosis in women at significant risk, nonestrogen treatment options should be considered. When used solely for the treatment of vulvar and vaginal atrophy, topical vaginal products should be considered.

Adverse Reactions

>10%:

- Central nervous system: Headache (11% to 68%), dizziness (11%), pain (11%)
- Endocrine & metabolic: Breast pain (29%), endometrial thickening (19%), metrorrhagia (14%)
- Gastrointestinal: Abdominal pain (9% to 28%), nausea (9% to 18%)
- Neuromuscular & skeletal: Paresthesia (8% to 33%), back pain (14%)
- Respiratory: Upper respiratory tract infection (13%)
- Miscellaneous: Infection (2% to 14%)

1% to 10%:

- Central nervous system: Anxiety (6%), fever (1%)
- Gastrointestinal: Dyspepsia (10%), vomiting (7%), constipation (6%), diarrhea (6%), weight gain (6%)
- Genitourinary: Vaginitis (8%)
- Neuromuscular & skeletal: Leg cramps (10%), hypertonia (6%)
- Respiratory: Rhinitis (6% to 8%), cough (6%)

In addition, the following have been reported with estrogen and/or progestin therapy:

- Cardiovascular: Edema, hypertension, MI, stroke, venous thromboembolism
- Central nervous system: Epilepsy exacerbation, irritability, mental depression, migraine, mood disturbances, nervousness
- Dermatologic: Angioedema, chloasma, erythema multiforme, erythema nodosum, hemorrhagic eruption, hirsutism, melasma, pruritus, rash, scalp hair loss, urticaria
- Endocrine & metabolic: Breast cancer, breast enlargement, breast tenderness, glucose tolerance impaired, HDL-cholesterol increased, hyper-/hypocalcemia, LDL-cholesterol decreased, libido changes, serum triglycerides/phospholipids increased, thyroid-binding globulin increased, total thyroid hormone (T_4) increased
- Gastrointestinal: Abdominal cramps, bloating, cholecystitis, cholelithiasis, gallbladder disease, pancreatitis, weight gain/loss

Genitourinary: Alterations in frequency and flow of menses, cervical secretion changes, endometrial cancer, endometrial hyperplasia, uterine leiomyomata size increased, vaginal candidiasis

Hematologic: Aggravation of porphyria, antithrombin III and antifactor Xa decreased, fibrinogen levels increased, platelet aggregability and platelet count increased; prothrombin and factors VII, VIII, IX, X increased

Hepatic: Cholestatic jaundice, hepatic hemangiomas enlarged

Neuromuscular & skeletal: Arthralgias, chorea, leg cramps

Local: Thrombophlebitis

Ocular: Contact lens intolerance, corneal curvature steepening, retinal vascular thrombosis

Respiratory: Asthma exacerbation, pulmonary thromboembolism

Miscellaneous: Anaphylactoid/anaphylactic reactions, carbohydrate intolerance

Drug Interactions

Metabolism/Transport Effects Based on estradiol and estrone: **Substrate** of CYP1A2 (major), 2A6 (minor), 2B6 (minor), 2C9 (minor), 2C19 (minor), 2D6 (minor), 2E1 (minor), 3A4 (major); **Inhibits** CYP1A2 (weak); **Induces** CYP3A4 (weak)

Avoid Concomitant Use There are no known interactions where it is recommended to avoid concomitant use.

Increased Effect/Toxicity

Estrogens (Conjugated A/Synthetic) may increase the levels/effects of: Corticosteroids (Systemic); Ropinirole; Tipranavir

The levels/effects of Estrogens (Conjugated A/Synthetic) may be increased by: Herbs (Estrogenic Properties)

Decreased Effect

Estrogens (Conjugated A/Synthetic) may decrease the levels/effects of: Maraviroc; Somatropin; Thyroid Products

The levels/effects of Estrogens (Conjugated A/Synthetic) may be decreased by: CYP1A2 Inducers (Strong); CYP3A4 Inducers (Strong); Deferasirox; Herbs (CYP3A4 Inducers); Tipranavir

Ethanol/Nutrition/Herb Interactions

Ethanol: Avoid ethanol (routine use increases estrogen level and risk of breast cancer).

Food: Grapefruit juice may increase estrogen levels, leading to increased adverse effects.

Herb/Nutraceutical: St John's wort may decrease levels. Herbs with estrogenic properties may enhance the adverse/toxic effect of estrogen derivatives; examples include alfalfa, black cohosh, bloodroot, hops, kudzu, licorice, red clover, saw palmetto, soybean, thyme, wild yam, yucca.

Stability Store at room temperature of 25°C (77°F).

Mechanism of Action Conjugated A/synthetic estrogens contain a mixture of 9 synthetic estrogen substances, including sodium estrone sulfate, sodium equilin sulfate, sodium 17 alpha-dihydroequilin, sodium 17 alpha-estradiol and sodium 17 beta-dihydroequilin. Estrogens are responsible for the development and maintenance of the female reproductive system and secondary sexual characteristics. Estradiol is the principle intracellular human estrogen and is more potent than estrone and estriol at the receptor level; it is the primary estrogen secreted prior to menopause. Following menopause, estrone and estrone sulfate are more highly produced. Estrogens modulate the pituitary secretion of gonadotropins, luteinizing hormone, and follicle-stimulating hormone through a negative feedback system; estrogen replacement reduces elevated levels of these hormones in postmenopausal women.

Pharmacodynamics/Kinetics

Absorption: Well absorbed over a period of several hours

Protein-binding: Sex hormone-binding globulin (SHBG) and albumin

Metabolism: Hepatic via CYP3A4; estradiol is converted to estrone and estriol; also undergoes enterohepatic recirculation; estrone sulfate is the main metabolite in postmenopausal women

Excretion: Urine (primarily estriol, also as estradiol, estrone, and conjugates)

Dosage The lowest dose that will control symptoms should be used; medication should be discontinued as soon as possible. Oral:

Adults:

Moderate-to-severe vasomotor symptoms: 0.45 mg/day; may be titrated up to 1.25 mg/day. Attempts to discontinue medication should be made at 3- to 6-month intervals.

Vulvar and vaginal atrophy: 0.3 mg/day

Elderly: Refer to adult dosing. A higher incidence of stroke and invasive breast cancer were observed in women >75 years in a WHI substudy using conjugated equine estrogen.

Monitoring Parameters Yearly physical examination that includes blood pressure and Papanicolaou smear, breast exam, mammogram. Monitor for signs of endometrial cancer in female patients with uterus. Adequate diagnostic measures, including endometrial sampling, if indicated, should be performed to rule out malignancy in all cases of undiagnosed abnormal vaginal bleeding. Monitor for loss of vision, sudden onset of proptosis, diplopia, migraine; signs and symptoms of thromboembolic disorders; glycemic control in patients with diabetes; lipid profiles in patients being treated for hyperlipidemias; thyroid function in patients on thyroid hormone replacement therapy.

Menopausal symptoms: Assess need for therapy at 3- to 6-month intervals

Test Interactions Pathologist should be advised of estrogen/progesterone therapy when specimens are submitted. Reduced response to metyrapone test observed with conjugated estrogens (equine).

Additional Information Not biologically equivalent to conjugated estrogens from equine source. Contains 9 unique estrogenic compounds (equine source contains at least 10 active estrogenic compounds).

Dosage Forms Excipient information presented when available (limited, particularly for generics); consult specific product labeling.

Tablet: 0.3 mg, 0.45 mg, 0.625 mg, 0.9 mg, 1.25 mg

Estrogens (Conjugated B/Synthetic)

(ES troe jenz, KON joo gate ed, bee, sin THET ik)

U.S. Brand Names Enjuvia™

Pharmacologic Category Estrogen Derivative

Use Treatment of moderate-to-severe vasomotor symptoms of menopause; treatment of vulvar and vaginal atrophy associated with menopause; treatment of moderate-to-severe vaginal dryness and pain with intercourse associated with menopause

Pregnancy Considerations Use during pregnancy is contraindicated.

Lactation Enters breast milk/use caution

Contraindications Hypersensitivity to estrogens or any component of the formulation; undiagnosed abnormal vaginal bleeding; history of or current thrombophlebitis or venous thromboembolic disorders (including DVT, PE); active or recent (within 1 year) arterial thromboembolic disease (eg, stroke, MI); carcinoma of the breast; estrogen-dependent tumor; hepatic dysfunction or disease; pregnancy

Warnings/Precautions

Cardiovascular-related considerations: **[U.S. Boxed Warning]: Estrogens with or without progestin should not be used to prevent coronary heart disease.** Use caution with cardiovascular disease or dysfunction. May increase the risks of hypertension, myocardial infarction (MI), stroke, pulmonary emboli (PE), and deep vein thrombosis; incidence of these effects was shown to be significantly increased in postmenopausal women using conjugated equine estrogens (CEE) in combination with medroxyprogesterone acetate (MPA). Nonfatal MI, PE, and thrombophlebitis have also been reported in males taking high doses of CEE (eg, for prostate cancer). Estrogen compounds are generally associated with lipid effects such as increased HDL-cholesterol and decreased LDL-cholesterol. Triglycerides may also be increased; use with caution in patients with familial defects of lipoprotein metabolism. Whenever possible, estrogens should be discontinued at least 4 weeks prior to and for 2 weeks following elective surgery associated with an increased risk of thromboembolism or during periods of prolonged immobilization.

Neurological considerations: **[U.S. Boxed Warning]: The risk of dementia may be increased in postmenopausal women;** increased incidence was observed in women ≥65 years of age taking CEE alone or in combination with MPA.

Cancer-related considerations: **[U.S. Boxed Warning]: Unopposed estrogens may increase the risk of endometrial carcinoma in postmenopausal women.** Estrogens may exacerbate endometriosis. Malignant transformation of residual endometrial implants has been reported posthysterectomy with estrogen only therapy. Consider adding a progestin in women with residual endometriosis posthysterectomy. Estrogens may increase the risk of breast cancer. An increased risk of invasive breast cancer was observed in postmenopausal women using CEE in combination with MPA; a smaller increase in risk was seen with estrogen therapy alone in observational studies. An increase in abnormal mammograms has also been reported with estrogen and progestin therapy. Estrogen use may lead to severe hypercalcemia in patients with breast cancer and bone metastases; discontinue estrogen if hypercalcemia occurs.

Estrogens may cause retinal vascular thrombosis; discontinue permanently if papilledema or retinal vascular lesions are observed on examination. Use with caution in patients with diseases which may be exacerbated by fluid retention, including asthma, epilepsy, migraine, diabetes or renal dysfunction. Use with caution in patients with a history of severe hypocalcemia, SLE, hepatic hemangiomas, porphyria, endometriosis, and gallbladder disease. Use caution with history of cholestatic jaundice associated with past estrogen use or pregnancy. Safety and efficacy in pediatric patients have not been established. Prior to puberty, estrogens may cause premature closure of the epiphyses, premature breast development in girls or gynecomastia in boys. Vaginal bleeding and vaginal cornification may also be induced in girls.

Before prescribing estrogen therapy to postmenopausal women, the risks and benefits must be weighed for each patient. Women should be informed of these risks and benefits, as well as possible effects of progestin when added to estrogen therapy. Estrogens with or without progestin should be used for shortest duration possible consistent with treatment goals. Conduct periodic risk: benefit assessments. When used solely for the treatment of vaginal dryness and pain with intercourse, or vulvar and vaginal atrophy, topical vaginal products should be considered.

Adverse Reactions

>10%:

- Central nervous system: Headache (15% to 25%), pain (10% to 19%)
- Endocrine & metabolic: Breast pain (up to 14%)
- Gastrointestinal: Abdominal pain (4% to 15%), nausea (7% to 12%)

1% to 10%:

- Central nervous system: Dizziness (1% to 7%)
- Endocrine & metabolic: Dysmenorrhea (1% to 8%)
- Gastrointestinal: Flatulence (4% to 7%)
- Genitourinary: Vaginitis (2% to 7%)
- Neuromuscular & skeletal: Paresthesia (up to 6%)
- Respiratory: Bronchitis (up to 7%), rhinitis (4% to 7%), sinusitis (3% to 7%)
- Miscellaneous: Flu-like syndrome (4% to 7%)

In addition, the following have been reported with estrogen and/or progestin therapy:

- Cardiovascular: Edema, hypertension, MI, stroke, venous thromboembolism
- Central nervous system: Epilepsy exacerbation, irritability, mental depression, migraine, mood disturbances, nervousness
- Dermatologic: Angioedema, chloasma, erythema multiforme, erythema nodosum, hemorrhagic eruption, hirsutism, loss of scalp hair, melasma, pruritus, rash, urticaria
- Endocrine & metabolic: Breast cancer, breast enlargement, breast tenderness, HDL-cholesterol increased, hyper-/hypocalcemia, impaired glucose tolerance, LDL-cholesterol decreased, libido (changes in), serum triglycerides/phospholipids increased, thyroid-binding globulin increased, total thyroid hormone (T_4) increased
- Gastrointestinal: Abdominal cramps, bloating, cholecystitis, cholelithiasis, gallbladder disease, pancreatitis, weight gain/loss
- Genitourinary: Alterations in frequency and flow of menses, changes in cervical secretions, endometrial cancer, endometrial hyperplasia, increased size of uterine leiomyomata, vaginal candidiasis
- Hematologic: Aggravation of porphyria; antithrombin III and antifactor Xa decreased; fibrinogen levels increased; platelet aggregability and platelet count increased; prothrombin and factors VII, VIII, IX, X increased
- Hepatic: Cholestatic jaundice, hepatic hemangiomas enlarged
- Local: Thrombophlebitis
- Neuromuscular & skeletal: Arthralgias, chorea, leg cramps
- Ocular: Contact lens intolerance, corneal curvature steepening, retinal vascular thrombosis
- Respiratory: Asthma exacerbation, pulmonary thromboembolism
- Miscellaneous: Anaphylactoid/anaphylactic reactions, carbohydrate intolerance

Drug Interactions

Metabolism/Transport Effects Based on estradiol and estrone: **Substrate** of CYP1A2 (major), 2A6 (minor), 2B6 (minor), 2C9 (minor), 2C19 (minor), 2D6 (minor), 2E1 (minor), 3A4 (major); **Inhibits** CYP1A2 (weak); **Induces** CYP3A4 (weak)

Avoid Concomitant Use There are no known interactions where it is recommended to avoid concomitant use.

Increased Effect/Toxicity

Estrogens (Conjugated B/Synthetic) may increase the levels/effects of: Corticosteroids (Systemic); Ropinirole; Tipranavir

The levels/effects of Estrogens (Conjugated B/Synthetic) may be increased by: Herbs (Estrogenic Properties)

Decreased Effect

Estrogens (Conjugated B/Synthetic) may decrease the levels/effects of: Somatropin; Thyroid Products

The levels/effects of Estrogens (Conjugated B/Synthetic) may be decreased by: CYP3A4 Inducers (Strong); Deferasirox; Herbs (CYP3A4 Inducers); Tipranavir

Ethanol/Nutrition/Herb Interactions

Ethanol: Avoid ethanol (routine use increases estrogen level and risk of breast cancer).

Food: Grapefruit juice may increase estrogen levels, leading to increased adverse effects.

Herb/Nutraceutical: St John's wort may decrease levels. Herbs with estrogenic properties may enhance the adverse/toxic effect of estrogen derivatives; examples include alfalfa, black cohosh, bloodroot, hops, kudzu, licorice, red clover, saw palmetto, soybean, thyme, wild yam, and yucca.

Stability Store at room temperature of 25°C (77°F).

Mechanism of Action Conjugated B/synthetic estrogens contain a mixture of 10 synthetic estrogen substances, including sodium estrone sulfate, sodium equilin sulfate, sodium 17-alpha-dihydroequilin, sodium 17-alpha-estradiol, and sodium 17-beta-dihydroequilin. Estrogens are responsible for the development and maintenance of the female reproductive system and secondary sexual characteristics. Estradiol is the principle intracellular human estrogen and is more potent than estrone and estriol at the receptor level; it is the primary estrogen secreted prior to menopause. Following menopause, estrone and estrone sulfate are more highly produced. Estrogens modulate the pituitary secretion of gonadotropins, luteinizing hormone, and follicle-stimulating hormone through a negative feedback system; estrogen replacement reduces elevated levels of these hormones in postmenopausal women.

Pharmacodynamics/Kinetics

Absorption: Well absorbed over a period of several hours

Protein-binding: Sex hormone-binding globulin (SHBG) and albumin

Metabolism: Hepatic via CYP3A4; estradiol is converted to estrone and estriol; also undergoes enterohepatic recirculation; estrone sulfate is the main metabolite in postmenopausal women

Half-life elimination: Conjugated estrone: 8-20 hours; conjugated equilin: 5-17 hours

Excretion: Urine (primarily estriol, also as estradiol, estrone, and conjugates)

Dosage The lowest dose that will control symptoms should be used; medication should be discontinued as soon as possible. Oral:

Adults:

Moderate-to-severe vasomotor symptoms associated with menopause: 0.3 mg/day; may be titrated up to 1.25 mg/day. Attempts to discontinue medication should be made at 3- to 6-month intervals.

Vaginal dryness/vulvar and vaginal atrophy associated with menopause: 0.3 mg/day. Attempts to discontinue medication should be made at 3- to 6-month intervals.

Elderly: A higher incidence of stroke and invasive breast cancer were observed in women >75 years in a WHI substudy using conjugated equine estrogen.

Monitoring Parameters Yearly physical examination that may include blood pressure and Papanicolaou smear, breast exam, mammogram. Monitor for signs of endometrial cancer in female patients with uterus. Adequate diagnostic measures, including endometrial sampling, if indicated, should be performed to rule out malignancy in all cases of undiagnosed abnormal vaginal bleeding. Monitor for loss of vision, sudden onset of proptosis, diplopia, migraine; signs and symptoms of thromboembolic disorders; glycemic control in patients with diabetes; lipid profiles in patients being treated for hyperlipidemias; thyroid function in patients on thyroid hormone replacement therapy.

Test Interactions Pathologist should be advised of estrogen/progesterone therapy when specimens are submitted. Reduced response to metyrapone test observed with conjugated estrogens (equine).

Additional Information Not biologically equivalent to conjugated estrogens from equine source. Contains 10 unique estrogenic compounds (equine source contains at least 10 active estrogenic compounds).

Dosage Forms Excipient information presented when available (limited, particularly for generics); consult specific product labeling.

Tablet:

Enjuvia™: 0.3 mg, 0.45 mg, 0.625 mg, 0.9 mg, 1.25 mg

Estrogens (Conjugated/Equine)

(ES troe jenz KON joo gate ed, EE kwine)

U.S. Brand Names Premarin®

Canadian Brand Names C.E.S.®; Premarin®

Index Terms C.E.S.; CE; CEE; Conjugated Estrogen; Estrogenic Substances, Conjugated

Pharmacologic Category Estrogen Derivative

Use Treatment of moderate-to-severe vasomotor symptoms associated with menopause; treatment of vulvar and vaginal atrophy; hypoestrogenism (due to hypogonadism, castration, or primary ovarian failure); prostatic cancer (palliation); breast cancer (palliation); osteoporosis (prophylaxis, postmenopausal women at significant risk only); abnormal uterine bleeding; moderate-to-severe dyspareunia (pain during intercourse) due to vaginal/vulvar atrophy of menopause

Unlabeled/Investigational Use Uremic bleeding

Pregnancy Considerations Estrogens are not indicated for use during pregnancy or immediately postpartum. In general, the use of estrogen and progestin as in combination hormonal contraceptives have not been associated with teratogenic effects when inadvertently taken early in pregnancy. These products are contraindicated for use during pregnancy. Use of the vaginal cream may weaken latex found in condoms, diaphragms or cervical caps.

Lactation Enters breast milk/use caution

Medication Safety Issues

Sound-alike/look-alike issues:

Premarin® may be confused with Primaxin®, Provera®, Remeron®

Contraindications Hypersensitivity to estrogens or any component of the formulation; undiagnosed abnormal vaginal bleeding; history of or current thrombophlebitis or venous thromboembolic disorders (including DVT, PE); active or recent (within 1 year) arterial thromboembolic disease (eg, stroke, MI); carcinoma of the breast (except in appropriately selected patients being treated for metastatic disease); estrogen-dependent tumor; hepatic dysfunction or disease; pregnancy

Warnings/Precautions

Cardiovascular-related considerations: **[U.S. Boxed Warning]: Estrogens with or without progestin should not be used to prevent cardiovascular disease.** Use caution with cardiovascular disease or dysfunction. May increase the risks of hypertension, myocardial infarction (MI), stroke, pulmonary emboli (PE), and deep vein thrombosis; incidence of these effects was shown to be significantly increased in postmenopausal women using conjugated estrogens (CE) alone or in combination with medroxyprogesterone acetate (MPA). Nonfatal MI, PE, and thrombophlebitis have also been reported in males taking high doses of CE (eg, for prostate cancer). Estrogen compounds are generally associated with lipid effects such as increased HDL-cholesterol and decreased LDL-cholesterol. Triglycerides may also be increased; use with caution in patients with familial defects of lipoprotein metabolism. Whenever possible, estrogens should be discontinued at least 4 weeks prior to and for 2 weeks following elective surgery associated with an increased risk of thromboembolism or during periods of prolonged immobilization.

Neurological considerations: **[U.S. Boxed Warning]: The risk of dementia may be increased in postmenopausal women;** increased incidence was observed in women ≥65 years of age taking CE alone or in combination with MPA.

Cancer-related considerations: **[U.S. Boxed Warning]: Adequate diagnostic measures, including endometrial sampling, if indicated, should be performed to rule out malignancy in all cases of undiagnosed abnormal vaginal bleeding. Unopposed estrogens may increase the risk of endometrial carcinoma in postmenopausal women with an intact uterus.** Risk appears to be associated with long-term use The use of a progestin should be considered when administering estrogens to postmenopausal women with an intact uterus. Estrogens may exacerbate endometriosis. Malignant transformation of residual endometrial implants has been reported posthysterectomy with estrogen only therapy. Consider adding a progestin in women with residual endometriosis posthysterectomy. Presentation of irregular, unresolving vaginal bleeding warrants further evaluation including endometrial sampling, if indicated, to rule out malignancy. Estrogens may increase the risk of breast cancer. An increased risk of invasive breast cancer was observed in postmenopausal women using CE in combination with MPA; a smaller increase in risk was seen with estrogen therapy alone in observational studies. An increase in abnormal mammograms has also been reported with estrogen and progestin therapy. Estrogen use may lead to severe hypercalcemia in patients with breast cancer and bone metastases; discontinue estrogen if hypercalcemia occurs.

Estrogens may cause retinal vascular thrombosis; discontinue permanently if papilledema or retinal vascular lesions are observed on examination. Use with caution in patients with diseases which may be exacerbated by fluid retention, including asthma, epilepsy, migraine, diabetes, heart failure, or renal dysfunction. Use with caution in patients with a history of severe hypocalcemia, SLE, hepatic hemangiomas, porphyria, endometriosis, and gallbladder disease. Use caution with history of cholestatic jaundice associated with past estrogen use or pregnancy. Safety and efficacy in pediatric patients have not been established. Prior to puberty, estrogens may cause premature closure of the epiphyses, premature breast development in girls or gynecomastia in boys. Vaginal bleeding and vaginal cornification may also be induced in girls.

[U.S. Boxed Warning]: Estrogens with or without progestin should be used for shortest duration possible at the lowest effective dose consistent with treatment goals. Before prescribing estrogen therapy to postmenopausal women, the risks and benefits must be weighed for each patient. Women should be informed of these risks and benefits, as well as possible effects of progestin when added to estrogen therapy. Estrogens with or without progestin should be used for shortest duration possible consistent with treatment goals. Conduct periodic risk:benefit assessments.

When used solely for prevention of osteoporosis in women at significant risk, nonestrogen treatment options should be considered. When used solely for the treatment of vulvar and vaginal atrophy, topical vaginal products should be considered. Use caution applying topical products to severely atrophic vaginal mucosa. Use of the vaginal cream may weaken latex found in condoms, diaphragms or cervical caps.

Adverse Reactions

Note: Percentages reported in postmenopausal women following oral use.

>10%:

- Central nervous system: Headache (26% to 32%; placebo 28%)
- Endocrine & metabolic: Breast pain (7% to 12%; placebo 9%)
- Gastrointestinal: Abdominal pain (15% to 17%)
- Genitourinary: Vaginal hemorrhage (2% to 14%)
- Neuromuscular & skeletal: Back pain (13% to 14%)

1% to 10%:

- Central nervous system: Nervousness (2% to 5%)
- Dermatologic: Pruritus (4% to 5%)
- Gastrointestinal: Flatulence (6% to 7%)
- Genitourinary: Vaginitis (5% to 7%), leukorrhea (4% to 7%), vaginal moniliasis (5% to 6%)
- Neuromuscular & skeletal: Weakness (7% to 8%), leg cramps (3% to 7%)

Additional adverse reactions reported with injection or vaginal cream; frequency not defined:

- Genitourinary: Cystis-like syndrome, genital pruritus, vulvovaginal discomfort
- Local: injection site: Edema, pain, phlebitis

In addition, the following have been reported with estrogen and/or progestin therapy:

Cardiovascular: DVT, edema, hypertension, MI, stroke, superficial venous thrombosis

Central nervous system: Dementia, dizziness, epilepsy exacerbation, headache, irritability, mental depression, migraine, mood disturbances, nervousness

Dermatologic: Angioedema, chloasma, erythema multiforme, erythema nodosum, hemorrhagic eruption, hirsutism, loss of scalp hair, melasma, pruritus, rash, urticaria

Endocrine & metabolic: Breast cancer, breast discharge, breast enlargement, breast tenderness, dysmenorrhea, fibrocystic breast changes, galactorrhea, glucose intolerance, HDL-cholesterol increased, hyper-/hypocalcemia, LDL-cholesterol decreased, libido (changes in), ovarian cancer, serum triglycerides/phospholipids increased, thyroid-binding globulin increased, total thyroid hormone (T_4) increased

Gastrointestinal: Abdominal cramps, bloating, cholecystitis, cholelithiasis, gallbladder disease, ischemic colitis, nausea, pancreatitis, vomiting, weight gain/loss

Genitourinary: Abnormal uterine bleeding/spotting, changes in cervical ectropion, changes in cervical secretions, endometrial cancer, endometrial hyperplasia, increased size of uterine leiomyomata, vaginal candidiasis

Hematologic: Aggravation of porphyria, antithrombin III and antifactor Xa decreased; factors II, II-VII-X complex, VII, VIII, VII-X complex, IX, X , and XII increased; increased beta-thromboglobulin, fibrinogen levels, plasminogen/plasminogen activity, platelet aggregability, platelet count, and prothrombin

Hepatic: Cholestatic jaundice, hepatic hemangiomas enlarged

Neuromuscular & skeletal: Arthralgias, chorea, leg cramps

Local: Thrombophlebitis

Ocular: Contact lens intolerance, corneal curvature steepening, retinal vascular thrombosis

Respiratory: Asthma exacerbation, pulmonary thromboembolism

Miscellaneous: Anaphylactoid/anaphylactic reactions, benign meningioma growth potentiation

Drug Interactions

Metabolism/Transport Effects

Based on estradiol and estrone: **Substrate** of CYP1A2 (major), 2A6 (minor), 2B6 (minor), 2C9 (minor), 2C19 (minor), 2D6 (minor), 2E1 (minor), 3A4 (major); Inhibits CYP1A2 (weak), 2C8 (weak); Induces CYP3A4 (weak)

Avoid Concomitant Use There are no known interactions where it is recommended to avoid concomitant use.

Increased Effect/Toxicity

Estrogens (Conjugated/Equine) may increase the levels/effects of: Corticosteroids (Systemic); Ropinirole; Tipranavir

The levels/effects of Estrogens (Conjugated/Equine) may be increased by: Herbs (Estrogenic Properties)

Decreased Effect

Estrogens (Conjugated/Equine) may decrease the levels/effects of: Maraviroc; Somatropin; Thyroid Products

The levels/effects of Estrogens (Conjugated/Equine) may be decreased by: CYP1A2 Inducers (Strong); CYP3A4 Inducers (Strong); Deferasirox; Herbs (CYP3A4 Inducers); Tipranavir

Ethanol/Nutrition/Herb Interactions

Ethanol: Avoid ethanol (routine use increases estrogen level and risk of breast cancer). Ethanol may also increase the risk of osteoporosis.

Food: Folic acid absorption may be decreased.

Herb/Nutraceutical: St John's wort may decrease levels. Herbs with estrogenic properties may enhance the adverse/toxic effect of estrogen derivatives; examples include alfalfa, black cohosh, bloodroot, hops, kudzu, licorice, red clover, saw palmetto, soybean, thyme, wild yam, yucca.

Stability

Injection: Refrigerate at 2°C to 8°C (36°F to 46°F) prior to reconstitution. Reconstitute with sterile water for injection; slowly inject diluent against side wall of the vial. Agitate gently; do not shake violently. Use immediately following reconstitution.

Tablets, vaginal cream: Store at room temperature 20°C to 25°C (68°F to 77°F).

Mechanism of Action Conjugated estrogens contain a mixture of estrone sulfate, equilin sulfate, 17 alpha-dihydroequilin, 17 alpha-estradiol and 17 beta-dihydroequilin. Estrogens are responsible for the development and maintenance of the female reproductive system and secondary sexual characteristics. Estradiol is the principle intracellular human estrogen and is more potent than estrone and estriol at the receptor level; it is the primary estrogen secreted prior to menopause. Following menopause, estrone and estrone sulfate are more highly produced. Estrogens modulate the pituitary secretion of gonadotropins, luteinizing hormone, and follicle-stimulating hormone through a negative feedback system; estrogen replacement reduces elevated levels of these hormones in postmenopausal women.

Pharmacodynamics/Kinetics

Absorption: Well absorbed

Protein binding: Binds to sex-hormone-binding globulin and albumin

Metabolism: Hepatic via CYP3A4; estradiol is converted to estrone and estriol; also undergoes enterohepatic recirculation (avoided with vaginal administration); estrone sulfite is the main metabolite in postmenopausal women

Half-life elimination: Total estrone: 27 hours

Time to peak, plasma: Total estrone: 7 hours

Excretion: Urine (primarily estriol, also as estradiol, estrone, and conjugates

Dosage Adults:

Male: Androgen-dependent prostate cancer palliation: Oral: 1.25-2.5 mg 3 times/day

Female:

Prevention of postmenopausal osteoporosis: Oral: Initial: 0.3 mg/day cyclically* or daily, depending on medical assessment of patient. Dose may be adjusted based on bone mineral density and clinical response. The lowest effective dose should be used.

Moderate-to-severe vasomotor symptoms associated with menopause: Oral: Initial: 0.3 mg/day, cyclically* or daily, depending on medical assessment of patient. The lowest dose that will control symptoms should be used. Medication should be discontinued as soon as possible.

Moderate-to-severe dyspareunia: Intravaginal: Vaginal cream: 0.5 g twice weekly (eg, Monday and Thursday) or once daily cyclically*

Vulvar and vaginal atrophy:

Oral: Initial: 0.3 mg/day; the lowest dose that will control symptoms should be used. May be given cyclically* or daily, depending on medical assessment of patient. Medication should be discontinued as soon as possible.

Vaginal cream: Intravaginal: 0.5-2 g/day given cyclically*

Abnormal uterine bleeding:

Acute/heavy bleeding:

Oral (unlabeled route): 1.25 mg, may repeat every 4 hours for 24 hours, followed by 1.25 mg once daily for 7-10 days

I.M., I.V.: 25 mg, may repeat in 6-12 hours if needed

Note: Treatment should be followed by a low-dose oral contraceptive; medroxyprogesterone acetate along with or following estrogen therapy can also be given

Nonacute/lesser bleeding: Oral (unlabeled route): 1.25 mg once daily for 7-10 days

Female hypogonadism: Oral: 0.3-0.625 mg/day given cyclically*; dose may be titrated in 6- to 12-month intervals; progestin treatment should be added to maintain bone mineral density once skeletal maturity is achieved.

Female castration, primary ovarian failure: Oral: 1.25 mg/day given cyclically*; adjust according to severity of symptoms and patient response. For maintenance, adjust to the lowest effective dose.

***Cyclic administration:** Either 3 weeks on, 1 week off **or** 25 days on, 5 days off

Male and Female:

Breast cancer palliation, metastatic disease in selected patients: Oral: 10 mg 3 times/day for at least 3 months

Uremic bleeding (unlabeled use): I.V.: 0.6 mg/kg/day for 5 days

Elderly: Refer to adult dosing; a higher incidence of stroke and invasive breast cancer was observed in women >75 years in a WHI substudy.

Dietary Considerations Ensure adequate calcium and vitamin D intake when used for the prevention of osteoporosis. Powder for reconstitution for injection (25 mg) contains lactose 200 mg.

Administration

Injection: May also be administered intramuscularly; when administered I.V., drug should be administered slowly to avoid the occurrence of a flushing reaction

Oral tablet: Administer at bedtime to minimize adverse effects. May be administered without regard to meals.

Vaginal cream: Administer at bedtime to minimize adverse effects. To clean applicator, remove plunger from barrel. Wash with mild soap and warm water; do not boil or use hot water.

Monitoring Parameters Routine physical examination that includes blood pressure and Papanicolaou smear, breast exam, mammogram. Monitor for signs of endometrial cancer in female patients with uterus. Adequate diagnostic measures, including endometrial sampling, if indicated, should be performed to rule out malignancy in all cases of undiagnosed abnormal vaginal bleeding. Monitor for loss of vision, sudden onset of proptosis, diplopia, migraine; signs and symptoms of thromboembolic disorders; glycemic control in patients with diabetes; lipid profiles in patients being treated for hyperlipidemias; thyroid function in patients on thyroid hormone replacement therapy.

Menopausal symptoms: Assess need for therapy at 3- to 6-month intervals

Prevention of osteoporosis: Bone density measurement

Uremic bleeding: Bleeding time

Reference Range

Children: <10 mcg/24 hours (SI: <35 μmol/day) (values at Mayo Medical Laboratories)

Adults:

Male: 15-40 mcg/24 hours (SI: 52-139 μmol/day)

Female:

Menstruating: 15-80 mcg/24 hours (SI: 52-277 μmol/day)

Postmenopausal: <20 mcg/24 hours (SI: <69 μmol/day)

Test Interactions Pathologist should be advised of estrogen/progesterone therapy when specimens are submitted. Reduced response to metyrapone test.

Dosage Forms Excipient information presented when available (limited, particularly for generics); consult specific product labeling.

Cream, vaginal:

Premarin®: 0.625 mg/g (42.5 g)

Injection, powder for reconstitution:

Premarin®: 25 mg [contains benzyl alcohol (in diluent), lactose 200 mg]

Tablet:

Premarin®: 0.3 mg, 0.45 mg, 0.625 mg, 0.9 mg, 1.25 mg

Estrogens (Conjugated/Equine) and Medroxyprogesterone

(ES troe jenz KON joo gate ed/EE kwine & me DROKS ee proe JES te rone)

U.S. Brand Names Premphase®; Prempro™

Canadian Brand Names Premphase®; Premplus®; Prempro™

Index Terms Medroxyprogesterone and Estrogens (Conjugated); MPA and Estrogens (Conjugated)

Pharmacologic Category Estrogen and Progestin Combination

Use Women with an intact uterus: Treatment of moderate-to-severe vasomotor symptoms associated with menopause; treatment of atrophic vaginitis; osteoporosis (prophylaxis)

Medication Safety Issues

Sound-alike/look-alike issues:

Premphase® may be confused with Prempro™

Prempro™ may be confused with Premphase®

Dosage Oral: Adults:

Treatment of moderate-to-severe vasomotor symptoms associated with menopause or treatment of atrophic vaginitis in females with an intact uterus. (The lowest dose that will control symptoms should be used; medication should be discontinued as soon as possible):

Premphase®: One maroon conjugated estrogen 0.625 mg tablet daily on days 1 through 14 and one light blue conjugated estrogen 0.625 mg/MPA 5 mg tablet daily on days 15 through 28; re-evaluate patients at 3- and 6-month intervals to determine if treatment is still necessary; monitor patients for signs of endometrial cancer; rule out malignancy if unexplained vaginal bleeding occurs

Prempro™: One conjugated estrogen 0.3 mg/MPA 1.5 mg tablet daily; re-evaluate at 3-and 6-month intervals to determine if therapy is still needed; dose may be increased to a maximum of one conjugated estrogen 0.625 mg/MPA 5 mg tablet daily in patients with bleeding or spotting, once malignancy has been ruled out

Osteoporosis prophylaxis in females with an intact uterus:

Premphase®: One maroon conjugated estrogen 0.625 tablet daily on days 1 through 14 and one light blue conjugated estrogen 0.625 mg/MPA 5 mg tablet daily on days 15 through 28; monitor patients for signs of endometrial cancer; rule out malignancy if unexplained vaginal bleeding occurs

Prempro™: One conjugated estrogen 0.3 mg/MPA 1.5 mg tablet daily; dose may be increased to one conjugated estrogen 0.625 mg/MPA 5 mg tablet daily; in patients with bleeding or spotting, once malignancy has been ruled out

Elderly: Refer to adult dosing; a higher incidence of stroke and invasive breast cancer was observed in women >75 years in a WHI substudy.

Additional Information Complete prescribing information for this medication should be consulted for additional detail.

Dosage Forms Excipient information presented when available (limited, particularly for generics); consult specific product labeling.

Tablet:

Premphase® [therapy pack contains 2 separate tablet formulations]: Conjugated estrogens 0.625 mg [14 maroon tablets] and conjugated estrogen 0.625 mg/medroxyprogesterone acetate 5 mg [14 light blue tablets] (28s)

Prempro™:

0.3/1.5: Conjugated estrogens 0.3 mg and medroxyprogesterone acetate 1.5 mg (28s)

0.45/1.5: Conjugated estrogens 0.45 mg and medroxyprogesterone acetate 1.5 mg (28s)

0.625/2.5: Conjugated estrogens 0.625 mg and medroxyprogesterone acetate 2.5 mg (28s)

0.625/5: Conjugated estrogens 0.625 mg and medroxyprogesterone acetate 5 mg (28s)

Estrogens (Esterified) (ES troe jenz, es TER i fied)

U.S. Brand Names Menest®

Canadian Brand Names Estratab®; Menest®

Index Terms Esterified Estrogens

Pharmacologic Category Estrogen Derivative

Use Treatment of moderate to severe vasomotor symptoms associated with menopause; treatment of vulvar and vaginal atrophy; hypoestrogenism (due to hypogonadism, castration, or primary ovarian failure); prostatic cancer (palliation); breast cancer (palliation); osteoporosis (prophylaxis, in women at significant risk only)

Pregnancy Risk Factor X

Pregnancy Considerations Increased risk of fetal reproductive tract disorders and other birth defects; do not use during pregnancy.

Lactation Enters breast milk/use caution

Medication Safety Issues

Sound-alike/look-alike issues:

Estratab® may be confused with Estratest®, Estratest® H.S.

Contraindications Hypersensitivity to estrogens or any component of the formulation; undiagnosed abnormal vaginal bleeding; history of or current thrombophlebitis or venous thromboembolic disorders (including DVT, PE); active or recent (within 1 year) arterial thromboembolic disease (eg, stroke, MI); carcinoma of the breast, except in appropriately selected patients being treated for metastatic disease; estrogen-dependent tumor; hepatic dysfunction or disease; pregnancy

Warnings/Precautions

Cardiovascular-related considerations: **[U.S. Boxed Warning]: Estrogens with or without progestin should not be used to prevent coronary heart disease.** Use caution with cardiovascular disease or dysfunction. May increase the risks of hypertension, myocardial infarction (MI), stroke, pulmonary emboli (PE), and deep vein thrombosis; incidence of these effects was shown to be significantly increased in postmenopausal women using conjugated equine estrogens (CEE) in combination with medroxyprogesterone acetate (MPA). Nonfatal MI, PE, and thrombophlebitis have also been reported in males taking high doses of CEE (eg, for prostate cancer). Estrogen compounds are generally associated with lipid effects such as increased HDL-cholesterol and decreased LDL-cholesterol. Triglycerides may also be increased; use with caution in patients with familial defects of lipoprotein metabolism. Whenever possible, estrogens should be discontinued at least 4 weeks prior to and for 2 weeks following elective surgery associated with an increased risk of thromboembolism or during periods of prolonged immobilization.

Neurological considerations: **[U.S. Boxed Warning]: The risk of dementia may be increased in postmenopausal women;** increased incidence was observed in women ≥65 years of age taking CEE alone or in combination with MPA.

Cancer-related considerations: **[U.S. Boxed Warning]: Unopposed estrogens may increase the risk of endometrial carcinoma in postmenopausal women.** Estrogens may exacerbate endometriosis. Malignant transformation of residual endometrial implants has been reported post-hysterectomy with estrogen only therapy. Consider adding a progestin in women with residual endometriosis post-hysterectomy. Estrogens may increase the risk of breast cancer. An increased risk of invasive breast cancer was observed in postmenopausal women using CEE in combination with MPA; a smaller increase in risk was seen with estrogen therapy alone in observational studies. An increase in abnormal mammograms has also been reported with estrogen and progestin therapy. Estrogen use may lead to severe hypercalcemia in patients with breast cancer and bone metastases; discontinue estrogen if hypercalcemia occurs.

Estrogens may cause retinal vascular thrombosis; discontinue permanently if papilledema or retinal vascular lesions are observed on examination. Use with caution in patients with diseases which may be exacerbated by fluid retention, including asthma, epilepsy, migraine, diabetes or renal dysfunction. Use with caution in patients with a history of severe hypocalcemia, SLE, hepatic hemangiomas, porphyria, endometriosis, and gallbladder disease. Use caution with history of cholestatic jaundice associated with past estrogen use or pregnancy. Safety and efficacy in pediatric patients have not been established. Prior to puberty, estrogens may cause premature closure of the epiphyses, premature breast development in girls or gynecomastia in boys. Vaginal bleeding and vaginal cornification may also be induced in girls.

Before prescribing estrogen therapy to postmenopausal women, the risks and benefits must be weighed for each patient. Women should be informed of these risks and benefits, as well as possible effects of progestin when added to estrogen therapy. Estrogens with or without progestin should be used for shortest duration possible consistent with treatment goals. Conduct periodic risk: benefit assessments.

When used solely for prevention of osteoporosis in women at significant risk, nonestrogen treatment options should be considered. When used solely for the treatment of vulvar and vaginal atrophy, topical vaginal products should be considered.

Adverse Reactions

Cardiovascular: Edema, hypertension, venous thromboembolism

Central nervous system: Dizziness, headache, mental depression, migraine

Dermatologic: Chloasma, erythema multiforme, erythema nodosum, hemorrhagic eruption, hirsutism, loss of scalp hair, melasma

Endocrine & metabolic: Breast enlargement, breast tenderness, libido (changes in), increased thyroid-binding globulin, increased total thyroid hormone (T_4), increased serum triglycerides/phospholipids, increased HDL-cholesterol, decreased LDL-cholesterol, impaired glucose tolerance, hypercalcemia

Gastrointestinal: Abdominal cramps, bloating, cholecystitis, cholelithiasis, gallbladder disease, nausea, pancreatitis, vomiting, weight gain/loss

Genitourinary: Alterations in frequency and flow of menses, changes in cervical secretions, endometrial cancer, increased size of uterine leiomyomata, vaginal candidiasis

Hematologic: Aggravation of porphyria, decreased antithrombin III and antifactor Xa, increased levels of fibrinogen, increased platelet aggregability and platelet count; increased prothrombin and factors VII, VIII, IX, X

Hepatic: Cholestatic jaundice

Neuromuscular & skeletal: Chorea

Ocular: Contact lens intolerance, corneal curvature steepening

Respiratory: Pulmonary thromboembolism

Miscellaneous: Carbohydrate intolerance

Drug Interactions

Metabolism/Transport Effects Based on estrone: **Substrate** of CYP1A2 (major), 2B6 (minor), 2C9 (minor), 2E1 (minor), 3A4 (major)

Avoid Concomitant Use There are no known interactions where it is recommended to avoid concomitant use.

Increased Effect/Toxicity

Estrogens (Esterified) may increase the levels/effects of: Corticosteroids (Systemic); Ropinirole; Tipranavir

The levels/effects of Estrogens (Esterified) may be increased by: Herbs (Estrogenic Properties)

Decreased Effect

Estrogens (Esterified) may decrease the levels/effects of: Somatropin; Thyroid Products

The levels/effects of Estrogens (Esterified) may be decreased by: CYP1A2 Inducers (Strong); CYP3A4 Inducers (Strong); Deferasirox; Herbs (CYP3A4 Inducers); Tipranavir

Ethanol/Nutrition/Herb Interactions

Ethanol: Avoid ethanol (routine use increases estrogen level and risk of breast cancer). Ethanol may also increase the risk of osteoporosis.

Food: Folic acid absorption may be decreased.

Herb/Nutraceutical: St John's wort may decrease levels. Herbs with estrogenic properties may enhance the adverse/toxic effect of estrogen derivatives; examples include alfalfa, black cohosh, bloodroot, hops, kudzu, licorice, red clover, saw palmetto, soybean, thyme, wild yam, yucca.

Stability Store below 30°C (86°F). Protect from moisture.

Mechanism of Action Esterified estrogens contain a mixture of estrogenic substances; the principle component is estrone. Preparations contain 75% to 85% sodium estrone sulfate and 6% to 15% sodium equilin sulfate such that the total is not <90%. Estrogens are responsible for the development and maintenance of the female reproductive system and secondary sexual characteristics. Estradiol is the principle intracellular human estrogen and is more potent than estrone and estriol at the receptor level; it is the primary estrogen secreted prior to menopause. In males and following menopause in females, estrone and estrone sulfate are more highly produced. Estrogens modulate the pituitary secretion of gonadotropins, luteinizing hormone, and follicle-stimulating hormone through a negative feedback system; estrogen replacement reduces elevated levels of these hormones.

Pharmacodynamics/Kinetics

Absorption: Readily

Metabolism: Rapidly hepatic to estrone sulfate, conjugated and unconjugated metabolites; first-pass effect

Excretion: Urine (as unchanged drug and as glucuronide and sulfate conjugates)

Dosage Oral: Adults:

Prostate cancer (palliation): 1.25-2.5 mg 3 times/day

Female hypogonadism: 2.5-7.5 mg of estrogen daily for 20 days followed by a 10-day rest period. Administer cyclically (3 weeks on and 1 week off). If bleeding does not occur by the end of the 10-day period, repeat the same dosing schedule; the number of courses is dependent upon the responsiveness of the endometrium. If bleeding occurs before the end of the 10-day period, begin an estrogen-progestin cyclic regimen of 2.5-7.5 mg esterified estrogens daily for 20 days. During the last 5 days of estrogen therapy, give an oral progestin. If bleeding occurs before regimen is concluded, discontinue therapy and resume on the fifth day of bleeding.

Moderate to severe vasomotor symptoms associated with menopause: 1.25 mg/day administered cyclically (3 weeks on and 1 week off). If patient has not menstruated within the last 2 months or more, cyclic administration is started arbitrary. If the patient is menstruating, cyclical administration is started on day 5 of the bleeding. For short-term use only and should be discontinued as soon as possible. Re-evaluate at 3- to 6-month intervals for tapering or discontinuation of therapy.

Atopic vaginitis and kraurosis vulvae: 0.3 to ≥1.25 mg/day, depending on the tissue response of the individual patient. Administer cyclically. For short-term use only and should be discontinued as soon as possible. Re-evaluate at 3- to 6-month intervals for tapering or discontinuation of therapy.

Breast cancer (palliation): 10 mg 3 times/day for at least 3 months

Osteoporosis in postmenopausal women: Initial: 0.3 mg/day and increase to a maximum daily dose of 1.25 mg/day; initiate therapy as soon as possible after menopause; cyclically or daily, depending on medical assessment of patient. Monitor patients with an intact uterus for signs of endometrial cancer; rule out malignancy if unexplained vaginal bleeding occurs

Female castration and primary ovarian failure: 1.25 mg/day, cyclically. Adjust dosage upward or downward, according to the severity of symptoms and patient response. For maintenance, adjust dosage to lowest level that will provide effective control.

Elderly: Refer to adult dosing. A higher incidence of stroke and invasive breast cancer were observed in women >75 years in a WHI substudy using conjugated equine estrogen.

Dosing adjustment in hepatic impairment:

Mild to moderate liver impairment: Dosage reduction of estrogens is recommended

Severe liver impairment: **Not recommended**

Dietary Considerations Should be taken with food at same time each day. Ensure adequate calcium and vitamin D intake when used for the prevention of osteoporosis.

Monitoring Parameters Yearly physical examination that includes blood pressure and Papanicolaou smear, breast exam, mammogram. Monitor for signs of endometrial cancer in female patients with uterus. Adequate diagnostic measures, including endometrial sampling, if indicated, should be performed to rule out malignancy in all cases of undiagnosed abnormal vaginal bleeding. Monitor for loss of vision, sudden onset of proptosis, diplopia, migraine; signs and symptoms of thromboembolic disorders; glycemic control in patients with diabetes; lipid profiles in patients being treated for hyperlipidemias; thyroid function in patients on thyroid hormone replacement therapy.

Menopausal symptoms: Assess need for therapy at 3- to 6-month intervals

Prevention of osteoporosis: Bone density measurement

Test Interactions Pathologist should be advised of estrogen/progesterone therapy when specimens are submitted. Reduced response to metyrapone test.

Dosage Forms Tablet: 0.3 mg, 0.625 mg, 1.25 mg, 2.5 mg

Estrogens (Esterified) and Methyltestosterone

(ES troe jenz es TER i fied & meth il tes TOS te rone)

U.S. Brand Names Covaryx™; Covaryx™ HS; E.E.M.T. D.S.; E.E.M.T. H.S.; Estratest®; Estratest® H.S.; Syntest D.S. [DSC]; Syntest H.S. [DSC]

Canadian Brand Names Estratest®

Index Terms Conjugated Estrogen and Methyltestosterone; Esterified Estrogen and Methyltestosterone

Pharmacologic Category Estrogen and Progestin Combination

Use Vasomotor symptoms of menopause

Pregnancy Risk Factor X

Medication Safety Issues

Sound-alike/look-alike issues:

Estratest® may be confused with Eskalith®, Estratab®, Estratest® H.S.

Estratest® H.S. may be confused with Eskalith®, Estratab®, Estratest®

Dosage Adults: Females: Oral: Lowest dose that will control symptoms should be chosen, normally given 3 weeks on and 1 week off

Additional Information Complete prescribing information for this medication should be consulted for additional detail.

Dosage Forms Excipient information presented when available (limited, particularly for generics); consult specific product labeling. [DSC] = Discontinued product

Tablet: Esterified estrogens 1.25 mg and methyltestosterone 2.5 mg [contains tartrazine]; esterified estrogen 0.625 mg and methyltestosterone 1.25 mg

Covaryx™: Esterified estrogens 1.25 mg and methyltestosterone 2.5 mg [contains tartrazine]

Covaryx™ H.S.: Esterified estrogens 1.25 mg and methyltestosterone 2.5 mg [contains tartrazine]

Estratest®: Esterified estrogen 1.25 mg and methyltestosterone 2.5 mg

Estratest® H.S.: Esterified estrogen 0.625 mg and methyltestosterone 1.25 mg

E.E.M.T. D.S., Syntest D.S. [DSC]: Esterified estrogen 1.25 mg and methyltestosterone 2.5 mg

E.E.M.T. H.S., Syntest H.S. [DSC]: Esterified estrogen 0.625 mg and methyltestosterone 1.25 mg

Estropipate (ES troe pih pate)

U.S. Brand Names Ogen®; Ortho-Est®

Canadian Brand Names Ogen®

Index Terms Ortho Est; Piperazine Estrone Sulfate

Pharmacologic Category Estrogen Derivative

Use Treatment of moderate to severe vasomotor symptoms associated with menopause; treatment of vulvar and vaginal atrophy; hypoestrogenism (due to hypogonadism, castration, or primary ovarian failure); osteoporosis (prophylaxis, in women at significant risk only)

Pregnancy Risk Factor X

Pregnancy Considerations Increased risk of fetal reproductive tract disorders and other birth defects; do not use during pregnancy.

Lactation Enters breast milk/use caution

Contraindications Hypersensitivity to estrogens or any component of the formulation; undiagnosed abnormal vaginal bleeding; history of or current thrombophlebitis or venous thromboembolic disorders (including DVT, PE);

active or recent (within 1 year) arterial thromboembolic disease (eg, stroke, MI); carcinoma of the breast, except in appropriately selected patients being treated for metastatic disease; estrogen-dependent tumor; hepatic dysfunction or disease; pregnancy

Warnings/Precautions Cardiovascular-related considerations: **[U.S. Boxed Warning]: Estrogens with or without progestin should not be used to prevent coronary heart disease.** Use caution with cardiovascular disease or dysfunction. May increase the risks of hypertension, myocardial infarction (MI), stroke, pulmonary emboli (PE), and deep vein thrombosis; incidence of these effects was shown to be significantly increased in postmenopausal women using conjugated equine estrogens (CEE) in combination with medroxyprogesterone acetate (MPA). Nonfatal MI, PE, and thrombophlebitis have also been reported in males taking high doses of CEE (eg, for prostate cancer). Estrogen compounds are generally associated with lipid effects such as increased HDL-cholesterol and decreased LDL-cholesterol. Triglycerides may also be increased; use with caution in patients with familial defects of lipoprotein metabolism. Whenever possible, estrogens should be discontinued at least 4 weeks prior to and for 2 weeks following elective surgery associated with an increased risk of thromboembolism or during periods of prolonged immobilization.

Neurological considerations: **[U.S. Boxed Warning]: The risk of dementia may be increased in postmenopausal women;** increased incidence was observed in women ≥65 years of age taking CEE alone or in combination with MPA.

Cancer-related considerations: **[U.S. Boxed Warning]: Unopposed estrogens may increase the risk of endometrial carcinoma in postmenopausal women.** Estrogens may exacerbate endometriosis. Malignant transformation of residual endometrial implants has been reported post-hysterectomy with estrogen only therapy. Consider adding a progestin in women with residual endometriosis post-hysterectomy. Estrogens may increase the risk of breast cancer. An increased risk of invasive breast cancer was observed in postmenopausal women using CEE in combination with MPA; a smaller increase in risk was seen with estrogen therapy alone in observational studies. An increase in abnormal mammograms has also been reported with estrogen and progestin therapy. Estrogen use may lead to severe hypercalcemia in patients with breast cancer and bone metastases; discontinue estrogen if hypercalcemia occurs.

Estrogens may cause retinal vascular thrombosis; discontinue permanently if papilledema or retinal vascular lesions are observed on examination. Use with caution in patients with diseases which may be exacerbated by fluid retention, including asthma, epilepsy, migraine, diabetes or renal dysfunction. Use with caution in patients with a history of severe hypocalcemia, SLE, hepatic hemangiomas, porphyria, endometriosis, and gallbladder disease. Use caution with history of cholestatic jaundice associated with past estrogen use or pregnancy. Safety and efficacy in pediatric patients have not been established. Prior to puberty, estrogens may cause premature closure of the epiphyses, premature breast development in girls or gynecomastia in boys. Vaginal bleeding and vaginal cornification may also be induced in girls.

Before prescribing estrogen therapy to postmenopausal women, the risks and benefits must be weighed for each patient. Women should be informed of these risks and benefits, as well as possible effects of progestin when added to estrogen therapy. Estrogens with or without progestin should be used for shortest duration possible consistent with treatment goals. Conduct periodic risk: benefit assessments.

When used solely for prevention of osteoporosis in women at significant risk, nonestrogen treatment options should be considered. When used solely for the treatment of vulvar and vaginal atrophy, topical vaginal products should be considered.

Adverse Reactions Frequency not defined.

Cardiovascular: Edema, hypertension, venous thromboembolism

Central nervous system: Dizziness, headache, mental depression, migraine

Dermatologic: Chloasma, erythema multiforme, erythema nodosum, hemorrhagic eruption, hirsutism, loss of scalp hair, melasma

Endocrine & metabolic: Breast enlargement, breast tenderness, libido (changes in), increased thyroid-binding globulin, increased total thyroid hormone (T_4), increased serum triglycerides/phospholipids, increased HDL-cholesterol, decreased LDL-cholesterol, impaired glucose tolerance, hypercalcemia

Gastrointestinal: Abdominal cramps, bloating, cholecystitis, cholelithiasis, gallbladder disease, nausea, pancreatitis, vomiting, weight gain/loss

Genitourinary: Alterations in frequency and flow of menses, changes in cervical secretions, endometrial cancer, increased size of uterine leiomyomata, vaginal candidiasis

Hematologic: Aggravation of porphyria, decreased antithrombin III and antifactor Xa, increased levels of fibrinogen, increased platelet aggregability and platelet count; increased prothrombin and factors VII, VIII, IX, X

Hepatic: Cholestatic jaundice

Neuromuscular & skeletal: Chorea

Ocular: Ocular: Contact lens intolerance, corneal curvature steepening

Respiratory: Pulmonary thromboembolism

Miscellaneous: Carbohydrate intolerance

Drug Interactions

Metabolism/Transport Effects Based on estrone: **Substrate** of CYP1A2 (major), 2B6 (minor), 2C9 (minor), 2E1 (minor), 3A4 (major)

Avoid Concomitant Use There are no known interactions where it is recommended to avoid concomitant use.

Increased Effect/Toxicity

Estropipate may increase the levels/effects of: Corticosteroids (Systemic); Ropinirole; Tipranavir

The levels/effects of Estropipate may be increased by: Herbs (Estrogenic Properties)

Decreased Effect

Estropipate may decrease the levels/effects of: Somatropin; Thyroid Products

The levels/effects of Estropipate may be decreased by: CYP1A2 Inducers (Strong); CYP3A4 Inducers (Strong); Deferasirox; Herbs (CYP3A4 Inducers); Tipranavir

Ethanol/Nutrition/Herb Interactions

Ethanol: Routine use increases estrogen level and risk of breast cancer; avoid ethanol. Ethanol may also increase the risk of osteoporosis.

Food: Folic acid absorption may be decreased.

Herb/Nutraceutical: St John's wort may decrease levels. Herbs with estrogenic properties may enhance the adverse/toxic effect of estrogen derivatives; examples include alfalfa, black cohosh, bloodroot, hops, kudzu, licorice, red clover, saw palmetto, soybean, thyme, wild yam, yucca.

Stability Tablet: Store below 25°C (77°F).

Mechanism of Action Estrogens are responsible for the development and maintenance of the female reproductive system and secondary sexual characteristics. Estradiol is the principle intracellular human estrogen and is more potent than estrone and estriol at the receptor level; it is the primary estrogen secreted prior to menopause. In males and following menopause in females, estrone and estrone sulfate are more highly produced. Estrogens modulate the pituitary secretion of gonadotropins, luteinizing hormone, and follicle-stimulating hormone through a negative feedback system; estrogen replacement reduces elevated levels of these hormones. Estropipate is prepared from purified crystalline estrone that has been solubilized as the sulfate and stabilized with piperazine.

Pharmacodynamics/Kinetics

Absorption: Well absorbed

Metabolism: Hepatic and in target tissues; first-pass effect

Dosage Adults:

Oral:

Moderate to severe vasomotor symptoms associated with menopause: Usual dosage range: 0.75-6 mg estropipate daily; use the lowest dose and regimen that will control symptoms, and discontinue as soon as possible. Attempt to discontinue or taper medication at 3- to 6-month intervals. If a patient with vasomotor symptoms has not menstruated within the last ≥2 months, start the cyclic administration arbitrarily. If the patient has menstruated, start cyclic administration on day 5 of bleeding.

Female hypogonadism: 1.5-9 mg estropipate daily for the first 3 weeks, followed by a rest period of 8-10 days; use the lowest dose and regimen that will control symptoms. Repeat if bleeding does not occur by the end of the rest period. The duration of therapy necessary to product the withdrawal bleeding will vary according to the responsiveness of the endometrium. If satisfactory withdrawal bleeding does not occur, give an oral progestin in addition to estrogen during the third week of the cycle.

Female castration or primary ovarian failure: 1.5-9 mg estropipate daily for the first 3 weeks of a theoretical cycle, followed by a rest period of 8-10 days; use the lowest dose and regimen that will control symptoms

Osteoporosis prophylaxis: 0.75 mg estropipate daily for 25 days of a 31-day cycle

Atrophic vaginitis or kraurosis vulvae: 0.75-6 mg estropipate daily; administer cyclically. Use the lowest dose and regimen that will control symptoms; discontinue as soon as possible.

Elderly: Refer to adult dosing. A higher incidence of stroke and invasive breast cancer were observed in women >75 years in a WHI substudy using conjugated equine estrogen.

Dosing adjustment in hepatic impairment:

Mild to moderate liver impairment: Dosage reduction of estrogens is recommended

Severe liver impairment: **Not recommended**

Dietary Considerations Ensure adequate calcium and vitamin D intake when used for the prevention of osteoporosis.

Monitoring Parameters Yearly physical examination that includes blood pressure and Papanicolaou smear, breast exam, mammogram. Monitor for signs of endometrial cancer in female patients with uterus. Adequate diagnostic measures, including endometrial sampling, if indicated, should be performed to rule out malignancy in all cases of undiagnosed abnormal vaginal bleeding. Monitor for loss of vision, sudden onset of proptosis, diplopia, migraine; signs and symptoms of thromboembolic disorders; glycemic control in patients with diabetes; lipid profiles in patients being treated for hyperlipidemias; thyroid function in patients on thyroid hormone replacement therapy.

Menopausal symptoms: Assess need for therapy at 3- to 6-month intervals

Prevention of osteoporosis: Bone density measurement

Test Interactions Pathologist should be advised of estrogen/progesterone therapy when specimens are submitted. Reduced response to metyrapone test.

Dosage Forms Excipient information presented when available (limited, particularly for generics); consult specific product labeling.

Tablet: 0.625 mg [estropipate 0.75 mg]; 1.25 mg [estropipate 1.5 mg]; 2.5 mg [estropipate 3 mg]

Ogen®: 0.625 mg [estropipate 0.75 mg]; 1.25 mg [estropipate 1.5 mg]; 2.5 mg [estropipate 3 mg]

Ortho-Est®: 0.625 mg [estropipate 0.75 mg]; 1.25 mg [estropipate 1.5 mg]

◆ **Estrostep® Fe** *see* Ethinyl Estradiol and Norethindrone *on page 581*

Eszopiclone (es zoe PIK lone)

U.S. Brand Names Lunesta®

Pharmacologic Category Hypnotic, Nonbenzodiazepine

Use Treatment of insomnia

Restrictions C-IV

An FDA-approved patient medication guide is available and must be distributed when dispensing an outpatient prescription (new or refill) where this medication is to be used without direct supervision of a healthcare provider. Medication guides are available at http://www.fda.gov/cder/Offices/ODS/medication_guides.htm.

Pregnancy Risk Factor C

Pregnancy Considerations No evidence of teratogenicity in animal models (high dose). There are no adequate or well-controlled studies in pregnant women; use only if clearly needed.

Lactation Excretion in breast milk unknown/use caution

Medication Safety Issues

Sound-alike/look-alike issues:

Lunesta® may be confused with Neulasta®

Contraindications There are no contraindications listed within the manufacturer's labeling.

Warnings/Precautions Symptomatic treatment of insomnia should be initiated only after careful evaluation of potential causes of sleep disturbance. Tolerance did not develop over 6 months of use. Use with caution in patients with depression or a history of drug dependence. Abrupt discontinuance may lead to withdrawal symptoms. Use with caution in patients receiving other CNS depressants or psychoactive medications. Hypnotics/sedatives have been associated with abnormal thinking and behavior changes including decreased inhibition, aggression, bizarre behavior, agitation, hallucinations, and depersonalization. These changes may occur unpredictably and may indicate previously unrecognized psychiatric disorders; evaluate appropriately. Amnesia may occur. May impair physical and mental capabilities. Postmarketing studies have indicated that the use of hypnotic/sedative agents for sleep has been associated with hypersensitivity reactions including anaphylaxis as well as angioedema. An increased risk for hazardous sleep-related activities such as sleep-driving; cooking and eating food, and making phone calls while asleep have also been noted. Use caution in patients with respiratory compromise, hepatic dysfunction, elderly or those taking strong CYP3A4 inhibitors. Because of the rapid onset of action, administer immediately prior to bedtime or after the patient has gone to bed and is having difficulty falling asleep. Safety and efficacy in children have not been established.

Adverse Reactions

>10%:

Central nervous system: Headache (15% to 21%)

Gastrointestinal: Unpleasant taste (8% to 34%)

1% to 10%:

Cardiovascular: Chest pain, peripheral edema

Central nervous system: Somnolence (8% to 10%), dizziness (5% to 7%), pain (4% to 5%), nervousness (up to 5%), depression (1% to 4%), confusion (up to

3%), hallucinations (1% to 3%), anxiety (1% to 3%), abnormal dreams (1% to 3%), migraine

Dermatologic: Rash (3% to 4%), pruritus (1% to 4%)

Endocrine & metabolic: Libido decreased (up to 3%), dysmenorrhea (up to 3%), gynecomastia (males up to 3%)

Gastrointestinal: Xerostomia (3% to 7%), dyspepsia (2% to 6%), nausea (4% to 5%), diarrhea (2% to 4%), vomiting (up to 3%)

Genitourinary: Urinary tract infection (up to 3%)

Neuromuscular & skeletal: Neuralgia (up to 3%)

Miscellaneous: Infection (5% to 10%), viral infection (3%), accidental injury (up to 3%)

<1% (Limited to important or life-threatening): Abnormal gait, agitation, alopecia, allergic reaction, amenorrhea, anaphylaxis, angioedema, anorexia, asthma, ataxia, breast enlargement, breast neoplasm, bronchitis, cholelithiasis, colitis; complex sleep-related behavior (sleep-driving, cooking or eating food, making phone calls); conjunctivitis, contact dermatitis, cystitis, dehydration, diaphoresis, dry eyes, dyspnea, dysphagia, dysuria, eczema, emotional lability, epistaxis, erythema multiforme, euphoria, facial edema, fever, gout, heat stroke, hematuria, hepatitis, hepatomegaly, herpes zoster, hostility, hypercholesterolemia, hypertension, hypokalemia, kidney calculus, kidney pain, liver damage, maculopapular rash, malaise, mastitis, melena, memory impairment, menorrhagia, myasthenia, mydriasis, myopathy, neck rigidity, neuritis, neuropathy, neurosis, nystagmus, oliguria, paresthesia, photophobia, photosensitivity, pyelonephritis, rectal hemorrhage, reflexes decreased, stomach ulcer, swelling, thrombophlebitis, tinnitus, tongue edema, tremor, twitching, ulcerative stomatitis, urinary frequency, urinary incontinence, urticaria, urethritis, vaginal hemorrhage, vaginitis, vestibular disorder, vertigo, vesiculobullous rash

Drug Interactions

Metabolism/Transport Effects **Substrate** of CYP2E1 (minor), 3A4 (major)

Avoid Concomitant Use There are no known interactions where it is recommended to avoid concomitant use.

Increased Effect/Toxicity

Eszopiclone may increase the levels/effects of: Alcohol (Ethyl); CNS Depressants

The levels/effects of Eszopiclone may be increased by: Antifungal Agents (Azole Derivatives, Systemic); CYP3A4 Inhibitors (Moderate); CYP3A4 Inhibitors (Strong); Dasatinib

Decreased Effect

The levels/effects of Eszopiclone may be decreased by: CYP3A4 Inducers (Strong); Deferasirox; Flumazenil; Herbs (CYP3A4 Inducers)

Ethanol/Nutrition/Herb Interactions

Ethanol: Use caution with concurrent use. Effects are additive and may decrease psychomotor function.

Food: Onset of action may be reduced if taken with or immediately after a heavy meal.

Herb/Nutraceutical: Avoid valerian, St John's wort, kava kava, gotu kola (may increase CNS depression).

Stability Store at controlled room temperature of 25°C (77°F).

Mechanism of Action May interact with GABA-receptor complexes at binding domains located close to or allosterically coupled to benzodiazepine receptors.

Pharmacodynamics/Kinetics

Absorption: Rapid; high-fat/heavy meal may delay absorption

Protein binding: 52% to 59%

Metabolism: Hepatic via oxidation and demethylation (CYP2E1, 3A4); 2 primary metabolites; one with activity less than parent.

Half-life elimination: ~6 hours; Elderly (≥65 years): ~9 hours

Time to peak, plasma: ~1 hour

Excretion: Urine (up to 75%, primarily as metabolites; <10% as parent drug)

Dosage Oral:

Adults: Insomnia: Initial: 2 mg immediately before bedtime (maximum dose: 3 mg)

Concurrent use with strong CYP3A4 inhibitor: 1 mg immediately before bedtime; if needed, dose may be increased to 2 mg

Elderly:

Difficulty **falling** asleep: Initial: 1 mg immediately before bedtime; maximum dose: 2 mg

Difficulty **staying** asleep: 2 mg immediately before bedtime

Dosage adjustment in renal impairment: None required

Dosage adjustment in hepatic impairment:

Mild-to-moderate: Use with caution; dosage adjustment unnecessary

Severe: Initial dose: 1 mg; maximum dose: 2 mg

Dietary Considerations Avoid taking after a heavy meal; may delay onset.

Administration Because of the rapid onset of action, eszopiclone should be administered immediately prior to bedtime or after the patient has gone to bed and is having difficulty falling asleep. Do not take with, or immediately following, a high-fat meal; do not crush or break tablet.

Dosage Forms Excipient information presented when available (limited, particularly for generics); consult specific product labeling.

Tablet: 1 mg, 2 mg, 3 mg

Etanercept (et a NER sept)

U.S. Brand Names Enbrel®

Canadian Brand Names Enbrel®

Pharmacologic Category Antirheumatic, Disease Modifying; Tumor Necrosis Factor (TNF) Blocking Agent

Use Treatment of moderately- to severely-active rheumatoid arthritis (RA); moderately- to severely-active polyarticular juvenile idiopathic arthritis (JIA); psoriatic arthritis; active ankylosing spondylitis (AS); moderate-to-severe chronic plaque psoriasis

Restrictions An FDA-approved patient medication guide is available and must be distributed when dispensing an outpatient prescription (new or refill) where this medication is to be used without direct supervision of a healthcare provider. Medication guides are available at http://www.fda.gov/cder/Offices/ODS/medication_guides.htm.

Pregnancy Risk Factor B

Pregnancy Considerations Developmental toxicity studies performed in animals have revealed no evidence of harm to the fetus. There are no studies in pregnant women; this drug should be used during pregnancy only if clearly needed. A pregnancy registry has been established to monitor outcomes of women exposed to etanercept during pregnancy (877-311-8972).

Lactation Excretion in breast milk unknown/not recommended

Contraindications Hypersensitivity to etanercept or any component of the formulation; patients with sepsis (mortality may be increased); active infections (including chronic or local infection)

Warnings/Precautions [U.S. Boxed Warning]: Serious and potentially fatal infections have been reported including bacterial sepsis and tuberculosis. Cases of unrecognized invasive fungal infections (eg, histoplasmosis, blastomycosis, coccidioidomycosis) have also been reported with anti-TNF agent use. Discontinue administration if patient develops a serious infection or sepsis. Caution should be exercised when considering the use in patients with chronic infection, history of recurrent infection, or predisposition to infection (eg, poorly-controlled diabetes or residence/travel from areas of endemic mycoses). Do not give to patients with an active chronic or localized infection. Patients should be educated about the symptoms of infection and closely monitored for signs and symptoms while undergoing treatment. **[U.S. Boxed Warning]: Tuberculosis (disseminated or extra-pulmonary) has been reported in patients receiving etanercept; both reactivation of latent infection and new infections have been reported.** Patients should be evaluated for latent tuberculosis infection with a tuberculin skin test prior to starting therapy. Treatment of latent tuberculosis should be initiated before therapy is used. Some patients who tested negative prior to therapy have developed active infection; monitor for signs and symptoms of tuberculosis in all patients. Rare reactivation of hepatitis B has occurred in chronic carriers of the virus; evaluate prior to initiation and during treatment in patients at risk for hepatitis B infection. Patients should be brought up to date with all immunizations before initiating therapy. Live vaccines should not be given concurrently. Patients with a significant exposure to varicella virus should temporarily discontinue etanercept. Treatment with varicella zoster immune globulin should be considered.

Impact on the development and course of malignancies is not fully defined. As compared to the general population, an increased risk of lymphoma has been noted in clinical trials; however, rheumatoid arthritis has been previously associated with an increased rate of lymphoma. Etanercept is not recommended for use in patients with Wegener's granulomatosis who are receiving immunosuppressive therapy. Treatment may result in the formation of autoimmune antibodies; cases of autoimmune disease have not been described. Non-neutralizing antibodies to etanercept may also be formed. Rarely, a reversible lupus-like syndrome has occurred. Safety and efficacy have not been established in children <2 years of age.

Use with caution in patients with pre-existing or recent onset CNS demyelinating disorders; rare cases of new onset or exacerbation of CNS demyelinating disorders have occurred; may present with mental status changes and some may be associated with permanent disability. Optic neuritis, transverse myelitis, multiple sclerosis, and new onset or exacerbation of seizures have been reported. Use with caution in patients with heart failure or decreased left ventricular function; worsening and new-onset heart failure has been reported. Use caution in patients with a history of significant hematologic abnormalities; has been associated with pancytopenia and aplastic anemia (rare). Discontinue if significant hematologic abnormalities are confirmed.

Due to higher incidence of serious infections, should not be used in combination with anakinra unless no satisfactory alternatives exist, and then only with extreme caution. Some dosage forms may contain dry natural rubber (latex).

Adverse Reactions Percentages reported for adults except where specified.

>10%:

- Central nervous system: Headache (17%; children 19%)
- Gastrointestinal: Abdominal pain (5%; children 19%), vomiting (3%; children 13%)
- Local: Injection site reaction (14% to 37%; erythema, itching, pain or swelling)
- Respiratory: Respiratory tract infection (upper; 12% to 29%), rhinitis (12% to 16%)
- Miscellaneous: Infection (35%; children 63%), positive ANA (11%), positive antidouble-stranded DNA antibodies (15% by RIA, 3% by *Crithidia luciliae* assay)

≥3% to 10%:

- Cardiovascular: Edema (2% to 8%)
- Central nervous system: Dizziness (7%)
- Dermatologic: Rash (5%)
- Gastrointestinal: Dyspepsia (4%), nausea (children 9%)
- Neuromuscular & skeletal: Weakness (5%)
- Respiratory: Pharyngitis (7%), respiratory disorder (5%), sinusitis (3%), cough (6%)

<3%, postmarketing, and/or case reports: Abscess, adenopathy, allergic reactions, alopecia, anemia, angioedema, anorexia, aplastic anemia, appendicitis, aseptic meningitis, bursitis, cerebral ischemia, chest pain, cholecystitis, coagulopathy; demyelinating CNS disorders (suggestive of multiple sclerosis, transverse myelitis, or optic neuritis); deep vein thrombosis, depression, diarrhea, dyspnea, erythema multiforme, fatigue, fever, flushing, flu-like syndrome, gastrointestinal hemorrhage, heart failure, hepatitis (autoimmune), hydrocephalus (with normal pressure), hyper-/hypotension; infections (bacterial, fungal, protozoal, viral); interstitial lung disease, intestinal perforation, joint pain, leukopenia, lupus-like syndrome, lymphadenopathy, malignancies (including lymphoma), membranous glomerulopathy, MI, mouth ulcer, multiple sclerosis, myocardial ischemia, neutropenia, ocular inflammation, optic neuritis, pancytopenia, pancreatitis, paresthesia, polymyositis, pruritus, psoriasis exacerbation, pulmonary disease, pulmonary embolism, renal calculus, sarcoidosis, seizure, stroke, Stevens-Johnson syndrome, subcutaneous nodules, taste disturbances, thrombocytopenia, thrombophlebitis, toxic epidermal necrolysis, transaminases increased, tuberculosis, tuberculous arthritis, urinary tract infection, urticaria, vasculitis (cutaneous), weight gain, xerophthalmia, xerostomia

Drug Interactions

Avoid Concomitant Use

Avoid concomitant use of Etanercept with any of the following: Anakinra; Natalizumab; Rilonacept; Vaccines (Live)

Increased Effect/Toxicity

Etanercept may increase the levels/effects of: Abatacept; Anakinra; Cyclophosphamide; Natalizumab; Rilonacept; Vaccines (Live)

The levels/effects of Etanercept may be increased by: Trastuzumab

Decreased Effect

Etanercept may decrease the levels/effects of: Vaccines (Inactivated)

The levels/effects of Etanercept may be decreased by: Echinacea

Ethanol/Nutrition/Herb Interactions Herb/Nutraceutical: Echinacea may decrease the therapeutic effects of etanercept (avoid concurrent use).

Stability Store prefilled syringes at 2°C to 8°C (36°F to 46°F); protect from light; do not freeze or shake. Powder for reconstitution must be refrigerated at 2°C to 8°C (36°F to 46°F). Do not freeze. Reconstitute lyophilized powder aseptically with 1 mL sterile bacteriostatic water for injection, USP (supplied); swirl gently, do not shake. Do not filter reconstituted solution during preparation or administration. Reconstituted vials of etanercept should be administered as soon as possible after reconstitution. If not administered immediately after reconstitution, etanercept may be stored in the vial at 2°C to 8°C (36°F to 46°F) for up to 14 days.

Mechanism of Action Etanercept is a recombinant DNA-derived protein composed of tumor necrosis factor receptor (TNFR) linked to the Fc portion of human IgG1. Etanercept binds tumor necrosis factor (TNF) and blocks its interaction with cell surface receptors. TNF plays an important role in the inflammatory processes and the resulting joint pathology of rheumatoid arthritis (RA), polyarticular-course juvenile idiopathic arthritis (JIA), ankylosing spondylitis (AS), and plaque psoriasis.

Pharmacodynamics/Kinetics

Onset of action: ~2-3 weeks; RA: 1-2 weeks

Half-life elimination: RA: SubQ: 72-132 hours

Time to peak: RA: SubQ: 35-103 hours

Excretion: Clearance: Children: 45.9 mL/hour/m^2; Adults: 89 mL/hour (52 mL/hour/m^2)

Dosage SubQ:

Children 2-17 years: Juvenile idiopathic arthritis:

Once-weekly dosing: 0.8 mg/kg (maximum: 50 mg/dose) once weekly

Twice-weekly dosing: 0.4 mg/kg (maximum: 25 mg/dose) twice weekly (individual doses should be separated by 72-96 hours)

Adults:

Rheumatoid arthritis, psoriatic arthritis, ankylosing spondylitis:

Once-weekly dosing: 50 mg once weekly

Twice weekly dosing: 25 mg given twice weekly (individual doses should be separated by 72-96 hours)

Plaque psoriasis:

Initial: 50 mg twice weekly, 3-4 days apart (starting doses of 25 or 50 mg once weekly have also been used successfully); maintain initial dose for 3 months

Maintenance dose: 50 mg once weekly

Elderly: Refer to adult dosing. Although greater sensitivity of some elderly patients cannot be ruled out, no overall differences in safety or effectiveness were observed.

Administration Administer subcutaneously. Rotate injection sites. New injections should be given at least one inch from an old site and never into areas where the skin is tender, bruised, red, or hard. **Note:** If the physician determines that it is appropriate, patients may self-inject after proper training in injection technique.

Powder for reconstitution: Follow package instructions carefully for reconstitution. The maximum amount injected at any single site should not exceed 25 mg.

Solution for injection: May be allowed to reach room temperature prior to injection.

Monitoring Parameters

Signs and symptoms of infection (prior to and during therapy); latent TB screening prior to therapy initiation

Dosage Forms Excipient information presented when available (limited, particularly for generics); consult specific product labeling.

Injection, powder for reconstitution:

Enbrel®: 25 mg [contains sucrose 10 mg; diluent contains benzyl alcohol]

Injection, solution [preservative free]:

Enbrel®: 50 mg/mL (0.51 mL, 0.98 mL) [contains sucrose 1%; natural rubber/natural latex in packaging]

◆ **Ethacrynate Sodium** *see* Ethacrynic Acid *on page 573*

Ethacrynic Acid (eth a KRIN ik AS id)

U.S. Brand Names Edecrin®; Sodium Edecrin®

Canadian Brand Names Edecrin®

Index Terms Ethacrynate Sodium

Pharmacologic Category Diuretic, Loop

Use Management of edema associated with congestive heart failure; hepatic cirrhosis or renal disease; short-term management of ascites due to malignancy, idiopathic edema, and lymphedema

Pregnancy Risk Factor B

Medication Safety Issues

Sound-alike/look-alike issues:

Edecrin® may be confused with Eulexin®, Ecotrin®

Dosage I.V. formulation should be diluted in D_5W or NS (1 mg/mL) and infused over several minutes.

Children: Oral: 1 mg/kg/dose once daily; increase at intervals of 2-3 days as needed, to a maximum of 3 mg/kg/day.

Adults:

Oral: 50-200 mg/day in 1-2 divided doses; may increase in increments of 25-50 mg at intervals of several days; doses up to 200 mg twice daily may be required with severe, refractory edema.

I.V.: 0.5-1 mg/kg/dose (maximum: 100 mg/dose); repeat doses not routinely recommended; however, if indicated, repeat doses every 8-12 hours.

Dosing adjustment/comments in renal impairment: Cl_{cr} <10 mL/minute: Avoid use.

Dialysis: Not removed by hemo- or peritoneal dialysis; supplemental dose is not necessary.

Additional Information Complete prescribing information for this medication should be consulted for additional detail.

Dosage Forms Excipient information presented when available (limited, particularly for generics); consult specific product labeling.

Injection, powder for reconstitution, as ethacrynate sodium:

Sodium Edecrin®: 50 mg

Tablet:

Edecrin®: 25 mg [scored]

Ethambutol (e THAM byoo tole)

U.S. Brand Names Myambutol®

Canadian Brand Names Etibi®

Index Terms Ethambutol Hydrochloride

Pharmacologic Category Antitubercular Agent

Additional Appendix Information

Antimicrobial Drugs of Choice *on page 1752*

Desensitization Protocols *on page 1691*

Guidelines for the Prevention of Opportunistic Infections in HIV Infected Persons *on page 1740*

Tuberculosis *on page 1776*

Use Treatment of tuberculosis and other mycobacterial diseases in conjunction with other antituberculosis agents

Pregnancy Risk Factor C

Pregnancy Considerations There are no adequate and well-controlled studies in pregnant women; teratogenic effects have been seen in animals. Ethambutol has been used safely during pregnancy.

Lactation Enters breast milk/use caution (AAP considers "compatible")

Medication Safety Issues

Sound-alike/look-alike issues:

Myambutol® may be confused with Nembutal®

Contraindications Hypersensitivity to ethambutol or any component of the formulation; optic neuritis; use in children, unconscious patients, or any other patient who may be unable to discern and report visual changes

Warnings/Precautions May cause optic neuritis, resulting in decreased visual acuity or other vision changes. Discontinue promptly in patients with changes in vision, color blindness, or visual defects (effects normally reversible, but reversal may require up to a year). Use only in children whose visual acuity can accurately be determined and monitored (not recommended for use in children <13 years of age unless the benefit outweighs the risk). Dosage modification is required in patients with renal insufficiency. Hepatic toxicity has been reported, possibly due to concurrent therapy.

Adverse Reactions Frequency not defined.

Cardiovascular: Myocarditis, pericarditis

Central nervous system: Headache, confusion, disorientation, malaise, mental confusion, fever, dizziness, hallucinations

Dermatologic: Rash, pruritus, dermatitis, exfoliative dermatitis

Endocrine & metabolic: Acute gout or hyperuricemia

Gastrointestinal: Abdominal pain, anorexia, nausea, vomiting
Hematologic: Leukopenia, thrombocytopenia, eosinophilia, neutropenia, lymphadenopathy
Hepatic: Abnormal LFTs, hepatotoxicity (possibly related to concurrent therapy), hepatitis
Neuromuscular & skeletal: Peripheral neuritis, arthralgia
Ocular: Optic neuritis; symptoms may include decreased acuity, scotoma, color blindness, or visual defects (usually reversible with discontinuation, irreversible blindness has been described)
Renal: Nephritis
Respiratory: Infiltrates (with or without eosinophilia), pneumonitis
Miscellaneous: Anaphylaxis, anaphylactoid reaction; hypersensitivity syndrome (rash, eosinophilia, and organ-specific inflammation)

Drug Interactions

Avoid Concomitant Use There are no known interactions where it is recommended to avoid concomitant use.

Increased Effect/Toxicity There are no known significant interactions involving an increase in effect.

Decreased Effect

The levels/effects of Ethambutol may be decreased by: Aluminum Hydroxide

Stability Store at controlled room temperature of 20°C to 25°C (68°F to 77°F).

Mechanism of Action Suppresses mycobacteria multiplication by interfering with RNA synthesis

Pharmacodynamics/Kinetics

Absorption: ~80%
Distribution: Widely throughout body; concentrated in kidneys, lungs, saliva, and red blood cells
Relative diffusion from blood into CSF: Adequate with or without inflammation (exceeds usual MICs)
CSF:blood level ratio: Normal meninges: 0%; Inflamed meninges: 25%
Protein binding: 20% to 30%
Metabolism: Hepatic (20%) to inactive metabolite
Half-life elimination: 2.5-3.6 hours; End-stage renal disease: 7-15 hours
Time to peak, serum: 2-4 hours
Excretion: Urine (~50%) and feces (20%) as unchanged drug

Dosage

Usual dosage range: Oral:
Children: 15-20 mg/kg/day (maximum: 1 g/day) **or** 50 mg/kg/dose twice weekly (maximum: 4 g/dose)
Adults: 15-25 mg/kg daily **or** 25-30 mg/kg/dose 3 times/week (maximum: 2.5 g/dose) **or** 50 mg/kg/dose twice weekly (maximum: 4 g/dose)

Indication-specific dosing: Oral:

Disseminated *Mycobacterium avium* complex (MAC) in patients with advanced HIV infection: Adults: 15 mg/kg ethambutol in combination with azithromycin 600 mg daily

Nontuberculous mycobacterium (*M. kansasii*) (unlabeled use; IDSA guidelines): Adults: 15 mg/kg/day for duration to include 12 months of culture-negative sputum; typically used in combination with rifampin and isoniazid; **Note:** Previous recommendations stated to use 25 mg/kg/day for the initial 2 months of therapy; however, IDSA guidelines state this may be unnecessary given the success of rifampin-based regimens with ethambutol 15 mg/kg/day or omitted altogether.

Tuberculosis, active: Note: Used as part of a multidrug regimen; treatment regimens consist of an initial 2 month phase, followed by a continuation phase of 4 or 7 additional months; frequency of dosing may differ depending on phase of therapy.

Children:
Daily therapy: 15-20 mg/kg/day (maximum: 1 g/day)
Twice weekly directly observed therapy (DOT): 50 mg/kg (maximum: 4 g/dose)

Adults (suggested doses by lean body weight):
Daily therapy: 15-25 mg/kg
40-55 kg: 800 mg
56-75 kg: 1200 mg
76-90 kg: 1600 mg (maximum dose regardless of weight)
Twice weekly directly observed therapy (DOT): 50 mg/kg
40-55 kg: 2000 mg
56-75 kg: 2800 mg
76-90 kg: 4000 mg (maximum dose regardless of weight)
Three times/week DOT: 25-30 mg/kg (maximum: 2.5 g)
40-55 kg: 1200 mg
56-75 kg: 2000 mg
76-90 kg: 2400 mg (maximum dose regardless of weight)

Dosing interval in renal impairment:
Cl_{cr} 10-50 mL/minute: Administer every 24-36 hours
Cl_{cr} <10 mL/minute: Administer every 48 hours
Hemodialysis: Slightly dialyzable (5% to 20%); Administer dose postdialysis
Peritoneal dialysis: Dose for Cl_{cr} <10 mL/minute
Continuous arteriovenous or venovenous hemofiltration: Administer every 24-36 hours

Dietary Considerations May be taken with food as absorption is not affected, may cause gastric irritation.

Monitoring Parameters Baseline and periodic (monthly) visual testing (each eye individually, as well as both eyes tested together) in patients receiving >15 mg/kg/day; baseline and periodic renal, hepatic, and hematopoietic tests

Dosage Forms Excipient information presented when available (limited, particularly for generics); consult specific product labeling.
Tablet, as hydrochloride: 100 mg, 400 mg

◆ **Ethambutol Hydrochloride** *see* Ethambutol *on page 573*

◆ **Ethamolin®** *see* Ethanolamine Oleate *on page 574*

◆ **Ethanoic Acid** *see* Acetic Acid *on page 35*

Ethanolamine Oleate (ETH a nol a meen OH lee ate)

U.S. Brand Names Ethamolin®

Index Terms Monoethanolamine

Pharmacologic Category Sclerosing Agent

Use Orphan drug: Sclerosing agent used for bleeding esophageal varices

Pregnancy Risk Factor C

Medication Safety Issues

Sound-alike/look-alike issues:
Ethamolin® may be confused with ethanol

Dosage Adults: 1.5-5 mL per varix, up to 20 mL total or 0.4 mL/kg for a 50 kg patient; doses should be decreased in patients with severe hepatic dysfunction and should receive less than recommended maximum dose

Additional Information Complete prescribing information for this medication should be consulted for additional detail.

Dosage Forms Excipient information presented when available (limited, particularly for generics); consult specific product labeling.
Injection, solution: 5% [50 mg/mL] (2 mL) [contains benzyl alcohol]

◆ **EtheDent™** *see* Fluoride *on page 635*

◆ **Ethezyme™ [DSC]** *see* Papain and Urea *on page 1142*

◆ **Ethezyme™ 650 [DSC]** *see* Papain and Urea *on page 1142*

◆ **Ethezyme™ 830 [DSC]** *see* Papain and Urea *on page 1142*

Ethinyl Estradiol and Desogestrel

(ETH in il es tra DYE ole & des oh JES trel)

U.S. Brand Names Apri®; Cesia™; Cyclessa®; Desogen®; Kariva™; Mircette®; Ortho-Cept®; Reclipsen™; Solia™; Velivet™

Canadian Brand Names Cyclessa®; Linessa®; Marvelon®; Ortho-Cept®

Index Terms Desogestrel and Ethinyl Estradiol; Ortho Cept

Pharmacologic Category Contraceptive; Estrogen and Progestin Combination

Use Prevention of pregnancy

Unlabeled/Investigational Use Treatment of hypermenorrhea (menorrhagia); pain associated with endometriosis; dysmenorrhea; dysfunctional uterine bleeding

Pregnancy Risk Factor X

Medication Safety Issues

Sound-alike/look-alike issues:

Apri® may be confused with Apriso™

Ortho-Cept® may be confused with Ortho-Cyclen®

Dosage Oral: Adults: Females: Contraception:

Schedule 1 (Sunday starter): Dose begins on first Sunday after onset of menstruation; if the menstrual period starts on Sunday, take first tablet that very same day. **With a Sunday start, an additional method of contraception should be used until after the first 7 days of consecutive administration.**

For 21-tablet package: Dosage is 1 tablet daily for 21 consecutive days, followed by 7 days off of the medication; a new course begins on the 8th day after the last tablet is taken.

For 28-tablet package: Dosage is 1 tablet daily without interruption.

Schedule 2 (Day 1 starter): Dose starts on first day of menstrual cycle taking 1 tablet daily.

For 21-tablet package: Dosage is 1 tablet daily for 21 consecutive days, followed by 7 days off of the medication; a new course begins on the 8th day after the last tablet is taken.

For 28-tablet package: Dosage is 1 tablet daily without interruption.

If all doses have been taken on schedule and one menstrual period is missed, continue dosing cycle. If two consecutive menstrual periods are missed, pregnancy test is required before new dosing cycle is started.

Missed doses **monophasic formulations** (refer to package insert for complete information):

One dose missed: Take as soon as remembered or take 2 tablets next day

Two consecutive doses missed in the first 2 weeks: Take 2 tablets as soon as remembered or 2 tablets next 2 days. **An additional method of contraception should be used for 7 days after missed dose.**

Two consecutive doses missed in week 3 or three consecutive doses missed at any time:

Schedule 1 (Sunday starter): Continue to take 1 tablet daily until Sunday, then discard the rest of the pack, and a new pack is started that same day.

Schedule 2 (Day 1 starter): Current pack should be discarded, and a new pack started that same day. **An additional method of contraception should be used for 7 days after missed dose.**

Missed doses **biphasic/triphasic formulations** (refer to package insert for complete information):

One dose missed: Take as soon as remembered or take 2 tablets next day.

Two consecutive doses missed in week 1 or week 2 of the pack: Take 2 tablets as soon as remembered and 2 tablets the next day. Resume taking 1 tablet daily until the pack is empty. **An additional method of contraception should be used for 7 days after a missed dose.**

Two consecutive doses missed in week 3 of the pack; **an additional method of contraception must be used for 7 days after a missed dose**:

Schedule 1 (Sunday starter): Take 1 tablet every day until Sunday. Discard the remaining pack and start a new pack of pills on the same day.

Schedule 2 (Day 1 starter): Discard the remaining pack and start a new pack the same day.

Three or more consecutive doses missed; **an additional method of contraception must be used for 7 days after a missed dose**:

Schedule 1 (Sunday starter): Take 1 tablet every day until Sunday; on Sunday, discard the pack and start a new pack.

Schedule 2 (Day 1 starter): Discard the remaining pack and begin new pack of tablets starting on the same day.

Dosage adjustment in renal impairment: Specific guidelines not available; use with caution and monitor blood pressure closely. Consider other forms of contraception.

Dosage adjustment in hepatic impairment: Contraindicated in patients with hepatic impairment

Additional Information Complete prescribing information for this medication should be consulted for additional detail.

Dosage Forms Excipient information presented when available (limited, particularly for generics); consult specific product labeling.

Tablet, low-dose formulations:

Kariva™:

Day 1-21: Ethinyl estradiol 0.02 mg and desogestrel 0.15 mg [21 white tablets]

Day 22-23: 2 inactive light green tablets

Day 24-28: Ethinyl estradiol 0.01 mg [5 light blue tablets] (28s)

Mircette®:

Day 1-21: Ethinyl estradiol 0.02 mg and desogestrel 0.15 mg [21 white tablets]

Day 22-23: 2 inactive green tablets

Day 24-28: Ethinyl estradiol 0.01 mg [5 yellow tablets] (28s)

Tablet, monophasic formulations:

Apri® 28: Ethinyl estradiol 0.03 mg and desogestrel 0.15 mg (28s) [21 rose tablets and 7 white inactive tablets]

Desogen®, Reclipsen™, Solia™: Ethinyl estradiol 0.03 mg and desogestrel 0.15 mg (28s) [21 white tablets and 7 green inactive tablets]

Ortho-Cept® 28: Ethinyl estradiol 0.03 mg and desogestrel 0.15 mg (28s) [21 orange tablets and 7 green inactive tablets]

Tablet, triphasic formulations:

Cesia™, Cyclessa®:

Day 1-7: Ethinyl estradiol 0.025 mg and desogestrel 0.1 mg [7 light yellow tablets]

Day 8-14: Ethinyl estradiol 0.025 mg and desogestrel 0.125 mg [7 orange tablets]

Day 14-21: Ethinyl estradiol 0.025 mg and desogestrel 0.15 mg [7 red tablets]

Day 21-28: 7 green inactive tablets (28s)

Velivet™:

Day 1-7: Ethinyl estradiol 0.025 mg and desogestrel 0.1 mg [7 beige tablets]

Day 8-14: Ethinyl estradiol 0.025 mg and desogestrel 0.125 mg [7 orange tablets]

Day 14-21: Ethinyl estradiol 0.025 mg and desogestrel 0.15 mg [7 pink tablets]
Day 21-28: 7 white inactive tablets (28s)

Ethinyl Estradiol and Drospirenone

(ETH in il es tra DYE ole & droh SPYE re none)

U.S. Brand Names Ocella™; Yasmin®; Yaz®
Canadian Brand Names Yasmin®
Index Terms Drospirenone and Ethinyl Estradiol
Pharmacologic Category Contraceptive; Estrogen and Progestin Combination
Use Females: Prevention of pregnancy; treatment of premenstrual dysphoric disorder (PMDD); treatment of acne
Unlabeled/Investigational Use Treatment of hypermenorrhea (menorrhagia); pain associated with endometriosis; dysmenorrhea; dysfunctional uterine bleeding
Pregnancy Risk Factor X
Dosage Oral:
Children ≥14 years and Adults: Females: Acne (Yaz®): Refer to dosing for contraception
Adults: Females: Contraception (Yasmin®, Yaz®), PMDD (Yaz®): Dosage is 1 tablet daily for 28 consecutive days. Dose should be taken at the same time each day, either after the evening meal or at bedtime. Dosing may be started on the first day of menstrual period (Day 1 starter) or on the first Sunday after the onset of the menstrual period (Sunday starter).

Day 1 starter: Dose starts on first day of menstrual cycle taking 1 tablet daily.
Sunday starter: Dose begins on first Sunday after onset of menstruation; if the menstrual period starts on Sunday, take first tablet that very same day. **With a Sunday start, an additional method of contraception should be used until after the first 7 days of consecutive administration.**
If all doses have been taken on schedule and one menstrual period is missed, continue dosing cycle. If two consecutive menstrual periods are missed, pregnancy test is required before new dosing cycle is started.
If doses have been missed during the first 3 weeks and the menstrual period is missed, pregnancy should be ruled out prior to continuing treatment.
Missed doses (monophasic formulations) (refer to package insert for complete information):
One dose missed: Take as soon as remembered or take 2 tablets next day
Two consecutive doses missed in the first 2 weeks: Take 2 tablets as soon as remembered or 2 tablets next 2 days. **An additional method of contraception should be used for 7 days after missed dose.**
Two consecutive doses missed in week 3 or three consecutive doses missed at any time: **An additional method of contraception must be used for 7 days after a missed dose.**
Day 1 starter: Current pack should be discarded, and a new pack should be started that same day.
Sunday starter: Continue dose of 1 tablet daily until Sunday, then discard the rest of the pack, and a new pack should be started that same day.
Any number of doses missed in week 4: Continue taking one pill each day until pack is empty; no back-up method of contraception is needed

Dosage adjustment in renal impairment: Contraindicated in patients with renal dysfunction (Cl_{cr} ≤50 mL/minute)
Dosage adjustment in hepatic impairment: Contraindicated in patients with hepatic dysfunction
Additional Information Complete prescribing information for this medication should be consulted for additional detail.

Dosage Forms Excipient information presented when available (limited, particularly for generics); consult specific product labeling.
Tablet:
Ocella™: Ethinyl estradiol 0.03 mg and drospirenone 3 mg (28s) [21 yellow active tablets and 7 white inactive tablets]
Yasmin®: Ethinyl estradiol 0.03 mg and drospirenone 3 mg (28s) [21 yellow active tablets and 7 white inactive tablets]
Yaz®: Ethinyl estradiol 0.02 mg and drospirenone 3 mg (28s) [24 light pink tablets and 4 white inactive tablets]

Ethinyl Estradiol and Ethynodiol Diacetate

(ETH in il es tra DYE ole & e thye noe DYE ole dye AS e tate)

U.S. Brand Names Kelnor™; Zovia®
Canadian Brand Names Demulen® 30
Index Terms Ethynodiol Diacetate and Ethinyl Estradiol
Pharmacologic Category Contraceptive; Estrogen and Progestin Combination
Use Prevention of pregnancy
Unlabeled/Investigational Use Treatment of hypermenorrhea (menorrhagia); pain associated with endometriosis; dysmenorrhea; dysfunctional uterine bleeding
Pregnancy Risk Factor X
Medication Safety Issues
Sound-alike/look-alike issues:
Demulen® may be confused with Dalmane®, Demerol®
Dosage Oral: Adults: Females: Contraception:
Schedule 1 (Sunday starter): Dose begins on first Sunday after onset of menstruation; if the menstrual period starts on Sunday, take first tablet that very same day. **With a Sunday start, an additional method of contraception should be used until after the first 7 days of consecutive administration.**
For 21-tablet package: 1 tablet/day for 21 consecutive days, followed by 7 days off of the medication; a new course begins on the 8th day after the last tablet is taken.
For 28-tablet package: 1 tablet/day without interruption.
Schedule 2 (Day 1 starter): Dose starts on first day of menstrual cycle taking 1 tablet daily.
For 21-tablet package: 1 tablet/day for 21 consecutive days, followed by 7 days off of the medication; a new course begins on the 8th day after the last tablet is taken.
For 28-tablet package: 1 tablet/day without interruption.
If all doses have been taken on schedule and one menstrual period is missed, continue dosing cycle. If two consecutive menstrual periods are missed, pregnancy test is required before new dosing cycle is started.
Missed doses **monophasic formulations** (refer to package insert for complete information):
One dose missed: Take as soon as remembered or take 2 tablets next day
Two consecutive doses missed in the first 2 weeks: Take 2 tablets as soon as remembered or 2 tablets next 2 days. **An additional method of contraception should be used for 7 days after missed dose.**
Two consecutive doses missed in week 3 or three consecutive doses missed at any time: **An additional method of contraception should be used for 7 days after missed dose:**
Schedule 1 (Sunday starter): Continue dose of 1 tablet daily until Sunday, then discard the rest of the pack, and a new pack should be started that same day.
Schedule 2 (Day 1 starter): Current package should be discarded, and a new pack should be started that same day.

Dosage adjustment in renal impairment: Specific guidelines not available; use with caution and monitor blood pressure closely. Consider other forms of contraception.

Dosage adjustment in hepatic impairment: Contraindicated in patients with hepatic impairment

Additional Information Complete prescribing information for this medication should be consulted for additional detail.

Dosage Forms Excipient information presented when available (limited, particularly for generics); consult specific product labeling.

Tablet, monophasic formulations:

Kelnor™ 1/35: Ethinyl estradiol 0.035 mg and ethynodiol diacetate 1 mg [21 light yellow tablets and 7 white inactive tablets] (28s)

Zovia® 1/35-28: Ethinyl estradiol 0.035 mg and ethynodiol diacetate 1 mg [21 light pink tablets and 7 white inactive tablets] (28s)

Zovia® 1/50-28: Ethinyl estradiol 0.05 mg and ethynodiol diacetate 1 mg [21 pink tablets and 7 white inactive tablets] (28s)

Ethinyl Estradiol and Etonogestrel

(ETH in il es tra DYE ole & et oh noe JES trel)

U.S. Brand Names NuvaRing®

Canadian Brand Names NuvaRing®

Index Terms Etonogestrel and Ethinyl Estradiol

Pharmacologic Category Contraceptive; Estrogen and Progestin Combination

Use Prevention of pregnancy

Unlabeled/Investigational Use Treatment of hypermenorrhea (menorrhagia); pain associated with endometriosis; dysmenorrhea; dysfunctional uterine bleeding

Pregnancy Risk Factor X

Dosage Vaginal: Adults: Females: Contraception: One ring, inserted vaginally and left in place for 3 consecutive weeks, then removed for 1 week. A new ring is inserted 7 days after the last was removed (even if bleeding is not complete) and should be inserted at approximately the same time of day the ring was removed the previous week.

Initial treatment should begin as follows (pregnancy should always be ruled out first):

No hormonal contraceptive use in the past month: Insert ring on the first day of menstrual cycle ("Day 1"). May also insert on days 2-5 even if bleeding is not complete, however, **a spermicide or barrier method of contraception should be used for the following 7 days.***

Switching from combination oral contraceptive: Ring can be inserted on any day within 7 days after the last **active** tablet in the cycle was taken and no later than the first day a new cycle of tablets would begin. Additional forms of contraception are not needed.

Switching from progestin-only contraceptive: **A spermicide or barrier method of contraception should be used for the following 7 days with any of the following.***

If previously using a progestin-only mini-pill, insert the ring on any day of the month; do not skip days between the last pill and insertion of the ring.

If previously using an implant, insert the ring on the same day of implant removal.

If previously using a progestin-containing IUD, insert the ring on day of IUD removal.

If previously using a progestin injection, insert the ring on the day the next injection would be given.

Following complete 1st trimester abortion: Insert ring within the first 5 days of abortion. If not inserted within 5 days, follow instructions for "No hormonal contraceptive use within the past month" and instruct patient to use a nonhormonal contraceptive in the interim.

Following delivery or 2nd trimester abortion: Insert ring 4 weeks postpartum (in women who are not breast-feeding) or following 2nd trimester abortion. **A spermicide or barrier method of contraception should be used for the following 7 days.***

If the ring is accidentally removed from the vagina at anytime during the 3-week period of use, it may be rinsed with cool or lukewarm water (not hot) and reinserted as soon as possible. If the ring is not reinserted within 3 hours, contraceptive effectiveness will be decreased. **A spermicide or barrier method of contraception should be used until the ring has been in place for 7 consecutive days.***

If the ring has been removed for longer than 1 week, pregnancy must be ruled out prior to restarting therapy. **A spermicide or barrier method of contraception should be used for the following 7 days.***

If the ring has been left in place for >3 weeks, a new ring should be inserted following a 1-week (ring-free) interval. Protection continues during week 4, however, if the ring is left in place >4 weeks, pregnancy must be ruled out prior to insertion and **a spermicide or barrier method of contraception should be used for the following 7 days.***

Disconnected ring: In the event the ring disconnects at the weld joint, discard and replace with a new ring.

***Note:** Diaphragms may interfere with proper ring placement, and therefore, are not recommended for use as an additional form of contraception.

Dosage adjustment in renal impairment: Specific guidelines not available; use with caution and monitor blood pressure closely. Consider other forms of contraception.

Dosage adjustment in hepatic impairment: Contraindicated in patients with hepatic impairment

Additional Information Complete prescribing information for this medication should be consulted for additional detail.

Dosage Forms Excipient information presented when available (limited, particularly for generics); consult specific product labeling.

Ring, vaginal:

NuvaRing®: Ethinyl estradiol 0.015 mg/day and etonogestrel 0.12 mg/day (1s) [3-week duration]

Ethinyl Estradiol and Levonorgestrel

(ETH in il es tra DYE ole & LEE voe nor jes trel)

U.S. Brand Names Alesse®; Aviane™; Enpresse™; Jolessa™; Lessina™; Levlen®; Levlite™; Levora®; Lutera™; Lybrel™; Nordette®; Portia™; Quasense™; Seasonale®; Seasonique™; Sronyx™; Triphasil®; Trivora®

Canadian Brand Names Alesse®; Aviane®; Min-Ovral®; Seasonale®; Triphasil®; Triquilar®

Index Terms Levonorgestrel and Ethinyl Estradiol

Pharmacologic Category Contraceptive; Estrogen and Progestin Combination

Use Prevention of pregnancy; postcoital contraception

Unlabeled/Investigational Use Treatment of hypermenorrhea (menorrhagia); pain associated with endometriosis; dysmenorrhea; dysfunctional uterine bleeding

Pregnancy Risk Factor X

Pregnancy Considerations Pregnancy should be ruled out prior to treatment and discontinued if pregnancy occurs. In general, the use of combination hormonal contraceptives when inadvertently taken early in pregnancy have not been associated with teratogenic effects. Due to increased risk of thromboembolism postpartum, combination hormonal contraceptives should not be started earlier than 4-6 weeks following delivery. Hormonal contraceptives may be less effective in obese patients. An increase in oral contraceptive failure was noted in women with a BMI >27.3. Similar findings were noted in patients weighing ≥90 kg (198 lb) using the contraceptive patch.

Lactation Enters breast milk/not recommended

Medication Safety Issues

Sound-alike/look-alike issues:

Alesse® may be confused with Aleve®
Nordette® may be confused with Nicorette®
PREVEN® may be confused with Prevnar®
Seasonale® may be confused with Seasonique™
Seasonique™ may be confused with Seasonale®
Tri-Levlen® may be confused with Trilafon®
Triphasil® may be confused with Tri-Norinyl®

Contraindications Hypersensitivity to ethinyl estradiol, levonorgestrel, or any component of the formulation; history of or current thrombophlebitis or venous thromboembolic disorders (including DVT, PE); active or recent (within 1 year) arterial thromboembolic disease (eg, stroke, MI); cerebral vascular disease, coronary artery disease, valvular heart disease with complications, severe/uncontrolled hypertension, thrombogenic rhythm disorders, hereditary or acquired thrombophilias; diabetes mellitus with vascular involvement; severe headache with focal neurological symptoms; known or suspected breast carcinoma, endometrial cancer, estrogen-dependent neoplasms, undiagnosed abnormal genital bleeding; hepatic dysfunction or tumor, cholestatic jaundice of pregnancy, jaundice with prior combination hormonal contraceptive use; major surgery with prolonged immobilization; heavy smoking (≥15 cigarettes/day) in patients >35 years of age; pregnancy

Canadian-labeling: Additional contraindication: Ocular lesions due to ophthalmic vascular disease including partial or complete loss of vision or defect in visual fields; severe dyslipoproteinemia; hereditary or acquired predisposition for venous or arterial thrombosis

Warnings/Precautions Combination hormonal contraceptives do not protect against HIV infection or other sexually-transmitted diseases. **[U.S. Boxed Warning]: The risk of cardiovascular side effects increases in women who smoke cigarettes, especially those who are >35 years of age; women who use combination hormonal contraceptives should be strongly advised not to smoke.** Combination hormonal contraceptives may lead to increased risk of myocardial infarction, use with caution in patients with risk factors for coronary artery disease. May increase the risk of thromboembolism. Whenever possible, combination hormonal contraceptives should be discontinued at least 4 weeks prior to and for 2 weeks following elective surgery associated with an increased risk of thromboembolism or during periods of prolonged immobilization. Combination hormonal contraceptives may have a dose-related risk of vascular disease, hypertension, and gallbladder disease and may worsen existing gallbladder disease. Women with hypertension or renal disease should be encouraged to use another form of contraception. The use of combination hormonal contraceptives has been associated with a slight increase in frequency of breast cancer, however, studies are not consistent. Combination hormonal contraceptives may cause glucose intolerance or effect serum triglyceride and lipoprotein levels. Retinal thrombosis has been reported (rarely). Use caution with conditions that may be aggravated by fluid retention, depression, or history of migraine. Not for use prior to menarche.

Presentation of irregular, unresolving vaginal bleeding warrants further evaluation including endometrial sampling, if indicated, to rule out malignancy; evaluate hypothalamic-pituitary-function in women with persistent (≥6 months) amenorrhea (especially associated with breast secretion) following discontinuation of therapy. Discontinue use with the onset of sudden enlargement, pain, or tenderness of fibroids (leiomyomata). Extremely rare hepatic adenomas and focal nodular hyperplasia resulting in fatal intra-abdominal hemorrhage have been reported in association with long-term oral contraceptive use; presentation of an abdominal mass, acute abdominal pain, or intra-abdominal bleeding warrants further evaluation to rule out source.

The minimum dosage combination of estrogen/progestin that will effectively treat the individual patient should be used. New patients should be started on products containing ≤0.035 mg of estrogen per tablet. Extended cycle regimen contraceptives provide more hormonal exposure per year than conventional monthly contraceptives.

Adverse Reactions The following reactions have been associated with oral contraceptive use:

Increased risk or evidence of association with use:

Cardiovascular: Arterial thromboembolism, cerebral hemorrhage, cerebral thrombosis, hypertension, mesenteric thrombosis, MI, venous thrombosis (with or without embolism)
Gastrointestinal: Gallbladder disease
Hepatic: Hepatic adenomas, liver tumors (benign)
Local: Thrombophlebitis
Ocular: Retinal thrombosis
Respiratory: Pulmonary embolism

Adverse reactions considered drug related:

Cardiovascular: Edema, varicose vein aggravation
Central nervous system: Depression, migraine, mood changes
Dermatologic: Chloasma, melasma, rash (allergic)
Endocrine & metabolic: Amenorrhea, breakthrough bleeding, breast changes (enlargement, pain, secretion, tenderness), carbohydrate tolerance decreased, fluid retention, infertility (temporary), lactation decreased (with use immediately postpartum), menstrual flow changes, spotting
Gastrointestinal: Abdominal bloating, abdominal cramps, abdominal pain, appetite changes, nausea, weight changes, vomiting
Genitourinary: Cervical ectropion, cervical secretion/erosion, endocervical hyperplasia, fibroid enlargement, vaginal candidiasis, vaginitis
Hematologic: Folate decreased, porphyria exacerbation
Hepatic: Cholestatic jaundice, focal nodular hyperplasia
Neuromuscular & skeletal: Chorea exacerbation
Ocular: Contact lens intolerance, corneal curvature changes (steepening)
Respiratory: Rhinitis
Miscellaneous: Anaphylactic/anaphylactoid reactions (including angioedema, circulatory collapse, respiratory collapse, urticaria), SLE exacerbation

Adverse reactions in which association is not confirmed or denied: Acne, auditory disturbances, Budd-Chiari syndrome, cataracts, cervical smear abnormal, colitis, cystitis-like syndrome, dizziness, dysmenorrhea, erythema multiforme, erythema nodosum, headache, hemolytic uremic syndrome, hemorrhagic eruption, hirsutism, libido changes, nervousness, optic neuritis (with or without partial or complete loss of vision), pancreatitis, premenstrual syndrome, renal function impaired, scalp hair loss

Drug Interactions

Metabolism/Transport Effects

Ethinyl estradiol: **Substrate** of CYP2C9 (minor), 3A4 (major), 3A5-7 (minor); **Inhibits** CYP1A2 (weak), 2B6 (weak), 2C8 (weak), 2C19 (weak), 3A4 (weak)
Levonorgestrel: **Substrate** of CYP3A4 (major)

Avoid Concomitant Use

Avoid concomitant use of Ethinyl Estradiol and Levonorgestrel with any of the following: Acitretin; Griseofulvin

Increased Effect/Toxicity

Ethinyl Estradiol and Levonorgestrel may increase the levels/effects of: Benzodiazepines (metabolized by oxidation); Corticosteroids (Systemic); Ropinirole; Selegiline; Tipranavir; TiZANidine; Voriconazole

The levels/effects of Ethinyl Estradiol and Levonorgestrel may be increased by: Herbs (Estrogenic Properties); Herbs (Progestogenic Properties); Voriconazole

Decreased Effect

Ethinyl Estradiol and Levonorgestrel may decrease the levels/effects of: LamoTRIgine; Protease Inhibitors; Thyroid Products; Vitamin K Antagonists

The levels/effects of Ethinyl Estradiol and Levonorgestrel may be decreased by: Acitretin; Aminoglutethimide; Aprepitant; Armodafinil; Barbiturates; CarBAMazepine; Colesevelam; CYP3A4 Inducers (Strong); Deferasirox; Felbamate; Fosaprepitant; Griseofulvin; Modafinil; Mycophenolate; Nafcillin; OXcarbazepine; Phenytoin; Protease Inhibitors; Retinoic Acid Derivatives; Rifamycin Derivatives; Rufinamide; St Johns Wort; Tipranavir; Topiramate

Ethanol/Nutrition/Herb Interactions

Food: CNS effects of caffeine may be enhanced if combination hormonal contraceptives are used concurrently with caffeine. Grapefruit juice increases ethinyl estradiol concentrations and would be expected to increase progesterone serum levels as well; clinical implications are unclear.

Herb/Nutraceutical: St John's wort may decrease levels. Herbs with estrogenic properties may enhance the adverse/toxic effect of estrogen derivatives; examples include alfalfa, black cohosh, bloodroot, hops, kudzu, licorice, red clover, saw palmetto, soybean, thyme, wild yam, yucca. Herbs with progestogenic properties may enhance the adverse/toxic effect of progestins; examples include bloodroot, chasteberry, damiana, oregano, yucca. Impaired folate metabolism and reduced serum levels of cyanocobalamin have been reported with oral contraceptive use; increased dietary intake or supplementation may be necessary.

Stability Store at controlled room temperature of 20°C to 25°C (68°F to 77°F).

Mechanism of Action Combination hormonal contraceptives inhibit ovulation via a negative feedback mechanism on the hypothalamus, which alters the normal pattern of gonadotropin secretion of a follicle-stimulating hormone (FSH) and luteinizing hormone by the anterior pituitary. The follicular phase FSH and midcycle surge of gonadotropins are inhibited. In addition, combination hormonal contraceptives produce alterations in the genital tract, including changes in the cervical mucus, rendering it unfavorable for sperm penetration even if ovulation occurs. Changes in the endometrium may also occur, producing an unfavorable environment for nidation. Combination hormonal contraceptive drugs may alter the tubal transport of the ova through the fallopian tubes. Progestational agents may also alter sperm fertility.

Pharmacodynamics/Kinetics

Absorption: Rapid

Distribution: Ethinyl estradiol: 4.3 L/kg; Levonorgestrel: 1.8 L/kg

Protein binding:

- Ethinyl estradiol: 95% to 97% to albumin
- Levonorgestrel: 97% to 99% primarily to sex hormone binding globulin (SHBG), lesser amounts to albumin

Metabolism:

- Ethinyl estradiol: Hepatic via CYP3A4; undergoes first-pass metabolism; forms metabolites
- Levonorgestrel: Forms conjugated in unconjugated metabolites

Bioavailability: Ethinyl estradiol: 38% to 48%; Levonorgestrel: 100%

Half-life elimination: Ethinyl estradiol: 12-23 hours; Levonorgestrel: 22-49 hours

Excretion:

- Ethinyl estradiol: Urine and feces
- Levonorgestrel: Urine (40% to 68%, parent drug and metabolites); feces (16% to 48% as metabolites)

Dosage Oral: Adults: Females:

Contraception, 28-day cycle:

Schedule 1 (Sunday starter): Dose begins on first Sunday after onset of menstruation; if the menstrual period starts on Sunday, take first tablet that very same day. With a Sunday start, an additional method of contraception should be used until after the first 7 days of consecutive administration:

- For 21-tablet package: 1 tablet/day for 21 consecutive days, followed by 7 days off of the medication; a new course begins on the 8th day after the last tablet is taken
- For 28-tablet package: 1 tablet/day without interruption

Schedule 2 (Day 1 starter): Dose starts on first day of menstrual cycle taking 1 tablet/day:

- For 21-tablet package: 1 tablet/day for 21 consecutive days, followed by 7 days off of the medication; a new course begins on the 8th day after the last tablet is taken
- For 28-tablet package: 1 tablet/day without interruption

If all doses have been taken on schedule and one menstrual period is missed, continue dosing cycle. If two consecutive menstrual periods are missed, pregnancy test is required before new dosing cycle is started.

Missed doses **monophasic formulations** (refer to package insert for complete information):

- One dose missed: Take as soon as remembered or take 2 tablets next day
- Two consecutive doses missed in the first 2 weeks: Take 2 tablets as soon as remembered or 2 tablets next 2 days. An additional method of contraception should be used for 7 days after missed dose.
- Two consecutive doses missed in week 3 or three consecutive doses missed at any time: An additional method of contraception must be used for 7 days after a missed dose:
  - Schedule 1 (Sunday starter): Continue dose of 1 tablet daily until Sunday, then discard the rest of the pack, and a new pack should be started that same day.
  - Schedule 2 (Day 1 starter): Current pack should be discarded, and a new pack should be started that same day.

Missed doses **biphasic/triphasic formulations** (refer to package insert for complete information):

- One dose missed: Take as soon as remembered or take 2 tablets next day.
- Two consecutive doses missed in week 1 or week 2 of the pack: Take 2 tablets as soon as remembered and 2 tablets the next day. Resume taking 1 tablet daily until the pack is empty. An additional method of contraception should be used for 7 days after a missed dose.
- Two consecutive doses missed in week 3 of the pack: An additional method of contraception must be used for 7 days after a missed dose.
  - Schedule 1 (Sunday starter): Take 1 tablet every day until Sunday. Discard the remaining pack and start a new pack of pills on the same day.
  - Schedule 2 (Day 1 starter): Discard the remaining pack and start a new pack the same day.
- Three or more consecutive doses missed: An additional method of contraception must be used for 7 days after a missed dose.
  - Schedule 1 (Sunday starter): Take 1 tablet every day until Sunday; on Sunday, discard the pack and start a new pack.

Schedule 2 (Day 1 starter): Discard the remaining pack and begin new pack of tablets starting on the same day.

Contraception, 91-day cycle (extended cycle regimen): Dose begins on first Sunday after onset of menstruation; if the menstrual period starts on Sunday, take first tablet that very same day. An additional method of contraception should be used until after the first 7 days of consecutive administration:

Seasonale®: One active tablet/day for 84 consecutive days, followed by 1 inactive tablet/day for 7 days; if all doses have been taken on schedule and one menstrual period is missed, pregnancy should be ruled out prior to continuing therapy.

Seasonique™: One active tablet/day for 84 consecutive days, followed by 1 low dose estrogen tablet/day for 7 days; if all doses have been taken on schedule and one menstrual period is missed, pregnancy should be ruled out prior to continuing therapy.

Missed doses:

One dose missed: Take as soon as remembered or take 2 tablets the next day

Two consecutive doses missed: Take 2 tablets as soon as remembered or 2 tablets the next 2 days. An additional nonhormonal method of contraception should be used for 7 consecutive days after the missed dose.

Three or more consecutive doses missed: Do not take the missed doses; continue taking 1 tablet/day until pack is complete. Bleeding may occur during the following week. An additional nonhormonal method of contraception should be used for 7 consecutive days after the missed dose.

Any number of pills during week 13: Throw away the missed pills and keep taking scheduled pills until the pack is finished. A back-up method of contraception is not needed

Contraception, continuous use (extended cycle regimen): Lybrel™: Take one tablet daily, at the same time each day, without a tablet-free interval. Therapy should be initiated as follows:

No previous contraception: Begin on the first day of menstrual cycle. Back-up contraception is not needed.

Previously taking a 21-day or 28-day combination hormonal contraceptive: Begin on day 1 of the withdrawal bleed (at the latest, 7 days after the last active tablet). Back-up contraception is not needed.

Previously using a progestin-only pill: Begin the day after taking a progestin only pill. Back-up contraception is needed for the first 7 days of therapy.

Previously using contraceptive implant: Begin the day of implant removal. Back-up contraception is needed for the first 7 days of therapy.

Previously using contraceptive injection: Begin when the next injection is due. Back-up contraception is needed for the first 7 days of therapy.

Missed doses:

One dose missed: Take as soon as remembered then take the next tablet at the regular time (2 tablets in 1 day). An additional nonhormonal method of contraception should also be used for 7 consecutive days.

Two consecutive doses missed: If remembered the day of the second missed tablet, take 2 tablets as soon as remembered, then 1 tablet the next day. If remembered the day after the second tablet is missed, take 2 tablets the day remembered, then 2 tablets the next day. An additional nonhormonal method of contraception should also be used for 7 consecutive days.

Three or more consecutive doses missed: Take 1 tablet daily and contact healthcare provider; do not take the missed pills. An additional nonhormonal method of contraception should also be used for 7 consecutive days.

Dosage adjustment in renal impairment: Specific guidelines not available; use with caution and monitor blood pressure closely. Consider other forms of contraception.

Dosage adjustment in hepatic impairment: Contraindicated in patients with hepatic impairment

Dietary Considerations Should be taken at the same time each day.

Administration Administer at the same time each day.

Monitoring Parameters Before starting therapy, a physical exam with reference to the breasts and pelvis are recommended, including a Papanicolaou smear. Exam may be deferred if appropriate; pregnancy should be ruled out prior to use. Monitor patient closely for loss of vision, sudden onset of proptosis, diplopia, migraine; blood pressure; signs and symptoms of thromboembolic disorders; signs or symptoms of depression; glycemic control in patients with diabetes; lipid profiles in patients being treated for hyperlipidemias. Adequate diagnostic measures, including endometrial sampling, if indicated, should be performed to rule out malignancy in all cases of undiagnosed abnormal vaginal bleeding.

Test Interactions Increased prothrombin and factors VII, VIII, IX, X; increased platelet aggregability, thyroid-binding globulin, total thyroid hormone (T4), serum triglycerides/phospholipids, AST, Alkaline Phosphatase, GGT; decreased serum folate concentration; pathologist should be advised of estrogen/progesterone therapy when specimens are submitted. Oral contraceptives suppress LH and FSH levels; wait at least 2 weeks after discontinuing use of contraceptive before measuring.

Additional Information Complete prescribing information for this medication should be consulted for additional detail.

Product Availability LoSeasonique™: FDA approved October 2008; availability anticipated during first quarter 2009

Dosage Forms Excipient information presented when available (limited, particularly for generics); consult specific product labeling. [DSC] = Discontinued product

Tablet, low-dose formulations:

Alesse® 28: Ethinyl estradiol 0.02 mg and levonorgestrel 0.1 mg (28s) [21 pink tablets and 7 light green inactive tablets]

Aviane™ 28: Ethinyl estradiol 0.02 mg and levonorgestrel 0.1 mg (28s) [21 orange tablets and 7 light green inactive tablets]

Lessina™ 28, Levlite™ 28: Ethinyl estradiol 0.02 mg and levonorgestrel 0.1 mg (28s) [21 pink tablets and 7 white inactive tablets]

Lutera™, Sronyx™: Ethinyl estradiol 0.02 mg and levonorgestrel 0.1 mg (28s) [21 white tablets and 7 peach inactive tablets]

Lybrel™: Ethinyl estradiol 0.02 mg and levonorgestrel 0.09 mg (28s) [28 yellow tablets]

Tablet, monophasic formulations:

Levlen® 28: Ethinyl estradiol 0.03 mg and levonorgestrel 0.15 mg (28s) [21 light orange tablets and 7 pink inactive tablets]

Levora® 28: Ethinyl estradiol 0.03 mg and levonorgestrel 0.15 mg (28s) [21 white tablets and 7 peach inactive tablets]

Nordette® 28: Ethinyl estradiol 0.03 mg and levonorgestrel 0.15 mg (28s) [21 light orange tablets and 7 pink inactive tablets]

Portia™ 28: Ethinyl estradiol 0.03 mg and levonorgestrel 0.15 mg (28s) [21 pink tablets and 7 white inactive tablets]

Tablet, monophasic formulations [extended cycle regimen]:
- Jolessa™, Seasonale®: Ethinyl estradiol 0.03 mg and levonorgestrel 0.15 mg (91s) [84 pink tablets and 7 white inactive tablets]
- Quasense™: Ethinyl estradiol 0.03 mg and levonorgestrel 0.15 mg (91s) [84 white tablets and 7 peach inactive tablets]
- Seasonique™: Ethinyl estradiol 0.03 mg and levonorgestrel 0.15 mg (91s) [84 light blue-green tablets] and ethinyl estradiol 0.01 mg [7 yellow tablets]

Tablet, triphasic formulations:
- Enpresse™:
  - Day 1-6: Ethinyl estradiol 0.03 mg and levonorgestrel 0.05 mg [6 pink tablets]
  - Day 7-11: Ethinyl estradiol 0.04 mg and levonorgestrel 0.075 mg [5 white tablets]
  - Day 12-21: Ethinyl estradiol 0.03 mg and levonorgestrel 0.125 mg [10 orange tablets]
  - Day 22-28: 7 light green inactive tablets (28s)
- Triphasil® 28:
  - Day 1-6: Ethinyl estradiol 0.03 mg and levonorgestrel 0.05 mg [6 brown tablets]
  - Day 7-11: Ethinyl estradiol 0.04 mg and levonorgestrel 0.075 mg [5 white tablets]
  - Day 12-21: Ethinyl estradiol 0.03 mg and levonorgestrel 0.125 mg [10 light yellow tablets]
  - Day 22-28: 7 light green inactive tablets (28s)
- Trivora® 28:
  - Day 1-6: Ethinyl estradiol 0.03 mg and levonorgestrel 0.05 mg [6 blue tablets]
  - Day 7-11: Ethinyl estradiol 0.04 mg and levonorgestrel 0.075 mg [5 white tablets]
  - Day 12-21: Ethinyl estradiol 0.03 mg and levonorgestrel 0.125 mg [10 pink tablets]
  - Day 22-28: 7 peach inactive tablets (28s)

◆ **Ethinyl Estradiol and NGM** *see* Ethinyl Estradiol and Norgestimate *on page 584*

Ethinyl Estradiol and Norelgestromin

(ETH in il es tra DYE ole & nor el JES troe min)

U.S. Brand Names Ortho Evra®

Canadian Brand Names Evra®

Index Terms Norelgestromin and Ethinyl Estradiol; Ortho-Evra

Pharmacologic Category Contraceptive; Estrogen and Progestin Combination

Use Prevention of pregnancy

Pregnancy Risk Factor X

Medication Safety Issues

Transdermal patch may contain conducting metal (eg, aluminum); remove patch prior to MRI.

Dosage Topical: Adults: Females:

Contraception: Apply one patch each week for 3 weeks (21 total days); followed by one week that is patch-free. Each patch should be applied on the same day each week ("patch change day") and only one patch should be worn at a time. No more than 7 days should pass during the patch-free interval.

Schedule 1 (Sunday starter): Dose begins on first Sunday after onset of menstruation; if the menstrual period starts on Sunday, apply one patch that very same day. **With a Sunday start, an additional method of contraception (nonhormonal) should be used until after the first 7 days of consecutive administration.** Each patch change will then occur on Sunday.

Schedule 2 (Day 1 starter): Dose starts on first day of menstrual cycle, applying one patch during the first 24 hours of menstrual cycle. No back-up method of contraception is needed as long as the patch is applied on the first day of cycle. Each patch change will then occur on that same day of the week.

Additional dosing considerations:

No bleeding during patch-free week/missed menstrual period: If patch has been applied as directed, continue treatment on usual "patch change day". If used correctly, no bleeding during patch-free week does not necessarily indicate pregnancy. However, if no withdrawal bleeding occurs for 2 consecutive cycles, pregnancy should be ruled out. If patch has not been applied as directed, and one menstrual period is missed, pregnancy should be ruled out prior to continuing treatment.

If a patch becomes partially or completely detached for <24 hours: Try to reapply to same place, or replace with a new patch immediately. Do not reapply if patch is no longer sticky, if it is sticking to itself or another surface, or if it has material sticking to it.

If a patch becomes partially or completely detached for >24 hours (or time period is unknown): Apply a new patch and use this day of the week as the new "patch change day" from this point on. **An additional method of contraception (nonhormonal) should be used until after the first 7 days of consecutive administration.**

Switching from oral contraceptives: Apply first patch on the first day of withdrawal bleeding. If there is no bleeding within 5 days of taking the last active tablet, pregnancy must first be ruled out. If patch is applied later than the first day of bleeding, **an additional method of contraception (nonhormonal) should be used until after the first 7 days of consecutive administration**

Use after childbirth: Therapy should not be started <4 weeks after childbirth. Pregnancy should be ruled out prior to treatment if menstrual periods have not restarted. **An additional method of contraception (nonhormonal) should be used until after the first 7 days of consecutive administration.**

Use after abortion or miscarriage: Therapy may be started immediately if abortion/miscarriage occur within the first trimester. If therapy is not started within 5 days, follow instructions for first time use. If abortion/miscarriage occur during the second trimester, therapy should not be started for at least 4 weeks. Follow directions for use after childbirth.

Dosage adjustment in renal impairment: Specific guidelines not available; use with caution and monitor blood pressure closely. Consider other forms of contraception.

Dosage adjustment in hepatic impairment: Contraindicated in patients with hepatic impairment

Additional Information Complete prescribing information for this medication should be consulted for additional detail.

Dosage Forms Excipient information presented when available (limited, particularly for generics); consult specific product labeling. [CAN] = Canadian brand name

Note: The formulation available in Canada differs from the U.S. product in both composition and the manufacturing process (although delivery rates appear similar).

Patch, transdermal:
- Ortho Evra®: Ethinyl estradiol 0.75 mg and norelgestromin 6 mg [releases ethinyl estradiol 20 mcg and norelgestromin 150 mcg per day] (1s, 3s)
- Evra® [CAN]: Ethinyl estradiol 0.6 mg and norelgestromin 6 mg [releases ethinyl estradiol 20 mcg and norelgestromin 150 mcg per day] (1s, 3s) [Not available in U.S.]

Ethinyl Estradiol and Norethindrone

(ETH in il es tra DYE ole & nor eth IN drone)

U.S. Brand Names Aranelle™; Balziva™; Brevicon®; Estrostep® Fe; Femcon™ Fe; femhrt®; Junel™; Junel™ Fe; Leena™; Loestrin®; Loestrin® 24 Fe; Loestrin® Fe; Microgestin™; Microgestin™ Fe; Modicon®; Necon® 0.5/35; Necon® 1/35; Necon® 10/11; Necon® 7/7/7; Norinyl®

1+35; Nortrel™; Nortrel™ 7/7/7; Ortho-Novum®; Ovcon®; Tilia™ Fe; Tri-Norinyl®; Zenchent™

Canadian Brand Names Brevicon® 0.5/35; Brevicon® 1/35; FemHRT®; Loestrin™ 1.5/30; Minestrin™ 1/20; Ortho® 0.5/35; Ortho® 1/35; Ortho® 7/7/7; Select™ 1/35; Synphasic®

Index Terms Norethindrone Acetate and Ethinyl Estradiol; Ortho Novum

Pharmacologic Category Contraceptive; Estrogen and Progestin Combination

Use Prevention of pregnancy; treatment of acne; moderate-to-severe vasomotor symptoms associated with menopause; prevention of osteoporosis (in women at significant risk only)

Unlabeled/Investigational Use Treatment of hypermenorrhea (menorrhagia); pain associated with endometriosis, dysmenorrhea; dysfunctional uterine bleeding

Pregnancy Risk Factor X

Medication Safety Issues

Sound-alike/look-alike issues:

femhrt® may be confused with Femara®

Modicon® may be confused with Mylicon®

Norinyl® may be confused with Nardil®

Tri-Norinyl® may be confused with Triphasil®

International issues:

Notrel™ may be confused with Nostril® which is a brand name for chlorhexidine and cetrimonium in France

Dosage Oral:

Adolescents ≥15 years and Adults: Females: Acne: Estrostep® Fe: Refer to dosing for contraception

Adults: Females:

Moderate-to-severe vasomotor symptoms associated with menopause: Initial: femhrt® 0.5/2.5: 1 tablet daily; patient should be re-evaluated at 3- to 6-month intervals to determine if treatment is still necessary; patient should be maintained at the lowest effective dose

Prevention of osteoporosis: Initial: femhrt® 0.5/2.5: 1 tablet daily; patient should be maintained on the lowest effective dose

Contraception:

Schedule 1 (Sunday starter): Dose begins on first Sunday after onset of menstruation; if the menstrual period starts on Sunday, take first tablet that very same day. With a Sunday start, an additional method of contraception should be used until after the first 7 days of consecutive administration.

For 21-tablet package: Dosage is 1 tablet daily for 21 consecutive days, followed by 7 days off of the medication; a new course begins on the 8th day after the last tablet is taken.

For 28-tablet package: Dosage is 1 tablet daily without interruption.

Schedule 2 (Day 1 starter): Dose starts on first day of menstrual cycle taking 1 tablet daily.

For 21-tablet package: Dosage is 1 tablet daily for 21 consecutive days, followed by 7 days off of the medication; a new course begins on the 8th day after the last tablet is taken.

For 28-tablet package: Dosage is 1 tablet daily without interruption.

If all doses have been taken on schedule and one menstrual period is missed, continue dosing cycle. If two consecutive menstrual periods are missed, pregnancy test is required before new dosing cycle is started.

Missed doses **monophasic formulations** (refer to package insert for complete information):

One dose missed: Take as soon as remembered or take 2 tablets next day Two consecutive doses missed in the first 2 weeks: Take 2 tablets as soon as remembered or 2 tablets next 2 days. An additional method of contraception should be used for 7 days after missed dose.

Two consecutive doses missed in week 3 or three consecutive doses missed at any time: An additional method of contraception must be used for 7 days after a missed dose.

Schedule 1 (Sunday starter): Continue dose of 1 tablet daily until Sunday, then discard the rest of the pack, and a new pack should be started that same day.

Schedule 2 (Day 1 starter): Current pack should be discarded, and a new pack should be started that same day.

Missed doses **biphasic/triphasic formulations** (refer to package insert for complete information):

One dose missed: Take as soon as remembered or take 2 tablets next day.

Two consecutive doses missed in week 1 or week 2 of the pack: Take 2 tablets as soon as remembered and 2 tablets the next day. Resume taking 1 tablet daily until the pack is empty. An additional method of contraception should be used for 7 days after a missed dose.

Two consecutive doses missed in week 3 of the pack: An additional method of contraception must be used for 7 days after a missed dose.

Schedule 1 (Sunday Starter): Take 1 tablet every day until Sunday. Discard the remaining pack and start a new pack of pills on the same day.

Schedule 2 (Day 1 starter): Discard the remaining pack and start a new pack the same day.

Three or more consecutive doses missed: An additional method of contraception must be used for 7 days after a missed dose.

Schedule 1 (Sunday Starter): Take 1 tablet every day until Sunday; on Sunday, discard the pack and start a new pack.

Schedule 2 (Day 1 Starter): Discard the remaining pack and begin new pack of tablets starting on the same day.

Dosage adjustment in renal impairment: Specific guidelines not available; use with caution and monitor blood pressure closely. Consider other forms of contraception.

Dosage adjustment in hepatic impairment: Contraindicated in patients with hepatic impairment.

Additional Information Complete prescribing information for this medication should be consulted for additional detail.

Dosage Forms Excipient information presented when available (limited, particularly for generics); consult specific product labeling.

Tablet:

femhrt® 1/5: Ethinyl estradiol 5 mcg and norethindrone acetate 1 mg [white tablets]

femhrt® 0.5/2.5: Ethinyl estradiol 2.5 mcg and norethindrone acetate 0.5 mg [white tablets]

Tablet, monophasic formulations:

Balziva™: Ethinyl estradiol 0.035 mg and norethindrone 0.4 mg (28s) [21 light peach tablets and 7 white inactive tablets]

Brevicon®: Ethinyl estradiol 0.035 mg and norethindrone 0.5 mg (28s) [21 blue tablets and 7 orange inactive tablets]

Junel™ 21 1/20: Ethinyl estradiol 0.02 mg and norethindrone acetate 1 mg (21s) [yellow tablets]

Junel™ 21 1.5/30: Ethinyl estradiol 0.03 mg and norethindrone acetate 1.5 mg (21s) [pink tablets]

Junel™ Fe 1/20: Ethinyl estradiol 0.02 mg and norethindrone acetate 1 mg (28s) [21 yellow tablets] and ferrous fumarate 75 mg [7 brown tablets]

Junel™ Fe 1.5/30: Ethinyl estradiol 0.03 mg and norethindrone acetate 1.5 mg (28s) [21 pink tablets] and ferrous fumarate 75 mg [7 brown tablets]

Loestrin® 21 1/20, Microgestin™ 1/20: Ethinyl estradiol 0.02 mg and norethindrone acetate 1 mg (21s) [white tablets]
Loestrin® 21 1.5/30, Microgestin™ 1.5/30: Ethinyl estradiol 0.03 mg and norethindrone acetate 1.5 mg (21s) [green tablets]
Loestrin® 24 Fe: 1/20: Ethinyl estradiol 0.02 mg and norethindrone acetate 1 mg (28s) [24 white tablets] and ferrous fumarate 75 mg [4 brown tablets]
Loestrin® Fe 1/20, Microgestin™ Fe 1/20: Ethinyl estradiol 0.02 mg and norethindrone acetate 1 mg (28s) [21 white tablets] and ferrous fumarate 75 mg [7 brown tablets]
Loestrin® Fe 1.5/30, Microgestin™ Fe 1.5/30: Ethinyl estradiol 0.03 mg and norethindrone acetate 1.5 mg (28s) [21 green tablets] and ferrous fumarate 75 mg [7 brown tablets]
Modicon® 28: Ethinyl estradiol 0.035 mg and norethindrone 0.5 mg (28s) [21 white tablets and 7 green inactive tablets]
Necon® 0.5/35-28: Ethinyl estradiol 0.035 mg and norethindrone 0.5 mg (28s) [21 light yellow tablets and 7 white inactive tablets]
Necon® 1/35-28: Ethinyl estradiol 0.035 mg and norethindrone 1 mg (28s) [21 dark yellow tablets and 7 white inactive tablets]
Norinyl® 1+35: Ethinyl estradiol 0.035 mg and norethindrone 1 mg (28s) [21 yellow-green tablets and 7 orange inactive tablets]
Nortrel™ 0.5/35 mg:
Ethinyl estradiol 0.035 mg and norethindrone 0.5 mg (21s) [light yellow tablets]
Ethinyl estradiol 0.035 mg and norethindrone 0.5 mg (28s) [21 light yellow tablets and 7 white inactive tablets]
Nortrel™ 1/35 mg:
Ethinyl estradiol 0.035 mg and norethindrone 1 mg (21s) [yellow tablets]
Ethinyl estradiol 0.035 mg and norethindrone 1 mg (28s) [21 yellow tablets and 7 white inactive tablets]
Ortho-Novum® 1/35 28: Ethinyl estradiol 0.035 mg and norethindrone 1 mg (28s) [21 peach tablets and 7 green inactive tablets]
Ovcon® 35 21-day: Ethinyl estradiol 0.035 mg and norethindrone 0.4 mg (21s) [peach tablets]
Ovcon® 35 28-day: Ethinyl estradiol 0.035 mg and norethindrone 0.4 mg (28s) [21 peach tablets and 7 green inactive tablets]
Ovcon® 50: Ethinyl estradiol 0.05 mg and norethindrone 1 mg (28s) [21 yellow tablets and 7 green inactive tablets]
Zenchent™: Ethinyl estradiol 0.035 mg and norethindrone 0.4 mg (28s) [21 light peach tablets and 7 white inactive tablets]

Tablet, chewable, monophasic formulations:
Femcon™ Fe: Ethinyl estradiol 0.035 mg and norethindrone 0.4 mg (28s) [21 white tablets and 7 brown inactive tablets] [spearmint flavor]

Tablet, biphasic formulations:
Necon® 10/11-28:
Day 1-10: Ethinyl estradiol 0.035 mg and norethindrone 0.5 mg [10 light yellow tablets]
Day 11-21: Ethinyl estradiol 0.035 mg and norethindrone 1 mg [11 dark yellow tablets]
Day 22-28: 7 white inactive tablets (28s)
Ortho-Novum® 10/11-28:
Day 1-10: Ethinyl estradiol 0.035 mg and norethindrone 0.5 mg [10 white tablets]
Day 11-21: Ethinyl estradiol 0.035 mg and norethindrone 1 mg [11 peach tablets]
Day 22-28: 7 green inactive tablets (28s)

Tablet, triphasic formulations:
Aranelle™:
Day 1-7: Ethinyl estradiol 0.035 mg and norethindrone 0.5 mg [7 light yellow tablets]
Day 8-16: Ethinyl estradiol 0.035 mg and norethindrone 1 mg [9 white tablets]
Day 17-21: Ethinyl estradiol 0.035 mg and norethindrone 0.5 mg [5 light yellow tablets]
Day 22-28: 7 peach inactive tablets (28s)
Estrostep® Fe:
Day 1-5: Ethinyl estradiol 0.02 mg and norethindrone acetate 1 mg [5 white triangular tablets]
Day 6-12: Ethinyl estradiol 0.03 mg and norethindrone acetate 1 mg [7 white square tablets]
Day 13-21: Ethinyl estradiol 0.035 mg and norethindrone acetate 1 mg [9 white round tablets]
Day 22-28: Ferrous fumarate 75 mg [7 brown tablets] (28s)
Leena™:
Day 1-7: Ethinyl estradiol 0.035 mg and norethindrone 0.5 mg [7 light blue tablets]
Day 8-16: Ethinyl estradiol 0.035 mg and norethindrone 1 mg [9 light yellow-green tablets]
Day 17-21: Ethinyl estradiol 0.035 mg and norethindrone 0.5 mg [5 light blue tablets]
Day 22-28: 7 orange inactive tablets (28s)
Necon® 7/7/7, Ortho-Novum® 7/7/7 28:
Day 1-7: Ethinyl estradiol 0.035 mg and norethindrone 0.5 mg [7 white tablets]
Day 8-14: Ethinyl estradiol 0.035 mg and norethindrone 0.75 mg [7 light peach tablets]
Day 15-21: Ethinyl estradiol 0.035 mg and norethindrone 1 mg [7 peach tablets]
Day 22-28: 7 green inactive tablets (28s)
Nortrel™ 7/7/7 28:
Day 1-7: Ethinyl estradiol 0.035 mg and norethindrone 0.5 mg [7 light yellow tablets]
Day 8-14: Ethinyl estradiol 0.035 mg and norethindrone 0.75 mg [7 blue tablets]
Day 15-21: Ethinyl estradiol 0.035 mg and norethindrone 1 mg [7 peach tablets]
Day 22-28: 7 white inactive tablets (28s)
Ortho-Novum® 7/7/7 28:
Day 1-7: Ethinyl estradiol 0.035 mg and norethindrone 0.5 mg [7 white tablets]
Day 8-14: Ethinyl estradiol 0.035 mg and norethindrone 0.75 mg [7 light peach tablets]
Day 15-21: Ethinyl estradiol 0.035 mg and norethindrone 1 mg [7 peach tablets]
Day 22-28: 7 green inactive tablets (28s)
Tilia™ Fe:
Day 1-5: Ethinyl estradiol 0.02 mg and norethindrone acetate 1 mg [5 white triangular tablets]
Day 6-12: Ethinyl estradiol 0.03 mg and norethindrone acetate 1 mg [7 white square tablets]
Day 13-21: Ethinyl estradiol 0.035 mg and norethindrone acetate 1 mg [9 white round tablets]
Day 22-28: Ferrous fumarate 75 mg [7 brown tablets] (28s)
Tri-Norinyl® 28:
Day 1-7: Ethinyl estradiol 0.035 mg and norethindrone 0.5 mg [7 blue tablets]
Day 8-16: Ethinyl estradiol 0.035 mg and norethindrone 1 mg [9 yellow-green tablets]
Day 17-21: Ethinyl estradiol 0.035 mg and norethindrone 0.5 mg [5 blue tablets]
Day 22-28: 7 orange inactive tablets (28s)

Ethinyl Estradiol and Norgestimate

(ETH in il es tra DYE ole & nor JES ti mate)

U.S. Brand Names MonoNessa®; Ortho Tri-Cyclen®; Ortho Tri-Cyclen® Lo; Ortho-Cyclen®; Previfem®; Sprintec®; Tri-Previfem®; Tri-Sprintec®; TriNessa®

Canadian Brand Names Cyclen®; Tri-Cyclen®; Tri-Cyclen® Lo

Index Terms Ethinyl Estradiol and NGM; Norgestimate and Ethinyl Estradiol; Ortho Cyclen; Ortho Tri Cyclen

Pharmacologic Category Contraceptive; Estrogen and Progestin Combination

Use Prevention of pregnancy; treatment of acne

Unlabeled/Investigational Use Treatment of hypermenorrhea (menorrhagia); pain associated with endometriosis; dysmenorrhea; dysfunctional uterine bleeding

Pregnancy Risk Factor X

Medication Safety Issues

Sound-alike/look-alike issues:

Ortho-Cyclen® may be confused with Ortho-Cept®

Dosage Oral:

Children ≥15 years and Adults: Females: Acne (Ortho Tri-Cyclen®): Refer to dosing for contraception

Adults: Females:

Contraception:

Schedule 1 (Sunday starter): Dose begins on first Sunday after onset of menstruation; if the menstrual period starts on Sunday, take first tablet that very same day. **With a Sunday start, an additional method of contraception should be used until after the first 7 days of consecutive administration.**

For 21-tablet package: Dosage is 1 tablet daily for 21 consecutive days, followed by 7 days off of the medication; a new course begins on the 8th day after the last tablet is taken.

For 28-tablet package: Dosage is 1 tablet daily without interruption.

Schedule 2 (Day 1 starter): Dose starts on first day of menstrual cycle taking 1 tablet daily.

For 21-tablet package: Dosage is 1 tablet daily for 21 consecutive days, followed by 7 days off of the medication; a new course begins on the 8th day after the last tablet is taken.

For 28-tablet package: Dosage is 1 tablet daily without interruption.

If all doses have been taken on schedule and one menstrual period is missed, continue dosing cycle. If two consecutive menstrual periods are missed, pregnancy test is required before new dosing cycle is started.

Missed doses **monophasic formulations** (refer to package insert for complete information):

One dose missed: Take as soon as remembered or take 2 tablets next day

Two consecutive doses missed in the first 2 weeks: Take 2 tablets as soon as remembered or 2 tablets next 2 days. **An additional method of contraception should be used for 7 days after missed dose.**

Two consecutive doses missed in week 3 or three consecutive doses missed at any time: **An additional method of contraception must be used for 7 days after a missed dose:**

Schedule 1 (Sunday starter): Continue dose of 1 tablet daily until Sunday, then discard the rest of the pack, and a new pack should be started that same day.

Schedule 2 (Day 1 starter): Current pack should be discarded, and a new pack should be started that same day.

Missed doses **biphasic/triphasic formulations** (refer to package insert for complete information):

One dose missed: Take as soon as remembered or take 2 tablets next day.

Two consecutive doses missed in week 1 or week 2 of the pack: Take 2 tablets as soon as remembered and 2 tablets the next day. Resume taking 1 tablet daily until the pack is empty. **An additional method of contraception must be used for 7 days after a missed dose.**

Two consecutive doses missed in week 3 of the pack. **An additional method of contraception must be used for 7 days after a missed dose.**

Schedule 1 (Sunday starter): Take 1 tablet every day until Sunday. Discard the remaining pack and start a new pack of pills on the same day.

Schedule 2 (Day 1 starter): Discard the remaining pack and start a new pack the same day.

Three or more consecutive doses missed. **An additional method of contraception must be used for 7 days after a missed dose.**

Schedule 1 (Sunday starter): Take 1 tablet every day until Sunday; on Sunday, discard the pack and start a new pack.

Schedule 2 (Day 1 starter): Discard the remaining pack and begin new pack of tablets starting on the same day.

Dosage adjustment in renal impairment: Specific guidelines not available; use with caution and monitor blood pressure closely. Consider other forms of contraception.

Dosage adjustment in hepatic impairment: Contraindicated in patients with hepatic impairment.

Additional Information Complete prescribing information for this medication should be consulted for additional detail.

Dosage Forms Excipient information presented when available (limited, particularly for generics); consult specific product labeling.

Tablet, monophasic formulations:

MonoNessa®, Ortho-Cyclen®: Ethinyl estradiol 0.035 mg and norgestimate 0.25 mg (28s) [21 blue tablets and 7 green inactive tablets]

Previfem®: Ethinyl estradiol 0.035 mg and norgestimate 0.25 mg (28s) [21 blue tablets and 7 teal inactive tablets]

Sprintec®: Ethinyl estradiol 0.035 mg and norgestimate 0.25 mg (28s) [21 blue tablets and 7 white inactive tablets]

Tablet, triphasic formulations:

Ortho Tri-Cyclen®, TriNessa®:

Day 1-7: Ethinyl estradiol 0.035 mg and norgestimate 0.18 mg [7 white tablets]

Day 8-14: Ethinyl estradiol 0.035 mg and norgestimate 0.215 mg [7 light blue tablets]

Day 15-21: Ethinyl estradiol 0.035 mg and norgestimate 0.25 mg [7 blue tablets]

Day 22-28: 7 green inactive tablets (28s)

Tri-Previfem®:

Day 1-7: Ethinyl estradiol 0.035 mg and norgestimate 0.18 mg [7 white tablets]

Day 8-14: Ethinyl estradiol 0.035 mg and norgestimate 0.215 mg [7 light blue tablets]

Day 15-21: Ethinyl estradiol 0.035 mg and norgestimate 0.25 mg [7 blue tablets]

Day 22-28: 7 teal inactive tablets (28s)

Tri-Sprintec®:

Day 1-7: Ethinyl estradiol 0.035 mg and norgestimate 0.18 mg [7 gray tablets]

Day 8-14: Ethinyl estradiol 0.035 mg and norgestimate 0.215 mg [7 light blue tablets]

Day 15-21: Ethinyl estradiol 0.035 mg and norgestimate 0.25 mg [7 blue tablets]

Day 22-28: 7 white inactive tablets (28s)

Ortho Tri-Cyclen® Lo:

Day 1-7: Ethinyl estradiol 0.025 mg and norgestimate 0.18 mg [7 white tablets]

Day 8-14: Ethinyl estradiol 0.025 mg and norgestimate 0.215 mg [7 light blue tablets]
Day 15-21: Ethinyl estradiol 0.025 mg and norgestimate 0.25 mg [7 dark blue tablets]
Day 22-28: 7 green inactive tablets (28s)

Ethinyl Estradiol and Norgestrel

(ETH in il es tra DYE ole & nor JES trel)

U.S. Brand Names Cryselle™; Lo/Ovral®; Low-Ogestrel®; Ogestrel®

Canadian Brand Names Ovral®

Index Terms Morning After Pill; Norgestrel and Ethinyl Estradiol

Pharmacologic Category Contraceptive; Estrogen and Progestin Combination

Use Prevention of pregnancy; postcoital contraceptive or "morning after" pill

Unlabeled/Investigational Use Treatment of hypermenorrhea (menorrhagia); pain associated with endometriosis; dysmenorrhea; dysfunctional uterine bleeding

Pregnancy Risk Factor X

Dosage Oral: Adults: Females:

Contraception:

Schedule 1 (Sunday starter): Dose begins on first Sunday after onset of menstruation; if the menstrual period starts on Sunday, take first tablet that very same day. **With a Sunday start, an additional method of contraception should be used until after the first 7 days of consecutive administration.**

For 21-tablet package: Dosage is 1 tablet daily for 21 consecutive days, followed by 7 days off of the medication; a new course begins on the 8th day after the last tablet is taken.

For 28-tablet package: Dosage is 1 tablet daily without interruption.

Schedule 2 (Day 1 starter): Dose starts on first day of menstrual cycle taking 1 tablet daily.

For 21-tablet package: Dosage is 1 tablet daily for 21 consecutive days, followed by 7 days off of the medication; a new course begins on the 8th day after the last tablet is taken.

For 28-tablet package: Dosage is 1 tablet daily without interruption.

If all doses have been taken on schedule and one menstrual period is missed, continue dosing cycle. If two consecutive menstrual periods are missed, pregnancy test is required before new dosing cycle is started.

Missed doses **monophasic formulations** (refer to package insert for complete information):

One dose missed: Take as soon as remembered or take 2 tablets next day

Two consecutive doses missed in the first 2 weeks: Take 2 tablets as soon as remembered or 2 tablets next 2 days. **An additional method of contraception should be used for 7 days after missed dose.**

Two consecutive doses missed in week 3 or three consecutive doses missed at any time:

Schedule 1 (Sunday starter): Continue to take 1 tablet daily until Sunday, then discard the rest of the pack, and a new pack is started that same day.

Schedule 2 (Day 1 starter): Current pack should be discarded, and a new pack started that same day. **An additional method of contraception should be used for 7 days after missed dose.**

Postcoital contraception:

Ethinyl estradiol 0.03 mg and norgestrel 0.3 mg formulation: 4 tablets within 72 hours of unprotected intercourse and 4 tablets 12 hours after first dose

Ethinyl estradiol 0.05 mg and norgestrel 0.5 mg formulation: 2 tablets within 72 hours of unprotected intercourse and 2 tablets 12 hours after first dose

Dosage adjustment in renal impairment: Specific guidelines not available; use with caution and monitor blood pressure closely. Consider other forms of contraception.

Dosage adjustment in hepatic impairment: Contraindicated in patients with hepatic impairment.

Additional Information Complete prescribing information for this medication should be consulted for additional detail.

Dosage Forms Excipient information presented when available (limited, particularly for generics); consult specific product labeling.

Tablet, monophasic formulations:

Cryselle™: Ethinyl estradiol 0.03 mg and norgestrel 0.3 mg [21 white tablets and 7 light green inactive tablets] (28s)

Low-Ogestrel® 28: Ethinyl estradiol 0.03 mg and norgestrel 0.3 mg [21 white tablets and 7 peach inactive tablets] (28s)

Lo/Ovral® 28: Ethinyl estradiol 0.03 mg and norgestrel 0.3 mg [21 white tablets and 7 pink inactive tablets] (28s)

Ogestrel® 28: Ethinyl estradiol 0.05 mg and norgestrel 0.5 mg [21 white tablets and 7 peach inactive tablets] (28s)

◆ **Ethiofos** *see* Amifostine *on page 82*

Ethionamide

(e thye on AM ide)

U.S. Brand Names Trecator®

Canadian Brand Names Trecator®

Pharmacologic Category Antitubercular Agent

Additional Appendix Information

Antimicrobial Drugs of Choice *on page 1752*
Tuberculosis *on page 1776*

Use Treatment of tuberculosis and other mycobacterial diseases, in conjunction with other antituberculosis agents, when first-line agents have failed or resistance has been demonstrated

Pregnancy Risk Factor C

Pregnancy Considerations Ethionamide crosses the placenta; teratogenic effects were observed in animal studies. Use during pregnancy is not recommended.

Lactation Excretion in breast milk unknown/use caution

Contraindications Hypersensitivity to ethionamide or any component of the formulation; severe hepatic impairment

Warnings/Precautions Use with caution in patients with diabetes mellitus or thyroid dysfunction; use with caution in patients receiving cycloserine or isoniazid. Use caution when switching patients from the sugar-coated tablet formulation (Trecator®-SC) to film-coated tablet (Trecator®); the dosage may need retitrated in order to avoid intolerance. Periodic eye exams are recommended.

Adverse Reactions Frequency not defined.

Cardiovascular: Postural hypotension

Central nervous system: Depression, dizziness, drowsiness, headache, psychiatric disturbances, restlessness, seizure

Dermatologic: Acne, alopecia, photosensitivity, purpura, rash

Endocrine & metabolic: Gynecomastia, hypoglycemia, hypothyroidism or goiter, pellagra-like syndrome

Gastrointestinal: Abdominal pain, anorexia, diarrhea, excessive salivation, metallic taste, nausea, stomatitis, vomiting, weight loss

Genitourinary: Impotence

Hematologic: Thrombocytopenia

Hepatic: Hepatitis, jaundice, liver function tests increased

Neuromuscular & skeletal: Peripheral neuritis, weakness (common)

Ocular: Blurred vision, diplopia, optic neuritis

Respiratory: Olfactory disturbances

Miscellaneous: Hypersensitivity reaction

Drug Interactions

Avoid Concomitant Use There are no known interactions where it is recommended to avoid concomitant use.

Increased Effect/Toxicity There are no known significant interactions involving an increase in effect.

Decreased Effect There are no known significant interactions involving a decrease in effect.

Ethanol/Nutrition/Herb Interactions

Ethanol: Avoid excessive ethanol ingestion; psychotic reaction may occur.

Mechanism of Action Inhibits peptide synthesis

Pharmacodynamics/Kinetics

Absorption: Rapid, complete

Distribution: Crosses placenta; V_d: 93.5 L

Protein binding: ~30%

Metabolism: Extensively hepatic to active and inactive metabolites

Bioavailability: 80%

Half-life elimination: 2-3 hours

Time to peak, serum: 1 hour

Excretion: Urine (<1% as unchanged drug; as active and inactive metabolites)

Dosage Oral:

Children: 15-20 mg/kg/day in 2-3 divided doses, not to exceed 1 g/day

Adults: 15-20 mg/kg/day; initiate dose at 250 mg/day for 1-2 days, then increase to 250 mg twice daily for 1-2 days, with gradual increases to highest tolerated dose; average adult dose: 750 mg/day (maximum: 1 g/day in 3-4 divided doses)

Dosing adjustment in renal impairment: Cl_{cr} <30 mL/minute: 250-500 mg/day

Dietary Considerations Healthcare provider may recommend an increase in dietary intake of pyridoxine to prevent neurotoxic effects of ethionamide. Avoid alcohol.

Administration Neurotoxic effects may be relieved by the administration of pyridoxine (6-100 mg daily, lower doses are more common). May be taken with or without meals. Gastrointestinal adverse effects may be decreased by administration at bedtime, decreased dose, or giving antiemetics.

Monitoring Parameters Initial and periodic serum ALT and AST; ophthalmic exams; thyroid function

Additional Information Neurotoxic effects may be relieved by the administration of pyridoxine.

Dosage Forms Excipient information presented when available (limited, particularly for generics); consult specific product labeling.

Tablet: 250 mg

◆ **Ethmozine® [DSC]** *see* Moricizine *on page* 1015

◆ **Ethmozine® (Can)** *see* Moricizine *on page* 1015

Ethosuximide (eth oh SUKS i mide)

U.S. Brand Names Zarontin®

Canadian Brand Names Zarontin®

Pharmacologic Category Anticonvulsant, Succinimide

Additional Appendix Information

Anticonvulsant Drugs of Choice *on page* 1637

Use Management of absence (petit mal) seizures

Medication Safety Issues

Sound-alike/look-alike issues:

Ethosuximide may be confused with methsuximide

Zarontin® may be confused with Xalatan®, Zantac®, Zaroxolyn®

Dosage Oral:

Children 3-6 years: Initial: 250 mg/day; increase every 4-7 days; usual maintenance dose: 20 mg/kg/day; maximum dose: 1.5 g/day in divided doses

Children >6 years and Adults: Initial: 500 mg/day; increase by 250 mg as needed every 4-7 days, up to 1.5 g/day in divided doses; usual maintenance dose for most pediatric patients is 20 mg/kg/day.

Dosing comment in renal/hepatic dysfunction: Use with caution.

Additional Information Complete prescribing information for this medication should be consulted for additional detail.

Dosage Forms Excipient information presented when available (limited, particularly for generics); consult specific product labeling.

Capsule: 250 mg

Zarontin®: 250 mg

Syrup: 250 mg/5 mL (473 mL)

Zarontin®: 250 mg/5 mL [contains sodium benzoate; raspberry flavor]

◆ **ETH-Oxydose™** *see* OxyCODONE *on page* 1120

◆ **Ethoxynaphthamido Penicillin Sodium** *see* Nafcillin *on page* 1033

◆ **Ethyl Aminobenzoate** *see* Benzocaine *on page* 183

◆ **Ethyl Esters of Omega-3 Fatty Acids** *see* Omega-3-Acid Ethyl Esters *on page* 1100

◆ **Ethynodiol Diacetate and Ethinyl Estradiol** *see* Ethinyl Estradiol and Ethynodiol Diacetate *on page* 576

◆ **Ethyol®** *see* Amifostine *on page* 82

◆ **Etibi® (Can)** *see* Ethambutol *on page* 573

Etidronate Disodium
(e ti DROE nate dye SOW dee um)

U.S. Brand Names Didronel®

Canadian Brand Names Didronel®; Gen-Etidronate

Index Terms EHDP; Sodium Etidronate

Pharmacologic Category Bisphosphonate Derivative

Use Symptomatic treatment of Paget's disease; prevention and treatment of heterotopic ossification due to spinal cord injury or after total hip replacement

Unlabeled/Investigational Use Postmenopausal osteoporosis

Pregnancy Risk Factor C

Medication Safety Issues

Sound-alike/look-alike issues:

Etidronate may be confused with etidocaine, etomidate, etretinate

Dosage Oral: Adults:

Paget's disease:

Initial: 5-10 mg/kg/day (not to exceed 6 months) or 11-20 mg/kg/day (not to exceed 3 months). Doses >20 mg/kg/day are **not** recommended.

Retreatment: Initiate only after etidronate-free period ≥90 days. Monitor patients every 3-6 months. Retreatment regimens are the same as for initial treatment.

Heterotopic ossification:

Caused by spinal cord injury: 20 mg/kg/day for 2 weeks, then 10 mg/kg/day for 10 weeks; total treatment period: 12 weeks

Complicating total hip replacement: 20 mg/kg/day for 1 month preoperatively then 20 mg/kg/day for 3 months postoperatively; total treatment period is 4 months

Postmenopausal osteoporosis (unlabeled use): Oral: 400 mg/day for 2 weeks, followed by 13-week period with no etidronate, then repeat cycle. Maintain adequate calcium and vitamin D intake during the entire 15-week treatment cycle

Dosing adjustment in renal impairment: Use with caution; specific guidelines are not available, however consider dose reduction.

Additional Information Complete prescribing information for this medication should be consulted for additional detail.

Dosage Forms Excipient information presented when available (limited, particularly for generics); consult specific product labeling.

Tablet: 200 mg, 400 mg

Etodolac (ee toe DOE lak)

Canadian Brand Names Apo-Etodolac®; Utradol™

Index Terms Etodolic Acid

Pharmacologic Category Nonsteroidal Anti-inflammatory Drug (NSAID), Oral

Additional Appendix Information

Nonsteroidal Anti-inflammatory Agents *on page 1669*

Use Acute and long-term use in the management of signs and symptoms of osteoarthritis; rheumatoid arthritis and juvenile rheumatoid arthritis; management of acute pain

Restrictions An FDA-approved medication guide must be distributed when dispensing an oral outpatient prescription (new or refill) where this medication is to be used without direct supervision of a healthcare provider. Medication guides are available at http://www.fda.gov/cder/Offices/ODS/medication_guides.htm.

Pregnancy Risk Factor C/D (3rd trimester)

Lactation Excretion in breast milk unknown/not recommended

Medication Safety Issues

Sound-alike/look-alike issues:

Lodine® may be confused with codeine, iodine, lopidine®, Lopid®

Contraindications Hypersensitivity to etodolac, aspirin, other NSAIDs, or any component of the formulation; perioperative pain in the setting of coronary artery bypass graft (CABG) surgery

Warnings/Precautions **[U.S. Boxed Warning]: NSAIDs are associated with an increased risk of adverse cardiovascular thrombotic events, including MI, stroke, and new onset or worsening of pre-existing hypertension.** Risk may be increased with duration of use or pre-existing cardiovascular risk factors or disease. Carefully evaluate individual cardiovascular risk profiles prior to prescribing. Use caution with fluid retention, heart failure, or hypertension. Concurrent administration of ibuprofen, and potentially other nonselective NSAIDs, may interfere with aspirin's cardioprotective effect. **[U.S. Boxed Warning]: Use is contraindicated for treatment of perioperative pain in the setting of coronary artery bypass graft (CABG) surgery.** Risk of MI and stroke may be increased with use following CABG surgery.

[U.S. Boxed Warning]: NSAIDs may increase risk of gastrointestinal irritation, inflammation, ulceration, bleeding, and perforation. These events may occur at any time during therapy and without warning. Use caution with a history of GI disease (bleeding or ulcers), concurrent therapy with aspirin, anticoagulants and/or corticosteroids, smoking, use of alcohol, the elderly or debilitated patients.

Platelet adhesion and aggregation may be decreased; may prolong bleeding time; patients with coagulation disorders or who are receiving anticoagulants should be monitored closely. Anemia may occur; patients on long-term NSAID therapy should be monitored for anemia. NSAID use may compromise existing renal function; dose-dependent decreases in prostaglandin synthesis may result from NSAID use, reducing renal blood flow which may cause renal decompensation. Patients with impaired renal function, dehydration, heart failure, liver dysfunction, those taking diuretics and ACE inhibitors, and the elderly are at greater risk for renal toxicity. Rehydrate patient before starting therapy; monitor renal function closely. Not recommended for use in patients with advanced renal disease. Long-term NSAID use may result in renal papillary necrosis.

Use the lowest effective dose for the shortest duration of time, consistent with individual patient goals, to reduce risk of cardiovascular or GI adverse events. Alternate therapies should be considered for patients at high risk.

NSAIDs may cause serious skin adverse events including exfoliative dermatitis, Stevens-Johnson syndrome (SJS), and toxic epidermal necrolysis (TEN); discontinue use at first sign of skin rash or hypersensitivity. Anaphylactoid reactions may occur, even without prior exposure; patients with "aspirin triad" (bronchial asthma, aspirin intolerance, rhinitis) may be at increased risk. Do not use in patients who experience bronchospasm, asthma, rhinitis, or urticaria with NSAID or aspirin therapy. Use caution in other forms of asthma.

Use with caution in patients with decreased hepatic function. Closely monitor patients with any abnormal LFT. Severe hepatic reactions (eg, fulminant hepatitis, liver failure) have occurred with NSAID use, rarely; discontinue if signs or symptoms of liver disease develop, or if systemic manifestations occur. The elderly are at increased risk for adverse effects (especially peptic ulceration, CNS effects, renal toxicity) from NSAIDs even at low doses.

Withhold for at least 4-6 half-lives prior to surgical or dental procedures. Safety and efficacy have not been established in children.

Use of extended release product consisting of a nondeformable matrix should be avoided in patients with stricture/narrowing of the GI tract; symptoms of obstruction have been associated with nondeformable products.

Adverse Reactions

1% to 10%:

Central nervous system: Dizziness (3% to 9 %), chills/fever (1% to 3%), depression (1% to 3%), nervousness (1% to 3%)

Dermatologic: Rash (1% to 3%), pruritus (1% to 3%)

Gastrointestinal: Abdominal cramps (3% to 9%), nausea (3% to 9%), vomiting (1% to 3%), dyspepsia (10%), diarrhea (3% to 9%), constipation (1% to 3%), flatulence (3% to 9%), melena (1% to 3%), gastritis (1% to 3%)

Genitourinary: Dysuria (1% to 3%)

Neuromuscular & skeletal: Weakness (3% to 9%)

Ocular: Blurred vision (1% to 3%)

Otic: Tinnitus (1% to 3%)

Renal: Polyuria (1% to 3%)

<1% (Limited to important or life-threatening): Agranulocytosis, allergic reaction, allergic/necrotizing vasculitis, alopecia, anaphylactic/anaphylactoid reactions, anemia, angioedema, anorexia, arrhythmia, aseptic meningitis, asthma, bleeding time increased, CHF, confusion, conjunctivitis, CVA, cystitis, duodenitis, dyspnea, ecchymosis, edema, erythema multiforme, esophagitis (+/- stricture or cardiospasm), exfoliative dermatitis, GI ulceration, hallucination, headache, hearing decreased, hematemesis, hematuria, hepatic failure, hepatitis, hyperglycemia (in controlled patients with diabetes), hyperpigmentation, hypertension, infection, insomnia, interstitial nephritis, irregular uterine bleeding, jaundice, LFTs increased, leukopenia, MI, palpitation, pancreatitis, pancytopenia, paresthesia, peptic ulcer (+/- bleeding/perforation), peripheral neuropathy, photophobia, photosensitivity, pulmonary infiltration (eosinophilia), rectal bleeding, renal calculus, renal failure, renal insufficiency, shock, Stevens-Johnson syndrome, syncope, thrombocytopenia, toxic epidermal necrolysis, ulcerative stomatitis, urticaria, vesiculobullous rash, renal papillary necrosis, visual disturbances

Drug Interactions

Avoid Concomitant Use

Avoid concomitant use of Etodolac with any of the following: Ketorolac

Increased Effect/Toxicity

Etodolac may increase the levels/effects of: Aminoglycosides; Anticoagulants; Antiplatelet Agents; Bisphosphonate Derivatives; CycloSPORINE; Desmopressin; Lithium; Methotrexate; Nonsteroidal Anti-Inflammatory Agents; Pemetrexed; Quinolone Antibiotics; Salicylates; Thrombolytic Agents; Vancomycin; Vitamin K Antagonists

The levels/effects of Etodolac may be increased by: Antidepressants (Tricyclic, Tertiary Amine); Corticosteroids (Systemic); Herbs (Anticoagulant/Antiplatelet Properties); Ketorolac; Probenecid; Selective Serotonin Reuptake Inhibitors; Serotonin/Norepinephrine Reuptake Inhibitors; Treprostinil

Decreased Effect

Etodolac may decrease the levels/effects of: ACE Inhibitors; Angiotensin II Receptor Blockers; Antiplatelet Agents; Beta-Blockers; Eplerenone; HydrALAZINE; Loop Diuretics; Salicylates; Thiazide Diuretics

The levels/effects of Etodolac may be decreased by: Bile Acid Sequestrants; Salicylates

Ethanol/Nutrition/Herb Interactions

Ethanol: Avoid ethanol (may enhance gastric mucosal irritation).

Food: Etodolac peak serum levels may be decreased if taken with food.

Herb/Nutraceutical: Avoid alfalfa, anise, bilberry, bladderwrack, bromelain, cat's claw, celery, chamomile, coleus, cordyceps, dong quai, evening primrose, fenugreek, feverfew, garlic, ginger, ginkgo biloba, ginseng (American, Panax, Siberian), grapeseed, green tea, guggul, horse chestnut seed, horseradish, licorice, prickly ash, red clover, reishi, SAMe (S-adenosylmethionine), sweet clover, turmeric, white willow (all have additional antiplatelet activity).

Stability Store at 20°C to 25°C (68°F to 77°F). Protect from moisture.

Mechanism of Action Reversibly inhibits cyclooxygenase-1 and 2 (COX-1 and 2) enzymes, which result in decreased formation of prostaglandin precursors; has antipyretic, analgesic, and anti-inflammatory properties

Pharmacodynamics/Kinetics

Onset of action: Analgesic: 2-4 hours; Maximum anti-inflammatory effect: A few days

Absorption: ≥80%

Distribution: V_d:

Immediate release: Adults:0.4 L/kg

Extended release: Adults: 0.57 L/kg; Children (6-16 years): 0 .08 L/kg

Protein binding: ≥99%, primarily albumin

Metabolism: Hepatic

Half-life elimination: Terminal: Adults: 5-8 hours

Extended release: Children (6-16 years): 12 hours

Time to peak, serum:

Immediate release: Adults: 1-2 hours

Extended release: Extended release: 5-7 hours, increased 1.4-3.8 hours with food

Excretion: Urine 73% (1% unchanged); feces 16%

Dosage Note: For chronic conditions, response is usually observed within 2 weeks.

Children 6-16 years: Oral: Juvenile rheumatoid arthritis (Lodine® XL):

20-30 kg: 400 mg once daily

31-45 kg: 600 mg once daily

46-60 kg: 800 mg once daily

>60 kg: 1000 mg once daily

Adults: Oral:

Acute pain: 200-400 mg every 6-8 hours, as needed, not to exceed total daily doses of 1000 mg

Rheumatoid arthritis, osteoarthritis: 400 mg 2 times/day **or** 300 mg 2-3 times/day **or** 500 mg 2 times/day (doses >1000 mg/day have not been evaluated)

Lodine® XL: 400-1000 mg once daily

Elderly: Refer to adult dosing; in patients ≥65 years, no dosage adjustment required based on pharmacokinetics. The elderly are more sensitive to antiprostaglandin effects and may need dosage adjustments.

Dosage adjustment in renal impairment:

Mild to moderate: No adjustment required

Severe: Use not recommended; use with caution

Hemodialysis: Not removed

Dosage adjustment in hepatic impairment: No adjustment required.

Dietary Considerations May be taken with food to decrease GI distress.

Monitoring Parameters Monitor CBC and chemistry profile, liver enzymes; in patients with an increased risk for renal failure (CHF or decreased renal function, taking ACE inhibitors or diuretics, elderly), monitor urine output and BUN/serum creatinine

Test Interactions False-positive for urinary bilirubin and ketone

Dosage Forms Excipient information presented when available (limited, particularly for generics); consult specific product labeling.

Capsule: 200 mg, 300 mg

Tablet: 400 mg, 500 mg

Tablet, extended release: 400 mg, 500 mg, 600 mg

◆ **Etodolic Acid** *see* Etodolac *on page* 587

Etomidate (e TOM i date)

U.S. Brand Names Amidate®

Canadian Brand Names Amidate®

Pharmacologic Category General Anesthetic

Use Induction and maintenance of general anesthesia

Unlabeled/Investigational Use Sedation for diagnosis of seizure foci

Pregnancy Risk Factor C

Medication Safety Issues

Sound-alike/look-alike issues:

Etomidate may be confused with etidronate

High alert medication: The Institute for Safe Medication Practices (ISMP) includes this medication among its list of drugs which have a heightened risk of causing significant patient harm when used in error.

Contraindications Hypersensitivity to etomidate or any component of the formulation

Warnings/Precautions Etomidate inhibits 11-B-hydroxylase, an enzyme important in adrenal steroid production. A single induction dose blocks the normal stress-induced increase in adrenal cortisol production for 4-8 hours, up to 24 hours in elderly and debilitated patients. Continuous infusion of etomidate for sedation in the ICU may increase mortality because patients may not be able to respond to stress. No increase in mortality has been identified with a single dose for induction of anesthesia. Consider exogenous corticosteroid replacement in patients undergoing severe stress. Safety and efficacy have not been established in children <10 years of age.

Adverse Reactions

>10%:

Gastrointestinal: Nausea, vomiting on emergence from anesthesia

Local: Pain at injection site (30% to 80%)

Neuromuscular & skeletal: Myoclonus (33%), transient skeletal movements, uncontrolled eye movements

1% to 10%: Hiccups

<1% (Limited to important or life-threatening): Apnea, arrhythmia, bradycardia, decreased cortisol synthesis, hypertension, hyperventilation, hypotension, hypoventilation, laryngospasm, tachycardia

Drug Interactions

Avoid Concomitant Use There are no known interactions where it is recommended to avoid concomitant use.

Increased Effect/Toxicity There are no known significant interactions involving an increase in effect.

Decreased Effect There are no known significant interactions involving a decrease in effect.

Stability Store at room temperature.

Mechanism of Action Ultrashort-acting nonbarbiturate hypnotic (benzylimidazole) used for the induction of anesthesia; chemically, it is a carboxylated imidazole which produces a rapid induction of anesthesia with minimal cardiovascular effects; produces EEG burst suppression at high doses

Pharmacodynamics/Kinetics

Onset of action: 30-60 seconds

Peak effect: 1 minute

Duration: 3-5 minutes; terminated by redistribution

Distribution: V_d: 2-4.5 L/kg

Protein binding: 76%;

Metabolism: Hepatic and plasma esterases

Half-life elimination: Terminal: 2.6 hours

Dosage Children >10 years and Adults: I.V.: Initial: 0.2-0.6 mg/kg over 30-60 seconds for induction of anesthesia; maintenance: 5-20 mcg/kg/minute

Administration Administer I.V. push over 30-60 seconds. Solution is highly irritating; avoid administration into small vessels; in some cases, preadministration of lidocaine may be considered.

Monitoring Parameters Cardiac monitoring and blood pressure required

Additional Information Etomidate decreases cerebral metabolism and cerebral blood flow while maintaining perfusion pressure. Premedication with opioids or benzodiazepines can decrease myoclonus. Etomidate can enhance somatosensory evoked potential recordings.

Dosage Forms Excipient information presented when available (limited, particularly for generics); consult specific product labeling.

Injection, solution: 2 mg/mL (10 mL, 20 mL) [contains propylene glycol 35% v/v]

Etonogestrel (e toe noe JES trel)

U.S. Brand Names Implanon™

Index Terms 3-Keto-desogestrel; ENG

Pharmacologic Category Contraceptive; Progestin

Use Prevention of pregnancy; for use in women who request long-acting (up to 3 years) contraception

Restrictions Only healthcare providers who have undergone training in the insertion and removal procedures will be able to order Implanon™.

Pregnancy Considerations Teratogenic effects were not observed in animal studies. Not for use during pregnancy; remove implant if pregnancy is detected. Ovulation may return within 1 week of implant removal; alternate forms of contraception may be required. In a multicenter clinical trial, 11 out of 46 women no longer using contraception became pregnant between 1 and 18 weeks following removal of the implant. Do not insert <21 days postpartum. Women weighing >130% of their ideal body weight were not included in clinical studies. With oral combination hormonal contraceptives, an increase in contraceptive failure was noted in women with a BMI >27.3. Similar findings were noted in patients weighing ≥90 kg (198 lb) using the contraceptive patch.

Lactation Enters breast milk/use caution

Contraindications Hypersensitivity to etonogestrel or any component of the formulation; undiagnosed abnormal uterine bleeding; active hepatic disease or malignant tumors; active thrombophlebitis or thromboembolic disorders (current or history of); known or suspected carcinoma of the breast; concomitant use with chronic potent hepatic enzyme inducers; pregnancy

Warnings/Precautions Use does not protect against HIV infection or other sexually-transmitted diseases. Improper insertion may lead to unintended pregnancy or may cause difficult or impossible removal. Failure to properly remove may lead to infertility, ectopic pregnancy, or continued adverse reactions. Menstrual bleeding patterns are likely to be altered; patients should be counseled prior to implant insertion. Abnormal bleeding should be evaluated as required to exclude pathologic conditions or pregnancy. Ectopic pregnancy (rare) may occur more commonly than in women using no contraception. Etonogestrel serum levels and contraceptive efficacy may be significantly decreased by potent hepatic enzyme inducers. The manufacturer does not recommend use in women chronically taking hepatic enzyme inducers. Use caution in overweight women; women >130% of ideal body weight were not included in clinical studies. Use caution with renal disease.

Additional warnings based on combination hormonal (estrogen and progestin) contraceptives: The risk of cardiovascular side effects increases in women who smoke cigarettes, especially those who are >35 years of age; women who use combination hormonal contraceptives should be strongly advised not to smoke. Combination hormonal contraceptives may lead to increased risk of myocardial infarction; use with caution in patients with risk factors for coronary artery disease. May increase the risk of thromboembolism (also reported with etonogestrel). Whenever possible, combination hormonal contraceptives should be discontinued at least 4 weeks prior to and for 2 weeks following elective surgery associated with an increased risk of thromboembolism or during periods of prolonged immobilization. Combination hormonal contraceptives may have a dose-related risk of vascular disease, hypertension, and gallbladder disease. Women with hypertension or renal disease should be encouraged to use another form of contraception. The use of combination hormonal contraceptives has been associated with a slight increase in frequency of breast cancer; however, studies are not consistent. Combination hormonal contraceptives may cause glucose intolerance or effect serum triglyceride and lipoprotein levels. Retinal thrombosis has been reported (rarely). Use caution with conditions that may be aggravated by fluid retention, depression, or history of migraine. Not for use prior to menarche.

Adverse Reactions

>10%:

Central nervous system: Headache (25%)

Dermatologic: Acne (14%)

Endocrine & metabolic: Infrequent menstrual bleeding (<3 episodes/90 days: 34%), amenorrhea (no bleeding in 90 days: 22%), prolonged menstrual bleeding (lasting >14 days: 18%), breast pain (13%), menstrual bleeding irregularities requiring discontinuation (11%)

Gastrointestinal: Weight gain (14%), abdominal pain (11%)

Genitourinary: Vaginitis (15%)

Respiratory: Upper respiratory tract infection (13%), pharyngitis (11%)

5% to 10%:

Central nervous system: Dizziness (7%), emotional lability (7%), depression (6%), nervousness (6%), pain (6%)

Endocrine & metabolic: Dysmenorrhea (7%), frequent menstrual bleeding (>5 episodes/90 days: 7%)

Gastrointestinal: Nausea (6%)

Genitourinary: Leukorrhea (10%)

Local: Insertion site pain (5%)

Neuromuscular & skeletal: Back pain (7%)

Respiratory: Sinusitis (6%)

Miscellaneous: Flu-like syndrome (8%)

<5% (Limited to important or life-threatening): Allergic reaction, alopecia, anorexia, anxiety, appetite increased, arthralgia, asthma, breast discharge, breast enlargement, breast fibroadenosis, cervical smear test positive, constipation, coughing, crying, diarrhea, dyspepsia, dysuria, edema, fatigue, fever, flatulence, gastritis, hot flushes, hypertension, hypoesthesia, injection site reaction, insomnia, lactation nonpuerperal, libido decreased, migraine, myalgia, otitis media, ovarian cyst, pelvic cramping, premenstrual tension, pruritus, rash, rhinitis, sexual function abnormal, skeletal pain, somnolence, vaginal discomfort, varicose vein, vision abnormal, vomiting, weakness, weight loss

Drug Interactions

Metabolism/Transport Effects **Substrate** of CYP3A4 (minor)

Avoid Concomitant Use

Avoid concomitant use of Etonogestrel with any of the following: Acitretin; Griseofulvin

Increased Effect/Toxicity

Etonogestrel may increase the levels/effects of: Benzodiazepines (metabolized by oxidation); Selegiline; Voriconazole

The levels/effects of Etonogestrel may be increased by: Herbs (Progestogenic Properties); Voriconazole

Decreased Effect

Etonogestrel may decrease the levels/effects of: Vitamin K Antagonists

The levels/effects of Etonogestrel may be decreased by: Acitretin; Aminoglutethimide; Aprepitant; Barbiturates; CarBAMazepine; Felbamate; Fosaprepitant; Griseofulvin; Mycophenolate; OXcarbazepine; Phenytoin; Retinoic Acid Derivatives; Rifamycin Derivatives; St Johns Wort

Ethanol/Nutrition/Herb Interactions

Herb/Nutraceutical: St John's wort (an enzyme inducer) may decrease serum levels of etonogestrel. Concomitant use is not recommended. Bloodroot, chasteberry, damiana, oregano, and yucca may enhance the adverse/toxic effect of progestins.

Stability Store at controlled room temperature 15°C to 30°C (59°F to 86°F); protect from light

Mechanism of Action Etonogestrel is the active metabolite of desogestrel. It prevents pregnancy by suppressing ovulation, increasing the viscosity of cervical mucous, and inhibiting endometrial proliferation.

Pharmacodynamics/Kinetics

Onset of action: Serum levels sufficient to inhibit ovulation: ≤8 hours of implant

Duration: Implant: Each rod maintains etonogestrel levels sufficient to inhibit ovulation for 3 years

Distribution: V_d: 201 L

Protein binding: Albumin (66%) and sex hormone-binding globulin (32%)

Metabolism: Hepatic via CYP3A4; forms metabolites (activity not known)

Bioavailability: Implant: 100%

Half-life, elimination: 25 hours

Excretion: Urine (primarily); feces

Dosage

Children: Not for use prior to menarche.

Adults: Contraception: Subdermal: Implant 1 rod in the inner side of the upper, nondominant arm. Remove no later than 3 years after the date of insertion. After ruling out pregnancy, timing of insertion is based on the patient's contraceptive history:

No hormonal contraceptives within the past month: Insert between days 1 through 5 of menstruation, even if woman is still bleeding

Switching from combination hormonal contraceptive:

Oral tablet: Insert anytime within 7 days after the last active tablet

Vaginal ring: Insert anytime during the 7-day ring-free period

Transdermal system: Insert anytime during the 7-day patch-free period

Switching from a progestin-only contraceptive:

Oral pill: Any day during the month; do not skip days between the last pill and implant insertion

Implant: Insert on same day as removal of implant

IUD: Insert on same day as removal of IUD

Injection: Insert on day next injection is due

First trimester abortion or miscarriage: Insert immediately. If not inserted within first 5 days follow directions for "no hormonal contraception within the past month"

Following delivery or second trimester abortion: May insert between 21 and 28 days (if not exclusively breast-feeding) or after 4 weeks (if exclusively breast-feeding). Patients should use a second form of contraception for the first 7 days if insertion occurs at >4 weeks.

Note: If following above insertion schedule, no back-up contraception needed. If deviating, use back-up method for 7 days postinsertion.

Elderly: Not for use after menopause

Dosage adjustment in renal impairment: Use with caution; formal studies have not been conducted

Dosage adjustment in hepatic impairment: Use is contraindicated

Administration Subdermal: For insertion under local anesthesia by healthcare providers trained in the insertion and removal procedure. Rod must be palpable after insertion. Deep insertion may require surgery to remove. If rod is impalpable, ultrasound should be used to locate the rod; MRI may also be useful if ultrasound is not successful. A pressure bandage should be applied and left in place for 24 hours after insertion to decrease bruising; a small bandage placed over the insertion site should remain in place for 3-5 days.

Monitoring Parameters Before starting therapy, a physical exam with reference to the breasts and pelvis are recommended, including a Papanicolaou smear. Exam may be deferred if appropriate; pregnancy should be ruled out prior to use. Monitor patient closely for loss of vision, sudden onset of proptosis, diplopia, migraine; blood pressure; signs and symptoms of thromboembolic disorders; signs or symptoms of depression; glycemic control in patients with diabetes; lipid profiles in patients being treated for hyperlipidemias. Adequate diagnostic measures, including endometrial sampling, if indicated, should be performed to rule out malignancy in all cases of undiagnosed abnormal vaginal bleeding.

Reference Range Etonogestrel: A release rate of 25-30 mcg/day is required to inhibit ovulation

Test Interactions

Sex hormone-binding globulin: Serum concentrations may be decreased for first 6 months following implantation.

Thyroxine: Serum concentrations may be slightly decreased initially.

Additional Information For subdermal insertion by healthcare providers trained on the insertion and removal procedure. For use in women who request long-acting (up to 3 years) contraception. A User Card (to give to the patient), consent form (to keep on file), and a medication guide (for the patient) are provided with the device.

The rod releases etonogestrel at a rate of 60-70 mcg/day, decreasing to 35-45 mcg/day after the first year, 30-40 mcg/day after the second year, and 25-30 mcg/day at the end of the third year. Following removal of rod, levels decrease rapidly and are less than the level of detection within 1 week.

Dosage Forms Excipient information presented when available (limited, particularly for generics); consult specific product labeling.

Rod, subdermal:

Implanon™: 68 mg [latex free]

- **Etonogestrel and Ethinyl Estradiol** *see* Ethinyl Estradiol and Etonogestrel *on page 577*
- **Etopophos®** *see* Etoposide Phosphate *on page 593*

Etoposide (e toe POE side)

U.S. Brand Names Toposar®; VePesid® [DSC]

Canadian Brand Names VePesid®

Index Terms Epipodophyllotoxin; VP-16; VP-16-213

Pharmacologic Category Antineoplastic Agent, Podophyllotoxin Derivative

Use Treatment of refractory testicular tumors; treatment of small cell lung cancer

Unlabeled/Investigational Use Treatment of lymphomas, acute nonlymphocytic leukemia (ANLL); lung, bladder, and prostate carcinoma; hepatoma, rhabdomyosarcoma, uterine carcinoma, neuroblastoma, mycosis fungoides, Kaposi's sarcoma, histiocytosis, gestational trophoblastic disease, Ewing's sarcoma, Wilms' tumor, brain tumors

Pregnancy Risk Factor D

Pregnancy Considerations Animal studies have demonstrated teratogenicity and fetal loss. There are no adequate and well-controlled studies in pregnant women. Women of childbearing potential should be advised to avoid pregnancy.

Lactation Enters breast milk/contraindicated

Medication Safety Issues

Sound-alike/look-alike issues:

Etoposide may be confused with teniposide

VePesid® may be confused with Versed

High alert medication: The Institute for Safe Medication Practices (ISMP) includes this medication among its list of drugs which have a heightened risk of causing significant patient harm when used in error.

Contraindications Hypersensitivity to etoposide or any component of the formulation; pregnancy

Warnings/Precautions Hazardous agent - use appropriate precautions for handling and disposal. **[U.S. Boxed Warning]: Severe myelosuppression with resulting infection or bleeding may occur.** Treatment should be withheld for platelets <50,000/mm^3 or absolute neutrophil count (ANC) <500/mm^3. May cause anaphylactic reaction manifested by chills, fever, tachycardia, bronchospasm, dyspnea, and hypotension. In children, the use of concentrations higher than recommended were associated with higher rates of anaphylactic-like reactions. Infusion should be interrupted and medications for the treatment of anaphylaxis should be available for immediate use. Must be diluted; do not give I.V. push, infuse over at least 30-60 minutes; hypotension is associated with rapid infusion. Dosage should be adjusted in patients with hepatic or renal impairment. **[U.S. Boxed Warning]: Should be administered under the supervision of an experienced cancer chemotherapy physician.** Injectable formula contains polysorbate 80; do not use in premature infants. May contain benzyl alcohol; do not use in newborn infants.

Adverse Reactions

>10%:

Dermatologic: Alopecia (8% to 66%)

Endocrine & metabolic: Ovarian failure (38%), amenorrhea

Gastrointestinal: Nausea/vomiting (31% to 43%), anorexia (10% to 13%), diarrhea (1% to 13%), mucositis/esophagitis (with high doses)

Hematologic: Leukopenia (60% to 91%; grade 4: 3% to 17%; onset: 5-7 days; nadir: 7-14 days; recovery: 21-28 days), thrombocytopenia (22% to 41%; grades 3/4: 1% to 20%; nadir 9-16 days), anemia (up to 33%)

1% to 10%:

Cardiovascular: Hypotension (1% to 2%; due to rapid infusion)

Gastrointestinal: Stomatitis (1% to 6%), abdominal pain (up to 2%)

Hepatic: Hepatic toxicity (up to 3%)

Neuromuscular & skeletal: Peripheral neuropathy (1% to 2%)

Miscellaneous: Anaphylactic-like reaction (I.V. infusion: 1% to 2%; including chills, fever, tachycardia, bronchospasm, dyspnea)

<1% (Limited to important or life-threatening): Anovulatory cycles, back pain; blindness (transient, cortical); CHF, constipation, cough, cyanosis, diaphoresis, dysphagia, erythema; extravasation (induration, necrosis, swelling); facial swelling, fatigue, fever, headache, hepatic toxicity, hepatitis, hyperpigmentation, hypersensitivity, hypersensitivity-associated apnea, hypomenorrhea, interstitial pneumonitis, laryngospasm, maculopapular rash, malaise, metabolic acidosis, MI, optic neuritis, perivasculitis, pruritus, pulmonary fibrosis, radiation-recall dermatitis, rash, seizure, somnolence, Stevens-Johnson syndrome, tachycardia, taste perversion, thrombophlebitis, tongue swelling, toxic epidermal necrolysis, urticaria, weakness

BMT:

Cardiovascular: Hypotension (infusion-related)

Dermatologic: Skin lesions resembling Stevens-Johnson syndrome, alopecia

Endocrine & metabolic: Metabolic acidosis

Gastrointestinal: Severe nausea and vomiting, mucositis

Hepatic: Hepatitis

Miscellaneous: Secondary malignancy, ethanol intoxication

Drug Interactions

Metabolism/Transport Effects Substrate of CYP1A2 (minor), 2E1 (minor), 3A4 (major); **Inhibits** CYP2C9 (weak), 3A4 (weak)

Avoid Concomitant Use

Avoid concomitant use of Etoposide with any of the following: Natalizumab; Vaccines (Live)

Increased Effect/Toxicity

Etoposide may increase the levels/effects of: Natalizumab; Vaccines (Live); Vitamin K Antagonists

The levels/effects of Etoposide may be increased by: CycloSPORINE; CYP3A4 Inhibitors (Moderate); CYP3A4 Inhibitors (Strong); Dasatinib; P-Glycoprotein Inhibitors; Trastuzumab

Decreased Effect

Etoposide may decrease the levels/effects of: Vaccines (Inactivated); Vitamin K Antagonists

The levels/effects of Etoposide may be decreased by: Barbiturates; CYP3A4 Inducers (Strong); Deferasirox; Echinacea; Herbs (CYP3A4 Inducers); P-Glycoprotein Inducers; Phenytoin

Ethanol/Nutrition/Herb Interactions

Ethanol: Avoid ethanol (may increase GI irritation).

Herb/Nutraceutical: Avoid concurrent St John's wort; may decrease etoposide levels.

Stability

Store intact vials of injection at 15°C to 30°C (59°F to 86°F). Protect from light. Store oral capsules at 2°C to 8°C (36°F to 46°F).

Etoposide should be diluted to a concentration of 0.2-0.4 mg/mL in D_5W or NS for administration. Diluted solutions have concentration-dependent stability; more concentrated solutions have shorter stability times. Precipitation may occur with concentrations >0.4 mg/mL.

Solutions for infusion, at room temperature, in D_5W or NS in polyvinyl chloride, the concentration is stable as follows:
0.2 mg/mL: 96 hours
0.4 mg/mL: 24 hours
Etoposide injection contains polysorbate 80 which may cause leaching of diethylhexyl phthalate (DEHP), a plasticizer contained in polyvinyl chloride (PVC) bags and tubing. Higher concentrations and longer storage time after preparation in PVC bags may increase DEHP leaching. Preparation in glass or polyolefin containers will minimize patient exposure to DEHP.
Etoposide injection diluted for oral use to 10 mg/mL in NS may be stored for 22 days in plastic oral syringes at room temperature. Mix with orange juice, apple juice, or lemonade to a concentration of ≤0.4 mg/mL, and use within a 3-hour period.

Mechanism of Action Etoposide has been shown to delay transit of cells through the S phase and arrest cells in late S or early G_2 phase. The drug may inhibit mitochondrial transport at the NADH dehydrogenase level or inhibit uptake of nucleosides into HeLa cells. It is a topoisomerase II inhibitor and appears to cause DNA strand breaks. Etoposide does not inhibit microtubular assembly.

Pharmacodynamics/Kinetics
Absorption: Oral: 25% to 75%; significant inter- and intrapatient variation
Distribution: Average V_d: 7-17 L/m^2; poor penetration across the blood-brain barrier; CSF concentrations <10% of plasma concentrations
Protein binding: 94% to 97%
Metabolism: Hepatic to hydroxy acid and cislactone metabolites
Bioavailability: Oral: ~50% (range 25% to 75%)
Half-life elimination: Terminal: 4-11 hours; Children: Normal renal/hepatic function: 6-8 hours
Time to peak, serum: Oral: 1-1.5 hours
Excretion:
Children: Urine (≤55% as unchanged drug)
Adults: Urine (42% to 67%; 8% to 35% as unchanged drug) within 24 hours; feces (up to 44%)

Dosage Refer to individual protocols:
Children (unlabeled uses): I.V.: 60-120 mg/m^2/day for 3-5 days every 3-6 weeks
AML:
Remission induction: 150 mg/m^2/day for 2-3 days for 2-3 cycles
Intensification or consolidation: 250 mg/m^2/day for 3 days, courses 2-5
Brain tumor: 150 mg/m^2/day on days 2 and 3 of treatment course
Neuroblastoma: 100 mg/m^2/day over 1 hour on days 1-5 of cycle; repeat cycle every 4 weeks
BMT conditioning regimen used in patients with rhabdomyosarcoma or neuroblastoma: I.V. continuous infusion: 160 mg/m^2/day for 4 days
Conditioning regimen for allogenic BMT: 60 mg/kg/dose as a single dose
Adults:
Small cell lung cancer (in combination with other approved chemotherapeutic drugs):
Oral: Due to poor bioavailability, oral doses should be twice the I.V. dose, rounded to the nearest 50 mg given once daily
I.V.: 35 mg/m^2/day for 4 days or 50 mg/m^2/day for 5 days every 3-4 weeks
IVPB: 60-100 mg/m^2/day for 3 days (with cisplatin)
CIV: 500 mg/m^2 over 24 hours every 3 weeks
Testicular cancer (in combination with other approved chemotherapeutic drugs):
IVPB: 50-100 mg/m^2/day for 5 days repeated every 3-4 weeks
I.V.: 100 mg/m^2 every other day for 3 doses repeated every 3-4 weeks
BMT/relapsed leukemia (unlabeled uses): I.V.: 2.4-3.5 g/m^2 or 25-70 mg/kg administered over 4-36 hours

Dosing adjustment in renal impairment:
The FDA-approved labeling recommends the following adjustments:
Cl_{cr} 15-50 mL/minute: Administer 75% of dose
Cl_{cr} <15 mL minute: Data not available; consider further dose reductions
The following guidelines have been used by some clinicians:
Aronoff, 2007:
Cl_{cr} 10-50 mL/minute: Children and Adults: Administer 75% of dose
Cl_{cr} <10 mL minute: Children and Adults: Administer 50% of dose
Hemodialysis:
Children: Administer 50% of dose
Adults: Supplemental dose is not necessary
Continuous ambulatory peritoneal dialysis (CAPD):
Children: Administer 50% of dose
Adults: Supplemental dose is not necessary
Continuous renal replacement therapy (CRRT): Children and Adults: Administer 75% of dose
Kintzel, 1995:
Cl_{cr} 46-60 mL/minute: Administer 85% of dose
Cl_{cr} 31-45 mL/minute: Administer 80% of dose
Cl_{cr} <30 mL/minute: Administer 75% of dose

Dosing adjustment in hepatic impairment: The FDA-approved labeling does not contain dosing adjustment guidelines. The following adjustments have been used by some clinicians:
Donelli, 1998: Liver dysfunction may reduce the metabolism and increase the toxicity of etoposide. Normal doses of I.V. etoposide should be given to patients with liver dysfunction (dose reductions may result in subtherapeutic concentrations); however, use caution with concomitant liver dysfunction (severe) and renal dysfunction as the decreased metabolic clearance cannot be compensated by increased renal clearance.
Floyd, 2006: Bilirubin 1.5-3 mg/dL or AST >3 times ULN: Administer 50% of dose
King, 2001: Bilirubin 1.5-3 mg/dL or ALT or AST >180 units/L: Administer 50% of dose
Koren, 1992: Bilirubin 1.5-3 mg/dL or AST >180 units/L: Administer 50% of dose
Perry, 1982:
Bilirubin 1.5-3 mg/dL or AST 60-180 units/L: Administer 50% of dose
Bilirubin >3 mg/dL or AST >180 units/L: Avoid use

Administration
Oral: Doses ≤400 mg/day as a single once daily dose; doses >400 mg should be given in 2-4 divided doses. If necessary, the injection may be used for oral administration.
I.V.: As a bolus or 24-hour continuous infusion; bolus infusions are usually administered over at least 45-60 minutes. Infusion of doses in ≤30 minutes greatly increases the risk of hypotension. Etoposide injection contains polysorbate 80 which may cause leaching of diethylhexyl phthalate (DEHP), a plasticizer contained in polyvinyl chloride (PVC) tubing. Administration through non-PVC (low sorbing) tubing will minimize patient exposure to DEHP. Concentrations >0.4 mg/mL are very unstable and may precipitate within a few minutes. For large doses, where dilution to ≤0.4 mg/mL is not feasible, consideration should be given to slow infusion of the undiluted drug through a running normal saline, dextrose or saline/dextrose infusion; or use of etoposide phosphate. Etoposide solutions of 0.1-0.4 mg/mL may be filtered through a 0.22 micron filter without damage to the filter or significant loss of drug.

Monitoring Parameters CBC with differential, platelet count, and hemoglobin, vital signs (blood pressure), bilirubin, and renal function tests

Dosage Forms Excipient information presented when available (limited, particularly for generics); consult specific product labeling. [DSC] = Discontinued product

Capsule, softgel: 50 mg

VePesid®: 50 mg [DSC]

Injection, solution: 20 mg/mL (5 mL, 25 mL, 50 mL)

Toposar®: 20 mg/mL (5 mL, 25 mL, 50 mL) [contains alcohol 33% and polysorbate 80]

Etoposide Phosphate (e toe POE side FOS fate)

U.S. Brand Names Etopophos®

Pharmacologic Category Antineoplastic Agent, Podophyllotoxin Derivative

Use Treatment of refractory testicular tumors; treatment of small cell lung cancer

Pregnancy Risk Factor D

Pregnancy Considerations Animal studies have demonstrated teratogenicity and fetal loss. There are no adequate and well-controlled studies in pregnant women. Women of childbearing potential should be advised to avoid pregnancy.

Lactation Enters breast milk/contraindicated

Medication Safety Issues

Sound-alike/look-alike issues:

Etoposide may be confused with teniposide

Etoposide phosphate is a prodrug of etoposide and is rapidly converted in the plasma to etoposide. To avoid confusion or dosing errors, **dosage should be expressed as the desired etoposide dose,** not as the etoposide phosphate dose (eg, etoposide phosphate equivalent to ____ mg etoposide).

High alert medication: The Institute for Safe Medication Practices (ISMP) includes this medication among its list of drugs which have a heightened risk of causing significant patient harm when used in error.

Contraindications Hypersensitivity to etoposide, etoposide phosphate, or any component of the formulation; pregnancy

Warnings/Precautions Hazardous agent - use appropriate precautions for handling and disposal. **[U.S. Boxed Warning]: Severe myelosuppression with resulting infection or bleeding may occur.** Treatment should be withheld for platelets <50,000/mm^3 or absolute neutrophil count (ANC) <500/mm^3. May cause anaphylactic reaction manifested by chills, fever, tachycardia, bronchospasm, dyspnea, and hypotension (higher concentrations were associated with higher rates of reactions in children). Infusion should be interrupted and medications for the treatment of anaphylaxis should be available for immediate use. Dosage should be adjusted in patients with hepatic or renal impairment. Use with caution in patients with low serum albumin; may increase risk for toxicities. Doses of etoposide phosphate >175 mg/m^2 have not been evaluated. Use caution in elderly patients (may be more likely to develop severe myelosuppression and/or GI effects. **[U.S. Boxed Warning]: Should be administered under the supervision of an experienced cancer chemotherapy physician.** Safety and efficacy in children have not been established.

Adverse Reactions Note: Also see adverse reactions for **etoposide**. Since etoposide phosphate is converted to etoposide, adverse reactions experienced with etoposide would also be expected with etoposide phosphate.

>10%:

Central nervous system: Chills/fever (24%)

Dermatologic: Alopecia (33% to 44%)

Gastrointestinal: Nausea/vomiting (37%), anorexia (16%), mucositis (11%)

Hematologic: Leukopenia (91%; grade 4: 17%), neutropenia (88%; grade 4: 37%), anemia (72%; grades 3/4: 19%), thrombocytopenia (23%; grade 4: 9%)

Neuromuscular & skeletal: Weakness/malaise (39%)

1% to 10%:

Cardiovascular: Hypotension (5%), hypertension (3%), facial flushing (2%)

Central nervous system: Dizziness (5%)

Dermatologic: Skin rash (3%)

Gastrointestinal: Constipation (8%), abdominal pain (7%), diarrhea (6%), taste perversion (6%)

Local: Extravasation/phlebitis (5%)

Miscellaneous: Anaphylactic-type reactions (3%; including chills, diaphoresis, fever, rigor, tachycardia, bronchospasm, dyspnea, pruritus)

<1% (Limited to important or life-threatening): Acute leukemia (with/without preleukemia phase), anaphylactic-like reactions, back pain, blindness (transient, cortical), cough, cyanosis, diaphoresis, dysphagia, erythema, facial swelling, hepatic toxicity, hyperpigmentation, hypersensitivity-associated apnea, infection, interstitial pneumonitis, laryngospasm, maculopapular rash, neutropenic fever, optic neuritis, perivasculitis, pruritus, pulmonary fibrosis, radiation recall dermatitis, seizure, Stevens-Johnson syndrome, taste perversion, tongue swelling, toxic epidermal necrolysis, urticaria

Drug Interactions

Metabolism/Transport Effects Substrate of CYP1A2 (minor), 2E1 (minor), 3A4 (major); **Inhibits** CYP2C9 (weak), 3A4 (weak)

Avoid Concomitant Use

Avoid concomitant use of Etoposide Phosphate with any of the following: Natalizumab; Vaccines (Live)

Increased Effect/Toxicity

Etoposide Phosphate may increase the levels/effects of: Natalizumab; Vaccines (Live)

The levels/effects of Etoposide Phosphate may be increased by: CycloSPORINE; CYP3A4 Inhibitors (Moderate); CYP3A4 Inhibitors (Strong); Dasatinib; P-Glycoprotein Inhibitors; Trastuzumab

Decreased Effect

Etoposide Phosphate may decrease the levels/effects of: Vaccines (Inactivated)

The levels/effects of Etoposide Phosphate may be decreased by: Barbiturates; CYP3A4 Inducers (Strong); Deferasirox; Echinacea; Herbs (CYP3A4 Inducers); P-Glycoprotein Inducers; Phenytoin

Ethanol/Nutrition/Herb Interactions

Ethanol: Avoid ethanol (may increase GI irritation).

Herb/Nutraceutical: Avoid St John's wort (may decrease etoposide levels).

Stability Store intact vials of injection under refrigeration 2°C to 8°C (36°F to 46°F). Protect from light. Reconstitute vials with 5 mL or 10 mL SWI, D_5W, NS, bacteriostatic SWI, or bacteriostatic NS to a concentration of 20 mg/mL or 10 mg/mL etoposide equivalent. These solutions may be administered without further dilution or may be diluted in 50-500 mL of D_5W or NS to a concentration as low as 0.1 mg/mL.

Reconstituted etoposide phosphate is stable refrigerated at 2°C to 8°C (36°F to 47°F) for 7 days. Undiluted solutions are stable for 24 hours at room temperature of 20°C to 25°C (68°F to 77°F) when reconstituted with SWI, D_5W or NS; and stable for 48 hours at room temperature when reconstituted with bacteriostatic SWI or NS. Further diluted solutions are stable at room temperature 20°C to 25°C (68°F to 77°F) or under refrigeration 2°C to 8°C (36°F to 47°F) for up to 24 hours.

Mechanism of Action Etoposide phosphate is converted *in vivo* to the active moiety, etoposide, by dephosphorylation. Etoposide inhibits mitotic activity; inhibits cells from entering prophase; inhibits DNA synthesis. Initially thought to be mitotic inhibitors similar to podophyllotoxin, but actually have no effect on microtubule assembly. However, later shown to induce DNA strand breakage and inhibition of topoisomerase II (an enzyme which breaks and repairs DNA); etoposide acts in late S or early G2 phases.

Pharmacodynamics/Kinetics

Distribution: Average V_d: 7-17 L/m^2; poor penetration across blood-brain barrier; concentrations in CSF being <10% that of plasma

Protein binding: 94% to 97%

Metabolism:

Etoposide phosphate: Rapidly and completely converted to etoposide in plasma

Etoposide: Hepatic, via CYP3A4, to hydroxy acid and cislactone metabolites

Half-life elimination: Terminal: 4-11 hours; Children: Normal renal/hepatic function: 6-8 hours

Excretion: Urine (56%; 45% as etoposide); feces (44% as etoposide and metabolites)

Children: I.V.: Urine (≤55% as etoposide)

Dosage Refer to individual protocols. Adults: **Note:** Etoposide phosphate is a prodrug of etoposide, doses should be expressed as the desired **ETOPOSIDE** dose; **not** as the etoposide phosphate dose. (eg, etoposide phosphate equivalent to ____ mg etoposide).

Small cell lung cancer (in combination with other approved chemotherapeutic drugs): I.V.: Etoposide 35 mg/m^2/day for 4 days to 50 mg/m^2/day for 5 days. Courses are repeated at 3- to 4-week intervals after adequate recovery from any toxicity.

Testicular cancer (in combination with other approved chemotherapeutic agents): I.V.: Etoposide 50-100 mg/m^2/day on days 1-5 to 100 mg/m^2/day on days 1, 3, and 5. Courses are repeated at 3- to 4-week intervals after adequate recovery from any toxicity.

Dosage adjustment in renal impairment:

Manufacturer recommended guidelines:

Cl_{cr} 15-50 mL/minute: Administer 75% of normal dose

Cl_{cr} <15 mL minute: Data are available; consider further dose reductions

Aronoff, 1999:

Cl_{cr} 10-50 mL/minute: Administer 75% of normal dose

Cl_{cr} <10 mL minute: Administer 50% of normal dose

Hemodialysis: Supplemental dose is not necessary

Peritoneal dialysis: Supplemental dose is not necessary

CAPD effects: Unknown

CAVH effects: Dose for Cl_{cr} 10-50 mL/minute (Aronoff, 1999)

Dosage adjustment in hepatic impairment:

Bilirubin 1.5-3 mg/dL or AST 60-180 units: Reduce dose by 50%

Bilirubin 3-5 mg/dL or AST >180 units: Reduce by 75%

Bilirubin >5 mg/dL: Do not administer

Administration Infuse over 5-210 minutes.

Monitoring Parameters CBC with differential, platelet count, bilirubin, renal function

Additional Information Etoposide phosphate 113.5 mg is equivalent to etoposide 100 mg. Dosages should always be expressed, and calculated, as the desired **etoposide** dose.

Dosage Forms Excipient information presented when available (limited, particularly for generics); consult specific product labeling.

Injection, powder for reconstitution:

Etopophos®: 100 mg

- **Etrafon® (Can)** *see* Amitriptyline and Perphenazine *on page 93*

Etravirine (et ra VIR een)

U.S. Brand Names Intelence™

Canadian Brand Names Intelence™

Index Terms TMC125

Pharmacologic Category Antiretroviral Agent, Reverse Transcriptase Inhibitor (Non-nucleoside)

Additional Appendix Information

Antiretroviral Therapy for HIV Infection: Adults and Adolescents *on page 1758*

Use Treatment of HIV-1 infection in combination with at least two additional antiretroviral agents in treatment-experienced patients exhibiting viral replication with documented non-nucleoside reverse transcriptase inhibitor (NNRTI) resistance

Pregnancy Risk Factor B

Dosage Oral: Adults: 200 mg twice daily after meals

Dosage adjustment in renal impairment: Due to minimal renal clearance, dose adjustment likely unnecessary in renal impairment.

Dosage adjustment in hepatic impairment: No adjustment required for mild-to-moderate (Child-Pugh class A/B) impairment; no data in severe impairment.

Additional Information Complete prescribing information for this medication should be consulted for additional detail.

Dosage Forms Excipient information presented when available (limited, particularly for generics); consult specific product labeling.

Tablet:

Intelence™: 100 mg

- **Eudal®-SR** *see* Guaifenesin and Pseudoephedrine *on page 713*
- **Euflex® (Can)** *see* Flutamide *on page 643*
- **Euflexxa™** *see* Hyaluronate and Derivatives *on page 734*
- **Euglucon® (Can)** *see* GlyBURIDE *on page 701*
- **Eulexin®** *see* Flutamide *on page 643*
- **Eurax®** *see* Crotamiton *on page 374*
- **Euro-Lithium (Can)** *see* Lithium *on page 897*
- **Euthyrox (Can)** *see* Levothyroxine *on page 881*
- **Evamist™** *see* Estradiol *on page 554*
- **Everone® 200 (Can)** *see* Testosterone *on page 1445*
- **Evista®** *see* Raloxifene *on page 1289*
- **Evoclin®** *see* Clindamycin *on page 344*
- **Evoxac®** *see* Cevimeline *on page 299*
- **Evra® (Can)** *see* Ethinyl Estradiol and Norelgestromin *on page 581*
- **Exactacain™** *see* Benzocaine, Butamben, and Tetracaine *on page 185*
- **Excedrin® Extra Strength [OTC]** *see* Acetaminophen, Aspirin, and Caffeine *on page 31*
- **Excedrin® Migraine [OTC]** *see* Acetaminophen, Aspirin, and Caffeine *on page 31*
- **Excedrin® P.M. [OTC]** *see* Acetaminophen and Diphenhydramine *on page 28*
- **ExeClear [DSC]** *see* Hydrocodone and Guaifenesin *on page 741*
- **ExeCof-XP [DSC]** *see* Hydrocodone and Guaifenesin *on page 741*
- **ExeFen** *see* Guaifenesin and Pseudoephedrine *on page 713*
- **ExeFen-DMX** *see* Guaifenesin, Pseudoephedrine, and Dextromethorphan *on page 715*

◆ **ExeFen-PD** *see* Guaifenesin and Phenylephrine *on page 712*
◆ **Exelderm®** *see* Sulconazole *on page 1405*
◆ **Exelon®** *see* Rivastigmine *on page 1331*

Exemestane (ex e MES tane)

U.S. Brand Names Aromasin®
Canadian Brand Names Aromasin®
Pharmacologic Category Antineoplastic Agent, Aromatase Inactivator
Use Treatment of advanced breast cancer in postmenopausal women whose disease has progressed following tamoxifen therapy; adjuvant treatment of postmenopausal estrogen receptor-positive early breast cancer following 2-3 years of tamoxifen (for a total of 5 years of adjuvant therapy)
Pregnancy Risk Factor D
Pregnancy Considerations Exemestane has been associated with prolonged gestation, abnormal or difficult labor, increased resorption, reduced number of live fetuses, decreased fetal weight, and retarded ossification in rats. It is not indicated for premenopausal women, but if exposure occurred during pregnancy, risk to the fetus and potential risk for loss of the pregnancy should be discussed.
Lactation Excretion in breast milk unknown/use caution
Medication Safety Issues
Sound-alike/look-alike issues:
Exemestane may be confused with estramustine.
Contraindications Hypersensitivity to exemestane or any component of the formulation; pregnancy
Warnings/Precautions Hazardous agent - use appropriate precautions for handling and disposal. Not indicated for premenopausal women; not to be given with estrogen-containing agents.
Adverse Reactions
>10%:
Cardiovascular: Hypertension (5% to 15%)
Central nervous system: Fatigue (8% to 22%), insomnia (11% to 14%), pain (13%), headache (7% to 13%), depression (6% to 13%)
Dermatological: Hyperhidrosis (4% to 18%), alopecia (15%)
Endocrine & metabolic: Hot flashes (13% to 21%)
Gastrointestinal: Nausea (9% to 18%), abdominal pain (6% to 11%)
Hepatic: Alkaline phosphatase increased (14% to 15%)
Neuromuscular & skeletal: Arthralgia (15% to 29%)
1% to 10%:
Cardiovascular: Edema (6% to 7%); cardiac ischemic events (2%: MI, angina, myocardial ischemia); chest pain
Central nervous system: Dizziness (8% to 10%), anxiety (4% to 10%), fever (5%), confusion, hypoesthesia
Dermatologic: Dermatitis (8%), itching, rash
Endocrine & metabolic: Weight gain (8%)
Gastrointestinal: Diarrhea (4% to 10%), vomiting (7%), anorexia (6%), constipation (5%), appetite increased (3%), dyspepsia
Genitourinary: Urinary tract infection
Hepatic: Bilirubin increased (5% to 7%)
Neuromuscular & skeletal: Back pain (9%), limb pain (9%), osteoarthritis (6%), weakness (6%), osteoporosis (5%), pathological fracture (4%), paresthesia (3%), carpal tunnel syndrome (2%), cramps (2%)
Ocular: Visual disturbances (5%)
Renal: Creatinine increased (6%)
Respiratory: Dyspnea (10%), cough (6%), bronchitis, pharyngitis, rhinitis, sinusitis, upper respiratory infection
Miscellaneous: Influenza-like symptoms (6%), diaphoresis (6%), lymphedema, infection
<1% (Limited to important or life-threatening): Cardiac failure, endometrial hyperplasia, GGT increased, neuropathy, osteochondrosis, thromboembolism, transaminases increased, trigger finger, uterine polyps

A dose-dependent decrease in sex hormone-binding globulin has been observed with daily doses of 25 mg or more. Serum luteinizing hormone and follicle-stimulating hormone levels have increased with this medicine.
Drug Interactions
Metabolism/Transport Effects **Substrate** of CYP3A4 (major)
Avoid Concomitant Use There are no known interactions where it is recommended to avoid concomitant use.
Increased Effect/Toxicity There are no known significant interactions involving an increase in effect.
Decreased Effect
Exemestane may decrease the levels/effects of: Maraviroc

The levels/effects of Exemestane may be decreased by: CYP3A4 Inducers (Strong); Deferasirox; Herbs (CYP3A4 Inducers); Rifampin
Ethanol/Nutrition/Herb Interactions
Food: Plasma levels increased by 40% when exemestane was taken with a fatty meal.
Herb/Nutraceutical: St John's wort may decrease exemestane levels. Avoid black cohosh, dong quai in estrogen-dependent tumors.
Stability Store at 25°C (77°F)
Mechanism of Action Exemestane is an irreversible, steroidal aromatase inactivator. It prevents conversion of androgens to estrogens by tying up the enzyme aromatase. In breast cancers where growth is estrogen-dependent, this medicine will lower circulating estrogens.
Pharmacodynamics/Kinetics
Absorption: Rapid and moderate (~42%) following oral administration; absorption increases ~40% following high-fat meal
Distribution: Extensive
Protein binding: 90%, primarily to albumin and α_1-acid glycoprotein
Metabolism: Extensively hepatic; oxidation (CYP3A4) of methylene group, reduction of 17-keto group with formation of many secondary metabolites; metabolites are inactive
Half-life elimination: 24 hours
Time to peak: Women with breast cancer: 1.2 hours
Excretion: Urine (<1% as unchanged drug, 39% to 45% as metabolites); feces (36% to 48%)
Dosage Adults: Oral: 25 mg once daily
Dosage adjustment with CYP3A4 inducers: 50 mg once daily when used with potent inducers (eg, rifampin, phenytoin)
Dosing adjustment in renal/hepatic impairment: Safety of chronic doses has not been studied
Dietary Considerations Take after a meal; patients on aromatase inhibitor therapy should receive vitamin D and calcium supplements.
Administration Administer after a meal.
Dosage Forms Excipient information presented when available (limited, particularly for generics); consult specific product labeling.
Tablet: 25 mg

Exenatide (ex EN a tide)

U.S. Brand Names Byetta®
Index Terms AC 2993; AC002993; Exendin-4 ; LY2148568
Pharmacologic Category Antidiabetic Agent, Incretin Mimetic
Use Management (adjunctive) of type 2 diabetes mellitus (noninsulin dependent, NIDDM) in patients receiving a

sulfonylurea, thiazolidinedione, or metformin (or a combination of these agents)

Pregnancy Risk Factor C

Pregnancy Considerations Due to adverse events observed in some animal studies, exenatide is classified as pregnancy category C. Based on *in vitro* data, exenatide has a low potential to cross the placenta. Maternal hyperglycemia can be associated with adverse effects in the fetus, including macrosomia, neonatal hyperglycemia, and hyperbilirubinemia; the risk of congenital malformations is increased when the Hb A_{1c} is above the normal range. Diabetes can also be associated with adverse effects in the mother. Poorly-treated diabetes may cause end-organ damage that may in turn negatively affect obstetric outcomes. Physiologic glucose levels should be maintained prior to and during pregnancy to decrease the risk of adverse events in the mother and the fetus. Until additional safety and efficacy data are obtained, the use of exenatide is generally not recommended in the routine management of diabetes mellitus during pregnancy. Insulin is the drug of choice for the control of diabetes mellitus during pregnancy. A registry has been established for women exposed to exenatide during pregnancy (1-800-633-9081).

Lactation Excretion in breast milk unknown/use caution

Contraindications Hypersensitivity to exenatide or any component of the formulation; type 1 diabetes; diabetic ketoacidosis

Warnings/Precautions Mechanism requires the presence of insulin, therefore use in type 1 diabetes (insulin dependent, IDDM) or diabetic ketoacidosis is not recommended; it is not a substitute for insulin in insulin-requiring patients. Concurrent use with other hypoglycemic agents and/or insulin therapy has not been evaluated. May increase the risk of hypoglycemia in patients receiving sulfonylurea therapy (risk of hypoglycemia was not increased when added to metformin monotherapy). Risk of hypoglycemia is related to the dosage of both exenatide and the sulfonylurea.

Exenatide is frequently associated with gastrointestinal adverse effects and is not recommended for use in patients with gastroparesis or severe gastrointestinal disease. Gastrointestinal effects may be dose-related and may decrease in frequency/severity with gradual titration and continued use. Cases of acute pancreatitis (including hemorrhagic and necrotizing with some fatalities) have been reported; monitor for unexplained severe abdominal pain and if pancreatitis suspected, discontinue use. Do not resume unless an alternative etiology of pancreatitis is confirmed. Consider alternative antidiabetic therapy in patients with a history of pancreatitis. Use may be associated with the development of anti-exenatide antibodies; low titers are not associated with a loss of efficacy, however high titers (observed in 6% of patients in clinical studies) may result in an attenuation of response. May be associated with weight loss (due to reduced intake) independent of the change in hemoglobin A_{1c}. Not recommended in severe renal impairment (Cl_{cr} <30 mL/minute). Safety and efficacy have not been established in children.

Adverse Reactions

>10%:

Endocrine & metabolic: Hypoglycemia (with concurrent sulfonylurea therapy 14% to 36%; frequency similar to placebo with metformin therapy)

Gastrointestinal: Nausea (44%), vomiting (13%), diarrhea (13%)

Miscellaneous: Anti-exenatide antibodies (low titers 38%, high titers 6%)

1% to 10%:

Central nervous system: Dizziness (9%), headache (9%)

Endocrine & metabolic: Appetite decreased (<5%)

Gastrointestinal: Dyspepsia (6%), GERD (<5%)

Neuromuscular & skeletal: Weakness (<5%)

Miscellaneous: Feeling jittery (9%), diaphoresis increased (<5%)

Postmarketing and/or case reports: Abdominal distension, abdominal pain, acute pancreatitis (including hemorrhagic and necrotizing), anaphylactic reaction, angioedema, chest pain, constipation, dysgeusia, eructation, flatulence, hypersensitivity pneumonitis, injection site reaction, macular or papular rash, pruritus, renal failure, serum creatinine increased, somnolence, urticaria

Drug Interactions

Avoid Concomitant Use There are no known interactions where it is recommended to avoid concomitant use.

Increased Effect/Toxicity There are no known significant interactions involving an increase in effect.

Decreased Effect There are no known significant interactions involving a decrease in effect.

Ethanol/Nutrition/Herb Interactions Ethanol: Caution with ethanol (may cause hypoglycemia)

Stability Prior to initial use, store under refrigeration at 2°C to 8°C (36°F to 46°F); after initial use, may be stored at a temperature ≤25° (≤77°F). Do not freeze (discard if freezing occurs). Protect from light. Pen should be discarded 30 days after initial use.

Mechanism of Action Exenatide is an analog of the hormone incretin (glucagon-like peptide 1 or GLP-1) which increases insulin secretion, increases B-cell growth/replication, slows gastric emptying, and may decrease food intake. When added to sulfonylureas, thiazolidinediones, and/or metformin, it results in additional lowering of hemoglobin A_{1c} by approximately 0.5% to 1%.

Pharmacodynamics/Kinetics

Distribution: V_d: 28.3 L

Metabolism: Minimal systemic metabolism; proteolytic degradation may occur following glomerular filtration

Half-life elimination: 2.4 hours

Time to peak, plasma: SubQ: 2.1 hours

Excretion: Urine (majority of dose)

Dosage SubQ: Adults: Initial: 5 mcg twice daily within 60 minutes prior to a meal; after 1 month, may be increased to 10 mcg twice daily (based on response)

Dosage adjustment in renal impairment:

Cl_{cr} ≥30 mL/minute: No adjustment necessary

Cl_{cr} <30 mL/minute: Not recommended

Administration Should be administered subcutaneously in the upper arm, thigh, or abdomen. Administer within 60 minutes prior to morning and evening meal (or prior to the 2 main meals of the day, approximately ≥6 hours apart). Set up each new pen before the first use by priming it. See pen user manual for further details. Dial the dose into the dose window before each administration.

Monitoring Parameters Serum glucose, hemoglobin A_{1c}, and renal function

Additional Information A dosing strategy which employs progressive dose escalation of exenatide (initiating at 0.02 mcg/kg 3 times daily and increasing in increments of 0.02 mcg/kg every 3 days) has been described, limiting the frequency and severity of gastrointestinal adverse effects. The complexity of this regimen may limit its clinical application.

In animal models, exenatide has been a useful adjunctive therapy when added to immunotherapy protocols, resulting in recovery of beta cell function and sustained remission.

Dosage Forms Excipient information presented when available (limited, particularly for generics); consult specific product labeling.

Injection, solution:

Byetta®: 250 mcg/mL (1.2 mL [5 mcg/0.02 mL; 60-dose pen]); (2.4 mL [10 mcg/0.04 mL; 60-dose pen])

◆ **Exendin-4** *see* Exenatide *on page* 595

- **ExeTuss [DSC]** *see* Guaifenesin and Phenylephrine *on page 712*
- **ExeTuss-GP** *see* Guaifenesin and Phenylephrine *on page 712*
- **Exforge®** *see* Amlodipine and Valsartan *on page 96*
- **Exjade®** *see* Deferasirox *on page 410*
- **ex-lax® Ultra [OTC]** *see* Bisacodyl *on page 198*
- **Extendryl®** *see* Chlorpheniramine, Phenylephrine, and Methscopolamine *on page 313*
- **Extendryl® GCP** *see* Carbetapentane, Guaifenesin, and Phenylephrine *on page 255*
- **Extendryl® HC [DSC]** *see* Hydrocodone and Guaifenesin *on page 741*
- **Extendryl® JR** *see* Chlorpheniramine, Phenylephrine, and Methscopolamine *on page 313*
- **Extendryl PSE** *see* Pseudoephedrine and Methscopolamine *on page 1267*
- **Extendryl® SR** *see* Chlorpheniramine, Phenylephrine, and Methscopolamine *on page 313*
- **Extina®** *see* Ketoconazole *on page 837*
- **Extraneal®** *see* Icodextrin *on page 764*
- **EYE001** *see* Pegaptanib *on page 1150*
- **EyeFlur** *see* Fluorescein and Benoxinate *on page 634*
- **Eyestil (Can)** *see* Hyaluronate and Derivatives *on page 734*
- **EZ-Char™ [OTC]** *see* Charcoal *on page 299*

Ezetimibe (ez ET i mibe)

U.S. Brand Names Zetia®

Canadian Brand Names Ezetrol®

Pharmacologic Category Antilipemic Agent, 2-Azetidinone

Additional Appendix Information

Hyperlipidemia Management *on page 1815*

Lipid-Lowering Agents *on page 1661*

Use Use in combination with dietary therapy for the treatment of primary hypercholesterolemia (as monotherapy or in combination with HMG-CoA reductase inhibitors); homozygous sitosterolemia; homozygous familial hypercholesterolemia (in combination with atorvastatin or simvastatin); mixed hyperlipidemia (in combination with fenofibrate)

Pregnancy Risk Factor C

Pregnancy Considerations Safety and efficacy have not been established; use during pregnancy only if the potential benefit to the mother outweighs the possible risk to the fetus.

Lactation Excretion in breast milk unknown/not recommended

Medication Safety Issues

Sound-alike/look-alike issues:

Zetia® may be confused with Zebeta®, Zestril®

Contraindications Hypersensitivity to ezetimibe or any component of the formulation; concomitant use with an HMG-CoA reductase inhibitor in patients with active hepatic disease, unexplained persistent elevations in serum transaminases; pregnancy; breast-feeding

Warnings/Precautions Secondary causes of hyperlipidemia should be ruled out prior to therapy. Use caution with severe renal (Cl_{cr} <30 mL/minute) or mild hepatic impairment (Child-Pugh class A); not recommended for use with moderate or severe hepatic impairment (Child-Pugh classes B and C). Concurrent use of ezetimibe and fibric acid derivatives may increase the risk of cholelithiasis. Safety and efficacy have not been established in patients <10 years of age.

Adverse Reactions

1% to 10%:

Central nervous system: Fatigue (2%)

Gastrointestinal: Diarrhea (4%)

Hepatic: Transaminases increased (with HMG-CoA reductase inhibitors) (≥3 x ULN, 1%)

Neuromuscular & skeletal: Arthralgia (3%), pain in extremity (3%)

Respiratory: Upper respiratory tract infection (4%), sinusitis (3%)

Miscellaneous: Influenza (2%)

Postmarketing and/or case reports: Anaphylaxis, angioedema, autoimmune hepatitis (Stolk, 2006), cholecystitis, cholelithiasis, cholestatic hepatitis (Stolk, 2006), CPK increased, depression, dizziness, hepatitis, hypersensitivity reactions, myalgia, myopathy, nausea, pancreatitis, paresthesia, rash, rhabdomyolysis, thrombocytopenia, urticaria

Drug Interactions

Avoid Concomitant Use There are no known interactions where it is recommended to avoid concomitant use.

Increased Effect/Toxicity

Ezetimibe may increase the levels/effects of: CycloSPORINE

The levels/effects of Ezetimibe may be increased by: CycloSPORINE; Eltrombopag; Fibric Acid Derivatives

Decreased Effect

The levels/effects of Ezetimibe may be decreased by: Bile Acid Sequestrants

Ethanol/Nutrition/Herb Interactions Food: Ezetimibe did not cause meaningful reductions in fat-soluble vitamin concentrations during a 2-week clinical trial. Effects of long-term therapy have not been evaluated.

Stability Store at controlled room temperature of 25°C (77°F). Protect from moisture.

Mechanism of Action Inhibits absorption of cholesterol at the brush border of the small intestine via the sterol transporter, Niemann-Pick C1-Like1 (NPC1L1). This leads to a decreased delivery of cholesterol to the liver, reduction of hepatic cholesterol stores and an increased clearance of cholesterol from the blood; decreases total C, LDL-cholesterol (LDL-C), ApoB, and triglycerides (TG) while increasing HDL-cholesterol (HDL-C).

Pharmacodynamics/Kinetics

Protein binding: >90% to plasma proteins

Metabolism: Undergoes glucuronide conjugation in the small intestine and liver; forms metabolite (active); may undergo enterohepatic recycling

Bioavailability: Variable

Half-life elimination: 22 hours (ezetimibe and metabolite)

Time to peak, plasma: 4-12 hours

Excretion: Feces (78%, 69% as ezetimibe); urine (11%, 9% as metabolite)

Dosage Oral:

Children ≥10 years and Adults: 10 mg/day

Elderly: Refer to adult dosing

Dosage adjustment in renal impairment: AUC increased with severe impairment (Cl_{cr} <30 mL/minute); no dosing adjustment recommended

Dosage adjustment in hepatic impairment: AUC increased with hepatic impairment

Mild impairment (Child-Pugh class A): No dosing adjustment necessary

Moderate-to-severe impairment (Child-Pugh classes B and C): Use of ezetimibe not recommended

Dietary Considerations May be taken without regard to meals. Before initiation of therapy, patients should be placed on a standard cholesterol-lowering diet for 6 weeks and the diet should be continued during drug therapy.

Administration May be administered without regard to meals. May be taken at the same time as HMG-CoA reductase inhibitors. Administer ≥2 hours before or ≥4 hours after bile acid sequestrants.

Monitoring Parameters Total cholesterol profile prior to therapy, and when clinically indicated and/or periodically thereafter. When used in combination with fenofibrate, monitor LFTs and signs and symptoms of cholelithiasis.

Additional Information When studied in combination with fenofibrate for mixed hyperlipidemia, the dose of fenofibrate was 160 mg daily.

Dosage Forms Excipient information presented when available (limited, particularly for generics); consult specific product labeling.

Tablet:

Zetia®: 10 mg

Ezetimibe and Simvastatin

(ez ET i mibe & SIM va stat in)

U.S. Brand Names Vytorin®

Index Terms Simvastatin and Ezetimibe

Pharmacologic Category Antilipemic Agent, 2-Azetidinone; Antilipemic Agent, HMG-CoA Reductase Inhibitor

Additional Appendix Information

Hyperlipidemia Management *on page 1815*

Lipid-Lowering Agents *on page 1661*

Use Used in combination with dietary modification for the treatment of primary hypercholesterolemia and homozygous familial hypercholesterolemia

Pregnancy Risk Factor X

Medication Safety Issues

Sound-alike/look-alike issues:

Vytorin® may be confused with Vyvanse™

Dosage Oral: Adults:

Homozygous familial hypercholesterolemia: Ezetimibe 10 mg and simvastatin 40 mg once daily or ezetimibe 10 mg and simvastatin 80 mg once daily in the evening. Dosing range: Ezetimibe 10 mg and simvastatin 10-80 mg once daily.

Hyperlipidemias: Initial: Ezetimibe 10 mg and simvastatin 20 mg once daily in the evening

Patients who require less aggressive reduction in LDL-C: Initial: Ezetimibe 10 mg and simvastatin 10 mg once daily

Patients who require >55% reduction in LDL-C: Initial: Ezetimibe 10 mg and simvastatin 40 mg once daily

Dosage adjustment with concomitant medications:

Amiodarone or verapamil: Dose should not exceed ezetimibe 10 mg and simvastatin 20 mg once daily.

Danazol or cyclosporine: Patient must first demonstrate tolerance to simvastatin ≥5 mg once daily. Dose should not exceed ezetimibe 10 mg and simvastatin 10 mg once daily.

Gemfibrozil: Although concurrent use is not recommended by manufacturer, dose should not exceed ezetimibe 10 mg and simvastatin 10 mg once daily.

Dosage adjustment in renal impairment: Dosage adjustment unnecessary in mild to moderate renal dysfunction. In severe dysfunction, start only if patient tolerates 5 mg daily of simvastatin; monitor closely.

Dosage adjustment in hepatic impairment: Dosage adjustment unnecessary in mild hepatic dysfunction.

Additional Information Complete prescribing information for this medication should be consulted for additional detail.

Dosage Forms Excipient information presented when available (limited, particularly for generics); consult specific product labeling.

Tablet:

10/10: Ezetimibe 10 mg and simvastatin 10 mg
10/20: Ezetimibe 10 mg and simvastatin 20 mg
10/40: Ezetimibe 10 mg and simvastatin 40 mg
10/80: Ezetimibe 10 mg and simvastatin 80 mg

◆ **Ezetrol® (Can)** *see* Ezetimibe *on page 597*

◆ **E•R•O [OTC]** *see* Carbamide Peroxide *on page 254*

◆ **F_3T** *see* Trifluridine *on page 1517*

◆ **Fabrazyme®** *see* Agalsidase Beta *on page 47*

◆ **Factive®** *see* Gemifloxacin *on page 688*

Factor VIIa (Recombinant)

(FAK ter SEV en aye ree KOM be nant)

U.S. Brand Names NovoSeven [DSC]; NovoSeven® RT

Canadian Brand Names Niastase®

Index Terms Coagulation Factor VIIa; Eptacog Alfa (Activated); rFVIIa

Pharmacologic Category Antihemophilic Agent; Blood Product

Use Treatment of bleeding episodes and prevention of bleeding in surgical interventions in patients with hemophilia A or B with inhibitors to factor VIII or factor IX, acquired hemophilia, and in patients with congenital factor VII deficiency

Unlabeled/Investigational Use Reduction of hematoma growth in patients with acute intracerebral hemorrhage, warfarin-related intracerebral hemorrhage

Pregnancy Risk Factor C

Pregnancy Considerations Animal studies have demonstrated fetal loss, but no evidence of teratogenic effects. There are no adequate and well-controlled studies in pregnant women. Use only if the potential benefit justifies the potential risk to the fetus.

Lactation Excretion in breast milk unknown/not recommended

Medication Safety Issues

Sound-alike/look-alike issues:

NovoSeven® may be confused with Novacet®

Contraindications There are no contraindications listed within the FDA-approved labeling.

Warnings/Precautions Use with caution in patients with known hypersensitivity to mouse, hamster, or bovine proteins, or factor VIIa, or any components of the product. Patients should be monitored for signs and symptoms of activation of the coagulation system or thrombosis. Thrombotic events may be increased in patients with disseminated intravascular coagulation (DIC), advanced atherosclerotic disease, sepsis, crush injury, or concomitant treatment with prothrombin complex concentrates. Decreased dosage or discontinuation is warranted in confirmed DIC. Efficacy with prolonged infusions and data evaluating this agent's long-term adverse effects are limited.

Adverse Reactions

1% to 10%:

Cardiovascular: Hypertension

Central nervous system: Fever

Hematologic: Hemorrhage, plasma fibrinogen decreased

Neuromuscular & skeletal: Hemarthrosis

<1% (Limited to important or life-threatening): Abnormal renal function, allergic reaction, anaphylactic reaction, arterial thrombosis, arthrosis, bradycardia, cerebral infarction and/or ischemia, coagulation disorder, consumptive coagulopathy, deep vein thrombosis, disseminated intravascular coagulation (DIC), edema, fibrinolysis increased, gastrointestinal bleeding, headache, hypersensitivity, hypotension, injection site reactions, intracranial hemorrhage, localized phlebitis, MI, myocardial ischemia, pain, pneumonia, prothrombin decreased, pruritus, pulmonary embolism, purpura, rash, splenic hematoma, therapeutic response decreased, thrombophlebitis, thrombosis, vomiting

Drug Interactions

Avoid Concomitant Use There are no known interactions where it is recommended to avoid concomitant use.

Increased Effect/Toxicity There are no known significant interactions involving an increase in effect.

Decreased Effect There are no known significant interactions involving a decrease in effect.

Stability Prior to reconstitution, bring vials to room temperature.

NovoSeven®: Store under refrigeration at 2°C to 8°C (36°F to 46°F). Protect from light. Add recommended diluent along wall of vial; do not inject directly onto powder. Gently swirl until dissolved. Reconstitute each vial to a final concentration of 0.6 mg/mL as follows:

1.2 mg vial: 2.2 mL sterile water

2.4 mg vial: 4.3 mL sterile water

4.8 mg vial: 8.5 mL sterile water

Reconstituted solutions may be stored at room temperature or under refrigeration, but must be infused within 3 hours of reconstitution. Do not freeze reconstituted solutions. Do not store reconstituted solutions in syringes.

NovoSeven® RT: Prior to reconstitution, store under refrigeration or between 2°C to 25°C (36°F to 77°F). Protect from light. Add recommended diluent along wall of vial; do not inject directly onto powder. Gently swirl until dissolved. Reconstitute each vial to a final concentration of 1 mg/mL using the provided histidine diluent as follows:

1 mg vial: 1.1 mL histidine diluent

2 mg vial: 2.1 mL histidine diluent

5 mg vial: 5.2 mL histidine diluent

Reconstituted solutions may be stored at room temperature or under refrigeration, but must be infused within 3 hours of reconstitution. Do not freeze reconstituted solutions. Do not store reconstituted solutions in syringes.

Mechanism of Action Recombinant factor VIIa, a vitamin K-dependent glycoprotein, promotes hemostasis by activating the extrinsic pathway of the coagulation cascade. It replaces deficient activated coagulation factor VII, which complexes with tissue factor and may activate coagulation factor X to Xa and factor IX to IXa. When complexed with other factors, coagulation factor Xa converts prothrombin to thrombin, a key step in the formation of a fibrin-platelet hemostatic plug.

Pharmacodynamics/Kinetics

Distribution: V_d: 103 mL/kg (78-139)

Half-life elimination: 2.3 hours (1.7-2.7)

Excretion: Clearance: 33 mL/kg/hour (27-49)

Dosage Children and Adults: I.V. administration only: Hemophilia A or B with inhibitors:

Bleeding episodes: 90 mcg/kg every 2 hours until hemostasis is achieved or until the treatment is judged ineffective. The dose and interval may be adjusted based upon the severity of bleeding and the degree of hemostasis achieved. For patients experiencing severe bleeds, dosing should be continued at 3- to 6-hour intervals after hemostasis has been achieved and the duration of dosing should be minimized.

Surgical interventions: 90 mcg/kg immediately before surgery; repeat at 2-hour intervals for the duration of surgery. Continue every 2 hours for 48 hours, then every 2-6 hours until healed for minor surgery; continue every 2 hours for 5 days, then every 4 hours until healed for major surgery.

Congenital factor VII deficiency: Bleeding episodes and surgical interventions: 15-30 mcg/kg every 4-6 hours until hemostasis. Doses as low as 10 mcg/kg have been effective.

Acquired hemophilia: 70-90 mcg/kg every 2-3 hours until hemostasis is achieved

Dietary Considerations Contains sodium 0.44 mEq/mg rFVIIa

Administration I.V. administration only; bolus over 2-5 minutes. Administer within 3 hours after reconstitution.

Monitoring Parameters Monitor for evidence of hemostasis; although the prothrombin time, aPTT, and factor VII clotting activity have no correlation with achieving hemostasis, these parameters may be useful as adjunct tests to evaluate efficacy and guide dose or interval adjustments

Dosage Forms Excipient information presented when available (limited, particularly for generics); consult specific product labeling. [DSC] = Discontinued product

Injection, powder for reconstitution [preservative free]:

NovoSeven®: 1.2 mg, 2.4 mg, 4.8 mg [contains sodium 0.44 mEq/mg rFVIIa, polysorbate 80] [DSC]

NovoSeven® RT:

1 mg [contains polysorbate 80, sodium 0.4 mEq/mg rFVIIa, sucrose 10 mg/vial]

2 mg [contains polysorbate 80, sodium 0.4 mEq/mg rFVIIa, sucrose 20 mg/vial]

5 mg [contains polysorbate 80, sodium 0.4 mEq/mg rFVIIa, sucrose 50 mg/vial]

◆ **Factor VIII (Human)** *see* Antihemophilic Factor (Human) *on page 120*

◆ **Factor VIII (Human)** *see* Antihemophilic Factor/von Willebrand Factor Complex (Human) *on page 122*

◆ **Factor VIII (Recombinant)** *see* Antihemophilic Factor (Recombinant) *on page 121*

Factor IX (FAK ter nyne)

U.S. Brand Names AlphaNine® SD; BeneFix®; Mononine®

Canadian Brand Names BeneFix®; Immunine® VH; Mononine®

Index Terms Factor IX Concentrate

Pharmacologic Category Antihemophilic Agent; Blood Product Derivative

Use Control bleeding in patients with factor IX deficiency (hemophilia B or Christmas disease)

Pregnancy Risk Factor C

Pregnancy Considerations Animal reproduction studies have not been conducted. Safety and efficacy in pregnant women have not been established. Use during pregnancy only if clearly needed. Parvovirus B19 or hepatitis A, which may be present in plasma-derived products, may affect a pregnant woman more seriously than a nonpregnant woman.

Contraindications Hypersensitivity to mouse protein (Mononine®) or hamster protein (BeneFix®)

Warnings/Precautions Hypersensitivity and anaphylactic reactions have been reported with use. Delayed reactions (up to 20 days after infusion) in previously untreated patients may also occur. Due to potential for allergic reactions, the initial ~10-20 administrations should be performed under appropriate medical supervision. The development of factor IX antibodies (or inhibitors) has been reported with factor IX therapy; the risk of severe hypersensitivity reactions occurring may be greater in these patients. Patients experiencing allergic reactions should be evaluated for factor IX inhibitors.

Observe closely for signs or symptoms of intravascular coagulation or thrombosis; risk is generally associated with the use of factor IX complex concentrates (containing therapeutic amounts of additional factors); however, potential risk exists with use of factor IX products (containing only factor IX). Use with caution when administering to patients with liver disease, postoperatively, neonates, or patients at risk of thromboembolic phenomena, disseminated intravascular coagulation or patients with signs of fibrinolysis due to the potential risk of thromboembolic complications.

Factor IX is **NOT INDICATED** for the treatment or reversal of coumarin-induced anticoagulation, hemophilia A patients with factor VIII inhibitors, or patients in a hemorrhagic state caused by reduced production of liver-dependent coagulation factors (eg, hepatitis, cirrhosis). AlphaNine® SD and Mononine® contain **nondetectable levels of factors II, VII, and X** and are, therefore, **NOT INDICATED** for replacement therapy of any of these clotting factors. AlphaNine® SD and Mononine® are products of human plasma and may potentially contain infectious agents which could transmit disease. Screening of donors, as well as testing and/or inactivation or removal of certain viruses, reduces the risk. Infections thought to be transmitted by this product should be reported to the manufacturer. Safety and efficacy have not been established with factor IX products in immune tolerance induction. Nephrotic syndrome has occurred following immune tolerance induction in patients with factor IX inhibitors and a history of allergic reactions to therapy.

Adverse Reactions Frequency not defined.

Cardiovascular: Cyanosis, flushing, hypotension, chest tightness, thrombosis

Central nervous system: Chills, dizziness, drowsiness, fever (including transient fever following rapid administration), headache, lethargy, lightheadedness, somnolence

Dermatologic: Angioedema, photosensitivity reaction, rash, urticaria

Gastrointestinal: Abnormal taste, diarrhea, nausea, vomiting

Hematologic: Disseminated intravascular coagulation (DIC)

Hepatic: Alkaline phosphatase increased, ALT increased, AST increased

Local: Injection site reactions: Cellulitis, discomfort, pain, phlebitis, stinging

Neuromuscular & skeletal: Neck tightness, paresthesia, rigors

Ocular: Visual disturbance

Respiratory: Allergic rhinitis, asthma, cough, dyspnea, hypoxia, laryngeal edema, lung disorder

Miscellaneous: Allergic reaction, anaphylaxis, burning sensation in jaw/skull, factor IX inhibitor development, hypersensitivity reaction

Postmarketing and/or case reports: HAV seroconversion, inadequate response/recovery, nephrotic syndrome (associated with immune tolerance induction), parvovirus B19 seroconversion, renal infarction

Drug Interactions

Avoid Concomitant Use

Avoid concomitant use of Factor IX with any of the following: Aminocaproic Acid

Increased Effect/Toxicity

The levels/effects of Factor IX may be increased by: Aminocaproic Acid

Decreased Effect There are no known significant interactions involving a decrease in effect.

Stability When stored at refrigerator temperature, 2°C to 8°C (36°F to 46°F), coagulation factor IX is stable for the period indicated by the expiration date on its label. Avoid freezing which may damage container for the diluent.

AlphaNine® SD: May also be stored at room temperature not to exceed 30°C (86°F) for up to 1 month,

BeneFix®: May also be stored at room temperature not to exceed 25°C (77°F) for up to 6 months. Reconstituted solution at room temperature should be used within 3 hours.

Mononine®: May also be stored at room temperature not to exceed 25°C (77°F) for up to 1 month.

Reconstitution: Refer to instructions for individual products. Diluent and factor IX complex should come to room temperature before combining.

Mechanism of Action Replaces deficient clotting factor IX. Hemophilia B, or Christmas disease, is an X-linked inherited disorder of blood coagulation characterized by insufficient or abnormal synthesis of the clotting protein factor IX. Factor IX is a vitamin K-dependent coagulation factor which is synthesized in the liver. Factor IX is activated by factor XIa in the intrinsic coagulation pathway. Activated factor IX (IXa), in combination with factor VII:C activates factor X to Xa, resulting ultimately in the conversion of prothrombin to thrombin and the formation of a fibrin clot. The infusion of exogenous factor IX to replace the deficiency present in hemophilia B temporarily restores hemostasis.

Pharmacodynamics/Kinetics Half-life elimination: IX component: Adults: 21-31 hours; children: 14-28 hours

Dosage Dosage is expressed in int. units of factor IX activity; dosing must be individualized based on severity of factor IX deficiency, extent and location of bleeding, and clinical status of patient. I.V.:

Formula for int. units required to raise blood level %:

AlphaNine® SD, Mononine®: Children and Adults:

Number of factor IX int. units required = body weight (in kg) x desired factor IX level increase (int. units/dL or % of normal) x 1 int. unit/kg

For example, for a 100% level a 70 kg patient who has an actual level of 20%: Number of factor IX int. units needed = 70 kg x 80% x 1 int. unit/kg = 5600 int. units

BeneFix®:

Children <15 years:

Number of factor IX int. units required = body weight (in kg) x desired factor IX level increase (int. units/dL or % of normal) x 1.4 int. units/kg

Children ≥15 years and Adults:

Number of factor IX int. units required = body weight (in kg) x desired factor IX level increase (int. units/dL or % of normal) x 1.3 int. units/kg

Guidelines: As a general rule, the level of factor IX required for treatment of different conditions is listed below:

Minor spontaneous hemorrhage, prophylaxis:

Desired levels of factor IX for hemostasis: 15% to 25%

Initial loading dose to achieve desired level: 20-30 int. units/kg

Frequency of dosing: Every 12-24 hours if necessary

Duration of treatment: 1-2 days

Moderate hemorrhage:

Desired levels of factor IX for hemostasis: 25% to 50%

Initial loading dose to achieve desired level: 25-50 int. units/kg

Frequency of dosing: Every 12-24 hours

Duration of treatment: 2-7 days

Major hemorrhage:

Desired levels of factor IX for hemostasis: >50%

Initial loading dose to achieve desired level: 30-50 int. units/kg

Frequency of dosing: Every 12-24 hours, depending on half-life and measured factor IX levels (after 3-5 days, maintain at least 20% activity)

Duration of treatment: 7-10 days, depending upon nature of insult

Surgery or major trauma:

Desired levels of factor IX for hemostasis: 50% to 100%

Initial loading dose to achieve desired level: 50-100 int. units/kg

Frequency of dosing: Every 12-24 hours or every 18-30 hours, depending on half-life and measured factor IX levels

Duration of treatment: 7-10 days, depending upon nature of insult

Administration Solution should be infused at room temperature

I.V. administration only: Should be infused **slowly**: The rate of administration should be determined by the response and comfort of the patient.

AlphaNine® SD: Administer I.V. at a rate not exceeding 10 mL/minute

BeneFix®: Administer I.V. over several minutes

Mononine®: Administer I.V. at a rate of ~2 mL/minute. Administration rates of up to 225 int. units/minute have been regularly tolerated without incident (when reconstituted as directed to ~100 int. units/mL).

Monitoring Parameters Levels of factors IX, PTT, BP, HR, signs of hypersensitivity reactions

Reference Range Average normal factor IX levels are 50% to 150%; patients with severe hemophilia will have levels <1%, often undetectable. Moderate forms of the disease have levels of 1% to 10% while some mild cases may have 11% to 49% of normal factor IX.

Maintain factor IX plasma level at least 20% until hemostasis achieved after acute joint or muscle bleeding.

In preparation for and following surgery:

Level to prevent spontaneous hemorrhage: 5%

Minimum level for hemostasis following trauma and surgery: 30% to 50%

Severe hemorrhage: >50%

Major surgery: ≥50% prior to procedure and for 48 hours after surgery, and 30% to 50% for 10 days thereafter

Dosage Forms Excipient information presented when available (limited, particularly for generics); consult specific product labeling.

Injection, powder for reconstitution (**Note:** Exact potency labeled on each vial):

BeneFix® [contains polysorbate 80; sucrose 0.8%; recombinant formulation; supplied with diluent]

Injection, powder for reconstitution [human derived] (**Note:** Exact potency labeled on each vial):

AlphaNine® SD [contains polysorbate 80; solvent detergent treated; virus filtered; contains nondetectable levels of factors II, VII, X; supplied with diluent]

Mononine® [contains polysorbate 80; monoclonal antibody purified; contains nondetectable levels of factors II, VII, X; supplied with diluent]

Factor IX Complex (Human)

(FAK ter nyne KOM pleks HYU man)

U.S. Brand Names Bebulin® VH; Profilnine® SD; Proplex® T [DSC]

Index Terms Prothrombin Complex Concentrate

Pharmacologic Category Antihemophilic Agent; Blood Product Derivative; Prothrombin Complex Concentrate (PCC)

Use Control bleeding in patients with factor IX deficiency (hemophilia B or Christmas disease) **Note:** Factor IX concentrate containing **only** factor IX is also available and preferable for this indication.

Unlabeled/Investigational Use Emergency correction of the coagulopathy of warfarin excess in critical situations. **Note:** Products contain low or nontherapeutic levels of factor VII component.

Pregnancy Risk Factor C

Contraindications Liver disease with signs of intravascular coagulation or fibrinolysis; not for use in factor VII deficiencies, patients undergoing elective surgery

Warnings/Precautions Use with caution in patients with liver dysfunction. Prepared from pooled human plasma - the risk of viral transmission is not totally eradicated. Thromboembolic complications rarely occur; more likely to occur during postoperative period or in patients with risk factors. Treatment should stop if respiratory distress or any changes in blood pressure or pulse rate occur.

Adverse Reactions

1% to 10%:

Central nervous system: Fever, headache, chills

Neuromuscular & skeletal: Tingling

Miscellaneous: Following rapid administration: Transient fever

<1% (Limited to important or life-threatening): Disseminated intravascular coagulation (DIC), flushing, nausea, somnolence, thrombosis (following high dosages because of presence of activated clotting factors), tightness in chest, tightness in neck, urticaria, vomiting

Drug Interactions

Avoid Concomitant Use

Avoid concomitant use of Factor IX Complex (Human) with any of the following: Aminocaproic Acid

Increased Effect/Toxicity

The levels/effects of Factor IX Complex (Human) may be increased by: Aminocaproic Acid

Decreased Effect There are no known significant interactions involving a decrease in effect.

Stability When stored at refrigerator temperature, 2°C to 8°C (36°F to 46°F), coagulation factor IX is stable for the period indicated by the expiration date on its label. Avoid freezing which may damage container for the diluent. Once diluted, should be used promptly; stable for up to 3 hours.

For reconstitution, refer to instructions for individual products. Diluent and factor IX complex should come to room temperature before combining. Diluent vial should be inverted over concentrate vial. After diluent is pulled, disconnect. The provided filter needle should be used to withdraw concentrate. Remove needle and attach to infusion set or replace needle for infusion.

Mechanism of Action Replaces deficient clotting factor including factor X; hemophilia B, or Christmas disease, is an X-linked recessively inherited disorder of blood coagulation characterized by insufficient or abnormal synthesis of the clotting protein factor IX. Factor IX is a vitamin K-dependent coagulation factor which is synthesized in the liver. Factor IX is activated by factor XIa in the intrinsic coagulation pathway. Activated factor IX (IXa), in combination with factor VII:C, activates factor X to Xa, resulting ultimately in the conversion of prothrombin to thrombin and the formation of a fibrin clot. The infusion of exogenous factor IX to replace the deficiency present in hemophilia B temporarily restores hemostasis.

Pharmacodynamics/Kinetics

Half-life elimination:

VII component: Initial: 4-6 hours; Terminal: 22.5 hours

IX component: 24 hours

Dosage Children and Adults: Dosage is expressed in units of factor IX activity and must be individualized. I.V. only:

Formula for units required to raise blood level %:

Total blood volume (mL blood/kg) = 70 mL/kg (adults), 80 mL/kg (children)

Plasma volume = total blood volume (mL) x [1 - Hct (in decimals)]

For example, for a 70 kg adult with a Hct = 40%: Plasma volume = [70 kg x 70 mL/kg] x [1 - 0.4] = 2940 mL

To calculate number of units needed to increase level to desired range (highly individualized and dependent on patient's condition): Number of units = desired level increase [desired level - actual level] x plasma volume (in mL)

For example, for a 100% level in the above patient who has an actual level of 20%: Number of units needed = [1 (for a 100% level) - 0.2] x 2940 mL = 2352 units

As a general rule, the level of factor IX required for treatment of different conditions is listed below:

Minor Spontaneous Hemorrhage, Prophylaxis:

Desired levels of factor IX for hemostasis: 15% to 25%

Initial loading dose to achieve desired level: <20-30 units/kg

Frequency of dosing: Once; repeated in 24 hours if necessary
Duration of treatment: Once; repeated if necessary

Major Trauma or Surgery:
Desired levels of factor IX for hemostasis: 25% to 50%
Initial loading dose to achieve desired level: <75 units/kg
Frequency of dosing: Every 18-30 hours, depending on half-life and measured factor IX levels
Duration of treatment: Up to 10 days, depending upon nature of insult

Anticoagulant overdosage (unlabeled use): I.V.: 15 units/kg

Administration I.V. administration only; should be infused **slowly**. Rate should not exceed 2 mL/minute for Bebulin® VH, 3 mL/minute for Proplex® T, or 10 mL/minute for Profilnine® SD.

Monitoring Parameters Levels of factors being replaced (eg, VII or IX), PT, PTT

Reference Range Average normal factor VII and factor IX levels are 50% to 150%; patients with severe hemophilia will have levels <1%, often undetectable. Moderate forms of the disease have levels of 1% to 10% while some mild cases may have 11% to 49% of normal factor IX.

Maintain factor IX plasma level at least 20% until hemostasis achieved after acute joint or muscle bleeding.
In preparation for and following surgery:
Level to prevent spontaneous hemorrhage: 5%
Minimum level for hemostasis following trauma and surgery: 30% to 50%
Severe hemorrhage: >60%
Major surgery: >60% prior to procedure, 30% to 50% for several days after surgery, and >20% for 7-10 days thereafter

Dosage Forms Excipient information presented when available (limited, particularly for generics); consult specific product labeling. [DSC] = Discontinued product

Injection, powder for reconstitution (**Note:** Exact potency labeled on each vial):
Bebulin® VH [single-dose vial; vapor heated; supplied with sterile water for injection]
Profilnine® SD [single-dose vial; solvent detergent treated]
Proplex® T [single-dose vial; heat treated; supplied with sterile water for injection] [DSC]

◆ **Factor IX Concentrate** *see* Factor IX *on page* 599

◆ **Factrel®** *see* Gonadorelin *on page* 704

Famciclovir (fam SYE kloe veer)

U.S. Brand Names Famvir®

Canadian Brand Names Apo-Famciclovir; Co-Famciclovir; Famvir®; PMS-Famciclovir; Sandoz-Famciclovir

Pharmacologic Category Antiviral Agent

Additional Appendix Information

Treatment of Sexually Transmitted Infections *on page 1773*

Use Treatment of acute herpes zoster (shingles); treatment and suppression of recurrent episodes of genital herpes in immunocompetent patients; treatment of herpes labialis (cold sores) in immunocompetent patients; treatment of recurrent mucocutaneous/genital herpes simplex in HIV-infected patients

Pregnancy Risk Factor B

Pregnancy Considerations Teratogenic effects were not observed in animal studies. There are no adequate and well-controlled studies in pregnant women. Use only if benefit outweighs risk. A registry has been established for women exposed to famciclovir during pregnancy (888-669-6682).

Lactation Excretion in breast milk unknown/use caution

Medication Safety Issues

Sound-alike/look-alike issues:
Famvir® may be confused with Femara®

Contraindications Hypersensitivity to famciclovir, penciclovir, or any component of the formulation

Warnings/Precautions Has not been studied in immunocompromised patients or patients with ophthalmic, disseminated zoster, or with initial episode of genital herpes. Dosage adjustment is required in patients with renal insufficiency. Tablets contain lactose; do not use with galactose intolerance, severe lactase deficiency, or glucose-galactose malabsorption syndromes. Safety and efficacy have not been established in children <18 years of age.

Adverse Reactions

Note: Frequencies vary with dose and duration. Single-dose treatment (herpes labialis) was associated only with headache (10%), diarrhea (2%), fatigue (1%), and dysmenorrhea (1%).

>10%:
Central nervous system: Headache (17% to 39%)
Gastrointestinal: Nausea (7% to 13%)

1% to 10%:
Central nervous system: Fatigue (4% to 6%), migraine (1% to 3%)
Dermatologic: Pruritus (1% to 4%), rash (<1% to 3%)
Endocrine & metabolic: Dysmenorrhea (up to 8%)
Gastrointestinal: Diarrhea (5% to 9%), flatulence (2% to 5%), vomiting (1% to 5%), abdominal pain (1% to 8%)
Hematologic: Neutropenia (3%), leukopenia (1%)
Hepatic: Transaminases increased (2% to 3%), bilirubin increased (2%)
Neuromuscular & skeletal: Paresthesia (1% to 3%)

Postmarketing and/or case reports: Confusion, delirium, disorientation, dizziness, erythema multiforme, hallucinations, jaundice, somnolence, thrombocytopenia, urticaria

Drug Interactions

Avoid Concomitant Use

Avoid concomitant use of Famciclovir with any of the following: Zoster Vaccine

Increased Effect/Toxicity There are no known significant interactions involving an increase in effect.

Decreased Effect

Famciclovir may decrease the levels/effects of: Zoster Vaccine

Ethanol/Nutrition/Herb Interactions Food: Rate of absorption and/or conversion to penciclovir and peak concentration are reduced with food, but bioavailability is not affected.

Stability Store at controlled room temperature.

Mechanism of Action Famciclovir undergoes rapid biotransformation to the active compound, penciclovir, which is phosphorylated by viral thymidine kinase in HSV-1, HSV-2, and VZV-infected cells to a monophosphate form; this is then converted to penciclovir triphosphate and competes with deoxyguanosine triphosphate to inhibit HSV-2 polymerase (eg, herpes viral DNA synthesis/replication is selectively inhibited)

Pharmacodynamics/Kinetics

Absorption: Food decreases maximum peak concentration and delays time to peak; AUC remains the same
Distribution: V_{dss}: 0.91-1.25 L/kg
Protein binding: ≤20%
Metabolism: Rapidly deacetylated and oxidized to penciclovir; not via CYP
Bioavailability: 69% to 85%
Half-life elimination: Penciclovir: 2-3 hours (10, 20, and 7 hours in HSV-1, HSV-2, and VZV-infected cells, respectively); prolonged with renal impairment
Time to peak: 0.9 hours; C_{max} and T_{max} are decreased and prolonged with noncompensated hepatic impairment

Excretion: Urine (73% primarily as penciclovir); feces (27%)

Dosage Adults: Oral:

Acute herpes zoster: 500 mg every 8 hours for 7 days (**Note:** Initiate therapy within 72 hours of rash onset.)

Recurrent genital herpes simplex in immunocompetent patients:

Initial: 1000 mg twice daily for 1 day (**Note:** Initiate therapy within 6 hours of symptoms/lesions.)

Suppressive therapy: 250 mg twice daily for up to 1 year

Recurrent herpes labialis (cold sores): 1500 mg as a single dose; initiate therapy at first sign or symptom such as tingling, burning, or itching (initiated within 1 hour in clinical studies)

Recurrent mucocutaneous/genital herpes simplex in HIV patients: 500 mg twice daily for 7 days

Dosing interval in renal impairment:

Herpes zoster:

Cl_{cr} 40-59 mL/minute: Administer 500 mg every 12 hours

Cl_{cr} 20-39 mL/minute: Administer 500 mg every 24 hours

Cl_{cr} <20 mL/minute: Administer 250 mg every 24 hours

Hemodialysis: Administer 250 mg after each dialysis session.

Recurrent genital herpes: Treatment (single day regimen):

Cl_{cr} 40-59 mL/minute: Administer 500 mg every 12 hours for 1 day

Cl_{cr} 20-39 mL/minute: Administer 500 mg as a single dose

Cl_{cr} <20 mL/minute: Administer 250 mg as a single dose

Hemodialysis: Administer 250 mg as a single dose after dialysis session.

Recurrent genital herpes: Suppression:

Cl_{cr} 20-39 mL/minute: Administer 125 mg every 12 hours

Cl_{cr} <20 mL/minute: Administer 125 mg every 24 hours

Hemodialysis: Administer 125 mg after each dialysis session.

Recurrent herpes labialis: Treatment (single dose regimen):

Cl_{cr} 40-59 mL/minute: Administer 750 mg as a single dose

Cl_{cr} 20-39 mL/minute: Administer 500 mg as a single dose

Cl_{cr} <20 mL/minute: Administer 250 mg as a single dose

Hemodialysis: Administer 250 mg as a single dose after dialysis session.

Recurrent orolabial or genital herpes in HIV-infected patients:

Cl_{cr} 20-39 mL/minute: Administer 500 mg every 12 hours

Cl_{cr} <20 mL/minute: Administer 250 mg every 24 hours

Hemodialysis: Administer 250 mg after each dialysis session.

Dietary Considerations May be taken with food or on an empty stomach.

Monitoring Parameters Periodic CBC during long-term therapy

Additional Information Most effective for herpes zoster if therapy is initiated within 48 hours of initial lesion. Resistance may occur by alteration of thymidine kinase, resulting in loss of or reduced penciclovir phosphorylation (cross-resistance occurs between acyclovir and famciclovir). When treatment for herpes labialis is initiated within 1 hour of symptom onset, healing time is reduced by ~2 days.

Dosage Forms Excipient information presented when available (limited, particularly for generics); consult specific product labeling.

Tablet: 125 mg, 250 mg, 500 mg

Famvir®: 125 mg, 250 mg, 500 mg

Famotidine (fa MOE ti deen)

U.S. Brand Names Pepcid®; Pepcid® AC Maximum Strength [OTC]; Pepcid® AC [OTC]

Canadian Brand Names Apo-Famotidine®; Apo-Famotidine® Injectable; Famotidine Omega; Gen-Famotidine; Novo-Famotidine; Nu-Famotidine; Pepcid®; Pepcid® AC; Pepcid® I.V.; ratio-Famotidine; Riva-Famotidine; Ulcidine

Pharmacologic Category Histamine H_2 Antagonist

Use Maintenance therapy and treatment of duodenal ulcer; treatment of gastroesophageal reflux, active benign gastric ulcer, and pathological hypersecretory conditions

OTC labeling: Relief of heartburn, acid indigestion, and sour stomach

Unlabeled/Investigational Use Part of a multidrug regimen for *H. pylori* eradication to reduce the risk of duodenal ulcer recurrence; stress ulcer prophylaxis in critically-ill patients; symptomatic relief in gastritis

Pregnancy Risk Factor B

Pregnancy Considerations Crosses the placenta. There are no adequate and well-controlled studies in pregnant women. Use only if clearly needed.

Lactation Enters breast milk/not recommended

Contraindications Hypersensitivity to famotidine, other H_2 antagonists, or any component of the formulation

Warnings/Precautions Modify dose in patients with moderate-to-severe renal impairment. Relief of symptoms does not preclude the presence of a gastric malignancy. Reversible confusional states, usually clearing within 3-4 days after discontinuation, have been linked to use. Increased age (>50 years) and renal or hepatic impairment are thought to be associated. Multidose vials for injection contain benzyl alcohol.

OTC labeling: When used for self-medication, patients should be instructed not to use if they have difficulty swallowing, are vomiting blood, or have bloody or black stools. Not for use with other acid reducers.

Adverse Reactions

Note: Agitation and vomiting have been reported in up to 14% of pediatric patients <1 year of age.

1% to 10%:

Central nervous system: Headache (5%), dizziness (1%)

Gastrointestinal: Diarrhea (2%), constipation (1%)

<1% (Limited to important or life-threatening): Abdominal discomfort, acne, agitation, agranulocytosis, allergic reaction, alopecia, anaphylaxis, angioedema, anorexia, anxiety, arrhythmia, arthralgia, AV block, bradycardia, bronchospasm, BUN/creatinine increased, cholestatic jaundice, confusion, depression, drowsiness, facial edema, fatigue, fever, flushing, hallucinations, injection site reactions, insomnia, interstitial pneumonia, jaundice, leukopenia, libido decreased, liver function tests increased, muscle cramps, nausea, palpitation, pancytopenia, paresthesia, proteinuria, pruritus, rash, seizure, somnolence, Stevens-Johnson syndrome, tinnitus, thrombocytopenia, toxic epidermal necrolysis, urticaria, vomiting, weakness, xerostomia

Drug Interactions

Avoid Concomitant Use

Avoid concomitant use of Famotidine with any of the following: Erlotinib; Mesalamine

Increased Effect/Toxicity

Famotidine may increase the levels/effects of: Saquinavir

Decreased Effect

Famotidine may decrease the levels/effects of: Antifungal Agents (Azole Derivatives, Systemic); Atazanavir; Cefpodoxime; Cefuroxime; Dasatinib; Erlotinib; Fosamprenavir; Indinavir; Iron Salts; Mesalamine; Nelfinavir

Ethanol/Nutrition/Herb Interactions

Ethanol: Avoid ethanol (may cause gastric mucosal irritation).

Food: Famotidine bioavailability may be increased if taken with food.

Stability

Oral:

Powder for oral suspension: Prior to mixing, dry powder should be stored at controlled room temperature of 25°C (77°F). Reconstituted oral suspension is stable for 30 days at room temperature; do not freeze.

Tablet: Store at controlled room temperature. Protect from moisture.

I.V.:

Solution for injection: Prior to use, store at 2°C to 8°C (36°F to 46°F). If solution freezes, allow to solubilize at controlled room temperature.

I.V. push: Dilute famotidine with NS (or another compatible solution) to a total of 5-10 mL (some centers also administer undiluted). Following preparation, solutions for I.V. push should be used immediately, or may be stored in refrigerator and used within 48 hours.

Infusion: Dilute with D_5W 100 mL or another compatible solution. Following preparation, the manufacturer states may be stored for up to 48 hours under refrigeration; however, solutions for infusion have been found to be physically and chemically stable for 7 days at room temperature.

Solution for injection, premixed bags: Store at controlled room temperature of 25°C (77°F). Avoid excessive heat.

Mechanism of Action Competitive inhibition of histamine at H_2 receptors of the gastric parietal cells, which inhibits gastric acid secretion

Pharmacodynamics/Kinetics

Onset of action: GI: Oral: Within 1-3 hour; I.V.: 30 minutes

Duration: 10-12 hours

Protein binding: 15% to 20%

Bioavailability: Oral: 40% to 45%

Half-life elimination: Injection, oral suspension, tablet: 2.5-3.5 hours; prolonged with renal impairment; Oliguria: >20 hours

Time to peak, serum: Oral: ~1-3 hours

Excretion: Urine (25% to 30% [oral], 65% to 70% [I.V.] as unchanged drug)

Dosage

Children: Treatment duration and dose should be individualized

Peptic ulcer: 1-16 years:

Oral: 0.5 mg/kg/day at bedtime or divided twice daily (maximum dose: 40 mg/day); doses of up to 1 mg/kg/day have been used in clinical studies

I.V.: 0.25 mg/kg every 12 hours (maximum dose: 40 mg/day); doses of up to 0.5 mg/kg have been used in clinical studies

GERD: Oral:

<3 months: 0.5 mg/kg once daily

3-12 months: 0.5 mg/kg twice daily

1-16 years: 1 mg/kg/day divided twice daily (maximum dose: 40 mg twice daily); doses of up to 2 mg/kg/day have been used in clinical studies

Children ≥12 years and Adults: Heartburn, indigestion, sour stomach: OTC labeling: Oral: 10-20 mg every 12 hours; dose may be taken 15-60 minutes before eating foods known to cause heartburn

Adults:

Duodenal ulcer: Oral: Acute therapy: 40 mg/day at bedtime for 4-8 weeks; maintenance therapy: 20 mg/day at bedtime

Helicobacter pylori eradication (unlabeled use): 40 mg once daily; requires combination therapy with antibiotics

Gastric ulcer: Oral: Acute therapy: 40 mg/day at bedtime

Hypersecretory conditions: Oral: Initial: 20 mg every 6 hours, may increase in increments up to 160 mg every 6 hours

GERD: Oral: 20 mg twice daily for 6 weeks

Esophagitis and accompanying symptoms due to GERD: Oral: 20 mg or 40 mg twice daily for up to 12 weeks

Patients unable to take oral medication: I.V.: 20 mg every 12 hours

Dosing adjustment in renal impairment: Cl_{cr} <50 mL/minute: Manufacturer recommendation: Administer 50% of dose **or** increase the dosing interval to every 36-48 hours (to limit potential CNS adverse effects).

Administration

Oral:

Suspension: Shake vigorously before use. May be taken with or without food.

Tablet: May be taken with or without food.

I.V.:

I.V. push: Inject over at least 2 minutes.

Solution for infusion: Administer over 15-30 minutes.

Dosage Forms Excipient information presented when available (limited, particularly for generics); consult specific product labeling.

Gelcap:

Pepcid® AC: 10 mg

Infusion [premixed in NS]: 20 mg (50 mL)

Pepcid®: 20 mg (50 mL)

Injection, solution: 10 mg/mL (4 mL, 20 mL, 50 mL)

Pepcid®: 10 mg/mL (20 mL) [contains benzyl alcohol]

Injection, solution [preservative free]: 10 mg/mL (2 mL)

Pepcid®: 10 mg/mL (2 mL)

Powder for oral suspension:

Pepcid®: 40 mg/5 mL (50 mL) [contains sodium benzoate; cherry-banana-mint flavor]

Tablet: 10 mg [OTC], 20 mg, 40 mg

Pepcid®: 20 mg, 40 mg

Pepcid® AC: 10 mg, 20 mg

Pepcid® AC Maximum Strength: 20 mg

Famotidine, Calcium Carbonate, and Magnesium Hydroxide

(fa MOE ti deen, KAL see um KAR bun ate, & mag NEE zhum hye DROKS ide)

U.S. Brand Names Pepcid® Complete [OTC]

Canadian Brand Names Pepcid® Complete [OTC]

Index Terms Calcium Carbonate, Magnesium Hydroxide, and Famotidine; Magnesium Hydroxide, Famotidine, and Calcium Carbonate

Pharmacologic Category Antacid; Histamine H_2 Antagonist

Use Relief of heartburn due to acid indigestion

Dosage Children ≥12 years and Adults: Relief of heartburn due to acid indigestion: Oral: Pepcid® Complete: 1 tablet as needed; no more than 2 tablets in 24 hours; do **not** swallow whole, chew tablet completely before swallowing; do not use for longer than 14 days

Additional Information Complete prescribing information for this medication should be consulted for additional detail.

Dosage Forms Excipient information presented when available (limited, particularly for generics); consult specific product labeling.

Tablet, chewable: Famotidine 10 mg, calcium carbonate 800 mg, and magnesium hydroxide 165 mg [berry blend and mint flavors]

◆ **Famotidine Omega (Can)** *see* Famotidine *on page* 603

◆ **Famvir®** *see* Famciclovir *on page* 602

◆ **Fansidar®** *see* Sulfadoxine and Pyrimethamine *on page* 1407

- **2F-ara-AMP** *see* Fludarabine *on page 628*
- **Fareston®** *see* Toremifene *on page 1493*
- **Faslodex®** *see* Fulvestrant *on page 675*
- **Fasturtec® (Can)** *see* Rasburicase *on page 1300*

Fat Emulsion (fat e MUL shun)

U.S. Brand Names Intralipid®; Liposyn® II; Liposyn® III
Canadian Brand Names Intralipid®; Liposyn® II
Index Terms Intravenous Fat Emulsion
Pharmacologic Category Caloric Agent
Use Source of calories and essential fatty acids for patients requiring parenteral nutrition of extended duration; prevention and treatment of essential fatty acid deficiency (EFAD)
Unlabeled/Investigational Use Local anesthetic-induced cardiac arrest unresponsive to conventional resuscitation
Pregnancy Risk Factor C
Dosage I.V.: **Note:** At the onset of therapy, the patient should be observed for any immediate allergic reactions.
Nutrition:
Premature infants: Initial dose: 0.25-0.5 g/kg/day, increase by 0.25-0.5 g/kg/day to a maximum of 3 g/kg/day depending on needs/nutritional goals; limit to 1 g/kg/day if on phototherapy; should be administered over 24 hours (A.S.P.E.N. guidelines)
Infants and Children: Initial dose: 0.5-1 g/kg/day, increase by 0.5 g/kg/day to a maximum of 3 g/kg/day depending on needs/nutritional goals; may administer over 24 hours (A.S.P.E.N. guidelines)
Note: Pediatric patients: Monitor triglycerides while receiving intralipids. If serum triglyceride levels >200 mg/dL, stop infusion and restart at 0.5-1g/kg/day. Intravenous heparin (1 unit/mL of parenteral nutrition) may enhance the clearance of lipid emulsions.
Adults: Initial dose: 1 g/kg/day, increase by 0.5-1 g/kg/day to a maximum of 2.5-3 g/kg/day
Prevention of essential fatty acid deficiency (EFAD): Adults: Administer 8% to 10% of total caloric intake as fat emulsion (may be higher in stressed patients with EFAD); may be given 2-3 times weekly to meet essential fatty acid requirements
Local anesthetic toxicity (unlabeled use): Adults: 20%: 1.5 mL/kg administered over 1 minute, followed immediately by an infusion of 0.25 mL/kg/minute. Continue chest compressions (lipid must circulate). Repeat bolus every 3-5 minutes up to 3 mL/kg total dose until circulation restored. Continue infusion until hemodynamic stability is restored. Increase the infusion rate to 0.5 mL/kg/minute if BP declines. A maximum total dose of 8 mL/kg is recommended.
Additional Information Complete prescribing information for this medication should be consulted for additional detail.
Dosage Forms Excipient information presented when available (limited, particularly for generics); consult specific product labeling.
Injection, emulsion:
Intralipid®: 20% (100 mL, 250 mL, 500 mL, 1000 mL) [contains aluminum, egg yolk phospholipids, and soybean oil]; 30% (500 mL) [contains aluminum, egg yolk phospholipids, and soybean oil]
Liposyn® II: 10% (500 mL) [contains aluminum, egg yolk phospholipids, safflower oil, and soybean oil]; 20% (500 mL) [contains aluminum, egg yolk phospholipids, safflower oil, and soybean oil]
Liposyn® III: 10% (200 mL, 500 mL) [contains aluminum, egg yolk phospholipids, and soybean oil] ; 20% (200 mL, 500 mL) [contains aluminum, egg yolk phospholipids, and soybean oil]; 30% (500 mL) [contains aluminum, egg yolk phospholipids, and soybean oil]

- **Father John's® Plus [OTC]** *see* Chlorpheniramine, Phenylephrine, and Dextromethorphan *on page 311*
- **FazaClo®** *see* Clozapine *on page 359*
- **5-FC** *see* Flucytosine *on page 627*
- **FC1157a** *see* Toremifene *on page 1493*
- **FE200486** *see* Degarelix *on page 413*
- **Feiba VH** *see* Anti-inhibitor Coagulant Complex *on page 123*
- **Feiba VH Immuno (Can)** *see* Anti-inhibitor Coagulant Complex *on page 123*

Felbamate (FEL ba mate)

U.S. Brand Names Felbatol®
Pharmacologic Category Anticonvulsant, Miscellaneous
Additional Appendix Information
Anticonvulsant Drugs of Choice *on page 1637*
Use Not as a first-line antiepileptic treatment; only in those patients who respond inadequately to alternative treatments and whose epilepsy is so severe that a substantial risk of aplastic anemia and/or liver failure is deemed acceptable in light of the benefits conferred by its use. Patient must be fully advised of risk and provide signed written informed consent. Felbamate can be used as either monotherapy or adjunctive therapy in the treatment of partial seizures (with and without generalization) and in adults with epilepsy. Used as adjunctive therapy in the treatment of partial and generalized seizures associated with Lennox-Gastaut syndrome in children.
Restrictions A patient "informed consent" form should be completed and signed by the patient and physician. Copies are available from Wallace Pharmaceuticals by calling 800-526-3840 or 609-655-6147.
Pregnancy Risk Factor C
Dosage Anticonvulsant:
Monotherapy: Children >14 years and Adults:
Initial: 1200 mg/day in divided doses 3 or 4 times/day; titrate previously untreated patients under close clinical supervision, increasing the dosage in 600 mg increments every 2 weeks to 2400 mg/day based on clinical response and thereafter to 3600 mg/day as clinically indicated
Conversion to monotherapy: Initiate at 1200 mg/day in divided doses 3 or 4 times/day, reduce the dosage of the concomitant anticonvulsant(s) by 20% to 33% at the initiation of felbamate therapy; at week 2, increase the felbamate dosage to 2400 mg/day while reducing the dosage of the other anticonvulsant(s) up to an additional 33% of their original dosage; at week 3, increase the felbamate dosage up to 3600 mg/day and continue to reduce the dosage of the other anticonvulsant(s) as clinically indicated
Adjunctive therapy: **Note:** Dose of concomitant carbamazepine, phenobarbital, phenytoin, or valproic acid should be decreased by 20% to 33% when initiating felbamate therapy. Further dosage reductions may be necessary as dose of felbamate is increased.
Children 2-14 years with Lennox-Gastaut syndrome: Initial: 15 mg/kg/day in divided doses 3 or 4 times/day; may increase once per week by 15 mg/kg/day increments up to 45 mg/kg/day in divided doses 3 or 4 times/day.
Children >14 years and Adults: Initial: 1200 mg/day in divided doses 3 or 4 times/day; may increase once per week by 1200 mg/day increments up to 3600 mg/day in divided doses 3 or 4 times/day.

Dosage adjustment in renal impairment: Use caution; reduce initial and maintenance doses by 50% (half-life prolonged by 9-15 hours)

Additional Information Complete prescribing information for this medication should be consulted for additional detail.

Dosage Forms Excipient information presented when available (limited, particularly for generics); consult specific product labeling.

Suspension, oral:

Felbatol®: 600 mg/5 mL (240 mL, 960 mL)

Tablet:

Felbatol®: 400 mg; 600 mg

◆ **Felbatol®** *see* Felbamate *on page 605*

◆ **Feldene®** *see* Piroxicam *on page 1201*

Felodipine (fe LOE di peen)

U.S. Brand Names Plendil®

Canadian Brand Names Plendil®; Renedil®

Pharmacologic Category Calcium Channel Blocker

Additional Appendix Information

Calcium Channel Blockers *on page 1651*

Use Treatment of hypertension

Unlabeled/Investigational Use Pediatric hypertension

Pregnancy Risk Factor C

Pregnancy Considerations Potentially, calcium channel blockers may prolong labor. There are no adequate or well-controlled studies in pregnant women.

Lactation Excretion in breast milk unknown/not recommended

Medication Safety Issues

Sound-alike/look-alike issues:

Plendil® may be confused with Isordil®, pindolol, Pletal®, Prilosec®, Prinivil®

Contraindications Hypersensitivity to felodipine, any component of the formulation, or other calcium channel blocker

Warnings/Precautions Increased angina and/or MI has occurred with initiation or dosage titration of dihydropyridine calcium channel blockers, reflex tachycardia may occur resulting in angina and/or MI in patients with obstructive coronary disease especially in the absence of concurrent beta-blockade. Use with extreme caution in patients with severe aortic stenosis. Use caution in patients with heart failure and/or hypertrophic cardiomyopathy with outflow tract obstruction. Elderly patients and patients with hepatic impairment should start off with a lower dose. Peripheral edema (dose dependent) is the most common side effect (occurs within 2-3 weeks of starting therapy). Symptomatic hypotension with or without syncope can rarely occur; blood pressure must be lowered at a rate appropriate for the patient's clinical condition. Safety and efficacy in children have not been established. Dosage titration should occur after 14 days on a given dose.

Adverse Reactions

>10%: Central nervous system: Headache (11% to 15%)

2% to 10%: Cardiovascular: Peripheral edema (2% to 17%), tachycardia (0.4% to 2.5%), flushing (4% to 7%)

<1% (Limited to important or life-threatening): Angina, angioedema, anxiety, arrhythmia, CHF, CVA, libido decreased, depression, dizziness, gingival hyperplasia, dyspnea, dysuria, gynecomastia, hypotension, impotence, insomnia, irritability, leukocytoclastic vasculitis, MI, nervousness, paresthesia, somnolence, syncope, urticaria, vomiting

Drug Interactions

Metabolism/Transport Effects **Substrate** of CYP3A4 (major); **Inhibits** CYP2C8 (moderate), 2C9 (weak), 2D6 (weak), 3A4 (weak)

Avoid Concomitant Use There are no known interactions where it is recommended to avoid concomitant use.

Increased Effect/Toxicity

Felodipine may increase the levels/effects of: Amifostine; CYP2C8 Substrates (High risk); Magnesium Salts; Neuromuscular-Blocking Agents (Nondepolarizing); Nitroprusside; Phenytoin; RiTUXimab; Tacrolimus

The levels/effects of Felodipine may be increased by: Alpha1-Blockers; Antifungal Agents (Azole Derivatives, Systemic); Calcium Channel Blockers (Nondihydropyridine); Cimetidine; CycloSPORINE; CYP3A4 Inhibitors (Moderate); CYP3A4 Inhibitors (Strong); Dasatinib; Diazoxide; Fluconazole; Grapefruit Juice; Herbs (Hypotensive Properties); Macrolide Antibiotics; Magnesium Salts; Prostacyclin Analogues; Protease Inhibitors; Quinupristin

Decreased Effect

Felodipine may decrease the levels/effects of: Clopidogrel

The levels/effects of Felodipine may be decreased by: Barbiturates; Calcium Salts; CarBAMazepine; CYP3A4 Inducers (Strong); Deferasirox; Herbs (CYP3A4 Inducers); Herbs (Hypertensive Properties); Methylphenidate; Nafcillin; Rifamycin Derivatives; Yohimbine

Ethanol/Nutrition/Herb Interactions

Ethanol: Increases felodipine's absorption; watch for a greater hypotensive effect.

Food: Increased therapeutic and vasodilator side effects, including severe hypotension and myocardial ischemia, may occur if felodipine is taken with grapefruit juice; avoid concurrent use. High-fat/carbohydrate meals will increase C_{max} by 60%; grapefruit juice will increase C_{max} by twofold.

Herb/Nutraceutical: St John's wort may decrease felodipine levels. Avoid dong quai if using for hypertension (has estrogenic activity). Avoid ephedra, yohimbe, ginseng (may worsen hypertension). Avoid garlic (may have increased antihypertensive effect).

Mechanism of Action Inhibits calcium ions from entering the "slow channels" or select voltage-sensitive areas of vascular smooth muscle and myocardium during depolarization, producing a relaxation of coronary vascular smooth muscle and coronary vasodilation; increases myocardial oxygen delivery in patients with vasospastic angina

Pharmacodynamics/Kinetics

Onset of action: Antihypertensive: 2-5 hours

Duration of antihypertensive effect: 24 hours

Absorption: 100%; Absolute: 20% due to first-pass effect

Protein binding: >99%

Metabolism: Hepatic; CYP3A4 substrate (major); extensive first-pass effect

Half-life elimination: Immediate release: 11-16 hours

Excretion: Urine (70% as metabolites); feces 10%

Dosage Oral: Hypertension:

Children (unlabeled use): Initial: 2.5 mg once daily; maximum: 10 mg/day

Adults: Oral: 2.5-10 mg once daily; usual initial dose: 5 mg; increase by 5 mg at 2-week intervals, as needed, to a maximum of 20 mg/day

Usual dose range (JNC 7) for hypertension: 2.5-20 mg once daily

Elderly: Begin with 2.5 mg/day

Dosing adjustment/comments in hepatic impairment: Initial: 2.5 mg/day; monitor blood pressure

Dietary Considerations Should be taken without food.

Administration Do not crush or chew extended release tablets; swallow whole.

Additional Information Felodipine maintains renal and mesenteric blood flow during hemorrhagic shock in animals.

Dosage Forms Excipient information presented when available (limited, particularly for generics); consult specific product labeling.

Tablet, extended release: 2.5 mg, 5 mg, 10 mg
Plendil®: 2.5 mg, 5 mg, 10 mg

- **Felodipine and Enalapril** *see* Enalapril and Felodipine *on page 518*
- **Femara®** *see* Letrozole *on page 865*
- **Fematrol [OTC]** *see* Bisacodyl *on page 198*
- **Femcon™ Fe** *see* Ethinyl Estradiol and Norethindrone *on page 581*
- **femhrt®** *see* Ethinyl Estradiol and Norethindrone *on page 581*
- **FemHRT® (Can)** *see* Ethinyl Estradiol and Norethindrone *on page 581*
- **Femilax™ [OTC]** *see* Bisacodyl *on page 198*
- **Femiron® [OTC]** *see* Ferrous Fumarate *on page 616*
- **Fem-Prin® [OTC]** *see* Acetaminophen, Aspirin, and Caffeine *on page 31*
- **Femring®** *see* Estradiol *on page 554*
- **Femstat® One (Can)** *see* Butoconazole *on page 231*
- **Femtrace®** *see* Estradiol *on page 554*
- **Fenesin DM IR** *see* Guaifenesin and Dextromethorphan *on page 710*
- **Fenesin IR** *see* GuaiFENesin *on page 709*
- **Fenesin PE IR** *see* Guaifenesin and Phenylephrine *on page 712*

Fenofibrate (fen oh FYE brate)

U.S. Brand Names Antara®; Fenoglide™; Lipofen®; Lofibra®; TriCor®; Triglide™

Canadian Brand Names Apo-Feno-Micro®; Apo-Fenofibrate®; Dom-Fenofibrate Supra; Feno-Micro-200; Fenomax; Gen-Fenofibrate Micro; Lipidil EZ®; Lipidil Micro®; Lipidil Supra®; Novo-Fenofibrate; Novo-Fenofibrate-S; Nu-Fenofibrate; PHL-Fenofibrate Supra; PMS-Fenofibrate Micro; Pro-Feno-Super; ratio-Fenofibrate MC; Riva-Fenofibrate Micro; Sandoz Fenofibrate S

Index Terms Procetofene; Proctofene

Pharmacologic Category Antilipemic Agent, Fibric Acid

Additional Appendix Information

Hyperlipidemia Management *on page 1815*
Lipid-Lowering Agents *on page 1661*

Use Adjunct to dietary therapy for the treatment of adults with elevations of serum triglyceride levels (types IV and V hyperlipidemia); adjunct to dietary therapy for the reduction of low density lipoprotein cholesterol (LDL-C), total cholesterol (total-C), triglycerides, and apolipoprotein B (apo B) in adult patients with primary hypercholesterolemia or mixed dyslipidemia (Fredrickson types IIa and IIb)

Pregnancy Risk Factor C

Pregnancy Considerations Animal studies have shown embryocidal and teratogenic effect. There are no adequate and well-controlled studies in pregnant women. Use should be avoided, if possible, in pregnant women since the neonatal glucuronide conjugation pathways are immature.

Lactation Excretion in breast milk unknown/not recommended

Medication Safety Issues

Sound-alike/look-alike issues:
TriCor® may be confused with Tracleer®

Contraindications Hypersensitivity to fenofibrate or any component of the formulation; hepatic dysfunction including primary biliary cirrhosis and unexplained persistent liver function abnormalities; severe renal dysfunction; pre-existing gallbladder disease; breast-feeding (only Fenoglide™)

Canadian labeling: Additional contraindications (not in U.S. labeling): Pregnancy; breast-feeding; known photoallergy or phototoxic reaction during treatment with fibrates or ketoprofen; allergy to soya lecithin or peanut or arachis oil

Warnings/Precautions Secondary causes of hyperlipidemia should be ruled out prior to therapy. Hepatic transaminases can become significantly elevated (dose-related); hepatocellular, chronic active, and cholestatic hepatitis have been reported. Regular monitoring of liver function tests is required. Increases in serum creatinine (>2 mg/dL) have been observed with use; monitor renal function in patients with renal impairment and consider monitoring patients with increased risk for developing renal impairment. May cause cholelithiasis. Use with caution in patient taking oral anticoagulants (eg, warfarin); adjustments in anticoagulation therapy may be required. Use caution with HMG-CoA reductase inhibitors (may lead to myopathy, rhabdomyolysis). In combination with HMG-CoA reductase inhibitors, fenofibrate is generally regarded as safer than gemfibrozil due to limited pharmacokinetic interaction with statins. Therapy should be withdrawn if an adequate response is not obtained after 2-3 months of therapy at the maximal daily dose. The occurrence of pancreatitis may represent a failure of efficacy in patients with severely elevated triglycerides. May cause mild-to-moderate decreases in hemoglobin, hematocrit, and WBC upon initiation of therapy which usually stabilizes with long-term therapy. Agranulocytosis and thrombocytopenia have rarely been reported. Periodic monitoring of blood counts is recommended during the first year of therapy.

Rare hypersensitivity reactions may occur. Use has been associated with pulmonary embolism (PE) and deep vein thrombosis (DVT). Use with caution in patients with risk factors for VTE. Dose adjustment is required for renal impairment and elderly patients. Safety and efficacy in children have not been established.

Adverse Reactions

>10%: Hepatic: Liver function tests increased (dose related; 3% to 13%)

1% to 10%:

Central nervous system: Headache (3%)
Gastrointestinal: Abdominal pain (5%), constipation (2%), nausea (2%)
Neuromuscular & skeletal: Back pain (3%), CPK increased (3%)
Respiratory: Respiratory disorder (6%), rhinitis (2%)

Postmarketing and/or case reports (limited to important or life-threatening): Abnormal vision, agranulocytosis, alkaline phosphatase decreased, allergic reaction, alopecia, amblyopia, anemia, angina pectoris, anorexia, anxiety, appetite increased, arrhythmia, arthralgia, arthritis, arthrosis, asthma, atrial fibrillation, bronchitis, bruising, bursitis, cataract, cholecystitis, cholelithiasis, cholestatic hepatitis, cirrhosis, colitis, conjunctivitis, contact dermatitis, cough, creatinine increased, cyst, cystitis, deep venous thrombosis, depression, diabetes mellitus, diaphoresis, diarrhea, dizziness, dyspepsia, dyspnea, dysuria, ear pain, eczema, edema, electrocardiogram abnormality, eosinophilia, esophagitis, extrasystoles, fatty liver deposits, fever, flatulence, fungal dermatitis, gastritis, gastroenteritis, gout, gynecomastia, hepatitis, herpes simplex, herpes zoster, hyper-/hypotension, hypersensitivity reaction, hypertonia, hyperuricemia, hypoglycemia, infection, insomnia, kidney function abnormality, laryngitis, leg cramps, leukopenia, libido decreased, lymphadenopathy, maculopapular rash, malaise, MI, migraine, myalgia, myasthenia, myopathy, myositis, nervousness, neuralgia, otitis media, pain, palpitation, pancreatitis, paresthesia, peptic ulcer, peripheral edema, peripheral vascular disorder, pharyngitis, phlebitis, photosensitivity reaction, pneumonia, pregnancy (unintended), prostate disorder, pruritus, pulmonary embolus, rash, rectal hemorrhage, refraction disorder, rhabdomyolysis, sinusitis, skin ulcer, somnolence, Stevens-Johnson syndrome, tachycardia, tenderness, tenosynovitis, thrombocytopenia, toxic epidermal necrolysis, urea in creased, urinary frequency, urolithiasis, urticaria, vaginal moniliasis, varicose veins, vasodilatation, vertigo, vomiting, weakness, weight gain/loss, xerostomia

Drug Interactions

Metabolism/Transport Effects **Substrate** of CYP3A4 (minor); **Inhibits** CYP2A6 (weak), 2C8 (weak), 2C9 (weak), 2C19 (weak)

Avoid Concomitant Use There are no known interactions where it is recommended to avoid concomitant use.

Increased Effect/Toxicity

Fenofibrate may increase the levels/effects of: Ezetimibe; HMG-CoA Reductase Inhibitors; Sulfonylureas; Vitamin K Antagonists; Warfarin

Decreased Effect

The levels/effects of Fenofibrate may be decreased by: Bile Acid Sequestrants

Stability Store at 15°C to 30°C (59°F to 86°F). Protect from light and moisture. Store tablets in moisture-protective container.

Mechanism of Action Fenofibric acid, an agonist for the nuclear transcription factor peroxisome proliferator-activated receptor-alpha (PPAR-alpha), downregulates apoprotein C-III (an inhibitor of lipoprotein lipase) and upregulates the synthesis of apolipoprotein A-I, fatty acid transport protein, and lipoprotein lipase resulting in an increase in VLDL catabolism, fatty acid oxidation, and elimination of triglyceride-rich particles; as a result of a decrease in VLDL levels, total plasma triglycerides are reduced by 30% to 60%; modest increase in HDL occurs in some hypertriglyceridemic patients.

Pharmacodynamics/Kinetics

Absorption: Increased when taken with meals

Distribution: Widely to most tissues

Protein binding: >99%

Metabolism: Tissue and plasma via esterases to active form, fenofibric acid; undergoes inactivation by glucuronidation hepatically or renally

Half-life elimination: Fenofibric acid: Mean: 20 hours (range: 10-35 hours)

Time to peak: 3-8 hours

Excretion: Urine (60% as metabolites); feces (25%); hemodialysis has no effect on removal of fenofibric acid from plasma

Dosage Oral:

Adults:

Hypertriglyceridemia: Initial:

Antara® (micronized): 43-130 mg/day; maximum dose: 130 mg/day

Fenoglide™: 40-120 mg/day; maximum dose: 120 mg/day

Lipidil EZ® [CAN; not available in U.S.]: 145 mg/day; maximum dose: 145 mg/day

Lipidil Micro® [CAN; not available in U.S.]: 200 mg/day; maximum dose: 200 mg/day

Lipidil Supra® [CAN; not available in U.S.]: 160 mg/day; maximum dose: 200 mg/day

Lipofen®: 50-150 mg/day; maximum dose: 150 mg/day

Lofibra® (micronized): 67-200 mg/day with meals; maximum dose: 200 mg/day

Lofibra® (tablets): 54-160 mg/day; maximum dose: 160 mg/day

TriCor®: 48-145 mg/day; maximum dose: 145 mg/day

Triglide™: 50-160 mg/day; maximum dose: 160 mg/day

Hypercholesterolemia or mixed hyperlipidemia:

Antara® (micronized): 130 mg/day

Fenoglide™: 120 mg/day

Lipidil EZ® [CAN; not available in U.S.]: 145 mg/day; maximum dose: 145 mg/day

Lipidil Micro® [CAN; not available in U.S.]: 200 mg/day; maximum dose: 200 mg/day

Lipidil Supra® [CAN; not available in U.S.]: 160 mg/day; maximum dose: 200 mg/day

Lipofen®: 150 mg/day

Lofibra® (micronized): 200 mg/day

Lofibra® (tablets): 160 mg/day

TriCor®: 145 mg/day

Triglide™: 160 mg/day

Elderly: Initial:

Antara® (micronized): 43 mg/day

Fenoglide™: Adjust dosage based on creatinine clearance

Lipidil EZ® [CAN; not available in U.S.]: 48 mg/day

Lipidil Micro® [CAN; not available in U.S.]: Adjust dosage based on creatinine clearance

Lipidil Supra® [CAN; not available in U.S.]: Adjust dosage based on creatinine clearance

Lipofen®: 50 mg/day

Lofibra® (micronized): 67 mg/day

Lofibra® (tablets): 54 mg/day

TriCor®: Adjust dosage based on creatinine clearance

Triglide™: 50 mg/day

Dosage adjustment/interval in renal impairment: Monitor renal function and lipid panel before adjusting. Decrease dose or increase dosing interval for patients with renal failure: **Note:** Use in severe renal impairment is contraindicated (see specific product labeling):

Antara® (micronized): 43 mg/day

Fenoglide™: Cl_{cr} 31-80 mL/minute: 40 mg/day

Lipidil EZ® [CAN; not available in U.S.]: Cl_{cr} ≥20-50 mL/minute: 48 mg/day

Lipidil Micro® [CAN; not available in U.S.]: Cl_{cr} ≥20-100 mL/minute: 67 mg/day; **Note:** Lipidil Micro® 67 mg capsules are discontinued in Canada. Micronized formulation at this dosage strength is available through other manufacturers in Canada.

Lipidil Supra® [CAN; not available in U.S.]: Cl_{cr} ≥20-100 mL/minute: 100 mg/day

Lipofen®: 50 mg/day

Lofibra® (micronized): 67 mg/day

Lofibra® (tablets): 54 mg/day

TriCor®: Cl_{cr} 31-80 mL/minute: 48 mg/day

Triglide™: 50 mg/day

Dietary Considerations

Fenoglide™, Lofibra® (capsules [micronized] and tablets), Lipofen®: Take with meals.

Antara®, TriCor®, Triglide™: May be taken with or without food.

Canadian products [not available in U.S.]:

Lipidil Micro®, Lipidil Supra®: Take with meals.

Lipidil EZ® : May be taken with or without food.

Administration 6-8 weeks of therapy is required to determine efficacy.

Fenoglide™, Lofibra® (capsules [micronized] and tablets), Lipofen®: Administer with meals.

Antara®, TriCor®: May be administered with or without food.

Triglide™: Do not consume chipped or broken tablets. May be administered with or without food.

Canadian products [not available in U.S.]:

Lipidil Micro®, Lipidil Supra®: Administer with meals.

Lipidil EZ® : May be administered with or without food.

Monitoring Parameters Periodic blood counts during first year of therapy. Total cholesterol, LDL-C, triglycerides, and HDL-C should be measured periodically; If only marginal changes are noted in 6-8 weeks, the drug should be discontinued. Monitor LFTs regularly and discontinue therapy if levels remain >3 times normal limits.

Dosage Forms Excipient information presented when available (limited, particularly for generics); consult specific product labeling. [DSC] = Discontinued product

Capsule:

Lipofen®: 50 mg; 100 mg [DSC]; 150 mg

Capsule [micronized]: 67 mg, 134 mg, 200 mg

Antara®: 43 mg, 130 mg

Lofibra®: 67 mg, 134 mg, 200 mg

Tablet: 54 mg, 160 mg

Fenoglide™: 40 mg, 120 mg

Lofibra®: 54 mg, 160 mg

TriCor®: 48 mg, 145 mg [contains soybean lecithin]

Triglide™: 50 mg, 160 mg [contains egg lecithin]

Fenofibric Acid (fen oh FYE brik AS id)

U.S. Brand Names TriLipix™

Index Terms ABT-335; Choline Fenofibrate

Pharmacologic Category Antilipemic Agent, Fibric Acid

Use Adjunct to dietary therapy for the treatment of severely elevated serum triglyceride levels; adjunct to dietary therapy for the reduction of low density lipoprotein cholesterol (LDL-C), total cholesterol (total-C), triglycerides, and apolipoprotein B (apo B) and to increase high density lipoprotein cholesterol (HDL-C) in patients with primary hypercholesterolemia or mixed dyslipidemia; adjunct to dietary therapy concomitantly with a statin to reduce triglyceride levels and increase HDL-C levels in patients with mixed dyslipidemia and coronary heart disease (CHD) or at risk for CHD

Restrictions An FDA-approved patient medication guide is available and must be distributed when dispensing an outpatient prescription (new or refill) where this medication is to be used without direct supervision of a healthcare provider. Medication guides are available at http://www.fda.gov/cder/Offices/ODS/medication_guides.htm.

Pregnancy Risk Factor C

Medication Safety Issues

Sound-alike/look-alike issues:

TriLipix™ may be confused with Trileptal®, TriLyte®

Dosage Oral:

Adults:

Mixed dyslipidemia (coadministered with a statin): 135 mg once daily (maximum: 135 mg/day)

Hypertriglyceridemia: Initial: 45-135 mg once daily; Maintenance: Individualize according to patient response (maximum: 135 mg/day)

Primary hypercholesterolemia or mixed dyslipidemia: 135 mg once daily (maximum: 135 mg/day)

Elderly: Dosage based on renal function

Dosage adjustment/interval in renal impairment:

Mild-to-moderate impairment (Cl_{cr} 30-80 mL/minute): Initial: 45 mg once daily; only increase once effects on lipids and renal function evaluated

Severe impairment(Cl_{cr} <30 mL/minute; with or without dialysis): Contraindicated

Additional Information Complete prescribing information for this medication should be consulted for additional detail.

Dosage Forms Excipient information presented when available (limited, particularly for generics); consult specific product labeling.

Capsule, delayed release:

TriLipix™: 45 mg, 135 mg

◆ **Fenoglide™** *see* Fenofibrate *on page 607*

Fenoldopam (fe NOL doe pam)

U.S. Brand Names Corlopam®

Canadian Brand Names Corlopam®

Index Terms Fenoldopam Mesylate

Pharmacologic Category Dopamine Agonist

Additional Appendix Information

Hypertension *on page 1820*

Use Treatment of severe hypertension (up to 48 hours in adults), including in patients with renal compromise; short-term (up to 4 hours) blood pressure reduction in pediatric patients

Pregnancy Risk Factor B

Pregnancy Considerations Fetal harm was not observed in animal studies; however, safety and efficacy have not been established for use during pregnancy. Use during pregnancy only if clearly needed. Fetal heart rate monitoring is recommended.

Lactation Excretion in breast milk unknown/use caution

Contraindications Hypersensitivity of fenoldopam or any component of the formulation

Warnings/Precautions Use caution in patients with glaucoma or intraocular hypertension. A dose-related tachycardia can occur, especially at infusion rates >0.1 mcg/kg/minute. Use caution in angina patients (can increase myocardial oxygen demand with tachycardia). Close monitoring of blood pressure is necessary (hypotension can occur). Monitor for hypokalemia at intervals of 6 hours during infusion. For continuous infusion only (no bolus doses). The effects of hemodialysis on the pharmacokinetics of fenoldopam have not been evaluated. Use caution with increased intracranial pressure. Contains sulfites; may cause allergic reaction in susceptible individuals.

Adverse Reactions Frequency not always defined.

Cardiovascular: Angina, asymptomatic T wave flattening on ECG, chest pain, edema, facial flushing (>5%), fibrillation (atrial), flutter (atrial), hypotension (>5%), tachycardia

Central nervous system: Dizziness, headache (>5%)

Endocrine & metabolic: Hypokalemia

Gastrointestinal: Abdominal pain/fullness, diarrhea, nausea (>5%), vomiting, xerostomia

Local: Injection site reactions

Ocular: Intraocular pressure (increased), blurred vision

Hepatic: Increases in portal pressure in cirrhotic patients

Drug Interactions

Avoid Concomitant Use There are no known interactions where it is recommended to avoid concomitant use.

Increased Effect/Toxicity There are no known significant interactions involving an increase in effect.

Decreased Effect There are no known significant interactions involving a decrease in effect.

Stability Store at 2°C to 30°C (35°F to 86°F). Must be diluted prior to infusion. Final dilution for children is 60 mcg/mL and for adults is 40 mcg/mL. Following dilution, store at room temperature and use solution within 24 hours.

Mechanism of Action A selective postsynaptic dopamine agonist (D_1-receptors) which exerts hypotensive effects by decreasing peripheral vasculature resistance with increased renal blood flow, diuresis, and natriuresis; 6 times as potent as dopamine in producing renal vasodilitation; has minimal adrenergic effects

Pharmacodynamics/Kinetics

Onset of action: I.V.: 10 minutes

Duration: I.V.: 1 hour

Distribution: V_d: 0.6 L/kg

Half-life elimination: I.V.: Children: 3-5 minutes; Adults: ~5 minutes

Metabolism: Hepatic via methylation, glucuronidation, and sulfation; the 8-sulfate metabolite may have some activity; extensive first-pass effect

Excretion: Urine (90%); feces (10%)

Dosage I.V.: Hypertension, severe:

Children: Initial: 0.2 mcg/kg/minute; may be increased to dosages of 0.3-0.5 mcg/kg/minute every 20-30 minutes (maximum dose: 0.8 mcg/kg/minute); limited to short-term (4 hours) use

Adults: Initial: 0.1-0.3 mcg/kg/minute (lower initial doses may be associated with less reflex tachycardia); may be increased in increments of 0.05-0.1 mcg/kg/minute every 15 minutes until target blood pressure is reached; the maximal infusion rate reported in clinical studies was 1.6 mcg/kg/minute

Dosing adjustment in renal impairment: None required

Dosing adjustment in hepatic impairment: None published

Administration For I.V. infusion using an infusion pump.

Monitoring Parameters Blood pressure, heart rate, ECG, renal/hepatic function tests

Reference Range Mean plasma fenoldopam levels after a 2 hour infusion (at 0.5 mcg/kg/minute) and a 100 mg dose is approximately 13 ng/mL and 50 ng/mL

Additional Information Suitable for use in patients whose condition is unstable or rapidly changing because the effects of the drug are predictable and easily reversible; it has been found to safely control blood pressure in patients with a variety of pre-existing conditions including kidney disease, liver disease, and heart failure. (Clinical benefit other than blood pressure reduction has not been established.) In none of these situations does the dose need to be adjusted, minimizing the risk of drug overdose in patients with these conditions. The drug is quickly metabolized into inactive substances before it is excreted; therefore, there are no toxic chemicals derived from the drug. Unlike the situation with some other intravenous antihypertensives, the adult patient does not need an arterial line for blood pressure monitoring; a blood pressure cuff is sufficient to monitor blood pressure lowering. Since the drug induces natriuresis, diuresis, and increased creatinine clearance, it may have an advantage over nitroprusside, especially in patients with severe renal insufficiency and in volume overloaded patients.

Dosage Forms Excipient information presented when available (limited, particularly for generics); consult specific product labeling.

Injection, solution: 10 mg/mL (1 mL, 2 mL) [contains sodium metabisulfite and propylene glycol]

◆ **Fenoldopam Mesylate** *see* Fenoldopam *on page 609*

◆ **Fenomax (Can)** *see* Fenofibrate *on page 607*

◆ **Feno-Micro-200 (Can)** *see* Fenofibrate *on page 607*

Fenoprofen (fen oh PROE fen)

U.S. Brand Names Nalfon®

Canadian Brand Names Nalfon®

Index Terms Fenoprofen Calcium

Pharmacologic Category Nonsteroidal Anti-inflammatory Drug (NSAID), Oral

Additional Appendix Information

Nonsteroidal Anti-inflammatory Agents *on page 1669*

Use Symptomatic treatment of acute and chronic rheumatoid arthritis and osteoarthritis; relief of mild to moderate pain

Restrictions An FDA-approved medication guide must be distributed when dispensing an oral outpatient prescription (new or refill) where this medication is to be used without direct supervision of a healthcare provider. Medication guides are available at http://www.fda.gov/cder/Offices/ODS/medication_guides.htm.

Pregnancy Risk Factor C/D (3rd trimester)

Medication Safety Issues

Sound-alike/look-alike issues:

Fenoprofen may be confused with flurbiprofen

Nalfon® may be confused with Naldecon®

Dosage Adults: Oral:

Rheumatoid arthritis, osteoarthritis: 300-600 mg 3-4 times/day; maximum dose: 3.2 g/day

Mild-to-moderate pain: 200 mg every 4-6 hours as needed; maximum dose: 3.2 g/day

Dosage adjustment in renal impairment: Not recommended in patients with advanced renal disease

Additional Information Complete prescribing information for this medication should be consulted for additional detail.

Dosage Forms Excipient information presented when available (limited, particularly for generics); consult specific product labeling.

Capsule, as calcium:

Nalfon®: 200 mg

Tablet, as calcium: 600 mg

◆ **Fenoprofen Calcium** *see* Fenoprofen *on page 610*

FentaNYL (FEN ta nil)

U.S. Brand Names Actiq®; Duragesic®; Fentora®; Sublimaze®

Canadian Brand Names Actiq®; Duragesic®; Fentanyl Citrate Injection, USP; RAN™-Fentanyl Transdermal System; ratio-Fentanyl

Index Terms Fentanyl Citrate; Fentanyl Hydrochloride; OTFC (Oral Transmucosal Fentanyl Citrate)

Pharmacologic Category Analgesic, Opioid; Anilidopiperidine Opioid; General Anesthetic

Use

Injection: Sedation, relief of pain, preoperative medication, adjunct to general or regional anesthesia

Transdermal patch (eg, Duragesic®): Management of persistent moderate-to-severe chronic pain

Transmucosal lozenge (eg, Actiq®), buccal tablet (Fentora®): Management of breakthrough cancer pain in opioid-tolerant patients

Restrictions C-II

An FDA-approved medication guide for buccal tablet (Fentora®), transmucosal lozenge (eg, Actiq®), and transdermal patch (eg, Duragesic®) must be distributed when dispensing an outpatient prescription (new or refill) where this medication is to be used without direct supervision of a healthcare provider. Medication guides are available at http://www.fda.gov/cder/Offices/ODS/medication_guides.htm.

Pregnancy Risk Factor C/D (prolonged use or high doses at term)

Pregnancy Considerations Fentanyl crosses the placenta and has been used safely during labor. Chronic use during pregnancy has shown detectable serum levels in the newborn with mild opioid withdrawal (case report). Transdermal patch, transmucosal lozenge, and buccal tablet (Fentora®) are not recommended for analgesia during labor and delivery.

Lactation Enters breast milk/not recommended (AAP rates "compatible")

Medication Safety Issues

Sound-alike/look-alike issues:

FentaNYL may be confused with alfentanil, SUFentanil

Dosing of transdermal fentanyl patches may be confusing. Transdermal fentanyl patches should always be prescribed in mcg/hour, not size. Patch dosage form of Duragesic®-12 actually delivers 12.5 mcg/hour of fentanyl. Use caution, as orders may be written as "Duragesic 12.5" which can be erroneously interpreted as a 125 mcg dose.

Fentora® and Actiq® are not interchangeable; do not substitute doses on a mcg-per-mcg basis.

High alert medication: The Institute for Safe Medication Practices (ISMP) includes this medication among its list of drug classes which have a heightened risk of causing significant patient harm when used in error.

Fentanyl transdermal system patches: Leakage of fentanyl gel from the patch has been reported; patch may be less effective; do not use. Thoroughly wash any skin surfaces coming into direct contact with gel with water (do not use soap).

Transdermal patch (eg, Duragesic®) does not contain any metal-based compounds; however, the printed ink used to indicate strength on the outer surface of the patch does contain titanium dioxide, but the amount is minimal.

Contraindications Hypersensitivity to fentanyl or any component of the formulation

Transdermal system: Severe respiratory disease or depression including acute asthma (unless patient is mechanically ventilated); paralytic ileus; patients requiring short-term therapy, management of intermittent pain

Transmucosal buccal tablets (Fentora®), lozenges (eg, Actiq®), and/or transdermal patches (eg, Duragesic®): Contraindicated in the management of acute or post-operative pain and in patients who are not opioid tolerant

Warnings/Precautions An opioid-containing analgesic regimen should be tailored to each patient's needs and based upon the type of pain being treated (acute versus chronic), the route of administration, degree of tolerance for opioids (naive versus chronic user), age, weight, and medical condition. The optimal analgesic dose varies widely among patients. Doses should be titrated to pain relief/prevention. When using with other CNS depressants, reduce dose of one or both agents. Fentanyl shares the toxic potentials of opiate agonists, and precautions of opiate agonist therapy should be observed; use with caution in patients with bradycardia or bradyarrhythmias; rapid I.V. infusion may result in skeletal muscle and chest wall rigidity leading to respiratory distress and/or apnea, bronchoconstriction, laryngospasm; inject slowly over 3-5 minutes. **[U.S. Boxed Warning]: Healthcare provider should be alert to problems of abuse, misuse, and diversion.** Tolerance or drug dependence may result from extended use. The elderly may be particularly susceptible to the CNS depressant and constipating effects of narcotics. Use extreme caution in patients with COPD or other chronic respiratory conditions. Use caution with head injuries, morbid obesity, renal impairment, or hepatic dysfunction. **[U.S. Boxed Warning]: Use with strong or moderate CYP3A4 inhibitors may result in increased effects and potential respiratory depression.** Concurrent use of agonist/antagonist analgesics may precipitate withdrawal symptoms and/or reduced analgesic efficacy in patients following prolonged therapy with mu opioid agonists. Abrupt discontinuation following prolonged use may also lead to withdrawal symptoms. Safety and efficacy have not been established in children <16 years of age for the lozenge and <18 years of age for the buccal tablet. **[U.S. Boxed Warning]: Safety and efficacy of the transdermal patch have been limited to children ≥2 years of age who are opioid-tolerant.**

[U.S. Boxed Warning] Actiq®, Duragesic®, Fentora®: May cause potentially life-threatening hypoventilation, respiratory depression, and/or death; Actiq®, Duragesic®, Fentora® should only be prescribed for opioid-tolerant patients. Risk of respiratory depression increased in elderly patients, debilitated patients, and patients with conditions associated with hypoxia or hypercapnia; usually occurs after administration of initial dose in nontolerant patients or when given with other drugs that depress respiratory function.

Transmucosal: Lozenge (eg, Actiq®), buccal tablet (Fentora®): **[U.S. Boxed Warning]: Should be used only for the care of opioid-tolerant cancer patients with breakthrough pain and is intended for use by specialists who are knowledgeable in treating cancer pain.** Not approved for use in management of acute or postoperative pain. **[U.S. Boxed Warning]: Buccal tablet and lozenge preparations contain an amount of medication that can be fatal to children. Keep all units out of the reach of children and discard any open units properly.** Patients and caregivers should be counseled on the dangers to children including the risk of exposure to partially-consumed units.

Transmucosal: Buccal tablet (Fentora®): **[U.S. Boxed Warning]: Due to the higher bioavailability of fentanyl in Fentora®, when converting patients from oral transmucosal fentanyl citrate (OTFC, Actiq®) to Fentora®, do not substitute Fentora®): on a mcg-per-mcg basis for any other fentanyl product. [U.S. Boxed Warning]: Fentora® is contraindicated in the management of acute or postoperative pain, including headache/migraine. Serious adverse events, including death, have been reported when used inappropriately (improper dose or patient selection). [U.S. Boxed Warning]: Patients using Fentora® who experience breakthrough pain may only take one additional dose using the same strength and must wait four hours before taking another dose.**

Transdermal patches (eg, Duragesic®): **[U.S. Boxed Warning]: Indicated for the management of persistent moderate-to-severe pain when around the clock pain control is needed for an extended time period. Should only be used in patients who are already receiving opioid therapy, are opioid tolerant, and who require a total daily dose equivalent to 25 mcg/hour transdermal patch. Contraindicated in patients who are not opioid tolerant, in the management of short-term analgesia, or in the management of postoperative pain. Should be applied only to intact skin. Use of a patch that has been cut, damaged, or altered in any way may result in overdosage.** Serum fentanyl concentrations may increase approximately one-third for patients with a body temperature of 40°C secondary to a temperature-dependent increase in fentanyl release from the patch and increased skin permeability. **[U.S. Boxed Warning]: Avoid exposure of application site and surrounding area to direct external heat sources.** Patients who experience fever or increase in core temperature should be monitored closely. Patients who experience adverse reactions should be monitored for at least 24 hours after removal of the patch. Transdermal patch does not contain any metal-based compounds; the printed ink used to indicate strength on the outer surface of the patch does contain titanium dioxide, but the amount is minimal; adverse events have not been reported while wearing during an MRI.

Adverse Reactions

>10%:

Cardiovascular: Bradycardia, edema

Central nervous system: CNS depression, confusion, dizziness, drowsiness, headache, sedation

Gastrointestinal: Nausea, vomiting, constipation, xerostomia

Local: Application-site reaction erythema

Neuromuscular & skeletal: Chest wall rigidity (high dose I.V.), muscle rigidity, weakness

Ocular: Miosis

Respiratory: Dyspnea, respiratory depression

Miscellaneous: Diaphoresis

1% to 10%:

Cardiovascular: Cardiac arrhythmia, chest pain, flushing, hyper-/hypotension, orthostatic hypotension, pallor, palpitation, peripheral edema, syncope, tachycardia, vasodilation

Central nervous system: Abnormal dreams, abnormal thinking, agitation, amnesia, anxiety, chills, depression, euphoria, fatigue, fever, hallucinations, hypoesthesia, insomnia, lethargy, migraine, nervousness, paranoid reaction, stupor, vertigo

Dermatologic: Alopecia, bruising, cellulitis, erythema, hyperhidrosis, papules, pruritus, rash

Endocrine & metabolic: Breast pain, dehydration, hyper-/hypocalcemia, hyper-/hypoglycemia, hypoalbuminemia, hypokalemia, hypomagnesemia

Gastrointestinal: Abdominal pain, abnormal taste, anorexia, biliary tract spasm, diarrhea, dyspepsia, dysphagia (buccal tablet), flatulence, GI hemorrhage, gingival pain (buccal tablet), gingivitis (lozenge), glossitis (lozenge), ileus, periodontal abscess (lozenge/buccal tablet), stomatitis (lozenge/buccal tablet), weight loss

Genitourinary: Dysuria, urinary incontinence, urinary retention, vaginitis, vaginal hemorrhage

Hematologic: Anemia, leukopenia, neutropenia, thrombocytopenia

Hepatic: Ascites, jaundice

Local: Application site pain, application site irritation

Neuromuscular & skeletal: Abnormal coordination, abnormal gait, arthralgia, back pain, myalgia, neuropathy, paresthesia, rigors, tremor

Renal: Renal failure

Respiratory: Apnea, asthma, bronchitis, cough, epistaxis, hemoptysis, hypoventilation, hypoxia, nasopharyngitis, pharyngolaryngeal pain, pharyngitis, pneumonia, rhinitis, sinusitis, upper respiratory infection, wheezing

Miscellaneous: Hiccups, flu-like syndrome, lymphadenopathy, speech disorder

<1% (Limited to important or life-threatening): Abdominal distention, amblyopia, allergic reaction, anaphylaxis, angina, anorgasmia, aphasia, bladder pain, blurred vision, bronchospasm, CNS excitation or delirium, cold/clammy skin, dental caries (lozenge), depersonalization, DVT, dysesthesia, ejaculatory difficulty, emotional lability, eructation, esophageal stenosis, exfoliative dermatitis, fecal impaction, flank pain, gum line erosion (lozenge), gum hemorrhage (lozenge), hematuria, hostility, hyper-/hypotonia, laryngospasm, libido decreased, moniliasis (lozenge/buccal tablet), mouth ulceration (lozenge/buccal tablet), myasthenia, nocturia, oliguria, pancytopenia, paradoxical dizziness, physical and psychological dependence with prolonged use, pleural effusion, polyuria, pustules, speech disorder, stertorous breathing, seizure, sputum increased, tooth loss (lozenge), urinary tract spasm, urticaria, vertigo

Drug Interactions

Metabolism/Transport Effects **Substrate** of CYP3A4 (major); **Inhibits** CYP3A4 (weak)

Avoid Concomitant Use There are no known interactions where it is recommended to avoid concomitant use.

Increased Effect/Toxicity

FentaNYL may increase the levels/effects of: Alcohol (Ethyl); Alvimopan; Beta-Blockers; Calcium Channel Blockers (Nondihydropyridine); CNS Depressants; Desmopressin; MAO Inhibitors; Selective Serotonin Reuptake Inhibitors

The levels/effects of FentaNYL may be increased by: Amphetamines; Antipsychotic Agents (Phenothiazines); CYP3A4 Inhibitors (Moderate); CYP3A4 Inhibitors (Strong); Dasatinib; Protease Inhibitors; Succinylcholine

Decreased Effect

FentaNYL may decrease the levels/effects of: Pegvisomant

The levels/effects of FentaNYL may be decreased by: Ammonium Chloride; Rifamycin Derivatives

Ethanol/Nutrition/Herb Interactions

Ethanol: Avoid ethanol (may increase CNS depression).

Herb/Nutraceutical: St John's wort may decrease fentanyl levels. Avoid valerian, St John's wort, kava kava, gotu kola (may increase CNS depression).

Stability

Injection formulation: Store at controlled room temperature of 20°C to 25°C (68°F to 77°F). Protect from light.

Transdermal patch: Do not store above 25°C (77°F).

Transmucosal (buccal tablets, lozenge): Store at controlled room temperature of 20°C to 25°C (68°F to 77°F). Protect from freezing and moisture.

Mechanism of Action Binds with stereospecific receptors at many sites within the CNS, increases pain threshold, alters pain reception, inhibits ascending pain pathways

Pharmacodynamics/Kinetics

Onset of action: Analgesic: I.M.: 7-8 minutes; I.V.: Almost immediate; Transmucosal: 5-15 minutes

Peak effect: Transmucosal: Analgesic: 15-30 minutes

Duration: I.M.: 1-2 hours; I.V.: 0.5-1 hour; Transmucosal: Related to blood level; respiratory depressant effect may last longer than analgesic effect

Absorption:

Transdermal: Initial application: Gradually absorbed for the first 12-24 hours, followed by a constant absorption for the remainder of the dosing interval

Transmucosal, buccal tablet: Rapid, ~50% from the buccal mucosa; remaining 50% swallowed with saliva and slowly absorbed from GI tract.

Transmucosal, lozenge: Rapid, ~25% from the buccal mucosa; 75% swallowed with saliva and slowly absorbed from GI tract

Distribution: 4-6 L/kg; Highly lipophilic, redistributes into muscle and fat

Protein binding: 80% to 85%

Metabolism: Hepatic, primarily via CYP3A4

Bioavailability: Total (transmucosal and GI absorption): Buccal: 65% (range: 45% to 85%); Lozenge: 47% (range: 37% to 57%)

Half-life elimination:

I.V.: 2-4 hours

Transdermal patch: 17 hours (13-22 hours, half-life is influenced by absorption rate)

Transmucosal: Lozenge: 7 hours; Buccal tablet: 100-200 mcg: 3-4 hours, 400-800 mcg: 11-12 hours

Time to peak: Buccal tablet: 20-240 minutes (median: 47 minutes); Lozenge: 20-480 minutes (median: 20-40 minutes); Transdermal patch: 24-72 hours, after several sequential 72-hour applications, steady state serum concentrations are reached

Excretion: Urine 75% (primarily as metabolites, <7% to 10% as unchanged drug); feces ~9%

Dosage Note: These are guidelines and do not represent the maximum doses that may be required in all patients. Doses and dosage intervals should be titrated to pain relief/prevention. Monitor vital signs routinely. Single I.M. doses have a duration of 1-2 hours, single I.V. doses last 0.5-1 hour.

Minor procedures/analgesia (unlabeled use): I.V.:

Children 1-12 years: 0.5-2 mcg/kg/dose given 3 minutes prior to procedure; may repeat every 1-2 hours

Children >12 years: 0.5-2 mcg/kg/dose (maximum 50 mcg/dose) given 3 minutes prior to procedure; may repeat in 5 minutes if necessary; if more than 2 doses are needed, repeat with a maximum of 25 mcg/dose up to 5 times

Surgery:

Children ≥2 years: Adjunct to anesthesia (induction and maintenance): Slow I.V.: 2-3 mcg/kg/dose every 1-2 hours as needed

Adults:

Premedication: I.M., slow I.V.: 50-100 mcg/dose 30-60 minutes prior to surgery

Adjunct to regional anesthesia: Slow I.V.: 25-100 mcg/dose over 1-2 minutes. **Note:** An I.V. should be in place with regional anesthesia so the I.M. route is rarely used but still maintained as an option in the package labeling.

Adjunct to general anesthesia: Slow I.V.:

Low dose: 0.5-2 mcg/kg/dose depending on the indication

Moderate dose: Initial: 2-20 mcg/kg/dose; Maintenance (bolus or infusion): 1-2 mcg/kg/hour. Discontinuing fentanyl infusion 30-60 minutes prior to the end of surgery will usually allow adequate ventilation upon emergence from anesthesia. For "fast-tracking" and early extubation following major surgery, total fentanyl doses are limited to 10-15 mcg/kg.

High-dose: 20-50 mcg/kg/dose; **Note:** Fentanyl is rarely used, but is still maintained in the package labeling.

Pain management:

Children (unlabeled use): I.V.: 0.5-2 mcg/kg/dose given every 1-2 hours as needed; continuous infusion: 0.5-2 mcg/kg/hour; titrate to desired effects

Adults:

I.V. (unlabeled use): Bolus at start of infusion: 1-2 mcg/kg **or** 25-100 mcg/dose; continuous infusion rate: 1-2 mcg/kg/hour **or** 25-200 mcg/hour

Severe: I.M, I.V. (unlabeled): 50-100 mcg/dose every 1-2 hours as needed; patients with prior opiate exposure may tolerate higher initial doses

Patient-controlled analgesia (PCA) (unlabeled use): I.V.: Usual concentration: 10 mcg/mL

Basal rate: ≤50 mcg/hour

Demand dose: Usual: 10 mcg; range: 10-50 mcg

Lockout interval: 5-10 minutes

Critically-ill patients (unlabeled dose): Slow I.V.: 25-100 mcg (based on ~70 kg patient) **or** 0.35-1.5 mcg/kg every 30-60 minutes as needed. **Note:** More frequent dosing may be needed (eg, mechanically-ventilated patients).

Continuous infusion: 50-700 mcg/hour (based on ~70 kg patient) **or** 0.7-10 mcg/kg/hour

Breakthrough cancer pain: For patients who are tolerant to and currently receiving opioid therapy for persistent cancer pain; dosing should be individually titrated to provide adequate analgesia with minimal side effects. Dose titration should be done if patient requires more than 1 dose/breakthrough pain episode for several consecutive episodes. Patients experiencing >4 breakthrough pain episodes/day should have the dose of their long-term opioid re-evaluated.

Children ≥16 years and Adults: Lozenge: Initial dose: 200 mcg; the second dose may be started 15 minutes after completion of the first dose. Consumption should be limited to ≤4 units/day. Additional requirements suggest need for improved baseline therapy.

Adults: Buccal tablet (Fentora®): Initial dose: 100 mcg; a second 100 mcg dose, if needed, may be started 30 minutes after the start of the first dose. **Note:** For patients previously using the transmucosal lozenge (Actiq®), the initial dose should be selected using the conversions listed below (maximum: 2 doses per breakthrough pain episode every 4 hours).

Dose titration, if required, should be done using multiples of the 100 mcg tablets. Patient can take two 100 mcg tablets (one on each side of mouth). If that dose is not successful, can use four 100 mcg tablets (two on each side of mouth). If titration requires >400 mcg/dose, then use 200 mcg tablets.

Conversion from lozenge to buccal tablet (Fentora®):

Lozenge dose 200-400 mcg, then buccal tablet 100 mcg

Lozenge dose 600-800 mcg, then buccal tablet 200 mcg

Lozenge dose 1200-1600 mcg, then buccal tablet 400 mcg

Note: Four 100 mcg buccal tablets deliver approximately 12% and 13% higher values of C_{max} and AUC, respectively, compared to one 400 mcg buccal tablet. To prevent confusion, patient should only have one strength available at a time. Using more than four buccal tablets at a time has not been studied.

Elderly >65 years: Transmucosal lozenge (eg, Actiq®): In clinical trials, patients who were >65 years of age were titrated to a mean dose that was 200 mcg less than that of younger patients.

Chronic pain management: Children ≥2 years and Adults (opioid-tolerant patients): Transdermal patch (eg, Duragesic®):

Initial: To convert patients from oral or parenteral opioids to transdermal patch, a 24-hour analgesic requirement should be calculated (based on prior opiate use). Using the tables, the appropriate initial dose can be determined. The initial fentanyl dosage may be approximated from the 24-hour morphine dosage equivalent and titrated to minimize adverse effects and provide analgesia. With the initial application, the absorption of transdermal fentanyl requires several hours to reach plateau; therefore transdermal fentanyl is inappropriate for management of acute pain. Change patch every 72 hours.

Conversion from continuous infusion of fentanyl: In patients who have adequate pain relief with a fentanyl infusion, fentanyl may be converted to transdermal dosing at a rate equivalent to the intravenous rate. A two-step taper of the infusion to be completed over 12 hours has been recommended (Kornick, 2001) after the patch is applied. The infusion is decreased to 50% of the original rate six hours after the application of the first patch, and subsequently discontinued twelve hours after application.

Titration: Short-acting agents may be required until analgesic efficacy is established and/or as supplements for "breakthrough" pain. The amount of supplemental doses should be closely monitored. Appropriate dosage increases may be based on daily supplemental dosage using the ratio of 45 mg/24 hours of oral morphine to a 12.5 mcg/hour increase in fentanyl dosage.

Frequency of adjustment: The dosage should not be titrated more frequently than every 3 days after the initial dose or every 6 days thereafter. Patients should wear a consistent fentanyl dosage through two applications (6 days) before dosage increase based on supplemental opiate dosages can be estimated. **Note:** Upon discontinuation, ~17 hours are required for a 50% decrease in fentanyl levels.

Frequency of application: The majority of patients may be controlled on every 72-hour administration; however, a small number of patients require every 48-hour administration.

Dose conversion guidelines for transdermal fentanyl[1] (see tables).

Recommended Initial Duragesic® Dose Based Upon Daily Oral Morphine Dose[1]

Oral 24-Hour Morphine (mg/d)	Duragesic® Dose (mcg/h)
60-134[2]	25
135-224	50
225-314	75
315-404	100
405-494	125
495-584	150
585-674	175
675-764	200
765-854	225
855-944	250
945-1034	275
1035-1124	300

[1]The table should NOT be used to convert from transdermal fentanyl (eg, Duragesic®) to other opioid analgesics. Rather, following removal of the patch, titrate the dose of the new opioid until adequate analgesia is achieved.

[2]Pediatric patients initiating therapy on a 25 mcg/hour Duragesic® system should be opioid-tolerant and receiving at least 60 mg oral morphine equivalents per day.

Dosing Conversion Guidelines[1,2]

Current Analgesic	Daily Dosage (mg/day)			
Morphine (I.M./I.V.)	10-22	23-37	38-52	53-67
Oxycodone (oral)	30-67	67.5-112	112.5-157	157.5-202
Oxycodone (I.M./I.V.)	15-33	33.1-56	56.1-78	78.1-101
Codeine (oral)	150-447	448-747	748-1047	1048-1347
Hydromorphone (oral)	8-17	17.1-28	28.1-39	39.1-51
Hydromorphone (I.V.)	1.5-3.4	3.5-5.6	5.7-7.9	8-10
Meperidine (I.M.)	75-165	166-278	279-390	391-503
Methadone (oral)	20-44	45-74	75-104	105-134
Methadone (I.M.)	10-22	23-37	38-52	53-67
Fentanyl transdermal recommended dose (mcg/h)	**25 mcg/h**	**50 mcg/h**	**75 mcg/h**	**100 mcg/h**

[1]The table should NOT be used to convert from transdermal fentanyl (eg, Duragesic®) to other opioid analgesics. Rather, following removal of the patch, titrate the dose of the new opioid until adequate analgesia is achieved.

[2]Duragesic® product insert, Janssen Pharmaceutica, Feb 2008.

Opioid Analgesics Initial Oral Dosing Commonly Used for Severe Pain

Drug	Equianalgesic Dose (mg)		Initial Oral Dose	
	Oral[1]	Parenteral[2]	Children (mg/kg)	Adults (mg)
Buprenorphine	—	0.4	—	—
Butorphanol	—	2	—	—
Hydromorphone	7.5	1.5	0.06	4-8
Levorphanol	Acute: 4 Chronic: 1	Acute: 2 Chronic: 1	0.04	2-4
Meperidine	300	75	Not recommended	
Methadone	10	5	0.2	5-10
Morphine	30	10	0.3	15-30
Nalbuphine	—	10	—	—
Pentazocine	50	30	—	—
Oxycodone	20	—	0.3	10-20
Oxymorphone	—	1	—	—

From "Principles of Analgesic Use in the Treatment of Acute Pain and Cancer Pain," *Am Pain Soc*, Fifth Ed.

[1]Elderly: Starting dose should be lower for this population group

[2]Standard parenteral doses for acute pain in adults; can be used to doses for I.V. infusions and repeated small I.V. boluses. Single I.V. boluses, use half the I.M. dose. Children >6 months: I.V. dose = parenteral equianalgesic dose x weight (kg)/100

Dosing adjustment in hepatic impairment: Actiq®: Although fentanyl kinetics may be altered in hepatic disease, Actiq® can be used successfully in the management of breakthrough cancer pain. Doses should be titrated to reach clinical effect with careful monitoring of patients with severe hepatic disease.

Dietary Considerations Transmucosal lozenge contains 2 g sugar per unit.

Administration

I.V.: Administer as slow I.V. infusion over 1-2 minutes. May also be administered as continuous infusion or PCA (unlabeled use) routes. Muscular rigidity may occur with rapid I.V. administration.

Transdermal patch (eg, Duragesic®): Apply to nonirritated and nonirradiated skin, such as chest, back, flank, or upper arm. Do not shave skin; hair at application site should be clipped. Prior to application, clean site with clear water and allow to dry completely. Do not use damaged, cut or leaking patches; patch may be less effective. Skin exposure from fentanyl gel leaking from patch may lead to serious adverse effects; thoroughly wash affected skin surfaces with water (do not use soap). Firmly press in place and hold for 30 seconds. Change patch every 72 hours. Do **not** use soap, alcohol, or other solvents to remove transdermal gel if it accidentally touches skin; use copious amounts of water. Avoid exposing application site to external heat sources (eg, heating pad, electric blanket, heat lamp, hot tub).

Lozenge: Foil overwrap should be removed just prior to administration. Place the unit in mouth and allow it to dissolve. Do not chew. Lozenge may be moved from one side of the mouth to the other. The unit should be consumed over a period of 15 minutes. Handle should be removed after it is consumed or if patient has achieved an adequate response and/or shows signs of respiratory depression.

Buccal tablet: Patient should not open blister until ready to administer. The blister backing should be peeled back to expose the tablet; tablet should not be pushed out through the blister. Immediately use tablet once removed from blister. Place entire tablet in the buccal cavity (above a rear molar, between the upper cheek and gum). Tablet should not be broken, sucked, chewed, or swallowed. Should dissolve in about 14-25 minutes when left between the cheek and the gum. If remnants remain they may be swallowed with water.

Monitoring Parameters Respiratory and cardiovascular status, blood pressure, heart rate; signs of misuse, abuse, or addiction

Transdermal patch: Monitor for 24 hours after application of first dose

Additional Information Fentanyl is 50-100 times as potent as morphine; morphine 10 mg I.M. is equivalent to fentanyl 0.1-0.2 mg I.M.; fentanyl has less hypotensive effects than morphine due to lack of histamine release. However, fentanyl may cause rigidity with high doses. If the patient has required high-dose analgesia or has used for a prolonged period (~7 days), taper dose to prevent withdrawal; monitor for signs and symptoms of withdrawal.

Transmucosal (oral lozenge): Disposal of lozenge units: After consumption of a complete unit, the handle may be disposed of in a trash container that is out of the reach of children. For a partially-consumed unit, or a unit that still has any drug matrix remaining on the handle, the handle should be placed under hot running tap water until the drug matrix has dissolved. Special child-resistant containers are available to temporarily store partially consumed units that cannot be disposed of immediately.

Transdermal patch (Duragesic®): Upon removal of the patch, ~17 hours are required before serum concentrations fall to 50% of their original values. Opioid withdrawal symptoms are possible. Gradual downward titration (potentially by the sequential use of lower-dose patches) is recommended. Keep transdermal patch (both used and unused) out of the reach of children. Do **not** use soap, alcohol, or other solvents to remove transdermal gel if it accidentally touches skin as they may increase transdermal absorption, use copious amounts of water. Avoid exposure of direct external heat sources (eg, heating pads, electric blankets, heat lamps, saunas, hot tubs, heated water beds) to application site.

Dosage Forms Excipient information presented when available (limited, particularly for generics); consult specific product labeling.

Note: Strengths expressed as base.

Injection, solution, as citrate [preservative free]: 0.05 mg/mL (2 mL, 5 mL, 10 mL, 20 mL; 30 mL [DSC]; 50 mL)

Sublimaze®: 0.05 mg/mL (2 mL, 5 mL, 10 mL [DSC], 20 mL)

Lozenge, oral, as citrate [transmucosal]: 200 mcg, 400 mcg, 600 mcg, 800 mcg, 1200 mcg, 1600 mcg

Actiq®: 200 mcg, 400 mcg, 600 mcg, 800 mcg, 1200 mcg, 1600 mcg [contains sugar 2 g/lozenge; berry flavor]

Powder, for prescription compounding, as citrate: USP (1 g)

Tablet, for buccal application, as citrate:

Fentora®: 100 mcg, 200 mcg, 300 mcg, 400 mcg, 600 mcg, 800 mcg

Transdermal system, topical, as base: 12 (5s) [delivers 12.5 mcg/hour; 3.13 cm^2]; 12 (5s) [delivers 12.5 mcg/hour; 5 cm^2]; 25 (5s) [delivers 25 mcg/hour; 10 cm^2]; 25 (5s) [delivers 25 mcg/hour; 6.25 cm^2]; 50 (5s) [delivers 50 mcg/hour; 12.5 cm^2]; 50 (5s) [delivers 50 mcg/hour; 20 cm^2]; 75 (5s) [delivers 75 mcg/hour; 18.75 cm^2]; 75 (5s) [delivers 75 mcg/hour; 30 cm^2]; 75 (5s) [delivers 75 mcg/hour; 32.1 cm^2]; 100 (5s) [delivers 100 mcg/hour; 25 cm^2]; 100 (5s) [delivers 100 mcg/hour; 40 cm^2]; 100 (5s) [delivers 100 mcg/hour; 42.8 cm^2]

Duragesic®: 12 (5s) [delivers 12.5 mcg/hour; 5 cm^2; contains ethanol 0.1 mL/10 cm^2]; 25 (5s) [delivers 25 mcg/hour; 10 cm^2; contains ethanol 0.1 mL/10 cm^2]; 50 (5s) [delivers 50 mcg/hour; 20 cm^2; contains ethanol 0.1 mL/10 cm^2]; 75 (5s) [delivers 75 mcg/hour; 30 cm^2; contains ethanol 0.1 mL/10 cm^2]; 100 (5s) [delivers 100 mcg/hour; 40 cm^2; contains ethanol 0.1 mL/10 cm^2]

◆ **Fentanyl Citrate** *see* FentaNYL *on page 610*

◆ **Fentanyl Citrate Injection, USP (Can)** *see* FentaNYL *on page 610*

◆ **Fentanyl Hydrochloride** *see* FentaNYL *on page 610*

◆ **Fentora®** *see* FentaNYL *on page 610*

◆ **Feosol® [OTC]** *see* Ferrous Sulfate *on page 617*

◆ **Feostat® [OTC] [DSC]** *see* Ferrous Fumarate *on page 616*

◆ **Feratab® [OTC]** *see* Ferrous Sulfate *on page 617*

◆ **Fer-Gen-Sol [OTC]** *see* Ferrous Sulfate *on page 617*

◆ **Fergon® [OTC]** *see* Ferrous Gluconate *on page 616*

◆ **Fer-In-Sol® [OTC]** *see* Ferrous Sulfate *on page 617*

◆ **Fer-In-Sol® (Can)** *see* Ferrous Sulfate *on page 617*

◆ **Fer-iron® [OTC]** *see* Ferrous Sulfate *on page 617*

◆ **Ferodan™ (Can)** *see* Ferrous Sulfate *on page 617*

◆ **Fero-Grad 500® [OTC]** *see* Ferrous Sulfate and Ascorbic Acid *on page 617*

◆ **Ferretts [OTC]** *see* Ferrous Fumarate *on page 616*

◆ **Ferrex 150 [OTC]** *see* Polysaccharide-Iron Complex *on page 1212*

◆ **Ferric (III) Hexacyanoferrate (II)** *see* Ferric Hexacyanoferrate *on page 615*

Ferric Gluconate (FER ik GLOO koe nate)

U.S. Brand Names Ferrlecit®

Canadian Brand Names Ferrlecit®

Index Terms Sodium Ferric Gluconate

Pharmacologic Category Iron Salt

Use Repletion of total body iron content in patients with iron-deficiency anemia who are undergoing hemodialysis in conjunction with erythropoietin therapy

Pregnancy Risk Factor B

Medication Safety Issues

Sound-alike/look-alike issues:

Ferrlecit® may be confused with Ferralet®

Dosage I.V.: Repletion of iron in hemodialysis patients:

Children ≥6 years: 1.5 mg/kg of elemental iron (maximum: 125 mg/dose) diluted in NS 25 mL, administered over 60 minutes at 8 sequential dialysis sessions

Adults: 125 mg elemental iron per 10 mL (either by I.V. infusion or slow I.V. injection). Most patients will require a cumulative dose of 1 g elemental iron over approximately 8 sequential dialysis treatments to achieve a favorable response.

Note: A test dose of 2 mL diluted in NS 50 mL administered over 60 minutes was previously recommended (not in current manufacturer labeling). Doses >125 mg are associated with increased adverse events.

Additional Information Complete prescribing information for this medication should be consulted for additional detail.

Dosage Forms Excipient information presented when available (limited, particularly for generics); consult specific product labeling.

Injection, solution:

Ferrlecit®: Elemental iron 12.5 mg/mL (5 mL) [contains benzyl alcohol and sucrose 20%]

Ferric Hexacyanoferrate

(FER ik hex a SYE an oh fer ate)

U.S. Brand Names Radiogardase®

Index Terms Ferric (III) Hexacyanoferrate (II); Insoluble Prussian Blue; Prussian Blue

Pharmacologic Category Antidote

Use Treatment of known or suspected internal contamination with radioactive cesium and/or radioactive or nonradioactive thallium

Pregnancy Risk Factor C

Dosage Oral: Internal contamination with radioactive cesium and/or radioactive or nonradioactive thallium:

Children 2-12 years: 1 g 3 times/day; treatment should begin as soon as possible following exposure, but is also effective if therapy is delayed

Children >12 years and Adults: 3 g 3 times/day; treatment should begin as soon as possible following exposure, but is also effective if therapy is delayed

Note: Cesium exposure: Once internal radioactivity is substantially decreased, dosage may be reduced to 1-2 g 3 times/day to improve gastrointestinal tolerance

Elderly: Refer to adult dosing

Dosage adjustment in renal impairment: Studies have not been conducted; however, ferric hexacyanoferrate is not renally eliminated.

Dosage adjustment in hepatic impairment: Studies have not been conducted; however, effectiveness may be decreased due to decreased bile excretion of cesium and thallium.

Additional Information Complete prescribing information for this medication should be consulted for additional detail.

Dosage Forms Excipient information presented when available (limited, particularly for generics); consult specific product labeling.

Capsule: 0.5 g

◆ **Ferrlecit®** *see* Ferric Gluconate *on page 615*

◆ **Ferro-Sequels® [OTC]** *see* Ferrous Fumarate *on page 616*

Ferrous Fumarate (FER us FYOO ma rate)

U.S. Brand Names Femiron® [OTC]; Feostat® [OTC] [DSC]; Ferretts [OTC]; Ferro-Sequels® [OTC]; Hemocyte® [OTC]; Ircon® [OTC]; Nephro-Fer® [OTC]

Canadian Brand Names Palafer®

Index Terms Iron Fumarate

Pharmacologic Category Iron Salt

Use Prevention and treatment of iron-deficiency anemias

Medication Safety Issues

Sound-alike/look-alike issues:

Feostat® may be confused with Feosol®

Dosage

Dietary Reference Intake: Dose is RDA presented as elemental iron unless otherwise noted:

0-6 months: 0.27 mg/day (adequate intake)

7-12 months: 11 mg/day

1-3 years: 7 mg/day

4-8 years: 10 mg/day

9-13 years: 8 mg/day

14-18 years: Male: 11 mg/day; Female: 15 mg/day; Pregnant female: 27 mg/day; Lactating female: 10 mg/day

19-50 years: Male: 8 mg/day; Female: 18 mg/day; Pregnant female: 27 mg/day; Lactating female: 9 mg/day

≥50 years: 8 mg/day

Doses expressed in terms of elemental iron; elemental iron content of ferrous fumarate is 33%. Oral:

Children:

Severe iron-deficiency anemia: 4-6 mg elemental iron/kg/day in 3 divided doses

Mild to moderate iron deficiency anemia: 3 mg elemental iron/kg/day in 1-2 divided doses

Prophylaxis: 1-2 mg elemental iron/kg/day

Adults:

Iron deficiency: Usual range: 150-200 mg elemental iron/day in divided doses; 60-100 mg elemental iron twice daily, up to 60 mg elemental iron 4 times/day

Prophylaxis: 60-100 mg elemental iron/day

To avoid GI upset, start with a single daily dose and increase by 1 tablet/day each week or as tolerated until desired daily dose is achieved

Elderly: 200 mg elemental iron 3-4 times/day

Additional Information Complete prescribing information for this medication should be consulted for additional detail.

Dosage Forms Excipient information presented when available (limited, particularly for generics); consult specific product labeling. [DSC] = Discontinued product

Tablet: 324 mg [elemental iron 106 mg]

Femiron®: 63 mg [elemental iron 20 mg]

Ferretts: 325 mg [elemental iron 106 mg]

Hemocyte®: 324 mg [elemental iron 106 mg]

Ircon®: 200 mg [elemental iron 66 mg]

Nephro-Fer®: 350 mg [elemental iron 115 mg; contains tartrazine]

Tablet, chewable (Feostat®): 100 mg [elemental iron 33 mg; chocolate flavor] [DSC]

Tablet, timed release (Ferro-Sequels®): 150 mg [elemental iron 50 mg; contains docusate sodium and sodium benzoate]

Ferrous Gluconate (FER us GLOO koe nate)

U.S. Brand Names Fergon® [OTC]

Canadian Brand Names Apo-Ferrous Gluconate®; Novo-Ferrogluc

Index Terms Iron Gluconate

Pharmacologic Category Iron Salt

Use Prevention and treatment of iron-deficiency anemias

Dosage Oral:

Dietary Reference Intake: Dose is RDA presented as elemental iron unless otherwise noted:

0-6 months: 0.27 mg/day (adequate intake)

7-12 months: 11 mg/day

1-3 years: 7 mg/day

4-8 years: 10 mg/day

9-13 years: 8 mg/day

14-18 years: Male: 11 mg/day; Female: 15 mg/day; Pregnant female: 27 mg/day; Lactating female: 10 mg/day

19-50 years: Male: 8 mg/day; Female: 18 mg/day; Pregnant female: 27 mg/day; Lactating female: 9 mg/day

≥50 years: 8 mg/day

Dose expressed in terms of elemental iron:

Children:

Severe iron-deficiency anemia: 4-6 mg Fe/kg/day in 3 divided doses

Mild to moderate iron deficiency anemia: 3 mg Fe/kg/day in 1-2 divided doses

Prophylaxis: 1-2 mg Fe/kg/day

Adults:

Iron deficiency: 60 mg twice daily up to 60 mg 4 times/day

Prophylaxis: 60 mg/day

Additional Information Complete prescribing information for this medication should be consulted for additional detail.

Dosage Forms Excipient information presented when available (limited, particularly for generics); consult specific product labeling. [DSC] = Discontinued product

Tablet: 246 mg [elemental iron 28 mg]; 300 mg [elemental iron 34 mg] [DSC]; 325 mg [elemental iron 36 mg]

Fergon®: 240 mg [elemental iron 27 mg]

Ferrous Sulfate (FER us SUL fate)

U.S. Brand Names Feosol® [OTC]; Fer-Gen-Sol [OTC]; Fer-In-Sol® [OTC]; Fer-iron® [OTC]; Feratab® [OTC]; MyKidz Iron 10™; Slow FE® [OTC]

Canadian Brand Names Apo-Ferrous Sulfate®; Fer-In-Sol®; Ferodan™

Index Terms $FeSO_4$; Iron Sulfate

Pharmacologic Category Iron Salt

Use Prevention and treatment of iron-deficiency anemias

Medication Safety Issues

Sound-alike/look-alike issues:

Feosol® may be confused with Feostat®, Fer-In-Sol®

Fer-In-Sol® may be confused with Feosol®

Slow FE® may be confused with Slow-K®

Dosage Oral:

Dietary Reference Intake: Dose is RDA presented as elemental iron unless otherwise noted:

0-6 months: 0.27 mg/day (adequate intake)

7-12 months: 11 mg/day

1-3 years: 7 mg/day

4-8 years: 10 mg/day

9-13 years: 8 mg/day

14-18 years: Male: 11 mg/day; Female: 15 mg/day; Pregnant female: 27 mg/day; Lactating female: 10 mg/day

19-50 years: Male: 8 mg/day; Female: 18 mg/day; Pregnant female: 27 mg/day; Lactating female: 9 mg/day

≥50 years: 8 mg/day

Children **(dose expressed in terms of elemental iron)**:

Severe iron-deficiency anemia: 4-6 mg Fe/kg/day in 3 divided doses

Mild-to-moderate iron-deficiency anemia: 3 mg Fe/kg/day in 1-2 divided doses

Prophylaxis: 1-2 mg Fe/kg/day up to a maximum of 15 mg/day

Adults **(dose expressed in terms of ferrous sulfate)**:

Iron deficiency: 300 mg twice daily up to 300 mg 4 times/day or 250 mg (extended release) 1-2 times/day

Prophylaxis: 300 mg/day

Additional Information Complete prescribing information for this medication should be consulted for additional detail.

Dosage Forms Excipient information presented when available (limited, particularly for generics); consult specific product labeling.

Elixir, oral: 220 mg/5 mL (480 mL) [elemental iron 44 mg/5 mL; contains alcohol]

Liquid, oral: 300 mg/5 mL (5 mL) [elemental iron ~60 mg/5 mL]

Liquid, oral [drops]: 75 mg/0.6 mL (50 mL) [elemental iron 15 mg/0.6 mL]

Fer-Gen-Sol: 75 mg/0.6 mL (50 mL) [elemental iron 15 mg/0.6 mL]

Fer-In-Sol®: 75 mg/1 mL (50 mL) [elemental iron 15 mg/1 mL; contains ethanol 0.2% and sodium bisulfite]

Fer-iron®: 75 mg/0.6 mL (50 mL) [elemental iron 15 mg/0.6 mL; contains ethanol 0.2%; lemon flavor]

Suspension, oral [drops]:

MyKidz Iron 10™: 75 mg/1.5 mL [elemental iron 15 mg/1.5 mL] (118 mL) [contains propylene glycol; ethanol free, dye free; strawberry-banana flavor]

Tablet, oral: 324 mg [elemental iron 65 mg]; 325 mg [elemental iron 65 mg]

Feratab®: 300 mg [elemental iron 60 mg]

Tablet, oral [exsiccated]: 200 mg [elemental iron 65 mg]

Feosol®: 200 mg [elemental iron 65 mg]

Tablet, oral [exsiccated, timed release]: 160 mg [elemental iron 50 mg]

Slow FE®: 160 mg [elemental iron 50 mg]

Tablet, oral, slow release: 160 mg [elemental iron 50 mg]

Ferrous Sulfate and Ascorbic Acid

(FER us SUL fate & a SKOR bik AS id)

U.S. Brand Names Fero-Grad 500® [OTC]; Vitelle™ Irospan® [OTC] [DSC]

Index Terms Ascorbic Acid and Ferrous Sulfate; Iron Sulfate and Vitamin C

Pharmacologic Category Iron Salt; Vitamin

Use Treatment of iron deficiency in nonpregnant adults; treatment and prevention of iron deficiency in pregnant adults

Dosage Adults: Oral: 1 tablet daily

Additional Information Complete prescribing information for this medication should be consulted for additional detail.

Dosage Forms Excipient information presented when available (limited, particularly for generics); consult specific product labeling. [DSC] = Discontinued product

Capsule, extended release (Vitelle™ Irospan®): Ferrous sulfate [elemental iron 65 mg] and ascorbic acid 150 mg [DSC]

Tablet, controlled release (Fero-Grad 500®): Ferrous sulfate 525 mg [elemental iron 105 mg] and ascorbic acid 500 mg

Tablet, extended release (Vitelle™ Irospan®): Ferrous sulfate [elemental iron 65 mg] and ascorbic acid 150 mg [DSC]

◆ **Fertinorm® H.P. (Can)** *see* Urofollitropin *on page* *1531*

◆ **FESO** *see* Fesoterodine *on page* *617*

◆ **$FeSO_4$** *see* Ferrous Sulfate *on page* *617*

Fesoterodine (fes oh TER oh deen)

U.S. Brand Names Toviaz™

Index Terms FESO; Fesoterodine Fumarate

Pharmacologic Category Anticholinergic Agent

Use Treatment of patients with an overactive bladder with symptoms of urinary frequency, urgency, or urge incontinence.

Pregnancy Risk Factor C

Pregnancy Considerations Teratogenic effects were observed in some animal studies. There are no adequate and well-controlled studies in pregnant women. Use during pregnancy only if the potential benefit to the mother outweighs the possible risk to the fetus.

Lactation Excretion in breast milk unknown/not recommended

Medication Safety Issues

Sound-alike/look-alike issues:

Fesoterodine may be confused with fexofenadine, tolterodine

Contraindications Hypersensitivity to fesoterodine or any component of the formulation; urinary retention; gastric retention; uncontrolled narrow-angle glaucoma

Warnings/Precautions May cause drowsiness and/or blurred vision, which may impair physical or mental abilities; patients must be cautioned about performing tasks which require mental alertness (eg, operating machinery or driving). Patients may experience decreased sweating; caution use in hot weather or during exercise. Use is not recommended in patients with severe hepatic impairment (Child-Pugh class C). Doses >4 mg are not recommended for patients with severe renal impairment (Cl_{cr} <30 mL/minute) or patients receiving concurrent therapy with potent CYP3A4 inhibitors. Use caution in patients with bladder flow obstruction, gastrointestinal obstructive disorders, myasthenia gravis, and treated narrow-angle glaucoma. Risk of adverse effects may be increased in elderly patients. Safety and efficacy have not been established in children.

Adverse Reactions

>10%: Gastrointestinal: Xerostomia (19% to 35%; dose related)

1% to 10%:

Central nervous system: Insomnia (1%)

Dermatological: Rash (1%)

Gastrointestinal: Constipation (4% to 6%), dyspepsia (2%), nausea (1% to 2%), abdominal pain (1%)

Genitourinary: Urinary tract infection (3% to 4%), dysuria (1% to 2%), urinary retention (1%)

Hepatic: ALT increased (1%), GGT increased (1%)

Neuromuscular & skeletal: Back pain (1% to 2%)

Ocular: Dry eyes (1% to 4%)

Respiratory: Upper respiratory tract infection (2% to 3%), cough (1% to 2%), dry throat (1% to 2%)

Miscellaneous: Peripheral edema (1%)

<1%: Angina, blurred vision, chest pain, diverticulitis, gastroenteritis, heart rate increased (dose related), heat prostration, irritable bowel syndrome, QT_c prolongation

Drug Interactions

Avoid Concomitant Use There are no known interactions where it is recommended to avoid concomitant use.

Increased Effect/Toxicity

Fesoterodine may increase the levels/effects of: Anticholinergics; Cannabinoids; Potassium Chloride

The levels/effects of Fesoterodine may be increased by: CYP2D6 Inhibitors; CYP3A4 Inhibitors (Moderate); CYP3A4 Inhibitors (Strong); Dasatinib; Pramlintide

Decreased Effect

Fesoterodine may decrease the levels/effects of: Acetylcholinesterase Inhibitors (Central); Secretin

The levels/effects of Fesoterodine may be decreased by: Acetylcholinesterase Inhibitors (Central); CYP3A4 Inducers (Strong); Deferasirox; Herbs (CYP3A4 Inducers)

Ethanol/Nutrition/Herb Interactions Ethanol: Adverse effects may be potentiated

Stability Store at 20°C to 25°C (68°F to 77°F); excursions permitted between 15°C to 30°C (59°F to 86°F). Protect from moisture.

Mechanism of Action Fesoterodine acts as a prodrug and is converted to an active metabolite, 5-hydroxymethyl tolterodine (5-HMT); 5-HMT is responsible for fesoterodine's antimuscarinic activity and acts as a competitive antagonist of muscarinic receptors.

Urinary bladder contractions are mediated by muscarinic receptors; fesoterodine inhibits the receptors in the bladder preventing symptoms of urgency and frequency.

Pharmacodynamics/Kinetics

Absorption: Well absorbed

Distribution: I.V.: 5-HMT: V_d: 169 L

Protein binding: 5-HMT: ~50% (primarily to albumin and $alpha_1$-acid glycoprotein)

Metabolism: Fesoterodine is rapidly and extensively metabolized to its active metabolite (5-hydroxymethyl tolterodine; 5-HMT) by nonspecific esterases; 5-HMT is further metabolized via CYP2D6 and CYP3A4 to inactive metabolites.

Bioavailability: 5-HMT: 52%

Half-life elimination: ~7 hours

Time to peak, plasma: 5-HMT: ~5 hours; C_{max} higher in poor CYP2D6 metabolizers

Excretion: Urine (~70%; 16% as 5-HMT, ~53% as inactive metabolites); feces (7%)

Dosage Oral: Adults: Overactive bladder: 4 mg once daily; dose may be increased to 8 mg once daily based on individual response and tolerability

Dosing adjustment for concomitant CYP3A4 inhibitors: Maximum dose: 4 mg/day when administered concomitantly with potent CYP3A4 inhibitors including (but not limited to) ketoconazole, itraconazole, and clarithromycin. Concurrent therapy of weak or moderate CYP3A4 inhibitors and fesoterodine should be limited to 4 mg/day and increased to 8 mg/day after assessing tolerability.

Dosing adjustment in renal impairment:

Mild-to-moderate renal impairment (Cl_{cr} 30-80 mL/minute): No dose adjustment is recommended

Severe renal impairment (Cl_{cr} <30 mL/minute): Maximum dose: 4 mg

Dosing adjustment in hepatic impairment:

Moderate hepatic impairment (Child-Pugh class B): No dose adjustment is recommended

Severe hepatic impairment (Child-Pugh class C): Use is not recommended; not studied in severe impairment

Dietary Considerations May be taken with or without food.

Administration May be administered with or without food. Swallow whole; do not chew, crush, or divide.

Product Availability Toviaz™: FDA approved November 2008; availability anticipated in the first half of 2009

Dosage Forms Excipient information presented when available (limited, particularly for generics); consult specific product labeling.

Tablet, extended release:

Toviaz™: 4 mg, 8 mg

◆ **Fesoterodine Fumarate** *see* Fesoterodine *on page 617*

◆ **FeverALL® [OTC]** *see* Acetaminophen *on page 25*

◆ **Fexmid™** *see* Cyclobenzaprine *on page 375*

Fexofenadine (feks oh FEN a deen)

U.S. Brand Names Allegra®; Allegra® ODT

Canadian Brand Names Allegra®

Index Terms Fexofenadine Hydrochloride

Pharmacologic Category Histamine H_1 Antagonist; Histamine H_1 Antagonist, Second Generation

Use Relief of symptoms associated with seasonal allergic rhinitis; treatment of chronic idiopathic urticaria

Pregnancy Risk Factor C

Pregnancy Considerations Decreased fetal weight gain and survival were observed in animal studies. There are no adequate and well-controlled studies in pregnant women; use during pregnancy only if potential benefit to mother outweighs possible risk to fetus.

Lactation Excretion in breast milk unknown/use caution (AAP rates "compatible")

Medication Safety Issues

Sound-alike/look-alike issues:

Fexofenadine may be confused with fesoterodine

Allegra® may be confused with Viagra®

International issues:

Allegra® may be confused with Allegro® which is a brand name for frovatriptan in Germany; a brand name for fluticasone in Israel

Contraindications Hypersensitivity to fexofenadine or any component of the formulation

Warnings/Precautions Use with caution in patients with renal impairment; dosage adjustment recommended. Safety and efficacy in children <6 months of age have not been established; orally disintegrating tablet not recommended for use in children <6 years of age. Orally disintegrating tablet contains phenylalanine.

Adverse Reactions

>10%:

Central nervous system: Headache (5% to 11%)

Gastrointestinal: Vomiting (children 6 months to 5 years: 4% to 12%)

1% to 10%:

Central nervous system: Fatigue (1% to 3%), somnolence (1% to 3%), dizziness (2%), fever (2%), pain (2%), drowsiness (1%)

Endocrine & metabolic: Dysmenorrhea (2%)

Gastrointestinal: Dyspepsia (1% to 2%), diarrhea (3% to 4%), nausea (2%)
Neuromuscular & skeletal: Myalgia (3%), back pain (2% to 3%), pain in extremities (2%)
Otic: Otitis media (2% to 4%)
Respiratory: Upper respiratory tract infection (3% to 4%), cough (2% to 4%), rhinorrhea (1% to 2%)
Miscellaneous: Viral infection (3%)

<1% (Limited to important or life-threatening): Hypersensitivity reactions (anaphylaxis, angioedema, chest tightness, dyspnea, flushing, pruritus, rash, urticaria); insomnia, nervousness, sleep disorders, paroniria

Drug Interactions

Metabolism/Transport Effects **Substrate** of CYP3A4 (minor); **Inhibits** CYP2D6 (weak)

Avoid Concomitant Use There are no known interactions where it is recommended to avoid concomitant use.

Increased Effect/Toxicity

Fexofenadine may increase the levels/effects of: Alcohol (Ethyl); Anticholinergics; CNS Depressants

The levels/effects of Fexofenadine may be increased by: Eltrombopag; Erythromycin; Ketoconazole; P-Glycoprotein Inhibitors; Pramlintide; Verapamil

Decreased Effect

Fexofenadine may decrease the levels/effects of: Acetylcholinesterase Inhibitors (Central); Betahistine

The levels/effects of Fexofenadine may be decreased by: Acetylcholinesterase Inhibitors (Central); Amphetamines; Antacids; Grapefruit Juice; P-Glycoprotein Inducers; Rifampin

Ethanol/Nutrition/Herb Interactions

Ethanol: Avoid ethanol (although limited with fexofenadine, may increase risk of sedation).
Food: Fruit juice (apple, grapefruit, orange) may decrease bioavailability of fexofenadine by ~36%.
Herb/Nutraceutical: St John's wort may decrease fexofenadine levels.

Stability Store at controlled room temperature of 20°C to 25°C (68°F to 77°F). Protect from excessive moisture.

Mechanism of Action Fexofenadine is an active metabolite of terfenadine and like terfenadine it competes with histamine for H_1-receptor sites on effector cells in the gastrointestinal tract, blood vessels and respiratory tract; it appears that fexofenadine does not cross the blood brain barrier to any appreciable degree, resulting in a reduced potential for sedation

Pharmacodynamics/Kinetics

Onset of action: 60 minutes
Duration: Antihistaminic effect: ≥12 hours
Protein binding: 60% to 70%, primarily albumin and $alpha_1$-acid glycoprotein
Metabolism: Minimal (~5%)
Half-life elimination: 14.4 hours (31% to 72% longer in renal impairment)
Time to peak, serum: ODT: 2 hours (4 hours with high-fat meal); Tablet: ~2.6 hours; Suspension: ~1 hour
Excretion: Feces (~80%) and urine (~11%) as unchanged drug

Dosage Oral:

Chronic idiopathic urticaria: Children 6 months to <2 years: 15 mg twice daily
Chronic idiopathic urticaria, seasonal allergic rhinitis:
Children 2-11 years: 30 mg twice daily
Children ≥12 years and Adults: 60 mg twice daily **or** 180 mg once daily
Elderly: Starting dose: 60 mg once daily; adjust for renal impairment

Dosing adjustment in renal impairment: Cl_{cr} <80 mL/minute:
Children 6 months to <2 years: Initial: 15 mg once daily
Children 2-11 years: Initial: 30 mg once daily
Children ≥12 years and Adults: Initial: 60 mg once daily

Dietary Considerations Allegra® ODT 30 mg contains phenylalanine 5.3 mg/tablet.

Administration

Suspension, tablet: Administer with water only; do not administer with fruit juices. Shake suspension well before use.
Orally disintegrating tablet: Take on an empty stomach. Do not remove from blister pack until administered. Using dry hands, place immediately on tongue. Tablet will dissolve within seconds, and may be swallowed with or without liquid. Do not split or chew.

Monitoring Parameters Relief of symptoms

Dosage Forms Excipient information presented when available (limited, particularly for generics); consult specific product labeling. [DSC] = Discontinued product

Suspension, oral, as hydrochloride:
Allegra®: 6 mg/mL (30 mL [DSC], 300 mL) [contains propylene glycol; raspberry cream]
Tablet, oral, as hydrochloride: 30 mg, 60 mg, 180 mg
Allegra®: 30 mg [DSC], 60 mg, 180 mg
Tablet, orally disintegrating, oral, as hydrochloride:
Allegra® ODT: 30 mg [contains phenylalanine 5.3 mg/tablet; orange cream flavor]

Fexofenadine and Pseudoephedrine

(feks oh FEN a deen & soo doe e FED rin)

U.S. Brand Names Allegra-D® 12 Hour; Allegra-D® 24 Hour

Canadian Brand Names Allegra-D®

Index Terms Pseudoephedrine and Fexofenadine

Pharmacologic Category Alpha/Beta Agonist; Histamine H_1 Antagonist; Histamine H_1 Antagonist, Second Generation

Use Relief of symptoms associated with seasonal allergic rhinitis in adults and children ≥12 years of age

Pregnancy Risk Factor C

Medication Safety Issues

Sound-alike/look-alike issues:
Allegra-D® may be confused with Viagra®

Dosage Oral: Children ≥12 years and Adults:

Allegra-D® 12 Hour: One tablet twice daily
Allegra-D® 24 Hour: One tablet once daily

Dosage adjustment in renal impairment:
Allegra-D® 12 Hour: Cl_{cr} <80 mL/minute (based on fexofenadine component): One tablet once daily
Allegra-D® 24 Hour: Avoid use.

Additional Information Complete prescribing information for this medication should be consulted for additional detail.

Dosage Forms Excipient information presented when available (limited, particularly for generics); consult specific product labeling.

Tablet, extended release:
Allegra-D® 12 Hour: Fexofenadine hydrochloride 60 mg [immediate release] and pseudoephedrine hydrochloride 120 mg [extended release]
Allegra-D® 24 Hour: Fexofenadine hydrochloride 180 mg [immediate release] and pseudoephedrine hydrochloride 240 mg [extended release]

◆ **Fexofenadine Hydrochloride** *see* Fexofenadine *on page 618*

◆ **Fiberall®** *see* Psyllium *on page 1268*

Fibrinogen Concentrate (Human)

(fi BRIN o gin KON suhn trate HYU man)

U.S. Brand Names RiaSTAP™

Index Terms Coagulation Factor I

Pharmacologic Category Blood Product Derivative

Use Treatment of acute bleeding episodes in patients with congenital fibrinogen deficiency (afibrinogenemia and hypofibrinogenemia)

Pregnancy Risk Factor C

Pregnancy Considerations Animal reproduction studies have not been conducted. Increased pregnancy loss is associated with untreated congenital fibrinogen disorders.

Contraindications Severe hypersensitivity reactions to fibrinogen concentrate or any component of the formulation

Warnings/Precautions
Hypersensitivity reactions (eg, urticaria, hives, wheezing, hypotension, anaphylaxis) may occur. In the event of hypersensitivity reactions, treatment should be discontinued immediately. Thrombosis may occur in patients with congenital fibrinogen deficiency with or without fibrinogen replacement therapy. Consider potential risk of thrombosis with use. Product of human plasma; may potentially contain infectious agents which could transmit disease. Screening of donors, as well as testing and/or inactivation or removal of certain viruses, reduces the risk. Infections thought to be transmitted by this product should be reported to the manufacturer. Not for the treatment of dysfibrinogenemia.

Adverse Reactions
>1%: Central nervous system: Fever, headache
Postmarketing and/or case reports: Allergic reactions, anaphylaxis, arterial thrombosis, chills, DVT, dyspnea, MI, nausea, pulmonary embolism, rash, thromboembolism, vomiting

Drug Interactions

Avoid Concomitant Use There are no known interactions where it is recommended to avoid concomitant use.

Increased Effect/Toxicity

Fibrinogen Concentrate (Human) may increase the levels/effects of: Antifibrinolytic Agents

The levels/effects of Fibrinogen Concentrate (Human) may be increased by: Antifibrinolytic Agents

Decreased Effect There are no known significant interactions involving a decrease in effect.

Stability Store at 2°C to 25°C (36°F to 77°F) in original carton; do not freeze. Protect from light. Transfer sterile water for injection 50 mL into vial. Gently swirl until dissolved; do not shake. Stable for 24 hours after reconstitution when stored at 20°C to 25°C (68°F to 77°F). Discard partially used vials.

Mechanism of Action Fibrinogen (coagulation factor I), a protein found in normal plasma, is required to clot blood. Fibrinogen concentrate made from pooled human plasma replaces this protein which is missing or reduced in patients with a congenital fibrinogen deficiency.

Pharmacodynamics/Kinetics
Distribution: V_d: 45-60 mL/kg (range 36-68 mL/kg)
Half-life elimination: 61-97 hours (range 56-117 hours); may be decreased in children <16 years of age

Dosage I.V.: Children and Adults: Congenital fibrinogen deficiency: **Note:** Adjust dose based on laboratory values and condition of patient. Maintain a target fibrinogen level of 100 mg/dL until hemostasis is achieved.
When baseline fibrinogen level is known:
Dose (mg/kg) = [Target level (mg/dL) - measured level (mg/dL)] **divided by** 1.7 (mg/dL per mg/kg body weight)
When baseline fibrinogen level is not known: 70 mg/kg

Administration For I.V. administration only; infuse at ≤5 mL/minute

Monitoring Parameters Signs and symptoms of hypersensitivity, thrombosis; fibrinogen level

Reference Range A target fibrinogen level of 100 mg/dL should be maintained until hemostasis occurs and wound healing is complete.
Normal fibrinogen levels: 200-450 mg/dL

Product Availability RiaSTAP™: FDA approved January 2009; availability currently undetermined

Dosage Forms Excipient information presented when available (limited, particularly for generics); consult specific product labeling. [DSC] = Discontinued product
Injection, powder for reconstitution:
RiaSTAP™: 900-1300 mg [contains albumin (human); exact potency labeled on vial]

◆ **Fibro-XL [OTC]** *see* Psyllium *on page* *1268*

◆ **Fibro-Lax [OTC]** *see* Psyllium *on page* *1268*

Filgrastim (fil GRA stim)

U.S. Brand Names Neupogen®

Canadian Brand Names Neupogen®

Index Terms G-CSF; Granulocyte Colony Stimulating Factor; NSC-614629

Pharmacologic Category Colony Stimulating Factor

Use Stimulation of granulocyte production in chemotherapy-induced neutropenia (nonmyeloid malignancies, acute myeloid leukemia, and bone marrow transplantation); severe chronic neutropenia (SCN); moblilization of hematopoietic progenitor cells in patients undergoing peripheral blood progenitor cell (PBPC) collection

Unlabeled/Investigational Use Treatment of anemia in myelodysplastic syndrome; treatment of drug-induced (nonchemotherapy) agranulocytosis in the elderly

Pregnancy Risk Factor C

Pregnancy Considerations Animal studies have demonstrated adverse effects and fetal loss. Filgrastim has been shown to cross the placenta in humans. There are no adequate and well-controlled studies in pregnant women. Use only if potential benefit to mother justifies risk to the fetus.

Lactation Excretion in breast milk unknown/use caution

Medication Safety Issues
Sound-alike/look-alike issues:
Neupogen® may be confused with Epogen®, Neumega®, Neupro®, Nutramigen®

Contraindications Hypersensitivity to filgrastim, *E. coli*-derived proteins, or any component of the formulation

Warnings/Precautions Do not use filgrastim in the period 24 hours before to 24 hours after administration of cytotoxic chemotherapy because of the potential sensitivity of rapidly dividing myeloid cells to cytotoxic chemotherapy. May potentially act as a growth factor for any tumor type, particularly myeloid malignancies; precaution should be exercised in the usage of filgrastim in any malignancy with myeloid characteristics. Increases circulating leukocytes when used in conjunction with plerixafor for stem cell mobilization; monitor WBC; use with caution in patients with neutrophil count >50,000/mm^3; tumor cells released from marrow could be collected in leukapheresis product; potential effect of tumor cell re-infusion is unknown. Reports of alveolar hemorrhage, manifested as pulmonary infiltrates and hemoptysis, have occurred in healthy donors undergoing PBPC collection (not FDA approved for use in healthy donors); hemoptysis resolved upon discontinuation. Safety and efficacy have not been established with patients receiving radiation therapy, or with chemotherapy associated with delayed myelosuppression (eg, nitrosoureas, mitomycin C).

Allergic-type reactions (rash, urticaria, wheezing, dyspnea, tachycardia and/or hypotension) have occurred with first or later doses. Reactions tended to occur more frequently with intravenous administration and within 30 minutes of administration. Rare cases of splenic rupture or acute respiratory distress syndrome have been reported in association with filgrastim; patients must be instructed to report left upper quadrant pain or shoulder tip pain or respiratory distress. Cutaneous vasculitis has been reported, generally occurring in SCN patients on long-term therapy; dose reductions may improve symptoms to allow for continued therapy. Use caution in patients with sickle cell diseases; sickle cell crises have been reported following filgrastim therapy. Cytogenetic abnormalities, transformation to AML and MDS have been observed in patients treated with filgrastim for congenital neutropenia; a longer duration of treatment and poorer ANC response appear to increase the risk. The packaging of some forms may contain latex.

Adverse Reactions

>10%:

Central nervous system: Fever (12%)

Dermatologic: Petechiae (17%), rash (12%)

Gastrointestinal: Splenomegaly (severe chronic neutropenia: 30%; rare in other patients)

Hepatic: Alkaline phosphatase increased (21%)

Neuromuscular & skeletal: Bone pain (22% to 33%), commonly in the lower back, posterior iliac crest, and sternum

Respiratory: Epistaxis (9% to 15%)

1% to 10%:

Cardiovascular: Hyper-/hypotension (4%), S-T segment depression (3%), myocardial infarction/arrhythmias (3%)

Central nervous system: Headache (7%)

Gastrointestinal: Nausea (10%), vomiting (7%), peritonitis (2%)

Hematologic: Leukocytosis (2%)

Miscellaneous: Transfusion reaction (10%)

<1% (Limited to important or life-threatening): Acute respiratory distress syndrome, allergic reactions, alopecia, alveolar hemorrhage, arthralgia, capillary leak syndrome, cerebral hemorrhage, cutaneous vasculitis, dyspnea, edema (facial), erythema nodosum, hematuria, hemoptysis, hepatomegaly, hypersensitivity reaction, injection site reaction, osteoporosis, pericarditis, proteinuria, psoriasis exacerbation, pulmonary infiltrates, renal insufficiency, sickle cell crisis, splenic rupture, Sweet's syndrome (acute febrile dermatosis), tachycardia, thrombocytopenia (in PBPC mobilization), thrombophlebitis, transient supraventricular arrhythmia, urticaria, wheezing

Drug Interactions

Avoid Concomitant Use There are no known interactions where it is recommended to avoid concomitant use.

Increased Effect/Toxicity

Filgrastim may increase the levels/effects of: Topotecan

Decreased Effect There are no known significant interactions involving a decrease in effect.

Stability Intact vials and prefilled syringes should be stored under refrigeration at 2°C to 8°C (36°F to 46°F) and protected from direct sunlight. Filgrastim should be protected from freezing and temperatures >30°C to avoid aggregation. If inadvertently frozen, thaw in a refrigerator and use within 24 hours; do not use if frozen >24 hours or frozen more than once. Do not shake.

Filgrastim vials and prefilled syringes are stable for 24 hours at 9°C to 30°C (47°F to 86°F).

Undiluted filgrastim is stable for 24 hours at 15°C to 30°C (59°F to 86°F) and for up to 14 days at 2°C to 8°C (36°F to 46°F) (data on file, Amgen Medical Information) in BD tuberculin syringes; however, sterility has only been assessed and maintained for up to 7 days when prepared under strict aseptic conditions (Singh, 1994; Jacobson, 1996). The manufacturer recommends using syringes within 24 hours due to the potential for bacterial contamination.

Do not dilute with saline at any time; product may precipitate. Filgrastim may be diluted with D_5W or with D_5W with albumin for I.V. infusion administration (5-15 mcg/mL; minimum concentration is 5 mcg/mL). This diluted solution is stable for 7 days at 2°C to 8°C (36°F to 46°F), however, should be used within 24 hours due to the possibility for bacterial contamination. Dilution to <5 mcg/mL is not recommended. Concentrations 5-15 mcg/mL require addition of albumin (final concentration of 2 mg/mL) to prevent adsorption to plastics.

Mechanism of Action Stimulates the production, maturation, and activation of neutrophils; filgrastim activates neutrophils to increase both their migration and cytotoxicity.

Pharmacodynamics/Kinetics

Onset of action: ~24 hours; plateaus in 3-5 days

Duration: ANC decreases by 50% within 2 days after discontinuing filgrastim; white counts return to the normal range in 4-7 days; peak plasma levels can be maintained for up to 12 hours

Absorption: SubQ: 100%

Distribution: V_d: 150 mL/kg; no evidence of drug accumulation over a 11- to 20-day period

Metabolism: Systemically degraded

Half-life elimination: 1.8-3.5 hours

Time to peak, serum: SubQ: 2-8 hours

Dosage Details concerning dosing in combination regimens and institution protocols should also be consulted.

Dosing, even in morbidly obese patients, should be based on actual body weight. Rounding doses to the nearest vial size often enhances patient convenience and reduces costs without compromising clinical response.

Children and Adults:

Chemotherapy-induced neutropenia: SubQ, I.V.: 5 mcg/kg/day; doses may be increased by 5 mcg/kg according to the duration and severity of the neutropenia; continue for up to 14 days or until the ANC reaches 10,000/mm^3

Bone marrow transplantation: SubQ, I.V.: 10 mcg/kg/day; adjust the dose according to the duration and severity of neutropenia; recommended steps based on neutrophil response:

When ANC >1000/mm^3 for 3 consecutive days: Reduce filgrastim dose to 5 mcg/kg/day

If ANC remains >1000/mm^3 for 3 more consecutive days: Discontinue filgrastim

If ANC decreases to <1000/mm^3: Resume at 5 mcg/kg/day

If ANC decreases <1000/mm^3 during the 5 mcg/kg/day dose, increase filgrastim to 10 mcg/kg/day and follow the above steps

Peripheral blood progenitor cell (PBPC) collection: SubQ: 10 mcg/kg daily in donors, usually for 6-7 days. Begin at least 4 days before the first leukopheresis and continue until the last leukopheresis; consider dose adjustment for WBC >100,000/mm^3

Hematopoietic stem cell mobilization (in combination with plerixafor, for autologous transplantation in patients with non-Hodgkin's lymphoma and multiple myeloma): SubQ: 10 mcg/kg once daily; begin 4 days before initiation of plerixafor; continue G-CSF on each day prior to apheresis

Severe chronic neutropenia: SubQ:

Congenital: 6 mcg/kg twice daily; adjust the dose based on ANC and clinical response

Idiopathic/cyclic: 5 mcg/kg/day; adjust the dose based on ANC and clinical response

Anemia in myelodysplastic syndrome (unlabeled use - in combination with epoetin): SubQ: 0.3-3 mcg/kg daily **or** 30-150 mcg daily **or** 1-2 mcg/kg 2-3 times weekly

Elderly: Refer to adult dosing.

Drug-induced agranulocytosis (nonchemotherapy) in the elderly (unlabeled use): SubQ: 300 mcg daily until ANC >1500/mm^3

Dietary Considerations Solution for injection contains sodium 0.035 mg/mL and sorbitol.

Administration May be administered undiluted by SubQ injection. May also be administered by I.V. bolus over

15-30 minutes in D_5W, or by continuous SubQ or I.V. infusion. Do not administer earlier than 24 hours after or in the 24 hours prior to cytotoxic chemotherapy.

Monitoring Parameters CBC with differential prior to treatment and twice weekly during filgrastim treatment for chemotherapy-induced neutropenia (3 times a week following marrow transplantation). For severe chronic neutropenia, monitor CBC with differential twice weekly during the first month of therapy and for 2 weeks following dose adjustments; monthly thereafter. In PBPC mobilization, monitor platelets.

Reference Range No clinical benefit seen with ANC >10,000/mm^3

Test Interactions May interfere with bone imaging studies; increased hematopoietic activity of the bone marrow may appear as transient positive bone imaging changes

Additional Information

Reimbursement Hotline: 1-800-272-9376

Professional Services [Amgen]: 1-800-77-AMGEN

Dosage Forms Excipient information presented when available (limited, particularly for generics); consult specific product labeling.

Injection, solution [preservative free]:

Neupogen®: 300 mcg/mL (1 mL, 1.6 mL) [vial; contains sodium 0.035 mg/mL and sorbitol]

Injection, solution [preservative free]:

Neupogen®: 600 mcg/mL (0.5 mL, 0.8 mL) [prefilled Singleject® syringe; contains sodium 0.035 mg/mL and sorbitol; needle cover contains latex]

◆ **Finacea®** *see* Azelaic Acid *on page* 165

Finasteride (fi NAS teer ide)

U.S. Brand Names Propecia®; Proscar®

Canadian Brand Names Propecia®; Proscar®

Pharmacologic Category 5 Alpha-Reductase Inhibitor

Use

Propecia®: Treatment of male pattern hair loss in **men only**. Safety and efficacy were demonstrated in men between 18-41 years of age.

Proscar®: Treatment of symptomatic benign prostatic hyperplasia (BPH); can be used in combination with an alpha-blocker, doxazosin

Unlabeled/Investigational Use Adjuvant monotherapy after radical prostatectomy in the treatment of prostatic cancer; female hirsutism

Pregnancy Risk Factor X

Pregnancy Considerations Abnormalities of external male genitalia were reported in animal studies. Pregnant women are advised to avoid contact with crushed or broken tablets.

Lactation Excretion in breast milk unknown/contraindicated

Medication Safety Issues

Sound-alike/look-alike issues:

Proscar® may be confused with ProSom®, Prozac®, Psorcon®

Contraindications Hypersensitivity to finasteride or any component of the formulation; pregnancy; not for use in children

Warnings/Precautions Hazardous agent - use appropriate precautions for handling and disposal. Other urological diseases including cancer should be ruled out before initiating. A minimum of 6 months of treatment may be necessary to determine whether an individual will respond to finasteride. Reduces prostate specific antigen (PSA) by 50%; in patients treated for ≥6 months the PSA should be doubled when comparing to normal ranges in untreated patients. Use with caution in those patients with hepatic dysfunction. Carefully monitor patients with a large residual urinary volume or severely diminished urinary flow for obstructive uropathy. These patients may not be candidates for finasteride therapy. Safety and efficacy have not been established in children.

Adverse Reactions Note: "Combination therapy" refers to finasteride and doxazosin.

>10%:

Endocrine & metabolic: Impotence (19%; combination therapy 23%), libido decreased (10%; combination therapy 12%)

Neuromuscular & skeletal: Weakness (5%; combination therapy 17%)

1% to 10%:

Cardiovascular: Postural hypotension (9%; combination therapy 18%), edema (1%, combination therapy 3%)

Central nervous system: Dizziness (7%; combination therapy 23%), somnolence (2%; combination therapy 3%)

Genitourinary: Ejaculation disturbances (7%; combination therapy 14%), decreased volume of ejaculate

Endocrine & metabolic: Gynecomastia (2%)

Respiratory: Dyspnea (1%; combination therapy 2%), rhinitis (1%; combination therapy 2%)

<1%, postmarketing and/or case reports: Hypersensitivity (pruritus, rash, urticaria, swelling of face/lips); breast tenderness, breast enlargement, breast cancer (males), prostate cancer (high grade), testicular pain

Drug Interactions

Metabolism/Transport Effects Substrate of CYP3A4 (minor)

Avoid Concomitant Use There are no known interactions where it is recommended to avoid concomitant use.

Increased Effect/Toxicity There are no known significant interactions involving an increase in effect.

Decreased Effect There are no known significant interactions involving a decrease in effect.

Ethanol/Nutrition/Herb Interactions

Herb/Nutraceutical: St John's wort may decrease finasteride levels. Avoid saw palmetto (concurrent use has not been adequately studied).

Stability Store below 30°C (86°F). Protect from light.

Mechanism of Action Finasteride is a competitive inhibitor of both tissue and hepatic 5-alpha reductase. This results in inhibition of the conversion of testosterone to dihydrotestosterone and markedly suppresses serum dihydrotestosterone levels

Pharmacodynamics/Kinetics

Onset of action: 3-6 months of ongoing therapy

Duration:

After a single oral dose as small as 0.5 mg: 65% depression of plasma dihydrotestosterone levels persists 5-7 days

After 6 months of treatment with 5 mg/day: Circulating dihydrotestosterone levels are reduced to castrate levels without significant effects on circulating testosterone; levels return to normal within 14 days of discontinuation of treatment

Distribution: V_{dss}: 76 L

Protein binding: 90%

Metabolism: Hepatic via CYP3A4; two active metabolites (<20% activity of finasteride)

Bioavailability: Mean: 63%

Half-life elimination, serum: Elderly: 8 hours; Adults: 6 hours (3-16)

Time to peak, serum: 2-6 hours

Excretion: Feces (57%) and urine (39%) as metabolites

Dosage Oral: Adults:

Male:

Benign prostatic hyperplasia (Proscar®): 5 mg/day as a single dose; clinical responses occur within 12 weeks to 6 months of initiation of therapy; long-term administration is recommended for maximal response

Male pattern baldness (Propecia®): 1 mg daily

Female hirsutism (unlabeled use): 5 mg/day

Dosing adjustment in renal impairment: No dosage adjustment is necessary

Dosing adjustment in hepatic impairment: Use with caution in patients with liver function abnormalities because finasteride is metabolized extensively in the liver

Administration Administration with food may delay the rate and reduce the extent of oral absorption. Women of childbearing age should not touch or handle broken tablets.

Monitoring Parameters Objective and subjective signs of relief of benign prostatic hyperplasia, including improvement in urinary flow, reduction in symptoms of urgency, and relief of difficulty in micturition

Dosage Forms Excipient information presented when available (limited, particularly for generics); consult specific product labeling.

Tablet: 5 mg

Propecia®: 1 mg

Proscar®: 5 mg

- **Fioricet®** *see* Butalbital, Acetaminophen, and Caffeine *on page 229*
- **Fiorinal®** *see* Butalbital, Aspirin, and Caffeine *on page 230*
- **First™-Progesterone VGS** *see* Progesterone *on page 1247*
- **First®-Testosterone** *see* Testosterone *on page 1445*
- **First®-Testosterone MC** *see* Testosterone *on page 1445*
- **Fisalamine** *see* Mesalamine *on page 949*
- **Fish Oil** *see* Omega-3-Acid Ethyl Esters *on page 1100*
- **FK506** *see* Tacrolimus *on page 1419*
- **Flagyl®** *see* MetroNIDAZOLE *on page 984*
- **Flagyl ER®** *see* MetroNIDAZOLE *on page 984*
- **Flamazine® (Can)** *see* Silver Sulfadiazine *on page 1370*
- **Flarex®** *see* Fluorometholone *on page 636*

Flavoxate (fla VOKS ate)

U.S. Brand Names Urispas®

Canadian Brand Names Apo-Flavoxate®; Urispas®

Index Terms Flavoxate Hydrochloride

Pharmacologic Category Antispasmodic Agent, Urinary

Use Antispasmodic to provide symptomatic relief of dysuria, nocturia, suprapubic pain, urgency, and incontinence due to detrusor instability and hyper-reflexia in elderly with cystitis, urethritis, urethrocystitis, urethrotrigonitis, and prostatitis

Pregnancy Risk Factor B

Medication Safety Issues

Sound-alike/look-alike issues:

Flavoxate may be confused with fluvoxamine

Urispas® may be confused with Urised®

Dosage Children >12 years and Adults: Oral: 100-200 mg 3-4 times/day; reduce the dose when symptoms improve

Additional Information Complete prescribing information for this medication should be consulted for additional detail.

Dosage Forms Excipient information presented when available (limited, particularly for generics); consult specific product labeling.

Tablet, as hydrochloride: 100 mg

- **Flavoxate Hydrochloride** *see* Flavoxate *on page 623*
- **Flebogamma®** *see* Immune Globulin (Intravenous) *on page 777*

Flecainide (fle KAY nide)

U.S. Brand Names Tambocor™

Canadian Brand Names Apo-Flecainide®; Tambocor™

Index Terms Flecainide Acetate

Pharmacologic Category Antiarrhythmic Agent, Class Ic

Use Prevention and suppression of documented life-threatening ventricular arrhythmias (eg, sustained ventricular tachycardia); controlling symptomatic, disabling supraventricular tachycardias in patients without structural heart disease in whom other agents fail

Pregnancy Risk Factor C

Lactation Enters breast milk/compatible

Medication Safety Issues

Sound-alike/look-alike issues:

Flecainide may be confused with fluconazole

Tambocor™ may be confused with tamoxifen

Contraindications Hypersensitivity to flecainide or any component of the formulation; pre-existing second- or third-degree AV block or with right bundle branch block when associated with a left hemiblock (bifascicular block) (except in patients with a functioning artificial pacemaker); cardiogenic shock; coronary artery disease (based on CAST study results); concurrent use of ritonavir or amprenavir

Warnings/Precautions **[U.S. Boxed Warning]: In the Cardiac Arrhythmia Suppression Trial (CAST), recent (>6 days but <2 years ago) myocardial infarction patients with asymptomatic, non-life-threatening ventricular arrhythmias did not benefit and may have been harmed by attempts to suppress the arrhythmia with flecainide or encainide.** An increased mortality or nonfatal cardiac arrest rate (7.7%) was seen in the active treatment group compared with patients in the placebo group (3%). The applicability of the CAST results to other populations is unknown. The risks of class 1C agents and the lack of improved survival make use in patients without life-threatening arrhythmias generally unacceptable. **[U.S. Boxed Warning]: Watch for proarrhythmic effects;** monitor and adjust dose to prevent QT_c prolongation. Not recommended for patients with chronic atrial fibrillation. **[U.S. Boxed Warning]: When treating atrial flutter, 1:1 atrioventricular conduction may occur; pre-emptive negative chronotropic therapy (eg, digoxin, beta-blockers) may lower the risk.** Pre-existing hypokalemia or hyperkalemia should be corrected before initiation (can alter drug's effect). A worsening or new arrhythmia may occur (proarrhythmic effect). Use caution in heart failure (may precipitate or exacerbate HF). Dose-related increases in PR, QRS, and QT intervals occur. Use with caution in sick sinus syndrome or with permanent pacemakers or temporary pacing wires (can increase endocardial pacing thresholds). Cautious use in significant hepatic impairment.

Adverse Reactions

>10%:

Central nervous system: Dizziness (19% to 30%)

Ocular: Visual disturbances (16%)

Respiratory: Dyspnea (~10%)

1% to 10%:

Cardiovascular: Palpitation (6%), chest pain (5%), edema (3.5%), tachycardia (1% to 3%), proarrhythmic (4% to 12%), sinus node dysfunction (1.2%), syncope

Central nervous system: Headache (4% to 10%), fatigue (8%), nervousness (5%) additional symptoms occurring at a frequency between 1% and 3%: fever, malaise, hypoesthesia, paresis, ataxia, vertigo, somnolence, tinnitus, anxiety, insomnia, depression

Dermatologic: Rash (1% to 3%)

Gastrointestinal: Nausea (9%), constipation (1%), abdominal pain (3%), anorexia (1% to 3%), diarrhea (0.7% to 3%)

Neuromuscular & skeletal: Tremor (5%), weakness (5%), paresthesia (1%)

Ocular: Diplopia (1% to 3%), blurred vision

<1% (Limited to important or life-threatening): Alopecia, alters pacing threshold, amnesia, angina, AV block, bradycardia, bronchospasm, CHF, corneal deposits, depersonalization, euphoria, exfoliative dermatitis, granulocytopenia, heart block, increased P-R, leukopenia, metallic taste, neuropathy, paradoxical increase in ventricular rate in atrial fibrillation/flutter, paresthesia, photophobia, pneumonitis, pruritus, QRS duration, swollen lips/tongue/mouth, tardive dyskinesia, thrombocytopenia, urinary retention, urticaria, ventricular arrhythmia

Drug Interactions

Metabolism/Transport Effects **Substrate** of CYP1A2 (minor), 2D6 (major); **Inhibits** CYP2D6 (weak)

Avoid Concomitant Use

Avoid concomitant use of Flecainide with any of the following: Nilotinib; Ritonavir; Tetrabenazine; Thioridazine; Tipranavir; Ziprasidone

Increased Effect/Toxicity

Flecainide may increase the levels/effects of: QTc-Prolonging Agents; Tetrabenazine; Thioridazine; Ziprasidone

The levels/effects of Flecainide may be increased by: Alfuzosin; Amiodarone; Carbonic Anhydrase Inhibitors; Ciprofloxacin; CYP2D6 Inhibitors (Moderate); CYP2D6 Inhibitors (Strong); Darunavir; Gadobutrol; Nilotinib; Ritonavir; Tipranavir

Decreased Effect There are no known significant interactions involving a decrease in effect.

Ethanol/Nutrition/Herb Interactions Food: Clearance may be decreased in patients following strict vegetarian diets due to urinary pH ≥8. Dairy products (milk, infant formula, yogurt) may interfere with the absorption of flecainide in infants; there is one case report of a neonate (GA 34 weeks PNA >6 days) who required extremely large doses of oral flecainide when administered every 8 hours with feedings ("milk feeds"); changing the feedings from "milk feeds" to 5% glucose feeds alone resulted in a doubling of the flecainide serum concentration and toxicity.

Mechanism of Action Class Ic antiarrhythmic; slows conduction in cardiac tissue by altering transport of ions across cell membranes; causes slight prolongation of refractory periods; decreases the rate of rise of the action potential without affecting its duration; increases electrical stimulation threshold of ventricle, His-Purkinje system; possesses local anesthetic and moderate negative inotropic effects

Pharmacodynamics/Kinetics

Absorption: Oral: Rapid

Distribution: Adults: V_d: 5-13.4 L/kg

Protein binding: $Alpha_1$ glycoprotein: 40% to 50%

Metabolism: Hepatic

Bioavailability: 85% to 90%

Half-life elimination: Infants: 11-12 hours; Children: 8 hours; Adults: 7-22 hours, increased with congestive heart failure or renal dysfunction; End-stage renal disease: 19-26 hours

Time to peak, serum: ~1.5-3 hours

Excretion: Urine (80% to 90%, 10% to 50% as unchanged drug and metabolites)

Dosage Oral:

Children:

Initial: 3 mg/kg/day or 50-100 mg/m^2/day in 3 divided doses

Usual: 3-6 mg/kg/day or 100-150 mg/m^2/day in 3 divided doses; up to 11 mg/kg/day or 200 mg/m^2/day for uncontrolled patients with subtherapeutic levels

Adults:

Life-threatening ventricular arrhythmias:

Initial: 100 mg every 12 hours

Increase by 50-100 mg/day (given in 2 doses/day) every 4 days; maximum: 400 mg/day.

Use of higher initial doses and more rapid dosage adjustments have resulted in an increased incidence of proarrhythmic events and congestive heart failure, particularly during the first few days. Do not use a loading dose. Use very cautiously in patients with history of congestive heart failure or myocardial infarction.

Prevention of paroxysmal supraventricular arrhythmias in patients with disabling symptoms but no structural heart disease: Initial: 50 mg every 12 hours; increase by 50 mg twice daily at 4-day intervals; maximum: 300 mg/day

Paroxysmal atrial fibrillation: Outpatient: "Pill-in-the-pocket" dose (unlabeled dose): 200 mg (weight <70 kg), 300 mg (weight ≥70 kg). May not repeat in ≤24 hours. **Note:** An initial inpatient conversion trial should have been successful before sending patient home on this approach. Patient must be taking an AV nodal-blocking agent (eg, beta-blocker, nondihydropyridine calcium channel blocker) prior to initiation of antiarrhythmic.

Dosing adjustment in severe renal impairment: GFR ≤50 mL/minute: Decrease dose by 50%; dose increases should be made cautiously at intervals >4 days and serum levels monitored frequently.

Hemodialysis: No supplemental dose recommended.

Peritoneal dialysis: No supplemental dose recommended.

Dosing adjustment/comments in hepatic impairment: Monitoring of plasma levels is recommended because of significantly increased half-life.

When transferring from another antiarrhythmic agent, allow for 2-4 half-lives of the agent to pass before initiating flecainide therapy.

Administration Administer around-the-clock to promote less variation in peak and trough serum levels

Monitoring Parameters ECG, blood pressure, pulse, periodic serum concentrations, especially in patients with renal or hepatic impairment

Reference Range Therapeutic: 0.2-1 mcg/mL; pediatric patients may respond at the lower end of the recommended therapeutic range

Dosage Forms Excipient information presented when available (limited, particularly for generics); consult specific product labeling.

Tablet, as acetate: 50 mg, 100 mg, 150 mg

Extemporaneous Preparations A 5 mg/mL suspension compounded from tablets and an oral flavored commercially available diluent (Roxane®) was stable for up to 45 days when stored at 5°C or 25°C in amber glass bottles. Flecainide 20 mg/mL was found stable for up to 60 days at 5°C and 25°C in a 1:1 preparation of Ora-Sweet® and Ora-Plus®, in Ora-Sweet® SF and Ora-Plus® and in cherry syrup

Allen LV and Erickson III MA, "Stability of Baclofen, Captopril, Diltiazem, Hydrochloride, Dipyridamole, and Flecainide Acetate in Extemporaneously Compounded Oral Liquids," *Am J Health Syst Pharm*, 53:2179-84.

Wiest DB, Garner SS, and Pagacz LR, "Stability of Flecainide Acetate in an Extemporaneously Compounded Oral Suspension," *Am J Hosp Pharm*, 1992, 49(6):1467-70.

◆ **Flecainide Acetate** *see* Flecainide *on page* 623

◆ **Flector®** *see* Diclofenac *on page* 437

◆ **Fleet® Bisacodyl [OTC]** *see* Bisacodyl *on page* 198

◆ **Fleet® Sof-Lax® [OTC]** *see* Docusate *on page* 473

- **Fleet® Stimulant Laxative [OTC]** *see* Bisacodyl *on page 198*
- **Flexbumin** *see* Albumin *on page 49*
- **Flexeril®** *see* Cyclobenzaprine *on page 375*
- **Flexitec (Can)** *see* Cyclobenzaprine *on page 375*
- **Flextra 650** *see* Acetaminophen and Phenyltoloxamine *on page 29*
- **Flextra-DS** *see* Acetaminophen and Phenyltoloxamine *on page 29*
- **Flolan®** *see* Epoprostenol *on page 534*
- **Flomax®** *see* Tamsulosin *on page 1426*
- **Flomax® CR (Can)** *see* Tamsulosin *on page 1426*
- **Flonase®** *see* Fluticasone *on page 644*
- **Florazole® ER (Can)** *see* MetroNIDAZOLE *on page 984*
- **Florical® [OTC]** *see* Calcium Carbonate *on page 238*
- **Florinef® [DSC]** *see* Fludrocortisone *on page 630*
- **Florinef® (Can)** *see* Fludrocortisone *on page 630*
- **Flovent® Diskus®** *see* Fluticasone *on page 644*
- **Flovent® HFA** *see* Fluticasone *on page 644*
- **Floxin®** *see* Ofloxacin *on page 1091*
- **Floxin Otic Singles** *see* Ofloxacin *on page 1091*
- **Fluarix®** *see* Influenza Virus Vaccine *on page 788*
- **Flubenisolone** *see* Betamethasone *on page 188*
- **Flucaine®** *see* Proparacaine and Fluorescein *on page 1254*

Fluconazole (floo KOE na zole)

U.S. Brand Names Diflucan®

Canadian Brand Names Apo-Fluconazole®; Co-Fluconazole; Diflucan®; Dom-Fluconazole; Fluconazole Injection; Fluconazole Omega; Gen-Fluconazole; GMD-Fluconazole; Novo-Fluconazole; PHL-Fluconazole; PMS-Fluconazole; Pro-Fluconazole; Riva-Fluconazole; Taro-Fluconazole; Zym-Fluconazole

Pharmacologic Category Antifungal Agent, Oral; Antifungal Agent, Parenteral

Additional Appendix Information

Antifungal Agents *on page 1640*

Guidelines for the Prevention of Opportunistic Infections in HIV Infected Persons *on page 1740*

Treatment of Sexually Transmitted Infections *on page 1773*

Use Treatment of candidiasis (vaginal, oropharyngeal, esophageal, urinary tract infections, peritonitis, pneumonia, and systemic infections); cryptococcal meningitis; antifungal prophylaxis in allogeneic bone marrow transplant recipients

Pregnancy Risk Factor C

Pregnancy Considerations When used in high doses, fluconazole is teratogenic in animal studies. Following exposure during the first trimester, case reports have noted similar malformations in humans when used in higher doses (400 mg/day) over extended periods of time. Use of lower doses (150 mg as a single dose or 200 mg/day) may have less risk; however, additional data is needed. Use during pregnancy only if the potential benefit to the mother outweighs any potential risk to the fetus.

Lactation Enters breast/not recommended (AAP rates "compatible")

Medication Safety Issues

Sound-alike/look-alike issues:

Fluconazole may be confused with flecainide

Diflucan® may be confused with diclofenac, Diprivan®, disulfiram

International issues:

Canesten® [Great Britain]: Brand name for clotrimazole in multiple international markets

Contraindications Hypersensitivity to fluconazole, other azoles, or any component of the formulation; concomitant administration with cisapride

Warnings/Precautions Should be used with caution in patients with renal and hepatic dysfunction or previous hepatotoxicity from other azole derivatives. Patients who develop abnormal liver function tests during fluconazole therapy should be monitored closely and discontinued if symptoms consistent with liver disease develop. Rare exfoliative skin disorders have been observed; monitor closely if rash develops. The manufacturer reports rare cases of QT_c prolongation and TdP associated with fluconazole use and advises caution in patients with concomitant medications or conditions which are arrhythmogenic. However, given the limited number of cases and the presence of multiple confounding variables, the likelihood that fluconazole causes conduction abnormalities appears remote.

Adverse Reactions Frequency not always defined.

Cardiovascular: Angioedema, pallor, QT prolongation (rare, case reports), torsade de pointes(rare, case reports)

Central nervous system: Headache (2% to 13%), seizure, dizziness

Dermatologic: Rash (2%), alopecia, toxic epidermal necrolysis, Stevens-Johnson syndrome

Endocrine & metabolic: Hypercholesterolemia, hypertriglyceridemia, hypokalemia

Gastrointestinal: Nausea (4% to 7%), abdominal pain (2% to 6%), diarrhea (2% to 3%), vomiting (2%), dyspepsia, taste perversion

Hematologic: Agranulocytosis, leukopenia, neutropenia, thrombocytopenia

Hepatic: Alkaline phosphatase increased, ALT increased, AST increased, cholestasis, hepatic failure (rare), hepatitis, jaundice

Respiratory: Dyspnea

Miscellaneous: Anaphylactic reactions (rare)

Drug Interactions

Metabolism/Transport Effects Inhibits CYP1A2 (weak), 2C9 (strong), 2C19 (strong), 3A4 (moderate)

Avoid Concomitant Use

Avoid concomitant use of Fluconazole with any of the following: Cisapride; Conivaptan; Dofetilide; Nilotinib; Pimozide; QuiNIDine; Ranolazine; Tetrabenazine; Thioridazine

Increased Effect/Toxicity

Fluconazole may increase the levels/effects of: Alfentanil; Aprepitant; Benzodiazepines (metabolized by oxidation); Bosentan; BusPIRone; Busulfan; Calcium Channel Blockers; CarBAMazepine; Cardiac Glycosides; Cilostazol; Cinacalcet; Cisapride; Conivaptan; Corticosteroids (Orally Inhaled); Corticosteroids (Systemic); CycloSPORINE; CYP2C19 Substrates; CYP2C9 Substrates (High risk); CYP3A4 Substrates; Docetaxel; Dofetilide; Eletriptan; Eplerenone; Erlotinib; Eszopiclone; FentaNYL; Fosaprepitant; Gefitinib; HMG-CoA Reductase Inhibitors; Imatinib; Irbesartan; Irinotecan; Losartan; Macrolide Antibiotics; Maraviroc; Methadone; Phenytoin; Phosphodiesterase 5 Inhibitors; Pimecrolimus; Pimozide; Protease Inhibitors; Proton Pump Inhibitors; QTc-Prolonging Agents; QuiNIDine; Ramelteon; Ranolazine; Repaglinide; Rifamycin Derivatives; Salmeterol; Sirolimus; Solifenacin; Sulfonylureas; Sunitinib; Tacrolimus; Temsirolimus; Tetrabenazine; Thioridazine; Tolterodine; VinCRIStine; Vitamin K Antagonists; Zidovudine; Ziprasidone; Zolpidem

The levels/effects of Fluconazole may be increased by: Alfuzosin; Ciprofloxacin; Gadobutrol; Macrolide Antibiotics; Nilotinib; Protease Inhibitors

Decreased Effect

Fluconazole may decrease the levels/effects of: Amphotericin B; Saccharomyces boulardii

The levels/effects of Fluconazole may be decreased by: Antacids; Didanosine; Grapefruit Juice; H2-Antagonists; Phenytoin; Rifamycin Derivatives; Sucralfate

Stability

Powder for oral suspension: Store dry powder at ≤30°C (86°F). Following reconstitution, store at 5°C to 30°C (41°F to 86°F). Discard unused portion after 2 weeks. Do not freeze.

Injection: Store injection in glass at 5°C to 30°C (41°F to 86°F). Store injection in Viaflex® at 5°C to 25°C (41°F to 77°F). Do not freeze. Do not unwrap unit until ready for use.

Mechanism of Action Interferes with fungal cytochrome P450 activity (lanosterol 14-α-demethylase), decreasing ergosterol synthesis (principal sterol in fungal cell membrane) and inhibiting cell membrane formation

Pharmacodynamics/Kinetics

Distribution: Widely throughout body with good penetration into CSF, eye, peritoneal fluid, sputum, skin, and urine

Relative diffusion blood into CSF: Adequate with or without inflammation (exceeds usual MICs)

CSF:blood level ratio: Normal meninges: 70% to 80%; Inflamed meninges: >70% to 80%

Protein binding, plasma: 11% to 12%

Bioavailability: Oral: >90%

Half-life elimination: Normal renal function: ~30 hours

Time to peak, serum: Oral: 1-2 hours

Excretion: Urine (80% as unchanged drug)

Dosage The daily dose of fluconazole is the same for oral and I.V. administration

Usual dosage ranges:

Neonates: First 2 weeks of life, especially premature neonates: Same dose as older children every 72 hours

Children: Loading dose: 6-12 mg/kg; maintenance: 3-12 mg/kg/day; duration and dosage depends on severity of infection

Adults: 200-800 mg/day; duration and dosage depends on severity of infection

Indication-specific dosing:

Children:

Candidiasis:

Oropharyngeal: Loading dose: 6 mg/kg; maintenance: 3 mg/kg/day for 2 weeks

Esophageal: Loading dose: 6 mg/kg; maintenance: 3-12 mg/kg/day for 21 days and at least 2 weeks following resolution of symptoms

Systemic infection: 6 mg/kg every 12 hours for 28 days

Meningitis, cryptococcal: Loading dose: 12 mg/kg; maintenance: 6-12 mg/kg/day for 10-12 weeks following negative CSF culture; relapse suppression (HIV-positive): 6 mg/kg/day

Adults:

Candidiasis:

Candidemia (neutropenic and non-neutropenic): 400-800 mg/day for 14 days after last positive blood culture and resolution of signs/symptoms

Chronic, disseminated: 400-800 mg/day for 3-6 months

Oropharyngeal (long-term suppression): 200 mg/day; chronic therapy is recommended in immunocompromised patients with history of oropharyngeal candidiasis (OPC)

Osteomyelitis: 400-800 mg/day for 6-12 months

Esophageal: 200 mg on day 1, then 100-200 mg/day for 2-3 weeks after clinical improvement

Prophylaxis in bone marrow transplant: 400 mg/day; begin 3 days before onset of neutropenia and continue for 7 days after neutrophils >1000 cells/mm^3

Urinary: 200 mg/day for 1-2 weeks

Vaginal: 150 mg as a single dose

Coccidiomycosis (unlabeled use, IDSA guideline): 400 mg/day; doses of 800-1000 mg/day have been used for meningeal disease; usual duration of therapy ranges from 3-6 months for primary uncomplicated infections and up to 1 year for pulmonary (chronic and diffuse) infection

Endocarditis, prosthetic valve, early (unlabeled use, IDSA guideline): 400-800 mg/day for 6 weeks after valve replacement; long-term suppression in absence of valve replacement: 200-400 mg/day

Endophthalmitis: 400-800 mg/day for 6-12 weeks after surgical intervention.

Meningitis, cryptococcal: Amphotericin 0.7-1 mg/kg +/- 5-FC for 2 weeks then fluconazole 400 mg/day for at least 10 weeks (consider life-long in HIV-positive); maintenance (HIV-positive): 200-400 mg/day life-long

Pneumonia, cryptococcal (mild-to-moderate) (unlabeled use, IDSA guideline): 200-400 mg/day for 6-12 months (consider life-long in HIV-positive patients)

Dosing adjustment/interval in renal impairment:

No adjustment for vaginal candidiasis single-dose therapy

For multiple dosing, administer usual load then adjust daily doses as follows:

Cl_{cr} ≤50 mL/minute (no dialysis): Administer 50% of recommended dose or administer every 48 hours.

Hemodialysis: 50% is removed by hemodialysis; administer 100% of daily dose (according to indication) after each dialysis treatment.

Continuous renal replacement therapy (CRRT): Drug clearance is highly dependent on the method of renal replacement, filter type, and flow rate. Appropriate dosing requires close monitoring of pharmacologic response, signs of adverse reactions due to drug accumulation, as well as drug levels in relation to target trough (if appropriate). The following are general recommendations only (based on dialysate flow/ultrafiltration rates of 1 L/hour) and should not supersede clinical judgment:

CVVH: 200-400 mg every 24 hours

CVVHD/CVVHDF: 400-800 mg every 24 hours

Note: Higher daily doses of 400 mg (CVVH) and 800 mg (CVVHD/CVVHDF) should be considered when treating resistant organisms and/or when employing combined ultrafiltration and dialysis flow rates of ≥2 L/hour for CVVHD/CVVHDF (Trotman, 2005).

Dietary Considerations Take with or without regard to food.

Administration

I.V.: Infuse over approximately 1-2 hours; do not exceed 200 mg/hour

Oral: May be administered with or without food

Monitoring Parameters Periodic liver function tests (AST, ALT, alkaline phosphatase) and renal function tests, potassium

Dosage Forms Excipient information presented when available (limited, particularly for generics); consult specific product labeling.

Infusion [premixed in sodium chloride or dextrose]: 200 mg (100 mL); 400 mg (200 mL)

Diflucan® [premixed in sodium chloride or dextrose]: 200 mg (100 mL); 400 mg (200 mL)

Powder for oral suspension: 10 mg/mL (35 mL); 40 mg/mL (35 mL)

Diflucan®: 10 mg/mL (35 mL); 40 mg/mL (35 mL) [contains sodium benzoate; orange flavor]

Tablet: 50 mg, 100 mg, 150 mg, 200 mg

Diflucan®: 50 mg, 100 mg, 150 mg, 200 mg

- **Fluconazole Injection (Can)** *see* Fluconazole *on page 625*
- **Fluconazole Omega (Can)** *see* Fluconazole *on page 625*

Flucytosine (floo SYE toe seen)

U.S. Brand Names Ancobon®

Canadian Brand Names Ancobon®

Index Terms 5-FC; 5-Fluorocytosine; 5-Flurocytosine

Pharmacologic Category Antifungal Agent, Oral

Additional Appendix Information

Antifungal Agents *on page 1640*

Use Adjunctive treatment of systemic fungal infections (eg, septicemia, endocarditis, UTI, meningitis, or pulmonary) caused by susceptible strains of *Candida* or *Cryptococcus*

Pregnancy Risk Factor C

Pregnancy Considerations Teratogenic in some animal studies, however, there are no adequate and well-controlled studies in pregnant women.

Lactation Excretion in breast milk unknown/not recommended

Medication Safety Issues

Sound-alike/look-alike issues:

Flucytosine may be confused with fluorouracil

Ancobon® may be confused with Oncovin®

High alert medication: The Institute for Safe Medication Practices (ISMP) includes this medication among its list of drugs which have a heightened risk of causing significant patient harm when used in error.

Contraindications Hypersensitivity to flucytosine or any component of the formulation

Warnings/Precautions [U.S. Boxed Warning]: Use with extreme caution in patients with renal dysfunction; dosage adjustment required. Avoid use as monotherapy; resistance rapidly develops. Use with caution in patients with bone marrow depression; patients with hematologic disease or who have been treated with radiation or drugs that suppress the bone marrow may be at greatest risk. Bone marrow toxicity can be irreversible. **[U.S. Boxed Warning]: Closely monitor hematologic, renal, and hepatic status.** Hepatotoxicity and bone marrow toxicity appear to be dose related; monitor levels closely and adjust dose accordingly. Safety and efficacy in children have not been established.

Adverse Reactions Frequency not defined.

Cardiovascular: Cardiac arrest, myocardial toxicity, ventricular dysfunction, chest pain

Central nervous system: Ataxia, confusion, dizziness, drowsiness, fatigue, hallucinations, headache, parkinsonism, psychosis, pyrexia, sedation, seizure, vertigo

Dermatologic: Rash, photosensitivity, pruritus, toxic epidermal necrolysis, urticaria

Endocrine & metabolic: Hypoglycemia, hypokalemia

Gastrointestinal: Abdominal pain, diarrhea, dry mouth, duodenal ulcer, hemorrhage, loss of appetite, nausea, ulcerative colitis, vomiting

Hematologic: Agranulocytosis, anemia, aplastic anemia, eosinophilia, leukopenia, pancytopenia, thrombocytopenia

Hepatic: Acute hepatic injury, bilirubin increased, hepatic dysfunction, jaundice, liver enzymes increased

Neuromuscular & skeletal: Paresthesia, peripheral neuropathy, weakness

Otic: Hearing loss

Renal: Azotemia, BUN increased, crystalluria, renal failure, serum creatinine increased

Respiratory: Dyspnea, respiratory arrest

Miscellaneous: Allergic reaction

Drug Interactions

Avoid Concomitant Use There are no known interactions where it is recommended to avoid concomitant use.

Increased Effect/Toxicity

The levels/effects of Flucytosine may be increased by: Amphotericin B

Decreased Effect

Flucytosine may decrease the levels/effects of: Saccharomyces boulardii

The levels/effects of Flucytosine may be decreased by: Cytarabine

Ethanol/Nutrition/Herb Interactions Food: Food decreases the rate, but not the extent of absorption.

Stability Store at room temperature of 15°C to 30°C (59°F to 86°F); protect from light.

Mechanism of Action Penetrates fungal cells and is converted to fluorouracil which competes with uracil interfering with fungal RNA and protein synthesis

Pharmacodynamics/Kinetics

Absorption: 76% to 89%

Distribution: Into CSF, aqueous humor, joints, peritoneal fluid, and bronchial secretions; V_d: 0.6 L/kg

Protein binding: 3% to 4%

Metabolism: Minimally hepatic; deaminated, possibly via gut bacteria, to 5-fluorouracil

Half-life elimination:

Normal renal function: 2-5 hours

Anuria: 85 hours (range: 30-250)

End stage renal disease: 75-200 hours

Time to peak, serum: ~1-2 hours

Excretion: Urine (>90% as unchanged drug)

Dosage

Usual dosage ranges: Children (unlabeled use) and Adults: Oral: 50-150 mg/kg/day in divided doses every 6 hours

Indication-specific dosing:

Children (unlabeled use) and Adults: Oral:

Endocarditis: 25-37.5 mg/kg every 6 hours (with amphotericin B) for at least 6 weeks after valve replacement

Meningoencephalitis, cryptococcal: Induction: 25 mg/kg/dose (with amphotericin B) every 6 hours for 2 weeks; if clinical improvement, may discontinue both amphotericin and flucytosine and follow with an extended course of fluconazole (400 mg/day); alternatively, may continue flucytosine for 6-10 weeks (with amphotericin B) without conversion to fluconazole treatment

Dosing interval in renal impairment: Use lower initial dose:

Cl_{cr} 20-40 mL/minute: Administer 37.5 mg/kg every 12 hours

Cl_{cr} 10-20 mL/minute: Administer 37.5 mg/kg every 24 hours

Cl_{cr} <10 mL/minute: Administer 37.5 mg/kg every 24-48 hours, but monitor drug concentrations frequently

Hemodialysis: Dialyzable (50% to 100%); administer dose posthemodialysis

Peritoneal dialysis: Adults: Administer 0.5-1 g every 24 hours

Continuous arteriovenous or venovenous hemodiafiltration effects: Change dosing frequency to every 12-24 hours (monitor serum concentrations and adjust)

Administration Administer around-the-clock to promote less variation in peak and trough serum levels. To avoid nausea and vomiting, administer a few capsules at a time over 15 minutes until full dose is taken.

Monitoring Parameters

Pretreatment: Electrolytes (especially potassium), CBC with differential, BUN, renal function, blood culture

During treatment: CBC with differential, and LFTs (eg, alkaline phosphatase, AST/ALT) frequently, serum flucytosine concentration, renal function

Reference Range

Therapeutic: Trough: 25–50 mcg/mL; peak: 50–100 mcg/mL; peak levels should not exceed 100 mcg/mL to avoid toxic bone marrow depressive and hepatic effects

Trough: Draw just prior to dose administration

Peak: Draw 2 hours after an oral dose administration

Test Interactions Flucytosine causes markedly false elevations in serum creatinine values when the Ektachem® analyzer is used. The Jaffé reaction is recommended for determining serum creatinine.

Dosage Forms Excipient information presented when available (limited, particularly for generics); consult specific product labeling.

Capsule: 250 mg, 500 mg

Extemporaneous Preparations Flucytosine oral liquid has been prepared by using the contents of ten 500 mg capsules triturated in a mortar and pestle with a small amount of distilled water; the mixture was transferred to a 500 mL volumetric flask; the mortar was rinsed several times with a small amount of distilled water and the fluid added to the flask; sufficient distilled water was added to make a total volume of 500 mL of a 10 mg/mL liquid; oral liquid was stable for 70 days when stored in glass or plastic prescription bottles at 4°C or for up to 14 days at room temperature.

Wintermeyer SM and Nahata MC, "Stability of Flucytosine in an Extemporaneously Compounded Oral Liquid," *Am J Health Syst Pharm*, 1996, 53:407-9.

◆ **Fludara®** *see* Fludarabine *on page* 628

Fludarabine (floo DARE a been)

U.S. Brand Names Fludara®

Canadian Brand Names Fludara®

Index Terms 2F-ara-AMP; Fludarabine Phosphate; NSC-312887

Pharmacologic Category Antineoplastic Agent, Antimetabolite (Purine Antagonist)

Use

U.S. labeling: Treatment of progressive or refractory B-cell chronic lymphocytic leukemia (CLL)

Canadian labeling: Second-line treatment of chronic lymphocytic leukemia (CLL); second-line treatment of low-grade, refractory non-Hodgkin's lymphoma (NHL)

Unlabeled/Investigational Use Treatment of non-Hodgkin's lymphoma (NHL); refractory acute leukemias and solid tumors (in pediatric patients); Waldenström's macroglobulinemia (WM); reduced-intensity conditioning regimens prior to allogeneic hematopoietic stem cell transplantation (generally administered in combination with busulfan and antithymocyte globulin or lymphocyte immune globulin, or in combination with melphalan and alemtuzumab)

Pregnancy Risk Factor D

Pregnancy Considerations Teratogenic effects were observed in animal studies. Effective contraception is recommended during and for 6 months after treatment for women and men of reproductive potential. The manufacturer recommends pregnant staff should not handle fludarabine injection.

Lactation Excretion in breast milk unknown/not recommended

Medication Safety Issues

Sound-alike/look-alike issues:

Fludarabine may be confused with cladribine, floxuridine, Flumadine®

Fludara® may be confused with FUDR®

High alert medication: The Institute for Safe Medication Practices (ISMP) includes this medication among its list of drug classes which have a heightened risk of causing significant patient harm when used in error.

Contraindications Hypersensitivity of fludarabine or any component of the formulation

Canadian labeling: Additional contraindications (not in U.S. labeling): Severe renal impairment (Cl_{cr} <30 mL/minute); decompensated hemolytic anemia; concurrent use with pentostatin; pregnancy

Warnings/Precautions Hazardous agent - use appropriate precautions for handling and disposal. Use with caution in patients with renal insufficiency (clearance of the primary metabolite 2-fluoro-ara-A is reduced); dosage modifications may be recommended; monitor closely. Use with caution in patients with pre-existing hematological disorders (particularly granulocytopenia) or pre-existing central nervous system disorder (epilepsy), spasticity, or peripheral neuropathy. **[U.S. Boxed Warning]: Higher than recommended doses are associated with severe neurologic toxicity (delayed blindness, coma, death);** symptoms of neurotoxicity appear from 21-60 days following the last fludarabine dose; similar toxicity was reported rarely at recommended doses. **[U.S. Boxed Warning]: Life-threatening (and sometimes fatal) autoimmune effects, including hemolytic anemia, autoimmune thrombocytopenia/thrombocytopenic purpura (ITP), Evans syndrome, and acquired hemophilia have occurred;** monitor closely for hemolysis; the hemolytic effects usually recur with fludarabine rechallenge. **[U.S. Boxed Warning]: Severe bone marrow suppression (anemia, thrombocytopenia, and neutropenia) may occur;** may be cumulative. Severe myelosuppression (trilineage bone marrow hypoplasia/aplasia) has been reported (rare); the duration of significant cytopenias in these cases may be prolonged (up to 1 year).

Use with caution in patients with documented infection or fever; prophylactic anti-infectives should be considered for patients with an increased risk for developing opportunistic infections. Progressive multifocal leukoencephalopathy (PML) due to JC virus (usually fatal) has been reported with use; usually in patients who had received prior and/or other concurrent chemotherapy; onset ranges from a few weeks to 1 year; evaluate any neurological change promptly. Avoid vaccination with live vaccines during and after fludarabine treatment. May cause tumor lysis syndrome; risk is increased in patients with large tumor burden prior to treatment. Patients receiving blood products should only receive irradiated blood products due to the potential for transfusion related GVHD. **[U.S. Boxed Warnings]: Do not use in combination with pentostatin; may lead to severe, even fatal pulmonary toxicity. Should be administered under the supervision of an experienced cancer chemotherapy physician.**

Adverse Reactions

>10%:

Cardiovascular: Edema (8% to 19%)

Central nervous system: Fever (11% to 69%), fatigue (10% to 38%), pain (5% to 22%), chills (11% to 19%)

Dermatologic: Rash (4% to 15%)

Gastrointestinal: Nausea/vomiting (1% to 38%), anorexia (≤34%), diarrhea (5% to 15%), gastrointestinal bleeding (3% to 13%)

Genitourinary: Urinary tract infection (2% to 15%)

Hematologic: Myelosuppression (nadir: 10-14 days; recovery: 5-7 weeks; dose-limiting toxicity), anemia (14% to 60%), neutropenia (grade 4: 37% to 59%; nadir: ~13 days), thrombocytopenia (17% to 55%; nadir: ~16 days)

Neuromuscular & skeletal: Weakness (9% to 65%), myalgia (4% to 16%), paresthesia (4% to 12%)

Ocular: Visual disturbance (3% to 15%)

Respiratory: Cough (≤44%), pneumonia (3% to 22%), dyspnea (1% to 22%), upper respiratory infection (2% to 16%), rhinitis (≤11%)

Miscellaneous: Infection (12% to 44%), diaphoresis (≤14%)

1% to 10%:

Cardiovascular: Peripheral edema (≤7%), angina (≤6%), chest pain (≤5%), CHF (≤3%), arrhythmia (≤3%), cerebrovascular accident (≤3%), MI (≤3%), supraventricular tachycardia (≤3%), deep vein thrombosis (1% to 3%), phlebitis (1% to 3%), aneurysm (≤1%), transient ischemic attack (≤1%)

Central nervous system: Headache (≤9%), malaise (6% to 8%), sleep disorder (1% to 3%), cerebellar syndrome (≤1%), depression (≤1%), mentation impaired (≤1%)

Dermatologic: Alopecia (≤3%), pruritus (1% to 3%), seborrhea (≤1%)

Endocrine & metabolic: Hyperglycemia (1% to 6%), LDH increased (≤6%), dehydration (≤1%)

Gastrointestinal: Abdominal pain (≤10%), stomatitis (≤9%), weight loss (≤6%), esophagitis (≤3%), constipation (1% to 3%), mucositis (≤2%), dysphagia (≤1%)

Genitourinary: Dysuria (3% to 4%), hesitancy (≤3%)

Hematologic: Hemorrhage (≤1%), myelodysplastic syndrome/acute myeloid leukemia (usually associated with prior or concurrent treatment with other anticancer agents)

Hepatic: Cholelithiasis (≤3%), liver function tests abnormal (1% to 3%), liver failure (≤1%)

Neuromuscular & skeletal: Back pain (≤9%), osteoporosis (≤2%), arthralgia (≤1%)

Otic: Hearing loss (2% to 6%)

Renal: Hematuria (2% to 3%), renal failure (≤1%), renal function test abnormal (≤1%), proteinuria (≤1%)

Respiratory: Bronchitis (≤9%), pharyngitis (≤9%), allergic pneumonitis (≤6%), hemoptysis (1% to 6%), sinusitis (≤5%), epistaxis (≤1%), hypoxia (≤1%)

Miscellaneous: Flu-like syndrome (5% to 8%), herpes simplex infection (≤8%), anaphylaxis (≤1%), tumor lysis syndrome (1%)

<1% (Limited to important or life-threatening): Acute respiratory distress syndrome, agitation, blindness, blurred vision, bone marrow fibrosis, coma, confusion, diplopia, eosinophilia, Epstein-Barr virus (EBV) associated lymphoproliferation, EBV reactivation, erythema multiforme, Evans syndrome, flank pain, hemolytic anemia (autoimmune), hemophilia (acquired), hemorrhagic cystitis, herpes zoster reactivation, hyperkalemia, hyperphosphatemia, hyperuricemia, hypocalcemia, interstitial pneumonitis, metabolic acidosis, opportunistic infection, optic neuritis, optic neuropathy, pancreatic enzymes abnormal, pancytopenia, pemphigus, pericardial effusion, peripheral neuropathy, photophobia (primarily with high doses), progressive multifocal leukoencephalopathy (PML), pulmonary fibrosis, pulmonary hemorrhage, pulmonary infiltrate, respiratory distress, respiratory failure, skin cancer (new onset or exacerbation), Stevens-Johnson syndrome, thrombocytopenia (autoimmune), thrombocytopenic purpura (autoimmune), toxic epidermal necrolysis, trilineage bone marrow aplasia, trilineage bone marrow hypoplasia, urate crystalluria, wrist drop

Also observed: Neurologic syndrome characterized by cortical blindness, coma, and paralysis [36% at doses >96 mg/m^2 for 5-7 days; <0.2% at doses <125 mg/m^2/cycle (onset of neurologic symptoms may be delayed for 3-4 weeks)]

Drug Interactions

Avoid Concomitant Use

Avoid concomitant use of Fludarabine with any of the following: Natalizumab; Vaccines (Live)

Increased Effect/Toxicity

Fludarabine may increase the levels/effects of: Natalizumab; Pentostatin; Vaccines (Live)

The levels/effects of Fludarabine may be increased by: Trastuzumab

Decreased Effect

Fludarabine may decrease the levels/effects of: Vaccines (Inactivated)

The levels/effects of Fludarabine may be decreased by: Echinacea

Ethanol/Nutrition/Herb Interactions Ethanol: Avoid ethanol (due to GI irritation).

Stability

I.V.: Store intact vials under refrigeration at 2°C to 8°C (36°F to 46°F). Reconstituted vials are stable for 16 days at room temperature of 15°C to 30°C (59°F to 86°F) or refrigerated, although the manufacturer recommends use within 8 hours. Solutions diluted in saline or dextrose are stable for 48 hours at room temperature or under refrigeration. Reconstitute vials with SWI, NS, or D_5W to a concentration of 10-25 mg/mL; standard I.V. dilution: 100-125 mL D_5W or NS.

Tablet: Store at 25°C (77°F); excursions permitted to 15°C to 30°C (59°F to 86°F); should be kept within packaging until use.

Mechanism of Action Fludarabine inhibits DNA synthesis by inhibition of DNA polymerase and ribonucleotide reductase; also inhibits DNA primase and DNA ligase I

Pharmacodynamics/Kinetics

Distribution: V_d: 38-96 L/m^2; widely with extensive tissue binding

Protein binding: 2-fluoro-ara-A: ~19% to 29%

Metabolism: I.V.: Fludarabine phosphate is rapidly dephosphorylated in the plasma to 2-fluoro-ara-A (active metabolite), which subsequently enters tumor cells and is phosphorylated by deoxycytidine kinase to the active triphosphate derivative (2-fluoro-ara-ATP)

Bioavailability: Oral: 2-fluoro-ara-A: 50% to 65%

Half-life elimination: 2-fluoro-ara-A: ~20 hours

Time to peak, plasma: Oral: 1-2 hours

Excretion: Urine (60%, 23% as 2-fluoro-ara-A) within 24 hours

Dosage Details concerning dosing in combination regimens should also be consulted.

Oral: Adults: CLL: 40 mg/m^2 once daily for 5 days every 28 days

I.V.:

Children (unlabeled use):

Refractory acute leukemia: 10 mg/m^2 bolus over 15 minutes followed by continuous infusion of 30.5 mg/m^2/day for 5 days **or**

10.5 mg/m^2 bolus over 15 minutes followed by 30.5 mg/m^2/day for 48 hours

Refractory solid tumors: 7 mg/m^2 bolus followed by 20 mg/m^2/day continuous infusion for 5 days

Adults:

CLL: 25 mg/m^2/day for 5 days every 28 days

Non-hodgkin's lymphoma, WM (unlabeled uses): 25 mg/m^2/day for 5 days every 28 days

Reduced-intensity conditioning regimens prior to allogeneic hematopoietic stem cell transplantation (unlabeled use): 120-150 mg/m^2 administered in divided doses over 4-5 days

Dosage adjustment for toxicity:

Hematologic or nonhematologic toxicity (other than neurotoxicity): Consider treatment delay or dosage reduction

Neurotoxicity: Consider treatment delay or discontinuation

Dosing in renal impairment:

FDA-approved labeling contains the following adjustment recommendations:

Cl_{cr} 30-70 mL/minute: Administer 80% of dose

Cl_{cr} <30 mL/minute:

I.V.: Avoid use

Oral: Administer 50% of dose

Canadian labeling contains the following adjustment recommendations:

Cl_{cr} 30-70 mL/minute: Administer 50% of dose

Cl_{cr} <30 mL/minute: Use is contraindicated

The following guidelines have been used by some clinicians:

Aronoff, 2007:

Children:

Cl_{cr} 30-50 mL/minute: Administer 80% of dose

Cl_{cr} <30 mL/minute: Not recommended

Hemodialysis: Administer 25% of dose

Continuous ambulatory peritoneal dialysis (CAPD): Not recommended

Continuous renal replacement therapy (CRRT): Administer 80% of dose

Adults:

Cl_{cr} 10-50 mL/minute: Administer 75% of dose

Cl_{cr} <10 mL/minute: Administer 50% of dose

Hemodialysis: Administer after dialysis

Continuous ambulatory peritoneal dialysis (CAPD): Administer 50% of dose

Continuous renal replacement therapy (CRRT): Administer 75% of dose

Kintzel, 1995:

Cl_{cr} 46-60 mL/minute: Administer 80% of dose

Cl_{cr} 31-45 mL/minute: Administer 75% of dose

Cl_{cr} <30 mL/minute: Administer 65% of dose

Dietary Considerations Tablet may be taken with or without food.

Administration

Oral: Tablet may be administered with or without food; should be swallowed whole with water; do not chew, break, or crush.

I.V.: Usually administered as a 30-minute infusion; continuous infusions are occasionally used

Monitoring Parameters CBC with differential, platelet count, AST, ALT, serum creatinine, serum albumin, uric acid; monitor for signs of infection and neurotoxicity

Product Availability Fludarabine oral formulation (brand name pending): FDA approved December 2008; availability currently undetermined

Dosage Forms Excipient information presented when available (limited, particularly for generics); consult specific product labeling. [CAN] = Canadian brand name

Injection, powder for reconstitution, as phosphate: 50 mg

Fludara®: 50 mg [contains mannitol 50 mg/vial]

Tablet, as phosphate: 10 mg

Fludara® [CAN]: 10 mg

◆ **Fludarabine Phosphate** *see* Fludarabine *on page 628*

Fludrocortisone (floo droe KOR ti sone)

U.S. Brand Names Florinef® [DSC]

Canadian Brand Names Florinef®

Index Terms 9α-Fluorohydrocortisone Acetate; Fludrocortisone Acetate; Fluohydrisone Acetate; Fluohydrocortisone Acetate

Pharmacologic Category Corticosteroid, Systemic

Additional Appendix Information

Corticosteroids *on page 1652*

Use Partial replacement therapy for primary and secondary adrenocortical insufficiency in Addison's disease; treatment of salt-losing adrenogenital syndrome

Pregnancy Risk Factor C

Pregnancy Considerations Animal reproduction studies have not been conducted with fludrocortisone; adverse events have been observed with corticosteroids in animal reproduction studies. Some studies have shown an association between first trimester systemic corticosteroid use and oral clefts; adverse events in the fetus/neonate have been noted in case reports following large doses of systemic corticosteroids during pregnancy.

Lactation Excretion in breast milk unknown/use caution

Medication Safety Issues

Sound-alike/look-alike issues:

Florinef® may be confused with Fioricet®, Fiorinal®

Contraindications Hypersensitivity to fludrocortisone or any component of the formulation; systemic fungal infections

Warnings/Precautions May cause hypercorticism or suppression of hypothalamic-pituitary-adrenal (HPA) axis, particularly in younger children or in patients receiving high doses for prolonged periods. HPA axis suppression may lead to adrenal crisis. Withdrawal and discontinuation of a corticosteroid should be done slowly and carefully. Fludrocortisone is primarily a mineralocorticoid agonist, but may also inhibit the HPA axis. May increase risk of infection and/or limit response to vaccinations; close observation is required in patients with latent tuberculosis and/or TB reactivity. Restrict use in active TB (only in conjunction with antituberculosis treatment). Use with caution in patients with sodium retention and potassium loss, hepatic impairment, myocardial infarction, osteoporosis, and/or renal impairment. Use with caution in the elderly. Withdraw therapy with gradual tapering of dose. Safety and efficacy have not been established in children.

Adverse Reactions Frequency not defined.

Cardiovascular: Hypertension, edema, CHF

Central nervous system: Convulsions, headache, dizziness

Dermatologic: Acne, rash, bruising

Endocrine & metabolic: Hypokalemic alkalosis, suppression of growth, hyperglycemia, HPA suppression

Gastrointestinal: Peptic ulcer

Neuromuscular & skeletal: Muscle weakness

Ocular: Cataracts

Miscellaneous: Diaphoresis, anaphylaxis (generalized)

Drug Interactions

Avoid Concomitant Use

Avoid concomitant use of Fludrocortisone with any of the following: Natalizumab; Vaccines (Live)

Increased Effect/Toxicity

Fludrocortisone may increase the levels/effects of: Acetylcholinesterase Inhibitors; Amphotericin B; CycloSPORINE; Loop Diuretics; Natalizumab; NSAID (COX-2 Inhibitor); NSAID (Nonselective); Thiazide Diuretics; Vaccines (Live); Warfarin

The levels/effects of Fludrocortisone may be increased by: Antifungal Agents (Azole Derivatives, Systemic); Aprepitant; Calcium Channel Blockers (Nondihydropyridine); CycloSPORINE; Estrogen Derivatives; Fluconazole; Fosaprepitant; Macrolide Antibiotics; Neuromuscular-Blocking Agents (Nondepolarizing); Quinolone Antibiotics; Salicylates; Trastuzumab

Decreased Effect

Fludrocortisone may decrease the levels/effects of: Antidiabetic Agents; Calcitriol; Corticorelin; Isoniazid; Salicylates; Vaccines (Inactivated)

The levels/effects of Fludrocortisone may be decreased by: Aminoglutethimide; Antacids; Barbiturates; Bile Acid Sequestrants; Echinacea; Primidone; Rifamycin Derivatives

Mechanism of Action Promotes increased reabsorption of sodium and loss of potassium from renal distal tubules

Pharmacodynamics/Kinetics
Absorption: Rapid and complete
Protein binding: 42%
Metabolism: Hepatic
Half-life elimination, plasma: 30-35 minutes; Biological: 18-36 hours
Time to peak, serum: ~1.7 hours

Dosage Oral:
Infants and Children: 0.05-0.1 mg/day
Adults: 0.1-0.2 mg/day with ranges of 0.1 mg 3 times/week to 0.2 mg/day
Addison's disease: Initial: 0.1 mg/day; if transient hypertension develops, reduce the dose to 0.05 mg/day. Preferred administration with cortisone (10-37.5 mg/day) or hydrocortisone (10-30 mg/day).
Salt-losing adrenogenital syndrome: 0.1-0.2 mg/day

Dietary Considerations Systemic use of mineralocorticoids/corticosteroids may require a diet with increased potassium, vitamins A, B_6, C, D, folate, calcium, zinc, and phosphorus, and decreased sodium. With fludrocortisone, a decrease in dietary sodium is often not required as the increased retention of sodium is usually the desired therapeutic effect.

Administration Administration in conjunction with a glucocorticoid is preferable

Monitoring Parameters Monitor blood pressure and signs of edema when patient is on chronic therapy; very potent mineralocorticoid with high glucocorticoid activity; monitor serum electrolytes, serum renin activity, and blood pressure; monitor for evidence of infection; stop treatment if a significant increase in weight or blood pressure, edema, or cardiac enlargement occurs

Additional Information In patients with salt-losing forms of congenital adrenogenital syndrome, use along with cortisone or hydrocortisone. Fludrocortisone 0.1 mg has sodium retention activity equal to DOCA® 1 mg.

Dosage Forms Excipient information presented when available (limited, particularly for generics); consult specific product labeling. [DSC] = Discontinued product
Tablet, as acetate: 0.1 mg
Florinef®: 0.1 mg [DSC]

◆ **Fludrocortisone Acetate** *see* Fludrocortisone *on page 630*

◆ **FluLaval™** *see* Influenza Virus Vaccine *on page 788*

◆ **Flumadine®** *see* Rimantadine *on page 1320*

Flumazenil (FLOO may ze nil)

U.S. Brand Names Romazicon®

Canadian Brand Names Anexate®; Flumazenil Injection; Flumazenil Injection, USP; Romazicon®

Pharmacologic Category Antidote

Use Benzodiazepine antagonist; reverses sedative effects of benzodiazepines used in conscious sedation and general anesthesia; treatment of benzodiazepine overdose

Pregnancy Risk Factor C

Pregnancy Considerations Teratogenic effects were not seen in animal studies. Embryocidal effects were seen at large doses. There are no adequate or well-controlled studies in pregnant women. Use only if clearly needed.

Lactation Excretion in breast milk unknown/use caution

Contraindications Hypersensitivity to flumazenil, benzodiazepines, or any component of the formulation; patients given benzodiazepines for control of potentially life-threatening conditions (eg, control of intracranial pressure or status epilepticus); patients who are showing signs of serious cyclic-antidepressant overdosage

Warnings/Precautions **[U.S. Boxed Warning]: Benzodiazepine reversal may result in seizures in some patients.** Patients who may develop seizures include patients on benzodiazepines for long-term sedation, tricyclic antidepressant overdose patients, concurrent major sedative-hypnotic drug withdrawal, recent therapy with repeated doses of parenteral benzodiazepines, myoclonic jerking or seizure activity prior to flumazenil administration. Flumazenil may not reliably reverse respiratory depression/hypoventilation. Flumazenil is not a substitute for evaluation of oxygenation; establishing an airway and assisting ventilation, as necessary, is always the initial step in overdose management. Resedation occurs more frequently in patients where a large single dose or cumulative dose of a benzodiazepine is administered along with a neuromuscular-blocking agent and multiple anesthetic agents. Flumazenil should be used with caution in the intensive care unit because of increased risk of unrecognized benzodiazepine dependence in such settings. Should not be used to diagnose benzodiazepine-induced sedation. Reverse neuromuscular blockade before considering use. Flumazenil does not antagonize the CNS effects of other GABA agonists (such as ethanol, barbiturates, or general anesthetics); nor does it reverse narcotics. Flumazenil does not consistently reverse amnesia; patient may not recall verbal instructions after procedure.

Use with caution in patients with a history of panic disorder; may provoke panic attacks. Use caution in drug and ethanol-dependent patients; these patients may also be dependent on benzodiazepines. Not recommended for treatment of benzodiazepine dependence. Use with caution in head injury patients. Use caution in patients with mixed drug overdoses; toxic effects of other drugs taken may emerge once benzodiazepine effects are reversed. Use caution in hepatic dysfunction and in patients relying on a benzodiazepine for seizure control. Safety and efficacy have not been established in children <1 year of age.

Adverse Reactions
>10%: Gastrointestinal: Vomiting, nausea
1% to 10%:
Cardiovascular: Vasodilation (1% to 3%), palpitation
Central nervous system: Headache (1% to 3%), agitation (3% to 9%), dizziness (10%), emotional lability (1% to 3%), fatigue (1% to 3%)
Gastrointestinal: Xerostomia
Local: Pain at injection site (3% to 9%)
Neuromuscular & skeletal: Tremor, weakness, paresthesia (1% to 3%)
Ocular: Abnormal vision, blurred vision (3% to 9%)
Respiratory: Dyspnea, hyperventilation (3% to 9%)
Miscellaneous: Diaphoresis
<1%: Abnormal hearing, altered blood pressure (increases and decreases), confusion, sensation of coldness, bradycardia, chest pain, generalized seizure, hiccups, hypertension, junctional tachycardia, shivering, somnolence, tachycardia, thick tongue, ventricular tachycardia, withdrawal syndrome

Drug Interactions

Avoid Concomitant Use There are no known interactions where it is recommended to avoid concomitant use.

Increased Effect/Toxicity There are no known significant interactions involving an increase in effect.

Decreased Effect
Flumazenil may decrease the levels/effects of: Hypnotics (Nonbenzodiazepine)

Stability Store at 15°C to 30°C (59°F to 86°F). For I.V. use only. Once drawn up in the syringe or mixed with solution use within 24 hours. Discard any unused solution after 24 hours.

Mechanism of Action Competitively inhibits the activity at the benzodiazepine receptor site on the GABA/benzodiazepine receptor complex. Flumazenil does not antagonize the CNS effect of drugs affecting GABA-ergic neurons by means other than the benzodiazepine receptor (ethanol, barbiturates, general anesthetics) and does not reverse the effects of opioids

Pharmacodynamics/Kinetics

Onset of action: 1-3 minutes; 80% response within 3 minutes

Peak effect: 6-10 minutes

Duration: Resedation: ~1 hour; duration related to dose given and benzodiazepine plasma concentrations; reversal effects of flumazenil may wear off before effects of benzodiazepine

Distribution: Initial V_d: 0.5 L/kg; V_{dss} 0.77-1.6 L/kg

Protein binding: 40% to 50%

Metabolism: Hepatic; dependent upon hepatic blood flow

Half-life elimination: Adults: Alpha: 7-15 minutes; Terminal: 41-79 minutes; Moderate hepatic dysfunction: 1.3 hours; severe hepatic impairment: 2.4 hours

Excretion: Feces; urine (0.2% as unchanged drug)

Dosage

Children and Adults: I.V.: See table.

Flumazenil

Pediatric Dosage	
Pediatric dosage for **reversal of conscious sedation and general anesthesia:**	
Initial dose	0.01 mg/kg over 15 seconds (maximum: 0.2 mg)
Repeat doses (maximum: 4 doses)	0.005-0.01 mg/kg (maximum: 0.2 mg) repeated at 1-minute intervals
Maximum total cumulative dose	1 mg or 0.05 mg/kg (whichever is lower)
Adult Dosage	
Adult dosage for **reversal of conscious sedation and general anesthesia:**	
Initial dose	0.2 mg intravenously over 15 seconds
Repeat doses (maximum: 4 doses)	If desired level of consciousness is not obtained, 0.2 mg may be repeated at 1-minute intervals.
Maximum total cumulative dose	1 mg (usual dose: 0.6-1 mg) **In the event of resedation:** Repeat doses may be given at 20-minute intervals with maximum of 1 mg/dose and 3 mg/hour.
Adult dosage for **suspected benzodiazepine overdose:**	
Initial dose	0.2 mg intravenously over 30 seconds; if the desired level of consciousness is not obtained, 0.3 mg can be given over 30 seconds
Repeat doses	0.5 mg over 30 seconds repeated at 1-minute intervals
Maximum total cumulative dose	3 mg (usual dose 1-3 mg) Patients with a partial response at 3 mg may require additional titration up to a total dose of 5 mg. If a patient has not responded 5 minutes after cumulative dose of 5 mg, the major cause of sedation is not likely due to benzodiazepines. **In the event of resedation:** May repeat doses at 20-minute intervals with maximum of 1 mg/dose and 3 mg/hour.

Resedation: Repeated doses may be given at 20-minute intervals as needed; repeat treatment doses of 1 mg (at a rate of 0.5 mg/minute) should be given at any time and no more than 3 mg should be given in any hour. After intoxication with high doses of benzodiazepines, the duration of a single dose of flumazenil is not expected to exceed 1 hour; if desired, the period of wakefulness may be prolonged with repeated low intravenous doses of flumazenil, or by an infusion of 0.1-0.4 mg/hour. Most patients with benzodiazepine overdose will respond to a cumulative dose of 1-3 mg and doses >3 mg do not reliably produce additional effects. Rarely, patients with a partial response at 3 mg may require additional titration up to a total dose of 5 mg. **If a patient has not responded 5 minutes after receiving a cumulative dose of 5 mg, the major cause of sedation is not likely to be due to benzodiazepines.**

Elderly: No differences in safety or efficacy have been reported. However, increased sensitivity may occur in some elderly patients.

Dosing in renal impairment: Not significantly affected by renal failure (Cl_{cr} <10 mL/minute) or hemodialysis beginning 1 hour after drug administration

Dosing in hepatic impairment: Use caution with initial and/or repeat doses in patients with liver disease

Administration I.V.: Administer in freely-running I.V. into large vein. Inject over 15 seconds for conscious sedation and general anesthesia and over 30 seconds for overdose.

Monitoring Parameters Monitor patients for return of sedation or respiratory depression

Dosage Forms Excipient information presented when available (limited, particularly for generics); consult specific product labeling.

Injection, solution: 0.1 mg/mL (5 mL, 10 mL)

Romazicon®: 0.1 mg/mL (5 mL, 10 mL) [contains edetate disodium]

◆ **Flumazenil Injection (Can)** *see* Flumazenil *on page 631*

◆ **Flumazenil Injection, USP (Can)** *see* Flumazenil *on page 631*

◆ **FluMist®** *see* Influenza Virus Vaccine *on page 788*

Flunisolide (floo NISS oh lide)

U.S. Brand Names AeroBid®; AeroBid®-M; Nasarel®

Canadian Brand Names Alti-Flunisolide; Apo-Flunisolide®; Nasalide®; PMS-Flunisolide; Rhinalar®

Pharmacologic Category Corticosteroid, Inhalant (Oral); Corticosteroid, Nasal

Additional Appendix Information

Asthma *on page 1793*

Use Steroid-dependent asthma; nasal solution is used for seasonal or perennial rhinitis

Pregnancy Risk Factor C

Medication Safety Issues

Sound-alike/look-alike issues:

Flunisolide may be confused with Flumadine®, fluocinonide

Nasarel® may be confused with Nizoral®

Dosage Note: AeroBid® and Aerospan™ are not interchangeable; dosing changes when switching from one to the other.

Oral inhalation: Asthma:

AeroBid®:

Children 6-15 years: 2 inhalations twice daily (morning and evening); up to 4 inhalations/day

Children ≥16 years and Adults: 2 inhalations twice daily (morning and evening); up to 8 inhalations/day maximum

NIH Asthma Guidelines (NIH, 2007) (administer in divided doses twice daily):

Children 5-11 years:

"Low" dose: 500-750 mcg/day

"Medium" dose: 1000-1250 mcg/day

"High" dose: >1250 mcg/day

Children ≥12 years and Adults:

"Low" dose: 500-1000 mcg/day

"Medium" dose: >1000-2000 mcg/day

"High" dose: >2000 mcg/day

Aerospan™:

Children 6-11 years: 1 inhalation twice daily; up to 4 inhalations/day

Children ≥12 years and Adults: 2 inhalations twice daily; up to 8 inhalations/day

NIH Asthma Guidelines (NIH, 2007) (administer in divided doses twice daily):

Children 5-11 years:

"Low" dose: 160 mcg/day

"Medium" dose: 320 mcg/day

"High" dose: ≥640 mcg/day

Children ≥12 years and Adults:

"Low" dose: 320 mcg/day

"Medium" dose: >320-640 mcg/day

"High" dose: >640 mcg/day

Intranasal: Rhinitis:

Children 6-14 years: 1 spray each nostril 3 times daily **or** 2 sprays in each nostril twice daily; not to exceed 4 sprays/day in each nostril (200 mcg/day)

Children ≥15 years and Adults: 2 sprays each nostril twice daily (morning and evening); may increase to 2 sprays 3 times daily; maximum dose: 8 sprays/day in each nostril (400 mcg/day)

Additional Information Complete prescribing information for this medication should be consulted for additional detail.

Dosage Forms Excipient information presented when available (limited, particularly for generics); consult specific product labeling.

Aerosol for oral inhalation:

AeroBid®: 250 mcg/actuation (7 g) [100 metered inhalations; contains chlorofluorocarbon]

AeroBid®-M: 250 mcg/actuation (7 g) [100 metered inhalations; contains chlorofluorocarbon; menthol flavor]

Solution, intranasal [spray]: 25 mcg/actuation (25 mL); 29 mcg/actuation (25 mL) [200 sprays]

Nasarel®: 29 mcg/actuation (25 mL) [200 sprays; contains benzalkonium chloride]

Fluocinolone (floo oh SIN oh lone)

U.S. Brand Names Capex®; Derma-Smoothe/FS®; DermOtic® ; Retisert®; Synalar® [DSC]

Canadian Brand Names Capex®; Derma-Smoothe/FS®; Synalar®

Index Terms Fluocinolone Acetonide

Pharmacologic Category Corticosteroid, Ophthalmic; Corticosteroid, Topical

Additional Appendix Information

Corticosteroids *on page 1652*

Use Relief of susceptible inflammatory dermatosis [low, medium corticosteroid]; dermatitis or psoriasis of the scalp; atopic dermatitis in adults and children ≥3 months of age

Ocular implant (Retisert®): Treatment of chronic, non-infectious uveitis affecting the posterior segment of the eye

Otic (DermOtic® Oil): Relief of chronic eczematous external otitis in adults and children ≥2 years of age.

Pregnancy Risk Factor C

Medication Safety Issues

Sound-alike/look-alike issues:

Fluocinolone may be confused with fluocinonide

Dosage

Ocular implant: Chronic uveitis: Children ≥12 years and Adults: One silicone-encased tablet (0.59 mg) surgically implanted into the posterior segment of the eye is designed to initially release 0.6 mcg/day, decreasing over 30 days to a steady-state release rate of 0.3-0.4 mcg/day for 30 months. Recurrence of uveitis denotes depletion of tablet, requiring reimplantation.

Otic: Chronic eczematous external otitis: Children ≥2 years and Adults: 5 drops into the affected ear twice daily for 1-2 weeks

Topical:

Atopic dermatitis (Derma-Smoothe/FS® body oil):

Children ≥3 months: Moisten skin; apply a thin film to affected area twice daily; do not use for longer than 4 weeks

Adults: Apply a thin film to affected area 3 times/day

Corticosteroid-responsive dermatoses: Children and Adults: Cream, ointment, solution: Apply a thin layer to affected area 2-4 times/day; may use occlusive dressings to manage psoriasis or recalcitrant conditions

Inflammatory and pruritic manifestations (dental use): Adults: Apply to oral lesion 4 times/day, after meals and at bedtime

Scalp psoriasis (Derma-Smoothe/FS® scalp oil): Adults: Massage thoroughly into wet or dampened hair/scalp; cover with shower cap. Leave on overnight (or for at least 4 hours). Remove by washing hair with shampoo and rinsing thoroughly.

Seborrheic dermatitis of the scalp (Capex®): Adults: Apply no more than 1 ounce to scalp once daily; work into lather and allow to remain on scalp for ~5 minutes. Remove from hair and scalp by rinsing thoroughly with water.

Additional Information Complete prescribing information for this medication should be consulted for additional detail.

Dosage Forms Excipient information presented when available (limited, particularly for generics); consult specific product labeling. [DSC] = Discontinued product

Cream, as acetonide: 0.01% (15 g, 60 g); 0.025% (15 g, 60 g)

Synalar®: 0.025% (15 g, 60 g) [DSC]

Implant, intravitreal, as acetonide:

Retisert®: 0.59 mg [enclosed in silicone elastomer]

Oil, as acetonide:

Derma-Smoothe/FS® [body oil]: 0.01% (120 mL) [contains peanut oil]

Derma-Smoothe/FS® [scalp oil]: 0.01% (120 mL) [contains peanut oil; packaged with shower caps]

DermaOtic® [otic drops]: 0.01% (20 mL) [contains peanut oil; packaged with dropper]

Ointment, as acetonide: 0.025% (15 g, 60 g)

Synalar®: 0.025% (15 g, 60 g) [DSC]

Shampoo, as acetonide:

Capex®: 0.01% (120 mL)

Solution, as acetonide: 0.01% (60 mL)

Synalar®: 0.01% (20 mL, 60 mL) [DSC]

◆ **Fluocinolone Acetonide** *see* Fluocinolone *on page 633*

Fluocinolone, Hydroquinone, and Tretinoin

(floo oh SIN oh lone, HYE droe kwin one, & TRET i noyn)

U.S. Brand Names Tri-Luma™

Index Terms Hydroquinone, Fluocinolone Acetonide, and Tretinoin; Tretinoin, Fluocinolone Acetonide, and Hydroquinone

Pharmacologic Category Corticosteroid, Topical; Depigmenting Agent; Retinoic Acid Derivative

Use Short-term treatment of moderate to severe melasma of the face

Pregnancy Risk Factor C

Dosage Topical: Adults: Melasma: Apply a thin film once daily to hyperpigmented areas of melasma (including 1/2 inch of normal-appearing surrounding skin). Apply 30 minutes prior to bedtime; not indicated for use beyond 8 weeks. Do not use occlusive dressings.

Additional Information Complete prescribing information for this medication should be consulted for additional detail.

Dosage Forms Excipient information presented when available (limited, particularly for generics); consult specific product labeling.

Cream, topical: Hydroquinone 4%, tretinoin 0.05%, fluocinolone acetonide 0.01% (30 g) [contains sodium metabisulfite]

Fluocinonide (floo oh SIN oh nide)

U.S. Brand Names Lidex-E® [DSC]; Lidex® [DSC]; Vanos™

Canadian Brand Names Lidemol®; Lidex®; Lyderm®; Tiamol®; Topsyn®

Pharmacologic Category Corticosteroid, Topical

Additional Appendix Information

Corticosteroids *on page 1652*

Use Anti-inflammatory, antipruritic; treatment of plaque-type psoriasis (up to 10% of body surface area) [high-potency topical corticosteroid]

Pregnancy Risk Factor C

Medication Safety Issues

Sound-alike/look-alike issues:

Fluocinonide may be confused with flunisolide, fluocinolone

Lidex® may be confused with Lasix®, Videx®, Wydase®

Dosage

Children and Adults: Pruritus and inflammation: Topical (0.05% cream): Apply thin layer to affected area 2-4 times/day depending on the severity of the condition. Therapy should be discontinued when control is achieved; if no improvement is seen, reassessment of diagnosis may be necessary.

Children ≥12 years and Adults: Plaque-type psoriasis (Vanos™): Topical (0.1% cream): Apply a thin layer once or twice daily to affected areas (limited to <10% of body surface area). **Note:** Not recommended for use >2 consecutive weeks or >60 g/week total exposure. Discontinue when control is achieved.

Additional Information Complete prescribing information for this medication should be consulted for additional detail.

Dosage Forms Excipient information presented when available (limited, particularly for generics); consult specific product labeling.

Cream, anhydrous, emollient: 0.05% (15 g, 30 g, 60 g, 120 g)

Lidex®: 0.05% (15 g, 30 g, 60 g) [DSC]

Cream, aqueous, emollient: 0.05% (15 g, 30 g, 60 g)

Lidex-E®: 0.05% (15 g, 30 g, 60 g) [DSC]

Cream:

Vanos™: 0.1% (30 g, 60 g)

Gel: 0.05% (15 g, 30 g, 60 g)

Lidex®: 0.05% (15 g, 30 g, 60 g) [DSC]

Ointment: 0.05% (15 g, 30 g, 60 g)

Lidex®: 0.05% (15 g, 30 g, 60 g) [DSC]

Solution: 0.05% (20 mL, 60 mL)

Lidex®: 0.05% (60 mL) [contains alcohol 35%] [DSC]

◆ **Fluohydrisone Acetate** *see* Fludrocortisone *on page 630*

◆ **Fluohydrocortisone Acetate** *see* Fludrocortisone *on page 630*

◆ **Fluoracaine® [DSC]** *see* Proparacaine and Fluorescein *on page 1254*

◆ **Flour-A-Day** *see* Fluoride *on page 635*

Fluorescein (FLURE e seen)

U.S. Brand Names AK-Fluor®; Angiofluor™; Angiofluor™ Lite; Fluorescite®; Fluorets®; Ful-Glo®

Canadian Brand Names Fluorescite®

Index Terms Fluorescein Sodium; Sodium Fluorescein; Soluble Fluorescein

Pharmacologic Category Diagnostic Agent

Use

Injection: Diagnostic aid in ophthalmic angiography and angioscopy

Topical: To stain the anterior segment of the eye for procedures (such as fitting contact lenses), disclosing corneal injury, and in applanation tonometry

Pregnancy Risk Factor C

Dosage

Ophthalmic: Strips: Children and Adults: Moisten strip with sterile water, saline or ophthalmic fluid. Touch conjunctiva or fornix with tip of strip until adequately stained. For best results, patient should blink several times after application.

Injection:

Children: 3.5 mg/lb (7.7 mg/kg) injected rapidly into antecubital vein

Adults: 500-750 mg injected rapidly into antecubital vein

Note: Prior to use, an intradermal test dose of 0.05 mL may be used if an allergy is suspected. Evaluate 30-60 minutes following intradermal injection.

Oral: Adults: 1 g of injection solution has been administered orally in patients with inaccessible veins and when early phases of an angiogram are not needed.

Dosage adjustment in renal impairment: Injection: Dialysis patients: Decrease dose by 50%

Additional Information Complete prescribing information for this medication should be consulted for additional detail.

Dosage Forms Excipient information presented when available (limited, particularly for generics); consult specific product labeling.

Injection, solution, as sodium: 10% (5 mL); 25% (2 mL)

AK-Fluor, Angiofluor™, Angiofluor™ Lite, Fluorescite®: 10% (5 mL); 25% (2 mL)

Strip, ophthalmic, as sodium: 1 mg

Fluorets®: 1 mg (100)

Ful-Glo®: 0.6 mg (300); 1 mg (300)

Fluorescein and Benoxinate
(FLURE e seen & ben OX i nate)

U.S. Brand Names EyeFlur; Fluress®; Flurox™

Index Terms Benoxinate Hydrochloride and Fluorescein Sodium

Pharmacologic Category Anesthetic, Topical; Diagnostic Agent; Ophthalmic Agent

Use For use in ophthalmic procedures when a topical disclosing agent is needed along with an anesthetic

Pregnancy Risk Factor C

Dosage Ophthalmic: Adults:

Removal of foreign bodies, sutures, or tonometry: Instill 1 or 2 drops (single instillations) into each eye before operating

Deep ophthalmic anesthesia: Instill 2 drops into each eye every 90 seconds up to 3 doses

Additional Information Complete prescribing information for this medication should be consulted for additional detail.

Dosage Forms Excipient information presented when available (limited, particularly for generics); consult specific product labeling.

Solution, ophthalmic: Fluorescein sodium 0.25% and benoxinate hydrochloride 0.4% (5 mL)

EyeFlur, Fluress®, Flurox™: Fluorescein sodium 0.25% and benoxinate hydrochloride 0.4% (5 mL)

◆ **Fluorescein and Proparacaine** *see* Proparacaine and Fluorescein *on page 1254*

◆ **Fluorescein Sodium** *see* Fluorescein *on page 634*

◆ **Fluorescite®** *see* Fluorescein *on page 634*

◆ **Fluorets®** *see* Fluorescein *on page 634*

Fluoride (FLOR ide)

U.S. Brand Names ACT® Plus [OTC]; ACT® x2™ [OTC]; ACT® [OTC]; CaviRinse™; ControlRx®; Denta 5000 Plus; DentaGel; EtheDent™; Fluor-A-Day; Fluorigard® [OTC]; Fluorinse®; Flura-Drops®; Gel-Kam® Rinse; Gel-Kam® [OTC]; Just for Kids™ [OTC]; Lozi-Flur™; Luride® Lozi-Tab®; Luride® [DSC]; NeutraCare®; NeutraGard® Advanced; NeutraGard® Plus; NeutraGard® [OTC]; Omnii Gel™ [OTC]; PerioMed™; Pharmaflur® 1.1 [DSC]; Pharmaflur® [DSC]; Phos-Flur®; Phos-Flur® Rinse [OTC]; PreviDent®; PreviDent® 5000 Plus™; StanGard®; StanGard® Perio; Stop®; Thera-Flur-N® [DSC]

Canadian Brand Names Fluor-A-Day

Index Terms Acidulated Phosphate Fluoride; Sodium Fluoride; Stannous Fluoride

Pharmacologic Category Nutritional Supplement

Use Prevention of dental caries

Pregnancy Risk Factor C

Medication Safety Issues

Sound-alike/look-alike issues:

Luride® may be confused with Lortab®

Phos-Flur® may be confused with PhosLo®

Thera-Flur-N® may be confused with Thera-Flu®

International issues:

Fluorex® [France] may be confused with Flarex® which is a brand name for fluorometholone in the U.S.

Dosage Oral:

The recommended daily dose of oral fluoride supplement (mg), based on fluoride ion content (ppm) in drinking water (2.2 mg of sodium fluoride is equivalent to 1 mg of fluoride ion): See table.

Fluoride Ion

Fluoride Content of Drinking Water	Daily Dose, Oral (mg)
<0.3 ppm	
Birth - 6 mo	None
6 mo - 3 y	0.25
3-6 y	0.5
6-16 y	1
0.3-0.6 ppm	
Birth - 6 mo	None
6 mo - 3 y	None
3-6 y	0.25
6-16 y	0.5

Adapted from Recommended Dosage Schedule of The American Dental Association, The American Academy of Pediatric Dentistry, and The American Academy of Pediatrics.

Cream: Children ≥6 years and Adults: Brush teeth with cream once daily regardless of fluoride content of drinking water

Dental rinse or gel:

Children 6-12 years: 5-10 mL rinse or apply to teeth and spit daily after brushing

Adults: 10 mL rinse or apply to teeth and spit daily after brushing

PreviDent® rinse: Children >6 years and Adults: Once weekly, rinse 10 mL vigorously around and between teeth for 1 minute, then spit; this should be done preferably at bedtime, after thoroughly brushing teeth; for maximum benefit, do not eat, drink, or rinse mouth for at least 30 minutes after treatment; do not swallow

Fluorinse®: Children >6 years and Adults: Once weekly, vigorously swish 5-10 mL in mouth for 1 minute, then spit

Lozenge (Lozi-Flur™): Adults: One lozenge daily regardless of fluoride content of drinking water

Additional Information Complete prescribing information for this medication should be consulted for additional detail.

Dosage Forms Excipient information presented when available (limited, particularly for generics); consult specific product labeling. [DSC] = Discontinued product

Cream, oral, as sodium [toothpaste]: 1.1% (51 g) [fluoride 2.5 mg/dose]

Denta 5000 Plus: 1.1% (51 g) [fluoride 2.5 mg/dose; spearmint flavor]

EtheDent™: 1.1% (51 g) [fluoride 2.5 mg/dose]

Gel-drops, as sodium fluoride:

Thera-Flur-N®: 1.1% (24 mL) [fluoride 0.5%; neutral pH; no artificial color or flavor] [DSC]

Gel, topical, as acidulated phosphate fluoride:

Phos-Flur®: 1.1% (60 g) [fluoride 0.5%; cherry and mint flavors]

Gel, topical, as sodium fluoride: 1.1% (56 g) [fluoride 2 mg/dose]

DentaGel, EtheDent™: 1.1% (56 g) [fluoride 2 mg/dose; fresh mint flavor]

NeutraCare®: 1.1% (60 g) [neutral pH; grape and mint flavors]

NeutraGard® Advanced: 1.1% (60 g) [cinnamon and mint flavors]

PreviDent®: 1.1% (60 g) [fluoride 2 mg/dose; berry and mint flavors]

Gel, topical, as stannous fluoride:

Gel-Kam®: 0.4% (129 g) [cinnamon, fruit/berry, and mint flavors]

Just for Kids™: 0.4% (122 g) [bubble gum, fruit punch, and grapey grape flavors]

Omnii Gel™: 0.4% (122 g) [cinnamon, grape, natural, mint, and raspberry flavors]

StanGard®: 0.4% (122 g) [bubble gum, cherry, mint, and raspberry flavors]

Stop®: 0.4% (120 g) [bubble gum, cinnamon, grape, and mint flavors]

Lozenge, as sodium:

Lozi-Flur™: 2.21 mg [fluoride 1 mg; cherry flavor]

Paste, oral, as sodium [toothpaste]:

ControlRx®: 1.1% (56 g) [vanilla mint flavor]

Solution, oral drops, as sodium: 1.1 mg/mL (50 mL) [fluoride 0.5 mg/mL]

Flura-Drops®: 0.55 mg/drop (24 mL) [fluoride 0.25 mg/drop; dye free, sugar free]

Luride®: 1.1 mg/mL (50 mL) [fluoride 0.5 mg/mL; sugar free] [DSC]

Solution, oral rinse, as sodium:

ACT®: 0.05% (530 mL) [fluoride 0.02%; bubble gum, cinnamon (contains tartrazine), and mint flavors]

ACT® Plus: 0.05% (530 mL) [fluoride 0.02%; alcohol free; icy cool mint flavor]

ACT® x2™: 0.5% (530 mL) [fluoride 0.02%; contains alcohol 11%; icy cool mint and spearmint flavors]

CaviRinse™: 0.2% (240 mL) [mint flavor]

Fluorigard®: 0.05% (480 mL) [alcohol free, sugar free; contains sodium benzoate and tartrazine; mint flavor]

Fluorinse®: 0.2% (480 mL) [alcohol free; cinnamon and mint flavors]

NeutraGard®: 0.05% (480 mL) [neutral pH; mint and tropical blast flavors]

NeutraGard® Plus: 0.2% (480 mL) [neutral pH; mint and tropical blast flavors]

Phos-Flur®: 0.44% (500 mL) [bubble gum, cherry, grape, and mint flavors]

PreviDent®: 0.2% (250 mL) [contains alcohol; mint flavor]

Solution, oral rinse concentrate, as stannous fluoride:
Gel-Kam®: 0.63% (300 mL) [fluoride 0.1%/dose; cinnamon and mint flavors]
PerioMed™: 0.63% (284 mL) [fluoride 7 mg/30 mL; alcohol free; cinnamon, mint and tropical fruit flavors]
StanGard® Perio: 0.63% (284 mL) [mint flavor]
Tablet, chewable, as sodium: 0.5 mg [fluoride 0.25 mg]; 1.1 mg [fluoride 0.5 mg]; 2.2 mg [fluoride 1 mg]
EtheDent™:
0.55 mg [fluoride 0.25 mg; sugar free; contains aspartame; vanilla flavor]
1.1 mg [fluoride 0.5 mg; sugar free; contains aspartame; grape flavor]
2.2 mg [fluoride 1 mg; sugar free; contains aspartame; cherry flavor]
Fluor-A-Day:
0.56 mg [fluoride 0.25 mg; raspberry flavor]
1.1 mg [fluoride 0.5 mg; raspberry flavor]
2.21 mg [fluoride 1 mg; raspberry flavor]
Luride® Lozi-Tab®:
0.55 mg [fluoride 0.25 mg; sugar free; vanilla flavor]
1.1 mg [fluoride 0.5 mg; sugar free; grape flavor]
2.2 mg [fluoride 1 mg; sugar free; cherry flavor] [DSC]
Pharmaflur®: 2.2 mg [fluoride 1 mg; dye free, sugar free; cherry flavor] [DSC]
Pharmaflur® 1.1: 1.1 mg [fluoride 0.5 mg; dye free, sugar free; grape flavor] [DSC]

◆ **Fluorigard® [OTC]** *see* Fluoride *on page* 635

◆ **Fluori-Methane®** *see* Dichlorodifluoromethane and Trichloromonofluoromethane *on page* 437

◆ **Fluorinse®** *see* Fluoride *on page* 635

◆ **5-Fluorocytosine** *see* Flucytosine *on page* 627

◆ **9α-Fluorohydrocortisone Acetate** *see* Fludrocortisone *on page* 630

Fluorometholone (flure oh METH oh lone)

U.S. Brand Names Flarex®; FML®; FML® Forte

Canadian Brand Names Flarex®; FML Forte®; FML®; PMS-Fluorometholone

Pharmacologic Category Corticosteroid, Ophthalmic

Use Treatment of steroid-responsive inflammatory conditions of the eye

Pregnancy Risk Factor C

Medication Safety Issues

International issues:
Flarex® may be confused with Flurets® which is a brand name for sodium fluoride in Australia
Flarex® may be confused with Fluarix® which is a brand name for influenza virus vaccine in the U.S. and in numerous international markets
Flarex® may be confused with Fluorex® which is a brand name for sodium fluoride in France
Fluor-Op® may be confused with Fluoron® which is a brand name for fluorine in Canada

Dosage Ophthalmic:

Children >2 years and Adults: Re-evaluate therapy if improvement is not seen within 2 days; use care not to discontinue prematurely; in chronic conditions, gradually decrease dosing frequency prior to discontinuing treatment
Ointment (FML®): Apply small amount (~1/2 inch ribbon) to conjunctival sac 1-3 times/day; may increase application to every 4 hours during the initial 24-48 hours
Suspension:
FML®: Instill 1 drop into conjunctival sac 2-4 times/day; may instill 1 drop every 4 hours during initial 24-48 hours
FML® Forte: Instill 1 drop into conjunctival sac 2-4 times/day

Adults: Suspension (Flarex®): Instill 1-2 drops into conjunctival sac 4 times/day; may increase application to 2 drops every 2 hours during initial 24-48 hours. Consult prescriber if no improvement after 14 days.

Additional Information Complete prescribing information for this medication should be consulted for additional detail.

Dosage Forms Excipient information presented when available (limited, particularly for generics); consult specific product labeling. [DSC] = Discontinued product

Ointment, ophthalmic, as base:
FML®: 0.1% (3.5 g)
Suspension, ophthalmic, as base: 0.1% (5 mL, 10 mL, 15 mL)
FML®: 0.1% (5 mL, 10 mL, 15 mL) [contains benzalkonium chloride]
FML® Forte: 0.25% (2 mL, 5 mL, 10 mL, 15 mL) [contains benzalkonium chloride]
Suspension, ophthalmic, as acetate:
Flarex®: 0.1% (5 mL) [contains benzalkonium chloride]

◆ **Fluoroplex®** *see* Fluorouracil *on page* 636

Fluorouracil (flure oh YOOR a sil)

U.S. Brand Names Adrucil®; Carac®; Efudex®; Fluoroplex®; Fluorouracil®

Canadian Brand Names Efudex®

Index Terms 5-Fluorouracil; 5-FU; FU

Pharmacologic Category Antineoplastic Agent, Antimetabolite (Pyrimidine Analog)

Use Treatment of carcinomas of the breast, colon, head and neck, pancreas, rectum, or stomach; topically for the management of actinic or solar keratoses and superficial basal cell carcinomas

Pregnancy Risk Factor D (injection); X (topical)

Pregnancy Considerations There are no adequate and well-controlled studies in pregnant women, however, fetal defects and miscarriages have been reported following use of topical and intravenous products. Use is contraindicated during pregnancy.

Lactation Excretion in breast milk unknown/not recommended

Medication Safety Issues

Sound-alike/look-alike issues:
Carac® may be confused with Kuric™
Fluorouracil may be confused with flucytosine
Efudex® may be confused with Efidac (Efidac 24®), Eurax®

High alert medication: The Institute for Safe Medication Practices (ISMP) includes this medication among its list of drugs which have a heightened risk of causing significant patient harm when used in error.

International issues:
Carac® may be confused with Carace® which is a brand name for lisinopril in Ireland and Great Britain

Contraindications Hypersensitivity to fluorouracil or any component of the formulation; dihydropyrimidine dehydrogenase (DPD) enzyme deficiency; pregnancy

Warnings/Precautions Hazardous agent - use appropriate precautions for handling and disposal. Use with caution in patients with impaired kidney or liver function. The drug should be discontinued if intractable vomiting or diarrhea, precipitous falls in leukocyte or platelet counts, stomatitis, hemorrhage, or myocardial ischemia occurs. Use with caution in patients who have had high-dose pelvic radiation or previous use of alkylating agents. Palmar-plantar erythrodysesthesia (hand-foot) syndrome has been associated with use. Safety and efficacy have not been established in pediatric patients.

Administration to patients with a genetic deficiency of dihydropyrimidine dehydrogenase (DPD) has been associated with increased toxicity following administration (diarrhea, neutropenia, and neurotoxicity). Systemic toxicity normally associated with parenteral administration has also been associated with topical use, particularly in patients with DPD. Discontinue if symptoms of DPD occur. **[U.S. Boxed Warning]: Should be administered under the supervision of an experienced cancer chemotherapy physician.**

Avoid topical application to mucous membranes due to potential for local inflammation and ulceration. The use of occlusive dressings with topical preparations may increase the severity of inflammation in nearby skin areas. Avoid exposure to ultraviolet rays during and immediately following therapy.

Adverse Reactions Toxicity depends on route and duration of treatment

I.V.:

Cardiovascular: Angina, myocardial ischemia, nail changes

Central nervous system: Acute cerebellar syndrome, confusion, disorientation, euphoria, headache, nystagmus

Dermatologic: Alopecia, dermatitis, dry skin, fissuring, palmar-plantar erythrodysesthesia syndrome, pruritic maculopapular rash, photosensitivity, vein pigmentations

Gastrointestinal: Anorexia, bleeding, diarrhea, esophagopharyngitis, nausea, sloughing, stomatitis, ulceration, vomiting

Hematologic: Agranulocytosis, anemia, leukopenia, pancytopenia, thrombocytopenia

Myelosuppression:

Onset: 7-10 days

Nadir: 9-14 days

Recovery: 21-28 days

Local: Thrombophlebitis

Ocular: Lacrimation, lacrimal duct stenosis, photophobia, visual changes

Respiratory: Epistaxis

Miscellaneous: Anaphylaxis, generalized allergic reactions, nail loss

Topical: Note: Systemic toxicity normally associated with parenteral administration (including neutropenia, neurotoxicity, and gastrointestinal toxicity) has been associated with topical use particularly in patients with a genetic deficiency of dihydropyrimidine dehydrogenase (DPD).

Central nervous system: Headache, insomnia, irritability

Dermatologic: Alopecia, photosensitivity, pruritus, rash, scarring, telangiectasia

Gastrointestinal: Medicinal taste, stomatitis

Hematologic: Leukocytosis, thrombocytopenia

Local: Application site reactions: Allergic contact dermatitis, burning, crusting, dryness, edema, erosion, erythema, hyperpigmentation, irritation, pain, soreness, ulceration

Ocular: Eye irritation (burning, watering, sensitivity, stinging, itching)

Miscellaneous: Birth defects, herpes simplex, miscarriage

Drug Interactions

Avoid Concomitant Use

Avoid concomitant use of Fluorouracil with any of the following: Natalizumab; Vaccines (Live)

Increased Effect/Toxicity

Fluorouracil may increase the levels/effects of: CYP2C9 Substrates (High risk); Natalizumab; Phenytoin; Vaccines (Live); Vitamin K Antagonists

The levels/effects of Fluorouracil may be increased by: Gemcitabine; Leucovorin-Levoleucovorin; Sorafenib; Trastuzumab

Decreased Effect

Fluorouracil may decrease the levels/effects of: Vaccines (Inactivated); Vitamin K Antagonists

The levels/effects of Fluorouracil may be decreased by: Echinacea; Sorafenib

Ethanol/Nutrition/Herb Interactions

Ethanol: Avoid ethanol (due to GI irritation).

Herb/Nutraceutical: Avoid black cohosh, dong quai in estrogen-dependent tumors.

Stability

Injection: Store intact vials at room temperature and protect from light; slight discoloration does not usually denote decomposition. Dilute in 50-1000 mL NS, D_5W, or bacteriostatic NS for infusion. If exposed to cold, a precipitate may form; **gentle** heating to 60°C will dissolve the precipitate without impairing the potency. Solutions in 50-1000 mL NS or D_5W, or undiluted solutions in syringes are stable for 72 hours at room temperature.

Topical: Store at controlled room temperature of 15°C to 30°C (59°F to 86°F).

Mechanism of Action A pyrimidine antimetabolite that interferes with DNA synthesis by blocking the methylation of deoxyuridylic acid; fluorouracil inhibits thymidylate synthetase (TS), or is incorporated into RNA. The reduced folate cofactor is required for tight binding to occur between the 5-FdUMP and TS.

Pharmacodynamics/Kinetics

Duration: ~3 weeks

Distribution: V_d: ~22% of total body water; penetrates extracellular fluid, CSF, and third space fluids (eg, pleural effusions and ascitic fluid)

Metabolism: Hepatic (90%); via a dehydrogenase enzyme; FU must be metabolized to be active

Bioavailability: <75%, erratic and undependable

Half-life elimination: Biphasic: Initial: 6-20 minutes; two metabolites, FdUMP and FUTP, have prolonged half-lives depending on the type of tissue

Excretion: Lung (large amounts as CO_2); urine (5% as unchanged drug) in 6 hours

Dosage Adults:

Refer to individual protocols:

I.V. bolus: 500-600 mg/m^2 every 3-4 weeks **or** 425 mg/m^2 on days 1-5 every 4 weeks

Continuous I.V. infusion: 1000 mg/m^2/day for 4-5 days every 3-4 weeks **or**

2300-2600 mg/m^2 on day 1 every week **or**

300-400 mg/m^2/day **or**

225 mg/m^2/day for 5-8 weeks (with radiation therapy)

Actinic keratoses: Topical:

Carac™: Apply thin film to lesions once daily for up to 4 weeks, as tolerated

Efudex®: Apply to lesions twice daily for 2-4 weeks; complete healing may not be evident for 1-2 months following treatment

Fluoroplex®: Apply to lesions twice daily for 2-6 weeks

Superficial basal cell carcinoma: Topical: Efudex® 5%: Apply to affected lesions twice daily for 3-6 weeks; treatment may be continued for up to 10-12 weeks

Dosage adjustment for renal impairment: The FDA-approved labeling does not contain specific dosing adjustment guidelines; however, it is stated that extreme caution should be used in patients with renal impairment.

Hemodialysis: Administer dose following hemodialysis.

Aronoff (2007): Recommends that dosage adjustment is not needed in adult patients with Cl_{cr} <50 mL/minute and patients receiving hemodialysis should be administered 50% of dose.

Dosage adjustment for hepatic impairment: The FDA-approved labeling does not contain specific dosing adjustment guidelines; however, it is stated that extreme caution should be used in patients with hepatic impairment. The following guidelines have been used by some clinicians:

Floyd, 2006: Bilirubin >5 mg/dL: Avoid use.

Koren, 1992: Hepatic impairment (degree not specified): Administer <50% of dose, then increase if toxicity does not occur.

Dietary Considerations Increase dietary intake of thiamine.

Administration

I.V.: I.V. bolus as a slow push or short (5-15 minutes) bolus infusion, or as a continuous infusion. Doses >1000 mg/m^2 are usually administered as a 24-hour infusion. Toxicity may be reduced by giving the drug as a constant infusion. Bolus doses may be administered by slow IVP or IVPB.

Note: I.V. formulation may be given orally mixed in water, grape juice, or carbonated beverage. It is generally best to drink undiluted solution, then rinse the mouth. CocaCola® has been recommended as the "best chaser" for oral fluorouracil.

Topical: Apply 10 minutes after washing, rinsing, and drying the affected area. Apply using fingertip (wash hands immediately after application) or nonmetal applicator. Do not cover area with an occlusive dressing. Wash hands immediately after topical application of the 5% cream. Topical preparations are for external use only; not for ophthalmic, oral, or intravaginal use.

Monitoring Parameters CBC with differential and platelet count, renal function tests, liver function tests

Dosage Forms Excipient information presented when available (limited, particularly for generics); consult specific product labeling.

Cream, topical:
- Carac™: 0.5% (30 g)
- Efudex®: 5% (40 g)
- Fluoroplex®: 1% (30 g) [contains benzyl alcohol]

Injection, solution: 50 mg/mL (10 mL, 20 mL, 50 mL, 100 mL)
- Adrucil®: 50 mg/mL (10 mL, 50 mL, 100 mL)

Solution, topical: 2% (10 mL); 5% (10 mL)
- Efudex®: 2% (10 mL); 5% (10 mL)
- Fluorouracil®: 5% (10 mL)

◆ **Fluorouracil®** *see* Fluorouracil *on page 636*

◆ **5-Fluorouracil** *see* Fluorouracil *on page 636*

FLUoxetine (floo OKS e teen)

U.S. Brand Names Prozac®; Prozac® Weekly™; Sarafem®; Selfemra™

Canadian Brand Names Apo-Fluoxetine®; CO Fluoxetine; Dom-Fluoxetine; Fluoxetine; FXT 40; Gen-Fluoxetine; Novo-Fluoxetine; Nu-Fluoxetine; PHL-Fluoxetine; PMS-Fluoxetine; PRO-Fluoxetine; Prozac®; ratio-Fluoxetine; Riva-Fluoxetine; Sandoz-Fluoxetine

Index Terms Fluoxetine Hydrochloride

Pharmacologic Category Antidepressant, Selective Serotonin Reuptake Inhibitor

Additional Appendix Information

Antidepressant Agents *on page 1638*

Selective Serotonin Reuptake Inhibitors (SSRIs) Pharmacokinetics *on page 1670*

Use Treatment of major depressive disorder (MDD); treatment of binge-eating and vomiting in patients with moderate-to-severe bulimia nervosa; obsessive-compulsive disorder (OCD); premenstrual dysphoric disorder (PMDD); panic disorder with or without agoraphobia

Unlabeled/Investigational Use Selective mutism; treatment of mild dementia-associated agitation in nonpsychotic patients

Restrictions An FDA-approved medication guide concerning the use of antidepressants in children, adolescents, and young adults must be distributed when dispensing an outpatient prescription (new or refill) where this medication is to be used without direct supervision of a healthcare provider. Medication guides are available at http://www.fda.gov/cder/Offices/ODS/medication_guides.htm. Dispense to parents or guardians of children and adolescents receiving this medication.

Pregnancy Risk Factor C

Pregnancy Considerations Due to adverse effects observed in animal studies, fluoxetine is classified as pregnancy category C. Fluoxetine and its metabolite cross the human placenta. Nonteratogenic effects in the newborn following SSRIs exposure late in the third trimester include respiratory distress, cyanosis, apnea, seizures, temperature instability, feeding difficulty, vomiting, hypoglycemia, hypo- or hypertonia, hyper-reflexia, jitteriness, irritability, constant crying, and tremor. An increased risk of low birth weight, lower APGAR scores, and blunted behavioral response to pain for a prolonged period after delivery have also been reported. Exposure to SSRIs after the twentieth week of gestation has been associated with persistent pulmonary hypertension of the newborn (PPHN). Adverse effects may be due to toxic effects of the SSRI or drug withdrawal without a taper. The long term effects of *in utero* SSRI exposure on infant development and behavior are not known.

Due to pregnancy-induced physiologic changes, women who are pregnant may require increased doses of fluoxetine to achieve euthymia. Women treated for major depression and who are euthymic prior to pregnancy are more likely to experience a relapse when medication is discontinued as compared to pregnant women who continue taking antidepressant medications. The ACOG recommends that therapy with SSRIs or SNRIs during pregnancy be individualized; treatment of depression during pregnancy should incorporate the clinical expertise of the mental health clinician, obstetrician, primary healthcare provider, and pediatrician. If treatment during pregnancy is required, consider tapering therapy during the third trimester in order to prevent withdrawal symptoms in the infant. If this is done and the woman is considered to be at risk of relapse from her major depressive disorder, the medication can be restarted following delivery, although the dose should be readjusted to that required before pregnancy.

Lactation Enters breast milk/not recommended (AAP rates "of concern")

Medication Safety Issues

Sound-alike/look-alike issues:
- FLUoxetine may be confused with DULoxetine, fluvastatin, fluvoxamine, PARoxetine
- Prozac® may be confused with Prilosec®, Prograf®, Proscar®, ProSom®, ProStep®
- Sarafem® may be confused with Serophene®

International issues:
- Fluoxin® [Czech Republic and Romania] may be confused with Floxin® which is a brand name for ofloxacin in the U.S.
- Prozac® may be confused with Prazac® a brand of prazosin in Denmark
- Reneuron® [Spain] may be confused with Remeron® a brand of mirtazapine in the U.S.

Contraindications Hypersensitivity to fluoxetine or any component of the formulation; patients currently receiving MAO inhibitors, pimozide, or thioridazine

Note: MAO inhibitor therapy must be stopped for 14 days before fluoxetine is initiated. Treatment with MAO inhibitors, thioridazine, or mesoridazine should not be initiated until 5 weeks after the discontinuation of fluoxetine.

Warnings/Precautions **[U.S. Boxed Warning]: Antidepressants increase the risk of suicidal thinking and behavior in children, adolescents, and young adults (18-24 years of age) with major depressive disorder (MDD) and other psychiatric disorders;** consider risk prior to prescribing. Short-term studies did not show an increased risk in patients >24 years of age and showed a decreased risk in patients ≥65 years. Closely monitor patients for clinical worsening, suicidality, or unusual changes in behavior, particularly during the initial 1-2 months of therapy or during periods of dosage adjustments (increases or decreases); the patient's family or caregiver should be instructed to closely observe the patient and communicate condition with healthcare provider. A medication guide concerning the use of antidepressants should be dispensed with each prescription. **Fluoxetine is FDA approved for the treatment of OCD in children ≥7 years of age and MDD in children ≥8 years of age.**

The possibility of a suicide attempt is inherent in major depression and may persist until remission occurs. Use caution in high-risk patients. Worsening depression and severe abrupt suicidality that are not part of the presenting symptoms may require discontinuation or modification of drug therapy. The patient's family or caregiver should be alerted to monitor patients for the emergence of suicidality and associated behaviors (such as agitation, irritability, hostility, impulsivity, and hypomania) and call healthcare provider.

May worsen psychosis in some patients or precipitate a shift to mania or hypomania in patients with bipolar disorder. Patients presenting with depressive symptoms should be screened for bipolar disorder. Monotherapy in patients with bipolar disorder should be avoided. **Fluoxetine is not FDA approved for the treatment of bipolar depression.** May cause insomnia, anxiety, nervousness, or anorexia. Use with caution in patients where weight loss is undesirable. May impair cognitive or motor performance; caution operating hazardous machinery or driving.

The potential for severe reactions exists when used with MAO inhibitors, SSRIs/SNRIs or triptans; serotonin syndrome (hyperthermia, muscular rigidity, mental status changes/agitation, autonomic instability) may occur. Concurrent use with MAO inhibitors is contraindicated. Fluoxetine may elevate plasma levels of thioridazine and increase the risk of QT_c interval prolongation. This may lead to serious ventricular arrhythmias, such as torsade de pointes-type arrhythmias, and sudden death. Fluoxetine use has been associated with occurrences of significant rash and allergic events, including vasculitis, lupus-like syndrome, laryngospasm, anaphylactoid reactions, and pulmonary inflammatory disease. Discontinue if underlying cause of rash cannot be identified.

Use caution in patients with a previous seizure disorder or condition predisposing to seizures such as brain damage, alcoholism, or concurrent therapy with other drugs which lower the seizure threshold. Use with caution in patients with hepatic or renal dysfunction and in elderly patients. May cause hyponatremia/SIADH (elderly at increased risk); volume depletion (diuretics may increase risk). May increase the risks associated with electroconvulsive treatment. Use caution with concomitant use of NSAIDs, ASA, or other drugs that affect coagulation; the risk of bleeding may be potentiated.Use caution with history of MI or unstable heart disease; use in these patients is limited. May alter glycemic control in patients with diabetes. Due to the long half-life of fluoxetine and its metabolites, the effects and interactions noted may persist for prolonged periods following discontinuation. May cause or exacerbate sexual dysfunction. Discontinuation symptoms (eg, dysphoric mood, irritability, agitation, confusion, anxiety, insomnia, hypomania) may occur upon abrupt discontinuation. Taper dose when discontinuing therapy.

Adverse Reactions Percentages listed for adverse effects as reported in placebo-controlled trials and were generally similar in adults and children; actual frequency may be dependent upon diagnosis and in some cases the range presented may be lower than or equal to placebo for a particular disorder.

>10%:

- Central nervous system: Insomnia (10% to 33%), headache (21%), anxiety (6% to 15%), nervousness (8% to 14%), somnolence (5% to 17%)
- Endocrine & metabolic: Libido decreased (1% to 11%)
- Gastrointestinal: Nausea (12% to 29%), diarrhea (8% to 18%), anorexia (4% to 11%), xerostomia (4% to 12%)
- Neuromuscular & skeletal: Weakness (7% to 21%), tremor (3% to 13%)
- Respiratory: Pharyngitis (3% to 11%), yawn (<1% to 11%)

1% to 10%:

- Cardiovascular: Vasodilation (1% to 5%), fever (2%), chest pain, hemorrhage, hypertension, palpitation
- Central nervous system: Dizziness (9%), dream abnormality (1% to 5%), thinking abnormality (2%), agitation, amnesia, chills, confusion, emotional lability, sleep disorder
- Dermatologic: Rash (2% to 6%), pruritus (4%)
- Endocrine & metabolic: Ejaculation abnormal (<1% to 7%), impotence (<1% to 7%)
- Gastrointestinal: Dyspepsia (6% to 10%), constipation (5%), flatulence (3%), vomiting (3%), weight loss (2%), appetite increased, taste perversion, weight gain
- Genitourinary: Urinary frequency
- Ocular: Vision abnormal (2%)
- Otic: Ear pain, tinnitus
- Respiratory: Sinusitis (1% to 6%)
- Miscellaneous: Flu-like syndrome (3% to 10%), diaphoresis (2% to 8%)

<1% (Limited to important or life-threatening): Allergies, alopecia, anaphylactoid reactions, angina, arrhythmia, asthma, cataract, CHF, cholelithiasis, cholestatic jaundice, colitis, dyskinesia, dysphagia, eosinophilic pneumonia, erythema nodosum, esophagitis, euphoria, exfoliative dermatitis, extrapyramidal symptoms (rare), gout, hallucinations, hepatic failure/necrosis, hemorrhage, hyperprolactinemia, hyponatremia (possibly in association with SIADH), immune-related hemolytic anemia, laryngospasm, lupus-like syndrome, MI, neuroleptic malignant syndrome (NMS), optic neuritis, pancreatitis, pancytopenia, photosensitivity reaction, postural hypotension, priapism, pulmonary embolism, pulmonary fibrosis, pulmonary hypertension, QT prolongation, renal failure, serotonin syndrome, Stevens-Johnson syndrome, syncope, thrombocytopenia, thrombocytopenic purpura, vasculitis, ventricular tachycardia (including torsade de pointes)

Drug Interactions

Metabolism/Transport Effects **Substrate** of CYP1A2 (minor), 2B6 (minor), 2C9 (major), 2C19 (minor), 2D6 (major), 2E1 (minor), 3A4 (minor); **Inhibits** CYP1A2 (moderate), 2B6 (weak), 2C9 (weak), 2C19 (moderate), 2D6 (strong), 3A4 (weak)

Avoid Concomitant Use

Avoid concomitant use of FLUoxetine with any of the following: Iobenguane I 123; MAO Inhibitors; Nilotinib; Pimozide; Sibutramine; Tamoxifen; Tetrabenazine; Thioridazine; Ziprasidone

Increased Effect/Toxicity

FLUoxetine may increase the levels/effects of: Alcohol (Ethyl); Alpha-/Beta-Blockers; Anticoagulants; Antidepressants (Serotonin Reuptake Inhibitor/Antagonist);

Antiplatelet Agents; Aspirin; Benzodiazepines (metabolized by oxidation); Beta-Blockers; BusPIRone; CarBAMazepine; Clozapine; CNS Depressants; CYP1A2 Substrates; CYP2C19 Substrates; CYP2D6 Substrates; Desmopressin; Dextromethorphan; Drotrecogin Alfa; Fesoterodine; Galantamine; Haloperidol; Ibritumomab; Lithium; Methadone; Mexiletine; NSAID (COX-2 Inhibitor); NSAID (Nonselective); Phenytoin; Pimozide; Propafenone; QTc-Prolonging Agents; QuiNIDine; Risperidone; Salicylates; Serotonin Modulators; Tamoxifen; Tetrabenazine; Thioridazine; Thrombolytic Agents; Tositumomab and Iodine I 131 Tositumomab; TraMADol; Tricyclic Antidepressants; Vitamin K Antagonists; Ziprasidone

The levels/effects of FLUoxetine may be increased by: Alfuzosin; Analgesics (Opioid); BusPIRone; Cimetidine; Ciprofloxacin; CYP2C9 Inhibitors (Moderate); CYP2C9 Inhibitors (Strong); CYP2D6 Inhibitors (Moderate); CYP2D6 Inhibitors (Strong); Darunavir; Dasatinib; Gadobutrol; Herbs (Anticoagulant/Antiplatelet Properties); Macrolide Antibiotics; MAO Inhibitors; Nilotinib; Omega-3-Acid Ethyl Esters; Pentosan Polysulfate Sodium; Prostacyclin Analogues; Sibutramine; TraMADol; Tryptophan

Decreased Effect

FLUoxetine may decrease the levels/effects of: Iobenguane I 123

The levels/effects of FLUoxetine may be decreased by: CarBAMazepine; CYP2C9 Inducers (Highly Effective); Cyproheptadine

Ethanol/Nutrition/Herb Interactions

Ethanol: Avoid ethanol (may increase CNS depression). Depressed patients should avoid/limit intake.

Herb/Nutraceutical: Avoid valerian, St John's wort, kava kava, gotu kola (may increase CNS depression).

Stability All dosage forms should be stored at controlled room temperature of 15°C to 30°C (50°F to 86°F). Oral liquid should be dispensed in a light-resistant container.

Mechanism of Action Inhibits CNS neuron serotonin reuptake; minimal or no effect on reuptake of norepinephrine or dopamine; does not significantly bind to alpha-adrenergic, histamine, or cholinergic receptors

Pharmacodynamics/Kinetics

Onset of action: Depression: The onset of action is within a week; however, individual response varies greatly and full response may not be seen until 8-12 weeks after initiation of treatment.

Absorption: Well absorbed; delayed 1-2 hours with weekly formulation

Distribution: V_d: 12-43 L/kg

Protein binding: 95% to albumin and $alpha_1$ glycoprotein

Metabolism: Hepatic, via CYP2C19 and 2D6, to norfluoxetine (activity equal to fluoxetine)

Half-life elimination: Adults:

Parent drug: 1-3 days (acute), 4-6 days (chronic), 7.6 days (cirrhosis)

Metabolite (norfluoxetine): 9.3 days (range: 4-16 days), 12 days (cirrhosis)

Time to peak, serum: 6-8 hours

Excretion: Urine (10% as norfluoxetine, 2.5% to 5% as fluoxetine)

Note: Weekly formulation results in greater fluctuations between peak and trough concentrations of fluoxetine and norfluoxetine compared to once-daily dosing (24% daily/164% weekly; 17% daily/43% weekly, respectively). Trough concentrations are 76% lower for fluoxetine and 47% lower for norfluoxetine than the concentrations maintained by 20 mg once-daily dosing. Steady-state fluoxetine concentrations are ~50% lower following the once-weekly regimen compared to 20 mg once daily. Average steady-state concentrations of once-daily dosing were highest in children ages 6 to <13 (fluoxetine 171 ng/mL; norfluoxetine 195 ng/mL), followed by adolescents ages 13 to <18 (fluoxetine 86 ng/mL; norfluoxetine 113 ng/mL); concentrations were considered to be within the ranges reported in adults (fluoxetine 91-302 ng/mL; norfluoxetine 72-258 ng/mL).

Dosage Oral: **Note:** Upon discontinuation of fluoxetine therapy, gradually taper dose. If intolerable symptoms occur following a dose reduction, consider resuming the previously prescribed dose and/or decrease dose at a more gradual rate.

Children:

Depression: 8-18 years: 10-20 mg/day; lower-weight children can be started at 10 mg/day, may increase to 20 mg/day after 1 week if needed

Obsessive-compulsive disorder: 7-18 years: Initial: 10 mg/day; in adolescents and higher-weight children, dose may be increased to 20 mg/day after 2 weeks. Range: 10-60 mg/day.

Selective mutism (unlabeled use):

<5 years: No dosing information available

5-18 years: Initial: 5-10 mg/day; titrate upwards as needed (usual maximum dose: 60 mg/day)

Adults: 20 mg/day in the morning; may increase after several weeks by 20 mg/day increments; maximum: 80 mg/day; doses >20 mg may be given once daily or divided twice daily. **Note:** Lower doses of 5-10 mg/day have been used for initial treatment.

Usual dosage range:

Bulimia nervosa: 60-80 mg/day

Depression: 20-40 mg/day; patients maintained on Prozac® 20 mg/day may be changed to Prozac® Weekly™ 90 mg/week, starting dose 7 days after the last 20 mg/day dose

Obsessive-compulsive disorder: 40-80 mg/day

Panic disorder: Initial: 10 mg/day; after 1 week, increase to 20 mg/day; may increase after several weeks; doses >60 mg/day have not been evaluated

Premenstrual dysphoric disorder (Sarafem™): 20 mg/day continuously, **or** 20 mg/day starting 14 days prior to menstruation and through first full day of menses (repeat with each cycle)

Elderly: Depression: Some patients may require an initial dose of 10 mg/day with dosage increases of 10 and 20 mg every several weeks as tolerated; should not be taken at night unless patient experiences sedation

Dosing adjustment in renal impairment:

Single dose studies: Pharmacokinetics of fluoxetine and norfluoxetine were similar among subjects with all levels of impaired renal function, including anephric patients on chronic hemodialysis

Chronic administration: Additional accumulation of fluoxetine or norfluoxetine may occur in patients with severely impaired renal function

Hemodialysis: Not removed by hemodialysis; use of lower dose or less frequent dosing is not usually necessary.

Dosing adjustment in hepatic impairment: Elimination half-life of fluoxetine is prolonged in patients with hepatic impairment; a lower or less frequent dose of fluoxetine should be used in these patients

Cirrhosis patients: Administer a lower dose or less frequent dosing interval

Compensated cirrhosis without ascites: Administer 50% of normal dose

Dietary Considerations May be taken with or without food.

Monitoring Parameters Mental status for depression, suicidal ideation (especially at the beginning of therapy or when doses are increased or decreased), anxiety, social functioning, mania, panic attacks; akathisia, sleep

Reference Range Therapeutic levels have not been well established

Therapeutic: Fluoxetine: 100-800 ng/mL (SI: 289-2314 nmol/L); Norfluoxetine: 100-600 ng/mL (SI: 289-1735 nmol/L)

Toxic: Fluoxetine plus norfluoxetine: >2000 ng/mL

Additional Information ECG may reveal S-T segment depression. Not shown to be teratogenic in rodents; 15-60 mg/day, buspirone and cyproheptadine, may be useful in treatment of sexual dysfunction during treatment with a selective serotonin reuptake inhibitor.

Weekly capsules are a delayed release formulation containing enteric-coated pellets of fluoxetine hydrochloride, equivalent to 90 mg fluoxetine. Therapeutic equivalence of weekly formulation with daily formulation for delaying time to relapse has not been established.

Dosage Forms Excipient information presented when available (limited, particularly for generics); consult specific product labeling. **Note:** Strength expressed as base unless otherwise noted. [DSC] = Discontinued product

Capsule: 10 mg, 20 mg, 40 mg
- Prozac®: 10 mg, 20 mg, 40 mg
- Sarafem®: 10 mg, 20 mg [DSC]
- Selfemra™: 10 mg, 20 mg [contains soya lecithin]

Capsule, delayed release, enteric coated pellets:
- Prozac® Weekly™: 90 mg

Solution, oral: 20 mg/5 mL (5 mL, 120 mL) [contains ethanol 0.23% and benzoic acid; mint flavor]
- Prozac®: 20 mg/5 mL (120 mL) [contains ethanol 0.23% and benzoic acid; mint flavor]

Tablet: 10 mg, 20 mg
- Prozac® [scored]: 10 mg [DSC]
- Sarafem®: 10 mg, 20 mg

Extemporaneous Preparations A 20 mg capsule may be mixed with 4 oz of water, apple juice, or Gatorade® to provide a solution that is stable for 14 days under refrigeration.

◆ **Fluoxetine (Can)** *see* FLUoxetine *on page 638*

◆ **Fluoxetine and Olanzapine** *see* Olanzapine and Fluoxetine *on page 1095*

◆ **Fluoxetine Hydrochloride** *see* FLUoxetine *on page 638*

Fluoxymesterone (floo oks i MES te rone)

U.S. Brand Names Androxy™

Pharmacologic Category Androgen

Use Replacement of endogenous testicular hormone; in females, palliative treatment of breast cancer

Unlabeled/Investigational Use Stimulation of erythropoiesis, angioneurotic edema

Restrictions C-III

Pregnancy Risk Factor X

Medication Safety Issues

Sound-alike/look-alike issues:
- Halotestin® may be confused with Haldol®, haloperidol, halothane

Dosage Adults: Oral:

Male:
- Hypogonadism: 5-20 mg/day
- Delayed puberty: 2.5-20 mg/day for 4-6 months

Female: Inoperable breast carcinoma: 10-40 mg/day in divided doses for 1-3 months

Additional Information Complete prescribing information for this medication should be consulted for additional detail.

Dosage Forms Excipient information presented when available (limited, particularly for generics); consult specific product labeling.

Tablet: 10 mg
- Androxy™: 10 mg

Fluphenazine (floo FEN a zeen)

Canadian Brand Names Apo-Fluphenazine Decanoate®; Apo-Fluphenazine®; Modecate®; Modecate® Concentrate; PMS-Fluphenazine Decanoate

Index Terms Fluphenazine Decanoate

Pharmacologic Category Antipsychotic Agent, Typical, Phenothiazine

Additional Appendix Information

Antipsychotic Agents *on page 1644*

Use Management of manifestations of psychotic disorders and schizophrenia; depot formulation may offer improved outcome in individuals with psychosis who are nonadherent with oral antipsychotics

Unlabeled/Investigational Use Pervasive developmental disorder; nonpsychotic patient, dementia behavior in the elderly; psychosis/agitation related to Alzheimer's dementia

Pregnancy Risk Factor C

Lactation Enters breast milk/not recommended

Medication Safety Issues

Sound-alike/look-alike issues:
- Prolixin® may be confused with Proloprim®

International issues:
- Prolixin® may be confused with Prolixan® which is a brand name for azapropazone in multiple international markets

Contraindications Hypersensitivity to fluphenazine or any component of the formulation (cross-reactivity between phenothiazines may occur); severe CNS depression; coma; subcortical brain damage; blood dyscrasias; hepatic disease

Warnings/Precautions May be sedating; use with caution in disorders where CNS depression is a feature. Use with caution in Parkinson's disease. Caution in patients with hemodynamic instability; predisposition to seizures; or severe cardiac, renal, or respiratory disease. Esophageal dysmotility and aspiration have been associated with antipsychotic use - use with caution in patients at risk of pneumonia (ie, Alzheimer's disease). Caution in breast cancer or other prolactin-dependent tumors (may elevate prolactin levels). May alter temperature regulation or mask toxicity of other drugs due to antiemetic effects. May alter cardiac conduction; life-threatening arrhythmias have occurred with therapeutic doses of phenothiazines. Hypotension may occur, particularly with I.M. administration. May cause orthostatic hypotension - use with caution in patients at risk of this effect or those who would tolerate transient hypotensive episodes (cerebrovascular disease, cardiovascular disease, or other medications which may predispose). Adverse effects of depot injections may be prolonged. Check blood counts periodically and discontinue at first signs of blood dyscrasias; use is contraindicated in patients with bone marrow suppression.

Due to anticholinergic effects, use caution in patients with decreased gastrointestinal motility, urinary retention, BPH, xerostomia, visual problems, narrow-angle glaucoma (screening is recommended), and myasthenia gravis. Relative to other antipsychotics, fluphenazine has a low potency of cholinergic blockade.

May cause extrapyramidal symptoms, including pseudoparkinsonism, acute dystonic reactions, akathisia, and tardive dyskinesia (risk of these reactions is high relative to other antipsychotics). Use caution in the elderly. May be associated with neuroleptic malignant syndrome (NMS) or pigmentary retinopathy.

Adverse Reactions Frequency not defined.

Cardiovascular: Tachycardia, fluctuations in blood pressure, hyper-/hypotension, arrhythmia, edema

Central nervous system: Parkinsonian symptoms, akathisia, dystonias, tardive dyskinesia, dizziness, hyperreflexia, headache, cerebral edema, drowsiness, lethargy, restlessness, excitement, bizarre dreams, EEG changes, depression, seizure, NMS, altered central temperature regulation

Dermatologic: Dermatitis, eczema, erythema, itching, photosensitivity, rash, seborrhea, skin pigmentation, urticaria

Endocrine & metabolic: Menstrual cycle changes, breast pain, amenorrhea, galactorrhea, gynecomastia, libido changes, prolactin increased, SIADH

Gastrointestinal: Weight gain, appetite loss, salivation, xerostomia, constipation, paralytic ileus, laryngeal edema

Genitourinary: Ejaculatory disturbances, impotence, polyuria, bladder paralysis, enuresis

Hematologic: Agranulocytosis, leukopenia, thrombocytopenia, nonthrombocytopenic purpura, eosinophilia, pancytopenia

Hepatic: Cholestatic jaundice, hepatotoxicity

Neuromuscular & skeletal: Trembling of fingers, SLE, facial hemispasm

Ocular: Pigmentary retinopathy, cornea and lens changes, blurred vision, glaucoma

Respiratory: Nasal congestion, asthma

Drug Interactions

Metabolism/Transport Effects Substrate of CYP2D6 (major); **Inhibits** CYP1A2 (weak), 2C9 (weak), 2D6 (weak), 2E1 (weak)

Avoid Concomitant Use There are no known interactions where it is recommended to avoid concomitant use.

Increased Effect/Toxicity

Fluphenazine may increase the levels/effects of: Alcohol (Ethyl); Analgesics (Opioid); Anticholinergics; Beta-Blockers; CNS Depressants

The levels/effects of Fluphenazine may be increased by: Acetylcholinesterase Inhibitors (Central); Antimalarial Agents; Beta-Blockers; CYP2D6 Inhibitors (Moderate); CYP2D6 Inhibitors (Strong); Darunavir; Lithium formulations; Pramlintide; Tetrabenazine

Decreased Effect

Fluphenazine may decrease the levels/effects of: Amphetamines; Anti-Parkinson's Agents (Dopamine Agonist)

The levels/effects of Fluphenazine may be decreased by: Antacids; Lithium formulations

Ethanol/Nutrition/Herb Interactions

Ethanol: Avoid ethanol (may increase CNS depression).

Herb/Nutraceutical: Avoid dong quai, St John's wort (may also cause photosensitization). Avoid kava kava, gotu kola, valerian, St John's wort (may increase CNS depression).

Stability Avoid freezing. Protect all dosage forms from light. Clear or slightly yellow solutions may be used. Should be dispensed in amber or opaque vials/bottles. Solutions may be diluted or mixed with fruit juices or other liquids, but must be administered immediately after mixing. Do not prepare bulk dilutions or store bulk dilutions.

Mechanism of Action Fluphenazine is a piperazine phenothiazine antipsychotic which blocks postsynaptic mesolimbic dopaminergic D_1 and D_2 receptors in the brain; depresses the release of hypothalamic and hypophyseal hormones; believed to depress the reticular activating system, thus affecting basal metabolism, body temperature, wakefulness, vasomotor tone, and emesis

Pharmacodynamics/Kinetics

Onset of action: I.M., SubQ (derivative dependent): Hydrochloride salt: ~1 hour

Peak effect: Neuroleptic: Decanoate: 48-96 hours

Duration: Hydrochloride salt: 6-8 hours; Decanoate: 24-72 hours

Absorption: Oral: Erratic and variable

Distribution: Crosses placenta; enters breast milk

Protein binding: 91% and 99%

Metabolism: Hepatic

Half-life elimination (derivative dependent): Hydrochloride: 33 hours; Decanoate: 163-232 hours

Excretion: Urine (as metabolites)

Dosage

Children: Oral: Childhood-onset pervasive developmental disorder (unlabeled use): 0.04 mg/kg/day

Adults: Psychoses:

Oral: 0.5-10 mg/day in divided doses at 6- to 8-hour intervals; some patients may require up to 40 mg/day

I.M.: 2.5-10 mg/day in divided doses at 6- to 8-hour intervals (parenteral dose is 1/3 to 1/2 the oral dose for the hydrochloride salts)

I.M. (decanoate): 12.5-37.5 mg every 2 weeks

Conversion from hydrochloride to decanoate I.M. 0.5 mL (12.5 mg) decanoate every 3 weeks is approximately equivalent to 10 mg hydrochloride/day; **Note:** Clinically, an every-2-week interval is frequently utilized

Elderly: Nonpsychotic patient, dementia behavior (unlabeled use): Oral: 1-2.5 mg/day; increase dose at 4- to 7-day intervals by 1-2.5 mg/day. Increase dosing intervals (bid, tid) as necessary to control response or side effects. Maximum daily dose: 20 mg; gradual increases (titration) may prevent some side effects or decrease their severity.

Hemodialysis: Not dialyzable (0% to 5%)

Administration Avoid contact of oral solution or injection with skin (contact dermatitis). Oral liquid should be diluted in the following **only**: Water, saline, homogenized milk, carbonated orange beverages, pineapple, apricot, prune, orange, tomato, and grapefruit juices. Do **not** dilute in beverages containing caffeine, tannics, or pectinate. Watch for hypotension when administering I.M.

Monitoring Parameters Vital signs; lipid profile, fasting blood glucose/Hgb A_{1c}; BMI; mental status, abnormal involuntary movement scale (AIMS), extrapyramidal symptoms (EPS)

Reference Range Therapeutic: 0.3-3 ng/mL (SI: 0.6-6.0 nmol/L); correlation of serum concentrations and efficacy is controversial; most often dosed to best response

Additional Information Less sedative and hypotensive effects than chlorpromazine.

Dosage Forms Excipient information presented when available (limited, particularly for generics); consult specific product labeling. [DSC] = Discontinued product

Elixir, as hydrochloride: 2.5 mg/5 mL (60 mL) [contains alcohol 14% and sodium benzoate] [DSC]

Injection, oil, as decanoate: 25 mg/mL (5 mL) [may contain benzyl alcohol, sesame oil]

Injection, solution, as hydrochloride: 2.5 mg/mL (10 mL)

Solution, oral concentrate, as hydrochloride: 5 mg/mL (120 mL) [contains alcohol 14%]

Tablet, as hydrochloride: 1 mg, 2.5 mg, 5 mg, 10 mg

◆ **Fluphenazine Decanoate** *see* Fluphenazine *on page 641*

◆ **Flura-Drops®** *see* Fluoride *on page 635*

Flurandrenolide (flure an DREN oh lide)

U.S. Brand Names Cordran®; Cordran® SP

Canadian Brand Names Cordran®

Index Terms Flurandrenolone

Pharmacologic Category Corticosteroid, Topical

Additional Appendix Information

Corticosteroids *on page 1652*

Use Inflammation of corticosteroid-responsive dermatoses [medium potency topical corticosteroid]

Pregnancy Risk Factor C

Medication Safety Issues

Sound-alike/look-alike issues:

Cordran® may be confused with Cardura®, codeine, Cordarone®

Dosage Topical: Therapy should be discontinued when control is achieved; if no improvement is seen, reassessment of diagnosis may be necessary.

Children:

Cream: Apply sparingly 1-2 times/day

Tape: Apply once daily

Adults: Cream, lotion: Apply sparingly 2-3 times/day

Additional Information Complete prescribing information for this medication should be consulted for additional detail.

Dosage Forms Excipient information presented when available (limited, particularly for generics); consult specific product labeling.

Cream, emulsified, as base (Cordran® SP): 0.05% (15 g, 30 g, 60 g)

Lotion (Cordran®): 0.05% (15 mL, 60 mL)

Tape, topical [roll] (Cordran®): 4 mcg/cm^2 (24 inch, 80 inch)

◆ **Flurandrenolone** *see* Flurandrenolide *on page 642*

Flurazepam (flure AZ e pam)

U.S. Brand Names Dalmane®

Canadian Brand Names Apo-Flurazepam®; Dalmane®; Som Pam

Index Terms Flurazepam Hydrochloride

Pharmacologic Category Hypnotic, Benzodiazepine

Additional Appendix Information

Benzodiazepines *on page 1646*

Use Short-term treatment of insomnia

Restrictions C-IV

Pregnancy Risk Factor X

Medication Safety Issues

Sound-alike/look-alike issues:

Flurazepam may be confused with temazepam

Dalmane® may be confused with Demulen®, Dialume®

Dosage Oral:

Children: Insomnia:

<15 years: Dose not established

≥15 years: 15 mg at bedtime

Adults: Insomnia: 15-30 mg at bedtime

Elderly: Insomnia: Oral: 15 mg at bedtime; avoid use if possible

Additional Information Complete prescribing information for this medication should be consulted for additional detail.

Dosage Forms Excipient information presented when available (limited, particularly for generics); consult specific product labeling.

Capsule, as hydrochloride: 15 mg, 30 mg

Dalmane®: 15 mg, 30 mg

◆ **Flurazepam Hydrochloride** *see* Flurazepam *on page 643*

Flurbiprofen (flure BI proe fen)

U.S. Brand Names Ocufen®

Canadian Brand Names Alti-Flurbiprofen; Ansaid®; Apo-Flurbiprofen®; Froben-SR®; Froben®; Novo-Flurprofen; Nu-Flurprofen; Ocufen®

Index Terms Flurbiprofen Sodium

Pharmacologic Category Nonsteroidal Anti-inflammatory Drug (NSAID), Ophthalmic; Nonsteroidal Anti-inflammatory Drug (NSAID), Oral

Additional Appendix Information

Nonsteroidal Anti-inflammatory Agents *on page 1669*

Use

Oral: Treatment of rheumatoid arthritis and osteoarthritis

Ophthalmic: Inhibition of intraoperative miosis

Restrictions An FDA-approved medication guide must be distributed when dispensing an oral outpatient prescription (new or refill) where this medication is to be used without direct supervision of a healthcare provider. Medication guides are available at http://www.fda.gov/cder/Offices/ODS/medication_guides.htm.

Pregnancy Risk Factor C/D (3rd trimester)

Medication Safety Issues

Sound-alike/look-alike issues:

Flurbiprofen may be confused with fenoprofen

Ansaid® may be confused with Asacol®, Axid®

Ocufen® may be confused with Ocuflox®, Ocupress®

Dosage

Oral:

Rheumatoid arthritis and osteoarthritis: 200-300 mg/day in 2, 3, or 4 divided doses; do not administer more than 100 mg for any single dose; maximum: 300 mg/day

Dental: Management of postoperative pain: 100 mg every 12 hours

Ophthalmic: Instill 1 drop every 30 minutes, beginning 2 hours prior to surgery (total of 4 drops in each affected eye)

Dosage adjustment in renal impairment: Not recommended in patients with advanced renal disease

Additional Information Complete prescribing information for this medication should be consulted for additional detail.

Dosage Forms Excipient information presented when available (limited, particularly for generics); consult specific product labeling.

Solution, ophthalmic, as sodium: 0.03% (2.5 mL)

Ocufen®: 0.03% (2.5 mL)

Tablet: 50 mg, 100 mg

◆ **Flurbiprofen Sodium** *see* Flurbiprofen *on page 643*

◆ **Fluress®** *see* Fluorescein and Benoxinate *on page 634*

◆ **5-Flurocytosine** *see* Flucytosine *on page 627*

◆ **Flurox™** *see* Fluorescein and Benoxinate *on page 634*

Flutamide (FLOO ta mide)

U.S. Brand Names Eulexin®

Canadian Brand Names Apo-Flutamide®; Euflex®; Eulexin®; Novo-Flutamide

Index Terms 4′-Nitro-3′-Trifluoromethylisobutyrantide; Niftolid; NSC-147834; SCH 13521

Pharmacologic Category Antineoplastic Agent, Antiandrogen

Use Treatment of metastatic prostatic carcinoma in combination therapy with LHRH agonist analogues

Unlabeled/Investigational Use Female hirsutism

Pregnancy Risk Factor D

Lactation Excretion in breast milk unknown/not recommended

Medication Safety Issues

Sound-alike/look-alike issues:

Flutamide may be confused with Flumadine®, thalidomide

Eulexin® may be confused with Edecrin®, Eurax®

Contraindications Hypersensitivity to flutamide or any component of the formulation; severe hepatic impairment; pregnancy

Warnings/Precautions Hazardous agent - use appropriate precautions for handling and disposal. **[U.S. Boxed Warning]: Hospitalization and, rarely, death due to liver failure have been reported in patients taking flutamide.** Elevated serum transaminase levels, jaundice, hepatic encephalopathy, and acute hepatic failure have been reported. Product labeling states flutamide is not for use in women, particularly for non-life-threatening conditions. In some patients, the toxicity reverses after discontinuation of therapy. About 50% of the cases occur within the first 3 months of treatment. Serum transaminase levels should be measured prior to starting treatment, monthly for 4 months, and periodically thereafter. Liver function tests should be obtained at the first suggestion of liver dysfunction (nausea, vomiting, abdominal pain, fatigue, anorexia, "flu-like" symptoms, hyperbilirubinuria, jaundice, or right upper quadrant tenderness). Flutamide should be immediately discontinued any time a patient has jaundice, and/or an ALT level greater than twice the upper limit of normal. Flutamide should not be used in patients whose ALT values are greater than twice the upper limit of normal.

Patients with glucose-6 phosphate dehydrogenase deficiency or hemoglobin M disease or smokers are at risk of toxicities associated with aniline exposure, including methemoglobinemia, hemolytic anemia, and cholestatic jaundice. Monitor methemoglobin levels.

Adverse Reactions

>10%:

Endocrine & metabolic: Gynecomastia, hot flashes, breast tenderness, galactorrhea (9% to 42%), impotence, libido decreased, tumor flare

Gastrointestinal: Nausea, vomiting (11% to 12%)

Hepatic: AST and LDH levels increased, transient, mild

1% to 10%:

Cardiovascular: Hypertension (1%), edema

Central nervous system: Drowsiness, confusion, depression, anxiety, nervousness, headache, dizziness, insomnia

Dermatologic: Pruritus, ecchymosis, photosensitivity

Gastrointestinal: Anorexia, appetite increased, constipation, indigestion, upset stomach (4% to 6%); diarrhea

Hematologic: Anemia (6%), leukopenia (3%), thrombocytopenia (1%)

Neuromuscular & skeletal: Weakness (1%)

Miscellaneous: Herpes zoster

<1% (Limited to important or life-threatening): Hepatic failure, hepatitis, hypersensitivity pneumonitis, jaundice, malignant breast neoplasm (male), MI, pulmonary embolism, sulfhemoglobinemia, thrombophlebitis, yellow discoloration of the urine

Drug Interactions

Metabolism/Transport Effects Substrate (major) of CYP1A2, 3A4; **Inhibits** CYP1A2 (weak)

Avoid Concomitant Use There are no known interactions where it is recommended to avoid concomitant use.

Increased Effect/Toxicity

The levels/effects of Flutamide may be increased by: CYP1A2 Inhibitors (Moderate); CYP1A2 Inhibitors (Strong); CYP3A4 Inhibitors (Moderate); CYP3A4 Inhibitors (Strong); Dasatinib

Decreased Effect

The levels/effects of Flutamide may be decreased by: CYP1A2 Inducers (Strong); CYP3A4 Inducers (Strong); Deferasirox; Herbs (CYP3A4 Inducers)

Ethanol/Nutrition/Herb Interactions

Food: No effect on bioavailability of flutamide.

Herb/Nutraceutical: St John's wort may decrease flutamide levels.

Stability Store at room temperature.

Mechanism of Action Nonsteroidal antiandrogen that inhibits androgen uptake or inhibits binding of androgen in target tissues

Pharmacodynamics/Kinetics

Absorption: Oral: Rapid and complete

Protein binding: Parent drug: 94% to 96%; 2-hydroxyflutamide: 92% to 94%

Metabolism: Extensively hepatic to more than 10 metabolites, primarily 2-hydroxyflutamide (active)

Half-life elimination: 5-6 hours (2-hydroxyflutamide)

Excretion: Primarily urine (as metabolites)

Dosage Oral: Adults:

Prostatic carcinoma: 250 mg 3 times/day; alternatively, once-daily doses of 0.5-1.5 g have been used (unlabeled dosing)

Female hirsutism (unlabeled use): 250 mg daily

Administration Usually administered orally in 3 divided doses. Contents of capsule may be opened and mixed with applesauce, pudding, or other soft foods. Mixing with a beverage is not recommended.

Monitoring Parameters Serum transaminase levels should be measured prior to starting treatment and should be repeated monthly for the first 4 months of therapy, and periodically thereafter. LFTs should be checked at the first sign or symptom of liver dysfunction (eg, nausea, vomiting, abdominal pain, fatigue, anorexia, flu-like symptoms, hyperbilirubinuria, jaundice, or right upper quadrant tenderness). Other parameters include tumor reduction, testosterone/estrogen, and phosphatase serum levels.

Dosage Forms Excipient information presented when available (limited, particularly for generics); consult specific product labeling.

Capsule: 125 mg

Fluticasone (floo TIK a sone)

U.S. Brand Names Cutivate®; Flonase®; Flovent® Diskus®; Flovent® HFA; Veramyst™

Canadian Brand Names Apo-Fluticasone; Avamys™; Cutivate™; Flonase®; Flovent® Diskus®; Flovent® HFA; ratio-Fluticasone

Index Terms Fluticasone Furoate; Fluticasone Propionate

Pharmacologic Category Corticosteroid, Inhalant (Oral); Corticosteroid, Nasal; Corticosteroid, Topical

Additional Appendix Information

Asthma *on page 1793*

Corticosteroids *on page 1652*

Use

Oral inhalation: Maintenance treatment of asthma as prophylactic therapy; also indicated for patients requiring oral corticosteroid therapy for asthma to assist in total discontinuation or reduction of total oral dose

Intranasal:

Flonase®: Management of seasonal and perennial allergic rhinitis and nonallergic rhinitis

Veramyst™: Management of seasonal and perennial allergic rhinitis

Avamys™ [CAN]: Management of seasonal allergic rhinitis

Topical: Relief of inflammation and pruritus associated with corticosteroid-responsive dermatoses; atopic dermatitis

Pregnancy Risk Factor C

Pregnancy Considerations Teratogenic events have been observed in some, but not all, animal studies. There are no adequate and well-controlled studies using inhaled fluticasone in pregnant women. Oral corticosteroid use has shown animals to be more prone to teratogenic effects than humans. Due to the natural increase in corticosteroid production during pregnancy, most women may require a lower steroid dose; use with caution.

Lactation Excretion in breast milk unknown/use caution

Medication Safety Issues

Sound-alike/look-alike issues:

Cutivate® may be confused with Ultravate®

International issues:

Allegro® [Israel] may be confused with Allegra® which is a brand name for fexofenadine in the U.S.

Allegro®: Brand name for frovatriptan in Germany

Flovent® may be confused with Flogen® which is a brand name for naproxen in Mexico

Contraindications Hypersensitivity to fluticasone or any component of the formulation; primary treatment of status asthmaticus or acute bronchospasm

Topical: Do not use if infection is present at treatment site, in the presence of skin atrophy, or for the treatment of rosacea or perioral dermatitis

Warnings/Precautions May cause hypercorticism or suppression of hypothalamic-pituitary-adrenal (HPA) axis, particularly in younger children or in patients receiving high doses for prolonged periods. HPA axis suppression may lead to adrenal crisis. Withdrawal and discontinuation of a corticosteroid should be done slowly and carefully. Particular care is required when patients are transferred from systemic corticosteroids to inhaled products due to possible adrenal insufficiency or withdrawal from steroids, including an increase in allergic symptoms. Patients receiving ≥20 mg per day of prednisone (or equivalent) may be most susceptible. Concurrent use of ritonavir (and potentially other strong inhibitors of CYP3A4) may increase fluticasone levels and effects on HPA suppression. Fatalities have occurred due to adrenal insufficiency in asthmatic patients during and after transfer from systemic corticosteroids to aerosol steroids; aerosol steroids do **not** provide the systemic steroid needed to treat patients having trauma, surgery, or infections.

Bronchospasm may occur with wheezing after inhalation; if this occurs, stop steroid and treat with a fast-acting bronchodilator. Supplemental steroids (oral or parenteral) may be needed during stress or severe asthma attacks. Corticosteroid use may cause psychiatric disturbances, including depression, euphoria, insomnia, mood swings, and personality changes. Pre-existing psychiatric conditions may be exacerbated by corticosteroid use. Prolonged use of corticosteroids may also increase the incidence of secondary infection, mask acute infection (including fungal infections), prolong or exacerbate viral infections, or limit response to vaccines. Exposure to chickenpox should be avoided; corticosteroids should not be used to treat ocular herpes simplex. Corticosteroids should not be used for cerebral malaria. Close observation is required in patients with latent tuberculosis and/or TB reactivity; restrict use in active TB (only in conjunction with antituberculosis treatment). Rare cases of vasculitis (Churg-Strauss syndrome) or other eosinophilic conditions can occur. Prolonged treatment with corticosteroids has been associated with the development of Kaposi's sarcoma (case reports); if noted, discontinuation of therapy should be considered.

Use with caution in patients with thyroid disease, hepatic impairment, renal impairment, cardiovascular disease, diabetes, glaucoma, cataracts, myasthenia gravis, patients at risk for osteoporosis, patients at risk for seizures, or GI diseases (diverticulitis, peptic ulcer, ulcerative colitis) due to perforation risk. Use caution following acute MI (corticosteroids have been associated with myocardial rupture). Because of the risk of adverse effects, systemic corticosteroids should be used cautiously in the elderly in the smallest possible effective dose for the shortest duration. Avoid nasal corticosteroid use in patients with recent nasal septal ulcers, nasal surgery, or nasal trauma until healing has occurred.

Orally-inhaled and intranasal corticosteroids may cause a reduction in growth velocity in pediatric patients (~1 centimeter per year [range 0.3-1.8 cm per year] and related to dose and duration of exposure). To minimize the systemic effects of orally-inhaled and intranasal corticosteroids, each patient should be titrated to the lowest effective dose. Growth should be routinely monitored in pediatric patients. Safety and efficacy have not been established in children <4 years of age.

Inhalation: Not to be used in status asthmaticus or for the relief of acute bronchospasm. Flovent® Diskus® contains lactose; very rare anaphylactic reactions have been reported in patients with severe milk protein allergy. There have been reports of systemic corticosteroid withdrawal symptoms (eg, joint/muscle pain, lassitude, depression) when withdrawing oral inhalation therapy. Local yeast infections (eg, oral pharyngeal candidiasis) may occur. Lower respiratory tract infections, including pneumonia, have been reported in patients with COPD with an even higher incidence in the elderly.

Topical: May also cause suppression of HPA axis, especially when used on large areas of the body, denuded areas, for prolonged periods of time, or with an occlusive dressing. Pediatric patients may be more susceptible to systemic toxicity.

Adverse Reactions

Oral inhalation (includes reactions from Flovent® HFA and Flovent® Diskus® trials):

>10%:

Central nervous system: Headache (2% to 14%)

Respiratory: Upper respiratory tract infection (14% to 21%), throat irritation (3% to 22%)

3% to 10%:

Central nervous system: Fever (1% to 7%)

Gastrointestinal: Oral candidiasis (≤9%), nausea/vomiting (1% to 8%), gastrointestinal infection (including viral; 1% to 5%), gastrointestinal discomfort/pain (1% to 4%)

Neuromuscular & skeletal: Musculoskeletal pain (2% to 5%), muscle injury (1% to 5%)

Respiratory: Sinusitis/sinus infection (4% to 10%), lower respiratory tract infections/pneumonia (1% to 7%; COPD diagnosis and age >65 years increase risk), cough (1% to 6%), bronchitis (≤8%), hoarseness/dysphonia (2% to 6%), upper respiratory tract inflammation (≤5%), viral respiratory infection (1% to 5%), rhinitis (1% to 4%)

Miscellaneous: Viral infection (≤5%)

1% to 3%:

Cardiovascular: Chest symptoms, edema, palpitation

Central nervous system: Cranial nerve paralysis, dizziness, fatigue, malaise, migraine, mood disorders, pain, sleep disorder

Dermatologic: Acne, dermatitis/dermatosis, eczema, folliculitis, photodermatitis, infection (fungal, viral), pruritus, rash, urticaria

Endocrine metabolic: Fluid disturbance, goiter, uric acid metabolism disturbance

Gastrointestinal: Abdominal discomfort/pain, appetite changes, dental discomfort/pain, diarrhea, dyspepsia, gastroenteritis, hyposalivation, oral discomfort/pain, oral erythema/rash, oral ulcerations, oropharyngeal plaques, tooth decay, weight gain

Genitourinary: Reproductive organ infections (bacterial), urinary tract infection

Hematologic: Hematoma

Hepatic: Cholecystitis

Neuromuscular & skeletal: Arthralgia, articular rheumatism, muscle cramps/spasms, muscle pain, muscle stiffness/tightness/rigidity, musculoskeletal inflammation

Ocular: Blepharoconjunctivitis, conjunctivitis, keratitis

Otic: Otitis

Respiratory: Epistaxis, hoarseness/dysphonia, laryngitis, nasal sinus disorder, pharyngitis/throat infection, rhinorrhea/postnasal drip, throat constriction

Miscellaneous: Infection (bacterial, fungal); injuries (including muscle, soft tissue); polyps (ear, nose, throat); tonsillitis

Postmarketing and/or case reports: Aggression, agitation, anaphylactic reaction (rare; Diskus®: some patients with severe milk allergy), angioedema, anxiety, aphonia, asthma exacerbation, behavioral changes (eg, hyperactivity and irritability in children; rare), bronchospasm (immediate and delayed), cataracts, chest tightness, Churg-Strauss syndrome, contusion, Cushingoid features, cutaneous hypersensitivity, depression, dyspnea, ecchymoses, eosinophilia, facial edema, growth velocity reduction in children/adolescents, HPA axis suppression, hyperglycemia, hypersensitivity reactions (immediate and delayed), oropharyngeal edema, osteoporosis, paradoxical bronchospasm, restlessness, throat soreness, vasculitis, wheeze

Nasal inhalation (includes reactions from Flonase®, Veramyst™, and Avamys™ [CAN] trials):

>10%: Central nervous system: Headache (7% to 16%)

1% to 10%:

- Central nervous system: Dizziness (1% to 3%), fever (1% to 5%)
- Gastrointestinal: Nausea/vomiting (3% to 5%), abdominal pain (1% to 3%), diarrhea (1% to 3%)
- Neuromuscular & skeletal: Back pain (1%)
- Respiratory: Pharyngitis (6% to 8%), epistaxis (4% to 7%), asthma symptoms (3% to 7%), cough (3% to 4%), pharyngolaryngeal pain (2% to 4%), blood in nasal mucous (1% to 3%), bronchitis (1% to 3%), runny nose (1% to 3%), nasal ulcer (1%)
- Miscellaneous: Aches and pains (1% to 3%), flu-like syndrome (1% to 3%)

<1% (Limited to important or life-threatening): Alteration or loss of sense of taste and/or smell, anaphylaxis/anaphylactoid reactions, angioedema, AST increased, AV block (second degree), blurred vision, bronchospasm, cataracts, conjunctivitis, dry/irritated eyes, dry throat, dyspnea, edema (face and tongue), glaucoma, hoarseness, hypersensitivity reactions, increased intraocular pressure, nasal candidiasis, nasal septal perforation (rare), palpitations, pruritus, psychomotor hyperactivity, sinus congestion, skin rash, sore throat, throat irritation, tremor, urticaria, vaginal candidiasis, voice changes, wheezing

Topical: Pruritus (3%), skin irritation (3%), exacerbation of eczema (2%), dryness (1%), numbness of fingers (1%)

Reported with other topical corticosteroids (in decreasing order of occurrence): Irritation, folliculitis, acneiform eruptions, hypopigmentation, perioral dermatitis, allergic contact dermatitis, secondary infection, skin atrophy, striae, miliaria, pustular psoriasis from chronic plaque psoriasis

Drug Interactions

Metabolism/Transport Effects Substrate of CYP3A4 (major)

Avoid Concomitant Use There are no known interactions where it is recommended to avoid concomitant use.

Increased Effect/Toxicity

Fluticasone may increase the levels/effects of: Amphotericin B; Loop Diuretics; Thiazide Diuretics

The levels/effects of Fluticasone may be increased by: Antifungal Agents (Azole Derivatives, Systemic); CYP3A4 Inhibitors (Moderate); CYP3A4 Inhibitors (Strong); Dasatinib; Protease Inhibitors

Decreased Effect

Fluticasone may decrease the levels/effects of: Antidiabetic Agents; Corticorelin

Ethanol/Nutrition/Herb Interactions Herb/Nutraceutical: In theory, St John's wort may decrease serum levels of fluticasone by inducing CYP3A4 isoenzymes.

Stability

Nasal spray:

- Flonase®: Store between 4°C to 30°C (39°F to 86°F).
- Veramyst™: Store between 15°C to 30°C (59°F to 86°F); do not refrigerate or freeze. Store in upright position with cap on.
- Avamys™ [CAN]: Store between 4°C to 30°C (39°F to 86°F); do not refrigerate or freeze. Store in upright position with cap on.

Oral inhalation:

- Flovent® HFA: Store at 15°C to 30°C (59°F to 86°F). Discard device when the dose counter reads "000". Store with mouthpiece down.
- Flovent® Diskus®: Store at 20°C to 25°C (68°F to 77°F) in a dry place away from direct heat or sunlight. Discard after 6 weeks from removal from protective foil pouch or when the dose counter reads "0" (whichever comes first); device is not reusable.

Topical, cream: Store at 15°C to 30°C (59°F to 86°F).

- Cutivate® lotion: Store at 15°C to 30°C (59°F to 86°F); do not refrigerate.
- Cutivate® cream, ointment: Store at 2°C to 30°C (36°F to 86°F).

Mechanism of Action Fluticasone belongs to a group of corticosteroids which utilizes a fluorocarbothioate ester linkage at the 17 carbon position; extremely potent vasoconstrictive and anti-inflammatory activity; has a weak HPA inhibitory potency when applied topically, which gives the drug a high therapeutic index. The effectiveness of inhaled fluticasone is due to its direct local effect. The mechanism of action for all topical corticosteroids is believed to be a combination of three important properties: anti-inflammatory activity, immunosuppressive properties, and antiproliferative actions.

Pharmacodynamics/Kinetics

Onset of action: Intranasal: Maximal benefit may take several days

- Flovent® HFA, Flovent® Diskus®: Maximal benefit may take 1-2 weeks or longer

Absorption:

- Topical cream: 5% (increased with inflammation)
- Oral inhalation: Absorbed systemically (Flovent® Diskus®: ~18%) primarily via lungs, minimal GI absorption (<1%) due to presystemic metabolism

Distribution: Propionate: 4.2 L/kg

Protein binding: 91% to 99%

Metabolism: Hepatic via CYP3A4 to 17β-carboxylic acid (negligible activity)

Bioavailability: Nasal: ≤2%; Oral inhalation: (~18% to 21%)

Excretion: Feces (as parent drug and metabolites); urine (<5% as metabolites)

Dosage

Children:

Asthma: Inhalation, oral:

Flovent® HFA:

- Children 4-11 years: 88 mcg twice daily
- Children ≥12 years: Refer to adult dosing.
- *NIH Asthma Guidelines (NIH, 2007)* (administer in divided doses twice daily):
  - "Low" dose:
    - 0-4 years: 176 mcg/day
    - 5-11 years: 88-176 mcg/day
    - ≥12 years: 88-264 mcg/day
  - "Medium" dose:
    - 0-4 years: >176-352 mcg/day
    - 5-11 years: >176-352 mcg/day
    - ≥12 years: >264-440 mcg/day
  - "High" dose:
    - 0-4 years: >352 mcg/day
    - 5-11 years: >352 mcg/day
    - ≥12 years: >440 mcg/day

Flovent® Diskus® *(U.S. labeling)*:

- Children 4-11 years: Usual starting dose: 50 mcg twice daily; may increase to 100 mcg twice daily in patients not adequately controlled after 2 weeks of therapy. Higher starting doses may be considered in patients with poorer asthma control or those requiring high ranges of inhaled corticosteroids. Titrate to the lowest effective dose once asthma stability is achieved (maximum dose: 100 mcg twice daily)

Children >11 years: Refer to adult dosing.

Flovent® Diskus® *(Canadian labeling)*:

Children 4-16 years: Usual starting dose: 50-100 mcg twice daily; may increase to 200 mcg twice daily in patients not adequately controlled; titrate to the lowest effective dose once asthma stability is achieved

Children ≥16 years: Refer to adult dosing.

Corticosteroid-responsive dermatoses: Topical: Children ≥3 months: Cream: Apply sparingly to affected area twice daily. If no improvement is seen within 2 weeks, reassessment of diagnosis may be necessary. **Note:** Safety and efficacy of treatment >4 weeks duration have not been established.

Atopic dermatitis: Topical:

Children ≥3 months: Cream: Apply sparingly to affected area 1-2 times/day. If no improvement is seen within 2 weeks, reassessment of diagnosis may be necessary.

Children ≥1 year: Lotion: Apply sparingly to affected area once daily

Note: Safety and efficacy of treatment >4 weeks duration have not been established.

Rhinitis: Intranasal:

Flonase® (fluticasone propionate): Children ≥4 years and Adolescents: Initial: 1 spray (50 mcg/spray) per nostril once daily; patients not adequately responding or patients with more severe symptoms may use 2 sprays (100 mcg) per nostril. Depending on response, dosage may be reduced to 100 mcg daily. Total daily dosage should not exceed 2 sprays in each nostril (200 mcg)/day. Dosing should be at regular intervals.

Veramyst™ (fluticasone furoate):

Children 2-11 years: Initial: 1 spray (27.5 mcg/spray) per nostril once daily (55 mcg/day); patients not adequately responding may use 2 sprays per nostril once daily (110 mcg/day). Once symptoms are controlled, dosage may be reduced to 55 mcg once daily. Total daily dosage should not exceed 2 sprays in each nostril (110 mcg)/day.

Children ≥12 years and Adolescents: Initial: 2 sprays (27.5 mcg/spray) per nostril once daily (110 mcg/day). Once symptoms are controlled, dosage may be reduced to 1 spray per nostril once daily (55 mcg/day). Total daily dosage should not exceed 2 sprays in each nostril (110 mcg)/day.

Avamys™ [CAN] (fluticasone furoate): Children ≥12 years: 2 sprays (27.5 mcg/spray) in each nostril once daily (110 mcg/day). Total daily dosage should not exceed 2 sprays in each nostril (110 mcg)/day.

Adults:

Asthma: Inhalation, oral: **Note:** Titrate to the lowest effective dose once asthma stability is achieved

Flovent® HFA: Manufacturers labeling: Dosing based on previous therapy

Bronchodilator alone: Recommended starting dose: 88 mcg twice daily; highest recommended dose: 440 mcg twice daily

Inhaled corticosteroids: Recommended starting dose: 88-220 mcg twice daily; highest recommended dose: 440 mcg twice daily; a higher starting dose may be considered in patients previously requiring higher doses of inhaled corticosteroids

Oral corticosteroids: Recommended starting dose: 440 mcg twice daily

Highest recommended dose: 880 mcg twice daily; starting dose is patient dependent. In patients on chronic oral corticosteroids therapy, reduce prednisone dose no faster than 2.5-5 mg/day on a weekly basis; begin taper after 1 week of fluticasone therapy.

NIH Asthma Guidelines (NIH, 2007) (administer in divided doses twice daily):

"Low" dose: 88-264 mcg/day

"Medium" dose: >264-440 mcg/day

"High" dose: >440 mcg/day

Flovent® Diskus® *(U.S. labeling)*: **Note:** May increase dose after 2 weeks of therapy in patients not adequately controlled. Higher starting doses may be considered in patients with poorer asthma control or those requiring high ranges of inhaled corticosteroids. Titrate to the lowest effective dose once asthma stability is achieved.

Bronchodilator alone: Recommended starting dose: 100 mcg twice daily; maximum recommended dose: 500 mcg twice daily

Inhaled corticosteroids: Recommended starting dose: 100-250 mcg twice daily; maximum recommended dose: 500 mcg twice daily

Oral corticosteroids: Recommended starting dose: 500-1000 mcg twice daily; maximum recommended dose: 1000 mcg twice daily. Starting dose is patient dependent. In patients on chronic oral corticosteroids therapy, reduce prednisone dose no faster than 2.5 mg/day on a weekly basis; begin taper after 1 week of fluticasone therapy.

Flovent® Diskus® *(Canadian labeling)*:

Mild asthma: 100-250 mcg twice daily

Moderate asthma: 250-500 mcg twice daily

Severe asthma: 500 mcg twice daily; may increase to 1000 mcg twice daily in very severe patients requiring high doses of corticosteroids

Corticosteroid-responsive dermatoses: Topical: Cream, lotion, ointment: Apply sparingly to affected area twice daily. If no improvement is seen within 2 weeks, reassessment of diagnosis may be necessary.

Atopic dermatitis: Topical: Cream, lotion: Apply sparingly to affected area once or twice daily. If no improvement is seen within 2 weeks, reassessment of diagnosis may be necessary.

Rhinitis: Intranasal:

Flonase® (fluticasone propionate): Initial: 2 sprays (50 mcg/spray) per nostril once daily; may also be divided into 100 mcg twice a day. After the first few days, dosage may be reduced to 1 spray per nostril once daily for maintenance therapy.

Veramyst™ (fluticasone furoate): Initial: 2 sprays (27.5 mcg/spray) per nostril once daily (110 mcg/day). Once symptoms are controlled, may reduce dosage to 1 spray per nostril once daily (55 mcg/day) for maintenance therapy.

Avamys™ [CAN] (fluticasone furoate): 2 sprays (27.5 mcg/spray) in each nostril once daily (110 mcg/day). Total daily dosage should not exceed 2 sprays in each nostril (110 mcg)/day.

Elderly: No differences in safety have been observed in the elderly when compared to younger patients. Based on current data, no dosage adjustment is needed based on age.

Dosage adjustment in hepatic impairment: Fluticasone is primarily cleared in the liver. Fluticasone plasma levels may be increased in patients with hepatic impairment, use with caution; monitor.

Dietary Considerations Flovent® Diskus® contains lactose; very rare anaphylactic reactions have been reported in patients with severe milk protein allergy.

Administration

Aerosol inhalation: Flovent® HFA: Shake container thoroughly before using. Take 3-5 deep breaths. Use inhaler on inspiration. Allow 1 full minute between inhalations. Rinse mouth with water after use to reduce aftertaste and incidence of candidiasis; do not swallow. Inhaler must be primed before first use, when not used for 7 days, or if dropped. To prime the first time, release

4 sprays into air; shake well before each spray and spray away from face. If dropped or not used for 7 days, prime by releasing a single test spray. Patient should contact pharmacy for refill when the dose counter reads "020". Discard device when the dose counter reads "000". Do not use "float" test to determine contents.

Nasal spray: Administer at regular intervals. Shake bottle gently before using. Blow nose to clear nostrils. Insert applicator into nostril, keeping bottle upright, and close off the other nostril. Breathe in through nose. While inhaling, press pump to release spray. Discard after labeled number of doses has been used, even if bottle is not completely empty.

Flonase®: Prime pump (press 6 times until fine spray appears) prior to first use or if spray unused for ≥7 days. Once weekly, nasal applicator may be removed and rinsed with warm water to clean.

Veramyst™, Avamys™ [CAN]: Prime pump (press 6 times until fine spray appears) prior to first use, if spray unused for ≥30 days, or if cap left off bottle for ≥5 days. After each use, nozzle should be wiped with a clean, dry tissue. Once weekly, inside of cap should be cleaned with a clean, dry tissue.

Powder for oral inhalation: Flovent® Diskus®: Do not use with a spacer device. Do not exhale into Diskus®. Do not wash or take apart. Use in horizontal position. Mouth should be rinsed with water after use (do not swallow). Discard after 6 weeks once removed from protective pouch or when the dose counter reads "0", whichever comes first (device is not reusable).

Topical cream, lotion, ointment: Apply sparingly in a thin film. Rub in lightly. Unless otherwise directed by healthcare professional, do not use with occlusive dressing; do not use on children's skin covered by diapers or plastic pants.

Monitoring Parameters Growth (adolescents and children); signs/symptoms of HPA axis suppression/adrenal insufficiency; possible eosinophilic conditions (including Churg-Strauss syndrome); FEV_1, peak flow, and/or other pulmonary function tests; asthma symptoms

Additional Information Effects of inhaled/intranasal steroids on growth have been observed in the absence of laboratory evidence of HPA axis suppression, suggesting that growth velocity is a more sensitive indicator of systemic corticosteroid exposure in pediatric patients than some commonly used tests of HPA axis function. The long-term effects of this reduction in growth velocity associated with orally-inhaled and intranasal corticosteroids, including the impact on final adult height, are unknown. The potential for "catch up" growth following discontinuation of treatment with inhaled corticosteroids has not been adequately studied. The product labeling notes that intranasal administration was not associated with a statistically-significant reduction in growth velocity (based on a small study conducted over 1 year).

In the United States, dosage for the metered dose inhaler (Flovent® HFA) is expressed as the amount of drug which leaves the actuater and is delivered to the patient. This differs from other countries, which express the dosage as the amount of drug which leaves the valve.

Dosage Forms Excipient information presented when available (limited, particularly for generics); consult specific product labeling. [CAN] = Canadian brand name

Aerosol for oral inhalation, as propionate [CFC free]:

Flovent® HFA: 44 mcg/inhalation (10.6 g) [120 metered actuations]

Flovent® HFA: 110 mcg/inhalation (12 g) [120 metered actuations]

Flovent® HFA: 220 mcg/inhalation (12 g) [120 metered actuations]

Cream, as propionate: 0.05% (15 g, 30 g, 60 g)

Cutivate®: 0.05% (30 g, 60 g)

Lotion, as propionate:

Cutivate®: 0.05% (120 mL)

Ointment, as propionate: 0.005% (15 g, 30 g, 60 g)

Cutivate®: 0.005% (30 g, 60 g)

Powder for oral inhalation, as propionate:

Flovent® Diskus® [U.S.]: 50 mcg (60s) [contains lactose; prefilled blister pack]

Flovent® Diskus® [CAN]: 50 mcg (28s, 60s) [contains lactose; prefilled blister pack] [not available in the U.S.]

Flovent® Diskus® [CAN]: 100 mcg (28s, 60s) [contains lactose; prefilled blister pack] [not available in the U.S.]

Flovent® Diskus® [CAN]: 250 mcg (28s, 60s) [contains lactose; prefilled blister pack] [not available in the U.S.]

Flovent® Diskus® [CAN]: 500 mcg (28s, 60s) [contains lactose; prefilled blister pack] [not available in the U.S.]

Suspension, intranasal, as furoate [spray]:

Avamys™ [CAN]: 27.5 mcg/inhalation (4.5 g) [30 metered actuations; contains benzalkonium chloride]; (10 g) [120 metered actuations; contains benzalkonium chloride] [not available in the U.S.]

Veramyst™: 27.5 mcg/inhalation (10 g) [120 metered actuations; contains benzalkonium chloride]

Suspension, intranasal, as propionate [spray]: 50 mcg/inhalation (16 g) [120 metered actuations]

Flonase®: 50 mcg/inhalation (16 g) [120 metered actuations; contains benzalkonium chloride]

Fluticasone and Salmeterol

(floo TIK a sone & sal ME te role)

U.S. Brand Names Advair Diskus®; Advair® HFA

Canadian Brand Names Advair Diskus®; Advair®

Index Terms Fluticasone Propionate and Salmeterol Xinafoate; Salmeterol and Fluticasone

Pharmacologic Category $Beta_2$-Adrenergic Agonist, Long-Acting; $Beta_2$-Adrenergic Agonist; Corticosteroid, Inhalant (Oral)

Use Maintenance treatment of asthma; maintenance treatment of COPD

Restrictions An FDA-approved medication guide must be distributed when dispensing an outpatient prescription (new or refill) where this medication is to be used without direct supervision of a healthcare provider. Medication guides are available at http://www.fda.gov/cder/Offices/ODS/medication_guides.htm.

Pregnancy Risk Factor C

Pregnancy Considerations See individual agents.

Lactation

Fluticasone: Excretion in breast milk unknown/use caution

Salmeterol: Enters breast milk/use caution

Medication Safety Issues

Sound-alike/look-alike issues:

Advair may be confused with Advicor®

Contraindications Hypersensitivity to fluticasone, salmeterol, or any component of the formulation; status asthmaticus; acute episodes of asthma or COPD

Warnings/Precautions See individual agents.

Adverse Reactions Percentages reported in patients with asthma; also see individual agents:

>10%:

Central nervous system: Headache (12% to 21%)

Respiratory: Upper respiratory tract infection (16% to 27%), pharyngitis (9% to 13%)

>3% to 10%:

Central nervous system: Dizziness (1% to 4%)

Endocrine & metabolic: Menstruation symptoms (3% to 5%)

Gastrointestinal: Nausea/vomiting (3% to 6%), diarrhea (2% to 4%), pain/discomfort (1% to 4%), oral candidiasis (1% to 4%), gastrointestinal infections (including viral, ≤4%)

Neuromuscular & skeletal: Musculoskeletal pain (2% to 7%), muscle pain (≤4%)

Respiratory: Throat irritation (7% to 9%), bronchitis (2% to 8%), upper respiratory tract inflammation (4% to 7%), lower respiratory tract infections/pneumonia (1% to 7%; COPD diagnosis and age >65 years increase risk), cough (3% to 6%), sinusitis (4% to 5%), hoarseness/dysphonia (1% to 5%), viral respiratory tract infection (3% to 5%)

1% to 3%:

Cardiovascular: Arrhythmia, chest symptoms, fluid retention, MI, palpitation, syncope, tachycardia

Central nervous system: Compressed nerve syndromes, hypnagogic effects, migraine, pain, sleep disorders, tremor

Dermatologic: Dermatitis, dermatosis, eczema, hives, skin flakiness, urticaria, viral skin infection

Endocrine & metabolic: Hypothyroidism

Gastrointestinal: Constipation, dental discomfort/pain, gastrointestinal infection, hemorrhoids, oral discomfort/pain, oral erythema/rash, oral ulcerations, unusual taste, weight gain

Genitourinary: Urinary tract infection

Hematologic: Contusions/hematomas

Hepatic: Abnormal liver function tests

Neuromuscular & skeletal: Arthralgia, articular rheumatism, bone/cartilage disorders, bone pain, cramps, fractures, muscle injuries (≤3%), muscle spasm, muscle stiffness, tightness/rigidity

Ocular: Conjunctivitis, edema, eye redness, keratitis, xerophthalmia

Respiratory: Blood in nasal mucosa, congestion, ear/nose/throat infection, epistaxis, laryngitis, lower respiratory hemorrhage, nasal irritation, rhinitis, rhinorrhea/postnasal drip, sneezing

Miscellaneous: Allergies/allergic reactions, bacterial infection, burns, candidiasis (≤3%), diaphoresis, sweat/sebum disorders, viral infection, wounds and lacerations

Postmarketing and/or case reports: Asthma exacerbation (serious and some fatal), abdominal pain, agitation, aggression, anaphylactic reaction (Diskus®: some in patients with severe milk allergy), angioedema, aphonia, atrial fibrillation, bronchospasm, cataracts, chest congestion, chest tightness, choking, contact dermatitis, Cushing syndrome, Cushingoid features, depression, dysmenorrhea, dyspepsia, dyspnea, earache, ecchymoses, edema (facial, oropharyngeal), eosinophilic conditions, glaucoma, growth velocity reduction in children/adolescents, hypercorticism, hyperglycemia, hypersensitivity reaction (immediate and delayed), hypertension, hypokalemia, hypothyroidism, influenza, intraocular pressure increased, laryngeal spasm/irritation, irregular menstruation, myositis, osteoporosis, pallor, paresthesia, paradoxical tracheitis, paranasal sinus pain, photodermatitis, PID, rash, restlessness, stridor, supraventricular tachycardia, syncope, vaginal candidiasis, vaginitis, vulvovaginitis, rare cases of vasculitis (Churg-Strauss syndrome), ventricular tachycardia, wheezing, xerostomia

Drug Interactions

Metabolism/Transport Effects Fluticasone: **Substrate** of CYP3A4 (major); Salmeterol: **Substrate** of CYP3A4 (major)

Avoid Concomitant Use

Avoid concomitant use of Fluticasone and Salmeterol with any of the following: CYP3A4 Inhibitors (Strong); Iobenguane I 123

Increased Effect/Toxicity

Fluticasone and Salmeterol may increase the levels/effects of: Amphotericin B; Loop Diuretics; Sympathomimetics; Thiazide Diuretics

The levels/effects of Fluticasone and Salmeterol may be increased by: Antifungal Agents (Azole Derivatives, Systemic); Atomoxetine; Cannabinoids; CYP3A4 Inhibitors (Moderate); CYP3A4 Inhibitors (Strong); Dasatinib; MAO Inhibitors; Protease Inhibitors; Tricyclic Antidepressants

Decreased Effect

Fluticasone and Salmeterol may decrease the levels/effects of: Antidiabetic Agents; Corticorelin; Iobenguane I 123

The levels/effects of Fluticasone and Salmeterol may be decreased by: Alpha-/Beta-Blockers; Beta-Blockers (Beta1 Selective); Beta-Blockers (Nonselective); Betahistine

Stability

Advair Diskus®: Store at controlled room temperature of 20°C to 25°C (68°F to 77°F). Store in a dry place out of direct heat or sunlight. Diskus® device should be discarded 1 month after removal from foil pouch, or when dosing indicator reads "0" (whichever comes first); device is not reusable.

Advair® HFA: Store at controlled room temperature of 25°C (77°F). Store with mouthpiece down. Discard after 120 inhalations. Discard device when the dose counter reads "000". Device is not reusable.

Mechanism of Action Combination of fluticasone (corticosteroid) and salmeterol (long-acting $beta_2$-agonist) designed to improve pulmonary function and control over what is produced by either agent when used alone. Because fluticasone and salmeterol act locally in the lung, plasma levels do not predict therapeutic effect.

Fluticasone: The mechanism of action for all topical corticosteroids is believed to be a combination of three important properties: Anti-inflammatory activity, immunosuppressive properties, and antiproliferative actions. Fluticasone has extremely potent vasoconstrictive and anti-inflammatory activity.

Salmeterol: Relaxes bronchial smooth muscle by selective action on $beta_2$-receptors with little effect on heart rate

Pharmacodynamics/Kinetics See individual agents.

Dosage Oral inhalation: **Note:** Do not use to transfer patients from systemic corticosteroid therapy.

COPD: Adults:

Advair Diskus®: Fluticasone 250 mcg/salmeterol 50 mcg twice daily, 12 hours apart. **Note:** This is the maximum dose.

Advair Diskus® [Canadian labeling; not in approved U.S. labeling]: Fluticasone 250 mcg/salmeterol 50 mcg **or** fluticasone 500 mcg/salmeterol 50 mcg twice daily, 12 hours apart.

Maximum dose: Fluticasone 500 mcg/salmeterol 50 mcg per inhalation (2 inhalations/day)

Asthma:

Children 4-11 years: Advair Diskus®: Fluticasone 100 mcg/salmeterol 50 mcg twice daily, 12 hours apart. **Note:** This is the maximum dose.

Children ≥12 and Adults:

Advair Diskus®: One inhalation twice daily, morning and evening, 12 hours apart

Maximum dose: Fluticasone 500 mcg/salmeterol 50 mcg per inhalation (2 inhalations/day)

Advair® HFA: Two inhalations twice daily, morning and evening, 12 hours apart

Maximum dose: Fluticasone 230 mcg/salmeterol 21 mcg per inhalation (4 inhalations/day)

Advair® 125 or Advair® 250 [Canadian labeling; not in approved U.S. labeling]: Two inhalations twice daily, morning and evening, 12 hours apart

Maximum dose: Fluticasone 250 mcg/salmeterol 25 mcg per inhalation (4 inhalations/day)

Note: Initial dose prescribed should be based upon previous dose of inhaled-steroid asthma therapy. Dose should be increased after 2 weeks if adequate response is not achieved. Patients should be titrated to lowest effective dose once stable. Each suggestion below specifies the product strength to use; remember to **use 1 inhalation for Diskus® and 2 inhalations for HFA.**

Patients not currently on inhaled corticosteroids:

Advair Diskus®: Fluticasone 100 mcg/salmeterol 50 mcg **or** fluticasone 250 mcg/salmeterol 50 mcg

Advair® HFA: Fluticasone 45 mcg/salmeterol 21 mcg **or** fluticasone 115 mcg/salmeterol 21 mcg

Patients currently using inhaled beclomethasone dipropionate:

≤160 mcg/day: Fluticasone 100 mcg/salmeterol 50 mcg **or** Advair® HFA: Fluticasone 45 mcg/salmeterol 21 mcg

320 mcg/day: Fluticasone 250 mcg/salmeterol 50 mcg **or** Advair® HFA: Fluticasone 115 mcg/salmeterol 21 mcg

640 mcg/day: Fluticasone 500 mcg/salmeterol 50 mcg **or** Advair® HFA: Fluticasone 230 mcg/salmeterol 21 mcg

Patients currently using inhaled budesonide:

≤400 mcg/day: Fluticasone 100 mcg/salmeterol 50 mcg **or** Advair® HFA: Fluticasone 45 mcg/salmeterol 21 mcg

800-1200 mcg/day: Fluticasone 250 mcg/salmeterol 50 mcg **or** Advair® HFA: Fluticasone 115 mcg/salmeterol 21mcg

1600 mcg/day: Fluticasone 500 mcg/salmeterol 50 mcg **or** Advair® HFA: Fluticasone 230 mcg/salmeterol 21 mcg

Patients currently using inhaled flunisolide CFC aerosol:

≤1000 mcg/day: Fluticasone 100 mcg/salmeterol 50 mcg **or** Advair® HFA: Fluticasone 45 mcg/salmeterol 21 mcg

1250-2000 mcg/day: Fluticasone 250 mcg/salmeterol 50 mcg **or** Advair® HFA: Fluticasone 115 mcg/salmeterol 21 mcg

Patients currently using inhaled flunisolide HFA inhalation aerosol:

≤320 mcg/day: Fluticasone 100 mcg/salmeterol 50 mcg **or** Advair® HFA: Fluticasone 45 mcg/salmeterol 21 mcg

640 mcg/day: Fluticasone 250 mcg/salmeterol 50 mcg **or** Advair® HFA: Fluticasone 115 mcg/salmeterol 21 mcg

Patients currently using inhaled fluticasone HFA aerosol:

≤176 mcg/day: Fluticasone 100 mcg/salmeterol 50 mcg **or** Advair® HFA: Fluticasone 45 mcg/salmeterol 21 mcg

440 mcg/day: Fluticasone 250 mcg/salmeterol 50 mcg **or** Advair® HFA: Fluticasone 115 mcg/salmeterol 21 mcg

660-880 mcg/day: Fluticasone 500 mcg/salmeterol 50 mcg **or** Advair® HFA: Fluticasone 230 mcg/salmeterol 21 mcg

Patients currently using inhaled fluticasone propionate powder:

≤200 mcg/day: Fluticasone 100 mcg/salmeterol 50 mcg **or** Advair® HFA: Fluticasone 45 mcg/salmeterol 21 mcg

500 mcg/day: Fluticasone 250 mcg/salmeterol 50 mcg **or** Advair® HFA: Fluticasone 115 mcg/salmeterol 21 mcg

1000 mcg/day: Fluticasone 500 mcg/salmeterol 50 mcg **or** Advair® HFA: Fluticasone 230 mcg/salmeterol 21 mcg

Patients currently using inhaled mometasone furoate powder:

220 mcg/day: Fluticasone 100 mcg/salmeterol 50 mcg **or** Advair® HFA: Fluticasone 45 mcg/salmeterol 21 mcg

440 mcg/day: Fluticasone 250 mcg/salmeterol 50 mcg **or** Advair® HFA: Fluticasone 115 mcg/salmeterol 21 mcg

880 mcg/day: Fluticasone 500 mcg/salmeterol 50 mcg **or** Advair® HFA: Fluticasone 230 mcg/salmeterol 21 mcg

Patients currently using inhaled triamcinolone acetonide:

≤1000 mcg/day: Fluticasone 100 mcg/salmeterol 50 mcg **or** Advair® HFA: Fluticasone 45 mcg/salmeterol 21 mcg

1100-1600 mcg/day: Fluticasone 250 mcg/salmeterol 50 mcg **or** Advair® HFA: Fluticasone 115 mcg/salmeterol 21 mcg

Elderly: No differences in safety or effectiveness have been seen in studies of patients ≥65 years of age. However, increased sensitivity may be seen in the elderly. Use with caution in patients with concomitant cardiovascular disease.

Dosage adjustment in renal impairment: Specific guidelines are not available

Dosage adjustment in hepatic impairment: No dosage adjustment required; manufacturer suggests close monitoring of patients with hepatic impairment.

Dietary Considerations Advair Diskus® powder for oral inhalation contains lactose; very rare anaphylactic reactions have been reported in patients with severe milk protein allergy.

Administration

Advair Diskus®: After removing from box and foil pouch, write the "Pouch opened" and "Use by" dates on the label on top of the Diskus®. The "Use by" date is 1 month from date of opening the pouch. Every time the lever is pushed back, a dose is ready to be inhaled. Do not close or tilt the Diskus® after the lever is pushed back. Do not play with the lever or move the lever more than once. The dose indicator tells you how many doses are left. When the numbers 5 to 0 appear in red, only a few doses remain. Discard device 1 month after you remove it from the foil pouch or when the dose counter reads "0" (whichever comes first). Rinse mouth with water after use to reduce risk of oral candidiasis.

Advair® HFA: Shake well for 5 seconds before each spray. Prime with 4 test sprays (into air and away from face) before using for the first time. If canister is dropped or not used for >4 weeks, prime with 2 sprays. Patient should contact pharmacy for refill when the dose counter reads "020". Discard device when the dose counter reads "000". Do not spray in eyes. Rinse mouth with water after use to reduce risk of oral candidiasis.

Monitoring Parameters FEV_1, peak flow, and/or other pulmonary function tests; blood pressure, heart rate; CNS stimulation. Monitor for increased use of short-acting $beta_2$-agonist inhalers; may be marker of a deteriorating asthma condition. The growth of pediatric patients receiving inhaled corticosteroids should be monitored routinely (eg, via stadiometry).

Additional Information Effects of inhaled/intranasal steroids on growth have been observed in the absence of laboratory evidence of HPA axis suppression, suggesting that growth velocity is a more sensitive indicator of systemic corticosteroid exposure in pediatric patients than some commonly used tests of HPA axis function. The long-term effects of this reduction in growth velocity associated with orally-inhaled and intranasal corticosteroids, including the impact on final adult height, are unknown. The potential for "catch up" growth following discontinuation of treatment with inhaled corticosteroids has not been adequately studied.

Advair® HFA: Salmeterol (base) 21 mcg is equivalent to 30.45 mcg of salmeterol xinafoate.

Dosage Forms Excipient information presented when available (limited, particularly for generics); consult specific product labeling. [DSC] = Discontinued product; [CAN] = Canadian brand name/formulation

Aerosol, for oral inhalation:
Advair® HFA:
45/21: Fluticasone propionate 45 mcg and salmeterol 21 mcg (12 g) [120 metered inhalations]
115/21: Fluticasone propionate 115 mcg and salmeterol 21 mcg (12 g) [120 metered inhalations]
230/21: Fluticasone propionate 230 mcg and salmeterol 21 mcg (12 g) [120 metered inhalations]
Advair® [CAN]:
125/25: Fluticasone propionate 125 mcg and salmeterol 25 mcg (12 g) [120 metered inhalations] [not available in the U.S.]
250/25: Fluticasone propionate 250 mcg and salmeterol 25 mcg (12 g) [120 metered inhalations] [not available in the U.S.]
Powder, for oral inhalation:
Advair Diskus®:
100/50: Fluticasone propionate 100 mcg and salmeterol 50 mcg (14s, 28s [DSC], 60s) [contains lactose; chlorofluorocarbon free]
250/50: Fluticasone propionate 250 mcg and salmeterol 50 mcg (14s [DSC], 60s) [contains lactose; chlorofluorocarbon free]
500/50: Fluticasone propionate 500 mcg and salmeterol 50 mcg (14s [DSC], 60s) [contains lactose; chlorofluorocarbon free]

◆ **Fluticasone Furoate** *see* Fluticasone *on page 644*

◆ **Fluticasone Propionate** *see* Fluticasone *on page 644*

◆ **Fluticasone Propionate and Salmeterol Xinafoate** *see* Fluticasone and Salmeterol *on page 648*

Fluvastatin (FLOO va sta tin)

U.S. Brand Names Lescol®; Lescol® XL
Canadian Brand Names Lescol®; Lescol® XL
Pharmacologic Category Antilipemic Agent, HMG-CoA Reductase Inhibitor
Additional Appendix Information
Hyperlipidemia Management *on page 1815*
Lipid-Lowering Agents *on page 1661*
Use To be used as a component of multiple risk factor intervention in patients at risk for atherosclerosis vascular disease due to hypercholesterolemia

Adjunct to dietary therapy to reduce elevated total cholesterol (total-C), LDL-C, triglyceride, and apolipoprotein B (apo-B) levels and to increase HDL-C in primary hypercholesterolemia and mixed dyslipidemia (Fredrickson types IIa and IIb); to slow the progression of coronary atherosclerosis in patients with coronary heart disease; reduce risk of coronary revascularization procedures in patients with coronary heart disease
Pregnancy Risk Factor X
Pregnancy Considerations Cholesterol biosynthesis may be important in fetal development. Contraindicated in pregnancy. Administer to women of childbearing potential only when conception is highly unlikely and patients have been informed of potential hazards.
Lactation Enters breast milk/contraindicated
Medication Safety Issues
Sound-alike/look-alike issues:
Fluvastatin may be confused with fluoxetine
Contraindications Hypersensitivity to fluvastatin or any component of the formulation; active liver disease; unexplained persistent elevations of serum transaminases; pregnancy; breast-feeding
Warnings/Precautions Secondary causes of hyperlipidemia should be ruled out prior to therapy. Liver function must be monitored by periodic laboratory assessment. Rhabdomyolysis with acute renal failure has occurred with fluvastatin and other HMG-CoA reductase inhibitors. Risk may be increased with concurrent use of other drugs which may cause rhabdomyolysis (including colchicine, gemfibrozil, fibric acid derivatives, or niacin at doses ≥1 g/day). Temporarily discontinue in any patient experiencing markedly elevated CPK levels, myopathy, or an acute/serious condition predisposing to renal failure secondary to rhabdomyolysis. Based upon current evidence, HMG-CoA reductase inhibitor therapy should be continued in the perioperative period unless risk outweighs cardioprotective benefit. Use with caution in patients with advanced age; these patients are predisposed to myopathy. Use caution in patients with previous liver disease or heavy ethanol use. Use caution in patients with concurrent medications or conditions which reduce steroidogenesis. Safety and efficacy in children <10 years of age have not been established.
Adverse Reactions As reported with fluvastatin capsules; in general, adverse reactions reported with fluvastatin extended release tablet were similar, but the incidence was less.

1% to 10%:
Central nervous system: Headache (9%), fatigue (3%), insomnia (3%)
Gastrointestinal: Dyspepsia (8%), diarrhea (5%), abdominal pain (5%), nausea (3%)
Genitourinary: Urinary tract infection (2%)
Neuromuscular & skeletal: Myalgia (5%)
Respiratory: Sinusitis (3%), bronchitis (2%)
<1% (Limited to important or life-threatening) including additional class-related events (not necessarily reported with fluvastatin therapy): Alopecia, anaphylaxis, angioedema, arthralgia, arthritis, cataracts, cholestatic jaundice, cirrhosis, CPK increased (>10x normal), depression, dermatomyositis, dyspnea, eosinophilia, erectile dysfunction, erythema multiforme, ESR increased, facial paresis, fatty liver, fever, fulminant hepatic necrosis, gynecomastia, hemolytic anemia, hepatitis, hepatoma, hypersensitivity reaction, impotence, leukopenia, memory loss, muscle cramps, myopathy, nodules, ophthalmoplegia, pancreatitis, paresthesia, peripheral nerve palsy, peripheral neuropathy, photosensitivity, polymyalgia rheumatica, positive ANA, pruritus, psychic disturbance, purpura, rash, renal failure (secondary to rhabdomyolysis), rhabdomyolysis, skin discoloration, Stevens-Johnson syndrome, systemic lupus erythematosus-like syndrome, taste alteration, thrombocytopenia, thyroid dysfunction, toxic epidermal necrolysis, transaminases increased, tremor, urticaria, vasculitis, vertigo
Drug Interactions
Metabolism/Transport Effects Substrate of CYP2C9 (major), 2C8 (minor), 2D6 (minor), 3A4 (minor); **Inhibits** CYP1A2 (weak), 2C8 (weak), 2C9 (moderate), 2D6 (weak), 3A4 (weak)
Avoid Concomitant Use There are no known interactions where it is recommended to avoid concomitant use.
Increased Effect/Toxicity
Fluvastatin may increase the levels/effects of: CYP2C9 Substrates (High risk); DAPTOmycin; Vitamin K Antagonists

The levels/effects of Fluvastatin may be increased by: Amiodarone; Colchicine; Eltrombopag; Fenofibrate; Fenofibric Acid; Fluconazole; Niacin; Niacinamide
Decreased Effect
The levels/effects of Fluvastatin may be decreased by: Etravirine; Phenytoin; Rifamycin Derivatives
Ethanol/Nutrition/Herb Interactions
Ethanol: Avoid excessive ethanol consumption (due to potential hepatic effects).
Food: Reduces rate but not the extent of absorption. Red yeast rice contains an estimated 2.4 mg lovastatin per 600 mg rice.
Stability Store at 15°C to 30°C (59°F to 86°F). Protect from light.

Mechanism of Action Acts by competitively inhibiting 3-hydroxyl-3-methylglutaryl-coenzyme A (HMG-CoA) reductase, the enzyme that catalyzes the reduction of HMG-CoA to mevalonate; this is an early rate-limiting step in cholesterol biosynthesis. HDL is increased while total, LDL, and VLDL cholesterols; apolipoprotein B; and plasma triglycerides are decreased.

Pharmacodynamics/Kinetics

Onset of action: Peak effect: Maximal LDL-C reductions achieved within 4 weeks

Distribution: V_d: 0.35 L/kg

Protein binding: >98%

Metabolism: To inactive and active metabolites (oxidative metabolism via CYP2C9 [75%], 2C8 [~5%], and 3A4 [~20%] isoenzymes); active forms do not circulate systemically; extensive (saturable) first-pass hepatic extraction

Bioavailability: Absolute: Capsule: 24%; Extended release tablet: 29%

Half-life elimination: Capsule: <3 hours; Extended release tablet: 9 hours

Time to peak: Capsule: 1 hour; Extended release tablet: 3 hours

Excretion: Feces (90%): urine (5%)

Dosage

Adolescents 10-16 years: Oral: Heterozygous familial hypercholesterolemia: Initial: 20 mg once daily; may increase every 6 weeks based on tolerability and response to a maximum recommended dose of 80 mg/day, given in 2 divided doses (immediate release capsule) or as a single daily dose (extended release tablet)

Note: Indicated only for adjunctive therapy when diet alone cannot reduce LDL-C below 190 mg/dL, or 160 mg/dL (with cardiovascular risk factors). Female patients must be 1 year postmenarche.

Adults: Oral:

Patients requiring ≥25% decrease in LDL-C: 40 mg capsule once daily in the evening, 80 mg extended release tablet once daily (anytime), or 40 mg capsule twice daily

Patients requiring <25% decrease in LDL-C: Initial: 20 mg capsule once daily in the evening; may increase based on tolerability and response to a maximum recommended dose of 80 mg/day, given in 2 divided doses (immediate release capsule) or as a single daily dose (extended release tablet)

Dosage adjustment in renal impairment: Less than 6% excreted renally; no dosage adjustment needed with mild-to-moderate renal impairment; use with caution in severe impairment

Dosage adjustment in hepatic impairment: Levels may accumulate in patients with liver disease (increased AUC and C_{max}); use caution with severe hepatic impairment or heavy ethanol ingestion; contraindicated in active liver disease or unexplained transaminase elevations; decrease dose and monitor effects carefully in patients with hepatic insufficiency

Elderly: No dosage adjustment necessary based on age

Dietary Considerations Generally, patients should be placed on a standard cholesterol-lowering diet and other lifestyle modifications for 3-6 months prior to the initiation of drug therapy. The diet should be continued during drug therapy. However, for patients with advanced risk factors (eg, known coronary heart disease), drug therapy may be initiated concurrently with diet modification. May be taken without regard to meals. Red yeast rice contains an estimated 2.4 mg lovastatin per 600 mg rice.

Administration Patient should be placed on a standard cholesterol-lowering diet before and during treatment. Fluvastatin may be taken without regard to meals. Adjust dosage as needed in response to periodic lipid determinations during the first 4 weeks after a dosage change; lipid-lowering effects are additive when fluvastatin is combined with a bile-acid binding resin or niacin, however, it must be administered at least 2 hours following these drugs. Do not break, chew, or crush extended release tablets; do not open capsules.

Monitoring Parameters Obtain baseline LFTs and total cholesterol profile; repeat tests at 12 weeks after initiation of therapy or elevation in dose, and periodically thereafter. Monitor LDL-C at intervals no less than 4 weeks.

Dosage Forms Excipient information presented when available (limited, particularly for generics); consult specific product labeling.

Capsule (Lescol®): 20 mg, 40 mg

Tablet, extended release (Lescol® XL): 80 mg

- **Fluviral S/F® (Can)** *see* Influenza Virus Vaccine *on page 788*
- **Fluvirin®** *see* Influenza Virus Vaccine *on page 788*

Fluvoxamine (floo VOKS a meen)

U.S. Brand Names Luvox® CR

Canadian Brand Names Alti-Fluvoxamine; Apo-Fluvoxamine®; Luvox®; Novo-Fluvoxamine; Nu-Fluvoxamine; PMS-Fluvoxamine; Rhoxal-Fluvoxamine; Riva-Fluvox; Sandoz-Fluvoxamine

Index Terms Luvox

Pharmacologic Category Antidepressant, Selective Serotonin Reuptake Inhibitor

Additional Appendix Information

Antidepressant Agents *on page 1638*

Selective Serotonin Reuptake Inhibitors (SSRIs) Pharmacokinetics *on page 1670*

Use Treatment of obsessive-compulsive disorder (OCD); treatment of social anxiety disorder

Unlabeled/Investigational Use Treatment of major depression; panic disorder; anxiety disorders in children; treatment of mild dementia-associated agitation in non-psychotic patients

Restrictions An FDA-approved medication guide concerning the use of antidepressants in children, adolescents, and young adults must be distributed when dispensing an outpatient prescription (new or refill) where this medication is to be used without direct supervision of a healthcare provider. Medication guides are available at http://www.fda.gov/cder/Offices/ODS/medication_guides.htm. Dispense to parents or guardians of children and adolescents receiving this medication.

Pregnancy Risk Factor C

Pregnancy Considerations Due to adverse effects observed in animal studies, fluvoxamine is classified as pregnancy category C. Fluvoxamine crosses the human placenta. Nonteratogenic effects in the newborn following SSRI exposure late in the third trimester include respiratory distress, cyanosis, apnea, seizures, temperature instability, feeding difficulty, vomiting, hypoglycemia, hypo- or hypertonia, hyper-reflexia, jitteriness, irritability, constant crying, and tremor. An increased risk of low birth weight and low APGAR scores has also been reported. Exposure to SSRIs after the twentieth week of gestation has been associated with persistent pulmonary hypertension of the newborn (PPHN). Adverse effects may be due to toxic effects of the SSRI or drug withdrawal due to discontinuation. The long-term effects of *in utero* SSRI exposure on infant development and behavior are not known.

Women treated for major depression and who are euthymic prior to pregnancy are more likely to experience a relapse when medication is discontinued as compared to pregnant women who continue taking antidepressant medications. The ACOG recommends that therapy with

SSRIs or SNRIs during pregnancy be individualized; treatment of depression during pregnancy should incorporate the clinical expertise of the mental health clinician, obstetrician, primary healthcare provider, and pediatrician (ACOG, 2007). If treatment during pregnancy is required, consider tapering therapy during the third trimester in order to prevent withdrawal symptoms in the infant. If this is done and the woman is considered to be at risk from her major depressive disorder, the medication can be restarted following delivery, although the dose should be readjusted to that required before pregnancy.

Lactation Enters breast milk/consider risk:benefit (AAP rates "of concern")

Medication Safety Issues

Sound-alike/look-alike issues:

Fluvoxamine may be confused with flavoxate, fluoxetine

Luvox may be confused with Lasix®, Levoxyl®, Lovenox®

Contraindications Hypersensitivity to fluvoxamine or any component of the formulation; concurrent use with alosetron, pimozide, thioridazine, or tizanidine; use with or within 14 days of MAO inhibitors

Warnings/Precautions [U.S. Boxed Warning]: Antidepressants increase the risk of suicidal thinking and behavior in children, adolescents, and young adults (18-24 years of age) with major depressive disorder (MDD) and other psychiatric disorders; consider risk prior to prescribing. Short-term studies did not show an increased risk in patients >24 years of age and showed a decreased risk in patients ≥65 years. Closely monitor patients for clinical worsening, suicidality, or unusual changes in behavior, particularly during the initial 1-2 months of therapy or during periods of dosage adjustments (increases or decreases); the patient's family or caregiver should be instructed to closely observe the patient and communicate condition with healthcare provider. A medication guide concerning the use of antidepressants should be dispensed with each prescription. **Fluvoxamine is FDA approved for the treatment of OCD in children ≥8 years of age; extended release capsules are not FDA approved for use in children.**

The possibility of a suicide attempt is inherent in major depression and may persist until remission occurs. Use caution in high-risk patients. Worsening depression and severe abrupt suicidality that are not part of the presenting symptoms may require discontinuation or modification of drug therapy. The patient's family or caregiver should be alerted to monitor patients for the emergence of suicidality and associated behaviors (such as agitation, irritability, hostility, impulsivity, and hypomania) and call healthcare provider.

May worsen psychosis in some patients or precipitate a shift to mania or hypomania in patients with bipolar disorder. Patients presenting with depressive symptoms should be screened for bipolar disorder. Monotherapy in patients with bipolar disorder should be avoided. **Fluvoxamine is not FDA approved for the treatment of bipolar depression.**

The potential for severe reaction exits when used with MAO inhibitors, SSRIs/SNRIs, or triptans; serotonin syndrome (hyperthermia, muscular rigidity, mental status changes/agitation, autonomic instability) may occur. Concurrent use with MAO inhibitors is contraindicated. Fluvoxamine has a low potential to impair cognitive or motor performance; caution operating hazardous machinery or driving. Use caution in patients with a previous seizure disorder or condition predisposing to seizures such as brain damage, alcoholism, or concurrent therapy with other drugs which lower the seizure threshold. Fluvoxamine may significantly increase alosetron concentrations; concurrent use **contraindicated.** Potential for QT_c prolongation and arrhythmia with thioridazine and pimozide; concurrent use of fluvoxamine with either of these agents is **contraindicated.** Concomitant use with tizanidine may cause a significant decrease in blood pressure and increase in drowsiness; concurrent use is **contraindicated.** Fluvoxamine levels may be lower in patients who smoke.

May increase the risks associated with electroconvulsive therapy. Use with caution in patients with hepatic dysfunction and in elderly patients. May cause hyponatremia/SIADH (elderly at increased risk); volume depletion (diuretics may increase risk). Use with caution in patients at risk of bleeding or receiving concurrent anticoagulant therapy, although not consistently noted, fluvoxamine may cause impairment in platelet function. May cause or exacerbate sexual dysfunction.

Adverse Reactions Frequency varies by dosage form and indication. Adverse reactions reported as a composite of all indications.

>10%:

Central nervous system: Headache (22% to 35%), insomnia (21% to 35%), somnolence (22% to 27%), dizziness (11% to 15%), nervousness (10% to 12%)

Gastrointestinal: Nausea (34% to 40%), diarrhea (11% to 18%), xerostomia (10% to 14%), anorexia (6% to 14%)

Genitourinary: Ejaculation abnormal (8% to 11%)

Neuromuscular & skeletal: Weakness (14% to 26%)

1% to 10%:

Cardiovascular: Chest pain (3%), palpitation (3%), vasodilation (2% to 3%), hypertension (1% to 2%), edema (≤1%), hypotension (≤1%), syncope (≤1%), tachycardia (≤1%)

Central nervous system: Pain (10%), anxiety (5% to 8%), abnormal dreams (3%), abnormal thinking (3%), agitation (2% to 3%), apathy (≥1% to 3%), chills (2%), CNS stimulation (2%), depression (2%), neurosis (2%), amnesia, malaise, manic reaction, psychotic reaction

Dermatologic: Bruising (4%), acne (2%)

Endocrine & metabolic: Libido decreased (2% to 10%; incidence higher in males), anorgasmia (2% to 5%), sexual function abnormal (2% to 4%), menorrhagia (3%)

Gastrointestinal: Dyspepsia (8% to 10%), constipation (4% to 10%), vomiting (4% to 6%), abdominal pain (5%), flatulence (4%), taste perversion (2% to 3%), tooth disorder (2% to 3%), dysphagia (2%), gingivitis (2%), weight loss (≤1% to 2%), weight gain

Genitourinary: Polyuria (2% to 3%), impotence (2%), urinary tract infection (2%), urinary retention (1%)

Hepatic: Liver function tests abnormal (≥1% to 2%)

Neuromuscular & skeletal: Tremor (5% to 8%), myalgia (5%), paresthesia (3%), hypertonia (2%), twitching (2%), hyper-/hypokinesia, myoclonus

Ocular: Amblyopia (2% to 3%)

Respiratory: Upper respiratory infection (9%), pharyngitis (6%), yawn (2% to 5%), laryngitis (3%), bronchitis (2%), dyspnea (2%), epistaxis (2%), cough increased, sinusitis

Miscellaneous: Diaphoresis (6% to 7%), flu-like syndrome (3%), viral infection (2%)

<1% (Limited to important or life-threatening): Acute renal failure, agranulocytosis, akinesia, allergic reaction, anaphylactic reaction, anemia, angina, angioedema, anuria, aplastic anemia, apnea, asthma, ataxia, AV block, bradycardia, bullous eruption, cardiomyopathy, cerebrovascular accident, cholecystitis, cholelithiasis, colitis, conduction delay, coronary artery disease, diplopia, dyskinesia, dystonia, extrapyramidal syndrome, embolus, GI bleeding, goiter, hallucinations, heart failure, hematemesis, hematuria, Henoch-Schönlein purpura, hepatitis, hemoptysis, hypercholesterolemia, hyper-/hypoglycemia, hypokalemia, hyponatremia, hypothyroidism, ileus, intestinal obstruction, jaundice, leukopenia, leukocytosis, lymphadenopathy, MI, myasthenia,

myopathy, neuralgia, neuroleptic malignant syndrome, neuropathy, pancreatitis, paralysis, pericarditis, porphyria, purpura, retinal detachment, serotonin syndrome, ST segment changes, seizure, Stevens-Johnson syndrome, suicidal tendencies, supraventricular extrasystoles, tardive dyskinesia, thrombocytopenia, toxic epidermal necrolysis, vasculitis, ventricular tachycardia (including torsade de pointes)

Drug Interactions

Metabolism/Transport Effects **Substrate** (major) of CYP1A2, 2D6; **Inhibits** CYP1A2 (strong), 2B6 (weak), 2C9 (weak), 2C19 (strong), 2D6 (weak), 3A4 (weak)

Avoid Concomitant Use

Avoid concomitant use of Fluvoxamine with any of the following: Alosetron; Iobenguane I 123; MAO Inhibitors; Pimozide; Ramelteon; Sibutramine; Thioridazine; TiZANidine

Increased Effect/Toxicity

Fluvoxamine may increase the levels/effects of: Alcohol (Ethyl); Alosetron; Anticoagulants; Antidepressants (Serotonin Reuptake Inhibitor/Antagonist); Antiplatelet Agents; Aspirin; Bendamustine; Benzodiazepines (metabolized by oxidation); BusPIRone; CarBAMazepine; Clozapine; CNS Depressants; CYP1A2 Substrates; CYP2C19 Substrates; Desmopressin; Drotrecogin Alfa; DULoxetine; Haloperidol; Ibritumomab; Lithium; Methadone; Mexiletine; NSAID (COX-2 Inhibitor); NSAID (Nonselective); OLANZapine; Phenytoin; Pimozide; Propranolol; QuiNIDine; Ramelteon; Ropivacaine; Salicylates; Serotonin Modulators; Tacrine; Theophylline Derivatives; Thioridazine; Thrombolytic Agents; TiZANidine; Tositumomab and Iodine I 131 Tositumomab; TraMADol; Tricyclic Antidepressants; Vitamin K Antagonists

The levels/effects of Fluvoxamine may be increased by: Analgesics (Opioid); BusPIRone; Cimetidine; CYP1A2 Inhibitors (Moderate); CYP1A2 Inhibitors (Strong); CYP2D6 Inhibitors (Moderate); CYP2D6 Inhibitors (Strong); Darunavir; Dasatinib; Herbs (Anticoagulant/Antiplatelet Properties); MAO Inhibitors; Omega-3-Acid Ethyl Esters; Pentosan Polysulfate Sodium; Prostacyclin Analogues; Sibutramine; TraMADol; Tryptophan

Decreased Effect

Fluvoxamine may decrease the levels/effects of: Iobenguane I 123

The levels/effects of Fluvoxamine may be decreased by: CarBAMazepine; CYP1A2 Inducers (Strong); Cyproheptadine

Ethanol/Nutrition/Herb Interactions

Ethanol: Avoid ethanol. Patients with depression should avoid/limit intake.

Food: The bioavailability of melatonin has been reported to be increased by fluvoxamine.

Herb/Nutraceutical: Avoid valerian, St John's wort, SAMe, kava kava (may increase risk of serotonin syndrome and/or excessive sedation). Avoid alfalfa, anise, bilberry, bladderwrack, bromelain, cat's claw, celery, chamomile, coleus, cordyceps, dong quai, evening primrose, fenugreek, feverfew, garlic, ginger, ginkgo biloba, ginseng (American), ginseng (Panax), ginseng (Siberian), grape seed, green tea, guggul, horse chestnuts, horseradish, licorice, prickly ash, red clover, reishi, SAMe (S-adenosylmethionine), sweet clover, turmeric, white willow (all have additional antiplatelet activity).

Stability Protect from high humidity and store at controlled room temperature 25°C (77°F).

Mechanism of Action Inhibits CNS neuron serotonin uptake; minimal or no effect on reuptake of norepinephrine or dopamine; does not significantly bind to alpha-adrenergic, histamine or cholinergic receptors

Pharmacodynamics/Kinetics

Onset of action: Depression: The onset of action is within a week; however, individual response varies greatly and full response may not be seen until 8-12 weeks after initiation of treatment.

Absorption: Steady-state plasma concentrations have been noted to be 2-3 times higher in children than those in adolescents; female children demonstrated a significantly higher AUC than males

Distribution: V_d: ~25 L/kg

Protein binding: ~80%, primarily to albumin

Metabolism: Extensively hepatic via oxidative demethylation and deamination

Bioavailability: Immediate release: 53%; not significantly affected by food

Half-life elimination: 15-16 hours; 17-26 hours in the elderly

Time to peak, plasma: 3-8 hours

Excretion: Urine (~85% as metabolites; ~2% as unchanged drug)

Dosage Oral:

Obsessive-compulsive disorder:

Children 8-17 years: Immediate release: Initial: 25 mg once daily at bedtime; may be increased in 25 mg increments at 4- to 7-day intervals, as tolerated, to maximum therapeutic benefit; usual dose range: 50-200 mg/day. **Note:** When total daily dose exceeds 50 mg, the dose should be given in 2 divided doses with larger portion administered at bedtime.

Maximum: Children: 8-11 years: 200 mg/day, adolescents: 300 mg/day; lower doses may be effective in female versus male patients

Adults:

Immediate release: Initial: 50 mg once daily at bedtime; may be increased in 50 mg increments at 4- to 7-day intervals, as tolerated; usual dose range: 100-300 mg/day; maximum dose: 300 mg/day. **Note:** When total daily dose exceeds 100 mg, the dose should be given in 2 divided doses with larger portion administered at bedtime.

Extended release: Initial: 100 mg once daily at bedtime; may be increased in 50 mg increments at intervals of at least 1 week; usual dosage range: 100-300 mg/day; maximum dose: 300 mg/day

Social anxiety disorder: Adults: Extended release: Initial: 100 mg once daily at bedtime; may be increased in 50 mg increments at intervals of at least 1 week; usual dosage range: 100-300 mg/day; maximum dose: 300 mg/day

Elderly: Reduce dose, titrate slowly

Dosage adjustment in hepatic impairment: Reduce dose, titrate slowly

Dietary Considerations May be taken with or without food.

Administration May be administered with or without food. Do not crush, open, or chew extended release capsules.

Monitoring Parameters Mental status for depression, suicidal ideation (especially at the beginning of therapy or when doses are increased or decreased), anxiety, social functioning, mania, panic attacks; akathisia, weight gain or loss, nutritional intake, sleep; liver function assessment prior to beginning drug therapy

Dosage Forms Excipient information presented when available (limited, particularly for generics); consult specific product labeling.

Tablet, as maleate: 25 mg, 50 mg, 100 mg

Capsule, extended release, as maleate:

Luvox® CR: 100 mg, 150 mg [gluten free]

- **Fluzone®** *see* Influenza Virus Vaccine *on page 788*
- **FML®** *see* Fluorometholone *on page 636*
- **FML® Forte** *see* Fluorometholone *on page 636*
- **FML Forte® (Can)** *see* Fluorometholone *on page 636*

Folic Acid (FOE lik AS id)

U.S. Brand Names Folacin-800 [OTC]

Canadian Brand Names Apo-Folic®

Index Terms Folacin; Folate; Pteroylglutamic Acid

Pharmacologic Category Vitamin, Water Soluble

Use Treatment of megaloblastic and macrocytic anemias due to folate deficiency; dietary supplement to prevent neural tube defects

Unlabeled/Investigational Use Adjunctive cofactor therapy in methanol toxicity (alternative to leucovorin)

Pregnancy Risk Factor A

Pregnancy Considerations Folic acid requirements are increased during pregnancy; a deficiency may result in fetal harm.

Lactation Enters breast milk/compatible

Medication Safety Issues

Sound-alike/look-alike issues:

Folic acid may be confused with folinic acid

Contraindications Hypersensitivity to folic acid or any component of the formulation

Warnings/Precautions Not appropriate for monotherapy with pernicious, aplastic, or normocytic anemias when anemia is present with vitamin B_{12} deficiency. Doses >0.1 mg/day may obscure pernicious anemia with continuing irreversible nerve damage progression. Resistance to treatment may occur with depressed hematopoiesis, alcoholism, and deficiencies of other vitamins. Injection contains benzyl alcohol (1.5%) as preservative (use care in administration to neonates).

Adverse Reactions Frequency not defined.

Allergic reaction, bronchospasm, flushing (slight), malaise (general), pruritus, rash

Drug Interactions

Avoid Concomitant Use

Avoid concomitant use of Folic Acid with any of the following: Raltitrexed

Increased Effect/Toxicity There are no known significant interactions involving an increase in effect.

Decreased Effect

Folic Acid may decrease the levels/effects of: PHENObarbital; Phenytoin; Primidone; Raltitrexed

Stability Do not use with oxidizing and reducing agents or heavy metal ions.

Mechanism of Action Folic acid is necessary for formation of a number of coenzymes in many metabolic systems, particularly for purine and pyrimidine synthesis; required for nucleoprotein synthesis and maintenance in erythropoiesis; stimulates WBC and platelet production in folate deficiency anemia. Folic acid enhances the elimination of formic acid, the toxic metabolite of methanol (unlabeled use).

Pharmacodynamics/Kinetics

Onset of action: Peak effect: Oral: 0.5-1 hour

Absorption: Proximal part of small intestine

Dosage

Oral, I.M., I.V., SubQ: Anemia:

Infants: 0.1 mg/day

Children <4 years: Up to 0.3 mg/day

Children >4 years and Adults: 0.4 mg/day

Pregnant and lactating women: 0.8 mg/day

Oral:

RDA: Expressed as dietary folate equivalents:

Children:

1-3 years: 150 mcg/day

4-8 years: 200 mcg/day

9-13 years: 300 mcg/day

Children ≥14 years and Adults: 400 mcg/day

Elderly: Vitamin B_{12} deficiency must be ruled out before initiating folate therapy due to frequency of combined nutritional deficiencies: RDA requirements (1999): 400 mcg/day (0.4 mg) minimum

Prevention of neural tube defects:

Females of childbearing potential: 400 mcg/day

Females at high risk or with family history of neural tube defects: 4 mg/day

Dietary Considerations As of January 1998, the FDA has required manufacturers of enriched flour, bread, corn meal, pasta, rice, and other grain products to add folic acid to their products. The intent is to help decrease the risk of neural tube defects by increasing folic acid intake. Other foods which contain folic acid include dark green leafy vegetables, citrus fruits and juices, and lentils.

Administration Oral preferred, but may also be administered by deep I.M., SubQ, or I.V. injection.

Reference Range Therapeutic: 0.005-0.015 mcg/mL

Test Interactions Falsely low serum concentrations may occur with the *Lactobacillus casei* assay method in patients on anti-infectives (eg, tetracycline)

Additional Information The RDA for folic acid is presented as dietary folate equivalents (DFE). DFE adjusts for the difference in bioavailability of folic acid from food as compared to dietary supplements.

Dosage Forms Excipient information presented when available (limited, particularly for generics); consult specific product labeling.

Injection, solution, as sodium folate: 5 mg/mL (10 mL) [contains benzyl alcohol, edetate disodium]

Tablet: 0.4 mg, 0.8 mg, 1 mg

Folacin-800: 0.8 mg

Extemporaneous Preparations A 1 mg/mL folic acid solution may be prepared by crushing fifty 1 mg tablets. Dissolve in a small amount of distilled water, then add sufficient distilled water to make a final volume of 50 mL. Adjust the pH to 8 with sodium hydroxide. It is stable for 42 days at room temperature.

Nahata MC and Hipple TF, *Pediatric Drug Formulations*, Harvey Whitney Books Company, 1992.

Folic Acid, Cyanocobalamin, and Pyridoxine

(FOE lik AS id, sye an oh koe BAL a min, & peer i DOKS een)

U.S. Brand Names AllanFol RX [DSC]; ComBgen™; Folamin™; Folbee; Folgard® RX; Folgard® [OTC]; Foltx®; Tricardio B

Index Terms Cyanocobalamin, Folic Acid, and Pyridoxine; Folacin, Vitamin B_{12}, and Vitamin B_6; Pyridoxine, Folic Acid, and Cyanocobalamin

Pharmacologic Category Vitamin

Use Nutritional supplement in end-stage renal failure, dialysis, hyperhomocysteinemia, homocystinuria, malabsorption syndromes, dietary deficiencies

Dosage Oral: Adults: One tablet daily

Additional Information Complete prescribing information for this medication should be consulted for additional detail.

Dosage Forms Excipient information presented when available (limited, particularly for generics); consult specific product labeling. [DSC] = Discontinued product

Tablet: Folic acid 0.8 mg, cyanocobalamin 1000 mcg, and pyridoxine hydrochloride 50 mg

AllanFol RX: Folic acid 2.2 mg, cyanocobalamin 1000 mcg, and pyridoxine hydrochloride 25 mg [DSC]

ComBgen™: Folic acid 2.2 mg, cyanocobalamin 500 mcg, and pyridoxine hydrochloride 25 mg

Folamin™: Folic acid 2.5 mg, cyanocobalamin 2000 mcg, and pyridoxine hydrochloride 25 mg

Folbee: Folic acid 2.5 mg, cyanocobalamin 1000 mcg, and pyridoxine hydrochloride 25 mg [dye free, lactose free, and sugar free]

Folgard®: Folic acid 0.8 mg, cyanocobalamin 115 mcg, and pyridoxine hydrochloride 10 mg

Folgard® RX: Folic acid 2.2 mg, cyanocobalamin 1000 mcg, and pyridoxine hydrochloride 25 mg

Foltx®: Folic acid 2.5 mg, cyanocobalamin 2000 mcg, and pyridoxine hydrochloride 25 mg

Tricardio B: Folic acid 0.4 mg, cyanocobalamin 250 mcg, and pyridoxine hydrochloride 25 mg

◆ **Folinic Acid (error prone synonym)** *see* Leucovorin Calcium *on page 866*

◆ **Follicle-Stimulating Hormone, Human** *see* Urofollitropin *on page 1531*

◆ **Follicle Stimulating Hormone, Recombinant** *see* Follitropin Alfa *on page 656*

◆ **Follicle Stimulating Hormone, Recombinant** *see* Follitropin Beta *on page 658*

◆ **Follistim® AQ** *see* Follitropin Beta *on page 658*

◆ **Follistim® AQ Cartridge** *see* Follitropin Beta *on page 658*

Follitropin Alfa (foe li TRO pin AL fa)

U.S. Brand Names Gonal-f® ; Gonal-f® RFF

Canadian Brand Names Gonal-f® ; Gonal-f® Pen

Index Terms Follicle Stimulating Hormone, Recombinant; FSH; rFSH-alpha; rhFSH-alpha

Pharmacologic Category Gonadotropin; Ovulation Stimulator

Use

Gonal-f®: Ovulation induction in patients in whom the cause of infertility is functional and not caused by primary ovarian failure; development of multiple follicles with Assisted Reproductive Technology (ART); spermatogenesis induction

Gonal-f® RFF: Ovulation induction in patients in whom the cause of infertility is functional and not caused by primary ovarian failure; development of multiple follicles with ART

Pregnancy Risk Factor X

Pregnancy Considerations Ectopic pregnancy, congenital abnormalities, spontaneous abortion, and multiple births have been reported. The incidence of congenital abnormality may be slightly higher after ART than with spontaneous conception; higher incidence may be related to parenteral characteristics (maternal age, sperm characteristics).

Lactation Excretion in breast milk unknown/not recommended

Contraindications Hypersensitivity to follitropins or any component of the formulation; high levels of FSH indicating primary gonadal failure (ovarian or testicular); uncontrolled thyroid or adrenal dysfunction; tumor of the ovary, breast, uterus, hypothalamus, testis, or pituitary gland; abnormal vaginal bleeding of undetermined origin; ovarian cysts or enlargement not due to polycystic ovary syndrome; pregnancy

Warnings/Precautions These medications should only be used by physicians who are thoroughly familiar with infertility problems and their management. To minimize risks, use only at the lowest effective dose. Monitor ovarian response with serum estradiol and vaginal ultrasound on a regular basis.

Ovarian enlargement, which may be accompanied by abdominal distention or abdominal pain, occurs in ~20% of those treated with urofollitropin and hCG, and generally regresses without treatment within 2-3 weeks. If ovaries are abnormally enlarged on the last day of treatment, withhold hCG to reduce the risk of ovarian hyperstimulation syndrome (OHSS). OHSS is reported in about 7% of patients; it is characterized by severe ovarian enlargement, abdominal pain/distention, nausea, vomiting, diarrhea, dyspnea, and oliguria, and may be accompanied by ascites, pleural effusion, hypovolemia, electrolyte imbalance, hemoperitoneum, and thromboembolic events. If hyperstimulation occurs, stop treatment and hospitalize patient. This syndrome develops rapidly within 24 hours to several days and generally occurs during the 7-10 days immediately following treatment. Hemoconcentration associated with fluid loss into the abdominal cavity has occurred and should be assessed by fluid intake and output, weight, hematocrit, serum and urinary electrolytes, urine specific gravity, BUN and creatinine, and abdominal girth. Determinations should be performed daily or more often if the need arises. Treatment is primarily symptomatic and consists of bedrest, fluid and electrolyte replacement, and analgesics. The ascitic, pleural, and pericardial fluids should not be removed unless needed to relieve symptoms of cardiopulmonary distress.

Serious pulmonary conditions (atelectasis, acute respiratory distress syndrome, and exacerbation of asthma) have been reported. Thromboembolic events, both in association with and separate from ovarian hyperstimulation syndrome, have been reported.

Multiple births may result from the use of these medications; advise patient of the potential risk of multiple births before starting the treatment. Safety and efficacy have not been established in children.

Adverse Reactions Percentage may vary by indication, product formulation

>10%:

Central nervous system: Headache

Endocrine & metabolic: Ovarian cyst

Gastrointestinal: Abdomen enlarged, abdominal pain, nausea

Miscellaneous: Upper respiratory infection

1% to 10%:

Central nervous system: Dizziness, emotional lability, fever, malaise, migraine, pain

Dermatologic: Acne

Endocrine & metabolic: Breast pain, cervix lesion, hot flashes, intermenstrual bleeding, menstrual disorder, ovarian disorder, ovarian hyperstimulation

Gastrointestinal: Constipation, diarrhea, dyspepsia, flatulence, pelvic pain, stomatitis (ulcerative), toothache, vomiting, weight gain

Genitourinary: Cystitis, leukorrhea, micturition frequency, urinary tract infection, uterine hemorrhage, vaginal hemorrhage

Local: Injection site bruising, edema, inflammation, pain, reaction

Neuromuscular & skeletal: Back pain

Respiratory: Cough, flu-like symptoms, pharyngitis, rhinitis, sinusitis

Miscellaneous: Infection, moniliasis

Postmarketing, case reports, or events reported with gonadotropins: Adnexal torsion, anaphylactoid reactions, hemoperitoneum, hypersensitivity reactions, ovarian enlargement, pulmonary complications, vascular complications

Drug Interactions

Avoid Concomitant Use There are no known interactions where it is recommended to avoid concomitant use.

Increased Effect/Toxicity There are no known significant interactions involving an increase in effect.

Decreased Effect There are no known significant interactions involving a decrease in effect.

Stability

Gonal-f®: Store powder refrigerated or at room temperature of 2°C to 25°C (36°F to 77°F). Protect from light. Dissolve the contents of vial by slowly injecting provided diluent; do not shake. If bubbles appear, allow to settle prior to use. Final concentration: 600 int. units/mL. Following reconstitution, multidose vials may be stored under refrigeration or at room temperature for up to 28 days. Protect from light.

Gonal-f® RFF:

Powder: Store at room temperature or under refrigeration of 2°C to 25°C (36°F to 77°F). Protect from light. Dissolve contents of one or more vials using diluent provided in prefilled syringe. (Total concentration should not exceed 450 int. units/mL.) Slowly inject diluent into vial, and gently rotate vial until powder is dissolved; do not shake vial. If bubbles appear, allow to settle prior to use. Use immediately after reconstitution.

Solution: Prior to dispensing, store under refrigeration at 2°C to 8°C (36°F to 46°F). Upon dispensing, patient may store under refrigeration until product expiration date or at room temperature of 20°C to 25°C (68°F to 77°F) for up to 3 months. Do not freeze. Protect from light. After first use, discard unused portion after 28 days.

Mechanism of Action Follitropin alfa is a human FSH preparation of recombinant DNA origin. Follitropins stimulate ovarian follicular growth in women who do not have primary ovarian failure, and stimulate spermatogenesis in men with hypogonadotrophic hypogonadism. FSH is required for normal follicular growth, maturation, gonadal steroid production, and spermatogenesis.

Pharmacodynamics/Kinetics

Onset of action: Peak effect:

Spermatogenesis, median: 6.8-12.4 months (range 2.7-15.7 months)

Follicle development: Within cycle

Absorption: I.M., SubQ: Absorption rate is slower than the elimination rate

Distribution: Mean V_d: 10 L with *in vitro* fertilization/embryo transfer patients

Bioavailability: ~66% to 76% in healthy female volunteers

Half-life elimination:

I.M.: 50 hours in healthy female volunteers

SubQ: 24 hours in healthy female volunteers; 32 hours with *in vitro* fertilization/embryo transfer patients; 32-41 hours in healthy male volunteers

Time to peak: In healthy volunteers:

Females: SubQ: 8-16 hours; I.M.: 25 hours

Males: SubQ: 11-20 hours

Excretion: Clearance: I.V.: 0.6 L/hour in healthy female volunteers

Dosage Adults: **Note:** Dose should be individualized. Use the lowest dose consistent with the expectation of good results. Over the course of treatment, doses may vary depending on individual patient response.

Gonal-f®, Gonal-f® RFF: Females:

Ovulation induction: SubQ: Initial: 75 int. units/day; incremental dose adjustments of up to 37.5 int. units may be considered after 14 days; further dose increases of the same magnitude can be made, if necessary, every 7 days (maximum dose: 300 int. units/day). If response to follitropin is appropriate, hCG is given 1 day following the last dose. Withhold hCG if serum estradiol is >2000 pg/mL, if the ovaries are abnormally enlarged, or if abdominal pain occurs. In general, therapy should not exceed 35 days.

ART: SubQ: Initiate therapy with follitropin alfa in the early follicular phase (cycle day 2 or day 3) at a dose of 150 int. units/day, until sufficient follicular development is attained. In most cases, therapy should not exceed 10 days. In patients ≥35 years whose endogenous gonadotropin levels are suppressed, initiate follitropin alfa at a dose of 225 int. units/day. Continue treatment until adequate follicular development is indicated as determined by ultrasound in combination with measurement of serum estradiol levels. Consider adjustments to dose after 5 days based on the patient's response; adjust subsequent dosage every 3-5 days by ≤75-150 int. units additionally at each adjustment. Doses >450 int. units/day are not recommended. Once adequate follicular development is evident, administer hCG to induce final follicular maturation in preparation for oocyte. Withhold hCG if the ovaries are abnormally enlarged.

Gonal-f®: Males: Spermatogenesis induction: SubQ: Therapy should begin with hCG pretreatment until serum testosterone is in normal range, then 150 int. units 3 times/week with hCG 3 times/week; continue with lowest dose needed to induce spermatogenesis (maximum dose: 300 int. units 3 times/week); may be given for up to 18 months

Administration Gonal-f®, Gonal-f® RFF: Administer SubQ. Contents of multidose vials should be administered using the calibrated syringes provided by the manufacturer. Do not shake solution; allow any bubbles to settle prior to administration.

Monitoring Parameters Monitor sufficient follicular maturation. This may be directly estimated by sonographic visualization of the ovaries and endometrial lining or measuring serum estradiol levels. The combination of both ultrasonography and measurement of estradiol levels is useful for monitoring for the growth and development of follicles and timing hCG administration.

The clinical evaluation of estrogenic activity (changes in vaginal cytology and changes in appearance and volume of cervical mucus) provides an indirect estimate of the estrogenic effect upon the target organs and, therefore, it should only be used adjunctively with more direct estimates of follicular development (ultrasonography and serum estradiol determinations).

The clinical confirmation of ovulation is obtained by direct and indirect indices of progesterone production. The indices most generally used are: rise in basal body temperature, increase in serum progesterone, and menstruation following the shift in basal body temperature.

Monitor for signs and symptoms of OHSS for at least 2 weeks following hCG administration.

Spermatogenesis: Monitor serum testosterone levels, sperm count

Additional Information The currently available recombinant follitropin products are structurally identical to native follicle-stimulating hormone. The "alpha" and "beta" nomenclature refers to their differences in purification and order of marketing. Follitropin alpha was marketed first, followed by follitropin beta. RFF for the Gonal-f® product signifies "revised formula female."

Dosage Forms Excipient information presented when available (limited, particularly for generics); consult specific product labeling.

Injection, powder for reconstitution [rDNA origin]:
Gonal-f®: 450 int. units [contains sucrose 30 mg; packaged with diluent and calibrated syringes; diluent contains benzyl alcohol]
Gonal-f® RFF: 75 int. units [contains sucrose 30 mg; packaged with diluent in prefilled syringe]
Injection, solution [rDNA origin]:
Gonal-f® RFF: 300 int. units/0.5 mL (0.5 mL) [contains sucrose 60 mg/mL]; 450 int. units/0.75 mL (0.75 mL) [contains sucrose 60 mg/mL]; 900 int. units/1.5 mL (1.5 mL) [contains sucrose 60 mg/mL]

Follitropin Beta (foe li TRO pin BAY ta)

U.S. Brand Names Follistim® AQ; Follistim® AQ Cartridge

Canadian Brand Names Puregon®

Index Terms Follicle Stimulating Hormone, Recombinant; FSH; rFSH-beta; rhFSH-beta

Pharmacologic Category Gonadotropin; Ovulation Stimulator

Use Ovulation induction in patients in whom the cause of infertility is functional and not caused by primary ovarian failure; development of multiple follicles with Assisted Reproductive Technology (ART)

Pregnancy Risk Factor X

Pregnancy Considerations Ectopic pregnancy, congenital abnormalities, and multiple births have been reported. The incidence of congenital abnormality may be slightly higher after ART than with spontaneous conception; higher incidence may be related to parenteral characteristics (maternal age, sperm characteristics).

Lactation Excretion in breast milk unknown/not recommended

Contraindications Hypersensitivity to follitropins or any component of the formulation; high levels of FSH indicating primary ovarian failure; uncontrolled thyroid or adrenal dysfunction; tumor of the ovary, breast, uterus, hypothalamus, or pituitary gland; abnormal vaginal bleeding of undetermined origin; ovarian cysts or enlargement not due to polycystic ovary syndrome; pregnancy

Warnings/Precautions These medications should only be used by physicians who are thoroughly familiar with infertility problems and their management. To minimize risks, use only at the lowest effective dose. Monitor ovarian response with serum estradiol and vaginal ultrasound on a regular basis.

Ovarian enlargement, which may be accompanied by abdominal distention or abdominal pain, occurs in ~20% of those treated with urofollitropin and hCG, and generally regresses without treatment within 2-3 weeks. If ovaries are abnormally enlarged on the last day of treatment, withhold hCG to reduce the risk of ovarian hyperstimulation syndrome (OHSS). OHSS is characterized by severe ovarian enlargement, abdominal pain/distention, nausea, vomiting, diarrhea, dyspnea, and oliguria, and may be accompanied by ascites, pleural effusion, hypovolemia, electrolyte imbalance, hemoperitoneum, and thromboembolic events. If hyperstimulation occurs, stop treatment and hospitalize patient. This syndrome develops rapidly within 24 hours to several days and generally occurs during the 7-10 days immediately following treatment. Hemoconcentration associated with fluid loss into the abdominal cavity has occurred and should be assessed by fluid intake and output, weight, hematocrit, serum and urinary electrolytes, urine specific gravity, BUN and creatinine, and abdominal girth. Determinations should be performed daily or more often if the need arises. Treatment is primarily symptomatic and consists of bedrest, fluid and electrolyte replacement, and analgesics. The ascitic, pleural, and pericardial fluids should not be removed unless needed to relieve symptoms of cardiopulmonary distress.

Serious pulmonary conditions (atelectasis, acute respiratory distress syndrome, and exacerbation of asthma) have been reported. Thromboembolic events, both in association with and separate from ovarian hyperstimulation syndrome, have been reported.

Multiple births may result from the use of these medications; advise patient of the potential risk of multiple births before starting the treatment. May contain trace amounts of neomycin or streptomycin. Safety and efficacy have not been established in children and the elderly.

Adverse Reactions Percentage may vary by indication, product formulation

>10%:
- Endocrine & metabolic: Breast pain
- Gastrointestinal: Abdominal pain, flatulence, nausea
- Miscellaneous: Miscarriage

1% to 10%:
- Central nervous system: Headache
- Endocrine & metabolic: Ovarian hyperstimulation syndrome, ovarian pain
- Gastrointestinal: Abdomen enlarged, constipation
- Local: Injection site reaction
- Neuromuscular & skeletal: Back pain
- Respiratory: Sinusitis, upper respiratory tract infection

Postmarketing, case reports, or events reported with gonadotropins: Acute respiratory distress syndrome, adnexal torsion, arterial occlusions, atelectasis, breast tenderness, chills, dizziness, dry skin, dyspnea, erythema, febrile reaction, fever, flu-like syndrome, hair loss, cerebral vascular occlusion, hemoperitoneum, hives, joint pain, malaise, musculoskeletal ache, ovarian neoplasm, pulmonary embolism, rash, tachycardia, tachypnea

Drug Interactions

Avoid Concomitant Use There are no known interactions where it is recommended to avoid concomitant use.

Increased Effect/Toxicity There are no known significant interactions involving an increase in effect.

Decreased Effect There are no known significant interactions involving a decrease in effect.

Stability Prior to dispensing, store refrigerated at 2°C to 8°C (36°F to 46°F). After dispensed, may be stored under refrigeration or ≤25°C (77°F) for up to 3 months. Once cartridge is pierced, must be stored in refrigerator and used within 28 days. Do not freeze. Protect from light.

Mechanism of Action Follitropin beta is a human FSH preparation of recombinant DNA origin. Follitropins stimulate ovarian follicular growth in women who do not have primary ovarian failure. FSH is required for normal follicular growth, maturation, gonadal steroid production, and spermatogenesis.

Pharmacodynamics/Kinetics

Onset of action: Peak effect: Follicle development: Within cycle

Absorption: I.M.: 76%; SubQ: 78%

Distribution: 8 L

Half-life elimination: I.M.: 44 hours (single dose), 27-30 hours (multiple doses); SubQ: 33 hours (single dose)

Time to peak: SubQ: 13 hours

Dosage Adults: Females: **Note:** Dose should be individualized. Use the lowest dose consistent with the expectation of good results. Over the course of treatment, doses may vary depending on individual patient response.

Ovulation induction:

Follistim® AQ: I.M., SubQ: Stepwise approach: Initiate therapy with 75 int. units/day for up to 14 days. Increase by 37.5 int. units at weekly intervals until follicular growth or serum estradiol levels indicate an adequate response. The maximum (individualized) daily dose that has been safely used for ovulation induction in patients during clinical trials is 300 int. units. If response to follitropin is appropriate, hCG is given 1 day following the last dose. Withhold hCG if the ovaries are abnormally enlarged, or if abdominal pain occurs.

Follistim® AQ Cartridge: SubQ: Stepwise approach: Initiate therapy with 75 int. units/day for up to 7 days. Increase by 25 or 50 int. units at weekly intervals until follicular growth or serum estradiol levels indicate an adequate response. The maximum (individualized) daily dose that has been safely used for ovulation induction in patients during clinical trials is 175 int. units. If response to follitropin is appropriate, hCG is given 1 day following the last dose. Withhold hCG if the ovaries are abnormally enlarged, or if abdominal pain occurs. See **"Note"** for dosage adjustment for this product.

ART:

Follistim® AQ: I.M., SubQ: A starting dose of 150-225 int. units is recommended for at least the first 4 days of treatment. The dose may be adjusted for the individual patient based upon their ovarian response. The usual maintenance dose was 75-300 int. units for 6-12 days; 375-600 int. units in patients who were poor responders. The maximum daily dose used in clinical studies is 600 int. units. When a sufficient number of follicles of adequate size are present, the final maturation of the follicles is induced by administering hCG. Oocyte retrieval is performed 34-36 hours later. Withhold hCG in cases where the ovaries are abnormally enlarged on the last day of follitropin beta therapy.

Follistim® AQ Cartridge: SubQ: A starting dose of 150-225 int. units is recommended for at least the first 5 days of treatment. The dose may be adjusted for the individual patient based upon their ovarian response. The maximum daily dose used in clinical studies is 450 int. units. When a sufficient number of follicles of adequate size are present, the final maturation of the follicles is induced by administering hCG. Oocyte retrieval is performed 34-36 hours later. Withhold hCG in cases where the ovaries are abnormally enlarged on the last day of follitropin beta therapy. See **"Note"** for dosage adjustment for this product.

Note: Dose adjustment for Follistim® AQ Cartridge: When administered using the Follistim Pen®, the Follistim® AQ Cartridge delivers 18% more follitropin beta when compared to dissolved lyophilized follitropin beta administered by a conventional syringe. If the above starting doses were previously used when administering a recombinant lyophilized gonadotropin product via a conventional syringe, lower starting and maintenance doses should be considered when switching to Follistim® AQ Cartridge. The following dose conversion may be used:

Follistim® AQ Dosing Conversion

Dose Administered Using Powder for Solution/Conventional Syringe	Follistim® AQ Dose Administered Using Follistim Pen®
75 int. units	50 int. units
150 int. units	125 int. units
225 int. units	175 int. units
300 int. units	250 int. units
375 int. units	300 int. units
450 int. units	375 int. units

Administration

Follistim® AQ: Administered by I.M. or SubQ injection

Follistim® AQ Cartridge: Follistim® AQ cartridge may be administered only by SubQ injection using the Follistim Pen® which can be set to deliver the appropriate dose.

Monitoring Parameters Monitor sufficient follicular maturation. This may be directly estimated by sonographic visualization of the ovaries and endometrial lining or measuring serum estradiol levels. The combination of both ultrasonography and measurement of estradiol levels is useful for monitoring for the growth and development of follicles and timing hCG administration.

The clinical evaluation of estrogenic activity (changes in vaginal cytology and changes in appearance and volume of cervical mucus) provides an indirect estimate of the estrogenic effect upon the target organs and, therefore, it should only be used adjunctively with more direct estimates of follicular development (ultrasonography and serum estradiol determinations).

The clinical confirmation of ovulation is obtained by direct and indirect indices of progesterone production. The indices most generally used are: rise in basal body temperature, increase in serum progesterone, and menstruation following the shift in basal body temperature.

Monitor for signs and symptoms of OHSS for at least 2 weeks following hCG administration.

Additional Information The currently available recombinant follitropin products are structurally identical to native follicle-stimulating hormone. The "alpha" and "beta" nomenclature refers to their differences in purification and order of marketing. Follitropin alpha was marketed first, followed by follitropin beta.

Dosage Forms Excipient information presented when available (limited, particularly for generics); consult specific product labeling.

Injection, solution [rDNA origin]:

Follistim® AQ Cartridge:

175 int. units/0.21 mL (0.21 mL) [delivers 150 int. units; contains benzyl alcohol and sucrose; may contain trace amounts of neomycin or streptomycin]

350 int. units/0.42 mL (0.42 mL) [delivers 300 int. units; contains benzyl alcohol and sucrose; may contain trace amounts of neomycin or streptomycin]

650 int. units/0.78 mL (0.78 mL) [delivers 600 int. units; contains benzyl alcohol and sucrose; may contain trace amounts of neomycin or streptomycin]

975 int. units/1.17 mL (1.17 mL) [delivers 900 int. units; contains benzyl alcohol and sucrose; may contain trace amounts of neomycin or streptomycin]

Injection, solution [rDNA origin; single-dose]:

Follistim® AQ:

75 int. units/0.5 mL (0.5mL) [contains sucrose; may contain trace amounts of neomycin or streptomycin]

150 int. units/0.5 mL (0.5 mL) [contains sucrose; may contain trace amounts of neomycin or streptomycin]

◆ **Foltx®** *see* Folic Acid, Cyanocobalamin, and Pyridoxine *on page 655*

Fomepizole (foe ME pi zole)

U.S. Brand Names Antizol®

Index Terms 4-Methylpyrazole; 4-MP

Pharmacologic Category Antidote

Use Treatment of methanol or ethylene glycol poisoning alone or in combination with hemodialysis

Unlabeled/Investigational Use Treatment of propylene glycol toxicity

Pregnancy Risk Factor C

Pregnancy Considerations Reproduction studies have not been conducted; use in pregnant women only if the benefits clearly outweigh the risks.

Lactation Excretion in breast milk unknown/not recommended

Contraindications Hypersensitivity to fomepizole, other pyrazoles, or any component of the formulation

Warnings/Precautions Should not be given undiluted or by bolus injection. Fomepizole is metabolized in the liver and excreted in the urine; use caution with hepatic or renal impairment. Hemodialysis should be used in patients with renal failure, significant or worsening metabolic acidosis, or ethylene glycol/methanol levels ≥50 mg/dL. Safety and efficacy in pediatric patients have not been established.

Adverse Reactions

>10%:

Central nervous system: Headache (14%)

Gastrointestinal: Nausea (11%)

1% to 10% (≤3% unless otherwise noted):

Cardiovascular: Bradycardia, facial flush, hypotension, shock, tachycardia

Central nervous system: Dizziness (6%), drowsiness increased (6%), agitation, anxiety, lightheadedness, seizure, vertigo

Dermatologic: Rash

Endocrine & metabolic: Liver function tests increased

Gastrointestinal: Bad/metallic taste (6%), abdominal pain, appetite decreased, diarrhea, heartburn, vomiting

Hematologic: Anemia, disseminated intravascular coagulation (DIC), eosinophilia, lymphangitis

Local: Application site reaction, injection site inflammation, pain during injection, phlebitis

Neuromuscular & skeletal: Backache

Ocular: Nystagmus, transient blurred vision, visual disturbances

Renal: Anuria

Respiratory: Abnormal smell, hiccups, pharyngitis

Miscellaneous: Multiorgan failure, speech disturbances

<1% (Limited to important or life-threatening): Mild allergic reactions (mild rash, eosinophilia)

Drug Interactions

Avoid Concomitant Use There are no known interactions where it is recommended to avoid concomitant use.

Increased Effect/Toxicity There are no known significant interactions involving an increase in effect.

Decreased Effect There are no known significant interactions involving a decrease in effect.

Ethanol/Nutrition/Herb Interactions Ethanol: Ethanol decreases the rate of fomepizole elimination by ~50%; conversely, fomepizole decreases the rate of elimination of ethanol by ~40%.

Stability Prior to administration, dilute in at least 100 mL 0.9% sodium chloride or dextrose 5% water for injection; diluted solution is stable for at least 24 hours when stored refrigerated or at room temperature. Although, it is chemically and physically stable when diluted as recommended, sterile precautions should be observed because diluents generally do not contain preservatives.

After dilution, do not use beyond 24 hours. Fomepizole solidifies at temperatures <25°C (77°F). If the fomepizole solution has become solid in the vial, the solution should carefully be warmed by running the vial under warm water or by holding in the hand. Solidification does not affect the efficacy, safety, or stability of the drug.

Mechanism of Action Fomepizole competitively inhibits alcohol dehydrogenase, an enzyme which catalyzes the metabolism of ethanol, ethylene glycol, and methanol to their toxic metabolites. Ethylene glycol is metabolized to glycoaldehyde, then oxidized to glycolate, glyoxylate, and oxalate. Glycolate and oxalate are responsible for metabolic acidosis and renal damage. Methanol is metabolized to formaldehyde, then oxidized to formic acid. Formic acid is responsible for metabolic acidosis and visual disturbances.

Pharmacodynamics/Kinetics

Onset of effect: Peak effect: Maximum: 1.5-2 hours

Absorption: Oral: Readily absorbed

Distribution: V_d: 0.6-1.02 L/kg; rapidly into total body water

Protein binding: Negligible

Metabolism: Hepatic to 4-carboxypyrazole (80% to 85% of dose), 4-hydroxymethylpyrazole, and their N-glucuronide conjugates; following multiple doses, induces its own metabolism via CYP oxidases after 30-40 hours

Half-life elimination: Has not been calculated; varies with dose

Excretion: Urine (1% to 3.5% as unchanged drug and metabolites)

Dosage Note: Fomepizole therapy should begin immediately upon suspicion of ethylene glycol or methanol ingestion.

Adults: Ethylene glycol and methanol toxicity: I.V.: A loading dose of 15 mg/kg should be administered, followed by doses of 10 mg/kg every 12 hours for 4 doses, then 15 mg/kg every 12 hours thereafter until ethylene glycol levels have been reduced <20 mg/dL and patient is asymptomatic with normal pH

Dosage adjustment in renal impairment: I.V.: The manufacturer provides the following dosage recommendations:

Dose at the beginning of hemodialysis:

If <6 hours since last fomepizole dose: Do not administer dose

If ≥6 hours since last fomepizole dose: Administer next scheduled dose

Dosing during hemodialysis: Dose every 4 hours

Dosing at the time hemodialysis is complete, based on time between last dose and the end of hemodialysis:

<1 hour: Do not administer dose at the end of hemodialysis

1-3 hours: Administer 1/2 of next scheduled dose

>3 hours: Administer next scheduled dose

Maintenance dose when off hemodialysis: Give next scheduled dose 12 hours from last dose administered.

Alternatively, a loading dose of 10-20 mg/kg followed by 1-1.5 mg/kg/hour continuous infusion during hemodialysis has been described in case reports (Jobard, 1996).

Dosage adjustment in hepatic impairment: Fomepizole is metabolized in the liver; specific dosage adjustments have not been determined in patients with hepatic impairment

Administration The appropriate dose of fomepizole should be drawn from the vial with a syringe and injected into at least 100 mL of sterile 0.9% sodium chloride injection or dextrose 5% injection. All doses should be administered as a slow intravenous infusion (IVPB) over 30 minutes.

Monitoring Parameters Fomepizole plasma levels should be monitored; response to fomepizole; monitor plasma/urinary ethylene glycol or methanol levels, urinary oxalate (ethylene glycol), plasma/urinary osmolality, renal/hepatic function, serum electrolytes, arterial blood gases; anion and osmolar gaps, resolution of clinical signs and symptoms of ethylene glycol or methanol intoxication

Reference Range The manufacturer recommends concentrations 100-300 µmol/L (8.2-24.6 mg/L) to achieve enzyme inhibition of alcohol dehydrogenase; according to practice guidelines, serum fomepizole concentrations of ≥0.8 mg/L provide constant inhibition of alcohol dehydrogenase

Additional Information Alternate therapies, including ethanol and hemodialysis, are difficult to use in children. Fomepizole's affinity for alcohol dehydrogenase is 8000 times greater than ethanol.

Dosage Forms Excipient information presented when available (limited, particularly for generics); consult specific product labeling.

Injection, solution [preservative free]: 1 g/mL (1.5 mL)

Antizol®: 1 g/mL (1.5 mL)

Fondaparinux (fon da PARE i nuks)

U.S. Brand Names Arixtra®

Canadian Brand Names Arixtra®

Index Terms Fondaparinux Sodium

Pharmacologic Category Factor Xa Inhibitor

Additional Appendix Information

Anticoagulants, Injectable *on page 1636*

Use Prophylaxis of deep vein thrombosis (DVT) in patients undergoing surgery for hip replacement, knee replacement, hip fracture (including extended prophylaxis following hip fracture surgery), or abdominal surgery (in patients at risk for thromboembolic complications); treatment of acute pulmonary embolism (PE); treatment of acute DVT without PE

Note: Additional Canadian approvals (not approved in U.S.): Unstable angina or non-ST segment elevation myocardial infarction (UA/NSTEMI) for the prevention of death and subsequent MI; ST segment elevation MI (STEMI) for the prevention of death and myocardial reinfarction

Unlabeled/Investigational Use Prophylaxis of DVT in patients with a history of heparin-induced thrombocytopenia (HIT)

Pregnancy Risk Factor B

Pregnancy Considerations Reproductive animal studies have not shown fetal harm. Based on case reports, small amounts of fondaparinux have been detected in the umbilical cord following multiple doses during pregnancy. There are no adequate and well-controlled studies in pregnant women; use only if clearly needed.

Lactation Excretion in breast milk unknown/use caution

Medication Safety Issues

High alert medication: The Institute for Safe Medication Practices (ISMP) includes this medication among its list of drugs which have a heightened risk of causing significant patient harm when used in error.

Contraindications Hypersensitivity to fondaparinux or any component of the formulation; severe renal impairment (Cl_{cr} <30 mL/minute); body weight <50 kg (prophylaxis); active major bleeding; bacterial endocarditis; thrombocytopenia associated with a positive *in vitro* test for antiplatelet antibody in the presence of fondaparinux

Warnings/Precautions [U.S. Boxed Warning]: Patients with recent or anticipated neuraxial anesthesia (epidural or spinal anesthesia) are at risk of spinal or epidural hematoma and subsequent paralysis. Not to be used interchangeably (unit-for-unit) with heparin, low molecular weight heparins (LMWHs), or heparinoids. Use caution in patients with moderate renal dysfunction (Cl_{cr} 30-50 mL/minute). Discontinue if severe dysfunction or labile function develops.

Use caution in congenital or acquired bleeding disorders; active ulcerative or angiodysplastic gastrointestinal disease; hemorrhagic stroke; shortly after brain, spinal, or ophthalmologic surgery; or in patients taking platelet inhibitors. Risk of major bleeding may be increased if initial dose is administered earlier then recommended (initiation recommended at 6-8 hours following surgery). Discontinue agents that may enhance the risk of hemorrhage if possible. Use caution in patients <50 kg who are being treated for DVT/PE. Use with caution in the elderly. Safety and efficacy in pediatric patients have not been established.

Canadian labeling warnings/precautions: The administration of fondaparinux is not recommended prior to and during primary percutaneous coronary intervention (PCI) for reperfusion in STEMI patients, due to an increased risk for guiding catheter thrombosis. UA/NSTEMI and STEMI patients undergoing any PCI should not receive fondaparinux as a sole anticoagulant agent. Use of an antithrombin regimen (eg, unfractionated heparin) is recommended as adjunctive therapy to PCI. Following sheath removal, fondaparinux therapy should not resume for at least 2 hours in UA/NSTEMI patients and 3 hours in STEMI patients. Use caution in UA/NSTEMI/STEMI patients <50 kg. Avoid administration 24 hours before and 48 hours after coronary artery bypass graft (CABG) surgery.

Adverse Reactions As with all anticoagulants, bleeding is the major adverse effect. Hemorrhage may occur at any site. Risk appears increased by a number of factors including renal dysfunction, age (>75 years), and weight (<50 kg).

>10%:

- Central nervous system: Fever (4% to 14%)
- Gastrointestinal: Nausea (11%)
- Hematologic: Anemia (20%)

1% to 10%:

- Cardiovascular: Edema (9%), hypotension (4%), thrombosis PCI catheter (without heparin 1%)
- Central nervous system: Insomnia (5%), dizziness (4%), headache (2% to 5%), confusion (3%), pain (2%)
- Dermatologic: Rash (8%), purpura (4%), bullous eruption (3%)
- Endocrine & metabolic: Hypokalemia (1% to 4%)
- Gastrointestinal: Constipation (5% to 9%), vomiting (6%), diarrhea (3%), dyspepsia (2%)
- Genitourinary: Urinary tract infection (4%), urinary retention (3%)
- Hematologic: Moderate thrombocytopenia (50,000-100,000/mm^3: 3%), major bleeding (1% to 3%), minor bleeding (2% to 4%), hematoma (3%); risk of major bleeding increased as high as 5% in patients receiving initial dose <6 hours following surgery
- Hepatic: ALT increased (3%), AST increased (2%)
- Local: Injection site reaction (bleeding, rash, pruritus)
- Miscellaneous: Wound drainage increased (5%)

<1% (Limited to important or life-threatening): Heparin-induced thrombocytopenia (1 case report), hepatic enzymes increased, severe thrombocytopenia (<50,000/mm^3)

Drug Interactions

Avoid Concomitant Use There are no known interactions where it is recommended to avoid concomitant use.

Increased Effect/Toxicity

Fondaparinux may increase the levels/effects of: Anticoagulants; Ibritumomab; Tositumomab and Iodine I 131 Tositumomab

The levels/effects of Fondaparinux may be increased by: Antiplatelet Agents; Dasatinib; Drotrecogin Alfa; Herbs (Anticoagulant/Antiplatelet Properties); Nonsteroidal Anti-Inflammatory Agents; Pentosan Polysulfate Sodium; Prostacyclin Analogues; Salicylates; Thrombolytic Agents

Decreased Effect There are no known significant interactions involving a decrease in effect.

Ethanol/Nutrition/Herb Interactions Herb/Nutraceutical: Avoid alfalfa, anise, bilberry, bladderwrack, bromelain, cat's claw, celery, coleus, cordyceps, dong quai, evening primrose oil, fenugreek, feverfew, garlic, ginger, ginkgo biloba, ginseng (American/Panax/Siberian), grapeseed, green tea, guggul, horse chestnut seed, horseradish, licorice, prickly ash, red clover, reishi, sweet clover, turmeric, white willow (all possess anticoagulant or antiplatelet activity and as such, may enhance the anticoagulant effects of fondaparinux).

Stability Store at 15°C to 30°C (59°F to 86°F).

Canadian labeling: For I.V. administration: May mix with 25 mL or 50 mL NS; manufacturer recommends immediate use once diluted in NS, but is stable for up to 24 hours at 15°C to 30°C (59°F to 86°F).

Mechanism of Action Fondaparinux is a synthetic pentasaccharide that causes an antithrombin III-mediated selective inhibition of factor Xa. Neutralization of factor Xa interrupts the blood coagulation cascade and inhibits thrombin formation and thrombus development.

Pharmacodynamics/Kinetics

Absorption: SubQ: Rapid and complete

Distribution: V_d: 7-11 L; mainly in blood

Protein binding: ≥94% to antithrombin III

Bioavailability: SubQ: 100%

Half-life elimination: 17-21 hours; prolonged with worsening renal impairment

Time to peak: SubQ: 2-3 hours

Excretion: Urine (as unchanged drug); decreased clearance in patients <50 kg

Dosage SubQ: Adults:

DVT prophylaxis: Adults ≥50 kg: 2.5 mg once daily. **Note:** Initiate dose after hemostasis has been established, 6-8 hours postoperatively.

DVT prophylaxis with history of HIT (unlabeled use): 2.5 mg once daily

Usual duration: 5-9 days (up to 10 days following abdominal surgery or up to 11 days following hip replacement or knee replacement)

Extended prophylaxis is recommended following hip fracture surgery (has been tolerated for up to 32 days).

Acute DVT/PE treatment: **Note:** Concomitant treatment with warfarin sodium should be initiated as soon as possible, usually within 72 hours:

<50 kg: 5 mg once daily

50-100 kg: 7.5 mg once daily

>100 kg: 10 mg once daily

Usual duration: 5-9 days (has been administered up to 26 days)

Canadian labeling only: Adults:

UA/NSTEMI: SubQ: 2.5 mg once daily; initiate as soon as possible after diagnosis; treat for up to 8 days or until hospital discharge.

STEMI: I.V.: 2.5 mg once; subsequent doses: SubQ: 2.5 mg once daily; treat for up to 8 days or until hospital discharge

Dosage adjustment in renal impairment:

Cl_{cr} 30-50 mL/minute: Use caution

Cl_{cr} <30 mL/minute: Contraindicated

Administration Do not administer I.M.; for SubQ administration only. Do not mix with other injections or infusions. Do not expel air bubble from syringe before injection. Administer according to recommended regimen; early initiation (before 6 hours after surgery) has been associated with increased bleeding.

Canadian labeling only: STEMI patients: I.V. push or mixed in 25-50 mL of NS and infused over 1-2 minutes. Flush tubing with NS after infusion to ensure complete administration of fondaparinux. Infusion bag should not be mixed with other agents.

Monitoring Parameters Periodic monitoring of CBC, serum creatinine, occult blood testing of stools recommended. Antifactor Xa activity of fondaparinux can be measured by the assay if fondaparinux is used as the calibrator. PT and aPTT are insensitive measures of fondaparinux activity.

Test Interactions International standards of heparin or LMWH are not the appropriate calibrators for antifactor Xa activity of fondaparinux.

Dosage Forms Excipient information presented when available (limited, particularly for generics); consult specific product labeling.

Injection, solution, as sodium [preservative free]: 2.5 mg/0.5 mL (0.5 mL); 5 mg/0.4 mL (0.4 mL); 7.5 mg/0.6 mL (0.6 mL); 10 mg/0.8 mL (0.8 mL) [prefilled syringe]

◆ **Fondaparinux Sodium** *see* Fondaparinux *on page 660*

◆ **Foradil® (Can)** *see* Formoterol *on page 662*

◆ **Foradil® Aerolizer®** *see* Formoterol *on page 662*

Formoterol (for MOH te rol)

U.S. Brand Names Foradil® Aerolizer®; Perforomist™

Canadian Brand Names Foradil®; Oxeze® Turbuhaler®

Index Terms Formoterol Fumarate; Formoterol Fumarate Dihydrate

Pharmacologic Category Beta2-Adrenergic Agonist, Long-Acting; Beta$_2$-Adrenergic Agonist

Additional Appendix Information

Bronchodilators *on page 1650*

Use Maintenance treatment of asthma and prevention of bronchospasm in patients ≥5 years of age with reversible obstructive airway disease, including patients with symptoms of nocturnal asthma, who require regular treatment with inhaled, short-acting beta$_2$-agonists; maintenance treatment of bronchoconstriction in patients with COPD; prevention of exercise-induced bronchospasm in patients ≥5 years of age

Note:

Oxeze® is also approved in Canada for acute relief of symptoms ("on demand" treatment) in patients ≥6 years of age.

Perforomist™ is only indicated for maintenance treatment of bronchoconstriction in patients with COPD.

Restrictions An FDA-approved medication guide must be distributed when dispensing an outpatient prescription (new or refill) where this medication is to be used without direct supervision of a healthcare provider. Medication guides are available at http://www.fda.gov/cder/Offices/ODS/medication_guides.htm.

Pregnancy Risk Factor C

Pregnancy Considerations When given orally to rats throughout organogenesis, formoterol caused delayed ossification and decreased fetal weight, but no malformations. There were no adverse events when given to pregnant rats in late pregnancy. Doses used were ≥70 times the recommended daily inhalation dose in humans. There are no adequate and well-controlled studies in pregnant women. Use only if benefit outweighs risk to the fetus. Beta-agonists interfere with uterine contractility so use during labor only if benefit outweighs risk to the fetus.

Lactation Excretion in breast milk unknown/use caution

Medication Safety Issues

Sound-alike/look-alike issues:

Foradil® may be confused with Toradol®

Foradil® capsules for inhalation are for administration via Aerolizer™ inhaler and are **not** for oral use.

International issues:

Foradil® may be confused with Theradol® which is a brand name for tramadol in the Netherlands.

Contraindications

Foradil®: Hypersensitivity to formoterol, or any component of the formulation

Oxeze®: Hypersensitivity to formoterol, inhaled lactose, or any component of the formulation; presence of tachyarrhythmias

Perforomist™: No contraindications listed in the product labeling

Warnings/Precautions [U.S. Boxed Warning]: Long-acting beta$_2$-agonists (LABAs) may increase the risk of asthma-related deaths. Formoterol for oral inhalation should only be used as adjuvant therapy in patients not adequately controlled on inhaled corticosteroids or whose disease requires two maintenance therapies. Foradil® should only be used as adjuvant therapy in patients not adequately controlled on other asthma medications (eg, low-to-medium dose inhaled corticosteroids) or whose disease warrants initiation of two maintenance therapies; should not be used as monotherapy for the treatment of asthma. Optimize anti-inflammatory treatment before initiating maintenance treatment with formoterol. Do not use as a component of chronic therapy without an anti-inflammatory agent. Corticosteroids should not be stopped or reduced at formoterol initiation. Patients using inhaled, short-acting beta$_2$-agonists should be instructed to discontinue routine use of these medications prior to beginning treatment; short-acting agents should still be provided to patients; however, use should be reserved for symptomatic relief of acute symptoms. Patient must be instructed to seek medical attention in cases where acute symptoms are not relieved by a rapid-onset beta-agonist or when a previous level of response is diminished. Treatment must not be delayed. Rarely, paradoxical bronchospasm may occur with use of inhaled bronchodilating agents; this should be distinguished from inadequate response. The safety and efficacy of Perforomist™ in the treatment of asthma have not been established.

Acute episodes should be treated with a rapid-onset beta$_2$-agonist. Oxeze® is a formulation of formoterol (available outside the U.S. [eg, Canada]) approved for acute treatment of asthmatic symptoms. The labelings for U.S. approved formulations (Foradil®, Perforomist™) state that formoterol is not meant to relieve acute asthmatic symptoms.

Because LABAs may disguise poorly controlled persistent asthma, frequent or chronic use of LABAs for exercise-induced bronchospasm is discouraged by the NIH Asthma Guidelines (NIH, 2007). Formoterol should not be used for the treatment of rapidly deteriorating COPD or for acute symptomatic COPD. Increased use and/or ineffectiveness of short-acting beta$_2$-agonists may indicate rapidly deteriorating disease and should prompt re-evaluation of the patient's condition.

Immediate hypersensitivity reactions (urticaria, angioedema, rash, bronchospasm) have been reported. Do not exceed recommended dose or frequency; serious adverse events (including serious asthma exacerbations and fatalities) have been associated with excessive use of inhaled sympathomimetics. Beta$_2$-agonists may increase risk of arrhythmias, decrease serum potassium, prolong QT_c interval, or increase serum glucose. These effects may be exacerbated in hypoxemia. Use caution in patients with cardiovascular disease (arrhythmia, coronary insufficiency, hypertension, or HF), seizures, diabetes, glaucoma, hyperthyroidism, or hypokalemia. Beta-agonists may cause elevation in blood pressure and heart rate, and result in CNS stimulation/excitation.

Powder for oral inhalation contains lactose; very rare anaphylactic reactions have been reported in patients with severe milk protein allergy. The contents of the Foradil® capsules are for inhalation via the Aerolizer™ device. There have been reports of incorrect administration (swallowing of the capsules).Safety and efficacy of Foradil® have not been established in children <5 years of age; safety and efficacy of Perforomist™ have not been established in children <18 years of age.

Adverse Reactions

1% to 10%:

Cardiovascular: Chest pain (2%), palpitation

Central nervous system: Anxiety (2%), dizziness (2%), fever (2%), insomnia (2%), dysphonia (1%), headache

Dermatologic: Rash (1%)

Gastrointestinal: Diarrhea (5%), nausea (5%), xerostomia (1% to 3%), vomiting (2%), abdominal pain, dyspepsia, gastroenteritis

Neuromuscular & skeletal: Tremor

Respiratory: Asthma exacerbation (age 5-12 years: 5% to 6%; age >12 years: <4%), bronchitis (5%), infection (3% to 7%), pharyngitis (3% to 4%), sinusitis (3%), dyspnea (2%), tonsillitis (1%)

<1% (Limited to important or life-threatening): Acute asthma deterioration, anaphylactic reactions (severe hypotension/angioedema), agitation, angina, arrhythmia, bronchospasm (paradoxical), fatigue, hyperglycemia, hypertension, hypokalemia, glucose intolerance, malaise, metabolic acidosis, muscle cramps, nervousness, tachycardia

Drug Interactions

Metabolism/Transport Effects **Substrate** (minor) of CYP2A6, 2C9, 2C19, 2D6

Avoid Concomitant Use

Avoid concomitant use of Formoterol with any of the following: Iobenguane I 123

Increased Effect/Toxicity

Formoterol may increase the levels/effects of: Sympathomimetics

The levels/effects of Formoterol may be increased by: Atomoxetine; Cannabinoids; MAO Inhibitors; Tricyclic Antidepressants

Decreased Effect

Formoterol may decrease the levels/effects of: Iobenguane I 123

The levels/effects of Formoterol may be decreased by: Alpha-/Beta-Blockers; Beta-Blockers (Beta1 Selective); Beta-Blockers (Nonselective); Betahistine

Stability

Foradil®: Prior to dispensing, store in refrigerator at 2°C to 8°C (36°F to 46°F). After dispensing, store at room temperature at 20°C to 25°C (68°F to 77°F). Protect from heat and moisture. Capsules should always be stored in the blister and only removed immediately before use. Always check expiration date. Use within 4 months of purchase date or product expiration date, whichever comes first.

Perforomist™: Prior to dispensing, store in refrigerator at 2°C to 8°C (36°F to 46°F). After dispensing, store at 2°C to 25°C (36°F to 77°F) for up to 3 months. Protect from heat. Unit-dose vials should always be stored in the foil pouch and only removed immediately before use.

Mechanism of Action Relaxes bronchial smooth muscle by selective action on beta$_2$ receptors with little effect on heart rate. Formoterol has a long-acting effect.

Pharmacodynamics/Kinetics

Onset of action: Within 3 minutes

Peak effect: 80% of peak effect within 15 minutes

Duration: Improvement in FEV_1 observed for 12 hours in most patients

Absorption: Rapidly into plasma

Protein binding: 61% to 64% *in vitro* at higher concentrations than achieved with usual dosing

Metabolism: Hepatic via direct glucuronidation and O-demethylation; CYP2D6, CYP2C8/9, CYP2C19, CYP2A6 involved in O-demethylation

Half-life elimination: Powder: ~10-14 hours; Nebulized solution: ~7 hours

Time to peak: Maximum improvement in FEV_1 in 1-3 hours

Excretion:

Children 5-12 years: Urine (7% to 9% as direct glucuronide metabolites, 6% as unchanged drug)

Adults: Urine (15% to 18% as direct glucuronide metabolites, 2% to 10% as unchanged drug)

Dosage

Asthma maintenance treatment: Children ≥5 years and Adults: Inhalation: **Note:** For long-term asthma control, long-acting beta$_2$-agonists (LABAs) should be used in combination with inhaled corticosteroids and **not** as monotherapy

Foradil®: 12 mcg capsule inhaled every 12 hours via Aerolizer™ device

Oxeze® (CAN): **Note:** Not labeled for use in the U.S.: Children ≥6 years and Adults: Inhalation: 6 mcg or 12 mcg every 12 hours. Maximum dose: Children: 24 mcg/day; Adults: 48 mcg/day

Prevention of exercise-induced bronchospasm: Children ≥5 years and Adults: Inhalation:

Foradil®:12 mcg capsule inhaled via Aerolizer™ device at least 15 minutes before exercise on an "as needed" basis; additional doses should not be used for another 12 hours. **Note:** If already using for asthma maintenance, then should not use additional doses for exercise-induced bronchospasm. Because LABAs may disguise poorly controlled persistent asthma, frequent or chronic use of LABAs for exercise-induced bronchospasm is discouraged by the NIH Asthma Guidelines (NIH, 2007).

Oxeze® (CAN): **Note:** Not labeled for use in the U.S.: Children ≥6 years and Adults: Inhalation: 6 mcg or 12 mcg at least 15 minutes before exercise.

COPD maintenance treatment: Adults: Inhalation:

Foradil®: 12 mcg capsule inhaled every 12 hours via Aerolizer™ device

Perforomist™: 20 mcg unit-dose vial twice daily (maximum dose: 40 mcg/day)

Additional indication for Oxeze® (approved in Canada): Acute ("on demand") relief of bronchoconstriction: Children ≥12 years and Adults: 6 mcg or 12 mcg as a single dose (maximum dose: 72 mcg in any 24-hour period). The prolonged use of high dosages (48 mcg/day for ≥3 consecutive days) may be a sign of suboptimal control, and should prompt the re-evaluation of therapy.

Administration

Foradil®: Remove capsule from foil blister **immediately** before use. Place capsule in the capsule-chamber in the base of the Aerolizer™ Inhaler. Must only use the Aerolizer™ Inhaler. Press both buttons **once only** and then release. Keep inhaler in a level, horizontal position. Exhale fully. Do not exhale into inhaler. Tilt head slightly back and inhale (rapidly, steadily, and deeply). Hold breath as long as possible. If any powder remains in capsule, exhale and inhale again. Repeat until capsule is empty. Throw away empty capsule; do not leave in inhaler. Do not use a spacer with the Aerolizer™ Inhaler. Always keep capsules and inhaler dry.

Perforomist™: Remove unit-dose vial from foil pouch **immediately** before use. Solution does not require dilution prior to administration; do not mix other medications with formoterol solution. Place contents of unit-dose vial into the reservoir of a standard jet nebulizer connected to an air compressor; assemble nebulizer based on the manufacturer's instructions and turn nebulizer on; breathe deeply and evenly until all of the medication has been inhaled. Discard any unused medication immediately; do not ingest contents of vial. Clean nebulizer after use.

Monitoring Parameters FEV_1, peak flow, and/or other pulmonary function tests; blood pressure, heart rate; CNS stimulation; serum glucose, serum potassium

Dosage Forms Excipient information presented when available (limited, particularly for generics); consult specific product labeling. [CAN] = Canadian brand name

Powder for oral inhalation, as fumarate:

Foradil® Aerolizer™ [capsule]: 12 mcg (12s, 60s) [contains lactose 25 mg]

Oxeze® Turbuhaler® [CAN]: 6 mcg/inhalation [delivers 60 metered doses; contains lactose 600 mcg/dose]; 12 mcg/inhalation [delivers 60 metered doses; contains lactose 600 mcg/dose] [not available in the U.S.]

Solution for nebulization, as fumarate dihydrate:

Perforomist™: 20 mcg/2 mL (2 mL)

◆ **Formoterol Fumarate** *see* Formoterol *on page 662*

◆ **Formoterol Fumarate Dihydrate** *see* Formoterol *on page 662*

◆ **Formoterol Fumarate Dihydrate and Budesonide** *see* Budesonide and Formoterol *on page 218*

◆ **Formulation R™ [OTC]** *see* Phenylephrine *on page 1183*

◆ **Formulex® (Can)** *see* Dicyclomine *on page 441*

◆ **5-Formyl Tetrahydrofolate** *see* Leucovorin Calcium *on page 866*

◆ **Fortamet®** *see* MetFORMIN *on page 954*

◆ **Fortaz®** *see* Ceftazidime *on page 282*

◆ **Forteo®** *see* Teriparatide *on page 1444*

◆ **Fortical®** *see* Calcitonin *on page 234*

◆ **Fosamax®** *see* Alendronate *on page 58*

◆ **Fosamax Plus D™** *see* Alendronate and Cholecalciferol *on page 60*

Fosamprenavir (FOS am pren a veer)

U.S. Brand Names Lexiva®

Canadian Brand Names Telzir®

Index Terms Fosamprenavir Calcium; GW433908G

Pharmacologic Category Antiretroviral Agent, Protease Inhibitor

Additional Appendix Information

Antiretroviral Therapy for HIV Infection: Adults and Adolescents *on page 1758*

Management of Healthcare Worker Exposures to HBV, HCV, and HIV *on page 1719*

Perinatal HIV Guidelines *on page 1730*

Use Treatment of HIV infections in combination with at least two other antiretroviral agents

Pregnancy Risk Factor C

Pregnancy Considerations Animal data showed some abortifacient and minor skeletal abnormalities with amprenavir. It is not known if amprenavir crosses the human placenta. There are no adequate and well-controlled studies in pregnant women. Pregnancy and protease inhibitors are both associated with an increased risk of hyperglycemia. Glucose levels should be closely monitored. Health professionals are encouraged to contact the antiretroviral pregnancy registry to monitor outcomes of pregnant women exposed to antiretroviral medications (1-800-258-4263 or www.APRegistry.com).

Lactation Excretion in breast milk unknown/contraindicated

Medication Safety Issues

Sound-alike/look-alike issues:

Lexiva® may be confused with Levitra®

Contraindications Clinically-significant hypersensitivity (eg, Stevens-Johnson syndrome) to fosamprenavir, amprenavir, or any component of the formulation; concurrent therapy with CYP3A4 substrates with a narrow therapeutic window; concomitant use with cisapride, delavirdine, ergot derivatives, lovastatin, midazolam, pimozide, rifampin, simvastatin, St John's wort, and triazolam; use of flecainide and propafenone with concomitant ritonavir therapy

The Canadian product labeling of fosamprenavir (Telzir®) indicates that this product is contraindicated in severe hepatic impairment; in addition, concurrent therapy with potent inducers of CYP3A4 including rifampin is specifically contraindicated

Warnings/Precautions Use with caution in patients taking strong CYP3A4 inhibitors, moderate or strong CYP3A4 inducers, and major CYP3A4 substrates (see Drug Interactions); consider alternative agents that avoid or lessen the potential for CYP-mediated interactions. Do not use with hormonal contraceptives.

Use with caution in patients with diabetes mellitus or sulfonamide allergy. Use caution with hepatic impairment (dosage adjustment required) or underlying hepatitis B or C. Redistribution of fat may occur (eg, buffalo hump, peripheral wasting, cushingoid appearance). Dosage adjustment is required for combination therapies (ritonavir and/or efavirenz); in addition, the risk of hyperlipidemia may be increased during concurrent therapy. Protease inhibitors have been associated with a variety of hypersensitivity events (some severe), including rash, anaphylaxis (rare), angioedema, bronchospasm, erythema multiforme, and/or Stevens-Johnson syndrome (rare). It is generally recommended to discontinue treatment if severe rash or moderate symptoms accompanied by other systemic symptoms occur. Acute hemolytic anemia has been reported in association with amprenavir use. Spontaneous bleeding has been reported in patients with hemophilia A or B following treatment with protease inhibitors; use caution. Immune reconstitution syndrome may develop resulting in the occurrence of an inflammatory response to an indolent or residual opportunistic infection; further evaluation and treatment may be necessary. Safety and efficacy have not been established in children <2 years of age.

Adverse Reactions Frequency not defined: Fat redistribution, immune reconstitution syndrome have been associated with protease inhibitor therapy.

>10%:

Dermatologic: Rash (up to 19%; onset ~11 days; duration ~13 days)

Endocrine & metabolic: Hypertriglyceridemia (>750 mg/dL: up to 11%)

Gastrointestinal: Diarrhea (moderate-to-severe; 5% to 13%)

1% to 10%:

Central nervous system: Headache (moderate-to-severe; 2% to 4%), fatigue (moderate-to-severe; 2% to 4%)

Dermatologic: Pruritus (7% to 8%)

Endocrine & metabolic: Hyperglycemia (>251 mg/dL: <1% to 2%)

Gastrointestinal: Serum lipase increased (>2 times ULN: 5% to 8%), nausea (moderate-to-severe; 3% to 7%, vomiting (moderate-to-severe; 2% to 6%), abdominal pain (moderate-to-severe; 1% to 2%)

Hematologic: Neutropenia (<750 cells/mm^3: 3%)

Hepatic: Transaminases increased (>5 times ULN: 4% to 8%)

<1% (Limited to important or life-threatening): Angioedema, Stevens-Johnson syndrome

Note: Spontaneous bleeding has been reported in patients with hemophilia A or B following treatment with protease inhibitors. Acute hemolytic anemia has been reported in association with amprenavir use.

Drug Interactions

Metabolism/Transport Effects As amprenavir: **Substrate** of CYP2C9 (minor), 3A4 (major); **Inhibits** CYP2C19 (weak), 3A4 (strong)

Avoid Concomitant Use

Avoid concomitant use of Fosamprenavir with any of the following: Alfuzosin; Amiodarone; Cisapride; Delavirdine; Eplerenone; Ergot Derivatives; Etravirine; Nilotinib; Nisoldipine; Pimozide; QuiNIDine; Ranolazine; Rivaroxaban; Salmeterol; Silodosin; St Johns Wort

Increased Effect/Toxicity

Fosamprenavir may increase the levels/effects of: Alfuzosin; Alosetron; Amiodarone; Antifungal Agents (Azole Derivatives, Systemic); Benzodiazepines (metabolized by oxidation); Calcium Channel Blockers (Dihydropyridine); Calcium Channel Blockers (Nondihydropyridine); CarBAMazepine; Ciclesonide; Cisapride; Clarithromycin; Corticosteroids (Orally Inhaled); CycloSPORINE; CYP3A4 Substrates; Digoxin; Enfuvirtide; Eplerenone; Ergot Derivatives; FentaNYL; Fesoterodine; Fusidic Acid; HMG-CoA Reductase Inhibitors; Ixabepilone; Maraviroc; Meperidine; Methadone; Nefazodone; Nilotinib; Nisoldipine; Phosphodiesterase 5 Inhibitors; Pimecrolimus; Pimozide; Protease Inhibitors; QuiNIDine; Ranolazine; Rifamycin Derivatives; Rivaroxaban; Salmeterol; Silodosin; Sirolimus; Sorafenib; Tacrolimus; Temsirolimus; Tenofovir; TraZODone; Tricyclic Antidepressants

The levels/effects of Fosamprenavir may be increased by: Antifungal Agents (Azole Derivatives, Systemic); Clarithromycin; CycloSPORINE; Delavirdine; Efavirenz; Enfuvirtide; Etravirine; Fusidic Acid; P-Glycoprotein Inhibitors; Phenytoin

Decreased Effect

Fosamprenavir may decrease the levels/effects of: Abacavir; Clarithromycin; Delavirdine; Meperidine; Oral Contraceptive (Estrogens); PARoxetine; Phenytoin; Valproic Acid; Zidovudine

The levels/effects of Fosamprenavir may be decreased by: Antacids; CarBAMazepine; CYP3A4 Inducers (Strong); Deferasirox; Efavirenz; Garlic; H2-Antagonists; Nevirapine; Oral Contraceptive (Estrogens); P-Glycoprotein Inducers; Rifamycin Derivatives; St Johns Wort; Tenofovir

Ethanol/Nutrition/Herb Interactions Herb/Nutraceutical: Amprenavir serum concentration may be decreased by St John's wort; concurrent use contraindicated.

Stability

Lexiva®: Store tablets at controlled room temperature of 25°C (77°F). Store oral suspension at 5°C to 30°C (41°F to 86°F). Do not freeze.

Telzir®: Store tablets 2°C to 30°C; do not freeze and discard 25 days after opening.

Mechanism of Action Fosamprenavir is rapidly and almost completely converted to amprenavir by cellular phosphatases *in vivo*. Amprenavir binds to the active site of HIV protease activity and inhibits cleavage of viral polyprotein precursors (eg, Gag and Gag-Pol) into individual functional proteins found in infectious HIV. Inhibition prevents cleavage of these polyproteins, resulting in the formation of immature, noninfectious viral particles.

Pharmacodynamics/Kinetics

Absorption: 63%

Protein-binding: >90% (to alpha$_1$-acid glycoprotein)

Metabolism: Fosamprenavir is rapidly and almost completely converted to amprenavir by cellular phosphatases in gut epithelium; amprenavir is hepatically metabolized via CYP isoenzymes (primarily CYP3A4)

Bioavailability: Not established; food does not have a significant effect on absorption of tablets. Administration of oral suspension with food reduced C_{max} by 46% and AUC by 28%.

Half-life elimination: ~7.7 hours (amprenavir)

Time to peak, plasma: 1.5-4 hours (median: 2.5 hours)

Excretion: Feces (75% as metabolites, <1% as unchanged drug); urine (14% as metabolites, <1% as unchanged drug)

Dosage Oral: HIV infection:

Children:

Antiretroviral therapy-naive patients:

Children 2-5 years of age: Fosamprenavir 30 mg/kg twice daily (not to exceed adult dosage of 1400 mg twice daily)

Children ≥6 years of age:

Unboosted regimen: Fosamprenavir 30 mg/kg twice daily (not to exceed adult dosage of 1400 mg twice daily)

Ritonavir-boosted regimen: Fosamprenavir 18 mg/kg twice daily plus ritonavir 3 mg/kg twice daily (not to exceed the adult dose of 700 mg plus ritonavir 100 mg twice daily)

Protease inhibitor-experienced patients: Children ≥6 years of age: Fosamprenavir 18 mg/kg plus ritonavir 3 mg/kg twice daily (not to exceed the adult dose of 700 mg plus ritonavir 100 mg twice daily)

Notes: The adult regimen of 1400 mg twice daily may be used for pediatric patients who weigh ≥47 kg. When combined with ritonavir, fosamprenavir tablets may be administered to children who weigh ≥39 kg while ritonavir capsules may be used for pediatric patients who weigh ≥33 kg.

Adults:

Antiretroviral therapy-naive patients:

Unboosted regimen: 1400 mg twice daily (without ritonavir)

Ritonavir-boosted regimens:

Once-daily regimen: Fosamprenavir 1400 mg plus ritonavir 100-200 mg once daily

Twice-daily regimen: Fosamprenavir 700 mg plus ritonavir 100 mg twice daily

Protease inhibitor-experienced patients: Fosamprenavir 700 mg plus ritonavir 100 mg twice daily. **Note:** Once-daily administration is not recommended in protease inhibitor-experienced patients.

Combination therapy with efavirenz (ritonavir-boosted regimen):

Once-daily regimen: Fosamprenavir 1400 mg daily plus ritonavir 300 mg once daily

Twice-daily regimen: No dosage adjustment recommended for twice-daily regimen

Combination therapy with nevirapine (ritonavir-boosted regimen): Fosamprenavir 700 mg plus ritonavir 100 mg twice daily

Dosage adjustment in renal impairment: No dosage adjustment required.

Dosage adjustment in hepatic impairment:

Mild impairment (Child-Pugh score 5-6): Reduce dosage of fosamprenavir to 700 mg twice daily without concurrent ritonavir (therapy naive) or fosamprenavir 700 mg twice daily plus ritonavir 100 mg once daily (therapy naive or PI experienced)

Moderate impairment (Child-Pugh score 7-9): Reduce dosage of fosamprenavir to 700 mg twice daily without concurrent ritonavir (therapy naive) or fosamprenavir 450 mg twice daily plus ritonavir 100 mg once daily (therapy naive or PI experienced)

Severe impairment (Child-Pugh score 10-12): Reduce dosage of fosamprenavir to 350 mg twice daily without concurrent ritonavir (therapy naive). No data concerning the use of fosamprenavir plus ritonavir are available in severe hepatic impairment.

Dietary Considerations Tablets may be taken with or without food. Adults should take oral suspension without food; however, children should take oral suspension with food.

Administration

Oral suspension: Administer **without** food to adults; administer **with** food to pediatric patients. Shake suspension vigorously prior to use.

Tablet: May be taken with or without food.

Monitoring Parameters Monitor viral load, CD4 count, triglycerides, cholesterol, glucose

Dosage Forms Excipient information presented when available (limited, particularly for generics); consult specific product labeling. [CAN] = Canadian brand name

Tablet, as calcium:

Lexiva®: 700 mg [equivalent to amprenavir ~600 mg)

Telzir® [CAN]: 700 mg [not available in the U.S.]

Suspension, oral, as calcium:

Lexiva®: 50 mg/mL (225 mL) [equivalent to amprenavir ~43 mg/mL; contains propylene glycol; grape-bubblegum-peppermint flavored]

Telzir® [CAN]: 50 mg/mL (225 mL) [not available in the U.S.]

◆ **Fosamprenavir Calcium** *see* Fosamprenavir *on page 664*

Fosaprepitant (fos a PRE pi tant)

U.S. Brand Names Emend® for Injection

Index Terms Aprepitant Injection; Fosaprepitant Dimeglumine; L-758,298; MK 0517

Pharmacologic Category Antiemetic; Substance P/ Neurokinin 1 Receptor Antagonist

Use Prevention of acute and delayed nausea and vomiting associated with moderately- and highly-emetogenic chemotherapy (in combination with other antiemetics)

Pregnancy Risk Factor B

Pregnancy Considerations Teratogenic effects were not observed in animal studies. There are no adequate and well-controlled studies in pregnant women; use only if clearly needed.

Lactation Excretion in breast milk unknown/not recommended

Medication Safety Issues

Sound-alike/look-alike issues:

Fosaprepitant may be confused with aprepitant, fosamprenavir, fospropofol

Emend® for injection (fosaprepitant) may be confused with Emend® (aprepitant) which is an oral capsule formulation.

Contraindications Hypersensitivity to fosaprepitant, aprepitant, polysorbate 80, or any component of the formulation; concurrent use with pimozide or cisapride

Warnings/Precautions Fosaprepitant is rapidly converted to aprepitant, which has a high potential for drug interactions. Use caution with agents primarily metabolized via CYP3A4; aprepitant is a 3A4 inhibitor. Effect on orally administered 3A4 substrates is greater than those administered intravenously. Use caution with hepatic impairment; has not been studied in patients with severe hepatic impairment (Child-Pugh class C). Not intended for treatment of existing nausea and vomiting or for chronic continuous therapy.

Adverse Reactions Adverse reactions reported with aprepitant and fosaprepitant (as part of a combination chemotherapy regimen) occurring at a higher frequency than standard therapy:

>10%:

Central nervous system: Fatigue (≤18%)

Gastrointestinal: Nausea (≤13%)

Neuromuscular & skeletal: Weakness (≤18%)

Miscellaneous: Hiccups (11%)

1% to 10%:

Central nervous system: Dizziness (≤7%), headache (≤3%)

Endocrine & metabolic: Dehydration (6%), hot flushing (3%)

Gastrointestinal: Diarrhea (≤10%), dyspepsia (≤8%), abdominal pain (5%), stomatitis (≤5%), epigastric discomfort (4%), gastritis (4%), throat pain (≤3%)

Hematologic: Neutropenia (≤9%)

Hepatic: ALT increased (≤6%), AST increased (≤3%)

Local: Injection site pain (8%), injection site induration (2%)

Renal: BUN increased (≤5%), proteinuria (≤7%)

>0.5% (Limited to important or life-threatening): Acid reflux, acne, alkaline phosphatase increased, anemia, anxiety, appetite decreased, arthralgia, back pain, candidiasis, confusion, conjunctivitis, cough, depression, diabetes mellitus, diaphoresis, DVT, dysphagia, dyspnea, dysuria, edema, eructation, erythrocyturia, flatulence, herpes simplex, hyper-/hypotension, hypokalemia,

hyponatremia, leukocytes increased, leukocyturia, malaise, MI, muscle weakness, musculoskeletal pain, myalgia, nasal secretion, obstipation, palpitation, pelvic pain, peripheral neuropathy, pharyngitis, pneumonitis, pulmonary embolism, rash, renal insufficiency, respiratory infection, respiratory insufficiency, rigors, salivation increased, sensory neuropathy, septic shock, swallowing disorder, tachycardia, taste disturbance, tremor, urinary tract infection, vocal disturbance, weight loss, xerostomia

Postmarketing and/or case reports (with fosaprepitant or aprepitant): Albumin decreased, angioedema, bilirubin increased, bradycardia, disorientation, duodenal ulcer (perforating), dysarthria, enterocolitis, fever, glycosuria, hematoma, hyperglycemia, hypoesthesia, hypothermia, hypovolemia, hypoxia, miosis, neutropenic sepsis, pneumonia, pruritus, sensory disturbance, sinus tachycardia, Stevens-Johnson syndrome, subileus, syncope, urticaria, visual acuity decreased, wheezing

Drug Interactions

Metabolism/Transport Effects **Substrate** of CYP1A2 (minor), 2C19 (minor), 3A4 (major); **Inhibits** CYP2C9 (weak), 2C19 (weak), 3A4 (moderate); **Induces** CYP2C9 (weak), 3A4 (weak)

Avoid Concomitant Use

Avoid concomitant use of Fosaprepitant with any of the following: Cisapride; Pimozide

Increased Effect/Toxicity

Fosaprepitant may increase the levels/effects of: Benzodiazepines (metabolized by oxidation); Cisapride; Corticosteroids (Systemic); CYP3A4 Substrates; Diltiazem; Eplerenone; FentaNYL; Maraviroc; Pimecrolimus; Pimozide; Ranolazine; Salmeterol

The levels/effects of Fosaprepitant may be increased by: Antifungal Agents (Azole Derivatives, Systemic); CYP3A4 Inhibitors (Moderate); CYP3A4 Inhibitors (Strong); Dasatinib; Diltiazem

Decreased Effect

Fosaprepitant may decrease the levels/effects of: Contraceptive (Progestins); Maraviroc; Oral Contraceptive (Estrogens); Warfarin

The levels/effects of Fosaprepitant may be decreased by: CYP3A4 Inducers (Strong); Deferasirox; Herbs (CYP3A4 Inducers); Rifampin

Ethanol/Nutrition/Herb Interactions

Food: Aprepitant serum concentration may be increased when taken with grapefruit juice; avoid concurrent use.

Herb/Nutraceutical: Avoid St John's wort (may decrease aprepitant levels).

Stability Store intact vials at 2°C to 8°C (36°F to 46°F). Reconstitute with 5 mL of sodium chloride 0.9%, directing diluent down side of vial to avoid foaming. Add reconstituted contents of vial to 110 mL sodium chloride 0.9%, resulting in a final concentration of 1 mg/mL; gently invert bag to mix. Solutions diluted for infusion are stable for 24 hours at room temperature of ≤25°C (≤77°F).

Mechanism of Action Fosaprepitant is a prodrug of aprepitant, which prevents acute and delayed vomiting by inhibiting the substance P/neurokinin 1 (NK1) receptor; augments the antiemetic activity of the 5-HT_3 receptor antagonist and corticosteroid activity and inhibits chemotherapy-induced emesis.

Pharmacodynamics/Kinetics

Distribution: Fosaprepitant: ~5 L; Aprepitant: V_d: ~70 L; crosses the blood brain barrier

Protein binding: Aprepitant: >95%

Metabolism:

Fosaprepitant: Hepatic and extrahepatic; rapidly converted to aprepitant (nearly complete conversion)

Aprepitant: Hepatic via CYP3A4 (major); CYP1A2 and CYP2C19 (minor); forms 7 weakly-active metabolites

Bioavailability: Fosaprepitant 115 mg I.V. is bioequivalent to aprepitant 125 mg orally.

Half-life elimination: Half-life elimination: Fosaprepitant: ~2 minutes; Aprepitant: ~9-13 hours

Time to peak, plasma: Fosaprepitant is converted to aprepitant within 30 minutes after the end of infusion

Excretion: Urine (57%); feces (45%)

Dosage I.V.: Adults: Prevention of chemotherapy-induced nausea/vomiting: 115 mg 30 minutes prior to chemotherapy on day 1 (followed by aprepitant 80 mg orally on days 2 and 3) in combination with other antiemetics

Dosage adjustment in renal impairment:

Mild, moderate, or severe impairment: No adjustment required

Dialysis-dependent end-stage renal disease (ESRD): No adjustment required

Dosage adjustment in hepatic impairment:

Child-Pugh class A and B: No adjustment required

Child-Pugh class C: Has not been evaluated

Administration Infuse over 15 minutes

Dosage Forms Excipient information presented when available (limited, particularly for generics); consult specific product labeling.

Injection, powder for reconstitution:

Emend® for Injection: 115 mg [contains edetate disodium; lactose; polysorbate 80]

◆ **Fosaprepitant Dimeglumine** *see* Fosaprepitant *on page 666*

◆ **Fosavance (Can)** *see* Alendronate and Cholecalciferol *on page 60*

Foscarnet (fos KAR net)

U.S. Brand Names Foscavir®

Canadian Brand Names Foscavir®

Index Terms PFA; Phosphonoformate; Phosphonoformic Acid

Pharmacologic Category Antiviral Agent

Additional Appendix Information

Guidelines for the Prevention of Opportunistic Infections in HIV Infected Persons *on page 1740*

Use Treatment of acyclovir-resistant mucocutaneous herpes simplex virus (HSV) infections in immunocompromised persons (eg, with advanced AIDS); treatment of CMV retinitis in persons with HIV

Unlabeled/Investigational Use Other CMV infections (eg, colitis, esophagitis, neurological disease); CMV prophylaxis for cancer patients receiving alemtuzumab therapy or allogeneic stem cell transplant

Pregnancy Risk Factor C

Pregnancy Considerations Associated with an increase in skeletal anomalies in animal studies at approximately the equivalent of 13% to 33% of the maximal daily human dose. There are no adequate and well controlled studies in pregnant women. A single case report of use during the third trimester with normal infant outcome was observed. Monitoring of amniotic fluid volumes by ultrasound is recommended weekly after 20 weeks of gestation to detect oligohydramnios.

Lactation Excretion in breast milk unknown/contraindicated

Contraindications Hypersensitivity to foscarnet or any component of the formulation

Warnings/Precautions Hazardous agent - use appropriate precautions for handling and disposal. **[U.S. Boxed Warning]: Indicated only for immunocompromised patients with CMV retinitis and mucocutaneous acyclovir-resistant HSV infection. [U.S. Boxed Warning]: Renal impairment occurs to some degree in the majority of patients treated with foscarnet;** renal impairment may occur at any time and is usually reversible within 1 week following dose adjustment or discontinuation of therapy, however, several patients have died with renal failure within 4 weeks of stopping foscarnet; therefore, renal function should be closely monitored. To reduce the risk of nephrotoxicity and the potential to administer a relative overdose, always calculate the creatine clearance even if serum creatinine is within the normal range. Adequate hydration may reduce the risk of nephrotoxicity; the manufacturer makes specific recommendations regarding this (see Administration).

Imbalance of serum electrolytes or minerals occurs in at least 15% of patients (hypocalcemia, low ionized calcium, hyper/hypophosphatemia, hypomagnesemia, or hypokalemia). Correct electrolytes before initiating therapy. Use caution when administering other medications that cause electrolyte imbalances. Patients who experience signs or symptoms of an electrolyte imbalance should be assessed immediately. **[U.S. Boxed Warning]: Seizures related to plasma electrolyte/mineral imbalance may occur;** incidence has been reported in up to 10% of HIV patients. Risk factors for seizures include impaired baseline renal function, low total serum calcium, and underlying CNS conditions. May cause anemia and granulocytopenia. May cause genital/vascular tissue irritation/ulceration; adequately hydrate and administer only into vein with adequate blood flow to minimize risk. Foscarnet is deposited in teeth and bone of young, growing animals; it has adversely affected tooth enamel development in rats.

Adverse Reactions

>10%:

Central nervous system: Fever (65%), headache (26%)

Endocrine & metabolic: Hypokalemia (16% to 48%), hypocalcemia (15% to 30%), hypomagnesemia (15% to 30%), hypophosphatemia (8% to 26%)

Gastrointestinal: Nausea (47%), diarrhea (30%), vomiting (26%)

Hematologic: Anemia (33%), granulocytopenia (17%)

Renal: Abnormal renal function/decreased creatinine clearance (12%; without adequate hydration 33%)

1% to 10%:

Cardiovascular: Chest pain (1% to 5%), edema (1% to 5%), facial edema (1% to 5%), flushing (1% to 5%), hyper-/hypotension (1% to 5%), palpitation (1% to 5%), ECG changes (1% to 5%)

Central nervous system: Seizure (includes grand mal; 8%), anxiety (≥5%), confusion (≥5%), depression (≥5%), dizziness (≥5%), fatigue (≥5%), hypoesthesia (≥5%), malaise (≥5%), pain (≥5%), aggressiveness (1% to 5%), agitation (1% to 5%), amnesia (1% to 5%), aphasia (1% to 5%), ataxia (1% to 5%), coordination abnormal (1% to 5%), dementia (1% to 5%), EEG abnormal (1% to 5%), hallucination (1% to 5%), insomnia (1% to 5%), meningitis (1% to 5%), nervousness (1% to 5%), somnolence (1% to 5%), stupor (1% to 5%)

Dermatologic: Rash (≥5%), erythematous rash (1% to 5%), maculopapular rash (1% to 5%), pruritus (1% to 5%), seborrhea (1% to 5%), skin discoloration (1% to 5%), skin ulceration (1% to 5%)

Endocrine & metabolic: Hyperphosphatemia (6%), acidosis (1% to 5%), hyponatremia (1% to 5%)

Gastrointestinal: Abdominal pain (≥5%), anorexia (≥5%), constipation (1% to 5%), dyspepsia (1% to 5%), dysphasia (1% to 5%), flatulence (1% to 5%), melena (1% to 5%), pancreatitis (1% to 5%), rectal hemorrhage (1% to 5%), taste perversion (1% to 5%), ulcerative stomatitis (1% to 5%), weight loss (1% to 5%), xerostomia (1% to 5%)

Genitourinary: Dysuria (1% to 5%), nocturia (1% to 5%), urinary retention (1% to 5%)

Hematologic: Leukopenia (≥5%), lymphadenopathy (1% to 5%), thrombocytopenia (1% to 5%), thrombosis (1% to 5%)

Hepatic: Alkaline phosphatase increased (1% to 5%), ALT increased (1% to 5%), AST increased (1% to 5%), hepatic function abnormal (1% to 5%), LDH increased (1% to 5%)

Local: Injection site pain/inflammation (1% to 5%)

Neuromuscular & skeletal: Paresthesia (≥5%), involuntary muscle contractions (≥5%), rigors (≥5%), neuropathy (peripheral; ≥5%), weakness (≥5%), arthralgia (1% to 5%), back pain (1% to 5%), leg cramps (1% to 5%), myalgia (1% to 5%), tremor (1% to 5%)

Ocular: Vision abnormalities (≥5%), conjunctivitis (1% to 5%), eye pain (1% to 5%)

Renal: Acute renal failure (1% to 5%), albuminuria (1% to 5%), BUN increased (1% to 5%), polyuria (1% to 5%), urinary tract infection (1% to 5%)

Respiratory: Cough (≥5%), dyspnea (≥5%), bronchospasm (1% to 5%), hemoptysis (1% to 5%), pharyngitis (1% to 5%), pneumonia (1% to 5%), pneumothorax (1% to 5%), rhinitis (1% to 5%), sinusitis (1% to 5%), stridor (1% to 5%)

Miscellaneous: Diaphoresis (≥5%), sepsis (≥5%), infection (includes bacterial and fungal; ≥5%), flu-like syndrome (1% to 5%), malignancies (lymphoma/sarcoma 1% to 5%), thirst (1% to 5%)

<1% (Limited to important or life-threatening): Amylase increased, cardiac arrest, coma, creatinine phosphokinase increased, dehydration, diabetes insipidus (usually nephrogenic), erythema multiforme, GGT increased muscle weakness, hematuria, hypoproteinemia, myopathy, myositis, neutropenia, pancytopenia, QT_c prolongation, renal calculus, rhabdomyolysis, Stevens-Johnson syndrome, syndrome of inappropriate antidiuretic hormone (SIADH), toxic epidermal necrolysis, ventricular arrhythmia, vesiculobullous eruptions

Drug Interactions

Avoid Concomitant Use

Avoid concomitant use of Foscarnet with any of the following: Nilotinib; Tetrabenazine; Thioridazine; Ziprasidone

Increased Effect/Toxicity

Foscarnet may increase the levels/effects of: QTc-Prolonging Agents; Tetrabenazine; Thioridazine; Ziprasidone

The levels/effects of Foscarnet may be increased by: Alfuzosin; Gadobutrol; Nilotinib

Decreased Effect There are no known significant interactions involving a decrease in effect.

Stability Foscarnet injection is a clear, colorless solution. Store intact bottles at room temperature of 15°C to 30°C (59°F to 86°F) and protect from temperatures >40°C and from freezing. Diluted solution is stable for 24 hours at room temperature or under refrigeration.

Foscarnet should be diluted in D_5W or NS. For peripheral line administration, foscarnet **must** be diluted to ≤12 mg/mL with D_5W or NS. For central line administration, foscarnet may be administered undiluted.

Mechanism of Action Pyrophosphate analogue which acts as a noncompetitive inhibitor of many viral RNA and DNA polymerases as well as HIV reverse transcriptase. Similar to ganciclovir, foscarnet is a virostatic agent. Foscarnet does not require activation by thymidine kinase.

Pharmacodynamics/Kinetics

Distribution: V_d: ~0.5 L/kg; up to 28% of cumulative I.V. dose may be deposited in bone

Protein binding: 14% to 17%

Metabolism: Biotransformation does not occur

Half-life elimination: Elimination: ~3-4 hours; terminal: ~88 hours (due to bone deposition)

Excretion: Urine (≤28% as unchanged drug)

Dosage

CMV retinitis: I.V.:

Induction treatment: 60 mg/kg/dose every 8 hours **or** 90 mg/kg every 12 hours for 14-21 days

Maintenance therapy: 90-120 mg/kg/day as a single daily infusion

Herpes simplex infections (acyclovir-resistant): Induction: I.V.: 40 mg/kg/dose every 8-12 hours for 14-21 days

Therapy of CMV infection in cancer patients (unlabeled use): I.V.:

Prophylaxis: 60 mg/kg every 8-12 hours for 7 days, followed by 90-120 mg/kg daily until day 100 after HSCT

Pre-emptive treatment: 60 mg/kg every 12 hours for 14 days; if CMV still detectable, continue with 90 mg/kg daily for 5 days/week for 2 additional weeks

Treatment: 90 mg/kg every 12 hours for 2 weeks, followed by 120 mg/kg daily for ≥2 weeks

Dosage adjustment in renal impairment: Induction and maintenance dosing schedules based on creatinine clearance (mL/minute/kg): See tables.

Induction Dosing of Foscarnet in Patients With Abnormal Renal Function

Cl_{cr} (mL/min/kg)	HSV Equivalent to 40 mg/kg q12h	HSV Equivalent to 40 mg/kg q8h	CMV Equivalent to 60 mg/kg q8h	CMV Equivalent to 90 mg/kg q12h
<0.4	Not recommended	Not recommended	Not recommended	Not recommended
≥0.4-0.5	20 mg/kg every 24 hours	35 mg/kg every 24 hours	50 mg/kg every 24 hours	50 mg/kg every 24 hours
>0.5-0.6	25 mg/kg every 24 hours	40 mg/kg every 24 hours	60 mg/kg every 24 hours	60 mg/kg every 24 hours
>0.6-0.8	35 mg/kg every 24 hours	25 mg/kg every 12 hours	40 mg/kg every 12 hours	80 mg/kg every 24 hours
>0.8-1.0	20 mg/kg every 12 hours	35 mg/kg every 12 hours	50 mg/kg every 12 hours	50 mg/kg every 12 hours
>1.0-1.4	30 mg/kg every 12 hours	30 mg/kg every 8 hours	45 mg/kg every 8 hours	70 mg/kg every 12 hours
>1.4	40 mg/kg every 12 hours	40 mg/kg every 8 hours	60 mg/kg every 8 hours	90 mg/kg every 12 hours

Maintenance Dosing of Foscarnet in Patients With Abnormal Renal Function

Cl_{cr} (mL/min/kg)	CMV Equivalent to 90 mg/kg q24h	CMV Equivalent to 120 mg/kg q24h
<0.4	Not recommended	Not recommended
≥0.4-0.5	50 mg/kg every 48 hours	65 mg/kg every 48 hours
>0.5-0.6	60 mg/kg every 48 hours	80 mg/kg every 48 hours
>0.6-0.8	80 mg/kg every 48 hours	105 mg/kg every 48 hours
>0.8-1.0	50 mg/kg every 24 hours	65 mg/kg every 24 hours
>1.0-1.4	70 mg/kg every 24 hours	90 mg/kg every 24 hours
>1.4	90 mg/kg every 24 hours	120 mg/kg every 24 hours

Hemodialysis:

Foscarnet is highly removed by hemodialysis (up to ~38% in 2.5 hours HD with high-flux membrane)

Doses of 50 mg/kg/dose posthemodialysis have been found to produce similar serum concentrations as doses of 90 mg/kg twice daily in patients with normal renal function

Doses of 60-90 mg/kg/dose loading dose (posthemodialysis) followed by 45-60 mg/kg/dose posthemodialysis (3 times/week) with the monitoring of weekly plasma concentrations to maintain peak plasma concentrations in the range of 400-800 μMolar have been recommended by some clinicians

Continuous arteriovenous or venovenous hemodiafiltration effects: Dose as for Cl_{cr} 10-50 mL/minute

Administration Foscarnet is administered by intravenous infusion, using an infusion pump, at a rate not exceeding 1 mg/kg/minute. Undiluted (24 mg/mL) solution can be administered without further dilution when using a central venous catheter for infusion. For peripheral vein administration, the solution **must** be diluted to a final concentration **not to exceed** 12 mg/mL. The manufacturer recommends 750-1000 mL of NS or D_5W be administered prior to first infusion to establish diuresis. With subsequent infusions of 90-120 mg/kg, this volume would be repeated. If the dose were 40-60 mg/kg, then the volume could be reduced to 500 mL. After the first dose, the hydration fluid should be administered concurrently with foscarnet.

Monitoring Parameters 24-hour creatinine clearance at baseline and periodically thereafter. During induction therapy: Obtain complete blood counts, and electrolytes (including serum creatinine, calcium, magnesium, potassium and phosphorus) twice weekly and then one weekly during maintenance therapy. More frequent monitoring may be required in some patients. Check hydration status before and after infusion.

Additional Information CMV retinitis maintenance treatment may be discontinued if immune reconstitution occurs as a result of ART.

Dosage Forms Excipient information presented when available (limited, particularly for generics); consult specific product labeling.

Injection, solution, as sodium [preservative-free]: 24 mg/mL (250 mL, 500 mL)

Foscavir®: 24 mg/mL (500 mL)

◆ **Foscavir®** *see* Foscarnet *on page 667*

Fosfomycin (fos foe MYE sin)

U.S. Brand Names Monurol®

Canadian Brand Names Monurol®

Index Terms Fosfomycin Tromethamine

Pharmacologic Category Antibiotic, Miscellaneous

Additional Appendix Information

Antimicrobial Drugs of Choice *on page 1752*

Use Single oral dose in the treatment of uncomplicated urinary tract infections in women due to susceptible strains of *E. coli* and *Enterococcus faecalis*

Unlabeled/Investigational Use Multiple doses have been investigated for complicated urinary tract infections in men

Pregnancy Risk Factor B

Medication Safety Issues

Sound-alike/look-alike issues:

Monurol® may be confused with Monopril®

Dosage Adults: Oral:

Females: Uncomplicated UTI: Single dose of 3 g in 3-4 oz (90-120 mL) of water

Males:

Complicated UTI (unlabeled): 3 g every 2-3 days for 3 doses

Prostatitis (unlabeled): 3 g every 3 days for a total of 21 days

Dosing adjustment in hepatic impairment: No dosage decrease needed

Additional Information Complete prescribing information for this medication should be consulted for additional detail.

Dosage Forms Excipient information presented when available (limited, particularly for generics); consult specific product labeling.

Powder for solution:

Monurol®: 3 g/sachet (3s) [orange flavor]

◆ **Fosfomycin Tromethamine** *see* Fosfomycin *on page 669*

Fosinopril (foe SIN oh pril)

U.S. Brand Names Monopril®

Canadian Brand Names Apo-Fosinopril®; Gen-Fosinopril; Monopril®; Novo-Fosinopril; PMS-Fosinopril; RAN-Fosinopril; Riva-Fosinopril

Index Terms Fosinopril Sodium

Pharmacologic Category Angiotensin-Converting Enzyme (ACE) Inhibitor

Additional Appendix Information

Angiotensin Agents *on page 1632*

Heart Failure (Systolic) *on page 1809*

Use Treatment of hypertension, either alone or in combination with other antihypertensive agents; treatment of heart failure (HF)

Pregnancy Risk Factor C (1st trimester); D (2nd and 3rd trimesters)

Pregnancy Considerations Due to adverse events observed in some animal studies, fosinopril is considered pregnancy category C during the first trimester. Based on human data, fosinopril is considered pregnancy category D if used during the second and third trimesters (per the manufacturer; however, one study suggests that fetal injury may occur at anytime during pregnancy). First trimester exposure to ACE inhibitors may cause major congenital malformations. An increased risk of cardiovascular and/or central nervous system malformations was observed in one study; however, an increased risk of teratogenic events was not observed in other studies. Second and third trimester use of an ACE inhibitor is associated with oligohydramnios. Oligohydramnios due to decreased fetal renal function may lead to fetal limb contractures, craniofacial deformation, and hypoplastic lung development. The use of ACE inhibitors during the second and third trimesters is also associated with anuria, hypotension, renal failure (reversible or irreversible), skull hypoplasia, and death in the fetus/neonate. Chronic maternal hypertension itself is also associated with adverse events in the fetus/infant. ACE inhibitors are not recommended during pregnancy to treat maternal hypertension or heart failure. Those who are planning a pregnancy should be considered for other medication options if an ACE inhibitor is currently prescribed or the ACE inhibitor should be discontinued as soon as possible once pregnancy is detected. The exposed fetus should be monitored for fetal growth, amniotic fluid volume, and organ formation. Infants exposed to an ACE inhibitor *in utero*, especially during the second and third trimester, should be monitored for hyperkalemia, hypotension, and oliguria.

[U.S. Boxed Warning]: Based on human data, ACE inhibitors can cause injury and death to the developing fetus when used in the second and third trimesters. ACE inhibitors should be discontinued as soon as possible once pregnancy is detected.

Lactation Enters breast milk/not recommended

Medication Safety Issues

Sound-alike/look-alike issues:

Fosinopril may be confused with lisinopril

Monopril® may be confused with Accupril®, minoxidil, moexipril, Monoket®, Monurol™, ramipril

Contraindications Hypersensitivity to fosinopril, any other ACE inhibitor, or any component of the formulation; angioedema related to previous treatment with an ACE inhibitor

Warnings/Precautions Anaphylactic reactions may occur rarely with ACE inhibitors. At any time during treatment (especially following first dose), angioedema may occur rarely with ACE inhibitors; it may involve the head and neck (potentially compromising airway) or the intestine (presenting with abdominal pain). African-Americans may be at an increased risk and patients with idiopathic or hereditary angioedema may be at an increased risk. Prolonged frequent monitoring may be required especially if tongue, glottis, or larynx are involved as they are associated with airway obstruction. Patients with a history of airway surgery may have a higher risk of airway obstruction. Aggressive early and appropriate management is critical. Use in patients with previous angioedema associated with ACE inhibitor therapy is contraindicated. Severe anaphylactoid reactions may be seen during hemodialysis (eg, CVVHD) with high-flux dialysis membranes (eg, AN69), and rarely, during low density lipoprotein apheresis with dextran sulfate cellulose. Rare cases of anaphylactoid reactions have been reported in patients undergoing sensitization treatment with hymenoptera (bee, wasp) venom while receiving ACE inhibitors.

Symptomatic hypotension with or without syncope can occur with ACE inhibitors (usually with the first several doses); effects are most often observed in volume-depleted patients; correct volume depletion prior to initiation; close monitoring of patient is required especially with initial dosing and dosing increases; blood pressure must be lowered at a rate appropriate for the patient's clinical condition. Initiation of therapy in patients with ischemic heart disease or cerebrovascular disease warrants close observation due to the potential consequences posed by falling blood pressure (eg, MI, stroke). Use with caution in hypertrophic cardiomyopathy with outflow tract obstruction, severe aortic stenosis, or before, during, or immediately after major surgery. **[U.S. Boxed Warning]: Based on human data, ACEIs can cause injury and death to the developing fetus when used in the second and third trimesters. ACEIs should be discontinued as soon as possible once pregnancy is detected.**

Hyperkalemia may occur with ACE inhibitors; risk factors include renal dysfunction, diabetes mellitus, concomitant use of potassium-sparing diuretics, potassium supplements, and/or potassium-containing salts. Use cautiously, if at all, with these agents and monitor potassium closely. Cough may occur with ACE inhibitors. Other causes of cough should be considered (eg, pulmonary congestion in patients with heart failure) and excluded prior to discontinuation.

May be associated with deterioration of renal function and/or increases in serum creatinine, particularly in patients with low renal blood flow (eg, renal artery stenosis, heart failure) whose glomerular filtration rate (GFR) is dependent on efferent arteriolar vasoconstriction by angiotensin II; deterioration may result in oliguria, acute renal failure, and progressive azotemia. Small increases in serum creatinine may occur following initiation; consider discontinuation only in patients with progressive and/or significant deterioration in renal function. Use with caution in patients with unstented unilateral/bilateral renal artery stenosis. When unstented bilateral renal artery stenosis is present, use is generally avoided due to the elevated risk of deterioration in renal function unless possible benefits outweigh risks.

Rare toxicities associated with ACE inhibitors include cholestatic jaundice (which may progress to fulminant hepatic necrosis), agranulocytosis, neutropenia or leukopenia with myeloid hypoplasia. Patients with collagen vascular diseases (especially with concomitant renal impairment) or renal impairment alone may be at increased risk for hematologic toxicity; periodically monitor CBC with differential in these patients.

Adverse Reactions Note: Frequency ranges include data from hypertension and heart failure trials. Higher rates of adverse reactions have generally been noted in patients with CHF. However, the frequency of adverse effects associated with placebo is also increased in this population.

>10%: Central nervous system: Dizziness (1.6% to 11.9%)

1% to 10%:

Cardiovascular: Orthostatic hypotension (1.4% to 1.9%), palpitation (1.4%)

Central nervous system: Dizziness (1% to 2%; up to 12% in CHF patients), headache (3.2%), fatigue (1% to 2%)

Endocrine & metabolic: Hyperkalemia (2.6%)

Gastrointestinal: Diarrhea (2.2%), nausea/vomiting (1.2% to 2.2%)

Hepatic: Transaminases increased

Neuromuscular & skeletal: Musculoskeletal pain (<1% to 3.3%), noncardiac chest pain (<1% to 2.2%), weakness (1.4%)

Renal: Serum creatinine increased, renal function worsening (in patients with bilateral renal artery stenosis or hypovolemia)

Respiratory: Cough (2.2% to 9.7%)

Miscellaneous: Upper respiratory infection (2.2%)

>1% but ≤ frequency in patients receiving placebo: Sexual dysfunction, fever, flu-like syndrome, dyspnea, rash, headache, insomnia

<1% (Limited to important or life-threatening): Anaphylactoid reaction, angina, angioedema, arthralgia, bronchospasm, cerebral infarction, cerebrovascular accident, gout, hepatitis, hepatomegaly, myalgia, MI, pancreatitis, paresthesia, photosensitivity, pleuritic chest pain, pruritus, rash, renal insufficiency, shock, sudden death, syncope, TIA, tinnitus, urticaria, vertigo. In a small number of patients, a symptom complex of cough, bronchospasm, and eosinophilia has been observed with fosinopril.

Other events reported with ACE inhibitors: Acute renal failure, agranulocytosis, anemia, aplastic anemia, bullous pemphigus, cardiac arrest, eosinophilic pneumonitis, exfoliative dermatitis, gynecomastia, hemolytic anemia, hepatic failure, jaundice, neutropenia, pancytopenia, Stevens-Johnson syndrome, symptomatic hyponatremia, thrombocytopenia. In addition, a syndrome which may include fever, myalgia, arthralgia, interstitial nephritis, vasculitis, rash, eosinophilia and positive ANA, and elevated ESR has been reported for other ACE inhibitors.

Drug Interactions

Avoid Concomitant Use There are no known interactions where it is recommended to avoid concomitant use.

Increased Effect/Toxicity

Fosinopril may increase the levels/effects of: Allopurinol; Amifostine; AzaTHIOprine; CycloSPORINE; Ferric Gluconate; Gold Sodium Thiomalate; Lithium; RiTUXimab

The levels/effects of Fosinopril may be increased by: Angiotensin II Receptor Blockers; Diazoxide; Eplerenone; Herbs (Hypotensive Properties); Loop Diuretics; Potassium Salts; Potassium-Sparing Diuretics; Prostacyclin Analogues; Sirolimus; Temsirolimus; Thiazide Diuretics; Trimethoprim

Decreased Effect

The levels/effects of Fosinopril may be decreased by: Antacids; Aprotinin; Herbs (Hypertensive Properties); Methylphenidate; Nonsteroidal Anti-Inflammatory Agents; Salicylates; Yohimbine

Ethanol/Nutrition/Herb Interactions Herb/Nutraceutical: Avoid bayberry, blue cohosh, cayenne, ephedra, ginger, ginseng (American), kola, licorice (may worsen hypertension). Avoid black cohosh, california poppy, coleus, golden seal, hawthorn, mistletoe, periwinkle, quinine, shepherd's purse (may have increased antihypertensive effect).

Stability Store at 25°C (77°F); excursions permitted to 15°C to 30°C (59°F to 86°F). Protect from moisture by keeping bottle tightly closed.

Mechanism of Action Competitive inhibitor of angiotensin-converting enzyme (ACE); prevents conversion of angiotensin I to angiotensin II, a potent vasoconstrictor; results in lower levels of angiotensin II which causes an increase in plasma renin activity and a reduction in aldosterone secretion; a CNS mechanism may also be involved in hypotensive effect as angiotensin II increases adrenergic outflow from CNS; vasoactive kallikreins may be decreased in conversion to active hormones by ACE inhibitors, thus reducing blood pressure

Pharmacodynamics/Kinetics

Onset of action: 1 hour

Duration: 24 hours

Absorption: 36%

Protein binding: 95%

Metabolism: Prodrug, hydrolyzed to its active metabolite fosinoprilat by intestinal wall and hepatic esterases

Bioavailability: 36%

Half-life elimination, serum (fosinoprilat): 12 hours

Time to peak, serum: ~3 hours

Excretion: Urine and feces (as fosinoprilat and other metabolites in roughly equal proportions, 45% to 50%)

Dosage Oral:

Children ≥6 years and >50 kg: Hypertension: Initial: 5-10 mg once daily (maximum: 40 mg/day)

Adults:

Hypertension: Initial: 10 mg/day; most patients are maintained on 20-40 mg/day (maximum: 80 mg/day). May need to divide the dose into two if trough effect is inadequate; discontinue the diuretic, if possible 2-3 days before initiation of therapy; resume diuretic therapy carefully, if needed.

Heart failure: Initial: 10 mg/day (5 mg if renal dysfunction present) and increase, as needed, to a maximum of 40 mg once daily over several weeks; usual dose: 20-40 mg/day. If hypotension, orthostasis, or azotemia occur during titration, consider decreasing concomitant diuretic dose, if any.

Dosing adjustment/comments in renal impairment: None needed since hepatobiliary elimination compensates adequately diminished renal elimination.

Hemodialysis: Moderately dialyzable (20% to 50%)

Dietary Considerations Should not take a potassium salt supplement without the advice of healthcare provider.

Monitoring Parameters Blood pressure; serum creatinine and potassium; if patient has collagen vascular disease and/or renal impairment, periodically monitor CBC with differential

Test Interactions Positive Coombs' [direct]; may cause false-positive results in urine acetone determinations using sodium nitroprusside reagent

Dosage Forms Excipient information presented when available (limited, particularly for generics); consult specific product labeling.

Tablet, as sodium: 10 mg, 20 mg, 40 mg

Monopril®: 10 mg, 20 mg, 40 mg

◆ **Fosinopril Sodium** *see* Fosinopril *on page* 670

Fosphenytoin (FOS fen i toyn)

U.S. Brand Names Cerebyx®

Canadian Brand Names Cerebyx®

Index Terms Fosphenytoin Sodium

Pharmacologic Category Anticonvulsant, Hydantoin

Additional Appendix Information

Status Epilepticus *on page* 1831

Use Used for the control of generalized convulsive status epilepticus and prevention and treatment of seizures occurring during neurosurgery; indicated for short-term parenteral administration when other means of phenytoin administration are unavailable, inappropriate, or deemed less advantageous (the safety and effectiveness of fosphenytoin in this use has not been systematically evaluated for more than 5 days)

Pregnancy Risk Factor D

Pregnancy Considerations Fosphenytoin is the prodrug of phenytoin. Refer to Phenytoin on page 1186 for additional information.

Lactation Excretion in breast milk unknown/not recommended

Medication Safety Issues

Sound-alike/look-alike issues:

Cerebyx® may be confused with Celebrex®, Celexa™, Cerezyme®

Fosphenytoin may be confused with fospropofol

Overdoses have occurred due to confusion between the **mg per mL concentration** of fosphenytoin (50 mg PE/mL) and **total drug content per vial** (either 100 mg PE/2 mL vial or 500 mg PE/10 mL vial). ISMP recommends that the total drug content per container is identified instead of the concentration in mg per mL to avoid confusion and potential overdosages. Additionally, since most errors have occurred with overdoses in children, they recommend that pediatric hospitals should consider stocking only the 2 mL vial.

Contraindications Hypersensitivity to phenytoin, other hydantoins, or any component of the formulation; patients with sinus bradycardia, sinoatrial block, second- and third-degree AV block, or Adams-Stokes syndrome; occurrence of rash during treatment (should not be resumed if rash is exfoliative, purpuric, or bullous); treatment of absence seizures

Warnings/Precautions Doses of fosphenytoin are expressed as their phenytoin sodium equivalent (PE). Antiepileptic drugs should not be abruptly discontinued. Hypotension may occur, especially after I.V. administration at high doses and high rates of administration. Administration of phenytoin has been associated with atrial and ventricular conduction depression and ventricular fibrillation. Careful cardiac monitoring is needed when administering I.V. loading doses of fosphenytoin. Acute hepatotoxicity associated with a hypersensitivity syndrome characterized by fever, skin eruptions, and lymphadenopathy has been reported to occur within the first 2 months of treatment. Discontinue if skin rash or lymphadenopathy occurs. A spectrum of hematologic effects have been reported with use (eg, neutropenia, leukopenia, thrombocytopenia, pancytopenia, and anemias). Use with caution in patients with hypotension, severe myocardial insufficiency, diabetes mellitus, porphyria, hypoalbuminemia, hypothyroidism, fever, or hepatic or renal dysfunction. Effects with other sedative drugs or ethanol may be potentiated. Safety and efficacy have not been established in children. Severe reactions, including toxic epidermal necrolysis and Stevens-Johnson syndromes, although rarely reported, have resulted in fatalities; drug should be discontinued if there are any signs of rash. Patients of Asian descent with the variant *HLA-B*1502* may be at an increased risk of developing Stevens-Johnson syndrome and/or toxic epidermal necrolysis.

Adverse Reactions The more important adverse clinical events caused by the I.V. use of fosphenytoin or phenytoin are cardiovascular collapse and/or central nervous system depression. Hypotension can occur when either drug is administered rapidly by the I.V. route. Do not exceed a rate of 150 mg phenytoin equivalent/minute when administering fosphenytoin.

The adverse clinical events most commonly observed with the use of fosphenytoin in clinical trials were nystagmus, dizziness, pruritus, paresthesia, headache, somnolence, and ataxia. Paresthesia and pruritus were seen more often following fosphenytoin (versus phenytoin) administration and occurred more often with I.V. fosphenytoin than with I.M. administration. These events were dose and rate related (doses ≥15 mg/kg at a rate of 150 mg/minute). These sensations, generally described as itching, burning, or tingling are usually not at the infusion site. The location of the discomfort varied with the groin mentioned most frequently. The paresthesia and pruritus were transient events that occurred within several minutes of the start of infusion and generally resolved within 10 minutes after completion of infusion.

Transient pruritus, tinnitus, nystagmus, somnolence, and ataxia occurred 2-3 times more often at doses ≥15 mg/kg and rates ≥150 mg/minute.

I.V. administration (maximum dose/rate):

>10%:

Central nervous system: Nystagmus, dizziness, somnolence, ataxia

Dermatologic: Pruritus

1% to 10%:

Cardiovascular: Hypotension, vasodilation, tachycardia

Central nervous system: Stupor, incoordination, paresthesia, extrapyramidal syndrome, tremor, agitation, hypoesthesia, dysarthria, vertigo, brain edema, headache

Gastrointestinal: Nausea, tongue disorder, dry mouth, vomiting

Neuromuscular & skeletal: Pelvic pain, muscle weakness, back pain

Ocular: Diplopia, amblyopia

Otic: Tinnitus, deafness

Miscellaneous: Taste perversion

I.M. administration (substitute for oral phenytoin):

1% to 10%:

Central nervous system: Nystagmus, tremor, ataxia, headache, incoordination, somnolence, dizziness, paresthesia, reflexes decreased

Dermatologic: Pruritus

Gastrointestinal: Nausea, vomiting

Hematologic/lymphatic: Ecchymosis

Neuromuscular & skeletal: Muscle weakness

<1% (Limited to important or life-threatening): Acidosis, acute hepatic failure, acute hepatotoxicity, alkalosis, anemia, atrial flutter, bundle branch block, cardiac arrest, cardiomegaly, cerebral hemorrhage, cerebral infarct, CHF, cyanosis, dehydration, hyperglycemia, hyperkalemia, hypertension, hypochromic anemia, hypokalemia, hypophosphatemia, ketosis, leukocytosis, leukopenia, lymphadenopathy, palpitation, postural hypotension, pulmonary embolus, QT interval prolongation, sinus bradycardia, syncope, Stevens-Johnson syndrome, thrombocytopenia, thrombophlebitis, toxic epidermal necrolysis, ventricular extrasystoles

Drug Interactions

Metabolism/Transport Effects As phenytoin: **Substrate** of CYP2C9 (major), 2C19 (major), 3A4 (minor); **Induces** CYP2B6 (strong), 2C8 (strong), 2C9 (strong), 2C19 (strong), 3A4 (strong)

Avoid Concomitant Use

Avoid concomitant use of Fosphenytoin with any of the following: Nilotinib; Nisoldipine; Ranolazine

Increased Effect/Toxicity

Fosphenytoin may increase the levels/effects of: Alcohol (Ethyl); CNS Depressants

The levels/effects of Fosphenytoin may be increased by: Carbonic Anhydrase Inhibitors; Chloramphenicol; Cimetidine; CYP2C19 Inhibitors (Moderate); CYP2C19 Inhibitors (Strong); CYP2C9 Inhibitors (Moderate); CYP2C9 Inhibitors (Strong)

Decreased Effect

Fosphenytoin may decrease the levels/effects of: Acetaminophen; Chloramphenicol; CYP2B6 Substrates;

CYP2C19 Substrates; CYP2C8 Substrates (High risk); CYP2C9 Substrates (High risk); CYP3A4 Substrates; Maraviroc; Nilotinib; Nisoldipine; Ranolazine; Sorafenib

The levels/effects of Fosphenytoin may be decreased by: Antacids; CYP2C19 Inducers (Strong); CYP2C9 Inducers (Highly Effective); Ketorolac; Mefloquine

Ethanol/Nutrition/Herb Interactions

Ethanol:

Acute use: Avoid or limit ethanol (inhibits metabolism of phenytoin); watch for sedation.

Chronic use: Avoid or limit ethanol (stimulates metabolism of phenytoin).

Stability Refrigerate at 2°C to 8°C (36°F to 46°F). Do not store at room temperature for more than 48 hours. Do not use vials that develop particulate matter. Must be diluted to concentrations of 1.5-25 mg PE/mL, in normal saline or D_5W, for I.V. infusion.

Mechanism of Action Diphosphate ester salt of phenytoin which acts as a water soluble prodrug of phenytoin; after administration, plasma esterases convert fosphenytoin to phosphate, formaldehyde, and phenytoin as the active moiety; phenytoin works by stabilizing neuronal membranes and decreasing seizure activity by increasing efflux or decreasing influx of sodium ions across cell membranes in the motor cortex during generation of nerve impulses

Pharmacodynamics/Kinetics Also refer to Phenytoin monograph for additional information.

Protein binding: Fosphenytoin: 95% to 99% to albumin; can displace phenytoin and increase free fraction (up to 30% unbound) during the period required for conversion of fosphenytoin to phenytoin

Metabolism: Fosphenytoin is rapidly converted via hydrolysis to phenytoin; phenytoin is metabolized in the liver and forms metabolites

Bioavailability: I.M.: Fosphenytoin: 100%

Half-life elimination:

Fosphenytoin: 15 minutes

Phenytoin: Variable (mean: 12-29 hours); kinetics of phenytoin are saturable

Time to peak: Conversion to phenytoin: Following I.V. administration (maximum rate of administration): 15 minutes; following I.M. administration, peak phenytoin levels are reached in 3 hours

Excretion: Phenytoin: Urine (as inactive metabolites)

Dosage The dose, concentration in solutions, and infusion rates for fosphenytoin are expressed as phenytoin sodium equivalents (PE); fosphenytoin should always be prescribed and dispensed in phenytoin sodium equivalents (PE)

Infants and Children (unlabeled use): I.V.:

Loading dose: 10-20 mg PE/kg for the treatment of generalized convulsive status epilepticus

Maintenance dosing: Phenytoin dosing guidelines in pediatric patients are used when dosing fosphenytoin using doses in PE equal to the phenytoin doses (ie, phenytoin 1 mg = fosphenytoin 1 PE); maintenance doses may be started 8-12 hours after a loading dose

Adults:

Status epilepticus: I.V.: Loading dose: 15-20 mg PE/kg I.V. administered at 100-150 mg PE/minute

Nonemergent loading and maintenance dosing: I.V. or I.M.:

Loading dose: 10-20 mg PE/kg I.V. or I.M. (maximum I.V. rate: 150 mg PE/minute)

Initial daily maintenance dose: 4-6 mg PE/kg/day I.V. or I.M.

I.M. or I.V. substitution for oral phenytoin therapy: May be substituted for oral phenytoin sodium at the same total daily dose; however, Dilantin® capsules are ~90% bioavailable by the oral route; phenytoin, supplied as fosphenytoin, is 100% bioavailable by both the I.M. and I.V. routes; for this reason, plasma phenytoin concentrations may increase when I.M. or I.V. fosphenytoin is substituted for oral phenytoin sodium therapy; in clinical trials, I.M. fosphenytoin was administered as a single daily dose utilizing either 1 or 2 injection sites; some patients may require more frequent dosing

Dosing adjustments in renal/hepatic impairment: Phenytoin clearance may be substantially reduced in cirrhosis and plasma level monitoring with dose adjustment advisable; free phenytoin levels should be monitored closely in patients with renal or hepatic disease or in those with hypoalbuminemia; furthermore, fosphenytoin clearance to phenytoin may be increased without a similar increase in phenytoin in these patients leading to increased frequency and severity of adverse events

Dietary Considerations Provides phosphate 0.0037 mmol/mg PE fosphenytoin

Administration

I.M.: May be administered as a single daily dose using either 1 or 2 injection sites.

I.V.: Rates of infusion:

Children: 1-3 mg PE/kg/minute

Adults: Should not exceed 150 mg PE/minute

Monitoring Parameters Continuous blood pressure, ECG, and respiratory function monitoring with loading dose and for 10-20 minutes following infusion; vital signs, CBC, liver function tests, plasma level monitoring (plasma levels should not be measured until conversion to phenytoin is complete, ~2 hours after an I.V. infusion or ~4 hours after an I.M. injection)

Reference Range

Therapeutic: 10-20 mcg/mL (SI: 40-79 μmol/L); toxicity is measured clinically, and some patients require levels outside the suggested therapeutic range

Toxic: 30-50 mcg/mL (SI: 120-200 μmol/L)

Lethal: >100 mcg/mL (SI: >400 μmol/L)

Manifestations of toxicity:

Nystagmus: 20 mcg/mL (SI: 79 μmol/L)

Ataxia: 30 mcg/mL (SI: 118.9 μmol/L)

Decreased mental status: 40 mcg/mL (SI: 159 μmol/L)

Coma: 50 mcg/mL (SI: 200 μmol/L)

Peak serum phenytoin level after a 375 mg I.M. fosphenytoin dose in healthy males: 5.7 mcg/mL

Peak serum fosphenytoin levels and phenytoin levels after a 1.2 g infusion (I.V.) in healthy subjects over 30 minutes were 129 mcg/mL and 17.2 mcg/mL, respectively

Test Interactions Increased glucose, alkaline phosphatase (S); decreased thyroxine (S), calcium (S); serum sodium increased in overdose setting

Additional Information 1.5 mg fosphenytoin is approximately equivalent to 1 mg phenytoin. Equimolar fosphenytoin dose is 375 mg (75 mg/mL solution) to phenytoin 250 mg (50 mg/mL).

Dosage Forms Excipient information presented when available (limited, particularly for generics); consult specific product labeling.

Injection, solution, as sodium: 75 mg/mL (2 mL, 10 mL) [equivalent to phenytoin sodium 50 mg/mL]

Cerebyx®: 75 mg/mL (2 mL, 10 mL) [equivalent to phenytoin sodium 50 mg/mL]

◆ **Fosphenytoin Sodium** *see* Fosphenytoin *on page* 671

Fospropofol (fos PROE po fole)

U.S. Brand Names Lusedra™

Index Terms Aquavan; Fospropofol Disodium; GPI 15715

Pharmacologic Category Sedative

Use Monitored anesthesia care (MAC) sedation in patients undergoing diagnostic or therapeutic procedures

Restrictions Pending information: Per the manufacturer, it is likely that fospropofol will be labeled as a C-II

Pregnancy Risk Factor B

Medication Safety Issues

Product availability: FDA approved December 2008; availability anticipated in April 2009

Sound-alike/look-alike issues:

Fospropofol may be confused with fosaprepitant, fosphenytoin, propofol

High alert medication: The Institute for Safe Medication Practices (ISMP) includes this medication among its list of drugs which have a heightened risk of causing significant patient harm when used in error.

Onset of action: The onset of action will be delayed due to need for conversion to the active metabolite, propofol. If supplemental doses are administered before full effect occurs, the risk of dose-stacking may be elevated resulting in deeper sedation than intended.

Dosage Monitored anesthesia care (MAC) sedation: I.V.: **Note: Onset of effect is delayed as compared to propofol-emulsion due to need for conversion to active component.** If <60 kg, base dosing on 60 kg; however, lower doses may be used to achieve lower levels of sedation. If >90 kg, base dosing on 90 kg.

Healthy adults <65 years or with mild systemic disease (ASA-PS1 or -PS2): *Standard dosing regimen:* Initial: 6.5 mg/kg (maximum initial dose: 577.5 mg or 16.5 mL), followed by supplemental doses of 1.6 mg/kg (maximum supplemental dose: 140 mg or 4 mL) no more frequently than every 4 minutes as needed to achieve desired level of sedation.

Elderly patients ≥65 years or patients with severe systemic disease (ASA-PS3 or -PS4): *Modified dosing regimen:* Initial: 4.9 mg/kg (maximum initial dose: 437.5 mg or 12.5 mL), followed by supplemental doses of 1.2 mg/kg (maximum supplemental dose: 105 mg or 3 mL) no more frequently than every 4 minutes as needed to achieve desired level of sedation.

Dosage adjustment in renal impairment: No dosage adjustment recommended. Use with caution in patients with severe renal impairment (Cl_{cr} <30 mL/minute); limited safety and efficacy data available in these patients.

Dosage adjustment in hepatic impairment: No dosage adjustment recommended. Use with caution in patients with hepatic impairment; has not been adequately studied in this population.

Additional Information Complete prescribing information for this medication should be consulted for additional detail.

Product Availability Lusedra™: FDA approved December 2008; availability anticipated in April 2009

Dosage Forms Excipient information presented when available (limited, particularly for generics); consult specific product labeling.

Injection [preservative-free]:

Lusedra ™: 35 mg/mL (30 mL)

- **Fospropofol Disodium** *see* Fospropofol *on page* 673
- **Fosrenol®** *see* Lanthanum *on page* 856
- **Fragmin®** *see* Dalteparin *on page* 392
- **Froben® (Can)** *see* Flurbiprofen *on page* 643
- **Froben-SR® (Can)** *see* Flurbiprofen *on page* 643
- **Frova®** *see* Frovatriptan *on page* 674

Frovatriptan (froe va TRIP tan)

U.S. Brand Names Frova®

Canadian Brand Names Frova®

Index Terms Frovatriptan Succinate

Pharmacologic Category Antimigraine Agent; Serotonin 5-$HT_{1B, 1D}$ Receptor Agonist

Additional Appendix Information

Antimigraine Drugs: 5-HT_1 Receptor Agonists *on page 1642*

Use Acute treatment of migraine with or without aura in adults

Pregnancy Risk Factor C

Pregnancy Considerations There are no adequate and well-controlled studies using frovatriptan in pregnant women. Use only if potential benefit to the mother outweighs the potential risk to the fetus.

Lactation Excretion in breast milk unknown/use caution

Medication Safety Issues

International issues:

Allegro® [Germany] may be confused with Allegra® which is a brand name for fexofenadine in the U.S.

Allegro®: Brand name for fluticasone in Israel

Contraindications Hypersensitivity to frovatriptan or any component of the formulation; patients with ischemic heart disease or signs or symptoms of ischemic heart disease (including Prinzmetal's angina, angina pectoris, myocardial infarction, silent myocardial ischemia); cerebrovascular syndromes (including strokes, transient ischemic attacks); peripheral vascular syndromes (including ischemic bowel disease); uncontrolled hypertension; use within 24 hours of ergotamine derivatives; use within 24 hours of another 5-HT_1 agonist; management of hemiplegic or basilar migraine; prophylactic treatment of migraine

Canadian labeling: Additional contraindications (not in U.S. labeling): Cardiac arrhythmias, valvular heart disease, congenital heart disease, atherosclerotic disease; management of ophthalmoplegic migraine; severe hepatic impairment

Warnings/Precautions Not intended for migraine prophylaxis, or treatment of cluster headaches, hemiplegic or basilar migraines. Rule out underlying neurologic disease in patients with atypical headache, migraine (with no prior history of migraine) or inadequate clinical response to initial dosing. Cardiac events (coronary artery vasospasm, transient ischemia, MI, ventricular tachycardia/fibrillation, cardiac arrest, and death), cerebral/subarachnoid hemorrhage, stroke, peripheral vascular ischemia, and colonic ischemia have been reported with 5-HT_1 agonist administration. May cause vasospastic reactions resulting in colonic, peripheral, or coronary ischemia. Do not give to patients with risk factors for CAD until a cardiovascular evaluation has been performed; if evaluation is satisfactory, the healthcare provider should administer the first dose and cardiovascular status should be periodically evaluated. Significant elevation in blood pressure, including hypertensive crisis, has also been reported on rare occasions in patients using other 5-HT_{1D} agonists with and without a history of hypertension. May lower seizure threshold, use caution in epilepsy or structural brain lesions. Symptoms of agitation, confusion, hallucinations, hyper-reflexia, myoclonus, shivering, and tachycardia (serotonin syndrome) may occur with concomitant proserotonergic drugs (ie, SSRIs/SNRIs or triptans) or agents which reduce frovatriptan's metabolism. Safety and efficacy in pediatric patients have not been established.

Adverse Reactions

1% to 10%:

Cardiovascular: Chest pain (2%), flushing (4%), palpitation (1%)

Central nervous system: Dizziness (8%), fatigue (5%), headache (4%), hot or cold sensation (3%), anxiety (1%), dysesthesia (1%), hypoesthesia (1%), insomnia (1%), pain (1%)

Gastrointestinal: Xerostomia (3%), dyspepsia (2%), abdominal pain (1%), diarrhea (1%), vomiting (1%)

Neuromuscular & skeletal: Paresthesia (4%), skeletal pain (3%)

Ocular: Vision abnormal (1%)
Otic: Tinnitus (1%)
Respiratory: Rhinitis (1%), sinusitis (1%)
Miscellaneous: Diaphoresis (1%)

<1% (Limited to important or life-threatening): Abnormal dreaming, abnormal gait, abnormal lacrimation, abnormal reflexes, abnormal urine, agitation, amnesia, arthralgia, arthrosis, ataxia, back pain, bradycardia, bullous eruption, cheilitis, concentration impaired, confusion, conjunctivitis, constipation, dehydration, depersonalization, depression, dysphagia, dyspnea, earache, ECG changes, emotional lability, epistaxis, eructation, esophagospasm, euphoria, eye pain, fever, gastroesophageal reflux, hiccup, hot flushes, hyperacusis, hyperesthesia, hypertonia, hyperventilation, hypocalcemia, hypoglycemia, hypotonia, involuntary muscle contractions, laryngitis, leg cramps, malaise, micturition, muscle weakness, myalgia, nervousness, nocturia, peptic ulcer, personality disorder, pharyngitis, polyuria, pruritus, purpura, renal pain, rigors, saliva increased, salivary gland pain, seizure, speech disorder, stomatitis, syncope, tachycardia, taste perversion, thirst, tongue paralysis, toothache, tremor, unspecified pain, urinary frequency, vertigo, weakness

Drug Interactions

Metabolism/Transport Effects **Substrate** of CYP1A2 (minor)

Avoid Concomitant Use

Avoid concomitant use of Frovatriptan with any of the following: Ergot Derivatives; Sibutramine

Increased Effect/Toxicity

Frovatriptan may increase the levels/effects of: Ergot Derivatives; Serotonin Modulators

The levels/effects of Frovatriptan may be increased by: Ergot Derivatives; Sibutramine

Decreased Effect There are no known significant interactions involving a decrease in effect.

Ethanol/Nutrition/Herb Interactions Food: Food does not affect frovatriptan bioavailability.

Stability Store at room temperature of 25°C (77°F); excursions permitted to 15°C to 30°C (59°F to 86°F). Protect from moisture and light.

Mechanism of Action Selective agonist for serotonin (5-HT_{1B} and 5-HT_{1D} receptor) in cranial arteries to cause vasoconstriction and reduces sterile inflammation associated with antidromic neuronal transmission correlating with relief of migraine.

Pharmacodynamics/Kinetics

Distribution: Male: 4.2 L/kg; Female: 3.0 L/kg
Protein binding: 15%
Metabolism: Primarily hepatic via CYP1A2
Bioavailability: 20% to 30%
Half-life elimination: 26 hours
Time to peak: 2-4 hours
Excretion: Feces (62%); urine (32%)

Dosage Oral: Adults: Migraine:

U.S. labeling: 2.5 mg; if headache recurs, a second dose may be given if first dose provided relief and at least 2 hours have elapsed since the first dose (maximum daily dose: 7.5 mg)

Canadian labeling: 2.5 mg; if headache recurs, a second dose may be given if first dose provided relief and at least 4 hours have elapsed since the first dose (maximum daily dose: 5 mg)

Dosage adjustment in renal impairment: No adjustment necessary

Dosage adjustment in hepatic impairment: No adjustment necessary in mild-to-moderate hepatic impairment; use with caution in severe impairment (has not been studied in severe impairment).

Canadian labeling (not in U.S. labeling): Use is contraindicated in severe hepatic impairment.

Administration Administer with fluids.

Dosage Forms Excipient information presented when available (limited, particularly for generics); consult specific product labeling.

Tablet, as base: 2.5 mg

- ◆ **Frovatriptan Succinate** *see* Frovatriptan *on page* 674
- ◆ **Frusemide** *see* Furosemide *on page* 676
- ◆ **FSH** *see* Follitropin Alfa *on page* 656
- ◆ **FSH** *see* Follitropin Beta *on page* 658
- ◆ **FSH** *see* Urofollitropin *on page* 1531
- ◆ **FTC** *see* Emtricitabine *on page* 513
- ◆ **FTC, TDF, and EFV** *see* Efavirenz, Emtricitabine, and Tenofovir *on page* 509
- ◆ **FU** *see* Fluorouracil *on page* 636
- ◆ **5-FU** *see* Fluorouracil *on page* 636
- ◆ **Ful-Glo®** *see* Fluorescein *on page* 634

Fulvestrant (fool VES trant)

U.S. Brand Names Faslodex®

Index Terms ICI-182,780; Zeneca 182,780; ZM-182,780

Pharmacologic Category Antineoplastic Agent, Estrogen Receptor Antagonist

Use Treatment of hormone receptor positive metastatic breast cancer in postmenopausal women with disease progression following antiestrogen therapy

Unlabeled/Investigational Use Endometriosis; uterine bleeding

Pregnancy Risk Factor D

Pregnancy Considerations Antiestrogenic compounds have been associated with embryotoxicity, abnormalities in fetal development, and failure to maintain pregnancy in animal models. Approved for use only in postmenopausal women.

Lactation Excretion in breast milk unknown/contraindicated

Contraindications Hypersensitivity to fulvestrant or any component of the formulation; contraindications to I.M. injections (bleeding diatheses, thrombocytopenia, or therapeutic anticoagulation); pregnancy

Warnings/Precautions Hazardous agent - use appropriate precautions for handling and disposal. Use caution in hepatic impairment. Safety and efficacy have not been established in children.

Adverse Reactions

>10%:

Cardiovascular: Vasodilation (18%)
Central nervous system: Pain (19%), headache (15%)
Endocrine & metabolic: Hot flushes (19% to 24%)
Gastrointestinal: Nausea (26%), vomiting (13%), constipation (13%), diarrhea (12%), abdominal pain (12%)
Local: Injection site reaction (11%)
Neuromuscular & skeletal: Weakness (23%), bone pain (16%), back pain (14%)
Respiratory: Pharyngitis (16%), dyspnea (15%)

1% to 10%:

Cardiovascular: Edema (9%), chest pain (7%)
Central nervous system: Dizziness (7%), insomnia (7%), paresthesia (6%), fever (6%), depression (6%), anxiety (5%)
Dermatologic: Rash (7%)
Gastrointestinal: Anorexia (9%), weight gain (1% to 2%)
Genitourinary: Pelvic pain (10%), urinary tract infection (6%), vaginitis (2% to 3%)
Hematologic: Anemia (5%)
Neuromuscular & skeletal: Arthritis (3%)
Respiratory: Cough (10%)
Miscellaneous: Diaphoresis increased (5%)

<1% (limited to important or life-threatening): Angioedema, hypersensitivity reactions, leukopenia, myalgia, thrombosis, urticaria, vaginal bleeding, vertigo

Drug Interactions

Metabolism/Transport Effects Substrate of CYP3A4 (minor)

Avoid Concomitant Use There are no known interactions where it is recommended to avoid concomitant use.

Increased Effect/Toxicity There are no known significant interactions involving an increase in effect.

Decreased Effect There are no known significant interactions involving a decrease in effect.

Stability Store under refrigeration at 2°C to 8°C (36°F to 46°F).

Mechanism of Action Steroidal compound which competitively binds to estrogen receptors on tumors and other tissue targets, producing a nuclear complex that decreases DNA synthesis and inhibits estrogen effects. Fulvestrant has no estrogen-receptor agonist activity. Causes down-regulation of estrogen receptors and inhibits tumor growth.

Pharmacodynamics/Kinetics

Duration: I.M.: Plasma levels maintained for at least 1 month

Distribution: V_d: 3-5 L/kg

Protein binding: 99%

Metabolism: Hepatic via multiple pathways (CYP3A4 substrate, relative contribution to metabolism unknown)

Bioavailability: Oral: Poor

Half-life elimination: ~40 days

Time to peak, plasma: I.M.: 7-9 days

Excretion: Feces (>90%); urine (<1%)

Dosage I.M.: Adults (postmenopausal women): 250 mg at 1-month intervals

Dosage adjustment in renal impairment: No adjustment required.

Dosage adjustment in hepatic impairment: Use in moderate-to-severe hepatic impairment has not been evaluated; use caution.

Administration I.M. injection into a relatively large muscle (ie, buttock); do not administer I.V., SubQ, or intra-arterially. May be administered as a single 5 mL injection or two concurrent 2.5 mL injections.

Dosage Forms Excipient information presented when available (limited, particularly for generics); consult specific product labeling.

Injection, solution:

Faslodex®: 50 mg/mL (2.5 mL, 5 mL) [contains alcohol, benzyl alcohol, benzyl stearate, castor oil]

◆ **FungiGuard [OTC]** *see* Tolnaftate *on page* 1487

◆ **Fungizone® (Can)** *see* Amphotericin B (Conventional) *on page* 104

◆ **Fungoid® Tincture [OTC]** *see* Miconazole *on page* 989

◆ **Furadantin®** *see* Nitrofurantoin *on page* 1072

◆ **Furazosin** *see* Prazosin *on page* 1229

Furosemide (fyoor OH se mide)

U.S. Brand Names Lasix®

Canadian Brand Names Apo-Furosemide®; Dom-Furosemide; Furosemide Injection, USP; Furosemide Special; Lasix®; Lasix® Special; Novo-Semide; Nu-Furosemide; PMS-Furosemide

Index Terms Frusemide

Pharmacologic Category Diuretic, Loop

Additional Appendix Information

Heart Failure (Systolic) *on page* 1809

Hemodynamic Support, Intravenous *on page* 1657

Sulfonamide Derivatives *on page* 1671

Use Management of edema associated with congestive heart failure and hepatic or renal disease; alone or in combination with antihypertensives in treatment of hypertension

Pregnancy Risk Factor C

Pregnancy Considerations Crosses the placenta. Increased fetal urine production, electrolyte disturbances reported. Generally, use of diuretics during pregnancy is avoided due to risk of decreased placental perfusion.

Lactation Enters breast milk/use caution

Medication Safety Issues

Sound-alike/look-alike issues:

Furosemide may be confused with torsemide

Lasix® may be confused with Esidrix®, Lanoxin®, Lidex®, Lomotil®, Luvox®, Luxiq®

International issues:

Urex® [Australia] may be confused with Eurax® which is a brand name for crotamiton in the U.S.

Urex® [Australia]: Brand name for methenamine in the U.S.

Contraindications Hypersensitivity to furosemide, any component, or sulfonylureas; anuria; patients with hepatic coma or in states of severe electrolyte depletion until the condition improves or is corrected

Warnings/Precautions Loop diuretics are potent diuretics; excess amounts can lead to profound diuresis with fluid and electrolyte loss; close medical supervision and dose evaluation are required. Watch for and correct electrolyte disturbances; adjust dose to avoid dehydration. In cirrhosis, avoid electrolyte and acid/base imbalances that might lead to hepatic encephalopathy. Coadministration of antihypertensives may increase the risk of hypotension.

Monitor fluid status and renal function in an attempt to prevent oliguria, azotemia, and reversible increases in BUN and creatinine; close medical supervision of aggressive diuresis is required. Rapid I.V. administration, renal impairment, excessive doses, and concurrent use of other ototoxins is associated with ototoxicity. Asymptomatic hyperuricemia has been reported with use.

Chemical similarities are present among sulfonamides, sulfonylureas, carbonic anhydrase inhibitors, thiazides, and loop diuretics (except ethacrynic acid). Use in patients with sulfonylurea allergy is specifically contraindicated in product labeling, however, a risk of cross-reaction exists in patients with allergy to any of these compounds; avoid use when previous reaction has been severe. Discontinue if signs of hypersensitivity are noted.

Adverse Reactions Frequency not defined.

Cardiovascular: Acute hypotension, chronic aortitis, necrotizing angiitis, orthostatic hypotension, thrombophlebitis, sudden death from cardiac arrest (with I.V. or I.M. administration)

Central nervous system: Blurred vision, dizziness, fever, headache, lightheadedness, restlessness, vertigo, xanthopsia

Dermatologic: Cutaneous vasculitis, erythema multiforme, exfoliative dermatitis, photosensitivity, pruritus, purpura, rash, urticaria

Endocrine & metabolic: Gout, hyperglycemia, hyperuricemia, hypocalcemia, hypochloremia, hypokalemia, hypomagnesemia, hyponatremia, metabolic alkalosis

Gastrointestinal: Anorexia, constipation, cramping, diarrhea, intrahepatic cholestatic jaundice, ischemia hepatitis, nausea, oral and gastric irritation, pancreatitis, vomiting

Genitourinary: Urinary bladder spasm, urinary frequency

Hematological: Agranulocytosis (rare), anemia, aplastic anemia (rare), hemolytic anemia, leukopenia, purpura, thrombocytopenia

Neuromuscular & skeletal: Muscle spasm, paresthesia, weakness

Otic: Hearing impairment (reversible or permanent with rapid I.V. or I.M. administration), reversible deafness (with rapid I.V. or I.M. administration), tinnitus

Renal: Allergic interstitial nephritis, fall in glomerular filtration rate and renal blood flow (due to overdiuresis), glycosuria, transient rise in BUN, vasculitis

Miscellaneous: Anaphylaxis (rare), exacerbate or activate systemic lupus erythematosus

Drug Interactions

Avoid Concomitant Use There are no known interactions where it is recommended to avoid concomitant use.

Increased Effect/Toxicity

Furosemide may increase the levels/effects of: ACE Inhibitors; Allopurinol; Amifostine; Aminoglycosides; Dofetilide; Neuromuscular-Blocking Agents; RiTUXimab

The levels/effects of Furosemide may be increased by: Corticosteroids (Orally Inhaled); Corticosteroids (Systemic); Diazoxide; Herbs (Hypotensive Properties); Prostacyclin Analogues

Decreased Effect

Furosemide may decrease the levels/effects of: Neuromuscular-Blocking Agents

The levels/effects of Furosemide may be decreased by: Aliskiren; Bile Acid Sequestrants; Herbs (Hypertensive Properties); Methylphenidate; Nonsteroidal Anti-Inflammatory Agents; Phenytoin; Yohimbine

Ethanol/Nutrition/Herb Interactions

Food: Furosemide serum levels may be decreased if taken with food.

Herb/Nutraceutical: Avoid dong quai if using for hypertension (has estrogenic activity). Avoid ephedra, yohimbe, and ginseng (may worsen hypertension). Limit intake of natural licorice. Avoid garlic (may have increased antihypertensive effect).

Stability Furosemide injection should be stored at controlled room temperature and protected from light. Exposure to light may cause discoloration; do not use furosemide solutions if they have a yellow color. Furosemide solutions are unstable in acidic media, but very stable in basic media Refrigeration may result in precipitation or crystallization, however, resolubilization at room temperature or warming may be performed without affecting the drug's stability.

I.V. infusion solution mixed in NS or D_5W solution is stable for 24 hours at room temperature. May also be diluted for infusion 1-2 mg/mL (maximum: 10 mg/mL) over 10-15 minutes (following infusion rate parameters).

Mechanism of Action Inhibits reabsorption of sodium and chloride in the ascending loop of Henle and distal renal tubule, interfering with the chloride-binding cotransport system, thus causing increased excretion of water, sodium, chloride, magnesium, and calcium

Pharmacodynamics/Kinetics

Onset of action: Diuresis: Oral: 30-60 minutes; I.M.: 30 minutes; I.V.: ~5 minutes

Peak effect: Oral: 1-2 hours

Duration: Oral: 6-8 hours; I.V.: 2 hours

Absorption: Oral: 60% to 67%

Protein binding: >98%

Metabolism: Minimally hepatic

Half-life elimination: Normal renal function: 0.5-1.1 hours; End-stage renal disease: 9 hours

Excretion: Urine (Oral: 50%, I.V.: 80%) within 24 hours; feces (as unchanged drug); nonrenal clearance prolonged in renal impairment

Dosage

Infants and Children:

Oral: 0.5-2 mg/kg/dose increased in increments of 1 mg/kg/dose with each succeeding dose until a satisfactory effect is achieved to a maximum of 6 mg/kg/dose no more frequently than 6 hours.

I.M., I.V.: 1 mg/kg/dose, increasing by each succeeding dose at 1 mg/kg/dose at intervals of 6-12 hours until a satisfactory response up to 6 mg/kg/dose.

Adults:

Oral: 20-80 mg/dose initially increased in increments of 20-40 mg/dose at intervals of 6-8 hours; usual maintenance dose interval is twice daily or every day; may be titrated up to 600 mg/day with severe edematous states.

Hypertension (JNC 7): 20-80 mg/day in 2 divided doses

I.M., I.V.: 20-40 mg/dose, may be repeated in 1-2 hours as needed and increased by 20 mg/dose until the desired effect has been obtained. Usual dosing interval: 6-12 hours; for acute pulmonary edema, the usual dose is 40 mg I.V. over 1-2 minutes. If not adequate, may increase dose to 80 mg. **Note:** ACC/AHA 2005 guidelines for chronic congestive heart failure recommend a maximum single dose of 160-200 mg.

Continuous I.V. infusion: Initial I.V. bolus dose 20-40 mg, followed by continuous I.V. infusion doses of 10-40 mg/hour. If urine output is <1 mL/kg/hour, double as necessary to a maximum of 80-160 mg/hour. The risk associated with higher infusion rates (80-160 mg/hour) must be weighed against alternative strategies. **Note:** ACC/AHA 2005 guidelines for chronic congestive heart failure recommend 40 mg I.V. load, then 10-40 mg/hour infusion.

Refractory heart failure: Oral, I.V.: Doses up to 8 g/day have been used.

Elderly: Oral, I.M., I.V.: Initial: 20 mg/day; increase slowly to desired response.

Dosing adjustment/comments in renal impairment: Acute renal failure: High doses (up to 1-3 g/day - oral/I.V.) have been used to initiate desired response; avoid use in oliguric states.

Dialysis: Not removed by hemo- or peritoneal dialysis; supplemental dose is not necessary.

Dosing adjustment/comments in hepatic disease: Diminished natriuretic effect with increased sensitivity to hypokalemia and volume depletion in cirrhosis; monitor effects, particularly with high doses.

Dietary Considerations May cause a potassium loss; potassium supplement or dietary changes may be required. Administer on an empty stomach. May be administered with food or milk if GI distress occurs. Do not mix with acidic solutions.

Administration

I.V.: I.V. injections should be given slowly. In adults, undiluted direct I.V. injections may be administered at a rate of 40 mg over 1-2 minutes; maximum rate of administration for IVPB or continuous infusion: 4 mg/minute. In children, a maximum rate of 0.5 mg/kg/minute has been recommended.

Oral: May be taken with or without food.

Monitoring Parameters Monitor weight and I & O daily; blood pressure, orthostasis, serum electrolytes, renal function; in high doses, monitor hearing

Dosage Forms Excipient information presented when available (limited, particularly for generics); consult specific product labeling.

Injection, solution: 10 mg/mL (2 mL, 4 mL, 10 mL)

Injection, solution [preservative free]: 10 mg/mL (2 mL, 4 mL, 10 mL)

Solution, oral: 10 mg/mL (60 mL, 120 mL) [orange flavor]; 40 mg/5 mL (5 mL, 500 mL) [pineapple-peach flavor]

Tablet: 20 mg, 40 mg, 80 mg

Lasix®: 20 mg

Lasix®: 40 mg, 80 mg [scored]

◆ **Furosemide Injection, USP (Can)** *see* Furosemide *on page 676*

◆ **Furosemide Special (Can)** *see* Furosemide *on page 676*

◆ **Fusilev™** *see* LEVOleucovorin *on page 878*

◆ **Fuzeon®** *see* Enfuvirtide *on page 518*

◆ **FVIII/vWF** *see* Antihemophilic Factor/von Willebrand Factor Complex (Human) *on page 122*

◆ **FXT 40 (Can)** *see* FLUoxetine *on page 638*

◆ **GAA** *see* Alglucosidase Alfa *on page 62*

Gabapentin (GA ba pen tin)

U.S. Brand Names Neurontin®

Canadian Brand Names Apo-Gabapentin®; CO-Gabapentin; DOM-Gabapentin; Gen-Gabapentin; Neurontin®; Novo-Gabapentin; Nu-Gabapentin; PHL-Gabapentin; PMS-Gabapentin; RATIO-Gabapentin; RIVA-Gabapentin

Pharmacologic Category Anticonvulsant, Miscellaneous

Additional Appendix Information

Anticonvulsant Drugs of Choice *on page 1637*

Use Adjunct for treatment of partial seizures with and without secondary generalized seizures in patients >12 years of age with epilepsy; adjunct for treatment of partial seizures in pediatric patients 3-12 years of age; management of postherpetic neuralgia (PHN) in adults

Unlabeled/Investigational Use Social phobia; chronic pain

Pregnancy Risk Factor C

Pregnancy Considerations Animal studies have documented teratogenic effects. There are no adequate and well-controlled studies in pregnant women. Use during pregnancy only if the potential benefit to the mother outweighs the potential risk to the fetus.

Lactation Enters breast milk/use caution

Medication Safety Issues

Sound-alike/look-alike issues:

Neurontin® may be confused with Neoral®, Noroxin®

Contraindications Hypersensitivity to gabapentin or any component of the formulation

Warnings/Precautions Avoid abrupt withdrawal, may precipitate seizures; use cautiously in patients with severe renal dysfunction; male rat studies demonstrated an association with pancreatic adenocarcinoma (clinical implication unknown). May cause CNS depression, which may impair physical or mental abilities. Patients must be cautioned about performing tasks which require mental alertness (eg, operating machinery or driving). Effects with other sedative drugs or ethanol may be potentiated. Pediatric patients (3-12 years of age) have shown increased incidence of CNS-related adverse effects, including emotional lability, hostility, thought disorder, and hyperkinesia. Safety and efficacy in children <3 years of age have not been established.

Adverse Reactions As reported in patients >12 years of age, unless otherwise noted in children (3-12 years)

>10%:

Central nervous system: Somnolence (20%; children 8%), dizziness (17% to 28%; children 3%), ataxia (13%), fatigue (11%)

Miscellaneous: Viral infection (children 11%)

1% to 10%:

Cardiovascular: Peripheral edema (2% to 8%), vasodilatation (1%)

Central nervous system: Fever (children 10%), hostility (children 8%), emotional lability (children 4%), fatigue (children 3%), headache (3%), ataxia (3%), abnormal thinking (2% to 3%; children 2%), amnesia (2%), depression (2%), dysarthria (2%), nervousness (2%), abnormal coordination (1% to 2%), twitching (1%), hyperesthesia (1%)

Dermatologic: Pruritus (1%), rash (1%)

Endocrine & metabolic: Hyperglycemia (1%)

Gastrointestinal: Diarrhea (6%), nausea/vomiting (3% to 4%; children 8%), abdominal pain (3%), weight gain (adults and children 2% to 3%), dyspepsia (2%), flatulence (2%), dry throat (2%), xerostomia (2% to 5%), constipation (2% to 4%), dental abnormalities (2%), appetite stimulation (1%)

Genitourinary: Impotence (2%)

Hematologic: Leukopenia (1%), decreased WBC (1%)

Neuromuscular & skeletal: Tremor (7%), weakness (6%), hyperkinesia (children 3%), abnormal gait (2%), back pain (2%), myalgia (2%), fracture (1%)

Ocular: Nystagmus (8%), diplopia (1% to 6%), blurred vision (3% to 4%), conjunctivitis (1%)

Otic: Otitis media (1%)

Respiratory: Rhinitis (4%), bronchitis (children 3%), respiratory infection (children 3%), pharyngitis (1% to 3%), cough (2%)

Miscellaneous: Infection (5%)

Postmarketing and additional clinical reports (limited to important or life-threatening): Acute renal failure, anemia, angina, angioedema, aphasia, arrhythmias (various), aspiration pneumonia, blindness, bradycardia, bronchospasm, cerebrovascular accident, CNS tumors, coagulation defect, colitis, Cushingoid appearance, dyspnea, encephalopathy, facial paralysis, fecal incontinence, glaucoma, glycosuria, heart block, hearing loss, hematemesis, hematuria, hemiplegia, hemorrhage, hepatitis, hepatomegaly, hyper-/hypotension, hyperlipidemia, hyper-/hypothyroidism, hyper-/hypoventilation, gastroenteritis, heart failure, leukocytosis, liver function tests increased, local myoclonus, lymphadenopathy, lymphocytosis, meningismus, MI, migraine, nephrosis, nerve palsy, non-Hodgkin's lymphoma, ovarian failure, pulmonary thrombosis, pericardial rub, pulmonary embolus, pericardial effusion, pericarditis, pancreatitis, peptic ulcer, purpura, paresthesia, palpitation, peripheral vascular disorder, pneumonia, psychosis, renal stone, retinopathy, skin necrosis, status epilepticus, subdural hematoma, suicidal behavior/ideation, syncope, tachycardia, thrombocytopenia, thrombophlebitis

Drug Interactions

Avoid Concomitant Use There are no known interactions where it is recommended to avoid concomitant use.

Increased Effect/Toxicity

Gabapentin may increase the levels/effects of: Alcohol (Ethyl); CNS Depressants

Decreased Effect

The levels/effects of Gabapentin may be decreased by: Ketorolac; Mefloquine

Ethanol/Nutrition/Herb Interactions

Ethanol: Avoid ethanol (may increase CNS depression).

Food: Does not change rate or extent of absorption.

Herb/Nutraceutical: Avoid evening primrose (seizure threshold decreased). Avoid valerian, St John's wort, kava kava, gotu kola (may increase CNS depression).

Stability Store at 25°C (77°F); excursions permitted to 15°C to 30°C (59°F to 86°F).

Mechanism of Action Gabapentin is structurally related to GABA. However, it does not bind to $GABA_A$ or $GABA_B$ receptors, and it does not appear to influence synthesis or uptake of GABA. High affinity gabapentin binding sites have been located throughout the brain; these sites correspond to the presence of voltage-gated calcium channels specifically possessing the alpha-2-delta-1 subunit. This channel appears to be located presynaptically, and may modulate the release of excitatory neurotransmitters which participate in epileptogenesis and nociception.

Pharmacodynamics/Kinetics

Absorption: 50% to 60% from proximal small bowel by L-amino transport system

Distribution: V_d: 0.6-0.8 L/kg

Protein binding: <3%

Bioavailability: Inversely proportional to dose due to saturable absorption:
900 mg/day: 60%
1200 mg/day: 47%
2400 mg/day: 34%
3600 mg/day: 33%
4800 mg/day: 27%
Half-life elimination: 5-7 hours; anuria 132 hours; during dialysis 3.8 hours
Excretion: Proportional to renal function; urine (as unchanged drug)

Dosage Oral:
Children: Anticonvulsant:
3-12 years: Initial: 10-15 mg/kg/day in 3 divided doses; titrate to effective dose over ~3 days; dosages of up to 50 mg/kg/day have been tolerated in clinical studies
3-4 years: Effective dose: 40 mg/kg/day in 3 divided doses
≥5-12 years: Effective dose: 25-35 mg/kg/day in 3 divided doses
See **"Note"** in adult dosing.
Children >12 years and Adults:
Anticonvulsant: Initial: 300 mg 3 times/day; if necessary the dose may be increased up to 1800 mg/day. Doses of up to 2400 mg/day have been tolerated in long-term clinical studies; up to 3600 mg/day has been tolerated in short-term studies.
Note: If gabapentin is discontinued or if another anticonvulsant is added to therapy, it should be done slowly over a minimum of 1 week
Pain (unlabeled use): 300-1800 mg/day given in 3 divided doses has been the most common dosage range
Adults: Postherpetic neuralgia or neuropathic pain: Day 1: 300 mg, Day 2: 300 mg twice daily, Day 3: 300 mg 3 times/day; dose may be titrated as needed for pain relief (range: 1800-3600 mg/day, daily doses >1800 mg do not generally show greater benefit)

Elderly: Studies in elderly patients have shown a decrease in clearance as age increases. This is most likely due to age-related decreases in renal function; dose reductions may be needed.

Dosing adjustment in renal impairment: Children ≥12 years and Adults: See table.
Hemodialysis: Dialyzable

Gabapentin Dosing Adjustments in Renal Impairment

Creatinine Clearance (mL/min)	Daily Dose Range
≥60	300-1200 mg tid
>30-59	200-700 mg bid
>15-29	200-700 mg daily
15[1]	100-300 mg daily
Hemodialysis[2]	125-350 mg

[1]Cl_{cr}<15 mL/minute: Reduce daily dose in proportion to creatinine clearance.

[2]Single supplemental dose administered after each 4 hours of hemodialysis.

Dietary Considerations May be taken without regard to meals.

Administration Administer first dose on first day at bedtime to avoid somnolence and dizziness. Dosage must be adjusted for renal function; when given 3 times daily, the maximum time between doses should not exceed 12 hours.

Monitoring Parameters Monitor serum levels of concomitant anticonvulsant therapy

Test Interactions False positives have been reported with the Ames N-Multistix SG® dipstick test for urine protein

Dosage Forms Excipient information presented when available (limited, particularly for generics); consult specific product labeling.
Capsule: 100 mg, 300 mg, 400 mg
Neurontin®: 100 mg, 300 mg, 400 mg
Solution, oral:
Neurontin®: 250 mg/5 mL (480 mL) [cool strawberry anise flavor]
Tablet: 100 mg, 300 mg, 400 mg, 600 mg, 800 mg
Neurontin®: 600 mg, 800 mg

Extemporaneous Preparations A 100 mg/mL suspension was stable for 91 days when refrigerated or 56 days when kept at room temperature when compounded as follows:
Triturate sixty-seven 300 mg tablets in a mortar, reduce to a fine powder, then add a small amount of one of the following vehicles to make a paste; then add the remaining vehicle in small quantities while mixing:
Vehicle 1. Methylcellulose 1% (100 mL) and Simple Syrup N.F. (100 mL) mixed together in a graduate, **or**
Vehicle 2. Ora-Sweet® (100 mL) and Ora-Plus® (100 mL) mixed together in a graduate
Shake well before using and keep in refrigerator
Nahata MC, Morosco RS, and Hipple TF, *Stability of Gabapentin in Extemporaneously Prepared Suspensions at Two Temperatures*, American Society of Health System Pharmacists Midyear Meeting, December 7-11, 1997.

◆ **Gabitril®** *see* TiaGABine *on page 1465*

Galantamine (ga LAN ta meen)

U.S. Brand Names Razadyne™; Razadyne™ ER; Reminyl® [DSC]

Canadian Brand Names Reminyl®; Reminyl® ER

Index Terms Galantamine Hydrobromide

Pharmacologic Category Acetylcholinesterase Inhibitor (Central)

Use Treatment of mild-to-moderate dementia of Alzheimer's disease

Unlabeled/Investigational Use Severe dementia associated with Alzheimer's disease; mild-to-moderate dementia associated with Parkinson's disease; Lewy body dementia

Pregnancy Risk Factor B

Pregnancy Considerations In animal studies, there was a slight increased in the incident of skeletal variations when given during organogenesis. Adequate, well-controlled studies in pregnant women do not exist. Should be used in pregnancy only if benefit outweighs potential risk to the fetus.

Lactation Excretion in breast milk unknown/not recommended

Medication Safety Issues
Sound-alike/look-alike issues:
Razedyne™ may be confused with Rozerem™
Reminyl® may be confused with Amaryl®
Due to patient safety concerns regarding prescribing and dispensing errors between Reminyl® and Amaryl®, Reminyl® (galantamine) is being renamed to Razadyne™ (immediate-release) and Razadyne™ ER (extended-release). The brand name Reminyl® was discontinued with the July, 2005 distribution of Razadyne™.

Contraindications Hypersensitivity to galantamine or any component of the formulation; severe liver dysfunction (Child-Pugh score 10-15); severe renal dysfunction (Cl_{cr} <9 mL/minute)

Warnings/Precautions Use caution in patients with supraventricular conduction delays (without a functional pacemaker in place); Alzheimer's treatment guidelines consider bradycardia to be a relative contraindication for use of centrally-active cholinesterase inhibitors. Use caution in patients taking medicines that slow conduction through SA or AV node. Use caution in peptic ulcer disease (or in patients at risk); seizure disorder; asthma; COPD; mild-to-moderate liver dysfunction; moderate renal dysfunction. May cause bladder outflow obstruction. May exaggerate neuromuscular blockade effects of succinylcholine and like agents. May cause nausea, vomiting, diarrhea, weight loss, and anorexia. Safety and efficacy in children have not been established.

Adverse Reactions

>10%: Gastrointestinal: Nausea (6% to 24%), vomiting (4% to 13%), diarrhea (6% to 12%)

1% to 10%:

Cardiovascular: Bradycardia (2% to 3%), syncope (0.4% to 2.2%: dose related), chest pain (≥1%)

Central nervous system: Dizziness (9%), headache (8%), depression (7%), fatigue (5%), insomnia (5%), somnolence (4%)

Gastrointestinal: Anorexia (7% to 9%), weight loss (5% to 7%), abdominal pain (5%), dyspepsia (5%), flatulence (≥1%)

Genitourinary: Urinary tract infection (8%), hematuria (<1% to 3%), incontinence (≥1%)

Hematologic: Anemia (3%)

Neuromuscular & skeletal: Tremor (3%)

Respiratory: Rhinitis (4%)

<1% (Limited to important or life-threatening): Aggression, alkaline phosphatase increased, aphasia, apraxia, ataxia, atrial fibrillation, AV block, bundle branch block, convulsions, dehydration, delirium, diverticulitis, dysphagia, epistaxis, esophageal perforation, fever, gastrointestinal bleeding, heart failure, hyper-/hypokinesia, hypokalemia, hypotension, malaise, melena, MI, palpitation, paranoid reaction, paresthesia, paroniria, postural hypotension, purpura, QT prolongation, rectal hemorrhage, renal calculi, renal failure (due to dehydration), stroke, suicide, supraventricular tachycardia, T-wave inversion, thrombocytopenia, TIA, ventricular tachycardia, vertigo, weakness

Drug Interactions

Metabolism/Transport Effects Substrate (minor) of CYP2D6, 3A4

Avoid Concomitant Use There are no known interactions where it is recommended to avoid concomitant use.

Increased Effect/Toxicity

Galantamine may increase the levels/effects of: Antipsychotics; Beta-Blockers; Cholinergic Agonists; Succinylcholine

The levels/effects of Galantamine may be increased by: Corticosteroids (Systemic); Ginkgo Biloba; Selective Serotonin Reuptake Inhibitors

Decreased Effect

Galantamine may decrease the levels/effects of: Anticholinergics; Neuromuscular-Blocking Agents (Nondepolarizing)

The levels/effects of Galantamine may be decreased by: Anticholinergics

Ethanol/Nutrition/Herb Interactions

Ethanol: Avoid ethanol (may increase CNS adverse events).

Herb/Nutraceutical: St John's wort may decrease galantamine serum levels; avoid concurrent use.

Stability Store at 15°C to 30°C (59°F to 86°F). Do not freeze oral solution; protect from light.

Mechanism of Action Centrally-acting cholinesterase inhibitor (competitive and reversible). It elevates acetylcholine in cerebral cortex by slowing the degradation of acetylcholine. Modulates nicotinic acetylcholine receptor to increase acetylcholine from surviving presynaptic nerve terminals. May increase glutamate and serotonin levels.

Pharmacodynamics/Kinetics

Duration: 3 hours; maximum inhibition of erythrocyte acetylcholinesterase ~40% at 1 hour post 8 mg oral dose; levels return to baseline at 30 hours

Absorption: Rapid and complete

Distribution: 175 L; levels in the brain are 2-3 times higher than in plasma

Protein binding: 18%

Metabolism: Hepatic; linear, CYP2D6 and 3A4; metabolized to epigalanthaminone and galanthaminone both of which have acetylcholinesterase inhibitory activity 130 times less than galantamine

Bioavailability: ~90%

Half-life elimination: 7 hours

Time to peak: Immediate release: 1 hour (2.5 hours with food); extended release: 4.5-5 hours

Excretion: Urine (25%)

Dosage Oral: Adults:

Note: Oral solution and tablet should be taken with breakfast and dinner; capsule should be taken with breakfast. If therapy is interrupted for ≥3 days, restart at the lowest dose and increase to current dose.

Immediate release tablet or solution: Mild-to-moderate dementia of Alzheimer's: Initial: 4 mg twice a day for 4 weeks; if tolerated, increase to 8 mg twice daily for ≥4 weeks; if tolerated, increase to 12 mg twice daily

Range: 16-24 mg/day in 2 divided doses

Extended-release capsule: Initial: 8 mg once daily for 4 weeks; if tolerated, increase to 16 mg once daily for ≥4 weeks; if tolerated, increase to 24 mg once daily

Range: 16-24 mg once daily

Conversion to galantamine from other cholinesterase inhibitors: Patients experiencing poor tolerability with donepezil or rivastigmine should wait until side effects subside or allow a 7-day washout period prior to beginning galantamine. Patients not experiencing side effects with donepezil or rivastigmine may begin galantamine therapy the day immediately following discontinuation of previous therapy (Morris, 2001).

Elderly: No dosage adjustment needed

Dosage adjustment in renal impairment:

Moderate renal impairment: Maximum dose: 16 mg/day.

Severe renal dysfunction (Cl_{cr} <9 mL/minute): Use is not recommended

Dosage adjustment in hepatic impairment:

Moderate liver dysfunction (Child-Pugh score 7-9): Maximum dose: 16 mg/day

Severe liver dysfunction (Child-Pugh score 10-15): Use is not recommended

Dietary Considerations Administration with food is preferred, but not required; should be taken with breakfast and dinner (tablet or solution) or with breakfast (capsule).

Administration Oral: Administer solution or tablet with breakfast and dinner; administer extended release capsule with breakfast. If therapy is interrupted for ≥3 days, restart at the lowest dose and increase to current dose. If using oral solution, mix dose with 3-4 ounces of any nonalcoholic beverage; mix well and drink immediately.

Monitoring Parameters Mental status

Dosage Forms Excipient information presented when available (limited, particularly for generics); consult specific product labeling.

Capsule, extended release, oral, as hydrobromide:

Razadyne™ ER: 8 mg, 16 mg, 24 mg [contains gelatin]

Solution, oral, as hydrobromide:

Razadyne™: 4 mg/mL (100 mL) [with calibrated pipette]

Tablet, as hydrobromide: 4 mg, 8 mg, 12 mg

Razadyne™: 4 mg, 8 mg, 12 mg

◆ **Galantamine Hydrobromide** *see* Galantamine *on page 679*
◆ **GamaSTAN™ S/D** *see* Immune Globulin (Intramuscular) *on page 776*
◆ **Gamimune® N (Can)** *see* Immune Globulin (Intravenous) *on page 777*
◆ **Gamma Benzene Hexachloride** *see* Lindane *on page 889*
◆ **Gamma E-Gems® [OTC]** *see* Vitamin E *on page 1566*
◆ **Gamma-E Plus [OTC]** *see* Vitamin E *on page 1566*
◆ **Gammagard Liquid** *see* Immune Globulin (Intravenous) *on page 777*
◆ **Gammagard S/D** *see* Immune Globulin (Intravenous) *on page 777*
◆ **Gamma Globulin** *see* Immune Globulin (Intramuscular) *on page 776*
◆ **Gamma Hydroxybutyric Acid** *see* Sodium Oxybate *on page 1384*
◆ **Gammaphos** *see* Amifostine *on page 82*
◆ **Gammar®-P I.V. [DSC]** *see* Immune Globulin (Intravenous) *on page 777*
◆ **Gamunex®** *see* Immune Globulin (Intravenous) *on page 777*

Ganciclovir (gan SYE kloe veer)

U.S. Brand Names Cytovene®; Vitrasert®

Canadian Brand Names Cytovene®; Vitrasert®

Index Terms DHPG Sodium; GCV Sodium; Nordeoxyguanosine

Pharmacologic Category Antiviral Agent

Additional Appendix Information

Guidelines for the Prevention of Opportunistic Infections in HIV Infected Persons *on page 1740*

Use

Parenteral: Treatment of CMV retinitis in immunocompromised individuals, including patients with acquired immunodeficiency syndrome; prophylaxis of CMV infection in transplant patients

Oral: Alternative to the I.V. formulation for maintenance treatment of CMV retinitis in immunocompromised patients, including patients with AIDS, in whom retinitis is stable following appropriate induction therapy and for whom the risk of more rapid progression is balanced by the benefit associated with avoiding daily I.V. infusions.

Implant: Treatment of CMV retinitis

Unlabeled/Investigational Use May be given in combination with foscarnet in patients who relapse after monotherapy with either drug

Pregnancy Risk Factor C

Pregnancy Considerations **[U.S. Boxed Warning]: Animal studies have demonstrated carcinogenic and teratogenic effects, and inhibition of spermatogenesis;** contraceptive precautions for female and male patients need to be followed during and for at least 90 days after therapy.

Lactation Excretion in breast milk unknown/contraindicated

Medication Safety Issues

Sound-alike/look-alike issues:

Cytovene® may be confused with Cytosar®, Cytosar-U®

Ganciclovir may be confused with acyclovir

Contraindications Hypersensitivity to ganciclovir, acyclovir, or any component of the formulation; absolute neutrophil count <500/mm^3; platelet count <25,000/mm^3

Warnings/Precautions Hazardous agent - use appropriate precautions for handling and disposal. **[U.S. Boxed Warning]: Granulocytopenia (neutropenia), anemia, and thrombocytopenia may occur.** Dosage adjustment or interruption of ganciclovir therapy may be necessary in patients with neutropenia and/or thrombocytopenia and patients with impaired renal function. **[U.S. Boxed Warning]: Animal studies have demonstrated carcinogenic and teratogenic effects, and inhibition of spermatogenesis;** contraceptive precautions for female and male patients need to be followed during and for at least 90 days after therapy with the drug; take care to administer only into veins with good blood flow. **[U.S. Boxed Warning]: Indicated only for treatment of CMV retinitis in the immunocompromised patient and CMV prevention in transplant patients at risk.**

Adverse Reactions

>10%:

Central nervous system: Fever (38% to 48%)

Dermatologic: Rash (15% oral, 10% I.V.)

Gastrointestinal: Abdominal pain (17% to 19%), diarrhea (40%), nausea (25%), anorexia (15%), vomiting (13%)

Hematologic: Anemia (20% to 25%), leukopenia (30% to 40%)

1% to 10%:

Central nervous system: Confusion, neuropathy (8% to 9%), headache (4%)

Dermatologic: Pruritus (5%)

Hematologic: Thrombocytopenia (6%), neutropenia with ANC <500/mm^3 (5% oral, 14% I.V.)

Neuromuscular & skeletal: Paresthesia (6% to 10%), weakness (6%)

Ocular: Retinal detachment (8% oral, 11% I.V.; relationship to ganciclovir not established)

Miscellaneous: Sepsis (4% oral, 15% I.V.)

<1% (Limited to important or life-threatening): Alopecia, arrhythmia, ataxia, bronchospasm, coma, dyspnea, encephalopathy, eosinophilia, exfoliative dermatitis, extrapyramidal symptoms, hemorrhage, nervousness, pancytopenia, psychosis, renal failure, seizure, SIADH, Stevens-Johnson syndrome, torsade de pointes, urticaria, visual loss

Drug Interactions

Avoid Concomitant Use

Avoid concomitant use of Ganciclovir with any of the following: Imipenem

Increased Effect/Toxicity

Ganciclovir may increase the levels/effects of: Imipenem; Mycophenolate; Reverse Transcriptase Inhibitors (Nucleoside); Tenofovir

The levels/effects of Ganciclovir may be increased by: Mycophenolate

Decreased Effect There are no known significant interactions involving a decrease in effect.

Stability Intact vials should be stored at room temperature and protected from temperatures >40°C Reconstitute powder with unpreserved sterile water **not** bacteriostatic water because parabens may cause precipitation; dilute in 250-1000 mL D_5W or NS to a concentration ≤10 mg/mL for infusion.

Reconstituted solution is stable for 12 hours at room temperature, however, conflicting data indicates that reconstituted solution is stable for 60 days under refrigeration (4°C). Stability of parenteral admixture at room temperature (25°C) and at refrigeration temperature (4°C) is 5 days.

Mechanism of Action Ganciclovir is phosphorylated to a substrate which competitively inhibits the binding of deoxyguanosine triphosphate to DNA polymerase resulting in inhibition of viral DNA synthesis

Pharmacodynamics/Kinetics

Distribution: V_d: 15.26 L/1.73 m^2; widely to all tissues including CSF and ocular tissue

Protein binding: 1% to 2%

Bioavailability: Oral: Fasting: 5%; Following food: 6% to 9%; Following fatty meal: 28% to 31%

Half-life elimination: 1.7-5.8 hours; prolonged with renal impairment; End-stage renal disease: 5-28 hours

Excretion: Urine (80% to 99% as unchanged drug)

Dosage

CMV retinitis: Slow I.V. infusion (dosing is based on total body weight):

Children >3 months and Adults:

Induction therapy: 5 mg/kg/dose every 12 hours for 14-21 days followed by maintenance therapy

Maintenance therapy: 5 mg/kg/day as a single daily dose for 7 days/week or 6 mg/kg/day for 5 days/week

CMV retinitis: Oral: 1000 mg 3 times/day with food **or** 500 mg 6 times/day with food

Prevention of CMV disease in patients with advanced HIV infection and normal renal function: Oral: 1000 mg 3 times/day with food

Prevention of CMV disease in transplant patients: Same initial and maintenance dose as CMV retinitis except duration of initial course is 7-14 days, duration of maintenance therapy is dependent on clinical condition and degree of immunosuppression

Intravitreal implant: One implant for 5- to 8-month period; following depletion of ganciclovir, as evidenced by progression of retinitis, implant may be removed and replaced

Elderly: Refer to adult dosing; in general, dose selection should be cautious, reflecting greater frequency of organ impairment

Dosing adjustment in renal impairment:

I.V. (Induction):

Cl_{cr} 50-69 mL/minute: Administer 2.5 mg/kg/dose every 12 hours

Cl_{cr} 25-49 mL/minute: Administer 2.5 mg/kg/dose every 24 hours

Cl_{cr} 10-24 mL/minute: Administer 1.25 mg/kg/dose every 24 hours

Cl_{cr} <10 mL/minute: Administer 1.25 mg/kg/dose 3 times/week following hemodialysis

I.V. (Maintenance):

Cl_{cr} 50-69 mL/minute: Administer 2.5 mg/kg/dose every 24 hours

Cl_{cr} 25-49 mL/minute: Administer 1.25 mg/kg/dose every 24 hours

Cl_{cr} 10-24 mL/minute: Administer 0.625 mg/kg/dose every 24 hours

Cl_{cr} <10 mL/minute: Administer 0.625 mg/kg/dose 3 times/week following hemodialysis

Oral:

Cl_{cr} 50-69 mL/minute: Administer 1500 mg/day or 500 mg 3 times/day

Cl_{cr} 25-49 mL/minute: Administer 1000 mg/day or 500 mg twice daily

Cl_{cr} 10-24 mL/minute: Administer 500 mg/day

Cl_{cr} <10 mL/minute: Administer 500 mg 3 times/week following hemodialysis

Hemodialysis effects: Dialyzable (50%) following hemodialysis; administer dose postdialysis. During peritoneal dialysis, dose as for Cl_{cr} <10 mL/minute. During continuous arteriovenous or venovenous hemofiltration, administer 2.5 mg/kg/dose every 24 hours.

Dietary Considerations Sodium content of 500 mg vial: 46 mg

Administration

Oral: Should be administered with food.

I.V.: Should not be administered by I.M., SubQ, or rapid IVP; administer by slow I.V. infusion over at least 1 hour

Monitoring Parameters CBC with differential and platelet count, serum creatinine, ophthalmologic exams

Dosage Forms Excipient information presented when available (limited, particularly for generics); consult specific product labeling.

Capsule: 250 mg, 500 mg

Implant, intravitreal:

Vitrasert®: 4.5 mg [released gradually over 5-8 months]

Injection, powder for reconstitution, as sodium:

Cytovene®: 500 mg

◆ **Ganidin NR** *see* GuaiFENesin *on page 709*

Ganirelix (ga ni REL ix)

Canadian Brand Names Orgalutran®

Index Terms Antagon; Ganirelix Acetate

Pharmacologic Category Gonadotropin Releasing Hormone Antagonist

Use Inhibits premature luteinizing hormone (LH) surges in women undergoing controlled ovarian hyperstimulation

Pregnancy Risk Factor X

Pregnancy Considerations Fetal resorption occurred in pregnant rats and rabbits. These effects are results of hormonal alterations and could result in fetal loss in humans. The drug should not be used in pregnant women.

Lactation Excretion in breast milk unknown/not recommended

Medication Safety Issues

International issues:

Antagon® (former U.S. brand name for ganirelix): Brand name for astemizole in Mexico; brand name for ranitidine in Brazil

Contraindications Hypersensitivity to ganirelix or any component of the formulation; hypersensitivity to gonadotropin-releasing hormone (GnRH) or any other GnRH analog; known or suspected pregnancy

Warnings/Precautions Should only be prescribed by fertility specialists. Hypersensitivity reactions, including anaphylactoid reactions, have been reported; may occur with the first dose. The packaging contains natural rubber latex (may cause allergic reactions). Pregnancy must be excluded before starting medication.

Adverse Reactions

1% to 10%:

Central nervous system: Headache (3%)

Endocrine & metabolic: Ovarian hyperstimulation syndrome (2%)

Gastrointestinal: Abdominal pain (1%), nausea (1%)

Genitourinary: Pelvic pain (5%), vaginal bleeding (2%)

Local: Injection site reaction (1%)

<1% (Limited to important or life-threatening): Anaphylactoid reaction, hypersensitivity

Drug Interactions

Avoid Concomitant Use There are no known interactions where it is recommended to avoid concomitant use.

Increased Effect/Toxicity There are no known significant interactions involving an increase in effect.

Decreased Effect There are no known significant interactions involving a decrease in effect.

Stability Store at controlled room temperature of 25°C (77°F); excursions permitted to 15°C to 30°C (59°F to 86°F). Protect from light.

Mechanism of Action Competitively blocks the gonadotropin-release hormone receptors on the pituitary gonadotroph and transduction pathway. This suppresses gonadotropin secretion and luteinizing hormone secretion preventing ovulation until the follicles are of adequate size.

Pharmacodynamics/Kinetics

Duration: <48 hours

Absorption: SubQ: Rapid

Distribution: Mean V_d: Single dose: 43.7 L; Multiple dosing: 76.5 L

Protein binding: 81.9%

Metabolism: Hepatic to two primary metabolites (1-4 and 1-6 peptide)

Bioavailability: SubQ: 91.1%

Half-life elimination: Single dose: 12.8 hours; Multiple dosing: 16.2 hours

Time to peak: 1.1 hours

Excretion: Feces (75%) within 288 hours; urine (22%) within 24 hours

Dosage Adult: SubQ: 250 mcg/day during the mid-to-late phase after initiating follicle-stimulating hormone on day 2 or 3 of cycle. Treatment should be continued daily until the day of chorionic gonadotropin administration.

Administration Administer SubQ in abdomen (around upper navel) or upper thigh; rotate injection site.

Monitoring Parameters Ultrasound to assess follicle size

Dosage Forms Excipient information presented when available (limited, particularly for generics); consult specific product labeling.

Injection, solution, as acetate: 250 mcg/0.5 mL [prefilled glass syringe with 27-gauge x 1/2 inch needle]

- ◆ **Ganirelix Acetate** *see* Ganirelix *on page 682*
- ◆ **Gani-Tuss DM NR** *see* Guaifenesin and Dextromethorphan *on page 710*
- ◆ **Gani-Tuss® NR** *see* Guaifenesin and Codeine *on page 710*
- ◆ **Gantrisin®** *see* SulfiSOXAZOLE *on page 1410*
- ◆ **GAR-936** *see* Tigecycline *on page 1469*
- ◆ **Garamycin® (Can)** *see* Gentamicin *on page 692*
- ◆ **Gardasil®** *see* Papillomavirus (Types 6, 11, 16, 18) Vaccine (Human, Recombinant) *on page 1142*
- ◆ **Gastrocrom®** *see* Cromolyn *on page 372*

Gatifloxacin (gat i FLOKS a sin)

U.S. Brand Names Zymar®

Canadian Brand Names Zymar®

Pharmacologic Category Antibiotic, Ophthalmic; Antibiotic, Quinolone

Additional Appendix Information

Antimicrobial Drugs of Choice *on page 1752*

Community-Acquired Pneumonia in Adults *on page 1766*

Use Treatment of bacterial conjunctivitis

Pregnancy Risk Factor C

Pregnancy Considerations Reports of arthropathy (observed in immature animals and reported rarely in humans) have limited the use of fluoroquinolones during pregnancy. Gatifloxacin has been show to be fetotoxic in animal studies. There are no adequate and well-controlled studies in pregnant women. Based on limited data, quinolones are not expected to be a major human teratogen. Although quinolone antibiotics should not be used as first-line agents during pregnancy, when considering treatment for life-threatening infection and/or prolonged duration of therapy, the potential risk to the fetus must be balanced against the severity of the potential illness.

Lactation Excretion in breast milk unknown/use caution

Contraindications Hypersensitivity to gatifloxacin, other quinolone antibiotics, or any component of the formulation

Warnings/Precautions Severe hypersensitivity reactions, including anaphylaxis, have occurred with systemic quinolone therapy. Reactions may present as typical allergic symptoms after a single dose, or may manifest as severe idiosyncratic dermatologic, vascular, pulmonary, renal, hepatic, and/or hematologic events, usually after multiple doses. Prompt discontinuation of drug should occur if skin rash or other symptoms arise. Prolonged use may result in fungal or bacterial superinfection. Do not inject ophthalmic solution subconjunctivally or introduce directly into the anterior chamber of the eye. Contact lenses should not be worn during treatment of ophthalmic infections. Safety and efficacy have not been established in children <1 year of age.

Adverse Reactions

5% to 10%: Ocular: Conjunctival irritation, keratitis, lacrimation increased, papillary conjunctivitis

1% to 4%:

Central nervous system: Headache

Gastrointestinal: Taste disturbance

Ocular: Chemosis, conjunctival hemorrhage, discharge, dry eye, edema, irritation, pain, visual acuity decreased

Drug Interactions

Avoid Concomitant Use

Avoid concomitant use of Gatifloxacin with any of the following: Nilotinib; Tetrabenazine; Thioridazine; Ziprasidone

Increased Effect/Toxicity

Gatifloxacin may increase the levels/effects of: Corticosteroids (Systemic); QTc-Prolonging Agents; Sulfonylureas; Tetrabenazine; Thioridazine; Vitamin K Antagonists; Ziprasidone

The levels/effects of Gatifloxacin may be increased by: Alfuzosin; Ciprofloxacin; Gadobutrol; Insulin; Nilotinib; Nonsteroidal Anti-Inflammatory Agents; Probenecid

Decreased Effect

Gatifloxacin may decrease the levels/effects of: Mycophenolate; Sulfonylureas; Typhoid Vaccine

The levels/effects of Gatifloxacin may be decreased by: Antacids; Calcium Salts; Didanosine; Iron Salts; Magnesium Salts; Quinapril; Sevelamer; Sucralfate; Zinc Salts

Stability Store between 15°C to 25°C (59°F to 77°F); do not freeze.

Mechanism of Action Gatifloxacin is a DNA gyrase inhibitor, and also inhibits topoisomerase IV. DNA gyrase (topoisomerase II) is an essential bacterial enzyme that maintains the superhelical structure of DNA. DNA gyrase is required for DNA replication and transcription, DNA repair, recombination, and transposition; inhibition is bactericidal.

Pharmacodynamics/Kinetics Absorption: Ophthalmic: Not measurable

Dosage Ophthalmic: Children ≥1 year and Adults:

Bacterial conjunctivitis:

Days 1 and 2: Instill 1 drop into affected eye(s) every 2 hours while awake (maximum: 8 times/day)

Days 3-7: Instill 1 drop into affected eye(s) up to 4 times/day while awake

Monitoring Parameters Signs of infection

Dosage Forms Excipient information presented when available (limited, particularly for generics); consult specific product labeling.

Solution, ophthalmic:

Zymar®: 0.3% (5 mL) [contains benzalkonium chloride]

- ◆ **Gaviscon® Extra Strength [OTC]** *see* Aluminum Hydroxide and Magnesium Carbonate *on page 75*
- ◆ **Gaviscon® Liquid [OTC]** *see* Aluminum Hydroxide and Magnesium Carbonate *on page 75*
- ◆ **Gaviscon® Tablet [OTC]** *see* Aluminum Hydroxide and Magnesium Trisilicate *on page 76*
- ◆ **G-CSF** *see* Filgrastim *on page 620*
- ◆ **G-CSF (PEG Conjugate)** *see* Pegfilgrastim *on page 1152*
- ◆ **GCV Sodium** *see* Ganciclovir *on page 681*
- ◆ **GD-Celecoxib (Can)** *see* Celecoxib *on page 290*
- ◆ **GD-Quinapril (Can)** *see* Quinapril *on page 1278*

Gefitinib (ge FI tye nib)

U.S. Brand Names IRESSA®

Index Terms NSC-715055; ZD1839

Pharmacologic Category Antineoplastic Agent, Tyrosine Kinase Inhibitor

Use

U.S. labeling: Treatment of locally advanced or metastatic nonsmall cell lung cancer after failure of platinum-based and docetaxel therapies. Treatment is limited to patients who are benefiting or have benefited from treatment with gefitinib.

Note: Due to the lack of improved survival data from clinical trials of gefitinib, and in response to positive survival data with another EGFR inhibitor, physicians are advised to use other treatment options in advanced nonsmall cell lung cancer patients following one or two prior chemotherapy regimens when they are refractory/intolerant to their most recent regimen.

Canada labeling: Approved indication is limited to NSCLC patients with epidermal growth factor receptor (EGFR) expression status positive or unknown.

Restrictions As of September 15, 2005, distribution will be limited to patients enrolled in the Iressa Access Program. Under this program, access to gefitinib will be limited to the following groups:

Patients who are currently receiving and benefitting from gefitinib (IRESSA®)

Patients who have previously received and benefited from gefitinib (IRESSA®)

Previously-enrolled patients or new patients in non-Investigational New Drug (IND) clinical trials involving gefitinib (IRESSA®) if these protocols were approved by an IRB prior to June 17, 2005

New patients may also receive Iressa if the manufacturer (AstraZeneca) decides to make it available under IND, and the patients meet the criteria for enrollment under the IND

Additional information on the IRESSA® Access Program, including enrollment forms, may be obtained by calling AstraZeneca at 1-800-601-8933 or via the web at www.Iressa-access.com

Pregnancy Risk Factor D

Pregnancy Considerations Animal studies have demonstrated fetal harm; there are no well-controlled studies in pregnant women. The risk of fetal harm should be carefully weighed. Women of childbearing potential should be advised to avoid pregnancy.

Lactation Excretion in breast milk unknown/not recommended

Medication Safety Issues

Sound-alike/look-alike issues:

Gefitinib may be confused with erlotinib

High alert medication: The Institute for Safe Medication Practices (ISMP) includes this medication among its list of drugs which have a heightened risk of causing significant patient harm when used in error.

Contraindications Hypersensitivity to gefitinib or any component of the formulation; pregnancy

Warnings/Precautions Hazardous agent - use appropriate precautions for handling and disposal. Rare, sometimes fatal, pulmonary toxicity (eg, alveolitis, interstitial pneumonia, pneumonitis) has occurred. Therapy should be interrupted in patients with acute onset or worsening pulmonary symptoms; discontinue gefitinib if interstitial pneumonitis is confirmed. Use caution in hepatic or severe renal impairment. May cause hepatic injury and elevation of transaminases; discontinue if elevations/changes are severe. Interruption of therapy may be required in patients with poorly tolerated diarrhea or adverse skin reactions. Eye pain should be promptly evaluated and therapy may be interrupted based on appropriate medical evaluation; may be reinitiated following resolution of symptoms and eye changes. Safety and efficacy in pediatric patients have not been established.

Adverse Reactions

>10%:

Dermatologic: Rash (43% to 54%), acne (25% to 33%), dry skin (13% to 26%)

Gastrointestinal: Diarrhea (48% to 76%), nausea (13% to 18%), vomiting (9% to 12%)

1% to 10%:

Cardiovascular: Peripheral edema (2%)

Dermatologic: Pruritus (8% to 9%)

Gastrointestinal: Anorexia (7% to 10%), weight loss (3% to 5%), mouth ulceration (1%)

Neuromuscular & skeletal: Weakness (4% to 6%)

Ocular: Amblyopia (2%), conjunctivitis (1%)

Respiratory: Dyspnea (2%), interstitial lung disease (1% to 2%)

<1%: Aberrant eyelash growth, angioedema, corneal erosion and membrane sloughing, epistaxis, erythema multiforme, eye pain, hematuria, hemorrhage, ocular hemorrhaging, ocular ischemia, pancreatitis, toxic epidermal necrolysis, urticaria

Postmarketing and/or case reports: CNS hemorrhage and death were reported in clinical trials of pediatric patients with primary CNS tumors

Drug Interactions

Metabolism/Transport Effects Substrate of CYP3A4 (major); **Inhibits** CYP2C19 (weak), 2D6 (weak)

Avoid Concomitant Use

Avoid concomitant use of Gefitinib with any of the following: Natalizumab; Vaccines (Live)

Increased Effect/Toxicity

Gefitinib may increase the levels/effects of: Natalizumab; Topotecan; Vaccines (Live); Vitamin K Antagonists

The levels/effects of Gefitinib may be increased by: Antifungal Agents (Azole Derivatives, Systemic); CYP3A4 Inhibitors (Moderate); CYP3A4 Inhibitors (Strong); Dasatinib; Trastuzumab

Decreased Effect

Gefitinib may decrease the levels/effects of: Cardiac Glycosides; Vaccines (Inactivated); Vitamin K Antagonists

The levels/effects of Gefitinib may be decreased by: CYP3A4 Inducers (Strong); Deferasirox; Echinacea; Herbs (CYP3A4 Inducers); Rifamycin Derivatives

Ethanol/Nutrition/Herb Interactions Food: Grapefruit juice may increase serum gefitinib concentrations; St John's wort may decrease serum gefitinib concentrations.

Stability Store tablets at controlled room temperature of 20°C to 25°C (68°F to 77°F).

Mechanism of Action The mechanism of antineoplastic action is not fully understood. Gefitinib inhibits tyrosine kinases (TK) associated with transmembrane cell surface receptors found on both normal and cancer cells. One such receptor is epidermal growth factor receptor. TK activity appears to be vitally important to cell proliferation and survival.

Pharmacodynamics/Kinetics

Absorption: Oral: slow

Distribution: I.V.: 1400 L

Protein binding: 90%, albumin and alpha$_1$-acid glycoprotein

Metabolism: Hepatic, primarily via CYP3A4; forms metabolites

Bioavailability: 60%

Half-life elimination: I.V.: 48 hours

Time to peak, plasma: Oral: 3-7 hours

Excretion: Feces (86%); urine (<4%)

Dosage Note: In response to the lack of improved survival data from the ISEL trial, AstraZeneca has temporarily suspended promotion of this drug.

Oral: Adults: 250 mg/day; consider 500 mg/day in patients receiving effective CYP3A4 inducers (eg, rifampin, phenytoin)

Dosage adjustment in renal/hepatic impairment: No adjustment necessary

Dosage adjustment for toxicity: Consider interruption of therapy in any patient with evidence of pulmonary decompensation or severe hepatic injury; discontinuation may be required if toxicity is confirmed. Poorly tolerated diarrhea or adverse skin reactions may be managed by a brief interruption of therapy (up to 14 days), followed by reinitiation of therapy at 250 mg/day. Eye pain should be promptly evaluated and therapy may be interrupted based on appropriate medical evaluation; may be reinitiated following resolution of symptoms and eye changes.

Dietary Considerations Food does not affect gefitinib absorption.

Administration May administer with or without food.

For patients unable to swallow tablets or for administration via NG tube: Tablets may be dispersed in noncarbonated drinking water. Drop whole tablet (do not crush) into 1/2 glass of water; stir until tablet is dispersed (~10 minutes). Drink immediately. Rinse with 1/2 glass of water and drink.

Monitoring Parameters Periodic liver function tests (asymptomatic increases in liver enzymes have occurred)

Dosage Forms Excipient information presented when available (limited, particularly for generics); consult specific product labeling.

Tablet: 250 mg

Gelatin, Pectin, and Methylcellulose

(JEL a tin, PEK tin, & meth il SEL yoo lose)

Index Terms Methylcellulose, Gelatin, and Pectin; Pectin, Gelatin, and Methylcellulose

Pharmacologic Category Topical Skin Product

Use Temporary relief from minor oral irritations

Dosage Press small dabs into place until the involved area is coated with a thin film; do not try to spread onto area; may be used as often as needed

Additional Information Complete prescribing information for this medication should be consulted for additional detail.

Dosage Forms Excipient information presented when available (limited, particularly for generics); consult specific product labeling.

◆ **Gel-Kam® [OTC]** *see* Fluoride *on page* 635

◆ **Gel-Kam® Rinse** *see* Fluoride *on page* 635

◆ **Gelnique™** *see* Oxybutynin *on page* 1119

◆ **Gelucast®** *see* Zinc Gelatin *on page* 1584

◆ **Gelusil® [OTC]** *see* Aluminum Hydroxide, Magnesium Hydroxide, and Simethicone *on page* 76

◆ **Gelusil® (Can)** *see* Aluminum Hydroxide, Magnesium Hydroxide, and Simethicone *on page* 76

◆ **Gelusil® Extra Strength (Can)** *see* Aluminum Hydroxide and Magnesium Hydroxide *on page* 76

Gemcitabine (jem SITE a been)

U.S. Brand Names Gemzar®

Canadian Brand Names Gemzar®

Index Terms Gemcitabine Hydrochloride; NSC-613327

Pharmacologic Category Antineoplastic Agent, Antimetabolite (Pyrimidine Analog)

Use Treatment of metastatic breast cancer; locally-advanced or metastatic nonsmall cell lung cancer (NSCLC) or pancreatic cancer; advanced, relapsed ovarian cancer

Unlabeled/Investigational Use Treatment of bladder cancer, acute leukemia

Pregnancy Risk Factor D

Pregnancy Considerations Embryotoxicity and fetal malformations (cleft palate, incomplete ossification, fused pulmonary artery, absence of gallbladder) have been reported in animal studies. There are no adequate and well-controlled studies in pregnant women. If patient becomes pregnant, she should be informed of risks.

Lactation Excretion in breast milk unknown/not recommended

Medication Safety Issues

Sound-alike/look-alike issues:

Gemcitabine may be confused with gemtuzumab

Gemzar® may be confused with Zinecard®

High alert medication: The Institute for Safe Medication Practices (ISMP) includes this medication among its list of drugs which have a heightened risk of causing significant patient harm when used in error.

Contraindications Hypersensitivity to gemcitabine or any component of the formulation; pregnancy

Warnings/Precautions Hazardous agent - use appropriate precautions for handling and disposal. Prolongation of the infusion time >60 minutes and more frequent than weekly dosing have been shown to increase toxicity. Gemcitabine can suppress bone marrow function (leukopenia, thrombocytopenia, and anemia); myelosuppression is usually the dose-limiting toxicity. Gemcitabine may cause fever in the absence of clinical infection. Pulmonary toxicity has occurred; discontinue if severe.

Hemolytic uremic syndrome has been reported; monitor for evidence of microangiopathic hemolysis (elevation of bilirubin or LDH, reticulocytosis, severe thrombocytopenia, and/or renal failure); use with caution in patients with preexisting renal impairment. Serious hepatotoxicity has been reported. Use caution with hepatic impairment (history of cirrhosis, hepatitis, or alcoholism) or in patients with hepatic metastases; may lead to exacerbation of hepatic impairment. Use caution with concurrent radiation therapy; radiation toxicity has been reported with concurrent and nonconcurrent administration; may have radiosensitizing activity when gemcitabine and radiation therapy are given ≤7 days apart; optimum regimen for combination therapy has not been determined for all tumor types. Use caution in the elderly; clearance is affected by age. Efficacy in children has not been established

Adverse Reactions

>10%:

Cardiovascular: Peripheral edema (20%), edema (13%)

Central nervous system: Pain (10% to 48%), fever (30% to 41%), somnolence (5% to 11%)

Dermatologic: Rash (24% to 30%), alopecia (15% to 18%), pruritus (13%)

Gastrointestinal: Nausea/vomiting (64% to 71%; grades 3/4: 1% to 13%), constipation (10% to 31%), diarrhea (19% to 30%), stomatitis (10% to 14%)

Hematologic: Anemia (65% to 73%; grade 4: 1% to 3%), leukopenia (62% to 71%; grade 4: ≤1%), neutropenia (61% to 63%; grade 4: 6% to 7%), thrombocytopenia (24% to 47%; grade 4: ≤1%), hemorrhage (4% to 17%; grades 3/4: <1% to 2%); myelosuppression is the dose-limiting toxicity

Hepatic: Transaminases increased (67% to 78%; grades 3/4: 1% to 12%), alkaline phosphatase increased (55% to 77%; grades 3/4: 2% to 16%), bilirubin increased (13% to 26%; grades 3/4: <1% to 6%)

Renal: Proteinuria (10% to 45%; grades 3/4: <1%), hematuria (13% to 35%; grades 3/4: <1%), BUN increased (8% to 16%; grades 3/4: 0%)

Respiratory: Dyspnea (6% to 23%)

Miscellaneous: Flu-like syndrome (19%), infection (8% to 16%; grades 3/4: <1% to 2%)

1% to 10%:

Local: Injection site reactions (4%)

Neuromuscular & skeletal: Paresthesia (2% to 10%)

Renal: Creatinine increased (2% to 8%)

Respiratory: Bronchospasm (<2%)

<1% (Limited to important or life-threatening; reported with single-agent use or with combination therapy, all reported rarely): Adult respiratory distress syndrome, anaphylactoid reaction, anorexia, arrhythmias, bullous skin ▶

eruptions, cellulitis, cerebrovascular accident, CHF, chills, cough, desquamation, diaphoresis, gangrene, GGT increased, headache, hemolytic uremic syndrome (HUS), hepatotoxic reaction (rare), hypertension, insomnia, interstitial pneumonitis, liver failure, malaise, MI, peripheral vasculitis, petechiae, pulmonary edema, pulmonary fibrosis, radiation recall, renal failure, respiratory failure, rhinitis, sepsis, supraventricular arrhythmia, weakness

Drug Interactions

Avoid Concomitant Use

Avoid concomitant use of Gemcitabine with any of the following: Natalizumab; Vaccines (Live)

Increased Effect/Toxicity

Gemcitabine may increase the levels/effects of: Bleomycin; Fluorouracil; Natalizumab; Vaccines (Live); Vitamin K Antagonists

The levels/effects of Gemcitabine may be increased by: Trastuzumab

Decreased Effect

Gemcitabine may decrease the levels/effects of: Vaccines (Inactivated); Vitamin K Antagonists

The levels/effects of Gemcitabine may be decreased by: Echinacea

Ethanol/Nutrition/Herb Interactions Ethanol: Avoid ethanol (due to GI irritation).

Stability Store intact vials at room temperature of 20°C to 25°C (68°F to 77°F). Reconstitute the 200 mg vial with preservative free 0.9% NaCl 5 mL or the 1000 mg vial with preservative free 0.9% NaCl 25 mL. Resulting solution is 38 mg/mL. Dilute with 50-500 mL 0.9% sodium chloride injection or D_5W to concentrations as low as 0.1 mg/mL. Reconstituted vials are stable for up to 35 days and infusion solutions diluted in 0.9% sodium chloride are stable up to 7 days at 23°C when protected from light; however, the manufacturer recommends use within 24 hours for both reconstituted vials and infusion solutions. Do not refrigerate.

Mechanism of Action A pyrimidine antimetabolite that inhibits DNA synthesis by inhibition of DNA polymerase and ribonucleotide reductase, specific for the S-phase of the cycle. Gemcitabine is phosphorylated intracellularly by deoxycytidine kinase to gemcitabine monophosphate, which is further phosphorylated to active metabolites gemcitabine diphosphate and gemcitabine triphosphate. Gemcitabine diphosphate inhibits DNA synthesis by inhibiting ribonucleotide reductase; gemcitabine triphosphate incorporates into DNA and inhibits DNA polymerase.

Pharmacodynamics/Kinetics

Distribution: Infusions <70 minutes: 50 L/m^2; Long infusion times: 370 L/m^2

Protein binding: Low

Metabolism: Metabolized intracellularly by nucleoside kinases to the active diphosphate (dFdCDP) and triphosphate (dFdCTP) nucleoside metabolites

Half-life elimination:

- Gemcitabine: Infusion time ≤1 hour: 42-94 minutes; infusion time 3-4 hours: 4-10.5 hours
- Metabolite (gemcitabine triphosphate), terminal phase: 1.7-19.4 hours

Time to peak, plasma: 30 minutes after completion of infusion

Excretion: Urine (92% to 98%; primarily as inactive uracil metabolite); feces (<1%)

Dosage Refer to individual protocols. **Note**: Prolongation of the infusion time >60 minutes and administration more frequently than once weekly have been shown to increase toxicity. I.V.:

Pancreatic cancer: Initial: 1000 mg/m^2 weekly for up to 7 weeks followed by 1 week rest; then weekly for 3 weeks out of every 4 weeks.

Dose adjustment: Patients who complete an entire cycle of therapy may have the dose in subsequent cycles increased by 25% as long as the absolute granulocyte count (AGC) nadir is >1500 x 10^6/L, platelet nadir is >100,000 x 10^6/L, and nonhematologic toxicity is less than WHO Grade 1. If the increased dose is tolerated (with the same parameters) the dose in subsequent cycles may again be increased by 20%.

Nonsmall cell lung cancer:

1000 mg/m^2 days 1, 8, and 15; repeat cycle every 28 days

or

1250 mg/m^2 days 1 and 8; repeat cycle every 21 days

Breast cancer: 1250 mg/m^2 days 1 and 8; repeat cycle every 21 days

Ovarian cancer: 1000 mg/m^2 days 1 and 8; repeat cycle every 21 days

Bladder cancer (unlabeled use):

- I.V.: 1000 mg/m^2 once weekly for 3 weeks; repeat cycle every 4 weeks
- Intravesicular instillation: 2000 mg (in 100 mL NS; retain for 1 hour) twice weekly for 3 weeks; repeat cycle every 4 weeks (for at least 2 cycles)

Dosing adjustment for toxicity:

Pancreatic cancer: Hematologic toxicity:

- AGC ≥1000 x 10^6/L and platelet count ≥100,000 x 10^6/L: Administer 100% of full dose
- AGC 500-999 x 10^6/L or platelet count 50,000-90,000 x 10^6/L: Administer 75% of full dose
- AGC <500 x 10^6/L or platelet count <50,000 x 10^6/L: Hold dose

Nonsmall cell lung cancer:

- Hematologic toxicity: Refer to guidelines for pancreatic cancer. Cisplatin dosage may also need adjusted.
- Severe (grades 3 or 4) nonhematologic toxicity (except alopecia, nausea and vomiting): Hold or decrease dose by 50%.

Breast cancer:

- Hematologic toxicity: Adjustments based on granulocyte and platelet counts on day 8:
  - AGC ≥1200 x 10^6/L and platelet count >75,000 x 10^6/L: Administer 100% of full dose
  - AGC 1000-1199 x 10^6/L or platelet count 50,000-75,000 x 10^6/L: Administer 75% of full dose
  - AGC 700-999 x 10^6/L and platelet count ≥50,000 x 10^6/L: Administer 50% of full dose
  - AGC <700 x 10^6/L or platelet count <50,000 x 10^6/L: Hold dose
- Severe (grades 3 or 4) nonhematologic toxicity (except alopecia, nausea, and vomiting): Hold or decrease dose by 50%. Paclitaxel dose may also need adjusted.

Ovarian cancer:

- Hematologic toxicity: Adjustments based on granulocyte and platelet counts on day 8:
  - AGC ≥1500 x 10^6/L and platelet count ≥100,000 x 10^6/L: Administer 100% of full dose
  - AGC 1000-1499 x 10^6/L and/or platelet count 75,000-99,999 x 10^6/L: Administer 50% of full dose
  - AGC <1000 x 10^6/L and/or platelet count <75,000 x 10^6/L: Hold dose
- Severe (grades 3 or 4) nonhematologic toxicity (except nausea and vomiting): Hold or decrease dose by 50%. Carboplatin dose may also need adjusted.
- Dose adjustment for subsequent cycles:
  - AGC < 500 x 10^6/L for >5 days, AGC <100 x 10^6/L for >3 days, febrile neutropenia, platelet count <25,000 x 10^6/L, cycle delay >1 week due to toxicity: Reduce gemcitabine to 800 mg/m2 on days 1 and 8.
  - For recurrence of any of the above toxicities after initial dose reduction: Administer gemcitabine 800 mg/m^2 on day 1 only for the subsequent cycle

Dosing adjustment in renal impairment: The FDA-approved labeling does not contain dosing adjustment guidelines; use caution. Gemcitabine has not been studied in patients with significant renal dysfunction.

Dosing adjustment in hepatic impairment: The FDA-approved labeling does not contain dosing adjustment guidelines; use caution. Gemcitabine has not been studied in patients with significant hepatic dysfunction. The following guidelines have been used by some clinicians (Floyd, 2006): Serum bilirubin >1.6 mg/dL: Use starting dose of 800 mg/m^2

Administration Infuse over 30 minutes. **Note**: Prolongation of the infusion time >60 minutes has been shown to increase toxicity. Gemcitabine is being investigated in clinical trials for fixed dose rate (FDR) infusion administration at doses from 1000 mg/m^2 to 2200 mg/m^2 at a rate of 10 mg/m^2/minute. Prolonged infusion times increase the accumulation of the active metabolite, gemcitabine triphosphate. Patients who receive gemcitabine FDR experience more grade 3/4 hematologic toxicity.

Monitoring Parameters CBC with differential and platelet count (prior to each dose); hepatic and renal function (prior to initiation of therapy and periodically, thereafter); monitor electrolytes, including potassium, magnesium, and calcium (when in combination therapy with cisplatin)

Dosage Forms Excipient information presented when available (limited, particularly for generics); consult specific product labeling.

Injection, powder for reconstitution:

Gemzar®: 200 mg, 1 g

◆ **Gemcitabine Hydrochloride** *see* Gemcitabine *on page 685*

Gemfibrozil (jem FI broe zil)

U.S. Brand Names Lopid®

Canadian Brand Names Apo-Gemfibrozil®; Gen-Gemfibrozil; GMD-Gemfibrozil; Lopid®; Novo-Gemfibrozil; Nu-Gemfibrozil; PMS-Gemfibrozil

Index Terms CI-719

Pharmacologic Category Antilipemic Agent, Fibric Acid

Additional Appendix Information

Hyperlipidemia Management *on page 1815*

Lipid-Lowering Agents *on page 1661*

Use Treatment of hypertriglyceridemia in types IV and V hyperlipidemia for patients who are at greater risk for pancreatitis and who have not responded to dietary intervention

Pregnancy Risk Factor C

Lactation Excretion in breast milk unknown/contraindicated

Medication Safety Issues

Sound-alike/look-alike issues:

Lopid® may be confused with Levbid®, Lodine®, Lorabid®, Slo-bid™

Contraindications Hypersensitivity to gemfibrozil or any component of the formulation; significant hepatic or renal dysfunction; primary biliary cirrhosis; pre-existing gallbladder disease

Warnings/Precautions Secondary causes of hyperlipidemia should be ruled out prior to therapy. Possible increased risk of malignancy and cholelithiasis. No evidence of cardiovascular mortality benefit. Anemia and leukopenia have been reported. Elevations in serum transaminases can be seen. Discontinue if lipid response not seen. Be careful in patient selection; this is not a first- or second-line choice. Other agents may be more suitable. Adjustments in warfarin therapy may be required with concurrent use. Has been associated with rare myositis or rhabdomyolysis; patients should be monitored closely. Patients should be instructed to report unexplained muscle pain, tenderness, weakness, or brown urine. Use caution when combining gemfibrozil with HMG-CoA reductase inhibitors (may lead to myopathy, rhabdomyolysis). Renal function deterioration has been seen when used in patients with a serum creatinine >2.0 mg/dL. Safety and efficacy in pediatric patients have not been established.

Adverse Reactions

>10%: Gastrointestinal: Dyspepsia (20%)

1% to 10%:

Central nervous system: Fatigue (4%), vertigo (2%), headache (1%)

Dermatologic: Eczema (2%), rash (2%)

Gastrointestinal: Abdominal pain (10%), diarrhea (7%), nausea/vomiting (3%), constipation (1%)

<1% (Limited to important or life-threatening): Alopecia, anaphylaxis, angioedema, bone marrow hypoplasia, cataracts, cholelithiasis, cholecystitis, depression, dermatomyositis/polymyositis, drug-induced lupus-like syndrome, eosinophilia, exfoliative dermatitis, hypokalemia, impotence, intracranial hemorrhage, jaundice, laryngeal edema, leukopenia, myasthenia, myopathy, nephrotoxicity, pancreatitis, paresthesia, peripheral neuritis, photosensitivity, positive ANA, rash, Raynaud's phenomenon, retinal edema, rhabdomyolysis, seizure, syncope, thrombocytopenia, urticaria, vasculitis

Drug Interactions

Metabolism/Transport Effects **Substrate** of CYP3A4 (minor); **Inhibits** CYP1A2 (moderate), 2C8 (strong), 2C9 (strong), 2C19 (strong)

Avoid Concomitant Use There are no known interactions where it is recommended to avoid concomitant use.

Increased Effect/Toxicity

Gemfibrozil may increase the levels/effects of: Antidiabetic Agents (Thiazolidinedione); CYP1A2 Substrates; CYP2C19 Substrates; CYP2C8 Substrates (High risk); CYP2C9 Substrates (High risk); Ezetimibe; HMG-CoA Reductase Inhibitors; Repaglinide; Sulfonylureas; Vitamin K Antagonists

Decreased Effect

The levels/effects of Gemfibrozil may be decreased by: Bile Acid Sequestrants

Ethanol/Nutrition/Herb Interactions Ethanol: Avoid ethanol to decrease triglycerides.

Mechanism of Action The exact mechanism of action of gemfibrozil is unknown, however, several theories exist regarding the VLDL effect; it can inhibit lipolysis and decrease subsequent hepatic fatty acid uptake as well as inhibit hepatic secretion of VLDL; together these actions decrease serum VLDL levels; increases HDL-cholesterol; the mechanism behind HDL elevation is currently unknown

Pharmacodynamics/Kinetics

Onset of action: May require several days

Absorption: Well absorbed

Protein binding: 99%

Metabolism: Hepatic via oxidation to two inactive metabolites; undergoes enterohepatic recycling

Half-life elimination: 1.4 hours

Time to peak, serum: 1-2 hours

Excretion: Urine (70% primarily as conjugated drug); feces (6%)

Dosage Adults: Oral: 1200 mg/day in 2 divided doses, 30 minutes before breakfast and dinner

Hemodialysis: Not removed by hemodialysis; supplemental dose is not necessary

Dietary Considerations Before initiation of therapy, patients should be placed on a standard cholesterol-lowering diet for 3-6 months and the diet should be continued during drug therapy.

Monitoring Parameters Serum cholesterol, LFTs

Dosage Forms Excipient information presented when available (limited, particularly for generics); consult specific product labeling.

Tablet, oral: 600 mg

Lopid®: 600 mg [scored]

Gemifloxacin (je mi FLOKS a sin)

U.S. Brand Names Factive®

Canadian Brand Names Factive®

Index Terms DW286; Gemifloxacin Mesylate; LA 20304a; SB-265805

Pharmacologic Category Antibiotic, Quinolone; Respiratory Fluoroquinolone

Additional Appendix Information

Community-Acquired Pneumonia in Adults *on page 1766*

Use Treatment of acute exacerbation of chronic bronchitis; treatment of community-acquired pneumonia (CAP), including pneumonia caused by multidrug-resistant strains of *S. pneumoniae* (MDRSP)

Unlabeled/Investigational Use Acute sinusitis

Restrictions An FDA-approved patient medication guide is available and must be distributed when dispensing an outpatient prescription (new or refill) where this medication is to be used without direct supervision of a healthcare provider. Medication guides are available at http://www.fda.gov/cder/Offices/ODS/medication_guides.htm.

Pregnancy Risk Factor C

Pregnancy Considerations Adverse events have been observed in some animal studies; therefore, the manufacturer classifies gemifloxacin as pregnancy category C. Quinolone exposure during human pregnancy has been reported with other agents (see Ciprofloxacin, Ofloxacin, and Norfloxacin monographs). To date, no specific teratogenic effect or increased pregnancy risk has been identified; however, because of concerns of cartilage damage in immature animals exposed to quinolones and the limited gemifloxacin specific data, gemifloxacin should only be used during pregnancy if a safer option is not available.

Lactation Excretion in breast milk unknown/not recommended

Contraindications Hypersensitivity to gemifloxacin, other fluoroquinolones, or any component of the formulation

Warnings/Precautions [U.S. Boxed Warning]: There have been reports of tendon inflammation and/or rupture with quinolone antibiotics; risk may be increased with concurrent corticosteroids, organ transplant recipients, and in patients >60 years of age. Rupture of the Achilles tendon sometimes requiring surgical repair has been reported most frequently; but other tendon sites (eg, rotator cuff, biceps) have also been reported. Strenuous physical activity, rheumatoid arthritis, and renal impairment may be an independent risk factor for tendonitis. Discontinue at first sign of tendon inflammation or pain. May occur even after discontinuation of therapy. Use with caution in patients with rheumatoid arthritis; may increase risk of tendon rupture. Fluoroquinolones may prolong QT_c interval; avoid use of gemifloxacin in patients with a history of QT_c prolongation, uncorrected hypokalemia, hypomagnesemia, or concurrent administration of other medications known to prolong the QT interval (including Class Ia and Class III antiarrhythmics, cisapride, erythromycin, antipsychotics, and tricyclic antidepressants). Use with caution in patients with significant bradycardia or acute myocardial ischemia. Use with caution in individuals at risk of seizures (CNS disorders or concurrent therapy with medications which may lower seizure threshold). Potential for seizures, although very rare, may be increased with concomitant NSAID therapy. Discontinue in patients who experience significant CNS adverse effects (dizziness, hallucinations, suicidal ideation or actions). Use caution in renal dysfunction; dosage adjustment required for Cl_{cr} ≤40 mL/minute.

Fluoroquinolones have been associated with the development of serious, and sometimes fatal, hypoglycemia, most often in elderly diabetics, but also in patients without diabetes. This occurred most frequently with gatifloxacin (no longer available systemically) but may occur at a lower frequency with other quinolones.

Severe hypersensitivity reactions, including anaphylaxis, have occurred with quinolone therapy. Reactions may present as typical allergic symptoms after a single dose, or may manifest as severe idiosyncratic dermatologic, vascular, pulmonary, renal, hepatic, and/or hematologic events, usually after multiple doses. May cause maculopapular rash, usually 8-10 days after treatment initiation; risk factors may include age <40 years, female gender (including postmenopausal women on HRT), and treatment duration >7 days. Prompt discontinuation of drug should occur if skin rash or other symptoms arise. Avoid excessive sunlight and take precautions to limit exposure (eg, loose fitting clothing, sunscreen); may cause moderate-to-severe phototoxicity reactions. Discontinue use if photosensitivity occurs. Prolonged use may result in fungal or bacterial superinfection, including *C. difficile*-associated diarrhea (CDAD) and pseudomembranous colitis; CDAD has been observed >2 months postantibiotic treatment. Peripheral neuropathy has been linked to the use of quinolones; these cases were rare. Hemolytic reactions may (rarely) occur with quinolone use in patients with latent or actual G6PD deficiency. Safety and effectiveness in pediatric patients (<18 years of age) have not been established.

Adverse Reactions

1% to 10%:

Central nervous system: Headache (4%), dizziness (2%)

Dermatologic: Rash (4%)

Gastrointestinal: Diarrhea (5%), nausea (4%), abdominal pain (2%), vomiting (2%)

Hematologic: Neutropenia/neutrophilia (1%), platelets increased (1%), thrombocythemia (1%)

Hepatic: Transaminases increased (1% to 4%), GGT increased (1%)

Neuromuscular & skeletal: CPK increased (1%)

<1% (Limited to important or life-threatening): Acute renal failure, alkaline phosphatase increased, anaphylactic reaction, anemia, anorexia, arthralgia, back pain, bilirubin increased, BUN increased, constipation, cramps (leg), dermatitis, dyspepsia, dyspnea, eczema, eosinophilia, erythema multiforme, facial edema, fatigue, flatulence, flushing, fungal infection, gastritis, gastroenteritis, genital moniliasis, granulocytopenia, hematocrit decreased/increased, hemoglobin decreased/increased, hemorrhage, hot flashes, hyperglycemia, hyper-/hypocalcemia, hyper-/hypokalemia, hyper-/hyponatremia, hypoalbuminemia, INR increased, insomnia, leukopenia, moniliasis, myalgia, nervousness, pain, pharyngitis, photosensitivity, pneumonia, pruritus, pseudomembranous colitis, QT_c prolongation, retinal hemorrhage, serum creatinine increased, skin exfoliation, somnolence, supraventricular tachycardia, syncope, taste perversion, tendonitis, tendon rupture, thrombocytopenia, TIA, tremor, urticaria, vaginitis, vertigo, vision abnormal, weakness, xerostomia

Important adverse effects reported with other agents in this drug class include (not reported for gemifloxacin): Allergic reactions, CNS stimulation, hepatic necrosis/failure, hepatitis, hypersensitivity, jaundice, pancytopenia, peripheral neuropathy, pneumonitis (eosinophilic), seizure, sensorimotor-axonal neuropathy (paresthesia, hypoesthesias, dysesthesias, weakness), serum sickness, severe dermatologic reactions (toxic epidermal necrolysis, Stevens-Johnson syndrome), thrombotic thrombocytopenia purpura, torsade de pointes, vasculitis

Drug Interactions

Avoid Concomitant Use There are no known interactions where it is recommended to avoid concomitant use.

Increased Effect/Toxicity

Gemifloxacin may increase the levels/effects of: Corticosteroids (Systemic); Sulfonylureas; Vitamin K Antagonists

The levels/effects of Gemifloxacin may be increased by: Insulin; Nonsteroidal Anti-Inflammatory Agents; Probenecid

Decreased Effect

Gemifloxacin may decrease the levels/effects of: Mycophenolate; Sulfonylureas; Typhoid Vaccine

The levels/effects of Gemifloxacin may be decreased by: Antacids; Calcium Salts; Didanosine; Iron Salts; Magnesium Salts; Quinapril; Sevelamer; Sucralfate; Zinc Salts

Ethanol/Nutrition/Herb Interactions Herb/Nutraceutical: Avoid dong quai, St John's wort (may also cause photosensitization).

Stability Store at 25°C (77°F). Protect from light.

Mechanism of Action Gemifloxacin is a DNA gyrase inhibitor and also inhibits topoisomerase IV. DNA gyrase (topoisomerase IV) is an essential bacterial enzyme that maintains the superhelical structure of DNA. DNA gyrase is required for DNA replication and transcription, DNA repair, recombination, and transposition; bactericidal

Pharmacodynamics/Kinetics

Absorption: Well absorbed from the GI tract

Distribution: V_{dss}: 4.2 L/kg

Bioavailability: ~71%

Metabolism: Hepatic (minor); forms metabolites (CYP isoenzymes are not involved)

Time to peak, plasma: 0.5-2 hours

Protein binding: ~60% to 70%

Half-life elimination: 7 hours (range 4-12 hours)

Excretion: Feces (61%); urine (36%)

Dosage

Usual dosage range:

Adults: Oral: 320 mg once daily

Indication-specific dosing:

Adults: Oral:

Acute exacerbations of chronic bronchitis: 320 mg once daily for 5 days

Community-acquired pneumonia (mild to moderate): 320 mg once daily for 5 or 7 days (decision to use 5- or 7-day regimen should be guided by initial sputum culture; 7 days are recommended for MDRSP, *Klebsiella*, or *M. catarrhalis* infection)

Sinusitis (unlabeled use): 320 mg once daily for 10 days

Elderly: Refer to adult dosing.

Dosage adjustment in renal impairment:

Cl_{cr} >40 mL/minute: No adjustment required

Cl_{cr} ≤40 mL/minute (or patients on hemodialysis/CAPD): 160 mg once daily (administer dose following hemodialysis)

Dosage adjustment in hepatic impairment: No adjustment required

Dietary Considerations May take tablets with or without food, milk, or calcium supplements. Gemifloxacin should be taken 3 hours before or 2 hours after supplements (including multivitamins) containing iron, zinc, or magnesium.

Administration May be administered with or without food, milk, or calcium supplements. Gemifloxacin should be taken 3 hours before or 2 hours after supplements (including multivitamins) containing iron, zinc, or magnesium.

Monitoring Parameters WBC, signs/symptoms of infection, renal function

Dosage Forms Excipient information presented when available (limited, particularly for generics); consult specific product labeling.

Tablet:

Factive®: 320 mg

◆ **Gemifloxacin Mesylate** *see* Gemifloxacin *on page 688*

Gemtuzumab Ozogamicin

(gem TOO zoo mab oh zog a MY sin)

U.S. Brand Names Mylotarg®

Canadian Brand Names Mylotarg®

Index Terms CMA-676; NSC-720568

Pharmacologic Category Antineoplastic Agent, Monoclonal Antibody

Use Treatment of relapsed CD33 positive acute myeloid leukemia (AML) in patients ≥60 years of age who are not candidates for cytotoxic chemotherapy

Unlabeled/Investigational Use Salvage therapy for acute promyelocytic leukemia (APL), relapsed/ refractory CD33 positive acute myeloid leukemia in children and adults <60 years

Pregnancy Risk Factor D

Pregnancy Considerations Animal studies have demonstrated teratogenic effects, fetal loss, and maternal toxicity. There are no adequate and well-controlled studies in pregnant women. May cause fetal harm when administered to a pregnant woman. Women of childbearing potential should avoid becoming pregnant while receiving treatment.

Lactation Excretion in breast milk unknown/not recommended

Medication Safety Issues

Sound-alike/look-alike issues:

Gemtuzumab may be confused with gemcitabine

High alert medication: The Institute for Safe Medication Practices (ISMP) includes this medication among its list of drug classes which have a heightened risk of causing significant patient harm when used in error.

Contraindications Hypersensitivity to gemtuzumab ozogamicin, calicheamicin derivatives, or any component of the formulation; patients with anti-CD33 antibody

Warnings/Precautions Hazardous agent - use appropriate precautions for handling and disposal.

[U.S. Boxed Warning]: Gemtuzumab has been associated with hepatotoxicity, including severe hepatic veno-occlusive disease (VOD). Symptoms of VOD include right upper quadrant pain, rapid weight gain, ascites, hepatomegaly, and bilirubin/transaminase elevations. Risk may be increased by combination chemotherapy, underlying hepatic disease, or hematopoietic stem cell transplant. Use with caution in patients with hepatic impairment; has not been studied in patients with serum bilirubin >2 mg/dL.

[U.S. Boxed Warning]: Severe hypersensitivity reactions (including anaphylaxis) and other infusion-related reactions may occur. Infusion-related events are common, generally reported to occur with the first dose after the end of the 2-hour intravenous infusion. These symptoms usually resolved after 2-4 hours with a supportive therapy of acetaminophen, diphenhydramine, and intravenous fluids. Other severe and potentially fatal infusion related pulmonary events (including dyspnea and hypoxia) have been reported infrequently. Symptomatic intrinsic lung disease or high peripheral blast counts may increase the risk of severe reactions. Fewer infusion-related events were observed after the second dose. Postinfusion reactions (may include fever, chills, hypotension, or dyspnea) may occur during the first 24 hours after administration. Consider discontinuation in patients who develop severe infusion-related reactions. In addition to infusion-related pulmonary events, gemtuzumab therapy is also associated with acute respiratory distress syndrome, pulmonary infiltrates, pleural effusion, noncardiogenic pulmonary edema, and pulmonary insufficiency.

[U.S. Boxed Warning]: Severe myelosuppression occurs in all patients at recommended dosages. Use caution in patients with renal impairment. Tumor lysis syndrome may occur as a consequence of leukemia treatment, adequate hydration and prophylactic allopurinol must be instituted prior to use. Other methods to lower WBC <30,000 cells/mm^3 may be considered (hydroxyurea or leukapheresis) to minimize the risk of tumor lysis syndrome, and/or severe infusion reactions. **[U.S. Boxed Warning]: Should be administered under the supervision of an experienced cancer chemotherapy physician. Should only be administered in facilities equipped to monitor and treat patients with leukemia. [U.S. Boxed Warning]: Safety and efficacy have not been established in combination with other chemotherapy agents,** in pediatric patients, or in patients with poor performance status. Gemtuzumab is not FDA-approved for use in children.

Adverse Reactions Adverse reactions reported for adults of all ages. **Note:** A postinfusion symptom complex (fever, chills, less commonly hypertension, and/or dyspnea) may occur within 24 hours of administration; the incidence of infusion-related events decreases with repeat administration.

>10%:

Cardiovascular: Hypotension (20%), hypertension (16%), peripheral edema (14%)

Central nervous system: Fever (82%), chills (66%), headache (37%), pain (18%), dizziness (12%), insomnia (12%)

Dermatologic: Petechiae (19%), rash (18%)

Endocrine & metabolic: Hypokalemia (26%)

Gastrointestinal: Nausea (68%), vomiting (58%), abdominal pain (32%), diarrhea (32%), anorexia (25%), mucositis/stomatitis (25%), constipation (23%)

Hematologic: Thrombocytopenia (grades 3/4: 49% to 99%; median recovery 36-51 days), neutropenia (grades 3/4: 98%; median recovery 40-51 days), leukopenia (grades 3/4: 46% to 96%), lymphopenia (grades 3/4: 94%), anemia/hemoglobin decreased (grades 3/4: 14% to 52%), neutropenic fever (17%), hemorrhage (11% to 13%)

Hepatic: Hyperbilirubinemia (grades 3/4: 29%), veno-occlusive disease (1% to 20%; higher frequency in patients with prior history of or subsequent hematopoietic stem cell transplant), AST increased (grades 3/4: 18%), LDH increased (16%)

Local: Local reaction (22%)

Neuromuscular & skeletal: Weakness (36%), back pain (14%)

Respiratory: Epistaxis (28%; grade 3/4: 3%), dyspnea (26%), cough (17%), pneumonia (13%; grades 3/4: 8%), pharyngitis (12%)

Miscellaneous: Infection (grades 3/4: 30%), sepsis (26%; grades 3/4: 17%), cutaneous herpes simplex (21%)

1% to 10%:

Cardiovascular: Tachycardia (10%), cerebral hemorrhage (2%)

Central nervous system: Depression (9%), anxiety (8%), intracranial hemorrhage (1%)

Dermatologic: Bruising (10%), pruritus (6%)

Endocrine & metabolic: Hyperglycemia (10%), hypocalcemia (10%), hypophosphatemia (8%) hypomagnesemia (6%)

Gastrointestinal: Dyspepsia (10%), gingival hemorrhage (9%), melena (1%)

Genitourinary: Vaginal hemorrhage (4%), vaginal bleeding (3%), hematuria (grade 3/4: 1%)

Hematologic: Disseminated intravascular coagulation (DIC) (1%)

Hepatic: ALT increased (grades 3/4: 9%), prothrombin time increased (grades 3/4: 9%), alkaline phosphatase increased (8%; grades 3/4: 4%), ascites (3%), PTT increased (grades 3/4: 2%)

Neuromuscular & skeletal: Arthralgia (10%), myalgia (6%)

Renal: Creatinine increased (2%)

Respiratory: Rhinitis (8%), hypoxia (5%)

<1% (Limited to important or life-threatening): Acute respiratory distress syndrome, anaphylaxis, bradycardia, Budd-Chiari syndrome, gastrointestinal hemorrhage, hepatic failure, hepatosplenomegaly, hypersensitivity reactions, jaundice, neutropenic sepsis, noncardiogenic pulmonary edema, portal vain thrombosis, pulmonary hemorrhage, renal impairment, renal failure (including renal failure secondary to tumor lysis syndrome)

Drug Interactions

Avoid Concomitant Use There are no known interactions where it is recommended to avoid concomitant use.

Increased Effect/Toxicity

The levels/effects of Gemtuzumab Ozogamicin may be increased by: Abciximab

Decreased Effect There are no known significant interactions involving a decrease in effect.

Ethanol/Nutrition/Herb Interactions Ethanol: Avoid ethanol (due to GI irritation).

Stability Light sensitive; protect from light (including direct and indirect sunlight, and unshielded fluorescent light). Store intact vials under refrigeration at 2°C to 8°C (36°F to 46°F). Reconstituted solutions may be stored for up to 2 hours at room temperature or under refrigeration. Following dilution for infusion, solutions are stable for up to 16 hours at room temperature. Administration requires 2 hours; therefore, the maximum elapsed time from initial reconstitution to completion of infusion should be 20 hours.

Reconstitution: Protect from light during preparation (and administration). Prepare in biologic safety hood with shielded fluorescent light; (some institutions prepare in a darkened room with the lights in the biologic safety cabinet turned off). Allow to warm to room temperature prior to reconstitution. Reconstitute vial with sterile water for injection to a concentration of 1 mg/mL. Dilute in 100 mL of 0.9% sodium chloride injection. The infusion container should be placed in a UV protectant bag immediately after preparation. Hazardous agent - use appropriate precautions for handling and disposal.

Mechanism of Action Antibody to CD33 antigen, which is expressed on leukemic blasts in 80% of AML patients. Binds to the CD33 antigen, resulting in internalization of the antibody-antigen complex. Following internalization, the calicheamicin derivative is released inside the myeloid cell. The calicheamicin derivative binds to DNA resulting in double strand breaks and cell death. Pluripotent stem cells and nonhematopoietic cells are not affected.

Pharmacodynamics/Kinetics

Distribution: V_{ss}: Adults: Initial dose: 21 L; Repeat dose: 10 L

Half-life elimination: Total calicheamicin: Initial: 41-45 hours, Repeat dose: 60-64 hours; Unconjugated: 100-143 hours (no change noted in repeat dosing)

Time to peak, plasma: Immediate; higher concentrations observed after repeat dose

Dosage I.V.:

Children: **Note:** Patients should receive diphenhydramine (1 mg/kg) 1 hour prior to infusion and acetaminophen 15 mg/kg 1 hour prior to infusion and every 4 hours for 2 additional doses.

AML (unlabeled use): 4-9 mg/m^2 infused over 2 hours every 2 weeks for a total of 1-3 doses per treatment course. Patients received the second and third doses

and/or dose escalation if no dose-limiting toxicities were observed. (**Note:** Higher incidences of liver toxicities were observed in children at the 9 mg/m^2 dose level.)
or
Children <3 years: 0.2 mg/kg infused over 2 hours every 2 weeks for a total of 2 doses
Children ≥3 years: 6 mg/m^2 infused over 2 hours every 2 weeks for a total of 2 doses

Adults: **Note:** Patients should receive diphenhydramine 50 mg orally and acetaminophen 650-1000 mg orally 1 hour prior to administration of each dose. Acetaminophen dosage should be repeated as needed every 4 hours for 2 additional doses. Pretreatment with methylprednisolone may ameliorate infusion-related symptoms.

AML:
≥60 years: 9 mg/m^2 infused over 2 hours. A full treatment course is a total of 2 doses administered with 14 days between doses. Full hematologic recovery is not necessary for administration of the second dose. There has been only limited experience with repeat courses of gemtuzumab ozogamicin.
<60 years (unlabeled use): 9 mg/m^2 infused over 2 hours. A full treatment course is a total of 2 doses administered with 14 days between doses.

APL (unlabeled use): 6 mg/m^2 infused over 2 hours. A full treatment course is a total of 2 doses administered with 15 days between doses.

Dosage adjustment with recent hematopoietic stem cell transplant (HSCT): Gemtuzumab use within 3-4 months of HSCT is associated with an increased risk of hepatic veno-occlusive disease, the National Comprehensive Cancer Network (NCCN) guidelines (AML, v.1.2009) recommend a 30% to 50% dosage reduction in this situation.

Dosage adjustment for toxicity:
Dyspnea or significant hypotension: Interrupt infusion; monitor
Anaphylaxis, pulmonary edema, acute respiratory distress syndrome: Strongly consider discontinuing treatment

Dosage adjustment in renal impairment: No recommendation (not studied)

Dosage adjustment in hepatic impairment: Use extra caution; has not been studied in patients with bilirubin >2 mg/dL

Administration Do not administer as I.V. push or bolus. Administer via I.V. infusion, over at least 2 hours through a low protein-binding (0.2-1.2 micron) in-line filter. Protect from light during infusion. Premedicate with acetaminophen and diphenhydramine prior to each infusion.

Monitoring Parameters Monitor vital signs during the infusion and for 4 hours following the infusion. Monitor for signs/symptoms of postinfusion reaction. Monitor electrolytes, liver function, CBC with differential and platelets frequently. Monitor for signs and symptoms of hepatic veno-occlusssive disease (weight gain, right upper quadrant abdominal pain, hepatomegaly, ascites).

Test Interactions None known

Additional Information Oncology Comment: In addition to the FDA-approved indication, the National Comprehensive Cancer Network (NCCN) Acute Myeloid Leukemia Guidelines (AML, v.1.2009) recommend gemtuzumab ozogamicin as salvage and/or post remission therapy for the treatment of acute promyelocytic leukemia (APL). Gemtuzumab has activity (single agent) in patients with persistent disease following postremission arsenic trioxide therapy in APL patients who are not candidates for allogeneic transplantation.

Dosage Forms Excipient information presented when available (limited, particularly for generics); consult specific product labeling.
Injection, powder for reconstitution [preservative free]:
Mylotarg®: 5 mg

◆ **Gemzar®** *see* Gemcitabine *on page* 685
◆ **Genac® [OTC]** *see* Triprolidine and Pseudoephedrine *on page* 1522
◆ **Gen-Acebutolol (Can)** *see* Acebutolol *on page* 25
◆ **Genaced™ [OTC]** *see* Acetaminophen, Aspirin, and Caffeine *on page* 31
◆ **Genacote™ [OTC]** *see* Aspirin *on page* 142
◆ **Gen-Acyclovir (Can)** *see* Acyclovir *on page* 40
◆ **Genahist® [OTC]** *see* DiphenhydrAMINE *on page* 456
◆ **Gen-Alendronate (Can)** *see* Alendronate *on page* 58
◆ **Gen-Alprazolam (Can)** *see* ALPRAZolam *on page* 68
◆ **Gen-Amilazide (Can)** *see* Amiloride and Hydrochlorothiazide *on page* 85
◆ **Gen-Amiodarone (Can)** *see* Amiodarone *on page* 87
◆ **Gen-Amoxicillin (Can)** *see* Amoxicillin *on page* 98
◆ **Gen-Anagrelide (Can)** *see* Anagrelide *on page* 115
◆ **Genapap™ [OTC]** *see* Acetaminophen *on page* 25
◆ **Genapap™ Children [OTC]** *see* Acetaminophen *on page* 25
◆ **Genapap™ Extra Strength [OTC]** *see* Acetaminophen *on page* 25
◆ **Genapap™ Infant [OTC]** *see* Acetaminophen *on page* 25
◆ **Genapap™ Sinus Maximum Strength [OTC] [DSC]** *see* Acetaminophen and Pseudoephedrine *on page* 30
◆ **Genaphed® [OTC]** *see* Pseudoephedrine *on page* 1265
◆ **Genasec™ [OTC]** *see* Acetaminophen and Phenyltoloxamine *on page* 29
◆ **Genasoft® [OTC]** *see* Docusate *on page* 473
◆ **Gen-Atenolol (Can)** *see* Atenolol *on page* 149
◆ **Genaton™ [OTC]** *see* Aluminum Hydroxide and Magnesium Carbonate *on page* 75
◆ **Genaton Tablet [OTC]** *see* Aluminum Hydroxide and Magnesium Trisilicate *on page* 76
◆ **Genatuss DM® [OTC]** *see* Guaifenesin and Dextromethorphan *on page* 710
◆ **Gen-Azathioprine (Can)** *see* AzaTHIOprine *on page* 163
◆ **Gen-Baclofen (Can)** *see* Baclofen *on page* 172
◆ **Gen-Beclo (Can)** *see* Beclomethasone *on page* 176
◆ **Gen-Bicalutamide (Can)** *see* Bicalutamide *on page* 197
◆ **Gen-Budesonide AQ (Can)** *see* Budesonide *on page* 215
◆ **Gen-Buspirone (Can)** *see* BusPIRone *on page* 226
◆ **Gen-Captopril (Can)** *see* Captopril *on page* 249
◆ **Gen-Carbamazepine CR (Can)** *see* CarBAMazepine *on page* 252
◆ **Gen-Cimetidine (Can)** *see* Cimetidine *on page* 326
◆ **Gen-Ciprofloxacin (Can)** *see* Ciprofloxacin *on page* 329
◆ **Gen-Citalopram (Can)** *see* Citalopram *on page* 337
◆ **Gen-Clarithromycin (Can)** *see* Clarithromycin *on page* 341
◆ **Gen-Clindamycin (Can)** *see* Clindamycin *on page* 344
◆ **Gen-Clobetasol (Can)** *see* Clobetasol *on page* 347
◆ **Gen-Clomipramine (Can)** *see* ClomiPRAMINE *on page* 350
◆ **Gen-Clonazepam (Can)** *see* ClonazePAM *on page* 352
◆ **Gen-Clozapine (Can)** *see* Clozapine *on page* 359
◆ **Gen-Combo Sterinebs (Can)** *see* Ipratropium and Albuterol *on page* 812

- ◆ **Gen-Cyclobenzaprine (Can)** *see* Cyclobenzaprine *on page 375*
- ◆ **Gen-Diltiazem (Can)** *see* Diltiazem *on page 450*
- ◆ **Gen-Diltiazem CD (Can)** *see* Diltiazem *on page 450*
- ◆ **Gen-Divalproex (Can)** *see* Valproic Acid and Derivatives *on page 1538*
- ◆ **Gen-Doxazosin (Can)** *see* Doxazosin *on page 483*
- ◆ **Genebs [OTC]** *see* Acetaminophen *on page 25*
- ◆ **Genebs Extra Strength [OTC]** *see* Acetaminophen *on page 25*
- ◆ **Gen-Enalapril (Can)** *see* Enalapril *on page 515*
- ◆ **Generlac** *see* Lactulose *on page 847*
- ◆ **Gen-Etidronate (Can)** *see* Etidronate Disodium *on page 586*
- ◆ **Genexa™ LA [DSC]** *see* Guaifenesin and Phenylephrine *on page 712*
- ◆ **Gen-Famotidine (Can)** *see* Famotidine *on page 603*
- ◆ **Gen-Fenofibrate Micro (Can)** *see* Fenofibrate *on page 607*
- ◆ **Genfiber™ [OTC]** *see* Psyllium *on page 1268*
- ◆ **Gen-Fluconazole (Can)** *see* Fluconazole *on page 625*
- ◆ **Gen-Fluoxetine (Can)** *see* FLUoxetine *on page 638*
- ◆ **Gen-Fosinopril (Can)** *see* Fosinopril *on page 670*
- ◆ **Gen-Gabapentin (Can)** *see* Gabapentin *on page 678*
- ◆ **Gen-Gemfibrozil (Can)** *see* Gemfibrozil *on page 687*
- ◆ **Gen-Glybe (Can)** *see* GlyBURIDE *on page 701*
- ◆ **Gengraf®** *see* CycloSPORINE *on page 379*
- ◆ **Gen-Hydroxychloroquine (Can)** *see* Hydroxychloroquine *on page 751*
- ◆ **Gen-Hydroxyurea (Can)** *see* Hydroxyurea *on page 753*
- ◆ **Gen-Indapamide (Can)** *see* Indapamide *on page 781*
- ◆ **Gen-Ipratropium (Can)** *see* Ipratropium *on page 811*
- ◆ **Gen-Lamotrigine (Can)** *see* LamoTRIgine *on page 850*
- ◆ **GEN-Leflunomide (Can)** *see* Leflunomide *on page 859*
- ◆ **Gen-Lisinopril (Can)** *see* Lisinopril *on page 894*
- ◆ **Gen-Lisinopril/Hctz (Can)** *see* Lisinopril and Hydrochlorothiazide *on page 896*
- ◆ **Gen-Lovastatin (Can)** *see* Lovastatin *on page 910*
- ◆ **Gen-Medroxy (Can)** *see* MedroxyPROGESTERone *on page 930*
- ◆ **Gen-Meloxicam (Can)** *see* Meloxicam *on page 935*
- ◆ **Gen-Metformin (Can)** *see* MetFORMIN *on page 954*
- ◆ **Gen-Metoprolol (Can)** *see* Metoprolol *on page 982*
- ◆ **Gen-Minocycline (Can)** *see* Minocycline *on page 999*
- ◆ **Gen-Mirtazapine (Can)** *see* Mirtazapine *on page 1002*
- ◆ **Gen-Nabumetone (Can)** *see* Nabumetone *on page 1030*
- ◆ **Gen-Naproxen EC (Can)** *see* Naproxen *on page 1041*
- ◆ **GEN-Nifedipine XL (Can)** *see* NIFEdipine *on page 1064*
- ◆ **Gen-Nitro (Can)** *see* Nitroglycerin *on page 1073*
- ◆ **Gen-Nizatidine (Can)** *see* Nizatidine *on page 1076*
- ◆ **Gen-Nortriptyline (Can)** *see* Nortriptyline *on page 1081*
- ◆ **Gen-Ondansetron (Can)** *see* Ondansetron *on page 1102*
- ◆ **Genotropin®** *see* Somatropin *on page 1388*
- ◆ **Genotropin Miniquick®** *see* Somatropin *on page 1388*
- ◆ **Gen-Oxybutynin (Can)** *see* Oxybutynin *on page 1119*
- ◆ **Gen-Pantoprazole (Can)** *see* Pantoprazole *on page 1140*
- ◆ **Gen-Paroxetine (Can)** *see* PARoxetine *on page 1146*
- ◆ **Gen-Pindolol (Can)** *see* Pindolol *on page 1194*
- ◆ **Gen-Pioglitazone (Can)** *see* Pioglitazone *on page 1195*
- ◆ **Gen-Piroxicam (Can)** *see* Piroxicam *on page 1201*
- ◆ **GEN-Pravastatin (Can)** *see* Pravastatin *on page 1227*
- ◆ **Genpril® [OTC] [DSC]** *see* Ibuprofen *on page 760*
- ◆ **Gen-Quetiapine (Can)** *see* QUEtiapine *on page 1275*
- ◆ **GEN-Ramipril (Can)** *see* Ramipril *on page 1292*
- ◆ **Gen-Ranidine (Can)** *see* Ranitidine *on page 1295*
- ◆ **Gen-Risperidone (Can)** *see* Risperidone *on page 1323*
- ◆ **Gen-Salbutamol (Can)** *see* Albuterol *on page 51*
- ◆ **Gen-Selegiline (Can)** *see* Selegiline *on page 1359*
- ◆ **Gen-Sertraline (Can)** *see* Sertraline *on page 1362*
- ◆ **Gen-Simvastatin (Can)** *see* Simvastatin *on page 1370*
- ◆ **Gen-Sotalol (Can)** *see* Sotalol *on page 1394*
- ◆ **Gen-Sumatriptan (Can)** *see* SUMAtriptan *on page 1414*
- ◆ **Gentak®** *see* Gentamicin *on page 692*

Gentamicin (jen ta MYE sin)

U.S. Brand Names Gentak®; Gentasol™

Canadian Brand Names Alcomicin®; Diogent®; Garamycin®; Gentamicin Injection, USP; SAB-Gentamicin

Index Terms Gentamicin Sulfate

Pharmacologic Category Antibiotic, Aminoglycoside; Antibiotic, Ophthalmic; Antibiotic, Topical

Additional Appendix Information

Aminoglycoside Dosing and Monitoring *on page 1630*
Antibiotic Treatment of Adults With Infective Endocarditis *on page 1748*
Antimicrobial Drugs of Choice *on page 1752*
Prevention of Infective Endocarditis *on page 1736*
Prevention of Wound Infection and Sepsis in Surgical Patients *on page 1738*
Treatment of Sexually Transmitted Infections *on page 1773*

Use Treatment of susceptible bacterial infections, normally gram-negative organisms including *Pseudomonas*, *Proteus*, *Serratia*, and gram-positive *Staphylococcus*; treatment of bone infections, respiratory tract infections, skin and soft tissue infections, as well as abdominal and urinary tract infections, and septicemia; treatment of infective endocarditis; used topically to treat superficial infections of the skin or ophthalmic infections caused by susceptible bacteria

Pregnancy Risk Factor C (ophthalmic, topical); D (injection)

Pregnancy Considerations Gentamicin crosses the placenta and produces detectable serum levels in the fetus. Because of several reports of total irreversible bilateral congenital deafness in children whose mothers received streptomycin during pregnancy, manufacturers classify gentamicin as pregnancy risk factor D. Renal toxicity has been observed in animals. Other than a single case report of renal cystic dysplasia, reports of fetal toxicity in humans have not been located. Adequate and well-controlled studies have not been conducted in pregnant women and it is not known whether gentamicin can cause fetal harm. Although manufacturers consider systemic gentamicin pregnancy risk factor D, gentamicin-specific clinical data would suggest a pregnancy risk factor C.

Due to pregnancy induced physiologic changes, some pharmacokinetic parameters of gentamicin may be altered. Pregnant women have an average-to-larger volume of distribution which may result in lower serum peak levels than for the same dose in nonpregnant women. Serum half-life is also shorter.

Lactation Enters breast milk (small amounts)/use caution (AAP rates "compatible")

Medication Safety Issues

Sound-alike/look-alike issues:

Garamycin® may be confused with kanamycin, Terramycin®

Gentamicin may be confused with gentian violet, kanamycin, vancomycin

High alert medication: The Institute for Safe Medication Practices (ISMP) includes this medication (intrathecal administration) among its list of drug classes which have a heightened risk of causing significant patient harm when used in error.

Contraindications Hypersensitivity to gentamicin or other aminoglycosides

Warnings/Precautions [U.S. Boxed Warning]: Aminoglycosides may cause neurotoxicity and/or nephrotoxicity; usual risk factors include pre-existing renal impairment, concomitant neuro-/nephrotoxic medications, advanced age and dehydration. Ototoxicity may be directly proportional to the amount of drug given and the duration of treatment; tinnitus or vertigo are indications of vestibular injury and impending hearing loss; renal damage is usually reversible. May cause neuromuscular blockade and respiratory paralysis; especially when given soon after anesthesia or muscle relaxants.

Not intended for long-term therapy due to toxic hazards associated with extended administration; use caution in pre-existing renal insufficiency, vestibular or cochlear impairment, myasthenia gravis, hypocalcemia, conditions which depress neuromuscular transmission. Dosage modification required in patients with impaired renal function. Prolonged use may result in fungal or bacterial superinfection, including *C. difficile*-associated diarrhea (CDAD) and pseudomembranous colitis; CDAD has been observed >2 months postantibiotic treatment.

Adverse Reactions

>10%:

Central nervous system: Neurotoxicity (vertigo, ataxia)

Neuromuscular & skeletal: Gait instability

Otic: Ototoxicity (auditory), ototoxicity (vestibular)

Renal: Nephrotoxicity, decreased creatinine clearance

1% to 10%:

Cardiovascular: Edema

Dermatologic: Skin itching, reddening of skin, rash

<1% (Limited to important or life-threatening): Agranulocytosis allergic reaction, anorexia, burning, drowsiness, dyspnea, enterocolitis erythema, granulocytopenia headache, LFTs increased, muscle cramps, nausea, photosensitivity, pseudomotor cerebri, salivation increased, stinging, thrombocytopenia, tremor, vomiting, weakness, weight loss

Drug Interactions

Avoid Concomitant Use

Avoid concomitant use of Gentamicin with any of the following: Gallium Nitrate

Increased Effect/Toxicity

Gentamicin may increase the levels/effects of: Bisphosphonate Derivatives; Botulinum Toxin Type A; Botulinum Toxin Type B; CARBOplatin; Colistimethate; CycloSPORINE; Gallium Nitrate; Neuromuscular-Blocking Agents

The levels/effects of Gentamicin may be increased by: Amphotericin B; Capreomycin; CISplatin; Loop Diuretics; Nonsteroidal Anti-Inflammatory Agents; Vancomycin

Decreased Effect

Gentamicin may decrease the levels/effects of: Typhoid Vaccine

The levels/effects of Gentamicin may be decreased by: Penicillins

Stability

Gentamicin is a colorless to slightly yellow solution which should be stored between 2°C to 30°C, but refrigeration is not recommended.

I.V. infusion solutions mixed in NS or D_5W solution are stable for 24 hours at room temperature and refrigeration.

Premixed bag: Manufacturer expiration date.

Out of overwrap stability: 30 days.

Mechanism of Action Interferes with bacterial protein synthesis by binding to 30S and 50S ribosomal subunits resulting in a defective bacterial cell membrane

Pharmacodynamics/Kinetics

Absorption:

Intramuscular: Rapid and complete

Oral: None

Distribution: Primarily into extracellular fluid (highly hydrophilic); high concentration in the renal cortex; minimal penetration to ocular tissues via I.V. route

V_d: Increased by edema, ascites, fluid overload; decreased with dehydration

Neonates: 0.4-0.6 L/kg

Children: 0.3-0.35 L/kg

Adults: 0.2-0.3 L/kg

Relative diffusion from blood into CSF: Minimal even with inflammation

CSF:blood level ratio: Normal meninges: Nil; Inflamed meninges: 10% to 30%

Protein binding: <30%

Half-life elimination:

Infants: <1 week: 3-11.5 hours; 1 week to 6 months: 3-3.5 hours

Adults: 1.5-3 hours; End-stage renal disease: 36-70 hours

Time to peak, serum: I.M.: 30-90 minutes; I.V.: 30 minutes after 30-minute infusion

Excretion: Urine (as unchanged drug)

Clearance: Directly related to renal function

Dosage Note: Dosage Individualization is **critical** because of the low therapeutic index.

Use of ideal body weight (IBW) for determining the mg/kg/dose appears to be more accurate than dosing on the basis of total body weight (TBW). In morbid obesity, dosage requirement may best be estimated using a dosing weight of IBW + 0.4 (TBW - IBW).

Initial and periodic plasma drug levels (eg, peak and trough with conventional dosing) should be determined, particularly in critically-ill patients with serious infections or in disease states known to significantly alter aminoglycoside pharmacokinetics (eg, cystic fibrosis, burns, or major surgery).

Usual dosage ranges:

Infants and Children <5 years: I.M., I.V.: 2.5 mg/kg/dose every 8 hours*

Children ≥5 years: I.M., I.V.: 2-2.5 mg/kg/dose every 8 hours*

***Note:** Higher individual doses and/or more frequent intervals (eg, every 6 hours) may be required in selected clinical situations (cystic fibrosis) or serum levels document the need

Children and Adults:

Ophthalmic:

Ointment: Instill 1/2" (1.25 cm) 2-3 times/day to every 3-4 hours

Solution: Instill 1-2 drops every 2-4 hours, up to 2 drops every hour for severe infections

Topical: Apply 3-4 times/day to affected area

Adults:

I.M., I.V.:

Conventional: 1-2.5 mg/kg/dose every 8-12 hours; to ensure adequate peak concentrations early in therapy, higher initial dosage may be considered in selected patients when extracellular water is increased (edema, septic shock, postsurgical, or trauma)

Once daily: 4-7 mg/kg/dose once daily; some clinicians recommend this approach for all patients with normal renal function; this dose is at least as efficacious with similar, if not less, toxicity than conventional dosing

Intrathecal: 4-8 mg/day

Indication-specific dosing:

Neonates: I.V.:

Meningitis:

0-7 days of age: <2000 g: 2.5 mg/kg every 18-24 hours; >2000 g: 2.5 mg/kg every 12 hours

8-28 days of age: <2000 g: 2.5 mg/kg every 8-12 hours; >2000 g: 2.5 mg/kg every 8 hours

Children and Adults: I.M., I.V.:

Brucellosis: 240 mg (I.M.) daily or 5 mg/kg (I.V.) daily for 7 days; either regimen recommended in combination with doxycycline

Cholangitis: 4-6 mg/kg once daily with ampicillin

Diverticulitis (complicated): 1.5-2 mg/kg every 8 hours (with ampicillin and metronidazole)

Endocarditis: Treatment: 3 mg/kg/day in 1-3 divided doses

Meningitis:

Enterococcus sp or *Pseudomonas aeruginosa*: Loading dose 2 mg/kg, then 1.7 mg/kg/dose every 8 hours (administered with another bacteriocidal drug)

Listeria: 5-7 mg/kg/day (with penicillin) for 1 week

Pelvic inflammatory disease: Loading dose: 2 mg/kg, then 1.5 mg/kg every 8 hours

Alternate therapy: 4.5 mg/kg once daily

Plague (*Yersinia pestis*): Treatment: 5 mg/kg/day, followed by postexposure prophylaxis with doxycycline

Pneumonia, hospital- or ventilator-associated: 7 mg/kg/day (with antipseudomonal beta-lactam or carbapenem)

Synergy (for gram-positive infections): 3 mg/kg/day in 1-3 divided doses (with ampicillin)

Tularemia: 5 mg/kg/day divided every 8 hours for 1-2 weeks

Urinary tract infection: 1.5 mg/kg/dose every 8 hours

Dosing interval in renal impairment:

Conventional dosing:

Cl_{cr} ≥60 mL/minute: Administer every 8 hours

Cl_{cr} 40-60 mL/minute: Administer every 12 hours

Cl_{cr} 20-40 mL/minute: Administer every 24 hours

Cl_{cr} <20 mL/minute: Loading dose, then monitor levels

High-dose therapy: Interval may be extended (eg, every 48 hours) in patients with moderate renal impairment (Cl_{cr} 30-59 mL/minute) and/or adjusted based on serum level determinations.

Hemodialysis: Dialyzable; removal by hemodialysis: 30% removal of aminoglycosides occurs during 4 hours of HD; administer dose after dialysis and follow levels

Removal by continuous ambulatory peritoneal dialysis (CAPD):

Administration via CAPD fluid:

Gram-negative infection: 4-8 mg/L (4-8 mcg/mL) of CAPD fluid

Gram-positive infection (eg, synergy): 3-4 mg/L (3-4 mcg/mL) of CAPD fluid

Administration via I.V., I.M. route during CAPD: Dose as for Cl_{cr} <10 mL/minute and follow levels

Removal via continuous arteriovenous or venovenous hemofiltration: Dose as for Cl_{cr} 10-40 mL/minute and follow levels

Dosing adjustment/comments in hepatic disease: Monitor plasma concentrations

Dietary Considerations Calcium, magnesium, potassium: Renal wasting may cause hypocalcemia, hypomagnesemia, and/or hypokalemia.

Administration

I.M.: Administer by deep I.M. route if possible. Slower absorption and lower peak concentrations, probably due to poor circulation in the atrophic muscle, may occur following I.M. injection; in paralyzed patients, suggest I.V. route.

Ophthalmic: Administer any other ophthalmics 10 minutes before or after gentamicin preparations.

Some penicillins (eg, carbenicillin, ticarcillin, and piperacillin) have been shown to inactivate aminoglycosides *in vitro*. This has been observed to a greater extent with tobramycin and gentamicin, while amikacin has shown greater stability against inactivation. Concurrent use of these agents may pose a risk of reduced antibacterial efficacy *in vivo*, particularly in the setting of profound renal impairment. However, definitive clinical evidence is lacking. If combination penicillin/aminoglycoside therapy is desired in a patient with renal dysfunction, separation of doses (if feasible), and routine monitoring of aminoglycoside levels, CBC, and clinical response should be considered.

Monitoring Parameters Urinalysis, urine output, BUN, serum creatinine; hearing should be tested before, during, and after treatment; particularly in those at risk for ototoxicity or who will be receiving prolonged therapy (>2 weeks)

Some penicillin derivatives may accelerate the degradation of aminoglycosides *in vitro*. This may be clinically-significant for certain penicillin (ticarcillin, piperacillin, carbenicillin) and aminoglycoside (gentamicin, tobramycin) combination therapy in patients with significant renal impairment. Close monitoring of aminoglycoside levels is warranted.

Reference Range

Timing of serum samples: Draw peak 30 minutes after 30-minute infusion has been completed or 1 hour after I.M. injection; draw trough immediately before next dose

Sample size: 0.5-2 mL blood (red top tube) or 0.1-1 mL serum (separated)

Therapeutic levels:

Peak:

Serious infections: 6-8 mcg/mL (12-17 μmol/L)

Life-threatening infections: 8-10 mcg/mL (17-21 μmol/L)

Urinary tract infections: 4-6 mcg/mL

Synergy against gram-positive organisms: 3-5 mcg/mL

Trough:

Serious infections: 0.5-1 mcg/mL

Life-threatening infections: 1-2 mcg/mL

The American Thoracic Society (ATS) recommends trough levels of <1 mcg/mL for patients with hospital-acquired pneumonia.

Obtain drug levels after the third dose unless renal dysfunction/toxicity suspected

Test Interactions

Some penicillin derivatives may accelerate the degradation of aminoglycosides *in vitro*, leading to a potential underestimation of aminoglycoside serum concentration.

Dosage Forms Excipient information presented when available (limited, particularly for generics); consult specific product labeling. [DSC] = Discontinued product

Cream, topical, as sulfate: 0.1% (15 g, 30 g)

Infusion, as sulfate [premixed in NS]: 40 mg (50 mL); 60 mg (50 mL, 100 mL); 70 mg (50 mL); 80 mg (50 mL, 100 mL); 90 mg (100 mL); 100 mg (50 mL, 100 mL); 120 mg (100 mL)

Injection, solution, as sulfate: 10 mg/mL (6 mL, 8 mL, 10 mL)

Injection, solution, as sulfate: 40 mg/mL (2 mL, 20 mL)

Injection, solution [pediatric], as sulfate: 10 mg/mL (2 mL)

Injection, solution [pediatric], as sulfate [preservative free]: 10 mg/mL (2 mL)
Ointment, ophthalmic, as sulfate (Gentak®): 0.3% [3 mg/g] (3.5 g)
Ointment, topical, as sulfate: 0.1% (15 g, 30 g)
Solution, ophthalmic, as sulfate: 0.3% (5 mL, 15 mL) [contains benzalkonium chloride]
Gentak®: 0.3% (5 mL; 15 mL [DSC]) [contains benzalkonium chloride]
Gentasol™: 0.3% (5 mL) [contains benzalkonium chloride]

- **Gentamicin and Prednisolone** *see* Prednisolone and Gentamicin *on page* 1232
- **Gentamicin Injection, USP (Can)** *see* Gentamicin *on page* 692
- **Gentamicin Sulfate** *see* Gentamicin *on page* 692
- **Gen-Tamoxifen (Can)** *see* Tamoxifen *on page* 1424
- **Gen-Tamsulosin (Can)** *see* Tamsulosin *on page* 1426
- **Gentasol™** *see* Gentamicin *on page* 692
- **Gen-Temazepam (Can)** *see* Temazepam *on page* 1432
- **Gen-Terbinafine (Can)** *see* Terbinafine *on page* 1441
- **Gentex LA [DSC]** *see* Guaifenesin and Phenylephrine *on page* 712
- **Gentex LQ** *see* Carbetapentane, Guaifenesin, and Phenylephrine *on page* 255

Gentian Violet (JEN shun VYE oh let)

Index Terms Crystal Violet; Methylrosaniline Chloride
Pharmacologic Category Antibiotic, Topical; Antifungal Agent, Topical
Use Treatment of cutaneous or mucocutaneous infections caused by *Candida albicans* and other superficial skin infections; external treatment of minor abrasions or cuts
Pregnancy Risk Factor C
Medication Safety Issues
Sound-alike/look-alike issues:
Gentian violet may be confused with gentamicin
Dosage Children and Adults: Topical: Apply to affected area once or twice daily. Solutions diluted to 0.25% to 0.5% may be less irritating. Solutions diluted to 0.01% have been recommended for use in closed cavities.
Additional Information Complete prescribing information for this medication should be consulted for additional detail.
Dosage Forms Excipient information presented when available (limited, particularly for generics); consult specific product labeling.
Solution, topical: 1% (59 mL); 2% (60 mL)

- **Gen-Ticlopidine (Can)** *see* Ticlopidine *on page* 1468
- **Gen-Timolol (Can)** *see* Timolol *on page* 1472
- **Gen-Tizanidine (Can)** *see* TiZANidine *on page* 1480
- **Gentlax® (Can)** *see* Bisacodyl *on page* 198
- **Gen-Topiramate (Can)** *see* Topiramate *on page* 1489
- **Gentran®** *see* Dextran *on page* 431
- **Gen-Trazodone (Can)** *see* TraZODone *on page* 1505
- **Gen-Triazolam (Can)** *see* Triazolam *on page* 1515
- **GEN-Venlafaxine XR (Can)** *see* Venlafaxine *on page* 1554
- **Gen-Verapamil (Can)** *see* Verapamil *on page* 1557
- **Gen-Verapamil SR (Can)** *see* Verapamil *on page* 1557
- **Gen-Warfarin (Can)** *see* Warfarin *on page* 1570
- **Geodon®** *see* Ziprasidone *on page* 1585
- **Geref® Diagnostic [DSC]** *see* Sermorelin Acetate *on page* 1362
- **German Measles Vaccine** *see* Rubella Virus Vaccine (Live) *on page* 1348
- **GF196960** *see* Tadalafil *on page* 1422
- **GG** *see* GuaiFENesin *on page* 709
- **GHB** *see* Sodium Oxybate *on page* 1384
- **GI87084B** *see* Remifentanil *on page* 1302
- **Gilphex TR®** *see* Guaifenesin and Phenylephrine *on page* 712
- **Glargine Insulin** *see* Insulin Glargine *on page* 794

Glatiramer Acetate (gla TIR a mer AS e tate)

U.S. Brand Names Copaxone®
Canadian Brand Names Copaxone®
Index Terms Copolymer-1
Pharmacologic Category Biological, Miscellaneous
Use Management of relapsing-remitting type multiple sclerosis
Pregnancy Risk Factor B
Pregnancy Considerations Adverse events were not observed in animal studies. There are no adequate and well-controlled studies in pregnant women. Use in pregnancy only if clearly necessary.
Lactation Excretion in breast milk unknown/use caution
Medication Safety Issues
Sound-alike/look-alike issues:
Copaxone® may be confused with Compazine®
Contraindications Hypersensitivity to glatiramer acetate, mannitol, or any component of the formulation
Warnings/Precautions For SubQ use only, **not for I.V. administration**. Glatiramer acetate is antigenic, and may possibly lead to the induction of untoward host responses. Immediate postinjection systemic reactions occur in a substantial percentage of patients (~10% in premarketing studies); symptoms may begin within minutes of injection and usually spontaneously resolve within 30 minutes. Most patients only have one reaction despite repeated administration. Safety and efficacy has not been established in patients with renal impairment, in the elderly, or in patients <18 years of age.
Adverse Reactions
>10%:
Cardiovascular: Vasodilation (27%), chest pain (21%), palpitation (17%)
Central nervous system: Pain (28%), anxiety (23%)
Dermatologic: Pruritus (18%), rash (18%)
Gastrointestinal: Nausea (22%), diarrhea (12%)
Local: Injection site reactions: Pain (73%), erythema (66%), inflammation (49%), pruritus (40%), mass (27%), induration (13%), welt (11%)
Neuromuscular & skeletal: Weakness (41%), arthralgia (24%), hypertonia (22%), back pain (16%)
Respiratory: Dyspnea (19%), rhinitis (14%)
Miscellaneous: Infection (50%), flu-like syndrome (19%), diaphoresis (15%), lymphadenopathy (12%)
1% to 10%:
Cardiovascular: Peripheral edema (7%), facial edema (6%), syncope (5%), tachycardia (5%), edema (3%), hypertension (1%)
Central nervous system: Fever (8%), vertigo (6%), migraine (5%), agitation (4%), chills (4%), confusion (2%), nervousness (2%), speech disorder (2%)
Dermatologic: Bruising (8%), erythema (4%), urticaria (4%), skin nodule (2%), eczema (1%), pustular rash (1%), skin atrophy (1%)
Endocrine & metabolic: Dysmenorrhea (6%)
Gastrointestinal: Anorexia (8%), vomiting (6%), gastrointestinal disorder (5%), gastroenteritis (3%), weight gain (3%), oral moniliasis (1%), salivary gland enlargement (1%), ulcerative stomatitis (1%)

Genitourinary: Urinary urgency (10%), vaginal moniliasis (8%), hematuria (1%)
Local: Injection site reactions: Hemorrhage (5%), urticaria (5%), edema (1%), atrophy (1%), abscess (1%), hypersensitivity (1%)
Neuromuscular & skeletal: Neck pain (8%), tremor (7%), foot drop (3%)
Ocular: Eye disorder (4%), nystagmus (2%)
Otic: Ear pain (7%)
Respiratory: Bronchitis (9%), laryngismus (5%)
Miscellaneous: Bacterial infection (5%), herpes simplex (4%), cyst (2%), herpes zoster (1%)

<1% (Limited to important or life-threatening): Allergic reaction, anaphylactoid reaction, angina, angioedema, aphasia, arrhythmia, atrial fibrillation, blindness; carcinoma (breast, bladder, lung); cardiomyopathy, CHF, cholecystitis, cholelithiasis, cirrhosis, CNS neoplasm, coma, corneal ulcer, effusion, esophageal ulcer, esophagitis, ethanol intolerance, gastrointestinal hemorrhage, GI carcinoma, glaucoma, gout, hallucination, hematemesis, hepatitis, hepatomegaly, hypotension, injection site abscess, injection site fibrosis, leukopenia, lupus erythematosus, manic reaction, meningitis, MI, neuralgia, optic neuritis, pancreatitis, pancytopenia, paraplegia, pericardial, photosensitivity reaction, postural hypotension, priapism, pulmonary embolism, rash, renal failure, rheumatoid arthritis, seizure, sepsis, serum sickness, splenomegaly, stomatitis, stroke, thrombocytopenia, thrombosis

Drug Interactions

Avoid Concomitant Use There are no known interactions where it is recommended to avoid concomitant use.

Increased Effect/Toxicity There are no known significant interactions involving an increase in effect.

Decreased Effect There are no known significant interactions involving a decrease in effect.

Stability Store in refrigerator at 2°C to 8°C (36°F to 46°F); excursions to room temperature for up to 1 month do not have a negative impact on potency. Avoid heat; protect from intense light.

Mechanism of Action Glatiramer is a mixture of random polymers of four amino acids; L-alanine, L-glutamic acid, L-lysine and L-tyrosine, the resulting mixture is antigenically similar to myelin basic protein, which is an important component of the myelin sheath of nerves; glatiramer is thought to induce and activate T-lymphocyte suppressor cells specific for a myelin antigen, it is also proposed that glatiramer interferes with the antigen-presenting function of certain immune cells opposing pathogenic T-cell function

Pharmacodynamics/Kinetics

Distribution: Small amounts of intact and partial hydrolyzed drug enter lymphatic circulation
Metabolism: SubQ: Large percentage hydrolyzed locally

Dosage Adults: SubQ: 20 mg daily

Administration For SubQ administration in the arms, abdomen, hips, or thighs; rotate injection sites to prevent lipoatrophy. Bring to room temperature prior to use. Visually inspect the solution; discard if solution is cloudy or contains any particulate matter.

Dosage Forms Excipient information presented when available (limited, particularly for generics); consult specific product labeling.

Injection, solution [preservative free]:
Copaxone®: 20 mg/mL (1 mL) [prefilled syringe; contains mannitol; packaged with alcohol pads]

◆ **Gleevec®** *see* Imatinib *on page* 768
◆ **Gliadel®** *see* Carmustine *on page* 262
◆ **Gliadel Wafer® (Can)** *see* Carmustine *on page* 262
◆ **Glibenclamide** *see* GlyBURIDE *on page* 701

Glimepiride (GLYE me pye ride)

U.S. Brand Names Amaryl®

Canadian Brand Names Amaryl®; Apo-Glimepiride; CO Glimepiride; Novo-Glimepiride; PMS-Glimepiride; ratio-Glimepiride; Rhoxal-glimepiride; Sandoz-Glimepiride

Pharmacologic Category Antidiabetic Agent, Sulfonylurea

Additional Appendix Information

Diabetes Mellitus Management, Adults *on page* 1801
Sulfonamide Derivatives *on page* 1671

Use Management of type 2 diabetes mellitus (noninsulin dependent, NIDDM) as an adjunct to diet and exercise to lower blood glucose; may be used in combination with metformin or insulin in patients whose hyperglycemia cannot be controlled by diet and exercise in conjunction with a single oral hypoglycemic agent

Pregnancy Risk Factor C

Pregnancy Considerations Adverse events have been observed in animal studies; therefore, glimepiride is classified as pregnancy category C. Severe hypoglycemia lasting 4-10 days has been noted in infants born to mothers taking a sulfonylurea at the time of delivery. The manufacturer recommends that patients be switched to insulin during pregnancy. Maternal hyperglycemia can be associated with adverse effects in the fetus, including macrosomia, neonatal hyperglycemia, and hyperbilirubinemia; the risk of congenital malformations is increased when the Hb A_{1c} is above the normal range. Diabetes can also be associated with adverse effects in the mother. Poorly-treated diabetes may cause end-organ damage that may in turn negatively affect obstetric outcomes. Physiologic glucose levels should be maintained prior to and during pregnancy to decrease the risk of adverse events in the mother and the fetus. Until additional safety and efficacy data are obtained, the use of oral agents is generally not recommended as routine management of GDM or type 2 diabetes mellitus during pregnancy. Insulin is the drug of choice for the control of diabetes mellitus during pregnancy.

Lactation Excretion in breast milk unknown/not recommended

Medication Safety Issues

Sound-alike/look-alike issues:
Glimepiride may be confused with glipiZIDE
Amaryl® may be confused with Altace®, Amerge®, Reminyl®

High alert medication: The Institute for Safe Medication Practices (ISMP) includes this medication among its list of drugs which have a heightened risk of causing significant patient harm when used in error.

Contraindications Hypersensitivity to glimepiride, any component of the formulation, or sulfonamides; diabetic ketoacidosis (with or without coma)

Warnings/Precautions All sulfonylurea drugs are capable of producing severe hypoglycemia. Hypoglycemia is more likely to occur when caloric intake is deficient, after severe or prolonged exercise, when ethanol is ingested, or when more than one glucose-lowering drug is used. It is also more likely in elderly patients, malnourished patients and in patients with impaired renal or hepatic function; use with caution.

Chemical similarities are present among sulfonamides, sulfonylureas, carbonic anhydrase inhibitors, thiazides, and loop diuretics (except ethacrynic acid). Use in patients with sulfonamide allergy is specifically contraindicated in product labeling, however, a risk of cross-reaction exists in patients with allergy to any of these compounds; avoid use when previous reaction has been severe.

Product labeling states oral hypoglycemic drugs may be associated with an increased cardiovascular mortality as compared to treatment with diet alone or diet plus insulin. Data to support this association are limited, and several studies, including a large prospective trial (UKPDS) have not supported an association.

It may be necessary to discontinue therapy and administer insulin if the patient is exposed to stress (fever, trauma, infection, surgery). Safety and efficacy have not been established in children.

Adverse Reactions

1% to 10%:

Central nervous system: Dizziness (2%), headache (2%)
Endocrine & metabolic: Hypoglycemia (1% to 2%)
Gastrointestinal: Nausea (1%)
Neuromuscular & skeletal: Weakness (2%)

<1% or frequency not defined: Agranulocytosis, anorexia, aplastic anemia, cholestatic jaundice, constipation, diarrhea, disulfiram-like reaction, diuretic effect, edema, epigastric fullness, gastrointestinal pain, erythema, heartburn, hemolytic anemia, hepatitis, hypoglycemia, hyponatremia, leukopenia, liver function tests abnormal, nausea, pancytopenia, photosensitivity, porphyria cutanea tarda, pruritus, rash (morbilliform or maculopapular), SIADH, thrombocytopenia, urticaria, vasculitis (allergic), visual accommodation changes (early treatment), vomiting

Drug Interactions

Metabolism/Transport Effects **Substrate** of CYP2C9 (major)

Avoid Concomitant Use There are no known interactions where it is recommended to avoid concomitant use.

Increased Effect/Toxicity

Glimepiride may increase the levels/effects of: Alcohol (Ethyl); CycloSPORINE

The levels/effects of Glimepiride may be increased by: Chloramphenicol; Cimetidine; Cyclic Antidepressants; CYP2C9 Inhibitors (Moderate); CYP2C9 Inhibitors (Strong); Fibric Acid Derivatives; Fluconazole; Herbs (Hypoglycemic Properties); Pegvisomant; Quinolone Antibiotics; Salicylates; Sulfonamide Derivatives

Decreased Effect

The levels/effects of Glimepiride may be decreased by: Corticosteroids (Orally Inhaled); Corticosteroids (Systemic); CYP2C9 Inducers (Highly Effective); Luteinizing Hormone-Releasing Hormone Analogs; Quinolone Antibiotics; Rifampin; Somatropin

Ethanol/Nutrition/Herb Interactions

Ethanol: Caution with ethanol (may cause hypoglycemia).
Herb/Nutraceutical: Caution with chromium, garlic, gymnema (may cause hypoglycemia).

Mechanism of Action Stimulates insulin release from the pancreatic beta cells; reduces glucose output from the liver; insulin sensitivity is increased at peripheral target sites

Pharmacodynamics/Kinetics

Onset of action: Peak effect: Blood glucose reductions: 2-3 hours
Duration: 24 hours
Absorption: 100%; delayed when given with food
Distribution: V_d: 8.8 L
Protein binding: >99.5%
Metabolism: Hepatic oxidation via CYP2C9 to M1 metabolite (~33% activity of parent compound); further oxidative metabolism to inactive M2 metabolite
Half-life elimination: 5-9 hours
Time to peak, plasma: 2-3 hours
Excretion: Urine (60%, 80% to 90% as M1 and M2); feces (40%, 70% as M1 and M2)

Dosage Oral:

Children 10-18 years (unlabeled use): Initial: 1 mg once daily; maintenance: 1-4 mg once daily

Adults: Initial: 1-2 mg once daily, administered with breakfast or the first main meal; usual maintenance dose: 1-4 mg once daily; after a dose of 2 mg once daily, increase in increments of 2 mg at 1- to 2-week intervals based upon the patient's blood glucose response to a maximum of 8 mg once daily. If inadequate response to maximal dose, combination therapy with metformin may be considered.

Combination with insulin therapy (fasting glucose level for instituting combination therapy is in the range of >150 mg/dL in plasma or serum depending on the patient): initial recommended dose: 8 mg once daily with the first main meal

After starting with low-dose insulin, upward adjustments of insulin can be done approximately weekly as guided by frequent measurements of fasting blood glucose. Once stable, combination-therapy patients should monitor their capillary blood glucose on an ongoing basis, preferably daily.

Conversion from therapy with long half-life agents: Observe patient carefully for 1-2 weeks when converting from a longer half-life agent (eg, chlorpropamide) to glimepiride due to overlapping hypoglycemic effects.

Dosing adjustment/comments in renal impairment: Cl_{cr} <22 mL/minute: Initial starting dose should be 1 mg and dosage increments should be based on fasting blood glucose levels

Dosing adjustment in hepatic impairment: No data available

Elderly: Initial: 1 mg/day; dose titration and maintenance dosing should be conservative to avoid hypoglycemia

Dietary Considerations Administer with breakfast or the first main meal of the day. Dietary modification based on ADA recommendations is a part of therapy. Decreases blood glucose concentration. Hypoglycemia may occur. Must be able to recognize symptoms of hypoglycemia (palpitations, sweaty palms, lightheadedness).

Administration Administer once daily with breakfast or first main meal of the day. Patients who are NPO may need to have their dose held to avoid hypoglycemia.

Monitoring Parameters Urine for glucose and ketones; monitor for signs and symptoms of hypoglycemia (fatigue, excessive hunger, profuse sweating, numbness of extremities), fasting blood glucose, hemoglobin A_{1c}, fructosamine

Reference Range Recommendations for glycemic control in adults with diabetes:

Hb A_{1c}: <7%
Preprandial capillary plasma glucose: 70-130 mg/dL
Peak postprandial capillary blood glucose: <180 mg/dL
Blood pressure: <130/80 mm Hg

Dosage Forms Excipient information presented when available (limited, particularly for generics); consult specific product labeling.

Tablet: 1 mg, 2 mg, 4 mg
Amaryl®: 1 mg, 2 mg, 4 mg

- **Glimepiride and Pioglitazone** *see* Pioglitazone and Glimepiride *on page 1197*
- **Glimepiride and Pioglitazone Hydrochloride** *see* Pioglitazone and Glimepiride *on page 1197*
- **Glimepiride and Rosiglitazone Maleate** *see* Rosiglitazone and Glimepiride *on page 1342*

GlipiZIDE (GLIP i zide)

U.S. Brand Names Glucotrol XL®; Glucotrol®

Index Terms Glydiazinamide

Pharmacologic Category Antidiabetic Agent, Sulfonylurea

Additional Appendix Information
Diabetes Mellitus Management, Adults *on page 1801*
Sulfonamide Derivatives *on page 1671*

Use Management of type 2 diabetes mellitus (noninsulin dependent, NIDDM)

Pregnancy Risk Factor C

Pregnancy Considerations Adverse events have been observed in animal studies; therefore, glipizide is classified as pregnancy category C. Glipizide crosses the placenta. Severe hypoglycemia lasting 4-10 days has been noted in infants born to mothers taking a sulfonylurea at the time of delivery. Maternal hyperglycemia can be associated with adverse effects in the fetus, including macrosomia, neonatal hyperglycemia, and hyperbilirubinemia; the risk of congenital malformations is increased when the Hb A_{1c} is above the normal range. Diabetes can also be associated with adverse effects in the mother. Poorly-treated diabetes may cause end-organ damage that may in turn negatively affect obstetric outcomes. Physiologic glucose levels should be maintained prior to and during pregnancy to decrease the risk of adverse events in the mother and the fetus. Until additional safety and efficacy data are obtained, the use of oral agents is generally not recommended as routine management of GDM or type 2 diabetes mellitus during pregnancy. The manufacturer recommends if glipizide is used during pregnancy it should be discontinued at least 1 month before the expected delivery date. Insulin is the drug of choice for the control of diabetes mellitus during pregnancy.

Lactation Excretion in breast milk unknown/not recommended

Medication Safety Issues
Sound-alike/look-alike issues:
GlipiZIDE may be confused with glimepiride, glyBURIDE
Glucotrol® may be confused with Glucophage®, Glucotrol® XL, glyBURIDE
Glucotrol® XL may be confused with Glucotrol®

High alert medication: The Institute for Safe Medication Practices (ISMP) includes this medication among its list of drugs which have a heightened risk of causing significant patient harm when used in error.

Contraindications Hypersensitivity to glipizide or any component of the formulation, other sulfonamides; type 1 diabetes mellitus (insulin dependent, IDDM); diabetic ketoacidosis

Warnings/Precautions All sulfonylurea drugs are capable of producing severe hypoglycemia. Hypoglycemia is more likely to occur when caloric intake is deficient, after severe or prolonged exercise, when ethanol is ingested, or when more than one glucose-lowering drug is used. It is also more likely in elderly patients, malnourished patients and in patients with impaired renal or hepatic function; use with caution.

Chemical similarities are present among sulfonamides, sulfonylureas, carbonic anhydrase inhibitors, thiazides, and loop diuretics (except ethacrynic acid). Use in patients with sulfonamide allergy is specifically contraindicated in product labeling, however, a risk of cross-reaction exists in patients with allergy to any of these compounds; avoid use when previous reaction has been severe.

Product labeling states oral hypoglycemic drugs may be associated with an increased cardiovascular mortality as compared to treatment with diet alone or diet plus insulin. Data to support this association are limited, and several studies, including a large prospective trial (UKPDS) have not supported an association.

Use with caution in patients with severe hepatic disease. It may be necessary to discontinue therapy and administer insulin if the patient is exposed to stress (fever, trauma, infection, surgery). Safety and efficacy have not been established in children.

Avoid use of extended release tablets (Glucotrol® XL) in patients with known stricture/narrowing of the GI tract.

Adverse Reactions Frequency not defined.
Cardiovascular: Edema, syncope
Central nervous system: Anxiety, depression, dizziness, drowsiness, headache, hypoesthesia, insomnia, nervousness, pain
Dermatologic: Eczema, erythema, maculopapular eruptions, morbilliform eruptions, photosensitivity, pruritus, rash, urticaria
Endocrine & metabolic: Disulfiram-like reaction, hypoglycemia, hyponatremia, SIADH (rare)
Gastrointestinal: Anorexia, constipation, diarrhea, epigastric fullness, flatulence, gastralgia, heartburn, nausea, vomiting
Hematologic: Agranulocytopenia, aplastic anemia, blood dyscrasias, hemolytic anemia, leukopenia, pancytopenia, porphyria cutanea tarda, thrombocytopenia
Hepatic: Cholestatic jaundice, hepatic porphyria
Neuromuscular & skeletal: Arthralgia, leg cramps, myalgia, paresthesia, tremor
Ocular: Blurred vision
Renal: Diuretic effect (minor)
Respiratory: Rhinitis
Miscellaneous: Diaphoresis

Postmarketing and/or case reports: Abdominal pain

Drug Interactions

Metabolism/Transport Effects Substrate of 2C9 (major)

Avoid Concomitant Use There are no known interactions where it is recommended to avoid concomitant use.

Increased Effect/Toxicity
GlipiZIDE may increase the levels/effects of: Alcohol (Ethyl); CycloSPORINE

The levels/effects of GlipiZIDE may be increased by: Chloramphenicol; Cimetidine; Cyclic Antidepressants; CYP2C9 Inhibitors (Moderate); CYP2C9 Inhibitors (Strong); Fibric Acid Derivatives; Fluconazole; Herbs (Hypoglycemic Properties); Pegvisomant; Quinolone Antibiotics; Salicylates; Sulfonamide Derivatives

Decreased Effect
The levels/effects of GlipiZIDE may be decreased by: Corticosteroids (Orally Inhaled); Corticosteroids (Systemic); CYP2C9 Inducers (Highly Effective); Luteinizing Hormone-Releasing Hormone Analogs; Quinolone Antibiotics; Rifampin; Somatropin

Ethanol/Nutrition/Herb Interactions
Ethanol: Caution with ethanol (may cause hypoglycemia or rare disulfiram reaction).
Food: A delayed release of insulin may occur if glipizide is taken with food. Immediate release tablets should be administered 30 minutes before meals to avoid erratic absorption.
Herb/Nutraceutical: Herbs with hypoglycemic properties may enhance the hypoglycemic effect of glipizide. This includes alfalfa, aloe, bilberry, bitter melon, burdock, celery, damiana, fenugreek, garcinia, garlic, ginger, ginseng (American), gymnema, marshmallow, stinging nettle

Mechanism of Action Stimulates insulin release from the pancreatic beta cells; reduces glucose output from the liver; insulin sensitivity is increased at peripheral target sites

Pharmacodynamics/Kinetics
Duration: 12-24 hours
Absorption: Rapid and complete; delayed with food
Distribution: 10-11 L
Protein binding: 98% to 99%; primarily to albumin
Bioavailability: 90% to 100%
Metabolism: Hepatic via CYP2C9; forms metabolites (inactive)
Half-life elimination: 2-5 hours

Time to peak: 1-3 hours; extended release tablets: 6-12 hours
Excretion: Urine (60% to 80%, 91% to 97% as metabolites); feces (11%)

Dosage Oral (allow several days between dose titrations):
Adults: Initial: 5 mg/day; adjust dosage at 2.5-5 mg daily increments as determined by blood glucose response at intervals of several days.
Immediate release tablet: Maximum recommended once-daily dose: 15 mg; maximum recommended total daily dose: 40 mg. Doses >15 mg/day should be administered in divided doses.
Extended release tablet (Glucotrol XL®): Maximum recommended dose: 20 mg
When transferring from insulin to glipizide:
Current insulin requirement ≤20 units: Discontinue insulin and initiate glipizide at usual dose
Current insulin requirement >20 units: Decrease insulin by 50% and initiate glipizide at usual dose; gradually decrease insulin dose based on patient response. Several days should elapse between dosage changes.
Elderly: Initial: 2.5 mg/day; increase by 2.5-5 mg/day at 1- to 2-week intervals

Dosing adjustment/comments in renal impairment: Cl_{cr} <10 mL/minute: Some investigators recommend not using

Dosing adjustment in hepatic impairment: Initial dosage should be 2.5 mg/day

Dietary Considerations Take immediate release tablets 30 minutes before meals; extended release tablets should be taken with breakfast. Dietary modification based on ADA recommendations is a part of therapy. Decreases blood glucose concentration. Hypoglycemia may occur. Must be able to recognize symptoms of hypoglycemia (palpitations, sweaty palms, lightheadedness).

Administration Administer immediate release tablets 30 minutes before a meal to achieve greatest reduction in postprandial hyperglycemia. Extended release tablets should be given with breakfast. Patients who are NPO may need to have their dose held to avoid hypoglycemia.

Monitoring Parameters Signs and symptoms of hypoglycemia (fatigue, excessive hunger, profuse sweating, numbness of extremities), blood glucose, hemoglobin A_{1c}

Reference Range Recommendations for glycemic control in adults with diabetes:
Hb A_{1c}: <7%
Preprandial capillary plasma glucose: 70-130 mg/dL
Peak postprandial capillary blood glucose: <180 mg/dL
Blood pressure: <130/80 mm Hg

Dosage Forms Excipient information presented when available (limited, particularly for generics); consult specific product labeling.
Tablet: 5 mg, 10 mg
Glucotrol®: 5 mg, 10 mg
Tablet, extended release: 2.5 mg, 5 mg, 10 mg
Glucotrol XL®: 2.5 mg, 5 mg, 10 mg

Glipizide and Metformin
(GLIP i zide & met FOR min)

U.S. Brand Names Metaglip™

Index Terms Glipizide and Metformin Hydrochloride; Metformin and Glipizide

Pharmacologic Category Antidiabetic Agent, Biguanide; Antidiabetic Agent, Sulfonylurea

Use Indicated as an adjunct to diet and exercise to improve glycemic control in adults with type 2 diabetes mellitus (noninsulin dependent, NIDDM)

Pregnancy Risk Factor C

Medication Safety Issues
High alert medication: The Institute for Safe Medication Practices (ISMP) includes this medication among its list of drugs which have a heightened risk of causing significant patient harm when used in error.

Dosage Oral: Type 2 diabetes:
Adults:
Patients inadequately controlled on diet and exercise alone: Initial dose: Glipizide 2.5 mg/metformin 250 mg once daily with a meal. In patients with fasting plasma glucose (FPG) 280-320 mg/dL, initiate therapy with glipizide 2.5 mg/metformin 500 mg twice daily.
Note: Increase dose by 1 tablet/day every 2 weeks (maximum daily dose: glipizide 10 mg/metformin 2000 mg in divided doses)
Patients inadequately controlled on a sulfonylurea and/or metformin: Initial dose: Glipizide 2.5 mg/metformin 500 mg or glipizide 5 mg/metformin 500 mg twice daily with morning and evening meals; starting dose should not exceed current daily dose of glipizide (or sulfonylurea equivalent) and/or metformin.
Note: Increase dose in increments of no more than glipizide 5 mg/metformin 500 mg (maximum daily dose: glipizide 20 mg/metformin 2000 mg)
Elderly: Conservative doses are recommended in the elderly due to potentially decreased renal function; **do not titrate to maximum dose**; should not be used in patients ≥80 years unless renal function is verified as normal

Dosage adjustment in renal impairment: Contraindicated in the presence of renal disease or renal dysfunction (serum creatinine ≥1.5 mg/dL [males], ≥1.4 mg/dL [females], or abnormal creatinine clearance)

Dosage adjustment in hepatic impairment: Avoid use in patients with impaired liver function

Additional Information Complete prescribing information for this medication should be consulted for additional detail.

Dosage Forms Excipient information presented when available (limited, particularly for generics); consult specific product labeling.
Tablet: 2.5/250: Glipizide 2.5 mg and metformin hydrochloride 250 mg; 2.5/500: Glipizide 2.5 mg and metformin hydrochloride 500 mg; 5/500: Glipizide 5 mg and metformin hydrochloride 500 mg
Metaglip™ 2.5/250: Glipizide 2.5 mg and metformin hydrochloride 250 mg
Metaglip™ 2.5/500: Glipizide 2.5 mg and metformin hydrochloride 500 mg
Metaglip™ 5/500: Glipizide 5 mg and metformin hydrochloride 500 mg

◆ **Glipizide and Metformin Hydrochloride** *see* Glipizide and Metformin *on page* 699
◆ **Glivec** *see* Imatinib *on page* 768
◆ **Gln** *see* Glutamine *on page* 700
◆ **GlucaGen®** *see* Glucagon *on page* 699
◆ **GlucaGen® Diagnostic Kit** *see* Glucagon *on page* 699
◆ **GlucaGen® HypoKit™** *see* Glucagon *on page* 699

Glucagon (GLOO ka gon)

U.S. Brand Names GlucaGen®; GlucaGen® Diagnostic Kit; GlucaGen® HypoKit™; Glucagon Emergency Kit

Index Terms Glucagon Hydrochloride

Pharmacologic Category Antidote; Diagnostic Agent

Use Management of hypoglycemia; diagnostic aid in radiologic examinations to temporarily inhibit GI tract movement

Unlabeled/Investigational Use Used with some success as a cardiac stimulant in management of severe cases of beta-adrenergic blocking agent overdosage; treatment of myocardial depression due to calcium channel blocker overdose

Pregnancy Risk Factor B

Lactation Excretion in breast milk unknown/compatible

Medication Safety Issues

Sound-alike/look-alike issues:

Glucagon may be confused with Glaucon®

Contraindications Hypersensitivity to glucagon or any component of the formulation; insulinoma; pheochromocytoma

Warnings/Precautions Use of glucagon is contraindicated in insulinoma; exogenous glucagon may cause an initial rise in blood glucose followed by rebound hypoglycemia. Use of glucagon is contraindicated in pheochromocytoma; exogenous glucagon may cause the release of catecholamines, resulting in an increase in blood pressure. Use caution with prolonged fasting, starvation, adrenal insufficiency or chronic hypoglycemia; levels of glucose stores in liver may be decreased. Supplemental carbohydrates should be given to patients who respond to glucagon for severe hypoglycemia to prevent secondary hypoglycemia. Monitor blood glucose levels closely. May contain lactose; avoid administration in hereditary galactose intolerance, Lapp lactase deficiency, or glucose-galactose malabsorption.

Adverse Reactions Frequency not defined.

Cardiovascular: Hypotension (up to 2 hours after GI procedures), hypertension, tachycardia

Gastrointestinal: Nausea, vomiting (high incidence with rapid administration of high doses)

Miscellaneous: Hypersensitivity reactions, anaphylaxis

Drug Interactions

Avoid Concomitant Use There are no known interactions where it is recommended to avoid concomitant use.

Increased Effect/Toxicity

Glucagon may increase the levels/effects of: Vitamin K Antagonists

Decreased Effect There are no known significant interactions involving a decrease in effect.

Ethanol/Nutrition/Herb Interactions Glucagon depletes glycogen stores.

Stability Prior to reconstitution, store at controlled room temperature of 20°C to 25°C (69°F to 77°F); do not freeze. Reconstitute powder for injection by adding 1 mL of sterile diluent to a vial containing 1 unit of the drug, to provide solutions containing 1 mg of glucagon/mL. Gently roll vial to dissolve. If dose to be administered is <2 mg of the drug, then use only the diluent provided by the manufacturer. If >2 mg, use sterile water for injection. Use immediately after reconstitution. May be kept at 5°C for up to 48 hours if necessary.

Mechanism of Action Stimulates adenylate cyclase to produce increased cyclic AMP, which promotes hepatic glycogenolysis and gluconeogenesis, causing a raise in blood glucose levels

Pharmacodynamics/Kinetics

Onset of action: Peak effect: Blood glucose levels:

Parenteral:

I.V.: 5-20 minutes

I.M.: 30 minutes

SubQ: 30-45 minutes

Duration: Glucose elevation:

SubQ: 60-90 minutes

I.V.: 30 minutes

Metabolism: Primarily hepatic; some inactivation occurring renally and in plasma

Half-life elimination, plasma: 8-18 minutes

Dosage

Hypoglycemia or insulin shock therapy: I.M., I.V., SubQ:

Children <20 kg: 0.5 mg or 20-30 mcg/kg/dose; repeated in 20 minutes as needed

Children ≥20 kg and Adults: 1 mg; may repeat in 20 minutes as needed

Note: I.V. dextrose should be administered as soon as it is available; if patient fails to respond to glucagon, I.V. dextrose must be given.

Beta-blocker overdose, calcium channel blocker overdose (unlabeled use): Adults: I.V.: 5-10 mg over 1 minutes followed by an infusion of 1-10 mg/hour. The following has also been reported for beta-blocker overdose: 3-10 mg or initially 0.5-5 mg bolus followed by continuous infusion 1-5 mg/hour

Diagnostic aid: Adults: I.M., I.V.: 0.25-2 mg 10 minutes prior to procedure

Dietary Considerations Administer carbohydrates to patient as soon as possible after response to treatment.

Administration I.V.: Bolus may be associated with nausea and vomiting. Continuous infusions may be used in beta-blocker overdose/toxicity.

Monitoring Parameters Blood pressure, blood glucose, ECG, heart rate, mentation

Additional Information 1 unit = 1 mg

Dosage Forms Excipient information presented when available (limited, particularly for generics); consult specific product labeling.

Injection, powder for reconstitution, as hydrochloride:

GlucaGen®: 1 mg [equivalent to 1 unit; contains lactose 107 mg]

GlucaGen® Diagnostic Kit: 1 mg [equivalent to 1 unit; contains lactose 107 mg; packaged with sterile water]

GlucaGen® HypoKit™: 1 mg [equivalent to 1 unit; contains lactose 107 mg; packaged with prefilled syringe containing sterile water]

Glucagon Emergency Kit: 1 mg [equivalent to 1 unit; contains lactose 49 mg; packaged with diluent syringe containing glycerin 12 mg/mL and water for injection]

- **Glucagon Emergency Kit** *see* Glucagon *on page* 699
- **Glucagon Hydrochloride** *see* Glucagon *on page* 699
- **Glucobay™ (Can)** *see* Acarbose *on page* 24
- **Glucocerebrosidase** *see* Alglucerase *on page* 62
- **GlucoNorm® (Can)** *see* Repaglinide *on page* 1303
- **Glucophage®** *see* MetFORMIN *on page* 954
- **Glucophage® XR** *see* MetFORMIN *on page* 954
- **Glucotrol®** *see* GlipiZIDE *on page* 697
- **Glucotrol XL®** *see* GlipiZIDE *on page* 697
- **Glucovance®** *see* Glyburide and Metformin *on page* 702
- **Glulisine Insulin** *see* Insulin Glulisine *on page* 794
- **Glumetza™** *see* MetFORMIN *on page* 954

Glutamine (GLOO ta meen)

U.S. Brand Names Enterex® Glutapak-10® [OTC]; NutreStore™; Resource® GlutaSolve® [OTC]; Sympt-X G.I. [OTC]; Sympt-X [OTC]

Index Terms Gln; L-Glutamine

Pharmacologic Category Amino Acid

Use Treatment of short bowel syndrome when used in combination with nutritional support and growth hormone therapy; a medical food used to promote GI tract healing and nutritional supplementation with GI disorders, HIV/AIDS, cancer, and other critical illnesses

Pregnancy Risk Factor C

Dosage Oral: Adults:

Nutritional supplement (Enterex® Glutapak-10®, Resource® GlutaSolve®, Sympt-X, Sympt-X G.I.): Average dose: 10 g 3 times/day; dosing range: 5-30 g/day

Short bowel syndrome (NutreStore™): 30 g/day administered as 5 g 6 times/day (every 2-3 hours while awake) for up to 16 weeks; to be used in combination with growth hormone and nutritional support

Additional Information Complete prescribing information for this medication should be consulted for additional detail.

Dosage Forms Excipient information presented when available (limited, particularly for generics); consult specific product labeling.

Powder for oral solution:

Enterex® Glutapak-10®: 10 g/packet (50s)

NutreStore™: 5 g/packet

Resource® GlutaSolve®: 15 g/packet (56s)

Sympt-X, Sympt-X G.I.: 10 g/packet (60s)

◆ **Glybenclamide** *see* GlyBURIDE *on page 701*

◆ **Glybenzcyclamide** *see* GlyBURIDE *on page 701*

GlyBURIDE (GLYE byoor ide)

U.S. Brand Names Diaβeta®; Glynase® PresTab®; Micronase®

Canadian Brand Names Albert® Glyburide; Apo-Glyburide®; Diaβeta®; Euglucon®; Gen-Glybe; Novo-Glyburide; Nu-Glyburide; PMS-Glyburide; ratio-Glyburide; Sandoz-Glyburide

Index Terms Diabeta; Glibenclamide; Glybenclamide; Glybenzcyclamide

Pharmacologic Category Antidiabetic Agent, Sulfonylurea

Additional Appendix Information

Diabetes Mellitus Management, Adults *on page 1801*

Sulfonamide Derivatives *on page 1671*

Use Management of type 2 diabetes mellitus (noninsulin dependent, NIDDM)

Unlabeled/Investigational Use Alternative to insulin in women for the treatment of gestational diabetes mellitus (GDM) (11-33 weeks gestation)

Pregnancy Risk Factor B/C (manufacturer dependent)

Pregnancy Considerations Reproduction studies differ by manufacturer labeling. Because adverse events were not observed in animal reproduction studies, one manufacturer classifies glyburide as pregnancy category B. Because adverse events were noted in animal studies during the period of lactation, another manufacturer classifies glyburide as pregnancy category C.

Glyburide was not found to significantly cross the placenta *in vitro* and was not found in the cord serum infants of mothers taking glyburide for gestational diabetes mellitus (GDM). Nonteratogenic effects such as hypoglycemia in the neonate have been associated with maternal glyburide use. Maternal hyperglycemia can be associated with adverse effects in the fetus, including macrosomia, neonatal hyperglycemia, and hyperbilirubinemia; the risk of congenital malformations is increased when the Hb A_{1c} is above the normal range. Diabetes can also be associated with adverse effects in the mother. Poorly-treated diabetes may cause end-organ damage that may in turn negatively affect obstetric outcomes. Physiologic glucose levels should be maintained prior to and during pregnancy to decrease the risk of adverse events in the mother and the fetus. The manufacturer recommends that if glyburide is used during pregnancy, it should be discontinued at least 2 weeks before the expected delivery date. Although studies have shown positive outcomes using glyburide for the treatment of GDM, use may not be appropriate for all women. Until additional safety and efficacy data are obtained, the use of oral agents is generally not recommended as routine management of type 2 diabetes mellitus during pregnancy. Insulin is considered the drug of choice for the control of diabetes mellitus during pregnancy.

Lactation Does not enter breast milk/use caution

Medication Safety Issues

Sound-alike/look-alike issues:

GlyBURIDE may be confused with glipiZIDE, Glucotrol®

Diaβeta® may be confused with Diabinese®, Zebeta®

Micronase® may be confused with microK®, miconazole, Micronor®, Microzide™

High alert medication: The Institute for Safe Medication Practices (ISMP) includes this medication among its list of drugs which have a heightened risk of causing significant patient harm when used in error.

Contraindications Hypersensitivity to glyburide, any component of the formulation, or other sulfonamides; type 1 diabetes mellitus (insulin dependent, IDDM), diabetic ketoacidosis; concurrent use with bosentan

Warnings/Precautions All sulfonylurea drugs are capable of producing severe hypoglycemia. Hypoglycemia is more likely to occur when caloric intake is deficient, after severe or prolonged exercise, when ethanol is ingested, or when more than one glucose-lowering drug is used. It is also more likely in elderly patients, malnourished patients and in patients with impaired renal or hepatic function; use with caution.

Elderly: Rapid and prolonged hypoglycemia (>12 hours) despite hypertonic glucose injections have been reported; age and hepatic and renal impairment are independent risk factors for hypoglycemia; dosage titration should be made at weekly intervals.

Chemical similarities are present among sulfonamides, sulfonylureas, carbonic anhydrase inhibitors, thiazides, and loop diuretics (except ethacrynic acid). Use in patients with sulfonamide allergy is specifically contraindicated in product labeling, however, a risk of cross-reaction exists in patients with allergy to any of these compounds; avoid use when previous reaction has been severe.

Product labeling states oral hypoglycemic drugs may be associated with an increased cardiovascular mortality as compared to treatment with diet alone or diet plus insulin. Data to support this association are limited, and several studies, including a large prospective trial (UKPDS) have not supported an association.

It may be necessary to discontinue therapy and administer insulin if the patient is exposed to stress (fever, trauma, infection, surgery). Safety and efficacy have not been established in children.

Adverse Reactions Frequency not defined.

Cardiovascular: Vasculitis

Central nervous system: Headache, dizziness

Dermatologic: Erythema, maculopapular eruptions, morbilliform eruptions, pruritus, purpura, rash, urticaria, photosensitivity reaction

Endocrine & metabolic: Disulfiram-like reaction, hypoglycemia, hyponatremia (SIADH reported with other sulfonylureas)

Gastrointestinal: Anorexia, constipation, diarrhea, epigastric fullness, heartburn, nausea

Genitourinary: Nocturia

Hematologic: Leukopenia, thrombocytopenia, hemolytic anemia, agranulocytosis, aplastic anemia, pancytopenia, porphyria cutanea tarda

Hepatic: Cholestatic jaundice, hepatitis, transaminase increased

Neuromuscular & skeletal: Arthralgia, myalgia, paresthesia

Ocular: Blurred vision

Renal: Diuretic effect (minor)

Miscellaneous: Allergic reaction

Drug Interactions

Metabolism/Transport Effects **Inhibits** CYP2C8 (weak), 3A4 (weak)

Avoid Concomitant Use

Avoid concomitant use of GlyBURIDE with any of the following: Bosentan

Increased Effect/Toxicity

GlyBURIDE may increase the levels/effects of: Alcohol (Ethyl); Bosentan; CycloSPORINE

The levels/effects of GlyBURIDE may be increased by: Chloramphenicol; Cimetidine; Cyclic Antidepressants; Fibric Acid Derivatives; Fluconazole; Herbs (Hypoglycemic Properties); Pegvisomant; Quinolone Antibiotics; Salicylates; Sulfonamide Derivatives

Decreased Effect

GlyBURIDE may decrease the levels/effects of: Bosentan

The levels/effects of GlyBURIDE may be decreased by: Bosentan; Colesevelam; Corticosteroids (Orally Inhaled); Corticosteroids (Systemic); Luteinizing Hormone-Releasing Hormone Analogs; Quinolone Antibiotics; Rifampin; Somatropin

Ethanol/Nutrition/Herb Interactions

Ethanol: Caution with ethanol (may cause hypoglycemia).

Herb/Nutraceutical: Herbs with hypoglycemic properties may enhance the hypoglycemic effect of glyburide. This includes alfalfa, aloe, bilberry, bitter melon, burdock, celery, damiana, fenugreek, garcinia, garlic, ginger, ginseng (American), gymnema, marshmallow, stinging nettle

Mechanism of Action Stimulates insulin release from the pancreatic beta cells; reduces glucose output from the liver; insulin sensitivity is increased at peripheral target sites

Pharmacodynamics/Kinetics

Onset of action: Serum insulin levels begin to increase 15-60 minutes after a single dose

Duration: ≤24 hours

Absorption: Significant within 1 hour

Distribution: 9-10 L

Protein binding, plasma: >99% primarily to albumin

Metabolism: Hepatic; forms metabolites (weakly active)

Half-life elimination: Diabeta®, Micronase®: 10 hours; Glynase® PresTab®: ~4 hours; may be prolonged with renal or hepatic impairment

Time to peak, serum: Adults: 2-4 hours

Excretion: Feces (50%) and urine (50%) as metabolites

Dosage Oral: Adults:

DiaBeta®, Micronase®:

Initial: 2.5-5 mg/day, administered with breakfast or the first main meal of the day. In patients who are more sensitive to hypoglycemic drugs, start at 1.25 mg/day.

Increase in increments of no more than 2.5 mg/day at weekly intervals based on the patient's blood glucose response

Maintenance: 1.25-20 mg/day given as single or divided doses; maximum: 20 mg/day

Elderly: Initial: 1.25-2.5 mg/day, increase by 1.25-2.5 mg/day every 1-3 weeks

Micronized tablets (Glynase® PresTab®): Adults:

Initial: 1.5-3 mg/day, administered with breakfast or the first main meal of the day in patients who are more sensitive to hypoglycemic drugs, start at 0.75 mg/day. Increase in increments of no more than 1.5 mg/day in weekly intervals based on the patient's blood glucose response.

Maintenance: 0.75-12 mg/day given as a single dose or in divided doses. Some patients (especially those receiving >6 mg/day) may have a more satisfactory response with twice-daily dosing. Maximum: 12 mg/day

Dosing adjustment/comments in renal impairment: Cl_{cr} <50 mL/minute: **Not recommended**

Dosing adjustment in hepatic impairment: Use conservative initial and maintenance doses and avoid use in severe disease

Dietary Considerations Should be taken with meals at the same time each day. Dietary modification based on ADA recommendations is a part of therapy. Decreases blood glucose concentration. Hypoglycemia may occur. Must be able to recognize symptoms of hypoglycemia (palpitations, sweaty palms, lightheadedness).

Administration Administer with meals at the same time each day. Patients who are anorexic or NPO may need to have their dose held to avoid hypoglycemia.

Monitoring Parameters Signs and symptoms of hypoglycemia, fasting blood glucose, hemoglobin A_{1c}

Reference Range Recommendations for glycemic control in adults with diabetes:

Hb A_{1c}: <7%

Preprandial capillary plasma glucose: 70-130 mg/dL

Peak postprandial capillary blood glucose: <180 mg/dL

Blood pressure: <130/80 mm Hg

Dosage Forms Excipient information presented when available (limited, particularly for generics); consult specific product labeling. [DSC] = Discontinued product

Tablet: 1.25 mg, 2.5 mg, 5 mg

DiaBeta®: 1.25 mg, 2.5 mg, 5 mg

Micronase®: 1.25 mg, 2.5 mg [DSC], 5 mg

Tablet, micronized: 1.5 mg, 3 mg, 6 mg

Glynase® PresTab®: 1.5 mg, 3 mg, 6 mg

Glyburide and Metformin

(GLYE byoor ide & met FOR min)

U.S. Brand Names Glucovance®

Index Terms Glyburide and Metformin Hydrochloride; Metformin and Glyburide

Pharmacologic Category Antidiabetic Agent, Biguanide; Antidiabetic Agent, Sulfonylurea

Use Adjunct to diet and exercise for the management of type 2 diabetes mellitus (noninsulin dependent, NIDDM)

Pregnancy Risk Factor B

Medication Safety Issues

Sound-alike/look-alike issues:

Glucovance may be confused with Vyvanse™

High alert medication: The Institute for Safe Medication Practices (ISMP) includes this medication among its list of drugs which have a heightened risk of causing significant patient harm when used in error.

Dosage Note: Dose must be individualized. Dosages expressed as glyburide/metformin components.

Adults: Oral:

Initial therapy (no prior treatment with sulfonylurea or metformin): 1.25 mg/250 mg once daily with a meal; patients with Hb A_{1c} >9% or fasting plasma glucose (FPG) >200 mg/dL may start with 1.25 mg/250 mg twice daily with meals. **Note:** Doses of 5 mg /500 mg should not be used as initial therapy, due to risk of hypoglycemia.

Dosage may be increased in increments of 1.25 mg/250 mg, at intervals of not less than 2 weeks; maximum daily dose: 10 mg/2000 mg (limited experience with higher doses)

Previously treated with a sulfonylurea or metformin alone: Initial: 2.5 mg/500 mg or 5 mg/500 mg twice daily with meals; increase in increments no greater than 5 mg/500 mg; maximum daily dose: 20 mg/2000 mg

When switching patients previously on a sulfonylurea and metformin together, do not exceed the daily dose of glyburide (or glyburide equivalent) or metformin.

Note: May combine with a thiazolidinedione in patients with an inadequate response to glyburide/metformin therapy (risk of hypoglycemia may be increased). When adding thiazolidinedione, continue glyburide and metformin at current dose and initiate thiazolidinedione at recommended starting dose.

Elderly: Oral: Conservative doses are recommended in the elderly due to potentially decreased renal function; **do not titrate to maximum dose**; should not be used in patients ≥80 years of age unless renal function is verified as normal

Dosage adjustment in renal impairment: Risk of lactic acidosis increases with degree of renal impairment; contraindicated in renal disease or renal dysfunction

Dosage adjustment in hepatic impairment: Use conservative initial and maintenance doses and avoid use in severe hepatic disease

Additional Information Complete prescribing information for this medication should be consulted for additional detail.

Dosage Forms Excipient information presented when available (limited, particularly for generics); consult specific product labeling.

Tablet: 1.25 mg/250 mg: Glyburide 1.25 mg and metformin hydrochloride 250 mg; 2.5 mg/500 mg: Glyburide 2.5 mg and metformin hydrochloride 500 mg; 5 mg/500 mg: Glyburide 5 mg and metformin hydrochloride 500 mg

Glucovance®: 1.25 mg/250 mg: Glyburide 1.25 mg and metformin hydrochloride 250 mg

Glucovance®: 2.5 mg/500 mg: Glyburide 2.5 mg and metformin hydrochloride 500 mg

Glucovance®: 5 mg/500 mg: Glyburide 5 mg and metformin hydrochloride 500 mg

◆ **Glyburide and Metformin Hydrochloride** *see* Glyburide and Metformin *on page 702*

◆ **Glycerol Guaiacolate** *see* GuaiFENesin *on page 709*

◆ **Glyceryl Trinitrate** *see* Nitroglycerin *on page 1073*

◆ **GlycoLax®** *see* Polyethylene Glycol 3350 *on page 1209*

◆ **Glycon (Can)** *see* MetFORMIN *on page 954*

Glycopyrrolate (glye koe PYE roe late)

U.S. Brand Names Robinul®; Robinul® Forte

Canadian Brand Names Glycopyrrolate Injection, USP

Index Terms Glycopyrronium Bromide

Pharmacologic Category Anticholinergic Agent

Use Inhibit salivation and excessive secretions of the respiratory tract preoperatively; reversal of neuromuscular blockade; control of upper airway secretions; adjunct in treatment of peptic ulcer

Pregnancy Risk Factor B

Pregnancy Considerations Teratogenic effects were not observed in animal studies. Small amounts of glycopyrrolate cross the human placenta.

Lactation Excretion in breast milk unknown/use caution

Contraindications Hypersensitivity to glycopyrrolate or any component of the formulation; severe ulcerative colitis, toxic megacolon complicating ulcerative colitis, paralytic ileus, obstructive disease of GI tract, intestinal atony in the elderly or debilitated patient; unstable cardiovascular status in acute hemorrhage; narrow-angle glaucoma; acute hemorrhage; tachycardia; obstructive uropathy; myasthenia gravis

Warnings/Precautions Diarrhea may be a sign of incomplete intestinal obstruction, treatment should be discontinued if this occurs. Use caution in elderly, patients with autonomic neuropathy, hepatic or renal disease, ulcerative colitis may precipitate/aggravate toxic megacolon, hyperthyroidism, CAD, CHF, arrhythmias, tachycardia, BPH, or hiatal hernia with reflux. Use of anticholinergics in gastric ulcer treatment may cause a delay in gastric emptying due to antral statis. Caution should be used in individuals demonstrating decreased pigmentation (skin and iris coloration, dark versus light) since there has been some evidence that these individuals have an enhanced sensitivity to the anticholinergic response. May cause drowsiness, eye sensitivity to light, or blurred vision; caution should be used when performing tasks which require mental alertness, such as driving. Thr risk of heat stroke with this medication may be increased during exercise or hot weather. Infants, patients with Down syndrome, and children with spastic paralysis or brain damage may be hypersensitive to antimuscarine effects. Injection contains benzyl alcohol (associated with gasping syndrome in neonates). Not recommended for use in children <12 years of age for the management of peptic ulcer or <16 years for preanesthetic use.

Adverse Reactions Frequency not defined. **Note:** Includes adverse effects which may occur as an extension of the pharmacologic action of anticholinergics (including glycopyrrolate) and adverse effects reported postmarketing with glycopyrrolate.

Cardiovascular: Arrhythmias, cardiac arrest, heart block, hyper-/hypotension, malignant hyperthermia, palpitation, QT_c interval prolongation, tachycardia

Central nervous system: Confusion, dizziness, drowsiness, excitement, headache, insomnia, nervousness, seizure

Dermatologic: Dry skin, pruritus, sensitivity to light increased

Endocrine & metabolic: Lactation suppression

Gastrointestinal: Bloated feeling, constipation, loss of taste, nausea, vomiting, xerostomia

Genitourinary: Impotence, urinary hesitancy, urinary retention

Local: Irritation at injection site

Neuromuscular & skeletal: Weakness

Ocular: Blurred vision, cycloplegia, mydriasis, ocular tension increased, photophobia, sensitivity to light increased

Respiratory: Respiratory depression

Miscellaneous: Anaphylactoid reactions, diaphoresis decreased, hypersensitivity reactions

Drug Interactions

Avoid Concomitant Use There are no known interactions where it is recommended to avoid concomitant use.

Increased Effect/Toxicity

Glycopyrrolate may increase the levels/effects of: Anticholinergics; Cannabinoids; Potassium Chloride

The levels/effects of Glycopyrrolate may be increased by: Pramlintide

Decreased Effect

Glycopyrrolate may decrease the levels/effects of: Acetylcholinesterase Inhibitors (Central); Secretin

The levels/effects of Glycopyrrolate may be decreased by: Acetylcholinesterase Inhibitors (Central)

Stability Store at 20°C to 25°C (68°F to 77°F).

Mechanism of Action Blocks the action of acetylcholine at parasympathetic sites in smooth muscle, secretory glands, and the CNS

Pharmacodynamics/Kinetics

Onset of action: Oral: 50 minutes; I.M.: 15-30 minutes; I.V.: ~1 minute

Peak effect: Oral: ~1 hour; I.M.: 30-45 minutes

Duration: Vagal effect: 2-3 hours; Inhibition of salivation: Up to 7 hours; Anticholinergic: Oral: 8-12 hours

Absorption: Oral: Poor and erratic

Distribution: V_d: 0.2-0.62 L/kg

Metabolism: Hepatic (minimal)

Bioavailability: ~10%

Half-life elimination: Infants: 22-130 minutes; Children 19-99 minutes; Adults: ~30-75 minutes

Excretion: Urine (as unchanged drug, I.M.: 80%, I.V.: 85%); bile (as unchanged drug)

Dosage

Children:

Reduction of secretions (preanesthetic):

Oral: 40-100 mcg/kg/dose 3-4 times/day

I.M., I.V.: 4-10 mcg/kg/dose every 3-4 hours; maximum: 0.2 mg/dose or 0.8 mg/24 hours

Intraoperative: I.V.: 4 mcg/kg not to exceed 0.1 mg; repeat at 2- to 3-minute intervals as needed

Preoperative: I.M.:

<2 years: 4-9 mcg/kg 30-60 minutes before procedure

>2 years: 4 mcg/kg 30-60 minutes before procedure

Children and Adults: Reverse neuromuscular blockade: I.V.: 0.2 mg for each 1 mg of neostigmine or 5 mg of pyridostigmine administered or 5-15 mcg/kg glycopyrrolate with 25-70 mcg/kg of neostigmine or 0.1-0.3 mg/kg of pyridostigmine (agents usually administered simultaneously, but glycopyrrolate may be administered first if bradycardia is present)

Adults:

Reduction of secretions:

Intraoperative: I.V.: 0.1 mg repeated as needed at 2- to 3-minute intervals

Preoperative: I.M.: 4 mcg/kg 30-60 minutes before procedure

Peptic ulcer:

Oral: 1-2 mg 2-3 times/day

I.M., I.V.: 0.1-0.2 mg 3-4 times/day

Administration For I.V. administration, glycopyrrolate may also be administered via the tubing of a running I.V. infusion of a compatible solution; may be administered in the same syringe with neostigmine or pyridostigmine.

Monitoring Parameters Heart rate; anticholinergic effects; bowel sounds

Dosage Forms Excipient information presented when available (limited, particularly for generics); consult specific product labeling. [DSC] = Discontinued product

Injection, solution: 0.2 mg/mL (1 mL, 2 mL, 5 mL, 20 mL)

Robinul®: 0.2 mg/mL (1 mL, 2 mL, 5 mL; 20 mL [DSC]) [contains benzyl alcohol]

Tablet: 1 mg, 2 mg

Robinul®: 1 mg

Robinul® Forte: 2 mg

- **Glycopyrrolate Injection, USP (Can)** *see* Glycopyrrolate *on page 703*
- **Glycopyrronium Bromide** *see* Glycopyrrolate *on page 703*
- **Glydiazinamide** *see* GlipiZIDE *on page 697*
- **Glynase® PresTab®** *see* GlyBURIDE *on page 701*
- **Gly-Oxide® [OTC]** *see* Carbamide Peroxide *on page 254*
- **Glyquin®** *see* Hydroquinone *on page 749*
- **Glyquin-XM™** *see* Hydroquinone *on page 749*
- **Glyquin® XM (Can)** *see* Hydroquinone *on page 749*
- **Glyset®** *see* Miglitol *on page 996*
- **GM-CSF** *see* Sargramostim *on page 1355*
- **GMD-Azithromycin (Can)** *see* Azithromycin *on page 166*
- **GMD-Fluconazole (Can)** *see* Fluconazole *on page 625*
- **GMD-Gemfibrozil (Can)** *see* Gemfibrozil *on page 687*
- **GMD-Sertraline (Can)** *see* Sertraline *on page 1362*
- **GnRH** *see* Gonadorelin *on page 704*
- **GnRH Agonist** *see* Histrelin *on page 732*

Gold Sodium Thiomalate
(gold SOW dee um thye oh MAL ate)

U.S. Brand Names Myochrysine®

Canadian Brand Names Myochrysine®

Index Terms Sodium Aurothiomalate

Pharmacologic Category Gold Compound

Use Treatment of progressive rheumatoid arthritis

Pregnancy Risk Factor C

Dosage I.M.:

Children: Initial: Test dose of 10 mg is recommended, followed by 1 mg/kg/week for 20 weeks; maintenance: 1 mg/kg/dose at 2- to 4-week intervals thereafter for as long as therapy is clinically beneficial and toxicity does not develop. Administration for 2-4 months is usually required before clinical improvement is observed.

Adults: 10 mg first week; 25 mg second week; then 25-50 mg/week until 1 g cumulative dose has been given; if improvement occurs without adverse reactions, administer 25-50 mg every 2-3 weeks for 2-20 weeks, then every 3-4 weeks indefinitely

Dosage adjustment for toxicity: If toxicity develops, gold sodium thiomalate should be discontinued immediately and symptomatic treatment may be given as required. Severe reactions are a contraindication to further gold therapy. If the reaction to gold therapy is not severe, therapy may be resumed, generally 2-3 weeks following resolution of the toxic reaction. A challenge dose of 5-10 mg of gold may be administered; if the "challenge dose" is tolerated, dosage may be cautiously increased by 5-10 mg in subsequent injections until usual dosage is achieved (25-50 mg).

Dosing adjustment in renal impairment:

Cl_{cr} 50-80 mL/minute: Administer 50% of normal dose

Cl_{cr} <50 mL/minute: Avoid use

Additional Information Complete prescribing information for this medication should be consulted for additional detail.

Dosage Forms Excipient information presented when available (limited, particularly for generics); consult specific product labeling.

Injection, solution:

Myochrysine®: 50 mg/mL (1 mL, 10 mL)

- **GoLYTELY®** *see* Polyethylene Glycol-Electrolyte Solution *on page 1209*

Gonadorelin (goe nad oh RELL in)

U.S. Brand Names Factrel®

Canadian Brand Names Lutrepulse™

Index Terms GnRH; Gonadorelin Acetate; Gonadorelin Hydrochloride; Gonadotropin Releasing Hormone; LHRH; LRH; Luteinizing Hormone Releasing Hormone

Pharmacologic Category Diagnostic Agent; Gonadotropin

Use Evaluation of functional capacity and response of gonadotrophic hormones; evaluate abnormal gonadotropin regulation as in precocious puberty and delayed puberty.

Orphan drug: Lutrepulse®: Induction of ovulation in females with hypothalamic amenorrhea

Pregnancy Risk Factor B

Lactation Excretion in breast milk unknown

Medication Safety Issues

Sound-alike/look-alike issues:

Gonadorelin may be confused with gonadotropin, guanadrel

Factrel® may be confused with Sectral®

Gonadotropin may be confused with gonadorelin

Contraindications Hypersensitivity to gonadorelin or any component of the formulation; women with any condition that could be exacerbated by pregnancy; patients who have ovarian cysts or causes of anovulation other than those of hypothalamic origin; any condition that may worsened by reproductive hormones

Warnings/Precautions Hypersensitivity and anaphylactic reactions have occurred following multiple-dose administration; multiple pregnancy is a possibility; use with caution in women in whom pregnancy could worsen pre-existing conditions (eg, pituitary prolactinemia). Multiple pregnancy is a possibility with Lutrepulse®.

Adverse Reactions 1% to 10%: Local: Pain at injection site

Drug Interactions

Avoid Concomitant Use There are no known interactions where it is recommended to avoid concomitant use.

Increased Effect/Toxicity There are no known significant interactions involving an increase in effect.

Decreased Effect There are no known significant interactions involving a decrease in effect.

Stability

Factrel®: Prepare immediately prior to use. After reconstitution, store at room temperature and use within 1 day. Discard unused portion.

Lutrepulse®: Store at room temperature. Reconstitute with diluent immediately prior to use and transfer to plastic reservoir. The solution will supply 90 minute pulsatile doses for 7 consecutive days (Lutrepulse® pump).

Mechanism of Action Stimulates the release of luteinizing hormone (LH) from the anterior pituitary gland

Pharmacodynamics/Kinetics

Onset of action: Peak effect: Maximal LH release: ~20 minutes

Duration: 3-5 hours

Half-life elimination: 4 minutes

Dosage

Diagnostic test: Children >12 years and Female Adults: I.V., SubQ hydrochloride salt: 100 mcg administered in women during early phase of menstrual cycle (day 1-7)

Primary hypothalamic amenorrhea: Female Adults: Acetate: I.V.: 5 mcg every 90 minutes via Lutrepulse® pump kit at treatment intervals of 21 days (pump will pulsate every 90 minutes for 7 days)

Administration

Factrel®: Dilute in 3 mL of normal saline; administer I.V. push over 30 seconds

Lutrepulse®: A presterilized reservoir bag with the infusion catheter set supplied with the kit should be filled with the reconstituted solution and administered I.V. using the Lutrepulse® pump. Set the pump to deliver 25-50 mL of solution, based upon the dose, over a pulse period of 1 minute and at a pulse frequency of 90 minutes.

Monitoring Parameters LH, FSH

Dosage Forms Excipient information presented when available (limited, particularly for generics); consult specific product labeling.

Injection, powder for reconstitution, as hydrochloride: 100 mcg [diluent contains benzyl alcohol]

- ◆ **Gonadorelin Acetate** *see* Gonadorelin *on page 704*
- ◆ **Gonadorelin Hydrochloride** *see* Gonadorelin *on page 704*
- ◆ **Gonadotropin Releasing Hormone** *see* Gonadorelin *on page 704*
- ◆ **Gonal-f®** *see* Follitropin Alfa *on page 656*
- ◆ **Gonal-f® Pen (Can)** *see* Follitropin Alfa *on page 656*
- ◆ **Gonal-f® RFF** *see* Follitropin Alfa *on page 656*
- ◆ **Goody's® Extra Strength Headache Powder [OTC]** *see* Acetaminophen, Aspirin, and Caffeine *on page 31*
- ◆ **Goody's® Extra Strength Pain Relief [OTC]** *see* Acetaminophen, Aspirin, and Caffeine *on page 31*
- ◆ **Goody's PM® [OTC]** *see* Acetaminophen and Diphenhydramine *on page 28*
- ◆ **Gordon Boro-Packs [OTC]** *see* Aluminum Sulfate and Calcium Acetate *on page 77*
- ◆ **Gormel® [OTC]** *see* Urea *on page 1530*

Goserelin (GOE se rel in)

U.S. Brand Names Zoladex®

Canadian Brand Names Zoladex®; Zoladex® LA

Index Terms D-Ser(Bu^t)^6,Azgly^{10}-LHRH; Goserelin Acetate; ICI-118630; NSC-606864

Pharmacologic Category Antineoplastic Agent, Gonadotropin-Releasing Hormone Agonist; Gonadotropin Releasing Hormone Agonist

Use Palliative treatment of advanced breast cancer and carcinoma of the prostate; treatment of endometriosis, including pain relief and reduction of endometriotic lesions; endometrial thinning agent as part of treatment for dysfunctional uterine bleeding

Pregnancy Risk Factor X (endometriosis, endometrial thinning); D (advanced breast cancer)

Pregnancy Considerations Goserelin has been found to be teratogenic and increases pregnancy loss in animal studies. Women of childbearing potential should avoid pregnancy. Pregnancy must be ruled out prior to treatment. Use of nonhormonal contraception should be used during therapy and following discontinuation until the return of menses (or for at least 12 weeks).

Lactation Enters breast milk/contraindicated

Contraindications Hypersensitivity to goserelin, LHRH, LHRH agonist analogues, or any component of the formulation; pregnancy (or potential to become pregnant); breast-feeding

Warnings/Precautions Hazardous agent - use appropriate precautions for handling and disposal. Transient worsening of signs and symptoms (tumor flare) may develop during the first few weeks of treatment. Urinary tract obstruction or spinal cord compression have been reported when used for prostate cancer; closely observe patients for weakness, paresthesias, and urinary tract obstruction in first few weeks of therapy. Decreased bone density has been reported in women and may be irreversible; use caution if other risk factors are present; evaluate and institute preventative treatment if necessary. Rare cases of pituitary apoplexy (frequently secondary to pituitary adenoma) have been observed with leuprolide administration (onset from 1 hour to usually <2 weeks); may present as sudden headache, vomiting, visual or mental status changes, and infrequently cardiovascular collapse; immediate medical attention required. Safety and efficacy have not been established in pediatric patients.

Adverse Reactions Percentages reported in males with prostatic carcinoma and females with endometriosis using the 1-month implant:

>10%:

Central nervous system: Headache (female 75%, male 1% to 5%), emotional lability (female 60%), depression (female 54%, male 1% to 5%), pain (female 17%, male 8%), insomnia (female 11%, male 5%)

Endocrine & metabolic: Hot flashes (female 96%, male 62%), sexual dysfunction (21%), erections decreased (18%), libido decreased (female 61%), breast enlargement (female 18%)

Genitourinary: Lower urinary symptoms (male 13%), vaginitis (75%), dyspareunia (female 14%)

Miscellaneous: Diaphoresis (female 45%, male 6%); infection (female 13%)

1% to 10%:

Cardiovascular: CHF (male 5%), arrhythmia, cerebrovascular accident, hypertension, MI, peripheral vascular disorder, chest pain, palpitation, tachycardia, edema

Central nervous system: Lethargy (male 8%), dizziness (female 6%, male 5%), abnormal thinking, anxiety, chills, fever, malaise, migraine, somnolence

Dermatologic: Rash (female >1%, male 6%), alopecia, bruising, dry skin, skin discoloration

Endocrine & metabolic: Breast pain (female 7%), breast swelling/tenderness (male 1% to 5%), dysmenorrhea, gout, hyperglycemia

Gastrointestinal: Anorexia (female >1%, male 5%), nausea (male 5%), constipation, diarrhea, flatulence, dyspepsia, ulcer, vomiting, weight increased, xerostomia

Genitourinary: Renal insufficiency, urinary frequency, urinary obstruction, urinary tract infection, vaginal hemorrhage

Hematologic: Anemia, hemorrhage

Neuromuscular & skeletal: Arthralgia, bone mineral density decreased (female; ~4% decrease in 6 months), joint disorder, paresthesia

Ocular: Amblyopia, dry eyes

Respiratory: Upper respiratory tract infection (male 7%), COPD (male 5%), pharyngitis (female 5%), bronchitis, cough, epistaxis, rhinitis, sinusitis

Miscellaneous: Allergic reaction

Postmarketing and/or case reports: Pituitary apoplexy

Drug Interactions

Avoid Concomitant Use There are no known interactions where it is recommended to avoid concomitant use.

Increased Effect/Toxicity There are no known significant interactions involving an increase in effect.

Decreased Effect

Goserelin may decrease the levels/effects of: Antidiabetic Agents

Stability Zoladex® should be stored at room temperature not to exceed 25°C or 77°F. Protect from light; should be dispensed in a lightproof bag.

Mechanism of Action Goserelin is a synthetic analog of luteinizing-hormone-releasing hormone (LHRH). Following an initial increase in luteinizing hormone (LH) and follicle stimulating hormone (FSH), chronic administration of goserelin results in a sustained suppression of pituitary gonadotropins. Serum testosterone falls to levels comparable to surgical castration. The exact mechanism of this effect is unknown, but may be related to changes in the control of LH or down-regulation of LH receptors.

Pharmacodynamics/Kinetics Note: Data reported using the 1-month implant.

Absorption: SubQ: Rapid and can be detected in serum in 10 minutes

Distribution: V_d: Male: 44.1 L; Female: 20.3 L

Time to peak, serum: SubQ: Male: 12-15 days, Female: 8-22 days

Half-life elimination: SubQ: Male: ~4 hours, Female: ~2 hours; Renal impairment: Male: 12 hours

Excretion: Urine (90%)

Dosage SubQ: Adults:

Prostate cancer:

Monthly implant: 3.6 mg injected into upper abdomen every 28 days

3-month implant: 10.8 mg injected into the upper abdominal wall every 12 weeks

Breast cancer, endometriosis, endometrial thinning: Monthly implant: 3.6 mg injected into upper abdomen every 28 days

Note: For breast cancer, treatment may continue indefinitely; for endometriosis, it is recommended that duration of treatment not exceed 6 months. Only 1-2 doses are recommended for endometrial thinning.

Dosing adjustment in renal/hepatic impairment: No adjustment is necessary

Administration Subcutaneous implant: Insert the hypodermic needle into the subcutaneous fat. Do not try to aspirate with the goserelin syringe. If the needle is in a large vessel, blood will immediately appear in the syringe chamber. Change the direction of the needle so it parallels the abdominal wall. Push the needle in until the barrel hub touches the patient's skin. Fully depress the plunger to discharge. Withdraw needle and bandage the site. Confirm discharge by ensuring tip of the plunger is visible within the tip of the needle.

Test Interactions Serum alkaline phosphatase, serum acid phosphatase, serum testosterone, serum LH and FSH, serum estradiol

Dosage Forms Excipient information presented when available (limited, particularly for generics); consult specific product labeling.

Implant, subcutaneous:

Zoladex®:

3.6 mg [1-month implant packaged with 16-gauge hypodermic needle]

10.8 mg [3-month implant packaged with 14-gauge hypodermic needle]

- ◆ **Goserelin Acetate** *see* Goserelin *on page 705*
- ◆ **GP 47680** *see* OXcarbazepine *on page 1116*
- ◆ **GPI 15715** *see* Fospropofol *on page 673*
- ◆ **GR38032R** *see* Ondansetron *on page 1102*
- ◆ **Gramicidin, Neomycin, and Polymyxin B** *see* Neomycin, Polymyxin B, and Gramicidin *on page 1052*

Granisetron (gra NI se tron)

U.S. Brand Names Granisol™; Kytril®; Sancuso®

Canadian Brand Names Kytril®

Index Terms BRL 43694

Pharmacologic Category Antiemetic; Selective 5-HT_3 Receptor Antagonist

Use Prophylaxis of nausea and vomiting associated with emetogenic chemotherapy and radiation therapy (including total body irradiation and fractionated abdominal radiation); prophylaxis and treatment of postoperative nausea and vomiting (PONV)

Transdermal patch: Prophylaxis of nausea and vomiting associated with moderate-to-high emetogenic chemotherapy regimens ≤5 days consecutive duration

Generally **not** recommended for treatment of existing chemotherapy-induced emesis (CIE) or for prophylaxis of nausea from agents with a low emetogenic potential.

Pregnancy Risk Factor B

Pregnancy Considerations There are no adequate or well-controlled studies in pregnant women. Teratogenic effects were not observed in animal studies. Injection (1 mg/mL strength) contains benzyl alcohol which may cross the placenta. Use only if benefit exceeds the risk.

Lactation Excretion in breast milk unknown/use caution

Medication Safety Issues

Sound-alike/look-alike issues:

Granisetron may be confused with dolasetron, ondansetron, palonosetron

Contraindications Hypersensitivity to granisetron or any component of the formulation

Warnings/Precautions Use with caution in patients with congenital long QT syndrome or other risk factors for QT prolongation (eg, medications known to prolong QT interval, electrolyte abnormalities, and cumulative high-dose anthracycline therapy). 5-HT_3 antagonists have been associated with a number of dose-dependent increases in ECG intervals (eg, PR, QRS duration, QT/QT_c, JT), usually occurring 1-2 hours after I.V. administration. In general, these changes are not clinically relevant, however, when used in conjunction with other agents that prolong these intervals, arrhythmia may occur. When used with agents that prolong the QT interval (eg, Class I and III antiarrhythmics), clinically relevant QT interval prolongation may occur resulting in torsade de pointes. I.V. formulations of 5-HT_3 antagonists have more association with ECG interval changes, compared to oral formulations.

For chemotherapy-related emesis, **granisetron should be used on a scheduled basis, not on an "as needed" (PRN) basis**, since data support the use of this drug in the prevention of nausea and vomiting and not in the rescue of nausea and vomiting. Granisetron should be used only in the first 24-48 hours of receiving chemotherapy or radiation. Data do not support any increased efficacy of granisetron in delayed nausea and vomiting.

Use with caution in patients allergic to other 5-HT_3 receptor antagonists; cross-reactivity has been reported. Routine prophylaxis for PONV is not recommended in patients where there is little expectation of nausea and vomiting postoperatively. In patients where nausea and vomiting must be avoided postoperatively, administer to all patients even when expected incidence of nausea and vomiting is low. Use caution following abdominal surgery or in chemotherapy-induced nausea and vomiting; may mask progressive ileus or gastric distention. Application site reactions, generally mild, have occurred with transdermal patch use; if skin reaction is severe or generalized, remove patch. Cover patch application site with clothing to protect from natural or artificial sunlight exposure while patch is applied and for 10 days following removal; granisetron may potentially be affected by natural or artificial sunlight. Do not apply patch to red, irritated, or damaged skin. Injection contains benzyl alcohol (1 mg/mL) and should not be used in neonates.

Adverse Reactions

>10%:

Central nervous system: Headache (3% to 21%; transdermal patch: 1%)

Gastrointestinal: Constipation (3% to 18%)

Neuromuscular & skeletal: Weakness (5% to 18%)

1% to 10%:

Cardiovascular: QT_c prolongation (1% to 3%), hypertension (1% to 2%)

Central nervous system: Pain (10%), fever (3% to 9%), dizziness (4% to 5%), insomnia (<2% to 5%), somnolence (1% to 4%), anxiety (2%), agitation (<2%), CNS stimulation (<2%)

Dermatologic: Rash (1%)

Gastrointestinal: Diarrhea (3% to 9%), abdominal pain (4% to 6%), dyspepsia (3% to 6%), taste perversion (2%)

Hepatic: Liver enzymes increased (5% to 6%)

Renal: Oliguria (2%)

Respiratory: Cough (2%)

Miscellaneous: Infection (3%)

<1% (Limited to important or life-threatening): Agitation, allergic reactions; anaphylaxis (including hypotension, dyspnea, urticaria); angina, application site reactions (transdermal patch), arrhythmias, atrial fibrillation, extrapyramidal syndrome, hot flashes, hypotension, hypersensitivity, syncope

Drug Interactions

Metabolism/Transport Effects Substrate of CYP3A4 (minor)

Avoid Concomitant Use

Avoid concomitant use of Granisetron with any of the following: Apomorphine

Increased Effect/Toxicity

Granisetron may increase the levels/effects of: Apomorphine

Decreased Effect There are no known significant interactions involving a decrease in effect.

Stability

I.V.: Store at 15°C to 30°C (59°F to 86°F). Stable when mixed in NS or D_5W for 7 days under refrigeration and for 3 days at room temperature. Protect from light. Do not freeze vials.

Oral: Store tablet or oral solution at 15°C to 30°C (59°F to 86°F). Protect from light.

Transdermal patch: Store at 20°C to 25°C (68°F to 77°F). Keep patch in original packaging until immediately prior to use.

Mechanism of Action Selective 5-HT_3-receptor antagonist, blocking serotonin, both peripherally on vagal nerve terminals and centrally in the chemoreceptor trigger zone

Pharmacodynamics/Kinetics

Duration: Oral, I.V.: Generally up to 24 hours

Absorption: Oral: Tablets and oral solution are bioequivalent; Transdermal patch: ~66% over 7 days

Distribution: V_d: 2-4 L/kg; widely throughout body

Protein binding: 65%

Metabolism: Hepatic via N-demethylation, oxidation, and conjugation; some metabolites may have 5-HT_3 antagonist activity

Half-life elimination: Oral: 6 hours; I.V.: 9 hours

Time to peak, plasma: Transdermal patch: Maximum systemic concentrations: ~48 hours after application (range: 24-168 hours)

Excretion: Urine (12% as unchanged drug, 48% to 49% as metabolites); feces (34% to 38% as metabolites)

Dosage

Oral: Adults:

Prophylaxis of chemotherapy-related emesis: 2 mg once daily up to 1 hour before chemotherapy or 1 mg twice daily; the first 1 mg dose should be given up to 1 hour before chemotherapy.

Prophylaxis of radiation therapy-associated emesis: 2 mg once daily given 1 hour before radiation therapy.

I.V.:

Children ≥2 years and Adults: Prophylaxis of chemotherapy-related emesis:

Within U.S.: 10 mcg/kg/dose (maximum: 1 mg/dose) given 30 minutes prior to chemotherapy; for some drugs (eg, carboplatin, cyclophosphamide) with a later onset of emetic action, 10 mcg/kg every 12 hours may be necessary

Outside U.S.: 40 mcg/kg/dose (or 3 mg/dose); maximum: 9 mg/24 hours

Breakthrough: Granisetron has not been shown to be effective in terminating nausea or vomiting once it occurs and should not be used for this purpose.

Adults: PONV:

Prevention: 1 mg given undiluted over 30 seconds; administer before induction of anesthesia or immediately before reversal of anesthesia

Treatment: 1 mg given undiluted over 30 seconds

Transdermal patch: Adults: Prophylaxis of chemotherapy-related emesis: Apply 1 patch at least 24 hours prior to chemotherapy; do not apply ≥48 hours before chemotherapy. Remove patch a minimum of 24 hours after chemotherapy completion. Maximum duration: Patch may be worn up to 7 days, depending on chemotherapy regimen duration.

Dosing interval in renal impairment: No dosage adjustment required.

Dosing interval in hepatic impairment: Kinetic studies in patients with hepatic impairment showed that total clearance was approximately halved, however, standard doses were very well tolerated, and dose adjustments are not necessary.

Administration

Oral: Doses should be given up to 1 hour prior to initiation of chemotherapy/radiation

I.V.: Administer I.V. push over 30 seconds or as a 5-10 minute-infusion

Prevention of PONV: Administer before induction of anesthesia or immediately before reversal of anesthesia.

Treatment of PONV: Administer undiluted over 30 seconds.

Transdermal (Sancuso®): Apply patch to clean, dry, intact skin on upper outer arm. Do not use on red, irritated or damaged skin. Remove patch from pouch immediately before application. Do not cut patch.

Dosage Forms Excipient information presented when available (limited, particularly for generics); consult specific product labeling. [DSC] = Discontinued product

Injection, solution: 1 mg/mL (1 mL, 4 mL)

Kytril®: 1 mg/mL (1 mL, 4 mL) [contains benzyl alcohol]

Injection, solution [preservative free]: 0.1 mg/mL (1 mL); 1 mg/mL (1 mL)

Kytril®: 0.1 mg/mL (1 mL)

Solution, oral:

Granisol™: 2 mg/10 mL (30 mL) [contains sodium benzoate; orange flavor]

Kytril®: 2 mg/10 mL (30 mL) [contains sodium benzoate; orange flavor] [DSC]

Tablet: 1 mg

Kytril®: 1 mg

Transdermal system, topical:

Sancuso®: 3.1 mg/24 hours (1s) [52 cm^2, total granisetron 34.3 mg]

◆ **Granisol™** *see* Granisetron *on page 706*

◆ **Granulex®** *see* Trypsin, Balsam Peru, and Castor Oil *on page 1526*

◆ **Granulocyte Colony Stimulating Factor** *see* Filgrastim *on page 620*

◆ **Granulocyte Colony Stimulating Factor (PEG Conjugate)** *see* Pegfilgrastim *on page 1152*

◆ **Granulocyte-Macrophage Colony Stimulating Factor** *see* Sargramostim *on page 1355*

◆ **Gravol® (Can)** *see* DimenhyDRINATE *on page 453*

◆ **Grifulvin® V** *see* Griseofulvin *on page 708*

Griseofulvin (gri see oh FUL vin)

U.S. Brand Names Grifulvin® V; Gris-PEG®

Index Terms Griseofulvin Microsize; Griseofulvin Ultramicrosize

Pharmacologic Category Antifungal Agent, Oral

Additional Appendix Information

Antifungal Agents *on page 1640*

Use Treatment of susceptible tinea infections of the skin, hair, and nails

Pregnancy Risk Factor C

Pregnancy Considerations Animal studies have shown decreased spermatogenesis, as well as embryotoxic and teratogenic effects with griseofulvin. There are no adequate and well-controlled studies in pregnant women. Use during pregnancy is contraindicated.

Lactation Excretion in breast milk unknown/use caution

Medication Safety Issues

Sound-alike/look-alike issues:

International issues: Fulvicin® (brand name used in international markets) may be confused with Furacin®

Contraindications Hypersensitivity to griseofulvin or any component of the formulation; severe liver disease; porphyria (interferes with porphyrin metabolism); pregnancy

Warnings/Precautions Safety and efficacy in children ≤2 years of age have not been established; during long-term therapy, periodic assessment of hepatic, renal, and hematopoietic functions should be performed; may cause fetal harm when administered to pregnant women; avoid exposure to intense sunlight to prevent photosensitivity reactions; hypersensitivity cross reaction between penicillins and griseofulvin is possible

Adverse Reactions Frequency not defined.

Central nervous system: Dizziness, fatigue, headache, insomnia, mental confusion

Dermatologic: Angioneurotic edema (rare), erythema multiforme-like drug reaction, photosensitivity, rash (most common), urticaria (most common),

Gastrointestinal: Nausea, vomiting, epigastric distress, diarrhea, GI bleeding

Genitourinary: Menstrual irregularities (rare)

Hematologic: Granulocytopenia, leukopenia

Hepatic: Hepatotoxicity

Neuromuscular & skeletal: Paresthesia (rare)

Renal: Nephrosis, proteinuria

Miscellaneous: Drug-induced lupus-like syndrome (rare), oral thrush

Drug Interactions

Metabolism/Transport Effects **Induces** CYP1A2 (weak), 2C8 (weak), 2C9 (weak), 3A4 (weak)

Avoid Concomitant Use

Avoid concomitant use of Griseofulvin with any of the following: Contraceptive (Progestins)

Increased Effect/Toxicity

Griseofulvin may increase the levels/effects of: Alcohol (Ethyl)

Decreased Effect

Griseofulvin may decrease the levels/effects of: Contraceptive (Progestins); CycloSPORINE; Maraviroc; Oral Contraceptive (Estrogens); *Saccharomyces boulardii;* Vitamin K Antagonists

The levels/effects of Griseofulvin may be decreased by: Barbiturates

Ethanol/Nutrition/Herb Interactions

Ethanol: Avoid ethanol (may increase CNS depression). Concomitant use with ethanol will cause "disulfiram"-type reaction consisting of tachycardia, flushing, headache, nausea, and in some patients, vomiting and chest and/or abdominal pain.

Food: Griseofulvin concentrations may be increased if taken with food, especially with high-fat meals.

Mechanism of Action Inhibits fungal cell mitosis at metaphase; binds to human keratin making it resistant to fungal invasion

Pharmacodynamics/Kinetics

Absorption: Ultramicrosize griseofulvin absorption is almost complete; absorption of microsize griseofulvin is variable (25% to 70% of an oral dose); enhanced by ingestion of a fatty meal (GI absorption of ultramicrosize is ~1.5 times that of microsize)

Distribution: Crosses placenta

Metabolism: Extensively hepatic

Half-life elimination: 9-22 hours

Excretion: Urine (<1% as unchanged drug); feces; perspiration

Dosage Oral:

Children >2 years:

Microsize: 10-20 mg/kg/day in single or 2 divided doses. In the treatment of tinea capitis, higher dosages (20-25 mg/kg/day for 8-12 weeks) have been recommended by some authors (unlabeled).

Ultramicrosize: Usual: 7.3 mg/kg/day in single dose or 2 divided doses; range: 5-15 mg/kg/day in single dose or 2 divided doses (maximum: 750 mg/day)

Adults:

Microsize: 500-1000 mg/day in single or divided doses

Ultramicrosize: 375 mg/day in single or divided doses; doses up to 750 mg/day have been used for infections more difficult to eradicate such as tinea unguium and tinea pedis

Duration of therapy depends on the site of infection:

Tinea corporis: 2-4 weeks

Tinea capitis: 4-6 weeks or longer (up to 8-12 weeks)

Tinea pedis: 4-8 weeks

Tinea unguium: 3-6 months or longer

Administration Oral: Administer with a fatty meal (peanuts or ice cream) to increase absorption, or with food or milk to avoid GI upset

Gris-PEG® tablets: May be swallowed whole or crushed and sprinkled onto 1 tablespoonful of applesauce and swallowed immediately without chewing.

Monitoring Parameters Periodic renal, hepatic, and hematopoietic function tests

Test Interactions False-positive urinary VMA levels

Dosage Forms Excipient information presented when available (limited, particularly for generics); consult specific product labeling.

Suspension, oral [microsize]: 125 mg/5mL (120 mL)

Grifulvin® V: 125 mg/5 mL (120 mL) [contains alcohol 0.2%]

Tablet, oral [microsize]:

Grifulvin® V: 500 mg

Tablet, oral [ultramicrosize]:

Gris-PEG®: 125 mg, 250 mg

- **Griseofulvin Microsize** *see* Griseofulvin *on page 708*
- **Griseofulvin Ultramicrosize** *see* Griseofulvin *on page 708*
- **Gris-PEG®** *see* Griseofulvin *on page 708*
- **Guaicon DM [OTC]** *see* Guaifenesin and Dextromethorphan *on page 710*
- **Guaicon DMS [OTC]** *see* Guaifenesin and Dextromethorphan *on page 710*
- **Guaifed®** *see* Guaifenesin and Phenylephrine *on page 712*
- **Guaifed-PD®** *see* Guaifenesin and Phenylephrine *on page 712*

GuaiFENesin (gwye FEN e sin)

U.S. Brand Names Allfen Jr; Diabetic Tussin® EX [OTC]; Fenesin IR; Ganidin NR; Guiatuss™ [OTC]; Mucinex® Maximum Strength [OTC]; Mucinex® [OTC]; Mucinex®, Children's Mini-Melts™ [OTC]; Mucinex®, Children's [OTC]; Mucinex®, Junior Mini-Melts™ [OTC]; Organidin® NR; Phanasin® Diabetic Choice [OTC]; Phanasin® [OTC]; Refenesen™ 400 [OTC]; Refenesen™ [OTC]; Robitussin® [OTC]; Scot-Tussin® Expectorant [OTC]; Siltussin DAS [OTC]; Siltussin SA [OTC]; Vicks® Casero™ Chest Congestion Relief [OTC]; XPECT™ [OTC]

Canadian Brand Names Balminil Expectorant; Benylin® E Extra Strength; Koffex Expectorant; Robitussin®

Index Terms GG; Glycerol Guaiacolate

Pharmacologic Category Expectorant

Use Help loosen phlegm and thin bronchial secretions to make coughs more productive

Pregnancy Risk Factor C

Pregnancy Considerations Reproduction studies have not been conducted.

Lactation Excretion in breast milk unknown/use caution

Medication Safety Issues

Sound-alike/look-alike issues:

GuaiFENesin may be confused with guanFACINE

Mucinex® may be confused with Mucomyst®

Naldecon® may be confused with Nalfon®

International issues:

Mucolex® [Hong Kong] may be confused with Mycelex® which is a brand name for clotrimazole in the U.S.

Contraindications Hypersensitivity to guaifenesin or any component of the formulation

Warnings/Precautions When used for self medication (OTC) notify healthcare provider if symptoms do not improve within 7 days, or are accompanied by fever, rash or persistent headache. Do not use for persistent or chronic cough (as with smoking, asthma, chronic bronchitis, emphysema) or if cough is accompanied b excessive phlegm unless directed to do so by healthcare provider. Not for OTC use in children <2 years of age. Some products may contain phenylalanine.

Adverse Reactions Frequency not defined.

Central nervous system: Dizziness, drowsiness, headache

Dermatologic: Rash

Endocrine & metabolic: Uric acid levels decreased

Gastrointestinal: Nausea, vomiting, stomach pain

Postmarketing and/or case reports: Kidney stone formation (with consumption of large quantities)

Drug Interactions

Avoid Concomitant Use There are no known interactions where it is recommended to avoid concomitant use.

Increased Effect/Toxicity There are no known significant interactions involving an increase in effect.

Decreased Effect There are no known significant interactions involving a decrease in effect.

Mechanism of Action Thought to act as an expectorant by irritating the gastric mucosa and stimulating respiratory tract secretions, thereby increasing respiratory fluid volumes and decreasing mucous viscosity

Pharmacodynamics/Kinetics

Absorption: Well absorbed

Half-life elimination: ~1 hour

Excretion: Urine (as unchanged drug and metabolites)

Dosage Oral:

Children:

6 months to 2 years: 25-50 mg every 4 hours, not to exceed 300 mg/day

2-5 years: 50-100 mg every 4 hours, not to exceed 600 mg/day

6-11 years: 100-200 mg every 4 hours, not to exceed 1.2 g/day

Children >12 years and Adults: 200-400 mg every 4 hours to a maximum of 2.4 g/day

Extended release tablet: 600-1200 mg every 12 hours, not to exceed 2.4 g/day

Dietary Considerations

Diabetic Tussin® EX contains phenylalanine 8.4 mg/5 mL.

Mucinex® Children's Mini-Melts™ 50 mg/packet contains phenylalanine 0.6 mg/packet; Mucinex® Junior Mini-Melts™ 100 mg/packet contains phenylalanine 1 mg/packet

Vicks® Casero™ contains phenylalanine 5.5 mg/12.5 mL and sodium 32 mg/12.5 mL.

Administration Do not crush, chew, or break extended release tablets; administer with a full glass of water

Test Interactions Possible color interference with determination of 5-HIAA and VMA; discontinue for 48 hours prior to test

Dosage Forms Excipient information presented when available (limited, particularly for generics); consult specific product labeling.

Caplet:

Fenesin IR, Refenesen™ 400: 400 mg

Granules, oral:

Mucinex® Children's Mini-Melts™: 50 mg/packet (12s) [contains phenylalanine 0.6 mg/packet and magnesium 6 mg/packet; grape flavor]

Mucinex® Junior Mini-Melts™: 100 mg/packet (12s) [contains phenylalanine 1 mg/packet and magnesium 10 mg/packet; bubble gum flavor]

Liquid: 100 mg/5 mL (120 mL, 480 mL)

Diabetic Tussin EX®: 100 mg/5 mL (120 mL) [alcohol free, sugar free, dye free; contains phenylalanine 8.4 mg/5 mL]

Ganidin NR: 100 mg/5 mL (480 mL) [raspberry flavor]

Mucinex® Children's: 100 mg/5 mL (120 mL) [alcohol free; grape flavor]

Organidin® NR: 100 mg/5 mL (480 mL) [contains sodium benzoate; raspberry flavor]

Siltussin DAS: 100 mg/5 mL (120 mL) [alcohol free, dye free, sugar free; strawberry flavor]
Syrup: 100 mg/5 mL (120 mL, 480 mL)
Guiatuss™: 100 mg/5 mL (120 mL, 480 mL) [alcohol free; fruit-mint flavor]
Phanasin®: 100 mg/5 mL (120 mL, 240 mL) [alcohol free, sugar free; mint flavor]
Phanasin® Diabetic Choice: 100 mg/5 mL (120 mL) [alcohol free, sugar free; mint flavor]
Robitussin®: 100 mg/5 mL (5 mL, 10 mL, 15 mL, 30 mL, 120 mL, 240 mL, 480 mL) [alcohol free; contains sodium benzoate]
Scot-Tussin® Expectorant: 100 mg/5 mL (120 mL) [alcohol free, dye free, sugar free; contains benzoic acid; grape flavor]
Siltussin SA: 100 mg/5 mL (120 mL, 240 mL, 480 mL) [alcohol free, sugar free; strawberry flavor]
Vicks® Casero™ Chest Congestion Relief: 100 mg/6.25 mL (120 mL, 240 mL) [contains phenylalanine 5.5 mg/12.5 mL, sodium 32 mg/12.5 mL, and sodium benzoate; honey menthol flavor]
Tablet: 200 mg
Allfen Jr: 400 mg [dye free]
Organidin® NR: 200 mg
Refenesen™: 200 mg
XPECT™: 400 mg
Tablet, extended release:
Mucinex®: 600 mg
Mucinex® Maximum Strength: 1200 mg

◆ **Guaifenesin AC** *see* Guaifenesin and Codeine *on page 710*

Guaifenesin and Codeine

(gwye FEN e sin & KOE deen)

U.S. Brand Names Brontex®; Cheracol®; Diabetic Tussin C®; Gani-Tuss® NR; Guaifenesin AC; Guaituss AC; Kolephrin® #1; Mytussin® AC; Robafen® AC; Romilar® AC; Tussi-Organidin® NR; Tussi-Organidin® S-NR; Tusso-C™

Index Terms Codeine and Guaifenesin

Pharmacologic Category Antitussive; Cough Preparation; Expectorant

Use Temporary control of cough due to minor throat and bronchial irritation

Restrictions C-V

Pregnancy Risk Factor C

Dosage Oral: **Note:** Also refer to specific product labeling:
Children:
2-6 years (Diabetic Tussin C® liquid, Tussi-Organidin® NR): Codeine 1 mg/kg/day in 4 divided doses
6-12 years (Diabetic Tussin C®, Kolephrin® #1, Romilar® AC, Tussi-Organidin® NR liquid): 5 mL every 4 hours; maximum 30 mL/24 hours
Children ≥12 years and Adults:
Brontex® tablets: 1 tablet every 4 hours; maximum 6 tablets/24 hours
Diabetic Tussin C®, Kolephrin® #1, Romilar® AC, Tussi-Organidin® NR liquid: 10 mL every 4 hours; maximum 60 mL/24 hours

Additional Information Complete prescribing information for this medication should be consulted for additional detail.

Dosage Forms Excipient information presented when available (limited, particularly for generics); consult specific product labeling.
Liquid: Guaifenesin 300 mg and codeine phosphate 10 mg per 5 mL (120 mL, 480 mL)
Brontex®: Guaifenesin 75 mg and codeine phosphate 2.5 mg per 5 mL (480 mL) [alcohol free; strawberry mint flavor]
Diabetic Tussin C®: Guaifenesin 200 mg and codeine phosphate 10 mg per 5 mL (480 mL) [contains phenylalanine 0.03 mcg/5 mL; cherry vanilla flavor]
Gani-Tuss® NR: Guaifenesin 100 mg and codeine phosphate 10 mg per 5 mL (480 mL) [raspberry flavor]
Guaifenesin AC: Guaifenesin 100 mg and codeine phosphate 10 mg per 5 mL (120 mL, 480 mL) [alcohol free, sugar free; raspberry flavor]
Kolephrin® #1: Guaifenesin 100 mg and codeine phosphate 10 mg per 5 mL (120 mL) [contains sodium 1.1 mg/5 mL and sodium benzoate]
Tussi-Organidin® NR: Guaifenesin 300 mg and codeine phosphate 10 mg per 5 mL (480 mL) [alcohol free, sugar free; contains sodium benzoate; raspberry flavor]
Tussi-Organidin® S-NR: Guaifenesin 300 mg and codeine phosphate 10 mg per 5 mL (120 mL) [alcohol free, sugar free; contains sodium benzoate; raspberry flavor]
Syrup:
Cheracol®: Guaifenesin 100 mg and codeine phosphate 10 mg per 5 mL (120 mL) [contains alcohol 4.75% and benzoic acid]
Guaituss AC: Guaifenesin 100 mg and codeine phosphate 10 mg per 5 mL (120 mL, 480 mL) [contains alcohol; sugar free; fruit-mint flavor]
Mytussin® AC: Guaifenesin 100 mg and codeine phosphate 10 mg per 5 mL (120 mL, 480 mL) [contains alcohol; sugar free; fruit flavor]
Robafen® AC: Guaifenesin 100 mg and codeine phosphate 10 mg per 5 mL (120 mL, 480 mL)
Romilar® AC: Guaifenesin 100 mg and codeine phosphate 10 mg per 5 mL (480 mL) [alcohol free, sugar free, dye free; contains benzoic acid and phenylalanine; grape flavor]
Tusso-C™: Guaifenesin 200 mg and codeine phosphate 10 mg per 5 mL (480 mL) [alcohol free, dye free, sugar free; contains phenylalanine 0.03 mcg/5 mL; cherry vanilla flavor]
Tablet: Guaifenesin 300 mg and codeine phosphate 10 mg
Brontex®: Guaifenesin 300 mg and codeine phosphate 10 mg

Guaifenesin and Dextromethorphan

(gwye FEN e sin & deks troe meth OR fan)

U.S. Brand Names Allfen-DM; Altarussin DM [OTC]; Cheracol® D [OTC]; Cheracol® Plus [OTC]; Coricidin HBP® Chest Congestion and Cough [OTC]; Diabetic Tussin® DM Maximum Strength [OTC]; Diabetic Tussin® DM [OTC]; Double Tussin DM [OTC]; Duratuss® DM; Fenesin DM IR; Gani-Tuss DM NR; Genatuss DM® [OTC]; Guaicon DM [OTC]; Guaicon DMS [OTC]; Guaifenex® DM [DSC]; Guia-D; Guiatuss-DM® [OTC]; Hydro-Tussin™ DM [DSC]; Kolephrin® GG/DM [OTC]; Mintab DM; Mucinex® Children's Cough [OTC]; Mucinex® DM Maximum Strength [OTC]; Mucinex® DM [OTC]; Phanatuss® DM [OTC]; Phlemex; Refenesen™ DM [OTC]; Respa-DM®; Robafen DM Clear [OTC]; Robafen DM [OTC]; Robitussin® Cough and Congestion [OTC]; Robitussin® DM Infant [OTC] [DSC]; Robitussin® DM [OTC]; Robitussin® Sugar Free Cough [OTC]; Safe Tussin® DM [OTC]; Scot-Tussin® Senior [OTC]; Silexin [OTC]; Siltussin DM DAS [OTC]; Siltussin DM [OTC]; Simuc-DM; Su-Tuss DM; Touro® DM; Tussi-Organidin® DM NR; Tussi-Organidin® DM-S NR; Vicks® 44E [OTC]; Vicks® Pediatric Formula 44E [OTC]; Z-Cof LA™

Canadian Brand Names Balminil DM E; Benylin® DM-E; Koffex DM-Expectorant; Robitussin® DM

Index Terms Dextromethorphan and Guaifenesin

Pharmacologic Category Antitussive; Cough Preparation; Expectorant

Use Temporary control of cough due to minor throat and bronchial irritation

Pregnancy Risk Factor C

Medication Safety Issues

Sound-alike/look-alike issues:

Benylin® may be confused with Benadryl®, Ventolin®

Dosage Oral:

Children 2-6 years:

General dosing guidelines: Guaifenesin 50-100 mg and dextromethorphan 2.5-5 mg every 4 hours (maximum dose: Guaifenesin 600 mg and dextromethorphan 30 mg per day)

Product-specific labeling:

Guaifenex® DM, Touro® DM: 1/2 tablet every 12 hours (maximum: 1 tablet/24 hour)

Robitussin® DM, Robitussin® Sugar Free Cough: 2.5 mL every 4 hours (maximum: 6 doses/24 hours)

Vicks® Pediatric Formula 44E: 7.5 mL every 4 hours (maximum: 6 doses/24 hours)

Children: 6-12 years:

General dosing guidelines: Guaifenesin 100-200 mg and dextromethorphan 5-10 mg every 4 hours (maximum dose: Guaifenesin 1200 mg and dextromethorphan 60 mg per day)

Product-specific labeling:

Guaifenex® DM, Touro® DM: 1 tablet every 12 hours (maximum: 2 tablets/24 hours)

Robitussin® DM, Robitussin® Sugar Free Cough: 5 mL every 4 hours (maximum: 6 doses/24 hours)

Vicks® 44E: 7.5 mL every 4 hours (maximum: 6 doses/24 hours)

Vicks® Pediatric Formula 44E: 15 mL every 4 hours (maximum: 6 doses/24 hours)

Z-Cof LA™: 1/2 tablet very 12 hours

Children ≥12 years and Adults:

General dosing guidelines: Guaifenesin 200-400 mg and dextromethorphan 10-20 mg every 4 hours (maximum dose: Guaifenesin 2400 mg and dextromethorphan 120 mg per day)

Product-specific labeling:

Guaifenex® DM, Mucinex® DM, Touro® DM: 1-2 tablets every 12 hours (maximum: 4 tablets/24 hours)

Robitussin® DM, Robitussin® Sugar Free Cough: 10 mL every 4 hours (maximum: 6 doses/24 hours)

Vicks® 44E: 15 mL every 4 hours (maximum: 6 doses/24 hours)

Vicks® Pediatric Formula 44E: 30 mL every 4 hours (maximum: 6 doses/24 hours)

Z-Cof LA™: 1 tablet every 12 hours

Additional Information Complete prescribing information for this medication should be consulted for additional detail.

Dosage Forms Excipient information presented when available (limited, particularly for generics); consult specific product labeling. [DSC] = Discontinued product

Caplet:

Fenesin DM IR: Guaifenesin 400 mg and dextromethorphan hydrobromide 15 mg

Refenesen™ DM: Guaifenesin 400 mg and dextromethorphan hydrobromide 20 mg

Capsule, softgel:

Coricidin HBP® Chest Congestion and Cough: Guaifenesin 200 mg and dextromethorphan hydrobromide 10 mg

Elixir:

Duratuss DM®: Guaifenesin 225 mg and dextromethorphan hydrobromide 25 mg per 5 mL (480 mL) [contains sodium benzoate; grape flavor]

Simuc-DM: Guaifenesin 225 mg and dextromethorphan hydrobromide 25 mg per 5 mL (480 mL) [grape flavor]

Su-Tuss DM: Guaifenesin 200 mg and dextromethorphan hydrobromide 20 mg per 5 mL (480 mL) [fruit flavor]

Liquid: Guaifenesin 100 mg and dextromethorphan hydrobromide 10 mg per 5 mL (480 mL); guaifenesin 300 mg and dextromethorphan hydrobromide 10 mg per 5 mL (120 mL, 480 mL)

Diabetic Tussin® DM: Guaifenesin 100 mg and dextromethorphan hydrobromide 10 mg per 5 mL (120 mL) [alcohol free, sugar free, dye free; contains phenylalanine 8.4 mg/5 mL]

Diabetic Tussin® DM Maximum Strength: Guaifenesin 200 mg and dextromethorphan hydrobromide 10 mg per 5 mL (120 mL) [alcohol free, sugar free, dye free; contains phenylalanine 8.4 mg/5 mL]

Double Tussin DM: Guaifenesin 300 mg and dextromethorphan hydrobromide 200 mg per 5 mL (120 mL, 480 mL) [alcohol free, dye free, sugar free]

Gani-Tuss® DM NR: Guaifenesin 100 mg and dextromethorphan hydrobromide 10 mg per 5 mL (480 mL) [raspberry flavor]

Hydro-Tussin™ DM: Guaifenesin 200 mg and dextromethorphan hydrobromide 20 mg per 5 mL (480 mL) [alcohol free, sugar free; contains sodium benzoate] [DSC]

Kolephrin® GG/DM: Guaifenesin 150 mg and dextromethorphan hydrobromide 10 mg per 5 mL (120 mL) [alcohol free; cherry flavor]

Mucinex® Children's Cough: Guaifenesin 100 mg and dextromethorphan hydrobromide 5 mg per 5 mL (120 mL) [contains sodium 3 mg/5 mL; cherry flavor]

Safe Tussin® DM: Guaifenesin 100 mg and dextromethorphan hydrobromide 15 mg per 5 mL (120 mL) [contains phenylalanine 4.2 mg/5 mL, benzoic acid, and propylene glycol; orange and mint flavors]

Scot-Tussin® Senior: Guaifenesin 200 mg and dextromethorphan hydrobromide 15 mg per 5 mL (120 mL) [alcohol free, sodium free, sugar free]

Tussi-Organidin® DM NR: Guaifenesin 300 mg and dextromethorphan hydrobromide 10 mg per 5 mL (480 mL) [alcohol free, sugar free; contains sodium benzoate; grape flavor]

Tussi-Organidin® DM-S NR: Guaifenesin 300 mg and dextromethorphan hydrobromide 10 mg per 5 mL (120 mL) [alcohol free, sugar free; contains sodium benzoate; grape flavor]

Vicks® 44E: Guaifenesin 200 mg and dextromethorphan hydrobromide 20 mg per 15 mL (120 mL, 235 mL) [contains sodium 31 mg/15 mL, alcohol, sodium benzoate]

Vicks® Pediatric Formula 44E: Guaifenesin 100 mg and dextromethorphan hydrobromide 10 mg per 15 mL (120 mL) [alcohol free; contains sodium 30 mg/15 mL, sodium benzoate; cherry flavor]

Liquid, oral [drops]:

Robitussin® DM Infant: Guaifenesin 100 mg and dextromethorphan hydrobromide 5 mg per 2.5 mL (30 mL) [alcohol free; contains sodium benzoate; fruit punch flavor] [DSC]

Syrup: Guaifenesin 100 mg and dextromethorphan hydrobromide 10 mg per 5 mL (120 mL, 480 mL)

Altarussin DM: Guaifenesin 100 mg and dextromethorphan hydrobromide 10 mg per 5 mL (120 mL, 240 mL, 480 mL, 3840 mL)

Cheracol® D: Guaifenesin 100 mg and dextromethorphan hydrobromide 10 mg per 5 mL (120 mL, 180 mL) [contains alcohol 4.75%, benzoic acid]

Cheracol® Plus: Guaifenesin 100 mg and dextromethorphan hydrobromide 10 mg per 5 mL (120 mL) [contains alcohol 4.75%, benzoic acid]

Genatuss DM®: Guaifenesin 100 mg and dextromethorphan hydrobromide 10 mg per 5 mL (120 mL)

Guiatuss® DM: Guaifenesin 100 mg and dextromethorphan hydrobromide 10 mg per 5 mL (120 mL, 480 mL, 3840 mL) [alcohol free; contains sodium benzoate]

Guaicon DM®: Guaifenesin 100 mg and dextromethorphan hydrobromide 10 mg per 5 mL (10 mL) [alcohol free]

Guaicon DMS®: Guaifenesin 100 mg and dextromethorphan hydrobromide 10 mg per 5 mL (10 mL) [alcohol free, sugar free]
Mintab DM: Guaifenesin 200 mg and dextromethorphan hydrobromide 10 mg per 5 mL (480 mL) [alcohol free, dye free; cherry vanilla flavor]
Phanatuss® DM: Guaifenesin 100 mg and dextromethorphan hydrobromide 10 mg per 5 mL (120 mL) [alcohol free, sugar free]
Robafen® DM: Guaifenesin 100 mg and dextromethorphan hydrobromide 10 mg per 5 mL (120 mL, 240 mL, 480 mL) [cherry flavor]
Robafen® DM Clear: Guaifenesin 100 mg and dextromethorphan hydrobromide 10 mg per 5 mL (120 mL)
Robitussin® Cough and Congestion: Guaifenesin 100 mg and dextromethorphan hydrobromide 10 mg per 5 mL (120 mL) [alcohol free; contains sodium benzoate]
Robitussin®-DM: Guaifenesin 100 mg and dextromethorphan hydrobromide 10 mg per 5 mL (5 mL, 120 mL, 340 mL, 360 mL) [alcohol free; contains sodium benzoate]
Robitussin® Sugar Free Cough: Guaifenesin 100 mg and dextromethorphan hydrobromide 10 mg per 5 mL (120 mL) [alcohol free, sugar free; contains sodium benzoate]
Silexin: Guaifenesin 100 mg and dextromethorphan hydrobromide 10 mg per 5 mL (45 mL) [alcohol free, sugar free)]
Siltussin DM: Guaifenesin 100 mg and dextromethorphan hydrobromide 10 mg per 5 mL (120 mL, 240 mL, 480 mL) [strawberry flavor]
Siltussin DM DAS: Guaifenesin 100 mg and dextromethorphan hydrobromide 10 mg per 5 mL (120 mL) [alcohol free, dye free, sugar free; strawberry flavor]

Tablet: Guaifenesin 1000 mg and dextromethorphan hydrobromide 60 mg; guaifenesin 1200 mg and dextromethorphan hydrobromide 60 mg
Silexin: Guaifenesin 100 mg and dextromethorphan hydrobromide 10 mg

Tablet, extended release: 800/30: Guaifenesin 800 mg and dextromethorphan hydrobromide 30 mg; 1200/20: Guaifenesin 1200 mg and dextromethorphan hydrobromide 20 mg
Guaifenex® DM: Guaifenesin 600 mg and dextromethorphan hydrobromide 30 mg [DSC]
Mucinex® DM, Respa-DM®: Guaifenesin 600 mg and dextromethorphan hydrobromide 30 mg
Mucophen® DM: Guaifenesin 1000 mg and dextromethorphan hydrobromide 60 mg
Mucinex® DM Maximum Strength: Guaifenesin 1200 mg and dextromethorphan hydrobromide 60 mg
Phlemex: Guaifenesin 1200 mg and dextromethorphan hydrobromide 20 mg
Touro® DM: Guaifenesin 575 mg and dextromethorphan hydrobromide 30 mg

Tablet, long-acting: Guaifenesin 1000 mg and dextromethorphan hydrobromide 60 mg
Z-Cof LA [scored]: Guaifenesin 650 mg and dextromethorphan hydrobromide 30 mg

Tablet, sustained release:
Allfen-DM: Guaifenesin 1000 mg and dextromethorphan hydrobromide 55 mg
Relacon LAX: Guaifenesin 835 mg and dextromethorphan hydrobromide 30 mg
Tussi-Bid®: Guaifenesin 1200 mg and dextromethorphan hydrobromide 60 mg

Tablet, timed release [scored]: Guaifenesin 1200 mg and dextromethorphan hydrobromide 60 mg
Guia-D: Guaifenesin 1000 mg and dextromethorphan hydrobromide 60 mg [dye free]

◆ **Guaifenesin and Dyphylline** *see* Dyphylline and Guaifenesin *on page 501*

◆ **Guaifenesin and Hydrocodone** *see* Hydrocodone and Guaifenesin *on page 741*

Guaifenesin and Phenylephrine

(gwye FEN e sin & fen il EF rin)

U.S. Brand Names Aldex™; Crantex LA; D-Phen 1000; Deconsal® II; Donatussin Drops; Duomax; Duratuss GP®; Duratuss®; ExeFen-PD; ExeTuss [DSC]; ExeTuss-GP; Fenesin PE IR; Genexa™ LA [DSC]; Gentex LA [DSC]; Gilphex TR®; Guaifed-PD®; Guaifed®; Guaiphen-D; Guaiphen-D 1200; Guaiphen-PD; Liquibid-D®; MyDex; Nasex-G; Nexphen PD; norel® EX; Pendex; PhenaVent™ D [DSC]; PhenaVent™ LA [DSC]; PhenaVent™ Ped [DSC]; PhenaVent™ [DSC]; Prolex®-D [DSC]; Prolex®-PD [DSC]; Refenesen™ PE [OTC]; Rescon GG [OTC]; Respa® PE [DSC]; Sil-Tex; Simuc [DSC]; Sina-12X; SINUvent® PE; XPECT-PE™ [DSC]

Index Terms Guaifenesin and Phenylephrine Tannate; Phenylephrine Hydrochloride and Guaifenesin

Pharmacologic Category Decongestant; Expectorant

Use Temporary relief of nasal congestion, sinusitis, rhinitis, and hay fever; temporary relief of cough associated with upper respiratory tract conditions, especially when associated with dry, nonproductive cough

Pregnancy Risk Factor C

Medication Safety Issues

Sound-alike/look-alike issues:
Endal® may be confused with Depen®, Intal®
Entex® may be confused with Tenex®
Entex® LA brand name represents a different product in the U.S. than it does in Canada. In the U.S., Entex® LA contains guaifenesin and phenylephrine, while in Canada the product bearing this brand name contains guaifenesin and pseudoephedrine.

Dosage Oral:

Children 3-6 months (Donatussin): 0.3-0.6 mL; may repeat every 4-6 hours as needed; maximum 4 doses/24 hours
Children 6 months to 1 year (Donatussin): 0.6-1 mL; may repeat every 4-6 hours as needed; maximum: 4 doses/24 hours
Children 1-2 years (Donatussin): 1-2 mL; may repeat every 4-6 hours as needed; maximum: 4 doses/24 hours
Children 2-6 years:
Rescon GG, Sil-Tex: 2.5 mL every 4-6 hours; maximum: 10 mL/24 hours
Sina-12X suspension: 2.5-5 mL every 12 hours
Children 6-12 years:
Aldex™, Crantex LA, Duomax, ExeTuss, Gentex LA, Liquibid-D®, PhenaVent™ D, Sina-12X tablet: One-half tablet every 12 hours; maximum: 1 tablet/24 hours
Deconsal® II: One capsule daily
Rescon GG: 5 mL every 4-6 hours; maximum: 20 mL/24 hours
ExeFen PD, Prolex®-D, Prolex®-PD: One-half to 1 tablet every 12 hours
Guaifed-PD®, PhenaVent™ Ped: One capsule every 12 hours
SINUvent® PE: One tablet every 12 hours; maximum: 2 tablets/24 hours
Sina-12X suspension: Refer to adult dosing.
Children ≥12 years:
Aldex™, Crantex LA, Deconsal® II, Duomax, ExeFen PD, ExeTuss, ExeTuss-GP, Gentex LA, Guaifed®, Guaifed-PD®, Liquibid-D®, PhenaVent™, PhenaVent™ D, PhenaVent™ LA, PhenaVent™ Ped, Prolex®-D, Prolex®-PD, Rescon GG, Sil-Tex, Sina-12X, SINUvent® PE: Refer to adult dosing
Adults:
Aldex™, Crantex LA, Duomax, ExeTuss, ExeTuss-GP, Gentex LA, XPECT-PE™, Liquibid-D®, PhenaVent™ D: One tablet every 12 hours

Deconsal® II: 1-2 capsules every 12 hours; maximum: 3 capsules/24 hours
Sil-Tex: 5-10 mL every 4-6 hours; maximum: 40 mL/24 hours
Guaifed-PD®, PhenaVent™ Ped: 1-2 capsules every 12 hours
Guaifed®, PhenaVent™, PhenaVent™ LA: One capsule every 12 hours; maximum: 2 capsules/24 hours
ExeFen PD, Prolex®-D, Prolex®-PD: 1-2 tablets every 12 hours
SINUvent® PE: Two tablets every 12 hours
Rescon GG: 10 mL every 4-6 hours; maximum: 40 mL/24 hours
Sina-12X suspension: 5-10 mL every 12 hours
Sina-12X tablet: 1-2 tablets every 12 hours; maximum: 4 tablets/24 hours

Additional Information Complete prescribing information for this medication should be consulted for additional detail.

Dosage Forms Excipient information presented when available (limited, particularly for generics); consult specific product labeling. [DSC] = Discontinued product

Caplet:
Fenesin PE IR, Refenesen™ PE: Guaifenesin 400 mg and phenylephrine hydrochloride 10 mg

Capsule:
Nexphen PD: Guaifenesin 200 mg and phenylephrine hydrochloride 7 mg

Capsule, variable release:
Deconsal® II: Guaifenesin 375 mg [immediate release] and phenylephrine hydrochloride 20 mg [extended release] [contains tartrazine]
Genexa™ LA [DSC], PhenaVent™ LA [DSC]: Guaifenesin 400 mg [immediate release] and phenylephrine hydrochloride 30 mg [extended release]
Guaifed®, PhenaVent™ [DSC]: Guaifenesin 400 mg [immediate release] and phenylephrine hydrochloride 15 mg [extended release]
Guaifed-PD®, PhenaVent™ Ped [DSC]: Guaifenesin 200 mg [immediate release] and phenylephrine hydrochloride 7.5 mg [extended release]

Liquid: Guaifenesin 100 mg and phenylephrine hydrochloride 7.5 mg per 5 mL (480 mL)
Sil-Tex: Guaifenesin 100 mg and phenylephrine hydrochloride 7.5 mg per 5 mL (480 mL) [alcohol free, dye-free, sugar free; punch flavor]
Rescon GG: Guaifenesin 100 mg and phenylephrine hydrochloride 5 mg per 5 mL (120 mL, 480 mL) [cherry orange-pineapple flavor]

Liquid [drops]:
Donatussin: Guaifenesin 20 mg and phenylephrine hydrochloride 1.5 mg (30 mL) [raspberry flavor]

Suspension:
Sina-12X: Guaifenesin 100 mg and phenylephrine tannate 5 mg per 5 mL (120 mL) [contains benzoic acid; grape flavor]

Tablet: Guaifenesin 900 mg and phenylephrine hydrochloride 30 mg
Sina-12X: Guaifenesin 200 mg and phenylephrine tannate 25 mg

Tablet, extended release: Guaifenesin 600 mg and phenylephrine hydrochloride 20 mg; guaifenesin 600 mg and phenylephrine hydrochloride 40 mg; guaifenesin 1200 mg and phenylephrine hydrochloride 40 mg
Aldex™: Guaifenesin 650 mg and phenylephrine hydrochloride 25 mg
D-Phen: Guaifenesin 1000 mg and phenylephrine hydrochloride 30 mg
Duomax: Guaifenesin 1200 mg and phenylephrine hydrochloride 40 mg [Duomatrix release]
ExeFen-PD: Guaifenesin 600 mg and phenylephrine hydrochloride 10 mg
Gentex LA: Guaifenesin 650 mg and phenylephrine hydrochloride 23.75 mg [DSC]
PhenaVent™ D: Guaifenesin 1200 mg and phenylephrine hydrochloride 40 mg [DSC]
Simuc: Guaifenesin 900 mg and phenylephrine hydrochloride 25 mg [DSC]
SINUvent® PE: Guaifenesin 600 mg and phenylephrine hydrochloride 15 mg

Tablet, long acting: Guaifenesin 900 mg and phenylephrine hydrochloride 25 mg; guaifenesin 1200 mg and phenylephrine hydrochloride 25 mg

Tablet, prolonged release: Guaifenesin 600 mg and phenylephrine hydrochloride 15 mg
Respa® PE: Guaifenesin 600 mg and phenylephrine hydrochloride 18 mg [DSC]

Tablet, sustained release: Guaifenesin 600 mg and phenylephrine hydrochloride 30 mg; guaifenesin 1200 mg and phenylephrine hydrochloride 30 mg
Crantex LA: Guaifenesin 600 mg and phenylephrine hydrochloride 30 mg [dye-free]
Duratuss®, ExeTuss [DSC]: Guaifenesin 900 mg and phenylephrine hydrochloride 25 mg
Duratuss GP®, ExeTuss-GP: Guaifenesin 1200 mg and phenylephrine hydrochloride 25 mg
MyDex: Guaifenesin 900 mg and phenylephrine hydrochloride 30 mg
Nasex-G: Guaifenesin 835 mg and phenylephrine hydrochloride 25 mg
Pendex, Prolex®-PD: Guaifenesin 600 mg and phenylephrine hydrochloride 10 mg
Prolex™-D: Guaifenesin 600 mg and phenylephrine hydrochloride 20 mg [dye-free] [DSC]
XPECT-PE™: Guaifenesin 1200 mg and phenylephrine hydrochloride 25 mg [DSC]

Tablet, timed release:
Gilphex TR®: Guaifenesin 600 mg and phenylephrine hydrochloride 25 mg [sugar free, dye free; scored]
Guaiphen-D: Guaifenesin 600 mg and phenylephrine hydrochloride 40 mg
Guaiphen-D 1200: Guaifenesin 1200 mg and phenylephrine hydrochloride 40 mg
Guaiphen-PD: Guaifenesin 275 mg and phenylephrine hydrochloride 25 mg

Tablet, variable release:
Liquibid-D®: Guaifenesin 400 mg and phenylephrine 10 mg [immediate release] and guaifenesin 800 mg and phenylephrine hydrochloride 30 mg [sustained release]
norel® EX: Guaifenesin 400 mg [immediate release] and guaifenesin 400 mg and phenylephrine hydrochloride 40 mg [extended release]

◆ **Guaifenesin and Phenylephrine Tannate** *see* Guaifenesin and Phenylephrine *on page* *712*

Guaifenesin and Pseudoephedrine

(gwye FEN e sin & soo doe e FED rin)

U.S. Brand Names Ambifed-G; Congestac® [OTC]; Dynex [DSC]; Entex® PSE; Eudal®-SR; ExeFen; Guaifenex® GP [DSC]; Guaifenex® PSE [DSC]; Guaimax-D®; Levall G; Maxifed-G®; Maxifed®; Medent LD; Mucinex® D Maximum Strength [OTC]; Mucinex®-D [OTC]; Nasatab® LA; Profen II® [DSC]; Pseudo GG TR; Pseudo Max; Pseudovent™ 400 [DSC]; Pseudovent™ [DSC]; Pseudovent™-Ped [DSC]; Refenesen Plus [OTC]; Respaire®-120 SR [DSC]; Respaire®-60 SR [DSC]; Respa®-1st; Rutuss Jr; Sinutab® Non-Drying [OTC]; SudaTex-G; Touro LA®

Canadian Brand Names Contac® Cold-Chest Congestion, Non Drowsy, Regular Strength; Entex® LA; Novahistex® Expectorant with Decongestant

Index Terms Pseudoephedrine and Guaifenesin

Pharmacologic Category Alpha/Beta Agonist; Expectorant

Use Temporary relief of nasal congestion and to help loosen phlegm and thin bronchial secretions in the treatment of cough

Pregnancy Risk Factor C

Medication Safety Issues

Sound-alike/look-alike issues:

Entex® may be confused with Tenex®

Entex® LA brand name represents a different product in the U.S. than it does in Canada. In the U.S., Entex® LA contains guaifenesin and phenylephrine, while in Canada the product bearing this brand name contains guaifenesin and pseudoephedrine.

Profen II® may be confused with Profen II DM®, Profen Forte®, Profen Forte™ DM

Profen Forte® may be confused with Profen II®, Profen II DM®, Profen Forte™ DM

Dosage Oral:

Children 2-6 years:

Guaifenex® PSE 60: One-half tablet every 12 hours (maximum: 1 tablet/12 hours)

Maxifed-G®: One-third to 1/2 tablet every 12 hours (maximum: 1 tablet/12 hours)

Children 6-12 years:

Ambifed-G, Dynex, Eudal®-SR, Guaimax-D®, Guaifenex® PSE 80, Guaifenex® PSE 120, Maxifed®, Nasatab® LA: One-half caplet or tablet every 12 hours (maximum: 1 tablet/24 hours)

Congestac®: One-half caplet every 4-6 hours (maximum: 2 caplets/24 hours)

Guaifenex® PSE 60, PanMist®-JR, Pseudovent™-Ped, Respaire®-60 SR: One tablet or capsule every 12 hours (maximum: 2 tablets or capsules every 24 hours)

Levall G: One capsule every 24 hours

Maxifed-G®: One-half to 1 tablet every 12 hours (maximum: 2 tablets/24 hours)

Children >12 years and Adults:

Ambifed-G, Dynex, Entex® PSE, Eudal®- SR, G-Phed, Guaifenex® GP, Guaifenex® PSE 120, Guaimax-D®, Levall G, Mucinex®-D 1200/120, Nasatab® LA, Pseudovent™, Respaire®-120 SR, Touro LA: One tablet or capsule every 12 hours (maximum: 2 tablets or capsules in 24 hours)

Congestac®: One caplet every 4-6 hours (maximum: 4 caplets in 24 hours)

Guaifenex® PSE 60, Maxifed-G®, Mucinex®-D 600/60, Pseudovent™-Ped, Respaire®-60 SR: 1-2 tablets or capsules every 12 hours (maximum: 4 tablets or capsules/24 hours)

Guaifenex® PSE 80: One tablet every twelve hours (maximum: 3 tablets/24 hours)

Guaifenex™ RX: 1-2 of the AM tablets every morning and 1-2 of the PM tablets 12 hours following morning dose

Maxifed®: One to 11/2 tablets every 12 hours (maximum: 3 tablets/24 hours)

Additional Information Complete prescribing information for this medication should be consulted for additional detail.

Dosage Forms Excipient information presented when available (limited, particularly for generics); consult specific product labeling. [DSC] = Discontinued product

Caplet:

Congestac®, Refenesen Plus: Guaifenesin 400 mg and pseudoephedrine hydrochloride 60 mg

Caplet, long acting:

Touro LA®: Guaifenesin 500 mg and pseudoephedrine hydrochloride 120 mg

Caplet, prolonged release:

Ambifed-G: Guaifenesin 1000 mg and pseudoephedrine hydrochloride 60 mg

Capsule, extended release:

Respaire®-60 SR: Guaifenesin 200 mg and pseudoephedrine hydrochloride 60 mg [DSC]

Respaire®-120 SR: Guaifenesin 250 mg and pseudoephedrine hydrochloride 120 mg [DSC]

Capsule, liquicap:

Sinutab® Non-Drying: Guaifenesin 200 mg and pseudoephedrine hydrochloride 30 mg

Capsule, variable release:

Entex® PSE: Guaifenesin 400 mg [immediate release] and pseudoephedrine hydrochloride 120 mg [extended release]

Levall G: Guaifenesin 400 mg [immediate release] and pseudoephedrine hydrochloride 90 mg [extended release]

Pseudovent™: Guaifenesin 250 mg [immediate release] and pseudoephedrine hydrochloride 120 mg [prolonged release] [DSC]

Pseudovent™-Ped: Guaifenesin 300 mg [immediate release] and pseudoephedrine hydrochloride 60 mg [prolonged release] [DSC]

Pseudovent™ 400: Guaifenesin 400 mg [immediate release] and pseudoephedrine hydrochloride 120 mg [extended release] [DSC]

Syrup: Guaifenesin 200 mg and pseudoephedrine hydrochloride 40 mg per 5 mL (480 mL)

Tablet:

ExeFen: Guaifenesin 780 mg and pseudoephedrine hydrochloride 80 mg

Rutuss Jr: 600/45: Guaifenesin 600 mg and pseudoephedrine hydrochloride 45 mg

Tablet, extended release:

Guaifenesin 550 mg and pseudoephedrine hydrochloride 60 mg

Guaifenesin 595 mg and pseudoephedrine hydrochloride 48 mg

Guaifenesin 600 mg and pseudoephedrine hydrochloride 120 mg

Guaifenesin 1200 mg and pseudoephedrine hydrochloride 50 mg

Guaifenesin 1200 mg and pseudoephedrine hydrochloride 75 mg

Guaifenesin 1200 mg and pseudoephedrine hydrochloride 120 mg

Guaifenex® GP: Guaifenesin 1200 mg and pseudoephedrine hydrochloride 120 mg [dye free] [DSC]

Guaifenex® PSE 60: Guaifenesin 600 mg and pseudoephedrine hydrochloride 60 mg [DSC]

Guaifenex® PSE 80: Guaifenesin 800 mg and pseudoephedrine hydrochloride 80 mg [DSC]

Guaifenex® PSE 85: Guaifenesin 795 mg and pseudoephedrine hydrochloride 85 mg [DSC]

Guaifenex® PSE 120: Guaifenesin 600 mg and pseudoephedrine hydrochloride 120 mg [dye free] [DSC]

Guaimax-D®: Guaifenesin 600 mg and pseudoephedrine hydrochloride 120 mg

Maxifed®: Guaifenesin 780 mg and pseudoephedrine hydrochloride 80 mg

Maxifed-G®: Guaifenesin 580 mg and pseudoephedrine hydrochloride 60 mg

Mucinex®-D 600/60: Guaifenesin 600 mg and pseudoephedrine hydrochloride 60 mg

Mucinex® D Maximum Strength [OTC]: Guaifenesin 1200 mg and pseudoephedrine hydrochloride 120 mg

Profen II®: Guaifenesin 800 mg and pseudoephedrine hydrochloride 45 mg [DSC]

Pseudo Max: Guaifenesin 700 mg and pseudoephedrine hydrochloride 80 mg

Tablet, long acting:

Dynex: Guaifenesin 1200 mg and pseudoephedrine hydrochloride 90 mg [DSC]

Medent LD: Guaifenesin 800 mg and pseudoephedrine hydrochloride 60 mg [dye free; scored]

Tablet, sustained release:

Nasatab® LA: Guaifenesin 500 mg and pseudoephedrine hydrochloride 120 mg

Respa®-1st: Guaifenesin 600 mg and pseudoephedrine hydrochloride 58 mg

SudaTex-G: Guaifenesin 580 mg and pseudoephedrine hydrochloride 60 mg [dye free; scored]

- ◆ **Guaifenesin and Theophylline** *see* Theophylline and Guaifenesin *on page 1457*
- ◆ **Guaifenesin, Carbetapentane Citrate, and Phenylephrine Hydrochloride** *see* Carbetapentane, Guaifenesin, and Phenylephrine *on page 255*
- ◆ **Guaifenesin, Chlorpheniramine, Phenylephrine, and Dextromethorphan** *see* Dextromethorphan, Chlorpheniramine, Phenylephrine, and Guaifenesin *on page 434*
- ◆ **Guaifenesin, Dihydrocodeine, and Pseudoephedrine** *see* Dihydrocodeine, Pseudoephedrine, and Guaifenesin *on page 448*
- ◆ **Guaifenesin, Hydrocodone, and Pseudoephedrine** *see* Hydrocodone, Pseudoephedrine, and Guaifenesin *on page 743*
- ◆ **Guaifenesin, Phenylephrine, and Chlorpheniramine** *see* Chlorpheniramine, Phenylephrine, and Guaifenesin *on page 312*

Guaifenesin, Pseudoephedrine, and Codeine

(gwye FEN e sin, soo doe e FED rin, & KOE deen)

U.S. Brand Names Guiatuss DAC; Mytussin® DAC; Nucofed® Expectorant [DSC]; Nucofed® Pediatric Expectorant [DSC]

Canadian Brand Names Benylin® 3.3 mg-D-E; Calmylin with Codeine

Index Terms Codeine, Guaifenesin, and Pseudoephedrine; Pseudoephedrine, Guaifenesin, and Codeine

Pharmacologic Category Antitussive/Decongestant/Expectorant

Use Temporarily relieves nasal congestion and controls cough associated with upper respiratory infections and related conditions (common cold, sinusitis, bronchitis, influenza)

Restrictions C-III; C-V

Pregnancy Risk Factor C

Dosage Oral:

Children 2-6 years:

Nucofed® Pediatric: 2.5 mL every 6 hours (maximum 10 mL/24 hours)

Nucofed®: 1.25 mL every 6 hours (maximum 5 mL/24 hours)

Children 6-12 years:

Guaituss DAC: 5 mL every 4 hours (maximum 20 mL/24 hours)

Nucofed® Pediatric: 5 mL every 6 hours (maximum 20 mL/24 hours)

Nucofed®: 2.5 mL every 6 hours (maximum 10 mL/24hours)

Children >12 years and Adults:

Guaituss DAC: 10 mL every 4 hours (maximum 40 mL/24 hours)

Nucofed® Pediatric: 10 mL every 6 hours (maximum 40 mL/24 hours)

Nucofed®: 5 mL every 6 hours (maximum 20 mL/24 hours)

Additional Information Complete prescribing information for this medication should be consulted for additional detail.

Dosage Forms Excipient information presented when available (limited, particularly for generics); consult specific product labeling. [DSC] = Discontinued product

Syrup:

Guiatuss DAC: Guaifenesin 100 mg, pseudoephedrine hydrochloride 30 mg, and codeine phosphate 10 mg per 5 mL (480 mL)

Mytussin® DAC: Guaifenesin 100 mg, pseudoephedrine hydrochloride 30 mg, and codeine phosphate 10 mg per 5 mL (120 mL, 480 mL) [sugar free; contains alcohol 1.7%; strawberry-raspberry flavor]

Nucofed® Expectorant: Guaifenesin 200 mg, pseudoephedrine hydrochloride 60 mg, and codeine phosphate 20 mg per 5 mL (480 mL) [contains alcohol 12.5%; cherry flavor] [DSC]

Nucofed® Pediatric Expectorant: Guaifenesin 100 mg, pseudoephedrine hydrochloride 30 mg, and codeine phosphate 10 mg per 5 mL (480 mL) [contains alcohol 6%; strawberry flavor] [DSC]

Guaifenesin, Pseudoephedrine, and Dextromethorphan

(gwye FEN e sin, soo doe e FED rin, & deks troe meth OR fan)

U.S. Brand Names Ambifed-G DM; Coldmist DM [DSC]; ExeFen-DMX; Maxifed DM; Maxifed DMX; Medent-DM; Profen Forte™ DM; Profen II DM®; Pseudo Max DMX; Pseudovent™ DM [DSC]; Relacon-DM NR; Robitussin® Cough and Cold CF [OTC]; Robitussin® Cough and Cold Infant CF [OTC]; Robitussin® Cough and Cold [OTC]; Ru-Tuss DM; SudaTex-DM; Touro® CC; Touro® CC-LD; Tri-Vent™ DM [DSC]; Trikof-D® [DSC]; Tusnel Liquid®; Tusnel Pediatric®; Tusnel-DM Pediatric®; Z-Cof™ 12DM

Canadian Brand Names Balminil DM + Decongestant + Expectorant; Benylin® DM-D-E; Koffex DM + Decongestant + Expectorant; Novahistex® DM Decongestant Expectorant; Novahistine® DM Decongestant Expectorant; Robitussin® Cough & Cold®

Index Terms Dextromethorphan, Guaifenesin, and Pseudoephedrine; Pseudoephedrine, Dextromethorphan, and Guaifenesin

Pharmacologic Category Antitussive/Decongestant/Expectorant

Use Temporarily relieves nasal congestion and controls cough due to minor throat and bronchial irritation; helps loosen phlegm and thin bronchial secretions to make coughs more productive

Pregnancy Risk Factor C

Medication Safety Issues

Sound-alike/look-alike issues:

Profen II DM® may be confused with Profen II®, Profen Forte®, Profen Forte™ DM

Profen Forte™ DM may be confused with Profen II®, Profen II DM®, Profen Forte®

Dosage Note: Also refer to specific product labeling.

Children 2-6 years:

Maxifed DM: 1/3 to 1/2 tablet every 12 hours, not to exceed 1 tablet/24 hours

Tri-Vent™ DM: 2.5 mL up to 3-4 times/day, not to exceed pseudoephedrine 4 mg/kg/day

Profen II DM (syrup): 1.25-2.5 mL every 4 hours, not to exceed 15 mL/24 hours

Robitussin® Pediatric Cough and Cold Infant: 2.5 mL every 4-6 hours, not to exceed 4 doses/24 hours

Touro® CC: 1/2 tablet every 12 hour, not to exceed 1 tablet/24 hours

Z-Cof™ DM: 2.5 mL 2-3 times/day, not to exceed 7.5 mL/24 hours

Children 6-12 years:

Ambifed-G DM, Profen Forte™ DM, Profen II DM®: 1/2 tablet every 12 hours not to exceed 1 tablet/24 hours

Maxifed DM: 1/2 to 1 tablet every 12 hours, not to exceed 2 tablets/24 hours

Tri-Vent™ DM: 5 mL up to 3-4 times/day, not to exceed pseudoephedrine 4 mg/kg/day

Touro® CC, Pseudovent™ DM: 1 tablet every 12 hours, not to exceed 2 tablets/24 hours
Profen II DM (syrup): 2.5-5 mL every 4 hours, not to exceed 30 mL/24 hours
Z-Cof™ DM: 5 mL 2-3 times/day, not to exceed 15 mL/24 hours

Children ≥12 years and Adults:
Ambifed-G DM, Aquatab® C, Profen Forte™ DM: 1 tablet every 12 hours not to exceed 2 tablets/24 hours
Maxifed DM, Touro® CC, Pseudovent™ DM: 1-2 tablets every 12 hours, not to exceed 4 tablets/24 hours
Tri-Vent™ DM: Up to 10 mL 3-4 times/day, not to exceed pseudoephedrine 240 mg/24 hours
Profen II DM (tablet): 1 to 1½ tablets every 12 hours, not to exceed 3 tablets/24 hours
Profen II DM (syrup): 5-10 mL every 4 hours, not to exceed 60 mL/24 hours
Z-Cof™ DM: 10 mL 2-3 times/day, not to exceed 30 mL/24 hours

Additional Information Complete prescribing information for this medication should be consulted for additional detail.

Dosage Forms Excipient information presented when available (limited, particularly for generics); consult specific product labeling. [DSC] = Discontinued product

Caplet, prolonged release:
Ambifed-G DM: Guaifenesin 1000 mg, pseudoephedrine hydrochloride 60 mg, and dextromethorphan hydrobromide 30 mg

Caplet, sustained release [scored]:
Touro® CC: Guaifenesin 575 mg, pseudoephedrine hydrochloride 60 mg, and dextromethorphan hydrobromide 30 mg [dye free]
Touro® CC-LD: Guaifenesin 575 mg, pseudoephedrine hydrochloride 25 mg, and dextromethorphan hydrobromide 30 mg

Capsule, softgel:
Robitussin® Cough and Cold: Guaifenesin 200 mg, pseudoephedrine hydrochloride 30 mg, and dextromethorphan hydrobromide 10 mg

Liquid: Guaifenesin 100 mg, pseudoephedrine hydrochloride 30 mg, and dextromethorphan hydrobromide 10 mg per 5 mL (120 mL)
Profen II DM®: Guaifenesin 200 mg, pseudoephedrine hydrochloride 15 mg, and dextromethorphan hydrobromide 10 mg per 5 mL (480 mL) [alcohol free, dye free, sugar free; cherry flavor]
Relacon-DM NR: Guaifenesin 200 mg, pseudoephedrine hydrochloride 32 mg, and dextromethorphan hydrobromide 15 mg (480 mL) [alcohol free, sugar free; grape flavor]
Tusnel Liquid®: Guaifenesin 200 mg, pseudoephedrine hydrochloride 30 mg, and dextromethorphan hydrobromide 15 mg per 5 mL (180 mL) [alcohol free, dye free, sugar free]
Tusnel Pediatric®: Guaifenesin 50 mg, pseudoephedrine hydrochloride 15 mg, and dextromethorphan hydrobromide 5 mg per 5 mL (120 mL) [alcohol free]

Liquid, oral [drops]:
Robitussin® Cough and Cold Infant CF: Guaifenesin 100 mg, pseudoephedrine hydrochloride 15 mg, and dextromethorphan hydrobromide 5 mg per 2.5 mL (30 mL) [alcohol free; contains sodium benzoate]
Tusnel-DM Pediatric®: Guaifenesin 25 mg, pseudoephedrine hydrochloride 5 mg, and dextromethorphan hydrobromide 5 mg per 1 mL (60 mL)

Suspension:
Z-Cof™ 12DM: Guaifenesin 175 mg, pseudoephedrine tannate (equivalent to pseudoephedrine hydrochloride 30 mg), and dextromethorphan tannate (equivalent to dextromethorphan hydrobromide 15 mg) per 5 mL (480 mL) [alcohol free; contains phenylalanine 25.26 mg/5 mL and sodium benzoate; grape flavor]

Syrup: Guaifenesin 100 mg, pseudoephedrine hydrochloride 45 mg, and dextromethorphan hydrobromide 15 mg per 5 mL (480 mL)
Robitussin® Cough and Cold CF: Guaifenesin 100 mg, pseudoephedrine hydrochloride 30 mg, and dextromethorphan hydrobromide 10 mg per 5 mL (120 mL, 240 mL, 360 mL) [alcohol free; contains sodium benzoate]
Ru-Tuss DM: Guaifenesin 100 mg, pseudoephedrine hydrochloride 45 mg, and dextromethorphan hydrobromide 15 mg per 5 mL (480 mL) [alcohol free, dye free, sugar free; strawberry flavor]
Tri-Vent™ DM: Guaifenesin 100 mg, pseudoephedrine hydrochloride 40 mg, and dextromethorphan hydrobromide 15 mg per 5 mL (480 mL) [alcohol free, dye free, sugar free; strawberry flavor] [DSC]

Tablet, extended release: Guaifenesin 100 mg, pseudoephedrine hydrochloride 30 mg, and dextromethorphan hydrobromide 10 mg; guaifenesin 800 mg, pseudoephedrine hydrochloride 60 mg, and dextromethorphan hydrobromide 30 mg; guaifenesin 1200 mg, pseudoephedrine hydrochloride 60 mg, and dextromethorphan hydrobromide 60 mg; guaifenesin 1200 mg, pseudoephedrine hydrochloride 120 mg, and dextromethorphan hydrobromide 60 mg; guaifenesin 800 mg, pseudoephedrine hydrochloride 90 mg, and dextromethorphan hydrobromide 60 mg; guaifenesin 550 mg, pseudoephedrine hydrochloride 60 mg, and dextromethorphan hydrobromide 30 mg; guaifenesin 595 mg, pseudoephedrine hydrochloride 48 mg, and dextromethorphan hydrobromide 32 mg; guaifenesin 600 mg, pseudoephedrine hydrochloride 60 mg, and dextromethorphan hydrobromide 30 mg
Coldmist DM: Guaifenesin 595 mg, pseudoephedrine hydrochloride 48 mg, and dextromethorphan hydrobromide 32 mg [DSC]
Profen Forte™ DM: Guaifenesin 800 mg, pseudoephedrine hydrochloride 90 mg, and dextromethorphan hydrobromide 60 mg
Profen II DM®: Guaifenesin 800 mg, pseudoephedrine hydrochloride 45 mg, and dextromethorphan hydrobromide 30 mg
Pseudovent™ DM: Guaifenesin 595 mg, pseudoephedrine hydrochloride 48 mg, and dextromethorphan hydrobromide 32 mg [DSC]

Tablet, long acting [scored]: Guaifenesin 800 mg, pseudoephedrine hydrochloride 60 mg, and dextromethorphan hydrobromide 30 mg
Medent-DM: Guaifenesin 800 mg, pseudoephedrine hydrochloride 60 mg, and dextromethorphan hydrobromide 30 mg [dye free]

Tablet, sustained release:
ExeFen-DMX: Guaifenesin 780 mg, pseudoephedrine hydrochloride 80 mg, and dextromethorphan hydrobromide 40 mg [dye free]
Maxifed DM, SudaTex-DM: Guaifenesin 580 mg, pseudoephedrine hydrochloride 60 mg, and dextromethorphan hydrobromide 30 mg [dye free; scored]
Maxifed DM: Guaifenesin 780 mg, pseudoephedrine hydrochloride 80 mg, and dextromethorphan hydrobromide 40 mg [dye free; scored]
Pseudo Max DMX: Guaifenesin 700 mg, pseudoephedrine hydrochloride 80 mg, and dextromethorphan hydrobromide 40 mg
Trikof-D®: Guaifenesin 600 mg, pseudoephedrine hydrochloride 50 mg, and dextromethorphan hydrobromide 30 mg [DSC]

◆ **Guaifenesin, Pyrilamine Tannate, and Phenylephrine Tannate** *see* Phenylephrine, Pyrilamine, and Guaifenesin *on page 1186*

◆ **Guaifenex® DM [DSC]** *see* Guaifenesin and Dextromethorphan *on page 710*

- **Guaifenex® GP [DSC]** *see* Guaifenesin and Pseudoephedrine *on page 713*
- **Guaifenex® PSE [DSC]** *see* Guaifenesin and Pseudoephedrine *on page 713*
- **Guaimax-D®** *see* Guaifenesin and Pseudoephedrine *on page 713*
- **Guaiphen-D** *see* Guaifenesin and Phenylephrine *on page 712*
- **Guaiphen-D 1200** *see* Guaifenesin and Phenylephrine *on page 712*
- **Guaiphen-PD** *see* Guaifenesin and Phenylephrine *on page 712*
- **Guaituss AC** *see* Guaifenesin and Codeine *on page 710*

Guanabenz (GWAHN a benz)

Canadian Brand Names Wytensin®

Index Terms Guanabenz Acetate

Pharmacologic Category $Alpha_2$-Adrenergic Agonist

Use Management of hypertension

Pregnancy Risk Factor C

Medication Safety Issues

Sound-alike/look-alike issues:

Guanabenz may be confused with guanadrel, guanfacine

Dosage Adults: Oral: Initial: 4 mg twice daily; increase in increments of 4-8 mg/day every 1-2 weeks to a maximum of 32 mg twice daily.

Dosing adjustment in hepatic impairment: Probably necessary

Additional Information Complete prescribing information for this medication should be consulted for additional detail.

Dosage Forms Excipient information presented when available (limited, particularly for generics); consult specific product labeling.

Tablet: 4 mg, 8 mg

- **Guanabenz Acetate** *see* Guanabenz *on page 717*

GuanFACINE (GWAHN fa seen)

U.S. Brand Names Tenex®

Canadian Brand Names Tenex®

Index Terms Guanfacine Hydrochloride

Pharmacologic Category $Alpha_2$-Adrenergic Agonist

Use Management of hypertension

Unlabeled/Investigational Use ADHD, tic disorder, aggression

Pregnancy Risk Factor B

Medication Safety Issues

Sound-alike/look-alike issues:

GuanFACINE may be confused with guaiFENesin, guanabenz, guanidine

Tenex® may be confused with Entex®, Ten-K®, Xanax®

International issues:

Tenex® may be confused with Kinex® which is a brand name for biperiden in Mexico

Dosage Oral: Adults:

Hypertension: 1 mg usually at bedtime, may increase if needed at 3- to 4-week intervals; usual dose range (JNC 7): 0.5-2 mg once daily

ADHD, tic disorder, aggression (unlabeled uses): Initial: 0.5 mg at bedtime; increase as tolerated (every 3-14 days) to usual dose range (1.5-3 mg/day) given in 3 divided doses (maximum: 4 mg/day)

Additional Information Complete prescribing information for this medication should be consulted for additional detail.

Dosage Forms Excipient information presented when available (limited, particularly for generics); consult specific product labeling.

Tablet: 1 mg, 2 mg

Tenex®: 1 mg, 2 mg

- **Guanfacine Hydrochloride** *see* GuanFACINE *on page 717*
- **Guia-D** *see* Guaifenesin and Dextromethorphan *on page 710*
- **Guiatuss™ [OTC]** *see* GuaiFENesin *on page 709*
- **Guiatuss DAC** *see* Guaifenesin, Pseudoephedrine, and Codeine *on page 715*
- **Guiatuss-DM® [OTC]** *see* Guaifenesin and Dextromethorphan *on page 710*
- **GW506U78** *see* Nelarabine *on page 1047*
- **GW433908G** *see* Fosamprenavir *on page 664*
- **GW572016** *see* Lapatinib *on page 856*
- **Gynazole-1®** *see* Butoconazole *on page 231*
- **Gyne-Lotrimin® 3 [OTC]** *see* Clotrimazole *on page 359*
- **Gyne-Lotrimin® 7 [OTC]** *see* Clotrimazole *on page 359*
- **Gynodiol® [DSC]** *see* Estradiol *on page 554*
- **Gynol II® [OTC]** *see* Nonoxynol 9 *on page 1077*
- **Gynol II® Extra Strength [OTC]** *see* Nonoxynol 9 *on page 1077*
- **H5N1 Influenza Vaccine** *see* Influenza Virus Vaccine (H5N1) *on page 791*
- **Habitrol** *see* Nicotine *on page 1062*
- **Habitrol® (Can)** *see* Nicotine *on page 1062*

Haemophilus b Conjugate and Hepatitis B Vaccine

(he MOF i lus bee KON joo gate & hep a TYE tis bee vak SEEN)

U.S. Brand Names Comvax®

Index Terms *Haemophilus* b (meningococcal protein conjugate) Conjugate Vaccine; Hepatitis B Vaccine (Recombinant); Hib Conjugate Vaccine

Pharmacologic Category Vaccine, Inactivated (Bacterial); Vaccine, Inactivated (Viral)

Use

Immunization against invasive disease caused by *H. influenzae* type b and against infection caused by all known subtypes of hepatitis B virus in infants 6 weeks to 15 months of age born of hepatitis B surface antigen (HB_sAg) negative mothers

Infants born of HB_sAg-positive mothers or mothers of unknown HB_sAg status should receive hepatitis B immune globulin and hepatitis B vaccine (recombinant) at birth and should complete the hepatitis B vaccination series given according to a particular schedule

Pregnancy Risk Factor C

Medication Safety Issues

Sound-alike/look-alike issues:

Comvax® may be confused with Recombivax [Recombivax HB®]

Dosage Infants: I.M.: 0.5 mL at 2, 4, and 12-15 months of age (total of 3 doses)

If the recommended schedule cannot be followed, the interval between the first two doses should be at least 6 weeks and the interval between the second and third dose should be as close as possible to 8-11 months. Minimum age for first dose is 6 weeks.

Modified Schedule: Children who receive one dose of hepatitis B vaccine at or shortly after birth may receive Comvax® on a schedule of 2, 4, and 12-15 months of age

Additional Information Complete prescribing information for this medication should be consulted for additional detail.

Dosage Forms Excipient information presented when available (limited, particularly for generics); consult specific product labeling.

Injection, suspension [preservative free]:

Comvax®: *Haemophilus* b capsular polysaccharide 7.5 mcg (bound to *Neisseria meningitides* OMPC 125 mcg) and hepatitis B surface antigen 5 mcg per 0.5 mL (0.5 mL) [contains aluminum; contains natural rubber/natural latex in packaging]

◆ ***Haemophilus* B Conjugate (Hib)** *see* Diphtheria and Tetanus Toxoids, Acellular Pertussis, Poliovirus and *Haemophilus* b Conjugate Vaccine *on page 462*

Haemophilus b Conjugate Vaccine

(he MOF fi lus bee KON joo gate vak SEEN)

U.S. Brand Names ActHIB®; PedvaxHIB®

Canadian Brand Names ActHIB®; PedvaxHIB®

Index Terms *Haemophilus* b Oligosaccharide Conjugate Vaccine; *Haemophilus* b Polysaccharide Vaccine; Diphtheria Toxoid Conjugate; HbCV; Hib Conjugate Vaccine; Hib Polysaccharide Conjugate; PRP-OMP; PRP-T

Pharmacologic Category Vaccine, Inactivated (Bacterial)

Additional Appendix Information

Immunization Recommendations *on page 1708*

Use Routine immunization of children against invasive disease caused by *H. influenzae* type b

The Advisory Committee on Immunization Practices (ACIP) recommends routine vaccination of all children through age 59 months. Efficacy data is not available for use in older children and adults with chronic conditions associated with an increased risk of Hib disease. However, a single dose may also be considered for older children, adolescents, and adults who did not receive the childhood series and who have had splenectomies or who have sickle cell disease, leukemia or HIV infection.

Pregnancy Risk Factor C

Pregnancy Considerations Reproduction studies have not been conducted.

Medication Safety Issues

Sound-alike/look-alike issues:

International issues:

Hiberix is also a brand name for influenza virus vaccine in multiple international markets

Contraindications Hypersensitivity to *Haemophilus* b polysaccharide vaccine or any component of the formulation

Warnings/Precautions If used in persons with malignancies or those receiving immunosuppressive therapy or who are otherwise immunocompromised, the expected immune response may not be obtained; may be used in patients with HIV infection. The decision to administer or delay vaccination because of current or recent febrile illness depends on the severity of symptoms and the etiology of the disease. Immunization should be delayed during the course of an acute febrile illness. Use caution in children with coagulation disorders (including thrombocytopenia) where intramuscular injections should not be used. Epinephrine 1:1000 should be readily available. Patients who develop symptoms suggestive of hypersensitivity after an injection should not receive further injections of the vaccine.

Children in whom DTP or DT vaccination is deferred: The carrier proteins used in PRP-T (but not PRP-OMP) are chemically and immunologically related to toxoids contained in DTP vaccine. Earlier or simultaneous vaccination with diphtheria or tetanus toxoids may be required to elicit an optimal anti-PRP antibody response. In contrast, the immunogenicity of PRP-OMP is not affected by vaccination with DTP. In infants in whom DTP or DT vaccination is deferred, PRP-OMP may be advantageous for *Haemophilus influenzae* type b vaccination.

In order to maximize vaccination rates, the ACIP recommends simultaneous administration of all age-appropriate vaccines (live or inactivated) for which a person is eligible at a single clinic visit, unless contraindications exist.

Packaging may contain latex.

Adverse Reactions All serious adverse reactions must be reported to the U.S. Department of Health and Human Services (DHHS) Vaccine Adverse Event Reporting System (VAERS) 1-800-822-7967. Frequency not defined:

Central nervous system: Crying (unusual, high pitched, prolonged), fever, irritability, pain, sleepiness

Dermatologic: Rash

Gastrointestinal: Anorexia, diarrhea, vomiting

Local: Injection site: Erythema, induration, pain, soreness, swelling, warmth

Otic: Otitis media

Respiratory: Upper respiratory tract infection

Postmarketing and/or case reports: Anaphylactoid reactions, angioedema, erythema multiforme, facial edema, febrile seizure, Guillain-Barré syndrome, headache, hypersensitivity, hyporesponsive episodes, hypotonia, inflammation, injection site abscess (sterile), lethargy, lymphadenopathy, malaise, mass, seizure, shock, skin discoloration, urticaria

Drug Interactions

Avoid Concomitant Use There are no known interactions where it is recommended to avoid concomitant use.

Increased Effect/Toxicity There are no known significant interactions involving an increase in effect.

Decreased Effect

The levels/effects of Haemophilus b Conjugate Vaccine may be decreased by: Immunosuppressants

Stability Store under refrigeration at 2°C to 8°C (36°F to 46°F); do not freeze.

ActHIB®: Use within 24 hours following reconstitution with saline. Use within 30 minutes following reconstitution with Tripedia®.

Mechanism of Action Stimulates production of anticapsular antibodies and provides active immunity to *Haemophilus influenzae* type b

Pharmacodynamics/Kinetics Seroconversion following one dose of Hib vaccine for children 18 months or 24 months of age or older is 75% to 90%, respectively.

Onset of action: Serum antibody response: 1-2 weeks

Duration: Immunity: 1.5 years

Dosage Children: I.M.: 0.5 mL as a single dose should be administered to previously unvaccinated children according to one of the following "brand-specific" schedules; number of doses in series is dependent upon age at first dose

ActHIB®: *Age at first dose:*

2 months of age: Immunization consists of 3 doses (0.5 mL/dose) administered at 2-, 4- and 6 months of age (may reconstitute with provided diluent or DTP vaccine). A booster dose is given at 15-18 months of age (may reconstitute with provided diluent or Tripedia® vaccine).

7-11 months of age: Two doses (0.5 mL/dose) administered 8 months apart, with a booster dose at 15-18 months of age

12-14 months of age: One dose (0.5 mL) followed by a booster dose 2 months later

PedvaxHIB®: *Age at first dose:*
2-10 months of age: Two doses (0.5 mL/dose) administered 2 months apart; booster dose at 12-15 months of age
11-14 months of age: Two doses (0.5 mL/dose) administered 1 months apart
15-71 months of age: One 0.5 mL dose

Administration For I.M. administration; do not inject I.V.

For patients at risk of hemorrhage following intramuscular injection, the ACIP recommends "it should be administered intramuscularly if, in the opinion of the physician familiar with the patients bleeding risk, the vaccine can be administered with reasonable safety by this route. If the patient receives antihemophilia or other similar therapy, intramuscular vaccination can be scheduled shortly after such therapy is administered. A fine needle (23 gauge or smaller) can be used for the vaccination and firm pressure applied to the site (without rubbing) for at least 2 minutes. The patient should be instructed concerning the risk of hematoma from the injection."

Administration with other vaccines:
Haemophilus b conjugate vaccine with live vaccines: May be given simultaneously or at any interval between doses.
Haemophilus b conjugate vaccine with other inactivated vaccines: May be given simultaneously or at any interval between doses.

Vaccine administration with antibody-containing products: *Haemophilus* b conjugate vaccine may ay be given simultaneously at different sites or at any interval between doses. Examples of antibody-containing products include I.M. and I.V. immune globulin, hepatitis B immune globulin, tetanus immune globulin, varicella zoster immune globulin, rabies immune globulin, whole blood, packed red cells, plasma, and platelet products

Test Interactions May interfere with interpretation of antigen detection tests; antigenuria may occur up to 2 weeks following immunization

Additional Information Federal law requires that the date of administration, the vaccine manufacturer, lot number of vaccine, and the administering person's name, title, and address be entered into the patient's permanent medical record.

The two conjugate vaccines currently available consist of *Haemophilus influenzae* type b (Hib) capsular polysaccharide (also referred to as PRP) linked to a carrier protein. PedvaxHIB® (PRP-OMP) is linked to the outer membrane protein complex from *Neisseria meningitidis*. ActHIB® (PRP-T) uses tetanus toxoid conjugate as the carrier protein.

Dosage Forms Excipient information presented when available (limited, particularly for generics); consult specific product labeling.
Injection, powder for reconstitution [preservative free]:
ActHIB® *Haemophilus* b capsular polysaccharide 10 mcg (bound to tetanus toxoid 24 mcg) per 0.5 mL [contains sucrose; may be reconstituted with provided diluent (forms solution; contains natural rubber/natural latex in packaging) or Tripedia® (forms suspension)]
Injection, suspension:
PedvaxHIB®: *Haemophilus* b capsular polysaccharide 7.5 mcg [bound to *Neisseria meningitidis* OMPC 125 mcg] per 0.5 mL (0.5 mL) [contains aluminum]

◆ ***Haemophilus* b (meningococcal protein conjugate) Conjugate Vaccine** *see Haemophilus* b Conjugate and Hepatitis B Vaccine *on page 717*

◆ ***Haemophilus* b Oligosaccharide Conjugate Vaccine** *see Haemophilus* b Conjugate Vaccine *on page 718*

◆ ***Haemophilus* B Polysaccharide** *see* Diphtheria and Tetanus Toxoids, Acellular Pertussis, Poliovirus and *Haemophilus* b Conjugate Vaccine *on page 462*

◆ ***Haemophilus* b Polysaccharide Vaccine** *see Haemophilus* b Conjugate Vaccine *on page 718*

◆ ***Haemophilus influenzae* b Conjugate Vaccine and Diphtheria, Tetanus Toxoids, and Acellular Pertussis Vaccine** *see* Diphtheria and Tetanus Toxoids, Acellular Pertussis, and *Haemophilus influenzae* b Conjugate Vaccine *on page 462*

Halcinonide (hal SIN oh nide)

U.S. Brand Names Halog®
Canadian Brand Names Halog®
Pharmacologic Category Corticosteroid, Topical
Additional Appendix Information
Corticosteroids *on page 1652*
Use Inflammation of corticosteroid-responsive dermatoses [high potency topical corticosteroid]
Pregnancy Risk Factor C
Medication Safety Issues
Sound-alike/look-alike issues:
Halcinonide may be confused with Halcion®
Halog® may be confused with Haldol®, Mycolog®
Dosage Children and Adults: Topical: Steroid-responsive dermatoses: Apply sparingly 1-3 times/day, occlusive dressing may be used for severe or resistant dermatoses; a thin film is effective; do not overuse. Therapy should be discontinued when control is achieved; if no improvement is seen, reassessment of diagnosis may be necessary.
Additional Information Complete prescribing information for this medication should be consulted for additional detail.
Dosage Forms Excipient information presented when available (limited, particularly for generics); consult specific product labeling.
Cream (Halog®): 0.1% (30 g, 60 g)
Ointment (Halog®): 0.1% (30 g, 60 g)

◆ **Halcion®** *see* Triazolam *on page 1515*

◆ **Haldol®** *see* Haloperidol *on page 720*

◆ **Haldol® Decanoate** *see* Haloperidol *on page 720*

◆ **Haley's M-O** *see* Magnesium Hydroxide and Mineral Oil *on page 916*

◆ **Halfprin® [OTC]** *see* Aspirin *on page 142*

Halobetasol (hal oh BAY ta sol)

U.S. Brand Names Ultravate®
Canadian Brand Names Ultravate®
Index Terms Halobetasol Propionate
Pharmacologic Category Corticosteroid, Topical
Additional Appendix Information
Corticosteroids *on page 1652*
Use Relief of inflammatory and pruritic manifestations of corticosteroid-response dermatoses [super high potency topical corticosteroid]
Pregnancy Risk Factor C
Medication Safety Issues
Sound-alike/look-alike issues:
Ultravate® may be confused with Cutivate®
Dosage Children ≥12 years and Adults: Topical:
Inflammatory and pruritic manifestations (dental use): Cream: Apply sparingly to lesion twice daily. Treatment should not exceed 2 consecutive weeks and total dosage should not exceed 50 g/week. Therapy should be discontinued when control is achieved; if no improvement is seen, reassessment of diagnosis may be necessary.

Steroid-responsive dermatoses: Apply sparingly to skin twice daily, rub in gently and completely; treatment should not exceed 2 consecutive weeks and total dosage should not exceed 50 g/week. Therapy should be discontinued when control is achieved; if no improvement is seen, reassessment of diagnosis may be necessary.

Additional Information Complete prescribing information for this medication should be consulted for additional detail.

Dosage Forms Excipient information presented when available (limited, particularly for generics); consult specific product labeling.

Cream, as propionate: 0.05% (15 g, 50 g)

Ointment, as propionate: 0.05% (15 g, 50 g)

◆ **Halobetasol Propionate** *see* Halobetasol *on page 719*

◆ **Halog®** *see* Halcinonide *on page 719*

Haloperidol (ha loe PER i dole)

U.S. Brand Names Haldol®; Haldol® Decanoate

Canadian Brand Names Apo-Haloperidol LA®; Apo-Haloperidol®; Haloperidol Injection, USP; Haloperidol Long Acting; Haloperidol-LA; Haloperidol-LA Omega; Novo-Peridol; Peridol; PMS-Haloperidol LA

Index Terms Haloperidol Decanoate; Haloperidol Lactate

Pharmacologic Category Antipsychotic Agent, Typical

Additional Appendix Information

Antipsychotic Agents *on page 1644*

Use Management of schizophrenia; control of tics and vocal utterances of Tourette's disorder in children and adults; severe behavioral problems in children

Unlabeled/Investigational Use Treatment of non-schizophrenia psychosis; may be used for the emergency sedation of severely-agitated or delirious patients; adjunctive treatment of ethanol dependence; antiemetic; psychosis/agitation related to Alzheimer's dementia

Pregnancy Risk Factor C

Lactation Enters breast milk/not recommended (AAP rates "of concern")

Medication Safety Issues

Sound-alike/look-alike issues:

Haloperidol may be confused Halotestin®

Haldol® may be confused with Halcion®, Halenol®, Halog®, Halotestin®, Stadol®

Contraindications Hypersensitivity to haloperidol or any component of the formulation; Parkinson's disease; severe CNS depression; bone marrow suppression; severe cardiac or hepatic disease; coma

Warnings/Precautions [U.S. Boxed Warning]: Elderly patients with dementia-related psychosis treated with antipsychotics are at an increased risk of death compared to placebo. An increased incidence of cerebrovascular adverse events (including fatalities) has been reported in elderly patients with dementia-related psychosis. Haloperidol is not approved for this indication. Hypotension may occur, particularly with parenteral administration. Although the short-acting form (lactate) is used clinically, the I.V. use of the injection is not an FDA-approved route of administration; the decanoate form should never be administered intravenously.

May alter cardiac conduction and prolong QT interval; life-threatening arrhythmias have occurred with therapeutic doses of antipsychotics but risk may be increased with doses exceeding recommendations and/or intravenous administration (unlabeled route). Use caution or avoid use in patients with electrolyte abnormalities (eg, hypokalemia, hypomagnesemia), hypothyroidism, familial long QT syndrome, concomitant medications which may augment QT prolongation, or any underlying cardiac abnormality which may also potentiate risk. Monitor ECG closely for dose-related QT effects. Adverse effects of decanoate may be prolonged. Avoid in thyrotoxicosis. Myelosuppression (eg, leukopenia, agranulocytosis) has been observed with antipsychotic use; check blood counts periodically and discontinue at first signs of blood dyscrasias; use is contraindicated in patients with bone marrow suppression. May be sedating, use with caution in disorders where CNS depression is a feature. Caution in patients with severe cardiovascular disease, predisposition to seizures, subcortical brain damage, renal or respiratory disease. Esophageal dysmotility and aspiration have been associated with antipsychotic use - use with caution in patients at risk of pneumonia (eg, Alzheimer's disease). Caution in breast cancer or other prolactin-dependent tumors (may elevate prolactin levels). May alter temperature regulation or mask toxicity of other drugs due to antiemetic effects. May cause orthostatic hypotension; use with caution in patients at risk of this effect or those who would tolerate transient hypotensive episodes (cerebrovascular disease, cardiovascular disease, or other medications which may predispose). Some tablets contain tartrazine.

May cause anticholinergic effects (confusion, agitation, constipation, xerostomia, blurred vision, urinary retention). Therefore, they should be used with caution in patients with decreased gastrointestinal motility, urinary retention, BPH, xerostomia, or visual problems. Conditions which also may be exacerbated by cholinergic blockade include narrow-angle glaucoma (screening is recommended) and worsening of myasthenia gravis. Relative to other neuroleptics, haloperidol has a low potency of cholinergic blockade.

May cause extrapyramidal symptoms (EPS), including pseudoparkinsonism, acute dystonic reactions, akathisia, and tardive dyskinesia (risk of these reactions is high relative to other neuroleptics). Risk of dystonia (and possibly other EPS) may be greater with increased doses, use of conventional antipsychotics, males, and younger patients. May be associated with neuroleptic malignant syndrome (NMS) or pigmentary retinopathy.

Adverse Reactions Frequency not defined.

Cardiovascular: Abnormal T waves with prolonged ventricular repolarization, arrhythmia, hyper-/hypotension, QT prolongation, sudden death, tachycardia, torsade de pointes

Central nervous system: Agitation, akathisia, altered central temperature regulation, anxiety, confusion, depression, drowsiness, dystonic reactions, euphoria, extrapyramidal reactions, headache, insomnia, lethargy, neuroleptic malignant syndrome (NMS), pseudoparkinsonian signs and symptoms, restlessness, seizure, tardive dyskinesia, tardive dystonia, vertigo

Dermatologic: Alopecia, contact dermatitis, hyperpigmentation, photosensitivity (rare), pruritus, rash

Endocrine & metabolic: Amenorrhea, breast engorgement, galactorrhea, gynecomastia, hyper-/hypoglycemia, hyponatremia, lactation, mastalgia, menstrual irregularities, sexual dysfunction

Gastrointestinal: Anorexia, constipation, diarrhea, dyspepsia, hypersalivation, nausea, vomiting, xerostomia

Genitourinary: Priapism, urinary retention

Hematologic: Cholestatic jaundice, obstructive jaundice

Ocular: Blurred vision

Respiratory: Bronchospasm, laryngospasm

Miscellaneous: Diaphoresis, heat stroke

Drug Interactions

Metabolism/Transport Effects Substrate of CYP1A2 (minor), 2D6 (major), 3A4 (major); **Inhibits** CYP2D6 (moderate), 3A4 (moderate)

Avoid Concomitant Use

Avoid concomitant use of Haloperidol with any of the following: Nilotinib; Thioridazine; Ziprasidone

Increased Effect/Toxicity

Haloperidol may increase the levels/effects of: Alcohol (Ethyl); Anticholinergics; ChlorproMAZINE; CNS Depressants; CYP2D6 Substrates; CYP3A4 Substrates; Eplerenone; FentaNYL; Fesoterodine; Maraviroc; Nebivolol; Pimecrolimus; QTc-Prolonging Agents; Ranolazine; Salmeterol; Tamoxifen; Thioridazine; Ziprasidone

The levels/effects of Haloperidol may be increased by: Acetylcholinesterase Inhibitors (Central); Alfuzosin; ChlorproMAZINE; Ciprofloxacin; CYP2D6 Inhibitors (Moderate); CYP2D6 Inhibitors (Strong); CYP3A4 Inhibitors (Moderate); CYP3A4 Inhibitors (Strong); Darunavir; Dasatinib; Gadobutrol; Lithium formulations; Nilotinib; Pramlintide; QuiNIDine; Selective Serotonin Reuptake Inhibitors; Tetrabenazine

Decreased Effect

Haloperidol may decrease the levels/effects of: Amphetamines; Anti-Parkinson's Agents (Dopamine Agonist); Codeine; TraMADol

The levels/effects of Haloperidol may be decreased by: CarBAMazepine; CYP3A4 Inducers (Strong); Deferasirox; Herbs (CYP3A4 Inducers); Lithium formulations

Ethanol/Nutrition/Herb Interactions

Ethanol: Avoid ethanol (may increase CNS depression).

Herb/Nutraceutical: Avoid valerian, St John's wort, kava kava, gotu kola (may increase CNS depression).

Stability

Protect oral dosage forms from light.

Haloperidol lactate injection should be stored at controlled room temperature; do not freeze or expose to temperatures >40°C. Protect from light; exposure to light may cause discoloration and the development of a grayish-red precipitate over several weeks.

Haloperidol lactate may be administered IVPB or I.V. infusion in D_5W solutions. NS solutions should not be used due to reports of decreased stability and incompatibility.

Standardized dose: 0.5-100 mg/50-100 mL D_5W.

Stability of standardized solutions is 38 days at room temperature (24°C).

Mechanism of Action Haloperidol is a butyrophenone antipsychotic which blocks postsynaptic mesolimbic dopaminergic D_1 and D_2 receptors in the brain; depresses the release of hypothalamic and hypophyseal hormones; believed to depress the reticular activating system thus affecting basal metabolism, body temperature, wakefulness, vasomotor tone, and emesis

Pharmacodynamics/Kinetics

Onset of action: Sedation: I.M., I.V.: 30-60 minutes

Duration: Decanoate: 2-4 weeks

Distribution: V_d: 8-18 L/kg; crosses placenta; enters breast milk

Protein binding: 90%

Metabolism: Hepatic to inactive compounds

Bioavailability: Oral: 60%

Half-life elimination: 18 hours; Decanoate: ~1 day

Time to peak, serum: Oral: 2-6 hours; I.M.: 20 minutes; Decanoate: 7 days

Excretion: Urine (33% to 40% as metabolites) within 5 days; feces (15%)

Clearance: 550 ± 133 mL/minute

Dosage

Children: 3-12 years (15-40 kg): Oral:

Initial: 0.05 mg/kg/day or 0.25-0.5 mg/day given in 2-3 divided doses; increase by 0.25-0.5 mg every 5-7 days; maximum: 0.15 mg/kg/day

Usual maintenance:

Agitation or hyperkinesia: 0.01-0.03 mg/kg/day once daily

Nonpsychotic disorders: 0.05-0.075 mg/kg/day in 2-3 divided doses

Psychotic disorders: 0.05-0.15 mg/kg/day in 2-3 divided doses

Children 6-12 years: Sedation/psychotic disorders: I.M. (as lactate): 1-3 mg/dose every 4-8 hours to a maximum of 0.15 mg/kg/day; change over to oral therapy as soon as able

Adults:

Psychosis:

Oral: 0.5-5 mg 2-3 times/day; usual maximum: 30 mg/day

I.M. (as lactate): 2-5 mg every 4-8 hours as needed

I.M. (as decanoate): Initial: 10-20 times the daily oral dose administered at 4-week intervals

Maintenance dose: 10-15 times initial oral dose; used to stabilize psychiatric symptoms

Delirium in the intensive care unit (unlabeled use, unlabeled route):

I.V.: 2-10 mg; may repeat bolus doses every 20-30 minutes until calm achieved then administer 25% of the maximum dose every 6 hours; monitor ECG and QT_c interval

Intermittent I.V.: 0.03-0.15 mg/kg every 30 minutes to 6 hours

Oral: Agitation: 5-10 mg

Continuous intravenous infusion (100 mg/100 mL D_5W): Rates of 3-25 mg/hour have been used

Rapid tranquilization of severely-agitated patient (unlabeled use): Administer every 30-60 minutes:

Oral: 5-10 mg

I.M. (as lactate): 5 mg

Average total dose (oral or I.M.) for tranquilization: 10-20 mg

Elderly: Nonpsychotic patient, dementia behavior (unlabeled use): Initial: Oral: 0.25-0.5 mg 1-2 times/day; increase dose at 4- to 7-day intervals by 0.25-0.5 mg/day; increase dosing intervals (twice daily, 3 times/day, etc) as necessary to control response or side effects

Hemodialysis/peritoneal dialysis: Supplemental dose is not necessary

Administration The decanoate injectable formulation should be administered I.M. only, **do not administer decanoate I.V.** Dilute the oral concentrate with water or juice before administration. Avoid skin contact with oral suspension or solution; may cause contact dermatitis.

Monitoring Parameters Vital signs; lipid profile, fasting blood glucose/Hgb A_{1c}; BMI; mental status, abnormal involuntary movement scale (AIMS), extrapyramidal symptoms (EPS); ECG (with off-label intravenous administration)

Reference Range

Therapeutic: 5-20 ng/mL (SI: 10-40 nmol/L) (psychotic disorders - less for Tourette's and mania)

Toxic: >42 ng/mL (SI: >84 nmol/L)

Dosage Forms Excipient information presented when available (limited, particularly for generics); consult specific product labeling. [DSC] = Discontinued product

Note: Strength expressed as base.

Injection, oil, as decanoate: 50 mg/mL (1 mL, 5 mL); 100 mg/mL (1 mL, 5 mL)

Haldol® Decanoate: 50 mg/mL (1 mL; 5 mL [DSC]); 100 mg/mL (1 mL; 5 mL [DSC]) [contains benzyl alcohol, sesame oil]

Injection, solution, as lactate: 5 mg/mL (1 mL, 10 mL)

Haldol®: 5 mg/mL (1 mL)

Solution, oral concentrate, as lactate: 2 mg/mL (15 mL, 120 mL)

Tablet: 0.5 mg, 1 mg, 2 mg, 5 mg, 10 mg, 20 mg

◆ **Haloperidol Decanoate** *see* Haloperidol *on page 720*

◆ **Haloperidol Injection, USP (Can)** *see* Haloperidol *on page 720*

◆ **Haloperidol-LA (Can)** *see* Haloperidol *on page 720*

◆ **Haloperidol Lactate** *see* Haloperidol *on page 720*

Heparin (HEP a rin)

U.S. Brand Names Hep-Lock U/P; Hep-Lock®; Hep-Flush®-10

Canadian Brand Names Hepalean®; Hepalean® Leo; Hepalean®-LOK

Index Terms Heparin Calcium; Heparin Lock Flush; Heparin Sodium

Pharmacologic Category Anticoagulant

Additional Appendix Information

Anticoagulants, Injectable *on page 1636*

Use Prophylaxis and treatment of thromboembolic disorders; as an anticoagulant for extracorporeal and dialysis procedures

Note: Heparin lock flush solution is intended only to maintain patency of I.V. devices and is **not** to be used for anticoagulant therapy.

Unlabeled/Investigational Use ST-elevation myocardial infarction (STEMI) - combination regimen of heparin (unlabeled dose), tenecteplase (half dose), and abciximab (full dose)

Pregnancy Risk Factor C

Pregnancy Considerations Animal reproduction studies have not been conducted. Heparin does not cross the placenta.

Lactation Does not enter breast milk/compatible

Medication Safety Issues

Sound-alike/look-alike issues:

Heparin may be confused with Hespan®

High alert medication: The Institute for Safe Medication Practices (ISMP) includes this medication among its list of drugs which have a heightened risk of causing significant patient harm when used in error.

Heparin sodium injection 10,000 units/mL and Hep-Lock U/P 10 units/mL have been confused with each other. Fatal medication errors have occurred between the two whose labels are both blue. **Never rely on color as a sole indicator to differentiate product identity.**

Heparin lock flush solution is intended only to maintain patency of I.V. devices and is **not** to be used for anticoagulant therapy.

Note: The 100 unit/mL concentration should not be used in neonates or infants <10 kg. The 10 unit/mL concentration may cause systemic anticoagulation in infants <1 kg who receive frequent flushes.

2009 National Patient Safety Goals: The Joint Commission on Accreditation of Healthcare Organizations requires healthcare organizations that provide anticoagulant therapy to have a process in place to reduce the risk of anticoagulant-associated patient harm. Patients receiving anticoagulants should receive individualized care through a defined process that includes standardized ordering, dispensing, administration, monitoring and education. This does not apply to routine short-term use of anticoagulants for prevention of venous thromboembolism when the expectation is that the patient's laboratory values will remain within or close to normal values (NPSG.03.05.01).

Contraindications Hypersensitivity to heparin or any component of the formulation (unless a life-threatening situation necessitates use and use of an alternative anticoagulant is not possible); severe thrombocytopenia; uncontrolled active bleeding except when due to disseminated intravascular coagulation (DIC); suspected intracranial hemorrhage; not for I.M. use; not for use when appropriate blood coagulation tests cannot be obtained at appropriate intervals (applies to full-dose heparin only)

Warnings/Precautions Hypersensitivity reactions can occur. Only in life-threatening situations when use of an alternative anticoagulant is not possible should heparin be cautiously used in patients with a documented hypersensitivity reaction. Hemorrhage is the most common complication. Monitor for signs and symptoms of bleeding. Certain patients are at increased risk of bleeding. Risk factors for bleeding include bacterial endocarditis; congenital or acquired bleeding disorders; active ulcerative or angiodysplastic GI diseases; continuous GI tube drainage; severe uncontrolled hypertension; history of hemorrhagic stroke; or use shortly after brain, spinal, or ophthalmology surgery; patient treated concomitantly with platelet inhibitors; conditions associated with increased bleeding tendencies (hemophilia, vascular purpura); recent GI bleeding; thrombocytopenia or platelet defects; severe liver disease; hypertensive or diabetic retinopathy; or in patients undergoing invasive procedures including spinal tap or spinal anesthesia. Many concentrations of heparin are available ranging from 1 unit/mL to 20,000 units/mL. Clinicians **must** carefully examine each prefilled syringe or vial prior to use ensuring that the correct concentration is chosen; fatal hemorrhages have occurred related to heparin overdose especially in pediatric patients. A higher incidence of bleeding has been reported in patients >60 years of age, particularly women. They are also more sensitive to the dose. Discontinue heparin if hemorrhage occurs; severe hemorrhage or overdosage may require protamine.

May cause thrombocytopenia; monitor platelet count closely. Patients who develop HIT may be at risk of developing a new thrombus (heparin-induced thrombocytopenia and thrombosis [HITT]). Discontinue therapy and consider alternatives if platelets are <100,000/mm^3 and/or thrombosis develops. HIT or HITT may be delayed and can occur up to several weeks after discontinuation of heparin. Osteoporosis may occur with prolonged use (>6 months) due to a reduction in bone mineral density. Monitor for hyperkalemia; can cause hyperkalemia by suppressing aldosterone production. Patients >60 years of age may require lower doses of heparin.

Some preparations contain benzyl alcohol as a preservative. In neonates, large amounts of benzyl alcohol (>100 mg/kg/day) have been associated with fatal toxicity (gasping syndrome). The use of preservative-free heparin is, therefore, recommended in neonates. Some preparations contain sulfite which may cause allergic reactions.

Heparin resistance may occur in patients with antithrombin deficiency, increased heparin clearance, elevations in heparin-binding proteins, elevations in factor VIII and/or fibrinogen; frequently encountered in patients with fever, thrombosis, thrombophlebitis, infections with thrombosing tendencies, MI, cancer, and in postsurgical patients; measurement of anticoagulant effects using antifactor Xa levels may be of benefit.

Adverse Reactions Frequency not defined.

Cardiovascular: Allergic vasospastic reaction (possibly related to thrombosis), chest pain, hemorrhagic shock, shock, thrombosis

Central nervous system: Chills, fever, headache

Dermatologic: Alopecia (delayed, transient), bruising (unexplained), cutaneous necrosis, dysesthesia pedis, erythematous plaques (case reports), eczema, urticaria, purpura,

Endocrine & metabolic: Adrenal hemorrhage, hyperkalemia (suppression of aldosterone synthesis), ovarian hemorrhage, rebound hyperlipidemia on discontinuation

Gastrointestinal: Constipation, hematemesis, nausea, tarry stools, vomiting

Genitourinary: Frequent or persistent erection

Hematologic: Bleeding from gums, epistaxis, hemorrhage, ovarian hemorrhage, retroperitoneal hemorrhage, thrombocytopenia (see note)

Hepatic: Liver enzymes increased

Local: Irritation, erythema, pain, hematoma, and ulceration have been rarely reported with deep SubQ injections; I.M. injection (not recommended) is associated with a high incidence of these effects

Neuromuscular & skeletal: Peripheral neuropathy, osteoporosis (chronic therapy effect)

Ocular: Conjunctivitis (allergic reaction), lacrimation

Renal: Hematuria

Respiratory: Asthma, bronchospasm (case reports), hemoptysis, pulmonary hemorrhage, rhinitis

Miscellaneous: Allergic reactions, anaphylactoid reactions, heparin resistance, hypersensitivity (including chills, fever, and urticaria)

Note: Thrombocytopenia has been reported to occur at an incidence between 0% and 30%. It is often of no clinical significance. However, immunologically mediated heparin-induced thrombocytopenia (HIT) has been estimated to occur in 1% to 2% of patients, and is marked by a progressive fall in platelet counts and, in some cases, thromboembolic complications (skin necrosis, pulmonary embolism, gangrene of the extremities, stroke or MI). For recommendations regarding platelet monitoring during heparin therapy, see Monitoring Parameters.

Drug Interactions

Avoid Concomitant Use

Avoid concomitant use of Heparin with any of the following: Corticorelin

Increased Effect/Toxicity

Heparin may increase the levels/effects of: Anticoagulants; Corticorelin; Drotrecogin Alfa; Ibritumomab; Tositumomab and Iodine I 131 Tositumomab

The levels/effects of Heparin may be increased by: Antiplatelet Agents; Aspirin; Dasatinib; Herbs (Anticoagulant/Antiplatelet Properties); Nonsteroidal Anti-Inflammatory Agents; Pentosan Polysulfate Sodium; Prostacyclin Analogues; Salicylates; Thrombolytic Agents

Decreased Effect

The levels/effects of Heparin may be decreased by: Nitroglycerin

Ethanol/Nutrition/Herb Interactions Herb/Nutraceutical: Avoid cat's claw, dong quai, evening primrose, feverfew, red clover, horse chestnut, garlic, green tea, ginseng, ginkgo (all have additional antiplatelet activity).

Stability

Heparin solutions are colorless to slightly yellow; minor color variations do not affect therapeutic efficacy.

Heparin should be stored at controlled room temperature. Protect from freezing and temperatures >40°C.

Stability at room temperature and refrigeration:

Prepared bag: 24 hours.

Premixed bag: After seal is broken, 4 days.

Out of overwrap stability: 30 days.

Standard concentration/diluent: 25,000 units/500 mL D_5W (premixed). If preparing solution, mix thoroughly prior to administration.

Minimum volume: 250 mL D_5W.

Mechanism of Action Potentiates the action of antithrombin III and thereby inactivates thrombin (as well as activated coagulation factors IX, X, XI, XII, and plasmin) and prevents the conversion of fibrinogen to fibrin; heparin also stimulates release of lipoprotein lipase (lipoprotein lipase hydrolyzes triglycerides to glycerol and free fatty acids)

Pharmacodynamics/Kinetics

Onset of action: Anticoagulation: I.V.: Immediate; SubQ: ~20-30 minutes

Absorption: Oral, rectal: Erratic at best from these routes of administration; SubQ absorption is also erratic, but considered acceptable for prophylactic use

Distribution: Does not cross placenta; does not enter breast milk

Metabolism: Hepatic; may be partially metabolized in the reticuloendothelial system

Half-life elimination: Mean: 1.5 hours; Range: 1-2 hours; affected by obesity, renal function, hepatic function, malignancy, presence of pulmonary embolism, and infections

Excretion: Urine (small amounts as unchanged drug)

Dosage Note: Many concentrations of heparin are available ranging from 1 unit/mL to 20,000 units/mL. Carefully examine each prefilled syringe or vial prior to use ensuring that the correct concentration is chosen. Heparin lock flush solution is intended only to maintain patency of I.V. devices and is not to be used for anticoagulant therapy.

Children >1 year:

Prophylaxis for cardiac catheterization (arterial approach): I.V.: Bolus: 100-150 units/kg (Monagle, 2008)

Systemic heparinization:

Intermittent I.V.: Initial: 50-100 units/kg, then 50-100 units/kg every 4 hours (**Note:** Continuous I.V. infusion is preferred)

I.V. infusion: Initial loading dose: 75 units/kg given over 10 minutes, then initial maintenance dose: 20 units/kg/hour; adjust dose to maintain aPTT of 60-85 seconds (assuming this reflects an antifactor Xa level of 0.35-0.7 units/mL); see table.

Pediatric Protocol For Systemic Heparin Adjustment

To be used after initial loading dose and maintenance I.V. infusion dose (see usual dosage listed above) to maintain aPTT of 60-85 seconds (assuming this reflects antifactor Xa level of 0.35-0.7 units/mL).

Obtain blood for aPTT 4 hours after heparin loading dose and 4 hours after every infusion rate change.

Obtain daily CBC and aPTT after aPTT is therapeutic.

aPTT (seconds)	Dosage Adjustment	Time to Repeat aPTT
<50	Give 50 units/kg bolus and increase infusion rate by 10%	4 h after rate change
50-59	Increase infusion rate by 10%	4 h after rate change
60-85	Keep rate the same	Next day
86-95	Decrease infusion rate by 10%	4 h after rate change
96-120	Hold infusion for 30 minutes and decrease infusion rate by 10%	4 h after rate change
>120	Hold infusion for 60 minutes and decrease infusion rate by 15%	4 h after rate change

Modified from Monagle P, Chalmers E, Chan A, et al, "Antithrombotic Therapy in Neonates and Children," *Chest*, 2008, 133(6 Suppl):887-968.

Adults:

Thromboprophylaxis (low-dose heparin): SubQ: 5000 units every 8-12 hours

Intermittent I.V.: Initial: 10,000 units, then 50-70 units/kg (5000-10,000 units) every 4-6 hours

I.V. infusion (weight-based dosing per institutional nomogram recommended):

Acute coronary syndromes:

STEMI: Fibrinolytic therapy:

Full-dose alteplase, reteplase, or tenecteplase with dosing as follows: Concurrent bolus of 60 units/kg (maximum: 4000 units), then 12 units/kg/hour (maximum: 1000 units/hour) as continuous infusion. Check aPTT every 4-6 hours; adjust to target of 1.5-2 times the upper limit of control (50-70 seconds in clinical trials); usual range 10-30 units/kg/hour. Duration of heparin therapy depends on concurrent therapy and the specific patient risks for systemic or venous thromboembolism.

Combination regimen (unlabeled): Half-dose tenecteplase (15-25 mg based on weight) and abciximab 0.25 mg/kg bolus then 0.125 mcg/kg/minute (maximum 10 mcg/minute) for 12 hours with heparin dosing as follows: Concurrent bolus of 40 units/kg (maximum 3000 units), then 7 units/kg/hour (maximum: 800 units/hour) as continuous infusion. Adjust to aPTT target of 50-70 seconds.

Percutaneous coronary intervention:

If no concurrent GPIIb/IIIa inhibitor: Initial bolus of 60-100 units/kg (target ACT 250-350 seconds)

or

If receiving GPIIb/IIIa inhibitor: Initial bolus of 50-70 units/kg (target ACT 200-250 seconds)

Treatment of unstable angina/non-ST-elevation myocardial infarction (NSTEMI): Initial bolus of 60 units/kg (maximum: 4000 units), followed by an initial infusion of 12 units/kg/hour (maximum: 1000 units/hour). The American College of Chest Physicians consensus conference has recommended dosage adjustments to correspond to a therapeutic range equivalent to heparin levels of 0.3-0.7 units/mL by antifactor Xa determinations.

Treatment of venous thromboembolism:

DVT/PE: I.V.: 80 units/kg (or 5000 units) I.V. push followed by continuous infusion of 18 units/kg/hour (or 1300 units/hour). The American College of Chest Physicians consensus conference has recommended dosage adjustments to correspond to a therapeutic range equivalent to heparin levels of 0.3-0.7 units/mL by antifactor Xa determinations.

DVT/PE: SubQ:

Monitored dosing regimen: Initial: 17,500 units or 250 units/kg then 250 units/kg every 12 hours. The American College of Chest Physicians consensus conference has recommended dosage adjustments to correspond to a therapeutic range equivalent to heparin levels of 0.3-0.7 units/mL by antifactor Xa determinations.

Unmonitored dosing regimen: Initial: 333 units/kg then 250 units/kg every 12 hours

Line flushing: When using daily flushes of heparin to maintain patency of single and double lumen central catheters, 10 units/mL is commonly used for younger infants (eg, <10 kg) while 100 units/mL is used for older infants, children, and adults. Capped PVC catheters and peripheral heparin locks require flushing more frequently (eg, every 6-8 hours). Volume of heparin flush is usually similar to volume of catheter (or slightly greater). Additional flushes should be given when stagnant blood is observed in catheter, after catheter is used for drug or blood administration, and after blood withdrawal from catheter.

Addition of heparin (0.5-3 unit/mL) to peripheral and central parenteral nutrition has not been shown to decrease catheter-related thrombosis. The final concentration of heparin used for TPN solutions may need to be decreased to 0.5 units/mL in small infants receiving larger amounts of volume in order to avoid approaching therapeutic amounts. Arterial lines are heparinized with a final concentration of 1 unit/mL.

Dosing adjustments in the elderly: Patients >60 years of age may have higher serum levels and clinical response (longer aPTTs) as compared to younger patients receiving similar dosages; lower dosages may be required

Administration SubQ: Inject in subcutaneous tissue only (not muscle tissue). Injection sites should be rotated (usually left and right portions of the abdomen, above iliac crest).

Do not administer I.M. due to pain, irritation, and hematoma formation; central venous catheters must be flushed with heparin solution when newly inserted, daily (at the time of tubing change), after blood withdrawal or transfusion, and after an intermittent infusion through an injectable cap. A volume of at least 10 mL of blood should be removed and discarded from a heparinized line before blood samples are sent for coagulation testing.

Monitoring Parameters Hemoglobin, hematocrit, signs of bleeding; fecal occult blood test; aPTT (or antifactor Xa activity levels) or ACT depending upon indication

Platelet counts should be routinely monitored when the risk of HIT is >0.1% (eg, receiving therapeutic dose heparin, postoperative antithrombotic prophylaxis), if the patient has received heparin or low molecular weight heparin (eg, enoxaparin) within the past 100 days, if preexposure history is uncertain, or if anaphylactoid reaction to heparin occurs. When the risk of HIT is <0.1% (eg, medical/obstetrical patients receiving heparin flushes), routine platelet count monitoring is not recommended (Hirsh, 2008).

For intermittent I.V. injections, aPTT is measured 3.5-4 hours after I.V. injection.

For SubQ injections, when used for treatment (eg, monitored dosing regimen), aPTT is measured 6 hours after injection.

Note: Continuous I.V. infusion is preferred over I.V. intermittent injections. For full-dose heparin (ie, nonlow-dose), the dose should be titrated according to aPTT results. For anticoagulation, an aPTT 1.5-2.5 times normal is usually desired. Because of variation among hospitals in the control aPTT values, nomograms should be established at each institution, designed to achieve aPTT values in the target range (eg, for a control aPTT of 30 seconds, the target range [1.5-2.5 times control] would be 45-75 seconds). Measurements should be made prior to heparin therapy, 6 hours (pediatric: 4 hours) after initiation, and 6 hours (pediatric: 4 hours) after any dosage change, and should be used to adjust the heparin infusion until the aPTT exhibits a therapeutic level. When two consecutive aPTT values are therapeutic, subsequent measurements may be made every 24 hours, and if necessary, dose adjustment carried out. In addition, a significant change in the patient's clinical condition (eg, recurrent ischemia, bleeding, hypotension) should prompt an immediate aPTT determination, followed by dose adjustment if necessary. In general, may increase or decrease infusion by 2-4 units/kg/hour dependent upon aPTT.

Heparin infusion dose adjustment: A number of dose-adjustment nomograms have been developed which target an aPTT range of 1.5-2.5 times control (Cruickshank, 1991; Flaker, 1994; Hull, 1992; Raschke, 1993). However, institution-specific and indication-specific nomograms should be consulted for dose adjustment. **Note:** aPTT values vary throughout the day with maximum values occurring during the night (Decousus, 1985).

Reference Range Heparin: 0.3-0.7 unit/mL (by anti-Xa chromogenic assay) or 0.2-0.4 unit/mL (by protamine titration); aPTT: 1.5-2.5 times **the patient's baseline**

Test Interactions Increased thyroxine (competitive protein binding methods); increased PT

Aprotinin significantly increases aPTT and celite Activated Clotting Time (ACT) which may not reflect the actual degree of anticoagulation by heparin. Kaolin-based ACTs are not affected by aprotinin to the same degree as celite ACTs. While institutional protocols may vary, a minimal celite ACT of 750 seconds or kaolin-ACT of 480 seconds is recommended in the presence of aprotinin. Consult the manufacturer's information on specific ACT test interpretation in the presence of aprotinin.

Dosage Forms Excipient information presented when available (limited, particularly for generics); consult specific product labeling.

Infusion, as sodium [premixed in NaCl 0.45%; porcine intestinal mucosa source]: 12,500 units (250 mL); 25,000 units (250 mL, 500 mL)

Infusion, as sodium [preservative free; premixed in D_5W; porcine intestinal mucosa source]: 10,000 units (100 mL) [contains sodium metabisulfite]; 12,500 units (250 mL) [contains sodium metabisulfite]; 20,000 units (500 mL) [contains sodium metabisulfite]; 25,000 units (250 mL, 500 mL) [contains sodium metabisulfite]

Infusion, as sodium [preservative free; premixed in NaCl 0.9%; porcine intestinal mucosa source]: 1000 units (500 mL); 2000 units (1000 mL)

Injection, solution, as sodium [lock flush preparation; porcine intestinal mucosa source; multidose vial]: 10 units/mL (1 mL, 10 mL, 30 mL) [contains parabens]; 100 units/mL (1 mL, 5 mL) [contains parabens]

Injection, solution, as sodium [lock flush preparation; porcine intestinal mucosa source; multidose vial]: 10 units/mL (10 mL, 30 mL); 100 units/mL (10 mL, 30 mL) [contains benzyl alcohol]

Hep-Lock®: 10 units/mL (1 mL, 2 mL, 10 mL, 30 mL); 100 units/mL (1 mL, 2 mL, 10 mL, 30 mL) [contains benzyl alcohol]

Injection, solution, as sodium [lock flush preparation; porcine intestinal mucosa source; prefilled syringe]: 10 units/mL (1 mL, 2 mL, 3 mL, 5 mL); 100 units/mL (1 mL, 2 mL, 3 mL, 5 mL) [contains benzyl alcohol]

Injection, solution, as sodium [preservative free; lock flush preparation; porcine intestinal mucosa source; prefilled syringe]: 1 unit/mL (2 mL, 3 mL, 5 mL); 2 units/mL (3 mL); 10 units/mL (2.5 mL, 3 mL, 5 mL, 10 mL); 100 units/mL (3 mL, 5 mL, 10 mL)

Injection, solution, as sodium [preservative free; lock flush preparation; porcine intestinal mucosa source; vial]:

HepFlush®-10: 10 units/mL (10 mL)

Hep-Lock U/P: 10 units/mL (1 mL); 100 units/mL (1 mL)

Injection, solution, as sodium [porcine intestinal mucosa source; multidose vial]: 1000 units/mL (1 mL, 10 mL, 30 mL) [contains benzyl alcohol]; 1000 units/mL (1 mL, 10 mL, 30 mL) [contains methylparabens]; 5000 units/mL (1 mL, 10 mL) [contains benzyl alcohol]; 5000 units/mL (1 mL) [contains methylparabens]; 10,000 units/mL (1 mL, 4 mL) [contains benzyl alcohol]; 10,000 units/mL (1 mL, 5 mL) [contains methylparabens]; 20,000 units/mL (1 mL) [contains methylparabens]

Injection, solution, as sodium [porcine intestinal mucosa source; prefilled syringe]: 5000 units/mL (1 mL) [contains benzyl alcohol]

Injection, solution, as sodium [preservative free; porcine intestinal mucosa source; prefilled syringe]: 10,000 units/mL (0.5 mL)

Injection, solution, as sodium [preservative free; porcine intestinal mucosa source; vial]: 1000 units/mL (2 mL); 2000 units/mL (5 mL); 2500 units/mL (10 mL)

◆ **Heparin Calcium** *see* Heparin *on page 722*

◆ **Heparin Cofactor I** *see* Antithrombin III *on page 124*

◆ **Heparin Lock Flush** *see* Heparin *on page 722*

◆ **Heparin Sodium** *see* Heparin *on page 722*

Hepatitis A and Hepatitis B Recombinant Vaccine

(hep a TYE tis aye & hep a TYE tis bee ree KOM be nant vak SEEN)

U.S. Brand Names Twinrix®

Canadian Brand Names Twinrix®

Index Terms Engerix-B® and Havrix®; Havrix® and Engerix-B®; Hepatitis B and Hepatitis A Vaccine

Pharmacologic Category Vaccine, Inactivated (Viral)

Use Active immunization against disease caused by hepatitis A virus and hepatitis B virus (all known subtypes) in populations desiring protection against or at high risk of exposure to these viruses.

Populations include travelers to areas of intermediate/high endemicity for **both** HAV and HBV; those at increased risk of HBV infection due to behavioral or occupational factors; patients with chronic liver disease; laboratory workers who handle live HAV and HBV; healthcare workers, police, and other personnel who render first-aid or medical assistance; workers who come in contact with sewage; employees of day care centers and correctional facilities; patients/staff of hemodialysis units; male homosexuals; patients frequently receiving blood products; military personnel; users of injectable illicit drugs; close household contacts of patients with hepatitis A and hepatitis B infection; residents of drug and alcohol treatment centers

Pregnancy Risk Factor C

Dosage I.M.: Adults: Primary immunization: Three doses (1 mL each) given on a 0-, 1-, and 6-month schedule

Alternative regimen: Accelerated regimen: Four doses (1 mL each) on day 0, 7, and 21-30, followed by a booster at 12 months

Additional Information Complete prescribing information for this medication should be consulted for additional detail.

Dosage Forms Excipient information presented when available (limited, particularly for generics); consult specific product labeling. [DSC] = Discontinued product

Injection, suspension [preservative free]:

Twinrix®: Hepatitis A virus antigen 720 ELISA units and hepatitis B surface antigen 20 mcg per mL (1 mL) [contains aluminum, yeast protein, and trace amounts of neomycin; prefilled syringe contains natural rubber/natural latex]

Hepatitis A Vaccine (hep a TYE tis aye vak SEEN)

U.S. Brand Names HAVRIX®; VAQTA®

Canadian Brand Names Avaxim®; Avaxim®-Pediatric; HAVRIX®; VAQTA®

Pharmacologic Category Vaccine, Inactivated (Viral)

Additional Appendix Information

Guidelines for the Prevention of Opportunistic Infections in HIV Infected Persons *on page 1740*

Immunization Recommendations *on page 1708*

Use

Active immunization against disease caused by hepatitis A virus (HAV)

The Advisory Committee on Immunization Practices (ACIP) recommends routine vaccination for:

- All children ≥12 months of age
- Travelers to countries with intermediate to high endemicity of HAV (a list of countries is available at http://wwwn.cdc.gov/travel/contentdiseases.aspx)
- Men who have sex with men
- Illegal drug users
- Patients with chronic liver disease
- Patients who receive clotting-factor concentrates
- Persons who work with HAV-infected primates or with HAV in a research laboratory setting

Pregnancy Risk Factor C

Pregnancy Considerations Reproduction studies have not been conducted. The safety of vaccination during pregnancy has not been determined, however, the theoretical risk to the infant is expected to be low.

Lactation Excretion in breast milk unknown/use caution

Contraindications Hypersensitivity to hepatitis A vaccine or any component of the formulation

Warnings/Precautions Use caution in patients on anticoagulants, with thrombocytopenia, or bleeding disorders (bleeding may occur following intramuscular injection). Treatment for anaphylactic reactions should be immediately available. Postpone vaccination with acute infection or febrile illness. May not prevent infection if adequate antibody titers are not achieved (including immunosuppressed patients, patients on immunosuppressant therapy). Packaging may contain natural latex rubber; some products may contain neomycin. In order to maximize vaccination rates, the ACIP recommends simultaneous administration of all age-appropriate vaccines (live or inactivated) for which a person is eligible at a single clinic visit, unless contraindications exist. Safety and efficacy have not been established in children <12 months of age.

Adverse Reactions All serious adverse reactions must be reported to the U.S. Department of Health and Human Services (DHHS) Vaccine Adverse Event Reporting System (VAERS) at 1-800-822-7967 or online at https://secure.vaers.org.

Frequency dependent upon age, product used, and concomitant vaccine administration. In general, injection site reactions were less common in younger children.

>10%:

Central nervous system: Irritability (11% to 36%), drowsiness (15% to 17%), headache (≤1% to 16%), fever ≥100.4°F (9% to 11%)

Gastrointestinal: Anorexia (1% to 19%)

Local: Injection site: Pain, soreness, tenderness (3% to 56%), erythema (1% to 22%), warmth (<1% to 17%), swelling (1% to 14%)

1% to 10%:

Central nervous system: Fever ≥102°F (3%)

Dermatologic: Rash (≤1% to 5%)

Endocrine & metabolic: Menstrual disorder (1%)

Gastrointestinal: Diarrhea (<1% to 6%), vomiting (<1% to 4%), nausea (2%), abdominal pain (<1% to 2%), anorexia (1%)

Local: Injection site bruising (1% to 2%)

Neuromuscular & skeletal: Weakness/fatigue (4%), myalgia (<1% to 2%), arm pain (1%), back pain (1%), stiffness (1%)

Ocular: Conjunctivitis (1%)

Otic: Otitis media (8%), otitis (2%)

Respiratory: Upper respiratory tract infection (<1% to 10%), rhinorrhea (6%), cough (1% to 5%), pharyngitis (<1% to 3%), respiratory congestion (2%), nasal congestion (1%), laryngotracheobronchitis (1%)

Miscellaneous: Crying (2%), viral exanthema (1%)

<1% (Limited to important or life threatening): Allergic reaction, anaphylaxis, angioedema, arthralgia, asthma, bronchial constriction, bronchiolitis, cerebellar ataxia, CK increased, dehydration, dermatitis, diabetes mellitus, dizziness, dyspnea, encephalitis, erythema multiforme, eosinophilia, eye irritation, gastroenteritis, Guillain-Barré syndrome, hepatitis, hyperhidrosis, hypertonic episode, injection site hematoma, injection site itching, injection site rash, insomnia, jaundice, Kawasaki's disease, liver function tests increased, lymphadenopathy, multiple sclerosis, myelitis, neuropathy, paresthesia, photophobia, pneumonia, pruritus, seizure, somnolence, syncope, taste disturbance, thrombocytopenia, urine protein increased, urticaria, vertigo, wheezing

Drug Interactions

Avoid Concomitant Use There are no known interactions where it is recommended to avoid concomitant use.

Increased Effect/Toxicity There are no known significant interactions involving an increase in effect.

Decreased Effect

The levels/effects of Hepatitis A Vaccine may be decreased by: Immunosuppressants

Stability Store under refrigeration at 2°C to 8°C (36°F to 46°F); do not freeze.

Mechanism of Action As an inactivated virus vaccine, hepatitis A vaccine offers active immunization against hepatitis A virus infection at an effective immune response rate in up to 99% of subjects

Pharmacodynamics/Kinetics

Onset of action (protection): 2-4 weeks after a single dose; 2 weeks after vaccine administration, 54% to 62% of patients develop neutralizing antibodies; this percentage increases to 94% to 100% at 1 month postvaccination (CDC, 2006)

Duration: Neutralizing antibodies have persisted for up to 8 years; based on kinetic models, antibodies may be present ≥14-20 years in children and ≥25 years in adults who receive the complete vaccination series (CDC, 2006; Van Damme, 2003).

Dosage I.M.: **Note:** When used for primary immunization, the vaccine should be given at least 2 weeks prior to expected HAV exposure. When used for post-exposure prophylaxis, the vaccine should be given as soon as possible.

HAVRIX®:

Children 12 months to 18 years: 720 ELISA units (0.5 mL) with a booster dose of 720 ELISA units to be given 6-12 months following primary immunization

Adults: 1440 ELISA units (1 mL) with a booster dose of 1440 ELISA units to be given 6-12 months following primary immunization

VAQTA®:

Children 12 months to 18 years: 25 units (0.5 mL) with 25 units (0.5 mL) booster dose of 25 units to be given 6-18 months after primary immunization (6-12 months if initial dose was with HAVRIX®)

Adults: 50 units (1 mL) with 50 units (1 mL) booster dose of 50 units to be given 6-18 months after primary immunization (6-12 months if initial dose was with HAVRIX®)

Administration The deltoid muscle is the preferred site for injection; gluteal administration may decrease efficacy. Do not administer intravenously, intradermally, or subcutaneously. Shake well prior to use; discard if the suspension is discolored or does not appear homogenous after shaking. When used for primary immunization, the vaccine should be given at least 2 weeks prior to expected HAV exposure. When used for post-exposure prophylaxis, the vaccine should be given as soon as possible. For patients at risk of hemorrhage following intramuscular injection, the ACIP recommends "it should be administered intramuscularly if, in the opinion of the physician familiar with the patients bleeding risk, the vaccine can be administered with reasonable safety by this route. If the patient receives antihemophilia or other similar therapy, intramuscular vaccination can be scheduled shortly after such therapy is administered. A fine needle (23 gauge or smaller) can be used for the vaccination and firm pressure applied to the site (without rubbing) for at least 2 minutes. The patient should be instructed concerning the risk of hematoma from the injection."

Administration with other vaccines:

Hepatitis A vaccine with live vaccines: May be given simultaneously or at any interval between doses.

Hepatitis A vaccine with other inactivated vaccines: May be given simultaneously or at any interval between doses.

Vaccine administration with antibody-containing products: Hepatitis A vaccine may be given simultaneously at different sites or at any interval between doses. Examples of antibody-containing products include I.M. and I.V. immune globulin, hepatitis B immune globulin, tetanus immune globulin, varicella zoster immune globulin, rabies immune globulin, whole blood, packed red cells, plasma, and platelet products.

Monitoring Parameters Liver function tests

Additional Information The ACIP currently recommends that older adults, the immunocompormised, or persons with underlying medical conditions (including chronic liver disease) that are vaccinated <2 weeks from departure to an area with a high risk of hepatitis A infection also receive immune globulin.

Federal law requires that the date of administration, the vaccine manufacturer, lot number of vaccine, and the administering person's name, title and address be entered into the patient's permanent medical record.

Dosage Forms Excipient information presented when available (limited, particularly for generics); consult specific product labeling.

Injection, suspension [adult formulation; preservative free]:

HAVRIX®: Hepatitis A virus antigen 1440 ELISA units/mL (1 mL) [contains aluminum, trace amounts of neomycin; prefilled syringe contains natural rubber/natural latex]

VAQTA®: Hepatitis A virus antigen 50 units/mL (1 mL) [contains aluminum, natural rubber/natural latex in packaging]

Injection, suspension [pediatric formulation; preservative free]:

HAVRIX®: Hepatitis A virus antigen 720 ELISA units/0.5 mL (0.5 mL) [contains aluminum, trace amounts of neomycin; prefilled syringe contains natural rubber/natural latex]

Injection, suspension [pediatric/adolescent formulation; preservative free]:

VAQTA®: Hepatitis A virus antigen 25 units/0.5 mL (0.5 mL) [contains aluminum, natural rubber/natural latex in packaging]

◆ **Hepatitis B and Hepatitis A Vaccine** *see* Hepatitis A and Hepatitis B Recombinant Vaccine *on page 725*

Hepatitis B Immune Globulin (Human)

(hep a TYE tis bee i MYUN GLOB yoo lin YU man)

U.S. Brand Names HepaGam B™; HyperHEP B™ S/D; Nabi-HB®

Canadian Brand Names HepaGam B™; HyperHep B®

Index Terms HBIG

Pharmacologic Category Immune Globulin

Additional Appendix Information

Immunization Recommendations *on page 1708*

Use

Passive prophylactic immunity to hepatitis B following: Acute exposure to blood containing hepatitis B surface antigen (HBsAg); perinatal exposure of infants born to HBsAg-positive mothers; sexual exposure to HBsAg-positive persons; household exposure to persons with acute HBV infection

Prevention of hepatitis B virus recurrence after liver transplantation in HBsAg-positive transplant patients

Note: Hepatitis B immune globulin is not indicated for treatment of active hepatitis B infection and is ineffective in the treatment of chronic active hepatitis B infection.

Pregnancy Risk Factor C

Pregnancy Considerations Reproduction studies have not been conducted.

Lactation Excretion in breast milk unknown/use caution

Medication Safety Issues

Sound-alike/look-alike issues:

HBIG may be confused with BabyBIG

Contraindications Hypersensitivity to hepatitis B immune globulin or any component of the formulation; severe allergy to gamma globulin or anti-immunoglobulin therapies

Warnings/Precautions Hypersensitivity and anaphylactic reactions can occur; immediate treatment (including epinephrine 1:1000) should be available. Use with caution in patients with previous systemic hypersensitivity to human immunoglobulins. Use with caution in patients with thrombocytopenia or coagulation disorders; I.M. injections may be contraindicated. Use with caution in patients with IgA deficiency. Product of human plasma; may potentially contain infectious agents which could transmit disease. Screening of donors, as well as testing and/or inactivation or removal of certain viruses, reduces the risk. Infections thought to be transmitted by this product should be reported to the manufacturer. Some products may contain maltose, which may result in falsely-elevated blood glucose readings.

Adverse Reactions Reported with postexposure prophylaxis. Adverse events reported in liver transplant patients included tremor and hypotension, were associated with a single infusion during the first week of treatment, and did not recur with additional infusions.

Central nervous system: Fainting, headache, lightheadedness, malaise

Dermatologic: Angioedema, bruising, urticaria

Gastrointestinal: Nausea, vomiting

Hematologic: WBC decreased

Hepatic: Alkaline phosphatase increased, AST increased
Local: Ache, erythema, pain, and/or tenderness at injection site
Neuromuscular & skeletal: Arthralgia, joint stiffness, myalgia
Renal: Creatinine increased
Respiratory: Cold symptoms
Miscellaneous: Anaphylaxis, flu-like syndrome

Drug Interactions

Avoid Concomitant Use There are no known interactions where it is recommended to avoid concomitant use.

Increased Effect/Toxicity There are no known significant interactions involving an increase in effect.

Decreased Effect

Hepatitis B Immune Globulin (Human) may decrease the levels/effects of: Vaccines (Live)

Stability Refrigerate at 2°C to 8°C (36°F to 46°F); do not freeze. Use within 6 hours of entering vial. Do not shake vial; avoid foaming.

Mechanism of Action Hepatitis B immune globulin (HBIG) is a nonpyrogenic sterile solution containing immunoglobulin G (IgG) specific to hepatitis B surface antigen (HB_sAg). HBIG differs from immune globulin in the amount of anti-HB_s. Immune globulin is prepared from plasma that is not preselected for anti-HB_s content. HBIG is prepared from plasma preselected for high titer anti-HB_s. In the U.S., HBIG has an anti-HB_s high titer >1:100,000 by IRA.

Pharmacodynamics/Kinetics

Duration: Postexposure prophylaxis: 3-6 months
Absorption: I.M.: Slow
Half-life: 17-25 days
Distribution: V_d: 7-15 L
Time to peak, serum: I.M.: 2-10 days

Dosage

I.M.:

Newborns: Perinatal exposure of infants born to HBsAg-positive mothers: 0.5 mL as soon after birth as possible (within 12 hours); active vaccination with hepatitis B vaccine may begin at the same time in a different site (if not contraindicated). If first dose of hepatitis B vaccine is delayed for as long as 3 months, dose may be repeated. If hepatitis B vaccine is refused, dose may be repeated at 3 and 6 months.

Infants <12 months: Household exposure prophylaxis: 0.5 mL (to be administered if mother or primary caregiver has acute HBV infection)

Children ≥12 months and Adults: Postexposure prophylaxis: 0.06 mL/kg as soon as possible after exposure (ie, within 24 hours of needlestick, ocular, or mucosal exposure or within 14 days of sexual exposure); usual dose: 3-5 mL; repeat at 28-30 days after exposure in nonresponders to hepatitis B vaccine or in patients who refuse vaccination

Note: HBIG may be administered at the same time (but at a different site) or up to 1 month preceding hepatitis B vaccination without impairing the active immune response

I.V.: Adults: Prevention of hepatitis B virus recurrence after liver transplantation (HepaGam B™): 20,000 int. units/dose according to the following schedule:

Anhepatic phase (Initial dose): One dose given with the liver transplant
Week 1 postop: One dose daily for 7 days (days 1-7)
Weeks 2-12 postop: One dose every 2 weeks starting day 14
Month 4 onward: One dose monthly starting on month 4
Dose adjustment: Adjust dose to reach anti-HBs levels of 500 int. units/L within the first week after transplantation. In patients with surgical bleeding, abdominal fluid drainage >500 mL or those undergoing plasmapheresis, administer 10,000 int. units/dose every 6 hours until target anti-HBs levels are reached.

Administration

I.M.: Postexposure prophylaxis: I.M. injection only in anterolateral aspect of upper thigh and deltoid muscle of upper arm; to prevent injury from injection, care should be taken when giving to patients with thrombocytopenia or bleeding disorders

I.V.:

HepaGam B™: Liver transplant: Administer at 2 mL/minute. Decrease infusion to ≤1 mL/minute for patient discomfort or infusion-related adverse events. Actual volume of infusion is dependant upon potency labeled on each individual vial.

Nabi-HB®: Although not an FDA-approved for this purpose, Nabi-HB® has been administered intravenously in hepatitis B-positive liver transplant patients

Monitoring Parameters Liver transplant: Serum HBsAg; infusion-related adverse events

Test Interactions

Glucose testing: HepaGam B™ contains maltose. Falsely-elevated blood glucose levels may occur when glucose monitoring devices and test strips utilizing the glucose dehydrogenase pyrroloquinolinequinone (GDH-PQQ) based methods are used.

Serological testing: Antibodies transferred following administration of immune globulins may provide misleading positive test results (eg, Coombs' test)

Additional Information Each vial contains anti-HB_s antibody equivalent to or exceeding the potency of anti-HB_s in a U.S. reference standard hepatitis B immune globulin (FDA). The U.S. reference standard has been tested against the WHO standard hepatitis B immune globulin with listed values between 207 int. units/mL and 220 int. units/mL (included in individual product information).

Dosage Forms Excipient information presented when available (limited, particularly for generics); consult specific product labeling.

Note: Potency expressed in international units (as compared to the WHO standard) is noted by individual lot on the vial label.

Injection, solution [preservative free]:

HyperHEP B™ S/D: Anti-HBs ≥220 int. units/mL (0.5 mL, 1 mL, 5 mL)
Nabi-HB®: Anti-HBs >312 int. units/mL (1 mL, 5 mL) [contains polysorbate 80]
HepaGam B™: Anti-HBs 312 int. units/mL (1 mL, 5 mL) [contains maltose and polysorbate 80]

◆ **Hepatitis B Inactivated Virus Vaccine (recombinant DNA)** *see* Hepatitis B Vaccine (Recombinant) *on page 728*

Hepatitis B Vaccine (Recombinant)

(hep a TYE tis bee vak SEEN ree KOM be nant)

U.S. Brand Names Engerix-B®; Recombivax HB®

Canadian Brand Names Engerix-B®; Recombivax HB®

Index Terms Hepatitis B Inactivated Virus Vaccine (recombinant DNA)

Pharmacologic Category Vaccine, Inactivated (Viral)

Additional Appendix Information

Guidelines for the Prevention of Opportunistic Infections in HIV Infected Persons *on page 1740*
Immunization Recommendations *on page 1708*

Use Immunization against infection caused by all known subtypes of hepatitis B virus (HBV), in individuals seeking protection from HBV infection and/or in the following individuals considered at high risk of potential exposure to hepatitis B virus or HBsAg-positive materials:

Workplace Exposure:

- Healthcare workers[1] (including students, custodial staff, lab personnel, etc)

- Police and fire personnel
- Military personnel
- Morticians and embalmers
- Clients/staff of institutions for the developmentally disabled

Lifestyle Factors:
- Homosexual men
- Heterosexually-active persons with multiple partners in a 6-month period or those with recently acquired sexually-transmitted disease
- Intravenous drug users

Specific Patient Groups:
- Those on hemodialysis[2], receiving transfusions[3], or in hematology/oncology units
- Adolescents
- Infants born of HBsAG-positive mothers
- Individuals with chronic liver disease
- Individual with HIV infection

Others:
- Prison inmates and staff of correctional facilities
- Household and sexual contacts of HBV carriers
- Residents, immigrants, adoptees, and refugees from areas with endemic HBV infection (eg, Alaskan Eskimos, Pacific Islanders, Indochinese, and Haitian descent)
- International travelers to areas of endemic HBV
- Children born after 11/21/1991

[1]The risk of hepatitis B virus (HBV) infection for healthcare workers varies both between hospitals and within hospitals. Hepatitis B vaccination is recommended for all healthcare workers with blood exposure.

[2]Hemodialysis patients often respond poorly to hepatitis B vaccination; higher vaccine doses or increased number of doses are required. A special formulation of one vaccine is now available for such persons (Recombivax HB®, 40 mcg/mL). The anti-HB_s (antibody to hepatitis B surface antigen) response of such persons should be tested after they are vaccinated, and those who have not responded should be revaccinated with 1-3 additional doses. Patients with chronic renal disease should be vaccinated as early as possible, ideally before they require hemodialysis. In addition, their anti-HB^s levels should be monitored at 6- to 12-month intervals to assess the need for revaccination.

[3]Patients with hemophilia should be immunized subcutaneously, not intramuscularly.

In addition, the Advisory Committee on Immunization Practices (ACIP) recommends vaccination for any persons who are wounded in bombings or similar mass casualty events who have penetrating injuries or nonintact skin exposure, or who have contact with mucous membranes (exception - superficial contact with intact skin), and who cannot confirm receipt of a hepatitis B vaccination.

Pregnancy Risk Factor C

Pregnancy Considerations Reproduction studies have not been conducted. The ACIP recommends HBsAg testing for all pregnant women. Based on limited data, there is no apparent risk to the fetus when the hepatitis B vaccine is administered during pregnancy. Pregnancy itself is not a contraindication to vaccination; vaccination should be considered if otherwise indicated.

Lactation Excretion in breast milk unknown/use caution

Medication Safety Issues

Sound-alike/look-alike issues:

Recombivax HB® may be confused with Comvax®

Contraindications Hypersensitivity to yeast, hepatitis B vaccine, or any component of the formulation

Warnings/Precautions Immediate treatment for anaphylactic/anaphylactoid reaction should be available during vaccine use. Consider delaying vaccination during acute, moderate-to-severe febrile illness. Use caution with decreased cardiopulmonary function Unrecognized hepatitis B infection may be present, immunization may not prevent infection in these patients. Patients >65 years may have lower response rates. Consider delaying vaccination for ≥3 months after receiving immunosuppressive therapy. Use caution in multiple sclerosis patients; rare exacerbations of symptoms have been observed. Some dosage forms contain dry natural latex rubber. In order to maximize vaccination rates, the ACIP recommends simultaneous administration of all age-appropriate vaccines (live or inactivated) for which a person is eligible at a single clinic visit, unless contraindications exist.

Adverse Reactions All serious adverse reactions must be reported to the U.S. Department of Health and Human Services (DHHS) Vaccine Adverse Event Reporting System (VAERS) 1-800-822-7967.

Frequency not defined. The most common adverse effects reported with both products included injection site reactions (>10%).

Cardiovascular: Flushing, hypotension

Central nervous system: Agitation, chills, dizziness, fatigue, fever (≥37.5°C / 100°F), headache, insomnia, irritability, lightheadedness, malaise, somnolence, vertigo

Dermatologic: Angioedema, petechiae, pruritus, rash, urticaria

Gastrointestinal: Abdominal pain, appetite decreased, constipation, cramps, diarrhea, dyspepsia, nausea, vomiting

Genitourinary: Dysuria

Local: Injection site reactions: Ecchymosis, erythema, induration, pain, nodule formation, soreness, swelling, tenderness, warmth

Neuromuscular & skeletal: Achiness, arthralgia, back pain, myalgia, neck pain, neck stiffness, paresthesia, shoulder pain, tingling, weakness

Otic: Earache

Respiratory: Cough, pharyngitis, rhinitis, upper respiratory tract infection

Miscellaneous: Diaphoresis, lymphadenopathy, flu-like syndrome

Postmarketing and/or case reports: Alopecia, anaphylaxis, arthritis, Bell's palsy, bronchospasm, conjunctivitis, eczema, encephalitis, erythema nodosum, erythema multiforme, erythrocyte sedimentation rate increased, febrile seizure, Guillain-Barré syndrome, herpes zoster, hypoesthesia, keratitis, liver enzymes increased, lupus-like syndrome, migraine, multiple sclerosis, muscle weakness, neuropathy, optic neuritis, palpitation, paresis, paresthesia, polyarteritis nodosa, purpura, seizure, serum-sickness like syndrome (may be delayed days to weeks), Stevens-Johnson syndrome, SLE, syncope, tachycardia, thrombocytopenia, tinnitus, transverse myelitis, vasculitis, visual disturbances, vertigo

Drug Interactions

Avoid Concomitant Use There are no known interactions where it is recommended to avoid concomitant use.

Increased Effect/Toxicity There are no known significant interactions involving an increase in effect.

Decreased Effect

The levels/effects of Hepatitis B Vaccine (Recombinant) may be decreased by: Immunosuppressants

Stability Refrigerate at 2°C to 8°C (36°F to 46°F); do not freeze.

Mechanism of Action Recombinant hepatitis B vaccine is a noninfectious subunit viral vaccine, which confers active immunity via formation of antihepatitis B antibodies. The vaccine is derived from hepatitis B surface antigen (HBsAg) produced through recombinant DNA techniques from yeast cells. The portion of the hepatitis B gene which codes for HBsAg is cloned into yeast which is then cultured to produce hepatitis B vaccine.

Pharmacodynamics/Kinetics Duration: Following a 3-dose series in children, up to 50% of patients will have low or undetectable anti-HB antibody 5-15 years postvaccination. However, anamnestic increases in anti-HB have been shown up to 23 years later suggesting a lifelong immune memory response.

Dosage I.M.:

Immunization regimen: Regimen consists of 3 doses (0, 1, and 6 months): First dose given on the elected date, second dose given 1 month later, third dose given 6 months after the first dose; see table.

When used for immediate prophylactic intervention (eg, administration to persons who are wounded in bombings or similar mass casualty events), vaccination should begin within 24 hours and no later than 7 days following the event.

Note: Infants born to mothers whose HBsAg status is unknown should follow the regimen for HBsAg-positive mothers, omitting the dose of HBIG.

Note: Preterm infants <2000 g and born to HBsAg-negative mothers should have the first dose delayed until 1 month after birth or hospital discharge due to decreased immune response in underweight infants.

Routine Immunization Regimen of Three I.M. Hepatitis B Vaccine Doses

Age	Initial		1 mo		2 mo	6 mo[1]	
	Recombivax HB® (mL)	Engerix-B® (mL)	Recombivax HB® (mL)	Engerix-B® (mL)	Engerix-B® (mL)	Recombivax HB® (mL)	Engerix-B® (mL)
Birth[2] to 19 y	0.5[3]	0.5[4]	0.5[3]	0.5[4]	–	0.5[3]	0.5[4]
≥20 y[5]	1[6]	1[7]	1[6]	1[7]	–	1[6]	1[7]
Dialysis or immunocompromised patients[8]	1[9]	2[10]	1[9]	2[10]	2[10]	1[9]	2[10]

[1]Final dose in series should not be administered before age of 24 weeks.

[2]Infants born of HBsAg **negative** mothers.

[3]5 mcg/0.5 mL pediatric/adolescent formulation.

[4]10 mcg/0.5 mL formulation.

[5]Alternately, doses may be administered at 0, 1, and 4 months **or** at 0, 2, and 4 months.

[6]10 mcg/mL adult formulation.

[7]20 mcg/mL formulation.

[8]Revaccinate if anti-HB_s <10 mIU/mL ≥1-2 months after third dose.

[9]40 mcg/mL dialysis formulation.

[10]Two 1 mL doses given at different sites using the 20 mcg/mL formulation.

Alternative dosing schedule for **Recombivax HB®:**

Children 11-15 years (10 mcg/mL adult formulation): First dose of 1 mL given on the elected date, second dose given 4-6 months later

Adults ≥20 years: Doses may be administered at 0, 1, and 4 months **or** at 0, 2, and 4 months

Alternative dosing schedules for **Engerix-B®:**

Children ≤10 years (10 mcg/0.5 mL formulation): High-risk children: 0.5 mL at 0, 1, 2, and 12 months; lower-risk children ages 5-10 who are candidates for an extended administration schedule may receive an alternative regimen of 0.5 mL at 0, 12, and 24 months. If booster dose is needed, revaccinate with 0.5 mL.

Adolescents 11-19 years (20 mcg/mL formulation): 1 mL at 0, 1, and 6 months. High-risk adolescents: 1 mL at 0, 1, 2, and 12 months; lower-risk adolescents 11-16 years who are candidates for an extended administration schedule may receive an alternative regimen of 0.5 mL (using the 10 mcg/0.5 mL) formulation at 0, 12, and 24 months. If booster dose is needed, revaccinate with 20 mcg.

Adults ≥20 years:

Doses may be administered at 0, 1, and 4 months **or** at 0, 2, and 4 months

High-risk adults (20 mcg/mL formulation): 1 mL at 0, 1, 2, and 12 months. If booster dose is needed, revaccinate with 1 mL.

Postexposure prophylaxis: **Note:** High-risk individuals may include children born of hepatitis B-infected mothers, those who have been or might be exposed or those who have traveled to high-risk areas. See table.

Postexposure Prophylaxis Recommended Dosage for Infants Born to HBsAg-Positive Mothers

Treatment	Birth ≤12 h	1 mo	6 mo
Engerix-B® (pediatric formulation 10 mcg/0.5 mL)[1]	0.5 mL[2]	0.5 mL	0.5 mL
Recombivax HB® (pediatric/adolescent formulation 5 mcg/0.5 mL)	0.5 mL[2]	0.5 mL	0.5 mL
Hepatitis B immune globulin	0.5 mL[2]	—	—

[1]An alternate regimen is administration of the vaccine at birth, and 1, 2, and 12 months later.

[2]The first dose of vaccine may be given at birth at the same time as HBIG, but give in the opposite anterolateral thigh. This may better ensure vaccine absorption. HBIG should be given immediately if mother is determined to be HBsAg-positive within 7 days of birth.

Administration It is possible to interchange the vaccines for completion of a series or for booster doses; the antibody produced in response to each type of vaccine is comparable, however, the quantity of the vaccine will vary

I.M. injection only; in adults, the deltoid muscle is the preferred site; the anterolateral thigh is the recommended site in infants and young children. Not for gluteal administration. Shake well prior to withdrawal and use.

For patients at risk of hemorrhage following intramuscular injection, hepatitis B vaccine may be administered subcutaneously although lower titers and/or increased incidence of local reactions may result. The ACIP recommends "it should be administered intramuscularly if, in the opinion of the physician familiar with the patients bleeding risk, the vaccine can be administered with reasonable safety by this route. If the patient receives antihemophilia or other similar therapy, intramuscular vaccination can be scheduled shortly after such therapy is administered. A fine needle (23 gauge or smaller) can be used for the vaccination and firm pressure applied to the site (without rubbing) for at least 2 minutes. The patient should be instructed concerning the risk of hematoma from the injection."

Administration with other vaccines:

Hepatitis B vaccine with live vaccines: May be given simultaneously or at any interval between doses.

Hepatitis B vaccine with other inactivated vaccines: May be given simultaneously or at any interval between doses.

Vaccine administration with antibody-containing products: Hepatitis B vaccine may be given simultaneously at different sites or at any interval between doses. Examples of antibody containing products include I.M. and I.V. immune globulin, hepatitis B immune globulin, tetanus immune globulin, varicella zoster immune globulin, rabies immune globulin, whole blood, packed red cells, plasma, and platelet products

Vaccination at the time of HBsAg testing: For persons in whom vaccination is recommended, the first dose of hepatitis B vaccine can be given after blood is drawn to test for HBsAg.

Additional Information Federal law requires that the date of administration, the vaccine manufacturer, lot number of vaccine, and the administering person's name, title, and address be entered into the patient's permanent medical record.

Dosage Forms Excipient information presented when available (limited, particularly for generics); consult specific product labeling.

Injection, suspension [adult; preservative free]:

Engerix-B®: Hepatitis B surface antigen 20 mcg/mL (1 mL) [contains aluminum, trace amounts of thimerosal; prefilled syringes contain natural rubber/natural latex]

Recombivax HB®: Hepatitis B surface antigen 10 mcg/mL (1 mL, 3 mL) [contains aluminum and yeast protein]

Injection, suspension [pediatric/adolescent; preservative free]:

Engerix-B®: Hepatitis B surface antigen 10 mcg/0.5 mL (0.5 mL) [contains aluminum, trace amounts of thimerosal; prefilled syringes contain natural rubber/natural latex]

Recombivax HB®: Hepatitis B surface antigen 5 mcg/0.5 mL (0.5 mL) [contains aluminum and yeast protein]

Injection, suspension [dialysis formulation; preservative free]:

Recombivax HB®: Hepatitis B surface antigen 40 mcg/mL (1 mL) [contains aluminum and yeast protein]

◆ **Hepatitis B Vaccine (Recombinant)** *see Haemophilus* b Conjugate and Hepatitis B Vaccine *on page 717*

◆ **HepFlush®-10** *see* Heparin *on page 722*

◆ **Hep-Lock®** *see* Heparin *on page 722*

◆ **Hep-Lock U/P** *see* Heparin *on page 722*

◆ **Hepsera™** *see* Adefovir *on page 45*

◆ **Heptovir® (Can)** *see* LamiVUDine *on page 848*

◆ **Herceptin®** *see* Trastuzumab *on page 1503*

◆ **HES** *see* Hetastarch *on page 731*

◆ **Hespan®** *see* Hetastarch *on page 731*

Hetastarch (HET a starch)

U.S. Brand Names Hespan®; Hextend®; Voluven®

Canadian Brand Names Hextend®; Voluven®

Index Terms HES; Hydroxyethyl Starch

Pharmacologic Category Plasma Volume Expander, Colloid

Use Blood volume expander used in treatment of hypovolemia; prevention of hypovolemia (Voluven®); adjunct in leukapheresis to improve harvesting and increase the yield of granulocytes by centrifugation (Hespan®)

Unlabeled/Investigational Use Hextend®: Priming fluid in pump oxygenators during cardiopulmonary bypass; plasma volume expansion during cardiopulmonary bypass

Pregnancy Risk Factor C

Medication Safety Issues

Sound-alike/look-alike issues:

Hespan® may be confused with heparin

Dosage I.V. infusion (requires an infusion pump):

Plasma volume expansion:

Children:

<2 years: Voluven®: Average dose: 7-25 mL/kg; titrate to individual colloid needs, hemodynamic and hydration status

2-12 years: Not studied

>12 years: Voluven®: Up to 50 mL/kg/day

Adults: 500-1000 mL (up to 1500 mL/day) or 20 mL/kg/day (up to 1500 mL/day); larger volumes (15,000 mL/24 hours) have been used safely in small numbers of patients

Voluven®: Up to 50 mL/kg/day

Leukapheresis (Hextend®): 250-700 mL; **Note:** Citrate anticoagulant is added before use.

Dosing adjustment in renal impairment: Cl_{cr} <10 mL/minute: Initial dose is the same but subsequent doses should be reduced by 20% to 50% of normal

Additional Information Complete prescribing information for this medication should be consulted for additional detail.

Dosage Forms Excipient information presented when available (limited, particularly for generics); consult specific product labeling.

Infusion [premixed in lactated electrolyte injection]:

Hextend®: 6% (500 mL)

Infusion, solution [premixed in NaCl 0.9%]: 6% (500 mL)

Hespan®, Voluven®: 6% (500 mL)

◆ **Hexachlorocyclohexane** *see* Lindane *on page 889*

Hexachlorophene (heks a KLOR oh feen)

U.S. Brand Names pHisoHex®

Canadian Brand Names pHisoHex®

Pharmacologic Category Antibiotic, Topical

Use Surgical scrub and as a bacteriostatic skin cleanser; control an outbreak of gram-positive infection when other procedures have been unsuccessful

Pregnancy Risk Factor C

Medication Safety Issues

Sound-alike/look-alike issues:

pHisoHex® may be confused with Fostex®, pHisoDerm®

Dosage Children and Adults: Topical: Apply 5 mL cleanser and water to area to be cleansed; lather and rinse thoroughly under running water

Additional Information Complete prescribing information for this medication should be consulted for additional detail.

Dosage Forms Excipient information presented when available (limited, particularly for generics); consult specific product labeling.

Liquid, topical: 3% (150 mL, 500 mL, 3840 mL)

◆ **Hexalen®** *see* Altretamine *on page 74*

◆ **Hexamethylenetetramine** *see* Methenamine *on page 961*

◆ **Hexamethylmelamine** *see* Altretamine *on page 74*

◆ **Hexit™ (Can)** *see* Lindane *on page 889*

◆ **HEXM** *see* Altretamine *on page 74*

◆ **Hextend®** *see* Hetastarch *on page 731*

◆ **hFSH** *see* Urofollitropin *on page 1531*

◆ **hGH** *see* Somatropin *on page 1388*

◆ **Hib Conjugate Vaccine** *see Haemophilus* b Conjugate and Hepatitis B Vaccine *on page 717*

◆ **Hib Conjugate Vaccine** *see Haemophilus* b Conjugate Vaccine *on page 718*

◆ **Hibiclens® [OTC]** *see* Chlorhexidine Gluconate *on page 305*

◆ **Hibidil® 1:2000 (Can)** *see* Chlorhexidine Gluconate *on page 305*

◆ **Hibistat® [OTC]** *see* Chlorhexidine Gluconate *on page 305*

◆ **Hib Polysaccharide Conjugate** *see Haemophilus* b Conjugate Vaccine *on page 718*

◆ **High Gamma Vitamin E Complete™ [OTC]** *see* Vitamin E *on page 1566*

◆ **High-Molecular-Weight Iron Dextran (DexFerrum®)** *see* Iron Dextran Complex *on page 817*

◆ **Hiprex®** *see* Methenamine *on page 961*

◆ **Hirulog** *see* Bivalirudin *on page 201*

◆ **Histade™ [DSC]** *see* Chlorpheniramine and Pseudoephedrine *on page 310*

◆ **Histantil (Can)** *see* Promethazine *on page 1249*

◆ **Histatab PH** *see* Chlorpheniramine, Phenylephrine, and Methscopolamine *on page 313*

◆ **Hista-Vent® DA [DSC]** *see* Chlorpheniramine, Phenylephrine, and Methscopolamine *on page 313*

◆ **Histex™** *see* Chlorpheniramine and Pseudoephedrine *on page 310*

◆ **Histex® SR** *see* Brompheniramine and Pseudoephedrine *on page 214*

Histrelin (his TREL in)

U.S. Brand Names Supprelin® LA; Vantas™

Canadian Brand Names Vantas™

Index Terms GnRH Agonist; Histrelin Acetate; LH-RH Agonist

Pharmacologic Category Gonadotropin Releasing Hormone Agonist

Use Palliative treatment of advanced prostate cancer; treatment of children with central precocious puberty (CPP)

Pregnancy Risk Factor X

Pregnancy Considerations Fetal harm and an increase in fetal mortalities have been noted in animal studies. Histrelin is contraindicated for use during pregnancy or in women who may become pregnant.

Lactation Excretion in breast milk unknown/contraindicated

Contraindications Hypersensitivity to histrelin acetate, GnRH, GnRH-agonist analogs, or any component of the formulation; pregnancy

Warnings/Precautions

CPP: Transient increases in estradiol serum levels (female) or testosterone levels (female and male) may occur during the first week of use. Worsening symptoms may occur, however, manifestations of puberty should decrease within 4 weeks. Safety and efficacy have not been established in children <2 years of age

Prostate cancer: Transient increases in testosterone serum levels occur during the first week of use (initial flare). Worsening symptoms such as bone pain, hematuria, neuropathy, ureteral or bladder outlet obstruction, and spinal cord compression have been reported. Spinal cord compression and ureteral obstruction may contribute to paralysis; close attention should be given during the first few weeks of therapy to both patients having metastatic vertebral lesions and/or urinary tract obstructions, and to any patients reporting weakness, paresthesias or poor urine output. Safety and efficacy have not been established in patients with hepatic dysfunction.

Adverse Reactions

CPP:

>10%: Local: Insertion site reaction (51%; includes bruising, discomfort, itching, pain, protrusion of implant area, soreness, swelling, tingling)

>2% to 10%:

Endocrine & metabolic: Metrorrhagia (4%)

Local: Keloid scar (6%), scar (6%), suture-related complication (6%), pain at the application site (4%), post procedural pain (4%)

≤2% (Limited to important or life-threatening): Amblyopia, breast tenderness, cold feeling, disease progression, dysmenorrhea, epistaxis, erythema, flu-like syndrome, gynecomastia, headache, infection at the implant site, menorrhagia, migraine, mood swings, pituitary adenoma, pruritus, weight increase

Prostate cancer:

>10%:

Endocrine & metabolic: Hot flashes (66%)

Local: Implant site reaction (6% to 14%; includes bruising, erythema, pain, soreness, swelling, tenderness)

2% to 10%:

Central nervous system: Fatigue (10%), headache (3%), insomnia (3%)

Endocrine & metabolic: Gynecomastia (4%), sexual dysfunction (4%), libido decreased (2%)

Gastrointestinal: Constipation (4%), weight gain (2%)

Genitourinary: Expected pharmacological consequence of testosterone suppression: Testicular atrophy (5%)

Renal: Renal impairment (5%)

<2% (Limited to important or life-threatening): Abdominal discomfort, alopecia, anemia, appetite increased, arthralgia, AST increased, back pain, bone density decreased, bone pain, breast pain, breast tenderness, cold feeling, contusion, craving food, creatinine increased, depression, diaphoresis, dizziness, dyspnea (exertional), dysuria, fluid retention, flushing, genital pruritus, hematoma, hematuria, hypercalcemia, hypercholesterolemia, hyperglycemia, irritability, LDH increased, lethargy, limb pain, liver disorder, malaise, muscle twitching, myalgia, nausea, neck pain, night sweats, palpitation, peripheral edema, prostatic acid phosphatase increased, pruritus, renal calculi, renal failure, stent occlusion, testosterone increased, tremor, urinary frequency, urinary retention, ventricular asystoles, weakness, weight loss

Drug Interactions

Avoid Concomitant Use There are no known interactions where it is recommended to avoid concomitant use.

Increased Effect/Toxicity

Histrelin may increase the levels/effects of: Vitamin K Antagonists

Decreased Effect

Histrelin may decrease the levels/effects of: Antidiabetic Agents; Cardiac Glycosides; Vitamin K Antagonists

Stability Supprelin® LA, Vantas™: Upon delivery, separate contents of implant carton. Store implant under refrigeration at 2°C to 8°C (36°F to 46°F), wrapped in the amber pouch for protection from light; do not freeze. The implantation kit does not require refrigeration.

Mechanism of Action Potent inhibitor of gonadotropin secretion; continuous administration results in, after an initiation phase, the suppression of luteinizing hormone (LH), follicle-stimulating hormone (FSH), and a subsequent decrease in testosterone (females and males) and estrogen (premenopausal females). Additionally, in patients with CPP, linear growth velocity is slowed (improves chance of attaining predicted adult height).

Pharmacodynamics/Kinetics

Onset of action: Prostate cancer: Chemical castration: 2-4 weeks; CPP: progression of sexual development stops and growth is decreased in ~1 month

Duration: 1 year

Distribution: Adults: V_d: ~58 L

Protein binding: Adults: 70% ± 9%

Metabolism: Hepatic via C-terminal dealkylation and hydrolysis

Bioavailability: Adults: 92%

Half-life elimination: Adults: Terminal: ~4 hours

Time to peak, serum: Adults: 12 hours

Dosage SubQ:

Children ≥2 years: CPP (Supprelin® LA): 50 mg implant surgically inserted every 12 months. Discontinue at the appropriate time for the onset of puberty.

Adults: Prostate cancer (Vantas™): 50 mg implant surgically inserted every 12 months

Elderly: See adult dosing

Dosage adjustment in renal impairment: Cl_{cr}: 15-60 mL/minute: Adjustment not needed

Administration SubQ: Surgical implantation into the inner portion of the upper arm requires the use of the implantation device provided. Use the patient's nondominant arm for placement. Removal must occur after 12 months; a replacement implant may be required. Palpate area of incision to locate implant for removal. If not readily palpated, ultrasound, CT or MRI may be used to locate implant; plain films are not recommended because the implant is not radiopaque.

Monitoring Parameters

CPP: LH, FSH, estradiol, or testosterone (after 1 month then every 6 months); height, bone age (every 6-12 months); tanner staging

Prostate cancer: LH and FSH levels, serum testosterone levels, prostate specific antigen (PSA), bone mineral density; weakness, paresthesias, and urinary tract obstruction (especially during first few weeks of therapy)

Reference Range Prostate cancer:

Testosterone level: Expected to rise during the first few days and decline to below initiation level by week 2 before reaching ≤50 ng/dL (castrate level)

PSA: Expected to decrease to normal levels after 6 months of therapy

Note: Lack of response (testosterone and PSA decreases) should prompt suspicion that the implant has been expelled.

Test Interactions Results of diagnostic test of pituitary gonadotropic and gonadal functions may be affected during and after therapy

Dosage Forms Excipient information presented when available (limited, particularly for generics); consult specific product labeling.

Implant, subcutaneous:

Supprelin® LA: 50 mg (1) [releases ~65 mcg/day over 12 months; packaged with implantation kit]

Vantas™: 50 mg (1) [releases 50-60 mcg/day over 12 months; packaged with implantation kit]

- ◆ **Histrelin Acetate** *see* Histrelin *on page 732*
- ◆ **hMG** *see* Menotropins *on page 941*
- ◆ **HMM** *see* Altretamine *on page 74*
- ◆ **HMR 3647** *see* Telithromycin *on page 1429*
- ◆ **HN_2** *see* Mechlorethamine *on page 927*

Homatropine (hoe MA troe peen)

U.S. Brand Names Isopto® Homatropine

Index Terms Homatropine Hydrobromide

Pharmacologic Category Anticholinergic Agent, Ophthalmic; Ophthalmic Agent, Mydriatic

Additional Appendix Information

Cycloplegic Mydriatics *on page 1655*

Use Producing cycloplegia and mydriasis for refraction; treatment of acute inflammatory conditions of the uveal tract; optical aid in axial lens opacities

Pregnancy Risk Factor C

Dosage Ophthalmic:

Children:

Mydriasis and cycloplegia for refraction: Instill 1 drop of 2% solution immediately before the procedure; repeat at 10-minute intervals as needed

Uveitis: Instill 1 drop of 2% solution 2-3 times/day

Adults:

Mydriasis and cycloplegia for refraction: Instill 1-2 drops of 2% solution or 1 drop of 5% solution before the procedure; repeat at 5- to 10-minute intervals as needed; maximum of 3 doses for refraction

Uveitis: Instill 1-2 drops of 2% or 5% 2-3 times/day up to every 3-4 hours as needed

Additional Information Complete prescribing information for this medication should be consulted for additional detail.

Dosage Forms Excipient information presented when available (limited, particularly for generics); consult specific product labeling.

Solution, ophthalmic, as hydrobromide:

Isopto® Homatropine: 2% (5 mL); 5% (5 mL, 15 mL) [contains benzalkonium chloride]

- ◆ **Homatropine and Hydrocodone** *see* Hydrocodone and Homatropine *on page 742*
- ◆ **Homatropine Hydrobromide** *see* Homatropine *on page 733*
- ◆ **Horse Antihuman Thymocyte Gamma Globulin** *see* Antithymocyte Globulin (Equine) *on page 124*
- ◆ **Hp-PAC® (Can)** *see* Lansoprazole, Amoxicillin, and Clarithromycin *on page 855*
- ◆ **HPV Vaccine** *see* Papillomavirus (Types 6, 11, 16, 18) Vaccine (Human, Recombinant) *on page 1142*
- ◆ **HTF919** *see* Tegaserod *on page 1428*
- ◆ **hu1124** *see* Efalizumab *on page 507*
- ◆ **Humalog®** *see* Insulin Lispro *on page 794*
- ◆ **Humalog® Mix 25 (Can)** *see* Insulin Lispro Protamine and Insulin Lispro *on page 795*
- ◆ **Humalog® Mix 50/50™** *see* Insulin Lispro Protamine and Insulin Lispro *on page 795*
- ◆ **Humalog® Mix 75/25™** *see* Insulin Lispro Protamine and Insulin Lispro *on page 795*
- ◆ **Human Antitumor Necrosis Factor Alpha** *see* Adalimumab *on page 43*
- ◆ **Human C1 Inhibitor** *see* C1 Inhibitor (Human) *on page 232*
- ◆ **Human Corticotrophin-Releasing Hormone, Analogue** *see* Corticorelin *on page 370*
- ◆ **Human Diploid Cell Cultures Rabies Vaccine** *see* Rabies Vaccine *on page 1287*
- ◆ **Human Growth Hormone** *see* Somatropin *on page 1388*
- ◆ **Humanized IgG1 Anti-CD52 Monoclonal Antibody** *see* Alemtuzumab *on page 56*
- ◆ **Human LFA-3/IgG(1) Fusion Protein** *see* Alefacept *on page 55*
- ◆ **Human Menopausal Gonadotropin** *see* Menotropins *on page 941*
- ◆ **Human Papillomavirus Vaccine** *see* Papillomavirus (Types 6, 11, 16, 18) Vaccine (Human, Recombinant) *on page 1142*
- ◆ **Human Rotavirus Vaccine, Attenuated (HRV)** *see* Rotavirus Vaccine *on page 1345*
- ◆ **Human Thyroid Stimulating Hormone** *see* Thyrotropin Alfa *on page 1465*
- ◆ **Humate-P®** *see* Antihemophilic Factor/von Willebrand Factor Complex (Human) *on page 122*
- ◆ **Humatin® [DSC]** *see* Paromomycin *on page 1146*
- ◆ **Humatin® (Can)** *see* Paromomycin *on page 1146*
- ◆ **Humatrope®** *see* Somatropin *on page 1388*
- ◆ **Humegon® (Can)** *see* Chorionic Gonadotropin (Human) *on page 320*
- ◆ **Humira®** *see* Adalimumab *on page 43*
- ◆ **Humist® [OTC]** *see* Sodium Chloride *on page 1381*
- ◆ **Humist® for Kids [OTC]** *see* Sodium Chloride *on page 1381*
- ◆ **Humulin® 20/80 (Can)** *see* Insulin NPH and Insulin Regular *on page 795*
- ◆ **Humulin® 50/50** *see* Insulin NPH and Insulin Regular *on page 795*
- ◆ **Humulin® 70/30** *see* Insulin NPH and Insulin Regular *on page 795*
- ◆ **Humulin® N** *see* Insulin NPH *on page 795*
- ◆ **Humulin® R** *see* Insulin Regular *on page 796*

- **Humulin® R U-500** *see* Insulin Regular *on page 796*
- **Hurricaine® [OTC]** *see* Benzocaine *on page 183*
- **HXM** *see* Altretamine *on page 74*
- **Hyalgan®** *see* Hyaluronate and Derivatives *on page 734*
- **Hyaluronan** *see* Hyaluronate and Derivatives *on page 734*

Hyaluronate and Derivatives

(hye al yoor ON ate & dah RIV ah tives)

U.S. Brand Names Biolon™ [DSC]; Bionect®; Euflexxa™; Healon GV®; Healon®; Healon®5; Hyalgan®; Hylaform®; Hylaform® Plus; Hylira™; IPM Wound Gel™ [OTC]; Juvederm™ 24HV; Juvederm™ 30; Juvederm™ 30HV; Orthovisc®; Perlane®; Provisc®; Restylane®; Supartz™; Synvisc®; Vitrax®

Canadian Brand Names Cystistat®; Durolane®; Eyestil; Healon GV®; Healon®; OrthoVisc®; Suplasyn®

Index Terms Hyaluronan; Hyaluronic Acid; Hylan Polymers; Sodium Hyaluronate

Pharmacologic Category Antirheumatic Miscellaneous; Ophthalmic Agent, Viscoelastic; Skin and Mucous Membrane Agent, Miscellaneous

Use

Intra-articular injection: Treatment of pain in osteoarthritis in knee in patients who have failed nonpharmacologic treatment and simple analgesics

Intradermal: Correction of moderate-to-severe facial wrinkles or folds

Ophthalmic: Surgical aid in cataract extraction, intraocular implantation, corneal transplant, glaucoma filtration, and retinal attachment surgery

Topical cream, gel, spray: Management of skin ulcers and wounds

Topical lotion: Treatment of xerosis (dry, scaly skin)

Unlabeled/Investigational Use Treatment of refractory interstitial cystitis

Pregnancy Risk Factor C

Pregnancy Considerations There are no adequate and well-controlled studies in pregnant women.

Lactation Excretion in breast milk unknown/not recommended

Medication Safety Issues

Sound-alike/look-alike issues:

Synvisc® may be confused with Synagis®

Contraindications Hypersensitivity to hyaluronate or any component of the formulation

Intradermal:

Hylaform®, Hylaform® Plus: Additional contraindications include hypersensitivity to avian proteins (egg products, feathers)

Juvederm™, Perlane®, Restylane®: Additional contraindications include history of or presence of multiple severe allergies; bleeding disorders; sensitivity to gram-positive bacterial proteins

Intra-articular: Knee joint infections, infections or skin diseases at the site of injection

Orthovisc®: Additional contraindications include hypersensitivity to avian proteins (egg products, feathers)

Warnings/Precautions Not for I.V. injection. Do not inject into blood vessels; may cause occlusion, infarction, embolism, or other systemic adverse events.

Intra-articular: Not for use in infected joints; do not use disinfectants containing quaternary salts for skin preparation (may cause precipitation of hyaluronate). Remove effusion, if present, prior to injection. Use with caution if venous or lymphatic stasis is present in the leg. Avoid strenuous activities for 48 hours after injection. Safety and efficacy have not been established in children.

Intradermal: Treatment may result in bruising/bleeding; use caution in patients receiving or recently exposed (≤3 weeks) to thrombolytics, anticoagulants, or platelet inhibitors. Do not inject into site of active inflammation or infection. Injection into a blood vessel may lead to localized superficial necrosis. Use in patients susceptible to keloid formation, hypertrophic scarring, or pigmentation disorders has not been studied; use cautiously. Use caution with immunosuppressive treatment. Use in patients with prior herpetic eruption may result in reactivation. Delayed inflammatory papules may result from injections, necessitating evaluation and treatment as soft tissue infection. Laser treatment or chemical peeling may cause acute inflammatory reaction. Patient must avoid exposure to ultraviolet rays (sun and UV lamp) or severe cold until swelling and redness is resolved. Treatment site reactions usually improve in <1 week. Strenuous exercise and ethanol consumption should be avoided for 24 hours following use. Supplemental "touch up" treatments may be required. Use in lip augmentation has not been established. Safety and efficacy in patients <18 years of age have not been established.

Ophthalmic: Do not overfill the anterior chamber; carefully monitor intraocular pressure

Topical: Bionect® products (cream, gel, spray): Do not use disinfectants containing quaternary ammonium salts for skin preparation (may cause precipitation of hyaluronate). IPM™ wound gel: Cleansing agents other than normal saline are not recommended. Hylira™ lotion: Avoid contact with eyes, lips, mucous membranes; discontinue if condition worsens.

Adverse Reactions Frequencies and/or type of local reaction may vary by formulation and site of application/injection.

>10%:

Local: Injection site (intradermal): Bruising (47% to 61%), erythema (58% to 93%), lumps/bumps (79% to 83%), pain (57% to 90%), swelling (81% to 89%); pruritus (28% to 36%), skin discoloration (31% to 34%)

Respiratory: Infection (12%)

1% to 10%:

Cardiovascular: Blood pressure increased (2% to 4%)

Central nervous system: Fatigue (1%)

Gastrointestinal: Nausea (≤2%)

Local: Dry skin (intradermal >1%), peeling (intradermal >1%)

Neuromuscular & skeletal: Back pain (<1% to 6%), tendonitis (2%), parasthesia (1%)

Respiratory: Rhinitis (3%)

Frequency not defined:

Cardiovascular: Edema, flushing, hypotension, tachycardia

Central nervous system: Dizziness, headache

Dermatologic: Rash, hyperpigmentation, exfoliation

Local: Injection site: Arthralgia, nodule

Neuromuscular & skeletal: Hypokinesia (knee)

Ocular (with ophthalmic formulation): Postoperative inflammatory reactions (iritis, hypopyon), corneal edema, corneal decompensation, transient postoperative increase in IOP

Miscellaneous: Abscess formation, allergic reactions, anaphylaxis, respiratory difficulties

Drug Interactions

Avoid Concomitant Use There are no known interactions where it is recommended to avoid concomitant use.

Increased Effect/Toxicity There are no known significant interactions involving an increase in effect.

Decreased Effect There are no known significant interactions involving a decrease in effect.

Stability

Bionect® products: Store at room temperature. Cream and gel may be stored up to 24 months; spray may be stored up to 36 months.

Euflexxa™: Store under refrigeration at 2°C to 8°C (36°F to 46°F) or at room temperature up to 25°C (77°F); do not freeze. Protect from light. If refrigerated, remove from refrigeration at least 20-30 minutes before use.

Healon® products, Provisc®: Store under refrigeration at 2°C to 8°C (36°F to 46°F); do not freeze. Protect from light.

Hylaform®, Hylaform® Plus: Store at room temperature of 2°C to 30°C; do not freeze. Do not use if gel separates or becomes cloudy.

Hyalgan®, Orthovisc®: Store below 25°C (77°F); do not freeze.

Hylira™ Lotion: Store at room temperature of 15°C to 30°C; do not freeze.

IPM Wound Gel™: Store below 35°C (95°F); do not freeze.

Juvederm™ (all formulations), Perlane®, Restylane®: Store at up to 25°C (77°F); do not freeze. Protect from light. Do not use if gel separates or becomes cloudy.

Synvisc®: Store at room temperature, below 30°C (86°C); do not freeze. Protect from light.

Mechanism of Action Sodium hyaluronate is a polysaccharide which is distributed widely in the extracellular matrix of connective tissue in man (vitreous and aqueous humor of the eye, synovial fluid, skin, and umbilical cord). Sodium hyaluronate and its derivatives form a viscoelastic solution in water (at physiological pH and ionic strength) which makes it suitable for aqueous and vitreous humor in ophthalmic surgery, and functions as a tissue and/or joint lubricant which plays an important role in modulating the interactions between adjacent tissues. Intradermal injection may decrease the depth of facial wrinkles.

Pharmacodynamics/Kinetics

Distribution: Intravitreous injection: Diffusion occurs slowly

Excretion: Ophthalmic: Via Canal of Schlemm

Dosage Adults:

Osteoarthritis of the knee: Intra-articular:

Eulexxa™: Inject 20 mg (2 mL) once weekly for 3 weeks

Hyalgan®: Inject 20 mg (2 mL) once weekly for 5 weeks; some patients may benefit with a total of 3 injections

Orthovisc®: Inject 30 mg (2 mL) once weekly for 3-4 weeks

Supartz™: Inject 25 mg (2.5 mL) once weekly for 5 weeks

Synvisc®: Inject 16 mg (2 mL) once weekly for 3 weeks (total of 3 injections)

Facial wrinkles: Intradermal:

Note: Formulations differ in terms of recommended injection depth: Juvederm™, Hylaform®, and Restylane® are intended for mid to deep intradermal injection; Perlane® is intended for injection into the deep dermis to superficial subcutis

Hylaform®, Hylaform® Plus: Inject as required for cosmetic result; typical treatment regimen requires <2 mL; limit injection to ≤1.5 mL per injection site; maximum: 20 mL/60 kg/year

Juvederm™ (all formulations): Inject as required for cosmetic result; typical treatment regimen requires <2 mL; limit injection to 1.6 mL per injection site; maximum: 20 mL/60 kg/year

Perlane®: Inject as required into deep dermis/superficial subcutis for cosmetic result; typical treatment regimen requires 1.9-4.6 mL; maximum 6 mL per treatment

Restylane®: Inject as required for cosmetic result; typical treatment regimen requires <2 mL; limit injection to ≤1.5 mL per injection site

Ophthalmic (Biolon™, Healon®, Provisc®, Vitrax®): Depends upon procedure (slowly introduce a sufficient quantity into eye)

Topical: Note: Formulations are used for different indications:

Bionect® cream, gel, and spray: Apply a thin layer to clean and disinfected wound or ulcer 2-3 times/day, and cover with sterile gauze pad. If needed, cover with elastic or compressive bandage.

IPM Wound Gel™: Apply to clean dry ulcer or wound, and cover with nonstick dressing; repeat daily. Discontinue if wound size increase after 3-4 applications.

Hylira™ lotion: Apply to affected area and rub in thoroughly 2-3 times daily. Discontinue if condition worsens.

Interstitial cystitis, refractory (unlabeled use): Intravesical (unlabeled route): 40 mg in 50 mL saline intravesically (retain in bladder for at least 30 minutes) once weekly for 4 weeks, then monthly for up to 1 year in patients showing an initial response

Administration

Intra-articular: Inject directly into the knee joint. Do not use disinfectants containing quaternary salts for skin cleansing prior to injection. Remove effusion, if present, prior to injection. If used for bilateral treatment, use a separate syringe for each injection site.

Intradermal: Do not inject into a blood vessel. May apply ice pack to injection site for a short period immediately after administration if treatment area swollen.

Juvederm™, Hylaform®, and Restylane® are intended for mid to deep intradermal injection

Perlane® is intended for injection into the deep dermis to superficial subcutis

Ophthalmic: Drug may become cloudy or form a slight precipitate after administration; clinical significance unknown, but cloudy or precipitated material should be removed by irrigation or aspiration

Topical:

Bionect® products: Clean and disinfect wound prior to use (do not use quaternary ammonium salts), and debride if necessary; apply a thin layer to wound or ulcer without extensive rubbing.

IPM Wound Gel™: Clean wound with normal saline; remove excess moisture with dry gauze; apply gel liberally to wound

Hylira™ lotion: Apply and rub in thoroughly into affected area. Avoid eyes, lips and mucous membranes.

Monitoring Parameters Intraocular pressure; intradermally administered products, signs and symptoms of excess local inflammation or infection

Additional Information Juvederm™ 24HV provides more versatility in contouring and volumizing of facial wrinkles. Juvederm™ 30 provides subtle correction for facial folds and wrinkles. Juvederm™ 30HV provides greater volumizing for correction of deeper folds and wrinkles. Perlane® differs from Restylane® in the size of its hyaluronate particles within the gel, allowing its use in deeper injections relative to other dermal fillers.

Dosage Forms Excipient information presented when available (limited, particularly for generics); consult specific product labeling. [DSC] = Discontinued product

Hylan B: Injection, gel:

Hylaform® [500 micron particle]: 5.5 mg/mL (0.75 mL) [prefilled syringe; derived from avian source]

Hylaform® Plus [700 micron particle]: 5.5 mg/mL (0.75 mL) [prefilled syringe; derived from avian source]

Hylan polymers A and B (Hylan G-F 20): Injection, solution, intra-articular (Synvisc®): 8 mg/mL (2 mL) [prefilled syringe; contains trace amounts of *Streptococcus*]

Sodium hyaluronate:

Cream, topical:

Bionect®: 0.2% (25 g)

Gel, topical:

Bionect®: 0.2% (30 g, 60 g)

IPM Wound Gel™: 2.5% (10 g)

Lotion, topical: 0.1% (340 g, 1000 g)
Hylira™: 0.1% (340 g, 1000 g)
Injection, gel, intradermal:
Juvederm™ 24HV, Juvederm™ 30, Juvederm™ 30HV: 24 mg/mL [prefilled syringe]
Perlane®: 20 mg/mL (1mL) [prefilled syringe]
Restylane®: 20 mg/mL [prefilled syringe]
Injection, solution, intra-articular:
Euflexxa™: 10 mg/mL (2 mL) [prefilled syringe; syringe contains latex]
Hyalgan®: 10 mg/mL (2 mL)
Orthovisc®: 15 mg/mL (2 mL) [prefilled syringe; derived from avian source]
Supartz™: 10 mg/mL (2.5 mL) [derived from avian source]
Synvisc®: 8 mg/mL (2 mL) [prefilled syringe; derived from avian source]
Injection, solution, intraocular:
Biolon™: 10 mg/mL (0.5 mL, 1 mL) [DSC]
Healon®: 10 mg/mL (0.4 mL, 0.55 mL, 0.85 mL, 2 mL)
Healon®5: 23 mg/mL
Healon GV®: 14 mg/mL (0.55 mL, 0.85 mL)
Provisc®: 10 mg/mL (0.4 mL, 0.55 mL, 0.8 mL) [prefilled syringe; contains lactose]
Vitrax®: 30 mg/mL (0.65 mL)
Solution, topical [spray]:
Bionect®: 0.2% (20 mL) [DSC]

- ◆ **Hyaluronic Acid** *see* Hyaluronate and Derivatives *on page 734*
- ◆ **Hycamptamine** *see* Topotecan *on page 1491*
- ◆ **Hycamtin®** *see* Topotecan *on page 1491*
- ◆ **hycet™** *see* Hydrocodone and Acetaminophen *on page 740*
- ◆ **Hycodan® [DSC]** *see* Hydrocodone and Homatropine *on page 742*
- ◆ **Hycort™ (Can)** *see* Hydrocortisone *on page 743*
- ◆ **Hycotuss® [DSC]** *see* Hydrocodone and Guaifenesin *on page 741*
- ◆ **Hydeltra T.B.A.® (Can)** *see* PrednisoLONE *on page 1230*
- ◆ **Hydergine [DSC]** *see* Ergoloid Mesylates *on page 539*
- ◆ **Hydergine® (Can)** *see* Ergoloid Mesylates *on page 539*
- ◆ **Hyderm (Can)** *see* Hydrocortisone *on page 743*

HydrALAZINE (hye DRAL a zeen)

Canadian Brand Names Apo-Hydralazine®; Apresoline®; Novo-Hylazin; Nu-Hydral

Index Terms Apresoline [DSC]; Hydralazine Hydrochloride

Pharmacologic Category Vasodilator

Additional Appendix Information

Heart Failure (Systolic) *on page 1809*
Hypertension *on page 1820*

Use Management of moderate to severe hypertension, congestive heart failure, hypertension secondary to pre-eclampsia/eclampsia; treatment of primary pulmonary hypertension

Pregnancy Risk Factor C

Pregnancy Considerations Crosses the placenta. One report of fetal arrhythmia; transient neonatal thrombocytopenia and fetal distress reported following late 3rd trimester use. A large amount of clinical experience with the use of this drug for management of hypertension during pregnancy is available. Available evidence suggests safe use during pregnancy.

Lactation Enters breast milk/compatible

Medication Safety Issues

Sound-alike/look-alike issues:
HydrALAZINE may be confused with hydrOXYzine

Contraindications Hypersensitivity to hydralazine or any component of the formulation; mitral valve rheumatic heart disease

Warnings/Precautions May cause a drug-induced lupus-like syndrome (more likely on larger doses, longer duration). Discontinue hydralazine in patients who develop SLE-like syndrome or positive ANA. Use with caution in patients with severe renal disease or cerebral vascular accidents or with known or suspected coronary artery disease; monitor blood pressure closely with I.V. use. Slow acetylators, patients with decreased renal function, and patients receiving >200 mg/day (chronically) are at higher risk for SLE. Titrate dosage cautiously to patient's response. Hypotensive effect after I.V. administration may be delayed and unpredictable in some patients. Usually administered with diuretic and a beta-blocker to counteract side effects of sodium and water retention and reflex tachycardia.

Adjust dose in severe renal dysfunction. Use with caution in CAD (increase in tachycardia may increase myocardial oxygen demand). Use with caution in pulmonary hypertension (may cause hypotension). Patients may be poorly compliant because of frequent dosing. Hydralazine-induced fluid and sodium retention may require addition or increased dosage of a diuretic.

Adverse Reactions Frequency not defined.

Cardiovascular: Tachycardia, angina pectoris, orthostatic hypotension (rare), dizziness (rare), paradoxical hypertension, peripheral edema, vascular collapse (rare), flushing
Central nervous system: Increased intracranial pressure (I.V., in patient with pre-existing increased intracranial pressure), fever (rare), chills (rare), anxiety*, disorientation*, depression*, coma*
Dermatologic: Rash (rare), urticaria (rare), pruritus (rare)
Gastrointestinal: Anorexia, nausea, vomiting, diarrhea, constipation, adynamic ileus
Genitourinary: Difficulty in micturition, impotence
Hematologic: Hemolytic anemia (rare), eosinophilia (rare), decreased hemoglobin concentration (rare), reduced erythrocyte count (rare), leukopenia (rare), agranulocytosis (rare), thrombocytopenia (rare)
Neuromuscular & skeletal: Rheumatoid arthritis, muscle cramps, weakness, tremor, peripheral neuritis (rare)
Ocular: Lacrimation, conjunctivitis
Respiratory: Nasal congestion, dyspnea
Miscellaneous: Drug-induced lupus-like syndrome (dose related; fever, arthralgia, splenomegaly, lymphadenopathy, asthenia, myalgia, malaise, pleuritic chest pain, edema, positive ANA, positive LE cells, maculopapular facial rash, positive direct Coombs' test, pericarditis, pericardial tamponade), diaphoresis
*Seen in uremic patients and severe hypertension where rapidly escalating doses may have caused hypotension leading to these effects.

Drug Interactions

Metabolism/Transport Effects Inhibits CYP3A4 (weak)

Avoid Concomitant Use There are no known interactions where it is recommended to avoid concomitant use.

Increased Effect/Toxicity

HydrALAZINE may increase the levels/effects of: Amifostine; RiTUXimab

The levels/effects of HydrALAZINE may be increased by: Diazoxide; Herbs (Hypotensive Properties); Prostacyclin Analogues

Decreased Effect

The levels/effects of HydrALAZINE may be decreased by: Herbs (Hypertensive Properties); Methylphenidate; Nonsteroidal Anti-Inflammatory Agents; Yohimbine

Ethanol/Nutrition/Herb Interactions

Ethanol: Avoid ethanol (may increase CNS depression).

Food: Food enhances bioavailability of hydralazine.
Herb/Nutraceutical: Avoid dong quai if using for hypertension (has estrogenic activity). Avoid ephedra, yohimbe, ginseng (may worsen hypertension). Avoid garlic (may have increased antihypertensive effect).

Stability Intact ampuls/vials of hydralazine should not be stored under refrigeration because of possible precipitation or crystallization. Hydralazine should be diluted in NS for IVPB administration due to decreased stability in D_5W. Stability of IVPB solution in NS is 4 days at room temperature.

Mechanism of Action Direct vasodilation of arterioles (with little effect on veins) with decreased systemic resistance

Pharmacodynamics/Kinetics
Onset of action: Oral: 20-30 minutes; I.V.: 5-20 minutes
Duration: Oral: Up to 8 hours; I.V.: 1-4 hours; **Note:** May vary depending on acetylator status of patient
Distribution: Crosses placenta; enters breast milk
Protein binding: 85% to 90%
Metabolism: Hepatically acetylated; extensive first-pass effect (oral)
Bioavailability: 30% to 50%; increased with food
Half-life elimination: Normal renal function: 2-8 hours; End-stage renal disease: 7-16 hours
Excretion: Urine (14% as unchanged drug)

Dosage
Children:
Oral: Initial: 0.75-1 mg/kg/day in 2-4 divided doses; increase over 3-4 weeks to maximum of 7.5 mg/kg/day in 2-4 divided doses; maximum daily dose: 200 mg/day
I.M., I.V.: 0.1-0.2 mg/kg/dose (not to exceed 20 mg) every 4-6 hours as needed, up to 1.7-3.5 mg/kg/day in 4-6 divided doses
Adults:
Oral:
Hypertension:
Initial dose: 10 mg 4 times/day for first 2-4 days; increase to 25 mg 4 times/day for the balance of the first week
Increase by 10-25 mg/dose gradually to 50 mg 4 times/day (maximum: 300 mg/day); usual dose range (JNC 7): 25-100 mg/day in 2 divided doses
Congestive heart failure:
Initial dose: 10-25 mg 3-4 times/day
Adjustment: Dosage must be adjusted based on individual response
Target dose: 225-300 mg/day in divided doses; use in combination with isosorbide dinitrate
I.M., I.V.:
Hypertension: Initial: 10-20 mg/dose every 4-6 hours as needed, may increase to 40 mg/dose; change to oral therapy as soon as possible.
Pre-eclampsia/eclampsia: 5 mg/dose then 5-10 mg every 20-30 minutes as needed.
Elderly: Oral: Initial: 10 mg 2-3 times/day; increase by 10-25 mg/day every 2-5 days.
Dosing interval in renal impairment:
Cl_{cr} 10-50 mL/minute: Administer every 8 hours.
Cl_{cr} <10 mL/minute: Administer every 8-16 hours in fast acetylators and every 12-24 hours in slow acetylators.
Hemodialysis: Supplemental dose is not necessary.
Peritoneal dialysis: Supplemental dose is not necessary.

Dietary Considerations Administer with meals.

Administration Inject over 1 minute. Hypotensive effect may be delayed and unpredictable in some patients.

Monitoring Parameters Blood pressure (monitor closely with I.V. use), standing and sitting/supine, heart rate, ANA titer

Dosage Forms Excipient information presented when available (limited, particularly for generics); consult specific product labeling.
Injection, solution, as hydrochloride: 20 mg/mL (1 mL)
Tablet, as hydrochloride: 10 mg, 25 mg, 50 mg, 100 mg

Extemporaneous Preparations An oral solution (20 mg/5 mL) has been made from 20 mL of the hydralazine injection (20 mg/mL), 8 mL of propylene glycol and purified water USP qs ad 100 mL; expected stability: 30 days if refrigerated

A flavored syrup (1.25 mg/mL) has been made using seventy-five hydralazine hydrochloride 50 mg tablets, dissolved in 250 mL of distilled water with 2250 g of Lycasin® (75% w/w maltitol syrup vehicle); edetate disodium 3 g and sodium saccharin 3 g dissolved in 50 mL distilled water was added; solution was preserved with 30 mL of a solution containing methylparaben 10% (w/v) and propylparaben 2% (w/v) in propylene glycol; flavored with 3 mL orange flavoring; qs ad to 3 L with distilled water and then pH adjusted to pH of 3.7 using glacial acetic acid; measured stability was 5 days at room temperature (25°C); less than 2% loss of hydralazine occurred at 2 weeks when syrup was stored at 5°C

Alexander KS, Pudipeddi M, and Parker GA, "Stability of Hydralazine Hydrochloride Syrup Compounded From Tablets," *Am J Hosp Pharm*, 1993, 50(4):683-6.
Nahata MC and Hipple TF, *Pediatric Drug Formulations*, 2nd ed, Cincinnati, OH: Harvey Whitney Books Co, 1992.

Hydralazine and Hydrochlorothiazide
(hye DRAL a zeen & hye droe klor oh THYE a zide)

Index Terms Apresazide [DSC]; Hydrochlorothiazide and Hydralazine

Pharmacologic Category Diuretic, Thiazide; Vasodilator, Direct-Acting

Use Management of moderate to severe hypertension and treatment of congestive heart failure

Pregnancy Risk Factor C

Dosage Adults: Oral: Hydralazine 25-100 mg/day and hydrochlorothiazide 25-50 mg/day in 2 divided doses (maximum: hydrochlorothiazide: 50 mg/day)

Additional Information Complete prescribing information for this medication should be consulted for additional detail.

Dosage Forms Excipient information presented when available (limited, particularly for generics); consult specific product labeling.
Capsule:
25/25: Hydralazine hydrochloride 25 mg and hydrochlorothiazide 25 mg
50/50: Hydralazine hydrochloride 50 mg and hydrochlorothiazide 50 mg
100/50: Hydralazine hydrochloride 100 mg and hydrochlorothiazide 50 mg

◆ **Hydralazine and Isosorbide Dinitrate** *see* Isosorbide Dinitrate and Hydralazine *on page 824*

◆ **Hydralazine Hydrochloride** *see* HydrALAZINE *on page 736*

◆ **Hydramine® [OTC]** *see* DiphenhydrAMINE *on page 456*

◆ **Hydrated Chloral** *see* Chloral Hydrate *on page 300*

◆ **Hydrea®** *see* Hydroxyurea *on page 753*

◆ **Hydro 40™** *see* Urea *on page 1530*

Hydrochlorothiazide (hye droe klor oh THYE a zide)

U.S. Brand Names Microzide®

Canadian Brand Names Apo-Hydro®; Novo-Hydrazide; PMS-Hydrochlorothiazide

Index Terms HCTZ (error-prone abbreviation)

Pharmacologic Category Diuretic, Thiazide

Additional Appendix Information
Sulfonamide Derivatives *on page 1671*

Use Management of mild to moderate hypertension; treatment of edema in congestive heart failure and nephrotic syndrome

Unlabeled/Investigational Use Treatment of lithium-induced diabetes insipidus

Pregnancy Risk Factor B (manufacturer); D (expert analysis)

Pregnancy Considerations Although there are no adequate and well-controlled studies using hydrochlorothiazide in pregnancy, thiazide diuretics may cause an increased risk of congenital defects. Hypoglycemia, hypokalemia, hyponatremia, jaundice, and thrombocytopenia are also reported as possible complications to the fetus or newborn.

Lactation Enters breast milk/use caution (AAP rates "compatible")

Medication Safety Issues
Sound-alike/look-alike issues:
- Esidrix may be confused with Lasix®
- HCTZ is an error-prone abbreviation (mistaken as hydrocortisone)
- Hydrochlorothiazide may be confused with hydrocortisone, hydroflumethiazide
- Microzide™ may be confused with Maxzide®, Micronase®

International issues:
- Microzide™ may be confused with Nitrobide® which is a brand name for isosorbide dinitrate in Japan
- Microzide™ may be confused with Mikrozid® which is a brand name for ethanol/propanol combination in Great Britain

Contraindications Hypersensitivity to hydrochlorothiazide or any component of the formulation, thiazides, or sulfonamide-derived drugs; anuria; renal decompensation; pregnancy

Warnings/Precautions Avoid in severe renal disease (ineffective as a diuretic). Electrolyte disturbances (hypokalemia, hypochloremic alkalosis, hyponatremia) can occur. Use with caution in severe hepatic dysfunction; hepatic encephalopathy can be caused by electrolyte disturbances. Gout may be precipitated in certain patients with a history of gout, a familial predisposition to gout, or chronic renal failure. Use with caution in patients with prediabetes and diabetes; may alter glucose control. May cause SLE exacerbation or activation. Use with caution in patients with moderate or high cholesterol concentrations. Photosensitization may occur. Correct hypokalemia before initiating therapy.

Chemical similarities are present among sulfonamides, sulfonylureas, carbonic anhydrase inhibitors, thiazides, and loop diuretics (except ethacrynic acid). Use in patients with sulfonamide allergy is specifically contraindicated in product labeling, however, a risk of cross-reaction exists in patients with allergy to any of these compounds; avoid use when previous reaction has been severe. Discontinue if signs of hypersensitivity are noted.

Adverse Reactions
1% to 10%:
- Cardiovascular: Orthostatic hypotension, hypotension
- Dermatologic: Photosensitivity
- Endocrine & metabolic: Hypokalemia
- Gastrointestinal: Anorexia, epigastric distress

<1% (Limited to important or life-threatening): Agranulocytosis, allergic myocarditis, allergic reactions (possibly with life-threatening anaphylactic shock), alopecia, aplastic anemia, eosinophilic pneumonitis, erythema multiforme, exfoliative dermatitis, hemolytic anemia, hepatic function impairment, hypercalcemia, interstitial nephritis, leukopenia, pancreatitis, renal failure, respiratory distress, Stevens-Johnson syndrome, thrombocytopenia, toxic epidermal necrolysis

Drug Interactions

Avoid Concomitant Use There are no known interactions where it is recommended to avoid concomitant use.

Increased Effect/Toxicity
Hydrochlorothiazide may increase the levels/effects of: ACE Inhibitors; Allopurinol; Amifostine; Calcitriol; Calcium Salts; Dofetilide; Lithium; RiTUXimab

The levels/effects of Hydrochlorothiazide may be increased by: Corticosteroids (Orally Inhaled); Corticosteroids (Systemic); Herbs (Hypotensive Properties); Prostacyclin Analogues

Decreased Effect
The levels/effects of Hydrochlorothiazide may be decreased by: Bile Acid Sequestrants; Herbs (Hypertensive Properties); Methylphenidate; Nonsteroidal Anti-Inflammatory Agents; Yohimbine

Ethanol/Nutrition/Herb Interactions
Food: Hydrochlorothiazide peak serum levels may be decreased if taken with food. This product may deplete potassium, sodium, and magnesium.
Herb/Nutraceutical: Avoid dong quai if using for hypertension (has estrogenic activity). Dong quai may also cause photosensitization. Avoid ephedra, ginseng, yohimbe (may worsen hypertension). Avoid garlic (may have increased antihypertensive effect).

Mechanism of Action Inhibits sodium reabsorption in the distal tubules causing increased excretion of sodium and water as well as potassium and hydrogen ions

Pharmacodynamics/Kinetics
Onset of action: Diuresis: ~2 hours
  Peak effect: 4-6 hours
Duration: 6-12 hours
Absorption: ~50% to 80%
Distribution: 3.6-7.8 L/kg
Protein binding: 68%
Metabolism: Not metabolized
Bioavailability: 50% to 80%
Half-life elimination: 5.6-14.8 hours
Time to peak: 1-2.5 hours
Excretion: Urine (as unchanged drug)

Dosage Oral (effect of drug may be decreased when used every day):
Children (in pediatric patients, chlorothiazide may be preferred over hydrochlorothiazide as there are more dosage formulations [eg, suspension] available): Edema, hypertension:
- <6 months: 1-3 mg/kg/day in 2 divided doses
- >6 months to 2 years: 1-3 mg/kg/day in 2 divided doses; maximum: 37.5 mg/day
- >2-17 years: Initial: 1 mg/kg/day; maximum: 3 mg/kg/day (50 mg/day)

Adults:
- Edema: 25-100 mg/day in 1-2 doses; maximum: 200 mg/day
- Hypertension: 12.5-50 mg/day; minimal increase in response and more electrolyte disturbances are seen with doses >50 mg/day

Elderly: 12.5-25 mg once daily

Dosing adjustment/comments in renal impairment: Cl_{cr} <10 mL/minute: Avoid use. Usually ineffective with GFR <30 mL/minute. Effective at lower GFR in combination with a loop diuretic.

Administration May be taken with food or milk. Take early in day to avoid nocturia. Take the last dose of multiple doses no later than 6 PM unless instructed otherwise.

Monitoring Parameters Assess weight, I & O reports daily to determine fluid loss; blood pressure, serum electrolytes, BUN, creatinine

Test Interactions Increased creatine phosphokinase [CPK] (S), ammonia (B), amylase (S), calcium (S), chloride

(S), cholesterol (S), glucose, increased acid (S), decreased chloride (S), magnesium, potassium (S), sodium (S); Tyramine and phentolamine tests, histamine tests for pheochromocytoma

Additional Information If given the morning of surgery it may render the patient volume depleted and blood pressure may be labile during general anesthesia. Effect of drug may be decreased when used every day.

Dosage Forms Excipient information presented when available (limited, particularly for generics); consult specific product labeling.

Capsule: 12.5 mg
  Microzide®: 12.5 mg
Tablet: 25 mg, 50 mg

- ◆ **Hydrochlorothiazide and Aliskiren** *see* Aliskiren and Hydrochlorothiazide *on page 64*
- ◆ **Hydrochlorothiazide and Amiloride** *see* Amiloride and Hydrochlorothiazide *on page 85*
- ◆ **Hydrochlorothiazide and Benazepril** *see* Benazepril and Hydrochlorothiazide *on page 181*
- ◆ **Hydrochlorothiazide and Bisoprolol** *see* Bisoprolol and Hydrochlorothiazide *on page 201*
- ◆ **Hydrochlorothiazide and Captopril** *see* Captopril and Hydrochlorothiazide *on page 251*
- ◆ **Hydrochlorothiazide and Cilazapril** *see* Cilazapril and Hydrochlorothiazide *on page 325*
- ◆ **Hydrochlorothiazide and Enalapril** *see* Enalapril and Hydrochlorothiazide *on page 518*
- ◆ **Hydrochlorothiazide and Eprosartan** *see* Eprosartan and Hydrochlorothiazide *on page 537*
- ◆ **Hydrochlorothiazide and Hydralazine** *see* Hydralazine and Hydrochlorothiazide *on page 737*
- ◆ **Hydrochlorothiazide and Irbesartan** *see* Irbesartan and Hydrochlorothiazide *on page 814*
- ◆ **Hydrochlorothiazide and Lisinopril** *see* Lisinopril and Hydrochlorothiazide *on page 896*
- ◆ **Hydrochlorothiazide and Losartan** *see* Losartan and Hydrochlorothiazide *on page 909*
- ◆ **Hydrochlorothiazide and Methyldopa** *see* Methyldopa and Hydrochlorothiazide *on page 971*
- ◆ **Hydrochlorothiazide and Metoprolol** *see* Metoprolol and Hydrochlorothiazide *on page 984*
- ◆ **Hydrochlorothiazide and Metoprolol Tartrate** *see* Metoprolol and Hydrochlorothiazide *on page 984*
- ◆ **Hydrochlorothiazide and Moexipril** *see* Moexipril and Hydrochlorothiazide *on page 1011*
- ◆ **Hydrochlorothiazide and Olmesartan Medoxomil** *see* Olmesartan and Hydrochlorothiazide *on page 1097*
- ◆ **Hydrochlorothiazide and Propranolol** *see* Propranolol and Hydrochlorothiazide *on page 1261*
- ◆ **Hydrochlorothiazide and Quinapril** *see* Quinapril and Hydrochlorothiazide *on page 1280*

Hydrochlorothiazide and Spironolactone

(hye droe klor oh THYE a zide & speer on oh LAK tone)

U.S. Brand Names Aldactazide®

Canadian Brand Names Aldactazide 25®; Aldactazide 50®; Novo-Spirozine

Index Terms Spironolactone and Hydrochlorothiazide

Pharmacologic Category Diuretic, Thiazide; Selective Aldosterone Blocker

Use Management of mild-to-moderate hypertension; treatment of edema in congestive heart failure and nephrotic syndrome, and cirrhosis of the liver accompanied by edema and/or ascites

Pregnancy Risk Factor C

Medication Safety Issues

Sound-alike/look-alike issues:
  Aldactazide® may be confused with Aldactone®

Dosage Oral:

Children: 1.5-3 mg/kg/day in 2-4 divided doses (maximum: 200 mg/day)

Adults: Hydrochlorothiazide 12.5-50 mg/day and spironolactone 12.5-50 mg/day; manufacturer labeling states hydrochlorothiazide maximum 200 mg/day, however, usual dose in JNC-7 is 12.5-50 mg/day

Additional Information Complete prescribing information for this medication should be consulted for additional detail.

Dosage Forms Excipient information presented when available (limited, particularly for generics); consult specific product labeling.

Tablet: Hydrochlorothiazide 25 mg and spironolactone 25 mg
  Aldactazide®:
    25/25: Hydrochlorothiazide 25 mg and spironolactone 25 mg
    50/50: Hydrochlorothiazide 50 mg and spironolactone 50 mg

- ◆ **Hydrochlorothiazide and Telmisartan** *see* Telmisartan and Hydrochlorothiazide *on page 1432*

Hydrochlorothiazide and Triamterene

(hye droe klor oh THYE a zide & trye AM ter een)

U.S. Brand Names Dyazide®; Maxzide®; Maxzide®-25

Canadian Brand Names Apo-Triazide®; Novo-Triamzide; Nu-Triazide; Penta-Triamterene HCTZ; Riva-Zide

Index Terms Triamterene and Hydrochlorothiazide

Pharmacologic Category Diuretic, Potassium-Sparing; Diuretic, Thiazide

Use Treatment of hypertension or edema (not recommended for initial treatment) when hypokalemia has developed on hydrochlorothiazide alone or when the development of hypokalemia must be avoided

Pregnancy Risk Factor C

Medication Safety Issues

Sound-alike/look-alike issues:
  Dyazide® may be confused with diazoxide, Dynacin®
  Maxzide® may be confused with Maxidex®, Microzide®

Dosage Oral: Adults:

Hydrochlorothiazide 25 mg and triamterene 37.5 mg: 1-2 tablets/capsules once daily

Hydrochlorothiazide 50 mg and triamterene 75 mg: 1/2-1 tablet daily

Additional Information Complete prescribing information for this medication should be consulted for additional detail.

Dosage Forms Excipient information presented when available (limited, particularly for generics); consult specific product labeling.

Capsule, oral: Hydrochlorothiazide 25 mg and triamterene 37.5 mg; hydrochlorothiazide 25 mg and triamterene 50 mg
  Dyazide®: Hydrochlorothiazide 25 mg and triamterene 37.5 mg
Tablet: Hydrochlorothiazide 25 mg and triamterene 37.5 mg; hydrochlorothiazide 50 mg and triamterene 75 mg
  Maxzide®: Hydrochlorothiazide 50 mg and triamterene 75 mg [scored]
  Maxzide®-25: Hydrochlorothiazide 25 mg and triamterene 37.5 mg [scored]

- ◆ **Hydrochlorothiazide and Valsartan** *see* Valsartan and Hydrochlorothiazide *on page 1544*
- ◆ **Hydrocil® Instant [OTC]** *see* Psyllium *on page 1268*

Hydrocodone and Acetaminophen

(hye droe KOE done & a seet a MIN oh fen)

U.S. Brand Names Co-Gesic® [DSC]; hycet™; Lorcet® 10/650; Lorcet® Plus; Lortab®; Margesic® H; Maxidone®; Norco®; Stagesic™; Vicodin®; Vicodin® ES; Vicodin® HP; Xodol® 10/300; Xodol® 5/300; Xodol® 7.5/300; Zamicet®; Zydone®

Index Terms Acetaminophen and Hydrocodone

Pharmacologic Category Analgesic Combination (Opioid)

Use Relief of moderate to severe pain

Restrictions C-III

Pregnancy Risk Factor C/D (prolonged use or high doses near term)

Medication Safety Issues

Sound-alike/look-alike issues:

Lorcet® may be confused with Fioricet®

Lortab® may be confused with Cortef®, Lorabid®, Luride®

Vicodin® may be confused with Hycodan®, Hycomine®, Indocin®, Uridon®

Zydone® may be confused with Vytone®

High alert medication: The Institute for Safe Medication Practices (ISMP) includes this medication among its list of drug classes which have a heightened risk of causing significant patient harm when used in error.

Duplicate therapy issues: This product contains acetaminophen, which may be a component of other combination products. Do not exceed the maximum recommended daily dose of acetaminophen.

Dosage Oral (doses should be titrated to appropriate analgesic effect): Analgesic:

Children 2-13 years or <50 kg: Hydrocodone 0.1-0.2 mg/kg/dose every 4-6 hours; do not exceed 6 doses/day or the maximum recommended dose of acetaminophen

Children and Adults ≥50 kg: Average starting dose in opioid naive patients: Hydrocodone 5-10 mg 4 times/day; the dosage of acetaminophen should be limited to ≤4 g/day (and possibly less in patients with hepatic impairment or ethanol use).

Dosage ranges (based on specific product labeling): Hydrocodone 2.5-10 mg every 4-6 hours; maximum: 60 mg hydrocodone/day (maximum dose of hydrocodone may be limited by the acetaminophen content of specific product)

Elderly: Doses should be titrated to appropriate analgesic effect; 2.5-5 mg of the hydrocodone component every 4-6 hours. Do not exceed 4 g/day of acetaminophen.

Dosage adjustment in hepatic impairment: Use with caution. Limited, low-dose therapy usually well tolerated in hepatic disease/cirrhosis; however, cases of hepatotoxicity at daily acetaminophen dosages <4 g/day have been reported. Avoid chronic use in hepatic impairment.

Additional Information Complete prescribing information for this medication should be consulted for additional detail.

Dosage Forms Excipient information presented when available (limited, particularly for generics); consult specific product labeling. [DSC] = Discontinued product

Capsule:

Margesic® H, Stagesic™: Hydrocodone bitartrate 5 mg and acetaminophen 500 mg

Elixir: Hydrocodone bitartrate 7.5 mg and acetaminophen 500 mg per 15 mL (480 mL)

Lortab®: Hydrocodone bitartrate 7.5 mg and acetaminophen 500 mg per 15 mL (480 mL) [contains ethanol 7%, propylene glycol; tropical fruit punch flavor]

Solution, oral: Hydrocodone bitartrate 7.5 mg and acetaminophen 500 mg per 15 mL (5 mL, 10 mL, 15 mL, 118 mL, 473 mL)

hycet™: Hydrocodone bitartrate 7.5 mg and acetaminophen 325 mg per 15 mL (473 mL) [contains ethanol 6.7%, propylene glycol; fruit flavor]

Zamicet™: Hydrocodone bitartrate 10 mg and acetaminophen 325 mg per 15 mL (473 mL) [contains ethanol 6.7%, propylene glycol; fruit flavor]

Tablet:

Hydrocodone bitartrate 2.5 mg and acetaminophen 500 mg

Hydrocodone bitartrate 5 mg and acetaminophen 325 mg

Hydrocodone bitartrate 5 mg and acetaminophen 500 mg

Hydrocodone bitartrate 7.5 mg and acetaminophen 325 mg

Hydrocodone bitartrate 7.5 mg and acetaminophen 500 mg

Hydrocodone bitartrate 7.5 mg and acetaminophen 650 mg

Hydrocodone bitartrate 7.5 mg and acetaminophen 750 mg

Hydrocodone bitartrate 10 mg and acetaminophen 325 mg

Hydrocodone bitartrate 10 mg and acetaminophen 500 mg

Hydrocodone bitartrate 10 mg and acetaminophen 650 mg

Hydrocodone bitartrate 10 mg and acetaminophen 660 mg

Hydrocodone bitartrate 10 mg and acetaminophen 750 mg

Co-Gesic® 5/500: Hydrocodone bitartrate 5 mg and acetaminophen 500 mg

Lorcet® 10/650: Hydrocodone bitartrate 10 mg and acetaminophen 650 mg

Lorcet® Plus: Hydrocodone bitartrate 7.5 mg and acetaminophen 650 mg

Lortab®:

5/500: Hydrocodone bitartrate 5 mg and acetaminophen 500 mg

7.5/500: Hydrocodone bitartrate 7.5 mg and acetaminophen 500 mg

10/500: Hydrocodone bitartrate 10 mg and acetaminophen 500 mg

Maxidone™: Hydrocodone bitartrate 10 mg and acetaminophen 750 mg

Norco®:

Hydrocodone bitartrate 5 mg and acetaminophen 325 mg

Hydrocodone bitartrate 7.5 mg and acetaminophen 325 mg

Hydrocodone bitartrate 10 mg and acetaminophen 325 mg

Vicodin®: Hydrocodone bitartrate 5 mg and acetaminophen 500 mg

Vicodin® ES: Hydrocodone bitartrate 7.5 mg and acetaminophen 750 mg

Vicodin® HP: Hydrocodone bitartrate 10 mg and acetaminophen 660 mg

Xodol®:

10/300: Hydrocodone bitartrate 10 mg and acetaminophen 300 mg

5/300: Hydrocodone bitartrate 5 mg and acetaminophen 300 mg

7/300: Hydrocodone bitartrate 7 mg and acetaminophen 300 mg

Zydone®:

Hydrocodone bitartrate 5 mg and acetaminophen 400 mg

Hydrocodone bitartrate 7.5 mg and acetaminophen 400 mg

Hydrocodone bitartrate 10 mg and acetaminophen 400 mg

Hydrocodone and Chlorpheniramine

(hye droe KOE done & klor fen IR a meen)

U.S. Brand Names TussiCaps™; Tussionex®

Index Terms Chlorpheniramine Maleate and Hydrocodone Bitartrate; Hydrocodone Polistirex and Chlorpheniramine Polistirex

Pharmacologic Category Alpha/Beta Agonist; Antitussive; Histamine H_1 Antagonist; Histamine H_1 Antagonist, First Generation

Use Symptomatic relief of cough and upper respiratory symptoms associated with cold and allergy

Restrictions C-III

Pregnancy Risk Factor C

Medication Safety Issues

Sound-alike/look-alike issues:

Tussionex® represents a different product in the U.S. than it does in Canada. In the U.S., Tussionex® contains hydrocodone and chlorpheniramine, while in Canada the product bearing this name contains hydrocodone and phenyltoloxamine.

Dosage Oral:

Children 6-12 years

TussiCaps™: 5 mg/4 mg: One capsule every 12 hours (maximum: 2 capsules/24 hours)

Tussionex®: 2.5 mL every 12 hours; do not exceed 5 mL/24 hours

Children >12 years and Adults:

TussiCaps™ 10 mg/8 mg: One capsule every 12 hours (maximum: 2 capsules/24 hours)

Tussionex®: 5 mL every 12 hours; do not exceed 10 mL/24 hours

Additional Information Complete prescribing information for this medication should be consulted for additional detail.

Dosage Forms Excipient information presented when available (limited, particularly for generics); consult specific product labeling.

Capsule, extended release:

TussiCaps™ 5 mg/4 mg: Hydrocodone polistirex [equivalent to hydrocodone bitartrate 5 mg] and chlorpheniramine polistirex [equivalent to chlorpheniramine maleate 4 mg]

TussiCaps™ 10 mg/8 mg: Hydrocodone polistirex [equivalent to hydrocodone bitartrate 10 mg] and chlorpheniramine polistirex [equivalent to chlorpheniramine maleate 8 mg]

Suspension, extended release:

Tussionex®: Hydrocodone polistirex [equivalent to hydrocodone bitartrate 10 mg] and chlorpheniramine polistirex [equivalent to chlorpheniramine maleate 8 mg] per 5 mL (480 mL)

Hydrocodone and Guaifenesin

(hye droe KOE done & gwye FEN e sin)

U.S. Brand Names Atuss® HX [DSC]; Codiclear® DH [DSC]; EndaCof [DSC]; EndaCof-XP [DSC]; ExeClear [DSC]; ExeCof-XP [DSC]; Extendryl® HC [DSC]; Hycotuss® [DSC]; Kwelcof® [DSC]; Maxi-Tuss HCG [DSC]; Pancof-XP [DSC]; Phanatuss® HC [DSC]; Pneumotussin® [DSC]; Touro® HC [DSC]; Tusso-DF® [DSC]; Vitussin [DSC]; Xpect-HC™ [DSC]; Ztuss™ ZT [DSC]

Index Terms Guaifenesin and Hydrocodone

Pharmacologic Category Antitussive/Expectorant

Use Symptomatic relief of nonproductive coughs associated with upper and lower respiratory tract congestion

Restrictions C-III

Pregnancy Risk Factor C

Dosage

Children:

<6 years (unlabeled): Hydrocodone 0.3 mg/kg/day in 4 divided doses

6-12 years:

Atuss® Hx: One capsule every 8 hours

Codiclear® DH, ExeClear, Hycotuss®, Kwelcof®, Maxi-Tuss HCG: 2.5-5 mL every 4 hours, after meals and at bedtime

Pneumotussin®: One tablet or 5 mL every 4-6 hours (maximum: 4 doses/24 hours)

>12 years:

Codiclear® DH, ExeClear, Hycotuss®, Kwelcof®, Maxi-Tuss HCG: 5-10 mL every 4 hours, after meals and at bedtime

Pneumotussin®: 1-2 tablets or 10 mL every 4-6 hours (maximum: 4 doses/24 hours)

Children ≥12 years and Adults (Atuss® HX): 1-2 capsules every 8 hours

Adults:

Atuss® HX: 1-2 capsules every 8 hours

Codiclear® DH, Kwelcof®, ExeClear, Hycotuss®: 5-15 mL every 4 hours, after meals and at bedtime (maximum: 30 mL/24 hours)

Maxi-Tuss HCG: 5-10 mL every 4 hours, after meals and at bedtime

Pneumotussin®: 1-2 tablets or 10 mL every 4-6 hours (maximum: 4 doses/24 hours)

Additional Information Complete prescribing information for this medication should be consulted for additional detail.

Dosage Forms Excipient information presented when available (limited, particularly for generics); consult specific product labeling. [DSC] = Discontinued product

Caplet:

Ztuss™ ZT: Hydrocodone bitartrate 5 mg and guaifenesin 300 mg [DSC]

Capsule, variable release:

Atuss® HX: Hydrocodone bitartrate 5 mg [immediate release] and guaifenesin 100 mg [sustained release] [DSC]

Liquid: Hydrocodone bitartrate 5 mg and guaifenesin 100 mg per 5 mL (480 mL, 960 mL) [DSC]

ExeCof-XP: Hydrocodone bitartrate 3 mg and guaifenesin 90 mg per 5 mL (3840 mL) [contains benzoic acid] [DSC]

Kwelcof®: Hydrocodone bitartrate 5 mg and guaifenesin 100 mg per 5 mL (480 mL) [alcohol free, dye free, sugar free; contains benzoic acid; apricot-pineapple flavor] [DSC]

Pancof-XP: Hydrocodone bitartrate 3 mg and guaifenesin 90 mg per 5 mL (3840 mL) [contains benzoic acid] [DSC]

Phanatuss® HC: Hydrocodone bitartrate 5 mg and guaifenesin 100 mg per 5 mL (480 mL) [alcohol free, sugar free; mint flavor] [DSC]

Vitussin: Hydrocodone bitartrate 5 mg and guaifenesin 100 mg per 5 mL (480 mL) [alcohol free, sugar free, dye free; cherry flavor] [DSC]

Syrup: Hydrocodone bitartrate 3.5 mg and guaifenesin 100 mg per 5 mL (120 mL, 480 mL); hydrocodone bitartrate 3.5 mg and guaifenesin 300 mg per 5 mL (120 mL, 480 mL); hydrocodone bitartrate 5 mg and guaifenesin 100 mg per 5 mL (480 mL) [DSC]

Codiclear® DH: Hydrocodone bitartrate 3.5 mg and guaifenesin 300 mg per 5 mL (120 mL, 480 mL) [alcohol free, dye free, sugar free; contains sodium benzoate; grape flavor] [DSC]

EndaCof-XP: Hydrocodone bitartrate 2.5 mg and guaifenesin 200 mg per 5 mL (480 mL) [alcohol free, dye free,

sugar free; contains phenylalanine; cherry punch flavor] [DSC]
ExeClear: Hydrocodone bitartrate 3.5 mg and guaifenesin 100 mg per 5 mL (480 mL) [DSC]
Hycotuss®: Hydrocodone bitartrate 5 mg and guaifenesin 100 mg per 5 mL (480 mL) [contains alcohol 10%; butterscotch flavor] [DSC]
Maxi-Tuss HCG: Hydrocodone bitartrate 6 mg and guaifenesin 200 mg per 5 mL (480 mL) [alcohol free, sugar free; contains aspartame; butterscotch flavor] [DSC]
Pneumotussin®: Hydrocodone bitartrate 2.5 mg and guaifenesin 200 mg per 5 mL (480 mL) [alcohol free, dye free, sugar free; cherry punch flavor] [DSC]
Tusso-DF®: Hydrocodone bitartrate 2.5 mg and guaifenesin 100 mg per 5 mL (480 mL) [cherry flavor] [DSC]
Tablet:
EndaCof: Hydrocodone bitartrate 2.5 mg and guaifenesin 300 mg [DSC]
Touro® HC: Hydrocodone bitartrate 5 mg and guaifenesin 575 mg [DSC]
Tablet, sustained release:
Extendryl® HC: Hydrocodone bitartrate 10 mg and guaifenesin 1000 mg [DSC]
Xpect-HC™: Hydrocodone bitartrate 5 mg and guaifenesin 600 mg [DSC]

Hydrocodone and Homatropine
(hye droe KOE done & hoe MA troe peen)

U.S. Brand Names Hycodan® [DSC]; Hydromet®; Tussigon®
Index Terms Homatropine and Hydrocodone
Pharmacologic Category Antitussive
Use Symptomatic relief of cough
Restrictions C-III
Pregnancy Risk Factor C
Medication Safety Issues
Sound-alike/look-alike issues:
Hycodan® may be confused with Hycomine®, Vicodin®
Dosage Oral:
Children 6-12 years: 1/2 tablet or 2.5 mL every 4-6 hours as needed (maximum: 3 tablets or 15 mL/24 hours)
Children ≥12 years and Adults: 1 tablet or 5 mL every 4-6 hours as needed (maximum: 6 tablets/24 hours or 30 mL/24 hours)
Additional Information Complete prescribing information for this medication should be consulted for additional detail.
Dosage Forms Excipient information presented when available (limited, particularly for generics); consult specific product labeling. [DSC] = Discontinued product
Syrup: Hydrocodone bitartrate 5 mg and homatropine methylbromide 1.5 mg per 5 mL (473 mL)
Hycodan® [DSC], Hydromet®: Hydrocodone bitartrate 5 mg and homatropine methylbromide 1.5 mg per 5 mL (480 mL) [cherry flavor]
Tablet: Hydrocodone bitartrate 5 mg and homatropine methylbromide 1.5 mg [DSC]
Hycodan® [DSC], Tussigon®: Hydrocodone bitartrate 5 mg and homatropine methylbromide 1.5 mg

Hydrocodone and Ibuprofen
(hye droe KOE done & eye byoo PROE fen)

U.S. Brand Names Ibudone™; Reprexain®; Vicoprofen®
Canadian Brand Names Vicoprofen®
Index Terms Hydrocodone Bitartrate and Ibuprofen; Ibuprofen and Hydrocodone
Pharmacologic Category Analgesic, Opioid; Nonsteroidal Anti-inflammatory Drug (NSAID), Oral
Use Short-term (generally <10 days) management of moderate to severe acute pain; is not indicated for treatment of such conditions as osteoarthritis or rheumatoid arthritis
Restrictions C-III; An FDA-approved medication guide for NSAIDs must be distributed when dispensing an oral outpatient prescription (new or refill) where this medication is to be used without direct supervision of a healthcare provider. Medication guides are available at http://www.fda.gov/cder/Offices/ODS/medication_guides.htm.
Pregnancy Risk Factor C/D (3rd trimester)
Medication Safety Issues
High alert medication: The Institute for Safe Medication Practices (ISMP) includes this medication among its list of drug classes which have a heightened risk of causing significant patient harm when used in error.
Dosage Oral:
Adults: 1 tablet every 4-6 hours as needed for pain; maximum: 5 tablets/day. **Note:** Short-term use is recommended (<10 days).
Elderly: Use with caution; consider reduced doses. Refer to dosing in individual monographs.
Additional Information Complete prescribing information for this medication should be consulted for additional detail.
Dosage Forms Excipient information presented when available (limited, particularly for generics); consult specific product labeling.
Tablet: Hydrocodone bitartrate 5 mg and ibuprofen 200 mg; hydrocodone bitartrate 7.5 mg and ibuprofen 200 mg
Ibudone™:
5/200: Hydrocodone bitartrate 5 mg and ibuprofen 200 mg
10/200: Hydrocodone bitartrate 10 mg and ibuprofen 200 mg
Reprexain®: Hydrocodone bitartrate 5 mg and ibuprofen 200 mg; hydrocodone bitartrate 7.5 mg and ibuprofen 200 mg
Vicoprofen®: Hydrocodone bitartrate 7.5 mg and ibuprofen 200 mg

Hydrocodone and Pseudoephedrine
(hye droe KOE done & soo doe e FED rin)

U.S. Brand Names Coughcold HCM [DSC]; P-V Tussin Tablet [DSC]; SymTan™ [DSC]
Index Terms Hydrocodone Tannate and Pseudoephedrine Tannate; Pseudoephedrine Hydrochloride and Hydrocodone Bitartrate
Pharmacologic Category Antitussive/Decongestant
Use Symptomatic relief of cough and nasal congestion
Restrictions C-III
Pregnancy Risk Factor C
Dosage Oral:
Children:
2-6 years: Coldcough HCM: 1.25-2.5 mL 4 times/day a needed
6-12 years:
Coldcough HCM: 2.5-5 mL 4 times/day as needed
SymTan™: 2.5 mL every 12 hours (maximum: 5 mL/day)
Children >12 years and Adults:
Coldcough HCM: 5-10 mL 4 times/day as needed
SymTan™: 5 mL every 12 hours (maximum: 10 mL/day)
Additional Information Complete prescribing information for this medication should be consulted for additional detail.
Dosage Forms Excipient information presented when available (limited, particularly for generics); consult specific product labeling. [DSC] = Discontinued product

Solution:
SymTan™: Hydrocodone tannate 10 mg and pseudoephedrine tannate 45 mg per 5 mL (480 mL) [contains aspartame, propylene glycol; cherry mint flavor] [DSC]
Syrup:
Coldcough HCM: Hydrocodone bitartrate 3 mg and pseudoephedrine hydrochloride 15 mg per 5 mL (480 mL) [alcohol, dye and sugar free; contains propylene glycol; grape flavor] [DSC]
Tablet:
P-V Tussin: Hydrocodone bitartrate 5 mg and pseudoephedrine hydrochloride 60 mg [DSC]

◆ **Hydrocodone Bitartrate and Ibuprofen** *see* Hydrocodone and Ibuprofen *on page* 742

◆ **Hydrocodone Bitartrate, Carbinoxamine Maleate, and Pseudoephedrine Hydrochloride** *see* Hydrocodone, Carbinoxamine, and Pseudoephedrine *on page* 743

Hydrocodone, Carbinoxamine, and Pseudoephedrine

(hye droe KOE done, kar bi NOKS a meen, & soo doe e FED rin)

U.S. Brand Names Tri-Vent™ HC [DSC]

Index Terms Carbinoxamine, Pseudoephedrine, and Hydrocodone; Hydrocodone Bitartrate, Carbinoxamine Maleate, and Pseudoephedrine Hydrochloride; Pseudoephedrine, Hydrocodone, and Carbinoxamine

Pharmacologic Category Alpha/Beta Agonist; Analgesic, Opioid; Antitussive; Histamine H_1 Antagonist; Histamine H_1 Antagonist, First Generation

Use Symptomatic relief of cough, congestion, and rhinorrhea associated with the common cold, influenza, bronchitis, or sinusitis

Restrictions C-III

Pregnancy Risk Factor C

Dosage Oral: Relief of cough, congestion, and runny nose:
Children:
2-10 years: Dosing based on hydrocodone content: 0.6 mg/kg/day given in 4 divided doses. Alternately, the following dosing may be used based on age:
2-4 years: 1.25 mL every 4-6 hours; maximum dose: 7.5 mL/24 hours
4-10 years: 2.5 mL every 4-6 hours; maximum dose: 15 mL/24 hours
>10 years: Refer to adult dosing
Adults: 5-10 mL every 4-6 hours; maximum dose: 30 mL/24 hours

Additional Information Complete prescribing information for this medication should be consulted for additional detail.

Dosage Forms Excipient information presented when available (limited, particularly for generics); consult specific product labeling. [DSC] = Discontinued product
Liquid:
Tri-Vent™ HC: Hydrocodone bitartrate 5 mg, carbinoxamine maleate 2 mg, and pseudoephedrine hydrochloride 30 mg per 5 mL (480 mL) [alcohol free, sugar free; peach flavor] [DSC]

◆ **Hydrocodone Polistirex and Chlorpheniramine Polistirex** *see* Hydrocodone and Chlorpheniramine *on page* 741

Hydrocodone, Pseudoephedrine, and Guaifenesin

(hye droe KOE done, soo doe e FED rin & gwye FEN e sin)

U.S. Brand Names Entex® HC [DSC]; Hydro-Tussin™ HD [DSC]; Hydro-Tussin™ XP [DSC]; Su-Tuss®-HD [DSC]; Ztuss™ Tablet [DSC]

Index Terms Guaifenesin, Hydrocodone, and Pseudoephedrine; Pseudoephedrine, Hydrocodone, and Guaifenesin

Pharmacologic Category Antitussive/Decongestant/Expectorant

Use Symptomatic relief of irritating, nonproductive cough associated with upper respiratory conditions and allergies

Restrictions C-III

Pregnancy Risk Factor C

Dosage Oral: Cough/congestion:
Children:
2-6 years: Hydro-Tussin™ XP: 1.25-2.5 mL 4 times/day as needed
6-12 years:
Hydro-Tussin™ XP: 2.5-5 mL 4 times/day as needed
Hydro-Tussin™ HD: 5 mL every 4-6 hours as needed
Ztuss™: One-half to 1 tablet every 4-6 hours (maximum: 6 tablets/24 hours)
Children ≥12 years and Adults:
Hydro-Tussin™ XP: 5-10 mL 4 times/day as needed
Hydro-Tussin™ HD: 10 mL every 4-6 hours as needed
Ztuss™: 1-1½ tablets every 4-6 hours (maximum: 8 tablets/24 hours)

Additional Information Complete prescribing information for this medication should be consulted for additional detail.

Dosage Forms Excipient information presented when available (limited, particularly for generics); consult specific product labeling.
Elixir:
Su-Tuss®-HD: Hydrocodone bitartrate 2.5 mg, pseudoephedrine hydrochloride 30 mg, and guaifenesin 100 mg per 5 mL (480 mL) [contains alcohol; fruit punch flavor] [DSC]
Liquid:
Entex® HC: Hydrocodone bitartrate 3.75 mg, pseudoephedrine hydrochloride 22.5 mg, and guaifenesin 50 mg per 5 mL (480 mL) [alcohol free, sugar free; contains propylene glycol; tropical fruit punch flavor] [DSC]
Hydro-Tussin™ HD: Hydrocodone bitartrate 2.5 mg, pseudoephedrine hydrochloride 30 mg, and guaifenesin 100 mg per 5 mL (480 mL) [alcohol free; contains sodium benzoate] [DSC]
Hydro-Tussin® XP: Hydrocodone bitartrate 3 mg, pseudoephedrine hydrochloride 15 mg, and guaifenesin 100 mg per 5 mL (480 mL) [alcohol free, dye free] [DSC]
Tablet:
Ztuss™: Hydrocodone bitartrate 5 mg, pseudoephedrine hydrochloride 30 mg, and guaifenesin 300 mg [sugar free] [DSC]

◆ **Hydrocodone Tannate and Pseudoephedrine Tannate** *see* Hydrocodone and Pseudoephedrine *on page* 742

Hydrocortisone (hye droe KOR ti sone)

U.S. Brand Names Anucort-HC®; Anusol-HC®; Anusol® HC-1 [OTC]; Aquanil™ HC [OTC]; Beta-HC®; Caldecort® [OTC]; Cetacort® [DSC]; Colocort®; Cortaid® Intensive Therapy [OTC]; Cortaid® Maximum Strength [OTC]; Cortaid® Sensitive Skin [OTC]; Cortef®; Cortenema®; Corticool® [OTC]; Cortifoam®; Cortizone®-10 Maximum Strength [OTC]; Cortizone®-10 Plus Maximum Strength [OTC]; Cortizone®-10 Quick Shot [OTC]; Dermarest Dricort® [OTC]; Dermtex® HC [OTC]; EarSol® HC; Encort™; Hemril®-30; Hydro-Rx; HydroZone Plus [OTC]; Hytone®; IvySoothe® [OTC]; Locoid Lipocream®; Locoid®; Nupercainal® Hydrocortisone Cream [OTC]; Nutracort®; Pandel®; Post Peel Healing Balm [OTC]; Preparation H® Hydrocortisone [OTC]; Procto-Kit™; Procto-Pak™; Proctocort®; ProctoCream® HC;

Proctosert; Proctosol-HC®; Proctozone-HC™; Sarnol®-HC [OTC]; Solu-Cortef®; Summer's Eve® SpecialCare™ Medicated Anti-Itch Cream [OTC] [DSC]; Texacort®; Tucks® Anti-Itch [OTC]; Westcort®

Canadian Brand Names Aquacort®; Cortamed®; Cortef®; Cortenema®; Cortifoam™; Emo-Cort®; Hycort™; Hyderm; HydroVal®; Locoid®; Prevex® HC; Sarna® HC; Solu-Cortef®; Westcort®

Index Terms A-hydroCort; Compound F; Cortisol; Hemorrhoidal HC; Hydrocortisone Acetate; Hydrocortisone Butyrate; Hydrocortisone Probutate; Hydrocortisone Sodium Succinate; Hydrocortisone Valerate

Pharmacologic Category Corticosteroid, Rectal; Corticosteroid, Systemic; Corticosteroid, Topical

Additional Appendix Information

Corticosteroids *on page 1652*

Use Management of adrenocortical insufficiency; relief of inflammation of corticosteroid-responsive dermatoses (low and medium potency topical corticosteroid); adjunctive treatment of ulcerative colitis

Unlabeled/Investigational Use Management of septic shock when blood pressure is poorly responsive to fluid resuscitation and vasopressor therapy

Pregnancy Risk Factor C

Pregnancy Considerations Adverse events have been observed with corticosteroids in animal reproduction studies. Hydrocortisone crosses the placenta. Some studies have shown an association between first trimester systemic corticosteroid use and oral clefts; adverse events in the fetus/neonate have been noted in case reports following large doses of systemic corticosteroids during pregnancy. Topical products are not recommended for extensive use, in large quantities, or for long periods of time in pregnant women.

Lactation Enters breast milk/use caution

Medication Safety Issues

Sound-alike/look-alike issues:

- Hydrocortisone may be confused with hydrocodone, hydroxychloroquine, hydrochlorothiazide
- Anusol® may be confused with Anusol-HC®, Aplisol®, Aquasol®
- Anusol-HC® may be confused with Anusol®
- Cortef® may be confused with Coreg®, Lortab®
- Cortizone® may be confused with cortisone
- HCT (occasional abbreviation for hydrocortisone) is an error-prone abbreviation (mistaken as hydrochlorothiazide)
- Hytone® may be confused with Vytone®
- Proctocort® may be confused with ProctoCream®
- ProctoCream® may be confused with Proctocort®
- Solu-Cortef® may be confused with Solu-Medrol®

International issues:

- Hytone® may be confused with Hysone® [Australia]
- Nutracort® may be confused with Nitrocor® which is a brand name of nitroglycerin in Chile and Italy

Contraindications Hypersensitivity to hydrocortisone or any component of the formulation; serious infections, except septic shock or tuberculous meningitis; viral, fungal, or tubercular skin lesions; I.M. administration contraindicated in idiopathic thrombocytopenia purpura

Rectal suspension: Systemic fungal infections; ileocolostomy during the immediate or early postoperative period

Warnings/Precautions Use with caution in patients with thyroid disease, hepatic impairment, renal impairment, heart failure, hypertension, diabetes, glaucoma, cataracts, myasthenia gravis, patients at risk for osteoporosis, patients at risk for seizures, or GI diseases (diverticulitis, peptic ulcer, ulcerative colitis) due to perforation risk. Use caution following acute MI (corticosteroids have been associated with myocardial rupture). Because of the risk of adverse effects, systemic corticosteroids should be used cautiously in the elderly in the smallest possible effective dose for the shortest duration. May affect growth velocity; growth should be routinely monitored in pediatric patients. Withdraw therapy with gradual tapering of dose.

May cause hypercorticism or suppression of hypothalamic-pituitary-adrenal (HPA) axis, particularly in younger children or in patients receiving high doses for prolonged periods. HPA axis suppression may lead to adrenal crisis. Withdrawal and discontinuation of a corticosteroid should be done slowly and carefully. Particular care is required when patients are transferred from systemic corticosteroids to inhaled products due to possible adrenal insufficiency or withdrawal from steroids, including an increase in allergic symptoms. Patients receiving >20 mg per day of prednisone (or equivalent) may be most susceptible. Fatalities have occurred due to adrenal insufficiency in asthmatic patients during and after transfer from systemic corticosteroids to aerosol steroids; aerosol steroids do not provide the systemic steroid needed to treat patients having trauma, surgery, or infections. Avoid use of topical preparations with occlusive dressings or on weeping or exudative lesions.

Acute myopathy has been reported with high dose corticosteroids, usually in patients with neuromuscular transmission disorders; may involve ocular and/or respiratory muscles; monitor creatine kinase; recovery may be delayed. Corticosteroid use may cause psychiatric disturbances, including depression, euphoria, insomnia, mood swings, and personality changes. Pre-existing psychiatric conditions may be exacerbated by corticosteroid use. Prolonged use of corticosteroids may also increase the incidence of secondary infection, mask acute infection (including fungal infections), prolong or exacerbate viral infections, or limit response to vaccines. Exposure to chickenpox should be avoided; corticosteroids should not be used to treat ocular herpes simplex. Corticosteroids should not be used for cerebral malaria or viral hepatitis. Close observation is required in patients with latent tuberculosis and/or TB reactivity; restrict use in active TB (only in conjunction with antituberculosis treatment). Prolonged treatment with corticosteroids has been associated with the development of Kaposi's sarcoma (case reports); if noted, discontinuation of therapy should be considered. High-dose corticosteroids should not be used to manage acute head injury.

Adverse Reactions

Systemic:

Frequency not defined:

- Cardiovascular: Edema, hypertension
- Central nervous system: Delirium, euphoria, hallucinations, headache, insomnia, nervousness, pseudotumor cerebri, psychoses, seizure, vertigo
- Dermatologic: Bruising, hyperpigmentation, skin atrophy
- Endocrine & metabolic: Adrenal suppression, alkalosis, amenorrhea, Cushing's syndrome, diabetes mellitus, glucose intolerance, growth suppression, hyperglycemia, hyperlipidemia, hypokalemia, pituitary-adrenal axis suppression, sodium and water retention
- Gastrointestinal: Abdominal distention, appetite increased, indigestion, nausea, pancreatitis, peptic ulcer, ulcerative esophagitis, vomiting
- Hematologic: Leukocytosis (transient)
- Neuromuscular & skeletal: Arthralgia, fractures, muscle weakness, osteoporosis
- Ocular: Cataracts, glaucoma
- Miscellaneous: Avascular necrosis, hypersensitivity reactions, infection, secondary malignancy

Topical:

- >10%: Dermatologic: Eczema (12.5%)
- 1% to 10%: Dermatologic: Pruritus (6%), stinging (2%), dry skin (2%)
- <1% (Limited to important or life-threatening): Allergic contact dermatitis, burning, dermal atrophy, folliculitis,

HPA axis suppression, hypopigmentation; metabolic effects (hyperglycemia, hypokalemia); striae

Drug Interactions

Metabolism/Transport Effects Substrate of CYP3A4 (minor); **Induces** CYP3A4 (weak)

Avoid Concomitant Use

Avoid concomitant use of Hydrocortisone with any of the following: Natalizumab; Vaccines (Live)

Increased Effect/Toxicity

Hydrocortisone may increase the levels/effects of: Acetylcholinesterase Inhibitors; Amphotericin B; CycloSPORINE; Loop Diuretics; Natalizumab; NSAID (COX-2 Inhibitor); NSAID (Nonselective); Thiazide Diuretics; Vaccines (Live); Warfarin

The levels/effects of Hydrocortisone may be increased by: Antifungal Agents (Azole Derivatives, Systemic); Aprepitant; Calcium Channel Blockers (Nondihydropyridine); CycloSPORINE; Estrogen Derivatives; Fluconazole; Fosaprepitant; Macrolide Antibiotics; Neuromuscular-Blocking Agents (Nondepolarizing); P-Glycoprotein Inhibitors; Quinolone Antibiotics; Salicylates; Trastuzumab

Decreased Effect

Hydrocortisone may decrease the levels/effects of: Antidiabetic Agents; Calcitriol; Corticorelin; Isoniazid; Maraviroc; Salicylates; Vaccines (Inactivated)

The levels/effects of Hydrocortisone may be decreased by: Aminoglutethimide; Antacids; Barbiturates; Bile Acid Sequestrants; Echinacea; P-Glycoprotein Inducers; Primidone; Rifamycin Derivatives

Ethanol/Nutrition/Herb Interactions

Ethanol: Avoid ethanol (may enhance gastric mucosal irritation).

Food: Hydrocortisone interferes with calcium absorption.

Herb/Nutraceutical: St John's wort may decrease hydrocortisone levels. Avoid cat's claw, echinacea (have immunostimulant properties).

Stability Store at controlled room temperature 20°C to 25°C (68°F to 77°F). Protect from light. Hydrocortisone sodium phosphate and hydrocortisone sodium succinate are clear, light yellow solutions which are heat labile.

Sodium succinate: Reconstitute 100 mg vials with bacteriostatic water (not >2 mL). Act-O-Vial (self-contained powder for injection plus diluent) may be reconstituted by pressing the activator to force diluent into the powder compartment. Following gentle agitation, solution may be withdrawn via syringe through a needle inserted into the center of the stopper. May be administered (I.V. or I.M.) without further dilution. After initial reconstitution, hydrocortisone sodium succinate solutions are stable for 3 days at room temperature or under refrigeration when protected from light. Stability of parenteral admixture (Solu-Cortef®) at room temperature (25°C) and at refrigeration temperature (4°C) is concentration-dependent:

Stability of concentration 1 mg/mL: 24 hours.

Stability of concentration 2 mg/mL to 60 mg/mL: At least 4 hours.

Solutions for I.V. infusion: Reconstituted solutions may be added to an appropriate volume of compatible solution for infusion. Concentration should generally not exceed 1 mg/mL. However, in cases where administration of a small volume of fluid is desirable, 100-3000 mg may be added to 50 mL of D_5W or NS (stability limited to 4 hours).

Mechanism of Action Decreases inflammation by suppression of migration of polymorphonuclear leukocytes and reversal of increased capillary permeability

Pharmacodynamics/Kinetics

Onset of action:

Hydrocortisone acetate: Slow

Hydrocortisone sodium succinate (water soluble): Rapid

Duration: Hydrocortisone acetate: Long

Absorption: Rapid by all routes, except rectally

Metabolism: Hepatic

Half-life elimination: Biologic: 8-12 hours

Excretion: Urine (primarily as 17-hydroxysteroids and 17-ketosteroids)

Dosage Dose should be based on severity of disease and patient response

Adrenal hyperplasia (congenital): Children: Oral: Initial: 10-20 mg/m^2/day in 3 divided doses; a variety of dosing schedules have been used. **Note:** Inconsistencies have occurred with liquid formulations; tablets may provide more reliable levels. Doses must be individualized by monitoring growth, bone age, and hormonal levels. Mineralocorticoid and sodium supplementation may be required based upon electrolyte regulation and plasma renin activity.

Adrenal insufficiency (acute): I.M., I.V.:

Infants and young Children: Succinate: 1-2 mg/kg/dose bolus, then 25-150 mg/day in divided doses every 6-8 hours

Older Children: Succinate: 1-2 mg/kg bolus then 150-250 mg/day in divided doses every 6-8 hours

Adults: Succinate: 100 mg I.V. bolus, then 300 mg/day in divided doses every 8 hours or as a continuous infusion for 48 hours; once patient is stable change to oral, 50 mg every 8 hours for 6 doses, then taper to 30-50 mg/day in divided doses

Adrenal insufficiency (chronic): Adults: Oral: 20-30 mg/day

Anti-inflammatory or immunosuppressive:

Infants and Children:

Oral: 2.5-10 mg/kg/day **or** 75-300 mg/m^2/day every 6-8 hours

I.M., I.V.: Succinate: 1-5 mg/kg/day **or** 30-150 mg/m^2/day divided every 12-24 hours

Adolescents and Adults: Oral, I.M., I.V.: Succinate: 15-240 mg every 12 hours

Physiologic replacement: Children:

Oral: 0.5-0.75 mg/kg/day **or** 20-25 mg/m^2/day every 8 hours

I.M.: Succinate: 0.25-0.35 mg/kg/day **or** 12-15 mg/m^2/day once daily

Rheumatic diseases: Adults:

Intralesional, intra-articular, soft tissue injection: Acetate:

Large joints: 25 mg (up to 37.5 mg)

Small joints: 10-25 mg

Tendon sheaths: 5-12.5 mg

Soft tissue infiltration: 25-50 mg (up to 75 mg)

Bursae: 25-37.5 mg

Ganglia: 12.5-25 mg

Septic shock (unlabeled use): I.V.: 50 mg every 6 hours (or 200-300 mg total daily dose) (Marik, 2008). Taper slowly (for total of 11 days) and do not stop abruptly. **Note:** Fludrocortisone is optional with use of hydrocortisone.

Shock: I.M., I.V.: Succinate:

Children: Initial: 50 mg/kg, then repeated in 4 hours and/or every 24 hours as needed

Adolescents and Adults: 500 mg to 2 g every 2-6 hours

Status asthmaticus: Children and Adults: I.V.: Succinate: 1-2 mg/kg/dose every 6 hours for 24 hours, then maintenance of 0.5-1 mg/kg every 6 hours

Stress dosing (surgery) in patients known to be adrenally-suppressed or on chronic systemic steroids: I.V.: Adults:

Minor stress (ie, inguinal herniorrhaphy): 25 mg/day for 1 day

Moderate stress (ie, joint replacement, cholecystectomy): 50-75 mg/day (25 mg every 8-12 hours) for 1-2 days

Major stress (pancreatoduodenectomy, esophagogastrectomy, cardiac surgery): 100-150 mg/day (50 mg every 8-12 hours) for 2-3 days

Dermatosis: Children >2 years and Adults: Topical: Apply to affected area 2-4 times/day (Buteprate: Apply once or twice daily). Therapy should be discontinued when control is achieved; if no improvement is seen, reassessment of diagnosis may be necessary.

Ulcerative colitis: Adults: Rectal: 10-100 mg 1-2 times/day for 2-3 weeks

Dietary Considerations Systemic use of corticosteroids may require a diet with increased potassium, vitamins A, B_6, C, D, folate, calcium, zinc, phosphorus, and decreased sodium. Sodium content of 1 g (sodium succinate injection): 47.5 mg (2.07 mEq)

Administration

Oral: Administer with food or milk to decrease GI upset

Parenteral: Hydrocortisone sodium succinate may be administered by I.M. or I.V. routes

I.V. bolus: Dilute to 50 mg/mL and administer over 30 seconds or over 10 minutes for doses ≥500 mg

I.V. intermittent infusion: Dilute to 1 mg/mL and administer over 20-30 minutes

Topical: Apply a thin film to clean, dry skin and rub in gently

Monitoring Parameters Blood pressure, weight, serum glucose, and electrolytes

Reference Range Therapeutic: AM: 5-25 mcg/dL (SI: 138-690 nmol/L), PM: 2-9 mcg/dL (SI: 55-248 nmol/L) depending on test, assay

Additional Information Hydrocortisone base topical cream, lotion, and ointments in concentrations of 0.25%, 0.5%, and 1% may be OTC or prescription depending on the product labeling.

Dosage Forms Excipient information presented when available (limited, particularly for generics); consult specific product labeling. [DSC] = Discontinued product

Aerosol, rectal, as acetate (Cortifoam®): 10% (15 g) [90 mg/applicator]

Cream, rectal, as acetate (Nupercainal® Hydrocortisone Cream): 1% (30 g) [strength expressed as base]

Cream, rectal, as base:

Cortizone®-10: 1% (30 g) [contains aloe]

Preparation H® Hydrocortisone: 1% (27 g)

Cream, topical, as acetate: 0.5% (9 g, 30 g, 60 g) [available with aloe]; 1% (30 g, 454 g) [available with aloe]

Cream, topical, as base: 0.5% (30 g); 1% (1.5 g, 30 g, 114 g, 454 g); 2.5% (20 g, 30 g, 454 g)

Anusol-HC®: 2.5% (30 g) [contains benzyl alcohol]

Caldecort®: 1% (30 g) [contains aloe vera gel]

Cortaid® Intensive Therapy: 1% (60 g)

Cortaid® Maximum Strength: 1% (15 g, 30 g, 40 g, 60 g) [contains aloe vera gel and benzyl alcohol]

Cortaid® Sensitive Skin: 0.5% (15 g) [contains aloe vera gel]

Cortizone®-10 Maximum Strength: 1% (15 g, 30 g, 60 g) [contains aloe]

Cortizone®-10 Plus Maximum Strength: 1% (30 g, 60 g) [contains vitamins A, D, E and aloe]

Dermarest® Dricort®: 1% (15 g, 30 g)

HydroZone Plus, Proctocort®, Procto-Pak™: 1% (30 g)

Hytone®: 2.5% (30 g, 60 g)

IvySoothe®: 1% (30 g) [contains aloe]

Post Peel Healing Balm: 1% (23 g)

ProctoCream® HC: 2.5% (30 g) [contains benzyl alcohol]

Procto-Kit™: 1% (30 g) [packaged with applicator tips and finger cots]; 2.5% (30 g) [packaged with applicator tips and finger cots]

Proctosol-HC®, Proctozone-HC™: 2.5% (30 g)

Summer's Eve® SpecialCare™ Medicated Anti-Itch Cream: 1% (30 g) [DSC]

Cream, topical, as butyrate (Locoid®, Locoid Lipocream®): 0.1% (15 g, 45 g)

Cream, topical, as probutate (Pandel®): 0.1% (15 g, 45 g, 80 g)

Cream, topical, as valerate (Westcort®): 0.2% (15 g, 45 g, 60 g)

Gel, topical, as base (Corticool®): 1% (45 g)

Injection, powder for reconstitution, as sodium succinate:

A-Hydrocort®: 100 mg [contains monobasic sodium phosphate 0.8 mg, anhydrous dibasic sodium phosphate 8.73 mg; strength expressed as base]

Solu-Cortef®: 100 mg, 250 mg, 500 mg, 1 g [diluent contains benzyl alcohol; strength expressed as base]

Lotion, topical, as base: 1% (120 mL); 2.5% (60 mL)

Aquanil™ HC: 1% (120 mL)

Beta-HC®, Cetacort® [DSC], Sarnol®-HC: 1% (60 mL)

HydroZone Plus: 1% (120 mL)

Hytone®: 2.5% (60 mL)

Nutracort®: 1% (60 mL, 120 mL); 2.5% (60 mL, 120 mL)

Lotion, topical, as butyrate:

Locoid®: 0.1% (60 mL)

Ointment, topical, as acetate: 1% (30 g) [strength expressed as base; available with aloe]

Anusol® HC-1: 1% (21 g) [strength expressed as base]

Cortaid® Maximum Strength: 1% (15 g, 30 g) [strength expressed as base]

Ointment, topical, as base: 0.5% (30 g); 1% (30 g, 454 g); 2.5% (20 g, 30 g, 454 g)

Cortizone®-10 Maximum Strength: 1% (30 g, 60 g)

Hytone®: 2.5% (30 g) [DSC]

Ointment, topical, as butyrate (Locoid®): 0.1% (15 g, 45 g)

Ointment, topical, as valerate (Westcort®): 0.2% (15 g, 45 g, 60 g)

Powder, for prescription compounding [micronized]:

Hydro-Rx: USP (10 g, 25 g, 50 g, 100 g)

Powder, for prescription compounding, as acetate [micronized]: USP (10 g, 25 g, 50 g)

Solution, otic, as base (EarSol® HC): 1% (30 mL) [contains alcohol 44%, benzyl benzoate, yerba santa]

Solution, topical, as base (Texacort®): 2.5% (30 mL) [contains ethanol 48%]

Solution, topical, as butyrate (Locoid®): 0.1% (20 mL, 60 mL) [contains alcohol 50%]

Solution, topical spray, as base:

Cortaid® Intensive Therapy: 1% (60 mL) [contains alcohol]

Cortizone®-10 Quick Shot: 1% (44 mL) [contains benzyl alcohol]

Dermtex® HC: 1% (52 mL) [contains menthol 1%]

Suppository, rectal, as acetate: 25 mg (12s, 24s, 100s)

Anucort-HC®, Tucks® Anti-Itch: 25 mg (12s, 24s, 100s) [strength expressed as base; Anucort-HC® *renamed* Tucks® Anti-Itch]

Anusol-HC®, Proctosol-HC®: 25 mg (12s, 24s)

Encort™, Proctocort®: 30 mg (12s)

Hemril®-30, Proctosert: 30 mg (12s, 24s)

Suspension, rectal, as base: 100 mg/60 mL (7s)

Colocort®, Cortenema®: 100 mg/60 mL (1s, 7s)

Tablet, as base: 20 mg

Cortef®: 5 mg, 10 mg, 20 mg

◆ **Hydrocortisone Acetate** *see* Hydrocortisone *on page 743*

◆ **Hydrocortisone, Acetic Acid, and Propylene Glycol Diacetate** *see* Acetic Acid, Propylene Glycol Diacetate, and Hydrocortisone *on page 35*

◆ **Hydrocortisone and Benzoyl Peroxide** *see* Benzoyl Peroxide and Hydrocortisone *on page 185*

◆ **Hydrocortisone and Ciprofloxacin** *see* Ciprofloxacin and Hydrocortisone *on page 333*

◆ **Hydrocortisone and Iodoquinol** *see* Iodoquinol and Hydrocortisone *on page 810*

◆ **Hydrocortisone and Pramoxine** *see* Pramoxine and Hydrocortisone *on page 1227*

◆ **Hydrocortisone and Urea** *see* Urea and Hydrocortisone *on page 1531*

◆ **Hydrocortisone, Bacitracin, Neomycin, and Polymyxin B** *see* Bacitracin, Neomycin, Polymyxin B, and Hydrocortisone *on page 172*

◆ **Hydrocortisone Butyrate** *see* Hydrocortisone *on page 743*

◆ **Hydrocortisone, Neomycin, and Polymyxin B** *see* Neomycin, Polymyxin B, and Hydrocortisone *on page 1052*

◆ **Hydrocortisone, Neomycin, Colistin, and Thonzonium** *see* Neomycin, Colistin, Hydrocortisone, and Thonzonium *on page 1051*

◆ **Hydrocortisone Probutate** *see* Hydrocortisone *on page 743*

◆ **Hydrocortisone Sodium Succinate** *see* Hydrocortisone *on page 743*

◆ **Hydrocortisone Valerate** *see* Hydrocortisone *on page 743*

◆ **Hydromet®** *see* Hydrocodone and Homatropine *on page 742*

◆ **Hydromorph Contin® (Can)** *see* HYDROmorphone *on page 747*

◆ **Hydromorph-IR® (Can)** *see* HYDROmorphone *on page 747*

HYDROmorphone (hye droe MOR fone)

U.S. Brand Names Dilaudid-HP®; Dilaudid®

Canadian Brand Names Dilaudid-HP-Plus®; Dilaudid-HP®; Dilaudid-XP®; Dilaudid®; Dilaudid® Sterile Powder; Hydromorph Contin®; Hydromorph-IR®; Hydromorphone HP; Hydromorphone HP® 10; Hydromorphone HP® 20; Hydromorphone HP® 50; Hydromorphone HP® Forte; Hydromorphone Hydrochloride Injection, USP; PMS-Hydromorphone

Index Terms Dihydromorphinone; Hydromorphone Hydrochloride

Pharmacologic Category Analgesic, Opioid

Additional Appendix Information

Narcotic / Opioid Analgesics *on page 1663*

Use Management of moderate-to-severe pain

Unlabeled/Investigational Use Antitussive

Restrictions C-II

Pregnancy Risk Factor C/D (prolonged use or high doses at term)

Pregnancy Considerations Hydromorphone was teratogenic in some, but not all, animal studies; however, maternal toxicity was also reported. Hydromorphone crosses the placenta. Chronic opioid use during pregnancy may lead to a withdrawal syndrome in the neonate. Symptoms include irritability, hyperactivity, loss of sleep pattern, abnormal crying, tremor, vomiting, diarrhea, weight loss, or failure to gain weight.

Lactation Excretion in breast milk unknown/not recommended

Medication Safety Issues

Sound-alike/look-alike issues:

Dilaudid® may be confused with Demerol®, Dilantin®

HYDROmorphone may be confused with morphine; significant overdoses have occurred when hydromorphone products have been inadvertently administered instead of morphine sulfate. Commercially available prefilled syringes of both products looks similar and are often stored in close proximity to each other. **Note:** Hydromorphone 1 mg oral is approximately equal to morphine 4 mg oral; hydromorphone 1 mg I.V. is approximately equal to morphine 5 mg I.V.

High alert medication: The Institute for Safe Medication Practices (ISMP) includes this medication among its list of drug classes which have a heightened risk of causing significant patient harm when used in error.

Dilaudid®, Dilaudid-HP®: Extreme caution should be taken to avoid confusing the highly-concentrated (Dilaudid-HP®) injection with the less-concentrated (Dilaudid®) injectable product.

Significant differences exist between oral and I.V. dosing. Use caution when converting from one route of administration to another.

Contraindications Hypersensitivity to hydromorphone, any component of the formulation; acute or severe asthma, severe respiratory depression (in absence of resuscitative equipment or ventilatory support); severe CNS depression; pregnancy (prolonged use or high doses at term); obstetrical analgesia

Warnings/Precautions Use with caution in patients with hypersensitivity reactions to other phenanthrene derivative opioid agonists (codeine, hydrocodone, levorphanol, oxycodone, oxymorphone). Hydromorphone shares toxic potential of opiate agonists, including CNS depression and respiratory depression. Precautions associated with opiate agonist therapy should be observed. May cause CNS depression, which may impair physical or mental abilities; patients must be cautioned about performing tasks which require mental alertness (eg, operating machinery or driving). Myoclonus and seizures have been reported with high doses. Critical respiratory depression may occur, even at therapeutic dosages, particularly in elderly or debilitated patients or in patients with pre-existing respiratory compromise (hypoxia and/or hypercapnia). Use caution in COPD or other obstructive pulmonary disease. Use with caution in patients with hypersensitivity to other phenanthrene opiates, kyphoscoliosis, biliary tract disease, acute pancreatitis, morbid obesity, adrenocortical insufficiency, hypothyroidism, acute alcoholism, toxic psychoses, prostatic hyperplasia and/or urinary stricture, or severe liver or renal failure. Use extreme caution in patients with head injury, intracranial lesions, or elevated intracranial pressure; exaggerated elevation of ICP may occur (in addition, hydromorphone may complicate neurologic evaluation due to pupillary dilation and CNS depressant effects). Use with caution in patients with depleted blood volume or drugs which may exaggerate hypotensive effects (including phenothiazines or general anesthetics). May obscure diagnosis or clinical course of patients with acute abdominal conditions.

[U.S. Boxed Warning]: Hydromorphone has a high potential for abuse. Those at risk for opioid abuse include patients with a history of substance abuse or mental illness. Tolerance or drug dependence may result from extended use; however, concerns for abuse should not prevent effective management of pain. In general, abrupt discontinuation of therapy in dependent patients should be avoided.

An opioid-containing analgesic regimen should be tailored to each patient's needs and based upon the type of pain being treated (acute versus chronic), the route of administration, degree of tolerance for opioids (naive versus chronic user), age, weight, and medical condition. The optimal analgesic dose varies widely among patients. Doses should be titrated to pain relief/prevention. I.M. use may result in variable absorption and a lag time to peak effect.

Dosage form specific warnings:

[U.S. Boxed Warning]: Dilaudid-HP®: Extreme caution should be taken to avoid confusing the highly-concentrated (Dilaudid-HP®) injection with the less-concentrated (Dilaudid®) injectable product. Dilaudid-HP® should only be used in patients who are opioid-tolerant.

Controlled release: Capsules should only be used when continuous analgesia is required over an extended period of time. Controlled release products are not to be used on an "as needed" (PRN) basis.

Some dosage forms contain trace amounts of sodium metabisulfite which may cause allergic reactions in susceptible individuals.

Adverse Reactions Frequency not defined.

Cardiovascular: Bradycardia, flushing of face, hyper-/hypotension, palpitation, peripheral vasodilation, syncope, tachycardia

Central nervous system: Agitation, chills, CNS depression, dizziness, drowsiness, dysphoria, euphoria, fatigue, hallucinations, headache, increased intracranial pressure, insomnia, lightheadedness, mental depression, nervousness, restlessness, sedation, seizure

Dermatologic: Pruritus, rash, urticaria

Endocrine & metabolic: Antidiuretic hormone release

Gastrointestinal: Anorexia, biliary tract spasm, constipation, diarrhea, nausea, paralytic ileus, stomach cramps, taste perversion, vomiting, xerostomia

Genitourinary: Ureteral spasm, urinary retention, urinary tract spasm, urination decreased

Hepatic: LFTs increased

Local: Pain at injection site (I.M.), wheal/flare over vein (I.V.)

Neuromuscular & skeletal: Myoclonus, paresthesia, trembling, tremor, weakness

Ocular: Blurred vision, diplopia, miosis, nystagmus

Respiratory: Apnea, bronchospasm, dyspnea, laryngospasm, respiratory depression

Miscellaneous: Diaphoresis, histamine release, physical and psychological dependence

Drug Interactions

Avoid Concomitant Use There are no known interactions where it is recommended to avoid concomitant use.

Increased Effect/Toxicity

HYDROmorphone may increase the levels/effects of: Alcohol (Ethyl); Alvimopan; CNS Depressants; Desmopressin; Selective Serotonin Reuptake Inhibitors

The levels/effects of HYDROmorphone may be increased by: Amphetamines; Antipsychotic Agents (Phenothiazines); Succinylcholine

Decreased Effect

HYDROmorphone may decrease the levels/effects of: Pegvisomant

The levels/effects of HYDROmorphone may be decreased by: Ammonium Chloride

Ethanol/Nutrition/Herb Interactions

Ethanol: Avoid ethanol (may increase CNS depression).

Herb/Nutraceutical: Avoid valerian, St John's wort, kava kava, gotu kola (may increase CNS depression).

Stability Store injection and oral dosage forms at 15°C to 30°C (59°F to 86°F). Protect tablets from light. A slightly yellowish discoloration has not been associated with a loss of potency.

Mechanism of Action Binds to opiate receptors in the CNS, causing inhibition of ascending pain pathways, altering the perception of and response to pain; causes cough supression by direct central action in the medulla; produces generalized CNS depression

Pharmacodynamics/Kinetics

Onset of action: Analgesic: Immediate release formulations:

Oral: 15-30 minutes

Peak effect: Oral: 30-60 minutes

Duration: Immediate release formulations: 4-5 hours

Absorption: I.M.: Variable and delayed

Distribution: V_d: 4 L/kg

Protein binding: ~8% to 19%

Metabolism: Hepatic via glucuronidation; to inactive metabolites

Bioavailability: 62%

Half-life elimination: Immediate release formulations: 1-3 hours

Excretion: Urine (primarily as glucuronide conjugates)

Dosage

Acute pain (moderate to severe): **Note:** These are guidelines and do not represent the maximum doses that may be required in all patients. Doses should be titrated to pain relief/prevention.

Children ≥6 months and <50 kg:

Oral: 0.03-0.08 mg/kg/dose every 3-4 hours as needed

I.V.: 0.015 mg/kg/dose every 3-6 hours as needed

Children >50 kg and Adults:

Oral: Initial: Opiate-naive: 2-4 mg every 3-6 hours as needed; elderly/debilitated patients may require lower doses; patients with prior opiate exposure may require higher initial doses; usual dosage range: 2-8 mg every 3-4 hours as needed

I.V.: Initial: Opiate-naive: 0.2-0.6 mg every 2-3 hours as needed; patients with prior opiate exposure may tolerate higher initial doses

Critically-ill patients (unlabeled dose): 0.7-2 mg (based on 70 kg patient) every 1-2 hours as needed. **Note:** More frequent dosing may be needed (eg, mechanically-ventilated patients).

Continuous infusion: Usual dosage range: 0.5-1 mg/hour (based on 70 kg patient) or 7-15 mcg/kg/hour

Patient-controlled analgesia (PCA): (Opiate-naive: Consider lower end of dosing range)

Usual concentration: 0.2 mg/mL

Demand dose: Usual: 0.1-0.2 mg; range: 0.05-0.5 mg

Lockout interval: 5-15 minutes

4-hour limit: 4-6 mg

Epidural:

Bolus dose: 1-1.5 mg

Infusion concentration: 0.05-0.075 mg/mL

Infusion rate: 0.04-0.4 mg/hour

Demand dose: 0.15 mg

Lockout interval: 30 minutes

I.M., SubQ: **Note:** I.M. use may result in variable absorption and a lag time to peak effect.

Initial: Opiate-naive: 0.8-1 mg every 4-6 hours as needed; patients with prior opiate exposure may require higher initial doses; usual dosage range: 1-2 mg every 3-6 hours as needed

Rectal: 3 mg every 4-8 hours as needed

Chronic pain: Adults: Oral: **Note:** Patients taking opioids chronically may become tolerant and require doses higher than the usual dosage range to maintain the desired effect. Tolerance can be managed by appropriate dose titration. There is no optimal or maximal dose for hydromorphone in chronic pain. The appropriate dose is one that relieves pain throughout its dosing interval without causing unmanageable side effects.

Controlled release formulation (Hydromorph Contin®, not available in U.S.): 3-30 mg every 12 hours. **Note:** A patient's hydromorphone requirement should be established using prompt release formulations; conversion to long acting products may be considered when chronic, continuous treatment is required. Higher dosages should be reserved for use only in opioid-tolerant patients.

Antitussive (unlabeled use): Oral:

Children 6-12 years: 0.5 mg every 3-4 hours as needed

Children >12 years and Adults: 1 mg every 3-4 hours as needed

Dosing adjustment in hepatic impairment: Should be considered

Administration

Parenteral: May be given SubQ or I.M.; vial stopper contains latex

I.V.: For IVP, must be given slowly over 2-3 minutes (rapid IVP has been associated with an increase in side effects, especially respiratory depression and hypotension)

Oral: Hydromorph Contin®: Capsule should be swallowed whole; do not crush or chew; contents may be sprinkled on soft food and swallowed

Monitoring Parameters Pain relief, respiratory and mental status, blood pressure

Test Interactions Some quinolones may produce a false-positive urine screening result for opiates using commercially-available immunoassay kits. This has been demonstrated most consistently for levofloxacin and ofloxacin, but other quinolones have shown cross-reactivity in certain assay kits. Confirmation of positive opiate screens by more specific methods should be considered.

Additional Information Equianalgesic doses: Morphine 10 mg I.M. = hydromorphone 1.5 mg I.M.

Dosage Forms Excipient information presented when available (limited, particularly for generics); consult specific product labeling. [CAN] = Canadian brand name

Capsule, controlled release:
- Hydromorph Contin® [CAN]: 3 mg, 6 mg, 12 mg, 18 mg, 24 mg, 30 mg [not available in U.S.]

Injection, powder for reconstitution, as hydrochloride:
- Dilaudid-HP®: 250 mg [may contain trace amounts of sodium bisulfite]

Injection, solution, as hydrochloride: 1 mg/mL (1 mL); 2 mg/mL (1 mL, 20 mL); 4 mg/mL (1 mL)
- Dilaudid®: 1 mg/mL (1 mL); 2 mg/mL (1 mL, 20 mL) [20 mL size contains edetate sodium; vial stopper contains latex]; 4 mg/mL (1 mL)

Injection, solution, as hydrochloride [preservative free]: 10 mg/mL (1 mL, 5 mL, 50 mL)
- Dilaudid-HP®: 10 mg/mL (1 mL, 5 mL) [contains sodium metabisulfate]
- Dilaudid-HP®: 10 mg/mL (50 mL) [contains natural rubber/natural latex in packaging, sodium metabisulfate]

Liquid, oral, as hydrochloride:
- Dilaudid®: 1 mg/mL (480 mL) [may contain trace amounts of sodium bisulfite]

Powder, for prescription compounding: 100% (15 grain)

Suppository, rectal, as hydrochloride: 3 mg
- Dilaudid®: 3 mg (6s)

Tablet, as hydrochloride: 2 mg, 4 mg, 8 mg
- Dilaudid®: 2 mg, 4 mg, 8 mg (8 mg tablets may contain trace amounts of sodium bisulfite)

- ◆ **Hydromorphone HP (Can)** *see* HYDROmorphone *on page 747*
- ◆ **Hydromorphone HP® 10 (Can)** *see* HYDROmorphone *on page 747*
- ◆ **Hydromorphone HP® 20 (Can)** *see* HYDROmorphone *on page 747*
- ◆ **Hydromorphone HP® 50 (Can)** *see* HYDROmorphone *on page 747*
- ◆ **Hydromorphone HP® Forte (Can)** *see* HYDROmorphone *on page 747*
- ◆ **Hydromorphone Hydrochloride** *see* HYDROmorphone *on page 747*
- ◆ **Hydromorphone Hydrochloride Injection, USP (Can)** *see* HYDROmorphone *on page 747*
- ◆ **Hydroquinol** *see* Hydroquinone *on page 749*

Hydroquinone (HYE droe kwin one)

U.S. Brand Names Aclaro PD™; Alphaquin HP®; Claripel™ [DSC]; Dermarest® Skin Correction Cream Plus [OTC]; Eldopaque Forte®; Eldopaque® [OTC]; Eldoquin Forte®; Eldoquin® [OTC]; EpiQuin™ Micro; Esoterica® Regular [OTC]; Glyquin-XM™; Glyquin®; Lustra-AF™; Lustra®; Melanex®; Melpaque HP®; Melquin HP®; Melquin-3®; NeoStrata® AHA [OTC]; Nuquin HP®; Palmer's® Skin Success Eventone® Fade Cream [OTC]; Solaquin Forte®; Solaquin® [OTC]

Canadian Brand Names Eldopaque®; Eldoquin®; Glyquin® XM; Lustra®; NeoStrata® HQ; Solaquin Forte®; Solaquin®; Ultraquin™

Index Terms Hydroquinol; Quinol

Pharmacologic Category Depigmenting Agent

Use Gradual bleaching of hyperpigmented skin conditions

Pregnancy Risk Factor C

Medication Safety Issues

Sound-alike/look-alike issues:
- Eldopaque® may be confused with Eldoquin®
- Eldoquin® may be confused with Eldopaque®
- Eldopaque Forte® may be confused with Eldoquin Forte®
- Eldoquin Forte® may be confused with Eldopaque Forte®

Dosage Children >12 years and Adults: Topical: Apply thin layer and rub in twice daily

Additional Information Complete prescribing information for this medication should be consulted for additional detail.

Dosage Forms Excipient information presented when available (limited, particularly for generics); consult specific product labeling. [DSC] = Discontinued product

Cream, topical: 4% (30 g) [may contain sodium metabisulfite]
- Alphaquin HP®: 4% (30 g, 60 g)
- Eldoquin®: 2% (15 g, 30 g)
- Eldoquin Forte®: 4% (30 g) [contains sodium metabisulfite]
- EpiQuin™ Micro: 4% (30 g) [contains benzyl alcohol and sodium metabisulfite]
- Esoterica® Regular: 2% (85 g) [contains sodium bisulfite]
- Lustra®: 4% (30 g) [contains sodium metabisulfite]
- Melquin HP®: 4% (15 g, 30 g) [contains sodium metabisulfite]

Cream, topical [with sunscreen]: 4% (30 g) [may contain sodium metabisulfite]
- Claripel™: 4% (30 g, 45 g) [contains sodium metabisulfite] [DSC]
- Dermarest® Skin Correcting Cream Plus: 2% (85 g) [contains aloe vera, sodium bisulfite]
- Eldopaque®: 2% (15 g, 30 g)
- Eldopaque Forte®: 4% (30 g) [contains sodium metabisulfite]
- Glyquin®: 4% (30 g)
- Glyquin-XM™: 4% (30 g)
- Lustra-AF™: 4% (30 g, 60 g) [contains sodium metabisulfite]
- Melpaque HP®: 4% (15 g, 30 g) [contains sodium metabisulfite; sunblocking cream base]
- Nuquin HP®: 4% (15 g, 30 g, 60 g) [contains sodium metabisulfite]
- Palmer's® Skin Success Eventone® Fade Cream: 2% (81 g, 132 g) [contains sodium sulfite; available in regular, oily skin, and dry skin formulas]
- Solaquin®: 2% (30 g)
- Solaquin Forte®: 4% (30 g) [contains sodium metabisulfite]

Emulsion, topical:
- Aclaro PD™: 4% (42.5 g) [contains benzyl alcohol; with sunscreen]

Gel, topical:
- NeoStrata® AHA: 2% (45 g) [contains glycolic acid 10%, sodium bisulfite, and sodium sulfite]

Gel, topical [with sunscreen]: 4% (30 g)
- Nuquin HP: 4% (15 g, 30 g) [contains sodium bisulfite]
- Solaquin Forte®: 4% (30 g) [contains sodium metabisulfite]

Solution, topical: 3% (30 mL) [DSC]
- Melanex®, Melquin-3®: 3% (30 mL) [contains alcohol]

Hydroxocobalamin (hye droks oh koe BAL a min)

U.S. Brand Names Cyanokit®

Index Terms Vitamin B_{12a}

Pharmacologic Category Antidote; Vitamin, Water Soluble

Use Treatment of pernicious anemia, vitamin B_{12} deficiency due to dietary deficiencies or malabsorption diseases, inadequate secretion of intrinsic factor, and inadequate utilization of B_{12} (eg, during neoplastic treatment); diagnostic agent for Schilling test

Cyanokit®: Treatment of cyanide poisoning (known or suspected)

Unlabeled/Investigational Use Neuropathies

Pregnancy Risk Factor C

Pregnancy Considerations Animal studies are insufficient to determine the effect, if any, on pregnancy or fetal development. There are no adequate and well-controlled studies in pregnant women. Data on the use of hydroxocobalamin in pregnancy for the treatment of cyanide poisoning and cobalamin defects are limited.

Lactation Excretion in breast milk unknown/use caution

Contraindications Hypersensitivity to hydroxocobalamin, cyanocobalamin, cobalt, or any component of the formulation

Warnings/Precautions

Solution for I.M. injection: Treatment of severe vitamin B_{12} megaloblastic anemia may result in thrombocytosis and severe hypokalemia, sometimes fatal, due to intracellular potassium shift upon anemia resolution. Use caution in folic acid deficient megaloblastic anemia; administration of vitamin B_{12} alone is not a substitute for folic acid and might mask true diagnosis. Vitamin B_{12} deficiency masks signs of polycythemia vera; vitamin B_{12} administration may unmask this condition. Neurologic manifestations of vitamin B_{12} deficiency will not be prevented with folic acid unless vitamin B_{12} is also given; spinal cord degeneration might also occur when folic acid is used as a substitute for vitamin B_{12} in anemia prevention. Blunted therapeutic response to vitamin B_{12} may occur in certain conditions (eg, infection, uremia, concurrent iron or folic acid deficiency) or in patients on medications with bone marrow suppressant properties (eg, chloramphenicol). Approved for use as I.M. injection only.

Cyanokit®: Use caution or consider alternatives in patients with known allergic reactions, including anaphylaxis, to hydroxocobalamin or cyanocobalamin. Increased blood pressure (≥180 mm Hg systolic or ≥110 mm Hg diastolic) is associated with infusion; elevations usually noted at beginning of infusion, peak toward the end of infusion and return to baseline within 4 hours of infusion. Collection of pretreatment blood cyanide concentrations does not preclude administration and should not delay administration in the emergency management of highly suspected or confirmed cyanide toxicity. Pretreatment levels may be useful as post infusion levels may be inaccurate. Treatment of cyanide poisoning should include decontamination and supportive therapy. Photosensitivity is a potential concern; avoid direct sunlight while skin remains discolored. Safety and efficacy have not been established in children.

Adverse Reactions

I.M. injection: Frequency not defined:

Dermatologic: Exanthema (transient), itching
Gastrointestinal: Diarrhea (mild, transient)
Local: Injection site pain
Miscellaneous: Anaphylaxis

I.V. infusion (Cyanokit®):

>10%:

Cardiovascular: Blood pressure increased (18% to 28%; systolic ≥180 mm Hg or diastolic ≥110 mm Hg)
Central nervous system: Headache (6% to 33%)
Dermatologic: Erythema (94% to 100%; may last up to 2 weeks), rash (predominantly acneiform; 20% to 44%; can appear 7-28 days after administration and usually resolves within a few weeks)
Gastrointestinal: Nausea (6% to 11%)
Genitourinary: Chromaturia (100%; may last up to 5 weeks after administration)
Hematologic: Lymphocytes decreased (8% to 17%)
Local: Infusion site reaction (6% to 39%)

Frequency not defined:

Cardiovascular: Chest discomfort, heart rate increased/decreased, hot flashes, peripheral edema
Central nervous system: Dizziness, memory impairment, restlessness
Dermatologic: Pruritus, urticaria
Gastrointestinal: Abdominal discomfort, diarrhea, dyspepsia, dysphagia, hematochezia, vomiting
Ocular: Irritation, redness, swelling
Respiratory: Dry throat, dyspnea, throat tightness
Miscellaneous: Allergic reaction (including anaphylaxis)

Postmarketing and/or case reports: Angioneurotic edema

Drug Interactions

Avoid Concomitant Use There are no known interactions where it is recommended to avoid concomitant use.

Increased Effect/Toxicity There are no known significant interactions involving an increase in effect.

Decreased Effect There are no known significant interactions involving a decrease in effect.

Stability

Solution for I.M. injection: Store at 20°C to 25°C (68°F to 77°F). Protect from light.

I.V. infusion (Cyanokit®): Prior to reconstitution, store at 15°C to 30°C (59°F to 86°F).

Temperature variation exposure allowed for transport of lyophilized form:

Usual transport: ≤15 days at 5°C to 40°C (41°F to 104°F)
Desert transport: ≤4 days at 5°C to 60°C (41°F to 140°F)
Freezing/defrosting cycles: ≤15 days at -20°C to 40°C (-4°F to 104°F)

Reconstitute each 2.5 g vial with 100 mL of NS using provided sterile transfer spike. If NS unavailable, may use LR or D_5W. Invert or rock each vial for at least 30 seconds prior to infusion; do not shake. Do not use if solution is **not** dark red. Following reconstitution, store up to 6 hours at ≤40°C (104°F); do not freeze. Discard any remaining solution after 6 hours.

Mechanism of Action Hydroxocobalamin (vitamin B_{12a}) is a precursor to cyanocobalamin (vitamin B_{12}). Cyanocobalamin acts as a coenzyme for various metabolic functions, including fat and carbohydrate metabolism and protein synthesis, used in cell replication and hematopoiesis. In the presence of cyanide, each hydroxocobalamin molecule can bind one cyanide ion by displacing it for the hydroxo ligand linked to the trivalent cobalt ion, forming cyanocobalamin.

Pharmacodynamics/Kinetics Following I.V. administration of Cyanokit®:

Protein binding: Significant; forms various cobalamin-(III) complexes

Half-life elimination: 26-31 hours

Excretion: Urine (50% to 60% within initial 72 hours)

Dosage

Vitamin B_{12} deficiency: I.M.:

Children: 100 mcg once daily for 2 or more weeks (total dose: 1-5 mg); maintenance: 30-50 mcg/month

Adults: 30 mcg/day for 5-10 days, followed by 100-200 mcg/month

Note: Larger doses may be required in critically-ill patients or if patient has neurologic disease, an infectious disease, or hyperthyroidism.

Schilling test: I.M.: Adults: 1000 mcg

Cyanide toxicity (Cyanokit®): I.V.: Adults: Initial: 5 g as single infusion; may repeat a second 5 g dose depending on severity of poisoning and clinical response. Maximum cumulative dose: 10 g. **Note:** If suspected, antidotal therapy must be given immediately.

Administration

Solution for I.M. injection: Administer 1000 mcg/mL solution I.M. only

Cyanokit®: Administer by I.V. infusion over 15 minutes; if repeat dose needed, administer second dose over 15 minutes to 2 hours

Monitoring Parameters Vitamin B_{12}, hematocrit, hemoglobin, reticulocyte count, red blood cell counts, folate and iron levels should be obtained prior to treatment and periodically during treatment.

Cyanide toxicity: Blood pressure and heart rate during and after infusion, serum lactate levels, venous-arterial PO_2 gradient. Pretreatment levels may be useful as post infusion levels may be inaccurate.

Megaloblastic anemia: In addition to normal hematological parameters, serum potassium and platelet counts should be monitored during therapy, particularly in the first 48 hours of treatment.

Reference Range Blood cyanide levels may be used for diagnosis confirmation; however, reliable levels require prompt testing and proper storage conditions.

Cyanide level:

Tachycardia/flushing: 0.5-1 mg/L

Obtundation: 1-2.5 mg/L

Coma: 2.5-3 mg/L

Death: >3 mg/L

Test Interactions The following values may be affected, *in vitro*, following hydroxocobalamin 5 g dose. Interference following hydroxocobalamin 10 g dose can be expected to last up to an additional 24 hours. **Note:** Extent and duration of interference dependant on analyzer used and patient variability.

Falsely elevated:

Basophils, hemoglobin, MCH, and MCHC [duration: 12-16 hours]

Albumin, alkaline phosphatase, cholesterol, creatinine, glucose, total protein, and triglycerides [duration: 24 hours]

Bilirubin [duration: up to 4 days]

Urinalysis: Glucose, protein, erythrocytes, leukocytes, ketones, bilirubin, urobilinogen, nitrite [duration: 2-8 days]

Falsely decreased: ALT and amylase [duration: 24 hours]

Unpredictable:

AST, CK, CKMB, LDH, phosphate, and uric acid [duration: 24 hours]

PT (quick or INR) and aPTT [duration: 24-48 hours]

Urine pH [duration: 2-8 days]

May also interfere with colorimetric tests

Additional Information Expert advice from a regional poison control center for appropriate use may be obtained (1-800-222-1222). Cyanide is a clear colorless gas or liquid with a faint bitter almond odor. Cyanide reacts with trivalent ions in cytochrome oxidase in the mitochondria leading to histotoxic hypoxia and lactic acidosis. Signs and symptoms of cyanide toxicity include headache, altered mental status, dyspnea, mydriasis, chest tightness, nausea, vomiting, tachycardia/hypertension (initially), bradycardia/hypotension (later), seizures, cardiovascular collapse, or coma.

Dosage Forms Excipient information presented when available (limited, particularly for generics); consult specific product labeling.

Injection, solution: 1000 mcg/mL (30 mL)

Injection, powder for reconstitution:

Cyanokit®: 2.5 g (2 vials) [provided in a kit which also contains one I.V. infusion set]

◆ **4-Hydroxybutyrate** *see* Sodium Oxybate *on page 1384*

◆ **Hydroxycarbamide** *see* Hydroxyurea *on page 753*

Hydroxychloroquine (hye droks ee KLOR oh kwin)

U.S. Brand Names Plaquenil®

Canadian Brand Names Apo-Hydroxyquine®; Gen-Hydroxychloroquine; Plaquenil®; Pro-Hydroxyquine

Index Terms Hydroxychloroquine Sulfate

Pharmacologic Category Aminoquinoline (Antimalarial)

Use Suppression and treatment of acute attacks of malaria; treatment of systemic lupus erythematosus (SLE) and rheumatoid arthritis

Unlabeled/Investigational Use Porphyria cutanea tarda, polymorphous light eruptions

Pregnancy Considerations Malaria infection in pregnant women may be more severe than in nonpregnant women. Therefore, pregnant women and women who are likely to become pregnant are advised to avoid travel to malaria-risk areas. Hydroxychloroquine is recommended as an alternative treatment of pregnant women for uncomplicated malaria in chloroquine-sensitive regions. Women exposed to hydroxychloroquine for the treatment of rheumatoid arthritis or systemic lupus erythematosus during pregnancy may be enrolled in the Organization of Teratology Information Specialists (OTIS) Autoimmune Diseases Study pregnancy registry (877-311-8972).

Lactation Enters breast milk (AAP considers "compatible")

Medication Safety Issues

Sound-alike/look-alike issues:

Hydroxychloroquine may be confused with hydrocortisone

Plaquenil® may be confused with Platinol®

Contraindications Hypersensitivity to hydroxychloroquine, 4-aminoquinoline derivatives, or any component of the formulation; retinal or visual field changes attributable to 4-aminoquinolines; long-term use in children

Warnings/Precautions May cause ophthalmic adverse effects or neuromyopathy; perform baseline and periodic (every 3 months) ophthalmologic examinations; test periodically for muscle weakness. Rare cardiomyopathy has been associated with long-term use of hydroxychloroquine. Aminoquinolines have been associated with rare hematologic reactions, including agranulocytosis, aplastic anemia, and thrombocytopenia; monitoring (CBC) is recommended in prolonged therapy. Use with caution in patients with hepatic disease, G6PD deficiency, psoriasis, and porphyria. Use caution in children due to increased sensitivity to adverse effects (long-term use in children is contraindicated). Not effective in the treatment of malaria caused by chloroquine resistant *P. falciparum*. **[U.S. Boxed Warning]: Should be prescribed by physicians familiar with its use.**

Adverse Reactions Frequency not defined.

Cardiovascular: Cardiomyopathy (rare, relationship to hydroxychloroquine unclear)

Central nervous system: Ataxia, dizziness, emotional changes, headache, irritability, lassitude, nervousness, nightmares, psychosis, seizure, vertigo

Dermatologic: Alopecia, angioedema, bleaching of hair, pigmentation changes (skin and mucosal; black-blue color), rash (acute generalized exanthematous pustulosis, erythema annulare centrifugum, exfoliative dermatitis, lichenoid, maculopapular, morbilliform, purpuric, Stevens-Johnson syndrome, urticarial), urticaria

Endocrine & metabolic: Weight loss

Gastrointestinal: Abdominal cramping, anorexia, diarrhea, nausea, vomiting

Hematologic: Agranulocytosis, aplastic anemia, hemolysis (in patients with glucose-6-phosphate deficiency), leukopenia, thrombocytopenia

Hepatic: Abnormal liver function/hepatic failure (isolated cases)

Neuromuscular & skeletal: Myopathy, palsy, or neuromyopathy leading to progressive weakness and atrophy of proximal muscle groups (may be associated with mild sensory changes, loss of deep tendon reflexes, and abnormal nerve conduction)

Ocular: Abnormal color vision, abnormal retinal pigmentation, atrophy, attenuation of retinal arterioles, decreased visual acuity, disturbance in accommodation, keratopathy, corneal changes/deposits (visual disturbances, blurred vision, photophobia [reversible on discontinuation]), macular edema, nystagmus, optic disc pallor/atrophy, pigmentary retinopathy, retinopathy (early changes reversible [may progress despite discontinuation if advanced]), scotoma

Otic: Deafness, tinnitus

Miscellaneous: Exacerbation of porphyria and nonlight sensitive psoriasis

Respiratory: Bronchospasm, respiratory failure (myopathy-related)

Drug Interactions

Avoid Concomitant Use

Avoid concomitant use of Hydroxychloroquine with any of the following: Mefloquine

Increased Effect/Toxicity

Hydroxychloroquine may increase the levels/effects of: Antipsychotic Agents (Phenothiazines); Beta-Blockers; Cardiac Glycosides; Mefloquine

The levels/effects of Hydroxychloroquine may be increased by: Mefloquine

Decreased Effect

Hydroxychloroquine may decrease the levels/effects of: Anthelmintics

Ethanol/Nutrition/Herb Interactions Ethanol: Avoid ethanol (due to GI irritation).

Mechanism of Action Interferes with digestive vacuole function within sensitive malarial parasites by increasing the pH and interfering with lysosomal degradation of hemoglobin; inhibits locomotion of neutrophils and chemotaxis of eosinophils; impairs complement-dependent antigen-antibody reactions

Pharmacodynamics/Kinetics

Onset of action: Rheumatic disease: May require 4-6 weeks to respond

Absorption: Rapid and complete

Protein binding: 55%

Metabolism: Hepatic

Half-life elimination: 32-50 days

Time to peak: Rheumatic disease: Several months

Excretion: Urine (as metabolites and unchanged drug); may be enhanced by urinary acidification

Dosage Note: Hydroxychloroquine sulfate 200 mg is equivalent to 155 mg hydroxychloroquine base and 250 mg chloroquine phosphate. Second-line alternative treatment (chloroquine is preferred). Oral:

Children:

Chemoprophylaxis of malaria: 5 mg/kg (base) once weekly; should not exceed the recommended adult dose; begin 2 weeks before exposure; continue for 4 weeks (per CDC guidelines) after leaving endemic area; if suppressive therapy is not begun prior to the exposure, double the initial dose and give in 2 doses, 6 hours apart and continue treatment for 8 weeks

Acute attack: 10 mg/kg (base) initially, followed by 5 mg/kg at 6, 24, and 48 hours

JRA or SLE (unlabeled use): 3-5 mg/kg/day divided 1-2 times/day; avoid exceeding 7 mg/kg/day

Adults:

Chemoprophylaxis of malaria: 310 mg (base) weekly on same day each week; begin 2 weeks before exposure; continue for 4 weeks (per CDC guidelines) after leaving endemic area; if suppressive therapy is not begun prior to the exposure, double the initial dose and give in 2 doses, 6 hours apart and continue treatment for 8 weeks

Acute attack: 620 mg (base) initially, followed by 310 mg (base) at 6, 24, and 48 hours

Rheumatoid arthritis: Initial: 310-465 mg/day (base) taken with food or milk; increase dose gradually until optimum response level is reached; usually after 4-12 weeks dose should be reduced by 1/2 to a maintenance dose of 155-310 mg/day (base)

Lupus erythematosus: 310 mg (base) every day or twice daily for several weeks-months depending on response; 155-310 mg/day (base) for prolonged maintenance therapy

Dietary Considerations May be taken with food or milk.

Administration Administer with food or milk

Monitoring Parameters Ophthalmologic exam at baseline and every 3 months during prolonged therapy (including visual acuity, slit-lamp, fundoscopic, and visual field exam); CBC at baseline and periodically; muscle strength (especially proximal, as a symptom of neuromyopathy) during long-term therapy

Dosage Forms Excipient information presented when available (limited, particularly for generics); consult specific product labeling.

Tablet, as sulfate: 200 mg [equivalent to 155 mg base]

Extemporaneous Preparations A 25 mg/mL hydroxychloroquine sulfate suspension is made by removing the coating off of fifteen 200 mg hydroxychloroquine sulfate tablets with a towel moistened with alcohol; tablets are ground to a fine powder and levigated to a paste with 15 mL of Ora-Plus® suspending agent; add an additional 45 mL of suspending agent and levigate until a uniform mixture is obtained; qs ad to 120 mL with sterile water for irrigation; a 30 day expiration date is recommended, although stability testing has not been performed

Pesko LJ, "Compounding: Hydroxychloroquine," *Am Druggist*, 1993, 207:57.

- **Hydroxychloroquine Sulfate** *see* Hydroxychloroquine *on page 751*
- **Hydroxydaunomycin Hydrochloride** *see* DOXOrubicin *on page 486*
- **1α-Hydroxyergocalciferol** *see* Doxercalciferol *on page 486*
- **Hydroxyethyl Starch** *see* Hetastarch *on page 731*
- **Hydroxyldaunorubicin Hydrochloride** *see* DOXOrubicin *on page 486*
- **9-hydroxy-risperidone** *see* Paliperidone *on page 1130*

Hydroxyurea (hye droks ee yoor EE a)

U.S. Brand Names Droxia®; Hydrea®; Mylocel™

Canadian Brand Names Apo-Hydroxyurea®; Gen-Hydroxyurea; Hydrea®

Index Terms Hydroxycarbamide

Pharmacologic Category Antineoplastic Agent, Antimetabolite

Use Treatment of melanoma, refractory chronic myelocytic leukemia (CML), relapsed and refractory metastatic ovarian cancer; radiosensitizing agent in the treatment of squamous cell head and neck cancer (excluding lip cancer); adjunct in the management of sickle cell patients who have had at least three painful crises in the previous 12 months (to reduce frequency of these crises and the need for blood transfusions)

Unlabeled/Investigational Use Treatment of HIV; treatment of psoriasis, treatment of hematologic conditions such as essential thrombocythemia, polycythemia vera, hypereosinophilia, and hyperleukocytosis due to acute leukemia; treatment of uterine, cervix and nonsmall cell lung cancers; radiosensitizing agent in the treatment of primary brain tumors; has shown activity against renal cell cancer and prostate cancer

Pregnancy Risk Factor D

Pregnancy Considerations Animal studies have demonstrated teratogenicity and embryotoxicity. There are no adequate and well-controlled studies in pregnant women. Women of childbearing potential should be advised to avoid pregnancy.

Lactation Enters breast milk/contraindicated

Medication Safety Issues

Sound-alike/look-alike issues:

Hydroxyurea may be confused with hydrOXYzine

High alert medication: The Institute for Safe Medication Practices (ISMP) includes this medication among its list of drugs which have a heightened risk of causing significant patient harm when used in error.

International issues:

Hydrea® may be confused with Hydra® which is a brand name for isoniazid in Japan

Contraindications Hypersensitivity to hydroxyurea or any component of the formulation; severe anemia; severe bone marrow suppression; WBC <2500/mm^3 or platelet count <100,000/mm^3 (neutrophils <2000/mm^3, platelets <80,000/mm^3, and hemoglobin <4.5 g/dL for sickle cell anemia); pregnancy

Warnings/Precautions Hazardous agent - use appropriate precautions for handling and disposal. Patients with a history of prior cytotoxic chemotherapy and radiation therapy are more likely to experience bone marrow depression. Patients with a history of radiation therapy are also at risk for exacerbation of post irradiation erythema. Megaloblastic erythropoiesis may be seen early in hydroxyurea treatment; plasma iron clearance may be delayed and the rate of utilization of iron by erythrocytes may be delayed. HIV-infected patients treated with hydroxyurea and antiretroviral agents (including didanosine) are at higher risk for potentially fatal pancreatitis, hepatotoxicity, hepatic failure, and severe peripheral neuropathy. **[U.S. Boxed Warning]: Hydroxyurea is mutagenic and clastogenic. Treatment of myeloproliferative disorders (polycythemia vera and thrombocythemia) with long-term hydroxyurea is associated with secondary leukemia**; it is unknown if this is drug-related or disease-related. Cutaneous vasculitic toxicities (vasculitic ulceration and gangrene) have been reported with hydroxyurea treatment, most often in patients with a history of or receiving concurrent interferon therapy; discontinue hydroxyurea and consider alternate cytoreductive therapy if cutaneous vasculitic toxicity develops. Use caution with renal dysfunction; may require dose reductions. **[U.S. Boxed Warning]: Should be administered under the supervision of a physician experienced in cancer chemotherapy or in the treatment of sickle cell anemia.**

Adverse Reactions Frequency not defined.

Cardiovascular: Edema

Central nervous system: Chills, disorientation, dizziness, drowsiness (dose-related), fever, hallucinations, headache, malaise, seizure

Dermatologic: Alopecia (rare), cutaneous vasculitic toxicities, dermatomyositis-like skin changes, dry skin, facial erythema, gangrene, hyperpigmentation, maculopapular rash, nail atrophy, nail pigmentation, peripheral erythema, scaling, skin atrophy, skin cancer, skin ulcer, vasculitis ulcerations, violet papules

Endocrine & metabolic: Hyperuricemia

Gastrointestinal: Anorexia, constipation, diarrhea, gastrointestinal irritation and mucositis, (potentiated with radiation therapy), nausea, pancreatitis, stomatitis, vomiting

Genitourinary: Dysuria (rare)

Hematologic: Myelosuppression (primarily leukopenia; onset: 24-48 hours; nadir: 10 days; recovery: 7 days after stopping drug; reversal of WBC count occurs rapidly but the platelet count may take 7-10 days to recover); thrombocytopenia and anemia, megaloblastic erythropoiesis, macrocytosis, hemolysis, serum iron decreased, persistent cytopenias, secondary leukemias (long-term use)

Hepatic: Hepatic enzymes increased, hepatotoxicity

Neuromuscular & skeletal: Peripheral neuropathy, weakness

Renal: BUN increased, creatinine increased

Respiratory: Acute diffuse pulmonary infiltrates (rare), dyspnea, pulmonary fibrosis (rare)

Drug Interactions

Avoid Concomitant Use

Avoid concomitant use of Hydroxyurea with any of the following: Natalizumab; Vaccines (Live)

Increased Effect/Toxicity

Hydroxyurea may increase the levels/effects of: Natalizumab; Vaccines (Live)

The levels/effects of Hydroxyurea may be increased by: Didanosine; Trastuzumab

Decreased Effect

Hydroxyurea may decrease the levels/effects of: Vaccines (Inactivated)

The levels/effects of Hydroxyurea may be decreased by: Echinacea

Stability Store at room temperature between 15°C and 30°C (59°F and 86°F).

Mechanism of Action Thought to interfere (unsubstantiated hypothesis) with synthesis of DNA, during the S phase of cell division, without interfering with RNA synthesis; inhibits ribonucleoside diphosphate reductase, preventing conversion of ribonucleotides to deoxyribonucleotides; cell-cycle specific for the S phase and may hold other cells in the G_1 phase of the cell cycle. In sickle cell anemia, hydroxyurea increases red blood cell (RBC) hemoglobin F levels, RBC water content, deformability of sickled cells, and alters adhesion of RBCs to endothelium.

Pharmacodynamics/Kinetics

Absorption: Readily (≥80%)

Distribution: Readily crosses blood-brain barrier; distributes into intestine, brain, lung, kidney tissues, effusions and ascites

Metabolism: 60% via hepatic and GI tract

Half-life elimination: 3-4 hours

Time to peak: 1-4 hours

Excretion: Urine (80%, 50% as unchanged drug, 30% as urea); exhaled gases (as CO_2)

Dosage Oral (refer to individual protocols): All doses should be based on ideal or actual body weight, whichever is less:

Children (unlabeled use):

No FDA-approved dosage regimens have been established; dosages of 1500-3000 mg/m^2 as a single dose in combination with other agents every 4-6 weeks have been used in the treatment of pediatric astrocytoma, medulloblastoma, and primitive neuroectodermal tumors

CML: Initial: 10-20 mg/kg/day once daily; adjust dose according to hematologic response

Adults: Dose should always be titrated to patient response and WBC counts; usual oral doses range from 10-30 mg/kg/day or 500-3000 mg/day; if WBC count falls to <2500 cells/mm^3, or the platelet count to <100,000/mm^3, therapy should be stopped for at least 3 days and resumed when values rise toward normal

Solid tumors:

Intermittent therapy: 80 mg/kg as a single dose every third day

Continuous therapy: 20-30 mg/kg/day given as a single dose/day

Concomitant therapy with irradiation: 80 mg/kg as a single dose every third day starting at least 7 days before initiation of irradiation

Resistant chronic myelocytic leukemia: Continuous therapy: 20-30 mg/kg once daily

HIV (unlabeled use; in combination with antiretroviral agents): 1000-1500 mg daily in a single dose or divided doses

Psoriasis (unlabeled use): 1000-1500 mg/day in a single dose or divided doses

Sickle cell anemia (moderate/severe disease): Initial: 15 mg/kg/day, increased by 5 mg/kg every 12 weeks if blood counts are in an acceptable range until the maximum tolerated dose of 35 mg/kg/day is achieved or the dose that does not produce toxic effects

Acceptable range:

Neutrophils ≥2500 cells/mm^3

Platelets ≥95,000/mm^3

Hemoglobin >5.3 g/dL, and

Reticulocytes ≥95,000/mm^3 if the hemoglobin concentration is <9 g/dL

Toxic range:

Neutrophils <2000 cells/mm^3

Platelets <80,000/mm^3

Hemoglobin <4.5 g/dL

Reticulocytes <80,000/mm^3 if the hemoglobin concentration is <9 g/dL

Monitor for toxicity every 2 weeks; if toxicity occurs, stop treatment until the bone marrow recovers; restart at 2.5 mg/kg/day less than the dose at which toxicity occurs; if no toxicity occurs over the next 12 weeks, then the subsequent dose should be increased by 2.5 mg/kg/day; reduced dosage of hydroxyurea alternating with erythropoietin may decrease myelotoxicity and increase levels of fetal hemoglobin in patients who have not been helped by hydroxyurea alone

Dosing adjustment in renal impairment:

The FDA-approved labeling recommends the following adjustment:

Sickle cell anemia: Cl_{cr} <60 mL/minute or ESRD: Reduce initial dose to 7.5 mg/kg; titrate to response/avoidance of toxicity (refer to usual dosing).

Other indications: It is recommended to reduce the initial dose; however, no specific guidelines are available.

The following guidelines have been used by some clinicians:

Aronoff, 2007: Adults:

Cl_{cr} 10-50 mL/minute: Administer 50% of dose

Cl_{cr} <10 mL/minute: Administer 20% of dose

Hemodialysis: Administer dose after dialysis on dialysis days; supplemental dose is not necessary. Hydroxyurea is a low molecular weight compound with high aqueous solubility that may be freely dialyzable, however, clinical studies confirming this hypothesis have not been performed.

Continuous renal replacement therapy (CRRT): Administer 50% of dose

Kintzel, 1995:

Cl_{cr} 46-60 mL/minute: Administer 85% of dose

Cl_{cr} 31-45 mL/minute: Administer 80% of dose

Cl_{cr} <30 mL/minute: Administer 75% of dose

Dosing adjustment in hepatic impairment: Specific guidelines are not available for dosage adjustment in hepatic impairment. The FDA-approved labeling recommends closely monitoring for bone marrow toxicity in patients with hepatic impairment.

Dietary Considerations In sickle cell patients, supplemental administration of folic acid is recommended; hydroxyurea may mask development of folic acid deficiency.

Administration Capsules may be opened and emptied into water (will not dissolve completely); observe proper handling procedures

Monitoring Parameters CBC with differential and platelets, renal function and liver function tests, serum uric acid

Sickle cell disease: Monitor for toxicity every 2 weeks. If toxicity occurs, stop treatment until the bone marrow recovers; restart at 2.5 mg/kg/day less than the dose at which toxicity occurs. If no toxicity occurs over the next 12 weeks, then the subsequent dose should be increased by 2.5 mg/kg/day. Reduced dosage of hydroxyurea alternating with erythropoietin may decrease myelotoxicity and increase levels of fetal hemoglobin in patients who have not been helped by hydroxyurea alone.

Acceptable range: Neutrophils ≥2500 cells/mm^3, platelets ≥95,000/mm^3, hemoglobin >5.3 g/dL, and reticulocytes ≥95,000/mm^3 if the hemoglobin concentration is <9 g/dL

Toxic range: Neutrophils <2000 cells/mm^3, platelets <80,000/mm^3, hemoglobin <4.5 g/dL, and reticulocytes <80,000/mm^3 if the hemoglobin concentration is <9 g/dL

Additional Information Although I.V. use is reported, no parenteral product is commercially available in the U.S.

If WBC decreases to <2500/mm^3 or platelet count to <100,000/mm^3 (neutrophils <2000/mm^3 and platelets <80,000/mm^3 for patients with sickle cell anemia), interrupt therapy until values rise significantly toward normal. Treat anemia with whole blood replacement; do not interrupt therapy (for sickle cell anemia patients, withhold treatment for hemoglobin <4.5 g/dL until recovery to >5.3 g/dL). Adequate trial period to determine the antineoplastic effectiveness is 6 weeks. Almost all patients receiving hydroxyurea in clinical trials needed to have their medication stopped for a time to allow their low blood count to return to acceptable levels.

Dosage Forms Excipient information presented when available (limited, particularly for generics); consult specific product labeling.

Capsule: 500 mg

Droxia®: 200 mg, 300 mg, 400 mg

Hydrea®: 500 mg

Tablet:

Mylocel™: 1000 mg

HydrOXYzine (hye DROKS i zeen)

U.S. Brand Names Vistaril®

Canadian Brand Names Apo-Hydroxyzine®; Atarax®; Hydroxyzine Hydrochloride Injection, USP; Novo-Hydroxyzin; PMS-Hydroxyzine; Vistaril®

Index Terms Hydroxyzine Hydrochloride; Hydroxyzine Pamoate

Pharmacologic Category Antiemetic; Histamine H_1 Antagonist; Histamine H_1 Antagonist, First Generation

Use Treatment of anxiety; preoperative sedative; antipruritic

Unlabeled/Investigational Use Antiemetic; ethanol withdrawal symptoms

Pregnancy Risk Factor C

Pregnancy Considerations Hydroxyzine-induced fetal abnormalities at high dosages in animal studies. Neonatal withdrawal symptoms have been reported following long-term maternal use or the use of large doses near term. Use in early pregnancy is contraindicated by the manufacturer.

Lactation Excretion in breast milk unknown/not recommended

Medication Safety Issues

Sound-alike/look-alike issues:

HydrOXYzine may be confused with hydrALAZINE, hydroxyurea

Atarax® may be confused with amoxicillin, Ativan®

Vistaril® may be confused with Restoril®, Versed, Zestril®

International issues:

Vistaril® may be confused with Vastarel® which is a brand name for trimetazidine in multiple international markets

Contraindications Hypersensitivity to hydroxyzine or any component of the formulation; early pregnancy; SubQ, intra-arterial, or I.V. administration of injection

Warnings/Precautions Causes sedation, caution must be used in performing tasks which require alertness (eg, operating machinery or driving). Sedative effects of CNS depressants or ethanol are potentiated. SubQ, I.V., and intra-arterial administration are contraindicated since tissue damage, intravascular hemolysis, thrombosis, and digital gangrene can occur. Use with caution with narrow-angle glaucoma, prostatic hyperplasia, bladder neck obstruction, asthma, or COPD.

Anticholinergic effects are not well tolerated in the elderly. Hydroxyzine may be useful as a short-term antipruritic, but it is not recommended for use as a sedative or anxiolytic in the elderly.

Adverse Reactions Frequency not defined.

Central nervous system: Dizziness, drowsiness, fatigue, hallucination, headache, nervousness, seizure

Dermatologic: Pruritus, rash, urticaria

Gastrointestinal: Xerostomia

Neuromuscular & skeletal: Involuntary movements, paresthesia, tremor

Ocular: Blurred vision

Respiratory: Thickening of bronchial secretions

Miscellaneous: Allergic reaction

Drug Interactions

Metabolism/Transport Effects **Inhibits** CYP2D6 (weak)

Avoid Concomitant Use There are no known interactions where it is recommended to avoid concomitant use.

Increased Effect/Toxicity

HydrOXYzine may increase the levels/effects of: Alcohol (Ethyl); Anticholinergics; CNS Depressants

The levels/effects of HydrOXYzine may be increased by: Pramlintide

Decreased Effect

HydrOXYzine may decrease the levels/effects of: Acetylcholinesterase Inhibitors (Central); Betahistine

The levels/effects of HydrOXYzine may be decreased by: Acetylcholinesterase Inhibitors (Central); Amphetamines

Ethanol/Nutrition/Herb Interactions

Ethanol: Avoid ethanol (may increase CNS depression).

Herb/Nutraceutical: Avoid valerian, St John's wort, kava kava, gotu kola (may increase CNS depression).

Stability Injection: Store at 15°C to 30°C. Protect from light.

Mechanism of Action Competes with histamine for H_1-receptor sites on effector cells in the gastrointestinal tract, blood vessels, and respiratory tract. Possesses skeletal muscle relaxing, bronchodilator, antihistamine, antiemetic, and analgesic properties.

Pharmacodynamics/Kinetics

Onset of action: Oral: 15-30 minutes

Duration: 4-6 hours

Absorption: Oral: Rapid

Metabolism: Forms metabolites

Half-life elimination: 3-7 hours

Time to peak: ~2 hours

Excretion: Urine

Dosage

Children:

Preoperative sedation:

Oral: 0.6 mg/kg/dose

I.M.: 0.5-1 mg/kg/dose

Pruritus, anxiety: Oral:

<6 years: 50 mg daily in divided doses

≥6 years: 50-100 mg daily in divided doses

Adults:

Antiemetic (unlabeled use): I.M.: 25-100 mg/dose every 4-6 hours as needed

Anxiety: Oral, I.M.: 50-100 mg 4 times/day

Preoperative sedation:

Oral: 50-100 mg

I.M.: 25-100 mg

Pruritus: Oral, I.M.: 25 mg 3-4 times/day

Dosing interval in hepatic impairment: Change dosing interval to every 24 hours in patients with primary biliary cirrhosis

Administration Do not administer SubQ or intra-arterially. Administer I.M. deep in large muscle. With I.V. administration, extravasation can result in sterile abscess and marked tissue induration.

Monitoring Parameters Relief of symptoms, mental status, blood pressure

Dosage Forms Excipient information presented when available (limited, particularly for generics); consult specific product labeling. [DSC] = Discontinued product

Capsule, as pamoate: 25 mg, 50 mg, 100 mg

Vistaril®: 25 mg, 50 mg

Injection, solution, as hydrochloride: 25 mg/mL (1 mL); 50 mg/mL (1 mL, 2 mL, 10 mL)

Suspension, oral, as pamoate:

Vistaril®: 25 mg/5 mL (120 mL, 480 mL) [lemon flavor] [DSC]

Syrup, as hydrochloride: 10 mg/5 mL (120 mL, 480 mL)

Tablet, as hydrochloride: 10 mg, 25 mg, 50 mg

- **Hydroxyzine Hydrochloride** *see* HydrOXYzine *on page 754*
- **Hydroxyzine Hydrochloride Injection, USP (Can)** *see* HydrOXYzine *on page 754*
- **Hydroxyzine Pamoate** *see* HydrOXYzine *on page 754*
- **HydroZone Plus [OTC]** *see* Hydrocortisone *on page 743*
- **Hyflex-DS® [DSC]** *see* Acetaminophen and Phenyltoloxamine *on page 29*
- **Hygroton** *see* Chlorthalidone *on page 318*
- **Hylaform®** *see* Hyaluronate and Derivatives *on page 734*
- **Hylaform® Plus** *see* Hyaluronate and Derivatives *on page 734*

Hyoscyamine (hye oh SYE a meen)

U.S. Brand Names Anaspaz®; Cystospaz®; Hyosyne; Levbid®; Levsin®; Levsin®/SL; NuLev™ [DSC]; Spacol T/S [DSC]; Spacol [DSC]; Symax SL; Symax SR

Canadian Brand Names Cystospaz®; Levsin®

Index Terms *l*-Hyoscyamine Sulfate; Hyoscyamine Sulfate

Pharmacologic Category Anticholinergic Agent

Use

Oral: Adjunctive therapy for peptic ulcers, irritable bowel, neurogenic bladder/bowel; treatment of infant colic, GI tract disorders caused by spasm; to reduce rigidity, tremors, sialorrhea, and hyperhidrosis associated with parkinsonism; as a drying agent in acute rhinitis

Injection: Preoperative antimuscarinic to reduce secretions and block cardiac vagal inhibitory reflexes; to improve radiologic visibility of the kidneys; symptomatic relief of biliary and renal colic; reduce GI motility to facilitate diagnostic procedures (ie, endoscopy, hypotonic duodenography); reduce pain and hypersecretion in pancreatitis, certain cases of partial heart block associated with vagal activity; reversal of neuromuscular blockade

Pregnancy Risk Factor C

Medication Safety Issues

Sound-alike/look-alike issues:

Anaspaz® may be confused with Anaprox®, Antispas®

Levbid® may be confused with Lithobid®, Lopid®, Lorabid®

Levsinex® may be confused with Lanoxin®

Levsin/SL® maybe confused with Levaquin®

Dosage

Oral: Children: Gastrointestinal disorders: Dose as listed, based on age and weight (kg) using 0.125 mg/mL drops; repeat dose every 4 hours as needed:

Children <2 years:

3.4 kg: 4 drops; maximum: 24 drops/24 hours

5 kg: 5 drops; maximum: 30 drops/24 hours

7 kg: 6 drops; maximum: 36 drops/24 hours

10 kg: 8 drops; maximum: 48 drops/24 hours

Oral, S.L.:

Children 2-12 years: Gastrointestinal disorders: Dose as listed, based on age and weight (kg); repeat dose every 4 hours as needed:

10 kg: 0.031-0.033 mg; maximum: 0.75 mg/24 hours

20 kg: 0.0625 mg; maximum: 0.75 mg/24 hours

40 kg: 0.0938 mg; maximum: 0.75 mg/24 hours

50 kg: 0.125 mg; maximum: 0.75 mg/24 hours

Children >12 years and Adults: Gastrointestinal disorders: 0.125-0.25 mg every 4 hours or as needed (before meals or food); maximum: 1.5 mg/24 hours

Cystospaz®: 0.15-0.3 mg up to 4 times/day

Oral (timed release): Children >12 years and Adults: Gastrointestinal disorders: 0.375-0.75 mg every 12 hours; maximum: 1.5 mg/24 hours

I.M., I.V., SubQ: Children >12 years and Adults: Gastrointestinal disorders: 0.25-0.5 mg; may repeat as needed up to 4 times/day, at 4-hour intervals

I.V.: Children >2 year and Adults: I.V.: Preanesthesia: 5 mcg/kg given 30-60 minutes prior to induction of anesthesia or at the time preoperative narcotics or sedatives are administered

I.V.: Adults: Diagnostic procedures: 0.25-0.5 mg given 5-10 minutes prior to procedure

To reduce drug-induced bradycardia during surgery: 0.125 mg; repeat as needed

To reverse neuromuscular blockade: 0.2 mg for every 1 mg neostigmine (or the physostigmine/pyridostigmine equivalent)

Additional Information Complete prescribing information for this medication should be consulted for additional detail.

Dosage Forms Excipient information presented when available (limited, particularly for generics); consult specific product labeling. [DSC] = Discontinued product

Capsule, timed release, as sulfate: 0.375 mg

Elixir, as sulfate: 0.125 mg/5 mL (480 mL)

Hyosyne: 0.125 mg/5 mL (480 mL) [contains ethanol 20% and sodium benzoate; orange flavor]

Levsin®: 0.125 mg/5 mL (480 mL) [contains ethanol 20%; orange flavor]

Injection, solution, as sulfate: 0.5 mg/mL (1 mL)

Levsin®: 0.5 mg/mL (1 mL)

Solution, oral, as sulfate [drops]: 0.125 mg/mL (15 mL)

Hyosyne: 0.125 mg/mL (15 mL) [contains ethanol 5% and sodium benzoate; orange flavor]

Levsin®: 0.125 mg/mL (15 mL) [contains ethanol 5%; orange flavor]

Tablet:

Cystospaz®: 0.15 mg [DSC]

Tablet, as sulfate: 0.125 mg

Anaspaz®: 0.125 mg

Levsin®: 0.125 mg

Tablet, extended release, as sulfate: 0.375 mg

Levbid®: 0.375 mg

Symax SR: 0.375 mg

Tablet, orally disintegrating, as sulfate: 0.125 mg

NuLev™: 0.125 mg [contains phenylalanine 1.7 mg/tablet, mint flavor] [DSC]

Tablet, sublingual, as sulfate: 0.125 mg

Levsin®/SL: 0.125 mg

Symax SL: 0.125 mg

Hyoscyamine, Atropine, Scopolamine, and Phenobarbital

(hye oh SYE a meen, A troe peen, skoe POL a meen, & fee noe BAR bi tal)

U.S. Brand Names Donnatal Extentabs®; Donnatal®

Index Terms Atropine, Hyoscyamine, Scopolamine, and Phenobarbital; Belladonna Alkaloids With Phenobarbital; Phenobarbital, Hyoscyamine, Atropine, and Scopolamine; Scopolamine, Hyoscyamine, Atropine, and Phenobarbital

Pharmacologic Category Anticholinergic Agent; Antispasmodic Agent, Gastrointestinal

Use Adjunct in treatment of irritable bowel syndrome, acute enterocolitis, duodenal ulcer

Pregnancy Risk Factor C

Medication Safety Issues

Sound-alike/look-alike issues:

Donnatal® may be confused with Donnagel®

Dosage Oral:

Children: Donnatal® elixir: To be given every 4-6 hours; initial dose based on weight:

4.5 kg: 0.5 mL every 4 hours **or** 0.75 mL every 6 hours

10 kg: 1 mL every 4 hours **or** 1.5 mL every 6 hours

14 kg: 1.5 mL every 4 hours **or** 2 mL every 6 hours

23 kg: 2.5 mL every 4 hours **or** 3.8 mL every 6 hours

34 kg: 3.8 mL every 4 hours **or** 5 mL every 6 hours

≥45 kg: 5 mL every 4 hours **or** 7.5 mL every 6 hours

Adults:

Donnatal®: 1-2 tablets or 5-10 mL of elixir 3-4 times/day

Donnatal Extentabs®: 1 tablet every 12 hours; may increase to 1 tablet every 8 hours if needed

Additional Information Complete prescribing information for this medication should be consulted for additional detail.

Dosage Forms Excipient information presented when available (limited, particularly for generics); consult specific product labeling.

Elixir:

Donnatal®: Hyoscyamine sulfate 0.1037 mg, atropine sulfate 0.0194 mg, scopolamine hydrobromide 0.0065 mg, and phenobarbital 16.2 mg per 5 mL (120 mL, 480 mL) [contains alcohol 95%; grape flavor]

Tablet: Hyoscyamine sulfate 0.1037 mg, atropine sulfate 0.0194 mg, scopolamine hydrobromide 0.0065 mg, and phenobarbital 16.2 mg

Donnatal®: Hyoscyamine sulfate 0.1037 mg, atropine sulfate 0.0194 mg, scopolamine hydrobromide 0.0065 mg, and phenobarbital 16.2 mg

Tablet, extended release:

Donnatal Extentabs®: Hyoscyamine sulfate 0.3111 mg, atropine sulfate 0.0582 mg, scopolamine hydrobromide 0.0195 mg, and phenobarbital 48.6 mg

- **Hyoscyamine, Methenamine, Benzoic Acid, Phenyl Salicylate, and Methylene Blue** *see* Methenamine, Phenyl Salicylate, Methylene Blue, Benzoic Acid, and Hyoscyamine *on page 962*
- **Hyoscyamine, Methenamine, Sodium Biphosphate, Phenyl Salicylate, and Methylene Blue** *see* Methenamine, Sodium Biphosphate, Phenyl Salicylate, Methylene Blue, and Hyoscyamine *on page 962*
- **Hyoscyamine Sulfate** *see* Hyoscyamine *on page 756*
- **Hyosyne** *see* Hyoscyamine *on page 756*
- **Hyperal** *see* Total Parenteral Nutrition *on page 1495*
- **Hyperalimentation** *see* Total Parenteral Nutrition *on page 1495*
- **HyperHep B® (Can)** *see* Hepatitis B Immune Globulin (Human) *on page 727*
- **HyperHEP B™ S/D** *see* Hepatitis B Immune Globulin (Human) *on page 727*
- **HyperRAB™ S/D** *see* Rabies Immune Globulin (Human) *on page 1286*
- **HyperRHO™ S/D Full Dose** *see* Rh_o(D) Immune Globulin *on page 1308*
- **HyperRHO™ S/D Mini Dose** *see* Rh_o(D) Immune Globulin *on page 1308*
- **Hyper-Sal™** *see* Sodium Chloride *on page 1381*
- **HyperTET™ S/D** *see* Tetanus Immune Globulin (Human) *on page 1448*
- **Hytakerol® [DSC]** *see* Dihydrotachysterol *on page 450*
- **Hytakerol® (Can)** *see* Dihydrotachysterol *on page 450*
- **Hytone®** *see* Hydrocortisone *on page 743*
- **Hytrin® (Can)** *see* Terazosin *on page 1440*
- **Hyzaar®** *see* Losartan and Hydrochlorothiazide *on page 909*
- **Hyzaar® DS (Can)** *see* Losartan and Hydrochlorothiazide *on page 909*
- **I^{123} Iobenguane** *see* Iobenguane I 123 *on page 810*
- **I-123 MIBG** *see* Iobenguane I 123 *on page 810*

Ibandronate (eye BAN droh nate)

U.S. Brand Names Boniva®

Canadian Brand Names Bondronat®

Index Terms Ibandronate Sodium; Ibandronic Acid; NSC-722623

Pharmacologic Category Bisphosphonate Derivative

Use Treatment and prevention of osteoporosis in postmenopausal females

Unlabeled/Investigational Use Hypercalcemia of malignancy; corticosteroid-induced osteoporosis; Paget's disease; reduce bone pain and skeletal complications from metastatic bone disease

Pregnancy Risk Factor C

Pregnancy Considerations Safety and efficacy have not been established in pregnant women. Bisphosphonates are incorporated into the bone matrix and are gradually released over time. Theoretically, there may be a risk of fetal harm when pregnancy follows the completion of therapy. Based on limited case reports with pamidronate, serum calcium levels in the newborn may be altered if administered during pregnancy.

Lactation Excretion in breast milk unknown/use caution

Contraindications Hypersensitivity to ibandronate, other bisphosphonates, or any component of the formulation; hypocalcemia; oral tablets are also contraindicated in patients unable to stand or sit upright for at least 60 minutes

Warnings/Precautions Hypocalcemia must be corrected before therapy initiation. Ensure adequate calcium and vitamin D intake. Bisphosphonate therapy has been associated with osteonecrosis, primarily of the jaw; this has been observed mostly in cancer patients, but also in patients with postmenopausal osteoporosis and other diagnoses. Dental exams and preventative dentistry should be performed prior to placing patients with risk factors on chronic bisphosphonate therapy. Invasive dental procedures should be avoided during treatment.

Infrequently, severe (and occasionally debilitating) bone, joint, and/or muscle pain have been reported during bisphosphonate treatment. The onset of pain ranged from a single day to several months. Symptoms usually resolve upon discontinuation. Some patients experienced recurrence when rechallenged with same drug or another bisphosphonate; avoid use in patients with a history of these symptoms in association with bisphosphonate therapy.

Oral bisphosphonates may cause dysphagia, esophagitis, esophageal or gastric ulcer; risk may increase in patients unable to comply with dosing instructions. Intravenous bisphosphonates may cause transient decreases in serum calcium and have also been associated with renal toxicity.

Use not recommended with severe renal impairment (Cl_{cr} <30 mL/minute or serum creatinine >2.3 mg/dL). Safety and efficacy have not been established in patients <18 years of age.

Adverse Reactions Percentages vary based on frequency of administration (daily vs monthly). Unless specified, percentages are reported with oral use.

>10%:

Gastrointestinal: Dyspepsia (6% to 12%)

Neuromuscular & skeletal: Back pain (4% to 14%)

1% to 10%:

Central nervous system: Headache (3% to 7%), dizziness (1% to 4%), insomnia (1% to 2%)

Dermatologic: Rash (1% to 2%)

Endocrine & metabolic: Hypercholesterolemia (5%)

Gastrointestinal: Abdominal pain (5% to 8%), diarrhea (4% to 7%), nausea (5%), tooth disorder (4%), constipation (3% to 4%), vomiting (3%)

Genitourinary: Urinary tract infection (2% to 6%)

Hepatic: Alkaline phosphatase decreased (frequency not defined)

Local: Injection site reaction (<2%)

Neuromuscular & skeletal: Pain in extremity (8%), myalgia (1% to 6%), joint disorder (4%), weakness (4%), muscle cramp (2%)

Respiratory: Bronchitis (3% to 10%), pneumonia (6%), pharyngitis/nasopharyngitis (3% to 4%), upper respiratory infection (2%)

Miscellaneous: Acute phase reaction (I.V. 10%; oral 4%), allergic reaction (3%), flu-like syndrome (1% to 3%)

Postmarketing and/or case reports: Incapacitating bone, joint or muscle pain, ocular inflammation, scleritis, uveitis

Drug Interactions

Avoid Concomitant Use There are no known interactions where it is recommended to avoid concomitant use.

Increased Effect/Toxicity

Ibandronate may increase the levels/effects of: Phosphate Supplements

The levels/effects of Ibandronate may be increased by: Aminoglycosides; Nonsteroidal Anti-Inflammatory Agents

Decreased Effect

The levels/effects of Ibandronate may be decreased by: Antacids; Calcium Salts; Iron Salts; Magnesium Salts

Ethanol/Nutrition/Herb Interactions

Ethanol: Avoid ethanol (may increase risk of osteoporosis).

Food: May reduce absorption; mean oral bioavailability is decreased up to 90% when given with food.

Stability Store at controlled room temperature of 15°C to 30°C (59°F to 86°F).

Mechanism of Action A bisphosphonate which inhibits bone resorption via actions on osteoclasts or on osteoclast precursors; decreases the rate of bone resorption, leading to an indirect increase in bone mineral density.

Pharmacodynamics/Kinetics

Distribution: Terminal V_d: 90 L; 40% to 50% of circulating ibandronate binds to bone

Protein binding: 85% to 99%

Bioavailability: Oral: Reduced by 90% following standard breakfast

Half-life elimination:

Oral: 150 mg dose: Terminal: 37-157 hours

I.V.: Terminal: ~5-25 hours

Time to peak, plasma: Oral: 0.5-2 hours

Excretion: Urine (50% to 60% of absorbed dose, excreted as unchanged drug); feces (unabsorbed drug)

Dosage

Oral:

Treatment of postmenopausal osteoporosis: 2.5 mg/day or 150 mg once a month

Prevention of postmenopausal osteoporosis: 2.5 mg/day; 150 mg once a month may be considered

Metastatic bone disease (unlabeled use): 50 mg once daily

I.V.:

Treatment of postmenopausal osteoporosis: 3 mg every 3 months

Hypercalcemia of malignancy (unlabeled use): 2-4 mg over 2 hours

Metastatic bone disease (unlabeled use): 6 mg over 1 hour every 3-4 weeks

Dosage adjustment in renal impairment:

Mild or moderate impairment: Dosing adjustment not needed

Severe impairment (Cl_{cr} <30 mL/minute): Use not recommended

Dose adjustment in renal impairment for oncologic uses (unlabeled): Severe impairment (Cl_{cr} <30 mL/minute):

Oral: 50 mg once weekly

I.V.: 2 mg over 1 hour every 3-4 weeks

Dosage adjustment in hepatic impairment: Dosing adjustment not needed

Dietary Considerations Supplemental calcium or vitamin D may be required if dietary intake is not adequate. Tablet should be taken with a full glass (6-8 oz) of plain water, at least 60 minutes prior to any food, beverages, or medications. Mineral water with a high calcium content should be avoided.

Administration

Oral: Should be administered 60 minutes before the first food or drink of the day (other than water). Ibandronate should be taken in an upright position with a full glass (6-8 oz) of plain water and the patient should avoid lying down for 60 minutes to minimize the possibility of GI side effects. Mineral water with a high calcium content should be avoided. The tablet should be swallowed whole; do not chew or suck.

Once-monthly dosing: The 150 mg tablet should be taken on the same date each month. In case of a missed dose, do not take two 150 mg tablets within the same week. If the next scheduled dose is 1-7 days away, wait until the next scheduled dose to take the tablet. If the next scheduled dose is >7 days away, take the dose the morning it is remembered, and then resume taking the once-monthly dose on the originally scheduled day.

I.V.: Administer as a 15-30 second bolus. Do not mix with calcium-containing solutions or other drugs. For osteoporosis, do not administer more frequently than every 3 months. Infuse over 1 hour for metastatic bone disease and over 2 hours for hypercalcemia of malignancy.

Monitoring Parameters Bone mineral density; serum creatinine prior to each I.V. dose

Test Interactions Bisphosphonates may interfere with diagnostic imaging agents such as technetium-99m-diphosphonate in bone scans.

Dosage Forms Excipient information presented when available (limited, particularly for generics); consult specific product labeling.

Injection, solution: 1 mg/mL (3 mL) [prefilled syringe]

Tablet: 2.5 mg [once-daily formulation]; 150 mg [once-monthly formulation]

◆ **Ibandronate Sodium** *see* Ibandronate *on page* 757

◆ **Ibandronic Acid** *see* Ibandronate *on page* 757

◆ **Ibidomide Hydrochloride** *see* Labetalol *on page* 845

Ibritumomab (ib ri TYOO mo mab)

U.S. Brand Names Zevalin®

Canadian Brand Names Zevalin®

Index Terms Ibritumomab Tiuxetan; IDEC-Y2B8; In-111 Ibritumomab; In-111 Zevalin; Y-90 Ibritumomab; Y-90 Zevalin

Pharmacologic Category Antineoplastic Agent, Monoclonal Antibody; Radiopharmaceutical

Use Treatment of relapsed or refractory low-grade or follicular B-cell non-Hodgkin's lymphoma

Pregnancy Risk Factor D

Pregnancy Considerations There are no adequate and well-controlled studies in pregnant women. Y-90 ibritumomab may cause fetal harm. Women of childbearing potential should avoid becoming pregnant during treatment with ibritumomab. Both males and females should use effective contraception for 12 months following treatment. The effect on future fertility is unknown.

Lactation Excretion in breast milk unknown/not recommended

Medication Safety Issues

High alert medication: The Institute for Safe Medication Practices (ISMP) includes this medication among its list of drug classes which have a heightened risk of causing significant patient harm when used in error.

Dosage maximum: Do not exceed the Y-90 Ibritumomab maximum allowable dose of 32 mCi, regardless of the patient's body weight.

Contraindications There are no contraindications listed within the manufacturer's labeling.

Warnings/Precautions Hazardous agent - use appropriate precautions for handling and disposal. **[U.S. Boxed Warning]: Severe cutaneous and mucocutaneous skin reactions have been reported (with fatalities) in postmarketing experience.** These include erythema multiforme, Stevens-Johnson syndrome, toxic epidermal necrolysis, bullous dermatitis, and exfoliative dermatitis. Onset may occur within days to 3-4 months following infusion. Patients experiencing severe cutaneous or mucocutaneous skin reactions should not receive any further component of the ibritumomab regimen.

To be used as part of the Zevalin® therapeutic regimen (in combination with rituximab). **[U.S. Boxed Warning]: Do not exceed the Y-90 Ibritumomab maximum allowable dose of 32 mCi; do not administer to patients with altered biodistribution.** Use should be reserved to physicians and other professionals qualified and experienced in the safe handling of radiopharmaceuticals, and in monitoring and emergency treatment of infusion reactions. The contents of the kit are not radioactive until radiolabeling occurs. During and after radiolabeling, adequate shielding should be used with this product, in accordance with institutional radiation safety practices.

[U.S. Boxed Warning]: Severe and potentially fatal infusion reactions (angioedema, bronchospasm, hypotension, hypoxia) have been reported, typically with the first rituximab infusion (during infusion or within 30-120 minutes of infusion). Severe reactions have also included acute respiratory distress syndrome, pulmonary infiltrates, urticaria, cardiogenic shock, MI, and ventricular fibrillation. Immediately stop infusion for severe infusion reaction; less severe reactions may be managed by slowing or interrupting infusion. Medications for the treatment of hypersensitivity reactions should be available for immediate use.

[U.S. Boxed Warning]: Delayed, prolonged, and severe cytopenias (thrombocytopenia and neutropenia) are common. Do not administer to patients with ≥25% lymphoma marrow involvement, patients with impaired bone marrow reserve (eg, prior myeloablative treatment, platelet count <100,000/mm^3, neutrophil count <1500/mm^3, hypocellular marrow), or to patients with prior stem cell collection failure. Hemorrhage may occur due to thrombocytopenia; use caution with patients taking anticoagulants or medications interfering with platelet function. Closely monitor patients for complications of cytopenias (eg, febrile neutropenia, hemorrhage) for up to 3 months after administration.

Secondary malignancies (acute myelogenous leukemia and/or myelodysplastic syndrome) have been reported following use; the median time to diagnosis (secondary malignancy) following ibritumomab treatment was 1.9 years (range: 0.4-6.3 years). Product contains albumin, which confers a theoretical risk of transmission of viral disease or Creutzfeldt-Jakob disease. The safety of immunization with live vaccines following ibritumomab therapy has not been studied; do not administer live viral vaccines to patients who have recently received ibritumomab treatment; the ability to generate a response to any vaccine after receiving treatment has not been studied. Safety and efficacy of repeated courses of the therapeutic regimen have not been established. Infusion site erythema and ulceration have been reported following extravasation; monitor infusion site; promptly terminate infusion with symptoms/signs of extravasation (restart in another limb). There is a case report of (delayed) erythema and ulceration, which is described as radiation necrosis following yttrium-90-ibritumomab extravasation (Williams, 2006). Delayed (up to 1 month) radiation injury has occurred in or near areas of lymphomatous involvement. Safety and efficacy have not been established in pediatric patients.

Adverse Reactions Severe, potentially life-threatening allergic reactions have occurred in association with infusions. Also refer to Rituximab monograph.

>10%:

- Central nervous system: Chills (24%), fever (17%), pain (13%), headache (12%)
- Gastrointestinal: Nausea (31%), abdominal pain (16%), vomiting (12%)
- Hematologic: Thrombocytopenia (95%; grades 3/4: 63%; nadir: 53 days), neutropenia (77%; grades 3/4: 60%; nadir: 62 days), anemia (61%; grades 3/4: 17%; nadir: 68 days), myelosuppression (nadir: 7-9 weeks; duration: 22-35 days)
- Neuromuscular & skeletal: Weakness (43%)
- Respiratory: Dyspnea (14%)
- Miscellaneous: Infection (29%)

1% to 10%:

- Cardiovascular: Peripheral edema (8%), flushing (6%), hypotension (6%)
- Central nervous system: Dizziness (10%), insomnia (5%), anxiety (4%)
- Dermatologic: Pruritus (9%), rash (8%), bruising (7%), angioedema (5%; grades 3/4: <1%), urticaria (4%), petechiae (3%)
- Gastrointestinal: Diarrhea (9%), anorexia (8%), abdominal distension (5%), constipation (5%), dyspepsia (4%), melena (2%; life threatening in 1%), gastrointestinal hemorrhage (severe: 1%)
- Hematologic: Pancytopenia (severe: 2%), secondary malignancies (2% to 6%; includes acute myelogenous leukemia and myelodysplastic syndrome)
- Neuromuscular & skeletal: Back pain (8%), arthralgia (7%), myalgia (7%)
- Respiratory: Cough (10%), throat irritation (10%), rhinitis (6%), bronchospasm (5%), epistaxis (3%), apnea (severe: 1%)
- Miscellaneous: Diaphoresis (4%), HAMA antibody formation (4%), allergic reaction (2%), infusion reaction (severe: 1%), tumor pain (severe: 1%)

<1% (Limited to important or life-threatening: Anaphylactic reactions, arthritis, cerebral hemorrhage, cytogenetic abnormalities, encephalopathy, hematemesis, hemorrhage, hypersensitivity; infusion site erythema/ulceration (following extravasation), radiation injury/complications (delayed; in tissues in or near areas of lymphomatous involvement), meningioma (benign), pulmonary edema, pulmonary embolism, radiation necrosis (following yttrium-90-ibritumomab extravasation), stroke (hemorrhagic), subdural hematoma, tachycardia, vaginal hemorrhage

Drug Interactions

Avoid Concomitant Use

Avoid concomitant use of Ibritumomab with any of the following: Natalizumab; Vaccines (Live)

Increased Effect/Toxicity

Ibritumomab may increase the levels/effects of: Natalizumab; Vaccines (Live); Vitamin K Antagonists

The levels/effects of Ibritumomab may be increased by: Anticoagulants; Antiplatelet Agents; Trastuzumab

Decreased Effect

Ibritumomab may decrease the levels/effects of: Cardiac Glycosides; Vaccines (Inactivated); Vitamin K Antagonists

The levels/effects of Ibritumomab may be decreased by: Echinacea

Ethanol/Nutrition/Herb Interactions Herb/Nutraceutical: Avoid echinacea (may diminish therapeutic effect). Avoid cat's claw, dong quai, evening primrose, feverfew, garlic, ginger, ginkgo, red clover, horse chestnut, green tea, ginseng (all have antiplatelet activity).

Stability Store at 2°C to 8°C (36°F to 46°F); do not freeze. Kit is not radioactive. To prepare radiolabeled injection, follow detailed preparation guidelines provided by manufacturer.

Mechanism of Action Ibritumomab is a monoclonal antibody directed against the CD20 antigen found on B lymphocytes (normal and malignant). Ibritumomab binding induces apoptosis in B lymphocytes *in vitro*. It is combined with the chelator tiuxetan, which acts as a specific chelation site for either Indium-111 (In-111) or Yttrium-90 (Y-90). The monoclonal antibody acts as a delivery system to direct the radioactive isotope to the targeted cells, however, binding has been observed in lymphoid cells throughout the body and in lymphoid nodules in organs such as the large and small intestines. Indium-111 is a gamma-emitter used to assess biodistribution of ibritumomab, while Y-90 emits beta particles. Beta-emission induces cellular damage through the formation of free radicals (in both target cells and surrounding cells).

Pharmacodynamics/Kinetics

Duration: Beta cell recovery begins in ~12 weeks; generally in normal range within 9 months

Distribution: To lymphoid cells throughout the body and in lymphoid nodules in organs such as the large and small intestines, spleen, testes, and liver

Metabolism: Has not been characterized; the product of yttrium-90 radioactive decay is zirconium-90 (nonradioactive); Indium-111 decays to cadmium-111 (nonradioactive)

Half-life elimination: Y-90 ibritumomab: 30 hours; Indium-111 decays with a physical half-life of 67 hours; Yttrium-90 decays with a physical half-life of 64 hours

Excretion: A median of 7.2% of the radiolabeled activity was excreted in urine over 7 days

Dosage I.V.: Adults: **Note:** Premedication with acetaminophen and diphenhydramine is recommended for rituximab infusions. Ibritumomab is administered **only** as part of the Zevalin® therapeutic regimen (a combined treatment regimen with rituximab). The regimen consists of two steps:

Day 1:

Rituximab infusion: 250 mg/m^2 at an initial rate of 50 mg/hour. If hypersensitivity or infusion-related events do not occur, increase infusion in increments of 50 mg/hour every 30 minutes, to a maximum of 400 mg/hour. Discontinue for severe infusion reaction. For less severe infusion reactions, temporarily slow or interrupt; the infusion may be resumed at one-half the previous rate upon improvement of symptoms.

In-111 ibritumomab infusion: Within 4 hours of the completion of rituximab infusion, inject 5 mCi (1.6 mg total antibody dose) over 10 minutes.

Biodistribution of In-111 ibritumomab should be assessed by imaging at 48-72 hours postinjection. Optional additional imaging may be performed to resolve ambiguities. If biodistribution is not acceptable, the patient should not proceed to Step 2.

Day 7, 8, or 9:

Rituximab infusion: 250 mg/m^2 at an initial rate of 100 mg/hour (50 mg/hour if infusion-related events occurred with the first infusion). If hypersensitivity or infusion-related events do not occur, increase infusion in increments of 100 mg/hour every 30 minutes, to a maximum of 400 mg/hour, as tolerated.

Y-90 ibritumomab infusion: Within 4 hours of the completion of rituximab infusion:

Platelet count ≥150,000 cells/mm^3: Inject 0.4 mCi/kg (14.8 MBq/kg actual body weight) over 10 minutes; maximum dose: 32 mCi (1184 MBq)

Platelet count between 100,000-149,000 cells/mm^3: Inject 0.3 mCi/kg (11.1 MBq/kg actual body weight) over 10 minutes; maximum dose: 32 mCi (1184 MBq)

Platelet count <100,000 cells/mm^3: Do **not** administer

Maximum dose: The prescribed, measured, and administered dose of Y-90 ibritumomab must not exceed 32 mCi (1184 MBq), regardless of the patient's body weight

Administration

Rituximab: Administer the first infusion of rituximab at an initial rate of 50 mg/hour. If hypersensitivity or infusion-related events do not occur, escalate the infusion rate in 50 mg/hour increments every 30 minutes, to a maximum of 400 mg/hour. Immediately stop infusion for severe infusion reaction (discontinue ibritumomab regimen); less severe reactions may be managed by slowing or interrupting infusion. For less severe reactions, infusion may continue at one-half the previous rate upon improvement of patient symptoms. Subsequent rituximab infusion can be administered at an initial rate of 100 mg/hour and increased in 100 mg/hour increments at 30-minute intervals, to a maximum of 400 mg/hour as tolerated.

In-111 and Y-90 ibritumomab: Inject slowly, over 10 minutes through a 0.22 micron low protein binding in-line filter. After injection, flush line with at least 10 mL normal saline. Y-90 ibritumomab: establish free-flowing I.V. line prior to administration; avoid extravasation.

Monitoring Parameters Patients must be monitored for infusion-related allergic reactions (typically within 30-120 minutes of administration). Obtain CBC with differential and platelet counts weekly. Platelet count must be obtained prior to Day 7, 8,or 9. Monitor for up to 3 months after use.

Biodistribution of In-111 ibritumomab should be assessed by imaging at 48-72 hours post injection. Optional additional imaging may be performed to resolve ambiguities. If biodistribution is not acceptable, the patient should not proceed to Day 7, 8, or 9.

Additional Information Ibritumomab tiuxetan is produced in Chinese hamster ovary cell cultures. Kit is not radioactive. Radiolabeling of ibritumomab with Yttrium-90 and Indium-111 (not included in kit) must be performed by appropriate personnel in a specialized facility.

Dosage Forms Excipient information presented when available (limited, particularly for generics); consult specific product labeling.

Each kit contains 4 vials for preparation of either In-111 or Y-90 conjugate (as indicated on container label)

Injection, solution:

Zevalin®: 1.6 mg/mL (2 mL) [supplied with sodium acetate solution, formulation buffer vial (includes albumin 750 mg), and an empty reaction vial]

◆ **Ibritumomab Tiuxetan** *see* Ibritumomab *on page* 758

◆ **Ibu®** *see* Ibuprofen *on page* 760

◆ **Ibu-200 [OTC]** *see* Ibuprofen *on page* 760

◆ **Ibudone™** *see* Hydrocodone and Ibuprofen *on page* 742

Ibuprofen (eye byoo PROE fen)

U.S. Brand Names Addaprin [OTC]; Advil® Children's [OTC]; Advil® Infants' [OTC]; Advil® Junior [OTC] [DSC]; Advil® Migraine [OTC]; Advil® [OTC]; Genpril® [OTC] [DSC]; I-Prin [OTC]; Ibu-200 [OTC]; Ibu®; Midol® Cramp and Body Aches [OTC]; Motrin® Children's [OTC]; Motrin® IB [OTC]; Motrin® Infants' [OTC]; Motrin® Junior [OTC]; Motrin® [DSC]; NeoProfen®; Proprinal [OTC]; Ultraprin [OTC]

Canadian Brand Names Advil®; Apo-Ibuprofen®; Motrin® (Children's); Motrin® IB; Novo-Profen; Nu-Ibuprofen

Index Terms *p*-Isobutylhydratropic Acid; Ibuprofen Lysine

Pharmacologic Category Nonsteroidal Anti-inflammatory Drug (NSAID), Oral; Nonsteroidal Anti-inflammatory Drug (NSAID), Parenteral

Additional Appendix Information

Nonsteroidal Anti-inflammatory Agents *on page 1669*

Use

Oral: Inflammatory diseases and rheumatoid disorders including juvenile rheumatoid arthritis, mild-to-moderate pain, fever, dysmenorrhea

Injection: Ibuprofen lysine is for use in premature infants weighing between 500-1500 g and who are ≤32 weeks gestational age (GA) to induce closure of a clinically-significant patent ductus arteriosus (PDA) when usual treatments are ineffective

Unlabeled/Investigational Use Cystic fibrosis, gout, ankylosing spondylitis, acute migraine headache

Restrictions An FDA-approved medication guide must be distributed when dispensing an oral outpatient prescription (new or refill) where this medication is to be used without direct supervision of a healthcare provider. Medication guides are available at http://www.fda.gov/cder/Offices/ODS/medication_guides.htm.

Pregnancy Risk Factor C/D (3rd trimester)

Lactation Enters breast milk/use caution (AAP rates "compatible")

Medication Safety Issues

Sound-alike/look-alike issues:

Haltran® may be confused with Halfprin®

Contraindications Hypersensitivity to ibuprofen, aspirin, other NSAIDs, or any component of the formulation; perioperative pain in the setting of coronary artery bypass graft (CABG) surgery

Ibuprofen lysine is contraindicated in preterm infants with untreated proven or suspected infection; congenital heart disease where patency of the PDA is necessary for pulmonary or systemic blood flow; bleeding (especially with active intracranial hemorrhage or GI bleed); thrombocytopenia; coagulation defects; proven or suspected necrotizing enterocolitis (NEC); significant renal dysfunction

Warnings/Precautions **[U.S. Boxed Warning]: NSAIDs are associated with an increased risk of adverse cardiovascular thrombotic events, including MI, stroke, and new onset or worsening of pre-existing hypertension.** Risk may be increased with duration of use or pre-existing cardiovascular risk factors or disease. Carefully evaluate individual cardiovascular risk profiles prior to prescribing. Use caution with fluid retention, heart failure, or hypertension. Concurrent administration of ibuprofen, and potentially other nonselective NSAIDs, may interfere with aspirin's cardioprotective effect. **[U.S. Boxed Warning]: Use is contraindicated for treatment of perioperative pain in the setting of coronary artery bypass graft (CABG) surgery.** Risk of MI and stroke may be increased with use following CABG surgery.

May increase the risk of aseptic meningitis, especially in patients with systemic lupus erythematosus (SLE) and mixed connective tissue disorders. Platelet adhesion and aggregation may be decreased; may prolong bleeding time; patients with coagulation disorders or who are receiving anticoagulants should be monitored closely. Anemia may occur; patients on long-term NSAID therapy should be monitored for anemia. NSAID use may compromise existing renal function; dose-dependent decreases in prostaglandin synthesis may result from NSAID use, reducing renal blood flow which may cause renal decompensation. Patients with impaired renal function, dehydration, heart failure, liver dysfunction, those taking diuretics, and ACE inhibitors, and the elderly are at greater risk of renal toxicity. Rehydrate patient before starting therapy; monitor renal function closely. Not recommended for use in patients with advanced renal disease. Long-term NSAID use may result in renal papillary necrosis.

NSAIDs may increase risk of gastrointestinal irritation, inflammation, ulceration, bleeding, and perforation. These events may occur at any time during therapy and without warning. Use caution with a history of GI disease (bleeding or ulcers), concurrent therapy with aspirin, anticoagulants and/or corticosteroids, smoking, use of alcohol, the elderly or debilitated patients.

Use the lowest effective dose for the shortest duration of time, consistent with individual patient goals, to reduce risk of cardiovascular or GI adverse events. Alternate therapies should be considered for patients at high risk.

NSAIDs may cause serious skin adverse events including exfoliative dermatitis, Stevens-Johnson Syndrome (SJS) and toxic epidermal necrolysis (TEN); discontinue use at first sign of skin rash or hypersensitivity. Anaphylactoid reactions may occur, even without prior exposure; patients with "aspirin triad" (bronchial asthma, aspirin intolerance, rhinitis) may be at increased risk. Do not use in patients who experience bronchospasm, asthma, rhinitis, or urticaria with NSAID or aspirin therapy. Use caution in other forms of asthma.

Use with caution in patients with decreased hepatic function. Closely monitor patients with any abnormal LFT. Severe hepatic reactions (eg, fulminant hepatitis, liver failure) have occurred with NSAID use, rarely; discontinue if signs or symptoms of liver disease develop, or if systemic manifestations occur.

The elderly are at increased risk for adverse effects (especially peptic ulceration, CNS effects, renal toxicity) from NSAIDs even at low doses.

Withhold for at least 4-6 half-lives prior to surgical or dental procedures. Some products may contain phenylalanine.

Injection: Hold second or third doses if urinary output is <0.6 mL/kg/hour. May alter signs of infection. May inhibit platelet aggregation; monitor for signs of bleeding. May displace bilirubin; use caution when total bilirubin is elevated. Long-term evaluations of neurodevelopment, growth, or diseases associated with prematurity following treatment have not been conducted. A second course of treatment, alternative pharmacologic therapy or surgery may be needed if the ductus arteriosus fails to close or reopens following the initial course of therapy.

Self medication (OTC use): Prior to self-medication, patients should contact healthcare provider if they have had recurring stomach pain or upset, ulcers, bleeding problems, high blood pressure, heart or kidney disease, other serious medical problems, are currently taking a diuretic, aspirin, anticoagulant, or are ≥60 years of age. If patients are using for migraines, they should also contact healthcare provider if they have not had a migraine diagnosis by healthcare provider, a headache that is different from usual migraine, worst headache of life, fever and neck stiffness, headache from head injury or coughing, first headache at ≥50 years of age, daily headache, or migraine requiring bed rest. Recommended dosages should not be exceeded, due to an increased risk of GI bleeding. Stop use and consult a healthcare provider if symptoms get worse, newly appear, fever lasts for >3 days or pain lasts >3 days (children) and >10 days (adults). Do not give for >10 days unless instructed by healthcare provider. Consuming ≥3 alcoholic beverages/day or taking longer than recommended may increase the risk of GI bleeding.

Adverse Reactions

Oral:

1% to 10%:

Cardiovascular: Edema (1% to 3%)

Central nervous system: Dizziness (3% to 9%), headache (1% to 3%), nervousness (1% to 3%)
Dermatologic: Rash (3% to 9%), itching (1% to 3%)
Endocrine & metabolic: Fluid retention (1% to 3%)
Gastrointestinal: Epigastric pain (3% to 9%), heartburn (3% to 9%), nausea (3% to 9%), abdominal pain/cramps/distress (1% to 3%), appetite decreased (1% to 3%), constipation (1% to 3%), diarrhea (1% to 3%), dyspepsia (1% to 3%), flatulence (1% to 3%), vomiting (1% to 3%)
Otic: Tinnitus (3% to 9%)

<1% (Limited to important or life-threatening): Acute renal failure, agranulocytosis, anaphylaxis, aplastic anemia, azotemia, blurred vision, bone marrow suppression, confusion, creatinine clearance decreased, duodenal ulcer, edema, eosinophilia, epistaxis, erythema multiforme, gastric ulcer, GI bleed, GI hemorrhage, GI ulceration, hallucinations, hearing decreased, hematuria, hematocrit decreased, hemoglobin decreased, hemolytic anemia, hepatitis, hypertension, inhibition of platelet aggregation, jaundice, liver function tests abnormal, leukopenia, melena, neutropenia, pancreatitis, photosensitivity, Stevens-Johnson syndrome, thrombocytopenia, toxic amblyopia, toxic epidermal necrolysis, urticaria, vesiculobullous eruptions, vision changes

Injection:

>10%:
Cardiovascular: Intraventricular hemorrhage (29%; grade 3/4: 15%)
Dermatologic: Skin irritation (16%)
Endocrine & metabolic: Hypocalcemia (12%), hypoglycemia (12%)
Gastrointestinal: GI disorders, non NEC (22%)
Hematologic: Anemia (32%)
Respiratory: Apnea (28%), respiratory infection (19%)
Miscellaneous: Sepsis (43%)

1% to 10%:
Cardiovascular: Edema (4%)
Endocrine & metabolic: Adrenal insufficiency (7%), hypernatremia (7%)
Genitourinary: Urinary tract infection (9%)
Renal: Urea increased (7%), renal impairment (6%), creatinine increased (3%), urine output decreased (3%; small decrease reported on days 2-6 with compensatory increase in output on day 9), renal failure (1%)
Respiratory: Respiratory failure (10%), atelectasis (4%)

Frequency not defined: Abdominal distension, cholestasis, feeding problems, gastritis, GI reflux, heart failure, hyperglycemia, hypotension, ileus, infection, inguinal hernia, injection site reaction, jaundice, neutropenia, seizure, tachycardia, thrombocytopenia

Postmarketing and/or case reports: GI perforation, necrotizing enterocolitis

Drug Interactions

Metabolism/Transport Effects **Substrate** (minor) of CYP2C9, 2C19; **Inhibits** CYP2C9 (strong)

Avoid Concomitant Use

Avoid concomitant use of Ibuprofen with any of the following: Ketorolac

Increased Effect/Toxicity

Ibuprofen may increase the levels/effects of: Aminoglycosides; Anticoagulants; Antiplatelet Agents; Bisphosphonate Derivatives; CycloSPORINE; CYP2C9 Substrates (High risk); Desmopressin; Lithium; Methotrexate; Nonsteroidal Anti-Inflammatory Agents; Pemetrexed; Quinolone Antibiotics; Salicylates; Thrombolytic Agents; Vancomycin; Vitamin K Antagonists

The levels/effects of Ibuprofen may be increased by: Antidepressants (Tricyclic, Tertiary Amine); Corticosteroids (Systemic); Herbs (Anticoagulant/Antiplatelet Properties); Ketorolac; Probenecid; Selective Serotonin Reuptake Inhibitors; Serotonin/Norepinephrine Reuptake Inhibitors; Treprostinil

Decreased Effect

Ibuprofen may decrease the levels/effects of: ACE Inhibitors; Angiotensin II Receptor Blockers; Antiplatelet Agents; Beta-Blockers; Eplerenone; HydrALAZINE; Loop Diuretics; Salicylates; Thiazide Diuretics

The levels/effects of Ibuprofen may be decreased by: Bile Acid Sequestrants; Salicylates

Ethanol/Nutrition/Herb Interactions

Ethanol: Avoid ethanol (may enhance gastric mucosal irritation).
Food: Ibuprofen peak serum levels may be decreased if taken with food.
Herb/Nutraceutical: Avoid alfalfa, anise, bilberry, bladderwrack, bromelain, cat's claw, celery, chamomile, coleus, cordyceps, dong quai, evening primrose, fenugreek, feverfew, garlic, ginger, ginkgo biloba, ginseng (American, Panax, Siberian), grapeseed, green tea, guggul, horse chestnut seed, horseradish, licorice, prickly ash, red clover, reishi, SAMe (S-adenosylmethionine), sweet clover, turmeric, white willow (all have additional antiplatelet activity).

Stability

Injection: Store at room temperature of 20°C to 25°C (68°F to 77°F). Protect from light. Dilute with dextrose or saline to an appropriate volume. Following dilution, administer within 30 minutes of preparation.
Suspension, tablet: Store at room temperature of 20°C to 25°C (68°F to 77°F).

Mechanism of Action Reversibly inhibits cyclooxygenase-1 and 2 (COX-1 and 2) enzymes, which result in decreased formation of prostaglandin precursors; has antipyretic, analgesic, and anti-inflammatory properties

Pharmacodynamics/Kinetics

Onset of action: Analgesic: 30-60 minutes; Anti-inflammatory: ≤7 days
Peak effect: 1-2 weeks
Duration: 4-6 hours
Absorption: Oral: Rapid (85%)
Distribution: Premature infants with ductal closure (highly variable between studies):
Day 3: 145-349 mL/kg
Day 5: 72-222 mL/kg
Protein binding: 90% to 99%
Metabolism: Hepatic via oxidation
Half-life elimination:
Premature infants (highly variable between studies):
Day 3: 35-51 hours
Day 5: 20-33 hours
Children 3 months to 10 years: 1.6 ± 0.7 hours
Adults: 2-4 hours; End-stage renal disease: Unchanged
Time to peak: ~1-2 hours
Excretion: Urine (80% as metabolites; 1% as unchanged drug); some feces

Dosage

I.V.: Infants between 500-1500 g and ≤32 weeks GA: Patent ductus arteriosus: Initial dose: Ibuprofen 10 mg/kg, followed by two doses of 5 mg/kg at 24 and 48 hours. Dose should be based on birth weight.

Oral:
Children:
Antipyretic: 6 months to 12 years: Temperature <102.5°F (39°C): 5 mg/kg/dose; temperature >102.5°F: 10 mg/kg/dose given every 6-8 hours (maximum daily dose: 40 mg/kg/day)
Juvenile rheumatoid arthritis: 30-50 mg/kg/24 hours divided every 8 hours; start at lower end of dosing range and titrate upward (maximum: 2.4 g/day)
Analgesic: 4-10 mg/kg/dose every 6-8 hours
Cystic fibrosis (unlabeled use): Chronic (>4 years) twice daily dosing adjusted to maintain serum levels of

50-100 mcg/mL has been associated with slowing of disease progression in younger patients with mild lung disease

OTC labeling (analgesic, antipyretic): **Note:** Treatment for >10 days is not recommended unless directed by healthcare provider.

Children 6 months to 11 years: See table; use of weight to select dose is preferred; doses may be repeated every 6-8 hours (maximum: 4 doses/day)

Children ≥12 years: 200 mg every 4-6 hours as needed (maximum: 1200 mg/24 hours)

Ibuprofen Dosing

Weight (lb)	Age	Dosage (mg)
12-17	6-11 mo	50
18-23	12-23 mo	75
24-35	2-3 y	100
36-47	4-5 y	150
48-59	6-8 y	200
60-71	9-10 y	250
72-95	11 y	300

Adults:

Inflammatory disease: 400-800 mg/dose 3-4 times/day (maximum dose: 3.2 g/day)

Analgesia/pain/fever/dysmenorrhea: 200-400 mg/dose every 4-6 hours (maximum daily dose: 1.2 g, unless directed by physician; under physician supervision daily doses ≤2.4 g may be used)

OTC labeling (analgesic, antipyretic): 200 mg every 4-6 hours as needed (maximum: 1200 mg/24 hours); treatment for >10 days is not recommended unless directed by healthcare provider.

Migraine: 2 capsules at onset of symptoms (maximum: 400 mg/24 hours unless directed by healthcare provider)

Dosing adjustment/comments in renal impairment: If anuria or oliguria evident, hold dose until renal function returns to normal

Dosing adjustment/comments in severe hepatic impairment: Avoid use

Dietary Considerations Should be taken with food. Chewable tablets may contain phenylalanine; amount varies by product, consult manufacturers labeling.

Administration

Oral: Administer with food

I.V.: For I.V. administration only; administration via umbilical arterial line has not been evaluated. Infuse over 15 minutes through port closest to insertion site. Avoid extravasation. Do not administer simultaneously via same line with TPN. If needed, interrupt TPN for 15 minutes prior to and after ibuprofen administration, keeping line open with dextrose or saline.

Monitoring Parameters CBC; occult blood loss and periodic liver function tests; monitor response (pain, range of motion, grip strength, mobility, ADL function), inflammation; observe for weight gain, edema; monitor renal function (urine output, serum BUN and creatinine); observe for bleeding, bruising; evaluate gastrointestinal effects (abdominal pain, bleeding, dyspepsia); mental confusion, disorientation; with long-term therapy, periodic ophthalmic exams

Injection: Renal function, signs of infection or bleeding, ECG

Reference Range Plasma concentrations >200 mcg/mL may be associated with severe toxicity

PDA: Minimum effective level: 10-12 mg/L

Dosage Forms Excipient information presented when available (limited, particularly for generics); consult specific product labeling. [DSC] = Discontinued product

Caplet: 200 mg [OTC]
Advil®: 200 mg [contains sodium benzoate]
Ibu-200, Motrin® IB: 200 mg
Motrin® Junior: 100 mg [scored]

Capsule, liquid-filled:
Advil®: 200 mg [solubilized ibuprofen; contains potassium 20 mg]
Advil® Migraine: 200 mg [solubilized ibuprofen; contains potassium 20 mg]

Gelcap:
Advil®: 200 mg [contains coconut oil]

Injection, solution, as lysine [preservative free]:
NeoProfen®: 17.1 mg/mL (2 mL) [equivalent to ibuprofen 10 mg/mL]

Suspension, oral: 100 mg/5 mL (5 mL, 10 mL, 120 mL, 240 mL, 480 mL)
Advil® Children's: 100 mg/5 mL (120 mL) [contains sodium benzoate, sodium, propylene glycol; blue raspberry, fruit, and grape flavors]
Motrin® Children's: 100 mg/5 mL (60 mL, 120 mL) [contains sodium benzoate; berry, dye free berry, bubble gum, and grape flavors]

Suspension, oral [concentrate, drops]: 40 mg/mL (15 mL)
Advil® Infants': 40 mg/mL (15 mL) [contains sodium benzoate; fruit, grape, and white grape flavors]
Motrin® Infants': 40 mg/mL (15 mL) [contains sodium benzoate; ethanol free; berry and dye-free berry flavors]

Tablet: 200 mg [OTC], 400 mg, 600 mg, 800 mg
Addaprin: 200 mg
Advil®: 200 mg [contains sodium benzoate]
Advil® Junior: 100 mg [contains sodium benzoate; coated tablets] [DSC]
Genpril® [DSC], I-Prin, Midol® Cramp and Body Aches, Motrin® IB, Proprinal, Ultraprin: 200 mg
Ibu®: 400 mg, 600 mg, 800 mg
Ibu-200: 200 mg
Motrin®: 400 mg, 600 mg, 800 mg [DSC]
Proprinal: 200 mg [contains sodium benzoate]
Ultraprin: 200 mg [sugar free]

Tablet, chewable:
Advil® Children's: 50 mg [contains phenylalanine 2.1 mg; grape flavors]
Advil® Junior: 100 mg [contains phenylalanine 4.2 mg; grape flavors] [DSC]
Motrin® Junior: 100 mg [contains phenylalanine 2.1 mg; grape and orange flavors]

◆ **Ibuprofen and Hydrocodone** *see* Hydrocodone and Ibuprofen *on page 742*

◆ **Ibuprofen and Oxycodone** *see* Oxycodone and Ibuprofen *on page 1123*

◆ **Ibuprofen and Pseudoephedrine** *see* Pseudoephedrine and Ibuprofen *on page 1267*

◆ **Ibuprofen Lysine** *see* Ibuprofen *on page 760*

Ibutilide (i BYOO ti lide)

U.S. Brand Names Corvert®

Index Terms Ibutilide Fumarate

Pharmacologic Category Antiarrhythmic Agent, Class III

Use Acute termination of atrial fibrillation or flutter of recent onset; the effectiveness of ibutilide has not been determined in patients with arrhythmias >90 days in duration

Pregnancy Risk Factor C

Pregnancy Considerations Teratogenic and embryocidal in rats; avoid use in pregnancy

Lactation Enters breast milk/contraindicated

Medication Safety Issues

High alert medication: The Institute for Safe Medication Practices (ISMP) includes this medication among its list

of drugs which have a heightened risk of causing significant patient harm when used in error.

Contraindications Hypersensitivity to ibutilide or any component of the formulation; QT_c >440 msec

Warnings/Precautions **[U.S. Boxed Warning]: Potentially fatal arrhythmias (eg, polymorphic ventricular tachycardia) can occur with ibutilide, usually in association with torsade de pointes (QT prolongation).** Studies indicate a 1.7% incidence of arrhythmias in treated patients. The drug should be given in a setting of continuous ECG monitoring and by personnel trained in treating arrhythmias particularly polymorphic ventricular tachycardia. **[U.S. Boxed Warning]: Patients with chronic atrial fibrillation may not be the best candidates for ibutilide since they often revert after conversion and the risks of treatment may not be justified when compared to alternative management.** Dosing adjustments are not required in patients with renal or hepatic dysfunction. Safety and efficacy in children have not been established. Use caution in elderly patients. Avoid concurrent use of any drug that can prolong QT interval. Correct hyperkalemia and hypomagnesemia before using. Monitor for heart block.

Adverse Reactions

1% to 10%:

Cardiovascular: Ventricular extrasystoles (5.1%), nonsustained monomorphic ventricular tachycardia (4.9%), nonsustained polymorphic ventricular tachycardia (2.7%), tachycardia/supraventricular tachycardia (2.7%), hypotension (2%), bundle branch block (1.9%), sustained polymorphic ventricular tachycardia (eg, torsade de pointes) (1.7%, often requiring cardioversion), AV block (1.5%), bradycardia (1.2%), QT segment prolongation, hypertension (1.2%), palpitation (1%)

Central nervous system: Headache (4%)

Gastrointestinal: Nausea (>1%)

<1% (Limited to important or life-threatening): CHF, erythematous bullous lesions, idioventricular rhythm, nodal arrhythmia, renal failure, supraventricular extrasystoles, sustained monomorphic ventricular tachycardia, syncope (0.3%, not > placebo)

Drug Interactions

Avoid Concomitant Use

Avoid concomitant use of Ibutilide with any of the following: Nilotinib; Tetrabenazine; Thioridazine; Ziprasidone

Increased Effect/Toxicity

Ibutilide may increase the levels/effects of: QTc-Prolonging Agents; Tetrabenazine; Thioridazine; Ziprasidone

The levels/effects of Ibutilide may be increased by: Alfuzosin; Ciprofloxacin; Gadobutrol; Nilotinib

Decreased Effect There are no known significant interactions involving a decrease in effect.

Stability Admixtures are chemically and physically stable for 24 hours at room temperature and for 48 hours at refrigerated temperatures. May be administered undiluted or diluted in 50 mL diluent (0.9% NS or D_5W).

Mechanism of Action Exact mechanism of action is unknown; prolongs the action potential in cardiac tissue

Pharmacodynamics/Kinetics

Onset of action: ~90 minutes after start of infusion (1/2 of conversions to sinus rhythm occur during infusion)

Distribution: V_d: 11 L/kg

Protein binding: 40%

Metabolism: Extensively hepatic; oxidation

Half-life elimination: 2-12 hours (average: 6 hours)

Excretion: Urine (82%, 7% as unchanged drug and metabolites); feces (19%)

Dosage I.V.: Initial:

Adults:

<60 kg: 0.01 mg/kg over 10 minutes

≥60 kg: 1 mg over 10 minutes

If the arrhythmia does not terminate within 10 minutes after the end of the initial infusion, a second infusion of equal strength may be infused over a 10-minute period

Elderly: Dose selection should be cautious, usually starting at the lower end of the dosing range.

Administration May be administered undiluted or diluted in 50 mL diluent (0.9% NS or D_5W); infuse over 10 minutes

Monitoring Parameters Observe patient with continuous ECG monitoring for at least 4 hours following infusion or until QT_c has returned to baseline; skilled personnel and proper equipment should be available during administration of ibutilide and subsequent monitoring of the patient

Dosage Forms Excipient information presented when available (limited, particularly for generics); consult specific product labeling.

Injection, solution, as fumarate: 0.1 mg/mL (10 mL)

◆ **Ibutilide Fumarate** *see* Ibutilide *on page 763*

◆ **ICI-182,780** *see* Fulvestrant *on page 675*

◆ **ICI-204,219** *see* Zafirlukast *on page 1575*

◆ **ICI-46474** *see* Tamoxifen *on page 1424*

◆ **ICI-118630** *see* Goserelin *on page 705*

◆ **ICI-176334** *see* Bicalutamide *on page 197*

◆ **ICI-D1033** *see* Anastrozole *on page 116*

◆ **ICL670** *see* Deferasirox *on page 410*

Icodextrin (eye KOE dex trin)

U.S. Brand Names Adept®; Extraneal®

Pharmacologic Category Adhesiolytic; Peritoneal Dialysate, Osmotic

Use

Adept®: Reduction of postsurgical adhesions in gynecologic laparoscopic procedures

Extraneal®: Daily exchange for the long dwell (8- to 16-hour) during continuous ambulatory peritoneal dialysis (CAPD) or automated peritoneal dialysis (APD) for the management of end-stage renal disease (ESRD); improvement of long-dwell ultrafiltration and clearance of creatinine and urea nitrogen (compared to 4.25% dextrose) in patients with high/average or greater transport characteristics as measured by peritoneal equilibration test (PET)

Pregnancy Risk Factor C

Medication Safety Issues

Special care is warranted in patients with diabetes: Due to potential interference by maltose, careful attention must be given to glucose monitoring; only glucose monitors and test strips which employ the glucose-specific method should be used. Innacurate methods (GDH-PQ or glucose-dye-oxidoreductase methods) can result in falsely-elevated readings. Inaccurate readings may mask recognition of true hypoglycemia, or may prompt the administration of insulin, potentially leading to life-threatening consequences.

Dosage Intraperitoneal: Adults:

CAPD or APD (Extraneal®): Given as a single daily exchange in CAPD or APD; dwell time of 8-16 hours is suggested

Laparoscopic gynecologic surgery (Adept®): Irrigate with at least 100 mL every 30 minutes during surgery; aspirate remaining fluid after surgery is completed, then instill 1 L into the cavity

Additional Information Complete prescribing information for this medication should be consulted for additional detail.

Dosage Forms Excipient information presented when available (limited, particularly for generics); consult specific product labeling.

Solution, intraperitoneal:

Adept®: 4% (1.5 L) [for laparoscopic surgery; contains sodium chloride 5.4 g/L, sodium lactate 4.5 g/L, calcium chloride 257 mg/L, magnesium chloride 51 mg/L]

Extraneal: 7.5% (1.5 L, 2 L, 2.5 L) [for peritoneal dialysis; contains sodium 132 mEq/L, calcium 3.5 mEq/L, magnesium 0.5 mEq/L, chloride 96 mEq/L, and lactate 40 mEq/L]

◆ **ICRF-187** *see* Dexrazoxane *on page 430*

◆ **Idamycin® (Can)** *see* IDArubicin *on page 765*

◆ **Idamycin PFS®** *see* IDArubicin *on page 765*

IDArubicin (eye da ROO bi sin)

U.S. Brand Names Idamycin PFS®

Canadian Brand Names Idamycin®

Index Terms 4-Demethoxydaunorubicin; 4-DMDR; Idarubicin Hydrochloride; IDR; IMI 30; NSC-256439; SC 33428

Pharmacologic Category Antineoplastic Agent, Anthracycline; Antineoplastic Agent, Antibiotic

Use Treatment of acute leukemias (AML, ANLL, ALL), accelerated phase or blast crisis of chronic myelogenous leukemia (CML), breast cancer

Unlabeled/Investigational Use Autologous hematopoietic stem cell transplantation

Pregnancy Risk Factor D

Lactation Excretion in breast milk unknown

Medication Safety Issues

Sound-alike/look-alike issues:

IDArubicin may be confused with DOXOrubicin, DAUNOrubicin, epirubicin

Idamycin PFS® may be confused with Adriamycin

High alert medication: The Institute for Safe Medication Practices (ISMP) includes this medication among its list of drugs which have a heightened risk of causing significant patient harm when used in error.

Contraindications Hypersensitivity to idarubicin, other anthracyclines, or any component of the formulation; bilirubin >5 mg/dL; pregnancy

Warnings/Precautions Hazardous agent - use appropriate precautions for handling and disposal. **[U.S. Boxed Warning]: May cause myocardial toxicity (HF, arrhythmias or cardiomyopathies) and is more common in patients who have previously received anthracyclines or have pre-existing cardiac disease.** The risk of myocardial toxicity is also increased in patients with concomitant or prior mediastinal/pericardial irradiation, patients with anemia, bone marrow depression, infections, leukemic pericarditis or myocarditis. Monitor cardiac function during treatment.

[U.S. Boxed Warnings]: May cause severe myelosuppression; use caution in patients with pre-existing myelosuppression from prior treatment or radiation. Use caution with renal or hepatic impairment; may required dosage reductions. For I.V. administration only; may cause severe local tissue damage and necrosis if extravasation occurs. Rapid lysis of leukemic cells may lead to hyperuricemia. Systemic infections should be managed prior to initiation of treatment. **[U.S. Boxed Warning]: Should be administered under the supervision of an experienced cancer chemotherapy physician. Safety and efficacy in children have not been established.**

Adverse Reactions

>10%:

Cardiovascular: Transient ECG abnormalities (supraventricular tachycardia, S-T wave changes, atrial or ventricular extrasystoles); generally asymptomatic and self-limiting. CHF, dose related. The relative cardiotoxicity of idarubicin compared to doxorubicin is unclear. Some investigators report no increase in cardiac toxicity at cumulative oral idarubicin doses up to 540 mg/m^2; other reports suggest a maximum cumulative intravenous dose of 150 mg/m^2.

Central nervous system: Headache

Dermatologic: Alopecia (25% to 30%), radiation recall, skin rash (11%), urticaria

Gastrointestinal: Nausea, vomiting (30% to 60%); diarrhea (9% to 22%); stomatitis (11%); GI hemorrhage (30%)

Emetic potential: Moderate (30% to 60%)

Genitourinary: Discoloration of urine (darker yellow)

Hematologic: Myelosuppression, primarily leukopenia; thrombocytopenia and anemia. Effects are generally less severe with oral dosing.

Nadir: 10-15 days

Recovery: 21-28 days

Hepatic: Bilirubin and transaminases increased (44%)

Local: Tissue necrosis upon extravasation, erythematous streaking

Vesicant chemotherapy

1% to 10%:

Central nervous system: Seizure

Neuromuscular & skeletal: Peripheral neuropathy

<1% (Limited to important or life-threatening): Hyperuricemia

Drug Interactions

Avoid Concomitant Use

Avoid concomitant use of IDArubicin with any of the following: Natalizumab; Vaccines (Live)

Increased Effect/Toxicity

IDArubicin may increase the levels/effects of: Natalizumab; Vaccines (Live)

The levels/effects of IDArubicin may be increased by: Bevacizumab; P-Glycoprotein Inhibitors; Taxane Derivatives; Trastuzumab

Decreased Effect

IDArubicin may decrease the levels/effects of: Cardiac Glycosides; Vaccines (Inactivated)

The levels/effects of IDArubicin may be decreased by: Cardiac Glycosides; Echinacea; P-Glycoprotein Inducers

Stability Store intact vials of solution under refrigeration (2°C to 8°C/36°F to 46°F). Protect from light. Solutions diluted in D_5W or NS for infusion are stable for 4 weeks at room temperature, protected from light. Syringe and IVPB solutions are stable for 72 hours at room temperature and 7 days under refrigeration.

Mechanism of Action Similar to doxorubicin and daunorubicin; inhibition of DNA and RNA synthesis by intercalation between DNA base pairs

Pharmacodynamics/Kinetics

Absorption: Oral: Variable (4% to 77%; mean: ~30%)

Distribution: V_d: 64 L/kg (some reports indicate 2250 L); extensive tissue binding; CSF

Protein binding: 94% to 97%

Metabolism: Hepatic to idarubicinol (pharmacologically active)

Half-life elimination: Oral: 14-35 hours; I.V.: 12-27 hours

Time to peak, serum: 1-5 hours

Excretion:

Oral: Urine (~5% of dose; 0.5% to 0.7% as unchanged drug, 4% as idarubicinol); hepatic (8%)

I.V.: Urine (13% as idarubicinol, 3% as unchanged drug); hepatic (17%)

Dosage Refer to individual protocols. I.V.:

Children:

Leukemia: 10-12 mg/m^2/day for 3 days every 3 weeks

Solid tumors: 5 mg/m^2/day for 3 days every 3 weeks

Adults:

Leukemia induction: 12 mg/m^2/day for 3 days

Leukemia consolidation: 10-12 mg/m^2/day for 2 days

Stem cell transplantation (unlabeled use): 20 mg/m^2/24 hours continuous I.V. infusion **or** 21 mg/m^2/24 hours continuous infusion for 48 hours (both with high-dose oral busulfan)

Dosing adjustment in renal impairment: The FDA-approved labeling does not contain specific dosing adjustment guidelines; however, it does reccomend that dosage reductions be made. Patients with S_{cr}: ≥2 mg/dL did not receive treatment in many clinical trials. The following guidelines have been used by some clinicians (Aronoff, 2007):

Children:

Cl_{cr} <50 mL/minute: Administer 75% of dose

Hemodialysis: Administer 75% of dose

Continuous ambulatory peritoneal dialysis (CAPD): Administer 75% of dose

Continuous renal replacement therapy (CRRT): Administer 75% of dose

Adults:

Cl_{cr} 10-50 mL/minute: Administer 75% of dose

Cl_{cr} <10 mL/minute: Administer 50% of dose

Hemodialysis/CAPD: Supplemental dose not needed

Dosing adjustment/comments in hepatic impairment:

Bilirubin 2.6-5 mg/dL: Administer 50% of dose

Bilirubin >5 mg/dL: Avoid use

Administration Do not administer I.M. or SubQ; administer as slow push over 3-5 minutes, preferably into the side of a freely-running saline or dextrose infusion **or** as intermittent infusion over 10-15 minutes into a free-flowing I.V. solution of NS or D_5W; also occasionally administered as a bladder lavage.

Extravasation management: Topical cooling may be achieved using ice packs or cooling pad with circulating ice water. Cooling of site for 24 hours as tolerated by the patient. Elevate and rest extremity 24-48 hours, then resume normal activity as tolerated. Application of cold inhibits vesicant's cytotoxicity. **Application of heat can be harmful and is contraindicated.** If pain, erythema, and/or swelling persist beyond 48 hours, refer patient immediately to plastic surgeon for consultation and possible debridement.

Monitoring Parameters CBC with differential, platelet count, cardiac function, serum electrolytes, creatinine, uric acid, ALT, AST, bilirubin, signs of extravasation

Dosage Forms Excipient information presented when available (limited, particularly for generics); consult specific product labeling.

Injection, solution, as hydrochloride [preservative free] (Idamycin PFS®): 1 mg/mL (5 mL, 10 mL, 20 mL)

- **Idarubicin Hydrochloride** *see* IDArubicin *on page 765*
- **IDEC-C2B8** *see* RiTUXimab *on page 1328*
- **IDEC-Y2B8** *see* Ibritumomab *on page 758*
- **IDR** *see* IDArubicin *on page 765*

Idursulfase (eye dur SUL fase)

U.S. Brand Names Elaprase™

Canadian Brand Names Elaprase™

Pharmacologic Category Enzyme

Use Replacement therapy in mucopolysaccharidosis II (MPS II, Hunter syndrome) for improvement of walking capacity

Pregnancy Risk Factor C

Medication Safety Issues

Sound-alike/look-alike issues:

Elaprase™ may be confused with Elspar®

Dosage I.V.: MPS II:

Children ≥5 years and Adults: 0.5 mg/kg once weekly

Elderly: Studies did not include patients ≥65 years

Additional Information Complete prescribing information for this medication should be consulted for additional detail.

Dosage Forms Excipient information presented when available (limited, particularly for generics); consult specific product labeling.

Injection, solution [preservative free]:

Elaprase™: 2 mg/mL (5 mL) [extractable volume: 3 mL]

- **Ifex®** *see* Ifosfamide *on page 766*
- **IFLrA** *see* Interferon Alfa-2a *on page 799*

Ifosfamide (eye FOSS fa mide)

U.S. Brand Names Ifex®

Canadian Brand Names Ifex®

Index Terms Isophosphamide; NSC-109724; Z4942

Pharmacologic Category Antineoplastic Agent, Alkylating Agent; Antineoplastic Agent, Alkylating Agent (Nitrogen Mustard)

Use Treatment of testicular cancer

Unlabeled/Investigational Use Treatment of bladder, breast, cervical, ovarian, pancreatic, and lung cancers; Hodgkin's and non-Hodgkin's lymphoma; acute lymphocytic leukemia; Ewing's sarcoma, osteosarcoma, and soft tissue sarcomas

Pregnancy Risk Factor D

Pregnancy Considerations Increased resorptions and embryotoxic effects have been observed in animal studies.

Lactation Enters breast milk/not recommended

Medication Safety Issues

Sound-alike/look-alike issues:

Ifosfamide may be confused with cyclophosphamide

High alert medication: The Institute for Safe Medication Practices (ISMP) includes this medication among its list of drugs which have a heightened risk of causing significant patient harm when used in error.

Contraindications Hypersensitivity to ifosfamide or any component of the formulation; patients with severely depressed bone marrow function

Warnings/Precautions Hazardous agent - use appropriate precautions for handling and disposal. **[U.S. Boxed Warning]: Urotoxic side effects, primarily hemorrhagic cystitis, may occur (dose-limiting toxicity).** Hydration (at least 2 L/day) and/or mesna administration will protect against hemorrhagic cystitis. **[U.S. Boxed Warning]: Severe bone marrow suppression may occur (dose-limiting toxicity);** use is contraindicated in patients with severely depressed bone marrow function. **[U.S. Boxed Warning]: May cause CNS toxicity, including confusion and coma;** usually reversible upon discontinuation of treatment. Encephalopathy, ranging from mild somnolence to hallucinations and/or coma may occur; risk factors may include hypoalbuminemia, renal dysfunction and prior history of ifosfamide-induced encephalopathy. Use with caution in patients with impaired renal function or those with compromised bone marrow reserve. May interfere with wound healing. **[U.S. Boxed Warning]: Should be administered under the supervision of an experienced cancer chemotherapy physician.** Safety and efficacy in children have not been established.

Adverse Reactions

>10%:

Central nervous system: CNS toxicity or encephalopathy (10% to 30%; includes somnolence, agitation, confusion, delirium, hallucinations, depressive psychosis, incontinence, palsy, diplopia, aphasia, or coma)

Dermatologic: Alopecia (83%)

Endocrine & metabolic: Metabolic acidosis (31%)

Gastrointestinal: Nausea/vomiting (58%), may be more common with higher doses or bolus infusion

Hematologic: Myelosuppression (onset: 7-14 days; nadir: 21-28 days; recovery: 21-28 days), leukopenia (50% to ≤100%; grade 4: ≤50%), thrombocytopenia (20%; grades 3/4: 8%)
Renal: Hematuria (6% to 92%; grade 2 [gross hematuria]: 8% to 12%)

1% to 10%:
Central nervous system: Fever
Hepatic: Bilirubin increased (3%), liver dysfunction (3%), transaminases increased (3%)
Local: Phlebitis (2%)
Renal: Renal impairment (6%)
Miscellaneous: Infection (8%)

<1% (Limited to important or life-threatening): Acidosis, acute renal failure, acute tubular necrosis, allergic reaction, anemia, anorexia, BUN increased, cardiotoxicity, chronic renal failure, coagulopathy, constipation, creatinine increased, dermatitis, diarrhea, Fanconi syndrome, fatigue, hyper-/hypotension, hyperpigmentation, malaise, nail banding/ridging, nonconvulsive status epilepticus, polyneuropathy, proteinuria, pulmonary fibrosis, renal rickets, renal tubular acidosis, salivation, SIADH, sterility, stomatitis

Drug Interactions

Metabolism/Transport Effects **Substrate** of CYP2A6 (major), 2B6 (minor), 2C8 (minor), 2C9 (minor), 2C19 (major), 3A4 (major); **Inhibits** CYP3A4 (weak); **Induces** CYP2C8 (weak), 2C9 (weak)

Avoid Concomitant Use

Avoid concomitant use of Ifosfamide with any of the following: Natalizumab; Vaccines (Live)

Increased Effect/Toxicity

Ifosfamide may increase the levels/effects of: Natalizumab; Vaccines (Live); Vitamin K Antagonists

The levels/effects of Ifosfamide may be increased by: CYP2A6 Inhibitors (Moderate); CYP2A6 Inhibitors (Strong); CYP2C19 Inhibitors (Moderate); CYP2C19 Inhibitors (Strong); CYP3A4 Inhibitors (Moderate); CYP3A4 Inhibitors (Strong); Dasatinib; Trastuzumab

Decreased Effect

Ifosfamide may decrease the levels/effects of: Vaccines (Inactivated); Vitamin K Antagonists

The levels/effects of Ifosfamide may be decreased by: CYP2A6 Inducers (Strong); CYP2C19 Inducers (Strong); CYP3A4 Inducers (Strong); Deferasirox; Echinacea; Herbs (CYP3A4 Inducers)

Ethanol/Nutrition/Herb Interactions Herb/Nutraceutical: St John's wort may decrease ifosfamide levels.

Stability Store intact vials of powder for injection at room temperature of 20°C to 25°C (68°F to 77°F). Store intact vials of solution under refrigeration at 2°C to 8°C (36°F to 46°F). Dilute powder with SWFI or bacteriostatic SWFI to a concentration of 50 mg/mL. Further dilution in 50-1000 mL D_5W or NS (to a final concentration of 0.6-20 mg/mL) is recommended for I.V. infusion. Reconstituted solutions may be stored under refrigeration for up to 21 days. Solutions diluted for administration are stable for 7 days at room temperature and for 6 weeks under refrigeration.

Mechanism of Action Causes cross-linking of strands of DNA by binding with nucleic acids and other intracellular structures; inhibits protein synthesis and DNA synthesis

Pharmacodynamics/Kinetics Pharmacokinetics are dose dependent

Distribution: V_d: 5.7-49 L; does penetrate CNS, but not in therapeutic levels
Protein binding: Negligible
Metabolism: Hepatic to active metabolites isofosforamide mustard, 4-hydroxy-ifosfamide, acrolein, and inactive dichloroethylated and carboxy metabolites; acrolein is the agent implicated in development of hemorrhagic cystitis
Half-life elimination:
High dose (3800-5000 mg/m^2): ~15 hours
Lower dose (1600-2400 mg/m^2): ~7 hours
Excretion:
High dose (5000 mg/m^2): Urine (70% to 86%; 61% as unchanged drug)
Lower dose (1600-2400 mg/m^2): Urine (12% to 18% as unchanged drug)

Dosage Refer to individual protocols. To prevent bladder toxicity, ifosfamide should be given with the urinary protector mesna and hydration of at least 2 L of oral or I.V. fluid per day.

Children (unlabeled use): I.V.
1200-1800 mg/m^2/day for 3-5 days every 21-28 days **or**
5 g/m^2 once every 21-28 days **or**
3 g/m^2/day for 2 days every 21-28 days

Adults: I.V.:
Testicular cancer: 1200 mg/m^2/day for 5 days every 3 weeks
Dose ranges used in other cancers (unlabeled uses):
4000-5000 mg/m^2/day for 1 day every 14-28 days **or**
1000-3000 mg/m^2/day for 2-5 days every 21-28 days

Dosing adjustment in renal impairment: The FDA-approved labeling does not contain dosage adjustment guidelines (has not been studied). The following guidelines have been used by some clinicians:
Aronoff, 2007:
Cl_{cr} <10 mL/minute: Children and Adults: Administer 75% of dose
Hemodialysis:
Children: 1 g/m^2 followed by hemodialysis 6-8 hours later
Adults: No supplemental dose needed
Kintzel, 1995:
Cl_{cr} 46-60 mL/minute: Administer 80% of dose
Cl_{cr} 31-45 mL/minute: Administer 75% of dose
Cl_{cr} <30 mL/minute: Administer 70% of dose

Dosing adjustment in hepatic impairment: The FDA-approved labeling does not contain dosage adjustment guidelines (has not been studied). The following guidelines have been used by some clinicians (Floyd, 2006): Bilirubin >3 mg/dL: Administer 25% of dose

Administration Administer I.V. over 30 minutes to several hours or continuous I.V. over 5 days

Monitoring Parameters CBC with differential, hemoglobin, and platelet count, urine output, urinalysis (prior to each dose), liver function, and renal function tests

Dosage Forms Excipient information presented when available (limited, particularly for generics); consult specific product labeling.
Injection, powder for reconstitution: 1 g
Ifex®: 1 g, 3 g
Injection, solution: 50 mg/mL (20 mL, 60 mL)

◆ **IG** *see* Immune Globulin (Intramuscular) *on page 776*

◆ **IgG4-Kappa Monoclonal Antibody** *see* Natalizumab *on page 1044*

◆ **IGIM** *see* Immune Globulin (Intramuscular) *on page 776*

◆ **IGIV** *see* Immune Globulin (Intravenous) *on page 777*

◆ **IL-1Ra** *see* Anakinra *on page 115*

◆ **IL-2** *see* Aldesleukin *on page 53*

◆ **IL-11** *see* Oprelvekin *on page 1106*

Iloprost (EYE loe prost)

U.S. Brand Names Ventavis®

Index Terms Iloprost Tromethamine; Prostacyclin PGI_2

Pharmacologic Category Prostacyclin; Prostaglandin; Vasodilator

Use Treatment of idiopathic pulmonary arterial hypertension in patients with NYHA Class III or IV symptoms

Pregnancy Risk Factor C

Dosage Inhalation: Adults: Initial: 2.5 mcg/dose; if tolerated, increase to 5 mcg/dose; administer 6-9 times daily (dosing at intervals ≥2 hours while awake according to individual need and tolerability); maintenance dose: 2.5-5 mcg/dose; maximum daily dose: 45 mcg

Dosage adjustment in renal impairment: Adjustments are not necessary. Use caution in dialysis patients; may be more susceptible to hypotension.

Dosage adjustment in hepatic impairment: Use caution

Additional Information Complete prescribing information for this medication should be consulted for additional detail.

Dosage Forms Excipient information presented when available (limited, particularly for generics); consult specific product labeling.

Solution for oral inhalation [preservative-free]:

Ventavis®: 10 mcg/mL (1 mL, 2 mL) [ampul]

◆ **Iloprost Tromethamine** *see* Iloprost *on page 767*

Imatinib (eye MAT eh nib)

U.S. Brand Names Gleevec®

Canadian Brand Names Gleevec®

Index Terms CGP-57148B; Glivec; Imatinib Mesylate; NSC-716051; STI-571

Pharmacologic Category Antineoplastic Agent, Tyrosine Kinase Inhibitor

Use Treatment of:

Gastrointestinal stromal tumors (GIST) kit-positive (CD117) unresectable and/or metastatic malignant

Philadelphia chromosome-positive (Ph+) chronic myeloid leukemia (CML) in chronic phase (newly-diagnosed)

Ph+ CML in chronic phase in pediatric patients recurring following stem cell transplant or who are resistant to interferon-alpha therapy (**not** an approved use in Canada)

Ph+ CML in blast crisis, accelerated phase, or chronic phase after failure of interferon therapy

Ph+ acute lymphoblastic leukemia (ALL) (relapsed or refractory)

Aggressive systemic mastocytosis (ASM) without D816V c-Kit mutation (or c-Kit mutation status unknown)

Dermatofibrosarcoma protuberans (DFSP) (unresectable, recurrent and/or metastatic)

Hypereosinophilic syndrome (HES) and/or chronic eosinophilic leukemia (CEL)

Myelodysplastic/myeloproliferative disease (MDS/MPD) associated with platelet-derived growth factor receptor (PDGFR) gene rearrangements

Note: The following use is approved in Canada (not an approved indication in the U.S.):

Ph+ ALL induction therapy (newly diagnosed)

Unlabeled/Investigational Use Treatment of desmoid tumors (soft tissue sarcoma)

Pregnancy Risk Factor D

Pregnancy Considerations There are no adequate and well-controlled studies in pregnant women. Animal studies have demonstrated teratogenic effects and fetal loss. Women of childbearing potential are advised not to become pregnant (female patients and female partners of male patients). Adequate contraception is recommended. Case reports of pregnancies while on therapy (both males and females) include reports of spontaneous abortion, minor abnormalities (hypospadias, pyloric stenosis, and small intestine rotation) at or shortly after birth, and other congenital abnormalities including skeletal malformations, hypoplastic lungs, exomphalos, kidney abnormalities, hydrocephalus, cerebellar hypoplasia, and cardiac defects.

Retrospective case reports of women with CML in complete hematologic response (CHR) with cytogenic response (partial or complete) who interrupted imatinib therapy due to pregnancy, demonstrated a loss of response in some patients while off treatment. At 18 months after treatment reinitiation following delivery, CHR was again achieved in all patients and cytogenic response was achieved in some patients. Cytogenetic response rates may not be at as high as compared to patients with 18 months of uninterrupted therapy (Ault, 2006; Pye, 2008).

Lactation Excretion in breast milk unknown/not recommended

Medication Safety Issues

High alert medication: The Institute for Safe Medication Practices (ISMP) includes this medication among its list of drug classes which have a heightened risk of causing significant patient harm when used in error.

Contraindications There are no contraindications listed within the FDA-approved manufacturer's labeling.

Canadian labeling: Hypersensitivity to imatinib or any component of the formulation

Warnings/Precautions Hazardous agent - use appropriate precautions for handling and disposal. Often associated with fluid retention, weight gain, and edema (probability increases with higher doses and age >65 years); occasionally leading to significant complications, including pleural effusion, pericardial effusion, pulmonary edema, and ascites. Use with caution in patients where fluid accumulation may be poorly tolerated, such as in cardiovascular disease (HF or hypertension) and pulmonary disease. Severe HF and left ventricular dysfunction (LVD) have been reported rarely, usually in patients with comorbidities and/or risk factors; carefully monitor patients with pre-existing cardiac disease or risk factors for heart failure. With initiation of imatinib treatment, cardiogenic shock and/or LVD have been reported in patients with hypereosinophilic syndrome and cardiac involvement (reversible with systemic steroids, circulatory support and temporary cessation of imatinib). Patients with high eosinophil levels and an abnormal echocardiogram or abnormal serum troponin level may benefit from prophylactic systemic steroids with the initiation of imatinib.

Severe bullous dermatologic reactions (including erythema multiforme and Stevens-Johnson syndrome) have been reported; reintroduction has been attempted following resolution. Successful resumption at a lower dose (with corticosteroids and/or antihistamine) has been described; however, some patients may experience recurrent reactions.

Hepatotoxicity may occur (may be severe); monitor; therapy interruption or dose reduction may be necessary; acute liver failure has also been reported. Use with caution in patients with pre-existing hepatic impairment; may require dosage adjustment. Use with caution in renal impairment; may require dosage adjustment.

May cause GI irritation, severe hemorrhage (grades 3 and 4; including gastrointestinal hemorrhage and/or tumor hemorrhage; hemorrhage incidence is higher in patients with GIST), or hematologic toxicity (anemia, neutropenia, and thrombocytopenia); median duration of neutropenia is 2-3 weeks; median duration of thrombocytopenia is 3-4 weeks. Hypothyroidism has been reported in thyroidectomy patients (receiving thyroid hormone replacement therapy) during imatinib therapy; monitor. Has been associated with development of opportunistic infections. Use with caution in patients receiving concurrent therapy with drugs which alter cytochrome P450 activity or require metabolism by these isoenzymes. Safety and efficacy in patients <2 years of age have not been established.

Adverse Reactions

>10%:

Cardiovascular: Edema/fluid retention (33% to 86%; grades 3/4: 3% to 13%; includes aggravated edema, anasarca, pericardial effusion, peripheral edema, pulmonary edema and superficial edema); facial edema (DFSP 17%), chest pain (CML 7% to 11%)

Central nervous system: Fatigue (29% to 75%), fever (13% to 41%), headache (20% to 37%), dizziness (10% to 19%), insomnia (10% to 19%), depression (≤15%), anxiety (7% to 12%), chills (≤11%)

Dermatologic: Rash (25% to 50%; grades 3/4: 3% to 9%), pruritus (8% to 19%), alopecia (GIST 12% to 15%)

Endocrine & metabolic: Hypokalemia (CML 6% to 13%)

Gastrointestinal: Nausea (42% to 73%), diarrhea (25% to 58%), vomiting (23% to 58%), abdominal pain (30% to 57%), anorexia (≤36%), weight gain (5% to 32%), dyspepsia (11% to 27%), constipation (9% to 16%), taste disturbance (GIST 3% to 15%), loose stools (GIST 10% to 12%)

Hematologic: Hemorrhage (12% to 53%; grades 3/4: 2% to 19%), neutropenia (grade 3: 7% to 27%; grade 4: 3% to 48%), thrombocytopenia (grade 3: 1% to 31%; grade 4: <1% to 33%), anemia (grade 3: 3% to 42%; grade 4: 1% to 11%), leukopenia (GIST 17% to 20%)

Hepatic: Ascites/pleural effusion (GIST 12% to 15%), hepatotoxicity (6% to 12%; grades 3/4: 3% to 8%)

Neuromuscular & skeletal: Muscle cramps (28% to 62%), musculoskeletal pain (adults 30% to 49%; children 21%), arthralgia (≤40%), joint pain (11% to 31%), myalgia (9% to 32%), back pain (GIST 23% to 26%), weakness (≤21%), rigors (10% to 12%), bone pain (≤11%)

Ocular: Periorbital edema (DFSP 33%; MPD 29%), lacrimation increased (DFSP 25%; GIST 16% to 18%)

Renal: Serum creatinine increased (≤11%; grade 3: ≤3%; DFSP: grade 4: 8%)

Respiratory: Nasopharyngitis (10% to 31%), cough (14% to 27%), dyspnea (≤21%), upper respiratory tract infection (3% to 21%), pharyngolaryngeal pain (7% to 18%), rhinitis (DFSP 17%), pharyngitis (CML 10% to 15%), pneumonia (CML 4% to 13%), sinusitis (4% to 11%)

Miscellaneous: Night sweats (CML 13% to 17%), infection without neutropenia (GIST 16% to 17%), influenza (1% to 14%), diaphoresis (GIST 9% to 13%)

1% to 10%:

Cardiovascular: Flushing

Central nervous system: CNS/cerebral hemorrhage (≤9%), hypoesthesia

Dermatologic: Dry skin, erythema, photosensitivity reaction

Endocrine & metabolic: Albumin decreased (grade 3: ≤4%)

Gastrointestinal: Flatulence (≤10%), stomatitis/mucositis (≤10%), gastrointestinal hemorrhage (2% to 8%), abdominal distension, gastritis, gastroesophageal reflux, mouth ulceration, weight loss, xerostomia

Hematologic: Lymphopenia (GIST 6% to 10%), neutropenic fever, pancytopenia

Hepatic: Alkaline phosphatase increased (grade 3: ≤6%; grade 4: <1%), ALT increased (grade 3: 2% to 7%; grade 4: <1%), AST increased (grade 3: 2% to 4%; grade 4: ≤3%), bilirubin increased (grade 3: 1% to 4%; grade 4: ≤3%)

Neuromuscular & skeletal: Joint swelling, paresthesia

Ocular: Blurred vision, conjunctival hemorrhage, conjunctivitis, dry eyes, eyelid edema

Respiratory: Epistaxis

Miscellaneous: Tumor hemorrhage (GIST 1% to 4%)

<1% (Limited to important or life-threatening): cute febrile neutropenic dermatosis (Sweet's syndrome), amylase increased, anaphylactic shock, angina, angioedema, aplastic anemia, arrhythmia, ascites, atrial fibrillation, avascular necrosis, blepharitis, breast enlargement, bullous eruption, cardiac arrest, cardiac failure, cardiac tamponade, cardiogenic shock, cataract, cellulitis, cerebral edema, cheilitis, CHF (severe), colitis, confusion, CPK increased, dehydration, diverticulitis, dysphagia, embolism, eosinophilia, erythema multiforme, esophagitis, exanthematous pustulosis (acute generalized), exfoliative dermatitis, fungal infection, gastric ulcer, gastroenteritis, gastrointestinal obstruction, gastrointestinal perforation, glaucoma, gout, hearing loss, hematoma, hematemesis, hematuria, hemolytic anemia, hepatic failure, hepatic necrosis, hepatitis, herpes simplex, herpes zoster, hip osteonecrosis, hypercalcemia, hyperglycemia, hyperkalemia, hyperuricemia, hyper-/hypotension, hypomagnesemia, hyponatremia, hypophosphatemia, ileus, inflammatory bowel disease, interstitial lung disease, interstitial pneumonitis, intracranial pressure increased, jaundice, LDH increased, left ventricular dysfunction, leukocytoclastic vasculitis, libido decreased, lichen planus, lichenoid keratosis, lymphadenopathy, macular edema, melena, memory impairment, menorrhagia, MI, migraine, optic neuritis, palpitation, pancreatitis, papilledema, pericarditis, peripheral neuropathy, petechiae, pleural effusion, pleuritic pain, pulmonary fibrosis, pulmonary hemorrhage, pulmonary hypertension, purpura, pustular rash, Raynaud's phenomenon, renal failure, respiratory failure, respiratory tract (lower) infection, retinal hemorrhage, sciatica, scleral hemorrhage, seizure, sepsis, sexual dysfunction, skin pigment changes, somnolence, Stevens-Johnson syndrome, syncope, tachycardia, thrombocythemia, thrombosis, tinnitus, toxic epidermal necrolysis, tremor, tumor necrosis, urinary tract infection, urticaria, vertigo, vesicular rash, vitreous hemorrhage

Drug Interactions

Metabolism/Transport Effects Substrate of CYP1A2 (minor), 2D6 (minor), 2C9 (minor), 2C19 (minor), 3A4 (major), **Inhibits** CYP2C9 (weak), 2D6 (moderate), 3A4 (strong)

Avoid Concomitant Use

Avoid concomitant use of Imatinib with any of the following: Alfuzosin; Eplerenone; Natalizumab; Nilotinib; Nisoldipine; Ranolazine; Rivaroxaban; Salmeterol; Silodosin; Thioridazine; Vaccines (Live)

Increased Effect/Toxicity

Imatinib may increase the levels/effects of: Acetaminophen; Alfuzosin; Alosetron; Ciclesonide; CycloSPORINE; CYP2D6 Substrates; CYP3A4 Substrates; Eplerenone; FentaNYL; Fesoterodine; Ixabepilone; Maraviroc; Natalizumab; Nebivolol; Nilotinib; Nisoldipine; Pimecrolimus; Ranolazine; Rivaroxaban; Salmeterol; Silodosin; Simvastatin; Sorafenib; Tamoxifen; Thioridazine; Topotecan; Vaccines (Live); Vitamin K Antagonists; Warfarin

The levels/effects of Imatinib may be increased by: Antifungal Agents (Azole Derivatives, Systemic); CYP3A4 Inhibitors (Moderate); CYP3A4 Inhibitors (Strong); Dasatinib; Lansoprazole; P-Glycoprotein Inhibitors; Trastuzumab

Decreased Effect

Imatinib may decrease the levels/effects of: Cardiac Glycosides; Codeine; TraMADol; Vaccines (Inactivated); Vitamin K Antagonists

The levels/effects of Imatinib may be decreased by: CYP3A4 Inducers (Strong); Deferasirox; Echinacea; P-Glycoprotein Inducers; Rifamycin Derivatives; St Johns Wort

Ethanol/Nutrition/Herb Interactions

Ethanol: Avoid ethanol.

Food: Food may reduce gastrointestinal irritation. Avoid grapefruit juice (may increase imatinib plasma concentration).

Herb/Nutraceutical: Avoid St John's wort (may increase metabolism and decrease imatinib plasma concentration).

Stability Store at 25°C (77°F); excursions permitted between 15°C to 30°C (59°F to 86°F). Protect from moisture.

Mechanism of Action Inhibits Bcr-Abl tyrosine kinase, the constitutive abnormal gene product of the Philadelphia chromosome in chronic myeloid leukemia (CML). Inhibition of this enzyme blocks proliferation and induces apoptosis in Bcr-Abl positive cell lines as well as in fresh leukemic cells in Philadelphia chromosome positive CML. Also inhibits tyrosine kinase for platelet-derived growth factor (PDGF), stem cell factor (SCF), c-Kit, and cellular events mediated by PDGF and SCF.

Pharmacodynamics/Kinetics

Absorption: Rapid

Protein binding: Parent drug and metabolite: ~95% to albumin and alpha$_1$-acid glycoprotein

Metabolism: Hepatic via CYP3A4 (minor metabolism via CYP1A2, CYP2D6, CYP2C9, CYP2C19); primary metabolite (active): N-demethylated piperazine derivative (CGP74588); severe hepatic impairment (bilirubin >3-10 times ULN) increases AUC by 45% to 55% for imatinib and its active metabolite, respectively

Bioavailability: 98%

Half-life elimination: Adults: Parent drug: ~18 hours; N-desmethyl metabolite: ~40 hours; Children: Parent drug: ~15 hours

Time to peak: 2-4 hours

Excretion: Feces (68% primarily as metabolites, 20% as unchanged drug); urine (13% primarily as metabolites, 5% as unchanged drug)

Dosage Oral: **Note:** For concurrent use with a strong CYP3A4 enzyme-inducing agent (eg, rifampin, phenytoin), imatinib dosage should be increased by at least 50%.

Children ≥2 years: **Note:** May be administered once daily or in 2 divided doses.

Ph+ CML (chronic phase, recurrent or resistant): 260 mg/m^2/day

Ph+ CML (chronic phase, newly diagnosed): 340 mg/m^2/day; maximum: 600 mg/day

Adults:

Ph+ CML:

Chronic phase: 400 mg once daily; may be increased to 600 mg/day, if tolerated, for disease progression, lack of hematologic response after 3 months, lack of cytogenetic response after 6-12 months, or loss of previous hematologic or cytogenetic response

Canadian labeling and NCCN CML guidelines (v.2.2009): Includes range up to 800 mg/day (400 mg twice daily)

Accelerated phase or blast crisis: 600 mg once daily; may be increased to 800 mg/day (400 mg twice daily), if tolerated, for disease progression, lack of hematologic response after 3 months, lack of cytogenetic response after 6-12 months, or loss of previous hematologic or cytogenetic response

Ph+ ALL (relapsed or refractory): 600 mg once daily

GIST: 400 mg once daily; may be increased up to 800 mg/day (400 mg twice daily), if tolerated, for disease progression

ASM with eosinophilia: Initiate at 100 mg once daily; titrate up to a maximum of 400 mg once daily (if tolerated) for insufficient response to lower dose

ASM without D816V c-Kit mutation or c-Kit mutation status unknown: 400 mg once daily

DFSP: 400 mg twice daily

HES/CEL: 400 mg once daily

HES/CEL with FIP1L1-PDGFRα fusion kinase: Initiate at 100 mg once daily; titrate up to a maximum of 400 mg once daily (if tolerated) if insufficient response to lower dose

MDS/MPD: 400 mg once daily

Ph+ ALL (induction, newly diagnosed): *Canadian labeling (not an approved use in the U.S.):* 600 mg once daily

Dosage adjustment with concomitant strong CYP3A4 inducers: Avoid concomitant use of strong CYP3A4 inducers (eg, dexamethasone, carbamazepine, phenobarbital, phenytoin, rifampin); if concomitant use can not be avoided, increase imatinib dose by at least 50% with careful monitoring.

Dosage adjustment for renal impairment:

Recommendation in the FDA-approved labeling:

Mild impairment (Cl_{cr} 40-59 mL/minute): Maximum recommended dose: 600 mg

Moderate impairment (Cl_{cr} 20-39 mL/minute): Decrease recommended starting dose by 50%; dose may be increased as tolerated; maximum recommended dose: 400 mg

Severe impairment (Cl_{cr} <20 mL/minute): Use caution; a dose of 100 mg/day has been tolerated in severe impairment (case reports)

Canadian labeling recommendation:

Mild impairment (Cl_{cr} 40-59 mL/minute): Use caution; usual minimum recommended effective dose: 400 mg once daily; titrate to efficacy and tolerability

Moderate impairment (Cl_{cr} 20-39 mL/minute): Use caution; usual minimum recommended effective dose: 400 mg once daily; titrate to efficacy and tolerability; the use of 800 mg dose is not recommended

Severe impairment (Cl_{cr} <20 mL/minute): Use is not recommended

Dosage adjustment for hepatic impairment:

Mild-to-moderate impairment: No adjustment necessary

Canadian labeling: GIST: Minimum effective dose: 400 mg once daily

Severe impairment: Reduce dose by 25%

Canadian labeling: GIST: 200 mg dose once daily with titration to 300 mg once daily in the absence of severe toxicity

Dosage adjustment for hepatotoxicity (during therapy) or other nonhematologic adverse reactions: Withhold treatment until toxicity resolves; may resume if appropriate (depending on initial severity of adverse event)

Hepatotoxicity (during therapy): If elevations of bilirubin >3 times upper limit of normal (ULN) or transaminases (ALT/AST) >5 times ULN occur, withhold treatment until bilirubin <1.5 times ULN or transaminases <2.5 times ULN. Resume treatment at a reduced dose as follows:

Children ≥2 years:

If current dose 260 mg/m^2/day, reduce dose to 200 mg/m^2/day

If current dose 340 mg/m^2/day, reduce dose to 260 mg/m^2/day

Adults:

If current dose 400 mg, reduce dose to 300 mg

If current dose 600 mg, reduce dose to 400 mg

If current dose 800 mg, reduce dose to 600 mg

Dosage adjustment for hematologic adverse reactions:

Chronic phase CML (initial dose 400 mg/day in adults or 260-340 mg/m^2/day in children), ASM, MDS/MPD, and HES/CEL (initial dose 400 mg/day), or GIST (initial dose 400 mg or 600 mg): If ANC <1 x 10^9/L and/or platelets <50 x 10^9/L: Withhold until ANC ≥1.5 x 10^9/L and platelets ≥75 x 10^9/L; resume treatment at original starting dose. For recurrent neutropenia or thrombocytopenia, withhold until recovery, and reinstitute treatment at a reduced dose as follows:

Children ≥2 years:

If initial dose 260 mg/m^2/day, reduce dose to 200 mg/m^2/day

If initial dose 340 mg/m^2/day, reduce dose to 260 mg/m^2/day
Adults:
If initial dose 400 mg, reduce dose to 300 mg
If initial dose 600 mg, reduce dose to 400 mg
CML (accelerated phase or blast crisis) and PH+ ALL: Adults (initial dose 600 mg): If ANC <0.5 x 10^9/L and/or platelets <10 x 10^9/L, establish whether cytopenia is related to leukemia (bone marrow aspirate or biopsy). If unrelated to leukemia, reduce dose to 400 mg. If cytopenia persists for an additional 2 weeks, further reduce dose to 300 mg. If cytopenia persists for 4 weeks and is still unrelated to leukemia, withhold treatment until ANC ≥1 x 10^9/L and platelets ≥20 x 10^9/L, then resume treatment at 300 mg.
ASM associated with eosinophilia and HES/CEL with FIP1L1-PDGFRα fusion kinase (starting dose 100 mg/day): If ANC <1 x 10^9/L and/or platelets <50 x 10^9/L: Withhold until ANC ≥1.5 x 10^9/L and platelets ≥75 x 10^9/L; resume treatment at previous dose.
DFSP (initial dose 800 mg/day): If ANC <1 x 10^9/L and/or platelets <50 x 10^9/L , withhold until ANC ≥1.5 x 10^9/L and platelets ≥75 x 10^9/L; resume treatment at reduced dose of 600 mg/day. If depression in neutrophils or platelets recurs, withhold until recovery, and reinstitute treatment with a further dose reduction to 400 mg/day.

Dietary Considerations Should be taken with food and a large glass of water to decrease gastrointestinal irritation.

Administration Should be administered with food and a large glass of water. Tablets may be dispersed in water or apple juice (using ~50 mL for 100 mg tablet, ~200 mL for 400 mg tablet); stir until dissolved and use immediately. For daily dosing ≥800 mg, the 400 mg tablets should be used in order to reduce iron exposure.

Monitoring Parameters CBC (weekly for first month, biweekly for second month, then periodically thereafter), liver function tests (at baseline and monthly or as clinically indicated), renal function, serum electrolytes (including calcium, phosphorus, potassium and sodium levels); thyroid function tests (in thyroidectomy patients); fatigue, weight, and edema/fluid status; consider echocardiogram and serum troponin levels in patients with HES/CEL, and in patients with MDS/MPD or ASM with high eosinophil levels; in pediatric patients, also monitor serum glucose and albumin

Monitor for signs/symptoms of CHF in patients with at risk for cardiac failure or patients with pre-existing cardiac disease. In Canada, a baseline evaluation of left ventricular ejection fraction is recommended prior to initiation of imatinib therapy in all patients with known underlying heart disease or in elderly patients.

Additional Information Patients with HES/CEL, MDS/MPD or ASM with an abnormal echocardiogram or abnormal serum troponin level may benefit from prophylactic systemic steroids (1-2 mg/kg for 1-2 weeks) with the initiation of imatinib.

Dosage Forms Excipient information presented when available (limited, particularly for generics); consult specific product labeling.
Tablet:
Gleevec®: 100 mg; 400 mg

◆ **Imatinib Mesylate** *see* Imatinib *on page 768*

◆ **IMC-C225** *see* Cetuximab *on page 297*

◆ **Imdur®** *see* Isosorbide Mononitrate *on page 824*

◆ **123I-Metaiodobenzylguanidine (MIBG)** *see* Iobenguane I 123 *on page 810*

◆ **Imferon** *see* Iron Dextran Complex *on page 817*

◆ **IMI 30** *see* IDArubicin *on page 765*

◆ **IMid-3** *see* Lenalidomide *on page 861*

◆ **Imidazole Carboxamide** *see* Dacarbazine *on page 388*

◆ **Imidazole Carboxamide Dimethyltriazene** *see* Dacarbazine *on page 388*

Imiglucerase (i mi GLOO ser ace)

U.S. Brand Names Cerezyme®

Canadian Brand Names Cerezyme®

Pharmacologic Category Enzyme

Use Long-term enzyme replacement therapy for patients with Type 1 Gaucher's disease

Pregnancy Risk Factor C

Medication Safety Issues
Sound-alike/look-alike issues:
Cerezyme® may be confused with Cerebyx®, Ceredase®

Dosage I.V.: Children ≥2 years and Adults: Initial: 30-60 units/kg every 2 weeks; dosing is individualized based on disease severity. Dosing range: 2.5 units/kg 3 times/week up to as much as 60 units/kg administered as frequently as once a week or as infrequently as every 4 weeks. Average dose: 60 units/kg administered every 2 weeks

Additional Information Complete prescribing information for this medication should be consulted for additional detail.

Dosage Forms Excipient information presented when available (limited, particularly for generics); consult specific product labeling.
Injection, powder for reconstitution:
Cerezyme®: 200 units, 400 units [derived from Chinese hamster cells; contains mannitol and polysorbate 80]

◆ **Imipemide** *see* Imipenem and Cilastatin *on page 771*

Imipenem and Cilastatin
(i mi PEN em & sye la STAT in)

U.S. Brand Names Primaxin®

Canadian Brand Names Primaxin®; Primaxin® I.V.

Index Terms Imipemide

Pharmacologic Category Antibiotic, Carbapenem

Additional Appendix Information
Antibiotic Treatment of Adults With Infective Endocarditis *on page 1748*
Antimicrobial Drugs of Choice *on page 1752*

Use Treatment of lower respiratory tract, urinary tract, intra-abdominal, gynecologic, bone and joint, skin and skin structure, and polymicrobic infections as well as bacterial septicemia and endocarditis. Antibacterial activity includes resistant gram-negative bacilli (*Pseudomonas aeruginosa* and *Enterobacter* sp), gram-positive bacteria (methicillin-sensitive *Staphylococcus aureus* and *Streptococcus* sp) and anaerobes.

Unlabeled/Investigational Use Hepatic abscess; neutropenic fever; melioidosis

Pregnancy Risk Factor C

Pregnancy Considerations With the exception of slightly decreased fetal weights at the highest doses in rats and an increase in embryonic loss in cynomolgus monkeys, most animal studies have not shown an increased fetal risk or teratogenic effects. However, due to the adverse events observed in some animal studies, imipenem/cilastatin is classified as pregnancy category C. No adequate and well-controlled studies have been conducted in pregnant women and it is not known whether imipenem can cause fetal harm. Due to pregnancy induced physiologic changes, some pharmacokinetic parameters of imipenem/cilastatin may be altered. Pregnant women have a larger volume of distribution resulting in lower serum peak levels than for the same dose in nonpregnant women. Clearance is also increased.

Lactation Enters breast milk/use caution

Medication Safety Issues

Sound-alike/look-alike issues:

Imipenem may be confused with ertapenem, meropenem

Primaxin® may be confused with Premarin®, Primacor®

Contraindications Hypersensitivity to imipenem/cilastatin or any component of the formulation

I.M. formulation (due to lidocaine diluent) additional contraindications: Hypersensitivity to amide-type anesthetics; severe shock or heart block

Warnings/Precautions Dosage adjustment required in patients with impaired renal function; elderly patients often require lower doses (adjust carefully to renal function). Prolonged use may result in fungal or bacterial superinfection, including *C. difficile*-associated diarrhea (CDAD) and pseudomembranous colitis; CDAD has been observed >2 months postantibiotic treatment. Has been associated with CNS adverse effects, including confusional states and seizures (myoclonic); use with caution in patients with a history of seizures or hypersensitivity to beta-lactams (including penicillins and cephalosporins); patients with impaired renal function are at increased risk of seizures if not properly dose adjusted. Not recommended in pediatric CNS infections due to seizure potential. Serious hypersensitivity reactions, including anaphylaxis, have been reported (some without a history of previous allergic reactions to beta-lactams). Doses for I.M. administration are mixed with lidocaine; consult information on lidocaine for associated warnings/precautions. Two different imipenem/cilastatin products are available; due to differences in formulation, the I.V. and I.M. preparations **cannot** be interchanged. Safety and efficacy of I.M. administration in children <12 years of age have not been established.

Adverse Reactions Adverse reactions reported with use for both I.V. and I.M. formulations in adults, except where noted.

1% to 10%:

Cardiovascular: Tachycardia (infants 2%; adults <1%)

Central nervous system: Seizure (infants 6%; adults <1%)

Dermatologic: Rash (≤1%, children 2%)

Gastrointestinal: Nausea (1% to 2%), diarrhea (children 3% to 4%; adults 1% to 2%), vomiting (≤2%)

Genitourinary: Oliguria/anuria (infants 2%; adults <1%)

Local: Phlebitis/thrombophlebitis (3%), pain at I.M. injection site (1.2%)

<1% (Limited to important or life-threatening): Abdominal pain, abnormal urinalysis, acute renal failure, alkaline phosphatase increased, anaphylaxis, anemia, angioneurotic edema, asthenia, bilirubin increased, bone marrow depression, BUN/creatinine increased, candidiasis, confusion, cyanosis, dizziness, drug fever, dyspnea, encephalopathy, eosinophilia, erythema multiforme, fever, flushing, gastroenteritis, glossitis, hallucinations, headache, hearing loss, hematocrit decreased, hemoglobin decreased, hemolytic anemia, hemorrhagic colitis, hepatitis (including fulminant onset), hepatic failure, hyperchloremia, hyperhidrosis, hyperkalemia, hypersensitivity, hyperventilation, hyponatremia, hypotension, injection site erythema, jaundice, lactate dehydrogenase increased, leukocytosis, leukopenia, myoclonus, neutropenia (including agranulocytosis), palpitation, pancytopenia, paresthesia, pharyngeal pain, polyarthralgia, polyuria, positive Coombs' test, prothrombin time increased, pruritus, pruritus vulvae, pseudomembranous colitis, psychic disturbances, rash, resistant *P. aeruginosa*, salivation increased, somnolence, staining of teeth, Stevens-Johnson syndrome, taste perversion, thoracic spine pain, thrombocythemia, thrombocytopenia, tinnitus, tongue/tooth discoloration, tongue papillar hypertrophy, toxic epidermal necrolysis, transaminases increased, tremor, urine discoloration, urticaria, vertigo

Drug Interactions

Avoid Concomitant Use

Avoid concomitant use of Imipenem and Cilastatin with any of the following: Ganciclovir

Increased Effect/Toxicity

The levels/effects of Imipenem and Cilastatin may be increased by: Ganciclovir; Uricosuric Agents

Decreased Effect

Imipenem and Cilastatin may decrease the levels/effects of: Typhoid Vaccine; Valproic Acid

Stability Imipenem/cilastatin powder for injection should be stored at <25°C (77°F).

I.M.: Prepare 500 mg vial with 2 mL 1% lidocaine (do not use lidocaine with epinephrine). The I.V. formulation does not form a stable suspension in lidocaine and cannot be used to prepare an I.M dose. The I.M. suspension should be used within 1 hour of reconstitution.

I.V.: Prior to use, dilute dose into 100-250 mL of an appropriate solution. Imipenem is inactivated at acidic or alkaline pH. Final concentration should not exceed 5 mg/mL. The I.M. formulation is not buffered and cannot be used to prepare I.V. solutions. Reconstituted I.V. solutions are stable for 4 hours at room temperature and 24 hours when refrigerated. Do not freeze.

Mechanism of Action Inhibits bacterial cell wall synthesis by binding to one or more of the penicillin binding proteins (PBPs); which in turn inhibits the final transpeptidation step of peptidoglycan synthesis in bacterial cell walls, thus inhibiting cell wall biosynthesis. Bacteria eventually lyse due to ongoing activity of cell wall autolytic enzymes (autolysins and murein hydrolases) while cell wall assembly is arrested. Cilastatin prevents renal metabolism of imipenem by competitive inhibition of dehydropeptidase along the brush border of the renal tubules.

Pharmacodynamics/Kinetics

Absorption: I.M.: Imipenem: 60% to 75%; cilastatin: 95% to 100%

Distribution: Rapidly and widely to most tissues and fluids including sputum, pleural fluid, peritoneal fluid, interstitial fluid, bile, aqueous humor, and bone; highest concentrations in pleural fluid, interstitial fluid, and peritoneal fluid; low concentrations in CSF

Protein binding: Imipenem: 20%; cilastatin: 40%

Metabolism: Imipenem is metabolized in the kidney by dehydropeptidase I; cilastatin prevents imipenem metabolism by this enzyme; cilastatin is partially metabolized renally

Half-life elimination: I.V.: Both drugs: 60 minutes; prolonged with renal impairment; I.M.: Imipenem: 2-3 hours

Time to peak: I.M.: 3.5 hours

Excretion: Both drugs: Urine (~70% as unchanged drug)

Dosage

Usual dosage ranges: Note: Dosage based on **imipenem** content:

Neonates ≤3 months and weight ≥1500 g: Non-CNS infections: I.V.:

<1 week: 25 mg/kg every 12 hours

1-4 weeks: 25 mg/kg every 8 hours

4 weeks to 3 months: 25 mg/kg every 6 hours

Children >3 months: Non-CNS infections: I.V.: 15-25 mg/kg every 6 hours; maximum dosage: Susceptible infections: 2 g/day; moderately-susceptible organisms: 4 g/day

Adults:

I.M.: 500-750 mg every 12 hours; maximum: 1500 mg/day

I.V.: Weight ≥70 kg: 250-1000 mg every 6-8 hours; maximum: 4 g/day. **Note:** For adults weighing <70 kg, refer to Dosing Adjustment in Renal Impairment:

Indication-specific dosing: Note: Doses based on imipenem content. I.M. administration is not intended for severe or life-threatening infections (eg, septicemia, endocarditis, shock), UTI, bone/joint or polymicrobic infections:

Children: I.V.:

Burkholderia mallei (melioidosis) (unlabeled use): 20 mg/kg every 8 hours for 10 days

Cystic fibrosis: Doses up to 90 mg/kg/day have been used

Adults:

Burkholderia mallei (melioidosis) (unlabeled use): I.V.: 20 mg/kg (up to 1 g) every 6-8 hours for 10 days

Intra-abdominal infections:

I.V.: Mild infection: 250-500 mg every 6 hours; severe: 500 mg every 6 hours

I.M.: Mild-to-moderate infection: 750 mg every 12 hours

Liver abscess (unlabeled use): I.V.: 500 mg every 6 hours for 2-3 weeks, then appropriate oral therapy for a total of 4-6 weeks

Lower respiratory tract, skin/skin structure, gynecologic infections: I.M.: Mild/moderate: 500-750 mg every 12 hours

Mild infection: Note: Rarely a suitable option in mild infections; normally reserved for moderate-severe cases:

I.M.: 500 mg every 12 hours

I.V.:

Fully-susceptible organisms: 250 mg every 6 hours

Moderately-susceptible organisms: 500 mg every 6 hours

Moderate infection:

I.M.: 750 mg every 12 hours

I.V.:

Fully-susceptible organisms: 500 mg every 6-8 hours

Moderately-susceptible organisms: 500 mg every 6 hours or 1 g every 8 hours

Neutropenic fever (unlabeled use): I.V.: 500 mg every 6 hours

***Pseudomonas* infections:** I.V.: 500 mg every 6 hours; **Note:** Higher doses may be required based on organism sensitivity.

Severe infection: I.V.:

Fully-susceptible organisms: 500 mg every 6 hours

Moderately-susceptible organisms: 1 g every 6-8 hours

Maximum daily dose should not exceed 50 mg/kg or 4 g/day, whichever is lower

Urinary tract infection: I.V.:

Uncomplicated: 250 mg every 6 hours

Complicated: 500 mg every 6 hours

Dosage adjustment in renal impairment: I.V.: **Note:** Adjustments have not been established for I.M. dosing:

Patients with a Cl_{cr} ≤5 mL/minute/1.73 m^2 should not receive imipenem/cilastatin unless hemodialysis is instituted within 48 hours.

Patients weighing <30 kg with impaired renal function should not receive imipenem/cilastatin.

Hemodialysis: Use the dosing recommendation for patients with a Cl_{cr} 6-20 mL/minute; administer dose after dialysis session and every 12 hours thereafter

Peritoneal dialysis: Dose as for Cl_{cr} 6-20 mL/minute

Continuous renal replacement therapy (CRRT): Drug clearance is highly dependent on the method of renal replacement, filter type, and flow rate. Appropriate dosing requires close monitoring of pharmacologic response, signs of adverse reactions due to drug accumulation, as well as drug levels in relation to target trough (if appropriate). The following are general recommendations only (based on dialysate flow/ultrafiltration rates of 1 L/hour) and should not supersede clinical judgment:

CVVH: 250 mg every 6 hours or 500 mg every 8 hours

CVVHD/CVVHDF: 250 mg every 6 hours or 500 mg every 6-8 hours

Note: Data suggest that 500 mg every 12 hours may provide sufficient T>MIC to cover organisms with MIC values ≤2 mg/L; however, a higher dose of 500 mg every 6 hours is recommended for resistant organisms (particularly *Pseudomonas*) with MIC ≥4 mg/L (Fish, 2005).

Dosage adjustment in hepatic impairment: Hepatic dysfunction may further impair cilastatin clearance; consider decreasing the dosing frequency.

See table.

Imipenem and Cilastatin Dosage in Renal Impairment

Reduced I.V. Dosage Regimen Based on Creatinine Clearance (mL/minute/1.73 m²) and/or Body Weight <70 kg					
	Body Weight (kg)				
	≥70	60	50	40	30
Total daily dose for normal renal function: 1 g/day					
Cl_{cr} ≥71	250 mg q6h	250 mg q8h	125 mg q6h	125 mg q6h	125 mg q8h
Cl_{cr} 41-70	250 mg q8h	125 mg q6h	125 mg q6h	125 mg q8h	125 mg q8h
Cl_{cr} 21-40	250 mg q12h	250 mg q12h	125 mg q8h	125 mg q12h	125 mg q12h
Cl_{cr} 6-20	250 mg q12h	125 mg q12h	125 mg q12h	125 mg q12h	125 mg q12h
Total daily dose for normal renal function: 1.5 g/day					
Cl_{cr} ≥71	500 mg q8h	250 mg q6h	250 mg q6h	250 mg q8h	125 mg q6h
Cl_{cr} 41-70	250 mg q6h	250 mg q8h	250 mg q8h	125 mg q6h	125 mg q8h
Cl_{cr} 21-40	250 mg q8h	250 mg q8h	250 mg q12h	125 mg q8h	125 mg q8h
Cl_{cr} 6-20	250 mg q12h	250 mg q12h	250 mg q12h	125 mg q12h	125 mg q12h
Total daily dose for normal renal function: 2 g/day					
Cl_{cr} ≥71	500 mg q6h	500 mg q8h	250 mg q6h	250 mg q6h	250 mg q8h
Cl_{cr} 41-70	500 mg q8h	250 mg q6h	250 mg q6h	250 mg q8h	125 mg q6h
Cl_{cr} 21-40	250 mg q6h	250 mg q8h	250 mg q8h	250 mg q12h	125 mg q8h
Cl_{cr} 6-20	250 mg q12h	250 mg q12h	250 mg q12h	250 mg q12h	125 mg q12h
Total daily dose for normal renal function: 3 g/day					
Cl_{cr} ≥71	1000 mg q8h	750 mg q8h	500 mg q6h	500 mg q8h	250 mg q6h
Cl_{cr} 41-70	500 mg q6h	500 mg q8h	500 mg q8h	250 mg q6h	250 mg q8h
Cl_{cr} 21-40	500 mg q8h	500 mg q8h	250 mg q6h	250 mg q8h	250 mg q8h
Cl_{cr} 6-20	500 mg q12h	500 mg q12h	250 mg q12h	250 mg q12h	250 mg q12h
Total daily dose for normal renal function: 4 g/day					
Cl_{cr} ≥71	1000 mg q6h	1000 mg q8h	750 mg q8h	500 mg q6h	500 mg q8h
Cl_{cr} 41-70	750 mg q8h	750 mg q8h	500 mg q6h	500 mg q8h	250 mg q6h
Cl_{cr} 21-40	500 mg q6h	500 mg q8h	500 mg q8h	250 mg q6h	250 mg q8h
Cl_{cr} 6-20	500 mg q12h	500 mg q12h	500 mg q12h	250 mg q12h	250 mg q12h

Dietary Considerations Sodium content of 500 mg injection:
I.M.: 32 mg (1.4 mEq)
I.V.: 37.5 mg (1.6 mEq)

Administration
I.M.: **Note:** I.M. administration is not intended for severe or life-threatening infections (eg, septicemia, endocarditis, shock). Administer by deep injection into a large muscle (gluteal or lateral thigh). **Only the I.M. formulation can be used for I.M. administration.**
I.V.: Do not administer I.V. push. Infuse doses ≤500 mg over 20-30 minutes; infuse doses ≥750 mg over 40-60 minutes. **Only the I.V. formulation can be used for I.V. administration.**

Monitoring Parameters Periodic renal, hepatic, and hematologic function tests; monitor for signs of anaphylaxis during first dose

Test Interactions Interferes with urinary glucose determination using Clinitest®

Dosage Forms Excipient information presented when available (limited, particularly for generics); consult specific product labeling.
Injection, powder for reconstitution [I.M.]:
Primaxin®: Imipenem 500 mg and cilastatin 500 mg [contains sodium 32 mg (1.4 mEq)]
Injection, powder for reconstitution [I.V.]:
Primaxin®: Imipenem 250 mg and cilastatin 250 mg [contains sodium 18.8 mg (0.8 mEq)]; imipenem 500 mg and cilastatin 500 mg [contains sodium 37.5 mg (1.6 mEq)]

Imipramine (im IP ra meen)

U.S. Brand Names Tofranil-PM®; Tofranil®

Canadian Brand Names Apo-Imipramine®; Novo-Pramine; Tofranil®

Index Terms Imipramine Hydrochloride; Imipramine Pamoate

Pharmacologic Category Antidepressant, Tricyclic (Tertiary Amine)

Additional Appendix Information
Antidepressant Agents *on page 1638*

Use Treatment of depression; treatment of nocturnal enuresis in children

Unlabeled/Investigational Use Analgesic for certain chronic and neuropathic pain; panic disorder; attention-deficit/hyperactivity disorder (ADHD)

Restrictions An FDA-approved medication guide concerning the use of antidepressants in children, adolescents, and young adults must be distributed when dispensing an outpatient prescription (new or refill) where this medication is to be used without direct supervision of a healthcare provider. Medication guides are available at http://www.fda.gov/cder/Offices/ODS/medication_guides.htm. Dispense to parents or guardians of children and adolescents receiving this medication.

Pregnancy Risk Factor D

Lactation Enters breast milk/not recommended (AAP rates "of concern")

Medication Safety Issues
Sound-alike/look-alike issues:
Imipramine may be confused with amitriptyline, desipramine, Norpramin®

Contraindications Hypersensitivity to imipramine (cross-reactivity with other dibenzodiazepines may occur) or any component of the formulation; concurrent use of MAO inhibitors (within 14 days); in a patient during acute recovery phase of MI; pregnancy

Warnings/Precautions **[U.S. Boxed Warning]: Antidepressants increase the risk of suicidal thinking and behavior in children, adolescents, and young adults (18-24 years of age) with major depressive disorder (MDD) and other psychiatric disorders;** consider risk prior to prescribing. Short-term studies did not show an increased risk in patients >24 years of age and showed a decreased risk in patients ≥65 years. Closely monitor for clinical worsening, suicidality, or unusual changes in behavior; the patient's family or caregiver should be instructed to closely observe the patient and communicate condition with healthcare provider. A medication guide should be dispensed with each prescription. **Imipramine is FDA approved for the treatment of nocturnal enuresis in children ≥6 years of age.**

The possibility of a suicide attempt is inherent in major depression and may persist until remission occurs. Monitor for worsening of depression or suicidality, especially during initiation of therapy (generally first 1-2 months) or with dose increases or decreases. Use caution in high-risk patients. Worsening depression and severe abrupt suicidality that are not part of the presenting symptoms may require discontinuation or modification of drug therapy. The patient's family or caregiver should be alerted to monitor patients for the emergence of suicidality and associated behaviors (such as agitation, irritability, hostility, impulsivity, and hypomania) and notify healthcare provider.

May worsen psychosis in some patients or precipitate a shift to mania or hypomania in patients with bipolar disorder. Patients presenting with depressive symptoms should be screened for bipolar disorder. Monotherapy in patients with bipolar disorder should be avoided. **Imipramine is not FDA approved for the treatment of bipolar depression.**

TCAs may rarely cause bone marrow suppression; monitor for any signs of infection and obtain CBC if symptoms (eg, fever, sore throat) evident. The degree of sedation, anticholinergic effects, orthostasis, and conduction abnormalities are high relative to other antidepressants. Imipramine often causes drowsiness/sedation, resulting in impaired performance of tasks requiring alertness (eg, operating machinery or driving). Sedative effects may be additive with other CNS depressants and/or ethanol. Use with caution in patients with a history of cardiovascular disease (including previous MI, stroke, tachycardia, or conduction abnormalities). Use with caution in patients with urinary retention, benign prostatic hyperplasia, narrow-angle glaucoma, xerostomia, visual problems, constipation, or a history of bowel obstruction.

Consider discontinuing, when possible, prior to elective surgery. Therapy should not be abruptly discontinued in patients receiving high doses for prolonged periods. May lower seizure threshold - use caution in patients with a previous seizure disorder or condition predisposing to seizures such as brain damage, alcoholism, or concurrent therapy with other drugs which lower the seizure threshold. May increase the risks associated with electroconvulsive therapy. Use with caution in hyperthyroid patients or those receiving thyroid supplementation. Use with caution in patients with diabetes mellitus; may alter glucose regulation. Use with caution in patients with hepatic or renal dysfunction and in elderly patients. Has been associated with photosensitization.

Adverse Reactions Reported for tricyclic antidepressants in general. Frequency not defined.
Cardiovascular: Arrhythmia, CHF, ECG changes, heart block, hypertension, MI, orthostatic hypotension, palpitation, stroke, tachycardia
Central nervous system: Agitation, anxiety, confusion, delusions, disorientation, dizziness, drowsiness, fatigue, hallucination, headache, hypomania, insomnia, nightmares, psychosis, restlessness, seizure
Dermatologic: Alopecia, itching, petechiae, photosensitivity, purpura, rash, urticaria

Endocrine & metabolic: Breast enlargement, galactorrhea, gynecomastia, increase or decrease in blood sugar, increase or decrease in libido, SIADH

Gastrointestinal: Abdominal cramps, anorexia, black tongue, constipation, diarrhea, epigastric disorders, ileus, nausea, stomatitis, taste disturbance, vomiting, weight gain/loss, xerostomia

Genitourinary: Impotence, testicular swelling, urinary retention

Hematologic: Agranulocytosis, eosinophilia, thrombocytopenia

Hepatic: Cholestatic jaundice, transaminases increased

Neuromuscular & skeletal: Ataxia, extrapyramidal symptoms, incoordination, numbness, paresthesia, peripheral neuropathy, tingling, tremor, weakness

Ocular: Blurred vision, disturbances of accommodation, mydriasis

Otic: Tinnitus

Miscellaneous: Diaphoresis, falling, hypersensitivity (eg, drug fever, edema)

Drug Interactions

Metabolism/Transport Effects Substrate of CYP1A2 (minor), 2B6 (minor), 2C19 (major), 2D6 (major), 3A4 (minor); **Inhibits** CYP1A2 (weak), 2C19 (weak), 2D6 (moderate), 2E1 (weak)

Avoid Concomitant Use

Avoid concomitant use of Imipramine with any of the following: Iobenguane I 123; MAO Inhibitors; Nilotinib; Sibutramine; Tetrabenazine; Thioridazine; Ziprasidone

Increased Effect/Toxicity

Imipramine may increase the levels/effects of: Alcohol (Ethyl); Alpha-/Beta-Agonists (Direct-Acting); Alpha1-Agonists; Amphetamines; Anticholinergics; Aspirin; Beta2-Agonists; CNS Depressants; CYP2D6 Substrates; Desmopressin; Fesoterodine; Nebivolol; NSAID (COX-2 Inhibitor); NSAID (Nonselective); QTc-Prolonging Agents; QuiNIDine; Serotonin Modulators; Sulfonylureas; Tamoxifen; Tetrabenazine; Thioridazine; TraMADol; Vitamin K Antagonists; Yohimbine; Ziprasidone

The levels/effects of Imipramine may be increased by: Alfuzosin; Altretamine; BuPROPion; Cimetidine; Cinacalcet; Ciprofloxacin; CYP2C19 Inhibitors (Moderate); CYP2C19 Inhibitors (Strong); CYP2D6 Inhibitors (Moderate); CYP2D6 Inhibitors (Strong); Darunavir; Dexmethylphenidate; DULoxetine; Gadobutrol; Lithium; MAO Inhibitors; Methylphenidate; Nilotinib; Pramlintide; Propoxyphene; Protease Inhibitors; QuiNIDine; Selective Serotonin Reuptake Inhibitors; Sibutramine; Terbinafine; Valproic Acid

Decreased Effect

Imipramine may decrease the levels/effects of: Acetylcholinesterase Inhibitors (Central); Alpha2-Agonists; Codeine; Iobenguane I 123

The levels/effects of Imipramine may be decreased by: Acetylcholinesterase Inhibitors (Central); Barbiturates; CarBAMazepine; CYP2C19 Inducers (Strong); St Johns Wort

Ethanol/Nutrition/Herb Interactions

Ethanol: Avoid ethanol (may increase CNS depression).

Herb/Nutraceutical: St John's wort may decrease imipramine levels. Avoid valerian, St John's wort, SAMe, kava kava (may increase risk of serotonin syndrome and/or excessive sedation).

Mechanism of Action Traditionally believed to increase the synaptic concentration of serotonin and/or norepinephrine in the central nervous system by inhibition of their reuptake by the presynaptic neuronal membrane. However, additional receptor effects have been found including desensitization of adenyl cyclase, down regulation of beta-adrenergic receptors, and down regulation of serotonin receptors.

Pharmacodynamics/Kinetics

Onset of action: Peak antidepressant effect: Usually after ≥2 weeks

Absorption: Well absorbed

Distribution: Crosses placenta

Metabolism: Hepatic, primarily via CYP2D6 to desipramine (active) and other metabolites; significant first-pass effect

Half-life elimination: 6-18 hours

Excretion: Urine (as metabolites)

Dosage Oral:

Children:

Depression (unlabeled use): 1.5 mg/kg/day with dosage increments of 1 mg/kg every 3-4 days to a maximum dose of 5 mg/kg/day in 1-4 divided doses; monitor carefully especially with doses ≥3.5 mg/kg/day

Enuresis: ≥6 years: Initial: 25 mg at bedtime, if inadequate response still seen after 1 week of therapy, increase by 25 mg/day; dose should not exceed 2.5 mg/kg/day or 50 mg at bedtime if 6-12 years of age or 75 mg at bedtime if ≥12 years of age

Adjunct in the treatment of cancer pain (unlabeled use): Initial: 0.2-0.4 mg/kg at bedtime; dose may be increased by 50% every 2-3 days up to 1-3 mg/kg/dose at bedtime

Adolescents: Depression: Initial: 25-50 mg/day; increase gradually; maximum: 100 mg/day in single or divided doses

Adults: Depression:

Outpatients: Initial: 75 mg/day; may increase gradually to 150 mg/day. May be given in divided doses or as a single bedtime dose; maximum: 200 mg/day

Inpatients: Initial: 100-150 mg/day; may increase gradually to 200 mg/day; if no response after 2 weeks, may further increase to 250-300 mg/day. May be given in divided doses or as a single bedtime dose; maximum: 300 mg/day.

Elderly: Depression: Initial: 25-50 mg at bedtime; may increase every 3 days for inpatients and weekly for outpatients if tolerated to a recommended maximum of 100 mg/day.

Monitoring Parameters Monitor blood pressure and pulse rate prior to and during initial therapy; ECG in older adults, with high doses, and/or in patients with pre-existing cardiovascular disease; evaluate mental status, suicidal ideation (especially at the beginning of therapy or when doses are increased or decreased); blood levels are useful for therapeutic monitoring

When used for the treatment of ADHD, thoroughly evaluate for cardiovascular risk. Monitor heart rate, blood pressure, and consider obtaining ECG prior to initiation (Vetter, 2008); ensure PR interval ≤200 ms, QRS duration ≤120 ms, and QT_c ≤460 ms.

Reference Range Therapeutic: Imipramine and desipramine: 150-250 ng/mL (SI: 530-890 nmol/L); desipramine: 150-300 ng/mL (SI: 560-1125 nmol/L); Toxic: >500 ng/mL (SI: 446-893 nmol/L); utility of serum level monitoring controversial

Dosage Forms Excipient information presented when available (limited, particularly for generics); consult specific product labeling.

Capsule, as pamoate: 75 mg, 100 mg, 125 mg, 150 mg

Tofranil-PM®: 75 mg, 100 mg, 125 mg, 150 mg

Tablet, as hydrochloride: 10 mg, 25 mg, 50 mg

Tofranil®): 10 mg, 25 mg, 50 mg

◆ **Imipramine Hydrochloride** *see* Imipramine *on page 774*

◆ **Imipramine Pamoate** *see* Imipramine *on page 774*

Imiquimod (i mi KWI mod)

U.S. Brand Names Aldara®

Canadian Brand Names Aldara®

Pharmacologic Category Skin and Mucous Membrane Agent; Topical Skin Product

Use Treatment of external genital and perianal warts/condyloma acuminata; nonhyperkeratotic, nonhypertrophic actinic keratosis on face or scalp; superficial basal cell carcinoma (sBCC) with a maximum tumor diameter of 2 cm located on the trunk, neck, or extremities (excluding hands or feet)

Unlabeled/Investigational Use Treatment of common warts

Pregnancy Risk Factor C

Medication Safety Issues

Sound-alike/look-alike issues:

Aldara™ may be confused with Alora®, Lialda™

Dosage Topical: **Note:** A rest period of several days may be taken if required by the patient's discomfort or severity of the local skin reaction. Treatment may resume once the reaction subsides.

Children ≥12 years and Adults: Perianal warts/condyloma acuminata: Apply a thin layer 3 times/week prior to bedtime and leave on skin for 6-10 hours. Remove with mild soap and water. Examples of 3 times/week application schedules are: Monday, Wednesday, Friday; or Tuesday, Thursday, Saturday. Continue imiquimod treatment until there is total clearance of the genital/perianal warts for ≤16 weeks.

Adults:

Actinic keratosis: Apply twice weekly for 16 weeks to a treatment area on face or scalp (but not both concurrently); apply prior to bedtime and leave on skin for 8 hours. Remove with mild soap and water.

Common oral warts (dental use): Apply once daily prior to bedtime

Common warts (unlabeled use): Apply once daily prior to bedtime

Superficial basal cell carcinoma: Apply once daily prior to bedtime, 5 days/week for 6 weeks. Treatment area should include a 1 cm margin of skin around the tumor. Leave on skin for 8 hours. Remove with mild soap and water.

Additional Information Complete prescribing information for this medication should be consulted for additional detail.

Dosage Forms Excipient information presented when available (limited, particularly for generics); consult specific product labeling.

Cream:

Aldara®: 5% (12s, 24s) [contains benzyl alcohol; single-dose packets]

◆ **Imitrex®** *see* SUMAtriptan *on page 1414*

◆ **Imitrex® DF (Can)** *see* SUMAtriptan *on page 1414*

◆ **Imitrex® Nasal Spray (Can)** *see* SUMAtriptan *on page 1414*

◆ **ImmuCyst® (Can)** *see* BCG Vaccine *on page 176*

Immune Globulin (Intramuscular)

(i MYUN GLOB yoo lin, IN tra MUS kyoo ler)

U.S. Brand Names GamaSTAN™ S/D

Canadian Brand Names BayGam®

Index Terms Gamma Globulin; IG; IGIM; Immune Serum Globulin; ISG

Pharmacologic Category Immune Globulin

Additional Appendix Information

Immunization Recommendations *on page 1708*

Use To provide passive immunity in susceptible individuals under the following circumstances:

Hepatitis A: Within 14 days of exposure and prior to manifestation of disease

Measles: For use within 6 days of exposure in an unvaccinated person, who has not previously had measles

Varicella: When Varicella Zoster Immune Globulin is not available

Rubella: Postexposure prophylaxis (within 72 hours) to reduce the risk of infection in exposed pregnant women who will not consider therapeutic abortion

Immunoglobulin deficiency: To help prevent serious infections

Pregnancy Risk Factor C

Pregnancy Considerations Reproduction studies have not been conducted with this product. Immune globulins cross the placenta in increased amounts after 30 weeks gestation.

Contraindications Hypersensitivity to immune globulin or any component of the formulation; IgA deficiency; severe thrombocytopenia or coagulation disorders where I.M. injections are contraindicated

Warnings/Precautions Hypersensitivity and anaphylactic reactions can occur; immediate treatment (including epinephrine 1:1000) should be available. Product of human plasma; may potentially contain infectious agents which could transmit disease. Screening of donors, as well as testing and/or inactivation or removal of certain viruses, reduces the risk. Infections thought to be transmitted by this product should be reported to the manufacturer. Skin testing should not be performed as local irritation can occur and be misinterpreted as a positive reaction. Not for I.V. administration.

Adverse Reactions Frequency not defined.

Cardiovascular: Flushing, angioedema

Central nervous system: Chills, lethargy, fever

Dermatologic: Urticaria, erythema

Gastrointestinal: Nausea, vomiting

Local: Pain, tenderness, muscle stiffness at I.M. site

Neuromuscular & skeletal: Myalgia

Miscellaneous: Hypersensitivity reactions

Drug Interactions

Avoid Concomitant Use There are no known interactions where it is recommended to avoid concomitant use.

Increased Effect/Toxicity There are no known significant interactions involving an increase in effect.

Decreased Effect

Immune Globulin (Intramuscular) may decrease the levels/effects of: Vaccines (Live)

Stability Store under refrigeration at 2°C to 8°C (36°F to 46°F).

Mechanism of Action Provides passive immunity by increasing the antibody titer and antigen-antibody reaction potential

Pharmacodynamics/Kinetics

Duration: Immune effect: Usually 3-4 weeks

Half-life elimination: 23 days

Time to peak, serum: I.M.: ~48 hours

Dosage I.M.: Children and Adults:

Hepatitis A:

Pre-exposure prophylaxis upon travel into endemic areas (hepatitis A vaccine preferred):

0.02 mL/kg for anticipated risk of exposure <3 months

0.06 mL/kg for anticipated risk of exposure ≥3 months

Repeat approximate dose every 5 months if exposure continues

Postexposure prophylaxis: 0.02 mL/kg given within 14 days of exposure. IG is not needed if at least 1 dose of hepatitis A vaccine was given at ≥1 month before exposure

Measles:

Prophylaxis, immunocompetent: 0.25 mL/kg/dose (maximum dose: 15 mL) given within 6 days of exposure followed by live attenuated measles vaccine in 5-6 months when indicated

Prophylaxis, immunocompromised: 0.5 mL/kg (maximum dose: 15 mL) immediately following exposure

Rubella: Prophylaxis during pregnancy: 0.55 mL/kg/dose within 72 hours of exposure

Varicella: Prophylaxis: 0.6-1.2 mL/kg (varicella zoster immune globulin preferred) within 72 hours of exposure

IgG deficiency: 0.66 mL/kg/dose every 3-4 weeks. A double dose may be given at onset of therapy; some patients may require more frequent injections.

Administration Not for I.V. administration

Administer I.M. in the anterolateral aspects of the upper thigh or deltoid muscle of the upper arm. Avoid gluteal region due to risk of injury to sciatic nerve; use upper outer quadrant only. Divide doses >10 mL.

For patients at risk of hemorrhage following intramuscular injection, the ACIP recommends "it should be administered intramuscularly if, in the opinion of the physician familiar with the patients bleeding risk, the vaccine can be administered with reasonable safety by this route. If the patient receives antihemophilia or other similar therapy, intramuscular vaccination can be scheduled shortly after such therapy is administered. A fine needle (23 gauge or smaller) can be used for the vaccination and firm pressure applied to the site (without rubbing) for at least 2 minutes. The patient should be instructed concerning the risk of hematoma from the injection."

Reference Range Immunoglobulin deficiency: Maintain circulating IgG levels ~200 mg/100 mL plasma to prevent serious infection

Test Interactions Skin tests should **not** be done

Additional Information When administering IG for hepatitis A prophylaxis, use should be considered for the following close contacts of persons with confirmed hepatitis A: unvaccinated household and sexual contacts, persons who have shared illicit drugs, regular babysitters, staff and attendees of child care centers, food handlers within the same establishment.

For travelers, IG is not an alternative to careful selection of foods and water; immune globulin can interfere with the antibody response to parenterally administered live virus vaccines. Frequent travelers should be tested for hepatitis A antibody, immune hemolytic anemia, and neutropenia (with ITP, I.V. route is usually used).

Dosage Forms Excipient information presented when available (limited, particularly for generics); consult specific product labeling.

Injection, solution [preservative free; solvent detergent-treated]:

GamaSTAN™ S/D: 15% to 18% (2 mL, 10 mL)

Immune Globulin (Intravenous)

(i MYUN GLOB yoo lin, IN tra VEE nus)

U.S. Brand Names Carimune® NF; Flebogamma®; Gammagard Liquid; Gammagard S/D; Gammar®-P I.V. [DSC]; Gamunex®; Octagam®; Panglobulin® NF [DSC]; Polygam® S/D [DSC]; Privigen™

Canadian Brand Names Gamimune® N; Gammagard Liquid; Gammagard S/D; Gamunex®

Index Terms IGIV; IV Immune Globulin; IVIG

Pharmacologic Category Immune Globulin

Additional Appendix Information

Immunization Recommendations *on page 1708*

Intravenous Immune Globulin *on page 1658*

Use

Treatment of primary immunodeficiency syndromes (congenital agammaglobulinemia, severe combined immunodeficiency syndromes [SCIDS], common variable immunodeficiency, X-linked immunodeficiency, Wiskott-Aldrich syndrome) (Carimune® NF, Flebogamma®, Gammagard Liquid, Gammagard S/D, Gammar®-P I.V., Gamunex®, Octagam®, Panglobulin® NF, Polygam® S/D, Privigen™)

Treatment of immune (idiopathic) thrombocytopenic purpura (ITP) (Carimune® NF, Gammagard S/D, Gamunex®, Panglobulin® NF, Polygam® S/D, Privigen™)

Prevention of coronary artery aneurysms associated with Kawasaki disease (in combination with aspirin) (Gammagard S/D, Polygam® S/D)

Prevention of bacterial infection in B-cell chronic lymphocytic leukemia (CLL) (Gammagard S/D, Polygam® S/D)

Treatment of chronic inflammatory demyelinating polyneuropathy (CIDP) (Gamunex®)

Unlabeled/Investigational Use Prevention of serious bacterial infections among HIV-infected children with hypogammaglobulinemia (IgG <400 mg/dL) (CDC guidelines); hematopoietic stem cell transplantation (HSCT), to prevent bacterial infections among allogeneic recipients with severe hypogammaglobulinemia (IgG <400 mg/dL) at <100 days post transplant (CDC guidelines); fetal-neonatal alloimmune thrombocytopenia; pregnancy-associated ITP; prevention of gastroenteritis in children; multiple sclerosis (relapsing, remitting when other therapies cannot be used); hemolytic disease of the newborn; HIV-associated thrombocytopenia; acquired hypogammaglobulinemia secondary to malignancy; myasthenia gravis; refractory dermatomyositis/polymyositis

Pregnancy Risk Factor C

Pregnancy Considerations Reproduction studies have not been conducted. Immune globulins cross the placenta in increased amounts after 30 weeks gestation. Intravenous immune globulin has been recommended for use in fetal-neonatal alloimmune thrombocytopenia and pregnancy-associated ITP.

Lactation Excretion in breast milk unknown

Medication Safety Issues

Sound-alike/look-alike issues:

Gamimune® N may be confused with CytoGam®

Immune globulin (intravenous) may be confused with hepatitis B immune globulin

Contraindications Hypersensitivity to immune globulin or any component of the formulation; selective IgA deficiency; hyperprolinemia (Privigen™)

Warnings/Precautions **[U.S. Boxed Warning]: Acute renal dysfunction (increased serum creatinine, oliguria, acute renal failure, osmotic nephrosis) can rarely occur; usually within 7 days of use (more likely with products stabilized with sucrose). Use with caution in the elderly, patients with renal disease, diabetes mellitus, volume depletion, sepsis, paraproteinemia, and nephrotoxic medications due to risk of renal dysfunction.** In patients at risk of renal dysfunction, the rate of infusion and concentration of solution should be minimized. discontinue if renal function deteriorates. High-dose regimens (1000 mg/kg for 1-2 days) are not recommended for individuals with fluid overload or where fluid volume may be of concern. Hypersensitivity and anaphylactic reactions can occur; immediate treatment (including epinephrine 1:1000) should be available; product of human plasma; may potentially contain infectious agents which could transmit disease. Screening of donors, as well as testing and/or inactivation or removal of certain viruses, reduces the risk. Infections thought to be transmitted by this product should be reported to the manufacturer. Aseptic meningitis may occur with high doses (≥2 g/kg); syndrome usually appears within several hours to 2 days following treatment; usually resolves within several days after IVIG is discontinued; patients with a migraine history may be at higher risk for AMS.

Intravenous immune globulin has been associated with antiglobulin hemolysis; monitor for signs of hemolytic anemia. Patients should be adequately hydrated prior to initiation of therapy. Hyperproteinemia, increased serum viscosity and hyponatremia may occur; distinguish hyponatremia from pseudohyponatremia to prevent volume depletion and further increase in serum viscosity. Use caution in patients with a history of thrombotic events or a history of atherosclerosis or cardiovascular disease or patients with known/suspected hyperviscosity; there is clinical evidence of a possible association between thrombotic events and administration of intravenous immune globulin. Consider a baseline assessment of blood viscosity in patients at risk for hyperviscosity. For intravenous administration only. Patients should be monitored for adverse events during and after the infusion. Stop administration with signs of infusion reaction (fever, chills, nausea, vomiting, and rarely shock). Risk may be increased with initial treatment, when switching brands of immune globulin, and with treatment interruptions of >8 weeks. Monitor for transfusion-related acute lung injury (TRALI); noncardiogenic pulmonary edema has been reported with intravenous immune globulin use. TRALI is characterized by severe respiratory distress, pulmonary edema, hypoxemia, and fever (in the presence of normal left ventricular function) and usually occurs within 1-6 hours after infusion. Response to live vaccinations may be impaired. Some products may contain maltose, which may result in falsely-elevated blood glucose readings. Some products may contain sucrose. Some products may contain sorbitol; do not use in patients with fructose intolerance. Privigen™ contains the stabilizer L-proline and is contraindicated in patients with hyperprolinemia. Packaging of some products may contain natural latex/ natural rubber.

Adverse Reactions Frequency not defined.

Cardiovascular: Chest tightness, edema, flushing of the face, hyper-/hypotension, palpitation, tachycardia

Central nervous system: Anxiety, aseptic meningitis syndrome, chills, dizziness, drowsiness, fatigue, fever, headache, irritability, lethargy, lightheadedness, malaise, migraine, pain

Dermatologic: Bruising, petechiae, pruritus, purpura, rash, urticaria

Gastrointestinal: Abdominal cramps, abdominal pain, diarrhea, discomfort, dyspepsia, nausea, sore throat, vomiting

Hematologic: Anemia, autoimmune hemolytic anemia, hematocrit decreased, hemolysis (mild), hemorrhage, thrombocytopenia

Hepatic: Bilirubin increased, LDH increased, liver function test increased

Local: Pain or irritation at the infusion site

Neuromuscular & skeletal: Arthralgia, back or hip pain, leg cramps, muscle cramps, myalgia, neck pain, weakness

Otic: Ear pain

Renal: Acute renal failure, acute tubular necrosis, anuria, BUN increased, creatinine increased, oliguria, proximal tubular nephropathy, osmotic nephrosis

Respiratory: Asthma aggravated, bronchitis, cough, dyspnea, epistaxis, nasal congestion, pharyngeal pain, pharyngitis, rhinitis, rhinorrhea, sinus headache, sinusitis, upper respiratory infection, wheezing

Miscellaneous: Anaphylaxis, diaphoresis, flu-like syndrome, hypersensitivity reactions, infusion reaction

Postmarketing and/or case reports: Apnea, ARDS, autoimmune pure red cell aplasia (PRCA) exacerbation, bronchopneumonia, bronchospasm, bullous dermatitis, cardiac arrest, chest pain, coma, Coombs' test positive, cyanosis, epidermolysis, erythema multiforme, hepatic dysfunction, hypoxemia, leukopenia, loss of consciousness, pancytopenia, papular rash, pulmonary edema, pulmonary embolism, rigors, seizure, Stevens-Johnson syndrome, thromboembolism, transfusion-related acute lung injury (TRALI), tremor, vascular collapse

Drug Interactions

Avoid Concomitant Use There are no known interactions where it is recommended to avoid concomitant use.

Increased Effect/Toxicity There are no known significant interactions involving an increase in effect.

Decreased Effect

Immune Globulin (Intravenous) may decrease the levels/ effects of: Vaccines (Live)

Stability Stability is dependent upon the manufacturer and brand. Do not freeze. Dilution is dependent upon the manufacturer and brand. Gently swirl; do not shake; avoid foaming. Do not mix products from different manufacturers together. Discard unused portion of vials.

Carimune® NF, Panglobulin® NF: Prior to reconstitution, store at or below 30°C (86°F). Reconstitute with NS, D_5W, or SWFI. Following reconstitution, store under refrigeration. Begin infusion within 24 hours.

Flebogamma®: Store at 2°C to 25°C (36°F to 77°F). Dilution is not recommended.

Gammagard Liquid: May dilute in D_5W only. Prior to use, store at 2°C to 8°C (36°F to 46°F) for up to 36 months; do not freeze. May store at room temperature of 25°C (77°F) within the first 24 months of manufacturing. Storage time at room temperature varies with length of time previously refrigerated; refer to product labeling for details.

Gammagard S/D, Polygam® S/D: Store at ≤25°C (≤77°F). Reconstitute with SWFI; may store diluted solution under refrigeration for up to 24 hours.

Gammar®-P I.V.: Store at ≤25°C (≤77°F). Reconstitute with SWFI.

Gamunex®: May be stored for up to 36 months at 2°C to 8°C (36°F to 46°F); may be stored at ≤25°C (≤77°F) for up to 6 months. Dilute in D_5W only.

Octagam®: Store at 2°C to 25°C (36°F to 77°F).

Privigen™: Store at ≤25°C (≤77°F); do not freeze (do not use if previously frozen). Protect from light. If necessary to further dilute, D_5W may be used.

Mechanism of Action Replacement therapy for primary and secondary immunodeficiencies; interference with F_c receptors on the cells of the reticuloendothelial system for autoimmune cytopenias and ITP; possible role of contained antiviral-type antibodies

Pharmacodynamics/Kinetics

Onset of action: I.V.: Provides immediate antibody levels

Duration: Immune effect: 3-4 weeks (variable)

Distribution: V_d: 0.09-0.13 L/kg

Intravascular portion (primarily): Healthy subjects: 41% to 57%; Patients with congenital humoral immunodeficiencies: ~70%

Half-life elimination: IgG (variable among patients): Healthy subjects: 14-24 days; Patients with congenital humoral immunodeficiencies: 26-40 days; hypermetabolism associated with fever and infection have coincided with a shortened half-life

Dosage Approved doses and regimens may vary between brands; check manufacturer guidelines. **Note:** Some clinicians dose IVIG on ideal body weight or an adjusted ideal body weight in morbidly-obese patients.

Children: I.V.: Pediatric HIV, prevention of infection (CDC guidelines): 400 mg/kg every 2-4 weeks

Children and Adults: I.V.:

Primary immunodeficiency disorders: **Note:** Adjust dose/ frequency based desired IgG levels and clinical response:

General dosing range: 200-800 mg/kg per month

Carimune® NF, Panglobulin® NF: 200 mg/kg every 4 weeks. May increase dose to 300 mg/kg every 4 weeks or may increase frequency based on patient response.

Flebogamma®, Gammagard Liquid, Gammagard S/D, Gamunex®, Octagam®, Polygam® S/D: 300-600 mg/ kg every 3-4 weeks; adjusted based on dosage and interval in conjunction with monitored serum IgG concentrations

Privigen™: 200-800 mg/kg every 3-4 weeks; adjusted based on dosage and interval in conjunction with monitored serum IgG concentrations

Gamma®-P I.V.:

Children and Adolescents: Initial dose: 200 mg/kg every 3-4 weeks

Adults: 200-400 mg/kg every 3-4 weeks

B-cell chronic lymphocytic leukemia (CLL) (Gammagard S/D, Polygam® S/D): 400 mg/kg/dose every 3-4 weeks

Immune (idiopathic) thrombocytopenic purpura (ITP):

Carimune® NF, Panglobulin® NF:

Acute: 400 mg/kg/day for 2-5 days

Chronic: 400 mg/kg as needed to maintain platelet count ≥30,000/mm^3 or to control significant bleeding; may increase dose if needed (range: 800-1000 mg/kg)

Gammagard S/D, Polygam® S/D: 1000 mg/kg; adjust additional doses based on patient response or platelet count. Up to 3 separate doses may be administered on alternate days if required.

Gamunex®: 1000 mg/kg/day for 1-2 days, **or** 400 mg/kg/day for 5 days

Privigen™: 1000 mg/kg/day for 2 consecutive days

Chronic inflammatory demyelinating polyneuropathy (CIDP): Gamunex®: Loading dose: 2000 mg/kg divided over 2-4 consecutive days; Maintenance: 1000 mg/kg/day for 1 day every 3 weeks **or** 500 mg/kg/day for 2 consecutive days every 3 weeks

Kawasaki disease: Initiate IVIG therapy within 10 days of disease onset: Must be used in combination with aspirin: 80-100 mg/kg/day in 4 divided doses for 14 days; when fever subsides, dose aspirin at 3-5 mg/kg once daily for ≥6-8 weeks

AHA guidelines: 2000 mg/kg as a single dose

Gammagard S/D, Polygam® S/D: 1000 mg/kg as a single dose administered over 10 hours, **or** 400 mg/kg/day for 4 days. Begin within 7 days of onset of fever.

Hematopoietic stem cell transplantation with hypogammaglobulinemia (CDC guidelines):

Children: 400 mg/kg per month; increase dose or frequency to maintain IgG levels >400 mg/dL

Adolescents and Adults: 500 mg/kg/week

Unlabeled uses:

Acquired hypogammaglobulinemia secondary to malignancy (unlabeled use): Adults: 400 mg/kg/dose every 3 weeks; reevaluate every 4-6 months

Guillain-Barré syndrome (unlabeled use): Children and Adults: Various regimens have been used, including:

400 mg/kg/day for 5 days

or

2000 mg/kg in divided doses administered over 2 days

HIV-associated thrombocytopenia (unlabeled use): Adults: 1000 mg/kg/day for 2 days

Multiple sclerosis (relapsing-remitting, when other therapies cannot be used) (unlabeled use): Adults: 1000 mg/kg per month, with or without an induction of 400 mg/kg/day for 5 days

Myasthenia gravis (severe exacerbation) (unlabeled use): Adults: Total dose of 2000 mg/kg over 2-5 days

Refractory dermatomyositis (unlabeled use): Adults: 2000 mg/kg per month administered over 2-5 days

Refractory polymyositis (unlabeled use): Adults: 2000 mg/kg per course administered over 2-5 days

Dosing adjustment/comments in renal impairment: Cl_{cr} <10 mL/minute: Avoid use; in patients at risk of renal dysfunction, consider infusion at a rate less than maximum.

Dietary Considerations Octagam® contains sodium 30 mmol/L

Administration I.V. infusion over 2-24 hours; for initial treatment, a lower concentration and/or a slower rate of infusion should be used. Administer in separate infusion line from other medications; if using primary line, flush with saline prior administration. Refrigerated product should be warmed to room temperature prior to infusion. Some products require filtration; refer to individual product labeling. Antecubital veins should be used, especially with concentrations ≥10% to prevent injection site discomfort. Decrease dose, rate and/or concentration of infusion in patients who may be at risk of renal failure. Decreasing the rate or stopping the infusion may help relieve some adverse effects (flushing, changes in pulse rate, changes in blood pressure). Epinephrine should be available during administration.

Monitoring Parameters Renal function, urine output, hemoglobin and hematocrit, platelets (in patients with ITP); infusion-related adverse reactions, anaphylaxis, signs and symptoms of hemolysis; blood viscosity (in patients at risk for hyperviscosity); presence of antineutrophil antibodies (if TRALI is suspected)

Test Interactions Octagam® contains maltose. Falsely-elevated blood glucose levels may occur when glucose monitoring devices and test strips utilizing the glucose dehydrogenase pyrroloquinolinequinone (GDH-PQQ) based methods are used. Glucose monitoring devices and test strips which utilize the glucose-specific method are recommended. Passively-transferred antibodies may yield false-positive serologic testing results; may yield false-positive direct and indirect Coombs' test.

Dosage Forms Excipient information presented when available (limited, particularly for generics); consult specific product labeling. [DSC] = Discontinued product

Injection, powder for reconstitution [preservative free]:

Gammar®-P I.V.: 5 g, 10 g [stabilized with human albumin and sucrose] [DSC]

Injection, powder for reconstitution [preservative free, nanofiltered]:

Carimune® NF: 3 g, 6 g, 12 g [contains sucrose]

Panglobulin® NF: 6 g, 12 g [contains sucrose] [DSC]

Injection, powder for reconstitution [preservative free, solvent detergent-treated]:

Gammagard S/D: 2.5 g, 5 g, 10 g [stabilized with human albumin, glycine, glucose, and polyethylene glycol; packaging may contain natural latex/natural rubber]

Polygam® S/D: 5 g, 10 g [stabilized with human albumin, glycine, glucose, and polyethylene glycol] [DSC]

Injection, solution [preservative free; solvent detergent-treated]:

Gammagard Liquid: 10% (10 mL, 25 mL, 50 mL, 100 mL, 200 mL) [latex free, sucrose free; stabilized with glycine]

Octagam®: 5% (20 mL, 50 mL, 100 mL, 200 mL) [sucrose free; contains sodium 30 mmol/L and maltose]

Injection, solution [preservative free]

Flebogamma®: 5% (10 mL, 50 mL, 100 mL, 200 mL) [contains polyethylene glycol and sorbitol]

Gamunex®: 10% (10 mL, 25 mL, 50 mL, 100 mL, 200 mL) [caprylate/chromatography purified]

Privigen™: 10% (50 mL, 100 mL, 200 mL) [sucrose free]

Immune Globulin (Subcutaneous)

(i MYUN GLOB yoo lin sub kyoo TAY nee us)

U.S. Brand Names Vivaglobin®

Index Terms Immune Globulin Subcutaneous (Human); SCIG

Pharmacologic Category Immune Globulin

Use Treatment of primary immune deficiency (PID)

Pregnancy Risk Factor C

Pregnancy Considerations Animal studies have not been conducted. There are no adequate and well-controlled studies in pregnant women. Use during pregnancy only if clearly needed.

Lactation Excretion in breast milk unknown/use caution

Contraindications Hypersensitivity to immune globulin or any component of the formulation; history of anaphylactic or severe systemic reaction to immune globulin preparations; selective IgA deficiency with known antibody against IgA

Warnings/Precautions For subcutaneous administration only; not for I.V. use. Hypersensitivity reactions and anaphylactic reactions can occur; use caution with initial treatment, when switching brands of immune globulin, and with treatment interruptions of >8 weeks. Patients should be monitored for adverse events during and after the first infusion. Stop infusion with signs of infusion reaction (fever, chills, nausea, vomiting, and rarely shock); medications for the treatment of hypersensitivity reactions should be available for immediate use. Use caution with IgA deficiency; sensitization to IgA may cause anaphylactic reaction. Product of human plasma; may potentially contain infectious agents which could transmit disease. Screening of donors, as well as testing and/or inactivation or removal of certain viruses, reduces the risk. Infections thought to be transmitted by this product should be reported to the manufacturer. Safety and effectiveness for children <2 years of age have not been established.

Adverse Reactions Adverse reactions can be expected to be similar to those experienced with other immune globulin products; percentages are reported as adverse events per patient; injection site reactions decreased with subsequent infusions

>10%:

Central nervous system: Headache (32% to 48%), fever (3% to 25%)

Dermatologic: Rash (6% to 17%)

Gastrointestinal: Gastrointestinal disorder (5% to 37%), nausea (11% to 18%), sore throat (17%)

Local: Injection site reactions (swelling, redness, itching; 92%)

Miscellaneous: Allergic reaction (11%)

1% to 10%:

Cardiovascular: Tachycardia (3%)

Central nervous system: Pain (10%)

Dermatologic: Skin disorder (3%)

Gastrointestinal: Diarrhea (10%)

Genitourinary: Urine abnormality (3%)

Neuromuscular & skeletal: Weakness (5%)

Respiratory: Cough (10%)

<1% (Limited to important or life-threatening): Abdominal pain, dyspnea, nervousness

Drug Interactions

Avoid Concomitant Use There are no known interactions where it is recommended to avoid concomitant use.

Increased Effect/Toxicity There are no known significant interactions involving an increase in effect.

Decreased Effect

Immune Globulin (Subcutaneous) may decrease the levels/effects of: Vaccines (Live)

Stability Store at 2°C to 8°C (36°F to 46°F); do not freeze. Do not shake. Store in original box until ready to use. Allow vial(s) to reach room temperature prior to use. The appearance of immune globulin (subcutaneous) may vary from colorless to light brown; do not use if cloudy or contains precipitate.

Mechanism of Action Immune globulin replacement therapy of IgG antibodies against bacteria and viral agents.

Pharmacodynamics/Kinetics

Bioavailability: 73% (compared to I.V.)

Time to peak, plasma: 2.5 days

Dosage Note: Consider premedicating with acetaminophen and diphenhydramine.

SubQ infusion: Children ≥2 years and Adults: 100-200 mg/kg weekly (maximum rate: 20 mL/hour; doses >15 mL should be divided between sites); adjust the dose over time to achieve desired clinical response or target IgG levels

Conversion from I.V. to SubQ: Multiply previous I.V. dose by 1.37, then divide into a weekly regimen by dividing by the previous I.V. dosing interval (eg, if the dosing interval was every 3 weeks, divide by 3); adjust the dose over time to achieve desired clinical response or target IgG levels. SubQ infusion administration should begin 1 week after the last I.V. dose.

Administration Subcutaneous: Initial dose should be administered in a healthcare setting capable of providing monitoring and treatment in the event of hypersensitivity. Using aseptic technique, follow the infusion device manufacturer's instructions for filling the reservoir and preparing the pump. Remove air from administration set and needle by priming. Inject via infusion pump into the abdomen, thigh, upper arm, and/or lateral hip. The maximum rate is 20 mL/hour and maximum volume per injection site is 15 mL (doses >15 mL should be divided and infused into several sites). Select the number of required infusion sites; multiple concurrent injection sites may be achieved with the use of Y-site connection tubing; injection sites must be at least 2 inches apart. After the sites are clean and dry, insert subcutaneous needle and prime administration set. Attach sterile needle to administration set, gently pull back on the syringe to assure a blood vessel has not been inadvertently accessed. Repeat for each injection site; infuse following instructions for the infusion device. Rotate the site(s) weekly. Treatment may be transitioned to the home/home care setting in the absence of adverse reactions.

Monitoring Parameters Infusion-related adverse reactions, anaphylaxis, IgG levels, clinical response

Reference Range Although the trough serum concentration of IgG has not been established, clinical experience has led to the use of 500 mg/dL as a guideline.

Test Interactions Passively-transferred antibodies may yield false-positive serologic testing results; may yield false-positive direct and indirect Coombs' test

Additional Information Serum IgG levels may be drawn at any time. Subcutaneous weekly treatments provide more constant levels rather than the more pronounced peak and trough patterns observed with I.V. monthly immune globulin treatments.

Dosage Forms Excipient information presented when available (limited, particularly for generics); consult specific product labeling.

Injection, solution [preservative free]: IgG 160 mg/mL (3 mL, 10 mL, 20 mL)

◆ **Immune Globulin Subcutaneous (Human)** *see* Immune Globulin (Subcutaneous) *on page* 779

◆ **Immune Serum Globulin** *see* Immune Globulin (Intramuscular) *on page* 776

◆ **Immunine® VH (Can)** *see* Factor IX *on page* 599

◆ **Imodium® (Can)** *see* Loperamide *on page* 900

◆ **Imodium® A-D [OTC]** *see* Loperamide *on page* 900

◆ **Imodium® Advanced** *see* Loperamide and Simethicone *on page* 901

◆ **Imogam® Rabies-HT** *see* Rabies Immune Globulin (Human) *on page* 1286

◆ **Imogam® Rabies Pasteurized (Can)** *see* Rabies Immune Globulin (Human) *on page* 1286

◆ **Imovax® Rabies** *see* Rabies Vaccine *on page* 1287

◆ **Implanon™** *see* Etonogestrel *on page* 589

◆ **Imuran®** *see* AzaTHIOprine *on page* 163

◆ **In-111 Ibritumomab** *see* Ibritumomab *on page* 758

◆ **In-111 Zevalin** *see* Ibritumomab *on page* 758

Inamrinone (eye NAM ri none)

Index Terms Amrinone Lactate

Pharmacologic Category Phosphodiesterase Enzyme Inhibitor

Use Short-term therapy in patients with intractable heart failure

Pregnancy Risk Factor C

Medication Safety Issues

Sound-alike/look-alike issues:

Amrinone may be confused with aMILoride, amiodarone

High alert medication: The Institute for Safe Medication Practices (ISMP) includes this medication among its list of drug classes which have a heightened risk of causing significant patient harm when used in error.

Dosage Dosage is based on clinical response (**Note:** Dose should not exceed 10 mg/kg/24 hours).

Infants (unlabeled population), Children (unlabeled population), and Adults: 0.75 mg/kg I.V. bolus over 2-3 minutes followed by maintenance infusion of 5-10 mcg/kg/minute; I.V. bolus may need to be repeated in 30 minutes.

Dosing adjustment in renal failure:

Infants and Children:

Cl_{cr} 30-50 mL/minute: Administer 100% of dose

Cl_{cr}10-29 mL/minute: Administer 50% of dose

Cl_{cr} <10 mL/minute: Administer 25% of dose

Intermittent hemodialysis or peritoneal dialysis: Administer 25% of dose

Adults:

Cl_{cr} ≥10 mL/minute: Administer 100% of dose

Cl_{cr} <10 mL/minute: Administer 50% to 75% of dose

Additional Information Complete prescribing information for this medication should be consulted for additional detail.

Dosage Forms Excipient information presented when available (limited, particularly for generics); consult specific product labeling.

Injection, solution, as lactate: 5 mg/mL (20 mL) [contains sodium metabisulfite]

◆ **Inapsine®** *see* Droperidol *on page 495*

◆ **Increlex™** *see* Mecasermin *on page 926*

Indapamide (in DAP a mide)

Canadian Brand Names Apo-Indapamide®; Dom-Indapamide; Gen-Indapamide; Lozide®; Lozol®; Novo-Indapamide; Nu-Indapamide; PHL-Indapamide; PMS-Indapamide; Pro-Indapamide; Riva-Indapamide

Pharmacologic Category Diuretic, Thiazide-Related

Additional Appendix Information

Sulfonamide Derivatives *on page 1671*

Use Management of mild to moderate hypertension; treatment of edema in congestive heart failure and nephrotic syndrome

Pregnancy Risk Factor B (manufacturer); D (expert analysis)

Lactation Excretion in breast milk unknown

Medication Safety Issues

Sound-alike/look-alike issues:

Indapamide may be confused with lopidine®

International issues:

Pretanix® [Hungary] may be confused with Protonix® which is a brand name for pantoprazole in the U.S.

Contraindications Hypersensitivity to indapamide or any component of the formulation, thiazides, or sulfonamide-derived drugs; anuria; renal decompensation; pregnancy (based on expert analysis)

Warnings/Precautions Use with caution in severe renal disease. Electrolyte disturbances (hypokalemia, hypochloremic alkalosis, hyponatremia) can occur. Use with caution in severe hepatic dysfunction; hepatic encephalopathy can be caused by electrolyte disturbances. Gout may be precipitated in certain patients with a history of gout, a familial predisposition to gout, or chronic renal failure. Use caution in patients with prediabetes or diabetes; may alter glucose control. I.V. use is generally not recommended (but is available). May cause SLE exacerbation or activation. Use with caution in patients with moderate or high cholesterol concentrations. Photosensitization may occur. Correct hypokalemia before initiating therapy.

Chemical similarities are present among sulfonamides, sulfonylureas, carbonic anhydrase inhibitors, thiazides, and loop diuretics (except ethacrynic acid). Use in patients with thiazide or sulfonamide allergy is specifically contraindicated in product labeling, however, a risk of cross-reaction exists in patients with allergy to any of these compounds; avoid use when previous reaction has been severe. Discontinue if signs of hypersensitivity are noted.

Adverse Reactions

1% to 10%:

Cardiovascular: Orthostatic hypotension, palpitation, flushing

Central nervous system: Dizziness, lightheadedness, vertigo, headache, weakness, restlessness, drowsiness, fatigue, lethargy, malaise, lassitude, anxiety, agitation, depression, nervousness

Gastrointestinal: Anorexia, gastric irritation, nausea, vomiting, abdominal pain, cramping, bloating, diarrhea, constipation, dry mouth, weight loss

Genitourinary: Nocturia, frequent urination, polyuria

Neuromuscular & skeletal: Muscle cramps, spasm

Ocular: Blurred vision

Respiratory: Rhinorrhea

<1% (Limited to important or life-threatening): Cutaneous vasculitis, glycosuria, hypercalcemia, hyperglycemia, hyperuricemia, impotency, necrotizing angiitis, pancreatitis, purpura, reduced libido, vasculitis

Drug Interactions

Avoid Concomitant Use

Avoid concomitant use of Indapamide with any of the following: Nilotinib; Tetrabenazine; Thioridazine; Ziprasidone

Increased Effect/Toxicity

Indapamide may increase the levels/effects of: ACE Inhibitors; Allopurinol; Amifostine; Calcitriol; Calcium Salts; Dofetilide; Lithium; QTc-Prolonging Agents; RiTUXimab; Tetrabenazine; Thioridazine; Ziprasidone

The levels/effects of Indapamide may be increased by: Alfuzosin; Ciprofloxacin; Corticosteroids (Orally Inhaled); Corticosteroids (Systemic); Gadobutrol; Herbs (Hypotensive Properties); Nilotinib; Prostacyclin Analogues

Decreased Effect

The levels/effects of Indapamide may be decreased by: Bile Acid Sequestrants; Herbs (Hypertensive Properties); Methylphenidate; Nonsteroidal Anti-Inflammatory Agents; Yohimbine

Ethanol/Nutrition/Herb Interactions Herb/Nutraceutical: Avoid dong quai if using for hypertension (has estrogenic activity). Avoid ephedra, yohimbe, ginseng (may worsen hypertension). Avoid garlic (may have increased antihypertensive effect).

Mechanism of Action Diuretic effect is localized at the proximal segment of the distal tubule of the nephron; it does not appear to have significant effect on glomerular filtration rate nor renal blood flow; like other diuretics, it enhances sodium, chloride, and water excretion by interfering with the transport of sodium ions across the renal tubular epithelium

Pharmacodynamics/Kinetics

Onset of action: 1-2 hours

Duration: ≤36 hours
Absorption: Complete
Protein binding, plasma: 71% to 79%
Metabolism: Extensively hepatic
Half-life elimination: 14-18 hours
Time to peak: 2-2.5 hours
Excretion: Urine (~60%) within 48 hours; feces (~16% to 23%)

Dosage Adults: Oral:
Edema: 2.5-5 mg/day. **Note:** There is little therapeutic benefit to increasing the dose >5 mg/day; there is, however, an increased risk of electrolyte disturbances
Hypertension: 1.25 mg in the morning, may increase to 5 mg/day by increments of 1.25-2.5 mg; consider adding another antihypertensive and decreasing the dose if response is not adequate

Dietary Considerations May be taken with food or milk to decrease GI adverse effects.

Administration May be taken with food or milk. Administer early in day to avoid nocturia. Administer the last dose of multiple doses no later than 6 PM unless instructed otherwise.

Monitoring Parameters Blood pressure (both standing and sitting/supine), serum electrolytes, renal function, assess weight, I & O reports daily to determine fluid loss

Dosage Forms Excipient information presented when available (limited, particularly for generics); consult specific product labeling.
Tablet: 1.25 mg, 2.5 mg

- **Inderal® [DSC]** *see* Propranolol *on page 1259*
- **Inderal® (Can)** *see* Propranolol *on page 1259*
- **Inderal® LA** *see* Propranolol *on page 1259*
- **Inderal®-LA (Can)** *see* Propranolol *on page 1259*
- **Inderide®** *see* Propranolol and Hydrochlorothiazide *on page 1261*

Indinavir (in DIN a veer)

U.S. Brand Names Crixivan®
Canadian Brand Names Crixivan®
Index Terms Indinavir Sulfate
Pharmacologic Category Antiretroviral Agent, Protease Inhibitor

Additional Appendix Information
Antiretroviral Therapy for HIV Infection: Adults and Adolescents *on page 1758*
Management of Healthcare Worker Exposures to HBV, HCV, and HIV *on page 1719*
Perinatal HIV Guidelines *on page 1730*

Use Treatment of HIV infection; should always be used as part of a multidrug regimen (at least three antiretroviral agents)

Pregnancy Risk Factor C

Pregnancy Considerations Plasma levels of indinavir were 74% lower at weeks 30-32 of gestation when compared to the same women at 14-28 weeks of gestation. Plasma levels were not measurable in some patients 8 hours post dose. It is not known if indinavir will exacerbate hyperbilirubinemia in neonates. Pregnancy and protease inhibitors are both associated with an increased risk of hyperglycemia. Glucose levels should be closely monitored. Until optimal dosing during pregnancy has been established, the manufacturer does not recommend indinavir use in pregnant patients. The AIDSinfo guidelines consider indinavir an alternative agent if lopinavir/ritonavir cannot be used, however, indinavir should be used in combination with low-dose ritonavir during pregnancy (optimal dosing is not known). Healthcare professionals are encouraged to contact the antiretroviral pregnancy registry to monitor outcomes of pregnant women exposed to antiretroviral medications (1-800-258-4263 or www.APRegistry.com).

Lactation Excretion in breast milk unknown/contraindicated

Medication Safety Issues
Sound-alike/look-alike issues:
Indinavir may be confused with Denavir™

Contraindications Hypersensitivity to indinavir or any component of the formulation; concurrent use of alprazolam, amiodarone, cisapride, triazolam, midazolam (oral), pimozide, or ergot alkaloids

Warnings/Precautions Because indinavir may cause nephrolithiasis/urolithiasis the drug should be discontinued if signs and symptoms occur. Adequate hydration is recommended. May cause tubulointerstitial nephritis (rare); severe asymptomatic leukocyturia may warrant evaluation. Use with caution in patients taking strong CYP3A4 inhibitors, moderate or strong CYP3A4 inducers and major CYP3A4 substrates (see Drug Interactions); consider alternative agents that avoid or lessen the potential for CYP-mediated interactions. Patients with hepatic insufficiency due to cirrhosis should have dose reduction. Warn patients about fat redistribution that can occur. Indinavir has been associated with hemolytic anemia (discontinue if diagnosed), hepatitis, hyperbilirubinemia, and hyperglycemia (exacerbation or new-onset diabetes). Treatment may result in immune reconstitution syndrome (acute inflammatory response to indolent or residual opportunistic infections). Use caution in patients with hemophilia; spontaneous bleeding has been reported.

Adverse Reactions
>10%:
Gastrointestinal: Abdominal pain (17%), nausea (12%)
Hepatic: Hyperbilirubinemia (14%; dose dependent)
Renal: Nephrolithiasis/urolithiasis, including flank pain with/without hematuria (29%, pediatric patients; 12% adult patients; dose dependent)

1% to 10%:
Central nervous system: Headache (5%), dizziness (3%), somnolence (2%), fever (2%), malaise (2%), fatigue (2%)
Dermatologic: Pruritus (4%), rash (1%)
Endocrine & metabolic: Hyperglycemia (1%)
Gastrointestinal: Vomiting (8%), diarrhea (3%), taste perversion (3%), acid reflux (3%), anorexia (3%), appetite increased (2%), dyspepsia (2%), serum amylase increased (2%)
Hematologic: Neutropenia (2%), anemia (1%), thrombocytopenia (1%)
Hepatic: Transaminases increased (4% to 5%), jaundice (2%)
Neuromuscular & skeletal: Back pain (8%), weakness (2%)
Renal: Dysuria (2%)
Respiratory: Cough (2%)

<1% (Limited to important or life-threatening): Abdominal distention, acute renal failure, alopecia, anaphylactoid reactions, angina, arthralgia, bleeding (spontaneous in patients with hemophilia A or B), cerebrovascular disorder, cholesterol increased, crystalluria, depression, dry skin, erythema multiforme, fat redistribution, hemolytic anemia, hepatic failure, hepatitis, hydronephrosis, hyperpigmentation, immune reconstitution syndrome, interstitial nephritis (with medullary calcification and cortical atrophy), leukocyturia (severe and asymptomatic), MI, new-onset diabetes, pancreatitis, paresthesia (oral), paronychia, pharyngitis, pyelonephritis, renal insufficiency, renal failure, Stevens-Johnson syndrome, triglycerides increased, upper respiratory infection, urticaria, vasculitis

Drug Interactions

Metabolism/Transport Effects Substrate of CYP2D6 (minor), 3A4 (major); **Inhibits** CYP2C9 (weak), 2C19 (weak), 2D6 (weak), 3A4 (strong)

Avoid Concomitant Use

Avoid concomitant use of Indinavir with any of the following: Alfuzosin; Amiodarone; Cisapride; Eplerenone; Ergot Derivatives; Nilotinib; Nisoldipine; Pimozide; QuiNIDine; Ranolazine; Rivaroxaban; Salmeterol; Silodosin; St Johns Wort

Increased Effect/Toxicity

Indinavir may increase the levels/effects of: Alfuzosin; Alosetron; Amiodarone; Antifungal Agents (Azole Derivatives, Systemic); Benzodiazepines (metabolized by oxidation); Calcium Channel Blockers (Dihydropyridine); Calcium Channel Blockers (Nondihydropyridine); CarBAMazepine; Ciclesonide; Cisapride; Clarithromycin; Corticosteroids (Orally Inhaled); CycloSPORINE; CYP3A4 Substrates; Digoxin; Enfuvirtide; Eplerenone; Ergot Derivatives; Etravirine; FentaNYL; Fesoterodine; Fusidic Acid; HMG-CoA Reductase Inhibitors; Ixabepilone; Maraviroc; Meperidine; Nefazodone; Nilotinib; Nisoldipine; Phosphodiesterase 5 Inhibitors; Pimecrolimus; Pimozide; Protease Inhibitors; QuiNIDine; Ranolazine; Rifamycin Derivatives; Rivaroxaban; Salmeterol; Silodosin; Sirolimus; Sorafenib; Tacrolimus; Temsirolimus; Tenofovir; TraZODone; Tricyclic Antidepressants

The levels/effects of Indinavir may be increased by: Antifungal Agents (Azole Derivatives, Systemic); Clarithromycin; CycloSPORINE; Delavirdine; Efavirenz; Enfuvirtide; Etravirine; Fusidic Acid; P-Glycoprotein Inhibitors

Decreased Effect

Indinavir may decrease the levels/effects of: Abacavir; Clarithromycin; Delavirdine; Etravirine; Meperidine; Oral Contraceptive (Estrogens); Theophylline Derivatives; Valproic Acid; Zidovudine

The levels/effects of Indinavir may be decreased by: Antacids; Atovaquone; CarBAMazepine; CYP3A4 Inducers (Strong); Deferasirox; Didanosine; Efavirenz; Garlic; H2-Antagonists; Nevirapine; Oral Contraceptive (Estrogens); P-Glycoprotein Inducers; Proton Pump Inhibitors; Rifamycin Derivatives; St Johns Wort; Tenofovir; Venlafaxine

Ethanol/Nutrition/Herb Interactions

Food: Indinavir bioavailability may be decreased if taken with food. Meals high in calories, fat, and protein result in a significant decrease in drug levels. Indinavir serum concentrations may be decreased by grapefruit juice.

Herb/Nutraceutical: Garlic may decrease the levels/effects of protease inhibitors. St John's wort *(Hypericum)* appears to induce CYP3A enzymes and has lead to 57% reductions in indinavir AUCs and 81% reductions in trough serum concentrations, which may lead to treatment failures; should not be used concurrently with indinavir.

Stability Medication should be stored at 15°C to 30°C (59°F to 86°F), and used in the original container and the desiccant should remain in the bottle. Capsules are sensitive to moisture.

Mechanism of Action Indinavir is a human immunodeficiency virus protease inhibitor, binding to the protease activity site and inhibiting the activity of this enzyme. HIV protease is an enzyme required for the cleavage of viral polyprotein precursors into individual functional proteins found in infectious HIV. Inhibition prevents cleavage of these polyproteins resulting in the formation of immature noninfectious viral particles.

Pharmacodynamics/Kinetics

Absorption: Administration with a high fat, high calorie diet resulted in a reduction in AUC and in maximum serum concentration (77% and 84% respectively); lighter meal resulted in little or no change in these parameters.

Protein binding, plasma: 60%

Metabolism: Hepatic via CYP3A4; seven metabolites of indinavir identified

Bioavailability: Good

Half-life elimination: 1.8 ± 0.4 hour; hepatic insufficiency: 2.8 ± 0.5 hour

Time to peak: 0.8 ± 0.3 hour

Excretion: Feces (83%; 19% as unchanged drug); urine (19%; 9% as unchanged drug)

Dosage

Children 4-15 years (investigational): 500 mg/m^2 every 8 hours

Adults: Oral:

Unboosted regimen: 800 mg every 8 hours

Ritonavir-boosted regimens:

Ritonavir 100-200 mg twice daily plus indinavir 800 mg twice daily **or**

Ritonavir 400 mg twice daily plus indinavir 400 mg twice daily

Dosage adjustments for indinavir when administered in combination therapy:

Delavirdine, itraconazole, or ketoconazole: Reduce indinavir dose to 600 mg every 8 hours

Efavirenz: Increase indinavir dose to 1000 mg every 8 hours

Lopinavir and ritonavir (Kaletra™): Indinavir 600 mg twice daily

Nelfinavir: Increase indinavir dose to 1200 mg twice daily

Nevirapine: Increase indinavir dose to 1000 mg every 8 hours

Rifabutin: Reduce rifabutin to 1/2 the standard dose plus increase indinavir to 1000 mg every 8 hours

Dosage adjustment in hepatic impairment: Mild-moderate impairment due to cirrhosis: 600 mg every 8 hours

Dietary Considerations Should be taken without food but with water 1 hour before or 2 hours after a meal. Administration with lighter meals (eg, dry toast, skim milk, corn flakes) resulted in little/no change in indinavir concentration. If taking with ritonavir, may take with food. Patient should drink at least 48 oz of water daily.

Administration Drink at least 48 oz of water daily. Administer with water, 1 hour before or 2 hours after a meal. May also be administered with other liquids (eg, skim milk, juice, coffee, tea) or a light meal (eg, toast, corn flakes). Administer around-the-clock to avoid significant fluctuation in serum levels. May be taken with food when administered in combination with ritonavir.

Monitoring Parameters Monitor viral load, CD4 count, triglycerides, cholesterol, glucose, liver function tests, CBC, urinalysis (severe leukocyturia should be monitored frequently).

Dosage Forms Excipient information presented when available (limited, particularly for generics); consult specific product labeling.

Capsule:

Crixivan®: 100 mg, 200 mg, 333 mg, 400 mg

- **Indinavir Sulfate** *see* Indinavir *on page 782*
- **Indocid® P.D.A. (Can)** *see* Indomethacin *on page 783*
- **Indocin®** *see* Indomethacin *on page 783*
- **Indocin® I.V.** *see* Indomethacin *on page 783*
- **Indo-Lemmon (Can)** *see* Indomethacin *on page 783*
- **Indometacin** *see* Indomethacin *on page 783*

Indomethacin (in doe METH a sin)

U.S. Brand Names Indocin®; Indocin® I.V.

Canadian Brand Names Apo-Indomethacin®; Indo-Lemmon; Indocid® P.D.A.; Indocin®; Indotec; Novo-Methacin; Nu-Indo; Rhodacine®

Index Terms Indometacin; Indomethacin Sodium Trihydrate

Pharmacologic Category Nonsteroidal Anti-inflammatory Drug (NSAID), Oral; Nonsteroidal Anti-inflammatory Drug (NSAID), Parenteral

Additional Appendix Information

Nonsteroidal Anti-inflammatory Agents *on page 1669*

Use Acute gouty arthritis, acute bursitis/tendonitis, moderate to severe osteoarthritis, rheumatoid arthritis, ankylosing spondylitis; I.V. form used as alternative to surgery for closure of patent ductus arteriosus in neonates

Restrictions An FDA-approved medication guide must be distributed when dispensing an oral outpatient prescription (new or refill) where this medication is to be used without direct supervision of a healthcare provider. Medication guides are available at http://www.fda.gov/cder/Offices/ODS/medication_guides.htm.

Pregnancy Risk Factor C/D (3rd trimester)

Lactation Enters breast milk/not recommended (AAP rates "compatible")

Medication Safety Issues

Sound-alike/look-alike issues:

Indocin® may be confused with Imodium®, Lincocin®, Minocin®, Vicodin®

International issues:

Flexin® [Great Britain] may be confused with Floxin® which is a brand name for ofloxacin in the U.S.

Flexin® [Great Britain]: Brand name for orphenadrine in Israel

Contraindications Hypersensitivity to indomethacin, aspirin, other NSAIDs, or any component of the formulation; perioperative pain in the setting of coronary artery bypass graft (CABG) surgery; patients with a history of proctitis or recent rectal bleeding (suppositories)

Neonates: Necrotizing enterocolitis; impaired renal function; active bleeding (including intracranial hemorrhage and gastrointestinal bleeding), thrombocytopenia, coagulation defects; untreated infection; congenital heart disease where patent ductus arteriosus is necessary

Warnings/Precautions [U.S. Boxed Warning]: NSAIDs are associated with an increased risk of adverse cardiovascular thrombotic events, including MI, stroke, and new onset or worsening of pre-existing hypertension. Risk may be increased with duration of use or pre-existing cardiovascular risk factors or disease. Use caution with fluid retention, heart failure, or hypertension. Concurrent administration of ibuprofen, and potentially other nonselective NSAIDs, may interfere with aspirin's cardioprotective effect. **[U.S. Boxed Warning]: Use is contraindicated for treatment of perioperative pain in the setting of coronary artery bypass graft (CABG) surgery.** Risk of MI and stroke may be increased with use following CABG surgery.

Platelet adhesion and aggregation may be decreased; may prolong bleeding time; patients with coagulation disorders or who are receiving anticoagulants should be monitored closely. Anemia may occur; patients on long-term NSAID therapy should be monitored for anemia. NSAID use may compromise existing renal function; dose-dependent decreases in prostaglandin synthesis may result from NSAID use, reducing renal blood flow which may cause renal decompensation. Patients with impaired renal function, dehydration, heart failure, liver dysfunction, those taking diuretics, and ACE inhibitors, and the elderly are at greater risk of renal toxicity. Rehydrate patient before starting therapy; monitor renal function closely. Not recommended for use in patients with advanced renal disease. Long-term NSAID use may result in renal papillary necrosis.

[U.S. Boxed Warning]: NSAIDs may increase risk of gastrointestinal irritation, inflammation, ulceration, bleeding, and perforation. Use caution with a history of GI disease (bleeding or ulcers), concurrent therapy with aspirin, anticoagulants and/or corticosteroids, smoking, use of alcohol, the elderly or debilitated patients.

Use the lowest effective dose for the shortest duration of time, consistent with individual patient goals, to reduce risk of cardiovascular or GI adverse events. Alternate therapies should be considered for patients at high risk.

NSAIDs may cause serious skin adverse events including exfoliative dermatitis, Stevens-Johnson syndrome (SJS) and toxic epidermal necrolysis (TEN); discontinue use at first sign of skin rash or hypersensitivity. Anaphylactoid reactions may occur, even without prior exposure; patients with "aspirin triad" (bronchial asthma, aspirin intolerance, rhinitis) may be at increased risk. Do not use in patients who experience bronchospasm, asthma, rhinitis, or urticaria with NSAID or aspirin therapy. Use caution in other forms of asthma.

Use with caution in patients with decreased hepatic function. Closely monitor patients with any abnormal LFT. Severe hepatic reactions (eg, fulminant hepatitis, liver failure) have occurred with NSAID use, rarely; discontinue if signs or symptoms of liver disease develop, or if systemic manifestations occur. The elderly are at increased risk for adverse effects (especially peptic ulceration, CNS effects, renal toxicity) from NSAIDs even at low doses. Prolonged use may cause corneal deposits and retinal disturbances; discontinue if visual changes are observed. Use caution with depression, epilepsy, or Parkinson's disease.

Withhold for at least 4-6 half-lives prior to surgical or dental procedures.

Oral: Safety and efficacy have not been established in children <14 years of age. Hepatotoxicity has been reported in younger children treated for JRA. Closely monitor if use is needed in children ≥2 years of age.

Adverse Reactions

>10%: Central nervous system: Headache (12%)

1% to 10%:

Central nervous system: Dizziness (3% to 9%), fatigue (<3%), vertigo (<3%), depression (<3%), malaise (<3%), somnolence (<3%)

Gastrointestinal: Nausea (3% to 9%), epigastric pain (3% to 9%), abdominal pain/cramps/distress (<3%), heartburn (3% to 9%), indigestion (3% to 9%), constipation (<3%), diarrhea (<3%), dyspepsia (3% to 9%), rectal irritation (suppository), tenesmus (suppository), vomiting

Otic: Tinnitus (<3%)

<1% (Limited to important or life-threatening): Acute respiratory distress, agranulocytosis, allergic rhinitis, anaphylaxis, anemia, angiitis, angioedema, aplastic anemia, arrhythmia, aseptic meningitis, asthma, bone marrow suppression, bronchospasm, chest pain, cholestatic jaundice, coma, confusion, CHF, cystitis, depersonalization, depression, diplopia, disseminated intravascular coagulation (DIC), dysarthria, dyspnea, ecchymosis, edema, epistaxis, erythema multiforme, erythema nodosum, exfoliative dermatitis, fluid retention, flushing, hair loss, gastric perforation (rare), gastritis, GI bleeding, GI ulceration, glucosuria, gynecomastia, hearing decreased, hematuria, hemolytic anemia, hepatitis (including fatal cases), hot flashes, hyperglycemia, hyperkalemia, hypersensitivity reactions, hyper-/hypotension, interstitial nephritis, intestinal strictures, involuntary muscle movements, leukopenia, lightheadedness, necrotizing fasciitis, nephrotic syndrome, oliguria, paresthesia, parkinson's exacerbation, peptic ulcer, peripheral neuropathy, proctitis, psychosis, pulmonary edema, purpura,

rectal bleeding, renal insufficiency, renal failure, retinal/macular disturbances, seizure exacerbation, shock, somnolence, Stevens-Johnson syndrome, stomatitis, syncope, thrombocytopenia, thrombocytopenic purpura, thrombophlebitis, toxic amblyopia, toxic epidermal necrolysis, ulcerative stomatitis

Drug Interactions

Metabolism/Transport Effects **Substrate** (minor) of CYP2C9, 2C19; **Inhibits** CYP2C9 (strong), 2C19 (weak)

Avoid Concomitant Use

Avoid concomitant use of Indomethacin with any of the following: Ketorolac

Increased Effect/Toxicity

Indomethacin may increase the levels/effects of: Aminoglycosides; Anticoagulants; Antiplatelet Agents; Bisphosphonate Derivatives; CycloSPORINE; CYP2C9 Substrates (High risk); Desmopressin; Lithium; Methotrexate; Nonsteroidal Anti-Inflammatory Agents; Pemetrexed; Quinolone Antibiotics; Salicylates; Thrombolytic Agents; Tiludronate; Triamterene; Vancomycin; Vitamin K Antagonists

The levels/effects of Indomethacin may be increased by: Antidepressants (Tricyclic, Tertiary Amine); Corticosteroids (Systemic); Herbs (Anticoagulant/Antiplatelet Properties); Ketorolac; Probenecid; Selective Serotonin Reuptake Inhibitors; Serotonin/Norepinephrine Reuptake Inhibitors; Treprostinil

Decreased Effect

Indomethacin may decrease the levels/effects of: ACE Inhibitors; Angiotensin II Receptor Blockers; Antiplatelet Agents; Beta-Blockers; Eplerenone; HydrALAZINE; Loop Diuretics; Salicylates; Thiazide Diuretics

The levels/effects of Indomethacin may be decreased by: Bile Acid Sequestrants; Salicylates

Ethanol/Nutrition/Herb Interactions

Ethanol: Avoid ethanol (may enhance gastric mucosal irritation).

Food: Food may decrease the rate but not the extent of absorption. Indomethacin peak serum levels may be delayed if taken with food.

Herb/Nutraceutical: Avoid alfalfa, anise, bilberry, bladderwrack, bromelain, cat's claw, celery, chamomile, coleus, cordyceps, dong quai, evening primrose, fenugreek, feverfew, garlic, ginger, ginkgo biloba, ginseng (American, Panax, Siberian), grapeseed, green tea, guggul, horse chestnut seed, horseradish, licorice, prickly ash, red clover, reishi, SAMe (S-adenosylmethionine), sweet clover, turmeric, white willow (all have additional antiplatelet activity).

Stability I.V.: Store below 30°C (86°F). Protect from light. Not stable in alkaline solution. Reconstitute with 1-2 mL preservative free NS or SWFI just prior to administration. Discard any unused portion. Do not use preservative-containing diluents for reconstitution.

Mechanism of Action Reversibly inhibits cyclooxygenase-1 and 2 (COX-1 and 2) enzymes, which result in decreased formation of prostaglandin precursors; has antipyretic, analgesic, and anti-inflammatory properties

Pharmacodynamics/Kinetics

Onset of action: ~30 minutes

Duration: 4-6 hours

Absorption: Oral: Immediate release: Prompt and extensive; Extended release: 90% over 12 hours

Distribution: V_d: 0.34-1.57 L/kg; crosses blood brain barrier and placenta; enters breast milk

Protein binding: 99%

Metabolism: Hepatic; significant enterohepatic recirculation

Bioavailability: 100%

Half-life elimination: 4.5 hours; prolonged in neonates

Time to peak: Oral: Immediate release: 2 hours

Excretion: Urine (60%, primarily as glucuronide conjugates); feces (33%, primarily as metabolites)

Dosage

Patent ductus arteriosus:

Neonates: I.V.: Initial: 0.2 mg/kg, followed by 2 doses depending on postnatal age (PNA):

PNA **at time of first dose** <48 hours: 0.1 mg/kg at 12- to 24-hour intervals

PNA **at time of first dose** 2-7 days: 0.2 mg/kg at 12- to 24-hour intervals

PNA **at time of first dose** >7 days: 0.25 mg/kg at 12- to 24-hour intervals

In general, may use 12-hour dosing interval if urine output >1 mL/kg/hour after prior dose; use 24-hour dosing interval if urine output is <1 mL/kg/hour but >0.6 mL/kg/hour; doses should be withheld if patient has oliguria (urine output <0.6 mL/kg/hour) or anuria

Inflammatory/rheumatoid disorders: Oral: Use lowest effective dose.

Children ≥2 years: 1-2 mg/kg/day in 2-4 divided doses; maximum dose: 4 mg/kg/day; not to exceed 150-200 mg/day

Adults: 25-50 mg/dose 2-3 times/day; maximum dose: 200 mg/day; extended release capsule should be given on a 1-2 times/day schedule (maximum dose for extended release: 150 mg/day). In patients with arthritis and persistent night pain and/or morning stiffness may give the larger portion (up to 100 mg) of the total daily dose at bedtime.

Bursitis/tendonitis: Oral: Adults: Initial dose: 75-150 mg/day in 3-4 divided doses **or** 1-2 divided doses for extended release; usual treatment is 7-14 days

Acute gouty arthritis: Oral: Adults: 50 mg 3 times daily until pain is tolerable then reduce dose; usual treatment <3-5 days

Elderly: Refer to adult dosing. Use lowest recommended dose and frequency in elderly to initiate therapy for indications listed in adult dosing.

Dosage adjustment in renal impairment: Not recommended in patients with advanced renal disease

Dietary Considerations May cause GI upset; take with food or milk to minimize

Administration

Oral: Administer with food, milk, or antacids to decrease GI adverse effects. Extended release capsules must be swallowed whole; do not crush.

I.V.: Administer over 20-30 minutes. Reconstitute I.V. formulation just prior to administration; discard any unused portion; avoid I.V. bolus administration or infusion via an umbilical catheter into vessels near the superior mesenteric artery as these may cause vasoconstriction and can compromise blood flow to the intestines. Do not administer intra-arterially.

Monitoring Parameters Monitor response (pain, range of motion, grip strength, mobility, ADL function), inflammation; observe for weight gain, edema; monitor renal function (serum creatinine, BUN); observe for bleeding, bruising; evaluate gastrointestinal effects (abdominal pain, bleeding, dyspepsia); mental confusion, disorientation, CBC, liver function tests (particularly with pediatric use); ophthalmologic exams with prolonged therapy

Test Interactions False-negative dexamethasone suppression test

Dosage Forms Excipient information presented when available (limited, particularly for generics); consult specific product labeling.

Capsule: 25 mg, 50 mg

Capsule, extended release, oral: 75 mg

Injection, powder for reconstitution:

Indocin® I.V.: 1 mg

Suppository, rectal: 50 mg (30s)

Suspension, oral:

Indocin®: 25 mg/5 mL (237 mL) [contains alcohol 1%; pineapple-coconut-mint flavor]

◆ **Indomethacin Sodium Trihydrate** *see* Indomethacin *on page 783*

◆ **Indotec (Can)** *see* Indomethacin *on page 783*

◆ **INF-alpha 2** *see* Interferon Alfa-2b *on page 801*

◆ **Infanrix®** *see* Diphtheria and Tetanus Toxoids, and Acellular Pertussis Vaccine *on page 463*

◆ **Infantaire [OTC]** *see* Acetaminophen *on page 25*

◆ **Infasurf®** *see* Calfactant *on page 243*

◆ **INFeD®** *see* Iron Dextran Complex *on page 817*

◆ **Infergen®** *see* Interferon Alfacon-1 *on page 805*

◆ **Inflamase® Mild (Can)** *see* PrednisoLONE *on page 1230*

InFLIXimab (in FLIKS e mab)

U.S. Brand Names Remicade®

Canadian Brand Names Remicade®

Index Terms Infliximab, Recombinant; NSC-728729

Pharmacologic Category Antirheumatic, Disease Modifying; Gastrointestinal Agent, Miscellaneous; Monoclonal Antibody; Tumor Necrosis Factor (TNF) Blocking Agent

Use Treatment of rheumatoid arthritis (moderate-to-severe, with methotrexate); treatment of Crohn's disease (moderate-to-severe with inadequate response to conventional therapy) for induction and maintenance of remission, and/or to reduce the number of draining enterocutaneous and rectovaginal fistulas, and to maintain fistula closure; treatment of psoriatic arthritis; treatment of plaque psoriasis (chronic severe); treatment of ankylosing spondylitis; treatment of and maintenance of healing of ulcerative colitis (moderately- to severely-active with inadequate response to conventional therapy)

Unlabeled/Investigational Use Acute graft-versus-host disease (GVHD), juvenile rheumatoid arthritis (JRA)

Restrictions An FDA-approved medication guide is available at www.fda.gov/cder/Offices/ODS/labeling.htm; distribute to each patient to whom this medication is dispensed.

Pregnancy Risk Factor B

Pregnancy Considerations Reproduction studies have not been conducted. Use during pregnancy only if clearly needed. A Rheumatoid Arthritis and Pregnancy Registry has been established for women exposed to infliximab during pregnancy (Organization of Teratology Information Services, 877-311-8972).

Lactation Excretion in breast milk unknown/not recommended

Medication Safety Issues

Sound-alike/look-alike issues:

Remicade® may be confused with Renacidin®, Rituxan®

InFLIXimab may be confused with riTUXimab

Contraindications Hypersensitivity to infliximab, murine proteins or any component of the formulation; doses >5 mg/kg in patients with moderate or severe congestive heart failure (NYHA Class III/IV)

Canadian labeling: Additional contraindications (not in U.S. labeling): Severe infections (eg, sepsis, abscesses, tuberculosis, and opportunistic infections)

Warnings/Precautions [U.S. Boxed Warning]: Opportunistic infections and/or reactivation of latent infections have been associated with infliximab therapy. Tuberculosis (may be disseminated or extrapulmonary) has been reactivated in patients previously exposed to TB while on infliximab. Most cases have been reported within the first 3-6 months of treatment. Other opportunistic infections (eg, invasive fungal infections, listeriosis, *Pneumocystis*) have occurred during therapy. Patients should be evaluated for latent tuberculosis infection with a tuberculin skin test prior to infliximab therapy. Treatment of latent tuberculosis should be initiated before infliximab is used. The risk/benefit ratio should be weighed in patients who have resided in regions where histoplasmosis is endemic.

Serious infections (including sepsis, pneumonia, and fatal infections) have been reported in patients receiving TNF-blocking agents. Cases of unrecognized invasive fungal infections (eg, histoplasmosis, blastomycosis, coccidioidomycosis) have also been reported with anti-TNF agent use. Many of the serious infections in patients treated with infliximab have occurred in patients on concomitant immunosuppressive therapy. Serious infections were reported when used in combination with anakinra or etanercept. Caution should be exercised when considering the use of infliximab in patients with a chronic infection, history of recurrent infection, or predisposition to infection (eg, diabetes or residence/travel from areas of endemic mycoses). Infliximab should not be given to patients with a clinically important, active infection. Patients who develop a new infection while undergoing treatment with infliximab should be monitored closely. If a patient develops a serious infection or sepsis, infliximab should be discontinued. Patients should be brought up to date with all immunizations before initiating therapy. Live vaccines should not be given concurrently; there is no data available concerning secondary transmission of live vaccines in patients receiving therapy. Rare reactivation of hepatitis B virus (HBV) has occurred in chronic virus carriers; use with caution; evaluate prior to initiation and during treatment.

[U.S. Boxed Warning]: Hepatosplenic T-cell lymphoma has been reported (rarely) in adolescent and young adults with Crohn's disease treated with infliximab and azathioprine or 6-mercaptopurine. The impact of infliximab on the development and course of malignancies is not fully defined, but may be dose dependent. As compared to the general population, an increased risk of lymphoma has been noted in clinical trials; however, rheumatoid arthritis alone has been previously associated with an increased rate of lymphoma. Use caution in patients with a history of COPD, higher rates of malignancy were reported in COPD patients treated with infliximab. Psoriasis patients with a history of phototherapy had a higher incidence of nonmelanoma skin cancers.

Severe hepatic reactions (including hepatitis, jaundice, acute hepatic failure, and cholestasis) have been reported during treatment; discontinue with jaundice or marked increase in liver enzymes (≥5 times ULN). Use caution with heart failure; if a decision is made to use with heart failure, monitor closely and discontinue if exacerbated or new symptoms occur. Doses >5 mg/kg should not be administered in patients with moderate to severe heart failure. Use caution with history of hematologic abnormalities; hematologic toxicities (eg, leukopenia, neutropenia, thrombocytopenia, pancytopenia) have been reported; discontinue if significant abnormalities occur. Autoimmune antibodies and a lupus-like syndrome have been reported. If antibodies to double-stranded DNA are confirmed in a patient with lupus-like symptoms, infliximab should be discontinued. Rare cases of optic neuritis and demyelinating disease have been reported; use with caution in patients with pre-existing or recent onset CNS demyelinating disorders, or seizures; discontinue if significant CNS adverse reactions develop.

Acute infusion reactions may occur. Hypersensitivity reaction may occur within 2 hours of infusion. Medication and equipment for management should be available for immediate use. Interruptions and/or reinstitution at a slower rate may be required (consult protocols).

Pretreatment may be considered, and may be warranted in all patients with prior infusion reactions. Serum sickness-like reactions have occurred; may be associated with a decreased response to treatment. Safety and efficacy for use in juvenile rheumatoid arthritis, pediatric plaque psoriasis, or pediatric ulcerative colitis have not been established. **Note:** For use in Crohn's disease: Safety and efficacy have not been established in children <6 years of age (U.S. labeling); safety and efficacy have not been established in children <9 years of age (Canadian labeling).

Adverse Reactions **Although profile is similar, frequency of adverse effects may vary with disease state. Except where noted, percentages reported in adults with rheumatoid arthritis:**

>10%:

Central nervous system: Headache (18%)
Gastrointestinal: Nausea (21%), diarrhea (12%), abdominal pain (12%, Crohn's 26%)
Hepatic: ALT increased (risk increased with concomitant methotrexate)
Respiratory: Upper respiratory tract infection (32%), sinusitis (14%), cough (12%), pharyngitis (12%)
Miscellaneous: Development of antinuclear antibodies (~50%), infection (36%), development of antibodies to double-stranded DNA (17%), infusion reactions (20%; severe <1%); Crohn's patients with fistulizing disease: Development of new abscess (15%)

5% to 10%:

Cardiovascular: Hypertension (7%)
Central nervous system: Fatigue (9%), pain (8%), fever (7%)
Dermatologic: Rash (1% to 10%), pruritus (7%)
Gastrointestinal: Dyspepsia (10%)
Genitourinary: Urinary tract infection (8%)
Neuromuscular & skeletal: Arthralgia (1% to 8%), back pain (8%)
Respiratory: Bronchitis (10%), rhinitis (8%), dyspnea (6%)
Miscellaneous: Moniliasis (5%)

<5%: Abscess, adult respiratory distress syndrome, allergic reaction, anemia, arrhythmia, basal cell carcinoma, biliary pain, bradycardia, brain infarction, breast cancer, cardiac arrest, cellulitis, cholecystitis, cholelithiasis, circulatory failure, confusion, constipation, dehydration, delayed hypersensitivity (plaque psoriasis), diaphoresis increased, dizziness, edema, gastrointestinal hemorrhage, heart failure, hemolytic anemia, hepatitis, hypersensitivity reactions, hypotension, ileus, intervertebral disk herniation, intestinal obstruction, intestinal perforation, intestinal stenosis, leukopenia, lupus-like syndrome, lymphadenopathy, lymphoma, malignancies, meningitis, menstrual irregularity, MI, myalgia, neuritis, pancreatitis, pancytopenia, peripheral neuropathy, peritonitis, pleural effusion, pleurisy, proctalgia, pulmonary edema, pulmonary embolism, renal calculus, renal failure, respiratory insufficiency, seizure, sepsis, serum sickness, suicide attempt, syncope, tachycardia, tendon disorder, thrombocytopenia, thrombophlebitis (deep), ulceration

The following adverse events were reported in children with Crohn's disease and were found more frequently in children than adults:

>10%:

Hepatic: Liver enzymes increased (18%; ≥5 times ULN: 1%)
Hematologic: Anemia (11%)
Miscellaneous: Infections (56%; more common with every 8-week versus every 12-week infusions)

1% to 10%:

Central nervous system: Flushing (9%)
Gastrointestinal: Blood in stool (10%)
Hematologic: Leukopenia (9%), neutropenia (7%)
Neuromuscular & skeletal: Bone fracture (7%)
Respiratory: Respiratory tract allergic reaction (6%)
Miscellaneous: Viral infection (8%), bacterial infection (6%), antibodies to infliximab (3%)

Postmarketing and/or case reports (adults or children): Agranulocytosis, anaphylactic reactions, anaphylactic shock, angina, angioedema, autoimmune hepatitis, bronchospasm, cholestasis, demyelinating disorders (eg, multiple sclerosis, optic neuritis); drug-induced lupus-like syndrome, erythema multiforme, Guillain-Barré syndrome, heart failure (worsening), hepatitis B reactivation, hepatocellular damage, hepatosplenic T-cell lymphoma (HSTCL), Hodgkin's disease, idiopathic thrombocytopenia purpura, interstitial fibrosis, interstitial pneumonitis, jaundice, laryngeal/pharyngeal edema, latent tuberculosis reactivation, liver failure, liver function tests increased, neuropathy, numbness, opportunistic infection, pericardial effusion, pneumonia, psoriasis, seizure, Stevens-Johnson syndrome, thrombotic thrombocytopenia purpura, taste abnormal, tingling, toxic epidermal necrolysis, transverse myelitis, tuberculosis, urticaria, vasculitis (systemic and cutaneous)

Drug Interactions

Avoid Concomitant Use

Avoid concomitant use of InFLIXimab with any of the following: Anakinra; Natalizumab; Rilonacept; Vaccines (Live)

Increased Effect/Toxicity

InFLIXimab may increase the levels/effects of: Abatacept; Anakinra; Natalizumab; Rilonacept; Vaccines (Live)

The levels/effects of InFLIXimab may be increased by: Abciximab; Trastuzumab

Decreased Effect

InFLIXimab may decrease the levels/effects of: Vaccines (Inactivated)

The levels/effects of InFLIXimab may be decreased by: Echinacea

Ethanol/Nutrition/Herb Interactions Herb/Nutraceutical: Avoid echinacea (may diminish the therapeutic effect of infliximab).

Stability Store vials at 2°C to 8°C (36°F to 46°F); do not freeze. Reconstitute vials with 10 mL sterile water for injection. Swirl vial gently to dissolve powder; do not shake. Allow solution to stand for 5 minutes. Total dose of reconstituted product should be further diluted to 250 mL of 0.9% sodium chloride injection to a final concentration of 0.4-4 mg/mL. Infusion of dose should begin within 3 hours of preparation.

Mechanism of Action Infliximab is a chimeric monoclonal antibody that binds to human tumor necrosis factor alpha (TNFα), thereby interfering with endogenous TNFα activity. Biological activities of TNFα include the induction of proinflammatory cytokines (interleukins), enhancement of leukocyte migration, activation of neutrophils and eosinophils, and the induction of acute phase reactants and tissue degrading enzymes. Animal models have shown TNFα expression causes polyarthritis, and infliximab can prevent disease as well as allow diseased joints to heal.

Pharmacodynamics/Kinetics

Onset of action: Crohn's disease: ~2 weeks

Distribution: V_d: 3-6 L

Half-life elimination: 7-12 days

Dosage I.V.: **Note:** Premedication with antihistamines (anti-H_1 and/or anti-H_2), acetaminophen and/or corticosteroids may be considered to prevent and/or manage infusion-related reactions:

Children: U.S. labeling ≥6 years, Canadian labeling ≥9 years:

Crohn's disease: 5 mg/kg at 0, 2, and 6 weeks, followed by a maintenance dose of 5 mg/kg every 8 weeks; if no response by week 14, consider discontinuing therapy

Juvenile rheumatoid arthritis (unlabeled use): 3-4 mg/kg at 0, 2, and 6 weeks, and then every 8 weeks thereafter

Adults:

Crohn's disease: Induction regimen: 5 mg/kg at 0, 2, and 6 weeks, followed by 5 mg/kg every 8 weeks thereafter; dose may be increased to 10 mg/kg in patients who respond but then lose their response. If no response by week 14, consider discontinuing therapy.

Psoriatic arthritis (with or without methotrexate): 5 mg/kg at 0, 2, and 6 weeks, then every 8 weeks

Rheumatoid arthritis (in combination with methotrexate therapy): 3 mg/kg at 0, 2, and 6 weeks, then every 8 weeks thereafter; doses have ranged from 3-10 mg/kg intravenous infusion repeated at 4- to 8-week intervals

Ankylosing spondylitis: 5 mg/kg at 0, 2, and 6 weeks, followed by 5 mg/kg every 6 weeks thereafter

Plaque psoriasis: 5 mg/kg at 0, 2, and 6 weeks, then every 8 weeks thereafter

Ulcerative colitis: 5 mg/kg at 0, 2, and 6 weeks, followed by 5 mg/kg every 8 weeks thereafter

Acute GVHD (unlabeled use): 10 mg/kg weekly for up to 8 weeks (median 4 weeks of treatment)

Dosage adjustment with CHF: Weigh risk versus benefits for individual patient:

NYHA Class III or IV: ≤5 mg/kg

Dosage adjustment in renal impairment: No specific adjustment is recommended

Dosage adjustment in hepatic impairment: No specific adjustment is recommended

Administration Infuse over at least 2 hours; do not infuse with other agents; use in-line low protein binding filter (≤1.2 micron). Temporarily discontinue or decrease infusion rate with infusion-related reactions. Antihistamines (anti-H_1 and/or anti-H_2), acetaminophen and/or corticosteroids may be used to manage reactions. Infusion may be reinitiated at a lower rate upon resolution of mild-to-moderate symptoms.

Canadian labeling (not approved in U.S. labeling): Infusion of doses ≤6 mg/kg over not less than 1 hour may be considered in patients treated for rheumatoid arthritis who have initially tolerated 3 infusions each over 2 hours. Safety of shortened infusion has not been studied with doses >6 mg/kg.

Guidelines for the treatment and prophylaxis of infusion reactions: (**Note:** Limited to dosages used in Crohn's; prospective information on other indications/ dosing such as in GVHD are not available).

Treatment of infusion reactions: Medications for the treatment of hypersensitivity reactions should be available for immediate use. A protocol for the treatment of acute infusion reactions, as well a prophylactic therapy for repeat infusions, has been published (Cheifetz, 2003). Decreasing the rate of infusion to 10 mL/hour (mild-to-moderate reactions) or a 20-minute interruption of the infusion (moderate-to-severe reactions) is recommended. Monitor vital signs every 10 minutes until normal. Administration of appropriate symptomatic treatment (acetaminophen and diphenhydramine, as well as hydrocortisone and epinephrine for severe reactions) should be instituted (consult institutional policies, if available). Following initial treatment, the infusion may be reinstituted at 10 mL/hour; then increased at 15-minute intervals, as tolerated (first to 20 mL/hour, then 40 mL/hour, then 80 mL/hour to completion).

Prophylaxis of infusion reactions: Premedication with acetaminophen and diphenhydramine 90 minutes prior to infusion may be considered in all patients with prior infusion reactions, and in patients with severe reactions corticosteroid administration is recommended (Cheifetz, 2003). Steroid dosing may be oral (prednisone 50 mg orally for 3 doses over a 24-hour period prior to infusion) or intravenous (a single dose of hydrocortisone 100 mg or methylprednisolone 20-240 mg administered 20 minutes prior to the infusion) (Cheifetz, 2003). On initiation of the infusion, a test dose (infusion at 10 mL/ hour for 15 minutes) may be considered. If tolerated, for patients with mild reactions, the infusion may be completed over 3 hours. For patients with prior moderate-to-severe reactions, the infusion may be increased at 15-minute intervals, as tolerated, to completion (first to 20 mL/hour, then 40 mL/hour, then 100 mL/hour, and finally 125 mL/hour to completion). A maximum rate of 100 mL/hour is recommended in patients who experienced prior severe reactions. In patients with cutaneous flushing, aspirin may be considered (Becker, 2004).

Monitoring Parameters During infusion, if reaction is noted, monitor vital signs every 10 minutes until normal. Follow-up monitoring includes monitoring for improvement of symptoms; signs of infection; LFTs (discontinue if >5 times ULN); place and read PPD before initiation. Psoriasis patients with history of phototherapy should be monitored for nonmelanoma skin cancer.

Dosage Forms Excipient information presented when available (limited, particularly for generics); consult specific product labeling.

Injection, powder for reconstitution [preservative free]:

Remicade®: 100 mg [contains sucrose 500 mg and polysorbate 80]

◆ **Infliximab, Recombinant** *see* InFLIXimab *on page 786*

Influenza Virus Vaccine

(in floo EN za VYE rus vak SEEN)

U.S. Brand Names Afluria®; Fluarix®; FluLaval™; FluMist®; Fluvirin®; Fluzone®

Canadian Brand Names Fluviral S/F®; Vaxigrip®

Index Terms Influenza Virus Vaccine (Purified Surface Antigen); Influenza Virus Vaccine (Split-Virus); Influenza Virus Vaccine (Trivalent, Live); Live Attenuated Influenza Vaccine (LAIV); Trivalent Inactivated Influenza Vaccine (TIV)

Pharmacologic Category Vaccine, Inactivated (Viral); Vaccine, Live (Viral)

Additional Appendix Information

Guidelines for the Prevention of Opportunistic Infections in HIV Infected Persons *on page 1740*

Immunization Recommendations *on page 1708*

Use Provide active immunity to influenza virus strains contained in the vaccine

Advisory Committee on Immunization Practices (ACIP) recommends annual vaccination for all children (6 months to 18 years) and adults. Target groups for vaccination (those at higher risk of complications from influenza infection and their close contacts) include the following:

- Persons ≥50 years of age
- Residents of nursing homes and other chronic-care facilities that house persons of any age with chronic medical conditions

- Adults and children with chronic disorders of the pulmonary or cardiovascular systems (except hypertension), including asthma
- Adults and children who have chronic metabolic diseases (including diabetes mellitus), hepatic disease, renal dysfunction, hematologic disorders, hemoglobinopathies, or immunosuppression (including immunosuppression caused by medications or HIV)
- Adults and children with conditions which may compromise respiratory function, the handling of respiratory secretions, or that can increase the risk of aspiration (eg, cognitive dysfunction, spinal; cord injuries, seizure disorders, other neuromuscular disorders)
- Children and adolescents (6 months to 18 years of age) who are receiving long-term aspirin therapy and therefore, may be at risk for developing Reye's syndrome after influenza
- Women who will be pregnant during the influenza season
- Children 6-59 months of age
- Healthcare personnel
- Household contacts and caregivers of children <5 years (particularly children <6 months) and adults ≥50 years
- Household contacts and caregivers of persons with medical conditions which put them at high risk of complications from influenza infection

Pregnancy Risk Factor C

Pregnancy Considerations Reproduction studies have not been conducted. Case reports and limited studies suggest pregnancy may increase the risk of serious medical complications from influenza infection. Vaccination is recommended regardless of stage of pregnancy. Vaccination with the injection during the third trimester of pregnancy has been shown to decrease the incidence of laboratory confirmed influenza and respiratory illness with fever in infants ≤6 months. The safety and efficacy of the nasal spray have not been studied in pregnant pregnant women; however, pregnant women do not need to avoid contact with persons recently vaccinated with LAIV.

Medication Safety Issues

Sound-alike/look-alike issues:

Fluarix® may be confused with Flarex®

Influenza virus vaccine may be confused with tetanus toxoid and tuberculin products. Medication errors have occurred when tuberculin skin tests (PPD) have been inadvertently administered instead of tetanus toxoid products and influenza virus vaccine. These products are refrigerated and often stored in close proximity to each other.

Influenza virus vaccine (human strain) may be confused with the avian strain (H5N1) of influenza virus vaccine

International issues:

Hiberix is also a brand name for *Haemophilus* b conjugate vaccine in Slovenia

Contraindications Hypersensitivity to influenza virus vaccine, or any component of the formulation; presence of acute respiratory disease or other active infections or febrile illnesses; active neurological disorder (immunization should be delayed)

In addition, for nasal spray: Children 2-17 years of age receiving aspirin therapy

Warnings/Precautions Antigenic response may not be as great as expected in patients requiring immunosuppressive drug therapy or HIV-infected persons with CD4 cells <100/mm^3 and with viral copies of HIV type 1 >30,000/mL. Some products contain thimerosal, neomycin, polymyxin, latex, or are manufactured with arginine, chicken egg protein, gelatin, and/or gentamicin; hypersensitivity reactions may occur. Influenza vaccines from previous seasons must not be used. Inactivated vaccine is preferred over live virus vaccine for household members, healthcare workers and others coming in close contact with severely-immunosuppressed persons requiring care in a protected environment. Use with caution in patients with history of Guillain-Barré (GBS); patients with history of GBS have a greater likelihood of developing GBS than those without. May consider avoiding vaccination in patients with a history of GBS and who are at low risk for severe influenza complications, and in patients known to have experienced GBS within 6 weeks following previous vaccination (consider influenza antiviral chemoprophylaxis in these patients). Immunization should be delayed during moderate-to-severe febrile illness; minor illnesses with or without fever generally do not preclude use of vaccine. Treatment for anaphylactic reactions (including epinephrine) should be readily available.

Injection (inactivated, split virus, TIV): For I.M. use only; use caution with thrombocytopenia or any coagulation disorder. Safety and efficacy for use in children <6 months of age have not been established. Immunization should be delayed during moderate-to-severe febrile illness; minor illnesses with or without fever generally do not preclude use of vaccine.

Nasal spray (live, attenuated virus; LAIV): For intranasal use only. **Avoid contact with severely immunocompromised individuals for at least 7 days following vaccination.** Use the nasal spray with caution in patients with asthma or children <5 years of age with recurrent wheezing; risk of wheezing following vaccination is increased. Patients with severe asthma or active wheezing were not included in clinical trials and use in these patients is not recommended. Children <24 months of age had increased wheezing and hospitalizations following administration in clinical trials; use of the nasal spray is not approved in this age group. Defer immunization if nasal congestion is present which may impede delivery of vaccine. Because safety and efficacy information is limited, the ACIP does not recommend the use of LAIV in patients with the following conditions: chronic metabolic diseases (including diabetes mellitus), hepatic disease, renal dysfunction, hematologic disorders, hemoglobinopathies, history of GBS, immunosuppression, chronic disorders of the pulmonary or cardiovascular systems (including asthma), pregnant women, or children and adolescents receiving long-term aspirin therapy. For use in healthy children and adults 2-49 years of age only; safety and efficacy for use in children <2 years or adults ≥50 years of age have not been established.

Adverse Reactions All serious adverse reactions must be reported to the U.S. Department of Health and Human Services (DHHS) Vaccine Adverse Event Reporting System (VAERS) 1-800-822-7967.

Injection:

Frequency not defined.

Cardiovascular: Chest tightness, facial edema

Central nervous system: Chills, fatigue, fever, headache, irritability, insomnia, and malaise (may start within 6-12 hours and last 1-2 days; incidence equal to placebo in adults; occurs more frequently than placebo in children); Guillain-Barré syndrome (GBS)

Dermatologic: Angioedema, bruising, rash, urticaria

Gastrointestinal: Sore throat

Local: Tenderness, redness, swelling, or induration at the site of injection (10% to 64%; may last up to 2 days); injection site pain

Neuromuscular & skeletal: Arthralgia, myalgia (may start within 6-12 hours and last 1-2 days; incidence equal to placebo in adults; occurs more frequently than placebo in children)

Ocular: Red eyes

Respiratory: Cough, nasopharyngitis

Miscellaneous: Allergic or anaphylactoid reactions (most likely to residual egg protein; includes allergic asthma, angioedema, hives, systemic anaphylaxis)

Postmarketing and/or case reports: Angioneurotic edema, arthritis, brachial neuritis, bronchospasm, cellulites, conjunctivitis, diaphoresis, dizziness, dysphagia, dysphonia, dyspnea, encephalopathy, eye pain, facial palsy (Bell's palsy), flushing, Henoch-Schönlein purpura, hypoesthesia, hypokinesia, limb paralysis, microscopic polyangiitis (vasculitis), paresthesia, laryngitis, lymphadenopathy, neuralgia, neuropathy, optic neuritis, pallor, pharyngitis, photophobia, periorbital edema, pruritus, rhinitis, seizure (rare; majority associated with fever), serum sickness, somnolence, Stevens-Johnson syndrome, syncope, tachycardia, throat tightness, transient thrombocytopenia, transverse myelitis, tremor, vasodilation, vasculitis (with transient renal involvement), vertigo, vomiting, weakness

Nasal spray: Frequency of events reported within 10 days

>10%:

Central nervous system: Headache (children 3% to 9%; adults 40%), irritability (children 12% to 21%), lethargy (children 6% to 14%)

Gastrointestinal: Appetite decreased (children 13% to 21%)

Neuromuscular & skeletal: Tiredness/weakness (adults 26%), muscle aches (children 2% to 6%; adults 17%)

Respiratory: Cough (adults 14%), nasal congestion/runny nose (children 51% to 58%; adults 9% to 44%), sore throat (children 5% to 11%; adults 28%)

1% to 10%:

Central nervous system: Chills (children 2% to 4%, adults 9%), fever (100°F to 101°F: children 6% to 9%; >101°F: children 1% to 4%)

Gastrointestinal: Abdominal pain (children 2%)

Otic: Otitis media (children 3%)

Respiratory: Sinusitis (adults 4%), sneezing (children 2%), wheezing (children 6-23 months 6%; children 24-59 months 2%)

Postmarketing and/or case reports: Anaphylactic reactions, asthma exacerbations, Bell's palsy, diarrhea, epistaxis, facial edema, Guillain-Barré syndrome, hypersensitivity reaction, mitochondrial encephalomyopathy (Leigh syndrome) exacerbation, nausea, rash, urticaria, vomiting

Drug Interactions

Avoid Concomitant Use

Avoid concomitant use of Influenza Virus Vaccine with any of the following: Immunosuppressants

Increased Effect/Toxicity

The levels/effects of Influenza Virus Vaccine may be increased by: Immunosuppressants

Decreased Effect

Influenza Virus Vaccine may decrease the levels/effects of: Tuberculin Tests

The levels/effects of Influenza Virus Vaccine may be decreased by: Antiviral Agents (Influenza A and B)

Stability

Injection: Store between 2°C to 8°C (36°F to 46°F). Potency is destroyed by freezing; do not use if product has been frozen.

Afluria®, FluLaval™: Discard 28 days after initial entry. Protect from light.

Fluarix®: Protect from light.

Fluzone®: Between uses, the multiple dose vial should be stored at 2°C to 8°C (36°F to 46°F).

Nasal spray: Store in refrigerator at 2°C to 8°C (36°F to 46°F). **Do not freeze.**

Mechanism of Action Promotes immunity to influenza virus by inducing specific antibody production. Each year the formulation is standardized according to the U.S. Public Health Service. Preparations from previous seasons must not be used.

Pharmacodynamics/Kinetics

Onset of action: Protective antibody titers achieved ~2 weeks after vaccination

Duration: Protective antibody titers persist approximately ≥6 months. Elderly: Protective antibody titers may fall ≤4 months after vaccination.

Dosage It is important to note that influenza seasons vary in their timing and duration from year to year. In general, the optimal time to receive vaccine is October-November, prior to exposure to influenza; however, vaccination should continue into December and throughout the influenza season as long as vaccine is available.

Note: Children <9 years who are not previously vaccinated or who received only 1 dose of vaccine during the previous season (if it was their first year of vaccination) should receive 2 doses, in order to achieve satisfactory antibody response per ACIP recommendations. Although products are licensed for use in specific ages, if a particular vaccine is inadvertently administered to a child in a nonapproved age group, it does not need to be repeated.

I.M.:

Fluzone®:

Children 6-35 months: 0.25 mL/dose (1 or 2 doses per season; see **Note**)

Children 3-8 years: 0.5 mL/dose (1 or 2 doses per season; see **Note**)

Children ≥9 years and Adults: 0.5 mL/dose (1 dose per season)

Fluvirin®:

Children 4-8 years: 0.5 mL/dose (1 or 2 doses per season; see **Note**)

Children ≥9 years and Adults: 0.5 mL/dose (1 dose per season)

Afluria®, Fluarix®, FluLaval™: Adults: 0.5 mL/dose (1 dose per season)

Intranasal (FluMist®):

Children 2-8 years, previously **not vaccinated** with influenza vaccine: Initial season: Two 0.2 mL doses separated by at least 4 weeks

Children 2-8 years, previously **vaccinated** with influenza vaccine: 0.2 mL/dose (1 or 2 doses separated by at least 4 weeks; see **Note**)

Children ≥9 years and Adults ≤49 years: 0.2 mL/dose (1 dose per season)

Administration

TIV: For I.M. administration only. Inspect for particulate matter and discoloration prior to administration. Adults and older children should be vaccinated in the deltoid muscle using a ≥1 inch needle length. Infants and young children <12 months of age should be vaccinated in the anterolateral aspect of the thigh using a 7/8 inch to 1 inch needle length. Young children with adequate deltoid muscle mass should be vaccinated using a 7/8 inch to 1.25 inch needle. Suspensions should be shaken well prior to use.

Note: For patients at risk of hemorrhage following intramuscular injection, the ACIP recommends "it should be administered intramuscularly if, in the opinion of the physician familiar with the patients bleeding risk, the vaccine can be administered with reasonable safety by this route. If the patient receives antihemophilia or other similar therapy, intramuscular vaccination can be scheduled shortly after such therapy is administered. A fine needle (23 gauge or smaller) can be used for the vaccination and firm pressure applied to the site (without rubbing) for at least 2 minutes. The patient should be instructed concerning the risk of hematoma from the injection."

LAIV: Intranasal: Half the dose (0.1 mL) is administered to each nostril; patient should be in upright position. A dose divider clip is provided. Severely-immunocompromised persons should not administer the live vaccine. If recipient sneezes following administration, the dose should not be repeated.

Administration with other vaccines:

Influenza virus vaccine (inactivated; TIV) with other inactivated vaccines: May be given simultaneously or at any interval between doses.

Influenza virus vaccine (inactivated; TIV) with live vaccines: May be given simultaneously or at any interval between doses

Influenza virus vaccine (live; LAIV) with other live vaccines:

Intranasal or injectable: If not given simultaneously, wait at least 4 weeks between administration

Oral: May be given simultaneously or at any interval between doses of live or inactivated injectable vaccines

Vaccine administration with antibody-containing products*:

Antibody-containing products and influenza virus vaccine (inactivated; TIV): May be given simultaneously at different sites or at any interval between doses

Antibody-containing products and influenza virus vaccine (live; LAIV): Influenza virus vaccine (live; LAIV) may be given at any time before, after or simultaneously with an antibody-containing product.

*Examples of antibody containing products include I.M. and I.V. immune globulin, hepatitis B immune globulin, tetanus immune globulin, varicella zoster immune globulin, rabies immune globulin, whole blood, packed red cells, plasma, and platelet products

Additional Information Pharmacies will stock the formulations(s) standardized according to the USPHS requirements for the season. Influenza vaccines from previous seasons must not be used. Federal law requires that the date of administration, the vaccine manufacturer, lot number of vaccine, and the administering person's name, title, and address be entered into the patient's permanent medical record.

The optimal time to receive vaccine is October-November, prior to exposure to influenza; however, vaccination should continue into December and later as long as vaccine is available. To avoid missed opportunities for vaccination, patients at risk for complications can be offered the vaccine during routine healthcare visits as early as September if vaccine is available. Avoid vaccination before October in older persons in nursing homes or similar housing facilities because antibody levels can decline more rapidly following vaccination. When vaccine is available, children aged 6 months to <9 years of age who have not been previously vaccinated, should receive their first dose in September so that both doses can be administered prior to the onset of influenza activity.

When vaccine supply is not limited, either TIV or LAIV can be used in healthy, nonpregnant persons aged 2-49 years of age.

When vaccine supply is limited, administration should focus on the ACIP target groups. When TIV vaccine is in short supply, administering LAIV to eligible persons is encouraged to increase available TIV to those patients in whom LAIV cannot be used. During periods of inactivated influenza vaccine (TIV) shortage, the CDC and ACIP have recommended vaccination be prioritized based on the following three tiers. The grouping is based on influenza associated mortality and hospitalization rates. Those listed in group 1 should be vaccinated first, followed by persons in group 2, and then group 3. If the vaccine supply is extremely limited, group 1 has also been subdivided in three tiers, where those in group 1A should be vaccinated first, followed by 1B, then 1C.

Priority groups for vaccination with inactivated influenza vaccine during periods of vaccine shortage:

Tier 1A:

- Persons ≥65 years with comorbid conditions
- Residents of long-term-care facilities

Tier 1B:

- Persons 2-64 years with comorbid conditions
- Persons ≥65 years without comorbid conditions
- Children 6-23 months
- Pregnant women

Tier 1C:

- Healthcare personnel
- Household contacts and out-of-home caregivers of children <6 months

Tier 2:

- Household contacts of children and adults at increased risk of influenza associated complications
- Healthy persons 50-64 years

Tier 3:

- Persons 2-49 years without high-risk conditions

Further information available at http://www.cdc.gov/mmwr/preview/mmwrhtml/mm5430a4.htm

Dosage Forms Excipient information presented when available (limited, particularly for generics); consult specific product labeling.

Injection, suspension [purified split-virus]:

Afluria®: 5 mL [TIV; contains chicken egg protein, thimerosal, neomycin (trace amounts), and polymyxin (trace amounts)]

FluLaval™: 5 mL [TIV; contains chicken egg protein and thimerosal]

Fluvirin®: 5 mL [TIV; contains chicken egg protein, thimerosal, neomycin (trace amounts), and polymyxin (trace amounts)]

Fluzone®: 5 mL [TIV; contains chicken egg protein and thimerosal]

Injection, suspension [purified split-virus; preservative free]:

Afluria®: 0.5 mL [TIV; contains chicken egg protein, neomycin (trace amounts), and polymyxin (trace amounts)]

Fluarix®: 0.5 mL [TIV; contains chicken egg protein, gentamicin (trace amounts), natural rubber/natural latex in packaging, polysorbate 80, and thimerosal (trace amounts)]

Fluvirin®: 0.5 mL [TIV; contains chicken egg protein, thimerosal (trace amounts), neomycin (trace amounts), and polymyxin (trace amounts)]

Fluzone®: 0.25 mL, 0.5 mL [TIV; contains chicken egg protein]

Solution, intranasal [preservative free; spray]:

FluMist®: 0.2 mL [trivalent, LAIV; contains arginine, chicken egg protein, gelatin, and gentamicin]

Influenza Virus Vaccine (H5N1)

(in floo EN za VYE rus vak SEEN H5N1)

Index Terms Avian Influenza Virus Vaccine; Bird Flu Vaccine; H5N1 Influenza Vaccine; Influenza Virus Vaccine (Monovalent)

Pharmacologic Category Vaccine

Additional Appendix Information

Guidelines for the Prevention of Opportunistic Infections in HIV Infected Persons *on page 1740*

Immunization Recommendations *on page 1708*

Use Active immunization of adults at increased risk of exposure to the H5N1 viral subtype of influenza

Restrictions Commercial distribution is not planned. The vaccine will be included as part of the U.S. Strategic National Stockpile. It will be distributed by public health officials if needed.

Pregnancy Risk Factor C

Pregnancy Considerations Reproduction studies have not been conducted. Vaccine should be given only if clearly needed.

Lactation Excretion in breast milk unknown/use caution

Medication Safety Issues

Sound-alike/look-alike issues:

Influenza virus vaccine (H5N1) may be confused with the nonavian strain of influenza virus vaccine

Contraindications Manufacturer states no contraindications

Warnings/Precautions Immediate treatment (including epinephrine 1:1000) for anaphylactoid and/or hypersensitivity reactions should be available during vaccine use. Use with caution in patients with a history of Guillain-Barré syndrome (GBS); these patients may have a greater likelihood of developing GBS. If recent occurrence of GBS (≤6 weeks), decision to administer vaccine should entail careful consideration of risk:benefit. Use with caution in severely immunocompromised patients (eg, patients receiving chemo/radiation therapy or other immunosuppressive therapy [including high-dose corticosteroids]); may have a reduced response to vaccination. Safety and efficacy in children and patients >64 years of age have not been established.

Adverse Reactions All serious adverse reactions must be reported to the U.S. Department of Health and Human Services (DHHS) Vaccine Adverse Event Reporting System (VAERS) 1-800-822-7967.

>10%:

Central nervous system: Headache (3% to 36%), malaise (22%)

Local: Pain (74%), tenderness (70%), erythema/redness (20%), induration/swelling (15%)

Neuromuscular & skeletal: Myalgia (16%)

1% to 10%:

Central nervous system: Fever (up to 7%)

Gastrointestinal: Nausea (10%), diarrhea (6%)

Respiratory: Nasopharyngitis (2%), upper respiratory infection (2%), nasal congestion (1%)

Additional reactions observed with other influenza vaccine formulations: Allergic reaction, anaphylaxis, angioedema, asthma, encephalopathy, facial paralysis, hives, GBS, neuropathy, optic neuritis, vasculitis

Drug Interactions

Avoid Concomitant Use There are no known interactions where it is recommended to avoid concomitant use.

Increased Effect/Toxicity There are no known significant interactions involving an increase in effect.

Decreased Effect

The levels/effects of Influenza Virus Vaccine (H5N1) may be decreased by: Immunosuppressants

Stability Store between 2°C to 8°C (36°F to 46°F). Potency is destroyed by freezing; do not use if product has been frozen. Protect from light.

Mechanism of Action A monovalent, split virus (inactivated) preparation of the H5N1 avian strain of influenza virus (A/Vietnam/1203/2004) which promotes active immunity to avian influenza.

Pharmacodynamics/Kinetics Onset of action: Four-fold increase in antibody titers occurred in up to 58% of patients 28 days after second dose.

Dosage I.M.: Adults 18-64 years: 1 mL, followed by second 1 mL dose given 28 days later (acceptable range: 21-35 days)

Administration For I.M. administration only. Inspect for particulate matter and discoloration prior to administration. Vaccinate in the deltoid muscle using a ≥1 inch needle length. Suspension should be shaken well prior to use. **Note:** For patients at risk of hemorrhage following intramuscular injection, the ACIP recommends "it should be administered intramuscularly if, in the opinion of the physician familiar with the patients bleeding risk, the vaccine can be administered with reasonable safety by this route. If the patient receives antihemophilia or other similar therapy, intramuscular vaccination can be scheduled shortly after such therapy is administered. A fine needle (23 gauge or smaller) can be used for the vaccination and firm pressure applied to the site (without rubbing) for at least 2 minutes. The patient should be instructed concerning the risk of hematoma from the injection."

Additional Information Federal law requires that the date of administration, the vaccine manufacturer, lot number of vaccine, and the administering person's name, title, and address be entered into the patient's permanent medical record.

The 2-dose regimen prompted antibody response consistent with a protective titer in up to 58% of patients. However, there are no clinical data evaluating whether vaccination protects patients against development of infection. Therefore, protection against a pandemic avian flu strain cannot be assured.

Healthcare workers involved in the care of patients with known or suspected H5N1 viral subtype influenza infection should be vaccinated with the most recent seasonal human influenza vaccine in order to reduce the risk of co-infection of human influenza A viruses.

Dosage Forms Injection, suspension [monovalent]: Hemagglutinin (H5N1 strain) 90 mcg/1 mL (5 mL) [contains thimerosal, and chicken, porcine, and egg proteins]

◆ **Influenza Virus Vaccine (Monovalent)** *see* Influenza Virus Vaccine (H5N1) *on page 791*

◆ **Influenza Virus Vaccine (Purified Surface Antigen)** *see* Influenza Virus Vaccine *on page 788*

◆ **Influenza Virus Vaccine (Split-Virus)** *see* Influenza Virus Vaccine *on page 788*

◆ **Influenza Virus Vaccine (Trivalent, Live)** *see* Influenza Virus Vaccine *on page 788*

◆ **Infufer® (Can)** *see* Iron Dextran Complex *on page 817*

◆ **Infumorph®** *see* Morphine Sulfate *on page 1016*

◆ **INH** *see* Isoniazid *on page 820*

◆ **Inhibace® Plus (Can)** *see* Cilazapril and Hydrochlorothiazide *on page 325*

◆ **Innohep®** *see* Tinzaparin *on page 1473*

◆ **InnoPran XL™** *see* Propranolol *on page 1259*

◆ **Insoluble Prussian Blue** *see* Ferric Hexacyanoferrate *on page 615*

◆ **Inspra™** *see* Eplerenone *on page 530*

◆ **Instat™** *see* Collagen Hemostat *on page 367*

◆ **Instat™ MCH** *see* Collagen Hemostat *on page 367*

Insulin Aspart (IN soo lin AS part)

U.S. Brand Names NovoLog®

Canadian Brand Names NovoRapid®

Index Terms Aspart Insulin

Pharmacologic Category Antidiabetic Agent, Insulin

Additional Appendix Information

Diabetes Mellitus Management, Adults *on page 1801*

Use Treatment of type 1 diabetes mellitus (insulin dependent, IDDM) and type 2 diabetes mellitus (noninsulin dependent, NIDDM) to improve glycemic control

Pregnancy Risk Factor B

Medication Safety Issues

Sound-alike/look-alike issues:

NovoLog® may be confused with Novolin®

NovoLog® Mix 70/30 may be confused with NovoLog®

High alert medication: The Institute for Safe Medication Practices (ISMP) includes this medication among its list

of drugs which have a heightened risk of causing significant patient harm when used in error. ***Due to the number of insulin preparations, it is essential to identify/clarify the type of insulin to be used.***

Cross-contamination may occur if insulin pens are shared among multiple patients. Steps should be taken to prohibit sharing of insulin pens.

Dosage Refer to Insulin Regular on page 796. Insulin aspart is a rapid-acting insulin analog which is normally administered as a premeal component of the insulin regimen. It is normally used along with a long-acting (basal) form of insulin or continuous basal administration of insulin via a SubQ infusion pump.

I.V.: Insulin aspart may be administered I.V. in selected clinical situations to control hyperglycemia. Appropriate medical supervision is required.

SubQ: When used in a meal-related treatment regimen, 50% to 70% of total daily insulin requirement may be provided by insulin aspart as divided premeal boluses and the remainder provided by an intermediate or long-acting insulin or continuous basal administration of insulin via a SubQ infusion pump. Due to rapid onset and short duration, some patients may require more basal insulin to prevent premeal hyperglycemia when using insulin aspart as opposed to regular insulin.

SubQ infusion pump: Initial programming of the pump may be based upon the total daily dose of insulin (TDD) given in the previous regimen with ~50% of the TDD given as divided premeal boluses and ~50% of TDD given as a basal infusion; adjust dose as necessary.

Dosing adjustment in renal impairment: Insulin requirements are reduced due to changes in insulin clearance or metabolism. Close monitoring of blood glucose and adjustment of therapy is required in renal impairment.

Dosing adjustment in hepatic impairment: Insulin requirements may be reduced. Close monitoring of blood glucose and adjustment of therapy is required in hepatic impairment.

Additional Information Complete prescribing information for this medication should be consulted for additional detail.

Dosage Forms Excipient information presented when available (limited, particularly for generics); consult specific product labeling.

Injection, solution:

NovoLog®: 100 units/mL (3 mL) [FlexPen® prefilled syringe or PenFill® prefilled cartridge]; (10 mL) [vial]

◆ **Insulin Aspart and Insulin Aspart Protamine** *see* Insulin Aspart Protamine and Insulin Aspart *on page 793*

Insulin Aspart Protamine and Insulin Aspart (IN soo lin AS part PROE ta meen & IN soo lin AS part)

U.S. Brand Names NovoLog® Mix 70/30

Canadian Brand Names NovoMix® 30

Index Terms Insulin Aspart and Insulin Aspart Protamine

Pharmacologic Category Antidiabetic Agent, Insulin

Use Treatment of type 1 diabetes mellitus (insulin dependent, IDDM) and type 2 diabetes mellitus (noninsulin dependent, NIDDM) to improve glycemic control

Pregnancy Risk Factor C

Medication Safety Issues

Sound-alike/look-alike issues:

NovoLog® Mix 70/30 may be confused with Novolin® 70/30

High alert medication: The Institute for Safe Medication Practices (ISMP) includes this medication among its list of drugs which have a heightened risk of causing significant patient harm when used in error. ***Due to the number of insulin preparations, it is essential to identify/clarify the type of insulin to be used.***

Cross-contamination may occur if insulin pens are shared among multiple patients. Steps should be taken to prohibit sharing of insulin pens.

Dosage Refer to Insulin Regular on page 796. Fixed ratio insulins (such as insulin aspart protamine and insulin aspart combination) are normally administered in 2 daily doses.

Dosing adjustment in renal impairment: Insulin requirements are reduced due to changes in insulin clearance or metabolism.

Additional Information Complete prescribing information for this medication should be consulted for additional detail.

Dosage Forms Excipient information presented when available (limited, particularly for generics); consult specific product labeling.

Injection, suspension:

NovoLog® Mix 70/30: Insulin aspart protamine suspension 70% [intermediate acting] and insulin aspart solution 30% [rapid acting]: 100 units/mL (3 mL) [FlexPen® prefilled syringe]; (10 mL) [vial]

Insulin Detemir (IN soo lin DE te mir)

U.S. Brand Names Levemir®

Canadian Brand Names Levemir®

Index Terms Detemir Insulin

Pharmacologic Category Antidiabetic Agent, Insulin

Additional Appendix Information

Diabetes Mellitus Management, Adults *on page 1801*

Use Treatment of type 1 diabetes mellitus (insulin dependent, IDDM) and type 2 diabetes mellitus (noninsulin dependent, NIDDM) to improve glycemic control

Pregnancy Risk Factor C

Medication Safety Issues

High alert medication: The Institute for Safe Medication Practices (ISMP) includes this medication among its list of drugs which have a heightened risk of causing significant patient harm when used in error. ***Due to the number of insulin preparations, it is essential to identify/clarify the type of insulin to be used.***

Note: Insulin detemir is a clear solution, but it is NOT intended for I.V. or I.M. administration.

Cross-contamination may occur if insulin pens are shared among multiple patients. Steps should be taken to prohibit sharing of insulin pens.

Dosage Also refer to Insulin Regular on page 796.

Notes: Duration is dose-dependent. Dosage must be carefully titrated (adjustment of dose and timing. Adjustment of concomitant antidiabetic treatment (short-acting insulins or oral antidiabetic agents) may be required. In Canada, insulin detemir is not approved for use in children.

SubQ: Children ≥6 years and Adults:

Basal insulin or basal-bolus (Type 1 or type 2 diabetes): May be substituted on a unit-per-unit basis. Adjust dose to achieve glycemic targets.

Insulin-naive patients (type 2 diabetes only): 0.1-0.2 units/kg once daily in the evening or 10 units once or twice daily. Adjust dose to achieve glycemic targets. **Note:**Canadian labeling recommends 10 units once daily (twice daily dosing is not included).

Dosage adjustment in renal impairment: Insulin requirements are reduced due to changes in insulin clearance or metabolism.

Additional Information Complete prescribing information for this medication should be consulted for additional detail.

Dosage Forms Excipient information presented when available (limited, particularly for generics); consult specific product labeling.

Injection, solution:

Levemir®: 100 units/mL (3 mL) [FlexPen® prefilled syringe]; (10 mL) [vial]

Insulin Glargine (IN soo lin GLAR jeen)

U.S. Brand Names Lantus®

Canadian Brand Names Lantus®; Lantus® OptiSet®

Index Terms Glargine Insulin

Pharmacologic Category Antidiabetic Agent, Insulin

Additional Appendix Information

Diabetes Mellitus Management, Adults *on page 1801*

Use Treatment of type 1 diabetes mellitus (insulin dependent, IDDM) and type 2 diabetes mellitus (noninsulin dependent, NIDDM) requiring basal (long-acting) insulin to improve glycemic control

Pregnancy Risk Factor C

Medication Safety Issues

Sound-alike/look-alike issues:

Insulin glargine may be confused with insulin glulisine
Lantus® may be confused with Lente®
Lente® may be confused with Lantus®

High alert medication: The Institute for Safe Medication Practices (ISMP) includes this medication among its list of drugs which have a heightened risk of causing significant patient harm when used in error. ***Due to the number of insulin preparations, it is essential to identify/clarify the type of insulin to be used.***

Dosage SubQ: Children ≥6 years and Adults:

Type 1 diabetes: As a basal component of combination insulin regimen, normally 50% to 75% of daily insulin requirement is administered as a long-acting form. More rapid acting forms are usually used in association with meals. Refer to Insulin Regular on page 796.

Type 2 diabetes:

Patient not already on insulin: 10 units once daily, adjusted according to patient response (range in clinical study: 2-100 units/day)

Patient already receiving insulin: In clinical studies, when changing to insulin glargine from once-daily NPH or Ultralente® insulin, the initial dose was not changed; when changing from twice-daily NPH to once-daily insulin glargine, the total daily dose was reduced by 20% and adjusted according to patient response

Dosage adjustment in renal impairment: Insulin requirements may be reduced due to changes in insulin clearance or metabolism.

Dosage adjustment in hepatic impairment: Insulin requirements may be reduced due to changes in glucose production and insulin metabolism.

Additional Information Complete prescribing information for this medication should be consulted for additional detail.

Dosage Forms Excipient information presented when available (limited, particularly for generics); consult specific product labeling.

Injection, solution:

Lantus®: 100 units/mL (3 mL) [OptiClik® prefilled cartridge or SoloStar® disposable insulin device]; (10 mL) [vial]

Insulin Glulisine (IN soo lin gloo LIS een)

U.S. Brand Names Apidra®

Canadian Brand Names Apidra®

Index Terms Glulisine Insulin

Pharmacologic Category Antidiabetic Agent, Insulin

Additional Appendix Information

Diabetes Mellitus Management, Adults *on page 1801*

Use Treatment of type 1 diabetes mellitus (insulin dependent, IDDM) and type 2 diabetes mellitus (noninsulin dependent, NIDDM) to improve glycemic control

Pregnancy Risk Factor C

Medication Safety Issues

Sound-alike/look-alike issues:

Insulin glulisine may be confused with insulin glargine

High alert medication: The Institute for Safe Medication Practices (ISMP) includes this medication among its list of drugs which have a heightened risk of causing significant patient harm when used in error. ***Due to the number of insulin preparations, it is essential to identify/clarify the type of insulin to be used.***

Dosage Refer to Insulin Regular on page 796. Insulin glulisine is equipotent to insulin regular, but has a more rapid onset. Insulin glulisine is normally administered as a premeal component of the insulin regimen. It is normally used along with a long-acting (basal) form of insulin or continuous basal administration of insulin via a SubQ infusion pump.

SubQ: When used in a meal-related treatment regimen, 50% to 70% of total daily insulin requirement may be provided by insulin glulisine (in divided doses) and the remainder provided by an intermediate- or long-acting insulin. Insulin glulisine may also be administered by external subcutaneous infusion pumps.

I.V.: Under close medical supervision, insulin glulisine may be administered by infusion.

Dosing adjustment in renal impairment: Insulin requirements are reduced due to changes in insulin clearance or metabolism. Close monitoring of blood glucose and adjustment of therapy is required in renal impairment.

Additional Information Complete prescribing information for this medication should be consulted for additional detail.

Dosage Forms Excipient information presented when available (limited, particularly for generics); consult specific product labeling.

Injection, solution:

Apidra®: 100 units/mL (3 mL [cartridge], 10 mL [vial])

Insulin Lispro (IN soo lin LYE sproe)

U.S. Brand Names Humalog®

Canadian Brand Names Humalog®

Index Terms Lispro Insulin

Pharmacologic Category Antidiabetic Agent, Insulin

Additional Appendix Information

Diabetes Mellitus Management, Adults *on page 1801*

Use Treatment of type 1 diabetes mellitus (insulin dependent, IDDM) and type 2 diabetes mellitus (noninsulin dependent, NIDDM) to improve glycemic control

Pregnancy Risk Factor B

Medication Safety Issues

Sound-alike/look-alike issues:

Humalog® may be confused with Humulin®, Humira®

High alert medication: The Institute for Safe Medication Practices (ISMP) includes this medication among its list of drugs which have a heightened risk of causing significant patient harm when used in error. ***Due to the number of insulin preparations, it is essential to identify/clarify the type of insulin to be used.***

Cross-contamination may occur if insulin pens are shared among multiple patients. Steps should be taken to prohibit sharing of insulin pens.

Dosage Refer to Insulin Regular on page 796. Insulin lispro is equipotent to insulin regular, but has a more rapid onset.

Dosing adjustment in renal impairment: Insulin requirements are reduced due to changes in insulin clearance or metabolism. Close monitoring of blood glucose and adjustment of therapy is required in renal impairment.

Additional Information Complete prescribing information for this medication should be consulted for additional detail.

Dosage Forms Excipient information presented when available (limited, particularly for generics); consult specific product labeling.

Injection, solution:

Humalog®: 100 units/mL (3 mL) [prefilled cartridge or prefilled disposable pen]; (10 mL) [vial]

◆ **Insulin Lispro and Insulin Lispro Protamine** *see* Insulin Lispro Protamine and Insulin Lispro *on page 795*

Insulin Lispro Protamine and Insulin Lispro

(IN soo lin LYE sproe PROE ta meen & IN soo lin LYE sproe)

U.S. Brand Names Humalog® Mix 50/50™; Humalog® Mix 75/25™

Canadian Brand Names Humalog® Mix 25

Index Terms Insulin Lispro and Insulin Lispro Protamine

Pharmacologic Category Antidiabetic Agent, Insulin

Additional Appendix Information

Diabetes Mellitus Management, Adults *on page 1801*

Use Treatment of type 1 diabetes mellitus (insulin dependent, IDDM) and type 2 diabetes mellitus (noninsulin dependent, NIDDM) to improve glycemic control

Pregnancy Risk Factor B

Medication Safety Issues

Sound-alike/look-alike issues:

Humalog® Mix 75/25™ may be confused with Humulin® 70/30.

High alert medication: The Institute for Safe Medication Practices (ISMP) includes this medication among its list of drugs which have a heightened risk of causing significant patient harm when used in error. ***Due to the number of insulin preparations, it is essential to identify/clarify the type of insulin to be used.***

Cross-contamination may occur if insulin pens are shared among multiple patients. Steps should be taken to prohibit sharing of insulin pens.

Dosage Refer to Insulin Regular on page 796. Fixed ratio insulins (such as insulin lispro protamine and insulin lispro) are normally administered in 2 daily doses.

Dosage adjustment in renal impairment: Insulin requirements are reduced due to changes in insulin clearance or metabolism.

Additional Information Complete prescribing information for this medication should be consulted for additional detail.

Dosage Forms Excipient information presented when available (limited, particularly for generics); consult specific product labeling.

Injection, suspension:

Humalog® Mix 50/50™: Insulin lispro protamine suspension 50% [intermediate acting] and insulin lispro solution 50% [rapid acting]: 100 units/mL (3 mL) [disposable pen]

Humalog® Mix 75/25™: Insulin lispro protamine suspension 75% [intermediate acting] and insulin lispro solution 25% [rapid acting]: 100 units/mL (3 mL) [disposable pen]; (10 mL) [vial]

Insulin NPH (IN soo lin N P H)

U.S. Brand Names Humulin® N; Novolin® N

Canadian Brand Names Humulin® N; Novolin® ge NPH

Index Terms Isophane Insulin; NPH Insulin

Pharmacologic Category Antidiabetic Agent, Insulin

Additional Appendix Information

Diabetes Mellitus Management, Adults *on page 1801*

Use Treatment of type 1 diabetes mellitus (insulin dependent, IDDM) and type 2 diabetes mellitus (noninsulin dependent, NIDDM) to improve glycemic control

Medication Safety Issues

Sound-alike/look-alike issues:

Humulin® may be confused with Humalog®, Humira®

Novolin® may be confused with NovoLog®

High alert medication: The Institute for Safe Medication Practices (ISMP) includes this medication among its list of drugs which have a heightened risk of causing significant patient harm when used in error. ***Due to the number of insulin preparations, it is essential to identify/clarify the type of insulin to be used.***

Cross-contamination may occur if insulin pens are shared among multiple patients. Steps should be taken to prohibit sharing of insulin pens.

Dosage Refer to Insulin Regular on page 796. Insulin NPH is usually administered 1-2 times daily.

Dosing adjustment in renal impairment: Insulin requirements are reduced due to changes in insulin clearance or metabolism.

Additional Information Complete prescribing information for this medication should be consulted for additional detail.

Dosage Forms Excipient information presented when available (limited, particularly for generics); consult specific product labeling. [CAN] = Canadian brand name

Injection, suspension:

Humulin® N: 100 units/mL (3 mL) [disposable pen]; (10 mL) [vial]

Novolin® ge NPH [CAN]: 100 units/mL (3 mL) [NovolinSet® prefilled syringe or PenFill® prefilled cartridge]; 10 mL [vial]

Novolin® N: 100 units/mL (3 mL) [InnoLet® prefilled syringe or PenFill® prefilled cartridge]; (10 mL) [vial]

Insulin NPH and Insulin Regular

(IN soo lin N P H & IN soo lin REG yoo ler)

U.S. Brand Names Humulin® 50/50; Humulin® 70/30; Novolin® 70/30

Canadian Brand Names Humulin® 20/80; Humulin® 70/30; Novolin® ge 30/70; Novolin® ge 40/60; Novolin® ge 50/50

Index Terms Insulin Regular and Insulin NPH; Isophane Insulin and Regular Insulin; NPH Insulin and Regular Insulin

Pharmacologic Category Antidiabetic Agent, Insulin

Use Treatment of type 1 diabetes mellitus (insulin dependent, IDDM) and type 2 diabetes mellitus (noninsulin dependent, NIDDM) to improve glycemic control

Medication Safety Issues

Sound-alike/look-alike issues:

Humulin® 70/30 may be confused with Humalog® Mix 75/25

Novolin® 70/30 may be confused with NovoLog® Mix 70/30

High alert medication: The Institute for Safe Medication Practices (ISMP) includes this medication among its list of drugs which have a heightened risk of causing significant patient harm when used in error. ***Due to the number of insulin preparations, it is essential to identify/clarify the type of insulin to be used.***

Cross-contamination may occur if insulin pens are shared among multiple patients. Steps should be taken to prohibit sharing of insulin pens.

Dosage Refer to Insulin Regular on page 796. Fixed ratio insulins are normally administered in 1-2 daily doses.

Additional Information Complete prescribing information for this medication should be consulted for additional detail.

Dosage Forms Excipient information presented when available (limited, particularly for generics); consult specific product labeling.

Injection, suspension:

Humulin® 50/50: Insulin NPH suspension 50% [intermediate acting] and insulin regular solution 50% [short acting]: 100 units/mL (10 mL) [vial]

Humulin® 70/30: Insulin NPH suspension 70% [intermediate acting] and insulin regular solution 30% [short acting]: 100 units/mL (3 mL) [disposable pen]; (10 mL) [vial]

Novolin® 70/30: Insulin NPH suspension 70% [intermediate acting] and insulin regular solution 30% [short acting]: 100 units/mL (3 mL) [InnoLet® prefilled syringe or PenFill® prefilled cartridge]; (10 mL) [vial]

Additional formulations available in Canada: Injection, suspension:

Humulin® 20/80: Insulin regular solution 20% [short acting] and insulin NPH suspension 80% [intermediate acting]: 100 units/mL (3 mL) [PenFill® prefilled cartridge]

Novolin® ge 30/70: Insulin regular solution 30% [short acting] and insulin NPH suspension 70% [intermediate acting]: 100 units/mL (3 mL) [prefilled syringe or PenFill® prefilled cartridge]; (10 mL) [vial]

Novolin® ge 40/60: Insulin regular solution 40% [short acting] and insulin NPH suspension 60% [intermediate acting]: 100 units/mL (3 mL) [PenFill® prefilled cartridge]

Novolin® ge 50/50: Insulin regular solution 50% [short acting] and insulin NPH suspension 50% [intermediate acting]: 100 units/mL (3 mL) [PenFill® prefilled cartridge]

Insulin Regular (IN soo lin REG yoo ler)

U.S. Brand Names Humulin® R; Humulin® R U-500; Novolin® R

Canadian Brand Names Humulin® R; Novolin® ge Toronto

Index Terms Regular Insulin

Pharmacologic Category Antidiabetic Agent, Insulin; Antidote

Additional Appendix Information

Desensitization Protocols *on page 1691*

Diabetes Mellitus Management, Adults *on page 1801*

Use Treatment of type 1 diabetes mellitus (insulin dependent, IDDM); type 2 diabetes mellitus (noninsulin dependent, NIDDM) unresponsive to treatment with diet and/or oral hypoglycemics, to improve glycemic control; adjunct to parenteral nutrition; diabetic ketoacidosis (DKA)

Unlabeled/Investigational Use Hyperkalemia (regular insulin only; use with glucose to shift potassium into cells to lower serum potassium levels)

Pregnancy Risk Factor B

Pregnancy Considerations Insulin has not been found to cross the placenta, but insulin bound to anti-insulin antibodies has been detected in cord blood. Maternal hyperglycemia can be associated with adverse effects in the fetus, including macrosomia, neonatal hyperglycemia, and hyperbilirubinemia; the risk of congenital malformations is increased when the Hb A_{1c} is above the normal range. Insulin requirements tend to fall during the first trimester of pregnancy and increase in the later trimesters, peaking at 28-32 weeks of gestation. Following delivery, insulin requirements decrease rapidly. Diabetes can be associated with adverse effects in the mother. Poorly-treated diabetes may cause end-organ damage that may in turn negatively affect obstetric outcomes. Physiologic glucose levels should be maintained prior to and during pregnancy to decrease the risk of adverse events in the fetus and the mother. Insulin is the drug of choice for the control of diabetes mellitus during pregnancy.

Lactation Excretion in breast milk unknown/compatible

Medication Safety Issues

Sound-alike/look-alike issues:

Humulin® may be confused with Humalog®, Humira®

Novolin® may be confused with NovoLog®

High alert medication: The Institute for Safe Medication Practices (ISMP) includes this medication among its list of drugs which have a heightened risk of causing significant patient harm when used in error. ***Due to the number of insulin preparations, it is essential to identify/clarify the type of insulin to be used.***

Concentrated solutions (eg, U-500) should not be available in patient care areas.

Cross-contamination may occur if insulin pens are shared among multiple patients. Steps should be taken to prohibit sharing of insulin pens.

Contraindications Hypersensitivity to any component of the formulation

Warnings/Precautions Hypoglycemia is the most common adverse effect of insulin. The timing of hypoglycemia differs among various insulin formulations. Hypoglycemia may result from increased work or exercise without eating; use of long-acting insulin preparations (insulin detemir, insulin glargine) may delay recovery from hypoglycemia. Profound and prolonged episodes of hypoglycemia may result in convulsions, unconsciousness, temporary or permanent brain damage or even death. Insulin requirements may be altered during illness, emotional disturbances or other stresses. Insulin may produce hypokalemia which, if left untreated, may result in respiratory paralysis, ventricular arrhythmia and even death. Use with caution in patients at risk for hypokalemia (eg, I.V. insulin use). Use with caution in renal or hepatic impairment.

Human insulin differs from animal-source insulin. Any change of insulin should be made cautiously; changing manufacturers, type, and/or method of manufacture may result in the need for a change of dosage.

Regular insulin is the only insulin to be used intravenously. Insulin aspart may also be administered I.V. in selected clinical situations to control hyperglycemia; close medical supervision is required.

The general objective of exogenous insulin therapy is to approximate the physiologic pattern of insulin secretion which is characterized by two distinct phases. Phase 1 insulin secretion suppresses hepatic glucose production and phase 2 insulin secretion occurs in response to carbohydrate ingestion; therefore, exogenous insulin therapy may consist of basal insulin (eg, intermediate- or long-acting insulin or continuous insulin infusion administered via an external SubQ insulin infusion pump) and/or preprandial insulin (eg, short- or rapid-acting insulin). Patients with type 1 diabetes do not produce endogenous insulin; therefore, these patients require both basal and preprandial insulin administration. Patients with type 2 diabetes retain some beta-cell function in the early stages of their disease; however, as the disease progresses, phase 1 insulin secretion may become completely impaired and phase 2 insulin secretion becomes delayed and/or inadequate in response to meals. Therefore, patients with type 2 diabetes may be treated with oral antidiabetic agents, basal insulin, and/or preprandial insulin depending on the stage of disease and current glycemic control. Since treatment regimens often consist of multiple agents, dosage adjustments must address the specific phase of insulin release that is primarily contributing to the patient's impaired glycemic control. Treatment and monitoring regimens must be individualized.

Adverse Reactions Frequency not defined.

Cardiovascular: Palpitation, pallor, tachycardia

Central nervous system: Fatigue, headache, hypothermia, loss of consciousness, mental confusion

Dermatologic: Urticaria, redness

Endocrine & metabolic: Hypoglycemia, hypokalemia

Gastrointestinal: Hunger, nausea, numbness of mouth, weight gain

Local: Atrophy or hypertrophy of SubQ fat tissue; edema, itching, pain or warmth at injection site; stinging

Neuromuscular & skeletal: Muscle weakness, paresthesia, tremor

Ocular: Transient presbyopia or blurred vision

Miscellaneous: Anaphylaxis, antibodies to insulin (no change in efficacy), diaphoresis, local allergy, systemic allergic symptoms

Drug Interactions

Metabolism/Transport Effects **Induces** CYP1A2 (weak)

Avoid Concomitant Use There are no known interactions where it is recommended to avoid concomitant use.

Increased Effect/Toxicity

Insulin Regular may increase the levels/effects of: Antidiabetic Agents (Thiazolidinedione); Quinolone Antibiotics

The levels/effects of Insulin Regular may be increased by: Beta-Blockers; Edetate CALCIUM Disodium; Edetate Disodium; Herbs (Hypoglycemic Properties); Pegvisomant

Decreased Effect

The levels/effects of Insulin Regular may be decreased by: Corticosteroids (Orally Inhaled); Corticosteroids (Systemic); Luteinizing Hormone-Releasing Hormone Analogs; Somatropin

Ethanol/Nutrition/Herb Interactions

Ethanol: Caution with ethanol (may increase hypoglycemia).

Food: Insulin shifts potassium from extracellular to intracellular space. Decreases potassium serum concentration.

Herb/Nutraceutical: Use caution with chromium, garlic, gymnema (may increase hypoglycemia).

Stability Insulin, regular (Humulin® R, Novolin® R): Store unopened containers in refrigerator at 2°C to 8°C (36°F to 46°F); do not freeze. Vial in use may be stored under refrigeration or at room temperature; store below 30°C (86°F) away from direct heat or light. Regular insulin should only be used if clear.

Note: Standard diluent for regular insulin: 100 units/100 mL NS; all bags should be prepared fresh; tubing should be flushed 30 minutes prior to administration to allow adsorption as time permits. Can be given as a more diluted solution (eg, 100 units/250 mL 0.45% NS).

Mechanism of Action Insulin acts via specific membrane-bound receptors on target tissues to regulate metabolism of carbohydrate, protein, and fats. Insulin facilitates entry of glucose into muscle, adipose, and other tissues via hexose transporters, including GLUT4. Insulin stimulates the cellular uptake of amino acids and increases cellular permeability to several ions, including potassium, magnesium, and phosphate. By activating sodium-potassium ATPases, insulin promotes the intracellular movement of potassium.

Target organs for insulin include the liver, skeletal muscle, and adipose tissue. Within the liver, insulin stimulates hepatic glycogen synthesis through the activation of the enzymes hexokinase, phosphofructokinase, and glycogen synthase as well as the inhibition of glucose-6 phosphatase. Insulin promotes hepatic synthesis of fatty acids, which are released into the circulation as lipoproteins. Skeletal muscle effects of insulin include increased protein synthesis and increased glycogen synthesis. Within adipose tissue, insulin stimulates the processing of circulating lipoproteins to provide free fatty acids, facilitating triglyceride synthesis and storage by adipocytes. Insulin also directly inhibits the hydrolysis of triglycerides.

Normally secreted by the pancreas, insulin products are manufactured for pharmacologic use through recombinant DNA technology using either *E. coli* or *Saccharomyces cerevisiae*. Insulins are categorized based on promptness and duration of effect, including rapid-, short-, intermediate-, and long-acting insulins.

Pharmacodynamics/Kinetics Note: Rate of absorption, onset, and duration of activity may be affected by site of injection, exercise, presence of lipodystrophy, local blood supply, and/or temperature.

Onset of action: 0.5 hours

Peak effect: 2.5-5 hours

Duration: 4-12 hours (may increase with dose)

Time to peak, plasma: 0.8-2 hours

Excretion: Urine

Dosage SubQ (regular insulin may also be administered I.V.): The number and size of daily doses, time of administration, and diet and exercise require continuous medical supervision. In addition, specific formulations may require distinct administration procedures.

Type 1 Diabetes Mellitus: Children and Adults: **Note:** Multiple daily doses guided by blood glucose monitoring are the standard of diabetes care. Combinations of insulin are commonly used.

Initial dose: 0.2-0.6 units/kg/day in divided doses. Conservative initial doses of 0.2-0.4 units/kg/day are often recommended to avoid the potential for hypoglycemia.

Division of daily insulin requirement: Generally, 50% to 75% of the daily insulin dose is given as an intermediate- or long-acting form of insulin (in 1-2 daily injections). The remaining portion of the 24-hour insulin requirement is divided and administered as a rapid-acting or short-acting form of insulin. These may be given with meals (before or at the time of meals depending on the form of insulin) or at the same time as injections of intermediate forms (some premixed combinations are intended for this purpose).

Adjustment of dose: Dosage must be titrated to achieve glucose control and avoid hypoglycemia. Adjust dose to maintain premeal and bedtime glucose of 80-140 mg/dL (children <5 years: 100-200 mg/dL). Since combinations of agents are frequently used, dosage adjustment must address the individual component of the insulin regimen which most directly influences the blood glucose value in question, based on the known onset and duration of the insulin component. Also see Additional Information.

Usual maintenance range: 0.5-1.2 units/kg/day in divided doses. An estimate of anticipated needs may be based on body weight and/or activity factors as follows:

Adolescents: May require ≤1.5 units/kg/day during growth spurts

Nonobese: 0.4-0.6 units/kg/day

Obese: 0.8-1.2 units/kg/day

Renal failure: Due to alterations in pharmacokinetics of insulin, may require <0.2 units/kg/day

Type 2 Diabetes Mellitus:

Augmentation therapy: Dosage must be carefully adjusted.

Insulins other than glargine: Initial dosage of 0.15-0.2 units/kg/day have been recommended

Insulin glargine: Initial dose: 10 units/day

Note: Administered when residual beta-cell function is present, as a supplemental agent when oral hypoglycemics have not achieved goal glucose control. Twice daily NPH, or an evening dose of NPH, lente, or glargine insulin may be added to oral therapy with metformin or a sulfonylurea. Augmentation to control postprandial glucose may be accomplished with regular, glulisine, aspart, or lispro insulin.

Monotherapy: Initial dose: Highly variable: See Augmentation therapy dosing.

Note: An empirically-defined scheme for dosage estimation based on fasting plasma glucose and degree of obesity has been published with recommended doses ranging from 6-77 units/day (Holman, 1995). In the setting of glucose toxicity (loss of beta-cell sensitivity to glucose concentrations), insulin therapy may be used for short-term management to restore sensitivity of beta-cells; in these cases, the dose may need to be rapidly reduced/withdrawn when sensitivity is re-established.

Diabetic ketoacidosis:

Children <20 years:

I.V.: Regular insulin infused at 0.1 units/kg/hour; continue until acidosis clears, then decrease to 0.05 units/kg/hour until SubQ replacement dosing can be initiated

SubQ, I.M.: If no I.V. infusion access, regular insulin 0.1 units/kg I.M. bolus followed by 0.1 units/kg/hour SubQ or I.M.; continue until acidosis clears, then decrease to 0.05 units/kg/hour until SubQ replacement dosing can be initiated

Adults:

I.V.: Regular insulin 0.15 units/kg initially followed by an infusion of 0.1 units/kg/hour

SubQ, I.M.: Regular insulin 0.4 units/kg given half as I.V. bolus and half as SubQ or I.M., followed by 0.1 units/kg/hour SubQ or I.M.

If serum glucose does not fall by 50-70 mg/dL in the first hour, double insulin dose hourly until glucose falls at an hourly rate of 50-70 mg/dL. Decrease dose to 0.05-0.1 units/kg/hour once serum glucose reaches 250 mg/dL.

Note: Newly-diagnosed patients with IDDM presenting in DKA and patients with blood sugars <800 mg/dL may be relatively "sensitive" to insulin and should receive loading and initial maintenance doses ~50% of those indicated.

Infusion should continue until reversal of acid-base derangement/ketonemia. Serum glucose is not a direct indicator of these abnormalities, and may decrease more rapidly than correction of the range of metabolic abnormalities.

Hyperkalemia (unlabeled use): Children and Adults: I.V.: Administer dextrose at 0.5-1 mL/kg and regular insulin 1 unit for every 4-5 g dextrose given

Dosing adjustment in renal impairment (regular): Insulin requirements are reduced due to changes in insulin clearance or metabolism. Close monitoring of blood glucose and adjustment of therapy is required in renal impairment.

Cl_{cr} 10-50 mL/minute: Administer at 75% of normal dose

Cl_{cr} <10 mL/minute: Administer at 25% to 50% of normal dose and monitor glucose closely

Hemodialysis: Because of a large molecular weight (6000 daltons), insulin is not significantly removed by either peritoneal or hemodialysis

Supplemental dose is not necessary

Peritoneal dialysis: Supplemental dose is not necessary

Continuous arteriovenous or venovenous hemofiltration effects: Supplemental dose is not necessary

Dietary Considerations Dietary modification based on ADA recommendations is a part of therapy.

Administration

SubQ administration: Cold injections should be avoided. SubQ administration is usually made into the thighs, arms, buttocks, or abdomen, with sites rotated. When mixing regular insulin with other preparations of insulin, regular insulin should be drawn into syringe first. Except for rapid-acting, short-acting, or insulin detemir or glargine, gently roll vial or pen in the palms of the hands to resuspend before using. When rapid-acting insulin is mixed with an intermediate- or long-acting insulin, it should be administered within 15 minutes before a meal.

Human regular insulin: Should be administered within 30-60 minutes before a meal; may be administered by SubQ, I.M., or I.V. routes.

I.V. administration (requires use of an infusion pump): May be administered I.V. with close monitoring of blood glucose and serum potassium.

I.V. infusions: To minimize adsorption problems to I.V. solution bag:

If new tubing is **not** needed: Wait a minimum of 30 minutes between the preparation of the solution and the initiation of the infusion.

If new tubing is needed: After receiving the insulin drip solution, the administration set should be attached to the I.V. container and the line should be flushed with the insulin solution. The nurse should wait 30 minutes, then flush the line again with the insulin solution prior to initiating the infusion.

If insulin is required prior to the availability of the insulin drip, regular insulin should be administered by I.V. push injection.

Because of adsorption, the actual amount of insulin being administered could be substantially less than the apparent amount. Therefore, adjustment of the insulin drip rate should be based on effect and not solely on the apparent insulin dose. Furthermore, the apparent dose should not be used as the basis for determining the subsequent insulin dose upon discontinuing the insulin drip. Dose requires continuous medical supervision.

Monitoring Parameters Urine sugar and acetone, serum glucose, electrolytes, Hb A_{1c}, lipid profile

DKA: Arterial blood gases, CBC with differential, urinalysis, serum glucose (baseline and every hour until reaches 250 mg/dL), BUN, creatinine, electrolytes, anion gap

Hyperkalemia: Serum potassium and glucose must be closely monitored to avoid hypoglycemia and/or hypokalemia.

Reference Range

Therapeutic, serum insulin (fasting): 5-20 μIU/mL (SI: 35-145 pmol/L)

Glucose, fasting:

Newborns: 60-110 mg/dL

Adults: 60-110 mg/dL

Elderly: 100-180 mg/dL

Recommendations for glycemic control, adults with type 1 diabetes:

Hb A_{1c}: <7%

Preprandial capillary plasma glucose: 70-130 mg/dL

Peak postprandial capillary blood glucose: <180 mg/dL

Blood pressure: <130/80 mm Hg

Criteria for diagnosis of DKA:

Serum glucose: >250 mg/dL

Arterial pH: <7.3

Bicarbonate: <15 mEq/L

Moderate ketonuria or ketonemia

Additional Information

Split-mixed or basal-bolus regimens: Combination regimens which exploit differences in the onset and duration of different insulin products are commonly used to approximate physiologic secretion. In split-mixed regimens, an intermediate-acting insulin (such as NPH insulin) is administered once or twice daily and supplemented by short-acting (regular) or rapid-acting (lispro, aspart, or glulisine) insulin. Blood glucose measurements are completed several times daily. Dosages are adjusted emphasizing the individual component of the regimen which most directly influences the blood sugar in question (either the intermediate-acting component or the shorter-acting component). Fixed-ratio formulations (eg, 70/30 mix) may be used as twice daily injections in this scenario; however, the ability to titrate the dosage of an individual component is limited. A example of a "split-mixed" regimen would be 21 units of NPH plus 9 units of regular insulin in the morning and an evening meal dose consisting of 14 units of NPH plus 6 units of regular insulin.

Basal-bolus regimens are designed to more closely mimic physiologic secretion. These employ a long-acting insulin (eg, glargine) to simulate basal insulin secretion. The basal component is frequently administered at bedtime or in the early morning. This is supplemented by multiple daily injections of very rapid-acting products (lispro or aspart) immediately prior to a meal, which provides insulin at the time when nutrients are absorbed. An example of a basal-bolus regimen would be 30 units of glargine at bedtime and 12 units of lispro insulin prior to each meal.

Estimation of the effect per unit: A "Rule of 1500" has been frequently used as a means to estimate the change in blood sugar relative to each unit of insulin administered. In fact, the recommended values used in these calculations may vary from 1500-2200 (a value of 1500 is generally recommended for regular insulin while 1800 is recommended for "rapid-acting insulins"). The higher values lead to more conservative estimates of the effect per unit of insulin, and therefore lead to more cautious adjustments. The effect per unit of insulin is approximated by dividing the selected numerical value (eg, 1500-2200) by the number of units/day received by the patient. This may be used as a crude approximation of the patient's insulin sensitivity as adjustments to individual components of the regimen are made. Each additional unit of insulin added to the corresponding insulin dose may be expected to lower the blood glucose by this amount.

To illustrate, in the "basal-bolus" regimen example presented above, the rule of 1800 would indicate an expected change of 27 mg/dL per unit of lispro insulin (the total daily insulin dose is 66 units; using the formula: 1800/66 = 27). A patient may be instructed to add additional insulin if the preprandial glucose is >125 mg/dL. For a prelunch glucose of 195 mg/dL, this would mean the patient would administer the scheduled 12 units of lispro along with an additional "correctional" 3 units for a total of 15 units prior to the meal. If correctional doses are required on a consistent basis, an adjustment of the patients diet and/or scheduled insulin dose may be necessary.

Dosage Forms Excipient information presented when available (limited, particularly for generics); consult specific product labeling.

Injection, solution:
- Humulin® R: 100 units/mL (10 mL)
- Novolin® R: 100 units/mL (3 mL) [InnoLet® prefilled syringe or PenFill® prefilled cartridge]; (10 mL) [vial]

Injection, solution [concentrate]:
- Humulin® R U-500: 500 units/mL (20 mL vial)

◆ **Insulin Regular and Insulin NPH** *see* Insulin NPH and Insulin Regular *on page 795*

◆ **Intal®** *see* Cromolyn *on page 372*

◆ **Integrilin®** *see* Eptifibatide *on page 537*

◆ **Intelence™** *see* Etravirine *on page 594*

◆ **α-2-interferon** *see* Interferon Alfa-2b *on page 801*

◆ **Interferon Alfa-2a (PEG Conjugate)** *see* Peginterferon Alfa-2a *on page 1153*

◆ **Interferon Alfa-2b and Ribavirin Combination Pack** *see* Interferon Alfa-2b and Ribavirin *on page 804*

◆ **Interferon Alfa-2b (PEG Conjugate)** *see* Peginterferon Alfa-2b *on page 1156*

Interferon Alfa-2a (in ter FEER on AL fa too aye)

U.S. Brand Names Roferon®-A [DSC]

Canadian Brand Names Roferon®-A

Index Terms IFLrA; Interferon Alpha-2a; NSC-367982; rIFN-A

Pharmacologic Category Interferon

Use

Patients >18 years of age: Treatment of hairy cell leukemia, chronic hepatitis C

Children and Adults: Treatment of Philadelphia chromosome-positive (Ph+) chronic myelogenous leukemia (CML) in chronic phase, within 1 year of diagnosis (limited experience in children)

Unlabeled/Investigational Use Adjuvant therapy for malignant melanoma; treatment of AIDS-related Kaposi's sarcoma, carcinoid tumors; bladder, cervical, and ovarian cancers; hemangioma; chronic hepatitis D; low-grade non-Hodgkin's lymphoma; multiple myeloma; renal cell carcinoma; basal and squamous cell skin cancer; cutaneous T-cell lymphoma

Restrictions An FDA-approved medication guide must be distributed when dispensing an outpatient prescription (new or refill) where this medication is to be used without direct supervision of a healthcare provider. Medication guides are available at http://www.fda.gov/cder/Offices/ODS/medication_guides.htm.

Pregnancy Risk Factor C

Pregnancy Considerations Animal studies have demonstrated abortifacient effects in large doses. Disruption of the normal menstrual cycle was also observed in animal studies; therefore, the manufacturer recommends that reliable contraception is used in women of childbearing potential. Alfa interferon is endogenous to normal amniotic fluid. *In vitro* administration studies have reported that when administered to the mother, it does not cross the placenta. Case reports of use in pregnant women are limited. The Perinatal HIV Guidelines Working Group does not recommend that interferon-alfa be used during pregnancy. Interferon alfa-2a should only be used in pregnancy when the potential benefit to the mother justifies the possible risk to the fetus.

Lactation Enters breast milk/not recommended (AAP rates "compatible")

Medication Safety Issues

Sound-alike/look-alike issues:
- Interferon alfa-2a may be confused with interferon alfa-2b, interferon alfa-n3, pegylated interferon alfa-2b
- Roferon-A® may be confused with Rocephin®

International issues:
- Interferon alfa-2a may be confused with interferon alpha multi-subtype which is available in international markets

Contraindications Hypersensitivity to interferon alfa or any component of the formulation; autoimmune hepatitis; hepatic decompensation (Child-Pugh class B or C)

Warnings/Precautions Hazardous agent - use appropriate precautions for handling and disposal.

[U.S. Boxed Warning]: May cause or aggravate fatal or life-threatening autoimmune disorders, neuropsychiatric symptoms (including depression and/or suicidal thoughts/behaviors), ischemic and/or infectious disorders; discontinue treatment for persistent severe or worsening symptoms.

Neuropsychiatric disorders: May cause severe psychiatric adverse events (eg, depression, psychosis, mania, suicidal behavior/ideation) in patients with and without previous psychiatric symptoms; use with extreme caution in patients with a history of depression. Careful neuropsychiatric monitoring is required during therapy. Patients developing severe depression may require discontinuation of treatment. Although dose reduction or discontinuation may resolve symptoms, depression may persist; suicides have been reported after therapy has been discontinued. Use with caution in patients with seizure disorders, brain metastases, or compromised CNS function. Higher doses in the elderly or in malignancies other than hairy cell leukemia may result in severe obtundation.

Hepatic disease: Transient liver abnormalities may occur when treating chronic hepatitis C with interferon alfa-2a; increased ascites, hepatic failure, and death may occur with poorly-compensated liver disease.

Bone marrow suppression: Causes bone marrow suppression, including potentially severe cytopenias, and very rarely, aplastic anemia. Use caution in patients with preexisting myelosuppression and/or with concomitant medications which cause myelosuppression.

Cardiovascular disease: Use caution and monitor closely in patients with history of cardiovascular disease; acute toxicities may exacerbate pre-existing cardiac conditions. MI has been observed (rarely) in patients receiving interferon alfa-2a; cardiomyopathy has been reported (rarely) in patients receiving interferon alfa.

Gastrointestinal disorders: Pancreatitis (occasionally fatal) has been observed; hypertriglyceridemia increases the risk for pancreatitis; consider discontinuing treatment in patients with pancreatitis. Hypertriglyceridemia has been reported; consider discontinuing with persistent elevations, particularly if combined with symptoms of pancreatitis. Gastrointestinal hemorrhage, ulcerative and hemorrhagic/ischemic colitis have been observed with interferon alfa treatment; may be severe and/or life-threatening; discontinue if symptoms (eg, abdominal pain, bloody diarrhea, and/or fever) develop.

Pulmonary disease: Dyspnea, pulmonary infiltrates, pneumonia, bronchiolitis obliterans, interstitial pneumonia, and sarcoidosis, resulting in potential fatal respiratory failure may occur with interferon alfa treatment. Discontinue with unexplained pulmonary infiltrates or evidence of impaired pulmonary function. Use caution in patients with a history of pulmonary disease.

Endocrine disorders: Thyroid disorders (hyper- or hypothyroidism) have been reported; use caution in patients with pre-existing thyroid disease. Hyperglycemia has been reported; use caution in patients with diabetes mellitus, may require adjustments in medications.

Autoimmune disorders: Avoid use in patients with history of autoimmune disorders. Development or exacerbation of autoimmune disorders (thrombocytopenic purpura, vasculitis, Raynaud's disease, rheumatoid arthritis, interstitial nephritis, thyroiditis, lupus erythematosus, and rhabdomyolysis) has been associated with interferon alfa. Monitor closely and consider discontinuing if autoimmune disease develops.

Ophthalmic disorders: Decreased/loss of vision, retinopathy (including macular edema), retinal artery or vein thrombosis, retinal hemorrhages, cotton wool spots, optic neuritis and papilledema have occurred in patients receiving interferon alfa. Use caution in patients with preexisting ophthalmic disorders; monitor closely and discontinue with new or worsening ophthalmic symptoms.

Infections: Commonly associated with flu-like symptoms, including fever; rule out other causes/infection with persistent or high fever. Serious and severe infections (bacterial, viral and fungal) have been reported in with treatment; evaluate and treat promptly; consider discontinuing interferon.

Renal disorders: Renal toxicities, some requiring dialysis, have been reported with interferon alfa (alone or in combination with interleukin-2). Use caution in patients with renal impairment (Cl_{cr} <50 mL/minute); monitor closely for signs/symptoms of toxicity.

Acute hypersensitivity reactions have been reported. **Due to differences in dosage, patients should not change brands of interferons without the concurrence of their healthcare provider.** Injection solution contains benzyl alcohol; do not use in neonates or infants. Safety and efficacy have not been established in children <18 years for uses other than Ph+ CML or in organ transplant recipients.

Adverse Reactions Note: A flu-like syndrome (fever, chills, tachycardia, malaise, myalgia, arthralgia, headache) occurs within 1-2 hours of administration; may last up to 24 hours and may be dose limiting.

>10%:

- Cardiovascular: Chest pain (<4% to 11%), edema (1% to 11%), hypertension (11%)
- Central nervous system: Fever (28% to 92%), fatigue (58% to 88%), headache (44% to 64%), chills (23% to 64%), depression (16% to 28%), pain (24%), dizziness (11% to 21%), mental status decreased (10% to 16%), irritability (15%), insomnia (14%), sleep disturbances (10% to 11%)
- Dermatologic: Rash (8% to 44%), alopecia (17% to 19%), pruritus (7% to 13%), dry skin (7% to 17%)
- Endocrine & metabolic: Hypocalcemia (28%), hypophosphatemia (22%)
- Gastrointestinal: Anorexia (14% to 48%), nausea (33% to 39%), vomiting (33% to 39%), diarrhea (20% to 37%), weight loss (33%), throat irritation (21%), abdominal pain (12%)
- Hematologic (often due to underlying disease): Myelosuppression (onset: 7-10 days; nadir 14 days [may be delayed 20-40 days in hairy cell leukemia], recovery: 21 days), neutropenia (≤68%; dose dependant); thrombocytopenia (5% to 62%), leukopenia (2% to 45%), anemia (≤31%)
- Hepatic: Alkaline phosphatase increased (≤50%), transaminases increased (≤50%)
- Local: Injection site reaction (29%)
- Neuromuscular & skeletal: Weakness (6% to 88%) myalgia (51% to 71%), arthralgia (47% to 51%), bone pain (25% to 47%), joint pain (25%), back pain (16%), numbness (12%), paresthesia (7% to 12%)
- Respiratory: Cough (1% to 19%), rhinorrhea/rhinitis (3% to 12%), dyspnea (1% to 12%), pneumonia (11%), sinusitis (11%)
- Miscellaneous: Flu-like syndrome (16% to 33%), diaphoresis (1% to 22%)

1% to 10%:

- Cardiovascular: Dysrhythmia (7%), hypotension (<5%), syncope (<5%), murmur (<5%), thrombophlebitis (<5%), palpitations (<3%), vasculitis (<3%), arrhythmia (1%)
- Central nervous system: Confusion (<4% to 7%), anxiety (5% to 6%), lethargy (1% to 6%), nervousness (<5%), vertigo (<5%), concentration impaired (4%), memory loss (<4%), seizure (<4%), behavior disturbances (3%), malaise (1%)
- Dermatologic: Bruising (<4%), skin lesions (1% to 3%)
- Endocrine & metabolic: Hyperphosphatemia (9%), diabetes (<5%), hyper-/hypothyroidism (<5%),

hypertriglyceridemia (<4%), libido changes (<4%), sexual dysfunction (1% to 3%), menstrual irregularity (2%)

Gastrointestinal: Colitis (<5%), gastrointestinal hemorrhage (<5%), pancreatitis (<5%), flatulence (3%), taste change (3% to <4%), stomatitis (1% to <5%), constipation (<3%), digestion impaired (2%), gingival bleeding (≤2%)

Genitourinary: Impotence (<4%), urinary tract infection (1% to 3%)

Hematologic: Coagulopathy (<4%), hemolytic anemia (<3%), hematoma (1%)

Hepatic: Liver pain (3%)

Neuromuscular & skeletal: Involuntary movements (7%), arthritis (≤5%), polyarthritis (5%), gait disturbance (<5%), leg cramps (3%), muscle cramps (1% to 3%)

Ocular: Visual disturbance (6%), conjunctivitis (4%), eye pain (1% to 3%)

Otic: Hearing alteration (<4%)

Renal: Proteinuria (≤10%)

Respiratory: Oropharynx dryness/inflammation (6%), pneumonitis (<5%), epistaxis (≤4%), bronchospasm (<4%), chest congestion (<3%)

Miscellaneous: Herpes virus reactivation (1% to 3%), lupus erythematosus syndrome (<3%)

<1% (Limited to important or life-threatening): Anaphylactic reaction, anaphylaxis, angioedema, aplastic anemia, ascites, autoimmune reaction with worsening of liver disease, bronchiolitis obliterans, BUN/creatinine increased, cardiomyopathy, coma, CHF, cutaneous eruptions, cyanosis, dysphasia, EEG abnormalities, encephalopathy, hallucinations, hearing loss, hemolytic anemia (Coombs' positive), hemorrhagic colitis, hepatic failure, hepatitis, hyperglycemia, hyperlipidemia, hypersensitivity, hyponatremia (SIADH), inflammation (injection site), macular edema, mania, idiopathic thrombocytopenia purpura, interstitial nephritis, interstitial pneumonitis, ischemic colitis, ischemic retinopathy, LDH increased, MI, myositis, nephrotic syndrome, obtundation, optic neuritis, petechiae, pneumonia, pneumonitis, presenile dementia, proteinuria, psoriasis, psychomotor retardation, psychotic episodes, pulmonary edema, pulmonary infiltrates, Raynaud's phenomenon, renal failure (acute), retinopathy, rhabdomyolysis, sarcoidosis, seizure, serum creatinine increased, somnolence, stroke, suicidal behavior/ideation, syncope, tachypnea, transient ischemic attacks, ulcerative colitis, uric acid increased, urticaria (injection site), vasculitis, visual acuity decreased

Drug Interactions

Metabolism/Transport Effects Inhibits CYP1A2 (weak)

Avoid Concomitant Use There are no known interactions where it is recommended to avoid concomitant use.

Increased Effect/Toxicity

Interferon Alfa-2a may increase the levels/effects of: Aldesleukin; Ribavirin; Theophylline Derivatives; Zidovudine

Decreased Effect There are no known significant interactions involving a decrease in effect.

Stability Refrigerate (2°C to 8°C/36°F to 46°F); do not freeze. Protect from light. Do not shake.

Mechanism of Action Following activation, multiple effects can be detected including induction of gene transcription. Inhibits cellular growth, alters the state of cellular differentiation, interferes with oncogene expression, alters cell surface antigen expression, increases phagocytic activity of macrophages, and augments cytotoxicity of lymphocytes for target cells

Pharmacodynamics/Kinetics

Distribution: V_d: 0.223-0.748 L/kg

Metabolism: Primarily renal; filtered through glomeruli and undergoes rapid proteolytic degradation during tubular reabsorption

Bioavailability: I.M.: 83%; SubQ: 90%

Half-life elimination: I.V.: 3.7-8.5 hours (mean ~5 hours)

Time to peak, serum: I.M., SubQ: ~4-7 hours

Dosage Refer to individual protocols

Children (limited data):

Ph+ chronic myelogenous leukemia (CML): I.M.: 2.5-5 million units/m^2/day; **Note:** In juveniles, higher dosages (30 million units/m^2/day) have been associated with severe adverse events, including death

Adults:

Hairy cell leukemia: SubQ: 3 million units/day for 16-24 weeks, then 3 million units 3 times/week for up to 6-24 months

Ph+ chronic myelogenous leukemia (CML): SubQ: 9 million units/day, continue treatment until disease progression **or** 3 million units/day for 3 days, followed by 6 million units/day for 3 days, followed by 9 million units daily until disease progression

AIDS-related Kaposi's sarcoma (unlabeled use): SubQ, I.M.: 36 million units/day for 10-12 weeks, then 36 million units 3 times/week; to minimize adverse reactions, can use escalating dose (3-, 9-, then 18 million units each day for 3 days, then 36 million units daily thereafter).

Chronic hepatitis C: SubQ: 3 million units 3 times/week for 12 months **or** 6 million units 3 times/week for 12 weeks followed by 3 million units 3 times/week for 36 weeks

Dosage adjustment in renal impairment: Not removed by hemodialysis

Administration

SubQ: For SubQ administration, rotate SubQ injection site.

I.M.: May also be administered I.M. (unlabeled route).

Monitoring Parameters CBC with differential and platelets, liver function, electrolytes, triglycerides. Baseline chest x-ray and ECG. Baseline ophthalmologic exam should be performed in all patients, with periodic reassessment in patients with impairment. Patients with thyroid dysfunction should be monitored by TSH levels at baseline and every 3 months during therapy.

Chronic hepatitis C: Monitor ALT (at baseline, after 2 weeks, and monthly thereafter) and HCV-RNA (particularly in first 3 months of therapy)

CML/hairy cell leukemia: Hematologic monitoring should be performed monthly

Dosage Forms Excipient information presented when available (limited, particularly for generics); consult specific product labeling. [DSC] = Discontinued product

Injection, solution:

Roferon®-A: 3 million units/0.5 mL (0.5 mL) [contains benzyl alcohol and polysorbate 80] [DSC]; 6 million units/0.5 mL (0.5 mL) [contains benzyl alcohol and polysorbate 80] [DSC]; 9 million units/0.5 mL (0.5 mL) [contains benzyl alcohol and polysorbate 80] [DSC]

Interferon Alfa-2b (in ter FEER on AL fa too bee)

U.S. Brand Names Intron® A

Canadian Brand Names Intron® A

Index Terms INF-alpha 2; Interferon Alpha-2b; NSC-377523; rLFN-α2; α-2-interferon

Pharmacologic Category Interferon

Use

Patients ≥1 year of age: Chronic hepatitis B

Patients ≥3 years of age: Chronic hepatitis C (in combination with ribavirin)

Patients ≥18 years of age: Condyloma acuminata, chronic hepatitis B, chronic hepatitis C, hairy cell leukemia, malignant melanoma, AIDS-related Kaposi's sarcoma, follicular non-Hodgkin's lymphoma

Unlabeled/Investigational Use AIDS-related thrombocytopenia, cutaneous ulcerations of Behçet's disease, neuroendocrine tumors (including carcinoid syndrome and islet cell tumor), cutaneous T-cell lymphoma, desmoid tumor, lymphomatoid granulomatosis, hepatitis D, chronic myelogenous leukemia (CML), non-Hodgkin's lymphomas (other than follicular lymphoma, see approved use), multiple myeloma, renal cell carcinoma, basal and squamous cell skin cancers, West Nile virus

Restrictions An FDA-approved medication guide is available at http://www.fda.gov/cder/Offices/ODS/labeling.htm; distribute to each patient to whom this medication is dispensed.

Pregnancy Risk Factor C / X in combination with ribavirin

Pregnancy Considerations Animal studies have demonstrated abortifacient effects. Disruption of the normal menstrual cycle was also observed in animal studies; therefore, the manufacturer recommends that reliable contraception is used in women of childbearing potential. Alfa interferon is endogenous to normal amniotic fluid. *In vitro* administration studies have reported that when administered to the mother, it does not cross the placenta. Case reports of use in pregnant women are limited. The Perinatal HIV Guidelines Working Group does not recommend that interferon-alfa be used during pregnancy. Interferon alfa-2b monotherapy should only be used in pregnancy when the potential benefit to the mother justifies the possible risk to the fetus. Combination therapy with ribavirin is contraindicated in pregnancy (refer to Ribavirin monograph); a pregnancy registry has been established for women inadvertently exposed to ribavirin while pregnant (800-593-2214).

Lactation Enters breast milk/not recommended (AAP rates "compatible")

Medication Safety Issues

Sound-alike/look-alike issues:

Interferon alfa-2b may be confused with interferon alfa-2a, interferon alfa-n3, pegylated interferon alfa-2b

Intron® A may be confused with PEG-Intron®

International issues:

Interferon alfa-2b may be confused with interferon alpha multi-subtype which is available in international markets

Contraindications Hypersensitivity to interferon alfa or any component of the formulation; decompensated liver disease; autoimmune hepatitis

Warnings/Precautions Hazardous agent - use appropriate precautions for handling and disposal.

[U.S. Boxed Warning]: May cause or aggravate fatal or life-threatening autoimmune disorders, neuropsychiatric symptoms (including depression and/or suicidal thoughts/behaviors), ischemic, and/or infectious disorders; discontinue treatment for persistent severe or worsening symptoms.

Neuropsychiatric disorders: May cause severe psychiatric adverse events (eg, depression, psychosis, mania, suicidal behavior/ideation) in patients with and without previous psychiatric symptoms, avoid use in patients with pre-existing psychiatric condition, severe psychiatric disorder or history of severe depression; careful neuropsychiatric monitoring is required during and for 6 months after therapy. Suicidal ideation or attempts may occur more frequently in pediatric patients when compared to adults. Discontinue in patients developing severe depression or psychiatric disorders. Higher doses in elderly patients, or diseases other than hairy cell leukemia, may result in increased CNS toxicity.

Hepatic disease: May cause hepatotoxicity; monitor closely if abnormal liver function tests develop. A transient increase in ALT (≥2 times baseline) may occur in patients treated with interferon alfa-2b for chronic hepatitis B. Therapy generally may continue; monitor. Worsening and potentially fatal liver disease, including jaundice, hepatic encephalopathy, and hepatic failure have been reported in patients receiving interferon alfa for chronic hepatitis B and C with decompensated liver disease, autoimmune hepatitis, history of autoimmune disease, and immunosuppressed transplant recipients; avoid use in these patients. Chronic hepatitis B or C patients with a history of autoimmune disease or who are immunosuppressed transplant recipients should not receive interferon alfa-2b. Discontinue treatment (if appropriate) in any patient developing signs or symptoms of liver failure.

Bone marrow suppression: Causes bone marrow suppression, including potentially severe cytopenias, and very rarely, aplastic anemia. Discontinue treatment for severe neutropenia (ANC <500/mm^3) or thrombocytopenia (platelets <25,000/mm^3). Hemolytic anemia (hemoglobin <10 g/dL) was observed when combined with ribavirin; anemia occurred within 1-2 weeks of initiation of therapy. Use caution in patients with pre-existing myelosuppression and in patients with concomitant medications which cause myelosuppression.

Autoimmune disorders: Avoid use in patients with history of autoimmune disorders; development of autoimmune disorders (thrombocytopenia, vasculitis, Raynaud's disease, rheumatoid arthritis, lupus erythematosus and rhabdomyolysis) has been associated with use. Monitor closely; consider discontinuing. Worsening of psoriasis and sarcoidosis (and the development of new sarcoidosis) have been reported; use caution.

Cardiovascular disease/coagulation disorders: Use caution and monitor closely in patients with cardiovascular disease (ischemic or thromboembolic), arrhythmias, hypertension, and in patients with a history of MI or prior therapy with cardiotoxic drugs. Patients with pre-existing cardiac disease and/or advanced cancer should have baseline and periodic ECGs. May cause hypotension (during administration or delayed), arrhythmia, tachycardia, cardiomyopathy (~2% in AIDS-related Kaposi's Sarcoma patients) and/or MI. Hemorrhagic cerebrovascular events have been observed with therapy. Use caution in patients with coagulation disorders.

Endocrine disorders: Thyroid disorders (possibly reversible) have been reported; use caution in patients with pre-existing thyroid disease. Discontinue use in patients who cannot maintain normal ranges with thyroid medication. Diabetes mellitus has been reported; discontinue if cannot effectively manage with medication. Use caution in patients with a history of diabetes mellitus, particularly if prone to DKA. Hypertriglyceridemia has been reported; discontinue if severe, and/or combined with symptoms of pancreatitis.

Pulmonary disease: Pulmonary infiltrates, pneumonitis and pneumonia have been reported with interferon alfa therapy; occurs more frequently in patients being treated for chronic hepatitis C. Patients with fever, cough, dyspnea or other respiratory symptoms should be evaluated with a chest x-ray; monitor closely and consider discontinuing treatment with evidence of impaired pulmonary function. Use with caution in patients with a history of pulmonary disease.

Ophthalmic disorders: Decreased/loss of vision, macular edema, optic neuritis, retinal hemorrhages, cotton wool spots, papilledema, and retinal artery or vein thrombosis have occurred (or been aggravated) in patients receiving alpha interferons. Use caution in patients with pre-existing eye disorders; monitor closely; discontinue with new or worsening ophthalmic disorders.

Commonly associated with fever and flu-like symptoms; rule out other causes/infection with persistent fever; use with caution in patients with debilitating conditions. Acute hypersensitivity reactions have been reported. Do not treat patients with visceral AIDS-related Kaposi's sarcoma associated with rapidly-progressing or life-threatening disease. Some formulations contain albumin, which may carry a remote risk of viral transmission. Due to differences in dosage, patients should not change brands of interferons without the concurrence of their healthcare provider. Safety and efficacy in children <1 year of age have not been established.

Adverse Reactions Note: In a majority of patients, a flu-like syndrome (fever, chills, tachycardia, malaise, myalgia, headache), occurs within 1-2 hours of administration; may last up to 24 hours and may be dose limiting.

>10%:

Cardiovascular: Chest pain (≤28%)

Central nervous system: Fatigue (8% to 96%), fever (34% to 94%), headache (21% to 62%), chills (≤54%), depression (3% to 40%; grades 3/4: 2%), somnolence (≤33%), dizziness (≤24%), irritability (≤22%), pain (≤18%), amnesia (≤14%), concentration impaired (≤14%), malaise (≤14%), confusion (≤12%), insomnia (≤12%)

Dermatologic: Alopecia (≤38%), rash (≤25%), pruritus (≤11%)

Endocrine & metabolic: Amenorrhea (≤12%)

Gastrointestinal: Anorexia (1% to 69%), nausea, (17% to 66%), diarrhea (2% to 45%), vomiting (2% to 32%), xerostomia (≤28%), taste alteration (≤24%), abdominal pain (1% to 23%), constipation (≤14%), gingivitis (≤14%), weight loss (<1% to 13%)

Hematologic: Neutropenia (≤92%; grade 4: 1% to 4%), leukopenia (≤68%), anemia (≤32%), thrombocytopenia (≤15%)

Hepatic: AST increased (≤63%; grades 3/4: 14%), ALT increased (≤15%), pain (upper right quadrant: up to 15%); alkaline phosphatase increased (≤13%)

Local: Injection site reaction (≤20%)

Neuromuscular & skeletal: Myalgia (28% to 75%), weakness (≤63%), rigors (≤42%), paresthesia (1% to 21%), skeletal pain (≤21%), arthralgia (≤19%), back pain (≤19%)

Renal: BUN increased (≤12%)

Respiratory: Dyspnea (≤34%), cough (≤31%), pharyngitis (≤31%), sinusitis (≤21%)

Miscellaneous: Flu-like syndrome (≤79%), diaphoresis (1% to 21%), moniliasis (≤17%)

5% to 10%:

Cardiovascular: Edema (≤10%), hypertension (≤9%)

Central nervous system: Hypoesthesia (≤10%), anxiety (≤9%), vertigo (≤8%), agitation (≤7%)

Dermatologic: Dry skin (≤10%), dermatitis (≤8%), purpura (≤5%)

Endocrine & metabolic: Libido decreased (≤5%)

Gastrointestinal: Loose stools (≤10%), dyspepsia (≤8%)

Genitourinary: Urinary tract infection (≤5%)

Renal: Polyuria (≤10%), serum creatinine increased (≤6%)

Respiratory: Bronchitis (≤10%), nasal congestion (≤10%), epistaxis (≤7%)

Miscellaneous: Infection (≤7%), herpes virus infections (≤5%)

<5% (Limited to important or life-threatening): Acute hypersensitivity reaction, aggression, albuminuria, alcohol intolerance, allergic reactions, anaphylaxis, angina, angioedema, aphasia, aplastic anemia (rarely), arrhythmia, ascites, asthma, ataxia, atrial fibrillation, bell's palsy, bilirubinemia, blurred vision, bradycardia, bronchoconstriction, bronchospasm, cardiac failure, cardiomegaly, cardiomyopathy, cellulitis, colitis, coma, conjunctivitis, coronary artery disorder, cotton wool spots, cyanosis, cystitis, dehydration, diabetes mellitus, dysphasia, dysuria, eczema, ejection fraction decreased, epidermal necrolysis, erythema, erythema multiforme, erythematous rash, esophagitis, extrapyramidal disorder, extrasystoles, gastrointestinal hemorrhage, granulocytopenia, hallucination, hearing loss/impairment, heart valve disorder, hematuria, hemolytic anemia, hemoptysis, hepatic encephalopathy, hepatic failure, hepatitis, hepatotoxicity, hot flashes, hyper-/hypothyroidism, hypercalcemia, hyperglycemia, hypertriglyceridemia, hypochromic anemia, hypotension, hypothermia, hypoventilation, impotence, incontinence, injection site necrosis, jaundice, lactate dehydrogenase increased, leukorrhea, liver function test abnormal, lupus erythematosus, lymphadenitis, lymphadenopathy, lymphocytosis, lymphopenia, maculopapular rash, macular edema, menorrhagia, MI, migraine, muscle atrophy, myositis, nephrotic syndrome, nervousness, neuralgia, neuropathy, neurosis, nystagmus, optic neuritis, palpitation, pancreatitis, papilledema, paranoia, peripheral ischemia, photophobia, photosensitivity, pleural effusion, pneumonitis, pneumothorax, proteinuria, psoriasis exacerbation, psychosis, pulmonary embolism, pulmonary fibrosis, pure red cell aplasia, raynaud's disease, renal failure, renal insufficiency, respiratory insufficiency, retinal artery thrombosis, retinal vein thrombosis, rhabdomyolysis, sarcoidosis exacerbation, sebaceous cyst, seizure, sepsis, sexual dysfunction, Stevens-Johnson syndrome, stomatitis, stroke, suicidal attempt/ideation, syncope, tachycardia, tendonitis, thrombocytopenia purpura (idiopathic and thrombotic), thrombosis, toxic epidermal necrolysis, upper respiratory tract infection, urticaria, uterine bleeding, vasculitis, wheezing

Drug Interactions

Metabolism/Transport Effects Inhibits CYP1A2 (weak)

Avoid Concomitant Use There are no known interactions where it is recommended to avoid concomitant use.

Increased Effect/Toxicity

Interferon Alfa-2b may increase the levels/effects of: Aldesleukin; Ribavirin; Theophylline Derivatives; Zidovudine

Decreased Effect There are no known significant interactions involving a decrease in effect.

Stability Store powder and solution for injection (vials and pens) under refrigeration at 2°C to 8°C (36°F to 46°F). Do not freeze. The manufacturer recommends reconstituting vial with the diluent provided (SWFI). To prepare solution for infusion, further dilute appropriate dose in NS 100 mL. Final concentration should be ≥10 million units/100 mL.

Powder for injection: Following reconstitution, should be used immediately, but may be stored under refrigeration for up to 24 hours.

Prefilled pens: After first use, discard unused portion after 4 weeks.

Mechanism of Action Following activation, multiple effects can be detected including induction of gene transcription. Inhibits cellular growth, alters the state of cellular differentiation, interferes with oncogene expression, alters cell surface antigen expression, increases phagocytic activity of macrophages, and augments cytotoxicity of lymphocytes for target cells

Pharmacodynamics/Kinetics

Distribution: V_d: 31 L; but has been noted to be much greater (370-720 L) in leukemia patients receiving continuous infusion IFN; IFN does not penetrate the CSF

Metabolism: Primarily renal

Bioavailability: I.M.: 83%; SubQ: 90%

Half-life elimination: I.V.: ~2 hours; I.M., SubQ: ~2-3 hours

Time to peak, serum: I.M., SubQ: ~3-12 hours

Dosage Details concerning dosing in combination regimens should also be consulted. **Note:** Withhold treatment for ANC <500/mm^3 or platelets <25,000/mm^3. Consider premedication with acetaminophen prior to administration to reduce the incidence of some adverse reactions. Not all dosage forms and strengths are appropriate for all indications; refer to product labeling for details.

Children 1-17 years: Chronic hepatitis B: SubQ: 3 million units/m^2 3 times/week for 1 week; then 6 million units/m^2 3 times/week; maximum: 10 million units 3 times/week; total duration of therapy 16-24 weeks

Children ≥3 years: Chronic hepatitis C: In combination with ribavirin (refer to Interferon Alfa-2b/Ribavirin combination pack monograph)

Adults:

Hairy cell leukemia: I.M., SubQ: 2 million units/m^2 3 times/week for up to 6 months (may continue treatment with continued treatment response)

Lymphoma (follicular): SubQ: 5 million units 3 times/week for up to 18 months

Malignant melanoma: Induction: 20 million units/m^2 I.V. for 5 consecutive days per week for 4 weeks, followed by maintenance dosing of 10 million units/m^2 SubQ 3 times/week for 48 weeks

AIDS-related Kaposi's sarcoma: I.M., SubQ: 30 million units/m^2 3 times/week

Chronic hepatitis B: I.M., SubQ: 5 million units/day or 10 million units 3 times/week for 16 weeks

Chronic hepatitis C: I.M., SubQ: 3 million units 3 times/week for 16 weeks. In patients with normalization of ALT at 16 weeks, continue treatment for 18-24 months; consider discontinuation if normalization does not occur at 16 weeks. **Note:** May be used in combination therapy with ribavirin in previously untreated patients or in patients who relapse following alpha interferon therapy.

Condyloma acuminata: Intralesionally: 1 million units/lesion (maximum: 5 lesions/treatment) 3 times/week (on alternate days) for 3 weeks; may administer a second course at 12-16 weeks

Dosage adjustment in renal impairment: Combination therapy with ribavirin (hepatitis C) should not be used in patients with reduced renal function (Cl_{cr} <50 mL/minute).

Dosage adjustment for toxicity: Manufacturer-recommended adjustments, listed according to indication:

Lymphoma (follicular):

Neutrophils >1000/mm^3 to <1500/mm^3: Reduce dose by 50%; may re-escalate to starting dose when neutrophils return to >1500/mm^3

Severe toxicity (neutrophils <1000/mm^3 or platelets <50,000/mm^3): Temporarily withhold

AST >5 times ULN or serum creatinine >2 mg/dL: Permanently discontinue

Hairy cell leukemia, chronic hepatitis C: Severe toxicity: Reduce dose by 50% or temporarily withhold and resume with 50% dose reduction; permanently discontinue if persistent or recurrent severe toxicity is noted

Chronic hepatitis B:

WBC <1500/mm^3, granulocytes <750/mm^3, or platelet count <50,000/mm^3, or other laboratory abnormality or severe adverse reaction: Reduce dose by 50%; may re-escalate to starting dose upon resolution of hematologic toxicity. Discontinue for persistent intolerance.

WBC <1000/mm^3, granulocytes <500/mm^3, or platelet count <25,000/mm^3: Permanently discontinue

Kaposi sarcoma: Severe toxicity: Reduce dose by 50% or temporarily withhold; may resume at reduced dose with toxicity resolution; permanently discontinue for persistent/recurrent toxicities

Malignant melanoma:

Severe toxicity (neutrophils >250/mm^3 to <500/mm^3 or ALT/AST >5-10 times ULN): Temporarily withhold; resume with a 50% dose reduction when adverse reaction abates

Neutrophils <250/mm^3, ALT/AST >10 times ULN, or severe/persistent adverse reactions: Permanently discontinue

Administration

I.M.: Administer in evening (if possible)

I.V.: Infuse over ~20 minutes

SubQ: Suggested for those who are at risk for bleeding or are thrombocytopenic. Rotate SubQ injection site. Administer in evening (if possible). Patient should be well hydrated. Reconstitute with recommended amount of SWFI and agitate gently; do not shake. **Note:** Different vial strengths require different amounts of diluent. Not every dosage form is appropriate for every indication; refer to manufacturer's labeling.

Monitoring Parameters Baseline chest x-ray, ECG; CBC with differential and platelets (baseline and routinely during treatment), liver function tests, serum creatinine, electrolytes, triglycerides, thyroid function tests (baseline and periodically during treatment); weight; ophthalmic exam (baseline and periodic, or with new ocular symptoms); patients with pre-existing cardiac abnormalities or in advanced stages of cancer should have ECGs taken before and during treatment

Dosage Forms Excipient information presented when available (limited, particularly for generics); consult specific product labeling. [DSC] = Discontinued product

Injection, powder for reconstitution [preservative free]:

Intron® A: 10 million units; 18 million units; 50 million units [contains human albumin]

Injection, solution [multidose prefilled pen]:

Intron® A:

Delivers 3 million units/0.2 mL (1.5 mL) [delivers 6 doses; 18 million units; contains polysorbate 80; edetate disodium]

Delivers 5 million units/0.2 mL (1.5 mL) [delivers 6 doses; 30 million units; contains polysorbate 80; edetate disodium]

Delivers 10 million units/0.2 mL (1.5 mL) [delivers 6 doses; 60 million units; contains polysorbate 80; edetate disodium]

Injection, solution [multidose vial]:

Intron® A: 6 million units/mL (3 mL); 10 million units/mL (2.5 mL) [contains polysorbate 80; edetate disodium]

Injection, solution [single-dose vial]:

Intron® A: 10 million units/ mL (1 mL) [DSC] [contains polysorbate 80; edetate disodium]

See also Interferon Alfa-2b and Ribavirin Combination Pack monograph.

Interferon Alfa-2b and Ribavirin

(in ter FEER on AL fa too bee & rye ba VYE rin)

U.S. Brand Names Rebetron®

Index Terms Interferon Alfa-2b and Ribavirin Combination Pack; Ribavirin and Interferon Alfa-2b Combination Pack

Pharmacologic Category Antiviral Agent; Interferon

Use Combination therapy for the treatment of chronic hepatitis C in patients with compensated liver disease previously untreated with alpha interferon or who have relapsed after alpha interferon therapy

Restrictions An FDA-approved medication guide must be distributed when dispensing an outpatient prescription (new or refill) for treatment of hepatitis C where this medication is to be used without direct supervision of a healthcare provider. Medication guides are available at http://www.fda.gov/cder/Offices/ODS/medication_guides.htm.

Pregnancy Risk Factor X

Dosage

Children ≥3 years: Chronic hepatitis C: **Note:** Treatment duration may vary. Consult current guidelines and literature. Combination therapy:

Intron® A: SubQ:

25-61 kg: 3 million int. units/m^2 3 times/week

>61 kg: Refer to adult dosing

Rebetol®: Oral: **Note:** Oral solution should be used in children 3-5 years of age, children ≤25 kg, or those unable to swallow capsules.

Capsule/solution: 15 mg/kg/day in 2 divided doses (morning and evening)

Capsule dosing recommendations:

26-36 kg: 400 mg/day (200 mg morning and evening)

37-49 kg: 600 mg/day (200 mg in the morning and two 200 mg capsules in the evening)

50-61 kg: 800 mg/day (two 200 mg capsules morning and evening)

>61 kg: Refer to adult dosing

Adults: Chronic hepatitis C: Recommended dosage of combination therapy:

Intron® A: SubQ: 3 million int. units 3 times/week **and**

Rebetol® capsule: Oral:

≤75 kg (165 lb): 1000 mg/day (two 200 mg capsules in the morning and three 200 mg capsules in the evening)

>75 kg: 1200 mg/day (three 200 mg capsules in the morning and three 200 mg capsules in the evening)

Note: Treatment duration may vary. Consult current guidelines and literature.

Dosing adjustment for toxicity: Note: Recommendations (per manufacturer labeling):

Anemia (RBC depression):

Patient **without** cardiac history:

Hemoglobin <10 g/dL:

Children: Decrease ribavirin dose by 1/2

Adults: Decrease ribavirin dose to 600 mg/day

Hemoglobin <8.5 g/dL: Permanently discontinue treatment

Patient **with** cardiac history:

Hemoglobin has ≥2 g/dL decrease during any 4-week period of treatment:

Children: Decrease ribavirin dose by 1/2 **and** decrease interferon alfa-2b to 1.5 million int. units 3 times/week

Adults: Decrease dose to ribavirin to 600 mg/day **and** decrease interferon-alfa 2b dose to 1.5 million int. units 3 times/week.

Hemoglobin <12 g/dL after 4 weeks of reduced dose: Permanently discontinue treatment

WBC, neutrophil, or platelet depression:

WBC <1500 cells/mm^3, neutrophils <750 cells/mm^3, or platelet count <50,000 cells/mm^3 (<80,000 cells/ mm^3 in children): Reduce interferon alfa-2b dose to 1.5 million int. units 3 times/week (50% reduction)

WBC <1000 cells/mm^3, neutrophils <500 cells/mm^3, or platelet count <25,000 cells/mm^3 (<50,000 cells/mm^3 in children): Permanently discontinue therapy

Dosage adjustment in renal impairment: Patients with Cl_{cr} <50 mL/minutes should not receive ribavirin.

Additional Information Complete prescribing information for this medication should be consulted for additional detail.

Dosage Forms Excipient information presented when available (limited, particularly for generics); consult specific product labeling.

Combination package:

For patients ≤75 kg [contains single-dose vials]:

Injection, solution: Interferon alfa-2b (Intron® A): 3 million int. units/0.5 mL (0.5 mL) [6 vials (3 million int. units/ vial), 6 syringes, and alcohol swabs]

Capsule: Ribavirin (Rebetol®): 200 mg (70s)

For patients ≤75 kg [contains multidose vials]:

Injection, solution: Interferon alfa-2b (Intron® A): 3 million int. units/0.5 mL (3.8 mL) [1 multidose vial (18 million int. units/vial), 6 syringes, and alcohol swabs]

Capsule: Ribavirin (Rebetol®): 200 mg (70s)

For patients ≤75 kg [contains multidose pen]:

Injection, solution: Interferon alfa-2b (Intron® A): 3 million int. units/0.2 mL (1.5 mL) [1 multidose pen (18 million int. units/pen), 6 needles, and alcohol swabs]

Capsule: Ribavirin (Rebetol®): 200 mg (70s)

For patients >75 kg [contains single-dose vials]:

Injection, solution: Interferon alfa-2b (Intron® A): 3 million int. units/0.5 mL (0.5 mL) [6 vials (3 million int. units/ vial), 6 syringes, and alcohol swabs]

Capsule: Ribavirin (Rebetol®): 200 mg (84s)

For patients >75 kg [contains multidose vials]:

Injection, solution: Interferon alfa-2b (Intron® A): 3 million int. units/0.5 mL (3.8 mL) [1 multidose vial (18 million int. units/vial), 6 syringes, and alcohol swabs]

Capsule: Ribavirin (Rebetol®): 200 mg (84s)

For patients >75 kg [contains multidose pen]:

Injection, solution: Interferon alfa-2b (Intron® A): 3 million int. units/0.2 mL (1.5 mL) [1 multidose pen (18 million int. units/pen), 6 needles, and alcohol swabs]

Capsule: Ribavirin (Rebetol®): 200 mg (84s)

For Rebetol® dose reduction [contains single-dose vials]:

Injection, solution: Interferon alfa-2b (Intron® A): 3 million int. units/0.5 mL (0.5 mL) [6 vials (3 million int. units/ vial), 6 syringes, and alcohol swabs]

Capsule: Ribavirin (Rebetol®): 200 mg (42s)

For Rebetol® dose reduction [contains multidose vials]:

Injection, solution: Interferon alfa-2b (Intron® A): 3 million int. units/0.5 mL (3.8 mL) [1 multidose vial (18 million int. units/vial), 6 syringes, and alcohol swabs]

Capsule: Ribavirin (Rebetol®): 200 mg (42s)

For Rebetol® dose reduction [contains multidose pen]:

Injection, solution: Interferon alfa-2b (Intron® A): 3 million int. units/0.2 mL (1.5 mL) [1 multidose pen (18 million int. units/pen), 6 needles, and alcohol swabs]

Capsule: Ribavirin (Rebetol®): 200 mg (42s)

Interferon Alfacon-1 (in ter FEER on AL fa con one)

U.S. Brand Names Infergen®

Pharmacologic Category Interferon

Use Treatment of chronic hepatitis C virus (HCV) infection in patients ≥18 years of age with compensated liver disease and anti-HCV serum antibodies or HCV RNA.

Restrictions An FDA-approved medication guide must be distributed when dispensing an outpatient prescription (new or refill) where this medication is to be used without direct supervision of a healthcare provider. Medication guides are available at http://www.fda.gov/cder/Offices/ODS/medication_guides.htm.

Pregnancy Risk Factor C

Medication Safety Issues

Sound-alike/look-alike issues:

Interferon alfacon-1 may be confused with interferon alfa-2a, interferon alfa-2b, interferon alfa-n3, peginterferon alfa-2b

International issues:

Interferon alfacon-1 may be confused with interferon alpha multi-subtype which is available in international markets

Dosage Adults ≥18 years: SubQ:

Chronic HCV infection: 9 mcg 3 times/week for 24 weeks; allow 48 hours between doses

Patients who have previously tolerated interferon therapy but did not respond or relapsed: 15 mcg 3 times/week for up to 48 weeks

Dose reduction for toxicity: Dose should be held in patients who experience a severe adverse reaction, and treatment should be stopped or decreased if the reaction does not become tolerable.

Doses were reduced from 9 mcg to 7.5 mcg in the pivotal study.

For patients receiving 15 mcg/dose, doses were reduced in 3 mcg decrements. Efficacy is decreased with doses <7.5 mcg

Dosage adjustment in renal impairment: No information available.

Dosage adjustment in hepatic impairment: Use in decompensated hepatic disease is contraindicated.

Elderly: No information available.

Additional Information Complete prescribing information for this medication should be consulted for additional detail.

Dosage Forms Excipient information presented when available (limited, particularly for generics); consult specific product labeling.

Injection, solution [preservative free]:

Infergen®: 30 mcg/mL (0.3 mL, 0.5 mL)

Interferon Alfa-n3 (in ter FEER on AL fa en three)

U.S. Brand Names Alferon® N

Canadian Brand Names Alferon® N

Pharmacologic Category Interferon

Use Patients ≥18 years of age: Intralesional treatment of refractory or recurring genital or venereal warts (condylomata acuminata)

Pregnancy Risk Factor C

Medication Safety Issues

Sound-alike/look-alike issues:

Alferon® may be confused with Alkeran®

Dosage Adults: Inject 250,000 units (0.05 mL) in each wart twice weekly for a maximum of 8 weeks; therapy should not be repeated for at least 3 months after the initial 8-week course of therapy

Additional Information Complete prescribing information for this medication should be consulted for additional detail.

Dosage Forms Excipient information presented when available (limited, particularly for generics); consult specific product labeling.

Injection, solution: 5 million int. units (1 mL) [contains albumin]

◆ **Interferon Alpha-2a** *see* Interferon Alfa-2a *on page 799*

◆ **Interferon Alpha-2b** *see* Interferon Alfa-2b *on page 801*

Interferon Beta-1a (in ter FEER on BAY ta won aye)

U.S. Brand Names Avonex®; Rebif®

Canadian Brand Names Avonex®; Rebif®

Index Terms rIFN beta-1a

Pharmacologic Category Interferon

Use Treatment of relapsing forms of multiple sclerosis (MS)

Restrictions An FDA-approved medication guide must be distributed when dispensing an outpatient prescription (new or refill) where this medication is to be used without direct supervision of a healthcare provider. Medication guides are available at http://www.fda.gov/cder/Offices/ODS/medication_guides.htm.

Pregnancy Risk Factor C

Pregnancy Considerations There are no adequate and well-controlled studies in pregnant women. Consideration should be given to discontinue treatment if a woman becomes pregnant, or plans to become pregnant during therapy. A dose-related abortifacient activity was reported in Rhesus monkeys.

Healthcare providers are encouraged to register pregnant women receiving Rebif® during pregnancy online at www.rebifpregnancyregistry.com or by telephone at MS LifeLines 1-877-44-REBIF. A registry has been established for women who become pregnant while receiving Avonex®. Women may be enrolled in the registry by calling 1-800-456-2255.

Lactation Excretion in breast milk unknown/not recommended

Medication Safety Issues

Sound-alike/look-alike issues:

Avonex® may be confused with Avelox®

Contraindications Hypersensitivity to natural or recombinant interferons, human albumin, or any other component of the formulation

Warnings/Precautions Interferons have been associated with severe psychiatric adverse events (psychosis, mania, depression, suicidal behavior/ideation) in patients with and without previous psychiatric symptoms, avoid use in severe psychiatric disorders and use caution in patients with a history of depression; patients exhibiting depressive symptoms should be closely monitored and discontinuation of therapy should be considered.

Autoimmune disorders including idiopathic thrombocytopenia, hyper- and hypothyroidism and rarely autoimmune hepatitis have been reported. Allergic reactions, including anaphylaxis, have been reported. Caution should be used in patients with hepatic impairment or in those who abuse alcohol. Rare cases of severe hepatic injury, including hepatic failure, have been reported in patients receiving interferon beta-1a; risk may be increased by ethanol use or concurrent therapy with hepatotoxic drugs. Treatment should be suspended if jaundice or symptoms of hepatic dysfunction occur. Transaminase elevations may be asymptomatic, so monitoring is important. Dose adjustment may be necessary with hepatic impairment. Hematologic effects, including pancytopenia (rare) and thrombocytopenia, have been reported. Associated with a high incidence of flu-like adverse effects; use of analgesics and/or antipyretics on treatment days may be helpful. Use caution in patients with pre-existing cardiovascular disease, including angina, HF, and/or arrythmia. Rare cases of new-onset cardiomyopathy and/or HF have been reported. Use caution in patients with seizure disorders, or myelosuppression. Safety and efficacy in patients with chronic progressive MS or in patients <18 years of age have not been established. Albumin is a component of some formulations (contraindicated in albumin-sensitive patients); rare risk of CJD or viral transmission.

Adverse Reactions Note: Adverse reactions reported as a composite of both commercially-available products. Spectrum and incidence of reactions is generally similar between products, but consult individual product labels for specific incidence.

>10%:

Central nervous system: Headache (58% to 70%), fatigue (33% to 41%), fever (20% to 28%), pain (23%), chills (19%), depression (18% to 25%), dizziness (14%)

Gastrointestinal: Nausea (23%), abdominal pain (8% to 22%)

Genitourinary: Urinary tract infection (17%)

Hematologic: Leukopenia (28% to 36%)

Hepatic: ALT increased (20% to 27%), AST increased (10% to 17%)

Local: Injection site reaction (3% to 92%)

Neuromuscular & skeletal: Myalgia (25% to 29%), back pain (23% to 25%), weakness (24%), skeletal pain (10% to 15%), rigors (6% to 13%)

Ocular: Vision abnormal (7% to 13%)

Respiratory: Sinusitis (14%), upper respiratory tract infection (14%)

Miscellaneous: Flu-like syndrome (49% to 59%), neutralizing antibodies (significance not known; Avonex® 5%; Rebif® 24%), lymphadenopathy (11% to 12%)

1% to 10%:

Cardiovascular: Chest pain (5% to 6%), vasodilation (2%)

Central nervous system: Migraine (5%), somnolence (4% to 5%), malaise (4% to 5%), seizure (1% to 5%)

Dermatologic: Erythematous rash (5% to 7%), maculopapular rash (4% to 5%), alopecia (4%), urticaria

Endocrine & metabolic: Thyroid disorder (4% to 6%)

Gastrointestinal: Xerostomia (1% to 5%), toothache (3%)

Genitourinary: Micturition frequency (2% to 7%), urinary incontinence (2% to 4%)

Hematologic: Thrombocytopenia (2% to 8%), anemia (3% to 5%)

Hepatic: Bilirubinemia (2% to 3%)

Local: Injection site pain (8%), injection site bruising (6%), injection site necrosis (1% to 3%), injection site inflammation

Neuromuscular & skeletal: Arthralgia (9%), hypertonia (6% to 7%), coordination abnormal (4% to 5%)

Ocular: Eye disorder (4%), xerophthalmia (1% to 3%)

Respiratory: Bronchitis (8%)

Miscellaneous: Infection (7%)

<1% (Limited to important and life-threatening): Anaphylaxis, autoimmune hepatitis, cardiomyopathy, CHF, hepatic failure, hepatitis, hyper-/hypothyroidism, idiopathic thrombocytopenia, injection site abscess/cellulitis, menorrhagia, metrorrhagia, pancytopenia, psychiatric disorders (new or worsening; including suicidal ideation), vesicular rash

Drug Interactions

Avoid Concomitant Use There are no known interactions where it is recommended to avoid concomitant use.

Increased Effect/Toxicity

Interferon Beta-1a may increase the levels/effects of: Theophylline Derivatives; Zidovudine

Decreased Effect There are no known significant interactions involving a decrease in effect.

Stability

Avonex®:

Prefilled syringe: Store at 2°C to 8°C (36°F to 46°F); do not freeze. Protect from light. Allow to warm to room temperature prior to use (do not use external heat source). If refrigeration is not available, product may be stored at ≤25°C (77°F) for up to 7 days.

Vial: Store unreconstituted vial at 2°C to 8°C (36°F to 46°F). If refrigeration is not available, may be stored at 25°C (77°F) for up to 30 days; do not freeze. Protect from light. Reconstitute with 1.1 mL of diluent and swirl gently to dissolve. Do not shake. The reconstituted product contains no preservative and is for single-use only; discard unused portion. Following reconstitution, use immediately, but may be stored up to 6 hours at 2°C to 8°C (36°F to 46°F); do not freeze.

Rebif®: Store at 2°C to 8°C (36°F to 46°F); do not freeze. Protect from light. May also be stored ≤25°C (77°F) for up to 30 days if protected from heat and light.

Mechanism of Action Interferon beta differs from naturally occurring human protein by a single amino acid substitution and the lack of carbohydrate side chains; alters the expression and response to surface antigens and can enhance immune cell activities. Properties of interferon beta that modify biologic responses are mediated by cell surface receptor interactions; mechanism in the treatment of MS is unknown.

Pharmacodynamics/Kinetics

Onset of action: Avonex®: 12 hours (based on biological response markers)

Duration: Avonex®: 4 days (based on biological response markers)

Half-life elimination: Avonex®: 10 hours; Rebif®: 69 hours

Time to peak, serum: Avonex® (I.M.): 3-15 hours; Rebif® (SubQ): 16 hours

Dosage Adults: **Note:** Analgesics and/or antipyretics may help decrease flu-like symptoms on treatment days:

I.M. (Avonex®): 30 mcg once weekly

SubQ (Rebif®): Doses should be separated by at least 48 hours:

Target dose 44 mcg 3 times/week:

Initial: 8.8 mcg (20 % of final dose) 3 times/week for 2 weeks

Titration: 22 mcg (50% of final dose) 3 times/week for 2 weeks

Final dose: 44 mcg 3 times/week

Target dose 22 mcg 3 times/week:

Initial: 4.4 mcg (20 % of final dose) 3 times/week for 2 weeks

Titration: 11 mcg (50% of final dose) 3 times/week for 2 weeks

Final dose: 22 mcg 3 times/week

Dosage adjustment in hepatic impairment: Rebif®: If liver function tests increase or in case of leukopenia: Decrease dose 20% to 50% until toxicity resolves

Administration

Avonex®: Must be administered by I.M. injection

Rebif®: Administer SubQ at the same time of day on the same 3 days each week (ie, late afternoon/evening Mon, Wed, Fri); rotate injection site

Monitoring Parameters Thyroid function tests, CBC with differential, transaminase levels, symptoms of autoimmune disorders, signs/symptoms of psychiatric disorder (including depression and/or suicidal ideation), signs/symptoms of new onset/worsening cardiovascular disease

Avonex®: Frequency of monitoring for patients receiving Avonex® has not been specifically defined; in clinical trials, monitoring was at 6-month intervals.

Rebif®: CBC and liver function testing at 1-, 3-, and 6 months, then periodically thereafter. Thyroid function every 6 months (in patients with pre-existing abnormalities and/or clinical indications)

Dosage Forms Excipient information presented when available (limited, particularly for generics); consult specific product labeling.

Combination package [preservative free] (Rebif® Titration Pack):

Injection, solution: 8.8 mcg/0.2 mL (0.2 mL) [6 prefilled syringes; contains albumin]

Injection, solution: 22 mcg/0.5 mL (0.5 mL) [6 prefilled syringes; contains albumin]

Injection, powder for reconstitution (Avonex®): 33 mcg [6.6 million units; provides 30 mcg/mL following reconstitution] [contains albumin; packaged with SWFI, alcohol wipes, and access pin and needle]

Injection, solution (Avonex®): 30 mcg/0.5 mL (0.5 mL) [albumin free; prefilled syringe; syringe cap contains latex; packaged with alcohol wipes, gauze pad, and adhesive bandages]

Injection, solution [preservative free] (Rebif®): 22 mcg/0.5 mL (0.5 mL) [prefilled syringe; contains albumin]; 44 mcg/0.5 mL (0.5 mL) [prefilled syringe; contains albumin]

Interferon Beta-1b (in ter FEER on BAY ta won bee)

U.S. Brand Names Betaseron®

Canadian Brand Names Betaseron®

Index Terms rIFN beta-1b

Pharmacologic Category Interferon

Use Treatment of relapsing forms of multiple sclerosis (MS); treatment of first clinical episode with MRI features consistent with MS

Restrictions An FDA-approved medication guide must be distributed when dispensing an outpatient prescription (new or refill) where this medication is to be used without direct supervision of a healthcare provider. Medication guide is available at http://www.berlex.com/html/products/pi/Betaseron_Medication_Guide.pdf.

Pregnancy Risk Factor C

Pregnancy Considerations A dose-related abortifacient activity was reported in Rhesus monkeys. There are no adequate and well-controlled studies in pregnant women. Treatment should be discontinued if a woman becomes pregnant, or plans to become pregnant during therapy.

Lactation Excretion in breast milk unknown/contraindicated

Contraindications Hypersensitivity to *E. coli*-derived products, natural or recombinant interferon beta, albumin human or any other component of the formulation

Warnings/Precautions Anaphylaxis has been reported rarely with use. Associated with a high incidence of flu-like adverse effects. Hepatotoxicity has been reported with beta interferons, including rare reports of hepatitis (autoimmune) and hepatic failure requiring transplant. Interferons have been associated with severe psychiatric adverse events (psychosis, mania, depression, suicidal behavior/ideation) in patients with and without previous psychiatric symptoms, avoid use in severe psychiatric disorders and use caution in patients with a history of depression; patients exhibiting symptoms of depression should be closely monitored and discontinuation of therapy should be considered. Use caution in patients with pre-existing cardiovascular disease, pulmonary disease, seizure disorders, renal impairment or hepatic impairment. Use caution in myelosuppression. Severe injection site reactions (necrosis) may occur, which may or may not heal with continued therapy; patient and/or caregiver competency in injection technique should be confirmed and periodically re-evaluated. Contains albumin, which may carry a remote risk of transmitting viral diseases. Safety and efficacy in patients <18 years of age have not been established.

Adverse Reactions Note: Flu-like syndrome (including at least two of the following - headache, fever, chills, malaise, diaphoresis, and myalgia) are reported in the majority of patients (60%) and decrease over time (average duration ~1 week).

>10%:

Cardiovascular: Peripheral edema (15%), chest pain (11%)

Central nervous system: Headache (57%), fever (36%), pain (51%), chills (25%), dizziness (24%), insomnia (24%)

Dermatologic: Rash (24%), skin disorder (12%)

Endocrine & metabolic: Metrorrhagia (11%)

Gastrointestinal: Nausea (27%), diarrhea (19%), abdominal pain (19%), constipation (20%), dyspepsia (14%)

Genitourinary: Urinary urgency (13%)

Hematologic: Lymphopenia (88%), neutropenia (14%), leukopenia (14%)

Local: Injection site reaction (85%), inflammation (53%), pain (18%)

Neuromuscular & skeletal: Weakness (61%), myalgia (27%), hypertonia (50%), myasthenia (46%), arthralgia (31%), incoordination (21%)

Miscellaneous: Flu-like syndrome (decreases over treatment course; 60%)

1% to 10%:

Cardiovascular: Palpitation (4%), vasodilation (8%), hypertension (7%), tachycardia (4%), peripheral vascular disorder (6%)

Central nervous system: Anxiety (10%), malaise (8%), nervousness (7%)

Dermatologic: Alopecia (4%)

Endocrine & metabolic: Menorrhagia (8%), dysmenorrhea (7%)

Gastrointestinal: Weight gain (7%)

Genitourinary: Impotence (9%), pelvic pain (6%), cystitis (8%), urinary frequency (7%), prostatic disorder (3%)

Hematologic: Lymphadenopathy (8%)

Hepatic: ALT increased >5x baseline (10%), AST increased >5x baseline (3%)

Local: Injection site necrosis (4% to 5%), edema (3%), mass (2%)

Neuromuscular & skeletal: Leg cramps (4%)

Respiratory: Dyspnea (7%)

Miscellaneous: Diaphoresis (8%), hypersensitivity (3%)

<1% (Limited to important or life-threatening): Anorexia, apnea, arrhythmia, ataxia, bronchospasm, capillary leak syndrome (in patients with pre-existing monoclonal gammopathy) , cardiac arrest, cardiomegaly, cardiomyopathy, cerebral hemorrhage, coma, confusion, delirium, depersonalization, depression, DVT, emotional lability, erythema nodosum, ethanol intolerance, exfoliative dermatitis, gamma GT increase, GI hemorrhage, hallucinations, heart failure, hematemesis, hepatic failure, hepatitis, hyperthyroidism, hyperuricemia, hypocalcemia, mania, MI, paresthesia, pericardial effusion, photosensitivity, pneumonia, pruritus, psychosis, pulmonary embolism, rash, seizure, sepsis, shock, skin discoloration, suicidal ideation, syncope, SIADH, thrombocytopenia, thyroid dysfunction, triglyceride increased, urinary tract infection, urosepsis, urticaria, vasculitis, vaginal hemorrhage, vomiting, weight loss

Drug Interactions

Avoid Concomitant Use There are no known interactions where it is recommended to avoid concomitant use.

Increased Effect/Toxicity

Interferon Beta-1b may increase the levels/effects of: Theophylline Derivatives; Zidovudine

Decreased Effect There are no known significant interactions involving a decrease in effect.

Stability Store at room temperature of 25°C (77°F); excursions permitted to 15°C to 30°C (59°F to 86°F). To reconstitute solution, inject 1.2 mL of diluent (provided); gently swirl to dissolve, do not shake. Reconstituted solution provides 0.25 mg/mL (8 million units). If not used immediately following reconstitution, refrigerate solution at 2°C to 8°C (36°F to 46°F) and use within 3 hours; do not freeze or shake solution.

Mechanism of Action Interferon beta-1b differs from naturally occurring human protein by a single amino acid substitution and the lack of carbohydrate side chains; mechanism in the treatment of MS is unknown; however, immunomodulatory effects attributed to interferon beta-1b include enhancement of suppressor T cell activity, reduction of proinflammatory cytokines, down-regulation of antigen presentation, and reduced trafficking of lymphocytes into the central nervous system. Improves MRI lesions, decreases relapse rate, and disease severity in patients with secondary progressive MS.

Pharmacodynamics/Kinetics Limited data due to small doses used

Half-life elimination: 8 minutes to 4.3 hours

Time to peak, serum: 1-8 hours

Dosage SubQ: **Note:** Gradual dose-titration, analgesics, and/or antipyretics may help decrease flu-like symptoms on treatment days:

Children <18 years: Not recommended

Adults: Initial: 0.0625 mg (2 million units; 0.25 mL) every other day; gradually increase dose by 0.0625 every 2 weeks

Target dose: 0.25 mg (8 million units; 1 mL) every other day

Administration Withdraw dose of reconstituted solution from the vial into a sterile syringe fitted with a 27-gauge needle and inject the solution subcutaneously; sites for self-injection include outer surface of the arms, abdomen, hips, and thighs. Rotate SubQ injection site. Patient should be well hydrated.

Monitoring Parameters Complete blood chemistries (including platelet count) and liver function tests are recommended at 1, 3, and 6 months following initiation of therapy and periodically thereafter. Thyroid function should be assessed every 6 months in patients with history of thyroid dysfunction.

Additional Information American Academy of Neurology and MS Council guidelines suggest that, based upon published data, 6 million units of Avonex® (interferon beta-1a) (30 mcg) is equivalent to approximately 7-9 million units of Betaseron® (220-280 mcg).

Dosage Forms Excipient information presented when available (limited, particularly for generics); consult specific product labeling.

Injection, powder for reconstitution [preservative free]:

Betaseron®: 0.3 mg [9.6 million units] [contains albumin; packaged with prefilled syringe containing diluent]

Interferon Gamma-1b

(in ter FEER on GAM ah won bee)

U.S. Brand Names Actimmune®

Canadian Brand Names Actimmune®

Pharmacologic Category Interferon

Use Reduce frequency and severity of serious infections associated with chronic granulomatous disease; delay time to disease progression in patients with severe, malignant osteopetrosis

Pregnancy Risk Factor C

Pregnancy Considerations Teratogenic effects were not observed in animal studies. A dose-related abortifacient activity was reported in Rhesus monkeys. Safety and efficacy in pregnant women has not been established.

Lactation Excretion in breast milk unknown/not recommended

Contraindications Hypersensitivity to interferon gamma, *E. coli* derived proteins, or any component of the formulation

Warnings/Precautions Hypersensitivity reactions have been reported (rarely). Transient cutaneous rashes may occur. Dose-related bone marrow toxicity has been reported; use caution in patients with myelosuppression. May cause hepatotoxicity and the incidence may be increased in children <1 year of age. Doses >10 times the weekly recommended dose (used in studies for unlabeled indications) have been associated with a different pattern/frequency of adverse effects. Flu-like symptoms which may exacerbate pre-existing cardiovascular disorders (including ischemia, HF, or arrhythmias) and the development of neurologic disorders have been noted at the higher doses. Caution should also be used in patients with seizure disorders or compromised CNS function.

Adverse Reactions Based on 50 mcg/m^2 dose administered 3 times weekly for chronic granulomatous disease

>10%:

Central nervous system: Fever (52%), headache (33%), chills (14%), fatigue (14%)

Dermatologic: Rash (17%)

Gastrointestinal: Diarrhea (14%), vomiting (13%)

Local: Injection site erythema or tenderness (14%)

1% to 10%:

Central nervous system: Depression (3%)

Gastrointestinal: Nausea (10%), abdominal pain (8%)

Neuromuscular & skeletal: Myalgia (6%), arthralgia (2%), back pain (2%)

Postmarketing and/or case reports: Alkaline phosphatase elevated, atopic dermatitis, granulomatous colitis, hepatomegaly, hypersensitivity reactions, hypokalemia, neutropenia, Stevens-Johnson syndrome

Additional adverse reactions noted at doses >100 mcg/m^2 administered 3 times weekly: ALT increased, AST increased, autoantibodies increased, bronchospasm, chest discomfort, confusion, dermatomyositis exacerbation, disorientation, DVT, gait disturbance, GI bleeding, hallucinations, heart block, heart failure, hepatic insufficiency, hyperglycemia, hypertriglyceridemia, hyponatremia, hypotension, interstitial pneumonitis, lupus-like syndrome, MI, neutropenia, pancreatitis (may be fatal), Parkinsonian symptoms, PE, proteinuria, renal insufficiency (reversible), seizure, syncope, tachyarrhythmia, tachypnea, thrombocytopenia, TIA

Drug Interactions

Metabolism/Transport Effects Inhibits CYP1A2 (weak), 2E1 (weak)

Avoid Concomitant Use There are no known interactions where it is recommended to avoid concomitant use.

Increased Effect/Toxicity

Interferon Gamma-1b may increase the levels/effects of: Theophylline Derivatives; Zidovudine

Decreased Effect There are no known significant interactions involving a decrease in effect.

Stability Store in refrigerator at 2°C to 8°C (36°F to 46°F); do not freeze. Do not shake. Discard if left unrefrigerated for >12 hours.

Mechanism of Action Interferon gamma participates in immunoregulation by enhancing the oxidative metabolism of macrophages; it also enhances antibody dependent cellular cytotoxicity, activates natural killer cells and has a role in the expression of Fc receptors and histocompatibility antigens. The exact mechanism of action for the treatment of chronic granulomatous disease or osteopetrosis has not been defined.

Pharmacodynamics/Kinetics

Absorption: I.M., SubQ: >89%

Half-life elimination: I.V.: 38 minutes; I.M.: ~3 hours, SubQ: ~6 hours

Time to peak, plasma: I.M.: 4 hours (1.5 ng/mL); SubQ: 7 hours (0.6 ng/mL)

Dosage If severe reactions occur, reduce dose by 50% or therapy should be interrupted until adverse reaction abates.

Children: Severe, malignant osteopetrosis: SubQ:

BSA ≤0.5 m^2: 1.5 mcg/kg/dose 3 times/week

BSA >0.5 m^2: 50 mcg/m^2 (1 million int. units/m^2) 3 times/week

Children and Adults: Chronic granulomatous disease: SubQ:

BSA ≤0.5 m^2: 1.5 mcg/kg/dose 3 times/week

BSA >0.5 m^2: 50 mcg/m^2 (1 million int. units/m^2) 3 times/week

Note: Previously expressed as 1.5 million units/m^2; 50 mcg is equivalent to 1 million int. units/m^2.

Administration Administer by SubQ injection into the right and left deltoid or anterior thigh.

Monitoring Parameters CBC with differential, platelets, LFTs (monthly in children <1 year), electrolytes, BUN, creatinine, and urinalysis prior to therapy and at 3-month intervals

Dosage Forms Excipient information presented when available (limited, particularly for generics); consult specific product labeling.

Injection, solution [preservative free]:

Actimmune®: 100 mcg [2 million int. units] (0.5 mL)

- **Interleukin-1 Receptor Antagonist** *see* Anakinra *on page 115*
- **Interleukin-2** *see* Aldesleukin *on page 53*
- **Interleukin-11** *see* Oprelvekin *on page 1106*
- **Intralipid®** *see* Fat Emulsion *on page 605*
- **Intrapleural Talc** *see* Talc (Sterile) *on page 1424*
- **Intravenous Fat Emulsion** *see* Fat Emulsion *on page 605*
- **Intrifiban** *see* Eptifibatide *on page 537*
- **Intron® A** *see* Interferon Alfa-2b *on page 801*

- **Intropin** *see* DOPamine *on page 479*
- **Invanz®** *see* Ertapenem *on page 543*
- **Invega®** *see* Paliperidone *on page 1130*
- **Inversine®** *see* Mecamylamine *on page 925*
- **Invirase®** *see* Saquinavir *on page 1353*

Iobenguane I 123

(eye oh BEN gwane eye one TWEN tee three)

U.S. Brand Names AdreView™

Index Terms 123 Meta-Iodobenzlyguanidine Sulfate; 123I-Metaiodobenzylguanidine (MIBG); I-123 MIBG; I^{123} Iobenguane; Iobenguane Sulfate I 123

Pharmacologic Category Radiopharmaceutical

Use As an adjunct to other diagnostic tests, in the detection of primary or metastatic pheochromocytoma or neuroblastoma

Pregnancy Risk Factor C

Dosage Note: Thyroid protective agents (SSKI, Lugol's solution or potassium iodide), should be given at least 1 hour prior to administration. Perform whole body planar scintigraphy imaging 18-30 hours after Iobenguane I 123 administration.

Radioimaging: I.V.:

Children 1 month to 16 years and <70 kg: Dose according to body weight; see table.

Children <16 years and ≥70 kg: 10 mCi (370 MBq)

Children ≥16 years and Adults: 10 mCi (370 MBq)

Iobenguane I 123 Pediatric Dosing by Body Weight

(Children 1 Month to 16 Years and <70 kg)

Weight (kg)	mCi Dose	MBq Dose
3	1	37
4	1.4	52
6	1.9	70
8	2.3	85.1
10	2.7	99.9
12	3.2	118.4
14	3.6	133.2
16	4	148
18	4.4	162.8
20	4.6	170.2
22	5	185
24	5.3	196.1
26	5.6	207.2
28	5.8	214.6
30	6.2	229.4
32	6.5	240.5
34	6.8	251.6
36	7.1	262.7
38	7.3	270.1
40	7.6	281.2
42	7.8	288.6
44	8	296
46	8.2	303.4
48	8.5	314.5
50	8.8	325.6
52-54	9	333
56-58	9.2	340.4
60-62	9.6	355.2
64-66	9.8	362.6
68	9.9	366.3

Additional Information Complete prescribing information for this medication should be consulted for additional detail.

Dosage Forms Excipient information presented when available (limited, particularly for generics); consult specific product labeling.

Injection, solution:

AdreView™: Iobenguane sulfate 0.08 mg and I 123 74 MBq (2 mCi) per mL (5 mL) [contains benzyl alcohol]

- **Iobenguane Sulfate I 123** *see* Iobenguane I 123 *on page 810*
- **Iodine I 131 Tositumomab and Tositumomab** *see* Tositumomab and Iodine I 131 Tositumomab *on page 1495*

Iodoquinol (eye oh doe KWIN ole)

U.S. Brand Names Yodoxin®

Canadian Brand Names Diodoquin®

Index Terms Diiodohydroxyquin

Pharmacologic Category Amebicide

Use Treatment of acute and chronic intestinal amebiasis; asymptomatic cyst passers; *Blastocystis hominis* infections; ineffective for amebic hepatitis or hepatic abscess

Pregnancy Risk Factor C

Dosage Oral:

Children: 30-40 mg/kg/day (maximum: 650 mg/dose) in 3 divided doses for 20 days; not to exceed 1.95 g/day

Adults: 650 mg 3 times/day after meals for 20 days; not to exceed 1.95 g/day

Additional Information Complete prescribing information for this medication should be consulted for additional detail.

Dosage Forms Excipient information presented when available (limited, particularly for generics); consult specific product labeling.

Tablet: 210 mg, 650 mg

Iodoquinol and Hydrocortisone

(eye oh doe KWIN ole & hye droe KOR ti sone)

U.S. Brand Names Alcortin™; Dermazene®; Vytone®

Index Terms Hydrocortisone and Iodoquinol

Pharmacologic Category Antifungal Agent, Topical; Corticosteroid, Topical

Use Treatment of eczema (including impetiginized, nuchal, and nummular); acne urticaria; anogenital pruritus, atopic dermatitis, chronic infectious dermatitis; chronic eczematoid otitis externa; folliculitis, intertrigo; lichen simplex chronicus; moniliasis; mycotic dermatoses; neurodermatitis (localized or systemic); pyoderma, stasis dermatitis

Pregnancy Risk Factor C

Medication Safety Issues

Sound-alike/look-alike issues:

Vytone® may be confused with Hytone®, Zydone®

Dosage Topical: Children ≥12 years and Adults: Apply 3-4 times/day

Additional Information Complete prescribing information for this medication should be consulted for additional detail.

Dosage Forms Excipient information presented when available (limited, particularly for generics); consult specific product labeling.

Cream: Iodoquinol 1% and hydrocortisone acetate 1% (30 g)

Dermazene®: Iodoquinol 1% and hydrocortisone acetate 1% (30 g, 45 g)

Vytone®: Iodoquinol 1% and hydrocortisone acetate 1% (30 g)

Gel, topical:
Alcortin™: Iodoquinol 1% and hydrocortisone 2% (2 g) [contains benzyl alcohol]

◆ **Ionamin®** *see* Phentermine *on page 1181*

◆ **Iopidine®** *see* Apraclonidine *on page 129*

◆ **Iosat™ [OTC]** *see* Potassium Iodide *on page 1218*

Ioxilan (eye OKS ee lan)

U.S. Brand Names Oxilan®

Canadian Brand Names Oxilan® 300; Oxilan® 350

Pharmacologic Category Iodinated Contrast Media; Radiological/Contrast Media, Nonionic (Low Osmolality)

Use

Intra-arterial: Ioxilan 300 mgI/mL is indicated for cerebral arteriography. Ioxilan 350 mgI/mL is indicated for coronary arteriography and left ventriculography, visceral angiography, aortography, and peripheral arteriography

Intravenous: Both products are indicated for excretory urography and contrast-enhanced computed tomographic (CECT) imaging of the head and body

Pregnancy Risk Factor B

Medication Safety Issues

High alert medication: The Institute for Safe Medication Practices (ISMP) includes this medication among its list of drugs which have a heightened risk of causing significant patient harm when used in error.

Dosage Adults:

Intra-arterial: Coronary arteriography and left ventriculography: For visualization of coronary arteries and left ventricle, ioxilan injection with a concentration of 350 mg iodine/mL is recommended

Usual injection volumes:

Left and right coronary: 2-10 mL (0.7-3.5 g iodine)

Left ventricle: 25-50 mL (8.75-17.5 g iodine)

Total doses should not exceed 250 mL; the injection rate of ioxilan should approximate the flow rate in the vessel injected

Cerebral arteriography: For evaluation of arterial lesions of the brain, a concentration of 300 mg iodine/mL is indicated

Recommended doses: 8-12 mL (2.4-3.6 g iodine)

Total dose should not exceed 150 mL

Additional Information Complete prescribing information for this medication should be consulted for additional detail.

Dosage Forms Excipient information presented when available (limited, particularly for generics); consult specific product labeling.

Injection, solution [preservative free]:

Oxilan® 300: 62% (50 mL, 100 mL, 150 mL, 200 mL) [provides organically-bound iodine 300 mg/mL; contains sodium 0.22 mg (0.01 mEq)/mL, edetate calcium disodium]

Oxilan® 350: 73% (50 mL, 100 mL, 150 mL, 200 mL) [provides organically- bound iodine 350 mg/mL; contains sodium 0.22 mg (0.01 mEq)/mL, edetate calcium disodium]

Ipecac Syrup (IP e kak SIR up)

Index Terms Syrup of Ipecac

Pharmacologic Category Antidote

Use Treatment of acute oral drug overdosage and in certain poisonings

Pregnancy Risk Factor C

Dosage Oral:

Children:

6-12 months: 5-10 mL followed by 10-20 mL/kg of water; repeat dose one time if vomiting does not occur within 20 minutes

1-12 years: 15 mL followed by 10-20 mL/kg of water; repeat dose one time if vomiting does not occur within 20 minutes

If emesis does not occur within 30 minutes after second dose, ipecac must be removed from stomach by gastric lavage

Adults: 15-30 mL followed by 200-300 mL of water; repeat dose one time if vomiting does not occur within 20 minutes

Additional Information Complete prescribing information for this medication should be consulted for additional detail.

Dosage Forms Excipient information presented when available (limited, particularly for generics); consult specific product labeling.

Syrup: 70 mg/mL (30 mL) [contains alcohol]

◆ **IPG-Citalopram (Can)** *see* Citalopram *on page 337*

◆ **Iplex™ [DSC]** *see* Mecasermin *on page 926*

◆ **IPM Wound Gel™ [OTC]** *see* Hyaluronate and Derivatives *on page 734*

◆ **IPOL®** *see* Poliovirus Vaccine (Inactivated) *on page 1207*

Ipratropium (i pra TROE pee um)

U.S. Brand Names Atrovent®; Atrovent® HFA

Canadian Brand Names Alti-Ipratropium; Apo-Ipravent®; Atrovent®; Atrovent® HFA; Gen-Ipratropium; Novo-Ipramide; Nu-Ipratropium; PMS-Ipratropium

Index Terms Ipratropium Bromide

Pharmacologic Category Anticholinergic Agent

Use

Oral inhalation: Anticholinergic bronchodilator used in bronchospasm associated with COPD, bronchitis, and emphysema

Nasal spray: Symptomatic relief of rhinorrhea associated with the common cold and allergic and nonallergic rhinitis

Unlabeled/Investigational Use Oral inhalation: Adjunct to short-acting beta-adrenergic agonists therapy in moderate-to-severe exacerbations of acute asthma in the emergency room

Pregnancy Risk Factor B

Pregnancy Considerations Teratogenic effects were not observed in animal studies.

Lactation Excretion in breast milk unknown/use caution

Medication Safety Issues

Sound-alike/look-alike issues:

Atrovent® may be confused with Alupent®, Serevent®

Contraindications Hypersensitivity to ipratropium, atropine (and its derivatives), or any component of the formulation

Warnings/Precautions Immediate hypersensitivity reactions (urticaria, angioedema, rash, bronchospasm) have been reported. Rarely, paradoxical bronchospasm may occur with use of inhaled bronchodilating agents; this should be distinguished from inadequate response. Not indicated for the initial treatment of acute episodes of bronchospasm where rescue therapy is required for rapid response. Should only be used in acute exacerbations of asthma in conjunction with short-acting beta-adrenergic agonists for acute episodes. Use with caution in patients with myasthenia gravis, narrow-angle glaucoma, benign prostatic hyperplasia (BPH), or bladder neck obstruction

Adverse Reactions

Inhalation aerosol and inhalation solution:

>10%: Respiratory: Upper respiratory tract infection (9% to 34%), bronchitis (10% to 23%), sinusitis (1% to 11%)

1% to 10%:

Cardiovascular: Chest pain (3%), palpitation

Central nervous system: Headache (6% to 7%), dizziness (2% to 3%)

Gastrointestinal: Dyspepsia (1% to 5%), nausea (4%), xerostomia (2% to 4%)

Genitourinary: Urinary tract infection (2% to 10%)

Neuromuscular & skeletal: Back pain (2% to 7%)

Respiratory: Dyspnea (7% to 10%), rhinitis (2% to 6%), cough (3% to 5%), pharyngitis (4%), bronchospasm (2%), sputum increased (1%)

Miscellaneous: Flu-like syndrome (4% to 8%)

<1% (Limited to important or life-threatening): Anaphylactic reaction, angioedema, arthritis, atrial fibrillation, bitter taste, constipation, diarrhea, eye pain (acute), glaucoma, hypersensitivity reactions, hypotension, insomnia, laryngospasm, mydriasis, nervousness, pruritus, rash, tachycardia (including supraventricular), tremor, urinary retention, urticaria

Nasal spray:

1% to 10%: Central nervous system: Headache (4% to 10%)

Gastrointestinal: Taste perversion (≤4%), xerostomia (1% to 4%), diarrhea (2%), nausea (2%)

Respiratory: Epistaxis (6% to 9%), pharyngitis (≤8%), upper respiratory tract infection (5% to 10%), nasal dryness (<1% to 5%), nasal irritation (2%), nasal congestion (1%)

<2% (Limited to important or life-threatening): Anaphylactic reaction, angioedema, blurred vision, conjunctivitis, cough, dizziness, hoarseness, laryngospasm, nasal burning, ocular irritation, palpitation, rash, tachycardia, thirst, tinnitus, urticaria, xerostomia

Drug Interactions

Avoid Concomitant Use There are no known interactions where it is recommended to avoid concomitant use.

Increased Effect/Toxicity

Ipratropium may increase the levels/effects of: Anticholinergics; Cannabinoids; Potassium Chloride

The levels/effects of Ipratropium may be increased by: Pramlintide

Decreased Effect

Ipratropium may decrease the levels/effects of: Acetylcholinesterase Inhibitors (Central); Secretin

The levels/effects of Ipratropium may be decreased by: Acetylcholinesterase Inhibitors (Central)

Stability

Oral inhalation aerosol and nasal spray: Store at controlled room temperature of 25°C (77°F). Do not store near heat or open flame.

Oral inhalation solution: Store at 15°C to 30°C (59°F to 86°F). Protect from light.

Mechanism of Action Blocks the action of acetylcholine at parasympathetic sites in bronchial smooth muscle causing bronchodilation; local application to nasal mucosa inhibits serous and seromucous gland secretions.

Pharmacodynamics/Kinetics

Onset of action: Bronchodilation: Within 15 minutes

Peak effect: 1-2 hours

Duration: 2-5 hours

Absorption: Negligible

Distribution: Inhalation: 15% of dose reaches lower airways

Protein Binding: ≤9%

Half-life elimination: 2 hours

Excretion: Urine

Dosage

Nebulization:

Children ≤12 years: Asthma exacerbation, acute (*NIH Asthma Guidelines, 2007*): 250-500 mcg every 20 minutes for 3 doses, then as needed. **Note:** Should be given in combination with a short-acting beta-adrenergic agonist.

Children >12 years and Adults:

Bronchodilator for COPD: 500 mcg (one unit-dose vial) 3-4 times/day with doses 6-8 hours apart

Asthma exacerbation, acute (*NIH Asthma Guidelines, 2007*): 500 mcg every 20 minutes for 3 doses, then as needed. **Note:** Should be given in combination with a short-acting beta-adrenergic agonist.

Oral inhalation: MDI:

Children ≤12 years: Asthma exacerbation, acute (*NIH Asthma Guidelines, 2007*): 4-8 inhalations every 20 minutes as needed for up to 3 hours. **Note:** Should be given in combination with a short-acting beta-adrenergic agonist.

Children >12 years and Adults:

Bronchodilator for COPD: 2 inhalations 4 times/day, up to 12 inhalations/24 hours

Asthma exacerbation, acute (*NIH Asthma Guidelines, 2007*): 8 inhalations every 20 minutes as needed for up to 3 hours. **Note:** Should be given in combination with a short-acting beta-adrenergic agonist.

Intranasal: Nasal spray:

Symptomatic relief of rhinorrhea associated with the common cold (safety and efficacy of use beyond 4 days in patients with the common cold have not been established):

Children 5-11 years: 0.06%: 2 sprays in each nostril 3 times/day

Children ≥12 years and Adults: 0.06%: 2 sprays in each nostril 3-4 times/day

Symptomatic relief of rhinorrhea associated with allergic/nonallergic rhinitis: Children ≥6 years and Adults: 0.03%: 2 sprays in each nostril 2-3 times/day

Symptomatic relief of rhinorrhea associated with seasonal allergic rhinitis (safety and efficacy of use beyond 3 weeks in patients with seasonal allergic rhinitis has not been established): Children ≥5 years and Adults: 0.06%: 2 sprays in each nostril 4 times/day

Administration Avoid spraying into the eyes.

Atrovent® HFA: Prior to initial use, prime inhaler by releasing 2 test sprays into the air. If the inhaler has not been used for >3 days, reprime.

Nasal spray: Prior to initial use, prime inhaler by releasing 7 test sprays into the air. If the inhaler has not been used for >24 hours, reprime by releasing 2 test sprays into the air.

Dosage Forms Excipient information presented when available (limited, particularly for generics); consult specific product labeling.

Aerosol for oral inhalation, as bromide:

Atrovent® HFA: 17 mcg/actuation (12.9 g)

Solution for nebulization, as bromide: 0.02% (2.5 mL)

Solution, intranasal, as bromide [spray]:

Atrovent®: 0.03% (30 mL); 0.06% (15 mL)

Ipratropium and Albuterol

(i pra TROE pee um & al BYOO ter ole)

U.S. Brand Names Combivent®; DuoNeb®

Canadian Brand Names CO Ipra-Sal; Combivent®; Gen-Combo Sterinebs; ratio-Ipra Sal UDV

Index Terms Albuterol and Ipratropium; Salbutamol and Ipratropium

Pharmacologic Category Bronchodilator

Use Treatment of COPD in those patients who are currently on a regular bronchodilator who continue to have bronchospasms and require a second bronchodilator

Pregnancy Risk Factor C

Medication Safety Issues

Sound-alike/look-alike issues:

Combivent® may be confused with Combivir®, Serevent®

International issues:

DuoNeb® may be confused with DuoTrav™ which is a brand name for travoprost/timolol combination product in Canada

Dosage Adults:

Aerosol for inhalation: 2 inhalations 4 times/day (maximum: 12 inhalations/24 hours)

Solution for nebulization: Initial: 3 mL every 6 hours (maximum: 3 mL every 4 hours)

Additional Information Complete prescribing information for this medication should be consulted for additional detail.

Dosage Forms Excipient information presented when available (limited, particularly for generics); consult specific product labeling.

Aerosol for oral inhalation:

Combivent®: Ipratropium bromide 18 mcg and albuterol sulfate 103 mcg per actuation (14.7 g) [contains chlorofluorocarbon, soya lecithin; 200 metered actuations]

Solution for nebulization: Ipratropium bromide 0.5 mg and albuterol base 2.5 mg per 3 mL (30s, 60s)

DuoNeb®: Ipratropium bromide 0.5 mg and albuterol base 2.5 mg per 3 mL (30s, 60s)

◆ **Ipratropium Bromide** *see* Ipratropium *on page 811*

◆ **I-Prin [OTC]** *see* Ibuprofen *on page 760*

◆ **Iproveratril Hydrochloride** *see* Verapamil *on page 1557*

◆ **IPV** *see* Poliovirus Vaccine (Inactivated) *on page 1207*

◆ **Iquix®** *see* Levofloxacin *on page 875*

Irbesartan (ir be SAR tan)

U.S. Brand Names Avapro®

Canadian Brand Names Avapro®

Pharmacologic Category Angiotensin II Receptor Blocker

Additional Appendix Information

Angiotensin Agents *on page 1632*

Use Treatment of hypertension alone or in combination with other antihypertensives; treatment of diabetic nephropathy in patients with type 2 diabetes mellitus (noninsulin dependent, NIDDM) and hypertension

Unlabeled/Investigational Use To slow the rate of progression of aortic-root dilation in pediatric patients with Marfan's syndrome

Pregnancy Risk Factor C (1st trimester); D (2nd and 3rd trimesters)

Pregnancy Considerations Medications which act on the renin-angiotensin system are reported to have the following fetal/neonatal effects: Hypotension, neonatal skull hypoplasia, anuria, renal failure, and death; oligohydramnios is also reported. These effects are reported to occur with exposure during the second and third trimesters. There are no adequate and well-controlled studies in pregnant women. **[U.S. Boxed Warning]: Based on human data, drugs that act on the angiotensin system can cause injury and death to the developing fetus when used in the second and third trimesters. Angiotensin receptor blockers should be discontinued as soon as possible once pregnancy is detected.**

Lactation Excretion in breast milk unknown/contraindicated

Medication Safety Issues

Sound-alike/look-alike issues:

Avapro® may be confused with Anaprox®

Contraindications Hypersensitivity to irbesartan or any component of the formulation

Warnings/Precautions **[U.S. Boxed Warning]: Based on human data, drugs that act on the angiotensin system can cause injury and death to the developing fetus when used in the second and third trimesters. Angiotensin receptor blockers should be discontinued as soon as possible once pregnancy is detected.** May cause hyperkalemia; avoid potassium supplementation unless specifically required by healthcare provider. May be associated with deterioration of renal function and/or increases in serum creatinine, particularly in patients with low renal blood flow (eg, renal artery stenosis, heart failure) whose glomerular filtration rate (GFR) is dependent on efferent arteriolar vasoconstriction by angiotensin II. Avoid use or use a much smaller dose in patients who are intravascularly volume-depleted; use caution in patients with unstented unilateral or bilateral renal artery stenosis. When unstented bilateral renal artery stenosis is present, use is generally avoided due to the elevated risk of deterioration in renal function unless possible benefits outweigh risks. AUCs of irbesartan (not the active metabolite) are about 50% greater in patients with Cl_{cr} <30 mL/minute and are doubled in hemodialysis patients. Safety and efficacy have not been established in pediatric patients <6 years of age.

Adverse Reactions Unless otherwise indicated, percentage of incidence is reported for patients with hypertension.

>10%: Endocrine & metabolic: Hyperkalemia (19%, diabetic nephropathy; rarely seen in HTN)

1% to 10%:

Cardiovascular: Orthostatic hypotension (5%, diabetic nephropathy)

Central nervous system: Fatigue (4%), dizziness (10%, diabetic nephropathy)

Gastrointestinal: Diarrhea (3%), dyspepsia (2%)

Respiratory: Upper respiratory infection (9%), cough (2.8% versus 2.7% in placebo)

<1% (Limited to important or life-threatening): Angina, angioedema, arrhythmia, cardiopulmonary arrest, conjunctivitis, depression, dyspnea, ecchymosis, edema, epistaxis, gout, heart failure, hepatitis, hypotension, jaundice, libido decreased, MI, orthostatic hypotension, paresthesia, sexual dysfunction, stroke, transaminases increased, urticaria. May be associated with worsening of renal function in patients dependent on renin-angiotensin-aldosterone system.

Drug Interactions

Metabolism/Transport Effects **Substrate** of CYP2C9 (minor); **Inhibits** CYP2C8 (moderate), 2C9 (moderate), 2D6 (weak), 3A4 (weak)

Avoid Concomitant Use There are no known interactions where it is recommended to avoid concomitant use.

Increased Effect/Toxicity

Irbesartan may increase the levels/effects of: ACE Inhibitors; Amifostine; CYP2C8 Substrates (High risk); CYP2C9 Substrates (High risk); Lithium; Potassium-Sparing Diuretics; RiTUXimab

The levels/effects of Irbesartan may be increased by: Diazoxide; Eplerenone; Fluconazole; Herbs (Hypotensive Properties); Potassium Salts; Prostacyclin Analogues; Trimethoprim

Decreased Effect

The levels/effects of Irbesartan may be decreased by: Herbs (Hypertensive Properties); Methylphenidate; Nonsteroidal Anti-Inflammatory Agents; Rifamycin Derivatives; Yohimbine

Ethanol/Nutrition/Herb Interactions Herb/Nutraceutical: Avoid dong quai if using for hypertension (has estrogenic activity). Avoid ephedra, yohimbe, ginseng (may worsen hypertension). Avoid garlic (may have increased antihypertensive effect).

Stability Store at room temperature of 15°C to 30°C (59°F to 86°F).

Mechanism of Action Irbesartan is an angiotensin receptor antagonist. Angiotensin II acts as a vasoconstrictor. In addition to causing direct vasoconstriction, angiotensin II also stimulates the release of aldosterone. Once aldosterone is released, sodium as well as water are reabsorbed. The end result is an elevation in blood pressure. Irbesartan binds to the AT1 angiotensin II receptor. This binding prevents angiotensin II from binding to the receptor thereby blocking the vasoconstriction and the aldosterone secreting effects of angiotensin II.

Pharmacodynamics/Kinetics

Onset of action: Peak effect: 1-2 hours
Duration: >24 hours
Distribution: V_d: 53-93 L
Protein binding, plasma: 90%
Metabolism: Hepatic, primarily CYP2C9
Bioavailability: 60% to 80%
Half-life elimination: Terminal: 11-15 hours
Time to peak, serum: 1.5-2 hours
Excretion: Feces (80%); urine (20%)

Dosage Oral:

Hypertension:
- Children:
  - <6 years: Safety and efficacy have not been established.
  - ≥6-12 years: Initial: 75 mg once daily; may be titrated to a maximum of 150 mg once daily
- Children ≥13 years and Adults: 150 mg once daily; patients may be titrated to 300 mg once daily
  - **Note:** Starting dose in volume-depleted patients should be 75 mg

Aortic-root dilation with Marfan's syndrome (unlabeled use): Children 14 months to 16 years: Initial: 1.4 mg/kg/day; can be increased to a maximum of 2 mg/kg/day (not to exceed adult maximum of 300 mg/day)

Nephropathy in patients with type 2 diabetes and hypertension: Adults: Target dose: 300 mg once daily

Dosage adjustment in renal impairment: No dosage adjustment necessary with mild to severe impairment unless the patient is also volume depleted.

Dietary Considerations May be taken with or without food.

Dosage Forms Excipient information presented when available (limited, particularly for generics); consult specific product labeling.

Tablet: 75 mg, 150 mg, 300 mg

Irbesartan and Hydrochlorothiazide
(ir be SAR tan & hye droe klor oh THYE a zide)

U.S. Brand Names Avalide®

Canadian Brand Names Avalide®

Index Terms Avapro® HCT; Hydrochlorothiazide and Irbesartan

Pharmacologic Category Angiotensin II Receptor Blocker; Diuretic, Thiazide

Use Combination therapy for the management of hypertension; may be used as initial therapy in patients likely to need multiple drugs to achieve blood pressure goals

Note: In Canada, this combination product is approved for initial therapy in severe, essential hypertension (sitting diastolic blood pressure [DBP] ≥110 mm Hg).

Pregnancy Risk Factor C/D (2nd and 3rd trimesters)

Medication Safety Issues

Sound-alike/look-alike issues:
- Avalide® may be confused with Avandia®

Dosage Oral: Adults:

Add-on therapy: Dose must be individualized. A patient who is not controlled with either agent alone may be switched to the combination product. Mean effect increases with the dose of each component. The lowest dosage available is irbesartan 150 mg/hydrochlorothiazide 12.5 mg. Dose increases should be made not more frequently than every 2-4 weeks.

Initial therapy: Irbesartan 150 mg/hydrochlorothiazide 12.5 mg once daily. If initial response is inadequate, may titrate dose after 2-4 weeks, to a maximum dose of irbesartan 300 mg/hydrochlorothiazide 25 mg once daily.

Dosing adjustment in renal impairment: Not recommended in patients with Cl_{cr} ≤30 mL/minute

Dosage adjustment in hepatic impairment: Use with caution

Additional Information Complete prescribing information for this medication should be consulted for additional detail.

Dosage Forms Excipient information presented when available (limited, particularly for generics); consult specific product labeling.

Tablet:
- Irbesartan 150 mg and hydrochlorothiazide 12.5 mg
- Irbesartan 300 mg and hydrochlorothiazide 12.5 mg
- Irbesartan 300 mg and hydrochlorothiazide 25 mg

◆ **Ircon® [OTC]** *see* Ferrous Fumarate *on page* 616

◆ **IRESSA®** *see* Gefitinib *on page* 683

Irinotecan (eye rye no TEE kan)

U.S. Brand Names Camptosar®

Canadian Brand Names Camptosar®; Irinotecan Hydrochloride Trihydrate

Index Terms Camptothecin-11; CPT-11; NSC-616348

Pharmacologic Category Antineoplastic Agent, Camptothecin; Antineoplastic Agent, Natural Source (Plant) Derivative

Use Treatment of metastatic carcinoma of the colon or rectum

Unlabeled/Investigational Use Lung cancer (small cell and nonsmall cell), cervical cancer, gastric cancer, pancreatic cancer, leukemia, lymphoma, breast cancer, brain tumors

Pregnancy Risk Factor D

Pregnancy Considerations Teratogenic effects were noted in animal studies. There are no adequate and well-controlled studies in pregnant women. Women of child-bearing potential should avoid becoming pregnant while receiving treatment.

Lactation Excretion in breast milk unknown/not recommended

Medication Safety Issues

High alert medication: The Institute for Safe Medication Practices (ISMP) includes this medication among its list of drug classes which have a heightened risk of causing significant patient harm when used in error.

Contraindications Hypersensitivity to irinotecan or any component of the formulation; concurrent use of ketoconazole, St John's wort

Warnings/Precautions Hazardous agent - use appropriate precautions for handling and disposal. Severe hypersensitivity reactions have occurred.

Patients with diarrhea should be carefully monitored and treated promptly. **[U.S. Boxed Warning]: Severe diarrhea may be dose-limiting and potentially fatal; two severe (life-threatening) forms of diarrhea may occur.** Early diarrhea occurs during or within 24 hours of receiving irinotecan and is characterized by cholinergic symptoms (eg, increased salivation, diaphoresis, abdominal cramping); it is usually responsive to atropine. Late diarrhea occurs more than 24 hours after treatment which may lead to dehydration, electrolyte imbalance, or sepsis; it should be promptly treated with loperamide. Colitis, complicated by ulceration, bleeding, ileus, and infection has been reported.

[U.S. Boxed Warning]: May cause severe myelosuppression. Deaths due to sepsis following severe myelosuppression have been reported. Therapy should be temporarily discontinued if neutropenic fever occurs or if the absolute neutrophil count is <1000/mm³. The dose of irinotecan should be reduced if there is a clinically significant decrease in the total WBC (<200/mm³), neutrophil count (<1500/mm³), hemoglobin (<8 g/dL), or platelet count (<100,000/mm³). Routine administration of a colony-stimulating factor is generally not necessary, but may be considered for patients experiencing significant neutropenia.

Patients with even modest elevations in total serum bilirubin levels (1-2 mg/dL) have a significantly greater likelihood of experiencing first-course grade 3 or 4 neutropenia than those with bilirubin levels that were <1 mg/dL. Patients with abnormal glucuronidation of bilirubin, such as those with Gilbert's syndrome, may also be at greater risk of myelosuppression when receiving therapy with irinotecan. Use caution when treating patients with known hepatic dysfunction or hyperbilirubinemia. Dosage adjustments should be considered.

Patients homozygous for the UGT1A1*28 allele are at increased risk of neutropenia; initial one-level dose reduction should be considered for both single-agent and combination regimens. Heterozygous carriers of the UGT1A1*28 allele may also be at increased risk; however, most patients have tolerated normal starting doses.

Renal impairment and acute renal failure have been reported, possibly due to dehydration secondary to diarrhea. Patients with bowel obstruction should not be treated with irinotecan until resolution of obstruction. Use caution in patients who previously received pelvic/abdominal radiation, elderly patients with comorbid conditions, or baseline performance status of 2; close monitoring and dosage adjustments are recommended. Contains sorbitol; do not use in patients with hereditary fructose intolerance. **[U.S. Boxed Warning]: Should be administered under the supervision of an experienced cancer chemotherapy physician.** Except as part of a clinical trial, use in combination with fluorouracil and leucovorin "Mayo Clinic" regimen is not recommended. Increased toxicity has also been noted in patients with a baseline performance status of 2 in other combination regimens containing irinotecan, leucovorin, and fluorouracil.

Adverse Reactions Frequency of adverse reactions reported for single-agent use of irinotecan only.

>10%:

Cardiovascular: Vasodilation (9% to 11%)

Central nervous system: Cholinergic toxicity (47% - includes rhinitis, increased salivation, miosis, lacrimation, diaphoresis, flushing and intestinal hyperperistalsis); fever (44% to 45%), pain (23% to 24%), dizziness (15% to 21%), insomnia (19%), headache (17%), chills (14%)

Dermatologic: Alopecia (46% to 72%), rash (13% to 14%)

Endocrine & metabolic: Dehydration (15%)

Gastrointestinal: Diarrhea, late (83% to 88%; grade 3/4: 5% to 31%), diarrhea, early (43% to 51%; grade 3/4: 6% to 22%), nausea (70% to 86%), abdominal pain (57% to 68%), vomiting (62% to 67%), cramps (57%), anorexia (44% to 55%), constipation (30% to 32%), mucositis (30%), weight loss (30%), flatulence (12%), stomatitis (12%)

Hematologic: Anemia (60% to 97%; grades 3/4: 5% to 22%), leukopenia (63% to 96%, grades 3/4: 14% to 28%), thrombocytopenia (96%, grades 3/4: 1% to 4%), neutropenia (30% to 96%; grades 3/4: 14% to 31%)

Hepatic: Bilirubin increased (84%), alkaline phosphatase increased (13%)

Neuromuscular & skeletal: Weakness (69% to 76%), back pain (14%)

Respiratory: Dyspnea (22%), cough (17% to 20%), rhinitis (16%)

Miscellaneous: Diaphoresis (16%), infection (14%)

1% to 10%:

Cardiovascular: Edema (10%), hypotension (6%), thromboembolic events (5%)

Central nervous system: Somnolence (9%), confusion (3%)

Gastrointestinal: Abdominal fullness (10%), dyspepsia (10%)

Hematologic: Neutropenic fever (grades 3/4: 2% to 6%), hemorrhage (grades 3/4: 1% to 5%), neutropenic infection (grades 3/4: 1% to 2%)

Hepatic: AST increased (10%), ascites and/or jaundice (grades 3/4: 9%)

Respiratory: Pneumonia (4%)

<1%, postmarketing, and/or case reports: ALT increased, amylase increased, anaphylactoid reaction, anaphylaxis, angina, arterial thrombosis, bleeding, bradycardia, cardiac arrest, cerebral infarct, cerebrovascular accident, circulatory failure, colitis, deep thrombophlebitis, dysrhythmia, embolus, gastrointestinal bleeding, gastrointestinal obstruction, hepatomegaly, hiccups, hyperglycemia, hypersensitivity, hyponatremia, ileus, interstitial lung disease, intestinal perforation, ischemic colitis, lipase increased, lymphocytopenia, megacolon, MI, muscle cramps, myocardial ischemia, pancreatitis, paresthesia, peripheral vascular disorder, pulmonary embolus; pulmonary toxicity (dyspnea, fever, reticulonodular infiltrates on chest x-ray); renal failure (acute), renal impairment, syncope, thrombophlebitis, thrombosis, typhlitis, ulceration, ulcerative colitis, vertigo

Note: In limited pediatric experience, dehydration (often associated with severe hypokalemia and hyponatremia) was among the most significant grade 3/4 adverse events, with a frequency up to 29%. In addition, grade 3/4 infection was reported in 24%.

Drug Interactions

Metabolism/Transport Effects Substrate (major) of CYP2B6, 3A4

Avoid Concomitant Use

Avoid concomitant use of Irinotecan with any of the following: Atazanavir; Natalizumab; St Johns Wort; Vaccines (Live)

Increased Effect/Toxicity

Irinotecan may increase the levels/effects of: Natalizumab; Vaccines (Live)

The levels/effects of Irinotecan may be increased by: Antifungal Agents (Azole Derivatives, Systemic); Atazanavir; Bevacizumab; CYP2B6 Inhibitors (Moderate); CYP2B6 Inhibitors (Strong); CYP3A4 Inhibitors (Moderate); CYP3A4 Inhibitors (Strong); Dasatinib; Eltrombopag; P-Glycoprotein Inhibitors; Sorafenib; Trastuzumab

Decreased Effect

Irinotecan may decrease the levels/effects of: Vaccines (Inactivated)

The levels/effects of Irinotecan may be decreased by: CYP2B6 Inducers (Strong); CYP3A4 Inducers (Strong); Deferasirox; Echinacea; P-Glycoprotein Inducers; Phenytoin; St Johns Wort

Ethanol/Nutrition/Herb Interactions Herb/Nutraceutical: Avoid St John's wort (decreases the efficacy of irinotecan).

Stability Store intact vials of injection at room temperature of 15°C to 30°C (59°F to 86°F). Protect from light. Doses should be diluted in 250-500 mL D_5W or NS to a final concentration of 0.12-2.8 mg/mL. Due to the relatively acidic pH, irinotecan appears to be more stable in D_5W than NS. Solutions diluted in D_5W are stable for 24 hours at room temperature or 48 hours under refrigeration at 2°C to 8°C. Solutions diluted in NS may precipitate if refrigerated. Do not freeze.

Mechanism of Action Irinotecan and its active metabolite (SN-38) bind reversibly to topoisomerase I-DNA complex preventing religation of the cleaved DNA strand. This results in the accumulation of cleavable complexes and double-strand DNA breaks. As mammalian cells cannot efficiently repair these breaks, cell death consistent with S-phase cell cycle specificity occurs, leading to termination of cellular replication.

Pharmacodynamics/Kinetics

Distribution: V_d: 33-150 L/m^2

Protein binding, plasma: Predominantly albumin; Parent drug: 30% to 68%, SN-38 (active metabolite): ~95%

Metabolism: Primarily hepatic to SN-38 (active metabolite) by carboxylesterase enzymes; SN-38 undergoes conjugation by UDP- glucuronosyl transferase 1A1 (UGT1A1) to form a glucuronide metabolite. Conversion of irinotecan to SN-38 is decreased and glucuronidation of SN-38 is increased patients who smoke cigarettes, resulting in lower levels of the metabolite and overall decreased systemic exposure. SN-38 is increased by UGT1A1*28 polymorphism (10% of North Americans are homozygous for UGT1A1*28 allele). The lactones of both irinotecan and SN-38 undergo hydrolysis to inactive hydroxy acid forms.

Half-life elimination: SN-38: Mean terminal: 10-20 hours

Time to peak: SN-38: Following 90-minute infusion: ~1 hour

Excretion: Within 24 hours: Urine: Irinotecan (11% to 20%), metabolites (SN-38 <1%, SN-38 glucuronide, 3%)

Dosage I.V. (Refer to individual protocols): **Note:** A reduction in the starting dose by one dose level should be considered for patients ≥65 years of age, prior pelvic/abdominal radiotherapy, performance status of 2, homozygosity for UGT1A1*28 allele, or increased bilirubin (dosing for patients with a bilirubin >2 mg/dL cannot be recommended based on lack of data per manufacturer).

Single-agent therapy:

125 mg/m^2 over 90 minutes on days 1, 8, 15, and 22 of a 6-week treatment cycle

Adjusted dose level -1: 100 mg/m^2

Adjusted dose level -2: 75 mg/m^2

Once-every-3-week regimen: 350 mg/m^2 over 90 minutes, once every 3 weeks

Adjusted dose level -1: 300 mg/m^2

Adjusted dose level -2: 250 mg/m^2

Depending on the patient's ability to tolerate therapy, doses should be adjusted in increments of 25-50 mg/m^2. Irinotecan doses may range from 50-150 mg/m^2 for the weekly regimen. Patients may be dosed as low as 200 mg/m^2 (in 50 mg/m^2 decrements) for the once-every-3-week regimen.

Combination therapy with fluorouracil and leucovorin:

Six-week (42-day) cycle:

Regimen 1: 125 mg/m^2 over 90 minutes on days 1, 8, 15, and 22; to be given in combination with bolus leucovorin and fluorouracil (leucovorin administered immediately following irinotecan; fluorouracil immediately following leucovorin)

Adjusted dose level -1: 100 mg/m^2

Adjusted dose level -2: 75 mg/m^2

Regimen 2: 180 mg/m^2 over 90 minutes on days 1, 15, and 29; to be given in combination with infusional leucovorin and bolus/infusion fluorouracil (leucovorin administered immediately following irinotecan; fluorouracil immediately following leucovorin)

Adjusted dose level -1: 150 mg/m^2

Adjusted dose level -2: 120 mg/m^2

Note: For all regimens: It is recommended that new courses begin only after the granulocyte count recovers to ≥1500/mm^3, the platelet count recovers to ≥100,000/mm^3, and treatment-related diarrhea has fully resolved. Treatment should be delayed 1-2 weeks to allow for recovery from treatment-related toxicities. If the patient has not recovered after a 2-week delay, consideration should be given to discontinuing irinotecan.

Dosing adjustment in renal impairment: Effects have not been evaluated; not recommended for use in patients on dialysis

Dosing adjustment in hepatic impairment: The manufacturer recommends that no change in dosage or administration be made for patients with liver metastases and normal hepatic function.

Consideration may be given to starting irinotecan at a lower dose (eg, 100 mg/m^2) if bilirubin is 1-2 mg/dL; for total serum bilirubin elevations >2 mg/dL, specific recommendations are not available in the FDA labeling. The following guidelines have been used by some clinicians:

Bilirubin 1.5-3 mg/dL: Administer 75% of dose (Floyd, 2006).

Dosage adjustment for toxicities: It is recommended that new courses begin only after the granulocyte count recovers to ≥1500/mm^3, the platelet counts recovers to ≥100,000/mm^3, and treatment-related diarrhea has fully resolved. Depending on the patient's ability to tolerate therapy, doses should be adjusted in increments of 25-50 mg/m^2. Treatment should be delayed 1-2 weeks to allow for recovery from treatment-related toxicities. If the patient has not recovered after a 2-week delay, consideration should be given to discontinuing irinotecan. See tables on next page.

Dietary Considerations Contains sorbitol; do not use in patients with hereditary fructose intolerance.

Administration Administer by I.V. infusion, usually over 90 minutes.

Monitoring Parameters CBC with differential, platelet count, and hemoglobin with each dose; bilirubin, electrolytes (with severe diarrhea); bowel movements and hydration status; monitor infusion site for signs of inflammation and avoid extravasation

Additional Information Patients who are homozygous for the UGT1A1*28 allele are at increased risk for neutropenia; a decreased dose is recommended. Clinical research of patients who are heterozygous for UGT1A1*28 have been variable for increased neutropenic risk and such patients have tolerated normal starting doses. An FDA-approved test (Invader® Molecular Assay) is available for clinical determination of UGT phenotype.

The recommended regimen to manage late diarrhea is loperamide 4 mg orally at onset of late diarrhea, followed by 2 mg every 2 hours (or 4 mg every 4 hours at night) until 12 hours have passed without a bowel movement. If diarrhea recurs, then repeat administration. Loperamide should not be used for more than 48 consecutive hours.

Dosage Forms Excipient information presented when available (limited, particularly for generics); consult specific product labeling.

Injection, solution, as hydrochloride: 20 mg/mL (2 mL, 5 mL)

Camptosar®: 20 mg/mL (2 mL, 5 mL) [contains sorbitol 45 mg/mL]

Single-Agent Schedule: Recommended Dosage Modifications[1]

Toxicity NCI Grade[2] (Value)	During a Cycle of Therapy	At Start of Subsequent Cycles of Therapy (After Adequate Recovery), Compared to Starting Dose in Previous Cycle[1]	
	Weekly	Weekly	Once Every 3 Weeks
No toxicity	Maintain dose level	↑ 25 mg/m^2 up to a maximum dose of 150 mg/m^2	Maintain dose level
Neutropenia			
1 (1500-1999/ mm^3)	Maintain dose level	Maintain dose level	Maintain dose level
2 (1000-1499/ mm^3)	↓ 25 mg/m^2	Maintain dose level	Maintain dose level
3 (500-999/ mm^3)	Omit dose until resolved to ≤ grade 2, then ↓ 25 mg/m^2	↓ 25 mg/m^2	↓ 50 mg/m^2
4 (<500/mm^3)	Omit dose until resolved to ≤ grade 2, then ↓ 50 mg/m^2	↓ 50 mg/m^2	↓ 50 mg/m^2
Neutropenic Fever (grade 4 neutropenia and ≥ grade 2 fever)	Omit dose until resolved, then ↓ 50 mg/m^2	↓ 50 mg/m^2	↓ 50 mg/m^2
Other Hematologic Toxicities	Dose modifications for leukopenia, thrombocytopenia, and anemia during a course of therapy and at the start of subsequent courses of therapy are also based on NCI toxicity criteria and are the same as recommended for neutropenia above.		
Diarrhea			
1 (2-3 stools/ day > pretreatment)	Maintain dose level	Maintain dose level	Maintain dose level
2 (4-6 stools/ day > pretreatment)	↓ 25 mg/m^2	Maintain dose level	Maintain dose level
3 (7-9 stools/ day > pretreatment)	Omit dose until resolved to ≤ grade 2, then ↓ 25 mg/m^2	↓ 25 mg/m^2	↓ 50 mg/m^2
4 (≥10 stools/ day > pretreatment)	Omit dose until resolved to ≤ grade 2, then ↓ 50 mg/m^2	↓ 50 mg/m^2	↓ 50 mg/m^2
Other Nonhematologic Toxicities[3]			
1	Maintain dose level	Maintain dose level	Maintain dose level
2	↓ 25 mg/m^2	↓ 25 mg/m^2	↓ 50 mg/m^2
3	Omit dose until resolved to ≤ grade 2, then ↓ 25 mg/m^2	↓ 25 mg/m^2	↓ 50 mg/m^2
4	Omit dose until resolved to ≤ grade 2, then ↓ 50 mg/m^2	↓ 50 mg/m^2	↓ 50 mg/m^2

[1]All dose modifications should be based on the worst preceding toxicity.

[2]National Cancer Institute Common Toxicity Criteria (version 1.0).

[3]Excludes alopecia, anorexia, asthenia.

Combination Schedules: Recommended Dosage Modifications[1]

Toxicity NCI[2] Grade (Value)	During a Cycle of Therapy	At the Start of Subsequent Cycles of Therapy (After Adequate Recovery), Compared to the Starting Dose in the Previous Cycle[1]
No toxicity	Maintain dose level	Maintain dose level
Neutropenia		
1 (1500-1999/ mm^3)	Maintain dose level	Maintain dose level
2 (1000-1499/ mm^3)	↓ 1 dose level	Maintain dose level
3 (500-999/ mm^3)	Omit dose until resolved to ≤ grade 2, then ↓ 1 dose level	↓ 1 dose level
4 (<500/mm^3)	Omit dose until resolved to ≤ grade 2, then ↓ 2 dose levels	↓ 2 dose levels
Neutropenic Fever (grade 4 neutropenia and ≥ grade 2 fever)	Omit dose until resolved, then ↓ 2 dose levels	
Other Hematologic Toxicities	Dose modifications for leukopenia or thrombocytopenia during a course of therapy and at the start of subsequent courses of therapy are also based on NCI toxicity criteria and are the same as recommended for neutropenia above.	
Diarrhea		
1 (2-3 stools/ day > pretreatment)	Delay dose until resolved to baseline, then give same dose	Maintain dose level
2 (4-6 stools/ day > pretreatment)	Omit dose until resolved to baseline, then ↓ 1 dose level	Maintain dose level
3 (7-9 stools/ day > pretreatment)	Omit dose until resolved to baseline, then ↓ by 1 dose level	↓ 1 dose level
4 (≥10 stools/ day > pretreatment)	Omit dose until resolved to baseline, then ↓ 2 dose levels	↓ 2 dose levels
Other Nonhematologic Toxicities[3]		
1	Maintain dose level	Maintain dose level
2	Omit dose until resolved to ≤ grade 1, then ↓ 1 dose level	Maintain dose level
3	Omit dose until resolved to ≤ grade 2, then ↓ 1 dose level	↓ 1 dose level
4	Omit dose until resolved to ≤ grade 2, then ↓ 2 dose levels	↓ 2 dose levels
Mucositis and/ or stomatitis	Decrease only 5-FU, not irinotecan	Decrease only 5-FU, not irinotecan

[1]All dose modifications should be based on the worst preceding toxicity.

[2]National Cancer Institute Common Toxicity Criteria (version 1.0).

[3]Excludes alopecia, anorexia, asthenia.

◆ **Irinotecan Hydrochloride Trihydrate (Can)** *see* Irinotecan *on page 814*

◆ **Iron Dextran** *see* Iron Dextran Complex *on page 817*

Iron Dextran Complex

(EYE ern DEKS tran KOM pleks)

U.S. Brand Names Dexferrum®; INFeD®

Canadian Brand Names Dexiron™; Infufer®

Index Terms High-Molecular-Weight Iron Dextran (DexFerrum®); Imferon; Iron Dextran; Low-Molecular-Weight Iron Dextran (INFeD®)

Pharmacologic Category Iron Salt

Use Treatment of iron deficiency in patients in whom oral administration is infeasible or ineffective

Pregnancy Risk Factor C

Pregnancy Considerations Adverse events have been observed in animal reproduction studies. It is not known if iron dextran (as iron dextran) crosses the placenta. It is recommended that pregnant women meet the dietary requirements of iron with diet and/or supplements in order to prevent adverse events associated with iron deficiency anemia in pregnancy. Treatment of iron deficiency anemia in pregnant women is the same as in nonpregnant women and in most cases, oral iron preparations may be used. Except in severe cases of maternal anemia, the fetus achieves normal iron stores regardless of maternal concentrations.

Lactation Enters breast milk/use caution

Medication Safety Issues

Sound-alike/look-alike issues:

Dexferrum® may be confused with Desferal®

Contraindications Hypersensitivity to iron dextran or any component of the formulation; any anemia not associated with iron deficiency

Warnings/Precautions [U.S. Boxed Warning]: Deaths associated with parenteral administration following anaphylactic-type reactions have been reported. Adverse events (including life-threatening) associated with iron dextran usually occur with the high-molecular-weight formulation (DexFerrum®), compared to low-molecular-weight (INFeD®) (Chertow, 2006). A test dose of 0.5 mL I.V. or I.M. should be given to observe for adverse reactions. Delayed (1-2 days) infusion reaction (including arthralgia, back pain, chills, dizziness, and fever) may occur with large doses (eg, total dose infusion) of I.V. iron dextran; usually subsides within 3-4 days. Delayed reaction may also occur (less commonly) with I.M. administration; subsiding within 3-7 days. Use with caution in patients with a history of significant allergies, asthma, serious hepatic impairment, pre-existing cardiac disease (may exacerbate cardiovascular complications), and rheumatoid arthritis (may exacerbate joint pain and swelling). Avoid use during acute kidney infection.

In patients with chronic kidney disease (CKD) requiring iron supplementation, the I.V. route is preferred for hemodialysis patients; either oral iron or I.V. iron may be used for nondialysis and peritoneal dialysis CKD patients. In patients with cancer-related anemia (either due to cancer or chemotherapy-induced) requiring iron supplementation, the I.V. route is superior to oral therapy; I.M. administration is not recommended for parenteral iron supplementation.

Use only in patients where the iron deficient state is not amenable to oral iron therapy. Discontinue oral iron prior to initiating parenteral iron therapy. Exogenous hemosiderosis may result from excess iron stores; patients with refractory anemias and/or hemoglobinopathies may be prone to iron overload with unwarranted iron supplementation. Anemia in the elderly is often caused by "anemia of chronic disease" or associated with inflammation rather than blood loss. Iron stores are usually normal or increased, with a serum ferritin >50 ng/mL and a decreased total iron binding capacity. I.V. administration of iron dextran is often preferred over I.M. in the elderly secondary to a decreased muscle mass and the need for daily injections. Intramuscular injections of iron-carbohydrate complexes may have a risk of delayed injection site tumor development. Not recommended in children <4 months of age. Intramuscular iron dextran use in neonates may be associated with an increased incidence of gram-negative sepsis.

Adverse Reactions Frequency not defined. **Note:** Adverse event risk is reported to be higher with the high-molecular-weight iron dextran formulation.

Cardiovascular: Arrhythmia, bradycardia, cardiac arrest, chest pain, chest tightness, cyanosis, flushing, hyper-/hypotension, shock, syncope, tachycardia

Central nervous system: Chills, disorientation, dizziness, fever, headache, malaise, seizure, unconsciousness, unresponsiveness

Dermatologic: Pruritus, purpura, rash, urticaria

Gastrointestinal: Abdominal pain, diarrhea, nausea, taste alteration, vomiting

Genitourinary: Discoloration of urine

Hematologic: Leukocytosis, lymphadenopathy

Local: Injection site reactions (cellulitis, inflammation, pain, phlebitis, soreness, swelling), muscle atrophy/fibrosis (with I.M. injection), skin/tissue staining (at the site of I.M. injection), sterile abscess

Neuromuscular & skeletal: Arthralgia, arthritis/arthritis exacerbation, back pain, myalgia, paresthesia, weakness

Respiratory: Bronchospasm, dyspnea, respiratory arrest, wheezing

Renal: Hematuria

Miscellaneous: Anaphylactic reactions (sudden respiratory difficulty, cardiovascular collapse), diaphoresis

Postmarketing and/or case reports: Angioedema, tumor formation (at former injection site)

Drug Interactions

Avoid Concomitant Use

Avoid concomitant use of Iron Dextran Complex with any of the following: Dimercaprol

Increased Effect/Toxicity

The levels/effects of Iron Dextran Complex may be increased by: Dimercaprol

Decreased Effect

Iron Dextran Complex may decrease the levels/effects of: Cefdinir; Eltrombopag; Phosphate Supplements; Trientine

The levels/effects of Iron Dextran Complex may be decreased by: Trientine

Stability Store at controlled room temperature. Solutions for infusion should be diluted in 250-1000 mL NS.

Mechanism of Action The released iron, from the plasma, eventually replenishes the depleted iron stores in the bone marrow where it is incorporated into hemoglobin

Pharmacodynamics/Kinetics

Onset of action: I.V.: Serum ferritin peak: 7-9 days after dose

Absorption:

I.M.: 50% to 90% is promptly absorbed, balance is slowly absorbed over month

I.V.: Uptake of iron by the reticuloendothelial system appears to be constant at about 10-20 mg/hour

Excretion: Urine and feces via reticuloendothelial system

Dosage I.M. (INFeD®; Z-track method should be used for I.M. injection), I.V. (Dexferrum®, INFeD®):

A 0.5 mL test dose (0.25 mL in infants) should be given prior to starting iron dextran therapy; total dose should be divided into a daily schedule for I.M., total dose may be given as a single continuous infusion. Individual doses of ≤2 mL may be administered daily until calculated total dose is received.

Iron-deficiency anemia:

Children 5-15 kg: Should not normally be given in the first 4 months of life:

Dose (mL) = 0.0442 (desired hemoglobin - observed hemoglobin) x W + (0.26 x W)

Desired hemoglobin: Usually 12 g/dL

W = Total body weight in kg

Children >15 kg and Adults:

Dose (mL) = 0.0442 (desired hemoglobin - observed hemoglobin) x LBW + (0.26 x LBW)

Desired hemoglobin: Usually 14.8 g/dL

LBW = Lean body weight in kg

Iron replacement therapy for blood loss: Replacement iron (mg) = blood loss (mL) x hematocrit

Cancer-associated anemia (NCCN guidelines v.3.2009): Adults: I.V.: Test dose: 25 mg slow I.V. slow push, followed 1 hour later by 100 mg over 5 minutes; larger doses (unlabeled), up to total dose infusion (over several hours) may be administered

Maximum daily dosage: Manufacturer's labeling: **Note:** Replacement of larger estimated iron deficits may be achieved by serial administration of smaller incremental dosages. Daily dosages should be limited to:

Children:

<5 kg: 25 mg iron (0.5 mL)

5-10 kg: 50 mg iron (1 mL)

Children ≥10 kg and Adults: 100 mg iron (2 mL)

Total dose infusion (unlabeled): The entire dose (estimated iron deficit) may be diluted and administered as a one-time I.V. infusion.

Administration Note: Test dose: A test dose should be given on the first day of therapy; patient should be observed for 1 hour for hypersensitivity reaction, then the remaining dose (dose minus test dose) should be given. Epinephrine should be available.

I.M. (INFeD®): Use Z-track technique (displacement of the skin laterally prior to injection); injection should be deep into the upper outer quadrant of buttock; alternate buttocks with subsequent injections. Administer test dose at same recommended site using the same technique.

I.V.: Test dose should be given gradually over at least 30 seconds (INFeD®) or 5 minutes (Dexferrum®). Subsequent dose(s) may be administered by I.V. bolus undiluted at a rate not to exceed 50 mg/minute or diluted in 250-1000 mL NS and infused over 1-6 hours (initial 25 mL should be given slowly and patient should be observed for allergic reactions); avoid dilutions with dextrose (increased incidence of local pain and phlebitis)

Monitoring Parameters Hemoglobin, hematocrit, reticulocyte count, serum ferritin, serum iron, TIBC; monitor for anaphylaxis/hypersensitivity reaction

Reference Range

Hemoglobin: Adults:

Males: 13.5-16.5 g/dL

Females: 12.0-15.0 g/dL

Serum iron: 40-160 mcg/dL

Total iron binding capacity: 230-430 mcg/dL

Transferrin: 204-360 mg/dL

Percent transferrin saturation: 20% to 50%

Test Interactions May cause falsely elevated values of serum bilirubin and falsely decreased values of serum calcium. Residual iron dextran may remain in reticuloendothelial cells; may affect accuracy of examination of bone marrow iron stores. Bone scans with 99m Tc-labeled bone seeking agents may show reduced bony uptake, marked renal activity, and excess blood pooling and soft tissue accumulation following I.V. iron dextran infusion or with high serum ferritin levels. Following I.M. iron dextran, bone scans with 99m Tc-diphosphonate may show dense activity in the buttocks.

Dosage Forms Excipient information presented when available (limited, particularly for generics); consult specific product labeling.

Note: Strength expressed as elemental iron

Injection, solution:

Dexferrum®: 50 mg/mL (1 mL, 2 mL) [high-molecular-weight iron dextran]

INFeD®: 50 mg/mL (2 mL) [low-molecular-weight iron dextran]

◆ **Iron Fumarate** *see* Ferrous Fumarate *on page 616*

◆ **Iron Gluconate** *see* Ferrous Gluconate *on page 616*

◆ **Iron-Polysaccharide Complex** *see* Polysaccharide-Iron Complex *on page 1212*

Iron Sucrose (EYE ern SOO krose)

U.S. Brand Names Venofer®

Canadian Brand Names Venofer®

Pharmacologic Category Iron Salt

Use Treatment of iron-deficiency anemia in chronic renal failure, including nondialysis-dependent patients (with or without erythropoietin therapy) and dialysis-dependent patients receiving erythropoietin therapy

Pregnancy Risk Factor B

Pregnancy Considerations Teratogenic effects were not observed in animal studies. There are no adequate and well-controlled studies in pregnant women. Based on limited data, iron sucrose may be effective for the treatment of iron-deficiency anemia in pregnancy. It is recommended that pregnant women meet the dietary requirements of iron with diet and/or supplements in order to prevent adverse events associated with iron deficiency anemia in pregnancy. Treatment of iron deficiency anemia in pregnant women is the same as in nonpregnant women and in most cases, oral iron preparations may be used. Except in severe cases of maternal anemia, the fetus achieves normal iron stores regardless of maternal concentrations.

Lactation Excretion in breast milk unknown/use caution

Contraindications Hypersensitivity to iron sucrose or any component of the formulation; evidence of iron overload; anemia not caused by iron deficiency

Warnings/Precautions Hypersensitivity reactions, including rare postmarketing anaphylactic and anaphylactoid reactions, have been reported. Hypotension has been reported frequently in hemodialysis-dependent patients. Hypotension has also been reported in peritoneal dialysis and nondialysis patients. Hypotension may be related to total dose or rate of administration (avoid rapid I.V. injection), follow recommended guidelines. Withhold iron in the presence of tissue iron overload; periodic monitoring of hemoglobin, hematocrit, serum ferritin, and transferrin saturation is recommended. Not FDA-approved for use in children.

Adverse Reactions

>10%:

Cardiovascular: Hypotension (1% to 7%; 39% in hemodialysis patients; may be related to total dose or rate of administration), peripheral edema (2% to 13%)

Central nervous system: Headache (3% to 13%)

Gastrointestinal: Nausea (1% to 15%)

Neuromuscular & skeletal: Muscle cramps (1% to 3%; 29% in hemodialysis patients)

1% to 10%:

Cardiovascular: Hypertension (6% to 8%), edema (1% to 7%), chest pain (1% to 6%), murmur (<1% to 3%), heart failure

Central nervous system: Dizziness (1% to 10%), fatigue (2% to 5%), fever (1% to 3%)

Dermatologic: Pruritus (1% to 7%), rash (≤1%)

Endocrine & metabolic: Gout (2% to 7%), hypoglycemia (<1% to 4%), hyperglycemia (3% to 4%), fluid overload (1% to 3%)

Gastrointestinal: Diarrhea (1% to 10%), vomiting (3% to 9%), taste perversion (1% to 9%), peritoneal infection (≤8%), constipation (1% to 7%), abdominal pain (1% to 4%), positive fecal occult blood (1% to 3%)

Genitourinary: Urinary tract infection (≤1%)

Local: Injection site reaction (2% to 4%), catheter site infection (≤4%)

Neuromuscular & skeletal: Muscle pain (1% to 7%), extremity pain (3% to 6%), arthralgia (1% to 4%), weakness (1% to 3%), back pain (1% to 3%)

Ocular: Conjunctivitis (<1% to 3%)

Otic: Ear pain (1% to 7%)

Respiratory: Dyspnea (1% to 10%), pharyngitis (<1% to 7%), cough (1% to 7%), sinusitis (1% to 4%), nasopharyngitis (≤3%), upper respiratory infection (1% to 3%), nasal congestion (1%), rhinitis (≤1%)

Miscellaneous: Graft complication (1% to 10%), sepsis

<1% (Limited to important or life-threatening): Anaphylactoid reactions, anaphylactic shock, bronchospasm (with dyspnea), collapse, facial rash, hypersensitivity (including wheezing),hypoesthesia, loss of consciousness, necrotizing enterocolitis (reported in premature infants, no causal relationship established), seizure, urticaria

Drug Interactions

Avoid Concomitant Use

Avoid concomitant use of Iron Sucrose with any of the following: Dimercaprol

Increased Effect/Toxicity

The levels/effects of Iron Sucrose may be increased by: Dimercaprol

Decreased Effect

Iron Sucrose may decrease the levels/effects of: Cefdinir; Eltrombopag; Phosphate Supplements; Trientine

The levels/effects of Iron Sucrose may be decreased by: Trientine

Stability Store vials at controlled room temperature of 25°C (77°F); do not freeze. May be administered via the dialysis line as an undiluted solution or by diluting 100 mg (5 mL) in a maximum of 100 mL normal saline. Doses ≥200mg should be diluted in a maximum of 250 mL normal saline. Following dilution, solutions are stable for 48 hours at room temperature or under refrigeration.

Mechanism of Action Iron sucrose is dissociated by the reticuloendothelial system into iron and sucrose. The released iron increases serum iron concentrations and is incorporated into hemoglobin.

Pharmacodynamics/Kinetics

Distribution: V_{dss}: Healthy adults: 7.9 L

Metabolism: Dissociated into iron and sucrose by the reticuloendothelial system

Half-life elimination: Healthy adults: 6 hours

Excretion: Healthy adults: Urine (5%) within 24 hours

Dosage Doses expressed in mg of **elemental** iron. **Note:** Test dose: Product labeling does not indicate need for a test dose in product-naive patients.

Children ≥2 years (unlabeled use): Iron-deficiency anemia in chronic renal disease (hemodialysis-dependent patients): I.V.:

Correction: 1 mg/kg/dose per dialysis session (maximum: 100 mg)

Maintenance therapy: 0.3 mg/kg/dose per dialysis session (maximum: 100 mg). **Note:** Dosing based on limited data from a study (Leijn, 2004); study used only 14 patients (2-14 years of age) with ESRD on hemodialysis. Study initially used an iron repletion dose of 3 mg/kg/dose per dialysis session which resulted in possible iron overload (ferritin >400 mcg/L); protocol dose subsequently lowered to 1 mg/kg/dose per dialysis session which resulted in a gradual increase in ferritin levels >100 mcg/L; maintenance therapy resulted in median ferritin levels between 193-250 mcg/L.

Adults: Iron-deficiency anemia in chronic renal disease: I.V.:

Hemodialysis-dependent patient: 100 mg over 2-5 minutes administered 1-3 times/week during dialysis; administer no more than 3 times/week to a cumulative total dose of 1000 mg (10 doses); may continue to administer at lowest dose necessary to maintain target hemoglobin, hematocrit, and iron storage parameters

Peritoneal dialysis-dependent patient: Slow intravenous infusion at the following schedule: Two infusions of 300 mg each over 1½ hours 14 days apart followed by a single 400 mg infusion over 2½ hours 14 days later (total cumulative dose of 1000 mg in 3 divided doses)

Nondialysis-dependent patient: 200 mg slow injection (over 2-5 minutes) on 5 different occasions within a 14-day period. Total cumulative dose: 1000 mg in 14-day period. **Note:** Dosage has also been administered as two infusions of 500 mg in a maximum of 250 mL 0.9% NaCl infused over 3.5-4 hours on day 1 and day 14 (limited experience)

Elderly: Insufficient data to identify differences between elderly and other adults; use caution

Administration Not for rapid I.V. injection; inject slowly over 2-5 minutes. Can be administered through dialysis line. Do not mix with other medications or parenteral nutrient solutions.

Slow I.V. injection: May administer undiluted by slow I.V. injection (100 mg over 2-5 minutes in hemodialysis-dependent patients **or** 200 mg over 2-5 minutes in nondialysis-dependent patients)

Infusion: Dilute 100 mg in maximum of 100 mL 0.9% NaCl; infuse over at least 15 minutes; 300 mg/250 mL should be infused over at least 1½ hours; 400 mg/250 mL should be infused over at least 2½ hours; 500 mg/250 mL should be infused over at least 3½ hours.

Monitoring Parameters Hematocrit, hemoglobin, serum ferritin, transferrin, percent transferrin saturation, TIBC; takes about 4 weeks of treatment to see increased serum iron and ferritin, and decreased TIBC. Serum iron concentrations should be drawn 48 hours after last dose.

Reference Range

Hemoglobin: Adults:

Males: 13.5-16.5 g/dL

Females: 12.0-15.0 g/dL

Serum iron: 40-160 mcg/dL

Total iron binding capacity: 230-430 mcg/dL

Transferrin: 204-360 mg/dL

Percent transferrin saturation: 20% to 50%

Dosage Forms Excipient information presented when available (limited, particularly for generics); consult specific product labeling.

Injection, solution [preservative free]:

Venofer®: 20 mg of elemental iron/mL (5 mL, 10 mL)

◆ **Iron Sulfate** *see* Ferrous Sulfate *on page 617*

◆ **Iron Sulfate and Vitamin C** *see* Ferrous Sulfate and Ascorbic Acid *on page 617*

◆ **ISD** *see* Isosorbide Dinitrate *on page 823*

◆ **ISDN** *see* Isosorbide Dinitrate *on page 823*

◆ **Isentress™** *see* Raltegravir *on page 1290*

◆ **ISG** *see* Immune Globulin (Intramuscular) *on page 776*

◆ **ISMN** *see* Isosorbide Mononitrate *on page 824*

◆ **Ismo®** *see* Isosorbide Mononitrate *on page 824*

◆ **Isoamyl Nitrite** *see* Amyl Nitrite *on page 114*

◆ **Isobamate** *see* Carisoprodol *on page 261*

◆ **Isochron™** *see* Isosorbide Dinitrate *on page 823*

◆ **Isometheptene, Acetaminophen, and Dichloralphenazone** *see* Acetaminophen, Isometheptene, and Dichloralphenazone *on page 34*

◆ **Isometheptene, Dichloralphenazone, and Acetaminophen** *see* Acetaminophen, Isometheptene, and Dichloralphenazone *on page 34*

Isoniazid (eye soe NYE a zid)

Canadian Brand Names Isotamine®; PMS-Isoniazid

Index Terms INH; Isonicotinic Acid Hydrazide

Pharmacologic Category Antitubercular Agent

Additional Appendix Information

Guidelines for the Prevention of Opportunistic Infections in HIV Infected Persons *on page 1740*

Tuberculosis *on page 1776*

Tyramine Content of Foods *on page 1850*

Use Treatment of susceptible tuberculosis infections; treatment of latent tuberculosis infection (LTBI)

Pregnancy Risk Factor C

Pregnancy Considerations Isoniazid was found to be embryocidal in animal studies; teratogenic effects were not noted. Isoniazid crosses the human placenta. Due to the risk of tuberculosis to the fetus, treatment is recommended when the probability of maternal disease is moderate to high. The CDC recommends isoniazid as part of the initial treatment regimen (CDC, 2003). Pyridoxine supplementation is recommended (25 mg/day).

Lactation Enters breast milk/compatible

Medication Safety Issues

International issues:

Hydra® [Japan] may be confused with Hydrea®

Contraindications Hypersensitivity to isoniazid or any component of the formulation; acute liver disease; previous history of hepatic damage during isoniazid therapy; previous severe adverse reaction (drug fever, chills, arthritis) to isoniazid

Warnings/Precautions Use with caution in patients with severe renal impairment and liver disease. **[U.S. Boxed Warning]: Severe and sometimes fatal hepatitis may occur; usually occurs within the first 3 months of treatment, although may develop even after many months of treatment.** The risk of developing hepatitis is age-related; daily ethanol consumption may also increase the risk. Patients must report any prodromal symptoms of hepatitis, such as fatigue, weakness, malaise, anorexia, nausea, or vomiting. Treatment with isoniazid for latent tuberculosis infection should be deferred in patients with acute hepatic diseases. Periodic ophthalmic examinations are recommended even when usual symptoms do not occur. Pyridoxine (10-50 mg/day) is recommended in individuals at risk for development of peripheral neuropathies (eg, HIV infection, nutritional deficiency, diabetes, pregnancy). Children with low milk and low meat intake should receive concomitant pyridoxine therapy. Multidrug regimens should be utilized for the treatment of active tuberculosis to prevent the emergence of drug resistance.

Adverse Reactions Frequency not defined.

Cardiovascular: Hypertension, palpitation, tachycardia, vasculitis

Central nervous system: Depression, dizziness, encephalopathy, fever, lethargy, memory impairment, psychosis, seizure, slurred speech

Dermatologic: Flushing, rash (morbilliform, maculopapular, pruritic, or exfoliative)

Endocrine & metabolic: Gynecomastia, hyperglycemia, metabolic acidosis, pellagra, pyridoxine deficiency

Gastrointestinal: Anorexia, nausea, vomiting, stomach pain

Hematologic: Agranulocytosis, anemia (sideroblastic, hemolytic, or aplastic), eosinophilia, thrombocytopenia

Hepatic: LFTs mildly increased (10% to 20%); hyperbilirubinemia, bilirubinuria, jaundice, hepatitis (may involve progressive liver damage; risk increases with age; 2.3% in patients >50 years), hepatic dysfunction

Neuromuscular & skeletal: Arthralgia, hyper-reflexia, peripheral neuropathy (dose-related incidence, 10% to 20% incidence with 10 mg/kg/day), weakness

Ocular: Blurred vision, loss of vision, optic neuritis and atrophy

Miscellaneous: Lupus-like syndrome, lymphadenopathy, rheumatic syndrome

Drug Interactions

Metabolism/Transport Effects Substrate of CYP2E1 (major); **Inhibits** CYP1A2 (weak), 2A6 (moderate), 2C9 (weak), 2C19 (strong), 2D6 (moderate), 2E1 (moderate), 3A4 (strong); **Induces** CYP2E1 (after discontinuation) (weak)

Avoid Concomitant Use

Avoid concomitant use of Isoniazid with any of the following: Alfuzosin; Eplerenone; Nilotinib; Nisoldipine; Ranolazine; Rivaroxaban; Salmeterol; Silodosin; Thioridazine

Increased Effect/Toxicity

Isoniazid may increase the levels/effects of: Acetaminophen; Alfuzosin; Alosetron; Benzodiazepines (metabolized by oxidation); CarBAMazepine; Chlorzoxazone; Ciclesonide; CYP2A6 Substrates; CYP2C19 Substrates; CYP2D6 Substrates; CYP2E1 Substrates; CYP3A4 Substrates; Eplerenone; FentaNYL; Fesoterodine; Ixabepilone; Maraviroc; Nebivolol; Nilotinib; Nisoldipine; Phenytoin; Pimecrolimus; Ranolazine; Rivaroxaban; Salmeterol; Silodosin; Sorafenib; Tamoxifen; Theophylline Derivatives; Thioridazine

The levels/effects of Isoniazid may be increased by: CycloSERINE; Rifamycin Derivatives

Decreased Effect

Isoniazid may decrease the levels/effects of: Codeine; TraMADol

The levels/effects of Isoniazid may be decreased by: Antacids; Corticosteroids (Systemic)

Ethanol/Nutrition/Herb Interactions

Ethanol: Avoid ethanol (increases the risk of hepatitis).

Food: Isoniazid should not be taken with food; serum levels may be decreased if taken with food. Has some ability to inhibit tyramine metabolism; several case reports of mild reactions (flushing, palpitations) after ingestion of cheese (with or without wine). Reactions resembling allergic symptoms following ingestion of fish high in histamine content have been reported. Isoniazid decreases folic acid absorption. Isoniazid alters pyridoxine metabolism.

Stability

Tablet: Store at 20°C to 25°C (68°F to 77°F). Protect from light.

Oral solution: Store at 15°C to 30°C (59°F to 86°F). Protect from light.

Mechanism of Action Unknown, but may include the inhibition of mycolic acid synthesis resulting in disruption of the bacterial cell wall

Pharmacodynamics/Kinetics

Absorption: Rapid and complete; rate can be slowed with food

Distribution: All body tissues and fluids including CSF; crosses placenta; enters breast milk

Protein binding: 10% to 15%

Metabolism: Hepatic with decay rate determined genetically by acetylation phenotype

Half-life elimination: Fast acetylators: 30-100 minutes; Slow acetylators: 2-5 hours; may be prolonged with hepatic or severe renal impairment

Time to peak, serum: 1-2 hours

Excretion: Urine (75% to 95%); feces; saliva

Dosage

Usual dosage ranges: Oral, I.M.:

Infants and Children: 10-15 mg/kg/day in 1-2 divided doses (maximum: 300 mg/day) or 20-40 mg/kg given 2-3 times per week (maximum: 900 mg/dose)

Adults: 5 mg/kg/day (usual: 300 mg/day) as a single daily dose or 15 mg/kg (maximum: 900 mg/dose) given 2-3 times per week

Indication-specific dosing: Oral, I.M.: Recommendations often change due to resistant strains and newly-developed information; consult *MMWR* for current CDC recommendations. Intramuscular injection is available for patients who are unable to either take or absorb oral therapy.

Infants and Children:

Tuberculosis, active:

Daily therapy: 10-15 mg/kg/day in 1-2 divided doses (maximum: 300 mg/day)

Twice weekly or 3 times/week directly observed therapy (DOT): 20-40 mg/kg (maximum: 900 mg)

Tuberculosis, latent infection (LTBI): 10 mg/kg/day as a single dose (maximum: 300 mg/day) **or** 20-30 mg/kg (maximum: 900 mg/dose) twice weekly for 9 months

Adults: **Note:** Concomitant administration of 10-50 mg/day pyridoxine is recommended in malnourished patients or those prone to neuropathy (eg, alcoholics, patients with diabetes).

Nontuberculous mycobacterium (*M. kansasii*) (unlabeled use): 5 mg/kg/day (maximum: 300 mg/day) for duration to include 12 months of culture-negative sputum; typically used in combination with ethambutol and rifampin

Tuberculosis, active:

Daily therapy: 5 mg/kg/day given daily (usual dose: 300 mg/day)

Twice weekly or 3 times/week directly observed therapy (DOT): 15 mg/kg (maximum: 900 mg). **Note:** CDC guidelines state that once-weekly therapy (15 mg/kg/dose) may be considered, but only after the first 2 months of initial therapy in HIV-negative patients, and only in combination with rifapentine.

Note: Treatment may be defined by the number of doses administered (eg, "six-month" therapy involves 182 doses of INH and rifampin, and 56 doses of pyrazinamide). Six months is the shortest interval of time over which these doses may be administered, assuming no interruption of therapy.

Tuberculosis, latent infection (LTBI): 300 mg/day or 900 mg twice weekly for 6-9 months in patients who do not have HIV infection (9 months is optimal, 6 months may be considered to reduce costs of therapy) and 9 months in patients who have HIV infection. Extend to 12 months of therapy if interruptions in treatment occur.

Dosing adjustment in renal impairment: No adjustment necessary

Hemodialysis: Dialyzable (50% to 100%); administer dose post dialysis

Dosing adjustment in hepatic impairment: No adjustment required, however, use with caution; may accumulate and additional liver damage may occur in patients with pre-existing liver disease. For ALT or AST >3 times the ULN: discontinue or temporarily withhold treatment. Treatment with isoniazid for latent tuberculosis infection should be deferred in patients with acute hepatic diseases.

Dietary Considerations Should be taken 1 hour before or 2 hours after meals on an empty stomach; increase dietary intake of folate, niacin, magnesium. Avoid tyramine-containing foods. Avoid histamine-containing foods.

Administration Should be administered 1 hour before or 2 hours after meals on an empty stomach.

Monitoring Parameters Baseline and periodic (more frequently in patients with higher risk for hepatitis) liver function tests (ALT and AST); sputum cultures monthly (until 2 consecutive negative cultures reported); monitoring for prodromal signs of hepatitis

Reference Range Therapeutic: 1-7 mcg/mL (SI: 7-51 µmol/L); Toxic: 20-710 mcg/mL (SI: 146-5176 µmol/L)

Test Interactions False-positive urinary glucose with Clinitest®

Additional Information The AAP recommends that pyridoxine supplementation (1-2 mg/kg/day) should be administered to malnourished patients, children or adolescents on meat or milk-deficient diets, breast-feeding infants, and those predisposed to neuritis to prevent peripheral neuropathy; administration of isoniazid syrup has been associated with diarrhea

Dosage Forms Excipient information presented when available (limited, particularly for generics); consult specific product labeling.

Injection, solution: 100 mg/mL (10 mL)

Oral solution: 50 mg/5 mL (473 mL) [orange flavor]

Tablet: 100 mg, 300 mg

Extemporaneous Preparations A 10 mg/mL oral suspension was stable for 21 days when refrigerated when compounded as follows:

Triturate ten 100 mg tablets in a mortar, reduce to a fine powder, then add 10 mL of purified water U.S.P. to make a paste; then transfer to a graduate and qs to 100 mL with sorbitol (do not use sugar-based solutions)

Shake well before using and keep in refrigerator

Nahata MC and Hipple TF, *Pediatric Drug Formulations*, 3rd ed, Cincinnati, OH: Harvey Whitney Books Co, 1997.

- ◆ **Isonicotinic Acid Hydrazide** *see* Isoniazid *on page 820*
- ◆ **Isonipecaine Hydrochloride** *see* Meperidine *on page 943*
- ◆ **Isophane Insulin** *see* Insulin NPH *on page 795*
- ◆ **Isophane Insulin and Regular Insulin** *see* Insulin NPH and Insulin Regular *on page 795*
- ◆ **Isophosphamide** *see* Ifosfamide *on page 766*

Isoproterenol (eye soe proe TER e nole)

U.S. Brand Names Isuprel®

Index Terms Isoproterenol Hydrochloride

Pharmacologic Category $Beta_1$- & $Beta_2$-Adrenergic Agonist Agent

Additional Appendix Information

Bronchodilators *on page 1650*

Use Ventricular arrhythmias due to AV nodal block; hemodynamically compromised bradyarrhythmias or atropine- and dopamine-resistant bradyarrhythmias (when transcutaneous/venous pacing is not available); temporary use in third-degree AV block until pacemaker insertion

Unlabeled/Investigational Use Pharmacologic overdrive pacing for torsade de pointes; diagnostic aid (vasovagal syncope)

Pregnancy Risk Factor C

Lactation Excretion in breast milk unknown

Medication Safety Issues

Sound-alike/look-alike issues:

Isuprel® may be confused with Disophrol®, Ismelin®, Isordil®

Contraindications Hypersensitivity to sulfites or isoproterenol, any component of the formulation, or other sympathomimetic amines; angina, pre-existing cardiac arrhythmias (ventricular); tachycardia or AV block caused by cardiac glycoside intoxication

Warnings/Precautions Use with extreme caution; not currently a treatment of choice; use with caution in elderly patients, patients with diabetes, renal or cardiovascular disease, seizure disorder, or hyperthyroidism; excessive or prolonged use may result in decreased effectiveness.

Adverse Reactions Frequency not defined.

Cardiovascular: Premature ventricular beats, bradycardia, hyper-/hypotension, chest pain, palpitation, tachycardia, ventricular arrhythmia, MI size increased

Central nervous system: Headache, nervousness or restlessness

Endocrine & metabolic: Serum glucose increased, serum potassium decreased, hypokalemia

Gastrointestinal: Nausea, vomiting

Respiratory: Dyspnea

Drug Interactions

Avoid Concomitant Use There are no known interactions where it is recommended to avoid concomitant use.

Increased Effect/Toxicity

The levels/effects of Isoproterenol may be increased by: COMT Inhibitors

Decreased Effect There are no known significant interactions involving a decrease in effect.

Ethanol/Nutrition/Herb Interactions Herb/Nutraceutical: Avoid ephedra, yohimbe (may cause CNS stimulation).

Stability Isoproterenol solution should be stored at room temperature. It should not be used if a color or precipitate is present. Exposure to air, light, or increased temperature may cause a pink to brownish pink color to develop. Stability of parenteral admixture at room temperature (25°C) or at refrigeration (4°C) is 24 hours.

Standard diluent: 2 mg/500 mL D_5W; 4 mg/500 mL D_5W.

Minimum volume: 1 mg/100 mL D_5W.

Mechanism of Action Stimulates $beta_1$- and $beta_2$-receptors resulting in relaxation of bronchial, GI, and uterine smooth muscle, increased heart rate and contractility, vasodilation of peripheral vasculature

Pharmacodynamics/Kinetics

Onset of action: Bronchodilation: I.V.: Immediate

Duration: I.V.: 10-15 minutes

Metabolism: Via conjugation in many tissues including hepatic and pulmonary

Half-life elimination: 2.5-5 minutes

Excretion: Urine (primarily as sulfate conjugates)

Dosage I.V.: Cardiac arrhythmias:

Children: Initial: 0.1 mcg/kg/minute (usual effective dose 0.2-2 mcg/kg/minute)

Adults: Initial: 2 mcg/minute; titrate to patient response (2-10 mcg/minute)

Administration I.V. infusion administration requires the use of an infusion pump. To prepare for infusion: 1 mg isoproterenol to 500 mL D_5W, final concentration 2 mcg/mL

Monitoring Parameters ECG, heart rate, respiratory rate, arterial blood gas, arterial blood pressure, CVP; serum glucose, serum potassium, serum magnesium

Dosage Forms Excipient information presented when available (limited, particularly for generics); consult specific product labeling.

Injection, solution, as hydrochloride:

Isuprel®: 0.2 mg/mL (1:5000) (1 mL, 5 mL) [contains sodium metabisulfite]

- **Isoproterenol Hydrochloride** *see* Isoproterenol *on page 822*
- **Isoptin® SR** *see* Verapamil *on page 1557*
- **Isopto® Atropine** *see* Atropine *on page 157*
- **Isopto® Carbachol** *see* Carbachol *on page 251*
- **Isopto® Carpine** *see* Pilocarpine *on page 1192*
- **Isopto® Eserine (Can)** *see* Physostigmine *on page 1190*
- **Isopto® Homatropine** *see* Homatropine *on page 733*
- **Isopto® Hyoscine** *see* Scopolamine Derivatives *on page 1356*
- **Isordil®** *see* Isosorbide Dinitrate *on page 823*

Isosorbide Dinitrate (eye soe SOR bide dye NYE trate)

U.S. Brand Names Dilatrate®-SR; Isochron™; Isordil®

Canadian Brand Names Apo-ISDN®; Cedocard®-SR; Coronex®; Novo-Sorbide; PMS-Isosorbide

Index Terms ISD; ISDN

Pharmacologic Category Vasodilator

Additional Appendix Information

Heart Failure (Systolic) *on page 1809*

Nitrates *on page 1668*

Use Prevention and treatment of angina pectoris; for congestive heart failure; to relieve pain, dysphagia, and spasm in esophageal spasm with GE reflux

Unlabeled/Investigational Use Esophageal spastic disorders

Pregnancy Risk Factor C

Lactation Excretion in breast milk unknown

Medication Safety Issues

Sound-alike/look-alike issues:

Isordil® may be confused with Inderal®, Isuprel®

International issues:

Nitrobide® [Japan] may be confused with Microzide® which is a brand name for hydrochlorothiazide in the U.S.

Contraindications Hypersensitivity to isosorbide dinitrate or any component of the formulation; hypersensitivity to organic nitrates; concurrent use with phosphodiesterase-5 (PDE-5) inhibitors (sildenafil, tadalafil, or vardenafil); angle-closure glaucoma (intraocular pressure may be increased); head trauma or cerebral hemorrhage (increase intracranial pressure); severe anemia

Warnings/Precautions Use with caution in patients with increased intracranial pressure, hypotension, hypovolemia, right ventricular infarctions, and glaucoma. Paradoxical bradycardia and increased angina pectoris can accompany hypotension. Postural hypotension may also occur; ethanol may potentiate this effect. Tolerance does develop to nitrates and appropriate dosing is needed to minimize this. Nitrates may aggravate angina caused by hypertrophic cardiomyopathy. Avoid concurrent use with PDE-5 inhibitors (eg, sildenafil, tadalafil, vardenafil). Safety and efficacy have not been established in children.- Sustained release products may be absorbed erratically in patients with GI hypermotility or malabsorption syndrome; do not crush or chew sublingual dosage form.

Adverse Reactions Frequency not defined.

Cardiovascular: Hypotension (infrequent), postural hypotension, crescendo angina (uncommon), rebound hypertension (uncommon), pallor, cardiovascular collapse, tachycardia, shock, flushing, peripheral edema, syncope (uncommon)

Central nervous system: Headache (most common), lightheadedness (related to blood pressure changes), dizziness, restlessness

Gastrointestinal: Nausea, vomiting, bowel incontinence, xerostomia

Genitourinary: Urinary incontinence

Hematologic: Methemoglobinemia (rare, overdose)

Neuromuscular & skeletal: Weakness

Ocular: Blurred vision

Miscellaneous: Cold sweat

The incidence of hypotension and adverse cardiovascular events may be increased when used in combination with sildenafil (Viagra®).

Drug Interactions

Metabolism/Transport Effects **Substrate** of CYP3A4 (major)

Avoid Concomitant Use

Avoid concomitant use of Isosorbide Dinitrate with any of the following: Phosphodiesterase 5 Inhibitors

Increased Effect/Toxicity

Isosorbide Dinitrate may increase the levels/effects of: Amifostine; RiTUXimab; Rosiglitazone

The levels/effects of Isosorbide Dinitrate may be increased by: CYP3A4 Inhibitors (Moderate); CYP3A4 Inhibitors (Strong); Dasatinib; Diazoxide; Herbs (Hypotensive Properties); Phosphodiesterase 5 Inhibitors; Prostacyclin Analogues

Decreased Effect

The levels/effects of Isosorbide Dinitrate may be decreased by: CYP3A4 Inducers (Strong); Deferasirox;

Herbs (CYP3A4 Inducers); Herbs (Hypertensive Properties); Methylphenidate; Yohimbine

Ethanol/Nutrition/Herb Interactions Ethanol: Caution with ethanol (may increase risk of hypotension).

Mechanism of Action Stimulation of intracellular cyclic-GMP results in vascular smooth muscle relaxation of both arterial and venous vasculature. Increased venous pooling decreases left ventricular pressure (preload) and arterial dilatation decreases arterial resistance (afterload). Therefore, this reduces cardiac oxygen demand by decreasing left ventricular pressure and systemic vascular resistance by dilating arteries. Additionally, coronary artery dilation improves collateral flow to ischemic regions; esophageal smooth muscle is relaxed via the same mechanism.

Pharmacodynamics/Kinetics

Onset of action: Sublingual tablet: 2-10 minutes; Chewable tablet: 3 minutes; Oral tablet: 45-60 minutes

Duration: Sublingual tablet: 1-2 hours; Chewable tablet: 0.5-2 hours; Oral tablet: 4-6 hours

Metabolism: Extensively hepatic to conjugated metabolites, including isosorbide 5-mononitrate (active) and 2-mononitrate (active)

Half-life elimination: Parent drug: 1-4 hours; Metabolite (5-mononitrate): 4 hours

Excretion: Urine and feces

Dosage Adults (elderly should be given lowest recommended daily doses initially and titrate upward): Oral:

Angina: 5-40 mg 4 times/day or 40 mg every 8-12 hours in sustained-release dosage form

Sublingual: 2.5-5 mg every 5-10 minutes for maximum of 3 doses in 15-30 minutes; may also use prophylactically 15 minutes prior to activities which may provoke an attack

Congestive heart failure:

Initial dose: 20 mg 3-4 times per day

Target dose: 120-160 mg/day in divided doses; use in combination with hydralazine

Esophageal spastic disorders (unlabeled use):

Oral: 5-10 mg before meals

Sublingual: 2.5 mg after meals

Tolerance to nitrate effects develops with chronic exposure: Dose escalation does not overcome this effect. Tolerance can only be overcome by short periods of nitrate absence from the body. Short periods (10-12 hours) of nitrate withdrawal help minimize tolerance. General recommendations are to take the last dose of short-acting agents no later than 7 PM; administer 2-3 times/day rather than 4 times/day. Sustained release preparations could be administered at times to allow a 15- to 17-hour interval between first and last daily dose. Example: Administer sustained release at 8 AM and 2 PM for a twice daily regimen.

Hemodialysis: During hemodialysis, administer dose postdialysis or administer supplemental 10-20 mg dose

Peritoneal dialysis: Supplemental dose is not necessary

Administration Do not administer around-the-clock; the first dose of nitrates should be administered in a physician's office to observe for maximal cardiovascular dynamic effects and adverse effects (orthostatic blood pressure drop, headache); when immediate release products are prescribed twice daily (recommend 7 AM and noon); for 3 times/day dosing (recommend 7 AM, noon, and 5 PM); when sustained-release products are indicated, suggest once a day in morning or via twice daily dosing at 8 AM and 2 PM. Do not crush sublingual tablets.

Monitoring Parameters Monitor for orthostasis

Test Interactions Decreased cholesterol (S)

Dosage Forms Excipient information presented when available (limited, particularly for generics); consult specific product labeling. [DSC] = Discontinued product

Capsule, sustained release (Dilatrate®-SR): 40 mg

Tablet: 5 mg, 10 mg, 20 mg, 30 mg

Isordil®: 5 mg, 10 mg [DSC], 20 mg [DSC], 30 mg [DSC], 40 mg

Tablet, extended release (Isochron™): 40 mg

Tablet, sublingual: 2.5 mg, 5 mg

Isordil®: 2.5 mg, 5 mg, 10 mg [DSC]

Isosorbide Dinitrate and Hydralazine

(eye soe SOR bide dye NYE trate & hye DRAL a zeen)

U.S. Brand Names BiDil®

Index Terms Hydralazine and Isosorbide Dinitrate

Pharmacologic Category Vasodilator

Use Treatment of heart failure, adjunct to standard therapy, in self-identified African-Americans

Pregnancy Risk Factor C

Dosage Oral: Adults: Initial: 1 tablet 3 times/day; titrate to a maximum dose of 2 tablets 3 times/day

Dosage adjustment for toxicity: If patient experiences persistent headache, adjust dosing to twice daily.

Additional Information Complete prescribing information for this medication should be consulted for additional detail.

Dosage Forms Excipient information presented when available (limited, particularly for generics); consult specific product labeling.

Tablet: Isosorbide dinitrate 20 mg and hydralazine 37.5 mg

Isosorbide Mononitrate

(eye soe SOR bide mon oh NYE trate)

U.S. Brand Names Imdur®; Ismo®; Monoket®

Canadian Brand Names Apo-ISMN®; Imdur®; PMS-ISMN; Pro-ISMN

Index Terms ISMN

Pharmacologic Category Vasodilator

Additional Appendix Information

Nitrates *on page 1668*

Use Long-acting metabolite of the vasodilator isosorbide dinitrate used for the prophylactic treatment of angina pectoris

Pregnancy Risk Factor C

Lactation Excretion in breast milk unknown

Medication Safety Issues

Sound-alike/look-alike issues:

Imdur® may be confused with Imuran®, Inderal LA®, K-Dur®

Monoket® may be confused with Monopril®

International issues:

Nitrex® [Italy] may be confused with Imitrex® which is a brand name for sumatriptan in the U.S.

Contraindications Hypersensitivity to isosorbide or any component of the formulation; hypersensitivity to organic nitrates; concurrent use with phosphodiesterase-5 (PDE-5) inhibitors (sildenafil, tadalafil, or vardenafil); angle-closure glaucoma (intraocular pressure may be increased); head trauma or cerebral hemorrhage (increase intracranial pressure); severe anemia

Warnings/Precautions Use with caution in volume depletion, hypotension, and right ventricular infarctions. Postural hypotension, transient episodes of weakness, dizziness, or syncope may occur even with small doses; ethanol accentuates these effects; tolerance and cross-tolerance to nitrate antianginal and hemodynamic effects may occur during prolonged isosorbide mononitrate therapy; (minimized by using the smallest effective dose, by alternating coronary vasodilators or offering drug-free intervals of as little as 12 hours). Excessive doses may result in severe headache, blurred vision, or xerostomia; increased anginal symptoms may be a result of dosage increases. Nitrates may aggravate angina caused by hypertrophic cardiomyopathy. Avoid concurrent use with

PDE-5 inhibitors (eg, sildenafil, tadalafil, vardenafil). Safety and efficacy have not been established in children.

Adverse Reactions

>10%: Central nervous system: Headache (19% to 38%)

1% to 10%:

Central nervous system: Dizziness (3% to 5%)

Gastrointestinal: Nausea/vomiting (2% to 4%)

<1% (Limited to important or life-threatening): Angina pectoris, arrhythmia, atrial fibrillation, impotence, methemoglobinemia (rare), pruritus, rash, supraventricular tachycardia, syncope, vomiting

The incidence of hypotension and adverse cardiovascular events may be increased when used in combination with sildenafil (Viagra®).

Drug Interactions

Metabolism/Transport Effects Substrate of CYP3A4 (major)

Avoid Concomitant Use

Avoid concomitant use of Isosorbide Mononitrate with any of the following: Phosphodiesterase 5 Inhibitors

Increased Effect/Toxicity

Isosorbide Mononitrate may increase the levels/effects of: Amifostine; RiTUXimab; Rosiglitazone

The levels/effects of Isosorbide Mononitrate may be increased by: CYP3A4 Inhibitors (Moderate); CYP3A4 Inhibitors (Strong); Dasatinib; Diazoxide; Herbs (Hypotensive Properties); Phosphodiesterase 5 Inhibitors; Prostacyclin Analogues

Decreased Effect

The levels/effects of Isosorbide Mononitrate may be decreased by: CYP3A4 Inducers (Strong); Deferasirox; Herbs (CYP3A4 Inducers); Herbs (Hypertensive Properties); Methylphenidate; Yohimbine

Ethanol/Nutrition/Herb Interactions Ethanol: Caution with ethanol (may increase risk of hypotension).

Stability Tablets should be stored in a tight container at room temperature of 15°C to 30°C (59°F to 86°F).

Mechanism of Action Prevailing mechanism of action for nitroglycerin (and other nitrates) is systemic venodilation, decreasing preload as measured by pulmonary capillary wedge pressure and left ventricular end diastolic volume and pressure; the average reduction in left ventricular end diastolic volume is 25% at rest, with a corresponding increase in ejection fractions of 50% to 60%. This effect improves congestive symptoms in heart failure and improves the myocardial perfusion gradient in patients with coronary artery disease.

Pharmacodynamics/Kinetics

Onset of action: 30-60 minutes

Absorption: Nearly complete and low intersubject variability in its pharmacokinetic parameters and plasma concentrations

Metabolism: Hepatic

Half-life elimination: Mononitrate: ~4 hours

Excretion: Urine and feces

Dosage Adults and Geriatrics (start with lowest recommended dose): Oral:

Regular tablet: 5-20 mg twice daily with the two doses given 7 hours apart (eg, 8 AM and 3 PM) to decrease tolerance development; then titrate to 10 mg twice daily in first 2-3 days.

Extended release tablet: Initial: 30-60 mg given in morning as a single dose; titrate upward as needed, giving at least 3 days between increases; maximum daily single dose: 240 mg

Dosing adjustment in renal impairment: Not necessary for elderly or patients with altered renal or hepatic function.

Tolerance to nitrate effects develops with chronic exposure. Dose escalation does not overcome this effect. Tolerance can only be overcome by short periods of nitrate absence from the body. Short periods (10-12 hours) of nitrate withdrawal help minimize tolerance. Recommended dosage regimens incorporate this interval. General recommendations are to take the last dose of short-acting agents no later than 7 PM; administer 2 times/day rather than 4 times/day. Administer sustained release tablet once daily in the morning.

Administration Do not administer around-the-clock; Monoket® and Ismo® should be scheduled twice daily with doses 7 hours apart (8 AM and 3 PM); Imdur® may be administered once daily. Extended release tablets should not be chewed or crushed. Should be swallowed with a half-glassful of fluid.

Monitoring Parameters Monitor for orthostasis, increased hypotension

Dosage Forms Excipient information presented when available (limited, particularly for generics); consult specific product labeling.

Tablet: 10 mg, 20 mg

Ismo®: 20 mg

Monoket®: 10 mg, 20 mg

Tablet, extended release: 30 mg, 60 mg, 120 mg

Imdur®: 30 mg, 60 mg, 120 mg

◆ **Isotamine® (Can)** *see* Isoniazid *on page 820*

Isotretinoin (eye soe TRET i noyn)

U.S. Brand Names Accutane®; Amnesteem™; Claravis™; Sotret®

Canadian Brand Names Accutane®; Clarus™; Isotrex®

Index Terms 13-*cis*-Retinoic Acid

Pharmacologic Category Acne Products; Retinoic Acid Derivative

Use Treatment of severe recalcitrant nodular acne unresponsive to conventional therapy

Unlabeled/Investigational Use Investigational: Treatment of children with metastatic neuroblastoma or leukemia that does not respond to conventional therapy

Restrictions All patients (male and female), prescribers, wholesalers, and dispensing pharmacists must register and be active in the iPLEDGE™ risk management program, designed to eliminate fetal exposures to isotretinoin. This program covers all isotretinoin products (brand and generic). The iPLEDGE™ program requires that all patients meet qualification criteria and monthly program requirements. Registration, activation, and additional information are provided at www.ipledgeprogram.com or by calling 866-495-0654.

An FDA-approved medication guide must be distributed when dispensing an outpatient prescription (new or refill) where this medication is to be used without direct supervision of a healthcare provider. Medication guides are available at http://www.fda.gov/cder/Offices/ODS/medication_guides.htm.

Pregnancy Risk Factor X

Pregnancy Considerations Major fetal abnormalities (both internal and external), spontaneous abortion, premature births and low IQ scores in surviving infants have been reported. **[U.S. Boxed Warning]: Because of the high likelihood of teratogenic effects, all patients (male and female), prescribers, wholesalers, and dispensing pharmacists must register and be active in the iPLEDGE™ risk management program; do not prescribe isotretinoin for women who are or who are likely to become pregnant while using the drug.** This medication is contraindicated in females of childbearing potential unless they are able to comply with the guidelines of the iPLEDGE™ pregnancy prevention program. Females of childbearing potential should not become pregnant during therapy or for 1 month following discontinuation of isotretinoin. Upon discontinuation of treatment, females of childbearing potential should have a pregnancy test after their last dose and again one month after their last dose. Two forms of contraception should be continued during this time. Any pregnancies should be reported to the iPLEDGE™ program (www.ipledgeprogram.com or 866-495-0654).

Lactation Excretion in breast milk unknown/contraindicated

Medication Safety Issues

Sound-alike/look-alike issues:

Accutane® may be confused with Accolate®, Accupril®

Claravis™ may be confused with Cleviprex™

Isotretinoin may be confused with tretinoin

Contraindications Hypersensitivity to isotretinoin or any component of the formulation; sensitivity to parabens, vitamin A, or other retinoids; pregnancy

Warnings/Precautions This medication should only be prescribed by prescribers competent in treating severe recalcitrant nodular acne, are experienced in the use of systemic retinoids. **[U.S. Boxed Warning]: Because of the high likelihood of teratogenic effects, all patients (male and female), prescribers, wholesalers, and dispensing pharmacists must register and be active in the iPLEDGE™ risk management program; do not prescribe isotretinoin for women who are or who are likely to become pregnant while using the drug (see Additional Information for details).** Women of childbearing potential must be capable of complying with effective contraceptive measures. Patients must select and commit to two forms of contraception. Therapy is begun after two negative pregnancy tests; effective contraception must be used for at least 1 month before beginning therapy, during therapy, and for 1 month after discontinuation of therapy. Prescriptions should be written for no more than a 30-day supply, and pregnancy testing and counseling should be repeated monthly.

May cause depression, psychosis, aggressive or violent behavior, and changes in mood; use with extreme caution in patients with psychiatric disorders. Rarely, suicidal thoughts and actions have been reported during isotretinoin usage. All patients should be observed closely for symptoms of depression or suicidal thoughts. Discontinuation of treatment alone may not be sufficient, further evaluation may be necessary. Cases of pseudotumor cerebri (benign intracranial hypertension) have been reported, some with concomitant use of tetracycline (avoid using together). Patients with papilledema, headache, nausea, vomiting, and visual disturbances should be referred to a neurologist and treatment with isotretinoin discontinued. Hearing impairment, which can continue after therapy is discontinued, may occur. Clinical hepatitis, elevated liver enzymes, inflammatory bowel disease, skeletal hyperostosis, premature epiphyseal closure, vision impairment, corneal opacities, and decreased night vision have also been reported with the use of isotretinoin.

Use with caution in patients with diabetes mellitus; impaired glucose control has been reported. Use caution in patients with hypertriglyceridemia; acute pancreatitis and fatal hemorrhagic pancreatitis (rare) have been reported. Bone mineral density may decrease; use caution in patients with a genetic predisposition to bone disorders (ie osteoporosis, osteomalacia) and with disease states or concomitant medications that can induce bone disorders. Patients may be at risk when participating in activities with repetitive impact (such as sports). Patients should be instructed not to donate blood during therapy and for 1 month following discontinuation of therapy due to risk of donated blood being given to a pregnant female. Safety of long-term use is not established and is not recommended. Safety and efficacy have not been established in children <12 years of age.

Adverse Reactions Frequency not defined.

Cardiovascular: Palpitation, tachycardia, vascular thrombotic disease, stroke, chest pain, syncope, flushing

Central nervous system: Edema, fatigue, pseudotumor cerebri, dizziness, drowsiness, headache, insomnia, lethargy, malaise, nervousness, paresthesia, seizure, stroke, suicidal ideation, suicide attempts, suicide, depression, psychosis, aggressive or violent behavior, emotional instability

Dermatologic: Cutaneous allergic reactions, purpura, acne fulminans, alopecia, bruising, cheilitis, dry mouth, dry nose, dry skin, epistaxis, eruptive xanthomas, fragility of skin, hair abnormalities, hirsutism, hyperpigmentation, hypopigmentation, peeling of palms, peeling of soles, photoallergic reactions, photosensitizing reactions, pruritus, rash, dystrophy, paronychia, facial erythema, seborrhea, eczema, increased sunburn susceptibility, diaphoresis, urticaria, abnormal wound healing

Endocrine & metabolic: Triglycerides increased (25%), abnormal menses, blood glucose increased, cholesterol increased, HDL decreased

Gastrointestinal: Weight loss, inflammatory bowel disease, regional ileitis, pancreatitis, bleeding and inflammation of the gums, colitis, nausea, nonspecific gastrointestinal symptoms

Genitourinary: Nonspecific urogenital findings

Hematologic: Anemia, thrombocytopenia, neutropenia, agranulocytosis, pyogenic granuloma

Hepatic: Hepatitis

Neuromuscular & skeletal: Skeletal hyperostosis, calcification of tendons and ligaments, premature epiphyseal closure, arthralgia, CPK elevations, arthritis, tendonitis, bone abnormalities, weakness, back pain (29% in pediatric patients), rhabdomyolysis (rare), bone mineral density decreased

Ocular: Corneal opacities, decreased night vision, cataracts, color vision disorder, conjunctivitis, dry eyes, eyelid inflammation, keratitis, optic neuritis, photophobia, visual disturbances

Otic: Hearing impairment, tinnitus

Renal: Vasculitis, glomerulonephritis

Respiratory: Bronchospasms, respiratory infection, voice alteration, Wegener's granulomatosis

Miscellaneous: Allergic reactions, anaphylactic reactions, lymphadenopathy, infection, disseminated herpes simplex, diaphoresis

Drug Interactions

Avoid Concomitant Use

Avoid concomitant use of Isotretinoin with any of the following: Tetracycline Derivatives

Increased Effect/Toxicity

The levels/effects of Isotretinoin may be increased by: Tetracycline Derivatives

Decreased Effect

Isotretinoin may decrease the levels/effects of: Oral Contraceptive (Estrogens); Oral Contraceptive (Progestins)

Ethanol/Nutrition/Herb Interactions

Ethanol: Avoid or limit ethanol (may increase triglyceride levels if taken in excess).

Food: Isotretinoin bioavailability increased if taken with food or milk.

Herb/Nutraceutical: Avoid dong quai, St John's wort (may also cause photosensitization and may decrease the effectiveness of oral contraceptives). Additional vitamin A supplements may lead to vitamin A toxicity (dry skin, irritation, arthralgias, myalgias, abdominal pain, hepatic changes); avoid use.

Stability Store at room temperature. Protect from light.

Mechanism of Action Reduces sebaceous gland size and reduces sebum production; regulates cell proliferation and differentiation

Pharmacodynamics/Kinetics

Distribution: Crosses placenta

Protein binding: 99% to 100%; primarily albumin

Metabolism: Hepatic via CYP2B6, 2C8, 2C9, 2D6, 3A4; forms metabolites; major metabolite: 4-oxo-isotretinoin (active)

Half-life elimination: Terminal: Parent drug: 21 hours; Metabolite: 21-24 hours

Time to peak, serum: 3-5 hours

Excretion: Urine and feces (equal amounts)

Dosage Oral:

Children: Maintenance therapy for neuroblastoma (investigational): 100-250 mg/m^2/day in 2 divided doses

Children 12-17 years and Adults: Severe recalcitrant nodular acne: 0.5-1 mg/kg/day in 2 divided doses (dosages as low as 0.05 mg/kg/day have been reported to be beneficial) for 15-20 weeks or until the total cyst count decreases by 70%, whichever is sooner. Adults with very severe disease/scarring or primarily involves the trunk may require dosage adjustment up to 2 mg/kg/day. A second course of therapy may be initiated after a period of ≥2 months off therapy.

Dosing adjustment in hepatic impairment: Dose reductions empirically are recommended in hepatitis disease

Dietary Considerations Should be taken with food. Limit intake of vitamin A; avoid use of other vitamin A products. Some formulations may contain soybean oil.

Administration Administer with food. Capsules should be swallowed whole with a full glass of water. For patients unable to swallow, the Accutane® capsule may be pierced with a large-gauge needle and the contents placed in food (cottage cheese, ice cream, pudding, or oatmeal with butter) for immediate consumption (Accutane® data on file, Roche Pharmaceuticals). Use appropriate precautions for handling teratogenic capsule contents.

Monitoring Parameters CBC with differential and platelet count, baseline sedimentation rate, glucose, CPK; signs of depression, mood alteration, psychosis, and agression

Pregnancy test (for all female patients of childbearing potential): Two negative tests with a sensitivity of at least 25 mIU/mL prior to beginning therapy (the second performed at least 19 days after the first test and performed during the first 5 days of the menstrual period immediately preceding the start of therapy); monthly tests to rule out pregnancy prior to refilling prescription.

Lipids: Prior to treatment and at weekly or biweekly intervals until response to treatment is established. Test should not be performed <36 hours after consumption of ethanol.

Liver function tests: Prior to treatment and at weekly or biweekly intervals until response to treatment is established.

Additional Information All patients (male and female), must be registered in the iPLEDGE™ risk management program. Females of childbearing potential must receive oral and written information reviewing the hazards of therapy and the effects that isotretinoin can have on a fetus. Therapy should not begin without two negative pregnancy tests at least 19 days apart. Two forms of contraception (a primary and secondary form as described in the iPLEDGE™ program materials) must be used simultaneously beginning 1 month prior to treatment, during treatment, and for 1 month after therapy is discontinued; limitations to their use must be explained. Prescriptions should be written for no more than a 30-day supply, and pregnancy testing and counseling should be repeated monthly. During therapy, pregnancy tests must be conducted by a CLIA-certified laboratory. Prescriptions must be filled and picked up from the pharmacy within 7 days of specimen collection for pregnancy test for women of childbearing potential. Prescriptions for males and females of non-childbearing potential must be filled and picked up within 30 days of prescribing.

Any cases of accidental pregnancy should be reported to the iPLEDGE™ program or FDA MedWatch. All patients (male and female) must read and sign the informed consent material provided in the pregnancy prevention program.

Dosage Forms Excipient information presented when available (limited, particularly for generics); consult specific product labeling.

Capsule:

Accutane®: 10 mg, 20 mg, 40 mg [contains soybean oil and parabens]

Amnesteem™: 10 mg, 20 mg, 40 mg [contains soybean oil]

Claravis™: 10 mg, 20 mg, 40 mg

Sotret®: 10 mg, 20 mg, 30 mg, 40 mg [contains soybean oil]

Extemporaneous Preparations

Alternate method of administration of Accutane® capsules, based on unpublished data (not recommended by manufacturer): An oral suspension using the entire capsule may be prepared by adding one 10 mg capsule to 15 mL warm (~37°C or 97°F) 2% reduced-fat milk (or 20 mg capsule to 30 mL, etc, so that the concentration is maintained). Stir until capsule shell dissolves and capsule contents are dispersed throughout solution (approximately 10-15 minutes). Suspension stable for ≤4 hours at controlled room temperature or under refrigeration. Use appropriate precautions for handling teratogenic capsule contents.

Accutane® data on file, Roche Pharmaceuticals

◆ **Isotrex® (Can)** *see* Isotretinoin *on page 825*

Isoxsuprine (eye SOKS syoo preen)

U.S. Brand Names Vasodilan® [DSC]

Index Terms Isoxsuprine Hydrochloride

Pharmacologic Category Vasodilator

Use Treatment of peripheral vascular diseases, such as arteriosclerosis obliterans and Raynaud's disease

Pregnancy Risk Factor C

Medication Safety Issues

Sound-alike/look-alike issues:

Vasodilan® may be confused with Vasocidin®

Dosage Oral: Adults: 10-20 mg 3-4 times/day; start with lower dose in elderly due to potential hypotension

Additional Information Complete prescribing information for this medication should be consulted for additional detail.

Dosage Forms Excipient information presented when available (limited, particularly for generics); consult specific product labeling.

Tablet, as hydrochloride: 10 mg, 20 mg

◆ **Isoxsuprine Hydrochloride** *see* Isoxsuprine *on page 827*

Isradipine (iz RA di peen)

U.S. Brand Names DynaCirc® CR

Canadian Brand Names DynaCirc®

Pharmacologic Category Calcium Channel Blocker

Additional Appendix Information

Calcium Channel Blockers *on page 1651*

Use Treatment of hypertension

Unlabeled/Investigational Use Pediatric hypertension

Pregnancy Risk Factor C

Pregnancy Considerations Teratogenic effects were not observed in animal studies. Isradipine crosses the human placenta. There are no adequate and well-controlled studies in pregnant women.

Lactation Excretion in breast milk unknown/not recommended

Medication Safety Issues

Sound-alike/look-alike issues:

DynaCirc® may be confused with Dynabac®, Dynacin®

Contraindications Hypersensitivity to isradipine or any component of the formulation; hypotension (<90 mm Hg systolic)

Warnings/Precautions Increased angina and/or MI has occurred with initiation or dosage titration of calcium channel blockers. The most common side effect is peripheral edema; occurs within 2-3 weeks of starting therapy. Reflex tachycardia may occur with use. Symptomatic hypotension with or without syncope can rarely occur; blood pressure must be lowered at a rate appropriate for the patient's clinical condition. Use cautiously in HF, hypertrophic cardiomyopathy (IHSS), and in hepatic dysfunction. Use controlled release tablets with caution in patients with severe GI narrowing. Safety and efficacy have not been established in pediatric patients. Adjust doses at 2- to 4-week intervals.

Adverse Reactions Percentages reported with capsule formulation.

>10%: Central nervous system: Headache (dose related 2% to 22%)

1% to 10%:

Cardiovascular: Edema (dose related 1% to 9%), palpitation (dose related 1% to 5%), flushing (dose related 1% to 5%), tachycardia (1% to 3%), chest pain (2% to 3%)

Central nervous system: Dizziness (2% to 8%), fatigue (dose related 1% to 9%)

Dermatologic: Rash (2%)

Gastrointestinal: Nausea (1% to 5%), abdominal discomfort (≤3%), vomiting (≤1%), diarrhea (≤3%)

Neuromuscular & skeletal: Weakness (≤1%)

Renal: Urinary frequency (1% to 3%)

Respiratory: Dyspnea (1% to 3%)

<1% (Limited to important or life-threatening): Angioedema, atrial fibrillation, back pain, constipation, cough, cramps of legs and feet, depression, drowsiness, drug fever, dry mouth, dysuria, epistaxis, gingival hyperplasia (incidence unknown), heart failure, hyperhidrosis, hypotension, impotence, insomnia, joint pain, leg pain, lethargy, leukopenia, libido decreased, liver function tests increased, MI, nasal congestion, nervousness, nocturia, numbness, paresthesia,pruritus, stroke, syncope, throat discomfort,transient ischemic attack, urticaria, ventricular fibrillation, visual disturbance, weight gain

Drug Interactions

Metabolism/Transport Effects **Substrate** of CYP3A4 (major); **Inhibits** CYP3A4 (weak)

Avoid Concomitant Use

Avoid concomitant use of Isradipine with any of the following: Nilotinib; Tetrabenazine; Thioridazine; Ziprasidone

Increased Effect/Toxicity

Isradipine may increase the levels/effects of: Amifostine; Magnesium Salts; Neuromuscular-Blocking Agents (Nondepolarizing); Nitroprusside; Phenytoin; QTc-Prolonging Agents; RiTUXimab; Tacrolimus; Tetrabenazine; Thioridazine; Ziprasidone

The levels/effects of Isradipine may be increased by: Alpha1-Blockers; Antifungal Agents (Azole Derivatives, Systemic); Calcium Channel Blockers (Nondihydropyridine); Cimetidine; Ciprofloxacin; CycloSPORINE; CYP3A4 Inhibitors (Moderate); CYP3A4 Inhibitors (Strong); Dasatinib; Diazoxide; Fluconazole; Gadobutrol; Grapefruit Juice; Herbs (Hypotensive Properties); Macrolide Antibiotics; Magnesium Salts; Nilotinib; Prostacyclin Analogues; Protease Inhibitors; Quinupristin

Decreased Effect

Isradipine may decrease the levels/effects of: Clopidogrel; QuiNIDine

The levels/effects of Isradipine may be decreased by: Barbiturates; Calcium Salts; CarBAMazepine; CYP3A4 Inducers (Strong); Deferasirox; Herbs (CYP3A4 Inducers); Herbs (Hypertensive Properties); Methylphenidate; Nafcillin; Rifamycin Derivatives; Yohimbine

Ethanol/Nutrition/Herb Interactions

Food: Administration with food delays absorption, but does not affect availability

Herb/Nutraceutical: St John's wort may decrease isradipine levels. Avoid dong quai if using for hypertension. Avoid bayberry, blue cohosh, cayenne, ephedra, ginger, ginseng (American), gotu kola, licorice (may worsen hypertension) Avoid garlic (may have increased antihypertensive effect).

Mechanism of Action Inhibits calcium ion from entering the "slow channels" or select voltage-sensitive areas of vascular smooth muscle and myocardium during depolarization, producing a relaxation of coronary vascular smooth muscle and coronary vasodilation; increases myocardial oxygen delivery in patients with vasospastic angina

Pharmacodynamics/Kinetics

Onset of action: Immediate release: 2-3 hours

Duration: Immediate release: >12 hours

Absorption: 90% to 95%

Distribution: V_d: 3 L/kg

Protein binding: 95%

Metabolism: Hepatic; CYP3A4 substrate (major); extensive first-pass effect; forms metabolites (inactive)

Bioavailability: 15% to 24%

Half-life elimination: Terminal: 8 hours

Time to peak, serum: 1-1.5 hours

Excretion: Urine (60% to 65% as metabolites); feces (25% to 30%)

Dosage Oral:

Children (unlabeled use): Capsule: Initial: 0.15-0.2 mg/kg/day in 2-3 divided doses; maximum 0.8 mg/kg/day, up to 20 mg/day. **Note:** Controlled release formulation is administered once daily or in 2 divided doses.

Adults:

Capsule: 2.5 mg twice daily; antihypertensive response occurs in 2-3 hours; maximal response in 2-4 weeks; increase dose at 2- to 4-week intervals at 2.5-5 mg increments; usual dose range (JNC 7): 2.5-10 mg/day in 2 divided doses. **Note:** Most patients show no improvement with doses >10 mg/day except adverse reaction rate increases; therefore, maximal dose in older adults should be 10 mg/day.

Controlled release tablet: 5 mg once daily; antihypertensive response occurs in 2 hours. Adjust dose in increments of 5 mg at 2-4 week intervals. Maximum dose 20 mg/day; adverse events are increased at doses >10 mg/day.

Elderly:

Capsule: Refer to adult dosing.

Controlled release tablet: Initial dose: 5 mg once daily

Dosage adjustment in renal impairment: Cl_{cr} 30-80 mL/minute: Bioavailability increased by 45%. Cl_{cr} <10 mL/minute on hemodialysis: Bioavailability decreased by 20% to 50%

Capsule: Refer to adult dosing.

Controlled release tablet: Initial dose: 5 mg once daily

Dosage adjustment in hepatic impairment: Peak serum concentrations are increased by 32% and bioavailability is increased by 52%

Capsule: Refer to adult dosing.

Controlled release tablet: Initial dose: 5 mg once daily

Dietary Considerations May be taken without regard to meals.

Administration Controlled release tablets should be swallowed whole; do not divide or chew

Monitoring Parameters Blood pressure; renal, hepatic dysfunction

Dosage Forms Excipient information presented when available (limited, particularly for generics); consult specific product labeling.

Capsule: 2.5 mg, 5 mg

Tablet, controlled release:

DynaCirc® CR: 5 mg, 10 mg

Extemporaneous Preparations A 1 mg/mL oral liquid was stable for 35 days when refrigerated when compounded as follows:

Dissolve the contents of ten 5 mg capsules in simple syrup, qs ad 50 mL

Shake well before using and keep in refrigerator

MacDonald JL, Johnson CE, and Jacobson P, "Stability of Isradipine in Extemporaneously Compounded Oral Liquids," *Am J Hosp Pharm*, 1994, 51(19):2409-11.

◆ **Istalol®** *see* Timolol *on page 1472*

◆ **Isuprel®** *see* Isoproterenol *on page 822*

Itraconazole (i tra KOE na zole)

U.S. Brand Names Sporanox®

Canadian Brand Names Sporanox®

Pharmacologic Category Antifungal Agent, Oral

Additional Appendix Information

Antifungal Agents *on page 1640*

Guidelines for the Prevention of Opportunistic Infections in HIV Infected Persons *on page 1740*

Use Treatment of susceptible fungal infections in immunocompromised and immunocompetent patients including blastomycosis and histoplasmosis; indicated for aspergillosis, and onychomycosis of the toenail; treatment of onychomycosis of the fingernail without concomitant toenail infection via a pulse-type dosing regimen; has activity against *Aspergillus*, *Candida*, *Coccidioides*, *Cryptococcus*, *Sporothrix*, tinea unguium

Oral: Useful in superficial mycoses including dermatophytoses (eg, tinea capitis), pityriasis versicolor, sebopsoriasis, vaginal and chronic mucocutaneous candidiases; systemic mycoses including candidiasis, meningeal and disseminated cryptococcal infections, paracoccidioidomycosis, coccidioidomycoses; miscellaneous mycoses such as sporotrichosis, chromomycosis, leishmaniasis, fungal keratitis, alternariosis, zygomycosis

Oral solution: Treatment of oral and esophageal candidiasis

Intravenous solution: Indicated in the treatment of blastomycosis, histoplasmosis (nonmeningeal), and aspergillosis (in patients intolerant or refractory to amphotericin B therapy); empiric therapy of febrile neutropenic fever

Pregnancy Risk Factor C

Pregnancy Considerations Should not be used to treat onychomycosis during pregnancy. Effective contraception should be used during treatment and for 2 months following treatment. Congenital abnormalities have been reported during postmarketing surveillance, but a causal relationship has not been established.

Lactation Enters breast milk/not recommended

Medication Safety Issues

Sound-alike/look-alike issues:

Sporanox® may be confused with Suprax®

Contraindications Hypersensitivity to itraconazole, any component of the formulation, or to other azoles; concurrent administration with cisapride, dofetilide, ergot derivatives, levomethadyl, lovastatin, midazolam, pimozide, quinidine, simvastatin, or triazolam; treatment of onychomycosis in patients with evidence of left ventricular dysfunction, CHF, or a history of CHF

Warnings/Precautions Discontinue if signs or symptoms of HF or neuropathy occur during treatment. **[U.S. Boxed Warning]: Rare cases of serious cardiovascular adverse events (including death), ventricular tachycardia, and torsade de pointes have been observed due to increased cisapride, pimozide, quinidine, dofetilide or levomethadyl concentrations induced by itraconazole; concurrent use contraindicated. Use with caution in patients with left ventricular dysfunction or a history of HF; not recommended for treatment of onychomycosis in these patients.** Not recommended for use in patients with active liver disease, elevated liver enzymes, or prior hepatotoxic reactions to other drugs. Itraconazole has been associated with rare cases of serious hepatotoxicity (including fatal cases and cases within the first week of treatment); treatment should be discontinued in patients who develop clinical symptoms of liver dysfunction or abnormal liver function tests during itraconazole therapy except in cases where expected benefit exceeds risk. Large differences in itraconazole pharmacokinetic parameters have been observed in cystic fibrosis patients receiving the solution; if a patient with cystic fibrosis does not respond to therapy, alternate therapies should be considered. Due to differences in bioavailability, oral capsules and oral solution **cannot be used interchangeably.** Intravenous formulation should be used with caution in renal impairment; consider conversion to oral therapy if renal dysfunction/toxicity is noted. Initiation of treatment with oral solution is not recommended in patients at immediate risk for systemic candidiasis (eg, patients with severe neutropenia).

Adverse Reactions Listed incidences are for higher doses appropriate for systemic fungal infection.

>10%: Gastrointestinal: Nausea (11%)

1% to 10%:

Cardiovascular: Edema (4%), hypertension (3%)

Central nervous system: Headache (4%), fatigue (2% to 3%), malaise (1%), fever (3%), dizziness (2%)

Dermatologic: Rash (9%), pruritus (3%)

Endocrine & metabolic: Decreased libido (1%), hypertriglyceridemia, hypokalemia (2%)

Gastrointestinal: Abdominal pain (2%), anorexia (1%), vomiting (5%), diarrhea (3%)

Hepatic: Abnormal LFTs (3%), hepatitis

Renal: Albuminuria (1%)

<1% (Limited to important or life-threatening): Adrenal suppression; allergic reactions (urticaria, angioedema); alopecia, anaphylactoid reactions, anaphylaxis, arrhythmia, CHF, constipation, gastritis, gynecomastia, hepatic failure, impotence, neutropenia, peripheral neuropathy, photosensitivity, pulmonary edema, somnolence, Stevens-Johnson syndrome, tinnitus

Drug Interactions

Metabolism/Transport Effects Substrate of CYP3A4 (major); **Inhibits** CYP3A4 (strong)

Avoid Concomitant Use

Avoid concomitant use of Itraconazole with any of the following: Alfuzosin; Cisapride; Conivaptan; Dabigatran Etexilate; Dofetilide; Nilotinib; Pimozide; QuiNIDine; Ranolazine; Rivaroxaban; Salmeterol; Silodosin; Topotecan

Increased Effect/Toxicity

Itraconazole may increase the levels/effects of: Alfentanil; Alfuzosin; Alosetron; Aprepitant; Benzodiazepines (metabolized by oxidation); Bosentan; BusPIRone; Busulfan; Calcium Channel Blockers; CarBAMazepine; Cardiac Glycosides; Ciclesonide; Cilostazol; Cisapride; Conivaptan; Corticosteroids (Orally Inhaled); Corticosteroids (Systemic); CycloSPORINE; CYP3A4 Substrates; Dabigatran Etexilate; Docetaxel; Dofetilide; Eletriptan;

Eplerenone; Erlotinib; Eszopiclone; FentaNYL; Fesoterodine; Fosaprepitant; Gefitinib; HMG-CoA Reductase Inhibitors; Imatinib; Irinotecan; Ixabepilone; Losartan; Macrolide Antibiotics; Maraviroc; Methadone; Nilotinib; Paliperidone; P-Glycoprotein Substrates; Phenytoin; Phosphodiesterase 5 Inhibitors; Pimecrolimus; Pimozide; Protease Inhibitors; QuiNIDine; Ramelteon; Ranolazine; Repaglinide; Rifamycin Derivatives; Rivaroxaban; Salmeterol; Silodosin; Sirolimus; Solifenacin; Sorafenib; Sunitinib; Tacrolimus; Temsirolimus; Tolterodine; Topotecan; VinBLAStine; VinCRIStine; Vitamin K Antagonists; Ziprasidone; Zolpidem

The levels/effects of Itraconazole may be increased by: Macrolide Antibiotics; Protease Inhibitors

Decreased Effect

Itraconazole may decrease the levels/effects of: Amphotericin B; Saccharomyces boulardii

The levels/effects of Itraconazole may be decreased by: Antacids; CYP3A4 Inducers (Strong); Deferasirox; Didanosine; Efavirenz; Grapefruit Juice; H2-Antagonists; Herbs (CYP3A4 Inducers); Phenytoin; Proton Pump Inhibitors; Rifamycin Derivatives; Sucralfate

Ethanol/Nutrition/Herb Interactions

Food:

Capsules: Enhanced by food and possibly by gastric acidity. Cola drinks have been shown to increase the absorption of the capsules in patients with achlorhydria or those taking H_2-receptor antagonists or other gastric acid suppressors. Avoid grapefruit juice.

Solution: Decreased by food, time to peak concentration prolonged by food.

Herb/Nutraceutical: St John's wort may decrease itraconazole levels.

Stability

Capsule: Store at room temperature, 15°C to 25°C (59°F to 77°F). Protect from light and moisture.

Oral solution: Store at ≤25°C (77°F); do not freeze.

Solution for injection: Store at ≤25°C (77°F); do not freeze. Protect from light. Dilute with 0.9% sodium chloride. Stable for 48 hours at room temperature or under refrigeration. A precise mixing ratio is required to maintain stability (3.33:1) and avoid precipitate formation. Add 25 mL (1 ampul) to 50 mL 0.9% sodium chloride. Mix and withdraw 15 mL of solution before infusing.

Mechanism of Action Interferes with cytochrome P450 activity, decreasing ergosterol synthesis (principal sterol in fungal cell membrane) and inhibiting cell membrane formation

Pharmacodynamics/Kinetics

Absorption: Requires gastric acidity; capsule better absorbed with food, solution better absorbed on empty stomach

Distribution: V_d (average): 796 ± 185 L or 10 L/kg; highly lipophilic and tissue concentrations are higher than plasma concentrations. The highest concentrations: adipose, omentum, endometrium, cervical and vaginal mucus, and skin/nails. Aqueous fluids (eg, CSF and urine) contain negligible amounts.

Protein binding, plasma: 99.9%; metabolite hydroxy-itraconazole: 99.5%

Metabolism: Extensively hepatic via CYP3A4 into >30 metabolites including hydroxy-itraconazole (major metabolite); appears to have *in vitro* antifungal activity. Main metabolic pathway is oxidation; may undergo saturation metabolism with multiple dosing.

Bioavailability: Variable, ~55% (oral solution) in 1 small study; **Note:** Oral solution has a higher degree of bioavailability (149% ± 68%) relative to oral capsules; should not be interchanged

Half-life elimination: Oral: After single 200 mg dose: 21 ± 5 hours; 64 hours at steady-state; I.V.: steady-state: 35 hours; steady-state concentrations are achieved in 13 days with multiple administration of itraconazole 100-400 mg/day.

Excretion: Feces (~3% to 18%); urine (~0.03% as parent drug, 40% as metabolites)

Dosage

Usual dosage ranges:

Children: Efficacy and safety have not been established; a small number of patients 3-16 years of age have been treated with 100 mg/day for systemic fungal infections with no serious adverse effects reported. A dose of 5 mg/kg once daily was used in a pharmacokinetic study using the oral solution in patients 6 months to 12 years; duration of study was 2 weeks.

Adults: Oral, I.V.: 100-400 mg/day; doses >200 mg/day are given in 2 divided doses; length of therapy varies from 1 day to >6 months depending on the condition and mycological response

Indication-specific dosing:

Adults:

Aspergillosis, invasive (salvage therapy): Duration of therapy should be a minimum of 6-12 weeks or throughout period of immunosuppression:

Oral: 200-400 mg/day; **Note:** 2008 IDSA guidelines recommend 600 mg/day for 3 days, followed by 400 mg/day

I.V.: 200 mg twice daily for 4 doses, followed by 200 mg daily

Appropriate use: Itraconazole should **NOT** be used for voriconazole-refractory aspergillosis since the same antifungal and/or resistance mechanism(s) may be shared by both agents. Itraconazole oral solution and capsule formulations are not bioequivalent or interchangeable. Due to variable bioavailability of oral preparations, therapeutic drug monitoring advisable.

Aspergillosis, allergic (ABPA, sinusitis): Oral: 200 mg/day; may be used in conjunction with corticosteroids

Blastomycosis/histoplasmosis:

Oral: 200 mg once daily, if no obvious improvement or there is evidence of progressive fungal disease, increase the dose in 100 mg increments to a maximum of 400 mg/day; doses >200 mg/day are given in 2 divided doses; length of therapy varies from 1 day to >6 months depending on the condition and mycological response

I.V.: 200 mg twice daily for 4 doses, followed by 200 mg/day

Brain abscess: Cerebral phaeohyphomycosis (dematiaceous): Oral: 200 mg twice daily for at least 6 months with amphotericin

Candidiasis:

Oropharyngeal: Oral solution: 200 mg once daily for 1-2 weeks; in patients unresponsive or refractory to fluconazole: 100 mg twice daily (clinical response expected in 1-2 weeks)

Esophageal: Oral solution: 100-200 mg once daily for a minimum of 3 weeks; continue dosing for 2 weeks after resolution of symptoms

Coccidioides: Oral: 200 mg twice daily

Infections, life-threatening:

Oral: 200 mg 3 times/day (600 mg/day) should be given for the first 3 days of therapy

I.V.: 200 mg twice daily for 4 doses, followed by 200 mg/day

Meningitis:

Coccidioides: Oral: 400-800 mg/day

Cryptococcal: HIV positive (unlabeled use): Induction: Oral: 400 mg/day for 10-12 weeks; maintenance: 200 mg twice daily lifelong

Onychomycosis: Oral: 200 mg once daily for 12 consecutive weeks; alternative "pulse-dosing" may be considering for fingernail involvement only: 200 mg twice daily for 1 week; repeat 1-week course after 3 week off-time

Pneumonia:

Coccidioides: Mild to moderate: Oral, I.V.: 200 mg twice daily

Cryptococcal: Mild to moderate (unlabeled use): 200-400 mg/day for 6-12 months (lifelong for HIV positive)

Protothecal infection: 200 mg once daily for 2 months

Sporotrichosis: Oral:

Lymphocutaneous: 100-200 mg/day for 3-6 months

Osteoarticular and pulmonary: 200 mg twice daily for 1-2 years (may use amphotericin B initially for stabilization)

Dosing adjustment in renal impairment: Not necessary; itraconazole injection is not recommended in patients with Cl_{cr} <30 mL/minute; hydroxypropyl-β-cyclodextrin (the excipient) is eliminated primarily by the kidneys.

Hemodialysis: Not dialyzable

Dosing adjustment in hepatic impairment: May be necessary, but specific guidelines are not available. Risk-to-benefit evaluation should be undertaken in patients who develop liver function abnormalities during treatment.

Dietary Considerations

Capsule: Administer with food.

Solution: Take without food, if possible.

Administration

Oral: Doses >200 mg/day are given in 2 divided doses; do not administer with antacids. Capsule and oral solution formulations are not bioequivalent and thus are not interchangeable. Capsule absorption is best if taken with food, therefore, it is best to administer itraconazole after meals; solution should be taken on an empty stomach. When treating oropharyngeal and esophageal candidiasis, solution should be swished vigorously in mouth, then swallowed.

I.V.: Infuse 60 mL of the dilute solution (3.33 mg/mL = 200 mg itraconazole, pH ~4.8) over 60 minutes; flush with 15-20 mL of 0.9% sodium chloride over 30 seconds to 15 minutes

Monitoring Parameters Liver function in patients with pre-existing hepatic dysfunction, and in all patients being treated for longer than 1 month; serum (trough) concentrations particularly for oral therapy (due to erratic bioavailability with capsule formulation)

Reference Range Trough serum concentrations may be performed to assure therapeutic levels, especially in the face of oral therapy. Trough concentration of itraconzole plus the metabolite hydroxyitraconazole should be at least 0.5 mcg/mL.

Additional Information Due to potential toxicity, the manufacturer recommends confirmation of diagnosis testing of nail specimens prior to treatment of onychomycosis.

Dosage Forms Excipient information presented when available (limited, particularly for generics); consult specific product labeling. [DSC] = Discontinued product

Capsule: 100 mg

Sporanox®: 100 mg

Injection, solution:

Sporanox®: 10 mg/mL (25 mL) [packaged in a kit containing sodium chloride 0.9% (50 mL); filtered infusion set (1)] [DSC]

Solution, oral:

Sporanox®: 100 mg/10 mL (150 mL) [cherry flavor]

Ivermectin (eye ver MEK tin)

U.S. Brand Names Stromectol®

Pharmacologic Category Anthelmintic

Use Treatment of the following infections: Strongyloidiasis of the intestinal tract due to the nematode parasite *Strongyloides stercoralis*. Onchocerciasis due to the nematode parasite *Onchocerca volvulus*. Ivermectin is only active against the immature form of *Onchocerca volvulus*, and the intestinal forms of *Strongyloides stercoralis*.

Unlabeled/Investigational Use Has been used for other parasitic infections including *Ascaris lumbricoides*, Bancroftian filariasis, *Brugia malayi*, scabies, *Enterobius vermicularis*, *Mansonella ozzardi*, *Gnathostomia spingerum*, *Mansonella ozzardi*, *Mansonella streptocera*, pediculosis pubis, *Trichuris trichiura*.

Pregnancy Risk Factor C

Pregnancy Considerations Teratogenic effects have been observed in animal studies. Safety has not been established in pregnant women. The manufacturer and the Centers for Disease Control and Prevention (CDC) do not recommend use in pregnant women.

Lactation Enters breast milk/not recommended

Contraindications Hypersensitivity to ivermectin or any component of the formulation

Warnings/Precautions Data have shown that antihelmintic drugs like ivermectin may cause cutaneous and/or systemic reactions (Mazzoti reaction) of varying severity including ophthalmological reactions in patients with onchocerciasis. These reactions are probably due to allergic and inflammatory responses to the death of microfilariae. Patients with hyper-reactive onchodermatitis may be more likely than others to experience severe adverse reactions, especially edema and aggravation of the onchodermatitis. Repeated treatment may be required in immunocompromised patients (eg, HIV); control of extraintestinal strongyloidiasis may necessitate suppressive (once monthly) therapy. Pretreatment assessment for *Loa loa* infection is recommended in any patient with significant exposure to endemic areas (West and Central Africa); serious and/or fatal encephalopathy has been reported (rarely) during treatment in patients with loiasis. Safety and efficacy in children <15 kg have not be established.

Adverse Reactions

>10%: Miscellaneous: Mazzotti-type reaction (with onchocerciasis): Pruritus (28%), fever (23%), skin involvement (including edema/urticarial rash [23%]), lymph node tenderness (1% to 14%), lymph node enlargement (3% to 13%), arthralgia/synovitis (9%)

1% to 10%:

Cardiovascular: Tachycardia (4%), peripheral edema (3%), facial edema (1%), orthostatic hypotension (1%)

Central nervous system: Dizziness (3%)

Dermatologic: Pruritus (3%)

Gastrointestinal: Diarrhea (2%), nausea (2%)

Hematologic: Eosinophilia (3%), leukocytes decreased (3%), hemoglobin increased (1%)

Hepatic: ALT increased (2%), AST increased (2%)

Ocular: Limbitis (4% to 6%), punctuate opacity (1% to 2%)

<1% (Limited to important or life-threatening): Abdominal pain, anemia, anorexia, anterior uveitis, asthma exacerbation, back pain, bilirubin increased, chest discomfort, chorioretinitis, choroiditis, coma, confusion, conjunctival hemorrhage, conjunctivitis, constipation, dyspnea, encephalopathy (rare; associated with loiasis), eyelid edema, eye sensation abnormal, fatigue, fecal incontinence, headache, hypotension, INR increased, keratitis, lethargy, leukopenia, mental status changes, myalgia,

neck pain, rash, red eye, seizure, somnolence, standing/walking difficulty, Stevens-Johnson syndrome, stupor, toxic epidermal necrolysis, tremor, urinary incontinence, urticaria, vertigo, vision loss (transient), weakness, vomiting

Drug Interactions

Metabolism/Transport Effects Substrate of CYP3A4 (minor)

Avoid Concomitant Use There are no known interactions where it is recommended to avoid concomitant use.

Increased Effect/Toxicity

Ivermectin may increase the levels/effects of: Vitamin K Antagonists

The levels/effects of Ivermectin may be increased by: P-Glycoprotein Inhibitors

Decreased Effect

Ivermectin may decrease the levels/effects of: Typhoid Vaccine

The levels/effects of Ivermectin may be decreased by: P-Glycoprotein Inducers

Ethanol/Nutrition/Herb Interactions

Food: Bioavailability is increased 2.5-fold when administered following a high-fat meal.

Stability Store at <30°C (86°F).

Mechanism of Action Ivermectin is a semisynthetic antihelminthic agent; it binds selectively and with strong affinity to glutamate-gated chloride ion channels which occur in invertebrate nerve and muscle cells. This leads to increased permeability of cell membranes to chloride ions then hyperpolarization of the nerve or muscle cell, and death of the parasite.

Pharmacodynamics/Kinetics

Onset of action: Peak effect in treatment of onchocerciasis: 3-6 months
Absorption: Well absorbed
Distribution: Does not cross blood-brain barrier
Half-life elimination: ~18 hours
Metabolism: Hepatic (>97%)
Bioavailability: Increased with high-fat meal
Time to peak, serum: ~4 hours
Excretion: Feces; urine (<1%)

Dosage Oral: Children ≥15 kg and Adults:

Onchocerciasis: 150 mcg/kg as a single dose; retreatment may be required every 3-12 months until the adult worms die

Weight-based dosage to provide ~150 mcg/kg:
15-25 kg: 3 mg
26-44 kg: 6 mg
45-64 kg: 9 mg
65-84 kg: 12 mg
≥85 kg: 150 mcg/kg

Strongyloidiasis: 200 mcg/kg as a single dose; perform follow-up stool examinations; CDC recommendations: 200 mcg/kg/day for 2 days

Weight-based dosage to provide ~200 mcg/kg:
15-24 kg: 3 mg
25-35 kg: 6 mg
36-50 kg: 9 mg
51-65 kg: 12 mg
66-79 kg: 15 mg
≥80 kg: 200 mcg/kg

Ascariasis due to *Ascaris lumbricoides* (unlabeled use): CDC recommendation: 150-200 mcg/kg as a single dose

Filariasis due to *Mansonella ozzardi* (unlabeled use): CDC recommendation: 200 mcg/kg as a single dose

Filariasis due to *Mansonella streptocera* (unlabeled use): CDC recommendation: 150 mcg/kg as a single dose

Gnathostomiasis due to *Gnathostomia spingerum* (unlabeled use): CDC recommendation: 200 mcg/kg/day for 2 days

Scabies due to *Sarcoptes scabiei* (unlabeled use): CDC recommendation: 200 mcg/kg as a single dose; repeat in 2 weeks

Dietary Considerations Take on an empty stomach with water.

Administration Administer on an empty stomach with water.

Monitoring Parameters Skin and eye microfilarial counts, periodic ophthalmologic exams; follow up stool examinations

Dosage Forms Excipient information presented when available (limited, particularly for generics); consult specific product labeling.

Tablet [scored]:
Stromectol®: 3 mg

◆ **IVIG** *see* Immune Globulin (Intravenous) *on page 777*

◆ **IV Immune Globulin** *see* Immune Globulin (Intravenous) *on page 777*

◆ **IvyBlock® [OTC]** *see* Bentoquatam *on page 183*

◆ **Ivy-Rid® [OTC]** *see* Benzocaine *on page 183*

◆ **IvySoothe® [OTC]** *see* Hydrocortisone *on page 743*

Ixabepilone (ix ab EP i lone)

U.S. Brand Names Ixempra™

Index Terms BMS-247550; NSC-710428

Pharmacologic Category Antineoplastic Agent, Antimicrotubular; Antineoplastic Agent, Epothilone B Analog

Use Treatment of metastatic or locally-advanced breast cancer (refractory or resistant)

Pregnancy Risk Factor D

Pregnancy Considerations In animal studies, ixabepilone caused maternal toxicity and embryo/fetal toxicity at doses ~1/10 the human dose. There are no adequate and well-controlled studies in pregnant women. Women of childbearing potential should be advised to use effective contraception during treatment.

Lactation Excretion in breast milk unknown/not recommended

Medication Safety Issues

High alert medication: The Institute for Safe Medication Practices (ISMP) includes this medication among its list of drug classes which have a heightened risk of causing significant patient harm when used in error.

Contraindications History of severe hypersensitivity to Cremophor® EL or its derivatives (eg, polyoxyethylated castor oil); neutrophil count <1500/mm^3 or platelet count <100,000mm^3; combination therapy with ixabepilone and capecitabine in patients with AST or ALT >2.5 times ULN or bilirubin >1 times ULN

Warnings/Precautions Hazardous agent - use appropriate precautions for handling and disposal. **[U.S. Boxed Warning]: Combination therapy with capecitabine is contraindicated in patients with AST or ALT >2.5 times ULN or bilirubin >1 times ULN;** the risk of toxicity and neutropenia-related death is increased. Use (as monotherapy) is not recommended if AST or ALT >10 times ULN or bilirubin >3 times ULN; use caution in patients with AST or ALT >5 times ULN. Toxicities and serious adverse reactions are increased (in mono- and combination therapy) with hepatic dysfunction; dosage reductions are necessary. Diluent contains Cremophor® EL, which is associated with hypersensitivity reactions; use is contraindicated in patients with a history of severe hypersensitivity to Cremophor® EL. Medications for the treatment of reaction should be available for immediate use; reactions may also be managed with a reduction of infusion rate. Premedicate with an H_1- and H_2-antagonist 1 hour prior to infusion; patients who experience hypersensitivity (eg, bronchospasm, dyspnea, flushing, rash) should also be premedicated with a corticosteroid for all subsequent cycles if treatment is continued.

Dose-dependent myelosuppression, particularly neutropenia, may occur with mono- or combination therapy. Neutropenic fever and infection have been reported with use. The risk for neutropenia is increased with hepatic dysfunction, especially when used in combination with capecitabine. Severe neutropenia and/or thrombocytopenia may require dosage adjustment and/or treatment delay. Peripheral (sensory and motor) neuropathy occurs commonly; may require dose reductions, treatment delays or discontinuation. Usually occurs during the first 3 cycles. Use with caution in patients with pre-existing neuropathy. Patients with diabetes may have an increased risk for severe peripheral neuropathy. Use with caution in patients with cardiovascular disease; the incidence of MI, ventricular dysfunction, and supraventricular arrhythmias is higher when ixabepilone is used in combination with capecitabine (as compared to capecitabine alone). Consider discontinuing ixabepilone in patients who develop cardiac ischemia or impaired cardiac function.

Due to the ethanol content in the diluent, may cause cognitive impairment; patients must be cautioned about performing tasks which require mental alertness (eg, operating machinery or driving). Toxicities or serious adverse events with combination therapy may be increased in the elderly. Safety and efficacy have not been established in children.

Adverse Reactions

Percentages reported with monotherapy:

>10%:

Central nervous system: Headache (11%)

Dermatologic: Alopecia (48%)

Gastrointestinal: Nausea (42%), vomiting (29%), mucositis/stomatitis (29%), diarrhea (22%), anorexia (19%), constipation (16%), abdominal pain (13%)

Hematologic: Leukopenia (36%; grade 4: 13%), neutropenia (31%; grade 4: 23%)

Neuromuscular & skeletal: Peripheral neuropathy (~75%; grades 3/4: 14%; median onset: cycle 4), sensory neuropathy (62%; grades 3/4: 14%), weakness (56%), myalgia/arthralgia (49%), musculoskeletal pain (20%)

1% to 10%:

Cardiovascular: Edema (9%), hot flush (6%), chest pain (5%)

Central nervous system: Fever (8%), pain (8%), dizziness (7%), insomnia (5%)

Dermatologic: Nail disorder (9%), rash (9%), palmar-plantar erythrodysesthesia/hand-and-foot syndrome (8%), pruritus (6%), skin exfoliation (2%), hyperpigmentation (2%)

Endocrine & metabolic: Dehydration (2%)

Gastrointestinal: Gastroesophageal reflux disease (6%), taste perversion (6%), weight loss (6%)

Hematologic: Anemia (6%; grade 4: 2%), neutropenic fever (3%; grade 3: 3%), thrombocytopenia (5%; grade 4: 2%)

Neuromuscular & skeletal: Motor neuropathy (10%; grade 3: 1%)

Ocular: Lacrimation increased (4%)

Respiratory: Dyspnea (9%), upper respiratory tract infection (6%), cough (2%)

Miscellaneous: Hypersensitivity (5%; grade 3: 1%), infection (5%)

Mono- and combination therapy: <1% (Limited to important or life-threatening): Alkaline phosphatase increased, angina, atrial flutter, autonomic neuropathy, cardiomyopathy, cerebral hemorrhage, coagulopathy, colitis, embolism, dysphagia, enterocolitis, erythema multiforme, gastrointestinal hemorrhage, gastroparesis, GGT increased, hemorrhage, hepatic failure (acute), hypokalemia, hyponatremia, hypotension, hypovolemia, hypovolemic shock, hypoxia, ileus, interstitial pneumonia, jaundice, left ventricular dysfunction, metabolic acidosis, MI, nephrolithiasis, neutropenic infection, orthostatic hypotension, pneumonia, pneumonitis, pulmonary edema (acute), renal failure, respiratory failure, sepsis, septic shock, supraventricular arrhythmia, syncope, thrombosis, transaminases increased, trismus, urinary tract infection, vasculitis

Drug Interactions

Metabolism/Transport Effects Substrate of CYP3A4 (major)

Avoid Concomitant Use There are no known interactions where it is recommended to avoid concomitant use.

Increased Effect/Toxicity

The levels/effects of Ixabepilone may be increased by: CYP3A4 Inhibitors (Moderate); CYP3A4 Inhibitors (Strong); Dasatinib

Decreased Effect

The levels/effects of Ixabepilone may be decreased by: CYP3A4 Inducers (Strong); Deferasirox; Herbs (CYP3A4 Inducers)

Ethanol/Nutrition/Herb Interactions Herb/Nutraceutical: Avoid St John's wort (may decrease ixabepilone levels).

Stability Store intact vials under refrigeration at 2°C to 8°C (36°F to 46°F); protect from light. Allow to reach room temperature for ~30 minutes prior to reconstitution. Diluent vial may contain a white precipitate which should dissolve upon reaching room temperature. **Reconstitute only with the provided diluent.** Dilute the 15 mg vial with 8 mL and the 45 mg vial with 23.5 mL (using provided diluent) to a concentration of 2 mg/mL (contains overfill). Gently swirl and invert vial until dissolved completely. Prior to administration, further dilute in lactated Ringer's (~250 mL) using a non-DEHP container (eg, glass, polypropylene or polyolefin), to a final concentration of 0.2-0.6 mg/mL. Reconstituted solution (in the vial) is stable for 1 hour at room temperature; infusion solution diluted in lactated Ringer's is stable for 6 hours at room temperature.

Mechanism of Action Epothilone B analog; binds to the beta-tubulin subunit of the microtubule, stabilizing microtubular function, thus arresting the cell cycle (at the G2/M phase) and inducing apoptosis

Pharmacodynamics/Kinetics

Distribution: >1000 L/m^2

Protein binding: 67% to 77%

Metabolism: Extensively hepatic, via CYP3A4; >30 metabolites (inactive) formed

Half-life elimination: ~52 hours

Time to peak, plasma: At the end of infusion (3 hours)

Excretion: Feces (65%; 2% as unchanged drug); urine (21%; 6% as unchanged drug)

Dosage Note: Premedicate with an oral H_1-antagonist (eg, diphenhydramine 50 mg) and an oral H_2-antagonist (eg, ranitidine 150-300 mg) 1 hour prior to infusion. Patients with a history of hypersensitivity should also be premedicated with corticosteroids (orally 1 hour before or I.V. 30 minutes before infusion). Body surface area (BSA) is capped at a maximum of 2.2 m^2.

I.V.: Adults: 40 mg/m^2 every 3 weeks (maximum dose: 88 mg)

Dosage adjustment with concurrent strong CYP3A4 inhibitor: If concurrent use can not be avoided, reduce ixabepilone dose to 20 mg/m^2. When a strong CYP3A4 inhibitor is discontinued, allow ~1 week to elapse prior to adjusting ixabepilone dose upward.

Ixabepilone dosage adjustments for toxicity for monotherapy or combination therapy:

Hematologic:

Neutrophils <500/mm^3 for ≥7 days: Reduce dose by 20%

Neutropenic fever: Reduce dose by 20%

Platelets <25,000/mm^3 (or <50,000/mm^3 with bleeding): Reduce dose by 20%

Nonhematologic:

Neuropathy:

Grade 2 (moderate) for ≥7 days: Reduce dose by 20%

Grade 3 (severe) for <7 days: Reduce dose by 20%

Grade 3 (severe or disabling) for ≥7 days: Discontinue treatment

Grade 3 toxicity (severe; other than neuropathy): Reduce dose by 20%

Grade 3 arthralgia/myalgia or fatigue (transient): Continue at current dose

Grade 3 hand-foot syndrome: Continue at current dose

Grade 4 toxicity (disabling): Discontinue treatment

Note: Adjust dosage at the start of a cycle are based on toxicities (hematologic and nonhematologic) from the previous cycle; delay new cycles until neutrophils have recovered to >1500/mm^3, platelets have recovered to >100,000/mm^3 and nonhematologic toxicities have resolved to at least grade 1. If toxicities persist despite initial dose reduction, reduce dose an additional 20%.

Capecitabine dosage adjustments for toxicity in combination therapy with ixabepilone:

Hematologic:

Neutrophils <500/mm^3 for ≥7 days or neutropenic fever: Hold for concurrent diarrhea or stomatitis until neutrophils recover to >1000/mm3, then continue at same dose

Platelets <25,000/mm^3 (or <50,000/mm^3 with bleeding): Hold for concurrent diarrhea or stomatitis until platelets recover to >50,000/mm^3, then continue at same dose

Nonhematologic: Refer to Capecitabine monograph.

Dosage adjustment in renal impairment: Pharmacokinetics (monotherapy) are not affected in patients with mild-to-moderate renal insufficiency (Cl_{cr} >30 mL/minute); monotherapy has not been studied in patients with serum creatinine >1.5 times ULN. Combination therapy with capecitabine has not been studied in patients with Cl_{cr} <50 mL/minute.

Dosage adjustment in hepatic impairment:

Ixabepilone monotherapy (initial cycle; adjust doses for subsequent cycles based on toxicity):

AST and ALT ≤2.5 times ULN and bilirubin ≤1 times ULN: No adjustment necessary

AST or ALT ≤10 times ULN and bilirubin ≤1.5 times ULN: Reduce dose to 32 mg/m^2

AST and ALT ≤10 times ULN and bilirubin >1.5 - ≤3 times ULN: Reduce dose to 20-30 mg/m^2

AST or ALT >10 times ULN or bilirubin >3 times ULN: Use is not recommended

Combination therapy of ixabepilone with capecitabine:

AST and ALT ≤2.5 times ULN and bilirubin ≤1 times ULN: No adjustment necessary

AST or ALT >2.5 times ULN or bilirubin >1 times ULN: Use is contraindicated

Dietary Considerations Avoid grapefruit juice.

Administration Infuse over 3 hours. Use non-DEHP administration set (eg, polyethylene); filter with a 0.2-1.2 micron inline filter.

Monitoring Parameters CBC with differential; hepatic function (ALT, AST, bilirubin); monitor for hypersensitivity

Dosage Forms Excipient information presented when available (limited, particularly for generics); consult specific product labeling.

Injection, powder for reconstitution:

Ixempra™: 15 mg, 45 mg [packaged with diluent; diluent contains alcohol and purified polyoxyethylated castor oil (Cremophor® EL)]

◆ **Ixempra™** *see* Ixabepilone *on page 832*

◆ **JAMP-Citalopram (Can)** *see* Citalopram *on page 337*

◆ **JAMP-Ondansetron (Can)** *see* Ondansetron *on page 1102*

◆ **Jamp® Travel Tablet (Can)** *see* DimenhyDRINATE *on page 453*

◆ **Jantoven®** *see* Warfarin *on page 1570*

◆ **Janumet™** *see* Sitagliptin and Metformin *on page 1376*

◆ **Januvia™** *see* SitaGLIPtin *on page 1375*

Japanese Encephalitis Virus Vaccine (Inactivated)

(jap a NEESE en sef a LYE tis VYE rus vak SEEN, in ak ti VAY ted)

U.S. Brand Names JE-VAX®

Canadian Brand Names JE-VAX®

Pharmacologic Category Vaccine

Use Active immunization against Japanese encephalitis

Pregnancy Risk Factor C

Pregnancy Considerations Reproduction studies have not been conducted. Risks of vaccine administration should be carefully considered and in general, pregnant women should only be vaccinated if they are at high risk for exposure. Infection from Japanese encephalitis during the 1st or 2nd trimesters of pregnancy may increase risk of abortion.

Contraindications Hypersensitivity to Japanese encephalitis virus vaccine, including serious adverse reaction (generalized urticaria or angioedema) to a prior dose; proven or suspected hypersensitivity to any component of the vaccine including proteins of rodent or neural origin; hypersensitivity to thimerosal

Warnings/Precautions Because of the potential for severe adverse reactions, Japanese encephalitis vaccine is not recommended for all persons traveling to or residing in Asia (also see Additional Information). Severe adverse reactions (generalized urticaria or angioedema) may occur within minutes to 17 days following vaccination; most occur within 10 days with the majority occurring within 48 hours. Immediate treatment for anaphylactic/anaphylactoid reaction should be available during vaccine use. Patients should be observed for 30 minutes after vaccination. Travel should not be started for ≥10 days following vaccination and patients should remain within ready access to medical care for 10 days and seek immediate medical attention at onset of any reaction.

Use caution with a significant history of urticaria following exposure to insect stings; risk of adverse events may be increased. Use caution with severe allergies to other medications. Avoid alcohol consumption within 48 hours of vaccination; may increase risk of hypersensitivity reactions.

Use of vaccine should also include other means to reduce the risk of mosquito exposure (bed nets, insect repellents, protective clothing, avoidance of travel in endemic areas, and avoidance of outdoor activity during twilight and evening periods).

In general, the decision to administer or delay vaccination because of current or recent febrile illness depends on the severity of symptoms and the etiology of the disease. Immunocompromised patients may have a reduced response to vaccines; information not available specific to this vaccine. Safety and efficacy have not been established for children <1 year of age.

Adverse Reactions Report allergic or unusual adverse reactions to the Vaccine Adverse Event Reporting System (VAERS) 1-800-822-7967. Percentage of adverse reactions may depend upon timing of vaccination. In general, adverse reactions occur more frequently following the first dose or when doses are administered closer together (abbreviated dosing schedule). However, reactions have been reported when previous doses were tolerated uneventfully.

>10%:

Central nervous system: Headache (<5% to 15%)

Local: Injection site reaction (<1% to 31%)

1% to 10%:

Central nervous system: Chills (~10%), dizziness (~10%), malaise (~10%), fever (<5% to 10%)

Dermatologic: Rash (≤10%)

Gastrointestinal: Abdominal pain (~10%), nausea (~10%), vomiting (~10%)

Neuromuscular & skeletal: Myalgia (~10%)

Miscellaneous: Flu-like syndrome (<5%)

<1%, frequency not defined, and/or case reports: Angioedema, behavior disorder, Bell's palsy, cerebellar ataxia, cranial nerve paresis, encephalopathy, erythema multiforme, erythema nodosum, facial swelling, Guillain-Barré syndrome, hepatitis, hives, hypotension, itching, joint swelling, myocarditis, optic neuritis, peripheral neuropathy, renal failure, respiratory distress, respiratory failure, seizure, transverse myelitis, urticaria (generalized), wheezing

Drug Interactions

Avoid Concomitant Use There are no known interactions where it is recommended to avoid concomitant use.

Increased Effect/Toxicity There are no known significant interactions involving an increase in effect.

Decreased Effect

The levels/effects of Japanese Encephalitis Virus Vaccine (Inactivated) may be decreased by: Immunosuppressants

Ethanol/Nutrition/Herb Interactions Ethanol: Alcohol consumption within 48 hours of vaccination may increase risk of hypersensitivity reactions.

Stability Prior to and following reconstitution, store under refrigeration at 2°C to 8°C (35°F to 46°F). Reconstitute with 1.3 mL of provided diluent. Shake well. Discard 8 hours after reconstitution. Do not freeze.

Dosage U.S. recommended primary immunization schedule:

Children 1-3 years: SubQ: Three 0.5 mL doses given on days 0, 7, and 30

Children >3 years and Adults: SubQ: Three 1 mL doses given on days 0, 7, and 30

Booster dose: Give after 2 years, or according to current recommendation

Abbreviated dosing schedule: Three recommended doses, given on days 0, 7, and 14 with the last dose given at least 10 days before travel. Alternately, two doses given 1 week apart provide immunity in ~80% of patients. Abbreviated schedules should be used only when necessary due to time constraints.

Elderly: Refer to adult dosing. Elderly may be at increased risk of developing neuroinvasive disease if infected with Japanese encephalitis virus.

Dietary Considerations Avoid alcohol for 48 hours following vaccination.

Administration The single-dose vial should only be reconstituted with the full 1.3 mL of diluent supplied. Administer 1 mL of the resulting liquid as one standard adult dose; discard the unused portion.

Additional Information Federal law requires that the date of administration, the vaccine manufacturer, lot number of vaccine, and the administering person's name, title, and address be entered into the patient's permanent medical record.

Because of the potential for severe adverse reactions, Japanese encephalitis vaccine is not recommended for all persons traveling to or residing in Asia. Risk of exposure to the Japanese encephalitis virus may vary from year to year for a particular area. In general, use should be limited to persons spending ≥1 month in endemic areas during transmission season. Under specific circumstances, the CDC notes that vaccination may also be considered for persons spending <30 days in endemic areas, such as:

- Travel to areas with epidemic transmission
- Travelers with high risk activities (eg, extensive outdoor activity in rural areas, adventure travelers)

The CDC also recommends vaccination for research laboratory workers who may be exposed to the Japanese encephalitis virus.

Dosage Forms Excipient information presented when available (limited, particularly for generics); consult specific product labeling.

Injection, powder for reconstitution:

JE-VAX®: [contains mouse serum protein, thimerosal, gelatin, polysorbate 80]

- ◆ **JE-VAX®** *see* Japanese Encephalitis Virus Vaccine (Inactivated) *on page 834*
- ◆ **Jolessa™** *see* Ethinyl Estradiol and Levonorgestrel *on page 577*
- ◆ **Jolivette™** *see* Norethindrone *on page 1078*
- ◆ **Junel™** *see* Ethinyl Estradiol and Norethindrone *on page 581*
- ◆ **Junel™ Fe** *see* Ethinyl Estradiol and Norethindrone *on page 581*
- ◆ **Just for Kids™ [OTC]** *see* Fluoride *on page 635*
- ◆ **Juvederm™ 24HV** *see* Hyaluronate and Derivatives *on page 734*
- ◆ **Juvederm™ 30** *see* Hyaluronate and Derivatives *on page 734*
- ◆ **Juvederm™ 30HV** *see* Hyaluronate and Derivatives *on page 734*
- ◆ **K-10® (Can)** *see* Potassium Chloride *on page 1216*
- ◆ **Kadian®** *see* Morphine Sulfate *on page 1016*
- ◆ **Kaletra®** *see* Lopinavir and Ritonavir *on page 901*

Kanamycin (kan a MYE sin)

U.S. Brand Names Kantrex®

Canadian Brand Names Kantrex®

Index Terms Kanamycin Sulfate

Pharmacologic Category Antibiotic, Aminoglycoside

Additional Appendix Information

Antimicrobial Drugs of Choice *on page 1752*

Tuberculosis *on page 1776*

Use Treatment of serious infections caused by susceptible strains of *E. coli*, *Proteus* species, *Enterobacter aerogenes*, *Klebsiella pneumoniae*, *Serratia marcescens*, and *Acinetobacter* species; second-line treatment of *Mycobacterium tuberculosis*

Pregnancy Risk Factor D

Medication Safety Issues

Sound-alike/look-alike issues:

Kanamycin may be confused with Garamycin®, gentamicin

Dosage Note: Dosing should be based on ideal body weight

Children: Infections: I.M., I.V.: 15 mg/kg/day in divided doses every 8-12 hours

Adults:

Infections: I.M., I.V.: 5-7.5 mg/kg/dose in divided doses every 8-12 hours (<15 mg/kg/day)

Intraperitoneal: After contamination in surgery: 500 mg

Irrigating solution: 0.25%; maximum 1.5 g/day (via all administration routes)

Aerosol: 250 mg 2-4 times/day

Dosing adjustment/interval in renal impairment:

Cl_{cr} 50-80 mL/minute: Administer 60% to 90% of dose or administer every 8-12 hours

Cl_{cr} 10-50 mL/minute: Administer 30% to 70% of dose or administer every 12 hours

Cl_{cr} <10 mL/minute: Administer 20% to 30% of dose or administer every 24-48 hours

Additional Information Complete prescribing information for this medication should be consulted for additional detail.

Dosage Forms Excipient information presented when available (limited, particularly for generics); consult specific product labeling.

Injection, solution, as sulfate: 1 g/3 mL (3 mL) [contains sodium bisulfate]

Ketamine (KEET a meen)

U.S. Brand Names Ketalar®

Canadian Brand Names Ketalar®; Ketamine Hydrochloride Injection, USP

Index Terms Ketamine Hydrochloride

Pharmacologic Category General Anesthetic

Use Induction and maintenance of general anesthesia

Unlabeled/Investigational Use Analgesia, sedation

Restrictions C-III

Pregnancy Considerations Adverse events have not been observed in animal reproduction studies. Ketamine crosses the placenta and can be detected in fetal tissue. Ketamine produces dose dependant increases in uterine contractions; effects may vary by trimester. The plasma clearance of ketamine is reduced during pregnancy. Dose related neonatal depression and decreased APGAR scores have been reported with large doses administered at delivery.

Medication Safety Issues

Sound-alike/look-alike issues:

Ketalar® may be confused with Kenalog®, ketorolac

High alert medication: The Institute for Safe Medication Practices (ISMP) includes this medication among its list of drugs which have a heightened risk of causing significant patient harm when used in error.

Contraindications Hypersensitivity to ketamine or any component of the formulation; conditions in which an increase in blood pressure would be hazardous

Warnings/Precautions Use with caution in patients with coronary artery disease, catecholamine depletion, hypertension, and tachycardia. Cardiac function should be continuously monitored in patients with increased blood pressure or cardiac decompensation. Postanesthetic emergence reactions which can manifest as vivid dreams, hallucinations, and/or frank delirium occur; these reactions are less common in patients >65 years of age and when given intramuscularly. Emergence reactions, confusion, or irrational behavior may occur up to 24 hours postoperatively and may be reduced by pretreatment with a benzodiazepine and the use of ketamine at the lower end of the dosing range. Rapid I.V. administration or overdose may cause respiratory depression, apnea, and enhanced pressor response. Resuscitative equipment should be available during use. Use with caution in patients with CSF pressure elevation, the chronic alcoholic or acutely alcohol-intoxicated. May cause dependence (withdrawal symptoms on discontinuation) and tolerance with prolonged use. May cause CNS depression, which may impair physical or mental abilities; patients must be cautioned about performing tasks which require mental alertness (eg, operating machinery or driving). When used on an outpatient basis, patient should be accompanied by a responsible adult. Should be administered under the supervision of a physician experienced in administering general anesthetics.

Adverse Reactions Frequency not always defined.

Cardiovascular: Arrhythmia, bradycardia, hyper-/hypotension, pulse rate increased

Central nervous system: CSF pressure increased

Dermatologic: Erythema (transient), morbilliform rash (transient)

Gastrointestinal: Anorexia, nausea, vomiting

Local: Pain at the injection site, exanthema at the injection site

Neuromuscular & skeletal: Skeletal muscle tone enhanced (tonic-clonic movements)

Ocular: Diplopia, intraocular pressure increased, nystagmus

Respiratory: Airway obstruction, apnea, respiratory depression or stimulation, laryngospasm

Miscellaneous: Anaphylaxis, dependence with prolonged use, emergence reactions (~12%; includes confusion, delirium, dreamlike state, excitement, hallucinations, irrational behavior, vivid imagery)

Drug Interactions

Metabolism/Transport Effects Substrate (major) of CYP2B6, 2C9, 3A4

Avoid Concomitant Use There are no known interactions where it is recommended to avoid concomitant use.

Increased Effect/Toxicity

The levels/effects of Ketamine may be increased by: CYP2B6 Inhibitors (Moderate); CYP2B6 Inhibitors (Strong); CYP2C9 Inhibitors (Moderate); CYP2C9 Inhibitors (Strong); CYP3A4 Inhibitors (Moderate); CYP3A4 Inhibitors (Strong); Dasatinib

Decreased Effect

The levels/effects of Ketamine may be decreased by: CYP2C9 Inducers (Highly Effective)

Stability Store at 20°C to 25°C (68°F to 77°F). Protect from light. The 50 mg/mL and 100 mg/mL vials may be further diluted in D_5W or NS to a final concentration of 1 mg/mL (or 2 mg/mL in patients with fluid restrictions). The 10 mg/mL vials are not recommended to be further diluted. Do not mix with barbiturates or diazepam (precipitation may occur).

Mechanism of Action Produces a cataleptic-like state in which the patient is dissociated from the surrounding environment by direct action on the cortex and limbic system. Releases endogenous catecholamines (epinephrine, norepinephrine) which maintain blood pressure and heart rate. Reduces polysynaptic spinal reflexes.

Pharmacodynamics/Kinetics

Onset of action:
- I.V.: Anesthetic effect: 30 seconds
- I.M.: Anesthetic effect: 3-4 minutes

Duration: Anesthetic effect: I.V.: 5-10 minutes; I.M.: 12-25 minutes

Metabolism: Hepatic via hydroxylation and N-demethylation; the metabolite norketamine is 33% as potent as parent compound

Half-life elimination: Alpha: 10-15 minutes; Beta: 2.5 hours

Excretion: Primarily urine

Dosage May be used in combination with anticholinergic agents to decrease hypersalivation.

Children: **Note:** Titrate dose for desired effect.
- Oral: Sedation (unlabeled use/route): 6-10 mg/kg for 1 dose (mixed in 0.2-0.3 mL/kg of cola or other beverage) given 30 minutes before the procedure
- I.M.: Sedation/analgesia (unlabeled use): 4-5 mg/kg/dose; doses up to 13 mg/kg have been reported
- I.V.: Sedation/analgesia (unlabeled use): 1-2 mg/kg/dose; titrate repeat doses for desired effect
- Continuous I.V. infusion: Sedation (unlabeled use): 5-20 mcg/kg/minute; titrate to reach desired level of sedation

Children ≥16 years and Adults:
- Induction of anesthesia:
  - I.M.: 6.5-13 mg/kg; usual dose to produce 12-25 minutes of anesthesia: 10 mg/kg
  - I.V.: 1-4.5 mg/kg; usual dose to produce 5-10 minutes of anesthesia: 2 mg/kg
  - I.V. infusion: 1-2 mg/kg infuse over 0.5 mg/kg/minute; may administer with diazepam to prevent emergence reactions
- Maintenance of anesthesia: Supplemental doses of 1/2 to the full induction dose; may also be maintained with a continuous infusion of 0.1-5 mg/minute

Administration

Oral: Use 100 mg/mL I.V. solution and mix the appropriate dose in 0.2-0.3 mL/kg of cola or other beverage.

Parenteral: I.V.: Do not exceed 0.5 mg/kg/minute or administer faster than 60 seconds. Solutions for infusion should not exceed final concentration of 2 mg/mL.

Monitoring Parameters Heart rate, blood pressure, respiratory rate, transcutaneous O_2 saturation, emergence reactions; cardiac function should be continuously monitored in patients with increased blood pressure or cardiac decompensation

Additional Information Produces emergence psychosis including auditory and visual hallucinations, restlessness, disorientation, vivid dreams, and irrational behavior in ~12% of patients; pretreatment with a benzodiazepine reduces incidence of psychosis by >50%. Spontaneous involuntary movements, nystagmus, hypertonus, and vocalizations are also commonly seen.

The analgesia outlasts the general anesthetic component. Bronchodilation is beneficial in asthmatic or COPD patients. Laryngeal reflexes may remain intact or may be obtunded. The direct myocardial depressant action of ketamine can be seen in stressed, catecholamine-deficient patients. Ketamine increases cerebral metabolism and cerebral blood flow while producing a noncompetitive block of the neuronal postsynaptic NMDA receptor. It lowers seizure threshold and stimulates salivary secretions (atropine/scopolamine treatment is recommended).

Dosage Forms Excipient information presented when available (limited, particularly for generics); consult specific product labeling.

Injection, solution: 50 mg/mL (10 mL); 100 mg/mL (5 mL)
- Ketalar®: 10 mg/mL (20 mL); 50 mg/mL (10 mL); 100 mg/mL (5 mL)

◆ **Ketamine Hydrochloride** *see* Ketamine *on page 836*

◆ **Ketamine Hydrochloride Injection, USP (Can)** *see* Ketamine *on page 836*

◆ **Ketek®** *see* Telithromycin *on page 1429*

Ketoconazole (kee toe KOE na zole)

U.S. Brand Names Extina®; Kuric™; Nizoral®; Nizoral® A-D [OTC]; Xolegel™

Canadian Brand Names Apo-Ketoconazole®; Ketoderm®; Novo-Ketoconazole; Xolegel™

Pharmacologic Category Antifungal Agent, Oral; Antifungal Agent, Topical

Additional Appendix Information

Antifungal Agents *on page 1640*

Guidelines for the Prevention of Opportunistic Infections in HIV Infected Persons *on page 1740*

Use

Systemic: Treatment of susceptible fungal infections, including candidiasis, oral thrush, blastomycosis, histoplasmosis, paracoccidioidomycosis, coccidioidomycosis, chromomycosis, candiduria, chronic mucocutaneous candidiasis, as well as certain recalcitrant cutaneous dermatophytoses

Topical:
- Cream: Treatment of tinea corporis, tinea cruris, tinea versicolor, cutaneous candidiasis, seborrheic dermatitis
- Foam, gel: Treatment of seborrheic dermatitis
- Shampoo: Treatment of dandruff, seborrheic dermatitis, tinea versicolor

Unlabeled/Investigational Use Tablet: Treatment of prostate cancer (androgen synthesis inhibitor)

Pregnancy Risk Factor C

Pregnancy Considerations

Teratogenic effects were noted in animal studies. There are no adequate and well-controlled studies in pregnant women.

Lactation Enters breast milk/not recommended

Medication Safety Issues

Sound-alike/look-alike issues:
- Kuric™ may be confused with Carac®
- Nizoral® may be confused with Nasarel®, Neoral®, Nitrol®

Contraindications Hypersensitivity to ketoconazole or any component of the formulation; CNS fungal infections (due to poor CNS penetration); coadministration with ergot derivatives or cisapride is contraindicated due to risk of potentially fatal cardiac arrhythmias

Warnings/Precautions [U.S. Boxed Warning]: Ketoconazole has been associated with hepatotoxicity, including some fatalities; use with caution in patients with impaired hepatic function and perform periodic liver function tests. **[U.S. Boxed Warning]: Concomitant use with cisapride is contraindicated due to the occurrence of ventricular arrhythmias.** High doses of ketoconazole may depress adrenocortical function.

Topical: Formulations may contain sulfites. Avoid exposure of gel to open flames during or immediately after application. Foam formulation contains alcohol and propane/butane; do not expose to open flame or smoking during or immediately after application; do not puncture or incinerate container.

Adverse Reactions

Oral:

1% to 10%:

Dermatologic: Pruritus (2%)

Gastrointestinal: Nausea/vomiting (3% to 10%), abdominal pain (1%)

<1% (Limited to important or life-threatening): Bulging fontanelles, chills, depression, diarrhea, dizziness, fever, gynecomastia, headache, hemolytic anemia, hepatotoxicity, impotence, leukopenia, photophobia, somnolence, thrombocytopenia

Topical cream/gel: Allergic reaction, contact dermatitis (possibly related to sulfites or propylene glycol), facial swelling, headache, impetigo, local burning, ocular irritation, paresthesia, pruritus, severe irritation, stinging (~5%)

Topical foam: Application site burning (10%), application site reaction (6%), contact sensitization, dryness, erythema, pruritus, rash

Shampoo: Abnormal hair texture, hair loss increase, irritation (<1%), itching, mild dryness of skin, oiliness/dryness of hair, scalp pustules

Drug Interactions

Metabolism/Transport Effects Substrate of CYP3A4 (major); **Inhibits** CYP1A2 (strong), 2A6 (moderate), 2B6 (weak), 2C8 (weak), 2C9 (strong), 2C19 (moderate), 2D6 (moderate), 3A4 (strong)

Avoid Concomitant Use

Avoid concomitant use of Ketoconazole with any of the following: Alfuzosin; Cisapride; Conivaptan; Dabigatran Etexilate; Dofetilide; Nilotinib; Pimozide; QuiNIDine; Ranolazine; Rivaroxaban; Salmeterol; Silodosin; Thioridazine; Topotecan

Increased Effect/Toxicity

Ketoconazole may increase the levels/effects of: Alfentanil; Alfuzosin; Aliskiren; Almotriptan; Alosetron; Aprepitant; Bendamustine; Benzodiazepines (metabolized by oxidation); Bosentan; BusPIRone; Busulfan; Calcium Channel Blockers; CarBAMazepine; Cardiac Glycosides; Ciclesonide; Cilostazol; Cinacalcet; Cisapride; Conivaptan; Corticosteroids (Orally Inhaled); Corticosteroids (Systemic); CycloSPORINE; CYP1A2 Substrates; CYP2A6 Substrates; CYP2C19 Substrates; CYP2C9 Substrates (High risk); CYP2D6 Substrates; CYP3A4 Substrates; Dabigatran Etexilate; Docetaxel; Dofetilide; Eletriptan; Eplerenone; Erlotinib; Eszopiclone; FentaNYL; Fesoterodine; Fexofenadine; Fosaprepitant; Gefitinib; HMG-CoA Reductase Inhibitors; Imatinib; Irinotecan; Ixabepilone; Losartan; Macrolide Antibiotics; Maraviroc; Methadone; Nebivolol; Nilotinib; P-Glycoprotein Substrates; Phenytoin; Phosphodiesterase 5 Inhibitors; Pimecrolimus; Pimozide; Praziquantel; Protease Inhibitors; Proton Pump Inhibitors; QuiNIDine; Ramelteon; Ranolazine; Repaglinide; Rifamycin Derivatives; Rivaroxaban; Salmeterol; Silodosin; Sirolimus; Solifenacin; Sorafenib; Sunitinib; Tacrolimus; Tamoxifen; Temsirolimus; Thioridazine; Tolterodine; Topotecan; VinCRIStine; Vitamin K Antagonists; Ziprasidone; Zolpidem

The levels/effects of Ketoconazole may be increased by: Macrolide Antibiotics; Protease Inhibitors

Decreased Effect

Ketoconazole may decrease the levels/effects of: Amphotericin B; Codeine; Saccharomyces boulardii; TraMADol

The levels/effects of Ketoconazole may be decreased by: Antacids; CYP3A4 Inducers (Strong); Deferasirox; Didanosine; Grapefruit Juice; H2-Antagonists; Herbs (CYP3A4 Inducers); Phenytoin; Proton Pump Inhibitors; Rifamycin Derivatives; Sucralfate

Ethanol/Nutrition/Herb Interactions

Food: Ketoconazole peak serum levels may be prolonged if taken with food.

Herb/Nutraceutical: St John's wort may decrease ketoconazole levels.

Stability

Cream: Store at <25°C (<77°F).

Foam: Store at 20°C to 25°C (68°F to 77°F). Do not refrigerate. Do not store in direct sunlight. Contents are flammable.

Gel: Store at 15°C to 30°C (59°F to 86°F).

Shampoo: Store between 2°C to 30°C (35°F to 86°F); protect from freezing. Protect from light.

Tablet: Store at 15°C to 25°C (59°F to 77°F).

Mechanism of Action Alters the permeability of the cell wall by blocking fungal cytochrome P450; inhibits biosynthesis of triglycerides and phospholipids by fungi; inhibits several fungal enzymes that results in a build-up of toxic concentrations of hydrogen peroxide; also inhibits androgen synthesis

Pharmacodynamics/Kinetics

Absorption: Oral: Rapid (~75%); Shampoo: None; Gel: Minimal

Distribution: Well into inflamed joint fluid, saliva, bile, urine, breast milk, sebum, cerumen, feces, tendons, skin and soft tissue, and testes; crosses blood-brain barrier poorly; only negligible amounts reach CSF

Protein binding: 93% to 96%

Metabolism: Partially hepatic via CYP3A4 to inactive compounds

Bioavailability: Decreases as gastric pH increases

Half-life elimination: Biphasic: Initial: 2 hours; Terminal: 8 hours

Time to peak, serum: 1-2 hours

Excretion: Feces (57%); urine (13%)

Dosage

Oral:

Fungal infections:

Children ≥2 years: 3.3-6.6 mg/kg/day as a single dose for 1-2 weeks for candidiasis, for at least 4 weeks in recalcitrant dermatophyte infections, and for up to 6 months for other systemic mycoses

Adults: 200-400 mg/day as a single daily dose for durations as stated above

Prostate cancer (unlabeled use): Adults: 400 mg 3 times/day

Shampoo: Seborrheic dermatitis, tinea versicolor: Children ≥12 years and Adults: Apply twice weekly for 4 weeks with at least 3 days between each shampoo

Topical:

Tinea infections: Adults: Cream: Rub gently into the affected area once daily. Duration of treatment: Tinea corporis, cruris: 2 weeks; tinea pedis: 6 weeks

Seborrheic dermatitis: Children ≥12 years and Adults:

Cream: Rub gently into the affected area twice daily for 4 weeks or until clinical response is noted

Foam: Apply to affected area twice daily for 4 weeks

Gel: Rub gently into the affected area once daily for 2 weeks

Dosing adjustment in hepatic impairment: Dose reductions should be considered in patients with severe liver disease

Hemodialysis: Not dialyzable (0% to 5%)

Dietary Considerations Tablet: May be taken with food or milk to decrease GI adverse effects.

Administration

Oral: Administer oral tablets 2 hours prior to antacids to prevent decreased absorption due to the high pH of gastric contents.

Cream, foam, gel, and shampoo are for external use only. Avoid exposure to flame or smoking immediately following application of gel or foam; do not apply directly to hands.

Monitoring Parameters Liver function tests

Dosage Forms Excipient information presented when available (limited, particularly for generics); consult specific product labeling.

Aerosol, topical [foam]:
Extina®: 2% (50 g, 100 g)
Cream, topical: 2% (15 g, 30 g, 60 g)
Kuric™: 2%: (75 g)
Gel, topical:
Xolegel™: 2% (15 g) [contains dehydrated alcohol 34%]
Shampoo, topical: 1% (120 mL), 2% (120 mL)
Nizoral®: 2% (120 mL)
Nizoral® A-D: 1% (120 mL, 210 mL)
Tablet: 200 mg

Extemporaneous Preparations A 20 mg/mL suspension may be made by pulverizing twelve 200 mg ketoconazole tablets to a fine powder; add 40 mL Ora-Plus® in small portions with thorough mixing; incorporate Ora-Sweet® to make a final volume of 120 mL and mix thoroughly; refrigerate (no stability information is available)

Allen LV, "Ketoconazole Oral Suspension," *US Pharm*, 1993, 18(2):98-9, 101.

◆ **Ketoderm® (Can)** *see* Ketoconazole *on page* 837

◆ **3-Keto-desogestrel** *see* Etonogestrel *on page* 589

Ketoprofen (kee toe PROE fen)

Canadian Brand Names Apo-Keto SR®; Apo-Keto-E®; Apo-Keto®; Novo-Keto; Novo-Keto-EC; Nu-Ketoprofen; Nu-Ketoprofen-E; Oruvail®; Rhodis SR™; Rhodis-EC™; Rhodis™

Pharmacologic Category Nonsteroidal Anti-inflammatory Drug (NSAID), Oral

Additional Appendix Information

Nonsteroidal Anti-inflammatory Agents *on page* 1669

Use Acute and long-term treatment of rheumatoid arthritis and osteoarthritis; primary dysmenorrhea; mild-to-moderate pain

Restrictions An FDA-approved medication guide must be distributed when dispensing an oral outpatient prescription (new or refill) where this medication is to be used without direct supervision of a healthcare provider. Medication guides are available at http://www.fda.gov/cder/Offices/ODS/medication_guides.htm.

Pregnancy Risk Factor C/D (3rd trimester)

Pregnancy Considerations Teratogenic effects were not observed in animal studies. Embryotoxicity was observed in some, but not all, animal studies. Renal insufficiency and pulmonary hypertension have been noted in premature infants (case reports). Accumulation of the active enantiomer of ketoprofen has also been reported in premature neonates with renal insufficiency. Exposure to NSAIDs late in pregnancy may lead to premature closure of the ductus arteriosus and may inhibit uterine contractions.

Lactation Excretion in breast milk unknown/not recommended

Medication Safety Issues

Sound-alike/look-alike issues:

Ketoprofen may be confused with ketotifen

Oruvail® may be confused with Clinoril®, Elavil®

Contraindications Hypersensitivity to ketoprofen, aspirin, other NSAIDs, or any component of the formulation; perioperative pain in the setting of coronary artery bypass graft (CABG) surgery

Warnings/Precautions [U.S. Boxed Warning]: NSAIDs are associated with an increased risk of adverse cardiovascular thrombotic events, including MI, stroke, and new onset or worsening of pre-existing hypertension. Risk may be increased with duration of use or pre-existing cardiovascular risk factors or disease. Carefully evaluate individual cardiovascular risk profiles prior to prescribing. Use caution with fluid retention, heart failure, or hypertension. Concurrent administration of ibuprofen, and potentially other nonselective NSAIDs, may interfere with aspirin's cardioprotective effect. **[U.S. Boxed Warning]: Use is contraindicated for treatment of perioperative pain in the setting of coronary artery bypass graft (CABG) surgery.** Risk of MI and stroke may be increased with use following CABG surgery.

NSAID use may compromise existing renal function; dose-dependent decreases in prostaglandin synthesis may result from NSAID use, reducing renal blood flow which may cause renal decompensation. Patients with impaired renal function, dehydration, heart failure, liver dysfunction, those taking diuretics, and ACE inhibitors, and the elderly are at greater risk of renal toxicity. Rehydrate patient before starting therapy; monitor renal function closely. Not recommended for use in patients with advanced renal disease. Long-term NSAID use may result in renal papillary necrosis.

[U.S. Boxed Warning]: NSAIDs may increase risk of gastrointestinal irritation, inflammation, ulceration, bleeding, and perforation. These events may occur at any time during therapy and without warning. Use caution with a history of GI disease (bleeding or ulcers), concurrent therapy with aspirin, anticoagulants and/or corticosteroids, smoking, use of alcohol, the elderly or debilitated patients. Platelet adhesion and aggregation may be decreased; may prolong bleeding time; patients with coagulation disorders or who are receiving anticoagulants should be monitored closely. Anemia may occur; patients on long-term NSAID therapy should be monitored for anemia.

Use the lowest effective dose for the shortest duration of time, consistent with individual patient goals, to reduce risk of cardiovascular or GI adverse events. Alternate therapies should be considered for patients at high risk.

NSAIDs may cause serious skin adverse events including exfoliative dermatitis, Stevens-Johnson syndrome (SJS), and toxic epidermal necrolysis (TEN); discontinue use at first sign of skin rash or hypersensitivity. Anaphylactoid reactions may occur, even without prior exposure; patients with "aspirin triad" (bronchial asthma, aspirin intolerance, rhinitis) may be at increased risk. Do not use in patients who experience bronchospasm, asthma, rhinitis, or urticaria with NSAID or aspirin therapy. Use caution in other forms of asthma.

Use with caution in patients with decreased hepatic function. Closely monitor patients with any abnormal LFT. Severe hepatic reactions (eg, fulminant hepatitis, liver failure) have occurred with NSAID use, rarely; discontinue if signs or symptoms of liver disease develop, or if systemic manifestations occur. The elderly are at increased risk for adverse effects (especially peptic ulceration, CNS effects, renal toxicity) from NSAIDs, even at low doses.

Withhold for at least 4-6 half-lives prior to surgical or dental procedures. Safety and efficacy have not been established in pediatric patients.

Adverse Reactions

>10%:

Gastrointestinal: Dyspepsia (11%)

Hepatic: Liver function test abnormal (≤15%)

1% to 10%:

Cardiovascular: Peripheral edema (2%)

Central nervous system: Headache (3% to 9%), depression, dizziness (>1%), dreams, insomnia, malaise, nervousness, somnolence

Dermatologic: Rash (>1%)

Gastrointestinal: Abdominal pain (3% to 9%), constipation (3% to 9%), diarrhea (3% to 9%), flatulence (3% to 9%), nausea (3% to 9%), gastrointestinal bleeding (>2%), peptic ulcer (>2%), anorexia (>1%), stomatitis (>1%), vomiting (>1%)

Genitourinary: Urinary tract irritation (>1%)

Ocular: Visual disturbances (>1%)

Otic: Tinnitus (>1%)

Renal: Renal dysfunction (3% to 9%)

<1% (Limited to important or life-threatening): Agranulocytosis, allergic reaction, allergic rhinitis, alopecia, anaphylaxis, anemia, angioedema, arrhythmia, aseptic meningitis, blurred vision, bone marrow suppression, bronchospasm, buccal necrosis, bullous rash, chills, cholestatic hepatitis, confusion, CHF, conjunctivitis, cystitis, diabetes mellitus (aggravated), drowsiness, dysphoria, dyspnea, eczema, edema, epistaxis, erythema multiforme, exfoliative dermatitis, facial edema, fecal occult blood, fluid retention, gastritis, gastrointestinal perforation, GI ulceration, gynecomastia, hallucinations, hearing decreased, hematemesis, hematuria, hemolytic anemia, hemoptysis, hepatic dysfunction, hepatitis, hot flashes, hypertension, hyponatremia, impotence, infection, interstitial nephritis, intestinal ulceration, jaundice, laryngeal edema, leukopenia, libido disturbance, melena, microvesicular steatosis, migraine, myocardial infarction, nephrotic syndrome, onycholysis, palpitation, pancreatitis, peptic ulcer, peripheral neuropathy, peripheral vascular disease, photosensitivity, polydipsia, polyuria, pruritus, purpura, purpuric rash, renal failure, renal papillary necrosis, retinal hemorrhage, septicemia, shock, Stevens-Johnson syndrome, tachycardia, thrombocytopenia, toxic amblyopia, toxic epidermal necrolysis, tubulopathy, ulcerative colitis, urticaria, vasodilation, xerostomia

Drug Interactions

Metabolism/Transport Effects Inhibits CYP2C9 (weak)

Avoid Concomitant Use

Avoid concomitant use of Ketoprofen with any of the following: Ketorolac

Increased Effect/Toxicity

Ketoprofen may increase the levels/effects of: Aminoglycosides; Anticoagulants; Antiplatelet Agents; Bisphosphonate Derivatives; CycloSPORINE; Desmopressin; Lithium; Methotrexate; Nonsteroidal Anti-Inflammatory Agents; Pemetrexed; Quinolone Antibiotics; Salicylates; Thrombolytic Agents; Vancomycin; Vitamin K Antagonists

The levels/effects of Ketoprofen may be increased by: Antidepressants (Tricyclic, Tertiary Amine); Corticosteroids (Systemic); Herbs (Anticoagulant/Antiplatelet Properties); Ketorolac; Probenecid; Selective Serotonin Reuptake Inhibitors; Serotonin/Norepinephrine Reuptake Inhibitors; Treprostinil

Decreased Effect

Ketoprofen may decrease the levels/effects of: ACE Inhibitors; Angiotensin II Receptor Blockers; Antiplatelet Agents; Beta-Blockers; Eplerenone; HydrALAZINE; Loop Diuretics; Salicylates; Thiazide Diuretics

The levels/effects of Ketoprofen may be decreased by: Bile Acid Sequestrants; Salicylates

Ethanol/Nutrition/Herb Interactions

Ethanol: Avoid ethanol (due to GI irritation).

Food: Food slows rate of absorption resulting in delayed and reduced peak serum concentrations; total bioavailability is not affected by food.

Herb/Nutraceutical: Avoid alfalfa, anise, bilberry, bladderwrack, bromelain, cat's claw, celery, chamomile, coleus, cordyceps, dong quai, evening primrose, fenugreek, feverfew, garlic, ginger, ginkgo biloba, ginseng (American, Panax, Siberian), grapeseed, green tea, guggul, horse chestnut seed, horseradish, licorice, prickly ash, red clover, reishi, SAMe (S-adenosylmethionine), sweet clover, turmeric, and white willow (all have additional antiplatelet activity).

Stability Store at room temperature of 25°C (77°F). Protect from light; avoid excessive heat and humidity.

Mechanism of Action Reversibly inhibits cyclooxygenase-1 and 2 (COX-1 and 2) enzymes, which result in decreased formation of prostaglandin precursors; has antipyretic, analgesic, and anti-inflammatory properties

Pharmacodynamics/Kinetics

Onset of action: Regular release: <30 minutes

Duration: Regular release: Up to 6 hours

Absorption: Almost complete

Protein binding: >99%, primarily to albumin; Hepatic impairment: Unbound fraction is approximately doubled

Metabolism: Hepatic via glucuronidation; metabolite can be converted back to parent compound; may have enterohepatic recirculation

Bioavailability: ~90%

Half-life elimination:

Regular release: 2-4 hours; Renal impairment: Mild: 3 hours; moderate-to-severe: 5-9 hours

Extended release: ~3-7.5 hours

Time to peak, serum:

Regular release: 0.5-2 hours

Extended release: 6-7 hours

Excretion: Urine (~80%, primarily as glucuronide conjugates)

Dosage Note: The extended release formulation is not recommended for the treatment of acute pain. Oral:

Adults:

Rheumatoid arthritis, osteoarthritis (lower doses may be used in small patients or in the elderly, or debilitated):

Regular release: 50 mg 4 times/day **or** 75 mg 3 times/day; up to a maximum of 300 mg/day

Extended release: 200 mg once daily

Dysmenorrhea, mild-to-moderate pain: Regular release: 25-50 mg every 6-8 hours up to a maximum of 300 mg/day

Elderly: Initial dose should be decreased in patients >75 years; use caution when dosage changes are made

Dosage adjustment in renal impairment: In general, NSAIDs are not recommended for use in patients with advanced renal disease, but the manufacturer of ketoprofen does provide some guidelines for adjustment in renal dysfunction:

Mild impairment: Maximum dose: 150 mg/day

Severe impairment: Cl_{cr} <25 mL/minute: Maximum dose: 100 mg/day

Dosage adjustment in hepatic impairment and serum albumin <3.5 g/dL: Maximum dose: 100 mg/day

Dietary Considerations In order to minimize gastrointestinal effects, ketoprofen can be prescribed to be taken with food or milk.

Administration May take with food to reduce GI upset. Do not crush or break extended release capsules.

Monitoring Parameters CBC, chemistry profile, occult blood loss, periodic liver function; renal function (urine output, serum BUN, creatinine)

Dosage Forms Excipient information presented when available (limited, particularly for generics); consult specific product labeling.

Capsule, regular release: 50 mg, 75 mg

Capsule, extended release: 200 mg

Ketorolac (KEE toe role ak)

U.S. Brand Names Acular LS™; Acular®; Acular® PF

Canadian Brand Names Acular LS™; Acular®; Apo-Ketorolac Injectable®; Apo-Ketorolac®; Ketorolac Tromethamine Injection, USP; Novo-Ketorolac; ratio-Ketorolac; Toradol®; Toradol® IM

Index Terms Ketorolac Tromethamine

Pharmacologic Category Nonsteroidal Anti-inflammatory Drug (NSAID), Ophthalmic; Nonsteroidal Anti-inflammatory Drug (NSAID), Oral; Nonsteroidal Anti-inflammatory Drug (NSAID), Parenteral

Additional Appendix Information

Nonsteroidal Anti-inflammatory Agents *on page 1669*

Use

Oral, injection: Short-term (≤5 days) management of moderate-to-severe acute pain requiring analgesia at the opioid level

Ophthalmic: Temporary relief of ocular itching due to seasonal allergic conjunctivitis; postoperative inflammation following cataract extraction; reduction of ocular pain and photophobia following incisional refractive surgery; reduction of ocular pain, burning, and stinging following corneal refractive surgery

Restrictions An FDA-approved medication guide must be distributed when dispensing an oral outpatient prescription (new or refill) where this medication is to be used without direct supervision of a healthcare provider. Medication guides are available at http://www.fda.gov/cder/Offices/ODS/medication_guides.htm.

Pregnancy Risk Factor C/D (3rd trimester)

Pregnancy Considerations **[U.S. Boxed Warning]: Ketorolac is contraindicated during labor and delivery (may inhibit uterine contractions and adversely affect fetal circulation).** Avoid the use of ketorolac (all dosage forms) during late pregnancy.

Lactation Enters breast milk/contraindicated

Medication Safety Issues

Sound-alike/look-alike issues:

Acular® may be confused with Acthar®, Ocular®

Ketorolac may be confused with Ketalar®

Toradol® may be confused with Foradil®, Inderal®, Tegretol®, Torecan®, traMADol, tromethamine

International issues:

Toradol® may be confused with Theradol® which is a brand name for tramadol in the Netherlands

Contraindications

Oral, injection: Hypersensitivity to ketorolac, aspirin, other NSAIDs, or any component of the formulation; active or history of peptic ulcer disease; recent or history of GI bleeding or perforation; patients with advanced renal disease or risk of renal failure (due to volume depletion); prophylaxis before major surgery; suspected or confirmed cerebrovascular bleeding; hemorrhagic diathesis, incomplete hemostasis, or high risk of bleeding; concurrent ASA or other NSAIDs; concomitant probenecid or pentoxifylline; epidural or intrathecal administration; perioperative pain in the setting of coronary artery bypass graft (CABG) surgery; labor and delivery; breast-feeding

Ophthalmic: Hypersensitivity to ketorolac or any component of the formulation

Warnings/Precautions **[U.S. Boxed Warning]: May inhibit platelet function; contraindicated in patients with cerebrovascular bleeding (suspected or confirmed), hemorrhagic diathesis, incomplete hemostasis and patients at high risk for bleeding.** Effects on platelet adhesion and aggregation may prolong bleeding time. Anemia may occur; patients on long-term NSAID therapy should be monitored for anemia.

[U.S. Boxed Warning]: NSAIDs are associated with an increased risk of adverse cardiovascular thrombotic events, including MI, stroke, and new onset or worsening of pre-existing hypertension. Risk may be increased with duration of use or pre-existing cardiovascular risk factors or disease. Carefully evaluate individual cardiovascular risk profiles prior to prescribing. Use caution with fluid retention, heart failure, or hypertension. Concurrent administration of ibuprofen, and potentially other nonselective NSAIDs, may interfere with aspirin's cardioprotective effect. **[U.S. Boxed Warning]: Use is contraindicated as prophylactic analgesic before any major surgery and is contraindicated for treatment of perioperative pain in the setting of coronary artery bypass graft (CABG) surgery.** Risk of MI and stroke may be increased with use following CABG surgery. Wound bleeding and postoperative hematomas have been associated with ketorolac use in the perioperative setting. Withhold for at least 4-6 half-lives prior to surgical or dental procedures.

[U.S. Boxed Warning]: Ketorolac is contraindicated in patients with advanced renal impairment and in patients at risk for renal failure due to volume depletion. NSAID use may compromise existing renal function; dose-dependent decreases in prostaglandin synthesis may result from NSAID use, reducing renal blood flow which may cause renal decompensation. Patients with impaired renal function, dehydration, heart failure, liver dysfunction, those taking diuretics and ACE inhibitors, and the elderly are at greater risk of renal toxicity. Use with caution in patients with impaired renal function or history of kidney disease; dosage adjustment is required in patients with moderate elevation in serum creatinine. Monitor renal function closely. Acute renal failure, interstitial nephritis, and nephrotic syndrome have been reported with ketorolac use; papillary necrosis and renal injury have been reported with the use of NSAIDs. Use of NSAIDs can compromise existing renal function. Rehydrate patient before starting therapy.

[U.S. Boxed Warning]: NSAIDs may increase risk of gastrointestinal irritation, inflammation, ulceration, bleeding, and perforation. These events may occur at any time during therapy and without warning. Use caution with a history of GI disease (bleeding, ulcers, inflammatory bowel disease), concurrent therapy with aspirin, anticoagulants and/or corticosteroids, smoking, use of alcohol, the elderly, or debilitated patients.

NSAIDs may cause serious skin adverse events including exfoliative dermatitis, Stevens-Johnson syndrome (SJS), and toxic epidermal necrolysis (TEN); discontinue use at first sign of skin rash or hypersensitivity. Hypersensitivity or anaphylactoid reactions may occur, even without prior exposure; patients with "aspirin triad" (bronchial asthma, aspirin intolerance, rhinitis) may be at increased risk. Do not use in patients who experience bronchospasm, asthma, rhinitis, or urticaria with NSAID or aspirin therapy. **[U.S. Boxed Warning]: Ketorolac injection is contraindicated in patients with prior hypersensitivity reaction to aspirin or NSAIDs.** Use caution in other forms of asthma.

Use with caution in patients with hepatic impairment or a history of liver disease. Closely monitor patients with any abnormal LFT. Rarely, severe hepatic reactions (eg, fulminant hepatitis, hepatic necrosis, liver failure) have occurred with NSAID use; discontinue if signs or symptoms of liver disease develop, or if systemic manifestations occur.

[U.S. Boxed Warning]: Dosage adjustment is required for patients ≥65 years of age. The elderly are at increased risk for adverse effects (especially peptic ulceration, CNS effects, renal toxicity) from NSAIDs, even at low doses. **[U.S. Boxed Warning]: Dosage adjustment is required for patients weighing <50 kg (<110 pounds). [U.S. Boxed Warning]: May inhibit uterine contractions and affect fetal circulation; inhibits prostaglandin synthesis in neonates; use is contraindicated in labor and delivery and breast-feeding women.** Avoid use in late pregnancy. **[U.S. Boxed Warning]: Concurrent use of ketorolac with aspirin or other NSAIDs is contraindicated due to the increased risk of adverse reactions.**

[U.S. Boxed Warning]: Contraindicated for epidural or intrathecal administration. [U.S. Boxed Warning]: Systemic ketorolac is indicated for short term (≤5 days) use in adults for treatment of moderately severe acute pain requiring opioid-level analgesia. Low doses of narcotics may be needed for breakthrough pain. **[U.S. Boxed Warning]: Oral therapy is only indicated for use as continuation treatment, following parenteral ketorolac and is not indicated for minor or chronic painful conditions. The maximum daily oral dose is 40 mg (adults); doses above 40 mg/day do not improve efficacy but may increase the risk of serious adverse effects.** The combined therapy duration (oral and parenteral) should not exceed 5 days. Use the lowest effective dose for the shortest duration of time, consistent with individual patient goals, to reduce risk of cardiovascular or GI adverse events. Alternate therapies should be considered for patients at high risk. **[U.S. Boxed Warning]: Oral ketorolac is not indicated for use in children.**

Ophthalmic: May increase bleeding time associated with ocular surgery. Use with caution in patients with known bleeding tendencies or those receiving anticoagulants. Healing time may be slowed or delayed. Corneal thinning, erosion, or ulceration have been reported with topical NSAIDs; discontinue if corneal epithelial breakdown occurs. Use caution with complicated ocular surgery, corneal denervation, corneal epithelial defects, diabetes, rheumatoid arthritis, ocular surface disease, or ocular surgeries repeated within short periods of time; risk of corneal epithelial breakdown may be increased. Use for >24 hours prior to or for >14 days following surgery also increases risk of corneal adverse effects. Do not administer while wearing soft contact lenses. Safety and efficacy in pediatric patients <3 years of age have not been established.

Adverse Reactions

Systemic (frequencies noted for parenteral administration):

>10%:

Central nervous system: Headache (17%)

Gastrointestinal: Gastrointestinal pain (13%), dyspepsia (12%), nausea (12%)

>1% to 10%:

Cardiovascular: Edema (4%), hypertension

Central nervous system: Dizziness (7%), drowsiness (6%)

Dermatologic: Pruritus, purpura, rash

Gastrointestinal: Diarrhea (7%), constipation, flatulence, GI bleeding, GI fullness, GI perforation, GI ulcer, heartburn, stomatitis, vomiting

Hematologic: Anemia, bleeding time increased

Hepatic: Liver enzymes increased

Local: Injection site pain (2%)

Otic: Tinnitus

Renal: Renal function abnormal

Miscellaneous: Diaphoresis

<1% (Limited to important or life-threatening): Abnormal thinking, acute pancreatitis, acute renal failure, agranulocytosis, alopecia, anaphylactoid reaction, anaphylaxis, angioedema, anxiety, aplastic anemia, arrhythmia, aseptic meningitis, asthma, azotemia, blurred vision, bradycardia, bronchospasm, bruising, chest pain, CHF, cholestatic jaundice, coma, confusion, conjunctivitis, cough, cystitis, depression, dyspnea, dysuria, eosinophilia, epistaxis, eructation, erythema multiforme, esophagitis, euphoria, excessive thirst, exfoliative dermatitis, extrapyramidal symptoms, fever, flank pain, flushing, gastritis, GI hemorrhage, glossitis, hallucinations, hearing loss, hematemesis, hematuria, hemolytic anemia, hemolytic uremic syndrome, hepatitis, hyperglycemia, hyperkalemia, hyperkinesis, hypersensitivity reactions, hyponatremia, hypotension, inability to concentrate, infection, infertility, inflammatory bowel disease exacerbation, insomnia, interstitial nephritis, jaundice, laryngeal edema, leukopenia, liver failure, Lyell's syndrome, lymphadenopathy, maculopapular rash, melena, MI, nephritis, nervousness, oliguria, pallor, palpitation, pancytopenia, paresthesia, photosensitivity, pneumonia, polyuria, proteinuria, psychosis, pulmonary edema, rectal bleeding, renal failure, respiratory depression, rhinitis, seizure, sepsis, somnolence, Stevens-Johnson syndrome, stomatitis (ulcerative), stupor, syncope, tachycardia, thrombocytopenia, tongue edema, toxic epidermal necrolysis, tremor, urinary frequency increased, urinary retention, urticaria, vasculitis, vertigo, weakness, weight gain, wound hemorrhage (postoperative), xerostomia

Ophthalmic solution:

>10%: Ocular: Transient burning/stinging (Acular®: 40%; Acular® PF: 20%)

>1% to 10%:

Central nervous system: Headache

Ocular: Conjunctival hyperemia, corneal infiltrates, iritis, ocular edema, ocular inflammation, ocular irritation, ocular pain, superficial keratitis, superficial ocular infection

Miscellaneous: Allergic reactions

≤1% (Limited to important or life-threatening): Blurred vision, corneal ulcer, corneal erosion, corneal perforation, corneal thinning, dry eyes, epithelial breakdown

Drug Interactions

Avoid Concomitant Use

Avoid concomitant use of Ketorolac with any of the following: Aspirin; Nonsteroidal Anti-Inflammatory Agents; Pentoxifylline; Probenecid

Increased Effect/Toxicity

Ketorolac may increase the levels/effects of: Aminoglycosides; Anticoagulants; Antiplatelet Agents; Aspirin; Bisphosphonate Derivatives; CycloSPORINE; Desmopressin; Lithium; Methotrexate; Neuromuscular-Blocking Agents (Nondepolarizing); Nonsteroidal Anti-Inflammatory Agents; Pemetrexed; Pentoxifylline; Quinolone Antibiotics; Salicylates; Thrombolytic Agents; Vancomycin; Vitamin K Antagonists

The levels/effects of Ketorolac may be increased by: Antidepressants (Tricyclic, Tertiary Amine); Corticosteroids (Systemic); Herbs (Anticoagulant/Antiplatelet Properties); Probenecid; Selective Serotonin Reuptake Inhibitors; Serotonin/Norepinephrine Reuptake Inhibitors; Treprostinil

Decreased Effect

Ketorolac may decrease the levels/effects of: ACE Inhibitors; Angiotensin II Receptor Blockers; Anticonvulsants; Antiplatelet Agents; Beta-Blockers; Eplerenone; HydrALAZINE; Latanoprost; Loop Diuretics; Salicylates; Thiazide Diuretics

The levels/effects of Ketorolac may be decreased by: Bile Acid Sequestrants; Salicylates

Ethanol/Nutrition/Herb Interactions

Ethanol: Avoid ethanol (may enhance gastric mucosal irritation).

Food: Oral: High-fat meals may delay time to peak (by ~1 hour) and decrease peak concentrations.

Herb/Nutraceuticals: Avoid alfalfa, anise, bilberry, bladderwrack, bromelain, cat's claw, celery, chamomile, coleus, cordyceps, dong quai, evening primrose, fenugreek, feverfew, garlic, ginger, ginkgo biloba, ginseng (American, Panax, Siberian), grapeseed, green tea, guggul, horse chestnut seed, horseradish, licorice, prickly ash, red clover, reishi, SAMe (S-adenosylmethionine), sweet clover, turmeric, and white willow (all have additional antiplatelet activity).

Stability

Injection: Store at room temperature of 15°C to 30°C (59°F to 86°F). Protect from light. Injection is clear and has a slight yellow color. Precipitation may occur at relatively low pH values.

Ophthalmic solution: Store at room temperature 15°C to 25°C (59°F to 77°F). Protect from light.

Tablet: Store at room temperature of 15°C to 30°C (59°F to 86°F).

Mechanism of Action Reversibly inhibits cyclooxygenase-1 and 2 (COX-1 and 2) enzymes, which result in decreased formation of prostaglandin precursors; has antipyretic, analgesic, and anti-inflammatory properties

Pharmacodynamics/Kinetics

Onset of action: Analgesic: I.M.: ~10 minutes

Peak effect: Analgesic: 2-3 hours

Duration: Analgesic: 6-8 hours

Absorption: Oral: Well absorbed (100%)

Distribution: ~13 L; poor penetration into CSF; crosses placenta

Protein binding: 99%

Metabolism: Hepatic

Half-life elimination: 2-6 hours; prolonged 30% to 50% in elderly; up to 19 hours in renal impairment

Time to peak, serum: I.M.: 30-60 minutes

Excretion: Urine (92%, ~60% as unchanged drug); feces ~6%

Dosage

Children 2-16 years (unlabeled use): Limited pediatric studies. The maximum combined duration of treatment (for parenteral and oral) is 5 days. **Do not exceed adult doses. Note:** The manufacturer warns that oral ketorolac is not indicated for children.

I.V.: Initial dose: 0.5 mg/kg, followed by 0.25-1 mg/kg every 6 hours for up to 48 hours (maximum daily dose: 90 mg)

Oral: 0.25 mg/kg every 6 hours

Children ≥16 years and Adults (pain relief usually begins within 10 minutes with parenteral forms): **Note:** The maximum combined duration of treatment (for parenteral and oral) is 5 days; do not increase dose or frequency; supplement with low-dose opioids if needed for breakthrough pain. For patients <50 kg and/or ≥65 years, see Elderly dosing.

I.M.: 60 mg as a single dose or 30 mg every 6 hours (maximum daily dose: 120 mg)

I.V.: 30 mg as a single dose or 30 mg every 6 hours (maximum daily dose: 120 mg)

Children ≥17 years and Adults: Oral: 20 mg, followed by 10 mg every 4-6 hours; do not exceed 40 mg/day; oral dosing is intended to be a continuation of I.M. or I.V. therapy only

Note: The maximum combined duration of treatment (for parenteral and oral) is 5 days; do not increase dose or frequency; supplement with low-dose opioids if needed for breakthrough pain. Therapy should not be initiated with oral formulation. For patients <50 kg and/or ≥65 years, see Elderly dosing.

Dosage adjustments in elderly (≥65 years), renal insufficiency, or low body weight (<50 kg): Note: These groups have an increased incidence of GI bleeding, ulceration, and perforation. The maximum combined duration of treatment (for parenteral and oral) is 5 days.

I.M.: 30 mg as a single dose or 15 mg every 6 hours (maximum daily dose: 60 mg)

I.V.: 15 mg as a single dose or 15 mg every 6 hours (maximum daily dose: 60 mg)

Oral: 10 mg, followed by 10 mg every 4-6 hours; do not exceed 40 mg/day; oral dosing is intended to be a continuation of I.M. or I.V. therapy only

Ophthalmic: Children ≥3 years and Adults:

Allergic conjunctivitis (relief of ocular itching) (Acular®): Instill 1 drop (0.25 mg) 4 times/day

Inflammation following cataract extraction (Acular®): Instill 1 drop (0.25 mg) to affected eye(s) 4 times/day beginning 24 hours after surgery; continue for 2 weeks

Pain and photophobia following incisional refractive surgery (Acular® PF): Instill 1 drop (0.25 mg) 4 times/day to affected eye for up to 3 days

Pain following corneal refractive surgery (Acular LS™): Instill 1 drop 4 times/day as needed to affected eye for up to 4 days

Dosage adjustment in renal impairment: Contraindicated in patients with advanced renal impairment. Patients with moderately-elevated serum creatinine should use half the recommended dose, not to exceed 60 mg/day I.M./I.V.

Dosage adjustment in hepatic impairment: Use with caution, may cause elevation of liver enzymes; discontinue if clinical signs and symptoms of liver disease develop

Dietary Considerations Administer tablet with food or milk to decrease gastrointestinal distress.

Administration

Oral: May take with food to reduce GI upset.

I.M.: Administer slowly and deeply into the muscle. Analgesia begins in 30 minutes and maximum effect within 2 hours.

I.V.: Administer I.V. bolus over a minimum of 15 seconds; onset within 30 minutes; peak analgesia within 2 hours.

Ophthalmic solution: Contact lenses should be removed before instillation.

Monitoring Parameters Monitor response (pain, range of motion, grip strength, mobility, ADL function), inflammation; observe for weight gain, edema; monitor renal function (serum creatinine, BUN, urine output); observe for bleeding, bruising; evaluate gastrointestinal effects (abdominal pain, bleeding, dyspepsia); mental confusion, disorientation, CBC and platelets, liver function tests

Reference Range Serum concentration: Therapeutic: 0.3-5 mcg/mL; Toxic: >5 mcg/mL

Additional Information First parenteral NSAID for analgesia; 30 mg provides the analgesia comparable to 12 mg of morphine or 100 mg of meperidine.

Dosage Forms Excipient information presented when available (limited, particularly for generics); consult specific product labeling.

Injection, solution, as tromethamine: 15 mg/mL (1 mL); 30 mg/mL (1 mL, 2 mL, 10 mL) [contains ethanol]

Solution, ophthalmic, as tromethamine:

Acular®: 0.5% (3 mL, 5 mL, 10 mL) [contains benzalkonium chloride]

Acular LS™: 0.4% (5 mL) [contains benzalkonium chloride]

Solution, ophthalmic, as tromethamine [preservative free]: Acular® P.F.: 0.5% (0.4 mL)

Tablet, as tromethamine: 10 mg

◆ **Ketorolac Tromethamine** *see* Ketorolac *on page 841*

◆ **Ketorolac Tromethamine Injection, USP (Can)** *see* Ketorolac *on page 841*

Ketotifen (kee toe TYE fen)

U.S. Brand Names Alaway™ [OTC]; Zaditor® [OTC]

Canadian Brand Names Novo-Ketotifen®; Nu-Ketotifen®; Zaditen®; Zaditor®

Index Terms Ketotifen Fumarate

Pharmacologic Category Histamine H_1 Antagonist; Histamine H_1 Antagonist, Second Generation; Mast Cell Stabilizer

Use

Ophthalmic: Temporary prevention of eye itching due to allergic conjunctivitis

Oral (Canadian use; not approved in U.S.): Adjunctive therapy in the chronic treatment of pediatric patients ≥6 months of age with mild, atopic asthma

Restrictions Oral formulation not available in U.S.

Pregnancy Risk Factor C

Medication Safety Issues

Sound-alike/look-alike issues:

Ketotifen may be confused with ketoprofen

Dosage

Ophthalmic: Allergic conjunctivitis: Children ≥3 years and Adults: Instill 1 drop into the affected eye(s) twice daily, every 8-12 hours

Oral (not approved in U.S.): Atopic asthma (**Note:** Not for acute attacks):

Children 6 months to 3 years: Initial: 0.025 mg/kg once daily or in 2 divided doses for 5 days; Maintenance: 0.05 mg/kg twice daily

Children >3 years: Initial: 0.5 mg once daily or in 2 divided doses for 5 days; Maintenance: 1 mg twice daily

Additional Information Complete prescribing information for this medication should be consulted for additional detail.

Dosage Forms Excipient information presented when available (limited, particularly for generics); consult specific product labeling. [CAN] = Canadian brand name

Solution, ophthalmic [drops]: 0.025% (5 mL)

Alaway™: 0.025% (10 mL) [contains benzalkonium chloride]

Zaditor®: 0.025% (5 mL) [contains benzalkonium chloride]

Syrup: 1 mg/5 mL (250 mL) [not available in U.S.]

Novo-Ketotifen® [CAN]: 1 mg/5 mL (250 mL) [not available in U.S.; contains alcohol, benzoate compounds; strawberry flavor]

Nu-Ketotifen® [CAN]: 1 mg/5 mL (250 mL) [not available in U.S.]

Zaditen® [CAN]: 1 mg/5 mL (250 mL) [not available in U.S.]

Tablet: 1 mg [not available in U.S.]

Novo-Ketotifen® [CAN]: 1 mg [not available in U.S.]

Zaditen® [CAN]: 1 mg [not available in U.S.]

◆ **Ketotifen Fumarate** *see* Ketotifen *on page 844*
◆ **Key-E® [OTC]** *see* Vitamin E *on page 1566*
◆ **Key-E® Kaps [OTC]** *see* Vitamin E *on page 1566*
◆ **Keygesic [OTC]** *see* Magnesium Salicylate *on page 917*
◆ **KI** *see* Potassium Iodide *on page 1218*
◆ **Kidkare Children's Cough and Cold [OTC]** *see* Chlorpheniramine, Pseudoephedrine, and Dextromethorphan *on page 315*
◆ **Kidkare Decongestant [OTC]** *see* Pseudoephedrine *on page 1265*
◆ **Kidrolase® (Can)** *see* Asparaginase *on page 140*
◆ **Kineret®** *see* Anakinra *on page 115*
◆ **Kinlytic™** *see* Urokinase *on page 1533*
◆ **Kinrix™** *see* Diphtheria and Tetanus Toxoids, Acellular Pertussis, and Poliovirus Vaccine *on page 462*
◆ **Kionex®** *see* Sodium Polystyrene Sulfonate *on page 1385*
◆ **Kivexa™ (Can)** *see* Abacavir and Lamivudine *on page 19*
◆ **Klaron®** *see* Sulfacetamide *on page 1405*
◆ **Klean-Prep® (Can)** *see* Polyethylene Glycol-Electrolyte Solution *on page 1209*
◆ **Klonopin®** *see* ClonazePAM *on page 352*
◆ **Klonopin® Wafers** *see* ClonazePAM *on page 352*
◆ **K-Lor®** *see* Potassium Chloride *on page 1216*
◆ **Klor-Con®** *see* Potassium Chloride *on page 1216*
◆ **Klor-Con® 8** *see* Potassium Chloride *on page 1216*
◆ **Klor-Con® 10** *see* Potassium Chloride *on page 1216*
◆ **Klor-Con®/25** *see* Potassium Chloride *on page 1216*
◆ **Klor-Con® M** *see* Potassium Chloride *on page 1216*
◆ **Klor-Con®/EF** *see* Potassium Bicarbonate and Potassium Citrate *on page 1216*
◆ **K-Lyte®** *see* Potassium Bicarbonate and Potassium Citrate *on page 1216*
◆ **K-Lyte/Cl® [DSC]** *see* Potassium Bicarbonate and Potassium Chloride *on page 1215*
◆ **K-Lyte®/Cl (Can)** *see* Potassium Chloride *on page 1216*
◆ **K-Lyte® DS** *see* Potassium Bicarbonate and Potassium Citrate *on page 1216*
◆ **KMD 3213** *see* Silodosin *on page 1370*
◆ **Koffex DM-D (Can)** *see* Pseudoephedrine and Dextromethorphan *on page 1266*
◆ **Koffex DM + Decongestant + Expectorant (Can)** *see* Guaifenesin, Pseudoephedrine, and Dextromethorphan *on page 715*
◆ **Koffex DM-Expectorant (Can)** *see* Guaifenesin and Dextromethorphan *on page 710*
◆ **Koffex Expectorant (Can)** *see* GuaiFENesin *on page 709*
◆ **Kogenate® (Can)** *see* Antihemophilic Factor (Recombinant) *on page 121*
◆ **Kogenate® FS** *see* Antihemophilic Factor (Recombinant) *on page 121*
◆ **Kolephrin® [OTC]** *see* Acetaminophen, Chlorpheniramine, and Pseudoephedrine *on page 31*
◆ **Kolephrin® #1** *see* Guaifenesin and Codeine *on page 710*
◆ **Kolephrin® GG/DM [OTC]** *see* Guaifenesin and Dextromethorphan *on page 710*
◆ **Konakion (Can)** *see* Phytonadione *on page 1191*
◆ **Konsyl® [OTC]** *see* Psyllium *on page 1268*
◆ **Konsyl-D™ [OTC]** *see* Psyllium *on page 1268*
◆ **Konsyl® Easy Mix™ [OTC]** *see* Psyllium *on page 1268*
◆ **Konsyl® Orange [OTC]** *see* Psyllium *on page 1268*
◆ **Konsyl® Original [OTC]** *see* Psyllium *on page 1268*
◆ **Kovia®** *see* Papain and Urea *on page 1142*
◆ **Koāte®-DVI** *see* Antihemophilic Factor (Human) *on page 120*
◆ **K-Pek II [OTC]** *see* Loperamide *on page 900*
◆ **K-Phos® MF** *see* Potassium Phosphate and Sodium Phosphate *on page 1222*
◆ **K-Phos® Neutral** *see* Potassium Phosphate and Sodium Phosphate *on page 1222*
◆ **K-Phos® No. 2** *see* Potassium Phosphate and Sodium Phosphate *on page 1222*

- ◆ **K-Phos® Original** *see* Potassium Acid Phosphate *on page 1215*
- ◆ **Kristalose®** *see* Lactulose *on page 847*
- ◆ **K-Tab®** *see* Potassium Chloride *on page 1216*
- ◆ **Kuric™** *see* Ketoconazole *on page 837*
- ◆ **Kuvan™** *see* Sapropterin *on page 1353*
- ◆ **ku-zyme® HP [DSC]** *see* Pancrelipase *on page 1136*
- ◆ **Kwelcof® [DSC]** *see* Hydrocodone and Guaifenesin *on page 741*
- ◆ **Kwellada-P™ (Can)** *see* Permethrin *on page 1176*
- ◆ **Kytril®** *see* Granisetron *on page 706*
- ◆ **L-749,345** *see* Ertapenem *on page 543*
- ◆ **L-758,298** *see* Fosaprepitant *on page 666*
- ◆ **L-M-X™ 4 [OTC]** *see* Lidocaine *on page 884*
- ◆ **L-M-X™ 5 [OTC]** *see* Lidocaine *on page 884*
- ◆ **L 754030** *see* Aprepitant *on page 129*
- ◆ **LA 20304a** *see* Gemifloxacin *on page 688*

Labetalol (la BET a lole)

U.S. Brand Names Trandate®

Canadian Brand Names Apo-Labetalol®; Labetalol Hydrochloride Injection, USP; Normodyne®; Trandate®

Index Terms Ibidomide Hydrochloride; Labetalol Hydrochloride

Pharmacologic Category Beta Blocker With Alpha-Blocking Activity

Additional Appendix Information

Beta-Blockers *on page 1648*

Hypertension *on page 1820*

Use Treatment of mild-to-severe hypertension; I.V. for severe hypertension (eg, hypertensive emergencies)

Unlabeled/Investigational Use Pediatric hypertension

Pregnancy Risk Factor C (manufacturer); D (2nd and 3rd trimesters - expert analysis)

Pregnancy Considerations Labetalol crosses the placenta. Beta-blockers have been associated with persistent bradycardia, hypotension, and IUGR; IUGR is probably related to maternal hypertension. Available evidence suggests beta-blockers are generally safe during pregnancy (JNC 7). Cases of neonatal hypoglycemia have been reported following maternal use of beta-blockers at parturition or during breast-feeding. Monitor breast-fed infant for symptoms of beta-blockade.

Lactation Enters breast milk/use caution (AAP rates "compatible")

Medication Safety Issues

Sound-alike/look-alike issues:

Labetalol may be confused with betaxolol, Hexadrol®, lamoTRIgine

Trandate® may be confused with traMADol, Trendar®, Trental®, Tridrate®

High alert medication: The Institute for Safe Medication Practices (ISMP) includes this medication among its list of drugs which have a heightened risk of causing significant patient harm when used in error.

Significant differences exist between oral and I.V. dosing. Use caution when converting from one route of administration to another.

Contraindications Hypersensitivity to labetalol or any component of the formulation; severe bradycardia; heart block greater than first degree (except in patients with a functioning artificial pacemaker); cardiogenic shock; bronchial asthma; uncompensated cardiac failure; conditions associated with severe and prolonged hypotension

Warnings/Precautions Consider pre-existing conditions such as sick sinus syndrome before initiating. Symptomatic hypotension with or without syncope may occur with labetalol; close monitoring of patient is required especially with initial dosing and dosing increases; blood pressure must be lowered at a rate appropriate for the patient's clinical condition. Initiation with a low dose and gradual up-titration may help to decrease the occurrence of hypotension or syncope. Patients should be advised to avoid driving or other hazardous tasks during initiation of therapy due to the risk of syncope. Orthostatic hypotension may occur with I.V. administration; patient should remain supine during and for up to 3 hours after I.V. administration. Use with caution in impaired hepatic function; bioavailability is increased due to decreased first-pass metabolism. Severe hepatic injury including some fatalities have also been rarely reported with use: periodically monitor LFTs with prolonged use. Use with caution in patients with diabetes mellitus; may potentiate hypoglycemia and/or mask signs and symptoms. May also reduce release of insulin in response to hyperglycemia; dosage of antidiabetic agents may need to be adjusted. Elimination of labetalol is reduced in elderly patients; lower maintenance doses may be required.

Use only with extreme caution in compensated heart failure and monitor for a worsening of the condition. Beta-blocker therapy should not be withdrawn abruptly (particularly in patients with CAD), but gradually tapered to avoid acute tachycardia, hypertension, and/or ischemia. Use caution with concurrent use of beta-blockers and either verapamil or diltiazem; bradycardia or heart block can occur. Patients with bronchospastic disease should not receive beta-blockers; if used at all, should be used cautiously with close monitoring. Use with caution in patients with myasthenia gravis, psychiatric disease (may cause or exacerbate CNS depression), or peripheral vascular disease. If possible, obtain diagnostic tests for pheochromocytoma prior to use. Labetalol has been shown to be effective in lowering blood pressure and relieving symptoms in patients with pheochromocytoma. However, some patients have experienced paradoxical hypertensive responses; use with caution in patients with pheochromocytoma. Additional alpha-blockade may be required during use of labetalol. Use caution with history of severe anaphylaxis to allergens; patients taking beta-blockers may become more sensitive to repeated challenges. Treatment of anaphylaxis (eg, epinephrine) in patients taking beta-blockers may be ineffective or promote undesirable effects. Use with caution in patients receiving anesthetic agents which decrease myocardial function.

Adverse Reactions

>10%:

Cardiovascular: Postural hypotension (I.V. use; ≤58%)

Central nervous system: Dizziness (1% to 20%), fatigue (1% to 11%)

Gastrointestinal: Nausea (≤19%)

1% to 10%:

Cardiovascular: Hypotension (1% to 5%), edema (≤2%), flushing (1%), ventricular arrhythmia (I.V. use; 1%)

Central nervous system: Somnolence (3%), headache (2%), vertigo (1% to 2%)

Dermatologic: Scalp tingling (≤7%), pruritus (1%), rash (1%)

Gastrointestinal: Dyspepsia (≤4%), vomiting (≤3%), taste disturbance (1%)

Genitourinary: Ejaculatory failure (≤5%), impotence (1% to 4%)

Hepatic: Transaminases increased (4%)

Neuromuscular & skeletal: Paresthesia (≤5%), weakness (1%)

Ocular: Vision abnormal (1%)

Renal: BUN increased (≤8%)

Respiratory: Nasal congestion (1% to 6%), dyspnea (2%)

Miscellaneous: Diaphoresis (≤4%)

<1% (Limited to important or life-threatening): Alopecia (reversible), anaphylactoid reaction, ANA positive, angioedema, bradycardia, bronchospasm, cholestatic jaundice, CHF, diabetes insipidus, heart block, hepatic necrosis, hepatitis, hypersensitivity, Peyronie's disease, Raynaud's syndrome, syncope, systemic lupus erythematosus, toxic myopathy, urinary retention, urticaria

Other adverse reactions noted with beta-adrenergic blocking agents include mental depression, catatonia, disorientation, short-term memory loss, emotional lability, clouded sensorium, intensification of pre-existing AV block, laryngospasm, respiratory distress, agranulocytosis, thrombocytopenic purpura, nonthrombocytopenic purpura, mesenteric artery thrombosis, and ischemic colitis.

Drug Interactions

Avoid Concomitant Use

Avoid concomitant use of Labetalol with any of the following: Methacholine

Increased Effect/Toxicity

Labetalol may increase the levels/effects of: Alpha-/Beta-Agonists (Direct-Acting); Alpha1-Blockers; Alpha2-Agonists; Amifostine; Antipsychotic Agents (Phenothiazines); Cardiac Glycosides; Insulin; Lidocaine; Methacholine; Midodrine; RiTUXimab

The levels/effects of Labetalol may be increased by: Acetylcholinesterase Inhibitors; Aminoquinolines (Antimalarial); Amiodarone; Anilidopiperidine Opioids; Antipsychotic Agents (Phenothiazines); Calcium Channel Blockers (Nondihydropyridine); Diazoxide; Dipyridamole; Disopyramide; Herbs (Hypotensive Properties); Propafenone; Propoxyphene; Prostacyclin Analogues; QuiNIDine; Reserpine; Selective Serotonin Reuptake Inhibitors

Decreased Effect

Labetalol may decrease the levels/effects of: Beta2-Agonists; Theophylline Derivatives

The levels/effects of Labetalol may be decreased by: Barbiturates; Herbs (Hypertensive Properties); Methylphenidate; Nonsteroidal Anti-Inflammatory Agents; Rifamycin Derivatives; Yohimbine

Ethanol/Nutrition/Herb Interactions

Food: Labetalol serum concentrations may be increased if taken with food.

Herb/Nutraceutical: Avoid dong quai if using for hypertension (has estrogenic activity). Avoid ephedra, yohimbe, ginseng (may worsen hypertension). Avoid natural licorice (causes sodium and water retention and increases potassium loss). Avoid garlic (may have increased antihypertensive effect).

Stability

Tablets: Store tablets at 2°C to 30°C (36°F to 86°F). Protect from light and excessive moisture.

Vials: Store unopened injectable vials at 20°C to 25°C (68°F to 77°F); do not freeze. Protect from light. The solution is clear to slightly yellow.

Parenteral admixture: Stability of parenteral admixture at room temperature (25°C) and refrigeration temperature (4°C): 3 days.

Standard concentration: 500 mg/250 mL D_5W.

Minimum volume: 250 mL D_5W.

Mechanism of Action Blocks alpha-, $beta_1$-, and $beta_2$-adrenergic receptor sites; elevated renins are reduced. The ratios of alpha- to beta-blockade differ depending on the route of administration: 1:3 (oral) and 1:7 (I.V.).

Pharmacodynamics/Kinetics

Onset of action: Oral: 20 minutes to 2 hours; I.V.: 2-5 minutes

Peak effect: Oral: 1-4 hours; I.V.: 5-15 minutes

Duration: Blood pressure response:

Oral: 8-12 hours (dose dependent)

I.V.: 2-18 hours (dose dependent; based on single and multiple sequential doses of 0.25-0.5 mg/kg with cumulative dosing up to 3.25 mg/kg)

Distribution: V_d: Adults: 3-16 L/kg; mean: <9.4 L/kg; moderately lipid soluble, therefore, can enter CNS; crosses placenta; small amounts enter breast milk

Protein binding: 50%

Metabolism: Hepatic, primarily via glucuronide conjugation; extensive first-pass effect

Bioavailability: Oral: 25%; increased with liver disease, elderly, and concurrent cimetidine

Half-life elimination: Oral: 6-8 hours; I.V.: ~5.5 hours

Excretion: Urine (55% to 60% as glucuronide conjugates, <5% as unchanged drug)

Clearance: Possibly decreased in neonates/infants

Dosage

Children: Due to limited documentation of its use, labetalol should be initiated cautiously in pediatric patients with careful dosage adjustment and blood pressure monitoring.

Oral: Hypertension (unlabeled use): Initial: 1-3 mg/kg/day, in 2 divided doses; maximum: 10-12 mg/kg/day, up to 1200 mg/day

I.V., intermittent bolus doses of 0.3-1 mg/kg/dose have been reported.

For treatment of pediatric hypertensive emergencies, initial continuous infusions of 0.4-1 mg/kg/hour with a maximum of 3 mg/kg/hour have been used. Administration requires the use of an infusion pump.

Adults:

Oral: Initial: 100 mg twice daily, may increase as needed every 2-3 days by 100 mg twice daily (titration increments not to exceed 200 mg twice daily) until desired response is obtained; usual dose: 200-400 mg twice daily; may require up to 2.4 g/day.

Usual dose range (JNC 7): 200-800 mg/day in 2 divided doses

I.V.: 20 mg (0.25 mg/kg for an 80 kg patient) I.V. push over 2 minutes; may administer 40-80 mg at 10-minute intervals, up to 300 mg total dose.

I.V. infusion (acute loading): Initial: 2 mg/minute; titrate to response up to 300 mg total dose, if needed. Administration requires the use of an infusion pump.

I.V. infusion (500 mg/250 mL D_5W) rates:

1 mg/minute: 30 mL/hour

2 mg/minute: 60 mL/hour

3 mg/minute: 90 mL/hour

4 mg/minute: 120 mL/hour

5 mg/minute: 150 mL/hour

6 mg/minute: 180 mL/hour

Note: Although loading infusions are well described in the product labeling, the labeling is silent in specific clinical situations, such as in the patient who has an initial response to labetalol infusions but cannot be converted to an oral route for subsequent dosing. There is limited documentation of prolonged continuous infusions. In rare clinical situations, higher continuous infusion dosages (up to 6 mg/minute) have been used in the critical care setting (eg, aortic dissection). At the other extreme, continuous infusions at relatively low doses (0.03-0.1 mg/minute) have been used in some settings (following loading infusion in patients who are unable to be converted to oral regimens or in some cases as a continuation of outpatient oral regimens). These prolonged infusions should not be confused with loading infusions. Because of wide variation in the use of infusions, an awareness of institutional policies and practices is extremely important. Careful clarification of orders and specific infusion rates/units is required to avoid confusion. Due to the prolonged duration of action, careful monitoring should be extended for the duration of the infusion and for several hours after the infusion. Excessive administration may result in prolonged hypotension and/or bradycardia.

Elderly: Initial dose: Refer to adult dosing. Usual maintenance: 100-200 mg twice daily

Dosage adjustment in renal impairment: Dialysis: Not removed by hemo- or peritoneal dialysis; supplemental dose is not necessary.

Dosage adjustment in hepatic impairment: Dosage reduction may be necessary.

Administration Bolus dose may be administered I.V. push at a rate of 10 mg/minute; may follow with continuous I.V. infusion

Monitoring Parameters Blood pressure, standing and sitting/supine, pulse, cardiac monitor and blood pressure monitor required for I.V. administration

Test Interactions False-positive urine catecholamines, vanillylmandelic acid (VMA) if measured by fluorometric or photometric methods; use HPLC or specific catecholamine radioenzymatic technique; false-positive amphetamine if measured by thin-layer chromatography or radioenzymatic assay (gas chromatographic-mass spectrometer technique should be used)

Dosage Forms Excipient information presented when available (limited, particularly for generics); consult specific product labeling.

Injection, solution, as hydrochloride: 5 mg/mL (4 mL, 8 mL, 20 mL, 40 mL)

Trandate®: 5 mg/mL (20 mL, 40 mL) [contains edetate disodium]

Tablet, as hydrochloride: 100 mg, 200 mg, 300 mg

Trandate®: 100 mg, 200 mg [contains sodium benzoate], 300 mg

Extemporaneous Preparations A 40 mg/mL suspension of labetalol hydrochloride can be made by first crushing sixteen 300 mg labetalol hydrochloride tablets into a fine powder. Using equal amounts of Ora-Sweet® and Ora-Plus® as a vehicle, add a small amount to make a paste; add additional amounts of the vehicle to qs to 120 mL. Suspension is stable for 60 days when stored in the refrigerator. Shake well before using.

Nahata MC and Hipple TF, *Pediatric Drug Formulations*, 4th ed, Cincinnati, OH: Harvey Whitney Books Co, 2000.

◆ **Labetalol Hydrochloride** *see* Labetalol *on page 845*

◆ **Labetalol Hydrochloride Injection, USP (Can)** *see* Labetalol *on page 845*

Lacosamide (la KOE sa mide)

U.S. Brand Names Vimpat®

Index Terms ADD 234037; Harkoseride; LCM; SPM 927

Pharmacologic Category Anticonvulsant, Miscellaneous

Additional Appendix Information

Anticonvulsant Drugs of Choice *on page 1637*

Use Adjunctive therapy in the treatment of partial-onset seizures

Restrictions An FDA-approved medication guide is available. Distribute to each patient to whom this medication is dispensed.

Pregnancy Risk Factor C

Medication Safety Issues

Sound-alike/look-alike issues:

Lacosamide may be confused with zonisamide

Dosage Oral, I.V.: Adolescents ≥17 years and Adults:

Partial onset seizure:

Initial: 50 mg twice daily; may be increased at weekly intervals by 100 mg/day

Maintenance dose: 200-400 mg/day

Note: When switching from oral to I.V. formulations, the total daily dose and frequency should be the same; I.V. therapy should only be used temporarily.

Dosing adjustment in renal impairment:

Mild-to-moderate renal impairment: No dose adjustment necessary

Severe renal impairment (Cl_{cr} ≤30 mL/minute): Maximum dose: 300 mg/day

Hemodialysis: Removed by hemodialysis; after 4-hour HD treatment, a supplemental dose of up to 50% should be considered.

Dosing adjustment in hepatic impairment:

Mild-to-moderate hepatic impairment: Maximum dose: 300 mg/day

Severe hepatic impairment: Use is not recommended

Additional Information Complete prescribing information for this medication should be consulted for additional detail.

Dosage Forms Excipient information presented when available (limited, particularly for generics); consult specific product labeling.

Injection, solution:

Vimpat®: 200 mg/20 mL

Tablet:

Vimpat®: 50 mg, 100 mg, 150 mg, 200 mg

◆ **Lactoflavin** *see* Riboflavin *on page 1313*

Lactulose (LAK tyoo lose)

U.S. Brand Names Constulose; Enulose; Generlac; Kristalose®

Canadian Brand Names Acilac; Apo-Lactulose®; Laxilose; PMS-Lactulose

Pharmacologic Category Ammonium Detoxicant; Laxative, Osmotic

Additional Appendix Information

Laxatives, Classification and Properties *on page 1660*

Use Adjunct in the prevention and treatment of portal-systemic encephalopathy; treatment of chronic constipation

Pregnancy Risk Factor B

Lactation Excretion in breast milk unknown

Medication Safety Issues

Sound-alike/look-alike issues:

Lactulose may be confused with lactose

Contraindications Hypersensitivity to lactulose or any component of the formulation; galactosemia (or patients requiring a low galactose diet)

Warnings/Precautions Use with caution in patients with diabetes mellitus; solution contains galactose and lactose; monitor periodically for electrolyte imbalance when lactulose is used >6 months or in patients predisposed to electrolyte abnormalities (eg, elderly); patients receiving lactulose and an oral anti-infective agent should be monitored for possible inadequate response to lactulose

Adverse Reactions Frequency not defined: Gastrointestinal: Flatulence, diarrhea (excessive dose), abdominal discomfort, nausea, vomiting, cramping

Drug Interactions

Avoid Concomitant Use There are no known interactions where it is recommended to avoid concomitant use.

Increased Effect/Toxicity There are no known significant interactions involving an increase in effect.

Decreased Effect There are no known significant interactions involving a decrease in effect.

Stability Keep solution at room temperature to reduce viscosity. Discard solution if cloudy or very dark.

Mechanism of Action The bacterial degradation of lactulose resulting in an acidic pH inhibits the diffusion of NH_3 into the blood by causing the conversion of NH_3 to NH_4+; also enhances the diffusion of NH_3 from the blood into the gut where conversion to NH_4+ occurs; produces an osmotic effect in the colon with resultant distention promoting peristalsis

Pharmacodynamics/Kinetics

Absorption: Not appreciable

Metabolism: Via colonic flora to lactic acid and acetic acid; requires colonic flora for drug activation

Excretion: Primarily feces and urine (~3%)

Dosage Diarrhea may indicate overdosage and responds to dose reduction

Prevention of portal systemic encephalopathy (PSE): Oral:

Infants: 2.5-10 mL/day divided 3-4 times/day; adjust dosage to produce 2-3 stools/day

Older Children: Daily dose of 40-90 mL divided 3-4 times/day; if initial dose causes diarrhea, then reduce it immediately; adjust dosage to produce 2-3 stools/day

Constipation: Oral:

Children: 5 g/day (7.5 mL) after breakfast

Adults: 15-30 mL/day increased to 60 mL/day in 1-2 divided doses if necessary

Acute PSE: Adults:

Oral: 20-30 g (30-45 mL) every 1-2 hours to induce rapid laxation; adjust dosage daily to produce 2-3 soft stools; doses of 30-45 mL may be given hourly to cause rapid laxation, then reduce to recommended dose; usual daily dose: 60-100 g (90-150 mL) daily

Rectal administration: 200 g (300 mL) diluted with 700 mL of H_2O or NS; administer rectally via rectal balloon catheter and retain 30-60 minutes every 4-6 hours

Dietary Considerations Contraindicated in patients on galactose-restricted diet; may be mixed with fruit juice, milk, water, or citrus-flavored carbonated beverages.

Administration Dilute lactulose in water, usually 60-120 mL, prior to administering through a gastric or feeding tube. Syrup formulation has been used in preparation of rectal solution.

Monitoring Parameters Blood pressure, standing/supine; serum potassium, bowel movement patterns, fluid status, serum ammonia

Dosage Forms Excipient information presented when available (limited, particularly for generics); consult specific product labeling.

Crystals for solution, oral:

Kristalose®: 10 g/packet (30s), 20 g/packet (30s)

Solution, oral: 10 g/15 mL (15 mL, 30 mL, 237 mL, 473 mL, 946 mL, 1890 mL)

Constulose: 10 g/15 mL (240 mL, 960 mL)

Enulose: 10 g/15 mL (480 mL)

Generlac: 10 g/15 mL (480 mL, 1920 mL)

Solution, oral/rectal: 10 g/15 mL (473 mL)

◆ **Ladakamycin** *see* AzaCITIDine *on page 161*

◆ **Lagesic™** *see* Acetaminophen and Phenyltoloxamine *on page 29*

◆ **L-All 12** *see* Carbetapentane and Phenylephrine *on page 255*

◆ **L-AmB** *see* Amphotericin B (Liposomal) *on page 107*

◆ **Lamictal®** *see* LamoTRIgine *on page 850*

◆ **Lamisil®** *see* Terbinafine *on page 1441*

◆ **Lamisil AT® [OTC]** *see* Terbinafine *on page 1441*

LamiVUDine (la MI vyoo deen)

U.S. Brand Names Epivir-HBV®; Epivir®

Canadian Brand Names 3TC®; Heptovir®

Index Terms 3TC

Pharmacologic Category Antiretroviral Agent, Reverse Transcriptase Inhibitor (Nucleoside)

Additional Appendix Information

Antiretroviral Therapy for HIV Infection: Adults and Adolescents *on page 1758*

Management of Healthcare Worker Exposures to HBV, HCV, and HIV *on page 1719*

Perinatal HIV Guidelines *on page 1730*

Use

Epivir®: Treatment of HIV infection when antiretroviral therapy is warranted; should always be used as part of a multidrug regimen (at least three antiretroviral agents)

Epivir-HBV®: Treatment of chronic hepatitis B associated with evidence of hepatitis B viral replication and active liver inflammation

Unlabeled/Investigational Use Postexposure prophylaxis for HIV exposure as part of a multidrug regimen

Pregnancy Risk Factor C

Pregnancy Considerations Lamivudine crosses the placenta. No increased risk of overall birth defects has been observed following 1st trimester exposure according to data collected by the antiretroviral pregnancy registry. The pharmacokinetics of lamivudine during pregnancy are not significantly altered and dosage adjustment is not required. The Perinatal HIV Guidelines Working Group recommends lamivudine for use during pregnancy; the combination of lamivudine with zidovudine is the recommended dual combination NRTI in pregnancy. It may also be used in combination with zidovudine in HIV-infected women who are in labor, but have had no prior antiretroviral therapy, in order to reduce the maternal-fetal transmission of HIV. Cases of lactic acidosis/hepatic steatosis syndrome have been reported in pregnant women receiving nucleoside analogues. It is not known if pregnancy itself potentiates this known side effect; however, pregnant women may be at increased risk of lactic acidosis and liver damage. Hepatic enzymes and electrolytes should be monitored frequently during the 3rd trimester of pregnancy in women receiving nucleoside analogues. Health professionals are encouraged to contact the antiretroviral pregnancy registry to monitor outcomes of pregnant women exposed to antiretroviral medications (1-800-258-4263 or www.APRegistry.com).

Lactation Enters breast milk/contraindicated

Medication Safety Issues

Sound-alike/look-alike issues:

LamiVUDine may be confused with lamoTRIgine

Epivir® may be confused with Combivir®

Contraindications Hypersensitivity to lamivudine or any component of the formulation

Warnings/Precautions Use caution with renal impairment; dosage reduction recommended. Use with extreme caution in children with history of pancreatitis or risk factors for development of pancreatitis. Pancreatitis has been reported, particularly in HIV-infected children with a history of nucleoside use. Do not use as monotherapy in treatment of HIV. Treatment of HBV in patients with unrecognized/untreated HIV may lead to rapid HIV resistance. In addition, treatment of HIV in patients with unrecognized/untreated HBV may lead to rapid HBV resistance. Use with caution in combination with interferon alfa with or without ribavirin in HIV/HBV coinfected patients; monitor closely for hepatic decompensation, anemia, or neutropenia; dose reduction or discontinuation of interferon and/or ribavirin may be required if toxicity evident. **[U.S. Boxed Warning]: Do not use Epivir-HBV® tablets or Epivir-HBV® oral solution for the treatment of HIV.**

[U.S. Boxed Warning]: Lactic acidosis and severe hepatomegaly with steatosis have been reported, including fatal cases. Use caution in hepatic impairment. Pregnancy, obesity, and/or prolonged therapy may increase the risk of lactic acidosis and liver damage.

Immune reconstitution syndrome may develop resulting in the occurrence of an inflammatory response to an indolent or residual opportunistic infection. May be associated with fat redistribution.

[U.S. Boxed Warning]: Monitor patients closely for several months following discontinuation of therapy for chronic hepatitis B; clinical exacerbations may occur.

Adverse Reactions Reported for treatment of HIV or HBV in adults. Incidence data includes patients on combination therapy with other antiretroviral agents.

>10%:

Central nervous system: Headache (21% to 35%), fatigue (24% to 27%), insomnia (11%)

Gastrointestinal: Nausea (15% to 33%), diarrhea (14% to 18%), pancreatitis (range: 0.3% to 18%; higher percentage in pediatric patients), abdominal pain (9% to 16%), vomiting (13% to 15%)

Hematologic: Neutropenia (7% to 15%)

Hepatic: Transaminases increased (2% to 11%)

Neuromuscular & skeletal: Myalgia (8% to 14%), neuropathy (12%), musculoskeletal pain (12%)

Respiratory: Nasal signs and symptoms (20%), cough (18%), sore throat (13%)

Miscellaneous: Infections (25%; includes ear, nose, and throat)

1% to 10%:

Central nervous system: Dizziness (10%), depression (9%), fever (7% to 10%), chills (7% to 10%)

Dermatologic: Rash (5% to 9%)

Gastrointestinal: Anorexia (10%), lipase increased (10%), abdominal cramps (6%), dyspepsia (5%), amylase increased (<1% to 4%), heartburn

Hematologic: Thrombocytopenia (1% to 4%), hemoglobinemia (2% to 3%)

Neuromuscular & skeletal: Creatine phosphokinase increased (9%), arthralgia (5% to 7%)

<1% (Limited to important or life-threatening): Alopecia, anaphylaxis, anemia, body fat redistribution, hepatitis B exacerbation, hepatomegaly, hyperbilirubinemia, hyperglycemia, immune reconstitution syndrome, lactic acidosis, lymphadenopathy, muscle weakness, paresthesia, peripheral neuropathy, pruritus, red cell aplasia, rhabdomyolysis, splenomegaly, steatosis, stomatitis, urticaria, weakness, wheezing

Drug Interactions

Avoid Concomitant Use

Avoid concomitant use of LamiVUDine with any of the following: Emtricitabine

Increased Effect/Toxicity

LamiVUDine may increase the levels/effects of: Emtricitabine

The levels/effects of LamiVUDine may be increased by: Ganciclovir-Valganciclovir; Ribavirin; Trimethoprim

Decreased Effect

LamiVUDine may decrease the levels/effects of: Zalcitabine

Ethanol/Nutrition/Herb Interactions Food: Food decreases the rate of absorption and C_{max}; however, there is no change in the systemic AUC. Therefore, may be taken with or without food.

Stability

Oral solution:

Epivir®: Store at 25°C (77°F) tightly closed.

Epivir-HBV®: Store at 20°C to 25°C (68°F to 77°F) tightly closed.

Tablet: Store at 25°C (77°F); excursions permitted to 15°C to 30°C (59°F to 86°F).

Mechanism of Action Lamivudine is a cytosine analog. After lamivudine is triphosphorylated, the principle mode of action is inhibition of HIV reverse transcription via viral DNA chain termination; inhibits RNA- and DNA-dependent DNA polymerase activities of reverse transcriptase. The monophosphate form of lamivudine is incorporated into the viral DNA by hepatitis B virus polymerase, resulting in DNA chain termination.

Pharmacodynamics/Kinetics

Absorption: Rapid

Distribution: V_d: 1.3 L/kg

Protein binding, plasma: <36%

Metabolism: 4.2% to trans-sulfoxide metabolite

Bioavailability: Absolute; Cp_{max} decreased with food although AUC not significantly affected

Children: 66%

Adults: 86% to 87%

Half-life elimination: Children: 2 hours; Adults: 5-7 hours

Time to peak, plasma: Fed: 3.2 hours; Fasted: 0.9 hours

Excretion: Primarily urine (as unchanged drug)

Dosage Oral: **Note:** The formulation and dosage of Epivir-HBV® are not appropriate for patients infected with both HBV and HIV. Use with at least two other antiretroviral agents when treating HIV

HIV:

Neonates <30 days (AIDSinfo guidelines): 2 mg/kg/dose twice daily

Infants 1-3 months (AIDSinfo guidelines): 4 mg/kg/dose twice daily

Infants and Children 3 months to 16 years: 4 mg/kg/dose twice daily (maximum: 150 mg/dose twice daily)

Alternate weight-based dosing using scored 150 mg tablets (AIDSinfo guidelines):

14-21 kg: 75 mg/dose twice daily (150 mg/day)

22-29 kg: 75 mg in the morning, 150 mg in the evening (225 mg/day)

≥30 kg: 150 mg/dose twice daily (300 mg/day)

Adults: 150 mg twice daily or 300 mg once daily

<50 kg (AIDSinfo guidelines): 4 mg/kg/dose twice daily (maximum: 150 mg/dose twice daily)

Treatment of hepatitis B (Epivir-HBV®): Note: Usual treatment duration is at least 1 year and varies with HBeAg status, consult current guidelines and literature.

Children 2-17 years: 3 mg/kg/dose once daily (maximum: 100 mg/day)

Adults: 100 mg/day

Postexposure prophylaxis for HIV exposure (unlabeled use): Adolescents and Adults: 150 mg twice daily (with zidovudine with or without a protease inhibitor, depending on risk)

Prevention of maternal-fetal HIV transmission (AIDS-info guidelines): Note: Lamivudine may be used in combination with zidovudine and nevirapine in select situations (eg, infants born to mothers with suboptimal viral suppression at delivery, infants born to mothers with only intrapartum therapy or no therapy, or infants born to mothers with known antiretroviral drug-resistant virus). Lamivudine is used in this situation to reduce the development of nevirapine resistant virus:

Mother: 150 mg twice daily starting at onset of labor and continuing through 1 week postpartum

Neonate: 2 mg/kg/dose twice daily given at birth through 1 week of age

Dosing adjustment in renal impairment: HIV:

Patients ≤16 years: Insufficient data; however, dose reduction should be considered.

Patients >16 years:

Cl_{cr} 30-49 mL/minute: Administer 150 mg once daily

Cl_{cr} 15-29 mL/minute: Administer 150 mg first dose, then 100 mg once daily

Cl_{cr} 5-14 mL/minute: Administer 150 mg first dose, then 50 mg once daily

Cl_{cr} <5 mL/minute: Administer 50 mg first dose, then 25 mg once daily

Dosing adjustment in renal impairment: Hepatitis B:

Adults:

Cl_{cr} 30-49: Administer 100 mg first dose then 50 mg once daily

Cl_{cr} 15-29: Administer 100 mg first dose then 25 mg once daily

Cl_{cr} 5-14: Administer 35 mg first dose then 15 mg once daily

Cl_{cr} <5: Administer 35 mg first dose then 10 mg once daily

Dialysis: Negligible amounts are removed by 4-hour hemodialysis or peritoneal dialysis. Supplemental dosing is not required.

Dietary Considerations May be taken with or without food. Each 5 mL of oral solution contains 1 g of sucrose.

Administration May be taken with or without food. Adjust dosage in renal failure.

Monitoring Parameters Amylase, bilirubin, liver enzymes, hematologic parameters, viral load, and CD4 count; signs and symptoms of pancreatitis

Additional Information Lamivudine has been well studied in the treatment of chronic hepatitis B infection. Potential compliance problems, frequency of administration, and adverse effects should be discussed with patients before initiating therapy to help prevent the emergence of resistance.

A high rate of early virologic nonresponse was observed when abacavir, lamivudine and tenofovir were used as the initial regimen in treatment-naive patients. A high rate of early virologic nonresponse was also observed when didanosine, lamivudine, and tenofovir were used as the initial regimen in treatment-naive patients. Use of either of these combinations is not recommended; patients currently on either of these regimens should be closely monitored for modification of therapy.

Dosage Forms Excipient information presented when available (limited, particularly for generics); consult specific product labeling.

Solution, oral:

Epivir®: 10 mg/mL (240 mL) [strawberry-banana flavor]

Epivir-HBV®: 5 mg/mL (240 mL) [strawberry-banana flavor]

Tablet:

Epivir®: 150 mg [scored], 300 mg

Epivir-HBV®: 100 mg

◆ **Lamivudine, Abacavir, and Zidovudine** *see* Abacavir, Lamivudine, and Zidovudine *on page 19*

◆ **Lamivudine and Abacavir** *see* Abacavir and Lamivudine *on page 19*

◆ **Lamivudine and Zidovudine** *see* Zidovudine and Lamivudine *on page 1583*

LamoTRIgine (la MOE tri jeen)

U.S. Brand Names Lamictal®

Canadian Brand Names Apo-Lamotrigine®; Gen-Lamotrigine; Lamictal®; Novo-Lamotrigine; PMS-Lamotrigine; ratio-Lamotrigine

Index Terms BW-430C; LTG

Pharmacologic Category Anticonvulsant, Miscellaneous

Additional Appendix Information

Anticonvulsant Drugs of Choice *on page 1637*

Use Adjunctive therapy in the treatment of generalized seizures of Lennox-Gastaut syndrome, primary generalized tonic-clonic seizures, and partial seizures in adults and children ≥2 years of age; conversion to monotherapy in adults with partial seizures who are receiving treatment with valproic acid or a single enzyme-inducing antiepileptic drug (specifically carbamazepine, phenytoin, phenobarbital or primidone); maintenance treatment of bipolar I disorder

Pregnancy Risk Factor C

Pregnancy Considerations Lamotrigine has been found to decrease folate concentrations in animal studies. Teratogenic effects in animals were not observed. Lamotrigine crosses the human placenta and can be measured in the plasma of exposed newborns. Preliminary data from the North American Antiepileptic Drug Pregnancy Registry (NAAED) suggest an increased incidence of cleft lip and/or cleft palate following first trimester exposure. Healthcare providers may enroll patients in the Lamotrigine Pregnancy Registry by calling (800) 336-2176. Patients may enroll themselves in the NAAED registry by calling (888) 233-2334. Dose of lamotrigine may need adjustment during pregnancy to maintain clinical response; lamotrigine serum levels may decrease during pregnancy and return to prepartum levels following delivery. Monitor frequently during pregnancy, following delivery, and when adding or discontinuing combination hormonal contraceptives.

Lactation Enters breast milk/not recommended (AAP rates "of concern")

Medication Safety Issues

Sound-alike/look-alike issues:

LamoTRIgine may be confused with labetalol, Lamisil®, lamiVUDine, Lomotil®, ludiomil

Lamictal® may be confused with Lamisil®, Lomotil®, ludiomil

Contraindications Hypersensitivity to lamotrigine or any component of the formulation

Warnings/Precautions [U.S. Boxed Warning]: Severe and potentially life-threatening skin rashes requiring hospitalization have been reported; risk may be increased by coadministration with valproic acid, higher than recommended starting doses, and rapid dose titration. The majority of cases occur in the first 8 weeks; however, isolated cases may occur after prolonged treatment. Discontinue at first sign of rash unless rash is clearly not drug related. Acute multiorgan failure has also been reported. A spectrum of hematologic effects have been reported with use (eg, neutropenia, leukopenia, thrombocytopenia, pancytopenia, and anemias); patients with a previous history of adverse hematologic reaction to any drug may be at increased risk. Early detection of hematologic change is important; advise patients of early signs and symptoms including fever, sore throat, mouth ulcers, infections, easy bruising, petechial or purpuric hemorrhage. May be associated with hypersensitivity syndrome. Use caution in patients with impaired renal, hepatic, or cardiac function. Avoid abrupt cessation, taper over at least 2 weeks if possible. May cause CNS depression, which may impair physical or mental abilities. Patients must be cautioned about performing tasks which require mental alertness (eg, operating machinery or driving). Effects with other sedative drugs or ethanol may be potentiated. Binds to melanin and may accumulate in the eye and other melanin-rich tissues; the clinical significance of this is not known. Safety and efficacy have not been established for use as initial monotherapy, conversion to monotherapy from antiepileptic drugs (AED) other than carbamazepine, phenytoin, phenobarbital, primidone or valproic acid or conversion to monotherapy from two or more AEDs. Patients treated for bipolar disorder should be monitored closely for clinical worsening or suicidality; prescriptions should be written for the smallest quantity consistent with good patient care. Hormonal contraceptives may cause a decrease in lamotrigine levels requiring dose adjustment.

Adverse Reactions Percentages reported in adults on monotherapy for epilepsy or bipolar disorder.

>10%: Gastrointestinal: Nausea (7% to 14%)

1% to 10%:

Cardiovascular: Chest pain (5%), peripheral edema (2% to 5%), edema (1% to 5%)

Central nervous system: Somnolence (9%), fatigue (8%), dizziness (7%), anxiety (5%), insomnia (5% to 10%), pain (5%), ataxia (2% to 5%), irritability (2% to 5%), suicidal ideation (2% to 5%), agitation (1% to 5%), amnesia (1% to 5%), depression (1% to 5%), dream abnormality (1% to 5%), emotional lability (1% to 5%), fever (1% to 5%), hypoesthesia (1% to 5%), migraine (1% to 5%), thought abnormality (1% to 5%), confusion (1%)

Dermatologic: Rash (nonserious: 7%), dermatitis (2% to 5%), dry skin (2% to 5%)

Endocrine & metabolic: Dysmenorrhea (5%), libido increased (2% to 5%)

Gastrointestinal: Vomiting (5% to 9%), dyspepsia (7%), abdominal pain (6%), xerostomia (2% to 6%), constipation (5%), weight loss (5%), anorexia (2% to 5%), peptic ulcer (2% to 5%), rectal hemorrhage (2% to 5%), flatulence (1% to 5%), weight gain (1% to 5%)

Genitourinary: Urinary frequency (1% to 5%)

Neuromuscular & skeletal: Back pain (8%), coordination abnormal (7%), weakness (2% to 5%), arthralgia (1% to 5%), myalgia (1% to 5%), neck pain (1% to 5%), paresthesia (1%)

Ocular: Nystagmus (2% to 5%), vision abnormal (2% to 5%), amblyopia (1%)

Respiratory: Rhinitis (7%), cough (5%), pharyngitis (5%), bronchitis (2% to 5%), dyspnea (2% to 5%), epistaxis (2% to 5%), sinusitis (1% to 5%)

Miscellaneous: Infection (5%), diaphoresis (2% to 5%), reflexes increased/decreased (2% to 5%), dyspraxia (1% to 5%)

<1%: Any indication (limited to important or life-threatening): Accommodation abnormality, acne, agranulocytosis, alcohol intolerance, allergic reaction, alopecia, anemia, angina, angioedema, aphasia, aplastic anemia, apnea, appetite increased, arthritis, atrial fibrillation, breast pain, bruising, cerebellar syndrome, cerebral sinus thrombosis, cerebrovascular accident, chills, choreoathetosis, CNS depression/stimulation, conjunctivitis, deafness, deep thrombophlebitis, delirium, delusions, dermatitis (exfoliative, fungal), disseminated intravascular coagulation, dry eyes, dysphagia, dysphoria, dystonia, ear pain, ECG abnormality, ejaculation abnormal, eructation, esophagitis, euphoria, extrapyramidal syndrome, faintness, flushing, gastritis, gingivitis, goiter, halitosis, hallucinations, hematuria, hemiplegia, hemolytic anemia, hemorrhage, hiccup, hirsutism, hot flashes, hyperalgesia, hyperglycemia, hypersensitivity reactions, hypertension, hyperventilation, hypokinesia, hypothyroidism, hypotonia, impotence, kidney failure (acute), leg cramps, leukopenia, liver function tests abnormal, lupus-like reaction, maculopapular rash, malaise, menorrhagia, MI, mouth ulceration, movement disorder, multiorgan failure, muscle spasm, myasthenia, neuralgia, neurosis, neutropenia, palpitation, pancreatitis, pancytopenia, paralysis, parkinsonian exacerbation, peripheral neuritis, photophobia, polyuria, postural hypotension, progressive immunosuppression, red cell aplasia, rhabdomyolysis, salivation increased, skin discoloration, Stevens-Johnson syndrome, suicide, syncope, tachycardia, taste loss/perversion, thrombocytopenia, tic, tinnitus, tongue edema, toxic epidermal necrolysis, twitching, urinary incontinence, urticaria, vasculitis, vasodilation, yawn

Also observed: Rash requiring hospitalization: Children <16 years 0.8% (epilepsy adjunctive therapy); Adults 0.3% (epilepsy adjunctive therapy), 0.13% (epilepsy monotherapy), 0.8% (bipolar disorder, monotherapy)

Drug Interactions

Avoid Concomitant Use There are no known interactions where it is recommended to avoid concomitant use.

Increased Effect/Toxicity

LamoTRIgine may increase the levels/effects of: Alcohol (Ethyl); CarBAMazepine; CNS Depressants; Desmopressin; OLANZapine

The levels/effects of LamoTRIgine may be increased by: Valproic Acid

Decreased Effect

The levels/effects of LamoTRIgine may be decreased by: Barbiturates; CarBAMazepine; Ketorolac; Mefloquine; Oral Contraceptive (Estrogens); Phenytoin; Primidone; Rifampin; Ritonavir

Ethanol/Nutrition/Herb Interactions

Ethanol: Avoid ethanol (may increase CNS depression).

Food: Has no effect on absorption.

Herb/Nutraceutical: Avoid evening primrose (seizure threshold decreased).

Stability Store at 25°C (77°F); excursions permitted to 15°C to 30°C (59°F to 86°F). Protect from light.

Mechanism of Action A triazine derivative which inhibits release of glutamate (an excitatory amino acid) and inhibits voltage-sensitive sodium channels, which stabilizes neuronal membranes. Lamotrigine has weak inhibitory effect on the 5-HT_3 receptor; *in vitro* inhibits dihydrofolate reductase.

Pharmacodynamics/Kinetics

Absorption: Rapid and complete

Distribution: V_d: ~1 L/kg

Protein binding: 55%

Metabolism: Hepatic and renal; metabolized by glucuronic acid conjugation to inactive metabolites

Bioavailability: 98%

Half-life elimination: Adults: 25-33 hours

Concomitant valproic acid therapy: 59-70 hours

Concomitant phenytoin or carbamazepine therapy: 13-14 hours

Chronic renal failure: 43 hours

Hemodialysis: 13 hours during dialysis; 57 hours between dialysis

Hepatic impairment: 26-148 hours

Time to peak, plasma: 1-5 hours

Excretion: Urine (94%, ~90% as glucuronide conjugates and ~10% unchanged); feces (2%)

Dosage Note: Only whole tablets should be used for dosing, round calculated dose down to the nearest whole tablet. Enzyme-inducing regimens specifically refer to those containing carbamazepine, phenytoin, phenobarbital, or primidone. Oral:

Children 2-12 years: Lennox-Gastaut (adjunctive), primary generalized tonic-clonic seizures (adjunctive), or partial seizures (adjunctive): **Note:** Children <30 kg will likely require maintenance doses to be increased as much as 50% based on clinical response regardless of regimen below:

Initial: 0.3 mg/kg/day in 1-2 divided doses for weeks 1 and 2, then increase to 0.6 mg/kg/day in 1-2 divided doses for weeks 3 and 4. Maintenance: Titrate dose to effect; after week 4, increase daily dose every 1-2 weeks by 0.6 mg/kg/day; usual maintenance: 4.5-7.5 mg/kg/day in 2 divided doses; maximum: 300 mg/day in 2 divided doses

Adjustment for AED regimens **containing** valproic acid (see **"Note"**): Initial: 0.15 mg/kg/day in 1-2 divided doses for weeks 1 and 2, then increase to 0.3 mg/kg/day in 1-2 divided doses for weeks 3 and 4. Maintenance: Titrate dose to effect; after week 4, increase daily dose every 1-2 weeks by 0.3 mg/kg/day; usual maintenance: 1-5 mg/kg/day in 2 divided doses; maximum: 200 mg/day in 1-2 divided doses

Note: For patients >6.7 kg and <14 kg, initial dosing should be 2 mg every other day for first 2 weeks, then increased to 2 mg daily for weeks 3-4. For patients taking lamotrigine with valproic acid alone, the usual maintenance dose is 1-3 mg/kg/day in 2 divided doses

Adjustment for **enzyme-inducing** AED regimens **without** valproic acid: Initial: 0.6 mg/kg/day in 2 divided doses for weeks 1 and 2, then increase to 1.2 mg/kg/day in 2 divided doses for weeks 3 and 4. Maintenance: Titrate dose to effect; after week 4, increase daily dose every 1-2 weeks by 1.2 mg/kg/day; usual maintenance: 5-15 mg/kg/day in 2 divided doses; maximum: 400 mg/day in 2 divided doses

Children >12 years: Lennox-Gastaut (adjunctive), primary generalized tonic-clonic seizures (adjunctive), or partial seizures (adjunctive): Refer to adult dosing.

Children ≥16 years: Conversion from adjunctive therapy with valproic acid or a single enzyme-inducing AED regimen to monotherapy with lamotrigine: Refer to adult dosing.

Adults:

Lennox-Gastaut (adjunctive), primary generalized tonic-clonic seizures (adjunctive) or partial seizures (adjunctive): Initial: 25 mg/day for weeks 1 and 2, then increase to 50 mg/day for weeks 3 and 4. Maintenance: Titrate dose to effect; after week 4 increase daily dose every 1-2 weeks by 50 mg/day; usual maintenance: 225-375 mg/day in 2 divided doses

Adjustment for AED regimens **containing** valproic acid (see **"Note"**): Initial: 25 mg every other day for weeks 1 and 2, then increase to 25 mg every day for weeks 3 and 4. Maintenance: Titrate dose to effect; after week 4 increase daily dose every 1-2 weeks by 25-50 mg/day; usual maintenance: 100-400 mg/day in 1 or 2 divided doses

Note: For patients taking lamotrigine with valproic acid alone, the usual maintenance dose is 100-200 mg/day

Adjustment for **enzyme-inducing** AED regimens **without** valproic acid: Initial: 50 mg/day for weeks 1 and 2, then increase to 100 mg/day in 2 divided doses for weeks 3 and 4. Maintenance: titrate dose to effect; after week 4 increase daily dose every 1-2 weeks by 100 mg/day; usual maintenance: 300-500 mg/day in 2 divided doses. Doses as high as 700 mg/day have been used, though additional benefit has not been established.

Conversion to monotherapy with lamotrigine:

Conversion from adjunctive therapy with valproic acid: Initiate and titrate as per recommendations to a lamotrigine dose of 200 mg/day. Then taper valproic acid dose in decrements of not >500 mg/day at intervals of 1 week (or longer) to a valproic acid dosage of 500 mg/day; this dosage should be maintained for 1 week. The lamotrigine dosage should then be increased to 300 mg/day while valproic acid is decreased to 250 mg/day; this dosage should be maintained for 1 week. Valproic acid may then be discontinued, while the lamotrigine dose is increased by 100 mg/day at weekly intervals to achieve a lamotrigine maintenance dose of 500 mg/day.

Conversion from adjunctive therapy with carbamazepine, phenytoin, phenobarbital, or primidone: Initiate and titrate as per recommendations to a lamotrigine dose of 500 mg/day. Concomitant enzyme-inducing AED should then be withdrawn by 20% decrements each week over a 4-week period. Patients should be monitored for rash.

Conversion from adjunctive therapy with AED other than carbamazepine, phenytoin, phenobarbital, primidone or valproic acid: No specific guidelines available

Bipolar disorder:

Initial: 25 mg/day for weeks 1 and 2, then increase to 50 mg/day for weeks 3 and 4, then increase to 100 mg/day for week 5; maintenance: increase dose to 200 mg/day beginning week 6

Adjustment for regimens **containing** valproic acid: Initial: 25 mg every other day for weeks 1 and 2, then increase to 25 mg every day for weeks 3 and 4, then increase to 50 mg/day for week 5; maintenance: 100 mg/day beginning week 6

Adjustment for **enzyme-inducing** regimens **without** valproic acid: Initial: 50 mg/day for weeks 1 and 2, then increase to 100 mg/day in divided doses for weeks 3 and 4, then increase to 200 mg/day in divided doses for week 5, then increase to 300 mg/day in divided dose for week 6; maintenance: 400 mg/day in divided doses beginning week 7

Adjustment following discontinuation of psychotropic medication:

Discontinuing valproic acid with current dose of lamotrigine 100 mg/day: 150 mg/day for week 1, then increase to 200 mg/day beginning week 2

Discontinuing carbamazepine, phenytoin, phenobarbital, primidone, or rifampin with current dose of lamotrigine 400 mg/day: 400 mg/day for week 1, then decrease to 300 mg/day for week 2, then decrease to 200 mg/day beginning week 3

Discontinuing therapy: Children and Adults: Decrease dose by ~50% per week, over at least 2 weeks unless safety concerns require a more rapid withdrawal. Discontinuing carbamazepine, phenytoin, phenobarbital, or primidone should prolong the half-life of lamotrigine; discontinuing valproic acid should shorten the half-life of lamotrigine

Restarting therapy after discontinuation: If lamotrigine has been withheld for >5 half-lives, consider restarting according to initial dosing recommendations.

Dosage adjustment with combination hormonal contraceptives: Follow initial dosing guidelines, maintenance dose should be adjusted as follows: Patients taking carbamazepine, phenytoin, phenobarbital, primidone or rifampin: No dosing adjustment required

Patients **not** taking carbamazepine, phenytoin, phenobarbital, primidone or rifampin: Maintenance dose may need increased by twofold over target dose. If already taking a stable dose of lamotrigine and starting contraceptive, maintenance dose may need increased by twofold. Dose increases should start when contraceptive is started and titrated to clinical response increasing no more rapidly than 50-100 mg/day every week. Gradual increases of lamotrigine plasma levels may occur during the inactive "pill-free" week and will be greater when dose increases are made the week before. If increased adverse events consistently occur during "pill-free" week, overall dose adjustments may be required. When discontinuing combination hormonal contraceptive, dose of lamotrigine may need decreased by as much as 50%; do not decrease by more than 25% of total daily dose over a 2-week period unless clinical response or plasma levels indicate otherwise. Dose adjustments during "pill-free" week are not recommended.

Dosage adjustment in renal impairment: Decreased dosage may be effective in patients with significant renal impairment; use with caution

Dosage adjustment in hepatic impairment:

Moderate-to-severe impairment without ascites: Decrease initial, escalation, and maintenance doses by ~25%

Moderate-to-severe impairment with ascites: Decrease initial, escalation, and maintenance doses by ~50%

Dietary Considerations Take without regard to meals; drug may cause GI upset.

Administration Doses should be rounded down to the nearest whole tablet. Dispersible tablets may be chewed, dispersed in water or diluted fruit juice, or swallowed whole. To disperse tablets, add to a small amount of liquid (just enough to cover tablet); let sit ~1 minute until dispersed; swirl solution and consume immediately. Do not administer partial amounts of liquid. If tablets are chewed, a small amount of water or diluted fruit juice should be used to aid in swallowing.

Monitoring Parameters Seizure, frequency and duration, serum levels of concurrent anticonvulsants, hypersensitivity reactions, especially rash

Reference Range A therapeutic serum concentration range has not been established for lamotrigine. Dosing should be based on therapeutic response. Lamotrigine plasma concentrations of 0.25-29.1 mcg/mL have been reported in the literature.

Dosage Forms Excipient information presented when available (limited, particularly for generics); consult specific product labeling.

Tablet: 25 mg, 100 mg, 150 mg, 200 mg
- Lamictal®: 25 mg, 100 mg, 150 mg, 200 mg

Tablet, combination package [each unit-dose starter kit contains]:
- Lamictal® (blue kit; for patients taking valproic acid):
  - Tablet: Lamotrigine 25 mg (35s)
- Lamictal® (green kit; for patients taking carbamazepine, phenytoin, phenobarbital, primidone, or rifampin and **not** taking valproic acid):
  - Tablet: Lamotrigine 25 mg (84s)
  - Tablet: Lamotrigine 100 mg (14s)
- Lamictal® (orange kit; for patients **not** taking carbamazepine, phenytoin, phenobarbital, primidone, rifampin, or valproic acid):
  - Tablet: Lamotrigine 25 mg (42s)
  - Tablet: Lamotrigine 100 mg (7s)

Tablet, dispersible/chewable: 5 mg, 25 mg
- Lamictal®: 2 mg, 5 mg, 25 mg [black currant flavor]

Extemporaneous Preparations A 1 mg/mL oral suspension may be compounded as follows: Crush one 100 mg tablet and reduce to a fine powder. Add small amount of Ora-Sweet® or Ora-Plus® and mix to uniform paste. Transfer to graduate and qs to 100 mL. Shake well before using and refrigerate. Suspension is stable for 91 days.

Nahata M, Morosco R, Hipple T. "Stability of Lamotrigine in Two Extemporaneously Prepared Oral Suspensions at 4 and 25°C," *Am J Health Syst Pharm*, 1999, 56:240-2.

◆ **Lanacane® [OTC]** *see* Benzocaine *on page* 183

◆ **Lanacane® Maximum Strength [OTC]** *see* Benzocaine *on page* 183

◆ **Lanaphilic® [OTC]** *see* Urea *on page* 1530

◆ **Lanoxicaps® [DSC]** *see* Digoxin *on page* 444

◆ **Lanoxicaps® (Can)** *see* Digoxin *on page* 444

◆ **Lanoxin®** *see* Digoxin *on page* 444

Lanreotide (lan REE oh tide)

U.S. Brand Names Somatuline® Depot

Canadian Brand Names Somatuline® Autogel®

Index Terms Lanreotide Acetate

Pharmacologic Category Somatostatin Analog

Use Long-term treatment of acromegaly in patients who are not candidates for or are unresponsive to surgery and/or radiotherapy

Canadian labeling: Also approved in Canada for relief of symptoms of acromegaly

Pregnancy Risk Factor C

Medication Safety Issues

Sound-alike/look-alike issues:
- Somatuline® may be confused with somatropin, SUMAtriptan

International issues:
- Somatuline® may be confused with Soma® which is a brand name for carisoprodol in the U.S.

Dosage SubQ: **Note: Differences in U.S. and Canadian labeled dosing:**

U.S. labeling: Adults: Acromegaly: 90 mg once every 4 weeks for 3 months; after initial 90 days of therapy, adjust dose based on clinical response of patient, growth hormone (GH) levels, and/or insulin-like growth factor 1 (IGF-1) levels as follows:
- GH ≤1 ng/mL, IGF-1 normal, symptoms stable:60 mg once every 4 weeks
- GH >1-2.5 ng/mL, IGF-1 normal, symptoms stable: 90 mg once every 4 weeks
- GH >2.5 ng/mL, IGF-1 elevated and/or uncontrolled symptoms: 120 mg once every 4 weeks

Canadian labeling: Children ≥16 years and Adults: Acromegaly: 90 mg once every 4 weeks for 3 months; after initial 90 days of therapy, adjust dose based on clinical response of patient, growth hormone (GH) levels, and/or insulin-like growth factor 1 (IGF-1) levels as follows:
- GH = 1 ng/mL, IGF-1 normal, symptoms stable: 60 mg once every 4 weeks
- GH >1-2.5 ng/mL, IGF-1 normal, symptoms stable: 90 mg once every 4 weeks
- GH >2.5 ng/mL, IGF-1 elevated and/or uncontrolled symptoms: 120 mg once every 4 weeks

Dosing adjustment in renal impairment:
- *U.S. labeling*: Moderate-to-severe impairment: Recommended starting dose: 60 mg
- *Canadian labeling:* No adjustment is necessary

Dosing adjustment in hepatic impairment:
- *U.S. labeling:* Moderate-to-severe impairment: Recommended starting dose: 60 mg
- *Canadian labeling:* No adjustment is necessary

Additional Information Complete prescribing information for this medication should be consulted for additional detail.

Dosage Forms Excipient information presented when available (limited, particularly for generics); consult specific product labeling. [CAN] = Canadian brand name

Injection, solution:
- Somatuline® Autogel® [CAN]: 60 mg/ 0.3 mL (0.3 mL); 90 mg/ 0.3 mL (0.3 mL); 120 mg/0.5 mL (0.5 mL) [packaging contains natural rubber/natural latex]
- Somatuline® Depot®: 60 mg/~0.4 mL (~0.4 mL); 90 mg/~0.4 mL (~0.4 mL); 120 mg/~0.5 mL (~0.5 mL) [packaging contains natural rubber/natural latex]

◆ **Lanreotide Acetate** *see* Lanreotide *on page* 853

Lansoprazole (lan SOE pra zole)

U.S. Brand Names Prevacid®; Prevacid® SoluTab™

Canadian Brand Names Prevacid®

Pharmacologic Category Proton Pump Inhibitor; Substituted Benzimidazole

Additional Appendix Information

Helicobacter pylori Treatment *on page* 1813

Use Short-term treatment of active duodenal ulcers; maintenance treatment of healed duodenal ulcers; as part of a multidrug regimen for *H. pylori* eradication to reduce the risk of duodenal ulcer recurrence; short-term treatment of active benign gastric ulcer; treatment of NSAID-associated gastric ulcer; to reduce the risk of NSAID-associated gastric ulcer in patients with a history of gastric ulcer who require an NSAID; short-term treatment of symptomatic GERD; short-term treatment for all grades of erosive esophagitis; to maintain healing of erosive esophagitis; long-term treatment of pathological hypersecretory conditions, including Zollinger-Ellison syndrome

Pregnancy Risk Factor B

Pregnancy Considerations Animal studies have not shown teratogenic effects to the fetus. However, there are no adequate and well-controlled studies in pregnant women; use during pregnancy only if clearly needed.

Lactation Excretion in breast milk unknown/not recommended

Medication Safety Issues

Sound-alike/look-alike issues:

Prevacid® may be confused with Pravachol®, Prevpac®, Prilosec®, Prinivil®

Contraindications Hypersensitivity to lansoprazole, substituted benzimidazoles (ie, esomeprazole, omeprazole, pantoprazole, rabeprazole), or any component of the formulation

Warnings/Precautions Use of proton pump inhibitors may increase the risk of gastrointestinal infections (eg, *Salmonella, Campylobacter*). Relief of symptoms does not preclude the presence of a gastric malignancy. Atrophic gastritis (by biopsy) has been noted with long-term omeprazole therapy; this may also occur with lansoprazole. No reports of enterochromaffin-like (ECL) cell carcinoids, dysplasia, or neoplasia have occurred. Severe liver dysfunction may require dosage reductions. Safety and efficacy have not been established in children <1 year of age.

Adverse Reactions

1% to 10%:

Central nervous system: Headache (children 1-11 years 3%, 12-17 years 7%)

Gastrointestinal: Abdominal pain (children 12-17 years 5%; adults 2%), constipation (children 1-11 years 5%; adults 1%), diarrhea (60 mg/day; adults 7%), nausea (children 12-17 years 3%; adults 1%)

<1% (Limited to important or life-threatening): Abnormal vision, agitation, allergic reaction, ALT increased, anaphylactoid reaction, anemia, angina, anxiety, aplastic anemia, arrhythmia, AST increased, chest pain, convulsion, depression, dizziness, dry eyes, dry mouth, erythema multiforme, esophagitis, gastrin levels increased, glucocorticoids increased, globulins increased, hemolysis, hemolytic anemia, hepatotoxicity, hyperglycemia, interstitial nephritis, LDH increased, maculopapular rash, myositis, pancreatitis, photophobia, rash, RBC abnormal, taste perversion, Stevens-Johnson syndrome, thrombocytopenia, tinnitus, toxic epidermal necrolysis, tremor, vertigo, visual field defect, vomiting, WBC abnormal

Drug Interactions

Metabolism/Transport Effects Substrate of CYP2C9 (minor), 2C19 (major), 3A4 (major); **Inhibits** CYP2C9 (weak), 2C19 (moderate), 2D6 (weak), 3A4 (weak); **Induces** CYP1A2 (weak)

Avoid Concomitant Use

Avoid concomitant use of Lansoprazole with any of the following: Erlotinib; Mesalamine; Nelfinavir

Increased Effect/Toxicity

Lansoprazole may increase the levels/effects of: CYP2C19 Substrates; Imatinib; Methotrexate; Saquinavir; Voriconazole

The levels/effects of Lansoprazole may be increased by: Fluconazole; Ketoconazole

Decreased Effect

Lansoprazole may decrease the levels/effects of: Atazanavir; Clopidogrel; Dabigatran Etexilate; Dasatinib; Erlotinib; Indinavir; Iron Salts; Itraconazole; Ketoconazole; Mesalamine; Mycophenolate; Nelfinavir

The levels/effects of Lansoprazole may be decreased by: CYP2C19 Inducers (Strong); CYP3A4 Inducers (Strong); Deferasirox; Herbs (CYP3A4 Inducers); Tipranavir

Ethanol/Nutrition/Herb Interactions

Ethanol: Avoid ethanol (may cause gastric mucosal irritation).

Food: Lansoprazole serum concentrations may be decreased if taken with food.

Herb/Nutraceutical: Avoid St John's wort (may decrease the levels/effect of lansoprazole).

Stability Store at 25°C (77°F); excursions permitted to 15°C to 30°C (59°F to 86°F).

Mechanism of Action Decreases acid secretion in gastric parietal cells through inhibition of (H+, K+)-ATPase enzyme system, blocking the final step in gastric acid production.

Pharmacodynamics/Kinetics

Duration: >1 day

Absorption: Rapid

Distribution: V_d: 14-18 L

Protein binding: 97%

Metabolism: Hepatic via CYP2C19 and 3A4, and in parietal cells to two active metabolites that are not present in systemic circulation

Bioavailability: 80%; decreased 50% to 70% if given 30 minutes after food

Half-life elimination: 1-2 hours; Elderly: 2-3 hours; Hepatic impairment: ≤7 hours

Time to peak, plasma: 1.7 hours

Excretion: Feces (67%); urine (33%)

Dosage Oral:

Children 1-11 years: GERD, erosive esophagitis:

≤30 kg: 15 mg once daily

>30 kg: 30 mg once daily

Note: Doses were increased in some pediatric patients if still symptomatic after 2 or more weeks of treatment (maximum dose: 30 mg twice daily)

Children 12-17 years:

Nonerosive GERD: 15 mg once daily for up to 8 weeks

Erosive esophagitis: 30 mg once daily for up to 8 weeks

Adults:

Duodenal ulcer: Short-term treatment: 15 mg once daily for 4 weeks; maintenance therapy: 15 mg once daily

Gastric ulcer: Short-term treatment: 30 mg once daily for up to 8 weeks

NSAID-associated gastric ulcer (healing): 30 mg once daily for 8 weeks; controlled studies did not extend past 8 weeks of therapy

NSAID-associated gastric ulcer (to reduce risk): 15 mg once daily for up to 12 weeks; controlled studies did not extend past 12 weeks of therapy

Symptomatic GERD: Short-term treatment: 15 mg once daily for up to 8 weeks

Erosive esophagitis: Short-term treatment: 30 mg once daily for up to 8 weeks; continued treatment for an additional 8 weeks may be considered for recurrence or for patients who do not heal after the first 8 weeks of therapy; maintenance therapy: 15 mg once daily

Hypersecretory conditions: Initial: 60 mg once daily; adjust dose based upon patient response and to reduce acid secretion to <10 mEq/hour (5 mEq/hour in patients with prior gastric surgery); doses of 90 mg twice daily have been used; administer doses >120 mg/day in divided doses

Helicobacter pylori eradication: Currently accepted recommendations (may differ from product labeling): Dose varies with regimen: 30 mg once daily or 60 mg/day in 2 divided doses; requires combination therapy with antibiotics

Elderly: No dosage adjustment is needed in elderly patients with normal hepatic function

Dosage adjustment in renal impairment: No dosage adjustment is needed

Dosing adjustment in hepatic impairment: Dose reduction is necessary for severe hepatic impairment

Dietary Considerations Should be taken before eating; best if taken before breakfast. Prevacid® SoluTab™ contains phenylalanine 2.5 mg per 15 mg tablet; phenylalanine 5.1 mg per 30 mg tablet.

Administration

Oral: Administer before food; best if taken before breakfast. The intact granules should not be chewed or crushed; however, several options are available for those patients unable to swallow capsules:

Capsules may be opened and the intact granules sprinkled on 1 tablespoon of applesauce, Ensure® pudding, cottage cheese, yogurt, or strained pears. The granules should then be swallowed immediately.

Capsules may be opened and emptied into ~60 mL orange juice, apple juice, or tomato juice; mix and swallow immediately. Rinse the glass with additional juice and swallow to assure complete delivery of the dose.

Orally-disintegrating tablets: Should not be swallowed whole or chewed. Place tablet on tongue; allow to dissolve (with or without water) until particles can be swallowed. Orally-disintegrating tablets may also be administered via an oral syringe: Place the 15 mg tablet in an oral syringe and draw up ~4 mL water, or place the 30 mg tablet in an oral syringe and draw up ~10 mL water. After tablet has dispersed, administer within 15 minutes. Refill the syringe with water (2 mL for the 15 mg tablet; 4 mL for the 30 mg tablet), shake gently, then administer any remaining contents.

Nasogastric tube administration:

Capsule: Capsule can be opened, the granules mixed (not crushed) with 40 mL of apple juice and then injected through the NG tube into the stomach, then flush tube with additional apple juice. Do not mix with other liquids.

Orally-disintegrating tablet: Nasogastric tube ≥8 French: Place a 15 mg tablet in a syringe and draw up ~4 mL water, or place the 30 mg tablet in a syringe and draw up ~10 mL water. After tablet has dispersed, administer within 15 minutes. Refill the syringe with ~5 mL water, shake gently, and then flush the nasogastric tube.

Monitoring Parameters Patients with Zollinger-Ellison syndrome should be monitored for gastric acid output, which should be maintained at ≤10 mEq/hour during the last hour before the next lansoprazole dose; lab monitoring should include CBC, liver function, renal function, and serum gastrin levels

Dosage Forms Excipient information presented when available (limited, particularly for generics); consult specific product labeling. [DSC] = Discontinued product

Capsule, delayed release:

Prevacid®: 15 mg, 30 mg

Tablet, delayed release, orally disintegrating:

Prevacid® SoluTab™: 15 mg [contains phenylalanine 2.5 mg; strawberry flavor]; 30 mg [contains phenylalanine 5.1 mg; strawberry flavor]

Extemporaneous Preparations A 3 mg/mL lansoprazole oral solution (Simplified Lansoprazole Solution) can be prepared with ten lansoprazole 30 mg capsules and 100 mL 8.4% sodium bicarbonate. Empty capsules into beaker. Add sodium bicarbonate solution. Gently stir (about 15 minutes) until dissolved. Transfer to amber-colored syringe or bottle. Stable for 8 hours at room temperature or for 14 days under refrigeration.

DiGiancinto JL, Olsen KM, Bergman KL, et al, "Stability of Suspension Formulations of Lansoprazole and Omeprazole Stored in Amber-Colored Plastic Oral Syringes," *Ann Pharmacother*, 2000, 34:600-5

Sharma V, "Comparison of 24-hour Intragastric pH Using Four Liquid Formulations of Lansoprazole and Omeprazole," *Am J Health Syst Pharm*, 1999, 56(Suppl 4): S18-21.

Sharma VK, Vasudeva R, and Howden CW, "Simplified Lansoprazole Suspension - Liquid Formulations of Lansoprazole - Effectively Suppresses Intragastric Acidity When Administered Through a Gastrostomy," *Am J Gastroenterol*, 1999, 94(7):1813-7.

Lansoprazole, Amoxicillin, and Clarithromycin

(lan SOE pra zole, a moks i SIL in, & kla RITH roe mye sin)

U.S. Brand Names Prevpac®

Canadian Brand Names Hp-PAC®; Prevpac®

Index Terms Amoxicillin, Lansoprazole, and Clarithromycin; Clarithromycin, Lansoprazole, and Amoxicillin

Pharmacologic Category Antibiotic, Macrolide Combination; Antibiotic, Penicillin; Gastrointestinal Agent, Miscellaneous

Use Eradication of *H. pylori* to reduce the risk of recurrent duodenal ulcer

Pregnancy Risk Factor C (clarithromycin)

Medication Safety Issues

Sound-alike/look-alike issues:

Prevpac® may be confused with Prevacid®

Dosage Oral: Adults: Lansoprazole 30 mg, amoxicillin 1 g, and clarithromycin 500 mg taken together twice daily for 10 or 14 days

Dosage adjustment in renal impairment: Cl_{cr} <30 mL/minute: Use is not recommended

Additional Information Complete prescribing information for this medication should be consulted for additional detail.

Dosage Forms Excipient information presented when available (limited, particularly for generics); consult specific product labeling.

Combination package [each administration card contains]:

Prevpac®:

Capsule: Amoxicillin 500 mg (4 capsules/day)

Capsule, delayed release (Prevacid®): Lansoprazole 30 mg (2 capsules/day)

Tablet (Biaxin®): Clarithromycin 500 mg (2 tablets/day)

Lansoprazole and Naproxen

(lan SOE pra zole & na PROKS en)

U.S. Brand Names Prevacid® NapraPAC™

Index Terms NapraPAC™; Naproxen and Lansoprazole

Pharmacologic Category Nonsteroidal Anti-inflammatory Drug (NSAID), Oral; Proton Pump Inhibitor

Use Reduction of the risk of NSAID-associated gastric ulcers in patients with history of gastric ulcer who require an NSAID for the treatment of rheumatoid arthritis, osteoarthritis, and ankylosing spondylitis

Restrictions An FDA-approved medication guide must be distributed when dispensing an oral outpatient prescription (new or refill) where this medication is to be used without direct supervision of a healthcare provider. Medication guides are available at http://www.fda.gov/cder/Offices/ODS/medication_guides.htm.

Pregnancy Risk Factor C (naproxen: D/third trimester)

Medication Safety Issues

Sound-alike/look-alike issues:

Prevacid® may be confused with Pravachol®, Prevpac®, Prilosec®, Prinivil®

Dosage Oral: Adults: Reduce NSAID-associated gastric ulcers during treatment for arthritis: Lansoprazole 15 mg once daily in the morning; naproxen 500 mg twice daily

Elderly: Naproxen: Dosing adjustment should be considered

Dosage adjustment in renal/hepatic impairment: Naproxen: Cl_{cr} <30 mL/minute: use is not recommended

Additional Information Complete prescribing information for this medication should be consulted for additional detail.

Dosage Forms Excipient information presented when available (limited, particularly for generics); consult specific product labeling. [DSC] = Discontinued product

Combination package:
Prevacid® NapraPAC™ 375 [each administration card contains] [DSC]:
Capsule, delayed release (Prevacid®): Lansoprazole 15 mg (7 capsules per card)
Tablet (Naprosyn®): Naproxen 375 mg (14 tablets per card)
Prevacid® NapraPAC™ 500 [each administration card contains]:
Capsule, delayed release (Prevacid®): Lansoprazole 15 mg (7 capsules per card)
Tablet (Naprosyn®): Naproxen 500 mg (14 tablets per card)

Lanthanum (LAN tha num)

U.S. Brand Names Fosrenol®
Canadian Brand Names Fosrenol®
Index Terms Lanthanum Carbonate
Pharmacologic Category Phosphate Binder
Use Reduction of serum phosphate in patients with stage 5 chronic kidney disease (end-stage renal disease [ESRD]; kidney failure: GFR <15 mL/minute/1.73 m^2 or dialysis)
Pregnancy Risk Factor C
Dosage Oral: Adults: Initial: 1500 mg/day divided and taken with meals; typical increases of 750 mg/day every 2-3 weeks are suggested as needed to bring the serum phosphate level <6 mg/dL; usual dosage range: 1500-3000 mg; doses of up to 3750 mg have been used
Additional Information Complete prescribing information for this medication should be consulted for additional detail.
Dosage Forms Excipient information presented when available (limited, particularly for generics); consult specific product labeling.
Tablet, chewable:
Fosrenol®: 500 mg, 750 mg, 1000 mg

◆ **Lanthanum Carbonate** *see* Lanthanum *on page 856*
◆ **Lantus®** *see* Insulin Glargine *on page 794*
◆ **Lantus® OptiSet® (Can)** *see* Insulin Glargine *on page 794*
◆ **Lanvis® (Can)** *see* Thioguanine *on page 1459*

Lapatinib (la PA ti nib)

U.S. Brand Names Tykerb®
Index Terms GW572016; Lapatinib Ditosylate; NSC-727989
Pharmacologic Category Antineoplastic Agent, Tyrosine Kinase Inhibitor; Epidermal Growth Factor Receptor (EGFR) Inhibitor
Use Treatment (in combination with capecitabine) of HER2/neu overexpressing advanced or metastatic breast cancer, in patients who have received prior therapy (with an anthracycline, a taxane, and trastuzumab)
Unlabeled/Investigational Use Treatment of head and neck cancers
Restrictions Lapatinib is available **only** at specialty pharmacies through a restricted-access program, Tykerb® CARES. Information is available at www.tykerbcares.com or 1-866-489-5372.
Pregnancy Risk Factor D
Pregnancy Considerations Increased pup deaths were demonstrated in animal studies. There are no adequate and well-controlled studies in pregnant women. Lapatinib may cause fetal harm if administered during pregnancy. Women of childbearing potential should be advised to avoid pregnancy during treatment.
Lactation Excretion in breast milk unknown/not recommended
Medication Safety Issues
Sound-alike/look-alike issues:
Lapatinib may be confused with dasatinib, erlotinib, imatinib

High alert medication: The Institute for Safe Medication Practices (ISMP) includes this medication among its list of drug classes which have a heightened risk of causing significant patient harm when used in error.
Contraindications There are no contraindications listed within the manufacturer's labeling.
Warnings/Precautions Hazardous agent - use appropriate precautions for handling and disposal.

Decreases in left ventricular ejection fraction (LVEF) have been reported; baseline and periodic LVEF evaluations are recommended; interrupt therapy or decrease dose with with decreased LVEF ≥ grade 2 or LVEF < LLN. QT_c prolongation has been observed; use caution in patients with a history of QT_c prolongation or with medications known to prolong the QT interval; a baseline and periodic 12-lead ECG should be considered; correct electrolyte (potassium, calcium and magnesium) abnormalities prior to and during treatment. Use caution in patients with a history of or predisposed (prior treatment with anthracyclines, chest wall irradiation) to left ventricular dysfunction. Interstitial lung disease (ILD) and pneumonitis have been reported (with lapatinib monotherapy and with combination chemotherapy); discontinue therapy for grade 3 (or higher) pulmonary symptoms indicative of ILD or pneumonitis (eg, dyspnea, dry cough).

[U.S. Boxed Warning]: Hepatotoxicity (ALT or AST >3 times ULN and total bilirubin >1.5 times ULN) has been reported with lapatinib; may be severe and/or fatal. Onset of hepatotoxicity may occur within days to several months after treatment initiation; monitor; discontinue with severe changes in liver function; do not retreat. Use caution in patients with hepatic dysfunction. Dose reductions should be considered in patients with severe (Child-Pugh class C) hepatic impairment. Avoid concurrent use with strong CYP3A4 inhibitors or inducers; if concomitant therapy cannot be avoided, lapatinib dosage adjustments should be considered. May cause diarrhea (may be severe); manage with antidiarrheal agents; severe diarrhea may require hydration, electrolytes, and or interruption of therapy. Safety and efficacy have not been established in children.
Adverse Reactions Percentages reported for combination chemotherapy.
>10%:
Central nervous system: Fatigue (10% to 18%)
Dermatologic: Palmar-plantar erythrodysesthesia (hand-and-foot syndrome) (53%; grade 3: 12%), rash (28%)
Gastrointestinal: Diarrhea (65%; grade 3: 13%; grade 4: 1%), nausea (44%), vomiting (26%), abdominal pain (15%), mucosal inflammation (15%), stomatitis (14%), dyspepsia (11%)
Hematologic: Anemia (56%; grade 3: <1%), neutropenia (22%; grade 3: 3%; grade 4: <1%), thrombocytopenia (18%; grade 3: <1%)
Hepatic: AST increased (49%; grade 3: 2%; grade 4: <1%), total bilirubin increased (45%; grade 3: 4%), ALT increased (37%; grade 3: 2%)
Neuromuscular & skeletal: Limb pain (12%), back pain (11%)
Respiratory: Dyspnea (12%)
1% to 10%:
Cardiovascular: LVEF decreased (grade 2: 2%; grade 3: <1%)
Central nervous system: Insomnia (10%)
Dermatologic: Dry skin (10%)
<1%, postmarketing, and/or case reports: Hepatotoxicity, interstitial lung disease, pneumonitis, Prinzmetal's angina, QT_c prolongation

Drug Interactions

Metabolism/Transport Effects Substrate of CYP2C8 (minor), 3A4 (major), P-glycoprotein (P-gp, ABCB1); **Inhibits** CYP2C8, 3A4

Avoid Concomitant Use

Avoid concomitant use of Lapatinib with any of the following: Dabigatran Etexilate; Nilotinib; Rivaroxaban; Silodosin; Tetrabenazine; Thioridazine; Topotecan; Ziprasidone

Increased Effect/Toxicity

Lapatinib may increase the levels/effects of: CYP2C8 Substrates (High risk); CYP3A4 Substrates; Dabigatran Etexilate; Eplerenone; FentaNYL; Maraviroc; P-Glycoprotein Substrates; Pimecrolimus; QTc-Prolonging Agents; Ranolazine; Rivaroxaban; Salmeterol; Silodosin; Tetrabenazine; Thioridazine; Topotecan; Ziprasidone

The levels/effects of Lapatinib may be increased by: Alfuzosin; Ciprofloxacin; CYP3A4 Inhibitors (Moderate); CYP3A4 Inhibitors (Strong); Dasatinib; Gadobutrol; Nilotinib; P-Glycoprotein Inhibitors

Decreased Effect

The levels/effects of Lapatinib may be decreased by: CYP3A4 Inducers (Strong); Deferasirox; Herbs (CYP3A4 Inducers); P-Glycoprotein Inducers

Ethanol/Nutrition/Herb Interactions

Food: Systemic exposure of lapatinib is increased when administered with food (AUC three- to fourfold higher). Avoid grapefruit juice (may increase the levels/effects of lapatinib).

Herb/Nutraceutical: Avoid St John's wort (may increase metabolism and decrease lapatinib concentrations).

Stability Store at room temperature of 25°C (77°F); excursions permitted between 15°C and 30°C (59°F and 86°F).

Mechanism of Action Tyrosine kinase (dual kinase) inhibitor; inhibitor of EGFR (ErbB1) and HER2 (ErbB2) by reversibly binding to tyrosine kinase, blocking phosphorylation and activation of downstream second messengers (Erk1/2 and Akt), regulating cellular proliferation and survival in ErbB- and ErbB2-expressing tumors.

Pharmacodynamics/Kinetics

Absorption: Incomplete and variable

Protein binding: >99% to albumin and alpha$_1$-acid glycoprotein

Metabolism: Hepatic; extensive via CYP3A4 and 3A5, and to a lesser extent via CYP2C19 and 2C8 to oxidized metabolites

Half-life elimination: ~24 hours

Time to peak, plasma: 3-6 hours

Excretion: Feces (27% as unchanged drug; range 3% to 67%); urine (<2%)

Dosage Details concerning dosing in combination regimens should also be consulted. **Note:** Dose reductions are likely to be needed when lapatinib is administered concomitantly with a strong CYP3A4 inhibitor (an alternate medication for CYP3A4 enzyme inhibitors should be investigated first).

Oral: Adults: 1250 mg once daily (in combination with capecitabine)

Dosage adjustment for concomitant CYP3A4 inhibitors/inducers:

CYP3A4 inhibitors: Dose reductions are likely to be needed when lapatinib is administered concomitantly with a strong CYP3A4 inhibitor (an alternate medication for CYP3A4 enzyme inhibitors should be investigated first); in the event that lapatinib must be administered concomitantly with a potent enzyme inhibitor, consider reducing lapatinib to 500 mg once daily with careful monitoring. (When a strong CYP3A4 inhibitor is discontinued; allow ~1 week to elapse prior to adjusting the lapatinib dose upward.)

CYP3A4 inducers: Concomitant administration with CYP3A4 inducers may require increased lapatinib doses (alternatives to the enzyme-inducing agent should be utilized first); consider titrating gradually up to 4500 mg/day, with careful monitoring. (If the strong CYP3A4 enzyme inducer is discontinued, reduce the lapatinib dose to the indicated dose.)

Dosage adjustment for toxicity:

Cardiac toxicity: Discontinue treatment for decreased LVEF ≥ grade 2 or LVEF < LLN; may be restarted after 2 weeks at 1000 mg once daily if LVEF recovers to normal and patient is asymptomatic

Other toxicities: Withhold for any toxicity (other than cardiac) ≥ grade 2 until toxicity resolves to ≤ grade 1; reduce dosage to 1000 mg once daily for persistent toxicity

Dosage adjustment in renal impairment: Not studied in renal dysfunction, however, due to the minimal renal elimination (<2%), dosage adjustments for renal dysfunction may not be necessary.

Dosage adjustment in hepatic impairment: Severe hepatic impairment (Child-Pugh Class C): Consider a dose reduction to 750 mg once daily.

Dietary Considerations Take on an empty stomach, 1 hour before or 1 hour after a meal. (**Note:** For combination with capecitabine treatment, capecitabine should be taken with food, or within 30 minutes after a meal.)

Administration Administer once daily, on an empty stomach, 1 hour before or 1 hour after a meal. Take at the same time each day; dividing doses is not recommended.

Monitoring Parameters LVEF (baseline and periodic), CBC with differential, liver function tests, including transaminases, bilirubin, and alkaline phosphatase (baseline and every 4-6 weeks during treatment); electrolytes including calcium, potassium, magnesium; monitor for fluid retention; ECG monitoring if at risk for QT_c prolongation; symptoms of ILD

Additional Information Oncology Comment: The National Comprehensive Cancer Network (NCCN) breast cancer guidelines list lapatinib (in combination with capecitabine) as an option for the treatment of HER2-positive breast cancer in patients who are refractory to anthracycline, taxane and trastuzumab treatment. In a randomized phase III study (Geyer, 2006) of lapatinib plus capecitabine versus capecitabine alone in HER2-positive advanced breast cancer, the addition of lapatinib was associated with a 51% reduction in the risk of disease progression in heavily pretreated patients. Lapatinib shows activity in HER2-positive metastatic breast cancer that has progressed after trastuzumab treatment.

Dosage Forms Excipient information presented when available (limited, particularly for generics); consult specific product labeling.

Tablet:

Tykerb®: 250 mg

◆ **Lapatinib Ditosylate** *see* Lapatinib *on page 856*

◆ **Largactil® (Can)** *see* ChlorproMAZINE *on page 316*

◆ **Lariam® [DSC]** *see* Mefloquine *on page 932*

◆ **Lariam® (Can)** *see* Mefloquine *on page 932*

Laronidase (lair OH ni days)

U.S. Brand Names Aldurazyme®

Canadian Brand Names Aldurazyme®

Index Terms Recombinant α-L-Iduronidase (Glycosaminoglycan α-L-Iduronohydrolase)

Pharmacologic Category Enzyme

Use Treatment of Hurler and Hurler-Scheie forms of mucopolysaccharidosis I (MPS I); treatment of Scheie form of MPS I in patients with moderate to severe symptoms

Pregnancy Risk Factor B

Pregnancy Considerations Teratogenic effects were not observed in animal studies; however, there are no adequate and well-controlled studies in pregnant women. Use during pregnancy only if clearly needed. Patients are encouraged to enroll in the MPS I registry.

Lactation Excretion in breast milk unknown/use caution

Contraindications There are no contraindications listed within the manufacturer's labeling.

Warnings/Precautions [U.S. Boxed Warning]: Anaphylactic reactions have been observed during infusion, immediate treatment for hypersensitivity reactions should be available during administration. Additional monitoring may be required in patients with compromised respiratory function or acute respiratory disease; may be at increased risk for acute exacerbation of respiratory symptoms due to infusion reaction. Patients with acute illness may also be at increased risk for infusion reactions. Reactions, which may include airway obstruction, bradycardia, bronchospasm, hypotension, hypoxia, respiratory distress/failure, stridor, tachypnea, and urticaria, may be severe and tend to occur during or within 3 hours after administration. Antipyretics and or antihistamines should be administered prior to infusion to reduce the incidence/severity of headache, fever, and/or flushing. In event of reaction, decrease the rate of infusion, temporarily discontinue the infusion, and/or administer additional antipyretics/antihistamines. Risks and benefits should be carefully considered prior to readministering following a severe hypersensitivity reaction. In the case of anaphylaxis, caution should be used if epinephrine is being considered; many patients with MPS I have preexisting heart disease.

Prepared infusions contain human albumin. Laronidase has not been studied in patients with mild symptoms of the Scheie form of MPS I. Not indicated for the CNS manifestations of the disorder. Studies did not include children <5 years of age. A patient registry has been established and all patients are encouraged to participate. Registry information may be obtained at www.MPSIregistry.com or by calling 800-745-4447.

Adverse Reactions Note: Percentages reported are from a placebo-controlled study (45 patients, 22 receiving laronidase).

>10%:

- Cardiovascular: Vein disorder (14%)
- Dermatologic: Rash (36%)
- Local: Injection site reaction (18%)
- Neuromuscular & skeletal: Hyper-reflexia (14%), paresthesia (14%)
- Respiratory: Upper respiratory tract infection (32%)
- Miscellaneous: Antibody development to laronidase (91%); infusion reactions (32%; may be severe; includes flushing [23%], fever, and headache; frequency decreased over time during open-label extension period)

1% to 10%:

- Cardiovascular: Chest pain (9%), edema (9%), facial edema (9%), hypotension (9%)
- Hematologic: Thrombocytopenia (9%)
- Hepatic: Bilirubinemia (9%)
- Local: Abscess (9%), injection site pain (9%)
- Ocular: Corneal opacity (9%)
- Miscellaneous: Allergic reaction (severe/serious: 1%)

<1% (Limited to important or life-threatening): Abdominal pain, airway obstruction, anaphylaxis, angioedema, arthralgia, bronchospasm, chills, cough, diarrhea, dyspnea, hypersensitivity, hypertension, nausea, oxygen saturation decreased, pruritus, tachycardia, urticaria, vomiting

Drug Interactions

Avoid Concomitant Use There are no known interactions where it is recommended to avoid concomitant use.

Increased Effect/Toxicity There are no known significant interactions involving an increase in effect.

Decreased Effect There are no known significant interactions involving a decrease in effect.

Stability Store vials under refrigeration at 2°C to 8°C (36°F to 46°F); do not freeze. Do not shake. Solution should be prepared based on body weight and should begin by making a solution of NS and albumin 0.1%.

≤20 kg: Using NS 100 mL PVC bag and albumin (human) [2 mL of albumin 5% or 0.4 mL of albumin 25%]:
Remove and discard a volume of NS equal to the amount of albumin to be added to the infusion bag. Add albumin; the total volume of this solution should equal 100 mL. From this bag, remove and discard an equal volume of the laronidase to be added (based on calculated dose). Slowly withdraw and add laronidase to the NS/albumin 0.1% solution; avoid excessive agitation, do not use filtered syringe. Gently rotate infusion bag to mix (do not shake).

>20 kg: Using NS 250 mL PVC bag and albumin (human) [5 mL of albumin 5% or 1 mL of albumin 25%]:
Remove and discard a volume of NS equal to the amount of albumin to be added to the infusion bag. Add albumin; the total volume of this solution should equal 250 mL. From this bag, remove and discard an equal volume of the laronidase to be added (based on calculated dose). Slowly withdraw and add laronidase to the NS/albumin 0.1% solution; avoid excessive agitation, do not use filtered syringe. Gently rotate infusion bag to mix (do not shake).

Following dilution, solution for infusion should be used immediately; however, if not used immediately, refrigerate. Infusion of solution should be completed within 36 hours of preparation.

Mechanism of Action Laronidase is a recombinant (replacement) form of α-L-iduronidase derived from Chinese hamster cells. α-L-iduronidase is an enzyme needed to break down endogenous glycosaminoglycans (GAGs) within lysosomes. A deficiency of α-L-iduronidase leads to an accumulation of GAGs, causing cellular, tissue, and organ dysfunction as seen in MPS I. Improved pulmonary function and walking capacity have been demonstrated with the administration of laronidase to patients with Hurler, Hurler-Scheie, or Scheie (with moderate to severe symptoms) forms of MPS.

Pharmacodynamics/Kinetics

Distribution: V_d: 0.24-0.6 L/kg

Half-life elimination: 1.5-3.6 hours

Excretion: Clearance: 1.7 to 2.7 mL/minute/kg; during the first 12 weeks of therapy the clearance of laronidase increases proportionally to the amount of antibodies a given patient develops against the enzyme. However, with long-term use (≥26 weeks) antibody titers have no effect on laronidase clearance.

Dosage Note: Premedicate with antipyretic and/or antihistamines 1 hour prior to start of infusion.

I.V.: Children ≥5 years and Adults: 0.58 mg/kg once weekly; dose should be rounded up to the nearest whole vial

Administration Administer using PVC container and PVC infusion set with in-line, low protein-binding 0.2 micrometer filter. Antipyretics and/or antihistamines should be administered prior to infusion. Volume and infusion rate are based on body weight. Vital signs should be monitored every 15 minutes, if stable; rate may be increased as follows:

≤20 kg: Total infusion volume: 100 mL
- 2 mL/hour for 15 minutes
- 4 mL/hour for 15 minutes
- 8 mL/hour for 15 minutes

16 mL/hour for 15 minutes
32 mL/hour for remainder of infusion
>20 kg: Total infusion volume: 250 mL
5 mL/hour for 15 minutes
10 mL/hour for 15 minutes
20 mL/hour for 15 minutes
40 mL/hour for 15 minutes
80 mL/hour for remainder of infusion

Note: In case of infusion-related reaction, decrease the rate of infusion, temporarily discontinue the infusion, and/ or administer additional antipyretics/antihistamines.

Monitoring Parameters Vital signs; injection site reactions, infusion reactions

Dosage Forms Excipient information presented when available (limited, particularly for generics); consult specific product labeling.

Injection, solution [preservative free]:
Aldurazyme®: 2.9 mg/5 mL (5 mL) [contains polysorbate 80; derived from Chinese hamster cells]

◆ **Lasix®** *see* Furosemide *on page 676*

◆ **Lasix® Special (Can)** *see* Furosemide *on page 676*

◆ **L-asparaginase** *see* Asparaginase *on page 140*

◆ **Lassar's Zinc Paste** *see* Zinc Oxide *on page 1584*

Latanoprost (la TA noe prost)

U.S. Brand Names Xalatan®

Canadian Brand Names Xalatan®

Pharmacologic Category Ophthalmic Agent, Antiglaucoma; Prostaglandin, Ophthalmic

Additional Appendix Information
Glaucoma Drug Therapy *on page 1808*

Use Reduction of elevated intraocular pressure in patients with open-angle glaucoma or ocular hypertension

Pregnancy Risk Factor C

Medication Safety Issues
Sound-alike/look-alike issues:
Xalatan® may be confused with Travatan®, Zarontin®

Dosage Adults: Ophthalmic: 1 drop (1.5 mcg) in the affected eye(s) once daily in the evening; do not exceed the once daily dosage because it has been shown that more frequent administration may decrease the IOP lowering effect

Note: A medication delivery device (Xal-Ease™) is available for use with Xalatan®.

Additional Information Complete prescribing information for this medication should be consulted for additional detail.

Dosage Forms Excipient information presented when available (limited, particularly for generics); consult specific product labeling.

Solution, ophthalmic: 0.005% (2.5 mL) [contains benzalkonium chloride]

◆ **Latisse™** *see* Bimatoprost *on page 198*

◆ **Laxilose (Can)** *see* Lactulose *on page 847*

◆ ***l*-Bunolol Hydrochloride** *see* Levobunolol *on page 873*

◆ **LCM** *see* Lacosamide *on page 847*

◆ **L-Deprenyl** *see* Selegiline *on page 1359*

◆ **LDP-341** *see* Bortezomib *on page 204*

◆ **Leena™** *see* Ethinyl Estradiol and Norethindrone *on page 581*

Leflunomide (le FLOO noh mide)

U.S. Brand Names Arava®

Canadian Brand Names Apo-Leflunomide®; Arava®; DOM-Leflunomide; GEN-Leflunomide; NOVO-Leflunomide; PHL-Leflunomide; PMS-Leflunomide; SANDOZ-Leflunomide

Pharmacologic Category Antirheumatic, Disease Modifying

Use Treatment of active rheumatoid arthritis; indicated to reduce signs and symptoms, and to retard structural damage and improve physical function

Orphan drug: Prevention of acute and chronic rejection in recipients of solid organ transplants

Unlabeled/Investigational Use Treatment of cytomegalovirus (CMV) disease

Pregnancy Risk Factor X

Pregnancy Considerations Has been associated with teratogenic and embryolethal effects in animal models at low doses. Leflunomide is contraindicated in pregnant women or women of childbearing potential who are not using reliable contraception. Pregnancy must be excluded prior to initiating treatment. **[U.S. Boxed Warning]: Women of childbearing potential should not receive therapy until pregnancy has been excluded, they have been counseled concerning fetal risk, and reliable contraceptive measures have been confirmed.** Following treatment, pregnancy should be avoided until undetectable plasma levels (<0.02 mcg/mL) are verified. This may be accomplished by an extended drug elimination procedure: Administer cholestyramine 8 g 3 times/day for 11 days (the 11 days do not need to be consecutive). Plasma levels <0.02 mg/L should be verified by two separate tests performed at least 14 days apart. If plasma levels are >0.02 mg/L, additional cholestyramine treatment should be considered. Pregnant women exposed to leflunomide should be registered with the pregnancy registry (877-311-8972).

Lactation Excretion in breast milk unknown/ contraindicated

Contraindications Hypersensitivity to leflunomide or any component of the formulation; pregnancy

Warnings/Precautions Leflunomide has been associated with rare reports of hepatotoxicity, hepatic failure, and death. Multiple risk factors for hepatotoxicity including hepatic disease (including seropositive hepatitis B or C patients) and/or concurrent exposure to other hepatotoxins may increase the risk of hepatotoxicity. Most severe cases occur within 6 months of initiation. Monitoring of hepatic function is required. Due to risk of toxicity, use in patients with hepatic impairment or evidence of hepatitis B or C is not recommended.

Not recommended for patients with severe immune deficiency, bone marrow dysplasia, or uncontrolled infection. Has been associated with rare pancytopenia, agranulocytosis, and thrombocytopenia, particularly when given in combination with methotrexate or other immunosuppressive agents. Monitoring of hematologic function is required. Use with caution in patients with a prior history of significant hematologic abnormalities. Discontinue if evidence of bone marrow suppression or severe dermatologic reaction occurs, and begin procedure to accelerate elimination (cholestyramine or activated charcoal). Interstitial lung disease has been associated (rarely) with leflunomide use. Discontinue in patients who develop new onset or worsening of pulmonary symptoms; accelerated elimination procedures should be considered if interstitial lung disease occurs; fatal outcomes have been reported. Consider interruption of therapy and accelerated elimination in patients who develop serious infections. The use of live vaccines is not recommended.

[U.S. Boxed Warning]: Women of childbearing potential should not receive leflunomide until pregnancy has been excluded. Patients have been counseled concerning fetal risk and reliable contraceptive measures have been confirmed. Caution in renal impairment. Leflunomide will increase uric acid excretion.

Immunosuppression may increase the risk of lymphoproliferative disorders or other malignancies. Safety and efficacy have not been established in children.

Adverse Reactions

>10%:

Gastrointestinal: Diarrhea (17%)

Respiratory: Respiratory tract infection (15%)

1% to 10%:

Cardiovascular: Hypertension (10%), chest pain (2%), palpitation, tachycardia, vasodilation, varicose vein, edema (peripheral)

Central nervous system: Headache (7%), dizziness (4%), pain (2%), fever, malaise, migraine, anxiety, depression, insomnia, sleep disorder

Dermatologic: Alopecia (10%), rash (10%), pruritus (4%), dry skin (2%), eczema (2%), acne, dermatitis, hair discoloration, hematoma, nail disorder, subcutaneous nodule, skin disorder/discoloration, skin ulcer, bruising

Endocrine & metabolic: Hypokalemia (1%), diabetes mellitus, hyperglycemia, hyperlipidemia, hyperthyroidism, menstrual disorder

Gastrointestinal: Nausea (9%), abdominal pain (5%), dyspepsia (5%), weight loss (4%), anorexia (3%), gastroenteritis (3%), stomatitis (3%), vomiting (3%), cholelithiasis, colitis, constipation, esophagitis, flatulence, gastritis, gingivitis, melena, candidiasis (oral), enlarged salivary gland, tooth disorder, xerostomia, taste disturbance

Genitourinary: Urinary tract infection (5%), albuminuria, cystitis, dysuria, hematuria, vaginal candidiasis, prostate disorder, urinary frequency

Hematologic: Anemia

Hepatic: Abnormal LFTs (5%)

Neuromuscular & skeletal: Back pain (5%), joint disorder (4%), weakness (3%), tenosynovitis (3%), synovitis (2%), paresthesia (2%), arthralgia (1%), muscle cramps (1%), neck pain, pelvic pain, CPK increased, arthrosis, bursitis, myalgia, bone necrosis, bone pain, tendon rupture, neuralgia, neuritis

Ocular: Blurred vision, cataract, conjunctivitis, eye disorder

Respiratory: Bronchitis (7%), cough (3%), pharyngitis (3%), pneumonia (2%), rhinitis (2%), sinusitis (2%), asthma, dyspnea, epistaxis

Miscellaneous: Accidental injury (5%), infection (4%), allergic reactions (2%), diaphoresis, herpes infection

<1% (Limited to important or life-threatening): Agranulocytosis, anaphylaxis, angioedema, cholestasis, cutaneous necrotizing vasculitis, eosinophilia, erythema multiforme; hepatotoxicity (rare, including hepatic necrosis and hepatic failure, some fatalities reported); interstitial lung disease, leukopenia, opportunistic infection, pancreatitis, pancytopenia, peripheral neuropathy, pneumonitis (interstitial), pulmonary fibrosis, sepsis, Stevens-Johnson syndrome, thrombocytopenia, toxic epidermal necrolysis, urticaria, vasculitis

Drug Interactions

Metabolism/Transport Effects Inhibits CYP2C9 (weak)

Avoid Concomitant Use There are no known interactions where it is recommended to avoid concomitant use.

Increased Effect/Toxicity

Leflunomide may increase the levels/effects of: Vitamin K Antagonists

The levels/effects of Leflunomide may be increased by: Methotrexate

Decreased Effect There are no known significant interactions involving a decrease in effect.

Ethanol/Nutrition/Herb Interactions Food: No interactions with food have been noted.

Stability Store at 25°C (77°F). Protect from light.

Mechanism of Action Inhibits pyrimidine synthesis, resulting in antiproliferative and anti-inflammatory effects. For CMV, may interfere with virion assembly.

Pharmacodynamics/Kinetics

Distribution: V_d: 0.13 L/kg

Metabolism: Hepatic to A77 1726 (MI) which accounts for nearly all pharmacologic activity; further metabolism to multiple inactive metabolites; undergoes enterohepatic recirculation

Bioavailability: 80%

Half-life elimination: Mean: 14-15 days; enterohepatic recycling appears to contribute to the long half-life of this agent, since activated charcoal and cholestyramine substantially reduce plasma half-life

Time to peak: 6-12 hours

Excretion: Feces (48%); urine (43%)

Dosage Oral:

Adults:

Rheumatoid arthritis: Loading dose: 100 mg/day for 3 days, followed by 20 mg/day; **Note:** May be omitted in patients at increased risk of hepatic or hematologic toxicity (eg, recent concomitant methotrexate). Dosage may be decreased to 10 mg/day in patients who have difficulty tolerating the 20 mg dose. Due to the long half-life of the active metabolite, plasma levels may require a prolonged period to decline after dosage reduction.

CMV (unlabeled use): Some authors recommend 200 mg/day for 7 days, followed by 40-60 mg/day, targeting blood levels of 100 mcg/mL. Others have utilized the standard arthritis dosing.

Elderly: Although hepatic function may decline with age, no specific dosage adjustment is recommended. Patients should be monitored closely for adverse effects which may require dosage adjustment.

Dosing adjustment in renal impairment: No specific dosage adjustment is recommended. There is no clinical experience in the use of leflunomide in patients with renal impairment. The free fraction of MI is doubled in dialysis patients. Patients should be monitored closely for adverse effects requiring dosage adjustment.

Dosing adjustment in hepatic impairment: No specific dosage adjustment is recommended; not recommended for use in patients with significant hepatic impairment. Since the liver is involved in metabolic activation and subsequent metabolism/elimination of leflunomide, patients with hepatic impairment should be monitored closely for adverse effects requiring dosage adjustment.

Dosing adjustment in hepatic toxicity: Guidelines for dosage adjustment or discontinuation based on the severity and persistence of ALT elevation secondary to leflunomide have been developed. If ALT elevations >2 times but ≤3 times ULN are noted, reduce dose to 10 mg/day, and monitor closely. If elevations persist or if elevations >3 times ULN are observed, discontinue leflunomide and initiate protocol to accelerate elimination. Cholestyramine (8 g 3 times/day for 1-3 days) or activated charcoal (50 g every 6 hours for 24 hours) may be administered to decrease leflunomide concentrations rapidly. If elevations >3 times ULN persist additional cholestyramine and/or activated charcoal may be required.

Dietary Considerations Administer without regard to meals.

Monitoring Parameters A complete blood count (WBC, hemoglobin, hematocrit, and platelet count), serum phosphate, as well as serum transaminase determinations should be monitored at baseline and monthly during the initial 6 months of treatment; if stable, monitoring frequency may be decreased to every 6-8 weeks thereafter (continue monthly when used in combination with other immunosuppressive agents). In addition, monitor for signs/symptoms of severe infection, abnormalities in hepatic function tests, or symptoms of hepatotoxicity. If coadministered with methotrexate, monthly transaminase and serum albumin levels are recommended.

Dosage Forms Excipient information presented when available (limited, particularly for generics); consult specific product labeling.

Tablet (Arava®): 10 mg, 20 mg

◆ **Legatrin PM® [OTC]** *see* Acetaminophen and Diphenhydramine *on page 28*

Lenalidomide (le na LID oh mide)

U.S. Brand Names Revlimid®

Canadian Brand Names Revlimid®

Index Terms CC-5013; IMid-3; NSC-703813

Pharmacologic Category Angiogenesis Inhibitor; Antineoplastic Agent; Immunomodulator, Systemic

Use Treatment of myelodysplastic syndrome (MDS) in patients with deletion 5q (del 5q) cytogenetic abnormality; treatment of multiple myeloma

Unlabeled/Investigational Use Treatment of metastatic malignant melanoma; treatment of myelofibrosis

Restrictions Lenalidomide is approved for marketing in the U.S. only under a Food and Drug Administration (FDA) approved, restricted distribution program called RevAssist[SM] (www.REVLIMID.com or 1-888-423-5436). In Canada, distribution is restricted through RevAid[SM] (www.RevAid.ca or 1-888-738-2431). Physicians, pharmacies, and patients must be registered; a maximum 28-day supply may be dispensed; a new prescription is required each time it is filled; pregnancy testing is required for females of childbearing potential.

An FDA-approved medication guide must be distributed when dispensing an outpatient prescription (new or refill) where this medication is to be used without direct supervision of a healthcare provider. Medication guides are available at http://www.fda.gov/cder/Offices/ODS/medication_guides.htm.

Pregnancy Risk Factor X

Pregnancy Considerations **[U.S. Boxed Warning]: Lenalidomide is an analogue of thalidomide (a human teratogen) and could potentially cause birth defects in humans.** Animal studies with lenalidomide are ongoing; there are no adequate and well-controlled studies in pregnant women. Women of childbearing potential should be treated only if they are able to comply with the conditions of the RevAssist[SM] program. Two forms of effective contraception are required beginning 4 weeks prior to, during, and for 4 weeks after therapy and during therapy interruptions. Pregnancy tests (sensitivity of at least 50 mIU/mL) should be performed 10-14 days and 24 hours prior to beginning therapy; weekly for the first 4 weeks and every 4 weeks (every 2 weeks if menstrual cycle irregular) thereafter and during therapy interruptions. Lenalidomide must be immediately discontinued and the patient referred to a reproductive toxicity specialist if pregnancy occurs during treatment. Males (even those vasectomized) should use a latex condom during any sexual contact with women of childbearing age. Risk to the fetus from semen of male patients is unknown. The parent or legal guardian for patients between 12 and 18 years of age must agree to ensure compliance with the required guidelines. Any suspected fetal exposure should be reported to the FDA via the MedWatch program (1-800-FDA-1088) and to Celgene Corporation (1-888-423-5436)

Lactation Excretion in breast milk unknown/not recommended

Medication Safety Issues

High alert medication: The Institute for Safe Medication Practices (ISMP) includes this medication among its list of drug classes which have a heightened risk of causing significant patient harm when used in error.

Contraindications Hypersensitivity to lenalidomide or any component of the formulation; pregnancy or women capable of becoming pregnant; patients unable to comply with the RevAssist[SM] program

Canadian labeling: Additional contraindications (not in U.S. labeling): Platelet count <50,000/mm^3; hypersensitivity to thalidomide; breast-feeding women

Warnings/Precautions Hazardous agent - use appropriate precautions for handling and disposal. **[U.S. Boxed Warning]: Hematologic toxicity (neutropenia and thrombocytopenia) occurs in a majority of patients (grade 3/4: 80%)** and may require dose reductions and/or delays; the use of blood product support and/or growth factors may be needed. **[U.S. Boxed Warning]: Lenalidomide has been associated with a significant increase in risk for thrombosis and embolism in multiple myeloma patients treated with combination therapy. Deep vein thrombosis (DVT) and pulmonary embolism (PE) have occurred;** monitor for signs and symptoms of thromboembolism (shortness of breath, chest pain, or arm or leg swelling) and seek prompt medical attention with development of these symptoms. Use caution in renal impairment; may experience an increased rate of toxicities.

[U.S. Boxed Warning]: Lenalidomide is an analogue of thalidomide (a human teratogen) and could potentially cause birth defects in humans. Patients should be advised not to donate blood during therapy and for 4 weeks following completion of therapy. May cause dizziness or fatigue; caution patients about performing tasks which require mental alertness (eg, operating machinery or driving). Formulation contains lactose; avoid use in patients with Lapp lactase deficiency, glucose-galactose malabsorption, or glucose intolerance. Distribution of lenalidomide is restricted; physicians, pharmacists, and patients must be registered with the RevAssist[SM] program. Safety and effectiveness in children <18 years of age have not been established.

Adverse Reactions

>10%:

Cardiovascular: Peripheral edema (8% to 21%)

Central nervous system: Fatigue (31% to 38%), insomnia (10% to 32%), pyrexia (21% to 23%), dizziness (20% to 21%), headache (20%)

Dermatologic: Pruritus (42%), rash (16% to 36%), dry skin (14%)

Endocrine & metabolic: Hyperglycemia (15%), hypokalemia (11%)

Gastrointestinal: Diarrhea (29% to 49%), constipation (24% to 39%), nausea (22% to 24%), weight loss (18%), dyspepsia (14%), anorexia (10% to 14%), taste perversion (6% to 13%), abdominal pain (8% to 12%)

Genitourinary: Urinary tract infection (11%)

Hematologic: Thrombocytopenia (17% to 62%; grades 3/4: 10% to 50%), neutropenia (28% to 59%; grades 3/4: 21% to 53%), anemia (12% to 24%; grades 3/4: 6% to 9%); myelosuppression is dose-dependent and reversible with treatment interruption and/or dose reduction

Neuromuscular & skeletal: Muscle cramp (18% to 30%), weakness (15% to 23%), arthralgia (10% to 22%), back pain (15% to 21%), tremor (20%), paresthesia (12%), limb pain (11%)

Ocular: Blurred vision (15%)

Respiratory: Nasopharyngitis (23%), cough (15% to 20%), dyspnea (7% to 20%), pharyngitis (16%), epistaxis (15%), upper respiratory infection (14% to 15%), pneumonia (11% to 12%)

1% to 10%:

Cardiovascular: Edema (10%), deep vein thrombosis (≤8%; grades 3/4: 7%), hypertension (6%), chest pain (5%), palpitation (5%), atrial fibrillation (grades 3/4: 3%), syncope (grade 3: 2%)

Central nervous system: Hypoesthesia (7%), pain (7%), depression (5%)

Dermatologic: Bruising (5% to 8%), cellulitis (5%), erythema (5%)

Endocrine & metabolic: Hypothyroidism (7%), hypomagnesemia (6%), hypocalcemia (grades 3/4: 4%)

Gastrointestinal: Vomiting (10%), xerostomia (7%), loose stools (6%)

Genitourinary: Dysuria (7%)

Hematologic: Leukopenia (8%; grade 3: 4%), febrile neutropenia (5%), lymphopenia (grade 3: 2%)

Hepatic: ALT increased (8%)

Neuromuscular & skeletal: Myalgia (9%), rigors (6%), neuropathy (peripheral 5%)

Respiratory: Sinusitis (8%), rhinitis (7%), bronchitis (6%), pulmonary embolism (≤3%; grades 3/4: 3%)

Miscellaneous: Night sweats (8%), diaphoresis increased (7%)

<1% (Limited to important or life-threatening): Acute febrile neutrophilic dermatosis, acute leukemia, acute myeloid leukemia (AML), adrenal insufficiency, angina, angioedema, aortic disorder, aphasia, azotemia, bacteremia, Basedow's disease, biliary obstruction, blindness, bone marrow depression, bradycardia, brain edema, C-reactive protein decreased, cardiac arrest, cardiac failure, cardiogenic shock, cardiomyopathy, cardiopulmonary arrest, cellulitis, cerebellar infarction, cerebral infarction, cerebrovascular accident, CHF, cholecystitis, chondrocalcinosis, chronic obstructive airway disease, circulatory collapse, coagulopathy, colonic polyp, dehydration, delirium, delusion, diabetes mellitus, diabetic ketoacidosis, diverticulitis, dysphagia, encephalitis, erythema multiforme, gait abnormal, gastritis, gastroenteritis, gastrointestinal hemorrhage, gout, hematuria, hemoglobin decreased, hemolysis, hemolytic anemia, hemorrhage, hepatitis, herpesvirus infection, hyperbilirubinemia, hypernatremia, hypersensitivity, hypoglycemia, hypotension, hypoxia, infection, INR increased, interstitial lung disease, intestinal perforation, intracranial hemorrhage, intracranial venous sinus thrombosis, irritable bowel syndrome, ischemia, ischemic colitis, leukoencephalopathy, liver failure, liver function tests abnormal, lung cancer, lung infiltration, lymphoma, melena, MI, migraine, myocardial ischemia, myopathy, neutropenic sepsis, orthostatic hypotension, pancreatitis, pancytopenia, performance status decreased, peripheral ischemia, phlebitis, post procedural hemorrhage, pseudomembraneous colitis, pulmonary edema, rectal hemorrhage, refractory anemia, renal calculus, renal failure, renal mass, renal tubular necrosis, respiratory failure, septic shock, sepsis, serum creatinine increased, skin desquamation, small bowel obstruction, somnolence, spinal cord compression, splenic infarction, Stevens-Johnson syndrome, stomatitis, subarachnoid hemorrhage, supraventricular arrhythmia, tachyarrhythmia, thrombophlebitis, thrombosis, toxic epidermal necrolysis, transient ischemic attack, troponin I increased, urinary retention, urosepsis, urticaria, ventricular dysfunction, wheezing

Drug Interactions

Avoid Concomitant Use

Avoid concomitant use of Lenalidomide with any of the following: Anakinra; Natalizumab; Rilonacept; Vaccines (Live)

Increased Effect/Toxicity

Lenalidomide may increase the levels/effects of: Abatacept; Anakinra; Natalizumab; Rilonacept; Vaccines (Live)

The levels/effects of Lenalidomide may be increased by: Dexamethasone; Trastuzumab

Decreased Effect

Lenalidomide may decrease the levels/effects of: Vaccines (Inactivated)

The levels/effects of Lenalidomide may be decreased by: Echinacea

Ethanol/Nutrition/Herb Interactions Herb/Nutraceutical: Avoid echinacea (has immunostimulant properties; consider therapy modifications).

Stability Store at controlled room temperature of 25°C (77°F); excursions permitted to 15°C and 30°C (59°F and 86°F).

Mechanism of Action Immunomodulatory, antiangiogenic, and antineoplastic characteristics via multiple mechanisms. Selectively inhibits secretion of proinflammatory cytokines (potent inhibitor of tumor necrosis factor-alpha secretion); enhances cell-mediated immunity by stimulating proliferation of anti-CD3 stimulated T cells (resulting in increased IL-2 and interferon gamma secretion); inhibits trophic signals to angiogenic factors in cells. Inhibits the growth of myeloma cells by inducing cell cycle arrest and cell death.

Pharmacodynamics/Kinetics

Absorption: Rapid

Protein binding: ~30%

Half-life elimination: ~3 hours

Time, to peak, plasma: Healthy volunteers: 0.6-1.5 hours; Myeloma patients: 0.5-4 hours

Excretion: Urine (~67% as unchanged drug)

Dosage Oral:

Adults:

Myelodysplastic syndrome (MDS): 10 mg once daily

Multiple myeloma: 25 mg once daily for 21 days of a 28-day treatment cycle (in combination with dexamethasone)

Metastatic malignant melanoma (unlabeled/investigational use): 10-25 mg once daily

Myelofibrosis (unlabeled/investigational use): 5-10 mg once daily

Elderly: Refer to adult dosing; due to the potential for decreased renal function in the elderly, select dose carefully and closely monitor renal function

Dosage adjustment in renal impairment: Select dose carefully and closely monitor renal function. The FDA-approved labeling does not contain renal dosing adjustment guidelines. Lenalidomide AUC is increased 56% in multiple myeloma patients with mild renal impairment. Consider dose reductions in patients with renal dysfunction. Lenalidomide use with renal dysfunction has been studied in a limited number of patients with the following initial dosage recommendations (Chen, 2007):

MDS:

Cl_{cr} 30-49 mL/minute: 5 mg once daily

Cl_{cr} <30 mL/minute (nondialysis dependent): 5 mg every 48 hours

Cl_{cr} <30 mL/minute (dialysis dependent): 5 mg 3 times/week (administer following dialysis)

Multiple myeloma:

Cl_{cr} 30-49 mL/minute: 10 mg once daily (may increase to 15 mg once daily for inadequate treatment response after 2 cycles)

Cl_{cr} <30 mL/minute (nondialysis dependent): 15 mg every 48 hours

Cl_{cr} <30 mL/minute (dialysis dependent): 15 mg 3 times/week (administer following dialysis)

Dosage adjustment for toxicity:

Adjustment for thrombocytopenia in MDS:

Thrombocytopenia developing within 4 weeks of beginning treatment at 10 mg/day:

Baseline platelets ≥100,000/mm^3:

If platelets <50,000/mm^3: Hold treatment

When platelets return to ≥50,000/mm^3: Resume treatment at 5 mg/day

Baseline platelets <100,000/mm^3:

If platelets fall to 50% of baseline: Hold treatment

If baseline ≥60,000/mm^3 and platelet level returns to ≥50,000/mm^3: Resume at 5 mg/day

If baseline <60,000/mm^3 and platelet level returns to ≥30,000/mm^3: Resume at 5 mg/day

Thrombocytopenia developing after 4 weeks of beginning treatment at 10 mg/day:

Platelets <30,000/mm^3 **or** <50,000/mm^3 with platelet transfusions: Hold treatment

Platelets ≥30,000/mm^3 (without hemostatic failure): Resume at 5 mg/day

Thrombocytopenia developing with treatment at 5 mg/day:

Platelets <30,000/mm^3 **or** <50,000/mm^3 with platelet transfusions: Hold treatment

Platelets ≥30,000/mm^3 (without hemostatic failure): Resume at 5 mg every other day day

Adjustment for neutropenia in MDS:

Neutropenia developing within 4 weeks of beginning treatment at 10 mg/day:

For baseline absolute neutrophil count (ANC) ≥1000/mm^3:

ANC <750/mm^3: Hold treatment

When ANC returns to ≥1000/mm^3: Resume at 5 mg/day

For baseline absolute neutrophil count (ANC) <1000/mm^3:

ANC <500/mm^3: Hold treatment

When ANC returns to ≥500/mm^3: Resume at 5 mg/day

Neutropenia developing after 4 weeks of beginning treatment at 10 mg/day:

ANC <500/mm^3 for ≥7 days or associated with fever: Hold treatment

When ≥500/mm^3: Resume at 5 mg/day

Neutropenia developing with treatment at 5 mg/day:

ANC <500/mm^3 for ≥7 days or associated with fever: Hold treatment

When ≥500/mm^3: Resume at 5 mg every other day

Adjustment for thrombocytopenia in multiple myeloma:

Platelets <30,000/mm^3: Hold treatment, check CBC weekly

When platelets ≥30,000/mm^3: Resume at 15 mg daily

Additional occurrence of platelets <30,000/mm^3: Hold treatment

When platelets ≥30,000/mm^3: Resume treatment at 5 mg below previous dose; do not dose below 5 mg daily

Adjustment for neutropenia in multiple myeloma:

ANC <1000/mm^3: Hold treatment, add G-CSF, check CBC weekly

When ≥1000/mm^3 (with neutropenia as only toxicity): Resume at 25 mg/day

When ≥1000/mm^3 (with additional toxicities): Resume at 15 mg/day

Additional occurrence of ANC <1000/mm^3: Hold treatment

When ≥1000/mm^3: Resume treatment at 5 mg below previous dose; do not dose below 5 mg daily.

Adjustment for other toxicities in multiple myeloma: For additional treatment-related grade 3/4 toxicities, hold treatment and restart at next dose level when toxicity has resolved to ≤ grade 2.

Administration Administer with water. Swallow capsule whole; do not break, open, or chew.

Monitoring Parameters CBC with differential (MDS: weekly for first 8 weeks; MM: every 2 weeks for the first 3 months), then monthly thereafter; serum creatinine, liver function tests, thyroid function tests; ECG when clinically indicated; monitor for signs and symptoms of thromboembolism

Women of childbearing potential: Pregnancy test 10-14 days **and** 24 hours prior to initiating therapy, then every 2-4 weeks through 4 weeks after therapy discontinued

Additional Information Pregnancy tests are required prior to beginning therapy, throughout treatment and during therapy interruptions for all women of childbearing age. The pregnancy test must be verified by the prescriber and the pharmacist prior to dispensing. Effective contraception with at least two reliable forms of contraception (IUD, hormonal contraception, tubal ligation or partner's vasectomy plus latex condom, diaphragm, or cervical cap) should be used for 4 weeks prior to beginning therapy, during therapy, and for 4 weeks following discontinuance of therapy. Women who have undergone a hysterectomy or have been postmenopausal for at least 24 consecutive months are the only exception. Do not prescribe, administer, or dispense to women of childbearing age or males who may have intercourse with women of childbearing age unless both female and male are capable of complying with contraceptive measures. Even males who have undergone vasectomy must acknowledge these risks in writing, and must use a latex condom during any sexual contact with women of childbearing age. Oral and written warnings concerning contraception and the hazards of thalidomide must be conveyed to females and males and they must acknowledge their understanding in writing. Parents or guardians must consent and sign acknowledgment for patients 12-18 years of age following therapy. A maximum 28-day supply should be dispensed.

Dosage Forms Excipient information presented when available (limited, particularly for generics); consult specific product labeling.

Capsule:

Revlimid®: 5 mg, 10 mg, 15 mg, 25 mg

Lepirudin (leh puh ROO din)

U.S. Brand Names Refludan®

Canadian Brand Names Refludan®

Index Terms Lepirudin (rDNA); Recombinant Hirudin

Pharmacologic Category Anticoagulant, Thrombin Inhibitor

Use Indicated for anticoagulation in patients with heparin-induced thrombocytopenia (HIT) and associated thromboembolic disease in order to prevent further thromboembolic complications

Unlabeled/Investigational Use Investigational: Prevention or reduction of ischemic complications associated with unstable angina

Pregnancy Risk Factor B

Pregnancy Considerations Lepirudin crosses the placenta in pregnant rats; however, it is not known if lepirudin crosses the placenta in humans.

Lactation Enters breast milk/consult prescriber

Medication Safety Issues

High alert medication: The Institute for Safe Medication Practices (ISMP) includes this medication among its list of drugs which have a heightened risk of causing significant patient harm when used in error.

Contraindications Hypersensitivity to hirudins or any component of the formulation

Warnings/Precautions Hemorrhagic events: Intracranial bleeding following concomitant thrombolytic therapy with rt-PA or streptokinase may be life threatening. For patients with an increased risk of bleeding, a careful assessment weighing the risk of lepirudin administration versus its anticipated benefit has to be made by the treating physician. In particular, this includes the following conditions: Recent puncture of large vessels or organ biopsy; anomaly of vessels or organs; recent cerebrovascular accident, stroke, intracerebral surgery, or other neuroaxial procedures; severe uncontrolled hypertension;

bacterial endocarditis; advanced renal impairment; hemorrhagic diathesis; recent major surgery; and recent major bleeding (eg, intracranial, gastrointestinal, intraocular, or pulmonary bleeding). With renal impairment, relative overdose might occur even with standard dosage regimen. The bolus dose and rate of infusion must be reduced in patients with known or suspected renal insufficiency.

Formation of antihirudin antibodies may increase the anticoagulant effect of lepirudin possibly due to delayed renal elimination of active lepirudin-antihirudin complexes. Therefore, strict monitoring of aPTT is necessary also during prolonged therapy. No evidence of neutralization of lepirudin or of allergic reactions associated with positive antibody test results was found. Allergic and hypersensitivity reactions, including anaphylaxis have been reported and may occur frequently in patients treated concomitantly with streptokinase; caution is warranted during re-exposure (anaphylaxis has been reported).

Serious liver injury (eg, liver cirrhosis) may enhance the anticoagulant effect of lepirudin due to coagulation defects secondary to reduced generation of vitamin K-dependent clotting factors.

Clinical trials have provided limited information to support any recommendations for re-exposure to lepirudin (anaphylaxis has been reported). Safety and efficacy have not been established in children.

Adverse Reactions As with all anticoagulants, bleeding is the most common adverse event associated with lepirudin. Hemorrhage may occur at virtually any site. Risk is dependent on multiple variables.

HIT patients:

>10%: Hematologic: Anemia (12%), bleeding from puncture sites (11%), hematoma (11%)

1% to 10%:
- Cardiovascular: Heart failure (3%), pericardial effusion (1%), ventricular fibrillation (1%)
- Central nervous system: Fever (7%)
- Dermatologic: Maculopapular rash (4%), eczema (3%)
- Gastrointestinal: GI bleeding/rectal bleeding (5%)
- Genitourinary: Vaginal bleeding (2%)
- Hepatic: Transaminases increased (6%)
- Renal: Hematuria (4%)
- Respiratory: Epistaxis (4%)

<1% (Limited to important or life-threatening): Allergic reactions, anaphylaxis, hemoperitoneum, hemoptysis, injection site reactions, intracranial bleeding, liver bleeding, mouth bleeding, pruritus, pulmonary bleeding, retroperitoneal bleeding, thrombocytopenia, urticaria

Non-HIT populations (including those receiving thrombolytics and/or contrast media):

1% to 10%: Respiratory: Bronchospasm/stridor/dyspnea/cough

<1% (Limited to important or life-threatening): Allergic reactions (unspecified), anaphylactoid reactions, anaphylaxis, angioedema, intracranial bleeding (0.6%), laryngeal edema, thrombocytopenia, tongue edema

Drug Interactions

Avoid Concomitant Use There are no known interactions where it is recommended to avoid concomitant use.

Increased Effect/Toxicity

Lepirudin may increase the levels/effects of: Anticoagulants; Ibritumomab; Tositumomab and Iodine I 131 Tositumomab

The levels/effects of Lepirudin may be increased by: Antiplatelet Agents; Dasatinib; Herbs (Anticoagulant/Antiplatelet Properties); Nonsteroidal Anti-Inflammatory Agents; Pentosan Polysulfate Sodium; Prostacyclin Analogues; Salicylates; Thrombolytic Agents

Decreased Effect There are no known significant interactions involving a decrease in effect.

Ethanol/Nutrition/Herb Interactions Herb/Nutraceutical: Avoid cat's claw, dong quai, evening primrose, feverfew, garlic, ginger, ginkgo, red clover, horse chestnut, green tea, ginseng (all have additional antiplatelet activity)

Stability

Intact vials should be stored at 2°C to 25°C (36°F to 77°F).

Intravenous bolus: Use a solution with a concentration of 5 mg/mL.

Preparation of a lepirudin solution with a concentration of 5 mg/mL: Reconstitute one vial (50 mg) of lepirudin with 1 mL of sterile water for injection or 0.9% sodium chloride injection. The final concentration of 5 mg/mL is obtained by transferring the contents of the vial into a sterile, single-use syringe (of at least 10 mL capacity) and diluting the solution to a total volume of 10 mL using sterile water for injection, 0.9% sodium chloride, or 5% dextrose in water.

Intravenous infusion: For continuous intravenous infusion, solutions with concentrations of 0.2 or 0.4 mg/mL may be used.

Preparation of a lepirudin solution with a concentration of 0.2 mg/mL or 0.4 mg/mL: Reconstitute 2 vials (50 mg each) of lepirudin with 1 mL each using either sterile water for injection or 0.9% sodium chloride injection. The final concentration of 0.2 mg/mL or 0.4 mg/mL is obtained by transferring the contents of both vials into an infusion bag containing 500 mL or 250 mL of 0.9% sodium chloride injection or 5% dextrose injection.

Reconstituted solutions of lepirudin are stable for 24 hours at room temperature. Manufacturer recommends using reconstituted solution immediately after preparation.

Mechanism of Action Lepirudin is a highly specific direct inhibitor of thrombin; lepirudin is a recombinant hirudin derived from yeast cells

Pharmacodynamics/Kinetics

Distribution: Two-compartment model; confined to extracellular fluids.

Metabolism: Via release of amino acids via catabolic hydrolysis of parent drug

Half-life elimination: Initial: ~10 minutes: Terminal: Healthy volunteers: 1.3 hours; Marked renal impairment (Cl_{cr} <15 mL/minute and on hemodialysis): ≤2 days

Excretion: Urine (~48%, 35% as unchanged drug and unchanged drug fragments of parent drug); systemic clearance is proportional to glomerular filtration rate or creatinine clearance

Dosage Note: Maximum infusion dose: Do not exceed 0.21 mg/kg/hour unless an evaluation of coagulation abnormalities limiting response has been completed.

Heparin-induced thrombocytopenia: Bolus dose: 0.4 mg/kg IVP (over 15-20 seconds), followed by continuous infusion at 0.15 mg/kg/hour (maximum initial bolus dose: 44 mg; maximum initial infusion dose: 16.5 mg/hour); bolus and infusion must be reduced in renal insufficiency

or

Alternate dosing regimen (unlabeled dose; Selleng, 2007; Warkentin, 2008): Bolus dose: 0.2 mg/kg (use only if life- or limb-threatening thrombosis present) followed by continuous infusion of 0.05-0.1 mg/kg/hour. Further dosage reduction may be required in patients with renal dysfunction. This alternate dosing regimen has been recommended due to higher rates of bleeding associated with the FDA-approved dosing regimen.

Concomitant use with thrombolytic therapy: Bolus dose: 0.2 mg/kg IVP (over 15-20 seconds), followed by continuous infusion at 0.1 mg/kg/hour

Dosing adjustments during infusions: Monitor first aPTT 4 hours after the start of the infusion. Subsequent determinations of aPTT should be obtained at least once daily during treatment. More frequent monitoring is recommended in renally- or hepatically-impaired patients.

Any aPTT ratio measurement out of range (1.5-2.5) should be confirmed prior to adjusting dose, unless a clinical need for immediate reaction exists. If the aPTT is below target range, increase infusion by 20%. If the aPTT is in excess of the target range, stop infusion for 2 hours and when restarted the infusion rate should be decreased by 50%. A repeat aPTT should be obtained 4 hours after any dosing change.

Use in patients scheduled for switch to oral anticoagulants: Once platelets normalize, reduce lepirudin dose gradually to reach aPTT ratio just above 1.5 before starting warfarin therapy. Monitor PT/INR closely until results stabilize in therapeutic range. When lepirudin is discontinued, there may be a small reduction in INR.

Dosing adjustment in renal impairment: All patients with a creatinine clearance of <60 mL/minute or a serum creatinine of >1.5 mg/dL require dosage reduction; there is only limited information on the therapeutic use of lepirudin in patients with HIT and significant renal impairment; the following dosage recommendations are mainly based on single-dose studies in a small number of patients with renal impairment. An alternate dosing regimen has also been recommended for patients with serum creatinine >1 mg/dL (Warkentin, 2008).

Initial: Bolus dose: 0.2 mg/kg IVP (over 15-20 seconds), followed by adjusted infusion based on renal function; refer to the following infusion rate adjustments based on creatinine clearance (mL/minute) and serum creatinine (mg/dL):

Note: Acute renal failure or hemodialysis: Infusion is to be avoided or stopped. Following the bolus dose, additional bolus doses of 0.1 mg/kg may be administered every other day only if aPTT falls below lower therapeutic limit (1.5-times patient baseline [or mean laboratory] aPTT).

Lepirudin infusion rates in patients with renal impairment: See tables.

Lepirudin Infusion Rates in Patients With Renal Impairment

Creatinine Clearance (mL/min)	Serum Creatinine (mg/dL)	Adjusted Infusion Rate: % of Standard Initial Infusion Rate	Adjusted Infusion Rate: mg/kg/h
45-60	1.6-2.0	50%	0.075
30-44	2.1-3.0	30%	0.045
15-29	3.1-6.0	15%	0.0225
<15	>6.0	***Avoid or STOP infusion***	

Alternate Dosing Regimen for Renal Impairment (based on *Chest* 2008 guidelines[1])

Serum Creatinine (mg/dL)	Adjusted Infusion Rate: % of Standard Initial Infusion Rate[2]	Adjusted Infusion Rate: mg/kg/h
1.0-1.6	50%	0.05
1.7-4.5	10%	0.01
>4.5-6.0	5%	0.005
>6.0	***Avoid or STOP infusion[3]***	

[1]Recommendation based on low or very low-quality evidence.

[2]Recommended standard initial infusion rate: 0.1 mg/kg/hour

[3]Recommendation based on manufacturer's labeling.

Note: The initial bolus should either be omitted, or in the case of perceived life- or limb-threatening thrombosis, be given at a reduced dose of 0.2 mg/kg.

Administration Administer **only** intravenously; administer I.V. bolus over 15-20 seconds

Monitoring Parameters Monitor aPTT levels; obtain baseline aPTT, then monitor first aPTT 4 hours after the start of the infusion and every 4 hours until steady state is reached (2 consecutive aPTTs in the same range) (Warkentin, 2008). Subsequent determinations of aPTT should be obtained at least once daily during treatment. More frequent monitoring is recommended in renally- or hepatically-impaired patients. Any aPTT ratio measurement out of range (1.5-2.5) should be confirmed prior to adjusting dose, unless a clinical need for immediate reaction exists

Reference Range aPTT 1.5 to 2.5 times the control value

Test Interactions PT/INR levels may become elevated in the absence of warfarin. If warfarin is initiated, initial PT/INR goals while on lepirudin may require modification.

Dosage Forms Excipient information presented when available (limited, particularly for generics); consult specific product labeling.

Injection, powder for reconstitution: 50 mg

◆ **Lepirudin (rDNA)** *see* Lepirudin *on page 863*

◆ **Lescol®** *see* Fluvastatin *on page 651*

◆ **Lescol® XL** *see* Fluvastatin *on page 651*

◆ **Lessina™** *see* Ethinyl Estradiol and Levonorgestrel *on page 577*

◆ **Letairis™** *see* Ambrisentan *on page 80*

Letrozole (LET roe zole)

U.S. Brand Names Femara®

Canadian Brand Names Femara®

Index Terms CGS-20267; NSC-719345

Pharmacologic Category Antineoplastic Agent, Aromatase Inhibitor

Use For use in postmenopausal women in the adjuvant treatment of hormone receptor positive early breast cancer, extended adjuvant treatment of early breast cancer after 5 years of tamoxifen, advanced breast cancer with disease progression following antiestrogen therapy, hormone receptor positive or hormone receptor unknown, locally-advanced, or metastatic breast cancer

Unlabeled/Investigational Use Treatment of ovarian (epithelial) cancer, endometrial cancer

Pregnancy Risk Factor D

Pregnancy Considerations Letrozole may cause fetal harm when administered to pregnant women. Animal studies have demonstrated embryotoxicity and fetotoxicity. There are no adequate and well-controlled studies in pregnant women. If used in pregnancy, or if patient becomes pregnant during treatment, the patient should be apprised of potential hazard to the fetus. Letrozole is FDA indicated for postmenopausal women only. Women who are perimenopausal or recently postmenopausal should use adequate contraception until postmenopausal status is fully established.

Lactation Excretion in breast milk unknown/use caution

Medication Safety Issues

Sound-alike/look-alike issues:

Femara® may be confused with Famvir®, femhrt®, Provera®

Letrozole may be confused with anastrozole

Contraindications Hypersensitivity to letrozole or any component of the formulation; women of premenopausal endocrine status

Warnings/Precautions Hazardous agent - use appropriate precautions for handling and disposal. Use caution with hepatic impairment; dose adjustment may be required. Increases in transaminases ≥5 times the upper limit of normal and in bilirubin ≥1.5 times the upper limit of normal were most often, but not always, associated with metastatic liver disease. May cause dizziness, fatigue, and somnolence; patients should be cautioned before performing tasks which require mental alertness (eg, operating machinery or driving). May increase total serum cholesterol. May cause decreases in bone mineral density. Safety and efficacy have not been established in children.

Adverse Reactions

>10%:

Cardiovascular: Edema (7% to 18%)

Central nervous system: Headache (4% to 20%), dizziness (2% to 14%), fatigue (6% to 13%)

Endocrine & metabolic: Hot flashes (5% to 50%), hypercholesterolemia (3% to 16%)

Gastrointestinal: Nausea (9% to 17%), constipation (2% to 11%), weight gain (2% to 11%)

Neuromuscular & skeletal: Weakness (4% to 34%), bone pain (22%), arthralgia (8% to 22%), arthritis (7% to 21%), back pain (5% to 18%)

Respiratory: Dyspnea (6% to 18%), cough (5% to 13%)

Miscellaneous: Diaphoresis (≤24%), night sweats (14%)

2% to 10%:

Cardiovascular: Chest pain (3% to 8%), hypertension (5% to 8%), peripheral edema (5%)

Central nervous system: Insomnia (6% to 7%), pain (5%), somnolence (2% to 3%), depression (<5%), anxiety (<5%), vertigo (<5%)

Dermatologic: Rash (4% to 5%), alopecia (<5%), pruritus (1% to 2%)

Endocrine & metabolic: Breast pain (7%), hypercalcemia (<5%)

Gastrointestinal: Diarrhea (5% to 8%), vomiting (3% to 7%), weight loss (7%), abdominal pain (5% to 6%), anorexia (3% to 5%), dyspepsia (3% to 4%)

Genitourinary: Urinary tract infection (6%), vaginal bleeding (5%), vaginal dryness (5%), vaginal hemorrhage (5%), vaginal irritation (4%)

Hepatic: Transaminases increased (≤3%)

Neuromuscular & skeletal: Limb pain (10%), myalgia (6% to 7%), bone fractures (≤6%), bone mineral density decreased/osteoporosis (2% to 7%)

Renal: Renal disorder (5%)

Respiratory: Pleural effusion (<5%)

Miscellaneous: Infection (7%), flu (6%), viral infection (5% to 6%)

<2% (Limited to important or life-threatening): Anaphylactic reaction, angina, angioedema, appetite increase, arterial thrombosis, bilirubin increased, blurred vision, cardiac ischemia, cardiac failure, cataract, coronary artery disease, dry skin, dysesthesia, endometrial cancer, endometrial proliferation disorder, eye irritation, fever, hemiparesis, hemorrhagic stroke, hypoesthesia, irritability, leukopenia, lymphopenia, MI, memory impairment, nervousness, palpitations, paresthesia, portal vein thrombosis, pulmonary embolism, secondary malignancy, stomatitis, tachycardia, taste disturbance, thirst, thrombocytopenia, thrombophlebitis, thromboembolic event, thrombotic stroke, transient ischemic attack, urinary frequency increased, urticaria, vaginal discharge, venous thrombosis, xerostomia

Drug Interactions

Metabolism/Transport Effects Substrate (minor) of CYP2A6, 3A4; **Inhibits** CYP2A6 (strong), 2C19 (weak)

Avoid Concomitant Use There are no known interactions where it is recommended to avoid concomitant use.

Increased Effect/Toxicity

Letrozole may increase the levels/effects of: CYP2A6 Substrates

Decreased Effect

The levels/effects of Letrozole may be decreased by: Tamoxifen

Stability Store at room temperature of 25°C (77°F); excursions permitted to 15°C to 30°C (59°F to 86°F).

Mechanism of Action Nonsteroidal competitive inhibitor of the aromatase enzyme system which binds to the heme group of aromatase, a cytochrome P450 enzyme which catalyzes conversion of androgens to estrogens (specifically, androstenedione to estrone and testosterone to estradiol). This leads to inhibition of the enzyme and a significant reduction in plasma estrogen (estrone, estradiol and estrone sulfate) levels. Does not affect synthesis of adrenal or thyroid hormones, aldosterone, or androgens.

Pharmacodynamics/Kinetics

Absorption: Rapid and well absorbed; not affected by food

Distribution: V_d: ~1.9 L/kg

Protein binding, plasma: Weak

Metabolism: Hepatic via CYP3A4 and 2A6 to an inactive carbinol metabolite

Half-life elimination: Terminal: ~2 days

Time to steady state, plasma: 2-6 weeks

Excretion: Urine (90%; 6% as unchanged drug, 75% as glucuronide carbinol metabolite, 9% as unidentified metabolites)

Dosage Oral: Adults: Females:

Breast cancer: 2.5 mg once daily

Ovarian (epithelial) cancer (unlabeled use): 2.5 mg once daily (Ramirez, 2008)

Elderly: No dosage adjustments required

Dosage adjustment in renal impairment: No dosage adjustment is required in patients with renal impairment if Cl_{cr} ≥10 mL/minute

Dosage adjustment in hepatic impairment:

Mild-to-moderate impairment (Child-Pugh class A and B): No adjustment recommended

Severe impairment (Child-Pugh class C): 2.5 mg every other day

Dietary Considerations May be taken without regard to meals. Calcium and vitamin D supplementation are recommended.

Administration Administer with or without food.

Monitoring Parameters Monitor periodically during therapy: Complete blood counts, thyroid function tests; serum electrolytes, cholesterol, transaminases, and creatinine; blood pressure; bone density

Dosage Forms Excipient information presented when available (limited, particularly for generics); consult specific product labeling.

Tablet:

Femara®: 2.5 mg

Leucovorin Calcium (loo koe VOR in KAL see um)

Index Terms 5-Formyl Tetrahydrofolate; Calcium Leucovorin; Citrovorum Factor; Folinic Acid (error prone synonym)

Pharmacologic Category Antidote; Chemotherapy Modulating Agent; Rescue Agent (Chemotherapy); Vitamin, Water Soluble

Additional Appendix Information

Guidelines for the Prevention of Opportunistic Infections in HIV Infected Persons *on page 1740*

Use Antidote for folic acid antagonists (methotrexate, trimethoprim, pyrimethamine) and rescue therapy following high-dose methotrexate; in combination with fluorouracil in the treatment of colon cancer; treatment of megaloblastic anemias when folate is deficient as in infancy, sprue, pregnancy, and nutritional deficiency when oral folate therapy is not possible

Unlabeled/Investigational Use I.T. administration following I.T. methotrexate overdose; adjunctive cofactor therapy in methanol toxicity

Pregnancy Risk Factor C

Pregnancy Considerations Animal reproduction studies have not been conducted. Leucovorin is a biologically active form of folic acid. Adequate amounts of folic acid are recommended during pregnancy. Refer to Folic Acid monograph.

Lactation Excretion in breast milk unknown/use caution

Medication Safety Issues

Sound-alike/look-alike issues:

Leucovorin may be confused with Leukeran®, Leukine®, LEVOleucovorin

Folinic acid may be confused with folic acid

Folinic acid is an error prone synonym and should not be used

Contraindications Pernicious anemia or vitamin B_{12}-deficient megaloblastic anemias

Warnings/Precautions When used for the treatment of accidental folic acid antagonist overdose, administer as soon as possible. When used for methotrexate rescue therapy, methotrexate serum concentrations should be monitored to determine dose and duration of leucovorin therapy. Dose may need increased or administration prolonged in situations where methotrexate excretion may be delayed (eg, ascites, pleural effusion, renal insufficiency, inadequate hydration). Combination of leucovorin and sulfamethoxazole-trimethoprim for the acute treatment of PCP in patients with HIV infection has been reported to cause increased rates of treatment failure. Leucovorin may increase the toxicity of 5-fluorouracil; dose of 5-fluorouracil may need decreased.

Powder for injection: When doses >10 mg/m^2 are required, reconstitute using sterile water for injection, not a solution containing benzyl alcohol.

Injection: Due to calcium content, do not administer I.V. solutions at a rate >160 mg/ minute. Not intended for intrathecal use.

Adverse Reactions Frequency not defined. Toxicities (especially gastrointestinal toxicity) of fluorouracil is higher when used in combination with leucovorin.

Dermatologic: Rash, pruritus, erythema, urticaria

Hematologic: Thrombocytosis

Respiratory: Wheezing

Miscellaneous: Allergic reactions, anaphylactoid reactions

Drug Interactions

Avoid Concomitant Use

Avoid concomitant use of Leucovorin Calcium with any of the following: Raltitrexed

Increased Effect/Toxicity

Leucovorin Calcium may increase the levels/effects of: Capecitabine; Fluorouracil

Decreased Effect

Leucovorin Calcium may decrease the levels/effects of: PHENobarbital; Phenytoin; Primidone; Raltitrexed; Trimethoprim

Stability

Powder for injection: Store at room temperature of 25°C (77°F). Protect from light. Reconstitute with SWFI or BWFI; dilute in 100-1000 mL NS, D_5W for infusion. When doses >10 mg/m^2 are required, reconstitute using sterile water for injection, not a solution containing benzyl alcohol. Solutions reconstituted with bacteriostatic water for injection U.S.P., must be used within 7 days. Solutions reconstituted with SWFI must be used immediately. Parenteral admixture is stable for 24 hours stored at room temperature (25°C) and for 4 days when stored under refrigeration (4°C).

Solution for injection: Prior to dilution, store vials under refrigeration at 2°C to 8°C (36°F to 46°F). Protect from light.

Tablet: Store at room temperature of 15°C to 30°C (59°F to 86°F).

Mechanism of Action A reduced form of folic acid, leucovorin supplies the necessary cofactor blocked by methotrexate, enters the cells via the same active transport system as methotrexate. Stabilizes the binding of 5-dUMP and thymidylate synthetase, enhancing the activity of fluorouracil.

Methanol toxicity treatment: Formic acid (methanol's toxic metabolite) is normally metabolized to carbon dioxide and water by 10-formyltetrahydrofolate dehydrogenase after being bound to tetrahydrofolate. Administering a source of tetrahydrofolate may aid the body in eliminating formic acid.

Pharmacodynamics/Kinetics

Absorption: Oral, I.M.: Well absorbed

Metabolism: Intestinal mucosa and hepatically to 5-methyltetrahydrofolate (5MTHF; active)

Bioavailability: Saturable at oral doses >25 mg; 25 mg (97%), 50 mg (75%), 100 mg (37%)

Half-life elimination: ~4-8 hours

Time to peak: Oral: ~2 hours; I.V.: Total folates: 10 minutes; 5MTHF: ~1 hour

Excretion: Urine (primarily); feces

Dosage

Children and Adults:

Treatment of folic acid antagonist overdosage: Oral: 5-15 mg/day

Folate-deficient megaloblastic anemia: I.M.: ≤1 mg/day

High-dose methotrexate-rescue dose: Initial: Oral, I.M., I.V.: 15 mg (~10 mg/m^2); start 24 hours after beginning methotrexate infusion; continue every 6 hours for 10 doses, until methotrexate level is <0.05 micromole/L. Adjust dose as follows:

Normal methotrexate elimination: Oral, I.M., I.V.: 15 mg every 6 hours

Delayed early methotrexate elimination: I.V.: 150 mg every 3 hours until methotrexate level is <1 micromole/L, then 15 mg every 3 hours until methotrexate level is <0.05 micromole/L

Adults:

Colorectal cancer (also refer to Combination Regimens): I.V.: 200 mg/m^2 over at least 3 minutes (used in combination with fluorouracil 370 mg/m^2)

or

I.V.: 20 mg/m^2 (used in combination with fluorouracil 425 mg/m^2)

Pemetrexed toxicity (unlabeled dose): I.V.: 100 mg/m^2 once, followed by 50 mg/m^2 every 6 hours for 8 days was used in clinical trial for CTC grade 4 leukopenia ≥3 days; CTC grade 4 neutropenia ≥3 days; immediately for CTC grade 4 thrombocytopenia, bleeding associated with grade 3 thrombocytopenia, or grade 3 or 4 mucositis

Cofactor therapy in methanol toxicity (unlabeled use): I.V.: 50 mg every 4-6 hours. Therapy should continue until methanol and formic acid have been completely eliminated.

Dietary Considerations Solutions for injection contain calcium 0.004 mEq per leucovorin 1 mg

Administration Due to calcium content, do not administer I.V. solutions at a rate >160 mg/ minute.

Refer to individual protocols. Should be administered I.M., I.V. push, or I.V. infusion (15 minutes to 2 hours). Leucovorin should not be administered concurrently with methotrexate. It is commonly initiated 24 hours after the start of methotrexate. Toxicity to normal tissues may be irreversible if leucovorin is not initiated by ~40 hours after the start of methotrexate.

As a rescue after folate antagonists: Administer by I.V. bolus, I.M., or orally.

Do not administer orally in the presence of nausea or vomiting. Doses >25 mg should be administered parenterally.

In combination with fluorouracil: Fluorouracil activity, the fluorouracil is usually given after, or at the midpoint, of the leucovorin infusion. Leucovorin is usually administered by I.V. bolus injection or short (10-120 minutes) I.V. ▶

infusion. Other administration schedules have been used; refer to individual protocols.

Monitoring Parameters

High-dose methotrexate therapy: Plasma methotrexate concentration; leucovorin is continued until the plasma methotrexate level <0.05 micromole/L. With 4- to 6-hour high-dose methotrexate infusions, plasma drug values in excess of 50 and 1 micromole/L at 24 and 48 hours after starting the infusion, respectively, are often predictive of delayed methotrexate clearance.

Fluorouracil therapy: CBC with differential and platelets, liver function tests, electrolytes

Dosage Forms Excipient information presented when available (limited, particularly for generics); consult specific product labeling. **Note:** Strength expressed as base

Injection, powder for reconstitution: 50 mg, 100 mg, 200 mg, 350 mg

Injection, solution [preservative free]: 10 mg/mL (50 mL)

Tablet: 5 mg, 10 mg, 15 mg, 25 mg

◆ **Leukeran®** *see* Chlorambucil *on page* 301

◆ **Leukine®** *see* Sargramostim *on page* 1355

Leuprolide (loo PROE lide)

U.S. Brand Names Eligard®; Lupron Depot-Ped®; Lupron Depot®; Lupron®; Viadur® [DSC]

Canadian Brand Names Eligard®; Lupron®; Lupron® Depot®; Viadur®

Index Terms Abbott-43818; Leuprolide Acetate; Leuprorelin Acetate; TAP-144

Pharmacologic Category Antineoplastic Agent, Gonadotropin-Releasing Hormone Agonist; Gonadotropin Releasing Hormone Agonist

Use Palliative treatment of advanced prostate cancer; management of endometriosis; treatment of anemia caused by uterine leiomyomata (fibroids); central precocious puberty

Unlabeled/Investigational Use Treatment of breast, ovarian, and endometrial cancer; infertility; prostatic hyperplasia

Pregnancy Risk Factor X

Pregnancy Considerations Pregnancy must be excluded prior to the start of treatment. Although leuprolide usually inhibits ovulation and stops menstruation, contraception is not ensured and a nonhormonal contraceptive should be used. Fetal abnormalities and increased fetal mortality have been noted in animal studies.

Lactation Excretion in breast milk unknown/contraindicated

Medication Safety Issues

Sound-alike/look-alike issues:

Lupron® may be confused with Nuprin®

Lupron Depot®-3 Month may be confused with Lupron Depot-Ped®

Contraindications Hypersensitivity to leuprolide, GnRH, GnRH-agonist analogs, or any component of the formulation; undiagnosed abnormal vaginal bleeding; pregnancy; breast-feeding

Lupron Depot®-4 month (30 mg) is not indicated for use in women

Eligard® and Viadur® are contraindicated in women and children

Warnings/Precautions Hazardous agent - use appropriate precautions for handling and disposal. Transient increases in testosterone serum levels occur at the start of treatment. Tumor flare, bone pain, neuropathy, urinary tract obstruction, and spinal cord compression have been reported when used for prostate cancer; closely observe patients for weakness, paresthesias, hematuria, and urinary tract obstruction in first few weeks of therapy. Observe patients with metastatic vertebral lesions or urinary obstruction closely. Exacerbation of endometriosis or uterine leiomyomata may occur initially. Decreased bone density has been reported when used for ≥6 months. Use caution in patients with a history of psychiatric illness; alteration in mood, memory impairment, and depression have been associated with use. Rare cases of pituitary apoplexy (frequently secondary to pituitary adenoma) have been observed with leuprolide administration (onset from 1 hour to usually <2 weeks); may present as sudden headache, vomiting, visual or mental status changes, and infrequently cardiovascular collapse; immediate medical attention required. Females treated for precocious puberty may experience menses or spotting during the first 2 months of treatment; notify healthcare provider if bleeding continues after the second month. Vehicle used in injectable (polylactide-co-glycolide microspheres) has rarely been associated with retinal artery occlusion in patients with abnormal arteriovenous anastomosis.

Adverse Reactions

Children:

2% to 10%:

Central nervous system: Pain (2%)

Dermatologic: Acne (2%), rash (2% including erythema multiforme), seborrhea (2%)

Genitourinary: Vaginitis (2%), vaginal bleeding (2%), vaginal discharge (2%)

Local: Injection site reaction (5%)

<2%: Alopecia, body odor, cervix disorder, dysphagia, emotional lability, epistaxis, fever, gingivitis, gynecomastia, headache, nausea, nervousness, peripheral edema, personality disorder, sexual maturity accelerated, skin striae, somnolence, syncope, urinary incontinence, vasodilation, vomiting, weight gain

Adults: Note: For prostate cancer treatment, an initial rise in serum testosterone concentrations may cause "tumor flare" or worsening of symptoms, including bone pain, neuropathy, hematuria, or ureteral or bladder outlet obstruction during the first 2 weeks. Similarly, an initial increase in estradiol levels, with a temporary worsening of symptoms, may occur in women treated with leuprolide.

Delayed release formulations:

10%:

Cardiovascular: Edema (≤14%)

Central nervous system: Headache (≤65%), pain (<2% to 33%), depression (≤31%), insomnia (≤31%), fatigue (≤17%), dizziness/vertigo (≤16%)

Dermatologic: Skin reaction (≤12%)

Endocrine & metabolic: Hot flashes (25% to 98%), testicular atrophy (≤20%), hyperlipidemia (≤12%), libido decreased (≤11%)

Gastrointestinal: Nausea/vomiting (≤25%), weight gain/loss (≤13%)

Genitourinary: Vaginitis (11% to 28%), urinary disorder (13% to 15%)

Local: Implant site bruising (35%), injection site burning/stinging (transient: ≤35%)

Neuromuscular & skeletal: Joint disorder (≤12%), weakness (≤12%)

Miscellaneous: Flu-like syndrome (≤12%)

1% to 10% (limited to important or life-threatening):

Cardiovascular: Angina (<5%), arrhythmia (<5%), atrial fibrillation (<5%), bradycardia (<5%), CHF (<5%), deep thrombophlebitis (<5%), hyper-/hypotension (<5%), palpitation (<5%), syncope (<5%), tachycardia (<5%)

Central nervous system: Nervousness (≤8%), anxiety (≤6%), confusion (<5%), delusions (<5%), dementia (<5%), fever (<5%), seizure (<5%)

Dermatologic: Acne (≤10%), alopecia (≤5%), bruising (≤5%), cellulitis (<5%), pruritus (≤3%), hirsutism (<2%), rash (<2%)

Endocrine & metabolic: Dehydration (≤8%), gynecomastia (≤7%), breast tenderness/pain (≤6%), bicarbonate decreased (≥5%), hyper-/hypocholesterolemia (≥5%), hyperglycemia (≥5%), hyperphosphatemia (≥5%), hyperuricemia (≥5%), hypoalbuminemia (≥5%), hypoproteinemia (≥5%), lactation (<5%), testicular pain (≤4%), menstrual disorder (≤2%)

Gastrointestinal: Dysphagia (<5%), gastrointestinal hemorrhage (<5%), intestinal obstruction (<5%), ulcer (<5%), gastroenteritis/colitis (≤3%), diarrhea (≤2%), constipation (≤2%)

Genitourinary: Prostatic acid phosphatase increased/decreased (≥5%), urine specific gravity increased/decreased (≥5%), impotence (≤5%), balanitis (<5%), incontinence (<5%), penile/testis disorder (<5%), urinary tract infection (<5%), nocturia (≤4%), polyuria (2% to 4%), bladder spasm (<2%), dysuria (<2%), erectile dysfunction (<2%), hematuria (<2%), urinary retention (<2%), urinary urgency (<2%)

Hematologic: Eosinophilia (≥5%), leukopenia (≥5%), platelets increased (≥5%), anemia

Hepatic: Liver function tests abnormal (≥5%), partial thromboplastin time increased (≥5%), prothrombin time increased (≥5%), hepatomegaly (<5%)

Local: Implant site reaction (persistent or delayed: 9% to 10%), implant site burning (6%), injection site pain (2% to 5%), injection site erythema (1% to 3%)

Neuromuscular & skeletal: Myalgia (≤8%), paresthesia (≤8%), neuropathy (<5%), paralysis (<5%), pathologic fracture (<5%), bone pain (<2%)

Renal: BUN increased (≥5%), creatinine increased (≥5%)

Respiratory: Emphysema (<5%), epistaxis (<5%), hemoptysis (<5%), pleural effusion (<5%), pulmonary edema (<5%), dyspnea (≤2%)

Miscellaneous: Diaphoresis (≤5%), allergic reaction (<5%), infection (5%), lymphadenopathy (<5%)

Immediate release formulation:

>10%:

Cardiovascular: ECG changes/ischemia (19%), peripheral edema (12%)

Central nervous system: Pain (13%)

Endocrine & metabolic: Hot flashes (55%)

1% to 10% (limited to important or life-threatening):

Cardiovascular: Hypertension (8%), murmur (3%), thrombosis/phlebitis (2%), CHF (1%), angina, arrhythmia, MI, syncope

Central nervous system: Headache (7%), insomnia (7%), dizziness/lightheadedness (5%), anxiety, depression, fatigue, fever, nervousness

Dermatologic: Dermatitis (5%), alopecia, bruising, itching, lesions, pigmentation

Endocrine & metabolic: Gynecomastia/breast tenderness/pain (7%), testicular size decreased (7%), diabetes, hypercalcemia, hypoglycemia, libido decreased, thyroid enlarged

Gastrointestinal: Constipation (7%), anorexia (6%), nausea/vomiting (5%), diarrhea, dysphagia, gastrointestinal bleeding, peptic ulcer, rectal polyps

Genitourinary: Urinary frequency/urgency (6%), impotence (4%), urinary tract infection (3%), bladder spasm, dysuria, incontinence, testicular pain, urinary obstruction

Hematologic: Anemia (5%)

Local: Injection site reaction

Neuromuscular & skeletal: Weakness (10%), bone pain (5%), peripheral neuropathy

Ocular: Blurred vision

Renal: Hematuria (6%), BUN increased, creatinine increased

Respiratory: Dyspnea (2%), cough, pneumonia, pulmonary embolus, pulmonary fibrosis

Miscellaneous: Infection, inflammation

Children and Adults: *Any formulations:* Postmarketing and/or case reports (limited to important or life-threatening): Anaphylactic/anaphylactoid reactions, asthmatic reactions, bone density decreased; fibromyalgia-like symptoms (arthralgia/myalgia, headaches, GI distress); hemoptysis, hepatic dysfunction, hypokalemia, hypoproteinemia, implant extrusion, implant migration, injection site induration/abscess, MI, pelvic fibrosis, penile swelling, photosensitivity; pituitary apoplexy (cardiovascular collapse, mental status altered, ophthalmoplegia, sudden headache, visual changes, vomiting); prostate pain, pulmonary embolism, pulmonary infiltrate, spinal fracture/paralysis, stroke, tenosynovitis-like symptoms, thrombocytopenia, transient ischemia attack, uric acid increased, urticaria, WBC increased

Drug Interactions

Avoid Concomitant Use There are no known interactions where it is recommended to avoid concomitant use.

Increased Effect/Toxicity There are no known significant interactions involving an increase in effect.

Decreased Effect

Leuprolide may decrease the levels/effects of: Antidiabetic Agents

Stability

Lupron®: Store unopened vials of injection in refrigerator. Vial in use can be kept at room temperature ≤30°C (86°F) for several months with minimal loss of potency. Protect from light and store vial in carton until use. Do not freeze.

Eligard®: Store at 2°C to 8°C (36°F to 46°C). Allow to reach room temperature prior to using. Once mixed, must be administered within 30 minutes. Eligard® is packaged in two syringes; one contains the Atrigel® polymer system and the second contains leuprolide acetate powder. Follow package instructions for mixing.

Lupron Depot® may be stored at room temperature of 15°C to 30°C (59°F to 86°F). Upon reconstitution, the suspension does not contain a preservative and should be used immediately. Reconstitute only with diluent provided.

Viadur® may be stored at room temperature of 15°C to 30°C (59°F and 86°F).

Mechanism of Action Leuprolide, is an agonist of luteinizing hormone-releasing hormone (LHRH). Acting as a potent inhibitor of gonadotropin secretion; continuous administration results in suppression of ovarian and testicular steroidogenesis due to decreased levels of LH and FSH with subsequent decrease in testosterone (male) and estrogen (female) levels. In males, testosterone levels are reduced to below castrate levels. Leuprolide may also have a direct inhibitory effect on the testes, and act by a different mechanism not directly related to reduction in serum testosterone.

Pharmacodynamics/Kinetics

Onset of action: Following transient increase, testosterone suppression occurs in ~2-4 weeks of continued therapy

Distribution: Males: V_d: 27 L

Protein binding: 43% to 49%

Metabolism: Major metabolite, pentapeptide (M-1)

Bioavailability: Oral: None; SubQ: 94%

Excretion: Urine (<5% as parent and major metabolite)

Dosage

Children: Precocious puberty (consider discontinuing by age 11 for females and by age 12 for males):

SubQ (Lupron®): Initial: 50 mcg/kg/day (per manufacturer, doses of 20-45 mcg/kg/day have also been reported); titrate dose upward by 10 mcg/kg/day if down-regulation is not achieved

I.M. (Lupron Depot-Ped®): 0.3 mg/kg/dose given every 28 days (minimum dose: 7.5 mg)

≤25 kg: 7.5 mg

>25-37.5 kg: 11.25 mg

>37.5 kg: 15 mg

Titrate dose upward in increments of 3.75 mg every 4 weeks if down-regulation is not achieved.

Adults:
Advanced prostate cancer:
SubQ:
Eligard®: 7.5 mg monthly **or** 22.5 mg every 3 months **or** 30 mg every 4 months **or** 45 mg every 6 months
Lupron®: 1 mg/day
Viadur®: 65 mg implanted subcutaneously every 12 months
I.M.:
Lupron Depot®: 7.5 mg/dose given monthly (every 28-33 days) **or**
Lupron Depot®-3: 22.5 mg every 3 months **or**
Lupron Depot®-4: 30 mg every 4 months
Breast cancer, premenopausal ovarian ablation (unlabeled use): I.M.:
Lupron Depot®: 3.75 mg every 28 days **or**
Lupron Depot®-3: 11.25 mg every 3 months
Endometriosis: I.M.: Initial therapy may be with leuprolide alone or in combination with norethindrone; if retreatment for an additional 6 months is necessary, norethindrone should be used. Retreatment is not recommended for longer than one additional 6-month course.
Lupron Depot®: 3.75 mg/month for up to 6 months **or**
Lupron Depot®-3: 11.25 mg every 3 months for up to 2 doses (6 months total duration of treatment)
Uterine leiomyomata (fibroids): I.M. (in combination with iron):
Lupron Depot®: 3.75 mg/month for up to 3 months **or**
Lupron Depot®-3: 11.25 mg as a single injection

Administration
I.M.: Lupron Depot®: Vary injection site periodically
SubQ:
Eligard®: Vary injection site; choose site with adequate subcutaneous tissue (eg, abdomen, upper buttocks)
Lupron®: Vary injection site; if an alternate syringe from the syringe provided is required, insulin syringes should be used
Implant (Viadur®): Requires surgical implantation (subcutaneous) and removal at 12-month intervals

Monitoring Parameters Bone mineral density
Precocious puberty: GnRH testing (blood LH and FSH levels), measurement of bone age every 6-12 months, testosterone in males and estradiol in females; Tanner staging
Prostatic cancer: LH and FSH levels, serum testosterone (2-4 weeks after initiation of therapy), PSA; weakness, paresthesias, and urinary tract obstruction in first few weeks of therapy

Test Interactions Interferes with pituitary gonadotropic and gonadal function tests during and up to 3 months after monthly administration of leuprolide therapy. Viadur®: Efficacy and stability of product not affected by MRI or radiographic exposure, although device will be visualized during these diagnostic procedures.

Additional Information
Eligard® Atrigel®: A nongelatin-based, biodegradable, polymer matrix
Viadur®: Leuprolide acetate implant containing 72 mg of leuprolide acetate, equivalent to 65 mg leuprolide free base. One Viadur® implant delivers 120 mcg of leuprolide/day over 12 months.
Oncology Comment: Guidelines from the American Society of Clinical Oncology (ASCO) for hormonal management of advanced prostate cancer which is androgen-sensitive (Loblaw, 2007) recommend either orchiectomy or luteinizing hormone-releasing hormone (LHRH) agonists as initial treatment for androgen deprivation.

Dosage Forms Excipient information presented when available (limited, particularly for generics); consult specific product labeling. [DSC] = Discontinued product
Implant, subcutaneous:
Viadur®: 65 mg [released over 12 months; packaged with administration kit] [DSC]
Injection, solution, as acetate: 5 mg/mL (2.8 mL)
Lupron®: 5 mg/mL (2.8 mL) [contains benzyl alcohol; packaged with syringes and alcohol swabs]
Injection, powder for reconstitution, as acetate [depot formulation]:
Eligard®:
7.5 mg [released over 1 month; contains polylactide-co-glycolide]
22.5 mg [released over 3 months; contains polylactide-co-glycolide]
30 mg [released over 4 months; contains polylactide-co-glycolide]
45 mg [released over 6 months; contains polylactide-co-glycolide]
Lupron Depot®: 3.75 mg, 7.5 mg [released over 1 month; contains polysorbate 80, polylactide-co-glycolide]
Lupron Depot®-3 Month: 11.25 mg, 22.5 mg [released over 3 months; contains polysorbate 80, polylactide-co-glycolide]
Lupron Depot®-4 Month: 30 mg [released over 4 months; contains polysorbate 80, polylactide-co-glycolide]
Lupron Depot-Ped®: 7.5 mg, 11.25 mg, 15 mg [released over 1 month; contains polysorbate 80, polylactide-co-glycolide]

◆ **Leuprolide Acetate** *see* Leuprolide *on page* 868
◆ **Leuprorelin Acetate** *see* Leuprolide *on page* 868
◆ **Leurocristine Sulfate** *see* VinCRIStine *on page* 1561
◆ **Leustatin®** *see* Cladribine *on page* 339

Levalbuterol (leve al BYOO ter ole)

U.S. Brand Names Xopenex HFA™; Xopenex®
Canadian Brand Names Xopenex®
Index Terms Levalbuterol Hydrochloride; Levalbuterol Tartrate; R-albuterol
Pharmacologic Category Beta$_2$-Adrenergic Agonist
Additional Appendix Information
Bronchodilators *on page* 1650
Use Treatment or prevention of bronchospasm in children and adults with reversible obstructive airway disease
Pregnancy Risk Factor C
Pregnancy Considerations Teratogenic effects were not observed in animal studies; however, racemic albuterol was teratogenic in some species. There are no adequate and well-controlled studies in pregnant women. This drug should be used during pregnancy only if benefit exceeds risk. Use caution if needed for bronchospasm during labor and delivery; has potential to interfere with uterine contractions.
Lactation Excretion in breast milk unknown/use caution
Medication Safety Issues
Sound-alike/look-alike issues:
Xopenex® may be confused with Xanax®
Contraindications Hypersensitivity to levalbuterol, albuterol, or any component of the formulation
Warnings/Precautions Optimize anti-inflammatory treatment before initiating maintenance treatment with levalbuterol. Do not use as a component of chronic therapy without an anti-inflammatory agent. Only the mildest form of asthma (Step 1 and/or exercise-induced) would not require concurrent use based upon asthma guidelines. Patient must be instructed to seek medical attention in cases where acute symptoms are not relieved or a previous level of response is diminished. The need to increase frequency of use may indicate deterioration of asthma, and treatment must not be delayed. A spacer device or valved holding chamber is recommended when using a metered-dose inhaler.

Use caution in patients with cardiovascular disease (arrhythmia or hypertension or HF), convulsive disorders, diabetes, glaucoma, hyperthyroidism, or hypokalemia. Beta-agonists may cause elevation in blood pressure, heart rate, and result in CNS stimulation/excitation. $Beta_2$-agonists may increase risk of arrhythmia, increase serum glucose, or decrease serum potassium.

Immediate hypersensitivity reactions (urticaria, angioedema, rash, bronchospasm) have been reported. Do not exceed recommended dose; serious adverse events including fatalities, have been associated with excessive use of inhaled sympathomimetics. Rarely, paradoxical bronchospasm may occur with use of inhaled bronchodilating agents; this should be distinguished from inadequate response. Use with caution during labor and delivery. Safety and efficacy have not been established in patients <4 years of age.

Adverse Reactions

>10%:

- Endocrine & metabolic: Serum glucose increased, serum potassium decreased
- Neuromuscular & skeletal: Tremor (≤7%)
- Respiratory: Rhinitis (3% to 11%)
- Miscellaneous: Viral infection (7% to 12%)

>2% to 10%:

- Central nervous system: Headache (8% to 12%), nervousness (3% to 10%), dizziness (1% to 3%), anxiety (≤3%), migraine (≤3%), weakness (3%)
- Cardiovascular: Tachycardia (~3%)
- Dermatologic: Rash (≤8%)
- Gastrointestinal: Diarrhea (2% to 6%), dyspepsia (1% to 3%)
- Neuromuscular & skeletal: Leg cramps (≤3%)
- Respiratory: Asthma (9%), pharyngitis (3% to 10%), cough (1% to 4%), sinusitis (1% to 4%), nasal edema (1% to 3%)
- Miscellaneous: Flu-like syndrome (1% to 4%), accidental injury (≤3%)

<2% (Limited to important or life-threatening): Abnormal ECG, acne, anaphylaxis, angina, angioedema, arrhythmia, atrial fibrillation, chest pain, chills, constipation, conjunctivitis, cough, diaphoresis, dysmenorrhea, dyspnea, epistaxis, extrasystole, gastroenteritis, hematuria, hyper-/hypotension, hypoesthesia (hand), hypokalemia, insomnia, itching eyes, lymphadenopathy, myalgia, nausea, oropharyngeal dryness, paresthesia, supraventricular arrhythmia, syncope, vaginal moniliasis, vertigo, vomiting, wheezing, xerostomia

Note: Immediate hypersensitivity reactions have occurred (including angioedema, oropharyngeal edema, urticaria, and anaphylaxis).

Drug Interactions

Avoid Concomitant Use

Avoid concomitant use of Levalbuterol with any of the following: Iobenguane I 123

Increased Effect/Toxicity

Levalbuterol may increase the levels/effects of: Sympathomimetics

The levels/effects of Levalbuterol may be increased by: Atomoxetine; Cannabinoids; MAO Inhibitors; Tricyclic Antidepressants

Decreased Effect

Levalbuterol may decrease the levels/effects of: Iobenguane I 123

The levels/effects of Levalbuterol may be decreased by: Alpha-/Beta-Blockers; Beta-Blockers (Beta1 Selective); Beta-Blockers (Nonselective); Betahistine

Stability

Aerosol: Store at room temperature of 20°C to 25°C (68°F to 77°F); protect from freezing and direct sunlight. Store with mouthpiece down. Discard after 200 actuations.

Solution for nebulization: Store in protective foil pouch at room temperature of 20°C to 25°C (68°F to 77°F). Protect from light and excessive heat. Vials should be used within 2 weeks after opening protective pouch. Use within 1 week and protect from light if removed from pouch. Vials of concentrated solution should be used immediately after removing from protective pouch. Concentrated solution should be diluted with 2.5 mL NS prior to use.

Mechanism of Action Relaxes bronchial smooth muscle by action on $beta_2$-receptors with little effect on heart rate

Pharmacodynamics/Kinetics

Onset of action (as measured by a 15% increase in FEV_1):
- Aerosol: 5.5-10.2 minutes
  - Peak effect: ~77 minutes
- Nebulization: 10-17 minutes
  - Peak effect: 1.5 hours

Duration (as measured by a 15% increase in FEV_1):
- Aerosol: 3-4 hours (up to 6 hours in some patients)
- Nebulization: 5-6 hours (up to 8 hours in some patients)

Absorption: A portion of inhaled dose is absorbed to systemic circulation

Half-life elimination: 3.3-4 hours

Time to peak, serum:
- Aerosol: Children: 0.8 hours, Adults: 0.5 hours
- Nebulization: Children: 0.3-0.6 hours, Adults: 0.2 hours

Dosage

Metered-dose inhaler (45 mcg/puff):
- Children 5-11 years:
  - Bronchospasm, quick relief: 1-2 puffs every 4-6 hours as needed
  - Exacerbation of asthma (acute, severe) *(NIH Guidelines, 2007)*: 4-8 puffs every 20 minutes for 3 doses, then every 1-4 hours as needed
- Children ≥12 years and Adults:
  - Bronchospasm, quick relief: 1-2 puffs every 4-6 hours
  - Exacerbation of asthma (acute, severe) *(NIH Guidelines, 2007)*: 4-8 puffs every 20 minutes for up to 4 hours, then every 1-4 hours as needed

Solution for nebulization:
- Children: ≤4 years:
  - Bronchospasm, quick relief *(NIH Guidelines, 2007)*: 0.31-1.25 mg every 4-6 hours as needed
  - Exacerbation of asthma (acute, severe) *(NIH Guidelines, 2007)*: 0.075 mg/kg (minimum: 1.25 mg) every 20 minutes for 3 doses, then 0.075-0.15 mg/kg (maximum: 5 mg) every 1-4 hours as needed
- Children 5-11 years:
  - Bronchospasm, quick relief: 0.31-0.63 mg every 8 hours as needed
  - Exacerbation of asthma (acute severe) *(NIH Guidelines, 2007)*: 0.075 mg/kg (minimum: 1.25 mg) every 20 minutes for 3 doses, then 0.075-0.15 mg/kg (maximum: 5 mg) every 1-4 hours as needed
- Children ≥12 years and Adults:
  - Bronchospasm, quick relief: 0.63-1.25 mg every 8 hours as needed
  - Exacerbation of asthma (acute, severe) *(NIH Guidelines, 2007)*: 1.25-2.5 mg every 20 minutes for 3 doses, then 1.25-5 mg every 1-4 hours as needed

Elderly: Only a small number of patients have been studied. Although greater sensitivity of some elderly patients cannot be ruled out, no overall differences in safety or effectiveness were observed. An initial dose of 0.63 mg should be used in all patients >65 years of age.

Administration Inhalation:

Metered-dose inhaler: Shake well before use; prime with 4 test sprays prior to first use or if inhaler has not been use of more than 3 days. Clean actuator (mouthpiece) weekly. A spacer device or valved holding chamber is recommended when using a metered-dose inhaler.

Solution for nebulization: Safety and efficacy were established when administered with the following nebulizers: PARI LC Jet™, PARI LC Plus™, as well as the following compressors: PARI Master®, Dura-Neb® 2000, and Dura-Neb® 3000. Concentrated solution should be diluted prior to use. Blow-by administration is not recommended, use a mask device if patient unable to hold mouthpiece in mouth for administration.

Monitoring Parameters Asthma symptoms; FEV_1, peak flow, and/or other pulmonary function tests; heart rate, blood pressure, CNS stimulation; arterial blood gases (if condition warrants); serum potassium, serum glucose (in selected patients)

Dosage Forms Excipient information presented when available (limited, particularly for generics); consult specific product labeling.

Note: Strength expressed as base.

Aerosol, for oral inhalation, as tartrate:

Xopenex HFA™: 45 mcg/actuation (15 g) [200 actuations; chlorofluorocarbon free]

Solution for nebulization, as hydrochloride [preservative free]:

Xopenex®: 0.31 mg/3 mL (24s); 0.63 mg/3 mL (24s); 1.25 mg/3 mL (24s)

Solution for nebulization, as hydrochloride [concentrate; preservative free]:

Xopenex®: 1.25 mg/0.5 mL (30s)

- ◆ **Levalbuterol Hydrochloride** *see* Levalbuterol *on page 870*
- ◆ **Levalbuterol Tartrate** *see* Levalbuterol *on page 870*
- ◆ **Levall™** *see* Carbetapentane, Guaifenesin, and Phenylephrine *on page 255*
- ◆ **Levall G** *see* Guaifenesin and Pseudoephedrine *on page 713*
- ◆ **Levaquin®** *see* Levofloxacin *on page 875*
- ◆ **Levarterenol Bitartrate** *see* Norepinephrine *on page 1077*
- ◆ **Levate® (Can)** *see* Amitriptyline *on page 90*
- ◆ **Levbid®** *see* Hyoscyamine *on page 756*
- ◆ **Levemir®** *see* Insulin Detemir *on page 793*

Levetiracetam (lee va tye RA se tam)

U.S. Brand Names Keppra XR™; Keppra®

Canadian Brand Names Apo-Levetiracetam; CO Levetiracetam; DOM-Levetiracetam; Keppra®; PHL-Levetiracetam; PMS-Levetiracetam

Pharmacologic Category Anticonvulsant, Miscellaneous

Additional Appendix Information

Anticonvulsant Drugs of Choice *on page 1637*

Use Adjunctive therapy in the treatment of partial onset, myoclonic, and/or primary generalized tonic-clonic seizures

Unlabeled/Investigational Use Bipolar disorder

Pregnancy Risk Factor C

Pregnancy Considerations Developmental toxicities were observed in animal studies. There are no adequate and well-controlled studies in pregnant women. Two registries are available for women exposed to levetiracetam during pregnancy:

Antiepileptic Drug Pregnancy Registry (888-233-2334 or http://www.mgh.harvard.edu/aed/)

Keppra® pregnancy registry (888-537-7734 or http://www.keppra.com)

Lactation Enters breast milk/not recommended

Medication Safety Issues

Sound-alike/look-alike issues:

Keppra® may be confused with Keppra XR™

Levetiracetam may be confused with levofloxacin

Potential for dispensing errors between Keppra® and Kaletra® (lopinavir/ritonavir)

Contraindications Hypersensitivity to levetiracetam or any component of the formulation

Warnings/Precautions Psychotic symptoms (psychosis, hallucinations) and behavioral symptoms (including aggression, anger, anxiety, depersonalization, depression, personality disorder) may occur; incidence may be increased in children. Dose reduction may be required. Levetiracetam should be withdrawn gradually to minimize the potential of increased seizure frequency. Use caution with renal impairment; dosage adjustment may be necessary. Weakness, dizziness, and somnolence occur mostly during the first month of therapy. Although rare, decreases in red blood cell counts, hemoglobin, hematocrit, white blood cell counts and neutrophils have been observed. Safety and efficacy in children <4 years of age (oral formulation) or <16 years (I.V. formulation and extended release tablets) have not been established.

Adverse Reactions

>10%:

Central nervous system: Behavioral symptoms (agitation, aggression, anger, anxiety, apathy, depersonalization, depression, emotional lability, hostility, hyperkinesias, irritability, nervousness, neurosis and personality disorder: adults 5% to 13%; children 5% to 38%), somnolence (8% to 23%), headache (14%), hostility (2% to 12%)

Gastrointestinal: Vomiting (15%), anorexia (3% to 13%)

Neuromuscular & skeletal: Weakness (9% to 15%)

Respiratory: Pharyngitis (6% to 14%), rhinitis (4% to 13%), cough (2% to 11%)

Miscellaneous: Accidental injury (17%), infection (2% to 13%)

1% to 10%:

Cardiovascular: Facial edema (2%)

Central nervous system: Fatigue (10%), nervousness (4% to 10%), dizziness (5% to 9%), personality disorder (8%), pain (6% to 7%), agitation (6%), irritability (6% to 7%), emotional lability (2% to 6%), mood swings (5%), depression (3% to 5%), vertigo (3% to 5%), ataxia (3%), amnesia (2%), anxiety (2%), confusion (2%)

Dermatologic: Bruising (4%), pruritus (2%), rash (2%), skin discoloration (2%)

Endocrine & metabolic: Dehydration (2%)

Gastrointestinal: Diarrhea (8%), nausea (5%), gastroenteritis (4%), constipation (3%)

Genitourinary: Urine abnormality (2%)

Hematologic: Leukocytes decreased (2% to 3%)

Neuromuscular & skeletal: Neck pain (2% to 8%), paresthesia (2%), reflexes increased (2%)

Ocular: Conjunctivitis (3%), diplopia (2%), amblyopia (2%)

Otic: Ear pain (2%)

Renal: Albuminuria (4%)

Respiratory: Influenza (5%), asthma (2%), sinusitis (2%)

Miscellaneous: Flu-like syndrome (3% to 8%), viral infection (2%)

<1% (Limited to important or life-threatening): Alopecia, anemia, catatonia, hematocrit decreased, hemoglobin decreased, hepatic failure, hepatitis, leukopenia, LFTs abnormal, neutropenia, pancreatitis, pancytopenia (with bone marrow suppression), psychotic symptoms, red blood cells decreased, suicide attempt, suicide behavior, suicide ideation, thrombocytopenia, weight loss

Drug Interactions

Avoid Concomitant Use There are no known interactions where it is recommended to avoid concomitant use.

Increased Effect/Toxicity

Levetiracetam may increase the levels/effects of: Alcohol (Ethyl); CNS Depressants

Decreased Effect

The levels/effects of Levetiracetam may be decreased by: Ketorolac; Mefloquine

Ethanol/Nutrition/Herb Interactions

Ethanol: Avoid ethanol (may increase CNS depression).

Food: Food may delay, but does not affect the extent of absorption.

Stability

Oral solution, tablets: Store at 25°C (77°F); excursions permitted to 15°C to 30°C (59°F to 86°F).

Injection solution: Store at 25°C (77°F); excursions permitted to 15°C to 30°C (59°F to 86°F). Must dilute dose in 100 mL of NS, LR, or D_5W. Admixed solution is stable for 24 hours in PVC bags kept at room temperature.

Mechanism of Action The precise mechanism by which levetiracetam exerts its antiepileptic effect is unknown. However, several studies have suggested the mechanism may involve one or more of the following central pharmacologic effects: inhibition of voltage-dependent N-type calcium channels; facilitation of GABA-ergic inhibitory transmission through displacement of negative modulators; reduction of delayed rectifier potassium current; and/or binding to synaptic proteins which modulate neurotransmitter release.

Pharmacodynamics/Kinetics

Absorption: Oral: Rapid and almost complete

Distribution: V_d: Similar to total body water

Protein binding: <10%

Metabolism: Not extensive; primarily by enzymatic hydrolysis; forms metabolites (inactive)

Bioavailability: 100%

Half-life elimination: ~6-8 hours; extended release tablet: ~7 hours; half-life increased in renal dysfunction

Time to peak, plasma: Oral: Immediate release: ~1 hour; Extended release: ~4 hours

Excretion: Urine (66% as unchanged drug)

Dosage

Oral:

Children 4-15 years: Partial onset seizures: Immediate release: 10 mg/kg/dose given twice daily; may increase every 2 weeks by 10 mg/kg/dose to a maximum of 30 mg/kg/dose twice daily

Children 6-15 years: Tonic-clonic seizures: Immediate release: Initial: 10 mg/kg dose given twice daily; may increase every 2 weeks by 10 mg/kg/dose to the recommended dose of 30 mg/kg twice daily. Efficacy of doses >60 mg/kg/day has not been established.

Children ≥12 years and Adults: Myoclonic seizures: Immediate release: Initial: 500 mg twice daily; may increase every 2 weeks by 500 mg/dose to the recommended dose of 1500 mg twice daily. Efficacy of doses >3000 mg/day has not been established.

Children ≥16 years and Adults:

Partial onset seizure:

Immediate release: Initial: 500 mg twice daily; may increase every 2 weeks by 500 mg/dose to a maximum of 1500 mg twice daily. Doses >3000 mg/day have been used in trials; however, there is no evidence of increased benefit.

Extended release: Initial: 1000 mg once daily; may increase every 2 weeks by 1000 mg/day to a maximum of 3000 mg once daily.

Tonic-clonic seizures: Immediate release: Initial: 500 mg twice daily; may increase every 2 weeks by 500 mg/dose to the recommended dose of 1500 mg twice daily. Efficacy of doses >3000 mg/day has not been established.

Bipolar disorder (unlabeled use): Immediate release: Initial: 500 mg twice daily; if tolerated, increase by 500 mg twice daily; dose may be increased every 3 days until target dose of 3000 mg/day is reached; maximum: 4000 mg/day

Adults: Loading dose (unlabeled): Immediate release: Initial doses of 1500-2000 mg have been well-tolerated (Koubeissi, 2008; Betts, 2000), although the necessity of a loading dose has not been established

I.V.: Children ≥16 years and Adults: Partial onset seizure: Initial: 500 mg twice daily; may increase every 2 weeks by 500 mg/dose to a maximum of 1500 mg twice daily. Doses >3000 mg/day have been used in trials; however, there is no evidence of increased benefit.

Note: When switching from oral to I.V. formulations, the total daily dose should be the same.

Dosing adjustment in renal impairment: Adults:

Immediate release and I.V. formulations:

Cl_{cr} >80 mL/minute: 500-1500 mg every 12 hours

Cl_{cr} 50-80 mL/minute: 500-1000 mg every 12 hours

Cl_{cr} 30-50 mL/minute: 250-750 mg every 12 hours

Cl_{cr} <30 mL/minute: 250-500 mg every 12 hours

End-stage renal disease patients using dialysis: 500-1000 mg every 24 hours; a supplemental dose of 250-500 mg following dialysis is recommended

Extended release tablets:

Cl_{cr} >80 mL/minute: 1000-3000 mg every 24 hours

Cl_{cr} 50-80 mL/minute: 1000-2000 mg every 24 hours

Cl_{cr} 30-50 mL/minute: 500-1500 mg every 24 hours

Cl_{cr} <30 mL/minute: 500-1000 mg every 24 hours

Dosing adjustment in hepatic impairment: No adjustment required

Dietary Considerations May be taken with or without food.

Administration

I.V.: Infuse over 15 minutes

Oral: May be taken with or without food.

Oral solution: Should be administered with a calibrated measuring device (not a household teaspoon or tablespoon)

Tablet (immediate release and extended release): Only administer as whole tablet; do not crush, break or chew.

Dosage Forms Excipient information presented when available (limited, particularly for generics); consult specific product labeling.

Injection, solution:

Keppra®: 100 mg/mL (5 mL)

Solution, oral:

Keppra®: 100 mg/mL (480 mL) [dye free; grape flavor]

Tablet: 250 mg, 500 mg, 750 mg

Keppra®: 250 mg, 500 mg, 750 mg, 1000 mg

Tablet, extended release:

Keppra XR™: 500 mg

◆ **Levitra®** *see* Vardenafil *on page 1547*

◆ **Levlen®** *see* Ethinyl Estradiol and Levonorgestrel *on page 577*

◆ **Levlite™** *see* Ethinyl Estradiol and Levonorgestrel *on page 577*

Levobunolol (lee voe BYOO noe lole)

U.S. Brand Names Betagan®

Canadian Brand Names Apo-Levobunolol®; Betagan®; Novo-Levobunolol; Optho-Bunolol®; PMS-Levobunolol; Sandoz-Levobunolol

Index Terms *l*-Bunolol Hydrochloride; Levobunolol Hydrochloride

Pharmacologic Category Beta-Adrenergic Blocker, Nonselective; Ophthalmic Agent, Antiglaucoma

Additional Appendix Information

Glaucoma Drug Therapy *on page 1808*

Use To lower intraocular pressure in chronic open-angle glaucoma or ocular hypertension

Pregnancy Risk Factor C

Medication Safety Issues

Sound-alike/look-alike issues:

Levobunolol may be confused with levocabastine

Betagan® may be confused with Betadine®, Betoptic® S

International issues:

Betagan® may be confused with Betagon® which is a brand name for mepindolol in Italy

Dosage Adults: Ophthalmic: Instill 1 drop in the affected eye(s) 1-2 times/day

Additional Information Complete prescribing information for this medication should be consulted for additional detail.

Dosage Forms Excipient information presented when available (limited, particularly for generics); consult specific product labeling.

Solution, ophthalmic, as hydrochloride: 0.25% (5 mL, 10 mL); 0.5% (5 mL, 10 mL, 15 mL) [contains benzalkonium chloride and sodium metabisulfite]

Betagan®: 0.25% (5 mL, 10 mL); 0.5% (2 mL, 5 mL, 10 mL, 15 mL) [contains benzalkonium chloride and sodium metabisulfite]

◆ **Levobunolol Hydrochloride** *see* Levobunolol *on page 873*

Levobupivacaine (LEE voe byoo PIV a kane)

U.S. Brand Names Chirocaine® [DSC]

Canadian Brand Names Chirocaine®

Pharmacologic Category Local Anesthetic

Use Production of local or regional anesthesia for surgery and obstetrics, and for postoperative pain management

Pregnancy Risk Factor B

Medication Safety Issues

High alert medication: The Institute for Safe Medication Practices (ISMP) includes this medication (epidural administration) among its list of drug classes which have a heightened risk of causing significant patient harm when used in error.

Dosage Adults: **Note:** Rapid injection of a large volume of local anesthetic solution should be avoided. Fractional (incremental) doses are recommended.

Guidelines (individual response varies): See table.

	Concentration	Volume	Dose	Motor Block
Surgical Anesthesia				
Epidural for surgery	0.5%-0.75%	10-20 mL	50-150 mg	Moderate to complete
Epidural for C-section	0.5%	20-30 mL	100-150 mg	Moderate to complete
Peripheral nerve	0.25%-0.5%	0.4 mL/kg (30 mL)	1-2 mg/kg (75-150 mg)	Moderate to complete
Ophthalmic	0.75%	5-15 mL	37.5-112.5 mg	Moderate to complete
Local infiltration	0.25%	60 mL	150 mg	Not applicable
Pain Management				
Levobupivacaine can be used epidurally with fentanyl or clonidine; dilutions for epidural administration should be made with preservative free 0.9% saline according to standard hospital procedures for sterility				
Labor analgesia (epidural bolus)	0.25%	10-20 mL	25-50 mg	Minimal to moderate
Postoperative pain (epidural infusion)	0.125%[1]-0.25%	4-10 mL/h	5-25 mg/h	Minimal to moderate

[1]0.125%: Adjunct therapy with fentanyl or clonidine.

Maximum dosage: Epidural doses up to 375 mg have been administered incrementally to patients during a surgical procedure.

Intraoperative block and postoperative pain: 695 mg in 24 hours

Postoperative epidural infusion over 24 hours: 570 mg

Single-fractionated injection for brachial plexus block: 300 mg

Additional Information Complete prescribing information for this medication should be consulted for additional detail.

Dosage Forms Excipient information presented when available (limited, particularly for generics); consult specific product labeling. [DSC] = Discontinued product

Injection, solution [preservative free]: 2.5 mg/mL (10 mL, 30 mL); 5 mg/mL (10 mL, 30 mL); 7.5 mg/mL (10 mL, 30 mL) [DSC]

Levocabastine (LEE voe kab as teen)

U.S. Brand Names Livostin® [DSC]

Canadian Brand Names Livostin®

Index Terms Levocabastine Hydrochloride

Pharmacologic Category Histamine H_1 Antagonist; Histamine H_1 Antagonist, Second Generation

Use Treatment of allergic conjunctivitis

Pregnancy Risk Factor C

Medication Safety Issues

Sound-alike/look-alike issues:

Levocabastine may be confused with levobunolol, levocarnitine

Livostin® may be confused with lovastatin

International issues:

Livostin® may be confused with Limoxin® which is a brand name for amoxicillin in Mexico

Livostin® may be confused with Lovastin® which is a brand name for lovastatin in Malaysia and Poland

Dosage Children ≥12 years and Adults: Instill 1 drop in affected eye(s) 4 times/day for up to 2 weeks

Additional Information Complete prescribing information for this medication should be consulted for additional detail.

Dosage Forms Excipient information presented when available (limited, particularly for generics); consult specific product labeling. [DSC] = Discontinued product

Suspension, ophthalmic: 0.05% (5 mL, 10 mL) [contains benzalkonium chloride] [DSC]

◆ **Levocabastine Hydrochloride** *see* Levocabastine *on page 874*

Levocetirizine (LEE vo se TI ra zeen)

U.S. Brand Names Xyzal®

Index Terms Levocetirizine Dihydrochloride

Pharmacologic Category Histamine H_1 Antagonist; Histamine H_1 Antagonist, Second Generation

Use Relief of symptoms of perennial and seasonal allergic rhinitis; treatment of skin manifestations (uncomplicated) of chronic idiopathic urticaria

Pregnancy Risk Factor B

Medication Safety Issues

Sound-alike/look-alike issues:

Levocetirizine may be confused with cetirizine

Dosage Oral: Allergic rhinitis, chronic urticaria:

Children 6-11 years: 2.5 mg once daily (in the evening); maximum: 2.5 mg/day

Children ≥12 years and Adults: 5 mg once daily (in the evening); some patients may experience relief of symptoms with 2.5 mg once daily

Elderly: Refer to adult dosing; dosing should begin at the lower end of the dosing range

Dosage adjustments in renal impairment:

Children 6-11 years with renal impairment: Contraindicated

Children ≥12 and Adults:

Cl_{cr} 50-80 mL/minute: 2.5 mg once daily

Cl_{cr} 30-50 mL/minute: 2.5 mg once every other day

Cl_{cr} 10-30 mL/minute: 2.5 mg twice weekly (every 3 or 4 days)

Cl_{cr} <10 mL/minute, hemodialysis patients: Contraindicated

Dosage adjustments in hepatic impairment: No adjustment required.

Additional Information Complete prescribing information for this medication should be consulted for additional detail.

Dosage Forms Excipient information presented when available (limited, particularly for generics); consult specific product labeling.

Solution, oral, as dihydrochloride:
Xyzal®: 0.5 mg/mL (150 mL)

Tablet, as dihydrochloride [scored]:
Xyzal®: 5 mg

◆ **Levocetirizine Dihydrochloride** *see* Levocetirizine *on page 874*

◆ **Levodopa and Carbidopa** *see* Carbidopa and Levodopa *on page 256*

Levodopa, Carbidopa, and Entacapone

(lee voe DOE pa, kar bi DOE pa, & en TA ka pone)

U.S. Brand Names Stalevo®

Canadian Brand Names Stalevo®

Index Terms Carbidopa, Levodopa, and Entacapone; Entacapone, Carbidopa, and Levodopa

Pharmacologic Category Anti-Parkinson's Agent, COMT Inhibitor; Anti-Parkinson's Agent, Dopamine Agonist

Additional Appendix Information

Antiparkinsonian Agents *on page 1643*

Use Treatment of idiopathic Parkinson's disease

Pregnancy Risk Factor C

Dosage Oral: Adults: Parkinson's disease:

Note: All strengths of Stalevo® contain a carbidopa/levodopa ratio of 1:4 plus entacapone 200 mg.

Dose should be individualized based on therapeutic response; doses may be adjusted by changing strength or adjusting interval. Fractionated doses are not recommended and only 1 tablet should be given at each dosing interval; maximum daily dose: 8 tablets of Stalevo® 50, 75, 100, 125, or 150, **or** 6 tablets of Stalevo® 200.

Patients previously treated with carbidopa/levodopa immediate release tablets (ratio of 1:4):

With current entacapone therapy: May switch directly to corresponding strength of combination tablet. No data available on transferring patients from controlled release preparations or products with a 1:10 ratio of carbidopa/levodopa.

Without entacapone therapy:

If current levodopa dose is >600 mg/day: Levodopa dose reduction may be required when adding entacapone to therapy; therefore, titrate dose using individual products first (carbidopa/levodopa immediate release with a ratio of 1:4 plus entacapone 200 mg); then transfer to combination product once stabilized.

If current levodopa dose is <600 mg without dyskinesias: May transfer to corresponding dose of combination product; monitor, dose reduction of levodopa may be required.

Dosage adjustment in renal impairment: Use caution with severe renal impairment; specific dosing recommendations not available

Dosage adjustment in hepatic impairment: Use with caution; specific dosing recommendations not available

Additional Information Complete prescribing information for this medication should be consulted for additional detail.

Dosage Forms Excipient information presented when available (limited, particularly for generics); consult specific product labeling.

Tablet:

Stalevo® 50: Levodopa 50 mg, carbidopa 12.5 mg, and entacapone 200 mg

Stalevo® 75: Levodopa 75 mg, carbidopa 18.75 mg, and entacapone 200 mg

Stalevo® 100: Levodopa 100 mg, carbidopa 25 mg, and entacapone 200 mg

Stelevo® 125: Levodopa 125 mg, carbidopa 31.25 mg, and entacapone 200 mg

Stalevo® 150: Levodopa 150 mg, carbidopa 37.5 mg, and entacapone 200 mg

Stalevo® 200: Levodopa 200 mg, carbidopa 50 mg, and entacapone 200 mg

◆ **Levo-Dromoran®** *see* Levorphanol *on page 881*

Levofloxacin (lee voe FLOKS a sin)

U.S. Brand Names Iquix®; Levaquin®; Quixin®

Canadian Brand Names Levaquin®; Novo-Levofloxacin

Pharmacologic Category Antibiotic, Quinolone; Respiratory Fluoroquinolone

Additional Appendix Information

Antimicrobial Drugs of Choice *on page 1752*

Community-Acquired Pneumonia in Adults *on page 1766*

Prevention of Wound Infection and Sepsis in Surgical Patients *on page 1738*

Treatment of Sexually Transmitted Infections *on page 1773*

Tuberculosis *on page 1776*

Use

Systemic: Treatment of community-acquired pneumonia, including multidrug resistant strains of *S. pneumoniae* (MDRSP); nosocomial pneumonia; chronic bronchitis (acute bacterial exacerbation); acute bacterial sinusitis; prostatitis, urinary tract infection (uncomplicated or complicated); acute pyelonephritis; skin or skin structure infections (uncomplicated or complicated); reduce incidence or disease progression of inhalational anthrax (postexposure)

Ophthalmic: Treatment of bacterial conjunctivitis caused by susceptible organisms (Quixin™ 0.5% ophthalmic solution); treatment of corneal ulcer caused by susceptible organisms (Iquix® 1.5% ophthalmic solution)

Unlabeled/Investigational Use Diverticulitis, enterocolitis (*Shigella* spp.), epididymitis (nongonococcal), gonococcal infections, Legionnaires' disease, peritonitis, PID

Note: As of April 2007, the CDC no longer recommends the use of fluoroquinolones for the treatment of gonococcal disease.

Restrictions An FDA-approved patient medication guide is available and must be distributed when dispensing an outpatient prescription (new or refill) where this medication is to be used without direct supervision of a healthcare provider. Medication guides are available at http://www.fda.gov/cder/Offices/ODS/medication_guides.htm.

Pregnancy Risk Factor C

Pregnancy Considerations Adverse events have been observed in some animal studies; therefore, the manufacturer classifies levofloxacin as pregnancy category C. Levofloxacin crosses the placenta. Quinolone exposure during human pregnancy has been reported with other agents (see Ciprofloxacin, Ofloxacin, and Norfloxacin monographs). To date, no specific teratogenic effect or increased pregnancy risk has been identified; however, because of concerns of cartilage damage in immature animals exposed to quinolones and the limited levofloxacin specific data, levofloxacin should only be used during pregnancy if a safer option is not available.

Lactation Enters breast milk/not recommended

Medication Safety Issues

Sound-alike/look-alike issues:

Levaquin® may be confused with Levoxyl®, Levsin/SL®, Lovenox®

Levofloxacin may be confused with levetiracetam, levodopa, levothyroxine

Contraindications Hypersensitivity to levofloxacin, any component of the formulation, or other quinolones

Warnings/Precautions

Systemic: [U.S. Boxed Warning]: There have been reports of tendon inflammation and/or rupture with quinolone antibiotics; risk may be increased with concurrent corticosteroids, organ transplant recipients, and in patients >60 years of age. Rupture of the Achilles tendon sometimes requiring surgical repair has been reported most frequently; but other tendon sites (eg, rotator cuff, biceps) have also been reported. Strenuous physical activity, rheumatoid arthritis, and renal impairment may be an independent risk factor for tendonitis. Discontinue at first sign of tendon inflammation or pain. May occur even after discontinuation of therapy. Use with caution in patients with rheumatoid arthritis; may increase risk of tendon rupture. Systemic use is only recommended in children <18 years of age for the prevention of inhalational anthrax (postexposure); increased incidence of musculoskeletal disorders (eg, arthralgia, tendon rupture) has been observed in children; CNS stimulation may occur (tremor, restlessness, confusion, and very rarely hallucinations or seizures). Potential for seizures, although very rare, may be increased with concomitant NSAID therapy. Use with caution in individuals at risk of seizures, with known or suspected CNS disorders or renal dysfunction. Avoid excessive sunlight and take precautions to limit exposure (eg, loose fitting clothing, sunscreen); may cause moderate-to-severe phototoxicity reactions. Discontinue use if photosensitivity occurs.

Rare cases of torsade de pointes have been reported in patients receiving levofloxacin. Use caution in patients with known prolongation of QT interval, bradycardia, hypokalemia, hypomagnesemia, or in those receiving concurrent therapy with Class Ia or Class III antiarrhythmics.

Severe hypersensitivity reactions, including anaphylaxis, have occurred with quinolone therapy. Reactions may present as typical allergic symptoms after a single dose, or may manifest as severe idiosyncratic dermatologic, vascular, pulmonary, renal, hepatic, and/or hematologic events, usually after multiple doses. Prompt discontinuation of drug should occur if skin rash or other symptoms arise. Prolonged use may result in fungal or bacterial superinfection, including *C. difficile*-associated diarrhea (CDAD) and pseudomembranous colitis; CDAD has been observed >2 months postantibiotic treatment. Peripheral neuropathies have been linked to levofloxacin use; discontinue if numbness, tingling, or weakness develops. Quinolones may exacerbate myasthenia gravis. Unrelated to hypersensitivity, severe hepatotoxicity (including acute hepatitis and fatalities) has been reported. Elderly patients may be at greater risk. Discontinue therapy immediately if signs and symptoms of hepatitis occur. Hemolytic reactions may (rarely) occur with quinolone use in patients with latent or actual G6PD deficiency.

Fluoroquinolones have been associated with the development of serious, and sometimes fatal, hypoglycemia, most often in elderly diabetics, but also in patients without diabetes. This occurred most frequently with gatifloxacin (no longer available systemically) but may occur at a lower frequency with other quinolones.

Ophthalmic solution: For topical use only. Do not inject subconjunctivally or introduce into anterior chamber of the eye. Contact lenses should not be worn during treatment for bacterial conjunctivitis. Safety and efficacy in children <1 year of age (Quixin™) or <6 years of age (Iquix®) have not been established. **Note:** Indications for ophthalmic solutions are product concentration-specific and should not be used interchangeably.

Adverse Reactions

1% to 10%:

Cardiovascular: Chest pain (1%), edema (1%)

Central nervous system: Headache (6%), insomnia (4%), dizziness (3%), fatigue (1%), pain (1%)

Dermatologic: Rash (2%), pruritus (1%)

Gastrointestinal: Taste disturbance (8% to 10% [ophthalmic]), nausea (7%), diarrhea (5%), constipation (3%), abdominal pain (2%), dyspepsia (2%), vomiting (2%)

Genitourinary: Vaginitis (1%)

Local: Injection site reaction (1%)

Ocular (with ophthalmic solution use): Decreased vision (transient), foreign body sensation, transient ocular burning, ocular pain or discomfort, photophobia

Respiratory: Pharyngitis (4%), dyspnea (1%)

Miscellaneous: Moniliasis (1%)

<1% (Limited to important or life-threatening):

Systemic: Acute renal failure, agitation, agranulocytosis; allergic reaction (including anaphylaxis, angioedema, pneumonitis rash, pneumonitis, and serum sickness); anaphylactoid reaction, arrhythmia (including atrial/ventricular tachycardia/fibrillation and torsade de pointes), aplastic anemia, arthralgia, ascites, bradycardia, bronchospasm, carcinoma, cardiac failure, cholecystitis, cholelithiasis, confusion, depression, EEG abnormalities, encephalopathy, eosinophilia, erythema multiforme, GI hemorrhage, granulocytopenia, hallucination, heart block, hemolytic anemia, hemoptysis, hepatic failure (some fatal), hepatitis, hyper-/hypoglycemia, hyperkalemia, hyperkinesias, hyper-/hypotension, infection, INR increased, intestinal obstruction, intracranial hypertension, involuntary muscle contractions, jaundice, leukocytosis, leukopenia, leukorrhea, lymphadenopathy, MI, migraine, multiple organ failure, myalgia, nephritis (interstitial), palpitation, pancreatitis, pancytopenia, paralysis, paresthesia, peripheral neuropathy, photosensitivity (<0.1%), pleural effusion, pneumonitis, postural hypotension, prothrombin time increased/decreased, pseudomembraneous colitis, psychosis, pulmonary edema, pulmonary embolism, purpura, QT_c prolongation, respiratory depression, rhabdomyolysis, seizure, skin disorder, somnolence, speech disorder, Stevens-Johnson syndrome, stupor, suicide attempt/ideation, syncope, tendonitis, tendon rupture, tongue edema, toxic epidermal necrolysis, transaminases increased, thrombocythemia, thrombocytopenia, tremor, urticaria, WBC abnormality

Ophthalmic solution: Allergic reaction, lid edema, ocular dryness, ocular itching

Drug Interactions

Avoid Concomitant Use

Avoid concomitant use of Levofloxacin with any of the following: Nilotinib; Tetrabenazine; Thioridazine; Ziprasidone

Increased Effect/Toxicity

Levofloxacin may increase the levels/effects of: Corticosteroids (Systemic); QTc-Prolonging Agents; Sulfonylureas; Tetrabenazine; Thioridazine; Vitamin K Antagonists; Ziprasidone

The levels/effects of Levofloxacin may be increased by: Alfuzosin; Ciprofloxacin; Gadobutrol; Insulin; Nilotinib; Nonsteroidal Anti-Inflammatory Agents; Probenecid

Decreased Effect

Levofloxacin may decrease the levels/effects of: Mycophenolate; Sulfonylureas; Typhoid Vaccine

The levels/effects of Levofloxacin may be decreased by: Antacids; Calcium Salts; Didanosine; Iron Salts; Magnesium Salts; Quinapril; Sevelamer; Sucralfate; Zinc Salts

Stability

Solution for injection:

Vial: Store at room temperature. Protect from light. When diluted to 5 mg/mL in a compatible I.V. fluid, solution is stable for 72 hours when stored at room temperature; stable for 14 days when stored under refrigeration. When frozen, stable for 6 months; do not refreeze. Do not thaw in microwave or by bath immersion.

Premixed: Store at ≤25°C (77°F); do not freeze. Brief exposure to 40°C (104°F) does not affect product. Protect from light.

Tablet, oral solution: Store at 25°C (77°F); excursions permitted to 15°C to 30°C (59°F to 86°F).

Ophthalmic solution: Store at 15°C to 25°C (59°F to 77°F).

Mechanism of Action As the S (-) enantiomer of the fluoroquinolone, ofloxacin, levofloxacin, inhibits DNA-gyrase in susceptible organisms thereby inhibits relaxation of supercoiled DNA and promotes breakage of DNA strands. DNA gyrase (topoisomerase II), is an essential bacterial enzyme that maintains the superhelical structure of DNA and is required for DNA replication and transcription, DNA repair, recombination, and transposition.

Pharmacodynamics/Kinetics

Absorption: Rapid and complete

Distribution: V_d: 74-112 L; CSF concentrations ~15% of serum levels; high concentrations are achieved in prostate, lung, and gynecological tissues, sinus, saliva

Protein binding: ~24% to 38%; primarily to albumin

Metabolism: Minimally hepatic

Bioavailability: ~99%

Half-life elimination: ~6-8 hours

Time to peak, serum: Oral: 1-2 hours

Excretion: Urine (~87% as unchanged drug, <5% as metabolites); feces (<4%)

Dosage Note: Sequential therapy (intravenous to oral) may be instituted based on prescriber's discretion.

Usual dosage range:

Children ≥1 year: Ophthalmic: 1-2 drops every 2-6 hours

Adults:

Ophthalmic: 1-2 drops every 2-6 hours

Oral, I.V.: 250-500 mg every 24 hours; severe or complicated infections: 750 mg every 24 hours

Indication-specific dosing:

Children ≥1 year and Adults: Ophthalmic:

Conjunctivitis (0.5% ophthalmic solution):

Treatment day 1 and day 2: Instill 1-2 drops into affected eye(s) every 2 hours while awake, up to 8 times/day

Treatment day 3 through day 7: Instill 1-2 drops into affected eye(s) every 4 hours while awake, up to 4 times/day

Children ≥6 years and Adults: Ophthalmic:

Corneal ulceration (1.5% ophthalmic solution):

Treatment day 1 through day 3: Instill 1-2 drops into affected eye(s) every 30 minutes to 2 hours while awake and 4-6 hours after retiring

Treatment day 4 through completion: Instill 1-2 drops into affected eye(s) every 1-4 hours while awake

Children ≥6 months and Adults: Oral, I.V.

Anthrax (inhalational, postexposure):

≤50 kg: 8 mg/kg every 12 hours for 60 days (do not exceed 250 mg/dose), beginning as soon as possible after exposure

>50 kg and Adults: 500 mg every 24 hours for 60 days, beginning as soon as possible after exposure

Adults: Oral, I.V.:

Chronic bronchitis (acute bacterial exacerbation): 500 mg every 24 hours for at least 7 days

Diverticulitis, peritonitis (unlabeled use): 750 mg every 24 hours for 7-10 days; use adjunctive metronidazole therapy

Dysenteric enterocolitis, *Shigella* spp. (unlabeled use): 500 mg every 24 hours for 3-5 days

Epididymitis, nongonococcal (unlabeled use): 500 mg once daily for 10 days

Gonococcal infection (unlabeled use):

Cervicitis, urethritis: 250 mg for one dose with azithromycin or doxycycline; **Note:** As of April 2007, the CDC no longer recommends the use of fluoroquinolones for the treatment of uncomplicated gonococcal disease.

Disseminated infection: 250 mg I.V. once daily; 24 hours after symptoms improve may change to 500 mg orally every 24 hours to complete total therapy of 7 days; **Note:** As of April 2007, the CDC no longer recommends the use of fluoroquinolones for the treatment of more serious gonococcal disease, unless no other options exist and susceptibility can be confirmed via culture.

Pelvic inflammatory disease (unlabeled use): 500 mg once daily for 14 days with or without adjunctive metronidazole; **Note:** The CDC recommends use only if standard cephalosporin therapy is not feasible and community prevalence of quinolone-resistant gonococcal organisms is low. Culture sensitivity must be confirmed.

Pneumonia:

Community-acquired: 500 mg every 24 hours for 7-14 days or 750 mg every 24 hours for 5 days (efficacy of 5-day regimen for MDRSP not established)

Nosocomial: 750 mg every 24 hours for 7-14 days

Prostatitis (chronic bacterial): 500 mg every 24 hours for 28 days

Sinusitis (acute bacterial): 500 mg every 24 hours for 10-14 days or 750 mg every 24 hours for 5 days

Skin and skin structure infections:

Uncomplicated: 500 mg every 24 hours for 7-10 days

Complicated: 750 mg every 24 hours for 7-14 days

Traveler's diarrhea (unlabeled use): 500 mg for one dose

Urinary tract infections:

Uncomplicated: 250 mg once daily for 3 days

Complicated, including pyelonephritis: 250 mg once daily for 10 days **or** 750 mg once daily for 5 days

Dosing adjustment in renal impairment:

Normal renal function dosing of 750 mg/day:

Cl_{cr} 20-49 mL/minute: Administer 750 mg every 48 hours

Cl_{cr} 10-19 mL/minute: Administer 750 mg initial dose, followed by 500 mg every 48 hours

Hemodialysis/CAPD: Administer 750 mg initial dose, followed by 500 mg every 48 hours

Normal renal function dosing of 500 mg/day:

Cl_{cr} 20-49 mL/minute: Administer 500 mg initial dose, followed by 250 mg every 24 hours

Cl_{cr} 10-19 mL/minute: Administer 500 mg initial dose, followed by 250 mg every 48 hours

Hemodialysis/CAPD: Administer 500 mg initial dose, followed by 250 mg every 48 hours

Normal renal function dosing of 250 mg/day:

Cl_{cr} 20-49 mL/minute: No dosage adjustment required

Cl_{cr} 10-19 mL/minute: Administer 250 mg every 48 hours (except in uncomplicated UTI, where no dosage adjustment is required)

Hemodialysis/CAPD: No information available

CRRT: **Note:** Clearance dependent on filter type, flow rates, and other variables.

CVVH/CVVHD/CVVHDF: Alternative recommendations exist:

500 mg every 48 hours **or**

250 mg every 24 hours (**Note:** This regimen has been shown to be equivalent to 500 mg/day in normal renal function. Appropriateness of this regimen for target dosing equal to 750 mg/day is not known.)

Dietary Considerations Tablets may be taken without regard to meals. Oral solution should be administered on an empty stomach (1 hour before or 2 hours after a meal). Take 2 hours before or 2 hours after multiple vitamins, antacids, or other products containing magnesium, aluminum, iron, or zinc.

Administration

Oral: Tablets may be administered without regard to meals. Oral solution should be administered 1 hour before or 2 hours after meals. Maintain adequate hydration of patient to prevent crystalluria.

I.V.: Infuse 250-500 mg I.V. solution over 60 minutes; infuse 750 mg I.V. solution over 90 minutes. Too rapid of infusion can lead to hypotension. Avoid administration through an intravenous line with a solution containing multivalent cations (eg, magnesium, calcium). Maintain adequate hydration of patient to prevent crystalluria.

Monitoring Parameters Evaluation of organ system functions (renal, hepatic, ophthalmologic, and hematopoietic) is recommended periodically during therapy; the possibility of crystalluria should be assessed; WBC and signs of infection

Test Interactions Some quinolones may produce a false-positive urine screening result for opiates using commercially-available immunoassay kits. This has been demonstrated most consistently for levofloxacin and ofloxacin, but other quinolones have shown cross-reactivity in certain assay kits. Confirmation of positive opiate screens by more specific methods should be considered.

Dosage Forms Excipient information presented when available (limited, particularly for generics); consult specific product labeling.

Infusion, premixed in D_5W [preservative free]:

Levaquin®: 250 mg (50 mL); 500 mg (100 mL); 750 mg (150 mL)

Injection, solution [preservative free]

Levaquin®: 25 mg/mL (20 mL, 30 mL)

Solution, ophthalmic [drops]:

Iquix®: 1.5% (5 mL)

Quixin®: 0.5% (5 mL) [contains benzalkonium chloride]

Solution, oral:

Levaquin®: 25 mg/mL (480 mL) [contains benzyl alcohol, propylene glycol]

Tablet, oral:

Levaquin®: 250 mg, 500 mg, 750 mg

Levaquin® Leva-Pak: 750 mg (5s)

◆ **Levo-folinic Acid** *see* LEVOleucovorin *on page 878*

LEVOleucovorin (lee voe loo koe VOR in)

U.S. Brand Names Fusilev™

Index Terms 6S-leucovorin; Calcium Levoleucovorin; L-leucovorin; Levo-folinic Acid; Levo-leucovorin; Levoleucovorin Calcium Pentahydrate; S-leucovorin

Pharmacologic Category Antidote; Rescue Agent (Chemotherapy)

Use Rescue agent after high-dose methotrexate therapy in osteosarcoma; antidote for impaired methotrexate elimination and for inadvertent overdosage of folic acid antagonists

Unlabeled/Investigational Use Treatment of colorectal cancer (in combination with fluorouracil)

Pregnancy Risk Factor C

Medication Safety Issues

Sound-alike/look-alike issues:

LEVOleucovorin may be confused with leucovorin calcium, Leukeran®, Leukine®

Dosage Note: Levoleucovorin is dosed at **one-half** the usual dose of the racemic form (leucovorin calcium):

High-dose methotrexate rescue: Children and Adults: I.V.: Usual dose: 7.5 mg (~5 mg/m^2) every 6 hours for 10 doses, beginning 24 hours after the start of the methotrexate infusion (based on a methotrexate dose of 12 g/m^2 I.V. over 4 hours). Levoleucovorin (and hydration and urinary alkalinization) should be continued and/or adjusted until the methotrexate level is <0.05 micromolar (5×10^{-8} M) as follows:

Normal methotrexate elimination (serum methotrexate levels ~10 micromolar at 24 hours post administration, 1 micromolar at 48 hours and <0.2 micromolar at 72 hours post infusion): 7.5 mg I.V. every 6 hours for 10 doses

Delayed late methotrexate elimination (serum methotrexate levels >0.2 micromolar at 72 hours and >0.05 micromolar at 96 hours post methotrexate infusion): Continue 7.5 mg I.V. every 6 hours until methotrexate level is <0.05 micromolar

Delayed early methotrexate elimination and/or evidence of acute renal injury (serum methotrexate level ≥50 micromolar at 24 hours, ≥5 micromolar at 48 hours or a doubling or more of the serum creatinine level at 24 hours post methotrexate infusion): 75 mg I.V. every 3 hours until methotrexate level is <1 micromolar, followed by 7.5 mg I.V. every 3 hours until methotrexate level is <0.05 micromolar

Significant clinical toxicity in the presence of less severe abnormalities in methotrexate elimination or renal function (as described above): Extend levoleucovorin treatment for an additional 24 hours (total of 14 doses) in subsequent treatment cycles.

Delayed methotrexate elimination due to third space fluid accumulation, renal insufficiency, or inadequate hydration: May require higher levoleucovorin doses or prolonged administration.

Methotrexate overdose (inadvertent): Children and Adults: I.V.: 7.5 mg (~5 mg/m^2) every 6 hours; continue until the methotrexate level is <0.01 micromolar (10^{-8} M). Initiate treatment as soon as possible after methotrexate overdose. Increase the levoleucovorin dose to 50 mg/m^2 I.V. every 3 hours if the 24 hour serum creatinine has increased 50% over baseline, or if the 24-hour methotrexate level is >5 micromolar (5×10^{-6} M), or if the 48-hour methotrexate level is >0.9 micromolar (9×10^{-7} M); continue levoleucovorin until the methotrexate level is <0.01 micromolar (10^{-8} M). Hydration (3 L/day) and urinary alkalinization (with sodium bicarbonate) should also be maintained.

Treatment of colorectal cancer (in combination with fluorouracil; unlabeled use): Adults: I.V.: Levoleucovorin is dosed at **one-half** the usual dose of the racemic form (leucovorin)

Additional Information Complete prescribing information for this medication should be consulted for additional detail.

Dosage Forms Excipient information presented when available (limited, particularly for generics); consult specific product labeling.

Note: Strength expressed as base.

Injection, powder for reconstitution:

Fusilev™: 50 mg

◆ **Levo-leucovorin** *see* LEVOleucovorin *on page 878*

◆ **Levoleucovorin Calcium Pentahydrate** *see* LEVOleucovorin *on page 878*

Levonorgestrel (LEE voe nor jes trel)

U.S. Brand Names Mirena®; Plan B® [RX/OTC]

Canadian Brand Names Mirena®; Norplant® Implant; Plan B™

Index Terms LNg 20

Pharmacologic Category Contraceptive; Progestin

Use

Intrauterine device (IUD): Prevention of pregnancy

Oral: Emergency contraception following unprotected intercourse or possible contraceptive failure

Unlabeled/Investigational Use IUD: Idiopathic menorrhagia; protection against endometrial hyperplasia in menopausal women using estrogen

Restrictions Plan B® is approved for OTC use by women ≥18 years of age and available by prescription only for women ≤17 years of age. Sales of Plan B® will be limited to pharmacies or healthcare clinics with a valid license to distribute prescription products. Because there will be one package for both OTC and prescription use, pharmacies are required to keep the product behind the counter.

Pregnancy Risk Factor X

Pregnancy Considerations Epidemiologic studies have not shown an increased risk of birth defects when used prior to pregnancy or inadvertently during early pregnancy, although rare reports of congenital anomalies have been reported. In doses larger than those used for oral contraception, progestins have been reported to increase the risk of masculinization of female genitalia.

Intrauterine device: Pregnancy should be ruled out prior to insertion. Women who become pregnant with an IUD in place risk septic abortion (septic shock and death may occur). Removal of the device is recommended, however, removal or manipulation of IUD may result in pregnancy loss. In addition, miscarriage, premature labor, and premature delivery may occur if pregnancy is continued with IUD in place. Following pregnancy, insertion of the device should not take place until 6 weeks postpartum or until involution of the uterus is complete. Consider waiting until 12 weeks postpartum if involution is substantially delayed. The device may be inserted immediately following a first trimester abortion. Following removal of the device, ~80% of women who wished to conceive became pregnant within 12 months.

Lactation Enters breast milk/use caution (AAP rates "compatible")

Contraindications Hypersensitivity to levonorgestrel or any component of the formulation; pregnancy

Additional product-specific contraindications:

Intrauterine device: Congenital or acquired uterine anomaly, acute pelvic inflammatory disease, history of pelvic inflammatory disease (unless there has been a subsequent intrauterine pregnancy), postpartum endometritis or infected abortion within past 3 months, known or suspected uterine or cervical neoplasia, unresolved/abnormal Pap smear, untreated acute cervicitis or vaginitis, conditions which increase susceptibility to pelvic infections, unremoved IUD, undiagnosed abnormal uterine bleeding, active hepatic disease or hepatic tumors, known or suspected carcinoma of the breast

Oral: It is not known if the same contraindications associated with long term progestin only contraceptives apply to the use of levonorgestrel and the emergency 2-dose regimen. A history of ectopic pregnancy is not a contraindication to use in emergency contraception.

Warnings/Precautions These products do not protect against HIV infection or other sexually-transmitted diseases. Menstrual bleeding patterns may be altered with use of the intrauterine device; the possibility of pregnancy should be considered if menstruation does not occur within 6 weeks of the previous menstrual period. If bleeding irregularities continue with prolonged use, appropriate diagnostic measures should be taken to rule out endometrial pathology. An increase in menstrual bleeding may indicate a partial or complete expulsion of the IUD. If expulsion occurs, device may be replaced within 7 days once pregnancy is ruled out. When using the oral tablet, the possibility of pregnancy should be considered if menstruation is delayed for >7 days of the expected menstrual period.

Patients taking progestin-only contraceptives and presenting with lower abdominal pain should be evaluated for follicular atresia and ectopic pregnancy. Use caution in patients with previous ectopic pregnancy. Women with history of ectopic pregnancy were excluded from clinical trials; women with previous ectopic pregnancy, tubal surgery, or pelvic infection may be at increased risk ectopic pregnancy. The possibility of ectopic pregnancy should be considered in patients with abdominal pain or vaginal bleeding in women with prior amenorrhea. Patients receiving hepatic enzyme-inducing medications should be evaluated for an alternative method of contraception. May have adverse effects on glucose tolerance; use caution in women with diabetes. Safety and efficacy for use in renal impairment has not been established. Not indicated for use in postmenopausal women.

The use of combination hormonal contraceptives has been associated with a slight increase in the frequency of breast cancer, however, studies are not consistent. Data is insufficient to determine if progestin only contraceptives also increase this risk. The risk of cardiovascular side effects increases in women using estrogen containing combined hormonal contraceptives and who smoke cigarettes, especially those who are >35 years of age. This risk relative to progestin-only contraceptives has not been established. Women who take contraceptives should be advised not to smoke

Additional formulation-specific warnings:

Intrauterine device: Insertion should be done by a trained healthcare provider. Increased incidence of group A streptococcal sepsis and pelvic inflammatory disease (may be asymptomatic). May perforate uterus or cervix; risk of perforation is increased in lactating women. Pregnancy may result if perforation occurs; delayed detection of perforation may result in migration of IUD outside of uterine cavity. Partial penetration or embedment in the myometrium may decrease effectiveness and lead to difficult removal. Use caution in patients with coagulopathy or receiving anticoagulants. Use caution in patients with congenital heart disease or other heart conditions which may increase the risk of infective endocarditis during insertion of the device (prophylactic antibiotics may be required at time of insertion). Bradycardia or syncope may occur during insertion or removal of the intrauterine device. The device should be removed for the following reasons: Bleeding which causes anemia; if the patient or her partner become HIV positive or acquire a sexually-transmitted disease; pelvic infection, endometritis, symptomatic genital actinomycosis; intractable pelvic pain, pain during intercourse; endometrial or cervical cancer; uterine or cervical perforation; pregnancy. Embedded devices should also be removed. Use caution with or consider removal of the intrauterine device if any of the following conditions occur for the first time during therapy: Migraine, severe headache, jaundice, marked increase in blood pressure, severe arterial disease (eg, stroke, MI). Use is contraindicated in patients with vaginitis or cervicitis. Postpone insertion until after treatment for infection is complete and cause of the cervicitis is proven not to be due to gonorrhea or chlamydia.

Oral tablet: Not intended to be used for routine contraception and will not terminate an existing pregnancy

Adverse Reactions

Intrauterine device:

>5%:

Cardiovascular: Hypertension

Central nervous system: Headache, depression, nervousness

Dermatologic: Acne

Endocrine & metabolic: Breast pain, dysmenorrhea, libido decreased, amenorrhea (20% at 1 year), enlarged follicles (12%), ovarian cysts

Gastrointestinal: Abdominal pain, nausea, weight gain

Genitourinary: Cervicitis, leukorrhea, pelvic pain, uterine/vaginal bleeding, vaginitis

Neuromuscular & skeletal: Back pain

<5%, postmarketing and/or case reports: Abdominal distension, alopecia, anemia, angioedema, device breakage, dyspareunia, eczema, edema, failed insertion, hirsutism, migraine, mood changes, pruritus, rash,sepsis, urticaria, vomiting

Oral tablets:

>10%:

Central nervous system: Fatigue (17%), headache (17%), dizziness (11%)

Endocrine & metabolic: Heavier menstrual bleeding (14%), lighter menstrual bleeding (12%), breast tenderness (11%)

Gastrointestinal: Nausea (23%), abdominal pain (18%)

1% to 10%: Gastrointestinal: Vomiting (6%), diarrhea (5%)

Drug Interactions

Metabolism/Transport Effects Substrate of CYP3A4 (major)

Avoid Concomitant Use

Avoid concomitant use of Levonorgestrel with any of the following: Acitretin; Griseofulvin

Increased Effect/Toxicity

Levonorgestrel may increase the levels/effects of: Benzodiazepines (metabolized by oxidation); Selegiline; Voriconazole

The levels/effects of Levonorgestrel may be increased by: Herbs (Progestogenic Properties); Voriconazole

Decreased Effect

Levonorgestrel may decrease the levels/effects of: Vitamin K Antagonists

The levels/effects of Levonorgestrel may be decreased by: Acitretin; Aminoglutethimide; Aprepitant; Barbiturates; CarBAMazepine; CYP3A4 Inducers (Strong); Deferasirox; Felbamate; Fosaprepitant; Griseofulvin; Mycophenolate; OXcarbazepine; Phenytoin; Retinoic Acid Derivatives; Rifamycin Derivatives; St Johns Wort

Ethanol/Nutrition/Herb Interactions Herb/Nutraceutical: St John's wort (an enzyme inducer) may decrease serum levels of levonorgestrel.

Stability Store at room temperature of 25°C (77°F).

Mechanism of Action Pregnancy may be prevented through several mechanisms: Thickening of cervical mucus, which inhibits sperm passage through the uterus and sperm survival; inhibition of ovulation, from a negative feedback mechanism on the hypothalamus, leading to reduced secretion of follicle stimulating hormone (FSH) and luteinizing hormone (LH); and inhibition of implantation. Levonorgestrel is not effective once the implantation process has begun.

Pharmacodynamics/Kinetics

Duration: Intrauterine device: Up to 5 years

Absorption: Oral: Rapid and complete

Protein binding: Highly bound to albumin (~50%) and sex hormone-binding globulin (~47%)

Metabolism: To inactive metabolites

Half-life elimination: Oral: ~24 hours

Excretion: Primarily urine

Dosage Adults: Females:

Long-term prevention of pregnancy: Intrauterine device: To be inserted into uterine cavity; should be inserted within 7 days of onset of menstruation or immediately after 1st trimester abortion; releases 20 mcg levonorgestrel/day over 5 years. May be removed and replaced with a new unit at anytime during menstrual cycle; do not leave any one system in place for >5 years

Emergency contraception: Oral tablet: One 0.75 mg tablet as soon as possible within 72 hours of unprotected sexual intercourse; a second 0.75 mg tablet should be taken 12 hours after the first dose; may be used at any time during menstrual cycle

Unlabeled dosing for emergency contraception: Two 0.75 mg tablets as a single dose **or** one 0.75 mg tablet followed by a second 0.75 mg tablet within 12-24 hours. Either regimen should be taken as soon as possible, but within 120 hours, following unprotected sexual intercourse.

Dosage adjustment in renal impairment: Safety and efficacy have not been established

Dosage adjustment in hepatic impairment: Safety and efficacy have not been established; use of the intrauterine device is contraindicated with active hepatic disease or hepatic tumor.

Elderly: Not indicated for use in postmenopausal women

Administration Intrauterine device: Inserted in the uterine cavity, to a depth of 6-9 cm, with the provided insertion device; should not be forced into the uterus

Monitoring Parameters IUD: Re-examine 4-12 weeks following insertion and then yearly. Threads should be visible; if length of thread has changed device may have become displaced, broken, perforated the uterus, or expelled. Transvaginal ultrasound may be used to check placement. Monitor for prolonged menstrual bleeding, amenorrhea, irregularity of menses, Pap smear, blood pressure, serum glucose in patients with diabetes, LDL levels in patients with hyperlipidemias; re-examine following first menses post-insertion of IUD. Patients presenting with lower abdominal pain should be evaluated for follicular atresia and ectopic pregnancy. Signs of infection following IUD insertion, especially in patients at increased risk (eg, patients on chronic corticosteroids, patients with type 1 diabetes mellitus).

Reference Range Intrauterine device: Plasma levels range from 150-200 pg/mL which are lower than those observed with other dosage forms of levonorgestrel

Test Interactions Decreased concentrations of sex hormone-binding globulin; decreased thyroxine concentrations (slight); increased triiodothyronine uptake

Additional Information Intrauterine device: The cumulative 5-year pregnancy rate is ~0.7 pregnancies/100 users. Over 70% of women in the trials had previously used IUDs. The reported pregnancy rate after 12 months was ≤0.2 pregnancies/100 users. Approximately 80% of women who wish to conceive have become pregnant within 12 months of device removal. The recommended patient profile for this product: A woman who has at least one child, is in a stable and mutually-monogamous relationship, no history of pelvic inflammatory disease, and no history of ectopic pregnancy or predisposition to ectopic pregnancy. Keep a copy of the consent form and record lot number of device.

Oral tablet: When used as directed for emergency contraception, the expected pregnancy rate is decreased from 8% to 1%. Approximately 87% of women have their next menstrual period at approximately the expected time. A rapid return to fertility following use is expected.

Dosage Forms Excipient information presented when available (limited, particularly for generics); consult specific product labeling.

Intrauterine device:
Mirena®: 52 mg/unit [releases levonorgestrel 20 mcg/day]
Tablet:
Plan B®: 0.75 mg

- **Levonorgestrel and Estradiol** *see* Estradiol and Levonorgestrel *on page 558*
- **Levonorgestrel and Ethinyl Estradiol** *see* Ethinyl Estradiol and Levonorgestrel *on page 577*
- **Levophed®** *see* Norepinephrine *on page 1077*
- **Levora®** *see* Ethinyl Estradiol and Levonorgestrel *on page 577*

Levorphanol (lee VOR fa nole)

U.S. Brand Names Levo-Dromoran®
Index Terms Levorphan Tartrate; Levorphanol Tartrate
Pharmacologic Category Analgesic, Opioid
Additional Appendix Information
Narcotic / Opioid Analgesics *on page 1663*
Use Relief of moderate to severe pain; also used parenterally for preoperative sedation and an adjunct to nitrous oxide/oxygen anesthesia
Restrictions C-II
Pregnancy Risk Factor B/D (prolonged use or high doses at term)
Medication Safety Issues
High alert medication: The Institute for Safe Medication Practices (ISMP) includes this medication among its list of drug classes which have a heightened risk of causing significant patient harm when used in error.
Dosage Adults: **Note:** These are guidelines and do not represent the maximum doses that may be required in all patients. Doses should be titrated to pain relief/prevention.
Acute pain (moderate to severe):
Oral: Initial: Opiate-naive: 2 mg every 6-8 hours as needed; patients with prior opiate exposure may require higher initial doses; usual dosage range: 2-4 mg every 6-8 hours as needed
I.M., SubQ: Initial: Opiate-naive: 1 mg every 6-8 hours as needed; patients with prior opiate exposure may require higher initial doses; usual dosage range: 1-2 mg every 6-8 hours as needed
Slow I.V.: Initial: Opiate-naive: Up to 1 mg/dose every 3-6 hours as needed; patients with prior opiate exposure may require higher initial doses
Chronic pain: Patients taking opioids chronically may become tolerant and require doses higher than the usual dosage range to maintain the desired effect. Tolerance can be managed by appropriate dose titration. **There is no optimal or maximal dose for levorphanol in chronic pain. The appropriate dose is one that relieves pain throughout its dosing interval without causing unmanageable side effects.**
Premedication: I.M., SubQ: 1-2 mg/dose 60-90 minutes prior to surgery; older or debilitated patients usually require less drug
Dosing adjustment in hepatic disease: Reduction is necessary in patients with liver disease
Additional Information Complete prescribing information for this medication should be consulted for additional detail.
Dosage Forms Excipient information presented when available (limited, particularly for generics); consult specific product labeling.
Injection, solution, as tartrate: 2 mg/mL (1 mL, 10 mL)
Tablet, as tartrate: 2 mg

- **Levorphanol Tartrate** *see* Levorphanol *on page 881*
- **Levorphan Tartrate** *see* Levorphanol *on page 881*
- **Levothroid®** *see* Levothyroxine *on page 881*

Levothyroxine (lee voe thye ROKS een)

U.S. Brand Names Levothroid®; Levoxyl®; Synthroid®; Unithroid®
Canadian Brand Names Eltroxin®; Euthyrox; Levothyroxine Sodium; Synthroid®
Index Terms *L*-Thyroxine Sodium; Levothyroxine Sodium; T_4
Pharmacologic Category Thyroid Product
Use Replacement or supplemental therapy in hypothyroidism; pituitary TSH suppression
Pregnancy Risk Factor A
Pregnancy Considerations Untreated maternal hypothyroidism may have adverse effects on fetal growth and development and is associated with higher rate of complications (spontaneous abortion, pre-eclampsia, stillbirth, premature delivery). Treatment should not be discontinued during pregnancy. TSH levels should be monitored during each trimester and 6-8 weeks postpartum. Increased doses may be needed during pregnancy.
Lactation Enters breast milk/compatible
Medication Safety Issues
Sound-alike/look-alike issues:
Levothyroxine may be confused with levofloxacin, liothyronine
Levoxyl® may be confused with Lanoxin®, Levaquin®, Luvox®
Synthroid® may be confused with Symmetrel®

To avoid errors due to misinterpretation of a decimal point, always express dosage in mcg (**not** mg).

Significant differences exist between oral and I.V. dosing. Use caution when converting from one route of administration to another.
Contraindications Hypersensitivity to levothyroxine sodium or any component of the formulation; recent MI or thyrotoxicosis; uncorrected adrenal insufficiency
Warnings/Precautions [U.S. Boxed Warning]: Ineffective and potentially toxic for weight reduction. High doses may produce serious or even life-threatening toxic effects particularly when used with some anorectic drugs. Use with caution and reduce dosage in patients with angina pectoris or other cardiovascular disease; decrease initial dose. Use cautiously in the elderly since they may be more likely to have compromised cardiovascular functions. Patients with adrenal insufficiency, myxedema, diabetes mellitus and insipidus may have symptoms exaggerated or aggravated. Chronic hypothyroidism predisposes patients to coronary artery disease. Long-term therapy can decrease bone mineral density. Levoxyl® may rapidly swell and disintegrate causing choking or gagging (should be administered with a full glass of water); use caution in patients with dysphagia or other swallowing disorders.
Adverse Reactions Frequency not defined.
Cardiovascular: Angina, arrhythmia, blood pressure increased, cardiac arrest, flushing, heart failure, MI, palpitation, pulse increased, tachycardia
Central nervous system: Anxiety, emotional lability, fatigue, fever, headache, hyperactivity, insomnia, irritability, nervousness, pseudotumor cerebri (children), seizure (rare)
Dermatologic: Alopecia
Endocrine & metabolic: Fertility impaired, menstrual irregularities
Gastrointestinal: Abdominal cramps, appetite increased, diarrhea, vomiting, weight loss
Hepatic: Liver function tests increased
Neuromuscular & skeletal: Bone mineral density decreased, muscle weakness, tremor, slipped capital femoral epiphysis (children)

Respiratory: Dyspnea
Miscellaneous: Diaphoresis, heat intolerance, hypersensitivity (to inactive ingredients, symptoms include urticaria, pruritus, rash, flushing, angioedema, GI symptoms, fever, arthralgia, serum sickness, wheezing)
Levoxyl®: Choking, dysphagia, gagging

Drug Interactions

Avoid Concomitant Use

Avoid concomitant use of Levothyroxine with any of the following: Sodium Iodide I131

Increased Effect/Toxicity

Levothyroxine may increase the levels/effects of: Vitamin K Antagonists

Decreased Effect

Levothyroxine may decrease the levels/effects of: Sodium Iodide I131; Theophylline Derivatives

The levels/effects of Levothyroxine may be decreased by: Bile Acid Sequestrants; CarBAMazepine; Estrogen Derivatives; Ferrous Sulfate; Orlistat; Phenytoin; Raloxifene; Rifampin; Sucralfate

Ethanol/Nutrition/Herb Interactions Food: Taking levothyroxine with enteral nutrition may cause reduced bioavailability and may lower serum thyroxine levels leading to signs or symptoms of hypothyroidism. Soybean flour (infant formula), cottonseed meal, walnuts, and dietary fiber may decrease absorption of levothyroxine from the GI tract.

Stability

Tablet: Store at room temperature of 15°C to 30°C (59°F to 86°F). Protect from light and moisture.
Injection: Store at room temperature of 15°C to 30°C (59°F to 86°F). Dilute vials for injection with 5 mL normal saline. Reconstituted concentrations for the 200 mcg and 500 mcg vials are 40 mcg/mL and 100 mcg/mL, respectively. Shake well. Reconstituted solutions should be used immediately and any unused portions discarded.

Mechanism of Action Exact mechanism of action is unknown; however, it is believed the thyroid hormone exerts its many metabolic effects through control of DNA transcription and protein synthesis; involved in normal metabolism, growth, and development; promotes gluconeogenesis, increases utilization and mobilization of glycogen stores, and stimulates protein synthesis, increases basal metabolic rate

Pharmacodynamics/Kinetics

Onset of action: Therapeutic: Oral: 3-5 days; I.V. 6-8 hours
Peak effect: I.V.: 24 hours
Absorption: Oral: Erratic (40% to 80%); may be decreased by age and specific foods and drugs
Protein binding: >99%
Metabolism: Hepatic to triiodothyronine (active)
Time to peak, serum: 2-4 hours
Half-life elimination: Euthyroid: 6-7 days; Hypothyroid: 9-10 days; Hyperthyroid: 3-4 days
Excretion: Urine and feces; decreases with age

Dosage Doses should be adjusted based on clinical response and laboratory parameters.

Oral:

Children: Hypothyroidism:

Newborns: Initial: 10-15 mcg/kg/day. Lower doses of 25 mcg/day should be considered in newborns at risk for cardiac failure. Newborns with T_4 levels <5 mcg/dL should be started at 50 mcg/day. Adjust dose at 4- to 6-week intervals.

Infants and Children: Dose based on body weight and age as listed below. Children with severe or chronic hypothyroidism should be started at 25 mcg/day; adjust dose by 25 mcg every 2-4 weeks. In older children, hyperactivity may be decreased by starting with 1/4 of the recommended dose and increasing by 1/4 dose each week until the full replacement dose is reached. Refer to adult dosing once growth and puberty are complete:
0-3 months: 10-15 mcg/kg/day
3-6 months: 8-10 mcg/kg/day
6-12 months: 6-8 mcg/kg/day
1-5 years: 5-6 mcg/kg/day
6-12 years: 4-5 mcg/kg/day
>12 years: 2-3 mcg/kg/day

Adults:

Hypothyroidism: 1.7 mcg/kg/day in otherwise healthy adults <50 years old, children in whom growth and puberty are complete, and older adults who have been recently treated for hyperthyroidism or who have been hypothyroid for only a few months. Titrate dose every 6 weeks. Average full replacement dose is 100-125 mcg/day for a 70 kg adult; usual doses are ≤200 mcg/day; doses ≥300 mcg/day are rare (consider poor compliance, malabsorption, and/or drug interactions). **Note:** For patients >50 years or patients with cardiac disease, refer to Elderly dosing.

Severe hypothyroidism: Initial: 12.5-25 mcg/day; adjust dose by 25 mcg/day every 2-4 weeks as appropriate; **Note:** Oral agents are not recommended for myxedema (see I.V. dosing).

Subclinical hypothyroidism (if treated): 1 mcg/kg/day

TSH suppression:

Well-differentiated thyroid cancer: Highly individualized; Doses >2 mcg/kg/day may be needed to suppress TSH to <0.1 mU/L. High-risk tumors may need a target level of <0.01 mU/L for TSH suppression.

Benign nodules and nontoxic multinodular goiter: Goal TSH suppression: 0.1-0.5 mU/L (benign nodules) and 0.5-1 mU/L (multinodular goiter)

Elderly: Hypothyroidism:

>50 years without cardiac disease **or** <50 years with cardiac disease: Initial: 25-50 mcg/day; adjust dose at 6- to 8-week intervals as needed

>50 years with cardiac disease: Initial: 12.5-25 mcg/day; adjust dose by 12.5-25 mcg increments at 4- to 6-week intervals. (**Note:** Many clinicians prefer to adjust at 6- to 8-week intervals.)

Note: Elderly patients may require <1 mcg/kg/day

I.M., I.V.: Children, Adults, Elderly: Hypothyroidism: 50% of the oral dose

I.V.:

Adults: Myxedema coma or stupor: 200-500 mcg, then 100-300 mcg the next day if necessary; smaller doses should be considered in patients with cardiovascular disease

Elderly: Myxedema coma: Refer to adult dosing; lower doses may be needed

Dietary Considerations Should be taken on an empty stomach, at least 30 minutes before food.

Administration

Oral: Administer in the morning on an empty stomach, at least 30 minutes before food. Tablets may be crushed and suspended in 1-2 teaspoonfuls of water; suspension should be used immediately. Levoxyl® should be administered with a full glass of water to prevent gagging (due to tablet swelling).

Parenteral: Dilute vial with 5 mL normal saline; use immediately after reconstitution; should not be admixed with other solutions

Monitoring Parameters Thyroid function test (serum thyroxine, thyrotropin concentrations), resin triiodothyronine uptake (rT_3U), free thyroxine index (FTI), T_4, TSH, heart rate, blood pressure, clinical signs of hypo- and hyperthyroidism; TSH is the most reliable guide for evaluating adequacy of thyroid replacement dosage. TSH may be elevated during the first few months of thyroid replacement despite patients being clinically euthyroid. In cases where T_4 remains low and TSH is within normal limits, an evaluation of "free" (unbound) T_4 is needed to evaluate further increase in dosage

Infants: Monitor closely for cardiac overload, arrhythmias, and aspiration from avid suckling

Infants/children: Monitor closely for under/overtreatment. Undertreatment may decrease intellectual development and linear growth, and lead to poor school performance due to impaired concentration and slowed mentation. Overtreatment may adversely affect brain maturation, accelerate bone age (leading to premature closure of the epiphyses and reduced adult height); craniosynostosis has been reported in infants. Treated children may experience a period of catch-up growth. Monitor TSH and total or free T_4 at 2 and 4 weeks after starting treatment; every 1-2 months for first year of life; every 2-3 months during years 1-3; every 3-12 months until growth completed.

Adults: Monitor TSH every 6-8 weeks until normalized; 8-12 weeks after dosage changes; every 6-12 months throughout therapy

Reference Range Pediatrics: Cord T_4 and values in the first few weeks are much higher, falling over the first months and years. ≥10 years: ~5.8-11 mcg/dL (SI: 75-142 nmol/L). Borderline low: ≤4.5-5.7 mcg/dL (SI: 58-73 nmol/L); low: ≤4.4 mcg/dL (SI: 57 nmol/L); results <2.5 mcg/dL (SI: <32 nmol/L) are strong evidence for hypothyroidism.

Approximate adult normal range: 4-12 mcg/dL (SI: 51-154 nmol/L). Borderline high: 11.1-13 mcg/dL (SI: 143-167 nmol/L); high: ≥13.1 mcg/dL (SI: 169 nmol/L). Normal range is increased in women on birth control pills (5.5-12 mcg/dL); normal range in pregnancy: ~5.5-16 mcg/dL (SI: ~71-206 nmol/L). TSH: 0.4-10 (for those ≥80 years) mIU/L; T_4: 4-12 mcg/dL (SI: 51-154 nmol/L); T_3 (RIA) (total T_3): 80-230 ng/dL (SI: 1.2-3.5 nmol/L); T_4 free (free T_4): 0.7-1.8 ng/dL (SI: 9-23 pmol/L).

Test Interactions Many drugs may have effects on thyroid function tests (see Additional Information). Pregnancy, infectious hepatitis, and acute intermittent porphyria may increase TBG concentrations; nephrosis, severe hypoproteinemia, severe liver disease, and acromegaly may decrease TBG concentrations.

Additional Information Equivalent doses: The following statement on relative potency of thyroid products is included in a joint statement by American Thyroid Association (ATA), American Association of Clinical Endocrinologists (AACE) and The Endocrine Society (TES): For purposes of conversion, levothyroxine sodium (T_4) 100 mcg is usually considered equivalent to desiccated thyroid 60 mg, thyroglobulin 60 mg, or liothyronine sodium (T_3) 25 mcg. However, these are rough guidelines only and do not obviate the careful re-evaluation of a patient when switching thyroid hormone preparations, including a change from one brand of levothyroxine to another. Joint position statement is available at http://www.thyroid.org/professionals/advocacy/04_12_08_thyroxine.html.

Note: Several medications have effects on thyroid production or conversion. The impact in thyroid replacement has not been specifically evaluated, but patient response should be monitored:

Methimazole: Decreases thyroid hormone secretion, while propylthiouracil decrease thyroid hormone secretion and decreases conversion of T_4 to T_3.

Beta-adrenergic antagonists: Decrease conversion of T_4 to T_3 (dose related, propranolol ≥160 mg/day); patients may be clinically euthyroid.

Iodide, iodine-containing radiographic contrast agents may decrease thyroid hormone secretion; may also increase thyroid hormone secretion, especially in patients with Graves' disease.

Other agents reported to impact on thyroid production/conversion include aminoglutethimide, amiodarone, chloral hydrate, diazepam, ethionamide, interferon-alpha, interleukin-2, lithium, lovastatin (case report), glucocorticoids (dose-related), mercaptopurine, sulfonamides, thiazide diuretics, and tolbutamide.

In addition, a number of medications have been noted to cause transient depression in TSH secretion, which may complicate interpretation of monitoring tests for levothyroxine, including corticosteroids, octreotide, and dopamine. Metoclopramide may increase TSH secretion

Dosage Forms Excipient information presented when available (limited, particularly for generics); consult specific product labeling.

Injection, powder for reconstitution, as sodium: 0.2 mg, 0.5 mg

Tablet, as sodium: 25 mcg, 50 mcg, 75 mcg, 88 mcg, 100 mcg, 112 mcg, 125 mcg, 137 mcg, 150 mcg, 175 mcg, 200 mcg, 300 mcg

- Levothroid®: 25 mcg, 50 mcg, 75 mcg, 88 mcg, 100 mcg, 112 mcg, 125 mcg, 137 mcg, 150 mcg, 175 mcg, 200 mcg, 300 mcg
- Levoxyl®: 25 mcg, 50 mcg, 75 mcg, 88 mcg, 100 mcg, 112 mcg, 125 mcg, 137 mcg, 150 mcg, 175 mcg, 200 mcg
- Synthroid®: 25 mcg, 50 mcg, 75 mcg, 88 mcg, 100 mcg, 112 mcg, 125 mcg, 137 mcg, 150 mcg, 175 mcg, 200 mcg, 300 mcg
- Unithroid®: 25 mcg, 50 mcg, 75 mcg, 88 mcg, 100 mcg, 112 mcg, 125 mcg, 150 mcg, 175 mcg, 200 mcg, 300 mcg

◆ **Levothyroxine Sodium** *see* Levothyroxine *on page 881*
◆ **Levoxyl®** *see* Levothyroxine *on page 881*
◆ **Levsin®** *see* Hyoscyamine *on page 756*
◆ **Levsin®/SL** *see* Hyoscyamine *on page 756*
◆ **Levulan® (Can)** *see* Aminolevulinic Acid *on page 86*
◆ **Levulan® Kerastick®** *see* Aminolevulinic Acid *on page 86*
◆ **Lexapro®** *see* Escitalopram *on page 547*
◆ **Lexiva®** *see* Fosamprenavir *on page 664*
◆ **Lexxel® [DSC]** *see* Enalapril and Felodipine *on page 518*
◆ **Lexxel® (Can)** *see* Enalapril and Felodipine *on page 518*
◆ **LFA-3/IgG(1) Fusion Protein, Human** *see* Alefacept *on page 55*
◆ **L-Glutamine** *see* Glutamine *on page 700*
◆ **LHRH** *see* Gonadorelin *on page 704*
◆ **LH-RH Agonist** *see* Histrelin *on page 732*
◆ ***l*-Hyoscyamine Sulfate** *see* Hyoscyamine *on page 756*
◆ **Lialda™** *see* Mesalamine *on page 949*
◆ **Librax® *[reformulation]* [DSC]** *see* Chlordiazepoxide and Methscopolamine *on page 305*
◆ **Librax® *[original formulation]*** *see* Clidinium and Chlordiazepoxide *on page 344*
◆ **Librax® (Can)** *see* Clidinium and Chlordiazepoxide *on page 344*
◆ **Librium®** *see* ChlordiazePOXIDE *on page 303*
◆ **Licide® [OTC]** *see* Pyrethrins and Piperonyl Butoxide *on page 1271*
◆ **LidaMantle®** *see* Lidocaine *on page 884*
◆ **Lidemol® (Can)** *see* Fluocinonide *on page 634*
◆ **Lidex® [DSC]** *see* Fluocinonide *on page 634*
◆ **Lidex® (Can)** *see* Fluocinonide *on page 634*
◆ **Lidex-E® [DSC]** *see* Fluocinonide *on page 634*

Lidocaine (LYE doe kane)

U.S. Brand Names Akten™; Anestacon®; Anestafoam™ [OTC]; Band-Aid® Hurt-Free™ Antiseptic Wash [OTC]; Burn Jel® [OTC]; Burn-O-Jel [OTC]; Burnamycin [OTC]; L-M-X™ 4 [OTC]; L-M-X™ 5 [OTC]; LidaMantle®; Lidoderm®; LTA® 360; Premjact® [OTC]; Solarcaine® Aloe Extra Burn Relief [OTC]; Topicaine® [OTC]; Unburn®; Xylocaine®; Xylocaine® MPF; Xylocaine® Viscous; Zilactin-L® [OTC]; Zingo™

Canadian Brand Names Betacaine®; Lidodan™; Lidoderm®; Xylocaine®; Xylocard®; Zilactin®

Index Terms Lidocaine Hydrochloride; Lignocaine Hydrochloride

Pharmacologic Category Analgesic, Topical; Antiarrhythmic Agent, Class Ib; Local Anesthetic; Local Anesthetic, Ophthalmic

Use Local anesthetic and acute treatment of ventricular arrhythmias (such as from myocardial infarction or cardiac manipulation)

Intradermal: To provide local anesthesia prior to venipuncture or peripheral I.V. cannulation

Ophthalmic: To provide local anesthesia to ocular surface during ophthalmologic procedures

Rectal: Temporary relief of pain and itching due to anorectal disorders

Topical: Local anesthetic for use in laser, cosmetic, and outpatient surgeries; minor burns, cuts, and abrasions of the skin

Lidoderm® Patch: Relief of allodynia (painful hypersensitivity) and chronic pain in postherpetic neuralgia

Unlabeled/Investigational Use ACLS guidelines (not considered drug of choice): Stable monomorphic VT (preserved ventricular function), polymorphic VT (preserved ventricular function), drug-induced monomorphic VT

Pregnancy Risk Factor B

Pregnancy Considerations Animal studies with lidocaine have not shown teratogenic effects. Use is not contraindicated during labor and delivery. Systemic exposure following use of the intradermal system is below the limit of detection.

Lactation Enters breast milk (small amounts)/use caution (AAP rates "compatible")

Medication Safety Issues

High alert medication: The Institute for Safe Medication Practices (ISMP) includes this medication (epidural administration; I.V. formulation) among its list of drugs which have a heightened risk of causing significant patient harm when used in error.

Transdermal patch may contain conducting metal (eg, aluminum); remove patch prior to MRI.

International issues:

Lidpen® may be confused with Linoten® which is a brand name for pamidronate in Spain

Contraindications Hypersensitivity to lidocaine or any component of the formulation; hypersensitivity to another local anesthetic of the amide type; Adam-Stokes syndrome; severe degrees of SA, AV, or intraventricular heart block (except in patients with a functioning artificial pacemaker); premixed injection may contain corn-derived dextrose and its use is contraindicated in patients with allergy to corn-related products

Warnings/Precautions Use caution in patients with severe hepatic dysfunction or pseudocholinesterase deficiency; may have increased risk of lidocaine toxicity.

Intravenous: Constant ECG monitoring is necessary during I.V. administration. Use cautiously in hepatic impairment, any degree of heart block, Wolff-Parkinson-White syndrome, HF, marked hypoxia, severe respiratory depression, hypovolemia, history of malignant hyperthermia, or shock. Increased ventricular rate may be seen when administered to a patient with atrial fibrillation. Correct electrolyte disturbances, especially hypokalemia or hypomagnesemia, prior to use and throughout therapy. Correct any underlying causes of ventricular arrhythmias. Monitor closely for signs and symptoms of CNS toxicity. The elderly may be prone to increased CNS and cardiovascular side effects. Reduce dose in hepatic dysfunction and CHF.

Injectable anesthetic: Follow appropriate administration techniques so as not to administer any intravascularly. Solutions containing antimicrobial preservatives should not be used for epidural or spinal anesthesia. Some solutions contain a bisulfite; avoid in patients who are allergic to bisulfite. Resuscitative equipment, medicine and oxygen should be available in case of emergency. Use products containing epinephrine cautiously in patients with significant vascular disease, compromised blood flow, or during or following general anesthesia (increased risk of arrhythmias). Adjust the dose for the elderly, pediatric, acutely ill, and debilitated patients.

Intradermal: For use on intact skin where adequate seal can be maintained. Do not apply to body orifices or mucous membranes. Use caution in patients with bleeding tendencies or platelet disorders; may have increased risk of superficial dermal bleeding. Safety and efficacy have not been established in children <3 years of age or adults.

Ophthalmic: For ophthalmic use only; not for injection. Prolonged use may cause permanent corneal ulceration and/or opacification with loss of vision.

Topical: Do not leave on large body areas for >2 hours. Potentially life threatening side effects (eg, irregular heart beat, seizures, coma, respiratory depression, death) have occurred when used prior to cosmetic procedures. Observe young children closely to prevent accidental ingestion. Not for ophthalmic use. Some products are not recommended for use on mucous membranes; consult specific product labeling.

Transdermal patch: Safety and efficacy have not been established in children.

Adverse Reactions Effects vary with route of administration. Many effects are dose related.

Frequency not defined.

Cardiovascular: Arrhythmia, bradycardia, arterial spasms, cardiovascular collapse, defibrillator threshold increased, edema, flushing, heart block, hypotension, sinus node supression, vascular insufficiency (periarticular injections)

Central nervous system: Agitation, anxiety, apprehension, coma, confusion, disorientation, dizziness, drowsiness, euphoria, hallucinations, headache, hyperesthesia, hypoesthesia, lethargy, lightheadedness, nervousness, psychosis, seizure, slurred speech, somnolence, unconsciousness

Dermatologic: Angioedema, bruising (transdermal system), contact dermatitis, depigmentation (transdermal system), edema of the skin, itching, petechia (transdermal system), pruritus, rash, urticaria

Gastrointestinal: Metallic taste, nausea, vomiting

Local: Burning (ophthalmic), irritation (transdermal system), thrombophlebitis

Neuromuscular & skeletal: Pain exacerbation (transdermal system), paresthesia, transient radicular pain (subarachnoid administration; up to 1.9%), tremor, twitching, weakness

Ocular: Conjunctival hyperemia (ophthalmic), corneal epithelial changes (ophthalmic), diplopia, visual changes

Otic: Tinnitus

Respiratory: Bronchospasm, dyspnea, respiratory depression or arrest

Miscellaneous: Allergic reactions, anaphylactoid reaction, sensitivity to temperature extremes

Intradermal system: Application site reactions: Erythema (53%), petechiae (44%), edema (8%), bruising/burning/contusion/hemorrhage/pain (4%), pruritus (1%; equal to placebo)

Following spinal anesthesia: Positional headache (3%), shivering (2%) nausea, peripheral nerve symptoms, respiratory inadequacy and double vision (<1%), hypotension, cauda equina syndrome

Postmarketing and/or case reports: ARDS (inhalation), asystole, disorientation, methemoglobinemia, skin reaction

Drug Interactions

Metabolism/Transport Effects Substrate of CYP1A2 (minor), 2A6 (minor), 2B6 (minor), 2C9 (minor), 2D6 (major), 3A4 (major); **Inhibits** CYP1A2 (strong), 2D6 (moderate), 3A4 (moderate)

Avoid Concomitant Use

Avoid concomitant use of Lidocaine with any of the following: Thioridazine

Increased Effect/Toxicity

Lidocaine may increase the levels/effects of: Bendamustine; CYP1A2 Substrates; CYP2D6 Substrates; CYP3A4 Substrates; Eplerenone; Fesoterodine; Maraviroc; Pimecrolimus; Ranolazine; Salmeterol; Tamoxifen; Thioridazine

The levels/effects of Lidocaine may be increased by: Amiodarone; Beta-Blockers; CYP2D6 Inhibitors (Moderate); CYP2D6 Inhibitors (Strong); CYP3A4 Inhibitors (Moderate); CYP3A4 Inhibitors (Strong); Darunavir; Dasatinib; Disopyramide; P-Glycoprotein Inhibitors

Decreased Effect

Lidocaine may decrease the levels/effects of: TraMADol

The levels/effects of Lidocaine may be decreased by: CYP3A4 Inducers (Strong); Deferasirox; Herbs (CYP3A4 Inducers); P-Glycoprotein Inducers

Ethanol/Nutrition/Herb Interactions Herb/Nutraceutical: St John's wort may decrease lidocaine levels; avoid concurrent use.

Stability

Injection: Stable at room temperature. Stability of parenteral admixture at room temperature (25°C) is the expiration date on premixed bag; out of overwrap stability is 30 days.

Standard concentration/diluent: 2 g/250 mL D_5W.

Ophthalmic: Store at 15°C to 25°C (59°F to 77°F). Protect from light. Discard after use.

Mechanism of Action Class Ib antiarrhythmic; suppresses automaticity of conduction tissue, by increasing electrical stimulation threshold of ventricle, His-Purkinje system, and spontaneous depolarization of the ventricles during diastole by a direct action on the tissues; blocks both the initiation and conduction of nerve impulses by decreasing the neuronal membrane's permeability to sodium ions, which results in inhibition of depolarization with resultant blockade of conduction

Pharmacodynamics/Kinetics

Onset of action: Single bolus dose: 45-90 seconds; Intradermal: 1-3 minutes; Ophthalmic: 20 seconds to 5 minutes (median: 40 seconds)

Duration: 10-20 minutes; Intradermal: Decreases after 10 minutes; Ophthalmic: 5-30 minutes (median: 15 minutes)

Absorption: Intradermal: Below limit of detection (<5 ng/mL)

Distribution: V_d: 1.1-2.1 L/kg; alterable by many patient factors; decreased in CHF and liver disease; crosses blood-brain barrier

Protein binding: 60% to 80% to $alpha_1$ acid glycoprotein

Metabolism: 90% hepatic; active metabolites monoethylglycinexylidide (MEGX) and glycinexylidide (GX) can accumulate and may cause CNS toxicity

Half-life elimination: Biphasic: Prolonged with congestive heart failure, liver disease, shock, severe renal disease; Initial: 7-30 minutes; Terminal: Infants, premature: 3.2 hours, Adults: 1.5-2 hours

Excretion: Urine (<10% as unchanged drug, ~90% as metabolites)

Dosage

Antiarrhythmic:

Children:

I.V., I.O.: **Note:** For use in pulseless VT or VF, give after defibrillation, CPR, and epinephrine:

Loading dose: 1 mg/kg (maximum 100 mg); follow with continuous infusion; may administer second bolus of 0.5-1 mg/kg if delay between bolus and start of infusion is >15 minutes

Continuous infusion: 20-50 mcg/kg/minute. Use 20 mcg/kg/minute in patients with shock, hepatic disease, cardiac arrest, mild CHF; moderate-to-severe CHF may require 1/2 loading dose and lower infusion rates to avoid toxicity.

E.T.: 2-3 mg/kg; flush with 5 mL of NS and follow with 5 assisted manual ventilations

Adults:

Ventricular fibrillation or pulseless ventricular tachycardia (after defibrillation, CPR, and vasopressor administration): I.V.: Initial: 1-1.5 mg/kg. Refractory ventricular tachycardia or ventricular fibrillation, a repeat 0.5-0.75 mg/kg bolus may be given every 5-10 minutes after initial dose for a maximum of 3 doses. Total dose should not exceed 3 mg/kg. Follow with continuous infusion (1-4 mg/minute) after return of perfusion. Reappearance of arrhythmia during constant infusion: 0.5 mg/kg bolus and reassessment of infusion.

E.T. (loading dose only): 2-2.5 times the recommended I.V. dose; dilute in 10 mL NS or distilled water. **Note:** Absorption is greater with distilled water, but causes more adverse effects on PaO_2.

Hemodynamically stable VT: 0.5-0.75 mg/kg followed by synchronized cardioversion

Note: Decrease dose in patients with CHF, shock, or hepatic disease.

Anesthesia, intradermal: Children 3-18 years: Zingo™: 0.5 mg to site of venipuncture or peripheral I.V. cannulation, 1-3 minutes prior to procedure. Procedure should be started within 10 minutes of application.

Anesthetic, local injectable: Children and Adults: Varies with procedure, degree of anesthesia needed, vascularity of tissue, duration of anesthesia required, and physical condition of patient; maximum: 4.5 mg/kg/dose; do not repeat within 2 hours.

Anesthesia, ocular: Children and Adults: Apply 2 drops to ocular surface in area where procedure will occur; may reapply to maintain effect.

Anesthesia, topical:

Cream:

LidaMantle®: Skin irritation: Children and Adults: Apply to affected area 2-3 times/day as needed

L-M-X™ 4: Children ≥2 years and Adults: Apply 1/4 inch thick layer to intact skin. Leave on until adequate anesthetic effect is obtained. Remove cream and cleanse area before beginning procedure.

L-M-X™ 5: Relief of anorectal pain and itching: Children ≥12 years and Adults: Rectal: Apply topically to clean, dry area **or** using applicator, insert rectally, up to 6 times/day

Gel, ointment, solution: Adults: Apply to affected area ≤3 times/day as needed (maximum dose: 4.5 mg/kg, not to exceed 300 mg)

Jelly:

Children ≥10 years: Dose varies with age and weight (maximum dose: 4.5 mg/kg)

Adults (maximum dose: 30 mL [600 mg] in any 12-hour period):

Anesthesia of male urethra: 5-30 mL

Anesthesia of female urethra: 3-5 mL

Lubrication of endotracheal tube: Apply a moderate amount to external surface only

Liquid: Cold sores and fever blisters: Children ≥5 years and Adults: Apply to affected area every 6 hours as needed

Patch: Postherpetic neuralgia: Adults: Apply patch to most painful area. Up to 3 patches may be applied in a single application. Patch may remain in place for up to 12 hours in any 24-hour period.

Dosage adjustment in renal impairment: Not dialyzable (0% to 5%) by hemo- or peritoneal dialysis; supplemental dose is not necessary.

Dosage adjustment in hepatic impairment: Reduce dose in acute hepatitis and decompensated cirrhosis by 50%.

Dietary Considerations Premixed injection may contain corn-derived dextrose and its use is contraindicated in patients with allergy to corn-related products.

Administration

Endotracheal: Dilute in NS or distilled water. Absorption is greater with distilled water, but causes more adverse effects on PaO_2. Pass catheter beyond tip of tracheal tube, stop compressions, spray drug quickly down tube. Follow immediately with several quick insufflations and continue chest compressions.

I.V.: Use microdrip (60 gtt/mL) or infusion pump to administer an accurate dose

Infusion rates: 2 g/250 mL D_5W (infusion pump should be used):

1 mg/minute: 7.5 mL/hour

2 mg/minute: 15 mL/hour

3 mg/minute: 22.5 mL/hour

4 mg/minute: 30 mL/hour

Buffered lidocaine for injectable local anesthetic: Add 2 mL of sodium bicarbonate 8.4% to 18 mL of lidocaine 1%

Topical:

Gel (Topicaine®): Avoid mucous membranes; remove prior to laser treatment.

Transdermal: Apply to painful area of skin immediately after removal from protective envelope. May be cut to appropriate size. After removal from skin, fold used transdermal systems so the adhesive side sticks to itself. Remove immediately if burning sensation occurs. Wash hands after application.

Intradermal (Zingo™): Apply to intact skin do not use on mucous membranes. When placing intradermal injection system on skin, hold device perpendicular to skin and seal to avoid gaps between system and skin which would impair drug delivery. A "popping" sound will indicate dose has been discharged. If needed, may apply at a new location following failed attempt at venous access; do not apply multiple times at the same site.

Reference Range

Therapeutic: 1.5-5.0 mcg/mL (SI: 6-21 μmol/L)

Potentially toxic: >6 mcg/mL (SI: >26 μmol/L)

Toxic: >9 mcg/mL (SI: >38 μmol/L)

Dosage Forms Excipient information presented when available (limited, particularly for generics); consult specific product labeling. [DSC] = Discontinued product

Aerosol, topical [foam]:

Anestafoam™: 4% (30 g) [contains benzalkonium chloride and benzyl alcohol]

Cream, rectal (L-M-X™ 5): 5% (15 g) [contains benzyl alcohol; packaged with applicator]; (30 g) [contains benzyl alcohol]

Cream, topical (L-M-X™ 4): 4% (5 g) [contains benzyl alcohol; packaged with Tegaderm™ dressing]; (15 g, 30 g) [contains benzyl alcohol]

Cream, topical, as hydrochloride: 3% (30 g)

LidaMantle®: 3% (30 g, 85 g)

Gel, ophthalmic:

Akten™: 3.5% (5 mL) [preservative free]

Gel, topical:

Burn-O-Jel: 0.5% (90 g)

Topicaine®: 4% (10 g, 30 g, 113 g) [contains alcohol 35%, benzyl alcohol, aloe vera, and jojoba]

Gel, topical, as hydrochloride:

Burn Jel®: 2% (3.5 g, 120 g)

Solarcaine® Aloe Extra Burn Relief: 0.5% (113 g, 226 g) [contains aloe vera gel and tartrazine]

Unburn®: 2.5% (3.5 g, 59 mL, 118 mL) [contains vitamin E]

Infusion, as hydrochloride [premixed in D_5W]: 0.4% [4 mg/mL] (250 mL, 500 mL); 0.8% [8 mg/mL] (250 mL, 500 mL)

Injection, solution, as hydrochloride: 0.5% [5 mg/mL] (50 mL); 1% [10 mg/mL] (2 mL, 10 mL, 20 mL, 30 mL, 50 mL); 2% [20 mg/mL] (2 mL, 5 mL, 20 mL, 50 mL)

Xylocaine®: 0.5% [5 mg/mL] (50 mL); 1% [10 mg/mL] (10 mL, 20 mL, 50 mL); 2% [20 mg/mL] (1.8 mL, 10 mL, 20 mL, 50 mL)

Injection, solution, as hydrochloride [preservative free]: 0.5% [5 mg/mL] (50 mL); 1% [10 mg/mL] (2 mL, 5 mL, 30 mL); 1.5% [15 mg/mL] (20 mL); 2% [20 mg/mL] (2 mL, 5 mL, 10 mL); 4% [40 mg/mL] (5 mL)

Xylocaine®: 10% [100 mg/mL] (5 mL) [for ventricular arrhythmias]

Xylocaine® MPF: 0.5% [5 mg/mL] (50 mL); 1% [10 mg/mL] (2 mL, 5 mL, 10 mL, 30 mL); 1.5% [15 mg/mL] (10 mL, 20 mL); 2% [20 mg/mL] (2 mL, 5 mL, 10 mL); 4% [40 mg/mL] (5 mL)

Injection, solution, as hydrochloride [premixed in $D_{7.5}W$, preservative free]: 5% (2 mL)

Xylocaine® MPF: 1.5% (2 mL) [DSC]

Jelly, topical, as hydrochloride: 2% (5 mL, 30 mL)

Anestacon®: 2% (15 mL) [contains benzalkonium chloride]

Xylocaine®: 2% (5 mL, 30 mL)

Liquid, topical (Zilactin®-L): 2.5% (7.5 mL)

Lotion, topical, as hydrochloride (LidaMantle®): 3% (177 mL)

Ointment, topical: 5% (37 g, 50 g)

Powder, intradermal, as hydrochloride:

Zingo™: 0.5 mg

Solution, topical, as hydrochloride: 4% [40 mg/mL] (50 mL)

Band-Aid® Hurt-Free™ Antiseptic Wash: 2% (180 mL)

LTA® 360: 4% [40 mg/mL] (4 mL) [packaged with cannula for laryngotracheal administration]

Xylocaine®: 4% [40 mg/mL] (50 mL)

Solution, viscous, as hydrochloride: 2% [20 mg/mL] (20 mL, 100 mL)

Xylocaine® Viscous: 2% [20 mg/mL] (100 mL, 450 mL)

Spray, topical:

Burnamycin: 0.5% (60 mL) [contains aloe vera gel and menthol]

Premjact®: 9.6% (13 mL)

Solarcaine® Aloe Extra Burn Relief: 0.5% (127 g) [contains aloe vera]

Transdermal system, topical (Lidoderm®): 5% (30s)

Lidocaine and Bupivacaine

(LYE doe kane & byoo PIV a kane)

U.S. Brand Names Duocaine™

Index Terms Bupivacaine and Lidocaine; Lidocaine Hydrochloride and Bupivacaine Hydrochloride

Pharmacologic Category Local Anesthetic

Use Local or regional anesthesia in ophthalmologic surgery by peripheral nerve block techniques such as peribulbar, retrobulbar, and facial blocks; may be used with or without epinephrine

Pregnancy Risk Factor C

Dosage Children ≥12 years and Adults: **Note:** Use lowest effective dose to limit toxic effects. Dosing based on lidocaine 1% and bupivacaine 0.375%

Retrobulbar injection: 2-5 mL; a portion of dose is injected retrobulbarly and remainder may be used to block the facial nerve

Peribulbar block: 6-12 mL

Maximum dose: 0.18 mL/kg or 12 mL; if used with epinephrine, the dose should not exceed 0.28 mL/kg or 20 mL

Dosage adjustment in renal impairment: Lidocaine: Accumulation of metabolites may increase with renal impairment

Dosage adjustment in hepatic impairment:

Lidocaine: Half-life of lidocaine is increased twofold with hepatic impairment

Bupivacaine: Toxicities may be increased with hepatic impairment

Additional Information Complete prescribing information for this medication should be consulted for additional detail.

Dosage Forms Excipient information presented when available (limited, particularly for generics); consult specific product labeling.

Injection, solution [preservative free]: Lidocaine hydrochloride 1% and bupivacaine hydrochloride 0.375% (10 mL)

Lidocaine and Epinephrine

(LYE doe kane & ep i NEF rin)

U.S. Brand Names LidoSite™; Lignospan® Forte; Lignospan® Standard; Xylocaine® MPF With Epinephrine; Xylocaine® With Epinephrine

Canadian Brand Names Xylocaine® With Epinephrine

Index Terms Epinephrine and Lidocaine

Pharmacologic Category Local Anesthetic

Use Local infiltration anesthesia; AVS for nerve block; topical local analgesia for superficial dermatologic procedures

Pregnancy Risk Factor B

Medication Safety Issues

Transdermal patch may contain conducting metal (eg, aluminum); remove patch prior to MRI.

Dosage Dosage varies with the anesthetic procedure, degree of anesthesia needed, vascularity of tissue, duration of anesthesia required, and physical condition of patient.

Dental anesthesia, infiltration, or conduction block:

Children <10 years: 20-30 mg (1-1.5 mL) of lidocaine hydrochloride as a 2% solution with epinephrine 1:100,000; maximum: 4-5 mg of lidocaine hydrochloride/kg of body weight or 100-150 mg as a single dose

Children >10 years and Adults: Do not exceed 6.6 mg/kg body weight or 300 mg of lidocaine hydrochloride and 3 mcg (0.003 mg) of epinephrine/kg of body weight or 0.2 mg epinephrine per dental appointment. The effective anesthetic dose varies with procedure, intensity of anesthesia needed, duration of anesthesia required, and physical condition of the patient. Always use the lowest effective dose along with careful aspiration.

For most routine dental procedures, lidocaine hydrochloride 2% with epinephrine 1:100,000 is preferred. When a more pronounced hemostasis is required, a 1:50,000 epinephrine concentration should be used.

Dermatologic procedure: Children ≥5 and Adults: Topical: Place 1 transdermal patch over area requiring analgesia; attach patch to iontophoretic controller and leave on for 10 minutes. Remove patch and perform procedure within 10-20 minutes of patch removal. Do not use another patch for 30 minutes.

Additional Information Complete prescribing information for this medication should be consulted for additional detail.

Dosage Forms Excipient information presented when available (limited, particularly for generics); consult specific product labeling.

Injection, solution:

0.5% / 1:200,000: Lidocaine hydrochloride 0.5% and epinephrine 1:200,000 (50 mL)

1% / 1:100,000: Lidocaine hydrochloride 1% and epinephrine 1:100,000 (20 mL, 30 mL, 50 mL)

1% / 1:200,000: Lidocaine hydrochloride 1% and epinephrine 1:200,000 (30 mL)

1.5% / 1:200,000: Lidocaine hydrochloride 1.5% and epinephrine 1:200,000 (30 mL)

2% / 1:50,000: Lidocaine hydrochloride 2% and epinephrine 1:50,000 (1.8 mL)

2% / 1:100,000: Lidocaine hydrochloride 2% and epinephrine 1:100,000 (1.8 mL, 30 mL, 50 mL)

2% / 1:200,000: Lidocaine hydrochloride 2% and epinephrine 1:200,000 (20 mL)

Lignospan® Forte: 2% / 1:50,000: Lidocaine hydrochloride 2% and epinephrine 1:50,000 (1.7 mL) [contains edetate disodium, potassium metabisulfite]

Lignospan® Standard: 2% / 1:100,000: Lidocaine hydrochloride 2% and epinephrine 1:100,000 (1.7 mL) [contains edetate disodium, potassium metabisulfite]

Xylocaine® with Epinephrine:

0.5% / 1:200,000: Lidocaine hydrochloride 0.5% and epinephrine 1:200,000 (50 mL) [contains methylparaben]

1% / 1:100,000: Lidocaine hydrochloride 1% and epinephrine 1:100,000 (10 mL, 20 mL, 50 mL) [contains methylparaben]

2% / 1:50,000: Lidocaine hydrochloride 2% and epinephrine 1:50,000 (1.8 mL) [contains sodium metabisulfite]

2% / 1:100,000: Lidocaine hydrochloride 2% and epinephrine 1:100,000 (1.8 mL) [contains sodium metabisulfite]; (10 mL, 20 mL, 50 mL) [contains methylparaben]

Xylocaine®-MPF with Epinephrine:

1% / 1:200,000: Lidocaine hydrochloride 1% and epinephrine 1:200,000 (5 mL, 10 mL, 30 mL) [contains sodium metabisulfite]

1.5% / 1:200,000: Lidocaine hydrochloride 1.5% and epinephrine 1:200,000 (5 mL, 10 mL, 30 mL) [contains sodium metabisulfite]

2% / 1:200,000: Lidocaine hydrochloride 2% and epinephrine 1:200,000 (5 mL, 10 mL, 20 mL) [contains sodium metabisulfite]

Transdermal system (LidoSite™): Lidocaine hydrochloride 10% and epinephrine 0.1% (25s) [contains sodium metabisulfite; for use only with LidoSite™ controller]

Lidocaine and Prilocaine

(LYE doe kane & PRIL oh kane)

U.S. Brand Names EMLA®; Oraquix®

Canadian Brand Names EMLA®

Index Terms Prilocaine and Lidocaine

Pharmacologic Category Local Anesthetic

Use Topical anesthetic for use on normal intact skin to provide local analgesia for minor procedures such as I.V.

cannulation or venipuncture; has also been used for painful procedures such as lumbar puncture and skin graft harvesting; for superficial minor surgery of genital mucous membranes and as an adjunct for local infiltration anesthesia in genital mucous membranes.

Pregnancy Risk Factor B

Dosage Although the incidence of systemic adverse effects with EMLA® is very low, caution should be exercised, particularly when applying over large areas and leaving on for >2 hours

Children (intact skin): EMLA® should **not** be used in neonates with a gestation age <37 weeks nor in infants <12 months of age who are receiving treatment with methemoglobin-inducing agents

Dosing is based on child's age and weight:

Age 0-3 months or <5 kg: Apply a maximum of 1 g over no more than 10 cm^2 of skin; leave on for no longer than 1 hour

Age 3 months to 12 months and >5 kg: Apply no more than a maximum 2 g total over no more than 20 cm^2 of skin; leave on for no longer than 4 hours

Age 1-6 years and >10 kg: Apply no more than a maximum of 10 g total over no more than 100 cm^2 of skin; leave on for no longer than 4 hours.

Age 7-12 years and >20 kg: Apply no more than a maximum 20 g total over no more than 200 cm^2 of skin; leave on for no longer than 4 hours.

Note: If a patient greater than 3 months old does not meet the minimum weight requirement, the maximum total dose should be restricted to the corresponding maximum based on patient weight.

Adults (intact skin):

EMLA® cream and EMLA® anesthetic disc: A thick layer of EMLA® cream is applied to intact skin and covered with an occlusive dressing, or alternatively, an EMLA® anesthetic disc is applied to intact skin

Minor dermal procedures (eg, I.V. cannulation or venipuncture): Apply 2.5 g of cream (1/2 of the 5 g tube) over 20-25 cm of skin surface area, or 1 anesthetic disc (1 g over 10 cm^2) for at least 1 hour. **Note:** In clinical trials, 2 sites were usually prepared in case there was a technical problem with cannulation or venipuncture at the first site.

Major dermal procedures (eg, more painful dermatological procedures involving a larger skin area such as split thickness skin graft harvesting): Apply 2 g of cream per 10 cm^2 of skin and allow to remain in contact with the skin for at least 2 hours.

Adult male genital skin (eg, pretreatment prior to local anesthetic infiltration): Apply a thick layer of cream (1 g/10 cm^2) to the skin surface for 15 minutes. Local anesthetic infiltration should be performed immediately after removal of EMLA® cream.

Note: Dermal analgesia can be expected to increase for up to 3 hours under occlusive dressing and persist for 1-2 hours after removal of the cream

Adult females: Genital mucous membranes: Minor procedures (eg, removal of condylomata acuminata, pretreatment for local anesthetic infiltration): Apply 5-10 g (thick layer) of cream for 5-10 minutes

Periodontal gel (Oraqix®): Adults: Apply on gingival margin around selected teeth using the blunt-tipped applicator included in package. Wait 30 seconds, then fill the periodontal pockets using the blunt-tipped applicator until gel becomes visible at the gingival margin. Wait another 30 seconds before starting treatment. Maximum recommended dose: One treatment session: 5 cartridges (8.5 g)

Additional Information Complete prescribing information for this medication should be consulted for additional detail.

Dosage Forms Excipient information presented when available (limited, particularly for generics); consult specific product labeling.

Cream, topical: Lidocaine 2.5% and prilocaine 2.5% (5 g, 30 g)

EMLA®: Lidocaine 2.5% and prilocaine 2.5% (5 g, 30 g) [each packaged with Tegaderm® dressings]

Disc, topical: Lidocaine 2.5% and prilocaine 2.5% per disc (2s, 10s) [each 1 g disc is 10 cm^2]

Gel, periodontal: Lidocaine 2.5% and prilocaine 2.5% (1.7 g) [cartridge]

Lidocaine and Tetracaine

(LYE doe kane & TET ra kane)

U.S. Brand Names Pliaglis™; Synera™

Index Terms Tetracaine and Lidocaine

Pharmacologic Category Analgesic, Topical; Local Anesthetic

Use Topical anesthetic for use on normal intact skin for minor procedures (eg, I.V. cannulation or venipuncture) and superficial dermatologic procedures

Pregnancy Risk Factor B

Dosage

Topical: Cream: Adults:

Superficial dermatological procedures (eg, dermal filler injection, facial laser ablation): Apply 20-30 minutes prior to procedure

Laser-assisted tattoo removal: Apply 60 minutes prior to procedure

Note: The amount of Pliaglis™ required is determined by the size of the treatment area. Use the ruler on the carton and in the packaging to measure out the proper amount (cm length of cream). Apply evenly and thinly (~1 mm or the thickness of a dime) over the area using a flat tool (eg, spatula, tongue depressor).

If surface area of treatment site:

10 cm^2: Apply 3 cm length Pliaglis™
20 cm^2: Apply 6 cm Pliaglis™
40 cm^2: Apply 12 cm Pliaglis™
80 cm^2: Apply 24 cm Pliaglis™
100 cm^2: Apply 30 cm Pliaglis™
150 cm^2: Apply 46 cm Pliaglis™
200 cm^2: Apply 61 cm Pliaglis™
250 cm^2: Apply 76 cm Pliaglis™
300 cm^2: Apply 91 cm Pliaglis™
350 cm^2: Apply 106 cm Pliaglis™
400 cm^2: Apply 121 cm Pliaglis™

After waiting the required application time, remove the Pliaglis™ by grasping a free edge and pulling it away from the skin.

Transdermal patch: Children ≥3 years and Adults:

Venipuncture or intravenous cannulation: Prior to procedure, apply to intact skin for 20-30 minutes; **Note:** Adults can use another patch at a new location to facilitate venous access after a failed attempt; remove previous patch.

Superficial dermatological procedures: Prior to procedure, apply to intact skin for 30 minutes

Dosage adjustment in hepatic impairment: Use caution in patients with severe hepatic dysfunction.

Additional Information Complete prescribing information for this medication should be consulted for additional detail.

Dosage Forms Excipient information presented when available (limited, particularly for generics); consult specific product labeling.

Cream, topical:

Pliaglis™: Lidocaine 7% and tetracaine 7% (30 g)

Transdermal system:

Synera™: Lidocaine 70 mg and tetracaine 70 mg (10s) [contains heating component; each patch is ~50 cm^2]

Lindane (LIN dane)

Canadian Brand Names Hexit™; PMS-Lindane

Index Terms Benzene Hexachloride; Gamma Benzene Hexachloride; Hexachlorocyclohexane

Pharmacologic Category Antiparasitic Agent, Topical; Pediculocide; Scabicidal Agent

Use Treatment of *Sarcoptes scabiei* (scabies), *Pediculus capitis* (head lice), and *Phthirus pubis* (crab lice); FDA recommends reserving lindane as a second-line agent or with inadequate response to other therapies

Restrictions An FDA-approved medication guide must be distributed when dispensing an outpatient prescription (new or refill) where this medication is to be used without direct supervision of a healthcare provider. Medication guides are available at http://www.fda.gov/cder/Offices/ODS/medication_guides.htm.

Pregnancy Risk Factor C

Pregnancy Considerations There are no well-controlled studies in pregnant women.

Lactation Enters breast milk/contraindicated

Contraindications Hypersensitivity to lindane or any component of the formulation; uncontrolled seizure disorders; crusted (Norwegian) scabies, acutely-inflamed skin or raw, weeping surfaces or other skin conditions which may increase systemic absorption

Warnings/Precautions **[U.S. Boxed Warning]: Not considered a drug of first choice; use only in patients who have failed first-line treatments, or in patients who cannot tolerate these agents.** Because of the potential for systemic absorption and CNS side effects, lindane should be used with caution; consider permethrin or crotamiton agent first. Oil-based hair dressing may increase toxic potential.

[U.S. Boxed Warning]: May be associated with severe neurologic toxicities (contraindicated in premature infants and uncontrolled seizure disorders). Seizures and death have been reported with use; use with caution in infants, small children, patients <50 kg, or patients with a history of seizures; use caution with conditions which may increase risk of seizures or medications which decrease seizure threshold; use caution with hepatic impairment; avoid contact with face, eyes, mucous membranes, and urethral meatus.

[U.S. Boxed Warning]: A lindane medication use guide must be given to all patients along with instructions for proper use. Patients should be informed that itching may occur following successful killing of lice and retreatment may not be indicated. Should be used as a part of an overall lice management program.

Adverse Reactions Frequency not defined (includes postmarketing and/or case reports).

Cardiovascular: Cardiac arrhythmia

Central nervous system: Ataxia, dizziness, headache, restlessness, seizure, pain

Dermatologic: Alopecia, contact dermatitis, skin and adipose tissue may act as repositories, eczematous eruptions, pruritus, urticaria

Gastrointestinal: Nausea, vomiting

Hematologic: Aplastic anemia

Hepatic: Hepatitis

Local: Burning and stinging

Neuromuscular & skeletal: Paresthesia

Renal: Hematuria

Respiratory: Pulmonary edema

Drug Interactions

Avoid Concomitant Use There are no known interactions where it is recommended to avoid concomitant use.

Increased Effect/Toxicity There are no known significant interactions involving an increase in effect.

Decreased Effect There are no known significant interactions involving a decrease in effect.

Mechanism of Action Directly absorbed by parasites and ova through the exoskeleton; stimulates the nervous system resulting in seizures and death of parasitic arthropods

Pharmacodynamics/Kinetics

Absorption: ≤13% systemically

Distribution: Stored in body fat; accumulates in brain; skin and adipose tissue may act as repositories

Metabolism: Hepatic

Half-life elimination: Children: 17-22 hours

Time to peak, serum: Children: 6 hours

Excretion: Urine and feces

Dosage Children and Adults: Topical:

Scabies: Apply a thin layer of lotion and massage it on skin from the neck to the toes; after 8-12 hours, bathe and remove the drug

Head lice, crab lice: Apply shampoo to dry hair and massage into hair for 4 minutes; add small quantities of water to hair until lather forms, then rinse hair thoroughly and comb with a fine tooth comb to remove nits. Amount of shampoo needed is based on length and density of hair; most patients will require 30 mL (maximum: 60 mL).

Administration For topical use only; never administer orally. Caregivers should apply with gloves (avoid natural latex, may be permeable to lindane). Rinse off with warm (not hot) water.

Lotion: Apply to dry, cool skin; do not apply to face or eyes. Wait at least 1 hour after bathing or showering (wet or warm skin increases absorption). Skin should be clean and free of any other lotions, creams, or oil prior to lindane application.

Shampoo: Apply to clean, dry hair. Wait at least 1 hour after washing hair before applying lindane shampoo. Hair should be washed with a shampoo not containing a conditioner; hair and skin of head and neck should be free of any lotions, oils, or creams prior to lindane application.

Dosage Forms Excipient information presented when available (limited, particularly for generics); consult specific product labeling.

Lotion, topical: 1% (60 mL)

Shampoo, topical: 1% (60 mL) [contains alcohol 0.5%]

Linezolid (li NE zoh lid)

U.S. Brand Names Zyvox®
Canadian Brand Names Zyvoxam®
Pharmacologic Category Antibiotic, Oxazolidinone
Additional Appendix Information

Antibiotic Treatment of Adults With Infective Endocarditis *on page 1748*
Antimicrobial Drugs of Choice *on page 1752*
Community-Acquired Pneumonia in Adults *on page 1766*

Use Treatment of vancomycin-resistant *Enterococcus faecium* (VRE) infections, nosocomial pneumonia caused by *Staphylococcus aureus* including MRSA or *Streptococcus pneumoniae* (including multidrug-resistant strains [MDRSP]), complicated and uncomplicated skin and skin structure infections (including diabetic foot infections without concomitant osteomyelitis), and community-acquired pneumonia caused by susceptible gram-positive organisms

Pregnancy Risk Factor C

Pregnancy Considerations Because adverse effects were observed in some animal studies, linezolid is classified pregnancy category C. There are no adequate and well-controlled studies in pregnant women.

Lactation Excretion in breast milk unknown/use caution

Medication Safety Issues

Sound-alike/look-alike issues:

Zyvox® may be confused with Ziox™, Zosyn®, Zovirax®

Contraindications Hypersensitivity to linezolid or any other component of the formulation; concurrent use or within 2 weeks of MAO inhibitors; patients with uncontrolled hypertension, pheochromocytoma, thyrotoxicosis, and/or taking sympathomimetics (eg, pseudoephedrine), vasopressive agents (eg, epinephrine, norepinephrine), or dopaminergic agents (eg, dopamine, dobutamine) unless closely monitored for increased blood pressure; patients with carcinoid syndrome and/or taking SSRIs, tricyclic antidepressants, serotonin 5-$HT_{1B,1D}$ receptor agonists, meperidine, or buspirone unless closely monitored for sign/symptoms of serotonin syndrome

Warnings/Precautions Myelosuppression has been reported and may be dependent on duration of therapy (generally >2 weeks of treatment); use with caution in patients with pre-existing myelosuppression, in patients receiving other drugs which may cause bone marrow suppression, or in chronic infection (previous or concurrent antibiotic therapy). Weekly CBC monitoring is recommended. Discontinue linezolid in patients developing myelosuppression (or in whom myelosuppression worsens during treatment).

Lactic acidosis has been reported with use. Linezolid exhibits mild MAO inhibitor properties and has the potential to have the same interactions as other MAO inhibitors; use with caution and monitor closely in patients with uncontrolled hypertension, pheochromocytoma, carcinoid syndrome, or untreated hyperthyroidism; use is contraindicated in the absence of close monitoring. Symptoms of agitation, confusion, hallucinations, hyper-reflexia, myoclonus, shivering, and tachycardia may occur with concomitant proserotonergic drugs (eg, SSRIs/SNRIs or triptans) or agents which reduce linezolid's metabolism; concurrent use with these medications if contraindicated unless patient is closely monitored for signs/symptoms of serotonin syndrome. Unnecessary use may lead to the development of resistance to linezolid; consider alternatives before initiating outpatient treatment.

Peripheral and optic neuropathy (with vision loss) has been reported and may occur primarily with extended courses of therapy >28 days; any symptoms of visual change or impairment warrant immediate ophthalmic evaluation and possible discontinuation of therapy. Seizures have been reported; use with caution in patients with a history of seizures. Prolonged use may result in fungal or bacterial superinfection, including *C. difficile*-associated diarrhea (CDAD) and pseudomembranous colitis; CDAD has been observed >2 months postantibiotic treatment.

Due to inconsistent concentrations in the CSF, empiric use in pediatric patients with CNS infections is not recommended by the manufacturer; however, there are multiple case reports describing successful treatment of documented VRE and *Staphylococcus aureus* CNS and shunt infections in the literature. Oral suspension contains phenylalanine.

Adverse Reactions Percentages as reported in adults; frequency similar in pediatric patients

>10%:

Central nervous system: Headache (<1% to 11%)
Gastrointestinal: Diarrhea (3% to 11%)

1% to 10%:

Central nervous system: Insomnia (3%), dizziness (≤2%), fever (2%)
Dermatologic: Rash (2%)
Gastrointestinal: Nausea (3% to 10%), vomiting (1% to 4%), pancreatic enzymes increased (≤4%), constipation (2%), taste alteration (1% to 2%), tongue discoloration (≤1%), oral moniliasis (≤1%), pancreatitis
Genitourinary: Vaginal moniliasis (1% to 2%)
Hematologic: Hemoglobin decreased (1% to 7%), thrombocytopenia (≤3%), anemia, leukopenia, neutropenia; **Note:** Myelosuppression (including anemia, leukopenia, pancytopenia, and thrombocytopenia; may be more common in patients receiving linezolid for >2 weeks)
Hepatic: Abnormal LFTs (≤10%), bilirubin increased (≤1%)
Renal: BUN increased (≤2%)
Miscellaneous: Fungal infection (0.1% to 2%), lactate dehydrogenase increased (<1% to 2%)

<1% or frequency not defined (limited to important or life-threatening): Anaphylaxis, angioedema, bullous skin disorders, *C. difficile*-related complications, dyspepsia, increased creatinine, hypertension, localized abdominal pain, pruritus, lactic acidosis, peripheral neuropathy, optic neuropathy, seizures, serotonin syndrome (with concurrent use of other serotonergic agents), Stevens-Johnson syndrome, vision loss

Drug Interactions

Avoid Concomitant Use

Avoid concomitant use of Linezolid with any of the following: Alpha-/Beta-Agonists (Indirect-Acting); Alpha1-Agonists; Alpha2-Agonists (Ophthalmic); Amphetamines; Atomoxetine; BuPROPion; BusPIRone; Cyclobenzaprine; Dexmethylphenidate; Dextromethorphan; MAO Inhibitors; Maprotiline; Meperidine; Methyldopa; Methylphenidate; Mirtazapine; Propoxyphene; Selective Serotonin Reuptake Inhibitors; Serotonin 5-HT1D Receptor Agonists; Serotonin/Norepinephrine Reuptake Inhibitors; Sibutramine; Tetrabenazine; Tricyclic Antidepressants

Increased Effect/Toxicity

Linezolid may increase the levels/effects of: Alpha-/Beta-Agonists (Direct-Acting); Alpha-/Beta-Agonists (Indirect-Acting); Alpha1-Agonists; Alpha2-Agonists (Ophthalmic); Amphetamines; Atomoxetine; Beta2-Agonists; BuPROPion; Dexmethylphenidate; Dextromethorphan; Lithium; Meperidine; Methyldopa; Methylphenidate; Mirtazapine; Rauwolfia Alkaloids; Selective Serotonin Reuptake Inhibitors; Serotonin 5-HT1D Receptor Agonists; Serotonin Modulators; Serotonin/Norepinephrine Reuptake Inhibitors; Tricyclic Antidepressants

The levels/effects of Linezolid may be increased by: Altretamine; Anilidopiperidine Opioids; BusPIRone;

COMT Inhibitors; Cyclobenzaprine; Levodopa; MAO Inhibitors; Maprotiline; Propoxyphene; Sibutramine; Tetrabenazine; TraMADol

Decreased Effect There are no known significant interactions involving a decrease in effect.

Ethanol/Nutrition/Herb Interactions

Ethanol: Avoid ethanol (based on CNS depressant effects and potential tyramine content)

Food: Concurrent ingestion of foods rich in tyramine may cause sudden and severe high blood pressure (hypertensive crisis). Avoid tyramine-containing foods with MAO-Is. Food's freshness is also an important concern; improperly stored or spoiled food can create an environment where tyramine concentrations may increase.

Herb/Nutraceutical: Avoid supplements containing caffeine, tyrosine, tryptophan or phenylalanine. Ingestion of large quantities may increase the risk of severe side effects (eg, hypertensive reactions, serotonin syndrome).

Stability

Infusion: Store at 25°C (77°F). Protect from light. Keep infusion bags in overwrap until ready for use. Protect infusion bags from freezing.

Oral suspension: Reconstitute with 123 mL of distilled water (in 2 portions); shake vigorously. Concentration is 100 mg/5 mL. Prior to administration mix gently by inverting bottle; do not shake. Following reconstitution, store at 25°C (77°F). Use reconstituted suspension within 21 days. Protect from light.

Tablet: Store at 25°C (77°F). Protect from light; protect from moisture.

Mechanism of Action Inhibits bacterial protein synthesis by binding to bacterial 23S ribosomal RNA of the 50S subunit. This prevents the formation of a functional 70S initiation complex that is essential for the bacterial translation process. Linezolid is bacteriostatic against enterococci and staphylococci and bactericidal against most strains of streptococci.

Pharmacodynamics/Kinetics

Absorption: Rapid and extensive

Distribution: V_{dss}: Adults: 40-50 L

Protein binding: Adults: 31%

Metabolism: Hepatic via oxidation of the morpholine ring, resulting in two inactive metabolites (aminoethoxyacetic acid, hydroxyethyl glycine); does not involve CYP

Bioavailability: Oral: ~100%

Half-life elimination: Children ≥1 week (full-term) to 11 years: 1.5-3 hours; Adults: 4-5 hours

Time to peak: Adults: Oral: 1-2 hours

Excretion: Urine (30% as parent drug, 50% as metabolites); feces (9% as metabolites)

Nonrenal clearance: ~65%; increased in children ≥1 week to 11 years

Dosage

Oral, I.V.:

VRE infections including concurrent bacteremia:

Preterm neonates (<34 weeks gestational age): 10 mg/kg every 12 hours; neonates with a suboptimal clinical response can be advanced to 10 mg/kg every 8 hours. By day 7 of life, all neonates should receive 10 mg/kg every 8 hours.

Infants (excluding preterm neonates <1 week) and Children ≤11 years: 10 mg/kg every 8 hours for 14-28 days

Children ≥12 years and Adults: 600 mg every 12 hours for 14-28 days

MRSA: Adults: 600 mg every 12 hours

Nosocomial pneumonia, complicated skin and skin structure infections, community acquired pneumonia including concurrent bacteremia: Oral, I.V.:

Preterm neonates (<34 weeks gestational age): 10 mg/kg every 12 hours; neonates with a suboptimal clinical response can be advanced to 10 mg/kg every 8 hours. By day 7 of life, all neonates should receive 10 mg/kg every 8 hours.

Infants (excluding preterm neonates <1 week) and Children ≤11 years: 10 mg/kg every 8 hours for 10-14 days

Children ≥12 years and Adults: 600 mg every 12 hours for 10-14 days

Uncomplicated skin and skin structure infections: Oral:

Preterm neonates (<34 weeks gestational age): 10 mg/kg every 12 hours; neonates with a suboptimal clinical response can be advanced to 10 mg/kg every 8 hours. By day 7 of life, all neonates should receive 10 mg/kg every 8 hours.

Infants (excluding preterm neonates <1 week) and Children <5 years: 10 mg/kg every 8 hours for 10-14 days

Children 5-11 years: 10 mg/kg every 12 hours for 10-14 days

Children ≥12-18 years: 600 mg every 12 hours for 10-14 days

Adults: 400 mg every 12 hours for 10-14 days

Note: 400 mg dose is recommended in the product labeling; however, 600 mg dose is commonly employed clinically

Elderly: No dosage adjustment required

Dosage adjustment in renal impairment: No adjustment is recommended. The two primary metabolites may accumulate in patients with renal impairment but the clinical significance is unknown. Weigh the risk of accumulation of metabolites versus the benefit of therapy. Monitor for hematopoietic (eg, anemia, leukopenia, thrombocytopenia) and neuropathic (eg, peripheral neuropathy) adverse events when administering for extended periods. Both linezolid and the two metabolites are eliminated by dialysis. Linezolid should be given after hemodialysis.

Continuous renal replacement therapy (CRRT): No adjustment needed.

Dosage adjustment in hepatic impairment: No dosage adjustment required for mild to moderate hepatic insufficiency (Child-Pugh Class A or B). Use in severe hepatic insufficiency has not been adequately evaluated.

Dietary Considerations Take with or without food. Avoid consuming large amounts of tyramine-containing foods/beverages. Some examples include aged or matured cheese, air-dried or cured meats (including sausages and salamis), fava or broad bean pods, tap/draft beers, Marmite concentrate, sauerkraut, soy sauce and other soybean condiments.

Suspension contains 20 mg phenylalanine per teaspoonful. Sodium content: 0.1 mEq/tablet; 0.4 mEq/5 mL; 1.7 mEq/100 mL infusion; 3.3 mEq/200 mL infusion; 5 mEq/300 mL infusion

Administration

I.V.: Administer intravenous infusion over 30-120 minutes. Do not mix or infuse with other medications. When the same intravenous line is used for sequential infusion of other medications, flush line with D_5W, NS, or LR before and after infusing linezolid. The yellow color of the injection may intensify over time without affecting potency.

Oral suspension: Invert gently to mix prior to administration, do not shake.

Monitoring Parameters Weekly CBC and platelet counts, particularly in patients at increased risk of bleeding, with pre-existing myelosuppression, on concomitant medications that cause bone marrow suppression, in those who require >2 weeks of therapy, or in those with chronic infection who have received previous or concomitant antibiotic therapy; visual function with extended therapy (≥3 months) or in patients with new onset visual symptoms, regardless of therapy length

Dosage Forms Excipient information presented when available (limited, particularly for generics); consult specific product labeling.

Infusion [premixed]:

Zyvox®: 200 mg (100 mL) [contains sodium 1.7 mEq]; 600 mg (300 mL) [contains sodium 5 mEq]

Powder for oral suspension:

Zyvox®: 20 mg/mL (150 mL) [contains phenylalanine 20 mg/5 mL, sodium benzoate, and sodium 0.4 mEq/5 mL; orange flavor]

Tablet:

Zyvox®: 600 mg [contains sodium 0.1 mEq/tablet]

◆ **Lin-Sotalol (Can)** *see* Sotalol *on page* 1394

◆ **Lioresal®** *see* Baclofen *on page* 172

◆ **Liotec (Can)** *see* Baclofen *on page* 172

Liothyronine (lye oh THYE roe neen)

U.S. Brand Names Cytomel®; Triostat®

Canadian Brand Names Cytomel®

Index Terms Liothyronine Sodium; Sodium *L*-Triiodothyronine; T_3 Sodium (error-prone abbreviation)

Pharmacologic Category Thyroid Product

Use

Oral: Replacement or supplemental therapy in hypothyroidism; management of nontoxic goiter; a diagnostic aid

I.V.: Treatment of myxedema coma/precoma

Pregnancy Risk Factor A

Medication Safety Issues

Sound-alike/look-alike issues:

Liothyronine may be confused with levothyroxine

T3 is an error-prone abbreviation (mistaken as acetaminophen and codeine [ie, Tylenol® #3])

Dosage Doses should be adjusted based on clinical response and laboratory parameters.

Children: Congenital hypothyroidism: Oral: 5 mcg/day increase by 5 mcg every 3-4 days until the desired response is achieved. Usual maintenance dose: 20 mcg/day for infants, 50 mcg/day for children 1-3 years of age, and adult dose for children >3 years.

Adults:

Hypothyroidism: Oral: 25 mcg/day increase by increments of 12.5-25 mcg/day every 1-2 weeks to a maximum of 100 mcg/day; usual maintenance dose: 25-75 mcg/day.

Patients with cardiovascular disease: Refer to Elderly dosing.

T_3 suppression test: Oral: 75-100 mcg/day for 7 days; use lowest dose for elderly

Myxedema: Oral: Initial: 5 mcg/day; increase in increments of 5-10 mcg/day every 1-2 weeks. When 25 mcg/day is reached, dosage may be increased at intervals of 5-25 mcg/day every 1-2 weeks. Usual maintenance dose: 50-100 mcg/day.

Myxedema coma: I.V.: 25-50 mcg

Patients with known or suspected cardiovascular disease: 10-20 mcg

Note: Normally, at least 4 hours should be allowed between doses to adequately assess therapeutic response and no more than 12 hours should elapse between doses to avoid fluctuations in hormone levels. Oral therapy should be resumed as soon as the clinical situation has been stabilized and the patient is able to take oral medication. If levothyroxine rather than liothyronine sodium is used in initiating oral therapy, the physician should bear in mind that there is a delay of several days in the onset of levothyroxine activity and that I.V. therapy should be discontinued gradually.

Simple (nontoxic) goiter: Oral: Initial: 5 mcg/day; increase by 5-10 mcg every 1-2 weeks; after 25 mcg/day is reached, may increase dose by 12.5-25 mcg. Usual maintenance dose: 75 mcg/day

Elderly: Oral: 5 mcg/day; increase by 5 mcg/day every 2 weeks

Additional Information Complete prescribing information for this medication should be consulted for additional detail.

Dosage Forms Excipient information presented when available (limited, particularly for generics); consult specific product labeling.

Injection, solution: 10 mcg/mL (1 mL)

Triostat®: 10 mcg/mL (1 mL) [contains ethanol 6.8%]

Tablet, oral:

Cytomel®: 5 mcg, 25 mcg, 50 mcg

◆ **Liothyronine Sodium** *see* Liothyronine *on page* 892

Liotrix (LYE oh triks)

U.S. Brand Names Thyrolar®

Canadian Brand Names Thyrolar®

Index Terms T_3/T_4 Liotrix

Pharmacologic Category Thyroid Product

Use Replacement or supplemental therapy in hypothyroidism (uniform mixture of T_4:T_3 in 4:1 ratio by weight); little advantage to this product exists and cost is not justified

Pregnancy Risk Factor A

Medication Safety Issues

Sound-alike/look-alike issues:

Liotrix may be confused with Klotrix®

Thyrolar® may be confused with Thyrogen®, Thytropar®

Dosage Oral:

Congenital hypothyroidism:

Children (dose of T_4 or levothyroxine/day):

0-6 months: 8-10 mcg/kg or 25-50 mcg/day

6-12 months: 6-8 mcg/kg or 50-75 mcg/day

1-5 years: 5-6 mcg/kg or 75-100 mcg/day

6-12 years: 4-5 mcg/kg or 100-150 mcg/day

>12 years: 2-3 mcg/kg or >150 mcg/day

Hypothyroidism (dose of thyroid equivalent):

Adults: 30 mg/day (15 mg/day if cardiovascular impairment), increasing by increments of 15 mg/day at 2- to 3-week intervals to a maximum of 180 mg/day (usual maintenance dose: 60-120 mg/day)

Elderly: Initial: 15 mg, adjust dose at 2- to 4-week intervals by increments of 15 mg

Additional Information Complete prescribing information for this medication should be consulted for additional detail.

Dosage Forms Excipient information presented when available (limited, particularly for generics); consult specific product labeling.

Tablet:

1/4 [levothyroxine sodium 12.5 mcg and liothyronine sodium 3.1 mcg]

1/2 [levothyroxine sodium 25 mcg and liothyronine sodium 6.25 mcg]

1 [levothyroxine sodium 50 mcg and liothyronine sodium 12.5 mcg]

2 [levothyroxine sodium 100 mcg and liothyronine sodium 25 mcg]

3 [levothyroxine sodium 150 mcg and liothyronine sodium 37.5 mcg]

◆ **Lipancreatin** *see* Pancrelipase *on page* 1136

◆ **Lipidil EZ® (Can)** *see* Fenofibrate *on page* 607

◆ **Lipidil Micro® (Can)** *see* Fenofibrate *on page* 607

◆ **Lipidil Supra® (Can)** *see* Fenofibrate *on page* 607

◆ **Lipitor®** *see* Atorvastatin *on page* 152

◆ **Lipofen®** *see* Fenofibrate *on page* 607

- ◆ **Liposomal DAUNOrubicin** *see* DAUNOrubicin Citrate (Liposomal) *on page 406*
- ◆ **Liposomal DOXOrubicin** *see* DOXOrubicin (Liposomal) *on page 488*
- ◆ **Liposyn® II** *see* Fat Emulsion *on page 605*
- ◆ **Liposyn® III** *see* Fat Emulsion *on page 605*
- ◆ **Lipram 4500 [DSC]** *see* Pancrelipase *on page 1136*
- ◆ **Lipram-CR [DSC]** *see* Pancrelipase *on page 1136*
- ◆ **Lipram-PN [DSC]** *see* Pancrelipase *on page 1136*
- ◆ **Lipram-UL [DSC]** *see* Pancrelipase *on page 1136*
- ◆ **Liqua-Cal [OTC]** *see* Calcium and Vitamin D *on page 238*
- ◆ **Liquadd™** *see* Dextroamphetamine *on page 431*
- ◆ **Liquibid-D®** *see* Guaifenesin and Phenylephrine *on page 712*
- ◆ **Liquid Antidote** *see* Charcoal *on page 299*

Lisdexamfetamine (lis dex am FET a meen)

U.S. Brand Names Vyvanse™

Index Terms Lisdexamfetamine Dimesylate; Lisdexamphetamine; NRP104

Pharmacologic Category Stimulant

Use Treatment of attention-deficit/hyperactivity disorder (ADHD)

Restrictions C-II

An FDA-approved medication guide must be distributed when dispensing an outpatient prescription (new or refill) where this medication is to be used without direct supervision of a healthcare provider. Medication guides are available at http://www.fda.gov/cder/Offices/ODS/medication_guides.htm.

Pregnancy Risk Factor C

Pregnancy Considerations Animal studies have shown that amphetamines may cause embryotoxic and teratogenic effects and that pre- or early postnatal exposure to amphetamines may lead to lasting changes in behavior, including impaired learning, memory, and motor skills, as well as changes to libido. There are no adequate and well-controlled studies in pregnant women. No reproductive studies have been performed with lisdexamfetamine. Infants born to mothers dependent on amphetamines are more likely to arrive prematurely with low birth weight and may experience withdrawal symptoms including irritation, restlessness, anxiousness, weakness, listlessness, or lethargy.

Lactation Enters breast milk/not recommended

Medication Safety Issues

Sound-alike/look-alike issues:

Vyvanse™ may be confused with Vytorin®, Glucovance®, Vivactil®

Contraindications Known hypersensitivity or idiosyncratic reaction sympathomimetic amines; advanced arteriosclerosis, symptomatic cardiovascular disease, moderate-to-severe hypertension; hyperthyroidism; glaucoma; agitated states; history of drug abuse; concurrent use or within 2 weeks of use of MAO inhibitors

Warnings/Precautions [U.S. Boxed Warning]: Use has been associated with serious cardiovascular events including sudden death in patients with pre-existing structural cardiac abnormalities or other serious heart problems (sudden death in children and adolescents; sudden death, stroke and MI in adults. Use of this product should be avoided in the patients with known serious structural cardiac abnormalities, cardiomyopathy, serious heart rhythm abnormalities, coronary artery disease (adults), or other serious cardiac problems that could increase the risk of sudden death that these conditions alone carry. Patients should be carefully evaluated for these cardiac disorders prior to initiation of therapy.

Use with caution in patients with psychiatric or seizure disorders. May exacerbate symptoms of behavior and thought disorder in psychotic patients. Stimulants may unmask tics in individuals with coexisting Tourette's syndrome. **[U.S. Boxed Warning]: Potential for drug dependency exists; prolonged use may lead to drug dependency.** Use is contraindicated is patients with history of ethanol or drug abuse. Prescriptions should be written for the smallest quantity consistent with good patient care to minimize the possibility of overdose. Abrupt discontinuation following high doses or for prolonged periods may result in symptoms for withdrawal. Recommended to be used as part of a comprehensive treatment program for attention deficit disorders. Safety and efficacy of long-term use have not yet been established. Safety and efficacy in children <6 years of age or children >12 years of age have not been established. Amphetamines are not recommended in children <3 years of age. Appetite suppression may occur; monitor weight during therapy, particularly in children. Use of stimulants has been associated with slowing of growth rate; monitor growth rate during treatment. Treatment interruption may be necessary in patients who are not growing or gaining weight as expected.

Adverse Reactions

>10%:

Central nervous system: Headache (children 12%), insomnia (19% to 27%; 4% [initially])

Gastrointestinal: Appetite decreased (27% to 39%), xerostomia (children 5%; adults 26%), abdominal pain (children 12%)

1% to 10%:

Cardiovascular: Blood pressure increased (adults 3%), heart rate increased (adults 2%)

Central nervous system: Irritability (children 10%), anxiety (adults 6%), dizziness (children 5%), jitteriness (adults 4%), affect lability (children 3%), agitation (adults 3%), restlessness (adults 3%), fever (children: 2%), somnolence (children 2%), tic (children 2%)

Dermatologic: Hyperhidrosis (adults 3%), rash (children 3%)

Gastrointestinal: Vomiting (children 9%), weight loss (children 9%), diarrhea (adults 7%), nausea (6% to 7%), anorexia (adult: 5%)

Neuromuscular & skeletal: Tremor (adults 2%)

Respiratory: Dyspnea (adults 2%)

Additional adverse reaction associated with amphetamines; frequency not defined.

Cardiovascular: Cardiomyopathy, hypertension, MI, palpitation, sudden death, tachycardia

Central nervous system: Depression, dyskinesia, dysphoria, euphoria, exacerbation of motor and phonic tics, Tourette's syndrome, overstimulation, psychotic episodes, seizure, stroke

Dermatologic: Angioedema, Stevens-Johnson syndrome, toxic epidermal necrolysis, urticaria

Endocrine & metabolic: Libido changes

Gastrointestinal: Abnormal taste, constipation

Genitourinary: Impotence

Miscellaneous: Anaphylaxis

Drug Interactions

Avoid Concomitant Use

Avoid concomitant use of Lisdexamfetamine with any of the following: Iobenguane I 123; MAO Inhibitors

Increased Effect/Toxicity

Lisdexamfetamine may increase the levels/effects of: Analgesics (Opioid); Sympathomimetics

The levels/effects of Lisdexamfetamine may be increased by: Alkalinizing Agents; Antacids;

Cannabinoids; Carbonic Anhydrase Inhibitors; MAO Inhibitors; Tricyclic Antidepressants

Decreased Effect

Lisdexamfetamine may decrease the levels/effects of: Antihistamines; Ethosuximide; Iobenguane I 123; PHEnobarbital; Phenytoin

The levels/effects of Lisdexamfetamine may be decreased by: Ammonium Chloride; Antipsychotics; Gastrointestinal Acidifying Agents; Lithium; Methenamine

Ethanol/Nutrition/Herb Interactions

Ethanol: Avoid ethanol (may increase CNS depression).

Food: High-fat meal prolongs T_{max} by ~1 hour.

Stability Store at controlled room temperature of 25°C (77°F) excursions permitted to 15°C to 30°C (59°F to 86°F). Protect from light.

Mechanism of Action Lisdexamfetamine dimesylate is a prodrug that is converted to the active component dextroamphetamine (a noncatecholamine, sympathomimetic amine); CNS stimulant effects are thought to result from the interference of norepinephrine and dopamine reuptake into presynaptic neurons as well as increasing their release from nerve terminals; inhibits the actions of monoamine oxidase; peripheral actions include increase in systolic and diastolic blood pressure as well as weak bronchodilator and respiratory stimulant action.

Pharmacodynamics/Kinetics

Absorption: Rapid

Distribution: Dextroamphetamine: V_d: Adults: 3.5-4.6 L/kg; distributes into CNS; mean CSF concentrations are 80% of plasma; enters breast milk

Metabolism: Non-CYP-mediated hepatic or intestinal metabolism to dextroamphetamine and l-lysine

Half-life elimination: Lisdexamfetamine: <1 hour; Dextroamphetamine: 10-13 hours

Time to peak, serum: T_{max}: Lisdexamfetamine: ~1 hour; Dextroamphetamine: ~3.5 hours

Excretion: Urine (96%, 42% as amphetamine-related compounds, 2% as lisdexamfetamine, 25% hippuric acid); feces (minimal)

Dosage Oral: Individualize dosage based on patient need and response to therapy. Administer at the lowest effective dose.

Children: 6-12 years and Adults: Initial: 30 mg once daily in the morning; may increase in increments of 10 mg or 20 mg/day at weekly intervals until optimal response is obtained; maximum: 70 mg/day

Dietary Considerations May be taken with or without food.

Administration Administer in the morning with or without food; swallow capsule whole, do not chew; capsule may be opened and the contents dissolved in glass of water; consume the resulting solution immediately; do not store solution.

Monitoring Parameters Cardiac evaluation should be completed on any patient who develops chest pain, unexplained syncope, and any symptom of cardiac disease during treatment with stimulants; growth and CNS activity in all patients

When used for the treatment of ADHD, thoroughly evaluate for cardiovascular risk. Monitor heart rate, blood pressure, and consider obtaining ECG prior to initiation (Vetter, 2008).

Test Interactions Amphetamines may interfere with urinary steroid determinations.

Dosage Forms

Capsule, as dimesylate:

Vyvanse™: 20 mg, 30 mg, 40 mg, 50 mg, 60 mg, 70 mg

◆ **Lisdexamfetamine Dimesylate** *see* Lisdexamfetamine *on page 893*

◆ **Lisdexamphetamine** *see* Lisdexamfetamine *on page 893*

Lisinopril (lyse IN oh pril)

U.S. Brand Names Prinivil®; Zestril®

Canadian Brand Names Apo-Lisinopril®; CO Lisinopril; Gen-Lisinopril; Novo-Lisinopril; PMS-Lisinopril; Prinivil®; Pro-Lisinopril; Ran-Lisinopril; ratio-Lisinopril; Riva-Lisinopril; Zestril®

Pharmacologic Category Angiotensin-Converting Enzyme (ACE) Inhibitor

Additional Appendix Information

Angiotensin Agents *on page 1632*

Heart Failure (Systolic) *on page 1809*

Use Treatment of hypertension, either alone or in combination with other antihypertensive agents; adjunctive therapy in treatment of heart failure (HF); treatment of acute myocardial infarction (MI) within 24 hours in hemodynamically-stable patients to improve survival

Pregnancy Risk Factor C (1st trimester); D (2nd and 3rd trimesters)

Pregnancy Considerations Due to adverse events observed in some animal studies, lisinopril is considered pregnancy category C during the first trimester. Based on human data, lisinopril is considered pregnancy category D if used during the second and third trimesters (per the manufacturer; however, one study suggests that fetal injury may occur at anytime during pregnancy). Lisinopril crosses the placenta. First trimester exposure to ACE inhibitors may cause major congenital malformations. An increased risk of cardiovascular and/or central nervous system malformations was observed in one study; however, an increased risk of teratogenic events was not observed in other studies. Second and third trimester use of an ACE inhibitor is associated with oligohydramnios. Oligohydramnios due to decreased fetal renal function may lead to fetal limb contractures, craniofacial deformation, and hypoplastic lung development. The use of ACE inhibitors during the second and third trimesters is also associated with anuria, hypotension, renal failure (reversible or irreversible), skull hypoplasia, and death in the fetus/neonate. Chronic maternal hypertension itself is also associated with adverse events in the fetus/infant. ACE inhibitors are not recommended during pregnancy to treat maternal hypertension or heart failure. Those who are planning a pregnancy should be considered for other medication options if an ACE inhibitor is currently prescribed or the ACE inhibitor should be discontinued as soon as possible once pregnancy is detected. The exposed fetus should be monitored for fetal growth, amniotic fluid volume, and organ formation. Infants exposed to an ACE inhibitor *in utero*, especially during the second and third trimester, should be monitored for hyperkalemia, hypotension, and oliguria.

[U.S. Boxed Warning]: Based on human data, ACE inhibitors can cause injury and death to the developing fetus when used in the second and third trimesters. ACE inhibitors should be discontinued as soon as possible once pregnancy is detected.

Lactation Excretion in breast milk unknown/not recommended

Medication Safety Issues

Sound-alike/look-alike issues:

Lisinopril may be confused with fosinopril, Lioresal®, Risperdal®

Prinivil® may be confused with Plendil®, Pravachol®, Prevacid®, Prilosec®, Proventil®

Zestril® may be confused with Desyrel®, Restoril®, Vistaril®, Zetia®, Zostrix®

International issues:

Acepril® [Denmark] may be confused with Accupril® which is a brand name for quinapril in the U.S.

Acepril®: Brand name for enalapril in Hungary and Switzerland; brand name for captopril in Great Britain

Carace® [Ireland; Great Britain] may be confused with Carac™ which is a brand name for fluorouracil in the U.S.

Zestril® may be confused with Nostril® which is a brand name for chlorhexidine/cetrimonium in France

Contraindications Hypersensitivity to lisinopril or any component of the formulation; angioedema related to previous treatment with an ACE inhibitor; patients with idiopathic or hereditary angioedema

Warnings/Precautions Anaphylactic reactions may occur rarely with ACE inhibitors. At any time during treatment (especially following first dose), angioedema may occur rarely with ACE inhibitors; it may involve the head and neck (potentially compromising airway) or the intestine (presenting with abdominal pain). African-Americans may be at an increased risk. Prolonged frequent monitoring may be required especially if tongue, glottis, or larynx are involved as they are associated with airway obstruction. Patients with a history of airway surgery may have a higher risk of airway obstruction. Aggressive early and appropriate management is critical. Use in patients with idiopathic or hereditary angioedema or previous angioedema associated with ACE inhibitor therapy is contraindicated. Severe anaphylactoid reactions may be seen during hemodialysis (eg, CVVHD) with high-flux dialysis membranes (eg, AN69), and rarely, during low density lipoprotein apheresis with dextran sulfate cellulose. Rare cases of anaphylactoid reactions have been reported in patients undergoing sensitization treatment with hymenoptera (bee, wasp) venom while receiving ACE inhibitors.

Symptomatic hypotension with or without syncope can occur with ACE inhibitors (usually with the first several doses); effects are most often observed in volume depleted patients; correct volume depletion prior to initiation; close monitoring of patient is required especially with initial dosing and dosing increases; blood pressure must be lowered at a rate appropriate for the patient's clinical condition. Initiation of therapy in patients with ischemic heart disease or cerebrovascular disease warrants close observation due to the potential consequences posed by falling blood pressure (eg, MI, stroke). Use with caution in hypertrophic cardiomyopathy with outflow tract obstruction, severe aortic stenosis, or before, during, or immediately after major surgery. **[U.S. Boxed Warning]: Based on human data, ACEIs can cause injury and death to the developing fetus when used in the second and third trimesters. ACEIs should be discontinued as soon as possible once pregnancy is detected.**

Hyperkalemia may occur with ACE inhibitors; risk factors include renal dysfunction, diabetes mellitus, concomitant use of potassium-sparing diuretics, potassium supplements, and/or potassium-containing salts. Use cautiously, if at all, with these agents and monitor potassium closely. Cough may occur with ACE inhibitors. Other causes of cough should be considered (eg, pulmonary congestion in patients with heart failure) and excluded prior to discontinuation.

May be associated with deterioration of renal function and/or increases in serum creatinine, particularly in patients with low renal blood flow (eg, renal artery stenosis, heart failure) whose glomerular filtration rate (GFR) is dependent on efferent arteriolar vasoconstriction by angiotensin II; deterioration may result in oliguria, acute renal failure, and progressive azotemia. Small increases in serum creatinine may occur following initiation; consider discontinuation only in patients with progressive and/or significant deterioration in renal function. Use with caution in patients with unstented unilateral/bilateral renal artery stenosis. When unstented bilateral renal artery stenosis is present, use is generally avoided due to the elevated risk of deterioration in renal function unless possible benefits outweigh risks.

Rare toxicities associated with ACE inhibitors include cholestatic jaundice (which may progress to fulminant hepatic necrosis), agranulocytosis, neutropenia, or leukopenia with myeloid hypoplasia. Patients with collagen vascular diseases (especially with concomitant renal impairment) or renal impairment alone may be at increased risk for hematologic toxicity; periodically monitor CBC with differential in these patients. Safety and efficacy have not been established in children <6 years of age or children with a Cl_{cr} ≤30 mL/minute.

Adverse Reactions Note: Frequency ranges include data from hypertension and heart failure trials. Higher rates of adverse reactions have generally been noted in patients with CHF. However, the frequency of adverse effects associated with placebo is also increased in this population.

1% to 10%:

- Cardiovascular: Orthostatic effects (1%), hypotension (1% to 4%)
- Central nervous system: Headache (4% to 6%), dizziness (5% to 12%), fatigue (3%)
- Dermatologic: Rash (1% to 2%)
- Endocrine & metabolic: Hyperkalemia (2% to 5%)
- Gastrointestinal: Diarrhea (3% to 4%), nausea (2%), vomiting (1%), abdominal pain (2%)
- Genitourinary: Impotence (1%)
- Hematologic: Decreased hemoglobin (small)
- Neuromuscular & skeletal: Chest pain (3%), weakness (1%)
- Renal: BUN increased (2%); deterioration in renal function (in patients with bilateral renal artery stenosis or hypovolemia); serum creatinine increased (often transient)
- Respiratory: Cough (4% to 9%), upper respiratory infection (1% to 2%)

<1% (Limited to important or life-threatening): Acute renal failure, alopecia, anaphylactoid reactions, angioedema, anuria, arrhythmia, arthralgia, arthritis, asthma, ataxia, azotemia, bilirubin increased, bone marrow suppression, bronchospasm, cardiac arrest, cutaneous pseudolymphoma, decreased libido, gout, hemolytic anemia, hepatic necrosis, hepatitis, hyponatremia, leukopenia, jaundice (cholestatic), MI, neutropenia, oliguria, orthostatic hypotension, pancreatitis, paresthesia, pemphigus, peripheral neuropathy, photosensitivity, pleural effusion, pulmonary embolism, pulmonary infiltrates, SIADH, Stevens-Johnson syndrome, stroke, syncope, systemic lupus erythematosus, thrombocytopenia, TIA, toxic epidermal necrolysis, transaminases increased, tremor, urticaria, vasculitis, vertigo, vision loss, volume overload, vomiting, weight gain/loss, wheezing, xerostomia

Drug Interactions

Avoid Concomitant Use There are no known interactions where it is recommended to avoid concomitant use.

Increased Effect/Toxicity

Lisinopril may increase the levels/effects of: Allopurinol; Amifostine; AzaTHIOprine; CycloSPORINE; Ferric Gluconate; Gold Sodium Thiomalate; Lithium; RiTUXimab

The levels/effects of Lisinopril may be increased by: Angiotensin II Receptor Blockers; Diazoxide; Eplerenone; Herbs (Hypotensive Properties); Loop Diuretics; Potassium Salts; Potassium-Sparing Diuretics; Prostacyclin Analogues; Sirolimus; Temsirolimus; Thiazide Diuretics; Trimethoprim

Decreased Effect

The levels/effects of Lisinopril may be decreased by: Antacids; Aprotinin; Herbs (Hypertensive Properties); Methylphenidate; Nonsteroidal Anti-Inflammatory Agents; Salicylates; Yohimbine

Ethanol/Nutrition/Herb Interactions

Food: Potassium-containing salt substitutes may increase risk of hyperkalemia.

Herb/Nutraceutical: Avoid bayberry, blue cohosh, cayenne, ephedra, ginger, ginseng (American), kola, licorice (may worsen hypertension). Avoid black cohosh, California poppy, coleus, golden seal, hawthorn, mistletoe, periwinkle, quinine, shepherd's purse (may have increased antihypertensive effect).

Mechanism of Action Competitive inhibitor of angiotensin-converting enzyme (ACE); prevents conversion of angiotensin I to angiotensin II, a potent vasoconstrictor; results in lower levels of angiotensin II which causes an increase in plasma renin activity and a reduction in aldosterone secretion; a CNS mechanism may also be involved in hypotensive effect as angiotensin II increases adrenergic outflow from CNS; vasoactive kallikreins may be decreased in conversion to active hormones by ACE inhibitors, thus reducing blood pressure

Pharmacodynamics/Kinetics

Onset of action: 1 hour

Peak effect: Hypotensive: Oral: ~6 hours

Duration: 24 hours

Absorption: Well absorbed; unaffected by food

Protein binding: 25%

Metabolism: Not metabolized

Bioavailability: Decreased with NYHA Class II-IV heart failure

Half-life elimination: 11-12 hours

Time to peak: ~7 hours

Excretion: Primarily urine (as unchanged drug)

Dosage Oral:

Hypertension:

Children ≥6 years: Initial: 0.07 mg/kg once daily (up to 5 mg); increase dose at 1- to 2-week intervals; doses >0.61 mg/kg or >40 mg have not been evaluated.

Adults: Usual dosage range (JNC 7): 10-40 mg/day

Not maintained on diuretic: Initial: 10 mg/day

Maintained on diuretic: Initial: 5 mg/day

Note: Antihypertensive effect may diminish toward the end of the dosing interval especially with doses of 10 mg/day. An increased dose may aid in extending the duration of antihypertensive effect. Doses up to 80 mg/day have been used, but do not appear to give greater effect.

Elderly: Initial: 2.5-5 mg/day; increase doses 2.5-5 mg/day at 1- to 2-week intervals; maximum daily dose: 40 mg

Patients taking diuretics should have them discontinued 2-3 days prior to initiating lisinopril if possible. Restart diuretic after blood pressure is stable if needed. If diuretic cannot be discontinued prior to therapy, begin with 5 mg with close supervision until stable blood pressure. In patients with hyponatremia (<130 mEq/L), start dose at 2.5 mg/day

Heart failure: Adults: Initial: 2.5-5 mg once daily; then increase by no more than 10 mg increments at intervals no less than 2 weeks to a maximum daily dose of 40 mg. Usual maintenance: 5-40 mg/day as a single dose. Target dose: 20-40 mg once daily (ACC/AHA 2005 Heart Failure Guidelines)

Note: If patient has hyponatremia (serum sodium <130 meq/L) or renal impairment (Cl_{cr} <30 mL/minute or creatinine >3 mg/dL), then initial dose should be 2.5 mg/day

Acute myocardial infarction (within 24 hours in hemodynamically stable patients): Oral: 5 mg immediately, then 5 mg at 24 hours, 10 mg at 48 hours, and 10 mg every day thereafter for 6 weeks. Patients should continue to receive standard treatments such as thrombolytics, aspirin, and beta-blockers.

Dosing adjustment in renal impairment:

Hypertension:

Adults: Initial doses should be modified and upward titration should be cautious, based on response (maximum: 40 mg/day)

Cl_{cr} >30 mL/minute: Initial: 10 mg/day

Cl_{cr} 10-30 mL/minute: Initial: 5 mg/day

Hemodialysis: Initial: 2.5 mg/day; dialyzable (50%)

Children: Use in not recommended in pediatric patients with GFR <30 mL/minute/1.73 m^2

Heart failure: Adults: Cl_{cr} <30 mL/minute or creatinine >3 mg/dL): Initial: 2.5 mg/day

Dietary Considerations Use potassium-containing salt substitutes cautiously in patients with diabetes, patients with renal dysfunction, or those maintained on potassium supplements or potassium-sparing diuretics.

Administration Watch for hypotensive effects within 1-3 hours of first dose or new higher dose.

Monitoring Parameters BUN, serum creatinine, renal function, WBC, and potassium; if patient has collagen vascular disease and/or renal impairment, periodically monitor CBC with differential

Test Interactions May cause false-positive results in urine acetone determinations using sodium nitroprusside reagent

Dosage Forms Excipient information presented when available (limited, particularly for generics); consult specific product labeling.

Tablet: 2.5 mg, 5 mg, 10 mg, 20 mg, 30 mg, 40 mg

Prinivil®: 5 mg, 10 mg, 20 mg

Zestril®: 2.5 mg, 5 mg, 10 mg, 20 mg, 30 mg, 40 mg

Extemporaneous Preparations Preparation of oral suspension (1 mg/mL): Note: Mix in a polyethylene terephthalate bottle. Add 10 mL of purified water (USP) to a bottle containing ten lisinopril 20 mg tablets (total 200 mg). Shake for at least 1 minute; then add 30 mL Bicitra® and 160 mL Ora-Sweet SF™ and shake gently to suspend contents. Store at 25°C (77°F); stable for up to 4 weeks.

Lisinopril and Hydrochlorothiazide

(lyse IN oh pril & hye droe klor oh THYE a zide)

U.S. Brand Names Prinzide®; Zestoretic®

Canadian Brand Names Apo-Lisinopril/Hctz; Gen-Lisinopril/Hctz; Novo-Lisinopril/Hctz; Prinzide®; Sandoz Lisinopril/Hctz; Zestoretic®

Index Terms Hydrochlorothiazide and Lisinopril

Pharmacologic Category Angiotensin-Converting Enzyme (ACE) Inhibitor; Diuretic, Thiazide

Use Treatment of hypertension

Pregnancy Risk Factor C/D (2nd and 3rd trimesters)

Dosage Adults: Oral: Dosage is individualized; see each component for appropriate dosing suggestions; doses >80 mg/day lisinopril or >50 mg/day hydrochlorothiazide are not recommended.

Additional Information Complete prescribing information for this medication should be consulted for additional detail.

Dosage Forms Excipient information presented when available (limited, particularly for generics); consult specific product labeling. [DSC] = Discontinued product

Tablet: 10/12.5: Lisinopril 10 mg and hydrochlorothiazide 12.5 mg; 20/12.5: Lisinopril 20 mg and hydrochlorothiazide 12.5 mg; 20/25: Lisinopril 20 mg and hydrochlorothiazide 25 mg

Prinizide®:

10/12.5: Lisinopril 10 mg and hydrochlorothiazide 12.5 mg

20/12.5: Lisinopril 20 mg and hydrochlorothiazide 12.5 mg [DSC]

20/25: Lisinopril 20 mg and hydrochlorothiazide 25 mg

Zestoretic®:
10/12.5: Lisinopril 10 mg and hydrochlorothiazide 12.5 mg
20/12.5: Lisinopril 20 mg and hydrochlorothiazide 12.5 mg
20/25: Lisinopril 20 mg and hydrochlorothiazide 25 mg

◆ **Lispro Insulin** *see* Insulin Lispro *on page 794*
◆ **Lithane™ (Can)** *see* Lithium *on page 897*

Lithium (LITH ee um)

U.S. Brand Names Eskalith CR® [DSC]; Eskalith® [DSC]; Lithobid®

Canadian Brand Names Apo-Lithium® Carbonate; Apo-Lithium® Carbonate SR; Carbolith™; Duralith®; Euro-Lithium; Lithane™; PMS-Lithium Carbonate; PMS-Lithium Citrate

Index Terms Lithium Carbonate; Lithium Citrate

Pharmacologic Category Antimanic Agent

Use Management of bipolar disorders; treatment of mania in individuals with bipolar disorder (maintenance treatment prevents or diminishes intensity of subsequent episodes)

Unlabeled/Investigational Use Potential augmenting agent for antidepressants; aggression, post-traumatic stress disorder, conduct disorder in children

Pregnancy Risk Factor D

Pregnancy Considerations Cardiac malformations in the infant, including Ebstein's anomaly, are associated with use of lithium during the first trimester of pregnancy. Nontoxic effects to the newborn include shallow respiration, hypotonia, lethargy, cyanosis, diabetes insipidus, thyroid depression, and nontoxic goiter when lithium is used near term. Efforts should be made to avoid lithium use during the first trimester; if an alternative therapy is not appropriate, the lowest possible dose of lithium should be used throughout the pregnancy. Fetal echocardiography and ultrasound to screen for anomalies should be conducted between 16-20 weeks of gestation. Lithium levels should be monitored in the mother and may need to be adjusted following delivery.

Lactation Enters breast milk/contraindicated

Medication Safety Issues

Sound-alike/look-alike issues:
Eskalith® may be confused with Estratest®
Lithobid® may be confused with Levbid®, Lithostat®

Do not confuse **mEq** (milliequivalent) with **mg** (milligram). **Note:** 8 mEq lithium carbonate equals 300 mg lithium carbonate. Dosage should be written in **mg** (milligrams) to avoid confusion. Check prescriptions for unusually high volumes of the syrup for dosing errors.

Contraindications Hypersensitivity to lithium or any component of the formulation; avoid use in patients with severe cardiovascular or renal disease, or with severe debilitation, dehydration, or sodium depletion; pregnancy

Warnings/Precautions [U.S. Boxed Warning]: Lithium toxicity is closely related to serum levels and can occur at therapeutic doses; serum lithium determinations are required to monitor therapy. Use with caution in patients with thyroid disease, mild-moderate renal impairment, or mild-moderate cardiovascular disease. Use caution in patients receiving medications which alter sodium excretion (eg, diuretics, ACE inhibitors, NSAIDs), or in patients with significant fluid loss (protracted sweating, diarrhea, or prolonged fever); temporary reduction or cessation of therapy may be warranted. Some elderly patients may be extremely sensitive to the effects of lithium, see Dosage and Reference Range. Chronic therapy results in diminished renal concentrating ability (nephrogenic DI); this is usually reversible when lithium is discontinued. Changes in renal function should be monitored, and re-evaluation of treatment may be necessary. Use caution in patients at risk of suicide (suicidal thoughts or behavior).

Use with caution in patients receiving neuroleptic medications - a syndrome resembling NMS has been associated with concurrent therapy. Lithium may impair the patient's alertness, affecting the ability to operate machinery or driving a vehicle. Neuromuscular-blocking agents should be administered with caution; the response may be prolonged.

Higher serum concentrations may be required and tolerated during an acute manic phase; however, the tolerance decreases when symptoms subside. Normal fluid and salt intake must be maintained during therapy.

Safety and efficacy have not been established in children <12 years of age.

Adverse Reactions Frequency not defined.

Cardiovascular: Cardiac arrhythmia, hypotension, sinus node dysfunction, flattened or inverted T waves (reversible), edema, bradycardia, syncope

Central nervous system: Dizziness, vertigo, slurred speech, blackout spells, seizure, sedation, restlessness, confusion, psychomotor retardation, stupor, coma, dystonia, fatigue, lethargy, headache, pseudotumor cerebri, slowed intellectual functioning, tics

Dermatologic: Dry or thinning of hair, folliculitis, alopecia, exacerbation of psoriasis, rash

Endocrine & metabolic: Euthyroid goiter and/or hypothyroidism, hyperthyroidism, hyperglycemia, diabetes insipidus

Gastrointestinal: Polydipsia, anorexia, nausea, vomiting, diarrhea, xerostomia, metallic taste, weight gain, salivary gland swelling, excessive salivation

Genitourinary: Incontinence, polyuria, glycosuria, oliguria, albuminuria

Hematologic: Leukocytosis

Neuromuscular & skeletal: Tremor, muscle hyperirritability, ataxia, choreoathetoid movements, hyperactive deep tendon reflexes, myasthenia gravis (rare)

Ocular: Nystagmus, blurred vision, transient scotoma

Miscellaneous: Coldness and painful discoloration of fingers and toes

Drug Interactions

Avoid Concomitant Use

Avoid concomitant use of Lithium with any of the following: Sibutramine

Increased Effect/Toxicity

Lithium may increase the levels/effects of: Antipsychotics; Neuromuscular-Blocking Agents; Serotonin Modulators; Tricyclic Antidepressants

The levels/effects of Lithium may be increased by: ACE Inhibitors; Angiotensin II Receptor Blockers; Calcium Channel Blockers (Nondihydropyridine); CarBAMazepine; Desmopressin; MAO Inhibitors; Methyldopa; Nonsteroidal Anti-Inflammatory Agents; Phenytoin; Potassium Iodide; Selective Serotonin Reuptake Inhibitors; Sibutramine; Thiazide Diuretics

Decreased Effect

Lithium may decrease the levels/effects of: Amphetamines; Antipsychotics; Desmopressin

The levels/effects of Lithium may be decreased by: Sodium Bicarbonate; Sodium Chloride; Theophylline Derivatives

Ethanol/Nutrition/Herb Interactions Food: Lithium serum concentrations may be increased if taken with food. Limit caffeine.

Mechanism of Action Alters cation transport across cell membrane in nerve and muscle cells and influences reuptake of serotonin and/or norepinephrine; second messenger systems involving the phosphatidylinositol cycle are inhibited; postsynaptic D2 receptor supersensitivity is inhibited

Pharmacodynamics/Kinetics

Absorption: Rapid and complete

Distribution: V_d: Initial: 0.3-0.4 L/kg; V_{dss}: 0.7-1 L/kg; crosses placenta; enters breast milk at 35% to 50% the concentrations in serum; distribution is complete in 6-10 hours

CSF, liver concentrations: 1/3 to 1/2 of serum concentration

Erythrocyte concentration: ~1/2 of serum concentration

Heart, lung, kidney, muscle concentrations: Equivalent to serum concentration

Saliva concentration: 2-3 times serum concentration

Thyroid, bone, brain tissue concentrations: Increase 50% over serum concentrations

Protein binding: Not protein bound

Metabolism: Not metabolized

Bioavailability: Not affected by food; Capsule, immediate release tablet: 95% to 100%; Extended release tablet: 60% to 90%; Syrup: 100%

Half-life elimination: 18-24 hours; can increase to more than 36 hours in elderly or with renal impairment

Time to peak, serum: Nonsustained release: ~0.5-2 hours; slow release: 4-12 hours; syrup: 15-60 minutes

Excretion: Urine (90% to 98% as unchanged drug); sweat (4% to 5%); feces (1%)

Clearance: 80% of filtered lithium is reabsorbed in the proximal convoluted tubules; therefore, clearance approximates 20% of GFR or 20-40 mL/minute

Dosage Oral: Monitor serum concentrations and clinical response (efficacy and toxicity) to determine proper dose

Children 6-12 years:

Bipolar disorder (unlabeled use): 15-60 mg/kg/day in 3-4 divided doses; dose not to exceed usual adult dosage

Conduct disorder (unlabeled use): 15-30 mg/kg/day in 3-4 divided doses; dose not to exceed usual adult dosage

Adults: Bipolar disorder: 900-2400 mg/day in 3-4 divided doses or 900-1800 mg/day (sustained release) in 2 divided doses

Elderly: Bipolar disorder: Initial dose: 300 mg once or twice daily; increase weekly in increments of 300 mg/day, monitoring levels; rarely need >900-1200 mg/day

Dosing adjustment in renal impairment:

Cl_{cr} 10-50 mL/minute: Administer 50% to 75% of normal dose

Cl_{cr} <10 mL/minute: Administer 25% to 50% of normal dose

Hemodialysis: Dialyzable (50% to 100%); 4-7 times more efficient than peritoneal dialysis

Dietary Considerations May be taken with meals to avoid GI upset; have patient drink 2-3 L of water daily.

Administration Administer with meals to decrease GI upset. Slow release tablets must be swallowed whole; do not crush or chew.

Monitoring Parameters Serum lithium every 4-5 days during initial therapy; draw lithium serum concentrations 8-12 hours postdose; renal, thyroid, and cardiovascular function; fluid status; serum electrolytes; CBC with differential, urinalysis; monitor for signs of toxicity; beta-hCG pregnancy test for all females not known to be sterile

Reference Range Levels should be obtained twice weekly until both patient's clinical status and levels are stable then levels may be obtained every 1-3 months

Timing of serum samples: Draw trough just before next dose (8-12 hours after previous dose)

Therapeutic levels:

Acute mania: 0.6-1.2 mEq/L (SI: 0.6-1.2 mmol/L)

Protection against future episodes in most patients with bipolar disorder: 0.8-1 mEq/L (SI: 0.8-1.0 mmol/L); a higher rate of relapse is described in subjects who are maintained at <0.4 mEq/L (SI: 0.4 mmol/L)

Elderly patients can usually be maintained at lower end of therapeutic range (0.6-0.8 mEq/L)

Toxic concentration: >1.5 mEq/L (SI: >2 mmol/L)

Adverse effect levels:

GI complaints/tremor: 1.5-2 mEq/L

Confusion/somnolence: 2-2.5 mEq/L

Seizures/death: >2.5 mEq/L

Dosage Forms Excipient information presented when available (limited, particularly for generics); consult specific product labeling. [DSC] = Discontinued product

Capsule, as carbonate: 150 mg, 300 mg, 600 mg

Eskalith®: 300 mg [contains benzyl alcohol] [DSC]

Solution, as citrate: 300 mg/5 mL (5 mL, 500 mL) [equivalent to amount of lithium in lithium carbonate]

Syrup, as citrate: 300 mg/5 mL (480 mL) [equivalent to amount of lithium in lithium carbonate]

Tablet, as carbonate: 300 mg

Tablet, controlled release, as carbonate: 450 mg

Eskalith CR®: 450 mg [DSC]

Tablet, slow release, as carbonate: 300 mg

Lithobid®: 300 mg

- **Lithium Carbonate** *see* Lithium *on page 897*
- **Lithium Citrate** *see* Lithium *on page 897*
- **Lithobid®** *see* Lithium *on page 897*
- **Little Colds® Multi-Symptom Cold Formula [OTC] [DSC]** *see* Acetaminophen, Dextromethorphan, and Phenylephrine *on page 32*
- **Little Fevers™ [OTC]** *see* Acetaminophen *on page 25*
- **Little Noses® Decongestant [OTC]** *see* Phenylephrine *on page 1183*
- **Little Noses® Saline [OTC]** *see* Sodium Chloride *on page 1381*
- **Little Noses® Stuffy Nose Kit [OTC]** *see* Sodium Chloride *on page 1381*
- **Little Teethers® [OTC]** *see* Benzocaine *on page 183*
- **Live Attenuated Influenza Vaccine (LAIV)** *see* Influenza Virus Vaccine *on page 788*
- **Live Smallpox Vaccine** *see* Smallpox Vaccine *on page 1377*
- **Livostin® [DSC]** *see* Levocabastine *on page 874*
- **Livostin® (Can)** *see* Levocabastine *on page 874*
- **L-leucovorin** *see* LEVOleucovorin *on page 878*
- **LM3100** *see* Plerixafor *on page 1202*
- **LMD®** *see* Dextran *on page 431*
- **LNg 20** *see* Levonorgestrel *on page 879*
- **Locoid®** *see* Hydrocortisone *on page 743*
- **Locoid Lipocream®** *see* Hydrocortisone *on page 743*
- **Lodosyn®** *see* Carbidopa *on page 256*

Lodoxamide (loe DOKS a mide)

U.S. Brand Names Alomide®

Canadian Brand Names Alomide®

Index Terms Lodoxamide Tromethamine

Pharmacologic Category Mast Cell Stabilizer

Use Treatment of vernal keratoconjunctivitis, vernal conjunctivitis, and vernal keratitis

Pregnancy Risk Factor B

Medication Safety Issues

International issues:

Thilomide® [Turkey] may be confused with Thalomid® which is a brand name for thalidomide in the U.S.

Dosage Ophthalmic: Instill 1-2 drops in eye(s) 4 times/day for up to 3 months

Additional Information Complete prescribing information for this medication should be consulted for additional detail.

Dosage Forms Excipient information presented when available (limited, particularly for generics); consult specific product labeling.

Solution, ophthalmic: 0.1% (10 mL) [contains benzalkonium chloride]

- **Lodoxamide Tromethamine** *see* Lodoxamide *on page 898*
- **Lodrane® [DSC]** *see* Brompheniramine and Pseudoephedrine *on page 214*
- **Lodrane® 12D** *see* Brompheniramine and Pseudoephedrine *on page 214*
- **Lodrane® 12 Hour** *see* Brompheniramine *on page 214*
- **Lodrane® 24** *see* Brompheniramine *on page 214*
- **Lodrane® 24D** *see* Brompheniramine and Pseudoephedrine *on page 214*
- **Lodrane® D** *see* Brompheniramine and Pseudoephedrine *on page 214*
- **Lodrane® XR** *see* Brompheniramine *on page 214*
- **Loestrin®** *see* Ethinyl Estradiol and Norethindrone *on page 581*
- **Loestrin™ 1.5/30 (Can)** *see* Ethinyl Estradiol and Norethindrone *on page 581*
- **Loestrin® 24 Fe** *see* Ethinyl Estradiol and Norethindrone *on page 581*
- **Loestrin® Fe** *see* Ethinyl Estradiol and Norethindrone *on page 581*
- **Lofibra®** *see* Fenofibrate *on page 607*
- **LoHist-12** *see* Brompheniramine *on page 214*
- **LoHist 12D** *see* Brompheniramine and Pseudoephedrine *on page 214*
- **LoHist-D** *see* Chlorpheniramine and Pseudoephedrine *on page 310*
- **LoHist LQ** *see* Brompheniramine and Pseudoephedrine *on page 214*
- **LoHist PD** *see* Brompheniramine and Pseudoephedrine *on page 214*
- **L-OHP** *see* Oxaliplatin *on page 1112*
- **LoKara™** *see* Desonide *on page 424*
- **Lomine (Can)** *see* Dicyclomine *on page 441*
- **Lomotil®** *see* Diphenoxylate and Atropine *on page 459*

Lomustine (loe MUS teen)

U.S. Brand Names CeeNU®

Canadian Brand Names CeeNU®

Index Terms CCNU; NSC-79037

Pharmacologic Category Antineoplastic Agent, Alkylating Agent

Use Treatment of brain tumors and Hodgkin's disease

Unlabeled/Investigational Use Non-Hodgkin's lymphoma, melanoma, renal carcinoma, lung cancer, colon cancer

Pregnancy Risk Factor D

Pregnancy Considerations Teratogenic effects and embryotoxicity have been observed in animal studies. There are no adequate and well-controlled studies in pregnant women. May cause fetal harm when administered to a pregnant woman. Women of childbearing potential should be advised to avoid pregnancy and should be advised of the potential harm to the fetus.

Lactation Enters breast milk/contraindicated

Medication Safety Issues

Sound-alike/look-alike issues:

Lomustine may be confused with carmustine

High alert medication: The Institute for Safe Medication Practices (ISMP) includes this medication among its list of drugs which have a heightened risk of causing significant patient harm when used in error.

Lomustine should only be administered as a single dose once every 6 weeks; serious errors have occurred when lomustine was inadvertently administered daily.

Contraindications Hypersensitivity to lomustine, any component of the formulation, or other nitrosoureas; pregnancy

Warnings/Precautions Hazardous agent - use appropriate precautions for handling and disposal. **[U.S. Boxed Warnings]: Bone marrow suppression, notably thrombocytopenia and leukopenia, may lead to bleeding and overwhelming infections in an already compromised patient;** will last for at least 6 weeks after a dose. Do not administer courses more frequently than every 6 weeks because the toxicity is delayed. Use with caution in patients with depressed platelet, leukocyte or erythrocyte counts, renal (may require dosage adjustment) or hepatic impairment. Bone marrow toxicity is cumulative; dose adjustments should be based on nadir counts from prior dose. May cause delayed pulmonary toxicity (infiltrates and/or fibrosis); usually related to cumulative doses >1100 mg/m^2. Long-term use may be associated with the development of secondary malignancies. **[U.S. Boxed Warning]: Should be administered under the supervision of an experienced cancer chemotherapy physician.**

Adverse Reactions

>10%:

Gastrointestinal: Nausea and vomiting, usually within 3-6 hours after oral administration. Administration of the dose at bedtime, with an antiemetic, significantly reduces both the incidence and severity of nausea.

Hematologic: Myelosuppression, common, dose-limiting, may be cumulative and irreversible; leukopenia (65%; nadir: 5-6 weeks; recovery 6-8 weeks); thrombocytopenia (nadir: 4 weeks; recovery 5-6 weeks)

Frequency not defined: Acute leukemia, alkaline phosphatase increased, alopecia, anemia, ataxia, azotemia (progressive), bilirubin increased, blindness, bone marrow dysplasia, disorientation, dysarthria, kidney size decreased, lethargy, optic atrophy, pulmonary fibrosis, pulmonary infiltrates, renal failure, stomatitis, transaminases increased, visual disturbances

Drug Interactions

Metabolism/Transport Effects Substrate of CYP2D6 (major); **Inhibits** CYP2D6 (weak), 3A4 (weak)

Avoid Concomitant Use

Avoid concomitant use of Lomustine with any of the following: Natalizumab; Vaccines (Live)

Increased Effect/Toxicity

Lomustine may increase the levels/effects of: Natalizumab; Vaccines (Live)

The levels/effects of Lomustine may be increased by: CYP2D6 Inhibitors (Moderate); CYP2D6 Inhibitors (Strong); Darunavir; Trastuzumab

Decreased Effect

Lomustine may decrease the levels/effects of: Vaccines (Inactivated)

The levels/effects of Lomustine may be decreased by: Echinacea

Ethanol/Nutrition/Herb Interactions Ethanol: Avoid ethanol (due to GI irritation).

Stability Store at 15°C to 30°C (59°F to 86°F).

Mechanism of Action Inhibits DNA and RNA synthesis via carbamylation of DNA polymerase, alkylation of DNA, and alteration of RNA, proteins, and enzymes

Pharmacodynamics/Kinetics

Duration: Marrow recovery: ~5-8 weeks

Absorption: Complete
Distribution: Crosses blood-brain barrier to a greater degree than BCNU; CNS concentrations are ≥50% of plasma concentrations
Metabolism: Rapidly hepatic via hydroxylation producing at least two active metabolites; enterohepatically recycled
Half-life elimination: Parent drug: 16-72 hours; Active metabolite: 16-48 hours
Time to peak, serum: Active metabolite: ~3 hours
Excretion: Urine (~50%); feces (<5%); expired air (<10%)

Dosage Oral (refer to individual protocols):
Children: 75-150 mg/m^2 as a single dose once every 6 weeks; subsequent doses are readjusted after initial treatment according to platelet and leukocyte counts
Adults: 100-130 mg/m^2 as a single dose once every 6 weeks; readjust after initial treatment according to platelet and leukocyte counts
With compromised marrow function: Initial dose: 100 mg/m^2 as a single dose once every 6 weeks
Repeat courses should only be administered after adequate recovery: Leukocytes >4000/mm^3 and platelet counts >100,000/mm^3

Subsequent dosing adjustment based on nadir:
Leukocytes 2000-2999/mm^3, platelets 25,000-74,999/mm^3: Administer 70% of prior dose
Leukocytes <2000/mm^3, platelets <25,000/mm^3: Administer 50% of prior dose

Dosage adjustment in renal impairment: The FDA-approved labeling does not contain renal dosing adjustment guidelines. The following guidelines have been used by some clinicians:
Aronoff, 2007: Adults:
Cl_{cr} 10-50 mL/minute: Administer 75% of dose
Cl_{cr} <10 mL/minute: Administer 25% to 50% of dose
Hemodialysis: Supplemental dose is not necessary
Continuous ambulatory peritoneal dialysis (CAPD): Administer 25% to 50% of dose
Kintzel, 1995:
Cl_{cr} 46-60 mL/minute: Administer 75% of normal dose
Cl_{cr} 31-45 mL/minute: Administer 70% of normal dose
Cl_{cr} ≤30 mL/minute: Avoid use

Dosage adjustment in hepatic impairment: The FDA-approved labeling does not contain hepatic adjustment guidelines; lomustine is hepatically metabolized and caution should be used in patients with hepatic dysfunction.

Dietary Considerations Should be taken with fluids on an empty stomach; no food or drink for 2 hours after administration to decrease nausea.

Administration Take with fluids on an empty stomach; no food or drink for 2 hours after administration.

Monitoring Parameters CBC with differential and platelet count (for at least 6 weeks after dose), hepatic and renal function tests (periodic), pulmonary function tests (baseline and periodic)

Test Interactions Liver function tests

Dosage Forms Excipient information presented when available (limited, particularly for generics); consult specific product labeling. [DSC] = Discontinued product
Capsule:
CeeNU®: 10 mg, 40 mg, 100 mg
Capsule [dose pack]:
CeeNU®: 10 mg (2s); 40 mg (2s); 100 mg (2s) [DSC]

◆ **Loniten® (Can)** *see* Minoxidil *on page 1001*

◆ **Lonox®** *see* Diphenoxylate and Atropine *on page 459*

◆ **Lo/Ovral®** *see* Ethinyl Estradiol and Norgestrel *on page 585*

◆ **Loperacap (Can)** *see* Loperamide *on page 900*

Loperamide (loe PER a mide)

U.S. Brand Names Diamode [OTC]; Imodium® A-D [OTC]; K-Pek II [OTC]; Kao-Paverin® [OTC]

Canadian Brand Names Apo-Loperamide®; Diarr-Eze; Dom-Loperamide; Imodium®; Loperacap; Novo-Loperamide; PMS-Loperamine; Rhoxal-Loperamide; Rho®-Loperamine; Riva-Loperamide; Sandoz-Loperamide

Index Terms Loperamide Hydrochloride

Pharmacologic Category Antidiarrheal

Use Treatment of chronic diarrhea associated with inflammatory bowel disease; acute nonspecific diarrhea; increased volume of ileostomy discharge
OTC labeling: Control of symptoms of diarrhea, including Traveler's diarrhea

Unlabeled/Investigational Use Cancer treatment-induced diarrhea (eg, irinotecan induced); chronic diarrhea caused by bowel resection

Pregnancy Risk Factor C

Pregnancy Considerations Teratogenic effects were not observed in animal studies.

Lactation Enters breast milk/not recommended.

Medication Safety Issues
Sound-alike/look-alike issues:
Imodium® A-D may be confused with Indocin®, Ionamin®

Contraindications Hypersensitivity to loperamide or any component of the formulation; abdominal pain without diarrhea; children <2 years
Avoid use as primary therapy in acute dysentery, acute ulcerative colitis, bacterial enterocolitis, pseudomembranous colitis

Warnings/Precautions Rare cases of anaphylaxis and anaphylactic shock have been reported. Should not be used if diarrhea is accompanied by high fever or blood in stool. Use caution in young children as response may be variable because of dehydration. Concurrent fluid and electrolyte replacement is often necessary in all age groups depending upon severity of diarrhea. Should not be used when inhibition of peristalsis is undesirable or dangerous. Discontinue if constipation, abdominal pain, or ileus develop. Use caution in treatment of AIDS patients; stop therapy at the sign of abdominal distention. Cases of toxic megacolon have occurred in this population. Loperamide is a symptom-directed treatment; if an underlying diagnosis is made, other disease-specific treatment may be indicated. Use caution in patients with hepatic impairment because of reduced first-pass metabolism; monitor for signs of CNS toxicity.

OTC labeling: If diarrhea lasts longer than 2 days, patient should stop taking loperamide and consult healthcare provider.

Adverse Reactions 1% to 10%:
Central nervous system: Dizziness (1%)
Gastrointestinal: Constipation (2% to 5%), abdominal cramping (<1% to 3%), nausea (<1% to 3%)
Postmarketing and/or case reports: Abdominal distention, abdominal pain, allergic reactions, anaphylactic shock, anaphylactoid reactions, angioedema, bullous eruption (rare), drowsiness, dry mouth, dyspepsia, erythema multiforme (rare), fatigue, flatulence, paralytic ileus, megacolon, pruritus, rash, Stevens-Johnson syndrome, toxic epidermal necrolysis, toxic megacolon, urinary retention, urticaria, vomiting

Drug Interactions
Metabolism/Transport Effects Substrate (minor) of CYP2B6
Avoid Concomitant Use There are no known interactions where it is recommended to avoid concomitant use.

Increased Effect/Toxicity
The levels/effects of Loperamide may be increased by: P-Glycoprotein Inhibitors

Decreased Effect
The levels/effects of Loperamide may be decreased by: P-Glycoprotein Inducers

Stability Store at 15°C to 25°C (59°F to 77°F).

Mechanism of Action Acts directly on circular and longitudinal intestinal muscles, through the opioid receptor, to inhibit peristalsis and prolong transit time; reduces fecal volume, increases viscosity, and diminishes fluid and electrolyte loss; demonstrates antisecretory activity. Loperamide increases tone on the anal sphincter

Pharmacodynamics/Kinetics
Absorption: Poor
Distribution: Poor penetration into brain; low amounts enter breast milk
Metabolism: Hepatic via oxidative N-demethylation
Half-life elimination: 7-14 hours
Time to peak, plasma: Liquid: 2.5 hours; Capsule: 5 hours
Excretion: Urine and feces (1% as metabolites, 30% to 40% as unchanged drug)

Dosage Oral:
Children:
Acute diarrhea: Initial doses (in first 24 hours):
2-5 years (13-20 kg): 1 mg 3 times/day
6-8 years (20-30 kg): 2 mg twice daily
8-12 years (>30 kg): 2 mg 3 times/day
Maintenance: After initial dosing, 0.1 mg/kg doses after each loose stool, but not exceeding initial dosage
Traveler's diarrhea:
6-8 years: 2 mg after first loose stool, followed by 1 mg after each subsequent stool (maximum dose: 4 mg/day)
9-11 years: 2 mg after first loose stool, followed by 1 mg after each subsequent stool (maximum dose: 6 mg/day)
≥12 years: See adult dosing.
Adults:
Acute diarrhea: Initial: 4 mg, followed by 2 mg after each loose stool, up to 16 mg/day
Chronic diarrhea: Initial: Follow acute diarrhea; maintenance dose should be slowly titrated downward to minimum required to control symptoms (typically, 4-8 mg/day in divided doses)
Traveler's diarrhea: Initial: 4 mg after first loose stool, followed by 2 mg after each subsequent stool (maximum dose: 8 mg/day)
Irinotecan-induced diarrhea (unlabeled use): 4 mg after first loose or frequent bowel movement, then 2 mg every 2 hours until 12 hours have passed without a bowel movement. If diarrhea recurs, then repeat administration

Dosage adjustment in hepatic impairment: No specific guidelines available.

Dietary Considerations
Imodium® A-D [new formulation] contains sodium 10 mg/30 mL.

Dosage Forms Excipient information presented when available (limited, particularly for generics); consult specific product labeling.
Caplet, as hydrochloride: 2 mg
Diamode, Imodium® A-D, Kao-Paverin®: 2 mg
Capsule, as hydrochloride: 2 mg
Liquid, oral, as hydrochloride: 1 mg/5 mL (5 mL, 10 mL, 120 mL)
Imodium® A-D: 1 mg/5 mL (60 mL, 120 mL) [contains alcohol, sodium benzoate, benzoic acid; cherry mint flavor]
Imodium® A-D [new formulation]: 1 mg/7.5 mL (60 mL, 120 mL, 360 mL) [contains sodium 10 mg/30 mL, sodium benzoate; creamy mint flavor]
Tablet, as hydrochloride: 2 mg
K-Pek II: 2 mg

Loperamide and Simethicone
(loe PER a mide & sye METH i kone)

U.S. Brand Names Imodium® Advanced

Index Terms Simethicone and Loperamide Hydrochloride

Pharmacologic Category Antidiarrheal; Antiflatulent

Use Control of symptoms of diarrhea and gas (bloating, pressure, and cramps)

Dosage Oral: Acute diarrhea (weight-based dosing is preferred):
Children:
6-8 years (48-59 lbs): 1 caplet or tablet after first loose stool, followed by 1/2 caplet/tablet with each subsequent loose stool (maximum: 2 caplets or tablets/24 hours)
9-11 years (60-95 lbs): 1 caplet or tablet after first loose stool, followed by 1/2 caplet or tablet with each subsequent loose stool (maximum: 3 caplets or tablets/24 hours)
Children >12 years and Adults: One caplet or tablet after first loose stool, followed by 1 caplet or tablet with each subsequent loose stool (maximum: 4 caplets or tablets/24 hours)

Additional Information Complete prescribing information for this medication should be consulted for additional detail.

Dosage Forms Excipient information presented when available (limited, particularly for generics); consult specific product labeling.
Caplet: Loperamide hydrochloride 2 mg and simethicone 125 mg
Tablet, chewable: Loperamide hydrochloride 2 mg and simethicone 125 mg [mint flavor]

◆ **Loperamide Hydrochloride** *see* Loperamide *on page 900*

◆ **Lopid®** *see* Gemfibrozil *on page 687*

Lopinavir and Ritonavir
(loe PIN a veer & rit ON uh veer)

U.S. Brand Names Kaletra®

Canadian Brand Names Kaletra®

Index Terms Ritonavir and Lopinavir

Pharmacologic Category Antiretroviral Agent, Protease Inhibitor

Additional Appendix Information
Antiretroviral Therapy for HIV Infection: Adults and Adolescents *on page 1758*
Management of Healthcare Worker Exposures to HBV, HCV, and HIV *on page 1719*
Perinatal HIV Guidelines *on page 1730*

Use Treatment of HIV infection in combination with other antiretroviral agents

Pregnancy Risk Factor C

Pregnancy Considerations Adverse events were not seen in animal studies, except at doses which were also maternally toxic. Safety and pharmacokinetic studies of the tablet in pregnant women are not completed. Preliminary information suggests increased dosage may be needed during pregnancy, although specific recommendations with the tablet formulation are not yet available. Once-daily dosing is not recommended during pregnancy. Lopinavir/ritonavir crosses the placenta, however, teratogenic effects have not been observed in humans. The Perinatal HIV Guidelines Working Group considers this a recommended combination for use during pregnancy. Pregnancy and protease inhibitors are both associated with an increased risk of hyperglycemia. Glucose levels should be closely monitored. Health professionals are encouraged to contact the antiretroviral pregnancy registry to monitor outcomes of pregnant women exposed to antiretroviral medications (1-800-258-4263 or www.APRegistry.com).

Lactation Excretion in breast milk unknown/contra-indicated

Medication Safety Issues

Sound-alike/look-alike issues:

Potential for dispensing errors between Kaletra™ and Keppra® (levetiracetam)

Administration issues:

Children's doses are based on weight and calculated by milligrams of lopinavir. Care should be taken to accurately calculate the dose. The oral solution contains lopinavir 80 mg and ritonavir 20 mg per one mL. Children <12 years of age (and ≤40 kg) who are not taking certain concomitant antiretroviral medications will receive <5 mL of solution per dose.

Contraindications Hypersensitivity (eg, Stevens-Johnson syndrome, erythema multiforme) to lopinavir, ritonavir, or any component of the formulation; coadministration with medications highly dependent upon CYP3A4 for clearance for which increased levels are associated with serious and/or life-threatening events; coadministration with strong CYP3A4 inducers, including cisapride, ergot alkaloids (eg, dihydroergotamine, ergonovine, ergotamine, methylergonovine), lovastatin, midazolam (oral), pimozide, rifampin, simvastatin, St John's wort, triazolam

Warnings/Precautions Use with caution in patients taking strong CYP3A4 inhibitors, moderate or strong CYP3A4 inducers and major CYP3A4 substrates (see Drug Interactions); contraindicated with certain CYP3A4 substrates and inducers (see Contraindications); consider alternative agents that avoid or lessen the potential for CYP-mediated interactions. Cases of pancreatitis, some fatal, have been associated with lopinavir/ritonavir; use caution in patients with a history of pancreatitis. Patients with signs or symptoms of pancreatitis should be evaluated and therapy suspended as clinically appropriate.

Changes in glucose tolerance, hyperglycemia, exacerbation of diabetes, DKA, and new-onset diabetes mellitus have been reported in patients receiving protease inhibitors. May cause hepatitis or exacerbate pre-existing hepatic dysfunction; use with caution in patients with hepatitis B or C and in hepatic disease; patients with hepatitis or elevations in transaminases prior to the start of therapy may be at increased risk for further increases in transaminases or hepatic dysfunction (rare fatalities reported in postmarketing). Large increases in total cholesterol and triglycerides have been reported; screening should be done prior to therapy and periodically throughout treatment. Increased bleeding may be seen in patients with hemophilia A or B who are taking protease inhibitors. Redistribution or accumulation of body fat has been observed in patients using antiretroviral therapy. An inflammatory response to indolent or residual opportunistic infections (referred to as immune reconstitution syndrome) has occurred with the use of combination retroviral therapy, including Kaletra®; further evaluation and treatment may be required. The oral solution is highly concentrated and contains large amounts of alcohol. Healthcare providers should pay special attention to accurate calculation, measurement, and administration of dose. Overdose in a child may lead to lethal alcohol toxicity. Once-daily dosing is not recommended in therapy-experienced patients, those receiving efavirenz, nevirapine, nelfinavir, amprenavir, or fosamprenavir, or in children <18 years of age. Safety and efficacy have not been established for children <14 days of age.

Adverse Reactions Data presented for short- and long-term combination antiretroviral therapy in both protease inhibitor experienced and naïve patients.

>10%:

Dermatologic: Rash (children 12%; adults up to 5%)

Endocrine & metabolic: Hypercholesterolemia (3% to 39%), triglycerides increased (4% to 36%)

Gastrointestinal: Diarrhea (5% to 28%), abnormal taste/taste perversion (children 22%; adults <2%), vomiting (children 21%; adults 2% to 6%), nausea (5% to 16%), abdominal pain (2% to 11%)

Hepatic: GGT increased (10% to 29%), ALT increased (grade 3/4: 3% to 11%)

2% to 10%:

Cardiovascular: Hypertension (up to 2%), vein distension (up to 3%)

Central nervous system: Headache (2% to 6%), insomnia (up to 3%), chills (up to 2%), depression (up to 2%), fever (2%)

Endocrine & metabolic: Amenorrhea (up to 5%), hyperglycemia (1% to 5%), hyperuricemia (up to 5%), sodium decreased or increased (3% children), hypogonadism (males: up to 2%), inorganic phosphorus decreased (1% to 2%), libido decreased (up to 2%)

Gastrointestinal: Amylase increased (3% to 8%), dyspepsia (up to 6%), flatulence (1% to 4%), weight loss (up to 3%), dysphagia (up to 2%), anorexia (up to 2%)

Hematologic: Platelets decreased (grade 3/4: 4% children), neutropenia (grade 3/4: 1% to 5%)

Hepatic: AST increased (grade 3/4: 2% to 10%), bilirubin increased (1%, children 3%)

Neuromuscular & skeletal: Weakness (up to 9%), myalgia (up to 2%), paresthesia (up to 2%)

Respiratory: Bronchitis (up to 2%)

<2% (Limited to important or life-threatening): Alopecia, amnesia, apathy, asthma, ataxia, atrial fibrillation, avitaminosis, bacterial infection, bone necrosis, bradyarrhythmia, breast enlargement, cerebral infarction, cholangitis, cholecystitis, cough, Cushing's syndrome, cyst, deep vein thrombosis, diabetes mellitus, dyskinesia, dyspnea, enteritis, erythema multiforme, extrapyramidal symptoms, facial paralysis, fatty deposits, flu-like syndrome, hemorrhagic colitis, hepatic dysfunction, hepatomegaly, hypertrophy, immune reconstitution syndrome, impotence, jaundice, joint disorder, lactic acidosis, liver tenderness, lung edema, maculopapular rash, MI, migraine, myasthenia, neoplasm, nephritis, neuropathy, pancreatitis, paresthesia, periodontitis, peripheral neuritis, pharyngitis, pulmonary edema, renal calculus, rhinitis, seborrhea, seizure, sinusitis, skin ulcer, somnolence, Stevens-Johnson syndrome, striae, tinnitus, varicose veins, vasculitis, xerostomia

Drug Interactions

Metabolism/Transport Effects

Lopinavir: **Substrate** of CYP3A4 (major); **Inhibits** P-glycoprotein

Ritonavir: **Substrate** of CYP1A2 (minor), 2B6 (minor), 2D6 (major), 3A4 (major); **Inhibits** CYP2C8 (strong), 2C9 (weak), 2C19 (weak), 2D6 (strong), 2E1 (weak), 3A4 (strong); **Induces** CYP1A2 (weak), 2C8 (weak), 2C9 (weak), 3A4 (weak)

Avoid Concomitant Use

Avoid concomitant use of Lopinavir and Ritonavir with any of the following: Alfuzosin; Amiodarone; Cisapride; Dabigatran Etexilate; Darunavir; Disulfiram; Eplerenone; Ergot Derivatives; Etravirine; Flecainide; Nilotinib; Nisoldipine; Pimozide; Propafenone; QuiNIDine; Ranolazine; Rivaroxaban; Salmeterol; Silodosin; St Johns Wort; Tamoxifen; Thioridazine; Topotecan; Voriconazole

Increased Effect/Toxicity

Lopinavir and Ritonavir may increase the levels/effects of: Alfuzosin; Alosetron; Amiodarone; Antifungal Agents (Azole Derivatives, Systemic); Benzodiazepines (metabolized by oxidation); Calcium Channel Blockers (Dihydropyridine); Calcium Channel Blockers (Nondihydropyridine); CarBAMazepine; Ciclesonide; Cisapride;

Clarithromycin; Corticosteroids (Orally Inhaled); CycloSPORINE; CYP2C8 Substrates (High risk); CYP2D6 Substrates; CYP3A4 Substrates; Dabigatran Etexilate; Digoxin; Dronabinol; Enfuvirtide; Eplerenone; Ergot Derivatives; FentaNYL; Fesoterodine; Flecainide; Fusidic Acid; HMG-CoA Reductase Inhibitors; Ixabepilone; Maraviroc; Meperidine; Methadone; Nebivolol; Nefazodone; Nilotinib; Nisoldipine; P-Glycoprotein Substrates; Phosphodiesterase 5 Inhibitors; Pimecrolimus; Pimozide; Propafenone; Protease Inhibitors; QuiNIDine; Ranolazine; Rifamycin Derivatives; Rivaroxaban; Salmeterol; Silodosin; Sirolimus; Sorafenib; Tacrolimus; Tamoxifen; Temsirolimus; Tenofovir; Tetrabenazine; Thioridazine; Topotecan; TraZODone; Tricyclic Antidepressants; VinBLAStine; VinCRIStine

The levels/effects of Lopinavir and Ritonavir may be increased by: Antifungal Agents (Azole Derivatives, Systemic); Clarithromycin; CycloSPORINE; Delavirdine; Disulfiram; Enfuvirtide; Fusidic Acid; P-Glycoprotein Inhibitors

Decreased Effect

Lopinavir and Ritonavir may decrease the levels/effects of: Abacavir; Atovaquone; BuPROPion; Clarithromycin; Codeine; CYP2C19 Substrates; Darunavir; Delavirdine; Didanosine; Etravirine; LamoTRIgine; Meperidine; Oral Contraceptive (Estrogens); Phenytoin; Theophylline Derivatives; TraMADol; Valproic Acid; Voriconazole; Warfarin; Zidovudine

The levels/effects of Lopinavir and Ritonavir may be decreased by: Antacids; CarBAMazepine; CYP3A4 Inducers (Strong); Deferasirox; Efavirenz; Garlic; Nevirapine; Oral Contraceptive (Estrogens); P-Glycoprotein Inducers; Phenytoin; Rifamycin Derivatives; St Johns Wort

Ethanol/Nutrition/Herb Interactions

Food: Moderate- to high-fat meals increase the C_{max} and AUC of lopinavir/ritonavir oral solution; no significant changes observed with oral tablets.

Herb/Nutraceutical: St John's wort may decrease levels of protease inhibitors and lead to possible resistance; concurrent use is contraindicated.

Stability

Oral solution: Store at 2°C to 8°C (36°F to 46°F). Avoid exposure to excessive heat. If stored at room temperature (25°C or 77°F), use within 2 months.

Tablet: Store at USP controlled room temperature of 20°C to 25°C (68°F to 77°F). Exposure to high humidity outside of the original container for >2 weeks is not recommended.

Mechanism of Action A coformulation of lopinavir and ritonavir. The lopinavir component is the active inhibitor of HIV protease. Lopinavir inhibits HIV protease and renders the enzyme incapable of processing polyprotein precursor which leads to production of noninfectious immature HIV particles. The ritonavir component inhibits the CYP3A metabolism of lopinavir, allowing increased plasma levels of lopinavir.

Pharmacodynamics/Kinetics

Ritonavir: See Ritonavir monograph.

Lopinavir:

Protein binding: 98% to 99%; decreased with mild-to-moderate hepatic dysfunction

Metabolism: Hepatic via CYP3A4; 13 metabolites identified

Half-life elimination: 5-6 hours

Time to peak, plasma: ~4 hours

Excretion: Feces (83%, 20% as unchanged drug); urine (10%; <3% as unchanged drug)

Dosage Oral:

Children: Dosage based on weight or body surface area (BSA), **presented based on lopinavir component** (maximum dose: Lopinavir 400 mg/ritonavir 100 mg).

14 days to 6 months: 16 mg/kg or 300 mg/m^2 twice daily

6 months to 18 years: **Note:** FDA-approved dose is approximately equivalent to lopinavir 230 mg/m^2 per dose.

<15 kg: 12 mg/kg twice daily

15-40 kg: 10 mg/kg twice daily

>40 kg: Lopinavir 400 mg/ritonavir 100 mg twice daily

Note: For therapy-experienced patients with suspected reduced susceptibility to lopinavir, refer to adult dosing.

Children >12 years: Therapy-naive: Lopinavir 400 mg/ritonavir 100 mg twice daily (AIDS Info guidelines). **Note:** For therapy-experienced patients with suspected reduced susceptibility to lopinavir, refer to adult dosing.

Adults:

Therapy-naive: Lopinavir 800 mg/ritonavir 200 mg once daily **or** lopinavir 400 mg/ritonavir 100 mg twice daily

Note: Once-daily dosing regimen should not be used with concurrent indinavir, maraviroc, saquinavir, phenytoin, carbamazepine, or phenobarbital therapy.

Therapy-experienced: Lopinavir 400 mg/ritonavir 100 mg twice daily

Note: For therapy-experienced patients receiving efavirenz or nevirapine, clinicians may use lopinavir 600 mg/ritonavir 150 mg twice daily **or** lopinavir 533 mg/ritonavir 133 mg solution twice daily (AIDS info guidelines)

Elderly: Initial studies did not include enough elderly patients to determine effects based on age. Use with caution due to possible decreased hepatic, renal, and cardiac function.

Dosage adjustment for combination therapy:

When taken with amprenavir, efavirenz, fosamprenavir, nelfinavir, or nevirapine: **Note:** Once-daily dosing regimen should not be used

Children 14 days to 6 months: Combination therapy with these agents is not recommended due to lack of data.

Children 6 months to 18 years: Solution or tablet (**based on mg of lopinavir component**): FDA-approved dose is approximately equivalent to lopinavir 300 mg/m^2 per dose:

<15 kg: 13 mg/kg twice daily (**Note:** Tablets are not recommended)

15-45 kg: 11 mg/kg twice daily

>45 kg: Refer to adult dosing

Children >45 kg and Adults: Therapy-naive and therapy-experienced patients:

Solution: Lopinavir 533 mg/ritonavir 133 mg (6.5 mL) twice daily

Tablet: Lopinavir 500 mg/ritonavir 125 mg twice daily

When taken with maraviroc (Selzentry™): Lopinavir 400 mg/ritonavir 100 mg twice daily

When taken with saquinavir (Invirase®): Lopinavir 400 mg/ritonavir 100 mg twice daily

Dosage adjustment in renal impairment: Has not been studied in patients with renal impairment; however, a decrease in clearance is not expected

Dosage adjustment in hepatic impairment: Lopinavir AUC may be increased ~30% in patients with mild-to-moderate hepatic impairment. No data available in patients with severe impairment.

Dietary Considerations Solution should be taken with food. Tablet may be taken with or without food

Administration Once-daily dosing is not recommended in therapy-experienced patients, those receiving efavirenz, nevirapine, nelfinavir, amprenavir, or fosamprenavir, or in children <18 years of age.

Solution: Administer with food; if using didanosine, take didanosine 1 hour before or 2 hours after lopinavir/ritonavir. Administer using calibrated dosing syringe.

Tablet: May be taken with or without food. Swallow whole, do not break, crush, or chew. May be taken with didanosine when taken without food. Tablets are not recommended in patients <15 kg.

Monitoring Parameters Triglycerides, cholesterol, LFTs, electrolytes, basic HIV monitoring, viral load and CD4 count, glucose

Dosage Forms Excipient information presented when available (limited, particularly for generics); consult specific product labeling.

Solution, oral:

Kaletra®: Lopinavir 80 mg and ritonavir 20 mg per mL (160 mL) [contains alcohol 42.4%]

Tablet:

Kaletra®:

Lopinavir 100 mg and ritonavir 25 mg

Lopinavir 200 mg and ritonavir 50 mg

◆ **Lopressor®** *see* Metoprolol *on page 982*

◆ **Lopressor HCT®** *see* Metoprolol and Hydrochlorothiazide *on page 984*

◆ **Loprox®** *see* Ciclopirox *on page 324*

◆ **Loradamed [OTC]** *see* Loratadine *on page 904*

Loratadine (lor AT a deen)

U.S. Brand Names Alavert™ Allergy Relief 24-Hour [OTC]; Alavert™ [OTC]; Allergy Relief [OTC]; Claritin® 24 Hour Allergy [OTC]; Claritin® Children's Allergy [OTC]; Claritin® Children's [OTC]; Claritin® Hives Relief [OTC]; Dimetapp® ND Children's [OTC]; Loradamed [OTC]; Tavist® ND ALLERGY [OTC]

Canadian Brand Names Apo-Loratadine®; Claritin®; Claritin® Kids

Pharmacologic Category Histamine H_1 Antagonist; Histamine H_1 Antagonist, Second Generation

Use Relief of nasal and non-nasal symptoms of seasonal allergic rhinitis; treatment of chronic idiopathic urticaria

Pregnancy Risk Factor B

Pregnancy Considerations Loratadine was not found to be teratogenic in animal studies. There are no adequate and well-controlled studies in pregnant woman; use during pregnancy only if clearly needed.

Lactation Enters breast milk/not recommended (AAP rates "compatible")

Medication Safety Issues

Sound-alike/look-alike issues:

Claritin® may be confused with clarithromycin

Contraindications Hypersensitivity to loratadine or any component of the formulation

Warnings/Precautions Use with caution in patients with liver or renal impairment; dosage adjustment recommended. Safety and efficacy in children <2 years of age have not been established. Some products may contain phenylalanine.

Adverse Reactions

Adults:

Central nervous system: Headache (12%), somnolence (8%), fatigue (4%)

Gastrointestinal: Xerostomia (3%)

Children:

Central nervous system: Nervousness (4% ages 6-12 years), fatigue (3% ages 6-12 years, 2% to 3% ages 2-5 years), malaise (2% ages 6-12 years)

Dermatologic: Rash (2% to 3% ages 2-5 years)

Gastrointestinal: Abdominal pain (2% ages 6-12 years), stomatitis (2% to 3% ages 2-5 years)

Neuromuscular & skeletal: Hyperkinesia (3% ages 6-12 years)

Ocular: Conjunctivitis (2% ages 6-12 years)

Respiratory: Wheezing (4% ages 6-12 years), dysphonia (2% ages 6-12 years), upper respiratory infection (2% ages 6-12 years), epistaxis (2% to 3% ages 2-5 years), pharyngitis (2% to 3% ages 2-5 years)

Miscellaneous: Flu-like syndrome (2% to 3% ages 2-5 years), viral infection (2% to 3% ages 2-5 years)

Adults and Children: <2% (Limited to important or life-threatening): Abnormal hepatic function, agitation, alopecia, altered lacrimation, altered micturition, altered salivation, altered taste, amnesia, anaphylaxis, angioneurotic edema, anorexia, arthralgia, back pain, blepharospasm, blurred vision, breast enlargement, breast pain, bronchospasm, chest pain, confusion, depression, dizziness, dysmenorrhea, dyspnea, erythema multiforme, hemoptysis, hepatic necrosis, hepatitis, hypotension, impaired concentration, impotence, insomnia, irritability, jaundice, menorrhagia, migraine, nausea, palpitation, paresthesia, paroniria, peripheral edema, photosensitivity, pruritus, purpura, rigors, seizure, supraventricular tachyarrhythmia, syncope, tachycardia, tremor, urinary discoloration, urticaria, thrombocytopenia, vaginitis, vertigo, vomiting, weight gain

Drug Interactions

Metabolism/Transport Effects Substrate (minor) of CYP2D6, 3A4; **Inhibits** CYP2C8 (weak), 2C19 (moderate), 2D6 (weak)

Avoid Concomitant Use There are no known interactions where it is recommended to avoid concomitant use.

Increased Effect/Toxicity

Loratadine may increase the levels/effects of: Alcohol (Ethyl); Anticholinergics; CNS Depressants

The levels/effects of Loratadine may be increased by: P-Glycoprotein Inhibitors; Pramlintide

Decreased Effect

Loratadine may decrease the levels/effects of: Acetylcholinesterase Inhibitors (Central); Betahistine

The levels/effects of Loratadine may be decreased by: Acetylcholinesterase Inhibitors (Central); Amphetamines; P-Glycoprotein Inducers

Ethanol/Nutrition/Herb Interactions

Ethanol: Avoid ethanol (although sedation is limited with loratadine, may increase risk of CNS depression).

Food: Increases bioavailability and delays peak.

Herb/Nutraceutical: St John's wort may decrease loratadine levels.

Stability Store at 2°C to 25°C (36°F to 77°F).

Rapidly-disintegrating tablets: Use within 6 months of opening foil pouch, and immediately after opening individual tablet blister. Store in a dry place.

Mechanism of Action Long-acting tricyclic antihistamine with selective peripheral histamine H_1-receptor antagonistic properties

Pharmacodynamics/Kinetics

Onset of action: 1-3 hours

Peak effect: 8-12 hours

Duration: >24 hours

Absorption: Rapid

Distribution: Significant amounts enter breast milk

Metabolism: Extensively hepatic via CYP2D6 and 3A4 to active metabolite

Half-life elimination: 12-15 hours

Excretion: Urine (40%) and feces (40%) as metabolites

Dosage Oral: Seasonal allergic rhinitis, chronic idiopathic urticaria:

Children 2-5 years: 5 mg once daily

Children ≥6 years and Adults: 10 mg once daily

Elderly: Peak plasma levels are increased; elimination half-life is slightly increased; specific dosing adjustments are not available

Dosage adjustment in renal impairment: Cl_{cr} ≤30 mL/minute:

Children 2-5 years: 5 mg every other day

Children ≥6 years and Adults: 10 mg every other day

Dosage adjustment in hepatic impairment: Elimination half-life increases with severity of disease

Children 2-5 years: 5 mg every other day

Children ≥6 years and Adults: 10 mg every other day

Dietary Considerations Take on an empty stomach. Alavert® and Dimetapp® Children's ND contain phenylalanine 8.4 mg per 10 mg tablet. Claritin® Children's Allergy 5 mg contains phenylalanine 1.4 mg per tablet.

Administration Take on an empty stomach.

Dosage Forms Excipient information presented when available (limited, particularly for generics); consult specific product labeling.

Solution, oral: 5 mg/5 mL (120 mL)

Syrup, oral: 1 mg/mL (120 mL)

Allergy Relief: 1 mg/mL (120 mL)

Claritin® Children's: 5 mg/5 mL (60 mL, 120 mL) [alcohol free, dye free, sugar free; contains propylene glycol, sodium benzoate, and sodium 6 mg/5 mL; grape flavor]

Claritin® Children's Allergy: 1 mg/mL (120 mL) [alcohol free, dye free; contains propylene glycol and sodium benzoate; fruit flavor]

Tablet, oral: 10 mg

Alavert™: 10 mg

Claritin® 24 Hour Allergy: 10 mg

Claritin® Hives Relief: 10 mg

Loradamed: 10 mg

Tavist® ND ALLERGY: 10 mg

Tablet, chewable, oral:

Claritin® Children's Allergy: 5 mg [contains phenylalanine 1.4 mg/tablet; grape flavor]

Tablet, orally disintegrating, oral:

Alavert™ Allergy Relief 24-Hour: 10 mg [contains phenylalanine 8.4 mg/tablet]

Dimetapp® ND Children's: 10 mg [contains phenylalanine 8.4 mg/tablet]

Loratadine and Pseudoephedrine

(lor AT a deen & soo doe e FED rin)

U.S. Brand Names Alavert™ Allergy and Sinus [OTC]; Claritin-D® 12 Hour Allergy & Congestion [OTC]; Claritin-D® 24 Hour Allergy & Congestion [OTC]

Canadian Brand Names Chlor-Tripolon ND®; Claritin® Extra; Claritin® Liberator

Index Terms Pseudoephedrine and Loratadine

Pharmacologic Category Alpha/Beta Agonist; Histamine H_1 Antagonist; Histamine H_1 Antagonist, Second Generation

Use Temporary relief of symptoms of seasonal allergic rhinitis, other upper respiratory allergies, or the common cold

Pregnancy Risk Factor B

Dosage Children ≥12 years and Adults: Oral:

Claritin-D® 12-Hour: 1 tablet every 12 hours

Alavert™ Allergy and Sinus, Claritin-D® 24-Hour: 1 tablet daily

Dosage adjustment in renal impairment: Cl_{cr} ≤30 mL/minute:

Claritin-D® 12-Hour: 1 tablet daily

Claritin-D® 24-Hour: 1 tablet every other day

Dosage adjustment in hepatic impairment: Should be avoided

Additional Information Complete prescribing information for this medication should be consulted for additional detail.

Dosage Forms Excipient information presented when available (limited, particularly for generics); consult specific product labeling.

Tablet, extended release: Loratadine 10 mg and pseudoephedrine sulfate 240 mg

Alavert™ Allergy and Sinus: Loratadine 5 mg and pseudoephedrine sulfate 120 mg

Claritin-D® 12 Hour Allergy & Congestion: Loratadine 5 mg and pseudoephedrine sulfate 120 mg [contains calcium 30 mg/tablet]

Claritin-D® 24 Hour Allergy & Congestion: Loratadine 10 mg and pseudoephedrine sulfate 240 mg [contains calcium 25 mg/tablet]

LORazepam (lor A ze pam)

U.S. Brand Names Ativan®; Lorazepam Intensol®

Canadian Brand Names Apo-Lorazepam®; Ativan®; Lorazepam Injection, USP; Novo-Lorazepam; Nu-Loraz; PHL-Lorazepam; PMS-Lorazepam; Riva-Lorazepam

Pharmacologic Category Benzodiazepine

Additional Appendix Information

Benzodiazepines *on page 1646*

Status Epilepticus *on page 1831*

Use

Oral: Management of anxiety disorders or short-term (≤4 months) relief of the symptoms of anxiety or anxiety associated with depressive symptoms

I.V.: Status epilepticus, preanesthesia for desired amnesia

Unlabeled/Investigational Use Ethanol detoxification; insomnia; psychogenic catatonia; partial complex seizures; agitation (I.V.); antiemetic adjunct

Restrictions C-IV

Pregnancy Risk Factor D

Pregnancy Considerations Teratogenic effects have been observed in some animal studies. Lorazepam crosses the human placenta. Respiratory depression, withdrawal symptoms, or hypotonia may occur if administered late in pregnancy or near the time of delivery.

Lactation Enters breast milk/not recommended (AAP rates "of concern")

Medication Safety Issues

Sound-alike/look-alike issues:

LORazepam may be confused with ALPRAZolam, clonazePAM, diazepam, temazepam

Ativan® may be confused with Atarax®, Atgam®, Avitene®

Injection dosage form contains propylene glycol. Monitor for toxicity when administering continuous lorazepam infusions.

Contraindications Hypersensitivity to lorazepam or any component of the formulation (cross-sensitivity with other benzodiazepines may exist); acute narrow-angle glaucoma; sleep apnea (parenteral); intra-arterial injection of parenteral formulation; severe respiratory insufficiency (except during mechanical ventilation)

Warnings/Precautions Use with caution in elderly or debilitated patients, patients with hepatic disease (including alcoholics) or renal impairment. Use with caution in patients with respiratory disease (COPD or sleep apnea) or limited pulmonary reserve, or impaired gag reflex. Initial doses in elderly or debilitated patients should be at the lower end of the dosing range. May worsen hepatic encephalopathy.

Causes CNS depression (dose-related) resulting in sedation, dizziness, confusion, or ataxia which may impair physical and mental capabilities. Patients must be cautioned about performing tasks which require mental alertness (eg, operating machinery or driving). Use with caution in patients receiving other CNS depressants or psychoactive agents. Effects with other sedative drugs or ethanol may be potentiated. Benzodiazepines have been associated with falls and traumatic injury and should be used with extreme caution in patients who are at risk of these events (especially the elderly).

Lorazepam may cause anterograde amnesia. Paradoxical reactions, including hyperactive or aggressive behavior have been reported with benzodiazepines, particularly in adolescent/pediatric or psychiatric patients. Does not have analgesic, antidepressant, or antipsychotic properties.

Use caution in patients with depression, particularly if suicidal risk may be present. Pre-existing depression may worsen or emerge during therapy. Not recommended for use in primary depressive or psychotic disorders. Use with caution in patients with a history of drug dependence, alcoholism, or significant personality disorders. Benzodiazepines have been associated with dependence and acute withdrawal symptoms on discontinuation or reduction in dose. Acute withdrawal, including seizures, may be precipitated after administration of flumazenil to patients receiving long-term benzodiazepine therapy.

As a hypnotic agent, should be used only after evaluation of potential causes of sleep disturbance. Failure of sleep disturbance to resolve after 7-10 days may indicate psychiatric or medical illness. A worsening of insomnia or the emergence of new abnormalities of thought or behavior may represent unrecognized psychiatric or medical illness and requires immediate and careful evaluation.

The parenteral formulation of lorazepam contains polyethylene glycol and propylene glycol which have resulted in toxicity during high dose and/or longer term infusions. Also contains benzyl alcohol; avoid in neonates.

Safety and efficacy have not been established in children <12 years of age.

Adverse Reactions

>10%:
- Central nervous system: Sedation
- Respiratory: Respiratory depression

1% to 10%:
- Cardiovascular: Hypotension
- Central nervous system: Akathisia, amnesia, ataxia, confusion, depression, disorientation, dizziness, headache
- Dermatologic: Dermatitis, rash
- Gastrointestinal: Changes in appetite, nausea, weight gain/loss
- Neuromuscular & skeletal: Weakness
- Ocular: Visual disturbances
- Respiratory: Apnea, hyperventilation, nasal congestion

<1% or frequency not defined (Limited to important or life-threatening): Asthenia, blood dyscrasias, disinhibition, euphoria, fatigue, increased salivation, menstrual irregularities, physical and psychological dependence (with prolonged use), reflex slowing, polyethylene glycol or propylene glycol poisoning (prolonged I.V. infusion), suicidal ideation, seizure, vertigo

Drug Interactions

Avoid Concomitant Use There are no known interactions where it is recommended to avoid concomitant use.

Increased Effect/Toxicity

LORazepam may increase the levels/effects of: Alcohol (Ethyl); Clozapine; CNS Depressants; Phenytoin

The levels/effects of LORazepam may be increased by: Loxapine; Probenecid; Valproic Acid

Decreased Effect

The levels/effects of LORazepam may be decreased by: Theophylline Derivatives; Yohimbine

Ethanol/Nutrition/Herb Interactions

Ethanol: Avoid or limit ethanol (may increase CNS depression).

Herb/Nutraceutical: Avoid valerian, St John's wort, kava kava, gotu kola (may increase CNS depression).

Stability

I.V.: Intact vials should be refrigerated. Protect from light. Do not use discolored or precipitate-containing solutions. May be stored at room temperature for up to 60 days. Parenteral admixture is stable at room temperature (25°C) for 24 hours. Dilute I.V. dose with equal volume of compatible diluent (D_5W, NS, SWI).

Infusion: Use 2 mg/mL injectable vial to prepare; there may be deceased stability when using 4 mg/mL vial. Dilute ≤1 mg/mL and mix in glass bottle. Precipitation may develop. Can also be administered undiluted via infusion.

Tablet: Store at room temperature.

Mechanism of Action Binds to stereospecific benzodiazepine receptors on the postsynaptic GABA neuron at several sites within the central nervous system, including the limbic system, reticular formation. Enhancement of the inhibitory effect of GABA on neuronal excitability results by increased neuronal membrane permeability to chloride ions. This shift in chloride ions results in hyperpolarization (a less excitable state) and stabilization.

Pharmacodynamics/Kinetics

Onset of action:
- Hypnosis: I.M.: 20-30 minutes
- Sedation: I.V.: 5-20 minutes
- Anticonvulsant: I.V.: 5 minutes, oral: 30-60 minutes

Duration: 6-8 hours

Absorption: Oral, I.M.: Prompt

Distribution:
- V_d: Neonates: 0.76 L/kg, Adults: 1.3 L/kg; crosses placenta; enters breast milk

Protein binding: 85%; free fraction may be significantly higher in elderly

Metabolism: Hepatic to inactive compounds

Bioavailability: Oral: 90%

Half-life elimination: Neonates: 40.2 hours; Older children: 10.5 hours; Adults: 12.9 hours; Elderly: 15.9 hours; End-stage renal disease: 32-70 hours

Time to peak: Oral: 2 hours

Excretion: Urine; feces (minimal)

Dosage

Antiemetic (unlabeled use):
- Children 2-15 years: I.V.: 0.05 mg/kg (up to 2 mg/dose) prior to chemotherapy
- Adults: Oral, I.V. (**Note:** May be administered sublingually; not a labeled route): 0.5-2 mg every 4-6 hours as needed

Anxiety and sedation (unlabeled in children except for oral use in children >12 years):
- Infants and Children: Oral, I.M., I.V.: Usual: 0.05 mg/kg/dose (range: 0.02-0.09 mg/kg) every 4-8 hours
  - I.V.: May use smaller doses (eg, 0.01-0.03 mg/kg) and repeat every 20 minutes, as needed to titrate to effect
- Adults: Oral: 1-10 mg/day in 2-3 divided doses; usual dose: 2-6 mg/day in divided doses
- Elderly: 0.5-4 mg/day; initial dose not to exceed 2 mg

Insomnia: Adults: Oral: 2-4 mg at bedtime

Preoperative: Adults:
- I.M.: 0.05 mg/kg administered 2 hours before surgery (maximum: 4 mg/dose)
- I.V.: 0.044 mg/kg 15-20 minutes before surgery (usual maximum: 2 mg/dose)

Preprocedural anxiety (dental use): Adults: Oral: 1-2 mg 1 hour before procedure

Operative amnesia: Adults: I.V.: Up to 0.05 mg/kg (maximum: 4 mg/dose)

Sedation (preprocedure): Infants and Children (unlabeled):
- Oral, I.M., I.V.: Usual: 0.05 mg/kg (range: 0.02-0.09 mg/kg)
  - I.V.: May use smaller doses (eg, 0.01-0.03 mg/kg) and repeat every 20 minutes, as needed to titrate to effect

Status epilepticus: I.V.:
- Infants and Children (unlabeled): 0.05-0.1 mg/kg slow I.V. over 2-5 minutes; do not exceed 4 mg/single dose; may repeat second dose of 0.05 mg/kg slow I.V. in 5-10 minutes if needed
- Adolescents: 0.07 mg/kg slow I.V. over 2-5 minutes; maximum: 4 mg/dose; may repeat in 5-10 minutes

Adults: 4 mg/dose slow I.V. over 2-5 minutes; may repeat in 5-10 minutes; usual maximum dose: 8 mg

Rapid tranquilization of agitated patient (administer every 30-60 minutes): Adults:

Oral: 1-2 mg

I.M.: 0.5-1 mg

Average total dose for tranquilization: Oral, I.M.: 4-8 mg

Agitation in the ICU patient (unlabeled): Adults:

I.V.: 0.02-0.06 mg/kg every 2-6 hours

I.V. infusion: 0.01-0.1 mg/kg/hour

Concurrent use of probenecid or valproic acid: Reduce lorazepam dose by 50%

Dosage adjustment in renal impairment: I.V.: Risk of propylene glycol toxicity. Monitor closely if using for prolonged periods of time or at high doses.

Dosage adjustment in hepatic impairment: Use cautiously.

Administration May be administered by I.M., I.V., or orally

I.M.: Should be administered deep into the muscle mass

I.V.: Do not exceed 2 mg/minute or 0.05 mg/kg over 2-5 minutes; dilute I.V. dose with equal volume of compatible diluent (D_5W, NS, SWI). Avoid intra-arterial administration. Monitor I.V. site for extravasation.

Monitoring Parameters Respiratory and cardiovascular status, blood pressure, heart rate, symptoms of anxiety

Reference Range Therapeutic: 50-240 ng/mL (SI: 156-746 nmol/L)

Additional Information Oral doses >0.09 mg/kg produced increased ataxia without increased sedative benefit vs lower doses; preferred anxiolytic when I.M. route needed. Abrupt discontinuation after sustained use (generally >10 days) may cause withdrawal symptoms.

Dosage Forms Excipient information presented when available (limited, particularly for generics); consult specific product labeling.

Injection, solution: 2 mg/mL (1 mL, 10 mL); 4 mg/mL (1 mL, 10 mL)

Ativan®: 2 mg/mL (1 mL, 10 mL); 4 mg/mL (1 mL, 10 mL) [contains benzyl alcohol, polyethylene glycol, and propylene glycol]

Solution, oral concentrate:

Lorazepam Intensol®: 2 mg/mL (30 mL) [alcohol free, dye free]

Tablet: 0.5 mg, 1 mg, 2 mg

Ativan®: 0.5 mg, 1 mg, 2 mg

◆ **Lorazepam Injection, USP (Can)** *see* LORazepam *on page 905*

◆ **Lorazepam Intensol®** *see* LORazepam *on page 905*

◆ **Lorcet® 10/650** *see* Hydrocodone and Acetaminophen *on page 740*

◆ **Lorcet® Plus** *see* Hydrocodone and Acetaminophen *on page 740*

◆ **Lortab®** *see* Hydrocodone and Acetaminophen *on page 740*

Losartan (loe SAR tan)

U.S. Brand Names Cozaar®

Canadian Brand Names Cozaar®

Index Terms DuP 753; Losartan Potassium; MK594

Pharmacologic Category Angiotensin II Receptor Blocker

Additional Appendix Information

Angiotensin Agents *on page 1632*

Heart Failure (Systolic) *on page 1809*

Use Treatment of hypertension (HTN); treatment of diabetic nephropathy in patients with type 2 diabetes mellitus (noninsulin dependent, NIDDM) and a history of hypertension; stroke risk reduction in patients with HTN and left ventricular hypertrophy (LVH)

Unlabeled/Investigational Use To slow the rate of progression of aortic-root dilation in pediatric patients with Marfan's syndrome

Pregnancy Risk Factor C (1st trimester); D (2nd and 3rd trimesters)

Pregnancy Considerations Medications which act on the renin-angiotensin system are reported to have the following fetal/neonatal effects: Hypotension, neonatal skull hypoplasia, anuria, renal failure, and death; oligohydramnios is also reported. These effects are reported to occur with exposure during the second and third trimesters. There are no adequate and well-controlled studies in pregnant women. **[U.S. Boxed Warning]: Based on human data, drugs that act on the angiotensin system can cause injury and death to the developing fetus when used in the second and third trimesters. Angiotensin receptor blockers should be discontinued as soon as possible once pregnancy is detected.**

Lactation Excretion in breast milk unknown/not recommended

Medication Safety Issues

Sound-alike/look-alike issues:

Cozaar® may be confused with Colace®, Coreg®, Hyzaar®, Zocor®

Losartan may be confused with valsartan

Contraindications Hypersensitivity to losartan or any component of the formulation

Warnings/Precautions **[U.S. Boxed Warning]: Based on human data, drugs that act on the angiotensin system can cause injury and death to the developing fetus when used in the second and third trimesters. Angiotensin receptor blockers should be discontinued as soon as possible once pregnancy is detected.** Avoid use or use a much smaller dose in patients who are volume-depleted; correct depletion first. Use with caution in patients with significant aortic/mitral stenosis. May cause hyperkalemia; avoid potassium supplementation unless specifically required by healthcare provider. May be associated with deterioration of renal function and/or increases in serum creatinine, particularly in patients with low renal blood flow (eg, renal artery stenosis, heart failure) whose glomerular filtration rate (GFR) is dependent on efferent arteriolar vasoconstriction by angiotensin II. Use caution in patients with unstented unilateral/bilateral renal artery stenosis. When unstented bilateral renal artery stenosis is present, use is generally avoided due to the elevated risk of deterioration in renal function unless possible benefits outweigh risks. Use with caution with pre-existing renal insufficiency. AUCs of losartan (not the active metabolite) are about 50% greater in patients with Cl_{cr} <30 mL/minute and are doubled in hemodialysis patients.

At any time during treatment (especially following first dose), angioedema may occur rarely; may involve the head and neck (potentially compromising airway) or the intestine (presenting with abdominal pain). Patients with idiopathic or hereditary angioedema or previous angioedema associated with ACE-inhibitor therapy may be at an increased risk. Prolonged frequent monitoring may be required, especially if tongue, glottis, or larynx are involved, as they are associated with airway obstruction. Patients with a history of airway surgery may have a higher risk of airway obstruction. Aggressive early management is critical; intramuscular (I.M.) administration of epinephrine may be necessary.

When used to reduce the risk of stroke in patients with HTN and LVH, may not be effective in African-American population. Use caution with hepatic dysfunction, dose adjustment may be needed. Safety and efficacy have not been established in children <6 years of age.

Adverse Reactions

Note: The incidence of some adverse reactions varied based on the underlying disease state. Notations are made, where applicable, for data derived from trials conducted in diabetic nephropathy and hypertensive patients, respectively.

>10%:

Cardiovascular: Chest pain (12% diabetic nephropathy)

Central nervous system: Fatigue (14% diabetic nephropathy)

Endocrine: Hypoglycemia (14% diabetic nephropathy)

Gastrointestinal: Diarrhea (2% hypertension to 15% diabetic nephropathy)

Genitourinary: Urinary tract infection (13% diabetic nephropathy)

Hematologic: Anemia (14% diabetic nephropathy)

Neuromuscular & skeletal: Weakness (14% diabetic nephropathy), back pain (2% hypertension to 12% diabetic nephropathy)

Respiratory: Cough (≤3% to 11%; similar to placebo; incidence higher in patients with previous cough related to ACE inhibitor therapy)

1% to 10%:

Cardiovascular: Hypotension (7% diabetic nephropathy), orthostatic hypotension (4% hypertension to 4% diabetic nephropathy), first-dose hypotension (dose related: <1% with 50 mg, 2% with 100 mg)

Central nervous system: Dizziness (4%), hypoesthesia (5% diabetic nephropathy), fever (4% diabetic nephropathy), insomnia (1%)

Dermatology: Cellulitis (7% diabetic nephropathy)

Endocrine: Hyperkalemia (<1% hypertension to 7% diabetic nephropathy)

Gastrointestinal: Gastritis (5% diabetic nephropathy), weight gain (4% diabetic nephropathy), dyspepsia (1% to 4%), abdominal pain (2%), nausea (2%)

Neuromuscular & skeletal: Muscular weakness (7% diabetic nephropathy), knee pain (5% diabetic nephropathy), leg pain (1% to 5%), muscle cramps (1%), myalgia (1%)

Respiratory: Bronchitis (10% diabetic nephropathy), upper respiratory infection (8%), nasal congestion (2%), sinusitis (1% hypertension to 6% diabetic nephropathy)

Miscellaneous: Infection (5% diabetic nephropathy), flu-like syndrome (10% diabetic nephropathy)

<1% (Limited to important or life-threatening): Acute psychosis with paranoid delusions, ageusia, allergic reaction, alopecia, anaphylactic reactions, anemia, angina, angioedema, anorexia, anxiety, arrhythmia, arthralgia, arthritis, ataxia, AV block (second degree), bilirubin increased, blurred vision, bradycardia, bronchitis, BUN increased, confusion, conjunctivitis, constipation, CVA, depression, dermatitis, dysgeusia, dyspnea, ecchymosis, epistaxis, erythroderma, erythema, facial edema, fever, flatulence, flushing, gastritis, gout, hematocrit decreased, hemoglobin decreased, Henoch-Schönlein purpura, hepatitis, hyperkalemia, hyponatremia, hypotension, impotence, joint swelling, maculopapular rash, myositis, memory impairment, MI, migraine, muscle weakness, nervousness, orthostatic effects, pancreatitis, paresthesia, peripheral neuropathy, pharyngitis, photosensitivity, pruritus, rash, rhabdomyolysis, rhinitis, serum creatinine increased, sleep disorder, somnolence, syncope, tachycardia, taste perversion, thrombocytopenia, tinnitus, transaminases increased, tremor, urinary frequency, urticaria, vasculitis, ventricular arrhythmia, vertigo, visual acuity decreased, vomiting, xerostomia

Drug Interactions

Metabolism/Transport Effects Substrate (major) of CYP2C9, 3A4; **Inhibits** CYP1A2 (weak), 2C8 (moderate), 2C9 (moderate), 2C19 (weak), 3A4 (weak)

Avoid Concomitant Use There are no known interactions where it is recommended to avoid concomitant use.

Increased Effect/Toxicity

Losartan may increase the levels/effects of: ACE Inhibitors; Amifostine; CYP2C8 Substrates (High risk); CYP2C9 Substrates (High risk); Lithium; Potassium-Sparing Diuretics; RiTUXimab

The levels/effects of Losartan may be increased by: Antifungal Agents (Azole Derivatives, Systemic); CYP2C9 Inhibitors (Moderate); CYP2C9 Inhibitors (Strong); Diazoxide; Eplerenone; Fluconazole; Herbs (Hypoglycemic Properties); Herbs (Hypotensive Properties); Potassium Salts; Prostacyclin Analogues; Trimethoprim

Decreased Effect

The levels/effects of Losartan may be decreased by: CYP2C9 Inducers (Highly Effective); CYP3A4 Inducers (Strong); Deferasirox; Herbs (CYP3A4 Inducers); Herbs (Hypertensive Properties); Methylphenidate; Nonsteroidal Anti-Inflammatory Agents; Rifamycin Derivatives; Yohimbine

Ethanol/Nutrition/Herb Interactions Herb/Nutraceutical: St John's wort may decrease levels of losartan. Avoid bayberry, blue cohosh, ginseng (American), kola, licorice (may worsen hypertension). Avoid black cohosh; california poppy; coleus; golden seal; hawthorn; mistletoe; periwinkle; quinine; shepherd's purse (may increase risk for hypotension). Hypoglycemic effects of losartan may be enhanced by alfalfa; aloe; bilberry; bitter melon; burdock; celery; damiana; fenugreek; garcinia; garlic; ginger; ginseng (American); gymnema; marshmallow; stinging nettle.

Stability Store at 15°C to 30°C (59°F to 86°F). Protect from light.

Mechanism of Action As a selective and competitive, nonpeptide angiotensin II receptor antagonist, losartan blocks the vasoconstrictor and aldosterone-secreting effects of angiotensin II; losartan interacts reversibly at the AT1 and AT2 receptors of many tissues and has slow dissociation kinetics; its affinity for the AT1 receptor is 1000 times greater than the AT2 receptor. Angiotensin II receptor antagonists may induce a more complete inhibition of the renin-angiotensin system than ACE inhibitors, they do not affect the response to bradykinin, and are less likely to be associated with nonrenin-angiotensin effects (eg, cough and angioedema). Losartan increases urinary flow rate and in addition to being natriuretic and kaliuretic, increases excretion of chloride, magnesium, uric acid, calcium, and phosphate.

Pharmacodynamics/Kinetics

Onset of action: 6 hours

Distribution: V_d: Losartan: 34 L; E-3174: 12 L; does not cross blood brain barrier

Protein binding, plasma: High

Metabolism: Hepatic (14%) via CYP2C9 and 3A4 to active metabolite, E-3174 (40 times more potent than losartan); extensive first-pass effect

Bioavailability: 25% to 33%; AUC of E-3174 is four times greater than that of losartan

Half-life elimination: Losartan: 1.5-2 hours; E-3174: 6-9 hours

Time to peak, serum: Losartan: 1 hour; E-3174: 3-4 hours

Excretion: Urine (4% as unchanged drug, 6% as active metabolite)

Clearance: Plasma: Losartan: 600 mL/minute; Active metabolite: 50 mL/minute

Dosage Oral:

Hypertension:

Children 6-16 years:

U.S. labeling: 0.7 mg/kg once daily (maximum: 50 mg/day); doses >1.4 mg/kg (maximum: 100 mg) have not been studied

Canadian labeling:

≥20 kg to <50 kg: 25 mg once daily (maximum: 50 mg once daily)

≥50 kg: 50 mg once daily (maximum: 100 mg once daily)

Adults: Usual starting dose: 50 mg once daily; can be administered once or twice daily with total daily doses ranging from 25-100 mg

Patients receiving diuretics or with intravascular volume depletion: Usual initial dose: 25 mg once daily

Aortic-root dilation with Marfan's syndrome (unlabeled use): Children 14 months to 16 years: Initial: 0.6 mg/kg/day; can be increased to a maximum of 1.4 mg/kg/day (not to exceed adult maximum of 100 mg/day)

Nephropathy in patients with type 2 diabetes and hypertension: Adults: Initial: 50 mg once daily; can be increased to 100 mg once daily based on blood pressure response

Stroke reduction (HTN with LVH): Adults: 50 mg once daily (maximum daily dose: 100 mg); may be used in combination with a thiazide diuretic

Dosing adjustment in renal impairment:

Children: Use is not recommended if GFR <30 mL/minute/1.73m^2

Adults: No adjustment necessary.

Dosing adjustment in hepatic impairment:

Children 6-16 years:

U.S. labeling: No specific dosing recommendations are provided in the approved labeling, however it may be advisable to initiate therapy at a reduced dosage.

Canadian labeling: Use is not recommended.

Adults: Reduce the initial dose to 25 mg/day

Dietary Considerations May be taken with or without food.

Administration May be administered with or without food.

Monitoring Parameters Supine blood pressure, electrolytes, serum creatinine, BUN, urinalysis, symptomatic hypotension and tachycardia, CBC

Dosage Forms Excipient information presented when available (limited, particularly for generics); consult specific product labeling.

Tablet, oral, as potassium:

Cozaar®: 25 mg [contains potassium 2.12 mg (0.054 mEq)]

Cozaar®: 50 mg [contains potassium 4.24 mg (0.108 mEq)]

Cozaar®: 100 mg [contains potassium 8.48 mg (0.216 mEq)]

Extemporaneous Preparations To prepare losartan suspension, combine 10 mL of purified water and ten (10) losartan 50 mg tablets in an 8 ounce bottle. Shake well for ≥2 minutes. Allow concentrate to stand for 1 hour then shake for 1 minute. Separately, prepare 190 mL of a 50/50 mixture of Ora-Plus™ and Ora-Sweet SF™. Add to tablet and water mixture; shake for 1 minute. Resulting 200 mL suspension will contain losartan 2.5 mg/mL. Store under refrigeration for up to 4 weeks; shake well before use.

Product information, October, 2004; Merck & Company, Inc

Losartan and Hydrochlorothiazide

(loe SAR tan & hye droe klor oh THYE a zide)

U.S. Brand Names Hyzaar®

Canadian Brand Names Hyzaar®; Hyzaar® DS

Index Terms Hydrochlorothiazide and Losartan

Pharmacologic Category Angiotensin II Receptor Blocker; Diuretic, Thiazide

Use Treatment of hypertension; stroke risk reduction in patients with HTN and left ventricular hypertrophy (LVH)

Pregnancy Risk Factor C/D (2nd and 3rd trimesters)

Medication Safety Issues

Sound-alike/look-alike issues:

Hyzaar® may be confused with Cozaar®

Dosage

Oral: Adults: Dose is individualized (combination substituted for individual components); dose may be titrated after 2-4 weeks of therapy

Hypertension/stroke reduction in hypertension (with LVH): Usual recommended starting dose of losartan: 50 mg once daily when used as monotherapy in patients who are not volume depleted

Dosage adjustment in renal impairment: Cl_{cr} ≤30 mL/minute: Use of combination formulation not recommended

Dosage adjustment in hepatic impairment: Use is not recommended

Additional Information Complete prescribing information for this medication should be consulted for additional detail.

Dosage Forms Excipient information presented when available (limited, particularly for generics); consult specific product labeling.

Tablet:

Hyzaar® 50-12.5: Losartan potassium 50 mg and hydrochlorothiazide 12.5 mg

Hyzaar® 100-12.5: Losartan potassium 100 mg and hydrochlorothiazide 12.5 mg

Hyzaar® 100-25: Losartan potassium 100 mg and hydrochlorothiazide 25 mg

- **Losartan Potassium** *see* Losartan *on page 907*
- **Losec® (Can)** *see* Omeprazole *on page 1100*
- **Losec MUPS® (Can)** *see* Omeprazole *on page 1100*
- **Lotemax®** *see* Loteprednol *on page 909*
- **Lotensin®** *see* Benazepril *on page 179*
- **Lotensin® HCT** *see* Benazepril and Hydrochlorothiazide *on page 181*

Loteprednol (loe te PRED nol)

U.S. Brand Names Alrex®; Lotemax®

Canadian Brand Names Alrex®; Lotemax®

Index Terms Loteprednol Etabonate

Pharmacologic Category Corticosteroid, Ophthalmic

Use

Suspension, 0.2% (Alrex®): Temporary relief of signs and symptoms of seasonal allergic conjunctivitis

Suspension, 0.5% (Lotemax®): Inflammatory conditions (treatment of steroid-responsive inflammatory conditions of the palpebral and bulbar conjunctiva, cornea, and anterior segment of the globe such as allergic conjunctivitis, acne rosacea, superficial punctate keratitis, herpes zoster keratitis, iritis, cyclitis, selected infective conjunctivitis, when the inherent hazard of steroid use is accepted to obtain an advisable diminution in edema and inflammation) and treatment of postoperative inflammation following ocular surgery

Pregnancy Risk Factor C

Medication Safety Issues

International issues:

Lotemax® may be confused with Lotanax® which is a brand name for terfenadine in the Czech Republic

Dosage Adults: Ophthalmic:

Suspension, 0.2% (Alrex®): Instill 1 drop into affected eye(s) 4 times/day

Suspension, 0.5% (Lotemax®):

Inflammatory conditions: Apply 1-2 drops into the conjunctival sac of the affected eye(s) 4 times/day. During the initial treatment within the first week, the dosing may be increased up to 1 drop every hour. Advise patients not to discontinue therapy prematurely.

If signs and symptoms fail to improve after 2 days, re-evaluate the patient.

Postoperative inflammation: Apply 1-2 drops into the conjunctival sac of the operated eye(s) 4 times/day beginning 24 hours after surgery and continuing throughout the first 2 weeks of the postoperative period

Additional Information Complete prescribing information for this medication should be consulted for additional detail.

Dosage Forms Excipient information presented when available (limited, particularly for generics); consult specific product labeling.

Suspension, ophthalmic, as etabonate:

Alrex®: 0.2% (5 mL, 10 mL) [contains benzalkonium chloride]

Lotemax®: 0.5% (2.5 mL, 5 mL, 10 mL, 15 mL) [contains benzalkonium chloride]

Loteprednol and Tobramycin

(loe te PRED nol & toe bra MYE sin)

U.S. Brand Names Zylet™

Index Terms Loteprednol Etabonate and Tobramycin; Tobramycin and Loteprednol Etabonate

Pharmacologic Category Antibiotic/Corticosteroid, Ophthalmic

Use Treatment of steroid-responsive ocular inflammatory conditions where either a superficial bacterial ocular infection or the risk of a superficial bacterial ocular infection exists

Pregnancy Risk Factor C

Dosage Ophthalmic: Adults: Instill 1-2 drops into the affected eye(s) every 4-6 hours; may increase frequency during the first 24-48 hours to every 1-2 hours. Interval should increase as signs and symptoms improve. Further evaluation should occur for use of greater than 20 mL.

Additional Information Complete prescribing information for this medication should be consulted for additional detail.

Dosage Forms Excipient information presented when available (limited, particularly for generics); consult specific product labeling.

Suspension, ophthalmic: Loteprednol 0.5% and tobramycin 0.3% (2.5 mL, 5 mL, 10 mL) [contains benzalkonium chloride]

- ◆ **Loteprednol Etabonate** *see* Loteprednol *on page 909*
- ◆ **Loteprednol Etabonate and Tobramycin** *see* Loteprednol and Tobramycin *on page 910*
- ◆ **Lotrel®** *see* Amlodipine and Benazepril *on page 95*
- ◆ **Lotriderm® (Can)** *see* Betamethasone and Clotrimazole *on page 190*
- ◆ **Lotrimin® AF Athlete's Foot Cream [OTC]** *see* Clotrimazole *on page 359*
- ◆ **Lotrimin® AF for Her [OTC]** *see* Clotrimazole *on page 359*
- ◆ **Lotrimin® AF Jock Itch Cream [OTC]** *see* Clotrimazole *on page 359*
- ◆ **Lotrimin® AF Jock Itch Powder Spray [OTC]** *see* Miconazole *on page 989*
- ◆ **Lotrimin® AF Powder/Spray [OTC]** *see* Miconazole *on page 989*
- ◆ **Lotrimin® Ultra™ [OTC]** *see* Butenafine *on page 230*
- ◆ **Lotrisone®** *see* Betamethasone and Clotrimazole *on page 190*

Lovastatin (LOE va sta tin)

U.S. Brand Names Altoprev®; Mevacor®

Canadian Brand Names Apo-Lovastatin®; CO Lovastatin; DOM-Lovastatin; Gen-Lovastatin; Mevacor®; Novo-Lovastatin; Nu-Lovastatin; PHL-Lovastatin; PMS-Lovastatin; PRO-Lovastatin; RAN™-Lovastatin; ratio-Lovastatin; Riva-Lovastatin; Sandoz-Lovastatin

Index Terms Mevinolin; Monacolin K

Pharmacologic Category Antilipemic Agent, HMG-CoA Reductase Inhibitor

Additional Appendix Information

Hyperlipidemia Management *on page 1815*

Lipid-Lowering Agents *on page 1661*

Use

Adjunct to dietary therapy to decrease elevated serum total and LDL-cholesterol concentrations in primary hypercholesterolemia

Primary prevention of coronary artery disease (patients without symptomatic disease with average to moderately elevated total and LDL-cholesterol and below average HDL-cholesterol); slow progression of coronary atherosclerosis in patients with coronary heart disease

Adjunct to dietary therapy in adolescent patients (10-17 years of age, females >1 year postmenarche) with heterozygous familial hypercholesterolemia having LDL >189 mg/dL, **or** LDL >160 mg/dL with positive family history of premature cardiovascular disease (CVD), **or** LDL >160 mg/dL with the presence of at least two other CVD risk factors

Pregnancy Risk Factor X

Pregnancy Considerations Cholesterol biosynthesis may be important in fetal development. Contraindicated in pregnancy. Administer to women of childbearing potential only when conception is highly unlikely and patients have been informed of potential hazards.

Lactation Excretion unknown/contraindicated

Medication Safety Issues

Sound-alike/look-alike issues:

Lovastatin may be confused with Leustatin®, Livostin®, Lotensin®

Mevacor® may be confused with Mivacron®

International issues:

Lovacol® [Chile and Finland] may be confused with Levatol® which is a brand name for penbutolol in the U.S.

Lovastin® [Poland] may be confused with Livostin® which is a brand name for levocabastine in the U.S.

Contraindications Hypersensitivity to lovastatin or any component of the formulation; active liver disease; unexplained persistent elevations of serum transaminases; pregnancy; breast-feeding

Warnings/Precautions Secondary causes of hyperlipidemia should be ruled out prior to therapy. Liver function must be monitored by periodic laboratory assessment. Rhabdomyolysis with or without acute renal failure has occurred. Risk is dose-related and is increased with concurrent use of lipid-lowering agents which may cause rhabdomyolysis (gemfibrozil, fibric acid derivatives, or niacin at doses ≥1 g/day) or during concurrent use with potent CYP3A4 inhibitors. Avoid concurrent use of azole antifungals, macrolide antibiotics, and protease inhibitors. Use caution/limit dose with amiodarone, cyclosporine, danazol, gemfibrozil (or other fibrates), lipid-lowering doses of niacin, or verapamil. Monitor closely if used with other drugs associated with myopathy (eg, colchicine). Patients should be instructed to report unexplained muscle pain or weakness; lovastatin should be discontinued if myopathy is suspected/confirmed. Temporarily discontinue in any patient experiencing an acute or serious condition predisposing to renal failure secondary to rhabdomyolysis. Based upon current evidence, HMG-CoA reductase inhibitor therapy should be continued in the perioperative period unless risk outweighs cardioprotective benefit. Use with caution in patients with advanced age, these patients are predisposed to myopathy. Use with caution in patients who consume large amounts of ethanol or have a history of liver disease. Safety and efficacy of the immediate release tablet have not been evaluated in prepubertal patients, patients <10 years of age, or doses >40 mg/day in appropriately-selected adolescents; extended release tablets have not been studied in patients <20 years of age.

Adverse Reactions Percentages as reported with immediate release tablets; similar adverse reactions seen with extended release tablets.

>10%: Neuromuscular & skeletal: Increased CPK (>2x normal) (11%)

1% to 10%:

Central nervous system: Headache (2% to 3%), dizziness (0.5% to 1%)

Dermatologic: Rash (0.8% to 1%)

Gastrointestinal: Abdominal pain (2% to 3%), constipation (2% to 4%), diarrhea (2% to 3%), dyspepsia (1% to 2%), flatulence (4% to 5%), nausea (2% to 3%)

Neuromuscular & skeletal: Myalgia (2% to 3%), weakness (1% to 2%), muscle cramps (0.6% to 1%)

Ocular: Blurred vision (0.8% to 1%)

<1% (Limited to important or life-threatening): Acid regurgitation, alopecia, arthralgia, chest pain, dermatomyositis, eye irritation, insomnia, leg pain, paresthesia, pruritus, vomiting, xerostomia

Additional class-related events or case reports (not necessarily reported with lovastatin therapy): Alkaline phosphatase increased, alopecia, alteration in taste, anaphylaxis, angioedema, anorexia, anxiety, arthritis, cataracts, chills, cholestatic jaundice, cirrhosis, CPK increased (>10x normal), depression, dryness of skin/mucous membranes, dyspnea, eosinophilia, erectile dysfunction, erythema multiforme, ESR increased, facial paresis, fatty liver, fever, flushing, fulminant hepatic necrosis, GGT increased, gynecomastia, hemolytic anemia, hepatitis, hepatoma, hyperbilirubinemia, hypersensitivity reaction, impaired extraocular muscle movement, impotence, leukopenia, libido decreased, malaise, memory loss, myopathy, nail changes, nodules, ophthalmoplegia, pancreatitis, paresthesia, peripheral nerve palsy, peripheral neuropathy, photosensitivity, polymyalgia rheumatica, positive ANA, pruritus, psychic disturbance, purpura, rash, renal failure (secondary to rhabdomyolysis), rhabdomyolysis, skin discoloration, Stevens-Johnson syndrome, systemic lupus erythematosus-like syndrome, thrombocytopenia, thyroid dysfunction, toxic epidermal necrolysis, transaminases increased, tremor, urticaria, vasculitis, vertigo, vomiting

Drug Interactions

Metabolism/Transport Effects **Substrate** of CYP3A4 (major); **Inhibits** CYP2C9 (weak), 2D6 (weak), 3A4 (weak)

Avoid Concomitant Use There are no known interactions where it is recommended to avoid concomitant use.

Increased Effect/Toxicity

Lovastatin may increase the levels/effects of: DAPTOmycin; Vitamin K Antagonists

The levels/effects of Lovastatin may be increased by: Amiodarone; Antifungal Agents (Azole Derivatives, Systemic); Calcium Channel Blockers (Nondihydropyridine); Colchicine; CycloSPORINE; CYP3A4 Inhibitors (Moderate); CYP3A4 Inhibitors (Strong); Danazol; Dasatinib; Fenofibrate; Fenofibric Acid; Fluconazole; Gemfibrozil; Grapefruit Juice; Macrolide Antibiotics; Nefazodone; Niacin; Niacinamide; P-Glycoprotein Inhibitors; Protease Inhibitors; Sildenafil

Decreased Effect

The levels/effects of Lovastatin may be decreased by: Bosentan; CYP3A4 Inducers (Strong); Deferasirox; Etravirine; P-Glycoprotein Inducers; Phenytoin; Rifamycin Derivatives; St Johns Wort

Ethanol/Nutrition/Herb Interactions

Ethanol: Avoid excessive ethanol consumption (due to potential hepatic effects).

Food: Food **decreases** the bioavailability of lovastatin extended release tablets and **increases** the bioavailability of lovastatin immediate release tablets. Lovastatin serum concentrations may be increased if taken with grapefruit juice; avoid concurrent intake of large quantities (>1 quart/day). Red yeast rice contains an estimated 2.4 mg lovastatin per 600 mg rice.

Herb/Nutraceutical: St John's wort may decrease lovastatin levels.

Stability

Tablet, immediate release: Store between 5°C to 30°C (41°F to 86°F). Protect from light

Tablet, extended release: Store between 20°C to 25°C (68°F to 77°F). Avoid excessive heat and humidity.

Mechanism of Action Lovastatin acts by competitively inhibiting 3-hydroxyl-3-methylglutaryl-coenzyme A (HMG-CoA) reductase, the enzyme that catalyzes the rate-limiting step in cholesterol biosynthesis

Pharmacodynamics/Kinetics

Onset of action: LDL-cholesterol reductions: 3 days

Absorption: 30%; increased with extended release tablets when taken in the fasting state

Protein binding: 95%

Metabolism: Hepatic; extensive first-pass effect; hydrolyzed to B-hydroxy acid (active)

Bioavailability: Increased with extended release tablets

Half-life elimination: 1.1-1.7 hours

Time to peak, serum: 2-4 hours

Excretion: Feces (~80% to 85%); urine (10%)

Dosage Oral:

Adolescents 10-17 years: Immediate release tablet:

LDL reduction <20%: Initial: 10 mg/day with evening meal

LDL reduction ≥20%: Initial: 20 mg/day with evening meal

Usual range: 10-40 mg with evening meal, then adjust dose at 4-week intervals

Adults: Initial: 20 mg with evening meal, then adjust at 4-week intervals; maximum dose: 80 mg/day immediate release tablet **or** 60 mg/day extended release tablet

Dosage modification/limits based on concurrent therapy:

Cyclosporine and other immunosuppressant drugs: Initial dose: 10 mg/day with a maximum recommended dose of 20 mg/day

Concurrent therapy with fibrates, danazol, and/or lipid-lowering doses of niacin (>1 g/day): Maximum recommended dose: 20 mg/day. Concurrent use with fibrates should be avoided unless risk to benefit favors use.

Concurrent therapy with amiodarone or verapamil: Maximum recommended dose: 40 mg/day of regular release or 20 mg/day with extended release.

Dosage adjustment in renal impairment: Cl_{cr} <30 mL/minute: Use doses >20 mg/day with caution.

Dietary Considerations Before initiation of therapy, patients should be placed on a standard cholesterol-lowering diet for 6 weeks and the diet should be continued during drug therapy. Avoid intake of large quantities of grapefruit juice (≥1 quart/day); may increase toxicity. Red yeast rice contains an estimated 2.4 mg lovastatin per 600 mg rice.

Administration Administer immediate release tablet with meals. Administer extended release tablet at bedtime; do not crush or chew.

Monitoring Parameters Obtain baseline LFTs and total cholesterol profile. LFTs should also be assessed prior to upwards dosage adjustment to ≥40 mg daily or when otherwise indicated clinically. Enzyme levels should be followed periodically thereafter as clinically warranted.

Reference Range NCEP classification of pediatric patients with familial history of hypercholesterolemia or premature CVD: Acceptable total cholesterol: <170 mg/dL, LDL: <110 mg/dL

Test Interactions Altered thyroid function tests

Dosage Forms Excipient information presented when available (limited, particularly for generics); consult specific product labeling.

Tablet: 10 mg, 20 mg, 40 mg

Mevacor®: 20 mg, 40 mg

Tablet, extended release:

Altoprev®: 20 mg, 40 mg, 60 mg

◆ **Lovastatin and Niacin** *see* Niacin and Lovastatin *on page 1059*

◆ **Lovaza®** *see* Omega-3-Acid Ethyl Esters *on page 1100*

◆ **Lovenox®** *see* Enoxaparin *on page 519*

◆ **Lovenox® HP (Can)** *see* Enoxaparin *on page 519*

◆ **Low-Molecular-Weight Iron Dextran (INFeD®)** *see* Iron Dextran Complex *on page 817*

◆ **Low-Ogestrel®** *see* Ethinyl Estradiol and Norgestrel *on page 585*

◆ **Loxapac® IM (Can)** *see* Loxapine *on page 912*

Loxapine (LOKS a peen)

U.S. Brand Names Loxitane®

Canadian Brand Names Apo-Loxapine®; Loxapac® IM; Nu-Loxapine; PMS-Loxapine

Index Terms Loxapine Succinate; Oxilapine Succinate

Pharmacologic Category Antipsychotic Agent, Typical

Additional Appendix Information

Antipsychotic Agents *on page 1644*

Use Management of psychotic disorders

Unlabeled/Investigational Use Psychosis/agitation related to Alzheimer's dementia

Pregnancy Risk Factor C

Medication Safety Issues

Sound-alike/look-alike issues:

Loxitane® may be confused with Lexapro®, Soriatane®

International issues:

Loxitane® may be confused with Lexotan® which is a brand name for bromazepam in multiple international markets

Dosage Oral:

Adults: 10 mg twice daily, increase dose until psychotic symptoms are controlled; usual dose range: 20-100 mg/day in divided doses 2-4 times/day; dosages >250 mg/day are not recommended

Elderly: 20-60 mg/day

Additional Information Complete prescribing information for this medication should be consulted for additional detail.

Dosage Forms Excipient information presented when available (limited, particularly for generics); consult specific product labeling.

Capsule, as succinate: 5 mg, 10 mg, 25 mg, 50 mg

◆ **Loxapine Succinate** *see* Loxapine *on page 912*

◆ **Loxitane®** *see* Loxapine *on page 912*

◆ **Lozide® (Can)** *see* Indapamide *on page 781*

◆ **Lozi-Flur™** *see* Fluoride *on page 635*

◆ **Lozol® (Can)** *see* Indapamide *on page 781*

◆ **L-PAM** *see* Melphalan *on page 936*

◆ **LRH** *see* Gonadorelin *on page 704*

◆ **L-Sarcolysin** *see* Melphalan *on page 936*

◆ **LTA® 360** *see* Lidocaine *on page 884*

◆ **LTG** *see* LamoTRIgine *on page 850*

◆ ***L*-Thyroxine Sodium** *see* Levothyroxine *on page 881*

◆ **Lu-26-054** *see* Escitalopram *on page 547*

Lubiprostone (loo bi PROS tone)

U.S. Brand Names Amitiza®

Index Terms RU 0211; SPI 0211

Pharmacologic Category Chloride Channel Activator; Gastrointestinal Agent, Miscellaneous

Use Treatment of chronic idiopathic constipation; treatment of irritable bowel syndrome with constipation in adult women

Pregnancy Risk Factor C

Dosage Oral:

Chronic idiopathic constipation: Adults: 24 mcg twice daily

Irritable bowel syndrome with constipation: Females ≥18 years: 8 mcg twice daily

Dosage adjustment for toxicity for chronic idiopathic constipation: May decrease dose to 24 mcg once daily in case of severe nausea

Dosage adjustment for renal/hepatic impairment: Has not been studied

Additional Information Complete prescribing information for this medication should be consulted for additional detail.

Dosage Forms Excipient information presented when available (limited, particularly for generics); consult specific product labeling.

Capsule, softgel:

Amitiza®: 8 mcg, 24 mcg

◆ **Lucentis®** *see* Ranibizumab *on page 1294*

◆ **Ludiomil** *see* Maprotiline *on page 921*

◆ **Lufyllin®-GG** *see* Dyphylline and Guaifenesin *on page 501*

◆ **Lugol's Solution** *see* Potassium Iodide and Iodine *on page 1220*

◆ **Lumigan®** *see* Bimatoprost *on page 198*

◆ **Luminal® Sodium** *see* PHENobarbital *on page 1179*

◆ **Lumitene™** *see* Beta-Carotene *on page 188*

◆ **Lunesta®** *see* Eszopiclone *on page 570*

◆ **Lupron®** *see* Leuprolide *on page 868*

◆ **Lupron Depot®** *see* Leuprolide *on page 868*

◆ **Lupron® Depot® (Can)** *see* Leuprolide *on page 868*

◆ **Lupron Depot-Ped®** *see* Leuprolide *on page 868*

◆ **Luride® [DSC]** *see* Fluoride *on page 635*

◆ **Luride® Lozi-Tab®** *see* Fluoride *on page 635*

◆ **Lusedra™** *see* Fospropofol *on page 673*

◆ **LuSonal™** *see* Phenylephrine *on page 1183*

◆ **Lustra®** *see* Hydroquinone *on page 749*

◆ **Lustra-AF™** *see* Hydroquinone *on page 749*

◆ **Luteinizing Hormone Releasing Hormone** *see* Gonadorelin *on page 704*

◆ **Lutera™** *see* Ethinyl Estradiol and Levonorgestrel *on page 577*

◆ **Lutrepulse™ (Can)** *see* Gonadorelin *on page 704*

Lutropin Alfa (LOO troe pin AL fa)

U.S. Brand Names Luveris®

Index Terms r-hLH; Recombinant Human Luteinizing Hormone

Pharmacologic Category Gonadotropin; Ovulation Stimulator

Use Stimulation of follicular development in infertile hypogonadotropic hypogonadal (HH) women with profound luteinizing hormone (LH) deficiency; to be used in combination with follitropin alfa

Pregnancy Risk Factor X

Pregnancy Considerations An increase in pre- and postimplantation loss was observed in animal studies. Lutropin alfa is contraindicated for use during pregnancy.

Lactation Excretion in breast milk unknown/use caution

Contraindications Hypersensitivity to lutropin alfa or any component of the formulation; primary ovarian failure; uncontrolled thyroid or adrenal dysfunction; uncontrolled organic intracranial lesion; abnormal uterine bleeding of undetermined origin; ovarian cyst or enlargement of undetermined origin; sex hormone-dependent tumors of the reproductive tract and accessory organs; pregnancy

Warnings/Precautions These medications should only be used by physicians who are thoroughly familiar with infertility problems and their management. May cause ovarian hyperstimulation syndrome (OHSS); if severe, treatment should be discontinued and patient should be hospitalized. OHSS results in a rapid (<24 hours to 7 days) accumulation of fluid in the peritoneal cavity, thorax, and possibly the pericardium, which may become more severe if pregnancy occurs; monitor for ovarian enlargement. Thromboembolic events have been reported. Patients should be advised of the potential risk for multiple births before beginning therapy. Safety and efficacy have not been established with hepatic or renal dysfunction. Not for use in children or postmenopausal women.

Adverse Reactions

1% to 10%:

Central nervous system: Headache (10%), fatigue (2% to 3%)

Endocrine & metabolic: Ovarian hyperstimulation (6%)

Gastrointestinal: Nausea (7%), constipation (2% to 3%), diarrhea (2% to 3%)

Adverse events reported with gonadotropin or menotropin therapy: Adnexal torsion, arterial thromboembolism, congenital abnormalities, ectopic pregnancy, hemoperitoneum, ovarian enlargement (mild-to-moderate), ovarian neoplasms (infrequent), postpartum fever, premature labor, pulmonary complications, spontaneous abortion, vascular complications

Drug Interactions

Avoid Concomitant Use There are no known interactions where it is recommended to avoid concomitant use.

Increased Effect/Toxicity There are no known significant interactions involving an increase in effect.

Decreased Effect There are no known significant interactions involving a decrease in effect.

Stability Store under refrigeration or at room temperature of 2°C to 25°C (36°F to 77°F). Protect from light. Reconstitute with SWFI. Mix gently, do not shake. Use immediately after reconstitution.

Mechanism of Action Lutropin alfa is a recombinant luteinizing hormone prepared using Chinese hamster cell ovaries. Administration leads to increased follicular estradiol secretion needed for follicle stimulating hormone induced follicular development.

Pharmacodynamics/Kinetics

Distribution: V_d: 10

Bioavailability: 56% ± 23%

Half-life elimination: Terminal: ~18 hours

Time to peak, serum: 4-16 hours

Excretion: Urine (<5% unchanged)

Dosage SubQ: Adults: Females: Infertility: 75 int. units daily until adequate follicular development is noted; maximum duration of treatment: 14 days; to be used concomitantly with follitropin alfa

Administration SubQ: Administer on the stomach, a few inches above or below the navel.

Monitoring Parameters

Prior to therapy: Baseline LH <1.2 int. units/L, FSH <5 int. units/L, negative progestin challenge test

During therapy: Signs and symptoms of OHSS, ovarian enlargement; follicular maturation (vaginal ultrasound, serum estradiol levels); ovulation (basal body temperature, serum progesterone, menstruation)

Dosage Forms Excipient information presented when available (limited, particularly for generics); consult specific product labeling.

Injection, powder for reconstitution:

Luveris®: 75 int. units [contains sucrose; packaged with SWFI]

◆ **Luveris®** *see* Lutropin Alfa *on page 912*

◆ **Luvox** *see* Fluvoxamine *on page 652*

◆ **Luvox® (Can)** *see* Fluvoxamine *on page 652*

◆ **Luvox® CR** *see* Fluvoxamine *on page 652*

◆ **Luxiq®** *see* Betamethasone *on page 188*

◆ **LY139603** *see* Atomoxetine *on page 150*

◆ **LY146032** *see* DAPTOmycin *on page 397*

◆ **LY170053** *see* OLANZapine *on page 1093*

◆ **LY231514** *see* Pemetrexed *on page 1159*

◆ **LY246736** *see* Alvimopan *on page 77*

◆ **LY248686** *see* DULoxetine *on page 498*

◆ **LY303366** *see* Anidulafungin *on page 117*

◆ **LY2148568** *see* Exenatide *on page 595*

◆ **Lybrel™** *see* Ethinyl Estradiol and Levonorgestrel *on page 577*

◆ **Lyderm® (Can)** *see* Fluocinonide *on page 634*

◆ **Lymphocyte Immune Globulin** *see* Antithymocyte Globulin (Equine) *on page 124*

◆ **Lymphocyte Mitogenic Factor** *see* Aldesleukin *on page 53*

◆ **Lyrica®** *see* Pregabalin *on page 1234*

◆ **Lysodren®** *see* Mitotane *on page 1006*

◆ **M-M-R® II** *see* Measles, Mumps, and Rubella Vaccines (Combined) *on page 923*

◆ **Maalox® [OTC]** *see* Aluminum Hydroxide, Magnesium Hydroxide, and Simethicone *on page 76*

◆ **Maalox® Max [OTC]** *see* Aluminum Hydroxide, Magnesium Hydroxide, and Simethicone *on page 76*

◆ **Maalox® Regular Chewable [OTC]** *see* Calcium Carbonate *on page 238*

◆ **Maalox® Total Stomach Relief® [OTC]** *see* Bismuth *on page 199*

◆ **MabCampath® (Can)** *see* Alemtuzumab *on page 56*

◆ **Macrobid®** *see* Nitrofurantoin *on page 1072*

◆ **Macrodantin®** *see* Nitrofurantoin *on page 1072*

◆ **Macugen®** *see* Pegaptanib *on page 1150*

Mafenide (MA fe nide)

U.S. Brand Names Sulfamylon®

Index Terms Mafenide Acetate

Pharmacologic Category Antibiotic, Topical

Additional Appendix Information

Sulfonamide Derivatives *on page 1671*

Use

Cream: Adjunctive antibacterial agent in the treatment of second- and third-degree burns

Solution: Adjunctive antibacterial agent for use under moist dressings over meshed autografts on excised burn wounds

Pregnancy Risk Factor C

Dosage Children and Adults: Topical:

Cream: Apply once or twice daily with a sterile-gloved hand; apply to a thickness of approximately 1/16 inch; the burned area should be covered with cream at all times

Solution: Cover graft area with 1 layer of fine mesh gauze. Wet an 8-ply burn dressing with mafenide solution and cover graft area. Keep dressing wet using syringe or irrigation tubing every 4 hours (or as necessary), or by moistening dressing every 6-8 hours (or as necessary). Irrigation dressing should be secured with bolster dressing and wrapped as appropriate. May leave dressings in place for up to 5 days.

Dosage adjustment for acidosis: Discontinuing treatment for 24-48 hours may aid in restoring acid-base balance

Additional Information Complete prescribing information for this medication should be consulted for additional detail.

Dosage Forms Excipient information presented when available (limited, particularly for generics); consult specific product labeling.

Cream, topical:
Sulfamylon®: 85 mg/g (60 g, 120 g, 454 g) [contains sodium metabisulfite]

Powder, for topical solution, as acetate:
Sulfamylon®: 50 g/packet (5s)

◆ **Mafenide Acetate** *see* Mafenide *on page 913*

◆ **Mag 64™ [OTC]** *see* Magnesium Chloride *on page 914*

Magaldrate and Simethicone

(MAG al drate & sye METH i kone)

U.S. Brand Names Riopan Plus® Double Strength [OTC] [DSC]; Riopan Plus® [OTC] [DSC]

Index Terms Simethicone and Magaldrate

Pharmacologic Category Antacid; Antiflatulent

Use Relief of hyperacidity associated with peptic ulcer, gastritis, peptic esophagitis, and hiatal hernia which are accompanied by symptoms of gas

Pregnancy Risk Factor C

Medication Safety Issues

Sound-alike/look-alike issues:
Riopan Plus® may be confused with Repan®

Dosage Adults: Oral: 5-10 mL (540-1080 mg magaldrate) between meals and at bedtime

Additional Information Complete prescribing information for this medication should be consulted for additional detail.

Dosage Forms Excipient information presented when available (limited, particularly for generics); consult specific product labeling. [DSC] = Discontinued product

Suspension, oral: Magaldrate 540 mg and simethicone 20 mg per 5 mL (360 mL)
Riopan Plus®: Magaldrate 540 mg and simethicone 20 mg per 5 mL (360 mL) [DSC]
Riopan Plus® Double Strength: Magaldrate 1080 mg and simethicone 40 mg per 5 mL (360 mL) [DSC]

◆ **Mag-Caps [OTC]** *see* Magnesium Oxide *on page 916*

◆ **Mag Delay® [OTC]** *see* Magnesium Chloride *on page 914*

◆ **Mag G® [OTC]** *see* Magnesium Gluconate *on page 915*

◆ **MagGel™ [OTC]** *see* Magnesium Oxide *on page 916*

◆ **Maginex™ [OTC]** *see* Magnesium L-aspartate Hydrochloride *on page 916*

◆ **Maginex™ DS [OTC]** *see* Magnesium L-aspartate Hydrochloride *on page 916*

◆ **Magnacet™** *see* Oxycodone and Acetaminophen *on page 1122*

◆ **Magnesia Magma** *see* Magnesium Hydroxide *on page 915*

◆ **Magnesium L-lactate Dihydrate** *see* Magnesium L-lactate *on page 916*

◆ **Magnesium Carbonate and Aluminum Hydroxide** *see* Aluminum Hydroxide and Magnesium Carbonate *on page 75*

Magnesium Chloride (mag NEE zhum KLOR ide)

U.S. Brand Names Chloromag®; Mag 64™ [OTC]; Mag Delay® [OTC]; Slow-Mag® [OTC]

Pharmacologic Category Electrolyte Supplement, Oral; Electrolyte Supplement, Parenteral; Magnesium Salt

Use Correction or prevention of hypomagnesemia; dietary supplement

Pregnancy Risk Factor C

Dosage Note: Serum magnesium is poor reflection of repletional status as the majority of magnesium is intracellular; serum levels may be transiently normal for a few hours after a dose is given; therefore, aim for consistently high normal serum levels in patients with normal renal function for most efficient repletion.

Dietary supplement: Adults: Oral (Mag 64™, Mag Delay®, Slow-Mag®): 2 tablets once daily

Parenteral nutrition supplementation: I.V. (elemental magnesium):
Children:
<50 kg: 0.3-0.5 mEq/kg/day
>50 kg: 10-30 mEq/day
Adults: 8-24 mEq/day

RDA (elemental magnesium):
Children:
1-3 years: 80 mg/day
4-8 years: 130 mg/day
9-13 years: 240 mg/day
14-18 years:
Female: 360 mg/day
Pregnant female: 400 mg/day
Male: 410 mg/day
Adults:
19-30 years:
Female: 310 mg/day
Pregnant female: 350 mg/day
Male: 400 mg/day
≥31 years:
Female: 320 mg/day
Pregnant female: 360 mg/day
Male: 420 mg/day

Dosage adjustment in renal impairment: Cl_{cr} <30 mL/minute: Use with caution; monitor for hypermagnesemia

Additional Information Complete prescribing information for this medication should be consulted for additional detail.

Dosage Forms Excipient information presented when available (limited, particularly for generics); consult specific product labeling.

Injection, solution: 200 mg/mL [1.97 mEq/mL] (50 mL)
Chloromag®: 200 mg/mL [1.97 mEq/mL] (50 mL)

Tablet [enteric coated]:
Slow-Mag®: Elemental magnesium 64 mg [contains elemental calcium 106 mg]

Tablet, delayed release:
Mag 64™, Mag Delay®: Magnesium chloride hexahydrate 535 mg [equivalent to elemental magnesium 64 mg; contains elemental calcium 110 mg]

Magnesium Citrate (mag NEE zhum SIT rate)

U.S. Brand Names Citroma® [OTC]

Canadian Brand Names Citro-Mag®

Index Terms Citrate of Magnesia

Pharmacologic Category Laxative, Saline; Magnesium Salt

Additional Appendix Information
Laxatives, Classification and Properties *on page 1660*

Use Evacuation of bowel prior to certain surgical and diagnostic procedures or overdose situations

Pregnancy Risk Factor B

Dosage Cathartic: Oral:
Children:
<6 years: 0.5 mL/kg up to a maximum of 200 mL repeated every 4-6 hours until stools are clear
6-12 years: 100-150 mL
Children ≥12 years and Adults: 1/2 to 1 full bottle (120-300 mL)

Additional Information Complete prescribing information for this medication should be consulted for additional detail.

Dosage Forms Excipient information presented when available (limited, particularly for generics); consult specific product labeling.
Solution, oral: 290 mg/5 mL (300 mL) [cherry and lemon flavors]
Citroma®: 290 mg/5 mL (300 mL) [contains magnesium 48 mg and potassium 13 mg per 5 mL; cherry and lemon flavors]; (300 mL) [contains magnesium 48 mg and sodium 7.5 mg per 5 mL; grape and lemony flavors]
Tablet: 100 mg [as elemental magnesium]

Magnesium Gluconate

(mag NEE zhum GLOO koe nate)

U.S. Brand Names Almora® [OTC]; Mag G® [OTC]; Magonate® [OTC]; Magtrate® [OTC]

Pharmacologic Category Electrolyte Supplement, Oral; Magnesium Salt

Use Dietary supplement

Dosage RDA (elemental magnesium):
Children:
1-3 years: 80 mg/day
4-8 years: 130 mg/day
9-13 years: 240 mg/day
14-18 years:
Female: 360 mg/day
Pregnant female: 400 mg/day
Male: 410 mg/day
Adults:
19-30 years:
Female: 310 mg/day
Pregnant female: 350 mg/day
Male: 400 mg/day
≥31 years:
Female: 320 mg/day
Pregnant female: 360 mg/day
Male: 420 mg/day

Dosing in renal impairment: Cl_{cr} <30 mL/minute: Use with caution; monitor for hypermagnesemia

Additional Information Complete prescribing information for this medication should be consulted for additional detail.

Dosage Forms Excipient information presented when available (limited, particularly for generics); consult specific product labeling.
Solution:
Magonate®: 1000 mg/5 mL (355 mL) [magnesium 4.8 mEq/5 mL; equivalent to elemental magnesium 54 mg/5 mL; contains sodium benzoate]
Tablet: 500 mg [magnesium 2.4 mEq; equivalent to elemental magnesium 27 mg]
Almora®, Mag G®, Magonate®, Magtrate®): 500 mg [magnesium 2.4 mEq; equivalent to elemental magnesium 27 mg]

Magnesium Hydroxide

(mag NEE zhum hye DROKS ide)

U.S. Brand Names Phillips'® Chews [OTC]; Phillips'® Milk of Magnesia [OTC]

Index Terms Magnesia Magma; Milk of Magnesia; MOM

Pharmacologic Category Antacid; Laxative; Magnesium Salt

Additional Appendix Information
Laxatives, Classification and Properties *on page 1660*

Use Short-term treatment of occasional constipation and symptoms of hyperacidity, laxative; dietary supplement

Dosage Oral:
Laxative:
Liquid:
Children: Magnesium hydroxide 400 mg/5 mL: 1-3 mL/kg/day; adjust dose to induce daily bowel movement
OTC labeling:
<2 years: Use not recommended
2-5 years: Magnesium hydroxide 400 mg/5 mL: 5-15 mL/day once daily at bedtime or in divided doses
6-11 years:
Magnesium hydroxide 400 mg/5 mL: 15-30 mL/day once daily at bedtime or in divided doses
Magnesium hydroxide 800 mg/5 mL: 7.5-15 mL/day once daily at bedtime or in divided doses
Children ≥12 years and Adults:
Magnesium hydroxide 400 mg/5 mL: 30-60 mL/day once daily at bedtime or in divided doses
Magnesium hydroxide 800 mg/5 mL: 15-30 mL/day once daily at bedtime or in divided doses
Tablet: OTC labeling:
Children:
<3 years: Use not recommended
3-5 years: Magnesium hydroxide 311 mg/tablet: 2 tablets/day once daily at bedtime or in divided doses
6-11 years: Magnesium hydroxide 311 mg/tablet: 4 tablets/day once daily at bedtime or in divided doses
Children ≥12 years and Adults: Magnesium hydroxide 311 mg/tablet: 8 tablets/day once daily at bedtime or in divided doses
Antacid: OTC labeling:
Liquid: Children ≥12 years and Adults: Magnesium hydroxide 400 mg/5 mL: 5-15 mL as needed up to 4 times/day
Tablet:
Children <12 years: Use not recommended
Children ≥12 years and Adults: Magnesium hydroxide 311 mg/tablet: 2-4 tablets every 4 hours up to 4 times/day
Dietary supplement: OTC labeling (Phillips'® Chews):
Children <12 years: Use not recommended
Children ≥12 years and Adults: Magnesium 500 mg: 2-4 tablets/day once daily at bedtime or in divided doses

Dosing in renal impairment: Patients in severe renal failure should not receive magnesium due to toxicity from accumulation. Patients with a Cl_{cr} <30 mL/minute receiving magnesium should be monitored by serum magnesium levels.

Additional Information Complete prescribing information for this medication should be consulted for additional detail.

Dosage Forms Excipient information presented when available (limited, particularly for generics); consult specific product labeling.
Liquid, oral: 400 mg/5 mL (360 mL, 480 mL, 960 mL, 3780 mL)
Phillips'® Milk of Magnesia: 400 mg/5 mL (120 mL, 360 mL, 780 mL) [contains magnesium 167 mg/5 mL, cherry flavor also contains sodium 2 mg/5 mL; original, cherry, and mint flavors]

Liquid, oral concentrate: 800 mg/5 mL (100 mL, 400 mL)
Phillips'® Milk of Magnesia [concentrate]: 800 mg/5 mL (240 mL) [strawberry flavor]
Tablet, chewable:
Phillips'® Chews: Magnesium 500 mg [contains sodium 10 mg/tablet, coconut oil and soybean oil; chocolate flavor]
Phillips'® Milk of Magnesia: 311 mg [contains magnesium 130 mg/tablet; mint flavor]

◆ **Magnesium Hydroxide, Aluminum Hydroxide, and Simethicone** *see* Aluminum Hydroxide, Magnesium Hydroxide, and Simethicone *on page* 76

◆ **Magnesium Hydroxide and Aluminum Hydroxide** *see* Aluminum Hydroxide and Magnesium Hydroxide *on page* 76

◆ **Magnesium Hydroxide and Calcium Carbonate** *see* Calcium Carbonate and Magnesium Hydroxide *on page* 239

Magnesium Hydroxide and Mineral Oil
(mag NEE zhum hye DROKS ide & MIN er al oyl)

U.S. Brand Names Phillips'® M-O [OTC]
Index Terms Haley's M-O; MOM/Mineral Oil Emulsion
Pharmacologic Category Laxative
Use Short-term treatment of occasional constipation
Dosage Oral: Laxative: OTC labeling:
Children <6 years: Use not recommended
Children 6-11 years: 20-30 mL at bedtime
Children ≥12 years and Adults: 45-60 mL at bedtime

Dosage adjustment in renal impairment: Patients in severe renal failure should not receive magnesium due to toxicity from accumulation. Patients with a Cl_{cr} <30 mL/minute should be monitored by serum magnesium levels.
Additional Information Complete prescribing information for this medication should be consulted for additional detail.
Dosage Forms Excipient information presented when available (limited, particularly for generics); consult specific product labeling.
Suspension, oral:
Phillips'® M-O: Magnesium hydroxide 300 mg and mineral oil 1.25 mL per 5 mL (360 mL, 780 mL) [contains magnesium 125 mg and sodium 1.5 mg per 5 mL mint flavors]

◆ **Magnesium Hydroxide, Famotidine, and Calcium Carbonate** *see* Famotidine, Calcium Carbonate, and Magnesium Hydroxide *on page* 604

Magnesium L-aspartate Hydrochloride
(mag NEE zhum el as PAR tate hye droe KLOR ide)

U.S. Brand Names Maginex™ DS [OTC]; Maginex™ [OTC]
Index Terms MAH
Pharmacologic Category Electrolyte Supplement, Oral; Magnesium Salt
Use Dietary supplement
Dosage
RDA (elemental magnesium):
Children:
1-3 years: 80 mg/day
4-8 years: 130 mg/day
9-13 years: 240 mg/day
14-18 years:
Female: 360 mg/day
Pregnant female: 400 mg/day
Male: 410 mg/day
Adults:
19-30 years:
Female: 310 mg/day
Pregnant female: 350 mg/day
Male: 400 mg/day
≥31 years:
Female: 320 mg/day
Pregnant female: 360 mg/day
Male: 420 mg/day
Dietary supplement: Adults: Oral: Magnesium-L-aspartate 1230 mg (magnesium 122 mg) up to 3 times/day

Dosage adjustment in renal impairment: Cl_{cr} <30 mL/minute: Use with caution; monitor for hypermagnesemia
Additional Information Complete prescribing information for this medication should be consulted for additional detail.
Dosage Forms Excipient information presented when available (limited, particularly for generics); consult specific product labeling.
Granules:
Maginex™ DS: 1230 mg/packet (30s) [magnesium 10 mEq; equivalent to magnesium 122 mg; lemon flavor]
Tablet [enteric coated]:
Maginex™: 615 mg [magnesium 5 mEq; equivalent to magnesium 61 mg]

Magnesium L-lactate (mag NEE zhum el LAK tate)

U.S. Brand Names Mag-Tab® SR
Index Terms Magnesium L-lactate Dihydrate
Pharmacologic Category Electrolyte Supplement; Magnesium Salt
Use Dietary supplement
Dosage
Dietary supplement: Oral: Adults: 1-2 caplets every 12 hours
RDA (elemental magnesium):
Children:
1-3 years: 80 mg/day
4-8 years: 130 mg/day
9-13 years: 240 mg/day
14-18 years:
Female: 360 mg/day
Pregnant female: 400 mg/day
Male: 410 mg/day
Adults:
19-30 years:
Female: 310 mg/day
Pregnant female: 350 mg/day
Male: 400 mg/day
≥31 years:
Female: 320 mg/day
Pregnant female: 360 mg/day
Male: 420 mg/day

Dosage adjustment in renal impairment: Cl_{cr} <30 mL/minute: Use with caution; monitor for hypermagnesemia
Additional Information Complete prescribing information for this medication should be consulted for additional detail.
Dosage Forms Excipient information presented when available (limited, particularly for generics); consult specific product labeling.
Caplet, sustained-release:
Mag-Tab® SR: Elemental magnesium 84 mg (7 mEq)

Magnesium Oxide (mag NEE zhum OKS ide)

U.S. Brand Names Mag-Caps [OTC]; Mag-Ox® 400 [OTC]; MagGel™ [OTC]; Uro-Mag® [OTC]
Pharmacologic Category Electrolyte Supplement, Oral; Magnesium Salt

Use Electrolyte replacement

Dosage

RDA (elemental magnesium):

Children:

1-3 years: 80 mg/day

4-8 years: 130 mg/day

9-13 years: 240 mg/day

14-18 years:

Female: 360 mg/day

Pregnant female: 400 mg/day

Male: 410 mg/day

Adults:

19-30 years:

Female: 310 mg/day

Pregnant female: 350 mg/day

Male: 400 mg/day

≥31 years:

Female: 320 mg/day

Pregnant female: 360 mg/day

Male: 420 mg/day

Dietary supplement: Adults: Oral:

Mag-Ox 400®: 2 tablets daily with food

Mag-Caps, Uro-Mag®: 4-5 capsules daily with food

Dosing in renal impairment: Cl_{cr} <30 mL/minute: Use with caution; monitor for hypermagnesemia

Additional Information Complete prescribing information for this medication should be consulted for additional detail.

Dosage Forms Excipient information presented when available (limited, particularly for generics); consult specific product labeling.

Caplet: 250 mg

Capsule:

Mag-Caps: Elemental magnesium 85 mg

Uro-Mag®: 140 mg [magnesium 7 mEq; equivalent to elemental magnesium 84.5 mg]

Capsule, softgel:

MagGel™: 600 mg [magnesium 28.64 mEq; equivalent to elemental magnesium 348 mg]

Tablet: 400 mg [magnesium 20 mEq; equivalent to elemental magnesium 242 mg], 500 mg

Mag-Ox® 400: 400 mg [magnesium 20 mEq; equivalent to elemental magnesium 242 mg]

Magnesium Salicylate (mag NEE zhum sa LIS i late)

U.S. Brand Names Doan's® Extra Strength [OTC]; Keygesic [OTC]; Momentum® [OTC]; Novasal™

Pharmacologic Category Salicylate

Use Mild-to-moderate pain, fever, various inflammatory conditions; relief of pain and inflammation of rheumatoid arthritis and osteoarthritis

Pregnancy Risk Factor C

Dosage Oral:

Children ≥12 years and Adults: Relief of mild-to-moderate pain:

Doan's® Extra Strength, Momentum®: Two caplets every 6 hours as needed (maximum: 8 caplets/24 hours)

Keygesic: One tablet every 4 hours as needed (maximum 4 tablets/24 hours)

Adults: Treatment of arthritis (Novasal™): Initial: 1 tablet 3-4 times/day. Maximum: 8 tablets/day

Elderly: Treatment of arthritis (Novasal™): Reduce adult dose to lowest effective dose; monitor for signs of toxicity

Additional Information Complete prescribing information for this medication should be consulted for additional detail.

Dosage Forms Excipient information presented when available (limited, particularly for generics); consult specific product labeling.

Caplet, as anhydrous: 467 mg

Doan's® Extra Strength: 467 mg

Momentum®: 467 mg

Tablet, chelated:

Keygesic: 650 mg

Tablet, as tetrahydrate [scored]:

Novasal™: 600 mg

Magnesium Sulfate (mag NEE zhum SUL fate)

Index Terms Epsom Salts; $MgSO_4$ (error-prone abbreviation)

Pharmacologic Category Anticonvulsant, Miscellaneous; Electrolyte Supplement, Parenteral; Magnesium Salt

Use Treatment and prevention of hypomagnesemia; prevention and treatment of seizures in severe pre-eclampsia or eclampsia, pediatric acute nephritis; torsade de pointes; treatment of cardiac arrhythmias (VT/VF) caused by hypomagnesemia; soaking aid

Unlabeled/Investigational Use

Asthma exacerbation (life-threatening)

Pregnancy Risk Factor A/C (manufacturer dependent)

Pregnancy Considerations Magnesium crosses the placenta; serum levels in the fetus correlate with those in the mother. Magnesium sulfate is used during pregnancy for the treatment of eclampsia and severe pre-eclampsia.

Lactation Enters breast milk/compatible

Medication Safety Issues

Sound-alike/look-alike issues:

Magnesium sulfate may be confused with manganese sulfate, morphine sulfate

$MgSO_4$ is an error-prone abbreviation (mistaken as morphine sulfate)

High alert medication: The Institute for Safe Medication Practices (ISMP) includes this medication (I.V. formulation) among its list of drugs which have a heightened risk of causing significant patient harm when used in error.

Contraindications Hypersensitivity to any component of the formulation; heart block; myocardial damage

Warnings/Precautions Use magnesium with caution in patients with impaired renal function (accumulation of magnesium may lead to magnesium intoxication). Use with extreme caution in patients with myasthenia gravis or other neuromuscular disease. Magnesium toxicity can lead to fatal cardiovascular arrest and/or respiratory paralysis; close monitoring of serum magnesium, respiratory rate, and presence of deep tendon reflex necessary during parenteral administration, particularly with repeated dosing. Vigilant monitoring and safe administration techniques (ISMP Medication Safety Alert, 2005) recommended to avoid potential for errors resulting in toxicity when used in obstetrics; monitor patient and fetal status, and serum magnesium levels closely. Solution for injection may contain aluminum; toxic levels may occur following prolonged administration in premature neonates or patients with renal dysfunction. Concurrent hypokalemia or hypocalcemia can accompany a magnesium deficit.

Adverse Reactions Adverse effects on neuromuscular function may occur at lower levels in patients with neuromuscular disease (eg, myasthenia gravis).

Frequency not defined:

Cardiovascular: Flushing (I.V.; dose related), hypotension (I.V.; rate related), vasodilation (I.V.; rate related)

Gastrointestinal: Diarrhea

Drug Interactions

Avoid Concomitant Use There are no known interactions where it is recommended to avoid concomitant use.

Increased Effect/Toxicity

Magnesium Sulfate may increase the levels/effects of: Alcohol (Ethyl); Calcium Channel Blockers; CNS Depressants; Neuromuscular-Blocking Agents

The levels/effects of Magnesium Sulfate may be increased by: Calcitriol; Calcium Channel Blockers

Decreased Effect

Magnesium Sulfate may decrease the levels/effects of: Bisphosphonate Derivatives; Eltrombopag; Mycophenolate; Phosphate Supplements; Quinolone Antibiotics; Tetracycline Derivatives; Trientine

The levels/effects of Magnesium Sulfate may be decreased by: Ketorolac; Mefloquine; Trientine

Ethanol/Nutrition/Herb Interactions Ethanol: Magnesium may enhance the CNS depressant effect of alcohol (ethyl).

Stability Prior to use, store at room temperature of 20°C to 25°C (68°F to 77°F). Refrigeration of solution may result in precipitation or crystallization.

Mechanism of Action When taken orally, magnesium promotes bowel evacuation by causing osmotic retention of fluid which distends the colon with increased peristaltic activity; parenterally, magnesium decreases acetylcholine in motor nerve terminals and acts on myocardium by slowing rate of S-A node impulse formation and prolonging conduction time. Magnesium is necessary for the movement of calcium, sodium, and potassium in and out of cells, as well as stabilizing excitable membranes.

Pharmacodynamics/Kinetics

Onset of action: Anticonvulsant: I.M.: 1 hour; I.V.: Immediate

Duration of anticonvulsant activity: I.M.: 3-4 hours; I.V.: 30 minutes

Distribution: Bone (50% to 60%); extracellular fluid (1% to 2%)

Protein binding: 30%, to albumin

Excretion: Urine (as magnesium)

Dosage Dose represented as magnesium sulfate unless stated otherwise. **Note:** Serum magnesium is poor reflection of repletional status as the majority of magnesium is intracellular; serum levels may be transiently normal for a few hours after a dose is given, therefore, aim for consistently high normal serum levels in patients with normal renal function for most efficient repletion.

Note: 1 g of magnesium sulfate = 98.6 mg elemental magnesium = 8.12 mEq elemental magnesium

Hypomagnesemia: Note: Treatment depends on severity and clinical status:

Children: I.V., I.O.: 25-50 mg/kg/dose over 10-20 minutes (faster in cardiac arrest); maximum single dose: 2000 mg

Adults:

Mild deficiency: I.M.: 1 g every 6 hours for 4 doses, or as indicated by serum magnesium levels

Severe deficiency:

I.M.: Up to 250 mg/kg within a 4-hour period

I.V.: Severe, non-life-threatening: 1-2 g/hour for 3-6 hours then 0.5-1 g/hour as needed to correct deficiency

Symptomatic deficiency: I.V.: 1-2 g over 5-60 minutes; maintenance infusion may be required to correct deficiency (0.5-1 g/hour).

Arrhythmia (ACLS guidelines, 2005), hypomagnesemia-induced (life-threatening): 1-2 g over 5-20 minutes (torsades with cardiac arrest) or over 5-60 minutes (symptomatic arrhythmias without cardiac arrest)

Seizures, hypomagnesemia-induced: I.V.: 2 g over 10 minutes; calcium administration may also be appropriate as many patients are also hypocalcemic.

Asthma (life-threatening or severe exacerbation after 1 hour of intensive conventional therapy; unlabeled use): I.V.:

Children: 25-75 mg/kg (maximum: 2 g)

Adults: 2 g

Eclampsia: Adults:

I.V.: 4-5 g infusion; followed by a 1-2 g/hour continous infusion; or may follow with I.M. doses of 4-5 g in each buttock every 4 hours. **Note:** Initial infusion may be given over 3-4 minutes if eclampsia is severe; maximum: 40 g/24 hours

ACOG Practice Bulletin 2002: 4-6 g over 15-20 minutes followed by 2 g/hour continuous infusion

Pre-eclampsia (severe): Adults: I.V. 4-5 g infusion; followed by a 1-2 g/hour continous infusion; or may follow with I.M. doses of 4-5 g in each buttock every 4 hours; maximum: 40 g/24 hour

Torsade de pointes: Adults: I.V.:

Pulseless: 1-2 g over 5-20 minutes

With pulse: 1-2 g over 5-60 minutes. **Note:** Slower administration preferable for stable patients.

Parenteral nutrition supplementation: I.V.:

Children:

<50 kg: 0.3-0.5 mEq elemental magnesium/kg/day

>50 kg: 10-30 mEq elemental magnesium/day

Adults: 8-24 mEq elemental magnesium/day

Soaking aid: Topical: Adults: Dissolve 2 cupfuls of powder per gallon of warm water

RDA:

Children:

1-3 years: 80 mg elemental magnesium/day

4-8 years: 130 mg elemental magnesium/day

9-13 years: 240 mg elemental magnesium/day

14-18 years:

Female: 360 mg elemental magnesium/day

Pregnant female: 400 mg elemental magnesium/day

Male: 410 mg elemental magnesium/day

Adults:

19-30 years:

Female: 310 mg elemental magnesium/day

Pregnant female: 350 mg elemental magnesium/day

Male: 400 mg elemental magnesium/day

≥31 years:

Female: 320 mg elemental magnesium/day

Pregnant female: 360 mg elemental magnesium/day

Male: 420 mg elemental magnesium/day

Dosage adjustment in renal impairment: Cl_{cr} <30 mL/minute: Use with caution; monitor for hypermagnesemia; do not exceed 20 g/48 hours as per manufacturer. Close monitoring is required.

Dietary Considerations Whole grains, legumes and dark-green leafy vegetables are dietary sources of magnesium.

10% elemental magnesium; 8.1 mEq magnesium/g; 4 mmol magnesium/g

500 mg magnesium sulfate = 4.06 mEq magnesium = 49.3 mg elemental magnesium

Administration

Injection: May be administered I.M. or I.V.

I.M.: A 25% or 50% concentration may be used for adults and dilution to a ≤20% solution is recommended for children

I.V.: Magnesium should be diluted to a ≤20% solution for I.V. infusion and may be administered IVP, IVPB or I.V.; when giving I.V. push, must dilute first and should not be given any faster than 150 mg/minute. Hypotension and asystole may occur with rapid administration.

Maximal rate of infusion: 2 g/hour to avoid hypotension; doses of 4 g/hour have been given in emergencies (eclampsia, seizures); optimally, should add magnesium to I.V. fluids, but bolus doses are also effective

Topical: Dissolve 2 cups of powder per gallon of warm water to use as a soaking aid. To make a compress, dissolve 2 cups of powder per 2 cups of hot water and use a towel to apply as a wet dressing.

Monitoring Parameters
I.V.: Rapid administration: ECG monitoring, vital signs, deep tendon reflexes; magnesium, calcium, and potassium levels; renal function during administration
Obstetrics: Patient status including vital signs, oxygen saturation, deep tendon reflexes, level of consciousness, fetal heart rate, maternal uterine activity.

Reference Range Serum magnesium: 1.5-2.5 mg/dL; slightly different ranges are reported by different laboratories

Dosage Forms Excipient information presented when available (limited, particularly for generics); consult specific product labeling.
Infusion [premixed in D_5W]: 10 mg/mL (100 mL); 20 mg/mL (500 mL)
Infusion [premixed in water for injection]: 40 mg/mL (100 mL, 500 mL, 1000 mL); 80 mg/mL (50 mL)
Injection, solution: 500 mg/mL (2 mL, 10 mL, 20 mL, 50 mL)
Powder, oral/topical: Magnesium sulfate USP (227 g, 454 g, 480 g, 1810 g, 1920 g, 2720 g)

- **Magnesium Trisilicate and Aluminum Hydroxide** *see* Aluminum Hydroxide and Magnesium Trisilicate *on page 76*
- **Magonate® [OTC]** *see* Magnesium Gluconate *on page 915*
- **Mag-Ox® 400 [OTC]** *see* Magnesium Oxide *on page 916*
- **Mag-Tab® SR** *see* Magnesium L-lactate *on page 916*
- **Magtrate® [OTC]** *see* Magnesium Gluconate *on page 915*
- **MAH** *see* Magnesium L-aspartate Hydrochloride *on page 916*
- **Malarone®** *see* Atovaquone and Proguanil *on page 154*
- **Malarone® Pediatric (Can)** *see* Atovaquone and Proguanil *on page 154*

Malathion (mal a THYE on)

U.S. Brand Names Ovide®

Pharmacologic Category Antiparasitic Agent, Topical; Pediculocide; Scabicidal Agent

Use Treatment of head lice and their ova

Pregnancy Risk Factor B

Dosage Sprinkle Ovide® lotion on dry hair and rub gently until the scalp is thoroughly moistened; pay special attention to the back of the head and neck. Allow to dry naturally - use no heat and leave uncovered. After 8-12 hours, the hair should be washed with a nonmedicated shampoo; rinse and use a fine-toothed comb to remove dead lice and eggs. If required, repeat with second application in 7-9 days. Further treatment is generally not necessary. Other family members should be evaluated to determine if infested and if so, receive treatment.

Additional Information Complete prescribing information for this medication should be consulted for additional detail.

Dosage Forms Excipient information presented when available (limited, particularly for generics); consult specific product labeling.
Lotion: 0.5% (59 mL) [contains isopropyl alcohol 78%]

- **Mandelamine® [DSC]** *see* Methenamine *on page 961*
- **Mandelamine® (Can)** *see* Methenamine *on page 961*
- **Mandrake** *see* Podophyllum Resin *on page 1207*

Manganese (MAN ga nees)

U.S. Brand Names Mangimin [OTC]

Index Terms Manganese Chloride; Manganese Sulfate

Pharmacologic Category Trace Element, Parenteral

Use Trace element added to total parenteral nutrition (TPN) solution to prevent manganese deficiency; orally as a dietary supplement

Pregnancy Risk Factor C

Medication Safety Issues
Sound-alike/look-alike issues:
Manganese sulfate may be confused with magnesium sulfate

Dosage
Oral: Adequate intake:
0-6 months: 0.003 mg/day
7-12 months: 0.6 mg/day
1-3 years: 1.2 mg/day
4-8 years: 1.5 mg/day
9 years to Adults, Male: 1.9-2.3 mg/day
9 years to Adults, Female: 1.6-1.8 mg/day
Pregnancy: 2 mg/day
Lactation: 2.6 mg/day
I.V.:
Children: 2-10 mcg/kg/day usually administered in TPN solutions
Note: Use caution in premature neonates; manganese chloride solution for injection contains aluminum
Adults: 150-800 mcg/day usually administered in TPN solutions
Dosage adjustment in renal impairment: Use caution; manganese chloride solution for injection contains aluminum
Dosage adjustment in hepatic impairment: Use caution; dose may need to be decreased or withheld

Additional Information Complete prescribing information for this medication should be consulted for additional detail.

Dosage Forms Excipient information presented when available (limited, particularly for generics); consult specific product labeling.
Injection, solution, as chloride [preservative free]: 0.1 mg/mL (10 mL) [contains aluminum ≤100 mcg/mL]
Injection, solution, as sulfate: 0.1 mg/mL (10 mL)
Tablet, as aspartate: 93 mg [equivalent to elemental manganese 25 mg]
Tablet, as gluconate: 5.7 mg [as elemental manganese]; 550 mg [equivalent to elemental manganese 30 mg]; 600 mg [equivalent to elemental manganese 50 mg]
Tablet, chelated: 50 mg [as elemental manganese]
Mangimin: 10 mg [as elemental manganese]

- **Manganese Chloride** *see* Manganese *on page 919*
- **Manganese Sulfate** *see* Manganese *on page 919*
- **Mangimin [OTC]** *see* Manganese *on page 919*

Mannitol (MAN i tole)

U.S. Brand Names Osmitrol®; Resectisol®

Canadian Brand Names Osmitrol®

Index Terms *D*-Mannitol

Pharmacologic Category Diuretic, Osmotic; Genitourinary Irrigant

Use Reduction of increased intracranial pressure associated with cerebral edema; promotion of diuresis in the prevention and/or treatment of oliguria or anuria due to acute renal failure; reduction of increased intraocular pressure; promoting urinary excretion of toxic substances; genitourinary irrigant in transurethral prostatic resection or other transurethral surgical procedures

Pregnancy Risk Factor C

Pregnancy Considerations Reproduction studies have not been conducted.

Lactation Excretion in breast milk unknown/use caution

Medication Safety Issues

Sound-alike/look-alike issues:

Osmitrol® may be confused with esmolol

Contraindications Hypersensitivity to mannitol or any component or the formulation; severe renal disease (anuria); severe dehydration; active intracranial bleeding except during craniotomy; progressive heart failure, pulmonary congestion, or renal dysfunction after mannitol administration; severe pulmonary edema or congestion

Warnings/Precautions Should not be administered until adequacy of renal function and urine flow is established; use 1-2 test doses to assess renal response. Excess amounts can lead to profound diuresis with fluid and electrolyte loss; close medical supervision and dose evaluation are required. Watch for and correct electrolyte disturbances; adjust dose to avoid dehydration. May cause renal dysfunction especially with high doses; use caution in patients taking other nephrotoxic agents, with sepsis or pre-existing renal disease. To minimize adverse renal effects, adjust to keep serum osmolality less than 320 mOsm/L. Discontinue if evidence of acute tubular necrosis.

In patients being treated for cerebral edema, mannitol may accumulate in the brain (causing rebound increases in intracranial pressure) if circulating for long periods of time as with continuous infusion; intermittent boluses preferred. Cardiovascular status should also be evaluated; do not administer electrolyte-free mannitol solutions with blood. If hypotension occurs monitor cerebral perfusion pressure to insure adequate.

Adverse Reactions Frequency not defined.

Cardiovascular: Chest pain, CHF, circulatory overload, hyper-/hypotension, tachycardia

Central nervous system: Chills, convulsions, dizziness, headache

Dermatologic: Rash, urticaria

Endocrine & metabolic: Fluid and electrolyte imbalance, dehydration and hypovolemia secondary to rapid diuresis, hyperglycemia, hypernatremia, hyponatremia (dilutional), hyperosmolality-induced hyperkalemia, metabolic acidosis (dilutional), osmolar gap increased, water intoxication

Gastrointestinal: Nausea, vomiting, xerostomia

Genitourinary: Dysuria, polyuria

Local: Pain, thrombophlebitis, tissue necrosis

Ocular: Blurred vision

Renal: Acute renal failure, acute tubular necrosis (>200 g/day; serum osmolality >320 mOsm/L)

Respiratory: Pulmonary edema, rhinitis

Miscellaneous: Allergic reactions

Drug Interactions

Avoid Concomitant Use There are no known interactions where it is recommended to avoid concomitant use.

Increased Effect/Toxicity

Mannitol may increase the levels/effects of: Amifostine; RiTUXimab

The levels/effects of Mannitol may be increased by: Diazoxide; Herbs (Hypotensive Properties); Prostacyclin Analogues

Decreased Effect

The levels/effects of Mannitol may be decreased by: Herbs (Hypertensive Properties); Methylphenidate; Yohimbine

Stability Should be stored at room temperature (15°C to 30°C); do not freeze. Crystallization may occur at low temperatures; do not use solutions that contain crystals. Heating in a hot water bath and vigorous shaking may be utilized for resolubilization. Cool solutions to body temperature before using.

Mechanism of Action Increases the osmotic pressure of glomerular filtrate, which inhibits tubular reabsorption of water and electrolytes and increases urinary output

Pharmacodynamics/Kinetics

Onset of action: Diuresis: Injection: 1-3 hours; Reduction in intracranial pressure: ~15-30 minutes

Duration: Reduction in intracranial pressure: 1.5-6 hours

Distribution: Remains confined to extracellular space (except in extreme concentrations); does not penetrate the blood-brain barrier (generally, penetration is low)

Metabolism: Minimally hepatic to glycogen

Half-life elimination: 1.1-1.6 hours

Excretion: Primarily urine (as unchanged drug)

Dosage

Children: I.V.:

Test dose (to assess adequate renal function): 200 mg/kg over 3-5 minutes to produce a urine flow of at least 1 mL/kg for 1-3 hours

Initial: 0.25-1 g/kg

Maintenance: 0.25-0.5 g/kg given every 4-6 hours

Adults:

I.V.:

Test dose (to assess adequate renal function): 12.5 g (200 mg/kg) over 3-5 minutes to produce a urine flow of at least 30-50 mL of urine per hour. If urine flow does not increase, a second test dose may be given. If test dose does not produce an acceptable urine output, then need to reassess management.

Initial: 0.5-1 g/kg

Maintenance: 0.25-0.5 g/kg every 4-6 hours; usual daily dose: 20-200 g/24 hours

Intracranial pressure: Cerebral edema: 0.25-1.5 g/kg/dose I.V. as a 15% to 20% solution over ≥30 minutes; maintain serum osmolality 310 to <320 mOsm/kg

Prevention of acute renal failure (oliguria): 50-100 g dose

Treatment of oliguria: 100 g dose

Preoperative for neurosurgery: 1.5-2 g/kg administered 1-1.5 hours prior to surgery

Reduction of intraocular pressure: 1.5-2 g/kg as a 15% to 20% solution; administer over 30 minutes

Topical: Transurethral irrigation: Use urogenital solution as required for irrigation

Elderly: Consider initiation at lower end of dosing range

Dosage adjustment in renal impairment: Contraindicated in severe renal impairment. If test dose does not produce adequate urine output reassess options. Use caution in patients with underlying renal disease.

Dosage adjustment in hepatic impairment: No adjustment required.

Administration Inspect for crystals prior to administration. If crystals present redissolve by warming solution. Use filter-type administration set; in-line 5-micron filter set should always be used for mannitol infusion with concentrations ≥20%; administer test dose (for oliguria) I.V. push over 3-5 minutes; avoid extravasation; for cerebral edema or elevated ICP, administer over 20-30 minutes; crenation and agglutination of red blood cells may occur if administered with whole blood.

Monitoring Parameters Renal function, daily fluid I & O, serum electrolytes, serum and urine osmolality; for treatment of elevated intracranial pressure, maintain serum osmolality 310 to <320 mOsm/kg.

Additional Information May autoclave or heat to redissolve crystals; mannitol 20% has an approximate osmolarity of 1100 mOsm/L and mannitol 25% has an approximate osmolarity of 1375 mOsm/L

Dosage Forms Excipient information presented when available (limited, particularly for generics); consult specific product labeling.

Injection, solution: 5% [50 mg/mL] (1000 mL); 10% [100 mg/mL] (500 mL, 1000 mL); 15% [150 mg/mL] (500 mL); 20% [200 mg/mL] (150 mL, 250 mL, 500 mL); 25% [250 mg/mL] (50 mL)

Osmitrol®: 5% [50 mg/mL] (1000 mL); 10% [100 mg/mL] (500 mL, 1000 mL); 15% [150 mg/mL] (500 mL); 20% [200 mg/mL] (250 mL, 500 mL)

Solution, urogenital (Resectisol®): 5% [50 mg/mL] (2000 mL, 4000 mL)

- **Mantoux** *see* Tuberculin Tests *on page 1527*
- **Mapap [OTC]** *see* Acetaminophen *on page 25*
- **Mapap Children's [OTC]** *see* Acetaminophen *on page 25*
- **Mapap Extra Strength [OTC]** *see* Acetaminophen *on page 25*
- **Mapap Infants [OTC]** *see* Acetaminophen *on page 25*
- **Mapap® Multi-Symptom Cold [OTC]** *see* Acetaminophen, Dextromethorphan, and Phenylephrine *on page 32*
- **Mapap® Sinus Congestion and Pain Daytime [OTC]** *see* Acetaminophen and Phenylephrine *on page 29*
- **Mapap Sinus Maximum Strength [OTC]** *see* Acetaminophen and Pseudoephedrine *on page 30*
- **Mapezine® (Can)** *see* CarBAMazepine *on page 252*

Maprotiline (ma PROE ti leen)

Canadian Brand Names Novo-Maprotiline

Index Terms Ludiomil; Maprotiline Hydrochloride

Pharmacologic Category Antidepressant, Tetracyclic

Additional Appendix Information

Antidepressant Agents *on page 1638*

Use Treatment of depression and anxiety associated with depression

Unlabeled/Investigational Use Bulimia; duodenal ulcers; enuresis; urinary symptoms of multiple sclerosis; pain; panic attacks; tension headache; cocaine withdrawal

Restrictions An FDA-approved medication guide concerning the use of antidepressants in children, adolescents, and young adults must be distributed when dispensing an outpatient prescription (new or refill) where this medication is to be used without direct supervision of a healthcare provider. Medication guides are available at http://www.fda.gov/cder/Offices/ODS/medication_guides.htm. Dispense to parents or guardians of children and adolescents receiving this medication.

Pregnancy Risk Factor B

Medication Safety Issues

Sound-alike/look-alike issues:

Ludiomil may be confused with Lamictal®, lamotrigine, Lomotil®

Dosage Oral:

Adults: Depression/anxiety: 75 mg/day to start, increase by 25 mg every 2 weeks up to 150-225 mg/day; given in 3 divided doses or in a single daily dose

Elderly: Depression/anxiety: Initial: 25 mg at bedtime, increase by 25 mg every 3 days for inpatients and weekly for outpatients if tolerated; usual maintenance dose: 50-75 mg/day, higher doses may be necessary in nonresponders

Additional Information Complete prescribing information for this medication should be consulted for additional detail.

Dosage Forms Excipient information presented when available (limited, particularly for generics); consult specific product labeling.

Tablet, as hydrochloride: 25 mg, 50 mg, 75 mg

- **Maprotiline Hydrochloride** *see* Maprotiline *on page 921*

Maraviroc (mah RAV er rock)

U.S. Brand Names Selzentry™

Canadian Brand Names Celsentri™

Index Terms UK-427,857

Pharmacologic Category Antiretroviral Agent, CCR5 Antagonist

Additional Appendix Information

Antiretroviral Therapy for HIV Infection: Adults and Adolescents *on page 1758*

Perinatal HIV Guidelines *on page 1730*

Use Treatment of CCR5-tropic HIV-1 infection, in combination with other antiretroviral agents in treatment-experienced patients with evidence of viral replication and HIV-1 strains resistant to multiple antiretroviral therapy

Restrictions An FDA-approved medication guide is available at http://www.selzentry.com/content/SELZENTRY_MedicationGuide.pdf; distribute to each patient to whom this medication is dispensed.

Pregnancy Risk Factor B

Pregnancy Considerations Adverse fetal effects were not observed in animal studies. There are no adequate and well-controlled studies in pregnant women and available data is insufficient to recommend use in pregnancy. An antiretroviral registry has been established to monitor maternal and fetal outcomes in women receiving antiretroviral drugs. Physicians are encouraged to register patients at 1-800-258-4263 or www.APRegistry.com.

Lactation Excretion in breast milk unknown/contraindicated

Contraindications There are no contraindications listed within the manufacturer's labeling.

Warnings/Precautions [U.S. Boxed Warning] Possible drug-induced hepatotoxicity with allergic type features has been reported; hepatotoxicity may be preceded by allergic type reactions (eg, pruritic rash, eosinophilia or increased IgE) and/or hepatic adverse events (transaminase increases or signs/symptoms of hepatitis). Consider discontinuation in any patient with possible hepatitis or with elevated transaminases combined with systemic allergic events. Patients may develop immune reconstitution syndrome resulting in the occurrence of an inflammatory response to an indolent or residual opportunistic infection; further evaluation and treatment may be required. Monitor closely for signs/symptoms of developing infections; associated with a small increase of certain upper respiratory tract infections and herpes virus infections during clinical trials. Use with caution in patients with cardiovascular disease or cardiac risk factors. During trials, a small increase in cardiovascular events (myocardial ischemia and/or infarction) occurred in treated patients compared to placebo, although a contributory relationship relative to therapy is unknown. Symptomatic postural hypotension has occurred; use caution in patients at risk for postural hypotension due to concomitant medication or history of condition.

Safety and efficacy has not been adequately studied in patients with hepatic impairment; use caution in patients with hepatic dysfunction or concomitant viral hepatitis B or C. Use with caution in patients taking strong CYP3A4/P-glycoprotein inhibitors and moderate or strong CYP3A4/P-glycoprotein inducers; may require dosage adjustments. Safety and efficacy not adequately studied in renal impairment; renal impairment may increase maraviroc concentrations. Concomitant therapy with CYP3A inhibitors in presence of renal impairment is expected to further increase levels and may lead to increased adverse events; therefore, avoid maraviroc in patients on concomitant CYP3A inhibitors with Cl_{cr} <50 mL/minute unless potential benefits outweighs potential risk. Prior to therapy, tropism testing should be performed for presence of CCR5-tropic HIV-1 infection. Therapy not recommended for use in patients with CXCR4- or dual/mixed tropic HIV-1 infection; efficacy not demonstrated in this population. Safety and efficacy have not been established in treatment-naive patients or in children <16 years of age.

Adverse Reactions

>10%:

Central nervous system: Fever (13%)

Respiratory: Upper respiratory tract infection (23%), cough (14%)

2% to 10%:

Cardiovascular: Vascular hypertensive disorder (3%)

Central nervous system: Dizziness (9%), insomnia (8%), anxiety (4%), consciousness disturbances (4%), depression (4%), pain (4%)

Dermatologic: Rash (11%), pruritus (4%), folliculitis (3%), skin neoplasms (benign; 3%), erythema (2%)

Endocrine & metabolic: Lipodystrophy (3%)

Gastrointestinal: Appetite disorders (8%), constipation (6%)

Genitourinary: Urinary tract/bladder symptoms (3% to 5%), genital warts (2%)

Hematologic: Neutropenia (grades 3/4: 4%)

Hepatic: Transaminases increased (grades 3/4: 2% to 5%), bilirubin increased (grades 3/4: 6%)

Neuromuscular & skeletal: Joint disorders (7%), paresthesia (5%), peripheral neuropathy (4%), sensory abnormality (4%), muscle pain (3%)

Ocular: Conjunctivitis (2%), infection/inflammation (2%)

Otic: Otitis media (2%)

Respiratory: Bronchitis (7%), sinusitis (7%), respiratory tract/sinus disorder (3% to 6%), breathing abnormality (4%)

Miscellaneous: Herpes infection (8%), sweat gland disturbances (5%), influenza (2%)

<2% (Limited to important or life-threatening): Acute cardiac failure, anal cancer, angina, basal cell carcinoma, bile duct neoplasm, bone marrow depression, cerebrovascular accident, cholestatic jaundice, coronary artery disease, coronary artery occlusion, creatine kinase increased, endocarditis, endocrine neoplasm, esophageal carcinoma, hepatic cirrhosis, hepatic failure, hepatotoxicity, hypoplastic anemia, liver metastases, lymphoma, MI, myocardial ischemia, myositis, osteonecrosis, pneumonia, portal vein thrombosis, rhabdomyolysis, seizure, septic shock, squamous cell carcinoma, syncope, T-cell lymphoma, tongue neoplasm, tremor, viral meningitis

Drug Interactions

Metabolism/Transport Effects Substrate of CYP3A4 (major), P-glycoprotein

Avoid Concomitant Use

Avoid concomitant use of Maraviroc with any of the following: St Johns Wort

Increased Effect/Toxicity

The levels/effects of Maraviroc may be increased by: CYP3A4 Inhibitors; Dasatinib; Lopinavir

Decreased Effect

The levels/effects of Maraviroc may be decreased by: CYP3A4 Inducers; Deferasirox; St Johns Wort

Ethanol/Nutrition/Herb Interactions Herb/Nutraceutical: St. John's wort may decrease maraviroc concentrations leading to loss of therapeutic efficacy and potentially increased risk of resistance; concomitant use not recommended.

Stability Store at 25°C (77°F); excursions permitted to 15°C to 30°C (59°F to 86°F).

Mechanism of Action Maraviroc, a CCR5 antagonist, selectively and reversibly binds to the chemokine (C-C motif receptor 5 [CCR5]) coreceptors located on human CD4 cells. CCR5 antagonism prevents interaction between the human CCR5 coreceptor and the gp120 subunit of the viral envelope glycoprotein, thereby inhibiting gp120 conformational change required for CCR5-tropic HIV-1 fusion with the CD4 cell and subsequent cell entry.

Pharmacodynamics/Kinetics

Distribution: V_d: ~194 L

Protein binding: ~76%

Metabolism: Hepatic, via CYP3A to inactive metabolites

Bioavailability: 23% to 33%

Half-life elimination: 14-18 hours

Time to peak, plasma: 0.5-4 hours

Excretion: Urine (~20%, 8% as unchanged drug); feces (76%, 25% as unchanged drug)

Dosage Oral: Adolescents ≥16 years and Adults: 300 mg twice daily

Dosage adjustment for concomitant CYP3A inhibitors/inducers:

CYP3A inhibitors (with or without a CYP3A inducer): 150 mg twice daily; dose recommended when maraviroc administered concomitantly with strong CYP3A inhibitors including (but not limited to) protease inhibitors (excluding tipranavir/ritonavir), delavirdine, ketoconazole, itraconazole, clarithromycin, nefazodone, and telithromycin.

CYP3A inducers (without a strong CYP3A inhibitor): 600 mg twice daily; dose recommended when maraviroc administered concomitantly with CYP3A inducers including (but not limited to) efavirenz, rifampin, carbamazepine, phenobarbital, and phenytoin

Dosage adjustment in renal impairment: Not studied in renal dysfunction; maraviroc levels may be increased.

Cl_{cr} <50 mL/minute (with concomitant CYP3A inhibitor): Not recommended; if no appropriate alternative exists, monitor for increased maraviroc adverse effects

Dosage adjustment in hepatic impairment: Use caution; not adequately studied in hepatic dysfunction

Administration Administer without regards to meals.

Monitoring Parameters Viral load, CD4 count, transaminases; signs/symptoms of infection, hepatitis and/or allergic reaction; postural hypotension; tropism testing (prior to initiation)

Dosage Forms Excipient information presented when available (limited, particularly for generics); consult specific product labeling.

Tablet:

Selzentry™: 150 mg, 300 mg

- ◆ **Marcaine®** *see* Bupivacaine *on page* 220
- ◆ **Marcaine® Spinal** *see* Bupivacaine *on page* 220
- ◆ **Margesic® H** *see* Hydrocodone and Acetaminophen *on page* 740
- ◆ **Marinol®** *see* Dronabinol *on page* 494
- ◆ **Mark 1™** *see* Atropine and Pralidoxime *on page* 159
- ◆ **Marvelon® (Can)** *see* Ethinyl Estradiol and Desogestrel *on page* 575
- ◆ **Matulane®** *see* Procarbazine *on page* 1242
- ◆ **3M™ Avagard™ [OTC]** *see* Chlorhexidine Gluconate *on page* 305
- ◆ **Mavik®** *see* Trandolapril *on page* 1499
- ◆ **Mavik™ (Can)** *see* Trandolapril *on page* 1499
- ◆ **Maxair™ Autohaler™** *see* Pirbuterol *on page* 1200
- ◆ **Maxalt®** *see* Rizatriptan *on page* 1333
- ◆ **Maxalt™ (Can)** *see* Rizatriptan *on page* 1333
- ◆ **Maxalt-MLT®** *see* Rizatriptan *on page* 1333
- ◆ **Maxalt RPD™ (Can)** *see* Rizatriptan *on page* 1333
- ◆ **Maxidex®** *see* Dexamethasone *on page* 425
- ◆ **Maxidone®** *see* Hydrocodone and Acetaminophen *on page* 740
- ◆ **Maxifed®** *see* Guaifenesin and Pseudoephedrine *on page* 713
- ◆ **Maxifed DM** *see* Guaifenesin, Pseudoephedrine, and Dextromethorphan *on page* 715

◆ **Maxifed DMX** *see* Guaifenesin, Pseudoephedrine, and Dextromethorphan *on page 715*
◆ **Maxifed-G®** *see* Guaifenesin and Pseudoephedrine *on page 713*
◆ **Maxipime®** *see* Cefepime *on page 273*
◆ **Maxitrol®** *see* Neomycin, Polymyxin B, and Dexamethasone *on page 1052*
◆ **Maxi-Tuss HCG [DSC]** *see* Hydrocodone and Guaifenesin *on page 741*
◆ **Maxzide®** *see* Hydrochlorothiazide and Triamterene *on page 739*
◆ **Maxzide®-25** *see* Hydrochlorothiazide and Triamterene *on page 739*
◆ **May Apple** *see* Podophyllum Resin *on page 1207*
◆ **MCH** *see* Collagen Hemostat *on page 367*
◆ **MCV** *see* Meningococcal Polysaccharide (Groups A / C / Y and W-135) Diphtheria Toxoid Conjugate Vaccine *on page 939*
◆ **MDL 73,147EF** *see* Dolasetron *on page 476*

Measles, Mumps, and Rubella Vaccines (Combined)

(MEE zels, mumpz & roo BEL a VYE rus vak SEEN)

U.S. Brand Names M-M-R® II

Canadian Brand Names M-M-R® II; Priorix™

Index Terms MMR; Mumps, Measles and Rubella Vaccines, Combined; Rubella, Measles and Mumps Vaccines, Combined

Pharmacologic Category Vaccine, Live (Viral)

Additional Appendix Information

Immunization Recommendations *on page 1708*

Use Measles, mumps, and rubella prophylaxis

The Advisory Committee on Immunization Practices (ACIP) recommends routine vaccination for the following:

- All children (first dose given at 12-15 months of age)
- Adults born 1957 or later (without evidence of immunity or documentation of vaccination).
- Adults at higher risk for exposure to and transmission of measles mumps and rubella should receive special consideration for vaccination. This includes international travelers, persons attending colleges and other post-high school education, persons working in healthcare facilities.

Pregnancy Risk Factor C

Medication Safety Issues

Sound-alike/look-alike issues:

MMR (measles, mumps and rubella virus vaccine) may be confused with MMRV (measles, mumps, rubella, and varicella) vaccine

Dosage SubQ:

Infants 6-11 months: Measles outbreak: If there is risk of exposure to measles, single-antigen measles vaccine should be administered. If single-antigen vaccine is not readily available, MMR is an acceptable alternative. Children should be revaccinated at ≥12 months with standard 2-dose series

Children ≥12 months:

Primary immunization: 12-15 months of age: 0.5 mL

Revaccination: 4-6 years of age: 0.5 mL; revaccination is recommended prior to elementary school. If the second dose was not received, the schedule should be completed by the 11- to 12-year old visit.

Mumps outbreak: During a mumps outbreak, children ages 1-4 years should consider a second dose of a live mumps virus vaccine; minimum interval between doses is 28 days

Measles outbreak: Revaccination with MMR is recommended for attendees and siblings of daycare facilities or schools if they cannot provide adequate documentation of 2 previous doses of a measles-containing vaccine after their first birthday or evidence of measles immunity.

Adults:

Birth year ≥1957 without evidence of immunity: 1 or 2 doses (0.5 mL/dose); minimum interval between doses is 28 days

Mumps outbreak:

Healthcare workers born <1957 without other evidence of immunity: Consider 2 doses of a live mumps virus vaccine; minimum interval between doses is 28 days

Low-risk adults: A second dose of a live mumps virus vaccine should be considered in adults who previously received 1 dose; minimum interval between doses is 28 days

Measles outbreak:

Students and personnel in affected schools and healthcare workers born <1957 without evidence of measles immunity: One dose of MMR vaccine

Students and personnel in affected schools and healthcare workers born ≥1957 without adequate documentation of 2 previous doses of a measles-containing vaccine after their first birthday or evidence of measles immunity: Two doses of MMR vaccine; minimum interval between doses is 28 days

Additional Information Complete prescribing information for this medication should be consulted for additional detail.

Dosage Forms Excipient information presented when available (limited, particularly for generics); consult specific product labeling.

Injection, powder for reconstitution [preservative free]:

M-M-R® II: Measles virus ≥1000 $TCID_{50}$, mumps virus ≥20,000 $TCID_{50}$, and , rubella virus ≥1000 $TCID_{50}$ [contains albumin (human), bovine serum, chicken egg protein, gelatin, neomycin, sorbitol, and sucrose 1.9 mg/vial]

Measles, Mumps, Rubella, and Varicella Virus Vaccine

(MEE zels, mumpz, roo BEL a, & var i SEL a VYE rus vak SEEN)

U.S. Brand Names ProQuad®

Index Terms MMR-V; MMRV; Mumps, Rubella, Varicella, and Measles Vaccine; Rubella, Varicella, Measles, and Mumps Vaccine; Varicella, Measles, Mumps, and Rubella Vaccine

Pharmacologic Category Vaccine, Live (Viral)

Use To provide simultaneous active immunization against measles, mumps, rubella, and varicella

Pregnancy Risk Factor C

Dosage SubQ: Children 12 months to 12 years: One dose (0.5 mL)

Administer on or after the first birthday, as soon as child becomes eligible for vaccination. It may be used whenever all components of the vaccine are needed in children within this age group. (Refer to current CDC Recommended Immunization Schedule)

Allow at least 1 month between administering a dose of a measles containing vaccine (eg, M-M-R® II) and ProQuad®.

Allow at least 3 months between administering a varicella containing vaccine (eg, Varivax®) and ProQuad®.

Additional Information Complete prescribing information for this medication should be consulted for additional detail.

Dosage Forms Excipient information presented when available (limited, particularly for generics); consult specific product labeling.

Injection, powder for reconstitution [preservative free]:

ProQuad®: Measles virus ≥3.00 log_{10} $TCID_{50}$, mumps virus ≥4.3 log_{10} $TCID_{50}$, rubella virus ≥3.00 log_{10}

$TCID_{50}$, and varicella virus ≥3.99 log_{10} PFU [contains albumin (human), bovine serum, chicken egg protein, gelatin, neomycin, sorbitol, and sucrose (≤21 mg/vial)]

Measles Virus Vaccine (Live)

(MEE zels VYE rus vak SEEN, live)

U.S. Brand Names Attenuvax®

Index Terms More Attenuated Enders Strain; Rubeola Vaccine

Pharmacologic Category Vaccine, Live (Viral)

Additional Appendix Information

Immunization Recommendations *on page 1708*

Use Active immunization against measles (rubeola)

Note: Trivalent measles - mumps - rubella (MMR) is the vaccine of choice if recipients are likely to be susceptible to rubella and/or mumps as well as to measles.

Pregnancy Risk Factor C

Pregnancy Considerations Reproduction studies have not been conducted. Vaccine should not be administered to pregnant women and the ACIP recommends that pregnancy be avoided for 28 days following vaccination. Infection with natural measles during pregnancy may increase the risk of spontaneous abortion, stillbirth, congenital defects and prematurity.

Lactation Excretion in breast milk unknown/use caution

Medication Safety Issues

Sound-alike/look-alike issues:

Attenuvax® may be confused with Meruvax®

Contraindications Hypersensitivity to measles vaccine or any component of the formulation; current febrile illness; patients receiving immunosuppressive therapy (not including steroid replacement); primary and acquired immunodeficiency states; blood dyscrasias, cancers affecting the bone marrow or lymphatic systems; pregnancy

Warnings/Precautions Use caution with history of cerebral injury, seizures, or other conditions where stress due to fever should be avoided. Immediate treatment for anaphylactic/anaphylactoid reaction should be available during vaccine use. Vaccine is produced in chick embryo cell culture; use extreme caution in patients with immediate-type hypersensitivity reactions to eggs. Vaccine also contains albumin, neomycin, and gelatin. A history of contact dermatitis to neomycin is not a contraindication to use, however, do not use with previous anaphylactic reaction to neomycin. Use caution in patients with thrombocytopenia and those who develop thrombocytopenia after first dose; thrombocytopenia may worsen. The manufacturer contraindicates use with febrile infections; however, the ACIP notes that patients with minor illnesses with or without fever (diarrhea, mild upper respiratory tract infection, otitis media) may receive vaccines.

Use is contraindicated in severely immunocompromised patients. However, leukemia patients who are in remission and who have not received chemotherapy for at least 3 months may be vaccinated; patients with HIV infection, who are asymptomatic and not severely immunosuppressed may be vaccinated. Therapy to treat tuberculosis should be started prior to administering vaccine to patients with untreated, active tuberculosis. Exposure to measles is not a contraindication to vaccine; use within 72 hours of exposure may provide some protection. Recent administration of immune globulins, blood, or blood products may interfere with immune response. Acceptable evidence of immunity is recommended for students entering institutions of higher learning, healthcare workers at time of employment, and for travelers to endemic areas. Safety and efficacy have not been established for children <6 months of age.

Adverse Reactions All serious adverse reactions must be reported to the U.S. Department of Health and Human Services (DHHS) Vaccine Adverse Event Reporting System (VAERS) 1-800-822-7967.

Frequency not defined.

Cardiovascular: Peripheral edema, syncope, vasculitis

Central nervous system: Ataxia, dizziness, encephalitis, encephalopathy, febrile seizure, fever, Guillain-Barré syndrome, headache, irritability, malaise, seizure

Dermatologic: Angioneurotic edema, erythema multiforme, panniculitis, purpura, rash, Stevens-Johnson syndrome, urticaria

Gastrointestinal: Diarrhea, nausea, vomiting

Hematologic: Leukocytosis, thrombocytopenia

Local: Injection site reactions: Burning, redness, stinging, swelling, vesiculation, wheal and flare

Neuromuscular & skeletal: Arthralgia, myalgia

Ocular: Conjunctivitis, ocular palsies, optic neuritis, papillitis, retinitis, retrobulbar neuritis

Otic: Nerve deafness, otitis media

Respiratory: Bronchial spasm, cough, pneumonitis, rhinitis

Miscellaneous: Anaphylaxis/anaphylactoid reactions, atypical measles, facial edema, lymphadenopathy, measles inclusion body encephalitis, subacute sclerosing pancephalitis

Drug Interactions

Avoid Concomitant Use

Avoid concomitant use of Measles Virus Vaccine (Live) with any of the following: Immunosuppressants

Increased Effect/Toxicity

The levels/effects of Measles Virus Vaccine (Live) may be increased by: Immunosuppressants

Decreased Effect

Measles Virus Vaccine (Live) may decrease the levels/effects of: Tuberculin Tests

The levels/effects of Measles Virus Vaccine (Live) may be decreased by: Immune Globulins

Stability During shipment, store at ≤10°C (50°F). Prior to and following reconstitution, refrigerate at 2°C to 8°C (36°F to 46°F). Protect from light at all times. Following reconstitution, use within 8 hours.

Mechanism of Action Promotes active immunity to measles virus by inducing specific measles IgG and IgM antibodies. Measles antibodies develop in ~95% of children vaccinated at 12 months of age and in 98% of children vaccinated at 15 months of age. Life-long immunity is induced in most persons completing vaccination schedule.

Dosage Note: Trivalent measles - mumps - rubella (MMR) vaccine should be used unless contraindicated in adults and children ≥12 months of age.

Children ≥6 months and Adults: SubQ: 0.5 mL in outer aspect of the upper arm

Primary vaccination recommended at 12-15 months of age and repeated at 4-6 years of age. Children requiring vaccination with measles virus vaccine prior to 12 months of age (eg, during local outbreak, international travel to endemic area) should receive another dose between 12-15 months and again prior to elementary school.

Adults born in or after 1957 without documentation of live vaccine on or after first birthday, without physician-diagnosed measles, or without laboratory evidence of immunity should be vaccinated, ideally with 2 doses of vaccine separated by no less than 1 month. For those previously vaccinated with 1 dose of measles vaccine, revaccination is recommended for students entering colleges and other institutions of higher education, for healthcare workers at the time of employment, and for international travelers who visit endemic areas. Persons vaccinated between 1963 and 1967 with a killed measles vaccine, followed by live vaccine within 3 months, or with a vaccine of unknown type should be revaccinated with live measles virus vaccine.

Administration Vaccine should not be administered I.V.; SubQ injection preferred with a 25-gauge 5/8" needle

Test Interactions May temporarily depress tuberculin skin test sensitivity; tuberculin test may be given simultaneously on the same day as vaccine or ≥4 weeks later.

Additional Information Federal law requires that the date of administration, the vaccine manufacturer, lot number of vaccine, and the administering person's name, title, and address be entered into the patient's permanent medical record.

Acceptable presumptive evidence of immunity includes one of the following:

1. Documentation of adequate vaccination. Adequate vaccination is defined as 1 dose of a live mumps virus vaccine for preschool children and adults not at high risk; 2 doses of a live mumps virus vaccine for school-aged children and high-risk adults. Healthcare workers, international travelers, and students in institutions of higher learning are considered high-risk adults.
2. Laboratory evidence of immunity
3. Birth prior to 1957
4. Documentation of physician-diagnosed disease

Dosage Forms Excipient information presented when available (limited, particularly for generics); consult specific product labeling.

Injection, powder for reconstitution [preservative free]:

Attenuvax®: ≥1000 $TCID_{50}$ [contains albumin (human), bovine serum, chicken egg protein, gelatin, neomycin, sorbitol, and sucrose (1.9 mg/vial)]

◆ **Mebaral®** *see* Mephobarbital *on page 944*

Mebendazole (me BEN da zole)

U.S. Brand Names Vermox® [DSC]

Canadian Brand Names Vermox®

Pharmacologic Category Anthelmintic

Use Treatment of pinworms (*Enterobius vermicularis*), whipworms (*Trichuris trichiura*), roundworms (*Ascaris lumbricoides*), and hookworms (*Ancylostoma duodenale*)

Pregnancy Risk Factor C

Lactation Excretion in breast milk unknown/use caution

Contraindications Hypersensitivity to mebendazole or any component of the formulation

Warnings/Precautions Pregnancy and children <2 years of age are relative contraindications since safety has not been established. Not effective for hydatid disease. Neutropenia and agranulocytosis have been reported with high doses and prolonged use.

Adverse Reactions Frequency not defined.

Cardiovascular: Angioedema

Central nervous system: Fever, dizziness, headache, seizure

Dermatologic: Rash, itching, alopecia (with high doses)

Gastrointestinal: Abdominal pain, diarrhea, nausea, vomiting

Hematologic: Neutropenia (sore throat, unusual fatigue)

Neuromuscular & skeletal: Unusual weakness

Drug Interactions

Avoid Concomitant Use There are no known interactions where it is recommended to avoid concomitant use.

Increased Effect/Toxicity

Mebendazole may increase the levels/effects of: MetroNIDAZOLE

Decreased Effect

The levels/effects of Mebendazole may be decreased by: Aminoquinolines (Antimalarial); CarBAMazepine; Phenytoin

Ethanol/Nutrition/Herb Interactions Food: Mebendazole serum levels may be increased if taken with food.

Mechanism of Action Selectively and irreversibly blocks glucose uptake and other nutrients in susceptible adult intestine-dwelling helminths

Pharmacodynamics/Kinetics

Absorption: 2% to 10%

Distribution: To serum, cyst fluid, liver, omental fat, and pelvic, pulmonary, and hepatic cysts; highest concentrations found in liver; relatively high concentrations found in muscle-encysted *Trichinella spiralis* larvae; crosses placenta

Protein binding: 95%

Metabolism: Extensively hepatic

Half-life elimination: 1-11.5 hours

Time to peak, serum: 2-4 hours

Excretion: Primarily feces; urine (5% to 10%)

Dosage Children ≥2 years and Adults: Oral:

Pinworms: 100 mg as a single dose; may need to repeat after 2 weeks; treatment should include family members in close contact with patient

Whipworms, roundworms, hookworms: One tablet twice daily, morning and evening on 3 consecutive days; if patient is not cured within 3-4 weeks, a second course of treatment may be administered

Capillariasis: 200 mg twice daily for 20 days

Dosing adjustment in hepatic impairment: Dosage reduction may be necessary in patients with liver dysfunction

Hemodialysis: Not dialyzable (0% to 5%)

Dietary Considerations Tablet can be crushed and mixed with food, swallowed whole, or chewed.

Administration Tablets may be chewed, swallowed whole, or crushed and mixed with food.

Monitoring Parameters Check for helminth ova in feces within 3-4 weeks following the initial therapy

Dosage Forms Excipient information presented when available (limited, particularly for generics); consult specific product labeling.

Tablet, chewable: 100 mg

Mecamylamine (mek a MIL a meen)

U.S. Brand Names Inversine®

Canadian Brand Names Inversine®

Index Terms Mecamylamine Hydrochloride

Pharmacologic Category Ganglionic Blocking Agent

Use Treatment of moderately severe to severe hypertension and in uncomplicated malignant hypertension

Unlabeled/Investigational Use Tourette's syndrome

Pregnancy Risk Factor C

Medication Safety Issues

Sound-alike/look-alike issues:

Mecamylamine may be confused with mesalamine

Contraindications Coronary insufficiency, pyloric stenosis, glaucoma, uremia, recent myocardial infarction, unreliable, uncooperative patients

Warnings/Precautions Use with caution in patients with impaired renal function, previous CNS abnormalities, prostatic hyperplasia, bladder obstruction, or urethral stricture. Do not abruptly discontinue.

Adverse Reactions Frequency not defined.

Cardiovascular: Postural hypotension

Central nervous system: Drowsiness, convulsions, confusion, mental depression

Endocrine & metabolic: Sexual ability decreased

Gastrointestinal: Xerostomia, loss of appetite, nausea, vomiting, bloating; frequent stools followed by severe constipation

Genitourinary: Dysuria

Neuromuscular & skeletal: Uncontrolled movements of hands, arms, legs, or face; trembling

Ocular: Blurred vision; enlarged pupils

Respiratory: Dyspnea

Drug Interactions

Avoid Concomitant Use There are no known interactions where it is recommended to avoid concomitant use.

Increased Effect/Toxicity There are no known significant interactions involving an increase in effect.

Decreased Effect There are no known significant interactions involving a decrease in effect.

Mechanism of Action Mecamylamine is a ganglionic blocker. This agent inhibits acetylcholine at the autonomic ganglia, causing a decrease in blood pressure. Mecamylamine also blocks central nicotinic cholinergic receptors, which inhibits the effects of nicotine and may suppress the desire to smoke.

Dosage Adults: Oral: 2.5 mg twice daily after meals for 2 days; increased by increments of 2.5 mg at intervals ≥2 days until desired blood pressure response is achieved; average daily dose: 25 mg (usually in 3 divided doses)

Note: Reduce dosage of other antihypertensives when combined with mecamylamine with exception of thiazide diuretics which may be maintained at usual dose while decreasing mecamylamine by 50%

Dosing adjustment/comments in renal impairment: Use with caution, if at all, although no specific guidelines are available

Dietary Considerations Should be taken after meals.

Monitoring Parameters Monitor for orthostatic hypotension; aid with ambulation

Dosage Forms Excipient information presented when available (limited, particularly for generics); consult specific product labeling.

Tablet, as hydrochloride: 2.5 mg

◆ **Mecamylamine Hydrochloride** *see* Mecamylamine *on page 925*

Mecasermin (mek a SER min)

U.S. Brand Names Increlex™; Iplex™ [DSC]

Index Terms Mecasermin (rDNA Origin) ; Mecasermin Rinfabate; Recombinant Human Insulin-Like Growth Factor-1; rhIGF-1; rhIGF-1/rhIGFBP-3

Pharmacologic Category Growth Hormone

Use Treatment of growth failure in children with severe primary insulin-like growth factor-1 deficiency (IGF-1 deficiency; primary IGFD), or with growth hormone (GH) gene deletions who have developed neutralizing antibodies to GH

Pregnancy Risk Factor C

Pregnancy Considerations Teratogenic effects were not observed in animal studies

Lactation Excretion in breast milk unknown/ use caution

Contraindications Hypersensitivity to mecasermin or any component of the formulation; patients with closed epiphyses; active or suspected neoplasia

Warnings/Precautions Correct thyroid or nutritional deficiencies prior to therapy. May cause hypoglycemic effects; patients should avoid high risk activities until a tolerated dose is established. Use with caution in patients with diabetes. Do not administer on days a patient cannot or will not eat. Increlex™ should be administered with a meal or a snack; patients using Iplex™ should avoid missing meals and maintain a balanced diet. Intracranial hypertension has been reported with growth hormone products and reverses after interruption of dosing; funduscopic examinations are recommended. Lymphoid hypertrophy has been reported and may lead to complications such as snoring, sleep apnea, and chronic middle-ear effusions. Progression of scoliosis and slipped capital epiphyses may occur in children experiencing rapid growth. Not intended for use in patients with secondary forms of IGF-1 deficiency (GH deficiency, malnutrition, hypothyroidism, chronic anti-inflammatory steroid therapy). Products may contain benzyl alcohol. Safety and efficacy have not been established in adults or in children <2 years of age (Increlex™) or <3 years of age (Iplex™).

Adverse Reactions

≥5%:

Cardiovascular: Cardiac murmur

Central nervous system: Convulsion, dizziness, headache (Iplex™: 22%)

Endocrine & metabolic: Hyper-/hypoglycemia (Increlex™: 42%; Iplex™ 31%), iron-deficiency anemia, ovarian cysts, thymus hypertrophy, thyromegaly

Gastrointestinal: Vomiting

Hepatic: Liver enzymes increased

Local: Injection site reactions: Erythema, bruising, hair growth, lipohypertrophy

Neuromuscular & skeletal: Arthralgia, bone pain, extremity pain, muscular atrophy

Ocular: Papilledema

Otic: Ear pain, hypoacusis, middle ear fluid, otitis media, serous otitis media, tympanometry abnormal

Renal: Hematuria

Respiratory: Snoring, tonsillar hypertrophy (Increlex™: 15%; Iplex™ 19%)

Miscellanous: Lymphadenopathy

<5% or frequency not defined: Hypoglycemic seizure, intracranial hypertension, loss of consciousness secondary to hypoglycemia, thickening of soft facial tissue

Drug Interactions

Avoid Concomitant Use There are no known interactions where it is recommended to avoid concomitant use.

Increased Effect/Toxicity There are no known significant interactions involving an increase in effect.

Decreased Effect There are no known significant interactions involving a decrease in effect.

Stability

Increlex™: Store under refrigeration at 2°C to 8°C (35°F to 46°F); do not freeze. Protect from direct light. After initial entry into vial, use within 30 days.

Iplex™: Must be kept frozen. Store at -70°C (-94°F) during distribution and at -20°C (-4°F) once in the patients home freezer. Transport to home freezer on dry ice. Do not use if product thaws during transportation or storage. If solution is cloudy, it may indicate that it has thawed during storage and should not bet used. May be stored up to 2 months at -20°C (-4°F). Prior to use, remove from freezer and allow to thaw at room temperature of 20°C to 25°C (68° to 77°F) for ~45 minutes. Use within 1 hour of reaching room temperature. Do not use if vial was kept at room temperature for >2 hours.

Mechanism of Action Mecasermin is an insulin-like growth factor (IGF-1) produced using recombinant DNA technology to replace endogenous IGF-1. Endogenous IGF-1 circulates predominately bound to insulin-like growth factor-binding protein-3 (IGFBP-3) and a growth hormone-dependent acid-labile subunit (ALS). Acting at receptors in the liver and other tissues, endogenous growth hormone (GH) stimulates the synthesis and secretion of IGF-1. In patients with primary severe IGF-1 deficiency, growth hormone receptors in the liver are unresponsive to GH, leading to reduced endogenous IGF-I concentrations and decreased growth (skeletal, cell, and organ). Endogenous IGF-1 also suppresses liver glucose production, stimulates peripheral glucose utilization and has an inhibitory effect on insulin secretion.

Mecasermin rinfabate is a complex of IGF-1 and IGFBP-3, both produced by recombinant DNA technology.

Pharmacodynamics/Kinetics

Distribution: V_d: Severe primary IGFD: 0.184-0.33 L/kg

Protein binding: >80% bound to IGFBP-3 and an acid-labile subunit (IGFBP-3 reduced with severe primary IGFD)

Metabolism: Hepatic and renal

Half-life elimination: Severe primary IGFD: Mecasermin: 5.8 hours; Mecasermin rinfabate: >12 hours

Dosage

Primary IGFD: SubQ:

Increlex™: Children ≥2 years: Initial: 0.04-0.08 mg/kg twice daily; if tolerated for 7 days, may increase by 0.04 mg/kg/dose (maximum dose: 0.12 mg/kg given twice daily). Must be administered within 20 minutes of a meal or snack; omit dose if patient is unable to eat. Reduce dose if hypoglycemia occurs despite adequate food intake.

Iplex™: Children ≥3 years: Initial: 0.5 mg/kg once daily; dose may be increased to 1-2 mg/kg/day, given once daily. Withhold dose if hypoglycemia is present.

Dietary Considerations Increlex™ must be administered within 20 minutes of a meal or snack. Patients using Iplex™ should avoid missing meals and maintain a balanced diet.

Administration For SubQ injection only; do not administer I.V. Omit dose and do not make up for omitted dose if patient is unable to eat. Rotate injection site.

Increlex™: Must be administered within 20 minutes of a meal or snack. May cause hypoglycemic effects; patients should avoid high-risk activities within 2-3 hours of dosing until a tolerated dose is established.

Iplex™: Prior to administration, gently swirl vial; do not shake. Do not use if solution is cloudy (may indicate thawing during storage); do not use if stored at room temperature >2 hours. Dose should be administered once daily, at the same time each day. May cause hypoglycemic effects; patients should avoid high risk activities for 3-5 days until a tolerated dose is established. Withhold dose if hypoglycemia is present.

Monitoring Parameters Preprandial glucose during treatment initiation and dose adjustment; facial features; lymphoid tissue; fundoscopic examination; growth; new onset of a limp or complaints of hip or knee pain. Monitor small children closely due to potentially erratic food intake.

Iplex™: Adjust dose based on IGF-1 level obtained 8-18 hours after previous dose.

Target treatment IGF-1 level: 0 to +2 SD score for age

Decrease dose for adverse events and/or IGF-1 levels ≥3 SD above normal

Reference Range Severe primary IGFD is defined as follows:

Height standard deviation score ≤ -3.0 **and**

Basal IGF-1 standard deviation score ≤ -3.0 **and**

Growth hormone: Normal or elevated

Dosage Forms Excipient information presented when available (limited, particularly for generics); consult specific product labeling.

Injection, solution:

Increlex™: 10 mg/mL (4 mL) [contains benzyl alcohol]

Injection, solution, as rinfabate [preservative free]:

Iplex™: 36 mg/0.6 mL (0.6 mL) [DSC]

◆ **Mecasermin (rDNA Origin)** *see* Mecasermin *on page 926*

◆ **Mecasermin Rinfabate** *see* Mecasermin *on page 926*

Mechlorethamine (me klor ETH a meen)

U.S. Brand Names Mustargen®

Canadian Brand Names Mustargen®

Index Terms Chlorethazine; Chlorethazine Mustard; HN_2; Mechlorethamine Hydrochloride; Mustine; Nitrogen Mustard; NSC-762

Pharmacologic Category Antineoplastic Agent, Alkylating Agent (Nitrogen Mustard)

Use Hodgkin's disease; non-Hodgkin's lymphoma; intracavitary injection for treatment of metastatic tumors; pleural and other malignant effusions; topical treatment of mycosis fungoides

Pregnancy Risk Factor D

Pregnancy Considerations Animal studies have demonstrated teratogenic effects. There are no adequate and well-controlled studies in pregnant women. Women of childbearing potential are advised not to become pregnant. Use only when potential benefit justifies potential risk to the fetus. **[U.S. Boxed Warning]: Avoid exposure during pregnancy.**

Lactation Excretion in breast milk unknown/not recommended

Medication Safety Issues

High alert medication: The Institute for Safe Medication Practices (ISMP) includes this medication among its list of drugs which have a heightened risk of causing significant patient harm when used in error.

Contraindications Hypersensitivity to mechlorethamine or any component of the formulation; pre-existing profound myelosuppression or infection

Warnings/Precautions [U.S. Boxed Warnings]: Hazardous agent - use appropriate precautions for handling and disposal. Avoid contact with skin or eyes; avoid exposure during pregnancy. Mechlorethamine is a potent vesicant; if extravasation occurs, severe tissue damage (leading to ulceration and necrosis) and pain may occur. Sodium thiosulfate should be available for treatment of extravasation. May cause lymphopenia, granulocytopenia, thrombocytopenia and anemia. Hyperuricemia may occur, especially with lymphomas; ensure adequate hydration. **[U.S. Boxed Warning]: Should be administered under the supervision of an experienced cancer chemotherapy physician.**

Adverse Reactions

>10%:

Endocrine & metabolic: Delayed menses, oligomenorrhea, temporary or permanent amenorrhea, impaired spermatogenesis; spermatogenesis may return in patients in remission several years after the discontinuation of chemotherapy, chromosomal abnormalities

Gastrointestinal: Nausea and vomiting usually occur in nearly 100% of patients and onset is within 30 minutes to 2 hours after administration

Emetic potential: Very high (>90%)

Time course of nausea/vomiting: Onset: 1-3 hours; duration 2-8 hours

Genitourinary: Azoospermia

Hematologic: Myelosuppressive: Leukopenia and thrombocytopenia can be severe; caution should be used with patients who are receiving radiotherapy, secondary leukemia

WBC: Severe

Platelets: Severe

Onset (days): 4-7

Nadir (days): 14

Recovery (days): 21

Otic: Ototoxicity

Miscellaneous: Precipitation of herpes zoster

1% to 10%:

Central nervous system: Fever, vertigo

Dermatologic: Alopecia

Endocrine & metabolic: Hyperuricemia

Gastrointestinal: Diarrhea, anorexia, metallic taste

Local: Thrombophlebitis/extravasation: May cause local vein discomfort which may be relieved by warm soaks and pain medication. A brown discoloration of veins may occur. Mechlorethamine is a strong vesicant and can cause tissue necrosis and sloughing.

Vesicant chemotherapy

Secondary malignancies: Have been reported after several years in 1% to 6% of patients treated

Neuromuscular & skeletal: Weakness

Otic: Tinnitus

Miscellaneous: Hypersensitivity, anaphylaxis

<1% (Limited to important or life-threatening): Hemolytic anemia, hepatotoxicity, myelosuppression, peripheral neuropathy

Drug Interactions

Avoid Concomitant Use

Avoid concomitant use of Mechlorethamine with any of the following: Natalizumab; Vaccines (Live)

Increased Effect/Toxicity

Mechlorethamine may increase the levels/effects of: Natalizumab; Vaccines (Live)

The levels/effects of Mechlorethamine may be increased by: Trastuzumab

Decreased Effect

Mechlorethamine may decrease the levels/effects of: Vaccines (Inactivated)

The levels/effects of Mechlorethamine may be decreased by: Echinacea

Ethanol/Nutrition/Herb Interactions Ethanol: Avoid ethanol (due to GI irritation).

Stability Store intact vials at room temperature (15°C to 30°C/59°F to 86°F). **Must be prepared immediately before use**; solution is stable for only 15-60 minutes after dilution. Dilute powder with 10 mL SWI to a final concentration of 1 mg/mL. May be diluted in up to 100 mL NS for intracavitary or topical administration. Extemporaneous formulations for topical use have been reported to retain biologic activity for 30 days.

Mechanism of Action Bifunctional alkylating agent that inhibits DNA and RNA synthesis via formation of carbonium ions; cross-links strands of DNA, causing miscoding, breakage, and failure of replication; produces interstrand and intrastrand cross-links in DNA resulting in miscoding, breakage, and failure of replication. Although not cell phase-specific *per se,* mechlorethamine effect is most pronounced in the S phase, and cell proliferation is arrested in the G_2 phase.

Pharmacodynamics/Kinetics

Duration: Unchanged drug is undetectable in blood within a few minutes

Absorption: Intracavitary administration: Incomplete secondary to rapid deactivation by body fluids

Metabolism: Rapid hydrolysis and demethylation, possibly in plasma

Half-life elimination: <1 minute

Excretion: Urine (50% as metabolites, <0.01% as unchanged drug)

Dosage Refer to individual protocols.

Children and Adults: I.V.: 6 mg/m^2 on days 1 and 8 of a 28-day cycle (MOPP regimen)

Adults:

I.V.: 0.4 mg/kg **or** 12-16 mg/m^2 for one dose **or** divided into 0.1 mg/kg/day for 4 days, repeated at 4- to 6-week intervals

Intracavitary: 0.2-0.4 mg/kg (10-20 mg) as a single dose; may be repeated if fluid continues to accumulate.

Intrapericardially: 0.2-0.4 mg/kg as a single dose; may be repeated if fluid continues to accumulate.

Topical: 0.01% to 0.02% solution, lotion, or ointment

Hemodialysis: Not removed; supplemental dosing is not required.

Peritoneal dialysis: Not removed; supplemental dosing is not required.

Administration I.V. as a slow push through the side of a freely-flowing saline or dextrose solution. Due to the limited stability of the drug, and the increased risk of phlebitis and venous irritation and blistering with increased contact time, infusions of the drug are not recommended.

Mechlorethamine may cause extravasation. Use within 1 hour of preparation. Avoid extravasation since mechlorethamine is a potent vesicant.

Monitoring Parameters CBC with differential, hemoglobin, and platelet count

Dosage Forms Excipient information presented when available (limited, particularly for generics); consult specific product labeling.

Injection, powder for reconstitution, as hydrochloride: 10 mg

◆ **Mechlorethamine Hydrochloride** *see* Mechlorethamine *on page 927*

Meclizine (MEK li zeen)

U.S. Brand Names Antivert®; Bonine® [OTC]; Dramamine® Less Drowsy Formula [OTC]; Medi-Meclizine [OTC]

Canadian Brand Names Bonamine™; Bonine®

Index Terms Meclizine Hydrochloride; Meclozine Hydrochloride

Pharmacologic Category Antiemetic; Histamine H_1 Antagonist; Histamine H_1 Antagonist, First Generation

Use Prevention and treatment of symptoms of motion sickness; management of vertigo with diseases affecting the vestibular system

Pregnancy Risk Factor B

Pregnancy Considerations No data available on crossing the placenta. Probably no effect on the fetus (insufficient data). Available evidence suggests safe use during pregnancy.

Lactation Excretion in breast milk unknown/not recommended

Medication Safety Issues

Sound-alike/look-alike issues:

Antivert® may be confused with Axert™

Contraindications Hypersensitivity to meclizine or any component of the formulation

Warnings/Precautions Use with caution in patients with asthma, angle-closure glaucoma, prostatic hyperplasia, pyloric or duodenal obstruction, or bladder neck obstruction. Elderly may be at risk for anticholinergic side effects such as glaucoma, prostatic hyperplasia, constipation, GI obstructive disease. If vertigo does not respond in 1-2 weeks, it is advised to discontinue use. May be sedating, use with caution in disorders where CNS depression is a feature; patients must be cautioned about performing tasks which require mental alertness (eg, operating machinery or driving). Effects may be potentiated when used with other sedative drugs or ethanol.

Adverse Reactions

>10%:

Central nervous system: Slight to moderate drowsiness

Respiratory: Thickening of bronchial secretions

1% to 10%:

Central nervous system: Headache, fatigue, nervousness, dizziness

Gastrointestinal: Appetite increase, weight gain, nausea, diarrhea, abdominal pain, dry mouth

Respiratory: Pharyngitis

<1% (Limited to important or life-threatening): Bronchospasm, hepatitis, hypotension, palpitation

Drug Interactions

Avoid Concomitant Use There are no known interactions where it is recommended to avoid concomitant use.

Increased Effect/Toxicity

Meclizine may increase the levels/effects of: Alcohol (Ethyl); Anticholinergics; CNS Depressants

The levels/effects of Meclizine may be increased by: Pramlintide

Decreased Effect

Meclizine may decrease the levels/effects of: Acetylcholinesterase Inhibitors (Central); Betahistine

The levels/effects of Meclizine may be decreased by: Acetylcholinesterase Inhibitors (Central); Amphetamines

Ethanol/Nutrition/Herb Interactions Ethanol: Avoid ethanol (may increase CNS depression).

Mechanism of Action Has central anticholinergic action by blocking chemoreceptor trigger zone; decreases excitability of the middle ear labyrinth and blocks conduction in the middle ear vestibular-cerebellar pathways

Pharmacodynamics/Kinetics

Onset of action: ~1 hour

Duration: 8-24 hours

Metabolism: Hepatic

Half-life elimination: 6 hours

Excretion: Urine (as metabolites); feces (as unchanged drug)

Dosage Children >12 years and Adults: Oral:

Motion sickness: 12.5-25 mg 1 hour before travel, repeat dose every 12-24 hours if needed; doses up to 50 mg may be needed

Vertigo: 25-100 mg/day in divided doses

Dosage Forms Excipient information presented when available (limited, particularly for generics); consult specific product labeling.

Tablet, as hydrochloride: 12.5 mg, 25 mg

Antivert®: 12.5 mg, 25 mg, 50 mg

Dramamine® Less Drowsy Formula: 25 mg

Medi-Meclizine: 25 mg

Tablet, chewable, as hydrochloride (Bonine®): 25 mg

◆ **Meclizine Hydrochloride** *see* Meclizine *on page 928*

Meclofenamate (me kloe fen AM ate)

Canadian Brand Names Meclomen®

Index Terms Meclofenamate Sodium

Pharmacologic Category Nonsteroidal Anti-inflammatory Drug (NSAID), Oral

Additional Appendix Information

Nonsteroidal Anti-inflammatory Agents *on page 1669*

Use Treatment of inflammatory disorders, arthritis, mild to moderate pain, dysmenorrhea

Restrictions An FDA-approved medication guide must be distributed when dispensing an oral outpatient prescription (new or refill) where this medication is to be used without direct supervision of a healthcare provider. Medication guides are available at http://www.fda.gov/cder/Offices/ODS/medication_guides.htm.

Pregnancy Risk Factor C/D (3rd trimester)

Pregnancy Considerations May cause premature closure of the ductus arteriosus in the 3rd trimester of pregnancy.

Lactation

Enters breast milk/not recommended

Contraindications Hypersensitivity to meclofenamate, aspirin, other NSAIDs, or any component of the formulation; perioperative pain in the setting of coronary artery bypass graft (CABG) surgery

Warnings/Precautions **[U.S. Boxed Warning]: NSAIDs are associated with an increased risk of adverse cardiovascular thrombotic events, including MI, stroke, and new onset or worsening of pre-existing hypertension.** Risk may be increased with duration of use or pre-existing cardiovascular risk factors or disease. Carefully evaluate individual cardiovascular risk profiles prior to prescribing. Use caution with fluid retention, heart failure, or hypertension. Concurrent administration of ibuprofen, and potentially other nonselective NSAIDs, may interfere with aspirin's cardioprotective effect. [U.S. Boxed Warning]: Use is contraindicated for treatment of perioperative pain in the setting of coronary artery bypass graft (CABG) surgery. Risk of MI and stroke may be increased with use following CABG surgery.

Platelet adhesion and aggregation may be decreased; may prolong bleeding time; patients with coagulation disorders or who are receiving anticoagulants should be monitored closely. Anemia may occur; patients on long-term NSAID therapy should be monitored for anemia. NSAID use may compromise existing renal function; dose-dependent decreases in prostaglandin synthesis may result from NSAID use, reducing renal blood flow which may cause renal decompensation. Patients with impaired renal function, dehydration, heart failure, liver dysfunction, those taking diuretics, and ACE inhibitors, and the elderly are at greater risk of renal toxicity. Rehydrate patient before starting therapy; monitor renal function closely. Not recommended for use in patients with advanced renal disease. Long-term NSAID use may result in renal papillary necrosis.

[U.S. Boxed Warning]: NSAIDs may increase risk of gastrointestinal irritation, inflammation, ulceration, bleeding, and perforation. These events may occur at any time during therapy and without warning. Use caution with a history of GI disease (bleeding or ulcers), concurrent therapy with aspirin, anticoagulants and/or corticosteroids, smoking, use of alcohol, the elderly or debilitated patients.

Use the lowest effective dose for the shortest duration of time, consistent with individual patient goals, to reduce risk of cardiovascular or GI adverse events. Alternate therapies should be considered for patients at high risk.

NSAIDs may cause serious skin adverse events including exfoliative dermatitis, Stevens-Johnson syndrome (SJS) and toxic epidermal necrolysis (TEN); discontinue use at first sign of skin rash or hypersensitivity. Anaphylactoid reactions may occur, even without prior exposure; patients with "aspirin triad" (bronchial asthma, aspirin intolerance, rhinitis) may be at increased risk. Do not use in patients who experience bronchospasm, asthma, rhinitis, or urticaria with NSAID or aspirin therapy. Use caution in other forms of asthma.

Use with caution in patients with decreased hepatic function. Closely monitor patients with any abnormal LFT. Severe hepatic reactions (eg, fulminant hepatitis, liver failure) have occurred with NSAID use, rarely; discontinue if signs or symptoms of liver disease develop, or if systemic manifestations occur.

The elderly are at increased risk for adverse effects (especially peptic ulceration, CNS effects, renal toxicity) from NSAIDs even at low doses

Withhold for at least 4-6 half-lives prior to surgical or dental procedures. Safety and efficacy have not been established in children <14 years of age.

Adverse Reactions

>10%:

Central nervous system: Dizziness

Dermatologic: Skin rash

Gastrointestinal: Abdominal cramps, heartburn, indigestion, nausea

1% to 10%:

Central nervous system: Headache, nervousness

Dermatologic: Itching

Endocrine & metabolic: Fluid retention

Gastrointestinal: Vomiting

Otic: Tinnitus

<1% (Limited to important or life-threatening): Acute renal failure, agranulocytosis, angioedema, arrhythmia, aseptic meningitis, bone marrow suppression, confusion, CHF, dyspnea, erythema multiforme, GI ulceration, hallucinations, hemolytic anemia, hepatitis, leukopenia, mental depression, peripheral neuropathy, somnolence, Stevens-Johnson syndrome, tachycardia, thrombocytopenia, toxic amblyopia, toxic epidermal necrolysis, urticaria

Drug Interactions

Avoid Concomitant Use

Avoid concomitant use of Meclofenamate with any of the following: Ketorolac

Increased Effect/Toxicity

Meclofenamate may increase the levels/effects of: Aminoglycosides; Anticoagulants; Antiplatelet Agents; Bisphosphonate Derivatives; CycloSPORINE; Desmopressin; Lithium; Methotrexate; Nonsteroidal Anti-Inflammatory Agents; Pemetrexed; Quinolone Antibiotics; Salicylates; Thrombolytic Agents; Vancomycin; Vitamin K Antagonists

The levels/effects of Meclofenamate may be increased by: Antidepressants (Tricyclic, Tertiary Amine); Corticosteroids (Systemic); Herbs (Anticoagulant/Antiplatelet Properties); Ketorolac; Probenecid; Selective Serotonin Reuptake Inhibitors; Serotonin/Norepinephrine Reuptake Inhibitors; Treprostinil

Decreased Effect

Meclofenamate may decrease the levels/effects of: ACE Inhibitors; Angiotensin II Receptor Blockers; Antiplatelet Agents; Beta-Blockers; Eplerenone; HydrALAZINE; Loop Diuretics; Salicylates; Thiazide Diuretics

The levels/effects of Meclofenamate may be decreased by: Bile Acid Sequestrants; Salicylates

Ethanol/Nutrition/Herb Interactions

Ethanol: Avoid ethanol (may enhance gastric mucosal irritation).

Herb/Nutraceutical: Avoid alfalfa, anise, bilberry, bladderwrack, bromelain, cat's claw, celery, chamomile, coleus, cordyceps, dong quai, evening primrose, fenugreek, feverfew, garlic, ginger, ginkgo biloba, ginseng (American, Panax, Siberian), grapeseed, green tea, guggul, horse chestnut seed, horseradish, licorice, prickly ash, red clover, reishi, SAMe (S-adenosylmethionine), sweet clover, turmeric, white willow (all have additional antiplatelet activity).

Mechanism of Action Reversibly inhibits cyclooxygenase-1 and 2 (COX-1 and 2) enzymes, which result in decreased formation of prostaglandin precursors; has antipyretic, analgesic, and anti-inflammatory properties

Pharmacodynamics/Kinetics

Duration: 2-4 hours

Distribution: Crosses placenta

Protein binding: 99%

Half-life elimination: 2-3.3 hours

Time to peak, serum: 0.5-1.5 hours

Excretion: Primarily urine and feces (as metabolites)

Dosage Children >14 years and Adults: Oral:

Mild to moderate pain: 50 mg every 4-6 hours; increases to 100 mg may be required; maximum dose: 400 mg

Rheumatoid arthritis and osteoarthritis: 50 mg every 4-6 hours; increase, over weeks, to 200-400 mg/day in 3-4 divided doses; do not exceed 400 mg/day; maximal benefit for any dose may not be seen for 2-3 weeks

Dietary Considerations May be taken with food, milk, or antacids.

Test Interactions Increased chloride (S), increased sodium (S)

Dosage Forms Excipient information presented when available (limited, particularly for generics); consult specific product labeling.

Capsule, as sodium: 50 mg, 100 mg

- ◆ **Meclofenamate Sodium** *see* Meclofenamate *on page 929*
- ◆ **Meclomen® (Can)** *see* Meclofenamate *on page 929*
- ◆ **Meclozine Hydrochloride** *see* Meclizine *on page 928*
- ◆ **Med-Diltiazem (Can)** *see* Diltiazem *on page 450*
- ◆ **Medent-DM** *see* Guaifenesin, Pseudoephedrine, and Dextromethorphan *on page 715*
- ◆ **Medent LD** *see* Guaifenesin and Pseudoephedrine *on page 713*
- ◆ **Medicinal Carbon** *see* Charcoal *on page 299*
- ◆ **Medicinal Charcoal** *see* Charcoal *on page 299*
- ◆ **Medicone® Suppositories [OTC]** *see* Phenylephrine *on page 1183*
- ◆ **Medigesic®** *see* Butalbital, Acetaminophen, and Caffeine *on page 229*
- ◆ **Medi-Meclizine [OTC]** *see* Meclizine *on page 928*
- ◆ **Medi-Phenyl [OTC]** *see* Phenylephrine *on page 1183*
- ◆ **Mediproxen [OTC]** *see* Naproxen *on page 1041*
- ◆ **Medi-Synal [OTC]** *see* Acetaminophen and Pseudoephedrine *on page 30*
- ◆ **MED-Metformin (Can)** *see* MetFORMIN *on page 954*
- ◆ **Medrol®** *see* MethylPREDNISolone *on page 976*

MedroxyPROGESTERone

(me DROKS ee proe JES te rone)

U.S. Brand Names Depo-Provera®; Depo-Provera® Contraceptive; depo-subQ provera 104™; Provera®

Canadian Brand Names Alti-MPA; Apo-Medroxy®; Depo-Prevera®; Depo-Provera®; Gen-Medroxy; Novo-Medrone; Provera-Pak; Provera®

Index Terms Acetoxymethylprogesterone; Medroxyprogesterone Acetate; Methylacetoxyprogesterone; MPA

Pharmacologic Category Contraceptive; Progestin

Use Endometrial carcinoma or renal carcinoma; secondary amenorrhea or abnormal uterine bleeding due to hormonal imbalance; reduction of endometrial hyperplasia in nonhysterectomized postmenopausal women receiving conjugated estrogens; prevention of pregnancy; management of endometriosis-associated pain

Pregnancy Risk Factor X

Pregnancy Considerations There is an increased risk of minor birth defects in children whose mothers take progesterones during the first 4 months of pregnancy. Hypospadias has been reported in male and mild masculinization of the external genitalia has been reported in female babies exposed during the first trimester. High doses are used to impair fertility. Low birth weight has been reported in neonates from unexpected pregnancies which occurred 1-2 months following injection of medroxyprogesterone (MPA) contraceptive. Ectopic pregnancies have been reported with use of the MPA contraceptive injection. When therapy is discontinued, fertility returns sooner in women of lower body weight. Median time to conception/return to ovulation following discontinuation of MPA contraceptive injection is 10 months following the last injection.

Lactation Enters breast milk/compatible

Medication Safety Issues

Sound-alike/look-alike issues:

MedroxyPROGESTERone may be confused with hydroxyprogesterone, methylPREDNISolone, methylTESTOSTERone

Provera® may be confused with Covera®, Femara®, Parlodel®, Premarin®

The injection dosage form is available in different formulations. Carefully review prescriptions to assure the correct formulation and route of administration.

Contraindications Hypersensitivity to medroxyprogesterone or any component of the formulation; history of or current thrombophlebitis or venous thromboembolic disorders (including DVT, PE); cerebral vascular disease; severe hepatic dysfunction or disease; carcinoma of the breast or genital organs, undiagnosed vaginal bleeding; missed abortion, diagnostic test for pregnancy, pregnancy

Warnings/Precautions [U.S. Boxed Warning]: Prolonged use of medroxyprogesterone contraceptive injection may result in a loss of bone mineral density (BMD). Loss is related to the duration of use, and may not be completely reversible on discontinuation of the drug. The impact on peak bone mass in adolescents should be considered in treatment decisions. **[U.S. Boxed Warning]: Long-term use (ie, >2 years) should be limited to situations where other birth control methods are inadequate.** Consider other methods of birth control in women with (or at risk for) osteoporosis.

Use caution with cardiovascular disease or dysfunction. MPA used in combination with estrogen may increase the risks of hypertension, myocardial infarction (MI), stroke, pulmonary emboli (PE), and deep vein thrombosis; incidence of these effects was shown to be significantly increased in postmenopausal women using conjugated equine estrogens (CEE) in combination with MPA. MPA in combination with estrogens should not be used to prevent coronary heart disease. Use with caution in patients with diabetes mellitus; may cause glucose intolerance.

The risk of dementia may be increased in postmenopausal women; increased incidence was observed in women ≥65 years of age taking MPA in combination with CEE. An increased risk of invasive breast cancer was observed in postmenopausal women using MPA in combination with CEE. An increase in abnormal mammograms has also been reported with estrogen and progestin therapy.

Discontinue pending examination in cases of sudden partial or complete vision loss, sudden onset of proptosis, diplopia, or migraine; discontinue permanently if papilledema or retinal vascular lesions are observed on examination. Use with caution in patients with diseases that may be exacerbated by fluid retention (including asthma, epilepsy, migraine, diabetes, or renal dysfunction). Use caution with history of depression. Whenever possible, progestins in combination with estrogens should be discontinued at least 4-6 weeks prior to surgeries associated with an increased risk of thromboembolism or during periods of prolonged immobilization. Progestins used in combination with estrogen should be used for shortest duration possible consistent with treatment goals. Conduct periodic risk:benefit assessments. Not for use prior to menarche.

Adverse Reactions Adverse effects as reported with any dosage form; percent ranges presented are noted with the MPA contraceptive injection:

>5%:

- Central nervous system: Dizziness, headache, nervousness
- Endocrine & metabolic: Libido decreased, menstrual irregularities (includes bleeding, amenorrhea, or both)
- Gastrointestinal: Abdominal pain/discomfort, weight changes (average: 3-5 pounds after 1 year, 8 pounds after 2 years)
- Neuromuscular & skeletal: Weakness

1% to 5%:

- Cardiovascular: Edema
- Central nervous system: Depression, fatigue, insomnia, irritability, pain
- Dermatologic: Acne, alopecia, rash
- Endocrine & metabolic: Anorgasmia, breast pain, hot flashes
- Gastrointestinal: Bloating, nausea
- Genitourinary: Cervical smear abnormal, leukorrhea, menometrorrhagia, menorrhagia, pelvic pain, urinary tract infection, vaginitis, vaginal infection, vaginal hemorrhage
- Local: Injection site atrophy, injection site reaction, injection site pain
- Neuromuscular & skeletal: Arthralgia, backache, leg cramp
- Respiratory: Respiratory tract infections

<1% (Limited to important or life-threatening): Allergic reaction, anaphylaxis, anaphylactoid reactions, anemia, angioedema, appetite changes, asthma, axillary swelling, blood dyscrasia, body odor, bone mineral density decreased, breast cancer, breast changes, cervical cancer, chest pain, chills, chloasma, convulsions, deep vein thrombosis, diaphoresis, drowsiness, dry skin, dysmenorrhea, dyspareunia, dyspnea, facial palsy, fever, galactorrhea, genitourinary infections, glucose tolerance decreased, hirsutism, hoarseness, jaundice, lack of return to fertility, lactation decreased, libido increased, melasma, nipple bleeding, osteoporosis, osteoporotic fractures, paralysis, paresthesia, pruritus, pulmonary embolus, rectal bleeding, scleroderma, sensation of pregnancy, somnolence, syncope, tachycardia, thirst, thrombophlebitis, uterine hyperplasia, vaginal cysts, varicose veins; residual lump, sterile abscess, or skin discoloration at the injection site

Drug Interactions

Metabolism/Transport Effects Substrate of CYP3A4 (major); **Induces** CYP3A4 (weak)

Avoid Concomitant Use

Avoid concomitant use of MedroxyPROGESTERone with any of the following: Acitretin; Griseofulvin

Increased Effect/Toxicity

The levels/effects of MedroxyPROGESTERone may be increased by: Herbs (Progestogenic Properties)

Decreased Effect

MedroxyPROGESTERone may decrease the levels/effects of: Maraviroc; Vitamin K Antagonists

The levels/effects of MedroxyPROGESTERone may be decreased by: Acitretin; Aminoglutethimide; Aprepitant; Barbiturates; CarBAMazepine; CYP3A4 Inducers (Strong); Deferasirox; Fosaprepitant; Griseofulvin; Phenytoin; Rifamycin Derivatives; St Johns Wort

Ethanol/Nutrition/Herb Interactions

Ethanol: Avoid ethanol (may increase risk of osteoporosis).

Food: Bioavailability of the oral tablet is increased when taken with food; half-life is unchanged.

Herb/Nutraceutical: St John's wort may diminish the therapeutic effect of progestin contraceptives (contraceptive failure is possible).

Stability Store at controlled room temperature.

Mechanism of Action Inhibits secretion of pituitary gonadotropins, which prevents follicular maturation and ovulation; causes endometrial thinning

Pharmacodynamics/Kinetics

Absorption: Oral: Well absorbed; I.M.: Slow

Protein binding: 86% to 90% primarily to albumin; does not bind to sex hormone-binding globulin

Metabolism: Extensively hepatic via hydroxylation and conjugation; forms metabolites

Time to peak: Oral: 2-4 hours

Half-life elimination: Oral: 12-17 hours; I.M. (Depo-Provera® Contraceptive): 50 days; SubQ: ~40 days

Excretion: Urine

Dosage

Adolescents and Adults:

- Amenorrhea: Oral: 5-10 mg/day for 5-10 days
- Abnormal uterine bleeding: Oral: 5-10 mg for 5-10 days starting on day 16 or 21 of cycle
- Contraception:
  - Depo-Provera® Contraceptive: I.M.: 150 mg every 3 months
  - depo-subQ provera 104™: SubQ: 104 mg every 3 months (every 12-14 weeks)
- Endometriosis: depo-subQ provera 104™: SubQ: 104 mg every 3 months (every 12-14 weeks)

Adults:

- Endometrial or renal carcinoma (Depo-Provera®): I.M.: 400-1000 mg/week

Accompanying cyclic estrogen therapy, postmenopausal: Oral: 5-10 mg for 12-14 consecutive days each month, starting on day 1 or day 16 of the cycle; lower doses may be used if given with estrogen continuously throughout the cycle

Dosing adjustment in hepatic impairment: Use is contraindicated with severe impairment. Consider lower dose or less frequent administration with mild-to-moderate impairment. Use of the contraceptive injection has not been studied in patients with hepatic impairment; consideration should be given to not readminister if jaundice develops

Dietary Considerations Ensure adequate calcium and vitamin D intake when used for the prevention of pregnancy

Administration

I.M.: Depo-Provera® Contraceptive: Administer first dose during the first 5 days of menstrual period, or within the first 5 days postpartum if not breast-feeding, or at the sixth week postpartum if breast feeding exclusively. Shake vigorously prior to administration. Administer by deep I.M. injection in the gluteal or deltoid muscle.

SubQ: depo-subQ provera 104™: Administer first dose during the first 5 days of menstrual period, or at the sixth week postpartum if breast-feeding. Shake vigorously prior to administration. Administer by SubQ injection in the upper thigh or abdomen; avoid boney areas and the umbilicus. Administer over 5-7 seconds. Do not rub the injection area. When switching from combined hormonal contraceptives (estrogen plus progestin), the first injection should be within 7 days after the last active pill, or removal of patch or ring. If switching from the I.M. to SubQ formulation, the next dose should be given within the prescribed dosing period for the I.M. injection.

Monitoring Parameters Before starting therapy, a physical exam with reference to the breasts and pelvis are recommended, including a Papanicolaou smear. Exam may be deferred if appropriate prior to administration of MPA contraceptive injection; pregnancy should be ruled out prior to use. Monitor patient closely for loss of vision; sudden onset of proptosis, diplopia, or migraine; signs and symptoms of thromboembolic disorders; signs or symptoms of depression; glucose in patients with diabetes; or blood pressure.

Test Interactions

The following tests may be decreased: Steroid levels (plasma and urinary), gonadotropin levels, SHBG concentration, T_3 uptake

The following tests may be increased: Protein-bound iodine, butanol extractable protein-bound iodine, Factors II, VII, VIII, IX, X

Pathologist should be advised of estrogen/progesterone therapy when specimens are submitted.

Dosage Forms Excipient information presented when available (limited, particularly for generics); consult specific product labeling.

Injection, suspension, as acetate: 150 mg/mL (1 mL)
 Depo-Provera®: 400 mg/mL (2.5 mL)
 Depo-Provera® Contraceptive: 150 mg/mL (1 mL) [prefilled syringe or vial]
 depo-subQ provera 104™: 104 mg/0.65 mL (0.65 mL) [prefilled syringe]

Tablet, as acetate: 2.5 mg, 5 mg, 10 mg
 Provera®: 2.5 mg, 5 mg, 10 mg

◆ **Medroxyprogesterone Acetate** *see* MedroxyPROGESTERone *on page* 930

◆ **Medroxyprogesterone and Estrogens (Conjugated)** *see* Estrogens (Conjugated/Equine) and Medroxyprogesterone *on page* 566

◆ **MED-Sotalol (Can)** *see* Sotalol *on page* 1394

◆ **Med-Verapamil (Can)** *see* Verapamil *on page* 1557

◆ **Mefenamic-250 (Can)** *see* Mefenamic Acid *on page* 932

Mefenamic Acid (me fe NAM ik AS id)

U.S. Brand Names Ponstel®

Canadian Brand Names Apo-Mefenamic®; Dom-Mefenamic Acid; Mefenamic-250; Nu-Mefenamic; PMS-Mefenamic Acid; Ponstan®

Pharmacologic Category Nonsteroidal Anti-inflammatory Drug (NSAID), Oral

Additional Appendix Information

Nonsteroidal Anti-inflammatory Agents *on page* 1669

Use Short-term relief of mild to moderate pain including primary dysmenorrhea

Restrictions An FDA-approved medication guide must be distributed when dispensing an oral outpatient prescription (new or refill) where this medication is to be used without direct supervision of a healthcare provider. Medication guides are available at http://www.fda.gov/cder/Offices/ODS/medication_guides.htm.

Pregnancy Risk Factor C/D (3rd trimester)

Medication Safety Issues

Sound-alike/look-alike issues:
 Ponstel® may be confused with Pronestyl®

Dosage Children >14 years and Adults: Oral: 500 mg to start then 250 mg every 4 hours as needed; maximum therapy: 1 week

Dosing adjustment/comments in renal impairment: Not recommended for use

Additional Information Complete prescribing information for this medication should be consulted for additional detail.

Dosage Forms Excipient information presented when available (limited, particularly for generics); consult specific product labeling.

Capsule: 250 mg
 Ponstel®: 250 mg

Mefloquine (ME floe kwin)

U.S. Brand Names Lariam® [DSC]

Canadian Brand Names Apo-Mefloquine®; Lariam®

Index Terms Mefloquine Hydrochloride

Pharmacologic Category Antimalarial Agent

Additional Appendix Information

Malaria Treatment *on page* 1770

Use Treatment of acute malarial infections and prevention of malaria

Restrictions An FDA-approved medication guide and wallet card must be distributed when dispensing an outpatient prescription (new or refill) to prevent malaria where this medication is to be used without direct supervision of a healthcare provider. Medication guides are available at http://www.fda.gov/cder/Offices/ODS/medication_guides.htm.

Pregnancy Risk Factor C

Pregnancy Considerations Mefloquine crosses the placenta and is teratogenic in animals. There are no adequate and well-controlled studies in pregnant women, however, clinical experience has not shown teratogenic or embryotoxic effects; use with caution during pregnancy if travel to endemic areas cannot be postponed. Nonpregnant women of childbearing potential are advised to use contraception and avoid pregnancy during malaria prophylaxis and for 3 months thereafter. In case of an unplanned pregnancy, treatment with mefloquine is not considered a reason for pregnancy termination.

Lactation Enters breast milk/not recommended

Contraindications Hypersensitivity to mefloquine, related compounds (eg, quinine and quinidine), or any component of the formulation; prophylactic use in patients with a history of seizures or severe psychiatric disorder (including active or recent history of depression, generalized anxiety disorder, psychosis, or schizophrenia)

Warnings/Precautions May cause a range of psychiatric symptoms (anxiety, paranoia, depression, hallucinations and psychosis). Occasionally, symptoms have been reported to persist long after mefloquine has been discontinued. Rare cases of suicidal ideation and suicide have been reported (no causal relationship established). The appearance of psychiatric symptoms such as acute anxiety, depression, restlessness or confusion may be considered a prodrome to more serious events. Use with caution in patients with a previous history of depression; prophylactic use is contraindicated in patients with active or recent history of psychiatric disorders. Discontinue if unexplained neuropsychiatric disturbances occur. Use caution in patients with significant cardiac disease, hepatic impairment, or seizure disorder. If mefloquine is to be used for a prolonged period, periodic evaluations including liver function tests and ophthalmic examinations should be performed. (Retinal abnormalities have not been observed with mefloquine in humans; however, it has with long-term administration to rats.)

In cases of life-threatening, serious, or overwhelming malaria infections due to *Plasmodium falciparum*, patients should be treated with intravenous antimalarial drug. Mefloquine may be given orally to complete the course. Dizziness, loss of balance, and other CNS disorders (eg, seizures) have been reported; due to long half-life, effects may persist after mefloquine is discontinued. Use caution in activities requiring alertness and fine motor coordination (eg, driving, piloting planes, operating machinery). Concurrent use with chloroquine and quinine derivatives may increase risk of seizures. Concurrent use with quininederivatives may increase risk of ECG abnormalities. Safety and efficacy have not been established in children <6 months of age. Early vomiting leading to treatment failure in children has been reported in some studies; consider alternate therapy if a second dose is not tolerated.

Adverse Reactions

1% to 10%:

Central nervous system: Chills, dizziness, fatigue, fever, headache

Dermatologic: Rash

Gastrointestinal: Vomiting (3%), abdominal pain, appetite decreased, diarrhea, nausea

Neuromuscular & skeletal: Myalgia

Otic: Tinnitus

<1% (Limited to important or life-threatening): Abnormal dreams, aggressive behavior, agitation, alopecia, anxiety, arthralgia, ataxia, AV block, bradycardia, cardiac arrest (with concomitant use of propranolol), chest pain, conduction abnormalities (transient), confusion, depression, diaphoresis (increased), dyspepsia, dyspnea, edema, emotional lability, encephalopathy, erythema, erythema multiforme, exanthema, extrasystoles, flushing, forgetfulness, hallucinations, hearing impairment, hematocrit decreased, hyper-/hypotension, insomnia, irregular pulse, leukocytosis, liver function tests increased, loss of balance, malaise, mood changes, muscle cramps/ weakness, palpitation, panic attacks, paranoia, paresthesia, pneumonitis (allergic etiology), pruritus, psychosis, restlessness, seizure, somnolence, Stevens-Johnson syndrome, suicidal ideation and behavior (causal relationship not established), syncope, tachycardia, thrombocytopenia, tremor, urticaria, vertigo, visual disturbances, weakness

Drug Interactions

Metabolism/Transport Effects **Substrate** of CYP3A4 (major); **Inhibits** CYP2D6 (weak), 3A4 (weak)

Avoid Concomitant Use

Avoid concomitant use of Mefloquine with any of the following: Aminoquinolines (Antimalarial); Dabigatran Etexilate; Halofantrine; Nilotinib; QuiNIDine; QuiNINE; Rivaroxaban; Silodosin; Tetrabenazine; Topotecan; Ziprasidone

Increased Effect/Toxicity

Mefloquine may increase the levels/effects of: Aminoquinolines (Antimalarial); Antipsychotic Agents (Phenothiazines); Dabigatran Etexilate; Halofantrine; P-Glycoprotein Substrates; QTc-Prolonging Agents; QuiNINE; Rivaroxaban; Silodosin; Tetrabenazine; Topotecan; Typhoid Vaccine; Ziprasidone

The levels/effects of Mefloquine may be increased by: Alfuzosin; Aminoquinolines (Antimalarial); Ciprofloxacin; CYP3A4 Inhibitors (Moderate); CYP3A4 Inhibitors (Strong); Dasatinib; Gadobutrol; Nilotinib; QuiNIDine; QuiNINE

Decreased Effect

Mefloquine may decrease the levels/effects of: Anticonvulsants

The levels/effects of Mefloquine may be decreased by: CYP3A4 Inducers (Strong); Deferasirox; Herbs (CYP3A4 Inducers)

Ethanol/Nutrition/Herb Interactions

Food: Food increases bioavailability by ~40%.

Herb/Nutraceutical: Mefloquine serum concentration may be decreased by St John's wort; avoid concurrent use.

Stability Store at controlled room temperature of 25°C (77°F); excursions permitted to 15°C to 30°C (59°F to 86°F).

Mechanism of Action Mefloquine is a quinoline-methanol compound structurally similar to quinine; mefloquine's effectiveness in the treatment and prophylaxis of malaria is due to the destruction of the asexual blood forms of the malarial pathogens that affect humans, *Plasmodium falciparum, P. vivax, P. malariae, P. ovale*

Pharmacodynamics/Kinetics

Absorption: Well absorbed

Distribution: V_d: ~20 L/kg; blood, urine, CSF, tissues; enters breast milk

Protein binding: 98%

Metabolism: Extensively hepatic to 2,8-bis-trifluoromethyl-4-quinoline carboxylic acid (inactive) and other metabolites

Bioavailability: Increased by food

Half-life elimination: ~3 weeks (range: 2-4 weeks)

Time to peak, plasma: 6-24 hours (median: ~17 hours)

Excretion: Primarily bile and feces; urine (9% as unchanged drug, 4% as primary metabolite)

Dosage Oral (dose expressed as mg of mefloquine hydrochloride):

Children ≥6 months and >5 kg:

Malaria treatment: 20-25 mg/kg in 2 divided doses, taken 6-8 hours apart (maximum: 1250 mg). If clinical improvement is not seen within 48-72 hours, an alternative therapy should be used for retreatment.

Malaria prophylaxis: 5 mg/kg/once weekly (maximum dose: 250 mg) starting 1 week before arrival in endemic area, continuing weekly during travel and for 4 weeks after leaving endemic area.

Adults:

Malaria treatment (mild to moderate infection): 5 tablets (1250 mg) as a single dose. If clinical improvement is not seen within 48-72 hours, an alternative therapy should be used for retreatment.

Malaria prophylaxis: 1 tablet (250 mg) weekly starting 1 week before arrival in endemic area, continuing weekly during travel and for 4 weeks after leaving endemic area

Dosage adjustment in renal impairment: No dosage adjustment needed in patients with renal impairment or on dialysis.

Dosage adjustment in hepatic impairment: Half-life may be prolonged and plasma levels may be higher. Specific dosing adjustments are not available.

Dietary Considerations Take with food and with at least 8 oz of water.

Administration Administer with food and with at least 8 oz of water. When used for malaria prophylaxis, dose should be taken once weekly on the same day each week. If vomiting occurs within 30 minutes after the dose, an additional full dose should be given; if it occurs within 30-60 minutes after dose, an additional half-dose should be given. Tablets may be crushed and suspended in a small amount of water, milk, or another beverage for persons unable to swallow tablets.

Monitoring Parameters When use is prolonged, periodic liver function tests and ocular examinations

Dosage Forms Excipient information presented when available (limited, particularly for generics); consult specific product labeling. [DSC] = Discontinued product

Tablet, as hydrochloride: 250 mg [equivalent to 228 mg base]

Lariam®: 250 mg [equivalent to 228 mg base] [DSC]

◆ **Mefloquine Hydrochloride** *see* Mefloquine *on page* 932

◆ **Megace®** *see* Megestrol *on page* 934

◆ **Megace® ES** *see* Megestrol *on page* 934

◆ **Megace® OS (Can)** *see* Megestrol *on page* 934

Megestrol (me JES trole)

U.S. Brand Names Megace®; Megace® ES

Canadian Brand Names Apo-Megestrol®; Megace®; Megace® OS; Nu-Megestrol

Index Terms 5071-1DL(6); Megestrol Acetate; NSC-71423

Pharmacologic Category Antineoplastic Agent, Hormone; Appetite Stimulant; Progestin

Use Palliative treatment of breast and endometrial carcinoma; treatment of anorexia, cachexia, or unexplained significant weight loss in patients with AIDS

Pregnancy Risk Factor D (tablet) / X (suspension)

Pregnancy Considerations Adverse effects were demonstrated in animal studies. Use during pregnancy is contraindicated (suspension).

Lactation Enters breast milk/not recommended

Medication Safety Issues

Sound-alike/look-alike issues:

Megace® may be confused with Reglan®

Contraindications Hypersensitivity to megestrol or any component of the formulation; pregnancy (suspension)

Warnings/Precautions Hazardous agent - use appropriate precautions for handling and disposal. May suppress hypothalamic-pituitary-adrenal (HPA) axis during chronic administration; consider the possibility of adrenal suppression in any patient receiving or being withdrawn from chronic therapy when signs/symptoms suggestive of hypoadrenalism are noted (during stress or in unstressed state). Laboratory evaluation and replacement/stress doses of rapid-acting glucocorticoid should be considered. New-onset diabetes and exacerbation of pre-existing diabetes have been reported with long-term use. Use with caution in patients with a history of thromboembolic disease. Vaginal bleeding or discharge may occur in females. Megace® ES suspension is not equivalent to other formulations on a mg per mg basis; Megace® ES suspension 625 mg/5 mL is equivalent to megestrol acetate suspension 800 mg/20 mL. Safety and efficacy in children have not been established.

Adverse Reactions

Frequency not always defined.

Cardiovascular: Hypertension (≤8%), cardiomyopathy (1% to 3%), chest pain (1% to 3%), edema (1% to 3%), palpitation (1% to 3%), peripheral edema (1% to 3%), heart failure

Central nervous system: Headache (≤10%), insomnia (≤6%), fever (1% to 6%), pain (≤6%, similar to placebo), abnormal thinking (1% to 3%), confusion (1% to 3%), depression (1% to 3%), hypoesthesia (1% to 3%), seizure (1% to 3%), mood changes, malaise, lethargy

Dermatologic: Rash (2% to 12%), alopecia (1% to 3%), pruritus (1% to 3%), vesiculobullous rash (1% to 3%)

Endocrine & metabolic: Hyperglycemia (≤6%), gynecomastia (1% to 3%), adrenal insufficiency, amenorrhea, breakthrough bleeding, cervical erosion and secretions (changes), breast tenderness increased, Cushing's syndrome, diabetes, glucose intolerance, HPA axis suppression, hot flashes, hypercalcemia, menstrual flow changes, spotting, vaginal bleeding pattern changes

Gastrointestinal: Diarrhea (6% to 15%, similar to placebo), flatulence (≤10%), vomiting (≤6%), nausea (≤5%), dyspepsia (≤4%), abdominal pain (1% to 3%), constipation (1% to 3%), salivation increased (1% to 3%), xerostomia (1% to 3%), weight gain (not attributed to edema or fluid retention)

Genitourinary: Impotence (4% to 14%), decreased libido (≤5%), urinary incontinence (1% to 3%), urinary tract infection (1% to 3%), urinary frequency (≤2%)

Hematologic: Anemia (≤5%), leukopenia (1% to 3%)

Hepatic: Hepatomegaly (1% to 3%), LDH increased (1% to 3%), cholestatic jaundice, hepatotoxicity

Neuromuscular & skeletal: Weakness (2% to 6%), neuropathy (1% to 3%), paresthesia (1% to 3%), carpal tunnel syndrome

Ocular: Amblyopia (1% to 3%)

Renal: Albuminuria (1% to 3%)

Respiratory: Dyspnea (1% to 3%), cough (1% to 3%), pharyngitis (1% to 3%), pneumonia (≤2%), hyperpnea

Miscellaneous: Diaphoresis (1% to 3%), herpes infection (1% to 3%), infection (1% to 3%), moniliasis (1% to 3%), tumor flare

Postmarketing and/or case reports: Thromboembolic phenomena (including deep vein thrombosis, pulmonary embolism, thrombophlebitis)

Drug Interactions

Avoid Concomitant Use There are no known interactions where it is recommended to avoid concomitant use.

Increased Effect/Toxicity

The levels/effects of Megestrol may be increased by: Herbs (Progestogenic Properties)

Decreased Effect

The levels/effects of Megestrol may be decreased by: Aminoglutethimide

Ethanol/Nutrition/Herb Interactions Herb/Nutraceutical: Avoid herbs with progestogenic properties (eg, bloodroot, chasteberry, damiana, oregano, and yucca); may enhance the adverse/toxic effect of megestrol.

Stability

Suspension: Store at 15°C to 25°C (59°F to 77°F); protect from heat.

Tablet: Store at 25°C (77°F); excursions permitted to 15°C to 30°C (59°F to 86°F); protect from heat (temperatures >40°C [>104°F])

Mechanism of Action A synthetic progestin with antiestrogenic properties which disrupt the estrogen receptor cycle. Megestrol interferes with the normal estrogen cycle and results in a lower LH titer. May also have a direct effect on the endometrium. Megestrol is an antineoplastic progestin thought to act through an antileutenizing effect mediated via the pituitary. May stimulate appetite by antagonizing the metabolic effects of catabolic cytokines.

Pharmacodynamics/Kinetics

Absorption: Well absorbed orally

Metabolism: Hepatic (to free steroids and glucuronide conjugates)

Half-life elimination: 13-105 hours

Time to peak, serum: 1-3 hours

Excretion: Urine (57% to 78%; 5% to 8% as metabolites); feces (8% to 30%)

Dosage Adults: Oral: **Note:** Megace® ES suspension is not equivalent to other formulations on a mg-per-mg basis:

Tablet: Females (refer to individual protocols):

Breast carcinoma: 40 mg 4 times/day

Endometrial carcinoma: 40-320 mg/day in divided doses; use for 2 months to determine efficacy; maximum doses used have been up to 800 mg/day

Suspension: Males/Females: HIV-related cachexia:

Megace®: Initial dose: 800 mg/day; daily doses of 400 and 800 mg/day were found to be clinically effective

Megace® ES: 625 mg/day

Dosing adjustment in renal impairment: No data available; however, the urinary excretion of megestrol acetate administered in doses of 4-90 mg ranged from 57% to 78% within 10 days

Administration Megestrol acetate (Megace®) oral suspension is compatible with water, orange juice, apple juice, or Sustacal H.C. for immediate consumption. Shake suspension well before use.

Monitoring Parameters Observe for signs of thromboembolic phenomena; blood pressure, weight; serum glucose

Test Interactions Altered thyroid and liver function tests

Dosage Forms Excipient information presented when available (limited, particularly for generics); consult specific product labeling.

Suspension, oral, as acetate: 40 mg/mL (10 mL, 20 mL, 240 mL, 480 mL)

Megace®: 40 mg/mL (240 mL) [contains ethanol 0.06% and sodium benzoate; lemon-lime flavor]

Megace® ES: 125 mg/mL (150 mL) [contains ethanol 0.06% and sodium benzoate; lemon-lime flavor]

Tablet, as acetate: 20 mg, 40 mg

◆ **Megestrol Acetate** *see* Megestrol *on page 934*

◆ **Melanex®** *see* Hydroquinone *on page 749*

◆ **Mellaril® (Can)** *see* Thioridazine *on page 1461*

Meloxicam (mel OKS i kam)

U.S. Brand Names Mobic®

Canadian Brand Names Apo-Meloxicam®; CO Meloxicam; Gen-Meloxicam; Mobicox®; Mobic®; Novo-Meloxicam; PMS-Meloxicam

Pharmacologic Category Nonsteroidal Anti-inflammatory Drug (NSAID), Oral

Additional Appendix Information

Nonsteroidal Anti-inflammatory Agents *on page 1669*

Use Relief of signs and symptoms of osteoarthritis, rheumatoid arthritis, and juvenile rheumatoid arthritis (JRA)

Restrictions An FDA-approved medication guide must be distributed when dispensing an oral outpatient prescription (new or refill) where this medication is to be used without direct supervision of a healthcare provider. Medication guides are available at http://www.fda.gov/cder/Offices/ODS/medication_guides.htm.

Pregnancy Risk Factor C/D (3rd trimester)

Pregnancy Considerations May cause premature closure of the ductus arteriosus in the 3rd trimester of pregnancy.

Lactation Excretion in breast milk unknown/not recommended

Contraindications Hypersensitivity (eg, asthma, urticaria, allergic-type reactions) to meloxicam, aspirin, other NSAIDs, or any component of the formulation; perioperative pain in the setting of coronary artery bypass graft (CABG) surgery

Warnings/Precautions [U.S. Boxed Warning]: NSAIDs are associated with an increased risk of adverse cardiovascular thrombotic events, including MI, stroke, and new onset or worsening of pre-existing hypertension. Risk may be increased with duration of use or pre-existing cardiovascular risk factors or disease. Carefully evaluate individual cardiovascular risk profiles prior to prescribing. Use caution with fluid retention, heart failure, or hypertension. Concurrent administration of ibuprofen, and potentially other nonselective NSAIDs, may interfere with aspirin's cardioprotective effect. **[U.S. Boxed Warning]: Use is contraindicated for treatment of perioperative pain in the setting of coronary artery bypass graft (CABG) surgery.** Risk of MI and stroke may be increased with use following CABG surgery.

Platelet adhesion and aggregation may be decreased; may prolong bleeding time; patients with coagulation disorders or who are receiving anticoagulants should be monitored closely. Anemia may occur; patients on long-term NSAID therapy should be monitored for anemia. NSAID use may compromise existing renal function; dose-dependent decreases in prostaglandin synthesis may result from NSAID use, reducing renal blood flow which may cause renal decompensation. Patients with impaired renal function, dehydration, heart failure, liver dysfunction, those taking diuretics, and ACE inhibitors, and the elderly are at greater risk of renal toxicity. Rehydrate patient before starting therapy; monitor renal function closely. Not recommended for use in patients with advanced renal disease. Long-term NSAID use may result in renal papillary necrosis.

[U.S. Boxed Warning]: NSAIDs may increase risk of gastrointestinal irritation, inflammation, ulceration, bleeding, and perforation. These events may occur at any time during therapy and without warning. Use caution with a history of GI disease (bleeding or ulcers), concurrent therapy with aspirin, anticoagulants and/or corticosteroids, smoking, use of alcohol, the elderly or debilitated patients.

Use the lowest effective dose for the shortest duration of time, consistent with individual patient goals, to reduce risk of cardiovascular or GI adverse events. Alternate therapies should be considered for patients at high risk.

NSAIDs may cause serious skin adverse events including exfoliative dermatitis, Stevens-Johnson syndrome (SJS) and toxic epidermal necrolysis (TEN); discontinue use at first sign of skin rash or hypersensitivity. Anaphylactoid reactions may occur, even without prior exposure; patients with "aspirin triad" (bronchial asthma, aspirin intolerance, rhinitis) may be at increased risk. Do not use in patients who experience bronchospasm, asthma, rhinitis, or urticaria with NSAID or aspirin therapy. Use caution in other forms of asthma.

Use with caution in patients with decreased hepatic function. Closely monitor patients with any abnormal LFT. Severe hepatic reactions (eg, fulminant hepatitis, liver failure) have occurred with NSAID use, rarely; discontinue if signs or symptoms of liver disease develop, or if systemic manifestations occur.

The elderly are at increased risk for adverse effects (especially peptic ulceration, CNS effects, renal toxicity) from NSAIDs even at low doses.

Withhold for at least 4-6 half-lives prior to surgical or dental procedures. Safety and efficacy have not been established in pediatric patients <2 years of age.

Adverse Reactions Percentages reported in adult patients; abdominal pain, diarrhea, fever, headache, pyrexia, and vomiting were reported more commonly in pediatric patients

2% to 10%:

Cardiovascular: Edema (≤5%)

Central nervous system: Headache (2% to 8%), pain (1% to 5%), dizziness (≤4%), insomnia (≤4%)

Dermatologic: Pruritus (≤2%), rash (≤3%)

Gastrointestinal: Dyspepsia (4% to 10%), diarrhea (2% to 8%), nausea (2% to 7%), abdominal pain (2% to 5%), constipation (≤3%), flatulence (≤3%), vomiting (≤3%)

Genitourinary: Urinary tract infection (≤7%), micturition (≤2%)

Hematologic: Anemia (≤4%)

Neuromuscular & skeletal: Arthralgia (≤5%), back pain (≤3%)

Respiratory: Upper respiratory infection (≤8%), cough (≤2%), pharyngitis (≤3%)

Miscellaneous: Flu-like syndrome (2% to 6%), falls (≤3%)

<2% (Limited to important or life-threatening): Abnormal dreams, abnormal vision, agranulocytosis, albuminuria, allergic reaction, alopecia, anaphylactoid reactions, angina, angioedema, anxiety, appetite increased, arrhythmia, asthma, bilirubinemia, bronchospasm, bullous eruption, BUN increased, cardiac failure, colitis, confusion, conjunctivitis, creatinine increased, dehydration, depression, diaphoresis, duodenal perforation, duodenal ulcer, dyspnea, edema (facial), eructation, erythema multiforme, esophagitis, exfoliative dermatitis, fatigue, fever, gastric perforation, gastric ulcer, gastritis, gastroesophageal reflux, gastrointestinal hemorrhage, GGT increased, hematemesis, hematuria, hepatic failure, hepatitis, hot flushes, hyper-/hypotension, interstitial nephritis, intestinal perforation, jaundice, leukopenia, malaise, melena, MI, mood alterations, nervousness, palpitation, pancreatitis, paresthesia, photosensitivity reaction, pruritus, purpura, renal failure, seizure, shock, somnolence, Stevens-Johnson syndrome, syncope, tachycardia, taste perversion, thrombocytopenia, tinnitus, toxic epidermal necrolysis, transaminases increased, tremor, ulcerative stomatitis, urinary retention (acute), urticaria, vasculitis, vertigo, xerostomia, weight gain/loss

Drug Interactions

Metabolism/Transport Effects **Substrate** (minor) of CYP2C9, 3A4; **Inhibits** CYP2C9 (weak)

Avoid Concomitant Use

Avoid concomitant use of Meloxicam with any of the following: Ketorolac

Increased Effect/Toxicity

Meloxicam may increase the levels/effects of: Aminoglycosides; Anticoagulants; Antiplatelet Agents; Bisphosphonate Derivatives; CycloSPORINE; Desmopressin; Lithium; Methotrexate; Nonsteroidal Anti-Inflammatory Agents; Pemetrexed; Quinolone Antibiotics; Salicylates; Thrombolytic Agents; Vancomycin; Vitamin K Antagonists

The levels/effects of Meloxicam may be increased by: Antidepressants (Tricyclic, Tertiary Amine); Corticosteroids (Systemic); Herbs (Anticoagulant/Antiplatelet Properties); Ketorolac; Probenecid; Selective Serotonin Reuptake Inhibitors; Serotonin/Norepinephrine Reuptake Inhibitors; Treprostinil

Decreased Effect

Meloxicam may decrease the levels/effects of: ACE Inhibitors; Angiotensin II Receptor Blockers; Antiplatelet Agents; Beta-Blockers; Eplerenone; HydrALAZINE; Loop Diuretics; Salicylates; Thiazide Diuretics

The levels/effects of Meloxicam may be decreased by: Bile Acid Sequestrants; Salicylates

Ethanol/Nutrition/Herb Interactions

Ethanol: Avoid ethanol (may enhance gastric mucosal irritation).

Herb/Nutraceutical: Avoid alfalfa, anise, bilberry, bladderwrack, bromelain, cat's claw, celery, chamomile, coleus, cordyceps, dong quai, evening primrose, fenugreek, feverfew, garlic, ginger, ginkgo biloba, ginseng (American, Panax, Siberian), grapeseed, green tea, guggul, horse chestnut seed, horseradish, licorice, prickly ash, red clover, reishi, SAMe (S-adenosylmethionine), sweet clover, turmeric, white willow (all have additional antiplatelet activity).

Stability Store at 25°C (77°F). Protect tablets from moisture.

Mechanism of Action Reversibly inhibits cyclooxygenase-1 and 2 (COX-1 and 2) enzymes, which result in decreased formation of prostaglandin precursors; has antipyretic, analgesic, and anti-inflammatory properties

Pharmacodynamics/Kinetics

Distribution: 10 L

Protein binding: ~99%, primarily to albumin

Metabolism: Hepatic via CYP2C9 and CYP3A4 (minor); forms 4 metabolites (inactive)

Bioavailability: 89%

Half-life elimination: Adults: 15-20 hours

Time to peak: Initial: 4-5 hours; Secondary: 12-14 hours

Excretion: Urine and feces (as inactive metabolites)

Dosage Oral:

Children ≥2 years: JRA: 0.125 mg/kg/day; maximum dose: 7.5 mg/day

Adults: Osteoarthritis, rheumatoid arthritis: Initial: 7.5 mg once daily; some patients may receive additional benefit from increasing dose to 15 mg once daily; maximum dose: 15 mg/day

Elderly: Increased concentrations may occur in elderly patients (particularly in females); however, no specific dosage adjustment is recommended

Dosage adjustment in renal impairment:

Mild-to-moderate impairment: No specific dosage recommendations

Significant impairment (Cl_{cr} ≤15 mL/minute): Patients with severe renal impairment have not been adequately studied; use not recommended.

Hemodialysis: Supplemental dose after dialysis not necessary.

Dosage adjustment in hepatic impairment:

Mild (Child-Pugh class A) to moderate (Child-Pugh class B) hepatic dysfunction: No dosage adjustment is necessary

Severe hepatic impairment: Patients with severe hepatic impairment have not been adequately studied

Dietary Considerations Should be taken with food or milk to minimize gastrointestinal irritation.

Monitoring Parameters Periodic CBC, serum chemistries, liver function, renal function (serum BUN, and creatinine) with long-term use; signs and symptoms of bleeding

Dosage Forms Excipient information presented when available (limited, particularly for generics); consult specific product labeling.

Suspension: 7.5 mg/5 mL (100 mL)

Mobic®: 7.5 mg/5 mL (100 mL) [contains sodium benzoate; raspberry flavor]

Tablet: 7.5 mg, 15 mg

Mobic®: 7.5 mg, 15 mg

◆ **Melpaque HP®** *see* Hydroquinone *on page 749*

Melphalan (MEL fa lan)

U.S. Brand Names Alkeran®

Canadian Brand Names Alkeran®

Index Terms L-PAM; L-Sarcolysin; NSC-8806; Phenylalanine Mustard

Pharmacologic Category Antineoplastic Agent, Alkylating Agent

Use Palliative treatment of multiple myeloma and nonresectable epithelial ovarian carcinoma

Unlabeled/Investigational Use Treatment of neuroblastoma, rhabdomyosarcoma, breast cancer; part of an induction regimen for marrow and stem cell transplantation

Pregnancy Risk Factor D

Pregnancy Considerations Animal studies have demonstrated embryotoxicity and teratogenicity. Therapy may suppress ovarian function leading to amenorrhea. There are no adequate and well-controlled studies in pregnant women. Women of childbearing potential should be advised to avoid pregnancy while on melphalan therapy.

Lactation Excretion in breast milk unknown/not recommended

Medication Safety Issues

Sound-alike/look-alike issues:

Melphalan may be confused with Mephyton®, Myleran®

Alkeran® may be confused with Alferon®, Leukeran®, Myleran®

High alert medication: The Institute for Safe Medication Practices (ISMP) includes this medication among its list of drugs which have a heightened risk of causing significant patient harm when used in error.

Contraindications Hypersensitivity to melphalan or any component of the formulation; severe bone marrow suppression; patients whose disease was resistant to prior melphalan therapy; pregnancy

Warnings/Precautions Hazardous agent - use appropriate precautions for handling and disposal. **[U.S. Boxed Warning]: Is potentially mutagenic, leukemogenic,** and carcinogenic. Suppresses ovarian function and produces amenorrhea; may also cause testicular suppression. **[U.S. Boxed Warning]: Bone marrow suppression is common.** Use with caution in patients with prior bone marrow suppression, impaired renal function (consider dose reduction), or who have received prior chemotherapy or irradiation. Toxicity to immunosuppressives is increased in elderly; start with lowest recommended adult doses. Signs of infection, such as fever and WBC rise, may not occur. Lethargy and confusion may be more prominent signs of infection. **[U.S. Boxed Warning]: Hypersensitivity has been reported with I.V. administration** and oral melphalan; may occur after multiple treatment cycles. **[U.S. Boxed Warning]: Should be administered under the supervision of an experienced cancer chemotherapy physician.** Safety and efficacy in children have not been established.

Adverse Reactions

>10%:

Gastrointestinal: Vomiting (oral low-dose: <10%; I.V.: 30% to 90%)

Hematologic: Myelosuppression, leukopenia (onset 7 days; nadir 14-35 days; recovery 28-56 days), thrombocytopenia (onset 7 days; nadir 14-35 days; recovery 28-56 days)

Miscellaneous: Secondary malignancy (<2% to 20%; cumulative dose and duration dependent)

1% to 10%: Miscellaneous: Hypersensitivity (I.V.: 2%)

Infrequent, frequency undefined, postmarketing, and/or case reports: Agranulocytosis, allergic reactions, alopecia, amenorrhea, anaphylaxis, anemia, bladder irritation, bone marrow failure (irreversible), diarrhea, hemolytic anemia, hemorrhagic cystitis, hemorrhagic necrotic enterocolitis, hepatic veno-occlusive disease (I.V. melphalan), hepatitis, interstitial pneumonitis, jaundice, nausea, ovarian suppression, pruritus, pulmonary fibrosis, radiation myelopathy, rash, secondary carcinoma, secondary leukemia, secondary myeloproliferative syndrome, SIADH, skin hypersensitivity, skin necrosis, skin ulceration (injection site), skin vesiculation, sterility, stomatitis, testicular suppression, transaminases increased, vasculitis

Drug Interactions

Avoid Concomitant Use

Avoid concomitant use of Melphalan with any of the following: Nalidixic Acid; Natalizumab; Vaccines (Live)

Increased Effect/Toxicity

Melphalan may increase the levels/effects of: CycloSPORINE; Natalizumab; Vaccines (Live); Vitamin K Antagonists

The levels/effects of Melphalan may be increased by: Nalidixic Acid; Trastuzumab

Decreased Effect

Melphalan may decrease the levels/effects of: Cardiac Glycosides; Vaccines (Inactivated); Vitamin K Antagonists

The levels/effects of Melphalan may be decreased by: Echinacea

Ethanol/Nutrition/Herb Interactions

Ethanol: Avoid ethanol (due to GI irritation).

Food: Food interferes with oral absorption.

Stability

Tablet: Store in refrigerator at 2°C to 8°C (36°F to 46°F). Protect from light.

Injection: Store at room temperature (15°C to 30°C). Protect from light. Must be prepared fresh. **The time between reconstitution/dilution and administration of parenteral melphalan must be kept to a minimum (manufacturer recommends <60 minutes) because reconstituted and diluted solutions are unstable.** Dissolve powder initially with 10 mL of diluent to a concentration of 5 mg/mL. Shake vigorously to dissolve. This solution is chemically and physically stable for at least 90 minutes when stored at 25°C (77°F). **Immediately** dilute dose in 250-500 mL NS to a concentration of 0.1-0.45 mg/mL. This solution is physically and chemically stable for at least 60 minutes at 25°C (77°F). Do not refrigerate solution; precipitation occurs.

Mechanism of Action Alkylating agent which is a derivative of mechlorethamine that inhibits DNA and RNA synthesis via formation of carbonium ions; cross-links strands of DNA; acts on both resting and rapidly dividing tumor cells.

Pharmacodynamics/Kinetics

Absorption: Oral: Variable and incomplete

Distribution: V_d: 0.5-0.6 L/kg throughout total body water

Protein binding: 60% to 90%; primarily to albumin, 20% to α_1-acid glycoprotein

Metabolism: Hepatic; chemical hydrolysis to monohydroxymelphalan and dihydroxymelphalan

Bioavailability: Unpredictable; 61% ± 26%, decreasing with repeated doses

Half-life elimination: Terminal: I.V.: 1.5 hours; oral: 1-1.25 hours

Time to peak, serum: ~1-2 hours

Excretion: Oral: Feces (20% to 50%); urine (10% to 30% as unchanged drug)

Dosage Refer to individual protocols.

Oral: Dose should always be adjusted to patient response and weekly blood counts:

Children (unlabeled use): 4-20 mg/m^2/day for 1-21 days

Adults:

Multiple myeloma (multiple regimens have been employed): **Note:** Response is gradual; may require repeated courses to realize benefit:

6 mg daily for 2-3 weeks initially, followed by up to 4 weeks rest, then a maintenance dose of 2 mg daily as hematologic recovery begins **or**

10 mg daily for 7-10 days; institute 2 mg daily maintenance dose after WBC >4000 cells/mm^3 and platelets >100,000 cells/mm^3 (~4-8 weeks); titrate maintenance dose to hematologic response **or**

0.15 mg/kg/day for 7 days, with a 2-6 week rest,

followed by a maintenance dose of ≤0.05 mg/kg/day as hematologic recovery begins **or**
0.25 mg/kg/day for 4 days (or 0.2 mg/kg/day for 5 days); repeat at 4- to 6-week intervals as ANC and platelet counts return to normal
Ovarian carcinoma: 0.2 mg/kg/day for 5 days, repeat every 4-5 weeks.
I.V.:
Children (unlabeled use):
Pediatric rhabdomyosarcoma: 10-35 mg/m^2/dose every 21-28 days
High-dose melphalan with bone marrow transplantation for neuroblastoma: I.V.: 100-220 mg/m^2 as a single dose or divided into 2-5 daily doses. Infuse over 20-60 minutes.
Adults: Multiple myeloma: 16 mg/m^2 administered at 2-week intervals for 4 doses, then administer at 4-week intervals after adequate hematologic recovery.

Dosing adjustment in renal impairment: The FDA-approved labeling contains the following adjustment recommendations based on route of administration:
Oral: Moderate-to-severe renal impairment: Consider a reduced dose initially
I.V.: BUN >30 mg/dL: Reduce dose by up to 50%
The following guidelines have been used by some clinicians:
Aronoff, 2007 (route of administration not specified):
Adults:
Cl_{cr} 10-50 mL/minute: Administer 75% of dose
Cl_{cr} <10 mL/minute: Administer 50% of dose
Hemodialysis: Administer dose after hemodialysis
Continuous ambulatory peritoneal dialysis (CAPD): Administer 50% of dose
Continuous renal replacement therapy (CRRT): Administer 75% of dose
Kintzel, 1995:
Oral: Adjust dose in the presence of hematologic toxicity
I.V.:
Cl_{cr} 46-60 mL/minute: Administer 85% of normal dose
Cl_{cr} 31-45 mL/minute: Administer 75% of normal dose
Cl_{cr} <30 mL/minute: Administer 70% of normal dose

Dosing adjustment in hepatic impairment: Melphalan is hepatically metabolized; however, dosage adjustment does not appear to be necessary (King, 2001).

Dietary Considerations Should be taken on an empty stomach (1 hour prior to or 2 hours after meals).

Administration
Oral: Administer on an empty stomach (1 hour prior to or 2 hours after meals)
Parenteral: Due to limited stability, complete administration of I.V. dose should occur within 60 minutes of reconstitution
I.V. infusion: Infuse over 15-20 minutes
I.V. bolus:
Central line: I.V. bolus doses of 17-200 mg/m^2 (reconstituted and not diluted) have been infused over 2-20 minutes
Peripheral line: I.V. bolus doses of 2-23 mg/m^2 (reconstituted and not diluted) have been infused over 1-4 minutes

Monitoring Parameters CBC with differential and platelet count, serum electrolytes, serum uric acid

Test Interactions False-positive Coombs' test [direct]

Dosage Forms Excipient information presented when available (limited, particularly for generics); consult specific product labeling.
Injection, powder for reconstitution: 50 mg [diluent contains ethanol and propylene glycol]
Tablet: 2 mg

◆ **Melquin-3®** *see* Hydroquinone *on page* 749

◆ **Melquin HP®** *see* Hydroquinone *on page* 749

Memantine (me MAN teen)

U.S. Brand Names Namenda™
Canadian Brand Names Ebixa®
Index Terms Memantine Hydrochloride
Pharmacologic Category N-Methyl-D-Aspartate Receptor Antagonist
Use Treatment of moderate-to-severe dementia of the Alzheimer's type
Unlabeled/Investigational Use Treatment of mild-to-moderate vascular dementia; mild cognitive impairment
Pregnancy Risk Factor B
Pregnancy Considerations Teratogenic effects were not observed in animal studies. There are no studies in pregnant women.
Lactation Excretion in breast milk unknown/use caution
Contraindications Hypersensitivity to memantine or any component of the formulation
Warnings/Precautions Use caution with seizure disorders or severe hepatic impairment. Caution with use in severe renal impairment; dose adjustment recommended. Clearance is significantly reduced by alkaline urine; use caution with medications, dietary changes, or patient conditions which may alter urine pH.

Adverse Reactions
1% to 10%:
Cardiovascular: Hypertension (4%), cardiac failure, syncope, cerebrovascular accident, transient ischemic attack
Central nervous system: Dizziness (7%), confusion (6%), headache (6%), hallucinations (3%), pain (3%), somnolence (3%), fatigue (2%), aggressive reaction, ataxia, vertigo
Dermatologic: Rash
Gastrointestinal: Constipation (5%), vomiting (3%), weight loss
Genitourinary: Micturition
Hematologic: Anemia
Hepatic: Alkaline phosphatase increased
Neuromuscular & skeletal: Back pain (3%), hypokinesia
Ocular: Cataract, conjunctivitis
Respiratory: Cough (4%), dyspnea (2%), pneumonia
<1% (Limited to important or life-threatening): Allergic reaction, AV block, cerebral infarction, dyskinesia, dysphagia, hepatic failure, hyperlipidemia, hypoglycemia, ileus, NMS, pancreatitis, renal failure, QT prolongation, seizure, Stevens-Johnson syndrome, sudden death, tardive dyskinesia, thrombocytopenia

Drug Interactions
Avoid Concomitant Use There are no known interactions where it is recommended to avoid concomitant use.
Increased Effect/Toxicity
Memantine may increase the levels/effects of: Trimethoprim

The levels/effects of Memantine may be increased by: Carbonic Anhydrase Inhibitors; Sodium Bicarbonate; Trimethoprim
Decreased Effect There are no known significant interactions involving a decrease in effect.

Stability Store at controlled room temperature of 15°C to 30°C (59°F to 86°F).

Mechanism of Action Glutamate, the primary excitatory amino acid in the CNS, may contribute to the pathogenesis of Alzheimer's disease (AD) by overstimulating various glutamate receptors leading to excitotoxicity and neuronal cell death. Memantine is an uncompetitive antagonist of the N-methyl-D-aspartate (NMDA) type of glutamate receptors, located ubiquitously throughout the brain. Under normal physiologic conditions, the (unstimulated) NMDA receptor ion channel is blocked by magnesium ions, which are displaced after agonist-induced depolarization.

Pathologic or excessive receptor activation, as postulated to occur during AD, prevents magnesium from reentering and blocking the channel pore resulting in a chronically open state and excessive calcium influx. Memantine binds to the intra-pore magnesium site, but with longer dwell time, and thus functions as an effective receptor blocker only under conditions of excessive stimulation; memantine does not affect normal neurotransmission.

Pharmacodynamics/Kinetics

Distribution: 9-11 L/kg

Protein binding: 45%

Metabolism: Forms 3 metabolites (minimal activity)

Half-life elimination: Terminal: 60-80 hours; severe renal impairment (Cl_{cr} 5-29 mL/minute): 117-156 hours

Time to peak, serum: 3-7 hours

Excretion: Urine (57% to 82% unchanged); excretion reduced by alkaline urine pH

Dosage Oral: Adults:

Alzheimer's disease: Initial: 5 mg/day; increase dose by 5 mg/day to a target dose of 20 mg/day; wait at least 1 week between dosage changes. Doses >5 mg/day should be given in 2 divided doses.

Suggested titration: 5 mg/day for ≥1 week; 5 mg twice daily for ≥1 week; 15 mg/day given in 5 mg and 10 mg separated doses for ≥1 week; then 10 mg twice daily

Mild-to-moderate vascular dementia (unlabeled use): 10 mg twice daily

Dosage adjustment in renal impairment:

Mild-to-moderate impairment: No adjustment required

Severe impairment: Cl_{cr} 5-29 mL/minute): 5 mg twice daily

Dietary Considerations May be taken with or without food.

Dosage Forms Excipient information presented when available (limited, particularly for generics); consult specific product labeling.

Solution, oral: 2 mg/mL (360 mL) [alcohol free, dye free, sugar free; peppermint flavor]

Tablet, as hydrochloride: 5 mg, 10 mg

Combination package [titration pack contains two separate tablet formulations]: Memantine hydrochloride 5 mg (28s) and memantine hydrochloride 10 mg (21s)

◆ **Memantine Hydrochloride** *see* Memantine *on page 938*

◆ **Menactra®** *see* Meningococcal Polysaccharide (Groups A / C / Y and W-135) Diphtheria Toxoid Conjugate Vaccine *on page 939*

◆ **Menest®** *see* Estrogens (Esterified) *on page 566*

◆ **Meningococcal Conjugate Vaccine** *see* Meningococcal Polysaccharide (Groups A / C / Y and W-135) Diphtheria Toxoid Conjugate Vaccine *on page 939*

Meningococcal Polysaccharide (Groups A / C / Y and W-135) Diphtheria Toxoid Conjugate Vaccine

(me NIN joe kok al pol i SAK a ride groops aye, see, why & dubl yoo won thur tee fyve dif THEER ee a TOKS oyds KON joo gate vak SEEN)

U.S. Brand Names Menactra®

Index Terms MCV; Meningococcal Conjugate Vaccine

Pharmacologic Category Vaccine, Inactivated (Bacterial)

Use Provide active immunization of children and adults (2-55 years of age) against invasive meningococcal disease caused by *N. meningitidis* serogroups A, C, Y, and W-135

The Advisory Committee on Immunization Practices (ACIP) recommends routine vaccination of all persons 11-18 years of age at the earliest opportunity. Adolescents should be vaccinated at the 11-12 year visit. For adolescents not previously vaccinated, vaccine should be administered prior to high school entry (~15 years of age).

The ACIP also recommends vaccination for persons at increased risk for meningococcal disease. (Meningococcal conjugate vaccine [MCV] is preferred for persons aged 2-55 years; meningococcal polysaccharide vaccine [MPSV] may be used if MCV is not available). Persons at increased risk include:

College freshmen living in dormitories

Microbiologists routinely exposed to isolates of *N. meningitides*

Military recruits

Persons traveling to or who reside in countries where *N. meningitides* is hyperendemic or epidemic, particularly if contact with local population will be prolonged

Persons with terminal complement component deficiencies

Persons with anatomic or functional asplenia

Use is also recommended during meningococcal outbreaks caused by vaccine preventable serogroups.

Pregnancy Risk Factor C

Pregnancy Considerations Animal reproduction studies have not been conducted. An isolated teratogenic effect was observed in an animal developmental toxicity study; not necessarily vaccine related. Carcinogenic or mutagenic studies have not been performed. There are no adequate and well-controlled studies in pregnant women. Patients should contact the Sanofi Pasteur Inc vaccine registry at 1-800-822-2463 if they are pregnant or become aware they were pregnant at the time of Menactra® vaccination.

Lactation Excretion in breast milk unknown/use caution

Medication Safety Issues

Administration issue:

Menactra® (MCV) should be administered by intramuscular (I.M.) injection only. Inadvertent subcutaneous (SubQ) administration has been reported; possibly due to confusion of this product with Menomume® (MPSV), also a meningococcal polysaccharide vaccine, which is administered by the SubQ route.

Contraindications Hypersensitivity to any component of the formulation, including diphtheria toxoid; latex hypersensitivity; history of Guillain-Barré syndrome

Warnings/Precautions Use with caution in patients with a history of bleeding disorders (including thrombocytopenia) and/or patients on anticoagulant therapy; bleeding/hematoma may occur from I.M. administration. May consider deferring administration in patients with moderate or severe acute illness (with or without fever); may administer to patients with mild acute illness (with or without fever). Menactra® is not to be used to treat meningococcal infections or to provide immunity against *N. meningitidis* serogroup B or diphtheria. Immunosuppressed patients may have a reduced response to vaccination. Risk of developing Guillain-Barré syndrome may be increased following vaccination with MCV. Persons previously diagnosed with Guillain-Barré syndrome should not be vaccinated with MCV. Vial stopper contains latex. Safety and efficacy have not been established in children <2 years of age or adults >55 years. Immediate treatment for anaphylactic reactions should be available. In order to maximize vaccination rates, the ACIP recommends simultaneous administration of all age-appropriate vaccines (live or inactivated) for which a person is eligible at a single clinic visit, unless contraindications exist.

Adverse Reactions All serious adverse reactions must be reported to the U.S. Department of Health and Human Services Vaccine Adverse Event Reporting System (VAERS) 1-800-822-7967 or www.vaers.org.

>10%:

Central nervous system: Pain (45% to 59%), headache (36% to 41%), fatigue (30% to 35%), malaise (22% to 24%), irritability (12%), drowsiness (11%)

Gastrointestinal: Diarrhea (11% to 16%), anorexia (8% to 12%)

Local: Redness (11% to 22%), swelling (11% to 17%), induration (16% to 19%)

Neuromuscular & skeletal: Arthralgia (7% to 20%)

1% to 10%:

Central nervous system: Chills (7% to 10%), fever (2% to 5%)

Gastrointestinal: Vomiting (2% to 3%)

Local: Rash (1% to 3%)

Postmarketing and/or case reports: Acute disseminated encephalomyelitis, anaphylactic/anaphylactoid reactions, breathing difficulties, erythema, facial palsy, Guillain-Barré syndrome, hypotension, myalgia, pruritus, transverse myelitis, upper airway swelling, urticaria, vasovagal syncope, wheezing

Drug Interactions

Avoid Concomitant Use There are no known interactions where it is recommended to avoid concomitant use.

Increased Effect/Toxicity There are no known significant interactions involving an increase in effect.

Decreased Effect

The levels/effects of Meningococcal Polysaccharide (Groups A / C / Y and W-135) Diphtheria Toxoid Conjugate Vaccine may be decreased by: Immunosuppressants

Stability Store between 2°C to 8°C (35°F to 46°F); do not freeze. Discard product exposed to freezing. Do not mix with other vaccines in the same syringe.

Mechanism of Action Induces immunity against meningococcal disease via the formation of bactericidal antibodies directed toward the polysaccharide capsular components of *Neisseria meningitidis* serogroups A, C, Y and W-135.

Dosage I.M.:

Children ≥2 years and Adults ≤55 years: 0.5 mL

Note: Revaccination: May be indicated in patients previously vaccinated with MPSV who remain at increased risk for infection. The ACIP recommends the use of MCV for revaccination; however, use of MPSV is also acceptable. The need for revaccination in patients previously vaccinated with MCV is currently under study. Children 2-10 years who received MPSV ≥3 years previously, or older children and adults who received MPSV ≥5 years previously, and who are still at increased risk for meningococcal disease should be revaccinated with MCV.

Elderly: Safety and efficacy not established in patients >55 years of age

Administration Administer by I.M. route, preferably into the upper deltoid region. Do not administer via I.V., SubQ or I.D. route. For patients at risk of hemorrhage, the ACIP recommends "it should be administered intramuscularly if, in the opinion of a physician familiar with the patient's bleeding risk, the vaccine can be administered with reasonable safety by this route. If the patient receives antihemophilia or other similar therapy, intramuscular vaccination can be scheduled shortly after such therapy is administered. A fine needle (≤23 gauge) can be used for the vaccination and firm pressure applied to the site (without rubbing) for at least 2 minutes. The patient or family should be instructed concerning the risk of hematoma from the injection."

For I.M. administration only. Based on limited data, inadvertent SubQ administration provides a lower serologic response, however, the response is still considered to be protective. If inadvertently administered by the SubQ route, revaccination is not necessary.

Administration with other vaccines:

MCV with other inactivated vaccines: May be given simultaneously or at any interval between doses. A one month interval between tetanus toxoid, reduced diphtheria toxoid, and reduced acellular pertussis vaccine and MCV is suggested if they are not administered simultaneously

MCV with live vaccines: May be given simultaneously or at any interval between doses

Vaccine administration with antibody-containing products: MCV may be given simultaneously at different sites or at any interval between doses with antibody-containing products. Examples of antibody containing products include I.M. and I.V. immune globulin, hepatitis B immune globulin, tetanus immune globulin, varicella zoster immune globulin, rabies immune globulin, whole blood, packed red cells, plasma, and platelet products.

Monitoring Parameters Monitor for syncope for ≥15 minutes following vaccination

Additional Information Federal law requires that the date of administration, the vaccine manufacturer, lot number of vaccine, and the administering person's name, title and address be entered into the patient's permanent medical record.

Dosage Forms Excipient information presented when available (limited, particularly for generics); consult specific product labeling.

Injection, solution [MCV; preservative free]:

Menactra®: 4 mcg each of polysaccharide antigen groups A, C, Y, and W-135 [bound to diphtheria toxoid 48 mcg] per 0.5 mL [contains natural rubber/natural latex in packaging of vials]

◆ **Meningococcal Polysaccharide Vaccine** *see* Meningococcal Polysaccharide Vaccine (Groups A / C / Y and W-135) *on page 940*

Meningococcal Polysaccharide Vaccine (Groups A / C / Y and W-135)

(me NIN joe kok al pol i SAK a ride vak SEEN groops aye, see, why & dubl yoo won thur tee fyve)

U.S. Brand Names Menomune®-A/C/Y/W-135

Index Terms Meningococcal Polysaccharide Vaccine; MPSV

Pharmacologic Category Vaccine, Inactivated (Bacterial)

Additional Appendix Information

Immunization Recommendations *on page 1708*

Use Provide active immunity to meningococcal serogroups contained in the vaccine

The Advisory Committee on Immunization Practices (ACIP) recommends routine vaccination for persons at increased risk for meningococcal disease. (Meningococcal conjugate vaccine [MCV] is preferred for persons aged 2-55 years; meningococcal polysaccharide vaccine [MPSV] may be used if MCV is not available.) Persons at increased risk include:

College freshmen living in dormitories

Microbiologists routinely exposed to isolates of *N. meningitides*

Military recruits

Persons traveling to or who reside in countries where *N. meningitides* is hyperendemic or epidemic, particularly if contact with local population will be prolonged

Persons with terminal complement component deficiencies

Persons with anatomic or functional asplenia

Use is also recommended during meningococcal outbreaks caused by vaccine preventable serogroups.

Pregnancy Risk Factor C

Pregnancy Considerations Animal studies have not been conducted. Based on limited data, teratogenic effects have not been reported when used during pregnancy. Pregnancy should not preclude vaccination with MPSV if indicated. Patients may contact the Sanofi Pasteur Inc vaccine registry at 1-800-822-2463 if they are pregnant or become aware they were pregnant at the time of vaccination.

Lactation Excretion in breast milk unknown/use caution

Medication Safety Issues

Administration issue:

Menomume® (MPSV) should be administered by subcutaneous (SubQ) injection. Menactra® (MCV), also a meningococcal polysaccharide vaccine, is to be administered by intramuscular (I.M.) injection only.

Contraindications Hypersensitivity to any component of the formulation; defer immunization during acute illness

Warnings/Precautions Immediate treatment (including epinephrine 1:1000) for anaphylactoid and/or hypersensitivity reactions should be available during vaccine use. Response may not be as great as desired in immunosuppressed patients. Not to be used to treat meningococcal infections or to provide immunity against *N. meningitidis* serogroup B. Use in pediatric patients <2 years of age is usually not recommended. Use with caution in patients with latex sensitivity; the stopper to the vial contains dry, natural latex rubber. Some dosage forms contain thimerosal. In order to maximize vaccination rates, the ACIP recommends simultaneous administration of all age-appropriate vaccines (live or inactivated) for which a person is eligible at a single clinic visit, unless contraindications exist.

Adverse Reactions All serious adverse reactions must be reported to the U.S. Department of Health and Human Services (DHHS) Vaccine Adverse Event Reporting System (VAERS) 1-800-822-7967. Percentages reported in adults; incidence of erythema, swelling, or tenderness may be higher in children

>10%: Local: Tenderness (9% to 36%)

1% to 10%:

Central nervous system: Headache (2% to 5%), malaise (2%), fever (100°F to 106°F: 3%), chills (2%)

Local: Pain at injection site (2% to 3%), erythema (1% to 4%), induration (1% to 4%)

Drug Interactions

Avoid Concomitant Use There are no known interactions where it is recommended to avoid concomitant use.

Increased Effect/Toxicity There are no known significant interactions involving an increase in effect.

Decreased Effect

The levels/effects of Meningococcal Polysaccharide Vaccine (Groups A / C / Y and W-135) may be decreased by: Immunosuppressants

Stability Prior to and following reconstitution, store at 2°C to 8°C (35°F to 46°F). Reconstitute using provided diluent; shake well. Use single-dose vial within 30 minutes of reconstitution. Use multidose vial within 35 days of reconstitution.

Mechanism of Action Induces the formation of bactericidal antibodies to meningococcal antigens; the presence of these antibodies is strongly correlated with immunity to meningococcal disease caused by *Neisseria meningitidis* groups A, C, Y and W-135.

Pharmacodynamics/Kinetics

Onset of action: Antibody levels: 7-10 days

Duration: Antibodies against group A and C polysaccharides decline markedly (to prevaccination levels) over the first 3 years following a single dose of vaccine, especially in children <4 years of age

Dosage SubQ:

Children <2 years: Not usually recommended. Two doses (0.5 mL/dose), 3 months apart, may be considered in children 3-18 months to elicit short-term protection against serogroup A disease. A single dose may be considered in children 19-23 months. (ACIP recommendations)

Children ≥2 years and Adults: 0.5 mL

Note: Revaccination: May be indicated in patients previously vaccinated with MPSV who remain at increased risk for infection. The ACIP recommends the use of MCV for revaccination; however, use of MPSV is also acceptable. Children 2-10 years who received MPSV ≥3 years previously, or older children and adults who received MPSV ≥5 years previously, and who are still at increased risk for meningococcal disease should be revaccinated with MCV.

Administration Administer by SubQ injection; do not administer intradermally, I.M., or I.V.

Administration with other vaccines:

MPSV with other inactivated vaccines: May be given simultaneously or at any interval between doses.

MPSV with live vaccines: May be given simultaneously or at any interval between doses.

Vaccine administration with antibody-containing products: MPSV may be given simultaneously at different sites or at any interval between doses with antibody-containing products. Examples of antibody-containing products include I.M. and I.V. immune globulin, hepatitis B immune globulin, tetanus immune globulin, varicella zoster immune globulin, rabies immune globulin, whole blood, packed red cells, plasma, and platelet products.

Monitoring Parameters Monitor for syncope for ≥15 minutes following vaccination.

Additional Information Federal law requires that the date of administration, the vaccine manufacturer, lot number of vaccine, and the administering person's name, title and address be entered into the patient's permanent medical record.

Dosage Forms Excipient information presented when available (limited, particularly for generics); consult specific product labeling.

Injection, powder for reconstitution [MPSV]:

Menomune®-A/C/Y/W-135: 50 mcg each of polysaccharide antigen groups A, C, Y, and W-135 per 0.5 mL dose [contains lactose 2.5-5 mg/0.5 mL, natural rubber/natural latex in packaging, thimerosal in diluent for multidose vial]

◆ **Menomune®-A/C/Y/W-135** *see* Meningococcal Polysaccharide Vaccine (Groups A / C / Y and W-135) *on page 940*

◆ **Menopur®** *see* Menotropins *on page 941*

◆ **Menostar®** *see* Estradiol *on page 554*

Menotropins (men oh TROE pins)

U.S. Brand Names Menopur®; Repronex®

Canadian Brand Names Menopur®; Repronex®

Index Terms hMG; Human Menopausal Gonadotropin

Pharmacologic Category Gonadotropin; Ovulation Stimulator

Use Female:

In conjunction with hCG to induce ovulation and pregnancy in infertile females experiencing oligoanovulation or anovulation when the cause of anovulation is functional and not caused by primary ovarian failure (Repronex®)

Stimulation of multiple follicle development in ovulatory patients as part of an assisted reproductive technology (ART) (Menopur®, Repronex®)

Unlabeled/Investigational Use Male: Stimulation of spermatogenesis in primary or secondary hypogonadotropic hypogonadism

Pregnancy Risk Factor X

Pregnancy Considerations Ectopic pregnancy and congenital abnormalities have been reported. The incidence of congenital abnormality is similar during natural conception.

Lactation Excretion in breast milk unknown/use caution

Medication Safety Issues

Sound-alike/look-alike issues:

Repronex® may be confused with Regranex®

Contraindications Hypersensitivity to menotropins or any component of the formulation; primary ovarian failure as indicated by a high follicle-stimulating hormone (FSH) level; uncontrolled thyroid and adrenal dysfunction; abnormal bleeding of undetermined origin; intracranial lesion (ie, pituitary tumor); ovarian cyst or enlargement not due to polycystic ovary syndrome; infertility due to any cause other than anovulation (except candidates for *in vitro* fertilization); sex hormone-dependent tumors of the reproductive tract and accessory organs; pregnancy

Warnings/Precautions These medications should only be used by physicians who are thoroughly familiar with infertility problems and their management. Advise patient of frequency and potential hazards of multiple pregnancy. May cause ovarian hyperstimulation syndrome (OHSS); if severe, treatment should be discontinued and patient should be hospitalized (may become more severe if pregnancy occurs). Monitor for ovarian enlargement; to minimize the hazard of abnormal ovarian enlargement, use the lowest possible dose. Serious pulmonary conditions (atelectasis, acute respiratory distress syndrome) and arterial thromboembolism have been reported. Safety and efficacy have not been established in renal or hepatic impairment, or in pediatric and geriatric patients. Use may lead to multiple births. Products may contain lactose.

Adverse Reactions Adverse effects may vary according to specific product, route, and/or dosage.

>10%:

Central nervous system: Headache (up to 34%)

Gastrointestinal: Abdominal pain (up to 18%), nausea (up to 12%)

Genitourinary: OHSS (up to 13%, dose related)

Local: Injection site reaction (4% to 12%)

1% to 10%:

Cardiovascular: Flushing

Central nervous system: Dizziness, malaise, migraine

Endocrine & metabolic: Breast tenderness, hot flashes, menstrual irregularities

Gastrointestinal: Abdominal cramping, abdominal fullness, constipation, diarrhea, enlarged abdomen, vomiting

Genitourinary: Ectopic pregnancy, ovarian disease, vaginal hemorrhage

Local: Injection site edema/pain

Neuromuscular & skeletal: Back pain

Respiratory: Cough increased, respiratory disorder

Miscellaneous: Infection, flu-like syndrome

Frequency not defined:

Cardiovascular: Stroke, tachycardia, thrombosis (venous or arterial)

Dermatologic: Angioedema, rash, urticaria

Genitourinary: Adnexal torsion, hemoperitoneum, ovarian enlargement

Neuromuscular & skeletal: Limb necrosis

Respiratory: Acute respiratory distress syndrome, atelectasis, dyspnea, embolism, laryngeal edema pulmonary infarction tachypnea

Miscellaneous: Allergic reactions, anaphylaxis

Drug Interactions

Avoid Concomitant Use There are no known interactions where it is recommended to avoid concomitant use.

Increased Effect/Toxicity There are no known significant interactions involving an increase in effect.

Decreased Effect There are no known significant interactions involving a decrease in effect.

Stability Lyophilized powder may be refrigerated or stored at room temperature. Protect from light. After reconstitution inject immediately; discard any unused portion.

Mechanism of Action Actions occur as a result of both follicle stimulating hormone (FSH) effects and luteinizing hormone (LH) effects; menotropins stimulate the development and maturation of the ovarian follicle (FSH), cause ovulation (LH), and stimulate the development of the corpus luteum (LH); in males it stimulates spermatogenesis (LH)

Pharmacodynamics/Kinetics Excretion: Urine (~10% as unchanged drug)

Dosage Adults:

Repronex®: I.M., SubQ:

Induction of ovulation in patients with oligoanovulation (Female): Initial: 150 int. units daily for the first 5 days of treatment. Adjustments should not be made more frequently than once every 2 days and should not exceed 75-150 int. units per adjustment. Maximum daily dose should not exceed 450 int. units and dosing beyond 12 days is not recommended. If patient's response is appropriate, hCG 5000-10,000 units should be given one day following the last dose of Repronex®. Hold dose if serum estradiol is >2000 pg/mL, if the ovaries are abnormally enlarged, or if abdominal pain occurs; the patient should also be advised to refrain from intercourse. May repeat process if follicular development is inadequate or if pregnancy does not occur.

Assisted reproductive technologies (Female): Initial (in patients who have received GnRH agonist or antagonist pituitary suppression): 225 int. units; adjustments in dose should not be made more frequently than once every 2 days and should not exceed more than 75-150 int. units per adjustment. The maximum daily doses of Repronex® given should not exceed 450 int. units and dosing beyond 12 days is not recommended. Once adequate follicular development is evident, hCG (5000-10,000 units) should be administered to induce final follicular maturation in preparation for oocyte retrieval. Withhold treatment when ovaries are abnormally enlarged on last day of therapy (to reduce chance of developing OHSS).

Menopur®: SubQ: *Assisted reproductive technologies (ART):* Initial (in patients who have received GnRH agonist for pituitary suppression): 225 int. units; adjustments in dose should not be made more frequently than once every 2 days and should not exceed more than 150 int. units per adjustment. The maximum daily dose given should not exceed 450 int. units and dosing beyond 20 days is not recommended. Once adequate follicular development is evident, hCG should be administered to induce final follicular maturation in preparation for oocyte retrieval. Withhold treatment when ovaries are abnormally enlarged on last day of therapy (to reduce chance of developing OHSS).

Spermatogenesis (Male) (unlabeled use): I.M.: Following pretreatment with hCG: 75 int. units 3 times/week and hCG 2000 units twice weekly until sperm is detected in the ejaculate (4-6 months); may then be increased to menotropins 150 int. units 3 times/week

Administration

Menopur®: SubQ: Administer to alternating sites of the abdomen; when administration to the lower abdomen is not possible, the injection may be given into the thigh.

Repronex®:

I.M.: Administer deep in a large muscle.

SubQ: Administer to alternating sites of the lower abdomen.

Monitoring Parameters hCG levels, serum estradiol; vaginal ultrasound; in cases of suspected OHSS, monitor fluid intake and output, weight, hematocrit, serum and urinary electrolytes, urine specific gravity, BUN and creatinine, and abdominal girth

Dosage Forms Excipient information presented when available (limited, particularly for generics); consult specific product labeling.

Injection, powder for reconstitution:

Menopur®: Follicle stimulating hormone activity 75 int. units and luteinizing hormone activity 75 int. units [packaged with diluent; contains lactose]

Repronex®: Follicle stimulating hormone activity 75 int. units and luteinizing hormone activity 75 int. units [packaged with diluent; contains lactose]

◆ **Mentax®** *see* Butenafine *on page 230*

◆ **292 MEP® (Can)** *see* Meprobamate and Aspirin *on page 946*

◆ **Mepergan** *see* Meperidine and Promethazine *on page 944*

Meperidine (me PER i deen)

U.S. Brand Names Demerol®

Canadian Brand Names Demerol®

Index Terms Isonipecaine Hydrochloride; Meperidine Hydrochloride; Pethidine Hydrochloride

Pharmacologic Category Analgesic, Opioid

Additional Appendix Information

Narcotic / Opioid Analgesics *on page 1663*

Use Management of moderate-to-severe pain; adjunct to anesthesia and preoperative sedation

Unlabeled/Investigational Use

Reduce postoperative shivering; reduce rigors from amphotericin

Restrictions C-II

Pregnancy Risk Factor C/D (prolonged use or high doses at term)

Pregnancy Considerations Meperidine is known to cross the placenta, which may result in respiratory or CNS depression in the newborn.

Lactation Enters breast milk/contraindicated (AAP rates "compatible")

Medication Safety Issues

Avoid the use of meperidine for pain control, especially in elderly and renally-compromised patients (Institute for Safe Medication Practices [ISMP], 2007)

Sound-alike/look-alike issues:

Meperidine may be confused with meprobamate

Demerol® may be confused with Demulen®, Desyrel®, dicumarol, Dilaudid®, Dymelor®, Pamelor®

High alert medication: The Institute for Safe Medication Practices (ISMP) includes this medication among its list of drug classes which have a heightened risk of causing significant patient harm when used in error.

Contraindications Hypersensitivity to meperidine or any component of the formulation; use with or within 14 days of MAO inhibitors; pregnancy (prolonged use or high doses near term)

Warnings/Precautions Oral meperidine is not recommended for acute/chronic pain management. Intravenous meperidine should be used cautiously for acute pain. The American Pain Society (2003) recommends that it not be used for more than 48 hours; in doses >600 mg/24 hours; or in patients with pre-existing CNS or renal dysfunction. The Institute for Safe Medication Practice recommends avoiding the use of meperidine for pain control, especially in the elderly and renally-impaired (ISMP, 2007). Normeperidine (an active metabolite and CNS stimulant) may accumulate and precipitate anxiety, tremors, or seizures; risk increases with renal dysfunction and cumulative dose. Effects may be potentiated when used with other sedative drugs or ethanol. May cause CNS depression, which may impair physical or mental abilities; patients must be cautioned about performing tasks which require mental alertness (eg, operating machinery or driving). Use only with extreme caution (if at all) in patients with head injury or increased intracranial pressure (ICP). Use caution with pulmonary, hepatic, or renal disorders, supraventricular tachycardias, acute abdominal conditions, hypothyroidism, toxic psychosis, kyphoscoliosis, morbid obesity, Addison's disease, BPH, or urethral stricture. Use with caution in patients with biliary tract dysfunction; acute pancreatitis may cause constriction of sphincter of Oddi. May cause hypotension; use with caution in patients with depleted blood volume or drugs which may exaggerate hypotensive effects (including phenothiazines or general anesthetics).

An opioid-containing analgesic regimen should be tailored to each patient's needs and based upon the type of pain being treated (acute versus chronic), the route of administration, degree of tolerance for opioids (naive versus chronic user), age, weight, and medical condition. The optimal analgesic dose varies widely among patients. Some preparations contain sulfites which may cause allergic reaction. Tolerance or drug dependence may result from extended use. Healthcare provider should be alert to problems of abuse, misuse, and diversion. Concurrent use of agonist/antagonist analgesics may precipitate withdrawal symptoms and/or reduced analgesic efficacy in patients following prolonged therapy with mu opioid agonists. Abrupt discontinuation following prolonged use may also lead to withdrawal symptoms. Avoid use in the elderly.

Adverse Reactions Frequency not defined.

Cardiovascular: Hypotension

Central nervous system: Fatigue, drowsiness, dizziness, nervousness, headache, restlessness, malaise, confusion, mental depression, hallucinations, paradoxical CNS stimulation, increased intracranial pressure, seizure (associated with metabolite accumulation), serotonin syndrome

Dermatologic: Rash, urticaria

Gastrointestinal: Nausea, vomiting, constipation, anorexia, stomach cramps, xerostomia, biliary spasm, paralytic ileus, sphincter of Oddi spasm

Genitourinary: Ureteral spasms, decreased urination

Local: Pain at injection site

Neuromuscular & skeletal: Weakness

Respiratory: Dyspnea

Miscellaneous: Histamine release, physical and psychological dependence

Drug Interactions

Metabolism/Transport Effects Substrate (minor) of CYP2B6, 2C19, 3A4

Avoid Concomitant Use

Avoid concomitant use of Meperidine with any of the following: MAO Inhibitors; Sibutramine

Increased Effect/Toxicity

Meperidine may increase the levels/effects of: Alcohol (Ethyl); Alvimopan; CNS Depressants; Desmopressin; Selective Serotonin Reuptake Inhibitors; Serotonin Modulators

The levels/effects of Meperidine may be increased by: Amphetamines; Antipsychotic Agents (Phenothiazines); Barbiturates; MAO Inhibitors; Protease Inhibitors; Sibutramine; Succinylcholine

Decreased Effect

Meperidine may decrease the levels/effects of: Pegvisomant

The levels/effects of Meperidine may be decreased by: Ammonium Chloride; Phenytoin; Protease Inhibitors

Ethanol/Nutrition/Herb Interactions

Ethanol: Avoid or limit ethanol (may increase CNS depression). Watch for sedation.

Herb/Nutraceutical: Avoid valerian, St John's wort, kava kava, gotu kola (may increase CNS depression).

Stability Meperidine injection should be stored at room temperature; do not freeze. Protect from light. Protect oral dosage forms from light.

Mechanism of Action Binds to opiate receptors in the CNS, causing inhibition of ascending pain pathways, altering the perception of and response to pain; produces generalized CNS depression

Pharmacodynamics/Kinetics

Onset of action: Analgesic: Oral, SubQ: 10-15 minutes; I.V.: ~5 minutes

Peak effect: SubQ.: ~1 hour; Oral: 2 hours

Duration: Oral, SubQ.: 2-4 hours

Absorption: I.M.: Erratic and highly variable

Distribution: Crosses placenta; enters breast milk

Protein binding: 65% to 75%

Metabolism: Hepatic; hydrolyzed to meperidinic acid (inactive) or undergoes N-demethylation to normeperidine (active; has 1/2 the analgesic effect and 2-3 times the CNS effects of meperidine)

Bioavailability: ~50% to 60%; increased with liver disease

Half-life elimination:

Parent drug: Terminal phase: Adults: 2.5-4 hours, Liver disease: 7-11 hours

Normeperidine (active metabolite): 15-30 hours; can accumulate with high doses (>600 mg/day) or with decreased renal function

Excretion: Urine (as metabolites)

Dosage Note: The American Pain Society (2003) and ISMP (2007) do not recommend meperidine's use as an analgesic.

Children: Pain: Oral, I.M., I.V., SubQ: 1-1.5 mg/kg/dose every 3-4 hours as needed; 1-2 mg/kg as a single dose preoperative medication may be used; maximum 100 mg/dose (**Note:** Oral route is not recommended for acute pain.)

Adults: Pain:

Oral: Initial: Opiate-naive: 50 mg every 3-4 hours as needed; usual dosage range: 50-150 mg every 2-4 hours as needed (manufacturers recommendation; oral route is not recommended for acute pain)

I.M., SubQ: Initial: Opiate-naive: 50-75 mg every 3-4 hours as needed; patients with prior opiate exposure may require higher initial doses

Slow I.V.: Initial: 5-10 mg every 5 minutes as needed

Preoperatively: 50-100 mg given 30-90 minutes before the beginning of anesthesia

Note: If use in acute pain (in patients without renal or CNS disease) cannot be avoided, treatment should be limited to ≤48 hours and doses should not exceed 600 mg/24 hours.

Elderly:

Oral: 50 mg every 4 hours

I.M.: 25 mg every 4 hours

Dosing adjustment in renal impairment: Avoid use in renal impairment

Dosing adjustment/comments in hepatic disease: Increased narcotic effect in cirrhosis; reduction in dose more important for oral than I.V. route

Administration Meperidine may be administered I.M., SubQ, or I.V.; I.V. push should be administered slowly, use of a 10 mg/mL concentration has been recommended. For continuous I.V. infusions, a more dilute solution (eg, 1 mg/mL) should be used.

Oral: Administer syrup diluted in 1/2 glass of water; undiluted syrup may exert topical anesthetic effect on mucous membranes

Monitoring Parameters Pain relief, respiratory and mental status, blood pressure; observe patient for excessive sedation, CNS depression, seizures, respiratory depression

Reference Range Therapeutic: 70-500 ng/mL (SI: 283-2020 nmol/L); Toxic: >1000 ng/mL (SI: >4043 nmol/L)

Test Interactions Increased amylase (S), increased BSP retention, increased CPK (I.M. injections)

Dosage Forms Excipient information presented when available (limited, particularly for generics); consult specific product labeling. [DSC] = Discontinued product

Injection, solution, as hydrochloride [ampul]: 25 mg/0.5 mL (0.5 mL); 25 mg/mL (1 mL); 50 mg/mL (1 mL, 1.5 mL, 2 mL); 75 mg/mL (1 mL); 100 mg/mL (1 mL)

Injection, solution, as hydrochloride [prefilled syringe]: 25 mg/mL (1 mL); 50 mg/mL (1 mL); 75 mg/mL (1 mL); 100 mg/mL (1 mL)

Injection, solution, as hydrochloride [for PCA pump]: 10 mg/mL (30 mL, 50 mL [DSC], 60 mL)

Injection, solution, as hydrochloride [vial]: 25 mg/mL (1 mL); 50 mg/mL (1 mL, 30 mL); 75 mg/mL (1 mL); 100 mg/mL (1 mL, 20 mL) [may contain sodium metabisulfite]

Solution, oral, as hydrochloride: 50 mg/5 mL (500 mL)

Syrup, as hydrochloride:

Demerol®: 50 mg/5 mL (480 mL) [contains benzoic acid; banana flavor] [DSC]

Tablet, as hydrochloride: 50 mg, 100 mg

Demerol®: 50 mg, 100 mg

Meperidine and Promethazine

(me PER i deen & proe METH a zeen)

Index Terms Mepergan; Promethazine and Meperidine

Pharmacologic Category Analgesic Combination (Opioid)

Use Management of moderate pain

Restrictions C-II

Medication Safety Issues

Sound-alike/look-alike issues:

Mepergan may be confused with meprobamate

High alert medication: The Institute for Safe Medication Practices (ISMP) includes this medication among its list of drug classes which have a heightened risk of causing significant patient harm when used in error.

Dosage Oral: Adults: One capsule every 4-6 hours as needed**Dosing adjustment/comment in renal impairment:** Repeated use in renal impairment **should be avoided** due to potential accumulation of neuroexcitatory meperidine metabolite.**Dosing adjustment/comments in hepatic disease:** Increased narcotic effect in cirrhosis

Additional Information Complete prescribing information for this medication should be consulted for additional detail.

Dosage Forms Excipient information presented when available (limited, particularly for generics); consult specific product labeling.

Capsule: Meperidine hydrochloride 50 mg and promethazine hydrochloride 25 mg

◆ **Meperidine Hydrochloride** *see* Meperidine *on page 943*

Mephobarbital (me foe BAR bi tal)

U.S. Brand Names Mebaral®

Canadian Brand Names Mebaral®

Index Terms Methylphenobarbital

Pharmacologic Category Barbiturate

Use Sedative; treatment of grand mal and petit mal epilepsy

Restrictions C-IV

Pregnancy Risk Factor D

Medication Safety Issues

Sound-alike/look-alike issues:

Mephobarbital may be confused with methocarbamol

Mebaral® may be confused with Medrol®, Mellaril®, Tegretol®

Dosage Oral:

Epilepsy:

Children: 6-12 mg/kg/day in 2-4 divided doses

Adults: 200-600 mg/day in 2-4 divided doses

Sedation:

Children:

<5 years: 16-32 mg 3-4 times/day

>5 years: 32-64 mg 3-4 times/day

Adults: 32-100 mg 3-4 times/day

Dosing adjustment in renal or hepatic impairment: Use with caution and reduce dosages

Additional Information Complete prescribing information for this medication should be consulted for additional detail.

Dosage Forms Excipient information presented when available (limited, particularly for generics); consult specific product labeling.

Tablet: 32 mg, 50 mg, 100 mg

◆ **Mephyton®** *see* Phytonadione *on page 1191*

Mepivacaine (me PIV a kane)

U.S. Brand Names Carbocaine®; Polocaine®; Polocaine® Dental; Polocaine® MPF; Scandonest® 3% Plain

Canadian Brand Names Carbocaine®; Polocaine®

Index Terms Mepivacaine Hydrochloride

Pharmacologic Category Local Anesthetic

Use Local or regional analgesia; anesthesia by local infiltration, peripheral and central neural techniques including epidural and caudal blocks; **not** for use in spinal anesthesia

Pregnancy Risk Factor C

Pregnancy Considerations Animal reproduction studies have not been conducted. Mepivacaine has been used in obstetrical analgesia.

Lactation Excretion in breast milk unknown/use caution

Medication Safety Issues

Sound-alike/look-alike issues:

Mepivacaine may be confused with bupivacaine

Polocaine® may be confused with prilocaine

High alert medication: The Institute for Safe Medication Practices (ISMP) includes this medication (epidural administration) among its list of drug classes which have a heightened risk of causing significant patient harm when used in error.

Contraindications Hypersensitivity to mepivacaine, other amide-type local anesthetics, or any component of the formulation

Warnings/Precautions Careful and constant monitoring of the patient's state of consciousness should be done following each local anesthetic injection; at such times, restlessness, anxiety, tinnitus, dizziness, blurred vision, tremors, depression, or drowsiness may be early warning signs of CNS toxicity. Treatment is primarily symptomatic and supportive. Use with caution in patients with cardiac disease, hepatic or renal disease, or hyperthyroidism. Local anesthetics have been associated with rare occurrences of sudden respiratory arrest; convulsions due to systemic toxicity leading to cardiac arrest have been reported presumably due to intravascular injection. A test dose is recommended prior to epidural administration and all reinforcing doses with continuous catheter technique. Do not use solutions containing preservatives for caudal or epidural block. Use caution in debilitated, elderly, or acutely-ill patients; dose reduction may be required. Resuscitative equipment, oxygen, and other resuscitative drugs should be available for immediate use.

Adverse Reactions Degree of adverse effects in the CNS and cardiovascular system is directly related to the blood levels of mepivacaine, route of administration, and physical status of the patient. The effects below are more likely to occur after systemic administration rather than infiltration.

Cardiovascular: Bradycardia, cardiac arrest, cardiac output decreased, heart block, hyper-/hypotension, myocardial depression, syncope, tachycardia, ventricular arrhythmias

Central nervous system: Anxiety, chills, convulsions, depression, dizziness, excitation, restlessness, tremors

Dermatologic: Angioneurotic edema, diaphoresis, erythema, pruritus, urticaria

Gastrointestinal: Fecal incontinence, nausea, vomiting

Genitourinary: Incontinence, urinary retention

Neuromuscular & skeletal: Paralysis

Ocular: Blurred vision, pupil constriction

Otic: Tinnitus

Respiratory: Apnea, hypoventilation, sneezing

Miscellaneous: Allergic reaction, anaphylactoid reaction

Drug Interactions

Avoid Concomitant Use There are no known interactions where it is recommended to avoid concomitant use.

Increased Effect/Toxicity There are no known significant interactions involving an increase in effect.

Decreased Effect There are no known significant interactions involving a decrease in effect.

Stability Store at controlled room temperature of 15°C to 30°C (59°F to 86°F). Brief exposure up to 40°C (104°F) does not adversely affect the product. Solutions may be sterilized. Dental solutions should be protected from light.

Mechanism of Action Mepivacaine is an amide local anesthetic similar to lidocaine; like all local anesthetics, mepivacaine acts by preventing the generation and conduction of nerve impulses

Pharmacodynamics/Kinetics

Onset of action (route and dose dependent): Range: 3-20 minutes

Duration (route and dose dependent): 2-2.5 hours

Protein binding: ~75%

Metabolism: Primarily hepatic via N-demethylation, hydroxylation, and glucuronidation

Half-life elimination: Neonates: 8.7-9 hours; Adults: 1.9-3 hours

Excretion: Urine (95% as metabolites)

Dosage

Injectable local anesthetic: Dose varies with procedure, degree of anesthesia needed, vascularity of tissue, duration of anesthesia required, and physical condition of patient. The smallest dose and concentration required to produce the desired effect should be used.

Children: Maximum dose: 5-6 mg/kg; only concentrations <2% should be used in children <3 years or <14 kg (30 lbs)

Adults: Maximum dose: 400 mg; do not exceed 1000 mg/24 hours

Cervical, brachial, intercostal, pudenal nerve block: 5-40 mL of a 1% solution (maximum: 400 mg) **or** 5-20 mL of a 2% solution (maximum: 400 mg). For pudenal block, inject 1/2 the total dose each side.

Transvaginal block (paracervical plus pudenal): Up to 30 mL (both sides) of a 1% solution (maximum: 300 mg). Inject 1/2 the total dose each side.

Paracervical block: Up to 20 mL (both sides) of a 1% solution (maximum: 200 mg). Inject 1/2 the total dose to each side. This is the maximum recommended dose per 90-minute procedure; inject slowly with 5 minutes between sides.

Caudal and epidural block (preservative free solutions only): 15-30 mL of a 1% solution (maximum: 300 mg) **or** 10-25 mL of a 1.5% solution (maximum: 375 mg) **or** 10-20 mL of a 2% solution (maximum: 400 mg)

Infiltration: Up to 40 mL of a 1% solution (maximum: 400 mg)

Therapeutic block (pain management): 1-5 mL of a 1% solution (maximum: 50 mg) **or** 1-5 mL of a 2% solution (maximum: 100 mg)

Dental anesthesia: Adults:

Single site in upper or lower jaw: 54 mg (1.8 mL) as a 3% solution

Infiltration and nerve block of entire oral cavity: 270 mg (9 mL) as a 3% solution. Manufacturer's maximum recommended dose is not more than 400 mg to normal healthy adults.

Administration Before injecting, withdraw syringe plunger to ensure injection is not into vein or artery

Monitoring Parameters Vital signs, state of consciousness; signs of CNS toxicity

Dosage Forms Excipient information presented when available (limited, particularly for generics); consult specific product labeling.

Injection, solution, as hydrochloride [contains methylparabens]:

Carbocaine®: 1% (50 mL); 2% (50 mL)

Polocaine®: 1% (50 mL); 2% (50 mL)

Scandonest® 3% Plain: 3% (1.7 mL) [dental cartridge]

Injection, solution, as hydrochloride [preservative free]:

Carbocaine®: 1% (30 mL); 1.5% (30 mL); 2% (20 mL); 3% (1.8 mL) [dental cartridge]

Polocaine® Dental: 3% (1.8 mL) [dental cartridge]

Polocaine® MPF: 1% (30 mL); 1.5% (30 mL); 2% (20 mL)

◆ **Mepivacaine Hydrochloride** *see* Mepivacaine *on page 945*

Meprobamate (me proe BA mate)

U.S. Brand Names Miltown® [DSC]

Canadian Brand Names Novo-Mepro

Index Terms Equanil

Pharmacologic Category Antianxiety Agent, Miscellaneous

Use Management of anxiety disorders

Unlabeled/Investigational Use Demonstrated value for muscle contraction, headache, premenstrual tension, external sphincter spasticity, muscle rigidity, opisthotonos-associated with tetanus

Restrictions C-IV

Pregnancy Risk Factor D

Medication Safety Issues

Sound-alike/look-alike issues:

Meprobamate may be confused with Mepergan, meperidine

Equanil may be confused with Elavil®

Dosage Oral:

Children 6-12 years: Anxiety: 100-200 mg 2-3 times/day

Adults: Anxiety: 400 mg 3-4 times/day, up to 2400 mg/day

Dosing interval in renal impairment:

Cl_{cr} 10-50 mL/minute: Administer every 9-12 hours

Cl_{cr} <10 mL/minute: Administer every 12-18 hours

Hemodialysis: Moderately dialyzable (20% to 50%)

Dosing adjustment in hepatic impairment: Probably necessary in patients with liver disease

Additional Information Complete prescribing information for this medication should be consulted for additional detail.

Dosage Forms Excipient information presented when available (limited, particularly for generics); consult specific product labeling. [DSC] = Discontinued product

Tablet: 200 mg, 400 mg [DSC]

Miltown®: 200 mg, 400 mg [DSC]

Meprobamate and Aspirin
(me proe BA mate & AS pir in)

U.S. Brand Names Equagesic®

Canadian Brand Names 292 MEP®

Index Terms Aspirin and Meprobamate

Pharmacologic Category Antianxiety Agent, Miscellaneous; Salicylate

Use Adjunct to the short-term treatment of pain in patients with skeletal-muscular disease exhibiting tension and/or anxiety

Restrictions C-IV

Pregnancy Risk Factor X

Dosage Oral: Children ≥12 years and Adults: 1-2 tablets 3-4 times/day for up to 10 days

Additional Information Complete prescribing information for this medication should be consulted for additional detail.

Dosage Forms Excipient information presented when available (limited, particularly for generics); consult specific product labeling.

Tablet:

Equagesic®: Meprobamate 200 mg and aspirin 325 mg

◆ **Mepron®** *see* Atovaquone *on page 153*

Mequinol and Tretinoin (ME kwi nole & TRET i noyn)

U.S. Brand Names Solagé®

Canadian Brand Names Solagé®

Index Terms Solage; Tretinoin and Mequinol

Pharmacologic Category Retinoic Acid Derivative; Vitamin A Derivative; Vitamin, Topical

Use Treatment of solar lentigines; the efficacy of using Solagé® daily for >24 weeks has not been established

Pregnancy Risk Factor X

Dosage Solar lentigines: Topical: Apply twice daily to solar lentigines using the applicator tip while avoiding application to the surrounding skin. Separate application by at least 8 hours or as directed by physician.

Additional Information Complete prescribing information for this medication should be consulted for additional detail.

Dosage Forms Excipient information presented when available (limited, particularly for generics); consult specific product labeling.

Liquid, topical:

Solagé®: Mequinol 2% and tretinoin 0.01% (30 mL) [contains alcohol 78%; dispensed in applicator bottle]

◆ **Mercaptoethane Sulfonate** *see* Mesna *on page 951*

Mercaptopurine (mer kap toe PYOOR een)

U.S. Brand Names Purinethol®

Canadian Brand Names Purinethol®

Index Terms 6-Mercaptopurine (error-prone abbreviation); 6-MP (error-prone abbreviation); NSC-755

Pharmacologic Category Antineoplastic Agent, Antimetabolite; Immunosuppressant Agent

Use Treatment (maintenance and induction) of acute lymphoblastic leukemia (ALL)

Unlabeled/Investigational Use Steroid-sparing agent for corticosteroid-dependent Crohn's disease (CD) and ulcerative colitis (UC); maintenance of remission in CD; fistulizing Crohn's disease

Pregnancy Risk Factor D

Lactation Enters breast milk/contraindicated

Medication Safety Issues

Sound-alike/look-alike issues:

Purinethol® may be confused with propylthiouracil

High alert medication: The Institute for Safe Medication Practices (ISMP) includes this medication among its list of drugs which have a heightened risk of causing significant patient harm when used in error.

To avoid potentially serious dosage errors, the terms "6-mercaptopurine" or "6-MP" should be avoided; use of these terms has been associated with sixfold overdosages.

Azathioprine is metabolized to mercaptopurine; concurrent use of these commercially-available products has resulted in profound myelosuppression.

Contraindications Hypersensitivity to mercaptopurine or any component of the formulation; patients whose disease showed prior resistance to mercaptopurine or thioguanine; severe liver disease, severe bone marrow suppression; pregnancy

Warnings/Precautions Hazardous agent - use appropriate precautions for handling and disposal. Consider adjusting dosage in patients with renal impairment or hepatic failure; use with caution in patients with prior bone marrow suppression. Toxicity to immunosuppressives is increased in elderly. Start with lowest recommended adult doses. Signs of infection, such as fever and WBC rise, may not occur. Lethargy and confusion may be more prominent signs of infection. Use caution with other hepatotoxic drugs or in dosages >2.5 mg/kg/day; hepatotoxicity may occur. Patients with genetic deficiency of thiopurine methyltransferase (TPMT) or concurrent therapy with drugs which may inhibit TPMT (eg, olsalazine) or xanthine oxidase (eg, allopurinol) may be sensitive to myelosuppressive effects. Azathioprine is metabolized to mercaptopurine; concomitant use may result in profound myelosuppression and should be avoided. Immune response to vaccines may be diminished.

To avoid potentially serious dosage errors, the terms "6-mercaptopurine" or "6-MP" should be avoided; use of these terms has been associated with sixfold overdosages.

Adverse Reactions

>10%:

Hematologic: Myelosuppression; leukopenia, thrombocytopenia, anemia

Onset: 7-10 days

Nadir: 14-16 days

Recovery: 21-28 days

Hepatic: Intrahepatic cholestasis and focal centralobular necrosis (40%), characterized by hyperbilirubinemia, increased alkaline phosphatase and AST, jaundice, ascites, encephalopathy; more common at doses >2.5 mg/kg/day. Usually occurs within 2 months of therapy but may occur within 1 week, or be delayed up to 8 years.

1% to 10%:

Central nervous system: Drug fever

Dermatologic: Hyperpigmentation, rash

Endocrine & metabolic: Hyperuricemia

Gastrointestinal: Nausea, vomiting, diarrhea, stomatitis, anorexia, stomach pain, mucositis

Renal: Renal toxicity

<1% (Limited to important or life-threatening): Alopecia, dry and scaling rash, glossitis, oligospermia, tarry stools

Drug Interactions

Avoid Concomitant Use

Avoid concomitant use of Mercaptopurine with any of the following: Natalizumab; Vaccines (Live)

Increased Effect/Toxicity

Mercaptopurine may increase the levels/effects of: Natalizumab; Vaccines (Live); Vitamin K Antagonists

The levels/effects of Mercaptopurine may be increased by: 5-ASA Derivatives; Allopurinol; AzaTHIOprine; Trastuzumab

Decreased Effect

Mercaptopurine may decrease the levels/effects of: Vaccines (Inactivated); Vitamin K Antagonists

The levels/effects of Mercaptopurine may be decreased by: Echinacea

Stability Store at room temperature of 15°C to 25°C (59°F to 77°F). Protect from moisture.

Mechanism of Action Purine antagonist which inhibits DNA and RNA synthesis; acts as false metabolite and is incorporated into DNA and RNA, eventually inhibiting their synthesis; specific for the S phase of the cell cycle

Pharmacodynamics/Kinetics

Absorption: Variable and incomplete (16% to 50%)

Distribution: V_d = total body water; CNS penetration is poor

Protein binding: 19%

Metabolism: Hepatic and in GI mucosa; hepatically via xanthine oxidase and methylation via TPMT to sulfate conjugates, 6-thiouric acid, and other inactive compounds; first-pass effect

Half-life elimination (age dependent): Children: 21 minutes; Adults: 47 minutes

Time to peak, serum: ~2 hours

Excretion: Urine (46% as mercaptopurine and metabolites)

Dosage Oral (refer to individual protocols):

Children: ALL:

Induction: 2.5-5 mg/kg/day **or** 70-100 mg/m²/day given once daily

Maintenance: 1.5-2.5 mg/kg/day **or** 50-75 mg/m²/day given once daily

Adults:

ALL:

Induction: 2.5-5 mg/kg/day (100-200 mg)

Maintenance: 1.5-2.5 mg/kg/day **or** 80-100 mg/m²/day given once daily

Reduction of steroid use in CD or UC, maintenance of remission in CD or fistulizing disease (unlabeled uses): Initial: 50 mg daily; may increase by 25 mg/day every 1-2 weeks as tolerated to target dose of 1-1.5 mg/kg/day

Dosage adjustment with concurrent allopurinol: Reduce mercaptopurine dosage to 1/4 to 1/3 the usual dose.

Dosage adjustment in TPMT-deficiency: Not established; substantial reductions are generally required only in homozygous deficiency.

Elderly: Due to renal decline with age, start with lower recommended doses for adults

Note: In ALL, administration in the evening (vs morning administration) may lower the risk of relapse.

Dosing adjustment in renal impairment: The FDA-approved labeling recommends starting with reduced doses in patients with renal impairment to avoid accumulation; however, specific guidelines are not available. The following guidelines have been used by some clinicians (Aronoff, 2007): Children:

Cl_{cr} <50 mL/minute: Administer every 48 hours

Hemodialysis: Administer every 48 hours

Continuous ambulatory peritoneal dialysis (CAPD): Administer every 48 hours

Continuous renal replacement therapy (CRRT): Administer every 48 hours

Dosing adjustment in hepatic impairment: The FDA-approved labeling recommends considering a reduced dose in patients with hepatic impairment; however, specific guidelines are not available.

Dietary Considerations Should not be administered with meals.

Administration Preferably on an empty stomach (1 hour before or 2 hours after meals)

Monitoring Parameters CBC with differential and platelet count, liver function tests, uric acid, urinalysis; TPMT genotyping may identify individuals at risk for toxicity

For use as immunomodulatory therapy in CD or UC, monitor CBC with differential weekly for 1 month, then biweekly for 1 month, followed by monitoring every 1-2 months throughout the course of therapy. LFTs should be assessed every 3 months.

Dosage Forms Excipient information presented when available (limited, particularly for generics); consult specific product labeling.

Tablet [scored]: 50 mg

Extemporaneous Preparations A 50 mg/mL oral suspension can be prepared by crushing thirty 50 mg tablets in a mortar, and then mixing in a small amount of vehicle (a 1:1 combination of methylcellulose 1% and syrup) to create a uniform paste. Add a sufficient quantity of vehicle to make 30 mL of suspension. Label "shake well." Room temperature stability is 14 days.

Dressman JB and Poust RI, "Stability of Allopurinol and of Five Antineoplastics in Suspension," *Am J Hosp Pharm*, 1983, 40:616-8.

Nahata MC, Morosco RS, and Hipple TF, 4th ed, *Pediatric Drug Formulations*, Cincinnati, OH: Harvey Whitney Books Co, 2000.

◆ **6-Mercaptopurine (error-prone abbreviation)** *see* Mercaptopurine *on page 946*

◆ **Mercapturic Acid** *see* Acetylcysteine *on page 36*

◆ **Meridia®** *see* Sibutramine *on page 1366*

Meropenem (mer oh PEN em)

U.S. Brand Names Merrem® I.V.

Canadian Brand Names Merrem®

Pharmacologic Category Antibiotic, Carbapenem

Additional Appendix Information

Antimicrobial Drugs of Choice *on page 1752*

Community-Acquired Pneumonia in Adults *on page 1766*

Use Treatment of intra-abdominal infections (complicated appendicitis and peritonitis); treatment of bacterial meningitis in pediatric patients ≥3 months of age caused by *S. pneumoniae, H. influenzae*, and *N. meningitidis*; treatment of complicated skin and skin structure infections caused by susceptible organisms

Unlabeled/Investigational Use *Burkholderia pseudomallei* (melioidosis), febrile neutropenia, liver abscess, meningitis (adults), otitis externa, pneumonia, urinary tract infections

Pregnancy Risk Factor B

Pregnancy Considerations Meropenem is classified as pregnancy category B because no evidence of impaired fertility or fetal harm has been found in animals. Adequate and well-controlled studies have not been conducted in pregnant women and it is not known whether meropenem can cause fetal harm.

Lactation Excretion in breast milk unknown/use caution

Medication Safety Issues

Sound-alike/look-alike issues:

Meropenem may be confused with ertapenem, imipenem, metronidazole.

Contraindications Hypersensitivity to meropenem, any component of the formulation, or other carbapenems (eg, imipenem); patients who have experienced anaphylactic reactions to other beta-lactams

Warnings/Precautions

Serious hypersensitivity reactions, including anaphylaxis, have been reported (some without a history of previous allergic reactions to beta-lactams). Has been associated with CNS adverse effects, including confusional states and seizures; use caution with CNS disorders (eg, brain lesions, history of seizures, or renal impairment). Prolonged use may result in fungal or bacterial superinfection, including *C. difficile*-associated diarrhea (CDAD) and pseudomembranous colitis; CDAD has been observed >2 months postantibiotic treatment. Use with caution in patients with renal impairment; dosage adjustment required in patients with moderate-to-severe renal dysfunction. Thrombocytopenia has been reported in patients with renal dysfunction. Lower doses (based upon renal function) are often required in the elderly.

Adverse Reactions

1% to 10%:

Cardiovascular: Peripheral vascular disorder

Central nervous system: Headache (2% to 8%), pain (≤5%)

Dermatologic: Rash (2% to 3%, includes diaper-area moniliasis in pediatrics), pruritus (1%)

Endocrine & metabolic: Hypoglycemia

Gastrointestinal: Diarrhea (4% to 7%), nausea/vomiting (1% to 8%), constipation (1% to 7%), oral moniliasis (up to 2% in pediatric patients), glossitis (1%)

Hematologic: Anemia (≤6%)

Local: Inflammation at the injection site (2%), phlebitis/thrombophlebitis (1%), injection site reaction (1%)

Respiratory: Apnea (1%), pharyngitis, pneumonia

Miscellaneous: Sepsis (2%), shock (1%)

<1% (Limited to important or life-threatening): Abdominal enlargement, abdominal pain, agitation/delirium, agranulocytosis, alkaline phosphatase increased, ALT increased, AST increased, anemia (hypochromic), angioedema, anorexia, anxiety, asthma, back pain, bilirubin increased, bradycardia, BUN increased, chest pain, chills, cholestatic jaundice/jaundice, confusion, cough, creatinine increased, depression, diaphoresis, dizziness, dyspepsia, dyspnea, dysuria, eosinophilia, epistaxis (0.2%), erythema multiforme, fever, flatulence, gastrointestinal hemorrhage (0.5%), hallucinations, heart failure, hemoglobin/hematocrit decreased, hemolytic anemia, hemoperitoneum (0.2%), hepatic failure, hyper-/hypotension, hypervolemia, hypokalemia, hypoxia, ileus, insomnia, intestinal obstruction, LDH increased, leukocytosis, leukopenia, melena (0.3%), MI, nervousness, neutropenia, paresthesia, pelvic pain, peripheral edema, platelets decreased/increased, pleural effusion, prothrombin time decreased, pulmonary edema, positive Coombs test, pulmonary embolism, renal failure, respiratory disorder, seizure, skin ulcer, somnolence, Stevens-Johnson syndrome, syncope, tachycardia, toxic epidermal necrolysis, urinary incontinence, urticaria, vaginal moniliasis, weakness, WBC decreased, whole body pain

Drug Interactions

Avoid Concomitant Use There are no known interactions where it is recommended to avoid concomitant use.

Increased Effect/Toxicity

The levels/effects of Meropenem may be increased by: Uricosuric Agents

Decreased Effect

Meropenem may decrease the levels/effects of: Typhoid Vaccine; Valproic Acid

Stability Dry powder should be stored at controlled room temperature 20°C to 25°C (68°F to 77°F). Meropenem infusion vials may be reconstituted with SWFI or a compatible diluent (eg, NS). The 500 mg vials should be reconstituted with 10 mL, and 1 g vials with 20 mL. May be further diluted with compatible solutions for infusion. Consult detailed reference/product labeling for compatibility.

Injection reconstitution: Stability in vial when constituted (up to 50 mg/mL) with:

SWFI: Stable for up to 2 hours at controlled room temperature of 15°C to 25°C (59°F to 77°F) or for up to 12 hours under refrigeration.

Sodium chloride: Stable for up to 2 hours at controlled room temperature of 15°C to 25°C (59°F to 77°F) or for up to 18 hours under refrigeration.

Dextrose 5% injection: Stable for 1 hour at controlled room temperature of 15°C to 25°C (59°F to 77°F) or for 8 hours under refrigeration.

Infusion admixture (1-20 mg/mL): Solution stability when diluted in NS is 4 hours at controlled room temperature of 15°C to 25°C (59°F to 77°F) or 24 hours under refrigeration. Stability in D_5W is 1 hour at controlled room temperature of 15°C to 25°C (59°F to 77°F) or 4 hours under refrigeration.

Mechanism of Action Inhibits bacterial cell wall synthesis by binding to several of the penicillin-binding proteins, which in turn inhibit the final transpeptidation step of peptidoglycan synthesis in bacterial cell walls, thus inhibiting cell wall biosynthesis; bacteria eventually lyse due to ongoing activity of cell wall autolytic enzymes (autolysins and murein hydrolases) while cell wall assembly is arrested

Pharmacodynamics/Kinetics

Distribution: V_d: Adults: ~0.3 L/kg, Children: 0.4-0.5 L/kg; penetrates well into most body fluids and tissues; CSF concentrations approximate those of the plasma

Protein binding: ~2%

Metabolism: Hepatic; metabolized to open beta-lactam form (inactive)

Half-life elimination:

Normal renal function: 1-1.5 hours

Cl_{cr} 30-80 mL/minute: 1.9-3.3 hours

Cl_{cr} 2-30 mL/minute: 3.82-5.7 hours

Time to peak, tissue: 1 hour following infusion

Excretion: Urine (~25% as inactive metabolites)

Dosage

Usual dosage ranges:

Neonates: I.V.:

Postnatal age 0-7 days: 20 mg/kg/dose every 12 hours

Postnatal age >7 days:

Weight 1200-2000 g: 20 mg/kg/dose every 12 hours

Weight >2000 g: 20 mg/kg/dose every 8 hours

Children ≥3 months: I.V.: 30-120 mg/kg/day divided every 8 hours (maximum dose: 6 g/day)

Adults: I.V.: 1.5-6 g/day divided every 8 hours

Indication-specific dosing:

Children ≥3 months (<50 kg): I.V.:

Febrile neutropenia (unlabeled use): 20 mg/kg every 8 hours (maximum dose: 1 g every 8 hours)

Intra-abdominal infections: 20 mg/kg every 8 hours (maximum dose: 1 g every 8 hours)

Meningitis: 40 mg/kg every 8 hours (maximum dose: 2 g every 8 hours)

Skin and skin structure infections (complicated): 10 mg/kg every 8 hours (maximum dose: 500 mg every 8 hours)

Children >50 kg and Adults: I.V.:

Burkholderia pseudomallei* (melioidosis) (unlabeled use), *Pseudomonas: 1 g every 8 hours

Cholangitis, intra-abdominal infections: 1 g every 8 hours

Febrile neutropenia, otitis externa, pneumonia (unlabeled uses): 1 g every 8 hours

Liver abscess (unlabeled use): 1 g every 8 hours for 2-3 weeks, then oral therapy for duration of 4-6 weeks

Meningitis (unlabeled use): 2 g every 8 hours

Mild-to-moderate infection, other severe infections (unlabeled use): 1.5-3 g/day divided every 8 hours

Skin and skin structure infections (complicated): 500 mg every 8 hours; diabetic foot: 1 g every 8 hours

Urinary tract infections, complicated (unlabeled use): 500 mg to 1 g every 8 hours

Dosing adjustment in renal impairment: Adults:

Cl_{cr} 26-50 mL/minute: Administer recommended dose based on indication every 12 hours

Cl_{cr} 10-25 mL/minute: Administer one-half recommended dose based on indication every 12 hours

Cl_{cr} <10 mL/minute: Administer one-half recommended dose based on indication every 24 hours

Dialysis: Meropenem and its metabolites are readily dialyzable; administer dose after dialysis

Continuous renal replacement therapy (CRRT): Drug clearance is highly dependent on the method of renal replacement, filter type, and flow rate. Appropriate dosing requires close monitoring of pharmacologic response, signs of adverse reactions due to drug accumulation, as well as drug levels in relation to target trough (if appropriate). The following are general recommendations only (based on dialysate flow/ultrafiltration rates of 1 L/hour) and should not supersede clinical judgment:

CVVH or CVVHD/CVVHDF: 1 g every 12 hours to achieve target trough of ~4 mg/L; 500 mg every 12 hours may be considered for highly sensitive organisms. **Note:** Substantial variability exists in various published recommendations, ranging from 1-3 g/day given in 2-3 divided doses.

Dietary Considerations 1 g of meropenem contains 90.2 mg of sodium as sodium carbonate (3.92 mEq)

Administration Administer I.V. infusion over 15-30 minutes; I.V. bolus injection over 3-5 minutes

Monitoring Parameters Perform culture and sensitivity testing prior to initiating therapy. Monitor for signs of anaphylaxis during first dose. During prolonged therapy, monitor renal function, liver function, CBC.

Dosage Forms Excipient information presented when available (limited, particularly for generics); consult specific product labeling.

Injection, powder for reconstitution:

Merrem® I.V: 500 mg [contains sodium 45.1 mg as sodium carbonate (1.96 mEq)]; 1 g [contains sodium 90.2 mg as sodium carbonate (3.92 mEq)]

◆ **Merrem® (Can)** *see* Meropenem *on page 948*

◆ **Merrem® I.V.** *see* Meropenem *on page 948*

◆ **Meruvax® II** *see* Rubella Virus Vaccine (Live) *on page 1348*

Mesalamine (me SAL a meen)

U.S. Brand Names Apriso™; Asacol®; Canasa®; Lialda™; Pentasa®; Rowasa®

Canadian Brand Names Asacol®; Asacol® 800; Mesasal®; Mezavant®; Novo-5 ASA; Pendo-5 ASA; Pentasa®; Quintasa®; Rowasa®; Salofalk®

Index Terms 5-Aminosalicylic Acid; 5-ASA; Fisalamine; Mesalazine

Pharmacologic Category 5-Aminosalicylic Acid Derivative

Use

Oral: Treatment and maintenance of remission of mildly- to moderately-active ulcerative colitis

Rectal: Treatment of active mild-to-moderate distal ulcerative colitis, proctosigmoiditis, or proctitis

Pregnancy Risk Factor B

Pregnancy Considerations Animal studies have not demonstrated teratogenicity or fertility impairment. There are no adequate and well-controlled studies in pregnant women. Mesalamine is known to cross the placenta.

Lactation Enters breast milk/use caution

Medication Safety Issues

Sound-alike/look-alike issues:

Mesalamine may be confused with mecamylamine, methenamine

Apriso™ may be confused with Apri®

Asacol® may be confused with Ansaid®, Os-Cal®

Lialda™ may be confused with Aldara®

Contraindications Hypersensitivity to mesalamine, aminosalicylates, salicylates, or any component of the formulation

Warnings/Precautions May cause an acute intolerance syndrome (cramping, acute abdominal pain, bloody diarrhea; sometimes fever, headache, rash); discontinue if this occurs. Use caution in patients with active peptic ulcers. Patients with pyloric stenosis may have prolonged gastric retention of tablets, delaying the release of mesalamine in the colon. Pericarditis or myocarditis should be considered in patients with chest pain; use with caution in patients predisposed to these conditions. Pancreatitis should be considered in patients with new abdominal discomfort. Symptomatic worsening of colitis/IBD may occur following initiation of therapy. Oligospermia (rare, reversible) has been reported in males. Use caution in patients with sulfasalazine hypersensitivity. Use caution in patients with impaired hepatic function; hepatic failure has been reported. Renal impairment (including minimal change nephropathy and acute/chronic interstitial nephritis) and failure have been reported; use caution in patients with renal impairment. Use caution with other medications converted to mesalamine. Postmarketing reports suggest an increased incidence of blood dyscrasias in patients >65 years of age. In addition, elderly may have difficulty administering and retaining rectal suppositories or may have decreased renal function; use with caution and monitor. Safety and efficacy in pediatric patients have not been established.

Apriso™ contains phenylalanine. Canasa® suppositories contain saturated vegetable fatty acid esters (contraindicated in patients with allergy to these components). Rowasa® enema contains potassium metabisulfite; may cause severe hypersensitivity reactions (ie, anaphylaxis) in patients with sulfite allergies.

Adverse Reactions Adverse effects vary depending upon dosage form. Incidence usually on lower end with enema and suppository dosage forms.

>10%:

Central nervous system: Headache (2% to 35%), pain (≤14%)

Gastrointestinal: Abdominal pain (1% to 18%), eructation (16%), nausea (3% to 13%)

Respiratory: Pharyngitis (11%)

1% to 10%:

Cardiovascular: Chest pain (3%), peripheral edema (3%)

Central nervous system: Dizziness (2% to 8%), fever (1% to 6%), chills (3%), malaise (2% to 3%), fatigue (<3%), vertigo (<3%), insomnia (2%)

Dermatologic: Rash (1% to 6%), pruritus (1% to 3%), alopecia (<3%), acne (1% to 2%)

Endocrine & metabolic: Triglyceride increased (<3%)

Gastrointestinal: Diarrhea (8%), dyspepsia (6%), flatulence (2% to 6%), constipation (5%), vomiting (1% to 5%), colitis exacerbation (1% to 3%), rectal bleeding (<3%), rectal pain (1% to 2%), hemorrhoids (1%)

Hematologic: Hematocrit/hemoglobin decreased (<3%)

Hepatic: Cholestatic hepatitis (<3%), transaminases increased (<3%), ALT increased (1%)

Local: Pain on insertion of enema tip (1%)

Neuromuscular & skeletal: Back pain (1% to 7%), arthralgia (≤5%), hypertonia (5%), myalgia (3%), arthritis (2%), leg/joint pain (2%)

Ocular: Conjunctivitis (2%)

Otic: Tinnitus (<3%)

Renal: Creatinine clearance decreased (<3%), hematuria (<3%)

Respiratory: Nasopharyngitis (4%), dyspnea (<3%), cough (2%)

Miscellaneous: Flu-like syndrome (3% to 5%), diaphoresis (3%), intolerance syndrome (3%)

<1% (Limited to important or life-threatening): Abdominal distention, agranulocytosis, albuminuria, alkaline phosphatase increased, amenorrhea, anxiety, anemia, angioedema, anorexia, aplastic anemia, asthma exacerbation, bilirubin increased, bloody diarrhea, bronchitis, BUN increased, cholestatic jaundice, cholecystitis, cramping, depression, disorientation, drug fever, dysphagia, dysuria, ear pain, edema, emotional lability, eosinophilia, eosinophilic pneumonia, epididymitis, erythema nodosum, eye pain, facial edema, fecal incontinence, fibrosing alveolitis, gastritis, gastroenteritis, gastrointestinal bleeding, GGT increased, gout, granulocytopenia, Guillain-Barré syndrome, hepatic failure, hepatic necrosis, hepatitis, hepatocellular damage, hepatotoxicity, hyperesthesia, hypersensitivity pneumonitis, hyper-/hypotension, indigestion, infertility, interstitial nephritis, interstitial pneumonia, jaundice, Kawasaki-like syndrome, LDH increased, leukopenia, libido decreased, lichen planus, lupus-like syndrome, lymphadenopathy, menorrhagia, metrorrhagia, migraine, minimal change nephrotic syndrome, myocarditis, neck pain, nephropathy, nephrotoxicity, neutropenia, oligospermia, oral moniliases, oral ulcers, palpitation, pancreatitis, pancytopenia, paresthesia, perforated peptic ulcer, pericardial effusion, pericarditis, peripheral neuropathy, pharyngolaryngeal pain, photosensitivity, pleuritis, pneumonitis, prurigo, psoriasis, pyoderma gangrenosum, rectal polyp, renal failure, rheumatoid arthritis, rhinitis, serum creatinine increased, somnolence, stomatitis, stool abnormalities, systemic lupus erythematosus, tachycardia, taste perversion, tenesmus, thrombocythemia, thrombocytopenia, transverse myelitis, tremor, T-wave abnormalities, urinary frequency, urinary urgency, urticaria, vasodilation, vision abnormalities, weakness, xerostomia

Drug Interactions

Avoid Concomitant Use

Avoid concomitant use of Mesalamine with any of the following: Antacids; H2-Antagonists; Proton Pump Inhibitors

Increased Effect/Toxicity

Mesalamine may increase the levels/effects of: Thiopurine Analogs; Varicella Virus-Containing Vaccines

Decreased Effect

Mesalamine may decrease the levels/effects of: Cardiac Glycosides

The levels/effects of Mesalamine may be decreased by: Antacids; H2-Antagonists; Proton Pump Inhibitors

Stability

Capsule:

Apriso™: Store at controlled room temperature of 20°C to 25°C (68°F to 77°F)

Pentasa®: Store at controlled room temperature of 15°C to 30°C (59°F to 86°F). Protect from light.

Enema: Store at controlled room temperature. Use promptly once foil wrap is removed. Contents may darken with time (do not use if dark brown).

Suppository: Store below 25°C (below 77°F). May store under refrigeration; do not freeze. Protect from direct heat, light, and humidity.

Tablet: Store at controlled room temperature:

Asacol®: 20°C to 25°C (68°F to 77°F)

Lialda™: 15°C to 30°C (59°F to 86°F)

Mezavant®: 15°C to 25°C (59°F to 77°F)

Mechanism of Action Mesalamine (5-aminosalicylic acid) is the active component of sulfasalazine; the specific mechanism of action of mesalamine is unknown; however, it is thought that it modulates local chemical mediators of the inflammatory response, especially leukotrienes, and is also postulated to be a free radical scavenger or an inhibitor of tumor necrosis factor (TNF); action appears topical rather than systemic

Pharmacodynamics/Kinetics

Absorption: Rectal: Variable and dependent upon retention time, underlying GI disease, and colonic pH; Oral: Tablet: ~21% to 28%, Capsule: ~20% to 40%

Distribution: ~18 L

Protein binding: 43%

Metabolism: Hepatic and via GI tract to N-acetyl-5-aminosalicylic acid

Half-life elimination: 5-ASA: 0.5-10 hours; N-acetyl-5-ASA: 2-15 hours

Time to peak, serum:

Capsule: Apriso™: ~4 hours; Pentasa®: 3 hours

Rectal: 4-7 hours

Tablet: Asacol®: 4-12 hours; Lialda™: 9-12 hours; Mezavant®: 8 hours

Excretion: Urine (primarily as metabolites, <8% as unchanged drug); feces (<2%)

Dosage Adults:

Oral:

Treatment of ulcerative colitis (usual course of therapy is 3-8 weeks):

Capsule: 1 g 4 times/day

Tablet: Initial:

Asacol®: 800 mg 3 times/day for 6 weeks

Lialda™, Mezavant®: 2.4-4.8 g once daily for up to 8 weeks

Maintenance of remission of ulcerative colitis:

Capsule:

Apriso™: 1.5 g once daily in the morning

Pentasa®: 1 g 4 times/day

Tablet (Asacol®): 1.6 g/day in divided doses; **Note:** Lialda™ and Mezavant® tablets are approved for treatment only.

Rectal:

Retention enema: 60 mL (4 g) at bedtime, retained overnight, approximately 8 hours

Rectal suppository (Canasa®): Insert one 1000 mg suppository in rectum daily at bedtime

Note: Suppositories should be retained for at least 1-3 hours to achieve maximum benefit.

Note: Some patients may require rectal and oral therapy concurrently.

Elderly: See adult dosing; use with caution

Dietary Considerations

Apriso™: Take with or without food; do not administer with antacids. Contains 0.56 mg phenylalanine per capsule.

Canasa® rectal suppository contains saturated vegetable fatty acid esters.

Administration

Oral: Swallow capsules or tablets whole, do not chew or crush.

Apriso™: Administer with or without food; do not administer with antacids

Asacol®: Do not break outer coating.

Lialda™: Do not break outer coating; should be administered once daily with a meal

Mezavant®: Do not break outer coating; should be administered once daily with a meal

Rectal enema: Shake bottle well. Retain enemas for 8 hours or as long as practical.

Suppository: Remove foil wrapper; avoid excessive handling. Should be retained for at least 1-3 hours to achieve maximum benefit.

Monitoring Parameters CBC and renal function, particularly in elderly patients

Dosage Forms Excipient information presented when available (limited, particularly for generics); consult specific product labeling. [CAN] = Canadian brand name

Capsule, controlled release:

Pentasa®: 250 mg, 500 mg

Capsule, extended release:

Apriso™: 0.375 g [contains phenylalanine 0.56 mg/capsule]

Suppository, rectal:

Canasa®: 1000 mg [contains saturated vegetable fatty acid esters]

Suspension, rectal: 4 g/60 mL (7s, 28s) [contains potassium metabisulfite and sodium benzoate]

Rowasa®: 4 g/60 mL (7s, 28s) [contains potassium metabisulfite and sodium benzoate]

Tablet, delayed release [enteric coated]:

Asacol®: 400 mg

Lialda™: 1.2 g

Tablet, delayed and extended release:

Mezavant® [CAN]: 1.2 g [not available in U.S.]

◆ **Mesalazine** *see* Mesalamine *on page* 949

◆ **Mesasal® (Can)** *see* Mesalamine *on page* 949

◆ **M-Eslon® (Can)** *see* Morphine Sulfate *on page* 1016

Mesna (MES na)

U.S. Brand Names Mesnex®

Canadian Brand Names Mesnex®; Uromitexan

Index Terms Mercaptoethane Sulfonate; Sodium 2-Mercaptoethane Sulfonate

Pharmacologic Category Antidote; Uroprotectant

Use Preventative agent to reduce the incidence of ifosfamide-induced hemorrhagic cystitis

Unlabeled/Investigational Use Preventative agent to reduce the incidence of cyclophosphamide-induced hemorrhagic cystitis with high-dose cyclophosphamide

Pregnancy Risk Factor B

Pregnancy Considerations Teratogenic effects were not observed in animal studies. There are no adequate and well-controlled studies in pregnant women. Use during pregnancy only if clearly needed.

Lactation Excretion in breast milk unknown/not recommended

Contraindications Hypersensitivity to mesna or other thiol compounds, or any component of the formulation

Warnings/Precautions Examine morning urine specimen for hematuria prior to ifosfamide or cyclophosphamide treatment; if hematuria (>50 RBC/HPF) develops, reduce the ifosfamide/cyclophosphamide dose or discontinue the drug; will not prevent or alleviate other toxicities associated with ifosfamide or cyclophosphamide and will not prevent hemorrhagic cystitis in all patients. Mesna will not reduce the risk of thrombocytopenia-related hematuria. Allergic reactions have been reported; symptoms ranged from mild hypersensitivity to systemic anaphylactic reactions; patients with autoimmune disorders receiving cyclophosphamide and mesna may be at increased risk. Patients should receive adequate hydration during treatment. I.V. formulation contains benzyl alcohol; do not use in neonates or infants (associated with "gasping syndrome").

Adverse Reactions

Mesna alone (frequency not defined):

Cardiovascular: Flushing

Central nervous system: Dizziness, fever, headache, hyperesthesia, somnolence

Dermatologic: Rash

Gastrointestinal: Anorexia, constipation, diarrhea, flatulence, nausea, taste alteration/bad taste (with oral administration), vomiting

Local: Injection site reactions

Neuromuscular: Arthralgia, back pain, rigors

Ocular: Conjunctivitis

Respiratory: Cough, pharyngitis, rhinitis

Miscellaneous: Flu-like syndrome

Mesna alone or in combination: Postmarketing and/or case reports: Allergic reaction, anaphylactic reaction, hypersensitivity, hyper-/hypotension, injection site erythema, injection site pain, limb pain, malaise, myalgia, platelets decreased, ST-segment increased, tachycardia, tachypnea, transaminases increased

Drug Interactions

Avoid Concomitant Use There are no known interactions where it is recommended to avoid concomitant use.

Increased Effect/Toxicity There are no known significant interactions involving an increase in effect.

Decreased Effect There are no known significant interactions involving a decrease in effect.

Stability Store intact vials and tablets at room temperature of 20°C to 25°C (68°F to 77°F). Opened multidose vials may be stored and used for up to 8 days after opening. Dilute injection in 50-1000 mL D_5W, NS, $D_5{}^1\!/\!_4NS$, $D_5{}^1\!/\!_3NS$, $D_5{}^1\!/\!_2NS$, or lactated Ringer's for infusion (the manufacturer recommends a final concentration of 20 mg/mL). Solutions diluted for infusion are stable for at least 24 hours at room temperature. Solutions in plastic syringes are stable for 9 days under refrigeration, or at room or body temperature. Solutions of mesna and ifosfamide in lactated Ringer's are stable for 7 days in a PVC ambulatory infusion pump reservoir. Solutions of mesna (0.5-3.2 mg/mL) and cyclophosphamide (1.8-10.8 mg/mL) in D_5W are stable for 48 hours refrigerated or 6 hours at room temperature (Menard, 2003). Mesna injection is stable for at least 7 days when diluted 1:2 or 1:5 with grape- and orange-flavored syrups or 11:1 to 1:100 in carbonated beverages for oral administration.

Mechanism of Action In blood, mesna is oxidized to dimesna which in turn is reduced in the kidney back to mesna, supplying a free thiol group which binds to and inactivates acrolein, the urotoxic metabolite of ifosfamide and cyclophosphamide

Pharmacodynamics/Kinetics

Distribution: No tissue penetration

Protein binding: 69% to 75%

Metabolism: Rapidly oxidized intravascularly to mesna disulfide (dimesna); dimesna is reduced in renal tubules back to mesna following glomerular filtration

Bioavailability: Oral: 45% to 79%

Half-life elimination:

I.V.: Mesna: ~22 minutes; Dimesna: ~70 minutes

I.V. followed by oral: 1-8 hours

Time to peak, plasma: 2-3 hours

Excretion: Urine (18% to 32% as mesna; 33% as dimesna)

Dosage

Children and Adults: **Note:** Details concerning dosing in combination regimens should also be consulted. Mesna dosing schedule should be repeated each day ifosfamide is received. If ifosfamide dose is adjusted, the mesna dose should also be modified to maintain the mesna-to-ifosfamide ratio.

I.V.: Prevention of ifosfamide-induced hemorrhagic cystitis:

Short infusion standard-dose ifosfamide (<2.5 g/m^2/day): Mesna dose is equal to 60% of the ifosfamide dose given in 3 divided doses (0, 4, and 8 hours after the start of ifosfamide)

Continuous infusion standard-dose ifosfamide (<2.5 g/m^2/day): ASCO guidelines: Mesna dose (as an I.V. bolus) is equal to 20% of the ifosfamide dose, followed by a continuous infusion of mesna at 40% of the ifosfamide dose, continue mesna infusion for 12-24 hours after completion of ifosfamide infusion (Hensley, 2008)

High-dose ifosfamide (>2.5 g/m^2/day): ASCO guidelines: Evidence for use is inadequate; more frequent and prolonged mesna administration regimens may be required.

I.V. followed by oral (for ifosfamide doses ≤2 g/m^2/day): Mesna dose is equal to 100% of the ifosfamide dose, given as 20% of the ifosfamide dose I.V. at hour 0, followed by 40% of the ifosfamide dose given orally 2 and 6 hours after start of ifosfamide

Administration

Oral: Administer orally in tablet formulation or parenteral solution diluted in water, milk, juice, or carbonated beverages; patients who vomit within 2 hours after taking oral mesna should repeat the dose or receive I.V. mesna

I.V.: Administer by short (15-30 minutes) infusion or continuous infusion (maintain continuous infusion for 12-24 after completion of ifosfamide infusion) (Hensley, 2008)

Monitoring Parameters Urinalysis

Test Interactions False-positive urinary ketones with Multistix® or Labstix®

Additional Information Oncology Comment: Guidelines from the American Society of Clinical Oncology (ASCO) for the use of chemotherapy and radiotherapy protectants (Schuchter, 2002; Hensley, 2008 [update]) recommend mesna to decrease the incidence of ifosfamide-induced urotoxicity associated with short infusion and continuous infusion standard-dose ifosfamide (<2.5 g/m^2/day). Although evidence is inadequate regarding mesna's uroprotective effects in high-dose ifosfamide (>2.5 g/m^2/day), the guidelines suggest more frequent and prolonged mesna administration times may be required. For prevention high-dose cyclophosphamide-induced urotoxicity (associated with stem cell transplantation), the guidelines recommend mesna in conjunction with saline diuresis (or forced saline diuresis alone).

Dosage Forms Excipient information presented when available (limited, particularly for generics); consult specific product labeling.

Injection, solution: 100 mg/mL (10 mL) [contains benzyl alcohol]

Mesnex®: 100 mg/mL (10 mL) [contains benzyl alcohol]

Tablet:

Mesnex®: 400 mg

- **Mesnex®** *see* Mesna *on page* *951*
- **Mestinon®** *see* Pyridostigmine *on page* *1272*
- **Mestinon®-SR (Can)** *see* Pyridostigmine *on page* *1272*
- **Mestinon® Timespan®** *see* Pyridostigmine *on page* *1272*
- **Mestranol and Norethindrone** *see* Norethindrone and Mestranol *on page* *1079*
- **Metacortandralone** *see* PrednisoLONE *on page* *1230*
- **Metadate® CD** *see* Methylphenidate *on page* *973*
- **Metadate® ER** *see* Methylphenidate *on page* *973*
- **Metadol™ (Can)** *see* Methadone *on page* *957*
- **Metaglip™** *see* Glipizide and Metformin *on page* *699*
- **123 Meta-Iodobenzlyguanidine Sulfate** *see* Iobenguane I 123 *on page* *810*
- **Metamucil® [OTC]** *see* Psyllium *on page* *1268*
- **Metamucil® (Can)** *see* Psyllium *on page* *1268*
- **Metamucil® Plus Calcium [OTC]** *see* Psyllium *on page* *1268*
- **Metamucil® Smooth Texture [OTC]** *see* Psyllium *on page* *1268*

Metaproterenol (met a proe TER e nol)

U.S. Brand Names Alupent® [DSC]

Canadian Brand Names Apo-Orciprenaline®; ratio-Orciprenaline®; Tanta-Orciprenaline®

Index Terms Metaproterenol Sulfate; Orciprenaline Sulfate

Pharmacologic Category Beta$_2$-Adrenergic Agonist

Additional Appendix Information

Bronchodilators *on page* *1650*

Use Bronchodilator in reversible airway obstruction due to asthma or COPD; because of its delayed onset of action (1 hour) and prolonged effect (4 or more hours), this may not be the drug of choice for assessing response to a bronchodilator

Pregnancy Risk Factor C

Pregnancy Considerations No data on crossing the placenta. Reported association with polydactyly in 1 study; may be secondary to severe maternal disease or chance.

Lactation Excretion in breast milk unknown

Medication Safety Issues

Sound-alike/look-alike issues:

Metaproterenol may be confused with metipranolol, metoprolol

Alupent® may be confused with Atrovent®

Contraindications Hypersensitivity to metaproterenol or any component of the formulation; pre-existing cardiac arrhythmias associated with tachycardia

Warnings/Precautions Optimize anti-inflammatory treatment before initiating maintenance treatment with metaproterenol. Do not use as a component of chronic therapy without an anti-inflammatory agent. Only the mildest form of asthma (Step 1 and/or exercise-induced) would not require concurrent use based upon asthma guidelines. Patient must be instructed to seek medical attention in cases where acute symptoms are not relieved or a previous level of response is diminished. The need to increase frequency of use may indicate deterioration of asthma, and treatment must not be delayed.

Use caution in patients with cardiovascular disease (arrhythmia or hypertension or HF), convulsive disorders, diabetes, glaucoma, hyperthyroidism, or hypokalemia. Beta-agonists may cause elevation in blood pressure, heart rate, and result in CNS stimulation/excitation. $Beta_2$-agonists may increase risk of arrhythmia, increase serum glucose, or decrease serum potassium.

Immediate hypersensitivity reactions (urticaria, angioedema, rash, bronchospasm) have been reported. Do not exceed recommended dose; serious adverse events including fatalities, have been associated with excessive use of inhaled sympathomimetics. Rarely, paradoxical bronchospasm may occur with use of inhaled bronchodilating agents; this should be distinguished from inadequate response. All patients should utilize a spacer device when using a metered-dose inhaler; additionally, a face mask should be used in children <4 years of age.

Metaproterenol has more $beta_1$ activity than $beta_2$-selective agents such as albuterol and, therefore, may no longer be the beta-agonist of first choice. Oral use should be avoided due to the increased incidence of adverse effects.

Adverse Reactions

>10%:

Cardiovascular: Tachycardia (<17%)

Central nervous system: Nervousness (3% to 14%)

Endocrine & metabolic: Serum glucose increased, serum potassium decreased

Neuromuscular & skeletal: Tremor (1% to 33%)

1% to 10%:

Cardiovascular: Palpitation (<4%)

Central nervous system: Headache (<4%), dizziness (1% to 4%), insomnia (2%)

Gastrointestinal: Nausea, vomiting, bad taste, heartburn (≥4%), xerostomia

Neuromuscular & skeletal: Trembling, muscle cramps, weakness (1%)

Respiratory: Coughing, pharyngitis (≤4%)

Miscellaneous: Diaphoresis (increased) (≤4%)

<1% (Limited to important or life-threatening): Angina, chest pain, diarrhea, drowsiness, hypertension, hypokalemia, paradoxical bronchospasm, taste change

Drug Interactions

Avoid Concomitant Use

Avoid concomitant use of Metaproterenol with any of the following: Iobenguane I 123

Increased Effect/Toxicity

Metaproterenol may increase the levels/effects of: Sympathomimetics

The levels/effects of Metaproterenol may be increased by: Atomoxetine; Cannabinoids; MAO Inhibitors; Tricyclic Antidepressants

Decreased Effect

Metaproterenol may decrease the levels/effects of: Iobenguane I 123

The levels/effects of Metaproterenol may be decreased by: Alpha-/Beta-Blockers; Beta-Blockers (Beta1 Selective); Beta-Blockers (Nonselective); Betahistine

Stability Store in tight, light-resistant container. Do not use if brown solution or contains a precipitate.

Mechanism of Action Relaxes bronchial smooth muscle by action on $beta_2$-receptors with very little effect on heart rate

Pharmacodynamics/Kinetics

Onset of action: Bronchodilation: Oral: ~15 minutes; Inhalation: ~60 seconds

Peak effect: Oral: ~1 hour

Duration: ~1-5 hours

Dosage

Oral:

Children:

<2 years: 0.4 mg/kg/dose given 3-4 times/day; in infants, the dose can be given every 8-12 hours

2-6 years: 1-2.6 mg/kg/day divided every 6 hours

6-9 years: 10 mg/dose 3-4 times/day

Children >9 years and Adults: 20 mg 3-4 times/day

Elderly: Initial: 10 mg 3-4 times/day, increasing as necessary up to 20 mg 3-4 times/day

Inhalation: Children >12 years and Adults: 2-3 inhalations every 3-4 hours, up to 12 inhalations in 24 hours

Nebulizer:

Infants and Children: 0.01-0.02 mL/kg of 5% solution; minimum dose: 0.1 mL; maximum dose: 0.3 mL diluted in 2-3 mL normal saline every 4-6 hours (may be given more frequently according to need)

Adolescents and Adults: 5-20 breaths of full strength 5% metaproterenol **or** 0.2 to 0.3 mL 5% metaproterenol in 2.5-3 mL normal saline until nebulized every 4-6 hours (can be given more frequently according to need)

Administration

Inhalation: Do not use solutions for nebulization if they are brown or contain a precipitate. Shake inhaler well before using.

Oral: Administer around-the-clock to promote less variation in peak and trough serum levels

Monitoring Parameters Assess lung sounds, heart rate, and blood pressure before administration and during peak of medication; observe patient for wheezing after administration, if this occurs, call physician; monitor respiratory rate, arterial or capillary blood gases if applicable; FEV_1, peak flow, and/or other pulmonary function tests; CNS stimulation; serum glucose, serum potassium

Test Interactions Increased potassium (S)

Additional Information Use with caution perioperatively due to $beta_1$ effect of agent. Hypertension and tachycardia are increased with exogenous sympathomimetics. During endotracheal intubation, $beta_2$-specific agent is more appropriate for perioperative use.

Dosage Forms Excipient information presented when available (limited, particularly for generics); consult specific product labeling. [DSC] = Discontinued product

Aerosol for oral inhalation, as sulfate:

Alupent®: 0.65 mg/inhalation (14 g) [contains chlorofluorocarbon; 200 doses] [DSC]

Solution for nebulization, as sulfate [preservative free]: 0.4% [4 mg/mL] (2.5 mL); 0.6% [6 mg/mL] (2.5 mL)
Syrup, as sulfate: 10 mg/5 mL (480 mL)
Tablet, as sulfate: 10 mg, 20 mg

◆ **Metaproterenol Sulfate** *see* Metaproterenol *on page 952*

◆ **Metastron®** *see* Strontium-89 *on page 1401*

Metaxalone (me TAKS a lone)

U.S. Brand Names Skelaxin®
Canadian Brand Names Skelaxin®
Pharmacologic Category Skeletal Muscle Relaxant
Use Relief of discomfort associated with acute, painful musculoskeletal conditions
Pregnancy Risk Factor C
Lactation Excretion in breast milk unknown/not recommended
Medication Safety Issues
Sound-alike/look-alike issues:
Metaxalone may be confused with metolazone
Contraindications Hypersensitivity to metaxalone or any component of the formulation; impaired hepatic or renal function, history of drug-induced hemolytic anemias or other anemias
Warnings/Precautions May cause CNS depression. CNS depressant effects may be augmented when used in conjunction with other depressants (eg, barbiturates, ethanol), when taken with food, or in the elderly. May impair mental and/or physical ability to perform hazardous tasks such as operating machinery or driving a motor vehicle. Use with caution in patients with impaired renal or hepatic function; routine monitoring of transaminases is recommended. An increase in bioavailability and half-life have been observed in female patients.
Adverse Reactions Frequency not defined.
Central nervous system: Dizziness, drowsiness, headache, irritability, paradoxical stimulation
Dermatologic: Rash (with or without pruritus)
Gastrointestinal: Gastrointestinal upset, nausea, vomiting
Hematologic: Hemolytic anemia, leukopenia
Hepatic: Jaundice
Miscellaneous: Hypersensitivity (including anaphylactoid reactions)
Drug Interactions
Avoid Concomitant Use There are no known interactions where it is recommended to avoid concomitant use.
Increased Effect/Toxicity
Metaxalone may increase the levels/effects of: Alcohol (Ethyl); CNS Depressants
Decreased Effect There are no known significant interactions involving a decrease in effect.
Ethanol/Nutrition/Herb Interactions
Ethanol: Avoid ethanol (may increase CNS depression).
Food: Bioavailability may be increased (may increase CNS depression).
Herb/Nutraceutical: Avoid valerian, St John's wort, kava kava, gotu kola (may increase CNS depression).
Stability Store at room temperature at 15°C to 30°C (59°F to 86°F).
Mechanism of Action Precise mechanism has not been established; however, efficacy appears to result from disruption of the spasm-pain-spasm cycle, probably by a general CNS depressant effect. Does not have a direct effect on skeletal muscle.
Pharmacodynamics/Kinetics
Onset of action: ~1 hour
Duration: ~4-6 hours
Metabolism: Hepatic
Bioavailability: Not established; food may increase
Half-life elimination: 9 hours
Time to peak: T_{max}: 3 hours
Excretion: Urine (as metabolites)
Dosage Children >12 years and Adults: Oral: 800 mg 3-4 times/day
Dietary Considerations Administration with food may increase serum concentrations.
Administration May be administered with or without food. However, serum concentrations may be increased when administered with food; clinical significance has not been established. Patients should be monitored.
Test Interactions False-positive Benedict's test
Dosage Forms Excipient information presented when available (limited, particularly for generics); consult specific product labeling. [DSC] = Discontinued product
Tablet: 400 mg [DSC], 800 mg

MetFORMIN (met FOR min)

U.S. Brand Names Fortamet®; Glucophage®; Glucophage® XR; Glumetza™; Riomet®
Canadian Brand Names Apo-Metformin®; CO-Metformin; DOM-Metformin; Gen-Metformin; Glucophage®; Glumetza™; Glycon; MED-Metformin; Novo-Metformin; Nu-Metformin; PHL-Metformin; PMS-Metformin; RAN™-Metformin; RATIO-Metformin; RHOXAL-Metformin; RIVA-Metformin; Sandoz-Metformin FC
Index Terms Metformin Hydrochloride
Pharmacologic Category Antidiabetic Agent, Biguanide
Additional Appendix Information
Diabetes Mellitus Management, Adults *on page 1801*
Hyperglycemia- or Hypoglycemia-Causing Drugs *on page 1814*
Use Management of type 2 diabetes mellitus (noninsulin dependent, NIDDM) as monotherapy when hyperglycemia cannot be managed with diet and exercise alone. In adults, may be used concomitantly with a sulfonylurea or insulin to improve glycemic control.
Unlabeled/Investigational Use Gestational diabetes mellitus (GDM); polycystic ovary syndrome (PCOS)
Pregnancy Risk Factor B
Pregnancy Considerations Adverse events have not been observed in animal studies; therefore, metformin is classified as pregnancy category B. Metformin has been found to cross the placenta in levels which may be comparable to those found in the maternal plasma. Pharmacokinetic studies suggest that clearance of metformin may be increased during pregnancy and dosing may need adjusted in some women when used during the third trimester.

Fetal, neonatal, and maternal outcomes have been evaluated following maternal use of metformin for the treatment of GDM and type 2 diabetes. Available information suggests that metformin use during pregnancy may be safe as long as good glycemic control is maintained; however, many studies used metformin during the second or third trimester only. Maternal hyperglycemia can be associated with adverse effects in the fetus, including macrosomia, neonatal hyperglycemia, and hyperbilirubinemia; the risk of congenital malformations is increased when the Hb A_{1c} is above the normal range. Diabetes can also be associated with adverse effects in the mother. Poorly-treated diabetes may cause end-organ damage that may negatively affect obstetric outcomes. Physiologic glucose levels should be maintained prior to and during pregnancy to decrease the risk of adverse events in the mother and the fetus. Until additional safety and efficacy data are obtained, the use of oral agents is generally not recommended as routine management of GDM or type 2 diabetes mellitus during pregnancy. Insulin is the drug of choice for the control of diabetes mellitus during pregnancy.

Metformin has also been evaluated for the treatment of PCOS, a syndrome which may exhibit oligomenorrhea and in some women, hyperinsulinemia. When used to treat infertility related to PCOS, current guidelines restrict the use of metformin to women with glucose intolerance.

Lactation Enters breast milk/not recommended

Medication Safety Issues

Sound-alike/look-alike issues:

MetFORMIN may be confused with metroNIDAZOLE

Glucophage® may be confused with Glucotrol®, Glutofac®

Contraindications Hypersensitivity to metformin or any component of the formulation; renal disease or renal dysfunction (serum creatinine ≥1.5 mg/dL in males or ≥1.4 mg/dL in females) or abnormal creatinine clearance from any cause, including shock, acute myocardial infarction, or septicemia; acute or chronic metabolic acidosis with or without coma (including diabetic ketoacidosis)

Note: Temporarily discontinue in patients undergoing radiologic studies in which intravascular iodinated contrast media are utilized.

Warnings/Precautions [U.S. Boxed Warning]: Lactic acidosis is a rare, but potentially severe consequence of therapy with metformin. Lactic acidosis should be suspected in any patient with diabetes receiving metformin with evidence of acidosis but without evidence of ketoacidosis. Discontinue metformin in clinical situations predisposing to hypoxemia, including conditions such as cardiovascular collapse, respiratory failure, acute myocardial infarction, acute congestive heart failure, and septicemia. Use caution in patients with congestive heart failure requiring pharmacologic management, particularly in patients with unstable or acute CHF; risk of lactic acidosis may be increased secondary to hypoperfusion.

Metformin is substantially excreted by the kidney. The risk of accumulation and lactic acidosis increases with the degree of impairment of renal function. Patients with renal function below the limit of normal for their age should not receive metformin. In elderly patients, renal function should be monitored regularly; should not be initiated in patients ≥80 years of age unless normal renal function is confirmed. Use of concomitant medications that may affect renal function (ie, affect tubular secretion) may also affect metformin disposition. Metformin should be withheld in patients with dehydration and/or prerenal azotemia. Therapy should be suspended for any surgical procedures (resume only after normal intake resumed and normal renal function is verified). Therapy should be temporarily discontinued prior to or at the time of intravascular administration of iodinated contrast media (potential for acute alteration in renal function). Metformin should be withheld for 48 hours after the radiologic study and restarted only after renal function has been confirmed as normal. It may be necessary to discontinue metformin and administer insulin if the patient is exposed to stress (fever, trauma, infection, surgery).

Avoid use in patients with impaired liver function. Patient must be instructed to avoid excessive acute or chronic ethanol use; ethanol may potentiate metformin's effect on lactate metabolism. Administration of oral antidiabetic drugs has been reported to be associated with increased cardiovascular mortality; metformin does not appear to share this risk. Safety and efficacy of metformin have been established for use in children ≥10 years of age; the extended release preparation is for use in patients ≥17 years of age.

Insoluble tablet shell of Glumetza™ 1000 mg extended release tablet may remain intact and be visible in the stool. Other extended released tablets (Fortamet®, Glucophage® XR, Glumetza™ 500 mg) may appear in the stool as a soft mass resembling the tablet.

Adverse Reactions

>10%:

Gastrointestinal: Diarrhea (10% to 53%), nausea/vomiting (7% to 26%), flatulence (12%)

Neuromuscular & skeletal: Weakness (9%)

1% to 10%:

Cardiovascular: Chest discomfort, flushing, palpitation

Central nervous system: Headache (6%), chills, dizziness, lightheadedness

Dermatologic: Rash

Endocrine & metabolic: Hypoglycemia

Gastrointestinal: Indigestion (7%), abdominal discomfort (6%), abdominal distention, abnormal stools, constipation, dyspepsia/ heartburn, taste disorder

Neuromuscular & skeletal: Myalgia

Respiratory: Dyspnea, upper respiratory tract infection

Miscellaneous: Decreased vitamin B_{12} levels (7%), increased diaphoresis, flu-like syndrome, nail disorder

<1% (Limited to important or life-threatening): Lactic acidosis, leukocytoclastic vasculitis, megaloblastic anemia, pneumonitis

Drug Interactions

Avoid Concomitant Use There are no known interactions where it is recommended to avoid concomitant use.

Increased Effect/Toxicity

The levels/effects of MetFORMIN may be increased by: Cephalexin; Cimetidine; Iodinated Contrast Agents; Pegvisomant

Decreased Effect

The levels/effects of MetFORMIN may be decreased by: Corticosteroids (Orally Inhaled); Corticosteroids (Systemic); Luteinizing Hormone-Releasing Hormone Analogs; Somatropin

Ethanol/Nutrition/Herb Interactions

Ethanol: Avoid or limit ethanol (incidence of lactic acidosis may be increased; may cause hypoglycemia).

Food: Food decreases the extent and slightly delays the absorption. May decrease absorption of vitamin B_{12} and/ or folic acid.

Herb/Nutraceutical: Caution with chromium, garlic, gymnema (may cause hypoglycemia).

Stability

Oral solution: Store at 15°C to 30°C (59°F to 86°F).

Tablets: Store at 20°C to 25°C (68°F to 77°F); excursion permitted to 15°C to 30°C (59°F to 86°F). Protect from light and moisture.

Mechanism of Action Decreases hepatic glucose production, decreasing intestinal absorption of glucose and improves insulin sensitivity (increases peripheral glucose uptake and utilization)

Pharmacodynamics/Kinetics

Onset of action: Within days; maximum effects up to 2 weeks

Distribution: V_d: 654 ± 358 L; partitions into erythrocytes

Protein binding: Negligible

Metabolism: Not metabolized by the liver

Bioavailability: Absolute: Fasting: 50% to 60%

Half-life elimination: Plasma: 4-9 hours

Time to peak, serum: Immediate release: 2-3 hours; Extended release: 7 hours (range: 4-8 hours)

Excretion: Urine (90% as unchanged drug; active secretion)

Dosage Type 2 diabetes management: **Note:** Allow 1-2 weeks between dose titrations: Generally, clinically significant responses are not seen at doses <1500 mg daily; however, a lower recommended starting dose and gradual increased dosage is recommended to minimize gastrointestinal symptoms.

Immediate release tablet or solution: Oral:

Children 10-16 years: Initial: 500 mg twice daily; increases in daily dosage should be made in increments of 500 mg at weekly intervals, given in divided doses, up to a maximum of 2000 mg/day

Chidlren ≥17 years and Adults: Initial: 500 mg twice daily **or** 850 mg once daily; increase dosage incrementally.

Incremental dosing recommendations based on dosage form:

500 mg tablet: One tablet/day at weekly intervals

850 mg tablet: One tablet/day every other week

Oral solution: 500 mg twice daily every other week

Doses of up to 2000 mg/day may be given twice daily. If a dose >2000 mg/day is required, it may be better tolerated in three divided doses. Maximum recommended dose 2550 mg/day.

Extended release tablet: Oral: **Note:** If glycemic control is not achieved at maximum dose, may divide dose and administer twice daily.

Children ≥17 years and Adults:

Fortamet®: Initial: 1000 mg once daily; dosage may be increased by 500 mg weekly; maximum dose: 2500 mg once daily

Glucophage® XR: Initial: 500 mg once daily; dosage may be increased by 500 mg weekly; maximum dose: 2000 mg once daily

Adults: Glumetza™: Initial: 1000 mg once daily; dosage may be increased by 500 mg weekly; maximum dose: 2000 mg once daily

Elderly: The initial and maintenance dosing should be conservative, due to the potential for decreased renal function. Generally, elderly patients should not be titrated to the maximum dose of metformin. Do not use in patients ≥80 years of age unless normal renal function has been established.

Transfer from other antidiabetic agents: No transition period is generally necessary except when transferring from chlorpropamide. When transferring from chlorpropamide, care should be exercised during the first 2 weeks because of the prolonged retention of chlorpropamide in the body, leading to overlapping drug effects and possible hypoglycemia.

Concomitant metformin and oral sulfonylurea therapy: If patients have not responded to 4 weeks of the maximum dose of metformin monotherapy, consider a gradual addition of an oral sulfonylurea, even if prior primary or secondary failure to a sulfonylurea has occurred. Continue metformin at the maximum dose. If adequate response has not occurred following 3 months of metformin and sulfonylurea combination therapy, consider switching to insulin with or without metformin.

Failed sulfonylurea therapy: Patients with prior failure on glyburide may be treated by gradual addition of metformin. Initiate with glyburide 20 mg and metformin 500 mg daily. Metformin dosage may be increased by 500 mg/day at weekly intervals, up to a maximum metformin dose (dosage of glyburide maintained at 20 mg/day).

Concomitant metformin and insulin therapy: Initial: 500 mg metformin once daily, continue current insulin dose; increase by 500 mg metformin weekly until adequate glycemic control is achieved

Maximum daily dose: Immediate release and solution: 2550 mg metformin; Extended release: 2000-2500 mg (varies by product)

Decrease insulin dose 10% to 25% when FPG <120 mg/dL; monitor and make further adjustments as needed

Dosing adjustment/comments in renal impairment: The plasma and blood half-life of metformin is prolonged and the renal clearance is decreased in proportion to the decrease in creatinine clearance. Per the manufacturer, metformin is contraindicated in the presence of renal dysfunction defined as a serum creatinine >1.5 mg/dL in males, or >1.4 mg/dL in females and in patients with abnormal clearance. Clinically, it has been recommended that metformin be avoided in patients with Cl_{cr} <60-70 mL/minute (DeFronzo, 1999).

Dosing adjustment in hepatic impairment: Avoid metformin; liver disease is a risk factor for the development of lactic acidosis during metformin therapy.

Dietary Considerations Drug may cause GI upset; take with food (to decrease GI upset). Take at the same time each day. Dietary modification based on ADA recommendations is a part of therapy. Monitor for signs and symptoms of vitamin B_{12} and/or folic acid deficiency; supplementation may be required.

Administration Extended release dosage form should be swallowed whole; do not crush, break, or chew; administer with food (to decrease GI upset). Administer Fortamet® with a glass of water.

Monitoring Parameters Urine for glucose and ketones, fasting blood glucose, and hemoglobin A_{1c}. Initial and periodic monitoring of hematologic parameters (eg, hemoglobin/hematocrit and red blood cell indices) and renal function should be performed, at least annually. Check vitamin B_{12} and folate if anemia is present.

Reference Range Recommendations for glycemic control in adults with diabetes:

Hb A_{1c}: <7%

Preprandial capillary plasma glucose: 70-130 mg/dL

Peak postprandial capillary blood glucose: <180 mg/dL

Blood pressure: <130/80 mm Hg

Dosage Forms Excipient information presented when available (limited, particularly for generics); consult specific product labeling.

Solution, oral, as hydrochloride:

Riomet®: 100 mg/mL (118 mL, 473 mL) [contains saccharin; cherry flavor]

Tablet, as hydrochloride: 500 mg, 850 mg, 1000 mg

Glucophage®: 500 mg, 850 mg, 1000 mg

Tablet, extended release, as hydrochloride: 500 mg, 750 mg

Fortamet®: 500 mg, 1000 mg

Glucophage® XR: 500 mg

Glumetza™: 500 mg, 1000 mg

◆ **Metformin and Glipizide** *see* Glipizide and Metformin *on page 699*

◆ **Metformin and Glyburide** *see* Glyburide and Metformin *on page 702*

◆ **Metformin and Repaglinide** *see* Repaglinide and Metformin *on page 1305*

◆ **Metformin and Rosiglitazone** *see* Rosiglitazone and Metformin *on page 1343*

◆ **Metformin and Sitagliptin** *see* Sitagliptin and Metformin *on page 1376*

◆ **Metformin Hydrochloride** *see* MetFORMIN *on page 954*

◆ **Metformin Hydrochloride and Pioglitazone Hydrochloride** *see* Pioglitazone and Metformin *on page 1198*

◆ **Metformin Hydrochloride and Rosiglitazone Maleate** *see* Rosiglitazone and Metformin *on page 1343*

Methacholine (meth a KOLE leen)

U.S. Brand Names Provocholine®

Canadian Brand Names Methacholine Omega; Provocholine®

Index Terms Methacholine Chloride

Pharmacologic Category Diagnostic Agent

Use Diagnosis of bronchial airway hyperactivity

Pregnancy Risk Factor C

Dosage Note: For inhalation only: Children ≥5 years and Adults:

Before inhalation challenge, perform baseline pulmonary function tests; the patient must have an FEV_1 of at least 70% of the predicted value. The following is a suggested schedule for administration of methacholine challenge. Calculate cumulative units by multiplying number of breaths by concentration given. Total cumulative units is the sum of cumulative units for each concentration given. See table.

Methacholine

Vial	Serial Concentration (mg/mL)	No. of Breaths	Cumulative Units per Concentration	Total Cumulative Units
E	0.025	5	0.125	0.125
D	0.25	5	1.25	1.375
C	2.5	5	12.5	13.88
B	10	5	50	63.88
A	25	5	125	188.88

Determine FEV_1 within 5 minutes of challenge, a positive challenge is a 20% reduction in FEV_1

Additional Information Complete prescribing information for this medication should be consulted for additional detail.

Dosage Forms Excipient information presented when available (limited, particularly for generics); consult specific product labeling.

Powder for reconstitution, for oral inhalation, as chloride:
Provocholine®: 100 mg

◆ **Methacholine Chloride** *see* Methacholine *on page 956*

◆ **Methacholine Omega (Can)** *see* Methacholine *on page 956*

Methadone (METH a done)

U.S. Brand Names Dolophine®; Methadone Diskets®; Methadone Intensol™; Methadose®

Canadian Brand Names Metadol™

Index Terms Methadone Hydrochloride

Pharmacologic Category Analgesic, Opioid

Additional Appendix Information

Narcotic / Opioid Analgesics *on page 1663*

Use Management of moderate-to-severe pain; detoxification and maintenance treatment of opioid addiction (if used for detoxification and maintenance treatment of narcotic addiction, it must be part of an FDA-approved program)

Restrictions C-II

When used for treatment of opioid addiction: May only be dispensed in accordance to guidelines established by the Substance Abuse and Mental Health Services Administration's (SAMHSA) Center for Substance Abuse Treatment (CSAT). Regulations regarding methadone use may vary by state and/or country. Obtain advice from appropriate regulatory agencies and/or consult with pain management/palliative care specialists.

Note: Regulatory Exceptions to the General Requirement to Provide Opioid Agonist Treatment (per manufacturer's labeling):

1. During inpatient care, when the patient was admitted for any condition other than concurrent opioid addiction, to facilitate the treatment of the primary admitting diagnosis.
2. During an emergency period of no longer than 3 days while definitive care for the addiction is being sought in an appropriately licensed facility.

Pregnancy Risk Factor C/D (prolonged use or high doses at term)

Pregnancy Considerations Teratogenic effects have been observed in some, but not all, animal studies. Data collected by the Teratogen Information System are complicated by maternal use of illicit drugs, nutrition, infection, and psychosocial circumstances. However, pregnant women in methadone treatment programs are reported to have improved fetal outcomes compared to pregnant women using illicit drugs. Methadone can be detected in the amniotic fluid, cord plasma, and newborn urine. Fetal growth, birth weight, length, and/or head circumference may be decreased in infants born to narcotic-addicted mothers treated with methadone during pregnancy. Growth deficits do not appear to persist; however, decreased performance on psychometric and behavioral tests has been found to continue into childhood. Abnormal fetal nonstress tests have also been reported. Withdrawal symptoms in the neonate may be observed up to 2-4 weeks after delivery. The manufacturer states that methadone should be used during pregnancy only if clearly needed. Because methadone clearance in pregnant women is increased and half-life is decreased during the 2nd and 3rd trimesters of pregnancy, withdrawal symptoms may be observed in the mother; dosage of methadone may need increased or dosing interval decreased during pregnancy.

Lactation Enters breast milk/not recommended (AAP rates "compatible")

Medication Safety Issues

Sound-alike/look-alike issues:

Methadone may be confused with dexmethylphenidate, Mephyton®, methylphenidate, Metadate® CD, and Metadate® ER

High alert medication: The Institute for Safe Medication Practices (ISMP) includes this medication among its list of drug classes which have a heightened risk of causing significant patient harm when used in error.

Contraindications Hypersensitivity to methadone or any component of the formulation; respiratory depression (in the absence of resuscitative equipment or in an unmonitored setting); acute bronchial asthma or hypercarbia; paralytic ileus; concurrent use of selegiline

Warnings/Precautions An opioid-containing analgesic regimen should be tailored to each patient's needs and based upon the type of pain being treated (acute versus chronic), the route of administration, degree of tolerance for opioids (naive versus chronic user), age, weight, and medical condition. The optimal analgesic dose varies widely among patients. Doses should be titrated to pain relief/prevention. Patients maintained on stable doses of methadone may need higher and/or more frequent doses in case of acute pain (eg, postoperative pain, physical trauma). Methadone is ineffective for the relief of anxiety.

[U.S. Boxed Warning]: May prolong the QT_c interval and increase risk for torsade de pointes. Patients should be informed of the potential arrhythmia risk, evaluated for any history of structural heart disease, arrhythmia, syncope, and for existence of potential drug interactions including drugs that possess QT_c interval-prolonging properties, promote hypokalemia, hypomagnesemia, or hypocalcemia, or reduce elimination of methadone (eg, CYP3A4 inhibitors). Obtain baseline ECG for all patients and risk stratify according to QT_c interval (see Monitoring Parameters). Use with caution in patients at risk for QT_c prolongation, with medications known to prolong the QT_c interval, promote electrolyte depletion, or inhibit CYP3A4, or history of conduction abnormalities. QT_c interval prolongation and torsade de pointes may be associated with doses >100 mg/day, but have also been observed with lower doses. May cause severe hypotension; use caution with severe volume depletion or other conditions which may compromise maintenance of normal blood pressure. Use caution with cardiovascular disease or patients predisposed to dysrhythmias.

[U.S. Boxed Warning]: May cause respiratory depression. Use caution in patients with respiratory disease or pre-existing respiratory conditions (eg, severe obesity, asthma, COPD, sleep apnea, CNS depression). Because the respiratory effects last longer than the analgesic effects, slow titration is required. Use extreme caution during treatment initiation, dose titration and conversion from other opioid agonists. Incomplete cross tolerance may occur; patients tolerant to other mu opioid agonists may not be tolerant to methadone. Abrupt cessation may precipitate withdrawal symptoms.

May cause CNS depression, which may impair physical or mental abilities. Patients must be cautioned about performing tasks which require mental alertness (eg, operating machinery or driving). Effects with other sedative drugs or ethanol may be potentiated. Use with caution in patients with depression or suicidal tendencies, or in patients with a history of drug abuse. Tolerance or psychological and physical dependence may occur with prolonged use.

Use with caution in patients with head injury or increased intracranial pressure. May obscure diagnosis or clinical course of patients with acute abdominal conditions. Elderly may be more susceptible to adverse effects (eg, CNS, respiratory, gastrointestinal). Decrease initial dose and use caution in the elderly or debilitated; with hyper/hypothyroidism, morbid obesity, adrenal insufficiency, prostatic hyperplasia, or urethral stricture; or with severe renal or hepatic failure. Use with caution in patients with biliary tract dysfunction; acute pancreatitis may cause constriction of sphincter of Oddi. Safety and efficacy have not been established in children. **[U.S. Boxed Warning]: For oral administration only;** excipients to deter use by injection are contained in tablets.

[U.S. Boxed Warning]: When used for treatment of narcotic addiction: May only be dispensed by opioid treatment programs certified by the Substance Abuse and Mental Health Services Administration (SAMHSA) and certified by the designated state authority. Exceptions include inpatient treatment of other conditions and emergency period (not >3 days) while definitive substance abuse treatment is being sought.

Adverse Reactions Frequency not defined. During prolonged administration, adverse effects may decrease over several weeks; however, constipation and sweating may persist.

Cardiovascular: Arrhythmia, bigeminal rhythms, bradycardia, cardiac arrest, cardiomyopathy, ECG changes, edema, extrasystoles, faintness, flushing, heart failure, hypotension, palpitation,peripheral vasodilation, phlebitis, orthostatic hypotension, QT interval prolonged, shock, syncope, tachycardia, torsade de pointes, T-wave inversion, ventricular fibrillation, ventricular tachycardia,

Central nervous system: Agitation, confusion, disorientation, dizziness, drowsiness, dysphoria, euphoria, hallucination, headache, insomnia, lightheadedness, sedation, seizure

Dermatologic: Hemorrhagic urticaria, pruritus, rash, urticaria

Endocrine & metabolic: Antidiuretic effect, amenorrhea, hypokalemia, hypomagnesemia, libido decreased

Gastrointestinal: Abdominal pain, anorexia, biliary tract spasm, constipation, glossitis, nausea, stomach cramps, vomiting, weight gain, xerostomia

Genitourinary: Impotence, urinary retention or hesitancy

Hematologic: Thrombocytopenia (reversible, reported in patients with chronic hepatitis)

Neuromuscular & skeletal: Weakness

Local: I.M./SubQ injection: Erythema, pain, swelling; I.V. injection: Hemorrhagic urticaria (rare), pruritus, urticaria, rash

Ocular: Miosis, visual disturbances

Respiratory: Pulmonary edema, respiratory depression, respiratory arrest

Miscellaneous: Death, diaphoresis, physical and psychological dependence

Drug Interactions

Metabolism/Transport Effects **Substrate** of CYP2C9 (minor), 2C19 (minor), 2D6 (minor), 3A4 (major); **Inhibits** CYP2D6 (moderate), 3A4 (weak)

Avoid Concomitant Use

Avoid concomitant use of Methadone with any of the following: Nilotinib; Tetrabenazine; Ziprasidone

Increased Effect/Toxicity

Methadone may increase the levels/effects of: Alcohol (Ethyl); Alvimopan; CNS Depressants; CYP2D6 Substrates; Desmopressin; Fesoterodine; Nebivolol; QTc-Prolonging Agents; Selective Serotonin Reuptake Inhibitors; Tamoxifen; Tetrabenazine; Zidovudine; Ziprasidone

The levels/effects of Methadone may be increased by: Alfuzosin; Amphetamines; Antifungal Agents (Azole Derivatives, Systemic); Antipsychotic Agents (Phenothiazines); Ciprofloxacin; CYP3A4 Inhibitors (Moderate); CYP3A4 Inhibitors (Strong); Dasatinib; Gadobutrol; Nilotinib; Protease Inhibitors; Selective Serotonin Reuptake Inhibitors; Succinylcholine

Decreased Effect

Methadone may decrease the levels/effects of: Codeine; Didanosine; Pegvisomant; TraMADol

The levels/effects of Methadone may be decreased by: Ammonium Chloride; Barbiturates; CarBAMazepine; CYP3A4 Inducers (Strong); Deferasirox; Etravirine; Herbs (CYP3A4 Inducers); Phenytoin; Reverse Transcriptase Inhibitors (Non-Nucleoside); Rifamycin Derivatives

Ethanol/Nutrition/Herb Interactions

Ethanol: Avoid ethanol (may increase CNS effects). Watch for sedation.

Herb/Nutraceutical: Avoid St John's wort (may decrease methadone levels; may increase CNS depression). Avoid valerian, kava kava, gotu kola (may increase CNS depression). Methadone is metabolized by CYP3A4 in the intestines; avoid concurrent use of grapefruit juice.

Stability

Injection: Store at controlled room temperature of 15°C to 30°C (59°F to 86°F). Protect from light.

Oral concentrate, oral solution, tablet: Store at controlled room temperature of 15°C to 30°C (59°F to 86°F).

Mechanism of Action Binds to opiate receptors in the CNS, causing inhibition of ascending pain pathways, altering the perception of and response to pain; produces generalized CNS depression

Pharmacodynamics/Kinetics

Onset of action: Oral: Analgesic: 0.5-1 hour; Parenteral: 10-20 minutes

Peak effect: Parenteral: 1-2 hours; Oral: continuous dosing: 3-5 days

Duration of analgesia: Oral: 4-8 hours, increases to 22-48 hours with repeated doses

Distribution: V_{dss}: 1-8 L/kg

Protein binding: 85% to 90%

Metabolism: Hepatic; N-demethylation primarily via CYP3A4, CYP2B6, and CYP2C19 to inactive metabolites

Bioavailability: Oral: 36% to 100%

Half-life elimination: 8-59 hours; may be prolonged with alkaline pH, decreased during pregnancy

Time to peak, plasma: 1-7.5 hours

Excretion: Urine (<10% as unchanged drug); increased with urine pH <6

Dosage Regulations regarding methadone use may vary by state and/or country. Obtain advice from appropriate regulatory agencies and/or consult with pain management/palliative care specialists. **Note:** These are guidelines and do not represent the maximum doses that may be required in all patients. Methadone accumulates with repeated doses and dosage may need reduction after 3-5 days to prevent CNS depressant effects. Some patients may benefit from every 8-12 hour dosing interval for chronic pain management. Doses should be titrated to appropriate effects.

Children (unlabeled use):

Pain (analgesia):

Oral: Initial: 0.1-0.2 mg/kg 4-8 hours initially for 2-3 doses, then every 6-12 hours as needed. Dosing interval may range from 4-12 hours during initial therapy; decrease in dose or frequency may be required (~days 2-5) due to accumulation with repeated doses (maximum dose: 5-10 mg)

I.V.: 0.1 mg/kg every 4-8 hours initially for 2-3 doses, then every 6-12 hours as needed. Dosing interval may range from 4-12 hours during initial therapy; decrease in dose or frequency may be required (~days 2-5) due to accumulation with repeated doses (maximum dose: 5-8 mg)

Iatrogenic narcotic dependency: Oral: General guidelines: Initial: 0.05-0.1 mg/kg/dose every 6 hours; increase by 0.05 mg/kg/dose until withdrawal symptoms are controlled; after 24-48 hours, the dosing interval can be lengthened to every 12-24 hours; to taper dose, wean by 0.05 mg/kg/day; if withdrawal symptoms recur, taper at a slower rate

Adults:

Acute pain (moderate-to-severe):

Oral: Opioid-naive: Initial: 2.5-10 mg every 8-12 hours; more frequent administration may be required during initiation to maintain adequate analgesia. Dosage interval may range from 4-12 hours, since duration of analgesia is relatively short during the first days of therapy, but increases substantially with continued administration.

Chronic pain (opioid-tolerant): **Conversion from oral morphine to oral methadone:**

Daily oral morphine dose <100 mg: Estimated daily oral methadone dose: 20% to 30% of total daily morphine dose

Daily oral morphine dose 100-300 mg: Estimated daily oral methadone dose: 10% to 20% of total daily morphine dose

Daily oral morphine dose 300-600 mg: Estimated daily oral methadone dose: 8% to 12% of total daily morphine dose

Daily oral morphine dose 600-1000 mg: Estimated daily oral methadone dose: 5% to 10% of total daily morphine dose.

Daily oral morphine dose >1000 mg: Estimated daily oral methadone dose: <5% of total daily morphine dose.

Note: The total daily methadone dose should then be divided to reflect the intended dosing schedule.

I.V.: Manufacturers labeling: Initial: 2.5-10 mg every 8-12 hours in opioid-naive patients; titrate slowly to effect; may also be administered by SubQ or I.M. injection

Conversion from oral methadone to parenteral methadone dose: Initial dose: Parenteral:Oral ratio: 1:2 (eg, 5 mg parenteral methadone equals 10 mg oral methadone)

Detoxification: Oral:

Initial: A single dose of 20-30 mg is generally sufficient to suppress symptoms. Should not exceed 30 mg; lower doses should be considered in patients with low tolerance at initiation (eg, absence of opioids ≥5 days); an additional 5-10 mg of methadone may be provided if withdrawal symptoms have not been suppressed or if symptoms reappear after 2-4 hours; total daily dose on the first day should not exceed 40 mg, unless the program physician documents in the patient's record that 40 mg did not control opiate abstinence symptoms.

Maintenance: Titrate to a dosage which attenuates craving, blocks euphoric effects of other opiates, and tolerance to sedative effect of methadone. Usual range: 80-120 mg/day (titration should occur cautiously)

Withdrawal: Dose reductions should be <10% of the maintenance dose, every 10-14 days

Detoxification (short-term): Oral:

Initial: Titrate to ~40 mg/day in divided doses to achieve stabilization, may continue 40 mg dose for 2-3 days

Maintenance: Titrate to a dosage which prevents/attenuates euphoric effects of self-administered opioids, reduces drug craving, and withdrawal symptoms are prevented for 24 hours.

Withdrawal: Requires individualization. Decrease daily or every other day, keeping withdrawal symptoms tolerable; hospitalized patients may tolerate a 20% reduction/day; ambulatory patients may require a slower reduction

Dosage adjustment during pregnancy: Methadone dose may need to be increased, or the dosing interval decreased; see Pregnancy Considerations - use should be reserved for cases where the benefits clearly outweigh the risks

Dosage adjustment for toxicity:

QT_c >450-499 msecs: Monitor QT_c more frequently

QT_c ≥500 msecs: Consider discontinuation or reducing methadone dose

Dosage adjustment in renal impairment: Cl_{cr} <10 mL/minute: Administer 50% to 75% of normal dose

Dosage adjustment in hepatic impairment: Avoid in severe liver disease

Administration Oral dose for detoxification and maintenance may be administered in fruit juice or water. Dispersible tablet should not be chewed or swallowed; add to liquid and allow to dissolve before administering. May rinse if residual remains.

Monitoring Parameters Obtain baseline ECG (evaluate QT_c interval), within 30 days of initiation, and then annually for all patients receiving methadone. Increase ECG monitoring if patient receiving >100 mg/day or if unexplained syncope or seizure occurs while on methadone (Krantz, 2008).

If before or at anytime during therapy:

QT_c >450-499 msecs: Discuss potential risks and benefits; monitor QT_c more frequently

QT_c ≥500 msecs: Consider discontinuation or reducing methadone dose **or** eliminate factors promoting QT_c prolongation (eg, potassium-wasting drugs) **or** use alternative therapy (eg, buprenorphine)

Pain relief, respiratory and mental status, blood pressure

Reference Range Prevention of opiate withdrawal: Therapeutic: 100-400 ng/mL (SI: 0.32-1.29 µmol/L); Toxic: >2 mcg/mL (SI: >6.46 µmol/L)

Test Interactions Some quinolones may produce a false-positive urine screening result for opiates using commercially-available immunoassay kits. This has been demonstrated most consistently for levofloxacin and ofloxacin, but other quinolones have shown cross-reactivity in certain assay kits. Confirmation of positive opiate screens by more specific methods should be considered.

Dosage Forms Excipient information presented when available (limited, particularly for generics); consult specific product labeling.

Injection, solution, as hydrochloride: 10 mg/mL (20 mL)

Solution, oral, as hydrochloride: 5 mg/5 mL (500 mL); 10 mg/5 mL (500 mL) [contains alcohol 8%; citrus flavor]

Solution, oral, as hydrochloride [concentrate]: 10 mg/mL (946 mL)

Methadone Intensol™: 10 mg/mL (30 mL)

Methadose®: 10 mg/mL (1000 mL) [cherry flavor]

Methadose®: 10 mg/mL (1000 mL) [dye free, sugar free, unflavored]

Tablet, as hydrochloride: 5 mg, 10 mg
Dolophine®: 5 mg, 10 mg
Methadose®: 5 mg, 10 mg [DSC]
Tablet, dispersible, as hydrochloride: 40 mg
Methadose®: 40 mg
Methadone Diskets®: 40 mg [orange-pineapple flavor]

- **Methadone Diskets®** *see* Methadone *on page 957*
- **Methadone Hydrochloride** *see* Methadone *on page 957*
- **Methadone Intensol™** *see* Methadone *on page 957*
- **Methadose®** *see* Methadone *on page 957*
- **Methaminodiazepoxide Hydrochloride** *see* ChlordiazePOXIDE *on page 303*

Methamphetamine (meth am FET a meen)

U.S. Brand Names Desoxyn®
Canadian Brand Names Desoxyn®
Index Terms Desoxyephedrine Hydrochloride; Methamphetamine Hydrochloride
Pharmacologic Category Anorexiant; Stimulant; Sympathomimetic
Use Treatment of attention-deficit/hyperactivity disorder (ADHD); exogenous obesity (short-term adjunct)
Unlabeled/Investigational Use Narcolepsy
Restrictions C-II

An FDA-approved medication guide must be distributed when dispensing an outpatient prescription (new or refill) where this medication is to be used without direct supervision of a healthcare provider. Medication guides are available at http://www.fda.gov/cder/drug/infopage/ADHD/default.htm.

Pharmacotherapy for weight loss is recommended only for obese patients with a body mass index ≥30 kg/m^2, or ≥27 kg/m^2 in the presence of other risk factors such as hypertension, diabetes, and/or dyslipidemia or a high waist circumference; therapy should be used in conjunction with a comprehensive weight management program. Rule out organic causes of obesity (eg, untreated hypothyroidism) prior to use.

Note: Methamphetamine is not approved for long-term use. The limited usefulness of medications in this class should be weighed against possible risks associated with their use. Consult weight loss guidelines for current pharmacotherapy recommendations.

Pregnancy Risk Factor C
Pregnancy Considerations Teratogenic and embryocidal effects have been observed in animal studies. Infants may deliver prematurely and suffer withdrawal symptoms. There are no adequate and well-controlled studies in pregnant women.
Lactation Enters breast milk/contraindicated
Medication Safety Issues
Sound-alike/look-alike issues:
Desoxyn® may be confused with digoxin
Contraindications Hypersensitivity to methamphetamine, any component of the formulation, or idiosyncrasy to amphetamines or other sympathomimetic amines; patients with advanced arteriosclerosis, symptomatic cardiovascular disease, moderate-to-severe hypertension, hyperthyroidism, glaucoma, agitated states; patients with a history of drug abuse; use during or within 14 days following MAO inhibitor therapy; stimulant medications are contraindicated for use in children with attention-deficit/hyperactivity disorders and concomitant Tourette's syndrome or tics
Warnings/Precautions Use has been associated with serious cardiovascular events including sudden death in patients with pre-existing structural cardiac abnormalities or other serious heart problems (sudden death in children and adolescents; sudden death, stroke and MI in adults). These products should be avoided in the patients with known serious structural cardiac abnormalities, cardiomyopathy, serious heart rhythm abnormalities, or other serious cardiac problems that could increase the risk of sudden death that these conditions alone carry. Patients should be carefully evaluated for cardiac disease prior to initiation of therapy. Use with caution in patients with hypertension and other cardiovascular conditions that might be exacerbated by increases in blood pressure or heart rate. Use is contraindicated in patients with moderate to severe hypertension. Amphetamines may impair the ability to engage in potentially hazardous activities. Difficulty in accommodation and blurred vision has been reported with the use of stimulants.

Use with caution in patients with psychiatric disorders, diabetes, or seizure disorders,. May exacerbate symptoms of behavior and thought disorder in psychotic patients. Stimulants may unmask tics in individuals with coexisting Tourette's syndrome **[U.S. Boxed Warning]: Potential for drug dependency exists; prolonged use may lead to drug dependency.** Use is contraindicated in patients with history of ethanol or drug abuse. Prescriptions should be written for the smallest quantity consistent with good patient care to minimize possibility of overdose. **[U.S. Boxed Warning]: Use in weight reduction programs only when alternative therapy has been ineffective.** Abrupt discontinuation following high doses or for prolonged periods may result in symptoms for withdrawal. Discontinue if satisfactory weight loss has not occurred within the first 4 weeks of treatment, or if tolerance develops. Safety and efficacy have not been established in children <12 years of age for obesity. Use of stimulants has been associated with suppression of growth; monitor growth rate during treatment.

Adverse Reactions Frequency not defined.
Cardiovascular: Hypertension, tachycardia, palpitation
Central nervous system: Restlessness, headache, exacerbation of motor and phonic tics and Tourette's syndrome, dizziness, psychosis, dysphoria, overstimulation, euphoria, insomnia
Dermatologic: Rash, urticaria
Endocrine & metabolic: Change in libido
Gastrointestinal: Diarrhea, nausea, vomiting, stomach cramps, constipation, anorexia, weight loss, xerostomia, unpleasant taste
Genitourinary: Impotence
Neuromuscular & skeletal: Tremor
Miscellaneous: Suppression of growth in children, tolerance and withdrawal with prolonged use

Drug Interactions
Metabolism/Transport Effects **Substrate** of CYP2D6 (major)
Avoid Concomitant Use
Avoid concomitant use of Methamphetamine with any of the following: Iobenguane I 123; MAO Inhibitors
Increased Effect/Toxicity
Methamphetamine may increase the levels/effects of: Analgesics (Opioid); Sympathomimetics

The levels/effects of Methamphetamine may be increased by: Alkalinizing Agents; Antacids; Cannabinoids; Carbonic Anhydrase Inhibitors; CYP2D6 Inhibitors (Moderate); CYP2D6 Inhibitors (Strong); Darunavir; MAO Inhibitors; Tricyclic Antidepressants
Decreased Effect
Methamphetamine may decrease the levels/effects of: Antihistamines; Ethosuximide; Iobenguane I 123; PHENobarbital; Phenytoin

The levels/effects of Methamphetamine may be decreased by: Ammonium Chloride; Antipsychotics; Gastrointestinal Acidifying Agents; Lithium; Methenamine

Ethanol/Nutrition/Herb Interactions
Ethanol: Avoid ethanol (may cause CNS depression).
Food: Amphetamine serum levels may be altered if taken with acidic food, juices, or vitamin C. Avoid caffeine.
Herb/Nutraceutical: Avoid ephedra (may cause hypertension or arrhythmias).

Stability Store below 30°C (86°F). Protect from light.

Mechanism of Action A sympathomimetic amine related to ephedrine and amphetamine with CNS stimulant activity; peripheral actions include elevation of systolic and diastolic blood pressure and weak bronchodilator and respiratory stimulant action

Pharmacodynamics/Kinetics
Absorption: Rapid from GI tract
Metabolism: Hepatic; forms metabolite
Half-life elimination: 4-5 hours
Excretion: Urine primarily (dependent on urine pH)

Dosage Oral:
Children ≥6 years and Adults: ADHD: 5 mg 1-2 times/day; may increase by 5 mg increments at weekly intervals until optimum response is achieved, usually 20-25 mg/day
Children ≥12 years and Adults: Exogenous obesity: 5 mg 30 minutes before each meal; treatment duration should not exceed a few weeks

Dietary Considerations Most effective when combined with a low calorie diet and behavior modification counseling.

Monitoring Parameters Heart rate, respiratory rate, blood pressure, CNS activity, body weight (BMI); growth rate in children

When used for the treatment of ADHD, thoroughly evaluate for cardiovascular risk. Monitor heart rate, blood pressure, and consider obtaining ECG prior to initiation (Vetter, 2008).

Reference Range
Adult classification of weight by BMI (kg/m^2):
Underweight: <18.5
Normal: 18.5-24.9
Overweight: 25-29.9
Obese, class I: 30-34.9
Obese, class II: 35-39.9
Extreme obesity (class III): ≥40
Waist circumference: In adults with a BMI of 25-34.9 kg/m^2, high-risk waist circumference is defined as:
Men >102 cm (>40 in)
Women >88 cm (>35 in)

Additional Information Illicit methamphetamine may contain lead; alkalinizing urine can result in longer methamphetamine half-life and elevated blood level; ephedrine is a precursor in the illicit manufacture of methamphetamine; ephedrine is extracted by dissolving ephedrine tablets in water or alcohol (50,000 tablets can result in 1 kg of ephedrine); conversion to methamphetamine occurs at a rate of 50% to 70% of the weight of ephedrine. 3,4-methylene dioxymethamphetamine (slang: XTC, Ecstasy, Adam) affects the serotonergic, dopaminergic, and noradrenergic pathways. As such, it can cause the serotonin syndrome associated with malignant hyperthermia and rhabdomyolysis.

Dosage Forms Excipient information presented when available (limited, particularly for generics); consult specific product labeling.
Tablet, as hydrochloride: 5 mg

◆ **Methamphetamine Hydrochloride** *see* Methamphetamine *on page 960*

Methazolamide (meth a ZOE la mide)

Canadian Brand Names Apo-Methazolamide®

Pharmacologic Category Carbonic Anhydrase Inhibitor; Diuretic, Carbonic Anhydrase Inhibitor; Ophthalmic Agent, Antiglaucoma

Additional Appendix Information
Glaucoma Drug Therapy *on page 1808*
Sulfonamide Derivatives *on page 1671*

Use Adjunctive treatment of open-angle or secondary glaucoma; short-term therapy of narrow-angle glaucoma when delay of surgery is desired

Pregnancy Risk Factor C

Medication Safety Issues
Sound-alike/look-alike issues:
Methazolamide may be confused with methenamine, metolazone
Neptazane® may be confused with Nesacaine®

Dosage Adults: Oral: 50-100 mg 2-3 times/day

Additional Information Complete prescribing information for this medication should be consulted for additional detail.

Dosage Forms Excipient information presented when available (limited, particularly for generics); consult specific product labeling.
Tablet: 25 mg, 50 mg

Methenamine (meth EN a meen)

U.S. Brand Names Hiprex®; Mandelamine® [DSC]; Urex™

Canadian Brand Names Dehydral®; Hiprex®; Mandelamine®; Urasal®; Urex™

Index Terms Hexamethylenetetramine; Methenamine Hippurate; Methenamine Mandelate

Pharmacologic Category Antibiotic, Miscellaneous

Use Prophylaxis or suppression of recurrent urinary tract infections; urinary tract discomfort secondary to hypermotility

Pregnancy Risk Factor C

Medication Safety Issues
Sound-alike/look-alike issues:
Methenamine may be confused with mesalamine, methazolamide, methionine
Urex® may be confused with Eurax®, Serax®

International issues:
Urex®: Brand name for furosemide in Australia

Dosage Oral:
Children:
>2-6 years: *Mandelate:* 50-75 mg/kg/day in 3-4 doses or 0.25 g/30 lb 4 times/day
6-12 years:
Hippurate: 0.5-1 g twice daily
Mandelate: 50-75 mg/kg/day in 3-4 doses or 0.5 g 4 times/day
>12 years and Adults:
Hippurate: 1 g twice daily
Mandelate: 1 g 4 times/day after meals and at bedtime
Dosing adjustment/comments in renal impairment: Cl_{cr} <50 mL/minute: Avoid use

Additional Information Complete prescribing information for this medication should be consulted for additional detail.

Dosage Forms Excipient information presented when available (limited, particularly for generics); consult specific product labeling. [DSC] = Discontinued product
Tablet, as hippurate: 1 g
Hiprex®, Urex™: 1 g [Hiprex® contains tartrazine dye]
Tablet, as mandelate: 500 mg [DSC], 1 g [DSC]
Mandelamine®: 500 mg [DSC], 1 g [DSC]

Methenamine and Sodium Acid Phosphate

(meth EN a meen & SOW dee um AS id FOS fate)

U.S. Brand Names Uroqid-Acid® No. 2

Index Terms Methenamine Mandelate and Sodium Acid Phosphate; Sodium Acid Phosphate and Methenamine

Pharmacologic Category Antibiotic, Miscellaneous

Use Prophylaxis or suppression of bacteriuria associated with recurrent urinary tract infections

Pregnancy Risk Factor C

Dosage Oral: Adults: Initial: 2 tablets 4 times daily; maintenance: 2-4 tablets daily in divided doses

Additional Information Complete prescribing information for this medication should be consulted for additional detail.

Dosage Forms Excipient information presented when available (limited, particularly for generics); consult specific product labeling.

Tablet: Methenamine mandelate 500 mg and sodium acid phosphate 500 mg [contains 83 mg sodium]

◆ **Methenamine Hippurate** *see* Methenamine *on page 961*

◆ **Methenamine Mandelate** *see* Methenamine *on page 961*

◆ **Methenamine Mandelate and Sodium Acid Phosphate** *see* Methenamine and Sodium Acid Phosphate *on page 962*

Methenamine, Phenyl Salicylate, Methylene Blue, Benzoic Acid, and Hyoscyamine

(meth EN a meen, fen nil sa LIS i late, METH i leen bloo, ben ZOE ik AS id & hye oh SYE a meen)

U.S. Brand Names Prosed®/DS

Index Terms Benzoic Acid, Methenamine, Methylene Blue, Phenyl Salicylate, and Hyoscyamine; Hyoscyamine, Methenamine, Benzoic Acid, Phenyl Salicylate, and Methylene Blue; Methylene Blue, Methenamine, Benzoic Acid, Phenyl Salicylate, and Hyoscyamine; Phenyl Salicylate, Methenamine, Methylene Blue, Benzoic Acid, and Hyoscyamine

Pharmacologic Category Antibiotic, Miscellaneous

Use Urinary tract discomfort secondary to hypermotility resulting from infection or diagnostic procedures

Pregnancy Risk Factor C

Dosage Oral:

Children >12 years: Dosage must be individualized

Adults: One tablet 4 times daily

Additional Information Complete prescribing information for this medication should be consulted for additional detail.

Dosage Forms Excipient information presented when available (limited, particularly for generics); consult specific product labeling.

Tablet, oral:

Prosed®/DS: Methenamine 81.6 mg, phenyl salicylate 36.2 mg, methylene blue 10.8 mg, benzoic acid 9 mg, hyoscyamine sulfate 0.12 mg

Methenamine, Sodium Biphosphate, Phenyl Salicylate, Methylene Blue, and Hyoscyamine

(meth EN a meen, SOW dee um bye FOS fate, fen nil sa LIS i late, METH i leen bloo, & hye oh SYE a meen)

U.S. Brand Names Urelle®; Urimar-T; Uta®; Utira™-C

Index Terms Hyoscyamine, Methenamine, Sodium Biphosphate, Phenyl Salicylate, and Methylene Blue; Methylene Blue, Methenamine, Sodium Biphosphate, Phenyl Salicylate, and Hyoscyamine; Phenyl Salicylate, Methenamine, Methylene Blue, Sodium Biphosphate, and Hyoscyamine; Sodium Biphosphate, Methenamine, Methylene Blue, Phenyl Salicylate, and Hyoscyamine

Pharmacologic Category Antibiotic, Miscellaneous

Use Treatment of symptoms of irritative voiding; relief of local symptoms associated with urinary tract infections; relief of urinary tract symptoms caused by diagnostic procedures

Pregnancy Risk Factor C

Lactation Enters breast milk/use caution

Contraindications Hypersensitivity to methenamine, hyoscyamine, methylene blue, or any component of the formulation

Warnings/Precautions Use caution in patients with a history of intolerance to belladonna alkaloids or salicylates. Use caution in patients with cardiovascular disease (cardiac arrhythmias, HF, coronary heart disease, mitral stenosis), gastrointestinal tract obstruction, glaucoma, myasthenia gravis, or obstructive uropathy (bladder neck obstruction or prostatic hyperplasia). Discontinue use immediately if tachycardia, dizziness, or blurred vision occur. Elderly may be more sensitive to anticholinergic effects of hyoscyamine; use caution. May cause urinary discoloration (blue). Prolonged use may result in fungal or bacterial superinfection, including *C. difficile*-associated diarrhea and pseudomembranous colitis. Safety and efficacy have not been established in children ≤6 years of age.

Adverse Reactions Frequency not defined.

Cardiovascular: Tachycardia, flushing

Central nervous system: Dizziness

Gastrointestinal: Xerostomia, nausea, vomiting

Genitourinary: Urinary retention (acute), micturition difficulty, discoloration of urine (blue)

Ocular: Blurred vision

Respiratory: Dyspnea

Drug Interactions

Avoid Concomitant Use There are no known interactions where it is recommended to avoid concomitant use.

Increased Effect/Toxicity

Methenamine, Sodium Biphosphate, Phenyl Salicylate, Methylene Blue, and Hyoscyamine may increase the levels/effects of: Anticholinergics; Cannabinoids; Potassium Chloride

The levels/effects of Methenamine, Sodium Biphosphate, Phenyl Salicylate, Methylene Blue, and Hyoscyamine may be increased by: Pramlintide

Decreased Effect

Methenamine, Sodium Biphosphate, Phenyl Salicylate, Methylene Blue, and Hyoscyamine may decrease the levels/effects of: Acetylcholinesterase Inhibitors (Central); Amphetamines; Secretin; Typhoid Vaccine

The levels/effects of Methenamine, Sodium Biphosphate, Phenyl Salicylate, Methylene Blue, and Hyoscyamine may be decreased by: Acetylcholinesterase Inhibitors (Central); Antacids; Carbonic Anhydrase Inhibitors

Stability Store at controlled room temperature of 15°C to 30°C (59°F to 86°F).

Dosage Oral:

Children >6 years: Dosage must be individualized

Adults: One tablet 4 times daily (followed by liberal fluid intake)

Dosage Forms Excipient information presented when available (limited, particularly for generics); consult specific product labeling.

Capsule, oral:

Uta®: Methenamine 120 mg, sodium biphosphate 40.8 mg, phenyl salicylate 36 mg, methylene blue 10 mg, hyoscyamine sulfate 0.12 mg

Tablet, oral:

Urelle®: Methenamine 81 mg, sodium biphosphate 40.8 mg, phenyl salicylate 32.4 mg, methylene blue 10.8 mg, hyoscyamine sulfate 0.12 mg

Urimar-T: Methenamine 81.6 mg, sodium biphosphate 40.8 mg, phenyl salicylate 36.2 mg, methylene blue 10.8 mg, hyoscyamine sulfate 0.12 mg

Utira™-C: Methenamine 81.6 mg, sodium biphosphate 40.8 mg, phenyl salicylate 36.2 mg, methylene blue 10.8 mg, hyoscyamine sulfate 0.12 mg

◆ **Methergine®** *see* Methylergonovine *on page* 971

Methimazole (meth IM a zole)

U.S. Brand Names Northyx™; Tapazole®

Canadian Brand Names Dom-Methimazole; PHL-Methimazole; Tapazole®

Index Terms Thiamazole

Pharmacologic Category Antithyroid Agent; Thioamide

Use Palliative treatment of hyperthyroidism, return the hyperthyroid patient to a normal metabolic state prior to thyroidectomy, and to control thyrotoxic crisis that may accompany thyroidectomy

Pregnancy Risk Factor D

Pregnancy Considerations Methimazole crosses the placenta and because adverse events may occur in the fetus following maternal use, it is classified as pregnancy category D. Rare cases of aplasia cutis congenital have been reported in the neonate, as well as a syndrome which includes choanal atresia, facial abnormalities, growth restriction and developmental abnormalities. Additional data is needed to determine any association of these adverse events with maternal methimazole use. Fetal thyroid function may also be transiently suppressed. Untreated hyperthyroidism may also cause adverse events in the mother (eg, heart failure, miscarriage, preeclampsia, thyroid storm); fetus (eg, goiter, growth restriction, hypo/hyperthyroidism, still birth); and neonate (eg, hyper-/hypothyroidism, neuropsychologic damage). The thioamides are treatment of choice for hyperthyroidism during pregnancy. In order to prevent adverse events to the fetus, the lowest effective dose should be used in order to achieve maternal levels of T_4 in the high euthyroid or low hyperthyroid range. Thyroid function should be monitored closely.

Lactation Enters breast milk/contraindicated (per manufacturer) (AAP rates "compatible")

Medication Safety Issues

Sound-alike/look-alike issues:

Methimazole may be confused with metolazone

Contraindications Hypersensitivity to methimazole or any component of the formulation; breast-feeding (per manufacturer; however, expert analysis and the AAP state this drug may be used in nursing mothers)

Warnings/Precautions Antithyroid agents have been associated (rarely) with significant bone marrow depression. The most severe manifestation is agranulocytosis. Aplastic anemia, thrombocytopenia, and leukopenia may also occur. Use with extreme caution in patients receiving other drugs known to cause myelosuppression particularly agranulocytosis, patients >40 years of age; avoid doses >40 mg/day (increased myelosuppression). Discontinue if significant bone marrow suppression occurs, particularly agranulocytosis or aplastic anemia.

Rare, severe hepatic reactions (hepatic necrosis, hepatitis) may occur. Symptoms suggestive of hepatic dysfunction should prompt evaluation. Discontinue in the presence of hepatitis (transaminase >3 times upper limit of normal). In addition, other rare hypersensitivity reactions to antithyroid agents have been reported, including the development of ANCA-positive vasculitis, drug fever, interstitial pneumonitis, exfoliative dermatitis, glomerulonephritis, leukocytoclastic vasculitis, and a lupus-like syndrome; prompt discontinuation is warranted in patients who develop symptoms consistent with a form of autoimmunity or other hypersensitivity during therapy. Minor dermatologic reactions may not require discontinuation, depending on severity.

May cause hypoprothrombinemia and bleeding; use with particular caution in patients >40 years of age.

Adverse Reactions Frequency not defined.

Cardiovascular: ANCA-positive vasculitis, edema, leukocytoclastic vasculitis, periarteritis

Central nervous system: CNS stimulation, depression, drowsiness, fever, headache, vertigo

Dermatologic: Alopecia, erythema nodosum, exfoliative dermatitis, pruritus, skin pigmentation, skin rash, urticaria

Endocrine & metabolic: Goiter

Gastrointestinal: Nausea, vomiting, stomach pain, abnormal taste, constipation, weight gain, salivary gland swelling

Hematologic: Agranulocytosis, aplastic anemia, granulocytopenia, hypoprothrombinemia, leukopenia, thrombocytopenia

Hepatic: Cholestatic jaundice, hepatitis, jaundice

Neuromuscular & skeletal: Arthralgia, paresthesia

Renal: Nephritis, nephrotic syndrome

Miscellaneous: SLE-like syndrome

Drug Interactions

Metabolism/Transport Effects Inhibits CYP1A2 (weak), 2A6 (weak), 2B6 (weak), 2C9 (weak), 2C19 (weak), 2D6 (moderate), 2E1 (weak), 3A4 (weak)

Avoid Concomitant Use

Avoid concomitant use of Methimazole with any of the following: Sodium Iodide I131

Increased Effect/Toxicity There are no known significant interactions involving an increase in effect.

Decreased Effect

Methimazole may decrease the levels/effects of: Sodium Iodide I131; Vitamin K Antagonists

Stability Protect from light.

Mechanism of Action Inhibits the synthesis of thyroid hormones by blocking the oxidation of iodine in the thyroid gland, blocking iodine's ability to combine with tyrosine to form thyroxine and triiodothyronine (T_3), does not inactivate circulating T_4 and T_3

Pharmacodynamics/Kinetics

Onset of action: Antithyroid: Oral: 12-18 hours

Duration: 36-72 hours

Distribution: Concentrated in thyroid gland; crosses placenta; enters breast milk (1:1)

Protein binding, plasma: None

Metabolism: Hepatic

Bioavailability: 80% to 95%

Half-life elimination: 4-13 hours

Excretion: Urine (80%)

Dosage Oral: Administer in 3 equally divided doses at approximately 8-hour intervals

Children: Initial: 0.4 mg/kg/day in 3 divided doses; maintenance: 0.2 mg/kg/day in 3 divided doses up to 30 mg/24 hours maximum

Alternatively: Initial: 0.5-0.7 mg/kg/day **or** 15-20 mg/m²/day in 3 divided doses

Maintenance: 1/3 to 2/3 of the initial dose beginning when the patient is euthyroid

Maximum: 30 mg/24 hours

Adults: Initial: 15 mg/day in 3 divided doses (approximately every 8 hours) for mild hyperthyroidism; 30-40 mg/day in moderately-severe hyperthyroidism; 60 mg/day in severe hyperthyroidism; maintenance: 5-15 mg/day (may be given as a single daily dose in many cases)

Adjust dosage as required to achieve and maintain serum T_3, T_4, and TSH levels in the normal range. An elevated T_3 may be the sole indicator of inadequate treatment. An elevated TSH indicates excessive antithyroid treatment.

Thyrotoxic crisis (recommendations vary widely and have not been evaluated in comparative trials): Dosages of 20-30 mg every 6-12 hours have been recommended for short-term initial therapy, followed by gradual reduction to a maintenance dosage (5-15 mg/day). Rectal administration has been described (Nabil, 1982).

Dosing adjustment in renal impairment: Adjustment is not necessary

Dietary Considerations Should be taken consistently in relation to meals every day.

Administration In thyroid storm, rectal administration has been attempted (Nabil, 1982).

Monitoring Parameters Monitor for signs of hypothyroidism, hyperthyroidism, T_4, T_3; CBC with differential, liver function (baseline and as needed), serum thyroxine, free thyroxine index

Dosage Forms Excipient information presented when available (limited, particularly for generics); consult specific product labeling.

Tablet: 5 mg, 10 mg, 20 mg

Northyx™: 5 mg, 10 mg, 15 mg, 20 mg

Tapazole®: 5 mg, 10 mg

◆ **Methitest™** *see* MethylTESTOSTERone *on page 979*

Methocarbamol (meth oh KAR ba mole)

U.S. Brand Names Robaxin®

Canadian Brand Names Robaxin®

Pharmacologic Category Skeletal Muscle Relaxant

Use Treatment of muscle spasm associated with acute painful musculoskeletal conditions; supportive therapy in tetanus

Pregnancy Risk Factor C

Pregnancy Considerations Animal reproduction studies have not been conducted. The manufacturer notes that fetal and congenital abnormalities have been rarely reported following *in utero* exposure. Use during pregnancy only if clearly needed.

Lactation Excretion in breast milk unknown/use caution

Medication Safety Issues

Sound-alike/look-alike issues:

Methocarbamol may be confused with mephobarbital

Robaxin® may be confused with ribavirin, Rubex®

Contraindications Hypersensitivity to methocarbamol or any component of the formulation; renal impairment (injection formulation)

Warnings/Precautions

May cause CNS depression, which may impair physical or mental abilities; patients must be cautioned about performing tasks which require mental alertness (eg, operating machinery or driving). Effects may be potentiated when used with other sedative drugs or ethanol.

Oral: Use caution with renal or hepatic impairment. Safety and efficacy of the oral formulation have not been established in children <16 years of age.

Injection: Rate of injection should not exceed 3 mL/minute; solution is hypertonic; avoid extravasation. Use with caution in patients with a history of seizures. Use caution with hepatic impairment. Vial stopper contains latex.

Adverse Reactions Frequency not defined.

Cardiovascular: Flushing of face, bradycardia, hypotension, syncope

Central nervous system: Drowsiness, dizziness, lightheadedness, convulsion, vertigo, headache, fever, amnesia, confusion, insomnia, sedation, coordination impaired (mild)

Dermatologic: Allergic dermatitis, urticaria, pruritus, rash, angioneurotic edema

Gastrointestinal: Nausea, vomiting, metallic taste, dyspepsia

Hematologic: Leukopenia

Hepatic: Jaundice

Local: Pain at injection site, thrombophlebitis

Ocular: Nystagmus, blurred vision, diplopia, conjunctivitis

Renal: Renal impairment

Respiratory: Nasal congestion

Miscellaneous: Allergic manifestations, anaphylactic reaction

Drug Interactions

Avoid Concomitant Use There are no known interactions where it is recommended to avoid concomitant use.

Increased Effect/Toxicity

Methocarbamol may increase the levels/effects of: Alcohol (Ethyl); CNS Depressants

Decreased Effect

Methocarbamol may decrease the levels/effects of: Pyridostigmine

Ethanol/Nutrition/Herb Interactions

Ethanol: Avoid ethanol (may increase CNS depression).

Herb/Nutraceutical: Avoid valerian, St John's wort, kava kava, gotu kola (may increase CNS depression).

Stability

Injection: Prior to dilution, store at controlled room temperature of 20°C to 25°C (68°F to 77°F). Injection when diluted to 4 mg/mL in sterile water, 5% dextrose, or 0.9% saline is stable for 6 days at room temperature. Do **not** refrigerate after dilution.

Tablet: Store at controlled room temperature of 20°C to 25°C (68°F to 77°F).

Mechanism of Action Causes skeletal muscle relaxation by general CNS depression

Pharmacodynamics/Kinetics

Onset of action: Muscle relaxation: Oral: ~30 minutes

Protein binding: 46% to 50%

Metabolism: Hepatic via dealkylation and hydroxylation

Half-life elimination: 1-2 hours

Time to peak, serum: ~2 hours

Excretion: Urine (as metabolites)

Dosage

Tetanus: I.V.:

Children: Recommended **only** for use in tetanus: 15 mg/kg/dose or 500 mg/m²/dose, may repeat every 6 hours if needed; maximum dose: 1.8 g/m²/day for 3 days only

Adults: Initial dose: 1-3 g; may repeat dose every 6 hours until oral dosing is possible; injection should not be used for more than 3 consecutive days

Muscle spasm: Children ≥16 years and Adults:

Oral: 1.5 g 4 times/day for 2-3 days (up to 8 g/day may be given in severe conditions), then decrease to 4-4.5 g/day in 3-6 divided doses

I.M., I.V.: 1 g every 8 hours if oral not possible; injection should not be used for more than 3 consecutive days. If condition persists, may repeat course of therapy after a drug-free interval of 48 hours.

Elderly: Muscle spasm: Oral: Initial: 500 mg 4 times/day; titrate to response

Dosing adjustment/comments in renal impairment: Do not administer parenteral formulation to patients with renal dysfunction.

Dosing adjustment in hepatic impairment: Specific dosing guidelines are not available; plasma protein binding and clearance are decreased; half-life is increased

Administration

Injection:

I.M.: A maximum of 5 mL can be administered into each gluteal region.

I.V.: Maximum rate: 3 mL/minute; should not be used for more than 3 consecutive days; may be administered undiluted. Monitor closely for extravasation. Administer I.V. while in recumbent position. Maintain position 15-30 minutes following infusion.

Tablet: May be crushed and mixed with food or liquid if needed. Avoid alcohol.

Test Interactions May cause color interference in certain screening tests for 5-HIAA using nitrosonaphthol reagent and in screening tests for urinary VMA using the Gitlow method.

Dosage Forms Excipient information presented when available (limited, particularly for generics); consult specific product labeling.

Injection, solution: 100 mg/mL (10 mL) [in polyethylene glycol; vial stopper contains latex]

Tablet: 500 mg, 750 mg

Methohexital (meth oh HEKS i tal)

U.S. Brand Names Brevital® Sodium

Canadian Brand Names Brevital®

Index Terms Methohexital Sodium

Pharmacologic Category Barbiturate; General Anesthetic

Use For induction of anesthesia prior to the use of other general anesthetic agents; as an adjunct to subpotent inhalational anesthetic agents for short surgical procedures; for short surgical, diagnostic, or therapeutic procedures associated with minimal painful stimuli

Additional indications for adults: For use with other parenteral agents, usually narcotic analgesics, to supplement subpotent inhalational anesthetic agents for longer surgical procedures; as an agent to induce a hypnotic state

Unlabeled/Investigational Use Wada test

Restrictions C-IV

Pregnancy Risk Factor B

Medication Safety Issues

Sound-alike/look-alike issues:

Brevital® may be confused with Brevibloc®

High alert medication: The Institute for Safe Medication Practices (ISMP) includes this medication among its list of drugs which have a heightened risk of causing significant patient harm when used in error.

Dosage Doses must be titrated to effect.

Infants <1 month: Safety and efficacy not established

Infants ≥1 month and Children:

Anesthesia induction:

I.M.: 6.6-10 mg/kg of a 5% solution

Rectal: Usual: 25 mg/kg of a 1% solution

I.V. (unlabeled dose): 1-2 mg/kg/dose of a 1% solution

Procedural sedation (unlabeled dose):

I.V.: Initial: 0.5 mg/kg given immediately prior to procedure; if sedation not adequate, repeat 0.5 mg/kg to a maximum total dose of 2 mg/kg

Rectal: 25 mg/kg of a 10% (100 mg/mL) solution given 5-15 minutes prior to procedure; maximum dose 500 mg

Adults: I.V.:

Induction: 1-1.5 mg/kg; maintenance: 50-120 mcg/kg/minute (or 20-40 mg every 4-7 minutes)

Wada test (unlabeled): 2-4 mg

Dosing adjustment/comments in hepatic impairment: Lower dosage and monitor closely

Additional Information Complete prescribing information for this medication should be consulted for additional detail.

Dosage Forms Excipient information presented when available (limited, particularly for generics); consult specific product labeling.

Injection, powder for reconstitution, as sodium:

Brevital® Sodium: 500 mg, 2.5 g

◆ **Methohexital Sodium** *see* Methohexital *on page* 965

Methotrexate (meth oh TREKS ate)

U.S. Brand Names Rheumatrex® Dose Pack®; Trexall™

Canadian Brand Names Apo-Methotrexate®; ratio-Methotrexate

Index Terms Amethopterin; Methotrexate Sodium; MTX (error-prone abbreviation); NSC-740

Pharmacologic Category Antineoplastic Agent, Antimetabolite (Antifolate); Antirheumatic, Disease Modifying

Use Treatment of trophoblastic neoplasms; leukemias; psoriasis; rheumatoid arthritis (RA), including polyarticular-course juvenile rheumatoid arthritis (JRA); breast, head and neck, and lung carcinomas; osteosarcoma; soft-tissue sarcomas; carcinoma of gastrointestinal tract, esophagus, testes; lymphomas

Unlabeled/Investigational Use Treatment and maintenance of remission in Crohn's disease; ectopic pregnancy

Pregnancy Risk Factor X (psoriasis, rheumatoid arthritis)

Pregnancy Considerations [U.S. Boxed Warning]: May cause fetal death or congenital abnormalities; do not use for psoriasis or RA treatment in pregnant women. Use for the treatment of neoplastic diseases only when the potential benefit to the mother outweighs the possible risk to the fetus. Pregnancy should be excluded prior to therapy in women of childbearing potential. Pregnancy should be avoided for ≥3 months following treatment in male patients and ≥1 ovulatory cycle in female patients.

Lactation Enters breast milk/contraindicated

Medication Safety Issues

Sound-alike/look-alike issues:

Methotrexate may be confused with metolazone, mitoxantrone

MTX is an error-prone abbreviation (mistaken as mitoxantrone)

High alert medication: The Institute for Safe Medication Practices (ISMP) includes this medication among its list of drugs which have a heightened risk of causing significant patient harm when used in error.

Errors have occurred (resulting in death) when methotrexate was administered as "daily" dose instead of the recommended "weekly" dose.

International issues:

Trexall™ may be confused with Truxal® which is a brand name for chlorprothixene in Belgium

Trexall™ may be confused with Trexol® which is a brand name for tramadol in Mexico

Contraindications Hypersensitivity to methotrexate or any component of the formulation; severe renal or hepatic impairment; pre-existing profound bone marrow suppression in patients with psoriasis or rheumatoid arthritis, alcoholic liver disease, AIDS, pre-existing blood dyscrasias; pregnancy (in patients with psoriasis or rheumatoid arthritis); breast-feeding

Warnings/Precautions Hazardous agent - use appropriate precautions for handling and disposal.

[U.S. Boxed Warning]: Methotrexate has been associated with acute (elevated transaminases) and potentially fatal chronic (fibrosis, cirrhosis) hepatotoxicity. Risk is related to cumulative dose and prolonged exposure. Monitor closely (with liver function tests, including serum albumin) for liver toxicities. Liver enzyme elevations may be noted, but may not be predictive of hepatic disease in long term treatment for psoriasis (but generally is predictive in rheumatoid arthritis [RA] treatment). With long-term use, liver biopsy may show histologic changes, fibrosis or cirrhosis; periodic liver biopsy is recommended with long-term use for psoriasis and for persistent abnormal liver function tests with RA;

discontinue methotrexate with moderate-to-severe change in liver biopsy. Ethanol abuse, obesity, advanced age, and diabetes may increase the risk of hepatotoxic reactions. Use caution with preexisting liver impairment; may require dosage reduction. Use caution when used with other hepatotoxic agents (azathioprine, retinoids, sulfasalazine). **[U.S. Boxed Warning]: Methotrexate elimination is reduced in patients with ascites;** may require dose reduction or discontinuation. Monitor closely for toxicity.

[U.S. Boxed Warning]: May cause renal damage leading to acute renal failure, especially with high-dose methotrexate; monitor renal function and methotrexate levels closely, maintain adequate hydration and urinary alkalinization. Use caution in osteosarcoma patients treated with high-dose methotrexate in combination with nephrotoxic chemotherapy (eg, cisplatin). **[U.S. Boxed Warning]: Methotrexate elimination is reduced in patients with renal impairment;** may require dose reduction or discontinuation; monitor closely for toxicity. **[U.S. Boxed Warning]: Tumor lysis syndrome may occur in patients with high tumor burden;** use appropriate prevention and treatment.

[U.S. Boxed Warning]: May cause potentially life-threatening pneumonitis (may occur at any time during therapy and at any dosage); monitor closely for pulmonary symptoms, particularly dry, nonproductive cough. Other potential symptoms include fever, dyspnea, hypoxemia, or pulmonary infiltrate. **[U.S. Boxed Warning]: Methotrexate elimination is reduced in patients with pleural effusions;** may require dose reduction or discontinuation. Monitor closely for toxicity.

[U.S. Boxed Warning]: Bone marrow suppression may occur, resulting in anemia, aplastic anemia, pancytopenia, leukopenia, neutropenia, and/or thrombocytopenia. Use caution in patients with pre-existing bone marrow suppression. Discontinue therapy in RA or psoriasis if a significant decrease in hematologic components is noted. **[U.S. Boxed Warning]: Use of low dose methotrexate has been associated with the development of malignant lymphomas;** may regress upon discontinuation of therapy; treat lymphoma appropriately if regression is not induced by cessation of methotrexate.

[U.S. Boxed Warning]: Diarrhea and ulcerative stomatitis may require interruption of therapy; death from hemorrhagic enteritis or intestinal perforation has been reported. Use with caution in patients with peptic ulcer disease, ulcerative colitis.

May cause neurotoxicity including seizures (usually in pediatric ALL patients), leukoencephalopathy (usually with concurrent cranial irradiation) and stroke-like encephalopathy (usually with high-dose regimens). Chemical arachnoiditis (headache, back pain, nuchal rigidity, fever), myelopathy and chronic leukoencephalopathy may result from intrathecal administration.

[U.S. Boxed Warning]: Any dose level or route of administration may cause severe and potentially fatal dermatologic reactions, including toxic epidermal necrolysis, Stevens-Johnson syndrome, exfoliative dermatitis, skin necrosis, and erythema multiforme. Radiation dermatitis and sunburn may be precipitated by methotrexate administration. Psoriatic lesions may be worsened by concomitant exposure to ultraviolet radiation.

[U.S. Boxed Warning]: Concomitant administration with NSAIDs may cause severe bone marrow suppression, aplastic anemia, and GI toxicity. Do not administer NSAIDs prior to or during high dose methotrexate therapy; may increase and prolong serum methotrexate levels. Doses used for psoriasis may still lead to unexpected toxicities; use caution when administering NSAIDs or salicylates with lower doses of methotrexate for RA. Methotrexate may increase the levels and effects of mercaptopurine; may require dosage adjustments. Vitamins containing folate may decrease response to systemic methotrexate; folate deficiency may increase methotrexate toxicity. **[U.S. Boxed Warning]: Concomitant methotrexate administration with radiotherapy may increase the risk of soft tissue necrosis and osteonecrosis.**

[U.S. Boxed Warnings]: Should be administered under the supervision of a physician experienced in the use of antimetabolite therapy; serious and fatal toxicities have occurred at all dose levels. Immune suppression may lead to potentially fatal opportunistic infections. For rheumatoid arthritis and psoriasis, immunosuppressive therapy should only be used when disease is active and less toxic, traditional therapy is ineffective. Methotrexate formulations and/or diluents containing preservatives should not be used for intrathecal or high-dose therapy. May cause fetal death or congenital abnormalities; do not use for psoriasis or RA treatment in pregnant women. May cause impairment of fertility, oligospermia, and menstrual dysfunction. Toxicity from methotrexate or any immunosuppressive is increased in the elderly. Methotrexate injection may contain benzyl alcohol and should not be used in neonates.

Adverse Reactions Note: Adverse reactions vary by route and dosage. Hematologic and/or gastrointestinal toxicities may be common at dosages used in chemotherapy; these reactions are much less frequent when used at typical dosages for rheumatic diseases.

>10%:
- Central nervous system (with I.T. administration or very high-dose therapy):
  - Arachnoiditis: Acute reaction manifested as severe headache, nuchal rigidity, vomiting, and fever; may be alleviated by reducing the dose
  - Subacute toxicity: 10% of patients treated with 12-15 mg/m^2 of I.T. methotrexate may develop this in the second or third week of therapy; consists of motor paralysis of extremities, cranial nerve palsy, seizure, or coma. This has also been seen in pediatric cases receiving very high-dose I.V. methotrexate.
  - Demyelinating encephalopathy: Seen months or years after receiving methotrexate; usually in association with cranial irradiation or other systemic chemotherapy
- Dermatologic: Reddening of skin
- Endocrine & metabolic: Hyperuricemia, defective oogenesis or spermatogenesis
- Gastrointestinal: Ulcerative stomatitis, glossitis, gingivitis, nausea, vomiting, diarrhea, anorexia, intestinal perforation, mucositis (dose dependent; appears in 3-7 days after therapy, resolving within 2 weeks)
- Hematologic: Leukopenia, thrombocytopenia
- Renal: Renal failure, azotemia, nephropathy
- Respiratory: Pharyngitis

1% to 10%:
- Cardiovascular: Vasculitis
- Central nervous system: Dizziness, malaise, encephalopathy, seizure, fever, chills
- Dermatologic: Alopecia, rash, photosensitivity, depigmentation or hyperpigmentation of skin
- Endocrine & metabolic: Diabetes
- Genitourinary: Cystitis
- Hematologic: Hemorrhage
- Myelosuppressive: This is the primary dose-limiting factor (along with mucositis) of methotrexate; occurs about 5-7 days after methotrexate therapy, and should resolve within 2 weeks
  - WBC: Mild
  - Platelets: Moderate
  - Onset: 7 days

Nadir: 10 days
Recovery: 21 days

Hepatic: Cirrhosis and portal fibrosis have been associated with chronic methotrexate therapy; acute elevation of liver enzymes are common after high-dose methotrexate, and usually resolve within 10 days.

Neuromuscular & skeletal: Arthralgia

Ocular: Blurred vision

Renal: Renal dysfunction: Manifested by an abrupt rise in serum creatinine and BUN and a fall in urine output; more common with high-dose methotrexate, and may be due to precipitation of the drug.

Respiratory: Pneumonitis: Associated with fever, cough, and interstitial pulmonary infiltrates; treatment is to withhold methotrexate during the acute reaction; interstitial pneumonitis has been reported to occur with an incidence of 1% in patients with RA (dose 7.5-15 mg/week)

<1% (Limited to important or life-threatening): Acute neurologic syndrome (at high dosages - symptoms include confusion, hemiparesis, transient blindness, and coma); anaphylaxis, alveolitis, cognitive dysfunction (has been reported at low dosage), decreased resistance to infection, erythema multiforme, hepatic failure, leukoencephalopathy (especially following craniospinal irradiation or repeated high-dose therapy), lymphoproliferative disorders, osteonecrosis and soft tissue necrosis (with radiotherapy), pericarditis, plaque erosions (psoriasis), seizure (more frequent in pediatric patients with ALL), Stevens-Johnson syndrome, thromboembolism

Drug Interactions

Avoid Concomitant Use

Avoid concomitant use of Methotrexate with any of the following: Acitretin; Natalizumab; Vaccines (Live)

Increased Effect/Toxicity

Methotrexate may increase the levels/effects of: CycloSPORINE; Leflunomide; Natalizumab; Vaccines (Live); Vitamin K Antagonists

The levels/effects of Methotrexate may be increased by: Acitretin; Ciprofloxacin; CycloSPORINE; Eltrombopag; Nonsteroidal Anti-Inflammatory Agents; Penicillins; P-Glycoprotein Inhibitors; Proton Pump Inhibitors; Salicylates; Sulfonamide Derivatives; Trastuzumab; Trimethoprim; Uricosuric Agents

Decreased Effect

Methotrexate may decrease the levels/effects of: Cardiac Glycosides; Sapropterin; Vaccines (Inactivated); Vitamin K Antagonists

The levels/effects of Methotrexate may be decreased by: Bile Acid Sequestrants; Echinacea; P-Glycoprotein Inducers

Ethanol/Nutrition/Herb Interactions

Ethanol: Avoid ethanol (may be associated with increased liver injury).

Food: Methotrexate peak serum levels may be decreased if taken with food. Milk-rich foods may decrease methotrexate absorption. Folate may decrease drug response.

Herb/Nutraceutical: Avoid echinacea (has immunostimulant properties).

Stability Store tablets and intact vials at room temperature (15°C to 25°C). Protect from light. Dilute powder with D_5W or NS to a concentration of ≤25 mg/mL (20 mg and 50 mg vials) and 50 mg/mL (1 g vial). Intrathecal solutions may be reconstituted to 2.5-5 mg/mL with NS, D_5W, lactated Ringer's, or Elliott's B solution. **Use preservative free preparations for intrathecal or high-dose administration.** Further dilution in D_5W or NS is stable for 24 hours at room temperature (21°C to 25°C). Reconstituted solutions with a preservative may be stored under refrigeration for up to 3 months, and up to 4 weeks at room temperature. Intrathecal dilutions are stable at room temperature for 7 days, but it is generally recommended that they be used within 4-8 hours.

Mechanism of Action Methotrexate is a folate antimetabolite that inhibits DNA synthesis. Methotrexate irreversibly binds to dihydrofolate reductase, inhibiting the formation of reduced folates, and thymidylate synthetase, resulting in inhibition of purine and thymidylic acid synthesis. Methotrexate is cell cycle specific for the S phase of the cycle.

The MOA in the treatment of rheumatoid arthritis is unknown, but may affect immune function. In psoriasis, methotrexate is thought to target rapidly proliferating epithelial cells in the skin.

In Crohn's disease, it may have immune modulator and anti-inflammatory activity.

Pharmacodynamics/Kinetics

Onset of action: Antirheumatic: 3-6 weeks; additional improvement may continue longer than 12 weeks

Absorption: Oral: Rapid; well absorbed at low doses (<30 mg/m^2), incomplete after large doses; I.M.: Complete

Distribution: Penetrates slowly into 3rd space fluids (eg, pleural effusions, ascites), exits slowly from these compartments (slower than from plasma); crosses placenta; small amounts enter breast milk; sustained concentrations retained in kidney and liver

Protein binding: 50%

Metabolism: <10%; degraded by intestinal flora to DAMPA by carboxypeptidase; hepatic aldehyde oxidase converts methotrexate to 7-OH methotrexate; polyglutamates are produced intracellularly and are just as potent as methotrexate; their production is dose- and duration-dependent and they are slowly eliminated by the cell once formed

Half-life elimination: Low dose: 3-10 hours; High dose: 8-12 hours

Time to peak, serum: Oral: 1-2 hours; I.M.: 30-60 minutes

Excretion: Urine (44% to 100%); feces (small amounts)

Dosage Refer to individual protocols.

Note: Doses between 100-500 mg/m^2 **may require** leucovorin rescue. Doses >500 mg/m^2 **require** leucovorin rescue: Oral, I.M., I.V.: Leucovorin 10-15 mg/m^2 every 6 hours for 8 or 10 doses, starting 24 hours after the start of methotrexate infusion. Continue until the methotrexate level is ≤0.1 micromolar (10^{-7} M). Some clinicians continue leucovorin until the methotrexate level is <0.05 micromolar (5×10^{-8} M) or 0.01 micromolar (10^{-8} M).

If the 48-hour methotrexate level is >1 micromolar (10^{-6} M) or the 72-hour methotrexate level is >0.2 micromolar (2×10^{-7} M): I.V., I.M, Oral: Leucovorin 100 mg/m^2 every 6 hours until the methotrexate level is ≤0.1 micromolar (10^{-7} M). Some clinicians continue leucovorin until the methotrexate level is <0.05 micromolar (5×10^{-8} M) or 0.01 micromolar (10^{-8} M).

Children:

Dermatomyositis: Oral: 15-20 mg/m^2/week as a single dose once weekly **or** 0.3-1 mg/kg/dose once weekly

Juvenile rheumatoid arthritis: Oral, I.M.: 10 mg/m^2 once weekly, then 5-15 mg/m^2/week as a single dose **or** as 3 divided doses given 12 hours apart

Antineoplastic dosage range:

Oral, I.M.: 7.5-30 mg/m^2/week **or** every 2 weeks

I.V.: 10-18,000 mg/m^2 bolus dosing **or** continuous infusion over 6-42 hours

Pediatric solid tumors (high-dose): I.V.:

<12 years: 12-25 g/m^2

≥12 years: 8 g/m^2

Acute lymphocytic leukemia (intermediate-dose): I.V.: Loading: 100 mg/m^2 bolus dose, followed by 900 mg/m^2/day infusion over 23-41 hours.

Meningeal leukemia: I.T.: 10-15 mg/m^2 (maximum dose: 15 mg) **or** an age-based dosing regimen; one possible system is:
≤3 months: 3 mg/dose
4-11 months: 6 mg/dose
1 year: 8 mg/dose
2 years: 10 mg/dose
≥3 years: 12 mg/dose

Adults: I.V.: Range is wide from 30-40 mg/m^2/week to 100-12,000 mg/m^2 with leucovorin rescue
Trophoblastic neoplasms:
Oral, I.M.: 15-30 mg/day for 5 days; repeat in 7 days for 3-5 courses
I.V.: 11 mg/m^2 days 1 through 5 every 3 weeks
Head and neck cancer: Oral, I.M., I.V.: 25-50 mg/m^2 once weekly
Mycosis fungoides (cutaneous T-cell lymphoma): Oral, I.M.: Initial (early stages):
5-50 mg once weekly **or**
15-37.5 mg twice weekly
Bladder cancer: I.V.:
30 mg/m^2 day 1 and 8 every 3 weeks **or**
30 mg/m^2 day 1, 15, and 22 every 4 weeks
Breast cancer: I.V.: 30-60 mg/m^2 days 1 and 8 every 3-4 weeks
Gastric cancer: I.V.: 1500 mg/m^2 every 4 weeks
Lymphoma, non-Hodgkin's: I.V.:
30 mg/m^2 days 3 and 10 every 3 weeks **or**
120 mg/m^2 day 8 and 15 every 3-4 weeks **or**
200 mg/m^2 day 8 and 15 every 3 weeks **or**
400 mg/m^2 every 4 weeks for 3 cycles **or**
1 g/m^2 every 3 weeks **or**
1.5 g/m^2 every 4 weeks
Sarcoma: I.V.: 8-12 g/m^2 weekly for 2-4 weeks
Rheumatoid arthritis: Oral: 7.5 mg once weekly **or** 2.5 mg every 12 hours for 3 doses/week, not to exceed 20 mg/week
Psoriasis:
Oral: 2.5-5 mg/dose every 12 hours for 3 doses given weekly **or**
Oral, I.M.: 10-25 mg/dose given once weekly
Ectopic pregnancy (unlabeled use): I.M.: 50 mg/m^2 as a single dose
Active Crohn's disease (unlabeled use): Induction of remission: I.M., SubQ: 15-25 mg once weekly; remission maintenance: 15 mg once weekly
Note: Oral dosing has been reported as effective but oral absorption is highly variable. If patient relapses after a switch to oral, may consider returning to injectable.

Elderly: Rheumatoid arthritis/psoriasis: Oral: Initial: 5-7.5 mg/week, not to exceed 20 mg/week

Dosing adjustment in renal impairment: The FDA-approved labeling does not contain dosage adjustment guidelines. The following guidelines have been used by some clinicians:
Cl_{cr} 61-80 mL/minute: Administer 75% of dose
Cl_{cr} 51-60 mL/minute: Administer 70% of dose
Cl_{cr} 10-50 mL/minute: Administer 30% to 50% of dose
Cl_{cr} <10 mL/minute: Avoid use
Hemodialysis: Not dialyzable (0% to 5%); supplemental dose is not necessary
Peritoneal dialysis effects: Supplemental dose is not necessary
CAVH effects: Unknown

Aronoff, 2007:
Children:
Cl_{cr} 10-50 mL/minute: Administer 50% of dose
Cl_{cr} <10 mL/minute: Administer 30% of dose
Hemodialysis: Administer 30% of dose
Continuous ambulatory peritoneal dialysis (CAPD): Administer 30% of dose
Continuous renal replacement therapy (CRRT): Administer 50% of dose
Adults:
Cl_{cr} 10-50 mL/minute: Administer 50% of dose
Cl_{cr} <10 mL/minute: Avoid use
Hemodialysis: Administer 50% of dose
Continuous renal replacement therapy (CRRT): Administer 50% of dose

Kintzel, 1995:
Cl_{cr} 46-60 mL/minute: Administer 65% of normal dose
Cl_{cr} 31-45 mL/minute: Administer 50% of normal dose
Cl_{cr} <30 mL/minute: Avoid use

Dosage adjustment in hepatic impairment: The FDA-approved labeling does not contain dosage adjustment guidelines. The following guidelines have been used by some clinicians (Floyd, 2006):
Bilirubin 3.1-5 mg/dL **or** transaminases >3 times ULN: Administer 75% of dose
Bilirubin >5 mg/dL: Avoid use

Dietary Considerations
Sodium content of 100 mg injection: 20 mg (0.86 mEq)
Sodium content of 100 mg (low sodium) injection: 15 mg (0.65 mEq)

Administration Methotrexate may be administered I.M., I.V., I.T., or SubQ; I.V. administration may be as slow push, short bolus infusion, or 24- to 42-hour continuous infusion

Specific dosing schemes vary, but high dose should be followed by leucovorin calcium to prevent toxicity; refer to Leucovorin calcium monograph on page 866

Monitoring Parameters For prolonged use (especially rheumatoid arthritis, psoriasis) a baseline liver biopsy, repeated at each 1-1.5 g cumulative dose interval, should be performed; WBC and platelet counts every 4 weeks; CBC and creatinine, LFTs every 3-4 months; chest x-ray

Reference Range Therapeutic levels: Variable; Toxic concentration: Variable; therapeutic range is dependent upon therapeutic approach.

High-dose regimens produce drug levels that are between 0.1-1 micromole/L 24-72 hours after drug infusion
Toxic: Low-dose therapy: >0.2 micromole/L; high-dose therapy: >1 micromole/L

Additional Information Latex-free products: 50 mg/2 mL, 100 mg/4 mL, and 250 mg/10 mL vials with and without preservatives by Immunex

Dosage Forms Excipient information presented when available (limited, particularly for generics); consult specific product labeling.
Injection, powder for reconstitution [preservative free]: 20 mg, 1 g
Injection, solution: 25 mg/mL (2 mL, 10 mL) [contains benzyl alcohol]
Injection, solution [preservative free]: 25 mg/mL (2 mL, 4 mL, 8 mL, 10 mL, 40 mL)
Tablet: 2.5 mg
Trexall™: 5 mg, 7.5 mg, 10 mg, 15 mg
Tablet, as sodium [dose pack] (Rheumatrex® Dose Pack): 2.5 mg (4 cards with 2, 3, 4, 5, or 6 tablets each)

◆ **Methotrexate Sodium** *see* Methotrexate *on page 965*

Methoxsalen (meth OKS a len)

U.S. Brand Names 8-MOP®; Oxsoralen-Ultra®; Oxsoralen®; Uvadex®
Canadian Brand Names Oxsoralen-Ultra®; Oxsoralen®; Ultramop™; Uvadex®
Index Terms 8-Methoxypsoralen; 8-MOP; Methoxypsoralen
Pharmacologic Category Psoralen

Use

Oral: Symptomatic control of severe, recalcitrant disabling psoriasis; repigmentation of idiopathic vitiligo; palliative treatment of skin manifestations of cutaneous T-cell lymphoma (CTCL)

Topical: Repigmentation of idiopathic vitiligo

Extracorporeal: Palliative treatment of skin manifestations of CTCL

Pregnancy Risk Factor C/D (Uvadex®)

Pregnancy Considerations Fetal toxicity has been observed in animal studies, however, there are no adequate and well-controlled studies in pregnant women. Use during pregnancy is not recommended. Women of childbearing potential should be advised to avoid pregnancy.

Lactation Excretion in breast milk unknown/not recommended

Medication Safety Issues

Sound-alike/look-alike issues:

Methoxsalen soft gelatin capsules (Oxsoralen-Ultra®) may be confused with methoxsalen hard gelatin capsules (8-MOP®, Oxsoralen®); bioavailability and photosensitization onset differ between the two products.

Contraindications Hypersensitivity to methoxsalen (psoralens) or any component of the formulation; diseases associated with photosensitivity (eg, albinism, lupus erythematosus, porphyria [cutanea tarda, erythropoietic and variegate], xeroderma pigmentosum); invasive squamous cell cancer; aphakia; melanoma or history of melanoma; children <12 years of age (Oxsoralen® lotion)

Warnings/Precautions [U.S. Boxed Warning]: Soft-gelatin capsule (Oxsoralen-Ultra®) and hard-gelatin capsule (8-MOP®, Oxsoralen®) are not interchangeable; retitration is required if the formulation is changed. Oxsoralen-Ultra® has a greater bioavailability and shorter photosensitization onset. Serious burns may occur from ultraviolet radiation or sunlight (even if exposed through glass) if recommended dose and/or exposure schedule is not maintained. Therapy may lead to increased risk of skin cancers (basal cell, melanoma and squamous cell); this risk may be increased with fair skin or prior exposure to prolonged tar and UVB treatment, ionizing radiation, or arsenic. Methoxsalen concentrates in the lens; eyes should be shielded from direct and indirect sunlight for 24 hours to prevent possible formation of cataracts. Use caution with basal cell carcinoma, hepatic, cardiac disease, or in the elderly. Use caution with other agents (systemic and topical) that may cause photosensitivity. Avoid sun (including sun lamp) exposure for 8 hours after methoxsalen ingestion. Protective clothing and sunscreen (do not apply sunscreen to psoriatic areas) should be used for 24 hours after combined methoxsalen/UVA therapy. Do not use in sunburned patients until they have fully recovered; pre-existing sunburn may obscure evaluation of response; advise patients to avoid sunbathing for 24 hours prior to treatment and for 48 hours after treatment. Use extreme caution in patients who have significant exposure to the sun through their occupation.

CTCL: For use only if inadequate response to other forms of therapy. Used in conjunction with long wave radiation of white blood cells using the UVAR® photopheresis system. Safety and efficacy in pediatric patients have not been established.

Psoriasis: For use only if inadequate response to other therapies when the diagnosis is biopsy proven. Administer only in conjunction with scheduled controlled doses of long wave ultraviolet (UVA) radiation (combination referred to as PUVA). Safety and efficacy in pediatric patients have not been established.

Vitiligo: Used in conjunction with controlled doses of long wave ultraviolet radiation or sunlight. Lotion should only be applied under direct supervision of prescriber and should not be dispensed to the patient. Safety and efficacy in children <12 years of age have not been established.

[U.S. Boxed Warning]: Should be administered under the supervision of an experienced physician with special competence in the diagnosis and treatment of dermatologic diseases.

Adverse Reactions Frequency not always defined.

Cardiovascular: Edema, hypotension

Central nervous system: Depression, dizziness, headache, insomnia, malaise, nervousness, vertigo

Dermatologic: Pruritus (10%), blistering (painful), bullae formation, burning, erythema, folliculitis, freckling, hypopigmentation, miliaria, peeling of skin, premature aging, rash, skin cancer, tenderness (cutaneous), urticaria, vesiculation

Gastrointestinal: Nausea (10%), gastrointestinal disturbance

Neuromuscular & skeletal: Loss of muscle coordination, leg cramps

Ocular: Cataract

Miscellaneous: Herpes simplex, infection

Drug Interactions

Metabolism/Transport Effects Substrate of CYP2A6 (minor); **Inhibits** CYP1A2 (strong), 2A6 (strong), 2C9 (weak), 2C19 (weak), 2D6 (weak), 2E1 (weak), 3A4 (weak)

Avoid Concomitant Use There are no known interactions where it is recommended to avoid concomitant use.

Increased Effect/Toxicity

Methoxsalen may increase the levels/effects of: Bendamustine; CYP1A2 Substrates; CYP2A6 Substrates

Decreased Effect There are no known significant interactions involving a decrease in effect.

Ethanol/Nutrition/Herb Interactions Food: Methoxsalen serum concentrations may be increased if taken with food. Avoid furocoumarin-containing foods (limes, figs, parsley, celery, cloves, lemon, mustard, carrots).

Mechanism of Action Bonds covalently to pyrimidine bases in DNA, inhibits the synthesis of DNA, and suppresses cell division. The augmented sunburn reaction involves excitation of the methoxsalen molecule by radiation in the long-wave ultraviolet light (UVA), resulting in transference of energy to the methoxsalen molecule producing an excited state ("triplet electronic state"). The molecule, in this "triplet state", then reacts with cutaneous DNA.

Pharmacodynamics/Kinetics

Protein binding: Reversibly bound to albumin

Metabolism: Hepatic; forms metabolites

Bioavailability: Bioavailability increased with soft-gelatin capsules (Oxsoralen-Ultra®) compared to hard-gelatin capsules (8-MOP®, Oxsoralen®); exposure using Uvadex® with the UVAR® photopheresis system is ~200 times less than with oral methoxsalen administration

Time to peak, serum:

Hard-gelatin capsules (8-MOP®, Oxsoralen®): 1.5-6 hours (peak photosensitivity: ~4 hours)

Soft-gelatin capsules (Oxsoralen-Ultra®): 0.5-4 hours (peak photosensitivity: 1.5-2 hours)

Half-life elimination: ~2 hours

Excretion: Urine (~95% as metabolites)

Dosage Note: Refer to treatment protocols for UVA exposure guidelines.

Children >12 years and Adults: Vitiligo: Topical (Oxsoralen®): Lotion is applied prior to UVA light exposure, usually no more than once weekly

Adults:
Psoriasis: Oral:
Initial: 10-70 mg 1.5-2 hours (Oxsoralen-Ultra®) or 2 hours (8-MOP®) before exposure to UVA light; dose may be repeated 2-3 times per week, based on UVA exposure; doses must be given at least 48 hours apart. Dosage is based upon patient's body weight and skin type:
<30 kg: 10 mg
30-50 kg: 20 mg
51-65 kg: 30 mg
66-80 kg: 40 mg
81-90 kg: 50 mg
91-115 kg: 60 mg
>115 kg: 70 mg
Note: Dosage may be increased (one time) by 10 mg after 15th treatment if minimal or no response.
Maintenance: When 95% psoriasis clearing achieved, may begin 1 treatment every week for at least 2 treatments; followed by 1 treatment every 2 weeks for at least 2 treatments; then every 3 weeks for at least 2 treatments then as needed to maintain response while minimizing UVA exposure.
Vitiligo:
Oral (8-MOP®): 20 mg 2-4 hours before exposure to UVA light; dose may be repeated based on erythema and tenderness of skin; do not give on 2 consecutive days
CTCL: Extracorporeal (Uvadex®): 200 mcg injected into the photoactivation bag during the collection cycle using the UVAR® photopheresis system (consult user's guide). Treatment schedule: Two consecutive days every 4 weeks for a minimum of 7 treatment cycles, may accelerate to two consecutive days every 2 weeks if skin score worsens (eg, increases from baseline) after assessment during the fourth treatment cycle. If skin score improves by 25% after 4 consecutive weeks of accelerated therapy, may resume regular treatment schedule. Maximum: 20 accelerated therapy cycles.

Dietary Considerations To reduce nausea, oral drug can be administered with food or milk or in 2 divided doses 30 minutes apart.

Administration Topical: Hands and fingers of person applying the lotion should be protected to prevent possible photosensitization and/or burns.

Monitoring Parameters CBC with differential (baseline and every 6-12 months), liver and renal function tests (baseline and every 6-12 months), antinuclear antibodies (baseline and every 6-12 months); ophthalmic exam (pretreatment and yearly)

Dosage Forms Excipient information presented when available (limited, particularly for generics); consult specific product labeling.
Capsule:
8-MOP®: 10 mg [hard-gelatin capsule]
Oxsoralen-Ultra®: 10 mg [soft-gelatin capsule]
Lotion (Oxsoralen®): 1% (30 mL) [contains alcohol 71%]
Solution, for extracorporeal administration (Uvadex®): 20 mcg/mL (10 mL) **[not for injection]**

◆ **Methoxypsoralen** *see* Methoxsalen *on page 968*

◆ **8-Methoxypsoralen** *see* Methoxsalen *on page 968*

◆ **Methscopolamine and Pseudoephedrine** *see* Pseudoephedrine and Methscopolamine *on page 1267*

◆ **Methscopolamine Nitrate and Chlordiazepoxide Hydrochloride** *see* Chlordiazepoxide and Methscopolamine *on page 305*

◆ **Methscopolamine Nitrate, Chlorpheniramine Maleate, and Phenylephrine Hydrochloride** *see* Chlorpheniramine, Phenylephrine, and Methscopolamine *on page 313*

Methsuximide (meth SUKS i mide)

U.S. Brand Names Celontin®
Canadian Brand Names Celontin®
Pharmacologic Category Anticonvulsant, Succinimide
Use Control of absence (petit mal) seizures that are refractory to other drugs
Unlabeled/Investigational Use Partial complex (psychomotor) seizures
Pregnancy Risk Factor C
Medication Safety Issues
Sound-alike/look-alike issues:
Methsuximide may be confused with ethosuximide
Dosage Oral:
Children: Anticonvulsant: Initial: 10-15 mg/kg/day in 3-4 divided doses; increase weekly up to maximum of 30 mg/kg/day
Adults: Anticonvulsant: 300 mg/day for the first week; may increase by 300 mg/day at weekly intervals up to 1.2 g/day in 2-4 divided doses/day
Additional Information Complete prescribing information for this medication should be consulted for additional detail.
Dosage Forms Excipient information presented when available (limited, particularly for generics); consult specific product labeling.
Capsule: 150 mg, 300 mg

Methyclothiazide (meth i kloe THYE a zide)

U.S. Brand Names Enduron® [DSC]
Canadian Brand Names Aquatensen®; Enduron®
Pharmacologic Category Diuretic, Thiazide
Additional Appendix Information
Sulfonamide Derivatives *on page 1671*
Use Management of mild to moderate hypertension; treatment of edema in congestive heart failure and nephrotic syndrome
Pregnancy Risk Factor B
Medication Safety Issues
Sound-alike/look-alike issues:
Enduron® may be confused with Empirin®, Imuran®, Inderal®
Dosage Adults: Oral:
Edema: 2.5-10 mg/day
Hypertension: 2.5-5 mg/day; may add another antihypertensive if 5 mg is not adequate after a trial of 8-12 weeks of therapy
Additional Information Complete prescribing information for this medication should be consulted for additional detail.
Dosage Forms Excipient information presented when available (limited, particularly for generics); consult specific product labeling.
Tablet: 5 mg

◆ **Methylacetoxyprogesterone** *see* MedroxyPROGESTERone *on page 930*

◆ **Methylcellulose, Gelatin, and Pectin** *see* Gelatin, Pectin, and Methylcellulose *on page 685*

Methyldopa (meth il DOE pa)

Canadian Brand Names Apo-Methyldopa®; Nu-Medopa
Index Terms Aldomet; Methyldopate Hydrochloride
Pharmacologic Category Alpha-Adrenergic Inhibitor; $Alpha_2$-Adrenergic Agonist
Additional Appendix Information
Hypertension *on page 1820*

Use Management of moderate to severe hypertension

Pregnancy Risk Factor B

Medication Safety Issues

Sound-alike/look-alike issues:

Methyldopa may be confused with L-dopa, levodopa

Dosage

Children:

Oral: Initial: 10 mg/kg/day in 2-4 divided doses; increase every 2 days as needed to maximum dose of 65 mg/kg/day; do not exceed 3 g/day.

I.V.: 5-10 mg/kg/dose every 6-8 hours up to a total dose of 65 mg/kg/24 hours or 3 g/24 hours

Adults:

Oral: Initial: 250 mg 2-3 times/day; increase every 2 days as needed (maximum dose: 3 g/day): usual dose range (JNC 7): 250-1000 mg/day in 2 divided doses

I.V.: 250-500 mg every 6-8 hours; maximum dose: 1 g every 6 hours

Dosing interval in renal impairment:

Cl_{cr} >50 mL/minute: Administer every 8 hours.

Cl_{cr} 10-50 mL/minute: Administer every 8-12 hours.

Cl_{cr} <10 mL/minute: Administer every 12-24 hours.

Hemodialysis: Slightly dialyzable (5% to 20%)

Additional Information Complete prescribing information for this medication should be consulted for additional detail.

Dosage Forms Excipient information presented when available (limited, particularly for generics); consult specific product labeling.

Injection, solution, as methyldopate hydrochloride: 50 mg/mL (5 mL) [contains sodium bisulfite]

Tablet: 250 mg, 500 mg

Methyldopa and Hydrochlorothiazide
(meth il DOE pa & hye droe klor oh THYE a zide)

U.S. Brand Names Aldoril®

Canadian Brand Names Apo-Methazide®

Index Terms Hydrochlorothiazide and Methyldopa

Pharmacologic Category $Alpha_2$-Adrenergic Agonist; Diuretic, Thiazide

Use Management of moderate-to-severe hypertension

Pregnancy Risk Factor C

Medication Safety Issues

Sound-alike/look-alike issues:

Aldoril® may be confused with Aldoclor®, Aldomet®, Elavil®

Dosage Oral: Dosage titrated on individual components, then switch to combination product; no more than methyldopa 3 g/day and/or hydrochlorothiazide 50 mg/day; maintain initial dose for first 48 hours, then decrease or increase at intervals of not less than 2 days until an adequate response is achieved

Methyldopa 250 mg and hydrochlorothiazide 15 mg: 2-3 times/day

Methyldopa 250 mg and hydrochlorothiazide 25 mg: Twice daily

Additional Information Complete prescribing information for this medication should be consulted for additional detail.

Dosage Forms Excipient information presented when available (limited, particularly for generics); consult specific product labeling.

Tablet:

Methyldopa 250 mg and hydrochlorothiazide 15 mg

Methyldopa 250 mg and hydrochlorothiazide 25 mg

Aldoril® 25: Methyldopa 250 mg and hydrochlorothiazide 25 mg

◆ **Methyldopate Hydrochloride** *see* Methyldopa *on page 970*

Methylene Blue (METH i leen bloo)

U.S. Brand Names Urolene Blue® [DSC]

Pharmacologic Category Antidote

Use Antidote for cyanide poisoning and drug-induced methemoglobinemia, indicator dye

Unlabeled/Investigational Use Treatment/prevention of ifosfamide-induced encephalopathy; topically, in conjunction with polychromatic light to photoinactivate viruses such as herpes simplex; alone or in combination with vitamin C for the management of chronic urolithiasis

Pregnancy Risk Factor C

Medication Safety Issues Due to potential toxicity (hemolytic anemia), do not use methylene blue to color enteral feedings to detect aspiration.

Dosage

Children: NADPH-methemoglobin reductase deficiency: Oral: 1-1.5 mg/kg/day (maximum: 300 mg/day) given with 5-8 mg/kg/day of ascorbic acid

Children and Adults: Methemoglobinemia: I.V.: 1-2 mg/kg or 25-50 mg/m^2 over several minutes; may be repeated in 1 hour if necessary

Adults:

Genitourinary antiseptic: Oral: 65-130 mg 3 times/day with a full glass of water (maximum: 390 mg/day)

Ifosfamide-induced encephalopathy (unlabeled use): Oral, I.V.:

Prevention: 50 mg every 6-8 hours

Treatment: 50 mg as a single dose or every 4-8 hours until symptoms resolve

Additional Information Complete prescribing information for this medication should be consulted for additional detail.

Dosage Forms Excipient information presented when available (limited, particularly for generics); consult specific product labeling.

Injection, solution: 10 mg/mL (1 mL, 10 mL)

Tablet:

Urolene Blue®: 65 mg [DSC]

◆ **Methylene Blue, Methenamine, Benzoic Acid, Phenyl Salicylate, and Hyoscyamine** *see* Methenamine, Phenyl Salicylate, Methylene Blue, Benzoic Acid, and Hyoscyamine *on page 962*

◆ **Methylene Blue, Methenamine, Sodium Biphosphate, Phenyl Salicylate, and Hyoscyamine** *see* Methenamine, Sodium Biphosphate, Phenyl Salicylate, Methylene Blue, and Hyoscyamine *on page 962*

◆ **Methylergometrine Maleate** *see* Methylergonovine *on page 971*

Methylergonovine (meth il er goe NOE veen)

U.S. Brand Names Methergine®

Canadian Brand Names Methergine®

Index Terms Methylergometrine Maleate; Methylergonovine Maleate

Pharmacologic Category Ergot Derivative

Use Prevention and treatment of postpartum and postabortion hemorrhage caused by uterine atony or subinvolution

Pregnancy Risk Factor C

Pregnancy Considerations Prolonged constriction of the uterine vessels and/or increased myometrial tone may lead to reduced placental blood flow. This has contributed to fetal growth retardation in animals. Methylergonovine is intended for use after delivery of the infant.

Lactation Enters breast milk/use caution

Medication Safety Issues

Sound-alike/look-alike issues:

Methylergonovine and terbutaline parenteral dosage forms look similar. Due to their contrasting indications, use care when administering these agents.

Contraindications Hypersensitivity to methylergonovine or any component of the formulation; ergot alkaloids are contraindicated with potent inhibitors of CYP3A4 (includes protease inhibitors, azole antifungals, and some macrolide antibiotics); hypertension; toxemia; pregnancy

Warnings/Precautions Use caution in patients with sepsis, obliterative vascular disease, cardiovascular disease, hepatic or renal involvement, or second stage of labor; administer with extreme caution if using intravenously. Pleural and peritoneal fibrosis have been reported with prolonged daily use of other ergot alkaloids. Cardiac valvular fibrosis has also been associated with ergot alkaloids. Ergot alkaloid use may result in ergotism (intense vasoconstriction) resulting in peripheral vascular ischemia and possible gangrene. Concomitant use with potent inhibitors of CYP3A4 (includes protease inhibitors, azole antifungals, and some macrolide antibiotics) and ergot alkaloids has been associated with acute ergot toxicity (ergotism); concurrent use of certain ergot alkaloids (eg, ergotamine and dihydroergotamine) are not recommended by the manufacturer. Use with caution in the elderly. Safety and efficacy have not been established in children.

Adverse Reactions Frequency not defined.

Cardiovascular: Acute MI, arterial spasm, bradycardia, hyper-/hypotension, palpitation, tachycardia, temporary chest pain

Central nervous system: Dizziness, hallucinations, headache, seizure

Dermatologic: Rash

Endocrine & metabolic: Water intoxication

Gastrointestinal: Diarrhea, foul taste, nausea, vomiting

Local: Thrombophlebitis

Neuromuscular & skeletal: Leg cramps

Otic: Tinnitus

Renal: Hematuria

Respiratory: Dyspnea, nasal congestion

Miscellaneous: Anaphylaxis, diaphoresis

Drug Interactions

Metabolism/Transport Effects Substrate of CYP3A4 (major)

Avoid Concomitant Use

Avoid concomitant use of Methylergonovine with any of the following: Efavirenz; Posaconazole; Protease Inhibitors; Serotonin 5-HT1D Receptor Agonists; Sibutramine; Voriconazole

Increased Effect/Toxicity

Methylergonovine may increase the levels/effects of: Serotonin 5-HT1D Receptor Agonists; Serotonin Modulators

The levels/effects of Methylergonovine may be increased by: CYP3A4 Inhibitors (Moderate); CYP3A4 Inhibitors (Strong); Dasatinib; Efavirenz; Macrolide Antibiotics; Posaconazole; Protease Inhibitors; Serotonin 5-HT1D Receptor Agonists; Sibutramine; Voriconazole

Decreased Effect There are no known significant interactions involving a decrease in effect.

Stability

Ampul: Store under refrigeration at 2°C to 8°C (36°F to 46°F). Protect from light.

Tablet: Store below 25°C (77°F).

Mechanism of Action Similar smooth muscle actions as seen with ergotamine; however, it affects primarily uterine smooth muscles producing sustained contractions and thereby shortens the third stage of labor and reduces blood loss.

Pharmacodynamics/Kinetics

Onset of action: Oxytocic: Oral: 5-10 minutes; I.M.: 2-5 minutes; I.V.: Immediately

Duration: Oral: ~3 hours; I.M.: ~3 hours; I.V.: 45 minutes

Absorption: Rapid

Distribution: V_d: 39-73 L

Rapid; primarily to plasma and extracellular fluid following I.V. administration; tissues

Metabolism: Hepatic

Bioavailability: Oral: 60%; I.M.: 78%

Half-life elimination: Biphasic: Initial: 1-5 minutes; Terminal: 0.5-2 hours

Time to peak, serum: Oral: 0.3-2 hours; I.M.: 0.2-0.6 hours

Excretion: Urine and feces

Dosage Adults:

Oral: 0.2 mg 3-4 times/day in the puerperium for 2-7 days

I.M., I.V.: 0.2 mg after delivery of anterior shoulder, after delivery of placenta, or during puerperium; may be repeated as required at intervals of 2-4 hours

Administration Administer over ≥60 seconds. Should not be routinely administered I.V. because of possibility of inducing sudden hypertension and cerebrovascular accident.

Dosage Forms Excipient information presented when available (limited, particularly for generics); consult specific product labeling.

Injection, solution, as maleate: 0.2 mg/mL (1 mL)

Methergine®: 0.2 mg/mL (1 mL)

Tablet, as maleate:

Methergine®: 0.2 mg

◆ **Methylergonovine Maleate** *see* Methylergonovine *on page 971*

◆ **Methylin®** *see* Methylphenidate *on page 973*

◆ **Methylin® ER** *see* Methylphenidate *on page 973*

◆ **Methylmorphine** *see* Codeine *on page 362*

Methylnaltrexone (meth il nal TREKS one)

U.S. Brand Names Relistor™

Canadian Brand Names Relistor™

Index Terms Methylnaltrexone Bromide; N-methylnaltrexone Bromide

Pharmacologic Category Gastrointestinal Agent, Miscellaneous; Opioid Antagonist, Peripherally-Acting

Use Treatment of opioid-induced constipation in patients with advanced illness receiving palliative care with inadequate response to conventional laxative regimens

Pregnancy Risk Factor B

Pregnancy Considerations Adverse effects were not observed in animal studies. There are no adequate and well-controlled studies in pregnant women.

Lactation Excretion in breast milk unknown/use caution

Medication Safety Issues

Sound-alike/look-alike issues:

Methylnaltrexone may be confused with naltrexone

Contraindications Known or suspected mechanical bowel obstruction

Warnings/Precautions Discontinue treatment for severe or persistent diarrhea. Use with caution in patients with renal impairment; dosage adjustment recommended for severe renal impairment (Cl_{cr} <30 mL/minute). Has not been studied in patients with end-stage renal impairment requiring dialysis. Discontinue methylnaltrexone if opioids are discontinued. Use has not been studied in patients with peritoneal catheters. Use beyond 4 months has not been studied. Safety and efficacy have not been established in children.

Adverse Reactions

>10%: Gastrointestinal: Abdominal pain (29%), flatulence (13%), nausea (12%)

1% to 10%:
Central nervous system: Dizziness (7%)
Gastrointestinal: Diarrhea (6%)
<1% (Limited to important or life-threatening): Abdominal cramps, body temperature increased, muscle spasm, syncope

Drug Interactions

Metabolism/Transport Effects **Inhibits** CYP2D6 (weak)

Avoid Concomitant Use There are no known interactions where it is recommended to avoid concomitant use.

Increased Effect/Toxicity There are no known significant interactions involving an increase in effect.

Decreased Effect There are no known significant interactions involving a decrease in effect.

Stability Store intact vials at room temperature of 20°C to 25°C (68°F to 77°F); excursions permitted to 15°C to 30°C (59°F to 86°F). Do not freeze, protect from light. Solution for injection is stable in a syringe for 24 hours at room temperature (protection from light during this 24 hours is not necessary).

Mechanism of Action An opioid receptor antagonist which blocks opioid binding at the mu receptor, methylnaltrexone is a quaternary derivative of naltrexone with ability to cross the blood-brain barrier restricted. It therefore functions as a peripheral acting opioid antagonist, including actions on the gastrointestinal tract to inhibit opioid-induced decreased gastrointestinal motility and delay in gastrointestinal transit time, decreasing opioid-induced constipation. Does not affect opioid analgesic effects or induce opioid withdrawal symptoms.

Pharmacodynamics/Kinetics
Onset of action: Usually within 30-60 minutes (in responding patients)
Absorption: SubQ: Rapid
Distribution: V_{ss}: 1.1 L/kg
Protein binding: 11% to 15%
Metabolism: Metabolized to methyl-6-naltrexol isomers, methylnaltrexone sulfate. and other minor metabolites
Half-life elimination: Terminal: ~8 hours
Time to peak, plasma: SubQ: 30 minutes
Excretion: Urine (~50%, primarily as unchanged drug); feces (<50%, primarily as unchanged drug)

Dosage SubQ: Adults: Opioid-induced constipation: Dosing is according to body weight: Administer 1 dose every other day as needed; maximum: 1 dose/24 hours
<38 kg: 0.15 mg/kg (round dose up to nearest 0.1 mL of volume)
38 to <62 kg: 8 mg
62-114 kg: 12 mg
>114 kg: 0.15 mg/kg (round dose up to nearest 0.1 mL of volume)

Dosage adjustment in renal impairment:
Mild-to-moderate renal impairment: No adjustment required
Severe renal impairment (Cl_{cr} <30 mL/minute): Administer 50% of normal dose
End-stage renal impairment (dialysis-dependent): Has not been studied

Dosage adjustment in hepatic impairment:
Mild-to-moderate hepatic impairment (Child-Pugh class A and B): No adjustment required
Severe hepatic impairment: Has not been studied

Administration SubQ: Administer subcutaneously into upper arm, abdomen, or thigh. Rotate injection site. Do not use tender, bruised, red, or hard areas.

Additional Information In some clinical trials, patients who received methylnaltrexone were on a palliative opioid therapy equivalent to a mean daily oral morphine dose of 172 mg, at a stable dose for ≥3 days. Constipation was defined as <3 bowel movements/week or no bowel movement for >2 days. Patients maintained their regular laxative regimen for at least 3 days prior to treatment and throughout the study.

Dosage Forms Excipient information presented when available (limited, particularly for generics); consult specific product labeling.
Injection, solution:
Relistor™: 12 mg/0.6 mL (0.6 mL) [contains edetate calcium disodium]

◆ **Methylnaltrexone Bromide** *see* Methylnaltrexone *on page 972*

Methylphenidate (meth il FEN i date)

U.S. Brand Names Concerta®; Daytrana™; Metadate® CD; Metadate® ER; Methylin®; Methylin® ER; Ritalin-SR®; Ritalin®; Ritalin® LA

Canadian Brand Names Apo-Methylphenidate®; Apo-Methylphenidate® SR; Biphentin®; Concerta®; PHL-Methylphenidate; PMS-Methylphenidate; RATIO-Methylphenidate; Riphenidate; Ritalin®; Ritalin® SR

Index Terms Methylphenidate Hydrochloride

Pharmacologic Category Central Nervous System Stimulant

Use Treatment of attention-deficit/hyperactivity disorder (ADHD); symptomatic management of narcolepsy

Unlabeled/Investigational Use Depression (especially elderly or medically ill)

Restrictions C-II

An FDA-approved medication guide must be distributed when dispensing an outpatient prescription (new or refill) where this medication is to be used without direct supervision of a healthcare provider. Medication guides are available at http://www.fda.gov/cder/Offices/ODS/medication_guides.htm.

Pregnancy Risk Factor C

Pregnancy Considerations Animal studies have shown teratogenic effects to the fetus. There are no adequate and well-controlled studies in pregnant women. Do not use in women of childbearing age unless the potential benefit outweighs the possible risk.

Lactation Enters breast milk/use caution

Medication Safety Issues
Sound-alike/look-alike issues:
Metadate® CD may be confused with Metadate® ER
Metadate® ER may be confused with Metadate® CD, methadone
Methylphenidate may be confused with methadone
Ritalin® may be confused with Ismelin®, Rifadin®, ritodrine

Contraindications Hypersensitivity to methylphenidate, any component of the formulation, or idiosyncratic reactions to sympathomimetic amines; marked anxiety, tension, and agitation; glaucoma; use during or within 14 days following MAO inhibitor therapy; family history or diagnosis of Tourette's syndrome or tics

Metadate® CD and Metadate® ER: Additional contraindications: Severe hypertension, heart failure, arrhythmia, hyperthyroidism, recent MI or angina; concomitant use of halogenated anesthetics

Warnings/Precautions CNS stimulant use has been associated with serious cardiovascular events including sudden death in patients with pre-existing structural cardiac abnormalities or other serious heart problems (sudden death in children and adolescents; sudden death, stroke, and MI in adults). These products should be avoided in patients with known serious structural cardiac abnormalities, cardiomyopathy, serious heart rhythm abnormalities, or other serious cardiac problems that could further increase their risk of sudden death. Patients should be carefully evaluated for cardiac disease prior to initiation of therapy. Use of stimulants can cause an increase in blood pressure (average 2-4 mm Hg) and increases in heart rate (average 3-6 bpm), although some patients may have larger than average increases. Use caution with hypertension, hyperthyroidism, or other cardiovascular conditions that might be exacerbated by increases in blood pressure or heart rate. Some products are contraindicated in patients with heart failure, arrhythmias, severe hypertension, hyperthyroidism, angina, or recent MI.

Has demonstrated value as part of a comprehensive treatment program for ADHD. Use with caution in patients with bipolar disorder (may induce mixed/manic episode). May exacerbate symptoms of behavior and thought disorder in psychotic patients; new onset psychosis or mania may occur with stimulant use; observe for symptoms of aggression and/or hostility. Use caution with seizure disorders (may reduce seizure threshold). Use caution in patients with history of ethanol or drug abuse. May exacerbate symptoms of behavior and thought disorder in psychotic patients. **[U.S. Boxed Warning]: Potential for drug dependency exists - avoid abrupt discontinuation in patients who have received for prolonged periods.** Visual disturbances have been reported (rare). Not labeled for use in children <6 years of age. Use of stimulants has been associated with suppression of growth in children; monitor growth rate during treatment.

Concerta® should not be used in patients with esophageal motility disorders or pre-existing severe gastrointestinal narrowing (small bowel disease, short gut syndrome, history of peritonitis, cystic fibrosis, chronic intestinal pseudo-obstruction, Meckel's diverticulum). Metadate® CD and Metadate® ER contain sucrose and lactose, respectively; avoid administration in hereditary galactose intolerance, Lapp lactase deficiency, or glucose-galactose malabsorption. Concomitant use with halogenated anesthetics is contraindicated; may cause sudden elevations in blood pressure; if surgery is planned, do not administer Metadate® CD or Metadate® ER on the day of surgery. Transdermal system may cause allergic contact sensitization, characterized by intense local reactions (edema, papules); sensitization may subsequently manifest systemically with other routes of methylphenidate administration; monitor closely. Avoid exposure of application site to any direct external heat sources (eg, hair dryers, heating pads, electric blankets); may increase risk of overdose. Efficacy of transdermal methylphenidate therapy for >7 weeks has not been established.

Adverse Reactions

Transdermal system: Frequency of adverse events as reported in trials of 7-week duration. Incidence of some events higher with extended use.

>10%:

- Central nervous system: Headache (long-term use in children: 28%), insomnia (13%; long-term use in children: 30%)
- Gastrointestinal: Appetite decreased (26%), nausea (12%)
- Miscellaneous: Viral infection (long-term use in children: 28%)

1% to 10%:

- Central nervous system: Tic (7%), emotional instability (6%)
- Gastrointestinal: Vomiting (10%), weight loss (9%), anorexia (5%; long-term use in children: 46%)
- Local: Application site reaction
- Respiratory: Nasal congestion (6%) nasopharyngitis (5%)

Postmarketing and/or case reports (limited to important or life-threatening): Allergic contact sensitization, anaphylaxis, angioedema, hallucinations, seizures

All dosage forms: Frequency not defined:

- Cardiovascular: Angina, cardiac arrhythmia, cerebral arteritis, cerebral occlusion, hyper-/hypotension, MI, murmur, palpitation, pulse increased/decreased, Raynaud's phenomenon, tachycardia
- Central nervous system: Aggression, agitation, anger, anxiety, confusional state, depression, dizziness, drowsiness, fatigue, fever, headache, hypervigilance, insomnia, irritability, lethargy, mood alterations, nervousness, neuroleptic malignant syndrome (NMS) (rare), restlessness, stroke, tension, Tourette's syndrome (rare), toxic psychosis, tremor, vertigo
- Dermatologic: Alopecia, erythema multiforme, exfoliative dermatitis, hyperhidrosis, rash, urticaria
- Endocrine & metabolic: Dysmenorrhea, growth retardation, libido decreased
- Gastrointestinal: Abdominal pain, anorexia, appetite decreased, bruxism, constipation, diarrhea, dyspepsia, nausea, vomiting, weight loss, xerostomia
- Genitourinary: Erectile dysfunction
- Hematologic: Anemia, leukopenia, pancytopenia, thrombocytopenic purpura, thrombocytopenia
- Hepatic: Bilirubin increased, liver function tests abnormal, hepatic coma, transaminases increased
- Neuromuscular & skeletal: Arthralgia, dyskinesia, muscle tightness, paresthesia
- Ocular: Blurred vision, dry eyes, mydriasis, visual accommodation disturbance
- Renal: Necrotizing vasculitis
- Respiratory: Cough increased, dyspnea, pharyngitis, pharyngolaryngeal pain, rhinitis, sinusitis, upper respiratory tract infection
- Miscellaneous: Accidental injury, hypersensitivity reactions
- Postmarketing and/or case reports: Alkaline phosphatase increased, angina pectoris, bradycardia, chest pain, diplopia, disorientation, extrasystole, mydriasis; hypersensitivity reactions (eg, angioedema, anaphylactic reactions, auricular swelling, bullous conditions, exfoliative conditions, urticaria, pruritus, rash, eruptions, exanthemas); muscle twitching, hallucinations, mania, erythema, seizure, supraventricular tachycardia, ventricular extrasystole

Drug Interactions

Metabolism/Transport Effects **Inhibits** CYP2D6 (weak)

Avoid Concomitant Use

Avoid concomitant use of Methylphenidate with any of the following: Inhalational Anesthetics; Iobenguane I 123; MAO Inhibitors

Increased Effect/Toxicity

Methylphenidate may increase the levels/effects of: CloNIDine; Inhalational Anesthetics; Phenytoin; Sympathomimetics; Tricyclic Antidepressants

The levels/effects of Methylphenidate may be increased by: Cannabinoids; MAO Inhibitors

Decreased Effect

Methylphenidate may decrease the levels/effects of: Antihypertensives; Iobenguane I 123

Ethanol/Nutrition/Herb Interactions

- Ethanol: Avoid ethanol (may cause CNS depression).
- Food: Food may increase oral absorption; Concerta® formulation is not affected. Food delays early peak and high-fat meals increase C_{max} and AUC of Metadate® CD formulation.
- Herb/Nutraceutical: Avoid ephedra (may cause hypertension or arrhythmias) and yohimbe (also has CNS stimulatory activity).

Stability

Capsule, *extended release:* Store at controlled room temperature of 20°C to 25°C (68°F to 77°F). Protect from light.

Solution: Store at controlled room temperature of 20°C to 25°C (68°F to 77°F).

Tablet:

Chewable: Store at controlled room temperature of 20°C to 25°C (68°F to 77°F). Protect from light and moisture.

Extended and sustained release: Store at controlled room temperature of 20°C to 25°C (68°F to 77°F). Protect from light and moisture.

Immediate release: Store at controlled room temperature of 20°C to 25°C (68°F to 77°F). Protect from light and moisture.

Osmotic controlled release (Concerta®): Store at controlled room temperature of 25°C; excursions permitted to 15°C to 30°C (59°F to 86°F). Protect from humidity.

Transdermal system: Store at controlled room temperature of 20°C to 25°C (68°F to 77°F). Keep patches stored in protective pouch. Once tray is opened, use patches within 2 months. Do not refrigerate or freeze.

Mechanism of Action Mild CNS stimulant; blocks the reuptake of norepinephrine and dopamine into presynaptic neurons; appears to stimulate the cerebral cortex and subcortical structures similar to amphetamines

Pharmacodynamics/Kinetics

Onset of action: Peak effect:

Immediate release tablet: Cerebral stimulation: ~2 hours

Extended release capsule (Metadate® CD): Biphasic; initial peak similar to immediate release product, followed by second rising portion (corresponding to extended release portion)

Sustained release tablet: 4-7 hours

Osmotic release tablet (Concerta®): Initial: 1-2 hours

Transdermal: ~2 hours; may be expedited by the application of external heat

Duration: Immediate release tablet: 3-6 hours; Sustained release tablet: 8 hours; Extended release tablet: Methylin® ER, Metadate® ER: 8 hours, Concerta®: 12 hours

Absorption:

Oral: Readily absorbed

Transdermal: Absorption increased when applied to inflamed skin or exposed to heat. Absorption is continuous for 9 hours after application.

Metabolism: Hepatic via de-esterification to minimally active metabolite

Half-life elimination: *d*-methylphenidate: 3-4 hours; *l*-methylphenidate: 1-3 hours

Time to peak: Concerta®: C_{max}: 6-8 hours; Daytrana™: 7.5-10.5 hours

Excretion: Urine (90% as metabolites and unchanged drug)

Dosage

ADHD:

Oral:

Immediate release products Children ≥6 years and Adults: Initial: 5 mg/dose (~0.3 mg/kg/dose) given twice daily before breakfast and lunch; increase by 5-10 mg/day (0.2 mg/kg/day) at weekly intervals; maximum dose: 60 mg/day (2 mg/kg/day). **Note:** Discontinue periodically to re-evaluate or if no improvement occurs within 1 month.

Extended release products:

Children ≥6 years and Adults:

Metadate® ER, Methylin® ER, Ritalin® SR: May be given in place of immediate release products, once the daily dose is titrated and the titrated 8-hour dosage corresponds to sustained or extended release tablet size; maximum: 60 mg/day

Metadate® CD, Ritalin® LA: Initial: 20 mg once daily; may be adjusted in 10-20 mg increments at weekly intervals; maximum: 60 mg/day

Children 6-12 years and Adolescents 13-17 years: *Concerta®:*

Patients not currently taking methylphenidate: Initial dose: 18 mg once daily in the morning

Patients currently taking methylphenidate: **Note:** Initial dose: Dosing based on current regimen and clinical judgment; suggested dosing listed below:

- Patients taking methylphenidate 5 mg 2-3 times/day: 18 mg once every morning
- Patients taking methylphenidate 10 mg 2-3 times/day: 36 mg once every morning
- Patients taking methylphenidate 15 mg 2-3 times/day: 54 mg once every morning

Dose adjustment: May increase dose in increments of 18 mg; dose may be adjusted at weekly intervals. A dosage strength of 27 mg is available for situations in which a dosage between 18-36 mg is desired. Maximum dose should not exceed 2 mg/kg/day **or** 54 mg/day in children 6-12 years or 72 mg/day in children 13-17 years.

Adults: *Concerta®:*

Patients not currently taking methylphenidate: Initial dose: 18-36 mg once daily in the morning

Patients currently taking methylphenidate: **Note:** Initial dose: Dosing based on current regimen and clinical judgment; suggested dosing listed below:

- Patients taking methylphenidate 5 mg 2-3 times/day: 18 mg once every morning
- Patients taking methylphenidate 10 mg 2-3 times/day: 36 mg once every morning
- Patients taking methylphenidate 15 mg 2-3 times/day: 54 mg once every morning
- Patients taking methylphenidate 20 mg 2-3 times/day: 72 mg once every morning

Dose adjustment: May increase dose in increments of 18 mg; dose may be adjusted at weekly intervals. A dosage strength of 27 mg is available for situations in which a dosage between 18-36 mg is desired. Maximum dose should not exceed 72 mg/day.

Transdermal (Daytrana™): Children ≥6 years: Initial: 10 mg patch once daily; remove up to 9 hours after application. Titrate based on response and tolerability; may increase to next transdermal dose no more frequently than every week. **Note:** Application should occur 2 hours prior to desired effect. Drug absorption may continue for a period of time after patch removal; patients converting from another formulation of methylphenidate should be initiated at 10 mg regardless of their previous dose and titrated as needed due to the differences in bioavailability of the transdermal formulation.

Narcolepsy: Oral: Adults: 10 mg 2-3 times/day, up to 60 mg/day

Depression (unlabeled use): Oral: Adults: Initial: 2.5 mg every morning before 9 AM; dosage may be increased by 2.5-5 mg every 2-3 days as tolerated to a maximum of 20 mg/day; may be divided (ie, 7 AM and 12 noon), but should not be given after noon; do not use sustained release product

Dietary Considerations Should be taken 30-45 minutes before meals. Concerta® is not affected by food and should be taken with water, milk, or juice. Metadate® CD should be taken before breakfast. Metadate® ER should be taken before breakfast and lunch. Methylin® chewable tablets contain phenylalanine 0.42 mg/methylphenidate 2.5 mg.

Administration

Oral: Do not crush or allow patient to chew sustained or extended release dosage form. To effectively avoid insomnia, dosing should be completed by noon.

Concerta®: Administer dose once daily in the morning. May be taken with or without food, but must be taken with water, milk, or juice.

Metadate® CD, Ritalin® LA: Capsules may be opened and the contents sprinkled onto a small amount (equal to 1 tablespoon) of applesauce. Swallow applesauce without chewing. Do not crush or chew capsule contents.

Methylin® chewable tablet: Administer with at least 8 ounces of water or other fluid.

Topical: Transdermal (Daytrana™): Apply to clean, dry, non-oily, intact skin to the hip area, avoiding the waistline. Apply at the same time each day to alternating hips. Press firmly for 30 seconds to ensure proper adherence. Avoid exposure of application site to external heat source, which may increase the amount of drug absorbed. Do not use a patch that has been damaged or torn; do not cut patch. If patch should dislodge, may replace with new patch (to different site) but total wear time should not exceed 9 hours; do not reapply with dressings, tape, or common adhesives. Patch may be removed early if a shorter duration of effect is desired or if late day side effects occur. Wash hands with soap and water after handling. Avoid touching the sticky side of the patch. If patch removal is difficult, an oil-based product (eg, petroleum jelly, olive oil) may be applied to the patch edges to aid removal; never apply acetone-based products (eg, nail polish remover) to patch. Dispose of used patch by folding adhesive side onto itself, and discard in toilet or appropriate lidded container.

Monitoring Parameters Blood pressure, heart rate, signs and symptoms of depression, aggression, or hostility; CBC, differential and platelet counts, liver function tests; growth rate in children, signs of central nervous system stimulation

Transdermal: Signs of worsening erythema, blistering or edema which does not improve within 24 hours of patch removal, or spreads beyond patch site.

When used for the treatment of ADHD, thoroughly evaluate for cardiovascular risk. Monitor heart rate, blood pressure, and consider obtaining ECG prior to initiation (Vetter, 2008).

Additional Information Treatment with methylphenidate may include "drug holidays" or periodic discontinuation in order to assess the patient's requirements and to decrease tolerance and limit suppression of linear growth and weight. Specific patients may require 3 doses/day for treatment of ADHD (ie, additional dose at 4 PM).

Concerta® is an osmotic controlled release formulation (OROS®) of methylphenidate. The tablet has an immediate-release overcoat that provides an initial dose of methylphenidate within 1 hour. The overcoat covers a trilayer core. The trilayer core is composed of two layers containing the drug and excipients, and one layer of osmotic components. As water from the gastrointestinal tract enters the core, the osmotic components expand and methylphenidate is released.

Metadate® CD capsules contain a mixture of immediate release and extended release beads, designed to release 30% of the dose immediately and 70% over an extended period.

Ritalin® LA uses a combination of immediate release and enteric coated, delayed release beads.

Dosage Forms Excipient information presented when available (limited, particularly for generics); consult specific product labeling. [DSC] = Discontinued product

Capsule, extended release, oral, as hydrochloride [bi-modal release]:

Metadate CD®: 10 mg [contains sucrose; 3 mg immediate release, 7 mg extended release]

Metadate CD®: 20 mg [contains sucrose; 6 mg immediate release, 14 mg extended release]

Metadate CD®: 30 mg [contains sucrose; 9 mg immediate release, 21 mg extended release]

Metadate CD®: 40 mg [contains sucrose; 12 mg immediate release, 28 mg extended release]

Metadate CD®: 50 mg [contains sucrose; 15 mg immediate release, 35 mg extended release]

Metadate CD®: 60 mg [contains sucrose; 18 mg immediate release, 42 mg extended release]

Ritalin LA®: 10 mg [5 mg immediate release, 5 mg extended release]

Ritalin LA®: 20 mg [10 mg immediate release, 10 mg extended release]

Ritalin LA®: 30 mg [15 mg immediate release, 15 mg extended release]

Ritalin LA®: 40 mg [20 mg immediate release, 20 mg extended release]

Solution, oral, as hydrochloride:

Methylin®: 5 mg/5 mL (500 mL) [grape flavor]; 10 mg/5 mL (500 mL) [grape flavor]

Tablet, as hydrochloride: 5 mg, 10 mg, 20 mg

Methylin®, Ritalin®: 5 mg, 10 mg, 20 mg

Tablet, chewable, as hydrochloride:

Methylin®: 2.5 mg [contains phenylalanine 0.42 mg; grape flavor]; 5 mg [contains phenylalanine 0.84 mg; grape flavor]; 10 mg [contains phenylalanine 1.68 mg; grape flavor]

Tablet, extended release, as hydrochloride: 20 mg

Metadate® ER: 10 mg [contains lactose]; 20 mg [contains lactose]

Methylin® ER: 10 mg, 20 mg

Tablet, extended release, as hydrochloride [bi-modal release]:

Concerta®: 18 mg [4 mg immediate release, 14 mg extended release]

Concerta®: 27 mg [6 mg immediate release, 21 mg extended release]

Concerta®: 36 mg [8 mg immediate release, 28 mg extended release]

Concerta®: 54 mg [12 mg immediate release, 42 mg extended release]

Tablet, sustained release, as hydrochloride: 20 mg

Ritalin-SR®: 20 mg [dye free]

Transdermal system [once-daily patch]:

Daytrana™: 10 mg/9 hours (10s [DSC], 30s) [12.5 cm^2, total methylphenidate 27.5 mg]

Daytrana™: 15 mg/9 hours (10s [DSC], 30s) [18.75 cm^2, total methylphenidate 41.3 mg]

Daytrana™: 20 mg/9 hours (10s [DSC], 30s) [25 cm^2, total methylphenidate 55 mg]

Daytrana™: 30 mg/9 hours (10s [DSC], 30s) [37.5 cm^2, total methylphenidate 82.5 mg]

◆ **Methylphenidate Hydrochloride** *see* Methylphenidate *on page 973*

◆ **Methylphenobarbital** *see* Mephobarbital *on page 944*

◆ **Methylphenoxy-Benzene Propanamine** *see* Atomoxetine *on page 150*

◆ **Methylphenyl Isoxazolyl Penicillin** *see* Oxacillin *on page 1111*

◆ **Methylphytyl Napthoquinone** *see* Phytonadione *on page 1191*

MethylPREDNISolone (meth il pred NIS oh lone)

U.S. Brand Names Depo-Medrol®; Medrol®; Solu-Medrol®

Canadian Brand Names Depo-Medrol®; Medrol®; Methylprednisolone Acetate; Solu-Medrol®

Index Terms 6-α-Methylprednisolone; A-Methapred; Methylprednisolone Acetate; Methylprednisolone Sodium Succinate

Pharmacologic Category Corticosteroid, Systemic

Additional Appendix Information

Contrast Media Reactions, Premedication for Prophylaxis *on page 1799*

Corticosteroids *on page 1652*

Use Primarily as an anti-inflammatory or immunosuppressant agent in the treatment of a variety of diseases including those of hematologic, allergic, inflammatory, neoplastic, and autoimmune origin. Prevention and treatment of graft-versus-host disease following allogeneic bone marrow transplantation.

Pregnancy Considerations Adverse events have been observed with corticosteroids in animal reproduction studies. Methylprednisolone crosses the placenta. Some studies have shown an association between first trimester systemic corticosteroid use and oral clefts; adverse events in the fetus/neonate have been noted in case reports following large doses of systemic corticosteroids during pregnancy. Pregnant women exposed to methylprednisolone for antirejection therapy following a transplant may contact the National Transplantation Pregnancy Registry (NTPR) at 215-955-4820. Women exposed to methylprednisolone during pregnancy for the treatment of an autoimmune disease may contact the OTIS Autoimmune Diseases Study at 877-311-8972.

Lactation Enters breast milk/use caution

Medication Safety Issues

Sound-alike/look-alike issues:

MethylPREDNISolone may be confused with medroxyPROGESTERone, predniSONE

Depo-Medrol® may be confused with Solu-Medrol®

Medrol® may be confused with Mebaral®

Solu-Medrol® may be confused with Depo-Medrol®, salmeterol, Solu-Cortef®

International issues:

Medor® may be confused with Medral® which is a brand name for omeprazole in Mexico

Contraindications Hypersensitivity to methylprednisolone or any component of the formulation; viral, fungal, or tubercular skin lesions; administration of live virus vaccines; serious infections, except septic shock or tuberculous meningitis. Methylprednisolone formulations containing benzyl alcohol preservative are contraindicated in infants. I.M. administration contraindicated in idiopathic thrombocytopenia purpura.

Warnings/Precautions Use with caution in patients with thyroid disease, hepatic impairment, renal impairment, cardiovascular disease, diabetes, glaucoma, cataracts, myasthenia gravis, patients at risk for osteoporosis, patients at risk for seizures, or GI diseases (diverticulitis, peptic ulcer, ulcerative colitis) due to perforation risk. Use caution following acute MI (corticosteroids have been associated with myocardial rupture). Because of the risk of adverse effects, systemic corticosteroids should be used cautiously in the elderly in the smallest possible effective dose for the shortest duration. May affect growth velocity; growth should be routinely monitored in pediatric patients. Withdraw therapy with gradual tapering of dose.

May cause hypercorticism or suppression of hypothalamic-pituitary-adrenal (HPA) axis, particularly in younger children or in patients receiving high doses for prolonged periods. HPA axis suppression may lead to adrenal crisis. Withdrawal and discontinuation of a corticosteroid should be done slowly and carefully. Particular care is required when patients are transferred from systemic corticosteroids to inhaled products due to possible adrenal insufficiency or withdrawal from steroids, including an increase in allergic symptoms. Patients receiving >20 mg per day of prednisone (or equivalent) may be most susceptible. Fatalities have occurred due to adrenal insufficiency in asthmatic patients during and after transfer from systemic corticosteroids to aerosol steroids; aerosol steroids do not provide the systemic steroid needed to treat patients having trauma, surgery, or infections.

Acute myopathy has been reported with high dose corticosteroids, usually in patients with neuromuscular transmission disorders; may involve ocular and/or respiratory muscles; monitor creatine kinase; recovery may be delayed. Corticosteroid use may cause psychiatric disturbances, including depression, euphoria, insomnia, mood swings, and personality changes. Pre-existing psychiatric conditions may be exacerbated by corticosteroid use. Prolonged use of corticosteroids may also increase the incidence of secondary infection, mask acute infection (including fungal infections), prolong or exacerbate viral infections, or limit response to vaccines. Exposure to chickenpox should be avoided; corticosteroids should not be used to treat ocular herpes simplex. Corticosteroids should not be used for cerebral malaria or viral hepatitis. Close observation is required in patients with latent tuberculosis and/or TB reactivity; restrict use in active TB (only in conjunction with antituberculosis treatment). Prolonged treatment with corticosteroids has been associated with the development of Kaposi's sarcoma (case reports); if noted, discontinuation of therapy should be considered. High-dose corticosteroids should not be used to manage acute head injury.

Adverse Reactions Frequency not defined.

Cardiovascular: Arrhythmia, edema, hypertension

Central nervous system: Delirium, euphoria, hallucinations, headache, insomnia, mood swings, nervousness, pseudotumor cerebri, psychosis, seizure, vertigo

Dermatologic: Acne, bruising, hirsutism, hyperpigmentation, skin atrophy

Endocrine & metabolic: Adrenal suppression, alkalosis, amenorrhea, Cushing's syndrome, diabetes mellitus, glucose intolerance, hyperglycemia, hyperlipidemia, hypokalemia, growth suppression, pituitary-adrenal axis suppression, sodium and water retention

Gastrointestinal: Abdominal distention, appetite Increased, indigestion, nausea, pancreatitis, peptic ulcer, ulcerative esophagitis, vomiting

Hematologic: Leukocytosis (transient)

Neuromuscular & skeletal: Arthralgia, fractures, muscle weakness, osteoporosis

Ocular: Cataracts, glaucoma

Miscellaneous: Avascular necrosis, hypersensitivity reactions, infection, intractable hiccups, secondary malignancy

Drug Interactions

Metabolism/Transport Effects Substrate of CYP3A4 (major); **Inhibits** CYP2C8 (weak), 3A4 (weak)

Avoid Concomitant Use

Avoid concomitant use of MethylPREDNISolone with any of the following: Natalizumab; Vaccines (Live)

Increased Effect/Toxicity

MethylPREDNISolone may increase the levels/effects of: Acetylcholinesterase Inhibitors; Amphotericin B; CycloSPORINE; Loop Diuretics; Natalizumab; NSAID (COX-2 Inhibitor); NSAID (Nonselective); Thiazide Diuretics; Vaccines (Live); Warfarin

The levels/effects of MethylPREDNISolone may be increased by: Antifungal Agents (Azole Derivatives, Systemic); Aprepitant; Calcium Channel Blockers (Nondihydropyridine); CycloSPORINE; Estrogen Derivatives; Fluconazole; Fosaprepitant; Macrolide Antibiotics; Neuromuscular-Blocking Agents (Nondepolarizing); Quinolone Antibiotics; Salicylates; Trastuzumab

Decreased Effect

MethylPREDNISolone may decrease the levels/effects of: Antidiabetic Agents; Calcitriol; Corticorelin; Isoniazid; Salicylates; Vaccines (Inactivated)

The levels/effects of MethylPREDNISolone may be decreased by: Aminoglutethimide; Antacids; Barbiturates; Bile Acid Sequestrants; Echinacea; Primidone; Rifamycin Derivatives

Ethanol/Nutrition/Herb Interactions

Ethanol: Avoid ethanol (may increase gastric mucosal irritation).

Food: Methylprednisolone interferes with calcium absorption. Limit caffeine.

Herb/Nutraceutical: St John's wort may decrease methylprednisolone levels. Avoid cat's claw, echinacea (have immunostimulant properties).

Stability

Intact vials of methylprednisolone sodium succinate should be stored at controlled room temperature of 20°C to 25°C (68°F to 77°F). Protect from light.

Reconstituted solutions of methylprednisolone sodium succinate should be stored at room temperature of 20°C to 25°C (68°F to 77°F), and used within 48 hours.

Stability of parenteral admixture at room temperature (25°C) and at refrigeration temperature (4°C) is 48 hours.

Standard diluent (Solu-Medrol®): 40 mg/50 mL D_5W; 125 mg/50 mL D_5W.

Minimum volume (Solu-Medrol®): 50 mL D_5W.

Mechanism of Action In a tissue-specific manner, corticosteroids regulate gene expression subsequent to binding specific intracellular receptors and translocation into the nucleus. Corticosteroids exert a wide array of physiologic effects including modulation of carbohydrate, protein, and lipid metabolism and maintenance of fluid and electrolyte homeostasis. Moreover cardiovascular, immunologic, musculoskeletal, endocrine, and neurologic physiology are influenced by corticosteroids. Decreases inflammation by suppression of migration of polymorphonuclear leukocytes and reversal of increased capillary permeability.

Pharmacodynamics/Kinetics

Onset of action: Peak effect (route dependent): Oral: 1-2 hours; I.M.: 4-8 days; Intra-articular: 1 week; methylprednisolone sodium succinate is highly soluble and has a rapid effect by I.M. and I.V. routes

Duration (route dependent): Oral: 30-36 hours; I.M.: 1-4 weeks; Intra-articular: 1-5 weeks; methylprednisolone acetate has a low solubility and has a sustained I.M. effect

Distribution: V_d: 0.7-1.5 L/kg

Half-life elimination: 3-3.5 hours; reduced in obese

Excretion: Clearance: Reduced in obese

Dosage Dosing should be based on the lesser of ideal body weight or actual body weight

Only sodium succinate may be given I.V.; methylprednisolone sodium succinate is highly soluble and has a rapid effect by I.M. and I.V. routes. Methylprednisolone acetate has a low solubility and has a sustained I.M. effect.

Children:

Acute spinal cord injury: I.V. (sodium succinate): 30 mg/kg over 15 minutes, followed in 45 minutes by a continuous infusion of 5.4 mg/kg/hour for 23 hours

Anti-inflammatory or immunosuppressive: Oral, I.M., I.V. (sodium succinate): 0.5-1.7 mg/kg/day **or** 5-25 mg/m²/day in divided doses every 6-12 hours; "Pulse" therapy: 15-30 mg/kg/dose over ≥30 minutes given once daily for 3 days

Asthma exacerbations, including status asthmaticus (emergency medical care or hospital doses) (NIH Asthma Guidelines, NAEPP, 2007): Children <12 years: Oral, I.V.: 1-2 mg/kg/day in 2 divided doses (maximum: 60 mg/day) until peak expiratory flow is 70% of predicted or personal best

Lupus nephritis: I.V. (sodium succinate): 30 mg/kg over ≥30 minutes every other day for 6 doses

Status asthmaticus: I.V. (sodium succinate): Previous NAEPP guidelines still encountered in clinical practice: Loading dose: 2 mg/kg/dose, then 0.5-1 mg/kg/dose every 6 hours for up to 5 days; **Note:** See new dosing guidelines for asthma exacerbations above.

Adults: **Only sodium succinate may be given I.V.;** methylprednisolone sodium succinate is highly soluble and has a rapid effect by I.M. and I.V. routes. Methylprednisolone acetate has a low solubility and has a sustained I.M. effect.

Acute spinal cord injury: I.V. (sodium succinate): 30 mg/kg over 15 minutes, followed in 45 minutes by a continuous infusion of 5.4 mg/kg/hour for 23 hours

Allergic conditions: Oral: Tapered-dosage schedule:

Day 1: 24 mg on day 1 administered as 8 mg before breakfast, 4 mg after lunch, 4 mg after supper, and 8 mg at bedtime **OR** 24 mg as a single dose or divided into 2 or 3 doses upon initiation (regardless of time of day)

Day 2: 20 mg on day 2 administered as 4 mg before breakfast, 4 mg after lunch, 4 mg after supper, and 8 mg at bedtime

Day 3: 16 mg on day 3 administered as 4 mg before breakfast, 4 mg after lunch, 4 mg after supper, and 4 mg at bedtime

Day 4: 12 mg on day 4 administered as 4 mg before breakfast, 4 mg after lunch, and 4 mg at bedtime

Day 5: 8 mg on day 5 administered as 4 mg before breakfast and 4 mg at bedtime

Day 6: 4 mg on day 6 administered as 4 mg before breakfast

Anti-inflammatory or immunosuppressive:

Oral: 2-60 mg/day in 1-4 divided doses to start, followed by gradual reduction in dosage to the lowest possible level consistent with maintaining an adequate clinical response.

I.M. (sodium succinate): 10-80 mg/day once daily

I.M. (acetate): 10-80 mg every 1-2 weeks

I.V. (sodium succinate): 10-40 mg over a period of several minutes and repeated I.V. or I.M. at intervals depending on clinical response; when high dosages are needed, give 30 mg/kg over a period ≥30 minutes and may be repeated every 4-6 hours for 48 hours.

Status asthmaticus: I.V. (sodium succinate): Loading dose: 2 mg/kg/dose, then 0.5-1 mg/kg/dose every 6 hours for up to 5 days

Lupus nephritis: High-dose "pulse" therapy: I.V. (sodium succinate): 1 g/day for 3 days

Aplastic anemia: I.V. (sodium succinate): 1 mg/kg/day or 40 mg/day (whichever dose is higher), for 4 days. After 4 days, change to oral and continue until day 10 or until symptoms of serum sickness resolve, then rapidly reduce over approximately 2 weeks.

Pneumocystis pneumonia in AIDs patients: I.V.: 30 mg twice daily for 5 days, then 30 mg once daily for 5 days, then 15 mg once daily for 11 days

Intra-articular (acetate): Administer every 1-5 weeks.

Large joints: 20-80 mg

Small joints: 4-10 mg

Intralesional (acetate): 20-60 mg every 1-5 weeks

Dietary Considerations Should be taken after meals or with food or milk; need diet rich in pyridoxine, vitamin C, vitamin D, folate, calcium, phosphorus, and protein.

Sodium content of 1 g sodium succinate injection: 2.01 mEq; 53 mg of sodium succinate salt is equivalent to 40 mg of methylprednisolone base

Methylprednisolone acetate: Depo-Medrol®

Methylprednisolone sodium succinate: Solu-Medrol®

Administration

Oral: Administer after meals or with food or milk

Parenteral: Methylprednisolone sodium succinate may be administered I.M. or I.V.; I.V. administration may be IVP over one to several minutes or IVPB or continuous I.V. infusion. **Acetate salt should not be given I.V.**

I.V.: Succinate:

Low dose: ≤1.8 mg/kg or ≤125 mg/dose: I.V. push over 3-15 minutes

Moderate dose: ≥2 mg/kg or 250 mg/dose: I.V. over 15-30 minutes

High dose: 15 mg/kg or ≥500 mg/dose: I.V. over ≥30 minutes

Doses >15 mg/kg or ≥1 g: Administer over 1 hour

Do **not** administer high-dose I.V. push; hypotension, cardiac arrhythmia, and sudden death have been reported in patients given high-dose methylprednisolone I.V. push (>0.5 g over <10 minutes); intermittent infusion over 15-60 minutes; maximum concentration: I.V. push 125 mg/mL

Monitoring Parameters Blood pressure, blood glucose, electrolytes

Test Interactions Interferes with skin tests

Additional Information Sodium content of 1 g sodium succinate injection: 2.01 mEq; 53 mg of sodium succinate salt is equivalent to 40 mg of methylprednisolone base

Methylprednisolone acetate: Depo-Medrol®

Methylprednisolone sodium succinate: Solu-Medrol®

Dosage Forms Excipient information presented when available (limited, particularly for generics); consult specific product labeling.

Injection, powder for reconstitution, as sodium succinate: 40 mg, 125 mg, 500 mg, 1 g [strength expressed as base]

Solu-Medrol®: 40 mg, 125 mg, 500 mg, 1 g, 2 g [contains benzyl alcohol (in diluent); strength expressed as base]

Solu-Medrol®: 500 mg, 1 g

Injection, suspension, as acetate: 40 mg/mL (5 mL, 10 mL); 80 mg/mL (5 mL)

Depo-Medrol®: 20 mg/mL (5 mL); 40 mg/mL (5 mL); 80 mg/mL (5 mL) [contains benzyl alcohol; strength expressed as base]

Depo-Medrol®: 40 mg/mL (1 mL); 80 mg/mL (1 mL)

Tablet: 4 mg

Medrol®: 2 mg, 4 mg, 8 mg, 16 mg, 32 mg

Tablet, dose-pack: 4 mg (21s)

Medrol® Dosepak™: 4 mg (21s)

◆ **6-α-Methylprednisolone** *see* MethylPREDNISolone *on page 976*

◆ **Methylprednisolone Acetate** *see* MethylPREDNISolone *on page 976*

◆ **Methylprednisolone Sodium Succinate** *see* MethylPREDNISolone *on page 976*

◆ **4-Methylpyrazole** *see* Fomepizole *on page 659*

◆ **Methylrosaniline Chloride** *see* Gentian Violet *on page 695*

MethylTESTOSTERone (meth il tes TOS te rone)

U.S. Brand Names Android®; Methitest™; Testred®; Virilon®

Pharmacologic Category Androgen

Use

Male: Hypogonadism; delayed puberty; impotence and climacteric symptoms

Female: Palliative treatment of metastatic breast cancer

Restrictions C-III

Pregnancy Risk Factor X

Medication Safety Issues

Sound-alike/look-alike issues:

MethylTESTOSTERone may be confused with medroxyPROGESTERone

Virilon® may be confused with Verelan®

Dosage Adults (buccal absorption produces twice the androgenic activity of oral tablets):

Male:

Hypogonadism, male climacteric and impotence: Oral: 10-40 mg/day

Androgen deficiency:

Oral: 10-50 mg/day

Buccal: 5-25 mg/day

Postpubertal cryptorchidism: Oral: 30 mg/day

Female:

Breast pain/engorgement:

Oral: 80 mg/day for 3-5 days

Buccal: 40 mg/day for 3-5 days

Breast cancer:

Oral: 50-200 mg/day

Buccal: 25-100 mg/day

Additional Information Complete prescribing information for this medication should be consulted for additional detail.

Dosage Forms Excipient information presented when available (limited, particularly for generics); consult specific product labeling.

Capsule (Android®, Testred®, Virilon®): 10 mg

Tablet (Methitest™): 10 mg

Metipranolol (met i PRAN oh lol)

U.S. Brand Names OptiPranolol®

Canadian Brand Names OptiPranolol®

Index Terms Metipranolol Hydrochloride

Pharmacologic Category Beta-Adrenergic Blocker, Nonselective; Ophthalmic Agent, Antiglaucoma

Additional Appendix Information

Glaucoma Drug Therapy *on page 1808*

Use Agent for lowering intraocular pressure in patients with chronic open-angle glaucoma

Pregnancy Risk Factor C

Medication Safety Issues

Sound-alike/look-alike issues:

Metipranolol may be confused with metaproterenol

International issues:

Betanol® [Monaco] may be confused with Beta-Val® which is a brand name for betamethasone in the U.S.

Betanol® [Monaco] may be confused with Patanol® which is a brand name for olopatadine in the U.S.

Betanol® [Monaco] may be confused with Betimol® which is a brand name for timolol in the U.S.

Dosage Ophthalmic: Adults: Instill 1 drop in the affected eye(s) twice daily

Additional Information Complete prescribing information for this medication should be consulted for additional detail.

Dosage Forms Excipient information presented when available (limited, particularly for generics); consult specific product labeling.

Solution, ophthalmic: 0.3% (5 mL, 10 mL) [contains benzalkonium chloride]

◆ **Metipranolol Hydrochloride** *see* Metipranolol *on page 979*

Metoclopramide (met oh KLOE pra mide)

U.S. Brand Names Reglan®

Canadian Brand Names Apo-Metoclop®; Metoclopramide Hydrochloride Injection; Nu-Metoclopramide

Pharmacologic Category Antiemetic; Gastrointestinal Agent, Prokinetic

Use

Oral: Symptomatic treatment of diabetic gastric stasis; gastroesophageal reflux

I.V., I.M.: Symptomatic treatment of diabetic gastric stasis; postpyloric placement of enteral feeding tubes; prevention and/or treatment of nausea and vomiting associated with chemotherapy, or postsurgery; to stimulate gastric emptying and intestinal transit of barium during radiological examination

Pregnancy Risk Factor B

Pregnancy Considerations Crosses the placenta; available evidence suggests safe use during pregnancy.

Lactation Enters breast milk/use caution

Medication Safety Issues

Sound-alike/look-alike issues:

Metoclopramide may be confused with metolazone

Reglan® may be confused with Megace®, Regonol®, Renagel®

Contraindications Hypersensitivity to metoclopramide or any component of the formulation; GI obstruction, perforation or hemorrhage; pheochromocytoma; history of seizures

Warnings/Precautions Use caution with a history of mental illness; has been associated with extrapyramidal symptoms (EPS) and depression. The frequency of EPS is higher in pediatric patients and adults <30 years of age; risk is increased at higher dosages. Extrapyramidal reactions typically occur within the initial 24-48 hours of treatment. Use caution with concurrent use of other drugs associated with EPS. Use caution in the elderly and with Parkinson's disease; may have increased risk of tardive dyskinesia. Neuroleptic malignant syndrome (NMS) has been reported (rarely) with metoclopramide. Use lowest recommended doses initially; may cause transient increase in serum aldosterone; use caution in patients who are at risk of fluid overload (HF, cirrhosis). Use caution in patients with hypertension or following surgical anastomosis/closure. Patients with NADH-cytochrome b5 reductase deficiency are at increased risk of methemoglobinemia and/or sulfhemoglobinemia. Abrupt discontinuation may (rarely) result in withdrawal symptoms (dizziness, headache, nervousness). Use caution and adjust dose in renal impairment.

Adverse Reactions Frequency not always defined.

Cardiovascular: AV block, bradycardia, CHF, fluid retention, flushing (following high I.V. doses), hyper-/hypotension, supraventricular tachycardia

Central nervous system: Drowsiness (~10% to 70%; dose related), acute dystonic reactions (<1% to 25%; dose and age related), fatigue (~10%), restlessness (~10%), akathisia, confusion, depression, dizziness, hallucinations (rare), headache, insomnia, neuroleptic malignant syndrome (rare), Parkinsonian-like symptoms, suicidal ideation, seizure, tardive dyskinesia

Dermatologic: Angioneurotic edema (rare), rash, urticaria

Endocrine & metabolic: Amenorrhea, galactorrhea, gynecomastia, impotence

Gastrointestinal: Diarrhea, nausea

Genitourinary: Incontinence, urinary frequency

Hematologic: Agranulocytosis, leukopenia, neutropenia, porphyria

Hepatic: Hepatotoxicity (rare)

Ocular: Visual disturbance

Respiratory: Bronchospasm, laryngeal edema (rare)

Miscellaneous: Allergic reactions, methemoglobinemia, sulfhemoglobinemia

Drug Interactions

Metabolism/Transport Effects Substrate (minor) of CYP1A2, 2D6; **Inhibits** CYP2D6 (weak)

Avoid Concomitant Use There are no known interactions where it is recommended to avoid concomitant use.

Increased Effect/Toxicity

Metoclopramide may increase the levels/effects of: CycloSPORINE; Sertraline; Venlafaxine

Decreased Effect

Metoclopramide may decrease the levels/effects of: Anti-Parkinson's Agents (Dopamine Agonist)

Ethanol/Nutrition/Herb Interactions Ethanol: Avoid ethanol (may increase CNS depression).

Stability

Injection: Store intact vial at controlled room temperature. Injection is photosensitive and should be protected from light during storage. Parenteral admixtures in D_5W or NS are stable for at least 24 hours and do not require light protection if used within 24 hours.

Tablet: Store at controlled room temperature.

Mechanism of Action Blocks dopamine receptors and (when given in higher doses) also blocks serotonin receptors in chemoreceptor trigger zone of the CNS; enhances the response to acetylcholine of tissue in upper GI tract causing enhanced motility and accelerated gastric emptying without stimulating gastric, biliary, or pancreatic secretions; increases lower esophageal sphincter tone

Pharmacodynamics/Kinetics

Onset of action: Oral: 0.5-1 hour; I.V.: 1-3 minutes; I.M.: 10-15 minutes

Duration: Therapeutic: 1-2 hours, regardless of route

Distribution: V_d: 2-4 L/kg

Protein binding: 30%

Bioavailability: Oral: 65% to 95%

Half-life elimination: Normal renal function: 4-6 hours (may be dose dependent)

Time to peak, serum: Oral: 1-2 hours

Excretion: Urine (~85%)

Dosage

Children:

Gastroesophageal reflux (unlabeled use): Oral: 0.1-0.2 mg/kg/dose 4 times/day

Antiemetic (chemotherapy-induced emesis) (unlabeled): I.V.: 1-2 mg/kg 30 minutes before chemotherapy and every 2-4 hours

Postpyloric feeding tube placement: I.V.:

<6 years: 0.1 mg/kg

6-14 years: 2.5-5 mg

>14 years: Refer to adult dosing.

Adults:

Gastroesophageal reflux: Oral: 10-15 mg/dose up to 4 times/day 30 minutes before meals or food and at bedtime; single doses of 20 mg are occasionally needed for provoking situations. Treatment >12 weeks has not been evaluated.

Diabetic gastric stasis:

Oral: 10 mg 30 minutes before each meal and at bedtime

I.M., I.V. (for severe symptoms): 10 mg over 1-2 minutes; 10 days of I.V. therapy may be necessary for best response

Chemotherapy-induced emesis:

I.V.: 1-2 mg/kg 30 minutes before chemotherapy and repeated every 2 hours for 2 doses, then every 3 hours for 3 doses (manufacturer labeling)

Alternate dosing (with or without diphenhydramine):

Moderate emetic risk chemotherapy: 0.5 mg/kg every 6 hours on days 2-4

Low and minimal risk chemotherapy: 1-2 mg/kg every 3-4 hours

Breakthrough treatment: 1-2 mg/kg every 3-4 hours

Oral (unlabeled use; with or without diphenhydramine):

Moderate emetic risk chemotherapy: 0.5 mg/kg every 6 hours or 20 mg 4 times/day on days 2-4

Low and minimal risk chemotherapy: 20-40 mg every 4-6 hours

Breakthrough treatment: 20-40 mg every 4-6 hours

Postoperative nausea and vomiting: I.M., I.V.: 10-20 mg near end of surgery

Postpyloric feeding tube placement, radiological exam: I.V.: 10 mg

Elderly:

Gastroesophageal reflux: Oral: 5 mg 4 times/day (30 minutes before meals or food and at bedtime); increase dose to 10 mg 4 times/day if no response at lower dose

Gastrointestinal hypomotility:

Oral: Initial: 5 mg 30 minutes before meals and at bedtime; increase if necessary to 10 mg doses

I.V.: Initiate at 5 mg over 1-2 minutes; increase to 10 mg if necessary

Postoperative nausea and vomiting: I.M., I.V.: 5 mg near end of surgery; may repeat dose if necessary

Dosing adjustment in renal impairment: Cl_{cr} <40 mL/minute: Administer at 50% of normal dose

Hemodialysis: Not dialyzable (0% to 5%); supplemental dose is not necessary

Administration Injection solution may be given I.M., direct I.V. push, short infusion (15-30 minutes), or continuous infusion; lower doses (≤10 mg) of metoclopramide can be given I.V. push undiluted over 1-2 minutes; higher doses to be given IVPB over at least 15 minutes; continuous SubQ infusion and rectal administration have been reported. **Note:** Rapid I.V. administration may be associated with a transient (but intense) feeling of anxiety and restlessness, followed by drowsiness.

Monitoring Parameters Dystonic reactions; signs of hypoglycemia in patients using insulin and those being treated for gastroparesis; agitation, and onfusion

Test Interactions Increased aminotransferase [ALT/AST] (S), increased amylase (S)

Dosage Forms Excipient information presented when available (limited, particularly for generics); consult specific product labeling.

Injection, solution [preservative free]: 5 mg/mL (2 mL)

Reglan®: 5 mg/mL (2 mL, 10 mL, 30 mL)

Solution, oral: 5 mg/5 mL (10 mL, 480 mL)

Tablet: 5 mg, 10 mg

Reglan®: 5 mg, 10 mg

◆ **Metoclopramide Hydrochloride Injection (Can)** *see* Metoclopramide *on page 979*

Metolazone (me TOLE a zone)

U.S. Brand Names Zaroxolyn®

Canadian Brand Names Zaroxolyn®

Pharmacologic Category Diuretic, Thiazide-Related

Additional Appendix Information

Heart Failure (Systolic) *on page 1809*

Sulfonamide Derivatives *on page 1671*

Use Management of mild to moderate hypertension; treatment of edema in congestive heart failure and nephrotic syndrome, impaired renal function

Pregnancy Risk Factor B (manufacturer); D (expert analysis)

Pregnancy Considerations Teratogenic effects were not observed in animal studies. Metolazone crosses the placenta and appears in cord blood. Hypoglycemia, hypokalemia, hyponatremia, jaundice, and thrombocytopenia are reported as complications to the fetus or newborn following maternal use of thiazide diuretics.

Lactation Enters breast milk/not recommended

Medication Safety Issues

Sound-alike/look-alike issues:

Metolazone may be confused with metaxalone, methazolamide, methimazole, methotrexate, metoclopramide, metoprolol, minoxidil

Zaroxolyn® may be confused with Zarontin®

Contraindications Hypersensitivity to metolazone, any component of the formulation, other thiazides, and sulfonamide derivatives; anuria; hepatic coma; pregnancy (expert analysis)

Warnings/Precautions Electrolyte disturbances (hypokalemia, hypochloremic alkalosis, hyponatremia) can occur. Large or prolonged fluid and electrolyte losses may occur with concomitant furosemide administration. Use with caution in severe hepatic dysfunction; hepatic encephalopathy can be caused by electrolyte disturbances. Gout can be precipitate in certain patients with a history of gout, a familial predisposition to gout, or chronic renal failure. Cautious use in patients with prediabetes or diabetes; may see a change in glucose control. Can cause SLE exacerbation or activation. Use caution in severe renal impairment. Use with caution in patients with moderate or high cholesterol concentrations. Photosensitization may occur.

Chemical similarities are present among sulfonamides, sulfonylureas, carbonic anhydrase inhibitors, thiazides, and loop diuretics (except ethacrynic acid). Use in patients with thiazide or sulfonamide allergy is specifically contraindicated in product labeling, however, a risk of cross-reaction exists in patients with allergy to any of these compounds; avoid use when previous reaction has been severe. Discontinue if signs of hypersensitivity are noted.

Adverse Reactions Frequency not defined.

Cardiovascular: Chest pain/discomfort, necrotizing angiitis, orthostatic hypotension, palpitation, syncope, venous thrombosis, vertigo, volume depletion

Central nervous system: chills, depression, dizziness, drowsiness, fatigue, headache, lightheadedness, restlessness

Dermatologic: Petechiae, photosensitivity, pruritus, purpura, rash, skin necrosis, Stevens-Johnson syndrome, toxic epidermal necrolysis, urticaria

Endocrine & metabolic: Gout attacks, hypercalcemia, hyperglycemia, hyperuricemia, hypochloremia, hypochloremic alkalosis, hypokalemia, hypomagnesemia, hyponatremia, hypophosphatemia

Gastrointestinal: Abdominal bloating, abdominal pain, anorexia, constipation, diarrhea, epigastric distress, nausea, pancreatitis, vomiting, xerostomia

Genitourinary: Impotence

Hematologic: Agranulocytosis, aplastic/hypoplastic anemia, hemoconcentration, leukopenia, thrombocytopenia

Hepatic: Cholestatic jaundice, hepatitis

Neuromuscular & skeletal: Joint pain, muscle cramps/spasm, neuropathy, paresthesia, weakness

Ocular: Blurred vision (transient)

Renal: BUN increased, glucosuria

Drug Interactions

Avoid Concomitant Use There are no known interactions where it is recommended to avoid concomitant use.

Increased Effect/Toxicity

Metolazone may increase the levels/effects of: ACE Inhibitors; Allopurinol; Amifostine; Calcitriol; Calcium Salts; Dofetilide; Lithium; RiTUXimab

The levels/effects of Metolazone may be increased by: Corticosteroids (Orally Inhaled); Corticosteroids (Systemic); Herbs (Hypotensive Properties); Prostacyclin Analogues

Decreased Effect

The levels/effects of Metolazone may be decreased by: Bile Acid Sequestrants; Herbs (Hypertensive Properties); Methylphenidate; Nonsteroidal Anti-Inflammatory Agents; Yohimbine

Ethanol/Nutrition/Herb Interactions

Ethanol: May potentiate hypotensive effect of metazolone.

Herb/Nutraceutical: Avoid dong quai if using for hypertension (has estrogenic activity). Avoid dong quai, St John's wort (may also cause photosensitization). Avoid ephedra, yohimbe, ginseng (may worsen hypertension). Avoid natural licorice. Avoid garlic (may have increased antihypertensive effect).

Mechanism of Action Inhibits sodium reabsorption in the distal tubules causing increased excretion of sodium and water, as well as, potassium and hydrogen ions

Pharmacodynamics/Kinetics
Onset of action: Diuresis: ~60 minutes
Duration: ≥24 hours
Absorption: Incomplete
Distribution: Crosses placenta; enters breast milk
Protein binding: 95%
Half-life elimination: 20 hours
Excretion: Urine (80%); bile (10%)

Dosage Oral:
Adults:
Edema: 2.5-20 mg/dose every 24 hours (ACC/AHA 2005 Heart Failure Guidelines)
Hypertension: 2.5-5 mg/dose every 24 hours
Elderly: Initial: 2.5 mg/day or every other day
Dosage adjustment in renal impairment: Dialysis: Not dialyzable (0% to 5%) via hemo- or peritoneal dialysis; supplemental dose is not necessary

Dietary Considerations Should be taken after breakfast; may require potassium supplementation

Administration May be taken with food or milk. Take early in day to avoid nocturia. Take the last dose of multiple doses no later than 6 PM unless instructed otherwise.

Monitoring Parameters Serum electrolytes (potassium, sodium, chloride, bicarbonate), renal function, blood pressure (standing, sitting/supine)

Additional Information Metolazone 5 mg is approximately equivalent to hydrochlorothiazide 50 mg.

Dosage Forms Excipient information presented when available (limited, particularly for generics); consult specific product labeling.
Tablet: 2.5 mg, 5 mg, 10 mg
Zaroxolyn®: 2.5 mg, 5 mg, 10 mg

Extemporaneous Preparations
A 1 mg/mL suspension may be made by crushing twelve 10 mg Zaroxolyn® tablets; add Ora-Sweet®, Ora-Sweet® SF, Ora-Plus®, or cherry syrup diluted 1:4 with simple syrup to total volume of 120 mL. Label "shake well"; stable 60 days refrigerated.
A 0.25 mg/mL suspension may be made by crushing one 2.5 mg tablet; add 1:1 mixture 1% methylcellulose:simple syrup mixture to a total volume of 10 mL; label "shake well"; refrigerate; stable 91 days refrigerated; 28 days at room temperature in plastic and 14 days at room temperature in glass.
Nahata, MC, Pai VB, and Hipple TF, *Pediatric Drug Formulations*, 5th ed, Cincinnati, OH: Harvey Whitney Books Co, 2004.

Metoprolol (me toe PROE lole)

U.S. Brand Names Lopressor®; Toprol-XL®

Canadian Brand Names Apo-Metoprolol®; Betaloc®; Betaloc® Durules®; Dom-Metoprolol; Gen-Metoprolol; Lopressor®; Metoprolol Tartrate Injection, USP; Metoprolol-25; Novo-Metoprolol; Nu-Metop; PHL-Metoprolol; PMS-Metoprolol; RIVA-Metoprolol ; Sandoz-Metoprolol; Toprol-XL®

Index Terms Metoprolol Succinate; Metoprolol Tartrate

Pharmacologic Category Beta Blocker, $Beta_1$ Selective

Additional Appendix Information
Beta-Blockers *on page 1648*
Heart Failure (Systolic) *on page 1809*

Use Treatment of angina pectoris, hypertension, or hemodynamically-stable acute myocardial infarction
Extended release: Treatment of angina pectoris or hypertension; to reduce mortality/hospitalization in patients with heart failure (stable NYHA Class II or III) already receiving ACE inhibitors, diuretics, and/or digoxin

Unlabeled/Investigational Use Treatment of ventricular arrhythmias, atrial ectopy; migraine prophylaxis, essential tremor, aggressive behavior (not recommended for dementia-associated aggression); prevention of myocardial infarction, atrial fibrillation, and atrial flutter; symptomatic treatment of hypertrophic obstructive cardiomyopathy

Pregnancy Risk Factor C (manufacturer); D (2nd and 3rd trimesters - expert analysis)

Pregnancy Considerations Teratogenic effects were not observed in animal studies. Metoprolol crosses the placenta. Maternal use of beta-blockers has been associated with fetal bradycardia, hypotension, and IUGR; IUGR is probably related to maternal hypertension. Available evidence suggests beta-blockers are generally safe during pregnancy (JNC 7). Cases of neonatal hypoglycemia have been reported following maternal use of beta-blockers at parturition. Information specific to metoprolol is limited.

Lactation Enters breast milk/use caution (AAP rates "compatible")

Medication Safety Issues
Sound-alike/look-alike issues:
Metoprolol may be confused with metaproterenol, metolazone, misoprostol
Toprol-XL® may be confused with Tegretol®, Tegretol®-XR, Topamax®

High alert medication: The Institute for Safe Medication Practices (ISMP) includes this medication among its list of drugs which have a heightened risk of causing significant patient harm when used in error.

Significant differences exist between oral and I.V. dosing. Use caution when converting from one route of administration to another.

Contraindications Note: Contraindications are indication-specific.
Hypersensitivity to metoprolol, any component of the formulation, or other beta-blockers; additionally:
Hypertension and angina: Sick sinus syndrome (except in patients with a functioning artificial pacemaker); severe peripheral arterial disease; pheochromocytoma (without alpha blockade)
Myocardial infarction: Severe sinus bradycardia (heart rate <45 beats/minute); significant first-degree heart block (P-R interval ≥0.24 seconds); second- and third-degree heart block; systolic blood pressure <100 mm Hg; moderate-to-severe cardiac failure; cardiogenic shock

Warnings/Precautions [U.S. Boxed Warning]: Beta-blocker therapy should not be withdrawn abruptly (particularly in patients with CAD), but gradually tapered over 1-2 weeks to avoid acute tachycardia, hypertension, and/or ischemia. Consider pre-existing conditions such as sick sinus syndrome before initiating. Metoprolol commonly produces mild first-degree heart block (P-R interval >0.2-0.24 sec). May also produce severe first- (P-R interval ≥0.26 sec), second-, or third-degree heart block. Patients with acute MI (especially right ventricular MI) have a high risk of developing heart block of varying degrees. If severe heart block occurs, metoprolol should be discontinued and measures to increase heart rate should be employed. Symptomatic hypotension may occur with use. Use caution in patients with PVD (can aggravate arterial insufficiency). Use caution with concurrent use of beta-blockers and either verapamil or diltiazem; bradycardia or heart block can occur; avoid concurrent I.V. use of both agents.

In general, beta-blockers should be avoided in patients with bronchospastic disease. Metoprolol, with B_1 selectivity, should be used cautiously in bronchospastic disease with close monitoring. Use cautiously in patients with diabetes because it can mask prominent hypoglycemic symptoms. Use caution in hyperthyroidism since beta-blockade may mask signs of thyrotoxicosis. Use caution with hepatic dysfunction. Use with caution in patients with myasthenia gravis or psychiatric disease (may cause CNS depression). Use caution with inhalation anesthetic agents which may decrease myocardial function. Use of beta-blockers may unmask cardiac failure in patients without a history of dysfunction. Adequate alpha-blockade is required prior to use of any beta-blocker for patients with untreated pheochromocytoma. Use caution with history of severe anaphylaxis to allergens; patients taking beta-blockers may become more sensitive to repeated allergen challenges. Treatment of anaphylaxis (eg, epinephrine) in patients taking beta-blockers may be ineffective or promote undesirable effects. Safety and efficacy have not been established in children <1 year of age.

Extended release: Use with caution in patients with compensated heart failure; monitor for a worsening of heart failure.

Adverse Reactions Frequency may not be defined.

Cardiovascular: Hypotension (1% to 27%), bradycardia (2% to 16%), first-degree heart block (P-R interval ≥0.26 sec; 5%), arterial insufficiency (usually Raynaud type; 1%), chest pain (1%), CHF (1%), edema (peripheral; 1%), palpitation (1%), syncope (1%)

Central nervous system: Dizziness (2% to 10%), fatigue (1% to 10%), depression (5%), confusion, hallucinations, headache, insomnia, memory loss (short-term), nightmares, sleep disturbances, somnolence, vertigo

Dermatology: Pruritus (5%), rash (5%), photosensitivity, psoriasis exacerbated

Endocrine & metabolic: Libido decreased, Peyronie's disease (<1%), diabetes exacerbated

Gastrointestinal: Diarrhea (5%), constipation (1%), flatulence (1%), gastrointestinal pain (1%), heartburn (1%), nausea (1%), xerostomia (1%), vomiting

Hematologic: Claudication

Neuromuscular & skeletal: Musculoskeletal pain

Ocular: Blurred vision, visual disturbances

Otic: Tinnitus

Respiratory: Dyspnea (1% to 3%), bronchospasm (1%), wheezing (1%), rhinitis

Miscellaneous: Cold extremities (1%)

Postmarketing and/or case reports: Agranulocytosis, alkaline phosphatase increased, alopecia (reversible), arthralgia, arthritis, anxiety, cardiogenic shock, diaphoresis increased, dry eyes, gangrene, hepatitis, HDL decreased, impotence, jaundice, lactate dehydrogenase increased, nervousness, paresthesia, retroperitoneal fibrosis, second-degree heart block, taste disturbance, third-degree heart block, thrombocytopenia, transaminases increased, triglycerides increased, urticaria, vomiting, weight gain

Other events reported with beta-blockers: Catatonia, emotional lability, fever, hypersensitivity reactions, laryngospasm, nonthrombocytopenic purpura, respiratory distress, thrombocytopenic purpura

Drug Interactions

Metabolism/Transport Effects **Substrate** of CYP2C19 (minor), 2D6 (major); **Inhibits** CYP2D6 (weak)

Avoid Concomitant Use

Avoid concomitant use of Metoprolol with any of the following: Methacholine

Increased Effect/Toxicity

Metoprolol may increase the levels/effects of: Alpha-/Beta-Agonists (Direct-Acting); Alpha1-Blockers; Alpha2-Agonists; Amifostine; Antipsychotic Agents (Phenothiazines); Cardiac Glycosides; Insulin; Lidocaine; Methacholine; Midodrine; RiTUXimab

The levels/effects of Metoprolol may be increased by: Acetylcholinesterase Inhibitors; Aminoquinolines (Antimalarial); Amiodarone; Anilidopiperidine Opioids; Antipsychotic Agents (Phenothiazines); Calcium Channel Blockers (Nondihydropyridine); CYP2D6 Inhibitors (Moderate); CYP2D6 Inhibitors (Strong); Darunavir; Diazoxide; Dipyridamole; Disopyramide; Herbs (Hypotensive Properties); Propafenone; Propoxyphene; Prostacyclin Analogues; QuiNIDine; Reserpine; Selective Serotonin Reuptake Inhibitors

Decreased Effect

Metoprolol may decrease the levels/effects of: Beta2-Agonists; Theophylline Derivatives

The levels/effects of Metoprolol may be decreased by: Barbiturates; Herbs (Hypertensive Properties); Methylphenidate; Nonsteroidal Anti-Inflammatory Agents; Rifamycin Derivatives; Yohimbine

Ethanol/Nutrition/Herb Interactions

Food: Food increases absorption. Metoprolol serum levels may be increased if taken with food.

Herb/Nutraceutical: Avoid bayberry, blue cohosh, cayenne, ephedra, ginger, ginseng (American), gotu kola, licorice, (may worsen hypertension). Avoid black cohosh, California poppy, coleus, golden seal, hawthorn, mistletoe, periwinkle, quinine, shepherd's purse (may have increased antihypertensive effect).

Stability

Injection: Store at controlled room temperature of 25°C (77°F). Protect from light.

Tablet: Store at controlled room temperature of 25°C (77°F). Protect from moisture.

Mechanism of Action Selective inhibitor of beta$_1$-adrenergic receptors; competitively blocks beta$_1$-receptors, with little or no effect on beta$_2$-receptors at doses <100 mg; does not exhibit any membrane stabilizing or intrinsic sympathomimetic activity

Pharmacodynamics/Kinetics

Onset of action: Peak effect: Oral: 1.5-4 hours; I.V.: 20 minutes (when infused over 10 minutes)

Duration: Oral: Immediate release: 10-20 hours, Extended release: ~24 hours; I.V.: 5-8 hours

Absorption: 95%, rapid and complete

Protein binding: 12% to albumin

Metabolism: Extensively hepatic via CYP2D6; significant first-pass effect (~50%)

Bioavailability: Oral: ~50%

Half-life elimination: 3-8 hours (dependent on rate of CYP2D6 metabolism)

Excretion: Urine (<5% to 10% as unchanged drug)

Dosage

Children: Hypertension: Oral:

1-17 years: Immediate release tablet: (National High Blood Pressure Education Program Working Group on High Blood Pressure in Children and Adolescents, 2004): Initial: 1-2 mg/kg/day; maximum 6 mg/kg/day (≤200 mg/day); administer in 2 divided doses

≥6 years: Extended release tablet: Initial: 1 mg/kg once daily (maximum initial dose: 50 mg/day). Adjust dose based on patient response (maximum: 2 mg/kg/day or 200 mg/day)

Adults:

Hypertension: Oral: 100-450 mg/day in 2-3 divided doses, begin with 50 mg twice daily and increase doses at weekly intervals to desired effect; usual dosage range (JNC 7): 50-100 mg/day

Extended release: Initial: 25-100 mg/day (maximum: 400 mg/day)

Angina, SVT, MI prophylaxis: Oral: 100-450 mg/day in 2-3 divided doses, begin with 50 mg twice daily and increase doses at weekly intervals to desired effect

Extended release: Initial: 100 mg/day (maximum: 400 mg/day)

Hypertension/ventricular rate control: I.V. (in patients having nonfunctioning GI tract): Initial: 1.25-5 mg every 6-12 hours; titrate initial dose to response. Initially, low doses may be appropriate to establish response;

however, up to 15 mg every 3-6 hours has been employed.

Congestive heart failure: Oral (extended release): Initial: 25 mg once daily (reduce to 12.5 mg once daily in NYHA class higher than class II); may double dosage every 2 weeks as tolerated (maximum: 200 mg/day)

Myocardial infarction (acute): I.V.: 5 mg every 2 minutes for 3 doses in early treatment of myocardial infarction; thereafter give 50 mg orally every 6 hours 15 minutes after last I.V. dose and continue for 48 hours; then administer a maintenance dose of 100 mg twice daily.

Elderly: Initiate at the lower end of the dosage range

Note: Switching dosage forms:

When switching from immediate release metoprolol to extended release, the same total daily dose of metoprolol should be used.

When switching between oral and intravenous dosage forms, equivalent beta-blocking effect is achieved when doses in a 2.5:1 (Oral:I.V.) ratio is used.

Dosing adjustment in renal impairment: No adjustment required.

Dosing adjustment in hepatic impairment: Reduced dose may be necessary

Dietary Considerations Regular tablets should be taken with food. Extended release tablets may be taken without regard to meals.

Administration

Oral: Extended release tablets may be divided in half; do not crush or chew.

I.V.: When administered acutely for cardiac treatment, monitor ECG and blood pressure. May administer by rapid infusion (I.V. push) over 1 minute or by slow infusion (ie, 5-10 mg of metoprolol in 50 mL of fluid) over ~30 minutes. Necessary monitoring for surgical patients who are unable to take oral beta-blockers (prolonged ileus) has not been defined. Some institutions require monitoring of baseline and postinfusion heart rate and blood pressure when a patient's response to beta-blockade has not been characterized (ie, the patient's initial dose or following a change in dose). Consult individual institutional policies and procedures.

Monitoring Parameters Acute cardiac treatment: Monitor ECG and blood pressure with I.V. administration; heart rate and blood pressure with oral administration

Dosage Forms Excipient information presented when available (limited, particularly for generics); consult specific product labeling.

Injection, solution, as tartrate: 1 mg/mL (5 mL)
Lopressor®: 1 mg/mL (5 mL)

Tablet, as tartrate: 25 mg, 50 mg, 100 mg
Lopressor®: 50 mg, 100 mg

Tablet, extended release, as succinate: 25 mg, 50 mg, 100 mg, 200 mg [expressed as mg equivalent to tartrate]
Toprol-XL®: 25 mg, 50 mg, 100 mg, 200 mg [expressed as mg equivalent to tartrate]

Extemporaneous Preparations To prepare a metoprolol 10 mg/mL liquid, crush 12 metoprolol tartrate 100 mg tablets into a fine powder. Add ~20 mL of either Ora-Sweet® and Ora-Plus® (1:1 preparation), or Ora-Sweet® SF and Ora-Plus® (1:1 preparation), or cherry syrup. Mix to a uniform paste. Continue to add the vehicle to bring the final volume to 120 mL. The preparation is stable for 60 days; shake well before using and protect from light.

Allen LV and Erickson III MA, "Stability of Labetalol Hydrochloride, Metoprolol Tartrate, Verapamil Hydrochloride, and Spironolactone With Hydrochlorothiazide in Extemporaneously Compounded Oral Liquids," *Am J Health Syst Pharm*, 1996, 53:2304-9.

◆ **Metoprolol-25 (Can)** *see* Metoprolol *on page 982*

Metoprolol and Hydrochlorothiazide

(me toe PROE lole & hye droe klor oh THYE a zide)

U.S. Brand Names Lopressor HCT®

Index Terms Hydrochlorothiazide and Metoprolol; Hydrochlorothiazide and Metoprolol Tartrate; Metoprolol Tartrate and Hydrochlorothiazide

Pharmacologic Category Beta Blocker, Beta$_1$ Selective; Diuretic, Thiazide

Use Treatment of hypertension (not recommended for initial treatment)

Pregnancy Risk Factor C/D (expert analysis)

Dosage Oral: Adults: Hypertension: Dosage should be determined by titration of the individual agents and the combination product substituted based upon the daily requirements.

Usual dose: Metoprolol 50-100 mg and hydrochlorothiazide 25-50 mg administered daily as single or divided doses (twice daily)

Note: Hydrochlorothiazide >50 mg/day is not recommended.

Concomitant therapy: It is recommended that if an additional antihypertensive agent is required, gradual titration should occur using 1/2 the usual starting dose of the other agent to avoid hypotension.

Additional Information Complete prescribing information for this medication should be consulted for additional detail.

Dosage Forms Excipient information presented when available (limited, particularly for generics); consult specific product labeling.

Tablet:

50/25: Metoprolol tartrate 50 mg and hydrochlorothiazide 25 mg

100/25: Metoprolol tartrate 100 mg and hydrochlorothiazide 25 mg

100/50: Metoprolol tartrate 100 mg and hydrochlorothiazide 50 mg

◆ **Metoprolol Succinate** *see* Metoprolol *on page 982*

◆ **Metoprolol Tartrate** *see* Metoprolol *on page 982*

◆ **Metoprolol Tartrate and Hydrochlorothiazide** *see* Metoprolol and Hydrochlorothiazide *on page 984*

◆ **Metoprolol Tartrate Injection, USP (Can)** *see* Metoprolol *on page 982*

◆ **MetroCream®** *see* MetroNIDAZOLE *on page 984*

◆ **MetroGel®** *see* MetroNIDAZOLE *on page 984*

◆ **Metrogel® (Can)** *see* MetroNIDAZOLE *on page 984*

◆ **MetroGel-Vaginal®** *see* MetroNIDAZOLE *on page 984*

◆ **MetroLotion®** *see* MetroNIDAZOLE *on page 984*

MetroNIDAZOLE

(met roe NYE da zole)

U.S. Brand Names Flagyl ER®; Flagyl®; MetroCream®; MetroGel-Vaginal®; MetroGel®; MetroLotion®; Noritate®; Vandazole™

Canadian Brand Names Apo-Metronidazole®; Flagyl®; Florazole® ER; MetroCream®; Metrogel®; Nidagel™; Noritate®; Trikacide

Index Terms Metronidazole Hydrochloride

Pharmacologic Category Amebicide; Antibiotic, Miscellaneous; Antibiotic, Topical; Antiprotozoal, Nitroimidazole

Additional Appendix Information

Antimicrobial Drugs of Choice *on page 1752*

Helicobacter pylori Treatment *on page 1813*

Prevention of Wound Infection and Sepsis in Surgical Patients *on page 1738*

Treatment of Sexually Transmitted Infections *on page 1773*

Use Treatment of susceptible anaerobic bacterial and protozoal infections in the following conditions: Amebiasis, symptomatic and asymptomatic trichomoniasis; skin and skin structure infections; CNS infections; intra-abdominal infections (as part of combination regimen); systemic anaerobic infections; treatment of antibiotic-associated pseudomembranous colitis (AAPC), bacterial vaginosis; as part of a multidrug regimen for *H. pylori* eradication to reduce the risk of duodenal ulcer recurrence

Topical: Treatment of inflammatory lesions and erythema of rosacea

Unlabeled/Investigational Use Crohn's disease

Pregnancy Risk Factor B (may be contraindicated in 1st trimester)

Pregnancy Considerations Crosses the placenta (carcinogenic in rats); contraindicated for the treatment of trichomoniasis during the first trimester of pregnancy, unless alternative treatment is inadequate. Until safety and efficacy for other indications have been established, use only during pregnancy when the benefit to the mother outweighs the potential risk to the fetus.

Lactation Enters breast milk/not recommended (AAP rates "of concern")

Medication Safety Issues

Sound-alike/look-alike issues:

MetroNIDAZOLE may be confused with meropenem, metFORMIN

Contraindications Hypersensitivity to metronidazole, nitroimidazole derivatives, or any component of the formulation; pregnancy (1st trimester - found to be carcinogenic in rats)

Warnings/Precautions Use with caution in patients with liver impairment due to potential accumulation, blood dyscrasias; history of seizures, CHF, or other sodium retaining states; reduce dosage in patients with severe liver impairment, CNS disease, and consider dosage reduction in longer-term therapy with severe renal failure (Cl_{cr} <10 mL/minute); if *H. pylori* is not eradicated in patients being treated with metronidazole in a regimen, it should be assumed that metronidazole-resistance has occurred and it should not again be used; seizures and neuropathies have been reported especially with increased doses and chronic treatment; if this occurs, discontinue therapy. **[U.S. Boxed Warning]: Possibly carcinogenic based on animal data.** Prolonged use may result in fungal or bacterial superinfection, including *C. difficile*-associated diarrhea (CDAD) and pseudomembranous colitis; CDAD has been observed >2 months postantibiotic treatment.

Adverse Reactions

Systemic: Frequency not defined:

Cardiovascular: Flattening of the T-wave, flushing

Central nervous system: Ataxia, confusion, coordination impaired, dizziness, fever, headache, insomnia, irritability, seizure, vertigo

Dermatologic: Erythematous rash, urticaria

Endocrine & metabolic: Disulfiram-like reaction, dysmenorrhea, libido decreased

Gastrointestinal: Nausea (~12%), anorexia, abdominal cramping, constipation, diarrhea, furry tongue, glossitis, proctitis, stomatitis, unusual/metallic taste, vomiting, xerostomia

Genitourinary: Cystitis, darkened urine (rare), dysuria, incontinence, polyuria, vaginitis

Hematologic: Neutropenia (reversible), thrombocytopenia (reversible, rare)

Neuromuscular & skeletal: Peripheral neuropathy, weakness

Respiratory: Nasal congestion, rhinitis, sinusitis, pharyngitis

Miscellaneous: Flu-like syndrome, moniliasis

Topical: Frequency not defined:

Central nervous system: Headache

Dermatologic: Burning, contact dermatitis, dryness, erythema, irritation, pruritus, rash

Gastrointestinal: Unusual/metallic taste, nausea, constipation

Local: Local allergic reaction

Neuromuscular & skeletal: Tingling/numbness of extremities

Ocular: Eye irritation

Vaginal:

>10%: Genitourinary: Vaginal discharge (12%)

1% to 10%:

Central nervous system: Headache (5%), dizziness (2%)

Gastrointestinal: Gastrointestinal discomfort (7%), nausea and/or vomiting (4%), unusual/metallic taste (2%), diarrhea (1%)

Genitourinary: Vaginitis (10%), vulva/vaginal irritation (9%), pelvic discomfort (3%)

Hematologic: WBC increased (2%)

<1%: Abdominal bloating, abdominal gas, darkened urine, depression, fatigue, itching, rash, thirst, xerostomia

Drug Interactions

Metabolism/Transport Effects Inhibits CYP2C9 (weak), 3A4 (moderate)

Avoid Concomitant Use

Avoid concomitant use of MetroNIDAZOLE with any of the following: Amprenavir

Increased Effect/Toxicity

MetroNIDAZOLE may increase the levels/effects of: Alcohol (Ethyl); Amprenavir; Busulfan; Calcineurin Inhibitors; CYP3A4 Substrates; Eplerenone; FentaNYL; Maraviroc; Pimecrolimus; Ranolazine; Salmeterol; Tipranavir; Vitamin K Antagonists

The levels/effects of MetroNIDAZOLE may be increased by: Disulfiram; Mebendazole

Decreased Effect

MetroNIDAZOLE may decrease the levels/effects of: Mycophenolate; Typhoid Vaccine

Ethanol/Nutrition/Herb Interactions

Ethanol: The manufacturer recommends to avoid all ethanol or any ethanol-containing drugs (may cause disulfiram-like reaction characterized by flushing, headache, nausea, vomiting, sweating, or tachycardia).

Food: Peak antibiotic serum concentration lowered and delayed, but total drug absorbed not affected.

Stability Metronidazole injection should be stored at 15°C to 30°C and protected from light. Product may be refrigerated but crystals may form. Crystals redissolve on warming to room temperature. Prolonged exposure to light will cause a darkening of the product. However, short-term exposure to normal room light does not adversely affect metronidazole stability. Direct sunlight should be avoided. Stability of parenteral admixture at room temperature (25°C): Out of overwrap stability: 30 days.

Standard diluent: 500 mg/100 mL NS.

Mechanism of Action After diffusing into the organism, interacts with DNA to cause a loss of helical DNA structure and strand breakage resulting in inhibition of protein synthesis and cell death in susceptible organisms

Pharmacodynamics/Kinetics

Absorption: Oral: Well absorbed; Topical: Concentrations achieved systemically after application of 1 g topically are 10 times less than those obtained after a 250 mg oral dose

Distribution: To saliva, bile, seminal fluid, breast milk, bone, liver, and liver abscesses, lung and vaginal secretions; crosses placenta and blood-brain barrier

CSF:blood level ratio: Normal meninges: 16% to 43%; Inflamed meninges: 100%

Protein binding: <20%

Metabolism: Hepatic (30% to 60%)

Half-life elimination: Neonates: 25-75 hours; Others: 6-8 hours, prolonged with hepatic impairment; End-stage renal disease: 21 hours

Time to peak, serum: Oral: Immediate release: 1-2 hours

Excretion: Urine (20% to 40% as unchanged drug); feces (6% to 15%)

Dosage

Infants and Children:

Amebiasis: Oral: 35-50 mg/kg/day in divided doses every 8 hours for 10 days

Trichomoniasis: Oral: 15-30 mg/kg/day in divided doses every 8 hours for 7 days

Anaerobic infections:

Oral: 15-35 mg/kg/day in divided doses every 8 hours

I.V.: 30 mg/kg/day in divided doses every 6 hours

Clostridium difficile (antibiotic-associated colitis): Oral: 20 mg/kg/day divided every 6 hours

Maximum dose: 2 g/day

Adults:

Anaerobic infections (diverticulitis, intra-abdominal, peritonitis, cholangitis, or abscess): Oral, I.V.: 500 mg every 6-8 hours, not to exceed 4 g/day

Acne rosacea: Topical:

0.75%: Apply and rub a thin film twice daily, morning and evening, to entire affected areas after washing. Significant therapeutic results should be noticed within 3 weeks. Clinical studies have demonstrated continuing improvement through 9 weeks of therapy.

1%: Apply thin film to affected area once daily

Amebiasis: Oral: 500-750 mg every 8 hours for 5-10 days

Antibiotic-associated pseudomembranous colitis: Oral: 250-500 mg 3-4 times/day for 10-14 days

Note: Due to the emergence of a new strain of *C. difficile*, some clinicians recommend converting to oral vancomycin therapy if the patient does not show a clear clinical response after 2 days of metronidazole therapy.

Giardiasis: 500 mg twice daily for 5-7 days

Helicobacter pylori eradication: Oral: 250-500 mg with meals and at bedtime for 14 days; requires combination therapy with at least one other antibiotic and an acid-suppressing agent (proton pump inhibitor or H_2 blocker)

Bacterial vaginosis or vaginitis due to *Gardnerella*, *Mobiluncus*:

Oral: 500 mg twice daily (regular release) or 750 mg once daily (extended release tablet) for 7 days

Vaginal: 1 applicatorful (~37.5 mg metronidazole) intravaginally once or twice daily for 5 days; apply once in morning and evening if using twice daily, if daily, use at bedtime

Trichomoniasis: Oral: 250 mg every 8 hours for 7 days **or** 375 mg twice daily for 7 days **or** 2 g as a single dose

Elderly: Use lower end of dosing recommendations for adults, do not administer as a single dose

Dosing adjustment in renal impairment: Cl_{cr} <10 mL/minute, but not on dialysis: Recommendations vary: To reduce possible accumulation in patients receiving multiple doses, consider reduction to 50% of dose or every 12 hours; **Note:** Dosage reduction is unnecessary in short courses of therapy. Clinical recommendations and practice vary. Some references do not recommend reduction at any level of renal impairment (Lamp, 1999).

Hemodialysis: Extensively removed by hemodialysis and peritoneal dialysis (50% to 100%); dosage reduction not recommended; administer full dose posthemodialysis

Peritoneal dialysis: Dose as for Cl_{cr} <10 mL/minute

Continuous arteriovenous or venovenous hemofiltration: Administer usual dose

Dosing adjustment/comments in hepatic disease: Unchanged in mild liver disease; reduce dosage in severe liver disease

Dietary Considerations Take on an empty stomach. Drug may cause GI upset; if GI upset occurs, take with food. Extended release tablets should be taken on an empty stomach (1 hour before or 2 hours after meals). Sodium content of 500 mg (I.V.): 322 mg (14 mEq). The manufacturer recommends that ethanol be avoided during treatment and for 3 days after therapy is complete.

Administration

Oral: May be taken with food to minimize stomach upset. Extended release tablets should be taken on an empty stomach (1 hour before or 2 hours after meals).

Topical: No disulfiram-like reactions have been reported after **topical** application, although metronidazole can be detected in the blood. Apply to clean, dry skin. Cosmetics may be used after application (wait at least 5 minutes after using lotion).

Test Interactions May interfere with AST, ALT, triglycerides, glucose, and LDH testing

Dosage Forms Excipient information presented when available (limited, particularly for generics); consult specific product labeling.

Capsule: 375 mg

Flagyl®: 375 mg

Cream, topical: 0.75% (45 g)

MetroCream®: 0.75% (45 g) [contains benzyl alcohol]

Noritate®: 1% (60 g)

Gel, topical: 0.75% (45 g)

MetroGel®: 1% (46 g, 60 g) [60 g tube also packaged in a kit with Cetaphil® skin cleanser]

Gel, vaginal: 0.75% (70 g)

MetroGel-Vaginal®, Vandazole™: 0.75% (70 g)

Infusion [premixed iso-osmotic sodium chloride solution]: 500 mg (100 mL)

Lotion, topical: 0.75% (60 mL)

MetroLotion®: 0.75% (60 mL) [contains benzyl alcohol]

Tablet: 250 mg, 500 mg

Flagyl®: 250 mg, 500 mg

Tablet, extended release:

Flagyl® ER: 750 mg

Extemporaneous Preparations A 20 mg/mL oral suspension can be prepared by crushing ten 250 mg tablets in a mortar, and then adding 10 mL purified water USP to create a uniform paste. Add a small quantity of syrup, then transfer to a graduate and add a sufficient quantity of syrup to make 125 mL. Label "shake well" and "refrigerate." Refrigerated stability is 10 days.

Irwin DB, Dupuis LL, Prober CG, et al, "The Acceptability, Stability, and Relative Bioavailability of an Extemporaneous Metronidazole Suspension," *Can J Hosp Pharm*, 1987, 40:42-6.

Nahata MC, Morosco RS, and Hipple TF, 4th ed, *Pediatric Drug Formulations*, Cincinnati, OH: Harvey Whitney Books Co, 2000.

- **Metronidazole, Bismuth Subcitrate Potassium, and Tetracycline** *see* Bismuth, Metronidazole, and Tetracycline *on page 199*
- **Metronidazole, Bismuth Subsalicylate, and Tetracycline** *see* Bismuth, Metronidazole, and Tetracycline *on page 199*
- **Metronidazole Hydrochloride** *see* MetroNIDAZOLE *on page 984*

Metyrosine (me TYE roe seen)

U.S. Brand Names Demser®

Canadian Brand Names Demser®

Index Terms AMPT; OGMT

Pharmacologic Category Tyrosine Hydroxylase Inhibitor

Use Short-term management of pheochromocytoma before surgery, long-term management when surgery is contraindicated or when chronic malignant pheochromocytoma exists

Pregnancy Risk Factor C

Medication Safety Issues

Sound-alike/look-alike issues:

Metyrosine may be confused with metyrapone

Dosage Children >12 years and Adults: Oral: Initial: 250 mg 4 times/day, increased by 250-500 mg/day up to 4 g/day; maintenance: 2-3 g/day in 4 divided doses; for preoperative preparation, administer optimum effective dosage for 5-7 days

Dosing adjustment in renal impairment: Adjustment should be considered

Additional Information Complete prescribing information for this medication should be consulted for additional detail.

Dosage Forms Excipient information presented when available (limited, particularly for generics); consult specific product labeling.

Capsule: 250 mg

◆ **Mevacor®** *see* Lovastatin *on page 910*

◆ **Mevinolin** *see* Lovastatin *on page 910*

◆ **Mexar™ [DSC]** *see* Sulfacetamide *on page 1405*

Mexiletine (meks IL e teen)

U.S. Brand Names Mexitil® [DSC]

Canadian Brand Names Novo-Mexiletine

Pharmacologic Category Antiarrhythmic Agent, Class Ib

Use Management of serious ventricular arrhythmias; suppression of PVCs

Unlabeled/Investigational Use Diabetic neuropathy

Pregnancy Risk Factor C

Lactation Enters breast milk/compatible

Contraindications Hypersensitivity to mexiletine or any component of the formulation; cardiogenic shock; second- or third-degree AV block (except in patients with a functioning artificial pacemaker)

Warnings/Precautions [U.S. Boxed Warning]: In the Cardiac Arrhythmia Suppression Trial (CAST), recent (>6 days but <2 years ago) myocardial infarction patients with asymptomatic, non-life-threatening ventricular arrhythmias did not benefit and may have been harmed by attempts to suppress the arrhythmia with flecainide or encainide. An increased mortality or nonfatal cardiac arrest rate (7.7%) was seen in the active treatment group compared with patients in the placebo group (3%). The applicability of the CAST results to other populations is unknown. Antiarrhythmic agents should be reserved for patients with life-threatening ventricular arrhythmias. Can be proarrhythmic. Electrolyte disturbances alter response; should be corrected before initiating therapy. Use cautiously in patients with first-degree block, pre-existing sinus node dysfunction, intraventricular conduction delays, significant hepatic dysfunction, hypotension, or severe HF. Alterations in urinary pH may change urinary excretion. Rare hepatic toxicity may occur; may cause acute hepatic injury.

Adverse Reactions

>10%:

Central nervous system: Lightheadedness (11% to 25%), dizziness (20% to 25%), nervousness (5% to 10%), incoordination (10%)

Gastrointestinal: GI distress (41%), nausea/vomiting (40%)

Neuromuscular & skeletal: Trembling, unsteady gait, tremor (13%), ataxia (10% to 20%)

1% to 10%:

Cardiovascular: Chest pain (3% to 8%), premature ventricular contractions (1% to 2%), palpitation (4% to 8%), angina (2%), proarrhythmia (10% to 15% in patients with malignant arrhythmia)

Central nervous system: Confusion, headache, insomnia (5% to 7%), depression (2%)

Dermatologic: Rash (4%)

Gastrointestinal: Constipation or diarrhea (4% to 5%), xerostomia (3%), abdominal pain (1%)

Neuromuscular & skeletal: Weakness (5%), numbness of fingers or toes (2% to 4%), paresthesia (2%), arthralgia (1%)

Ocular: Blurred vision (5% to 7%), nystagmus (6%)

Otic: Tinnitus (2% to 3%)

Respiratory: Dyspnea (3%)

<1% (Limited to important or life-threatening): Agranulocytosis, alopecia, AV block, cardiogenic shock, CHF, dysphagia, exfoliative dermatitis, hallucinations, hepatic necrosis, hepatitis, hypotension, impotence, leukopenia, myelofibrosis, pancreatitis (rare), psychosis, pulmonary fibrosis, seizure, sinus arrest, SLE syndrome, Stevens-Johnson syndrome, syncope, thrombocytopenia, torsade de pointes, upper GI bleeding, urinary retention, urticaria

Drug Interactions

Metabolism/Transport Effects Substrate (major) of CYP1A2, 2D6; **Inhibits** CYP1A2 (strong)

Avoid Concomitant Use There are no known interactions where it is recommended to avoid concomitant use.

Increased Effect/Toxicity

Mexiletine may increase the levels/effects of: Bendamustine; CYP1A2 Substrates; Theophylline Derivatives

The levels/effects of Mexiletine may be increased by: CYP1A2 Inhibitors (Moderate); CYP1A2 Inhibitors (Strong); CYP2D6 Inhibitors (Moderate); CYP2D6 Inhibitors (Strong); Darunavir; Selective Serotonin Reuptake Inhibitors

Decreased Effect

The levels/effects of Mexiletine may be decreased by: CYP1A2 Inducers (Strong); Phenytoin

Ethanol/Nutrition/Herb Interactions Food: Food may decrease the rate, but not the extent of oral absorption; diets which affect urine pH can increase or decrease excretion of mexiletine. Avoid dietary changes that alter urine pH.

Mechanism of Action Class IB antiarrhythmic, structurally related to lidocaine, which inhibits inward sodium current, decreases rate of rise of phase 0, increases effective refractory period/action potential duration ratio

Pharmacodynamics/Kinetics

Absorption: Elderly have a slightly slower rate, but extent of absorption is the same as young adults

Distribution: V_d: 5-7 L/kg

Protein binding: 50% to 70%

Metabolism: Hepatic; low first-pass effect

Half-life elimination: Adults: 10-14 hours (average: elderly: 14.4 hours, younger adults: 12 hours); prolonged with hepatic impairment or heart failure

Time to peak: 2-3 hours

Excretion: Urine (10% to 15% as unchanged drug); urinary acidification increases excretion, alkalinization decreases excretion

Dosage Adults: Oral: Initial: 200 mg every 8 hours (may load with 400 mg if necessary); adjust dose every 2-3 days; usual dose: 200-300 mg every 8 hours; maximum dose: 1.2 g/day (some patients respond to every 12-hour dosing). When switching from another antiarrhythmic, initiate a 200 mg dose 6-12 hours after stopping former agents, 3-6 hours after stopping procainamide.

Dosage adjustment in hepatic impairment: Reduce dose to 25% to 30% of usual dose

Administration Administer around-the-clock rather than 3 times/day to promote less variation in peak and trough serum levels; administer with food

Reference Range Therapeutic range: 0.5-2 mcg/mL; potentially toxic: >2 mcg/mL

Test Interactions Abnormal liver function test, positive ANA, thrombocytopenia

Dosage Forms Excipient information presented when available (limited, particularly for generics); consult specific product labeling. [DSC] = Discontinued product

Capsule, as hydrochloride: 150 mg, 200 mg, 250 mg

Mexitil®: 150 mg, 200 mg, 250 mg [DSC]

- **Mexitil® [DSC]** *see* Mexiletine *on page 987*
- **Mezavant® (Can)** *see* Mesalamine *on page 949*
- **$MgSO_4$ (error-prone abbreviation)** *see* Magnesium Sulfate *on page 917*
- **Miacalcin®** *see* Calcitonin *on page 234*
- **Miacalcin® NS (Can)** *see* Calcitonin *on page 234*
- **Mi-Acid [OTC]** *see* Aluminum Hydroxide, Magnesium Hydroxide, and Simethicone *on page 76*
- **Mi-Acid™ Double Strength [OTC]** *see* Calcium Carbonate and Magnesium Hydroxide *on page 239*
- **Mi-Acid Maximum Strength [OTC]** *see* Aluminum Hydroxide, Magnesium Hydroxide, and Simethicone *on page 76*
- **Micaderm® [OTC]** *see* Miconazole *on page 989*

Micafungin (mi ka FUN gin)

U.S. Brand Names Mycamine®

Canadian Brand Names Mycamine®

Index Terms Micafungin Sodium

Pharmacologic Category Antifungal Agent, Parenteral; Echinocandin

Additional Appendix Information

Antifungal Agents *on page 1640*

Use Treatment of esophageal candidiasis; *Candida* prophylaxis in patients undergoing hematopoietic stem cell transplant (HSCT); treatment of candidemia, acute disseminated candidiasis, and other *Candida* infections (peritonitis and abscesses)

Unlabeled/Investigational Use Treatment of infections due to *Aspergillus* spp; prophylaxis of HIV-related esophageal candidiasis

Pregnancy Risk Factor C

Pregnancy Considerations Visceral teratogenic and abortifacient effects were noted in animal studies. There are no adequate and well-controlled studies in pregnant women. Use only if benefit outweighs risk.

Lactation Excretion in breast milk unknown/use caution

Contraindications Hypersensitivity to micafungin, other echinocandins, or any component of the formulation

Warnings/Precautions Anaphylactic reactions, including shock, have been reported. New onset or worsening hepatic failure has been reported; use caution in pre-existing mild-moderate hepatic impairment; safety in severe liver failure has not been evaluated. Hemolytic anemia and hemoglobinuria have been reported. Increased BUN, serum creatinine, renal dysfunction, and/or acute renal failure has been reported; use with caution in patients with pre-existing renal impairment and monitor closely. Safety and efficacy in pediatric patients have not been established.

Adverse Reactions Percentages reflect incidence across all approved indications (prophylaxis and treatment); however, in general, a higher frequency of adverse reactions was observed in studies with HSCT patients.

>10%:

Central nervous system: Fever (20%), headache (16%)

Endocrine & metabolic: Hypokalemia (18%), hypomagnesemia (13%)

Gastrointestinal: Diarrhea (23%), nausea (22%), vomiting (22%), mucosal inflammation (14%), constipation (11%)

Hematologic: Thrombocytopenia (15%), neutropenia (14%)

1% to 10%:

Cardiovascular: Hypotension (9%), tachycardia (8%), hypertension (7%), peripheral edema (7%), phlebitis (6%), edema (5%)

Central nervous system: Insomnia (10%), anxiety (6%), fatigue (6%)

Dermatologic: Rash (9%), pruritus (6%)

Endocrine & metabolic: Hypocalcemia (7%), hyperglycemia (6%)

Gastrointestinal: Abdominal pain (10%), anorexia (6%), dyspepsia (6%)

Hematologic: Anemia (10%), febrile neutropenia (6%)

Hepatic: AST increased (6%), ALT increased (5%), serum alkaline phosphatase increased (5%)

Neuromuscular & skeletal: Rigors (9%), back pain (5%)

Respiratory: Cough (8%), dyspnea (6%), epistaxis (6%)

Miscellaneous: Bacteremia (6%), sepsis (5%)

<1% (Limited to important or life-threatening) or frequency not defined: Acidosis, acute renal failure, anuria, apnea, arrhythmia, arthralgia, atrial fibrillation, BUN increased, cardiac arrest, coagulopathy, creatinine increased, cyanosis, deep vein thrombosis, delirium, hypoxia, encephalopathy, erythema multiforme, facial edema, hemoglobinuria, hemolysis, hemolytic anemia, hepatic dysfunction, hepatic failure, hepatocellular damage, hepatomegaly, hiccups, hyperbilirubinemia, hyponatremia, hypoxia, infection, injection site necrosis, injection site thrombosis, intracranial hemorrhage, jaundice, MI, mucosal inflammation, oliguria, pancytopenia, pneumonia, pulmonary embolism, renal impairment, renal tubular necrosis, seizure, shock, skin necrosis, thrombotic thrombocytopenia purpura, thrombophlebitis, urticaria, vasodilatation, WBC decreased

Drug Interactions

Metabolism/Transport Effects Substrate of CYP3A4 (minor); **Inhibits** CYP3A4 (weak)

Avoid Concomitant Use There are no known interactions where it is recommended to avoid concomitant use.

Increased Effect/Toxicity There are no known significant interactions involving an increase in effect.

Decreased Effect

Micafungin may decrease the levels/effects of: Saccharomyces boulardii

Stability Store at controlled room temperature of 25°C (77°F). Reconstituted and diluted solutions are stable for 24 hours at room temperature. Protect from light. Aseptically add 5 mL of NS (preservative-free) to each 50 or 100 mg vial. Swirl to dissolve; do not shake. Further dilute 50-150 mg in 100 mL NS. Protect from light. Alternatively, D_5W may be used for reconstitution and dilution.

Mechanism of Action Concentration-dependent inhibition of 1,3-beta-D-glucan synthase resulting in reduced formation of 1,3-beta-D-glucan, an essential polysaccharide comprising 30% to 60% of *Candida* cell walls (absent in mammalian cells); decreased glucan content leads to osmotic instability and cellular lysis

Pharmacodynamics/Kinetics

Distribution: 0.28-0.5 L/kg

Protein binding: >99%; primarily to albumin

Metabolism: Hepatic; forms M-1 (catechol) and M-2 (methoxy) metabolites (activity unknown)

Half-life elimination: 11-21 hours

Excretion: Primarily feces (71%); urine (<15%)

Dosage I.V.: Adults:

Candidemia, acute disseminated candidiasis, and *Candida* peritonitis and abscesses: 100 mg daily; mean duration of therapy (from clinical trials) was 15 days (range: 10-47 days)

Esophageal candidiasis: 150 mg daily; mean duration of therapy (from clinical trials) was 15 days (range: 10-30 days)

Prophylaxis of *Candida* infection in hematopoietic stem cell transplantation: 50 mg daily

Dosing adjustment in renal impairment: No adjustment required

Dosing adjustment in hepatic impairment: No dosage adjustment required for moderate hepatic impairment (Child-Pugh score 7-9). Patients with severe hepatic dysfunction have not been studied.

Administration For intravenous use only; infuse over 1 hour. Flush line with NS prior to administration.

Monitoring Parameters Liver function tests

Dosage Forms Excipient information presented when available (limited, particularly for generics); consult specific product labeling.

Injection, powder for reconstitution, as sodium [preservative-free]:

Mycamine®: 50 mg, 100 mg [contains lactose]

- **Micafungin Sodium** *see* Micafungin *on page 988*
- **Micanol® (Can)** *see* Anthralin *on page 118*
- **Micardis®** *see* Telmisartan *on page 1431*
- **Micardis® HCT** *see* Telmisartan and Hydrochlorothiazide *on page 1432*
- **Micardis® Plus (Can)** *see* Telmisartan and Hydrochlorothiazide *on page 1432*
- **Micatin® (Can)** *see* Miconazole *on page 989*
- **Micatin® Athlete's Foot [OTC]** *see* Miconazole *on page 989*
- **Micatin® Jock Itch [OTC]** *see* Miconazole *on page 989*

Miconazole (mi KON a zole)

U.S. Brand Names Aloe Vesta® 2-n-1 Antifungal [OTC]; Baza® Antifungal [OTC]; Carrington Antifungal [OTC]; Critic-Aid® Clear AF [OTC]; DermaFungal [OTC]; Dermagran® AF [OTC]; DiabetAid™ Antifungal Foot Bath [OTC]; Fungoid® Tincture [OTC]; Lotrimin® AF Jock Itch Powder Spray [OTC]; Lotrimin® AF Powder/Spray [OTC]; Micaderm® [OTC]; Micatin® Athlete's Foot [OTC]; Micatin® Jock Itch [OTC]; Micro-Guard® [OTC]; Mitrazol™ [OTC]; Monistat-Derm® [DSC]; Monistat® 1 Combination Pack [OTC]; Monistat® 3 Combination Pack [OTC]; Monistat® 3 [OTC]; Monistat® 7 [OTC]; Neosporin® AF [OTC]; Podactin Cream [OTC]; Secura® Antifungal [OTC]; Zeasorb®-AF [OTC]

Canadian Brand Names Dermazole; Micatin®; Micozole; Monistat®; Monistat® 3

Index Terms Miconazole Nitrate

Pharmacologic Category Antifungal Agent, Topical; Antifungal Agent, Vaginal

Additional Appendix Information

Antifungal Agents *on page 1640*

Treatment of Sexually Transmitted Infections *on page 1773*

Use Treatment of vulvovaginal candidiasis and a variety of skin and mucous membrane fungal infections

Pregnancy Risk Factor C

Lactation Excretion in breast milk unknown/use caution

Medication Safety Issues

Sound-alike/look-alike issues:

Miconazole may be confused with Micronase®, Micronor®

Lotrimin® may be confused with Lotrisone®, Otrivin®

Micatin® may be confused with Miacalcin®

Contraindications Hypersensitivity to miconazole or any component of the formulation

Warnings/Precautions For topical use only; avoid contact with eyes. Discontinue if sensitivity or irritation develop. Petrolatum-based vaginal products may damage rubber or latex condoms or diaphragms. Separate use by 3 days. Consult with healthcare provider prior to self-medication (OTC use) of vaginal products if experiencing vaginal itching/discomfort, lower abdominal pain, back or shoulder pain, chills, nausea, vomiting, foul-smelling discharge, if this is the first vaginal yeast infection, or if exposed to HIV. Contact healthcare provider if symptoms do not begin to improve after 3 days or last longer than 7 days. Topical products are not for self-medication (OTC use) in children <2 years of age; vaginal products are not for OTC use in children <12 years of age.

Fungoid® tincture: Patients with diabetes, circulatory problems, renal or hepatic dysfunction should contact healthcare provider prior to self-medication (OTC use).

Adverse Reactions Frequency not defined.

Topical: Allergic contact dermatitis, burning, maceration

Vaginal: Abdominal cramps, burning, irritation, itching

Drug Interactions

Metabolism/Transport Effects Substrate of CYP3A4 (major); **Inhibits** CYP1A2 (moderate), 2A6 (strong), 2B6 (weak), 2C9 (strong), 2C19 (strong), 2D6 (strong), 2E1 (moderate), 3A4 (strong)

Avoid Concomitant Use

Avoid concomitant use of Miconazole with any of the following: Alfuzosin; Cisapride; Conivaptan; Dofetilide; Nilotinib; Pimozide; QuiNIDine; Ranolazine; Rivaroxaban; Salmeterol; Silodosin; Tamoxifen; Thioridazine

Increased Effect/Toxicity

Miconazole may increase the levels/effects of: Alfentanil; Alfuzosin; Alosetron; Aprepitant; Benzodiazepines (metabolized by oxidation); Bosentan; BusPIRone; Busulfan; Calcium Channel Blockers; CarBAMazepine; Ciclesonide; Cilostazol; Cinacalcet; Cisapride; Conivaptan; Corticosteroids (Orally Inhaled); Corticosteroids (Systemic); CycloSPORINE; CYP1A2 Substrates; CYP2A6 Substrates; CYP2B6 Substrates; CYP2C19 Substrates; CYP2C9 Substrates (High risk); CYP2D6 Substrates; CYP2E1 Substrates; CYP3A4 Substrates; Docetaxel; Dofetilide; Eletriptan; Eplerenone; Erlotinib; Eszopiclone; FentaNYL; Fesoterodine; Fosaprepitant; Gefitinib; HMG-CoA Reductase Inhibitors; Imatinib; Irinotecan; Ixabepilone; Losartan; Macrolide Antibiotics; Maraviroc; Methadone; Nebivolol; Nilotinib; Phosphodiesterase 5 Inhibitors; Pimecrolimus; Pimozide; QuiNIDine; Ramelteon; Ranolazine; Repaglinide; Rivaroxaban; Salmeterol; Silodosin; Sirolimus; Solifenacin; Sorafenib; Sunitinib; Tamoxifen; Temsirolimus; Tetrabenazine; Thioridazine; Tolterodine; VinCRIStine; Vitamin K Antagonists; Ziprasidone

The levels/effects of Miconazole may be increased by: Macrolide Antibiotics

Decreased Effect

Miconazole may decrease the levels/effects of: Amphotericin B; Codeine; Saccharomyces boulardii; TraMADol

The levels/effects of Miconazole may be decreased by: CYP3A4 Inducers (Strong); Deferasirox; Herbs (CYP3A4 Inducers)

Ethanol/Nutrition/Herb Interactions Herb/Nutraceutical: St John's wort may decrease miconazole levels.

Mechanism of Action Inhibits biosynthesis of ergosterol, damaging the fungal cell wall membrane, which increases permeability causing leaking of nutrients

Pharmacodynamics/Kinetics

Absorption: Topical: Negligible

Distribution: Widely to body tissues; penetrates well into inflamed joints, vitreous humor of eye, and peritoneal cavity, but poorly into saliva and sputum; crosses blood-brain barrier but only to a small extent

Protein binding: 91% to 93%
Metabolism: Hepatic
Half-life elimination: Multiphasic: Initial: 40 minutes; Secondary: 126 minutes; Terminal: 24 hours
Excretion: Feces (~50%); urine (<1% as unchanged drug)

Dosage

Topical: Children and Adults: **Note:** Not for OTC use in children <2 years:
- Tinea corporis: Apply twice daily for 4 weeks
- Tinea pedis: Apply twice daily for 4 weeks
  - Effervescent tablet: Dissolve 1 tablet in ~1 gallon of water; soak feet for 15-30 minutes; pat dry
- Tinea cruris: Apply twice daily for 2 weeks

Vaginal: Children ≥12 years and Adults: Vulvovaginal candidiasis:
- Cream, 2%: Insert 1 applicatorful at bedtime for 7 days
- Cream, 4%: Insert 1 applicatorful at bedtime for 3 days
- Suppository, 100 mg: Insert 1 suppository at bedtime for 7 days
- Suppository, 200 mg: Insert 1 suppository at bedtime for 3 days
- Suppository, 1200 mg: Insert 1 suppository (a one-time dose); may be used at bedtime or during the day

Note: Many products are available as a combination pack, with a suppository for vaginal instillation and cream to relieve external symptoms. External cream may be used twice daily, as needed, for up to 7 days.

Dosage Forms Excipient information presented when available (limited, particularly for generics); consult specific product labeling. [DSC] = Discontinued product

Combination products: Miconazole nitrate vaginal suppository 200 mg (3s) and miconazole nitrate external cream 2%
- Monistat® 1 Combination Pack: Miconazole nitrate vaginal insert 1200 mg (1) and miconazole nitrate external cream 2% (5 g) [Note: Do not confuse with 1-Day™ (formerly Monistat® 1) which contains tioconazole]
- Monistat® 3 Combination Pack:
  - Miconazole nitrate vaginal insert 200 mg (3s) and miconazole nitrate external cream 2%
  - Miconazole nitrate vaginal cream 4% and miconazole nitrate external cream 2%
- Monistat® 7 Combination Pack:
  - Miconazole nitrate vaginal suppository 100 mg (7s) and miconazole nitrate external cream 2%
  - Miconazole nitrate vaginal cream 2% (7 prefilled applicators) and miconazole nitrate external cream 2%

Cream, topical, as nitrate: 2% (15 g, 30 g, 45 g)
- Baza® Antifungal: 2% (4 g, 57 g, 142 g) [zinc oxide based formula]
- Carrington Antifungal: 2% (150 g)
- Micaderm®, Neosporin® AF, Podactin: 2% (30 g)
- Micatin® Athlete's Foot, Micatin® Jock Itch: 2% (15 g)
- Micro-Guard®, Mitrazol™: 2% (60 g)
- Monistat-Derm®: 2% (15 g, 30 g, 85 g) [DSC]
- Secura® Antifungal: 2% (60 g, 98 g)

Cream, vaginal, as nitrate [prefilled or refillable applicator]: 2% (45 g)
- Monistat® 3: 4% (15 g, 25 g)
- Monistat® 7: 2% (45 g)

Gel, topical, as nitrate:
- Zeasorb®-AF: 2% (24 g)

Liquid, spray, topical, as nitrate:
- Micatin® Athlete's Foot: 2% (90 mL) [contains alcohol]
- Neosporin AF®: 2% (105 mL)

Lotion, powder, as nitrate:
- Zeasorb®-AF: 2% (56 g) [contains alcohol 36%] [DSC]

Ointment, topical, as nitrate:
- Aloe Vesta® 2-n-1 Antifungal: 2% (60 g, 150 g)
- Critic-Aid® Clear AF: 2% (4 g, 57 g, 142 g)
- DermaFungal: 2% (113 g)
- Dermagran® AF: (113 g) [contains vitamin A and zinc]

Powder, topical, as nitrate:
- Lotrimin® AF: 2% (160 g)
- Micro-Guard®: 2% (90 g)
- Mitrazol™: 2% (30 g)
- Zeasorb®-AF: 2% (70 g)

Powder spray, topical, as nitrate:
- Lotrimin® AF, Lotrimin® AF Jock Itch: 2% (140 g)
- Micatin® Athlete's Foot, Micatin® Jock Itch: 2% (90 g) [contains alcohol]
- Neosporin® AF: 2% (85 g)

Suppository, vaginal, as nitrate: 100 mg (7s); 200 mg (3s)
- Monistat® 3: 200 mg (3s)
- Monistat® 7: 100 mg (7s)

Tablet, for solution, topical, as nitrate [effervescent]:
- DiabetAid™ Antifungal Foot Bath: 2% (10s)

Tincture, topical, as nitrate (Fungoid®): 2% (30 mL, 473 mL) [contains isopropyl alcohol 30%]; 30 mL size also available in a treatment kit which contains nail scrub and nail brush]

Miconazole and Zinc Oxide

(mi KON a zole & zink OKS ide)

U.S. Brand Names Vusion®

Index Terms Zinc Oxide and Miconazole Nitrate

Pharmacologic Category Antifungal Agent, Topical

Use Adjunctive treatment of diaper dermatitis complicated by *Candida albicans* infection

Pregnancy Risk Factor C

Dosage Diaper dermatitis: Topical: Children ≥4 weeks: Apply to affected area with each diaper change for 7 days. Treatment should continue for 7 days, even with initial improvement. Do not use for >7 days.

Additional Information Complete prescribing information for this medication should be consulted for additional detail.

Dosage Forms Excipient information presented when available (limited, particularly for generics); consult specific product labeling. [DSC] = Discontinued product

Ointment, topical:
- Vusion®: Miconazole nitrate 0.25% and zinc oxide 15% (30 g [DSC]; 60 g)

- ◆ **Miconazole Nitrate** *see* Miconazole *on page* 989
- ◆ **Micozole (Can)** *see* Miconazole *on page* 989
- ◆ **MICRhoGAM®** *see* Rh_o(D) Immune Globulin *on page* 1308
- ◆ **Microfibrillar Collagen Hemostat** *see* Collagen Hemostat *on page* 367
- ◆ **Microgestin™** *see* Ethinyl Estradiol and Norethindrone *on page* 581
- ◆ **Microgestin™ Fe** *see* Ethinyl Estradiol and Norethindrone *on page* 581
- ◆ **Micro-Guard® [OTC]** *see* Miconazole *on page* 989
- ◆ **microK®** *see* Potassium Chloride *on page* 1216
- ◆ **microK® 10** *see* Potassium Chloride *on page* 1216
- ◆ **Micro-K Extencaps® (Can)** *see* Potassium Chloride *on page* 1216
- ◆ **Micronase®** *see* GlyBURIDE *on page* 701
- ◆ **Micronor® (Can)** *see* Norethindrone *on page* 1078
- ◆ **Microzide®** *see* Hydrochlorothiazide *on page* 737

Midazolam (MID aye zoe lam)

Canadian Brand Names Apo-Midazolam®; Midazolam Injection

Index Terms Midazolam Hydrochloride; Versed

Pharmacologic Category Benzodiazepine

Additional Appendix Information

Benzodiazepines *on page 1646*

Status Epilepticus *on page 1831*

Use Preoperative sedation and provides conscious sedation prior to diagnostic or radiographic procedures; ICU sedation (continuous infusion); intravenous anesthesia (induction); intravenous anesthesia (maintenance)

Unlabeled/Investigational Use Anxiety, status epilepticus

Restrictions C-IV

Pregnancy Risk Factor D

Pregnancy Considerations Midazolam has been found to cross the placenta; not recommended for use during pregnancy.

Lactation Enters breast milk/not recommended (AAP rates "of concern")

Medication Safety Issues

Sound-alike/look-alike issues:

Versed may be confused with VePesid®, Vistaril®

High alert medication: The Institute for Safe Medication Practices (ISMP) includes this medication among its list of drugs which have a heightened risk of causing significant patient harm when used in error.

Contraindications Hypersensitivity to midazolam or any component of the formulation, including benzyl alcohol (cross-sensitivity with other benzodiazepines may exist); parenteral form is not for intrathecal or epidural injection; narrow-angle glaucoma; concurrent use of potent inhibitors of CYP3A4 (amprenavir, atazanavir, or ritonavir); pregnancy

Warnings/Precautions [U.S. Boxed Warning]: May cause severe respiratory depression, respiratory arrest, or apnea. Use with extreme caution, particularly in noncritical care settings. Appropriate resuscitative equipment and qualified personnel must be available for administration and monitoring. Initial dosing must be cautiously titrated and individualized, particularly in elderly or debilitated patients, patients with hepatic impairment (including alcoholics), or in renal impairment, particularly if other CNS depressants (including opiates) are used concurrently. **[U.S. Boxed Warning]: Initial doses in elderly or debilitated patients should be conservative; as little as 1 mg, but not to exceed 2.5 mg.** Use with caution in patients with respiratory disease or impaired gag reflex. Use during upper airway procedures may increase risk of hypoventilation. Prolonged responses have been noted following extended administration by continuous infusion (possibly due to metabolite accumulation) or in the presence of drugs which inhibit midazolam metabolism.

Causes CNS depression (dose-related) resulting in sedation, dizziness, confusion, or ataxia which may impair physical and mental capabilities. Patients must be cautioned about performing tasks which require mental alertness (eg, operating machinery or driving). A minimum of 1 day should elapse after midazolam administration before attempting these tasks. Use with caution in patients receiving other CNS depressants or psychoactive agents. Effects with other sedative drugs or ethanol may be potentiated. Benzodiazepines have been associated with falls and traumatic injury and should be used with extreme caution in patients who are at risk of these events (especially the elderly).

May cause hypotension - hemodynamic events are more common in pediatric patients or patients with hemodynamic instability. Hypotension and/or respiratory depression may occur more frequently in patients who have received opioid analgesics. Use with caution in obese patients, chronic renal failure, and HF. Does not protect against increases in heart rate or blood pressure during intubation. Should not be used in shock, coma, or acute alcohol intoxication. **[U.S. Boxed Warning]: Parenteral form contains benzyl alcohol; avoid rapid injection in neonates or prolonged infusions.** Avoid intra-arterial administration or extravasation of parenteral formulation.

Midazolam causes anterograde amnesia. Paradoxical reactions, including hyperactive or aggressive behavior have been reported with benzodiazepines, particularly in adolescent/pediatric or psychiatric patients. Does not have analgesic, antidepressant, or antipsychotic properties.

Benzodiazepines have been associated with dependence and acute withdrawal symptoms on discontinuation or reduction in dose. Acute withdrawal, including seizures, may be precipitated after administration of flumazenil to patients receiving long-term benzodiazepine therapy.

Adverse Reactions As reported in adults unless otherwise noted:

>10%: Respiratory: Decreased tidal volume and/or respiratory rate decrease, apnea (3% children)

1% to 10%:

Cardiovascular: Hypotension (3% children)

Central nervous system: Drowsiness (1%), oversedation, headache (1%), seizure-like activity (1% children)

Gastrointestinal: Nausea (3%), vomiting (3%)

Local: Pain and local reactions at injection site (4% I.M., 5% I.V.; severity less than diazepam)

Ocular: Nystagmus (1% children)

Respiratory: Cough (1%)

Miscellaneous: Physical and psychological dependence with prolonged use, hiccups (4%, 1% children), paradoxical reaction (2% children)

<1% (Limited to important or life-threatening): Agitation, amnesia, bigeminy, bronchospasm, emergence delirium, euphoria, hallucinations, laryngospasm, rash

Drug Interactions

Metabolism/Transport Effects Substrate of CYP2B6 (minor), 3A4 (major); **Inhibits** CYP2C8 (weak), 2C9 (weak), 3A4 (weak)

Avoid Concomitant Use

Avoid concomitant use of Midazolam with any of the following: Efavirenz

Increased Effect/Toxicity

Midazolam may increase the levels/effects of: Alcohol (Ethyl); Clozapine; CNS Depressants; Phenytoin

The levels/effects of Midazolam may be increased by: Antifungal Agents (Azole Derivatives, Systemic); Aprepitant; Atorvastatin; Calcium Channel Blockers (Nondihydropyridine); Cimetidine; CYP3A4 Inhibitors (Moderate); CYP3A4 Inhibitors (Strong); Dasatinib; Disulfiram; Efavirenz; Fluconazole; Fosaprepitant; Grapefruit Juice; Isoniazid; Macrolide Antibiotics; Nefazodone; Oral Contraceptive (Estrogens); Oral Contraceptive (Progestins); Protease Inhibitors; Proton Pump Inhibitors; Selective Serotonin Reuptake Inhibitors

Decreased Effect

The levels/effects of Midazolam may be decreased by: CarBAMazepine; CYP3A4 Inducers (Strong); Deferasirox; Rifamycin Derivatives; St Johns Wort; Theophylline Derivatives; Yohimbine

Ethanol/Nutrition/Herb Interactions

Ethanol: Avoid ethanol (may increase CNS depression).

Food: Grapefruit juice may increase serum concentrations of midazolam; avoid concurrent use with oral form.

Herb/Nutraceutical: Avoid concurrent use with St John's wort (may decrease midazolam levels, may increase CNS depression). Avoid concurrent use with valerian, kava kava, gotu kola (may increase CNS depression).

Stability The manufacturer states that midazolam, at a final concentration of 0.5 mg/mL, is stable for up to 24 hours when diluted with D_5W or NS. A final concentration of 1 mg/mL in NS has been documented to be stable for up to 10 days (McMullen, 1995). Admixtures do not require protection from light for short-term storage.

Mechanism of Action Binds to stereospecific benzodiazepine receptors on the postsynaptic GABA neuron at several sites within the central nervous system, including the limbic system, reticular formation. Enhancement of the inhibitory effect of GABA on neuronal excitability results by increased neuronal membrane permeability to chloride ions. This shift in chloride ions results in hyperpolarization (a less excitable state) and stabilization.

Pharmacodynamics/Kinetics

Onset of action: I.M.: Sedation: ~15 minutes; I.V.: 1-5 minutes

Peak effect: I.M.: 0.5-1 hour

Duration: I.M.: Up to 6 hours; Mean: 2 hours

Absorption: Oral: Rapid

Distribution: V_d: 0.8-2.5 L/kg; increased with congestive heart failure (CHF) and chronic renal failure

Protein binding: 95%

Metabolism: Extensively hepatic via CYP3A4

Bioavailability: Mean: 45%

Half-life elimination: 1-4 hours; prolonged with cirrhosis, congestive heart failure, obesity, and elderly

Excretion: Urine (as glucuronide conjugated metabolites); feces (~2% to 10%)

Dosage The dose of midazolam needs to be individualized based on the patient's age, underlying diseases, and concurrent medications. Decrease dose (by ~30%) if narcotics or other CNS depressants are administered concomitantly. **Personnel and equipment needed for standard respiratory resuscitation should be immediately available during midazolam administration.**

Children <6 years may require higher doses and closer monitoring than older children; calculate dose on ideal body weight

Conscious sedation for procedures or preoperative sedation:

Oral: 0.25-0.5 mg/kg as a single dose preprocedure, up to a maximum of 20 mg; administer 30-45 minutes prior to procedure. Children <6 years or less cooperative patients may require as much as 1 mg/kg as a single dose; 0.25 mg/kg may suffice for children 6-16 years of age.

Intranasal (not an approved route): 0.2 mg/kg (up to 0.4 mg/kg in some studies), to a maximum of 15 mg; may be administered 30-45 minutes prior to procedure

I.M.: 0.1-0.15 mg/kg 30-60 minutes before surgery or procedure; range 0.05-0.15 mg/kg; doses up to 0.5 mg/kg have been used in more anxious patients; maximum total dose: 10 mg

I.V.:

Infants <6 months: Limited information is available in nonintubated infants; dosing recommendations not clear; infants <6 months are at higher risk for airway obstruction and hypoventilation; titrate dose in small increments to desired effect; monitor carefully

Infants 6 months to Children 5 years: Initial: 0.05-0.1 mg/kg; titrate dose carefully; total dose of 0.6 mg/kg may be required; usual maximum total dose: 6 mg

Children 6-12 years: Initial: 0.025-0.05 mg/kg; titrate dose carefully; total doses of 0.4 mg/kg may be required; usual maximum total dose: 10 mg

Children 12-16 years: Dose as adults; usual maximum total dose: 10 mg

Conscious sedation during mechanical ventilation: Children: Loading dose: 0.05-0.2 mg/kg, followed by initial continuous infusion: 0.06-0.12 mg/kg/hour (1-2 mcg/kg/minute); titrate to the desired effect; usual range: 0.4-6 mcg/kg/minute

Status epilepticus refractory to standard therapy (unlabeled use): Infants >2 months and Children: Loading dose: 0.15 mg/kg followed by a continuous infusion of 0.06 mg/kg/hour; titrate dose upward every 5 minutes until clinical seizure activity is controlled; mean infusion rate required in 24 children was 0.14 mg/kg/hour (2.3 mcg/kg/minute) with a range of 0.06-1.1 mg/kg/hour

Adults:

Preoperative sedation:

I.M.: 0.07-0.08 mg/kg 30-60 minutes prior to surgery/procedure; usual dose: 5 mg; **Note:** Reduce dose in patients with COPD, high-risk patients, patients ≥60 years of age, and patients receiving other narcotics or CNS depressants

I.V.: 0.02-0.04 mg/kg; repeat every 5 minutes as needed to desired effect or up to 0.1-0.2 mg/kg

Intranasal (not an approved route): 0.2 mg/kg (up to 0.4 mg/kg in some studies); administer 30-45 minutes prior to surgery/procedure

Conscious sedation: I.V.: Initial: 0.5-2 mg slow I.V. over at least 2 minutes; slowly titrate to effect by repeating doses every 2-3 minutes if needed; usual total dose: 2.5-5 mg; use decreased doses in elderly

Healthy Adults <60 years: Some patients respond to doses as low as 1 mg; no more than 2.5 mg should be administered over a period of 2 minutes. Additional doses of midazolam may be administered after a 2-minute waiting period and evaluation of sedation after each dose increment. A total dose >5 mg is generally not needed. If narcotics or other CNS depressants are administered concomitantly, the midazolam dose should be reduced by 30%.

Anesthesia: I.V.:

Induction:

Unpremedicated patients: 0.3-0.35 mg/kg (up to 0.6 mg/kg in resistant cases)

Premedicated patients: 0.15-0.35 mg/kg

Maintenance: 0.05-0.3 mg/kg as needed, or continuous infusion 0.25-1.5 mcg/kg/minute

Sedation in mechanically-ventilated patients: I.V. continuous infusion: 100 mg in 250 mL D_5W or NS (if patient is fluid-restricted, may concentrate up to a maximum of 0.5 mg/mL); initial dose: 0.02-0.08 mg/kg (~1 mg to 5 mg in 70 kg adult) initially and either repeated at 5-15 minute intervals until adequate sedation is achieved or continuous infusion rates of 0.04-0.2 mg/kg/hour and titrate to reach desired level of sedation

Refractory status epilepticus (unlabeled use): I.V.: Initial: 0.2 mg/kg bolus, then 0.05-0.6 mg/kg/hour

Elderly: I.V.: Conscious sedation: Initial: 0.5 mg slow I.V.; give no more than 1.5 mg in a 2-minute period; if additional titration is needed, give no more than 1 mg over 2 minutes, waiting another 2 or more minutes to evaluate sedative effect; a total dose of >3.5 mg is rarely necessary

Dosage adjustment in renal impairment:

Hemodialysis: Supplemental dose is not necessary

Peritoneal dialysis: Significant drug removal is unlikely based on physiochemical characteristics

Dietary Considerations Injection: Sodium content of 1 mL: 0.14 mEq

Administration

Intranasal: Administer using a 1 mL needleless syringe into the nostrils over 15 seconds; use the 5 mg/mL injection; 1/2 of the dose may be administered to each nostril

Oral: Do not mix with any liquid (such as grapefruit juice) prior to administration

Parenteral:

I.M.: Administer deep I.M. into large muscle.

I.V.: Administer by slow I.V. injection over at least 2-5 minutes at a concentration of 1-5 mg/mL or by I.V. infusion. Continuous infusions should be administered via an infusion pump.

Monitoring Parameters Respiratory and cardiovascular status, blood pressure, blood pressure monitor required during I.V. administration

Additional Information Abrupt discontinuation after sustained use (generally >10 days) may cause withdrawal symptoms. For neonates, since both concentrations of the injection contain 1% benzyl alcohol, use the 5 mg/mL injection and dilute to 0.5 mg/mL with SWI without preservatives to decrease the amount of benzyl alcohol delivered to the neonate; with continuous infusion, midazolam may accumulate in peripheral tissues; use lowest effective infusion rate to reduce accumulation effects; midazolam is 3-4 times as potent as diazepam; paradoxical reactions associated with midazolam use in children (eg, agitation, restlessness, combativeness) have been successfully treated with flumazenil (Massanari, 1997).

Dosage Forms Excipient information presented when available (limited, particularly for generics); consult specific product labeling.

Injection, solution: 1 mg/mL (2 mL, 5 mL, 10 mL); 5 mg/mL (1 mL, 2 mL, 5 mL, 10 mL) [contains benzyl alcohol 1%]

Injection, solution [preservative free]: 1 mg/mL (2 mL, 5 mL); 5 mg/mL (1 mL, 2 mL)

Syrup: 2 mg/mL (118 mL) [contains sodium benzoate; cherry flavor]

◆ **Midazolam Hydrochloride** *see* Midazolam *on page 990*

◆ **Midazolam Injection (Can)** *see* Midazolam *on page 990*

Midodrine (MI doe dreen)

U.S. Brand Names ProAmatine®

Canadian Brand Names Amatine®; Apo-Midodrine®

Index Terms Midodrine Hydrochloride

Pharmacologic Category Alpha$_1$ Agonist

Use Orphan drug: Treatment of symptomatic orthostatic hypotension

Unlabeled/Investigational Use Investigational: Management of urinary incontinence

Pregnancy Risk Factor C

Pregnancy Considerations Increased rate of embryo resorption and decreased fetal weight were observed in animal studies. Use during pregnancy should be avoided unless the potential benefit outweighs the risk to the fetus.

Lactation Excretion in breast milk is unknown/use caution

Medication Safety Issues

Sound-alike/look-alike issues:

ProAmatine® may be confused with protamine

Contraindications Hypersensitivity to midodrine or any component of the formulation; severe organic heart disease; urinary retention; pheochromocytoma; thyrotoxicosis; persistent and significant supine hypertension

Warnings/Precautions [U.S. Boxed Warning]: Indicated for patients for whom orthostatic hypotension significantly impairs their daily life despite standard clinical care. May cause hypertension. Use is not recommended with supine hypertension. Caution should be exercised in patients with diabetes, visual problems (especially if receiving fludrocortisone), urinary retention (reduce initial dose), or hepatic dysfunction; monitor renal and hepatic function prior to and periodically during therapy; safety and efficacy have not been established in children.

Adverse Reactions

>10%:

Cardiovascular: Supine hypertension (7% to 13%)

Dermatologic: Piloerection (13%), pruritus (12%)

Genitourinary: Urinary urgency, retention, or polyuria, dysuria (up to 13%)

Neuromuscular & skeletal: Paresthesia (18%)

1% to 10%:

Central nervous system: Chills (5%), pain (5%)

Dermatologic: Rash (2%)

Gastrointestinal: Abdominal pain

<1% (Limited to important or life-threatening): Anxiety, canker sore, confusion, dizziness, dry skin, erythema multiforme, facial flushing, flushing, headache, hyperesthesia, insomnia, ICP increased, nausea, somnolence, weakness, xerostomia

Drug Interactions

Avoid Concomitant Use

Avoid concomitant use of Midodrine with any of the following: Iobenguane I 123; MAO Inhibitors

Increased Effect/Toxicity

Midodrine may increase the levels/effects of: Sympathomimetics

The levels/effects of Midodrine may be increased by: Beta-Blockers; Calcium Channel Blockers (Nondihydropyridine); Cannabinoids; Cardiac Glycosides; MAO Inhibitors; Tricyclic Antidepressants

Decreased Effect

Midodrine may decrease the levels/effects of: Iobenguane I 123

Mechanism of Action Midodrine forms an active metabolite, desglymidodrine, that is an alpha$_1$-agonist. This agent increases arteriolar and venous tone resulting in a rise in standing, sitting, and supine systolic and diastolic blood pressure in patients with orthostatic hypotension. See table.

Causes of Orthostatic Hypotension

Primary Autonomic Causes
Pure autonomic failure (Bradbury-Eggleston syndrome, idiopathic orthostatic hypotension)
Autonomic failure with multiple system atrophy (Shy-Drager syndrome)
Familial dysautonomia (Riley-Day syndrome)
Dopamine beta-hydroxylase deficiency
Secondary Autonomic Causes
Chronic alcoholism
Parkinson's disease
Diabetes mellitus
Porphyria
Amyloidosis
Various carcinomas
Vitamin B_1 or B_{12} deficiency
Nonautonomic Causes
Hypovolemia (such as associated with hemorrhage, burns, or hemodialysis) and dehydration
Diminished homeostatic regulation (such as associated with aging, pregnancy, fever, or prolonged bedrest)
Medications (eg, antihypertensives, insulin, tricyclic antidepressants)

Pharmacodynamics/Kinetics

Onset of action: ~1 hour

Duration: 2-3 hours

Absorption: Rapid

Distribution: V_d (desglymidodrine): <1.6 L/kg; poorly across membrane (eg, blood brain barrier)

Protein binding: Minimal

Metabolism: Hepatic; midodrine is a prodrug which undergoes rapid deglycination to desglymidodrine (active metabolite); metabolism occurs in many tissues and plasma

Bioavailability: Desglymidodrine: 93%

Half-life elimination: Desglymidodrine: ~3-4 hours; Midodrine: 25 minutes

Time to peak, serum: Desglymidodrine: 1-2 hours; Midodrine: 30 minutes

Excretion: Urine (2% to 4%)

Clearance: Desglymidodrine: 385 mL/minute (predominantly by renal secretion)

Dosage Adults: Oral: 10 mg 3 times/day during daytime hours (every 3-4 hours) when patient is upright (maximum: 40 mg/day)

Dosing adjustment in renal impairment: 2.5 mg 3 times/day, gradually increasing as tolerated

Hemodialysis: Dialyzable

Administration Doses may be given in approximately 3- to 4-hour intervals (eg, shortly before or upon rising in the morning, at midday, in the late afternoon not later than 6 PM). Avoid dosing after the evening meal or within 4 hours of bedtime. Continue therapy only in patients who appear to attain symptomatic improvement during initial treatment. Standing systolic blood pressure may be elevated 15-30 mm Hg at 1 hour after a 10 mg dose. Some effect may persist for 2-3 hours.

Monitoring Parameters Blood pressure, renal and hepatic parameters

Dosage Forms Excipient information presented when available (limited, particularly for generics); consult specific product labeling.

Tablet, as hydrochloride: 2.5 mg, 5 mg, 10 mg

ProAmatine®: 2.5 mg, 5 mg, 10 mg [scored]

- ◆ **Midodrine Hydrochloride** *see* Midodrine *on page 993*
- ◆ **Midol® Cramp and Body Aches [OTC]** *see* Ibuprofen *on page 760*
- ◆ **Midol® Extended Relief** *see* Naproxen *on page 1041*
- ◆ **Midol Teen Formula [OTC]** *see* Acetaminophen and Pamabrom *on page 28*
- ◆ **Midrin®** *see* Acetaminophen, Isometheptene, and Dichloralphenazone *on page 34*
- ◆ **Mifeprex®** *see* Mifepristone *on page 994*

Mifepristone (mi FE pris tone)

U.S. Brand Names Mifeprex®

Index Terms RU-38486; RU-486

Pharmacologic Category Abortifacient; Antineoplastic Agent, Hormone Antagonist; Antiprogestin

Use Medical termination of intrauterine pregnancy, through day 49 of pregnancy. Patients may need treatment with misoprostol and possibly surgery to complete therapy

Unlabeled/Investigational Use Treatment of unresectable meningioma; has been studied in the treatment of breast cancer, ovarian cancer, and adrenal cortical carcinoma

Restrictions Investigators wishing to obtain the agent for use in oncology patients must apply for a patient-specific IND from the FDA. Mifepristone will be supplied only to licensed physicians who sign and return a "Prescriber's Agreement." Distribution of mifepristone will be subject to specific requirements imposed by the distributor. Mifepristone will **not** be available to the public through licensed pharmacies. An FDA-approved medication guide must be distributed when dispensing an outpatient prescription (new or refill) where this medication is to be used without direct supervision of a healthcare provider. Medication guides are available at http://www.fda.gov/cder/Offices/ODS/medication_guides.htm.

Not available in Canada

Pregnancy Risk Factor X

Pregnancy Considerations This medication is used to terminate pregnancy; there are no approved treatment indications for its use during pregnancy. Prostaglandins (including mifepristone and misoprostol) may have teratogenic effects when used during pregnancy. If treatment fails, there is a risk of fetal malformation. In sexually active women, pregnancy can occur prior to the first menstrual period following treatment. Appropriate contraception can be started as soon as termination of pregnancy is confirmed or before sexual intercourse is resumed.

Lactation Excretion in breast milk unknown/contraindicated

Medication Safety Issues

Sound-alike/look-alike issues:

Mifeprex® may be confused with Mirapex®

Mifepristone may be confused with misoprostol

High alert medication: The Institute for Safe Medication Practices (ISMP) includes this medication among its list of drug classes which have a heightened risk of causing significant patient harm when used in error.

Contraindications Hypersensitivity to mifepristone, misoprostol, other prostaglandins, or any component of the formulation; chronic adrenal failure; porphyrias; hemorrhagic disorder or concurrent anticoagulant therapy; pregnancy termination >49 days; intrauterine device (IUD) in place; ectopic pregnancy or undiagnosed adnexal mass; concurrent long-term corticosteroid therapy; inadequate or lack of access to emergency medical services; inability to understand effects and/or comply with treatment

Warnings/Precautions [U.S. Boxed Warning]: Patient must be instructed of the treatment procedure and expected effects. A signed agreement form must be kept in the patient's file. Physicians may obtain patient agreement forms, physician enrollment forms, and medical consultation directly from Danco Laboratories at 1-877-432-7596. Adverse effects (including blood transfusions, hospitalization, ongoing pregnancy, and other major complications) must be reported in writing to the medication distributor. To be administered only by physicians who can date pregnancy, diagnose ectopic pregnancies, provide access to surgical abortion (if needed), and can provide access to emergency care. Medication will be distributed directly to these physicians following signed agreement with the distributor. Must be administered under supervision by the qualified physician. Pregnancy is dated from day 1 of last menstrual period (presuming a 28-day cycle, ovulation occurring midcycle). Pregnancy duration can be determined using menstrual history and clinical examination. Ultrasound should be used if an ectopic pregnancy is suspected or if duration of pregnancy is uncertain. Ultrasonography may not identify all ectopic pregnancies, and healthcare providers should be alert for signs and symptoms which may be related to undiagnosed ectopic pregnancy in any patient who receives mifepristone

[U.S. Boxed Warning]: Patients should be counseled to seek medical attention in cases of excessive bleeding. Bleeding occurs and should be expected (average 9-16 days, may be ≥30 days). In some cases, bleeding may be prolonged and heavy, potentially leading to hypovolemic shock; the manufacturer cites soaking through two thick sanitary pads per hour for two consecutive hours as an example of excessive bleeding. Bleeding may require blood transfusion (rare), curettage, saline infusions, and/or vasoconstrictors. Use caution in patients with severe anemia. Confirmation of pregnancy termination by clinical exam or ultrasound must be made 14 days following treatment. Manufacturer recommends surgical termination of pregnancy when medical termination fails or is not complete. Prescriber should determine in advance whether they will provide such care themselves or through other providers. Preventative measures to prevent rhesus immunization must be taken prior to surgical abortion. Prescriber should also give the patient clear instructions on whom to call and what to do in the event of an emergency following administration of mifepristone.

[U.S. Boxed Warning]: Bacterial infections have been reported following use of this product. In rare cases, these infections may be serious and/or fatal, with septic shock as a potential complication. A causal relationship has not been established. Sustained fever, abdominal pain, or pelvic tenderness should prompt evaluation; however, healthcare professionals are warned that atypical presentations of serious infection without these symptoms have also been noted. Patients presenting with nausea, vomiting, diarrhea, or weakness, with or without abdominal pain or fever, should be evaluated for serious bacterial infection when symptoms occur >24 hours after taking misoprostol. Treatment with antibiotics, including coverage for anaerobic bacteria (eg, *Clostridium sordellii*) should be initiated. **[U.S. Boxed Warning]: Patients undergoing treatment with mifepristone should be instructed to bring their Medication Guide with them when an obtaining treatment from an emergency room or healthcare provider that did not prescribe the medication initially in order to identify that they are undergoing a medical abortion.**

Safety and efficacy have not been established for use in women with chronic cardiovascular, hypertensive, hepatic, respiratory, or renal disease, insulin-dependent diabetes mellitus, severe anemia, or heavy smokers. Women >35 years of age and smokers (>10 cigarettes/day) were excluded from clinical trials. Safety and efficacy in pediatric patients have not been established.

Adverse Reactions Vaginal bleeding and uterine cramping are expected to occur when this medication is used to terminate a pregnancy; 90% of women using this medication for this purpose also report adverse reactions. Bleeding or spotting occurs in most women for a period of 9-16 days. Up to 8% of women will experience some degree of bleeding or spotting for 30 days or more. In some cases, bleeding may be prolonged and heavy, potentially leading to hypovolemic shock.

>10%:

- Central nervous system: Headache (2% to 31%), dizziness (1% to 12%)
- Gastrointestinal: Abdominal pain (cramping) (96%), nausea (43% to 61%), vomiting (18% to 26%), diarrhea (12% to 20%)
- Genitourinary: Uterine cramping (83%)

1% to 10%:

- Cardiovascular: Syncope (1%)
- Central nervous system: Fatigue (10%), fever (4%), insomnia (3%), anxiety (2%), fainting (2%)
- Gastrointestinal: Dyspepsia (3%)
- Genitourinary: Uterine hemorrhage (5%), vaginitis (3%), pelvic pain (2%), endometriosis/salpingitis/pelvic inflammatory disease (1%)
- Hematologic: Decreased hemoglobin >2 g/dL (6%), anemia (2%), leukorrhea (2%)
- Neuromuscular & skeletal: Back pain (9%), rigors (3%), leg pain (2%), weakness (2%)
- Respiratory: Sinusitis (2%)
- Miscellaneous: Viral infection (4%)

<1% (Limited to important or life-threatening): Adult respiratory distress syndrome (ADRS), allergic reaction including urticaria and hives, bacterial infection (including an ectopic bacteria such as *Clostridium sordellii*), Crohn's disease (exacerbation), disseminated intravascular coagulopathy (DIC), dyspnea, hypotension, lightheadedness, loss of consciousness, MI, pancreatitis (acute), postabortal infection, QT prolongation, ruptured ectopic pregnancy, sepsis, septic shock, sickle cell crisis (exacerbation), tachycardia, toxic shock syndrome

In trials for unresectable meningioma, the most common adverse effects included fatigue, hot flashes, gynecomastia or breast tenderness, hair thinning, and rash. In premenopausal women, vaginal bleeding may be seen shortly after beginning therapy and cessation of menses is common. Thyroiditis and effects related to antiglucocorticoid activity have also been noted.

Drug Interactions

Metabolism/Transport Effects Substrate of CYP3A4 (minor); **Inhibits** CYP2D6 (weak), 3A4 (weak)

Avoid Concomitant Use There are no known interactions where it is recommended to avoid concomitant use.

Increased Effect/Toxicity There are no known significant interactions involving an increase in effect.

Decreased Effect There are no known significant interactions involving a decrease in effect.

Ethanol/Nutrition/Herb Interactions

Food: Do not take with grapefruit juice; grapefruit juice may inhibit mifepristone metabolism leading to increased levels.

Herb/Nutraceutical: Avoid St John's wort (may induce mifepristone metabolism, leading to decreased levels).

Stability Store at room temperature of 25°C (77°F).

Mechanism of Action Mifepristone, a synthetic steroid, competitively binds to the intracellular progesterone receptor, blocking the effects of progesterone. When used for the termination of pregnancy, this leads to contraction-inducing activity in the myometrium. In the absence of progesterone, mifepristone acts as a partial progesterone agonist. Mifepristone also has weak antiglucocorticoid and antiandrogenic properties; it blocks the feedback effect of cortisol on corticotropin secretion.

Pharmacodynamics/Kinetics

Absorption: Oral: rapid

Protein binding: 98% to albumin and α_1-acid glycoprotein

Metabolism: Hepatic via CYP3A4 to three metabolites (may possess some antiprogestin and antiglucocorticoid activity)

Bioavailability: Oral: 69%

Half-life elimination: Terminal: 18 hours following a slower phase where 50% eliminated between 12-72 hours

Time to peak: Oral: 90 minutes

Excretion: Feces (83%); urine (9%)

Dosage Oral:

Adults:

Termination of pregnancy: Treatment consists of three office visits by the patient; the patient must read medication guide and sign patient agreement prior to treatment:

- Day 1: 600 mg (three 200 mg tablets) taken as a single dose under physician supervision
- Day 3: Patient must return to the healthcare provider 2 days following administration of mifepristone; unless abortion has occurred (confirmed using ultrasound or clinical examination): 400 mcg (two 200 mcg tablets) of misoprostol; patient may need treatment for cramps or gastrointestinal symptoms at this time
- Day 14: Patient must return to the healthcare provider ~14 days after administration of mifepristone; confirm complete termination of pregnancy by ultrasound or clinical exam. Surgical termination is recommended to manage treatment failures.

Meningioma (unlabeled use): Refer to individual protocols. The dose used in meningioma is usually 200 mg/day, continued based on toxicity and response.

Elderly: Safety and efficacy have not been established

Dosage adjustment in renal impairment: Safety and efficacy have not been established

Dosage adjustment in hepatic impairment: Safety and efficacy have not been established; use with caution due to CYP3A4 metabolism

Monitoring Parameters Clinical exam and/or ultrasound to confirm complete termination of pregnancy; hemoglobin, hematocrit, and red blood cell count in cases of heavy bleeding. Consider CBC in any patient who reports nausea, vomiting, or diarrhea and weakness with or without abdominal pain, and without fever or other signs of infection more than 24 hours after administration of misoprostol.

Test Interactions hCG levels will not be useful to confirm pregnancy termination until at least 10 days following mifepristone treatment

Additional Information Medication will be distributed directly to qualified physicians following signed agreement with the distributor, Danco Laboratories. It will not be available through pharmacies. Major adverse reactions (hospitalization, blood transfusion, ongoing pregnancy, etc) should be reported to Danco Laboratories.

Dosage Forms Excipient information presented when available (limited, particularly for generics); consult specific product labeling.

Tablet: 200 mg

Miglitol (MIG li tol)

U.S. Brand Names Glyset®

Canadian Brand Names Glyset®

Pharmacologic Category Antidiabetic Agent, Alpha-Glucosidase Inhibitor

Additional Appendix Information

Diabetes Mellitus Management, Adults *on page 1801*

Use Type 2 diabetes mellitus (noninsulin-dependent, NIDDM):

Monotherapy adjunct to diet to improve glycemic control in patients with type 2 diabetes mellitus (noninsulin-dependent, NIDDM) whose hyperglycemia cannot be managed with diet alone

Combination therapy with a sulfonylurea when diet plus either miglitol or a sulfonylurea alone do not result in adequate glycemic control. The effect of miglitol to enhance glycemic control is additive to that of sulfonylureas when used in combination.

Pregnancy Risk Factor B

Pregnancy Considerations Adverse events have not been reported in animal reproduction studies; therefore, miglitol is classified as pregnancy category B. Information specific to the use of miglitol during pregnancy has not been located. Maternal hyperglycemia can be associated with adverse effects in the fetus, including macrosomia, neonatal hyperglycemia, and hyperbilirubinemia; the risk of congenital malformations is increased when the Hb A_{1c} is above the normal range. Diabetes can also be associated with adverse effects in the mother. Poorly-treated diabetes may cause end-organ damage that may in turn negatively affect obstetric outcomes. Physiologic glucose levels should be maintained prior to and during pregnancy to decrease the risk of adverse events in the mother and the fetus. Until additional safety and efficacy data are obtained, the use of oral agents is generally not recommended as routine management of GDM or type 2 diabetes mellitus during pregnancy. Insulin is the drug of choice for the control of diabetes mellitus during pregnancy.

Lactation Enters breast milk (small amounts)/not recommended

Contraindications Hypersensitivity to miglitol or any of component of the formulation; diabetic ketoacidosis; inflammatory bowel disease; colonic ulceration; partial intestinal obstruction or predisposition to intestinal obstruction; chronic intestinal diseases associated with marked disorders of digestion or absorption or with conditions that may deteriorate as a result of increased gas formation in the intestine

Warnings/Precautions GI symptoms are the most common reactions. The incidence of abdominal pain and diarrhea tend to diminish considerably with continued treatment. Long-term clinical trials in patients with diabetes with significant renal dysfunction (serum creatinine >2 mg/dL) have not been conducted. Treatment of these patients is not recommended. In combination with a sulfonylurea will cause a further lowering of blood glucose and may increase the hypoglycemic potential of the sulfonylurea. It may be necessary to discontinue miglitol and administer insulin if the patient is exposed to stress (ie, fever, trauma, infection, surgery). Safety and efficacy have not been established in children.

Adverse Reactions

>10%: Gastrointestinal: Flatulence (41.5%), diarrhea (28.7%), abdominal pain (11.7%)

1% to 10%: Dermatologic: Rash (4.3%)

Drug Interactions

Avoid Concomitant Use There are no known interactions where it is recommended to avoid concomitant use.

Increased Effect/Toxicity

The levels/effects of Miglitol may be increased by: Herbs (Hypoglycemic Properties); Pegvisomant

Decreased Effect

The levels/effects of Miglitol may be decreased by: Corticosteroids (Orally Inhaled); Corticosteroids (Systemic); Luteinizing Hormone-Releasing Hormone Analogs; Somatropin

Mechanism of Action In contrast to sulfonylureas, miglitol does not enhance insulin secretion; the antihyperglycemic action of miglitol results from a reversible inhibition of membrane-bound intestinal alpha-glucosidases which hydrolyze oligosaccharides and disaccharides to glucose and other monosaccharides in the brush border of the small intestine. In patients with diabetes, this enzyme inhibition results in delayed glucose absorption and lowering of postprandial hyperglycemia.

Pharmacodynamics/Kinetics

Absorption: Saturable at high doses: 25 mg dose: Completely absorbed; 100 mg dose: 50% to 70% absorbed

Distribution: V_d: 0.18 L/kg

Protein binding: <4%

Metabolism: None

Half-life elimination: ~2 hours

Time to peak: 2-3 hours

Excretion: Urine (as unchanged drug)

Dosage Adults: Oral: 25 mg 3 times/day with the first bite of food at each meal; the dose may be increased to 50 mg 3 times/day after 4-8 weeks; maximum recommended dose: 100 mg 3 times/day

Dosing adjustment in renal impairment: Miglitol is primarily excreted by the kidneys; there is little information of miglitol in patients with a Cl_{cr} <25 mL/minute

Dosing adjustment in hepatic impairment: No adjustment necessary

Administration Should be taken orally at the start (with the first bite) of each main meal

Monitoring Parameters Monitor therapeutic response by periodic blood glucose tests; measurement of glycosylated hemoglobin is recommended for the monitoring of long-term glycemic control

Reference Range Recommendations for glycemic control in adults with diabetes:

Hb A_{1c}: <7%

Preprandial capillary plasma glucose: 70-130 mg/dL

Peak postprandial capillary blood glucose: <180 mg/dL

Blood pressure: <130/80 mm Hg

Dosage Forms Excipient information presented when available (limited, particularly for generics); consult specific product labeling.

Tablet: 25 mg, 50 mg, 100 mg

Miglustat (MIG loo stat)

U.S. Brand Names Zavesca®

Canadian Brand Names Zavesca®

Index Terms OGT-918

Pharmacologic Category Enzyme Inhibitor

Use Treatment of mild-to-moderate type 1 Gaucher disease when enzyme replacement therapy is not a therapeutic option

Pregnancy Risk Factor X

Dosage Oral: Adults: Type 1 Gaucher disease: 100 mg 3 times/day; dose may be reduced to 100 mg 1-2 times/day in patients with adverse effects (ie, tremor, GI distress)

Dosage adjustment in renal impairment:

Cl_{cr} 50-75 mL/minute: 100 mg twice daily

Cl_{cr} 30-50 mL/minute: 100 mg once daily

Cl_{cr} <30 mL/minute: Not recommended

Additional Information Complete prescribing information for this medication should be consulted for additional detail.

Dosage Forms Excipient information presented when available (limited, particularly for generics); consult specific product labeling.

Capsule:

Zavesca®: 100 mg

◆ **Migquin [DSC]** *see* Acetaminophen, Isometheptene, and Dichloralphenazone *on page* 34

◆ **Migranal®** *see* Dihydroergotamine *on page* 449

◆ **Migratine** *see* Acetaminophen, Isometheptene, and Dichloralphenazone *on page* 34

◆ **Migrazone® [DSC]** *see* Acetaminophen, Isometheptene, and Dichloralphenazone *on page* 34

◆ **Migrin-A [DSC]** *see* Acetaminophen, Isometheptene, and Dichloralphenazone *on page* 34

◆ **Mild-C® [OTC]** *see* Ascorbic Acid *on page* 139

◆ **Milk of Magnesia** *see* Magnesium Hydroxide *on page* 915

◆ **Millipred™** *see* PrednisoLONE *on page* 1230

Milnacipran (mil NAY ci pran)

U.S. Brand Names Savella™

Pharmacologic Category Antidepressant, Serotonin/Norepinephrine Reuptake Inhibitor

Use Management of fibromyalgia

Restrictions An FDA-approved medication guide is available. Distribute to each patient to whom this medication is dispensed.

Pregnancy Risk Factor C

Pregnancy Considerations There are no adequate and well-controlled studies in pregnant women. Use during pregnancy only if the potential benefits justify the risks.

Nonteratogenic effects in the newborn following SSRI/SNRI exposure late in the third trimester include respiratory distress, cyanosis, apnea, seizures, temperature instability, feeding difficulty, vomiting, hypoglycemia, hyper- or hypotonia, hyper-reflexia, jitteriness, irritability, constant crying, and tremor. The long-term effects on neurobehavior have not been studied.

Lactation Excretion in breast milk unknown/not recommended

Medication Safety Issues

Sound-alike/look-alike issues:

Savella™ may be confused with cevimeline, sevelamer

Contraindications Concomitant use or within 2 weeks of MAO inhibitors; uncontrolled narrow-angle glaucoma

Warnings/Precautions

[U.S. Boxed Warning]: Antidepressants increase the risk of suicidal thinking and behavior in children, adolescents, and young adults (18-24 years of age) with major depressive disorder (MDD) and other psychiatric disorders; consider risk prior to prescribing. Short-term studies did not show an increased risk in patients >24 years of age and showed a decreased risk in patients ≥65 years. Closely monitor for clinical worsening, suicidality, or unusual changes in behavior; the patient's family or caregiver should be instructed to closely observe the patient and communicate condition with healthcare provider. A medication guide should be dispensed with each prescription. **Milnacipran is not FDA approved for the treatment of major depressive disorder or for use in children.**The possibility of a suicide attempt is inherent in major depression and may persist until remission occurs. Monitor for worsening of depression or suicidality, especially during initiation of therapy (generally first 1-2 months) or with dose increases or decreases. Use caution in high-risk patients. Worsening depression and severe abrupt suicidality that are not part of the presenting symptoms may require discontinuation or modification of drug therapy. The patient's family or caregiver should be alerted to monitor patients for the emergence of suicidality and associated behaviors (such as agitation, irritability, hostility, impulsivity, and hypomania) and call healthcare provider. May worsen psychosis in some patients or precipitate a shift to mania or hypomania in patients with bipolar disorder. Patients presenting with depressive symptoms should be screened for bipolar disorder. Monotherapy in patients with bipolar disorder should be avoided. **Milnacipran is not FDA approved for the treatment of bipolar depression.** The potential for severe reactions exists when used with MAO inhibitors, proserotoneric drugs (myoclonus, diaphoresis, hyperthermia, NMS features, seizures, and death). May cause sustained increase in blood pressure or heart rate. Control preexisting hypertension and cardiovascular disease prior to initiation of milnacipran. Use caution in patients with renal impairment; dose reduction required in severe renal impairment. Use caution in patients with hepatic impairment. Avoid ethanol use. May cause hyponatremia/SIADH (elderly at increased risk); volume depletion (diuretics may increase risk). Safety and efficacy have not been established in children <17 years of age.Use cautiously in patients with a history of seizures. May impair platelet aggregation, resulting in bleeding. May cause increased urinary resistance. Use caution in patients with controlled narrow-angle glaucoma. Milnacipran tablets contain tartrazine (FD&C Yellow No. 5); allergic reactions may result in susceptible patients.Abrupt discontinuation or dosage reduction after extended therapy may lead to agitation, dysphoria, anxiety, and other symptoms. When discontinuing therapy, dosage should be tapered gradually. If intolerable symptoms occur following a decrease in dosage or upon discontinuation of therapy, then resuming the previous dose with a more gradual taper should be considered.

Adverse Reactions

>10%:

Central nervous system: Headache (18%), insomnia (12%)

Endocrine & metabolic: Hot flashes (12%)

Gastrointestinal: Nausea (37%), constipation (16%)

1% to 10%:

Cardiovascular: Palpitation (7%), heart rate increased (6%), hypertension (5%), flushing (3%), blood pressure increased (3%), tachycardia (2%), peripheral edema (≥1%)

Central nervous system: Dizziness (10%), migraine (5%), chills (2%), tremor (2%), depression (≥1%), fatigue (≥1%), fever (≥1%), irritability (≥1%), somnolence (≥1%)

Dermatologic: Hyperhidrosis (9%), rash (3%)

Endocrine & metabolic: Hypercholesterolemia (≥1%)

Gastrointestinal: Vomiting (7%), xerostomia (5%), abdominal pain (3%), appetite decreased (2%), abdominal distension (≥1%), abnormal taste (≥1%), diarrhea (≥1%), dyspepsia (≥1%), flatulence (≥1%), gastroesophageal reflux disease (≥1%)

Genitourinary: Dysuria (≥2%), ejaculation disorder/failure (≥2%), erectile dysfunction (≥2%), libido decreased

(≥2%), prostatitis (≥2%), scrotal pain (≥2%), testicular pain (≥2%), testicular swelling (≥2%), urethral pain (≥2%), urinary hesitation (≥2%), urinary retention (≥2%), urine flow decreased (≥2%), cystitis (≥1%), urinary tract infection (≥1%)

Neuromuscular & skeletal: Falling (≥1%)

Ocular: Blurred vision (2%)

Respiratory: Dyspnea (2%)

Miscellaneous: Night sweats (≥1%)

<1% (Limited to important or life-threatening): Accommodation disorder, acute renal failure, anorexia, delirium, erythema multiforme, galactorrhea, hallucination, hepatitis, hyperprolactinemia, hypertensive crisis, hyponatremia, leukopenia, loss of consciousness, neuroleptic malignant syndrome, neutropenia, parkinsonism, rhabdomyolysis, seizures, serotonin syndrome, Stevens-Johnson syndrome, supraventricular tachycardia, thrombocytopenia

Drug Interactions

Avoid Concomitant Use

Avoid concomitant use of Milnacipran with any of the following: Iobenguane I 123; MAO Inhibitors; Sibutramine

Increased Effect/Toxicity

Milnacipran may increase the levels/effects of: Alcohol (Ethyl); Alpha-/Beta-Agonists; Aspirin; CNS Depressants; Digoxin; NSAID (Nonselective); Serotonin Modulators

The levels/effects of Milnacipran may be increased by: ClomiPRAMINE; MAO Inhibitors; Sibutramine

Decreased Effect

Milnacipran may decrease the levels/effects of: Alpha2-Agonists; Iobenguane I 123

Ethanol/Nutrition/Herb Interactions

Ethanol: Avoid ethanol use.

Herb/Nutraceutical: Avoid valerian, St John's wort, SAMe, kava kava, tryptophan (may increase risk of serotonin syndrome and/or excessive sedation).

Stability Store at 25°C (77°F); excursions permitted between 15°C to 30°C (59°F to 86°F).

Mechanism of Action Potent inhibitor of norepinephrine and serotonin reuptake (3:1). Milnacipran has no significant activity for serotonergic, alpha- and beta-adrenergic, muscarinic, histaminergic, dopaminergic, opiate, benzodiazepine, and GABA receptors. It does not possess MAO-inhibitory activity.

Pharmacodynamics/Kinetics

Absorption: Well absorbed

Distribution: I.V: V_d: ~400 L

Protein binding: 13%

Metabolism: Hepatic to inactive metabolites

Bioavailability: 85% to 90%

Half-life elimination: 6-8 hours

Time to peak, plasma: Oral: 2-4 hours

Excretion: Urine (55% as unchanged drug)

Dosage Oral: Adults: 50 mg twice daily (maximum dose: 200 mg/day)

Note: Recommended titration schedule: 12.5 mg once on day one, then 12.5 mg twice daily on days 2-3, 25 mg twice daily on days 4-7, then 50 mg twice daily thereafter.

Dosing adjustment in renal impairment:

Mild renal impairment: No dose adjustment is recommended

Moderate renal impairment: Use with caution

Severe renal impairment (Cl_{cr} ≤29 mL/minute): Reduce maintenance dose to 25 mg twice daily; dose may be increased to 50 mg twice daily, based on individual tolerance

End-stage renal disease (ESRD): Use not recommended

Dosing adjustment in hepatic impairment:

Mild-to-moderate hepatic impairment: No dose adjustment is recommended

Severe hepatic impairment: Use with caution

Dietary Considerations May be taken with or without food; food may improve tolerability.

Administration May be administered with or without food; food may improve tolerability.

Monitoring Parameters Blood pressure and heart rate should be regularly monitored; renal function should be monitored for dosing purposes; mental status for suicidal ideation (especially at the beginning of therapy or when doses are increased or decreased); intraocular pressure should be monitored in those with baseline elevations or a history of glaucoma

Product Availability Savella™: FDA approved January 2009; availability anticipated in March 2009

Dosage Forms Excipient information presented when available (limited, particularly for generics); consult specific product labeling.

Tablet:

Savella™: 12.5 mg, 25 mg, 50 mg, 100 mg

◆ **Milophene® (Can)** *see* ClomiPHENE *on page 349*

Milrinone (MIL ri none)

U.S. Brand Names Primacor®

Canadian Brand Names Milrinone Lactate Injection; Primacor®

Index Terms Milrinone Lactate

Pharmacologic Category Phosphodiesterase Enzyme Inhibitor

Additional Appendix Information

Hemodynamic Support, Intravenous *on page 1657*

Use Short-term I.V. therapy of acutely-decompensated heart failure

Unlabeled/Investigational Use Inotropic therapy for patients unresponsive to other acute heart failure therapies (eg, dobutamine); outpatient inotropic therapy for heart transplant candidates; palliation of symptoms in end-stage heart failure patients who cannot otherwise be discharged from the hospital and are not transplant candidates

Pregnancy Risk Factor C

Lactation Excretion in breast milk unknown/use caution

Medication Safety Issues

Sound-alike/look-alike issues:

Primacor® may be confused with Primaxin®

High alert medication: The Institute for Safe Medication Practices (ISMP) includes this medication among its list of drugs which have a heightened risk of causing significant patient harm when used in error.

Contraindications Hypersensitivity to milrinone, inamrinone, or any component of the formulation; concurrent use of inamrinone

Warnings/Precautions Monitor closely for hypotension. Avoid in severe obstructive aortic or pulmonic valvular disease. Milrinone may aggravate outflow tract obstruction in hypertrophic subaortic stenosis. Supraventricular and ventricular arrhythmias have developed in high-risk patients. Ensure that ventricular rate controlled in atrial fibrillation/flutter prior to initiating milrinone. Not recommended for use in acute MI patients. Monitor and correct fluid and electrolyte problems. Adjust dose in renal dysfunction. Discontinue therapy if dose-related elevations in LFTs and clinical symptoms of hepatotoxicity occur.

Adverse Reactions

>10%: Cardiovascular: Ventricular arrhythmia (ectopy 9%, NSVT 3%, sustained ventricular tachycardia 1%, ventricular fibrillation <1%)

1% to 10%:

Cardiovascular: Supraventricular arrhythmia (4%), hypotension (3%), angina/chest pain (1%)

Central nervous system: Headache (3%)

<1% (Limited to important or life-threatening): Anaphylaxis, atrial fibrillation, bronchospasm, hypokalemia, injection

site reaction, liver function abnormalities, MI, rash, thrombocytopenia, torsade de pointes, tremor, ventricular fibrillation

Drug Interactions

Avoid Concomitant Use There are no known interactions where it is recommended to avoid concomitant use.

Increased Effect/Toxicity There are no known significant interactions involving an increase in effect.

Decreased Effect There are no known significant interactions involving a decrease in effect.

Stability Store at 15°C to 30°C (59°F to 86°F). Avoid freezing. Stable at 0.2 mg/mL in 1/2NS, NS, or D_5W for 72 hours at room temperature in normal light.

Standard dilution: For a final concentration of 0.2 mg/mL: Dilute Primacor® 1 mg/mL (20 mL) with 80 mL diluent (final volume: 100 mL). May also dilute 1 mg/mL (10 mL) with 40 mL diluent (final volume: 50 mL).

Mechanism of Action A selective phosphodiesterase inhibitor in cardiac and vascular tissue, resulting in vasodilation and inotropic effects with little chronotropic activity.

Pharmacodynamics/Kinetics

Onset of action: I.V.: 5-15 minutes

Distribution: V_{dss}: 0.32-0.45 L/kg

Protein binding, plasma: ~70%

Metabolism: Hepatic (12%)

Half-life elimination: ~2.5 hours

Excretion: Urine (85% as unchanged drug) within 24 hours; active tubular secretion is a major elimination pathway for milrinone

Dosage Adults: I.V.: Loading dose (optional): 50 mcg/kg administered over 10 minutes followed by a maintenance dose titrated according to the hemodynamic and clinical response; Maintenance dose: I.V. infusion: 0.375-0.75 mcg/kg/minute.

Dosing adjustment in renal impairment:

Cl_{cr} 50 mL/minute: Administer 0.43 mcg/kg/minute

Cl_{cr} 40 mL/minute: Administer 0.38 mcg/kg/minute

Cl_{cr} 30 mL/minute: Administer 0.33 mcg/kg/minute

Cl_{cr} 20 mL/minute: Administer 0.28 mcg/kg/minute

Cl_{cr} 10 mL/minute: Administer 0.23 mcg/kg/minute

Cl_{cr} 5 mL/minute: Administer 0.2 mcg/kg/minute

Administration Infuse via infusion pump

Monitoring Parameters Platelet count, CBC, electrolytes (especially potassium and magnesium), liver function and renal function tests; ECG, CVP, SBP, DBP, heart rate; infusion site

If pulmonary artery catheter is in place, monitor cardiac index, stroke volume, systemic vascular resistance, pulmonary capillary wedge pressure and pulmonary vascular resistance.

Dosage Forms Excipient information presented when available (limited, particularly for generics); consult specific product labeling. [DSC] = Discontinued product

Infusion [premixed in D_5W]: 200 mcg/mL (100 mL, 200 mL)

Primacor®: 200 mcg/mL (200 mL)

Injection, solution: 1 mg/mL (10 mL, 20 mL, 50 mL)

◆ **Milrinone Lactate** *see* Milrinone *on page 998*

◆ **Milrinone Lactate Injection (Can)** *see* Milrinone *on page 998*

◆ **Miltown® [DSC]** *see* Meprobamate *on page 946*

◆ **Minestrin™ 1/20 (Can)** *see* Ethinyl Estradiol and Norethindrone *on page 581*

◆ **Minipress®** *see* Prazosin *on page 1229*

◆ **Minirin® (Can)** *see* Desmopressin *on page 421*

◆ **Minitran™** *see* Nitroglycerin *on page 1073*

◆ **Minocin® (Can)** *see* Minocycline *on page 999*

◆ **Minocin® PAC** *see* Minocycline *on page 999*

Minocycline (mi noe SYE kleen)

U.S. Brand Names Dynacin®; Minocin® PAC; myrac™; Solodyn™

Canadian Brand Names Alti-Minocycline; Apo-Minocycline®; Gen-Minocycline; Minocin®; Novo-Minocycline; PMS-Minocycline; Rhoxal-minocycline; Sandoz-Minocycline

Index Terms Minocycline Hydrochloride

Pharmacologic Category Antibiotic, Tetracycline Derivative

Additional Appendix Information

Antimicrobial Drugs of Choice *on page 1752*

Use Treatment of susceptible bacterial infections of both gram-negative and gram-positive organisms; treatment of anthrax (inhalational, cutaneous, and gastrointestinal); moderate-to-severe acne; meningococcal (asymptomatic) carrier state; Rickettsial diseases (including Rocky Mountain spotted fever, Q fever); nongonococcal urethritis, gonorrhea; acute intestinal amebiasis

Extended release (Solodyn™): Only indicated for treatment of inflammatory lesions of non-nodular moderate-to-severe acne

Unlabeled/Investigational Use Rheumatoid arthritis (patients with low disease activity of short duration)

Pregnancy Risk Factor D

Pregnancy Considerations Tetracyclines, including minocycline, cross the placenta, enter fetal circulation, and may cause permanent discoloration of teeth if used during the second or third trimester. Congenital anomalies after minocycline use have been reported postmarketing. Because use during pregnancy may cause fetal harm, minocycline is classified as pregnancy category D.

Lactation Enters breast milk/not recommended

Medication Safety Issues

Sound-alike/look-alike issues:

Dynacin® may be confused with Dyazide®, Dynabac®, DynaCirc®, Dynapen®

Minocin® may be confused with Indocin®, Lincocin®, Minizide®, Mithracin®, niacin

Contraindications Hypersensitivity to minocycline, other tetracyclines, or any component of the formulation

Warnings/Precautions May be associated with increases in BUN secondary to antianabolic effects; use caution in patients with renal impairment (Cl_{cr} <80 mL/minute). Hepatotoxicity has been reported; use caution in patients with hepatic insufficiency. Autoimmune syndromes (eg, lupus-like, hepatitis, and vasculitis) have been reported; discontinue if symptoms. CNS effects (lightheadedness, vertigo) may occur; patients must be cautioned about performing tasks which require mental alertness (eg, operating machinery or driving). Pseudotumor cerebri has been (rarely) reported with tetracycline use; usually resolves with discontinuation. May cause photosensitivity; discontinue if skin erythema occurs. Prolonged use may result in fungal or bacterial superinfection, including *C. difficile*-associated diarrhea (CDAD) and pseudomembranous colitis; CDAD has been observed >2 months postantibiotic treatment. May cause tissue hyperpigmentation, enamel hypoplasia, or permanent tooth discoloration; use of tetracyclines should be avoided during tooth development (children ≤8 years of age) unless other drugs are not likely to be effective or are contraindicated. However, recommended in treatment of anthrax exposure. Do not use during pregnancy. In addition to affecting tooth development, tetracycline use has been associated with retardation of skeletal development and reduced bone growth.

Adverse Reactions Frequency not defined.

Cardiovascular: Myocarditis, pericarditis, vasculitis

Central nervous system: Bulging fontanels, dizziness, fatigue, fever, headache, hypoesthesia, malaise, mood changes, paresthesia, pseudotumor cerebri, sedation, seizure, somnolence, vertigo

Dermatologic: Alopecia, angioedema, erythema multiforme, erythema nodosum, erythematous rash, exfoliative dermatitis, hyperpigmentation of nails, maculopapular rash, photosensitivity, pigmentation of the skin and mucous membranes, pruritus, Stevens-Johnson syndrome, toxic epidermal necrolysis, urticaria

Endocrine & metabolic: Thyroid discoloration, thyroid dysfunction

Gastrointestinal: Anorexia, diarrhea, dyspepsia, dysphagia, enamel hypoplasia, enterocolitis, esophageal ulcerations, esophagitis, glossitis, inflammatory lesions (oral/anogenital), moniliasis, nausea, oral cavity discoloration, pancreatitis, pseudomembranous colitis, stomatitis, tooth discoloration, vomiting, xerostomia

Genitourinary: Balanitis, vulvovaginitis

Hematologic: Agranulocytosis, eosinophilia, hemolytic anemia, leukopenia, neutropenia, pancytopenia, thrombocytopenia

Hepatic: Hepatic cholestasis, hepatic failure, hepatitis, hyperbilirubinemia, jaundice, liver enzyme increases

Neuromuscular & skeletal: Arthralgia, arthritis, bone discoloration, joint stiffness, joint swelling, myalgia

Otic: Hearing loss, tinnitus

Renal: Acute renal failure, BUN increased, interstitial nephritis

Respiratory: Asthma, bronchospasm, cough, dyspnea, pneumonitis, pulmonary infiltrate (with eosinophilia)

Miscellaneous: Anaphylaxis, hypersensitivity, lupus erythematosus, lupus-like syndrome, serum sickness

Drug Interactions

Avoid Concomitant Use

Avoid concomitant use of Minocycline with any of the following: Retinoic Acid Derivatives

Increased Effect/Toxicity

Minocycline may increase the levels/effects of: Neuromuscular-Blocking Agents; Retinoic Acid Derivatives; Vitamin K Antagonists

Decreased Effect

Minocycline may decrease the levels/effects of: Penicillins; Typhoid Vaccine

The levels/effects of Minocycline may be decreased by: Antacids; Bile Acid Sequestrants; Bismuth; Bismuth Subsalicylate; Iron Salts; Magnesium Salts; Quinapril; Zinc Salts

Ethanol/Nutrition/Herb Interactions

Food: Minocycline serum concentrations are not significantly altered if taken with food or dairy products.

Herb/Nutraceutical: Avoid dong quai, St John's wort (may also cause photosensitization).

Stability

Capsule (including pellet-filled), tablet: Store at 20°C to 25°C (68°F to 77°F); protect from heat. Protect from light and moisture.

Extended release tablet: Store at 15°C to 30°C (59°F to 86°F); protect from heat. Protect from light and moisture.

Mechanism of Action Inhibits bacterial protein synthesis by binding with the 30S and possibly the 50S ribosomal subunit(s) of susceptible bacteria; cell wall synthesis is not affected

Rheumatoid arthritis: The mechanism of action of minocycline in rheumatoid arthritis is not completely understood. It is thought to have antimicrobial, antiinflammatory, immunomodulatory, and chondroprotective effects. More specifically, it is thought to be a potent inhibitor of metalloproteinases, which are active in rheumatoid arthritis joint destruction.

Pharmacodynamics/Kinetics

Absorption: Well absorbed

Protein binding: 70% to 75%

Metabolism: Hepatic to inactive metabolites

Half-life elimination: 16 hours (range: 11-22 hours)

Time to peak: Capsule, pellet filled: 1-4 hours; Extended release tablet: 3.5-4 hours

Excretion: Urine, feces

Dosage

Usual dosage range:

Capsule or immediate release tablet:

Children >8 years: Oral: Initial: 4 mg/kg, followed by 2 mg/kg/dose every 12 hours

Adults: Oral: Initial: 200 mg, followed by 100 mg every 12 hours; more frequent dosing intervals may be used (100-200 mg initially, followed by 50 mg 4 times daily)

Extended release tablet (Solodyn™): Children ≥12 years and Adults (≥45 kg): Oral: 45-135 mg once daily (weight based)

Indication-specific dosing:

Children ≥12 years: Oral: **Acne** *(inflammatory, non-nodular, moderate-to-severe)* (Solodyn™):

45-59 kg: 45 mg once daily

60-90 kg: 90 mg once daily

91-136 kg: 135 mg once daily

Note: Therapy should be continued for 12 weeks. Higher doses do not confer greater efficacy, and safety of use beyond 12 weeks has not been established.

Adults: Oral:

Acne: Capsule or immediate-release tablet: 50-100 mg twice daily

Inflammatory, non-nodular, moderate-to-severe (Solodyn™):

45-59 kg: 45 mg once daily

60-90 kg: 90 mg once daily

91-136 kg: 135 mg once daily

Note: Therapy should be continued for 12 weeks. Higher doses do not confer greater efficacy, and safety of use beyond 12 weeks has not been established.

Chlamydial or *Ureaplasma urealyticum* infection, uncomplicated: Urethral, endocervical, or rectal: 100 mg every 12 hours for at least 7 days

Gonococcal infection, uncomplicated (males):

Without urethritis or anorectal infection: Initial: 200 mg, followed by 100 mg every 12 hours for at least 4 days (cultures 2-3 days post-therapy)

Urethritis: 100 mg every 12 hours for 5 days

Meningococcal carrier state: 100 mg every 12 hours for 5 days

Mycobacterium marinum: 100 mg every 12 hours for 6-8 weeks

Nocardiosis, cutaneous (non-CNS): 100 mg every 12 hours

Rheumatoid arthritis (unlabeled use): 100 mg twice daily (O'Dell, 2001)

Syphilis: Initial: 200 mg, followed by 100 mg every 12 hours for 10-15 days

Elderly: Refer to adult dosing.

Dosage adjustment in renal impairment: Use with caution; monitor BUN and creatinine clearance. Consider decreasing dose or increasing dosing interval (extended release).

Dietary Considerations May be taken with or without food.

Administration May be taken with or without food. Administer with adequate fluid to decrease the risk of esophageal irritation and ulceration. Swallow pellet-filled capsule and extended release tablet whole; do not chew, crush, or split.

Monitoring Parameters Culture and sensitivity testing prior to initiating therapy; LFTs, BUN, renal function with long-term treatment; if symptomatic for autoimmune disorder, include ANA, CBC

Test Interactions May cause interference with fluorescence test for urinary catecholamines (false elevations)

Dosage Forms Excipient information presented when available (limited, particularly for generics); consult specific product labeling. [DSC] = Discontinued product

Capsule: 50 mg, 75 mg, 100 mg

Dynacin®: 75 mg [DSC], 100 mg [DSC]

Capsule, pellet filled: 50 mg, 100 mg

Minocin® PAC: 50 mg, 100 mg [packaged with wipes, serum, and masque]

Tablet: 50 mg, 75 mg, 100 mg

Dynacin®, myrac™: 50 mg, 75 mg, 100 mg

Tablet, extended release:

Solodyn™: 45 mg, 90 mg, 135 mg

◆ **Minocycline Hydrochloride** *see* Minocycline *on page 999*

◆ **Min-Ovral® (Can)** *see* Ethinyl Estradiol and Levonorgestrel *on page 577*

◆ **Minox (Can)** *see* Minoxidil *on page 1001*

Minoxidil (mi NOKS i dil)

U.S. Brand Names Rogaine® Extra Strength for Men [OTC]; Rogaine® for Men [OTC]; Rogaine® for Women [OTC]

Canadian Brand Names Apo-Gain®; Loniten®; Minox; Rogaine®

Pharmacologic Category Topical Skin Product; Vasodilator, Direct-Acting

Additional Appendix Information

Hypertension *on page 1820*

Use Management of severe hypertension (usually in combination with a diuretic and beta-blocker); treatment (topical formulation) of alopecia androgenetica in males and females

Pregnancy Risk Factor C

Pregnancy Considerations Adverse events were observed in some animal studies. There are no adequate and well-controlled studies in pregnant women.

Lactation Enters breast milk/not recommended

Medication Safety Issues

Sound-alike/look-alike issues:

Minoxidil may be confused with metolazone, midodrine, Minipress®, Minocin®, Monopril®, Noxafil®

International issues:

Noxidil® [Thailand] may be confused with Noxafil® which is a brand name for posaconazole in the U.S.

Contraindications Hypersensitivity to minoxidil or any component of the formulation; pheochromocytoma

Warnings/Precautions [U.S. Boxed Warning]: Minoxidil may cause pericarditis and pericardial effusion that may progress to tamponade; patients with renal impairment not on dialysis may be at higher risk. Observe patients closely. **[U.S. Boxed Warning]: May increase oxygen demand and exacerbate angina pectoris;** concomitant use with a beta-blocker (if no contraindication exists may help reduce the effect. Use with caution in patients with pulmonary hypertension, significant renal failure, or HF; use with caution in patients with coronary artery disease or recent myocardial infarction; renal failure or dialysis patients may require smaller doses; usually used with a beta-blocker (to treat minoxidil-induced tachycardia) and a diuretic (for treatment of water retention/edema. Compared to placebo minoxidil increased the frequency of clinical events, including increased need for diuretics, angina, ventricular arrhythmias, worsening heart failure and death (Franciosa, 1984). Use with caution in the elderly; initiate at the low end of the dosage range and monitor closely.

[U.S. Boxed Warning]: Maximum therapeutic doses of a diuretic and two antihypertensives should be used before this drug is ever added. Should be given with a diuretic to minimize fluid gain and a beta-blocker (if no contraindications) to prevent tachycardia. Anyone with malignant hypertension should be hospitalized with close medical supervision to ensure blood pressure is reducing and to prevent too rapid of a reduction in blood pressure. Inform patients of excessive hair growth before initiating therapy; may take 1-6 months for hypertrichosis to reverse itself after discontinuation of the drug.

Adverse Reactions

Oral: Incidence of reactions not always reported.

Cardiovascular: ECG changes (T-wave changes 60%), peripheral edema (7%), pericardial effusion with tamponade (3%), pericardial effusion without tamponade (3%), angina pectoris, heart failure, pericarditis, rebound hypertension (in children after a gradual withdrawal), sodium and water retention, tachycardia

Dermatologic: Hypertrichosis (common; 80%), bullous eruption (rare), rash, Stevens-Johnson syndrome (rare)

Endocrine & metabolic: Breast tenderness (rare; <1%)

Gastrointestinal: Nausea, vomiting, weight gain

Hematologic: Leukopenia (rare), thrombocytopenia (rare), transient decreased erythrocyte count (hemodilution), transient decreased hematocrit/hemoglobin (hemodilution)

Hepatic: Increased alkaline phosphatase

Renal: Transient increase in serum BUN and creatinine

Respiratory: Pulmonary edema

Topical: Incidence of adverse events is not always reported.

Cardiovascular: Blood pressure increased/decreased, cardiac output increased, chest pain (transient), edema, left ventricular mass increased, left ventricular end-diastolic volume increased, palpitation, tachycardia

Central nervous system: Anxiety (rare), dizziness, faintness, headache, mental depression (rare), taste alterations

Dermatologic: Allergic contact dermatitis (7.4%), alopecia, dryness, eczema, exacerbation of hair loss, flushing, folliculitis; hair growth increased outside the area of application (face, beard, eyebrows, ear, arm); hypertrichosis, local erythema, papular rash, pruritus, scaling/flaking, seborrhea

Endocrine & metabolic: Menstrual changes

Gastrointestinal: Diarrhea, nausea

Genitourinary: Urinary tract infection (rare), renal calculi (rare), urethritis (rare), prostatitis (rare), epididymitis (rare), impotence (rare)

Hematologic: Lymphadenopathy, thrombocytopenia

Neuromuscular & skeletal: Fractures, back pain, retrosternal chest pain of muscular origin, tendonitis (2.6%), weakness

Ocular: Conjunctivitis, visual disturbances, decreased visual acuity

Respiratory: Bronchitis, upper respiratory infection

Drug Interactions

Avoid Concomitant Use There are no known interactions where it is recommended to avoid concomitant use.

Increased Effect/Toxicity

Minoxidil may increase the levels/effects of: Amifostine; RiTUXimab

The levels/effects of Minoxidil may be increased by: CycloSPORINE; Diazoxide; Herbs (Hypotensive Properties); Prostacyclin Analogues

Decreased Effect

The levels/effects of Minoxidil may be decreased by: Herbs (Hypertensive Properties); Methylphenidate; Yohimbine

Ethanol/Nutrition/Herb Interactions Herb/Nutraceutical: Bayberry, blue cohosh, cayenne, ephedra, ginger, ginseng (American), kola, licorice may diminish the antihypertensive effects of minoxidil. Black cohosh, California poppy, coleus, golden seal, hawthorn, mistletoe, periwinkle, quinine, shepherd's purse may enhance the hypotensive effects of minoxidil.

Stability Store at controlled room temperature of 15°C to 30°C (59°F to 86°F).

Mechanism of Action Produces vasodilation by directly relaxing arteriolar smooth muscle, with little effect on veins; effects may be mediated by cyclic AMP; stimulation of hair growth is secondary to vasodilation, increased cutaneous blood flow and stimulation of resting hair follicles

Pharmacodynamics/Kinetics

Onset of action: Hypotensive: Oral: ~30 minutes
Peak effect: 2-8 hours
Duration: 2-5 days
Protein binding: None
Metabolism: 88%, primarily via glucuronidation
Bioavailability: Oral: 90%
Half-life elimination: Adults: 3.5-4.2 hours
Excretion: Urine (12% as unchanged drug)

Dosage

Children <12 years: Hypertension: Oral: Initial: 0.1-0.2 mg/kg once daily; maximum: 5 mg/day; increase gradually every 3 days; usual dosage range: 0.25-1 mg/kg/day in 1-2 divided doses; maximum: 50 mg/day

Children ≥12 years and Adults: Hypertension: Oral: Initial: 5 mg once daily, increase gradually every 3 days (maximum: 100 mg/day); usual dosage range (JNC 7): 2.5-80 mg/day in 1-2 divided doses

Note: Dosage adjustment is needed when added to concomitant therapy.

Adults: Alopecia: Topical: Apply twice daily; 4 months of therapy may be necessary for hair growth.

Elderly: Hypertension: Oral: Initial: 2.5 mg once daily; increase gradually.

Dosing adjustment in renal impairment: Patient with renal failure and/or receiving dialysis may require dosage reduction.

Supplemental dose is not necessary after hemo- or peritoneal dialysis.

Monitoring Parameters Blood pressure, standing and sitting/supine; fluid and electrolyte balance and body weight should be monitored. Any tests that are abnormal at the time of initiation (including, renal function tests, ECG, echocardiogram, chest x-ray) should be repeated initially every 1-3 months then every 6-12 months once stable.

Dosage Forms Excipient information presented when available (limited, particularly for generics); consult specific product labeling. [DSC] = Discontinued product

Aerosol, topical [foam]:
Rogaine for Men®: 5% (60 g)
Solution, topical: 2% (60 mL); 5% (60 mL)
Rogaine® for Men: (60 mL) [DSC] [supplied with dropper applicator]
Rogaine® for Women: 2% (60 mL) [supplied with dropper applicator]
Rogaine® Extra Strength for Men: 5% (60 mL) [supplied with dropper applicator]
Tablet: 2.5 mg, 10 mg

- ◆ **Mintab DM** *see* Guaifenesin and Dextromethorphan *on page* *710*
- ◆ **Mint-Citalopram (Can)** *see* Citalopram *on page* *337*
- ◆ **Mintezol®** *see* Thiabendazole *on page* *1457*
- ◆ **MINT-Ondansetron (Can)** *see* Ondansetron *on page* *1102*
- ◆ **Mintox Extra Strength [OTC]** *see* Aluminum Hydroxide, Magnesium Hydroxide, and Simethicone *on page* *76*
- ◆ **Mintox Plus [OTC]** *see* Aluminum Hydroxide, Magnesium Hydroxide, and Simethicone *on page* *76*
- ◆ **Mintuss DR** *see* Chlorpheniramine, Phenylephrine, and Dextromethorphan *on page* *311*
- ◆ **Miochol®-E** *see* Acetylcholine *on page* *35*
- ◆ **Miostat®** *see* Carbachol *on page* *251*
- ◆ **MiraLax® [OTC]** *see* Polyethylene Glycol 3350 *on page* *1209*
- ◆ **Mirapex®** *see* Pramipexole *on page* *1224*
- ◆ **Mircette®** *see* Ethinyl Estradiol and Desogestrel *on page* *575*
- ◆ **Mirena®** *see* Levonorgestrel *on page* *879*

Mirtazapine (mir TAZ a peen)

U.S. Brand Names Remeron SolTab®; Remeron®

Canadian Brand Names Apo-Mirtazapine; CO Mirtazapine; DOM-Mirtazapine; Gen-Mirtazapine; Novo-Mirtazapine; PHL-Mirtazapine; PMS-Mirtazapine; PRO-Mirtazapine; ratio-Mirtazapine; Remeron®; Remeron® RD; Riva-Mirtazapine; Sandoz-Mirtazapine; Sandoz-Mirtazapine FC

Pharmacologic Category Antidepressant, Alpha-2 Antagonist

Additional Appendix Information

Antidepressant Agents *on page* *1638*

Use Treatment of depression

Restrictions An FDA-approved medication guide concerning the use of antidepressants in children, adolescents, and young adults must be distributed when dispensing an outpatient prescription (new or refill) where this medication is to be used without direct supervision of a healthcare provider. Medication guides are available at http://www.fda.gov/cder/Offices/ODS/medication_guides.htm. Dispense to parents or guardians of children and adolescents receiving this medication.

Pregnancy Risk Factor C

Pregnancy Considerations Adverse events were observed in some animal studies; therefore, the manufacturer classifies mirtazapine as pregnancy category C. A significant increase in major teratogenic effects has not been observed in humans following exposure to mirtazapine during pregnancy; however, some nonteratogenic adverse events (similar to those observed with SSRI agents) have been reported. Mirtazapine was found to cross the placenta following a maternal overdose. Pregnancy itself does not provide "protection" against depression. Women treated for major depression and who are euthymic prior to pregnancy are more likely to experience a relapse when medication is discontinued as compared to pregnant women who continue taking antidepressant medications. The ACOG recommends that therapy with antidepressants during pregnancy be individualized. According to their recommendations, treatment of depression during pregnancy should incorporate the clinical expertise of the mental health clinician, obstetrician, primary care provider, and pediatrician. If treatment during pregnancy is required, consider tapering therapy during the third trimester in order to prevent withdrawal symptoms in the infant. If this is done, and the woman is considered to be at risk of relapse from her major depressive disorder, the medication can be restarted following delivery, although the dose should be readjusted to that required before pregnancy.

Lactation Excreted in breast milk/use caution

Medication Safety Issues

Sound-alike/look-alike issues:
Remeron® may be confused with Premarin®, ramelteon, Rozerem®, Zemuron®

International issues:
Avanza® [Australia] may be confused with Albenza® which is a brand name for albendazole in the U.S.
Avanza® [Australia] may be confused with Avandia® which is a brand name for rosiglitazone in the U.S.

Remeron® my be confused with Reneuron® which is a brand name for fluoxetine in Spain

Contraindications Hypersensitivity to mirtazapine or any component of the formulation; use of MAO inhibitors within 14 days

Warnings/Precautions [U.S. Boxed Warning]: Antidepressants increase the risk of suicidal thinking and behavior in children, adolescents, and young adults (18-24 years of age) with major depressive disorder (MDD) and other psychiatric disorders; consider risk prior to prescribing. Short-term studies did not show an increased risk in patients >24 years of age and showed a decreased risk in patients ≥65 years. Closely monitor for clinical worsening, suicidality, or unusual changes in behavior; the patient's family or caregiver should be instructed to closely observe the patient and communicate condition with healthcare provider. A medication guide should be dispensed with each prescription. **Mirtazapine is not FDA approved for use in children.**

The possibility of a suicide attempt is inherent in major depression and may persist until remission occurs. Monitor for worsening of depression or suicidality, especially during initiation of therapy (generally first 1-2 months) or with dose increases or decreases. Use caution in high-risk patients. Worsening depression and severe abrupt suicidality that are not part of the presenting symptoms may require discontinuation or modification of drug therapy. The patient's family or caregiver should be alerted to monitor patients for the emergence of suicidality and associated behaviors (such as agitation, irritability, hostility, impulsivity, and hypomania) and call healthcare provider.

May worsen psychosis in some patients or precipitate a shift to mania or hypomania in patients with bipolar disorder. Patients presenting with depressive symptoms should be screened for bipolar disorder. Monotherapy in patients with bipolar disorder should be avoided. **Mirtazapine is not FDA approved for the treatment of bipolar depression.**

Discontinue immediately if signs and symptoms of neutropenia/agranulocytosis occur. May cause sedation, resulting in impaired performance of tasks requiring alertness (eg, operating machinery or driving). Sedative effects may be additive with other CNS depressants and/or ethanol. The degree of sedation is moderate-high relative to other antidepressants. The risks of orthostatic hypotension or anticholinergic effects are low relative to other antidepressants. The incidence of sexual dysfunction with mirtazapine is generally lower than with SSRIs. Potential for severe reaction when used with MAO inhibitors; autonomic instability, coma, death, delirium, diaphoresis, hyperthermia, mental status changes/agitation, muscular rigidity, myoclonus, neuroleptic malignant syndrome features, and seizures may occur.

May increase appetite and stimulate weight gain. Weight gain of >7% of body weight reported in 7.5% of patients treated with mirtazapine compared to 0% for placebo; 8% of patients receiving mirtazapine discontinued treatment due to the weight gain. In an 8-week pediatric clinical trial, 49% of mirtazapine-treated patients had a weight gain of at least 7% (mean increase 4 kg) as compared to 5.7% of placebo-treated patients (mean increase 1 kg). May increase serum cholesterol and triglyceride levels.

Use caution in patients with a previous seizure disorder or condition predisposing to seizures such as brain damage, alcoholism, or concurrent therapy with other drugs which lower the seizure threshold. Use with caution in patients with hepatic or renal dysfunction and in elderly patients. SolTab® formulation contains phenylalanine.

Adverse Reactions

>10%:

Central nervous system: Somnolence (54%)

Endocrine & metabolic: Cholesterol increased

Gastrointestinal: Constipation (13%), xerostomia (25%), appetite increased (17%), weight gain (12%; weight gain of >7% reported in 8% of adults, ≤49% of pediatric patients)

1% to 10%:

Cardiovascular: Hypertension, vasodilatation, peripheral edema (2%), edema (1%)

Central nervous system: Dizziness (7%), abnormal dreams (4%), abnormal thoughts (3%), confusion (2%), malaise

Endocrine & metabolic: Triglycerides increased

Gastrointestinal: Vomiting, anorexia, abdominal pain

Genitourinary: Urinary frequency (2%)

Neuromuscular & skeletal: Myalgia (2%), back pain (2%), arthralgia, tremor (2%), weakness (8%)

Respiratory: Dyspnea (1%)

Miscellaneous: Flu-like syndrome (5%), thirst (<1%)

<1% (Limited to important or life-threatening): Agranulocytosis, dehydration, liver function test increases, lymphadenopathy, neutropenia, orthostatic hypotension, seizure (1 case reported), torsade de pointes (1 case reported), weight loss

Drug Interactions

Metabolism/Transport Effects Substrate of CYP1A2 (major), 2C9 (minor), 2D6 (major), 3A4 (major); **Inhibits** CYP1A2 (weak), 3A4 (weak)

Avoid Concomitant Use

Avoid concomitant use of Mirtazapine with any of the following: MAO Inhibitors; Sibutramine

Increased Effect/Toxicity

Mirtazapine may increase the levels/effects of: Alcohol (Ethyl); CNS Depressants; Serotonin Modulators

The levels/effects of Mirtazapine may be increased by: CYP1A2 Inhibitors (Moderate); CYP1A2 Inhibitors (Strong); CYP2D6 Inhibitors (Moderate); CYP2D6 Inhibitors (Strong); CYP3A4 Inhibitors (Moderate); CYP3A4 Inhibitors (Strong); Darunavir; Dasatinib; MAO Inhibitors; Sibutramine

Decreased Effect

Mirtazapine may decrease the levels/effects of: Alpha2-Agonists

The levels/effects of Mirtazapine may be decreased by: CYP1A2 Inducers (Strong); CYP3A4 Inducers (Strong); Deferasirox; Herbs (CYP3A4 Inducers)

Ethanol/Nutrition/Herb Interactions

Ethanol: Avoid ethanol (may increase CNS depression).

Herb/Nutraceutical: Avoid St John's wort (may decrease mirtazapine levels). Avoid valerian, St John's wort, SAMe, kava kava (may increase CNS depression).

Stability Store at controlled room temperature.

SolTab®: Protect from light and moisture. Use immediately upon opening tablet blister.

Mechanism of Action Mirtazapine is a tetracyclic antidepressant that works by its central presynaptic alpha$_2$-adrenergic antagonist effects, which results in increased release of norepinephrine and serotonin. It is also a potent antagonist of 5-HT$_2$ and 5-HT$_3$ serotonin receptors and H1 histamine receptors and a moderate peripheral alpha$_1$-adrenergic and muscarinic antagonist; it does not inhibit the reuptake of norepinephrine or serotonin.

Pharmacodynamics/Kinetics

Absorption: Rapid and complete

Distribution: 4.5 L/kg

Protein binding: 85%

Metabolism: Extensively hepatic via CYP1A2, 2C9, 2D6, 3A4 and via demethylation (forms demethylmirtazapine,

an active metabolite) and hydroxylation (forms inactive metabolites)
Bioavailability: 50%
Half-life elimination: 20-40 hours; hampered with renal or hepatic impairment
Time to peak, serum: 2 hours
Excretion: Urine (75%) and feces (15%) as metabolites

Dosage

Treatment of depression: Adults: Oral: Initial: 15 mg nightly, titrate up to 15-45 mg/day with dose increases made no more frequently than every 1-2 weeks; there is an inverse relationship between dose and sedation

Elderly: Decreased clearance seen (40% males, 10% females); no specific dosage adjustment recommended by manufacturer

Alzheimer's dementia-related depression: Initial: 7.5 mg at bedtime; may increase at 7.5-15 mg increments to 45-60 mg/day

Dosage adjustment in renal impairment:
Cl_{cr} 11-39 mL/minute: 30% decreased clearance
Cl_{cr} <10 mL/minute: 50% decreased clearance

Dosage adjustment in hepatic impairment: Clearance decreased by 30%

Dietary Considerations Remeron SolTab® contains phenylalanine: 2.6 mg per 15 mg tablet; 5.2 mg per 30 mg tablet; 7.8 mg per 45 mg tablet

Administration SolTab®: Open blister pack and place tablet on the tongue. Do not split tablet. Tablet is formulated to dissolve on the tongue without water.

Monitoring Parameters Patients should be monitored for signs of agranulocytosis or severe neutropenia such as sore throat, stomatitis or other signs of infection or a low WBC; mental status for depression, suicidal ideation (especially at the beginning of therapy or when doses are increased or decreased), anxiety, social functioning, mania, panic attacks; lipid profile

Additional Information Note: At least 14 days should elapse between discontinuation of an MAO inhibitor and initiation of therapy with mirtazapine; at least 14 days should be allowed after discontinuing mirtazapine before starting an MAO inhibitor.

Dosage Forms Excipient information presented when available (limited, particularly for generics); consult specific product labeling.

Tablet: 7.5 mg, 15 mg, 30 mg, 45 mg
Remeron®: 15 mg, 30 mg, 45 mg
Tablet, orally disintegrating: 15 mg, 30 mg
Remeron SolTab®:
15 mg [contains phenylalanine 2.6 mg/tablet; orange flavor]
30 mg [contains phenylalanine 5.2 mg/tablet; orange flavor]
45 mg [contains phenylalanine 7.8 mg/tablet; orange flavor]

Misoprostol (mye soe PROST ole)

U.S. Brand Names Cytotec®

Canadian Brand Names Apo-Misoprostol®; Novo-Misoprostol

Pharmacologic Category Prostaglandin

Use Prevention of NSAID-induced gastric ulcers; medical termination of pregnancy of ≤49 days (in conjunction with mifepristone)

Unlabeled/Investigational Use Cervical ripening and labor induction; NSAID-induced nephropathy; fat malabsorption in cystic fibrosis

Pregnancy Risk Factor X

Pregnancy Considerations [U.S. Boxed Warning]: Not to be used in women of childbearing potential unless woman is capable of complying with effective contraceptive measures; therapy is normally begun on the second or third day of next normal menstrual period. Misoprostol is an abortifacient. During pregnancy, use to prevent NSAID-induced ulcers is contraindicated. Reports of fetal death, congenital anomalies, uterine perforation, and abortion have been received after the use of misoprostol in pregnancy.

Lactation Excretion in breast milk unknown/contraindicated

Medication Safety Issues

Sound-alike/look-alike issues:
Cytotec® may be confused with Cytoxan®, Sytobex®
Misoprostol may be confused with metoprolol, mifepristone

Contraindications Hypersensitivity to misoprostol, prostaglandins, or any component of the formulation; pregnancy (when used to reduce NSAID-induced ulcers)

Warnings/Precautions Safety and efficacy have not been established in children <18 years of age; use with caution in patients with renal impairment, cardiovascular disease and the elderly. **[U.S. Boxed Warning]: Not to be used in pregnant women or women of childbearing potential unless woman is capable of complying with effective contraceptive measures;** therapy is normally begun on the second or third day of next normal menstrual period. Uterine perforation and/or rupture have been reported in association with intravaginal use to induce labor or with combined oral/intravaginal use to induce abortion. Should not be used as a cervical-ripening agent for induction of labor. However, The American College of Obstetricians and Gynecologists (ACOG) continues to support this off-label use.

Adverse Reactions

>10%: Gastrointestinal: Diarrhea, abdominal pain
1% to 10%:
Central nervous system: Headache
Gastrointestinal: Constipation, flatulence, nausea, dyspepsia, vomiting
<1% (Limited to important or life-threatening): Anaphylaxis, anxiety, appetite changes, arrhythmia, arterial thrombosis, bronchospasm, confusion, cramps, depression, drowsiness, edema, fetal or infant death (when used during pregnancy), fever, GI bleeding, GI inflammation, gingivitis, gout, hyper-/hypotension, impotence, loss of libido, MI, neuropathy, neurosis, pulmonary embolism, purpura, rash, reflux, rigors, thrombocytopenia, uterine rupture, weakness, weight changes

Drug Interactions

Avoid Concomitant Use There are no known interactions where it is recommended to avoid concomitant use.

Increased Effect/Toxicity

Misoprostol may increase the levels/effects of: Oxytocin

Decreased Effect There are no known significant interactions involving a decrease in effect.

Ethanol/Nutrition/Herb Interactions Food: Misoprostol peak serum concentrations may be decreased if taken with food (not clinically significant).

Stability Store at or below 25°C (77°F).

Mechanism of Action Misoprostol is a synthetic prostaglandin E_1 analog that replaces the protective prostaglandins consumed with prostaglandin-inhibiting therapies (eg, NSAIDs); has been shown to induce uterine contractions

Pharmacodynamics/Kinetics

Absorption: Rapid
Metabolism: Hepatic; rapidly de-esterified to misoprostol acid (active)
Half-life elimination: Metabolite: 20-40 minutes
Time to peak, serum: Active metabolite: Fasting: 15-30 minutes
Excretion: Urine (64% to 73%) and feces (15%) within 24 hours

Dosage
Oral:
Children 8-16 years: Fat absorption in cystic fibrosis (unlabeled use): 100 mcg 4 times/day
Adults:
Prevention of NSAID-induced gastric ulcers: 200 mcg 4 times/day with food; if not tolerated, may decrease dose to 100 mcg 4 times/day with food or 200 mcg twice daily with food; last dose of the day should be taken at bedtime
Medical termination of pregnancy: Refer to Mifepristone monograph.
Intravaginal: Adults: Labor induction or cervical ripening (unlabeled uses): 25 mcg (1/4 of 100 mcg tablet); may repeat at intervals no more frequent than every 3-6 hours. Do not use in patients with previous cesarean delivery or prior major uterine surgery.

Dietary Considerations Should be taken with food; incidence of diarrhea may be lessened by having patient take dose right after meals.

Administration Incidence of diarrhea may be lessened by having patient take dose right after meals. Therapy is usually begun on the second or third day of the next normal menstrual period.

Dosage Forms Excipient information presented when available (limited, particularly for generics); consult specific product labeling.
Tablet: 100 mcg, 200 mcg

◆ **Misoprostol and Diclofenac** *see* Diclofenac and Misoprostol *on page 440*

Mitomycin (mye toe MYE sin)

Canadian Brand Names Mutamycin®

Index Terms Mitomycin-C; Mitomycin-X; MTC; NSC-26980

Pharmacologic Category Antineoplastic Agent, Antibiotic

Use Treatment of adenocarcinoma of stomach or pancreas, bladder cancer, breast cancer, or colorectal cancer

Unlabeled/Investigational Use Prevention of excess scarring in glaucoma filtration procedures in patients at high risk of bleb failure

Pregnancy Risk Factor D

Pregnancy Considerations Mitomycin can cause fetal harm in humans. Animal studies show delayed fetal development, fetal external anomalies, and neonatal anomalies.

Lactation Enters breast milk/contraindicated

Medication Safety Issues
Sound-alike/look-alike issues:
Mitomycin may be confused with mithramycin, mitotane, mitoxantrone

High alert medication: The Institute for Safe Medication Practices (ISMP) includes this medication among its list of drugs which have a heightened risk of causing significant patient harm when used in error.

Contraindications Hypersensitivity to mitomycin or any component of the formulation; thrombocytopenia; coagulation disorders, increased bleeding tendency; pregnancy

Warnings/Precautions Hazardous agent - use appropriate precautions for handling and disposal. **[U.S. Boxed Warning]: May cause bone marrow suppression (thrombocytopenia and leukopenia);** monitor for infections. Use with caution in patients who have received radiation therapy or in the presence of hepatobiliary dysfunction; reduce dosage in patients who are receiving radiation therapy simultaneously. Monitor for renal toxicity; do not administer if serum creatinine is >1.7 mg/dL. **[U.S. Boxed Warning]: Hemolytic-uremic syndrome, potentially fatal, has been reported;** is correlated with total dose (single doses ≥60 mg or cumulative doses ≥50 mg/m^2) and total duration of therapy (>5-11 months). Bladder fibrosis/contraction has been reported with intravesical administration. **Mitomycin is a potent vesicant, may cause ulceration, necrosis, cellulitis, and tissue sloughing if infiltrated.** Shortness of breath and bronchospasm have been reported in patients receiving vinca alkaloids in combination with or after mitomycin; may be managed with bronchodilators, steroids and/or oxygen. Safety and efficacy in children have not been established. **[U.S. Boxed Warning]: Should be administered under the supervision of an experienced cancer chemotherapy physician.**

Adverse Reactions
>10%:
Cardiovascular: CHF (3% to 15%) (doses >30 mg/m^2)
Central nervous system: Fever (14%)
Dermatologic: Alopecia, nail banding/discoloration
Gastrointestinal: Nausea, vomiting and anorexia (14%)
Hematologic: Anemia (19% to 24%); myelosuppression, common, dose limiting, delayed
Onset: 3 weeks
Nadir: 4-6 weeks
Recovery: 6-8 weeks
1% to 10%:
Dermatologic: Rash
Gastrointestinal: Stomatitis
Neuromuscular: Paresthesia
Renal: Creatinine increase (2%)
Respiratory: Interstitial pneumonitis, infiltrates, dyspnea, cough (7%)
<1% (Limited to important or life-threatening): Extravasation reactions, hemolytic uremic syndrome, malaise, pruritus, renal failure, bladder fibrosis/contraction (intravesical administration)

Drug Interactions

Avoid Concomitant Use
Avoid concomitant use of Mitomycin with any of the following: Natalizumab; Vaccines (Live)

Increased Effect/Toxicity
Mitomycin may increase the levels/effects of: Natalizumab; Vaccines (Live)

The levels/effects of Mitomycin may be increased by: Antineoplastic Agents (Vinca Alkaloids); P-Glycoprotein Inhibitors; Trastuzumab

Decreased Effect
Mitomycin may decrease the levels/effects of: Vaccines (Inactivated)

The levels/effects of Mitomycin may be decreased by: Echinacea; P-Glycoprotein Inducers

Ethanol/Nutrition/Herb Interactions Herb/Nutraceutical: Avoid black cohosh, dong quai in estrogen-dependent tumors.

Stability Store intact vials at controlled room temperature. Dilute powder with SWFI or 0.9% sodium chloride to a concentration of 0.5-1 mg/mL. Solution is stable for 7 days at room temperature and 14 days when refrigerated if protected from light. Solution of 0.5 mg/mL in a syringe is stable for 7 days at room temperature and 14 days when refrigerated and protected from light.
Further dilution to 20-40 mcg/mL:
In normal saline: Stable for 12 hours at room temperature.
In sodium lactate: Stable for 24 hours at room temperature.

Mechanism of Action Acts like an alkylating agent and produces DNA cross-linking (primarily with guanine and cytosine pairs); cell-cycle nonspecific; inhibits DNA and RNA synthesis; degrades preformed DNA, causes nuclear lysis and formation of giant cells. While not phase-specific *per se*, mitomycin has its maximum effect against cells in late G and early S phases.

Pharmacodynamics/Kinetics

Distribution: V_d: 22 L/m^2; high drug concentrations found in kidney, tongue, muscle, heart, and lung tissue; probably not distributed into the CNS

Metabolism: Hepatic

Half-life elimination: 23-78 minutes; Terminal: 50 minutes

Excretion: Urine (<10% as unchanged drug), with elevated serum concentrations

Dosage Refer to individual protocols. Children (unlabeled use) and Adults:

Single agent therapy: I.V.: 20 mg/m^2 every 6-8 weeks

Combination therapy: I.V.: 10 mg/m^2 every 6-8 weeks

Bladder carcinoma: Intravesicular instillation (unapproved route): 20-40 mg instilled into the bladder and retained for 3 hours up to 3 times/week for up to 20 procedures per course

Glaucoma surgery (unlabeled use): 0.2-0.5 mg (0.2-0.5 mg/mL solution)

Dosage adjustment in renal impairment: The FDA-approved labeling states to avoid use in patients with serum creatine >1.7 mg/dL, but offers no other dosage adjustment guidelines. The following guidelines have been used by some clinicians (Aronoff, 2007): Adults:

Cl_{cr} <10 mL/minute: Administer 75% of dose

Continuous ambulatory peritoneal dialysis (CAPD): Administer 75% of dose

Dosage adjustment in hepatic impairment: Although some mitomycin may be excreted in the bile, no specific guidelines regarding dosage adjustment in hepatic impairment are available.

Administration

I.V.: Administer slow I.V. push or by slow (15-30 minute) infusion via a freely-running dextrose or saline infusion. Consider using a central venous catheter.

Intravesicular (unlabeled route): Instill into bladder for up to 3 hours (rotate patient every 15-30 minutes)

Glaucoma surgery (unlabeled route): Apply to pledget and place in contact with surgical wound for 2-5 minutes (doses and techniques may vary)

Monitoring Parameters Platelet count, CBC with differential, hemoglobin, prothrombin time, renal and pulmonary function tests

Dosage Forms Excipient information presented when available (limited, particularly for generics); consult specific product labeling.

Injection, powder for reconstitution: 5 mg, 20 mg, 40 mg

- **Mitomycin-X** *see* Mitomycin *on page* 1005
- **Mitomycin-C** *see* Mitomycin *on page* 1005

Mitotane (MYE toe tane)

U.S. Brand Names Lysodren®

Canadian Brand Names Lysodren®

Index Terms NSC-38721; o,p'-DDD

Pharmacologic Category Antineoplastic Agent, Miscellaneous

Use Treatment of adrenocortical carcinoma

Unlabeled/Investigational Use Treatment of Cushing's syndrome

Pregnancy Risk Factor C

Pregnancy Considerations Animal studies have not been conducted. There are no adequate and well-controlled studies in pregnant women. Use during pregnancy only if clearly needed.

Lactation Excretion in breast milk unknown/not recommended

Medication Safety Issues

Sound-alike/look-alike issues:

Mitotane may be confused with mitomycin

High alert medication: The Institute for Safe Medication Practices (ISMP) includes this medication among its list of drugs which have a heightened risk of causing significant patient harm when used in error.

Contraindications Hypersensitivity to mitotane or any component of the formulation

Warnings/Precautions Hazardous agent - use appropriate precautions for handling and disposal. Steroid replacement with glucocorticoid, and sometimes mineralocorticoid, is necessary. It has been recommended that replacement therapy be initiated at the start of therapy, rather than waiting for evidence of adrenal insufficiency. Because mitotane can increase the metabolism of hydrocortisone, higher than usual replacement doses of the latter may be required. Surgically remove tumor tissues from metastatic masses prior to initiation of treatment; rapid cytotoxic effect may cause tumor hemorrhage. Observe patients for neurotoxicity with long-term (>2 years) use. Use caution with hepatic impairment; metabolism may be decreased. **[U.S. Boxed Warnings]: Acute adrenal insufficiency may occur in the face of shock, trauma, or infection. Mitotane should be discontinued temporarily in this setting and appropriate steroid coverage should be administered. Should be administered under the supervision of an experienced cancer chemotherapy physician.** Safety and efficacy in children have not been established.

Adverse Reactions

>10%:

Central nervous system: CNS depression (32%), somnolence (25%), dizziness/vertigo (15%)

Dermatologic: Skin rash (15%)

Gastrointestinal: Anorexia (24%), nausea (39%), vomiting (37%), diarrhea (13%)

Neuromuscular & skeletal: Weakness (12%)

1% to 10%:

Central nervous system: Headache (5%), confusion (3%)

Neuromuscular & skeletal: Muscle tremor (3%)

<1% and/or frequency not defined: Albuminuria, blurred vision, diplopia, flushing, hematuria, hemorrhagic cystitis, hypertension, hyperpyrexia, lens opacity, myalgia, orthostatic hypotension, protein bound iodine decreased, toxic retinopathy

Drug Interactions

Avoid Concomitant Use There are no known interactions where it is recommended to avoid concomitant use.

Increased Effect/Toxicity

Mitotane may increase the levels/effects of: Vitamin K Antagonists

Decreased Effect

Mitotane may decrease the levels/effects of: Vitamin K Antagonists

The levels/effects of Mitotane may be decreased by: Potassium-Sparing Diuretics

Ethanol/Nutrition/Herb Interactions Ethanol: Avoid ethanol (may increase CNS depression).

Stability Store at room temperature.

Mechanism of Action Causes adrenal cortical atrophy; drug affects mitochondria in adrenal cortical cells and decreases production of cortisol; also alters the peripheral metabolism of steroids

Pharmacodynamics/Kinetics

Absorption: Oral: ~35% to 40%

Distribution: Stored mainly in fat tissue but is found in all body tissues

Metabolism: Hepatic and other tissues

Half-life elimination: 18-159 days

Time to peak, serum: 3-5 hours

Excretion: Urine (10% as metabolites) and feces (1% to 17% as metabolites)

Dosage Adrenocortical carcinoma: Oral:
Children (unlabeled use): 1-2 g/day in divided doses, increasing gradually to a maximum of 5-7 g/day
Adults: Start at 2-6 g/day in 3-4 divided doses, then increase incrementally to 9-10 g/day in 3-4 divided doses (maximum daily dose: 18 g)
Dosing adjustment in hepatic impairment: Dose may need to be decreased in patients with liver disease

Monitoring Parameters Adrenal function; neurologic assessments with chronic (>2 years) use

Dosage Forms Excipient information presented when available (limited, particularly for generics); consult specific product labeling.
Tablet [scored]:
Lysodren®: 500 mg

Mitoxantrone (mye toe ZAN trone)

U.S. Brand Names Novantrone®

Canadian Brand Names Mitoxantrone Injection®; Novantrone®

Index Terms CL-232315; DHAD; DHAQ; Dihydroxyanthracenedione Dihydrochloride; Mitoxantrone Hydrochloride; Mitozantrone; NSC-301739

Pharmacologic Category Antineoplastic Agent, Anthracenedione

Use Treatment of acute nonlymphocytic leukemias, prostate cancer, lymphoma, secondary progressive or relapsing-remitting multiple sclerosis (MS)

Unlabeled/Investigational Use Treatment of pediatric acute leukemias, pediatric sarcoma

Pregnancy Risk Factor D

Pregnancy Considerations Adverse effects were noted in animal studies. May cause fetal harm if administered to a pregnant woman. There are no adequate and well-controlled studies in pregnant women. Pregnancy should be avoided while on treatment. Women with multiple sclerosis and who are biologically capable of becoming pregnant should have a pregnancy test prior to each dose.

Lactation Enters breast milk/contraindicated

Medication Safety Issues
Sound-alike/look-alike issues:
Mitoxantrone may be confused with methotrexate, mitomycin, Mutamycin®

High alert medication: The Institute for Safe Medication Practices (ISMP) includes this medication among its list of drug classes which have a heightened risk of causing significant patient harm when used in error.

Contraindications Hypersensitivity to mitoxantrone or any component of the formulation; multiple sclerosis with left ventricular ejection fraction (LVEF) <50% or clinically significant decrease in LVEF

Warnings/Precautions Hazardous agent - use appropriate precautions for handling and disposal.

[U.S. Boxed Warning]: Do not use if baseline neutrophil count <1500 cells/mm^3 (except for treatment of ANLL). Treatment may lead to severe myelosuppression; use with caution in patients with pre-existing myelosuppression.

[U.S. Boxed Warning]: May cause myocardial toxicity and potentially-fatal CHF; risk increases with cumulative dosing. Effects may be delayed. Predisposing factors for mitoxantrone-induced cardiotoxicity include prior anthracycline therapy, prior cardiovascular disease, concomitant use of cardiotoxic drugs, and mediastinal/pericardial irradiation. Not recommended for use when left ventricular ejection fraction (LVEF) <50%, or baseline LVEF below the lower limit of normal (LLN) for MS patients. Use in MS should be limited to a cumulative dose of ≤140 mg/m^2, and discontinued if LVEF falls below LLN or a significant decrease in LVEF is observed; decreases in LVEF and heart failure have been observed in patients with MS who have received cumulative doses <100 mg/m^2. Patients with MS should undergo annual LVEF evaluation following discontinuation of therapy to monitor for delayed cardiotoxicity.

[U.S. Boxed Warnings]: For I.V. administration only; may cause severe local tissue damage if extravasation occurs. Do not administer intrathecally; may cause serious and permanent neurologic damage. May cause urine, saliva, tears, and sweat to turn blue-green for 24 hours postinfusion. Whites of eyes may have blue-green tinge. **[U.S. Boxed Warning]: Has been associated with the development of secondary acute myelogenous leukemia and myelodysplasia.**

[U.S. Boxed Warning]: Should be administered under the supervision of an experienced cancer chemotherapy physician. Dosage should be reduced in patients with impaired hepatobiliary function; not for treatment of multiple sclerosis in patients with concurrent hepatic impairment. Not for treatment of primary progressive multiple sclerosis. Safety and efficacy in children have not been established.

Adverse Reactions Includes events reported with any indication; incidence varies based on treatment/dose
>10%:
Cardiovascular: Arrhythmia (3% to 18%), edema (10% to 31%), ECG changes (11%)
Central nervous system: Pain (8% to 41%), fatigue (up to 39%), fever (6% to 78%), headache (6% to 13%)
Dermatologic: Alopecia (20% to 61%), nail bed changes (11%)
Endocrine & metabolic: Amenorrhea (28% to 53%), menstrual disorder (26% to 61%), hyperglycemia (10% to 31%)
Gastrointestinal: Abdominal pain (9% to 15%), anorexia (22% to 25%), nausea (26% to 76%), constipation (10% to 16%), diarrhea (14% to 47%), GI bleeding (2% to 16%), mucositis (10% to 29%), stomatitis (8% to 29%), dyspepsia (5% to 14%), vomiting (6% to 11%), weight gain/loss (13% to 17%)
Genitourinary: Abnormal urine (6% to 11%), urinary tract infection (7% to 32%)
Hematologic: Neutropenia (79% to 100%), leukopenia (9% to 100%), lymphopenia (72% to 95%), anemia (5% to 75%), hemoglobin decreased (43%), thrombocytopenia (33% to 39%), petechiae/bruising (6% to 11%); myelosuppression (WBC: mild; platelets: mild; onset: 7-10 days; nadir: 14 days; recovery: 21 days)
Hepatic: Alkaline phosphatase increased (37%), transaminases increased (5% to 20%), GGT increased (3% to 15%)
Neuromuscular & skeletal: Weakness (24%)
Renal: BUN increased (22%), creatinine increased (13%), hematuria (11%)
Respiratory: Cough (5% to 13%), dyspnea (6% to 18%), upper respiratory tract infection (7% to 53%)
Miscellaneous: Fungal infection (9% to 15%), infection (4% to 18%), sepsis (ANLL 31% to 34%)
1% to 10%:
Cardiovascular: Ischemia (5%), LVEF decreased (≤5%), hypertension (4%), CHF (2% to 5%)
Central nervous system: Chills (5%), anxiety (5%), depression (5%), seizure (2% to 4%)
Dermatologic: Skin infection
Endocrine & metabolic: Hypocalcemia (10%), hypokalemia (7% to 10%), hyponatremia (9%), menorrhagia (7%)
Gastrointestinal: Aphthosis (10%)
Genitourinary: Impotence (7%), sterility (5%)
Hematologic: Granulocytopenia (6%), hemorrhage (6%)
Hepatic: Jaundice (3% to 7%)

Neuromuscular & skeletal: Back pain (8%), myalgia (5%), arthralgia (5%)
Ocular: Conjunctivitis (5%), blurred vision (3%)
Renal: Renal failure (8%), proteinuria (6%)
Respiratory: Rhinitis (10%), pneumonia (9%), sinusitis (6%)
Miscellaneous: Systemic infection, diaphoresis (9%), development of secondary leukemia (~1% to 2%)

<1% or frequency not defined (Limited to important or life-threatening): Acute leukemia, allergic reaction, anaphylactoid reactions, anaphylaxis, extravasation and phlebitis at the infusion site, interstitial pneumonitis (has occurred during combination chemotherapy), irritant chemotherapy with blue skin discoloration, rash, tachycardia

Drug Interactions

Metabolism/Transport Effects **Inhibits** CYP3A4 (weak)

Avoid Concomitant Use

Avoid concomitant use of Mitoxantrone with any of the following: Natalizumab; Vaccines (Live)

Increased Effect/Toxicity

Mitoxantrone may increase the levels/effects of: Natalizumab; Vaccines (Live)

The levels/effects of Mitoxantrone may be increased by: Trastuzumab

Decreased Effect

Mitoxantrone may decrease the levels/effects of: Vaccines (Inactivated)

The levels/effects of Mitoxantrone may be decreased by: Echinacea

Ethanol/Nutrition/Herb Interactions Herb/Nutraceutical: Avoid echinacea (may diminish the immunosuppressant effect).

Stability Store intact vials at 15°C to 25°C (59°F to 77°F); do not freeze. Opened vials may be stored at room temperature for 7 days or under refrigeration for up to 14 days. Dilute in at least 50 mL of NS or D_5W. Solutions diluted for administration are stable for 7 days at room temperature or under refrigeration.

Mechanism of Action Analogue of the anthracyclines, mitoxantrone intercalates DNA; binds to nucleic acids and inhibits DNA and RNA synthesis by template disordering and steric obstruction; replication is decreased by binding to DNA topoisomerase II and seems to inhibit the incorporation of uridine into RNA and thymidine into DNA; active throughout entire cell cycle

Pharmacodynamics/Kinetics

Absorption: Oral: Poor
Distribution: V_d: 14 L/kg; distributes into pleural fluid, kidney, thyroid, liver, heart, and red blood cells
Protein binding: >95%, 76% to albumin
Metabolism: Hepatic; pathway not determined
Half-life elimination: Terminal: 23-215 hours; may be prolonged with hepatic impairment
Excretion: Urine (6% to 11%; 65% as unchanged drug); feces (25%; 65% as unchanged drug)

Dosage Details concerning dosing in combination regimens should also be consulted. I.V. (dilute in D_5W or NS):

Acute leukemias:
Children ≤2 years (unlabeled use): 0.4 mg/kg/day once daily for 3-5 days
Children >2 years (unlabeled use): 8-12 mg/m^2/day once daily for 4-5 days
Adults:
Induction: 12 mg/m^2 once daily for 3 days; for incomplete response, may repeat at 12 mg/m^2 once daily for 2 days
Consolidation: 12 mg/m^2 once daily for 2 days, repeat in 4 weeks

Solid tumors:
Children (unlabeled use): 18-20 mg/m^2 every 3-4 weeks **or** 5-8 mg/m^2 every week
Adults: 12-14 mg/m^2 every 3-4 weeks **or** 2-4 mg/m^2/day for 5 days every 4 weeks

Hormone-refractory prostate cancer: Adults: 12-14 mg/m^2 every 3 weeks

Multiple sclerosis: Adults: 12 mg/m^2 every 3 months (maximum lifetime cumulative dose: 140 mg/m^2; discontinue use with LVEF <50% or clinically significant reduction in LVEF)

Dosing adjustment in renal impairment: Safety and efficacy have not been established
Hemodialysis: Supplemental dose is not necessary
Peritoneal dialysis: Supplemental dose is not necessary
Elderly: Clearance is decreased in elderly patients; use with caution

Dosing adjustment in hepatic impairment: Official dosage adjustment recommendations have not been established. Clearance is reduced in hepatic dysfunction; patients with severe hepatic dysfunction (bilirubin >3.4 mg/dL) have an AUC of 3 times greater than patients with normal hepatic function. Consider dose adjustments. **Note:** MS patients with hepatic impairment should not receive mitoxantrone.

Administration Avoid extravasation. Administered as a short (5-30 minutes) I.V. infusion; continuous 24-hour infusions are occasionally used. Although not generally recommended, mitoxantrone has been given as a rapid bolus over 1-3 minutes. High doses for bone marrow transplant are usually given as 1- to 4-hour infusions.

Monitoring Parameters CBC, serum uric acid (for treatment of leukemia), liver function tests; signs and symptoms of cardiac disease; evaluate ECG and LVEF prior to start of therapy and regularly during treatment, especially with the development of signs and symptoms of heart failure. In addition, for the treatment of multiple sclerosis, obtain pregnancy test and monitor LVEF prior to each dose and annually after completion of therapy (to monitor for delayed cardiotoxicity).

Dosage Forms Excipient information presented when available (limited, particularly for generics); consult specific product labeling. [DSC] = Discontinued product

Injection, solution [concentrate; preservative free]: 2 mg/mL (10 mL, 12.5 mL, 15 mL, 20 mL)
Novantrone®: 2 mg/mL (10 mL, 15 mL [DSC])

◆ **Mitoxantrone Hydrochloride** *see* Mitoxantrone *on page 1007*

◆ **Mitoxantrone Injection® (Can)** *see* Mitoxantrone *on page 1007*

◆ **Mitozantrone** *see* Mitoxantrone *on page 1007*

◆ **Mitrazol™ [OTC]** *see* Miconazole *on page 989*

◆ **MK383** *see* Tirofiban *on page 1478*

◆ **MK-0431** *see* SitaGLIPtin *on page 1375*

◆ **MK462** *see* Rizatriptan *on page 1333*

◆ **MK 0517** *see* Fosaprepitant *on page 666*

◆ **MK-0518** *see* Raltegravir *on page 1290*

◆ **MK594** *see* Losartan *on page 907*

◆ **MK0826** *see* Ertapenem *on page 543*

◆ **MK 869** *see* Aprepitant *on page 129*

◆ **MLN341** *see* Bortezomib *on page 204*

◆ **MMF** *see* Mycophenolate *on page 1026*

◆ **MMR** *see* Measles, Mumps, and Rubella Vaccines (Combined) *on page 923*

◆ **MMR-V** *see* Measles, Mumps, Rubella, and Varicella Virus Vaccine *on page 923*

- **MMRV** *see* Measles, Mumps, Rubella, and Varicella Virus Vaccine *on page 923*
- **Moban®** *see* Molindone *on page 1012*
- **Mobic®** *see* Meloxicam *on page 935*
- **Mobicox® (Can)** *see* Meloxicam *on page 935*

Modafinil (moe DAF i nil)

U.S. Brand Names Provigil®

Canadian Brand Names Alertec®; APO-Modafinil

Pharmacologic Category Stimulant

Use Improve wakefulness in patients with excessive daytime sleepiness associated with narcolepsy and shift work sleep disorder (SWSD); adjunctive therapy for obstructive sleep apnea/hypopnea syndrome (OSAHS)

Unlabeled/Investigational Use Attention-deficit/hyperactivity disorder (ADHD); treatment of fatigue in MS and other disorders

Restrictions C-IV

Pregnancy Risk Factor C

Pregnancy Considerations Embryotoxic effects have been observed in some, but not all animal studies. There are no adequate and well-controlled studies in pregnant women; use only when the potential risk of drug therapy is outweighed by the drug's benefits. Efficacy of steroidal contraceptives may be decreased; alternate means of contraception should be considered during therapy and for 1 month after modafinil is discontinued.

Lactation Excretion in breast milk unknown/use caution

Contraindications Hypersensitivity to modafinil, armodafinil, or any component of the formulation

Warnings/Precautions For use following complete evaluation of sleepiness and in conjunction with other standard treatments (eg, CPAP). The degree of sleepiness should be reassessed frequently; some patients may not return to a normal level of wakefulness. Use is not recommended with a history of angina, cardiac ischemia, recent history of myocardial infarction, left ventricular hypertrophy, or patients with mitral valve prolapse who have developed mitral valve prolapse syndrome with previous CNS stimulant use.

Serious and life-threatening rashes (including Stevens-Johnson syndrome and toxic epidermal necrolysis) have been reported with modafinil. Most cases have occurred within the first 5 weeks of therapy, however rare cases have occurred after long-term use. No risk factors have been identified to predict occurrence or severity. Patients should be advised to discontinue at first sign of rash. In addition, rare cases of multiorgan hypersensitivity reactions in association with modafinil use, and lone cases of angioedema and anaphylactoid reactions with armodafinil, have been reported. Signs and symptoms are diverse, reflecting the involvement of specific organs. Patients typically present with fever and rash associated with organ-system dysfunction. Patients should be advised to report any signs and symptoms related to these effects; discontinuation of therapy is recommended.

Caution should be exercised when modafinil is given to patients with a history of psychosis; may impair the ability to engage in potentially hazardous activities. Stimulants may unmask tics in individuals with coexisting Tourette's syndrome. Use caution with renal or hepatic impairment (dosage adjustment in hepatic dysfunction is recommended). Safety and efficacy have not been established in children <16 years of age (U.S. labeling) or <18 years of age (Canadian labeling).

Adverse Reactions

>10%:

Central nervous system: Headache (34%, dose related)

Gastrointestinal: Nausea (11%)

1% to 10%:

Cardiovascular: Chest pain (3%), hypertension (3%), palpitation (2%), tachycardia (2%), vasodilation (2%), edema (1%)

Central nervous system: Nervousness (7%), dizziness (5%), depression (2%), anxiety (5%; dose related), insomnia (5%), somnolence (2%), chills (1%), agitation (1%), confusion (1%), emotional lability (1%), vertigo (1%)

Dermatologic: Rash (1%; includes some severe cases requiring hospitalization)

Gastrointestinal: Diarrhea (6%), dyspepsia (5%), xerostomia (4%), anorexia (4%), constipation (2%), flatulence (1%), mouth ulceration (1%), taste perversion (1%)

Genitourinary: Abnormal urine (1%), hematuria (1%), pyuria (1%)

Hematologic: Eosinophilia (1%)

Hepatic: LFTs abnormal (2%)

Neuromuscular & skeletal: Back pain (6%), paresthesia (2%), dyskinesia (1%), hyperkinesia (1%), hypertonia (1%), neck rigidity (1%), tremor (1%)

Ocular: Amblyopia (1%), eye pain (1%), vision abnormal (1%)

Respiratory: Pharyngitis (4%), rhinitis (7%), lung disorder (2%), asthma (1%), epistaxis (1%)

Miscellaneous: Diaphoresis

Postmarketing and/or case reports: Agranulocytosis, anaphylactic reaction, angioedema, DRESS syndrome, erythema multiforme, hypersensitivity syndrome (multi-organ), mania, psychosis, Stevens-Johnson syndrome, toxic epidermal necrolysis

Drug Interactions

Metabolism/Transport Effects **Substrate** of CYP3A4 (major); **Inhibits** CYP1A2 (weak), 2A6 (weak), 2C9 (weak), 2C19 (strong), 2E1 (weak), 3A4 (weak); **Induces** CYP1A2 (weak), 2B6 (weak), 3A4 (weak)

Avoid Concomitant Use

Avoid concomitant use of Modafinil with any of the following: Iobenguane I 123

Increased Effect/Toxicity

Modafinil may increase the levels/effects of: CYP2C19 Substrates; Sympathomimetics

The levels/effects of Modafinil may be increased by: Cannabinoids; CYP3A4 Inhibitors (Moderate); CYP3A4 Inhibitors (Strong); Dasatinib

Decreased Effect

Modafinil may decrease the levels/effects of: Iobenguane I 123; Maraviroc; Oral Contraceptive (Estrogens)

The levels/effects of Modafinil may be decreased by: CYP3A4 Inducers (Strong); Deferasirox; Herbs (CYP3A4 Inducers)

Ethanol/Nutrition/Herb Interactions

Ethanol: Avoid or limit ethanol.

Food: Delays absorption, but does not affect bioavailability.

Mechanism of Action The exact mechanism of action is unclear, it does not appear to alter the release of dopamine or norepinephrine, it may exert its stimulant effects by decreasing GABA-mediated neurotransmission, although this theory has not yet been fully evaluated; several studies also suggest that an intact central alpha-adrenergic system is required for modafinil's activity; the drug increases high-frequency alpha waves while decreasing both delta and theta wave activity, and these effects are consistent with generalized increases in mental alertness

Pharmacodynamics/Kinetics Modafinil is a racemic compound (10% *d*-isomer and 90% *l*-isomer at steady state) whose enantiomers have different pharmacokinetics

Distribution: V_d: 0.9 L/kg

Protein binding: 60%, primarily to albumin

Metabolism: Hepatic; multiple pathways including CYP3A4

Half-life elimination: Effective half-life: 15 hours; Steady-state: 2-4 days
Time to peak, serum: 2-4 hours
Excretion: Urine (as metabolites, <10% as unchanged drug)

Dosage Oral:
Children: ADHD (unlabeled use): 50-100 mg once daily
Adults:
ADHD (unlabeled use): 100-300 mg once daily
Narcolepsy, obstructive sleep apnea/hypopnea syndrome (OSAHS): Initial: 200 mg as a single daily dose in the morning
Shift work sleep disorder (SWSD): Initial: 200 mg as a single dose taken ~1 hour prior to start of work shift
Note: Doses of 400 mg/day, given as a single dose, have been well tolerated, but there is no consistent evidence that this dose confers additional benefit.
Elderly: Elimination of modafinil and its metabolites may be reduced as a consequence of aging and as a result, consider initiating dose at 100 mg once daily.
Dosing adjustment in renal impairment: Safety and efficacy have not been established in severe renal impairment.
Dosing adjustment in hepatic impairment: Dose should be reduced to one-half of that recommended for patients with normal liver function.

Monitoring Parameters Levels of sleepiness; blood pressure in patients with hypertension

When used for the treatment of ADHD, thoroughly evaluate for cardiovascular risk. Monitor heart rate, blood pressure, and consider obtaining ECG prior to initiation (Vetter, 2008).

Dosage Forms Excipient information presented when available (limited, particularly for generics); consult specific product labeling.
Tablet:
Provigil®: 100 mg, 200 mg

◆ **Modecate® (Can)** *see* Fluphenazine *on page 641*

◆ **Modecate® Concentrate (Can)** *see* Fluphenazine *on page 641*

◆ **Modicon®** *see* Ethinyl Estradiol and Norethindrone *on page 581*

◆ **Modified Dakin's Solution** *see* Sodium Hypochlorite Solution *on page 1384*

◆ **Modified Shohl's Solution** *see* Sodium Citrate and Citric Acid *on page 1383*

◆ **Moduret (Can)** *see* Amiloride and Hydrochlorothiazide *on page 85*

Moexipril (mo EKS i pril)

U.S. Brand Names Univasc®

Index Terms Moexipril Hydrochloride

Pharmacologic Category Angiotensin-Converting Enzyme (ACE) Inhibitor

Additional Appendix Information
Angiotensin Agents *on page 1632*

Use Treatment of hypertension, alone or in combination with thiazide diuretics

Pregnancy Risk Factor C (1st trimester); D (2nd and 3rd trimesters)

Pregnancy Considerations Due to adverse events observed in some animal studies, moexipril is considered pregnancy category C during the first trimester. Based on human data, moexipril is considered pregnancy category D if used during the second and third trimesters (per the manufacturer; however, one study suggests that fetal injury may occur at anytime during pregnancy). First trimester exposure to ACE inhibitors may cause major congenital malformations. An increased risk of cardiovascular and/or central nervous system malformations was observed in one study; however, an increased risk of teratogenic events was not observed in other studies. Second and third trimester use of an ACE inhibitor is associated with oligohydramnios. Oligohydramnios due to decreased fetal renal function may lead to fetal limb contractures, craniofacial deformation, and hypoplastic lung development. The use of ACE inhibitors during the second and third trimesters is also associated with anuria, hypotension, renal failure (reversible or irreversible), skull hypoplasia, and death in the fetus/neonate. Chronic maternal hypertension itself is also associated with adverse events in the fetus/infant. ACE inhibitors are not recommended during pregnancy to treat maternal hypertension or heart failure. Those who are planning a pregnancy should be considered for other medication options if an ACE inhibitor is currently prescribed or the ACE inhibitor should be discontinued as soon as possible once pregnancy is detected. The exposed fetus should be monitored for fetal growth, amniotic fluid volume, and organ formation. Infants exposed to an ACE inhibitor *in utero*, especially during the second and third trimester, should be monitored for hyperkalemia, hypotension, and oliguria

[U.S. Boxed Warning]: Based on human data, ACE inhibitors can cause injury and death to the developing fetus when used in the second and third trimesters. ACE inhibitors should be discontinued as soon as possible once pregnancy is detected.

Lactation Excretion in breast milk unknown/use caution

Medication Safety Issues
Sound-alike/look-alike issues:
Moexipril may be confused with Monopril®

Contraindications Hypersensitivity to moexipril or any component of the formulation; angioedema related to previous treatment with an ACE inhibitor

Warnings/Precautions Anaphylactic reactions may occur rarely with ACE inhibitors. At any time during treatment (especially following first dose) angioedema may occur rarely with ACE inhibitors; it may involve the head and neck (potentially compromising airway) or the intestine (presenting with abdominal pain). African-Americans and patients with idiopathic or hereditary angioedema may be at an increased risk. Prolonged frequent monitoring may be required especially if tongue, glottis, or larynx are involved as they are associated with airway obstruction. Patients with a history of airway surgery may have a higher risk of airway obstruction. Aggressive early and appropriate management is critical. Use in patients with previous angioedema associated with ACE inhibitor therapy is contraindicated. Severe anaphylactoid reactions may be seen during hemodialysis (eg, CVVHD) with high-flux dialysis membranes (eg, AN69), and rarely, during low density lipoprotein apheresis with dextran sulfate cellulose. Rare cases of anaphylactoid reactions have been reported in patients undergoing sensitization treatment with hymenoptera (bee, wasp) venom while receiving ACE inhibitors.

Symptomatic hypotension with or without syncope can occur with ACE inhibitors (usually with the first several doses); effects are most often observed in volume depleted patients; correct volume depletion prior to initiation; close monitoring of patient is required especially with initial dosing and dosing increases; blood pressure must be lowered at a rate appropriate for the patient's clinical condition. Initiation of therapy in patients with ischemic heart disease or cerebrovascular disease warrants close observation due to the potential consequences posed by falling blood pressure (eg, MI, stroke). Use with caution in hypertrophic cardiomyopathy with outflow tract obstruction, severe aortic stenosis, or before, during, or immediately after major surgery. **[U.S. Boxed Warning]: Based on human data, ACEIs can cause injury and death to the developing fetus when used in the second and third trimesters. ACEIs should be discontinued as soon as possible once pregnancy is detected.**

Hyperkalemia may occur with ACE inhibitors; risk factors include renal dysfunction, diabetes mellitus, concomitant use of potassium-sparing diuretics, potassium supplements, and/or potassium-containing salts. Use cautiously, if at all, with these agents and monitor potassium closely. Cough may occur with ACE inhibitors. Other causes of cough should be considered (eg, pulmonary congestion in patients with heart failure) and excluded prior to discontinuation.

May be associated with deterioration of renal function and/or increases in serum creatinine, particularly in patients with low renal blood flow (eg, renal artery stenosis, heart failure) whose glomerular filtration rate (GFR) is dependent on efferent arteriolar vasoconstriction by angiotensin II; deterioration may result in oliguria, acute renal failure, and progressive azotemia. Small increases in serum creatinine may occur following initiation; consider discontinuation only in patients with progressive and/or significant deterioration in renal function. Use with caution in patients with unstented unilateral/bilateral renal artery stenosis. When unstented bilateral renal artery stenosis is present, use is generally avoided due to the elevated risk of deterioration in renal function unless possible benefits outweigh risks.

Rare toxicities associated with ACE inhibitors include cholestatic jaundice (which may progress to fulminant hepatic necrosis), agranulocytosis, neutropenia, or leukopenia with myeloid hypoplasia. Patients with collagen vascular diseases (especially with concomitant renal impairment) or renal impairment alone may be at increased risk for hematologic toxicity; periodically monitor CBC with differential in these patients. Safety and efficacy have not been established in children.

Adverse Reactions

1% to 10%:

- Cardiovascular: Hypotension, peripheral edema
- Central nervous system: Headache, dizziness, fatigue
- Dermatologic: Flushing, rash
- Endocrine & metabolic: Hyperkalemia, hyponatremia
- Gastrointestinal: Diarrhea, nausea, heartburn
- Genitourinary: Polyuria
- Neuromuscular & skeletal: Myalgia
- Renal: Reversible increases in creatinine or BUN
- Respiratory: Cough, pharyngitis, upper respiratory infection, sinusitis

<1% (Limited to important or life-threatening): Alopecia, anemia, angioedema, arrhythmia, bronchospasm, cerebrovascular accident, chest pain, dyspnea, elevated LFTs, eosinophilic pneumonitis, hepatitis, hypercholesterolemia, MI, oliguria, orthostatic hypotension, palpitation, proteinuria, syncope

Drug Interactions

Avoid Concomitant Use There are no known interactions where it is recommended to avoid concomitant use.

Increased Effect/Toxicity

Moexipril may increase the levels/effects of: Allopurinol; Amifostine; AzaTHIOprine; CycloSPORINE; Ferric Gluconate; Gold Sodium Thiomalate; Lithium; RiTUXimab

The levels/effects of Moexipril may be increased by: Angiotensin II Receptor Blockers; Diazoxide; Eplerenone; Herbs (Hypotensive Properties); Loop Diuretics; Potassium Salts; Potassium-Sparing Diuretics; Prostacyclin Analogues; Sirolimus; Temsirolimus; Thiazide Diuretics; Trimethoprim

Decreased Effect

The levels/effects of Moexipril may be decreased by: Antacids; Aprotinin; Herbs (Hypertensive Properties); Methylphenidate; Nonsteroidal Anti-Inflammatory Agents; Salicylates; Yohimbine

Ethanol/Nutrition/Herb Interactions

Food: Food may delay and reduce peak serum levels.

Herb/Nutraceutical: Avoid bayberry, blue cohosh, cayenne, ephedra, ginger, ginseng (American), kola, licorice (may worsen hypertension). Avoid black cohosh, California poppy, coleus, golden seal, hawthorn, mistletoe, periwinkle, quinine, shepherd's purse (may have increased antihypertensive effect).

Mechanism of Action Competitive inhibitor of angiotensin-converting enzyme (ACE); prevents conversion of angiotensin I to angiotensin II, a potent vasoconstrictor; results in lower levels of angiotensin II which causes an increase in plasma renin activity and a reduction in aldosterone secretion

Pharmacodynamics/Kinetics

Absorption: Incomplete

Onset of action: Peak effect: 1-2 hours

Duration: >24 hours

Distribution: V_d (moexiprilat): 180 L

Protein binding, plasma: Moexipril: 90%; Moexiprilat: 50% to 70%

Metabolism: Parent drug: Hepatic and via GI tract to moexiprilat, 1000 times more potent than parent

Bioavailability: Moexiprilat: 13%; reduced with food (AUC decreased by ~40%)

Half-life elimination: Moexipril: 1 hour; Moexiprilat: 2-9 hours

Time to peak: 1.5 hours

Excretion: Feces (50%)

Dosage Adults: Oral: Initial: 7.5 mg once daily (in patients **not** receiving diuretics), 1 hour prior to a meal **or** 3.75 mg once daily (when combined with thiazide diuretics); maintenance dose: 7.5-30 mg/day in 1 or 2 divided doses 1 hour before meals

Dosing adjustment in renal impairment: Cl_{cr} ≤40 mL/minute: Patients may be cautiously placed on 3.75 mg once daily, then upwardly titrated to a maximum of 15 mg/day.

Dietary Considerations Administer on an empty stomach.

Monitoring Parameters Blood pressure; serum creatinine and potassium; if patient has collagen vascular disease and/or renal impairment, periodically monitor CBC with differential

Test Interactions Increases BUN, creatinine, potassium, positive Coombs' [direct]; decreases cholesterol (S); may cause false-positive results in urine acetone determinations using sodium nitroprusside reagent

Dosage Forms Excipient information presented when available (limited, particularly for generics); consult specific product labeling.

Tablet, as hydrochloride [scored]: 7.5 mg, 15 mg

Univasc®: 7.5 mg, 15 mg

Moexipril and Hydrochlorothiazide

(mo EKS i pril & hye droe klor oh THYE a zide)

U.S. Brand Names Uniretic®

Canadian Brand Names Uniretic®

Index Terms Hydrochlorothiazide and Moexipril

Pharmacologic Category Angiotensin-Converting Enzyme (ACE) Inhibitor; Diuretic, Thiazide

Use Treatment of hypertension; not indicated for initial treatment of hypertension

Pregnancy Risk Factor C/D (2nd and 3rd trimesters)

Dosage Adults: Oral: 7.5-30 mg of moexipril, taken either in a single or divided dose one hour before meals; hydrochlorothiazide dose should be ≤50 mg/day

Additional Information Complete prescribing information for this medication should be consulted for additional detail.

Dosage Forms Excipient information presented when available (limited, particularly for generics); consult specific product labeling.

Tablet [scored]:

7.5/12.5: Moexipril hydrochloride 7.5 mg and hydrochlorothiazide 12.5 mg

15/12.5: Moexipril hydrochloride 15 mg and hydrochlorothiazide 12.5 mg

15/25: Moexipril hydrochloride 15 mg and hydrochlorothiazide 25 mg

Uniretic®:

7.5/12.5: Moexipril hydrochloride 7.5 mg and hydrochlorothiazide 12.5 mg

15/12.5: Moexipril hydrochloride 15 mg and hydrochlorothiazide 12.5 mg

15/25: Moexipril hydrochloride 15 mg and hydrochlorothiazide 25 mg

◆ **Moexipril Hydrochloride** *see* Moexipril *on page 1010*

Molindone (moe LIN done)

U.S. Brand Names Moban®

Canadian Brand Names Moban®

Index Terms Molindone Hydrochloride

Pharmacologic Category Antipsychotic Agent, Typical

Additional Appendix Information

Antipsychotic Agents *on page 1644*

Use Management of schizophrenia

Unlabeled/Investigational Use Management of psychotic disorders; behavioral symptoms associated with dementia (elderly); psychosis/agitation related to Alzheimer's dementia

Pregnancy Risk Factor C

Medication Safety Issues

Sound-alike/look-alike issues:

Molindone may be confused with Mobidin®

Moban® may be confused with Mobidin®, Modane®

Dosage Oral:

Children: Schizophrenia/psychoses (unlabeled use):

3-5 years: 1-2.5 mg/day in 4 divided doses

5-12 years: 0.5-1 mg/kg/day in 4 divided doses

Adults: Schizophrenia/psychoses:

Initial: 50-75 mg/day, may increase to 100 mg/day in 3-4 days; may further increase dose gradually to maximum of 225 mg/day

Maintenance: 5-15 mg (mild symptoms) or 10-25 mg (moderate symptoms) 3-4 times/day (up to 225 mg/day may be required in severe cases)

Elderly: Behavioral symptoms associated with dementia (unlabeled use): Initial: 5-10 mg 1-2 times/day; increase at 4- to 7-day intervals by 5-10 mg/day; increase dosing intervals (bid, tid, etc) as necessary to control response or side effects.

Additional Information Complete prescribing information for this medication should be consulted for additional detail.

Dosage Forms Excipient information presented when available (limited, particularly for generics); consult specific product labeling.

Tablet, as hydrochloride: 5 mg, 10 mg, 25 mg, 50 mg

◆ **Molindone Hydrochloride** *see* Molindone *on page 1012*

◆ **MOM** *see* Magnesium Hydroxide *on page 915*

◆ **Momentum® [OTC]** *see* Magnesium Salicylate *on page 917*

Mometasone (moe MET a sone)

U.S. Brand Names Asmanex® Twisthaler®; Elocon®; Nasonex®

Canadian Brand Names Elocom®; Nasonex®; PMS-Mometasone; ratio-Mometasone; Taro-Mometasone

Index Terms Mometasone Furoate

Pharmacologic Category Corticosteroid, Inhalant (Oral); Corticosteroid, Nasal; Corticosteroid, Topical

Additional Appendix Information

Corticosteroids *on page 1652*

Use Relief of the inflammatory and pruritic manifestations of corticosteroid-responsive dermatoses (medium potency topical corticosteroid); treatment of nasal symptoms of seasonal and perennial allergic rhinitis; prevention of nasal symptoms associated with seasonal allergic rhinitis; treatment of nasal polyps in adults; maintenance treatment of asthma as prophylactic therapy or as a supplement in asthma patients requiring oral corticosteroids for the purpose of decreasing or eliminating the oral corticosteroid requirement

Pregnancy Risk Factor C

Pregnancy Considerations There are no adequate and well-controlled studies using topical or inhaled mometasone during pregnancy. However, teratogenicity and intrauterine growth retardation has been reported in animal studies with some topical steroids. Avoid use of large amounts for long periods of time during pregnancy. Hypoadrenalism may occur in infants born to women receiving corticosteroids during pregnancy. Monitor these infants closely after birth. Following oral inhalation, <1% of a single 400 mcg dose is available systemically in the mother; inhaled corticosteroids are considered first-line agents for the treatment of persistent of asthma during pregnancy.

Lactation Excretion in breast milk unknown/use caution

Medication Safety Issues

Sound-alike/look-alike issues:

Elocon® lotion may be confused with ophthalmic solutions. Manufacturer's labeling emphasizes the product is **NOT** for use in the eyes.

Contraindications Hypersensitivity to mometasone or any component of the formulation; treatment of acute bronchospasm (oral inhaler)

Warnings/Precautions May cause hypercorticism or suppression of hypothalamic-pituitary-adrenal (HPA) axis, particularly in younger children or in patients receiving high doses for prolonged periods. HPA axis suppression may lead to adrenal crisis. Withdrawal and discontinuation of a corticosteroid should be done slowly and carefully. Particular care is required when patients are transferred from systemic corticosteroids to inhaled products due to possible adrenal insufficiency or withdrawal from steroids, including an increase in allergic symptoms. Patients receiving >20 mg per day of prednisone (or equivalent) may be most susceptible. Fatalities have occurred due to adrenal insufficiency in asthmatic patients during and after transfer from systemic corticosteroids to aerosol steroids; aerosol steroids do not provide the systemic steroid needed to treat patients having trauma, surgery, or infections. When transferring to oral inhaler, previously-suppressed allergic conditions (rhinitis, conjunctivitis, eczema) may be unmasked.

Bronchospasm may occur with wheezing after inhalation; if this occurs stop steroid and treat with a fast-acting bronchodilator. Supplemental steroids (oral or parenteral) may be needed during stress or severe asthma attacks. Not to be used in status asthmaticus or for the relief of acute bronchospasm. Corticosteroid use may cause psychiatric disturbances, including depression, euphoria, insomnia, mood swings, and personality changes. Pre-existing psychiatric conditions may be exacerbated by corticosteroid use. Prolonged use of corticosteroids may also increase the incidence of secondary infection, mask acute infection (including fungal infections), prolong or exacerbate viral infections, or limit response to vaccines. Exposure to chickenpox should be avoided; corticosteroids should not be used to treat ocular herpes simplex. Corticosteroids should not be used for cerebral malaria or viral hepatitis. Close observation is required in patients with latent tuberculosis and/or TB reactivity; restrict use in active TB (only in conjunction with antituberculosis treatment). Prolonged treatment with corticosteroids has been associated with the development of Kaposi's sarcoma (case reports); if noted, discontinuation of therapy should be considered.

Use with caution in patients with thyroid disease, hepatic impairment, renal impairment, cardiovascular disease, diabetes, glaucoma, cataracts, myasthenia gravis, patients with or who are at risk for osteoporosis, patients at risk for seizures, or GI diseases (diverticulitis, peptic ulcer, ulcerative colitis) due to perforation risk. Use caution following acute MI (corticosteroids have been associated with myocardial rupture). Because of the risk of adverse effects, systemic corticosteroids should be used cautiously in the elderly in the smallest possible effective dose for the shortest duration. Avoid nasal corticosteroid use in patients with recent nasal septal ulcers, nasal surgery or nasal trauma until healing has occurred.

Orally-inhaled and intranasal corticosteroids may cause a reduction in growth velocity in pediatric patients (~1 centimeter per year [range: 0.3-1.8 cm per year] and related to dose and duration of exposure). To minimize the systemic effects of orally-inhaled and intranasal corticosteroids, each patient should be titrated to the lowest effective dose. Growth should be routinely monitored in pediatric patients. Prior to use, the dose and duration of treatment should be based on the risk versus benefit for each individual patient. In general, use the smallest effective dose for the shortest duration of time to minimize adverse events. A gradual tapering of dose may be required prior to discontinuing therapy. There have been reports of systemic corticosteroid withdrawal symptoms (eg, joint/muscle pain, lassitude, depression) when withdrawing inhalation therapy.

Adverse Reactions

Nasal/oral inhalation:

>10%:

- Central nervous system: Headache (17% to 26%), fatigue (oral inhalation 1% to 13%), depression (oral inhalation 11%)
- Neuromuscular & skeletal: Musculoskeletal pain (1% to 22%), arthralgia (oral inhalation 13%)
- Respiratory: Rhinitis (2% to 20%), upper respiratory infection (5% to 15%), pharyngitis (8% to 13%), cough (nasal inhalation 7% to 13%), epistaxis (1% to 11%)
- Miscellaneous: Viral infection (nasal inhalation 8% to 14%), oral candidiasis (oral inhalation 4% to 22%)

1% to 10%:

- Cardiovascular: Chest pain
- Central nervous system: Pain
- Gastrointestinal: Abdominal pain, anorexia, dry throat (oral inhalation), diarrhea, dyspepsia, flatulence, gastroenteritis, nausea, vomiting
- Genitourinary: Dysmenorrhea
- Neuromuscular & skeletal: Back pain, myalgia
- Ocular: Conjunctivitis
- Otic: Earache, otitis media
- Respiratory: Asthma, bronchitis, dysphonia, nasal irritation, sinusitis, wheezing
- Miscellaneous: Accidental injury, flu-like syndrome

<1% (Limited to important or life-threatening): Anaphylaxis, angioedema, growth suppression, nasal candidiasis, nasal burning and irritation, nasal septal perforation, nasal ulcers, oral candidiasis (nasal inhalation), smell disturbance (rare), taste disturbance (rare)

Topical:

1% to 10%: Dermatologic: Bacterial skin infection, burning, furunculosis, pruritus, skin atrophy, tingling/stinging

<1% (Limited to important or life-threatening): Folliculitis, glucocorticoid levels decreased (pediatric patients), moniliasis, paresthesia, rosacea, skin depigmentation, skin atrophy

Cataract formation, reduction in growth velocity, and HPA axis suppression have been reported with other corticosteroids

Drug Interactions

Metabolism/Transport Effects **Substrate** of CYP3A4 (minor)

Avoid Concomitant Use There are no known interactions where it is recommended to avoid concomitant use.

Increased Effect/Toxicity There are no known significant interactions involving an increase in effect.

Decreased Effect

Mometasone may decrease the levels/effects of: Corticorelin

Stability

Cream: Store between 2°C to 25°C (36°F to 77°F).

Lotion: Store between 2°C to 30°C (36°F to 86°F).

Nasal spray: Store at room temperature of 15°C to 30°C (59°F to 86°F). Protect from light.

Ointment: Store at room temperature of 15°C to 30°C (59°F to 86°F).

Oral Inhaler: Store at room temperature of 25°C (77°F). Discard when oral dose counter reads "00" (or 45 days after opening the foil pouch).

Mechanism of Action May depress the formation, release, and activity of endogenous chemical mediators of inflammation (kinins, histamine, liposomal enzymes, prostaglandins). Leukocytes and macrophages may have to be present for the initiation of responses mediated by the above substances. Inhibits the margination and subsequent cell migration to the area of injury, and also reverses the dilatation and increased vessel permeability in the area resulting in decreased access of cells to the sites of injury.

Pharmacodynamics/Kinetics

Absorption:

- Nasal inhalation: Mometasone furoate monohydrate: Undetectable in plasma
- Ointment: 0.7%; increased by occlusive dressings
- Oral inhalation: Systemic absorption <1%

Protein binding: Mometasone furoate: 98% to 99%

Metabolism: Mometasone furoate: Hepatic via CYP3A4; forms metabolite

Half-life elimination: Oral inhalation: 5 hours

Excretion: Feces, bile, urine

Dosage

Oral inhalation:

- Children 4-11 years: 110 mcg once daily in the evening (maximum 110 mcg/day)
- Children ≥12 years and Adults: Previous therapy:
  - Bronchodilators or inhaled corticosteroids: Initial: 1 inhalation (220 mcg) daily (maximum 2 inhalations or 440 mcg/day); may be given in the evening or in divided doses twice daily
  - Oral corticosteroids: Initial: 440 mcg twice daily (maximum 880 mcg/day); prednisone should be reduced no faster than 2.5 mg/day on a weekly basis, beginning after at least 1 week of mometasone furoate use

NIH Asthma Guidelines (NIH, 2007): Children ≥12 years and Adults:
"Low" dose: 220 mcg/day
"Medium" dose: 440 mcg/day
"High" dose: >440 mcg/day
Note: Maximum effects may not be evident for 1-2 weeks or longer; dose should be titrated to effect, using the lowest possible dose
Nasal spray:
Allergic rhinitis:
Children 2-11 years: 1 spray (50 mcg) in each nostril daily
Children ≥12 years and Adults: 2 sprays (100 mcg) in each nostril daily; when used for the prevention of allergic rhinitis, treatment should begin 2-4 weeks prior to pollen season
Nasal polyps: Adults: 2 sprays (100 mcg) in each nostril twice daily; 2 sprays (100 mcg) once daily may be effective in some patients
Topical: Apply sparingly, do not use occlusive dressings. Therapy should be discontinued when control is achieved; if no improvement is seen in 2 weeks, reassessment of diagnosis may be necessary.
Cream, ointment: Children ≥2 years and Adults: Apply a thin film to affected area once daily; do not use in pediatric patients for longer than 3 weeks
Lotion: Children ≥12 years and Adults: Apply a few drops to affected area once daily

Dietary Considerations Asmanex® Twisthaler® contains lactose.

Administration
Nasal spray: Prior to first use, prime pump by actuating 10 times or until fine spray appears; may store for a maximum of 1 week without repriming. Spray should be administered once or twice daily, at a regular interval. Shake well prior to use.
Oral inhalation: Exhale fully prior to bringing the Twisthaler® up to the mouth. Place between lips and inhale quickly and deeply. Do not breathe out through the inhaler. Remove inhaler and hold breath for 10 seconds if possible.
Topical: Apply sparingly; avoid eyes, face, underarms, and groin. Do not wrap or bandage affected area.

Monitoring Parameters HPA axis suppression
Asthma: FEV_1, peak flow, and/or other pulmonary function tests

Dosage Forms Excipient information presented when available (limited, particularly for generics); consult specific product labeling.
Cream, topical, as furoate: 0.1% (15 g, 45 g)
Elocon®: 0.1% (15 g, 45 g)
Lotion, topical, as furoate: 0.1% (30 mL, 60 mL)
Elocon®: 0.1% (30 mL, 60 mL) [contains isopropyl alcohol 40%]
Ointment, topical, as furoate: 0.1% (15 g, 45 g)
Elocon®: 0.1% (15 g, 45 g)
Powder for oral inhalation, as furoate:
Asmanex® Twisthaler®: 110 mcg (30 units) [contains lactose; delivers 100 mcg/actuation]; 220 mcg (14 units, 30 units, 60 units, 120 units) [contains lactose; delivers 200 mcg/actuation]
Suspension, intranasal, as furoate [spray]:
Nasonex®: 50 mcg/spray (17 g) [delivers 120 sprays; contains benzalkonium chloride]

◆ **Mometasone Furoate** *see* Mometasone *on page 1012*
◆ **MOM/Mineral Oil Emulsion** *see* Magnesium Hydroxide and Mineral Oil *on page 916*
◆ **Monacolin K** *see* Lovastatin *on page 910*
◆ **Monarc-M™** *see* Antihemophilic Factor (Human) *on page 120*
◆ **Monistat® (Can)** *see* Miconazole *on page 989*
◆ **Monistat® 1 Combination Pack [OTC]** *see* Miconazole *on page 989*
◆ **Monistat® 3 [OTC]** *see* Miconazole *on page 989*
◆ **Monistat® 3 (Can)** *see* Miconazole *on page 989*
◆ **Monistat® 3 Combination Pack [OTC]** *see* Miconazole *on page 989*
◆ **Monistat® 7 [OTC]** *see* Miconazole *on page 989*
◆ **Monistat-Derm® [DSC]** *see* Miconazole *on page 989*
◆ **Monitan® (Can)** *see* Acebutolol *on page 25*
◆ **Monoclate-P®** *see* Antihemophilic Factor (Human) *on page 120*
◆ **Monoclonal Antibody** *see* Muromonab-CD3 *on page 1024*
◆ **Monocor® (Can)** *see* Bisoprolol *on page 200*
◆ **Monodox®** *see* Doxycycline *on page 491*
◆ **Monoethanolamine** *see* Ethanolamine Oleate *on page 574*
◆ **Monoket®** *see* Isosorbide Mononitrate *on page 824*
◆ **MonoNessa®** *see* Ethinyl Estradiol and Norgestimate *on page 584*
◆ **Mononine®** *see* Factor IX *on page 599*
◆ **Monopril®** *see* Fosinopril *on page 670*

Montelukast (mon te LOO kast)

U.S. Brand Names Singulair®
Canadian Brand Names Singulair®
Index Terms Montelukast Sodium
Pharmacologic Category Leukotriene-Receptor Antagonist
Use Prophylaxis and chronic treatment of asthma; relief of symptoms of seasonal allergic rhinitis and perennial allergic rhinitis; prevention of exercise-induced bronchospasm
Unlabeled/Investigational Use Acute asthma
Pregnancy Risk Factor B
Pregnancy Considerations Montelukast was not teratogenic in animal studies, however, there are no adequate and well-controlled studies in pregnant women. Use during pregnancy only if clearly needed. Based on limited data, structural defects have been reported in neonates exposed to montelukast *in utero*, however, a specific pattern and relationship to montelukast has not been established. Healthcare providers should report any prenatal exposures to the montelukast pregnancy registry at (800) 986-8999.
Lactation Excretion in breast milk unknown/use caution
Medication Safety Issues
Sound-alike/look-alike issues:
Singulair® may be confused with Sinequan®
Contraindications Hypersensitivity to montelukast or any component of the formulation
Warnings/Precautions Montelukast is not FDA approved for use in the reversal of bronchospasm in acute asthma attacks, including status asthmaticus; some clinicians, however, support its use (Cylly, 2003; Camargo, 2003; Ferreira, 2001). Advise patients to have appropriate rescue medication available. Appropriate clinical monitoring and caution are recommended when systemic corticosteroid reduction is considered in patients receiving montelukast. Inform phenylketonuric patients that the chewable tablet contains phenylalanine. Safety and efficacy in children <6 months of age have not been established.

In rare cases, patients on therapy with montelukast may present with systemic eosinophilia, sometimes presenting with clinical features of vasculitis consistent with Churg-Strauss syndrome, a condition which is often treated with systemic corticosteroid therapy. Healthcare providers should be alert to eosinophilia, vasculitic rash, worsening pulmonary symptoms, cardiac complications, and/or neuropathy presenting in their patients. A causal association between montelukast and these underlying conditions has not been established. Montelukast will not interrupt bronchoconstrictor response to aspirin or other NSAIDs; aspirin sensitive asthmatics should continue to avoid these agents.

Adverse Reactions (As reported in adults)

1% to 10%:

Central nervous system: Dizziness (2%), fatigue (2%), fever (2%)

Dermatologic: Rash (2%)

Gastrointestinal: Abdominal pain (3%), dyspepsia (2%), dental pain (2%), gastroenteritis (2%)

Hepatic: AST increased (2%)

Neuromuscular & skeletal: Weakness (2%)

Respiratory: Cough (3%), nasal congestion (2%)

<1% (Limited to important or life-threatening): Aggression, agitation, anaphylaxis, angioedema, arthralgia, behavior/mood changes, bleeding tendency, bruising, cholestasis (rare), Churg-Strauss syndrome (rare), depression, diarrhea, dream abnormalities, drowsiness, dyspepsia, edema, eosinophilia (systemic; rare), erythema nodosum, hallucinations, hepatic eosinophilic infiltration (rare); hepatitis (mixed pattern, hepatocellular, and cholestatic); hypersensitivity, hypoesthesia, insomnia, irritability, muscle cramps, myalgia, nausea, palpitation, pancreatitis (rare), paresthesia, pruritus, psychomotor hyperactivity, restlessness, seizure (rare), suicidal thinking/behavior (suicidality), suicide, tremor, urticaria, vasculitis (rare), vomiting

Drug Interactions

Metabolism/Transport Effects Substrate (major) of CYP2C9, 3A4; **Inhibits** CYP2C8 (weak), 2C9 (weak)

Avoid Concomitant Use There are no known interactions where it is recommended to avoid concomitant use.

Increased Effect/Toxicity

The levels/effects of Montelukast may be increased by: CYP2C9 Inhibitors (Moderate); CYP2C9 Inhibitors (Strong)

Decreased Effect

The levels/effects of Montelukast may be decreased by: CYP2C9 Inducers (Highly Effective); CYP3A4 Inducers (Strong); Deferasirox; Herbs (CYP3A4 Inducers)

Ethanol/Nutrition/Herb Interactions Herb/Nutraceutical: St John's wort may decrease montelukast levels.

Stability Store at room temperature of 15°C to 30°C (59°F to 86°F). Protect from moisture and light.

Granules: Use within 15 minutes of opening packet.

Mechanism of Action Selective leukotriene receptor antagonist that inhibits the cysteinyl leukotriene receptor. Cysteinyl leukotrienes and leukotriene receptor occupation have been correlated with the pathophysiology of asthma, including airway edema, smooth muscle contraction, and altered cellular activity associated with the inflammatory process, which contribute to the signs and symptoms of asthma. Cysteinyl leukotrienes are also released from the nasal mucosa following allergen exposure leading to symptoms associated with allergic rhinitis.

Pharmacodynamics/Kinetics

Duration: >24 hours

Absorption: Rapid

Distribution: V_d: 8-11 L

Protein binding, plasma: >99%

Metabolism: Extensively hepatic via CYP3A4 and 2C9

Bioavailability: Tablet: 10 mg: Mean: 64%; 5 mg: 63% to 73%

Half-life elimination, plasma: Mean: 2.7-5.5 hours

Time to peak, serum: Tablet: 10 mg: 3-4 hours; 5 mg: 2-2.5 hours; 4 mg: 2 hours

Excretion: Feces (86%); urine (<0.2%)

Dosage Oral:

Children:

6-11 months: Asthma (unlabeled use): 4 mg (oral granules) once daily, taken in the evening

6-23 months: Perennial allergic rhinitis: 4 mg (oral granules) once daily

12-23 months: Asthma: 4 mg (oral granules) once daily, taken in the evening

2-5 years: Asthma, seasonal or perennial allergic rhinitis: 4 mg (chewable tablet or oral granules) once daily, taken in the evening

6-14 years: Asthma, seasonal or perennial allergic rhinitis: 5 mg (chewable tablet) once daily, taken in the evening

Children ≥15 years and Adults:

Asthma, seasonal or perennial allergic rhinitis: 10 mg/day, taken in the evening

Asthma, acute (unlabeled use): 10 mg as a single dose administered with first-line therapy

Bronchoconstriction, exercise-induced (prevention): 10 mg at least 2 hours prior to exercise; additional doses should not be administered within 24 hours. Daily administration to prevent exercise-induced bronchoconstriction has not been evaluated.

Dosing adjustment in renal impairment: No adjustment necessary

Dosing adjustment in hepatic impairment: Mild-to-moderate: No adjustment necessary. Patients with severe hepatic disease were **not** studied.

Dietary Considerations Tablet, chewable: 4 mg strength contains phenylalanine 0.674 mg; 5 mg strength contains phenylalanine 0.842 mg

Administration When treating asthma, administer dose in the evening. Patients with allergic rhinitis may individualize administration time. Granules may be administered directly in the mouth or mixed with applesauce, carrots, rice, ice cream, baby formula, or breast milk; do not add to any other liquids. Administer within 15 minutes of opening packet.

Monitoring Parameters Mood or behavior changes, including suicidal thinking/behavior

Dosage Forms Excipient information presented when available (limited, particularly for generics); consult specific product labeling.

Granules:

Singulair®: 4 mg/packet (30s)

Tablet:

Singulair®: 10 mg

Tablet, chewable:

Singulair®: 4 mg [contains phenylalanine 0.674 mg; cherry flavor]; 5 mg [contains phenylalanine 0.842 mg; cherry flavor]

◆ **Montelukast Sodium** *see* Montelukast *on page 1014*

◆ **Monurol®** *see* Fosfomycin *on page 669*

◆ **8-MOP** *see* Methoxsalen *on page 968*

◆ **8-MOP®** *see* Methoxsalen *on page 968*

◆ **More Attenuated Enders Strain** *see* Measles Virus Vaccine (Live) *on page 924*

Moricizine (mor I siz een)

U.S. Brand Names Ethmozine® [DSC]

Canadian Brand Names Ethmozine®

Index Terms Moricizine Hydrochloride

Pharmacologic Category Antiarrhythmic Agent, Class I

Use Treatment of ventricular tachycardia and life-threatening ventricular arrhythmias

Unlabeled/Investigational Use PVCs, complete and nonsustained ventricular tachycardia, atrial arrhythmias

Pregnancy Risk Factor B

Lactation Enters breast milk/not recommended

Medication Safety Issues

Sound-alike/look-alike issues:

Ethmozine® may be confused with Erythrocin®, erythromycin

Contraindications Hypersensitivity to moricizine or any component of the formulation; pre-existing second- or third-degree AV block (except in patients with a functioning artificial pacemaker); right bundle branch block when associated with left hemiblock or bifascicular block (unless functional pacemaker in place); cardiogenic shock

Warnings/Precautions Considering the known proarrhythmic properties and lack of evidence of improved survival for any antiarrhythmic drug in patients without life-threatening arrhythmias, it is prudent to reserve the use for patients with life-threatening ventricular arrhythmias. **[U.S. Boxed Warning]: The CAST II trial demonstrated a trend towards decreased survival for patients treated with moricizine.** Avoid use in CAD, previous history of MI, HF, and cardiomegaly. Use with caution in patients with sick-sinus syndrome, hepatic, and renal impairment; correct electrolyte disturbances, especially hypokalemia or hypomagnesemia, prior to use and throughout therapy; safety and efficacy have not been established in pediatric patients

Adverse Reactions

>10%: Central nervous system: Dizziness

1% to 10%:

Cardiovascular: Proarrhythmia, palpitation, cardiac death, ECG abnormalities, CHF

Central nervous system: Headache, fatigue, insomnia

Endocrine & metabolic: Decreased libido

Gastrointestinal: Nausea, diarrhea, ileus

Ocular: Blurred vision, periorbital edema

Respiratory: Dyspnea

<1% (Limited to important or life-threatening): Apnea, cardiac chest pain, hyper-/hypotension, MI, supraventricular arrhythmia, syncope, ventricular tachycardia

Drug Interactions

Metabolism/Transport Effects Substrate of CYP3A4 (major); **Induces** CYP1A2 (weak), 3A4 (weak)

Avoid Concomitant Use There are no known interactions where it is recommended to avoid concomitant use.

Increased Effect/Toxicity

The levels/effects of Moricizine may be increased by: Cimetidine; CYP3A4 Inhibitors (Moderate); CYP3A4 Inhibitors (Strong); Dasatinib

Decreased Effect

Moricizine may decrease the levels/effects of: Maraviroc; Theophylline Derivatives

The levels/effects of Moricizine may be decreased by: CYP3A4 Inducers (Strong); Deferasirox; Herbs (CYP3A4 Inducers)

Ethanol/Nutrition/Herb Interactions Food: Moricizine peak serum concentrations may be decreased if taken with food.

Mechanism of Action Class I antiarrhythmic agent; reduces the fast inward current carried by sodium ions, shortens Phase I and Phase II repolarization, resulting in decreased action potential duration and effective refractory period

Pharmacodynamics/Kinetics

Protein binding, plasma: 95%

Metabolism: Significant first-pass effect; some enterohepatic recycling

Bioavailability: 38%

Half-life elimination: Healthy volunteers: 3-4 hours; Cardiac disease: 6-13 hours

Excretion: Feces (56%); urine (39%)

Dosage Adults: Oral: 200-300 mg every 8 hours, adjust dosage at 150 mg/day at 3-day intervals.

Recommendations for transferring patients from other antiarrhythmic agents to Ethmozine®: See table.

Moricizine

Transferred From	Start Ethmozine®
Encainide, propafenone, tocainide, or mexiletine	8-12 hours after last dose
Flecainide	12-24 hours after last dose
Procainamide	3-6 hours after last dose
Quinidine, disopyramide	6-12 hours after last dose

Dosing interval in renal or hepatic impairment: Start at 600 mg/day or less.

Dietary Considerations Best if taken on an empty stomach.

Dosage Forms Excipient information presented when available (limited, particularly for generics); consult specific product labeling. [DSC] = Discontinued product

Tablet, as hydrochloride:

Ethmozine®: 200 mg, 250 mg, 300 mg [DSC]

◆ **Moricizine Hydrochloride** *see* Moricizine *on page 1015*

◆ **Morning After Pill** *see* Ethinyl Estradiol and Norgestrel *on page 585*

◆ **Morphine HP® (Can)** *see* Morphine Sulfate *on page 1016*

◆ **Morphine LP® Epidural (Can)** *see* Morphine Sulfate *on page 1016*

Morphine Sulfate (MOR feen SUL fate)

U.S. Brand Names Astramorph/PF™; Avinza®; DepoDur®; Duramorph®; Infumorph®; Kadian®; MS Contin®; Oramorph SR®; Roxanol™

Canadian Brand Names Doloral; Kadian®; M-Eslon®; M.O.S.-SR®; M.O.S.-Sulfate®; M.O.S.® 10; M.O.S.® 20; M.O.S.® 30; Morphine HP®; Morphine LP® Epidural; MS Contin®; MS-IR®; Novo-Morphine SR; PMS-Morphine Sulfate SR; Ratio-Morphine; Ratio-Morphine SR; Statex®; Zomorph®

Index Terms MS (error-prone abbreviation and should not be used) ; MSO_4 (error-prone abbreviation and should not be used)

Pharmacologic Category Analgesic, Opioid

Additional Appendix Information

Narcotic / Opioid Analgesics *on page 1663*

Use Relief of moderate to severe acute and chronic pain; relief of pain of myocardial infarction; relief of dyspnea of acute left ventricular failure and pulmonary edema; preanesthetic medication

DepoDur®: Epidural (lumbar) single-dose management of surgical pain

Infumorph®: Used in continuous microinfusion devices for intrathecal or epidural administration in treatment of intractable chronic pain

Controlled, extended, or sustained release products: Only intended/indicated for use when repeated doses for an extended period of time are required. The 100 mg and 200 mg tablets or capsules of Kadian®, MS Contin®, and morphine sulfate controlled-release tablets and the 60 mg, 90 mg, and 120 mg capsules of Avinza® should only be used in opioid-tolerant patients.

Restrictions C-II

Pregnancy Risk Factor C/D (prolonged use or high doses at term)

Pregnancy Considerations Morphine crosses the placenta. The frequency of congenital malformations has not been reported to be greater than expected in children from mothers treated with morphine during pregnancy. Reduced growth and behavioral abnormalities in offspring have been observed in animal studies. Neonates born to mothers receiving chronic opioids during pregnancy should be monitored for neonatal withdrawal syndrome.

DepoDur® may be used in women undergoing cesarean section following clamping of the umbilical cord; not for use in vaginal labor and delivery.

Lactation Enters breast milk/use caution (AAP rates "compatible")

Medication Safety Issues

Sound-alike/look-alike issues:

Morphine may be confused with HYDROmorphone

Morphine sulfate may be confused with magnesium sulfate

MS Contin® may be confused with Oxycontin®

MSO_4 and MS are error-prone abbreviations (mistaken as magnesium sulfate)

Avinza® may be confused with Evista®, Invanz®

Roxanol™ may be confused with OxyFast®, Roxicet™, Roxicodone®

High alert medication: The Institute for Safe Medication Practices (ISMP) includes this medication (I.V. formulation) among its list of drug classes which have a heightened risk of causing significant patient harm when used in error.

Use care when prescribing and/or administering morphine solutions. These products are available in different concentrations. Always prescribe dosage in mg; **not** by volume (mL).

Use caution when selecting a morphine formulation for use in neurologic infusion pumps (eg, Medtronic delivery systems). The product should be appropriately labeled as "preservative-free" and suitable for intraspinal use via continuous infusion. In addition, the product should be formulated in a pH range that is compatible with the device operation specifications.

Significant differences exist between oral and I.V. dosing. Use caution when converting from one route of administration to another.

Contraindications Note: Some contraindications are product specific. For details, please see detailed product prescribing information.

Hypersensitivity to morphine sulfate or any component of the formulation; severe respiratory depression (without resuscitative equipment); acute or severe asthma; known or suspected paralytic ileus; sustained release products are not recommended with gastrointestinal obstruction or in acute/postoperative pain; pregnancy (prolonged use or high doses at term). Oral solutions contraindicated in patients with heart failure due to chronic lung disease, cardiac arrhythmias, head injuries, brain tumors, acute alcoholism, deliriums tremens, seizure disorders, Injectable solution contraindicated during labor when a premature birth is anticipated. Some products contraindicated in patients with head injuries or increased intracranial pressure. DepoDur® contraindicated in circulatory shock and upper airway obstruction. MS Contin® and Kadian® contraindicated in patients with hypercarbia. Some immediate release formulations (tablets and solution) contraindicated in post biliary tract surgery, suspected surgical abdomen, surgical anastomosis, MAO inhibitor use (concurrent or within 14 days), general CNS depression.

Warnings/Precautions An opioid-containing analgesic regimen should be tailored to each patient's needs and based upon the type of pain being treated (acute versus chronic), the route of administration, degree of tolerance for opioids (naive versus chronic user), age, weight, and medical condition. The optimal analgesic dose varies widely among patients. Doses should be titrated to pain relief/prevention. When used as an epidural injection, monitor for delayed sedation. **[U.S. Boxed Warning]: Healthcare provider should be alert to problems of abuse, misuse, and diversion.**

May cause respiratory depression; use with caution in patients (particularly elderly or debilitated) with impaired respiratory function, morbid obesity, adrenal insufficiency, prostatic hyperplasia, urinary stricture, renal impairment, or severe hepatic dysfunction and in patients with hypersensitivity reactions to other phenanthrene derivative opioid agonists (codeine, hydrocodone, hydromorphone, levorphanol, oxycodone, oxymorphone). Use with caution in patients with biliary tract dysfunction; acute pancreatitis may cause constriction of sphincter of Oddi. Some preparations contain sulfites which may cause allergic reactions; infants <3 months of age are more susceptible to respiratory depression, use with caution and generally in reduced doses in this age group.

May cause CNS depression, which may impair physical or mental abilities; patients must be cautioned about performing tasks which require mental alertness (eg, operating machinery or driving). Effects may be potentiated when used with other sedative drugs or ethanol. May cause hypotension in patients with acute myocardial infarction, volume depletion, or concurrent drug therapy which may exaggerate vasodilation. Use with extreme caution in patients with head injury, intracranial lesions, or elevated intracranial pressure; exaggerated elevation of ICP may occur. May cause seizures if high doses are used; use with caution in patients with seizure disorders. Tolerance or drug dependence may result from extended use. Concurrent use of agonist/antagonist analgesics may precipitate withdrawal symptoms and/or reduced analgesic efficacy in patients following prolonged therapy with mu opioid agonists. Abrupt discontinuation following prolonged use may also lead to withdrawal symptoms. Elderly may be particularly susceptible to adverse effects of narcotics. May obscure diagnosis or clinical course of patients with acute abdominal conditions.

Extended or sustained-release formulations:

[U.S. Boxed Warning]: Extended or sustained release dosage forms should not be crushed or chewed. Controlled-, extended-, or sustained-release products are not intended for "as needed (PRN)" use. **MS Contin® 100 or 200 mg tablets and Kadian® 100 mg or 200 mg capsules are for use only in opioid-tolerant patients.** Avinza®, Kadian®, MS Contin®: **[U.S. Boxed Warning]: Indicated for the management of moderate-to-severe pain when around the clock pain control is needed for an extended time period.**

[U.S. Boxed Warning]: Avinza®: Do not administer with alcoholic beverages or ethanol-containing products, which may disrupt extended-release characteristic of product.

Injections: Note: Products are designed for administration by specific routes (I.V., intrathecal, epidural). Use caution when prescribing, dispensing, or administering to use formulations only by intended route(s).

[U.S. Boxed Warning]: Duramorph®: Due to the risk of severe and/or sustained cardiopulmonary depressant effects of Duramorph® must be administered in a fully equipped and staffed environment. Naloxone injection should be immediately available. Patient should remain in this environment for at least 24 hours following the initial dose.

[U.S. Boxed Warning]: Intrathecal dosage is usually 1/10 that of epidural dosage.

Infumorph® solutions are **for use in microinfusion devices only**; not for I.V., I.M., or SubQ administration, or for single-dose administration.

When used as an epidural injection, monitor for delayed sedation.

DepoDur®: **For lumbar administration only.** Intrathecal administration has resulted in prolonged respiratory depression. Freezing may adversely affect modified-release mechanism of drug; check freeze indicator within carton prior to administration.

Adverse Reactions Note: Individual patient differences are unpredictable, and percentage may differ in acute pain (surgical) treatment. Reactions may be dose, formulation, and/or route dependent.

Frequency not defined:

- Cardiovascular: Circulatory depression, flushing, shock
- Central nervous system: Physical and psychological dependence, sedation
- Endocrine & metabolic: Antidiuretic hormone release

>10%:

- Cardiovascular: Bradycardia, hypotension
- Central nervous system: Drowsiness (9% to 48%; tolerance usually develops to drowsiness with regular dosing for 1-2 weeks), dizziness (6% to 20%), fever (<3% to >10%), confusion, headache (following epidural or intrathecal use)
- Dermatologic: Pruritus (may be dose related)
- Gastrointestinal: Xerostomia (78%), constipation (9% to 40%; tolerance develops very slowly if at all), nausea (7% to 28%; tolerance usually develops to nausea and vomiting with chronic use), vomiting
- Genitourinary: Urinary retention (16%; may be prolonged, up to 20 hours, following epidural or intrathecal use)
- Hematologic: Anemia (following intrathecal use)
- Local: Pain at injection site
- Neuromuscular & skeletal: Weakness
- Respiratory: Oxygen saturation decreased
- Miscellaneous: Histamine release

1% to 10%:

- Cardiovascular: Atrial fibrillation (<3%), chest pain (<3%), edema, hypertension, palpitation, peripheral edema, syncope, tachycardia, vasodilation
- Central nervous system: Amnesia, agitation, anxiety, apathy, ataxia, chills, coma, delirium, depression, dream abnormalities, euphoria, false sense of well being, hallucination, hypoesthesia, insomnia, lethargy, malaise, nervousness, restlessness, seizure, slurred speech, somnolence, vertigo
- Dermatologic: Dry skin, rash, urticaria
- Endocrine & metabolic: Gynecomastia (<3%), hypokalemia, hyponatremia, libido decreased
- Gastrointestinal: Abdominal distension, abdominal pain, anorexia, biliary colic, diarrhea, dyspepsia, dysphagia, flatulence, gastroenteritis, GERD, GI irritation, paralytic ileus, rectal disorder, taste perversion, weight loss
- Genitourinary: Bladder spasm, dysuria, ejaculation abnormal, impotence, urination decreased
- Hematologic: Leukopenia (<3%), thrombocytopenia (<3%), hematocrit decreased
- Hepatic: Liver function tests increased
- Neuromuscular & skeletal: Arthralgia, back pain, bone pain, foot drop, gait abnormalities, paresthesia, rigors, skeletal muscle rigidity, tremor
- Ocular: Amblyopia, conjunctivitis, eye pain, vision problems/disturbance
- Renal: Oliguria
- Respiratory: Asthma, atelectasis, dyspnea, hiccups, hypercapnia, hypoxia, pulmonary edema (noncardiogenic), respiratory depression, rhinitis
- Miscellaneous: Diaphoresis, flu-like syndrome, infection, thirst, voice alteration, withdrawal syndrome

<1% (Limited to important or life-threatening): Amenorrhea, anaphylaxis, apnea, biliary tract spasm, blurred vision, bronchospasm, cardiac arrest, cough reflex decreased, dehydration, diplopia, disorientation, hemorrhagic urticaria, intestinal obstruction, intracranial pressure increased, laryngospasm, menstrual irregularities, miosis, myoclonus, nystagmus, paradoxical CNS stimulation, respiratory arrest, sepsis, urinary tract spasm, thermal dysregulation, toxic psychoses

Drug Interactions

Metabolism/Transport Effects Substrate of CYP2D6 (minor)

Avoid Concomitant Use There are no known interactions where it is recommended to avoid concomitant use.

Increased Effect/Toxicity

Morphine Sulfate may increase the levels/effects of: Alcohol (Ethyl); Alvimopan; CNS Depressants; Desmopressin; Selective Serotonin Reuptake Inhibitors

The levels/effects of Morphine Sulfate may be increased by: Amphetamines; Antipsychotic Agents (Phenothiazines); Succinylcholine

Decreased Effect

Morphine Sulfate may decrease the levels/effects of: Pegvisomant; Trovafloxacin

The levels/effects of Morphine Sulfate may be decreased by: Ammonium Chloride; Rifamycin Derivatives

Ethanol/Nutrition/Herb Interactions

Ethanol: Avoid ethanol, including alcoholic beverages or ethanol-containing products (may increase CNS depression).

Avinza®: Alcoholic beverages or ethanol-containing products may disrupt extended-release formulation resulting in rapid release of entire morphine dose.

Food: Administration of oral morphine solution with food may increase bioavailability (ie, a report of 34% increase in morphine AUC when morphine oral solution followed a high-fat meal). The bioavailability of Avinza®, Oramorph SR®, or Kadian® does not appear to be affected by food.

Herb/Nutraceutical: Avoid valerian, St John's wort, kava kava, gotu kola (may increase CNS depression).

Stability

Capsule, sustained release (Avinza®, Kadian®): Store at 25°C (77°F); excursions permitted to 15°C to 30°C (59°F to 86°F). Protect from light and moisture.

Injection: Store at controlled room temperature of 20°C to 25°C (68°F to 77°F); do not freeze. Protect from light. Degradation depends on pH and presence of oxygen; relatively stable in pH ≤4; darkening of solutions indicate degradation. Usual concentration for continuous I.V. infusion: 0.1-1 mg/mL in D_5W.

DepoDur®: Store under refrigeration at 2°C to 8°C (36°F to 46°F); keep vials in carton during refrigeration; do not freeze. Check freeze indicator before administration; do not administer if bulb is pink or purple. May store at room temperature for up to 30 days in sealed, unopened vials. DepoDur® may be diluted in preservative-free NS to a volume of 5 mL. Gently invert to suspend particles prior to removal from vial. Once vial is opened, use within 4 hours.

Oral solution: Store at controlled room temperature of 25°C (68°F to 77°F). Do not freeze.

Suppositories: Store at controlled room temperature 25°C (77°F). Protect from light.

Tablet, extended release: Store at controlled room temperature of 25°C (77°F).

Tablet, immediate release: Store at controlled room temperature of 25°C (77°F). Protect from moisture.

Mechanism of Action Binds to opiate receptors in the CNS, causing inhibition of ascending pain pathways, altering the perception of and response to pain; produces generalized CNS depression

Pharmacodynamics/Kinetics

Onset of action (patient dependent; dosing must be individualized): Oral (immediate release): ~30 minutes; I.V.: 5-10 minutes

Duration (patient dependent; dosing must be individualized): Pain relief:

Immediate release formulations: 4 hours

Extended release capsule and tablet: 8-24 hours (formulation dependent)

Extended release epidural injection (DepoDur®): >48 hours

Absorption: Variable

Distribution: V_d: 3-4 L/kg; binds to opioid receptors in the CNS and periphery (eg, GI tract)

Protein binding: 30% to 35%

Metabolism: Hepatic via conjugation with glucuronic acid primarily to morphine-6-glucoronide (active analgesic) morphine-3-glucuronide (inactive as analgesic); minor metabolites include morphine-3-6-diglucuronide; other minor metabolites include normorphine (active) and morphine 3-ethereal sulfate

Bioavailability: Oral: 17% to 33% (first-pass effect limits oral bioavailability; oral:parenteral effectiveness reportedly varies from 1:6 in opioid naive patients to 1:3 with chronic use)

Half-life elimination: Adults: 2-4 hours (immediate release forms)

Time to peak, plasma: Avinza®: 30 minutes (maintained for 24 hours); Kadian®: ~10 hours; Oramorph® SR: ~4 hours

Excretion: Urine (primarily as morphine-3-glucuronide, ~2% to 12% excreted unchanged); feces (~7% to 10%). It has been suggested that accumulation of morphine-6-glucuronide might cause toxicity with renal insufficiency. All of the metabolites (ie, morphine-3-glucuronide, morphine-6-glucuronide, and normorphine) have been suggested as possible causes of neurotoxicity (eg, myoclonus).

Dosage Note: These are guidelines and do not represent the doses that may be required in all patients. Doses and dosage intervals should be titrated to pain relief/prevention.

Children >6 months and <50 kg: Acute pain (moderate-to-severe):

Oral (immediate release formulations): 0.15-0.3 mg/kg every 3-4 hours as needed

I.M., I.V.: 0.1-0.2 mg/kg every 3-4 hours as needed

I.V. infusion: Range: 10-60 mcg/kg/hour

Adults:

Acute pain (moderate-to-severe):

Oral (immediate release formulations): Opiate-naive: Initial: 10 mg every 4 hours as needed; patients with prior opiate exposure may require higher initial doses: usual dosage range: 10-30 mg every 4 hours as needed

I.M., SubQ: **Note:** Repeated SubQ administration causes local tissue irritation, pain, and induration.

Initial: Opiate-naive: 5-10 mg every 4 hours as needed; patients with prior opiate exposure may require higher initial doses; usual dosage range: 5-20 mg every 4 hours as needed

Rectal: 10-20 mg every 3-4 hours

I.V.: Initial: Opiate-naive: 2.5-5 mg every 3-4 hours; patients with prior opiate exposure may require higher initial doses. **Note:** Repeated doses (up to every 5 minutes if needed) in small increments (eg, 1-4 mg) may be preferred to larger and less frequent doses.

Acute myocardial infarction, analgesia (ACC/AHA 2004 guidelines): Initial management: 2-4 mg, give 2-8 mg every 5-15 minutes as needed.

Critically-ill patients (unlabeled dose): 0.7-10 mg (based on 70 kg patient) **or** 0.01-0.15 mg/kg every 1-2 hours as needed. **Note:** More frequent dosing may be needed (eg, mechanically-ventilated patients).

I.V., SubQ continuous infusion: 0.8-10 mg/hour; usual range: Up to 80 mg/hour

Continuous infusion: Usual dosage range: 5-35 mg/hour (based on 70 kg patient) **or** 0.07-0.5 mg/kg/hour

Patient-controlled analgesia (PCA): (Opiate-naive: Consider lower end of dosing range):

Usual concentration: 1 mg/mL

Demand dose: Usual: 1 mg; range: 0.5-2.5 mg

Lockout interval: 5-10 minutes

Intrathecal (I.T.): **Note:** Administer with extreme caution and in reduced dosage to geriatric or debilitated patients. I.T. dose is usually 1/10 that of epidural dosage.

Opioid-naive: 0.2-1 mg/dose (may provide adequate relief for 24 hours); repeat doses are **not** recommended

Continuous microinfusion (Infumorph®): Initial: 0.2-1 mg/day

Opioid-tolerant: 1-10 mg/day

Continuous microinfusion (Infumorph®): Initial: 1-10 mg/day, titrate to effect; usual maximum is ~20 mg/day

Epidural: Pain management: **Note:** Administer with extreme caution and in reduced dosage to geriatric or debilitated patients. Vigilant monitoring is particularly important in these patients.

Single-dose (Astromorph/PF™, Duramorph®): Initial: 5 mg, if pain relief not achieved in 1 hour, careful administration of 1-2 mg at intervals sufficient to assess effectiveness may be given; maximum: 10 mg/24 hours

Infusion: Bolus dose: 1-6 mg; infusion rate: 0.1-0.2 mg/hour; maximum dose: 10 mg/24 hours

Continuous microinfusion (Infumorph®):

Opioid-naive: Initial: 0.2-1 mg/day

Opioid-tolerant: Initial: 1-10 mg/day, titrate to effect; usual maximum is ~20 mg/day

Surgical anesthesia: Epidural: Single-dose (extended release, DepoDur®): Lumbar epidural only; not recommended in patients <18 years of age:

Cesarean section: 10 mg (after clamping umbilical cord)

Lower abdominal/pelvic surgery: 10-15 mg

Major orthopedic surgery of lower extremity: 15 mg

For DepoDur®: To minimize the pharmacokinetic interaction resulting in higher peak serum concentrations of morphine, administer the test dose of the local anesthetic at least 15 minutes prior to DepoDur® administration. Use of DepoDur® with epidural local anesthetics has not been studied. Other medications should not be administered into the epidural space for at least 48 hours after administration of DepoDur®.

Note: Some patients may benefit from a 20 mg dose; however, the incidence of adverse effects may be increased.

Chronic pain: Note: Patients taking opioids chronically may become tolerant and require doses higher than the usual dosage range to maintain the desired effect. Tolerance can be managed by appropriate dose titration. There is no optimal or maximal dose for morphine in chronic pain. The appropriate dose is one that relieves pain throughout its dosing interval without causing unmanageable side effects.

Oral: Controlled-, extended-, or sustained-release formulations: A patient's morphine requirement should be established using prompt-release formulations. Conversion to long-acting products may be considered when chronic, continuous treatment is required. Higher dosages should be reserved for use only in opioid-tolerant patients.

Capsules, extended release (Avinza®): Daily dose administered once daily (for best results, administer at same time each day)

Capsules, sustained release (Kadian®): Daily dose administered once daily or in 2 divided doses daily (every 12 hours)

Tablets, controlled release (MS Contin®), sustained release (Oramorph SR®), or extended release: Daily dose divided and administered every 8 or every 12 hours

Elderly or debilitated patients: Use with caution; may require dose reduction

Dosing adjustment in renal impairment:

Cl_{cr} 10-50 mL/minute: Children and Adults: Administer at 75% of normal dose

Cl_{cr} <10 mL/minute: Children and Adults: Administer at 50% of normal dose

Intermittent HD:

Children: Administer 50% of normal dose

Adults: No dosage adjustment necessary

Peritoneal dialysis: Children: Administer 50% of normal dose

CRRT: Children and Adults: Administer 75% of normal dose, titrate

Dosing adjustment/comments in hepatic disease: Unchanged in mild liver disease; substantial extrahepatic metabolism may occur; excessive sedation may occur in cirrhosis

Dietary Considerations Morphine may cause GI upset; take with food if GI upset occurs. Be consistent when taking morphine with or without meals.

Administration

Oral: Do not crush controlled release drug product, swallow whole. Kadian® and Avinza® can be opened and sprinkled on applesauce; do not crush or chew the beads. Contents of Kadian® capsules may be opened and sprinkled over 10 mL water and flushed through prewetted 16F gastrostomy tube; do not administer Kadian® through nasogastric tube.

I.V.: When giving morphine I.V. push, it is best to first dilute in 4-5 mL of sterile water, and then to administer slowly (eg, 15 mg over 3-5 minutes)

Epidural: Use preservative-free solutions

Epidural, extended release liposomal suspension (DepoDur®): Intended for lumbar administration only. Thoracic administration has not been studied. May be administered undiluted or diluted up to 5 mL total volume in preservative-free NS. Do not use an in-line filter during administration. Not for I.V., I.M., or intrathecal administration.

Resedation may occur following epidural administration; this may be delayed ≥48 hours in patients receiving extended-release (DepoDur®) injections.

Administration of an epidural test dose (lidocaine 1.5% and epinephrine 1:200,000) may affect the release of morphine from the liposomal preparation. Delaying the dose for an interval of at least 15 minutes following the test dose minimizes this pharmacokinetic interaction. Except for a test dose, other epidural local anesthetics or medications should not be administered epidurally before or after this product for a minimum of 48 hours.

Intrathecal: Use preservative-free solutions

Monitoring Parameters Pain relief, respiratory and mental status, blood pressure

Astromorph/PF™, Duramorph®, Infumorph®: Patients should be observed in a fully-equipped and staffed environment for at least 24 hours following initiation, and as appropriate for the first several days after catheter implantation.

DepoDur®: Patient should be monitored for at least 48 hours following administration.

Reference Range Therapeutic: Surgical anesthesia: 65-80 ng/mL (SI: 227-280 nmol/L); Toxic: 200-5000 ng/mL (SI: 700-17,500 nmol/L)

Test Interactions Some quinolones may produce a false-positive urine screening result for opiates using commercially-available immunoassay kits. This has been demonstrated most consistently for levofloxacin and ofloxacin, but other quinolones have shown cross-reactivity in certain assay kits. Confirmation of positive opiate screens by more specific methods should be considered.

Dosage Forms Excipient information presented when available (limited, particularly for generics); consult specific product labeling. [DSC] = Discontinued product; [CAN] Canadian brand name

Capsule, extended release:

Avinza®: 30 mg, 60 mg, 90 mg, 120 mg

Kadian®: 10 mg, 20 mg, 30 mg, 50 mg, 60 mg, 80 mg, 100 mg, 200 mg

Infusion [premixed in D_5W]: 1 mg/mL (100 mL, 250 mL)

Injection, extended release liposomal suspension [lumbar epidural injection, preservative free]:

DepoDur®: 10 mg/mL (1 mL, 1.5 mL, 2 mL)

Injection, solution: 2 mg/mL (1 mL); 4 mg/mL (1 mL); 5 mg/mL (1 mL); 8 mg/mL (1 mL); 10 mg/0.7 mL (0.7 mL); 10 mg/mL (1 mL, 10 mL); 15 mg/mL (1 mL, 20 mL); 25 mg/mL (4 mL, 10 mL, 20 mL, 40 mL, 50 mL, 100 mL, 250 mL); 50 mg/mL (20 mL, 40 mL) [some preparations contain sodium metabisulfite]

Injection, solution [epidural, intrathecal, or I.V. infusion; preservative free]:

Astramorph/PF™: 0.5 mg/mL (2 mL, 10 mL); 1 mg/mL (2 mL, 10 mL)

Duramorph®: 0.5 mg/mL (10 mL); 1 mg/mL (10 mL)

Injection, solution [epidural or intrathecal infusion via microinfusion device; preservative free]:

Infumorph®: 10 mg/mL (20 mL); 25 mg/mL (20 mL)

Injection, solution [I.V. infusion via PCA pump]: 0.5 mg/mL (30 mL); 1 mg/mL (30 mL, 50 mL); 2 mg/mL (30 mL); 5 mg/mL (30 mL, 50 mL)

Injection, solution [preservative free]: 0.5 mg/mL (10 mL); 1 mg/mL (10 mL); 25 mg/mL (4 mL, 10 mL, 20 mL)

Solution, oral: 10 mg/5 mL (5 mL, 100 mL, 500 mL); 20 mg/5 mL (100 mL, 500 mL); 20 mg/mL (30 mL, 120 mL, 240 mL)

Doloral [CAN]: 1 mg/mL (10 mL, 250 mL, 500 mL); 5 mg/mL (10 mL, 250 mL, 500 mL) [not available in U.S.]

Solution, oral [concentrate]: 5 mg/0.25 mL (0.25 mL) [DSC]; 10 mg/0.5 mL (0.5 mL) [DSC]; 20 mg/mL (1 mL [DSC], 15 ml, 30 mL, 120 mL, 240 mL)

Roxanol™: 20 mg/mL (30 mL, 120 mL); 100 mg/5 mL (240 mL)

Suppository, rectal: 5 mg (12s), 10 mg (12s), 20 mg (12s), 30 mg (12s)

Tablet: 10 mg [DSC], 15 mg, 30 mg

Tablet, controlled release:

MS Contin®: 15 mg, 30 mg, 60 mg, 100 mg, 200 mg

Tablet, extended release: 15 mg, 30 mg, 60 mg, 100 mg, 200 mg

Tablet, sustained release:

Oramorph SR®: 15 mg, 30 mg, 60 mg, 100 mg

Morrhuate Sodium (MOR yoo ate SOW dee um)

U.S. Brand Names Scleromate®

Pharmacologic Category Sclerosing Agent

Use Treatment of small, uncomplicated varicose veins of the lower extremities

Pregnancy Risk Factor C

Dosage Adults: I.V.: 50-250 mg, repeated at 5- to 7-day intervals (50-100 mg for small veins, 150-250 mg for large veins)

Additional Information Complete prescribing information for this medication should be consulted for additional detail.

Dosage Forms Excipient information presented when available (limited, particularly for generics); consult specific product labeling.

Injection, solution: 50 mg/mL (30 mL)

- ◆ **M.O.S.® 10 (Can)** *see* Morphine Sulfate *on page 1016*
- ◆ **M.O.S.® 20 (Can)** *see* Morphine Sulfate *on page 1016*
- ◆ **M.O.S.® 30 (Can)** *see* Morphine Sulfate *on page 1016*
- ◆ **M.O.S.-SR® (Can)** *see* Morphine Sulfate *on page 1016*
- ◆ **M.O.S.-Sulfate® (Can)** *see* Morphine Sulfate *on page 1016*
- ◆ **Motofen® [DSC]** *see* Difenoxin and Atropine *on page 443*
- ◆ **Motrin® [DSC]** *see* Ibuprofen *on page 760*
- ◆ **Motrin® Children's [OTC]** *see* Ibuprofen *on page 760*
- ◆ **Motrin® (Children's) (Can)** *see* Ibuprofen *on page 760*
- ◆ **Motrin® IB [OTC]** *see* Ibuprofen *on page 760*
- ◆ **Motrin® IB (Can)** *see* Ibuprofen *on page 760*
- ◆ **Motrin® Infants' [OTC]** *see* Ibuprofen *on page 760*
- ◆ **Motrin® Junior [OTC]** *see* Ibuprofen *on page 760*
- ◆ **MoviPrep®** *see* Polyethylene Glycol-Electrolyte Solution *on page 1209*
- ◆ **Moxatag®** *see* Amoxicillin *on page 98*

Moxifloxacin (moxs i FLOKS a sin)

U.S. Brand Names Avelox®; Avelox® I.V.; Vigamox™

Canadian Brand Names Avelox®; Avelox® I.V.; Vigamox™

Index Terms Moxifloxacin Hydrochloride

Pharmacologic Category Antibiotic, Ophthalmic; Antibiotic, Quinolone; Respiratory Fluoroquinolone

Additional Appendix Information

Antimicrobial Drugs of Choice *on page 1752*
Community-Acquired Pneumonia in Adults *on page 1766*
Prevention of Wound Infection and Sepsis in Surgical Patients *on page 1738*

Use Treatment of mild-to-moderate community-acquired pneumonia, including multidrug-resistant *Streptococcus pneumoniae* (MDRSP); acute bacterial exacerbation of chronic bronchitis; acute bacterial sinusitis; complicated and uncomplicated skin and skin structure infections; complicated intra-abdominal infections; bacterial conjunctivitis (ophthalmic formulation)

Unlabeled/Investigational Use *Legionella*

Restrictions An FDA-approved patient medication guide is available and must be distributed when dispensing an outpatient prescription (new or refill) where this medication is to be used without direct supervision of a healthcare provider. Medication guides are available at http://www.fda.gov/cder/Offices/ODS/medication_guides.htm.

Pregnancy Risk Factor C

Pregnancy Considerations Adverse events have been observed in some animal studies; therefore, the manufacturer classifies moxifloxacin as pregnancy category C. Quinolone exposure during human pregnancy has been reported with other agents (see Ciprofloxacin, Ofloxacin, and Norfloxacin monographs). To date, no specific teratogenic effect or increased pregnancy risk has been identified; however, because of concerns of cartilage damage in immature animals exposed to quinolones and the limited moxifloxacin specific data, moxifloxacin should only be used during pregnancy if a safer option is not available.

Lactation Excretion in breast milk unknown/not recommended

Medication Safety Issues

Sound-alike/look-alike issues:

Avelox® may be confused with Avonex®

International issues:

Vigamox™ may be confused with Fisamox® which is a brand name for amoxicillin in Australia

Contraindications Hypersensitivity to moxifloxacin, other quinolone antibiotics, or any component of the formulation

Warnings/Precautions [U.S. Boxed Warning]: There have been reports of tendon inflammation and/or rupture with quinolone antibiotics; risk may be increased with concurrent corticosteroids, organ transplant recipients, and in patients >60 years of age. Rupture of the Achilles tendon sometimes requiring surgical repair has been reported most frequently; but other tendon sites (eg, rotator cuff, biceps) have also been reported. Strenuous physical activity, rheumatoid arthritis, and renal impairment may be an independent risk factor for tendonitis. Discontinue at first sign of tendon inflammation or pain. Tendon rupture may occur even after discontinuation of therapy. Use with caution in patients with rheumatoid arthritis or renal impairment; may increase risk of tendon rupture.

Use with caution in patients with significant bradycardia or acute myocardial ischemia. Moxifloxacin causes a concentration-dependent QT prolongation. Do not exceed recommended dose or infusion rate. Avoid use with uncorrected hypokalemia, with other drugs that prolong the QT interval or induce bradycardia, or with class Ia or III antiarrhythmic agents. Use with caution in individuals at risk of seizures (CNS disorders or concurrent therapy with medications which may lower seizure threshold). Potential for seizures, although very rare, may be increased with concomitant NSAID therapy. Discontinue in patients who experience significant CNS adverse effects (dizziness, hallucinations, suicidal ideation or actions). Use with caution in patients with mild, moderate, or severe hepatic impairment or liver cirrhosis; may increase the risk of QT prolongation. Use with caution in diabetes; glucose regulation may be altered.

Fluoroquinolones have been associated with the development of serious, and sometimes fatal, hypoglycemia, most often in elderly diabetics, but also in patients without diabetes. This occurred most frequently with gatifloxacin (no longer available systemically) but may occur at a lower frequency with other quinolones.

Severe hypersensitivity reactions, including anaphylaxis, have occurred with quinolone therapy. Reactions may present as typical allergic symptoms after a single dose, or may manifest as severe idiosyncratic dermatologic, vascular, pulmonary, renal, hepatic, and/or hematologic events, usually after multiple doses. Prompt discontinuation of drug should occur if skin rash or other symptoms arise. Avoid excessive sunlight and take precautions to limit exposure (eg, loose fitting clothing, sunscreen); may cause moderate-to-severe phototoxicity reactions. Discontinue use if photosensitivity occurs. Prolonged use may result in fungal or bacterial superinfection, including *C. difficile*-associated diarrhea (CDAD) and pseudomembranous colitis; CDAD has been observed >2 months postantibiotic treatment. Quinolones may exacerbate myasthenia gravis. Peripheral neuropathy may rarely occur. Hemolytic reactions may (rarely) occur with quinolone use in patients with latent or actual G6PD deficiency. Adverse effects (eg, tendon rupture, QT changes) may be increased in the elderly. Some quinolones may exacerbate myasthenia gravis, use with caution (rare, potentially life-threatening weakness of respiratory muscles may occur). Safety and efficacy of systemically administered moxifloxacin (oral, intravenous) in patients <18 years of age have not been established.

Ophthalmic: Eye drops should not be injected subconjunctivally or introduced directly into the anterior chamber of the eye. Contact lenses should not be worn during therapy.

Adverse Reactions

Systemic:

2% to 10%:

Central nervous system: Dizziness (2%)

Endocrine & metabolic: Serum chloride increased (≥2%), serum ionized calcium increased (≥2%), serum glucose decreased (≥2%)

Gastrointestinal: Nausea (6%), diarrhea (5%), amylase decreased (≥2%)

Hematologic: Decreased serum levels of the following (≥2%): Basophils, eosinophils, hemoglobin, RBC, neutrophils; increased serum levels of the following (≥2%): MCH, neutrophils, WBC

Hepatic: Bilirubin decreased/increased (≥2%)

Renal: Serum albumin increased (≥2%)

Respiratory: PO_2 decreased (≥2%)

0.1% to <2%:

Cardiovascular: Cardiac arrhythmias, palpitation, QT_c prolongation, tachycardia, vasodilation

Central nervous system: Anxiety, headache, insomnia, malaise, nervousness, pain, somnolence, vertigo

Dermatologic: Pruritus, rash (maculopapular, purpuric, pustular), urticaria

Gastrointestinal: Abdominal pain, amylase increased, anorexia, constipation, dyspepsia, flatulence, glossitis, lactic dehydrogenase increased, stomatitis, taste perversion, vomiting, xerostomia

Genitourinary: Vaginal moniliasis, vaginitis

Hematologic: Eosinophilia, leukopenia, prothrombin time prolonged, increased INR, thrombocythemia

Hepatic: GGTP increased, liver function test abnormal

Local: Injection site reaction

Neuromuscular & skeletal: Arthralgia, myalgia, tremor, weakness

Respiratory: Pharyngitis, pneumonia, rhinitis, sinusitis

Miscellaneous: Allergic reaction, infection, diaphoresis, oral moniliasis

<0.1% (Limited to important or life-threatening): Abnormal dreams, abnormal gait, agitation, amblyopia, amnesia, anaphylactic reaction, anaphylactic shock, anemia, angioedema, aphasia, arthritis, asthma, atrial fibrillation, back pain, *C. difficile*-positive diarrhea, chest pain, cholestasis, confusion, depersonalization, depression, dysphagia, dyspnea, ECG abnormalities, emotional lability, face edema, gastritis, hallucinations, hepatic failure, hepatitis, hyperglycemia, hyperlipidemia, hyper-/hypotension, hypertonia, hyperuricemia, hypoesthesia, incoordination, INR decreased, jaundice (cholestatic), laryngeal edema, leg pain, nightmares, paresthesia, parosmia, pelvic pain, peripheral edema, peripheral neuropathy, photosensitivity/toxicity, prothrombin time decreased, pseudomembranous colitis, psychotic reaction, renal dysfunction, renal failure, seizure, sleep disorder, speech disorder, Stevens-Johnson syndrome, supraventricular tachycardia, syncope, taste loss, tendonitis, tendon rupture, thinking abnormal, thrombocytopenia, thromboplastin decreased, tinnitus, tongue discoloration, toxic epidermal necrolysis, ventricular tachyarrhythmias (including torsade de pointes and cardiac arrest [usually in patients with concurrent, severe proarrhythmic conditions]), vision abnormalities

Additional reactions with **ophthalmic** preparation: 1% to 6%: Conjunctivitis, dry eye, ocular discomfort, ocular hyperemia, ocular pain, ocular pruritus, subconjunctival hemorrhage, tearing, visual acuity decreased

Drug Interactions

Avoid Concomitant Use

Avoid concomitant use of Moxifloxacin with any of the following: Nilotinib; Tetrabenazine; Thioridazine; Ziprasidone

Increased Effect/Toxicity

Moxifloxacin may increase the levels/effects of: Corticosteroids (Systemic); QTc-Prolonging Agents; Sulfonylureas; Tetrabenazine; Thioridazine; Vitamin K Antagonists; Ziprasidone

The levels/effects of Moxifloxacin may be increased by: Alfuzosin; Ciprofloxacin; Gadobutrol; Insulin; Nilotinib; Nonsteroidal Anti-Inflammatory Agents; Probenecid

Decreased Effect

Moxifloxacin may decrease the levels/effects of: Mycophenolate; Sulfonylureas; Typhoid Vaccine

The levels/effects of Moxifloxacin may be decreased by: Antacids; Didanosine; Iron Salts; Magnesium Salts; Quinapril; Sevelamer; Sucralfate; Zinc Salts

Ethanol/Nutrition/Herb Interactions Food: Absorption is not affected by administration with a high-fat meal or yogurt.

Stability Store at controlled room temperature of 25°C (77°F). Do not refrigerate infusion solution.

Mechanism of Action Moxifloxacin is a DNA gyrase inhibitor, and also inhibits topoisomerase IV. DNA gyrase (topoisomerase II) is an essential bacterial enzyme that maintains the superhelical structure of DNA. DNA gyrase is required for DNA replication and transcription, DNA repair, recombination, and transposition; inhibition is bactericidal.

Pharmacodynamics/Kinetics

Absorption: Well absorbed; not affected by high-fat meal or yogurt

Distribution: V_d: 1.7 to 2.7 L/kg; tissue concentrations often exceed plasma concentrations in respiratory tissues, alveolar macrophages, abdominal tissues/fluids, and sinus tissues

Protein binding: ~30% to 50%

Metabolism: Hepatic (~52% of dose) via glucuronide (~14%) and sulfate (~38%) conjugation

Bioavailability: ~90%

Half-life elimination: Single dose: Oral: 12-16 hours; I.V.: 8-15 hours

Excretion: Urine (as unchanged drug [20%] and glucuronide conjugates); feces (as unchanged drug [25%] and sulfate conjugates)

Dosage

Usual dosage range:

Children ≥1 year and Adults: Ophthalmic: Instill 1 drop into affected eye(s) 3 times/day for 7 days

Adults: Oral, I.V.: 400 mg every 24 hours

Indication-specific dosing:

Children ≥1 year and Adults: Ophthalmic:

Bacterial conjunctivitis: Instill 1 drop into affected eye(s) 3 times/day for 7 days

Adults: Oral, I.V.:

Acute bacterial sinusitis: 400 mg every 24 hours for 10 days

Chronic bronchitis, acute bacterial exacerbation: 400 mg every 24 hours for 5 days

Intra-abdominal infections (complicated): 400 mg every 24 hours for 5-14 days (initiate with I.V.)

Pneumonia, community-acquired (including MDRSP): 400 mg every 24 hours for 7-14 days

Skin and skin structure infections:

Complicated: 400 mg every 24 hours for 7-21 days

Uncomplicated: 400 mg every 24 hours for 7 days

Elderly: No dosage adjustments are required based on age

Dosage adjustment in renal impairment: No dosage adjustment is required, including patients on hemodialysis, CRRT, or CAPD.

Dosage adjustment in hepatic impairment: No dosage adjustment is required in mild, moderate, or severe hepatic insufficiency (Child-Pugh class A, B, or C); however, use with caution in this patient population secondary to the risk of QT prolongation.

Dietary Considerations May be taken with or without food. Take 4 hours before or 8 hours after multiple vitamins, antacids, or other products containing magnesium, aluminum, iron, or zinc.

Avelox® I.V. infusion (premixed in sodium chloride 0.8%) contains sodium 34.2 mEq (~787mg)/250 mL.

Administration I.V.: Infuse over 60 minutes; do not infuse by rapid or bolus intravenous infusion

Monitoring Parameters WBC, signs of infection

Test Interactions Some quinolones may produce a false-positive urine screening result for opiates using commercially-available immunoassay kits. This has been demonstrated most consistently for levofloxacin and ofloxacin, but other quinolones have shown cross-reactivity in certain assay kits. Confirmation of positive opiate screens by more specific methods should be considered.

Dosage Forms Excipient information presented when available (limited, particularly for generics); consult specific product labeling.

Infusion [premixed in sodium chloride 0.8%]:

Avelox® I.V.: 400 mg (250 mL) [contains sodium ~787mg (34.2 mEq)/250 mL]

Solution, ophthalmic:

Vigamox™: 0.5% (3 mL)

Tablet:

Avelox®: 400 mg

Avelox® ABC Pack [unit-dose pack]: 400 mg (5s)

- ◆ **Moxifloxacin Hydrochloride** *see* Moxifloxacin *on page 1021*
- ◆ **Mozobil™** *see* Plerixafor *on page 1202*
- ◆ **4-MP** *see* Fomepizole *on page 659*
- ◆ **MPA** *see* MedroxyPROGESTERone *on page 930*
- ◆ **MPA** *see* Mycophenolate *on page 1026*
- ◆ **MPA and Estrogens (Conjugated)** *see* Estrogens (Conjugated/Equine) and Medroxyprogesterone *on page 566*
- ◆ **6-MP (error-prone abbreviation)** *see* Mercaptopurine *on page 946*
- ◆ **MPSV** *see* Meningococcal Polysaccharide Vaccine (Groups A / C / Y and W-135) *on page 940*
- ◆ **MS Contin®** *see* Morphine Sulfate *on page 1016*
- ◆ **MS (error-prone abbreviation and should not be used)** *see* Morphine Sulfate *on page 1016*
- ◆ **MS-IR® (Can)** *see* Morphine Sulfate *on page 1016*
- ◆ **MSO_4 (error-prone abbreviation and should not be used)** *see* Morphine Sulfate *on page 1016*
- ◆ **MTC** *see* Mitomycin *on page 1005*
- ◆ **MTX (error-prone abbreviation)** *see* Methotrexate *on page 965*
- ◆ **Mucinex® [OTC]** *see* GuaiFENesin *on page 709*
- ◆ **Mucinex®-D [OTC]** *see* Guaifenesin and Pseudoephedrine *on page 713*
- ◆ **Mucinex® D Maximum Strength [OTC]** *see* Guaifenesin and Pseudoephedrine *on page 713*
- ◆ **Mucinex®, Children's [OTC]** *see* GuaiFENesin *on page 709*
- ◆ **Mucinex® Children's Cough [OTC]** *see* Guaifenesin and Dextromethorphan *on page 710*
- ◆ **Mucinex®, Children's Mini-Melts™ [OTC]** *see* GuaiFENesin *on page 709*
- ◆ **Mucinex® DM [OTC]** *see* Guaifenesin and Dextromethorphan *on page 710*
- ◆ **Mucinex® DM Maximum Strength [OTC]** *see* Guaifenesin and Dextromethorphan *on page 710*
- ◆ **Mucinex®, Junior Mini-Melts™ [OTC]** *see* GuaiFENesin *on page 709*
- ◆ **Mucinex® Maximum Strength [OTC]** *see* GuaiFENesin *on page 709*
- ◆ **Mucomyst** *see* Acetylcysteine *on page 36*
- ◆ **Mucomyst® (Can)** *see* Acetylcysteine *on page 36*
- ◆ **Multitargeted Antifolate** *see* Pemetrexed *on page 1159*
- ◆ **Mumps, Measles and Rubella Vaccines, Combined** *see* Measles, Mumps, and Rubella Vaccines (Combined) *on page 923*
- ◆ **Mumps, Rubella, Varicella, and Measles Vaccine** *see* Measles, Mumps, Rubella, and Varicella Virus Vaccine *on page 923*
- ◆ **Mumpsvax®** *see* Mumps Virus Vaccine *on page 1023*

Mumps Virus Vaccine (mumpz VYE rus vak SEEN)

U.S. Brand Names Mumpsvax®

Pharmacologic Category Vaccine

Additional Appendix Information

Immunization Recommendations *on page 1708*

Use Mumps prophylaxis by promoting active immunity

Note: Trivalent measles-mumps-rubella (MMR) vaccine is the preferred agent for most children and many adults; persons born prior to 1957 are generally considered immune and need not be vaccinated

Pregnancy Risk Factor C

Pregnancy Considerations Reproduction studies have not been conducted. Rates of spontaneous abortion may be increased if mumps infection occurs during the first trimester. Although mumps vaccine virus can infect the placenta and fetus, there is not good evidence that it causes congenital malformations. Pregnancy should be avoided for 3 months following vaccination.

Lactation Excretion in breast milk unknown/use caution

Contraindications

Hypersensitivity to mumps vaccine or any component of the formulation, including gelatin; febrile respiratory illness or active febrile infection; immunosuppressant therapy; primary or acquired immunodeficiency states; blood dyscrasias, leukemia, lymphoma or other malignant neoplasm affecting bone marrow or lymphatic systems; untreated tuberculosis; pregnancy

Warnings/Precautions Use caution with hypersensitivity to eggs or neomycin; patients with history of anaphylactic reaction may be at increased risk of immediate-type hypersensitivity reaction. Patients with minor illnesses (diarrhea, mild upper respiratory tract infection with or without low grade fever or other illnesses with low-grade fever) may receive vaccine. Leukemia patients who are in remission and who have not received chemotherapy for at least 3 months may be vaccinated. Patients with a history of congenital or hereditary immunodeficiency should not receive immunization until immune competence is demonstrated. Do not administer to severely immunocompromised persons with the exception of asymptomatic children with HIV. Corticosteroid replacement therapy is not a contraindication for vaccination. Use caution in patients with thrombocytopenia and those who develop thrombocytopenia after first dose; thrombocytopenia may worsen. Immediate treatment for anaphylactic/anaphylactoid reaction should be available during vaccine use. Safety and efficacy in children <12 months of age have not been established.

Adverse Reactions All serious adverse reactions must be reported to the U.S. Department of Health and Human Services (DHHS) Vaccine Adverse Event Reporting System (VAERS) 1-800-822-7967.

Frequency not defined.

Cardiovascular: Syncope, vasculitis

Central nervous system: Encephalitis, febrile seizure, fever, Guillain-Barré syndrome, irritability

Dermatologic: Angioneurotic edema, erythema multiforme, purpura, Stevens-Johnson syndrome, urticaria

Endocrine & metabolic: Diabetes mellitus, parotitis

Gastrointestinal: Diarrhea, pancreatitis

Genitourinary: Orchitis

Hematologic: Leukocytosis, thrombocytopenia

Local: Burning/stinging at injection site, wheal and flare at injection site

Ocular: Conjunctivitis, ocular palsies, optic neuritis, papillitis, retrobulbar neuritis

Otic: Nerve deafness, otitis media

Respiratory: Bronchial spasm, cough, rhinitis

Miscellaneous: Anaphylaxis, anaphylactoid reactions, lymphadenopathy

Drug Interactions

Avoid Concomitant Use

Avoid concomitant use of Mumps Virus Vaccine with any of the following: Immunosuppressants

Increased Effect/Toxicity

The levels/effects of Mumps Virus Vaccine may be increased by: Immunosuppressants

Decreased Effect

Mumps Virus Vaccine may decrease the levels/effects of: Tuberculin Tests

The levels/effects of Mumps Virus Vaccine may be decreased by: Immune Globulins

Stability Product is shipped at ≤10°C (50°F). Prior to reconstitution, vaccine must be stored at ≤2°C to 8°C (36°F to 46°F). Reconstitute using entire contents of one vial of provided preservative free diluent. Following reconstitution, use as soon as possible, but may be stored at 2°C to 8°C (36°F to 46°F) for up to 8 hours. Protect from light prior to and after reconstitution.

Mechanism of Action Promotes active immunity to mumps virus by inducing specific antibodies.

Dosage Children ≥12-15 months and Adults: SubQ: 0.5 mL as a single dose

Administration For SubQ administration in outer aspect of the upper arm using a 25G 5/8" needle

Test Interactions Temporary suppression of tuberculosis skin test

Additional Information Federal law requires that the date of administration, the vaccine manufacturer, lot number of vaccine, and the administering person's name, title, and address be entered into the patient's permanent medical record.

Acceptable presumptive evidence of immunity includes one of the following:

1. Documentation of adequate vaccination. Adequate vaccination for mumps is defined as 1 dose of a live mumps virus vaccine for preschool children and adults not at high risk; 2 doses of a live mumps virus vaccine for school-aged children and high-risk adults. Healthcare workers, international travelers, and students in institutions of higher learning are considered high-risk adults.
2. Laboratory evidence of immunity to mumps
3. Birth prior to 1957
4. Documentation of physician-diagnosed mumps

During a mumps outbreak, additional doses of a mumps virus vaccine may need to be considered. MMR vaccine is recommended; refer to Measles, Mumps, and Rubella Vaccine (Combined) monograph. Minimum interval between doses is 28 days.

Dosage Forms Excipient information presented when available (limited, particularly for generics); consult specific product labeling.

Injection, powder for reconstitution [preservative free]:

Mumpsvax®: ≥20,000 $TCID_{50}$ [contains albumin (human), bovine serum, chicken egg protein, gelatin, sorbitol, and sucrose (1.9 mg/vial)]

Mupirocin (myoo PEER oh sin)

U.S. Brand Names Bactroban®; Bactroban® Nasal; Centany™ [DSC]

Canadian Brand Names Bactroban®

Index Terms Mupirocin Calcium; Pseudomonic Acid A

Pharmacologic Category Antibiotic, Topical

Use

Intranasal: Eradication of nasal colonization with MRSA in adult patients and healthcare workers

Topical: Treatment of impetigo or secondary infected traumatic skin lesions due to *S. aureus* and *S. pyogenes*

Unlabeled/Investigational Use Intranasal: Surgical prophylaxis to prevent wound infections

Pregnancy Risk Factor B

Medication Safety Issues

Sound-alike/look-alike issues:

Bactroban® may be confused with bacitracin, baclofen, Bactrim™

Dosage

Intranasal: Children ≥12 years and Adults: Eradication of nasal MRSA: Approximately one-half of the ointment from the single-use tube should be applied into one nostril and the other half into the other nostril twice daily for 5 days

Topical:

Children ≥2 months and Adults: Impetigo: Ointment: Apply to affected area 3 times/day; re-evaluate after 3-5 days if no clinical response

Children ≥3 months and Adults: Secondary skin infections: Cream: Apply to affected area 3 times/day for 10 days; re-evaluate after 3-5 days if no clinical response

Additional Information Complete prescribing information for this medication should be consulted for additional detail.

Dosage Forms Excipient information presented when available (limited, particularly for generics); consult specific product labeling. [DSC] = Discontinued product

Note: Strength expressed as base

Cream, topical, as calcium:

Bactroban®: 2% (15 g, 30 g) [contains benzyl alcohol]

Ointment, intranasal, as calcium:

Bactroban® Nasal: 2% (1 g) [single-use tube]

Ointment, topical: 2% (0.9 g, 22 g)

Bactroban®: 2% (22 g) [contains polyethylene glycol]

Centany™: 2% (15 g) [DSC]

◆ **Mupirocin Calcium** *see* Mupirocin *on page* 1024

◆ **Murine® Ear Wax Removal System [OTC]** *see* Carbamide Peroxide *on page* 254

◆ **Muro 128® [OTC]** *see* Sodium Chloride *on page* 1381

◆ **Murocoll-2®** *see* Phenylephrine and Scopolamine *on page* 1185

Muromonab-CD3 (myoo roe MOE nab see dee three)

U.S. Brand Names Orthoclone OKT® 3

Canadian Brand Names Orthoclone OKT® 3

Index Terms Monoclonal Antibody; OKT3

Pharmacologic Category Immunosuppressant Agent

Use Treatment of acute allograft rejection in renal transplant patients; treatment of acute hepatic, and kidney rejection episodes resistant to conventional treatment

Unlabeled/Investigational Use Treatment of acute pancreas rejection episodes resistant to conventional treatment

Pregnancy Risk Factor C

Lactation Excretion in breast milk unknown/contraindicated

Contraindications Hypersensitivity to OKT3 or any murine product; patients with uncompensated heart failure or uncontrolled hypertension, in fluid overload or those with >3% weight gain within 1 week prior to start of OKT3; mouse antibody titers >1:1000; history of seizures; known or suspected pregnancy; breast-feeding

Warnings/Precautions It is imperative, especially prior to the first few doses, that there be no clinical evidence of volume overload, uncontrolled hypertension, or uncompensated heart failure, including a clear chest x-ray and weight restriction of ≤3% above the patient's minimum weight during the week prior to injection.

Risk of development of lymphoproliferative disorders (particularly of the skin) is increased. May result in an increased susceptibility to infection; dosage of concomitant immunosuppressants should be reduced during OKT3 therapy; cyclosporine should be decreased to 50% usual maintenance dose and maintenance therapy resumed about 4 days before stopping OKT3.

Severe pulmonary edema has occurred in patients with fluid overload. Seizures, encephalopathy, cerebral edema, aseptic meningitis, and headache have been reported following muromonab-CD3. Contraindicated for use in patients with a history of seizures or those who are predisposed to seizures. Arterial, venous, and capillary thrombosis of allografts and other vascular beds have been reported with use; use with caution in patients with history of thrombosis or underlying vascular disease.

[U.S. Boxed Warning]: Anaphylactic and anaphylactoid reactions may occur after administration of any dose of muromonab-CD3; acute hypersensitivity reactions may be characterized by cardiovascular collapse, cardiorespiratory arrest, loss of consciousness, shock, tachycardia, tingling, angioedema, airway obstruction, bronchospasm, dyspnea, urticaria, and pruritus. These reactions may be difficult to differentiate from the cytokine release syndrome associated with use; however, hypersensitivity reactions are more likely to occur within the first 10 minutes after administration. Cytokine release syndrome may occur in a significant proportion of patients following the first couple of doses of muromonab-CD3; symptoms usually begin 30-60 minutes after administration of dose and may persist for several hours; symptoms range from a mild, self-limiting "flu-like reaction" to severe, life-threatening shock-like reaction. Patients at higher risk for serious complications include those with unstable angina, recent MI or ischemic heart disease, heart failure, pulmonary edema, COPD, intravascular volume overload or depletion, cerebrovascular disease, patients with advanced symptomatic vascular disease or neuropathy, history of seizures, and septic shock. Pretreatment with corticosteroids may decrease serum levels of cytokines and manifestations of the syndrome, but it is not known if this decreases organ damage and sequelae associated with it.

Cardiopulmonary resuscitation may be needed. If the patient's temperature is >37.8°C, reduce before administering OKT3. **[U.S. Boxed Warning]: Should be administered under the supervision of a physician experienced in immunosuppressive therapy in a facility appropriate for monitoring and resuscitation.**

Adverse Reactions Note: Signs and symptoms of cytokine release syndrome (characterized by pyrexia, chills, dyspnea, nausea, vomiting, chest pain, diarrhea, tremor, wheezing, headache, tachycardia, rigor, hypertension, pulmonary edema and/or other cardiorespiratory manifestations) occurs in a significant proportion of patients following the first couple of doses of muromonab-CD3. See Warnings/Precautions. Additionally, some patients have experienced immediate hypersensitivity reactions to muromonab-CD3 (characterized by cardiovascular collapse, cardiorespiratory arrest, loss of consciousness, hypotension/shock, tachycardia, tingling, angioedema (including laryngeal, pharyngeal, or facial edema), airway obstruction, bronchospasm, dyspnea, urticaria, and/or pruritus) upon initial exposure and reexposure.

>10%:

- Cardiovascular: Tachycardia (26%), hypotension (25%), hypertension (19%), edema (12%)
- Central nervous system: Pyrexia (77%), chills (43%), headache (28%)
- Dermatologic: Rash (14%; erythematous 2%)
- Gastrointestinal: Diarrhea (37%), nausea (32%), vomiting (25%)
- Respiratory: Dyspnea (16%)

1% to 10%:

- Cardiovascular: Chest pain (9%), vasodilation (7%), arrhythmia (4%), bradycardia (4%), vascular occlusion (2%)
- Central nervous system: Fatigue (9%), confusion (6%), dizziness (6%), lethargy (6%), pain trunk (6%), malaise (5%), nervousness (5%), depression (3%), somnolence (2%), meningitis (1%), seizure (1%)
- Dermatologic: Pruritus (7%)
- Gastrointestinal: Gastrointestinal pain (7%), abdominal pain (6%), anorexia (4%)
- Hematologic: Leukopenia (7%), anemia (2%), thrombocytopenia (2%), leukocytosis (1%)
- Neuromuscular & skeletal: Weakness (10%), arthralgia (7%), myalgia (1%), tremor (14%)
- Ocular: Photophobia (1%)
- Otic: Tinnitus (1%)
- Renal: Renal dysfunction (3%)
- Respiratory: Abnormal chest sound (10%), hyperventilation (7%), wheezing (6%), respiratory congestion (4%), pulmonary edema (2%), hypoxia (1%), pneumonia (1%)
- Miscellaneous: Diaphoresis (7%), infections (various)

<1% (Limited to important or life-threatening): ALT increased, AST increased, angina, anuria, apnea, cardiac arrest, coagulation disorder, coma, conjunctivitis, encephalopathy, epilepsy, GI hemorrhage, hallucinations, hearing decreased, heart failure, hepatitis, hypotonia, lymphadenopathy, lymphopenia, MI, mood changes, neoplasms (various), oliguria, paranoia, pneumonitis, psychosis, shock, thrombosis

Drug Interactions

Avoid Concomitant Use

Avoid concomitant use of Muromonab-CD3 with any of the following: Natalizumab; Vaccines (Live)

Increased Effect/Toxicity

Muromonab-CD3 may increase the levels/effects of: Natalizumab; Vaccines (Live)

The levels/effects of Muromonab-CD3 may be increased by: Trastuzumab

Decreased Effect

Muromonab-CD3 may decrease the levels/effects of: Vaccines (Inactivated)

The levels/effects of Muromonab-CD3 may be decreased by: Echinacea

Stability Refrigerate; do not freeze. Do not shake. Stable in Becton Dickinson syringe for 16 hours at room temperature or refrigeration.

Mechanism of Action Reverses graft rejection by binding to T cells and interfering with their function by binding T-cell receptor-associated CD3 glycoprotein

Pharmacodynamics/Kinetics

Duration: 7 days after discontinuation

Time to peak: Steady-state: Trough: 3-14 days

Dosage I.V. (refer to individual protocols):

Children <30 kg: 2.5 mg/day once daily for 7-14 days

Children >30 kg: 5 mg/day once daily for 7-14 days

OR

Children <12 years: 0.1 mg/kg/day once daily for 10-14 days

Children ≥12 years and Adults: 5 mg/day once daily for 10-14 days

Hemodialysis: Molecular size of OKT3 is 150,000 daltons; not dialyzed by most standard dialyzers; however, may be dialyzed by high flux dialysis; OKT3 will be removed by plasmapheresis; administer following dialysis treatments

Peritoneal dialysis: Significant drug removal is unlikely based on physiochemical characteristics

Note: Suggested prevention/treatment of muromonab-CD3 first-dose effects (grouped by adverse reaction):

Severe pulmonary edema:

- Effective prevention or palliation: Clear chest x-ray within 24 hours preinjection; weight restriction to ≤3% gain over 7days preinjection
- Supportive treatment: Prompt intubation and oxygenation; 24 hours close observation

Fever, chills:

- Effective prevention or palliation: 15 mg/kg methylprednisolone sodium succinate 1 hour preinjection; fever reduction to <37.8°C (100°F) 1 hour preinjection; acetaminophen (1 g orally) and diphenhydramine (50 mg orally) 1 hour preinjection
- Supportive treatment: Cooling blanket; acetaminophen as needed

Respiratory effects:

- Effective prevention or palliation: 100 mg hydrocortisone sodium succinate 30 minutes postinjection
- Supportive treatment: Additional 100 mg hydrocortisone sodium succinate as needed for wheezing; if respiratory distress, give epinephrine 1:1000 (0.3 mL SubQ)

Dietary Considerations Injection solution contains sodium 43 mg/5 mL.

Administration Not for I.M. administration. Filter each dose through a low protein-binding 0.22 micron filter (Millex GV) before administration; administer I.V. push over <1 minute at a final concentration of 1 mg/mL

Children and Adults:

Methylprednisolone sodium succinate 15 mg/kg I.V. administered prior to first muromonab-CD3 administration and I.V. hydrocortisone sodium succinate 50-100 mg given 30 minutes after administration are strongly recommended to decrease the incidence of reactions to the first dose

Patient temperature should not exceed 37.8°C (100°F) at time of administration

Monitoring Parameters Chest x-ray, weight gain, CBC with differential, temperature, vital signs (blood pressure, temperature, pulse, respiration); immunologic monitoring of T cells, serum levels of OKT3

Reference Range

OKT3 serum concentrations:

Serum level monitoring should be performed in conjunction with lymphocyte subset determinations; Trough concentration sampling best correlates with clinical outcome. Serial monitoring may provide a better early indicator of inadequate dosing during induction or rejection.

Mean serum trough levels rise during the first 3 days, then average 0.9 mcg/mL on days 3-14

Circulating levels ≥0.8 mcg/mL block the function of cytotoxic T cells *in vitro* and *in vivo*

Several recent analysis have suggested appropriate dosage adjustments of OKT3 induction course are better determined with OKT3 serum levels versus lymphocyte subset determination; however, no prospective controlled trials have been performed to validate the equivalency of these tests in predicting clinical outcome.

Lymphocyte subset monitoring: CD3+ cells: Trough sample measurement is preferable and reagent utilized defines reference range.

OKT3-FITC: <10-50 cells/mm^3 or <3% to 5%

CD3(IgG1)-FITC: similar to OKT3-FITC

Leu-4a: Higher number of CD3+ cells appears acceptable

Dosage adjustments should be made in conjunction with clinical response and based upon trends over several consecutive days

Dosage Forms Excipient information presented when available (limited, particularly for generics); consult specific product labeling.

Injection, solution: 1 mg/mL (5 mL) [contains sodium 43 mg/5 mL]

◆ **Muse®** *see* Alprostadil *on page 70*

◆ **Muse® Pellet (Can)** *see* Alprostadil *on page 70*

◆ **Mustargen®** *see* Mechlorethamine *on page 927*

◆ **Mustine** *see* Mechlorethamine *on page 927*

◆ **Mutamycin® (Can)** *see* Mitomycin *on page 1005*

◆ **Myambutol®** *see* Ethambutol *on page 573*

◆ **Mycamine®** *see* Micafungin *on page 988*

◆ **Mycelex®** *see* Clotrimazole *on page 359*

◆ **Mycinaire™ [OTC] [DSC]** *see* Sodium Chloride *on page 1381*

◆ **Mycinettes® [OTC]** *see* Benzocaine *on page 183*

◆ **Mycobutin®** *see* Rifabutin *on page 1314*

◆ **Mycocide® NS [OTC]** *see* Tolnaftate *on page 1487*

◆ **Mycolog®-II [DSC]** *see* Nystatin and Triamcinolone *on page 1087*

Mycophenolate (mye koe FEN oh late)

U.S. Brand Names CellCept®; Myfortic®

Canadian Brand Names CellCept®; Myfortic®

Index Terms MMF; MPA; Mycophenolate Mofetil; Mycophenolate Sodium; Mycophenolic Acid

Pharmacologic Category Immunosuppressant Agent

Use Prophylaxis of organ rejection concomitantly with cyclosporine and corticosteroids in patients receiving allogeneic renal (CellCept®, Myfortic®), cardiac (CellCept®), or hepatic (CellCept®) transplants

Unlabeled/Investigational Use Treatment of rejection in liver transplant patients unable to tolerate tacrolimus or cyclosporine due to neurotoxicity; mild rejection in heart transplant patients; treatment of moderate-severe psoriasis; treatment of proliferative lupus nephritis; treatment of myasthenia gravis; prevention and treatment of graft-versus-host disease (GVHD)

Pregnancy Risk Factor D

Pregnancy Considerations **[U.S. Boxed Warning]: Mycophenolate is associated with an increased risk of congenital malformations and spontaneous abortions when used during pregnancy.** Adverse events have been reported in animal studies at doses less than the equivalent recommended human dose. Data from the National Transplantation Pregnancy Registry (NTPR) have observed an increase in structural malformations (including ear malformations) in infants born to mothers taking mycophenolate during pregnancy. Spontaneous abortions have also been noted. Females of childbearing potential should have a negative pregnancy test within 1 week prior to beginning therapy. Two reliable forms of contraception should be used beginning 4 weeks prior to, during, and for 6 weeks after therapy. The effectiveness of hormonal contraceptive agents may be affected by mycophenolate.

The National Transplantation Pregnancy Registry (NTPR, Temple University) is a registry for pregnant women taking immunosuppressants following any solid organ transplant. The NTPR encourages reporting of all immunosuppressant exposures during pregnancy in transplant recipients at 877-955-6877.

Lactation Excretion in breast milk unknown/not recommended

Contraindications Hypersensitivity to mycophenolate mofetil, mycophenolic acid, mycophenolate sodium, or any component of the formulation; intravenous formulation is contraindicated in patients who are allergic to polysorbate 80

Warnings/Precautions Hazardous agent - use appropriate precautions for handling and disposal. **[U.S. Boxed Warning]: Risk for infection and development of lymphoma and skin malignancy is increased.** Patients should be monitored appropriately, instructed to limit exposure to sunlight/UV light, and given supportive treatment should these conditions occur. Progressive multifocal leukoencephalopathy (PML) may occur rarely particularly in immunosuppressed patients or those receiving immunosuppressant therapy; monitor for signs of neurologic impairment (eg, apathy, ataxia, cognitive deficiencies, confusion, and hemiparesis); may require dosage reduction. Severe neutropenia may occur, requiring interruption of treatment (risk greater from day 31-180 post-transplant). Use caution with active peptic ulcer disease; may be associated with GI bleeding and/or perforation. Use caution in renal impairment as toxicity may be increased; may require dosage adjustment in severe impairment. Patients may be at increased risk of infection.

[U.S. Boxed Warning]: Mycophenolate is associated with an increased risk of congenital malformations and spontaneous abortions when used during pregnancy. Females of childbearing potential should have a negative pregnancy test within 1 week prior to beginning therapy. Two reliable forms of contraception should be used beginning 4 weeks prior to, during, and for 6 weeks after therapy. Because mycophenolate mofetil has demonstrated teratogenic effects in rats and rabbits, tablets should not be crushed, and capsules should not be opened or crushed. Avoid inhalation or direct contact with skin or mucous membranes of the powder contained in the capsules and the powder for oral suspension. Caution should be exercised in the handling and preparation of solutions of intravenous mycophenolate. Avoid skin contact with the intravenous solution and reconstituted suspension. If such contact occurs, wash thoroughly with soap and water, rinse eyes with plain water.

Theoretically, use should be avoided in patients with the rare hereditary deficiency of hypoxanthine-guanine phosphoribosyltransferase (such as Lesch-Nyhan or Kelley-Seegmiller syndrome). Intravenous solutions should be given over at least 2 hours; **never** administer intravenous solution by rapid or bolus injection. **[U.S. Boxed Warning]: Should be administered under the supervision of a physician experienced in immunosuppressive therapy.**

Note: CellCept® and Myfortic® dosage forms should not be used interchangeably due to differences in absorption. Some dosage forms may contain phenylalanine.

Adverse Reactions As reported in adults following oral dosing of CellCept® alone in renal, cardiac, and hepatic allograft rejection studies. In general, lower doses used in renal rejection patients had less adverse effects than higher doses. Rates of adverse effects were similar for each indication, except for those unique to the specific organ involved. The type of adverse effects observed in pediatric patients was similar to those seen in adults; abdominal pain, anemia, diarrhea, fever, hypertension, infection, pharyngitis, respiratory tract infection, sepsis, and vomiting were seen in higher proportion; lymphoproliferative disorder was the only type of malignancy observed. Percentages of adverse reactions were similar in studies comparing CellCept® to Myfortic® in patients following renal transplant.

>20%:

- Cardiovascular: Hypertension (28% to 77%), hypotension (up to 33%), peripheral edema (27% to 64%), edema (27% to 28%), tachycardia (20% to 22%)
- Central nervous system: Pain (31% to 76%), headache (16% to 54%), insomnia (41% to 52%), fever (21% to 52%), dizziness (up to 29%), anxiety (28%)
- Dermatologic: Rash (up to 22%)
- Endocrine & metabolic: Hyperglycemia (44% to 47%), hypercholesterolemia (41%), hypokalemia (32% to 37%), hypocalcemia (up to 30%), hypomagnesemia (up to 39%), hyperkalemia (up to 22%)
- Gastrointestinal: Abdominal pain (25% to 62%), nausea (20% to 54%), diarrhea (31% to 52%), constipation (18% to 41%), vomiting (33% to 34%), anorexia (up to 25%), dyspepsia (22%)
- Genitourinary: Urinary tract infection (37%)
- Hematologic: Leukopenia (23% to 46%), leukocytosis (22% to 40%), hypochromic anemia (26% to 43%), thrombocytopenia (24% to 36%)
- Hepatic: Liver function tests abnormal (up to 25%), ascites (24%)
- Neuromuscular & skeletal: Back pain (35% to 47%), weakness (35% to 43%), tremor (24% to 34%), paresthesia (21%)
- Renal: BUN increased (up to 35%), creatinine increased (up to 39%)
- Respiratory: Dyspnea (31% to 37%), respiratory tract infection (22% to 37%), cough (31%), lung disorder (22% to 30%)
- Miscellaneous: Infection (18% to 27%), *Candida* (11% to 22%), herpes simplex (10% to 21%)

3% to <20%:

- Cardiovascular: Angina, arrhythmia, arterial thrombosis, atrial fibrillation, atrial flutter, bradycardia, cardiac arrest, cardiac failure, CHF, extrasystole, facial edema, hypervolemia, pallor, palpitation, pericardial effusion, peripheral vascular disorder, postural hypotension, supraventricular extrasystoles, supraventricular tachycardia, syncope, thrombosis, vasodilation, vasospasm, venous pressure increased, ventricular extrasystole, ventricular tachycardia
- Central nervous system: Agitation, chills with fever, confusion, convulsion, delirium, depression, emotional lability, hallucinations, hypoesthesia, malaise, nervousness, psychosis, somnolence, thinking abnormal, vertigo
- Dermatologic: Acne, alopecia, bruising, cellulitis, hirsutism, petechia, pruritus, skin carcinoma, skin hypertrophy, skin ulcer, vesiculobullous rash
- Endocrine & metabolic: Acidosis, Cushing's syndrome, dehydration, diabetes mellitus, gout, hypercalcemia, hyperlipemia, hyperphosphatemia, hyperuricemia, hypochloremia, hypoglycemia, hyponatremia,

hypoproteinemia, hypothyroidism, parathyroid disorder, weight gain/loss

Gastrointestinal: Abdomen enlarged, dry mouth, dysphagia, esophagitis, flatulence, gastritis, gastroenteritis, gastrointestinal hemorrhage, gastrointestinal moniliasis, gingivitis, gum hyperplasia, ileus, melena, mouth ulceration, oral moniliasis, stomach disorder, stomatitis

Genitourinary: Impotence, nocturia, pelvic pain, prostatic disorder, scrotal edema, urinary frequency, urinary incontinence, urinary retention, urinary tract disorder

Hematologic: Coagulation disorder, hemorrhage, neutropenia, pancytopenia, polycythemia, prothrombin time increased, thromboplastin increased

Hepatic: Alkaline phosphatase increased, alkalosis, bilirubinemia, cholangitis, cholestatic jaundice, GGT increased, hepatitis, jaundice, liver damage, transaminases increased

Local: Abscess

Neuromuscular & skeletal: Arthralgia, hypertonia, joint disorder, leg cramps, myalgia, myasthenia, neck pain, neuropathy, osteoporosis

Ocular: Amblyopia, cataract, conjunctivitis, eye hemorrhage, lacrimation disorder, vision abnormal

Otic: Deafness, ear disorder, ear pain, tinnitus

Renal: Albuminuria, creatinine increased, dysuria, hematuria, hydronephrosis, kidney failure, kidney tubular necrosis, oliguria

Respiratory: Apnea, asthma, atelectasis, bronchitis, epistaxis, hemoptysis, hiccup, hyperventilation, hypoxia, respiratory acidosis, lung edema, pharyngitis, pleural effusion, pneumonia, pneumothorax, pulmonary hypertension, respiratory moniliasis, rhinitis, sinusitis, sputum increased, voice alteration

Miscellaneous: *Candida* (mucocutaneous 15% to 18%), CMV viremia/syndrome (12% to 14%), CMV tissue invasive disease (6% to 11%), herpes zoster cutaneous disease (4% to 10%), cyst, diaphoresis, flu-like syndrome, fungal dermatitis, healing abnormal, hernia, ileus infection, lactic dehydrogenase increased, peritonitis, pyelonephritis, thirst

Postmarketing and/or case reports: Atypical mycobacterial infection, colitis, gastrointestinal perforation, gastrointestinal ulcers, infectious endocarditis, interstitial lung disorder, intestinal villous atrophy, meningitis, pancreatitis, progressive multifocal leukoencephalopathy, pulmonary fibrosis (fatal), tuberculosis

Drug Interactions

Avoid Concomitant Use

Avoid concomitant use of Mycophenolate with any of the following: Cholestyramine Resin; Natalizumab; Rifamycin Derivatives; Vaccines (Live)

Increased Effect/Toxicity

Mycophenolate may increase the levels/effects of: Acyclovir-Valacyclovir; Ganciclovir-Valganciclovir; Natalizumab; Vaccines (Live)

The levels/effects of Mycophenolate may be increased by: Acyclovir-Valacyclovir; Ganciclovir-Valganciclovir; Probenecid; Trastuzumab

Decreased Effect

Mycophenolate may decrease the levels/effects of: Oral Contraceptive (Estrogens); Oral Contraceptive (Progestins); Vaccines (Inactivated)

The levels/effects of Mycophenolate may be decreased by: Antacids; Cholestyramine Resin; CycloSPORINE; Echinacea; Magnesium Salts; MetroNIDAZOLE; Proton Pump Inhibitors; Quinolone Antibiotics; Rifamycin Derivatives; Sevelamer

Ethanol/Nutrition/Herb Interactions

Food: Decreases C_{max} of MPA by 40% following CellCept® administration and 33% following Myfortic® use; the extent of absorption is not changed

Herb/Nutraceutical: Avoid cat's claw, echinacea (have immunostimulant properties)

Stability

Capsules: Store at room temperature of 15°C to 39°C (59°F to 86°F).

Tablets: Store at room temperature of 15°C to 39°C (59°F to 86°F). Protect from light.

Oral suspension: Store powder for oral suspension at room temperature of 15°C to 39°C (59°F to 86°F). Should be constituted prior to dispensing to the patient and **not** mixed with any other medication. Add 47 mL of water to the bottle and shake well for ~1 minute. Add another 47 mL of water to the bottle and shake well for an additional minute. Final concentration is 200 mg/mL of mycophenolate mofetil. Once reconstituted, the oral solution may be stored at room temperature or under refrigeration. Do not freeze. The mixed suspension is stable for 60 days.

I.V.: Store intact vials at room temperature 15°C to 30°C (59°F to 86°F). Reconstitute the contents of each vial with 14 mL of 5% dextrose injection; dilute the contents of a vial with 5% dextrose in water to a final concentration of 6 mg mycophenolate mofetil per mL. Begin infusion within 4 hours of reconstitution. **Note:** Vial is vacuum-sealed; if a lack of vacuum is noted during preparation, the vial should not be used. Store solutions at 15°C to 30°C (59°F to 86°F).

Mechanism of Action MPA exhibits a cytostatic effect on T and B lymphocytes. It is an inhibitor of inosine monophosphate dehydrogenase (IMPDH) which inhibits *de novo* guanosine nucleotide synthesis. T and B lymphocytes are dependent on this pathway for proliferation.

Pharmacodynamics/Kinetics

Onset of action: Peak effect: Correlation of toxicity or efficacy is still being developed, however, one study indicated that 12-hour AUCs >40 mcg/mL/hour were correlated with efficacy and decreased episodes of rejection

T_{max}: Oral: MPA:

CellCept®: 1-1.5 hours

Myfortic®: 1.5-2.5 hours

Absorption: AUC values for MPA are lower in the early post-transplant period versus later (>3 months) post-transplant period. The extent of absorption in pediatrics is similar to that seen in adults, although there was wide variability reported.

Oral: Myfortic®: 93%

Distribution:

CellCept®: MPA: Oral: 4 L/kg; I.V.: 3.6 L/kg

Myfortic®: MPA: Oral: 54 L (at steady state); 112 L (elimination phase)

Protein binding: MPA: 97%, MPAG 82%

Metabolism: Hepatic and via GI tract; CellCept® is completely hydrolyzed in the liver to mycophenolic acid (MPA; active metabolite); enterohepatic recirculation of MPA may occur; MPA is glucuronidated to MPAG (inactive metabolite)

Bioavailability: Oral: CellCept®: 94%; Myfortic®: 72%

Half-life elimination:

CellCept®: MPA: Oral: 18 hours; I.V.: 17 hours

Myfortic®: MPA: Oral: 8-16 hours; MPAG: 13-17 hours

Excretion:

CellCept®: MPA: Urine (<1%), feces (6%); MPAG: Urine (87%)

Myfortic®: MPA: Urine (3%), feces; MPAG: Urine (>60%)

Dosage

Children: Renal transplant: Oral:

CellCept® suspension: 600 mg/m^2/dose twice daily; maximum dose: 1 g twice daily

Alternatively, may use solid dosage forms according to BSA as follows:

BSA 1.25-1.5 m^2: 750 mg capsule twice daily

BSA >1.5 m^2: 1 g capsule or tablet twice daily

Myfortic®: 400 mg/m^2/dose twice daily; maximum dose: 720 mg twice daily
BSA <1.19 m^2: Use of this formulation is not recommended
BSA 1.19-1.58 m^2: 540 mg twice daily (maximum: 1080 mg/day)
BSA >1.58 m^2: 720 mg twice daily (maximum: 1440 mg/day)

Adults: **Note:** May be used I.V. for up to 14 days; transition to oral therapy as soon as tolerated.
Renal transplant:
CellCept®:
Oral: 1 g twice daily. Doses >2 g/day are not recommended.
I.V.: 1 g twice daily
Myfortic®: Oral: 720 mg twice daily (1440 mg/day)
Cardiac transplantation:
Oral (CellCept®): 1.5 g twice daily
I.V. (CellCept®): 1.5 g twice daily
Hepatic transplantation:
Oral (CellCept®): 1.5 g twice daily
I.V. (CellCept®): 1 g twice daily
Myasthenia gravis (unlabeled use): Oral (CellCept®): 1 g twice daily (range 1-3 g/day)

Dosing adjustment in renal impairment:
Renal transplant: GFR <25 mL/minute in patients outside the immediate post-transplant period:
CellCept®: Doses of >1 g administered twice daily should be avoided; patients should also be carefully observed; no dose adjustments are needed in renal transplant patients experiencing delayed graft function postoperatively
Myfortic®: Cl_{cr} <25 mL/minute: Monitor carefully
Cardiac or liver transplant: No data available; mycophenolate may be used in cardiac or hepatic transplant patients with severe chronic renal impairment if the potential benefit outweighs the potential risk

Hemodialysis: Not removed; supplemental dose is not necessary

Peritoneal dialysis: Supplemental dose is not necessary

Dosage adjustment in hepatic impairment: No dosage adjustment is recommended for renal patients with severe hepatic parenchymal disease; however, it is not currently known whether dosage adjustments are necessary for hepatic disease with other etiologies

Elderly: Dosage is the same as younger patients, however, dosing should be cautious due to possibility of increased hepatic, renal or cardiac dysfunction; elderly patients may be at an increased risk of certain infections, gastrointestinal hemorrhage, and pulmonary edema, as compared to younger patients

Dosing adjustment for toxicity (neutropenia): ANC <1.3 x 10^3/µL: Dosing should be interrupted or the dose reduced, appropriate diagnostic tests performed and patients managed appropriately

Dietary Considerations Oral dosage formulations should be taken on an empty stomach to avoid variability in MPA absorption. However, in stable renal transplant patients, may be administered with food if necessary. Oral suspension contains 0.56 mg phenylalanine/mL; use caution if administered to patients with phenylketonuria.

Administration

Oral dosage formulations (tablet, capsule, suspension) should be administered on an empty stomach to avoid variability in MPA absorption. The oral solution may be administered via a nasogastric tube (minimum 8 French, 1.7 mm interior diameter); oral suspension should not be mixed with other medications. Delayed release tablets should not be crushed, cut, or chewed.

Intravenous solutions should be administered over at least 2 hours (either peripheral or central vein); do **not** administer intravenous solution by rapid or bolus injection.

Monitoring Parameters Complete blood count; signs and symptoms of infection; pregnancy test (prior to initiation in females of childbearing potential)

Dosage Forms Excipient information presented when available (limited, particularly for generics); consult specific product labeling.
Capsule, as mofetil:
CellCept®: 250 mg
Injection, powder for reconstitution, as mofetil hydrochloride:
CellCept®: 500 mg [contains polysorbate 80]
Powder for oral suspension, as mofetil:
CellCept®: 200 mg/mL (225 mL) [provides 175 mL suspension following reconstitution; contains phenylalanine 0.56 mg/mL; mixed fruit flavor]
Tablet, as mofetil:
CellCept®: 500 mg [may contain ethyl alcohol]
Tablet, delayed release, as mycophenolic acid:
Myfortic®: 180 mg, 360 mg [formulated as a sodium salt]

- ◆ **Mycophenolate Mofetil** *see* Mycophenolate *on page 1026*
- ◆ **Mycophenolate Sodium** *see* Mycophenolate *on page 1026*
- ◆ **Mycophenolic Acid** *see* Mycophenolate *on page 1026*
- ◆ **Mycostatin®** *see* Nystatin *on page 1087*
- ◆ **MyDex** *see* Guaifenesin and Phenylephrine *on page 712*
- ◆ **Mydfrin®** *see* Phenylephrine *on page 1183*
- ◆ **Mydral™** *see* Tropicamide *on page 1525*
- ◆ **Mydriacyl®** *see* Tropicamide *on page 1525*
- ◆ **Myfortic®** *see* Mycophenolate *on page 1026*
- ◆ **MyHist-PD** *see* Chlorpheniramine, Pyrilamine, and Phenylephrine *on page 315*
- ◆ **MyKidz Iron 10™** *see* Ferrous Sulfate *on page 617*
- ◆ **Mylanta™ (Can)** *see* Aluminum Hydroxide and Magnesium Hydroxide *on page 76*
- ◆ **Mylanta® Children's [OTC]** *see* Calcium Carbonate *on page 238*
- ◆ **Mylanta® Double Strength (Can)** *see* Aluminum Hydroxide, Magnesium Hydroxide, and Simethicone *on page 76*
- ◆ **Mylanta® Extra Strength (Can)** *see* Aluminum Hydroxide, Magnesium Hydroxide, and Simethicone *on page 76*
- ◆ **Mylanta® Gelcaps® [OTC]** *see* Calcium Carbonate and Magnesium Hydroxide *on page 239*
- ◆ **Mylanta® Liquid [OTC]** *see* Aluminum Hydroxide, Magnesium Hydroxide, and Simethicone *on page 76*
- ◆ **Mylanta® Maximum Strength Liquid [OTC]** *see* Aluminum Hydroxide, Magnesium Hydroxide, and Simethicone *on page 76*
- ◆ **Mylanta® Regular Strength (Can)** *see* Aluminum Hydroxide, Magnesium Hydroxide, and Simethicone *on page 76*
- ◆ **Mylanta® Supreme [OTC]** *see* Calcium Carbonate and Magnesium Hydroxide *on page 239*
- ◆ **Mylanta® Ultra [OTC]** *see* Calcium Carbonate and Magnesium Hydroxide *on page 239*
- ◆ **Myleran®** *see* Busulfan *on page 227*
- ◆ **Mylocel™** *see* Hydroxyurea *on page 753*
- ◆ **Mylotarg®** *see* Gemtuzumab Ozogamicin *on page 689*
- ◆ **Myobloc®** *see* Botulinum Toxin Type B *on page 210*
- ◆ **Myochrysine®** *see* Gold Sodium Thiomalate *on page 704*
- ◆ **Myozyme®** *see* Alglucosidase Alfa *on page 62*
- ◆ **myrac™** *see* Minocycline *on page 999*

- **Mysoline®** *see* Primidone *on page 1238*
- **Mytussin® AC** *see* Guaifenesin and Codeine *on page 710*
- **Mytussin® DAC** *see* Guaifenesin, Pseudoephedrine, and Codeine *on page 715*
- **N-9** *see* Nonoxynol 9 *on page 1077*
- **N-0923** *see* Rotigotine *on page 1346*
- **Na_2EDTA** *see* Edetate Disodium *on page 505*
- **NAAK** *see* Atropine and Pralidoxime *on page 159*
- **Nabi-HB®** *see* Hepatitis B Immune Globulin (Human) *on page 727*
- **nab-Paclitaxel** *see* Paclitaxel (Protein Bound) *on page 1129*

Nabumetone (na BYOO me tone)

Canadian Brand Names Apo-Nabumetone®; Gen-Nabumetone; Novo-Nabumetone; Relafen®; Rhoxal-nabumetone; Sandoz-Nabumetone

Index Terms Relafen

Pharmacologic Category Nonsteroidal Anti-inflammatory Drug (NSAID), Oral

Additional Appendix Information

Nonsteroidal Anti-inflammatory Agents *on page 1669*

Use Management of osteoarthritis and rheumatoid arthritis

Unlabeled/Investigational Use Moderate pain

Restrictions An FDA-approved medication guide must be distributed when dispensing an oral outpatient prescription (new or refill) where this medication is to be used without direct supervision of a healthcare provider. Medication guides are available at http://www.fda.gov/cder/Offices/ODS/medication_guides.htm.

Pregnancy Risk Factor C/D (3rd trimester)

Lactation Excretion in breast milk unknown/not recommended

Contraindications Hypersensitivity to nabumetone, aspirin, other NSAIDs, or any component of the formulation; perioperative pain in the setting of coronary artery bypass graft (CABG) surgery

Warnings/Precautions **[U.S. Boxed Warning]: NSAIDs are associated with an increased risk of adverse cardiovascular thrombotic events, including MI, stroke, and new onset or worsening of pre-existing hypertension.** Risk may be increased with duration of use or pre-existing cardiovascular risk factors or disease. Carefully evaluate individual cardiovascular risk profiles prior to prescribing. Use caution with fluid retention, heart failure, or hypertension. Concurrent administration of ibuprofen, and potentially other nonselective NSAIDs, may interfere with aspirin's cardioprotective effect. **[U.S. Boxed Warning]: Use is contraindicated for treatment of perioperative pain in the setting of coronary artery bypass graft (CABG) surgery.** Risk of MI and stroke may be increased with use following CABG surgery.

Platelet adhesion and aggregation may be decreased; may prolong bleeding time; patients with coagulation disorders or who are receiving anticoagulants should be monitored closely. Anemia may occur; patients on long-term NSAID therapy should be monitored for anemia. NSAID use may compromise existing renal function; dose-dependent decreases in prostaglandin synthesis may result from NSAID use, reducing renal blood flow which may cause renal decompensation. Patients with impaired renal function, dehydration, heart failure, liver dysfunction, those taking diuretics, and ACE inhibitors, and the elderly are at greater risk of renal toxicity. Rehydrate patient before starting therapy; monitor renal function closely. Not recommended for use in patients with advanced renal disease. Long-term NSAID use may result in renal papillary necrosis.

[U.S. Boxed Warning]: NSAIDs may increase risk of gastrointestinal irritation, inflammation, ulceration, bleeding, and perforation. These events may occur at any time during therapy and without warning. Use caution with a history of GI disease (bleeding or ulcers), concurrent therapy with aspirin, anticoagulants and/or corticosteroids, smoking, use of alcohol, the elderly or debilitated patients.

Use the lowest effective dose for the shortest duration of time, consistent with individual patient goals, to reduce risk of cardiovascular or GI adverse events. Alternate therapies should be considered for patients at high risk.

NSAIDs may cause serious skin adverse events including exfoliative dermatitis, Stevens-Johnson syndrome (SJS) and toxic epidermal necrolysis (TEN); discontinue use at first sign of skin rash or hypersensitivity. Anaphylactoid reactions may occur, even without prior exposure; patients with "aspirin triad" (bronchial asthma, aspirin intolerance, rhinitis) may be at increased risk. Do not use in patients who experience bronchospasm, asthma, rhinitis, or urticaria with NSAID or aspirin therapy. Use caution in other forms of asthma.

Use with caution in patients with decreased hepatic function. Closely monitor patients with any abnormal LFT. Severe hepatic reactions (eg, fulminant hepatitis, liver failure) have occurred with NSAID use, rarely; discontinue if signs or symptoms of liver disease develop, or if systemic manifestations occur.

The elderly are at increased risk for adverse effects (especially peptic ulceration, CNS effects, renal toxicity) from NSAIDs even at low doses.

Withhold for at least 4-6 half-lives prior to surgical or dental procedures. May cause photosensitivity reactions. Safety and efficacy have not been established in pediatric patients.

Adverse Reactions

>10%: Gastrointestinal: Abdominal pain (12%), diarrhea (14%), dyspepsia (13%)

1% to 10%:

Cardiovascular: Edema (3% to 9%)

Central nervous system: Dizziness (3% to 9%), headache (3% to 9%), fatigue (1% to 3%), insomnia (1% to 3%), nervousness (1% to 3%), somnolence (1% to 3%)

Dermatologic: Pruritus (3% to 9%), rash (3% to 9%)

Gastrointestinal: Constipation (3% to 9%), flatulence (3% to 9%), guaiac positive (3% to 9%), nausea (3% to 9%), gastritis (1% to 3%), stomatitis (1% to 3%), vomiting (1% to 3%), xerostomia (1% to 3%)

Otic: Tinnitus

Miscellaneous: Diaphoresis (1% to 3%)

<1% (Limited to important or life-threatening): Abnormal vision, acne, agitation, albuminuria, alopecia, anaphylactoid reaction, anaphylaxis, anemia, angina, angioneurotic edema, anorexia, anxiety, arrhythmia, asthma, azotemia, bilirubinemia duodenitis, bullous eruptions, CHF, chills, confusion, cough, depression, duodenal ulcer, dysphagia, dyspnea, dysuria, eosinophilic pneumonia, eructation, erythema multiforme, fever, gallstones, gastric ulcer, gastroenteritis, gingivitis, GI bleeding, glossitis, granulocytopenia, hematuria, hepatic failure, hyperglycemia, hypersensitivity pneumonitis, hypertension, hyperuricemia, hypokalemia, impotence, interstitial nephritis, interstitial pneumonitis, jaundice, leukopenia, liver function abnormalities, malaise, melena, MI, nephrotic syndrome, nightmares, palpitation, pancreatitis, paresthesia, photosensitivity, pseudoporphyria cutanea tarda, rectal bleeding, renal failure, renal stones, Stevens-Johnson syndrome, syncope, taste disorder, thrombocytopenia, thrombophlebitis, toxic epidermal necrolysis, tremor, urticaria, vasculitis, vertigo, weakness, weight gain/loss

Drug Interactions

Avoid Concomitant Use

Avoid concomitant use of Nabumetone with any of the following: Ketorolac

Increased Effect/Toxicity

Nabumetone may increase the levels/effects of: Aminoglycosides; Anticoagulants; Antiplatelet Agents; Bisphosphonate Derivatives; CycloSPORINE; Desmopressin; Lithium; Methotrexate; Nonsteroidal Anti-Inflammatory Agents; Pemetrexed; Quinolone Antibiotics; Salicylates; Thrombolytic Agents; Vancomycin; Vitamin K Antagonists

The levels/effects of Nabumetone may be increased by: Antidepressants (Tricyclic, Tertiary Amine); Corticosteroids (Systemic); Herbs (Anticoagulant/Antiplatelet Properties); Ketorolac; Probenecid; Selective Serotonin Reuptake Inhibitors; Serotonin/Norepinephrine Reuptake Inhibitors; Treprostinil

Decreased Effect

Nabumetone may decrease the levels/effects of: ACE Inhibitors; Angiotensin II Receptor Blockers; Antiplatelet Agents; Beta-Blockers; Eplerenone; HydrALAZINE; Loop Diuretics; Salicylates; Thiazide Diuretics

The levels/effects of Nabumetone may be decreased by: Bile Acid Sequestrants; Salicylates

Ethanol/Nutrition/Herb Interactions

Ethanol: Avoid ethanol (may enhance gastric mucosal irritation).

Food: Nabumetone peak serum concentrations may be increased if taken with food or dairy products.

Herb/Nutraceutical: Avoid alfalfa, anise, bilberry, bladderwrack, bromelain, cat's claw, celery, chamomile, coleus, cordyceps, dong quai, evening primrose, fenugreek, feverfew, garlic, ginger, ginkgo biloba, ginseng (American, Panax, Siberian), grapeseed, green tea, guggul, horse chestnut seed, horseradish, licorice, prickly ash, red clover, reishi, SAMe (S-adenosylmethionine), sweet clover, turmeric, white willow (all have additional antiplatelet activity).

Mechanism of Action Reversibly inhibits cyclooxygenase-1 and 2 (COX-1 and 2) enzymes, which result in decreased formation of prostaglandin precursors; has antipyretic, analgesic, and anti-inflammatory properties

Pharmacodynamics/Kinetics

Onset of action: Several days

Distribution: Diffusion occurs readily into synovial fluid

V_d: 6MNA: 29-82 L

Protein binding: 6MNA: >99%

Metabolism: Prodrug, rapidly metabolized in the liver to an active metabolite [6-methoxy-2-naphthylacetic acid (6MNA)] and inactive metabolites; extensive first-pass effect

Half-life elimination: 6MNA: ~24 hours

Time to peak, serum: 6MNA: Oral: 2.5-4 hours; Synovial fluid: 4-12 hours

Excretion: 6MNA: Urine (80%) and feces (9%)

Dosage Adults: Oral: 1000 mg/day; an additional 500-1000 mg may be needed in some patients to obtain more symptomatic relief; may be administered once or twice daily (maximum dose: 2000 mg/day)

Note: Patients <50 kg are less likely to require doses >1000 mg/day.

Dosage adjustment in renal impairment: In general, NSAIDs are not recommended for use in patients with advanced renal disease, but the manufacturer of nabumetone does provide some guidelines for adjustment in renal dysfunction:

Moderate impairment (Cl_{cr} 30-49 mL/minute): Initial dose: 750 mg/day; maximum dose: 1500 mg/day

Severe impairment (Cl_{cr} <30 mL/minute): Initial dose: 500 mg/day; maximum dose: 1000 mg/day

Monitoring Parameters Patients with renal insufficiency: Baseline renal function followed by repeat test within weeks (to determine if renal function has deteriorated)

Dosage Forms Excipient information presented when available (limited, particularly for generics); consult specific product labeling. [DSC] = Discontinued product

Tablet: 500 mg, 750 mg

Relafen®: 500 mg, 750 mg [DSC]

- **NAC** *see* Acetylcysteine *on page 36*
- ***N*-Acetyl-L-cysteine** *see* Acetylcysteine *on page 36*
- ***N*-Acetylcysteine** *see* Acetylcysteine *on page 36*
- **N-Acetyl-P-Aminophenol** *see* Acetaminophen *on page 25*
- **NaCl** *see* Sodium Chloride *on page 1381*

Nadolol (NAY doe lol)

U.S. Brand Names Corgard®

Canadian Brand Names Alti-Nadolol; Apo-Nadol®; Corgard®; Novo-Nadolol

Pharmacologic Category Beta-Adrenergic Blocker, Nonselective

Additional Appendix Information

Beta-Blockers *on page 1648*

Use Treatment of hypertension and angina pectoris; prophylaxis of migraine headaches

Unlabeled/Investigational Use Primary and secondary prophylaxis of variceal hemorrhage

Pregnancy Risk Factor C

Pregnancy Considerations No data available on crossing the placenta. Beta-blockers have been associated with bradycardia, hypotension, and IUGR; IUGR is probably related to maternal hypertension. Alternative beta-blockers are preferred for use during pregnancy due to limited data and prolonged half-life. Cases of neonatal hypoglycemia have been reported following maternal use of beta-blockers at parturition or during breast-feeding. Monitor breast-fed infant for symptoms of beta-blockade.

Lactation Enters breast milk/use caution (AAP rates "compatible")

Medication Safety Issues

Sound-alike/look-alike issues:

Nadolol may be confused with Mandol®

Corgard® may be confused with Cognex®, Coreg®

Contraindications Hypersensitivity to nadolol or any component of the formulation; bronchial asthma; sinus bradycardia; sinus node dysfunction; heart block greater than first degree (except in patients with a functioning artificial pacemaker); cardiogenic shock; uncompensated cardiac failure

Warnings/Precautions Consider pre-existing conditions such as sick sinus syndrome before initiating. Administer only with extreme caution in patients with compensated heart failure, monitor for a worsening of the condition. Efficacy in heart failure has not been established for nadolol. **[U.S. Boxed Warning]: Beta-blocker therapy should not be withdrawn abruptly (particularly in patients with CAD), but gradually tapered to avoid acute tachycardia, hypertension, and/or ischemia.** Use caution with concurrent use of beta-blockers and either verapamil or diltiazem; bradycardia or heart block can occur. In general, patients with bronchospastic disease should not receive beta-blockers. Nadolol, if used at all, should be used cautiously in bronchospastic disease with close monitoring. Use cautiously in diabetics because it can mask prominent hypoglycemic symptoms. Use cautiously in the renally impaired (dosage adjustments are required). Use with caution in patients with myasthenia gravis, peripheral vascular disease, or psychiatric disease (may cause CNS depression). Use care with anesthetic agents which decrease myocardial function. Adequate alpha-blockade is required prior to use of any beta-blocker for patients with untreated pheochromocytoma. Use caution with history of severe anaphylaxis to allergens; patients taking beta-blockers may become more sensitive to repeated challenges. Treatment of anaphylaxis (eg, epinephrine) in patients taking beta-blockers may be ineffective or promote undesirable effects. Safety and efficacy have not been established in children.

Adverse Reactions

>10%:

Central nervous system: Drowsiness, insomnia

Endocrine & metabolic: Decreased sexual ability

1% to 10%:

Cardiovascular: Bradycardia, palpitation, edema, CHF, reduced peripheral circulation

Central nervous system: Mental depression

Gastrointestinal: Diarrhea or constipation, nausea, vomiting, stomach discomfort

Respiratory: Bronchospasm

Miscellaneous: Cold extremities

<1% (Limited to important or life-threatening): Arrhythmias, chest pain, confusion (especially in the elderly), depression, dyspnea, hallucinations, leukopenia, orthostatic hypotension, thrombocytopenia

Drug Interactions

Avoid Concomitant Use

Avoid concomitant use of Nadolol with any of the following: Methacholine

Increased Effect/Toxicity

Nadolol may increase the levels/effects of: Alpha-/Beta-Agonists (Direct-Acting); Alpha1-Blockers; Alpha2-Agonists; Amifostine; Cardiac Glycosides; Insulin; Lidocaine; Methacholine; Midodrine; RiTUXimab

The levels/effects of Nadolol may be increased by: Acetylcholinesterase Inhibitors; Amiodarone; Anilidopiperidine Opioids; Calcium Channel Blockers (Nondihydropyridine); Diazoxide; Dipyridamole; Disopyramide; Herbs (Hypotensive Properties); P-Glycoprotein Inhibitors; Prostacyclin Analogues; Reserpine

Decreased Effect

Nadolol may decrease the levels/effects of: Beta2-Agonists; Theophylline Derivatives

The levels/effects of Nadolol may be decreased by: Herbs (Hypertensive Properties); Methylphenidate; Nonsteroidal Anti-Inflammatory Agents; P-Glycoprotein Inducers; Yohimbine

Ethanol/Nutrition/Herb Interactions Herb/Nutraceutical: Avoid dong quai if using for hypertension (has estrogenic activity). Avoid ephedra, garlic, yohimbe, ginseng (may worsen hypertension). Avoid natural licorice (causes sodium and water retention and increases potassium loss).

Mechanism of Action Competitively blocks response to $beta_1$- and $beta_2$-adrenergic stimulation; does not exhibit any membrane stabilizing or intrinsic sympathomimetic activity. Nonselective beta-adrenergic blockers (propranolol, nadolol) reduce portal pressure by producing splanchnic vasoconstriction ($beta_2$ effect) thereby reducing portal blood flow.

Pharmacodynamics/Kinetics

Duration: 17-24 hours

Absorption: 30% to 40%

Distribution: Concentration in human breast milk is 4.6 times higher than serum

Protein binding: 28%

Half-life elimination: Adults: 10-24 hours; prolonged with renal impairment; End-stage renal disease: 45 hours

Time to peak, serum: 2-4 hours

Excretion: Urine (as unchanged drug)

Dosage Oral:

Adults: Initial: 40 mg/day, increase dosage gradually by 40-80 mg increments at 3- to 7-day intervals until optimum clinical response is obtained with profound slowing of heart rate; doses up to 160-240 mg/day in angina and 240-320 mg/day in hypertension may be necessary.

Hypertension: Usual dosage range (JNC 7): 40-120 mg once daily

Variceal hemorrhage prophylaxis (unlabeled use; Garcia-Tsao, 2007):

Primary prophylaxis: Initial: 40 mg once daily; adjust to maximal tolerated dose. **Note:** Risk factors for hemorrhage include Child-Pugh class B/C or variceal red wale markings on endoscopy.

Secondary prophylaxis: Initial: 40 mg once daily; adjust to maximal tolerated dose

Elderly: Initial: 20 mg/day; increase doses by 20 mg increments at 3- to 7-day intervals; usual dosage range: 20-240 mg/day.

Dosing adjustment in renal impairment:

Cl_{cr} 31-40 mL/minute: Administer every 24-36 hours or administer 50% of normal dose.

Cl_{cr} 10-30 mL/minute: Administer every 24-48 hours or administer 50% of normal dose.

Cl_{cr} <10 mL/minute: Administer every 40-60 hours or administer 25% of normal dose.

Hemodialysis: Moderately dialyzable (20% to 50%); administer dose postdialysis or administer 40 mg supplemental dose.

Peritoneal dialysis: Supplemental dose is not necessary.

Dosing adjustment/comments in hepatic disease: Reduced dose probably necessary.

Dietary Considerations May be taken without regard to meals.

Dosage Forms Excipient information presented when available (limited, particularly for generics); consult specific product labeling. [DSC] = Discontinued product

Tablet: 20 mg, 40 mg, 80 mg

Corgard®: 20 mg, 40 mg, 80 mg, 120 mg [DSC], 160 mg [DSC]

Nafarelin (naf a REL in)

U.S. Brand Names Synarel®

Canadian Brand Names Synarel®

Index Terms Nafarelin Acetate

Pharmacologic Category Gonadotropin Releasing Hormone Agonist

Use Treatment of endometriosis, including pain and reduction of lesions; treatment of central precocious puberty (CPP; gonadotropin-dependent precocious puberty) in children of both sexes

Pregnancy Risk Factor X

Pregnancy Considerations Major fetal abnormalities have been reported in some animal studies; a dose-related increase in fetal mortality and decrease in fetal weight was also observed. Ovulation is inhibited and menstruation is stopped when used appropriately for the treatment of endometriosis, however contraception is not assured. Nonhormonal contraception is recommended. Pregnancy should be excluded prior to initiating treatment. There is no evidence that pregnancy rates are enhanced or adversely affected by use.

Lactation Excretion in breast milk unknown/contraindicated

Medication Safety Issues

Sound-alike/look-alike issues:

Nafarelin may be confused with Anafranil®, enalapril

Contraindications Hypersensitivity to gonadotropin-releasing hormone (GnRH), GnRH-agonist analogs, or any component of the formulation; undiagnosed abnormal vaginal bleeding; pregnancy; breast-feeding

Warnings/Precautions Hazardous agent - use appropriate precautions for handling and disposal. Use with caution in patients with risk factors for decreased bone mineral density, nafarelin therapy may pose an additional risk. Ovarian cysts may occur within the first 2 months of therapy and may occur more commonly in women with polycystic ovarian disease. When used for the treatment of CPP, some signs of puberty (eg vaginal bleeding, breast enlargement) may occur but should resolve within the first 2 months of therapy.

Adverse Reactions Note: Adverse events may be more frequent in the first 6 weeks of treatment due to stimulation of the pituitary-gonadal axis. Sensitivity reactions included chest pain, pruritus, shortness of breath, rash.

CPP: 1% to 10%:

Central nervous system: Emotional lability (6%)
Dermatologic: Acne (10%), seborrhea (3%)
Endocrine & metabolic: Breast enlargement (8%; transient), vaginal bleeding (8%), hot flashes (3%; transient), vaginal discharge (3%)
Respiratory: Rhinitis (5%)
Miscellaneous: Pubic hair increased (5%; transient), body odor (4%), sensitivity reactions (3%)

Endometriosis:

>10%:

Central nervous system: Headache, emotional lability
Dermatologic: Acne
Endocrine & metabolic: Hot flashes (90%), hyperphosphatemia, hypertriglyceridemia, hypocalcemia, libido decreased
Genitourinary: Vaginal dryness
Hematologic: Leukopenia

1% to 10%:

Cardiovascular: Edema
Central nervous system: Depression, insomnia
Dermatologic: Hirsutism, seborrhea
Endocrine & metabolic: Breast size reduced, cholesterol increased, hyperlipidemia, libido increased
Gastrointestinal: Weight gain/loss
Neuromuscular & skeletal: Bone mineral density decreased, myalgia
Respiratory: Nasal irritation

<1% (Limited to important or life-threatening): Arthralgia, breast engorgement, chloasma, eye pain, lactation, maculopapular rash, palpitation, paresthesia, sensitivity reactions, weakness

Postmarketing and/or case reports (any indication): ALT increased, AST increased, pituitary apoplexy, pituitary gland changes

Drug Interactions

Avoid Concomitant Use There are no known interactions where it is recommended to avoid concomitant use.

Increased Effect/Toxicity There are no known significant interactions involving an increase in effect.

Decreased Effect

Nafarelin may decrease the levels/effects of: Antidiabetic Agents

Stability Store at room temperature of 15°C to 30°C (59°F to 86°F). Protect from light.

Mechanism of Action Potent synthetic decapeptide analogue of gonadotropin-releasing hormone (GnRH; LHRH) which is approximately 200 times more potent than GnRH in terms of pituitary release of luteinizing hormone (LH) and follicle-stimulating hormone (FSH). Effects on the pituitary gland and sex hormones are dependent upon its length of administration. After acute administration, an initial stimulation of the release of LH and FSH from the pituitary is observed; an increase in androgens and estrogens subsequently follows. Continued administration of nafarelin, however, suppresses gonadotrope responsiveness to endogenous GnRH resulting in reduced secretion of LH and FSH and, secondarily, decreased ovarian and testicular steroid production.

Pharmacodynamics/Kinetics

Protein binding, plasma: 80%
Metabolism: Degraded by peptidase; forms metabolites
Bioavailability: ~1% to 6%
Half-life elimination: ~3 hours; Metabolites: ~86 hours
Time to peak, serum: 10-45 minutes
Excretion: Urine (44% to 55%, ~3% as unchanged drug); feces (19% to 44%)

Dosage Intranasal:

Endometriosis: Adults: Female: 1 spray (200 mcg) in 1 nostril each morning and the other nostril each evening starting on days 2-4 of menstrual cycle (total: 2 sprays/day). Dose may be increased to 2 sprays (400 mcg; 1 spray in each nostril) in the morning and evening if amenorrhea is not achieved (total: 8 sprays [1600 mcg]/day). Total duration of therapy should not exceed 6 months due to decreases in bone mineral density; retreatment is not recommended by the manufacturer.

Central precocious puberty: Children: Male/Female: 2 sprays (400 mcg) into each nostril in the morning and 2 sprays (400 mcg) into each nostril in the evening (total: 8 sprays [1600 mcg]/day). If inadequate suppression, may increase dose to 3 sprays (600 mcg) into alternating nostrils 3 times/day (total: 9 sprays [1800 mcg]/day).

Administration Nasal spray: Do not use topical nasal decongestant for at least 2 hours after nafarelin use. Allow ~30 seconds to elapse between sprays. Sneezing during or immediately after dosing should be avoided (may decrease drug absorption).

Monitoring Parameters

CPP: Bone mineral density, GnRH testing (blood LH and FSH levels), measurement of bone age, Tanner staging
Endometriosis: Menstruation, vaginal bleeding or spotting which persists after 2 months of treatment

Test Interactions Diagnostic tests of pituitary gonadotropic and gonadal functions during and up to 4-8 weeks after discontinuing treatment may be misleading.

Dosage Forms Excipient information presented when available (limited, particularly for generics); consult specific product labeling.

Solution, intranasal [spray]:

Synarel®: 2 mg/mL (8 mL) [200 mcg/spray: 60 metered sprays; contains benzalkonium chloride]

◆ **Nafarelin Acetate** *see* Nafarelin *on page 1032*

Nafcillin (naf SIL in)

Canadian Brand Names Nallpen®; Unipen®

Index Terms Ethoxynaphthamido Penicillin Sodium; Nafcillin Sodium; Nallpen; Sodium Nafcillin

Pharmacologic Category Antibiotic, Penicillin

Additional Appendix Information

Antibiotic Treatment of Adults With Infective Endocarditis *on page 1748*

Use Treatment of infections such as osteomyelitis, septicemia, endocarditis, and CNS infections caused by susceptible strains of staphylococci species

Pregnancy Risk Factor B

Pregnancy Considerations Adverse events have not been observed in animal studies; therefore, nafcillin is classified as pregnancy category B. There is no available data on the placental transfer of nafcillin. Human experience with the penicillins during pregnancy has not shown any positive evidence of adverse effects on the fetus.

Lactation Enters breast milk/use caution

Contraindications Hypersensitivity to nafcillin, or any component of the formulation, or penicillins; premixed injection may contain corn-derived dextrose and its use is contraindicated in patients with allergy to corn-related products

Warnings/Precautions Serious and occasionally severe or fatal hypersensitivity (anaphylactoid) reactions have been reported in patients on penicillin therapy, especially with a history of beta-lactam hypersensitivity, history of sensitivity to multiple allergens, or previous IgE-mediated reactions (eg, anaphylaxis, angioedema, urticaria). Use with caution in asthmatic patients. Extravasation of I.V. infusions should be avoided. Modification of dosage is necessary in patients with both severe renal and hepatic impairment. Elimination rate will be slow in neonates. Prolonged use may result in fungal or bacterial superinfection, including *C. difficile*-associated diarrhea (CDAD) and pseudomembranous colitis; CDAD has been observed >2 months postantibiotic treatment.

Adverse Reactions Frequency not defined.

Central nervous system: Neurotoxicity (high doses)

Gastrointestinal: Pseudomembranous colitis

Hematologic: Agranulocytosis, bone marrow depression, neutropenia

Local: Inflammation, pain, phlebitis, skin sloughing, swelling, and thrombophlebitis at the injection site; oxacillin (less likely to cause phlebitis) is often preferred in pediatric patients; tissue necrosis with sloughing (SubQ extravasation)

Renal: Interstitial nephritis (rare), renal tubular damage (rare)

Miscellaneous: Anaphylaxis, hypersensitivity reactions (immediate and delayed; general incidence of 1% to 10% for penicillins), serum sickness

Drug Interactions

Metabolism/Transport Effects Induces CYP3A4 (strong)

Avoid Concomitant Use

Avoid concomitant use of Nafcillin with any of the following: Nilotinib; Ranolazine

Increased Effect/Toxicity

Nafcillin may increase the levels/effects of: Methotrexate

The levels/effects of Nafcillin may be increased by: Uricosuric Agents

Decreased Effect

Nafcillin may decrease the levels/effects of: Calcium Channel Blockers; CycloSPORINE; CYP3A4 Substrates; Maraviroc; Nilotinib; Oral Contraceptive (Estrogens); Ranolazine; Sorafenib; Typhoid Vaccine; Vitamin K Antagonists

The levels/effects of Nafcillin may be decreased by: Fusidic Acid; Tetracycline Derivatives

Stability

Premixed infusions: Store in a freezer at -20°C (4°F). Thaw at room temperature or under refrigeration only. Thawed bags are stable for 21 days under refrigeration or 72 hours at room temperature. Do not refreeze.

Vials: Reconstituted parenteral solution is stable for 3 days at room temperature and 7 days when refrigerated or 12 weeks when frozen. For I.V. infusion in NS or D_5W, solution is stable for 24 hours at room temperature and 96 hours when refrigerated.

Mechanism of Action Interferes with bacterial cell wall synthesis during active multiplication, causing cell wall death and resultant bactericidal activity against susceptible bacteria

Pharmacodynamics/Kinetics

Distribution: Widely distributed; CSF penetration is poor but enhanced by meningeal inflammation

Protein binding: ~90%; primarily to albumin

Metabolism: Primarily hepatic; undergoes enterohepatic recirculation

Half-life elimination:

- Neonates: <3 weeks: 2.2-5.5 hours; 4-9 weeks: 1.2-2.3 hours
- Children 3 months to 14 years: 0.75-1.9 hours
- Adults: Normal renal/hepatic function: 30-60 minutes

Time to peak, serum: I.M.: 30-60 minutes

Excretion: Primarily feces; urine (10% to 30% as unchanged drug)

Dosage

Usual dosage range:

Neonates: I.M., I.V.:

- 1200-2000 g, <7 days: 50 mg/kg/day divided every 12 hours
- >2000 g, <7 days: 75 mg/kg/day divided every 8 hours
- 1200-2000 g, ≥7 days: 75 mg/kg/day divided every 8 hours
- >2000 g, ≥7 days: 100-140 mg/kg/day divided every 6 hours

Children:

- I.M.: 25 mg/kg twice daily
- I.V.: 50-200 mg/kg/day in divided doses every 4-6 hours (maximum: 12 g/day)

Adults:

- I.M.: 500 mg every 4-6 hours
- I.V.: 500-2000 mg every 4-6 hours

Indication-specific dosing:

Children:

Mild-to-moderate infections: I.M., I.V.: 50-100 mg/kg/day in divided doses every 6 hours

Severe infections: I.M., I.V.: 100-200 mg/kg/day in divided doses every 4-6 hours (maximum dose: 12 g/day)

Staphylococcal endocarditis: I.V.:

Native valve: 200 mg/kg/day in divided doses every 4-6 hours for 6 weeks

Prosthetic valve: 200 mg/kg/day in divided doses every 4-6 hours for ≥6 weeks (use with rifampin and gentamicin)

Adults: I.V.:

Endocarditis: MSSA:

Native valve: 12 g/24 hours in 4-6 divided doses for 6 weeks

Prosthetic valve: 12 g/24 hours in 6 divided doses for ≥6 weeks (use with rifampin and gentamicin)

Joint:

Bursitis, septic: 2 g every 4 hours

Prosthetic: 2 g every 4-6 hours with rifampin for 6 weeks

***Staphylococcus aureus*, methicillin-susceptible infections, including brain abscess, empyema, erysipelas, mastitis, myositis, orbital cellulitis, osteomyelitis, pneumonia, splenic abscess, toxic shock, urinary tract (perinephric abscess):** 2 g every 4 hours

Dosing adjustment in renal impairment: Not necessary unless renal impairment is in the setting of concomitant hepatic impairment

Dialysis: Not dialyzable (0% to 5%) via hemodialysis; supplemental dosage not necessary with hemo- or peritoneal dialysis or continuous arteriovenous or venovenous hemofiltration

Dosing adjustment in hepatic impairment: In patients with both hepatic and renal impairment, modification of dosage may be necessary; no data available.

Dietary Considerations Premixed injection may contain corn-derived dextrose and its use is contraindicated in patients with allergy to corn-related products. Sodium content of 1 g: 76.6 mg (3.33 mEq).

Administration

I.M.: Rotate injection sites

I.V.: Vesicant. Administer around-the-clock to promote less variation in peak and trough serum levels; infuse over 30-60 minutes

Extravasation management: Use cold packs. Hyaluronidase: Add 1 mL NS to 150 unit vial to make 150 units/mL of concentration; mix 0.1 mL of above with 0.9 mL NS in 1 mL syringe to make final concentration = 15 units/mL.

Monitoring Parameters Baseline and periodic CBC with differential; periodic urinalysis, BUN, serum creatinine,

AST and ALT; observe for signs and symptoms of anaphylaxis during first dose

Test Interactions Positive Coombs' test (direct), false-positive urinary and serum proteins; may inactivate aminoglycosides *in vitro*

Dosage Forms Excipient information presented when available (limited, particularly for generics); consult specific product labeling.

Infusion [premixed iso-osmotic dextrose solution]: 1 g (50 mL); 2 g (100 mL)

Injection, powder for reconstitution, as sodium: 1 g, 2 g, 10 g

◆ **Nafcillin Sodium** *see* Nafcillin *on page 1033*

Naftifine (NAF ti feen)

U.S. Brand Names Naftin®

Index Terms Naftifine Hydrochloride

Pharmacologic Category Antifungal Agent, Topical

Use Topical treatment of tinea cruris (jock itch), tinea corporis (ringworm), and tinea pedis (athlete's foot)

Pregnancy Risk Factor B

Dosage Adults: Topical: Apply cream once daily and gel twice daily (morning and evening) for up to 4 weeks

Additional Information Complete prescribing information for this medication should be consulted for additional detail.

Dosage Forms Excipient information presented when available (limited, particularly for generics); consult specific product labeling.

Cream, as hydrochloride:

Naftin®: 1% (15 g, 30 g, 60 g, 90 g) [contains benzyl alcohol]

Gel, as hydrochloride:

Naftin®: 1% (20 g, 40 g, 60 g, 90 g) [contains alcohol 52%]

◆ **Naftifine Hydrochloride** *see* Naftifine *on page 1035*

◆ **Naftin®** *see* Naftifine *on page 1035*

◆ **$NaHCO_3$** *see* Sodium Bicarbonate *on page 1380*

Nalbuphine (NAL byoo feen)

U.S. Brand Names Nubain®

Index Terms Nalbuphine Hydrochloride

Pharmacologic Category Analgesic, Opioid

Additional Appendix Information

Narcotic / Opioid Analgesics *on page 1663*

Use Relief of moderate to severe pain; preoperative analgesia, postoperative and surgical anesthesia, and obstetrical analgesia during labor and delivery

Unlabeled/Investigational Use Opioid-induced pruritus

Pregnancy Risk Factor B/D (prolonged use or high doses at term)

Pregnancy Considerations Severe fetal bradycardia has been reported following use in labor/delivery. Fetal bradycardia may occur when administered earlier in pregnancy (not documented). Use only if clearly needed, with monitoring to detect and manage possible adverse fetal effects. Naloxone has been reported to reverse bradycardia. Newborn should be monitored for respiratory depression or bradycardia following nalbuphine use in labor.

Lactation Enters breast milk/use caution

Medication Safety Issues

Sound-alike/look-alike issues:

Nubain® may be confused with Navane®, Nebcin®

High alert medication: The Institute for Safe Medication Practices (ISMP) includes this medication among its list of drug classes which have a heightened risk of causing significant patient harm when used in error.

Contraindications Hypersensitivity to nalbuphine or any component of the formulation

Warnings/Precautions Use caution in CNS depression. Sedation and psychomotor impairment are likely, and are additive with other CNS depressants or ethanol. May cause respiratory depression. Ambulatory patients must be cautioned about performing tasks which require mental alertness (eg, operating machinery or driving). Effects may be potentiated when used with other sedative drugs or ethanol. Use with caution in patients with recent myocardial infarction, biliary tract impairment, morbid obesity, thyroid dysfunction, head trauma, or increased intracranial pressure. Use caution in patients with prostatic hyperplasia and/or urinary stricture, adrenal insufficiency, decreased hepatic or renal function. Use with caution in patients with pre-existing respiratory compromise (hypoxia and/or hypercapnia), COPD or other obstructive pulmonary disease; critical respiratory depression may occur, even at therapeutic dosages. May cause hypotension; use with caution in patients with hypovolemia, cardiovascular disease (including acute MI), or drugs which may exaggerate hypotensive effects (including phenothiazines or general anesthetics). May obscure diagnosis or clinical course of patients with acute abdominal conditions. May result in tolerance and/or drug dependence with chronic use; use with caution in patients with a history of drug dependence. Abrupt discontinuation following prolonged use may lead to withdrawal symptoms. May precipitate withdrawal symptoms in patients following prolonged therapy with mu opioid agonists. Use with caution in pregnancy (close neonatal monitoring required when used in labor and delivery). Use with caution in the elderly and debilitated patients; may be more sensitive to adverse effects. Safety and efficacy in children have not been established.

Adverse Reactions

>10%: Central nervous system: Sedation (36%)

1% to 10%:

Central nervous system: Dizziness (5%), headache (3%)

Gastrointestinal: Nausea/vomiting (6%), xerostomia (4%)

Miscellaneous: Clamminess (9%)

<1% (Limited to important or life-threatening): Abdominal pain, agitation, allergic reaction, anaphylaxis, anaphylactoid reaction, anxiety, asthma, bitter taste, blurred vision, bradycardia, cardiac arrest, confusion, crying, delusion, depersonalization, depression, diaphoresis, dreams (abnormal), dyspepsia, dysphoria, dyspnea, euphoria, faintness, fever, floating sensation, flushing, gastrointestinal cramps, hallucinations, hostility, hypertension, hypotension, injection site reactions (pain, swelling, redness, burning); laryngeal edema, loss of consciousness, nervousness, numbness, pruritus, pulmonary edema, rash, respiratory depression, respiratory distress, restlessness, seizure, sensation of warmth/burning, somnolence, speech disorder, stridor, tachycardia, tingling, tremor, unreality, urinary urgency, urticaria

Drug Interactions

Avoid Concomitant Use There are no known interactions where it is recommended to avoid concomitant use.

Increased Effect/Toxicity

Nalbuphine may increase the levels/effects of: Alcohol (Ethyl); Alvimopan; CNS Depressants; Desmopressin; Selective Serotonin Reuptake Inhibitors

The levels/effects of Nalbuphine may be increased by: Amphetamines; Antipsychotic Agents (Phenothiazines); Succinylcholine

Decreased Effect

Nalbuphine may decrease the levels/effects of: Pegvisomant

The levels/effects of Nalbuphine may be decreased by: Ammonium Chloride

Ethanol/Nutrition/Herb Interactions

Ethanol: Avoid ethanol (may increase CNS depression).

Herb/Nutraceutical: Avoid valerian, St John's wort, kava kava, gotu kola (may increase CNS depression).

Stability Store at room temperature of 15°C to 30°C (59°F to 86°F). Protect from light.

Mechanism of Action Agonist of kappa opiate receptors and partial antagonist of mu opiate receptors in the CNS, causing inhibition of ascending pain pathways, altering the perception of and response to pain; produces generalized CNS depression

Pharmacodynamics/Kinetics

Onset of action: Peak effect: SubQ, I.M.: <15 minutes; I.V.: 2-3 minutes

Metabolism: Hepatic

Half-life elimination: 5 hours

Excretion: Feces; urine (~7% as metabolites)

Dosage

Children ≥1 year (unlabeled use): Pain management: I.M., I.V., SubQ: 0.1-0.2 mg/kg every 3-4 hours as needed; maximum: 20 mg/dose and/or 160 mg/day

Adults:

Pain management: I.M., I.V., SubQ: 10 mg/70 kg every 3-6 hours; maximum single dose in nonopioid-tolerant patients: 20 mg; maximum daily dose: 160 mg

Surgical anesthesia supplement: I.V.: Induction: 0.3-3 mg/kg over 10-15 minutes; maintenance doses of 0.25-0.5 mg/kg may be given as required

Opioid-induced pruritus (unlabeled use): I.V. 2.5-5 mg; may repeat dose

Dosing adjustment in renal impairment: Use with caution and reduce dose; monitor.

Dosing adjustment in hepatic impairment: Use with caution and reduce dose.

Administration Administer I.M., SubQ, or I.V.

Monitoring Parameters Relief of pain, respiratory and mental status, blood pressure

Dosage Forms Excipient information presented when available (limited, particularly for generics); consult specific product labeling. [DSC] = Discontinued product

Injection, solution, as hydrochloride: 10 mg/mL (10 mL); 20 mg/mL (10 mL)

Nubain®: 10 mg/mL (10 mL) [DSC]; 20 mg/mL (10 mL)

Injection, solution, as hydrochloride [preservative free]: 10 mg/mL (1 mL); 20 mg/mL (1 mL)

Nubain®: 10 mg/mL (1 mL); 20 mg/mL (1 mL)

- **Nalbuphine Hydrochloride** *see* Nalbuphine *on page* 1035
- **Nalcrom® (Can)** *see* Cromolyn *on page* 372
- **Nalex®-A** *see* Chlorpheniramine, Phenylephrine, and Phenyltoloxamine *on page* 314
- **Nalex A 12** *see* Chlorpheniramine, Pyrilamine, and Phenylephrine *on page* 315
- **Nalfon®** *see* Fenoprofen *on page* 610
- **Nallpen** *see* Nafcillin *on page* 1033
- **Nallpen® (Can)** *see* Nafcillin *on page* 1033
- ***N*-allylnoroxymorphine Hydrochloride** *see* Naloxone *on page* 1037

Nalmefene (NAL me feen)

U.S. Brand Names Revex® [DSC]

Index Terms Nalmefene Hydrochloride

Pharmacologic Category Antidote; Opioid Antagonist

Use Complete or partial reversal of opioid drug effects, including respiratory depression induced by natural or synthetic opioids; reversal of postoperative opioid depression; management of known or suspected opioid overdose

Pregnancy Risk Factor B

Pregnancy Considerations Animal studies have not demonstrated fetal harm or fertility impairment. There are no adequate and well-controlled studies in pregnant women. Use only if clearly needed.

Lactation Excretion in breast milk unknown/use caution

Medication Safety Issues

Sound-alike/look-alike issues:

Revex® may be confused with Nimbex®, ReVia®, Rubex®

Color-coded ampuls denote indication-specific concentrations:

Blue-labeled ampul (for postoperative use) contains 1 mL (100 mcg/mL)

Green-labeled ampul (for overdose management) contains 2 mL (1 mg/mL)

International issues:

Revex® may be confused with Brivex® which is a brand name for brivudine in Switzerland

Revex® may be confused with Rubex® which is a brand name for ascorbic acid in Ireland

Contraindications Hypersensitivity to nalmefene or any component of the formulation

Warnings/Precautions May induce symptoms of acute withdrawal in opioid-dependent patients; recurrence of respiratory depression is possible if the opioid involved is long-acting; observe patients until there is no reasonable risk of recurrent respiratory depression. Nalmefene is structurally similar to both naltrexone and naloxone; patients with hypersensitivity to these agents may also react to nalmefene. Concurrent use of flumazenil and nalmefene may increase the risk of seizures. Safety and efficacy have not been established in children. Avoid abrupt reversal of opioid effects in patients of high cardiovascular risk or who have received potentially cardiotoxic drugs. Pulmonary edema and cardiovascular instability have been reported in association with abrupt reversal with other narcotic antagonists. Animal studies indicate nalmefene may not completely reverse buprenorphine-induced respiratory depression. Use caution with renal impairment. Excessive dosages should be avoided after use of opiates in surgery. Abrupt postoperative reversal may result in nausea, vomiting, sweating, tachycardia, hypertension, seizures, and other cardiovascular events (including pulmonary edema and arrhythmias). Discharged patients who are opioid-dependent may attempt to override the narcotic-blocking effect of nalmefene. Patients are at a greater risk of overdose when nalmefene wears off if megadosing of opiates has occurred. Adequate duration of monitoring should be provided.

Two products are available at different concentrations. A blue-labeled ampul contains a 100 mcg/mL solution of nalmefene and is intended for postoperative use. A green-labeled ampul contains a 1 mg/mL (**10** times as concentrated; **20** times as much drug) and is intended to be used for the management of an overdose.

Adverse Reactions

>10%: Gastrointestinal: Nausea (18%)

1% to 10%:

Cardiovascular: Tachycardia (5%), hypertension (5%), hypotension (1%), vasodilation (1%)

Central nervous system: Fever (3%), dizziness (3%), headache (1%), chills (1%)

Gastrointestinal: Vomiting (9%)

Miscellaneous: Postoperative pain (4%)

<1% (Limited to important or life-threatening): Agitation, arrhythmia, AST increased, bradycardia, confusion, depression, diarrhea, myoclonus, nervousness, pharyngitis, pruritus, pulmonary edema, somnolence, tremor, urinary retention, withdrawal syndrome, xerostomia

Drug Interactions

Avoid Concomitant Use There are no known interactions where it is recommended to avoid concomitant use.

Increased Effect/Toxicity There are no known significant interactions involving an increase in effect.

Decreased Effect There are no known significant interactions involving a decrease in effect.

Stability Store at controlled room temperature.

Mechanism of Action As a 6-methylene analog of naltrexone, nalmefene acts as a competitive antagonist at opioid receptor sites, preventing or reversing the respiratory depression, sedation, and hypotension induced by opiates; no pharmacologic activity of its own (eg, opioid agonist activity) has been demonstrated

Pharmacodynamics/Kinetics

Onset of action: I.M., SubQ: 5-15 minutes

Distribution: V_d: 8.6 L/kg; rapid

Protein binding: 45%

Metabolism: Hepatic via glucuronide conjugation to metabolites with little or no activity

Bioavailability: I.M., SubQ: 100%

Half-life elimination: 10.8 hours

Time to peak, serum: Serum: I.M.: 2.3 hours; I.V.: <2 minutes; SubQ: 1.5 hours

Excretion: Feces (17%); urine (<5% as unchanged drug)

Clearance: 0.8 L/hour/kg

Dosage I.M., I.V., SubQ:

Reversal of postoperative opioid depression: Blue-labeled product (100 mcg/mL): Titrate to reverse the undesired effects of opioids; initial dose for nonopioid dependent patients: 0.25 mcg/kg followed by 0.25 mcg/kg incremental doses at 2- to 5-minute intervals; after a total dose >1 mcg/kg, further therapeutic response is unlikely

Note: In patients with increased cardiovascular risks, dilute 1:1 in NS or SWFI, and initiate/titrate with 0.1 mcg/kg doses.

Management of known/suspected opioid overdose: **Note:** I.V. route is preferred. Green-labeled product (1 mg/mL): Adults:

Nonopioid-dependent patients: 0.5 mg/70 kg; may repeat with 1 mg/70 kg in 2-5 minutes; further increase beyond a total dose of 1.5 mg/70 kg will not likely result in improved response and may result in cardiovascular stress and precipitated withdrawal syndrome

Opioid-dependent patients: Administer a challenge dose of 0.1 mg/70 kg; if no withdrawal symptoms are observed in 2 minutes, give 0.5 mg/70 kg; may repeat with 1 mg/70 kg in 2-5 minutes; further increase beyond a total dose of 1.5 mg/70 kg will not likely result in improved response and may result in cardiovascular stress and precipitated withdrawal syndrome

Note: If recurrence of respiratory depression is noted, dose may again be titrated to clinical effect using incremental doses.

Note: If I.V. access is lost or not readily obtainable, a single SubQ or I.M. dose of 1 mg may be effective in 5-15 minutes.

Dosing adjustment in renal impairment: Not necessary with single use, however, slow administration (over 60 seconds) of incremental doses is recommended to minimize hypertension and dizziness

Dosing adjustment in hepatic impairment: No adjustment necessary with single use.

Administration Check dosage strength carefully before use to avoid error. Slow administration (over 60 seconds) of incremental doses is recommended to minimize hypertension and dizziness in renal patients. Dilute drug (1:1) with diluent and use smaller doses in patients known to be at increased cardiovascular risk. May be administered via I.M. or SubQ routes if I.V. access is not feasible. A single SubQ or I.M. dose of 1 mg may be effective in 5-15 minutes.

Monitoring Parameters Symptoms of withdrawal; neurological status, oxygenation, pain, vital signs

Additional Information Proper steps should be used to prevent use of the incorrect dosage strength. The goal of treatment in the postoperative setting is to achieve reversal of excessive opioid effects without inducing a complete reversal and acute pain.

If opioid dependence is suspected, nalmefene should only be used in opioid overdose if the likelihood of overdose is high based on history or the clinical presentation of respiratory depression with concurrent pupillary constriction is present.

Dosage Forms Excipient information presented when available (limited, particularly for generics); consult specific product labeling.

Injection, solution:

Revex®: 100 mcg/mL (1 mL) [blue label]; 1 mg/mL (2 mL) [green label] [DSC]

◆ **Nalmefene Hydrochloride** *see* Nalmefene *on page 1036*

Naloxone (nal OKS one)

Canadian Brand Names Naloxone Hydrochloride Injection®

Index Terms *N*-allylnoroxymorphine Hydrochloride; Naloxone Hydrochloride; Narcan

Pharmacologic Category Antidote; Opioid Antagonist

Use

Complete or partial reversal of opioid depression, including respiratory depression, induced by natural and synthetic opioids, including heroin, morphine, propoxyphene, methadone, and certain mixed agonist-antagonist analgesics: nalbuphine, pentazocine, and butorphanol

Diagnosis of suspected opioid dependence or acute opioid overdose

Adjunctive agent to increase blood pressure in the management of septic shock

Unlabeled/Investigational Use Opioid-induced pruritus

Pregnancy Risk Factor C

Pregnancy Considerations Consider benefit to the mother and the risk to the fetus before administering to a pregnant woman who is known or suspected to be opioid dependent. May precipitate withdrawal in both the mother and fetus.

Lactation Excretion in breast milk unknown/not recommended

Medication Safety Issues

Sound-alike/look-alike issues:

Naloxone may be confused with naltrexone

Narcan® may be confused with Marcaine®, Norcuron®

International issues:

Narcan® may be confused with Marcen® which is a brand name for ketazolam in Spain

Contraindications Hypersensitivity to naloxone or any component of the formulation

Warnings/Precautions Due to an association between naloxone and acute pulmonary edema, use with caution in patients with cardiovascular disease or in patients receiving medications with potential adverse cardiovascular effects (eg, hypotension, pulmonary edema, or arrhythmias). Administration of naloxone causes the release of catecholamines; may precipitate acute withdrawal or unmask pain in those who regularly take opioids. Excessive dosages should be avoided after use of opiates in surgery. Abrupt postoperative reversal may result in nausea, vomiting, sweating, tachycardia, hypertension, seizures, and other cardiovascular events (including pulmonary edema and arrhythmias). May precipitate withdrawal symptoms in patients addicted to opiates, including pain, hypertension, sweating, agitation, irritability; in neonates: shrill cry, failure to feed; carefully titrate dose to reverse hypoventilation; do not fully awaken patient or reverse analgesic effect (postoperative patient). Use caution in patients with history of seizures; avoid use in treatment of meperidine-induced seizures. Recurrence of respiratory depression is possible if the opioid involved is long-acting; observe patients until there is no reasonable risk of recurrent respiratory depression.

Adverse Reactions Adverse reactions are related to reversing dependency and precipitating withdrawal. Withdrawal symptoms are the result of sympathetic excess. Adverse events occur secondarily to reversal (withdrawal) of narcotic analgesia and sedation.

Central nervous system: Narcotic withdrawal

Drug Interactions

Avoid Concomitant Use There are no known interactions where it is recommended to avoid concomitant use.

Increased Effect/Toxicity There are no known significant interactions involving an increase in effect.

Decreased Effect There are no known significant interactions involving a decrease in effect.

Stability Store at 25°C (77°F). Protect from light. Stable in 0.9% sodium chloride and D_5W at 4 mcg/mL for 24 hours.

Mechanism of Action Pure opioid antagonist that competes and displaces narcotics at opioid receptor sites

Pharmacodynamics/Kinetics

Onset of action: Endotracheal, I.M., SubQ: 2-5 minutes; I.V.: ~2 minutes

Duration: ~30-120 minutes depending on route of administration; I.V. has a shorter duration of action than I.M. administration; since naloxone's action is shorter than that of most opioids, repeated doses are usually needed

Distribution: Crosses placenta

Metabolism: Primarily hepatic via glucuronidation

Half-life elimination: Neonates: 3-4 hours; Adults: 0.5-1.5 hours

Excretion: Urine (as metabolites)

Dosage Note: I.M., I.V. (preferred), and SubQ routes are available. Endotracheal administration is the least desirable and is supported by only anecdotal evidence (case report) (ACLS guidelines, 2005):

Infants and Children: Postoperative reversal: 0.01 mg/kg; may repeat every 2-3 minutes as needed based on response (adequate ventilation without significant pain)

Children:

Opioid intoxication: Respiratory depression:

I.V.:

Birth (including premature infants) to 5 years or <20 kg: Initial: 0.1 mg/kg (maximum dose: 2 mg); repeat every 2-3 minutes if needed (*Drugs for Pediatric Emergencies*, 1998)

>5 years or ≥20 kg: 2 mg/dose; if no response, repeat every 2-3 minutes (*Drugs for Pediatric Emergencies*, 1998)

Continuous infusion: I.V.: If continuous infusion is required, calculate dosage/hour based on effective intermittent dose used and duration of adequate response seen **or** use 2/3 of the initial effective naloxone bolus on an hourly basis; titrate dose (typically 0.04-0.16 mg/kg/hour for 2-5 days in children); 1/2 of the initial bolus dose should be readministered 15 minutes after initiation of the continuous infusion to prevent a drop in naloxone levels; increase infusion rate as needed to assure adequate ventilation and prevent withdrawal symptoms

Adults:

Opioid intoxication: Respiratory depression: I.V.: 0.4-2 mg; may need to repeat doses every 2-3 minutes; after reversal, may need to readminister dose(s) at a later interval (ie, 20-60 minutes) depending on type/duration of opioid. If no response is observed after 10 mg, consider other causes of respiratory depression. **Note:** Opioid-dependent patients may require lower doses (0.1 mg) titrated incrementally to avoid precipitating acute withdrawal.

Continuous infusion: I.V.: Calculate dosage/hour based on effective intermittent dose used and duration of adequate response seen **or** use 2/3 of the initial effective naloxone bolus on an hourly basis (typically 0.25-6.25 mg/hour); 1/2 of the initial bolus dose should be readministered 15 minutes after initiation of the continuous infusion to prevent a drop in naloxone levels; adjust infusion rate as needed to assure adequate ventilation and prevent withdrawal symptoms

Opioid-dependent patients being treated for cancer pain (unlabeled; NCCN guidelines, 2008): I.V.: 0.04-0.08 mg (40-80 mcg) slow I.V. push; administer every 30-60 seconds until improvement in symptoms, if no response is observed after total naloxone dose 1 mg, consider other causes of respiratory depression. **Note:** May dilute 0.4 mg/mL (1 mL) ampule into 9 mL of normal saline for a total volume of 10 mL to achieve a 0.04 mg/mL (40 mcg/mL) concentration.

Postoperative reversal: I.V.: 0.1-0.2 mg every 2-3 minutes until desired response (adequate ventilation and alertness without significant pain). **Note:** Repeat doses may be needed within 1-2 hour intervals depending on type, dose, and timing of the last dose of opioid administered.

Opioid-induced pruritus (unlabeled use): I.V. infusion: 0.25 mcg/kg/hour; **Note:** Monitor pain control; verify that the naloxone is not reversing analgesia.

Administration

Endotracheal: There is only anecdotal support for this route of administration. May require a slightly higher dose than used in other routes. Dilute to 1-2 mL with normal saline; flush with 5 cc of saline and then administer 5 ventilations

Intratracheal: Dilute to 1-2 mL with normal saline

I.V. push: Administer over 30 seconds as undiluted preparation **or** (unlabeled) administer as diluted preparation slow I.V. push by diluting 0.4 mg (1 mL) ampul with 9 mL of normal saline for a total volume of 10 mL to achieve a concentration of 0.04 mg/mL

I.V. continuous infusion: Dilute to 4 mcg/mL in D_5W or normal saline

Monitoring Parameters Respiratory rate, heart rate, blood pressure, temperature, level of consciousness, ABGs or pulse oximetry

Additional Information May contain methyl and propylparabens

Dosage Forms Excipient information presented when available (limited, particularly for generics); consult specific product labeling.

Injection, solution, as hydrochloride: 0.4 mg/mL (1 mL, 10 mL)

Injection, solution, as hydrochloride [preservative free]: 0.4 mg/mL (1 mL); 1 mg/mL (2 mL)

- ◆ **Naloxone and Buprenorphine** *see* Buprenorphine and Naloxone *on page 223*
- ◆ **Naloxone Hydrochloride** *see* Naloxone *on page 1037*
- ◆ **Naloxone Hydrochloride and Pentazocine Hydrochloride** *see* Pentazocine *on page 1169*
- ◆ **Naloxone Hydrochloride Dihydrate and Buprenorphine Hydrochloride** *see* Buprenorphine and Naloxone *on page 223*
- ◆ **Naloxone Hydrochloride Injection® (Can)** *see* Naloxone *on page 1037*

Naltrexone (nal TREKS one)

U.S. Brand Names Depade®; ReVia®; Vivitrol™
Canadian Brand Names ReVia®
Index Terms Naltrexone Hydrochloride
Pharmacologic Category Antidote; Opioid Antagonist
Use Treatment of ethanol dependence; blockade of the effects of exogenously administered opioids
Pregnancy Risk Factor C
Pregnancy Considerations Evidence of early fetal loss has been observed in animal studies with oral naltrexone. There are no adequate and well-controlled studies in pregnant women.
Lactation Enters breast milk/not recommended
Medication Safety Issues
Sound-alike/look-alike issues:
Naltrexone may be confused with methylnaltrexone, naloxone
ReVia® may be confused with Revatio®, Revex®

Administration issues: Vivitrol™: For intramuscular (I.M.) gluteal injection only
Contraindications Hypersensitivity to naltrexone or any component of the formulation; narcotic dependence or current use of opioid analgesics; acute opioid withdrawal; failure to pass Narcan® challenge or positive urine screen for opioids; acute hepatitis; liver failure
Warnings/Precautions
[U.S. Boxed Warning]: Dose-related hepatocellular injury is possible; the margin of separation between the apparent safe and hepatotoxic doses appears to be ≤ fivefold.

May precipitate withdrawal symptoms in patients addicted to opiates; patients should be opioid-free for a minimum of 7-10 days; use naloxone challenge test to confirm. Use with caution in patients with hepatic or renal impairment. Patients may respond to lower opioid doses than previously used. This could result in potentially life-threatening opioid intoxication. Use of naltrexone does not eliminate or diminish withdrawal symptoms. Warn patients that attempts to overcome opioid blockade could lead to fatal overdose. Suicidal thoughts and depression have been reported; monitor closely. Cases of eosinophilic pneumonia have been reported; monitor for hypoxia and dyspnea. Use with caution in patients with a history of bleeding disorders (including thrombocytopenia) and/or patients on anticoagulant therapy; bleeding/hematoma may occur from I.M. administration. Serious injection site reactions (eg, cellulitis, induration, hematoma, abscess, necrosis) have been reported with use. Patients should report injection site pain, swelling, bruising, pruritus, or redness that does not improve (or worsens) within 2 weeks; consider surgical consult for worsening reactions. For I.M. use only; do not administer I.V., SubQ, or into fatty tissue; may increase the risk of injection site reactions. Vehicle used in injectable (polylactide-co-glycolide microspheres) has rarely been associated with retinal artery occlusion in patients with abnormal arteriovenous anastomosis. Safety and efficacy in children have not been established.
Adverse Reactions Combined reporting of adverse events from oral and injectable formulations:
>10%:
Cardiovascular: Syncope (13%)
Central nervous system: Headache (25%), insomnia (14%), dizziness (13%), anxiety (12%), somnolence (4%), nervousness, fatigue
Gastrointestinal: Nausea (33%), vomiting (14%), appetite decreased (14%), diarrhea (13%), abdominal pain (11%), abdominal cramping
Local: Injection site reaction (69%; includes bruising, induration, nodules, pain, pruritus, swelling, tenderness)
Neuromuscular & skeletal: Arthralgia (12%), CPK increased (11%)
Respiratory: Upper respiratory tract infection (13%), pharyngitis (11%)
1% to 10%:
Central nervous system: Depression (8%), suicidal thoughts (1%), energy increased, feeling down
Dermatologic: Rash (6%)
Endocrine & metabolic: Polydipsia
Gastrointestinal: Dry mouth (5%)
Genitourinary: Delayed ejaculation, impotency
Hepatic: AST increased (2%)
Neuromuscular & skeletal: Muscle cramps (8%), back pain (6%)
<1% (Limited to important or life-threatening): ALT increased, angina, atrial fibrillation, blood pressure increased, cerebral aneurysm, chest pain, chest tightness, CHF, cholecystitis, cholelithiasis, colitis, COPD, dehydration, delirium, disorientation, DVT, dyspnea, eosinophilic pneumonia, euphoria, GI hemorrhage, hallucinations, hypercholesterolemia, hypersensitivity reaction (includes angioedema and urticaria), hypertension, influenza, ischemic stroke, leukocytosis, lymphadenopathy, MI, narcotic withdrawal, palpitation, paralytic ileus, paranoia, PE, perirectal abscess, pneumonia, pyrexia, rigors, seizure, suicide attempts, tachycardia, thrombocytopenia, tooth abscess, UTI
Drug Interactions
Avoid Concomitant Use There are no known interactions where it is recommended to avoid concomitant use.
Increased Effect/Toxicity There are no known significant interactions involving an increase in effect.
Decreased Effect There are no known significant interactions involving a decrease in effect.
Stability
Injection: Store unopened kit at 2°C to 8°C (36°F to 46°F). Kit may be kept at room temperature of ≤25°C (77°F) for ≤7 days prior to use; do not freeze.
Tablet: Store at 20°C to 25°C (68°F to 77°F).
Mechanism of Action Naltrexone (a pure opioid antagonist) is a cyclopropyl derivative of oxymorphone similar in structure to naloxone and nalorphine (a morphine derivative); it acts as a competitive antagonist at opioid receptor sites, showing the highest affinity for mu receptors.
Pharmacodynamics/Kinetics
Duration: Oral: 50 mg: 24 hours; 100 mg: 48 hours; 150 mg: 72 hours; I.M.: 4 weeks
Absorption: Oral: Almost complete
Distribution: V_d: 19 L/kg; widely throughout the body but considerable interindividual variation exists
Protein binding: 21%
Metabolism: Noncytochrome-mediated dehydrogenase conversion to 6-beta-naltrexol and related minor metabolites; Oral: Extensive first-pass effect
Half-life elimination: Oral: 4 hours; 6-beta-naltrexol: 13 hours; I.M.: naltrexone and 6-beta-naltrexol: 5-10 days
Time to peak, serum: Oral: ~60 minutes; I.M.: Biphasic: 2 hours (first peak), 2-3 days (second peak)
Excretion: Primarily urine (as metabolites and unchanged drug)
Dosage Adults: Do not give until patient is opioid-free for 7-10 days as determined by urinalysis
Oral: Alcohol dependence, opioid antidote: 25 mg; if no withdrawal signs within 1 hour give another 25 mg; maintenance regimen is flexible, variable and individualized (50 mg/day to 100-150 mg 3 times/week for 12 weeks); up to 800 mg/day has been tolerated in a small number of healthy adults without an adverse effect
I.M.: Alcohol dependence: 380 mg once every 4 weeks

Dosage adjustment in renal impairment: Use caution. No adjustment needed in mild impairment. Not adequately studied in moderate-to-severe renal impairment.

Dosage adjustment in hepatic impairment: Use caution. An increase in naltrexone AUC of approximately five- and 10-fold in patients with compensated or decompensated liver cirrhosis respectively, compared with normal liver function has been reported No adjustment required with mild-to-moderate hepatic impairment. Not adequately studied in severe hepatic impairment.

Administration If there is any question of occult opioid dependence, perform a naloxone challenge test; do not attempt treatment until naloxone challenge is negative.

Oral: To minimize adverse gastrointestinal effects, administer with food or antacids or after meals; advise patient not to self-administer opiates while receiving naltrexone therapy.

I.M.: Vivitrol™: Administer I.M. into the upper outer quadrant of the gluteal area; use provided 1.5 inch 20-gauge needle for administration. Avoid inadvertent injection into a blood vessel; do not administer I.V., SubQ, or into fatty tissue (the risk of serious injection site reaction is increased if given SubQ or into fatty tissue. Injection should alternate between the two buttocks. Do not substitute any components of the dose-pack.

Monitoring Parameters For narcotic withdrawal; liver function tests; injection site reactions

Test Interactions May cause cross-reactivity with some opioid immunoassay methods.

Dosage Forms Excipient information presented when available (limited, particularly for generics); consult specific product labeling.

Injection, microspheres for suspension, extended release:
- Vivitrol™: 380 mg [contains polylactide-co-glycolide; packaged with diluent, syringe, needles, and safety device]

Tablet, as hydrochloride: 50 mg
- Depade®: 25 mg, 50 mg, 100 mg
- ReVia®: 50 mg

◆ **Naltrexone Hydrochloride** *see* Naltrexone *on page 1039*

◆ **Namenda™** *see* Memantine *on page 938*

Nandrolone (NAN droe lone)

Canadian Brand Names Deca-Durabolin®; Durabolin®

Index Terms Nandrolone Decanoate; Nandrolone Phenpropionate

Pharmacologic Category Androgen

Use Control of metastatic breast cancer; management of anemia of renal insufficiency

Restrictions C-III

Pregnancy Risk Factor X

Dosage Deep I.M. (into gluteal muscle):

Children 2-13 years (decanoate): 25-50 mg every 3-4 weeks

Adults:

Male:
- Breast cancer (phenpropionate): 50-100 mg/week
- Anemia of renal insufficiency (decanoate): 100-200 mg/week

Female: 50-100 mg/week
- Breast cancer (phenpropionate): 50-100 mg/week
- Anemia of renal insufficiency (decanoate): 50-100 mg/week

Additional Information Complete prescribing information for this medication should be consulted for additional detail.

Dosage Forms Excipient information presented when available (limited, particularly for generics); consult specific product labeling.

Injection, solution, as decanoate [in sesame oil]: 100 mg/mL (2 mL); 200 mg/mL (1 mL) [contains benzyl alcohol] [DSC]

◆ **Nandrolone Decanoate** *see* Nandrolone *on page 1040*

◆ **Nandrolone Phenpropionate** *see* Nandrolone *on page 1040*

◆ **NAPA and NABZ** *see* Sodium Phenylacetate and Sodium Benzoate *on page 1384*

Naphazoline (naf AZ oh leen)

U.S. Brand Names AK-Con™; Albalon® [DSC]; Clear eyes® for Dry Eyes and ACR Relief [OTC]; Clear eyes® for Dry Eyes and Redness Relief [OTC]; Clear eyes® Redness Relief [OTC]; Clear eyes® Seasonal Relief [OTC]; Naphcon® [OTC]; Privine® [OTC]

Canadian Brand Names Naphcon Forte®; Vasocon®

Index Terms Naphazoline Hydrochloride

Pharmacologic Category Alpha$_1$ Agonist; Imidazoline Derivative; Ophthalmic Agent, Vasoconstrictor

Use Topical ocular vasoconstrictor; temporary relief of nasal congestion associated with the common cold, upper respiratory allergies or sinusitis; relief of redness of the eye due to minor irritation

Pregnancy Risk Factor C

Dosage

Nasal: Children ≥12 years and Adults: 0.05% instill 1-2 drops or sprays every 6 hours if needed; therapy should not exceed 3 days

Ophthalmic: Adults:
- 0.1% (prescription): 1-2 drops into conjuctival sac every 3-4 hours as needed
- 0.012% or 0.025% (OTC): 1-2 drops into affected eye(s) up to 4 times a day; therapy should not exceed 3 days

Additional Information Complete prescribing information for this medication should be consulted for additional detail.

Dosage Forms Excipient information presented when available (limited, particularly for generics); consult specific product labeling.

Solution, intranasal, as hydrochloride [drops]:
- Privine®: 0.05% (25 mL)

Solution, intranasal, as hydrochloride [spray]:
- Privine®: 0.05% (20 mL)

Solution, ophthalmic, as hydrochloride:
- AK-Con™, Albalon® [DSC]: 0.1% (15 mL) [contains benzalkonium chloride]
- Clear eyes® for Dry Eyes and ACR Relief: 0.025% (15 mL) [contains hypromellose, and zinc sulfate]
- Clear eyes® for Dry Eyes and Redness Relief: 0.012% (15 mL) [contains hypromellose, glycerin and benzalkonium chloride]
- Clear eyes® Redness Relief: 0.012% (6 mL, 15 mL, 30 mL) [contains glycerin and benzalkonium chloride]
- Clear eyes® Seasonal Relief: 0.012% (15 mL, 30 mL) [contains glycerin, zinc sulfate and benzalkonium chloride]
- Naphcon®: 0.012% (15 mL) [contains benzalkonium chloride]

Naphazoline and Pheniramine
(naf AZ oh leen & fen NIR a meen)

U.S. Brand Names Naphcon-A® [OTC]; Opcon-A® [OTC]; Visine-A® [OTC]

Canadian Brand Names Naphcon-A®; Visine® Advanced Allergy

Index Terms Pheniramine and Naphazoline

Pharmacologic Category Histamine H_1 Antagonist; Histamine H_1 Antagonist, First Generation; Ophthalmic Agent, Vasoconstrictor

Use Treatment of ocular congestion, irritation, and itching

Pregnancy Risk Factor C

Medication Safety Issues

Sound-alike/look-alike issues:

Visine® may be confused with Visken®

Dosage Ophthalmic: Children ≥6 years and Adults: 1-2 drops up to 4 times/day

Additional Information Complete prescribing information for this medication should be consulted for additional detail.

Dosage Forms Excipient information presented when available (limited, particularly for generics); consult specific product labeling.

Solution, ophthalmic:

Naphcon-A®: Naphazoline hydrochloride 0.025% and pheniramine maleate 0.3% (5 mL) [contains benzalkonium chloride; 2 bottles/box], (15 mL) [contains benzalkonium chloride]

Opcon-A®: Naphazoline hydrochloride 0.027% and pheniramine maleate 0.3% (15 mL) [contains benzalkonium chloride]

Visine-A®: Naphazoline hydrochloride 0.025% and pheniramine maleate 0.3% (15 mL) [contains benzalkonium chloride]

◆ **Naphazoline Hydrochloride** *see* Naphazoline *on page 1040*

◆ **Naphcon® [OTC]** *see* Naphazoline *on page 1040*

◆ **Naphcon-A® [OTC]** *see* Naphazoline and Pheniramine *on page 1040*

◆ **Naphcon-A® (Can)** *see* Naphazoline and Pheniramine *on page 1040*

◆ **Naphcon Forte® (Can)** *see* Naphazoline *on page 1040*

◆ **NapraPAC™** *see* Lansoprazole and Naproxen *on page 855*

◆ **Naprelan®** *see* Naproxen *on page 1041*

◆ **Naprosyn®** *see* Naproxen *on page 1041*

Naproxen (na PROKS en)

U.S. Brand Names Aleve® [OTC]; Anaprox®; Anaprox® DS; EC-Naprosyn®; Mediproxen [OTC]; Midol® Extended Relief; Naprelan®; Naprosyn®; Pamprin® Maximum Strength All Day Relief [OTC]

Canadian Brand Names Anaprox®; Anaprox® DS; Apo-Napro-Na DS®; Apo-Napro-Na®; Apo-Naproxen EC®; Apo-Naproxen SR®; Apo-Naproxen®; Gen-Naproxen EC; Naprosyn®; Naxen®; Naxen® EC; Novo-Naproc EC; Novo-Naprox; Novo-Naprox Sodium; Novo-Naprox Sodium DS; Novo-Naprox SR; Nu-Naprox; PMS-Naproxen EC; Pro-Naproxen EC; Riva-Naproxen; Sab-Naproxen

Index Terms Naproxen Sodium

Pharmacologic Category Nonsteroidal Anti-inflammatory Drug (NSAID), Oral

Additional Appendix Information

Nonsteroidal Anti-inflammatory Agents *on page 1669*

Use Management of ankylosing spondylitis, osteoarthritis, and rheumatoid disorders (including juvenile rheumatoid arthritis); acute gout; mild-to-moderate pain; tendonitis, bursitis; dysmenorrhea; fever

Restrictions An FDA-approved medication guide must be distributed when dispensing an oral outpatient prescription (new or refill) where this medication is to be used without direct supervision of a healthcare provider. Medication guides are available at http://www.fda.gov/cder/Offices/ODS/medication_guides.htm.

Pregnancy Risk Factor C/D (3rd trimester)

Lactation Enters breast milk/not recommended (AAP rates "compatible")

Medication Safety Issues

Sound-alike/look-alike issues:

Naproxen may be confused with Natacyn®, Nebcin®

Aleve® may be confused with Alesse®

Anaprox® may be confused with Anaspaz®, Avapro®

Naprelan® may be confused with Naprosyn®

Naprosyn® may be confused with Naprelan®, Natacyn®, Nebcin®

International issues:

Flogen® [Mexico] may be confused with Flovent® which is a brand name for fluticasone in the U.S.

Flogen® [Mexico] may be confused with Floxin® which is a brand name for ofloxacin in the U.S.

Contraindications Hypersensitivity to naproxen, aspirin, other NSAIDs, or any component of the formulation; perioperative pain in the setting of coronary artery bypass graft (CABG) surgery

Warnings/Precautions [U.S. Boxed Warning]: NSAIDs are associated with an increased risk of adverse cardiovascular thrombotic events, including MI, stroke, and new onset or worsening of pre-existing hypertension. Risk may be increased with duration of use or pre-existing cardiovascular risk factors or disease. Carefully evaluate individual cardiovascular risk profiles prior to prescribing. Use caution with fluid retention, heart failure, or hypertension. Use the lowest effective dose for the shortest duration of time, consistent with individual patient goals, to reduce risk of cardiovascular or GI adverse events. Alternate therapies should be considered for patients at high risk. Concurrent administration of ibuprofen, and potentially other nonselective NSAIDs, may interfere with aspirin's cardioprotective effect. **[U.S. Boxed Warning]: Use is contraindicated for treatment of perioperative pain in the setting of coronary artery bypass graft (CABG) surgery.** Risk of MI and stroke may be increased with use following CABG surgery.

[U.S. Boxed Warning]: NSAIDs may increase risk of gastrointestinal irritation, inflammation, ulceration, bleeding, and perforation. These events may occur at any time during therapy and without warning. Use caution with a history of GI disease (bleeding or ulcers), concurrent therapy with aspirin, anticoagulants and/or corticosteroids, smoking, use of alcohol, the elderly or debilitated patients.

May increase the risk of aseptic meningitis, especially in patients with systemic lupus erythematosus (SLE) and mixed connective tissue disorders. Platelet adhesion and aggregation may be decreased; may prolong bleeding time; patients with coagulation disorders or who are receiving anticoagulants should be monitored closely. Anemia may occur; patients on long-term NSAID therapy should be monitored for anemia. NSAID use may compromise existing renal function; dose-dependent decreases in prostaglandin synthesis may result from NSAID use, reducing renal blood flow which may cause renal decompensation. Patients with impaired renal function, dehydration, heart failure, liver dysfunction, those taking diuretics, and ACE inhibitors, and the elderly are at greater risk of renal toxicity. Rehydrate patient before starting therapy; monitor renal function closely. Not recommended for use in patients with advanced renal disease. Long-term NSAID use may result in renal papillary necrosis.

NSAIDs may cause serious skin adverse events including exfoliative dermatitis, Stevens-Johnson Syndrome (SJS) and toxic epidermal necrolysis (TEN); discontinue use at first sign of skin rash or hypersensitivity. Anaphylactoid reactions may occur, even without prior exposure; patients with "aspirin triad" (bronchial asthma, aspirin intolerance, rhinitis) may be at increased risk. Do not use in patients who experience bronchospasm, asthma, rhinitis, or urticaria with NSAID or aspirin therapy. Use caution in other forms of asthma.

Use with caution in patients with decreased hepatic function. Closely monitor patients with any abnormal LFT. Severe hepatic reactions (eg, fulminant hepatitis, liver failure) have occurred with NSAID use, rarely; discontinue if signs or symptoms of liver disease develop, or if systemic manifestations occur.

The elderly are at increased risk for adverse effects (especially peptic ulceration, CNS effects, renal toxicity) from NSAIDs even at low doses.

Withhold for at least 4-6 half-lives prior to surgical or dental procedures. Safety and efficacy have not been established in children <2 years of age.

OTC labeling: Prior to self-medication, patients should contact healthcare provider if they have had recurring stomach pain or upset, ulcers, bleeding problems, high blood pressure, heart or kidney disease, other serious medical problems, are currently taking a diuretic, or are ≥60 years of age. Recommended dosages should not be exceeded, due to an increased risk of GI bleeding. Consuming ≥3 alcoholic beverages/day or taking longer than recommended may increase the risk of GI bleeding. Not for self-medication (OTC use) in children <12 years of age.

Adverse Reactions

1% to 10%:

Cardiovascular: Edema (3% to 9%), palpitations (<3%)

Central nervous system: Dizziness (3% to 9%), drowsiness (3% to 9%), headache (3% to 9%), lightheadedness (<3%), vertigo (<3%)

Dermatologic: Pruritus (3% to 9%), skin eruption (3% to 9%), ecchymosis (3% to 9%), purpura (<3%), rash

Endocrine & metabolic: Fluid retention (3% to 9%)

Gastrointestinal: Abdominal pain (3% to 9%), constipation (3% to 9%), nausea (3% to 9%), heartburn (3% to 9%), diarrhea (<3%), dyspepsia (<3%), stomatitis (<3%), flatulence, gross bleeding/perforation, indigestion, ulcers, vomiting

Genitourinary: Abnormal renal function

Hematologic: Hemolysis (3% to 9%), ecchymosis (3% to 9%), anemia, bleeding time increased

Hepatic: LFTs increased

Ocular: Visual disturbances (<3%)

Otic: Tinnitus (3% to 9%), hearing disturbances (<3%)

Respiratory: Dyspnea (3% to 9%)

Miscellaneous: Diaphoresis (<3%), thirst (<3%)

<1% (Limited to important or life-threatening): Agranulocytosis, alopecia, anaphylactic/anaphylactoid reaction, angioneurotic edema, arrhythmia, aseptic meningitis, asthma, blurred vision, cognitive dysfunction, colitis, coma, confusion, CHF, conjunctivitis, cystitis, depression, dream abnormalities, dysuria, eosinophilia, eosinophilic pneumonitis, erythema multiforme, exfoliative dermatitis, glossitis, granulocytopenia, hallucinations, hematemesis, hepatitis, hyper-/hypoglycemia, hyper-/hypotension, infection, interstitial nephritis, melena, jaundice, leukopenia, liver failure, lymphadenopathy, menstrual disorders, malaise, MI, muscle weakness, myalgia, oliguria, pancreatitis, pancytopenia, paresthesia, photosensitivity, pneumonia, polyuria, proteinuria, pyrexia, rectal bleeding, renal failure, renal papillary necrosis, respiratory depression, sepsis, Stevens-Johnson syndrome, tachycardia, seizure, syncope, thrombocytopenia, toxic epidermal necrolysis ulcerative stomatitis, vasculitis

Drug Interactions

Metabolism/Transport Effects Substrate (minor) of CYP1A2, 2C9

Avoid Concomitant Use

Avoid concomitant use of Naproxen with any of the following: Ketorolac

Increased Effect/Toxicity

Naproxen may increase the levels/effects of: Aminoglycosides; Anticoagulants; Antiplatelet Agents; Bisphosphonate Derivatives; CycloSPORINE; Desmopressin; Lithium; Methotrexate; Nonsteroidal Anti-Inflammatory Agents; Pemetrexed; Quinolone Antibiotics; Salicylates; Thrombolytic Agents; Vancomycin; Vitamin K Antagonists

The levels/effects of Naproxen may be increased by: Antidepressants (Tricyclic, Tertiary Amine); Corticosteroids (Systemic); Herbs (Anticoagulant/Antiplatelet Properties); Ketorolac; Probenecid; Selective Serotonin Reuptake Inhibitors; Serotonin/Norepinephrine Reuptake Inhibitors; Treprostinil

Decreased Effect

Naproxen may decrease the levels/effects of: ACE Inhibitors; Angiotensin II Receptor Blockers; Antiplatelet Agents; Beta-Blockers; Eplerenone; HydrALAZINE; Loop Diuretics; Salicylates; Thiazide Diuretics

The levels/effects of Naproxen may be decreased by: Bile Acid Sequestrants; Salicylates

Ethanol/Nutrition/Herb Interactions

Ethanol: Avoid ethanol (may enhance gastric mucosal irritation).

Food: Naproxen absorption rate/levels may be decreased if taken with food.

Herb/Nutraceutical: Avoid alfalfa, anise, bilberry, bladderwrack, bromelain, cat's claw, celery, chamomile, coleus, cordyceps, dong quai, evening primrose, fenugreek, feverfew, garlic, ginger, ginkgo biloba, ginseng (American, Panax, Siberian), grapeseed, green tea, guggul, horse chestnut seed, horseradish, licorice, prickly ash, red clover, reishi, SAMe (S-adenosylmethionine), sweet clover, turmeric, white willow (all have additional antiplatelet activity).

Stability Store oral suspension and tablet at 15°C to 30°C (59°F to 86°F).

Mechanism of Action Reversibly inhibits cyclooxygenase-1 and 2 (COX-1 and 2) enzymes, which result in decreased formation of prostaglandin precursors; has antipyretic, analgesic, and anti-inflammatory properties

Pharmacodynamics/Kinetics

Onset of action: Analgesic: 1 hour; Anti-inflammatory: ~2 weeks

Peak effect: Anti-inflammatory: 2-4 weeks

Duration: Analgesic: ≤7 hours; Anti-inflammatory: ≤12 hours

Absorption: Almost 100%

Protein binding: >99%; increased free fraction in elderly

Half-life elimination: Normal renal function: 12-17 hours; End-stage renal disease: No change

Time to peak, serum: 1-4 hours

Excretion: Urine (95%)

Dosage Note: Dosage expressed as naproxen base; 200 mg naproxen base is equivalent to 220 mg naproxen sodium.

Oral:

Children >2 years: Juvenile arthritis: 10 mg/kg/day in 2 divided doses

Adults:

Gout, acute: Initial: 750 mg, followed by 250 mg every 8 hours until attack subsides. **Note:** EC-Naprosyn® is not recommended.

Migraine, acute (unlabeled use): Initial: 500-750 mg.; an additional 250-500 mg may be given if needed (maximum: 1250 mg in 24 hours). **Note:** EC-Naprosyn® is not recommended.

Pain (mild-to-moderate), dysmenorrhea, acute tendonitis, bursitis: Initial: 500 mg, then 250 mg every 6-8 hours; maximum: 1250 mg/day naproxen base

Rheumatoid arthritis, osteoarthritis, and ankylosing spondylitis: 500-1000 mg/day in 2 divided doses; may increase to 1.5 g/day of naproxen base for limited time period

OTC labeling: Pain/fever:

Children ≥12 years and Adults ≤65 years: 200 mg naproxen base every 8-12 hours; if needed, may take 400 mg naproxen base for the initial dose; maximum: 600 mg naproxen base/24 hours

Adults >65 years: 200 mg naproxen base every 12 hours

Dosing adjustment in renal impairment: Cl_{cr} <30 mL/minute: use is not recommended

Dietary Considerations Drug may cause GI upset, bleeding, ulceration, perforation; take with food or milk to minimize GI upset.

Administration Administer with food, milk, or antacids to decrease GI adverse effects

Suspension: Shake suspension well before administration.

Tablet, extended release: Swallow tablet whole; do not break, crush, or chew.

Monitoring Parameters Occult blood loss, periodic liver function test, CBC, BUN, serum creatinine; urine output

Test Interactions Naproxen may interfere with 5-HIAA urinary assays; due to an interaction with m-dinitrobenzene, naproxen should be discontinued 72 hours before adrenal function testing if the Porter-Silber test is used.

Dosage Forms Excipient information presented when available (limited, particularly for generics); consult specific product labeling.

Caplet, as sodium: 220 mg [equivalent to naproxen 200 mg and sodium 20 mg]

Aleve®, Midol® Extended Relief, Pamprin® Maximum Strength All Day Relief: 220 mg [equivalent to naproxen 200 mg and sodium 20 mg]

Capsule, liquid gel, as sodium:

Aleve®: 220 mg [equivalent to naproxen 200 mg and sodium 20 mg]

Gelcap, as sodium:

Aleve®: 220 mg [equivalent to naproxen 200 mg and sodium 20 mg]

Suspension, oral: 125 mg/5 mL (500 mL)

Naprosyn®: 125 mg/5 mL (480 mL) [contains sodium 39 mg (1.5 mEq/5 mL); orange-pineapple flavor]

Tablet: 250 mg, 375 mg, 500 mg

Naprosyn®: 250 mg, 375 mg, 500 mg

Tablet, as sodium: 220 mg [equivalent to naproxen 200 mg and sodium 20 mg]; 275 mg [equivalent to naproxen 250 mg and sodium 25 mg]; 550 mg [equivalent to naproxen 500 mg and sodium 50 mg]

Aleve®: 220 mg [equivalent to naproxen 200 mg and sodium 20 mg]

Anaprox®: 275 mg [equivalent to naproxen 250 mg and sodium 25 mg]

Anaprox® DS: 550 mg [equivalent to naproxen 500 mg and sodium 50 mg]

Mediproxen: 220 mg [equivalent to naproxen 200 mg and sodium 20 mg]

Tablet, controlled release, as sodium: 550 mg [equivalent to naproxen 500 mg and sodium 50 mg]

Naprelan®: 412.5 mg [equivalent to naproxen 375 mg and sodium 37.5 mg]; 550 mg [equivalent to naproxen 500 mg and sodium 50 mg]

Tablet, delayed release, enteric coated: 375 mg, 500 mg

EC-Naprosyn®: 375 mg, 500 mg

Tablet, extended release, as sodium: 550 mg [equivalent to naproxen 500 mg and sodium 50 mg]

◆ **Naproxen and Lansoprazole** *see* Lansoprazole and Naproxen *on page 855*

Naproxen and Pseudoephedrine

(na PROKS en & soo doe e FED rin)

U.S. Brand Names Aleve® Cold & Sinus [OTC] [DSC]; Aleve® Sinus & Headache [OTC] [DSC]; Aleve®-D Sinus & Cold [OTC]; Aleve®-D Sinus & Headache [OTC]

Index Terms Naproxen Sodium and Pseudoephedrine; Pseudoephedrine and Naproxen

Pharmacologic Category Decongestant/Analgesic

Use Temporary relief of cold, sinus, and flu symptoms (including nasal congestion, sinus congestion/pressure, headache, minor body aches and pains, and fever)

Dosage Oral: Children ≥12 years and Adults: Aleve®-D Cold & Sinus, Aleve®-D Sinus & Headache: One caplet every 12 hours (maximum dose: 2 caplets/24 hours); treatment for >10 days is not recommended unless directed by healthcare provider.

Additional Information Complete prescribing information for this medication should be consulted for additional detail.

Dosage Forms Excipient information presented when available (limited, particularly for generics); consult specific product labeling. [DSC] = Discontinued product

Caplet, extended release:

Aleve® Cold & Sinus [DSC], Aleve® Sinus & Headache [DSC], Aleve®-D Sinus & Cold, Aleve®-D Sinus & Headache: Naproxen sodium 220 mg [equivalent to naproxen 200 mg and sodium 20 mg] and pseudoephedrine hydrochloride 120 mg

◆ **Naproxen and Sumatriptan** *see* Sumatriptan and Naproxen *on page 1415*

◆ **Naproxen Sodium** *see* Naproxen *on page 1041*

◆ **Naproxen Sodium and Pseudoephedrine** *see* Naproxen and Pseudoephedrine *on page 1043*

◆ **Naproxen Sodium and Sumatriptan** *see* Sumatriptan and Naproxen *on page 1415*

◆ **Naproxen Sodium and Sumatriptan Succinate** *see* Sumatriptan and Naproxen *on page 1415*

Naratriptan (NAR a trip tan)

U.S. Brand Names Amerge®

Canadian Brand Names Amerge®

Index Terms Naratriptan Hydrochloride

Pharmacologic Category Antimigraine Agent; Serotonin $5\text{-}HT_{1B,\ 1D}$ Receptor Agonist

Additional Appendix Information

Antimigraine Drugs: $5\text{-}HT_1$ Receptor Agonists *on page 1642*

Use Treatment of acute migraine headache with or without aura

Pregnancy Risk Factor C

Pregnancy Considerations There are no adequate and well-controlled studies using naratriptan in pregnant women. Use only if potential benefit to the mother outweighs the potential risk to the fetus. A pregnancy registry has been established to monitor outcomes of women exposed to naratriptan during pregnancy (800-336-2176). In animal studies, administration was associated with embryolethality, fetal abnormalities, and pup mortality and growth retardation. Tremors were observed in the offspring of female rats when exposed to naratriptan late in gestation.

Lactation Excretion in breast milk unknown/use caution

Medication Safety Issues

Sound-alike/look-alike issues:

Amerge® may be confused with Altace®, Amaryl®

Contraindications Hypersensitivity to naratriptan or any component of the formulation; cerebrovascular, peripheral vascular disease (ischemic bowel disease), ischemic heart disease (angina pectoris, history of myocardial infarction, or proven silent ischemia); or in patients with symptoms consistent with ischemic heart disease, coronary artery vasospasm, or Prinzmetal's angina; uncontrolled hypertension or patients who have received within 24 hours another 5-HT agonist (sumatriptan, zolmitriptan) or ergotamine-containing product; patients with known risk factors associated with coronary artery disease; patients with severe hepatic or renal disease (Cl_{cr} <15 mL/minute); do not administer naratriptan to patients with hemiplegic or basilar migraine

Warnings/Precautions Use only if there is a clear diagnosis of migraine. Do not give to patients with risk factors for CAD until a cardiovascular evaluation has been performed; if evaluation is satisfactory, the healthcare provider should administer the first dose and cardiovascular status should be periodically re-evaluated. Cardiac events (coronary artery vasospasm, transient ischemia, myocardial infarction, ventricular tachycardia/fibrillation, cardiac arrest, and death), cerebral/subarachnoid hemorrhage, stroke, peripheral vascular ischemia, and colonic ischemia have been reported with 5-HT_1 agonist administration. Significant elevation in blood pressure, including hypertensive crisis, has also been reported on rare occasions in patients with and without a history of hypertension. If the patient does not respond to the first dose, re-evaluate the diagnosis of migraine before trying a second dose. Safety and efficacy have not been established in children <18 years of age.

Adverse Reactions

1% to 10%:

Central nervous system: Dizziness, drowsiness, malaise/fatigue

Gastrointestinal: Nausea, vomiting

Neuromuscular & skeletal: Paresthesia

Miscellaneous: Pain or pressure in throat or neck

<1% (Limited to important or life-threatening): Allergic reaction, atrial fibrillation, atrial flutter, coronary artery vasospasm, hallucinations, MI, PR prolongation, premature ventricular contractions, QT_c prolongation, seizure, ventricular fibrillation, ventricular tachycardia

Drug Interactions

Avoid Concomitant Use

Avoid concomitant use of Naratriptan with any of the following: Ergot Derivatives; Sibutramine

Increased Effect/Toxicity

Naratriptan may increase the levels/effects of: Ergot Derivatives; Serotonin Modulators

The levels/effects of Naratriptan may be increased by: Ergot Derivatives; Sibutramine

Decreased Effect There are no known significant interactions involving a decrease in effect.

Mechanism of Action The therapeutic effect for migraine is due to serotonin agonist activity

Pharmacodynamics/Kinetics

Onset of action: 30 minutes

Absorption: Well absorbed

Protein binding, plasma: 28% to 31%

Metabolism: Hepatic via CYP

Bioavailability: 70%

Time to peak: 2-3 hours

Excretion: Urine

Dosage

Adults: Oral: 1-2.5 mg at the onset of headache; it is recommended to use the lowest possible dose to minimize adverse effects. If headache returns or does not fully resolve, the dose may be repeated after 4 hours; do not exceed 5 mg in 24 hours.

Elderly: Not recommended for use in the elderly

Dosing in renal impairment:

Cl_{cr} 18-39 mL/minute: Initial: 1 mg; do not exceed 2.5 mg in 24 hours

Cl_{cr} <15 mL/minute: Do not use

Dosing in hepatic impairment: Contraindicated in patients with severe liver failure; maximum dose: 2.5 mg in 24 hours for patients with mild or moderate liver failure; recommended starting dose: 1 mg

Administration Do **not** crush or chew tablet; swallow whole with water.

Dosage Forms Excipient information presented when available (limited, particularly for generics); consult specific product labeling.

Tablet: 1 mg, 2.5 mg

◆ **Naratriptan Hydrochloride** *see* Naratriptan *on page 1043*

◆ **Narcan** *see* Naloxone *on page 1037*

◆ **Nardil®** *see* Phenelzine *on page 1177*

◆ **Naropin®** *see* Ropivacaine *on page 1339*

◆ **Nasacort® AQ** *see* Triamcinolone *on page 1510*

◆ **NasalCrom® [OTC]** *see* Cromolyn *on page 372*

◆ **Nasalide® (Can)** *see* Flunisolide *on page 632*

◆ **Nasal Moist® Saline [OTC]** *see* Sodium Chloride *on page 1381*

◆ **Nasal Spray [OTC]** *see* Sodium Chloride *on page 1381*

◆ **Nasarel®** *see* Flunisolide *on page 632*

◆ **Nasatab® LA** *see* Guaifenesin and Pseudoephedrine *on page 713*

◆ **Nascobal®** *see* Cyanocobalamin *on page 374*

◆ **Nasex-G** *see* Guaifenesin and Phenylephrine *on page 712*

◆ **Nasofed™** *see* Pseudoephedrine *on page 1265*

◆ **Nasonex®** *see* Mometasone *on page 1012*

◆ **Nasop12™** *see* Phenylephrine *on page 1183*

◆ **Natacyn®** *see* Natamycin *on page 1045*

Natalizumab (na ta LIZ u mab)

U.S. Brand Names Tysabri®

Canadian Brand Names Tysabri®

Index Terms AN100226; Anti-4 Alpha Integrin; IgG4-Kappa Monoclonal Antibody

Pharmacologic Category Gastrointestinal Agent, Miscellaneous; Monoclonal Antibody, Selective Adhesion-Molecule Inhibitor

Use

U.S. labeling: Monotherapy for the treatment of relapsing forms of multiple sclerosis; treatment of moderately- to severely-active Crohn's disease

Canada labeling: Treatment of relapsing forms of multiple sclerosis

Restrictions Patients must be enrolled in the Tysabri® Outreach Unified Commitment to Health (TOUCH™) Prescribing Program (800-456-2255) to receive natalizumab (MS-TOUCH™ for multiple sclerosis or CD-TOUCH™ for Crohn's disease). Healthcare providers must also register with the program in order to prescribe, dispense or administer natalizumab. Treatment must be reauthorized every 6 months. Natalizumab is available only through infusion centers registered with the TOUCH™ program; infusion center information is available at 1-800-456-2255.

Medication guides are available at http://www.fda.gov/cder/Offices/ODS/MG/natalizumabMG.pdf and should be provided to every patient prior to initiation of therapy.

Pregnancy Risk Factor C

Dosage I.V.: Adults:

Multiple sclerosis: 300 mg infused over 1 hour every 4 weeks

Crohn's disease: 300 mg infused over 1 hour every 4 weeks; discontinue if therapeutic benefit is not observed within initial 12 weeks of therapy

Concomitant use with corticosteroids: For patients who begin treatment while on chronic oral corticosteroids, begin tapering oral steroids when the onset of natalizumab therapeutic benefit is observed; discontinue use if patient cannot be tapered off of oral corticosteroids within 6 months of therapy initiation. If additional concomitant corticosteroids are required and exceed 3 months/year (in addition to initial corticosteroid taper), consider discontinuing therapy.

Dosage adjustment in renal impairment: Not studied

Dosage adjustment in hepatic impairment: Not studied. Discontinue use with jaundice or signs/symptoms of hepatic injury.

Additional Information Complete prescribing information for this medication should be consulted for additional detail.

Dosage Forms Excipient information presented when available (limited, particularly for generics); consult specific product labeling.

Injection, solution [preservative free]:

Tysabri®: 300 mg/15 mL (15 mL) [contains polysorbate-80]

Natamycin (na ta MYE sin)

U.S. Brand Names Natacyn®

Canadian Brand Names Natacyn®

Index Terms Pimaricin

Pharmacologic Category Antifungal Agent, Ophthalmic

Use Treatment of blepharitis, conjunctivitis, and keratitis caused by susceptible fungi (*Aspergillus*, *Candida*, *Cephalosporium*, *Fusarium*, and *Penicillium*)

Pregnancy Risk Factor C

Medication Safety Issues

Sound-alike/look-alike issues:

Natacyn® may be confused with Naprosyn®

Dosage Adults: Ophthalmic:

Fungal keratitis: Instill 1 drop in conjunctival sac every 1-2 hours, after 3-4 days reduce to one drop 6-8 times/day; usual course of therapy is 2-3 weeks or until resolution of active fungal keratitis (may be useful to gradually reduce dosage at 4-7 day intervals to assure elimination of organism)

Fungal blepharitis or conjunctivitis: Instill 1 drop in conjunctival sac every 4-6 hours

Additional Information Complete prescribing information for this medication should be consulted for additional detail.

Dosage Forms Excipient information presented when available (limited, particularly for generics); consult specific product labeling.

Suspension, ophthalmic:

Natacyn®: 5% (15 mL) [contains benzalkonium chloride]

Nateglinide (na te GLYE nide)

U.S. Brand Names Starlix®

Canadian Brand Names Starlix®

Pharmacologic Category Antidiabetic Agent, Meglitinide Derivative

Additional Appendix Information

Diabetes Mellitus Management, Adults *on page 1801*

Use Management of type 2 diabetes mellitus (noninsulin dependent, NIDDM) as monotherapy when hyperglycemia cannot be managed by diet and exercise alone; in combination with metformin or a thiazolidinedione to lower blood glucose in patients whose hyperglycemia cannot be controlled by exercise, diet, or a single agent alone

Pregnancy Risk Factor C

Pregnancy Considerations Adverse events have been observed in animal reproduction studies; therefore, nateglinide is classified as pregnancy category C. Information describing the effects of nateglinide on pregnancy outcomes is limited. Maternal hyperglycemia can be associated with adverse effects in the fetus, including macrosomia, neonatal hyperglycemia, and hyperbilirubinemia; the risk of congenital malformations is increased when the Hb A_{1c} is above the normal range. Diabetes can also be associated with adverse effects in the mother. Poorly-treated diabetes may cause end-organ damage that may in turn negatively affect obstetric outcomes. Physiologic glucose levels should be maintained prior to and during pregnancy to decrease the risk of adverse events in the mother and the fetus. Until additional safety and efficacy data are obtained, the use of oral agents is generally not recommended as routine management of GDM or type 2 diabetes mellitus during pregnancy. Insulin is the drug of choice for the control of diabetes mellitus during pregnancy.

Lactation Excretion in breast milk unknown/not recommended

Medication Safety Issues

High alert medication: The Institute for Safe Medication Practices (ISMP) includes this medication among its list of drug classes which have a heightened risk of causing significant patient harm when used in error.

Contraindications Hypersensitivity to nateglinide or any component of the formulation; diabetic ketoacidosis, with or without coma (treat with insulin); type 1 diabetes mellitus (insulin dependent, IDDM)

Warnings/Precautions Use with caution in patients with moderate-to-severe hepatic impairment. Use caution in severe renal dysfunction, elderly, malnourished, or patients with adrenal/pituitary dysfunction; may be more susceptible to glucose-lowering effects. All oral hypoglycemic agents are capable of producing hypoglycemia. Proper patient selection, dosage, and instructions to the patients are important to avoid hypoglycemic episodes. It may be necessary to discontinue nateglinide and administer insulin if the patient is exposed to stress (ie, fever, trauma, infection, surgery). Indicated for adjunctive therapy with metformin; not to be used as a substitute for metformin monotherapy. Combination treatment with sulfonylureas is not recommended (no additional benefit). Patients not adequately controlled on oral agents which stimulate insulin release (eg, glyburide) should not be switched to nateglinide or have nateglinide added to therapy. Safety and efficacy in pediatric patients have not been established.

Adverse Reactions As reported with nateglinide monotherapy:

1% to 10%:

Central nervous system: Dizziness (4%)

Endocrine & metabolic: Hypoglycemia (2%), increased uric acid

Gastrointestinal: Weight gain

Neuromuscular & skeletal: Arthropathy (3%)

Respiratory: Upper respiratory infection (10%)

Miscellaneous: Flu-like syndrome (4%)

Postmarketing and/or case reports: Cholestatic hepatitis, jaundice, liver enzymes increased, rash, pruritus, urticaria

Drug Interactions

Metabolism/Transport Effects Substrate (major) of CYP2C9, 3A4; **Inhibits** CYP2C9 (weak)

Avoid Concomitant Use There are no known interactions where it is recommended to avoid concomitant use.

Increased Effect/Toxicity

The levels/effects of Nateglinide may be increased by: CYP2C9 Inhibitors (Moderate); CYP2C9 Inhibitors (Strong); CYP3A4 Inhibitors (Moderate); CYP3A4

Inhibitors (Strong); Dasatinib; Eltrombopag; Herbs (Hypoglycemic Properties); Pegvisomant

Decreased Effect

The levels/effects of Nateglinide may be decreased by: Corticosteroids (Orally Inhaled); Corticosteroids (Systemic); CYP2C9 Inducers (Highly Effective); CYP3A4 Inducers (Strong); Deferasirox; Herbs (CYP3A4 Inducers); Luteinizing Hormone-Releasing Hormone Analogs; Somatropin

Ethanol/Nutrition/Herb Interactions

Ethanol: Avoid ethanol (increased risk of hypoglycemia).

Food: Rate of absorption is decreased and time to T_{max} is delayed when taken with food. Food does not affect AUC. Multiple peak plasma concentrations may be observed if fasting. Not affected by composition of meal.

Herb/Nutraceutical: Avoid alfalfa, aloe, bilberry, bitter melon, burdock, celery, damiana, fenugreek, garcinia, garlic, ginger, ginseng (American), gymnema, marshmallow, and stinging nettle (may enhance the hypoglycemic effects of antidiabetic agents). St. John's wort may decrease the levels/effect of nateglinide.

Stability Store at 25°C (77°F).

Mechanism of Action A phenylalanine derivative, nonsulfonylurea hypoglycemic agent used in the management of type 2 diabetes mellitus (noninsulin dependent, NIDDM); stimulates insulin release from the pancreatic beta cells to reduce postprandial hyperglycemia; amount of insulin release is dependent upon existing glucose levels

Pharmacodynamics/Kinetics

Onset of action: Insulin secretion: ~20 minutes

Peak effect: 1 hour

Duration: 4 hours

Absorption: Rapid

Distribution: 10 L

Protein binding: 98%, primarily to albumin

Metabolism: Hepatic via hydroxylation followed by glucuronide conjugation via CYP2C9 (70%) and CYP3A4 (30%) to metabolites

Bioavailability: 73%

Half-life elimination: 1.5 hours

Time to peak: ≤1 hour

Excretion: Urine (83%, 16% as unchanged drug); feces (10%)

Dosage

Adults: Management of type 2 diabetes mellitus: Oral: Initial and maintenance dose: 120 mg 3 times/day, 1-30 minutes before meals; may be given alone or in combination with metformin or a thiazolidinedione; patients close to Hb A_{1c} goal may be started at 60 mg 3 times/day

Elderly: No changes in safety and efficacy were seen in patients ≥65 years; however, some elderly patients may show increased sensitivity to dosing

Dosage adjustment in renal impairment: No specific dosage adjustment is recommended for patients with mild-to-severe renal disease; patients on dialysis showed reduced medication exposure and plasma protein binding. Patients with severe renal dysfunction are more susceptible to glucose-lowering effect; use with caution.

Dosage adjustment in hepatic impairment: Increased serum levels seen with mild hepatic insufficiency; no dosage adjustment is needed. Has not been studied in patients with moderate to severe liver disease; use with caution.

Dietary Considerations Nateglinide should be taken 1-30 minutes prior to meals. Scheduled dose should not be taken if meal is missed. Dietary modification based on ADA recommendations is a part of therapy. Decreases blood glucose concentration. Hypoglycemia may occur. Must be able to recognize symptoms of hypoglycemia (palpitations, sweaty palms, lightheadedness).

Administration Patients who are anorexic or NPO will need to have their dose held to avoid hypoglycemia.

Monitoring Parameters Glucose and Hb A_{1c} levels, weight, lipid profile

Reference Range Recommendations for glycemic control in adults with diabetes:

Hb A_{1c}: <7%

Preprandial capillary plasma glucose: 70-130 mg/dL

Peak postprandial capillary blood glucose: <180 mg/dL

Blood pressure: <130/80 mm Hg

Additional Information An increase in weight was seen in nateglinide monotherapy, which was not seen when used in combination with metformin.

Dosage Forms Excipient information presented when available (limited, particularly for generics); consult specific product labeling.

Tablet:

Starlix®: 60 mg, 120 mg

◆ **Natrecor®** *see* Nesiritide *on page 1054*

◆ **Natriuretic Peptide** *see* Nesiritide *on page 1054*

◆ **Natulan® (Can)** *see* Procarbazine *on page 1242*

◆ **Natural Fiber Therapy [OTC]** *see* Psyllium *on page 1268*

◆ **Natural Fiber Therapy Smooth Texture [OTC]** *see* Psyllium *on page 1268*

◆ **Natural Lung Surfactant** *see* Beractant *on page 187*

◆ **Nature-Throid™** *see* Thyroid, Desiccated *on page 1464*

◆ **Nauseatol (Can)** *see* DimenhyDRINATE *on page 453*

◆ **Navane®** *see* Thiothixene *on page 1463*

◆ **Navelbine®** *see* Vinorelbine *on page 1563*

◆ **Naxen® (Can)** *see* Naproxen *on page 1041*

◆ **Naxen® EC (Can)** *see* Naproxen *on page 1041*

◆ **Na-Zone® [OTC]** *see* Sodium Chloride *on page 1381*

◆ **NC-722665** *see* Bicalutamide *on page 197*

◆ ***n*-Docosanol** *see* Docosanol *on page 473*

Nebivolol (ne BIV oh lole)

U.S. Brand Names Bystolic™

Index Terms Nebivolol Hydrochloride

Pharmacologic Category Beta Blocker, $Beta_1$ Selective

Use Treatment of hypertension, alone or in combination with other agents

Unlabeled/Investigational Use Heart failure

Pregnancy Risk Factor C (manufacturer); D (2nd and 3rd trimesters - expert analysis)

Dosage Oral:

Adults:

Hypertension: Initial: 5 mg once daily; if initial response is inadequate, may be increased at 2-week intervals to a maximum dose of 40 mg once daily

Heart failure (unlabeled use): Adults ≥70 years: Initial: 1.25 mg once daily; if tolerated, may increase by 2.5 mg at 1- to 2-week intervals to a maximum dose of 10 mg once daily

Elderly: Refer to adult dosing.

Dosing adjustment in renal impairment: Severe impairment (Cl_{cr} <30 mL/minute): Initial: 2.5 mg/day; increase cautiously

Dosage adjustment in hepatic impairment: Moderate impairment (Child-Pugh class B): Initial: 2.5 mg/day; increase cautiously

Additional Information Complete prescribing information for this medication should be consulted for additional detail.

Dosage Forms Excipient information presented when available (limited, particularly for generics); consult specific product labeling.

Tablet:

Bystolic™: 2.5 mg, 5 mg, 10 mg

- ◆ **Nebivolol Hydrochloride** *see* Nebivolol *on page 1046*
- ◆ **NebuPent®** *see* Pentamidine *on page 1168*
- ◆ **Necon® 0.5/35** *see* Ethinyl Estradiol and Norethindrone *on page 581*
- ◆ **Necon® 1/35** *see* Ethinyl Estradiol and Norethindrone *on page 581*
- ◆ **Necon® 1/50** *see* Norethindrone and Mestranol *on page 1079*
- ◆ **Necon® 7/7/7** *see* Ethinyl Estradiol and Norethindrone *on page 581*
- ◆ **Necon® 10/11** *see* Ethinyl Estradiol and Norethindrone *on page 581*

Nedocromil (ne doe KROE mil)

U.S. Brand Names Alocril®; Tilade® [DSC]

Canadian Brand Names Alocril®; Tilade®

Index Terms Nedocromil Sodium

Pharmacologic Category Mast Cell Stabilizer

Additional Appendix Information

Asthma *on page 1793*

Use

Aerosol: Maintenance therapy in patients with mild to moderate bronchial asthma

Ophthalmic: Treatment of itching associated with allergic conjunctivitis

Pregnancy Risk Factor B

Dosage

Inhalation: Children ≥6 years and Adults: 2 inhalations 4 times/day; may reduce dosage to 2-3 times/day once desired clinical response to initial dose is observed. Drug has no known therapeutic systemic activity when delivered by inhalation.

Ophthalmic: Children ≥3 years and Adults: 1-2 drops in each eye twice daily

Additional Information Complete prescribing information for this medication should be consulted for additional detail.

Dosage Forms Excipient information presented when available (limited, particularly for generics); consult specific product labeling. [DSC] = Discontinued product

Aerosol for oral inhalation, as sodium:

Tilade®: 1.75 mg/activation (16.2 g; at least 104 inhalations) [DSC]

Solution, ophthalmic, as sodium:

Alocril®: 2% (5 mL) [contains benzalkonium chloride]

- ◆ **Nedocromil Sodium** *see* Nedocromil *on page 1047*

Nefazodone (nef AY zoe done)

Index Terms Nefazodone Hydrochloride; Serzone

Pharmacologic Category Antidepressant, Serotonin Reuptake Inhibitor/Antagonist

Additional Appendix Information

Antidepressant Agents *on page 1638*

Use Treatment of depression

Unlabeled/Investigational Use Post-traumatic stress disorder

Restrictions An FDA-approved medication guide concerning the use of antidepressants in children, adolescents, and young adults must be distributed when dispensing an outpatient prescription (new or refill) where this medication is to be used without direct supervision of a healthcare provider. Medication guides are available at http://www.fda.gov/cder/Offices/ODS/medication_guides.htm. Dispense to parents or guardians of children and adolescents receiving this medication.

Pregnancy Risk Factor C

Medication Safety Issues

Sound-alike/look-alike issues:

Serzone® may be confused with selegiline, Serentil®, Seroquel®, sertraline

Dosage Oral:

Children and Adolescents (unlabeled use): Depression: Target dose: 300-400 mg/day (mean: 3.4 mg/kg)

Adults: Depression: 200 mg/day, administered in 2 divided doses initially, with a range of 300-600 mg/day in 2 divided doses thereafter

Additional Information Complete prescribing information for this medication should be consulted for additional detail.

Dosage Forms Excipient information presented when available (limited, particularly for generics); consult specific product labeling.

Tablet, as hydrochloride: 50 mg, 100 mg, 150 mg, 200 mg, 250 mg

- ◆ **Nefazodone Hydrochloride** *see* Nefazodone *on page 1047*

Nelarabine (nel AY re been)

U.S. Brand Names Arranon®

Canadian Brand Names Atriance™

Index Terms 2-Amino-6-Methoxypurine Arabinoside; 506U78; GW506U78

Pharmacologic Category Antineoplastic Agent, Antimetabolite

Use Treatment of relapsed or refractory T-cell acute lymphoblastic leukemia (ALL) and T-cell lymphoblastic lymphoma

Unlabeled/Investigational Use CML (Philadelphia chromosome positive) T-Cell blast phase

Pregnancy Risk Factor D

Pregnancy Considerations Teratogenic effects were observed in animal studies. There are no adequate and well-controlled studies in pregnant women. Women of childbearing potential should be advised to use effective contraception and avoid becoming pregnant during therapy.

Lactation Excretion in breast milk unknown/not recommended

Medication Safety Issues

High alert medication: The Institute for Safe Medication Practices (ISMP) includes this medication among its list of drugs which have a heightened risk of causing significant patient harm when used in error.

Contraindications Hypersensitivity to nelarabine or any component of the formulation

Warnings/Precautions Hazardous agent - use appropriate precautions for handling and disposal. **[U.S. Boxed Warning]: Neurotoxicity is the dose-limiting toxicity;** observe closely for signs and symptoms of neurotoxicity (somnolence, confusion, convulsions, ataxia, paresthesia, hypoesthesia, coma, status epilepticus, craniospinal demyelination, or ascending neuropathy). Risk of neurotoxicity may increase in patients with concurrent or previous intrathecal chemotherapy or history of craniospinal irradiation. Appropriate measures must be taken to prevent hyperuricemia and tumor lysis syndrome; use extreme caution in patients with increased uric acid, gout, and history of uric acid stones; monitor, consider allopurinol and hydrate accordingly. Bone marrow suppression is common. Avoid administration of live vaccines. Use caution in patients with renal impairment; ara-G clearance may be reduced with renal dysfunction. Use caution with severe hepatic impairment; risk of adverse reactions may be higher with hepatic dysfunction.

[U.S. Boxed Warning]: Should be administered under the supervision of an experienced cancer chemotherapy physician.

Adverse Reactions Note: Pediatric adverse reactions fell within a range similar to adults except where noted.

>10%:

Cardiovascular: Peripheral edema (15%), edema (11%)

Central nervous system: Fatigue (50%), fever (23%), somnolence (7% to 23%; grades 2-4: 1% to 6%), dizziness (21%; grade 2: 8% adults), headache (15% to 17%; grades 2-4: 4% to 8%), hypoesthesia (6% to 17%; grades 2-4: children 5%, adults 12%), pain (11%)

Dermatologic: Petechiae (12%)

Endocrine & metabolic: Hypokalemia (11%)

Gastrointestinal: Nausea (41%), diarrhea (22%), vomiting (10% to 22%), constipation (21%)

Hematologic: Anemia (95% to 99%; grade 4: 10% to 14%), neutropenia (81% to 94%; grade 4: children 62%, adults 49%), thrombocytopenia (86% to 88%; grade 4: 22% to 32%), leukopenia (38%; grade 4: 7%), febrile neutropenia (12%; grade 4: 1%)

Hepatic: Transaminases increased (12%)

Neuromuscular & skeletal: Peripheral neuropathy (12% to 21%; grades 2-4: 11% to 14%), weakness (6% to 17%; grade 4: 1%), paresthesia (4% to 15%; grades 2-4: 3% to 4%), myalgia (13%)

Respiratory: Cough (25%), dyspnea (7% to 20%)

1% to 10%:

Cardiovascular: Hypotension (8%), tachycardia (8%), chest pain (5%)

Central nervous system: Ataxia (2% to 9%; grades 2-4: children 1%, adults 8%), confusion (8%), insomnia (7%), depressed level of consciousness (6%; grades 2-4: 2%), depression (6%), seizure (grade 3: 1% adults; grade 4: 6% children), motor dysfunction (4%; grades 2-4: 2%), amnesia (3%; grades 2-4: 1%), balance disorder (2%; grades 2-4: 1%), nerve paralysis (2%), sensory loss (1% to 2%), aphasia (1%), cerebral hemorrhage (1%), coma (1%), encephalopathy (1%), hemiparesis (1%), hydrocephalus (1%), lethargy (1%), leukoencephalopathy (1%), loss of consciousness (1%), mental impairment (1%), neuropathic pain (1%), nerve palsy (1%), nystagmus (1%), paralysis (1%), sciatica (1%), sensory disturbance (1%), speech disorder (1%), demyelination, ascending peripheral neuropathy

Endocrine & Metabolic: Hypocalcemia (8%), dehydration (7%), hyper-/hypoglycemia (6%), hypomagnesemia (6%)

Gastrointestinal: Abdominal pain (9%), anorexia (9%), stomatitis (8%), abdominal distension (6%), taste perversion (3%)

Hepatic: Albumin decreased (10%), bilirubin increased (10%), AST increased (6%)

Neuromuscular & skeletal: Arthralgia (9%), back pain (8%), muscle weakness (8%), rigors (8%), limb pain (7%), abnormal gait (6%), noncardiac chest pain (5%), tremor (4% to 5%; grades 2-4: 2% to 3%), dysarthria (1%), hyporeflexia (1%), hypertonia (1%), incoordination (1%)

Ocular: Blurred vision (4%)

Renal: Creatinine increased (6%)

Respiratory: Pleural effusion (10%), epistaxis (8%), pneumonia (8%), sinusitis (7%), wheezing (5%), sinus headache (1%)

Miscellaneous: Infection (5% to 9%)

Postmarketing and/or case reports: Tumor lysis syndrome

Drug Interactions

Avoid Concomitant Use

Avoid concomitant use of Nelarabine with any of the following: Natalizumab; Vaccines (Live)

Increased Effect/Toxicity

Nelarabine may increase the levels/effects of: Natalizumab; Vaccines (Live)

The levels/effects of Nelarabine may be increased by: Trastuzumab

Decreased Effect

Nelarabine may decrease the levels/effects of: Vaccines (Inactivated)

The levels/effects of Nelarabine may be decreased by: Echinacea

Stability Store unopened vials at 15°C to 30°C (59°F to 86°F). Reconstitution is not required; the appropriate dose should be added to empty plastic bag or glass container. Stable in plastic or glass containers for up to 8 hours at room temperature.

Mechanism of Action Nelarabine, a prodrug of ara-G, is demethylated by adenosine deaminase to ara-G and then converted to ara-GTP. Ara-GTP is incorporated into the DNA of the leukemic blasts, leading to inhibition of DNA synthesis and inducing apoptosis. Ara-GTP appears to accumulate at higher levels in T-cells, which correlates to clinical response.

Pharmacodynamics/Kinetics

Distribution: V_{ss}:

Nelarabine: Children: ~213 L/m^2; Adults: ~197 L/m^2

Ara-G: Children: ~50 L/m^2; Adults: ~33 L/m^2

Protein binding: Nelarabine and ara-G: <25%

Metabolism: Hepatic; demethylated by adenosine deaminase to form ara-G (active); also hydrolyzed to form methylguanine. Both ara-G and methylguanine metabolized to guanine. Guanine is deaminated into xanthine, which is further oxidized to form uric acid, which is then oxidized to form allantoin.

Half-life elimination: Nelarabine: 30 minutes; ara-G: 3 hours

Time to peak: Ara-G: 3-25 hours

Excretion: Urine (nelarabine 7%, ara-G 27%) within 24 hours of infusion on day 1

Dosage I.V.: T-cell ALL, T-cell lymphoblastic lymphoma:

Children: 650 mg/m^2/day on days 1 through 5; repeat every 21 days

Adults: 1500 mg/m^2/day on days 1, 3, and 5; repeat every 21 days

Dosage adjustment for toxicity:

Neurologic toxicity ≥ grade 2: Discontinue treatment.

Hematologic or other (non-neurologic) toxicity: Consider treatment delay.

Dosage adjustment in renal impairment:

Cl_{cr} ≥50 mL/minute: No adjustment recommended

Cl_{cr} <50 mL/minute: Safety has not been established

Cl_{cr} <30 mL/minute: Closely monitor

Dosage adjustment in hepatic impairment: Safety has not been established; closely monitor with severe impairment (bilirubin >3 mg/dL)

Administration Adequate I.V. hydration recommended to prevent tumor lysis syndrome; allopurinol may be used if hyperuricemia is anticipated.

Children: Infuse over 1 hour daily for 5 consecutive days

Adults: Infuse over 2 hours on days 1, 3, and 5

Monitoring Parameters Closely monitor for neurologic toxicity (severe somnolence, seizure, peripheral neuropathy, confusion, ataxia, paresthesia, hypoesthesia, coma, or craniospinal demyelination); signs and symptoms of tumor lysis syndrome; hydration status; CBC with platelet counts, liver and kidney function

Dosage Forms Excipient information presented when available (limited, particularly for generics); consult specific product labeling. [CAN] = Canadian brand name

Injection, solution:

Arranon®: 5 mg/mL (50 mL)

Atriance™ [CAN]: 5 mg/ml (50 mL)

Nelfinavir (nel FIN a veer)

U.S. Brand Names Viracept®

Canadian Brand Names Viracept®

Index Terms NFV

Pharmacologic Category Antiretroviral Agent, Protease Inhibitor

Additional Appendix Information

Antiretroviral Therapy for HIV Infection: Adults and Adolescents *on page 1758*

Desensitization Protocols *on page 1691*

Management of Healthcare Worker Exposures to HBV, HCV, and HIV *on page 1719*

Perinatal HIV Guidelines *on page 1730*

Use In combination with other antiretroviral therapy in the treatment of HIV infection

Pregnancy Risk Factor B

Pregnancy Considerations Adverse events were not observed in animal studies and no increased risk of overall birth defects has been observed following 1st trimester exposure in humans according to data collected by the antiretroviral pregnancy registry. Nelfinavir crosses the placenta. The Perinatal HIV Guidelines Working Group recommends nelfinavir as an alternative PI in combination regimens during pregnancy with HAART for perinatal prophylaxis. A dose of 1250 mg twice daily has been shown to provide adequate plasma concentrations although lower and variable levels may occur late in pregnancy. Pregnancy and protease inhibitors are both associated with an increased risk of hyperglycemia. Glucose levels should be closely monitored. Health professionals are encouraged to contact the antiretroviral pregnancy registry to monitor outcomes of pregnant women exposed to antiretroviral medications (1-800-258-4263 or www.APRegistry.com).

Lactation Excretion in breast milk unknown/contraindicated

Medication Safety Issues

Sound-alike/look-alike issues:

Nelfinavir may be confused with nevirapine

Viracept® may be confused with Viramune®

Contraindications Hypersensitivity to nelfinavir or any component of the formulation; concurrent therapy with amiodarone, ergot derivatives, midazolam, pimozide, quinidine, triazolam

Warnings/Precautions Use with caution in patients taking strong CYP3A4 inhibitors, moderate or strong CYP3A4 inducers and major CYP3A4 substrates (see Drug Interactions); consider alternative agents that avoid or lessen the potential for CYP-mediated interactions. Not recommended for use with rifampin, St John's wort, lovastatin, simvastatin, phosphodiesterase-5 (PDE-5) inhibitors, or proton pump inhibitors (based on omeprazole data). Use caution with hepatic impairment; use not recommended with moderate-to-severe impairment. Warn patients that redistribution of body fat can occur. New-onset diabetes mellitus, exacerbation of diabetes, and hyperglycemia have been reported in HIV-infected patients receiving protease inhibitors. Use with caution in patients with hemophilia A or B; increased bleeding during protease inhibitor therapy has been reported. Immune reconstitution syndrome has been reported; may require additional evaluation and treatment. The oral powder contains phenylalanine. Safety and efficacy have not been established in children <2 years of age.

Adverse Reactions Data presented on experience in adults, unless otherwise noted.

>10%: Gastrointestinal: Diarrhea (14% to 20%; children: 39% to 47%)

2% to 10%:

Dermatologic: Rash (1% to 3%)

Gastrointestinal: Nausea (3% to 7%), flatulence (1% to 5%)

Hematologic: Lymphocytes decreased (1% to 6%), neutrophils decreased (1% to 5%)

<2% (Limited to important or life-threatening): Abdominal pain, acute iritis, alkaline phosphatase increased, allergic reaction, amylase increased, anemia, anorexia, anxiety, arthralgia, arthritis, back pain, bilirubinemia, body fat redistribution/accumulation, cramps, creatinine phosphokinase increased, dehydration, depression, dermatitis, diaphoresis, dizziness, dyspepsia, dyspnea, emotional lability, epigastric pain, eye disorder, fever, folliculitis, fungal dermatitis, gastrointestinal bleeding, GGTP increased, headache, hepatitis, hyperkinesia, hyper-/hypoglycemia, hyperlipemia; hypersensitivity reaction (bronchospasm, rash, edema); hyperuricemia, immune reconstitution syndrome, insomnia, jaundice, kidney calculus, lactic dehydrogenase increased, leukopenia, lipoatrophy, lipodystrophy, liver function tests abnormal, maculopapular rash, malaise, metabolic acidosis, migraine, mouth ulceration, myalgia, myasthenia, myopathy, pain, pancreatitis, paresthesia, pharyngitis, pruritus, QT_c prolongation, rhinitis, seizure, sexual dysfunction, sinusitis, sleep disorder, somnolence, suicidal ideation, thrombocytopenia, torsade de pointes, transaminases increased, urine abnormality, urticaria, vomiting, weakness

Drug Interactions

Metabolism/Transport Effects Substrate of CYP2C9 (minor), 2C19 (major), 2D6 (minor), 3A4 (major); **Inhibits** CYP1A2 (weak), 2B6 (weak), 2C9 (weak), 2C19 (weak), 2D6 (weak), 3A4 (strong)

Avoid Concomitant Use

Avoid concomitant use of Nelfinavir with any of the following: Alfuzosin; Amiodarone; Cisapride; Dabigatran Etexilate; Eplerenone; Ergot Derivatives; Nilotinib; Nisoldipine; Pimozide; Proton Pump Inhibitors; QuiNIDine; Ranolazine; Rivaroxaban; Salmeterol; Silodosin; St Johns Wort; Topotecan

Increased Effect/Toxicity

Nelfinavir may increase the levels/effects of: Alfuzosin; Alosetron; Amiodarone; Antifungal Agents (Azole Derivatives, Systemic); Azithromycin; Benzodiazepines (metabolized by oxidation); Calcium Channel Blockers (Dihydropyridine); Calcium Channel Blockers (Nondihydropyridine); CarBAMazepine; Ciclesonide; Cisapride; Clarithromycin; Corticosteroids (Orally Inhaled); CycloSPORINE; CYP3A4 Substrates; Dabigatran Etexilate; Digoxin; Enfuvirtide; Eplerenone; Ergot Derivatives; Etravirine; FentaNYL; Fesoterodine; Fusidic Acid; HMG-CoA Reductase Inhibitors; Ixabepilone; Maraviroc; Meperidine; Methadone; Nefazodone; Nilotinib; Nisoldipine; P-Glycoprotein Substrates; Phosphodiesterase 5 Inhibitors; Pimecrolimus; Pimozide; Protease Inhibitors; QuiNIDine; Ranolazine; Rifamycin Derivatives; Rivaroxaban; Salmeterol; Silodosin; Sirolimus; Sorafenib; Tacrolimus; Temsirolimus; Tenofovir; Topotecan; TraZODone; Tricyclic Antidepressants

The levels/effects of Nelfinavir may be increased by: Antifungal Agents (Azole Derivatives, Systemic); Clarithromycin; CycloSPORINE; Delavirdine; Efavirenz; Enfuvirtide; Etravirine; Fusidic Acid; P-Glycoprotein Inhibitors

Decreased Effect

Nelfinavir may decrease the levels/effects of: Abacavir; Clarithromycin; Delavirdine; Etravirine; Meperidine; Oral Contraceptive (Estrogens); Theophylline Derivatives; Valproic Acid; Zidovudine

The levels/effects of Nelfinavir may be decreased by: Antacids; CarBAMazepine; CYP2C19 Inducers (Strong); CYP3A4 Inducers (Strong); Deferasirox; Efavirenz; Garlic; H2-Antagonists; Nevirapine; Oral Contraceptive (Estrogens); P-Glycoprotein Inducers; Proton Pump Inhibitors; Rifamycin Derivatives; St Johns Wort; Tenofovir

Ethanol/Nutrition/Herb Interactions

Food: Nelfinavir taken with food increases plasma concentration time curve (AUC) by two- to threefold. Do not administer with acidic food or juice (orange juice, apple juice, or applesauce) since the combination may have a bitter taste.

Herb/Nutraceutical: St John's wort may decrease the levels/effects of protease inhibitors; concurrent use should probably be avoided.

Stability Store at room temperature of 15°C to 30°C (59°F to 86°F). Oral powder (or dissolved tablets) diluted in nonacidic liquid is stable for 6 hours under refrigeration.

Mechanism of Action Inhibits the HIV-1 protease; inhibition of the viral protease prevents cleavage of the gag-pol polyprotein resulting in the production of immature, noninfectious virus

Pharmacodynamics/Kinetics

Absorption: Food increases AUC of nelfinavir by two- to fivefold

Distribution: V_d: 2-7 L/kg

Protein binding: >98%

Metabolism: Hepatic via CYP2C19 and 3A4; major metabolite has activity comparable to parent drug

Half-life elimination: 3.5-5 hours

Time to peak, serum: 2-4 hours

Excretion: Feces (98% to 99%, 78% as metabolites, 22% as unchanged drug); urine (1% to 2%)

Dosage Oral:

Children 2-13 years: 45-55 mg/kg twice daily **or** 25-35 mg/kg 3 times/day (maximum: 2500 mg/day). If tablets are unable to be taken, use oral powder in small amount of water, milk, formula, or dietary supplements; do not use acidic food/juice or store for >6 hours.

Adults: 750 mg 3 times/day or 1250 mg twice daily with meals in combination with other antiretroviral therapies

Dosing adjustment in renal impairment: No pharmacokinetic data in patients with renal impairment. However, <2% of dose excreted in urine; no dose adjustment is needed.

Dosing adjustment in hepatic impairment: No dose adjustment necessary in mild impairment (Child-Pugh class A); not recommended in patients with moderate-to-severe impairment (Child-Pugh class B or C)

Dietary Considerations Should be taken as scheduled with a meal. Oral powder contains phenylalanine 11.2 mg/g.

Administration

Oral powder: Administer with a meal. Mix powder in a small amount of water, milk, formula, soy milk, soy formula, pudding, ice cream, or dietary supplement. Do not reconstitute the oral powder in its original container. Be sure entire contents is consumed to receive full dose. Do not use acidic food/juice to dilute due to bitter taste. Once mixed, solution should be used immediately, but may be stored for up to 6 hours if refrigerated.

Tablets: Administer with a meal. If unable to swallow tablets, may dissolve tablets in a small amount of water; mix cloudy liquid well and consume immediately. Rinse glass with water to ensure receiving full dose. Tablets may also be crushed and mixed with pudding.

Monitoring Parameters Liver function tests, viral load, CD4 count, triglycerides, cholesterol, blood glucose, CBC with differential

Additional Information A patient package insert (PPI), including a list of medications that should not be taken with nelfinavir, is available and should be dispensed with medication.

Dosage Forms Excipient information presented when available (limited, particularly for generics); consult specific product labeling.

Powder, oral:

Viracept®: 50 mg/g (144 g) [contains phenylalanine 11.2 mg/g]

Tablet:

Viracept®: 250 mg, 625 mg

- ◆ **Nembutal®** *see* PENTobarbital *on page 1170*
- ◆ **Nembutal® Sodium (Can)** *see* PENTobarbital *on page 1170*
- ◆ **Neo DM** *see* Chlorpheniramine, Phenylephrine, and Dextromethorphan *on page 311*
- ◆ **Neo-Fradin™** *see* Neomycin *on page 1050*
- ◆ **Neofrin™** *see* Phenylephrine *on page 1183*

Neomycin (nee oh MYE sin)

U.S. Brand Names Neo-Fradin™; Neo-Rx

Index Terms Neomycin Sulfate

Pharmacologic Category Ammonium Detoxicant; Antibiotic, Aminoglycoside; Antibiotic, Topical

Additional Appendix Information

Prevention of Wound Infection and Sepsis in Surgical Patients *on page 1738*

Use Orally to prepare GI tract for surgery; topically to treat minor skin infections; treatment of diarrhea caused by *E. coli*; adjunct in the treatment of hepatic encephalopathy; bladder irrigation; ocular infections

Pregnancy Risk Factor D

Pregnancy Considerations Neomycin crosses the placenta. Because neomycin has limited maternal absorption, the portion of an orally administered maternal dose available to cross the placenta is very low. Because of several reports of total irreversible bilateral congenital deafness in children whose mothers received streptomycin during pregnancy, the manufacturer classifies neomycin as pregnancy risk factor D. There have been no reports of fetal toxicity in humans from neomycin. No adequate and well-controlled studies have been conducted in pregnant women and it is not known whether neomycin can cause fetal harm. Although the manufacturer considers neomycin pregnancy risk factor D, neomycin-specific clinical data would suggest a pregnancy risk factor C.

Lactation Excretion in breast milk unknown

Contraindications Hypersensitivity to neomycin or any component of the formulation, or other aminoglycosides; intestinal obstruction

Warnings/Precautions [U.S. Boxed Warning]: May cause neurotoxicity, nephrotoxicity, and/or neuromuscular blockade and respiratory paralysis; usual risk factors include pre-existing renal impairment, concomitant neuro-/nephrotoxic medications, advanced age and dehydration. The drug's neurotoxicity can result in respiratory paralysis from neuromuscular blockade, especially when the drug is given soon after anesthesia or muscle relaxants. Use with caution in patients with renal impairment, pre-existing hearing impairment, neuromuscular disorders; neomycin is more toxic than other aminoglycosides when given parenterally; **do not administer parenterally**; topical neomycin is a contact sensitizer with sensitivity occurring in 5% to 15% of patients treated with the drug; symptoms include itching, reddening, edema, and failure to heal; **do not use as peritoneal lavage** due to significant systemic adsorption of the drug. Prolonged use may result in fungal or bacterial superinfection, including *C. difficile*-associated diarrhea (CDAD) and pseudomembranous colitis; CDAD has been observed >2 months postantibiotic treatment.

Adverse Reactions

Oral:

>10%: Gastrointestinal: Nausea, diarrhea, vomiting, irritation or soreness of the mouth or rectal area

<1% (Limited to important or life-threatening): Dyspnea, eosinophilia, nephrotoxicity, neurotoxicity, ototoxicity (auditory), ototoxicity (vestibular)

Topical: >10%: Dermatologic: Contact dermatitis

Drug Interactions

Avoid Concomitant Use

Avoid concomitant use of Neomycin with any of the following: Gallium Nitrate

Increased Effect/Toxicity

Neomycin may increase the levels/effects of: Bisphosphonate Derivatives; Botulinum Toxin Type A; Botulinum Toxin Type B; CARBOplatin; Colistimethate; CycloSPORINE; Gallium Nitrate; Neuromuscular-Blocking Agents

The levels/effects of Neomycin may be increased by: Amphotericin B; Capreomycin; CISplatin; Loop Diuretics; Nonsteroidal Anti-Inflammatory Agents; Vancomycin

Decreased Effect

Neomycin may decrease the levels/effects of: Cardiac Glycosides

The levels/effects of Neomycin may be decreased by: Penicillins

Mechanism of Action Interferes with bacterial protein synthesis by binding to 30S ribosomal subunits

Pharmacodynamics/Kinetics

Absorption: Oral, percutaneous: Poor (3%)

Distribution: 97% of an orally administered dose remains in the GI tract. Absorbed neomycin distributes to tissues and concentrates in the renal cortex. With repeated doses, accumulation also occurs in the inner ear.

V_d: 0.36 L/kg

Protein binding: 0% to 30%

Metabolism: Slightly hepatic

Half-life elimination (age and renal function dependent): 3 hours

Time to peak, serum: Oral: 1-4 hours

Excretion: Feces (97% of oral dose as unchanged drug); urine (30% to 50% of absorbed drug as unchanged drug)

Dosage

Children: Oral:

Preoperative intestinal antisepsis: 90 mg/kg/day divided every 4 hours for 2 days; or 25 mg/kg at 1 PM, 2 PM, and 11 PM on the day preceding surgery as an adjunct to mechanical cleansing of the intestine and in combination with erythromycin base

Hepatic encephalopathy: 50-100 mg/kg/day in divided doses every 6-8 hours or 2.5-7 g/m^2/day divided every 4-6 hours for 5-6 days not to exceed 12 g/day

Children and Adults: Topical: Topical solutions containing 0.1% to 1% neomycin have been used for irrigation

Adults: Oral:

Preoperative intestinal antisepsis: 1 g each hour for 4 doses then 1 g every 4 hours for 5 doses; or 1 g at 1 PM, 2 PM, and 11 PM on day preceding surgery as an adjunct to mechanical cleansing of the bowel and oral erythromycin; or 6 g/day divided every 4 hours for 2-3 days

Hepatic encephalopathy: 500-2000 mg every 6-8 hours or 4-12 g/day divided every 4-6 hours for 5-6 days

Chronic hepatic insufficiency: 4 g/day for an indefinite period

Monitoring Parameters Renal function tests, audiometry in symptomatic patients

Dosage Forms Excipient information presented when available (limited, particularly for generics); consult specific product labeling.

Powder, micronized, as sulfate [for prescription compounding] (Neo-Rx): (10 g, 100 g)

Solution, oral, as sulfate (Neo-Fradin™): 125 mg/5 mL (60 mL, 480 mL) [contains benzoic acid; cherry flavor]

Tablet, as sulfate: 500 mg

Neomycin and Polymyxin B

(nee oh MYE sin & pol i MIKS in bee)

U.S. Brand Names Neosporin® G.U. Irrigant

Canadian Brand Names Neosporin® Irrigating Solution

Index Terms Polymyxin B and Neomycin

Pharmacologic Category Antibiotic, Topical; Genitourinary Irrigant

Use Short-term as a continuous irrigant or rinse in the urinary bladder to prevent bacteriuria and gram-negative rod septicemia associated with the use of indwelling catheters; to help prevent infection in minor cuts, scrapes, and burns

Pregnancy Risk Factor C/D (for G.U. irrigant)

Dosage Children and Adults: Bladder irrigation: **Not for injection**; add 1 mL irrigant to 1 L isotonic saline solution and connect container to the inflow of lumen of 3-way catheter. Continuous irrigant or rinse in the urinary bladder for up to a maximum of 10 days with administration rate adjusted to patient's urine output; usually no more than 1 L of irrigant is used per day.

Additional Information Complete prescribing information for this medication should be consulted for additional detail.

Dosage Forms Excipient information presented when available (limited, particularly for generics); consult specific product labeling.

Solution, irrigation: Neomycin 40 mg and polymyxin B 200,000 units per mL (1 mL, 20 mL)

Neosporin® G.U. Irrigant: Neomycin 40 mg and polymyxin B 200,000 units per mL (1 mL, 20 mL)

◆ **Neomycin, Bacitracin, and Polymyxin B** *see* Bacitracin, Neomycin, and Polymyxin B *on page 171*

◆ **Neomycin, Bacitracin, Polymyxin B, and Hydrocortisone** *see* Bacitracin, Neomycin, Polymyxin B, and Hydrocortisone *on page 172*

Neomycin, Colistin, Hydrocortisone, and Thonzonium

(nee oh MYE sin, koe LIS tin, hye droe KOR ti sone, & thon ZOE nee um)

U.S. Brand Names Coly-Mycin® S; Cortisporin®-TC

Index Terms Colistin, Neomycin, Hydrocortisone, and Thonzonium; Hydrocortisone, Neomycin, Colistin, and Thonzonium; Thonzonium, Neomycin, Colistin, and Hydrocortisone

Pharmacologic Category Antibiotic/Corticosteroid, Otic

Use Treatment of superficial and susceptible bacterial infections of the external auditory canal; for treatment of susceptible bacterial infections of mastoidectomy and fenestration cavities

Dosage Otic:

Calibrated dropper:

Children: 4 drops in affected ear 3-4 times/day

Adults: 5 drops in affected ear 3-4 times/day

Dropper bottle:

Children: 3 drops in affected ear 3-4 times/day

Adults: 4 drops in affected ear 3-4 times/day

Note: Alternatively, a cotton wick may be inserted in the ear canal and saturated with suspension every 4 hours; wick should be replaced at least every 24 hours

Additional Information Complete prescribing information for this medication should be consulted for additional detail.

Dosage Forms Excipient information presented when available (limited, particularly for generics); consult specific product labeling.

Suspension, otic [drops]:

Coly-Mycin® S: Neomycin 0.33%, colistin 0.3%, hydrocortisone acetate 1%, and thonzonium bromide 0.05% (5 mL) [contains thimerosal; packaged with dropper]

Cortisporin®-TC: Neomycin 0.33%, colistin 0.3%, hydrocortisone acetate 1%, and thonzonium bromide 0.05% (10 mL) [contains thimerosal; packaged with dropper]

Neomycin, Polymyxin B, and Dexamethasone

(nee oh MYE sin, pol i MIKS in bee, & deks a METH a sone)

U.S. Brand Names AK-Trol® [DSC]; Maxitrol®; Poly-Dex™

Canadian Brand Names Dioptrol®; Maxitrol®

Index Terms Dexamethasone, Neomycin, and Polymyxin B; Polymyxin B, Neomycin, and Dexamethasone

Pharmacologic Category Antibiotic/Corticosteroid, Ophthalmic

Use Steroid-responsive inflammatory ocular conditions in which a corticosteroid is indicated and where bacterial infection or a risk of bacterial infection exists

Pregnancy Risk Factor C

Medication Safety Issues

Sound-alike/look-alike issues:

AK-Trol® may be confused with AKTob®

Dosage Children and Adults: Ophthalmic:

Ointment: Place a small amount (~1/2") in the affected eye 3-4 times/day or apply at bedtime as an adjunct with drops

Suspension: Instill 1-2 drops into affected eye(s) every 3-4 hours; in severe disease, drops may be used hourly and tapered to discontinuation

Additional Information Complete prescribing information for this medication should be consulted for additional detail.

Dosage Forms Excipient information presented when available (limited, particularly for generics); consult specific product labeling. [DSC] = Discontinued product

Ointment, ophthalmic (Maxitrol®, Poly-Dex™): Neomycin 3.5 mg, polymyxin B sulfate 10,000 units, and dexamethasone 0.1% per g (3.5 g)

Suspension, ophthalmic (AK-Trol® [DSC], Maxitrol®, Poly-Dex™): Neomycin 3.5 mg, polymyxin B sulfate 10,000 units, and dexamethasone 0.1% per mL (5 mL) [contains benzalkonium chloride]

Neomycin, Polymyxin B, and Gramicidin

(nee oh MYE sin, pol i MIKS in bee, & gram i SYE din)

U.S. Brand Names Neosporin® Ophthalmic Solution

Canadian Brand Names Neosporin®; Optimyxin Plus®

Index Terms Gramicidin, Neomycin, and Polymyxin B; Polymyxin B, Neomycin, and Gramicidin

Pharmacologic Category Antibiotic, Ophthalmic

Use Treatment of superficial ocular infection

Pregnancy Risk Factor C

Dosage Children and Adults: Ophthalmic: Instill 1-2 drops 4-6 times/day or more frequently as required for severe infections

Additional Information Complete prescribing information for this medication should be consulted for additional detail.

Dosage Forms Excipient information presented when available (limited, particularly for generics); consult specific product labeling.

Solution, ophthalmic: Neomycin 1.75 mg, polymyxin B 10,000 units, and gramicidin 0.025 mg per 1 mL (10 mL)

Neosporin® Ophthalmic Solution: Neomycin 1.75 mg, polymyxin B 10,000 units, and gramicidin 0.025 mg per 1 mL (10 mL)

Neomycin, Polymyxin B, and Hydrocortisone

(nee oh MYE sin, pol i MIKS in bee, & hye droe KOR ti sone)

U.S. Brand Names Cortisporin® Cream; Cortisporin® Ophthalmic [DSC]; Cortisporin® Otic; PediOtic®

Canadian Brand Names Cortimyxin®; Cortisporin® Otic

Index Terms Hydrocortisone, Neomycin, and Polymyxin B; Polymyxin B, Neomycin, and Hydrocortisone

Pharmacologic Category Antibiotic, Ophthalmic; Antibiotic, Otic; Antibiotic, Topical; Corticosteroid, Ophthalmic; Corticosteroid, Otic; Corticosteroid, Topical

Use Steroid-responsive inflammatory condition for which a corticosteroid is indicated and where bacterial infection or a risk of bacterial infection exists

Pregnancy Risk Factor C

Dosage Note: Duration of use of ophthalmic and otic preparations should be limited to 10 days unless otherwise directed by the healthcare provider.

Ophthalmic:

Children (unlabeled use): Instill 1-2 drops 2-4 times/day, or more frequently as required for severe infections

Adults: Instill 1-2 drops 2-4 times/day, or more frequently as required for severe infections

Otic: Otic solution is used **only** for bacterial infections of external auditory canal (eg, swimmer's ear).

Children 6 months to 2 years (unlabeled use): Instill 3 drops into affected ear 3-4 times/day

Children ≥2 years: Instill 3 drops into affected ear 3-4 times/day

Adults: Instill 4 drops into affected ear 3-4 times/day; otic suspension is the preferred otic preparation

Topical:

Children (unlabeled use): Apply a thin layer 1-4 times/day. Therapy should be discontinued when control is achieved; if no improvement is seen, reassessment of diagnosis may be necessary.

Adults: Apply a thin layer 1-4 times/day. Therapy should be discontinued when control is achieved; if no improvement is seen, reassessment of diagnosis may be necessary.

Additional Information Complete prescribing information for this medication should be consulted for additional detail.

Dosage Forms Excipient information presented when available (limited, particularly for generics); consult specific product labeling.

Cream, topical (Cortisporin®): Neomycin 3.5 mg, polymyxin B 10,000 units, and hydrocortisone acetate 5 mg per g (7.5 g)

Solution, otic (Cortisporin®): Neomycin 3.5 mg, polymyxin B 10,000 units, and hydrocortisone 10 mg per mL (10 mL) [contains potassium metabisulfite]

Suspension, ophthalmic (Cortisporin® [DSC]): Neomycin 3.5 mg, polymyxin B 10,000 units, and hydrocortisone 10 mg per mL (7.5 mL) [contains thimerosal]

Suspension, otic: Neomycin 3.5 mg, polymyxin B 10,000 units, and hydrocortisone 10 mg per mL (10 mL)

Cortisporin®: Neomycin 3.5 mg, polymyxin B 10,000 units, and hydrocortisone 10 mg per mL (10 mL) [contains thimerosal]

PediOtic®: Neomycin 3.5 mg, polymyxin B 10,000 units, and hydrocortisone 10 mg per mL (7.5 mL) [contains thimerosal]

Neomycin, Polymyxin B, and Prednisolone

(nee oh MYE sin, pol i MIKS in bee, & pred NIS oh lone)

U.S. Brand Names Poly-Pred®

Index Terms Polymyxin B, Neomycin, and Prednisolone; Prednisolone, Neomycin, and Polymyxin B

Pharmacologic Category Antibiotic/Corticosteroid, Ophthalmic

Use Steroid-responsive inflammatory ocular condition in which bacterial infection or a risk of bacterial ocular infection exists

Pregnancy Risk Factor C

Dosage Children and Adults: Ophthalmic: Instill 1-2 drops every 3-4 hours; acute infections may require every 30-minute instillation initially with frequency of administration reduced as the infection is brought under control. To treat the lids: Instill 1-2 drops every 3-4 hours, close the eye and rub the excess on the lids and lid margins.

Additional Information Complete prescribing information for this medication should be consulted for additional detail.

Dosage Forms Excipient information presented when available (limited, particularly for generics); consult specific product labeling.

Suspension, ophthalmic: Neomycin 0.35%, polymyxin B 10,000 units per mL, and prednisolone acetate 0.5% (5 mL; 10 mL [DSC]) [contains thimerosal]

- ◆ **Neomycin Sulfate** *see* Neomycin *on page* 1050
- ◆ **NeoProfen®** *see* Ibuprofen *on page* 760
- ◆ **Neoral®** *see* CycloSPORINE *on page* 379
- ◆ **Neo-Rx** *see* Neomycin *on page* 1050
- ◆ **Neosar** *see* Cyclophosphamide *on page* 376
- ◆ **Neosporin® (Can)** *see* Neomycin, Polymyxin B, and Gramicidin *on page* 1052
- ◆ **Neosporin® AF [OTC]** *see* Miconazole *on page* 989
- ◆ **Neosporin® G.U. Irrigant** *see* Neomycin and Polymyxin B *on page* 1051
- ◆ **Neosporin® Irrigating Solution (Can)** *see* Neomycin and Polymyxin B *on page* 1051
- ◆ **Neosporin® Neo To Go® [OTC]** *see* Bacitracin, Neomycin, and Polymyxin B *on page* 171
- ◆ **Neosporin® Ophthalmic Ointment [DSC]** *see* Bacitracin, Neomycin, and Polymyxin B *on page* 171
- ◆ **Neosporin® Ophthalmic Ointment (Can)** *see* Bacitracin, Neomycin, and Polymyxin B *on page* 171
- ◆ **Neosporin® Ophthalmic Solution** *see* Neomycin, Polymyxin B, and Gramicidin *on page* 1052
- ◆ **Neosporin® Topical [OTC]** *see* Bacitracin, Neomycin, and Polymyxin B *on page* 171

Neostigmine (nee oh STIG meen)

U.S. Brand Names Prostigmin®

Canadian Brand Names Prostigmin®

Index Terms Neostigmine Bromide; Neostigmine Methylsulfate

Pharmacologic Category Acetylcholinesterase Inhibitor

Use Diagnosis and treatment of myasthenia gravis; prevention and treatment of postoperative bladder distention and urinary retention; reversal of the effects of nondepolarizing neuromuscular-blocking agents after surgery

Pregnancy Risk Factor C

Lactation Excretion in breast milk unknown/not recommended

Medication Safety Issues

Sound-alike/look-alike issues:

Prostigmin® may be confused with physostigmine

Contraindications Hypersensitivity to neostigmine, bromides, or any component of the formulation; GI or GU obstruction

Warnings/Precautions Does **not** antagonize and may prolong the Phase I block of depolarizing muscle relaxants (eg, succinylcholine). Use with caution in patients with epilepsy, asthma, bradycardia, hyperthyroidism, cardiac arrhythmias, or peptic ulcer; not generally recommended for use in patients with vagotonia. Adequate facilities should be available for cardiopulmonary resuscitation when testing and adjusting dose for myasthenia gravis. Have atropine and epinephrine ready to treat hypersensitivity reactions. Overdosage may result in cholinergic crisis, this must be distinguished from myasthenic crisis. Anticholinesterase insensitivity can develop for brief or prolonged periods.

Adverse Reactions Frequency not defined.

Cardiovascular: Arrhythmias (especially bradycardia), hypotension, tachycardia, AV block, nodal rhythm, nonspecific ECG changes, cardiac arrest, syncope, flushing

Central nervous system: Convulsions, dysarthria, dysphonia, dizziness, loss of consciousness, drowsiness, headache

Dermatologic: Skin rash, thrombophlebitis (I.V.), urticaria

Gastrointestinal: Hyperperistalsis, nausea, vomiting, salivation, diarrhea, stomach cramps, dysphagia, flatulence

Genitourinary: Urinary urgency

Neuromuscular & skeletal: Weakness, fasciculations, muscle cramps, spasms, arthralgia

Ocular: Small pupils, lacrimation

Respiratory: Increased bronchial secretions, laryngospasm, bronchiolar constriction, respiratory muscle paralysis, dyspnea, respiratory depression, respiratory arrest, bronchospasm

Miscellaneous: Diaphoresis (increased), anaphylaxis, allergic reactions

Drug Interactions

Avoid Concomitant Use There are no known interactions where it is recommended to avoid concomitant use.

Increased Effect/Toxicity

Neostigmine may increase the levels/effects of: Beta-Blockers; Cholinergic Agonists; Succinylcholine

The levels/effects of Neostigmine may be increased by: Corticosteroids (Systemic); Ginkgo Biloba

Decreased Effect

Neostigmine may decrease the levels/effects of: Neuromuscular-Blocking Agents (Nondepolarizing)

Mechanism of Action Inhibits destruction of acetylcholine by acetylcholinesterase which facilitates transmission of impulses across myoneural junction

Pharmacodynamics/Kinetics

Onset of action: I.M.: 20-30 minutes; I.V.: 1-20 minutes

Duration: I.M.: 2.5-4 hours; I.V.: 1-2 hours

Absorption: Oral: Poor, <2%

Metabolism: Hepatic

Half-life elimination: Normal renal function: 0.5-2.1 hours; End-stage renal disease: Prolonged

Excretion: Urine (50% as unchanged drug)

Dosage

Myasthenia gravis: Diagnosis: I.M.:

Children: 0.04 mg/kg as a single dose

Adults: 0.02 mg/kg as a single dose

Myasthenia gravis: Treatment:

Children:

Oral: 2 mg/kg/day divided every 3-4 hours

I.M., I.V., SubQ: 0.01-0.04 mg/kg every 2-4 hours

Adults:

Oral: 15 mg/dose every 3-4 hours up to 375 mg/day maximum; interval between doses must be individualized to maximal response

I.M., I.V., SubQ: 0.5-2.5 mg every 1-3 hours up to 10 mg/24 hours maximum

Reversal of nondepolarizing neuromuscular blockade after surgery in conjunction with atropine (must administer atropine several minutes prior to neostigmine): I.V.:

Infants: 0.025-0.1 mg/kg/dose

Children: 0.025-0.08 mg/kg/dose

Adults: 0.5-2.5 mg; total dose not to exceed 5 mg

Bladder atony: Adults: I.M., SubQ:

Prevention: 0.25 mg every 4-6 hours for 2-3 days

Treatment: 0.5-1 mg every 3 hours for 5 doses after bladder has emptied

Dosing adjustment in renal impairment:

Cl_{cr} 10-50 mL/minute: Administer 50% of normal dose

Cl_{cr} <10 mL/minute: Administer 25% of normal dose

Administration May be administered undiluted by slow I.V. injection over several minutes

Additional Information In the diagnosis of myasthenia gravis, all anticholinesterase medications should be discontinued for at least 8 hours before administering neostigmine.

Dosage Forms Excipient information presented when available (limited, particularly for generics); consult specific product labeling.

Injection, solution, as methylsulfate: 0.5 mg/mL (1 mL, 10 mL); 1 mg/mL (10 mL)

Tablet, as bromide: 15 mg

- ◆ **Neostigmine Bromide** *see* Neostigmine *on page 1053*
- ◆ **Neostigmine Methylsulfate** *see* Neostigmine *on page 1053*
- ◆ **NeoStrata® AHA [OTC]** *see* Hydroquinone *on page 749*
- ◆ **NeoStrata® HQ (Can)** *see* Hydroquinone *on page 749*
- ◆ **Neo-Synephrine® (Can)** *see* Phenylephrine *on page 1183*
- ◆ **Neo-Synephrine® Extra Strength [OTC]** *see* Phenylephrine *on page 1183*
- ◆ **Neo-Synephrine® Injection** *see* Phenylephrine *on page 1183*
- ◆ **Neo-Synephrine® Mild [OTC]** *see* Phenylephrine *on page 1183*
- ◆ **Neo-Synephrine® Regular Strength [OTC]** *see* Phenylephrine *on page 1183*

Nepafenac (ne pa FEN ak)

U.S. Brand Names Nevanac™

Canadian Brand Names Nevanac™

Pharmacologic Category Nonsteroidal Anti-inflammatory Drug (NSAID), Ophthalmic

Use Treatment of pain and inflammation associated with cataract surgery

Pregnancy Risk Factor C/D (3rd trimester)

Dosage Ophthalmic: Children ≥10 years and Adults: Instill 1 drop into affected eye(s) 3 times/day, beginning 1 day prior to surgery, the day of surgery, and through the first 2 weeks of the postoperative period

Additional Information Complete prescribing information for this medication should be consulted for additional detail.

Dosage Forms Excipient information presented when available (limited, particularly for generics); consult specific product labeling.

Suspension, ophthalmic: 0.1% (3 mL) [contains benzalkonium chloride]

- ◆ **Nephro-Calci® [OTC]** *see* Calcium Carbonate *on page 238*
- ◆ **Nephro-Fer® [OTC]** *see* Ferrous Fumarate *on page 616*
- ◆ **Nerve Agent Antidote Kit** *see* Atropine and Pralidoxime *on page 159*
- ◆ **Nesacaine®** *see* Chloroprocaine *on page 306*
- ◆ **Nesacaine®-CE (Can)** *see* Chloroprocaine *on page 306*
- ◆ **Nesacaine®-MPF** *see* Chloroprocaine *on page 306*

Nesiritide (ni SIR i tide)

U.S. Brand Names Natrecor®

Canadian Brand Names Natrecor®

Index Terms B-type Natriuretic Peptide (Human); hBNP; Natriuretic Peptide

Pharmacologic Category Natriuretic Peptide, B-Type, Human; Vasodilator

Additional Appendix Information

Hemodynamic Support, Intravenous *on page 1657*

Use Treatment of acutely decompensated congestive heart failure (CHF) in patients with dyspnea at rest or with minimal activity

Pregnancy Risk Factor C

Lactation Excretion in breast milk unknown/use caution

Medication Safety Issues

High alert medication: The Institute for Safe Medication Practices (ISMP) includes this medication among its list of drugs which have a heightened risk of causing significant patient harm when used in error.

International issues:

Natrecor® may be confused with Nitrocor® which is a brand name for nitroglycerin in Chile and Italy

Contraindications Hypersensitivity to natriuretic peptide or any component of the formulation; cardiogenic shock (when used as primary therapy); hypotension (systolic blood pressure <90 mm Hg)

Warnings/Precautions May cause hypotension; administer in clinical situations when blood pressure may be closely monitored. Use caution in patients systolic blood pressure <100 mm Hg (contraindicated if <90 mm Hg); more likely to experience hypotension. Effects may be additive with other agents capable of causing hypotension. Hypotensive effects may last for several hours.

Should not be used in patients with low cardiac filling pressures, or in patients with conditions which depend on venous return including significant valvular stenosis, restrictive or obstructive cardiomyopathy, constrictive pericarditis, and pericardial tamponade. May be associated with development of azotemia; use caution in patients with renal impairment or in patients where renal perfusion is dependent on renin-angiotensin-aldosterone system; avoid initiation at doses higher than recommended.

Monitor for allergic or anaphylactic reactions. Use caution with prolonged infusions; limited experience for infusions >48 hours. Safety and efficacy in pediatric patients have not been established.

Adverse Reactions Note: Frequencies cited below were recorded in VMAC trial at dosages similar to approved labeling. Higher frequencies have been observed in trials using higher dosages of nesiritide. The percentages marked with an asterisk (*) indicate frequency less than or equal to placebo or other standard therapy.

>10%:

Cardiovascular: Hypotension (total: 11%; symptomatic 4% at recommended dose, up to 17% at higher doses)

Renal: Increased serum creatinine (28% with >0.5 mg/dL increase over baseline)

1% to 10%:
Cardiovascular: Ventricular tachycardia (3%)*, ventricular extrasystoles (3%)*, angina (2%)*, bradycardia (1%), tachycardia, atrial fibrillation, AV node conduction abnormalities
Central nervous system: Headache (8%)*, dizziness (3%)*, insomnia (2%)*, anxiety (3%), fever, confusion, paresthesia, somnolence, tremor
Dermatologic: Pruritus, rash
Gastrointestinal: Nausea (4%)*, abdominal pain (1%)*, vomiting (1%)*
Hematologic: Anemia
Local: Injection site reaction
Neuromuscular & skeletal: Back pain (4%), leg cramps
Ocular: Amblyopia
Respiratory: Cough (increased), hemoptysis, apnea
Miscellaneous: Increased diaphoresis
Postmarketing and/or case reports: Hypersensitivity reactions (rare)

Drug Interactions

Avoid Concomitant Use There are no known interactions where it is recommended to avoid concomitant use.

Increased Effect/Toxicity

Nesiritide may increase the levels/effects of: Amifostine; RiTUXimab

The levels/effects of Nesiritide may be increased by: Diazoxide; Herbs (Hypotensive Properties); Prostacyclin Analogues

Decreased Effect

The levels/effects of Nesiritide may be decreased by: Herbs (Hypertensive Properties); Methylphenidate; Yohimbine

Ethanol/Nutrition/Herb Interactions Herb/Nutraceutical: Avoid bayberry, blue cohosh, cayenne, ephedra, ginger, ginseng (American), kola, and licorice (may increase blood pressure). Avoid black cohosh, California poppy, coleus, golden seal, hawthorn, mistletoe, periwinkle, quinine, and shepherd's purse (may enhance decreased blood pressure).

Stability Vials may be stored below 25°C (77°F); do not freeze. Protect from light. Following reconstitution, vials are stable at 2°C to 25°C (36°F to 77°F) for up to 24 hours. Use reconstituted solution within 24 hours.

Reconstitute 1.5 mg vial with 5 mL of diluent removed from a prefilled 250 mL plastic I.V. bag (compatible with D_5W, $D_5{}^1/_2NS$, $D_5{}^1/_4NS$, NS). Do not shake vial to dissolve (roll gently). Withdraw entire contents of vial and add to 250 mL I.V. bag. Invert several times to mix. Resultant concentration of solution is ~6 mcg/mL.

Mechanism of Action Binds to guanylate cyclase receptor on vascular smooth muscle and endothelial cells, increasing intracellular cyclic GMP, resulting in smooth muscle cell relaxation. Has been shown to produce dose-dependent reductions in pulmonary capillary wedge pressure (PCWP) and systemic arterial pressure.

Pharmacodynamics/Kinetics

Onset of action: 15 minutes (60% of 3-hour effect achieved)
Duration: >60 minutes (up to several hours) for systolic blood pressure; hemodynamic effects persist longer than serum half-life would predict
Distribution: V_{ss}: 0.19 L/kg
Metabolism: Proteolytic cleavage by vascular endopeptidases and proteolysis following receptor binding and cellular internalization
Half-life elimination: Initial (distribution) 2 minutes; Terminal: 18 minutes
Time to peak: 1 hour
Excretion: Urine

Dosage Adults: I.V.: Initial: 2 mcg/kg (bolus); followed by continuous infusion at 0.01 mcg/kg/minute. **Note:** Should not be initiated at a dosage higher than initial recommended dose. There is limited experience with increasing the dose >0.01 mcg/kg/minute; in one trial, a limited number of patients received higher doses that were increased no faster than every 3 hours by 0.005 mcg/kg/minute (preceded by a bolus of 1 mcg/kg), up to a maximum of 0.03 mcg/kg/minute. Increases beyond the initial infusion rate should be limited to selected patients and accompanied by close hemodynamic and renal function monitoring.

Patients experiencing hypotension during the infusion: Infusion dose should be reduced or discontinued. Other measures to support blood pressure should be initiated (eg, I.V. fluids, Trendelenburg position). May attempt to restart at a lower dose (reduce previous infusion dose by 30% and omit bolus).

Dosage adjustment in renal impairment: No adjustment required, but use cautiously in patients with renal impairment or those patients who rely on the renin-angiotensin-aldosterone system for renal perfusion. Monitor renal function closely.

Dosage adjustment in hepatic impairment: No dosage adjustment recommended.

Administration Do not administer through a heparin-coated catheter (concurrent administration of heparin via a separate catheter is acceptable, per manufacturer).

Prime I.V. tubing with 5 mL of infusion prior to connection with vascular access port and prior to administering bolus or starting the infusion. Withdraw bolus from the prepared infusion bag and administer over 60 seconds. Begin infusion immediately following administration of the bolus.

Monitoring Parameters Blood pressure, hemodynamic responses (PCWP, RAP, CI), BUN, creatinine; urine output

Additional Information The duration of symptomatic improvement with nesiritide following discontinuation of the infusion has been limited (generally lasting several days). Atrial natriuretic peptide, which is related to nesiritide, has been associated with increased vascular permeability. This has not been observed in clinical trials with nesiritide, but patients should be monitored for this effect.

Dosage Forms Excipient information presented when available (limited, particularly for generics); consult specific product labeling.

Injection, powder for reconstitution:
Natrecor®: 1.5 mg

- **Neulasta®** *see* Pegfilgrastim *on page* *1152*
- **Neumega®** *see* Oprelvekin *on page* *1106*
- **Neupogen®** *see* Filgrastim *on page* *620*
- **Neupro® [DSC]** *see* Rotigotine *on page* *1346*
- **Neurontin®** *see* Gabapentin *on page* *678*
- **Neut®** *see* Sodium Bicarbonate *on page* *1380*
- **NeutraCare®** *see* Fluoride *on page* *635*
- **NeutraGard® [OTC]** *see* Fluoride *on page* *635*
- **NeutraGard® Advanced** *see* Fluoride *on page* *635*
- **NeutraGard® Plus** *see* Fluoride *on page* *635*
- **Neutra-Phos® [OTC] [DSC]** *see* Potassium Phosphate and Sodium Phosphate *on page* *1222*
- **Neutra-Phos®-K [OTC] [DSC]** *see* Potassium Phosphate *on page* *1220*
- **NeuTrexin® [DSC]** *see* Trimetrexate *on page* *1520*
- **Nevanac™** *see* Nepafenac *on page* *1054*

Nevirapine (ne VYE ra peen)

U.S. Brand Names Viramune®
Canadian Brand Names Viramune®
Index Terms NVP

Pharmacologic Category Antiretroviral Agent, Reverse Transcriptase Inhibitor (Non-nucleoside)

Additional Appendix Information

Antiretroviral Therapy for HIV Infection: Adults and Adolescents *on page 1758*

Management of Healthcare Worker Exposures to HBV, HCV, and HIV *on page 1719*

Perinatal HIV Guidelines *on page 1730*

Use In combination therapy with other antiretroviral agents for the treatment of HIV-1

Restrictions An FDA-approved medication guide must be distributed when dispensing an outpatient prescription (new or refill) where this medication is to be used without direct supervision of a healthcare provider. Medication guides are available at http://www.fda.gov/cder/Offices/ODS/medication_guides.htm.

Pregnancy Risk Factor B

Pregnancy Considerations Nevirapine crosses the placenta. No increased risk of overall birth defects has been observed following 1st trimester exposure according to data collected by the antiretroviral pregnancy registry. Pharmacokinetics are not altered during pregnancy and dose adjustment is not needed. The Perinatal HIV Guidelines Working Group recommends nevirapine as the NNRTI for use during pregnancy. When used to prevent perinatal transmission in women who do not need therapy for their own health, use is not recommended if $CD4^+$ lymphocyte counts >250/mm^3 (monitor for liver toxicity during first 18 weeks of therapy). It may also be used in combination with zidovudine in HIV-infected women who are in labor, but have had no prior antiretroviral therapy, in order to reduce the maternal-fetal transmission of HIV; consider adding intrapartum and postpartum zidovudine and lamivudine to reduce nevirapine resistance. Health professionals are encouraged to contact the antiretroviral pregnancy registry to monitor outcomes of pregnant women exposed to antiretroviral medications (1-800-258-4263 or www.APRegistry.com).

Lactation Enters breast milk/contraindicated

Medication Safety Issues

Sound-alike/look-alike issues:

Nevirapine may be confused with nelfinavir

Viramune® may be confused with Viracept®

Contraindications Hypersensitivity to nevirapine or any component of the formulation; moderate-to-severe hepatic impairment (Child-Pugh class B or C)

Warnings/Precautions [U.S. Boxed Warning]: Severe hepatotoxic reactions may occur (fulminant and cholestatic hepatitis, hepatic necrosis) and, in some cases, have resulted in hepatic failure and death. The greatest risk of these reactions is within the initial 6 weeks of treatment. Patients with a history of chronic hepatitis (B or C) or increased baseline transaminase levels may be at increased risk of hepatotoxic reactions. Female gender and patients with increased $CD4^+$-cell counts may be at substantially greater risk of hepatic events (often associated with rash). Therapy should not be started with elevated $CD4^+$-cell counts unless the benefit of therapy outweighs the risk of serious hepatotoxicity (females: $CD4^+$-cell counts >250 cells/mm^3; males: $CD4^+$-cell counts >400 cells/mm^3). **[U.S. Boxed Warning]: Severe life-threatening skin reactions (eg, Stevens-Johnson syndrome, toxic epidermal necrolysis, hypersensitivity reactions with rash and organ dysfunction) have occurred; intensive monitoring is required during the initial 18 weeks of therapy to detect potentially life-threatening dermatologic, hypersensitivity, and hepatic reactions.** Nevirapine must be initiated with a 14-day lead-in dosing period to decrease the incidence of adverse effects. The lead-in dosing can be extended up to 28 days if necessary, but an alternative regimen is necessary if >28 days is required. If a severe dermatologic or hypersensitivity reaction occurs, or if signs and symptoms of hepatitis occur, nevirapine should be permanently discontinued. These events may include a severe rash, or a rash associated with fever, blisters, oral lesions, conjunctivitis, facial edema, muscle or joint aches, transaminase elevations, general malaise, hepatitis, eosinophilia, granulocytopenia, lymphadenopathy, or renal dysfunction.

May cause redistribution of fat (eg, buffalo hump, peripheral wasting with increased abdominal girth, cushingoid appearance). Patients may develop immune reconstitution syndrome resulting in the occurrence of an inflammatory response to an indolent or residual opportunistic infection; further evaluation and treatment may be required. Rhabdomyolysis has been observed in conjunction with skin and/or hepatic adverse events during postmarketing surveillance. Termination of therapy is warranted with evidence of severe skin or liver toxicity.

Use with caution in patients taking strong CYP3A4 inhibitors, moderate or strong CYP3A4 inducers and major CYP3A4 substrates (see Drug Interactions); consider alternative agents that avoid or lessen the potential for CYP-mediated interactions. Consider alteration of antiretroviral therapies if disease progression occurs while patients are receiving nevirapine.

Adverse Reactions Note: Potentially life-threatening nevirapine-associated adverse effects may present with the following symptoms: Abrupt onset of flu-like symptoms, abdominal pain, jaundice, or fever with or without rash; may progress to hepatic failure with encephalopathy. Skin rash is present in ~50% of cases.

Percentages of adverse effects vary by clinical trial:

>10%:

Dermatologic: Rash (grade 1/2: 13%; grade 3/4: 1.5%) is the most common toxicity; occurs most frequently within the first 6 weeks of therapy; women may be at higher risk than men

Hepatic: ALT >250 units/L (5% to 14%); symptomatic hepatic events (4%, range: up to 11%) are more common in women, women with $CD4^+$ cell counts >250 cells/mm^3, and men with $CD4^+$ cell counts >400 cells/mm^3

1% to 10%:

Central nervous system: Headache (1% to 4%), fatigue (up to 5%)

Gastrointestinal: Nausea (<1% to 9%), abdominal pain (<1% to 2%), diarrhea (up to 2%)

Hepatic: AST >250 units/L (4% to 8%); coinfection with hepatitis B or C and/or increased liver function tests at the beginning of therapy are associated with a greater risk of asymptomatic transaminase elevations (ALT or AST >5 times ULN: 6%, range: up to 9%) or symptomatic events occurring ≥6 weeks after beginning treatment

Postmarketing and/or case reports: Allergic reactions, anaphylaxis, anemia, angioedema, arthralgia, blisters, bullous eruptions, conjunctivitis, eosinophilia, facial edema, fever, fulminant and cholestatic hepatitis, granulocytopenia, hepatic failure, hepatic necrosis, hypersensitivity syndrome, jaundice, lymphadenopathy, malaise, neutropenia, oral lesions, paresthesia, redistribution/accumulation of body fat, renal dysfunction, rhabdomyolysis, Stevens-Johnson syndrome, somnolence, toxic epidermal necrolysis, ulcerative stomatitis, urticaria, vomiting

Drug Interactions

Metabolism/Transport Effects Substrate of CYP2B6 (minor), 2D6 (minor), 3A4 (major); **Inhibits** CYP1A2 (weak), 2D6 (weak), 3A4 (weak); **Induces** CYP2B6 (strong), 3A4 (strong)

Avoid Concomitant Use

Avoid concomitant use of Nevirapine with any of the following: Etravirine; Nilotinib; Nisoldipine; Ranolazine

Increased Effect/Toxicity

Nevirapine may increase the levels/effects of: Etravirine; Rifabutin

The levels/effects of Nevirapine may be increased by: Voriconazole

Decreased Effect

Nevirapine may decrease the levels/effects of: Caspofungin; CYP2B6 Substrates; CYP3A4 Substrates; Etravirine; Maraviroc; Methadone; Nilotinib; Nisoldipine; Protease Inhibitors; Ranolazine; Rifabutin; Sorafenib; Voriconazole

The levels/effects of Nevirapine may be decreased by: CYP3A4 Inducers (Strong); Deferasirox; Herbs (CYP3A4 Inducers); Rifabutin; Rifampin

Ethanol/Nutrition/Herb Interactions Herb/Nutraceutical: Nevirapine serum concentration may be decreased by St John's wort; avoid concurrent use.

Stability Store at 25°C (77°F); excursion permitted to 15°C to 30°C (59°F to 86°F).

Mechanism of Action As a non-nucleoside reverse transcriptase inhibitor, nevirapine has activity against HIV-1 by binding to reverse transcriptase. It consequently blocks the RNA-dependent and DNA-dependent DNA polymerase activities including HIV-1 replication. It does not require intracellular phosphorylation for antiviral activity.

Pharmacodynamics/Kinetics

Absorption: >90%

Distribution: Widely; V_d: 1.2-1.4 L/kg; CSF penetration approximates 40% to 50% of plasma

Protein binding, plasma: 60%

Metabolism: Extensively hepatic via CYP3A4 (hydroxylation to inactive compounds); may undergo enterohepatic recycling

Half-life elimination: Decreases over 2- to 4-week time with chronic dosing due to autoinduction (ie, half-life = 45 hours initially and decreases to 25-30 hours)

Time to peak, serum: 2-4 hours

Excretion: Urine (~81%, primarily as metabolites, <3% as unchanged drug); feces (~10%)

Dosage Oral:

HIV infection:

Infants ≥15 days and Children: 150 mg/m^2 once daily for first 14 days (maximum dose: 200 mg/day); increase dose to 150 mg/m^2 twice daily if no rash or untoward effects (maximum dose: ≤400 mg/day). Children ≤8 years of age: May require 200 mg/m^2 twice daily.

Adolescents and Adults: Initial: 200 mg once daily for first 14 days; maintenance: 200 mg twice daily (in combination with an additional antiretroviral agent) if there is no rash or other adverse event

Note: If patient experiences a rash during the 14-day lead-in period, dose should not be increased until the rash has resolved. Lead-in period should not exceed 28 days; alternative treatment should be considered at that point. Discontinue if severe rash, rash with constitutional symptoms, or rash with elevated hepatic transaminases is noted. Use of prednisone to prevent nevirapine-associated rash is not recommended. Permanently discontinue if symptomatic hepatic events occur. If therapy is interrupted for >7 days, restart with initial dose for 14 days.

Prevention of maternal-fetal HIV transmission (AIDSinfo guidelines): Note: Nevirapine is used in combination with zidovudine (and possibly lamivudine) in select situations (eg, infants born to mothers with suboptimal viral suppression at delivery, infants born to mothers with only intrapartum therapy or no therapy, or infants born to mothers with known antiretroviral drug-resistant virus)

Mother: 200 mg as a single dose at onset of labor

Neonate: 2 mg/kg as a single dose between birth and 72 hours if mother received intrapartum dose of nevirapine. If maternal dose was given ≤2 hours prior to delivery, administer infant dose as soon as possible following birth.

Dosage adjustment in renal impairment:

Cl_{cr} ≥20 mL/minute: No adjustment required

Hemodialysis: An additional 200 mg dose is recommended following dialysis.

Dosage adjustment in hepatic impairment: Use is contraindicated with moderate-to-severe hepatic impairment. Permanently discontinue if symptomatic hepatic events occur.

Administration Oral: May be administered with or without food; may be administered with an antacid or didanosine; shake suspension gently prior to administration

Monitoring Parameters Monitor CBC and viral load. Baseline liver function tests should be obtained prior to nevirapine's initiation. AIDS guidelines recommend serum transaminase monitoring every 2 weeks for the first 4 weeks of therapy, then monthly for 3 months, followed by every 3-4 months. Assess/evaluate AST/ALT immediately in any patients with a rash. Permanently discontinue if patient experiences severe rash, constitutional symptoms associated with rash, rash with elevated AST/ALT, or clinical hepatitis, Mild-to-moderate rash without AST/ALT elevation may continue treatment per discretion of prescriber. If mild-to-moderate urticarial rash, do not restart if treatment is interrupted.

Additional Information Potential compliance problems, frequency of administration, and adverse effects should be discussed with patients before initiating therapy to help prevent the emergence of resistance. Early virologic failure was observed with tenofovir and didanosine delayed release capsules, plus either efavirenz or nevirapine; use caution in treatment-naive patients with high baseline viral loads.

Dosage Forms Excipient information presented when available (limited, particularly for generics); consult specific product labeling.

Suspension, oral:

Viramune®: 50 mg/5 mL (240 mL)

Tablet:

Viramune®: 200 mg

- **New-Fill®** *see* Poly-L-Lactic Acid *on page* 1210
- **Nexavar®** *see* Sorafenib *on page* 1392
- **Nexium®** *see* Esomeprazole *on page* 551
- **Nexphen PD** *see* Guaifenesin and Phenylephrine *on page* 712
- **NFV** *see* Nelfinavir *on page* 1049

Niacin (NYE a sin)

U.S. Brand Names Niacin-Time®; Niacor®; Niaspan®; Slo-Niacin® [OTC]

Canadian Brand Names Niaspan®

Index Terms Nicotinic Acid; Vitamin B_3

Pharmacologic Category Antilipemic Agent, Miscellaneous; Vitamin, Water Soluble

Additional Appendix Information

Hyperlipidemia Management *on page* 1815

Lipid-Lowering Agents *on page* 1661

Use Adjunctive treatment of dyslipidemias (types IIa and IIb or primary hypercholesterolemia) to lower the risk of recurrent MI and/or slow progression of coronary artery disease, including combination therapy with other antidyslipidemic agents when additional triglyceride-lowering or HDL-increasing effects are desired; treatment of hypertriglyceridemia in patients at risk of pancreatitis;

treatment of peripheral vascular disease and circulatory disorders; treatment of pellagra; dietary supplement

Pregnancy Risk Factor A/C (dose exceeding RDA recommendation)

Pregnancy Considerations Animal reproduction studies have not been conducted. It is unknown whether or not niacin at lipid-lowering doses is harmful to the developing fetus. If a woman becomes pregnant while receiving niacin for primary hypercholesterolemia, niacin should be discontinued. If a woman becomes pregnant while receiving niacin for hypertriglyceridemia, the benefits and risks of continuing niacin should be assessed on an individual basis.

Lactation Enters breast milk/consult prescriber

Medication Safety Issues

Sound-alike/look-alike issues:

Niacin may be confused with Minocin®, Niaspan®, Nispan®

Niaspan® may be confused with niacin

Nicobid® may be confused with Nitro-Bid®

International issues:

Niacor® may be confused with Nacor® which is a brand name for enalapril in Spain

Contraindications Hypersensitivity to niacin, niacinamide, or any component of the formulation; active hepatic disease or significant or unexplained hepatic dysfunction; active peptic ulcer; arterial hemorrhage

Warnings/Precautions Use caution in heavy ethanol users, unstable angina or MI, diabetes (may interfere with glucose control), renal disease, active gallbladder disease (can exacerbate), gout, past history of hepatic disease, or with anticoagulants (may slightly increase prothrombin time). Rare cases of rhabdomyolysis have occurred during concomitant use with HMG-CoA reductase inhibitors. With concurrent use or if symptoms suggestive of myopathy occur, monitor creatinine phosphokinase (CPK) and potassium. Immediate and extended or sustained release products are not interchangeable. Cases of severe hepatotoxicity have occurred when immediate release (crystalline) niacin products have been substituted with sustained-release (modified release, timed-release) niacin products at equivalent doses. Patients should be initiated with low doses (eg, 500 mg at bedtime) with titration to achieve desired response. Flushing is common and can be attenuated with a gradual increase in dose, and/or by taking aspirin or an NSAID 30-60 minutes before dosing. Compliance is enhanced with twice-daily dosing. Prior to initiation, secondary causes for hypercholesterolemia (eg, poorly controlled diabetes mellitus, hypothyroidism) should be excluded; management with diet and other nonpharmacologic measures (eg, exercise or weight reduction) should be attempted prior to initiation.

Adverse Reactions Frequency not defined.

Cardiovascular: Arrhythmias, atrial fibrillation, edema, flushing, hypotension, orthostasis, palpitation, syncope (rare), tachycardia

Central nervous system: Chills, dizziness, headache, insomnia, migraine, nervousness, pain

Dermatologic: Acanthosis nigricans, dry skin, hyperpigmentation, maculopapular rash, pruritus, rash, urticaria

Endocrine & metabolic: Glucose tolerance decreased, gout, phosphorous levels decreased, hyperuricemia

Gastrointestinal: Abdominal pain, diarrhea, dyspepsia, eructation, flatulence, nausea, peptic ulcers, vomiting

Hematologic: Platelet counts decreased

Hepatic: Hepatic necrosis (rare), jaundice, transaminases increased (dose-related), prothrombin time increased

Neuromuscular & skeletal: Leg cramps, myalgia, myasthenia, myopathy (with concurrent HMG-CoA reductase inhibitor), paresthesia, rhabdomyolysis (with concurrent HMG-CoA reductase inhibitor; rare), weakness

Ocular: Cystoid macular edema, toxic amblyopia

Respiratory: Dyspnea

Miscellaneous: Diaphoresis, hypersensitivity reactions (rare)

Drug Interactions

Avoid Concomitant Use There are no known interactions where it is recommended to avoid concomitant use.

Increased Effect/Toxicity

Niacin may increase the levels/effects of: HMG-CoA Reductase Inhibitors

Decreased Effect

The levels/effects of Niacin may be decreased by: Bile Acid Sequestrants

Ethanol/Nutrition/Herb Interactions Ethanol: Avoid heavy use; avoid use around niacin dose.

Stability

Niaspan®: Store at room temperature of 20°C to 25°C (68°F to 77°F).

Niacor®: Store at controlled room temperature of 15°C to 30°C (59°F to 86°F).

Mechanism of Action Component of two coenzymes which is necessary for tissue respiration, lipid metabolism, and glycogenolysis; inhibits the synthesis of very low density lipoproteins (VLDL) and low density lipoproteins (LDL); may also increase the rate of chylomicron triglyceride removal from plasma.

Pharmacodynamics/Kinetics

Absorption: Rapid and extensive (60% to 76%)

Distribution: Mainly to hepatic, renal, and adipose tissue

Metabolism: Extensive first-pass effects; converted to nicotinamide adenine dinucleotide, nicotinuric acid, and other metabolites

Half-life elimination: 20-45 minutes

Time to peak, serum: Immediate release formulation: 30-60 minutes; extended release formulation: 4-5 hours

Excretion: Urine 60% to 88% (unchanged drug and metabolites)

Dosage Note: Formulations of niacin (regular release versus extended release) are not interchangeable.

Children: Oral:

Pellagra: 50-100 mg/dose 3 times/day

Recommended daily allowances:

0-0.5 years: 5 mg/day

0.5-1 year: 6 mg/day

1-3 years: 9 mg/day

4-6 years: 12 mg/day

7-10 years: 13 mg/day

Children and Adolescents: Recommended daily allowances:

Male:

11-14 years: 17 mg/day

15-18 years: 20 mg/day

19-24 years: 19 mg/day

Female: 11-24 years: 15 mg/day

Adults: Oral:

Recommended daily allowances:

Male: 25-50 years: 19 mg/day; >51 years: 15 mg/day

Female: 25-50 years: 15 mg/day; >51 years: 13 mg/day

Hyperlipidemia: Usual target dose: Regular release: 1.5-6 g/day in 3 divided doses with or after meals using a dosage titration schedule. Extended release: 500 mg to 2 g once daily at bedtime.

Regular release formulation (Niacor®): Initial: 250 mg once daily (with evening meal); increase frequency and/or dose every 4-7 days to desired response or first-level therapeutic dose (1.5-2 g/day in 2-3 divided doses); after 2 months, may increase at 2- to 4-week intervals to 3 g/day in 3 divided doses (maximum dose: 6 g/day in 3 divided doses)

Extended release formulation (Niaspan®): Initial: 500 mg at bedtime for 4 weeks, then 1 g at bedtime for 4 weeks; adjust dose to response and tolerance; can increase to a maximum of 2 g/day, but only at 500 mg/day at 4-week intervals

With lovastatin: Recommended initial dose: 20 mg/day; Maximum lovastatin dose: 40 mg/day
Pellagra: 50-100 mg 3-4 times/day, maximum: 500 mg/day
Niacin deficiency: 10-20 mg/day, maximum: 100 mg/day

Dosage adjustment in renal impairment: Use with caution

Dosage adjustment in hepatic impairment: Contraindicated in patients with significant or unexplained hepatic dysfunction, active liver disease or unexplained transaminase elevations.

Dosage adjustment for hepatic toxicity: Transaminases rise ≥3 times ULN, either persistent or if symptoms of nausea, fever, and/or malaise occur: Discontinue therapy.

Dietary Considerations Should be taken with meal; low-fat meal if treating hyperlipidemia. Avoid hot drinks around the time of niacin dose.

Administration Administer with food. Administer Niaspan® at bedtime. Niaspan® tablet strengths are not interchangeable. When switching from immediate release tablet, initiate Niaspan® at lower dose and titrate. Long-acting forms should not be crushed, broken, or chewed. Do not substitute long-acting forms for immediate release ones.

Monitoring Parameters Blood glucose (in diabetic patients); CPK and serum potassium (if on concurrent HMG-CoA reductase inhibitor); liver function tests pretreatment, every 6-12 weeks for first year, then periodically (approximately every 6 months), monitor liver function more frequently if history of transaminase elevation with prior use; lipid profile; platelets; PT (if on anticoagulants); uric acid (if predisposed to gout); phosphorus (if predisposed to hypophosphatemia)

Test Interactions False elevations in some fluorometric determinations of plasma or urinary catecholamines; false-positive urine glucose (Benedict's reagent)

Dosage Forms Excipient information presented when available (limited, particularly for generics); consult specific product labeling.
Capsule, extended release: 125 mg, 250 mg, 400 mg, 500 mg
Capsule, timed release: 250 mg, 500 mg
Tablet: 50 mg, 100 mg, 250 mg, 500 mg
Niacor®: 500 mg
Tablet, controlled release (Slo-Niacin®): 250 mg, 500 mg, 750 mg
Tablet, extended release (Niaspan®): 500 mg, 750 mg, 1000 mg
Tablet, timed release: 250 mg, 500 mg, 750 mg, 1000 mg
Niacin-Time®: 500 mg

Niacinamide (nye a SIN a mide)

U.S. Brand Names Nicomide-T™

Index Terms Nicotinamide; Nicotinic Acid Amide; Vitamin B_3

Pharmacologic Category Vitamin, Water Soluble

Use
Oral: Prophylaxis and treatment of pellagra
Topical: Improve the appearance of acne and decrease visible inflammation and irritation caused by acne medications

Pregnancy Risk Factor A/C (dose exceeding RDA recommendation)

Medication Safety Issues
Sound-alike/look-alike issues:
Niacinamide may be confused with niCARdipine

Dosage
Pellagra: Oral:
Children: 100-300 mg/day in divided doses
Adults: 300-500 mg/day
Acne: Topical: Adults: Apply to affected area on face twice daily

Additional Information Complete prescribing information for this medication should be consulted for additional detail.

Dosage Forms Excipient information presented when available (limited, particularly for generics); consult specific product labeling.
Cream (Nicomide-T™): 4% (30 g) [contains benzyl alcohol]
Gel (Nicomide-T™): 4% (30 g) [contains alcohol]
Tablet: 100 mg, 250 mg, 500 mg

Niacin and Lovastatin (NYE a sin & LOE va sta tin)

U.S. Brand Names Advicor®

Canadian Brand Names Advicor®

Index Terms Lovastatin and Niacin

Pharmacologic Category Antilipemic Agent, HMG-CoA Reductase Inhibitor; Antilipemic Agent, Miscellaneous

Additional Appendix Information
Hyperlipidemia Management *on page 1815*
Lipid-Lowering Agents *on page 1661*

Use For use when treatment with both extended-release niacin and lovastatin is appropriate in combination with a standard cholesterol-lowering diet:
Extended-release niacin: Adjunctive treatment of dyslipidemias (types IIa and IIb or primary hypercholesterolemia) to lower the risk of recurrent MI and/or slow progression of coronary artery disease, including combination therapy with other antidyslipidemic agents when additional triglyceride-lowering or HDL-increasing effects are desired; treatment of hypertriglyceridemia in patients at risk of pancreatitis
Lovastatin: Treatment of primary hypercholesterolemia (Frederickson types IIa and IIb); primary and secondary prevention of cardiovascular disease

Pregnancy Risk Factor X

Medication Safety Issues
Sound-alike/look-alike issues:
Advicor® may be confused with Advair, Altocor™

Dosage Dosage forms are a fixed combination of niacin and lovastatin.
Oral: Adults: Lowest dose: Niacin 500 mg/lovastatin 20 mg; may increase by not more than 500 mg (niacin) at 4-week intervals (maximum dose: Niacin 2000 mg/lovastatin 40 mg daily); should be taken at bedtime with a low-fat snack. **Note:** If therapy is interrupted for >7 days, reinstitution of therapy should begin with the lowest dose followed by retitration as needed.
Not for use as initial therapy of dyslipidemias. May be substituted for equivalent dose of Niaspan®, however, manufacturer does not recommend direct substitution with other niacin products.

Dosage adjustment in renal impairment:
Mild-to-moderate impairment: No dosage adjustment required
Cl_{cr} <30 mL/minute: Use doses of lovastatin >20 mg/day with caution

Dosage adjustment in hepatic impairment: Do not use in active liver disease or unexplained persistent elevations of serum transaminases.

Additional Information Complete prescribing information for this medication should be consulted for additional detail.

Dosage Forms Excipient information presented when available (limited, particularly for generics); consult specific product labeling.
Tablet, variable release (Advicor®):
500/20: Niacin 500 mg [extended release] and lovastatin 20 mg [immediate release] [contains polysorbate 80]

750/20: Niacin 750 mg [extended release] and lovastatin 20 mg [immediate release] [contains polysorbate 80]
1000/20: Niacin 1000 mg [extended release] and lovastatin 20 mg [immediate release] [contains polysorbate 80]
1000/40: Niacin 1000 mg [extended release] and lovastatin 40 mg [immediate release] [contains polysorbate 80]

Niacin and Simvastatin (NYE a sin & sim va STAT in)

U.S. Brand Names Simcor®

Index Terms Simvastatin and Niacin

Pharmacologic Category Antilipemic Agent, HMG-CoA Reductase Inhibitor; Antilipemic Agent, Miscellaneous

Additional Appendix Information

Hyperlipidemia Management *on page 1815*
Lipid-Lowering Agents *on page 1661*

Use Treatment of primary hypercholesterolemia, mixed dyslipidemia (types IIa and IIb), or hypertriglyceridemia (type IV hyperlipidemia) in combination with standard cholesterol-lowering diet when simvastatin or niacin monotherapy is inadequate

Pregnancy Risk Factor X

Medication Safety Issues

International issue:
Simcor® is also a brand name for simvastatin in Indonesia.

Dosage Dosage forms are a fixed combination of niacin extended-release and simvastatin.

Oral: Adults:
Lowest dose (initiate in patients naïve to niacin therapy or those currently receiving niacin immediate-release): Niacin 500 mg/simvastatin 20 mg once daily at bedtime with a low-fat snack; may increase by not more than 500 mg (niacin) at 4-week intervals
Maintenance dose: Niacin 1000 mg/simvastatin 20 mg to niacin 2000 mg/simvastatin 40 mg once daily (maximum: Niacin 2000 mg/simvastatin 40 mg once daily)

Note: If therapy is interrupted for >7 days, reinstitution of therapy should begin with the lowest dose followed by retitration as tolerated. Not for use as initial therapy of dyslipidemias. May be substituted for equivalent dose of niacin extended-release, however, manufacturer does not recommend direct substitution with immediate-release preparations.

Dosage adjustment for toxicity: Discontinue therapy if transaminases >3 times ULN persist or are accompanied by symptoms (nausea, fever, malaise).

Dosage adjustment in renal impairment:
Mild-to-moderate impairment: No dosage adjustment required; use caution
Severe renal impairment: Use with extreme caution or avoid unless patient already tolerating simvastatin doses ≥10 mg

Dosage adjustment in hepatic impairment: Contraindicated in active liver disease or unexplained persistent elevations of serum transaminases

Additional Information Complete prescribing information for this medication should be consulted for additional detail.

Dosage Forms Excipient information presented when available (limited, particularly for generics); consult specific product labeling.

Tablet, variable release:
Simcor®:
500/20: Niacin 500 mg [extended release] and simvastatin 20 mg [immediate release]
750/20: Niacin 750 mg [extended release] and simvastatin 20 mg [immediate release]
1000/20: Niacin 1000 mg [extended release] and simvastatin 20 mg [immediate release]

◆ **Niacin-Time®** *see* Niacin *on page 1057*

◆ **Niacor®** *see* Niacin *on page 1057*

◆ **Niaspan®** *see* Niacin *on page 1057*

◆ **Niastase® (Can)** *see* Factor VIIa (Recombinant) *on page 598*

NiCARdipine (nye KAR de peen)

U.S. Brand Names Cardene®; Cardene® I.V.; Cardene® SR

Index Terms Nicardipine Hydrochloride

Pharmacologic Category Calcium Channel Blocker

Additional Appendix Information

Calcium Channel Blockers *on page 1651*
Hypertension *on page 1820*

Use Chronic stable angina (immediate-release product only); management of hypertension (immediate and sustained release); parenteral only for short-term use when oral treatment is not feasible

Unlabeled/Investigational Use Congestive heart failure, control of blood pressure in acute ischemic stroke and spontaneous intracranial hemorrhage, postoperative hypertension associated with carotid endarterectomy, perioperative hypertension, prevention of migraine headaches, subarachnoid hemorrhage associated cerebral vasospasm

Pregnancy Risk Factor C

Pregnancy Considerations Crosses the placenta; may exhibit tocolytic effect

Lactation Enters breast milk/not recommended

Medication Safety Issues

Sound-alike/look-alike issues:
NiCARdipine may be confused with niacinamide, NIFEdipine, niMODipine
Cardene® may be confused with Cardizem®, Cardura®, codeine

International issues:
Cardene® may be confused with Cardem® which is a brand name for celiprolol in Spain
Cardene® may be confused with Cardin® which is a brand name for methyldopa in Brazil and a brand name for simvastatin in Poland

Significant differences exist between oral and I.V. dosing. Use caution when converting from one route of administration to another.

Contraindications Hypersensitivity to nicardipine or any component of the formulation; advanced aortic stenosis

Warnings/Precautions Symptomatic hypotension with or without syncope can rarely occur; blood pressure must be lowered at a rate appropriate for the patient's clinical condition. Reflex tachycardia may occur resulting in angina and/or MI in patients with obstructive coronary disease especially in the absence of concurrent beta blockade. The most common side effect is peripheral edema (dose-dependent); occurs within 2-3 weeks of starting therapy. Use with caution in CAD (can cause increase in angina), HF (can worsen heart failure symptoms), aortic stenosis (may reduce coronary perfusion resulting in ischemia), and hypertrophic cardiomyopathy with outflow tract obstruction. Peripheral infusion sites (for I.V. therapy) should be changed every 12 hours. Titrate I.V. dose cautiously in patients with HF, renal or hepatic dysfunction. Use the I.V. form cautiously in patients with portal hypertension (can cause increase in hepatic pressure gradient). Initiate at the low end of the dosage range in the elderly. Concurrent use of fentanyl anesthesia may result in hypotension. Abrupt withdrawal may cause rebound angina in patients with CAD. Safety and efficacy have not been established in pediatric patients.

Adverse Reactions

1% to 10%:

Cardiovascular: Cardiovascular: Flushing (6% to 10%), peripheral edema (dose related; 6% to 8%), hypotension (I.V. 6%), increased angina (dose related; 6%), palpitation (3% to 4%), tachycardia (1% to 4%), vasodilation (1% to 5%), chest pain (I.V. 1%), ECG abnormal (I.V. 1%), extrasystoles (I.V. 1%), hemopericardium (I.V. 1%), hypertension (I.V. 1%), orthostasis (1%), supraventricular tachycardia (I.V. 1%), syncope (1%), ventricular extrasystoles (I.V. 1%), ventricular tachycardia (I.V. 1%)

Central nervous system: Headache (6% to 15%), dizziness (1% to 7%), hypoesthesia (1%), intracranial hemorrhage (1%) pain (1%), somnolence (1%)

Dermatologic: Rash (1%)

Endocrine & metabolic: Hypokalemia (I.V. 1%)

Gastrointestinal: Nausea (2% to 5%), vomiting (I.V. 5%), dyspepsia (oral 2%), abdominal pain (I.V. 1%), dry mouth (1%)

Genitourinary: Polyuria (1%)

Local: Injection site pain (I.V. 1%), injection site reaction (I.V. 1%)

Neuromuscular & skeletal: Weakness (1% to 6%), myalgia (1%), paresthesia (1%)

Renal: Hematuria (1%)

Respiratory: Dyspnea (1%)

Miscellaneous: Diaphoresis (1%)

<1% (Limited to important or life-threatening): Allergic reaction, confusion, constipation, deep vein thrombophlebitis; ECG effects (AV block, inverted T wave, ST segment depression); gingival hyperplasia, hypertonia, hypophosphatemia, insomnia, malaise, nervousness, nocturia, parotitis, thrombocytopenia, tinnitus, tremor

Drug Interactions

Metabolism/Transport Effects Substrate of CYP1A2 (minor), 2C9 (minor), 2D6 (minor), 2E1 (minor), 3A4 (major); **Inhibits** CYP2C9 (strong), 2C19 (moderate), 2D6 (moderate), 3A4 (strong)

Avoid Concomitant Use

Avoid concomitant use of NiCARdipine with any of the following: Dabigatran Etexilate; Eplerenone; Nilotinib; Nisoldipine; Ranolazine; Rivaroxaban; Salmeterol; Thioridazine; Topotecan

Increased Effect/Toxicity

NiCARdipine may increase the levels/effects of: Alosetron; Amifostine; Ciclesonide; CYP2C19 Substrates; CYP2C9 Substrates (High risk); CYP2D6 Substrates; CYP3A4 Substrates; Dabigatran Etexilate; Eplerenone; FentaNYL; Fesoterodine; Ixabepilone; Magnesium Salts; Maraviroc; Neuromuscular-Blocking Agents (Nondepolarizing); Nilotinib; Nisoldipine; Nitroprusside; P-Glycoprotein Substrates; Phenytoin; Pimecrolimus; Ranolazine; RiTUXimab; Rivaroxaban; Salmeterol; Sorafenib; Tacrolimus; Tamoxifen; Thioridazine; Topotecan

The levels/effects of NiCARdipine may be increased by: Alpha1-Blockers; Antifungal Agents (Azole Derivatives, Systemic); Calcium Channel Blockers (Nondihydropyridine); CycloSPORINE; CYP3A4 Inhibitors (Moderate); CYP3A4 Inhibitors (Strong); Dasatinib; Diazoxide; Fluconazole; Grapefruit Juice; Herbs (Hypotensive Properties); Macrolide Antibiotics; Magnesium Salts; P-Glycoprotein Inhibitors; Prostacyclin Analogues; Protease Inhibitors; Quinupristin

Decreased Effect

NiCARdipine may decrease the levels/effects of: Clopidogrel; Codeine; QuiNIDine; TraMADol

The levels/effects of NiCARdipine may be decreased by: Barbiturates; Calcium Salts; CarBAMazepine; CYP3A4 Inducers (Strong); Deferasirox; Herbs (CYP3A4 Inducers); Herbs (Hypertensive Properties); Methylphenidate; Nafcillin; P-Glycoprotein Inducers; Rifamycin Derivatives; Yohimbine

Ethanol/Nutrition/Herb Interactions

Ethanol: Avoid ethanol (may increase CNS depression).

Food: Nicardipine average peak concentrations may be decreased if taken with food. Serum concentrations/toxicity of nicardipine may be increased by grapefruit juice; avoid concurrent use.

Herb/Nutraceutical: St John's wort may decrease levels. Avoid bayberry, blue cohosh, cayenne, ephedra, ginger, ginseng (American), kola, licorice (may worsen hypertension). Avoid black cohosh, California poppy, coleus, golden seal, hawthorn, mistletoe, periwinkle, quinine, shepherd's purse (may have increased antihypertensive effect).

Stability

I.V.:

Premixed bags: Store at controlled room temperature of 20°C to 25°C (68°F to 77°F) . Protect from light and excessive heat. Do not freeze.

Vials: Store at controlled room temperature of 20°C to 25°C (68°F to 77°F). Diluted solutions are stable for 24 hours at room temperature. Protect from light. Dilute 25 mg ampul with 240 mL of compatible solution to provide a 250 mL total volume solution and a final concentration of 0.1 mg/mL.

Oral (Cardene®, Cardene SR®): Store at 15°C to 30°C (59°F to 86°F). Protect from light. Freezing does not affect stability.

Mechanism of Action Inhibits calcium ion from entering the "slow channels" or select voltage-sensitive areas of vascular smooth muscle and myocardium during depolarization, producing a relaxation of coronary vascular smooth muscle and coronary vasodilation; increases myocardial oxygen delivery in patients with vasospastic angina

Pharmacodynamics/Kinetics

Onset of action: Oral: 0.5-2 hours; I.V.: 10 minutes; Hypotension: ~20 minutes

Duration:

I.V.: ≤8 hours

Oral: Immediate release capsules: ≤8 hours; Sustained release capsules: 8-12 hours

Absorption: Oral: ~100%

Protein binding: >95%

Metabolism: Hepatic; CYP3A4 substrate (major); extensive first-pass effect (saturable)

Bioavailability: 35%

Half-life elimination: 2-4 hours

Time to peak, serum: Oral: Immediate release: 30-120 minutes; Sustained release: 60-240 minutes

Excretion: Urine (49% to 60% as metabolites); feces (43% as metabolites)

Dosage

Adults:

Oral:

Immediate release: Initial: 20 mg 3 times/day; usual: 20-40 mg 3 times/day (allow 3 days between dose increases)

Sustained release: Initial: 30 mg twice daily, titrate up to 60 mg twice daily

Note: The total daily dose of immediate-release product may not automatically be equivalent to the daily sustained-release dose; use caution in converting.

I.V.:

Acute hypertension: Initial: 5 mg/hour increased by 2.5 mg/hour every 15 minutes to a maximum of 15 mg/hour; consider reduction to 3 mg/hour after response is achieved. Monitor and titrate to lowest dose necessary to maintain stable blood pressure.

Substitution for oral therapy (approximate equivalents): 20 mg every 8 hours oral, equivalent to 0.5 mg/hour I.V. infusion

30 mg every 8 hours oral, equivalent to 1.2 mg/hour I.V. infusion

40 mg every 8 hours oral, equivalent to 2.2 mg/hour I.V. infusion

Elderly: Initiate at the low end of the dosage range. Specific guidelines for adjustment of nicardipine are not available, but careful monitoring is warranted and adjustment may be necessary.

Dosing adjustment in renal impairment: Titrate dose beginning with 20 mg 3 times/day (immediate release capsule) or 30 mg twice daily (sustained release capsule). Specific guidelines for adjustment of nicardipine are not available, but careful monitoring is warranted and adjustment may be necessary.

Dosing adjustment in hepatic impairment: Starting dose: 20 mg twice daily (immediate release) with titration. Specific guidelines for adjustment of nicardipine are not available, but careful monitoring is warranted and adjustment may be necessary.

Administration

Oral: The total daily dose of immediate-release product may not automatically be equivalent to the daily sustained-release dose; use caution in converting. Do not chew or crush the sustained release formulation, swallow whole. Do not open or cut capsules.

I.V.:

Ampuls must be diluted before use. Administer as a slow continuous infusion.

Premixed bags: No further dilution needed. For single use only, discard any unused portion. Use only if solution is clear; the manufacturer recommends not to admix or run in the same line as other medications.

Dosage Forms Excipient information presented when available (limited, particularly for generics); consult specific product labeling.

Capsule, oral, as hydrochloride: 20 mg, 30 mg
Cardene®: 20 mg, 30 mg

Capsule, sustained release, oral, as hydrochloride:
Cardene® SR: 30 mg, 45 mg, 60 mg

Infusion, premixed in iso-osmotic dextrose, as hydrochloride:
Cardene® IV: 20 mg (200 mL); 40 mg (200 mL)

Infusion, premixed in iso-osmotic sodium chloride, as hydrochloride:
Cardene® IV: 20 mg (200 mL); 40 mg (200 mL)

Injection, solution, as hydrochloride: 2.5 mg/mL (10 mL)
Cardene® IV: 2.5 mg/mL (10 mL)

- ◆ **Nicardipine Hydrochloride** *see* NiCARdipine *on page 1060*
- ◆ **Nicoderm® (Can)** *see* Nicotine *on page 1062*
- ◆ **NicoDerm® CQ® [OTC]** *see* Nicotine *on page 1062*
- ◆ **Nicomide-T™** *see* Niacinamide *on page 1059*
- ◆ **Nicorette® [OTC]** *see* Nicotine *on page 1062*
- ◆ **Nicorette® (Can)** *see* Nicotine *on page 1062*
- ◆ **Nicorette® Plus (Can)** *see* Nicotine *on page 1062*
- ◆ **Nicotinamide** *see* Niacinamide *on page 1059*

Nicotine (nik oh TEEN)

U.S. Brand Names Commit® [OTC]; NicoDerm® CQ® [OTC]; Nicorette® [OTC]; Nicotrol® Inhaler; Nicotrol® NS; Thrive™ [OTC]

Canadian Brand Names Habitrol®; Nicoderm®; Nicorette®; Nicorette® Plus; Nicotrol®

Index Terms Habitrol

Pharmacologic Category Smoking Cessation Aid

Use Treatment to aid smoking cessation for the relief of nicotine withdrawal symptoms (including nicotine craving)

Unlabeled/Investigational Use Management of ulcerative colitis (transdermal)

Pregnancy Risk Factor D (nasal)

Pregnancy Considerations Nicotine is teratogenic in animal studies. Nicotine exposure via cigarette smoke may cause increased ectopic pregnancy, low birth weight, increased risk of spontaneous abortion, increased perinatal mortality; increased aortic blood flow, increased heart rate, decreased uterine blood flow, and decreased breathing have been reported in the fetus. Smoking during pregnancy is associated with sudden infant death syndrome (SIDS), an increased risk of asthma, infantile colic, and childhood obesity. Women who are pregnant should be encouraged not to smoke. The use of nicotine replacement products to aid in smoking cessation has not been adequately studied in pregnant women (amount of nicotine exposure is varied). Nonpharmacologic treatments are recommended. If the benefits of nicotine replacement therapy outweigh the unknown risks, products with intermittent dosing are suggested to be tried first. If a patch is used, it is suggested to remove it overnight while sleeping to decrease fetal exposure.

Lactation Excretion in breast milk unknown/use caution

Medication Safety Issues

Sound-alike/look-alike issues:
NicoDerm® may be confused with Nitroderm
Nicorette® may be confused with Nordette®

Transdermal patch may contain conducting metal (eg, aluminum); remove patch prior to MRI.

Contraindications Hypersensitivity to nicotine or any component of the formulation; patients who are smoking during the postmyocardial infarction period; patients with life-threatening arrhythmias, or severe or worsening angina pectoris; active temporomandibular joint disease (gum); pregnancy; not for use in nonsmokers

Warnings/Precautions Use caution in patients with hyperthyroidism, pheochromocytoma, or insulin-dependent diabetes. Use with caution in oropharyngeal inflammation and in patients with history of esophagitis, peptic ulcer, coronary artery disease, serious cardiac arrhythmias, vasospastic disease, angina, hypertension, hyperthyroidism, pheochromocytoma, diabetes, severe renal dysfunction, and hepatic dysfunction. The inhaler should be used with caution in patients with bronchospastic disease (other forms of nicotine replacement may be preferred). Use of nasal product is not recommended with chronic nasal disorders (eg, allergy, rhinitis, nasal polyps, and sinusitis). Transdermal patch may contain conducting metal (eg, aluminum); remove patch prior to MRI. Cautious use of topical nicotine in patiens with certain skin diseases. Hypersensitivity to the topical products can occur. Dental problems may be worsened by chewing the gum. Urge patients to stop smoking completely when initiating therapy. Safety and efficacy have not been established in pediatric patients.

Adverse Reactions

Nasal spray/inhaler:

>10%:

Central nervous system: Headache (18% to 26%)

Gastrointestinal: Inhaler: Mouth/throat irritation (66%), dyspepsia (18%)

Respiratory: Inhaler: Cough (32%), rhinitis (23%)

1% to 10%:

Dermatologic: Acne (3%)

Endocrine & metabolic: Dysmenorrhea (3%)

Gastrointestinal: Flatulence (4%), gum problems (4%), diarrhea, hiccup, nausea, taste disturbance, tooth disorder

Neuromuscular & skeletal: Back pain (6%), arthralgia (5%), jaw/neck pain

Respiratory: Sinusitis

Miscellaneous: Withdrawal symptoms

<1% (Limited to important or life-threatening): Allergy, amnesia, aphasia, bronchitis, bronchospasm, edema, migraine, numbness, pain, purpura, rash, sputum increased, vision abnormalities, xerostomia

Adverse events previously reported in prescription labeling for chewing gum, lozenge and/or transdermal systems. Frequency not defined; may be product or dose specific:

Central nervous system: Concentration impaired, depression, dizziness, headache, insomnia, nervousness, pain

Gastrointestinal: Aphthous stomatitis, constipation, cough, diarrhea, dyspepsia, flatulence, gingival bleeding, glossitis, hiccups, jaw pain, nausea, salivation increased, stomatitis, taste perversion, tooth disorder, ulcerative stomatitis, xerostomia

Dermatologic: Rash

Local: Application site reaction, local edema, local erythema

Neuromuscular & skeletal: Arthralgia, myalgia, paresthesia

Respiratory: Cough, sinusitis

Miscellaneous: Allergic reaction, diaphoresis

Drug Interactions

Metabolism/Transport Effects **Substrate** (minor) of CYP1A2, 2A6, 2B6, 2C9, 2C19, 2D6, 2E1, 3A4; **Inhibits** CYP2A6 (weak), 2E1 (weak)

Avoid Concomitant Use There are no known interactions where it is recommended to avoid concomitant use.

Increased Effect/Toxicity

Nicotine may increase the levels/effects of: Adenosine

The levels/effects of Nicotine may be increased by: Cimetidine

Decreased Effect There are no known significant interactions involving a decrease in effect.

Ethanol/Nutrition/Herb Interactions Food: Lozenge: Acidic foods/beverages decrease absorption of nicotine.

Stability Nicotrol®: Store inhaler cartridge at room temperature not to exceed 30°C (86°F). Protect cartridges from light.

Mechanism of Action Nicotine is one of two naturally-occurring alkaloids which exhibit their primary effects via autonomic ganglia stimulation. The other alkaloid is lobeline which has many actions similar to those of nicotine but is less potent. Nicotine is a potent ganglionic and central nervous system stimulant, the actions of which are mediated via nicotine-specific receptors. Biphasic actions are observed depending upon the dose administered. The main effect of nicotine in small doses is stimulation of all autonomic ganglia; with larger doses, initial stimulation is followed by blockade of transmission. Biphasic effects are also evident in the adrenal medulla; discharge of catecholamines occurs with small doses, whereas prevention of catecholamines release is seen with higher doses as a response to splanchnic nerve stimulation. Stimulation of the central nervous system (CNS) is characterized by tremors and respiratory excitation. However, convulsions may occur with higher doses, along with respiratory failure secondary to both central paralysis and peripheral blockade to respiratory muscles.

Pharmacodynamics/Kinetics

Onset of action: Intranasal: More closely approximate the time course of plasma nicotine levels observed after cigarette smoking than other dosage forms

Duration: Transdermal: 24 hours

Absorption: Transdermal: Slow

Metabolism: Hepatic, primarily to cotinine (1/5 as active)

Half-life elimination: 4 hours

Time to peak, serum: Transdermal: 8-9 hours

Excretion: Urine

Clearance: Renal: pH dependent

Dosage

Smoking deterrent: Patients should be advised to completely stop smoking upon initiation of therapy.

Oral:

Gum: Chew 1 piece of gum when urge to smoke, up to 24 pieces/day. Patients who smoke <25 cigarettes/day should start with 2-mg strength; patients smoking ≥25 cigarettes/day should start with the 4-mg strength. Use according to the following 12-week dosing schedule:

Weeks 1-6: Chew 1 piece of gum every 1-2 hours; to increase chances of quitting, chew at least 9 pieces/day during the first 6 weeks

Weeks 7-9: Chew 1 piece of gum every 2-4 hours

Weeks 10-12: Chew 1 piece of gum every 4-8 hours

Inhaler: Usually 6 to 16 cartridges per day; best effect was achieved by frequent continuous puffing (20 minutes); recommended duration of treatment is 3 months, after which patients may be weaned from the inhaler by gradual reduction of the daily dose over 6-12 weeks

Lozenge: Patients who smoke their first cigarette within 30 minutes of waking should use the 4 mg strength; otherwise the 2 mg strength is recommended. Use according to the following 12-week dosing schedule:

Weeks 1-6: One lozenge every 1-2 hours

Weeks 7-9: One lozenge every 2-4 hours

Weeks 10-12: One lozenge every 4-8 hours

Note: Use at least 9 lozenges/day during first 6 weeks to improve chances of quitting; do not use more than one lozenge at a time (maximum: 5 lozenges every 6 hours, 20 lozenges/day)

Topical:

Transdermal patch: Apply new patch every 24 hours to nonhairy, clean, dry skin on the upper body or upper outer arm; each patch should be applied to a different site. **Note:** Adjustment may be required during initial treatment (move to higher dose if experiencing withdrawal symptoms; lower dose if side effects are experienced).

NicoDerm CQ®:

Patients smoking ≥10 cigarettes/day: Begin with **step 1** (21 mg/day) for 6 weeks, followed by **step 2** (14 mg/day) for 2 weeks; finish with **step 3** (7 mg/day) for 2 weeks

Patients smoking <10 cigarettes/day: Begin with **step 2** (14 mg/day) for 6 weeks, followed by **step 3** (7 mg/day) for 2 weeks

Note: Patients receiving >600 mg/day of cimetidine: Decrease to the next lower patch size

Note: Benefits of use of nicotine transdermal patches beyond 3 months have not been demonstrated.

Ulcerative colitis (unlabeled use): Transdermal: Titrated to 22-25 mg/day

Nasal: Spray: 1-2 sprays/hour; do not exceed more than 5 doses (10 sprays) per hour [maximum: 40 doses/day (80 sprays); each dose (2 sprays) contains 1 mg of nicotine]

Dietary Considerations

Commit®: Each lozenge contains phenylalanine 3.4 mg and sodium 18 mg.

Nicorette®: Fresh mint and fruit chill flavors: The 2-mg strength contains calcium 94 mg/gum and sodium 11 mg/gum. The 4-mg strength contains calcium 94 mg/gum and sodium 13 mg/gum.

Administration

Gum: Should be chewed slowly to avoid jaw ache and to maximize benefit. Chew slowly until it tingles, then park gum between cheek and gum until tingle is gone; repeat process until most of tingle is gone (~30 minutes).

Lozenge: Should not be chewed or swallowed; allow to dissolve slowly (~20-30 minutes)

Transdermal patch: Do not cut patch; causes rapid evaporation, rendering the patch useless

Monitoring Parameters Heart rate and blood pressure periodically during therapy; discontinue therapy if signs of nicotine toxicity occur (eg, severe headache, dizziness, mental confusion, disturbed hearing and vision, abdominal pain; rapid, weak and irregular pulse; salivation, nausea, vomiting, diarrhea, cold sweat, weakness); therapy should be discontinued if rash develops; discontinuation may be considered if other adverse effects of patch occur such as myalgia, arthralgia, abnormal dreams, insomnia, nervousness, dry mouth, sweating

Additional Information A cigarette has 10-25 mg nicotine.

Dosage Forms Excipient information presented when available (limited, particularly for generics); consult specific product labeling.

Gum, chewing, as polacrilex: 2 mg (20s, 50s, 110s); 4 mg (20s, 50s, 110s)

Nicorette®:

2 mg (48s, 50s, 108s, 110s, 168s, 170s, 192s, 200s, 216s) [original and mint flavors]; (48s, 108s, 110s) [orange flavor]; (40s, 100s) [contains calcium 94 mg/gum and sodium 11 mg/gum; fresh mint and fruit chill flavors]

4 mg (48s, 50s, 108s, 110s, 168s, 170s, 192s, 200s, 216s) [original and mint flavors]; (48s, 108s, 110s) [orange flavor]; (40s, 100s) [contains calcium 94 mg/gum and sodium 13 mg/gum; fresh mint and fruit chill flavors]

Thrive™:

2 mg (40s) [gluten free, sucrose free; mint flavor]

4 mg (40s) [gluten free, sucrose free; mint flavor]

Lozenge, as polacrilex:

Commit®:

2 mg (48s, 72s, 84s, 168s) [contains phenylalanine 3.4 mg/lozenge, sodium 18 mg/lozenge; mint flavor]; (108s) [contains phenylalanine 3.4 mg/lozenge, sodium 18 mg/lozenge; original flavor]

4 mg (48s, 72s, 84s, 168s, 192s) [contains phenylalanine 3.4 mg/lozenge, sodium 18 mg/lozenge; mint flavor]; (108s) [contains phenylalanine 3.4 mg/lozenge, sodium 18 mg/lozenge; original flavor]

Oral inhalation system:

Nicotrol® Inhaler: 10 mg cartridge (168s) [cartridge delivers nicotine 4 mg; each unit consists of 5 mouthpieces, 28 storage trays each containing 6 cartridges, and 1 storage case]

Solution, intranasal [spray]:

Nicotrol® NS: 10 mg/mL (10 mL) [delivers 0.5 mg/spray; 200 sprays]

Transdermal system, topical: 7 mg/24 (30s); 14 mg/24 hours (30s); 21 mg/24 hours (30s)

NicoDerm® CQ®: 7 mg/24 hours (14s) [step 3; available in tan or clear patch]; 14 mg/24 hours (14s) [step 2; available in tan or clear patch]; 21 mg/24 hours (7s, 14s) [step 1; available in tan or clear patch]

- **Nicotinic Acid** *see* Niacin *on page 1057*
- **Nicotinic Acid Amide** *see* Niacinamide *on page 1059*
- **Nicotrol® (Can)** *see* Nicotine *on page 1062*
- **Nicotrol® Inhaler** *see* Nicotine *on page 1062*
- **Nicotrol® NS** *see* Nicotine *on page 1062*
- **Nidagel™ (Can)** *see* MetroNIDAZOLE *on page 984*
- **Nifediac™ CC** *see* NIFEdipine *on page 1064*
- **Nifedical™ XL** *see* NIFEdipine *on page 1064*

NIFEdipine (nye FED i peen)

U.S. Brand Names Adalat® CC; Afeditab™ CR; Nifediac™ CC; Nifedical™ XL; Procardia XL®; Procardia®

Canadian Brand Names Adalat® XL®; Apo-Nifed PA®; Apo-Nifed®; GEN-Nifedipine XL; Nifedipine PA; Novo-Nifedin; Nu-Nifed; Nu-Nifedipine-PA; PMS-Nifedipine; Procardia®

Pharmacologic Category Calcium Channel Blocker

Additional Appendix Information

Calcium Channel Blockers *on page 1651*

Use Angina and hypertension (sustained release only), pulmonary hypertension

Pregnancy Risk Factor C

Pregnancy Considerations Use in pregnancy only when clearly needed and when the benefits outweigh the potential hazard to the fetus. No data on crossing the placenta. Hypotension, IUGR reported. IUGR probably related to maternal hypertension. May exhibit tocolytic effects. Available evidence suggests safe use during pregnancy.

Lactation Enters breast milk/compatible

Medication Safety Issues

Sound-alike/look-alike issues:

NIFEdipine may be confused with niCARdipine, niMODipine, nisoldipine

Procardia XL® may be confused with Cartia® XT

International issues:

Nipin® [Italy and Singapore] may be confused with Nipent® which is a brand name for pentostatin in the U.S.

Contraindications Hypersensitivity to nifedipine or any component of the formulation; immediate release preparation for treatment of urgent or emergent hypertension; acute MI

Warnings/Precautions Symptomatic hypotension with or without syncope can rarely occur; blood pressure must be lowered at a rate appropriate for the patient's clinical condition. **The use of sublingual short-acting nifedipine in hypertensive emergencies and urgencies is neither safe nor effective and SHOULD BE ABANDONED!** Serious adverse events (eg, cerebrovascular ischemia, syncope, stroke, acute myocardial infarction, and fetal distress) have been reported in relation to such use.

Blood pressure lowering should be done at a rate appropriate for the patient's condition. Rapid drops in blood pressure can lead to arterial insufficiency. Increased angina and/or MI has occurred with initiation or dosage titration of calcium channel blockers. Severe hypotension may occur in patients taking immediate release concurrently with beta-blockers when undergoing CABG with high dose fentanyl anesthesia. When considering surgery with high dose fentanyl, may consider withdrawing nifedipine (>36 hours) before surgery if possible.

The most common side effect is peripheral edema; occurs within 2-3 weeks of starting therapy. Reflex tachycardia may occur with use. Use with caution in HF or severe aortic stenosis (especially with concomitant beta-adrenergic blocker), severe left ventricular dysfunction, renal impairment, hypertrophic cardiomyopathy (especially obstructive), concomitant therapy with beta-blockers or digoxin, and edema. Use caution in patients with severe hepatic impairment (may need dosage adjustment). Mild and transient elevations in liver function enzymes may be apparent within 8 weeks of therapy initiation. Abrupt withdrawal may cause rebound angina in patients with CAD. The elderly may be more susceptible to adverse effects. Avoid use of extended release tablets (Procardia XL®) in patients with known stricture/narrowing of the GI tract.

Adverse Reactions

>10%:

Cardiovascular: Flushing (10% to 25%), peripheral edema (dose related 7% to 10%; up to 50%)

Central nervous system: Dizziness/lightheadedness/ giddiness (10% to 27%), headache (10% to 23%)
Gastrointestinal: Nausea/heartburn (10% to 11%)
Neuromuscular & skeletal: Weakness (10% to 12%)

≥1% to 10%:

Cardiovascular: Palpitation (≤2% to 7%), transient hypotension (dose related 5%), CHF (2%)
Central nervous system: Nervousness/mood changes (≤2% to 7%), shakiness (≤2%), jitteriness (≤2%), sleep disturbances (≤2%), difficulties in balance (≤2%), fever (≤2%), chills (≤2%)
Dermatologic: Dermatitis (≤2%), pruritus (≤2%), urticaria (≤2%)
Endocrine & metabolic: Sexual difficulties (≤2%)
Gastrointestinal: Diarrhea (≤2%), constipation (≤2%), cramps (≤2%), flatulence (≤2%), gingival hyperplasia (≤10%)
Neuromuscular & skeletal: Muscle cramps/tremor (≤2% to 8%), inflammation (≤2%), joint stiffness (≤2%)
Ocular: Blurred vision (≤2%)
Respiratory: Cough/wheezing (6%), nasal congestion/ sore throat (≤2% to 6%), chest congestion (≤2%), dyspnea (≤2%)
Miscellaneous: Diaphoresis (≤2%)

<1% (Limited to important or life-threatening): Agranulocytosis, allergic hepatitis, angina, angioedema, aplastic anemia, arthritis with positive ANA, bezoars (sustained-release preparations), cerebral ischemia, depression, erythema multiforme, erythromelalgia, exfoliative dermatitis, extrapyramidal symptoms, fever, gingival hyperplasia, gynecomastia, leukopenia, memory dysfunction, paranoid syndrome, photosensitivity, purpura, Stevens-Johnson syndrome, syncope, thrombocytopenia, tinnitus, transient blindness

Reported with use of sublingual short-acting nifedipine: Acute MI, cerebrovascular ischemia, ECG changes, fetal distress, heart block, severe hypotension, sinus arrest, stroke, syncope

Drug Interactions

Metabolism/Transport Effects Substrate of CYP2D6 (minor), 3A4 (major); **Inhibits** CYP1A2 (moderate), 2C9 (weak), 2D6 (weak), 3A4 (weak)

Avoid Concomitant Use There are no known interactions where it is recommended to avoid concomitant use.

Increased Effect/Toxicity

NIFEdipine may increase the levels/effects of: Amifostine; CYP1A2 Substrates; Magnesium Salts; Neuromuscular-Blocking Agents (Nondepolarizing); Nitroprusside; Phenytoin; RiTUXimab; Tacrolimus; VinCRIStine

The levels/effects of NIFEdipine may be increased by: Alcohol (Ethyl); Alpha1-Blockers; Antifungal Agents (Azole Derivatives, Systemic); Calcium Channel Blockers (Nondihydropyridine); Cimetidine; Cisapride; CycloSPORINE; CYP3A4 Inhibitors (Moderate); CYP3A4 Inhibitors (Strong); Dasatinib; Diazoxide; Fluconazole; Grapefruit Juice; Herbs (Hypotensive Properties); Macrolide Antibiotics; Magnesium Salts; Prostacyclin Analogues; Protease Inhibitors; Quinupristin

Decreased Effect

NIFEdipine may decrease the levels/effects of: Clopidogrel; QuiNIDine

The levels/effects of NIFEdipine may be decreased by: Barbiturates; Calcium Salts; CarBAMazepine; CYP3A4 Inducers (Strong); Deferasirox; Herbs (CYP3A4 Inducers); Herbs (Hypertensive Properties); Methylphenidate; Nafcillin; Rifamycin Derivatives; Yohimbine

Ethanol/Nutrition/Herb Interactions

Ethanol: Avoid ethanol (may increase CNS depression and may increase the effects of nifedipine). Monitor.

Food: Nifedipine serum levels may be decreased if taken with food. Food may decrease the rate but not the extent of absorption of Procardia XL®. Increased therapeutic and vasodilator side effects, including severe hypotension and myocardial ischemia, may occur if nifedipine is taken by patients ingesting grapefruit.

Herb/Nutraceutical: St John's wort may decrease nifedipine levels. Avoid dong quai if using for hypertension (has estrogenic activity). Avoid ephedra, yohimbe, ginseng (may worsen hypertension). Avoid garlic (may have increased antihypertensive effect).

Mechanism of Action Inhibits calcium ion from entering the "slow channels" or select voltage-sensitive areas of vascular smooth muscle and myocardium during depolarization, producing a relaxation of coronary vascular smooth muscle and coronary vasodilation; increases myocardial oxygen delivery in patients with vasospastic angina

Pharmacodynamics/Kinetics

Onset of action: Immediate release: ~20 minutes
Protein binding (concentration dependent): 92% to 98%
Metabolism: Hepatic to inactive metabolites
Bioavailability: Capsule: 40% to 77%; Sustained release: 65% to 89% relative to immediate release capsules
Half-life elimination: Adults: Healthy: 2-5 hours, Cirrhosis: 7 hours; Elderly: 6.7 hours
Excretion: Urine (as metabolites)

Dosage Oral:

Children:

Hypertrophic cardiomyopathy: 0.6-0.9 mg/kg/24 hours in 3-4 divided doses
Hypertension: Children 1-17 years: Extended release tablet: Initial: 0.25-0.5 mg/kg/day once daily or in 2 divided doses; maximum: 3 mg/kg/day up to 120 mg/day

Adults: (**Note:** When switching from immediate release to sustained release formulations, total daily dose will start the same)

Initial: 30 mg once daily as sustained release formulation, or if indicated, 10 mg 3 times/day as capsules
Usual dose: 10-30 mg 3 times/day as capsules or 30-60 mg once daily as sustained release
Maximum dose: 120-180 mg/day
Increase sustained release at 7- to 14-day intervals

Hemodialysis: Supplemental dose is not necessary.

Peritoneal dialysis effects: Supplemental dose is not necessary.

Dosing adjustment in hepatic impairment: Reduce oral dose by 50% to 60% in patients with cirrhosis.

Dietary Considerations Avoid grapefruit juice with all products.

Immediate release: Capsule is rapidly absorbed orally if it is administered without food, but may result in vasodilator side effects; if flushing is problematic, administration with low-fat meals may decrease. In general, can take with or without food.

Extended release: Adalat®CC, Afeditab™ CR, Nifediac™ CC: Take on an empty stomach (manufacturer recommendation). Other extended release products may not have this recommendation; consult product labeling.

Administration

Immediate release: In general, may be administered with or without food.

Extended release: Tablets should be swallowed whole; do not crush or chew.

Adalat®CC, Afeditab™ CR, Nifediac™ CC: Administer on an empty stomach (per manufacturer). Other extended release products may not have this recommendation; consult product labeling.

Monitoring Parameters Heart rate, blood pressure, signs and symptoms of CHF, peripheral edema

Additional Information When measuring smaller doses from the liquid-filled capsules, consider the following concentrations (for Procardia®) 10 mg capsule = 10 mg/0.34 mL; 20 mg capsule = 20 mg/0.45 mL; may be used preoperative to treat hypertensive urgency.

Considerable attention has been directed to potential increases in mortality and morbidity when short-acting nifedipine is used in treating hypertension. The rapid reduction in blood pressure may precipitate adverse cardiovascular events. At this time, there is no indication for the use of short-acting calcium channel blocker therapy. Nifedipine also has potent negative inotropic effects and can worsen heart failure.

Dosage Forms Excipient information presented when available (limited, particularly for generics); consult specific product labeling.

Capsule, softgel: 10 mg, 20 mg
  Procardia®: 10 mg
Tablet, extended release: 30 mg, 60 mg, 90 mg
  Adalat® CC, Procardia XL®: 30 mg, 60 mg, 90 mg
  Afeditab™ CR, Nifedical™ XL: 30 mg, 60 mg
  Nifediac™ CC: 30 mg, 60 mg, 90 mg [90 mg tablet contains tartrazine]

◆ **Nifedipine PA (Can)** *see* NIFEdipine *on page 1064*

◆ **Niferex® [OTC]** *see* Polysaccharide-Iron Complex *on page 1212*

◆ **Niftolid** *see* Flutamide *on page 643*

◆ **Nilandron®** *see* Nilutamide *on page 1068*

Nilotinib (nye LOE ti nib)

U.S. Brand Names Tasigna®

Canadian Brand Names Tasigna®

Index Terms AMN107; Nilotinib Hydrochloride Monohydrate

Pharmacologic Category Antineoplastic Agent, Tyrosine Kinase Inhibitor

Use Treatment of Philadelphia chromosome-positive chronic myelogenous leukemia (Ph+ CML) in chronic and accelerated phase (refractory or intolerant to prior therapy, including imatinib)

Unlabeled/Investigational Use Treatment of Ph+ acute lymphoblastic leukemia (ALL), systemic mastocytosis (with c-kit activation), hypereosinophilic syndrome

Pregnancy Risk Factor D

Pregnancy Considerations Animal studies have demonstrated embryo-fetal toxicity and maternal toxicity. There are no adequate and well-controlled studies in pregnant women. Women of childbearing potential should be advised to use effective contraception during treatment.

Lactation Excretion in breast milk unknown/not recommended

Medication Safety Issues

Sound-alike/look-alike issues:
  Nilotinib may be confused with nilutamide

High alert medication: The Institute for Safe Medication Practices (ISMP) includes this medication among its list of drug classes which have a heightened risk of causing significant patient harm when used in error.

Contraindications Use in patients with hypokalemia, hypomagnesemia, or long QT syndrome

Warnings/Precautions Hazardous agent - use appropriate precautions for handling and disposal. **[U.S. Boxed Warning]: May prolong the QT interval; sudden deaths have been reported.** Sudden deaths appear to be related to dose-dependent ventricular repolarization abnormalities. Prolonged QT interval may result in torsade de pointes, which may cause syncope, seizure, and/or death. Use in patients with hypokalemia, hypomagnesemia, or long QT syndrome is contraindicated. Electrolyte abnormalities may occur during treatment, including hypophosphatemia, hyper-/hypokalemia, hypocalcemia, and hyponatremia. Correct electrolyte abnormalities prior to treatment initiation; monitor ECG. Concurrent use with other drugs which may prolong QT interval may increase the risk of potentially-fatal arrhythmias. Concurrent use with CYP3A4 inhibitors/inducers is not recommended; dosage adjustments are recommended if concurrent use cannot be avoided. Patients with uncontrolled or significant cardiovascular disease were excluded from studies.

[U.S. Boxed Warning]: Use with caution in patients with hepatic impairment; nilotinib metabolism is primarily hepatic; carefully monitor for QT prolongation. Nilotinib use in patients with ALT and/or AST >2.5 times ULN (>5 times ULN if disease-related) and/or bilirubin >1.5 times ULN has not been studied. May cause hepatotoxicity, including dose-limiting elevations in bilirubin, transaminases, and alkaline phosphatase; monitor liver function.

Reversible myelosuppression, including grades 3 and 4 thrombocytopenia, neutropenia, and anemia may occur; may require dose reductions and/or treatment delay. **[U.S. Boxed Warning]: Administer on an empty stomach, at least 1 hour before and 2 hours after food.** Use with caution in patients with a history of pancreatitis, may cause dose-limiting elevations of serum lipase and amylase; monitor. Capsules contain lactose; do not use with galactose intolerance, severe lactase deficiency, or glucose-galactose malabsorption syndromes. Safety and efficacy have not been established in children.

Adverse Reactions Frequency not always defined.

10%:
  Cardiovascular: Peripheral edema (11%)
  Central nervous system: Headache (21% to 31%), fatigue (16% to 28%), fever (14% to 24%)
  Dermatologic: Rash (28% to 33%), pruritus (20% to 29%)
  Endocrine & metabolic: Hyperglycemia (grades 3/4: 4% to 11%)
  Gastrointestinal: Nausea (18% to 31%), diarrhea (19% to 22%), constipation (18% to 21%), vomiting (10% to 21%), lipase increased (grades 3/4: 15% to 17%), abdominal pain (11% to 13%)
  Hematologic: Neutropenia (grades 3/4: 28% to 37%; median duration: 15 days), thrombocytopenia (grade 3: 7% to 11%; grade 4: 17% to 30%; median duration: 22 days), anemia (grades 3/4: 8% to 23%)
  Neuromuscular & skeletal: Arthralgia (16% to 18%), limb pain (13% to 16%), myalgia (14%), weakness (12% to 14%), muscle spasm (11% to 14%), bone pain (11% to 13%), back pain (10% to 12%)
  Respiratory: Cough (13% to 17%), nasopharyngitis (11% to 16%), dyspnea (8% to 11%)

1% to 10%:
  Cardiovascular: Flushing, hypertension, palpitation, QT interval prolonged
  Central nervous system: Dizziness, dysphonia, insomnia, vertigo
  Dermatologic: Alopecia, dry skin, eczema, erythema, hyperhidrosis, urticaria
  Endocrine & metabolic: Hypophosphatemia (grades 3/4: 10%), hypokalemia (grades 3/4: 1% to 5%), hyperkalemia (grades 3/4: 3% to 4%), hypocalcemia (grades 3/4: 1% to 4%), hyponatremia (grades 3/4: 3%), albumin decreased (grades 3/4: 1%), hypomagnesemia
  Gastrointestinal: Abdominal discomfort, amylase increased, anorexia, dyspepsia, flatulence, pancreatitis (≤1%)
  Hematologic: Neutropenic fever, pancytopenia
  Hepatic: Hyperbilirubinemia (grades 3/4: 9% to 10%), ALT increased (grades 3/4: 2% to 4%), alkaline phosphatase increased (grades 3/4: 1% to 3%), AST increased (grades 3/4: 1%), GGT increased
  Neuromuscular & skeletal: Musculoskeletal pain, paresthesia
  Respiratory: Dyspnea (exertional), pleural effusion (≤1%)
  Miscellaneous: Night sweats

<1% (Limited to important or life-threatening): Angina, atrial fibrillation, blurred vision, bradycardia, brain edema,

bruising, BUN increased, candidiasis, cardiac failure, cardiac flutter, cardiac murmur, cardiomegaly, chest pain, confusion, coronary artery disease, creatinine elevated, depression, diabetes mellitus, diplopia, dysuria, epistaxis, erectile dysfunction, erythema nodosum, exfoliative rash, extrasystoles, eye hemorrhage, facial edema, gastroenteritis, gastrointestinal hemorrhage, gastrointestinal ulcer perforation, gynecomastia, hematemesis, hematoma, hematuria, hemorrhagic shock, hepatitis, hepatomegaly, hepatotoxicity, herpes simplex, hypercalcemia, hyper-/hypothyroidism, hyperphosphatemia, hypertensive crisis, hypoglycemia, hypotension, influenza-like illness, interstitial lung disease, intracranial hemorrhage, jaundice, joint swelling, lactic dehydrogenase increased, leukocytosis, loss of consciousness, melena, MI, migraine, mouth ulceration, optic neuritis, papilledema, pericardial effusion, pericarditis, periorbital edema, peripheral neuropathy, petechiae, pneumonia, pulmonary edema, pulmonary hypertension, renal failure, retroperitoneal hemorrhage, sepsis, stomatitis, subileus, thrombocytosis, thrombosis, thyroiditis, troponin increased, ulcerative esophagitis, urinary tract infection, ventricular dysfunction, visual acuity decreased

Drug Interactions

Metabolism/Transport Effects **Substrate** of CYP3A4 (major), P-glycoprotein (P-gp, ABCB1); **Inhibits** CYP3A4, 2C8, 2C9, 2D6, UGT1A1, P-glycoprotein (P-gp, ABCB1); **Induces** CYP2B6, 2C8, 2C9

Avoid Concomitant Use

Avoid concomitant use of Nilotinib with any of the following: CYP3A4 Inducers (Strong); CYP3A4 Inhibitors (Strong); Dabigatran Etexilate; Natalizumab; QTc-Prolonging Agents; Rivaroxaban; Silodosin; Tetrabenazine; Thioridazine; Topotecan; Vaccines (Live); Ziprasidone

Increased Effect/Toxicity

Nilotinib may increase the levels/effects of: CYP2C8 Substrates (High risk); CYP2C9 Substrates (High risk); CYP2D6 Substrates; Dabigatran Etexilate; Fesoterodine; Natalizumab; Nebivolol; P-Glycoprotein Substrates; QTc-Prolonging Agents; Rivaroxaban; Silodosin; Tamoxifen; Tetrabenazine; Thioridazine; Topotecan; Vaccines (Live); Vitamin K Antagonists; Ziprasidone

The levels/effects of Nilotinib may be increased by: Alfuzosin; Ciprofloxacin; CYP3A4 Inhibitors (Moderate); CYP3A4 Inhibitors (Strong); Dasatinib; Gadobutrol; Trastuzumab

Decreased Effect

Nilotinib may decrease the levels/effects of: Cardiac Glycosides; Codeine; TraMADol; Vaccines (Inactivated); Vitamin K Antagonists

The levels/effects of Nilotinib may be decreased by: CYP3A4 Inducers (Strong); Deferasirox; Echinacea; Herbs (CYP3A4 Inducers)

Ethanol/Nutrition/Herb Interactions Herb/Nutraceutical: Avoid St John's wort (may decrease nilotinib levels).

Stability Store at 15°C to 30°C (59°F to 86°F).

Mechanism of Action Selective tyrosine kinase inhibitor that targets BCR-ABL kinase, c-KIT and platelet derived growth factor receptor (PDGFR); does not have activity against the SRC family. Inhibits BCR-ABL mediated proliferation of leukemic cell lines by binding to the ATP-binding site of BCR-ABL and inhibiting tyrosine kinase activity. Nilotinib has activity in imatinib-resistant BCR-ABL kinase mutations.

Pharmacodynamics/Kinetics

Protein binding: ~98%

Metabolism: Hepatic; oxidation and hydroxylation, via CYP3A4 to primarily inactive metabolites

Bioavailability: Increased 82% when administered 30 minutes after a high-fat meal

Half-life elimination: ~15-17 hours

Time to peak: 3 hours

Excretion: Feces (93%; 69% as parent drug)

Dosage Oral: Adults: 400 mg twice daily (continue treatment until disease progression or unacceptable toxicity)

Dosage adjustment for concomitant CYP3A4 inhibitors/inducers:

CYP3A4 inhibitors: The concomitant use of a strong CYP3A4 inhibitor with nilotinib is not recommended. If a strong CYP3A4 inhibitor is required, interruption of nilotinib treatment is recommended; if therapy cannot be interrupted and concurrent use can not be avoided, consider reducing the nilotinib dose by 50%, to 400 mg once daily, with careful monitoring, especially of the QT interval. When a strong CYP3A4 inhibitor is discontinued, allow a washout period prior to adjusting nilotinib dose upward.

CYP3A4 inducers: The concomitant use of a strong CYP3A4 inducer with nilotinib is not recommended. If a strong CYP3A4 inducer is required, the nilotinib dose may need to be increased, with careful monitoring. When the strong CYP3A4 inducer is discontinued, reduce nilotinib to the indicated dose.

Dosage adjustment in renal impairment: Not studied in patients with serum creatinine >1.5 times ULN, however, nilotinib and its metabolites have minimal renal excretion; dosage adjustments for renal dysfunction may not be needed.

Dosage adjustment in hepatic impairment: Not studied in patients with hepatic impairment; nilotinib metabolism is primarily hepatic, use caution.

For hepatotoxicity during treatment:

If bilirubin >3 times ULN (≥ grade 3): Withhold treatment, monitor bilirubin, resume treatment at 400 mg once daily when bilirubin returns to ≤1.5 times ULN (≤ grade 1)

If ALT or AST >5 times ULN (≥ grade 3): Withhold treatment, monitor transaminases, resume treatment at 400 mg once daily when ALT or AST returns to ≤2.5 times ULN (≤ grade 1)

Dosage adjustment for hematologic toxicity:

ANC <1000/mm^3 and/or platelets <50,000/mm^3: Withhold treatment, monitor blood counts

If ANC >1000/mm^3 and platelets >50,000/mm^3 within 2 weeks: Continue at 400 mg twice daily

If ANC <1000/mm^3 and/or platelets <50,000/mm^3 for >2 weeks: Reduce dose to 400 mg once daily

Dosage adjustment for nonhematologic toxicity:

Amylase or lipase ≥2 times ULN (≥ grade 3): Withhold treatment, monitor serum amylase or lipase, resume treatment at 400 mg once daily when lipase or amylase returns to ≤1.5 times ULN (≤ grade 1)

Clinically-significant moderate or severe nonhematologic toxicity: Withhold treatment, upon resolution of toxicity, resume at 400 mg once daily; may escalate back to 400 mg twice daily if clinically appropriate.

Dosage adjustment for QT prolongation:

QT_c >480 msec: Withhold treatment, monitor and correct potassium and magnesium levels.

If within 2 weeks:

QT_cF returns to <450 msec and to within 20 msec of baseline within 2 weeks: Continue at 400 mg twice daily

QT_cF returns to 450-480 msec: Reduce dose to 400 mg once daily

If QT_cF >480 msec after dosage reduction to 400 mg once daily, discontinue therapy.

Dietary Considerations The bioavailability of nilotinib is increased with food. Take on an empty stomach, at least 1 hour before or 2 hours after food. Avoid grapefruit juice.

Administration Administer twice daily, ~12 hours apart. Swallow capsules whole with water. Administer on an empty stomach, at least 1 hour before or 2 hours after food.

Monitoring Parameters CBC with differential (every 2 weeks for first 2 months, then monthly); electrolytes (including potassium and magnesium; baseline and periodic); hepatic function (ALT/AST, bilirubin, alkaline phosphatase; baseline and periodic); serum lipase (baseline and periodic); bone marrow assessments; ECG (baseline, 7 days after treatment initiation or dosage adjustments, and periodically thereafter)

Additional Information If clinically indicated, may be administered in combination with hematopoietic growth factors (eg, erythropoietin, filgrastim) and with hydroxyurea or anagrelide.

Dosage Forms Excipient information presented when available (limited, particularly for generics); consult specific product labeling.

Capsule:

Tasigna®: 200 mg

◆ **Nilotinib Hydrochloride Monohydrate** *see* Nilotinib *on page 1066*

◆ **Nilstat (Can)** *see* Nystatin *on page 1087*

Nilutamide (ni LOO ta mide)

U.S. Brand Names Nilandron®

Canadian Brand Names Anandron®

Index Terms NSC-684588; RU-23908

Pharmacologic Category Antiandrogen; Antineoplastic Agent, Antiandrogen

Use Treatment of metastatic prostate cancer

Pregnancy Risk Factor C

Pregnancy Considerations Not indicated for use in women

Lactation Not indicated for use in women

Medication Safety Issues

Sound-alike/look-alike issues:

Nilutamide may be confused with nilotinib

Contraindications Hypersensitivity to nilutamide or any component of the formulation; severe hepatic impairment; severe respiratory insufficiency

Warnings/Precautions Hazardous agent - use appropriate precautions for handling and disposal. **[U.S. Boxed Warning]: Interstitial pneumonitis has been reported in 2% of patients exposed to nilutamide.** Patients typically experienced progressive exertional dyspnea, and possibly cough, chest pain and fever. X-rays showed interstitial or alveolo-interstitial changes. The suggestive signs of pneumonitis most often occurred within the first 3 months of nilutamide treatment.

Hepatitis or marked increases in liver enzymes leading to drug discontinuation occurred in 1% of nilutamide patients. Rare cases of elevated hepatic enzymes followed by death have been reported.

13% to 57% of patients receiving nilutamide reported a delay in adaptation to the dark, ranging from seconds to a few minutes. This effect sometimes does not abate as drug treatment is continued. Caution patients who experience this effect about driving at night or through tunnels. This effect can be alleviated by wearing tinted glasses.

Adverse Reactions

>10%:

Central nervous system: Headache, insomnia

Endocrine & metabolic: Hot flashes (30% to 67%), gynecomastia (10%)

Gastrointestinal: Nausea (mild - 10% to 32%), abdominal pain (10%), constipation, anorexia

Genitourinary: Testicular atrophy (16%), libido decreased

Hepatic: Transaminases increased (8% to 13%; transient)

Ocular: Impaired dark adaptation (13% to 57%), usually reversible with dose reduction, may require discontinuation of the drug in 1% to 2% of patients

Respiratory: Dyspnea (11%)

1% to 10%:

Cardiovascular: Chest pain, edema, heart failure, hypertension, syncope

Central nervous system: Dizziness, drowsiness, malaise, hypoesthesia, depression

Dermatologic: Pruritus, alopecia, dry skin, rash

Endocrine & metabolic: Disulfiram-like reaction (hot flashes, rash) (5%); flu-like syndrome, fever

Gastrointestinal: Vomiting, diarrhea, dyspepsia, GI hemorrhage, melena, weight loss, xerostomia

Genitourinary: Hematuria, nocturia

Hematologic: Anemia

Hepatic: Hepatitis (1%)

Neuromuscular & skeletal: Arthritis, paresthesia

Ocular: Chromatopsia (9%), abnormal vision (6% to 7%), cataracts, photophobia

Respiratory: Interstitial pneumonitis (2% - typically exertional dyspnea, cough, chest pain, and fever; most often occurring within the first 3 months of treatment); rhinitis

Miscellaneous: Diaphoresis

<1% (Limited to important or life-threatening): Aplastic anemia

Drug Interactions

Metabolism/Transport Effects Substrate of CYP2C19 (major); **Inhibits** CYP2C19 (weak)

Avoid Concomitant Use There are no known interactions where it is recommended to avoid concomitant use.

Increased Effect/Toxicity

The levels/effects of Nilutamide may be increased by: CYP2C19 Inhibitors (Moderate); CYP2C19 Inhibitors (Strong)

Decreased Effect

The levels/effects of Nilutamide may be decreased by: CYP2C19 Inducers (Strong)

Ethanol/Nutrition/Herb Interactions

Ethanol: Avoid ethanol. Up to 5% of patients may experience a systemic reaction (flushing, hypotension, malaise) when combined with nilutamide.

Herb/Nutraceutical: St John's wort may decrease nilutamide levels.

Stability Store at room temperature of 15°C to 30°C (59°F to 86°F). Protect from light.

Mechanism of Action Nonsteroidal antiandrogen that inhibits androgen uptake or inhibits binding of androgen in target tissues. It specifically blocks the action of androgens by interacting with cytosolic androgen receptor F sites in target tissue

Pharmacodynamics/Kinetics

Absorption: Rapid and complete

Protein binding: 72% to 85%

Metabolism: Hepatic, forms active metabolites

Half-life elimination: Terminal: 23-87 hours; Metabolites: 35-137 hours

Excretion: Urine (up to 78% at 120 hours; <1% as unchanged drug); feces (1% to 7%)

Dosage Refer to individual protocols.

Adults: Oral: 300 mg daily for 30 days starting the same day or day after surgical castration, then 150 mg/day

Dietary Considerations May be taken without regard to food.

Monitoring Parameters Obtain a chest x-ray if a patient reports dyspnea; if there are findings suggestive of interstitial pneumonitis, discontinue treatment with nilutamide. Measure serum hepatic enzyme levels at baseline and at regular intervals (3 months); if transaminases increase over 2-3 times the upper limit of normal, discontinue treatment. Perform appropriate laboratory testing at the first symptom/sign of liver injury (eg, jaundice, dark urine, fatigue, abdominal pain or unexplained GI symptoms).

Dosage Forms Excipient information presented when available (limited, particularly for generics); consult specific product labeling.

Tablet: 150 mg

◆ **Nimbex®** *see* Cisatracurium *on page* 334

NiMODipine (nye MOE di peen)

U.S. Brand Names Nimotop® [DSC]

Canadian Brand Names Nimotop®

Pharmacologic Category Calcium Channel Blocker

Additional Appendix Information

Calcium Channel Blockers *on page* 1651

Use Spasm following subarachnoid hemorrhage from ruptured intracranial aneurysms regardless of the patients neurological condition postictus (Hunt and Hess grades I-V)

Pregnancy Risk Factor C

Pregnancy Considerations Use in pregnancy only when clearly needed and when the benefits outweigh the potential hazard to the fetus. Teratogenic and embryotoxic effects have been demonstrated in small animals. No well-controlled studies have been conducted in pregnant women.

Lactation Enters breast milk/not recommended

Medication Safety Issues

Sound-alike/look-alike issues:

NiMODipine may be confused with niCARdipine, NIFEdipine, nisoldipine

Administration issues: **For oral administration only.** For patients unable to swallow a capsule, the drug should be dispensed in an oral syringe labeled **"for oral use only."** Nimodipine has inadvertently been administered I.V. when withdrawn from capsules into a syringe for subsequent nasogastric administration. Severe cardiovascular adverse events, including fatalities, have resulted. Employ precautions against such an event.

Contraindications Hypersensitivity to nimodipine or any component of the formulation

Warnings/Precautions Increased angina and/or MI has occurred with initiation or dosage titration of calcium channel blockers. The most common side effect is peripheral edema; occurs within 2-3 weeks of starting therapy. Reflex tachycardia may occur with use. Symptomatic hypotension with or without syncope can rarely occur; blood pressure must be lowered at a rate appropriate for the patient's clinical condition. Use caution in hepatic impairment. Intestinal pseudo-obstruction and ileus have been reported during the use of nimodipine. Use caution in patients with decreased GI motility of a history of bowel obstruction. Use caution when treating patients with hypertrophic cardiomyopathy. Safety and efficacy have not been established in children.

[U.S. Boxed Warning]: Nimodipine has inadvertently been administered I.V. when withdrawn from capsules into a syringe for subsequent nasogastric administration. Severe cardiovascular adverse events, including fatalities, have resulted; precautions should be employed against such an event.

Adverse Reactions

1% to 10%:

Cardiovascular: Reductions in systemic blood pressure (1% to 8%)

Central nervous system: Headache (1% to 4%)

Dermatologic: Rash (1% to 2%)

Gastrointestinal: Diarrhea (2% to 4%), abdominal discomfort (2%)

<1% (Limited to important or life-threatening): Anemia, CHF, deep vein thrombosis, depression, disseminated intravascular coagulation, dyspnea, ECG abnormalities, GI hemorrhage, hemorrhage, hepatitis, jaundice, neurological deterioration, rebound vasospasm, thrombocytopenia, vomiting

Drug Interactions

Metabolism/Transport Effects Substrate of CYP3A4 (major)

Avoid Concomitant Use There are no known interactions where it is recommended to avoid concomitant use.

Increased Effect/Toxicity

NiMODipine may increase the levels/effects of: Amifostine; Magnesium Salts; Neuromuscular-Blocking Agents (Nondepolarizing); Nitroprusside; Phenytoin; RiTUXimab; Tacrolimus

The levels/effects of NiMODipine may be increased by: Alpha1-Blockers; Antifungal Agents (Azole Derivatives, Systemic); Calcium Channel Blockers (Nondihydropyridine); Cimetidine; CycloSPORINE; CYP3A4 Inhibitors (Moderate); CYP3A4 Inhibitors (Strong); Dasatinib; Diazoxide; Fluconazole; Grapefruit Juice; Herbs (Hypotensive Properties); Macrolide Antibiotics; Magnesium Salts; Prostacyclin Analogues; Protease Inhibitors; Quinupristin

Decreased Effect

NiMODipine may decrease the levels/effects of: Clopidogrel; QuiNIDine

The levels/effects of NiMODipine may be decreased by: Barbiturates; Calcium Salts; CarBAMazepine; CYP3A4 Inducers (Strong); Deferasirox; Herbs (CYP3A4 Inducers); Herbs (Hypertensive Properties); Methylphenidate; Nafcillin; Rifamycin Derivatives; Yohimbine

Ethanol/Nutrition/Herb Interactions

Food: Nimodipine has shown a 1.5-fold increase in bioavailability when taken with grapefruit juice; avoid concurrent use.

Herb/Nutraceutical: St John's wort may decrease levels. Avoid dong quai if using for hypertension (has estrogenic activity). Avoid ephedra, yohimbe, ginseng (may worsen hypertension). Avoid garlic (may have increased antihypertensive effect).

Mechanism of Action Nimodipine shares the pharmacology of other calcium channel blockers; animal studies indicate that nimodipine has a greater effect on cerebral arterials than other arterials; this increased specificity may be due to the drug's increased lipophilicity and cerebral distribution as compared to nifedipine; inhibits calcium ion from entering the "slow channels" or select voltage sensitive areas of vascular smooth muscle and myocardium during depolarization

Pharmacodynamics/Kinetics

Protein binding: >95%

Metabolism: Extensively hepatic

Bioavailability: 13%

Half-life elimination: 1-2 hours; prolonged with renal impairment

Time to peak, serum: ~1 hour

Excretion: Urine (50%) and feces (32%) within 4 days

Dosage Note: Capsules and contents are for oral administration **ONLY.**

Adults: Oral: 60 mg every 4 hours for 21 days, start therapy within 96 hours after subarachnoid hemorrhage.

Dialysis: Not removed by hemo- or peritoneal dialysis; supplemental dose is not necessary.

Dosing adjustment in hepatic impairment: Reduce dosage to 30 mg every 4 hours in patients with liver failure.

Administration For oral administration **ONLY.** If the capsules cannot be swallowed, the liquid may be removed by making a hole in each end of the capsule with an 18-gauge needle and extracting the contents into a syringe. If administered via NG tube, follow with a flush of 30 mL NS.

Dosage Forms Excipient information presented when available (limited, particularly for generics); consult specific product labeling. [DSC] = Discontinued product

Capsule, liquid filled: 30 mg

Nimotop®: 30 mg [DSC]

◆ **Nimotop® [DSC]** *see* NiMODipine *on page 1069*

◆ **Nimotop® (Can)** *see* NiMODipine *on page 1069*

◆ **Nipent®** *see* Pentostatin *on page 1171*

◆ **Niravam™** *see* ALPRAZolam *on page 68*

Nisoldipine (nye SOL di peen)

U.S. Brand Names Sular®

Pharmacologic Category Calcium Channel Blocker

Additional Appendix Information

Calcium Channel Blockers *on page 1651*

Use Management of hypertension, alone or in combination with other antihypertensive agents

Pregnancy Risk Factor C

Pregnancy Considerations Animal studies have demonstrated fetotoxic but not teratogenic effects. There are no adequate and well-controlled studies in pregnant women. Use during pregnancy only if potential benefit to the mother outweighs potential risk to the fetus.

Lactation Excretion in breast milk unknown/not recommended

Medication Safety Issues

Sound-alike/look-alike issues:

Nisoldipine may be confused with NIFEdipine, niMODipine

Contraindications Hypersensitivity to nisoldipine, any component of the formulation, or other dihydropyridine calcium channel blockers

Warnings/Precautions With initiation or dosage titration of dihydropyridine calcium channel blockers, reflex tachycardia may occur resulting in angina and/or MI in patients with obstructive coronary disease especially in the absence of concurrent beta-blockade. Use with caution in patients with severe aortic stenosis, HF, and hypertrophic cardiomyopathy with outflow tract obstruction. Use with caution in hepatic impairment; lower starting dose required. The most common side effect is peripheral edema; occurs within 2-3 weeks of starting therapy. Symptomatic hypotension with or without syncope can rarely occur; blood pressure must be lowered at a rate appropriate for the patient's clinical condition. Contains tartrazine, which may cause allergic reactions in certain individuals (eg, aspirin hypersensitivity). Use with caution in patients >65 years of age; lower starting dose recommended. Safety and efficacy have not been established in children.

Adverse Reactions

>10%:

Cardiovascular: Peripheral edema (dose related; 7% to 27%)

Central nervous system: Headache (22%)

1% to 10%:

Cardiovascular: Vasodilation (4%), palpitation (3%), angina exacerbation (2%), chest pain (2%)

Central nervous system: Dizziness (3% to 7%)

Dermatologic: Rash (2%)

Gastrointestinal: Nausea (2%)

Respiratory: Pharyngitis (5%), sinusitis (3%)

<1% (Limited to important or life-threatening): Alopecia, amblyopia, amnesia, anemia, angina, anxiety, arthralgia, arthritis, asthma, ataxia, atrial fibrillation, blepharitis, BUN increased, bruising, cellulitis, cerebral ischemia, chills, colitis, confusion, conjunctivitis, cough, creatinine increased, creatine kinase increased, CVA, depression, diabetes mellitus, diaphoresis, diarrhea, dyspepsia, dysphagia, dyspnea, dysuria, end inspiratory wheeze, epistaxis, exfoliative dermatitis, facial edema, fever, first-degree AV block, flu-like syndrome, fungal dermatitis, gastritis, gastrointestinal hemorrhage, gingival hyperplasia, glaucoma, glossitis, gout, gynecomastia, heart failure, hematuria, hepatomegaly, herpes simplex, herpes zoster; hypersensitivity reaction (eg, angioedema, shortness of breath, tachycardia, chest tightness, hypotension, and rash); hyper-/hypotension, hypertonia, hypoesthesia, hypokalemia, jugular venous distention, keratoconjunctivitis, laryngitis, leg cramps, leukopenia, libido decreased, liver function tests abnormal, maculopapular rash, malaise, melena, migraine, mouth ulceration, myalgia, myasthenia, MI, myositis, nervousness, nocturia, nonprotein nitrogen increased, otitis media, paresthesia, petechiae, photosensitivity, pleural effusion, postural hypotension, pruritus, pustular rash, rales, retinal detachment, skin discoloration, skin ulcer, somnolence, supraventricular tachycardia, syncope, systolic ejection murmur, temporary unilateral loss of vision, tenosynovitis, thyroiditis, tinnitus, tremor; T-wave abnormalities on ECG (flattening, inversion, nonspecific changes); urinary frequency, urticaria, vaginal hemorrhage, vaginitis, venous insufficiency, ventricular extrasystoles, vertigo, vision abnormal, vitreous floater, weight gain/loss, xerostomia

Drug Interactions

Metabolism/Transport Effects Substrate of CYP3A4 (major); **Inhibits** CYP1A2 (weak), 3A4 (weak)

Avoid Concomitant Use

Avoid concomitant use of Nisoldipine with any of the following: CYP3A4 Inducers (Strong); CYP3A4 Inhibitors (Strong)

Increased Effect/Toxicity

Nisoldipine may increase the levels/effects of: Amifostine; Magnesium Salts; Neuromuscular-Blocking Agents (Nondepolarizing); Nitroprusside; Phenytoin; RiTUXimab; Tacrolimus

The levels/effects of Nisoldipine may be increased by: Alpha1-Blockers; Antifungal Agents (Azole Derivatives, Systemic); Calcium Channel Blockers (Nondihydropyridine); Cimetidine; CycloSPORINE; CYP3A4 Inhibitors (Moderate); CYP3A4 Inhibitors (Strong); Dasatinib; Diazoxide; Fluconazole; Grapefruit Juice; Herbs (Hypotensive Properties); Macrolide Antibiotics; Magnesium Salts; Prostacyclin Analogues; Protease Inhibitors; Quinupristin

Decreased Effect

Nisoldipine may decrease the levels/effects of: Clopidogrel

The levels/effects of Nisoldipine may be decreased by: Barbiturates; Calcium Salts; CarBAMazepine; CYP3A4 Inducers (Strong); Deferasirox; Herbs (CYP3A4 Inducers); Herbs (Hypertensive Properties); Methylphenidate; Nafcillin; Rifamycin Derivatives; Yohimbine

Ethanol/Nutrition/Herb Interactions

Food: Nisoldipine bioavailability may be increased if taken with high-lipid foods or with grapefruit juice. Avoid grapefruit products before and after dosing.

Herb/Nutraceutical: Avoid St John's wort (may decrease nisoldipine levels). Avoid bayberry, blue cohosh, cayenne, ephedra, ginger, ginseng (American), kola, licorice (may worsen hypertension). Avoid black cohosh, California poppy, coleus, golden seal, hawthorn, mistletoe, periwinkle, quinine, shepherd's purse (may have increased antihypertensive effect).

Stability Store at controlled room temperature of 20°C to 25°C (68°F to 77°F). Protect from light; protect from moisture.

Mechanism of Action As a dihydropyridine calcium channel blocker, structurally similar to nifedipine, nisoldipine impedes the movement of calcium ions into vascular smooth muscle and cardiac muscle. Dihydropyridines are potent vasodilators and are not as likely to suppress cardiac contractility and slow cardiac conduction as other calcium antagonists such as verapamil and diltiazem; nisoldipine is 5-10 times as potent a vasodilator as nifedipine.

Pharmacodynamics/Kinetics

Duration: >24 hours

Absorption: Well absorbed

Protein binding: >99%

Metabolism: Extensively hepatic; 1 active metabolite (10% of parent); first-pass effect

Bioavailability: ~5%

Half-life elimination: 9-18 hours

Time to peak: 4-14 hours

Excretion: Urine (as metabolites)

Dosage Oral:

Adults: Initial: 17 mg once daily, then increase by 8.5 mg/week (or longer intervals) to attain adequate control of blood pressure; usual dose range: 17-34 mg once daily; doses >34 mg once daily are not recommended.

Elderly: Initial dose: 8.5 mg/day, increase by 8.5 mg/week (or longer intervals) to attain adequate blood pressure control

Dosage adjustment in hepatic impairment: A starting dose not exceeding 8.5 mg/day is recommended.

Dietary Considerations Take on an empty stomach (1 hour before or 2 hours after a meal).

Administration Administer at the same time each day to ensure minimal fluctuation of serum levels. Avoid high-fat diet. Administer on an empty stomach (1 hour before or 2 hours after a meal). Swallow whole; do not crush, break, split, or chew.

Monitoring Parameters Blood pressure, heart rate

Dosage Forms Excipient information presented when available (limited, particularly for generics); consult specific product labeling.

Tablet, extended release [original formulation]: 20 mg, 30 mg, 40 mg

Sular®: 10 mg, 20 mg, 30 mg 40 mg [DSC]

Tablet, extended release [Geomatrix® delivery system]:

Sular®: 8.5 mg; 17 mg [contains tartrazine]; 25.5 mg, 34 mg

◆ **Nitalapram** *see* Citalopram *on page* 337

Nitazoxanide (nye ta ZOX a nide)

U.S. Brand Names Alinia®

Index Terms NTZ

Pharmacologic Category Antiprotozoal

Use Treatment of diarrhea caused by *Cryptosporidium parvum* or *Giardia lamblia*

Pregnancy Risk Factor B

Pregnancy Considerations Teratogenic effects were not observed in animal studies. There are no adequate and well-controlled studies in pregnant women.

Lactation Excretion in breast milk unknown/use caution

Contraindications Hypersensitivity to nitazoxanide or any component of the formulation

Warnings/Precautions Use caution with renal or hepatic impairment. Safety and efficacy have not been established with HIV infection, immunodeficiency, or in children <1 year of age (suspension) and <12 years of age (tablet).

Adverse Reactions Rates of adverse effects were similar to those reported with placebo.

1% to 10%:

Central nervous system: Headache (1% to 3%)

Gastrointestinal: Abdominal pain (7% to 8%), diarrhea (2% to 4%), nausea (3%), vomiting (1%)

<1% (Limited to important or life-threatening): Allergic reaction, ALT increased, anemia, anorexia, appetite increased, creatinine increased, diaphoresis, dizziness, eye discoloration (pale yellow), fever, flatulence, hypertension, infection, malaise, nausea, pruritus, rhinitis, salivary glands enlarged, tachycardia, urine discoloration

Drug Interactions

Avoid Concomitant Use There are no known interactions where it is recommended to avoid concomitant use.

Increased Effect/Toxicity There are no known significant interactions involving an increase in effect.

Decreased Effect There are no known significant interactions involving a decrease in effect.

Ethanol/Nutrition/Herb Interactions Food: Food increases AUC.

Stability

Suspension: Prior to and following reconstitution, store at room temperature of 15°C to 30°C (59°F to 86°F). For preparation at time of dispensing, add 48 mL incrementally to 60 mL bottle; shake vigorously. Resulting suspension is 20 mg/mL (100 mg per 5 mL). Following reconstitution, discard unused portion of suspension after 7 days.

Tablet: Store at room temperature.

Mechanism of Action Nitazoxanide is rapidly metabolized to the active metabolite tizoxanide *in vivo*. Activity may be due to interference with the pyruvate:ferredoxin oxidoreductase (PFOR) enzyme-dependent electron transfer reaction which is essential to anaerobic metabolism. *In vitro*, nitazoxanide and tizoxanide inhibit the growth of sporozoites and oocysts of *Cryptosporidium parvum* and trophozoites of *Giardia lamblia*.

Pharmacodynamics/Kinetics

Protein binding: Tizoxanide: >99%

Bioavailability: Relative bioavailability of suspension compared to tablet: 70%

Metabolism: Hepatic, to an active metabolite, tizoxanide. Tizoxanide undergoes conjugation to form tizoxanide glucuronide. Nitazoxanide is not detectable in the serum following oral administration.

Time to peak, plasma: Tizoxanide and tizoxanide glucuronide: 1-4 hours

Excretion: Tizoxanide: Urine, bile, and feces; Tizoxanide glucuronide: Urine and bile

Dosage Diarrhea caused by *Cryptosporidium parvum* or *Giardia lamblia*:

Children 1-3 years: 100 mg every 12 hours for 3 days

Children 4-11 years: 200 mg every 12 hours for 3 days

Children ≥12 years and Adults: 500 mg every 12 hours for 3 days

Dosage adjustment in renal/hepatic impairment: Specific recommendations are not available; use with caution

Dietary Considerations Should be taken with food. Suspension contains sucrose 1.48 g/5 mL.

Administration Administer with food. Shake suspension well prior to administration.

Dosage Forms Excipient information presented when available (limited, particularly for generics); consult specific product labeling.

Powder for suspension, oral: 100 mg/5 mL (60 mL) [contains sucrose 1.48 g/5 mL, sodium benzoate; strawberry flavor]

Tablet: 500 mg

Alinia® 3-Day Therapy Packs™ [unit-dose pack]: 500 mg (6s)

Nitisinone (ni TIS i known)

U.S. Brand Names Orfadin®

Pharmacologic Category 4-Hydroxyphenylpyruvate Dioxygenase Inhibitor

Use Treatment of hereditary tyrosinemia type 1 (HT-1); to be used with dietary restriction of tyrosine and phenylalanine

Restrictions Distributed by Rare Disease Therapeutics, Inc (contact 615-399-0700)

Pregnancy Risk Factor C

Dosage Oral: **Note:** Must be used in conjunction with a low protein diet restricted in tyrosine and phenylalanine.

Infants: See dosing for Children and Adults; infants may require maximal dose once liver function has improved

Children and Adults: Initial: 1 mg/kg/day in divided doses, given in the morning and evening, 1 hour before meals; doses do not need to be divided evenly

Dose adjustment: If biochemical parameters are not normalized within in 1-month period, dose may be increased to 1.5 mg/kg/day (maximum dose: 2 mg/kg/day).

Additional Information Complete prescribing information for this medication should be consulted for additional detail.

Dosage Forms Excipient information presented when available (limited, particularly for generics); consult specific product labeling.

Capsule: 2 mg, 5 mg, 10 mg

- **Nitoman™ (Can)** *see* Tetrabenazine *on page 1450*
- **Nitrek® [DSC]** *see* Nitroglycerin *on page 1073*
- **4′-Nitro-3′-Trifluoromethylisobutyrantide** *see* Flutamide *on page 643*
- **Nitro-Bid®** *see* Nitroglycerin *on page 1073*
- **Nitro-Dur®** *see* Nitroglycerin *on page 1073*

Nitrofurantoin (nye troe fyoor AN toyn)

U.S. Brand Names Furadantin®; Macrobid®; Macrodantin®

Canadian Brand Names Apo-Nitrofurantoin®; Macrobid®; Macrodantin®; Novo-Furantoin

Pharmacologic Category Antibiotic, Miscellaneous

Additional Appendix Information

Antimicrobial Drugs of Choice *on page 1752*

Use Prevention and treatment of urinary tract infections caused by susceptible strains of *E. coli*, *S. aureus*, *Enterococcus*, *Klebsiella*, and *Enterobacter*

Pregnancy Risk Factor B (contraindicated at term)

Pregnancy Considerations Teratogenic effects have not been observed in animal studies, however, may cause hemolytic anemia in infants. Use of nitrofurantoin is contraindicated at term (38-42 weeks gestation), during labor and delivery, or when the onset of labor is imminent.

Lactation Enters breast milk/not recommended (infants <1 month); AAP rates "compatible"

Medication Safety Issues

International issues:

Macrobid® may be confused with Mikrozid® which is a brand name for ethanol/propanol combination in Great Britain

Contraindications Hypersensitivity to nitrofurantoin or any component of the formulation; renal impairment (anuria, oliguria, significantly elevated serum creatinine, or Cl_{cr} <60 mL/minute); infants <1 month (due to the possibility of hemolytic anemia); pregnancy at term (38-42 weeks gestation), during labor and delivery, or when the onset of labor is imminent

Warnings/Precautions Use with caution in patients with G6PD deficiency or in patients with anemia. Therapeutic concentrations of nitrofurantoin are not attained in urine of patients with Cl_{cr} <60 mL/minute. Use with caution if prolonged therapy is anticipated due to possible pulmonary toxicity. Acute, subacute, or chronic (usually after 6 months of therapy) pulmonary reactions have been observed in patients treated with nitrofurantoin; if these occur, discontinue therapy immediately; monitor closely for malaise, dyspnea, cough, fever, radiologic evidence of diffuse interstitial pneumonitis or fibrosis. Rare, but severe hepatic reactions have been associated with nitrofurantoin (onset may be insidious); discontinue immediately if hepatitis occurs. Has been associated with peripheral neuropathy (rare); risk may be increased by renal impairment, diabetes, vitamin B deficiency, or electrolyte imbalance; use caution. Prolonged use may result in fungal or bacterial superinfection, including *C. difficile*-associated diarrhea (CDAD) and pseudomembranous colitis; CDAD has been observed >2 months postantibiotic treatment. Safety and efficacy have not been established in children <1 month of age.

Adverse Reactions Frequency not defined.

Cardiovascular: Chest pain, cyanosis, ECG changes

Central nervous system: Bulging fontanels (infants), chills, confusion, depression, dizziness, drowsiness, fever, headache, malaise, pseudotumor cerebri, psychotic reaction, vertigo

Dermatologic: Alopecia, angioedema, erythema multiforme, exfoliative dermatitis, pruritus, rash (eczematous, erythematous, maculopapular), Stevens-Johnson syndrome, urticaria

Gastrointestinal: Abdominal pain, *C. difficile* colitis, constipation, diarrhea, dyspepsia, flatulence, nausea, pancreatitis, sialadenitis, vomiting

Hematologic: Agranulocytosis, eosinophilia, granulocytopenia, hemolytic anemia, leukopenia, megaloblastic anemia, thrombocytopenia

Hepatic: Cholestasis, hepatitis, hepatic necrosis, transaminases increased, jaundice (cholestatic)

Neuromuscular & skeletal: Arthralgia, myalgia, numbness, paresthesia, peripheral neuropathy, weakness

Ocular: Amblyopia, nystagmus, optic neuritis

Respiratory: Cough, dyspnea, pneumonitis, pulmonary fibrosis (with long-term use), pulmonary infiltration

Miscellaneous: Anaphylaxis, hypersensitivity (including acute pulmonary hypersensitivity), lupus-like syndrome

Drug Interactions

Avoid Concomitant Use

Avoid concomitant use of Nitrofurantoin with any of the following: Norfloxacin

Increased Effect/Toxicity There are no known significant interactions involving an increase in effect.

Decreased Effect

Nitrofurantoin may decrease the levels/effects of: Norfloxacin; Typhoid Vaccine

Ethanol/Nutrition/Herb Interactions

Ethanol: Avoid ethanol (may increase CNS depression).

Food: Nitrofurantoin serum concentrations may be increased if taken with food.

Stability Store at room temperature 15°C to 30°C (59°F to 86°F).

Mechanism of Action Inhibits several bacterial enzyme systems including acetyl coenzyme A interfering with metabolism and possibly cell wall synthesis

Pharmacodynamics/Kinetics

Absorption: Well absorbed; macrocrystalline form absorbed more slowly due to slower dissolution (causes less GI distress)

Distribution: V_d: 0.8 L/kg; crosses placenta; enters breast milk

Protein binding: 60% to 90%

Metabolism: Body tissues (except plasma) metabolize 60% of drug to inactive metabolites

Bioavailability: Increased with food

Half-life elimination: 20-60 minutes; prolonged with renal impairment

Excretion:

Suspension: Urine (40%) and feces (small amounts) as metabolites and unchanged drug

Macrocrystals: Urine (20% to 25% as unchanged drug)

Dosage Oral:

Children >1 month:

UTI treatment (Furadantin®, Macrodantin®): 5-7 mg/kg/day in divided doses every 6 hours; maximum: 400 mg/day. Administer for 7 days or at least 3 days after obtaining sterile urine

UTI prophylaxis (Furadantin®, Macrodantin®): 1-2 mg/kg/day in divided doses every 12-24 hours; maximum: 100 mg/day

Children >12 years: UTI treatment (Macrobid®): 100 mg twice daily for 7 days

Adults:

UTI treatment:

Furadantin®, Macrodantin®: 50-100 mg/dose every 6 hours; administer for 7 days or at least 3 days after obtaining sterile urine

Macrobid®: 100 mg twice daily for 7 days

UTI prophylaxis (Furadantin®, Macrodantin®): 50-100 mg/dose at bedtime

Dosing adjustment in renal impairment: Cl_{cr} <60 mL/minute: Contraindicated

Contraindicated in hemo- and peritoneal dialysis and continuous arteriovenous or venovenous hemofiltration

Administration Administer with meals to improve absorption and decrease adverse effects; suspension may be mixed with water, milk, fruit juice, or infant formula. Shake suspension well before use.

Monitoring Parameters Signs of pulmonary reaction, signs of numbness or tingling of the extremities, periodic liver function tests

Test Interactions False-positive urine glucose (Benedict's and Fehling's methods); no false positives with enzymatic tests

Dosage Forms Excipient information presented when available (limited, particularly for generics); consult specific product labeling.

Capsule [macrocrystal]: 50 mg, 100 mg

Macrodantin®: 25 mg, 50 mg, 100 mg

Capsule [macrocrystal/monohydrate]: 100 mg [nitrofurantoin macrocrystal 25% and nitrofurantoin monohydrate 75%]

Macrobid®: 100 mg [nitrofurantoin macrocrystal 25% and nitrofurantoin monohydrate 75%]

Suspension, oral:

Furadantin®: 25 mg/5 mL (470 mL)

◆ **Nitrogen Mustard** *see* Mechlorethamine *on page 927*

Nitroglycerin (nye troe GLI ser in)

U.S. Brand Names Minitran™; Nitrek® [DSC]; Nitro-Bid®; Nitro-Dur®; Nitrolingual®; NitroQuick®; Nitrostat®; NitroTime®

Canadian Brand Names Gen-Nitro; Minitran™; Nitro-Dur®; Nitroglycerin Injection, USP; Nitrol®; Nitrostat™; Rho®-Nitro; Transderm-Nitro®; Trinipatch® 0.2; Trinipatch® 0.4; Trinipatch® 0.6

Index Terms Glyceryl Trinitrate; Nitroglycerol; NTG

Pharmacologic Category Vasodilator

Additional Appendix Information

Hemodynamic Support, Intravenous *on page 1657*

Hypertension *on page 1820*

Nitrates *on page 1668*

Use Treatment of angina pectoris; I.V. for congestive heart failure (especially when associated with acute myocardial infarction); pulmonary hypertension; hypertensive emergencies occurring perioperatively (especially during cardiovascular surgery)

Unlabeled/Investigational Use Esophageal spastic disorders (sublingual)

Pregnancy Risk Factor C

Lactation Excretion in breast milk unknown/use caution

Medication Safety Issues

Sound-alike/look-alike issues:

Nitroglycerin may be confused with nitroprusside

Nitro-Bid® may be confused with Nicobid®

Nitroderm may be confused with NicoDerm®

Nitrol® may be confused with Nizoral®

Nitrostat® may be confused with Nilstat®, nystatin

Nitroglycerin transdermal patches should be removed prior to defibrillation or MRI study.

International issues:

Nitrocor® [Chile and Italy] may be confused with Natrecor® which is a brand name for nesiritide in the U.S.

Nitrocor® [Chile and Italy] may be confused with Nutracort® which is a brand name for hydrocortisone in the U.S.

Nitro-Dur® may be confused with Nitrocor® [Chile and Italy]

Contraindications Hypersensitivity to organic nitrates; hypersensitivity to isosorbide, nitroglycerin, or any component of the formulation; concurrent use with phosphodiesterase-5 (PDE-5) inhibitors (sildenafil, tadalafil, or vardenafil); angle-closure glaucoma (intraocular pressure may be increased); head trauma or cerebral hemorrhage (increase intracranial pressure); severe anemia; allergy to adhesive (transdermal product)

Additional contraindications for I.V. product: Hypotension; uncorrected hypovolemia; inadequate cerebral circulation; constrictive pericarditis; pericardial tamponade

Warnings/Precautions Severe hypotension can occur. Use with caution in volume depletion, hypotension, and right ventricular infarctions. Paradoxical bradycardia and increased angina pectoris can accompany hypotension. Orthostatic hypotension can also occur. Ethanol can accentuate this. Tolerance does develop to nitrates and appropriate dosing is needed to minimize this (drug-free interval). Avoid use of long-acting agents in acute MI or HF; cannot easily reverse. Nitrate may aggravate angina caused by hypertrophic cardiomyopathy. Nitroglycerin transdermal patches should be removed prior to defibrillation or MRI study. Avoid concurrent use with PDE-5 inhibitors. Safety and efficacy have not been established in children.

Adverse Reactions

Frequency not always defined:

Cardiovascular: Hypotension (4%), postural hypotension, crescendo angina (2%), tachycardia, flushing, peripheral edema

Central nervous system: Headache (most common; 50% to 63%), lightheadedness (6%), syncope (4%), dizziness

Gastrointestinal: Nausea, vomiting, bowel incontinence, xerostomia

Genitourinary: Urinary incontinence

Ocular: Blurred vision

Miscellaneous: Diaphoresis

<1% (Limited to important or life-threatening): Allergic reactions, application site irritation (patch), cardiovascular collapse, exfoliative dermatitis, methemoglobinemia (rare; overdose), pallor, palpitation, rash, rebound hypertension, restlessness, shock, vertigo, weakness

Drug Interactions

Avoid Concomitant Use

Avoid concomitant use of Nitroglycerin with any of the following: Phosphodiesterase 5 Inhibitors

Increased Effect/Toxicity

Nitroglycerin may increase the levels/effects of: Amifostine; RiTUXimab; Rosiglitazone

The levels/effects of Nitroglycerin may be increased by: Diazoxide; Herbs (Hypotensive Properties); Phosphodiesterase 5 Inhibitors; Prostacyclin Analogues

Decreased Effect

Nitroglycerin may decrease the levels/effects of: Alteplase; Heparin

The levels/effects of Nitroglycerin may be decreased by: Herbs (Hypertensive Properties); Methylphenidate; Yohimbine

Ethanol/Nutrition/Herb Interactions

Ethanol: Avoid ethanol (may increase the hypotensive effects of nitroglycerin). Monitor.

Herb/Nutraceutical: Avoid bayberry, blue cohosh, cayenne, ephedra, ginger, ginseng (american), kola, licorice (may worsen hypertension). Avoid black cohosh, California poppy, coleus, golden seal, hawthorn, mistletoe, periwinkle, quinine, shepherd's purse (may cause hypotension).

Stability Doses should be made in glass bottles, Excell® or PAB® containers. Adsorption occurs to soft plastic (ie, PVC).

Nitroglycerin diluted in D_5W or NS in glass containers is physically and chemically stable for 48 hours at room temperature and 7 days under refrigeration. In D_5W or NS in Excell®/PAB® containers it is physically and chemically stable for 24 hours at room temperature and 14 days under refrigeration.

Premixed bottles are stable according to the manufacturer's expiration dating.

Standard diluent: 50 mg/250 mL D_5W; 50 mg/500 mL D_5W.

Minimum volume: 100 mg/250 mL D_5W; concentration should not exceed 400 mcg/mL.

Store sublingual tablets and ointment in tightly closed containers at 15°C to 30°C. Store spray and transdermal patch at 25°C; excursions permitted to 15°C to 30°C (59°F to 86°F).

Mechanism of Action Works by relaxation of smooth muscle, producing a vasodilator effect on the peripheral veins and arteries with more prominent effects on the veins. Primarily reduces cardiac oxygen demand by decreasing preload (left ventricular end-diastolic pressure); may modestly reduce afterload; dilates coronary arteries and improves collateral flow to ischemic regions

Pharmacodynamics/Kinetics

Onset of action: Sublingual tablet: 1-3 minutes; Translingual spray: 2 minutes; Sustained release: 20-45 minutes; Topical: 15-60 minutes; Transdermal: 40-60 minutes; I.V. drip: Immediate

Peak effect: Sublingual tablet: 4-8 minutes; Translingual spray: 4-10 minutes; Sustained release: 45-120 minutes; Topical: 30-120 minutes; Transdermal: 60-180 minutes; I.V. drip: Immediate

Duration: Sublingual tablet: 30-60 minutes; Translingual spray: 30-60 minutes; Sustained release: 4-8 hours; Topical: 2-12 hours; Transdermal: 18-24 hours; I.V. drip: 3-5 minutes

Protein binding: 60%

Metabolism: Extensive first-pass effect

Half-life elimination: 1-4 minutes

Excretion: Urine (as inactive metabolites)

Dosage Note: Hemodynamic and antianginal tolerance often develop within 24-48 hours of continuous nitrate administration. Nitrate-free interval (10-12 hours/day) is recommended to avoid tolerance development; gradually decrease dose in patients receiving NTG for prolonged period to avoid withdrawal reaction.

Children: Pulmonary hypertension: Continuous infusion: Start 0.25-0.5 mcg/kg/minute and titrate by 1 mcg/kg/minute at 20- to 60-minute intervals to desired effect; usual dose: 1-3 mcg/kg/minute; maximum: 5 mcg/kg/minute

Adults:

Oral: 2.5-9 mg 2-4 times/day (up to 26 mg 4 times/day)

I.V.: 5 mcg/minute, increase by 5 mcg/minute every 3-5 minutes to 20 mcg/minute; if no response at 20 mcg/minute increase by 10 mcg/minute every 3-5 minutes, up to 200 mcg/minute

Ointment: 1/2" upon rising and 1/2" 6 hours later; the dose may be doubled and even doubled again as needed

Patch, transdermal: Initial: 0.2-0.4 mg/hour, titrate to doses of 0.4-0.8 mg/hour; tolerance is minimized by using a patch-on period of 12-14 hours and patch-off period of 10-12 hours

Sublingual: 0.2-0.6 mg every 5 minutes for maximum of 3 doses in 15 minutes; may also use prophylactically 5-10 minutes prior to activities which may provoke an attack

Esophageal spastic disorders (unlabeled use): 0.3-0.4 mg 5 minutes before meals

Translingual: 1-2 sprays into mouth under tongue every 3-5 minutes for maximum of 3 doses in 15 minutes, may also be used 5-10 minutes prior to activities which may provoke an attack prophylactically

Hemodialysis: Supplemental dose is not necessary

Peritoneal dialysis: Supplemental dose is not necessary

Elderly: In general, dose selection should be cautious, usually starting at the low end of the dosing range

Administration

I.V.: I.V. must be prepared in glass bottles; use special sets intended for nitroglycerin. Glass I.V. bottles and administration sets provided by manufacturer.

Sublingual: Do not crush sublingual product (tablet). Place under tongue and allow to dissolve.

Translingual spray: Do not shake container. Release spray onto or under tongue. Do not rinse the mouth for at least 5-10 minutes. Priming sprays should be directed away from patient and others. The end of the pump should be covered by the fluid in the bottle.

Nitrolingual®: Prime prior to first use (5 sprays into the air). If unused for 6 weeks, a single priming spray should be completed.

Monitoring Parameters Blood pressure, heart rate

Additional Information I.V. preparations contain alcohol and/or propylene glycol; may need to use nitrate-free interval (10-12 hours/day) to avoid tolerance development. Tolerance may possibly be reversed with acetylcysteine; gradually decrease dose in patients receiving NTG for prolonged period to avoid withdrawal reaction.

Concomitant use of sildenafil (Viagra®) or other phosphodiesterase-5 enzyme inhibitors (PDE-5) may precipitate acute hypotension, myocardial infarction, or death. Nitrates used in right ventricular infarction may induce acute hypotension. Nitrate use in severe pericardial effusion may reduce cardiac filling pressure and precipitate cardiac tamponade. In the management of heart failure, the combination of isosorbide dinitrate and hydralazine confers beneficial effects on disease progression and cardiac outcomes.

Dosage Forms Excipient information presented when available (limited, particularly for generics); consult specific product labeling.

Capsule, extended release: 2.5 mg, 6.5 mg, 9 mg

Nitro-Time®: 2.5 mg, 6.5 mg, 9 mg

Infusion [premixed in D_5W]: 25 mg (250 mL) [0.1 mg/mL]; 50 mg (250 mL) [0.2 mg/mL]; 50 mg (500 mL) [0.1 mg/mL]; 100 mg (250 mL) [0.4 mg/mL]; 200 mg (500 mL) [0.4 mg/mL]

Injection, solution: 5 mg/mL (5 mL, 10 mL) [contains ethanol and propylene glycol]

Ointment, topical:

Nitro-Bid®: 2% [20 mg/g] (1 g, 30 g, 60 g)

Solution, translingual [spray]:
Nitrolingual®: 0.4 mg/metered spray (4.9 g) [contains ethanol 20%; 60 metered sprays]; (12 g) [contains ethanol 20%; 200 metered sprays]; (16.9 g) [contains ethanol 20%; 260 metered sprays]
Tablet, sublingual: 0.3 mg, 0.4 mg, 0.6 mg
NitroQuick®, Nitrostat®: 0.3 mg, 0.4 mg, 0.6 mg
Transdermal system [once-daily patch]: 0.1 mg/hour (30s); 0.2 mg/hour (30s); 0.4 mg/hour (30s); 0.6 mg/hour (30s)
Minitran™: 0.1 mg/hour (30s); 0.2 mg/hour (30s); 0.4 mg/hour (30s); 0.6 mg/hour (30s)
Nitrek®: 0.2 mg/hour (30s); 0.4 mg/hour (30s); 0.6 mg/hour (30s) [DSC]
Nitro-Dur®: 0.1 mg/hour (30s); 0.2 mg/hour (30s); 0.3 mg/hour (30s); 0.4 mg/hour (30s); 0.6 mg/hour (30s); 0.8 mg/hour (30s)

◆ **Nitroglycerin Injection, USP (Can)** *see* Nitroglycerin *on page 1073*

◆ **Nitroglycerol** *see* Nitroglycerin *on page 1073*

◆ **Nitrol® (Can)** *see* Nitroglycerin *on page 1073*

◆ **Nitrolingual®** *see* Nitroglycerin *on page 1073*

◆ **Nitropress®** *see* Nitroprusside *on page 1075*

Nitroprusside (nye troe PRUS ide)

U.S. Brand Names Nitropress®

Index Terms Nitroprusside Sodium; Sodium Nitroferricyanide; Sodium Nitroprusside

Pharmacologic Category Vasodilator

Additional Appendix Information

Hemodynamic Support, Intravenous *on page 1657*
Hypertension *on page 1820*

Use Management of hypertensive crises; congestive heart failure; used for controlled hypotension to reduce bleeding during surgery

Pregnancy Risk Factor C

Lactation Excretion in breast milk unknown

Medication Safety Issues

Sound-alike/look-alike issues:
Nitroprusside may be confused with nitroglycerin

High alert medication: The Institute for Safe Medication Practices (ISMP) includes this medication among its list of drugs which have a heightened risk of causing significant patient harm when used in error.

Contraindications Hypersensitivity to nitroprusside or any component of the formulation; treatment of compensatory hypertension (aortic coarctation, arteriovenous shunting); high output failure; congenital optic atrophy or tobacco amblyopia

Warnings/Precautions [U.S. Boxed Warning]: Continuous blood pressure monitoring is needed. Except when used briefly or at low (<2 mcg/kg/minute) infusion rates, nitroprusside gives rise to large cyanide quantities. Do not use the maximum dose for more than 10 minutes; if blood pressure not controlled then discontinue infusion. Monitor for cyanide toxicity via acid-base balance and venous oxygen concentration. Use with extreme caution in patients with elevated intracranial pressure (head trauma, cerebral hemorrhage), severe renal impairment, hepatic failure, hypothyroidism. Use the lowest end of the dosage range with renal impairment. Cyanide toxicity may occur in patients with decreased liver function. Thiocyanate toxicity occurs in patients with renal impairment or those on prolonged infusions. **[U.S. Boxed Warning]: Should not be administered by direct injection; must be further diluted with 5% dextrose in water.**

Adverse Reactions 1% to 10%:

Cardiovascular: Excessive hypotensive response, palpitation, substernal distress
Central nervous system: Disorientation, psychosis, headache, restlessness
Endocrine & metabolic: Thyroid suppression
Gastrointestinal: Nausea, vomiting
Neuromuscular & skeletal: Weakness, muscle spasm
Otic: Tinnitus
Respiratory: Hypoxia
Miscellaneous: Diaphoresis, thiocyanate toxicity

Drug Interactions

Avoid Concomitant Use There are no known interactions where it is recommended to avoid concomitant use.

Increased Effect/Toxicity

Nitroprusside may increase the levels/effects of: Amifostine; RiTUXimab

The levels/effects of Nitroprusside may be increased by: Calcium Channel Blockers; Diazoxide; Herbs (Hypotensive Properties); Prostacyclin Analogues

Decreased Effect

The levels/effects of Nitroprusside may be decreased by: Herbs (Hypertensive Properties); Methylphenidate; Yohimbine

Stability

Nitroprusside sodium should be reconstituted freshly by diluting 50 mg in 250-1000 mL of D_5W.

Use only clear solutions; solutions of nitroprusside exhibit a color described as brownish, brown, brownish-pink, light orange, and straw. Solutions are highly sensitive to light. Exposure to light causes decomposition, resulting in a highly colored solution of orange, dark brown or blue. **A blue color indicates almost complete degradation and breakdown to cyanide.**

Solutions should be wrapped with aluminum foil or other opaque material to protect from light (do as soon as possible).

Stability of parenteral admixture at room temperature (25°C) and at refrigeration temperature (4°C) is 24 hours.

Mechanism of Action Causes peripheral vasodilation by direct action on venous and arteriolar smooth muscle, thus reducing peripheral resistance; will increase cardiac output by decreasing afterload; reduces aortal and left ventricular impedance

Pharmacodynamics/Kinetics

Onset of action: BP reduction <2 minutes
Duration: 1-10 minutes
Metabolism: Nitroprusside is converted to cyanide ions in the bloodstream; decomposes to prussic acid which in the presence of sulfur donor is converted to thiocyanate (hepatic and renal rhodanase systems)
Half-life elimination: Parent drug: <10 minutes; Thiocyanate: 2.7-7 days
Excretion: Urine (as thiocyanate)

Dosage Administration requires the use of an infusion pump. Average dose: 5 mcg/kg/minute.

Children: Pulmonary hypertension: I.V.: Initial: 1 mcg/kg/minute by continuous I.V. infusion; increase in increments of 1 mcg/kg/minute at intervals of 20-60 minutes; titrating to the desired response; usual dose: 3 mcg/kg/minute, rarely need >4 mcg/kg/minute; maximum: 5 mcg/kg/minute.

Adults: I.V. Initial: 0.3-0.5 mcg/kg/minute; increase in increments of 0.5 mcg/kg/minute, titrating to the desired hemodynamic effect or the appearance of headache or nausea; usual dose: 3 mcg/kg/minute; rarely need >4 mcg/kg/minute; maximum: 10 mcg/kg/minute. When administered by prolonged infusion faster than 2 mcg/kg/minute, cyanide is generated faster than an unaided patient can handle.

Administration I.V. infusion only, not for direct injection

Monitoring Parameters Blood pressure, heart rate; monitor for cyanide and thiocyanate toxicity; monitor acid-base status as acidosis can be the earliest sign of cyanide toxicity; monitor thiocyanate levels if requiring prolonged infusion (>3 days) or dose ≥4 mcg/kg/minute or patient has renal dysfunction; monitor cyanide blood levels in patients with decreased hepatic function; cardiac monitor and blood pressure monitor required

Reference Range Monitor thiocyanate levels if requiring prolonged infusion (>4 days) or ≥4 mcg/kg/minute; not to exceed 100 mcg/mL (or 10 mg/dL) plasma thiocyanate

Thiocyanate:
- Therapeutic: 6-29 mcg/mL
- Toxic: 35-100 mcg/mL
- Fatal: >200 mcg/mL

Cyanide: Normal <0.2 mcg/mL; normal (smoker): <0.4 mcg/mL
- Toxic: >2 mcg/mL
- Potentially lethal: >3 mcg/mL

Dosage Forms Excipient information presented when available (limited, particularly for generics); consult specific product labeling.

Injection, solution, as sodium: 25 mg/mL (2 mL)

◆ **Nitroprusside Sodium** *see* Nitroprusside *on page* 1075

◆ **NitroQuick®** *see* Nitroglycerin *on page* 1073

◆ **Nitrostat®** *see* Nitroglycerin *on page* 1073

◆ **Nitrostat™ (Can)** *see* Nitroglycerin *on page* 1073

◆ **NitroTime®** *see* Nitroglycerin *on page* 1073

◆ **Nix® [OTC]** *see* Permethrin *on page* 1176

◆ **Nix® (Can)** *see* Permethrin *on page* 1176

Nizatidine (ni ZA ti deen)

U.S. Brand Names Axid®; Axid® AR [OTC]

Canadian Brand Names Apo-Nizatidine®; Axid®; Gen-Nizatidine; Novo-Nizatidine; Nu-Nizatidine; PMS-Nizatidine

Pharmacologic Category Histamine H_2 Antagonist

Use Treatment and maintenance of duodenal ulcer; treatment of benign gastric ulcer; treatment of gastroesophageal reflux disease (GERD); OTC tablet used for the prevention of meal-induced heartburn, acid indigestion, and sour stomach

Unlabeled/Investigational Use Part of a multidrug regimen for *H. pylori* eradication to reduce the risk of duodenal ulcer recurrence

Pregnancy Risk Factor B

Pregnancy Considerations Teratogenic effects were not observed in animal studies.

Lactation Enters breast milk/may be compatible

Medication Safety Issues

Sound-alike/look-alike issues:
- Axid® may be confused with Ansaid®

International issues:
- Tazac® [Australia] may be confused with Tiazac® which is a brand name for diltiazem in the U.S.

Contraindications Hypersensitivity to nizatidine or any component of the formulation; hypersensitivity to other H_2 antagonists (cross-sensitivity has been observed)

Warnings/Precautions Relief of symptoms does not preclude the presence of a gastric malignancy. Use with caution in children <12 years of age. Use with caution in patients with liver and renal impairment. Dosage modification required in patients with renal impairment

Adverse Reactions

>10%: Central nervous system: Headache (16%)

1% to 10%:
- Central nervous system: Anxiety, dizziness, fever (reported in children), insomnia, irritability (reported in children), somnolence, nervousness
- Dermatologic: Pruritus, rash
- Gastrointestinal: Abdominal pain, anorexia, constipation, diarrhea, dry mouth, flatulence, heartburn, nausea, vomiting
- Respiratory: Reported in children: Cough, nasal congestion, nasopharyngitis

<1% (Limited to important or life-threatening): Alkaline phosphatase increased, ALT increased, anaphylaxis, anemia, AST increased, bronchospasm, confusion, eosinophilia, exfoliative dermatitis, gynecomastia, hepatitis, jaundice, laryngeal edema, serum-sickness like reactions, thrombocytopenia, thrombocytopenic purpura, vasculitis, ventricular tachycardia

Drug Interactions

Metabolism/Transport Effects Inhibits 3A4 (weak)

Avoid Concomitant Use

Avoid concomitant use of Nizatidine with any of the following: Erlotinib; Mesalamine

Increased Effect/Toxicity

Nizatidine may increase the levels/effects of: Saquinavir

Decreased Effect

Nizatidine may decrease the levels/effects of: Antifungal Agents (Azole Derivatives, Systemic); Atazanavir; Cefpodoxime; Cefuroxime; Dasatinib; Erlotinib; Fosamprenavir; Indinavir; Iron Salts; Mesalamine; Nelfinavir

Ethanol/Nutrition/Herb Interactions

Ethanol: Avoid ethanol (may cause gastric mucosal irritation).

Food: Administration with apple juice may decrease absorption.

Mechanism of Action Competitive inhibition of histamine at H_2-receptors of the gastric parietal cells resulting in reduced gastric acid secretion, gastric volume and hydrogen ion concentration reduced. In healthy volunteers, nizatidine suppresses gastric acid secretion induced by pentagastrin infusion or food.

Pharmacodynamics/Kinetics

Distribution: V_d: 0.8-1.5 L/kg

Protein binding: 35% to α_1-acid glycoprotein

Metabolism: Partially hepatic; forms metabolites

Bioavailability: >70%

Half-life elimination: 1-2 hours; prolonged with renal impairment

Time to peak, plasma: 0.5-3.0 hours

Excretion: Urine (90%; ~60% as unchanged drug); feces (<6%)

Dosage Oral:

Children:
- <12 years: GERD (unlabeled use): 10 mg/kg/day in divided doses given twice daily; may not be as effective in children <12 years
- ≥12 years:
  - GERD: Refer to adult dosing
  - Meal-induced heartburn, acid indigestion and sour stomach: Refer to adult dosing

Adults:
- Duodenal ulcer:
  - Treatment of active ulcer: 300 mg at bedtime or 150 mg twice daily
  - Maintenance of healed ulcer: 150 mg/day at bedtime
- Gastric ulcer: 150 mg twice daily or 300 mg at bedtime
- GERD: 150 mg twice daily
- Meal-induced heartburn, acid indigestion, and sour stomach: 75 mg tablet [OTC] twice daily, 30 to 60 minutes prior to consuming food or beverages
- *Helicobacter pylori* eradication (unlabeled use): 150 mg twice daily; requires combination therapy

Dosing adjustment in renal impairment:

Active treatment:
- Cl_{cr} 20-50 mL/minute: 150 mg/day
- Cl_{cr} <20 mL/minute: 150 mg every other day

Maintenance treatment:
- Cl_{cr} 20-50 mL/minute: 150 mg every other day
- Cl_{cr} <20 mL/minute: 150 mg every 3 days

Test Interactions False-positive urine protein using Multistix®, gastric acid secretion test, skin tests allergen extracts, serum creatinine and serum transaminase concentrations, urine protein test

Additional Information Giving dose at 6 PM (rather than 10 PM) may better suppress nocturnal acid secretion

Dosage Forms Excipient information presented when available (limited, particularly for generics); consult specific product labeling.

Capsule:
Axid®: 150 mg, 300 mg [DSC]

Solution, oral:
Axid®: 15 mg/mL (120 mL, 480 mL) [bubble gum flavor]

Tablet:
Axid® AR: 75 mg

◆ **Nizoral®** *see* Ketoconazole *on page 837*

◆ **Nizoral® A-D [OTC]** *see* Ketoconazole *on page 837*

◆ **N-Methylhydrazine** *see* Procarbazine *on page 1242*

◆ **N-methylnaltrexone Bromide** *see* Methylnaltrexone *on page 972*

◆ **No Doz® Maximum Strength [OTC]** *see* Caffeine *on page 232*

◆ **NoHist** *see* Chlorpheniramine and Phenylephrine *on page 309*

◆ **NoHist-A** *see* Chlorpheniramine, Phenylephrine, and Phenyltoloxamine *on page 314*

◆ **Nolvadex® (Can)** *see* Tamoxifen *on page 1424*

◆ **Nolvadex®-D (Can)** *see* Tamoxifen *on page 1424*

Nonoxynol 9 (non OKS i nole nine)

U.S. Brand Names Advantage-S® [OTC]; Conceptrol® [OTC]; Delfen® [OTC]; Encare® [OTC]; Gynol II® Extra Strength [OTC] ; Gynol II® [OTC]; Today® [OTC]; VCF™ [OTC]

Index Terms N-9

Pharmacologic Category Contraceptive; Spermicide

Use Prevention of pregnancy

Medication Safety Issues

Sound-alike/look-alike issues:
Delfen® may be confused with Delsym®

Dosage Adolescents and Adults: **Note:** Prior to use, refer to specific product labeling for complete instructions.

Prevention of pregnancy: Vaginal:
Advantage-S®, Conceptrol®: Insert 1 applicatorful vaginally up to 1 hour prior to intercourse
Encare®: Unwrap and insert 1 suppository vaginally at least 10 minutes prior to intercourse; effective for 1 hour
Today® Sponge: Insert 1 sponge vaginally prior to intercourse; allow to remain in place for 6 hours after intercourse before removing; effective for use up to 24 continuous hours. Do not leave in place for >30 hours.
VCF®:
Film: Insert 1 film vaginally at least 15 minutes, but no more than 3 hours, prior to intercourse. Insert new film for each act of intercourse or if more than 3 hours have elapsed.
Foam: Insert 1 applicatorful at least 15 minutes prior to intercourse; effective for up to 1 hour

Additional Information Complete prescribing information for this medication should be consulted for additional detail.

Dosage Forms Excipient information presented when available (limited, particularly for generics); consult specific product labeling.

Aerosol, vaginal [foam]:
Delfen®: 12.5% (18 g) [contains benzoic acid]
VCF™: 12.5% (40 g)

Film, vaginal:
VCF™: 28% (3s, 6s,12s)

Gel, vaginal:
Advantage-S®: 3.5% (1.5 g) [packaged in 3s or with 6 prefilled applicators]; (30g) [packaged with reusable applicator]
Conceptrol®: 4% (2.7 g) [packaged in 6s and 10s with disposable applicators]
Gynol II®: 2% (85 g, 114 g)
Gynol II® Extra Strength: 3% (85.5 g)

Sponge, vaginal:
Today®: 1 g (3s, 6s, 12s) [contains benzoic acid, sodium metabisulfite]

Suppository, vaginal:
Encare®: 100 mg (12s, 18s)

◆ **Nora-BE™** *see* Norethindrone *on page 1078*

◆ **Noradrenaline** *see* Norepinephrine *on page 1077*

◆ **Noradrenaline Acid Tartrate** *see* Norepinephrine *on page 1077*

◆ **Norco®** *see* Hydrocodone and Acetaminophen *on page 740*

◆ **Norcuron® [DSC]** *see* Vecuronium *on page 1553*

◆ **Norcuron® (Can)** *see* Vecuronium *on page 1553*

◆ **Nordeoxyguanosine** *see* Ganciclovir *on page 681*

◆ **Nordette®** *see* Ethinyl Estradiol and Levonorgestrel *on page 577*

◆ **Norditropin®** *see* Somatropin *on page 1388*

◆ **Norditropin® NordiFlex®** *see* Somatropin *on page 1388*

◆ **Norel DM™** *see* Chlorpheniramine, Phenylephrine, and Dextromethorphan *on page 311*

◆ **norel® EX** *see* Guaifenesin and Phenylephrine *on page 712*

◆ **Norelgestromin and Ethinyl Estradiol** *see* Ethinyl Estradiol and Norelgestromin *on page 581*

Norepinephrine (nor ep i NEF rin)

U.S. Brand Names Levophed®

Canadian Brand Names Levophed®

Index Terms Levarterenol Bitartrate; Noradrenaline; Noradrenaline Acid Tartrate; Norepinephrine Bitartrate

Pharmacologic Category Alpha/Beta Agonist

Additional Appendix Information

Hemodynamic Support, Intravenous *on page 1657*

Use Treatment of shock which persists after adequate fluid volume replacement

Pregnancy Risk Factor C

Lactation Excretion in breast milk unknown

Medication Safety Issues

High alert medication: The Institute for Safe Medication Practices (ISMP) includes this medication among its list of drugs which have a heightened risk of causing significant patient harm when used in error.

Contraindications Hypersensitivity to norepinephrine, bisulfites (contains metabisulfite), or any component of the formulation; hypotension from hypovolemia except as an emergency measure to maintain coronary and cerebral perfusion until volume could be replaced; mesenteric or peripheral vascular thrombosis unless it is a lifesaving procedure; during anesthesia with cyclopropane or halothane anesthesia (risk of ventricular arrhythmias)

Warnings/Precautions Assure adequate circulatory volume to minimize need for vasoconstrictors. Avoid hypertension; monitor blood pressure closely and adjust infusion rate. Use with extreme caution in patients taking MAO-Inhibitors. Avoid extravasation; infuse into a large vein if possible. Avoid infusion into leg veins. Watch I.V. site closely. **[U.S. Boxed Warning]: If extravasation occurs, infiltrate the area with diluted phentolamine (5-10 mg in 10-15 mL of saline) with a fine hypodermic**

needle. Phentolamine should be administered as soon as possible after extravasation is noted. Product may contain sodium metasulfite.

Adverse Reactions Frequency not defined.

Cardiovascular: Bradycardia, arrhythmia, peripheral (digital) ischemia

Central nervous system: Headache (transient), anxiety

Local: Skin necrosis (with extravasation)

Respiratory: Dyspnea, respiratory difficulty

Drug Interactions

Avoid Concomitant Use

Avoid concomitant use of Norepinephrine with any of the following: Iobenguane I 123

Increased Effect/Toxicity

Norepinephrine may increase the levels/effects of: Bromocriptine; Sympathomimetics

The levels/effects of Norepinephrine may be increased by: Antacids; Beta-Blockers; Cannabinoids; Carbonic Anhydrase Inhibitors; COMT Inhibitors; MAO Inhibitors; Serotonin/Norepinephrine Reuptake Inhibitors; Tricyclic Antidepressants

Decreased Effect

Norepinephrine may decrease the levels/effects of: Iobenguane I 123

Stability Readily oxidized. Protect from light. Do not use if brown coloration. Dilute with D_5W or D_5NS, but not recommended to dilute in normal saline. Stability of parenteral admixture at room temperature (25°C) is 24 hours.

Mechanism of Action Stimulates $beta_1$-adrenergic receptors and alpha-adrenergic receptors causing increased contractility and heart rate as well as vasoconstriction, thereby increasing systemic blood pressure and coronary blood flow; clinically alpha effects (vasoconstriction) are greater than beta effects (inotropic and chronotropic effects)

Pharmacodynamics/Kinetics

Onset of action: I.V.: Very rapid-acting

Duration: vasopressor: 1-2 minutes

Metabolism: Via catechol-o-methyltransferase (COMT) and monoamine oxidase (MAO)

Excretion: Urine (84% to 96% as inactive metabolites)

Dosage Administration requires the use of an infusion pump!

Note: Norepinephrine dosage is stated in terms of norepinephrine base and intravenous formulation is norepinephrine bitartrate

Norepinephrine bitartrate 2 mg = Norepinephrine base 1 mg

Continuous I.V. infusion:

Children: Initial: 0.05-0.1 mcg/kg/minute; titrate to desired effect; maximum dose: 1-2 mcg/kg/minute

Adults: Initial: 0.5-1 mcg/minute and titrate to desired response; 8-30 mcg/minute is usual range; range used in clinical trials: 0.01-3 mcg/kg/minute; ACLS dosage range: 0.5-30 mcg/minute

Administration Administer into large vein to avoid the potential for extravasation; potent drug, must be diluted prior to use; do not administer $NaHCO_3$ through an I.V. line containing norepinephrine.

Dosage Forms Excipient information presented when available (limited, particularly for generics); consult specific product labeling.

Injection, solution, as bitartrate: 1 mg/mL (4 mL) [contains sodium metabisulfite]

◆ **Norepinephrine Bitartrate** *see* Norepinephrine *on page 1077*

Norethindrone (nor ETH in drone)

U.S. Brand Names Aygestin®; Camila™; Errin™; Jolivette™; Nor-QD®; Nora-BE™; Ortho Micronor®

Canadian Brand Names Micronor®; Norlutate®

Index Terms Norethindrone Acetate; Norethisterone

Pharmacologic Category Contraceptive; Progestin

Use Treatment of amenorrhea; abnormal uterine bleeding; endometriosis; prevention of pregnancy

Pregnancy Risk Factor X

Pregnancy Considerations First trimester exposure may cause genital abnormalities including hypospadias in male infants and mild virilization of external female genitalia. Significant adverse events related to growth and development have not been observed (limited studies). Use is contraindicated during pregnancy. May be started immediately postpartum if not breast-feeding.

Lactation Enters breast milk/use caution

Medication Safety Issues

Sound-alike/look-alike issues:

Micronor® may be confused with miconazole, Micronase®

Contraindications Hypersensitivity to norethindrone or any component of the formulation; history of or current thrombophlebitis or venous thromboembolic disorders (including DVT, PE); hepatic dysfunction or tumor; known or suspected breast carcinoma; undiagnosed vaginal bleeding; pregnancy; missed abortion or as a diagnostic test for pregnancy

Warnings/Precautions Progestin only contraceptives do not protect against HIV infection or other sexually-transmitted diseases. Irregular menstrual bleeding patterns are common with progestin-only contraceptives; nonpharmacologic causes of abnormal bleeding should be ruled out. Progestin use has been associated with retinal vascular lesions; discontinue pending examination in case of sudden vision loss, complete loss of vision, sudden onset of proptosis, diplopia or migraine. May have adverse effects on glucose tolerance; use caution in women with diabetes. May have adverse effects on lipid metabolism; use caution in women with hyperlipidemias. Use with caution in patients with depression.

Use with caution in patients with diseases which may be exacerbated by fluid retention, including asthma, epilepsy, migraine, cardiac or renal dysfunction. Use caution in patients at increased risk of thromboembolism; includes elective surgery associated with an increased risk of thromboembolism or during periods of prolonged immobilization. The use of combination hormonal contraceptives has been associated with a slight increase in the frequency of breast cancer, however studies are not consistent. Data is insufficient to determine if progestin-only contraceptives also increase this risk. The risk of cardiovascular side effects increases in women using estrogen containing combined hormonal contraceptives and who smoke cigarettes, especially those who are >35 years of age. This risk relative to progestin-only contraceptives has not been established. Extremely rare hepatic adenomas and focal nodular hyperplasia resulting in fatal intra-abdominal hemorrhage have been reported in association with long-term combination oral contraceptive use. Data is insufficient to determine if progestin-only contraceptives also increase this risk. Not for use prior to menarche.

Adverse Reactions Frequency not defined.

Cardiovascular: Cerebral embolism, cerebral thrombosis, DVT, edema

Central nervous system: Depression, dizziness, headache, insomnia, migraine, mood swings

Dermatologic: Acne, chloasma, hirsutism, melasma, pruritus, rash, urticaria

Endocrine & metabolic: Amenorrhea, breakthrough bleeding, breast enlargement/tenderness, menstrual flow changes, spotting
Gastrointestinal: Nausea, weight gain/loss
Genitourinary: Cervical erosion changes, cervical secretion changes
Hepatic: Cholestatic jaundice, liver function test abnormalities
Ocular: Optic neuritis (with or without vision loss), retinal vascular thrombosis
Respiratory: Pulmonary embolism
Miscellaneous: Anaphylactic/anaphylactoid reactions

Drug Interactions

Metabolism/Transport Effects Substrate of CYP3A4 (major); **Induces** CYP2C19 (weak)

Avoid Concomitant Use

Avoid concomitant use of Norethindrone with any of the following: Acitretin; Griseofulvin

Increased Effect/Toxicity

Norethindrone may increase the levels/effects of: Benzodiazepines (metabolized by oxidation); Selegiline; Voriconazole

The levels/effects of Norethindrone may be increased by: Herbs (Progestogenic Properties); Voriconazole

Decreased Effect

Norethindrone may decrease the levels/effects of: Vitamin K Antagonists

The levels/effects of Norethindrone may be decreased by: Acitretin; Aminoglutethimide; Aprepitant; Barbiturates; CarBAMazepine; Colesevelam; CYP3A4 Inducers (Strong); Darunavir; Deferasirox; Felbamate; Fosaprepitant; Griseofulvin; Mycophenolate; OXcarbazepine; Phenytoin; Retinoic Acid Derivatives; Rifamycin Derivatives; Rufinamide; St Johns Wort

Ethanol/Nutrition/Herb Interactions Herb/Nutraceutical: Avoid bloodroot, chasteberry, damiana, oregano, and yucca; may enhance the adverse/toxic effect of progestins. Avoid St John's wort; may diminish the therapeutic effect of progestin contraceptives; contraceptive failure is possible.

Stability Store at controlled room temperature of 25°C (77°F).

Mechanism of Action Inhibits secretion of pituitary gonadotropin (LH) which prevents follicular maturation and ovulation

Pharmacodynamics/Kinetics

Absorption: Oral: Rapidly absorbed
Distribution: V_d: 4 L/kg
Protein binding: 61% to albumin; 36% to sex hormone-binding globulin (SHBG); SHBG capacity affected by plasma ethinyl estradiol levels
Metabolism: Oral: Hepatic via reduction and conjugation; first-pass effect
Bioavailability: 64%
Half-life elimination: ~8 hours
Time to peak: 1-2 hours
Excretion: Urine (>50% as metabolites); feces (20% to 40% as metabolites)

Dosage Oral: Adolescents and Adults: Female:

Contraception: Progesterone only: Norethindrone 0.35 mg every day (no missed days)
  Initial dose: Start on first day of menstrual period or the day after a miscarriage or abortion. If switching from a combined oral contraceptive, begin the day after finishing the last active combined tablet.
  Missed dose: Take as soon as remembered. A back up method of contraception should be used for 48 hours if dose is taken ≥3 hours late.
Amenorrhea and abnormal uterine bleeding: Norethindrone acetate: 2.5-10 mg/day for 5-10 days during the second half of the menstrual cycle
Endometriosis: Norethindrone acetate: 5 mg/day for 14 days; increase at increments of 2.5 mg/day every 2 weeks to reach 15 mg/day; continue for 6-9 months or until breakthrough bleeding demands temporary termination

Dietary Considerations Should be taken at same time each day.

Administration

Administer at the same time each day. When used for the prevention of pregnancy, a back up method of contraception should be used for 48 hours if dose is missed or taken ≥3 hours late.

Monitoring Parameters Contraception: Before starting therapy, a physical exam with reference to the breasts and pelvis are recommended, including a Papanicolaou smear. Exam may be deferred if appropriate; pregnancy should be ruled out prior to use. Monitor patient closely for loss of vision, sudden onset of proptosis, diplopia, migraine; blood pressure; signs and symptoms of thromboembolic disorders; signs or symptoms of depression; glycemic control in patients with diabetes; lipid profiles in patients being treated for hyperlipidemias. Adequate diagnostic measures, including endometrial sampling, if indicated, should be performed to rule out malignancy in all cases of undiagnosed abnormal vaginal bleeding.

Test Interactions May increase prothrombin, factors VII, VIII, IX and X, PBI, and BEI. May decrease T_3 uptake; may decrease sex hormone-binding globulin (SHBG); may have a reduced response to metyrapone test.

Dosage Forms Excipient information presented when available (limited, particularly for generics); consult specific product labeling.

Tablet:
  Camila™, Errin™, Jolivette™, Ortho Micronor®, Nora-BE™, Nor-QD®: 0.35 mg
Tablet, as acetate:
  Aygestin®: 5 mg

◆ **Norethindrone Acetate** *see* Norethindrone *on page 1078*

◆ **Norethindrone Acetate and Ethinyl Estradiol** *see* Ethinyl Estradiol and Norethindrone *on page 581*

◆ **Norethindrone and Estradiol** *see* Estradiol and Norethindrone *on page 558*

Norethindrone and Mestranol

(nor eth IN drone & MES tra nole)

U.S. Brand Names Necon® 1/50; Norinyl® 1+50; Ortho-Novum® 1/50 [DSC]

Canadian Brand Names Ortho-Novum® 1/50

Index Terms Mestranol and Norethindrone; Ortho Novum 1/50

Pharmacologic Category Contraceptive; Estrogen and Progestin Combination

Use Prevention of pregnancy

Unlabeled/Investigational Use Treatment of hypermenorrhea (menorrhagia); pain associated with endometriosis; dysmenorrhea; dysfunctional uterine bleeding

Pregnancy Risk Factor X

Medication Safety Issues

Sound-alike/look-alike issues:
  Norinyl® may be confused with Nardil®

Dosage Oral: Adults: Female: Contraception:

Schedule 1 (Sunday starter): Dose begins on first Sunday after onset of menstruation; if the menstrual period starts on Sunday, take first tablet that very same day. **With a Sunday start, an additional method of contraception should be used until after the first 7 days of consecutive administration.**
  For 21-tablet package: Dosage is 1 tablet daily for 21 consecutive days, followed by 7 days off of the

medication; a new course begins on the 8th day after the last tablet is taken.

For 28-tablet package: Dosage is 1 tablet daily without interruption.

Schedule 2 (Day 1 starter): Dose starts on first day of menstrual cycle taking 1 tablet daily.

For 21-tablet package: Dosage is 1 tablet daily for 21 consecutive days, followed by 7 days off of the medication; a new course begins on the 8th day after the last tablet is taken.

For 28-tablet package: Dosage is 1 tablet daily without interruption.

If all doses have been taken on schedule and one menstrual period is missed, continue dosing cycle. If two consecutive menstrual periods are missed, pregnancy test is required before new dosing cycle is started.

Missed doses **monophasic formulations** (refer to package insert for complete information):

One dose missed: Take as soon as remembered or take 2 tablets next day

Two consecutive doses missed in the first 2 weeks: Take 2 tablets as soon as remembered or 2 tablets next 2 days. **An additional method of contraception should be used for 7 days after missed dose.**

Two consecutive doses missed in week 3 or three consecutive doses missed at any time: **An additional method of contraception must be used for 7 days after a missed dose:**

Schedule 1 (Sunday starter): Continue dose of 1 tablet daily until Sunday, then discard the rest of the pack, and a new pack should be started that same day.

Schedule 2 (Day 1 starter): Current pack should be discarded, and a new pack should be started that same day.

Dosage adjustment in renal impairment: Specific guidelines not available; use with caution and monitor blood pressure closely. Consider other forms of contraception.

Dosage adjustment in hepatic impairment: Contraindicated in patients with hepatic impairment

Additional Information Complete prescribing information for this medication should be consulted for additional detail.

Dosage Forms Excipient information presented when available (limited, particularly for generics); consult specific product labeling.

Tablet, monophasic formulations:

Necon® 1/50: Norethindrone 1 mg and mestranol 0.05 mg [21 light blue tablets and 7 white inactive tablets] (28s)

Norinyl® 1+50: Norethindrone 1 mg and mestranol 0.05 mg [21 white tablets and 7 orange inactive tablets] (28s)

Ortho-Novum® 1/50: Norethindrone 1 mg and mestranol 0.05 mg [21 yellow tablets and 7 green inactive tablets] (28s) [DSC]

- **Norethisterone** *see* Norethindrone *on page 1078*
- **Norflex™** *see* Orphenadrine *on page 1108*

Norfloxacin (nor FLOKS a sin)

U.S. Brand Names Noroxin®

Canadian Brand Names Apo-Norflox®; CO Norfloxacin; Norfloxacine®; Noroxin®; Novo-Norfloxacin; PMS-Norfloxacin; Riva-Norfloxacin

Pharmacologic Category Antibiotic, Quinolone

Use Uncomplicated and complicated urinary tract infections caused by susceptible gram-negative and gram-positive bacteria; sexually-transmitted disease (eg, uncomplicated urethral and cervical gonorrhea) caused by *N. gonorrhoeae*; prostatitis due to *E. coli*

Note: As of April 2007, the CDC no longer recommends the use of fluoroquinolones for the treatment of gonococcal disease.

Restrictions An FDA-approved patient medication guide is available and must be distributed when dispensing an outpatient prescription (new or refill) where this medication is to be used without direct supervision of a healthcare provider. Medication guides are available at http://www.fda.gov/cder/Offices/ODS/medication_guides.htm.

Pregnancy Risk Factor C

Medication Safety Issues

Sound-alike/look-alike issues:

Norfloxacin may be confused with Norflex™, Noroxin®

Noroxin® may be confused with Neurontin®, Norflex™, norfloxacin

Dosage

Usual dosage range:

Adults: Oral: 400 mg every 12 hours (maximum: 800 mg/day)

Indication-specific dosing:

Adults: Oral:

Dysenteric enterocolitis *(Shigella* unlabeled use): 400 mg twice daily for 5 days

Prostatitis: 400 mg every 12 hours for 4-6 weeks

Traveler's diarrhea (unlabeled use): 400 mg twice daily for 3 days, single dose may also be effective

Uncomplicated gonorrhea: 800 mg as a single dose. **Note:** As of April 2007, the CDC no longer recommends the use of fluoroquinolones for the treatment of uncomplicated gonococcal disease.

Urinary tract infections:

Uncomplicated due to *E. coli, K. pneumoniae, P. mirabilis*: 400 mg twice daily for 3 days

Uncomplicated due to other organisms: 400 mg twice daily for 7-10 days

Complicated: 400 mg twice daily for 10-21 days

Dosing interval in renal impairment: Cl_{cr} ≤30 mL/minute/1.73 m^2: Administer 400 mg every 24 hours

Additional Information Complete prescribing information for this medication should be consulted for additional detail.

Dosage Forms Excipient information presented when available (limited, particularly for generics); consult specific product labeling.

Tablet:

Noroxin®: 400 mg

- **Norfloxacine® (Can)** *see* Norfloxacin *on page 1080*
- **Norgesic™ [DSC]** *see* Orphenadrine, Aspirin, and Caffeine *on page 1108*
- **Norgesic™ (Can)** *see* Orphenadrine, Aspirin, and Caffeine *on page 1108*
- **Norgesic™ Forte [DSC]** *see* Orphenadrine, Aspirin, and Caffeine *on page 1108*
- **Norgesic™ Forte (Can)** *see* Orphenadrine, Aspirin, and Caffeine *on page 1108*
- **Norgestimate and Ethinyl Estradiol** *see* Ethinyl Estradiol and Norgestimate *on page 584*
- **Norgestrel and Ethinyl Estradiol** *see* Ethinyl Estradiol and Norgestrel *on page 585*
- **Norinyl® 1+35** *see* Ethinyl Estradiol and Norethindrone *on page 581*
- **Norinyl® 1+50** *see* Norethindrone and Mestranol *on page 1079*
- **Noritate®** *see* MetroNIDAZOLE *on page 984*
- **Norlutate® (Can)** *see* Norethindrone *on page 1078*
- **Normal Human Serum Albumin** *see* Albumin *on page 49*
- **Normal Saline** *see* Sodium Chloride *on page 1381*

Nortriptyline (nor TRIP ti leen)

U.S. Brand Names Pamelor®

Canadian Brand Names Alti-Nortriptyline; Apo-Nortriptyline®; Aventyl®; Gen-Nortriptyline; Norventyl; Novo-Nortriptyline; Nu-Nortriptyline; PMS-Nortriptyline

Index Terms Nortriptyline Hydrochloride

Pharmacologic Category Antidepressant, Tricyclic (Secondary Amine)

Additional Appendix Information

Antidepressant Agents *on page 1638*

Use Treatment of symptoms of depression

Unlabeled/Investigational Use Chronic pain, anxiety disorders, enuresis, attention-deficit/hyperactivity disorder (ADHD); adjunctive therapy for smoking cessation

Restrictions An FDA-approved medication guide concerning the use of antidepressants in children, adolescents, and young adults must be distributed when dispensing an outpatient prescription (new or refill) where this medication is to be used without direct supervision of a healthcare provider. Medication guides are available at http://www.fda.gov/cder/Offices/ODS/medication_guides.htm. Dispense to parents or guardians of children and adolescents receiving this medication.

Lactation Enters breast milk/contraindicated (AAP rates "of concern")

Medication Safety Issues

Sound-alike/look-alike issues:

Aventyl® HCl may be confused with Bentyl®

Nortriptyline may be confused with amitriptyline, desipramine, Norpramin®

Pamelor® may be confused with Demerol®, Dymelor®, Panlor® DC

Contraindications Hypersensitivity to nortriptyline and similar chemical class, or any component of the formulation; use of MAO inhibitors within 14 days; use in a patient during the acute recovery phase of MI

Warnings/Precautions [U.S. Boxed Warning]: Antidepressants increase the risk of suicidal thinking and behavior in children, adolescents, and young adults (18-24 years of age) with major depressive disorder (MDD) and other psychiatric disorders; consider risk prior to prescribing. Short-term studies did not show an increased risk in patients >24 years of age and showed a decreased risk in patients ≥65 years. Closely monitor for clinical worsening, suicidality, or unusual changes in behavior; the patient's family or caregiver should be instructed to closely observe the patient and communicate condition with healthcare provider. A medication guide should be dispensed with each prescription. **Nortriptyline is not FDA approved for use in children.**

The possibility of a suicide attempt is inherent in major depression and may persist until remission occurs. Monitor for worsening of depression or suicidality, especially during initiation of therapy (generally first 1-2 months) or with dose increases or decreases. Use caution in high-risk patients. Worsening depression and severe abrupt suicidality that are not part of the presenting symptoms may require discontinuation or modification of drug therapy. The patient's family or caregiver should be alerted to monitor patients for the emergence of suicidality and associated behaviors (such as agitation, irritability, hostility, impulsivity, and hypomania) and call healthcare provider.

May worsen psychosis in some patients or precipitate a shift to mania or hypomania in patients with bipolar disorder. Patients presenting with depressive symptoms should be screened for bipolar disorder. Monotherapy in patients with bipolar disorder should be avoided. **Nortriptyline is not FDA approved for the treatment of bipolar depression.**

TCAs may rarely cause bone marrow suppression; monitor for any signs of infection and obtain CBC if symptoms (eg, fever, sore throat) evident. The risk of sedation and orthostatic effects are low relative to other antidepressants. However, nortriptyline may result in impaired performance of tasks requiring alertness (eg, operating machinery or driving). Sedative effects may be additive with other CNS depressants and/or ethanol. The degree of anticholinergic blockade produced by this agent is moderate relative to other cyclic antidepressants, however, caution should still be used in patients with urinary retention, benign prostatic hyperplasia, narrow-angle glaucoma, xerostomia, visual problems, constipation, or history of bowel obstruction. May cause orthostatic hypotension (risk is low relative to other antidepressants) or conduction disturbances. Use with caution in patients with a history of cardiovascular disease (including previous MI, stroke, tachycardia, or conduction abnormalities). The risk conduction abnormalities with this agent is moderate relative to other antidepressants.

Consider discontinuing, when possible, prior to elective surgery. Therapy should not be abruptly discontinued in patients receiving high doses for prolonged periods. May alter glucose regulation - use caution in patients with diabetes. Use caution in patients with a previous seizure disorder or condition predisposing to seizures such as brain damage, alcoholism, or concurrent therapy with other drugs which lower the seizure threshold. May increase the risks associated with electroconvulsive therapy. Use with caution in hyperthyroid patients or those receiving thyroid supplementation. Use with caution in patients with hepatic or renal dysfunction and in elderly patients.

Adverse Reactions Frequency not defined.

Cardiovascular: Arrhythmia, flushing, heart block, hypertension, MI, palpitation, postural hypotension, tachycardia

Central nervous system: Agitation, anxiety, ataxia, confusion, delirium, delusions, disorientation, dizziness, drowsiness, EEG changes, exacerbation of psychosis, extrapyramidal symptoms, fatigue, hallucinations, headache, hypomania, incoordination, insomnia, nightmares, panic, restlessness, seizure

Dermatologic: Alopecia, itching, petechiae, photosensitivity, rash, urticaria

Endocrine & metabolic: Blood sugar increases/decreases, breast enlargement, galactorrhea, gynecomastia, increase or decrease in libido, sexual dysfunction, SIADH

Gastrointestinal: Abdominal cramps, anorexia, black tongue, constipation, diarrhea, epigastric distress, nausea, paralytic ileus, stomatitis, taste disturbance, vomiting, weight gain/loss, xerostomia

Genitourinary: Delayed micturition, impotence, nocturia, polyuria, testicular edema, urinary retention

Hematologic: Agranulocytosis (rare), eosinophilia, purpura, thrombocytopenia

Hepatic: Cholestatic jaundice, transaminases increased

Neuromuscular & skeletal: Numbness, paresthesia, peripheral neuropathy, tingling, tremor, weakness

Ocular: Blurred vision, disturbances in accommodation, eye pain, mydriasis

Otic: Tinnitus

Miscellaneous: Allergic reactions (eg, general edema or of the face/tongue), diaphoresis (excessive), withdrawal symptoms

Drug Interactions

Metabolism/Transport Effects Substrate of CYP1A2 (minor), 2C19 (minor), 2D6 (major), 3A4 (minor); **Inhibits** CYP2D6 (weak), 2E1 (weak)

Avoid Concomitant Use

Avoid concomitant use of Nortriptyline with any of the following: Iobenguane I 123; MAO Inhibitors; Nilotinib; Sibutramine; Tetrabenazine; Thioridazine; Ziprasidone

Increased Effect/Toxicity

Nortriptyline may increase the levels/effects of: Alcohol (Ethyl); Alpha-/Beta-Agonists (Direct-Acting); Alpha1-Agonists; Amphetamines; Anticholinergics; Beta2-Agonists; CNS Depressants; Desmopressin; QTc-Prolonging Agents; QuiNIDine; Serotonin Modulators; Sulfonylureas; Tetrabenazine; Thioridazine; TraMADol; Vitamin K Antagonists; Yohimbine; Ziprasidone

The levels/effects of Nortriptyline may be increased by: Alfuzosin; Altretamine; BuPROPion; Cimetidine; Cinacalcet; Ciprofloxacin; CYP2D6 Inhibitors (Moderate); CYP2D6 Inhibitors (Strong); Darunavir; Dexmethylphenidate; DULoxetine; Gadobutrol; Lithium; MAO Inhibitors; Methylphenidate; Nilotinib; Pramlintide; Propoxyphene; Protease Inhibitors; QuiNIDine; Selective Serotonin Reuptake Inhibitors; Sibutramine; Terbinafine; Valproic Acid

Decreased Effect

Nortriptyline may decrease the levels/effects of: Acetylcholinesterase Inhibitors (Central); Alpha2-Agonists; Iobenguane I 123

The levels/effects of Nortriptyline may be decreased by: Acetylcholinesterase Inhibitors (Central); Barbiturates; CarBAMazepine; St Johns Wort

Ethanol/Nutrition/Herb Interactions

Ethanol: Avoid ethanol (may increase CNS depression).

Herb/Nutraceutical: Avoid valerian, St John's wort, SAMe, kava kava (may increase risk of serotonin syndrome and/or excessive sedation).

Stability Store at 20°C to 25°C (68°F to 77°F). Protect from light.

Mechanism of Action Traditionally believed to increase the synaptic concentration of serotonin and/or norepinephrine in the central nervous system by inhibition of their reuptake by the presynaptic neuronal membrane. However, additional receptor effects have been found including desensitization of adenyl cyclase, down regulation of beta-adrenergic receptors, and down regulation of serotonin receptors.

Pharmacodynamics/Kinetics

Onset of action: Therapeutic: 1-3 weeks

Distribution: V_d: 21 L/kg

Protein binding: 93% to 95%

Metabolism: Primarily hepatic; extensive first-pass effect

Half-life elimination: 28-31 hours

Time to peak, serum: 7-8.5 hours

Excretion: Urine (as metabolites and small amounts of unchanged drug); feces (small amounts)

Dosage Oral:

Nocturnal enuresis: Children (unlabeled use): 10-20 mg/day; titrate to a maximum of 40 mg/day

Depression: Children (unlabeled use): 1-3 mg/kg/day

Depression:

Adults: 25 mg 3-4 times/day up to 150 mg/day; doses may be given once daily

Elderly: Initial: 30-50 mg/day, given as a single daily dose or in divided doses. **Note:** Nortriptyline is one of the best tolerated TCAs in the elderly)

Myofascial pain, neuralgia, burning mouth syndrome (dental use): Adults: Initial: 10-25 mg at bedtime; dosage may be increased by 25 mg/day weekly, if tolerated; usual maintenance dose: 75 mg as a single bedtime dose or 2 divided doses

Chronic urticaria, angioedema, nocturnal pruritus (unlabeled use): Adults: Oral: 75 mg/day

Smoking cessation (unlabeled use): Adults: 25-75 mg/day beginning 10-14 days before "quit" day; continue therapy for ≥12 weeks after "quit" day

Dosing adjustment in hepatic impairment: Lower doses and slower titration dependent on individualization of dosage is recommended

Monitoring Parameters Blood pressure and pulse rate (ECG, cardiac monitoring) prior to and during initial therapy in older adults; weight; blood levels are useful for therapeutic monitoring; suicidal ideation (especially at the beginning of therapy or when doses are increased or decreased)

Reference Range

Plasma levels do not always correlate with clinical effectiveness

Therapeutic: 50-150 ng/mL (SI: 190-570 nmol/L)

Toxic: >500 ng/mL (SI: >1900 nmol/L)

Dosage Forms Excipient information presented when available (limited, particularly for generics); consult specific product labeling.

Capsule: 10 mg, 25 mg, 50 mg, 75 mg

Pamelor®: 10 mg, 25 mg, 50 mg, 75 mg [may contain benzyl alcohol; 50 mg may also contain sodium bisulfite]

Solution:

Pamelor®: 10 mg/5 mL (473 mL) [contains ethanol 4% and benzoic acid]

- **Nortriptyline Hydrochloride** *see* Nortriptyline *on page 1081*
- **Norvasc®** *see* AmLODIPine *on page 93*
- **Norventyl (Can)** *see* Nortriptyline *on page 1081*
- **Norvir®** *see* Ritonavir *on page 1326*
- **Norvir® SEC (Can)** *see* Ritonavir *on page 1326*
- **Notuss®-DC** *see* Pseudoephedrine and Codeine *on page 1266*
- **Novahistex® DM Decongestant (Can)** *see* Pseudoephedrine and Dextromethorphan *on page 1266*
- **Novahistex® DM Decongestant Expectorant (Can)** *see* Guaifenesin, Pseudoephedrine, and Dextromethorphan *on page 715*
- **Novahistex® Expectorant with Decongestant (Can)** *see* Guaifenesin and Pseudoephedrine *on page 713*
- **Novahistine DH** *see* Dihydrocodeine, Chlorpheniramine, and Phenylephrine *on page 448*
- **Novahistine® DM Decongestant (Can)** *see* Pseudoephedrine and Dextromethorphan *on page 1266*
- **Novahistine® DM Decongestant Expectorant (Can)** *see* Guaifenesin, Pseudoephedrine, and Dextromethorphan *on page 715*
- **Novamilor (Can)** *see* Amiloride and Hydrochlorothiazide *on page 85*
- **Novamoxin® (Can)** *see* Amoxicillin *on page 98*

◆ **Nu-Verap (Can)** *see* Verapamil *on page 1557*
◆ **Nuvigil™** *see* Armodafinil *on page 136*
◆ **NVP** *see* Nevirapine *on page 1055*
◆ **Nyaderm (Can)** *see* Nystatin *on page 1087*
◆ **Nyamyc™** *see* Nystatin *on page 1087*

Nystatin (nye STAT in)

U.S. Brand Names Bio-Statin®; Mycostatin®; Nyamyc™; Nystat-Rx®; Nystop®; Paddock Nystatin™; Pedi-Dri®

Canadian Brand Names Candistatin®; Nilstat; Nyaderm; PMS-Nystatin

Pharmacologic Category Antifungal Agent, Oral Nonabsorbed; Antifungal Agent, Topical; Antifungal Agent, Vaginal

Additional Appendix Information

Antifungal Agents *on page 1640*

Treatment of Sexually Transmitted Infections *on page 1773*

Use Treatment of susceptible cutaneous, mucocutaneous, and oral cavity fungal infections normally caused by the *Candida* species

Pregnancy Risk Factor B/C (oral)

Lactation Does not enter breast milk/compatible (not absorbed orally)

Medication Safety Issues

Sound-alike/look-alike issues:

Nystatin may be confused with Nilstat®, Nitrostat®

Nilstat may be confused with Nitrostat®, nystatin

Contraindications Hypersensitivity to nystatin or any component of the formulation

Adverse Reactions

Frequency not defined: Dermatologic: Contact dermatitis, Stevens-Johnson syndrome

1% to 10%: Gastrointestinal: Nausea, vomiting, diarrhea, stomach pain

<1% (Limited to important or life-threatening): Hypersensitivity reactions

Drug Interactions

Avoid Concomitant Use There are no known interactions where it is recommended to avoid concomitant use.

Increased Effect/Toxicity There are no known significant interactions involving an increase in effect.

Decreased Effect

Nystatin may decrease the levels/effects of: Saccharomyces boulardii

Stability

Vaginal insert: Store in refrigerator. Protect from temperature extremes, moisture, and light.

Oral tablet, ointment, topical powder, and oral suspension: Store at controlled room temperature of 15°C to 25°C (59°F to 77°F).

Mechanism of Action Binds to sterols in fungal cell membrane, changing the cell wall permeability allowing for leakage of cellular contents

Pharmacodynamics/Kinetics

Onset of action: Symptomatic relief from candidiasis: 24-72 hours

Absorption: Topical: None through mucous membranes or intact skin; Oral: Poorly absorbed

Excretion: Feces (as unchanged drug)

Dosage

Oral candidiasis:

Suspension (swish and swallow orally):

Premature infants: 100,000 units 4 times/day

Infants: 200,000 units 4 times/day or 100,000 units to each side of mouth 4 times/day

Children and Adults: 400,000-600,000 units 4 times/day

Powder for compounding: Children and Adults: 1/8 teaspoon (500,000 units) to equal approximately 1/2 cup of water; give 4 times/day

Mucocutaneous infections: Children and Adults: Topical: Apply 2-3 times/day to affected areas; very moist topical lesions are treated best with powder

Intestinal infections: Adults: Oral: 500,000-1,000,000 units every 8 hours

Vaginal infections: Adults: Vaginal tablets: Insert 1 tablet/day at bedtime for 2 weeks

Administration Suspension: Shake well before using. Should be swished about the mouth and retained in the mouth for as long as possible (several minutes) before swallowing.

Dosage Forms Excipient information presented when available (limited, particularly for generics); consult specific product labeling. [DSC] = Discontinued product

Capsule:

Bio-Statin®: 500,000 units, 1 million units

Cream: 100,000 units/g (15 g, 30 g)

Mycostatin®: 100,000 units/g (30 g)

Ointment, topical: 100,000 units/g (15 g, 30 g)

Powder, for prescription compounding: 50 million units (10 g); 150 million units (30 g); 500 million units (100 g); 2 billion units (400 g)

Nystat-Rx®: 50 million units (10 g); 150 million units (30 g); 500 million units (100 g); 1 billion units (190 g); 2 billion units (350 g)

Powder, for prescription compounding: 1 billion units (190 g); 150 million units (30 g); 2 billion units (350 g); 50 million units (10 g); 500 million units (100 g)

Bio-Statin®: 2 billion units (30 g)

Powder for suspension, oral [preservative free]:

Paddock Nystatin™: 150 million units (30 g); 2 billion units (400 g); 50 million units (10 g); 500 million units (100 g) [sugar free]

Powder, topical:

Mycostatin®: 100,000 units/g (15 g) [contains talc] [DSC]

Nyamyc™: 100,000 units/g (15 g, 30 g) [contains talc]

Nystop®: 100,000 units/g (15 g, 30 g, 60 g) [contains talc]

Pedi-Dri®: 100,000 units/g (56.7 g) [contains talc]

Suspension, oral: 100,000 units/mL (5 mL, 60 mL, 480 mL)

Tablet: 500,000 units

Tablet, vaginal: 100,000 units (15s) [packaged with applicator]

Nystatin and Triamcinolone
(nye STAT in & trye am SIN oh lone)

U.S. Brand Names Mycolog®-II [DSC]

Index Terms Triamcinolone and Nystatin

Pharmacologic Category Antifungal Agent, Topical; Corticosteroid, Topical

Use Treatment of cutaneous candidiasis

Pregnancy Risk Factor C

Medication Safety Issues

Sound-alike/look-alike issues:

Mycolog®-II may be confused with Halog®

Dosage Children and Adults: Topical: Apply sparingly 2-4 times/day. Therapy should be discontinued when control is achieved; if no improvement is seen, reassessment of diagnosis may be necessary.

Additional Information Complete prescribing information for this medication should be consulted for additional detail.

Dosage Forms Excipient information presented when available (limited, particularly for generics); consult specific product labeling. [DSC] = Discontinued product

Cream (Mycolog®-II [DSC]): Nystatin 100,000 units and triamcinolone acetonide 0.1% (15 g, 30 g, 60 g)

Ointment: Nystatin 100,000 units and triamcinolone acetonide 0.1% (15 g, 30 g, 60 g)

Mycolog®-II: Nystatin 100,000 units and triamcinolone acetonide 0.1% (15 g, 30 g, 60 g) [DSC]

◆ **Nystat-Rx®** *see* Nystatin *on page 1087*

◆ **Nystop®** *see* Nystatin *on page 1087*

◆ **Nytol® (Can)** *see* DiphenhydrAMINE *on page 456*

◆ **Nytol® Extra Strength (Can)** *see* DiphenhydrAMINE *on page 456*

◆ **Nytol® Quick Caps [OTC]** *see* DiphenhydrAMINE *on page 456*

◆ **Nytol® Quick Gels [OTC]** *see* DiphenhydrAMINE *on page 456*

◆ **NāSal™ [OTC]** *see* Sodium Chloride *on page 1381*

◆ **NāSop™ [DSC]** *see* Phenylephrine *on page 1183*

◆ **OCBZ** *see* OXcarbazepine *on page 1116*

◆ **Ocean® [OTC]** *see* Sodium Chloride *on page 1381*

◆ **Ocean® for Kids [OTC]** *see* Sodium Chloride *on page 1381*

◆ **Ocella™** *see* Ethinyl Estradiol and Drospirenone *on page 576*

◆ **Octagam®** *see* Immune Globulin (Intravenous) *on page 777*

◆ **Octostim® (Can)** *see* Desmopressin *on page 421*

Octreotide (ok TREE oh tide)

U.S. Brand Names Sandostatin LAR®; Sandostatin®

Canadian Brand Names Octreotide Acetate Injection; Octreotide Acetate Omega; Sandostatin LAR®; Sandostatin®

Index Terms NSC-671663; Octreotide Acetate

Pharmacologic Category Antidiarrheal; Antidote; Somatostatin Analog

Use Control of symptoms in patients with metastatic carcinoid and vasoactive intestinal peptide-secreting tumors (VIPomas); treatment of acromegaly

Unlabeled/Investigational Use AIDS-associated secretory diarrhea (including *Cryptosporidiosis*); control of bleeding of esophageal varices; second-line treatment for thymic malignancies; Cushing's syndrome (ectopic); insulinomas; glucagonoma; small bowel fistulas; pancreatic tumors; gastrinoma; postgastrectomy dumping syndrome; chemotherapy-induced diarrhea; graft-versus-host disease (GVHD) induced diarrhea; Zollinger-Ellison syndrome; congenital hyperinsulinism; hypothalamic obesity; treatment of hypoglycemia secondary to sulfonylurea poisoning (as an adjunct to dextrose)

Pregnancy Risk Factor B

Pregnancy Considerations Teratogenic effects were not observed in animal studies. Octreotide crosses the human placenta; data concerning use in pregnancy is limited. Women of childbearing potential should use adequate contraception during treatment with octreotide; normalization of IGF-1 and GH may restore fertility in women with acromegaly. In case reports of acromegalic women who received normal doses of octreotide during pregnancy, no congenital malformations were reported.

Lactation Excretion in breast milk unknown/use caution

Medication Safety Issues

Sound-alike/look-alike issues:

Sandostatin® may be confused with Sandimmune®, Sandostatin LAR®, sargramostim, simvastatin

Contraindications Hypersensitivity to octreotide or any component of the formulation

Warnings/Precautions May impair gallbladder function; monitor patients for cholelithiasis. Use with caution in patients with renal and/or hepatic impairment; dosage adjustment is required in patients receiving dialysis and in patients with established cirrhosis. Somatostatin analogs may affect glucose regulation. In type I diabetes, severe hypoglycemia may occur; in type II diabetes or patients without diabetes, hyperglycemia may occur. Insulin and other hypoglycemic medication requirements may change. Do not use depot formulation for the treatment of sulfonylurea-induced hypoglycemia. Bradycardia, conduction abnormalities, and arrhythmia have been observed in acromegalic and carcinoid syndrome patients; use caution with CHF or concomitant medications that alter heart rate or rhythm. Cardiovascular medication requirements may change. Octreotide may enhance the adverse/toxic effects of other QT_c-prolonging agents. May alter absorption of dietary fats; monitor for pancreatitis. May reduce excessive fluid loss in patients with conditions that cause such loss; monitor for elevations in zinc levels in such patients that are maintained on total parenteral nutrition (TPN). Chronic treatment has been associated with abnormal Schillings test; monitor vitamin B_{12} levels. Suppresses secretion of TSH; monitor for hypothyroidism. Therapy may restore fertility; females of childbearing potential should use adequate contraception. Dosage adjustment may be necessary in the elderly; significant increases in elimination half-life have been observed in older adults. Vehicle used in depot injection (polylactide-co-glycolide microspheres) has rarely been associated with retinal artery occlusion in patients with abnormal arteriovenous anastomosis.

Adverse Reactions Adverse reactions vary by route of administration and dosage form. Frequency of cardiac, endocrine, and gastrointestinal adverse reactions was generally higher in acromegalics.

>16%:

Cardiovascular: Sinus bradycardia (19% to 25%), chest pain (≤20%; non-depot formulations)

Central nervous system: Fatigue (1% to 32%), headache (6% to 30%), malaise (16% to 20%), fever (16% to 20%), dizziness (5% to 20%)

Dermatologic: Pruritus (≤18%)

Endocrine & metabolic: Hyperglycemia (2% to 27%)

Gastrointestinal: Abdominal pain (5% to 61%), loose stools (5% to 61%), nausea (5% to 61%), diarrhea (34% to 58%), flatulence (≤38%), cholelithiasis (13% to 38%; length of therapy dependent), biliary sludge (24%; length of therapy dependent), constipation (9% to 21%), vomiting (4% to 21%), biliary duct dilatation (12%)

Local: Injection site pain (2% to 50%; dose and formulation related)

Neuromuscular & skeletal: Back pain (1% to 27%), arthropathy (8% to 19%), myalgia (≤18%)

Respiratory: Upper respiratory infection (10% to 23%), dyspnea (≤20%; non-depot formulations)

Miscellaneous: Antibodies to octreotide (up to 25%; no efficacy change), flu symptoms (1% to 20%)

5% to 15%:

Cardiovascular: Hypertension (≤13%), conduction abnormalities (9% to 10%), arrhythmia (3% to 9%), palpitation, peripheral edema

Central nervous system: Pain (4% to 15%), anxiety, confusion, hypoesthesia, insomnia

Dermatologic: Rash (15%; depot formulation), alopecia (≤13%)

Endocrine & metabolic: Hypothyroidism (≤12%; non-depot formulations), goiter (≤8%; non-depot formulations)

Gastrointestinal: Anorexia, cramping, tenesmus (4% to 6%), dyspepsia (4% to 6%), steatorrhea (4% to 6%), feces discoloration (4% to 6%)

Hematologic: Anemia (≤15%; non-depot formulations: <1%)

Neuromuscular & skeletal: Arthralgia, myalgia, paresthesia, rigors, weakness

Otic: Earache

Renal: Renal calculus

Respiratory: Cough, pharyngitis, sinusitis, rhinitis

Miscellaneous: Allergy, diaphoresis

1% to 4%:

Cardiovascular: Angina, cardiac failure, edema, flushing, hematoma, phlebitis

Central nervous system: Abnormal gait, amnesia, depression, dysphonia, hallucinations, nervousness, neuralgia, somnolence, vertigo

Dermatologic: Acne, bruising, cellulitis

Endocrine & metabolic: Hypoglycemia (2% to 4%), hypokalemia, hypoproteinemia, gout, cachexia, breast pain, impotence

Gastrointestinal: Colitis, diverticulitis, dysphagia, fat malabsorption, gastritis, gastroenteritis, gingivitis, glossitis, melena, stomatitis, taste perversion, xerostomia

Genitourinary: Incontinence, pollakuria (non-depot formulations), urinary tract infection

Local: Injection site hematoma

Neuromuscular & skeletal: Hyperkinesia, hypertonia, joint pain, neuropathy, tremor

Ocular: Blurred vision, visual disturbance

Otic: Tinnitus

Renal: Albuminuria, renal abscess

Respiratory: Bronchitis, epistaxis

Miscellaneous: Bacterial infection, cold symptoms, moniliasis

<1% (Limited to important or life-threatening): Anaphylactic shock, anaphylactoid reaction, aneurysm, aphasia, appendicitis, arthritis, ascending cholangitis, ascites, atrial fibrillation, basal cell carcinoma, Bell's palsy, biliary obstruction, breast carcinoma, cardiac arrest, cerebral vascular disorder, CHF, cholestatic hepatitis, CK increased, creatinine increased, deafness, diabetes insipidus, diabetes mellitus, facial edema, fatty liver, galactorrhea, gallbladder polyp, GI bleeding, GI hemorrhage, GI ulcer, glaucoma, gynecomastia, hearing loss, hematuria, hemiparesis, hemorrhoids, hepatitis, hyperesthesia, hypertensive reaction, hypoadrenalism, intestinal obstruction, intracranial hemorrhage, intraocular pressure increased, ischemia, jaundice, joint effusion, lactation, LFTs increased, libido decreased, malignant hyperpyrexia, menstrual irregularities, MI, migraine, nephrolithiasis, neuritis, orthostatic hypotension, pancreatitis, pancytopenia, paresis, petechiae, pituitary apoplexy, pleural effusion, pneumonia, pneumothorax, pulmonary embolism, pulmonary hypertension, pulmonary nodule, Raynaud's syndrome, rectal bleeding, renal failure, renal insufficiency, retinal vein thrombosis, scotoma, seizure, status asthmaticus, suicide attempt, syncope, tachycardia, thrombocytopenia, thrombophlebitis, thrombosis, urticaria, visual field defect, weight loss, wheal/erythema

Drug Interactions

Avoid Concomitant Use

Avoid concomitant use of Octreotide with any of the following: Nilotinib; Tetrabenazine; Thioridazine; Ziprasidone

Increased Effect/Toxicity

Octreotide may increase the levels/effects of: Codeine; Pegvisomant; QTc-Prolonging Agents; Tetrabenazine; Thioridazine; Ziprasidone

The levels/effects of Octreotide may be increased by: Alfuzosin; Ciprofloxacin; Gadobutrol; Herbs (Hypoglycemic Properties); Nilotinib

Decreased Effect

Octreotide may decrease the levels/effects of: CycloSPORINE

Ethanol/Nutrition/Herb Interactions

Herb/Nutraceutical: Avoid hypoglycemic herbs, including alfalfa, aloe, bilberry, bitter melon, burdock, celery, damiana, fenugreek, garcinia, garlic, ginger, ginseng (American), gymnema, marshmallow, and stinging nettle (may enhance the hypoglycemic effect of octreotide).

Stability

Solution: Octreotide is a clear solution and should be stored at refrigerated temperatures between 2°C and 8°C (36°F and 46°F). Protect from light. May be stored at room temperature of 20°C to 30°C (70°F and 86°F) for up to 14 days when protected from light. Stability of parenteral admixture is stable in NS for 96 hours at room temperature (25°C) and in D_5W for 24 hours. Discard multidose vials within 14 days after initial entry.

Suspension: Prior to dilution, store at refrigerated temperatures between 2°C and 8°C (36°F and 46°F) and protect from light. Depot drug product kit may be at room temperature for 30-60 minutes prior to use. Use suspension immediately after preparation.

Mechanism of Action Mimics natural somatostatin by inhibiting serotonin release, and the secretion of gastrin, VIP, insulin, glucagon, secretin, motilin, and pancreatic polypeptide. Decreases growth hormone and IGF-1 in acromegaly. Octreotide provides more potent inhibition of growth hormone, glucagon, and insulin as compared to endogenous somatostatin. Also suppresses LH response to GnRH, secretion of thyroid-stimulating hormone and decreases splanchnic blood flow.

Pharmacodynamics/Kinetics

Duration: SubQ: 6-12 hours

Absorption: SubQ: Rapid and complete; I.M. (depot formulation): Released slowly (via microsphere degradation in the muscle)

Distribution: V_d: 14 L (13-30 L in acromegaly)

Protein binding: 65%, mainly to lipoprotein (41% in acromegaly)

Metabolism: Extensively hepatic

Bioavailability: SubQ: 100%; I.M: 60% to 63% of SubQ dose

Half-life elimination: 1.7-1.9 hours; Increased in elderly patients; Cirrhosis: Up to 3.7 hours; Fatty liver disease: Up to 3.4 hours; Renal impairment: Up to 3.1 hours

Time to peak, plasma: SubQ: 0.4 hours (0.7 hours acromegaly); I.M.: 1 hour

Excretion: Urine (32% as unchanged drug)

Dosage

Acromegaly: Adults:

SubQ, I.V.: Initial: 50 mcg 3 times/day; titrate to achieve growth hormone levels <5 ng/mL or IGF-I (somatomedin C) levels <1.9 units/mL in males and <2.2 units/mL in females. Usual effective dose 100-200 mcg 3 times/day; range 300-1500 mcg/day. **Note:** Should be withdrawn yearly for a 4-week interval (8 weeks for depot injection) in patients who have received irradiation. Resume if levels increase and signs/symptoms recur.

I.M. depot injection: Patients must be stabilized on subcutaneous octreotide for at least 2 weeks before switching to the long-acting depot. Upon switch: 20 mg I.M. intragluteally every 4 weeks for 3 months, then the dose may be modified based upon response.

Dosage adjustment for acromegaly: After 3 months of depot injections, the dosage may be continued or modified as follows:

GH ≤1 ng/mL, IGF-1 normal, and symptoms controlled: Reduce octreotide LAR® to 10 mg I.M. every 4 weeks

GH ≤2.5 ng/mL, IGF-1 normal, and symptoms controlled: Maintain octreotide LAR® at 20 mg I.M. every 4 weeks

GH >2.5 ng/mL, IGF-1 elevated, and/or symptoms uncontrolled: Increase octreotide LAR® to 30 mg I.M. every 4 weeks

Note: Patients not adequately controlled at a dose of 30 mg may increase dose to 40 mg every 4 weeks. Dosages >40 mg are not recommended.

Carcinoid tumors: Adults:

SubQ, I.V.: Initial 2 weeks: 100-600 mcg/day in 2-4 divided doses; usual range 50-750 mcg/day (some patients may require up to 1500 mcg/day)

I.M. depot injection: Patients must be stabilized on subcutaneous octreotide for at least 2 weeks before switching to the long-acting depot. Upon switch: 20 mg I.M. intragluteally every 4 weeks for 2 months, then the dose may be modified based upon response.

Note: Patients should continue to receive their SubQ injections for the first 2 weeks at the same dose in order to maintain therapeutic levels (some patients may require 3-4 weeks of continued SubQ injections). Patients who experience periodic exacerbations of symptoms may require temporary SubQ injections in addition to depot injections (at their previous SubQ dosing regimen) until symptoms have resolved.

Dosage adjustment: See dosing adjustment for VIPomas.

VIPomas: Adults:

SubQ, I.V.: Initial 2 weeks: 200-300 mcg/day in 2-4 divided doses; titrate dose based on response/tolerance. Range: 150-750 mcg/day (doses >450 mcg/day are rarely required)

I.M. depot injection: Patients must be stabilized on subcutaneous octreotide for at least 2 weeks before switching to the long-acting depot. Upon switch: 20 mg I.M. intragluteally every 4 weeks for 2 months, then the dose may be modified based upon response.

Note: Patients receiving depot injection should continue to receive their SubQ injections for the first 2 weeks at the same dose in order to maintain therapeutic levels (some patients may require 3-4 weeks of continued SubQ injections). Patients who experience periodic exacerbations of symptoms may require temporary SubQ injections in addition to depot injections (at their previous SubQ dosing regimen) until symptoms have resolved.

Dosage adjustment for carcinoid tumors and VIPomas: After 2 months of depot injections, the dosage may be continued or modified as follows:

Increase to 30 mg I.M. every 4 weeks if symptoms are inadequately controlled

Decrease to 10 mg I.M. every 4 weeks, for a trial period, if initially responsive to 20 mg dose

Dosage >30 mg is not recommended

Congenital hyperinsulinism (unlabeled use): Infants and Children: SubQ: Doses of 3-40 mcg/kg/day have been used

Diarrhea (unlabeled use):

Infants and Children: I.V., SubQ: Doses of 1-10 mcg/kg every 12 hours have been used in children beginning at the low end of the range and increasing by 0.3 mcg/kg/dose at 3-day intervals. Suppression of growth hormone (animal data) is of concern when used as long-term therapy.

Adults: I.V.: Initial: 50-100 mcg every 8 hours; increase by 100 mcg/dose at 48-hour intervals; maximum dose: 500 mcg every 8 hours

Esophageal varices bleeding (unlabeled use): Adults: I.V. bolus: 25-50 mcg followed by continuous I.V. infusion of 25-50 mcg/hour

Hypoglycemia in sulfonylurea poisoning (unlabeled use): Note: SubQ is the preferred route of administration; repeat dosing or initiation of a continuous infusion may be required in patients who experience recurrent hypoglycemia. Duration of treatment may exceed 24 hours. Optimal care decisions should be made based upon patient-specific details:

Children: SubQ: 1-1.5 mcg/kg (maximum dose: 50 mcg); repeat in 6-12 hours as needed based upon blood glucose concentrations

Adults:

SubQ (preferred route of administration): 50-100 mcg; repeat in 6-12 hours as needed based upon blood glucose concentrations

I.V.: Doses up to 100-125 mcg/hour have been used successfully

Elderly: Elimination half-life is increased by 46% and clearance is decreased by 26%; dose adjustment may be required. Dosing should generally begin at the lower end of dosing range.

Dosage adjustment in renal impairment:

Nondialysis-dependent renal impairment: No dosage adjustment required

Dialysis-dependent renal impairment: Depot injection: Initial dose: 10 mg I.M. every 4 weeks; titrate based upon response (clearance is reduced by ~50%)

Dosage adjustment in hepatic impairment: Patients with established cirrhosis of the liver: Depot injection: Initial dose: 10 mg I.M. every 4 weeks; titrate based upon response

Dietary Considerations Schedule injections between meals to decrease GI effects. May alter absorption of dietary fats.

Administration

Regular injection formulation (do not use if solution contains particles or is discolored): Administer SubQ or I.V.; I.V. administration may be IVP, IVPB, or continuous I.V. infusion (unlabeled route):

IVP should be administered undiluted over 3 minutes

IVPB should be administered over 15-30 minutes

Continuous I.V. infusion rates have ranged from 25-50 mcg/hour for the treatment of esophageal variceal bleeding (unlabeled route/use); continuous I.V. infusion rates of 100-125 mcg/hour have been used for the treatment of sulfonylurea-induced hypoglycemia (unlabeled use).

SubQ: Use the concentration with smallest volume to deliver dose to reduce injection site pain. Rotate injection site; may bring to room temperature prior to injection.

Depot formulation: Administer I.M. intragluteal (avoid deltoid administration); alternate gluteal injection sites to avoid irritation. Do not administer Sandostatin LAR® intravenously or subcutaneously; must be administered immediately after mixing.

Monitoring Parameters

Acromegaly: Growth hormone, somatomedin C (IGF-1)

Carcinoid: 5-HIAA, plasma serotonin and plasma substance P

VIPomas: Vasoactive intestinal peptide

Chronic therapy: Thyroid function (baseline and periodic), vitamin B_{12} level, blood glucose, cardiac function (heart rate, EKG), zinc level (patients with excessive fluid loss maintained on TPN)

Reference Range Vasoactive intestinal peptide: <75 ng/L; levels vary considerably between laboratories

Dosage Forms Excipient information presented when available (limited, particularly for generics); consult specific product labeling.

Injection, microspheres for suspension, as acetate [depot formulation]:

Sandostatin LAR®: 10 mg, 20 mg, 30 mg [contains polylactide-co-glycolide; packaged with diluent and syringe]

Injection, solution, as acetate: 0.2 mg/mL (5 mL); 1 mg/mL (5 mL)

Sandostatin®: 0.2 mg/mL (5 mL); 1 mg/mL (5 mL)

Injection, solution, as acetate [preservative free]: 0.05 mg/mL (1 mL); 0.1 mg/mL (1 mL); 0.5 mg/mL (1 mL)

Sandostatin®: 0.05 mg/mL (1 mL); 0.1 mg/mL (1 mL); 0.5 mg/mL (1 mL)

◆ **Octreotide Acetate** *see* Octreotide *on page* 1088

Ofloxacin (oh FLOKS a sin)

U.S. Brand Names Floxin®; Ocuflox®

Canadian Brand Names Apo-Ofloxacin®; Apo-Oflox®; Floxin®; Novo-Ofloxacin; Ocuflox®; PMS-Ofloxacin

Index Terms Floxin Otic Singles

Pharmacologic Category Antibiotic, Quinolone

Additional Appendix Information

Antimicrobial Drugs of Choice *on page 1752*

Prevention of Wound Infection and Sepsis in Surgical Patients *on page 1738*

Treatment of Sexually Transmitted Infections *on page 1773*

Tuberculosis *on page 1776*

Use Quinolone antibiotic for the treatment of acute exacerbations of chronic bronchitis, community-acquired pneumonia, skin and skin structure infections (uncomplicated), urethral and cervical gonorrhea (acute, uncomplicated), urethritis and cervicitis (nongonococcal), mixed infections of the urethra and cervix, pelvic inflammatory disease (acute), cystitis (uncomplicated), urinary tract infections (complicated), prostatitis

Note: As of April 2007, the CDC no longer recommends the use of fluoroquinolones for the treatment of gonococcal disease.

Ophthalmic: Treatment of superficial ocular infections involving the conjunctiva or cornea due to strains of susceptible organisms

Otic: Otitis externa, chronic suppurative otitis media, acute otitis media

Unlabeled/Investigational Use Epididymitis (nongonococcal), leprosy, Traveler's diarrhea

Restrictions An FDA-approved patient medication guide is available and must be distributed when dispensing an outpatient prescription (new or refill) where this medication is to be used without direct supervision of a healthcare provider. Medication guides are available at http://www.fda.gov/cder/Offices/ODS/medication_guides.htm.

Pregnancy Risk Factor C

Pregnancy Considerations Adverse events have been observed in some animal studies; therefore, the manufacturer classifies ofloxacin as pregnancy category C. Ofloxacin crosses the placenta and produces measurable concentrations in the amniotic fluid. An increased risk of teratogenic effects has not been observed in animals or humans following ofloxacin use during pregnancy; however, because of concerns of cartilage damage in immature animals, ofloxacin should only be used during pregnancy if a safer option is not available. Serum concentrations of ofloxacin may be lower during pregnancy than in nonpregnant patients.

Lactation Enters breast milk/not recommended (AAP rates "compatible")

Medication Safety Issues

Sound-alike/look-alike issues:

Floxin® may be confused with Flexeril®

Ocuflox® may be confused with Occlusal®-HP, Ocufen®

International issues:

Floxin® may be confused with Flogen® which is a brand name for naproxen in Mexico

Floxin® may be confused with Fluoxin® which is a brand name for fluoxetine in the Czech Republic and Romania

Floxin® may be confused with Flexin® which is a brand name for orphenadrine in Israel and indomethacin in Great Britain

Contraindications Hypersensitivity to ofloxacin or other members of the quinolone group, such as nalidixic acid, oxolinic acid, cinoxacin, norfloxacin, and ciprofloxacin; hypersensitivity to any component of the formulation

Warnings/Precautions [U.S. Boxed Warning]: There have been reports of tendon inflammation and/or rupture with quinolone antibiotics; risk may be increased with concurrent corticosteroids, organ transplant recipients, and in patients >60 years of age. Rupture of the Achilles tendon sometimes requiring surgical repair has been reported most frequently; but other tendon sites (eg, rotator cuff, biceps) have also been reported. Strenuous physical activity, rheumatoid arthritis, and renal impairment may be an independent risk factor for tendonitis. Discontinue at first sign of tendon inflammation or pain. May occur even after discontinuation of therapy. Use with caution in patients with rheumatoid arthritis; may increase risk of tendon rupture. Use with caution in patients with epilepsy or other CNS diseases which could predispose seizures; potential for seizures, although very rare, may be increased with concomitant NSAID therapy. Tremor, restlessness, confusion, and very rarely hallucinations or seizures may occur; use with caution in patients with known or suspected CNS disorder. Discontinue in patients who experience significant CNS adverse effects (eg, dizziness, hallucinations, suicidal ideations or actions). Use with caution in patients with renal or hepatic impairment. Peripheral neuropathies have been linked to ofloxacin use; discontinue if numbness, tingling, or weakness develops.

Fluoroquinolones have been associated with the development of serious, and sometimes fatal, hypoglycemia, most often in elderly diabetics, but also in patients without diabetes. This occurred most frequently with gatifloxacin (no longer available systemically) but may occur at a lower frequency with other quinolones.

Rare cases of torsade de pointes have been reported in patients receiving ofloxacin and other quinolones. Risk may be minimized by avoiding use in patients with known prolongation of the QT interval, bradycardia, hypokalemia, hypomagnesemia, cardiomyopathy, or in those receiving concurrent therapy with Class Ia or Class III antiarrhythmics.

Severe hypersensitivity reactions, including anaphylaxis, have occurred with quinolone therapy. Reactions may present as typical allergic symptoms after a single dose, or may manifest as severe idiosyncratic dermatologic, vascular, pulmonary, renal, hepatic, and/or hematologic events, usually after multiple doses. Prompt discontinuation of drug should occur if skin rash or other symptoms arise. Prolonged use may result in fungal or bacterial superinfection, including *C. difficile*-associated diarrhea (CDAD) and pseudomembranous colitis; CDAD has been observed >2 months postantibiotic treatment. Quinolones may exacerbate myasthenia gravis. Avoid excessive sunlight and take precautions to limit exposure (eg, loose fitting clothing, sunscreen); may cause moderate-to-severe phototoxicity reactions. Discontinue use if photosensitivity occurs. Since ofloxacin is ineffective in the treatment of syphilis and may mask symptoms, all patients should be tested for syphilis at the time of gonorrheal diagnosis and 3 months later. Hemolytic reactions may (rarely) occur with quinolone use in patients with latent or actual G6PD deficiency. Safety and efficacy have not been established in children.

Adverse Reactions

Systemic:

1% to 10%:

Cardiovascular: Chest pain (1% to 3%)

Central nervous system: Headache (1% to 9%), insomnia (3% to 7%), dizziness (1% to 5%), fatigue (1% to 3%), somnolence (1% to 3%), sleep disorders (1% to 3%), nervousness (1% to 3%), pyrexia (1% to 3%)

Dermatologic: Rash/pruritus (1% to 3%)

Gastrointestinal: Diarrhea (1% to 4%), vomiting (1% to 4%), GI distress (1% to 3%), abdominal cramps (1% to 3%), flatulence (1% to 3%), abnormal taste (1% to 3%), xerostomia (1% to 3%), appetite decreased (1% to 3%), nausea (3% to 10%), constipation (1% to 3%)

Genitourinary: Vaginitis (1% to 5%), external genital pruritus in women (1% to 3%)

Ocular: Visual disturbances (1% to 3%)

Respiratory: Pharyngitis (1% to 3%)

Miscellaneous: Trunk pain

<1%, postmarketing, and/or case reports (limited to important or life-threatening): Anaphylaxis reactions, anxiety, blurred vision, chills, cognitive change, cough, depression, dream abnormality, ecchymosis, edema, erythema nodosum, euphoria, extremity pain, hallucinations, hearing acuity decreased, hepatic dysfunction, hepatic failure (some fatal), hepatitis, hyper-/hypoglycemia, hypertension, interstitial nephritis, lightheadedness, malaise, myasthenia gravis exacerbation, palpitation, paresthesia, peripheral neuropathy, photophobia, photosensitivity, pneumonitis, psychotic reactions, rhabdomyolysis, seizure, Stevens-Johnson syndrome, syncope, tendonitis and tendon rupture, thirst, tinnitus, torsade de pointes, Tourette's syndrome, toxic epidermal necrolysis, vasculitis, vasodilation, vertigo, weakness, weight loss

Ophthalmic: Frequency not defined:

Central nervous system: Dizziness

Gastrointestinal: Nausea

Ocular: Blurred vision, burning, chemical conjunctivitis/keratitis, discomfort, dryness, edema, eye pain, foreign body sensation, itching, photophobia, redness, stinging, tearing

Otic:

>10%: Local: Application site reaction (<1% to 17%)

1% to 10%:

Central nervous system: Dizziness (≤1%), vertigo (≤1%)

Dermatologic: Pruritus (1% to 4%), rash (1%)

Gastrointestinal: Taste perversion (7%)

Neuromuscular & skeletal: Paresthesia (1%)

<1% (Limited to important or life-threatening): Diarrhea, fever, headache, hearing loss (transient), hypertension, nausea, otorrhagia, tinnitus, transient neuropsychiatric disturbances, tremor, vomiting, xerostomia

Drug Interactions

Metabolism/Transport Effects **Inhibits** CYP1A2 (strong)

Avoid Concomitant Use There are no known interactions where it is recommended to avoid concomitant use.

Increased Effect/Toxicity

Ofloxacin may increase the levels/effects of: Bendamustine; Corticosteroids (Systemic); CYP1A2 Substrates; Sulfonylureas; Theophylline Derivatives; Vitamin K Antagonists

The levels/effects of Ofloxacin may be increased by: Insulin; Nonsteroidal Anti-Inflammatory Agents; Probenecid

Decreased Effect

Ofloxacin may decrease the levels/effects of: Mycophenolate; Sulfonylureas; Typhoid Vaccine

The levels/effects of Ofloxacin may be decreased by: Antacids; Calcium Salts; Didanosine; Iron Salts; Magnesium Salts; Quinapril; Sevelamer; Sucralfate; Zinc Salts

Ethanol/Nutrition/Herb Interactions

Food: Ofloxacin average peak serum concentrations may be decreased by 20% if taken with food.

Herb/Nutraceutical: Avoid dong quai, St John's wort (may also cause photosensitization).

Stability

Ophthalmic and otic solution: Store at 15°C to 25°C (59°F to 77°F).

Otic Singles™: Store at 15°C to 30°C (59°F to 86°F). Store in pouch to protect from light.

Tablet: Store below 30°C (86°F).

Mechanism of Action Ofloxacin is a DNA gyrase inhibitor. DNA gyrase is an essential bacterial enzyme that maintains the superhelical structure of DNA. DNA gyrase is required for DNA replication and transcription, DNA repair, recombination, and transposition; bactericidal

Pharmacodynamics/Kinetics

Absorption: Well absorbed; food causes only minor alterations

Distribution: V_d: 2.4-3.5 L/kg

Protein binding: 32%

Bioavailability: Oral: 98%

Half-life elimination: Biphasic: 4-5 hours and 20-25 hours (accounts for <5%); prolonged with renal impairment

Excretion: Primarily urine (as unchanged drug)

Dosage

Usual dosage range:

Children ≥6 months: Otic: 5 drops daily

Children >1 year: Ophthalmic: 1-2 drops every 30 minutes to 4 hours initially, decreasing to every 4-6 hours

Children >12 years: Otic: 10 drops once or twice daily

Adults:

Ophthalmic: 1-2 drops every 30 minutes to 4 hours initially, decreasing to every 4-6 hours

Oral: 200-400 mg every 12 hours

Otic: 10 drops once or twice daily

Indication-specific dosing:

Children 6 months to 13 years: Otic:

Otitis externa: Instill 5 drops (or the contents of 1 single-dose container) into affected ear(s) once daily for 7 days

Children 1-12 years: Otic:

Acute otitis media with tympanostomy tubes: Instill 5 drops (or the contents of 1 single-dose container) into affected ear(s) twice daily for 10 days

Children >1 year and Adults: Ophthalmic:

Conjunctivitis: Instill 1-2 drops in affected eye(s) every 2-4 hours for the first 2 days, then use 4 times/day for an additional 5 days

Corneal ulcer: Instill 1-2 drops every 30 minutes while awake and every 4-6 hours after retiring for the first 2 days; beginning on day 3, instill 1-2 drops every hour while awake for 4-6 additional days; thereafter, 1-2 drops 4 times/day until clinical cure.

Children >12 years and Adults: Otic:

Otitis media, chronic suppurative with perforated tympanic membranes: Instill 10 drops (or the contents of 2 single-dose containers) into affected ear twice daily for 14 days

Children ≥13 years and Adults: Otic:

Otitis externa: Instill 10 drops (or the contents of 2 single-dose containers) into affected ear(s) once daily for 7 days

Adults: Oral:

Cervicitis/urethritis:

Nongonococcal: 300 mg every 12 hours for 7 days

Gonococcal (acute, uncomplicated): 400 mg as a single dose; **Note:** As of April 2007, the CDC no longer recommends the use of fluoroquinolones for the treatment of uncomplicated gonococcal disease.

Chronic bronchitis (acute exacerbation), community-acquired pneumonia, skin and skin structure infections (uncomplicated): 400 mg every 12 hours for 10 days

Epididymitis, nongonococcal (unlabeled use): 300 mg twice daily for 10 days

Leprosy (unlabeled use): 400 mg once daily

Pelvic inflammatory disease (acute): 400 mg every 12 hours for 10-14 days with or without metronidazole; **Note:** The CDC recommends use only if standard cephalosporin therapy is not feasible and community prevalence of quinolone-resistant gonococcal organisms is low. Culture sensitivity must be confirmed.

Prostatitis:

Acute: 400 mg for 1 dose, then 300 mg twice daily for 10 days

Chronic: 200 mg every 12 hours for 6 weeks

Traveler's diarrhea (unlabeled use): 300 mg twice daily for 3 days

UTI:

Uncomplicated: 200 mg every 12 hours for 3-7 days

Complicated: 200 mg every 12 hours for 10 days

Dosing adjustment/interval in renal impairment: Adults:

Oral: After a normal initial dose, adjust as follows:

Cl_{cr} 20-50 mL/minute: Administer usual dose every 24 hours

Cl_{cr} <20 mL/minute: Administer half the usual dose every 24 hours

Continuous arteriovenous or venovenous hemodiafiltration effects: Administer 300 mg every 24 hours

Dosing adjustment in hepatic impairment: Severe impairment: Maximum dose: 400 mg/day

Administration

Ophthalmic: For ophthalmic use only; avoid touching tip of applicator to eye or other surfaces.

Oral: Do not take within 2 hours of food or any antacids which contain zinc, magnesium, or aluminum.

Otic: Prior to use, warm solution by holding container in hands for 1-2 minutes. Patient should lie down with affected ear upward and medication instilled. Pump tragus 4 times to ensure penetration of medication. Patient should remain in this position for 5 minutes.

Test Interactions Some quinolones may produce a false-positive urine screening result for opiates using commercially-available immunoassay kits. This has been demonstrated most consistently for levofloxacin and ofloxacin, but other quinolones have shown cross-reactivity in certain assay kits. Confirmation of positive opiate screens by more specific methods should be considered.

Dosage Forms Excipient information presented when available (limited, particularly for generics); consult specific product labeling.

Solution, ophthalmic [drops]: 0.3% (5 mL, 10 mL)

Ocuflox®: 0.3% (5 mL) [contains benzalkonium chloride]

Solution, otic [drops]: 0.3% (5 mL, 10 mL)

Floxin®: 0.3% (5 mL, 10 mL) [contains benzalkonium chloride]

Floxin® Otic Singles™: 0.3% (0.25 mL) [contains benzalkonium chloride; packaged as 2 single-dose containers per pouch, 10 pouches per carton, total net volume 5 mL]

Tablet: 200 mg, 300 mg, 400 mg

◆ **Ogen®** *see* Estropipate *on page 568*

◆ **Ogestrel®** *see* Ethinyl Estradiol and Norgestrel *on page 585*

◆ **OGMT** *see* Metyrosine *on page 986*

◆ **OGT-918** *see* Miglustat *on page 996*

◆ **9-OH-risperidone** *see* Paliperidone *on page 1130*

◆ **OKT3** *see* Muromonab-CD3 *on page 1024*

OLANZapine (oh LAN za peen)

U.S. Brand Names Zyprexa®; Zyprexa® Zydis®

Canadian Brand Names Novo-Olanzapine; Zyprexa®; Zyprexa® Zydis®

Index Terms LY170053; Zyprexa Zydis

Pharmacologic Category Antimanic Agent; Antipsychotic Agent, Atypical

Additional Appendix Information

Antipsychotic Agents *on page 1644*

Use Treatment of the manifestations of schizophrenia; treatment of acute or mixed mania episodes associated with Bipolar I Disorder (as monotherapy or in combination with lithium or valproate); maintenance treatment of bipolar disorder; acute agitation (patients with schizophrenia or bipolar mania)

Unlabeled/Investigational Use Treatment of psychosis/schizophrenia in children or adolescents; chronic pain; prevention of chemotherapy-associated delayed nausea or vomiting; psychosis/agitation related to Alzheimer's dementia

Pregnancy Risk Factor C

Pregnancy Considerations No evidence of teratogenicity reported in animal studies. However, fetal toxicity and prolonged gestation have been observed. There are no adequate and well-controlled studies in pregnant women. Healthcare providers are encouraged to enroll women 18-45 years of age exposed to olanzapine during pregnancy in the Atypical Antipsychotics Pregnancy Registry (1-866-961-2388).

Lactation Enters breast milk/not recommended

Medication Safety Issues

Sound-alike/look-alike issues:

OLANZapine may be confused with olsalazine, QUEtiapine

Zyprexa® may be confused with Celexa™, Zyrtec®

Contraindications Hypersensitivity to olanzapine or any component of the formulation

Warnings/Precautions [U.S. Boxed Warning]: Elderly patients with dementia-related psychosis treated with atypical antipsychotics are at an increased risk of death compared to placebo. An increased incidence of cerebrovascular adverse events (including fatalities) has been reported in elderly patients with dementia-related psychosis. Olanzapine is not approved for this indication.

Moderate to highly sedating, use with caution in disorders where CNS depression is a feature; patients must be cautioned about performing tasks which require mental alertness (eg, operating machinery or driving). Use caution in patients with cardiac disease. Use with caution in Parkinson's disease, predisposition to seizures, or severe hepatic or renal disease. Life-threatening arrhythmias have occurred with therapeutic doses of some neuroleptics. May induce orthostatic hypotension; use caution with history of cardiovascular disease. Esophageal dysmotility and aspiration have been associated with antipsychotic use; use with caution in patients at risk of aspiration pneumonia. Caution in breast cancer or other prolactin-dependent tumors (elevates prolactin levels). Significant weight gain (>7% of baseline weight) may occur; monitor waist circumference and BMI. Impaired core body temperature regulation may occur; caution with strenuous exercise, heat exposure, dehydration, and concomitant medication possessing anticholinergic effects.

May cause anticholinergic effects; use with caution in patients with decreased gastrointestinal motility, urinary retention, BPH, xerostomia, glaucoma, or myasthenia gravis. Relative to other neuroleptics, olanzapine has a moderate potency of cholinergic blockade. May cause extrapyramidal symptoms (EPS), although risk of these reactions is lower relative to other neuroleptics. Risk of dystonia (and probably other EPS) may be greater with increased doses, use of conventional antipsychotics, males, and younger patients. May be associated with neuroleptic malignant syndrome (NMS). May cause extreme and life-threatening hyperglycemia; use with caution in patients with diabetes or other disorders of glucose regulation; monitor. Olanzapine levels may be lower in patients who smoke, requiring dosage adjustment.

The possibility of a suicide attempt is inherent in psychotic illness or bipolar disorder; use caution in high-risk patients during initiation of therapy. Prescriptions should be written for the smallest quantity consistent with good patient care. Safety and efficacy in pediatric patients have not been established.

Intramuscular administration: Patients should remain recumbent if drowsy/dizzy until hypotension, bradycardia, and/or hypoventilation has been ruled out. Concurrent use of I.M./I.V. benzodiazepines is not recommended (fatalities have been reported, though causality not determined).

Adverse Reactions

>10%:

Central nervous system: Somnolence (6% to 39% dose dependent), extrapyramidal symptoms (15% to 32% dose dependent), insomnia (up to 12%), dizziness (4% to 18%)

Gastrointestinal: Dyspepsia (7% to 11%), constipation (9% to 11%), weight gain (5% to 6%, has been reported as high as 40%), xerostomia (9% to 22% dose dependent)

Neuromuscular & skeletal: Weakness (2% to 20% dose dependent)

Miscellaneous: Accidental injury (12%)

1% to 10%:

Cardiovascular: Postural hypotension (1% to 5%), tachycardia (up to 3%), peripheral edema (up to 3%), chest pain (up to 3%), hyper-/hypotension (up to 2%)

Central nervous system: Personality changes (8%), speech disorder (7%), fever (up to 6%), abnormal dreams, euphoria, amnesia, delusions, emotional lability, mania, schizophrenia

Dermatologic: Bruising (up to 5%)

Endocrine & metabolic: Cholesterol increased, prolactin increased

Gastrointestinal: Nausea (up to 9% dose dependent), appetite increased (3% to 6%), vomiting (up to 4%), flatulence, salivation increased, thirst

Genitourinary: Incontinence (up to 2%), UTI (up to 2%), vaginitis

Hepatic: ALT increased (2%)

Local: Injection site pain (I.M. administration)

Neuromuscular & skeletal: Tremor (1% to 7% dose dependent), abnormal gait (6%), back pain (up to 5%), joint/extremity pain (up to 5%), akathisia (3% to 5% dose dependent), hypertonia (up to 3%), articulation impairment (up to 2%), falling (particularly in older patients), joint stiffness, paresthesia, twitching

Ocular: Amblyopia (up to 3%), conjunctivitis

Respiratory: Rhinitis (up to 7%), cough (up to 6%), pharyngitis (up to 4%), dyspnea

Miscellaneous: Dental pain, diaphoresis, flu-like syndrome

<1% (Limited to important or life-threatening): Acidosis, akinesia, albuminuria, anaphylactoid reaction, anemia, angioedema, apnea, arteritis, asthma, ataxia, atelectasis, atrial fibrillation, AV block, cerebrovascular accident, coma, confusion, congestive heart failure, deafness, diabetes mellitus, diabetic acidosis, diabetic coma, dyskinesia, dysphagia, dystonia, dysuria, encephalopathy, facial paralysis, glaucoma, gynecomastia, heart arrest, heart block, heart failure, hematuria, hemoptysis, hemorrhage (eye, rectal, subarachnoid, vaginal), hepatitis, hyper-/hypoglycemia, hyper-/hypokalemia, hyperlipemia, hyper-/hyponatremia, hyperuricemia, hyper-/hypoventilation, hypoesthesia, hypokinesia, hypoproteinemia, hypoxia, jaundice, ileus, ketosis, leukocytosis (eosinophilia), leukopenia, liver damage (cholestatic or mixed), liver fatty deposit, lung edema, lymphadenopathy, menstrual irregularities, migraine, myasthenia, myopathy, neuralgia, neuroleptic malignant syndrome, neuropathy, neutropenia, osteoporosis, pancreatitis, paralysis, priapism, pulmonary embolus, rhabdomyolysis, seizure, stridor, sudden death, suicide attempt, syncope, tardive dyskinesia, thrombocythemia, thrombocytopenia, tongue edema, venous thrombotic events, vomiting, withdrawal syndrome

Drug Interactions

Metabolism/Transport Effects Substrate of CYP1A2 (major), 2D6 (minor); **Inhibits** CYP1A2 (weak), 2C9 (weak), 2C19 (weak), 2D6 (weak), 3A4 (weak)

Avoid Concomitant Use There are no known interactions where it is recommended to avoid concomitant use.

Increased Effect/Toxicity

OLANZapine may increase the levels/effects of: Alcohol (Ethyl); Anticholinergics; CNS Depressants

The levels/effects of OLANZapine may be increased by: Acetylcholinesterase Inhibitors (Central); CYP1A2 Inhibitors (Moderate); CYP1A2 Inhibitors (Strong); Fluvoxamine; LamoTRIgine; Lithium formulations; Pramlintide; Tetrabenazine

Decreased Effect

OLANZapine may decrease the levels/effects of: Amphetamines; Anti-Parkinson's Agents (Dopamine Agonist)

The levels/effects of OLANZapine may be decreased by: CYP1A2 Inducers (Strong); Lithium formulations

Ethanol/Nutrition/Herb Interactions

Ethanol: Avoid ethanol (may increase CNS depression).

Herb/Nutraceutical: Avoid dong quai, St John's wort (may also cause photosensitization). Avoid kava kava, gotu kola, valerian, St John's wort (may increase CNS depression).

Stability

Injection, powder for reconstitution: Store at room temperature 15°C to 30°C (59°F to 86°F); do not freeze. Protect from light. Reconstitute 10 mg vial with 2.1 mL SWFI. Resulting solution is ~5 mg/mL. Use immediately (within 1 hour) following reconstitution. Discard any unused portion.

Tablet and orally-disintegrating tablet: Store at room temperature of 15°C to 30°C (59°F to 86°F). Protect from light and moisture.

Mechanism of Action Olanzapine is a second generation thienobenzodiazepine antipsychotic which displays potent antagonism of serotonin $5\text{-}HT_{2A}$ and $5\text{-}HT_{2C}$, dopamine D_{1-4}, histamine H_1 and alpha$_1$-adrenergic receptors. Olanzapine shows moderate antagonism of $5\text{-}HT_3$ and muscarinic M_{1-5} receptors, and weak binding to GABA-A, BZD, and beta-adrenergic receptors. Although the precise mechanism of action in schizophrenia and bipolar disorder is not known, the efficacy of olanzapine is thought to be mediated through combined antagonism of dopamine and serotonin type 2 receptor sites.

Pharmacodynamics/Kinetics

Absorption:

I.M.: Rapidly absorbed

Oral: Well absorbed; not affected by food; tablets and orally-disintegrating tablets are bioequivalent

Distribution: V_d: Extensive, 1000 L

Protein binding, plasma: 93% bound to albumin and alpha$_1$-glycoprotein

Metabolism: Highly metabolized via direct glucuronidation and cytochrome P450 mediated oxidation (CYP1A2, CYP2D6); 40% removed via first pass metabolism

Bioavailability: >57%

Half-life elimination: 21-54 hours; ~1.5 times greater in elderly

Time to peak, plasma: Maximum plasma concentrations after I.M. administration are 5 times higher than maximum plasma concentrations produced by an oral dose.

I.M.: 15-45 minutes

Oral: ~6 hours

Excretion: Urine (57%, 7% as unchanged drug); feces (30%)

Clearance: 40% increase in olanzapine clearance in smokers; 30% decrease in females

Dosage

Children: Schizophrenia/bipolar disorder (unlabeled use): Oral: Initial: 2.5 mg/day; titrate as necessary to 20 mg/day (0.12-0.29 mg/kg/day)

Adults:

Schizophrenia: Oral: Initial: 5-10 mg once daily (increase to 10 mg once daily within 5-7 days); thereafter, adjust by 5 mg/day at 1-week intervals, up to a recommended maximum of 20 mg/day. Maintenance: 10-20 mg once daily. **Note:** Doses of 30-50 mg/day have been used; however, doses >10 mg/day have not demonstrated better efficacy, and safety and efficacy of doses >20 mg/day have not been evaluated.

Bipolar I acute mixed or manic episodes: Oral:

Monotherapy: Initial: 10-15 mg once daily; increase by 5 mg/day at intervals of not less than 24 hours. Maintenance: 5-20 mg/day; recommended maximum dose: 20 mg/day.

Combination therapy (with lithium or valproate): Initial: 10 mg once daily; dosing range: 5-20 mg/day

Agitation (acute, associated with bipolar I mania or schizophrenia): I.M.: Initial dose: 5-10 mg (a lower dose of 2.5 mg may be considered when clinical factors warrant); additional doses (2.5-10 mg) may be considered; however, 2-4 hours should be allowed between doses to evaluate response (maximum total daily dose: 30 mg, per manufacturer's recommendation)

Prevention of chemotherapy-associated delayed nausea or vomiting (unlabeled use; in combination with a corticosteroid and serotonin [$5HT_3$] antagonist): Oral: 10 mg once daily for 3-5 days, beginning on day 1 of chemotherapy **or** 5 mg once daily for 2 days before chemotherapy, followed by 10 mg once daily (beginning on the day of chemotherapy) for 3-8 days

Elderly: Oral, I.M.: Consider lower starting dose of 2.5-5 mg/day for elderly or debilitated patients; may increase as clinically indicated and tolerated with close monitoring of orthostatic blood pressure

Psychosis/agitation related to Alzheimer's dementia (unlabeled use): Initial: 1.25-5 mg/day; if necessary, gradually increase as tolerated not to exceed 10 mg/day

Dosage adjustment in renal impairment: No adjustment required. Not removed by dialysis.

Dosage adjustment in hepatic impairment: Dosage adjustment may be necessary, however, there are no specific recommendations. Monitor closely.

Dietary Considerations Tablets may be taken with or without food. Zyprexa® Zydis®: 5 mg tablet contains phenylalanine 0.34 mg; 10 mg tablet contains phenylalanine 0.45 mg; 15 mg tablet contains phenylalanine 0.67 mg; 20 mg tablet contains phenylalanine 0.9 mg.

Administration

Injection: For I.M. administration only; do not administer injection intravenously; inject slowly, deep into muscle. If dizziness and/or drowsiness are noted, patient should remain recumbent until examination indicates postural hypotension and/or bradycardia are not a problem. Concurrent use of I.M/I.V. benzodiazepines is not recommended (fatalities have been reported, though causality not determined).

Tablet: May be administered with or without food.

Orally-disintegrating: Remove from foil blister by peeling back (do not push tablet through the foil); place tablet in mouth immediately upon removal; tablet dissolves rapidly in saliva and may be swallowed with or without liquid. May be administered with or without food/meals.

Monitoring Parameters Vital signs; fasting lipid profile and fasting blood glucose/Hgb A_{1c} (prior to treatment, at 3 months, then annually); periodic assessment of hepatic transaminases (in patients with hepatic disease); BMI, personal/family history of obesity, waist circumference; orthostatic blood pressure; mental status, abnormal involuntary movement scale (AIMS), extrapyramidal symptoms (EPS). Weight should be assessed prior to treatment, at 4 weeks, 8 weeks, 12 weeks, and then at quarterly intervals. Consider titrating to a different antipsychotic agent for a weight gain ≥5% of the initial weight.

Dosage Forms Excipient information presented when available (limited, particularly for generics); consult specific product labeling.

Injection, powder for reconstitution (Zyprexa® IntraMuscular): 10 mg [contains lactose 50 mg]

Tablet (Zyprexa®): 2.5 mg, 5 mg, 7.5 mg, 10 mg, 15 mg, 20 mg

Tablet, orally disintegrating (Zyprexa® Zydis®): 5 mg [contains phenylalanine 0.34 mg/tablet], 10 mg [contains phenylalanine 0.45 mg/tablet], 15 mg [contains phenylalanine 0.67 mg/tablet], 20 mg [contains phenylalanine 0.9 mg/tablet]

Olanzapine and Fluoxetine

(oh LAN za peen & floo OKS e teen)

U.S. Brand Names Symbyax®

Index Terms Fluoxetine and Olanzapine; Olanzapine and Fluoxetine Hydrochloride

Pharmacologic Category Antidepressant, Selective Serotonin Reuptake Inhibitor; Antipsychotic Agent, Atypical

Use Treatment of depressive episodes associated with bipolar disorder

Restrictions An FDA-approved medication guide concerning the use of antidepressants in children, adolescents, and young adults must be distributed when dispensing an outpatient prescription (new or refill) where this medication is to be used without direct supervision of a healthcare provider. Medication guides are available at http://www.fda.gov/cder/Offices/ODS/medication_guides.htm. Dispense to parents or guardians of children and adolescents receiving this medication.

Pregnancy Risk Factor C

Dosage Oral:

Adults: Depression associated with bipolar disorder: Initial: Olanzapine 3-6 mg/fluoxetine 25 mg once daily in the evening. Dosing range: Olanzapine 6-12 mg/fluoxetine 25-50 mg. Lower doses (olanzapine 3 mg/fluoxetine 25 mg) should be used in patients predisposed to hypotension, in hepatic impairment, with combined factors for reduced metabolism (females, the elderly, nonsmokers), or enhanced sensitivity to olanzapine; use caution in dose adjustments in these patients. Safety of daily doses of olanzapine >18 mg/fluoxetine >75 mg have not been evaluated.

Elderly: Initial: Olanzapine 3-6 mg/fluoxetine 25 mg once daily in the evening; use caution adjusting dose (metabolism may be decreased). Safety and efficacy have not been established in patients >65 years of age.

Dosage adjustment in hepatic impairment: Initial: Olanzapine 6 mg/fluoxetine 25 mg once daily in the evening; use caution adjusting dose (metabolism may be decreased).

Additional Information Complete prescribing information for this medication should be consulted for additional detail.

Dosage Forms Excipient information presented when available (limited, particularly for generics); consult specific product labeling.

Capsule:

Symbyax® 3/25: Olanzapine 3 mg and fluoxetine 25 mg
Symbyax® 6/25: Olanzapine 6 mg and fluoxetine 25 mg
Symbyax® 6/50: Olanzapine 6 mg and fluoxetine 50 mg
Symbyax® 12/25: Olanzapine 12 mg and fluoxetine 25 mg
Symbyax® 12/50: Olanzapine 12 mg and fluoxetine 50 mg

◆ **Olanzapine and Fluoxetine Hydrochloride** *see* Olanzapine and Fluoxetine *on page 1095*

◆ **Oleovitamin A** *see* Vitamin A *on page 1565*

Olmesartan (ole me SAR tan)

U.S. Brand Names Benicar®

Canadian Brand Names Olmetec®

Index Terms Olmesartan Medoxomil

Pharmacologic Category Angiotensin II Receptor Blocker

Additional Appendix Information

Angiotensin Agents *on page 1632*

Use Treatment of hypertension with or without concurrent use of other antihypertensive agents

Pregnancy Risk Factor C (1st trimester); D (2nd and 3rd trimesters)

Pregnancy Considerations Medications which act on the renin-angiotensin system are reported to have the following fetal/neonatal effects: Hypotension, neonatal skull hypoplasia, anuria, renal failure, and death; oligohydramnios is also reported. These effects are reported to occur with exposure during the second and third trimesters. There are no adequate and well-controlled studies in pregnant women. **[U.S. Boxed Warning]: Based on human data, drugs that act on the angiotensin system can cause injury and death to the developing fetus when used in the second and third trimesters. Angiotensin receptor blockers should be discontinued as soon as possible once pregnancy is detected.**

Lactation Excretion in breast milk unknown/contraindicated

Contraindications Hypersensitivity to olmesartan or any component of the formulation

Warnings/Precautions [U.S. Boxed Warning]: Based on human data, drugs that act on the angiotensin system can cause injury and death to the developing fetus when used in the second and third trimesters. Angiotensin receptor blockers should be discontinued as soon as possible once pregnancy is detected. May cause hyperkalemia; avoid potassium supplementation unless specifically required by healthcare provider. Avoid use or use a smaller dose in patients who are volume depleted; correct depletion first. May be associated with deterioration of renal function and/or increases in serum creatinine, particularly in patients with low renal blood flow (eg, renal artery stenosis, heart failure) whose glomerular filtration rate (GFR) is dependent on efferent arteriolar vasoconstriction by angiotensin II. Use with caution in unstented unilateral/bilateral renal artery stenosis. When unstented bilateral renal artery stenosis is present, use is generally avoided due to the elevated risk of deterioration in renal function unless possible benefits outweigh risks. Use with caution with pre-existing renal insufficiency; significant aortic/mitral stenosis. Safety and efficacy in pediatric patients have not been established.

Adverse Reactions

1% to 10%:

Central nervous system: Dizziness (3%), headache
Endocrine & metabolic: Hyperglycemia, hypertriglyceridemia
Gastrointestinal: Diarrhea
Neuromuscular & skeletal: Back pain, CPK increased
Renal: Hematuria
Respiratory: Bronchitis, pharyngitis, rhinitis, sinusitis
Miscellaneous: Flu-like syndrome

<1% (Limited to important or life-threatening): Abdominal pain, acute renal failure, alopecia, angioedema, arthralgia, arthritis, bilirubin increased, chest pain, dyspepsia, facial edema, fatigue, gastroenteritis, hypercholesterolemia, hyperkalemia, hyperlipidemia, hyperuricemia, insomnia, liver enzymes increased, myalgia, nausea, pain, peripheral edema, pruritus, rash, rhabdomyolysis, serum creatinine increased, skeletal pain, tachycardia, urinary tract infection, urticaria, vertigo, vomiting

Drug Interactions

Avoid Concomitant Use There are no known interactions where it is recommended to avoid concomitant use.

Increased Effect/Toxicity

Olmesartan may increase the levels/effects of: ACE Inhibitors; Amifostine; Lithium; Potassium-Sparing Diuretics; RiTUXimab

The levels/effects of Olmesartan may be increased by: Diazoxide; Eltrombopag; Eplerenone; Herbs (Hypotensive Properties); Potassium Salts; Prostacyclin Analogues; Trimethoprim

Decreased Effect

The levels/effects of Olmesartan may be decreased by: Herbs (Hypertensive Properties); Methylphenidate; Nonsteroidal Anti-Inflammatory Agents; Yohimbine

Ethanol/Nutrition/Herb Interactions

Food: Does not affect olmesartan bioavailability.

Herb/Nutraceutical: Avoid bayberry, blue cohosh, cayenne, ephedra, ginger, ginseng (American), kola, licorice (may worsen hypertension). Avoid black cohosh, California poppy, coleus, golden seal, hawthorn, mistletoe, periwinkle, quinine, shepherd's purse (may have increased antihypertensive effect).

Stability Store at 20°C to 25°C (68°F to 77°F).

Mechanism of Action As a selective and competitive, nonpeptide angiotensin II receptor antagonist, olmesartan blocks the vasoconstrictor and aldosterone-secreting effects of angiotensin II; olmesartan interacts reversibly at the AT1 and AT2 receptors of many tissues and has slow dissociation kinetics; its affinity for the AT1 receptor is 12,500 times greater than the AT2 receptor. Angiotensin II receptor antagonists may induce a more complete inhibition of the renin-angiotensin system than ACE inhibitors, they do not affect the response to bradykinin, and are less likely to be associated with nonrenin-angiotensin effects (eg, cough and angioedema). Olmesartan increases urinary flow rate and, in addition to being natriuretic and kaliuretic, increases excretion of chloride, magnesium, uric acid, calcium, and phosphate.

Pharmacodynamics/Kinetics

Distribution: 17 L; does not cross the blood-brain barrier (animal studies)

Protein binding: 99%

Metabolism: Olmesartan medoxomil is hydrolyzed in the GI tract to active olmesartan. No further metabolism occurs.

Bioavailability: 26%

Half-life elimination: Terminal: 13 hours

Time to peak: 1-2 hours

Excretion: All as unchanged drug: Feces (50% to 65%); urine (35% to 50%)

Dosage Oral:

Adults: Initial: Usual starting dose is 20 mg once daily; if initial response is inadequate, may be increased to 40 mg once daily after 2 weeks. May administer with other antihypertensive agents if blood pressure inadequately controlled with olmesartan. Consider lower starting dose in patients with possible depletion of intravascular volume (eg, patients receiving diuretics).

Elderly: No dosage adjustment necessary

Dosage adjustment in renal impairment: No specific guidelines for dosage adjustment; patients undergoing hemodialysis have not been studied.

Dosage adjustment in hepatic impairment: No adjustment necessary.

Dietary Considerations May be taken with or without food.

Administration May be administered with or without food.

Monitoring Parameters Blood pressure, serum potassium

Dosage Forms Excipient information presented when available (limited, particularly for generics); consult specific product labeling.

Tablet, as medoxomil:

Benicar®: 5 mg, 20 mg, 40 mg

- ◆ **Olmesartan and Amlodipine** *see* Amlodipine and Olmesartan *on page 95*

Olmesartan and Hydrochlorothiazide

(ole me SAR tan & hye droe klor oh THYE a zide)

U.S. Brand Names Benicar HCT®

Canadian Brand Names Olmetec Plus®

Index Terms Hydrochlorothiazide and Olmesartan Medoxomil; Olmesartan Medoxomil and Hydrochlorothiazide

Pharmacologic Category Angiotensin II Receptor Blocker; Diuretic, Thiazide

Use Treatment of hypertension (not recommended for initial treatment)

Pregnancy Risk Factor C/D (2nd and 3rd trimesters)

Dosage Oral: Adults: One tablet daily; dosage must be individualized (see below). May be titrated at 2- to 4-week intervals.

Replacement therapy: May be substituted for previously titrated dosages of the individual components.

Patients not controlled with single-agent therapy: Initiate by adding the lowest available dose of the alternative component (hydrochlorothiazide 12.5 mg or olmesartan 20 mg). Titrate to effect (maximum daily hydrochlorothiazide dose: 25 mg; maximum daily olmesartan dose: 40 mg).

Dosage adjustment in renal impairment: Not recommended in patients with Cl_{cr} <30 mL/minute

Additional Information Complete prescribing information for this medication should be consulted for additional detail.

Dosage Forms Excipient information presented when available (limited, particularly for generics); consult specific product labeling.

Tablet:

20/12.5: Olmesartan medoxomil 20 mg and hydrochlorothiazide 12.5 mg

40/12.5: Olmesartan medoxomil 40 mg and hydrochlorothiazide 12.5 mg

40/25: Olmesartan medoxomil 40 mg and hydrochlorothiazide 25 mg

- ◆ **Olmesartan Medoxomil** *see* Olmesartan *on page 1096*
- ◆ **Olmesartan Medoxomil and Hydrochlorothiazide** *see* Olmesartan and Hydrochlorothiazide *on page 1097*
- ◆ **Olmetec® (Can)** *see* Olmesartan *on page 1096*
- ◆ **Olmetec Plus® (Can)** *see* Olmesartan and Hydrochlorothiazide *on page 1097*

Olopatadine (oh la PAT a deen)

U.S. Brand Names Pataday™; Patanase®; Patanol®

Canadian Brand Names Patanol®

Index Terms Olopatadine Hydrochloride

Pharmacologic Category Histamine H_1 Antagonist; Histamine H_1 Antagonist, Second Generation

Use

Nasal spray: Treatment of the symptoms of seasonal allergic rhinitis

Ophthalmic: Treatment of the signs and symptoms of allergic conjunctivitis

Pregnancy Risk Factor C

Pregnancy Considerations Teratogenic effects were not observed in animal studies; however, a decrease in fetal weight and a decrease in live births were observed. There are no adequate and well-controlled studies in pregnant women.

Lactation Excretion in breast milk unknown/use caution

Medication Safety Issues

Sound-alike/look-alike issues:

Patanol® may be confused with Platinol®

International issues:

Patanol® may be confused with Betanol® which is a brand name for metipranolol in Monaco and a brand name for atenolol in Bangladesh

Contraindications Hypersensitivity to olopatadine hydrochloride or any component of the formulation

Warnings/Precautions

Nasal spray: May cause drowsiness in some patients; instruct patient to use caution when driving or operating machinery. Effects may be additive with CNS depressants and/or ethanol. Periodically examine nasal mucosa for ulceration and consider discontinuing if ulceration occurs. Safety and efficacy have not been established in children <12 years of age.

Ophthalmic: Not for use to treat contact lens-related irritation. Solution contains benzalkonium chloride; remove lens prior to administration and wait at least 10 minutes before reinserting. Do not use contact lenses if eyes are red. Safety and efficacy have not been established in children <3 years of age.

Adverse Reactions

Nasal spray:

>10%: Gastrointestinal: Bitter taste (13%)

1% to 10%:

Central nervous system: Somnolence (1%)

Gastrointestinal: Xerostomia (1%)

Genitourinary: Urinary tract infection (1%)

Neuromuscular & skeletal: CPK increased (1%)

Respiratory: Nasal ulceration (9%), epistaxis (3%), pharyngolaryngeal pain (2%), postnasal drip (2%), cough (1%), throat irritation (1%)

Miscellaneous: Influenza (1%)

<1% (Limited to important or life-threatening): Weight gain

Ophthalmic:

>5%:

Central nervous system: Cold syndrome (up to 10%), headache (up to 7%)

Respiratory: Pharyngitis (up to 10%)

≤5%:

Gastrointestinal: Nausea, taste perversion

Neuromuscular & skeletal: Back pain, weakness

Ocular: Blurred vision, burning, conjunctivitis, dry eyes, eye pain, eyelid edema, foreign body sensation, hyperemia, itching, keratitis, ocular pruritus, stinging

Respiratory: Cough, rhinitis, sinusitis

Miscellaneous: Flu-like syndrome, hypersensitivity, infection

Drug Interactions

Avoid Concomitant Use There are no known interactions where it is recommended to avoid concomitant use.

Increased Effect/Toxicity

Olopatadine may increase the levels/effects of: Anticholinergics; CNS Depressants

The levels/effects of Olopatadine may be increased by: Pramlintide

Decreased Effect

Olopatadine may decrease the levels/effects of: Acetylcholinesterase Inhibitors (Central)

The levels/effects of Olopatadine may be decreased by: Acetylcholinesterase Inhibitors (Central); Amphetamines

Ethanol/Nutrition/Herb Interactions Ethanol: Avoid ethanol (may cause increased somnolence or fatigue).

Stability

Nasal spray: Store at 4°C to 25°C (39°F to 77°F).

Ophthalmic solution: Store at 2°C to 25°C (36°F to 77°F).

Mechanism of Action

Selective histamine H_1-antagonist; inhibits release of histamine from mast cells. Inhibits histamine induced effects on conjunctival epithelial cells and the respiratory tract. Has no effect on alpha-adrenergic, dopaminergic, and muscarinic type 1 and 2 receptors.

Pharmacodynamics/Kinetics

Onset of action: Intranasal: 30 minutes in seasonal allergy patients

Absorption: Ophthalmic: Low systemic absorption

Protein binding: ~55% (primarily albumin)

Metabolism: Not extensively metabolized

Bioavailability: Intranasal: 57%

Half-life elimination: Ophthalmic: ~3 hours; Intranasal: 8-12 hours

Time to peak, serum: Intranasal: 15 minutes to 2 hours

Excretion: Urine (60% to 70%, mostly as unchanged drug); feces (17%)

Dosage

Intranasal (Patanase®): Children ≥12 years and Adults: 2 sprays into each nostril twice daily

Ophthalmic: Children ≥3 years and Adults:

Patanol®: Instill 1 drop into affected eye(s) twice daily (allowing 6-8 hours between doses); results from an environmental study demonstrated that olopatadine was effective when dosed twice daily for up to 6 weeks

Pataday™: Instill 1 drop into affected eye(s) once daily

Administration

Inhalation (Patanase®): For intranasal use only. Before initial use of the nasal spray, the delivery system should be primed with 5 sprays or until a fine mist appears. If 7 or more days have elapsed since last use, the delivery system should be reprimed with 2 sprays or until a fine mist appears. Blow nose to clear nostrils. Keep head tilted downward when spraying. Insert applicator into nostril, keeping bottle upright, and close off the other nostril. Breathe in through nose. While inhaling, press pump to release spray. Alternate sprays between nostrils. After each use, wipe the spray tip with a clean tissue or cloth.

Ophthalmic (Patanol®, Pataday™): For topical ophthalmic use only. After instilling drops, wait at least 10 minutes before inserting contact lenses. Do not insert contacts if eyes are red.

Monitoring Parameters Observe patients periodically for adverse nasal effects (eg, ulceration, perforation)

Dosage Forms Excipient information presented when available (limited, particularly for generics); consult specific product labeling.

Solution, intranasal [spray]:

Patanase®: 0.6% (30.5 g) [contains benzalkonium chloride; equivalent to olopatadine hydrochloride 665 mcg/100 microliters; 240 metered sprays]

Solution, ophthalmic:

Patanol®: 0.1% (5 mL) [contains benzalkonium chloride]

Pataday™: 0.2% (2.5 mL) [contains benzalkonium chloride]

◆ **Olopatadine Hydrochloride** *see* Olopatadine *on page 1097*

Olsalazine (ole SAL a zeen)

U.S. Brand Names Dipentum®

Canadian Brand Names Dipentum®

Index Terms Olsalazine Sodium

Pharmacologic Category 5-Aminosalicylic Acid Derivative

Use Maintenance of remission of ulcerative colitis in patients intolerant to sulfasalazine

Pregnancy Risk Factor C

Pregnancy Considerations Animal studies have demonstrated fetal developmental toxicities. There are no well-controlled studies in pregnant women. Use during pregnancy only if clearly necessary.

Lactation Enters breast milk/not recommended

Medication Safety Issues

Sound-alike/look-alike issues:

Olsalazine may be confused with OLANZapine

Dipentum® may be confused with Dilantin®

Contraindications Hypersensitivity to olsalazine, salicylates, or any component of the formulation

Warnings/Precautions Diarrhea is a common adverse effect of olsalazine. May exacerbate symptoms of colitis. Use with caution in patients with renal or hepatic impairment. Use with caution in elderly patients. Use with caution in patients with severe allergies or asthma. Safety and efficacy have not been established in children.

Adverse Reactions

>10%: Gastrointestinal: Diarrhea (11% to 17%; dose related)

1% to 10%:

Central nervous system: Headache (5%), depression (2%). fatigue (2%), vertigo (1%)

Dermatologic: Rash (2%), pruritus (1%)

Gastrointestinal: Abdominal pain/cramps (10%), heartburn (2%), nausea (5%), stomatitis (1%), vomiting (1%)

Neuromuscular & skeletal: Arthralgia (4%)

Respiratory: Upper respiratory infection (2%)

Postmarketing and/or case reports: Alopecia, angioedema, aplastic anemia, bilirubin increase, blood dyscrasias, blood in stool, blurred vision, bronchospasm, cholestatic jaundice, chills, cirrhosis, dyspnea, dysuria, eosinophilia, erythema, erythema nodosum, fever, heart block (second degree), hematuria, hemolytic anemia, hepatitis, hepatic failure, hepatic necrosis, hypertension, impotence, interstitial nephritis, interstitial pneumonia, jaundice, Kawasaki-like syndrome, leukopenia, lymphopenia, menorrhagia, muscle cramps, myalgia, myocarditis, nephritic syndrome, neutropenia, orthostatic hypotension, pancreatitis, pancytopenia, paresthesia, pericarditis, peripheral edema, photosensitivity, proteinuria, rectal bleeding, rigors, tachycardia, thrombocytopenia, tinnitus, transaminase increase, tremor, urinary frequency, xerostomia

Drug Interactions

Avoid Concomitant Use There are no known interactions where it is recommended to avoid concomitant use.

Increased Effect/Toxicity

Olsalazine may increase the levels/effects of: Thiopurine Analogs; Varicella Virus-Containing Vaccines

Decreased Effect
Olsalazine may decrease the levels/effects of: Cardiac Glycosides

Mechanism of Action Mesalamine (5-aminosalicylic acid) is the active component of olsalazine; the specific mechanism of action of mesalamine is unknown; however, it is thought that it modulates local chemical mediators of the inflammatory response, especially leukotrienes, and is also postulated to be a free radical scavenger or an inhibitor of tumor necrosis factor (TNF); action appears topical rather than systemic.

Pharmacodynamics/Kinetics
Absorption: <3%; very little intact olsalazine is systemically absorbed
Protein binding, plasma: >99%
Metabolism: Primarily via colonic bacteria to active drug, 5-aminosalicylic acid
Half-life elimination: 56 minutes
Time to peak: ~1 hour
Excretion: Primarily feces

Dosage Adults: Oral: 1 g/day in 2 divided doses

Dietary Considerations Take with food, increases residence of drug in body.

Administration Administer with food in evenly divided doses.

Monitoring Parameters CBC, hepatic function, renal function; stool frequency

Test Interactions Increased ALT, AST (S), GGT, LDH, alkaline phosphatase, bilirubin

Dosage Forms Excipient information presented when available (limited, particularly for generics); consult specific product labeling.
Capsule, as sodium: 250 mg

- **Olsalazine Sodium** *see* Olsalazine *on page 1098*
- **Olux®** *see* Clobetasol *on page 347*
- **Olux-E™** *see* Clobetasol *on page 347*
- **Omacor® [DSC]** *see* Omega-3-Acid Ethyl Esters *on page 1100*

Omalizumab (oh mah lye ZOO mab)

U.S. Brand Names Xolair®

Canadian Brand Names Xolair®

Index Terms rhuMAb-E25

Pharmacologic Category Monoclonal Antibody, Anti-Asthmatic

Use Treatment of moderate-to-severe, persistent allergic asthma not adequately controlled with inhaled corticosteroids

Restrictions An FDA-approved medication guide is available at http://www.fda.gov/cder/Offices/ODS/medication_guides.htm; distribute to each patient to whom this medication is dispensed.

Pregnancy Risk Factor B

Pregnancy Considerations Teratogenic effects were not observed in animal studies. There are no adequate and well-controlled studies in pregnant women. IgG molecules are known to cross the placenta; use during pregnancy only if clearly needed. A registry has been established to monitor outcomes of women exposed to omalizumab during pregnancy or within 8 weeks prior to pregnancy (866-496-5247).

Lactation Excretion in breast milk unknown/use caution

Contraindications Hypersensitivity to omalizumab or any component of the formulation; acute bronchospasm, status asthmaticus

Warnings/Precautions [U.S. Boxed Warning]: Anaphylaxis, including delayed-onset anaphylaxis, has been reported following administration; reactions usually occur within 2 hours of administration, but may occur up to 24 hours and in some cases >1 year after initiation of regular treatment. Patients should receive treatment only under direct medical supervision and be observed for a minimum of 2 hours following administration; appropriate medications for the treatment of anaphylactic reactions should be available. Hypersensitivity reactions may occur following any dose, even during chronic therapy; discontinue therapy following any severe reaction.

For use in patients with a documented reactivity to a perennial aeroallergen and with symptoms uncontrolled using inhaled corticosteroids; not used to control acute asthma symptoms. Dosing is based on pretreatment IgE serum levels and body weight. IgE levels remain elevated up to 1 year following treatment, therefore, levels taken during treatment cannot be used as a dosage guide. Corticosteroid therapy should be tapered gradually, do not discontinue abruptly. Malignant neoplasms have been reported with use in short-term studies; impact of long-term use is not known. Use caution with and monitor patients at risk for parasitic (helminth) infections (risk of infection may be increased). Safety and efficacy in children <12 years of age have not been established.

Adverse Reactions
>10%:
Central nervous system: Headache (15%)
Local: Injection site reaction (45%; placebo 43%; severe 12%). Most reactions occurred within 1 hour, lasted <8 days, and decreased in frequency with additional dosing.
Respiratory: Upper respiratory tract infection (20%), sinusitis (16%), pharyngitis (11%)
Miscellaneous: Viral infection (23%)
1% to 10%:
Central nervous system: Pain (7%), fatigue (3%), dizziness (3%)
Dermatologic: Dermatitis (2%), pruritus (2%)
Neuromuscular & skeletal: Arthralgia (8%), leg pain (4%), arm pain (2%), fracture (2%)
Otic: Earache (2%)
<1% (Limited to important or life-threatening): Alopecia; anaphylaxis (angioedema of the throat or tongue, bronchospasm, chest tightness, cough, cutaneous angioedema, dyspnea, hypotension, generalized pruritus, syncope, and urticaria); antibody formation to omalizumab, hot flushes, malignancy (0.5%; placebo 0.2%), throat edema, thrombocytopenia, tongue edema, urticaria, wheezing

Drug Interactions
Avoid Concomitant Use There are no known interactions where it is recommended to avoid concomitant use.
Increased Effect/Toxicity There are no known significant interactions involving an increase in effect.
Decreased Effect There are no known significant interactions involving a decrease in effect.

Stability Prior to reconstitution, store under refrigeration at 2°C to 8°C (36°F to 46°F); product may be shipped at room temperature. Prepare using SWFI, USP only; add SWFI 1.4 mL to upright vial and swirl gently for 5-10 seconds every 5 minutes until dissolved; may take >20 minutes to dissolve completely. Resulting solution is 150 mg/1.2 mL. Do not use if powder takes >40 minutes to dissolve. Following reconstitution, protect from direct sunlight. May be stored for up to 8 hours if refrigerated or 4 hours if stored at room temperature.

Mechanism of Action Omalizumab is an IgG monoclonal antibody (recombinant DNA derived) which inhibits IgE binding to the high-affinity IgE receptor on mast cells and basophils. By decreasing bound IgE, the activation and release of mediators in the allergic response (early and late phase) is limited. Serum-free IgE levels and the number of high-affinity IgE receptors are decreased. Long-term treatment in patients with allergic asthma showed a decrease in asthma exacerbations and corticosteroid usage.

Pharmacodynamics/Kinetics

Absorption: Slow following SubQ injection

Distribution: V_d: 78 ± 32 mL/kg

Metabolism: Hepatic; IgG degradation by reticuloendothelial system and endothelial cells

Bioavailability: 62%

Half-life elimination: 26 days

Time to peak: 7-8 days

Excretion: Primarily via hepatic degradation; intact IgG may be secreted in bile

Dosage SubQ: Children ≥12 years and Adults: Asthma: Dose is based on pretreatment IgE serum levels and body weight. Dosing should not be adjusted based on IgE levels taken during treatment or <1 year following discontinuation of therapy; doses should be adjusted during treatment for significant changes in body weight.

IgE ≥30-100 int. units/mL:
- 30-90 kg: 150 mg every 4 weeks
- >90-150 kg: 300 mg every 4 weeks

IgE >100-200 int. units/mL:
- 30-90 kg: 300 mg every 4 weeks
- >90-150 kg: 225 mg every 2 weeks

IgE >200-300 int. units/mL:
- 30-60 kg: 300 mg every 4 weeks
- >60-90 kg: 225 mg every 2 weeks
- >90-150 kg: 300 mg every 2 weeks

IgE >300-400 int. units/mL:
- 30-70 kg: 225 mg every 2 weeks
- >70-90 kg: 300 mg every 2 weeks
- >90 kg: Do not administer dose

IgE >400-500 int. units/mL:
- 30-70 kg: 300 mg every 2 weeks
- >70-90 kg: 375 mg every 2 weeks
- >90 kg: Do not administer dose

IgE >500-600 int. units/mL:
- 30-60 kg: 300 mg every 2 weeks
- >60-70 kg: 375 mg every 2 weeks
- >70 kg: Do not administer dose

IgE >600-700 int. units/mL:
- 30-60 kg: 375 mg every 2 weeks
- >60 kg: Do not administer dose

Administration For SubQ injection only; doses >150 mg should divided over more than one site. Injections may take 5-10 seconds to administer. Administer only under direct medical supervision and observe patient for a minimum of 2 hours following administration of any dose given.

Monitoring Parameters Anaphylactic/hypersensitivity reactions, baseline IgE; FEV_1, peak flow, and/or other pulmonary function tests; monitor for signs of infection

Test Interactions Total IgE levels are elevated for up to 1 year following treatment. Total serum IgE may be retested after interruption of therapy for 1 year or more.

Dosage Forms Excipient information presented when available (limited, particularly for generics); consult specific product labeling.

Injection, powder for reconstitution [preservative free]:

Xolair®: 150 mg [contains sucrose 145.5 g]

Omega-3-Acid Ethyl Esters

(oh MEG a three AS id ETH il ES ters)

U.S. Brand Names Lovaza®; Omacor® [DSC]

Index Terms Ethyl Esters of Omega-3 Fatty Acids; Fish Oil

Pharmacologic Category Antilipemic Agent, Miscellaneous

Use Lovaza®: Adjunct to diet therapy in the treatment of hypertriglyceridemia (≥500 mg/dL)

Note: A number of OTC formulations containing omega-3 fatty acids are marketed as nutritional supplements; these do not have FDA-approved indications and may not contain the same amounts of the active ingredient.

Unlabeled/Investigational Use Lovaza®: Treatment of IgA nephropathy

Pregnancy Risk Factor C

Medication Safety Issues

Sound-alike/look-alike issues:

Omacor® may be confused with Amicar®

Dosage Oral: Adults:

Hypertriglyceridemia: 4 g/day as a single daily dose or in 2 divided doses

Treatment of IgA nephropathy (unlabeled use): 4 g/day

Dosage adjustment in renal impairment: No dosage adjustment required.

Additional Information Complete prescribing information for this medication should be consulted for additional detail.

Dosage Forms Excipient information presented when available (limited, particularly for generics); consult specific product labeling. [DSC] = Discontinued product

Capsule:

Lovaza®, Omacor® [DSC]: 1 g [contains EPA ~465 mg and DHA ~375 mg]

Omeprazole (oh MEP ra zole)

U.S. Brand Names Prilosec OTC™ [OTC]; Prilosec®

Canadian Brand Names Apo-Omeprazole®; Losec MUPS®; Losec®; PMS-Omeprazole DR; ratio-Omeprazole; Sandoz Omeprazole

Pharmacologic Category Proton Pump Inhibitor; Substituted Benzimidazole

Additional Appendix Information

Antimicrobial Drugs of Choice *on page* 1752

Helicobacter pylori Treatment *on page* 1813

Use Short-term (4-8 weeks) treatment of active duodenal ulcer disease or active benign gastric ulcer; treatment of heartburn and other symptoms associated with gastroesophageal reflux disease (GERD); short-term (4-8 weeks) treatment of endoscopically-diagnosed erosive esophagitis; maintenance healing of erosive esophagitis; long-term treatment of pathological hypersecretory conditions; as part of a multidrug regimen for *H. pylori* eradication to reduce the risk of duodenal ulcer recurrence

OTC labeling: Short-term treatment of frequent, uncomplicated heartburn occurring ≥2 days/week

Unlabeled/Investigational Use Healing NSAID-induced ulcers; prevention of NSAID-induced ulcer; stress-ulcer prophylaxis in the critically-ill

Pregnancy Risk Factor C

Pregnancy Considerations Crosses the placenta; congenital abnormalities have been reported sporadically following omeprazole use during pregnancy. Based on data collected by the Teratogen Information System (TERIS), it was concluded that therapeutic doses used during pregnancy would be unlikely to pose a substantial teratogenic risk (quantity/quality of data: fair). Because the possibility of harm still exists, the manufacturer recommends use during pregnancy only if the potential benefit to the mother outweighs the possible risk to the fetus.

Lactation Enters breast milk/not recommended

Medication Safety Issues

Sound-alike/look-alike issues:

Prilosec® may be confused with Plendil®, Prevacid®, predniSONE, prilocaine, Prinivil®, Proventil®, Prozac®

International issues:

Norpramin®: Brand name for desipramine in the U.S.

Contraindications Hypersensitivity to omeprazole, substituted benzimidazoles (ie, esomeprazole, lansoprazole, pantoprazole, rabeprazole), or any component of the formulation

Warnings/Precautions Use of proton pump inhibitors may increase the risk of gastrointestinal infections (eg, *Salmonella, Campylobacter*). Relief of symptoms does not preclude the presence of a gastric malignancy. Atrophic gastritis (by biopsy) has been noted with long-term omeprazole therapy. In long-term (2-year) studies in rats, omeprazole produced a dose-related increase in gastric carcinoid tumors. While available endoscopic evaluations and histologic examinations of biopsy specimens from human stomachs have not detected a risk from short-term exposure to omeprazole, further human data on the effect of sustained hypochlorhydria and hypergastrinemia are needed to rule out the possibility of an increased risk for the development of tumors in humans receiving long-term therapy. Bioavailability may be increased in the elderly, Asian population, and with hepatic dysfunction; consider dosage reductions. Safety and efficacy have not been established in children <1 year of age. When used for self-medication (OTC), do not use for >14 days. Treatment should not be repeated more often than every 4 months. OTC use is not approved for children <18 years of age.

Adverse Reactions

1% to 10%:

Central nervous system: Headache (3% to 7%), dizziness (2%)

Dermatologic: Rash (2%)

Gastrointestinal: Diarrhea (3% to 4%), abdominal pain (2% to 5%), nausea (2% to 4%), vomiting (2% to 3%), flatulence (≤3%), acid regurgitation (2%), constipation (1% to 2%), taste perversion

Neuromuscular & skeletal: Back pain (1%), weakness (1%)

Respiratory: Upper respiratory infection (2%), cough (1%)

1% (Limited to important or life-threatening; adverse event occurrence may vary based on formulation): Abdominal swelling, abnormal dreams, aggression, agitation, agranulocytosis, alkaline phosphatase increased, allergic reactions, alopecia, ALT increased, AST increased, anaphylaxis, anemia, angina, angioedema, anorexia, anxiety, apathy, atrophic gastritis, benign gastric polyps, bilirubin increased, blurred vision, bradycardia, bronchospasm, chest pain, cholestatic hepatitis, confusion, creatinine increased, depression, diaphoresis, double vision, dry skin, epistaxis, erythema multiforme, esophageal candidiasis, fatigue, fecal discoloration, fever, gastroduodenal carcinoids, GGT increased, glycosuria, gynecomastia, hallucinations, hematuria, hemifacial dysesthesia, hemolytic anemia, hepatic encephalopathy, hepatic failure, hepatic necrosis, hepatitis, hepatocellular hepatitis, hyperhidrosis, hypersensitivity, hypertension, hypoglycemia, hyponatremia, insomnia, interstitial nephritis, irritable colon, jaundice, joint pain, leg pain, leukocytosis, leukopenia, liver disease (hepatocellular, cholestatic, mixed), malaise, microscopic pyuria, mucosal atrophy (tongue), muscle cramps, muscle weakness, myalgia, nervousness, neutropenia, ocular irritation, optic atrophy, optic neuritis, optic neuropathy (anterior ischemic), pain, palpitation, pancreatitis, pancytopenia, paresthesia, peripheral edema, petechiae, pharyngeal pain, photosensitivity, pneumothorax, proteinuria, pruritus, psychic disturbance, purpura, skin inflammation, sleep disturbance, somnolence, Stevens-Johnson syndrome, stomatitis, tachycardia, testicular pain, thrombocytopenia, tinnitus, toxic epidermal necrolysis, tremor, urinary frequency, urinary tract infection, urticaria, vertigo, weight gain, xerophthalmia, xerostomia

Drug Interactions

Metabolism/Transport Effects Substrate of CYP2A6 (minor), 2C9 (minor), 2C19 (major), 2D6 (minor), 3A4 (major); **Inhibits** CYP1A2 (weak), 2C9 (moderate), 2C19 (strong), 2D6 (weak), 3A4 (weak); **Induces** CYP1A2 (weak)

Avoid Concomitant Use

Avoid concomitant use of Omeprazole with any of the following: Erlotinib; Mesalamine; Nelfinavir

Increased Effect/Toxicity

Omeprazole may increase the levels/effects of: Benzodiazepines (metabolized by oxidation); Cilostazol; Clozapine; CYP2C19 Substrates; CYP2C9 Substrates (High risk); Methotrexate; Phenytoin; Saquinavir; Voriconazole; Warfarin

The levels/effects of Omeprazole may be increased by: Fluconazole; Ketoconazole

Decreased Effect

Omeprazole may decrease the levels/effects of: Atazanavir; Clopidogrel; Clozapine; Dabigatran Etexilate; Dasatinib; Erlotinib; Indinavir; Iron Salts; Itraconazole; Ketoconazole; Mesalamine; Mycophenolate; Nelfinavir

The levels/effects of Omeprazole may be decreased by: CYP2C19 Inducers (Strong); Tipranavir

Ethanol/Nutrition/Herb Interactions

Ethanol: Avoid ethanol (may cause gastric mucosal irritation).

Food: Food delays absorption.

Stability Store at 15°C to 30°C (59°F to 86°F). Protect from light and moisture.

Mechanism of Action Proton pump inhibitor; suppresses gastric basal and stimulated acid secretion by inhibiting the parietal cell H+/K+ ATP pump

Pharmacodynamics/Kinetics

Onset of action: Antisecretory: ~1 hour

Peak effect: Within 2 hours

Duration: Up to 72 hours; 50% of maximum effect at 24 hours

Absorption: Rapid

Protein binding: ~95%

Metabolism: Extensively hepatic by cytochrome P450 system to inactive metabolites

Bioavailability: Oral: ~30% to 40%; increased in Asian patients and patients with hepatic dysfunction

Half-life elimination: Delayed release capsule: 0.5-1 hour; hepatic impairment: ~3 hours

Time to peak, plasma: 0.5-3.5 hours

Excretion: Urine (77% as metabolites, very small amount as unchanged drug); feces

Dosage Oral:

Children 1-16 years: GERD or other acid-related disorders:

5 kg to <10 kg: 5 mg once daily

10 kg to <20 kg: 10 mg once daily

≥20 kg: 20 mg once daily

Adults:

Active duodenal ulcer: 20 mg/day for 4-8 weeks

Gastric ulcers: 40 mg/day for 4-8 weeks

Symptomatic GERD (without esophageal lesions): 20 mg/day for up to 4 weeks

Erosive esophagitis: 20 mg/day for 4-8 weeks; maintenance of healing: 20 mg/day for up to 12 months total therapy (including treatment period of 4-8 weeks)

Helicobacter pylori eradication: Dose varies with regimen: 40 mg/day as single dose or in 2 divided doses; requires combination therapy with antibiotics for 10-14 days; may require an additional 14-18 days of Prilosec® 20 mg/day (monotherapy) after combination treatment complete if ulcer is present

Pathological hypersecretory conditions: Initial: 60 mg once daily; doses up to 120 mg 3 times/day have been administered; administer daily doses >80 mg in divided doses

Stress-ulcer prophylaxis (ICU patients; unlabeled use): 40 mg once daily; periodically evaluate patient for continued need.

Frequent heartburn (OTC labeling): 20 mg/day for 14 days; treatment may be repeated after 4 months if needed

Dosage adjustment in hepatic impairment: Bioavailability is increased with chronic liver disease. Consider dosage adjustment for maintenance of erosive esophagitis ulcer healing. Specific guidelines are not available.

Dietary Considerations Should be taken on an empty stomach; best if taken before breakfast.

Administration Best if taken before breakfast.

Capsule: Should be swallowed whole; do not chew or crush. Delayed release capsule may be opened and contents added to 1 tablespoon of applesauce (use immediately after adding to applesauce). Administration via NG tube should be in an acidic juice.

Tablet: Should be swallowed whole; do not crush or chew.

Dosage Forms Excipient information presented when available (limited, particularly for generics); consult specific product labeling.

Capsule, delayed release: 10 mg, 20 mg, 40 mg

Prilosec®: 10 mg, 20 mg, 40 mg

Tablet, delayed release: 20 mg

Prilosec OTC™: 20 mg

Extemporaneous Preparations A 2 mg/mL oral omeprazole solution (Simplified Omeprazole Solution) can be prepared with five omeprazole 20 mg delayed release capsules and 50 mL 8.4% sodium bicarbonate. Empty capsules into beaker. Add sodium bicarbonate solution. Gently stir (about 15 minutes) until a white suspension is formed. Transfer to amber-colored syringe or bottle. Stable for 14 days at room temperature or for 30 days under refrigeration.

DiGiancinto JL, Olsen KM, Bergman KL, et al, "Stability of Suspension Formulations of Lansoprazole and Omeprazole Stored in Amber-Colored Plastic Oral Syringes," *Ann Pharmacother*, 2000, 34:600-5.

Quercia R, Fan C, Liu X, et al, "Stability of Omeprazole in an Extemporaneously Prepared Oral Liquid," *Am J Health Syst Pharm*, 1997, 54:1833-6.

Sharma V, "Comparison of 24-hour Intragastric pH Using Four Liquid Formulations of Lansoprazole and Omeprazole," *Am J Health Syst Pharm*, 1999, 56(Suppl 4): S18-21.

Extemporaneous preparation for NG administration (Prilosec®): The manufacturer recommends the use of an acidic juice for preparation to administer via nasogastric (NG) tube. Alternative methods have been described as follows. NG tube administration for the prevention of stress-related mucosal damage in ventilated, critically-ill patients. The manufacturer makes no judgment regarding the safety or efficacy of these practices.

The contents of one or two 20 mg omeprazole delayed release capsules were poured into a syringe; 10-20 mL of an 8.4% sodium bicarbonate solution was withdrawn in the syringe; 30 minutes were allowed for the enteric-coated omeprazole granules to break down. The resulting milky substance was shaken prior to administration. The NG tube was then flushed with 5-10 mL of water and then clamped for at least 1 hour. Patients received omeprazole 40 mg once, then 40 mg 6-8 hours later, then 20 mg once daily using this technique.

Another study used a different technique. The omeprazole delayed release capsule (20 mg or 40 mg) was opened; then the intact granules were poured into a container holding 30 mL of water. With the plunger removed, 1/3 to 1/2 of the granules were then poured into a 30 mL syringe which was attached to a nasogastric tube (NG). The plunger was replaced with 1 cm of air between the granules and the plunger top while the plunger was depressed. This process was repeated until all the granules were flushed, then a final 15 mL of water was flushed through the tube. Patients who received omeprazole 40 mg in this manner had a more predictable increase in intragastric pH than patients who received omeprazole 20 mg.

Omeprazole and Sodium Bicarbonate

(oh MEP ra zole & SOW dee um bye KAR bun ate)

U.S. Brand Names Zegerid®

Pharmacologic Category Proton Pump Inhibitor; Substituted Benzimidazole

Use Short-term (4-8 weeks) treatment of active duodenal ulcer disease or active benign gastric ulcer; treatment of heartburn and other symptoms associated with gastroesophageal reflux disease (GERD); short-term (4-8 weeks) treatment of endoscopically-diagnosed erosive esophagitis; maintenance healing of erosive esophagitis; reduction of risk of upper gastrointestinal bleeding in critically-ill patients

Pregnancy Risk Factor C

Dosage Oral: Adults:

Active duodenal ulcer: 20 mg/day for 4-8 weeks

Gastric ulcers: 40 mg/day for 4-8 weeks

Symptomatic GERD: 20 mg/day for up to 4 weeks

Erosive esophagitis: 20 mg/day for 4-8 weeks; maintenance of healing: 20 mg/day for up to 12 months total therapy (including treatment period of 4-8 weeks)

Risk reduction of upper GI bleeding in critically-ill patients (Zegerid® powder for oral suspension):

Loading dose: Day 1: 40 mg every 6-8 hours for two doses

Maintenance dose: 40 mg/day for up to 14 days; therapy >14 days has not been evaluated

Dosage adjustment in renal impairment: No adjustment necessary

Dosage adjustment in hepatic impairment: Specific guidelines are not available; bioavailability is increased with chronic liver disease

Additional Information Complete prescribing information for this medication should be consulted for additional detail.

Dosage Forms Excipient information presented when available (limited, particularly for generics); consult specific product labeling.

Capsule, immediate release:

Zegerid®: 20 mg, 40 mg [both strengths contain sodium bicarbonate 1100 mg, equivalent to sodium 300 mg (13 mEq) per capsule]

Powder for oral suspension:

Zegerid®: 20 mg/packet (30s), 40 mg/packet (30s) [both strengths contain sodium bicarbonate 1680 mg, equivalent to sodium 460 mg per packet]

◆ **Omnaris™** *see* Ciclesonide *on page* 322

◆ **Omnicef®** *see* Cefdinir *on page* 271

◆ **OMNIhist® II L.A.** *see* Chlorpheniramine, Phenylephrine, and Methscopolamine *on page* 313

◆ **Omnii Gel™ [OTC]** *see* Fluoride *on page* 635

◆ **Omnipred™** *see* PrednisoLONE *on page* 1230

◆ **Omnitrope™** *see* Somatropin *on page* 1388

◆ **Oncaspar®** *see* Pegaspargase *on page* 1151

◆ **Oncotice™ (Can)** *see* BCG Vaccine *on page* 176

◆ **Oncovin** *see* VinCRIStine *on page* 1561

Ondansetron (on DAN se tron)

U.S. Brand Names Zofran®; Zofran® ODT

Canadian Brand Names Apo-Ondansetron®; DOM-Ondansetron; Gen-Ondansetron; JAMP-Ondansetron; MINT-Ondansetron; Novo-Ondansetron; Ondansetron Injection; Ondansetron-Omega; PHL-Ondansetron; PMS-Ondansetron; RAN-Ondansetron; RATIO-Ondansetron; Sandoz-Ondansetron; Zofran®; Zofran® ODT

Index Terms GR38032R; Ondansetron Hydrochloride

Pharmacologic Category Antiemetic; Selective 5-HT_3 Receptor Antagonist

Use Prevention of nausea and vomiting associated with moderately- to highly-emetogenic cancer chemotherapy; radiotherapy in patients receiving total body irradiation or fractions to the abdomen; prevention of postoperative nausea and vomiting (PONV); treatment of PONV if no prophylactic dose received

Unlabeled/Investigational Use Treatment of early-onset alcoholism; hyperemesis gravidarum

Pregnancy Risk Factor B

Pregnancy Considerations Teratogenic effects were not observed in animal studies; however, there are no adequate and well-controlled studies in pregnant women. Use of ondansetron for the treatment of nausea and vomiting of pregnancy (NVP) has been evaluated. Additional studies are needed to determine safety to the fetus, particularly during the first trimester. Based on preliminary data, use is generally reserved for severe NVP (hyperemesis gravidarum) or when conventional treatments are not effective.

Lactation Excretion in breast milk unknown/use caution

Medication Safety Issues

Sound-alike/look-alike issues:

Ondansetron may be confused with dolasetron, granisetron, palonosetron

Zofran® may be confused with Zantac®, Zosyn®

Contraindications Hypersensitivity to ondansetron, other selective 5-HT_3 antagonists, or any component of the formulation

Warnings/Precautions **Ondansetron should be used on a scheduled basis, not on an "as needed" (PRN) basis,** since data support the use of this drug only in the prevention of nausea and vomiting (due to antineoplastic therapy) and not in the rescue of nausea and vomiting. Ondansetron should only be used in the first 24-48 hours of chemotherapy. Data do not support any increased efficacy of ondansetron in delayed nausea and vomiting. Does not stimulate gastric or intestinal peristalsis; may mask progressive ileus and/or gastric distension. Use with caution in patients allergic to other 5-HT_3 receptor antagonists; cross-reactivity has been reported.

Use with caution in patients with congenital long QT syndrome or other risk factors for QT prolongation (eg, medications known to prolong QT interval, electrolyte abnormalities, and cumulative high-dose anthracycline therapy). 5-HT_3 antagonists have been associated with a number of dose-dependent increases in ECG intervals (eg, PR, QRS duration, QT/QT_c, JT), usually occurring 1-2 hours after I.V. administration. In general, these changes are not clinically relevant, however, when used in conjunction with other agents that prolong these intervals, arrhythmia may occur. When used with agents that prolong the QT interval (eg, Class I and III antiarrhythmics), clinically relevant QT interval prolongation may occur resulting in torsade de pointes. I.V. formulations of 5-HT_3 antagonists have more association with ECG interval changes, compared to oral formulations.

Orally-disintegrating tablets contain phenylalanine. Safety and efficacy for children <1 month of age have not been established.

Adverse Reactions Note: Percentages reported in adult patients.

>10%:

Central nervous system: Headache (9% to 27%), malaise/fatigue (9% to 13%)

Gastrointestinal: Constipation (6% to 11%)

1% to 10%:

Central nervous system: Drowsiness (8%), fever (2% to 8%), dizziness (4% to 7%), anxiety (6%), cold sensation (2%)

Dermatologic: Pruritus (2% to 5%), rash (1%)

Gastrointestinal: Diarrhea (2% to 7%)

Genitourinary: Gynecological disorder (7%), urinary retention (5%)

Hepatic: ALT increased (1% to 5%), AST increased (1% to 5%)

Local: Injection site reaction (4%; pain, redness, burning)

Neuromuscular & skeletal: Paresthesia (2%)

Respiratory: Hypoxia (9%)

<1% (Limited to important or life-threatening): Anaphylactoid reactions, anaphylaxis, angina, angioedema, arrhythmia, blindness (transient/following infusion; lasting ≤48 hours), blurred vision (transient/following infusion), bradycardia, bronchospasm, cardiopulmonary arrest, dyspnea, dystonic reaction, ECG changes, electrocardiographic alterations (second-degree heart block and ST-segment depression), extrapyramidal symptoms, flushing, grand mal seizure, hiccups, hypersensitivity reaction, hypokalemia, hypotension, laryngeal edema, laryngospasm, oculogyric crisis, palpitation, premature ventricular contractions (PVC), QT interval increased, shock, stridor, supraventricular tachycardia, syncope, tachycardia, urticaria, vascular occlusive events, ventricular arrhythmia

Drug Interactions

Metabolism/Transport Effects **Substrate** of CYP1A2 (minor), 2C9 (minor), 2D6 (minor), 2E1 (minor), 3A4 (major); **Inhibits** CYP1A2 (weak), 2C9 (weak), 2D6 (weak)

Avoid Concomitant Use

Avoid concomitant use of Ondansetron with any of the following: Apomorphine

Increased Effect/Toxicity

Ondansetron may increase the levels/effects of: Apomorphine

The levels/effects of Ondansetron may be increased by: P-Glycoprotein Inhibitors

Decreased Effect

The levels/effects of Ondansetron may be decreased by: CYP3A4 Inducers (Strong); Deferasirox; Herbs (CYP3A4 Inducers); P-Glycoprotein Inducers; Rifamycin Derivatives

Ethanol/Nutrition/Herb Interactions

Food: Food increases the extent of absorption. The C_{max} and T_{max} do not change much.

Herb/Nutraceutical: St John's wort may decrease ondansetron levels.

Stability

Oral solution: Store between 15°C and 30°C (59°F and 86°F). Protect from light.

Premixed bag: Store between 2°C and 30°C (36°F and 86°F). Protect from light.

Tablet: Store between 2°C and 30°C (36°F and 86°F).

Vial: Store between 2°C and 30°C (36°F and 86°F). Protect from light. Prior to I.V. infusion, dilute in 50 mL D_5W or NS. Solution is stable for 48 hours at room temperature.

Mechanism of Action Selective 5-HT_3-receptor antagonist, blocking serotonin, both peripherally on vagal nerve terminals and centrally in the chemoreceptor trigger zone

Pharmacodynamics/Kinetics

Onset of action: ~30 minutes

Distribution: V_d: Children: 1.7-3.7 L/kg; Adults: 2.2-2.5 L/kg

Protein binding, plasma: 70% to 76%

Metabolism: Extensively hepatic via hydroxylation, followed by glucuronide or sulfate conjugation; CYP1A2, CYP2D6, and CYP3A4 substrate; some demethylation occurs

Bioavailability: Oral: 56% to 71%; Rectal: 58% to 74%

Half-life elimination: Children <15 years: 2-7 hours; Adults: 3-6 hours

Mild-to-moderate hepatic impairment: Adults: 12 hours

Severe hepatic impairment (Child-Pugh C): Adults: 20 hours

Time to peak: Oral: ~2 hours

Excretion: Urine (44% to 60% as metabolites, 5% to 10% as unchanged drug); feces (~25%)

Dosage Note: Studies in adults have shown a single daily dose of 8-12 mg I.V. or 8-24 mg orally to be as effective as mg/kg dosing, and should be considered for **all** patients whose mg/kg dose exceeds 8-12 mg I.V.; oral solution and ODT formulations are bioequivalent to corresponding doses of tablet formulation

Children:

I.V.:

Prevention of chemotherapy-induced emesis: 6 months to 18 years: 0.15 mg/kg/dose administered 30 minutes prior to chemotherapy, 4 and 8 hours after the first dose **or** 0.45 mg/kg/day as a single dose

Prevention of postoperative nausea and vomiting: 1 month to 12 years:

≤40 kg: 0.1 mg/kg as a single dose

>40 kg: 4 mg as a single dose

Oral: Prevention of chemotherapy-induced emesis:

4-11 years: 4 mg 30 minutes before chemotherapy; repeat 4 and 8 hours after initial dose, then 4 mg every 8 hours for 1-2 days after chemotherapy completed

≥12 years: Refer to adult dosing.

Adults:

I.V.:

Prevention of chemotherapy-induced emesis:

0.15 mg/kg 3 times/day beginning 30 minutes prior to chemotherapy **or**

0.45 mg/kg once daily **or**

8-10 mg 1-2 times/day **or**

24 mg or 32 mg once daily

Treatment of hyperemesis gravidum (unlabeled use): 8 mg administered over 15 minutes every 12 hours **or** 1 mg/hour infused continuously for up to 24 hours

I.M., I.V.: Postoperative nausea and vomiting: 4 mg as a single dose approximately 30 minutes before the end of anesthesia, or as treatment if vomiting occurs after surgery

Note: Repeat doses given in response to inadequate control of nausea/vomiting from preoperative doses are generally ineffective.

Oral:

Chemotherapy-induced emesis:

Highly-emetogenic agents/single-day therapy: 24 mg given 30 minutes prior to the start of therapy

Moderately-emetogenic agents: 8 mg every 12 hours beginning 30 minutes before chemotherapy, continuously for 1-2 days after chemotherapy completed

Total body irradiation: 8 mg 1-2 hours before daily each fraction of radiotherapy

Single high-dose fraction radiotherapy to abdomen: 8 mg 1-2 hours before irradiation, then 8 mg every 8 hours after first dose for 1-2 days after completion of radiotherapy

Daily fractionated radiotherapy to abdomen: 8 mg 1-2 hours before irradiation, then 8 mg 8 hours after first dose for each day of radiotherapy

Postoperative nausea and vomiting: 16 mg given 1 hour prior to induction of anesthesia

Treatment of hyperemesis gravidum (unlabeled use): 8 mg every 12 hours

Elderly: No dosing adjustment required

Dosage adjustment in renal impairment: No dosing adjustment required

Dosage adjustment in hepatic impairment: Severe liver disease (Child-Pugh C): Maximum daily dose: 8 mg

Dietary Considerations Take without regard to meals. Orally-disintegrating tablet contains <0.03 mg phenylalanine

Administration

Oral: Oral dosage forms should be administered 30 minutes prior to chemotherapy; 1-2 hours before radiotherapy; 1 hour prior to the induction of anesthesia.

Orally-disintegrating tablets: Do not remove from blister until needed. Peel backing off the blister, do not push tablet through. Using dry hands, place tablet on tongue and allow to dissolve. Swallow with saliva.

I.M.: Should be administered undiluted.

I.V.:

IVPB: Dilute in 50 mL D_5W or NS. Infuse over 15-30 minutes; 24-hour continuous infusions have been reported, but are rarely used.

Chemotherapy-induced nausea and vomiting: Give first dose 30 minutes prior to beginning chemotherapy.

I.V. push: Prevention of postoperative nausea and vomiting: Single doses may be administered I.V. injection over 2-5 minutes as undiluted solution.

Monitoring Parameters Closely monitor patients <4 months of age

Dosage Forms Excipient information presented when available (limited, particularly for generics); consult specific product labeling. [DSC] = Discontinued product

Infusion, premixed in D_5 [preservative free]: 32 mg (50 mL)

Zofran®: 32 mg (50 mL) [DSC]

Injection, solution: 2 mg/mL (2 mL, 20 mL)

Zofran®: 2 mg/mL (2 mL, 20 mL)

Injection, solution [preservative free]: 2 mg/mL (2 mL)

Solution, oral: 4 mg/5 mL (50 mL)

Zofran®: 4 mg/5 mL (50 mL) [contains sodium benzoate; strawberry flavor]

Tablet: 4 mg; 8 mg

Zofran®: 4 mg; 8 mg

Tablet, orally disintegrating: 4 mg; 8 mg

Zofran® ODT: 4 mg, 8 mg [each strength contains phenylalanine <0.03 mg/tablet; strawberry flavor]

Extemporaneous Preparations A 0.8 mg/mL syrup may be made by crushing ten 8 mg tablets; flaking of the tablet coating occurs. Mix thoroughly with 50 mL of the suspending vehicle, Ora-Plus® (Paddock), in 5 mL increments. Add sufficient volume of any of the following syrups: Cherry syrup USP, Syrpalta® (Humco), Ora-Sweet® (Paddock), or Ora-Sweet® Sugar-Free (Paddock) to make a final volume of 100 mL. Stability is 42 days refrigerated.

Trissel LA, "Trissel's Stability of Compounded Formulations," American Pharmaceutical Association, 1996.

Rectal suppositories: Calibrate a suppository mold for the base being used. Determine the displacement factor (DF) for ondansetron for the base being used (Fattibase® = 1.1; Polybase® = 0.6). Weigh the ondansetron tablet. Divide the tablet weight by the DF. Subtract the weight of base displaced from the calculated weight of base required for each suppository. Grind the ondansetron tablets to a fine powder in a mortar. Weigh out the appropriate weight of suppository base. Melt the base over a water bath (<55°C). Add the ondansetron powder to the suppository base and mix well. Pour the mixture into the suppository mold and cool. Stable for at least 30 days under refrigeration.

Allen LV, "Ondansetron Suppositories," *US Pharm*, 20 (7):84-6.

- ◆ **Ondansetron Hydrochloride** *see* Ondansetron *on page 1102*
- ◆ **Ondansetron Injection (Can)** *see* Ondansetron *on page 1102*
- ◆ **Ondansetron-Omega (Can)** *see* Ondansetron *on page 1102*
- ◆ **One Gram C [OTC]** *see* Ascorbic Acid *on page 139*
- ◆ **ONTAK®** *see* Denileukin Diftitox *on page 417*
- ◆ **Onxol®** *see* Paclitaxel *on page 1127*

- ◆ **Opana®** *see* Oxymorphone *on page 1124*
- ◆ **Opana® ER** *see* Oxymorphone *on page 1124*
- ◆ **OPC-13013** *see* Cilostazol *on page 325*
- ◆ **OPC-14597** *see* Aripiprazole *on page 134*
- ◆ **Opcon-A® [OTC]** *see* Naphazoline and Pheniramine *on page 1040*
- ◆ **Operand® [OTC]** *see* Povidone-Iodine *on page 1222*
- ◆ **Operand® Chlorhexidine Gluconate [OTC]** *see* Chlorhexidine Gluconate *on page 305*
- ◆ **Ophthetic®** *see* Proparacaine *on page 1253*
- ◆ **Ophtho-Dipivefrin™ (Can)** *see* Dipivefrin *on page 466*
- ◆ **Ophtho-Tate® (Can)** *see* PrednisoLONE *on page 1230*
- ◆ **Opium and Belladonna** *see* Belladonna and Opium *on page 178*

Opium Tincture (OH pee um TING chur)

Index Terms DTO (error-prone abbreviation); Opium Tincture, Deodorized

Pharmacologic Category Analgesic, Opioid; Antidiarrheal

Use Treatment of diarrhea or relief of pain

Restrictions C-II

Pregnancy Risk Factor B/D (prolonged use or high doses at term)

Lactation Enters breast milk/use caution

Medication Safety Issues

Sound-alike/look-alike issues:

Opium tincture may be confused with camphorated tincture of opium (paregoric)

High alert medication: The Institute for Safe Medication Practices (ISMP) includes this medication among its list of drugs which have a heightened risk of causing significant patient harm when used in error.

Use care when prescribing opium tincture; each mL contains the equivalent of morphine 10 mg; paregoric contains the equivalent of morphine 0.4 mg/mL

DTO is an error-prone abbreviation (mistaken as Diluted Tincture of Opium; dose equivalency of paregoric)

Contraindications Hypersensitivity to morphine sulfate or any component of the formulation; increased intracranial pressure; severe respiratory depression; severe hepatic or renal insufficiency; pregnancy (prolonged use or high dosages near term)

Warnings/Precautions May cause CNS depression, which may impair physical or mental abilities; patients must be cautioned about performing tasks which require mental alertness (eg, operating machinery or driving). Effects may be potentiated when used with other sedative drugs or ethanol. Opium shares the toxic potential of opiate agonists, and usual precautions of opiate agonist therapy should be observed; use with caution in patients with CNS depression or coma, morbid obesity, adrenal insufficiency, hepatic impairment, head trauma, thyroid dysfunction, prostatic hyperplasia/urinary stricture, respiratory disease, or a history of drug abuse. Use with caution in patients with biliary tract dysfunction; acute pancreatitis may cause constriction of sphincter of Oddi. May cause hypotension; use with caution in patients with hypovolemia, cardiovascular disease (including acute MI), or with drugs which may exaggerate hypotensive effects (including phenothiazines or general anesthetics). May obscure diagnosis or clinical course of patients with acute abdominal conditions. Concurrent use of agonist/antagonist analgesics may precipitate withdrawal symptoms and/or reduced analgesic efficacy in patients following prolonged therapy with mu opioid agonists. Abrupt discontinuation following prolonged use may also lead to withdrawal symptoms. Use with caution in the elderly and debilitated patients; may be more sensitive to adverse effects. Some preparations contain sulfites which may cause allergic reactions. Infants <3 months of age are more susceptible to respiratory depression; use with caution and generally in reduced doses in this age group. This is **not** paregoric, dose accordingly.

Adverse Reactions Frequency not defined.

Cardiovascular: Palpitation, hypotension, bradycardia, peripheral vasodilation

Central nervous system: Drowsiness, dizziness, restlessness, headache, malaise, CNS depression, intracranial pressure increased, insomnia, mental depression

Gastrointestinal: Nausea, vomiting, constipation, anorexia, stomach cramps, biliary tract spasm

Genitourinary: Urination decreased, urinary tract spasm

Neuromuscular & skeletal: Weakness

Ocular: Miosis

Respiratory: Respiratory depression

Miscellaneous: Histamine release, physical and psychological dependence

Drug Interactions

Avoid Concomitant Use There are no known interactions where it is recommended to avoid concomitant use.

Increased Effect/Toxicity

Opium Tincture may increase the levels/effects of: Alcohol (Ethyl); Alvimopan; CNS Depressants; Desmopressin; Selective Serotonin Reuptake Inhibitors

The levels/effects of Opium Tincture may be increased by: Amphetamines; Antipsychotic Agents (Phenothiazines); Succinylcholine

Decreased Effect

Opium Tincture may decrease the levels/effects of: Pegvisomant

The levels/effects of Opium Tincture may be decreased by: Ammonium Chloride

Ethanol/Nutrition/Herb Interactions Ethanol: Avoid ethanol (may increase CNS depression).

Stability Protect from light.

Mechanism of Action Contains many narcotic alkaloids including morphine; its mechanism for gastric motility inhibition is primarily due to this morphine content; it results in a decrease in digestive secretions, an increase in GI muscle tone, and therefore a reduction in GI propulsion

Pharmacodynamics/Kinetics

Duration: 4-5 hours

Absorption: Variable

Metabolism: Hepatic

Excretion: Urine

Dosage Oral: **Note:** Opium tincture 10% contains morphine 10 mg/mL. Use caution in ordering, dispensing, and/or administering.

Children:

Diarrhea: 0.005-0.01 mL/kg/dose every 3-4 hours for a maximum of 6 doses/24 hours

Analgesia: 0.01-0.02 mL/kg/dose every 3-4 hours

Adults:

Diarrhea: 0.3-1 mL/dose every 2-6 hours to maximum of 6 mL/24 hours

Analgesia: 0.6-1.5 mL/dose every 3-4 hours

Monitoring Parameters Observe patient for excessive sedation, respiratory depression, implement safety measures, assist with ambulation

Test Interactions Increased aminotransferase [ALT/AST] (S)

Dosage Forms Excipient information presented when available (limited, particularly for generics); consult specific product labeling.

Liquid: 10% (120 mL, 480 mL) [0.6 mL equivalent to morphine 6 mg; contains alcohol 19%]

◆ **Opium Tincture, Deodorized** *see* Opium Tincture *on page 1105*

Oprelvekin (oh PREL ve kin)

U.S. Brand Names Neumega®

Index Terms IL-11; Interleukin-11; NSC-722848; Recombinant Human Interleukin-11; Recombinant Interleukin-11; rhIL-11; rIL-11

Pharmacologic Category Biological Response Modulator; Human Growth Factor

Use Prevention of severe thrombocytopenia; reduce the need for platelet transfusions following myelosuppressive chemotherapy

Pregnancy Risk Factor C

Pregnancy Considerations Animal studies have demonstrated adverse fetal effects. There are no adequate and well-controlled studies in pregnant women. Use during pregnancy only if the potential benefits outweigh the potential risk to the fetus.

Lactation Excretion in breast milk unknown/not recommended

Medication Safety Issues

Sound-alike/look-alike issues:

Oprelvekin may be confused with aldesleukin, Proleukin®

Neumega® may be confused with Neulasta®, Neupogen®

Contraindications Hypersensitivity to oprelvekin or any component of the formulation

Warnings/Precautions [U.S. Boxed Warning]: Allergic or hypersensitivity reactions, including anaphylaxis have been reported. May occur with the first or with subsequent doses. Permanently discontinue in any patient developing an allergic reaction. May cause serious fluid retention; use cautiously in patients with conditions where expansion of plasma volume should be avoided (eg, left ventricular dysfunction, HF, hypertension). Closely monitor fluid and electrolytes in patient on chronic diuretic therapy; severe hypokalemia contributing to sudden death have been reported in these patients. Arrhythmia, pulmonary edema, and cardiac arrest have been reported; use in patients with a history of atrial arrhythmia only if the potential benefit exceeds possible risks. Patients experiencing arrhythmia may be at risk for stroke; use caution in patients with a history of transient ischemic attack or stroke. Ventricular arrhythmia has also been reported, occurring within 2-7 days of treatment initiation. Use caution in patients with conduction defects, respiratory disease; history of thromboembolic problems; pre-existing pericardial effusions or ascites. Use with caution in hepatic or renal dysfunction. Not indicated following myeloablative chemotherapy; increased toxicities were reported when used following myeloablative therapy. Efficacy has not been established with chemotherapy regimens >5 days duration or with regimens associated with delayed myelosuppression (eg, nitrosoureas, mitomycin C). Safety and efficacy have not been established with chronic administration. Papilledema, more frequently associated with use in children, has occurred; use caution in patients with pre-existing papilledema or with tumors involving the central nervous system. Papilledema is dose limiting. Patients experiencing oprelvekin-related papilledema may be at risk for visual acuity changes, including blurred vision or blindness. Although used in children in clinical trials, safety and efficacy have not been established in pediatric patients.

Adverse Reactions

>10%:

Cardiovascular: Tachycardia (children 84%; adults 20%), edema (59%), palpitation (14%), cardiomegaly (children 21%), vasodilation (19%), syncope (13%), atrial arrhythmia (12%)

Central nervous system: Headache (41%), dizziness (38%), fever (36%), insomnia (33%), fatigue (30%)

Dermatologic: Rash (25%)

Endocrine & metabolic: Fluid retention

Gastrointestinal: Nausea/vomiting (77%), diarrhea (43%), oral moniliasis (14%)

Hematologic: Anemia (dilutional); appears within 3 days of initiation of therapy, resolves in about 1 week after cessation of oprelvekin

Neuromuscular & skeletal: Weakness (severe 14%), arthralgia, periostitis (children 11%)

Ocular: Conjunctival injection/redness/swelling (children 57%; adults 19%), papilledema (children 16%; adults 1%)

Respiratory: Dyspnea (48%), rhinitis (42%), cough (29%), pharyngitis (25%)

1% to 10%:

Gastrointestinal: Weight gain (5%)

Respiratory: Pleural effusion (10%)

Postmarketing and/or case reports: Allergic reaction, amblyopia, anaphylaxis/anaphylactoid reactions, blindness, blurred vision, capillary leak syndrome, CHF, dehydration, exfoliative dermatitis, eye hemorrhage, facial edema, fibrinogen increased, fluid overload, hypoalbuminemia, hypocalcemia, hypotension, injection site reactions (dermatitis, pain, discoloration), optic neuropathy, paresthesia, pericardial effusion, pulmonary edema, renal failure, skin discoloration, stroke, ventricular arrhythmia

Drug Interactions

Avoid Concomitant Use There are no known interactions where it is recommended to avoid concomitant use.

Increased Effect/Toxicity There are no known significant interactions involving an increase in effect.

Decreased Effect There are no known significant interactions involving a decrease in effect.

Stability Store vials under refrigeration between 2°C to 8°C (36°F to 46°F); do not freeze. Protect from light. Reconstitute to a final concentration of 5 mg/mL with SWFI; swirl gently, do not shake. Use reconstituted oprelvekin within 3 hours of reconstitution and store in the vial at either 2°C to 8°C (36°F to 46°F) or room temperature of ≤25°C (77°F). Do not freeze or shake reconstituted solution.

Mechanism of Action Oprelvekin is a growth factor which stimulates multiple stages of megakaryocytopoiesis and thrombopoiesis, resulting in proliferation of megakaryocyte progenitors and megakaryocyte maturation, or increased platelet production.

Pharmacodynamics/Kinetics

Bioavailability: >80%

Half-life elimination: Terminal: 5-9 hours

Time to peak, serum: 1-6 hours

Excretion: Urine (primarily as metabolites)

Dosage SubQ: Administer first dose ~6-24 hours after the end of chemotherapy. Discontinue at least 48 hours before beginning the next cycle of chemotherapy.

Children (unlabeled use): 75-100 mcg/kg once daily for 10-21 days (until postnadir platelet count ≥50,000 cells/μL)

Note: A safe and effective dose for use in children has not been established by the manufacturer.

Adults: 50 mcg/kg once daily for ~10-21 days (until postnadir platelet count ≥50,000 cells/μL)

Dosage adjustment in renal impairment: Cl_{cr} <30 mL/minute: 25 mcg/kg once daily

Administration Subcutaneously in the abdomen, thigh, hip, or upper arm.

Monitoring Parameters Monitor electrolytes and fluid balance during therapy; obtain a CBC at regular intervals during therapy; monitor platelet counts until adequate recovery has occurred

Test Interactions Decrease in hemoglobin concentration, serum concentration of albumin and other proteins (result of expansion of plasma volume)

Dosage Forms Excipient information presented when available (limited, particularly for generics); consult specific product labeling.

Injection, powder for reconstitution:

Neumega®: 5 mg [packaged with diluent]

- **Optase™** *see* Trypsin, Balsam Peru, and Castor Oil *on page 1526*
- **Optho-Bunolol® (Can)** *see* Levobunolol *on page 873*
- **Opticrom® (Can)** *see* Cromolyn *on page 372*
- **Optimyxin® (Can)** *see* Bacitracin and Polymyxin B *on page 171*
- **Optimyxin Plus® (Can)** *see* Neomycin, Polymyxin B, and Gramicidin *on page 1052*
- **OptiPranolol®** *see* Metipranolol *on page 979*
- **Optison™** *see* Perflutren Protein Type A *on page 1174*
- **Optivar®** *see* Azelastine *on page 165*
- **o,p'-DDD** *see* Mitotane *on page 1006*
- **Orabase® with Benzocaine [OTC]** *see* Benzocaine *on page 183*
- **Oracea™** *see* Doxycycline *on page 491*
- **Oracit®** *see* Sodium Citrate and Citric Acid *on page 1383*
- **Oracort (Can)** *see* Triamcinolone *on page 1510*
- **Orajel® Baby Daytime and Nighttime [OTC]** *see* Benzocaine *on page 183*
- **Orajel® Baby Teething [OTC]** *see* Benzocaine *on page 183*
- **Orajel® Baby Teething Nighttime [OTC]** *see* Benzocaine *on page 183*
- **Orajel® Denture Plus [OTC]** *see* Benzocaine *on page 183*
- **Orajel® Maximum Strength [OTC]** *see* Benzocaine *on page 183*
- **Orajel® Medicated Toothache [OTC]** *see* Benzocaine *on page 183*
- **Orajel® Mouth Sore [OTC]** *see* Benzocaine *on page 183*
- **Orajel® Multi-Action Cold Sore [OTC]** *see* Benzocaine *on page 183*
- **Orajel® Perioseptic® Spot Treatment [OTC]** *see* Carbamide Peroxide *on page 254*
- **Orajel PM® Maximum Strength [OTC]** *see* Benzocaine *on page 183*
- **Orajel® Ultra Mouth Sore [OTC]** *see* Benzocaine *on page 183*
- **Oramorph SR®** *see* Morphine Sulfate *on page 1016*
- **Oranyl [OTC]** *see* Pseudoephedrine *on page 1265*
- **Oranyl Plus [OTC]** *see* Acetaminophen and Pseudoephedrine *on page 30*
- **Orap®** *see* Pimozide *on page 1194*
- **Orapred®** *see* PrednisoLONE *on page 1230*
- **Orapred ODT™** *see* PrednisoLONE *on page 1230*
- **Oraquix®** *see* Lidocaine and Prilocaine *on page 887*
- **OraVerse™** *see* Phentolamine *on page 1182*
- **Orazinc® [OTC]** *see* Zinc Sulfate *on page 1584*
- **Orciprenaline Sulfate** *see* Metaproterenol *on page 952*
- **Orencia®** *see* Abatacept *on page 20*
- **Orfadin®** *see* Nitisinone *on page 1071*
- **ORG 946** *see* Rocuronium *on page 1334*
- **Orgalutran® (Can)** *see* Ganirelix *on page 682*
- **Organidin® NR** *see* GuaiFENesin *on page 709*
- **ORG NC 45** *see* Vecuronium *on page 1553*

Orlistat (OR li stat)

U.S. Brand Names Alli™ [OTC]; Xenical®

Canadian Brand Names Xenical®

Pharmacologic Category Lipase Inhibitor

Use Management of obesity, including weight loss and weight management, when used in conjunction with a reduced-calorie and low-fat diet; reduce the risk of weight regain after prior weight loss; indicated for obese patients with an initial body mass index (BMI) ≥30 kg/m^2 or ≥27 kg/m^2 in the presence of other risk factors

Pregnancy Risk Factor B

Pregnancy Considerations There are no adequate and well-controlled studies of orlistat in pregnant women. Because animal reproductive studies are not always predictive of human response, orlistat is not recommended for use during pregnancy. Teratogenicity studies were conducted in rats and rabbits at doses up to 800 mg/kg/day. Neither study showed embryotoxicity or teratogenicity. This dose is 23 and 47 times the daily human dose calculated on a body surface area basis for rats and rabbits, respectively.

Lactation Excretion in breast milk unknown/not recommended

Medication Safety Issues

Sound-alike/look-alike issues:

Xenical® may be confused with Xeloda®

Contraindications Hypersensitivity to orlistat or any component of the formulation; chronic malabsorption syndrome or cholestasis

Warnings/Precautions Patients should be advised to adhere to dietary guidelines; gastrointestinal adverse events may increase if taken with a diet high in fat (>30% total daily calories from fat). The daily intake of fat should be distributed over three main meals. If taken with any one meal very high in fat, the possibility of gastrointestinal effects increases. Patients should be counseled to take a multivitamin supplement that contains fat-soluble vitamins to ensure adequate nutrition because orlistat has been shown to reduce the absorption of some fat-soluble vitamins and beta-carotene. Some patients may develop increased levels of urinary oxalate following treatment; caution should be exercised when prescribing it to patients with a history of hyperoxaluria or calcium oxalate nephrolithiasis. As with any weight-loss agent, the potential exists for misuse in appropriate patient populations (eg, patients with anorexia nervosa or bulimia). Safety and efficacy have not been established in children <12 years of age. Safety and efficacy with >4 years of use have not been established.

OTC labeling: Prior to use, patients should contact their healthcare provider if they have ever had kidney stones, gall bladder disease, or pancreatitis. Patients taking medications for diabetes or thyroid disease, anticoagulants, or other weight-loss products should consult their healthcare provider or pharmacist. Patients who have had an organ transplant should not use orlistat. If severe and/or continuous abdominal pain occurs, use should be discontinued and healthcare provider consulted.

Adverse Reactions

>10%:

Central nervous system: Headache (31%)

Gastrointestinal: Oily spotting (27%), abdominal pain/discomfort (26%), flatus with discharge (24%), fecal urgency (22%), fatty/oily stool (20%), oily evacuation (12%), defecation increased (11%)

Neuromuscular & skeletal: Back pain (14%)

Respiratory: Upper respiratory infection (38%)

1% to 10%:

Central nervous system: Fatigue (7%), anxiety (5%), sleep disorder (4%)

Dermatologic: Dry skin (2%)

Endocrine & metabolic: Menstrual irregularities (10%)

Gastrointestinal: Fecal incontinence (8%), nausea (8%), infectious diarrhea (5%), rectal pain/discomfort (5%), vomiting (4%)

Neuromuscular & skeletal: Arthritis (5%), myalgia (4%)

Otic: Otitis (4%)

<1% (Limited to important or life-threatening): Abdominal distension, allergic reactions, anaphylaxis, angioedema, bronchitis, bronchospasm, bullous eruption, cholelithiasis (may be caused by weight loss), hepatitis (causal relationship not established), hypoglycemia (in patients with diabetes), pancreatitis, pruritus, rash, transaminases increased, urticaria

Drug Interactions

Avoid Concomitant Use There are no known interactions where it is recommended to avoid concomitant use.

Increased Effect/Toxicity

Orlistat may increase the levels/effects of: Warfarin

Decreased Effect

Orlistat may decrease the levels/effects of: Amiodarone; Levothyroxine

Ethanol/Nutrition/Herb Interactions

Fat-soluble vitamins: Absorption of vitamins A, D, E, and K may be decreased by orlistat. A multivitamin containing the fat-soluble vitamins (A, D, E, and K) should be administered once daily at least 2 hours before or after orlistat.

Stability Store at 15°C to 30°C (59°F to 86°F).

Mechanism of Action A reversible inhibitor of gastric and pancreatic lipases, thus inhibiting absorption of dietary fats by 30% (at doses of 120 mg 3 times/day).

Pharmacodynamics/Kinetics

Onset of action: 24-48 hours

Duration: 48-72 hours

Absorption: Minimal

Metabolism: Metabolized within the gastrointestinal wall; forms inactive metabolites

Excretion: Feces (97%, 83% as unchanged drug); urine (<2%)

Dosage Oral:

Children ≥12 years and Adults (Xenical®): 120 mg 3 times/day with each main meal containing fat (during or up to 1 hour after the meal); omit dose if meal is occasionally missed or contains no fat.

Adults (Alli™): OTC labeling: 60 mg 3 times/day with each main meal containing fat

Dietary Considerations Multivitamin supplements that contain fat-soluble vitamins should be taken once daily at least 2 hours before or after the administration of orlistat (ie, bedtime). Distribute the daily intake of fat over 3 main meals. Gastrointestinal effects of orlistat may increase if taken with any 1 meal very high in fat.

Dosage Forms Excipient information presented when available (limited, particularly for generics); consult specific product labeling.

Capsule:

Alli™: 60 mg

Xenical®: 120 mg

◆ **Ornex® [OTC]** *see* Acetaminophen and Pseudoephedrine *on page* 30

◆ **Ornex® Maximum Strength [OTC]** *see* Acetaminophen and Pseudoephedrine *on page* 30

◆ **ORO-Clense (Can)** *see* Chlorhexidine Gluconate *on page* 305

◆ **Orphenace® (Can)** *see* Orphenadrine *on page* 1108

Orphenadrine (or FEN a dreen)

U.S. Brand Names Norflex™

Canadian Brand Names Norflex™; Orphenace®; Rhoxal-orphendrine

Index Terms Orphenadrine Citrate

Pharmacologic Category Anti-Parkinson's Agent, Anticholinergic; Skeletal Muscle Relaxant

Use Treatment of muscle spasm associated with acute painful musculoskeletal conditions

Pregnancy Risk Factor C

Medication Safety Issues

Sound-alike/look-alike issues:

Norflex™ may be confused with norfloxacin, Noroxin®

International issues:

Flexin® [Israel] may be confused with Floxin® which is a brand name for ofloxacin in the U.S.

Flexin® [Israel]: Brand name for indomethacin in Great Britain

Dosage

Adults:

Oral: 100 mg twice daily

I.M., I.V.: 60 mg every 12 hours

Elderly: Use caution; generally not recommended for use in the elderly

Additional Information Complete prescribing information for this medication should be consulted for additional detail.

Dosage Forms Excipient information presented when available (limited, particularly for generics); consult specific product labeling.

Injection, solution, as citrate: 30 mg/mL (2 mL)

Norflex™: 30 mg/mL (2 mL) [contains sodium bisulfite]

Tablet, extended release, as citrate: 100 mg

Orphenadrine, Aspirin, and Caffeine

(or FEN a dreen, AS pir in, & KAF een)

U.S. Brand Names Norgesic™ Forte [DSC]; Norgesic™ [DSC]; Orphengesic Forte [DSC]; Orphengesic [DSC]

Canadian Brand Names Norgesic™; Norgesic™ Forte

Index Terms Aspirin, Orphenadrine, and Caffeine; Caffeine, Orphenadrine, and Aspirin

Pharmacologic Category Skeletal Muscle Relaxant

Use Relief of discomfort associated with skeletal muscular conditions

Pregnancy Risk Factor D

Medication Safety Issues

Sound-alike/look-alike issues:

Norgesic™ Forte may be confused with Norgesic 40®

Dosage Oral: 1-2 tablets 3-4 times/day

Additional Information Complete prescribing information for this medication should be consulted for additional detail.

Dosage Forms Excipient information presented when available (limited, particularly for generics); consult specific product labeling. [DSC] = Discontinued product

Tablet: Orphenadrine citrate 25 mg, aspirin 385 mg, and caffeine 30 mg; orphenadrine citrate 50 mg, aspirin 770 mg, and caffeine 60 mg

Norgesic™, Orphengesic: Orphenadrine citrate 25 mg, aspirin 385 mg, and caffeine 30 mg [DSC]

Norgesic™ Forte, Orphengesic Forte: Orphenadrine citrate 50 mg, aspirin 770 mg, and caffeine 60 mg [DSC]

◆ **Orphenadrine Citrate** *see* Orphenadrine *on page* 1108

◆ **Orphengesic [DSC]** *see* Orphenadrine, Aspirin, and Caffeine *on page* 1108

◆ **Orphengesic Forte [DSC]** *see* Orphenadrine, Aspirin, and Caffeine *on page* 1108

◆ **Ortho® 0.5/35 (Can)** *see* Ethinyl Estradiol and Norethindrone *on page 581*

◆ **Ortho® 1/35 (Can)** *see* Ethinyl Estradiol and Norethindrone *on page 581*

◆ **Ortho® 7/7/7 (Can)** *see* Ethinyl Estradiol and Norethindrone *on page 581*

◆ **Ortho Cept** *see* Ethinyl Estradiol and Desogestrel *on page 575*

◆ **Ortho-Cept®** *see* Ethinyl Estradiol and Desogestrel *on page 575*

◆ **Orthoclone OKT® 3** *see* Muromonab-CD3 *on page 1024*

◆ **Ortho Cyclen** *see* Ethinyl Estradiol and Norgestimate *on page 584*

◆ **Ortho-Cyclen®** *see* Ethinyl Estradiol and Norgestimate *on page 584*

◆ **Ortho Est** *see* Estropipate *on page 568*

◆ **Ortho-Est®** *see* Estropipate *on page 568*

◆ **Ortho-Evra** *see* Ethinyl Estradiol and Norelgestromin *on page 581*

◆ **Ortho Evra®** *see* Ethinyl Estradiol and Norelgestromin *on page 581*

◆ **Ortho Micronor®** *see* Norethindrone *on page 1078*

◆ **Ortho Novum** *see* Ethinyl Estradiol and Norethindrone *on page 581*

◆ **Ortho-Novum®** *see* Ethinyl Estradiol and Norethindrone *on page 581*

◆ **Ortho Novum 1/50** *see* Norethindrone and Mestranol *on page 1079*

◆ **Ortho-Novum® 1/50 [DSC]** *see* Norethindrone and Mestranol *on page 1079*

◆ **Ortho-Novum® 1/50 (Can)** *see* Norethindrone and Mestranol *on page 1079*

◆ **Ortho Tri Cyclen** *see* Ethinyl Estradiol and Norgestimate *on page 584*

◆ **Ortho Tri-Cyclen®** *see* Ethinyl Estradiol and Norgestimate *on page 584*

◆ **Ortho Tri-Cyclen® Lo** *see* Ethinyl Estradiol and Norgestimate *on page 584*

◆ **Orthovisc®** *see* Hyaluronate and Derivatives *on page 734*

◆ **OrthoVisc® (Can)** *see* Hyaluronate and Derivatives *on page 734*

◆ **Oruvail® (Can)** *see* Ketoprofen *on page 839*

◆ **Os-Cal® (Can)** *see* Calcium Carbonate *on page 238*

◆ **Os-Cal® 500 [OTC] [DSC]** *see* Calcium Carbonate *on page 238*

◆ **Os-Cal® 500+D [OTC]** *see* Calcium and Vitamin D *on page 238*

Oseltamivir (oh sel TAM i vir)

U.S. Brand Names Tamiflu®

Canadian Brand Names Tamiflu®

Pharmacologic Category Antiviral Agent; Neuraminidase Inhibitor

Additional Appendix Information

Community-Acquired Pneumonia in Adults *on page 1766*

Guidelines for the Prevention of Opportunistic Infections in HIV Infected Persons *on page 1740*

Use Treatment of uncomplicated acute illness due to influenza (A or B) infection in children ≥1 year of age and adults who have been symptomatic for no more than 2 days; prophylaxis against influenza (A or B) infection in children ≥1 year of age and adults

The Advisory Committee on Immunization Practices (ACIP) recommends that **treatment** be considered for the following:

- Persons hospitalized with laboratory confirmed influenza (may also have benefit if started >48 hours after onset of illness).
- Persons with laboratory confirmed influenza pneumonia.
- Persons with laboratory confirmed influenza and bacterial infections.
- Persons with laboratory confirmed influenza and who are at higher risk for influenza complications.
- Persons presenting for care within 48 hours of laboratory confirmed influenza onset and who want to decrease duration and/or severity of their symptoms or decrease the risk of transmission to those at high risk for complications.

The ACIP recommends that **prophylaxis** be considered for the following:

- Persons at high risk for influenza infection during the first 2 weeks following vaccination (eg, children <9 years and not previously vaccinated) if the virus is circulating in the community.
- Persons at high risk for influenza infection, but the vaccination is contraindicated.
- Unvaccinated family members or healthcare providers with prolonged exposure to or close contact with high-risk persons, unvaccinated persons, or infants <6 months of age.
- Persons at high risk for influenza infection, their family members and close contacts, and healthcare workers when the circulating strain of influenza is not matched with the vaccine.
- Persons with immune deficiency or those who may not respond to vaccination.
- Unvaccinated staff and persons during response to an outbreak in a closed institutional setting that has patients at high risk for infection (eg, extended care facilities).

Pregnancy Risk Factor C

Pregnancy Considerations There are insufficient human data to determine the risk to a pregnant woman or developing fetus. Studies evaluating the effects on embryo-fetal development in rats and rabbits showed a dose-dependent increase in the rates of minor skeleton abnormalities in exposed offspring. The rate of each abnormality remained within the background rate of occurrence in the species studied.

Lactation Enters breast milk/not recommended

Medication Safety Issues

Sound-alike/look-alike issues:

Tamiflu® may be confused with Thera-Flu®

Contraindications Hypersensitivity to oseltamivir or any component of the formulation

Warnings/Precautions Oseltamivir is not a substitute for the influenza virus vaccine. Use caution with renal impairment; dosage adjustment is required for creatinine clearance <30 mL/minute. Also consider primary or concomitant bacterial infections. Safety and efficacy for use in severe hepatic impairment or for treatment or prophylaxis in immunocompromised patients have not been established. Efficacy has not been established if treatment begins >40 hours after the onset of symptoms or in the treatment of patients with chronic cardiac and/or respiratory disease. Rare but severe hypersensitivity reactions (anaphylaxis, severe dermatologic reactions) have been associated with use. Rare occurrences of neuropsychiatric events (including confusion, delirium, hallucinations, and/or self-injury) have been reported from postmarketing surveillance (primarily in pediatric patients); direct causation is difficult to establish (influenza infection may also be associated with behavioral and neurologic changes). Monitor closely for signs of any unusual ▶

behavior. Safety and efficacy in children (<1 year of age) have not been established.

Adverse Reactions

>10%: Gastrointestinal: Vomiting (2% to 15%)

1% to 10%: Gastrointestinal: Nausea (3% to 10%), abdominal pain (2% to 5%)

<1% (Limited to important or life-threatening): Allergy, anaphylactic/anaphylactoid reaction, arrhythmia, confusion, dermatitis, diabetes aggravation, eczema, erythema multiforme, hepatitis, liver function tests abnormal, neuropsychiatric events (self-injury, confusion, delirium), rash, seizure, Stevens-Johnson syndrome, swelling of face or tongue, toxic epidermal necrolysis, urticaria

Drug Interactions

Avoid Concomitant Use There are no known interactions where it is recommended to avoid concomitant use.

Increased Effect/Toxicity There are no known significant interactions involving an increase in effect.

Decreased Effect

Oseltamivir may decrease the levels/effects of: Influenza Virus Vaccine

Stability

Capsules: Store at 25°C (77°F).

Oral suspension: Store powder for suspension at 25°C (77°F). Reconstitute with 23 mL of water (to make 25 mL total suspension). Once reconstituted, store suspension under refrigeration at 2°C to 8°C (36°F to 46°F); do not freeze. Use within 10 days of preparation.

Mechanism of Action Oseltamivir, a prodrug, is hydrolyzed to the active form, oseltamivir carboxylate (OC). OC inhibits influenza virus neuraminidase, an enzyme known to cleave the budding viral progeny from its cellular envelope attachment point (neuraminic acid) just prior to release.

Pharmacodynamics/Kinetics

Absorption: Well absorbed

Distribution: V_d: 23-26 L (oseltamivir carboxylate)

Protein binding, plasma: Oseltamivir carboxylate: 3%; Oseltamivir: 42%

Metabolism: Hepatic (90%) to oseltamivir carboxylate; neither the parent drug nor active metabolite has any effect on the cytochrome P450 system

Bioavailability: 75% as oseltamivir carboxylate

Half-life elimination: Oseltamivir: 1-3 hours; Oseltamivir carboxylate: 6-10 hours

Excretion: Urine (>90% as oseltamivir carboxylate); feces

Dosage Oral:

Treatment: Initiate treatment within 2 days of onset of symptoms; duration of treatment: 5 days:

- Children: 1-12 years:
  - ≤15 kg: 30 mg twice daily
  - >15 kg to ≤23 kg: 45 mg twice daily
  - >23 kg to ≤40 kg: 60 mg twice daily
  - >40 kg: 75 mg twice daily
- Adolescents ≥13 years and Adults: 75 mg twice daily

Prophylaxis: Initiate treatment within 2 days of contact with an infected individual; duration of treatment: 10 days

- Children: 1-12 years:
  - ≤15 kg: 30 mg once daily
  - >15 kg to ≤23 kg: 45 mg once daily
  - >23 kg to ≤40 kg: 60 mg once daily
  - >40 kg: 75 mg once daily
- Adolescents ≥13 years and Adults: 75 mg once daily. During community outbreaks, dosing is 75 mg once daily. May be used for up to 6 weeks; duration of protection lasts for length of dosing period

Dosage adjustment in renal impairment: Adults:

Cl_{cr} 10-30 mL/minute:

Treatment: Reduce dose to 75 mg once daily for 5 days

Prophylaxis: 75 mg every other day or 30 mg once daily

CAPD (unlabeled dose): 30 mg once weekly (Robson, 2006)

Hemodialysis (unlabeled dose): 30 mg after every other session (Robson, 2006)

Dosage adjustment in hepatic impairment: No adjustment required in mild-to-moderate hepatic impairment. Safety and kinetics in patients with severe hepatic impairment have not been evaluated.

Dietary Considerations Take with or without food; take with food to improve tolerance.

Administration Capsules may be opened and mixed with sweetened liquid (eg, chocolate syrup).

Monitoring Parameters Signs or symptoms of unusual behavior, including attempts at self-injury, confusion, and/or delirium

Additional Information In clinical studies of the influenza virus, 1.3% of post-treatment isolates in adults and adolescents and 8.6% of isolates in children had decreased neuraminidase susceptibility *in vitro* to oseltamivir carboxylate.

Dosage Forms Excipient information presented when available (limited, particularly for generics); consult specific product labeling.

Capsule, as phosphate:

Tamiflu®: 30 mg, 45 mg, 75 mg

Powder for oral suspension:

Tamiflu®: 12 mg/mL (25 mL) [contains sodium benzoate; tutti-frutti flavor]

Extemporaneous Preparations

If the commercially prepared oral suspension is not available, the manufacturer provides the following compounding information to prepare a **15 mg/mL** suspension in emergency situations. **Note:** The strength and dosing instructions differ from that of the commercially prepared product (see chart on next page).

1. Calculate the total volume needed by patient weight (refer to chart on next page).
2. Calculate the number of capsules and required volume of vehicle (refer to chart on next page). **Note:** Acceptable vehicles are cherry syrup or Ora-Sweet®SF.
3. Transfer contents of capsules into mortar and triturate granules into a fine powder.
4. Add ~1/3 of vehicle and triturate into a uniform suspension.
5. Add another 1/3 of vehicle and triturate, transfer to amber prescription bottle.
6. Add remaining vehicle to prescription bottle; shake well.

Suspension is stable for 35 days under refrigeration at 2°C to 8°C (36°F to 46°F) or 5 days at room temperature of 25°C (77°F). Shake gently prior to use. Do **not** dispense with dosing device provided with commercially-available product.

Preparation of Oseltamivir 15 mg/mL Suspension

Body Weight	Total Volume per Patient[1]	# of 75 mg Capsules[2]	Required Volume of Vehicle[2,3]	Treatment Dose (wt based)[4]	Prophylactic Dose (wt based)[4]
≤15 kg	30 mL	6	29 mL	2 mL (30 mg) twice daily for 5 days	2 mL (30 mg) once daily for 10 days
16-23 kg	40 mL	8	38.5 mL	3 mL (45 mg) twice daily for 5 days	3 mL (45 mg) once daily for 10 days
24-40 kg	50 mL	10	48 mL	4 mL (60 mg) twice daily for 5 days	4 mL (60 mg) once daily for 10 days
≥41 kg	60 mL	12	57 mL	5 mL (75 mg) twice daily for 5 days	5 mL (75 mg) once daily for 10 days

[1]Entire course of therapy.

[2]Based on total volume per patient.

[3]Acceptable vehicles are cherry syrup or Ora-Sweet® SF.

[4]Using 15 mg/mL suspension.

- **OSI-774** *see* Erlotinib *on page 541*
- **Osmitrol®** *see* Mannitol *on page 919*
- **Osteocit® (Can)** *see* Calcium Citrate *on page 241*
- **Ostoforte® (Can)** *see* Ergocalciferol *on page 538*
- **OTFC (Oral Transmucosal Fentanyl Citrate)** *see* FentaNYL *on page 610*
- **Otix® [OTC]** *see* Carbamide Peroxide *on page 254*
- **Outgro® [OTC]** *see* Benzocaine *on page 183*
- **Ovace®** *see* Sulfacetamide *on page 1405*
- **Ovace® Plus** *see* Sulfacetamide *on page 1405*
- **Ovcon®** *see* Ethinyl Estradiol and Norethindrone *on page 581*
- **Ovide®** *see* Malathion *on page 919*
- **Ovidrel®** *see* Chorionic Gonadotropin (Recombinant) *on page 321*
- **Ovine Corticotrophin-Releasing Hormone** *see* Corticorelin *on page 370*
- **Ovral® (Can)** *see* Ethinyl Estradiol and Norgestrel *on page 585*

Oxacillin (oks a SIL in)

Index Terms Methylphenyl Isoxazolyl Penicillin; Oxacillin Sodium

Pharmacologic Category Antibiotic, Penicillin

Additional Appendix Information

Antibiotic Treatment of Adults With Infective Endocarditis *on page 1748*

Use Treatment of infections such as osteomyelitis, septicemia, endocarditis, and CNS infections caused by susceptible strains of *Staphylococcus*

Pregnancy Risk Factor B

Pregnancy Considerations Adverse events have not been observed in animal studies; therefore, oxacillin is classified as pregnancy category B. Oxacillin is distributed into the amniotic fluid and is detected in cord blood. There was not an increased risk of teratogenic effects with oxacillin observed in an epidemiologic study.

Lactation Enters breast milk/use caution

Contraindications Hypersensitivity to oxacillin or other penicillins or any component of the formulation

Warnings/Precautions Elimination rate will be slow in neonates. Modify dosage in patients with renal impairment and in the elderly. Serious and occasionally severe or fatal hypersensitivity (anaphylactoid) reactions have been reported in patients on penicillin therapy, especially with a history of beta-lactam hypersensitivity, history of sensitivity to multiple allergens, or previous IgE-mediated reactions (eg, anaphylaxis, angioedema, urticaria). Use with caution in asthmatic patients. Prolonged use may result in fungal or bacterial superinfection, including *C. difficile*-associated diarrhea (CDAD) and pseudomembranous colitis; CDAD has been observed >2 months postantibiotic treatment.

Adverse Reactions Frequency not defined.

Central nervous system: Fever

Dermatologic: Rash

Gastrointestinal: Nausea, diarrhea, vomiting

Hematologic: Eosinophilia, leukopenia, neutropenia, thrombocytopenia, agranulocytosis

Hepatic: Hepatotoxicity, AST increased

Renal: Acute interstitial nephritis, hematuria

Miscellaneous: Serum sickness-like reactions

Drug Interactions

Avoid Concomitant Use There are no known interactions where it is recommended to avoid concomitant use.

Increased Effect/Toxicity

Oxacillin may increase the levels/effects of: Methotrexate

The levels/effects of Oxacillin may be increased by: Uricosuric Agents

Decreased Effect

Oxacillin may decrease the levels/effects of: Typhoid Vaccine

The levels/effects of Oxacillin may be decreased by: Fusidic Acid; Tetracycline Derivatives

Stability Reconstituted parenteral solution is stable for 3 days at room temperature and 7 days when refrigerated. For I.V. infusion in NS or D_5W, solution is stable for 24 hours at room temperature.

Mechanism of Action Inhibits bacterial cell wall synthesis by binding to one or more of the penicillin-binding proteins (PBPs); which in turn inhibits the final transpeptidation step of peptidoglycan synthesis in bacterial cell walls, thus inhibiting cell wall biosynthesis. Bacteria eventually lyse due to ongoing activity of cell wall autolytic enzymes (autolysins and murein hydrolases) while cell wall assembly is arrested.

Pharmacodynamics/Kinetics

Distribution: Into bile, synovial and pleural fluids, bronchial secretions; also distributes to peritoneal and pericardial fluids; penetrates the blood-brain barrier only when meninges are inflamed

Protein binding: ~94%

Metabolism: Hepatic to active metabolites

Half-life elimination: Children 1 week to 2 years: 0.9-1.8 hours; Adults: 23-60 minutes; prolonged in neonates and with renal impairment

Time to peak, serum: I.M.: 30-60 minutes

Excretion: Urine and feces (small amounts as unchanged drug and metabolites)

Dosage

Usual dosage range:

Infants and Children: I.M., I.V.: 100-200 mg/kg/day in divided doses every 6 hours (maximum: 12 g/day)

Adults: I.M., I.V.: 250-2000 mg every 4-6 hours

Indication-specific dosing:

Children:

Arthritis (septic): I.V.: 37 mg/kg every 6 hours

Epiglottitis: I.V.: 150-200 mg/kg/day divided every 6 hours

Mild-to-moderate infections: I.M., I.V.: 100-150 mg/kg/day in divided doses every 6 hours (maximum: 4 g/day)

Severe infections: I.M., I.V.: 150-200 mg/kg/day in divided doses every 6 hours (maximum: 12 g/day)

Staphylococcal scalded-skin syndrome: I.V.: 150 mg/kg/day divided every 6 hours for 5-7 days

Adults:

Endocarditis: I.V.: 2 g every 4 hours with gentamicin

Mild-to-moderate infections: I.M., I.V.: 250-500 mg every 4-6 hours

Prosthetic joint infection: I.V.: 2 g every 4 hours with rifampin

Severe infections: I.M., I.V.: 1-2 g every 4-6 hours

***Staphylococcus aureus*, methicillin-susceptible infections, including brain abscess, bursitis, erysipelas, mastitis, mastoiditis, osteomyelitis, perinephric abscess, pneumonia, pyomyositis, scalded skin syndrome, toxic shock syndrome:** I.V.: 2 g every 4 hours

Dosing adjustment in renal impairment: Cl_{cr} <10 mL/minute: Clinical practice varies; some clinicians recommend adjustment to the lower range of the usual dosage as based on severity of infection.

Hemodialysis: Not dialyzable (0% to 5%)

Dietary Considerations Sodium content of 1 g: 92.4 mg (4.02 mEq)

Administration Administer around-the-clock to promote less variation in peak and trough serum levels. Administer IVP over 10 minutes. Administer IVPB over 30 minutes.

Monitoring Parameters Observe for signs and symptoms of anaphylaxis during first dose; monitor periodic CBC, urinalysis, BUN, serum creatinine, AST and ALT

Test Interactions May interfere with urinary glucose tests using cupric sulfate (Benedict's solution, Clinitest®); may inactivate aminoglycosides *in vitro*; false-positive urinary and serum proteins

Dosage Forms Excipient information presented when available (limited, particularly for generics); consult specific product labeling.

Infusion [premixed iso-osmotic dextrose solution]: 1 g (50 mL); 2 g (50 mL)

Injection, powder for reconstitution: 1 g, 2 g, 10 g

◆ **Oxacillin Sodium** *see* Oxacillin *on page 1111*

Oxaliplatin (ox AL i pla tin)

U.S. Brand Names Eloxatin®

Canadian Brand Names Eloxatin®

Index Terms Diaminocyclohexane Oxalatoplatinum; L-OHP; NSC-266046

Pharmacologic Category Antineoplastic Agent, Alkylating Agent; Antineoplastic Agent, Platinum Analog

Use Treatment of stage III colon cancer and advanced colorectal cancer

Unlabeled/Investigational Use Treatment of esophageal cancer, gastric cancer, head and neck cancer, non-Hodgkin's lymphoma, ovarian cancer, pancreatic cancer

Pregnancy Risk Factor D

Pregnancy Considerations Decreased fetal weight, decreased ossification, and increased fetal deaths were observed in animal studies at one-tenth the equivalent human dose. There are no adequate and well-controlled studies in pregnant women. Women of childbearing potential should be advised to avoid pregnancy and use effective contraception during treatment.

Canadian labeling: Use in pregnant women is contraindicated in the Canadian labeling. Males should be advised not to father children during and for up to 6 months following therapy. May cause permanent infertility in males. Prior to initiating therapy, advise males desiring to father children, to seek counseling on sperm storage.

Lactation Excretion in breast milk unknown/not recommended

Medication Safety Issues

Sound-alike/look-alike issues:

Oxaliplatin may be confused with Aloxi®, carboplatin

High alert medication: The Institute for Safe Medication Practices (ISMP) includes this medication among its list of drug classes which have a heightened risk of causing significant patient harm when used in error.

Contraindications Hypersensitivity to oxaliplatin, other platinum-containing compounds, or any component of the formulation

Canadian labeling: Additional contraindications (not in U.S. labeling): Pregnancy, breast-feeding; severe renal impairment (Cl_{cr} <30 mL/minute)

Warnings/Precautions Hazardous agent - use appropriate precautions for handling and disposal. **[U.S. Boxed Warning]: Anaphylactic/anaphylactoid reactions may occur within minutes of oxaliplatin administration; symptoms may be managed with epinephrine, corticosteroids, and antihistamines.** Allergic reactions may occur with any cycle and may include bronchospasm (rare), erythema, hypotension (rare), pruritus, rash, and/or urticaria.

Two different types of peripheral sensory neuropathy may occur: First, an acute (within first 2 days), reversible (resolves within 14 days), with primarily peripheral symptoms that are often exacerbated by cold (may include pharyngolaryngeal dysesthesia); may recur with subsequent doses; avoid mucositis prophylaxis with ice chips during oxaliplatin infusion. Secondly, a more persistent (>14 days) presentation that often interferes with daily activities (eg, writing, buttoning, swallowing), these symptoms may improve upon discontinuing treatment.

May cause pulmonary fibrosis; withhold treatment for unexplained pulmonary symptoms (eg, crackles, dyspnea, nonproductive cough, pulmonary infiltrates) until interstitial lung disease or pulmonary fibrosis are excluded. Hepatotoxicity (including hepatic failure and hepatitis) has been observed with use; the presence of hepatic vascular disorders (including veno-occlusive disease) should be considered, especially in individuals developing portal hypertension or who present with increased liver function tests. Use caution with renal dysfunction; increased toxicity may occur. When administered as sequential infusions, taxane derivatives (docetaxel, paclitaxel) should be administered before platinum derivatives (carboplatin, cisplatin, oxaliplatin) to limit myelosuppression and enhance efficacy. Concomitant use with 5-FU may increase risk for adverse hematologic or GI effects. Elderly patients are more sensitive to some adverse events including diarrhea, dehydration, hypokalemia, leukopenia, fatigue and syncope. Safety and efficacy in children have not been established.

Adverse Reactions Percentages reported with monotherapy.

>10%:

Central nervous system: Fatigue (61%), fever (25%), pain (14%), headache (13%), insomnia (11%)

Gastrointestinal: Nausea (64%), diarrhea (46%), vomiting (37%), abdominal pain (31%), constipation (31%), anorexia (20%), stomatitis (14%)

Hematologic: Anemia (64%; grades 3/4: 1%), thrombocytopenia (30%; grades 3/4: 3%), leukopenia (13%)

Hepatic: AST increased (54%; grades 3/4: 4%), ALT increased (36%; grades 3/4: 1%), total bilirubin increased (13%; grades 3/4: 5%)

Neuromuscular & skeletal: Peripheral neuropathy (may be dose limiting; 76%; acute 65%; grades 3/4: 5%; persistent 43%; grades 3/4: 3%), back pain (11%)

Respiratory: Dyspnea (13%), cough (11%)

1% to 10%:

Cardiovascular: Edema (10%), chest pain (5%), peripheral edema (5%), flushing (3%), thromboembolism (2%)

Central nervous system: Dizziness (7%)
Dermatologic: Rash (5%), alopecia (3%), hand-foot syndrome (1%)
Endocrine & metabolic: Dehydration (5%), hypokalemia (3%)
Gastrointestinal: Dyspepsia (7%), taste perversion (5%), flatulence (3%), mucositis (2%), gastroesophageal reflux (1%), dysphagia (acute 1% to 2%)
Genitourinary: Dysuria (1%)
Hematologic: Neutropenia (7%)
Local: Injection site reaction (9%; redness/swelling/pain)
Neuromuscular & skeletal: Rigors (9%), arthralgia (7%)
Ocular: Abnormal lacrimation (1%)
Renal: Serum creatinine increased (5% to 10%)
Respiratory: URI (7%), rhinitis (6%), epistaxis (2%), pharyngitis (2%), pharyngolaryngeal dysesthesia (grades 3/4: 1% to 2%)
Miscellaneous: Allergic reactions (3%); hypersensitivity (includes urticaria, pruritus, facial flushing, shortness of breath, bronchospasm, diaphoresis, hypotension, syncope: grades 3/4: 2% to 3%); hiccup (2%)

<1% (Limited to important or life-threatening; reported with mono- and combination therapy): Acute renal failure, alkaline phosphatase increased, anaphylactic/anaphylactoid reactions, anaphylactic shock, angioedema, aphonia, ataxia, colitis, cranial nerve palsies, deep tendon reflex loss, deafness, diplopia, dysarthria, dysphonia, eosinophilic pneumonia, extravasation (including necrosis), fasciculations, gait abnormal, hemolysis, hemolytic anemia (immuno-allergic), hemolytic uremia syndrome, hepatic failure, hepatitis, hepatotoxicity, hypertension, hypomagnesemia, ileus, INR increased, interstitial lung diseases, interstitial nephritis (acute), intestinal obstruction, Lhermittes' sign, metabolic acidosis, muscle spasm, myoclonus, necrosis (following extravasation), neutropenic fever, optic neuritis, pancreatitis, perisinusoidal fibrosis, prothrombin time increased, ptosis, pulmonary fibrosis, rhabdomyolysis, seizure, thrombocytopenia (immuno-allergic), trigeminal neuralgia, tubular necrosis (acute), veno-occlusive liver disease (sinusoidal obstruction syndrome and perisinusoidal fibrosis), visual acuity decreased, visual field disturbance

Drug Interactions

Avoid Concomitant Use

Avoid concomitant use of Oxaliplatin with any of the following: Natalizumab; Vaccines (Live)

Increased Effect/Toxicity

Oxaliplatin may increase the levels/effects of: Natalizumab; Taxane Derivatives; Topotecan; Vaccines (Live); Vitamin K Antagonists

The levels/effects of Oxaliplatin may be increased by: Trastuzumab

Decreased Effect

Oxaliplatin may decrease the levels/effects of: Cardiac Glycosides; Vaccines (Inactivated); Vitamin K Antagonists

The levels/effects of Oxaliplatin may be decreased by: Echinacea

Stability Store intact vials at room temperature of 25°C (77°F); excursions permitted to 15°C to 30°C (59°F to 86°F); do not freeze. Protect concentrated solution from light (store in original outer carton). According to the manufacturer, solutions diluted for infusion are stable up to 6 hours at room temperature of 20°C to 25°C (68°F to 77°F) or up to 24 hours under refrigeration at 2°C to 8°C (36°F to 46°F). Oxaliplatin solution diluted with D_5W to a final concentration of 0.7 mg/mL (polyolefin container) has been shown to retain >90% of it's original concentration for up to 30 days when stored at room temperature or refrigerated; artificial light did not affect the concentration (Andre, 2007). As this study did not examine sterility, refrigeration would be preferred to limit microbial growth.

Aqueous solution: **Do not prepare using a chloride-containing solution (eg, NaCl).** Dilution with D_5W (250 or 500 mL) is required prior to administration. Infusion solutions do not require protection from light. Use appropriate precautions for handling and disposal.

Lyophilized powder [CAN; not available in U.S.]: **Do not prepare using a chloride-containing solution (eg, NaCl).** Use only water for injection or D_5W to reconstitute powder. To obtain final concentration of 5 mg/mL add 10 mL of diluent to 50 mg vial or 20 mL diluent to 100 mg vial. Gently swirl vial to dissolve powder. Dilution with D_5W (250 or 500 mL) is required prior to administration. Infusion solutions do not require protection from light. Discard unused portion of vial. Use appropriate precautions for handling and disposal.

Mechanism of Action Oxaliplatin, a platinum derivative, is an alkylating agent. Following intracellular hydrolysis, the platinum compound binds to DNA forming cross-links which inhibit DNA replication and transcription, resulting in cell death. Cytotoxicity is cell-cycle nonspecific.

Pharmacodynamics/Kinetics

Distribution: V_d: 440 L
Protein binding: >90% primarily albumin and gamma globulin (irreversible binding to platinum)
Metabolism: Nonenzymatic (rapid and extensive), forms active and inactive derivatives
Half-life elimination: Terminal: 391 hours; Distribution: Alpha phase: 0.4 hours, Beta phase: 16.8 hours
Excretion: Primarily urine (~54%); feces (~2%)

Dosage Details concerning dosing in combination regimens should also be consulted.

Adults: Stage III colon cancer and colorectal cancer: I.V.: 85 mg/m^2 every 2 weeks **or**
Unlabeled doses:
20-25 mg/m^2 days 1-5 every 3 weeks **or**
100-130 mg/m^2 every 2-3 weeks

Elderly: No dosing adjustment recommended

Dosage adjustments for toxicity: Acute toxicities: Longer infusion times may mitigate acute toxicities.
Neurosensory events:
Persistent (>7 days) grade 2 neurosensory events: Consider oxaliplatin dose reduction if symptoms do not resolve:
Stage III colon cancer: Reduce dose to 75 mg/m^2
Advanced colorectal cancer: Reduce dose to 65 mg/m^2
Consider withholding oxaliplatin for grade 2 neuropathy lasting >7 days despite dose reduction.
Persistent grade 3 neurosensory events: Consider discontinuing oxaliplatin
Other toxicities (grade 3/4 gastrointestinal toxicity, grade 4 neutropenia, or grade 3/4 thrombocytopenia): After recovery from toxicity, oxaliplatin dose reductions are recommended:
Stage III colon cancer: Reduce dose to 75 mg/m^2; delay next dose until neutrophils recover to ≥1500/mm^3 and platelets recover to ≥75,000/mm^3
Advanced colorectal cancer: Reduce dose to 65 mg/m^2; delay next dose until neutrophils recover to ≥1500/mm^3 and platelets recover to ≥75,000/mm^3

Dosage adjustment in renal impairment: The FDA-approved labeling does not contain renal dosing adjustment guidelines. Oxaliplatin is primarily eliminated renally; in patients with Cl_{cr} <30 mL/minute, the AUC is increased ~190%. Oxaliplatin use has been studied in 25 patients with renal dysfunction; treatment was well-tolerated in patients with mild-to-moderate impairment (Cl_{cr} 20-59 mL/minute), suggesting that dose reduction is not necessary in this patient population (Takimoto, 2003). Patients with severe renal impairment (Cl_{cr} <20 mL/minute) have not been adequately studied; consider omitting dose or changing chemotherapy regimen if Cl_{cr} <20 mL/minute.

Note: Canadian labeling: Use in patients with Cl_{cr} <30 mL/minute is contraindicated in Canadian labeling.

Dosage adjustment in hepatic impairment: Mild, moderate, or severe hepatic impairment: Dosage adjustment not necessary (Synold, 2007; Doroshow, 2003)

Administration Administer as I.V. infusion over 2-6 hours. Flush infusion line with D_5W prior to administration of any concomitant medication. Patients should receive an antiemetic premedication regimen. Avoid mucositis prophylaxis with ice chips during oxaliplatin infusion.

Monitoring Parameters CBC with differential, serum creatinine, liver function tests (including ALT, AST and bilirubin); INR and prothrombin time (in patients on oral anticoagulant therapy); signs of neuropathy, hypersensitivity, and/or respiratory effects; delay dosage until recovery of neutrophils ≥1.5 x 10^9/L and platelets ≥75 x 10^9/L

Additional Information Cold temperature may exacerbate acute neuropathy. Do not use ice for mucositis prophylaxis.

Dosage Forms Excipient information presented when available (limited, particularly for generics); consult specific product labeling. [CAN] = Canadian availability; not available in U.S.

Injection, solution [preservative free]:
Eloxatin®: 5 mg/mL (10 mL, 20 mL, 40 mL)

Injection, powder for reconstitution [preservative free]:
Eloxatin® [CAN]: 50 mg [contains lactose], 100 mg [contains lactose] [not available in U.S.]

◆ **Oxandrin®** *see* Oxandrolone *on page* 1114

Oxandrolone (oks AN droe lone)

U.S. Brand Names Oxandrin®

Pharmacologic Category Androgen

Use Adjunctive therapy to promote weight gain after weight loss following extensive surgery, chronic infections, or severe trauma, and in some patients who, without definite pathophysiologic reasons, fail to gain or to maintain normal weight; to offset protein catabolism with prolonged corticosteroid administration; relief of bone pain associated with osteoporosis

Restrictions C-III

Pregnancy Risk Factor X

Pregnancy Considerations Masculinization of the fetus has been reported.

Lactation Excretion in breast milk unknown/not recommended

Contraindications Hypersensitivity to oxandrolone or any component of the formulation; nephrosis; carcinoma of breast or prostate; hypercalcemia; pregnancy

Warnings/Precautions [U.S. Boxed Warning]: Anabolic steroids may cause peliosis hepatis or liver cell tumors which may not be apparent until liver failure or intra-abdominal hemorrhage develops. Discontinue in case of cholestatic hepatitis with jaundice or abnormal liver function tests. Use caution with concomitant warfarin therapy; warfarin dose may need significantly decreased. **[U.S. Boxed Warning]: May cause blood lipid changes with increased risk of arteriosclerosis.** Use with caution in elderly patients, they may be at greater risk for prostatic hyperplasia, fluid retention, and transaminase elevations. Use with caution in patients with cardiac, renal, or hepatic disease; COPD; diabetes; or epilepsy. Use with caution in patients with breast cancer; may cause hypercalcemia by stimulating osteolysis. Discontinue with evidence of mild virilization in women. May accelerate bone maturation without producing compensatory gain in linear growth in children; in prepubertal children perform radiographic examination of the hand and wrist every 6 months to determine the rate of bone maturation and to assess the effect of treatment on the epiphyseal centers.

Adverse Reactions Frequency not defined.

Cardiovascular: Edema

Central nervous system: Depression, excitation, insomnia

Dermatologic: Acne (females and prepubertal males)
Also reported in females: Hirsutism, male-pattern baldness

Endocrine & metabolic: Electrolyte imbalances, glucose intolerance, gonadotropin secretion inhibited, gynecomastia, HDL decreased, LDL increased
Also reported in females: Clitoral enlargement, menstrual irregularities

Genitourinary:
Prepubertal males: Increased or persistent erections, penile enlargement
Postpubertal males: Bladder irritation, epididymitis, impotence, oligospermia, priapism (chronic), testicular atrophy, testicular function

Hepatic: Alkaline phosphatase increased, ALT increased, AST increased, bilirubin increased, cholestatic jaundice, hepatic necrosis (rare), hepatocellular neoplasms, peliosis hepatis (with long-term therapy)

Neuromuscular & skeletal: CPK increased, premature closure of epiphyses (in children)

Renal: Creatinine excretion increased

Miscellaneous: Bromsulfophthalein retention, habituation, voice alteration (deepening, in females)

Drug Interactions

Avoid Concomitant Use There are no known interactions where it is recommended to avoid concomitant use.

Increased Effect/Toxicity
Oxandrolone may increase the levels/effects of: CycloSPORINE; Vitamin K Antagonists

Decreased Effect There are no known significant interactions involving a decrease in effect.

Mechanism of Action Synthetic testosterone derivative with similar androgenic and anabolic actions

Pharmacodynamics/Kinetics Half-life elimination: 10-13 hours

Dosage

Children: Total daily dose: ≤0.1 mg/kg **or** ≤0.045 mg/lb

Adults: 2.5-20 mg in divided doses 2-4 times/day based on individual response; a course of therapy of 2-4 weeks is usually adequate. This may be repeated intermittently as needed.

Elderly: 5 mg twice daily

Dosing adjustment in renal impairment: Caution is recommended because of the propensity of oxandrolone to cause edema and water retention

Dosing adjustment in hepatic impairment: Caution is advised but there are not specific guidelines for dosage reduction

Monitoring Parameters Liver function tests, cholesterol profile, hemoglobin/hematocrit; INR/PT in patients on anticoagulant therapy

Children: Radiographs of left wrist every 6 months (to assess bone maturation)

Adult females: Signs of virilization (deepening voice, hirsutism, acne, clitoromegaly); urine and serum calcium in women with breast cancer

Test Interactions May suppress factors II, V, VII, and X; may increase PT; may decrease thyroxine-binding globulin and radioactive iodine uptake

Dosage Forms Excipient information presented when available (limited, particularly for generics); consult specific product labeling.

Tablet: 2.5 mg, 10 mg
Oxandrin®: 2.5 mg, 10 mg

Oxaprozin (oks a PROE zin)

U.S. Brand Names Daypro®

Canadian Brand Names Apo-Oxaprozin®; Daypro®

Pharmacologic Category Nonsteroidal Anti-inflammatory Drug (NSAID), Oral

Additional Appendix Information

Nonsteroidal Anti-inflammatory Agents *on page 1669*

Use Acute and long-term use in the management of signs and symptoms of osteoarthritis and rheumatoid arthritis; juvenile rheumatoid arthritis

Restrictions An FDA-approved medication guide must be distributed when dispensing an oral outpatient prescription (new or refill) where this medication is to be used without direct supervision of a healthcare provider. Medication guides are available at http://www.fda.gov/cder/Offices/ODS/medication_guides.htm.

Pregnancy Risk Factor C/D (3rd trimester)

Pregnancy Considerations Safety and efficacy in pregnant women have not been established. Exposure late in pregnancy may lead to premature closure of the ductus arteriosus and may inhibit uterine contractions.

Lactation Excretion in breast milk unknown/not recommended

Medication Safety Issues

Sound-alike/look-alike issues:

Daypro® may be confused with Diupres®

Oxaprozin may be confused with oxazepam

Contraindications Hypersensitivity to oxaprozin, aspirin, other NSAIDs, or any component of the formulation; perioperative pain in the setting of coronary artery bypass graft (CABG) surgery

Warnings/Precautions **[U.S. Boxed Warning]: NSAIDs are associated with an increased risk of adverse cardiovascular thrombotic events, including MI, stroke, and new onset or worsening of pre-existing hypertension.** Risk may be increased with duration of use or pre-existing cardiovascular risk factors or disease. Carefully evaluate individual cardiovascular risk profiles prior to prescribing. Use caution with fluid retention, heart failure, or hypertension. Concurrent administration of ibuprofen, and potentially other nonselective NSAIDs, may interfere with aspirin's cardioprotective effect. **[U.S. Boxed Warning]: Use is contraindicated for treatment of perioperative pain in the setting of coronary artery bypass graft (CABG) surgery.** Risk of MI and stroke may be increased with use following CABG surgery.

Platelet adhesion and aggregation may be decreased; may prolong bleeding time; patients with coagulation disorders or who are receiving anticoagulants should be monitored closely. Anemia may occur; patients on long-term NSAID therapy should be monitored for anemia. NSAID use may compromise existing renal function; dose-dependent decreases in prostaglandin synthesis may result from NSAID use, reducing renal blood flow which may cause renal decompensation. Patients with impaired renal function, dehydration, heart failure, liver dysfunction, those taking diuretics, and ACE inhibitors, and the elderly are at greater risk of renal toxicity. Rehydrate patient before starting therapy; monitor renal function closely. Not recommended for use in patients with advanced renal disease. Long-term NSAID use may result in renal papillary necrosis.

[U.S. Boxed Warning]: NSAIDs may increase risk of gastrointestinal irritation, inflammation, ulceration, bleeding, and perforation. These events may occur at any time during therapy and without warning. Use caution with a history of GI disease (bleeding or ulcers); concurrent therapy with aspirin, anticoagulants, and/or corticosteroids; smoking; use of alcohol; and the elderly or debilitated patients.

Use the lowest effective dose for the shortest duration of time, consistent with individual patient goals, to reduce risk of cardiovascular or GI adverse events. Alternate therapies should be considered for patients at high risk.

NSAIDs may cause serious skin adverse events including exfoliative dermatitis, Stevens-Johnson syndrome (SJS), and toxic epidermal necrolysis (TEN); discontinue use at first sign of skin rash or hypersensitivity. Anaphylactoid reactions may occur, even without prior exposure; patients with "aspirin triad" (bronchial asthma, aspirin intolerance, rhinitis) may be at increased risk. Do not use in patients who experience bronchospasm, asthma, rhinitis, or urticaria with NSAID or aspirin therapy. Use caution in other forms of asthma.

Use with caution in patients with decreased hepatic function. Closely monitor patients with any abnormal LFT. Severe hepatic reactions (eg, fulminant hepatitis, liver failure) have occurred with NSAID use, rarely; discontinue if signs or symptoms of liver disease develop, or if systemic manifestations occur.

The elderly are at increased risk for adverse effects (especially peptic ulceration, CNS effects, renal toxicity) from NSAIDs even at low doses.

Withhold for at least 4-6 half-lives prior to surgical or dental procedures. May cause mild photosensitivity reactions. Safety and efficacy have not been established in children <6 years of age.

Adverse Reactions

1% to 10%:

Cardiovascular: Edema

Central nervous system: Confusion, depression, dizziness, headache, sedation, sleep disturbance, somnolence

Dermatologic: Pruritus, rash

Gastrointestinal: Abdominal distress, abdominal pain, anorexia, constipation, diarrhea, flatulence, gastrointestinal ulcer, gross bleeding with perforation, heartburn, nausea, vomiting

Hematologic: Anemia, bleeding time increased

Hepatic: Liver enzyme elevation

Otic: Tinnitus

Renal: Dysuria, renal function abnormal, urinary frequency

<1% (Limited to important or life-threatening; effects reported with oxaprozin or other NSAIDs): Acute interstitial nephritis, acute renal failure, agranulocytosis, anaphylaxis, angioedema, asthma, bruising, CHF, erythema multiforme, exfoliative dermatitis, gastritis, gastrointestinal bleeding, hearing decreased, hematemesis, hematuria, hemorrhoidal bleeding, hepatitis, hypersensitivity reaction, hypertension, jaundice, leukopenia, nephrotic syndrome, pancreatitis, peptic ulcer, photosensitivity, rectal bleeding, renal insufficiency, Stevens-Johnson syndrome, toxic epidermal necrolysis, thrombocytopenia

Drug Interactions

Avoid Concomitant Use

Avoid concomitant use of Oxaprozin with any of the following: Ketorolac

Increased Effect/Toxicity

Oxaprozin may increase the levels/effects of: Aminoglycosides; Anticoagulants; Antiplatelet Agents; Bisphosphonate Derivatives; CycloSPORINE; Desmopressin; Lithium; Methotrexate; Nonsteroidal Anti-Inflammatory Agents; Pemetrexed; Quinolone Antibiotics; Salicylates; Thrombolytic Agents; Vancomycin; Vitamin K Antagonists

The levels/effects of Oxaprozin may be increased by: Antidepressants (Tricyclic, Tertiary Amine); Corticosteroids (Systemic); Herbs (Anticoagulant/Antiplatelet Properties); Ketorolac; Probenecid; Selective Serotonin Reuptake Inhibitors; Serotonin/Norepinephrine Reuptake Inhibitors; Treprostinil

Decreased Effect

Oxaprozin may decrease the levels/effects of: ACE Inhibitors; Angiotensin II Receptor Blockers; Antiplatelet Agents; Beta-Blockers; Eplerenone; HydrALAZINE; Loop Diuretics; Salicylates; Thiazide Diuretics

The levels/effects of Oxaprozin may be decreased by: Bile Acid Sequestrants; Salicylates

Ethanol/Nutrition/Herb Interactions

Ethanol: Avoid ethanol (may enhance gastric mucosal irritation).

Herb/Nutraceutical: Avoid alfalfa, anise, bilberry, bladderwrack, bromelain, cat's claw, celery, chamomile, coleus, cordyceps, dong quai, evening primrose, fenugreek, feverfew, garlic, ginger, ginkgo biloba, ginseng (American, Panax, Siberian), grapeseed, green tea, guggul, horse chestnut seed, horseradish, licorice, prickly ash, red clover, reishi, SAMe (S-adenosylmethionine), sweet clover, turmeric, white willow (all have additional antiplatelet activity).

Stability Store at 25°C (77°F). Protect from light; keep bottle tightly closed.

Mechanism of Action Reversibly inhibits cyclooxygenase-1 and 2 (COX-1 and 2) enzymes, which result in decreased formation of prostaglandin precursors; has antipyretic, analgesic, and anti-inflammatory properties

Pharmacodynamics/Kinetics

Absorption: Almost complete

Protein binding: >99%

Metabolism: Hepatic via oxidation and glucuronidation; no active metabolites

Half-life elimination: 40-50 hours

Time to peak: 2-4 hours

Excretion: Urine (5% unchanged, 65% as metabolites); feces (35% as metabolites)

Dosage Oral (individualize dosage to lowest effective dose to minimize adverse effects):

Children 6-16 years: Juvenile rheumatoid arthritis:
- 22-31 kg: 600 mg once daily
- 32-54 kg: 900 mg once daily
- ≥55 kg: 1200 mg once daily

Adults:
- Osteoarthritis: 600-1200 mg once daily; patients should be titrated to lowest dose possible; patients with low body weight should start with 600 mg daily
- Rheumatoid arthritis: 1200 mg once daily; a one-time loading dose of up to 1800 mg/day or 26 mg/kg (whichever is lower) may be given
- Maximum doses:
  - Patient <50 kg: Maximum: 1200 mg/day
  - Patient >50 kg with normal renal/hepatic function and low risk of peptic ulcer: Maximum: 1800 mg or 26 mg/kg (whichever is lower) in divided doses

Dosing adjustment in renal impairment: In general, NSAIDs are not recommended for use in patients with advanced renal disease but the manufacturer of oxaprozin does provide some guidelines for adjustment in renal dysfunction.

Severe renal impairment or on dialysis: 600 mg once daily; may increase cautiously to 1200 mg/day with close monitoring

Dosing adjustment in hepatic impairment: Use caution in patients with severe dysfunction

Monitoring Parameters Monitor CBC; hepatic, renal, and ocular function

Test Interactions False-positive urine immunoassay screening tests for benzodiazepines have been reported and may occur several days after discontinuing oxaprozin.

Dosage Forms Excipient information presented when available (limited, particularly for generics); consult specific product labeling.

Tablet: 600 mg

Oxazepam (oks A ze pam)

U.S. Brand Names Serax®

Canadian Brand Names Apo-Oxazepam®; Bio-Oxazepam; Novoxapram®; Oxpam®; Oxpram®; PMS-Oxazepam; Riva-Oxazepam

Pharmacologic Category Benzodiazepine

Additional Appendix Information

Benzodiazepines *on page 1646*

Use Treatment of anxiety; management of ethanol withdrawal

Unlabeled/Investigational Use Anticonvulsant in management of simple partial seizures; hypnotic

Restrictions C-IV

Pregnancy Risk Factor D

Medication Safety Issues

Sound-alike/look-alike issues:
- Oxazepam may be confused with oxaprozin, quazepam
- Serax® may be confused with Eurax®, Urex®, Zyrtec®

International issues:
- Murelax® [Australia] may be confused with Miralax™ which is a brand name for polyethylene glycol 3350 in the U.S.

Dosage Oral:

Adults:
- Anxiety: 10-30 mg 3-4 times/day
- Ethanol withdrawal: 15-30 mg 3-4 times/day
- Hypnotic: 15-30 mg

Elderly: Oral: Anxiety: 10 mg 2-3 times/day; increase gradually as needed to a total of 30-45 mg/day. Dose titration should be slow to evaluate sensitivity.

Hemodialysis: Not dialyzable (0% to 5%)

Additional Information Complete prescribing information for this medication should be consulted for additional detail.

Dosage Forms Excipient information presented when available (limited, particularly for generics); consult specific product labeling.

Capsule: 10 mg, 15 mg, 30 mg

Tablet: 15 mg [contains tartrazine]

OXcarbazepine (ox car BAZ e peen)

U.S. Brand Names Trileptal®

Canadian Brand Names Trileptal®

Index Terms GP 47680; OCBZ

Pharmacologic Category Anticonvulsant, Miscellaneous

Additional Appendix Information

Anticonvulsant Drugs of Choice *on page 1637*

Use Monotherapy or adjunctive therapy in the treatment of partial seizures in adults and children ≥4 years of age with epilepsy; adjunctive therapy in the treatment of partial seizures in children ≥2 years of age with epilepsy

Unlabeled/Investigational Use Bipolar disorder; treatment of neuropathic pain

Pregnancy Risk Factor C

Pregnancy Considerations Oxcarbazepine crosses the human placenta. Teratogenic effects have been observed in animal studies. There are no adequate and well-controlled studies in pregnant women; however, oxcarbazepine is structurally related to carbamazepine (teratogenic in humans); use during pregnancy only if the benefit to the mother outweighs the potential risk to the fetus. Nonhormonal forms of contraception should be used during therapy.

Lactation Enters breast milk/not recommended

Medication Safety Issues

Sound-alike/look-alike issues:
- OXcarbazepine may be confused with carBAMazepine
- Trileptal® may be confused with TriLipix™

Contraindications Hypersensitivity to oxcarbazepine or any component of the formulation

Warnings/Precautions Clinically-significant hyponatremia (sodium <125 mmol/L) can develop during oxcarbazepine use. Rare cases of anaphylaxis and angioedema have been reported, even after initial dosing; permanently discontinue should symptoms occur. Use caution in patients with previous hypersensitivity to carbamazepine (cross-sensitivity occurs in 25% to 30%). Potentially serious, sometimes fatal, dermatologic reactions (eg, Stevens-Johnson, toxic epidermal necrolysis) and multi-organ hypersensitivity reactions have been reported in adults and children; monitor for signs and symptoms of skin reactions and possible disparate manifestations associated with lymphatic, hepatic, renal, and/or hematologic organ systems; discontinuation and conversion to alternate therapy may be required. As with all antiepileptic drugs, oxcarbazepine should be withdrawn gradually to minimize the potential of increased seizure frequency. Use of oxcarbazepine has been associated with CNS-related adverse events, most significant of these were cognitive symptoms including psychomotor slowing, difficulty with concentration, speech or language problems, somnolence or fatigue, and coordination abnormalities, including ataxia and gait disturbances. Effects with other sedative drugs or ethanol may be potentiated. Single-dose studies show that half-life of the primary active metabolite is prolonged 3-4 fold and AUC is doubled in patients with Cl_{cr} <30 mL/minute; dose adjustment required in these patients. May reduce the efficacy of oral contraceptives (nonhormonal contraceptive measures are recommended). Safety and efficacy in children <2 years of age have not been established.

Adverse Reactions As reported in adults with doses of up to 2400 mg/day (includes patients on monotherapy, adjunctive therapy, and those not previously on AEDs); incidence in children was similar.

>10%:

- Central nervous system: Dizziness (22% to 49%), somnolence (20% to 36%), headache (13% to 32%), ataxia (5% to 31%), fatigue (12% to 15%), vertigo (6% to 15%)
- Gastrointestinal: Vomiting (7% to 36%), nausea (15% to 29%), abdominal pain (10% to 13%)
- Neuromuscular & skeletal: Abnormal gait (5% to 17%), tremor (3% to 16%)
- Ocular: Diplopia (14% to 40%), nystagmus (7% to 26%), abnormal vision (4% to 14%)

1% to 10%:

- Cardiovascular: Hypotension (1% to 2%), leg edema (1% to 2%)
- Central nervous system: Nervousness (2% to 5%), amnesia (4%), abnormal thinking (2% to 4%), insomnia (2% to 4%), speech disorder (1% to 3%), EEG abnormalities (2%), abnormal feelings (1% to 2%), agitation (1% to 2%), confusion (1% to 2%)
- Dermatologic: Rash (4%), acne (1% to 2%)
- Endocrine & metabolic: Hyponatremia (1% to 3%)
- Gastrointestinal: Diarrhea (5% to 7%), dyspepsia (5% to 6%), constipation (2% to 6%), gastritis (1% to 2%), weight gain (1% to 2%)
- Neuromuscular & skeletal: Weakness (3% to 6%), back pain (4%), falling down (4%), abnormal coordination (1% to 4%), dysmetria (1% to 3%), sprains/strains (2%), muscle weakness (1% to 2%)
- Ocular: Abnormal accommodation (2%)
- Respiratory: Upper respiratory tract infection (7%), rhinitis (2% to 5%), chest infection (4%), epistaxis (4%), sinusitis (4%)

Postmarketing and/or case reports (limited to important or life-threatening): Aggressive reaction, amylase increased, anaphylaxis, angioedema, aphasia, asthma, aura, biliary pain, blood in stool, bradycardia, bruising, cardiac failure, cataract, cerebral hemorrhage, chest pain, cholelithiasis, colitis, conjunctival hemorrhage, consciousness decreased, convulsions aggravated, delirium, delusion, duodenal ulcer, dysphagia, dysphonia, dyspnea, dystonia, dysuria, emotional lability, enteritis, erythema multiforme, erythematosus rash, esophagitis, eye edema, extrapyramidal disorder, facial rash, gastric ulcer, GGT increased, gingival bleeding, hematuria, hemianopia, hemiplegia, hematemesis, hot flushes, hyper-/hypoglycemia, hyper-/hypokinesia, hyper-/hyporeflexia, hypersensitivity reaction, hyper-/hypotonia, hypertension, hypocalcemia, hypochondrium pain, hypoesthesia, hypokalemia, hysteria, intermenstrual bleeding, laryngismus, leukopenia, leukorrhea, lipase increased, liver enzymes elevated, maculopapular rash, manic reaction, migraine, menorrhagia, multiorgan hypersensitivity (eosinophilia, arthralgia, rash, fever, lymphadenopathy), muscle contractions (involuntary), mydriasis, neuralgia, oculogyric crisis, otitis externa, palpitation, pancreatitis, panic disorder, paralysis, paroniria, photophobia, photosensitivity reaction, pleurisy, postural hypotension, priapism, purpura, psychosis, ptosis, rectal hemorrhage, renal calculus, renal pain, rigors, scotoma, sialoadenitis, Stevens-Johnson syndrome, stupor, suicidal behavior/ideation, syncope, systemic lupus erythematosus, tachycardia, tetany, thrombocytopenia, toxic epidermal necrolysis, ulcerative stomatitis, urinary tract pain, urticaria, vitiligo, weight loss, xerophthalmia

Drug Interactions

Metabolism/Transport Effects **Inhibits** CYP2C19 (weak); **Induces** CYP3A4 (strong)

Avoid Concomitant Use

Avoid concomitant use of OXcarbazepine with any of the following: Nilotinib; Nisoldipine; Ranolazine

Increased Effect/Toxicity

OXcarbazepine may increase the levels/effects of: Phenytoin

Decreased Effect

OXcarbazepine may decrease the levels/effects of: CYP3A4 Substrates; Maraviroc; Nilotinib; Nisoldipine; Oral Contraceptive (Estrogens); Oral Contraceptive (Progestins); Ranolazine; Sorafenib

The levels/effects of OXcarbazepine may be decreased by: PHENobarbital; Phenytoin; Valproic Acid

Ethanol/Nutrition/Herb Interactions

Ethanol: Avoid ethanol (may increase CNS depression).

Herb/Nutraceutical: St John's wort may decrease oxcarbazepine levels. Avoid evening primrose (seizure threshold decreased). Avoid valerian, St John's wort, kava kava, gotu kola.

Stability Store tablets and suspension at 25°C (77°F). Use suspension within 7 weeks of first opening container.

Mechanism of Action Pharmacological activity results from both oxcarbazepine and its monohydroxy metabolite (MHD). Precise mechanism of anticonvulsant effect has not been defined. Oxcarbazepine and MHD block voltage-sensitive sodium channels, stabilizing hyperexcited neuronal membranes, inhibiting repetitive firing, and decreasing the propagation of synaptic impulses. These actions are believed to prevent the spread of seizures. Oxcarbazepine and MHD also increase potassium conductance and modulate the activity of high-voltage activated calcium channels.

Pharmacodynamics/Kinetics

Absorption: Complete; food has no affect on rate or extent

Distribution: MHD: V_d: 49 L

Protein binding, serum: MHD: 40%

Metabolism: Hepatic to 10-monohydroxy metabolite (MHD; active); MHD is further glucuronidated or oxidized to a 10,11-dihydroxy metabolite (DHD; inactive)

Bioavailability: Decreased in children <8 years; increased in elderly >60 years

Half-life elimination: Parent drug: 2 hours; MHD: 9 hours; renal impairment (Cl_{cr} 30 mL/minute): MHD: 19 hours

Clearance of MHD is increased in younger children (~80% in children 2-4 years of age) and approaches that of adults by ~13 years of age

Time to peak, serum (median): Tablets: 4.5 hours; oral suspension: 6 hours

Excretion: Urine (95%, <1% as unchanged oxcarbazepine, 27% as unchanged MHD, 49% as MHD glucuronides); feces (<4%)

Dosage Oral:

Children 2-3 years:

Adjunctive therapy: 8-10 mg/kg/day, not to exceed 600 mg/day, given in 2 divided daily doses. Maintenance dose should be achieved over 2 weeks, and is dependent upon patient weight.

<20 kg: Consider initiating dose at 16-20 mg/kg/day; maximum maintenance dose should be achieved over 2-4 weeks and should not exceed 60 mg/kg/day

Children 4-16 years:

Adjunctive therapy: 8-10 mg/kg/day, not to exceed 600 mg/day, given in 2 divided daily doses. Maintenance dose should be achieved over 2 weeks, and is dependent upon patient weight, according to the following:

20-29 kg: 900 mg/day in 2 divided doses

29.1-39 kg: 1200 mg/day in 2 divided doses

>39 kg: 1800 mg/day in 2 divided doses

Children 4-16 years:

Conversion to monotherapy: Oxcarbazepine 8-10 mg/kg/day in twice daily divided doses, while simultaneously initiating the reduction of the dose of the concomitant antiepileptic drug; the concomitant drug should be withdrawn over 3-6 weeks. Oxcarbazepine dose may be increased by a maximum of 10 mg/kg/day at weekly intervals. See below for recommended total daily dose by weight.

Initiation of monotherapy: Oxcarbazepine should be initiated at 8-10 mg/kg/day in twice daily divided doses; doses may be titrated by 5 mg/kg/day every third day. See below for recommended total daily dose by weight.

Range of maintenance doses by weight during monotherapy:

20 kg: 600-900 mg/day

25-30 kg: 900-1200 mg/day

35-40 kg: 900-1500 mg/day

45 kg: 1200-1500 mg/day

50-55 kg: 1200-1800 mg/day

60-65 kg: 1200-2100 mg/day

70 kg: 1500-2100 mg/day

Adults:

Adjunctive therapy: Initial: 300 mg twice daily; dose may be increased by as much as 600 mg/day at weekly intervals; recommended daily dose: 1200 mg/day in 2 divided doses. Although daily doses >1200 mg/day were somewhat more efficacious, most patients were unable to tolerate 2400 mg/day (due to CNS effects).

Conversion to monotherapy: Oxcarbazepine 600 mg/day in twice daily divided doses while simultaneously initiating the reduction of the dose of the concomitant antiepileptic drug. The concomitant dosage should be withdrawn over 3-6 weeks, while the maximum dose of oxcarbazepine should be reached in about 2-4 weeks. Recommended daily dose: 2400 mg/day.

Initiation of monotherapy: Oxcarbazepine should be initiated at a dose of 600 mg/day in twice daily divided doses; doses may be titrated upward by 300 mg/day every third day to a final dose of 1200 mg/day given in 2 daily divided doses

Dosing adjustment in renal impairment: Cl_{cr} <30 mL/minute: Therapy should be initiated at one-half the usual starting dose (300 mg/day in adults) and increased slowly to achieve the desired clinical response

Dosing adjustment in hepatic impairment: Adjustment not needed for mild-to-moderate impairment. No data in patients with severe impairment.

Dietary Considerations May be taken with or without food.

Administration Suspension: Prior to using for the first time, firmly insert the plastic adapter provided with the bottle. Cover adapter with child-resistant cap when not in use. Shake bottle for at least 10 seconds, remove child-resistant cap, and insert the oral dosing syringe provided to withdraw appropriate dose. Dose may be taken directly from oral syringe or may be mixed in a small glass of water immediately prior to swallowing. Rinse syringe with warm water after use and allow to dry thoroughly. Discard any unused portion after 7 weeks of first opening bottle.

Monitoring Parameters Seizure frequency, serum sodium (particularly during first 3 months of therapy), symptoms of CNS depression (dizziness, headache, somnolence). Additional serum sodium monitoring recommended during maintenance treatment in patients receiving other medications known to decrease sodium levels, in patients with signs/symptoms of hyponatremia, and in patients with an increase in seizure frequency or severity

Test Interactions Thyroid function tests may depress serum T_4 without affecting T_3 levels or TSH.

Dosage Forms Excipient information presented when available (limited, particularly for generics); consult specific product labeling.

Suspension, oral:

Trileptal®: 300 mg/5 mL (250 mL) [contains ethanol; packaged with oral syringe]

Tablet: 150 mg, 300 mg, 600 mg

Trileptal®: 150 mg, 300 mg, 600 mg

◆ **Oxeze® Turbuhaler® (Can)** *see* Formoterol *on page* 662

Oxiconazole (oks i KON a zole)

U.S. Brand Names Oxistat®

Canadian Brand Names Oxistat®

Index Terms Oxiconazole Nitrate

Pharmacologic Category Antifungal Agent, Topical

Use Treatment of tinea pedis (athlete's foot), tinea cruris (jock itch), tinea corporis (ringworm), and tinea (pityriasis) versicolor

Pregnancy Risk Factor B

Dosage Topical: Children and Adults:

Tinea corporis/tinea cruris: Cream, lotion: Apply to affected areas 1-2 times daily for 2 weeks

Tinea pedis: Cream, lotion: Apply to affected areas 1-2 times daily for 1 month

Tinea versicolor: Cream: Apply to affected areas once daily for 2 weeks

Additional Information Complete prescribing information for this medication should be consulted for additional detail.

Dosage Forms Excipient information presented when available (limited, particularly for generics); consult specific product labeling.

Cream:

Oxistat®: 1% (15 g, 30 g, 60 g) [contains benzoic acid]

Lotion:

Oxistat®: 1% (30 mL) [contains benzoic acid]

◆ **Oxiconazole Nitrate** *see* Oxiconazole *on page* 1118

◆ **Oxilan®** *see* Ioxilan *on page* 811

◆ **Oxilan® 300 (Can)** *see* Ioxilan *on page* 811

◆ **Oxilan® 350 (Can)** *see* Ioxilan *on page* 811

◆ **Oxilapine Succinate** *see* Loxapine *on page* 912

◆ **Oxistat®** *see* Oxiconazole *on page* 1118

◆ **Oxpam® (Can)** *see* Oxazepam *on page* 1116

◆ **Oxpentifylline** *see* Pentoxifylline *on page 1173*
◆ **Oxpram® (Can)** *see* Oxazepam *on page 1116*
◆ **Oxsoralen®** *see* Methoxsalen *on page 968*
◆ **Oxsoralen-Ultra®** *see* Methoxsalen *on page 968*

Oxybutynin (oks i BYOO ti nin)

U.S. Brand Names Ditropan®; Ditropan® XL; Gelnique™; Oxytrol®

Canadian Brand Names Apo-Oxybutynin®; Ditropan®; Ditropan® XL; Gen-Oxybutynin; Novo-Oxybutynin; Nu-Oxybutyn; Oxytrol®; PMS-Oxybutynin; Riva-Oxybutynin; Uromax®

Index Terms Oxybutynin Chloride

Pharmacologic Category Antispasmodic Agent, Urinary

Use Antispasmodic for neurogenic bladder (urgency, frequency, urge incontinence)

Pregnancy Risk Factor B

Pregnancy Considerations Teratogenic effects were not observed in animal studies. There are no adequate and well-controlled studies in pregnant women; use during pregnancy only if clearly needed.

Lactation Excretion in breast milk unknown/use caution

Medication Safety Issues

Sound-alike/look-alike issues:

Oxybutynin may be confused with OxyContin®

Ditropan® may be confused with Detrol®, diazepam, Diprivan®, dithranol

Transdermal patch may contain conducting metal (eg, aluminum); remove patch prior to MRI.

Contraindications Hypersensitivity to oxybutynin or any component of the formulation; untreated glaucoma; urinary retention; gastric retention or conditions with severely decreased GI motility

Warnings/Precautions Use with caution in patients with bladder outflow obstruction, angle-closure glaucoma (treated), hyperthyroidism, reflux esophagitis (including concurrent therapy with oral bisphosphonates or drugs which may increase the risk of esophagitis), heart disease, hepatic or renal disease, prostatic hyperplasia, autonomic neuropathy, ulcerative colitis (may cause ileus and toxic megacolon), hypertension, hiatal hernia, myasthenia gravis, dementia, ulcerative colitis, or intestinal atony. Caution should be used in elderly due to anticholinergic activity (eg, confusion, constipation, blurred vision, and tachycardia). May increase the risk of heat prostration. May cause anticholinergic effects (agitation, confusion, hallucinations, somnolence) which may require dose reduction or discontinuation of therapy. May cause CNS depression, which may impair physical or mental abilities; patients must be cautioned about performing tasks which require mental alertness (eg, operating machinery or driving).

The extended release formulation consists of drug within a nondeformable matrix; following drug release/absorption, the matrix/shell is expelled in the stool. The use of nondeformable products in patients with known stricture/narrowing of the GI tract has been associated with symptoms of obstruction. Transdermal patch may contain conducting metal (eg, aluminum); remove patch prior to MRI.

Adverse Reactions

Oral:

>10%:

Central nervous system: Dizziness (4% to 17%), somnolence (2% to 14%)

Gastrointestinal: Xerostomia (29% to 71%; dose related), constipation (7% to 15%), nausea (2% to 12%)

5% to 10%:

Central nervous system: Headache (6% to 10%), pain (4% to 7%), nervousness (1% to 7%), insomnia (1% to 6%)

Gastrointestinal: Diarrhea (7% to 9%), dyspepsia (6% to 7%)

Genitourinary: Urinary hesitation (9%), urinary tract infection (5% to 7%), urinary retention (6%)

Neuromuscular & skeletal: Weakness (3% to 7%)

Ocular: Blurred vision (1% to 10%), dry eyes (3% to 6%)

Respiratory: Rhinitis (2% to 6%)

1% to <5% (Limited to important or life-threatening): Abdominal pain, agitation, aptyalism, arrhythmia, arthralgia, asthma, back pain, bronchitis, confusion, convulsion, cough, cycloplegia, cystitis, depression, dry skin, dry throat, dysgeusia, dysphagia, dysuria, edema, eructation, extremity pain, eye irritation, fatigue, flank pain, flatulence, fluid retention, flushing, fungal infection, gastrointestinal reflux disease, GI motility decreased, hallucination, hoarseness, hyperglycemia, hyper-/hypotension, impotence, keratoconjunctivitis sicca, loose stools, mydriasis, nasal congestion, nasal dryness, nasopharyngitis, pain, palpitation, pharyngolaryngeal pain, pollakiuria, pruritus, psychotic disorder, rash, sinus congestion, sinus headache, sweating decreased, tachycardia, thirst, tongue coated, upper respiratory tract infection, vomiting

Transdermal:

>10%: Local: Application site reaction (17%), pruritus (14%)

1% to 10%:

Gastrointestinal: Xerostomia (4% to 10%), diarrhea (3%), constipation (3%)

Genitourinary: Dysuria (2%)

Local: Erythema (6% to 8%), vesicles (3%), rash (3%)

Ocular: Vision changes (3%)

Postmarketing and/or case reports: Cardiac arrhythmia, cycloplegia, hallucinations, lactation suppressed, myocarditis, impotence, seizure, sweating decreased, tachycardia

Drug Interactions

Metabolism/Transport Effects Substrate of CYP3A4 (minor); **Inhibits** CYP2C8 (weak), 2D6 (weak), 3A4 (weak)

Avoid Concomitant Use There are no known interactions where it is recommended to avoid concomitant use.

Increased Effect/Toxicity

Oxybutynin may increase the levels/effects of: Anticholinergics; Cannabinoids; Potassium Chloride

The levels/effects of Oxybutynin may be increased by: Pramlintide

Decreased Effect

Oxybutynin may decrease the levels/effects of: Acetylcholinesterase Inhibitors (Central); Secretin

The levels/effects of Oxybutynin may be decreased by: Acetylcholinesterase Inhibitors (Central)

Ethanol/Nutrition/Herb Interactions Ethanol: Use ethanol with caution (may increase CNS depression and toxicity). Watch for sedation.

Stability Store at controlled room temperature. Protect syrup from light. Keep transdermal patch in sealed pouch.

Mechanism of Action Direct antispasmodic effect on smooth muscle, also inhibits the action of acetylcholine on smooth muscle (exhibits 1/5 the anticholinergic activity of atropine, but is 4-10 times the antispasmodic activity); does not block effects at skeletal muscle or at autonomic ganglia; increases bladder capacity, decreases uninhibited contractions, and delays desire to void, therefore, decreases urgency and frequency

Pharmacodynamics/Kinetics

Onset of action: Oral: 30-60 minutes

Peak effect: 3-6 hours

Duration: 6-10 hours (up to 24 hours for extended release oral formulation)
Absorption: Oral: Rapid and well absorbed; Transdermal: High
Distribution: I.V.: V_d: 193 L
Metabolism: Hepatic via CYP3A4; Oral: High first-pass metabolism (not with I.V. or transdermal use); forms active and inactive metabolites
Bioavailability: Oral: ~6%
Half-life elimination: I.V.: ~2 hours (parent drug), 7-8 hours (metabolites)
Time to peak, serum: Oral: ~60 minutes; Transdermal: 24-48 hours
Excretion: Urine, as metabolites and unchanged drug (<0.1%)

Dosage
Oral:
Children:
1-5 years (unlabeled use): 0.2 mg/kg/dose 2-4 times/day
>5 years: 5 mg twice daily, up to 5 mg 3 times/day maximum
>6 years: Extended release: 5 mg once daily; adjust dose in 5 mg increments; maximum dose: 20 mg/day
Adults: 5 mg 2-3 times/day up to 5 mg 4 times/day maximum
Extended release: Initial: 5-10 mg once daily, adjust dose in 5 mg increments at weekly intervals; maximum: 30 mg daily
Elderly: Regular release: Initial dose: 2.5 mg 2-3 times/day; increase as needed to 5 mg 2-3 times/day
Transdermal: Adults: Apply one 3.9 mg/day patch twice weekly (every 3-4 days)

Note: Should be discontinued periodically to determine whether the patient can manage without the drug and to minimize resistance to the drug

Dietary Considerations Food causes a slight delay in the absorption of the oral solution and bioavailability is increased by ~25%. Absorption of the extended release tablet is not affected by food.

Administration
Oral: Immediate release tablets and solution should be administered on an empty stomach with water. Extended release tablets may be taken with or without food and must be swallowed whole; do not crush, divide, or chew.
Transdermal: Apply to clean, dry skin on abdomen, hip, or buttock. Select a new site for each new system (avoid reapplication to same site within 7 days).

Monitoring Parameters Incontinence episodes, postvoid residual (PVR)

Test Interactions May suppress the wheal and flare reactions to skin test antigens.

Product Availability
Gelnique™: FDA approved January 2009; anticipated availability in second quarter 2009
Gelnique™ is a topical gel for the treatment of overactive bladder.

Dosage Forms Excipient information presented when available (limited, particularly for generics); consult specific product labeling.
Syrup, as chloride: 5 mg/5 mL (473 mL)
Ditropan®: 5 mg/5 mL (473 mL)
Tablet, as chloride: 5 mg
Ditropan®: 5 mg
Tablet, extended release, as chloride: 5 mg, 10 mg, 15 mg
Ditropan® XL: 5 mg, 10 mg, 15 mg
Transdermal system:
Oxytrol®: 3.9 mg/day (8s) [39 cm^2; total oxybutynin 36 mg]

◆ **Oxybutynin Chloride** *see* Oxybutynin *on page 1119*

◆ **Oxycocet® (Can)** *see* Oxycodone and Acetaminophen *on page 1122*

◆ **Oxycodan® (Can)** *see* Oxycodone and Aspirin *on page 1123*

OxyCODONE (oks i KOE done)

U.S. Brand Names ETH-Oxydose™; OxyContin®; Oxy-Fast®; OxyIR®; Roxicodone®

Canadian Brand Names Oxy.IR®; OxyContin®; PMS-Oxycodone; Supeudol®

Index Terms Dihydrohydroxycodeinone; Oxycodone Hydrochloride

Pharmacologic Category Analgesic, Opioid

Additional Appendix Information
Narcotic / Opioid Analgesics *on page 1663*

Use Management of moderate-to-severe pain, normally used in combination with nonopioid analgesics

OxyContin® is indicated for around-the-clock management of moderate-to-severe pain when an analgesic is needed for an extended period of time.

Restrictions C-II

Pregnancy Risk Factor B/D (prolonged use or high doses at term)

Pregnancy Considerations Should be used in pregnancy only if clearly needed. Use of narcotics during pregnancy may produce physical dependence in the neonate; respiratory depression may occur in the newborn if narcotics are used prior to delivery (especially high doses).

Lactation Enters breast milk/use caution

Medication Safety Issues
Sound-alike/look-alike issues:
OxyCODONE may be confused with HYDROcodone, OxyContin®, oxymorphone
OxyContin® may be confused with MS Contin®, oxybutynin
OxyFast® may be confused with Roxanol™
Roxicodone® may be confused with Roxanol™

High alert medication: The Institute for Safe Medication Practices (ISMP) includes this medication among its list of drug classes which have a heightened risk of causing significant patient harm when used in error.

Contraindications Hypersensitivity to oxycodone or any component of the formulation; significant respiratory depression; hypercarbia; acute or severe bronchial asthma; OxyContin® is also contraindicated in paralytic ileus (known or suspected); pregnancy (prolonged use or high doses at term)

Warnings/Precautions May cause CNS depression, which may impair physical or mental abilities; patients must be cautioned about performing tasks which require mental alertness (eg, operating machinery or driving). Effects may be potentiated when used with other sedative drugs or ethanol. Use with caution in patients with hypersensitivity reactions to other phenanthrene derivative opioid agonists (morphine, hydrocodone, hydromorphone, levorphanol, oxymorphone), respiratory diseases including asthma, emphysema, or COPD. Use with caution in pancreatitis or biliary tract disease, acute alcoholism (including delirium tremens), morbid obesity, adrenocortical insufficiency, history of seizure disorders, CNS depression/coma, kyphoscoliosis (or other skeletal disorder which may alter respiratory function), hypothyroidism (including myxedema), prostatic hyperplasia, urethral stricture, and toxic psychosis. May obscure diagnosis or clinical course of patients with acute abdominal conditions.

Use with caution in the elderly, debilitated, severe hepatic or renal function. Hemodynamic effects (hypotension, orthostasis) may be exaggerated in patients with hypovolemia, concurrent vasodilating drugs, or in patients with head injury. Respiratory depressant effects and capacity to elevate CSF pressure may be exaggerated in presence of head injury, other intracranial lesion, or pre-existing intracranial pressure.

Use the oral concentrate formulation with caution in patients with latex sensitivity; dropper dispenser contains dry, natural rubber. Concurrent use of agonist/antagonist analgesics may precipitate withdrawal symptoms and/or reduced analgesic efficacy in patients following prolonged therapy with mu opioid agonists. Abrupt discontinuation following prolonged use may also lead to withdrawal symptoms.

[U.S. Boxed Warning]: Healthcare provider should be alert to problems of abuse, misuse, and diversion. Tolerance or drug dependence may result from extended use.

Controlled-release formulations:

[U.S. Boxed Warning]: OxyContin® is not intended for use as an "as needed" analgesic or for immediately-postoperative pain management (should be used postoperatively only if the patient has received it prior to surgery or if severe, persistent pain is anticipated). **[U.S. Boxed Warning]: Do NOT crush, break, or chew controlled-release tablets;** 60 mg, 80 mg, and 160 mg strengths are for use only in opioid-tolerant patients.

Adverse Reactions

>10%:

Central nervous system: Somnolence (23% to 24%), dizziness (13% to 16%)

Dermatologic: Pruritus (12% to 13%)

Gastrointestinal: Nausea (23% to 27%), constipation (23% to 26%), vomiting (12% to 14%)

1% to 10%:

Cardiovascular: Postural hypotension (1% to 5%)

Central nervous system: Headache (7% to 8%), abnormal dreams (1% to 5%), anxiety (1% to 5%), chills (1% to 5%), confusion (1% to 5%), euphoria (1% to 5%), fever (1% to 5%), insomnia (1% to 5%), nervousness (1% to 5%), thought abnormalities (1% to 5%)

Dermatologic: Rash (1% to 5%)

Gastrointestinal: Xerostomia (6% to 7%), abdominal pain (1% to 5%), anorexia (1% to 5%), diarrhea (1% to 5%), dyspepsia (1% to 5%), gastritis (1% to 5%)

Neuromuscular & skeletal: Weakness (6% to 7%), twitching (1% to 5%)

Respiratory: Dyspnea (1% to 5%), hiccups (1% to 5%)

Miscellaneous: Diaphoresis (5% to 6%)

<1% (Limited to important or life-threatening): Agitation, amenorrhea, amnesia, anaphylaxis, anaphylactoid reaction, appetite increased, chest pain, cough, dehydration, depression, dysphagia, dysuria, edema, emotional lability, eructation, exfoliative dermatitis, facial edema, hallucinations, hematuria, histamine release, hyperkinesia, hypoesthesia, hyponatremia, hypotonia, ileus, impotence, intracranial pressure increased, libido decreased, malaise, migraine, paradoxical CNS stimulation, paralytic ileus, paresthesia, pharyngitis, physical dependence, polyuria, psychological dependence, seizure, SIADH, speech disorder, ST segment depression, stomatitis, stupor, syncope, tablet in stool (OxyCodone®), taste perversion, thirst, tinnitus, tremor, urinary retention, urticaria, vasodilation, vertigo, vision change, voice alteration, withdrawal syndrome

Drug Interactions

Metabolism/Transport Effects Substrate (minor) of CYP2D6, 3A

Avoid Concomitant Use There are no known interactions where it is recommended to avoid concomitant use.

Increased Effect/Toxicity

OxyCODONE may increase the levels/effects of: Alcohol (Ethyl); Alvimopan; CNS Depressants; Desmopressin; Selective Serotonin Reuptake Inhibitors

The levels/effects of OxyCODONE may be increased by: Amphetamines; Antipsychotic Agents (Phenothiazines); Succinylcholine

Decreased Effect

OxyCODONE may decrease the levels/effects of: Pegvisomant

The levels/effects of OxyCODONE may be decreased by: Ammonium Chloride

Ethanol/Nutrition/Herb Interactions

Ethanol: Avoid ethanol (may increase CNS depression).

Food: When taken with a high-fat meal, peak concentration is 25% greater following a single OxyContin® 160 mg tablet as compared to two 80 mg tablets.

Herb/Nutraceutical: Avoid valerian, St John's wort, kava kava, gotu kola (may increase CNS depression).

Stability Store at 15°C to 30°C (59°F to 86°F). Protect from light.

Mechanism of Action Binds to opiate receptors in the CNS, causing inhibition of ascending pain pathways, altering the perception of and response to pain; produces generalized CNS depression

Pharmacodynamics/Kinetics

Onset of action: Pain relief: 10-15 minutes

Peak effect: 0.5-1 hour

Duration: Immediate release: 3-6 hours; Controlled release: ≤12 hours

Distribution: V_d: 2.6 L/kg; distributed to skeletal muscle, liver, intestinal tract, lungs, spleen, brain, and breast milk

Protein binding: ~45%

Metabolism: Hepatically via CYP3A4 to noroxycodone (has weak analgesic), noroxymorphone, and alpha- and beta-noroxycodol. CYP2D6 mediated metabolism produces oxymorphone (has analgesic activity; low plasma concentrations), alpha- and beta-oxymorphol.

Bioavailability: Controlled release, immediate release: 60% to 87%

Half-life elimination: Immediate release: 2-3 hours; controlled release: ~5 hours

Excretion: Urine (~19% as parent; >64% as metabolites)

Dosage Oral:

Children: Immediate release:

6-12 years: 1.25 mg every 6 hours as needed

>12 years: 2.5 mg every 6 hours as needed

Adults:

Immediate release: 5 mg every 6 hours as needed

Controlled release:

Opioid naive: 10 mg every 12 hours

Concurrent CNS depressants: Reduce usual dose by $^1/_3$ to $^1/_2$

Conversion from transdermal fentanyl: For each 25 mcg/hour transdermal dose, substitute 10 mg controlled release oxycodone every 12 hours; should be initiated 18 hours after the removal of the transdermal fentanyl patch

Currently on opioids: Use standard conversion chart to convert daily dose to oxycodone equivalent. Divide daily dose in 2 (for twice-daily dosing, usually every 12 hours) and round down to nearest dosage form.

Note: 60 mg, 80 mg, or 160 mg tablets are for use **only** in opioid-tolerant patients. Special safety considerations must be addressed when converting to OxyContin® doses ≥160 mg every 12 hours. Dietary caution must be taken when patients are initially titrated to 160 mg tablets. Using different strengths to obtain the same daily dose is equivalent (eg, four 40 mg tablets, two 80 mg tablets, one 160 mg tablet); all produce similar blood levels.

Multiplication factors for converting the daily dose of current oral opioid to the daily dose of oral oxycodone:

Current opioid mg/day dose x factor = Oxycodone mg/day dose

Codeine mg/day oral dose **x** 0.15 = Oxycodone mg/day dose

Hydrocodone mg/day oral dose **x** 0.9 = Oxycodone mg/day dose

Hydromorphone mg/day oral dose **x** 4 = Oxycodone mg/day dose

Levorphanol mg/day oral dose **x** 7.5 = Oxycodone mg/day dose

Meperidine mg/day oral dose **x** 0.1 = Oxycodone mg/day dose

Methadone mg/day oral dose **x** 1.5 = Oxycodone mg/day dose

Morphine mg/day oral dose **x** 0.5 = Oxycodone mg/day dose

Note: Divide the oxycodone mg/day dose into the appropriate dosing interval for the specific form being used.

Dosing adjustment in hepatic impairment: Reduce dosage in patients with severe liver disease

Dietary Considerations Instruct patient to avoid high-fat meals when taking OxyContin® 160 mg tablets.

Administration Do not crush, break, or chew controlled-release tablets; 60 mg, 80 mg, and 160 mg tablets are for use **only** in opioid-tolerant patients. Do not administer OxyContin® 160 mg tablet with a high-fat meal. Controlled release tablets are not indicated for rectal administration; increased risk of adverse events due to better rectal absorption.

Monitoring Parameters Pain relief, respiratory and mental status, blood pressure

Reference Range Blood level of 5 mg/L associated with fatality

Test Interactions Some quinolones may produce a false-positive urine screening result for opiates using commercially-available immunoassay kits. This has been demonstrated most consistently for levofloxacin and ofloxacin, but other quinolones have shown cross-reactivity in certain assay kits. Confirmation of positive opiate screens by more specific methods should be considered.

Additional Information Prophylactic use of a laxative should be considered. OxyContin® 60 mg, 80 mg, and 160 mg tablets are for use in opioid-tolerant patients only.

Dosage Forms Excipient information presented when available (limited, particularly for generics); consult specific product labeling.

Capsule, immediate release, as hydrochloride: 5 mg

OxyIR®: 5 mg

Liquid, oral, as hydrochloride [concentrate]:

Roxicodone®: 20 mg/mL (30 mL) [contains sodium benzoate]

Solution, oral, as hydrochloride: 5 mg/5 mL (500 mL)

Roxicodone®: 5 mg/5 mL (5 mL, 500 mL) [contains ethanol]

Solution, oral, as hydrochloride [concentrate]: 20 mg/mL (30 mL)

ETH-Oxydose™: 20 mg/mL (1 mL, 30 mL) [contains sodium benzoate; berry flavor]

OxyFast®: 20 mg/mL (30 mL) [contains natural rubber/natural latex in packaging and sodium benzoate]

Tablet, as hydrochloride: 5 mg, 10 mg, 15 mg, 20 mg, 30 mg

Roxicodone®: 5 mg, 15 mg, 30 mg

Tablet, controlled release, as hydrochloride:

OxyContin®: 10 mg, 15 mg, 20 mg, 30 mg, 40 mg, 60 mg, 80 mg, 160 mg

Tablet, extended release, as hydrochloride: 10 mg, 20 mg, 40 mg, 80 mg [DSC]

Oxycodone and Acetaminophen

(oks i KOE done & a seet a MIN oh fen)

U.S. Brand Names Endocet®; Magnacet™; Percocet®; Primalev™; Roxicet™; Roxicet™ 5/500; Tylox®

Canadian Brand Names Endocet®; Oxycocet®; Percocet®; Percocet®-Demi; PMS-Oxycodone-Acetaminophen

Index Terms Acetaminophen and Oxycodone

Pharmacologic Category Analgesic, Opioid

Use Management of moderate-to-severe pain

Restrictions C-II

Pregnancy Risk Factor C/D (prolonged periods or high doses at term)

Medication Safety Issues

Sound-alike/look-alike issues:

Endocet® may be confused with Indocid®

Percocet® may be confused with Fioricet®, Percodan®

Roxicet™ may be confused with Roxanol™

Tylox® may be confused with Trimox®, Tylenol®, Wymox®, Xanax®

High alert medication: The Institute for Safe Medication Practices (ISMP) includes this medication among its list of drug classes which have a heightened risk of causing significant patient harm when used in error.

Duplicate therapy issues: This product contains acetaminophen, which may be a component of other combination products. Do not exceed the maximum recommended daily dose of acetaminophen.

Dosage Oral: Doses should be given every 4-6 hours as needed and titrated to appropriate analgesic effects. **Note:** Initial dose is based on the **oxycodone** content; however, the maximum daily dose is based on the **acetaminophen** content.

Children: Maximum acetaminophen dose: Children <45 kg: 90 mg/kg/day; children >45 kg: 4 g/day

Mild-to-moderate pain: Initial dose, **based on oxycodone content:** 0.05-0.1 mg/kg/dose

Severe pain: Initial dose, **based on oxycodone content:** 0.3 mg/kg/dose

Adults:

Mild-to-moderate pain: Initial dose, **based on oxycodone content:** 2.5-5 mg

Severe pain: Initial dose, **based on oxycodone content:** 10-30 mg. Do not exceed acetaminophen 4 g/day.

Elderly: Doses should be titrated to appropriate analgesic effects: Initial dose, **based on oxycodone content:** 2.5-5 mg every 6 hours. Do not exceed acetaminophen 4 g/day.

Dosage adjustment in hepatic impairment: Dose should be reduced in patients with severe liver disease.

Additional Information Complete prescribing information for this medication should be consulted for additional detail.

Dosage Forms Excipient information presented when available (limited, particularly for generics); consult specific product labeling.

Caplet:

Roxicet™ 5/500: Oxycodone hydrochloride 5 mg and acetaminophen 500 mg

Capsule: 5/500: Oxycodone hydrochloride 5 mg and acetaminophen 500 mg

Tylox®: 5/500: Oxycodone hydrochloride 5 mg and acetaminophen 500 mg [contains sodium benzoate and sodium metabisulfite]

Solution, oral:

Roxicet™: Oxycodone hydrochloride 5 mg and acetaminophen 325 mg per 5 mL (5 mL, 500 mL) [contains alcohol <0.5%]

Tablet: 2.5/325: Oxycodone hydrochloride 2.5 mg and acetaminophen 325 mg; 5/325: Oxycodone hydrochloride 5 mg and acetaminophen 325 mg; 7.5/325: Oxycodone hydrochloride 7.5 mg and acetaminophen

325 mg; 7.5/500: Oxycodone hydrochloride 7.5 mg and acetaminophen 500 mg; 10/325: Oxycodone hydrochloride 10 mg and acetaminophen 325 mg; 10/650: Oxycodone hydrochloride 10 mg and acetaminophen 650 mg

Endocet® 5/325 [scored]: Oxycodone hydrochloride 5 mg and acetaminophen 325 mg

Endocet® 7.5/325: Oxycodone hydrochloride 7.5 mg and acetaminophen 325 mg

Endocet® 7.5/500: Oxycodone hydrochloride 7.5 mg and acetaminophen 500 mg

Endocet® 10/325: Oxycodone hydrochloride 10 mg and acetaminophen 325 mg

Endocet® 10/650: Oxycodone hydrochloride 10 mg and acetaminophen 650 mg

Magnacet™ 2.5/400: Oxycodone hydrochloride 2.5 mg and acetaminophen 400 mg

Magnacet™ 5/400: Oxycodone hydrochloride 5 mg and acetaminophen 400 mg

Magnacet™ 7.5/400: Oxycodone hydrochloride 7.5 mg and acetaminophen 400 mg

Magnacet™ 10/400: Oxycodone hydrochloride 10 mg and acetaminophen 400 mg

Percocet® 2.5/325: Oxycodone hydrochloride 2.5 mg and acetaminophen 325 mg

Percocet® 5/325 [scored]: Oxycodone hydrochloride 5 mg and acetaminophen 325 mg

Percocet® 7.5/325: Oxycodone hydrochloride 7.5 mg and acetaminophen 325 mg

Percocet® 7.5/500: Oxycodone hydrochloride 7.5 mg and acetaminophen 500 mg

Percocet® 10/325: Oxycodone hydrochloride 10 mg and acetaminophen 325 mg

Percocet® 10/650: Oxycodone hydrochloride 10 mg and acetaminophen 650 mg

Primalev™ 2.5/300: Oxycodone hydrochloride 2.5 mg and acetaminophen 300 mg

Primalev™ 5/300: Oxycodone hydrochloride 5 mg and acetaminophen 300 mg

Primalev™ 7.5/300: Oxycodone hydrochloride 7.5 mg and acetaminophen 300 mg

Primalev™ 10/300: Oxycodone hydrochloride 10 mg and acetaminophen 300 mg

Roxicet™ [scored]: Oxycodone hydrochloride 5 mg and acetaminophen 325 mg

Oxycodone and Aspirin (oks i KOE done & AS pir in)

U.S. Brand Names Endodan®; Percodan®

Canadian Brand Names Endodan®; Oxycodan®; Percodan®

Index Terms Aspirin and Oxycodone

Pharmacologic Category Analgesic, Opioid

Use Management of moderate-to-severe pain

Restrictions C-II

Pregnancy Risk Factor D

Medication Safety Issues

Sound-alike/look-alike issues:

Percodan® may be confused with Decadron®, Percocet®, Percogesic®, Periactin®

High alert medication: The Institute for Safe Medication Practices (ISMP) includes this medication among its list of drug classes which have a heightened risk of causing significant patient harm when used in error.

Dosage Oral (based on oxycodone combined salts):

Children: Maximum oxycodone: 5 mg/dose; maximum aspirin dose should not exceed 4 g/day. Doses should be given every 6 hours as needed.

Mild-to-moderate pain: Initial dose, **based on oxycodone content:** 0.05-0.1 mg/kg/dose

Severe pain: Initial dose, **based on oxycodone content**: 0.3 mg/kg/dose

Adults: Percodan®: 1 tablet every 6 hours as needed for pain; maximum aspirin dose should not exceed 4 g/day.

Dosing adjustment in hepatic impairment: Dose should be reduced in patients with severe liver disease.

Additional Information Complete prescribing information for this medication should be consulted for additional detail.

Dosage Forms Excipient information presented when available (limited, particularly for generics); consult specific product labeling.

Tablet: Oxycodone hydrochloride 4.5 mg, oxycodone terephthalate 0.38 mg, and aspirin 325 mg

Endodan®, Percodan®: Oxycodone hydrochloride 4.8355 mg and aspirin 325 mg

Oxycodone and Ibuprofen

(oks i KOE done & eye byoo PROE fen)

U.S. Brand Names Combunox™

Index Terms Ibuprofen and Oxycodone

Pharmacologic Category Analgesic, Opioid; Nonsteroidal Anti-inflammatory Drug (NSAID), Oral

Use Short-term (≤7 days) management of acute, moderate-to-severe pain

Restrictions C-II

A medication guide should be dispensed with each prescription for oral administration. A template for the required MedGuide can be found on the FDA website at http://www.fda.gov/cder/drug/infopage/COX2/NSAIDmedguide.htm

Pregnancy Risk Factor C/D (3rd trimester)

Medication Safety Issues

High alert medication: The Institute for Safe Medication Practices (ISMP) includes this medication among its list of drug classes which have a heightened risk of causing significant patient harm when used in error.

Dosage Oral: Adults: Pain: Take 1 tablet every 6 hours as needed (maximum: 4 tablets/24 hours); do not take for longer than 7 days

Additional Information Complete prescribing information for this medication should be consulted for additional detail.

Dosage Forms Excipient information presented when available (limited, particularly for generics); consult specific product labeling.

Tablet: Oxycodone 5 mg and ibuprofen 400 mg

Combunox™: 5/400: Oxycodone 5 mg and ibuprofen 400 mg

◆ **Oxycodone Hydrochloride** *see* OxyCODONE *on page 1120*

◆ **OxyContin®** *see* OxyCODONE *on page 1120*

◆ **OxyFast®** *see* OxyCODONE *on page 1120*

◆ **OxyIR®** *see* OxyCODONE *on page 1120*

◆ **Oxy.IR® (Can)** *see* OxyCODONE *on page 1120*

Oxymetholone (oks i METH oh lone)

U.S. Brand Names Anadrol®-50

Pharmacologic Category Anabolic Steroid

Use Treatment of anemias caused by deficient red cell production

Restrictions C-III

Pregnancy Risk Factor X

Medication Safety Issues

Sound-alike/look-alike issues:

Oxymetholone may be confused with oxymetazoline, oxymorphone

Dosage Children and Adults: Erythropoietic effects: Oral: 1-5 mg/kg/day in one daily dose; usual effective dose: 1-2 mg/kg/day; give for a minimum trial of 3-6 months because response may be delayed

Dosing adjustment in hepatic impairment:

Mild-to-moderate hepatic impairment: Oxymetholone should be used with caution in patients with liver dysfunction because of its hepatotoxic potential

Severe hepatic impairment: Oxymetholone should **not** be used

Additional Information Complete prescribing information for this medication should be consulted for additional detail.

Dosage Forms Excipient information presented when available (limited, particularly for generics); consult specific product labeling.

Tablet:

Anadrol®-50: 50 mg

Oxymorphone (oks i MOR fone)

U.S. Brand Names Opana®; Opana® ER

Index Terms Oxymorphone Hydrochloride

Pharmacologic Category Analgesic, Opioid

Additional Appendix Information

Narcotic / Opioid Analgesics *on page 1663*

Use

Parenteral: Management of moderate-to-severe pain and preoperatively as a sedative and/or supplement to anesthesia

Oral, regular release: Management of moderate-to-severe pain

Oral, extended release: Management of moderate-to-severe pain in patients requiring around-the-clock opioid treatment for an extended period of time

Restrictions C-II

Pregnancy Risk Factor C/D (prolonged use or high doses at term)

Pregnancy Considerations Teratogenic effects were not observed in animal studies, however, decreased fetal weight, decreased litter size, increased stillbirths, and increased neonatal death were noted. Chronic opioid use during pregnancy may lead to a withdrawal syndrome in the neonate. Symptoms include irritability, hyperactivity, loss of sleep pattern, abnormal crying, tremor, vomiting, diarrhea, weight loss, or failure to gain weight. Opioid analgesics are considered pregnancy risk factor D if used for prolonged periods or in larger doses near term.

Lactation Excretion in breast milk unknown/use caution

Medication Safety Issues

Sound-alike/look-alike issues:

Oxymorphone may be confused with oxycodone, oxymetholone

High alert medication: The Institute for Safe Medication Practices (ISMP) includes this medication among its list of drug classes which have a heightened risk of causing significant patient harm when used in error.

Contraindications Hypersensitivity to oxymorphone, other morphine analogs (phenanthrene derivatives), or any component of the formulation; paralytic ileus (known or suspected); increased intracranial pressure; moderate-to-severe hepatic impairment; severe respiratory depression (unless in monitored setting with resuscitative equipment); acute/severe bronchial asthma; hypercarbia; pregnancy (prolonged use or high doses at term).

Note: Injection formulation is also contraindicated in the treatment of upper airway obstruction and pulmonary edema due to a chemical respiratory irritant.

Warnings/Precautions An opioid-containing analgesic regimen should be tailored to each patient's needs and based upon the type of pain being treated (acute versus chronic), the route of administration, degree of tolerance for opioids (naive versus chronic user), age, weight, and medical condition. The optimal analgesic dose varies widely among patients. Doses should be titrated to pain relief/prevention.

May cause CNS depression, which may impair physical or mental abilities; patients must be cautioned about performing tasks which require mental alertness (eg, operating machinery or driving). Effects may be potentiated when used with other sedative drugs or ethanol. Use with caution in patients with hypersensitivity reactions to other phenanthrene-derivative opioid agonists (codeine, hydrocodone, hydromorphone, levorphanol, oxycodone). May cause respiratory depression. Use extreme caution in patients with COPD or other chronic respiratory conditions characterized by hypoxia, hypercapnia, or diminished respiratory reserve (myxedema, cor pulmonale, kyphoscoliosis, obstructive sleep apnea, severe obesity). Use with caution in patients (particularly elderly or debilitated) with impaired respiratory function, adrenal disease, morbid obesity, thyroid dysfunction, prostatic hyperplasia, or renal impairment. Use caution in mild hepatic dysfunction; use is contraindicated in moderate-to-severe hepatic impairment. Use only with extreme caution (if at all) in patients with head injury or increased intracranial pressure (ICP); potential to elevate ICP and/or blunt papillary response may be greatly exaggerated in these patients. Use with caution in biliary tract disease or acute pancreatitis (may cause constriction of sphincter of Oddi). May obscure diagnosis or clinical course of patients with acute abdominal conditions.

Oxymorphone shares the toxic potential of opiate agonists and usual precautions of opiate agonist therapy should be observed; may cause hypotension in patients with acute myocardial infarction, volume depletion, or concurrent drug therapy which may exaggerate vasodilation. The elderly may be particularly susceptible to adverse effects of narcotics. Safety and efficacy have not been established in children <18 years of age.

[U.S. Boxed Warning]: Healthcare provider should be alert to problems of abuse, misuse, and diversion. Tolerance or drug dependence may result from extended use. Use caution in patients with a history of drug dependence or abuse. Abrupt discontinuation may precipitate withdrawal syndrome.

Extended release formulation:

[U.S. Boxed Warnings]: Opana® ER is an extended release oral formulation of oxymorphone and is not suitable for use as an "as needed" analgesic. Tablets should not be broken, chewed, dissolved, or crushed; tablets should be swallowed whole. Opana® ER is intended for use in long-term, continuous management of moderate to severe chronic pain. It is not indicated for use in the immediate postoperative period (12-24 hours). **[U.S. Boxed Warning]: The coingestion of ethanol or ethanol-containing medications with Opana® ER may result in accelerated release of drug from the dosage form, abruptly increasing plasma levels, which may have fatal consequences.**

Adverse Reactions Frequency not defined.

Cardiovascular: Bradycardia, cardiac shock, flushing, hypotension, orthostatic hypotension, palpitation, peripheral vasodilation, shock, tachycardia

Central nervous system: Agitation, amnesia, anorexia, anxiety, CNS depression, coma, confusion, convulsion, dizziness, drowsiness, dysphoria, euphoria, fatigue, fever, hallucinations, headache, insomnia, intracranial pressure increased, malaise, mental depression, mental impairment, nervousness, restlessness, paradoxical CNS stimulation

Dermatologic: Pruritus, urticaria, rash

Endocrine & metabolic: Antidiuretic hormone release, weight loss

Gastrointestinal: Abdominal pain, appetite depression, biliary tract spasm, constipation, dehydration, dry mouth, dyspepsia, flatulence, nausea, paralytic ileus, stomach cramps, vomiting, xerostomia

Genitourinary: Urination decreased, urinary retention, urinary tract spasm

Local: Pain/reaction at injection site

Neuromuscular & skeletal: Weakness

Ocular: Blurred vision, diplopia, miosis

Renal: Oliguria

Respiratory: Apnea, bronchospasm, cyanosis, dyspnea, hypoventilation, laryngeal edema, laryngeal spasm, respiratory depression

Miscellaneous: Diaphoresis, histamine release, physical and psychological dependence

Drug Interactions

Avoid Concomitant Use There are no known interactions where it is recommended to avoid concomitant use.

Increased Effect/Toxicity

Oxymorphone may increase the levels/effects of: Alcohol (Ethyl); Alvimopan; CNS Depressants; Desmopressin; Selective Serotonin Reuptake Inhibitors

The levels/effects of Oxymorphone may be increased by: Amphetamines; Antipsychotic Agents (Phenothiazines); Succinylcholine

Decreased Effect

Oxymorphone may decrease the levels/effects of: Pegvisomant

The levels/effects of Oxymorphone may be decreased by: Ammonium Chloride

Ethanol/Nutrition/Herb Interactions

Ethanol: Avoid ethanol (may increase CNS depression). Ethanol ingestion with extended-release tablets is specifically contraindicated due to possible accelerated release and potentially fatal overdose.

Food: When taken orally with a high-fat meal, peak concentration is 38% to 50% greater. Both immediate-release and extended-release tablets should be taken 1 hour before or 2 hours after eating.

Herb/Nutraceutical: Avoid valerian, St John's wort, kava kava, gotu kola (may increase CNS depression).

Stability Injection solution, tablet: Store at 15°C to 30°C (59°F to 86°F).

Mechanism of Action Oxymorphone hydrochloride (Numorphan®) is a potent narcotic analgesic with uses similar to those of morphine. The drug is a semisynthetic derivative of morphine (phenanthrene derivative) and is closely related to hydromorphone chemically (Dilaudid®).

Pharmacodynamics/Kinetics

Onset of action: Parenteral: 5-10 minutes

Duration: Analgesic: Parenteral: 3-6 hours

Distribution: V_d: I.V.: 1.94-4.22 L/kg

Protein binding: 10% to 12%

Metabolism: Hepatic via glucuronidation to active and inactive metabolites

Bioavailability: Oral: 10%

Half-life elimination: Oral: Immediate release: 7-9 hours; Extended release: 9-11 hours

Excretion: Urine (<1% as unchanged drug); feces

Dosage Adults: **Note:** Dosage must be individualized.

I.M., SubQ: Initial: 1-1.5 mg; may repeat every 4-6 hours as needed

Labor analgesia: I.M.: 0.5-1 mg

I.V.: Initial: 0.5 mg

Oral:

Immediate release:

Opioid-naive: 10-20 mg every 4-6 hours as needed. Initial dosages as low as 5 mg may be considered in selected patients and/or patients with renal impairment. Dosage adjustment should be based on level of analgesia, side effects, and pain intensity. Initiation of therapy with initial dose >20 mg is **not** recommended.

Currently on stable dose of parenteral oxymorphone: ~10 times the daily parenteral requirement. The calculated amount should be divided and given in 4-6 equal doses.

Currently on other opioids: Use standard conversion chart to convert daily dose to oxymorphone equivalent. Generally start with 1/2 the calculated daily oxymorphone dosage and administered in divided doses every 4-6 hours.

Extended release (Opana® ER):

Opioid-naive: Initial: 5 mg every 12 hours. Supplemental doses of immediate-release oxymorphone may be used as "rescue" medication as dosage is titrated.

Note: Continued requirement for supplemental dosing may be used to titrate the dose of extended-release continuous therapy. Adjust therapy incrementally, by 5-10 mg every 12 hours at intervals of every 3-7 days. Ideally, basal dosage may be titrated to generally mild pain or no pain with the regular use of fewer than 2 supplemental doses per 24 hours.

Currently on stable dose of parenteral oxymorphone: Approximately 10 times the daily parenteral requirement. The calculated amount should be given in 2 divided doses (every 12 hours).

Currently on opioids: Use conversion chart (see Note below) to convert daily dose to oxymorphone equivalent. Generally start with 1/2 the calculated daily oxymorphone dosage. Divide daily dose in 2 (for every 12-hour dosing) and round down to nearest dosage form. **Note:** Per manufacturer, the following approximate oral dosages are equivalent to oxymorphone 10 mg:

Hydrocodone 20 mg

Oxycodone 20 mg

Methadone 20 mg

Morphine 30 mg

Conversion of stable dose of immediate-release oxymorphone to extended-release oxymorphone: Administer 1/2 of the daily dose of immediate-release oxymorphone (Opana®) as the extended-release formulation (Opana® ER) every 12 hours

Elderly: Initiate dosing at the lower end of the dosage range

Dosing adjustment in renal impairment: Cl_{cr} <50 mL/minute: Reduce initial dosage of oral formulations (bioavailability increased 57% to 65%). Begin therapy at lowest dose and titrate carefully.

Dosing adjustment in hepatic impairment: Generally, contraindicated for use in patients with moderate-to-severe liver disease. Initiate with lowest possible dose and titrate slowly in mild impairment.

Dietary Considerations Immediate release and extended release tablets should be taken 1 hour before or 2 hours after eating.

Administration Administer immediate release and extended release tablets 1 hour before or 2 hours after eating. Opana® ER tablet should be swallowed; do not break, crush, or chew.

Monitoring Parameters Respiratory rate, heart rate, blood pressure, CNS activity

Test Interactions Some quinolones may produce a false-positive urine screening result for opiates using commercially-available immunoassay kits. This has been demonstrated most consistently for levofloxacin and ofloxacin, but other quinolones have shown cross-reactivity in certain assay kits. Confirmation of positive opiate screens by more specific methods should be considered. May cause elevation in amylase (due to constriction of the sphincter of Oddi).

Dosage Forms Excipient information presented when available (limited, particularly for generics); consult specific product labeling.

Injection, solution, as hydrochloride:

Opana®: 1 mg/mL (1 mL)

Tablet, as hydrochloride:

Opana®: 5 mg, 10 mg

Tablet, extended release, as hydrochloride:

Opana®: ER: 5 mg, 7.5 mg, 10 mg, 15 mg, 20 mg, 30 mg, 40 mg

◆ **Oxymorphone Hydrochloride** *see* Oxymorphone *on page 1124*

Oxytocin (oks i TOE sin)

U.S. Brand Names Pitocin®

Canadian Brand Names Pitocin®; Syntocinon®

Index Terms Pit

Pharmacologic Category Oxytocic Agent

Use Induction of labor at term; control of postpartum bleeding; adjunctive therapy in management of abortion

Pregnancy Risk Factor X

Pregnancy Considerations [U.S. Boxed Warning]: To be used for medical rather than elective induction of labor. Reproduction studies have not been conducted. When used as indicated, teratogenic effects would not be expected. Nonteratogenic adverse reactions are reported in the neonate as well as the mother.

Lactation Excretion in breast milk unknown/use caution

Medication Safety Issues

Sound-alike/look-alike issues:

Pitocin® may be confused with Pitressin®

High alert medication: The Institute for Safe Medication Practices (ISMP) includes this medication among its list of drugs which have a heightened risk of causing significant patient harm when used in error.

Contraindications Hypersensitivity to oxytocin or any component of the formulation; significant cephalopelvic disproportion; unfavorable fetal positions; fetal distress; hypertonic or hyperactive uterus; contraindicated vaginal delivery (invasive cervical cancer, active genital herpes, prolapse of the cord, cord presentation, total placenta previa, or vasa previa)

Warnings/Precautions [U.S. Boxed Warning]: To be used for medical rather than elective induction of labor. May produce antidiuretic effect (ie, water intoxication and excess uterine contractions). High doses or hypersensitivity to oxytocin may cause uterine hypertonicity, spasm, tetanic contraction, or rupture of the uterus. Severe water intoxication with convulsions, coma, and death is associated with a slow oxytocin infusion over 24 hours.

Adverse Reactions Frequency not defined.

Fetus or neonate:

Cardiovascular: Arrhythmias (including premature ventricular contractions), bradycardia

Central nervous system: Brain or CNS damage (permanent), neonatal seizure

Hepatic: Neonatal jaundice

Ocular: Neonatal retinal hemorrhage

Miscellaneous: Fetal death, low Apgar score (5 minute)

Mother:

Cardiovascular: Arrhythmias, hypertensive episodes, premature ventricular contractions

Gastrointestinal: Nausea, vomiting

Genitourinary: Pelvic hematoma, postpartum hemorrhage, uterine hypertonicity, tetanic contraction of the uterus, uterine rupture, uterine spasm

Hematologic: Afibrinogenemia (fatal)

Miscellaneous: Anaphylactic reaction, subarachnoid hemorrhage

Drug Interactions

Avoid Concomitant Use There are no known interactions where it is recommended to avoid concomitant use.

Increased Effect/Toxicity

The levels/effects of Oxytocin may be increased by: Dinoprostone; Misoprostol

Decreased Effect There are no known significant interactions involving a decrease in effect.

Stability Store oxytocin at 2°C to 8°C (36°F to 46°F); do not freeze. Pitocin® may also be stored at 15°C to 25°C (59°F to 77°F) for up to 30 days. Reconstitution: I.V.:

Induction or stimulation of labor: Add oxytocin 10 units to NS or LR 1000 mL to yield a solution containing oxytocin 10 milliunits/mL. Rotate solution to mix.

Postpartum uterine bleeding: Add oxytocin 10-40 units to running I.V. infusion; maximum: 40 units/1000 mL.

Adjunctive management of abortion: Add oxytocin 10 units to 500 mL of a physiologic saline solution or D_5W.

Mechanism of Action Produces the rhythmic uterine contractions characteristic to delivery

Pharmacodynamics/Kinetics

Onset of action: Uterine contractions: I.M.: 3-5 minutes; I.V.: ~1 minute

Duration: I.M.: 2-3 hour; I.V.: 1 hour

Metabolism: Rapidly hepatic and via plasma (by oxytocinase) and to a smaller degree the mammary gland

Half-life elimination: 1-5 minutes

Excretion: Urine

Dosage I.V. administration requires the use of an infusion pump. Adults:

Induction of labor: I.V.: 0.5-1 milliunits/minute; gradually increase dose in increments of 1-2 milliunits/minute until desired contraction pattern is established; dose may be decreased after desired frequency of contractions is reached and labor has progressed to 5-6 cm dilation. Infusion rates of 6 milliunits/minute provide oxytocin levels similar to those at spontaneous labor; rates >9-10 milliunits/minute are rarely required.

Postpartum bleeding:

I.M.: Total dose of 10 units after delivery

I.V.: 10-40 units by I.V. infusion in 1000 mL of intravenous fluid at a rate sufficient to control uterine atony

Adjunctive treatment of abortion: I.V.: 10-20 milliunits/minute; maximum total dose: 30 units/12 hours

Administration I.V.: Refer to Stability (reconstitution) for dilution information; an infusion pump is required for administration

Monitoring Parameters Fluid intake and output during administration; fetal monitoring

Dosage Forms Excipient information presented when available (limited, particularly for generics); consult specific product labeling.

Injection, solution: 10 units/mL (1 mL, 10 mL, 30 mL)

Pitocin®: 10 units/mL (1 mL, 10 mL)

◆ **Oxytrol®** *see* Oxybutynin *on page 1119*

◆ **Oysco D [OTC]** *see* Calcium and Vitamin D *on page 238*

◆ **Oysco 500 [OTC]** *see* Calcium Carbonate *on page 238*

◆ **Oysco 500+D [OTC]** *see* Calcium and Vitamin D *on page 238*

◆ **Oyst-Cal-D [OTC]** *see* Calcium and Vitamin D *on page 238*

◆ **Oyst-Cal 500 [OTC]** *see* Calcium Carbonate *on page 238*

◆ **Oyst-Cal-D 500 [OTC]** *see* Calcium and Vitamin D *on page 238*

◆ **P-V Tussin Tablet [DSC]** *see* Hydrocodone and Pseudoephedrine *on page 742*

◆ **P-071** *see* Cetirizine *on page 295*

◆ **Pacerone®** *see* Amiodarone *on page 87*

◆ **Pacis™ (Can)** *see* BCG Vaccine *on page 176*

Paclitaxel (pac li TAKS el)

U.S. Brand Names Onxol® ; Taxol®

Canadian Brand Names Abraxane® For Injectable Suspension; Apo-Paclitaxel®; Taxol®

Index Terms NSC-125973; NSC-673089

Pharmacologic Category Antineoplastic Agent, Antimicrotubular; Antineoplastic Agent, Natural Source (Plant) Derivative; Antineoplastic Agent, Taxane Derivative

Use Treatment of breast, nonsmall cell lung, and ovarian cancers; treatment of AIDS-related Kaposi's sarcoma (KS)

Unlabeled/Investigational Use Treatment of bladder, cervical, prostate, small cell lung, and head and neck cancers; treatment of (unknown primary) adenocarcinoma

Pregnancy Risk Factor D

Pregnancy Considerations Animal studies have demonstrated embryotoxicity, fetal toxicity, and maternal toxicity. There are no adequate and well-controlled studies in pregnant women. Women of childbearing potential should be advised to avoid becoming pregnant.

Lactation Excretion in breast milk unknown/contraindicated

Medication Safety Issues

Sound-alike/look-alike issues:

Paclitaxel may be confused with paroxetine, Paxil®

Paclitaxel (conventional) may be confused with paclitaxel (protein-bound)

Taxol® may be confused with Abraxane®, Paxil®, Taxotere®

High alert medication: The Institute for Safe Medication Practices (ISMP) includes this medication among its list of drugs which have a heightened risk of causing significant patient harm when used in error.

Contraindications Hypersensitivity to paclitaxel, Cremophor® EL (polyoxyethylated castor oil), or any component of the formulation

Warnings/Precautions Hazardous agent - use appropriate precautions for handling and disposal. **[U.S. Boxed Warning]: Severe hypersensitivity reactions have been reported;** premedication may minimize this effect. Stop infusion and do not rechallenge for severe hypersensitivity reactions (hypotension requiring treatment, dyspnea requiring bronchodilators, angioedema, urticaria). Minor hypersensitivity reactions (flushing, skin reactions, dyspnea, hypotension, or tachycardia) do not require interruption of treatment. **[U.S. Boxed Warning]: Bone marrow suppression is the dose-limiting toxicity; do not administer if baseline absolute neutrophil count (ANC) is <1500 cells/mm^3 (<1000 cells/mm^3 for patients with AIDS-related KS);** reduce future doses by 20% for severe neutropenia (<500 cells/mm^3 for 7 days or more) and consider the use of supportive therapy, including growth factor treatment.

Use extreme caution with hepatic dysfunction (myelotoxicity may be worsened); dose reductions are recommended. Peripheral neuropathy may occur; patients with pre-existing neuropathies from chemotherapy or coexisting conditions (eg, diabetes mellitus) may be at a higher risk; reduce dose by 20% for severe neuropathy. Paclitaxel formulations contain dehydrated alcohol; may cause adverse CNS effects. Infusion-related hypotension, bradycardia, and/or hypertension may occur; frequent monitoring of vital signs is recommended, especially during the first hour of the infusion. Rare but severe conduction abnormalities have been reported; conduct cardiac monitoring during subsequent infusions for these patients. When administered as sequential infusions, taxane derivatives (docetaxel, paclitaxel) should be administered before platinum derivatives (carboplatin, cisplatin) to limit myelosuppression. Elderly patients have an increased risk of toxicity (neutropenia, neuropathy). **[U.S. Boxed Warning]: Should be administered under the supervision of an experienced cancer chemotherapy physician.** Safety and efficacy in children have not been established.

Adverse Reactions Percentages reported with single-agent therapy. **Note:** Myelosuppression is dose related, schedule related, and infusion-rate dependent (increased incidences with higher doses, more frequent doses, and longer infusion times) and, in general, rapidly reversible upon discontinuation.

>10%:

Cardiovascular: Flushing (28%), ECG abnormal (14% to 23%), edema (21%), hypotension (4% to 12%)

Dermatologic: Alopecia (87%), rash (12%)

Gastrointestinal: Nausea/vomiting (52%), diarrhea (38%), mucositis (17% to 35%; grades 3/4: up to 3%), stomatitis (15%; most common at doses >390 mg/m^2), abdominal pain (with intraperitoneal paclitaxel)

Hematologic: Neutropenia (78% to 98%; grade 4: 14% to 75%; onset 8-10 days, median nadir 11 days, recovery 15-21 days), leukopenia (90%; grade 4: 17%), anemia (47% to 90%; grades 3/4: 2% to 16%), thrombocytopenia (4% to 20%; grades 3/4: 1% to 7%), bleeding (14%)

Hepatic: Alkaline phosphatase increased (22%), AST increased (19%)

Local: Injection site reaction (erythema, tenderness, skin discoloration, swelling: 13%)

Neuromuscular & skeletal: Peripheral neuropathy (42% to 70%; grades 3/4: up to 7%), arthralgia/myalgia (60%), weakness (17%)

Renal: Creatinine increased (observed in KS patients only: 18% to 34%; severe: 5% to 7%)

Miscellaneous: Hypersensitivity reaction (31% to 45%; grades 3/4: up to 2%), infection (15% to 30%)

1% to 10%:

Cardiovascular: Bradycardia (3%), tachycardia (2%), hypertension (1%), rhythm abnormalities (1%), syncope (1%), venous thrombosis (1%)

Dermatologic: Nail changes (2%)

Hematologic: Febrile neutropenia (2%)

Hepatic: Bilirubin increased (7%)

Respiratory: Dyspnea (2%)

<1% (Limited to important or life-threatening): Anaphylaxis, ataxia, atrial fibrillation, AV block, back pain, cardiac conduction abnormalities, cellulitis, CHF, chills, conjunctivitis, dehydration, enterocolitis, extravasation recall, hepatic encephalopathy, hepatic necrosis, induration, intestinal obstruction, intestinal perforation, interstitial pneumonia, ischemic colitis, lacrimation increased, maculopapular rash, malaise, MI, necrotic changes and ulceration following extravasation, neuroencephalopathy, neutropenic enterocolitis, ototoxicity (tinnitus and hearing loss), pancreatitis, paralytic ileus, phlebitis, pruritus, pulmonary embolism, pulmonary fibrosis, radiation recall, radiation pneumonitis, pruritus, renal insufficiency, seizure, skin exfoliation, skin fibrosis, skin necrosis, Stevens-Johnson syndrome, supraventricular tachycardia, toxic epidermal necrolysis, ventricular tachycardia (asymptomatic), visual disturbances (scintillating scotomata)

Drug Interactions

Metabolism/Transport Effects Substrate (major) of CYP2C8, 3A4; **Induces** CYP3A4 (weak)

Avoid Concomitant Use

Avoid concomitant use of Paclitaxel with any of the following: Natalizumab; Vaccines (Live)

Increased Effect/Toxicity

Paclitaxel may increase the levels/effects of: Antineoplastic Agents (Anthracycline); DOXOrubicin; Natalizumab; Trastuzumab; Vaccines (Live); Vinorelbine

The levels/effects of Paclitaxel may be increased by: CYP2C8 Inhibitors (Moderate); CYP2C8 Inhibitors (Strong); CYP2C9 Inhibitors (Moderate); CYP2C9

Inhibitors (Strong); CYP3A4 Inhibitors (Moderate); CYP3A4 Inhibitors (Strong); Dasatinib; P-Glycoprotein Inhibitors; Platinum Derivatives; Trastuzumab

Decreased Effect

Paclitaxel may decrease the levels/effects of: Maraviroc; Vaccines (Inactivated)

The levels/effects of Paclitaxel may be decreased by: CYP2C8 Inducers (Highly Effective); CYP2C9 Inducers (Highly Effective); CYP3A4 Inducers (Strong); Deferasirox; Echinacea; Herbs (CYP3A4 Inducers); P-Glycoprotein Inducers; Trastuzumab

Ethanol/Nutrition/Herb Interactions Herb/Nutraceutical: Avoid black cohosh, dong quai in estrogen-dependent tumors. Avoid valerian, St John's wort (may decrease paclitaxel levels), kava kava, gotu kola (may increase CNS depression).

Stability Store intact vials at room temperature of 20°C to 25°C (68°F to 77°F) and protect from light. Dilute in 250-1000 mL D_5W, D_5LR, D_5NS, or NS to a concentration of 0.3-1.2 mg/mL. Solutions in D_5W and NS are stable for up to 3 days at room temperature (25°C). Chemotherapy dispensing devices (eg, Chemo Dispensing Pin™) should not be used to withdraw paclitaxel from the vial.

Paclitaxel should be dispensed in either glass or non-PVC containers (eg, Excel™/PAB™). Use **nonpolyvinyl** (non-PVC) tubing (eg, polyethylene) to minimize leaching. Formulated in a vehicle known as Cremophor® EL (polyoxyethylated castor oil). Cremophor® EL has been found to leach the plasticizer DEHP from polyvinyl chloride infusion bags or administration sets. Contact of the undiluted concentrate with plasticized polyvinyl chloride (PVC) equipment or devices is not recommended.

Mechanism of Action Paclitaxel promotes microtubule assembly by enhancing the action of tubulin dimers, stabilizing existing microtubules, and inhibiting their disassembly, interfering with the late G_2 mitotic phase, and inhibiting cell replication. In addition, the drug can distort mitotic spindles, resulting in the breakage of chromosomes. Paclitaxel may also suppress cell proliferation and modulate immune response.

Pharmacodynamics/Kinetics

Distribution:

V_d: Widely distributed into body fluids and tissues; affected by dose and duration of infusion

V_{dss}:

1- to 6-hour infusion: 67.1 L/m^2

24-hour infusion: 227-688 L/m^2

Protein binding: 89% to 98%

Metabolism: Hepatic via CYP2C8 and 3A4; forms metabolites (primarily 6α-hydroxypaclitaxel)

Half-life elimination:

1- to 6-hour infusion: Mean (beta): 6.4 hours

3-hour infusion: Mean (terminal): 13.1-20.2 hours

24-hour infusion: Mean (terminal): 15.7-52.7 hours

Excretion: Feces (~70%, 5% as unchanged drug); urine (14%)

Clearance: Mean: Total body: After 1- and 6-hour infusions: 5.8-16.3 L/hour/m^2; After 24-hour infusions: 14.2-17.2 L/hour/m^2

Dosage Premedication with dexamethasone (20 mg orally or I.V. at 12 and 6 hours **or** 14 and 7 hours before the dose; reduce dexamethasone dose to 10 mg orally with advanced HIV disease), diphenhydramine (50 mg I.V. 30-60 minutes prior to the dose), and cimetidine, famotidine, or ranitidine (I.V. 30-60 minutes prior to the dose) is recommended.

Adults: I.V.: Refer to individual protocols

Ovarian carcinoma: 135-175 mg/m^2 over 3 hours every 3 weeks **or**

135 mg/m^2 over 24 hours every 3 weeks **or**

50-80 mg/m^2 over 1-3 hours weekly **or**

1.4-4 mg/m^2/day continuous infusion for 14 days every 4 weeks

Metastatic breast cancer: 175-250 mg/m^2 over 3 hours every 3 weeks **or**

50-80 mg/m^2 weekly **or**

1.4-4 mg/m^2/day continuous infusion for 14 days every 4 weeks

Nonsmall cell lung carcinoma: 135 mg/m^2 over 24 hours every 3 weeks

AIDS-related Kaposi's sarcoma: 135 mg/m^2 over 3 hours every 3 weeks **or**

100 mg/m^2 over 3 hours every 2 weeks

Intraperitoneal (unlabeled route): Ovarian carcinoma: 60 mg/m^2 on day 8 of a 21-day treatment cycle for 6 cycles, in combination with I.V. paclitaxel and intraperitoneal cisplatin. **Note:** Administration of intraperitoneal paclitaxel should include the standard paclitaxel premedication regimen.

Dosage modification for toxicity (solid tumors, including ovary, breast, and lung carcinoma): Courses of paclitaxel should not be repeated until the neutrophil count is ≥1500 cells/mm^3 and the platelet count is ≥100,000 cells/mm^3; reduce dosage by 20% for patients experiencing severe peripheral neuropathy or severe neutropenia (neutrophil <500 cells/mm^3 for a week or longer)

Dosage modification for immunosuppression in advanced HIV disease: Paclitaxel should not be given to patients with HIV if the baseline or subsequent neutrophil count is <1000 cells/mm^3. Additional modifications include: Reduce dosage of dexamethasone in premedication to 10 mg orally; reduce dosage by 20% in patients experiencing severe peripheral neuropathy or severe neutropenia (neutrophil <500 cells/mm^3 for a week or longer); initiate concurrent hematopoietic growth factor (G-CSF) as clinically indicated

Dosage adjustment in renal impairment: There are no FDA-approved labeling guidelines for dosage adjustment in patients with renal impairment. Arnoff (2007) recommends no dosage adjustment necessary for adults with Cr_{cl} <50 mL/minute.

Dosage adjustment in hepatic impairment: Note: The FDA-approved labeling recommendations are based upon the patient's first course of therapy where the usual dose would be 135 mg/m^2 dose over 24 hours or the 175 mg/m^2 dose over 3 hours in patients with normal hepatic function. Dosage in subsequent courses should be based upon individual tolerance. Adjustments for other regimens are not available.

24-hour infusion:

Transaminases <2 times upper limit of normal (ULN) and bilirubin level ≤1.5 mg/dL: 135 mg/m^2

Transaminases 2-<10 times ULN and bilirubin level ≤1.5 mg/dL: 100 mg/m^2

Transaminases <10 times ULN and bilirubin level 1.6-7.5 mg/dL: 50 mg/m^2

Transaminases ≥10 times ULN **or** bilirubin level >7.5 mg/dL: Avoid use

3-hour infusion:

Transaminases <10 times ULN and bilirubin level ≤1.25 times ULN: 175 mg/m^2

Transaminases <10 times ULN and bilirubin level 1.26-2 times ULN: 135 mg/m^2

Transaminases <10 times ULN and bilirubin level 2.01-5 times ULN: 90 mg/m^2

Transaminases ≥10 times ULN **or** bilirubin level >5 times ULN: Avoid use

Administration

I.V.: Infuse over 1-96 hours. When administered as sequential infusions, taxane derivatives should be administered before platinum derivatives (cisplatin, carboplatin) to limit myelosuppression and to enhance efficacy.

Premedication with dexamethasone (20 mg orally or I.V. at 12 and 6 hours **or** 14 and 7 hours before the dose; reduce to 10 mg with advanced HIV disease), diphenhydramine (50 mg I.V. 30-60 minutes prior to the dose), and cimetidine 300 mg, famotidine 20 mg, or ranitidine 50 mg (I.V. 30-60 minutes prior to the dose) is recommended.

Administer I.V. infusion over 1-24 hours; infuse through a 0.22 micron in-line filter and nonsorbing administration set.

Intraperitoneal: 1-2 hour infusion

Monitoring Parameters CBC with differential; monitor for hypersensitivity reactions, vital signs (frequently during the first hour of infusion), continuous cardiac monitoring (patients with conduction abnormalities)

Reference Range Mean maximum serum concentrations: 435-802 ng/mL following 24-hour infusions of 200-275 mg/m^2 and were approximately 10% to 30% of those following 6-hour infusions of equivalent doses

Additional Information Sensory neuropathy is almost universal at doses >250 mg/m^2; motor neuropathy is uncommon at doses <250 mg/m^2. Myopathic effects are common with doses >200 mg/m^2, generally occur within 2-3 days of treatment, and resolve over 5-6 days. Intraperitoneal administration of paclitaxel is associated with a higher incidence of chemotherapy related toxicity.

Dosage Forms Excipient information presented when available (limited, particularly for generics); consult specific product labeling.

Injection, solution: 6 mg/mL (5 mL, 16.7 mL, 25 mL, 50 mL) [contains ethanol and purified Cremophor® EL (polyoxyethylated castor oil)]

Onxol® : 6 mg/mL (5 mL, 25 mL, 50 mL) [contains ethanol and purified Cremophor® EL (polyoxyethylated castor oil)]

Taxol®: 6 mg/mL (5 mL [DSC], 16.7 mL, 50 mL) [contains ethanol and purified Cremophor® EL (polyoxyethylated castor oil)]

Paclitaxel (Protein Bound)

(pac li TAKS el PROE teen bownd)

U.S. Brand Names Abraxane®

Index Terms ABI-007; Albumin-Bound Paclitaxel; nab-Paclitaxel; NSC-736631; Protein-Bound Paclitaxel

Pharmacologic Category Antineoplastic Agent, Antimicrotubular; Antineoplastic Agent, Natural Source (Plant) Derivative; Antineoplastic Agent, Taxane Derivative

Use Treatment of relapsed or refractory breast cancer

Pregnancy Risk Factor D

Medication Safety Issues

Sound-alike/look-alike issues:

Paclitaxel (protein bound) may be confused with paclitaxel (conventional)

Abraxane® may be confused with Paxil®, Taxol®, Taxotere®

High alert medication: The Institute for Safe Medication Practices (ISMP) includes this medication among its list of drug classes which have a heightened risk of causing significant patient harm when used in error.

Dosage I.V.: Adults: Breast cancer: 260 mg/m^2 every 3 weeks **or** alternate weekly schedule (unlabeled): 100-150 mg/m^2 on days 1, 8, and 15 of a 28-day cycle

Dosage adjustment for toxicity:

Severe neutropenia (<500 cells/mm^3) ≥1 week: Reduce dose to 220 mg/m^2 for subsequent courses

Recurrent severe neutropenia: Reduce dose to 180 mg/m^2

Sensory neuropathy, grade 3: Hold treatment until resolved to grade 1 or 2, then resume with reduced dose

Severe sensory neuropathy: Reduce dose to 220 mg/m^2 for subsequent courses

Recurrent severe sensory neuropathy: Reduce dose to 180 mg/m^2

Dosage adjustment in renal impairment: Safety not established for serum creatinine >2 mg/dL; use with caution

Dosage adjustment in hepatic impairment: Effects of hepatic dysfunction (serum bilirubin >1.5 mg/dL) unknown; dosage adjustment recommendations are not available

Additional Information Complete prescribing information for this medication should be consulted for additional detail.

Dosage Forms Excipient information presented when available (limited, particularly for generics); consult specific product labeling.

Injection, powder for reconstitution:

Abraxane®: 100 mg [contains albumin (human)]

◆ **Paddock Nystatin™** *see* Nystatin *on page 1087*

◆ **Pain Eze [OTC]** *see* Acetaminophen *on page 25*

◆ **Pain-Off [OTC]** *see* Acetaminophen, Aspirin, and Caffeine *on page 31*

◆ **Palafer® (Can)** *see* Ferrous Fumarate *on page 616*

◆ **Palcaps [DSC]** *see* Pancrelipase *on page 1136*

◆ **Palgic®** *see* Carbinoxamine *on page 257*

◆ **Palgic®-D [DSC]** *see* Carbinoxamine and Pseudoephedrine *on page 258*

◆ **Palgic®-DS [DSC]** *see* Carbinoxamine and Pseudoephedrine *on page 258*

Palifermin (pal ee FER min)

U.S. Brand Names Kepivance®

Index Terms AMJ 9701; rhKGF; rhu Keratinocyte Growth Factor; rHu-KGF

Pharmacologic Category Keratinocyte Growth Factor

Use Decrease the incidence and severity of severe oral mucositis associated with hematologic malignancies in patients receiving myelotoxic therapy requiring hematopoietic stem cell support

Pregnancy Risk Factor C

Pregnancy Considerations Palifermin has been shown to be embryotoxic in animal studies at doses also associated with maternal toxicity. There are no adequate and well-controlled studies in pregnant women.

Lactation Excretion in breast milk unknown/use caution

Contraindications Hypersensitivity to palifermin, *E. coli*-derived proteins, or any component of the formulation

Warnings/Precautions Edema, erythema, pruritus, rash, oral/perioral dysesthesia, taste alteration, tongue discoloration, and tongue thickening may occur; instruct patients to report mucocutaneous effects. Safety and efficacy have not been established with nonhematologic malignancies; effect on the growth of nonhematopoietic human tumors is not known. Palifermin has been shown to enhance epithelial tumor cell lines *in vitro*. Palifermin should be administered prior to and following, but not with, chemotherapy. If administered during or within 24 hours of (before or after) chemotherapy, palifermin may increase the severity and duration of mucositis due to the increased sensitivity of rapidly-dividing epithelial cells. Safety and efficacy have not been established in children.

Adverse Reactions

>10%:

Cardiovascular: Edema (28%), hypertension (7% to 14%)

Central nervous system: Fever (39%); pain (16%); dysesthesia (oral hyperesthesia, hypoesthesia, and paresthesia 12%)

Dermatologic: Rash (62%; grade 3: 3%), pruritus (35%), erythema (32%)
Gastrointestinal: Serum amylase increased (grades 3/4: 38%), mouth/tongue discoloration or thickness (17%), taste alteration (16%), serum lipase increased (grades 3/4: 11%)
Renal: Proteinuria (17%)
Respiratory: Cough (32%), rhinitis (16%)

1% to 10%:
Neuromuscular & skeletal: Arthralgia (10%)
Miscellaneous: Antibody formation (2%)

<1% (Limited to important or life-threatening): Flexural hyperpigmentation

Drug Interactions

Avoid Concomitant Use There are no known interactions where it is recommended to avoid concomitant use.

Increased Effect/Toxicity There are no known significant interactions involving an increase in effect.

Decreased Effect There are no known significant interactions involving a decrease in effect.

Stability Store intact vials under refrigeration at 2°C to 8°C (36°F to 46°F). Protect from light. To reconstitute, slowly add 1.2 mL SWFI, to a final concentration of 5 mg/mL. Swirl gently; do not shake or vigorously agitate. Do not filter during preparation or administration. Protect reconstituted solution from light. Reconstituted vials are stable for up to 72 hours refrigerated and should not be used if left at room temperature >2 hours (data on file). The product labeling, however, indicates that reconstituted vials are stable for up to 24 hours refrigerated and should not be used if left at room temperature >1 hour. Do not freeze reconstituted product.

Mechanism of Action Palifermin is a recombinant keratinocyte growth factor (KGF) produced in *E. coli*. Endogenous KGF is produced by mesenchymal cells in response to epithelial tissue injury. KGF binds to the KGF receptor resulting in proliferation, differentiation and migration of epithelial cells in multiple tissues, including (but not limited to) the tongue, buccal mucosa, esophagus, and salivary gland.

Pharmacodynamics/Kinetics
Onset of action: Epithelial cell proliferation (dose-dependent): 48 hours
Half-life elimination: 4.5 hours (range: 3.3-5.7 hours)

Dosage I.V.: Adults: 60 mcg/kg/day for 3 consecutive days before and after myelotoxic therapy; total of 6 doses

Note: Administer first 3 doses prior to myelotoxic therapy, with the 3rd dose given 24-48 hours before therapy begins. The last 3 doses should be administered after myelotoxic therapy, with the first of these doses after but on the same day as hematopoietic stem cell infusion and at least 4 days after the most recent dose of palifermin.

Dosage adjustment in renal impairment: No adjustment necessary

Administration Administer by I.V. bolus. If heparin is used to maintain the patency of the I.V. line, flush line with saline prior to and after palifermin administration. Do not administer palifermin during or within 24 hours before or after chemotherapy. Allow solution to reach room temperature prior to administration; do not use if at room temperature >1 hour. Do not filter.

Additional Information Oncology Comment: The Multinational Association of Supportive Care in Cancer and the International Society for Oral Oncology (MASCC/ISOO) guidelines for the prevention and treatment of mucositis recommend palifermin (at the FDA-approved dose) for the prevention of oral mucositis in patients with hematologic malignancies who are receiving high-dose chemotherapy and total body irradiation with autologous stem cell transplantation (Keefe, 2007).

Guidelines from the American Society of Clinical Oncology (ASCO) for the use of chemotherapy and radiotherapy protectants (Hensley, 2008) recommend the use of palifermin to decrease the incidence of severe mucositis in patients undergoing autologous stem-cell transplantation with a total body irradiation (TBI) conditioning regimen. According to the ASCO guidelines, data are insufficient to recommend palifermin when the conditioning regimen is chemotherapy only. Palifermin may be considered in patients undergoing myeloablative allogeneic stem-cell transplantation with a TBI conditioning regimen, however data are again insufficient to recommend palifermin when the conditioning regimen is chemotherapy only. Due to a lack of appropriate data, the guidelines also do not recommend palifermin use in non-stem-cell transplantation treatment regimens or for use when treating solid tumors.

Dosage Forms Excipient information presented when available (limited, particularly for generics); consult specific product labeling.

Injection, powder for reconstitution [preservative free]:
Kepivance®: 6.25 mg [contains mannitol 50 mg, sucrose 25 mg]

Paliperidone (pal ee PER i done)

U.S. Brand Names Invega®

Canadian Brand Names Invega®

Index Terms 9-hydroxy-risperidone; 9-OH-risperidone

Pharmacologic Category Antipsychotic Agent, Atypical

Additional Appendix Information
Antipsychotic Agents *on page 1644*

Use Treatment of schizophrenia

Unlabeled/Investigational Use Psychosis/agitation related to Alzheimer's dementia

Pregnancy Risk Factor C

Pregnancy Considerations Animal studies with risperidone indicate an increase in fetal mortality. There are no adequate and well-controlled studies in pregnant women. Reversible EPS symptoms were noted in neonates following maternal use of risperidone during the last trimester. Healthcare providers are encouraged to enroll women 18-45 years of age exposed to paliperidone during pregnancy in the Atypical Antipsychotics Pregnancy Registry (1-866-961-2388).

Lactation Enters breast milk/use caution

Contraindications Hypersensitivity to paliperidone, risperidone, or any component of the formulation

Warnings/Precautions [U.S. Boxed Warning]: Elderly patients with dementia-related psychosis treated with atypical antipsychotics are at an increased risk of death compared to placebo. An increased incidence of cerebrovascular adverse events (including fatalities) has been reported in elderly patients with dementia-related psychosis. Paliperidone has not been studied in this clinical population and is not approved for the treatment of dementia-related psychosis.

Compared with risperidone, paliperidone is low to moderately sedating; use with caution in disorders where CNS depression is a feature. Use caution in patients with predisposition to seizures. Use with caution in renal dysfunction; dose reduction recommended. Esophageal dysmotility and aspiration have been associated with antipsychotic use; use with caution in patients at risk of aspiration pneumonia (eg, Alzheimer's disease). Elevates prolactin levels; use with caution in breast cancer or other prolactin-dependent tumors. May alter temperature regulation. May mask toxicity of other drugs or conditions (eg intestinal obstruction, Reyes syndrome, brain tumor) due to antiemetic effects.

May cause orthostasis. Use with caution in patients with cardiovascular diseases (eg, heart failure, history of myocardial infarction or ischemia, cerebrovascular disease, conduction abnormalities). Use caution in patients receiving medications for hypertension (orthostatic effects may be exacerbated) or in patients with hypovolemia or dehydration. May alter cardiac conduction; life-threatening arrhythmias have occurred with therapeutic doses of neuroleptics. Avoid use in combination with QT_c-prolonging drugs. Avoid use in patients with congenital long-QT syndrome and in patients with history of cardiac arrhythmia.

May cause extrapyramidal symptoms (EPS), including pseudoparkinsonism, acute dystonic reactions, akathisia, and tardive dyskinesia (risk of these reactions is low relative to other neuroleptics, and is dose dependent). Risk of dystonia (and probably other EPS) may be greater with increased doses, use of conventional antipsychotics, males, and younger patients. Risk of neuroleptic malignant syndrome (NMS) may be increased in patients with Parkinson's disease or Lewy body dementia; monitor for symptoms of confusion, obtundation, postural instability and extrapyramidal symptoms. May cause hyperglycemia; in some cases may be extreme and associated with ketoacidosis, hyperosmolar coma, or death. Use with caution in patients with diabetes (or risk factors) or other disorders of glucose regulation; monitor for worsening of glucose control. Significant weight gain has been observed with antipsychotic therapy; incidence varies with product. Monitor waist circumference and BMI.

The possibility of a suicide attempt is inherent in psychotic illness or bipolar disorder; use caution in high-risk patients during initiation of therapy. Prescriptions should be written for the smallest quantity consistent with good patient care.

Formulation consists of drug within a nonabsorbable shell that is expelled and may be visible in the stool. Use is not recommended in patients with pre-existing severe gastrointestinal narrowing disorders. Patients with upper GI tract alterations in transit time may have increased or decreased bioavailability of paliperidone. Do not use in patients unable to swallow the tablet whole.

Safety and efficacy have not been established in patients <18 years of age.

Adverse Reactions

>10%:

- Cardiovascular: Tachycardia (12% to 14%)
- Central nervous system: Headache (11% to 14%), somnolence (6% to 11% dose dependent)

1% to 10%:

- Cardiovascular: Orthostatic hypotension (1% to 4% dose dependent), bundle branch block (<1% to 3%), AV block (first degree ≤2%), arrhythmia (≤2%)
- Central nervous system: Akathisia (3% to 10% dose dependent), EPS (2% to 7% dose dependent), parkinsonism (≤7% dose dependent), dizziness (4% to 6%), dystonia (1% to 5% dose dependent), hypertonia (1% to 4% dose dependent), fatigue (1% to 2%)
- Endocrine & metabolic: Weight gain (6% to 9% dose dependent)
- Gastrointestinal: Salivation increased (≤4% dose dependent), xerostomia (1% to 3%), abdominal pain (1% to 3%)
- Neuromuscular & skeletal: Hyperkinesia (3% to 10% dose dependent), dyskinesia (3% to 9% dose dependent), tremor (3% to 4%), weakness (≤2%)

<1% (Limited to important or life-threatening): Anaphylactic reaction, bradycardia, edema, hyperglycemia, ischemia, neuroleptic malignant syndrome, palpitation, prolactin increased, QT_c interval prolongation, sedation, seizure, syncope, tardive dyskinesia, tongue swelling

Drug Interactions

Avoid Concomitant Use There are no known interactions where it is recommended to avoid concomitant use.

Increased Effect/Toxicity

Paliperidone may increase the levels/effects of: Alcohol (Ethyl); CNS Depressants

The levels/effects of Paliperidone may be increased by: Acetylcholinesterase Inhibitors (Central); Itraconazole; Lithium formulations; P-Glycoprotein Inhibitors; Tetrabenazine

Decreased Effect

Paliperidone may decrease the levels/effects of: Amphetamines; Anti-Parkinson's Agents (Dopamine Agonist)

The levels/effects of Paliperidone may be decreased by: CarBAMazepine; Lithium formulations; P-Glycoprotein Inducers

Ethanol/Nutrition/Herb Interactions

Ethanol: Avoid ethanol (may increase CNS depression).

Herb/Nutraceutical: Avoid kava kava, gotu kola, valerian, St John's wort (may increase CNS depression).

Stability Store at controlled room temperature of ≤25°C (77°F); excursions permitted to 15°C to 30°C (59°F to 86°F). Protect from moisture.

Mechanism of Action Paliperidone is considered a benzisoxazole atypical antipsychotic as it is the primary active metabolite of risperidone. As with other atypical antipsychotics, it's therapeutic efficacy is believed to result from mixed central serotonergic and dopaminergic antagonism. The addition of serotonin antagonism to dopamine antagonism (classic neuroleptic mechanism) is thought to improve negative symptoms of psychoses and reduce the incidence of extrapyramidal side effects. Similar to risperidone, paliperidone demonstrates high affinity to α_1, D_2, H_1, and $5\text{-}HT_{2C}$ receptors, and low affinity for muscarinic and $5\text{-}HT_{1A}$ receptors. In contrast to risperidone, paliperidone displays nearly 10-fold lower affinity for α_2 and $5\text{-}HT_{2A}$ receptors, and nearly three- to fivefold less affinity for $5\text{-}HT_{1A}$ and $5\text{-}HT_{1D}$, respectively.

Pharmacodynamics/Kinetics

Distribution: V_d: 487 L

Protein binding: 74%

Metabolism: Hepatic via CYP2D6 and 3A4 (limited role in elimination); minor metabolism (<10% each) via dealkylation, hydroxylation, dehydrogenation, and benzisoxazole scission

Bioavailability: 28%

Half-life elimination: 23 hours; 24-51 hours with renal impairment (Cl_{cr} <80 mL/minute)

Time to peak, plasma: ~24 hours

Excretion: Urine (80%); feces (11%)

Dosage Oral:

Adults: Schizophrenia: Usual: 6 mg once daily in the morning; titration not required, though some may benefit from higher or lower doses. If exceeding 6 mg/day, increases of 3 mg/day are recommended no more frequently than every 5 days, up to a maximum of 12 mg/day. Some patients may require only 3 mg/day.

Dosage adjustment in renal impairment:

Mild impairment (Cl_{cr} 50 to <80 mL/minute): Initial: 3 mg once daily; may increase to maximal dose of 6 mg/day if needed

Moderate-to-severe impairment (Cl_{cr} 10-49 mL/minute): Initial: 1.5 mg once daily; may increase to maximal dose of 3 mg/day if needed

Severe impairment (Cl_{cr} <10 mL/minute): Has not been studied; not recommended

Dosage adjustment in hepatic impairment: No adjustment necessary for mild-to-moderate (Child-Pugh class A and B) impairment. Not studied in severe impairment.

Dietary Considerations May be taken with or without food.

Administration May be administered with or without food. Extended release tablets should be swallowed whole with liquids; do not crush, chew, or divide.

Monitoring Parameters Vital signs; fasting lipid profile and fasting blood glucose/Hgb A_{1c} (prior to treatment, at 3 months, then annually), prolactin levels; BMI, personal/family history of obesity, diabetes, waist circumference; blood pressure; mental status, abnormal involuntary movement scale (AIMS), extrapyramidal symptoms; orthostatic blood pressure changes for 3-5 days after starting or increasing dose. Weight should be assessed prior to treatment, at 4 weeks, 8 weeks, 12 weeks, and then at quarterly intervals. Consider titrating to a different antipsychotic agent for a weight gain ≥5% of the initial weight.

Additional Information Invega® is an extended release tablet based on the OROS® osmotic delivery system. Water from the GI tract enters through a semipermeable membrane coating the tablet, solubilizing the drug into a gelatinous form which, through hydrophilic expansion, is then expelled through laser-drilled holes in the coating.

Dosage Forms Excipient information presented when available (limited, particularly for generics); consult specific product labeling. [CAN] = Canadian availability; not available in U.S.

Tablet, extended-release:

Invega®: 1.5 mg, 3 mg, 6 mg, 9 mg [osmotic controlled release]

Invega® [CAN]: 12 mg [osmotic controlled release, not available in the U.S.]

Palivizumab (pah li VIZ u mab)

U.S. Brand Names Synagis®

Canadian Brand Names Synagis®

Pharmacologic Category Monoclonal Antibody

Use Prevention of serious lower respiratory tract disease caused by respiratory syncytial virus (RSV) in infants and children at high risk of RSV disease

Pregnancy Risk Factor C

Pregnancy Considerations Not for adult use; reproduction studies have not been conducted

Medication Safety Issues

Sound-alike/look-alike issues:

Synagis® may be confused with Synalgos®-DC, Synvisc®

Contraindications History of severe prior reaction to palivizumab or any component of the formulation

Warnings/Precautions Very rare cases of anaphylaxis have been observed following palivizumab. Rare cases of severe acute hypersensitivity reactions have also been reported. Use with caution after mild hypersensitivity reaction; permanently discontinue for severe hypersensitivity reaction. Safety and efficacy of palivizumab have not been demonstrated in the treatment of established RSV disease. Use with caution in patients with thrombocytopenia or any coagulation disorder. Safety and efficacy have been established in infants with chronic lung disease, infants with a history of premature birth (≤35 weeks gestational age), and children with hemodynamically-significant congenital heart disease (CHD).

Adverse Reactions The incidence of adverse events was similar between the palivizumab and placebo groups.

>1%:

Cardiovascular: Arrhythmia, cyanosis

Central nervous system: Fever, nervousness

Dermatologic: Rash

Gastrointestinal: Diarrhea, gastroenteritis, vomiting

Hepatic: ALT increase

Otic: Otitis media

Respiratory: Cough, rhinitis, upper respiratory infection, wheezing

<1% (Limited to important or life-threatening): Anaphylaxis (very rare - includes angioedema, dyspnea, hypotonia, pruritus, respiratory failure, unresponsiveness, urticaria); antibody development, hypersensitivity reactions, injection site reactions, thrombocytopenia

Drug Interactions

Avoid Concomitant Use There are no known interactions where it is recommended to avoid concomitant use.

Increased Effect/Toxicity

The levels/effects of Palivizumab may be increased by: Abciximab

Decreased Effect There are no known significant interactions involving a decrease in effect.

Stability Store in refrigerator at a temperature between 2°C to 8°C (35.6°F to 46.4°F) in original container; do not freeze. Do not shake, vigorously agitate, or dilute the solution.

Mechanism of Action Exhibits neutralizing and fusion-inhibitory activity against RSV; these activities inhibit RSV replication in laboratory and clinical studies

Pharmacodynamics/Kinetics

Half-life elimination: Children <24 months: 20 days

Time to peak, serum: 48 hours

Dosage I.M.: Infants and Children <2 years:

Prevention of RSV: 15 mg/kg of body weight, monthly throughout RSV season (first dose administered prior to commencement of RSV season)

Note: Cardiopulmonary bypass patients: Administer a dose as soon as possible after cardiopulmonary bypass procedure, even if <1 month from previous dose.

Administration Injection should (preferably) be in the anterolateral aspect of the thigh; gluteal muscle should not be used routinely; injection volume over 1 mL should be administered as divided doses

Monitoring Parameters Monitor for anaphylaxis or acute hypersensitivity reactions

Additional Information RSV prophylaxis should be initiated at the onset of the RSV season. In most areas of the United States, onset of RSV outbreaks is October to December, and termination is March to May, but regional differences occur.

Dosage Forms Excipient information presented when available (limited, particularly for generics); consult specific product labeling.

Injection, solution [preservative free]:

Synagis®: 100 mg/mL (0.5 mL, 1 mL)

- **Palmer's® Skin Success Eventone® Fade Cream [OTC]** *see* Hydroquinone *on page* 749
- **Palmitate-A® [OTC]** *see* Vitamin A *on page* 1565

Palonosetron (pal oh NOE se tron)

U.S. Brand Names Aloxi®

Index Terms Palonosetron Hydrochloride; RS-25259; RS-25259-197

Pharmacologic Category Antiemetic; Selective 5-HT_3 Receptor Antagonist

Use

I.V.: Prevention of chemotherapy-associated nausea and vomiting; indicated for prevention of acute (highly-emetogenic therapy) as well as acute and delayed (moderately-emetogenic therapy) nausea and vomiting; prevention of postoperative nausea and vomiting (PONV)

Oral: Prevention of chemotherapy-associated nausea and vomiting (moderately-emetogenic therapy)

Pregnancy Risk Factor B

Pregnancy Considerations Teratogenic effects were not observed in animal studies. There are no adequate and well-controlled studies in pregnant women; use during pregnancy only if clearly needed.

Lactation Excretion in breast milk unknown/not recommended

Medication Safety Issues

Sound-alike/look-alike issues:

Aloxi® may be confused with Eloxatin®, oxaliplatin

Palonosetron may be confused with dolasetron, granisetron, ondansetron

Contraindications Hypersensitivity to palonosetron or any component of the formulation

Warnings/Precautions Hypersensitivity has been observed rarely with I.V. palonosetron. Use caution in patients allergic to other 5-HT_3 receptor antagonists; cross-reactivity is possible. Some selective 5-HT_3 receptor antagonists have been associated with dose-dependent increases in ECG intervals (eg, PR, QRS duration, QT/QT_c, JT), usually occurring 1-2 hours after I.V. administration. In general, these changes are not clinically relevant, however, when these agents are used in conjunction with other agents that prolong these intervals, arrhythmia may occur. When used with agents that prolong the QT interval (eg, Class I and III antiarrhythmics), clinically relevant QT interval prolongation could result in torsade de pointes. A number of trials have shown that 5-HT_3 antagonists produce QT interval prolongation to variable degrees. Use with caution in patients at risk of QT prolongation and/or ventricular arrhythmia. Reduction in heart rate may also occur with the 5-HT_3 antagonists. Use with caution in patients with congenital long QT syndrome or other risk factors for QT prolongation (eg, medications known to prolong QT interval, electrolyte abnormalities, and cumulative high dose anthracycline therapy).

Not intended for treatment of nausea and vomiting or for chronic continuous therapy. **For chemotherapy, should be used on a scheduled basis, not on an "as needed" (PRN) basis,** since data support the use of this drug only in the prevention of nausea and vomiting (due to antineoplastic therapy) and not in the rescue of nausea and vomiting. For PONV, may use for low expectation of PONV if it is essential to avoid nausea and vomiting in the postoperative period; use is not recommended if there is little expectation of nausea and vomiting. Safety and efficacy in children have not been established.

Adverse Reactions Adverse events may vary according to indication. In general, adverse reactions similar between I.V. and oral dosage forms.

1% to 10%:

Cardiovascular: QT prolongation (chemotherapy-associated <1%; PONV 1% to 5%), bradycardia (chemotherapy-associated 1%; PONV 4%), hypotension (≤1%), sinus bradycardia (≤1%), tachycardia (nonsustained) (≤1%)

Central nervous system: Headache (chemotherapy-associated 4% to 9%; PONV 3%), anxiety (1%), dizziness (≤1%), fatigue (≤1%)

Dermatologic: Pruritus (≤1%)

Endocrine & metabolic: Hyperkalemia (1%)

Gastrointestinal: Constipation (1% to 5%), diarrhea (≤1%), flatulence (≤1%)

Genitourinary: Urinary retention (≤1%)

Hepatic: ALT increased (≤1%; transient), AST increased (≤1%; transient)

Neuromuscular & skeletal: Weakness (1%)

<1% (Limited to important or life-threatening): Abdominal pain, abnormal taste, allergic dermatitis, alopecia, amblyopia, anemia, anorexia, appetite decreased, arrhythmia, arthralgia, atrioventricular block (first and second degree), bilirubin increased (transient), chills, dyspepsia, dyspnea, edema (generalized), electrolyte fluctuations, epistaxis, erythema, euphoric mood, extrasystoles, eye irritation/edema, fever, flu-like syndrome, gastritis, glycosuria, hiccups, hot flash, hyperglycemia, hypersensitivity (rare), hypersomnia, hypertension, hypokalemia, hypoventilation, injection site reactions (burning/discomfort/induration/pain; rare), insomnia, intestinal hypomotility, joint stiffness, laryngospasm, metabolic acidosis, motion sickness, myalgia, myocardial ischemia, pain in extremities, paresthesia, platelets decreased, rash, salivation increased, sinus arrhythmia, sinus tachycardia, sinusitis, somnolence, supraventricular extrasystoles, tinnitus, T-wave amplitude decreased, vein discoloration, vein distention, ventricular extrasystoles, xerostomia

Drug Interactions

Metabolism/Transport Effects **Substrate** (minor) of CYP1A2, 2D6, 3A4

Avoid Concomitant Use

Avoid concomitant use of Palonosetron with any of the following: Apomorphine

Increased Effect/Toxicity

Palonosetron may increase the levels/effects of: Apomorphine

Decreased Effect There are no known significant interactions involving a decrease in effect.

Stability

Capsule: Store at room temperature of 25°C (77°F); excursions permitted to 15°C to 30°C (59°F to 86°F). Protect from light.

Injection: Store intact vials at room temperature of 20°C to 25°C (68°F to 77°F); excursions permitted to 15°C to 30°C (59°F to 86°F); do not freeze. Protect from light. Solutions of 5 mcg/mL and 30 mcg/mL in NS, D_5W, $D_5$1/2NS, and D_5LR injection are stable for 48 hours at room temperature and 14 days under refrigeration.

Mechanism of Action Selective 5-HT_3 receptor antagonist, blocking serotonin, both on vagal nerve terminals in the periphery and centrally in the chemoreceptor trigger zone

Pharmacodynamics/Kinetics

Absorption: Well absorbed

Distribution: V_d: 8.3 ± 2.5 L/kg

Protein binding: ~62%

Metabolism: ~50% metabolized via CYP enzymes (and likely other pathways) to relatively inactive metabolites (N-oxide-palonosetron and 6-S-hydroxy-palonosetron); CYP1A2, 2D6, and 3A4 contribute to its metabolism

Bioavailability: Oral: 97%

Half-life elimination: I.V.: Terminal: ~40 hours; Oral: 29-45 hours (healthy patients), 38-62 hours (cancer patients)

Time to peak, plasma: Oral: 3-7 hours (healthy patients); ~5 hours (cancer patients)

Excretion: Urine (80% to 93%, 40% as unchanged drug); feces (5% to 8%)

Dosage Adults:

Chemotherapy-associated nausea and vomiting:

I.V.: 0.25 mg 30 minutes prior to the start of chemotherapy administration, day 1 of each cycle

Oral: 0.5 mg 1 hour prior to the start of chemotherapy

Breakthrough: Palonosetron has not been shown to be effective in terminating nausea or vomiting once it occurs and should not be used for this purpose.

PONV: I.V.: 0.075 mg immediately prior to anesthesia induction

Elderly: No dosage adjustment necessary

Dosage adjustment in renal/hepatic impairment: No dosage adjustment necessary

Dietary Considerations Capsule: May be taken with or without meals.

Administration

I.V.: Flush I.V. line with NS prior to and following administration.

Chemotherapy-associated nausea and vomiting: Infuse over 30 seconds, 30 minutes prior to the start of chemotherapy

PONV: Infuse over 10 seconds immediately prior to anesthesia induction

Oral: May administer with or without meals.

Product Availability Aloxi® capsules: FDA approved August 2008; availability anticipated in the first quarter of 2009

Dosage Forms Excipient information presented when available (limited, particularly for generics); consult specific product labeling.

Capsule:

Aloxi®: 0.5 mg

Injection, solution:

Aloxi®: 0.05 mg/mL (1.5 mL, 5 mL) [contains edetate disodium]

◆ **Palonosetron Hydrochloride** *see* Palonosetron *on page 1132*

◆ **2-PAM** *see* Pralidoxime *on page 1223*

◆ **Pamabrom and Acetaminophen** *see* Acetaminophen and Pamabrom *on page 28*

◆ **Pamelor®** *see* Nortriptyline *on page 1081*

Pamidronate (pa mi DROE nate)

U.S. Brand Names Aredia®

Canadian Brand Names Aredia®; Pamidronate Disodium®; Rhoxal-pamidronate

Index Terms Pamidronate Disodium

Pharmacologic Category Antidote; Bisphosphonate Derivative

Use Treatment of hypercalcemia associated with malignancy; treatment of osteolytic bone lesions associated with multiple myeloma or metastatic breast cancer; moderate to severe Paget's disease of bone

Unlabeled/Investigational Use Treatment of pediatric osteoporosis, treatment of osteogenesis imperfecta

Pregnancy Risk Factor D

Pregnancy Considerations Pamidronate has been shown to cross the placenta and cause nonteratogenic embryo/fetal effects in animals. There are no adequate and well-controlled studies in pregnant women; manufacturer states pamidronate should not be used in pregnancy. Based on limited case reports, serum calcium levels in the newborn may be altered if pamidronate is administered during pregnancy. Bisphosphonates are incorporated into the bone matrix and gradually released over time. Theoretically, there may be a risk of fetal harm when pregnancy follows the completion of therapy. Women of childbearing potential should be advised to use effective contraception and avoid becoming pregnant during therapy.

Lactation Excretion in breast milk unknown/use caution

Medication Safety Issues

Sound-alike/look-alike issues:

Aredia® may be confused with Adriamycin, Meridia®

International issues:

Linoten® [Spain] may be confused with Lidopen® which is a brand name for lidocaine in the U.S.

Contraindications Hypersensitivity to pamidronate, other bisphosphonates, or any component of the formulation

Warnings/Precautions Bisphosphonate therapy has been associated with osteonecrosis, primarily of the jaw; this has been observed mostly in cancer patients, but also in patients with postmenopausal osteoporosis and other diagnoses. Dental exams and preventative dentistry should be performed prior to placing patients with risk factors on chronic bisphosphonate therapy. Invasive dental procedures should be avoided during treatment.

Infrequently, severe (and occasionally debilitating) bone, joint, and/or muscle pain have been reported during bisphosphonate treatment. The onset of pain ranged from a single day to several months. Symptoms usually resolve upon discontinuation. Some patients experienced recurrence when rechallenged with same drug or another bisphosphonate; avoid use in patients with a history of these symptoms in association with bisphosphonate therapy.

Initial or single doses have been associated with renal deterioration, progressing to renal failure and dialysis. Withhold pamidronate treatment (until renal function returns to baseline) in patients with evidence of renal deterioration. Glomerulosclerosis (focal segmental) with or without nephrotic syndrome has also been reported. Longer infusion times (>2 hours) may reduce the risk for renal toxicity, especially in patients with pre-existing renal insufficiency. Single pamidronate doses should not exceed 90 mg. Patients with serum creatinine >3 mg/dL were not studied in clinical trials; limited data is available in patients with Cl_{cr} <30 mL/minute. Evaluate serum creatinine prior to each treatment. For the treatment of bone metastases, use is not recommended in patients with severe renal impairment; for renal impairment in indications other than bone metastases, use clinical judgment to determine if benefits outweigh potential risks.

Use has been associated with asymptomatic electrolyte abnormalities (including hypophosphatemia, hypokalemia, hypomagnesemia, and hypocalcemia). Rare cases of symptomatic hypocalcemia, including tetany have been reported. Patients with a history of thyroid surgery may have relative hypoparathyroidism; predisposing them to pamidronate-related hypocalcemia. Leukopenia has been observed with oral pamidronate and monitoring of white blood cell counts is suggested. Patients with pre-existing anemia, leukopenia, or thrombocytopenia should be closely monitored during the first 2 weeks of treatment.

Adequate hydration is required during treatment (urine output ~2 L/day); avoid overhydration, especially in patients with heart failure. Vein irritation and thrombophlebitis may occur with infusions. Women of childbearing potential should be advised to use effective contraception and avoid becoming pregnant during therapy.

Adverse Reactions Note: Actual percentages may vary by indication; treatment for multiple myeloma is associated with higher percentage.

>10%:

Central nervous system: Fatigue (≤37%), fever (18% to 39%), headache (≤26%), insomnia (≤22%)

Endocrine & metabolic: Hypophosphatemia (≤18%), hypokalemia (4% to 18%), hypomagnesemia (4% to 12%), hypocalcemia (≤12%)

Gastrointestinal: Nausea (≤54%), vomiting (≤36%), anorexia (≤26%), abdominal pain (≤23%), dyspepsia (≤23%)

Genitourinary: Urinary tract infection (≤19%)

Hematologic: Anemia (≤43%), granulocytopenia (≤20%)

Local: Infusion site reaction (≤18%; includes induration, pain, redness and swelling)

Neuromuscular & skeletal: Weakness (≤22%), myalgia (≤26%), arthralgia (≤14%), osteonecrosis of the jaw (cancer patients: 1% to 11%)

Renal: Serum creatinine increased (≤19%)

Respiratory: Dyspnea (≤30%), cough (≤26%), upper respiratory tract infection (≤24%), sinusitis (≤16%), pleural effusion (≤11%)

1% to 10%:

Cardiovascular: Atrial fibrillation (≤6%), hypertension (≤6%), syncope (≤6%), tachycardia (≤6%), atrial flutter (≤1%), cardiac failure (≤1%), edema (≤1%)

Central nervous system: Somnolence (≤6%), psychosis (≤4%)

Endocrine & metabolic: Hypothyroidism (≤6%)

Gastrointestinal: Constipation (≤6%), gastrointestinal hemorrhage (≤6%), diarrhea (≤1%), stomatitis (≤1%)

Hematologic: Leukopenia (≤4%), neutropenia (≤1%), thrombocytopenia (≤1%)

Neuromuscular & skeletal: Back pain (≤5%), bone pain (≤5%)
Renal: Uremia (≤4%)
Respiratory: Rales (≤6%), rhinitis (≤6%)
Miscellaneous: Moniliasis (≤6%)

<1% (Limited to important or life-threatening): Acute renal failure, adult respiratory distress syndrome, allergic reaction, anaphylactic shock, angioedema, bronchospasm, CHF, confusion, conjunctivitis, electrolyte/mineral abnormality, episcleritis, fluid overload, flu-like syndrome, focal segmental glomerulosclerosis (including collapsing variant), hallucinations (visual), hematuria, herpes virus reactivation, hyperkalemia, hypernatremia, hypotension, injection site phlebitis/thrombophlebitis, interstitial pneumonitis, iridocyclitis, iritis, joint and/or muscle pain (sometimes severe and/or incapacitating), left ventricular failure, lymphocytopenia, malaise, nephrotic syndrome, osteonecrosis (other than jaw), paresthesia, pruritus, rash, renal deterioration, scleritis, seizure, tetany, uveitis, xanthopsia

Drug Interactions

Avoid Concomitant Use There are no known interactions where it is recommended to avoid concomitant use.

Increased Effect/Toxicity

Pamidronate may increase the levels/effects of: Phosphate Supplements

The levels/effects of Pamidronate may be increased by: Aminoglycosides; Nonsteroidal Anti-Inflammatory Agents; Thalidomide

Decreased Effect There are no known significant interactions involving a decrease in effect.

Stability

Powder for injection: Store below 30°C (86°F). Reconstitute by adding 10 mL of SWFI to each vial of lyophilized pamidronate disodium powder; the resulting solution will be 30 mg/10 mL or 90 mg/10 mL. The reconstituted solution is stable for 24 hours stored under refrigeration at 2°C to 8°C (36°F to 46°F).

Solution for injection: Store at 20°C to 25°C (68°f to 77°F).

Pamidronate may be further diluted in 250-1000 mL of 0.45% or 0.9% sodium chloride or 5% dextrose. (The manufacturer recommends dilution in 1000 mL for hypercalcemia of malignancy, 500 mL for Paget's disease and bone metastases of myeloma, and 250 mL for bone metastases of breast cancer.) Pamidronate solution for infusion is stable at room temperature for up to 24 hours.

Mechanism of Action A bisphosphonate which inhibits bone resorption via actions on osteoclasts or on osteoclast precursors. Does not appear to produce any significant effects on renal tubular calcium handling and is poorly absorbed following oral administration (high oral doses have been reported effective); therefore, I.V. therapy is preferred.

Pharmacodynamics/Kinetics

Onset of action: 24-48 hours
Peak effect: Maximum: 5-7 days
Absorption: Poor; pharmacokinetic studies lacking
Metabolism: Not metabolized
Half-life elimination: 21-35 hours
Excretion: Biphasic; urine (30% to 62% as unchanged drug; lower in patients with renal dysfunction) within 120 hours

Dosage Dilute prior to administration and infuse intravenously slowly over at least 2 hours. Single doses should not exceed 90 mg. I.V.: Adults:

Hypercalcemia of malignancy:

Moderate cancer-related hypercalcemia (corrected serum calcium: 12-13.5 mg/dL): 60-90 mg, as a single dose over 2-24 hours

Severe cancer-related hypercalcemia (corrected serum calcium: >13.5 mg/dL): 90 mg, as a single dose over 2-24 hours

A period of 7 days should elapse before the use of second course; repeat infusions every 2-3 weeks have been suggested, however, could be administered every 2-3 months according to the degree and of severity of hypercalcemia and/or the type of malignancy.

Osteolytic bone lesions with multiple myeloma: 90 mg over 2-4 hours monthly

Osteolytic bone lesions with metastatic breast cancer: 90 mg over 2 hours repeated every 3-4 weeks

Paget's disease: 30 mg over 4 hours daily for 3 consecutive days

Elderly: Begin at lower end of adult dosing range.

Dosing adjustment in renal impairment: Safety and efficacy have not been established in patients with serum creatinine >5 mg/dL; studies are limited in multiple myeloma patients with serum creatinine ≥3 mg/dL

The manufacturer recommends the following guidelines:

Treatment of bone metastases: Use is not recommended in patients with severe renal impairment.

Renal impairment in indications other than bone metastases: Use clinical judgment to determine if benefits outweigh potential risks.

American Society of Clinical Oncology (ASCO) guidelines for bisphosphonate use in multiple myeloma (Kyle, 2007) recommend considering a reduced initial dose in patients with pre-existing renal impairment.

Dosing adjustment in renal toxicity: In patients with bone metastases, treatment should be withheld for deterioration in renal function (increase of serum creatinine ≥0.5 mg/dL in patients with normal baseline or ≥1.0 mg/dL in patients with abnormal baseline). Resumption of therapy may be considered when serum creatinine returns to within 10% of baseline.

Dosage in hepatic impairment: No adjustment required in patients with mild-to-moderate hepatic impairment; not studied in patients with severe hepatic impairment.

Dietary Considerations Multiple myeloma or metastatic bone lesions from solid tumors or Paget's disease: Take adequate daily calcium and vitamin D supplement

Administration I.V. infusion over 2-24 hours. Longer infusion times (>2 hours) may reduce the risk for renal toxicity, especially in patients with pre-existing renal insufficiency. The manufacturer recommends infusing over 2-24 hours for hypercalcemia of malignancy; over 2 hours for osteolytic bone lesions with metastatic breast cancer; and over 4 hours for Paget's disease and for osteolytic bone lesions with multiple myeloma. The ASCO guidelines for bisphosphonate use in multiple myeloma recommend infusing pamidronate over at least 2 hours; if therapy is withheld due to renal toxicity, infuse over at least 4 hours upon reintroduction of treatment after renal recovery.

Monitoring Parameters Serum creatinine (prior to each treatment); serum electrolytes, including calcium, phosphate, magnesium and potassium; CBC with differential; monitor for hypocalcemia for at least 2 weeks after therapy; dental exam and preventative dentistry for patients at risk for osteonecrosis; patients with pre-existing anemia, leukopenia, or thrombocytopenia should be closely monitored during the first 2 weeks of treatment

Reference Range Calcium (total): Adults: 9.0-11.0 mg/dL (SI: 2.05-2.54 mmol/L), may slightly decrease with aging; Phosphorus: 2.5-4.5 mg/dL (SI: 0.81-1.45 mmol/L)

Test Interactions Bisphosphonates may interfere with diagnostic imaging agents such as technetium-99m-diphosphonate in bone scans.

Dosage Forms Excipient information presented when available (limited, particularly for generics); consult specific product labeling.

Injection, powder for reconstitution, as disodium: 30 mg, 90 mg

Aredia®: 30 mg, 90 mg

Injection, solution: 3 mg/mL (10 mL); 6 mg/mL (10 mL); 9 mg/mL (10 mL)

- ◆ **Pamidronate Disodium** *see* Pamidronate *on page 1134*
- ◆ **Pamidronate Disodium® (Can)** *see* Pamidronate *on page 1134*
- ◆ **p-Aminoclonidine** *see* Apraclonidine *on page 129*
- ◆ **Pamprin® Maximum Strength All Day Relief [OTC]** *see* Naproxen *on page 1041*
- ◆ **Panafil®** *see* Chlorophyllin, Papain, and Urea *on page 306*
- ◆ **Panafil® SE** *see* Chlorophyllin, Papain, and Urea *on page 306*
- ◆ **Pancof®-EXP** *see* Dihydrocodeine, Pseudoephedrine, and Guaifenesin *on page 448*
- ◆ **Pancof-XP [DSC]** *see* Hydrocodone and Guaifenesin *on page 741*
- ◆ **Pancrease® (Can)** *see* Pancrelipase *on page 1136*
- ◆ **Pancrease® MT** *see* Pancrelipase *on page 1136*
- ◆ **Pancrecarb MS®** *see* Pancrelipase *on page 1136*

Pancrelipase (pan kre LYE pase)

U.S. Brand Names Creon®; ku-zyme® HP [DSC]; Lipram 4500 [DSC]; Lipram-CR [DSC]; Lipram-PN [DSC]; Lipram-UL [DSC]; Palcaps [DSC]; Pancrease® MT; Pancrecarb MS®; Pangestyme™ CN; Pangestyme™ EC; Pangestyme™ MT; Pangestyme™ UL; Panocaps MT [DSC]; Panocaps [DSC]; Panokase® 16 [DSC]; Panokase® [DSC]; Plaretase® 8000; Ultracaps MT [DSC]; Ultrase®; Ultrase® MT; Viokase®

Canadian Brand Names Cotazym®; Creon®; Pancrease®; Pancrease® MT; Ultrase®; Ultrase® MT; Viokase®

Index Terms Lipancreatin

Pharmacologic Category Enzyme

Use Replacement therapy in symptomatic treatment of malabsorption syndrome caused by pancreatic insufficiency

Unlabeled/Investigational Use Treatment of occluded feeding tubes

Pregnancy Risk Factor B/C (product specific)

Lactation Excretion in breast milk unknown/use caution

Contraindications Hypersensitivity to pork protein or any component of the formulation; acute pancreatitis or acute exacerbations of chronic pancreatic disease

Warnings/Precautions Pancrelipase is inactivated by acids; do not crush or chew, some capsules may be opened and sprinkled on food. Fibrotic strictures in the colon, some requiring surgery, have been reported with high doses; use caution, especially in children with cystic fibrosis. Use caution when adjusting doses or changing brands. Avoid inhalation of powder; may cause nasal and respiratory tract irritation.

Adverse Reactions Frequency not defined; occurrence of events may be dose related.

Central nervous system: Pain

Dermatologic: Rash

Endocrine & metabolic: Hyperuricemia

Gastrointestinal: Nausea, cramps, constipation, diarrhea, perianal irritation/inflammation (large doses), irritation of the mouth, abdominal pain, intestinal obstruction, vomiting, flatulence, melena, weight loss, fibrotic strictures, greasy stools

Ocular: Lacrimation

Renal: Hyperuricosuria

Respiratory: Sneezing, dyspnea, bronchospasm

Miscellaneous: Allergic reactions

Drug Interactions

Avoid Concomitant Use There are no known interactions where it is recommended to avoid concomitant use.

Increased Effect/Toxicity There are no known significant interactions involving an increase in effect.

Decreased Effect There are no known significant interactions involving a decrease in effect.

Ethanol/Nutrition/Herb Interactions Food: Avoid placing contents of opened capsules on alkaline food (pH >5.5); pancrelipase may impair absorption of oral iron and folic acid.

Stability Store between 15°C to 25°C (59°F to 77°F); do not refrigerate. Keep in a dry place.

Mechanism of Action Pancrelipase is a natural product harvested from the hog pancreas. It contains a combination of lipase, amylase, and protease. Products are formulated to dissolve in the more basic pH of the duodenum so that they may act locally to break down fats, protein, and starch.

Pharmacodynamics/Kinetics

Absorption: None; acts locally in GI tract

Excretion: Feces

Dosage Oral:

Powder: Actual dose depends on the condition being treated and the digestive requirements of the patient

Children <1 year: Start with 1/8 teaspoonful with feedings

Adults: 0.7 g (1/4 teaspoonful) with meals

Capsules/tablets: The following dosage recommendations are only an approximation for initial dosages. The actual dosage will depend on the condition being treated and the digestive requirements of the individual patient. Adjust dose based on body weight and stool fat content. Total daily dose reflects ~3 meals/day and 2-3 snacks/day, with half the mealtime dose given with a snack. Older patients may need less units/kg due to increased weight, but decreased ingestion of fat/kg. Maximum dose: 2500 units of lipase/kg/meal (10,000 units of lipase/kg/day)

Children:

<1 year: 2000 units of lipase with meals

1-6 years: 4000-8000 units of lipase with meals and 4000 units with snacks

7-12 years: 4000-12,000 units of lipase with meals and snacks

Adults: 4000-48,000 units of lipase with meals and with snacks

Occluded feeding tubes: One tablet of Viokase® crushed with one 325 mg tablet of sodium bicarbonate (to activate the Viokase®) in 5 mL of water can be instilled into the nasogastric tube and clamped for 5 minutes; then, flushed with 50 mL of tap water

Dietary Considerations Should be used as part of a high-calorie diet, appropriate for age and clinical status. Administer with meals or snacks and swallow whole with a generous amount of liquid. Do not crush or chew. Delayed-release capsules containing enteric coated microspheres or microtablets may also be opened and the contents sprinkled on soft food with a low pH such as applesauce, gelatin; apricot, banana, or sweet potato baby food; baby formula. Dairy products such as milk, custard or ice cream may have a high pH and should be avoided.

Administration Oral: Administer with meals or snacks and swallow whole with a generous amount of liquid. Do not crush or chew; retention in the mouth before swallowing may cause mucosal irritation and stomatitis. Delayed-release capsules containing enteric-coated microspheres or microtablets may also be opened and the contents sprinkled on soft food with a low pH that does not require chewing, such as applesauce, gelatin; apricot, banana, or sweet potato baby food; baby formula. Dairy products such as milk, custard, or ice cream may have a high pH and should be avoided. Avoid inhalation of powder, may cause nasal and respiratory tract irritation.

Monitoring Parameters Abdominal symptoms, nutritional intake, growth (in children), stool character, fecal fat

Dosage Forms Excipient information presented when available (limited, particularly for generics); consult specific product labeling. [DSC] = Discontinued product

Capsule:
- ku-zyme® HP: Lipase 8000 units, protease 30,000 units, and amylase 30,000 units [DSC]

Capsule, delayed release, enteric coated granules:
- Pangestyme™ CN-10: Lipase 10,000 units, protease 37,500 units, amylase 33,200 units
- Pangestyme™ CN-20: Lipase 20,000 units, protease 75,000 units, amylase 66,400 units
- Pangestyme™ EC: Lipase 4500 units, protease 25,000 units, and amylase 20,000 units
- Pangestyme™ MT16: Lipase 16,000 units, protease 48,000 units, and amylase 48,000 units
- Pangestyme™ UL 12: Lipase 12,000 units, protease 39,000 units, and amylase 39,000 units
- Pangestyme™ UL 18: Lipase 18,000 units, protease 58,500 units, and amylase 58,500 units
- Pangestyme™ UL 20: Lipase 20,000 units, protease 65,000 units, and amylase 65,000 units

Capsule, delayed release, enteric coated microspheres: Lipase 4500 units, protease 25,000 units, and amylase 20,000 units
- Creon® 5: Lipase 5000 units, protease 18,750 units, and amylase 16,600 units
- Creon® 10, Palcaps 10: Lipase 10,000 units, protease 37,500 units, and amylase 33,200 units
- Creon® 20, Palcaps 20: Lipase 20,000 units, protease 75,000 units, and amylase 66,400 units
- Lipram 4500, Panocaps: Lipase 4500 units, protease 25,000 units, and amylase 20,000 units [DSC]
- Lipram-CR10: Lipase 10,000 units, protease 37,500 units, and amylase 33,200 units [DSC]
- Lipram-CR20: Lipase 20,000 units, protease 75,000 units, and amylase 66,400 units [DSC]
- Lipram-PN10: Lipase 10,000 units, protease 30,000 units, and amylase 30,000 units [DSC]
- Lipram-PN16, Panocap MT 16: Lipase 16,000 units, protease 48,000 units, and amylase 48,000 units [DSC]
- Lipram-PN20, Panocap MT 20: Lipase 20,000 units, protease 44,000 units, and amylase 56,000 units [DSC]
- Lipram-UL20, Ultracaps MT 20: Lipase 20,000 units, protease 65,000 units, and amylase 65,000 units [DSC]
- Pancrecarb MS-4®: Lipase 4000 units, protease 25,000 units, and amylase 25,000 units [buffered]
- Pancrecarb MS-8®: Lipase 8000 units, protease 45,000 units, and amylase 40,000 units [buffered]
- Pancrecarb MS-16® Lipase 16,000 units, protease 52,000 units, and amylase 52,000 units [buffered]

Capsule, enteric coated microspheres:
- Ultrase®: Lipase 4500 units, protease 25,000 units, and amylase 20,000 units

Capsule, enteric coated microtablets:
- Pancrease® MT 4: Lipase 4000 units, protease 12,000 units, and amylase 12,000 units
- Pancrease® MT 10: Lipase 10,000 units, protease 30,000 units, and amylase 30,000 units
- Pancrease® MT 16: Lipase 16,000 units, protease 48,000 units, and amylase 48,000 units
- Pancrease® MT 20: Lipase 20,000 units, protease 44,000 units, and amylase 56,000 units

Capsule, enteric coated minitablets:
- Ultrase® MT12: Lipase 12,000 units, protease 39,000 units, and amylase 39,000 units
- Ultrase® MT18: Lipase 18,000 units, protease 58,500 units, and amylase 58,500 units
- Ultrase® MT20: Lipase 20,000 units, protease 65,000 units, and amylase 65,000 units

Powder (Viokase®): Lipase 16,800 units, protease 70,000 units, and amylase 70,000 units per 0.7 g (227 g)

Tablet: Lipase 8000 units, protease 30,000 units, and amylase 30,000 units
- Panokase®: Lipase 8000 units, protease 30,000 units, and amylase 30,000 units [DSC]
- Panokase® 16: Lipase 16,000 units, protease 60,000 units, and amylase 60,000 units [DSC]
- Plaretase™ 8000: Lipase 8000 units, protease 30,000 units, and amylase 30,000 units
- Viokase® 8: Lipase 8000 units, protease 30,000 units, and amylase 30,000 units
- Viokase® 16: Lipase 16,000 units, protease 60,000 units, and amylase 60,000 units

Pancuronium (pan kyoo ROE nee um)

Canadian Brand Names Pancuronium Bromide®

Index Terms Pancuronium Bromide; Pavulon [DSC]

Pharmacologic Category Neuromuscular Blocker Agent, Nondepolarizing

Additional Appendix Information

Neuromuscular-Blocking Agents *on page 1665*

Use Adjunct to general anesthesia to facilitate endotracheal intubation and to relax skeletal muscles during surgery; to facilitate mechanical ventilation in ICU patients; does not relieve pain or produce sedation

Drug of choice for neuromuscular blockade except in patients with renal failure, hepatic failure, or cardiovascular instability or in situations not suited for pancuronium's long duration of action

Pregnancy Risk Factor C

Lactation Excretion in breast milk unknown/not recommended

Medication Safety Issues

Sound-alike/look-alike issues:
- Pancuronium may be confused with pipecuronium

High alert medication: The Institute for Safe Medication Practices (ISMP) includes this medication among its list of drugs which have a heightened risk of causing significant patient harm when used in error.

Contraindications Hypersensitivity to pancuronium, bromide, or any component of the formulation

Warnings/Precautions Ventilation must be supported during neuromuscular blockade; use with caution in patients with renal and/or hepatic impairment (adjust dose appropriately); certain clinical conditions may result in potentiation or antagonism of neuromuscular blockade:
- Potentiation: Electrolyte abnormalities, severe hyponatremia, severe hypocalcemia, severe hypokalemia, hypermagnesemia, neuromuscular diseases, acidosis, acute intermittent porphyria, renal failure, hepatic failure
- Antagonism: Alkalosis, hypercalcemia, demyelinating lesions, peripheral neuropathies, diabetes mellitus

Increased sensitivity in patients with myasthenia gravis, Eaton-Lambert syndrome; resistance in burn patients (>30% of body) for period of 5-70 days postinjury; resistance in patients with muscle trauma, denervation, immobilization, infection. Cross-sensitivity with other neuromuscular-blocking agents may occur; use extreme caution in patients with previous anaphylactic reactions. Use caution in the elderly. **[U.S. Boxed Warning]: Should be administered by adequately trained individuals familiar with its use.**

Adverse Reactions Frequency not defined.
- Cardiovascular: Elevation in pulse rate, elevated blood pressure and cardiac output, tachycardia, edema, skin flushing, circulatory collapse
- Dermatologic: Rash, itching, erythema, burning sensation along the vein
- Gastrointestinal: Excessive salivation
- Neuromuscular & skeletal: Profound muscle weakness
- Respiratory: Wheezing, bronchospasm

Miscellaneous: Hypersensitivity reaction

Postmarketing and/or case reports: Acute quadriplegic myopathy syndrome (prolonged use), myositis ossificans (prolonged use)

Drug Interactions

Avoid Concomitant Use There are no known interactions where it is recommended to avoid concomitant use.

Increased Effect/Toxicity

Pancuronium may increase the levels/effects of: Botulinum Toxin Type A; Botulinum Toxin Type B; Cardiac Glycosides; Corticosteroids (Systemic)

The levels/effects of Pancuronium may be increased by: Aminoglycosides; Calcium Channel Blockers; Capreomycin; Colistimethate; Inhalational Anesthetics; Ketorolac; Lincosamide Antibiotics; Lithium; Loop Diuretics; Magnesium Salts; Polymyxin B; Procainamide; QuiNIDine; Tetracycline Derivatives; Vancomycin

Decreased Effect

The levels/effects of Pancuronium may be decreased by: Acetylcholinesterase Inhibitors; Loop Diuretics

Stability Refrigerate; however, stable for up to 6 months at room temperature.

Mechanism of Action Blocks neural transmission at the myoneural junction by binding with cholinergic receptor sites

Pharmacodynamics/Kinetics

Onset of effect: Peak effect: I.V.: 2-3 minutes

Duration (dose dependent): 60-100 minutes

Metabolism: Hepatic (30% to 45%); active metabolite 3-hydroxypancuronium (1/3 to 1/2 the activity of parent drug)

Half-life elimination: 110 minutes

Excretion: Urine (55% to 70% as unchanged drug)

Dosage Administer I.V.; dose to effect; doses will vary due to interpatient variability; use ideal body weight for obese patients

Surgery:

Neonates <1 month:

Test dose: 0.02 mg/kg to measure responsiveness

Initial: 0.03 mg/kg/dose repeated twice at 5- to 10-minute intervals as needed; maintenance: 0.03-0.09 mg/kg/dose every 30 minutes to 4 hours as needed

Infants >1 month, Children, and Adults: Initial: 0.06-0.1 mg/kg or 0.05 mg/kg after initial dose of succinylcholine for intubation; maintenance dose: 0.01 mg/kg 60-100 minutes after initial dose and then 0.01 mg/kg every 25-60 minutes

Pretreatment/priming: 10% of intubating dose given 3-5 minutes before initial dose

ICU: 0.05-0.1 mg/kg bolus followed by 0.8-1.7 mcg/kg/minute once initial recovery from bolus observed or 0.1-0.2 mg/kg every 1-3 hours

Dosing adjustment in renal impairment: Elimination half-life is doubled, plasma clearance is reduced and rate of recovery is sometimes much slower

Cl_{cr} 10-50 mL/minute: Administer 50% of normal dose

Cl_{cr} <10 mL/minute: Do not use

Dosing adjustment/comments in hepatic/biliary tract disease: Elimination half-life is doubled, plasma clearance is reduced, recovery time is prolonged, volume of distribution is increased (50%) and results in a slower onset, higher total initial dosage and prolongation of neuromuscular blockade

Administration May be administered undiluted by rapid I.V. injection

Monitoring Parameters Heart rate, blood pressure, assisted ventilation status; cardiac monitor, blood pressure monitor, and ventilator required

Additional Information Pancuronium is classified as a long-duration neuromuscular-blocking agent. Neuromuscular blockade will be prolonged in patients with decreased renal function. Pancuronium does not relieve pain or produce sedation. It may produce cumulative effect on duration of blockade. It produces tachycardia secondary to vagolytic activity and sympathetic stimulation.

Dosage Forms Excipient information presented when available (limited, particularly for generics); consult specific product labeling.

Injection, solution, as bromide: 1 mg/mL (10 mL); 2 mg/mL (2 mL, 5 mL) [may contain benzyl alcohol]

- **Pancuronium Bromide** *see* Pancuronium *on page 1137*
- **Pancuronium Bromide® (Can)** *see* Pancuronium *on page 1137*
- **Pandel®** *see* Hydrocortisone *on page 743*
- **Pangestyme™ CN** *see* Pancrelipase *on page 1136*
- **Pangestyme™ EC** *see* Pancrelipase *on page 1136*
- **Pangestyme™ MT** *see* Pancrelipase *on page 1136*
- **Pangestyme™ UL** *see* Pancrelipase *on page 1136*
- **Panglobulin® NF [DSC]** *see* Immune Globulin (Intravenous) *on page 777*

Panitumumab (pan i TOOM yoo mab)

U.S. Brand Names Vectibix®

Canadian Brand Names Vectibix®

Index Terms ABX-EGF; NSC-742319; rHuMAb-EGFr

Pharmacologic Category Antineoplastic Agent, Monoclonal Antibody; Epidermal Growth Factor Receptor (EGFR) Inhibitor

Use Monotherapy in treatment of refractory metastatic colorectal cancer

Pregnancy Risk Factor C

Pregnancy Considerations Animal reproductive studies have demonstrated adverse fetal effects. Based on animal studies, panitumumab may disrupt normal menstrual cycles. There are no adequate and well-controlled studies in pregnant women. IgG is known to cross the placenta; therefore, it is possible the developing fetus may be exposed to panitumumab. Because panitumumab inhibits epidermal growth factor (EGF), a component of fetal development, adverse effects on pregnancy would be expected. Panitumumab should only be given to a pregnant woman if the potential benefit justifies the potential risk to the fetus. Women of childbearing potential should use effective contraception during and for 6 months after treatment. Women who become pregnant during panitumumab treatment are encouraged to enroll in Amgen's Pregnancy Surveillance Program (1-800-772-6436).

Lactation Excretion in breast milk unknown/not recommended

Contraindications There are no contraindications listed in manufacturer's labeling.

Warnings/Precautions [U.S. Boxed Warning]: Dermatologic toxicities have been reported in ~90% of patients (severe in 12% of patients); may include dermatitis acneiform, pruritus, erythema, rash, skin exfoliation, paronychia, dry skin and skin fissures. Severe skin toxicities may be complicated by infection, sepsis, or abscesses. The median time to development of skin (or ocular) toxicity was 2 weeks, with resolution ~7 weeks after discontinuation. Withhold treatment (and monitor) for severe or life-threatening dermatologic toxicities; may require dose reduction or permanent discontinuation. The severity of dermatologic toxicity is predictive for response; grades 2-4 skin toxicity correlates with improved progression free survival and overall survival, compared to grade 1 skin toxicity (Van Cutsem, 2007). Patients should minimize sunlight exposure; may exacerbate skin reactions. Gastric mucosal, ocular and nail toxicities have also been reported.

[U.S. Boxed Warning]: Severe infusion reactions (anaphylactic reaction, bronchospasm, fever, chills, and hypotension) have been reported in ~1% of patients. Discontinue infusion for severe reactions; permanently discontinue in patients with persistent severe infusion reactions. Appropriate medical support for the management of infusion reactions should be readily available. Mild to moderate infusion reactions are managed by slowing the infusion rate.

Pulmonary fibrosis has been reported (rarely); permanently discontinue treatment if interstitial lung disease, pneumonitis or lung infiltrates develop. Use caution with lung disease; patients with underlying lung disease were excluded from clinical trials. May cause diarrhea; the incidence and severity of chemotherapy-induced diarrhea and other toxicities (rash, electrolyte abnormalities, stomatitis) is increased with combination chemotherapy; combined use with chemotherapy regimens is not recommended. In addition to increased toxicity, studies using panitumumab in combination with chemotherapy (with or without bevacizumab) resulted in decreased progression-free survival compared to regimens without panitumumab; therefore, not indicated for use in combination with chemotherapy. Electrolyte depletion may occur during treatment and after treatment is discontinued; monitor for hypomagnesemia and hypocalcemia. Safety and efficacy in children have not been established.

Adverse Reactions

>10%:

Cardiovascular: Peripheral edema (12%)

Central nervous system: Fatigue (26%)

Dermatologic: Skin toxicity (90%; grades 3/4: 16%), erythema (65%; grades 3/4: 5%), acneiform rash (57%; grades 3/4: 7%), pruritus (57%; grades 3/4: 2%), exfoliation (25%; grades 3/4: 2%), paronychia (25%), rash (22%; grades 3/4: 1%), fissures (20%; grades 3/4: 1%), acne (13%; grades 3/4: 1%)

Endocrine & metabolic: Hypomagnesemia (38%; grades 3/4: 4%)

Gastrointestinal: Abdominal pain (25%), nausea (23%), diarrhea (21%; grades 3/4: 2%), constipation (21%), vomiting (19%)

Respiratory: Cough (14%)

1% to 10%:

Dermatologic: Dry skin (10%), nail disorder (other than paronychia: 9%)

Gastrointestinal: Stomatitis (7%), mucositis (6%)

Ocular: Eyelash growth (6%), conjunctivitis (4%), ocular hyperemia (3%), lacrimation increased (2%), eye/eye lid irritation (1%)

Miscellaneous: Antibody formation (≤5%), infusion reactions (3%; grades 3/4: 1%)

<1% (Limited to important or life-threatening): Allergic reaction, anaphylactoid reaction, chills, dyspnea, fever, hypocalcemia, hypoxia, pulmonary embolism, pulmonary fibrosis, pulmonary infiltrate

Drug Interactions

Avoid Concomitant Use There are no known interactions where it is recommended to avoid concomitant use.

Increased Effect/Toxicity There are no known significant interactions involving an increase in effect.

Decreased Effect There are no known significant interactions involving a decrease in effect.

Stability Store unopened vials under refrigeration at 2°C to 8°C (36°F to 46°F). Do not freeze; do not shake; protect from light. Dilute in 100-150 mL of normal saline to a final concentration of ≤10 mg/mL. Do not shake, invert gently to mix. Preparations in infusion containers are stable for 24 hours under refrigeration at 2°C to 8°C (36°F to 46°F) or for 6 hours at room temperature (do not freeze).

Mechanism of Action Recombinant human IgG2 monoclonal antibody which binds specifically to the epidermal growth factor receptor (EGFR, HER1, c-ErbB-1) and competitively inhibits the binding of epidermal growth factor (EGF) and other ligands. Binding to the EGFR blocks phosphorylation and activation of intracellular tyrosine kinases, resulting in inhibition of cell survival, growth, proliferation and transformation.

Pharmacodynamics/Kinetics Half-life elimination: ~7.5 days (range: 4-11 days)

Dosage I.V.: Adults: Metastatic colorectal cancer: 6 mg/kg every 2 weeks

Dosing adjustment for toxicity:

Infusion reactions, mild-to-moderate (grade 1 or 2): Reduce the infusion rate by 50% for the duration of infusion

Infusion reactions, severe (grade 3 or 4): Immediately and permanently discontinue treatment

Dermatologic toxicity (grade 3 or 4, or intolerable): Withhold treatment; if skin toxicity does not improve to ≤ grade 2 within 1 month, permanently discontinue. If skin toxicity improves to ≤ grade 2 within 1 month (with patient missing ≤2 doses), resume treatment at 50% of the original dose. Dose may be increased in increments of 25% of the original dose (up to 6 mg/kg) if skin toxicities do not recur. For recurrent skin toxicity, permanently discontinue.

Dosage adjustment in renal impairment: Has not been studied

Dosage adjustment in hepatic impairment: Has not been studied

Administration Doses ≤1000 mg, infuse over 1 hour; doses >1000 mg, infuse over 90 minutes; reduce infusion rate by 50% for mild-to-moderate infusion reactions; discontinue for severe infusion reactions. Administer through a low protein-binding 0.2 or 0.22 micrometer in-line filter. Flush with NS before and after infusion.

Monitoring Parameters KRAS genotyping of tumor tissue. Monitor serum electrolytes, including magnesium and calcium (periodically during and for at least 8 weeks after therapy). Monitor vital signs and temperature before, during, and after infusion. Monitor for skin toxicity.

Additional Information Oncology Comment: The National Comprehensive Cancer Network® (NCCN) guidelines for colon cancer (v.4.2008) recommend genotyping tumor tissue for KRAS mutation in all patients with metastatic colorectal cancer (genotyping may be done on archived specimens). Patients with known codon 12 or 13 KRAS gene mutations are unlikely to respond to EGFR inhibitors and should not receive panitumumab. Favorable progression-free survival and higher response rates have been demonstrated with panitumumab in patients with KRAS wild-type; patients with the KRAS mutation did not respond to panitumumab (Amado, 2008). Because EGFR testing in colorectal tumors does not correlate with response, the NCCN guidelines do not recommend routine EGFR testing in colorectal cancer. Severity of dermatologic toxicity associated with panitumumab is predictive for response; grades 2-4 skin toxicity correlates with improved progression free survival and overall survival, compared to patients with grade 1 skin toxicity (Van Cutsem, 2007). The NCCN guidelines do not recommend the use of panitumumab after failure of cetuximab therapy.

Dosage Forms Excipient information presented when available (limited, particularly for generics); consult specific product labeling.

Injection, solution [preservative free]:

Vectibix®: 20 mg/mL (5 mL, 10 mL, 20 mL)

- **Panocaps [DSC]** *see* Pancrelipase *on page 1136*
- **Panocaps MT [DSC]** *see* Pancrelipase *on page 1136*
- **Panokase® [DSC]** *see* Pancrelipase *on page 1136*
- **Panokase® 16 [DSC]** *see* Pancrelipase *on page 1136*
- **Panretin®** *see* Alitretinoin *on page 64*
- **Panto™ I.V. (Can)** *see* Pantoprazole *on page 1140*

- **Pantoloc® (Can)** *see* Pantoprazole *on page 1140*
- **Pantoloc® M (Can)** *see* Pantoprazole *on page 1140*

Pantoprazole (pan TOE pra zole)

U.S. Brand Names Protonix®

Canadian Brand Names Apo-Pantoprazole; Co-Pantoprazole; Gen-Pantoprazole; Novo-Pantoprazole; Pantoloc®; Pantoloc® M; Panto™ I.V.; PMS-Pantoprazole; Protonix®; Ran-Pantoprazole; Ratio-Pantoprazole; Riva-Pantoprazole; Sandoz-Pantoprazole; Tecta™

Pharmacologic Category Proton Pump Inhibitor; Substituted Benzimidazole

Use

Oral: Treatment and maintenance of healing of erosive esophagitis associated with GERD; reduction in relapse rates of daytime and nighttime heartburn symptoms in GERD; hypersecretory disorders associated with Zollinger-Ellison syndrome or other GI hypersecretory disorders

I.V.: Short-term treatment (7-10 days) of patients with gastroesophageal reflux disease (GERD) and a history of erosive esophagitis; hypersecretory disorders associated with Zollinger-Ellison syndrome or other neoplastic disorders

Unlabeled/Investigational Use Peptic ulcer disease, active ulcer bleeding (parenteral formulation); adjunct treatment with antibiotics for *Helicobacter pylori* eradication; stress-ulcer prophylaxis in the critically-ill

Pregnancy Risk Factor B

Pregnancy Considerations Teratogenic effects were not observed in animal studies. There are no adequate and well-controlled studies in pregnant women. Use in pregnancy only if clearly needed.

Lactation Enters breast milk/not recommended

Medication Safety Issues

Sound-alike/look-alike issues:

Protonix® may be confused with Lotronex®, Lovenox®, protamine

Vials containing Protonix® I.V. for injection are not recommended for use with spiked I.V. system adaptors. Nurses and pharmacists have reported breakage of the glass vials during attempts to connect spiked I.V. system adaptors, which may potentially result in injury to healthcare professionals.

International issues:

Protonix® may be confused with Pretanix® which is a brand name for indapamide in Hungary

Contraindications Hypersensitivity to pantoprazole, substituted benzamidazoles (eg, esomeprazole, lansoprazole, omeprazole, rabeprazole), or any component of the formulation

Warnings/Precautions Use of proton pump inhibitors may increase the risk of gastrointestinal infections (eg, *Salmonella, Campylobacter*). Relief of symptoms does not preclude the presence of a gastric malignancy. Long-term pantoprazole therapy (especially in patients who were *H. pylori* positive) has caused biopsy-proven atrophic gastritis. No reports of enterochromaffin-like (ECL) cell carcinoids, dysplasia, or neoplasia such as those seen in rodent studies have occurred in humans. Not indicated for maintenance therapy; safety and efficacy for use beyond 16 weeks have not been established. Prolonged treatment (typically >3 years) may lead to vitamin B_{12} malabsorption and subsequent deficiency. Intravenous preparation contains edetate sodium (EDTA); use caution in patients who are at risk for zinc deficiency if other EDTA-containing solutions are coadministered.

Adverse Reactions

≥1%:

Cardiovascular: Chest pain

Central nervous system: Headache (2% to 9%), insomnia (≤1%), anxiety, dizziness, migraine, pain

Dermatologic: Rash (≤2%)

Endocrine & metabolic: Hyperglycemia (≤1%), hyperlipidemia

Gastrointestinal: Diarrhea (2% to 6%), flatulence (2% to 4%), abdominal pain (1% to 4%), nausea (≤2%), vomiting (≤2%), eructation (≤1%), constipation, dyspepsia, gastroenteritis, rectal disorder

Genitourinary: Urinary frequency, UTI

Hepatic: Liver function tests abnormal (≤2%)

Local: Injection site reaction (includes thrombophlebitis and abscess)

Neuromuscular & skeletal: Arthralgia, back pain, hypertonia, neck pain, weakness

Respiratory: Bronchitis, cough, dyspnea, pharyngitis, rhinitis, sinusitis, upper respiratory tract infection

Miscellaneous: Flu syndrome, infection

<1% (Limited to important or life-threatening): Abnormal dreams, acne, albuminuria, alkaline phosphatase increased, allergic reaction, alopecia, anaphylaxis, anemia, angioedema, angina pectoris, anorexia, aphthous stomatitis, appetite increased, arrhythmia, asthma exacerbation, atrial fibrillation/flutter, atrophic gastritis, balanitis, biliary pain, blurred vision, bone pain, breast pain, bursitis, cataract, CHF, chills, cholecystitis, cholelithiasis, CPK increased, colitis, confusion, contact dermatitis, creatinine increased, cystitis, deafness, decreased reflexes, dehydration, depression, diabetes mellitus, diaphoresis, diplopia, duodenitis, dysarthria, dysmenorrhea, dysphagia, dysuria, ecchymosis, ECG abnormality, eczema, eosinophilia, epididymitis, epistaxis, erythema multiforme, esophagitis, extraocular palsy, facial edema, fever, fungal dermatitis, gastrointestinal carcinoma, gastrointestinal hemorrhage, gastrointestinal moniliasis, generalized edema, GGT increased, gingivitis, glaucoma, glossitis, glycosuria, goiter, gout, halitosis, hallucinations, heat stroke, hematemesis, hematuria, hemorrhage, hepatic failure, hepatitis, hernia, herpes simplex, herpes zoster, hiccup, hyperbilirubinemia, hyperesthesia, hyper-/hypotension, hyperkinesia, hyperuricemia, hypokinesia, impaired urination, impotence, interstitial nephritis, jaundice, kidney calculus, kidney pain, laryngitis, leg cramps, leukocytosis, leukopenia, libido decreased, lichenoid dermatitis, maculopapular rash, malaise, melena, mouth ulceration, myalgia, myocardial infarction, myocardial ischemia, neoplasm, nervousness, neuralgia, neuritis, nocturia, optic neuropathy (including anterior ischemic), otitis externa, palpitation, pancreatitis, pancytopenia, paresthesia, periodontal abscess, periodontitis, photosensitivity, pneumonia, pruritus, pyelonephritis, rectal hemorrhage, retinal vascular disorder, rhabdomyolysis, salivation increased, scrotal edema, seizure, skin ulcer, somnolence, Stevens-Johnson syndrome, stomach ulcer, stomatitis, syncope, tachycardia, taste perversion, tenosynovitis, thrombocytopenia, thrombosis, tinnitus, tongue discoloration, toxic epidermal necrolysis, tremor, urethral pain, urethritis, urticaria, vaginitis, vasodilation, vertigo, vision abnormal, weight changes, xerostomia

Drug Interactions

Metabolism/Transport Effects Substrate of CYP2C19 (major), 2C9 (minor), 2D6 (minor), 3A4 (minor); **Inhibits** 2C9 (weak); **Induces** CYP1A2 (weak), 3A4 (weak)

Avoid Concomitant Use

Avoid concomitant use of Pantoprazole with any of the following: Erlotinib; Mesalamine; Nelfinavir

Increased Effect/Toxicity

Pantoprazole may increase the levels/effects of: Methotrexate; Saquinavir; Topotecan; Voriconazole

The levels/effects of Pantoprazole may be increased by: Fluconazole; Ketoconazole

Decreased Effect

Pantoprazole may decrease the levels/effects of: Atazanavir; Clopidogrel; Dabigatran Etexilate; Dasatinib; Erlotinib; Indinavir; Iron Salts; Itraconazole; Ketoconazole; Mesalamine; Mycophenolate; Nelfinavir

The levels/effects of Pantoprazole may be decreased by: CYP2C19 Inducers (Strong); Tipranavir

Ethanol/Nutrition/Herb Interactions

Ethanol: Avoid ethanol (may cause gastric mucosal irritation).

Herb/Nutraceutical: Prolonged treatment (typically >3 years) may lead to vitamin B_{12} malabsorption and subsequent deficiency.

Stability

Oral: Store tablet and oral suspension at controlled room temperature of 20°C to 25°C (68°F to 77°F).

I.V.: Prior to reconstitution, store at controlled room temperature of 20°C to 25°C (68°F to 77°F). Protect from light. Reconstitute with 10 mL NS (final concentration 4 mg/mL). Reconstituted solution may be given intravenously (over 2 minutes) or may be added to 100 mL D_5W, NS, or LR (for 15-minute infusion). When reconstituted, solution is stable up to 96 hours at room temperature (Johnson, 2005). The preparation should be stored at 3°C to 5°C (37°F to 41°F) if it is stored beyond 48 hours to minimize discoloration. If further diluting in 100 mL of D_5W, LR, or NS, dilute within 6 hours of reconstitution. Diluted solution is stable at room temperature for up to 24 hours from the time of initial reconstitution; protection from light is not required.

Mechanism of Action Suppresses gastric acid secretion by inhibiting the parietal cell H^+/K^+ ATP pump

Pharmacodynamics/Kinetics

Absorption: Rapid, well absorbed

Distribution: V_d: 11-24 L

Protein binding: 98%, primarily to albumin

Metabolism: Extensively hepatic; CYP2C19 (demethylation), CYP3A4; no evidence that metabolites have pharmacologic activity

Bioavailability: 77%

Half-life elimination: 1 hour; increased to 3.5-10 hours with CYP2C19 deficiency

Time to peak: Oral: 2.5 hours

Excretion: Urine (71%); feces (18%)

Dosage

Oral:

Children ≥5 years (unlabeled use): GERD, erosive esophagitis associated with GERD: 20-40 mg once daily

Adults:

Erosive esophagitis associated with GERD:

Treatment: 40 mg once daily for up to 8 weeks; an additional 8 weeks may be used in patients who have not healed after an 8-week course

Maintenance of healing: 40 mg once daily

Note: Lower doses (20 mg once daily) have been used successfully in mild GERD treatment and maintenance of healing

Hypersecretory disorders (including Zollinger-Ellison): Initial: 40 mg twice daily; adjust dose based on patient needs; doses up to 240 mg/day have been administered

Helicobacter pylori eradication (unlabeled use): Doses up to 40 mg twice daily have been used as part of combination therapy

I.V.:

Erosive esophagitis associated with GERD: 40 mg once daily for 7-10 days

Hypersecretory disorders: 80 mg twice daily; adjust dose based on acid output measurements; 160-240 mg/day in divided doses has been used for a limited period (up to 7 days)

Prevention of rebleeding in peptic ulcer bleed (unlabeled use): 80 mg, followed by 8 mg/hour infusion for 72 hours. **Note:** A daily infusion of 40 mg does not raise gastric pH sufficiently to enhance coagulation in active GI bleeds.

Elderly: Dosage adjustment not required

Dosage adjustment in renal impairment: Not required; pantoprazole is not removed by hemodialysis

Dosage adjustment in hepatic impairment: Not required

Dietary Considerations

Oral: May be taken with or without food; best if taken before breakfast.

I.V.: Due to EDTA in preparation, zinc supplementation may be needed in patients prone to zinc deficiency.

Administration

I.V.: Flush I.V. line before and after administration. In-line filter not required.

2-minute infusion: The volume of reconstituted solution (4 mg/mL) to be injected may be administered intravenously over at least 2 minutes.

15-minute infusion: Infuse over 15 minutes at a rate not to exceed 7 mL/minute (3 mg/minute).

Oral:

Tablet: Should be swallowed whole, do not crush or chew. Best if taken before breakfast.

Delayed-release oral suspension: Should only be administered in apple juice or applesauce and taken ~30 minutes before a meal. Do not administer with any other liquid (eg, water) or foods.

Oral administration in **applesauce**: Sprinkle intact granules on 1 tablespoon of applesauce and swallow within 10 minutes of preparation.

Oral administration in **apple juice**: Empty intact granules into 5 mL of apple juice (~1 teaspoonful), stir for 5 seconds, and swallow immediately after preparation. Rinse container once or twice with apple juice and swallow immediately.

Nasogastric tube administration: Separate the plunger from the barrel of a 60 mL catheter tip syringe and connect to a ≥16 French nasogastric tube. Holding the syringe attached to the tubing as high as possible, empty the contents of the packet into barrel of the syringe, add 10 mL of apple juice and gently tap/shake the barrel of the syringe to help empty the syringe. Add an additional 10 mL of apple juice and gently tap/shake the barrel to help rinse. Repeat rinse with at least 2 -10 mL aliquots of apple juice. No granules should remain in the syringe.

Monitoring Parameters Hypersecretory disorders: Acid output measurements, target level <10 mEq/hour (<5 mEq/hour if prior gastric acid-reducing surgery)

Test Interactions False-positive urine screening tests for tetrahydrocannabinol (THC) have been noted in patients receiving proton pump inhibitors, including pantoprazole.

Dosage Forms Excipient information presented when available (limited, particularly for generics); consult specific product labeling. [CAN] = Canadian brand name

Note: Strength expressed as base

Granules for suspension, delayed release, enteric coated, as sodium, oral:

Protonix®: 40 mg/packet (30s)

Injection, powder for reconstitution, as sodium:

Protonix®: 40 mg [contains edetate sodium 1 mg]

Tablet, delayed release, as sodium: 20 mg, 40 mg

Protonix®: 20 mg, 40 mg

Tablet, enteric coated, as magnesium:

Pantoloc® M [CAN]: 40 mg [not available in the U.S.]

Extemporaneous Preparations A 2 mg/mL pantoprazole oral liquid can be prepared with twenty pantoprazole 40 mg tablets, 340 mL sterile water, and 33.6 g of sodium bicarbonate powder. Remove the Protonix® imprint from each of the tablets on a paper towel dampened with ethanol (improves the look of product). Let tablets air dry.

Grind the tablets into a coarse powder, transfer to a 600 mL beaker and add 340 mL of sterile water for irrigation and place beaker on a magnetic stirrer. Add 16.8 g of sodium bicarbonate powder and stir for about 20 minutes until the tablet remnants have disintegrated. While stirring, add another 16.8 g of sodium bicarbonate powder and stir for about 5 minutes until powder has dissolved. Add enough sterile water for irrigation to bring the final volume to 400 mL. Mix well. Transfer to amber-colored bottle. Stable for 62 days under refrigeration. Shake well before use.

Dentinger PJ, Swenson CF, and Anaizi NH, "Stability of Pantoprazole in an Extemporaneously Compounded Oral Liquid," *Am J Health Syst Pharm*, 2002, 59:953-6.

◆ **Pantothenyl Alcohol** *see* Dexpanthenol *on page 430*

Papain and Urea (pa PAY in & yoor EE a)

U.S. Brand Names Accuzyme®; Accuzyme® SE; AllanEnzyme; Ethezyme™ 650 [DSC]; Ethezyme™ 830 [DSC]; Ethezyme™ [DSC]; Kovia®; Paptase™

Pharmacologic Category Enzyme, Topical Debridement

Use Debridement of necrotic tissue and liquefaction of slough in acute and chronic lesions such as pressure ulcers, varicose and diabetic ulcers, burns, postoperative wounds, pilonidal cyst wounds, carbuncles, and miscellaneous traumatic or infected wounds

Dosage Topical: Adults: Apply with each dressing change. Daily or twice daily dressing changes are preferred, but may be every 2-3 days. Cover with dressing following application.

Ointment: Apply 1/8-inch thickness over the wound with clean applicator.

Spray: Completely cover the wound site so that the wound is not visible.

Additional Information Complete prescribing information for this medication should be consulted for additional detail.

Dosage Forms Excipient information presented when available (limited, particularly for generics); consult specific product labeling. [DSC] = Discontinued product

Aerosol, topical:

Paptase™: Papain 8.3 x 10^5 units/g and urea 10% (45 g)

Emulsion, topical [spray]:

Accuzyme® SE: Papain 8.3 x 10^5 units/g and urea 10% (34 mL)

Ointment, topical:

Accuzyme®: Papain 8.3 x 10^5 units/g and urea 10% (6 g, 30 g)

AllanEnzyme: Papain 8.3 x 10^5 units/g and urea 10% (30 g)

Ethezyme™: Papain 1.1 x 10^6 units and urea 10% (30 g) [DSC]

Ethezyme™ 650: Papain 6.5 x 10^5 units/g and urea 10% (30 g) [DSC]

Ethezyme™ 830: Papain 8.3 x 10^5 units/g and urea 10% (30 g) [DSC]

Kovia®: Papain 8.3 x 10^5 units/g and urea 10% (3.5 g) [single-dose packet]; 30 g

Solution, topical [spray]:

AllanEnzyme: Papain 8.3 x 10^5 units/g and urea 10% (33 mL)

◆ **Papain, Urea, and Chlorophyllin** *see* Chlorophyllin, Papain, and Urea *on page 306*

Papaverine (pa PAV er een)

U.S. Brand Names Para-Time SR®

Index Terms Papaverine Hydrochloride; Pavabid [DSC]

Pharmacologic Category Vasodilator

Use Oral: Relief of peripheral and cerebral ischemia associated with arterial spasm and myocardial ischemia complicated by arrhythmias

Unlabeled/Investigational Use Investigational: Parenteral: Various vascular spasms associated with muscle spasms as in myocardial infarction, angina, peripheral and pulmonary embolism, peripheral vascular disease, angiospastic states, and visceral spasm (ureteral, biliary, and GI colic); testing for impotence

Pregnancy Risk Factor C

Dosage

I.M., I.V.:

Children: 6 mg/kg/day in 4 divided doses

Adults: 30-65 mg (rarely up to 120 mg); may repeat every 3 hours

Oral, sustained release: Adults: 150-300 mg every 12 hours; in difficult cases: 150 mg every 8 hours

Additional Information Complete prescribing information for this medication should be consulted for additional detail.

Dosage Forms Excipient information presented when available (limited, particularly for generics); consult specific product labeling.

Capsule, sustained release, as hydrochloride: 150 mg

Para-Time SR®: 150 mg

Injection, solution, as hydrochloride: 30 mg/mL (2 mL, 10 mL)

◆ **Papaverine Hydrochloride** *see* Papaverine *on page 1142*

◆ **Papfyll™** *see* Chlorophyllin, Papain, and Urea *on page 306*

Papillomavirus (Types 6, 11, 16, 18) Vaccine (Human, Recombinant)

(pap ih LO ma VYE rus typs six e LEV en SIX teen AYE teen vak SEEN YU man ree KOM be nant)

U.S. Brand Names Gardasil®

Canadian Brand Names Gardasil®

Index Terms HPV Vaccine; Human Papillomavirus Vaccine; Papillomavirus Vaccine, Recombinant; Quadrivalent Human Papillomavirus Vaccine

Pharmacologic Category Vaccine, Inactivated (Viral)

Additional Appendix Information

Immunization Recommendations *on page 1708*

Use Females: Prevention of cervical, vulvar, and vaginal cancer, genital warts, cervical adenocarcinoma *in situ*, and vulvar, vaginal, or cervical intraepithelial neoplasia caused by human papillomavirus (HPV) types 6, 11, 16, 18

The Advisory Committee on Immunization Practices (ACIP) recommends routine vaccination for females 11-12 years of age; catch-up vaccination is recommended for females 13-26 years of age

Pregnancy Risk Factor B

Pregnancy Considerations Teratogenic effects were not observed in animal studies. Administration of the vaccine in pregnancy is not recommended. In clinical trials, women who were found to be pregnant before the completion of the 3-dose regimen were instructed to defer any remaining dose until pregnancy resolution. Pregnancies detected within 30 days of vaccination had a higher rate of congenital anomalies (pyloric stenosis, congenital megacolon, congenital hydronephrosis, hip dysplasia, club foot) than the placebo group. Pregnancies with onset beyond 30 days of vaccination had a rate of congenital anomalies consistent with the general population. Overall, the type of teratogenic events were the same as those generally observed for this age group. A registry has been established for women exposed to the HPV vaccine during pregnancy (1-800-986-8999).

Lactation Excretion in breast milk unknown/use caution

Contraindications Hypersensitivity to papillomavirus recombinant vaccine or any component of the formulation

Warnings/Precautions Immediate treatment for anaphylactoid reaction should be available during vaccine use. There is no evidence that individuals already infected with HPV will be protected; those already infected with 1 or more HPV types were protected from disease in the remaining HPV types. Not for the treatment of active disease; will not protect against diseases not caused by human papillomavirus (HPV) vaccine types 6, 11, 16, and 18. May administer with mild concurrent febrile illness; consider deferring vaccination with serious illness. Immunocompromised patients may have a reduced response to vaccination. Administered I.M., therefore use caution in patients at risk for bleeding. The entire 3-dose regimen should be completed for maximum efficacy. Not recommended for use during pregnancy. Syncope may occur following vaccination; observe for 15 minutes following administration. Safety and efficacy in girls <9 years of age or women >26 years have not been established. Safety and efficacy have not been established in males. Product may contain yeast. In order to maximize vaccination rates, the ACIP recommends simultaneous administration of all age-appropriate vaccines (live or inactivated) for which a person is eligible at a single clinic visit, unless contraindications exist.

Adverse Reactions All serious adverse reactions must be reported to the U.S. Department of Health and Human Services (DHHS) Vaccine Adverse Event Reporting System (VAERS) 1-800-822-7967.

>10%:

Central nervous system: Fever (13%)

Local: Injection site: Pain (84%), swelling (25%), erythema (25%)

1% to 10%:

Central nervous system: Dizziness (4%), malaise (1%), insomnia (1%)

Gastrointestinal: Nausea (7%), diarrhea (4%), vomiting (2%), toothache (2%)

Local: Injection site: Bruising (3%), pruritus (3%)

Neuromuscular & skeletal: Arthralgia (1%)

Respiratory: Cough (2%), nasal congestion (1%)

<1% (Limited to important or life-threatening): Anaphylactic/anaphylactoid reaction, appendicitis, arrhythmia, arthritis, asthma, autoimmune hemolytic anemia, bronchospasm, DVT, fatigue, gastroenteritis, Guillain-Barré syndrome, headache, hypersensitivity reaction, hyperthyroidism, JRA, lymphadenopathy, motor neuron disease, myalgia, pancreatitis, paralysis, pelvic inflammatory disease, pulmonary embolus, RA, renal failure (acute), seizure, sepsis, syncope, transverse myelitis, urticaria, weakness

Drug Interactions

Avoid Concomitant Use There are no known interactions where it is recommended to avoid concomitant use.

Increased Effect/Toxicity There are no known significant interactions involving an increase in effect.

Decreased Effect

The levels/effects of Papillomavirus (Types 6, 11, 16, 18) Vaccine (Human, Recombinant) may be decreased by: Immunosuppressants

Stability Store at 2°C to 8°C (36°F to 46°F); do not freeze. Protect from light.

Mechanism of Action Contains inactive human papillomavirus (HPV) proteins HPV 6 L1, HPV 11 L1, HPV 16 L1, and HPV 18 L1 which produce neutralizing antibodies to prevent cervical cancer, cervical adenocarcinoma, cervical, vaginal and vulvar neoplasia and genital warts caused by HPV.

Dosage I.M.: Females: Children ≥9 years and Adults ≤26 years: 0.5 mL followed by 0.5 mL at 2 and 6 months after initial dose

CDC recommended immunization schedule: Administer first dose to females at age 11-12 years; begin series in females aged 13-26 years if not previously vaccinated. Minimum interval between first and second doses is 4 weeks; the minimum interval between first and third doses is 24 weeks.

Administration Shake suspension well before use. Inject I.M. into the deltoid region of the upper arm or higher anterolateral thigh area. Observe for syncope for 15 minutes following administration.

Administration with other vaccines:

Papillomavirus (Types 6, 11, 16, 18) Recombinant vaccine with other inactivated vaccines: May be given simultaneously or at any interval between doses.

Papillomavirus (Types 6, 11, 16, 18) Recombinant vaccine with live vaccines: May be given simultaneously or at any interval between doses

Vaccine administration with antibody-containing products: Papillomavirus (Types 6, 11, 16, 18) Recombinant vaccine may be given simultaneously at different sites or at any interval between doses. Examples of antibody-containing products include I.M. and I.V. immune globulin, hepatitis B immune globulin, tetanus immune globulin, varicella zoster immune globulin, rabies immune globulin, whole blood, packed red cells, plasma, and platelet products

For patients at risk of hemorrhage following intramuscular injection, the ACIP recommends "it should be administered intramuscularly if, in the opinion of the physician familiar with the patients bleeding risk, the vaccine can be administered with reasonable safety by this route. If the patient receives antihemophilia or other similar therapy, intramuscular vaccination can be scheduled shortly after such therapy is administered. A fine needle (23 gauge or smaller) can be used for the vaccination and firm pressure applied to the site (without rubbing) for at least 2 minutes. The patient should be instructed concerning the risk of hematoma from the injection."

Monitoring Parameters Gynecologic screening exam, papillomavirus test; observe for syncope/fainting for ~15 minutes after administration of vaccine

Additional Information Federal law requires that the date of administration, the vaccine manufacturer, lot number of vaccine, and the administering person's name, title and address be entered into the patient's permanent medical record. Ideally, administration of vaccine should occur prior to potential HPV exposure. Benefits of vaccine decrease once infected with ≥1 of the HPV vaccine types.

Dosage Forms Excipient information presented when available (limited, particularly for generics); consult specific product labeling.

Injection, suspension [preservative free]:

Gardasil®: HPV 6 L1 protein 20 mcg, HPV 11 L1 protein 40 mcg, HPV 16 L1 protein 40 mcg, and HPV 18 L1 protein 20 mcg per 0.5 mL (0.5 mL) [contains aluminum, polysorbate 80; manufactured using *S. cerevisiae* (baker's yeast)]

- **Papillomavirus Vaccine, Recombinant** *see* Papillomavirus (Types 6, 11, 16, 18) Vaccine (Human, Recombinant) *on page 1142*
- **Paptase™** *see* Papain and Urea *on page 1142*
- **Para-Aminosalicylate Sodium** *see* Aminosalicylic Acid *on page 86*
- **Paracetamol** *see* Acetaminophen *on page 25*
- **Parafon Forte® (Can)** *see* Chlorzoxazone *on page 318*
- **Parafon Forte® DSC** *see* Chlorzoxazone *on page 318*
- **Paraplatin-AQ (Can)** *see* CARBOplatin *on page 258*
- **Parathyroid Hormone (1-34)** *see* Teriparatide *on page 1444*
- **Para-Time SR®** *see* Papaverine *on page 1142*

◆ **Parcaine™** *see* Proparacaine *on page 1253*

◆ **Parcopa™** *see* Carbidopa and Levodopa *on page 256*

Paregoric (par e GOR ik)

Index Terms Camphorated Tincture of Opium (error-prone synonym)

Pharmacologic Category Analgesic, Opioid

Use Treatment of diarrhea or relief of pain; neonatal opiate withdrawal

Restrictions C-III

Pregnancy Risk Factor B/D (prolonged use or high doses)

Lactation Enters breast milk/use caution

Medication Safety Issues

Sound-alike/look-alike issues:

Camphorated tincture of opium is an error-prone synonym (mistaken as opium tincture)

Paregoric may be confused with Percogesic®

High alert medication: The Institute for Safe Medication Practices (ISMP) includes this medication among its list of drug classes which have a heightened risk of causing significant patient harm when used in error.

Use care when prescribing opium tincture; each mL contains the equivalent of morphine 10 mg; paregoric contains the equivalent of morphine 0.4 mg/mL

Contraindications Hypersensitivity to opium or any component of the formulation; diarrhea caused by poisoning until the toxic material has been removed; pregnancy (prolonged use or high doses)

Warnings/Precautions May cause CNS depression, which may impair physical or mental abilities; patients must be cautioned about performing tasks which require mental alertness (eg, operating machinery or driving). Effects may be potentiated when used with other sedative drugs or ethanol. Use with caution in patients with respiratory, hepatic or renal dysfunction, adrenal insufficiency, morbid obesity, severe prostatic hyperplasia, urinary stricture, head trauma, thyroid dysfunction, seizure disorder, CNS depression/coma or history of narcotic abuse. Use with caution in patients with biliary tract dysfunction; acute pancreatitis may cause constriction of sphincter of Oddi. May obscure diagnosis or clinical course of patients with acute abdominal conditions. Opium shares the toxic potential of opiate agonists, and usual precautions of opiate agonist therapy should be observed; some preparations contain sulfites which may cause allergic reactions; infants <3 months of age are more susceptible to respiratory depression, use with caution and generally in reduced doses in this age group; tolerance or drug dependence may result from extended use. Concurrent use of agonist/antagonist analgesics may precipitate withdrawal symptoms and/or reduced analgesic efficacy in patients following prolonged therapy with mu opioid agonists. Abrupt discontinuation following prolonged use may also lead to withdrawal symptoms. Use with caution in the elderly and debilitated patients; may be more sensitive to adverse effects.

Adverse Reactions Frequency not defined.

Cardiovascular: Hypotension, peripheral vasodilation

Central nervous system: Drowsiness, dizziness, insomnia, CNS depression, mental depression, increased intracranial pressure, restlessness, headache, malaise

Gastrointestinal: Constipation, anorexia, stomach cramps, nausea, vomiting, biliary tract spasm

Genitourinary: Ureteral spasms, decreased urination, urinary tract spasm

Hepatic: Increased liver function tests

Neuromuscular & skeletal: Weakness

Ocular: Miosis

Respiratory: Respiratory depression

Miscellaneous: Physical and psychological dependence, histamine release

Drug Interactions

Avoid Concomitant Use There are no known interactions where it is recommended to avoid concomitant use.

Increased Effect/Toxicity

Paregoric may increase the levels/effects of: Alcohol (Ethyl); Alvimopan; CNS Depressants; Desmopressin; Selective Serotonin Reuptake Inhibitors

The levels/effects of Paregoric may be increased by: Amphetamines; Antipsychotic Agents (Phenothiazines); Succinylcholine

Decreased Effect

Paregoric may decrease the levels/effects of: Pegvisomant

The levels/effects of Paregoric may be decreased by: Ammonium Chloride

Ethanol/Nutrition/Herb Interactions Ethanol: Avoid ethanol (may increase CNS depression).

Stability Store in light-resistant, tightly-closed container.

Mechanism of Action Increases smooth muscle tone in GI tract, decreases motility and peristalsis, diminishes digestive secretions

Pharmacodynamics/Kinetics In terms of opium:

Metabolism: Hepatic

Excretion: Urine (primarily as morphine glucuronide conjugates and unchanged drug - morphine, codeine, papaverine, etc)

Dosage Oral:

Neonatal opiate withdrawal: 3-6 drops every 3-6 hours as needed, or initially 0.2 mL every 3 hours; increase dosage by approximately 0.05 mL every 3 hours until withdrawal symptoms are controlled; it is rare to exceed 0.7 mL/dose. Stabilize withdrawal symptoms for 3-5 days, then gradually decrease dosage over a 2- to 4-week period.

Children: 0.25-0.5 mL/kg 1-4 times/day

Adults: 5-10 mL 1-4 times/day

Additional Information Contains morphine 0.4 mg/mL and alcohol 45%. Do **not** confuse this product with opium tincture which is 25 times **more** potent; each 5 mL of paregoric contains 2 mg morphine equivalent, 0.02 mL anise oil, 20 mg benzoic acid, 20 mg camphor, 0.2 mL glycerin and alcohol; final alcohol content 45%; paregoric also contains papaverine and noscapine; because all of these additives may be harmful to neonates, **a 25-fold dilution of opium tincture** is often preferred for treatment of neonatal abstinence syndrome (opiate withdrawal).

Dosage Forms Excipient information presented when available (limited, particularly for generics); consult specific product labeling.

Liquid, oral: Morphine equivalent 2 mg/5 mL (473 mL) [equivalent to opium 20 mg powder; contains alcohol 45% and benzoic acid]

◆ **Parenteral Nutrition** *see* Total Parenteral Nutrition *on page 1495*

Paricalcitol (pah ri KAL si tole)

U.S. Brand Names Zemplar®

Canadian Brand Names Zemplar®

Pharmacologic Category Vitamin D Analog

Use

I.V.: Prevention and treatment of secondary hyperparathyroidism associated with stage 5 chronic kidney disease (CKD)

Oral: Prevention and treatment of secondary hyperparathyroidism associated with stage 3 and 4 CKD

Pregnancy Risk Factor C

Pregnancy Considerations

Teratogenic effects were not observed in animal studies. There are no adequate and well-controlled studies in pregnant women.

Lactation Excretion in breast milk unknown/not recommended

Contraindications Hypersensitivity to paricalcitol or any component of the formulation; patients with evidence of vitamin D toxicity; hypercalcemia

Warnings/Precautions Excessive administration may lead to over suppression of PTH, hypercalcemia, hypercalciuria, hyperphosphatemia and adynamic bone disease. Acute hypercalcemia may increase risk of cardiac arrhythmias and seizures; use caution with cardiac glycosides as digitalis toxicity may be increased. Chronic hypercalcemia may lead to generalized vascular and other soft-tissue calcification. Phosphate and vitamin D (and its derivatives) should be withheld during therapy to avoid hypercalcemia. Safety and efficacy have not been established in children for the oral formulation or in children <5 years of age for the I.V. formulation.

Adverse Reactions

>10%: Gastrointestinal: Nausea (6% to 13%)

1% to 10%:

Cardiovascular: Edema (7%), hypertension (7%), hypotension (5%), palpitation (3%), chest pain (3%), syncope (3%), cardiomyopathy (2%), MI (2%), postural hypotension (2%)

Central nervous system: Pain (8%), chills (5%), dizziness (5%), headache (5%), lightheadedness (5%), vertigo (5%), fever (3% to 5%), depression (3%), insomnia (2%)

Dermatologic: Rash (2% to 6%), skin ulcer (3%), pruritus (3%), skin hypertrophy (2%)

Endocrine & metabolic: Dehydration (3%), acidosis (2%), hypokalemia (2%)

Gastrointestinal: Vomiting (6% to 8%), diarrhea (7%), GI bleeding (5%), abdominal pain (4%), xerostomia (3%), constipation (4%), gastroenteritis (3%), dyspepsia (2%), gastritis (2%), rectal disorder (2%)

Genitourinary: Urinary tract infection (3%), kidney function abnormal (2%)

Neuromuscular & skeletal: Arthritis (5%), back pain (4%), leg cramps (3%), weakness (3%), neuropathy (2%)

Ocular: Amblyopia (2%), retinal disorder (2%)

Respiratory: Pneumonia (2% to 5%), rhinitis (5%), sinusitis (3%), bronchitis (3%), cough (3%), epistaxis (2%)

Miscellaneous: Infection (bacterial, fungal, viral: 2% to 8%); allergic reaction (6%), flu-like syndrome (2% to 5%), sepsis (5%), cyst (2%)

Postmarketing and/or case reports: Facial edema, oral edema, taste perversion (metallic), urticaria

Drug Interactions

Metabolism/Transport Effects

Substrate of CYP3A4 (major)

Avoid Concomitant Use There are no known interactions where it is recommended to avoid concomitant use.

Increased Effect/Toxicity There are no known significant interactions involving an increase in effect.

Decreased Effect There are no known significant interactions involving a decrease in effect.

Mechanism of Action Decreased renal conversion of vitamin D to its primary active metabolite (1,25-hydroxyvitamin D) in chronic renal failure leads to reduced activation of vitamin D receptor (VDR), which subsequently removes inhibitory suppression of parathyroid hormone (PTH) release; increased serum PTH (secondary hyperparathyroidism) reduces calcium excretion and enhances bone resorption. Paricalcitol is a synthetic vitamin D analog which binds to and activates the VDR in kidney, parathyroid gland, intestine and bone, thus reducing PTH levels and improving calcium and phosphate homeostasis.

Pharmacodynamics/Kinetics

Distribution: V_d:

Healthy subjects: Oral: 34 L; I.V.: 24 L

Stage 3 and 4 CKD: Oral: 44-46 L

Stage 5 CKD: I.V.: 31-35 L

Protein binding: >99%

Metabolism: Hydroxylation and glucuronidation via hepatic and nonhepatic enzymes, including CYP24, CYP3A4, UGT1A4; forms metabolites (at least one active)

Bioavailability: Oral: ~72% in healthy subjects

Half-life elimination:

Healthy subjects: Oral: 4-6 hours

Stage 3 and 4 CKD: Oral: 17-20 hours

Stage 5 CKD: I.V.: 14-15 hours

Excretion: Healthy subjects: Feces (oral: 70% to 74%; I.V.: 63%); urine (oral: 16% to 18%, I.V.: 19%); 51% to 59% as metabolites

Dosage Note: If hypercalcemia or Ca x P >75 is observed, reduce or interrupt dosing until parameters are normalized.

Secondary hyperparathyroidism associated with chronic renal failure (stage 5 CKD): Children ≥5 years and Adults: I.V.: 0.04-0.1 mcg/kg (2.8-7 mcg) given as a bolus dose no more frequently than every other day at any time during dialysis; dose may be increased by 2-4 mcg every 2-4 weeks; doses as high as 0.24 mcg/kg (16.8 mcg) have been administered safely; the dose of paricalcitol should be adjusted based on serum intact PTH (iPTH) levels, as follows:

Same or increasing iPTH level: Increase paricalcitol dose

iPTH level decreased by <30%: Increase paricalcitol dose

iPTH level decreased by >30% and <60%: Maintain paricalcitol dose

iPTH level decrease by >60%: Decrease paricalcitol dose

iPTH level 1.5-3 times upper limit of normal: Maintain paricalcitol dose

Secondary hyperparathyroidism associated with stage 3 and 4 CKD: Adults: Oral: Initial dose based on baseline serum iPTH:

iPTH ≤500 pg/mL: 1 mcg/day or 2 mcg 3 times/week

iPTH >500 pg/mL: 2 mcg/day or 4 mcg 3 times/week

Dosage adjustment based on iPTH level relative to baseline, adjust dose at 2-4 week intervals:

iPTH same or increased: Increase paricalcitol dose by 1 mcg/day or 2 mcg 3 times/week

iPTH decreased by <30%: Increase paricalcitol dose by 1 mcg/day or 2 mcg 3 times//week

iPTH decreased by ≥30% or ≤60%: Maintain paricalcitol dose

iPTH decreased by >60%: Decrease paricalcitol dose by 1 mcg/day* or 2 mcg 3 times/week

iPTH <60 pg/mL: Decrease paricalcitol dose by 1 mcg/day* or 2 mcg 3 times/week

*If patient is taking the lowest dose on a once-daily regimen, but further dose reduction is needed, decrease dose to 1 mcg 3 times/week. If further dose reduction is required, withhold drug as needed and restart at a lower dose. If applicable, calcium-phosphate binder dosing may also be adjusted or withheld, or switch to noncalcium-based binder.

Dosage adjustment in hepatic impairment: Adjustment not needed for mild-to-moderate impairment. Paricalcitol has not been evaluated in severe hepatic impairment.

Dietary Considerations The capsules may contain coconut or palm kernel oil.

Administration

Oral: May be administered with or without food. With the 3 times/week dosing schedule, doses should not be given more frequently than every other day.

I.V.: Administered as a bolus dose at anytime during dialysis. Doses should not be administered more often than every other day.

Monitoring Parameters

Signs and symptoms of vitamin D intoxication

Serum calcium and phosphorus:

I.V.: Twice weekly during initial phase, then at least monthly once dose established

Oral: At least every 2 weeks for 3 months or following dose adjustment, then monthly for 3 months, then every 3 months

Serum or plasma intact PTH (iPTH):

I.V.: Every 3 months

Oral: At least every 2 weeks for 3 months or following dose adjustment, then monthly for 3 months, then every 3 months

In trials, a mean PTH level reduction of 30% was achieved within 6 weeks with I.V. administration

Reference Range

CKD (definition of stages; chronic disease is kidney damage or GFR <60 mL/minute/1.73 m^2 for ≥3 months)

Stage 3: GFR 30-59 mL/minute/1.73 m^2 (moderate decrease GFR)

Stage 4: GFR 15-29 mL/minute/1.73 m^2 (severe decreased GFR)

Stage 5: GFR <15 mL/minute/1.73 m^2 or dialysis (kidney failure)

Target range for iPTH:

Stage 3 CKD: 35-70 pg/mL

Stage 4 CKD: 70-110 pg/mL

Stage 5 CKD: 150-300 pg/mL

Serum phosphorous:

Stage 3 and 4 CKD: ≥2.7 to <4.6 mg/dL

Stage 5 CKD: 3.5-5.5 mg/dL

Dosage Forms Excipient information presented when available (limited, particularly for generics); consult specific product labeling.

Capsule, gelatin: 1 mcg, 2 mcg, 4 mcg [contains alcohol and coconut or palm kernel oil]

Injection, solution: 2 mcg/mL (1 mL); 5 mcg/mL (1 mL, 2 mL) [contains alcohol 20% v/v and propylene glycol 30% v/v]

◆ **Pariet® (Can)** *see* Rabeprazole *on page 1285*

◆ **Pariprazole** *see* Rabeprazole *on page 1285*

◆ **Parlodel®** *see* Bromocriptine *on page 213*

◆ **Parlodel® SnapTabs®** *see* Bromocriptine *on page 213*

◆ **Parnate®** *see* Tranylcypromine *on page 1501*

Paromomycin (par oh moe MYE sin)

U.S. Brand Names Humatin® [DSC]

Canadian Brand Names Humatin®

Index Terms Paromomycin Sulfate

Pharmacologic Category Amebicide

Use Treatment of acute and chronic intestinal amebiasis; hepatic coma

Unlabeled/Investigational Use Treatment of cryptosporidiosis

Pregnancy Risk Factor C

Lactation Does not enter breast milk/compatible

Contraindications Hypersensitivity to paromomycin or any component of the formulation; intestinal obstruction

Warnings/Precautions Use with caution in patients with impaired renal function or possible or proven ulcerative bowel lesions. Prolonged use may result in fungal or bacterial superinfection, including *C. difficile*-associated diarrhea (CDAD) and pseudomembranous colitis; CDAD has been observed >2 months postantibiotic treatment.

Adverse Reactions

1% to 10%: Gastrointestinal: Diarrhea, abdominal cramps, nausea, vomiting, heartburn

<1% (Limited to important or life-threatening): Eosinophilia, exanthema, headache, ototoxicity, pruritus, rash, secondary enterocolitis, steatorrhea, vertigo

Drug Interactions

Avoid Concomitant Use There are no known interactions where it is recommended to avoid concomitant use.

Increased Effect/Toxicity There are no known significant interactions involving an increase in effect.

Decreased Effect There are no known significant interactions involving a decrease in effect.

Ethanol/Nutrition/Herb Interactions Food: Paromomycin may cause malabsorption of xylose, sucrose, and fats.

Mechanism of Action Acts directly on ameba; has antibacterial activity against normal and pathogenic organisms in the GI tract; interferes with bacterial protein synthesis by binding to 30S ribosomal subunits

Pharmacodynamics/Kinetics

Absorption: None

Excretion: Feces (100% as unchanged drug)

Dosage Oral:

Intestinal amebiasis: Children and Adults: 25-35 mg/kg/day in 3 divided doses for 5-10 days

Dientamoeba fragilis: Children and Adults: 25-30 mg/kg/day in 3 divided doses for 7 days

Cryptosporidium (unlabeled use): Adults with AIDS: 1.5-2.25 g/day in 3-6 divided doses for 10-14 days (occasionally courses of up to 4-8 weeks may be needed)

Tapeworm (fish, dog, bovine, porcine):

Children: 11 mg/kg every 15 minutes for 4 doses

Adults: 1 g every 15 minutes for 4 doses

Hepatic coma: Adults: 4 g/day in 2-4 divided doses for 5-6 days

Dwarf tapeworm: Children and Adults: 45 mg/kg/dose every day for 5-7 days

Dosage Forms Excipient information presented when available (limited, particularly for generics); consult specific product labeling. [DSC] = Discontinued product

Capsule: 250 mg

Humatin®: 250 mg [DSC]

◆ **Paromomycin Sulfate** *see* Paromomycin *on page 1146*

PARoxetine (pa ROKS e teen)

U.S. Brand Names Paxil CR®; Paxil®; Pexeva®

Canadian Brand Names Apo-Paroxetine®; CO Paroxetine; Gen-Paroxetine; Novo-Paroxetine; Paxil CR®; Paxil®; PMS-Paroxetine; ratio-Paroxetine; Rhoxal-paroxetine; Sandoz-Paroxetine

Index Terms Paroxetine Hydrochloride; Paroxetine Mesylate

Pharmacologic Category Antidepressant, Selective Serotonin Reuptake Inhibitor

Additional Appendix Information

Antidepressant Agents *on page 1638*

Selective Serotonin Reuptake Inhibitors (SSRIs) Pharmacokinetics *on page 1670*

Use Treatment of major depressive disorder (MDD); treatment of panic disorder with or without agoraphobia; obsessive-compulsive disorder (OCD); social anxiety disorder (social phobia); generalized anxiety disorder (GAD); post-traumatic stress disorder (PTSD); premenstrual dysphoric disorder (PMDD)

Unlabeled/Investigational Use May be useful in eating disorders, impulse control disorders, self-injurious behavior; vasomotor symptoms of menopause; treatment of depression and obsessive-compulsive disorder (OCD) in children; treatment of mild dementia-associated agitation in nonpsychotic patients

Restrictions An FDA-approved medication guide concerning the use of antidepressants in children, adolescents, and young adults must be distributed when dispensing an outpatient prescription (new or refill) where this medication is to be used without direct supervision of a healthcare provider. Medication guides are available at http://www.fda.gov/cder/Offices/ODS/medication_guides.htm. Dispense to parents or guardians of children and adolescents receiving this medication.

Pregnancy Risk Factor D

Pregnancy Considerations Due to adverse events observed in human studies, paroxetine is classified as pregnancy category D. Paroxetine crosses the placenta. The risk of cardiovascular and other congenital malformations may be higher with paroxetine than with other antidepressants. Nonteratogenic effects in the newborn following SSRI exposure late in the third trimester include respiratory distress, cyanosis, apnea, seizures, temperature instability, feeding difficulty, vomiting, hypoglycemia, hypo- or hypertonia, hyper-reflexia, jitteriness, irritability, constant crying, and tremor. An increased risk of low birth weight, lower APGAR scores, and blunted behavioral response to pain for a prolonged period after delivery has also been reported. Exposure to SSRIs after the twentieth week of gestation has been associated with persistent pulmonary hypertension of the newborn (PPHN). Adverse effects may be due to toxic effects of the SSRI or drug withdrawal due to discontinuation. The long-term effects of *in utero* SSRI exposure on infant development and behavior are not known.

Due to pregnancy-induced physiologic changes, women who are pregnant may require increased doses of paroxetine to achieve euthymia. Women treated for major depression and who are euthymic prior to pregnancy are more likely to experience a relapse when medication is discontinued as compared to pregnant women who continue taking antidepressant medications. The ACOG recommends that therapy with SSRIs or SNRIs during pregnancy be individualized; treatment of depression during pregnancy should incorporate the clinical expertise of the mental health clinician, obstetrician, primary healthcare provider, and pediatrician (ACOG, 2007). The ACOG also recommend that therapy with paroxetine be avoided during pregnancy if possible and that fetuses exposed in early pregnancy be assessed with a fetal echocardiography. If treatment during pregnancy is required, consider tapering therapy during the third trimester in order to prevent withdrawal symptoms in the infant. If this is done and the woman is considered to be at risk from her major depressive disorder, the medication can be restarted following delivery, although the dose should be readjusted to that required before pregnancy.

Lactation Enters breast milk/use caution (AAP rates "of concern")

Medication Safety Issues

Sound-alike/look-alike issues:

PARoxetine may be confused with FLUoxetine, paclitaxel, pyridoxine

Paxil® may be confused with Doxil®, paclitaxel, Plavix®, Taxol®

Contraindications Hypersensitivity to paroxetine or any component of the formulation; use with or within 14 days of MAO inhibitors; concurrent use with thioridazine or pimozide

Warnings/Precautions [U.S. Boxed Warning]: Antidepressants increase the risk of suicidal thinking and behavior in children, adolescents, and young adults (18-24 years of age) with major depressive disorder (MDD) and other psychiatric disorders; consider risk prior to prescribing. Short-term studies did not show an increased risk in patients >24 years of age and showed a decreased risk in patients ≥65 years. Closely monitor patients for clinical worsening, suicidality, or unusual changes in behavior, particularly during the initial 1-2 months of therapy or during periods of dosage adjustments (increases or decreases); the patient's family or caregiver should be instructed to closely observe the patient and communicate condition with healthcare provider. A medication guide concerning the use of antidepressants should be dispensed with each prescription. **Paroxetine is not FDA approved for use in children.**

The possibility of a suicide attempt is inherent in major depression and may persist until remission occurs. Patients treated with antidepressants (for any indication) should be observed for clinical worsening and suicidality, especially during the initial few months of a course of drug therapy, or at times of dose changes, either increases or decreases. Use caution in high-risk patients. Worsening depression and severe abrupt suicidality that are not part of the presenting symptoms may require discontinuation or modification of drug therapy. The patient's family or caregiver should be alerted to monitor patients for the emergence of suicidality and associated behaviors (such as agitation, irritability, hostility, impulsivity, and hypomania) and call healthcare provider.

May worsen psychosis in some patients or precipitate a shift to mania or hypomania in patients with bipolar disorder. Patients presenting with depressive symptoms should be screened for bipolar disorder. Monotherapy in patients with bipolar disorder should be avoided. **Paroxetine is not FDA approved for the treatment of bipolar depression.**

Potential for severe reaction when used with MAO inhibitors, SSRIs/SNRIs or triptans; serotonin syndrome (hyperthermia, muscular rigidity, mental status changes/agitation, autonomic instability) may occur; concurrent use with MAO inhibitors contraindicated. May increase the risks associated with electroconvulsive therapy. Has a low potential to impair cognitive or motor performance - caution operating hazardous machinery or driving. Symptoms of agitation and/or restlessness may occur during initial few weeks of therapy. Low potential for sedation or anticholinergic effects relative to cyclic antidepressants.

Use caution in patients with a previous seizure disorder or condition predisposing to seizures such as brain damage, alcoholism, or concurrent therapy with other drugs which lower the seizure threshold. Use with caution in patients with hepatic dysfunction and in elderly patients. May cause hyponatremia/SIADH (elderly at increased risk); volume depletion (diuretics may increase risk). Use caution with concomitant use of NSAIDs, ASA, or other drugs that affect coagulation; the risk of bleeding may be potentiated. Use with caution in patients with renal insufficiency or other concurrent illness (due to limited experience); dose reduction recommended with severe renal impairment. May cause or exacerbate sexual dysfunction. Use caution in patients with narrow-angle glaucoma. Avoid use in the first trimester of pregnancy.

Upon discontinuation of paroxetine therapy, gradually taper dose and monitor for discontinuation symptoms (eg, dizziness, dysphoric mood, irritability, agitation, confusion, paresthesias). If intolerable symptoms occur following a decrease in dosage or upon discontinuation of therapy, then resuming the previous dose with a more gradual taper should be considered. Safety and efficacy in children have not been established.

Adverse Reactions Frequency varies by dose and indication. Adverse reactions reported as a composite of all indications.

>10%:

Central nervous system: Somnolence (15% to 24%), insomnia (11% to 24%), headache (17% to 18%), dizziness (6% to 14%)

Endocrine & metabolic: Libido decreased (3% to 15%)

Gastrointestinal: Nausea (19% to 26%), xerostomia (9% to 18%), constipation (5% to 16%), diarrhea (9% to 12%)

Genitourinary: Ejaculatory disturbances (10% to 28%)

Neuromuscular & skeletal: Weakness (12% to 22%), tremor (4% to 11%)

Miscellaneous: Diaphoresis (5% to 14%)

1% to 10%:

Cardiovascular: Vasodilation (2% to 4%), chest pain (3%), palpitation (2% to 3%), hypertension (≥1%), tachycardia (≥1%)

Central nervous system: Nervousness (4% to 9%), anxiety (5%), agitation (3% to 5%), abnormal dreams (3% to 4%), concentration impaired (3% to 4%), yawning (2% to 4%), depersonalization (up to 3%), amnesia (2%), emotional lability (≥1%), vertigo (≥1%), confusion (1%), chills (2%)

Dermatologic: Rash (2% to 3%), pruritus (≥1%)

Endocrine & metabolic: Orgasmic disturbance (2% to 9%), dysmenorrhea (5%)

Gastrointestinal: Anorexia, appetite decreased (5% to 9%), dyspepsia (2% to 5%), flatulence (4%), abdominal pain (4%), appetite increased (2% to 4%), vomiting (2% to 3%), taste perversion (2%), weight gain (≥1%)

Genitourinary: Impotence (2% to 9%), genital disorder (female 2% to 9%), urinary frequency (2% to 3%), urinary tract infection (2%)

Neuromuscular & skeletal: Paresthesia (4%), myalgia (2% to 4%), back pain (3%), myoclonus (2% to 3%), myopathy (2%), myasthenia (1%), arthralgia (≥1%)

Ocular: Blurred vision (4%), abnormal vision (2% to 4%)

Otic: Tinnitus (≥1%)

Respiratory: Respiratory disorder (up to 7%), pharyngitis (4%), sinusitis (up to 4%), rhinitis (3%)

Miscellaneous: Infection (5% to 6%)

<1%, postmarketing, and/or case reports (limited to important or life-threatening): Acute renal failure, adrenergic syndrome, akinesia, alkaline phosphatase increased, allergic reaction, anaphylaxis, anemias (various), angina pectoris, angioedema, aphasia, aphthous stomatitis, arrhythmias (atrial and ventricular), arthrosis, asthma, behavioral disturbances (various), bilirubinemia, bleeding time increased, blood dyscrasias, bloody diarrhea, bradycardia, bronchitis, bulimia, BUN increased, bundle branch block, cardiospasm, cataract, cellulitis, cerebral ischemia, cerebrovascular accident, cholelithiasis, colitis, congestive heart failure, creatinine phosphokinase increased, deafness, dehydration, delirium, diabetes mellitus, drug dependence, dyskinesia, dysphagia, dyspnea, dystonia, ecchymosis, eclampsia, electrolyte abnormalities, emphysema, erythema, exfoliative dermatitis, extrapyramidal syndrome, fecal impactions, fungal dermatitis, gamma globulins increased, gastroenteritis, glaucoma, goiter, Guillain-Barré syndrome, hallucinations, hematemesis, hematoma, hemorrhage, hemoptysis, hepatic necrosis, hepatitis, hypercholesteremia, hyper-/hypoglycemia, hyper-/hypothyroidism, hypotension, ileus, intestinal obstruction, jaundice, ketosis, lactic dehydrogenase increased, liver function tests abnormal, low cardiac output, lung fibrosis, lymphadenopathy, meningitis, MI, migraine, myelitis, myocardial ischemia, neuroleptic malignant syndrome, neuropathy, osteoporosis, pancreatitis, pancytopenia, peptic ulcer, peritonitis, phlebitis, pneumonia, platelet count abnormalities, pulmonary edema, pulmonary embolus, pulmonary hypertension, seizure, sepsis, serotonin syndrome, status epilepticus, suicidal tendencies, syncope, tetany, thrombophlebitis, thrombosis, tongue edema, torsade de pointes, toxic epidermal necrolysis, vasculitic syndrome

Drug Interactions

Metabolism/Transport Effects Substrate of CYP2D6 (major); **Inhibits** CYP1A2 (weak), 2B6 (moderate), 2C9 (weak), 2C19 (weak), 2D6 (strong), 3A4 (weak)

Avoid Concomitant Use

Avoid concomitant use of PARoxetine with any of the following: Iobenguane I 123; MAO Inhibitors; Pimozide; Sibutramine; Tamoxifen; Thioridazine

Increased Effect/Toxicity

PARoxetine may increase the levels/effects of: Alcohol (Ethyl); Alpha-/Beta-Blockers; Anticoagulants; Antidepressants (Serotonin Reuptake Inhibitor/Antagonist); Antiplatelet Agents; Aspirin; Atomoxetine; Beta-Blockers; BusPIRone; CarBAMazepine; Clozapine; CNS Depressants; CYP2B6 Substrates; CYP2D6 Substrates; Desmopressin; Dextromethorphan; Drotrecogin Alfa; DULoxetine; Fesoterodine; Galantamine; Haloperidol; Ibritumomab; Lithium; Methadone; Mexiletine; NSAID (COX-2 Inhibitor); NSAID (Nonselective); Pimozide; Propafenone; Risperidone; Salicylates; Serotonin Modulators; Tamoxifen; Tetrabenazine; Thioridazine; Thrombolytic Agents; Tositumomab and Iodine I 131 Tositumomab; TraMADol; Tricyclic Antidepressants; Vitamin K Antagonists

The levels/effects of PARoxetine may be increased by: Analgesics (Opioid); BusPIRone; Cimetidine; CYP2D6 Inhibitors (Moderate); CYP2D6 Inhibitors (Strong); Dasatinib; Herbs (Anticoagulant/Antiplatelet Properties); MAO Inhibitors; Omega-3-Acid Ethyl Esters; Pentosan Polysulfate Sodium; Prostacyclin Analogues; Sibutramine; TraMADol; Tryptophan

Decreased Effect

PARoxetine may decrease the levels/effects of: Iobenguane I 123

The levels/effects of PARoxetine may be decreased by: Amprenavir; CarBAMazepine; Cyproheptadine; Darunavir; Fosamprenavir

Ethanol/Nutrition/Herb Interactions

Ethanol: Avoid ethanol (may increase CNS depression).

Food: Peak concentration is increased, but bioavailability is not significantly altered by food.

Herb/Nutraceutical: Avoid valerian, St John's wort, SAMe, kava kava.

Stability

Suspension: Store at ≤25°C (≤77°F).

Tablet: Store at 15°C to 30°C (59°F to 86°F).

Mechanism of Action Paroxetine is a selective serotonin reuptake inhibitor, chemically unrelated to tricyclic, tetracyclic, or other antidepressants; presumably, the inhibition of serotonin reuptake from brain synapse stimulated serotonin activity in the brain

Pharmacodynamics/Kinetics

Onset of action: Depression: The onset of action is within a week; however, individual response varies greatly and full response may not be seen until 8-12 weeks after initiation of treatment.

Absorption: Completely absorbed following oral administration

Distribution: V_d: 8.7 L/kg (3-28 L/kg)

Protein binding: 93% to 95%

Metabolism: Extensively hepatic via CYP2D6 enzymes; primary metabolites are formed via oxidation and methylation of parent drug, with subsequent glucuronide/sulfate conjugation; nonlinear pharmacokinetics (via 2D6 saturation) may be seen with higher doses and longer duration of therapy. Metabolites exhibit ~2% potency of parent compound. C_{min} concentrations are 70% to 80% greater in the elderly compared to nonelderly patients; clearance is also decreased.

Half-life elimination: 21 hours (3-65 hours)

Time to peak: Immediate release: 5.2 hours; controlled release: 6-10 hours

Excretion: Urine (64%, 2% as unchanged drug); feces (36% primarily via bile, <1% as unchanged drug)

Dosage Oral:

Children:

Depression (unlabeled use; not recommended by FDA): Initial: 10 mg/day and adjusted upward on an individual basis to 20 mg/day

Obsessive-compulsive disorder (unlabeled use): Initial: 10 mg/day and titrate up as necessary to 60 mg/day

Self-injurious behavior (unlabeled use): 20 mg/day

Social anxiety disorder (unlabeled use): 2.5-15 mg/day

Adults:

Major depressive disorder:

Paxil®, Pexeva®: Initial: 20 mg once daily, preferably in the morning; increase if needed by 10 mg/day increments at intervals of at least 1 week; maximum dose: 50 mg/day

Paxil CR®: Initial: 25 mg once daily; increase if needed by 12.5 mg/day increments at intervals of at least 1 week; maximum dose: 62.5 mg/day

Generalized anxiety disorder (Paxil®, Pexeva®): Initial: 20 mg once daily, preferably in the morning (if dose is increased, adjust in increments of 10 mg/day at 1-week intervals); doses of 20-50 mg/day were used in clinical trials, however, no greater benefit was seen with doses >20 mg.

Obsessive-compulsive disorder (Paxil®, Pexeva™): Initial: 20 mg once daily, preferably in the morning; increase if needed by 10 mg/day increments at intervals of at least 1 week; recommended dose: 40 mg/day; range: 20-60 mg/day; maximum dose: 60 mg/day

Panic disorder:

Paxil®, Pexeva®: Initial: 10 mg once daily, preferably in the morning; increase if needed by 10 mg/day increments at intervals of at least 1 week; recommended dose: 40 mg/day; range: 10-60 mg/day; maximum dose: 60 mg/day

Paxil CR®: Initial: 12.5 mg once daily; increase if needed by 12.5 mg/day at intervals of at least 1 week; maximum dose: 75 mg/day

Premenstrual dysphoric disorder (Paxil CR®): Initial: 12.5 mg once daily in the morning; may be increased to 25 mg/day; dosing changes should occur at intervals of at least 1 week. May be given daily throughout the menstrual cycle or limited to the luteal phase.

Post-traumatic stress disorder (Paxil®): Initial: 20 mg once daily, preferably in the morning; increase if needed by 10 mg/day increments at intervals of at least 1 week; range: 20-50 mg. Limited data suggest doses of 40 mg/day were not more efficacious than 20 mg/day.

Social anxiety disorder:

Paxil®: Initial: 20 mg once daily, preferably in the morning; recommended dose: 20 mg/day; range: 20-60 mg/day; doses >20 mg may not have additional benefit

Paxil CR®: Initial: 12.5 mg once daily, preferably in the morning; may be increased by 12.5 mg/day at intervals of at least 1 week; maximum dose: 37.5 mg/day

Vasomotor symptoms of menopause (unlabeled use, Paxil CR®): 12.5-25 mg/day

Elderly:

Paxil®, Pexeva®: Initial: 10 mg/day; increase if needed by 10 mg/day increments at intervals of at least 1 week; maximum dose: 40 mg/day

Paxil CR®; Initial: 12.5 mg/day; increase if needed by 12.5 mg/day increments at intervals of at least 1 week; maximum dose: 50 mg/day

Note: Upon discontinuation of paroxetine therapy, gradually taper dose:

Paxil®, Pexeva®: 10 mg/day at weekly intervals; when 20 mg/day dose is reached, continue for 1 week before treatment is discontinued. Some patients may need to be titrated to 10 mg/day for 1 week before discontinuation.

Paxil CR®: Patients receiving 37.5 mg/day in clinical trials had their dose decreased by 12.5 mg/day to a dose of 25 mg/day and remained at a dose of 25 mg/day for 1 week before treatment was discontinued.

Dosage adjustment in renal impairment: Adults:

Cl_{cr} <30 mL/minute: Mean plasma concentration is ~4 times that seen in normal function.

Cl_{cr} 30-60 mL/minute: Plasma concentration is 2 times that seen in normal function.

Paxil®, Pexeva®: Initial: 10 mg/day; increase if needed by 10 mg/day increments at intervals of at least 1 week; maximum dose: 40 mg/day

Paxil CR®: Initial: 12.5 mg/day; increase if needed by 12.5 mg/day increments at intervals of at least 1 week; maximum dose: 50 mg/day

Dosage adjustment in severe hepatic impairment: Adults: In hepatic dysfunction, plasma concentration is 2 times that seen in normal function.

Paxil®, Pexeva®: Initial: 10 mg/day; increase if needed by 10 mg/day increments at intervals of at least 1 week; maximum dose: 40 mg/day

Paxil CR®: Initial: 12.5 mg/day; increase if needed by 12.5 mg/day increments at intervals of at least 1 week; maximum dose: 50 mg/day

Dietary Considerations May be taken with or without food.

Administration May be administered with or without food. Do not crush, break, or chew controlled release tablets.

Monitoring Parameters Mental status for depression, suicidal ideation (especially at the beginning of therapy or when doses are increased or decreased), anxiety, social functioning, mania, panic attacks; akathisia

Additional Information Paxil CR® incorporates a degradable polymeric matrix (Geomatrix™) to control dissolution rate over a period of 4-5 hours. An enteric coating delays the start of drug release until tablets have left the stomach.

Dosage Forms Excipient information presented when available (limited, particularly for generics); consult specific product labeling.

Note: Strength expressed as base:

Suspension, oral, as hydrochloride: 10 mg/5 mL (250 mL)

Paxil®: 10 mg/5 mL (250 mL) [orange flavor]

Tablet, as hydrochloride: 10 mg, 20 mg, 30 mg, 40 mg

Paxil®: 10 mg, 20 mg, 30 mg, 40 mg

Tablet, as mesylate:

Pexeva®: 10 mg, 20 mg, 30 mg, 40 mg

Tablet, controlled release, as hydrochloride: 37.5 mg

Paxil CR®: 12.5 mg, 25 mg, 37.5 mg

Tablet, extended release, as hydrochloride: 12.5 mg, 25 mg

◆ **Paroxetine Hydrochloride** *see* PARoxetine *on page 1146*

◆ **Paroxetine Mesylate** *see* PARoxetine *on page 1146*

◆ **Parvolex® (Can)** *see* Acetylcysteine *on page 36*

◆ **PAS** *see* Aminosalicylic Acid *on page 86*

◆ **Paser®** *see* Aminosalicylic Acid *on page 86*

◆ **Pataday™** *see* Olopatadine *on page 1097*

◆ **Patanase®** *see* Olopatadine *on page 1097*

◆ **Patanol®** *see* Olopatadine *on page 1097*

◆ **Pathocil® (Can)** *see* Dicloxacillin *on page 440*

◆ **Pavabid [DSC]** *see* Papaverine *on page 1142*

◆ **Pavulon [DSC]** *see* Pancuronium *on page 1137*

◆ **Paxil®** *see* PARoxetine *on page 1146*

◆ **Paxil CR®** *see* PARoxetine *on page 1146*

Pegademase Bovine (peg A de mase BOE vine)

U.S. Brand Names Adagen®

Canadian Brand Names Adagen®

Pharmacologic Category Enzyme

Use Enzyme replacement therapy for adenosine deaminase (ADA) deficiency in patients with severe combined immunodeficiency disease (SCID) who are not candidates for or who have failed bone marrow transplant

Pregnancy Risk Factor C

Dosage Note: Dose should be individualized based on monitoring of plasma ADA activity levels and dATP content.Infants and Children: I.M.: Dose given every 7 days, 10 units/kg the first dose, 15 units/kg the second dose, and 20 units/kg the third dose; maintenance dose: 20 units/kg/week is recommended depending on patient's ADA level; maximum single dose: 30 units/kg

Additional Information Complete prescribing information for this medication should be consulted for additional detail.

Dosage Forms Excipient information presented when available (limited, particularly for generics); consult specific product labeling.

Injection, solution [preservative free]:
  Adagen®: 250 units/mL (1.5 mL)

Pegaptanib (peg AP ta nib)

U.S. Brand Names Macugen®

Canadian Brand Names Macugen®

Index Terms EYE001; Pegaptanib Sodium

Pharmacologic Category Ophthalmic Agent; Vascular Endothelial Growth Factor (VEGF) Inhibitor

Use Treatment of neovascular (wet) age-related macular degeneration (AMD)

Pregnancy Risk Factor B

Pregnancy Considerations Teratogenic effects were not reported in animal studies. There are no adequate and well-controlled studies in pregnant women.

Lactation Excretion in breast milk unknown/use caution

Contraindications Hypersensitivity to pegaptanib or any component of the formulation; ocular or periocular infection

Warnings/Precautions Intravitreous injections may be associated with endophthalmitis; patients should be instructed to report any signs of infection immediately. Intraocular pressure may increase following injection. Safety and efficacy for administration into both eyes concurrently have not been studied. Safety and efficacy have not been established with hepatic impairment, or in patients requiring hemodialysis. Rare hypersensitivity reactions (including anaphylaxis) have been associated with pegaptanib, occurring within several hours of use; monitor closely. Equipment and appropriate personnel should be available for monitoring and treatment of anaphylaxis. Safety and efficacy have not been established in children.

Adverse Reactions

10% to 40%:

Cardiovascular: Hypertension

Ocular: Anterior chamber inflammation, blurred vision, cataract, conjunctival hemorrhage, corneal edema, eye discharge, eye irritation, eye pain, intraocular pressure increased, ocular discomfort, punctate keratitis, visual acuity decreased, visual disturbance, vitreous floaters, vitreous opacities

1% to 10%:

Cardiovascular: Carotid artery occlusion (1% to 5%), cerebrovascular accident (1% to 5%), chest pain (1% to 5%), transient ischemic attack (1% to 5%)

Central nervous system: Dizziness (6% to 10%), headache (6% to 10%), vertigo (1% to 5%)

Dermatologic: Contact dermatitis (1% to 5%)

Endocrine & metabolic: Diabetes mellitus (1% to 5%)

Gastrointestinal: Diarrhea (6% to 10%), nausea (6% to 10%), dyspepsia (1% to 5%), vomiting (1% to 5%)

Genitourinary: Urinary retention (1% to 5%)

Neuromuscular & skeletal: Arthritis (1% to 5%), bone spur (1% to 5%)

Ocular: Blepharitis (6% to 10%), conjunctivitis (6% to 10%), photopsia (6% to 10%), vitreous disorder (6% to 10%), allergic conjunctivitis (1% to 5%), conjunctival edema (1% to 5%), corneal abrasion (1% to 5%), corneal deposits (1% to 5%), corneal epithelium disorder (1% to 5%), endophthalmitis (1% to 5%), eye inflammation (1% to 5%), eye swelling (1% to 5%), eyelid irritation (1% to 5%), meibomianitis (1% to 5%), mydriasis (1% to 5%), periorbital hematoma (1% to 5%), retinal edema (1% to 5%), vitreous hemorrhage (1% to 5%)

Otic: Hearing loss (1% to 5%)

Renal: Urinary tract infection (6% to 10%)

Respiratory: Bronchitis (6% to 10%), pleural effusion (1% to 5%)

Miscellaneous: Contusion (1% to 5%)

<1% (Limited to important or life-threatening): Anaphylaxis, anaphylactoid reaction, angioedema, hypersensitivity, iatrogenic traumatic cataract, endophthalmitis, retinal detachment

Drug Interactions

Avoid Concomitant Use There are no known interactions where it is recommended to avoid concomitant use.

Increased Effect/Toxicity There are no known significant interactions involving an increase in effect.

Decreased Effect There are no known significant interactions involving a decrease in effect.

Stability Store under refrigeration at 2°C to 8°C (36°F to 46°F); do not freeze. Do not shake vigorously.

Mechanism of Action Pegaptanib is an apatamer, an oligonucleotide covalently bound to polyethylene glycol, which can adopt a three-dimensional shape and bind to vascular endothelial growth factor (VEGF). Pegaptanib binds to extracellular VEGF, inhibiting VEGF from binding to its receptors and thereby suppressing neovascularization and slowing vision loss.

Pharmacodynamics/Kinetics

Absorption: Slow systemic absorption following intravitreous injection

Metabolism: Metabolized by endo- and exonucleases

Half-life elimination: Plasma: 6-14 days

Dosage Intravitreous injection: Adults: AMD: 0.3 mg into affected eye every 6 weeks

Dosage adjustment in renal impairment: Adjustment not required with renal impairment; information not available for patients requiring hemodialysis

Administration For intravitreous injection only; adequate anesthesia and a broad spectrum antibiotic should be administered prior to injection

pH: 6-7

Monitoring Parameters Intraocular pressure (within 30 minutes and 2-7 days after injection); endophthalmitis

Dosage Forms Excipient information presented when available (limited, particularly for generics); consult specific product labeling.

Injection, solution [preservative free]: 0.3 mg/90 µL (90 µL) [prefilled syringe]

◆ **Pegaptanib Sodium** *see* Pegaptanib *on page 1150*

Pegaspargase (peg AS par jase)

U.S. Brand Names Oncaspar®

Index Terms NSC-644954; PEG-L-asparaginase

Pharmacologic Category Antineoplastic Agent, Miscellaneous

Use Treatment of acute lymphocytic leukemia (ALL); treatment of ALL with previous hypersensitivity to native L-asparaginase

Pregnancy Risk Factor C

Pregnancy Considerations Reproduction studies have not been conducted with pegaspargase.

Lactation Excretion in breast milk unknown/not recommended

Medication Safety Issues

Sound-alike/look-alike issues:

Pegaspargase may be confused with asparaginase

High alert medication: The Institute for Safe Medication Practices (ISMP) includes this medication among its list of drugs which have a heightened risk of causing significant patient harm when used in error.

Contraindications Hypersensitivity to pegaspargase or any component of the formulation; history of serious thrombosis with previous L-asparaginase treatment; pancreatitis or a history of pancreatitis; previous serious allergic reactions (urticaria, bronchospasm, laryngeal edema, hypotension) or other unacceptable adverse reactions to pegaspargase; previous hemorrhagic event with L-asparaginase

Warnings/Precautions Hazardous agent - use appropriate precautions for handling and disposal. Monitor for severe allergic reactions; may be used cautiously in patients who have had hypersensitivity reactions to *E. coli* asparaginase; however, up to 32% of patients who have an allergic reaction to *E. coli* asparaginase will also react to pegaspargase; immediate treatment for hypersensitivity reactions should be available during administration. Thrombotic events may occur; discontinue with serious thrombotic event. Discontinue if pancreatitis occurs during treatment. May cause (possibly irreversible) glucose intolerance. Coagulopathy has been reported; monitor coagulation parameters. Use cautiously in patients with an underlying coagulopathy or previous hematologic complications from asparaginase, hepatic dysfunction, concomitant hepatotoxic medications, hyperglycemia, or diabetes.

Adverse Reactions In general, pegaspargase toxicities tend to be less frequent and appear somewhat later than comparable toxicities of asparaginase. Intramuscular rather than intravenous injection may decrease the incidence of coagulopathy; GI, hepatic, and renal toxicity. Except for hypersensitivity reactions, adults tend to have a higher incidence than children.

>5%:

Cardiovascular: Edema

Central nervous system: Fever, malaise

Dermatologic: Rash (1% to >5%)

Gastrointestinal: Nausea, vomiting

Hematologic: Coagulopathy (7%; grades 3/4: 2%)

Hepatic: Transaminases increased (11%; grades 3/4: 3%), ALT increased

Miscellaneous: Allergic reactions (including bronchospasm, chills, dyspnea, edema, erythema, fever, rash, urticaria: 1% to 10%; 32% in patients with prior hypersensitivity to asparaginase products)

1% to 5%:

Cardiovascular: Hypotension, peripheral edema, tachycardia, thrombosis (4%)

Central nervous system: Chills, CNS thrombosis/hemorrhage (2%), headache, seizure

Dermatologic: Lip edema, urticaria

Endocrine & metabolic: Hyperglycemia (3% to 5%), hyperuricemia, hypoglycemia, hypoproteinemia

Gastrointestinal: Abdominal pain, anorexia, diarrhea, pancreatitis (1% to 2%; grades 3/4: 2%)

Hematologic: Anticoagulant effect decreased, disseminated intravascular coagulation (DIC), fibrinogen decreased, hemolytic anemia, leukopenia, pancytopenia, thrombocytopenia, thromboplastin increased, myelosuppression (mild to moderate; onset: 7 days; nadir: 14 days; recovery: 21 days)

Hepatic: Liver function tests abnormal (5%), hyperbilirubinemia, jaundice, AST increased

Local: Injection site hypersensitivity, pain or reaction

Neuromuscular & skeletal: Arthralgia, limb pain, myalgia, paresthesia

Respiratory: Dyspnea

Miscellaneous: Anaphylactic reactions, night sweats

<1% (Limited to important or life-threatening): Abnormal renal function, alopecia, amylase increased, anemia, antithrombin III decreased, appetite increased, ascites,

bone pain, bronchospasm, bruising, BUN increased, chest pain, coagulation disorder, coagulation time increased, colitis, coma, confusion, constipation, cough, creatinine increased, dizziness, DVT, emotional lability, endocarditis, epistaxis, erythema, excessive thirst, face edema, fatigue, fatty liver deposits, flatulence, gastrointestional pain, glucose intolerance, hematuria, hemorrhagic cystitis, hepatomegaly, hyperammonemia, hypertension, hypoalbuminemia, hyponatremia, joint disorder, lesional edema, lipase increased, liver failure, metabolic acidosis, mucositis, petechial rash, polyuria, proteinuria, prothrombin time increased, pruritus, purpura, renal failure, sagittal sinus thrombosis, sepsis, septic shock, somnolence, subacute bacterial endocarditis, superficial venous thrombosis, thirst, upper respiratory infection, uric acid nephropathy, urinary frequency, weight loss

Drug Interactions

Avoid Concomitant Use

Avoid concomitant use of Pegaspargase with any of the following: Natalizumab; Vaccines (Live)

Increased Effect/Toxicity

Pegaspargase may increase the levels/effects of: Natalizumab; Vaccines (Live)

The levels/effects of Pegaspargase may be increased by: Trastuzumab

Decreased Effect

Pegaspargase may decrease the levels/effects of: Vaccines (Inactivated)

The levels/effects of Pegaspargase may be decreased by: Echinacea

Stability Refrigerate at 2°C to 8°C (36°F to 46°F); do not freeze. Do not use product if it is known to have been frozen. Do not use if stored at room temperature for >48 hours. Avoid excessive agitation; do **not** shake. Do not use if cloudy or if precipitate is present.

Standard I.M. dilution: Usually not more than 2 mL/injection site.

Standard I.V. dilution: Dilute in 100 mL NS or D_5W; stable for 48 hours at room temperature.

Mechanism of Action Pegaspargase is a modified version of asparaginase. Leukemic cells, especially lymphoblasts, require exogenous asparagine; normal cells can synthesize asparagine. Asparaginase contains L-asparaginase amidohydrolase type EC-2 which inhibits protein synthesis by deaminating asparagine to aspartic acid and ammonia in the plasma and extracellular fluid and therefore deprives tumor cells of the amino acid for protein synthesis. Asparaginase is cycle-specific for the G_1 phase of the cell cycle.

Pharmacodynamics/Kinetics

Duration: Asparaginase was measurable for at least 20 days following initial treatment with pegaspargase

Distribution: V_d: 4-5 L/kg; 70% to 80% of plasma volume; does not penetrate the CSF

Metabolism: Systemically degraded

Half-life elimination: 5.8 days; unaffected by age, renal or hepatic function; half life decreased to 3.2 days in patients with previous hypersensitivity to native L-asparaginase

Excretion: Urine (trace amounts)

Dosage Usually administered as part of a combination chemotherapy regimen.

I.M. administration is **preferred** over I.V. administration due to lower incidence of hepatotoxicity, coagulopathy, gastrointestinal and renal disorders with I.M. administration.

Children: I.M., I.V.:

Body surface area <0.6 m^2: 82.5 int. units/kg every 14 days

Body surface area ≥0.6 m^2: 2500 int. units/m^2 every 14 days

Adults: I.M., I.V.: 2500 int. units/m^2 every 14 days

Hemodialysis: Significant drug removal is unlikely based on physiochemical characteristics

Peritoneal dialysis: Significant drug removal is unlikely based on physiochemical characteristics

Administration

I.M.: Must only be administered as a deep intramuscular injection into a large muscle; if I.M. injection volume is >2 mL, use multiple injection sites.

I.V.: May be administered as a 1 - to 2-hour I.V. infusion; **do not administer I.V. push**.

Monitoring Parameters Vital signs during administration, CBC with differential, platelets, amylase, liver enzymes, fibrinogen, PT, PTT, renal function tests, urine dipstick for glucose, blood glucose; monitor for onset of abdominal pain and mental status changes

Dosage Forms Excipient information presented when available (limited, particularly for generics); consult specific product labeling.

Injection, solution [preservative free]:

Oncaspar®: 750 units/mL (5 mL)

◆ **Pegasys®** *see* Peginterferon Alfa-2a *on page* 1153

Pegfilgrastim (peg fil GRA stim)

U.S. Brand Names Neulasta®

Canadian Brand Names Neulasta®

Index Terms G-CSF (PEG Conjugate); Granulocyte Colony Stimulating Factor (PEG Conjugate); NSC-725961; SD/01

Pharmacologic Category Colony Stimulating Factor

Use To decrease the incidence of infection, by stimulation of granulocyte production, in patients with nonmyeloid malignancies receiving myelosuppressive therapy associated with a significant risk of febrile neutropenia

Pregnancy Risk Factor C

Pregnancy Considerations Animal studies have demonstrated adverse effects and fetal loss. There are no adequate and well-controlled studies in pregnant women; use only if potential benefit to mother justifies the potential risk to the fetus.

Lactation Excretion in breast milk unknown/use caution

Medication Safety Issues

Sound-alike/look-alike issues:

Neulasta® may be confused with Neumega® and Lunesta™

Contraindications Hypersensitivity to pegfilgrastim, filgrastim, *E. coli*-derived proteins, or any component of the formulation

Warnings/Precautions Do not use pegfilgrastim in the period 14 days before to 24 hours after administration of cytotoxic chemotherapy because of the potential sensitivity of rapidly dividing myeloid cells to cytotoxic chemotherapy. Pegfilgrastim can potentially act as a growth factor for any tumor type, particularly myeloid malignancies. Caution should be exercised in the usage of pegfilgrastim in any malignancy with myeloid characteristics. Tumors of nonhematopoietic origin may have surface receptors for pegfilgrastim. Pegfilgrastim has not been evaluated with patients receiving radiation therapy, or with chemotherapy associated with delayed myelosuppression (nitrosoureas, mitomycin C). Safety and efficacy have not been evaluated for peripheral blood progenitor cell (PBPC) mobilization.

Allergic-type reactions (anaphylaxis, erythema, skin rash, urticaria) have occurred primarily with the initial dose and may recur after discontinuation; close follow up for several days and permanent discontinuation are recommended for severe reactions. Rare cases of splenic rupture have been reported; patients must be instructed to report left upper quadrant pain or shoulder tip pain. Acute respiratory distress syndrome (ARDS) has been associated with use; evaluate patients with pulmonary symptoms such as fever, lung infiltrates, or respiratory distress; discontinue or withhold pegfilgrastim if ARDS occurs. May precipitate sickle cell crises in patients with sickle cell disease; carefully evaluate potential risks and benefits. The packaging (needle cover) contains latex. Safety and efficacy in pediatric patients have not been established. The 6 mg fixed dose should not be used in adolescents weighing <45 kg.

Adverse Reactions

>10%:

Cardiovascular: Peripheral edema (12%)

Central nervous system: Headache (16%)

Gastrointestinal: Vomiting (13%)

Neuromuscular & skeletal: Bone pain (31% to 57%), myalgia (21%), arthralgia (16%), weakness (13%)

1% to 10%: Gastrointestinal: Constipation (10%)

<1% (Limited to important or life-threatening): Acute respiratory distress syndrome (ARDS), allergic reaction, anaphylaxis, fever, hyperleukocytosis, hypoxia, leukocytosis, rash, sickle cell crisis, splenic rupture, Sweet's syndrome (acute febrile dermatosis), urticaria. Cytopenias resulting from an antibody response to exogenous growth factors have been reported on rare occasions in patients treated with other recombinant growth factors.

Drug Interactions

Avoid Concomitant Use There are no known interactions where it is recommended to avoid concomitant use.

Increased Effect/Toxicity There are no known significant interactions involving an increase in effect.

Decreased Effect There are no known significant interactions involving a decrease in effect.

Stability Store under refrigeration 2°C to 8°C (36°F to 46°F); do not freeze. If inadvertently frozen, allow to thaw in refrigerator; discard if frozen more than one time. Protect from light. Do not shake. Allow to reach room temperature prior to injection. May be kept at room temperature for up to 48 hours.

Mechanism of Action Stimulates the production, maturation, and activation of neutrophils, pegfilgrastim activates neutrophils to increase both their migration and cytotoxicity. Pegfilgrastim has a prolonged duration of effect relative to filgrastim and a reduced renal clearance.

Pharmacodynamics/Kinetics Half-life elimination: SubQ: 15-80 hours

Dosage SubQ: Adolescents >45 kg and Adults: 6 mg once per chemotherapy cycle; do not administer in the period between 14 days before and 24 hours after administration of cytotoxic chemotherapy; do not use in infants, children, and smaller adolescents weighing <45 kg

Dosage adjustment in renal impairment: No adjustment necessary

Administration Do not use 6 mg fixed dose in infants, children, or adolescents <45 kg. Engage/activate needle guard following use to prevent accidental needlesticks.

Monitoring Parameters Complete blood count (with differential) and platelet count should be obtained prior to chemotherapy. Leukocytosis (white blood cell counts 100,000/mm^3) has been observed in <1% of patients receiving pegfilgrastim. Monitor platelets and hematocrit regularly. Evaluate fever, pulmonary infiltrates, and respiratory distress; evaluate for left upper abdominal pain, shoulder tip pain, or splenomegaly. Monitor for sickle cell crisis (in patients with sickle cell anemia).

Test Interactions May interfere with bone imaging studies; increased hematopoietic activity of the bone marrow may appear as transient positive bone imaging changes

Dosage Forms Excipient information presented when available (limited, particularly for generics); consult specific product labeling.

Injection, solution [preservative free]:

Neulasta®: 10 mg/mL (0.6 mL) [prefilled syringe; needle cover contains latex]

Peginterferon Alfa-2a

(peg in ter FEER on AL fa too aye)

U.S. Brand Names Pegasys®

Canadian Brand Names Pegasys®

Index Terms Interferon Alfa-2a (PEG Conjugate); Pegylated Interferon Alfa-2a

Pharmacologic Category Interferon

Use Treatment of chronic hepatitis C (CHC), alone or in combination with ribavirin, in patients with compensated liver disease and histological evidence of cirrhosis (Child-Pugh class A) and patients with clinically-stable HIV disease; treatment of patients with HBeAg positive and HBeAg negative chronic hepatitis B with compensated liver disease and evidence of viral replication and liver inflammation

Restrictions An FDA-approved medication guide must be distributed when dispensing an outpatient prescription (new or refill) where this medication is to be used without direct supervision of a healthcare provider. Medication guides are available at http://www.fda.gov/cder/Offices/ODS/medication_guides.htm.

Pregnancy Risk Factor C / X in combination with ribavirin

Pregnancy Considerations Reproduction studies with pegylated interferon alfa have not been conducted. Animal studies with nonpegylated interferon alfa-2b have demonstrated abortifacient effects. Disruption of the normal menstrual cycle was also observed in animal studies; therefore, the manufacturer recommends that reliable contraception is used in women of childbearing potential. Alfa interferon is endogenous to normal amniotic fluid. *In vitro* administration studies have reported that when administered to the mother, it does not cross the placenta. Case reports of use in pregnant women are limited. The Perinatal HIV Guidelines Working Group does not recommend that peginterferon-alfa be used during pregnancy. Peginterferon monotherapy should only be used in pregnancy when the potential benefit to the mother justifies the possible risk to the fetus. Combination therapy with ribavirin is contraindicated in pregnancy (refer to Ribavirin monograph); a pregnancy registry has been established for women inadvertently exposed to ribavirin while pregnant (800-593-2214).

Lactation Excretion in breast milk unknown/not recommended

Contraindications Hypersensitivity to polyethylene glycol (PEG), interferon alfa, or any component of the formulation; autoimmune hepatitis; decompensated liver disease in cirrhotic patients (Child-Pugh score >6); decompensated liver disease (Child-Pugh score ≥6, class B and C) in CHC coinfected with HIV; neonates and infants

Warnings/Precautions Hazardous agent: Use appropriate precautions for handling and disposal.

[U.S. Boxed Warning]: May cause or aggravate fatal or life threatening autoimmune disorders, neuropsychiatric symptoms (including depression and/or suicidal thoughts/behaviors), ischemic (including radiographic changes or worsening hepatic function) and/or infectious disorders; discontinue treatment for persistent severe or worsening symptoms.

Neuropsychiatric disorders: Severe psychiatric adverse effects (including depression, suicidal ideation, and suicide attempt) may occur. Avoid use in severe psychiatric disorders; use with extreme caution in patients with a history of depression. Patients who experience dizziness, confusion, somnolence or fatigue should use caution when performing tasks which require mental alertness (eg, operating machinery or driving).

Bone marrow suppression: May cause myelosuppression (including neutropenia, thrombocytopenia, lymphopenia, aplastic anemia). Use caution with baseline neutrophil count <1500/mm^3, platelet count <90,000/mm^3 or hemoglobin <10 g/dL. Discontinue therapy (at least temporarily) if ANC <500/mm^3 or platelet count <25,000/mm^3. Use with caution in patients with an increased risk for severe anemia (eg, spherocytosis, history of GI bleeding).

Hepatic disease: Hepatic decompensation and death have been associated with the use of alpha interferons including Pegasys®, in cirrhotic chronic hepatitis C patients; patients coinfected with HIV and receiving highly active antiretroviral therapy have shown an increased risk. Monitor hepatic function; discontinue if decompensation occurs (Child-Pugh score >6) in monoinfected patients and (Child-Pugh score ≥6, class B and C) in patients coinfected with HIV. In hepatitis B patients, flares (transient and potentially severe increases in serum ALT) may occur during or after treatment; more frequent monitoring of LFTs and a dose reduction are recommended. Discontinue if ALT elevation continues despite dose reduction or if increased bilirubin or hepatic decompensation occur.

Gastrointestinal disorders: Gastrointestinal hemorrhage, ulcerative and hemorrhagic/ischemic colitis have been observed with interferon alfa treatment; may be severe and/or life-threatening; discontinue if symptoms of colitis (eg, abdominal pain, bloody diarrhea, and/or fever) develop. Discontinue therapy if known or suspected pancreatitis develops.

Dermatologic disorders: Serious cutaneous reactions, including vesiculobullous eruptions, Stevens-Johnson syndrome and exfoliative dermatitis, have been reported (rarely) with use, with or without ribavirin therapy; discontinue with signs or symptoms of severe skin reactions.

Ophthalmic disease: Discontinue if new or worsening ophthalmologic disorders occur including retinal hemorrhages, cotton wool spots, and retinal artery or vein obstruction; visual exams are recommended in these instances, at the initiation of therapy, and periodically during therapy.

Pulmonary disorders: Dyspnea, pulmonary infiltrates, pneumonia, bronchiolitis obliterans, interstitial pneumonia, and sarcoidosis, resulting in potentially fatal respiratory failure may occur with treatment. Discontinue with unexplained pulmonary infiltrates or evidence of impaired pulmonary function. Use caution in patients with a history of pulmonary disease.

Endocrine disorders: Use with caution in patients with diabetes mellitus; hyper- or hypoglycemia have been reported which may require adjustments in medications. Use with caution in patients with pre-existing thyroid disease; thyroid disorders (hyper- or hypothyroidism) or exacerbations have been reported.

Severe acute hypersensitivity reactions have occurred rarely; prompt discontinuation is advised. Commonly associated with flu-like symptoms, including fever; rule out other causes/infection with persistent or high fever. Serious and severe infections (bacterial, viral and fungal) have been reported with treatment. Use with caution in patients with renal dysfunction (Cl_{cr} <50 mL/minute); monitor for signs/symptoms of toxicity (dosage adjustment required if toxicity occurs). Use with caution in patients with pulmonary dysfunction, prior cardiovascular disease, or autoimmune disease. Use with caution in the elderly. Safety and efficacy have not been established in children. **Due to differences in dosage, patients should not change brands of interferon without the concurrence of their healthcare provider.** Safety and efficacy have not been established in patients who have failed other alpha interferon therapy, received organ transplants, been coinfected with HBV and HCV or HIV; or with HCV and HIV with a CD4+ cell count <100 cells/microL, or been treated for >48 weeks. **[U.S. Boxed Warning]: Combination treatment with ribavirin may cause birth defects and/or fetal mortality; hemolytic anemia (which may worsen cardiac disease), genotoxicity, mutagenicity, and may possibly be carcinogenic.**

Adverse Reactions Note: Percentages are reported for peginterferon alfa-2a in chronic hepatitis C (CHC) patients. Other percentages indicated as "with ribavirin" or "in HIV/CHC" are those which significantly exceed incidence reported for peginterferon monotherapy in CHC patients.

>10%:

Central nervous system: Headache (54%), fatigue (56%), pyrexia (37%; 41% with ribavirin; 54% in hepatitis B), insomnia (19%; 30% with ribavirin), depression (18%), dizziness (16%), irritability/anxiety/nervousness (19%; 33% with ribavirin), pain (11%)

Dermatologic: Alopecia (23%; 28% with ribavirin), pruritus (12%; 19% with ribavirin), dermatitis (16% with ribavirin)

Gastrointestinal: Nausea/vomiting (24%), anorexia (17%; 24% with ribavirin), diarrhea (16%), weight loss (16% in HIV/CHC), abdominal pain (15%)

Hematologic: Neutropenia (21%; 27% with ribavirin; 40% in HIV/CHC), lymphopenia (14% with ribavirin), anemia (11% with ribavirin; 14% in HIV/CHC)

Hepatic: ALT increases 5-10 x ULN during treatment (25% to 27% in hepatitis B); ALT increases >10 x ULN during treatment (12% to 18% in hepatitis B); ALT increases 5-10 x ULN after treatment (13% to 16% in hepatitis B); ALT increases >10 x ULN after treatment (7% to 12% in hepatitis B)

Local: Injection site reaction (22%)

Neuromuscular & skeletal: Weakness (56%; 65% with ribavirin), myalgia (37%), rigors (35%; 25% to 27% in hepatitis B), arthralgia (28%)

Respiratory: Dyspnea (13% with ribavirin)

1% to 10%:

Central nervous system: Concentration impaired (8%), memory impaired (5%), mood alteration (3%; 9% in HIV/CHC)

Dermatologic: Dermatitis (8%), rash (5%), dry skin (4%; 10% with ribavirin), eczema (1%; 5% with ribavirin)

Endocrine & metabolic: Hypothyroidism (3% to 4%), hyperthyroidism (≤1%)

Gastrointestinal: Xerostomia (6%), dyspepsia (<1%; 6% with ribavirin), weight loss (4%; 10% with ribavirin)

Hematologic: Thrombocytopenia (5%; 8% in HIV/CHC), lymphopenia (3%), anemia (2%)

Hepatic: Hepatic decompensation (2% in CHC/HIV)

Neuromuscular & skeletal: Back pain (9%)

Ocular: Blurred vision (4%)

Respiratory: Cough (4%; 10% with ribavirin), dyspnea (4%), exertional dyspnea (4% with ribavirin)

Miscellaneous: Diaphoresis (6%), bacterial infection (3%; 5% in HIV/CHC)

≤1% (Limited to important or life-threatening): Aggression, anaphylaxis, angioedema, angina, aplastic anemia, arrhythmia, autoimmune disorders, bronchiolitis obliterans, bronchoconstriction, cerebral hemorrhage, chest pain, cholangitis, colitis, coma, corneal ulcer, cotton wool spots, diabetes mellitus, endocarditis, erythema multiforme major, exertional dyspnea, exfoliative dermatitis, fatty liver, gastrointestinal bleeding, hallucination, hearing impairment, hearing loss, hemoglobin decreased, hematocrit decreased, hepatic dysfunction, hepatic decompensation, hyper-/hypoglycemia, hypersensitivity reactions, hypertension, influenza, interstitial pneumonitis, MI, myositis, optic neuritis, papilledema, pancreatitis, peptic ulcer, peripheral neuropathy, pneumonia, psychiatric disorder, psychosis, pulmonary embolism, pulmonary infiltrates, retinal hemorrhage, retinopathy, rheumatoid arthritis, sarcoidosis, Stevens-Johnson syndrome, substance overdose, suicidal ideation, suicide, supraventricular arrhythmia, systemic lupus erythematosus, thrombotic thrombocytopenic purpura, urticaria, vesiculobullous eruptions, vision decreased/loss

Drug Interactions

Metabolism/Transport Effects **Inhibits** CYP1A2 (weak)

Avoid Concomitant Use There are no known interactions where it is recommended to avoid concomitant use.

Increased Effect/Toxicity

Peginterferon Alfa-2a may increase the levels/effects of: Aldesleukin; Ribavirin; Theophylline Derivatives; Zidovudine

Decreased Effect There are no known significant interactions involving a decrease in effect.

Ethanol/Nutrition/Herb Interactions Ethanol: Avoid use in patients with hepatitis C virus.

Stability Store in refrigerator at 2°C to 8°C (36°F to 46°F); do not freeze or shake. Protect from light. Discard unused solution.

Mechanism of Action Alpha interferons are a family of proteins, produced by nucleated cells, that have antiviral, antiproliferative, and immune-regulating activity. There are 16 known subtypes of alpha interferons. Interferons interact with cells through high affinity cell surface receptors. Following activation, multiple effects can be detected including induction of gene transcription. Inhibits cellular growth, alters the state of cellular differentiation, interferes with oncogene expression, alters cell surface antigen expression, increases phagocytic activity of macrophages, and augments cytotoxicity of lymphocytes for target cells.

Pharmacodynamics/Kinetics

Half-life elimination: Terminal: 50-160 hours; increased with renal dysfunction

Time to peak, serum: 72-96 hours

Dosage SubQ: Adults:

Chronic hepatitis C (monoinfection or coinfection with HIV):

Monotherapy: 180 mcg once weekly for 48 weeks

Combination therapy with ribavirin: Recommended dosage: 180 mcg once/week with ribavirin (Copegus®)

Duration of therapy: Monoinfection (based on genotype):

Genotype 1,4: 48 weeks

Genotype 2,3: 24 weeks

Duration of therapy: Coinfection with HIV: 48 weeks

Chronic hepatitis B: 180 mcg once weekly for 48 weeks

Dose modifications for adverse reactions/toxicity:

For moderate-to-severe adverse reactions: Initial: 135 mcg/week; may need decreased to 90 mcg/week in some cases

Based on hematologic parameters:

ANC <750/mm^3: 135 mcg/week

ANC <500/mm^3: Suspend therapy until >1000/mm^3, then restart at 90 mcg/week; monitor ANC

Platelet count <50,000/mm^3: 90 mcg/week

Platelet count <25,000/mm^3: Discontinue therapy

Depression (severity based on DSM-IV criteria):

Mild depression: No dosage adjustment required; evaluate once weekly by visit/phone call. If depression remains stable, continue weekly visits. If depression improves, resume normal visit schedule

Moderate depression: Decrease interferon dose to 90-135 mcg once/week; evaluate once weekly with an office visit at least every other week. If depression remains stable, consider psychiatric evaluation and continue with reduced dosing. If symptoms improve and remain stable for 4 weeks, resume normal visit schedule; continue reduced dosing or return to normal dose.

Severe depression: Discontinue interferon permanently. Obtain immediate psychiatric consultation. Discontinue ribavirin if using concurrently.

Dosage adjustment in renal impairment:

Cl_{cr} <50 mL/minute: Use caution; monitor for toxicity

End-stage renal disease requiring hemodialysis: 135 mcg/week; monitor for toxicity

Dosage adjustment in hepatic impairment:

HCV: ALT progressively rising above baseline: Decrease dose to 135 mcg/week. If ALT continues to rise or is accompanied by increased bilirubin or hepatic decompensation, discontinue therapy immediately.

HBV:

ALT >5 x ULN: Monitor LFTs more frequently; consider decreasing dose to 135 mcg/week or temporarily discontinuing (may resume after ALT flare subsides).

ALT >10 x ULN: Consider discontinuing.

Dietary Considerations Avoid ethanol use in patients with hepatitis C virus.

Administration SubQ: Administer in the abdomen or thigh. Rotate injection site. Do not use if solution contains particulate matter or is discolored. Discard unused solution. Administration should be done on the same day and at approximately the same time each week.

Monitoring Parameters Prior to treatment, pregnancy screening should occur for women of childbearing age who are receiving treatment or who have male partners who are receiving treatment. In combination therapy with ribavirin, pregnancy tests should continue monthly up to 6 months after discontinuation of therapy. Standard hematological tests should be performed prior to therapy, at week 2, and periodically. Standard biochemical tests should be performed prior to therapy, at week 4, and periodically. Evaluate for depression and other psychiatric symptoms before and during therapy; baseline eye examination and periodically in patients with baseline disorders; baseline echocardiogram in patients with cardiac disease; serum HCV RNA levels after 12 weeks of treatment. Consider discontinuing treatment if virologic tests indicate no response by week 12.

Clinical studies tested as follows: CBC (including hemoglobin, WBC, and platelets) and chemistries (including liver function tests and uric acid) measured at weeks 1, 2, 4, 6, and 8, and then every 4-6 weeks (more frequently if abnormal) weeks; TSH measured every 12 weeks

In addition, the following baseline values were used as entrance criteria:

Platelet count ≥90,000/mm^3 (as low as 75,000/mm^3 in patients with cirrhosis or transition to cirrhosis)

ANC ≥1500/mm^3

Serum creatinine <1.5 times ULN

TSH and T_4 within normal limits or adequately controlled

$CD4^+$ cell count ≥200 cells/microL or $CD4^+$ cell count ≥100 cells/ microL, but <200 cells/ microL and HIV-1 RNA <5000 copies/mL in CHC patients coinfected with HIV

Hemoglobin ≥12 g/dL for women and ≥13 g/dL for men in CHC monoinfected patients

Hemoglobin ≥11 g/dL for women and ≥12 g/dL for men in CHC patients coinfected with HIV

Dosage Forms Excipient information presented when available (limited, particularly for generics); consult specific product labeling.

Injection solution:

Pegasys®

180 mcg/0.5 mL (0.5 mL) [prefilled syringe; contains benzyl alcohol and polysorbate 80; packaged with needles and alcohol swabs]

180 mcg/mL (1 mL) [vial; contains benzyl alcohol and polysorbate 80]

Peginterferon Alfa-2b

(peg in ter FEER on AL fa too bee)

U.S. Brand Names PegIntron™

Canadian Brand Names PegIntron™

Index Terms Interferon Alfa-2b (PEG Conjugate); Pegylated Interferon Alfa-2b

Pharmacologic Category Interferon

Use Treatment of chronic hepatitis C (in combination with ribavirin) in patients who have never received alfa interferons and have compensated liver disease; treatment of chronic hepatitis C (as monotherapy) in adult patients who have never received alfa interferons

Unlabeled/Investigational Use Treatment of advanced melanoma

Restrictions An FDA-approved medication guide must be distributed when dispensing an outpatient prescription (new or refill) where this medication is to be used without direct supervision of a healthcare provider. Medication guides are available at http://www.fda.gov/cder/Offices/ODS/medication_guides.htm.

Pregnancy Risk Factor C / X in combination with ribavirin

Pregnancy Considerations Reproduction studies with pegylated interferon alfa have not been conducted. Animal studies with nonpegylated interferon alfa-2b have demonstrated abortifacient effects. Disruption of the normal menstrual cycle was also observed in animal studies; therefore, the manufacturer recommends that reliable contraception is used in women of childbearing potential. Alfa interferon is endogenous to normal amniotic fluid. *In vitro* administration studies have reported that when administered to the mother, it does not cross the placenta. Case reports of use in pregnant women are limited. The Perinatal HIV Guidelines Working Group does not recommend that peginterferon-alfa be used during pregnancy. Peginterferon alfa-2b monotherapy should only be used in pregnancy when the potential benefit to the mother justifies the possible risk to the fetus. **[U.S. Boxed Warning]: Combination therapy with ribavirin may cause birth defects; avoid pregnancy in females and female partners of male patients;** combination therapy with ribavirin is contraindicated in pregnancy. A pregnancy registry has been established for women inadvertently exposed to ribavirin while pregnant (800-593-2214).

Lactation Excretion in breast milk unknown/not recommended

Medication Safety Issues

Sound-alike/look-alike issues:

Peginterferon alfa-2b may be confused with interferon alfa-2a, interferon alfa-2b, interferon alfa-n3, peginterferon alfa-2a

PegIntron™ may be confused with Intron® A

International issues:

Peginterferon alfa-2b may be confused with interferon alpha multi-subtype which is available in international markets

Contraindications Hypersensitivity (including urticaria, angioedema, bronchoconstriction, anaphylaxis, Stevens Johnson syndrome and toxic epidermal necrolysis) to interferons, or any component of the formulation; autoimmune hepatitis; decompensated liver disease (Child-Pugh score >6, classes B and C) in cirrhotic chronic hepatitis C (prior to or during treatment)

Combination therapy with peginterferon alfa-2b and ribavirin is also contraindicated in pregnancy, women who may become pregnant, males with pregnant partners; hemoglobinopathies (eg, thalassemia major, sickle-cell anemia); renal dysfunction (Cl_{cr} <50 mL/minute)

Warnings/Precautions Hazardous agent - use appropriate precautions for handling and disposal.

[U.S. Boxed Warning]: May cause or aggravate fatal or life-threatening autoimmune disorders, neuropsychiatric symptoms (including depression and/or suicidal thoughts/behaviors), infectious disorders, ischemic disorders, and/or hemorrhagic cerebrovascular events; discontinue treatment for persistent severe or worsening symptoms.

Neuropsychiatric disorders: Neuropsychiatric effects may occur in patients with and without a history of psychiatric disorder; addiction relapse, aggression, depression, homicidal ideation and suicidal behavior/ideation have been observed with peginterferon alfa-2b; bipolar disorder, hallucinations, mania, and psychosis have been observed with other alfa interferons. Use with extreme caution in patients with a history of psychiatric disorders, including depression. Monitor all patients for evidence of depression; patients who develop psychiatric disorders should be monitored during and for 6 months after completion of therapy; discontinue treatment if psychiatric symptoms persist, worsen, or if suicidal behavior develops. Higher doses may be associated with the development of encephalopathy (higher risk in elderly patients).

Bone marrow suppression: Causes bone marrow suppression, including potentially severe cytopenias; alfa interferons may (rarely) cause aplastic anemia. Use with caution in patients who are chronically immunosuppressed, with low peripheral blood counts or myelosuppression, including concurrent use of myelosuppressive therapy. Dosage modification may be necessary for hematologic toxicity. Combination therapy with ribavirin may potentiate the neutropenic effects of alfa interferons. When used in combination with ribavirin, an increased incidence of anemia was observed when using ribavirin weight-based dosing, as compared to flat-dose ribavirin.

Hepatic disease: Discontinue treatment immediately with hepatic decompensation (Child Pugh score >6). Patients with chronic hepatitis C (CHC) with cirrhosis receiving peginterferon alfa-2b are at risk for hepatic decompensation. CHC patients coinfected with human immunodeficiency virus (HIV) are at increased risk for hepatic decompensation when receiving highly active antiretroviral therapy (HAART); monitor closely. A transient increase in ALT (2-5 times above baseline) which is not associated with deterioration of liver function may occur with peginterferon alfa-2b use; therapy generally may continue with monitoring.

Gastrointestinal disorders: Pancreatitis has been observed with alfa interferon therapy; discontinue therapy if known or suspected pancreatitis develops. Ulcerative or hemorrhagic/ischemic colitis has been observed with alfa interferons; discontinue therapy if signs of colitis (abdominal pain, bloody diarrhea, fever) develop.

Autoimmune disorders: Thyroiditis, thrombotic thrombocytopenic purpura, idiopathic thrombocytopenic purpura, rheumatoid arthritis, interstitial nephritis, systemic lupus erythematosus, and psoriasis have been reported with therapy; use with caution in patients with autoimmune disorders.

Cardiovascular disease: Use with caution in patients with cardiovascular disease or a history of cardiovascular disease; hypotension, arrhythmia, tachycardia, cardiomyopathy, angina pectoris and MI have been observed with treatment. Patients with pre-existing cardiac abnormalities should have baseline ECGs prior to combination treatment with ribavirin; patients with a history of significant or unstable cardiac disease should not receive combination treatment with ribavirin.

Endocrine disorders: Diabetes mellitus, hyperglycemia, and thyroid disorders have been reported; discontinue peginterferon alfa-2b if cannot be effectively managed with medication. Use caution in patients with a history of diabetes mellitus, particularly if prone to DKA. Use with caution in patients with thyroid disorders; may cause or aggravate hyper- or hypothyroidism.

Pulmonary disease: May cause or aggravate dyspnea, pulmonary infiltrates, pneumonia, bronchiolitis obliterans, interstitial pneumonitis and sarcoidosis which may result in respiratory failure; may recur upon rechallenge with treatment; monitor closely.

Ophthalmic disorders: Ophthalmologic disorders (including decreased/loss of vision, macular edema, retinal hemorrhages, optic neuritis, papilledema, cotton wool spots, and retinal artery or vein thrombosis) have occurred with peginterferon alfa-2b and/or with other alfa interferons. Prior to start of therapy, ophthalmic exams are recommended for all patients; patients with diabetic or hypertensive retinopathy should have periodic ophthalmic exams during treatment. Discontinue treatment with new or worsening ophthalmic disorder.

[U.S. Boxed Warning]: Combination treatment with ribavirin may cause birth defects and/or fetal mortality (avoid pregnancy in females and female partners of male patients); hemolytic anemia (which may worsen cardiac disease), genotoxicity, mutagenicity, and may possibly be carcinogenic. Interferon therapy is commonly associated with flu-like symptoms, including fever; rule out other causes/infection with persistent or high fever. Acute hypersensitivity reactions and cutaneous reactions have been reported (rarely) with alfa interferons; prompt discontinuation is recommended; transient rashes do not require interruption of therapy. Hypertriglyceridemia has been reported with use; discontinue if severe (triglycerides >1000 mg/dL), particularly if combined with symptoms of pancreatitis. Use with caution in patients with renal impairment (Cl_{cr} <50 mL/minute); monitor closely; dosage adjustments are recommended with monotherapy in patients with moderate to severe impairment; do not use combination therapy with ribavirin in adult patients renal dysfunction (Cl_{cr} <50 mL/minute); discontinue if serum creatinine >2 mg/dL in children. Serum creatinine increases have been reported in patients with renal insufficiency. Use with caution in the elderly; the potential adverse effects may be more pronounced in the elderly. Dental/periodontal disorders have been reported with combination therapy; dry mouth may affect teeth and mucous membranes; instruct patients to brush teeth twice daily; encourage regular dental exams.

Combination therapy with ribavirin is preferred over monotherapy for the treatment of chronic hepatitis C. Safety and efficacy have not been established in patients who have failed other alpha interferon therapy, received organ transplants, coinfected with HIV or hepatitis B, or received treatment for >1 year. Safety and efficacy have not been established in children <3 years of age. Growth velocity (height and weight) was decreased in children on combination treatment, particularly during the first 6 months of treatment. **[U.S. Boxed Warning]: Combination therapy with ribavirin is contraindicated in pregnancy.** Due to differences in dosage, patients should not change brands of interferon.

Adverse Reactions Note: Percentages reported for adults receiving monotherapy unless noted:

>10%:

Central nervous system: Headache (56%), fatigue (52%), depression (16% to 29%; may be severe), anxiety/emotional liability/irritability (28%), insomnia (23%), fever (22%), dizziness (12%)

Dermatologic: Alopecia (22%), pruritus (12%), dry skin (11%)

Gastrointestinal: Nausea (26%), anorexia (20%), diarrhea (18%), abdominal pain (8% to 15%), weight loss (11%)

Hematologic: Neutropenia (6% to 70%; grade 4: 1%), thrombocytopenia (7% to 20%; grades 3/4: <4%), anemia (in combination with ribavirin: 12% to 47%)

Local: Injection site inflammation/reaction (23% to 47%)

Neuromuscular & skeletal: Myalgia (54%), weakness (52%), musculoskeletal pain (28%), arthralgia (23%), rigors (23%)

Miscellaneous: Viral infection (11%)

>1% to 10%:

Cardiovascular: Chest pain (6%), flushing (6%)

Central nervous system: Concentration impaired (10%), malaise (7%), nervousness (4%), agitation (2%), suicidal behavior (ideation/attempt/suicide ≤2%)

Dermatologic: Rash (6%)

Endocrine & metabolic: Hypothyroidism (5%), menstrual disorder (4%), hyperthyroidism (3%)

Gastrointestinal: Vomiting (7%), dyspepsia (6%), xerostomia (6%), constipation (1%)

Hepatic: Transaminases increased (10%; transient), hepatomegaly (6%)

Local: Injection site pain (2% to 3%)

Ocular: Conjunctivitis (4%), blurred vision (2%)

Respiratory: Pharyngitis (10%), cough (8%), sinusitis (7%), dyspnea (4%), rhinitis (2%)

Miscellaneous: Diaphoresis (6%), neutralizing antibodies (2%)

≤1% (Limited to important and life-threatening): Abscess, addiction (drug) relapse, aggressive behavior, anaphylaxis, angina, angioedema, aphthous stomatitis, aplastic anemia, arrhythmia, autoimmune thrombocytopenia (with or without purpura), bronchiolitis obliterans, bronchoconstriction, cardiomyopathy, cellulitis, cerebral hemorrhage, cerebral ischemia, cotton wool spots, cytopenia, diabetes mellitus, drug overdose, emphysema, encephalopathy, erythema multiforme, fungal infection, gastroenteritis, gout, hallucinations, hearing impairment/loss, hemorrhagic colitis, homicidal ideation, hyperglycemia, hypersensitivity reactions, hypertriglyceridemia, hypotension, injection site necrosis, interstitial nephritis, interstitial pneumonia, ischemic colitis, leukopenia, loss of consciousness, lupus-like syndrome, macular edema, memory loss, MI, migraine, myositis, nerve palsy (facial/oculomotor), optic neuritis, pancreatitis, papilledema, pericardial effusion, peripheral neuropathy, phototoxicity, pleural effusion, pneumonia, pneumonitis, polyneuropathy, psoriasis, psychosis, pulmonary infiltrates, pure red cell aplasia, renal insufficiency, renal failure, retinal artery or vein thrombosis, retinal hemorrhage, retinal ischemia, rhabdomyolysis, rheumatoid arthritis, sarcoidosis, seizure, sepsis, serum creatinine increased, Stevens-Johnson syndrome, supraventricular arrhythmia, tachycardia, thrombotic thrombocytopenic purpura, thyroiditis, toxic epidermal necrolysis, transient ischemic attack, ulcerative colitis, urticaria, vasculitis, vertigo, vision decrease/loss, visual acuity decreased

Drug Interactions

Metabolism/Transport Effects Inhibits CYP1A2 (weak)

Avoid Concomitant Use There are no known interactions where it is recommended to avoid concomitant use.

Increased Effect/Toxicity

Peginterferon Alfa-2b may increase the levels/effects of: Aldesleukin; Ribavirin; Theophylline Derivatives; Zidovudine

Decreased Effect There are no known significant interactions involving a decrease in effect.

Ethanol/Nutrition/Herb Interactions Ethanol: Avoid use in patients with hepatitis C virus.

Stability Prior to reconstitution, store Redipen™ at 2°C to 8°C (36°F to 46°F). Store vials at 25°C (77°F); excursions permitted to 15°C to 30°C (59°F to 86°F).

Redipen™: Hold cartridge upright and press the two halves together until there is a "click". Gently invert to mix; do not shake.

Vial: Add 0.7 mL of sterile water for injection, USP (supplied diluent) to the vial. Gently swirl. Do not re-enter vial after dose removed. Discard unused portion.

Once reconstituted each product should be used immediately or may be stored for ≤24 hours at 2°C to 8°C (36°F to 46°F); do not freeze. Products do not contain preservative.

Mechanism of Action Alpha interferons are a family of proteins, produced by nucleated cells, that have antiviral, antiproliferative, and immune-regulating activity. There are 16 known subtypes of alpha interferons. Interferons interact with cells through high affinity cell surface receptors. Following activation, multiple effects can be detected including induction of gene transcription. Inhibits cellular growth, alters the state of cellular differentiation, interferes with oncogene expression, alters cell surface antigen expression, increases phagocytic activity of macrophages, and augments cytotoxicity of lymphocytes for target cells.

Pharmacodynamics/Kinetics

Bioavailability: Increases with chronic dosing

Half-life elimination: ~40 hours (range: 22-60 hours)

Time to peak: 15-44 hours

Excretion: Urine (30%)

Dosage SubQ:

Children ≥3 years: Chronic hepatitis C: Combination therapy with ribavirin: 60 mcg/m^2 once weekly (in combination with ribavirin 15 mg/kg/day in 2 divided doses); **Note:** Children who reach their 18th birthday during treatment should remain on the pediatric regimen. Discontinue combination therapy at 12 weeks if HCV-RNA decreases <2 $\log_{10}$ (compared to pretreatment) or if detectable HCV-RNA at 24 weeks.

Adults:

Chronic hepatitis C: Administer dose once weekly; **Note:** Treatment duration may vary. Consult current guidelines and literature. Discontinue after 6 months of treatment if HCV viral levels remain detectable.

Monotherapy: Initial: 1 mcg/kg/week
- ≤45 kg: 40 mcg once weekly
- 46-56 kg: 50 mcg once weekly
- 57-72 kg: 64 mcg once weekly
- 73-88 kg: 80 mcg once weekly
- 89-106 kg: 96 mcg once weekly
- 107-136 kg: 120 mcg once weekly
- 137-160 kg: 150 mcg once weekly

Combination therapy with ribavirin: Initial: 1.5 mcg/kg/week
- <40 kg: 50 mcg once weekly (with ribavirin 800 mg/day)
- 40-50 kg: 64 mcg once weekly (with ribavirin 800 mg/day)
- 51-60 kg: 80 mcg once weekly (with ribavirin 800 mg/day)
- 61-65 kg: 96 mcg once weekly (with ribavirin 800 mg/day)
- 66-75 kg: 96 mcg once weekly (with ribavirin 1000 mg/day)
- 76-85 kg: 120 mcg once weekly (with ribavirin 1000 mg/day)
- 86-105 kg: 150 mcg once weekly (with ribavirin 1200 mg/day)
- >105 kg: 150 mcg once weekly (with ribavirin 1400 mg/day)

Advanced melanoma (unlabeled use): 6 mcg/kg weekly for 8 weeks, followed by 3 mcg/kg weekly for a total of 5 years (Eggermont, 2008).

Elderly: May require dosage reduction based upon renal dysfunction, but no established guidelines are available.

Dosage adjustment for toxicity: For serious adverse reaction during treatment, modify dosage or discontinue; discontinue for persistent serious adverse reaction:

Dosage adjustment for depression (severity based upon DSM-IV criteria):

Mild depression: No dosage adjustment required; evaluate once weekly by visit/phone call. If depression remains stable, continue weekly visits. If depression improves, resume normal visit schedule.

Moderate depression: Adults: Decrease peginterferon alfa-2b dose by 50%; Children: Decrease peginterferon alfa-2b dose to 40 mcg/m^2/week, may further decrease to 20 mcg/m^2/week if needed. Evaluate once weekly with an office visit at least every other week. If depression remains stable, consider psychiatric evaluation and continue with reduced dosing. If symptoms improve and remain stable for 4 weeks, resume normal visit schedule; continue reduced dosing or return to normal dose.

Severe depression: Discontinue peginterferon alfa-2b and ribavirin permanently. Obtain immediate psychiatric consultation.

Dosage adjustment in hematologic toxicity:

Children:

Hemoglobin decrease ≥2 g/dL in any 4-week period in patients with pre-existing cardiac disease: Monitor and evaluate weekly

Hemoglobin <10 g/dL: Decrease ribavirin dose to 12 mg/kg/day; may further reduce to 8 mg/kg/day

WBC <1.5 x 10^9/L, neutrophils <0.75 x 10^9/L, or platelets <70 x 10^9/L: Reduce peginterferon alfa-2b dose to 40 mcg/m^2/week; may further reduce to 20 mcg/m^2/week.

Hemoglobin <8.5 g/dL, WBC <1.0 x 10^9/L, neutrophils <0.5 x 10^9/L, or platelets <50 x 10^9/L: Permanently discontinue peginterferon alfa-2b and ribavirin

Adults:

Hemoglobin decrease >2 g/dL in any 4-week period and stable cardiac disease: Decrease peginterferon alfa-2b dose by 50%; decrease ribavirin dose by 200 mg/day. Hemoglobin <12 g/dL after dose reductions: Permanently discontinue both peginterferon alfa-2b and ribavirin.

Hemoglobin <10 g/dL in patients with cardiac disease: Reduce peginterferon alfa-2b dose by 50%; decrease ribavirin dose by 200 mg/day.

WBC <1.5 x 10^9/L, neutrophils <0.75 x 10^9/L, or platelets <80 x 10^9/L: Reduce peginterferon alfa-2b dose by 50%.

Hemoglobin <8.5 g/dL, WBC <1.0 x 10^9/L, neutrophils <0.5 x 10^9/L, or platelets <50 x 10^9/L: Permanently discontinue peginterferon alfa-2b and ribavirin.

Dosage adjustment in renal impairment:

Peginterferon alfa-2b monotherapy:
- Cl_{cr} 30-50 mL/minute: Reduce dose by 25%
- Cl_{cr} 10-29 mL/minute: Reduce dose by 50%
- Hemodialysis: Reduce dose by 50%
- Discontinue use if renal function declines during treatment.

Peginterferon alfa-2b combination with ribavirin:
- Children: Serum creatinine >2 mg/dL: Discontinue treatment
- Adults: Cl_{cr} <50 mL/minute: Combination therapy with ribavirin is not recommended

Dosage adjustment in hepatic impairment: Contraindicated in decompensated liver disease

Administration For SubQ administration; rotate injection site; thigh, outer surface of upper arm, and abdomen are preferred injection sites; do not inject near navel or waistline; patients who are thin should only use thigh or upper arm. Do not inject into bruised, infected, irritated, red, or scarred skin.

Monitoring Parameters Baseline and periodic TSH, hematology (including CBC with differential, platelets), chemistry (including LFTs) testing, renal function, triglycerides. Evaluate for depression and other psychiatric symptoms before and after initiation of therapy; baseline ophthalmic eye examination; periodic ophthalmic exam in patients with diabetic or hypertensive retinopathy; baseline echocardiogram in patients with cardiac disease; serum HCV RNA levels, serum glucose or Hb A_{1c} (for patients with diabetes mellitus).

In combination therapy with ribavirin, pregnancy tests (for women of childbearing age who are receiving treatment or who have male partners who are receiving treatment), continue monthly up to 6 months after discontinuation of therapy.

Reference Range

Early viral response (EVR): >2 log decrease in HCV RNA after 12 weeks of treatment

End of treatment response (ETR): Absence of detectable HCV RNA at end of the recommended treatment period

Sustained treatment response (STR): Absence of HCV RNA in the serum 6 months following completion of full treatment course

Dosage Forms Excipient information presented when available (limited, particularly for generics); consult specific product labeling.

Injection, powder for reconstitution [preservative free]:

PegIntron™: 50 mcg, 80 mcg, 120 mcg, 150 mcg [contains polysorbate 80 and sucrose]

PegIntron™ Redipen®: 50 mcg, 80 mcg, 120 mcg, 150 mcg [contains polysorbate 80 and sucrose]

◆ **PegIntron™** *see* Peginterferon Alfa-2b *on page 1156*

◆ **PegLyte® (Can)** *see* Polyethylene Glycol-Electrolyte Solution *on page 1209*

Pegvisomant (peg VI soe mant)

U.S. Brand Names Somavert®

Canadian Brand Names Somavert®

Index Terms B2036-PEG

Pharmacologic Category Growth Hormone Receptor Antagonist

Use Treatment of acromegaly in patients resistant to or unable to tolerate other therapies

Pregnancy Risk Factor B

Dosage SubQ: Adults: Initial loading dose: 40 mg; maintenance dose: 10 mg once daily; doses may be adjusted by 5 mg increments in 4- to 6-week intervals based on IGF-I concentrations (maximum maintenance dose: 30 mg/day)

Dosage adjustment in hepatic impairment:

At initiation of therapy:

Normal liver function test (LFT): Initiate therapy; monitor LFT monthly for first 6 months, quarterly for next 6 months, then biannually the following year.

Baseline LFT elevated but ≤3 x ULN: May initiate therapy with monthly evaluation of LFT for 1 year then biannually the following year.

Baseline LFT >3 x ULN: Do not initiate treatment without comprehensive work-up to determine cause; monitor closely if treatment is started.

With ongoing therapy:

LFT ≥3 x but <5 x ULN without signs/symptoms of hepatitis, hepatic injury, or increase in total bilirubin: Continue treatment, but monitor LFT weekly for further increases; perform comprehensive hepatic work-up to rule out alternative cause of hepatic dysfunction

LFT ≥5 x ULN or transaminase ≥3 x ULN associated with any increase in total bilirubin: Discontinue immediately and perform comprehensive hepatic work-up. If LFTs return to normal, may cautiously consider restarting therapy with frequent LFT monitoring.

Signs or symptoms of hepatitis or hepatic injury: Discontinue therapy immediately and perform comprehensive hepatic work-up; discontinue permanently if liver injury is confirmed.

Additional Information Complete prescribing information for this medication should be consulted for additional detail.

Dosage Forms Excipient information presented when available (limited, particularly for generics); consult specific product labeling.

Injection, powder for reconstitution [preservative free]:

Somavert®: 10 mg, 15 mg, 20 mg [vial stopper contains latex; packaged with SWFI]

◆ **Pegylated DOXOrubicin Liposomal** *see* DOXOrubicin (Liposomal) *on page 488*

◆ **Pegylated Interferon Alfa-2a** *see* Peginterferon Alfa-2a *on page 1153*

◆ **Pegylated Interferon Alfa-2b** *see* Peginterferon Alfa-2b *on page 1156*

◆ **Pegylated Liposomal DOXOrubicin** *see* DOXOrubicin (Liposomal) *on page 488*

◆ **PE-Hist DM** *see* Chlorpheniramine, Phenylephrine, and Dextromethorphan *on page 311*

Pemetrexed (pem e TREKS ed)

U.S. Brand Names Alimta®

Canadian Brand Names Alimta®

Index Terms LY231514; Multitargeted Antifolate; NSC-698037; Pemetrexed Disodium

Pharmacologic Category Antineoplastic Agent, Antimetabolite; Antineoplastic Agent, Antimetabolite (Antifolate)

Use Treatment of malignant pleural mesothelioma; treatment of locally advanced or metastatic nonsquamous nonsmall cell lung cancer (NSCLC)

Unlabeled/Investigational Use Treatment of bladder cancer

Pregnancy Risk Factor D

Pregnancy Considerations Adverse events were observed in animal reproduction studies. There are no adequate and well-controlled trials in pregnant women. Women of childbearing potential should avoid becoming pregnant during treatment.

Lactation Excretion in breast milk unknown/not recommended

Medication Safety Issues

High alert medication: The Institute for Safe Medication Practices (ISMP) includes this medication among its list of drug classes which have a heightened risk of causing significant patient harm when used in error.

Contraindications Severe hypersensitivity to pemetrexed or any component of the formulation

Warnings/Precautions Hazardous agent - use appropriate precautions for handling and disposal. May cause bone marrow suppression (anemia, neutropenia, thrombocytopenia and/or pancytopenia); may require dose reductions in subsequent cycles. Prophylactic folic acid and vitamin B_{12} supplements are necessary to reduce hematologic and gastrointestinal toxicity and should be started 1 week before the first dose of pemetrexed. Pretreatment with corticosteroids reduces the incidence and severity of cutaneous reactions. Effects of third space fluid on drug disposition is unknown; consider draining effusion(s) prior to treatment. Use caution with hepatic dysfunction not due to metastases; may require dose adjustment.

Decreased renal function results in increased toxicity. Use caution in patients receiving concurrent nephrotoxins; may result in delayed pemetrexed clearance. NSAIDs may reduce the clearance of pemetrexed; patients with Cl_{cr} 45-79 mL/minute should avoid NSAIDs with short elimination half-lives (eg, ibuprofen, indomethacin, ketoprofen, ketorolac) for 2 days before, the day of, and 2 days following a dose of pemetrexed; all patients should avoid NSAIDs with long half-lives (eg, nabumetone, naproxen, oxaprozin, piroxicam) for 5 days before, the day of, and 2 days following a dose of pemetrexed. The manufacturer does not recommend use for Cl_{cr} <45 mL/minute. Safety and efficacy in children have not been established.

Adverse Reactions Note: Reported for monotherapy in patients who received folate and B_{12} supplementation.

>10%:

- Central nervous system: Fatigue (34%; dose-limiting)
- Dermatologic: Rash/desquamation (14%)
- Gastrointestinal: Nausea (31%), anorexia (22%), vomiting (16%), stomatitis (15%), diarrhea (13%)
- Hematologic: Anemia (19%; grades 3/4: 4%), leukopenia (12%; grades 3/4: 4%), neutropenia (11%; grades 3/4: 5%; nadir: 8-10 days; recovery: 12-17 days; dose-limiting)
- Respiratory: Pharyngitis (15%)

1% to 10%:

- Cardiovascular: Edema (5%)
- Central nervous system: Fever (8%)
- Dermatologic: Pruritus (7%), alopecia (6%), erythema multiforme
- Gastrointestinal: Constipation (6%), weight loss (1%), abdominal pain
- Hematologic: Thrombocytopenia (8%; grades 3/4: 2%; dose-limiting), febrile neutropenia (grades 3/4: 2%)
- Hepatic: ALT increased (8%; grades 3/4: 2%), AST increased (7%; grades 3/4: 1%)
- Neuromuscular & skeletal: Neuropathy (sensory and motor)
- Renal: Creatinine increased
- Miscellaneous: Allergic reaction/hypersensitivity, infection

<1% (Limited to important or life-threatening; mono- or combination therapy): Colitis, interstitial pneumonitis, pancytopenia, radiation recall (median onset: 6 days; range: 1-35 days), renal failure, supraventricular arrhythmia

Drug Interactions

Avoid Concomitant Use There are no known interactions where it is recommended to avoid concomitant use.

Increased Effect/Toxicity

The levels/effects of Pemetrexed may be increased by: NSAID (Nonselective)

Decreased Effect There are no known significant interactions involving a decrease in effect.

Ethanol/Nutrition/Herb Interactions Lower ANC nadirs occur in patients with elevated baseline cystathionine or homocysteine concentrations. Levels of these substances can be reduced by folic acid and vitamin B_{12} supplementation.

Stability Store intact vials at room temperature of 25°C (77°F); excursions permitted to 15°C to 30°C (59°F to 86°F). Reconstitute with NS (preservative free); add 4.2 mL to the 100 mg vial and 20 mL to the 500 mg vial, resulting in a 25 mg/mL concentration. Gently swirl. Solution may be colorless to green-yellow. Further dilute in 100 mL NS for infusion. Use appropriate precautions for handling and disposal. Reconstituted and infusion solutions are stable for 24 hours when refrigerated at 2°C to 8°C (36°F to 46°F) or stored at room temperature of 15°C to 30°C (59°F to 86°F). Concentrations at 25 mg/mL are stable in polypropylene syringes for 2 days at room temperature (23°C) (Zhang, 2005).

Mechanism of Action Inhibits thymidylate synthase (TS), dihydrofolate reductase (DHFR), glycinamide ribonucleotide formyltransferase (GARFT), and aminoimidazole carboxamide ribonucleotide formyltransferase (AICARFT), the enzymes involved in folate metabolism and DNA synthesis, resulting in inhibition of purine and thymidine nucleotide and protein synthesis.

Pharmacodynamics/Kinetics

Duration: V_{dss}: 16.1 L

Protein binding: ~73% to 81%

Metabolism: Minimal

Half-life elimination: Normal renal function: 3.5 hours; Cl_{cr} 40-59 mL/minute: 5.3-5.8 hours

Excretion: Urine (70% to 90% as unchanged drug)

Dosage Details concerning dosing in combination regimens should also be consulted. **Note:** Start vitamin supplements 1 week before initial dose of pemetrexed: Folic acid 350-1000 mcg/day orally (must be taken at least 5 out of 7 days prior to treatment initiation; continue for 21 days after last pemetrexed dose) and vitamin B_{12} 1000 mcg I.M. during the week prior to treatment initiation and then every 3 cycles. Give dexamethasone 4 mg orally twice daily for 3 days, beginning the day before treatment to minimize cutaneous reactions. New treatment cycles should not begin unless ANC ≥1500/mm^3, platelets ≥100,000/mm^3, and Cl_{cr} ≥45 mL/minute.

I.V.: Adults:

- Nonsmall cell lung cancer: 500 mg/m^2 on day 1 of each 21-day cycle (in combination with cisplatin for initial treatment; monotherapy in patients who have received prior treatment)
- Malignant pleural mesothelioma: 500 mg/m^2 on day 1 of each 21-day cycle (in combination with cisplatin)

Dosage adjustments for toxicities:

Toxicity: Discontinue if patient develops grade 3 or 4 toxicity after two dose reductions (except grade 3 transaminase elevations) or immediately if grade 3 or 4 neurotoxicity develops

Hematologic toxicity: Upon recovery, reinitiate therapy

- Nadir ANC <500/mm^3 and nadir platelets ≥50,000/mm^3: Reduce dose to 75% of previous dose of pemetrexed (and cisplatin)
- Nadir platelets <50,000/mm^3 **without bleeding** (regardless of nadir ANC): Reduce dose to 75% of previous dose of pemetrexed (and cisplatin)
- Nadir platelets <50,000/mm^3 **with bleeding** (regardless of nadir ANC): Reduce dose to 50% of previous dose of pemetrexed (and cisplatin)

Nonhematologic toxicity (excluding neurotoxicity or grade 3 transaminase elevations): Withhold treatment until recovery to baseline; upon recovery, reinitiate therapy as follows:

- Grade 3 or 4 toxicity (excluding mucositis or grade 3 transaminase elevations): Reduce dose to 75% of previous dose of pemetrexed (and cisplatin)
- Grade 3 or 4 diarrhea or any diarrhea requiring hospitalization: Reduce dose to 75% of previous dose of pemetrexed (and cisplatin)
- Grade 3 or 4 mucositis: Reduce pemetrexed dose to 50% of previous dose (continue cisplatin at 100% of previous dose)

Neurotoxicity:

- Common Toxicity Criteria (CTC) Grade 0-1: Continue at 100% of previous dose of pemetrexed (and cisplatin)
- CTC Grade 2: Continue pemetrexed at previous dose; reduce cisplatin dose to 50% of previous dose

Dosage adjustment in renal impairment:

Cl_{cr} ≥45 mL/minute: No dosage adjustment required.

Cl_{cr} <45 mL/minute: No dosage adjustment guidelines are available; manufacturer recommends not using the drug.

Dosage adjustment in hepatic impairment: Grade 4 transaminase elevation (>20 times ULN): Reduce dose to 75% of previous dose

Dietary Considerations Initiate folic acid supplementation 1 week before first dose of pemetrexed, continue for full course of therapy, and for 21 days after last dose. Institute vitamin B_{12} 1 week before the first dose; administer every 9 weeks thereafter.

Administration I.V.: Infuse over 10 minutes.

Monitoring Parameters CBC with differential and platelets (before each dose); serum creatinine, total bilirubin, ALT, AST (day 1 of each, or every other, cycle)

Dosage Forms Excipient information presented when available (limited, particularly for generics); consult specific product labeling.

Injection, powder for reconstitution:

Alimta®: 100 mg, 500 mg

◆ **Pemetrexed Disodium** *see* Pemetrexed *on page 1159*

Pemirolast (pe MIR oh last)

U.S. Brand Names Alamast®

Canadian Brand Names Alamast®

Pharmacologic Category Mast Cell Stabilizer; Ophthalmic Agent, Miscellaneous

Use Prevention of itching of the eye due to allergic conjunctivitis

Pregnancy Risk Factor C

Dosage Children >3 years and Adults: 1-2 drops instilled in affected eye(s) 4 times/day

Additional Information Complete prescribing information for this medication should be consulted for additional detail.

Dosage Forms Excipient information presented when available (limited, particularly for generics); consult specific product labeling.

Solution, ophthalmic, as potassium: 0.1% (10 mL) [contains lauralkonium chloride]

Penciclovir (pen SYE kloe veer)

U.S. Brand Names Denavir®

Pharmacologic Category Antiviral Agent

Use Topical treatment of herpes simplex labialis (cold sores)

Pregnancy Risk Factor B

Medication Safety Issues

Sound-alike/look-alike issues:

Denavir® may be confused with indinavir

Dosage Children ≥12 years and Adults: Topical: Apply cream at the first sign or symptom of cold sore (eg, tingling, swelling); apply every 2 hours during waking hours for 4 days

Additional Information Complete prescribing information for this medication should be consulted for additional detail.

Dosage Forms Excipient information presented when available (limited, particularly for generics); consult specific product labeling.

Cream: 1% (1.5 g)

◆ **Pendex** *see* Guaifenesin and Phenylephrine *on page 712*

◆ **Pendo-5 ASA (Can)** *see* Mesalamine *on page 949*

Penicillamine (pen i SIL a meen)

U.S. Brand Names Cuprimine®; Depen®

Canadian Brand Names Cuprimine®; Depen®

Index Terms D-3-Mercaptovaline; D-Penicillamine; β,β-Dimethylcysteine

Pharmacologic Category Chelating Agent

Use Treatment of Wilson's disease, cystinuria; adjunctive treatment of rheumatoid arthritis

Unlabeled/Investigational Use Chelation therapy for the treatment of lead poisoning (third-line agent); treatment of arsenic poisoning

Pregnancy Risk Factor D

Pregnancy Considerations Birth defects, including congenital cutix laxa and associated defects, have been reported in infants following penicillamine exposure during pregnancy. Use for the treatment of rheumatoid arthritis during pregnancy is contraindicated. Use for the treatment of cystinuria only if the possible benefits to the mother outweigh the potential risks to the fetus. Continued treatment of Wilson's disease during pregnancy protects the mother against relapse. Discontinuation has detrimental maternal and fetal effects. Daily dosage should be limited to 750 mg. For planned cesarean section, reduce dose to 250 mg/day for the last 6 weeks of pregnancy, and continue at this dosage until wound healing is complete.

Lactation Excretion in breast milk unknown/contraindicated

Medication Safety Issues

Sound-alike/look-alike issues:

Penicillamine may be confused with penicillin

Depen® may be confused with Endal®

International issues:

Depen® may be confused with Depon® which is a brand name for acetaminophen in Greece

Depen® may be confused with Dipen® which is a brand name for diltiazem in Greece

Pemine® [Italy] may be confused with Pamine® which is a brand name for methscopolamine in the U.S.

Contraindications Hypersensitivity to penicillamine or any component of the formulation; renal insufficiency (in patients with rheumatoid arthritis); patients with previous penicillamine-related aplastic anemia or agranulocytosis; breast-feeding; pregnancy (in patients with rheumatoid arthritis)

Warnings/Precautions Patients with a penicillin allergy may theoretically have cross-sensitivity to penicillamine; however, the possibility has been eliminated now that penicillamine is produced synthetically and no longer contains trace amounts of penicillin. Once instituted for Wilson's disease or cystinuria, continue treatment on a daily basis; interruptions of even a few days have been followed by hypersensitivity with reinstitution of therapy. Penicillamine has been associated with fatalities due to agranulocytosis, aplastic anemia, thrombocytopenia, Goodpasture's syndrome, and myasthenia gravis. **[U.S. Boxed Warning]: Patients should be warned to report promptly any symptoms suggesting toxicity (fever, sore throat, chills, bruising, or bleeding);** approximately 33% of patients will experience an allergic reaction; toxicity may be dose related, use caution in the elderly. Use caution with other hematopoietic-depressant drugs (eg, gold, immunosuppressants, antimalarials, phenylbutazone); hematologic and renal adverse reactions are similar. Proteinuria or hematuria may develop; monitor for membranous glomerulopathy which can lead to nephrotic syndrome. In rheumatoid arthritis patients, discontinue if gross hematuria or persistent microscopic hematuria develop. Monitor liver function tests periodically due to rare reports of intrahepatic cholestasis or toxic hepatitis. **[U.S. Boxed Warning]: Should be administered under the close supervision of a physician familiar with the toxicity and dosage considerations.**

Lead poisoning: Investigate, identify, and remove sources of lead exposure prior to treatment. Penicillamine is considered to be a third-line agent for the treatment of lead poisoning in children due to the overall toxicity associated with its use; penicillamine should only be used when unacceptable reactions have occurred with edetate CALCIUM disodium and succimer. Primary care providers should consult experts in chemotherapy of lead toxicity before using chelation drug therapy.

Adverse Reactions Frequency not defined, may vary by indication. Adverse effects requiring discontinuation of treatment have been reported in 20% to 30% of patients with Wilson's disease.

Cardiovascular: Vasculitis

Central nervous system: Anxiety, agitation, fever, hyperpyrexia, psychiatric disturbances; worsening neurologic symptoms (10% to 50% patients with Wilson's disease)

Dermatologic: Alopecia, cheilosis, dermatomyositis, exfoliative dermatitis, lichen planus, rash (early and late 5%), pemphigus, pruritus, skin friability increased, toxic epidermal necrolysis, urticaria, wrinkling (excessive), yellow nail syndrome

Endocrine & metabolic: Hypoglycemia, thyroiditis

Gastrointestinal: Anorexia, diarrhea (17%), epigastric pain, gingivostomatitis, glossitis, nausea, oral ulcerations, pancreatitis, peptic ulcer reactivation, taste alteration (12%), vomiting

Hematologic: Eosinophilia, hemolytic anemia, leukocytosis, leukopenia (2% to 5%), monocytosis, red cell aplasia, thrombocytopenia (4% to 5%), thrombotic thrombocytopenia purpura, thrombocytosis

Hepatic: Alkaline phosphatase increased, hepatic failure, intrahepatic cholestasis, toxic hepatitis

Local: Thrombophlebitis, white papules at venipuncture and surgical sites

Neuromuscular & skeletal: Arthralgia, dystonia, myasthenia gravis, muscle weakness, neuropathies, polyarthralgia (migratory, often with objective synovitis), polymyositis

Ocular: Diplopia, extraocular muscle weakness, optic neuritis, ptosis, visual disturbances

Otic: Tinnitus

Renal: Goodpasture's syndrome, hematuria, nephrotic syndrome, proteinuria (6%), renal failure, renal vasculitis

Respiratory: Asthma, interstitial pneumonitis, pulmonary fibrosis, obliterative bronchiolitis

Miscellaneous: Allergic alveolitis, anetoderma, elastosis perforans serpiginosa, lupus-like syndrome, lactic dehydrogenase increased, lymphadenopathy, mammary hyperplasia, positive ANA test

Drug Interactions

Avoid Concomitant Use There are no known interactions where it is recommended to avoid concomitant use.

Increased Effect/Toxicity There are no known significant interactions involving an increase in effect.

Decreased Effect

Penicillamine may decrease the levels/effects of: Digoxin

The levels/effects of Penicillamine may be decreased by: Antacids; Iron Salts

Ethanol/Nutrition/Herb Interactions

Ethanol: Avoid or limit ethanol.

Food: Penicillamine serum levels may be decreased if taken with food. Do not administer with milk.

Stability Store in tight, well-closed containers.

Mechanism of Action Chelates with lead, copper, mercury and other heavy metals to form stable, soluble complexes that are excreted in urine; depresses circulating IgM rheumatoid factor, depresses T-cell but not B-cell activity; combines with cystine to form a compound which is more soluble, thus cystine calculi are prevented

Pharmacodynamics/Kinetics

Onset of action: Rheumatoid arthritis: 2-3 months; Wilson's disease: 1-3 months

Absorption: 40% to 70%

Protein binding: 80% to albumin and ceruloplasmin

Metabolism: Hepatic (small amounts metabolized to s-methyl-d-penicillamine)

Half-life elimination: 1.7-3.2 hours

Time to peak, serum: ~2 hours

Excretion: Urine (30% to 60% as unchanged drug)

Dosage Oral:

Rheumatoid arthritis:

Children (unlabeled use): Initial: 3 mg/kg/day (≤250 mg/day) for 3 months, then 6 mg/kg/day (≤500 mg/day) in divided doses twice daily for 3 months to a maximum of 10 mg/kg/day in 3-4 divided doses; maximum dose: 750 mg/day

Adults: 125-250 mg/day, may increase dose at 1- to 3-month intervals up to 1-1.5 g/day; maximum in older adults: 750 mg/day

Wilson's disease (doses titrated to maintain urinary copper excretion >2 mg/day); decrease dose for surgery and during last trimester of pregnancy

Children <12 years: 20 mg/kg/day in 2-3 divided doses, round off to the nearest 250 mg dose; maximum 1 g/day

Adults: 250 mg 4 times/day (maximum in older adults: 750 mg/day)

Cystinuria: **Note:** Adjust dose to limit cystine excretion to 100-200 mg/day (<100 mg/day with history of stone formation)

Children: 30 mg/kg/day in 4 divided doses

Lead poisoning (unlabeled use): Children: 20-30 mg/kg/day, administered in 3-4 divided doses; initiating treatment at 25% of this dose and gradually increasing to the full dose over 2-3 weeks may minimize adverse reactions. Doses of 15 mg/kg/day may also be effective and have less adverse effects (Shannon 2000). **Note:** For the treatment of high blood lead levels in children, the CDC recommends chelation treatment when blood lead levels are >45 mcg/dL (CDC, 2002). Children with blood lead levels >70 mcg/dL or symptomatic lead poisoning should be treated with parenteral agents (AAP, 2005).

Arsenic poisoning (unlabeled use):

Children: 100 mg/kg/day in divided doses every 6 hours for 5 days; maximum: 1 g/day

Adults: 500 mg 4 times/day for 5 days

Dosing adjustment/comments in renal impairment: Cl_{cr} <50 mL/minute: Avoid use

Hemodialysis: Dialyzable; a dosing decrease from 250 mg/day to 250 mg 3 times/week after dialysis has been suggested in the treatment of rheumatoid arthritis.

Dietary Considerations Should be taken at least 1 hour before a meal on an empty stomach. Iron may decrease drug action. Patients with Wilson's disease or cystinuria should receive pyridoxine supplementation 25 mg/day. For Wilson's disease, decrease copper in diet to <1-2 mg/day and omit chocolate, nuts, shellfish, mushrooms, liver, raisins, broccoli, copper-enriched cereal, multivitamins with copper, and molasses. For lead poisoning, decrease calcium in diet. For cystinuria, increase daily fluid intake including 1 pint of fluid prior to bedtime and 1 additional pint during the night.

Administration For patients who cannot swallow, contents of capsules may be administered in 15-30 mL of chilled puréed fruit or fruit juice. Give on an empty stomach (1 hour before meals and at bedtime).

Cystinuria: If administering 4 equal doses is not feasible, administer the larger dose at bedtime.

Rheumatoid arthritis: Doses ≤500 mg/day may be given as a single dose; >500 mg administer in divided doses

Monitoring Parameters Urinalysis, CBC with differential, platelet count, skin, lymph nodes, and body temperature twice weekly during the first month of therapy, then every 2 weeks for 5 months, then monthly; LFTs every 6 months

Cystinuria: Urinary cystine, annual X-ray for renal stones

Lead poisoning: Serum lead concentration (baseline and 7-21 days after completing chelation therapy); hemoglobin or hematocrit, iron status, free erythrocyte protoporphyrin or zinc protoporphyrin; neurodevelopmental changes

Wilson's disease: Serum copper, 24-hour urinary copper excretion, LFTs every 3 months during the first year of treatment

CBC: WBC <3500/mm^3, neutrophils <2000/mm^3, or monocytes >500/mm^3 indicate need to stop therapy immediately; platelet counts <100,000/mm^3 indicate need to stop therapy until numbers of platelets increase

Urinalysis: Monitor for proteinuria and hematuria. A quantitative 24-hour urine protein at 1- to 2-week intervals initially (first 2-3 months) is recommended if proteinuria develops; in patients with rheumatoid arthritis, discontinue or decrease dose with proteinuria >1 g/24 hours, progressively increasing proteinuria or hematuria.

Dosage Forms Excipient information presented when available (limited, particularly for generics); consult specific product labeling.

Capsule:

Cuprimine®: 250 mg

Tablet:

Depen®: 250 mg

Extemporaneous Preparations A 50 mg/mL suspension may be made by mixing twenty 250 mg capsules with 1 g carboxymethylcellulose, 50 g sucrose, 100 mg citric acid, parabens, and purified water to a total volume of 100 mL; cherry flavor may be added. Stability is 30 days refrigerated.

Nahata MC and Hipple TF, *Pediatric Drug Formulations*, 1st ed, Cincinnati, OH: Harvey Whitney Books Co, 1990.

Penicillin G Benzathine

(pen i SIL in jee BENZ a theen)

U.S. Brand Names Bicillin® L-A

Canadian Brand Names Bicillin® L-A

Index Terms Benzathine Benzylpenicillin; Benzathine Penicillin G; Benzylpenicillin Benzathine

Pharmacologic Category Antibiotic, Penicillin

Additional Appendix Information

Treatment of Sexually Transmitted Infections *on page 1773*

Use Active against some gram-positive organisms, few gram-negative organisms such as *Neisseria gonorrhoeae*, and some anaerobes and spirochetes; used in the treatment of syphilis; used only for the treatment of mild to moderately severe infections caused by organisms susceptible to low concentrations of penicillin G or for prophylaxis of infections caused by these organisms

Pregnancy Risk Factor B

Pregnancy Considerations Adverse events have not been observed in animal studies; therefore, penicillin G is classified as pregnancy category B. Penicillin crosses the placenta and distributes into amniotic fluid. There is no evidence of adverse fetal effects after penicillin use during pregnancy in humans. Penicillin G is the drug of choice for treatment of syphilis during pregnancy.

Lactation Enters breast milk/compatible

Medication Safety Issues

Sound-alike/look-alike issues:

Penicillin may be confused with penicillamine

Bicillin® may be confused with Wycillin®

Bicillin® C-R (penicillin G benzathine and penicillin G procaine) may be confused with Bicillin® L-A (penicillin G benzathine). Penicillin G benzathine is the only product currently approved for the treatment of syphilis. Administration of penicillin G benzathine and penicillin G procaine combination instead of Bicillin® L-A may result in inadequate treatment response.

Penicillin G benzathine may only be administered by deep intramuscular injection; intravenous administration of penicillin G benzathine has been associated with cardiopulmonary arrest and death.

Contraindications Hypersensitivity to penicillin or any component of the formulation

Warnings/Precautions Use with caution in patients with impaired renal function, seizure disorder, or history of hypersensitivity to other beta-lactams; CDC and AAP do not currently recommend the use of penicillin G benzathine to treat congenital syphilis or neurosyphilis due to reported treatment failures and lack of published clinical data on its efficacy. Prolonged use may result in fungal or bacterial superinfection, including *C. difficile*-associated diarrhea (CDAD) and pseudomembranous colitis; CDAD has been observed >2 months postantibiotic treatment. Extended duration of therapy or use associated with high serum concentrations may be associated with an increased risk for some adverse reactions.

Adverse Reactions Frequency not defined.

Central nervous system: Convulsions, confusion, drowsiness, myoclonus, fever

Dermatologic: Rash

Endocrine & metabolic: Electrolyte imbalance

Hematologic: Positive Coombs' reaction, hemolytic anemia

Local: Pain, thrombophlebitis

Renal: Acute interstitial nephritis

Miscellaneous: Anaphylaxis, hypersensitivity reactions, Jarisch-Herxheimer reaction

Drug Interactions

Avoid Concomitant Use There are no known interactions where it is recommended to avoid concomitant use.

Increased Effect/Toxicity

Penicillin G Benzathine may increase the levels/effects of: Methotrexate

The levels/effects of Penicillin G Benzathine may be increased by: Uricosuric Agents

Decreased Effect

Penicillin G Benzathine may decrease the levels/effects of: Typhoid Vaccine

The levels/effects of Penicillin G Benzathine may be decreased by: Fusidic Acid; Tetracycline Derivatives

Stability Refrigerate

Mechanism of Action Interferes with bacterial cell wall synthesis during active multiplication, causing cell wall death and resultant bactericidal activity against susceptible bacteria

Pharmacodynamics/Kinetics

Duration: 1-4 weeks (dose dependent); larger doses result in more sustained levels

Distribution: Highest levels in the kidney; lesser amounts in liver, skin, intestines

Protein Binding: ~60%

Absorption: I.M.: Slow

Time to peak, serum: 12-24 hours

Dosage Note: Administer undiluted injection; higher doses result in more sustained rather than higher levels. Use a penicillin G benzathine-penicillin G procaine combination to achieve early peak levels in acute infections.

Usual dosage range:

Children: I.M.: 25,000-50,000 units/kg as a single dose (maximum: 2.4 million units)

Adults: I.M.: 1.2-2.4 million units as a single dose

Indication-specific dosing:

Neonates >1200 g: I.M.:

Congenital syphilis (asymptomatic): 50,000 units/kg as a single dose

Infants and Children: I.M.:

Group A streptococcal upper respiratory infection: 25,000-50,000 units/kg as a single dose (maximum: 1.2 million units)

Prophylaxis of recurrent rheumatic fever: 25,000-50,000 units/kg every 3-4 weeks (maximum: 1.2 million units/dose)

Syphilis:

Early: 50,000 units/kg as a single injection (maximum: 2.4 million units)

More than 1-year duration: 50,000 units/kg every week for 3 doses (maximum: 2.4 million units/dose)

Adults: I.M.:

Group A streptococcal upper respiratory infection: 1.2 million units as a single dose

Prophylaxis of recurrent rheumatic fever: 1.2 million units every 3-4 weeks or 600,000 units twice monthly

Syphilis:

Early: 2.4 million units as a single dose in 2 injection sites

More than 1-year duration: 2.4 million units in 2 injection sites once weekly for 3 doses

Neurosyphilis: Not indicated as single-drug therapy, but may be given once weekly for 3 weeks following I.V. treatment; refer to Penicillin G (Parenteral/Aqueous) monograph for dosing

Administration Administer by deep I.M. injection in the upper outer quadrant of the buttock do **not** administer I.V., intra-arterially, or SubQ; in children <2 years of age, I.M. injections should be made into the midlateral muscle of the thigh, not the gluteal region; when doses are repeated, rotate the injection site

Monitoring Parameters Observe for signs and symptoms of anaphylaxis during first dose

Test Interactions Positive Coombs' [direct], false-positive urinary and/or serum proteins; false-positive or negative urinary glucose using Clinitest®

Dosage Forms Excipient information presented when available (limited, particularly for generics); consult specific product labeling.

Injection, suspension [prefilled syringe]: 600,000 units/mL (1 mL, 2 mL, 4 mL)

Penicillin G Benzathine and Penicillin G Procaine

(pen i SIL in jee BENZ a theen & pen i SIL in jee PROE kane)

U.S. Brand Names Bicillin® C-R; Bicillin® C-R 900/300

Index Terms Penicillin G Procaine and Benzathine Combined

Pharmacologic Category Antibiotic, Penicillin

Use May be used in specific situations in the treatment of streptococcal infections

Pregnancy Risk Factor B

Medication Safety Issues

Bicillin® C-R (penicillin G benzathine and penicillin G procaine) may be confused with Bicillin® L-A (penicillin G benzathine). Penicillin G benzathine is the only product currently approved for the treatment of syphilis. Administration of penicillin G benzathine and penicillin G procaine combination instead of Bicillin® L-A may result in inadequate treatment response.

Penicillin G benzathine may only be administered by deep intramuscular injection; intravenous administration of penicillin G benzathine has been associated with cardiopulmonary arrest and death.

Sound-alike/look-alike issues:

Penicillin may be confused with penicillamine

Bicillin® may be confused with Wycillin®

Dosage

Usual dosage range and indication-specific dosing:

Streptococcal infections:

Children: I.M.:

<14 kg: 600,000 units in a single dose

14-27 kg: 900,000 units to 1.2 million units in a single dose

Children >27 kg and Adults: 2.4 million units in a single dose

Additional Information Complete prescribing information for this medication should be consulted for additional detail.

Dosage Forms Excipient information presented when available (limited, particularly for generics); consult specific product labeling. [DSC] = Discontinued product

Injection, suspension [prefilled syringe]:

Bicillin® C-R:

600,000 units: Penicillin G benzathine 300,000 units and penicillin G procaine 300,000 units per 1 mL (1 mL) [DSC]

1,200,000 units: Penicillin G benzathine 600,000 units and penicillin G procaine 600,000 units per 2 mL (2 mL)

2,400,000 units: Penicillin G benzathine 1,200,000 units and penicillin G procaine 1,200,000 units per 4 mL (4 mL) [DSC]

Bicillin® C-R 900/300: 1,200,000 units: Penicillin G benzathine 900,000 units and penicillin G procaine 300,000 units per 2 mL (2 mL)

Penicillin G (Parenteral/Aqueous)

(pen i SIL in jee, pa REN ter al, AYE kwee us)

U.S. Brand Names Pfizerpen®

Canadian Brand Names Crystapen®

Index Terms Benzylpenicillin Potassium; Benzylpenicillin Sodium; Crystalline Penicillin; Penicillin G Potassium; Penicillin G Sodium

Pharmacologic Category Antibiotic, Penicillin

Additional Appendix Information

Antibiotic Treatment of Adults With Infective Endocarditis *on page 1748*

Antimicrobial Drugs of Choice *on page 1752*

Desensitization Protocols *on page 1691*

Treatment of Sexually Transmitted Infections *on page 1773*

Use Treatment of infections (including sepsis, pneumonia, pericarditis, endocarditis, meningitis, anthrax) caused by susceptible organisms; active against some gram-positive organisms, generally not *Staphylococcus aureus*; some gram-negative organisms such as *Neisseria gonorrhoeae*, and some anaerobes and spirochetes

Pregnancy Risk Factor B

Pregnancy Considerations Adverse events have not been observed in animal studies; therefore, penicillin G is classified as pregnancy category B. Penicillin crosses the placenta and distributes into amniotic fluid. There is no evidence of adverse fetal effects after penicillin use during pregnancy in humans. Penicillin G is the drug of choice for treatment of syphilis during pregnancy and penicillin G (parenteral/aqueous) is the drug of choice for the prevention of early-onset Group B Streptococcal (GBS) disease in newborns.

Lactation Enters breast milk/compatible

Medication Safety Issues

Sound-alike/look-alike issues:

Penicillin may be confused with penicillamine

Contraindications Hypersensitivity to penicillin or any component of the formulation

Warnings/Precautions Avoid intra-arterial administration or injection into or near major peripheral nerves or blood vessels since such injections may cause severe and/or permanent neurovascular damage; use with caution in patients with renal impairment (dosage reduction required), concomitant renal and hepatic impairment (further dosage adjustment may be required), pre-existing seizure disorders, or with a history of hypersensitivity to cephalosporins. Prolonged use may result in fungal or bacterial superinfection, including *C. difficile*-associated diarrhea (CDAD) and pseudomembranous colitis; CDAD has been observed >2 months postantibiotic treatment.

Serious and occasionally severe or fatal hypersensitivity (anaphylactoid) reactions have been reported in patients on penicillin therapy, especially with a history of beta-lactam hypersensitivity, history of sensitivity to multiple allergens, or previous IgE-mediated reactions (eg, anaphylaxis, angioedema, urticaria). Use with caution in asthmatic patients. Extended duration of therapy or use associated with high serum concentrations may be associated with an increased risk for some adverse reactions. Neonates may have decreased renal clearance of penicillin and require frequent dosage adjustments depending on age. Product contains sodium and potassium; high doses of I.V. therapy may alter serum levels.

Adverse Reactions Frequency not defined.

Central nervous system: Coma (high doses), hyperreflexia (high doses), seizures (high doses)

Dermatologic: Contact dermatitis, rash

Endocrine & metabolic: Electrolyte imbalance (high doses)

Gastrointestinal: Pseudomembranous colitis

Hematologic: Neutropenia, positive Coombs' hemolytic anemia (rare, high doses)

Local: Injection site reaction, phlebitis, thrombophlebitis

Neuromuscular & skeletal: Myoclonus (high doses)

Renal: Acute interstitial nephritis (high doses), renal tubular damage (high doses)

Miscellaneous: Anaphylaxis, hypersensitivity reactions (immediate and delayed), Jarisch-Herxheimer reaction, serum sickness

Drug Interactions

Avoid Concomitant Use There are no known interactions where it is recommended to avoid concomitant use.

Increased Effect/Toxicity

Penicillin G (Parenteral/Aqueous) may increase the levels/effects of: Methotrexate

The levels/effects of Penicillin G (Parenteral/Aqueous) may be increased by: Uricosuric Agents

Decreased Effect

Penicillin G (Parenteral/Aqueous) may decrease the levels/effects of: Typhoid Vaccine

The levels/effects of Penicillin G (Parenteral/Aqueous) may be decreased by: Fusidic Acid; Tetracycline Derivatives

Stability

Penicillin G potassium powder for injection should be stored below 86°F (30°C). Following reconstitution, solution may be stored for up to 7 days under refrigeration. Premixed bags for infusion should be stored in the freezer (-20°C to -4°F); frozen bags may be thawed at room temperature or in refrigerator. Once thawed, solution is stable for 14 days if stored in refrigerator or for 24 hours when stored at room temperature. Do not refreeze once thawed.

Penicillin G sodium powder for injection should be stored at controlled room temperature. Reconstituted solution may be stored under refrigeration for up to 3 days.

Mechanism of Action Interferes with bacterial cell wall synthesis during active multiplication, causing cell wall death and resultant bactericidal activity against susceptible bacteria

Pharmacodynamics/Kinetics

Distribution: Poor penetration across blood-brain barrier, despite inflamed meninges

Relative diffusion from blood into CSF: Poor unless meninges inflamed (exceeds usual MICs)

CSF:blood level ratio: Normal meninges: <1%; Inflamed meninges: 2% to 6%

Protein binding: 65%

Metabolism: Hepatic (30%) to penicilloic acid

Half-life elimination:

Neonates: <6 days old: 3.2-3.4 hours; 7-13 days old: 1.2-2.2 hours; >14 days old: 0.9-1.9 hours

Children and Adults: Normal renal function: 30-50 minutes

End-stage renal disease: 3.3-5.1 hours

Time to peak, serum: I.M.: ~30 minutes; I.V.: ~1 hour

Excretion: Urine (58% to 85% as unchanged drug)

Dosage

Usual dosage range:

Infants >1 month and Children: I.M., I.V.: 100,000-400,000 units/kg/day in divided doses every 4-6 hours (maximum dose: 24 million units/day)

Adults: I.M., I.V.: 2-30 million units/day in divided doses every 4-6 hours depending on sensitivity of the organism and severity of the infection

Indication-specific dosing:

Infants >1 month and Children:

***Meningitis* (gonococcal):** I.V.: 250,000 units/kg/day in 4 divided doses

Moderate infections: I.M., I.V.: 100,000-250,000 units/kg/day in 4 divided doses

Severe infections: I.M., I.V.: 250,000-400,000 units/kg/day in divided doses every 4-6 hours (maximum dose: 24 million units/day)

Syphilis (congenital): Infants: I.V.: 50,000 units/kg every 4-6 hours for 10 days

Adults:

***Actinomyces* species:** I.V.: 10-20 million units/day in divided doses every 4-6 hours for 4-6 weeks

Clostridium perfringens: I.V.: 24 million units/day in divided doses every 4-6 hours with clindamycin

Corynebacterium diphtheriae: I.V.: 2-3 million units/day in divided doses every 4-6 hours for 10-12 days

Erysipelas: I.V.: 1-2 million units every 4-6 hours

Erysipelothrix: I.V.: 2-4 million units every 4 hours

Fascial space infections: I.V.: 2-4 million units every 4-6 hours with metronidazole

Leptospirosis: I.V.: 1.5 million units every 6 hours for 7 days

Listeria: I.V.: 15-20 million units/day in divided doses every 4-6 hours for 2 weeks (meningitis) or 4 weeks (endocarditis)

Lyme disease (meningitis): I.V.: 20 million units/day in divided doses

Neurosyphilis: I.V.: 18-24 million units/day in divided doses every 4 hours (or by continuous infusion) for 10-14 days

Streptococcus:

Brain abscess: I.V.: 18-24 million units/day in divided doses every 4 hours with metronidazole

Endocarditis or osteomyelitis: I.V.: 3-4 million units every 4 hours for at least 4 weeks

Pregnancy (prophylaxis GBS): I.V.: 5 million units x 1 dose, then 2.5 million units every 4 hours until delivery (AGOG, 2002; CDC, 2002)

Skin and soft tissue: I.V.: 3-4 million units every 4 hours for 10 days

Toxic shock: I.V.: 24 million units/day in divided doses with clindamycin

Streptococcal pneumonia: I.V.: 2-3 million units every 4 hours

Whipple's disease: I.V.: 2 million units every 4 hours for 2 weeks, followed by oral trimethoprim/sulfamethoxazole or doxycycline for 1 year

Relapse or CNS involvement: 4 million units every 4 hours for 4 weeks

Dosing interval in renal impairment:

Uremic patients with Cl_{cr} >10 mL/minute/1.73 m^2: Administer full loading dose followed by 1/2 of the loading dose given every 4-5 hours

Cl_{cr} <10 mL/minute/1.73 m^2: Administer full loading dose followed by 1/2 of the loading dose given every 8-10 hours

Dietary Considerations

Injection powder for reconstitution as potassium contains sodium 6.8 mg (0.3 mEq) and potassium 65.6 mg (1.68 mEq) per 1 million units

Injection solution (premixed) as a potassium contains sodium 23.5 mg (1.02 mEq) and potassium 66.5 mg (1.7 mEq) per 1 million units

Administration Administer I.M. by deep injection in the upper outer quadrant of the buttock

Monitoring Parameters Periodic electrolyte, hepatic, renal, cardiac and hematologic function tests during prolonged/high-dose therapy; observe for signs and symptoms of anaphylaxis during first dose

Test Interactions False-positive or negative urinary glucose determination using Clinitest®; positive Coombs' [direct]; false-positive urinary and/or serum proteins

Additional Information 1 million units is approximately equal to 625 mg.

Dosage Forms Excipient information presented when available (limited, particularly for generics); consult specific product labeling.

Infusion, as potassium [premixed iso-osmotic dextrose solution, frozen]: 1 million units (50 mL), 2 million units (50 mL), 3 million units (50 mL) [contains sodium 1.02 mEq and potassium 1.7 mEq per 1 million units]

Injection, powder for reconstitution, as potassium (Pfizerpen®): 5 million units, 20 million units [contains sodium 6.8 mg (0.3 mEq) and potassium 65.6 mg (1.68 mEq) per 1 million units]

Injection, powder for reconstitution, as sodium: 5 million units [contains sodium 1.68 mEq per 1 million units]

◆ **Penicillin G Potassium** *see* Penicillin G (Parenteral/Aqueous) *on page 1164*

Penicillin G Procaine (pen i SIL in jee PROE kane)

Canadian Brand Names Pfizerpen-AS®; Wycillin®

Index Terms APPG; Aqueous Procaine Penicillin G; Procaine Benzylpenicillin; Procaine Penicillin G; Wycillin [DSC]

Pharmacologic Category Antibiotic, Penicillin

Additional Appendix Information

Treatment of Sexually Transmitted Infections *on page 1773*

Use Treatment of moderately-severe infections due to *Treponema pallidum* and other penicillin G-sensitive microorganisms that are susceptible to low, but prolonged serum penicillin concentrations; anthrax due to *Bacillus anthracis* (postexposure) to reduce the incidence or progression of disease following exposure to aerolized *Bacillus anthracis*

Pregnancy Risk Factor B

Pregnancy Considerations Adverse events have not been observed in animal studies; therefore, penicillin G is classified as pregnancy category B. Penicillin crosses the placenta and distributes into amniotic fluid. There is no evidence of adverse fetal effects after penicillin use during pregnancy in humans.

Lactation Enters breast milk/compatible

Medication Safety Issues

Sound-alike/look-alike issues:

Penicillin G procaine may be confused with penicillin V potassium

Wycillin® may be confused with Bicillin®

Contraindications Hypersensitivity to penicillin, procaine, or any component of the formulation

Warnings/Precautions May need to modify dosage in patients with severe renal impairment or seizure disorders; avoid I.V., intravascular, or intra-arterial administration of penicillin G procaine since severe and/or permanent neurovascular damage may occur. Serious and occasionally severe or fatal hypersensitivity (anaphylactoid) reactions have been reported in patients on penicillin therapy, especially with a history of beta-lactam hypersensitivity, history of sensitivity to multiple allergens, or previous IgE-mediated reactions (eg, anaphylaxis, angioedema, urticaria). Use with caution in asthmatic patients. Extended duration of therapy or use associated with high serum concentrations may be associated with an increased risk for some adverse reactions. Prolonged use may result in fungal or bacterial superinfection, including *C. difficile*-associated diarrhea (CDAD) and pseudomembranous colitis; CDAD has been observed >2 months postantibiotic treatment.

Adverse Reactions Frequency not defined.

Cardiovascular: Myocardial depression, vasodilation, conduction disturbances

Central nervous system: Confusion, drowsiness, myoclonus, CNS stimulation, seizure

Hematologic: Positive Coombs' reaction, hemolytic anemia, neutropenia

Local: Pain at injection site, thrombophlebitis, sterile abscess at injection site

Renal: Interstitial nephritis

Miscellaneous: Pseudoanaphylactic reactions, hypersensitivity reactions, Jarisch-Herxheimer reaction, serum sickness

Drug Interactions

Avoid Concomitant Use There are no known interactions where it is recommended to avoid concomitant use.

Increased Effect/Toxicity

Penicillin G Procaine may increase the levels/effects of: Methotrexate

The levels/effects of Penicillin G Procaine may be increased by: Uricosuric Agents

Decreased Effect

Penicillin G Procaine may decrease the levels/effects of: Typhoid Vaccine

The levels/effects of Penicillin G Procaine may be decreased by: Fusidic Acid; Tetracycline Derivatives

Stability Refrigerate

Mechanism of Action Inhibits bacterial cell wall synthesis by binding to one or more of the penicillin binding proteins (PBPs); which in turn inhibits the final transpeptidation step of peptidoglycan synthesis in bacterial cell walls, thus inhibiting cell wall biosynthesis. Bacteria eventually lyse due to ongoing activity of cell wall autolytic enzymes (autolysins and murein hydrolases) while cell wall assembly is arrested.

Pharmacodynamics/Kinetics

Duration: Therapeutic: 15-24 hours

Absorption: I.M.: Slow

Distribution: Penetration across the blood-brain barrier is poor, despite inflamed meninges

Protein binding: 65%

Metabolism: ~30% hepatically inactivated

Time to peak, serum: 1-4 hours

Excretion: Urine (60% to 90% as unchanged drug)

Clearance: Renal: Delayed in neonates, young infants, and with impaired renal function

Dosage

Usual dosage range:

Infants and Children: I.M.: 25,000-50,000 units/kg/day in divided doses 1-2 times/day; (maximum: 4.8 million units/day)

Adults: I.M.: 0.6-4.8 million units/day in divided doses every 12-24 hours

Indication-specific dosing:

Children: I.M.:

Anthrax, inhalational (postexposure prophylaxis): 25,000 units/kg every 12 hours (maximum: 1,200,000 units every 12 hours); see "Note" in adult dosing

Syphilis (congenital): 50,000 units/kg/day for 10 days; if more than 1 day of therapy is missed, the entire course should be restarted

Adults: I.M.:

Anthrax:

Inhalational (postexposure prophylaxis): 1,200,000 units every 12 hours

Note: Overall treatment duration should be 60 days. Available safety data suggest continued administration of penicillin G procaine for longer than 2 weeks may incur additional risk for adverse reactions. Clinicians may consider switching to effective alternative treatment for completion of therapy beyond 2 weeks.

Cutaneous (treatment): 600,000-1,200,000 units/day; alternative therapy is recommended in severe cutaneous or other forms of anthrax infection

Endocarditis caused by susceptible viridans *Streptococcus* (when used in conjunction with an aminoglycoside): 1.2 million units every 6 hours for 2-4 weeks

Gonorrhea (uncomplicated): 4.8 million units as a single dose divided in 2 sites given 30 minutes after probenecid 1 g orally

Neurosyphilis: 2.4 million units/day with 500 mg probenecid by mouth 4 times/day for 10-14 days; **Note: Penicillin G aqueous I.V. is the preferred agent**

Whipple's disease: 1.2 million units/day (with streptomycin) for 10-14 days, followed by oral trimethoprim/sulfamethoxazole or doxycycline for 1 year

Hemodialysis: Moderately dialyzable (20% to 50%)

Administration Procaine suspension for deep I.M. injection only; do not inject in gluteal muscle in children <2 years of age; rotate the injection site; avoid I.V., intravascular, or intra-arterial administration of penicillin G procaine since severe and/or permanent neurovascular damage may occur

Monitoring Parameters Periodic renal and hematologic function tests with prolonged therapy; fever, mental status, WBC count

Test Interactions Positive Coombs' [direct], false-positive urinary and/or serum proteins

Dosage Forms Excipient information presented when available (limited, particularly for generics); consult specific product labeling.

Injection, suspension: 600,000 units/mL (1 mL, 2 mL)

◆ **Penicillin G Procaine and Benzathine Combined** *see* Penicillin G Benzathine and Penicillin G Procaine *on page 1164*

◆ **Penicillin G Sodium** *see* Penicillin G (Parenteral/Aqueous) *on page 1164*

Penicillin V Potassium

(pen i SIL in vee poe TASS ee um)

Canadian Brand Names Apo-Pen VK®; Novo-Pen-VK; Nu-Pen-VK

Index Terms Pen VK; Phenoxymethyl Penicillin

Pharmacologic Category Antibiotic, Penicillin

Additional Appendix Information

Antimicrobial Drugs of Choice *on page 1752*

Desensitization Protocols *on page 1691*

Use Treatment of infections caused by susceptible organisms involving the respiratory tract, otitis media, sinusitis, skin, and urinary tract; prophylaxis in rheumatic fever

Pregnancy Risk Factor B

Pregnancy Considerations Adverse events have not been observed in animal studies; therefore, penicillin V is classified as pregnancy category B. Penicillin crosses the placenta and distributes into amniotic fluid. There is no evidence of adverse fetal effects after penicillin use during pregnancy in humans. Due to pregnancy-induced physiologic changes, some pharmacokinetic parameters of penicillin V may be altered in the second and third trimester. Higher doses or increased dosing frequency may be required.

Lactation Enters breast milk/compatible

Medication Safety Issues

Sound-alike/look-alike issues:

Penicillin V procaine may be confused with penicillin G potassium

Contraindications Hypersensitivity to penicillin or any component of the formulation

Warnings/Precautions Use with caution in patients with severe renal impairment (modify dosage) or history of seizures. Serious and occasionally severe or fatal hypersensitivity (anaphylactoid) reactions have been reported in patients on penicillin therapy, especially with a history of beta-lactam hypersensitivity, history of sensitivity to multiple allergens, or previous IgE-mediated reactions (eg, anaphylaxis, angioedema, urticaria). Use with caution in asthmatic patients. Extended duration of therapy or use associated with high serum concentrations may be associated with an increased risk for some adverse reactions. Prolonged use may result in fungal or bacterial superinfection, including *C. difficile*-associated diarrhea (CDAD) and pseudomembranous colitis; CDAD has been observed >2 months postantibiotic treatment.

Adverse Reactions

>10%: Gastrointestinal: Mild diarrhea, vomiting, nausea, oral candidiasis

<1% (Limited to important or life-threatening): Acute interstitial nephritis, convulsions, hemolytic anemia, positive Coombs' reaction

Drug Interactions

Avoid Concomitant Use There are no known interactions where it is recommended to avoid concomitant use.

Increased Effect/Toxicity

Penicillin V Potassium may increase the levels/effects of: Methotrexate

The levels/effects of Penicillin V Potassium may be increased by: Uricosuric Agents

Decreased Effect

Penicillin V Potassium may decrease the levels/effects of: Typhoid Vaccine

The levels/effects of Penicillin V Potassium may be decreased by: Fusidic Acid; Tetracycline Derivatives

Ethanol/Nutrition/Herb Interactions Food: Decreases drug absorption rate; decreases drug serum concentration.

Stability Refrigerate suspension after reconstitution; discard after 14 days

Mechanism of Action Inhibits bacterial cell wall synthesis by binding to one or more of the penicillin binding proteins (PBPs); which in turn inhibits the final transpeptidation step of peptidoglycan synthesis in bacterial cell walls, thus inhibiting cell wall biosynthesis. Bacteria eventually lyse due to ongoing activity of cell wall autolytic enzymes (autolysins and murein hydrolases) while cell wall assembly is arrested.

Pharmacodynamics/Kinetics

Absorption: 60% to 73%

Distribution: Widely distributed to kidneys, liver, skin, tonsils, and into synovial, pleural, and pericardial fluids

Protein binding, plasma: 80%

Half-life elimination: 30 minutes; prolonged with renal impairment

Time to peak, serum: 0.5-1 hour

Excretion: Urine (as unchanged drug and metabolites)

Dosage

Usual dosage range:

Children <12 years: Oral: 25-50 mg/kg/day in divided doses every 6-8 hours (maximum dose: 3 g/day)

Children ≥12 years and Adults: Oral: 125-500 mg every 6-8 hours

Indication-specific dosing:

Children: Oral:

Pharyngitis (streptococcal): 250 mg 2-3 times/day for 10 days

Prophylaxis of pneumococcal infections:

Children <5 years: 125 mg twice daily

Children ≥5 years: 250 mg twice daily

Prophylaxis of recurrent rheumatic fever:

Children <5 years: 125 mg twice daily

Children ≥5 years: 250 mg twice daily

Adults: Oral:

Acintomycosis:

Mild: 2-4 g/day in 4 divided doses for 8 weeks

Surgical: 2-4 g/day in 4 divided doses for 6-12 months (after I.V. penicillin G therapy of 4-6 weeks)

Erysipelas: 500 mg 4 times/day

Periodontal infections: 250-500 mg every 6 hours for 5-7 days

Note: Efficacy of antimicrobial therapy in periapical abscess is questionable; the American Academy of Periodontology recommends use of antibiotic therapy only when systemic symptoms (eg, fever, lymphadenopathy) are present or in immunocompromised patients.

Pharyngitis (streptococcal): 500 mg 3-4 times/day for 10 days

Prophylaxis of pneumococcal or recurrent rheumatic fever infections: 250 mg twice daily

Dosing interval in renal impairment: Cl_{cr} <10 mL/minute: Administer 250 mg every 6 hours

Dietary Considerations Take on an empty stomach 1 hour before or 2 hours after meals.

Administration Administer on an empty stomach to increase oral absorption

Monitoring Parameters Periodic renal and hematologic function tests during prolonged therapy; monitor for signs of anaphylaxis during first dose

Test Interactions False-positive or negative urinary glucose determination using Clinitest®; positive Coombs' [direct]; false-positive urinary and/or serum proteins

Additional Information 0.7 mEq of potassium per 250 mg penicillin V; 250 mg equals 400,000 units of penicillin

Dosage Forms Excipient information presented when available (limited, particularly for generics); consult specific product labeling.

Note: 250 mg = 400,000 units

Powder for oral solution: 125 mg/5 mL (100 mL, 200 mL); 250 mg/5 mL (100 mL, 200 mL)

Tablet: 250 mg, 500 mg

- **Penicilloyl-polylysine** *see* Benzylpenicilloyl-polylysine *on page* 186
- **Penlac®** *see* Ciclopirox *on page* 324
- **Pennsaid® (Can)** *see* Diclofenac *on page* 437
- **Pentacel®** *see* Diphtheria and Tetanus Toxoids, Acellular Pertussis, Poliovirus and *Haemophilus* b Conjugate Vaccine *on page* 462
- **Pentahydrate** *see* Sodium Thiosulfate *on page* 1386
- **Pentam-300®** *see* Pentamidine *on page* 1168

Pentamidine (pen TAM i deen)

U.S. Brand Names NebuPent®; Pentam-300®

Canadian Brand Names Pentamidine Isetionate for Injection

Index Terms Pentamidine Isethionate

Pharmacologic Category Antibiotic, Miscellaneous

Additional Appendix Information

Guidelines for the Prevention of Opportunistic Infections in HIV Infected Persons *on page* 1740

Use Treatment and prevention of pneumonia caused by *Pneumocystis carinii* (PCP)

Unlabeled/Investigational Use Treatment of trypanosomiasis and visceral leishmaniasis

Pregnancy Risk Factor C

Lactation Excretion in breast milk unknown/contraindicated

Contraindications Hypersensitivity to pentamidine isethionate or any component of the formulation (inhalation and injection)

Warnings/Precautions Use with caution in patients with diabetes mellitus, renal or hepatic dysfunction; cardiovascular disease, pancreatitis; leukopenia, thrombocytopenia, asthma, hypo/hyperglycemia. Severe hypotension (some fatalities) has been observed, even after a single dose; more common with rapid I.V. administration. Prolonged use may result in fungal or bacterial superinfection, including *C. difficile*-associated diarrhea (CDAD) and pseudomembranous colitis; CDAD has been observed >2 months postantibiotic treatment.

Adverse Reactions

Inhalation:

>10%:

Cardiovascular: Chest pain

Dermatologic: Rash

Respiratory: Wheezing, dyspnea, cough, pharyngitis

1% to 10%: Gastrointestinal: Bitter or metallic taste

<1% (Limited to important or life-threatening): Hypoglycemia, renal insufficiency

Systemic:

>10%:

Cardiovascular: Hypotension

Dermatologic: Rash

Endocrine & metabolic: Hyperglycemia or hypoglycemia

Gastrointestinal: Nausea, vomiting, anorexia, diarrhea

Hematologic: Leukopenia or neutropenia, thrombocytopenia

Hepatic: Elevated LFTs

Renal: Nephrotoxicity

1% to 10%:

Cardiovascular: Cardiac arrhythmia

Gastrointestinal: Pancreatitis, metallic taste

Hematologic: Anemia

Local: Local reactions at injection site

<1% (Limited to important or life-threatening): Arrhythmias

Drug Interactions

Metabolism/Transport Effects Substrate of CYP2C19 (major); **Inhibits** CYP2C8/9 (weak), 2C19 (weak), 2D6 (weak), 3A4 (weak)

Avoid Concomitant Use

Avoid concomitant use of Pentamidine with any of the following: Nilotinib; Tetrabenazine; Thioridazine; Ziprasidone

Increased Effect/Toxicity

Pentamidine may increase the levels/effects of: QTc-Prolonging Agents; Tetrabenazine; Thioridazine; Ziprasidone

The levels/effects of Pentamidine may be increased by: Alfuzosin; Ciprofloxacin; CYP2C19 Inhibitors (Moderate); CYP2C19 Inhibitors (Strong); Gadobutrol; Nilotinib

Decreased Effect

Pentamidine may decrease the levels/effects of: Typhoid Vaccine

The levels/effects of Pentamidine may be decreased by: CYP2C19 Inducers (Strong)

Ethanol/Nutrition/Herb Interactions Ethanol: Avoid ethanol (may increase CNS depression or aggravate hypoglycemia).

Stability Store intact vials at controlled room temperature and protect from light. Do not refrigerate due to the possibility of crystallization. Powder for inhalation should be reconstituted with SWFI. Powder for injection may be reconstituted with SWFI or D_5W. Precipitation may occur if products are reconstituted with NS. Following reconstitution, solution for injection may be diluted. Solutions for injection (1-2.5 mg/mL) in D_5W are stable for at least 24 hours at room temperature. The manufacturer's labeling recommends D_5W, however stability in NS has also been documented; in addition, light protection is recommended by the manufacturer, but stability has been documented without protection from light.

Mechanism of Action Interferes with RNA/DNA, phospholipids and protein synthesis, through inhibition of oxidative phosphorylation and/or interference with incorporation of nucleotides and nucleic acids into RNA and DNA, in protozoa

Pharmacodynamics/Kinetics

Absorption: I.M.: Well absorbed; Inhalation: Limited systemic absorption

Half-life elimination: Terminal: 6.4-9.4 hours; may be prolonged with severe renal impairment

Excretion: Urine (33% to 66% as unchanged drug)

Dosage

Children:

Treatment of PCP pneumonia: I.M., I.V. (I.V. preferred): 4 mg/kg/day once daily for 10-14 days

Prevention of PCP pneumonia:

I.M., I.V.: 4 mg/kg monthly or every 2 weeks

Inhalation (aerosolized pentamidine in children ≥5 years): 300 mg/dose given every 3-4 weeks via Respirgard® II inhaler (8 mg/kg dose has also been used in children <5 years)

Treatment of trypanosomiasis (unlabeled use): I.V.: 4 mg/kg/day once daily for 10 days

Adults:

Treatment: I.M., I.V. (I.V. preferred): 4 mg/kg/day once daily for 14-21 days

Prevention: Inhalation: 300 mg every 4 weeks via Respirgard® II nebulizer

Dialysis: Not removed by hemo or peritoneal dialysis or continuous arteriovenous or venovenous hemofiltration; supplemental dosage is not necessary

Dosing adjustment in renal impairment: Adults: I.V.:

Cl_{cr} 10-50 mL/minute: Administer 4 mg/kg every 24-36 hours

Cl_{cr} <10 mL/minute: Administer 4 mg/kg every 48 hours

Administration

Inhalation: Deliver until nebulizer is gone (30-45 minutes)

I.V.: Infuse slowly over a period of at least 60 minutes or administer deep I.M.

Monitoring Parameters Liver function tests, renal function tests, blood glucose, serum potassium and calcium, ECG, blood pressure

Additional Information Virtually undetectable amounts are transferred to healthcare personnel during aerosol administration.

Dosage Forms Excipient information presented when available (limited, particularly for generics); consult specific product labeling.

Injection, powder for reconstitution, as isethionate [preservative free]:

Pentam-300®: 300 mg

Powder for solution, for nebulization, as isethionate [preservative free]:

NebuPent®: 300 mg

- **Pentamidine Isethionate** *see* Pentamidine *on page 1168*
- **Pentamidine Isetionate for Injection (Can)** *see* Pentamidine *on page 1168*
- **Pentamycetin® (Can)** *see* Chloramphenicol *on page 302*
- **Pentasa®** *see* Mesalamine *on page 949*
- **Pentasodium Colistin Methanesulfonate** *see* Colistimethate *on page 366*
- **Penta-Triamterene HCTZ (Can)** *see* Hydrochlorothiazide and Triamterene *on page 739*
- **Pentavalent Human-Bovine Reassortant Rotavirus Vaccine (PRV)** *see* Rotavirus Vaccine *on page 1345*

Pentazocine (pen TAZ oh seen)

U.S. Brand Names Talwin®; Talwin® Nx

Canadian Brand Names Talwin®

Index Terms Naloxone Hydrochloride and Pentazocine Hydrochloride; Pentazocine Hydrochloride; Pentazocine Hydrochloride and Naloxone Hydrochloride; Pentazocine Lactate

Pharmacologic Category Analgesic, Opioid

Additional Appendix Information

Narcotic / Opioid Analgesics *on page 1663*

Use

Talwin®: Relief of moderate-to-severe pain; has also been used as a sedative prior to surgery and as a supplement to surgical anesthesia

Talwin® Nx: Relief of moderate-to-severe pain; indicated for oral use only

Restrictions C-IV

Pregnancy Risk Factor C/D (prolonged use or high doses at term)

Medication Safety Issues

High alert medication: The Institute for Safe Medication Practices (ISMP) includes this medication among its list of drug classes which have a heightened risk of causing significant patient harm when used in error.

Dosage

Preoperative/preanesthetic: Children 1-16 years: I.M.: 0.5 mg/kg

Analgesia:

Children: I.M.:

5-8 years: 15 mg

8-14 years: 30 mg

Children >12 years and Adults: Oral: 50 mg every 3-4 hours; may increase to 100 mg/dose if needed, but should not exceed 600 mg/day (maximum: 12 tablets/day)

Adults:

I.M., SubQ: 30-60 mg every 3-4 hours; do not exceed 60 mg/dose (maximum: 360 mg/day)

I.V.: 30 mg every 3-4 hours; do not exceed 30 mg/dose (maximum: 360 mg/day)

Elderly: Elderly patients may be more sensitive to the analgesic and sedating effects. The elderly may also have impaired renal function. If needed, dosing should be started at the lower end of dosing range and adjust dose for renal function.

Dosing adjustment in renal impairment:

Cl_{cr} 10-50 mL/minute: Administer 75% of normal dose

Cl_{cr} <10 mL/minute: Administer 50% of normal dose

Dosing adjustment in hepatic impairment: Reduce dose or avoid use in patients with liver disease

Additional Information Complete prescribing information for this medication should be consulted for additional detail.

Dosage Forms Excipient information presented when available (limited, particularly for generics); consult specific product labeling.

Injection, solution:
Talwin®: 30 mg/mL (1 mL, 10 mL) [10 mL size contains sodium bisulfite]
Tablet: Pentazocine 50 mg and naloxone 0.5 mg
Talwin® Nx: Pentazocine 50 mg and naloxone 0.5 mg

- **Pentazocine Hydrochloride** *see* Pentazocine *on page 1169*
- **Pentazocine Hydrochloride and Naloxone Hydrochloride** *see* Pentazocine *on page 1169*
- **Pentazocine Lactate** *see* Pentazocine *on page 1169*

PENTobarbital (pen toe BAR bi tal)

U.S. Brand Names Nembutal®

Canadian Brand Names Nembutal® Sodium

Index Terms Pentobarbital Sodium

Pharmacologic Category Anticonvulsant, Barbiturate; Barbiturate

Additional Appendix Information

Status Epilepticus *on page 1831*

Use Sedative/hypnotic; preanesthetic; high-dose barbiturate coma for treatment of increased intracranial pressure or status epilepticus unresponsive to other therapy

Restrictions C-II

Pregnancy Risk Factor D

Lactation Enters breast milk/contraindicated

Medication Safety Issues

Sound-alike/look-alike issues:
PENTobarbital may be confused with PHENobarbital
Nembutal® may be confused with Myambutol®

Contraindications Hypersensitivity to barbiturates or any component of the formulation; marked hepatic impairment; dyspnea or airway obstruction; porphyria; pregnancy

Warnings/Precautions Tolerance to hypnotic effect can occur; do not use for >2 weeks to treat insomnia. Potential for drug dependency exists, abrupt cessation may precipitate withdrawal, including status epilepticus in epileptic patients. Do not administer to patients in acute pain. Use caution in elderly, debilitated, renally impaired, hepatic dysfunction, or pediatric patients. May cause paradoxical responses, including agitation and hyperactivity, particularly in acute pain and pediatric patients. Use with caution in patients with depression or suicidal tendencies, or in patients with a history of drug abuse. Tolerance, psychological and physical dependence may occur with prolonged use.

May cause CNS depression, which may impair physical or mental abilities. Patients must be cautioned about performing tasks which require mental alertness (eg, operating machinery or driving). Effects with other sedative drugs or ethanol may be potentiated. Use of this agent as a hypnotic in the elderly is not recommended due to its long half-life and potential for physical and psychological dependence.

May cause respiratory depression or hypotension, particularly when administered intravenously. Use with caution in hemodynamically unstable patients or patients with respiratory disease. High doses (loading doses of 15-35 mg/kg given over 1-2 hours) have been utilized to induce pentobarbital coma, but these higher doses often cause hypotension requiring vasopressor therapy.

Adverse Reactions Frequency not defined.

Cardiovascular: Bradycardia, hypotension, syncope
Central nervous system: Drowsiness, lethargy, CNS excitation or depression, impaired judgment, "hangover" effect, confusion, somnolence, agitation, hyperkinesia, ataxia, nervousness, headache, insomnia, nightmares, hallucinations, anxiety, dizziness
Dermatologic: Rash, exfoliative dermatitis, Stevens-Johnson syndrome
Gastrointestinal: Nausea, vomiting, constipation
Hematologic: Agranulocytosis, thrombocytopenia, megaloblastic anemia
Local: Pain at injection site, thrombophlebitis with I.V. use
Renal: Oliguria
Respiratory: Laryngospasm, respiratory depression, apnea (especially with rapid I.V. use), hypoventilation
Miscellaneous: Gangrene with inadvertent intra-arterial injection

Drug Interactions

Metabolism/Transport Effects **Induces** CYP2A6 (strong), 3A4 (strong)

Avoid Concomitant Use

Avoid concomitant use of PENTobarbital with any of the following: Nilotinib; Ranolazine

Increased Effect/Toxicity

PENTobarbital may increase the levels/effects of: Alcohol (Ethyl); CNS Depressants; Meperidine

The levels/effects of PENTobarbital may be increased by: Carbonic Anhydrase Inhibitors; Chloramphenicol; Felbamate; Primidone; Valproic Acid

Decreased Effect

PENTobarbital may decrease the levels/effects of: Acetaminophen; Beta-Blockers; Calcium Channel Blockers; Chloramphenicol; Contraceptive (Progestins); Corticosteroids (Systemic); CycloSPORINE; CYP2A6 Substrates; CYP3A4 Substrates; Disopyramide; Doxycycline; Etoposide; Etoposide Phosphate; Griseofulvin; LamoTRIgine; Maraviroc; Methadone; Nilotinib; Oral Contraceptive (Estrogens); Propafenone; QuiNIDine; Ranolazine; Sorafenib; Teniposide; Theophylline Derivatives; Tricyclic Antidepressants; Valproic Acid; Vitamin K Antagonists

The levels/effects of PENTobarbital may be decreased by: Ketorolac; Mefloquine; Pyridoxine; Rifamycin Derivatives

Ethanol/Nutrition/Herb Interactions Ethanol: Avoid ethanol (may increase CNS depression).

Stability Protect from freezing. Aqueous solutions are not stable; a commercially available vehicle (containing propylene glycol) is more stable. When mixed with an acidic solution, precipitate may form. Use only clear solution.

Mechanism of Action Short-acting barbiturate with sedative, hypnotic, and anticonvulsant properties. Barbiturates depress the sensory cortex, decrease motor activity, alter cerebellar function, and produce drowsiness, sedation, and hypnosis. In high doses, barbiturates exhibit anticonvulsant activity; barbiturates produce dose-dependent respiratory depression.

Pharmacodynamics/Kinetics

Onset of action: I.M.: 10-15 minutes; I.V.: ~1 minute
Duration: I.V.: 15 minutes
Distribution: V_d: Children: 0.8 L/kg; Adults: 1 L/kg
Protein binding: 35% to 55%
Metabolism: Extensively hepatic via hydroxylation and oxidation pathways
Half-life elimination: Terminal: Children: 25 hours; Adults: Healthy: 22 hours (range: 15-50 hours)
Excretion: Urine (<1% as unchanged drug)

Dosage

Children:
Hypnotic: I.M.: 2-6 mg/kg; maximum: 100 mg/dose
Preoperative/preprocedure sedation: ≥6 months:
Note: Limited information is available for infants <6 months of age.
I.M.: 2-6 mg/kg; maximum: 100 mg/dose
I.V.: 1-3 mg/kg to a maximum of 100 mg until asleep
Conscious sedation prior to a procedure: Children 5-12 years: I.V.: 2 mg/kg 5-10 minutes before procedures, may repeat one time

Adolescents: Conscious sedation: I.V.: 100 mg prior to a procedure

Children and Adults: Barbiturate coma in head injury patients: I.V.: Loading dose: 5-10 mg/kg given slowly over 1-2 hours; monitor blood pressure and respiratory rate; Maintenance infusion: Initial: 1 mg/kg/hour; may increase to 2-3 mg/kg/hour; maintain burst suppression on EEG

Status epilepticus: I.V.: **Note**: Intubation required; monitor hemodynamics

Children: Loading dose: 5-15 mg/kg given slowly over 1-2 hours; maintenance infusion: 0.5-5 mg/kg/hour

Adults: Loading dose: 10-20 mg/kg given slowly over 1-2 hours; maintenance infusion: 0.5-3 mg/kg/hour

Adults:

Hypnotic:

I.M.: 150-200 mg

I.V.: Initial: 100 mg, may repeat every 1-3 minutes up to 200-500 mg total dose

Preoperative sedation: I.M.: 150-200 mg

Dosing adjustment in hepatic impairment: Reduce dosage in patients with severe liver dysfunction

Administration Pentobarbital may be administered by deep I.M. or slow I.V. injection.

I.M.: No more than 5 mL (250 mg) should be injected at any one site because of possible tissue irritation.

I.V.: I.V. push doses can be given undiluted, but should be administered no faster than 50 mg/minute; parenteral solutions are highly alkaline; avoid extravasation; avoid rapid I.V. administration >50 mg/minute; avoid intra-arterial injection

Monitoring Parameters Respiratory status (for conscious sedation, includes pulse oximetry), cardiovascular status, CNS status; cardiac monitor and blood pressure monitor required

Reference Range

Therapeutic:

Hypnotic: 1-5 mcg/mL (SI: 4-22 μmol/L)

Coma: 10-50 mcg/mL (SI: 88-221 μmol/L)

Toxic: >10 mcg/mL (SI: >44 μmol/L)

Dosage Forms Excipient information presented when available (limited, particularly for generics); consult specific product labeling.

Injection, solution, as sodium: 50 mg/mL (20 mL, 50 mL) [contains alcohol 10% and propylene glycol 40%]

◆ **Pentobarbital Sodium** *see* PENTobarbital *on page 1170*

Pentosan Polysulfate Sodium

(PEN toe san pol i SUL fate SOW dee um)

U.S. Brand Names Elmiron®

Canadian Brand Names Elmiron®

Index Terms PPS

Pharmacologic Category Analgesic, Urinary

Use Orphan drug: Relief of bladder pain or discomfort due to interstitial cystitis

Pregnancy Risk Factor B

Medication Safety Issues

Sound-alike/look-alike issues:

Pentosan may be confused with pentostatin

Elmiron® may be confused with Imuran®

Dosage Adults: Oral: 100 mg 3 times/day taken with water 1 hour before or 2 hours after meals

Patients should be evaluated at 3 months and may be continued an additional 3 months if there has been no improvement and if there are no therapy-limiting side effects. **The risks and benefits of continued use beyond 6 months in patients who have not responded is not yet known.**

Additional Information Complete prescribing information for this medication should be consulted for additional detail.

Dosage Forms Excipient information presented when available (limited, particularly for generics); consult specific product labeling.

Capsule: 100 mg

Pentostatin (pen toe STAT in)

U.S. Brand Names Nipent®

Canadian Brand Names Nipent®

Index Terms 2′-Deoxycoformycin; Co-Vidarabine; dCF; Deoxycoformycin; NSC-218321

Pharmacologic Category Antineoplastic Agent, Antibiotic; Antineoplastic Agent, Antimetabolite (Purine Antagonist)

Use Treatment of hairy cell leukemia

Unlabeled/Investigational Use Treatment of cutaneous T-cell lymphoma, chronic lymphocytic leukemia (CLL), and acute and chronic graft-versus-host-disease (GVHD)

Pregnancy Risk Factor D

Pregnancy Considerations Animal studies have demonstrated teratogenicity, maternal toxicity, and fetal loss. There are no adequate and well-controlled studies in pregnant women. Women of childbearing potential should be advised to avoid becoming pregnant.

Lactation Excretion in breast milk unknown/not recommended

Medication Safety Issues

Sound-alike/look-alike issues:

Pentostatin may be confused with pentamidine, pentosan

High alert medication: The Institute for Safe Medication Practices (ISMP) includes this medication among its list of drug classes which have a heightened risk of causing significant patient harm when used in error.

International issues:

Nipent® may be confused with Nipin® which is a brand name for nifedipine in Italy and Singapore

Contraindications Hypersensitivity to pentostatin or any component of the formulation

Warnings/Precautions Hazardous agent - use appropriate precautions for handling and disposal. **[U.S. Boxed Warnings]: Severe renal, liver, pulmonary and CNS toxicities have occurred with doses higher than recommended; do not exceed the recommended dose. Do not administer concurrently with fludarabine; concomitant use has resulted in serious or fatal pulmonary toxicity.** Bone marrow suppression may occur, primarily early in treatment; if neutropenia persists beyond early cycles, evaluate for disease status. In patients who present with infections prior to treatment, infections should be resolved, if possible, prior to initiation of treatment; treatment should be temporarily withheld for active infections during therapy. Use cautiously in patients with renal dysfunction (the half-life is prolonged); appropriate dosing guidelines in renal insufficiency have not been determined. May cause elevations (reversible) in liver function tests. Withhold treatment for CNS toxicity or severe rash. Fatal pulmonary edema and hypotension have been reported in patients treated with pentostatin in combination with carmustine, etoposide, or high-dose cyclophosphamide as part of a myeloablative regimen for bone marrow transplant. **[U.S. Boxed Warning]: Should be administered under the supervision of an experienced cancer chemotherapy physician.** Safety and efficacy in children have not been established.

Adverse Reactions

>10%:

Central nervous system: Fever (42% to 46%), fatigue (29% to 42%), pain (8% to 20%), chills (11% to 19%), headache (13% to 17%), CNS toxicity (1% to 11%)

Dermatologic: Rash (26% to 43%), pruritus (10% to 21%), skin disorder (4% to 17%)

Gastrointestinal: Nausea/vomiting (22% to 63%), diarrhea (15% to 17%), anorexia (13% to 16%), abdominal pain (4% to 16%), stomatitis (5% to 12%)

Hematologic: Myelosuppression (nadir: 7 days; recovery: 10-14 days), leukopenia (22% to 60%), anemia (8% to 35%), thrombocytopenia (6% to 32%)

Hepatic: Transaminases increased (2% to 19%)

Neuromuscular & skeletal: Myalgia (11% to 19%), weakness (10% to 12%)

Respiratory: Cough (17% to 20%), upper respiratory infection (13% to 16%), rhinitis (10% to 11%), dyspnea (8% to 11%)

Miscellaneous: Infection (7% to 36%), allergic reaction (2% to 11%)

1% to 10%:

Cardiovascular: Chest pain (3% to 10%), facial edema (3% to 10%), hypotension (3% to 10%), peripheral edema (3% to 10%), angina (<3%), arrhythmia (<3%), AV block (<3%), bradycardia (<3%), cardiac arrest (<3%), deep thrombophlebitis (<3%), heart failure (<3%), hypertension (<3%), pericardial effusion (<3%), sinus arrest (<3%), syncope (<3%), tachycardia (<3%), vasculitis (<3%), ventricular extrasystoles (<3%)

Central nervous system: Anxiety (3% to 10%), confusion (3% to 10%), depression (3% to 10%), dizziness (3% to 10%), insomnia (3% to 10%), nervousness (3% to 10%), somnolence (3% to 10%), abnormal dreams/thinking (<3%), amnesia (<3%), ataxia (<3%), emotional lability (<3%), encephalitis (<3%), hallucination (<3%), hostility (<3%), meningism (<3%), neuritis (<3%), neurosis (<3%), seizure (<3%), vertigo (<3%)

Dermatologic: Cellulitis (6%), furunculosis (4%), dry skin (3% to 10%), urticaria (3% to 10%), acne (<3%), alopecia (<3%), eczema (<3%), petechial rash (<3%), photosensitivity (<3%), abscess (2%)

Endocrine & metabolic: Amenorrhea (<3%), hypercalcemia (<3%), hyponatremia (<3%), gout (<3%), libido decreased/loss (<3%)

Gastrointestinal: Dyspepsia (3% to 10%) flatulence (3% to 10%), gingivitis (3% to 10%), constipation (<3%), dysphagia (<3%), glossitis (<3%), ileus (<3%), taste perversion (<3%), oral moniliasis (2%)

Genitourinary: Urinary tract infection (3%), impotence (<3%)

Hematologic: Agranulocytosis (3% to 10%), hemorrhage (3% to 10%), acute leukemia (<3%), aplastic anemia (<3%), hemolytic anemia (<3%)

Local: Phlebitis (<3%)

Neuromuscular & skeletal: Arthralgia (3% to 10%), paresthesia (3% to 10%), arthritis (<3%), dysarthria (<3%), hyperkinesia (<3%), neuralgia (<3%), neuropathy (<3%), paralysis (<3%), twitching (<3%), osteomyelitis (1%)

Ocular: Conjunctivitis (4%), amblyopia (<3%), eyes nonreactive (<3%), lacrimation disorder (<3%), photophobia (<3%), retinopathy (<3%), vision abnormal (<3%), watery eyes (<3%), xerophthalmia (<3%)

Otic: Deafness (<3%), earache (<3%), labyrinthitis (<3%), tinnitus (<3%)

Renal: Creatinine increased (3% to 10%), nephropathy (<3%), renal failure (<3%), renal insufficiency (<3%), renal function abnormal (<3%), renal stone (<3%)

Respiratory: Pharyngitis (8% to 10%), sinusitis (6%), pneumonia (5%), asthma (3% to 10%), bronchitis (3%), bronchospasm (<3%), laryngeal edema (<3%), pulmonary embolus (<3%)

Miscellaneous: Diaphoresis (8% to 10%), herpes zoster (8%), viral infection (≤8%), bacterial infection (5%), herpes simplex (4%), sepsis (3%), flu-like syndrome (<3%)

<1% (Limited to important or life-threatening): Dysuria, fungal infection (skin), hematuria, lethargy, pulmonary edema, pulmonary toxicity (fatal; in combination with fludarabine), uveitis/vision loss

Drug Interactions

Avoid Concomitant Use

Avoid concomitant use of Pentostatin with any of the following: Natalizumab; Pegademase Bovine; Vaccines (Live)

Increased Effect/Toxicity

Pentostatin may increase the levels/effects of: Cyclophosphamide; Natalizumab; Vaccines (Live)

The levels/effects of Pentostatin may be increased by: Fludarabine; Trastuzumab

Decreased Effect

Pentostatin may decrease the levels/effects of: Pegademase Bovine; Vaccines (Inactivated)

The levels/effects of Pentostatin may be decreased by: Echinacea; Pegademase Bovine

Stability Store intact vials under refrigeration at 2°C to 8°C (36°F to 46°F); reconstituted vials, or further dilutions, are stable at room temperature for 8 hours in D_5W or 48 hours in NS. Reconstitute with 5 mL SWFI to a concentration of 2 mg/mL. The solution may be further diluted in 25-50 mL NS or D_5W for infusion.

Mechanism of Action Pentostatin is a purine antimetabolite that inhibits adenosine deaminase, preventing the deamination of adenosine to inosine. Accumulation of deoxyadenosine (dAdo) and deoxyadenosine 5′-triphosphate (dATP) results in a reduction of purine metabolism and DNA synthesis and cell death.

Pharmacodynamics/Kinetics

Distribution: I.V.: V_d: 36.1 L (20.1 L/m^2); rapidly to body tissues

Protein binding: ~4%

Half-life elimination: Distribution half-life: 11-85 minutes; Terminal: 3-7 hours; renal impairment (Cl_{cr} <50 mL/minute): 4-18 hours

Excretion: Urine (~50% to 96%) within 24 hours (30% to 90% as unchanged drug)

Dosage I.V.: Adults (refer to individual protocols):

Hairy cell leukemia: 4 mg/m^2 every 2 weeks

CLL (unlabeled use): 4 mg/m^2 weekly for 3 weeks, then every 2 weeks

Cutaneous T-cell lymphoma (unlabeled use): 3.75-5 mg/m^2 daily for 3 days every 3 weeks

Acute GVHD (unlabeled use): 1.5 mg/m^2 daily for 3 days; may repeat after 2 weeks if needed

Chronic GVHD (unlabeled use): 4 mg/m^2 every 2 weeks for 12 doses; then 4 mg/m^2 every 3-4 weeks (if still improving)

Dosage adjustment in renal impairment: The FDA-approved labeling does not contain renal dosage adjustment guidelines; use with caution in patients with Cl_{cr} <60 mL/minute. Two patients with Cl_{cr} 50-60 mL/minute achieved responses when treated with 2 mg/m^2/dose. The following guidelines have been used by some clinicians:

Kintzel, 1995:

- Cl_{cr} 46-60 mL/minute: Administer 70% of dose
- Cl_{cr} 31-45 mL/minute: Administer 60% of dose
- Cl_{cr} <30 mL/minute: Consider use of alternative drug

Lathia, 2002:

- Cl_{cr} 40-59 mL/minute: Administer 3 mg/m^2/dose
- Cl_{cr} 20-39 mL/minute: Administer 2 mg/m^2/dose

Administration Administer I.V. 20- to 30-minute infusion or I.V. bolus over 5 minutes. Hydrate with 500-1000 mL fluid prior to infusion and 500 mL after infusion.

Monitoring Parameters CBC with differential, platelet count, liver function, serum uric acid, renal function (creatinine clearance), bone marrow evaluation

Dosage Forms Excipient information presented when available (limited, particularly for generics); consult specific product labeling.

Injection, powder for reconstitution [preservative free]: 10 mg [contains mannitol 50 mg]

Nipent®: 10 mg [contains mannitol 50 mg]

◆ **Pentothal®** *see* Thiopental *on page 1460*

Pentoxifylline (pen toks IF i lin)

U.S. Brand Names Pentoxil®; Trental®

Canadian Brand Names Albert® Pentoxifylline; Apo-Pentoxifylline SR®; Nu-Pentoxifylline SR; ratio-Pentoxifylline; Trental®

Index Terms Oxpentifylline

Pharmacologic Category Blood Viscosity Reducer Agent

Use Treatment of intermittent claudication on the basis of chronic occlusive arterial disease of the limbs; may improve function and symptoms, but not intended to replace more definitive therapy

Unlabeled/Investigational Use AIDS patients with increased TNF, CVA, cerebrovascular diseases, diabetic atherosclerosis, diabetic neuropathy, gangrene, hemodialysis shunt thrombosis, vascular impotence, cerebral malaria, septic shock, sickle cell syndromes, vasculitis, and venous leg ulcers

Pregnancy Risk Factor C

Pregnancy Considerations Teratogenic effects were not observed in animal studies. There are no adequate and well-controlled studies in pregnant women.

Lactation Enters breast milk/not recommended

Medication Safety Issues

Sound-alike/look-alike issues:

Pentoxifylline may be confused with tamoxifen

Trental® may be confused with Bentyl®, Tegretol®, Trandate®

Contraindications Hypersensitivity to pentoxifylline, xanthines (eg, caffeine, theophylline), or any component of the formulation; recent cerebral and/or retinal hemorrhage

Warnings/Precautions Start with lower doses in elderly patients and monitor renal function. Safety and efficacy in pediatric patients have not been established.

Adverse Reactions

1% to 10%: Gastrointestinal: Nausea (2%), vomiting (1%)

<1% (Limited to important or life-threatening): Anaphylactoid reaction, angioedema, angina, anorexia, anxiety, aplastic anemia, arrhythmia, aseptic meningitis, bloating, blurred vision, brittle fingernails, chest pain, cholecystitis, confusion, conjunctivitis, constipation, depression, dyspnea, earache, edema, epistaxis, eructation, fibrinogen decreased (serum), flatus, flu-like syndrome, hallucinations, hepatitis, hypotension, jaundice, laryngitis, leukemia, leukopenia, liver enzymes increased, malaise, nasal congestion, pancytopenia, pruritus, purpura, rash, scotoma, seizure, sialism, sore throat, taste perversion, tachycardia, thrombocytopenia, tremor, urticaria, weight change, xerostomia

Drug Interactions

Metabolism/Transport Effects **Inhibits** CYP1A2 (weak)

Avoid Concomitant Use

Avoid concomitant use of Pentoxifylline with any of the following: Ketorolac

Increased Effect/Toxicity

Pentoxifylline may increase the levels/effects of: Theophylline Derivatives

The levels/effects of Pentoxifylline may be increased by: Ciprofloxacin; Ketorolac

Decreased Effect There are no known significant interactions involving a decrease in effect.

Ethanol/Nutrition/Herb Interactions Food: Food may decrease rate but not extent of absorption. Pentoxifylline peak serum levels may be decreased if taken with food.

Stability Store between 15°C to 30°C (59°F to 86°F).

Mechanism of Action Reduces blood viscosity via increased leukocyte and erythrocyte deformability and decreased neutrophil adhesion/activation; improves peripheral tissue oxygenation presumably through enhanced blood flow.

Pharmacodynamics/Kinetics

Absorption: Well absorbed

Metabolism: Hepatic and via erythrocytes; extensive first-pass effect

Half-life elimination: Parent drug: 24-48 minutes; Metabolites: 60-96 minutes

Time to peak, serum: 2-4 hours

Excretion: Primarily urine (active metabolites); feces (4%)

Dosage Adults: Oral: 400 mg 3 times/day with meals; maximal therapeutic benefit may take 2-4 weeks to develop; recommended to maintain therapy for at least 8 weeks. May reduce to 400 mg twice daily if GI or CNS side effects occur.

Dietary Considerations May be taken with meals or food.

Administration Tablets should be swallowed whole; do not chew, break, or crush.

Test Interactions Decreased calcium (S), magnesium (S); false-positive theophylline levels

Dosage Forms Excipient information presented when available (limited, particularly for generics); consult specific product labeling.

Tablet, controlled release:

Trental®: 400 mg

Tablet, extended release: 400 mg

Pentoxil®: 400 mg

◆ **Pentoxil®** *see* Pentoxifylline *on page 1173*

◆ **Pen VK** *see* Penicillin V Potassium *on page 1167*

◆ **Pepcid®** *see* Famotidine *on page 603*

◆ **Pepcid® AC [OTC]** *see* Famotidine *on page 603*

◆ **Pepcid® AC (Can)** *see* Famotidine *on page 603*

◆ **Pepcid® AC Maximum Strength [OTC]** *see* Famotidine *on page 603*

◆ **Pepcid® Complete [OTC]** *see* Famotidine, Calcium Carbonate, and Magnesium Hydroxide *on page 604*

◆ **Pepcid® I.V. (Can)** *see* Famotidine *on page 603*

◆ **Peptic Relief [OTC]** *see* Bismuth *on page 199*

◆ **Pepto-Bismol® [OTC]** *see* Bismuth *on page 199*

◆ **Pepto-Bismol® Maximum Strength [OTC]** *see* Bismuth *on page 199*

◆ **Pepto Relief [OTC]** *see* Bismuth *on page 199*

◆ **Percocet®** *see* Oxycodone and Acetaminophen *on page 1122*

◆ **Percocet®-Demi (Can)** *see* Oxycodone and Acetaminophen *on page 1122*

◆ **Percodan®** *see* Oxycodone and Aspirin *on page 1123*

◆ **Percogesic® [OTC]** *see* Acetaminophen and Phenyltoloxamine *on page 29*

◆ **Percogesic® Extra Strength [OTC]** *see* Acetaminophen and Diphenhydramine *on page 28*

Perflutren Protein Type A

(per FLOO tren PRO teen typ aye)

U.S. Brand Names Optison™

Pharmacologic Category Diagnostic Agent

Use Opacification of left ventricular chamber and improvement of delineation of the left ventricular endocardial border in patients with suboptimal echocardiograms

Pregnancy Risk Factor C

Dosage I.V.: Adults: 0.5 mL via peripheral vein; flush with D_5W or NS following dose; may repeat in increments of 0.5 mL up to 5 mL cumulatively in 10 minutes (maximum total dose: 8.7 mL in any one patient study)

Additional Information Complete prescribing information for this medication should be consulted for additional detail.

Dosage Forms Excipient information presented when available (limited, particularly for generics); consult specific product labeling.

Injection, suspension [preservative free]:

Optison™: Perflutren 0.11-0.33 mg and protein-type A microspheres 5-8 x 10^8 per mL (3 mL) [contains human albumin 10 mg/mL]

◆ **Perforomist™** *see* Formoterol *on page 662*

◆ **Periactin** *see* Cyproheptadine *on page 383*

◆ **Peri-Colace® [OTC]** *see* Docusate and Senna *on page 474*

◆ **Peridex®** *see* Chlorhexidine Gluconate *on page 305*

◆ **Peridex® Oral Rinse (Can)** *see* Chlorhexidine Gluconate *on page 305*

◆ **Peridol (Can)** *see* Haloperidol *on page 720*

Perindopril Erbumine (per IN doe pril er BYOO meen)

U.S. Brand Names Aceon®

Canadian Brand Names Apo-Perindopril®; Coversyl®

Pharmacologic Category Angiotensin-Converting Enzyme (ACE) Inhibitor

Additional Appendix Information

Angiotensin Agents *on page 1632*

Heart Failure (Systolic) *on page 1809*

Use Treatment of hypertension; reduction of cardiovascular mortality or nonfatal myocardial infarction in patients with stable coronary artery disease

Unlabeled/Investigational Use To delay the progression of nephropathy and reduce risks of cardiovascular events in hypertensive patients with type 1 or 2 diabetes mellitus

Pregnancy Risk Factor D

Pregnancy Considerations Due to adverse events observed in humans, perindopril is considered pregnancy category D. Perindopril crosses the placenta. First trimester exposure to ACE inhibitors may cause major congenital malformations. An increased risk of cardiovascular and/or central nervous system malformations was observed in one study; however, an increased risk of teratogenic events was not observed in other studies. Second and third trimester use of an ACE inhibitor is associated with oligohydramnios. Oligohydramnios due to decreased fetal renal function may lead to fetal limb contractures, craniofacial deformation, and hypoplastic lung development. The use of ACE inhibitors during the second and third trimesters is also associated with anuria, hypotension, renal failure (reversible or irreversible), skull hypoplasia, and death in the fetus/neonate. Chronic maternal hypertension itself is also associated with adverse events in the fetus/infant. ACE inhibitors are not recommended during pregnancy to treat maternal hypertension or heart failure. Those who are planning a pregnancy should be considered for other medication options if an ACE inhibitor is currently prescribed or the ACE inhibitor should be discontinued as soon as possible once pregnancy is detected. The exposed fetus should be monitored for fetal growth, amniotic fluid volume, and organ formation. Infants exposed to an ACE inhibitor *in utero*, especially during the second and third trimester, should be monitored for hyperkalemia, hypotension, and oliguria.

[U.S. Boxed Warning]: Based on human data, ACE inhibitors can cause injury and death to the developing fetus. ACE inhibitors should be discontinued as soon as possible once pregnancy is detected.

Lactation Excretion in breast milk unknown/use caution

Contraindications Hypersensitivity to perindopril, any other ACE inhibitor, or any component of the formulation; angioedema related to previous treatment with an ACE inhibitor

Warnings/Precautions Anaphylactic reactions may occur rarely with ACE inhibitors. At any time during treatment (especially following first dose), angioedema may occur rarely with ACE inhibitors; it may involve the head and neck (potentially compromising airway) or the intestine (presenting with abdominal pain). African-Americans and patients with idiopathic or hereditary angioedema may be at an increased risk. Prolonged frequent monitoring may be required especially if tongue, glottis, or larynx are involved as they are associated with airway obstruction. Patients with a history of airway surgery may have a higher risk of airway obstruction. Aggressive early and appropriate management is critical. Use in patients with previous angioedema associated with ACE inhibitor therapy is contraindicated. Severe anaphylactoid reactions may be seen during hemodialysis (eg, CVVHD) with high-flux dialysis membranes (eg, AN69), and rarely, during low density lipoprotein apheresis with dextran sulfate cellulose. Rare cases of anaphylactoid reactions have been reported in patients undergoing sensitization treatment with hymenoptera (bee, wasp) venom while receiving ACE inhibitors.

Symptomatic hypotension with or without syncope can occur with ACE inhibitors (usually with the first several doses); effects are most often observed in volume-depleted patients; correct volume depletion prior to initiation; close monitoring of patient is required especially with initial dosing and dosing increases; blood pressure must be lowered at a rate appropriate for the patient's clinical condition. Initiation of therapy in patients with ischemic heart disease or cerebrovascular disease warrants close observation due to the potential consequences posed by falling blood pressure (eg, MI, stroke). Use with caution in hypertrophic cardiomyopathy with outflow tract obstruction, severe aortic stenosis, or before, during, or immediately after major surgery. **[U.S. Boxed Warning]: Based on human data, ACEIs can cause injury and death to the developing fetus when used in the second and third trimesters. ACEIs should be discontinued as soon as possible once pregnancy is detected.**

Hyperkalemia may occur with ACE inhibitors; risk factors include renal dysfunction, diabetes mellitus, concomitant use of potassium-sparing diuretics, potassium supplements, and/or potassium-containing salts. Use cautiously, if at all, with these agents and monitor potassium closely. Cough may occur with ACE inhibitors. Other causes of cough should be considered (eg, pulmonary congestion in patients with heart failure) and excluded prior to discontinuation.

May be associated with deterioration of renal function and/or increases in serum creatinine, particularly in patients with low renal blood flow (eg, renal artery stenosis, heart failure) whose glomerular filtration rate (GFR) is dependent on efferent arteriolar vasoconstriction by angiotensin II;

deterioration may result in oliguria, acute renal failure, and progressive azotemia. Small increases in serum creatinine may occur following initiation; consider discontinuation only in patients with progressive and/or significant deterioration in renal function. Use with caution in patients with unstented unilateral/bilateral renal artery stenosis. When unstented bilateral renal artery stenosis is present, use is generally avoided due to the elevated risk of deterioration in renal function unless possible benefits outweigh risks.

Rare toxicities associated with ACE inhibitors include cholestatic jaundice (which may progress to fulminant hepatic necrosis), agranulocytosis, neutropenia or leukopenia with myeloid hypoplasia. Patients with collagen vascular diseases (especially with concomitant renal impairment) or renal impairment alone may be at increased risk for hematologic toxicity; periodically monitor CBC with differential in these patients. Safety and efficacy have not been established in children.

Adverse Reactions

>10%:

Central nervous system: Headache (24%)

Respiratory: Cough (incidence is higher in women, 3:1) (12%)

1% to 10%:

Cardiovascular: Edema (4%), chest pain (2%), ECG abnormal (2%), palpitation (1%)

Central nervous system: Dizziness (8%, less than placebo), sleep disorders (3%), depression (2%), fever (2%), nervousness (1%), somnolence (1%)

Dermatologic: Rash (2%)

Endocrine & metabolic: Hyperkalemia (1%, less than placebo), triglycerides increased (1%), menstrual disorder (1%)

Gastrointestinal: Diarrhea (4%), abdominal pain (3%), nausea (2%), vomiting (2%), dyspepsia (2%), flatulence (1%)

Genitourinary: Urinary tract infection (3%), sexual dysfunction (male 1%)

Hepatic: ALT increased (2%)

Neuromuscular & skeletal: Weakness (8%), back pain (6%), lower extremity pain (5%), upper extremity pain (3%), hypertonia (3%), paresthesia (2%), joint pain (1%), myalgia (1%), arthritis (1%), neck pain (1%)

Renal: Proteinuria (2%)

Respiratory: Upper respiratory tract infection (9%), sinusitis (5%), rhinitis (5%), pharyngitis (3%)

Otic: Tinnitus (2%), ear infection (1%)

Miscellaneous: Viral infection (3%), seasonal allergy (2%)

Note: Some reactions occurred at an incidence >1% but ≤ placebo.

<1% (Limited to important or life-threatening): Amnesia, anaphylaxis, angioedema, anxiety, AST increased, dyspnea, erythema, fluid retention, gout, leukopenia, migraine, MI, nephrolithiasis, neutropenia, orthostatic hypotension, pruritus, psychosocial disorder, pulmonary fibrosis, purpura, stroke, syncope, urinary retention, vertigo

Additional adverse effects that have been reported with **ACE inhibitors** include agranulocytosis (especially in patients with renal impairment or collagen vascular disease), neutropenia, anemia, bullous pemphigoid, cardiac arrest, eosinophilic pneumonitis, exfoliative dermatitis, falls, hepatic failure, hyponatremia, jaundice, pancreatitis (acute), pancytopenia, pemphigus, psoriasis, thrombocytopenia; decreases in creatinine clearance in some elderly hypertensive patients or those with chronic renal failure, and worsening of renal function in patients with bilateral renal artery stenosis or hypovolemic patients (diuretic therapy). In addition, a syndrome which may include fever, myalgia, arthralgia, interstitial nephritis, vasculitis, rash, eosinophilia and positive ANA, and elevated ESR has been reported with ACE inhibitors.

Drug Interactions

Avoid Concomitant Use There are no known interactions where it is recommended to avoid concomitant use.

Increased Effect/Toxicity

Perindopril Erbumine may increase the levels/effects of: Allopurinol; Amifostine; AzaTHIOprine; CycloSPORINE; Ferric Gluconate; Gold Sodium Thiomalate; Lithium; RiTUXimab

The levels/effects of Perindopril Erbumine may be increased by: Angiotensin II Receptor Blockers; Diazoxide; Eplerenone; Herbs (Hypotensive Properties); Loop Diuretics; Potassium Salts; Potassium-Sparing Diuretics; Prostacyclin Analogues; Sirolimus; Temsirolimus; Thiazide Diuretics; Trimethoprim

Decreased Effect

The levels/effects of Perindopril Erbumine may be decreased by: Antacids; Aprotinin; Herbs (Hypertensive Properties); Methylphenidate; Nonsteroidal Anti-Inflammatory Agents; Salicylates; Yohimbine

Ethanol/Nutrition/Herb Interactions

Food: Perindopril active metabolite concentrations may be lowered if taken with food.

Herb/Nutraceutical: Avoid bayberry, blue cohosh, cayenne, ephedra, ginger, ginseng (American), kola, licorice (may worsen hypertension). Avoid black cohosh, California poppy, coleus, golden seal, hawthorn, mistletoe, periwinkle, quinine, shepherd's purse (may have increased antihypertensive effect).

Stability Store at room temperature of 20°C to 25°C (68°F to 77°F). Protect from moisture.

Mechanism of Action Perindopril is a prodrug for perindoprilat, which acts as a competitive inhibitor of angiotensin-converting enzyme (ACE); prevents conversion of angiotensin I to angiotensin II, a potent vasoconstrictor; results in lower levels of angiotensin II which, in turn, causes an increase in plasma renin activity and a reduction in aldosterone secretion

Pharmacodynamics/Kinetics

Onset of action: Peak effect: 1-2 hours

Protein binding: Perindopril: 60%; Perindoprilat: 10% to 20%

Metabolism: Hepatically hydrolyzed to active metabolite, perindoprilat (~17% to 20% of a dose) and other inactive metabolites

Bioavailability: Perindopril: 75%; Perindoprilat ~25% (~16% with food)

Half-life elimination: Parent drug: 1.5-3 hours; Metabolite: Effective: 3-10 hours, Terminal: 30-120 hours

Time to peak: Chronic therapy: Perindopril: 1 hour; Perindoprilat: 3-7 hours (maximum perindoprilat serum levels are 2-3 times higher and T_{max} is shorter following chronic therapy); CHF: Perindoprilat: 6 hours

Excretion: Urine (75%, 4% to 12% as unchanged drug)

Dosage Oral:

Adults:

Hypertension: Initial: 4 mg/day but may be titrated to response; usual range: 4-8 mg/day (may be given in 2 divided doses); increase at 1- to 2-week intervals (maximum: 16 mg/day)

Concomitant therapy with diuretics: To reduce the risk of hypotension, discontinue diuretic, if possible, 2-3 days prior to initiating perindopril. If unable to stop diuretic, initiate perindopril at 2-4 mg/day and monitor blood pressure closely for the first 2 weeks of therapy, and after any dose adjustment of perindopril or diuretic.

Stable coronary artery disease: Initial: 4 mg once daily for 2 weeks; increase as tolerated to 8 mg once daily.

Heart failure (unlabeled use): Initial: 2 mg once daily; increase at 1- to 2-week intervals; target dose: 8-16 mg once daily (ACC/AHA 2005 Heart Failure Guidelines)

Elderly:

Hypertension: >65 years of age: Initial: 4 mg/day; maintenance: 8 mg/day; experience with doses >8 mg/day is limited

Stable coronary artery disease: >70 years of age: Initial: 2 mg/day for 1 week; increase as tolerated to 4 mg/day for 1 week; then increase as tolerated to 8 mg/day; experience with doses >8 mg/day is limited

Dosing adjustment in renal impairment:

Cl_{cr} >30 mL/minute: Initial: 2 mg/day; maintenance dosing not to exceed 8 mg/day

Cl_{cr} <30 mL/minute: Safety and efficacy not established.

Hemodialysis: Perindopril and its metabolites are dialyzable

Dosing adjustment in hepatic impairment: No adjustment necessary

Monitoring Parameters Blood pressure; serum creatinine and potassium; if patient has collagen vascular disease and/or renal impairment, periodically monitor CBC with differential

Dosage Forms Excipient information presented when available (limited, particularly for generics); consult specific product labeling.

Tablet: 2 mg, 4 mg, 8 mg

◆ **PerioChip®** *see* Chlorhexidine Gluconate *on page 305*

◆ **PerioGard®** *see* Chlorhexidine Gluconate *on page 305*

◆ **PerioMed™** *see* Fluoride *on page 635*

◆ **Periostat®** *see* Doxycycline *on page 491*

◆ **Perlane®** *see* Hyaluronate and Derivatives *on page 734*

Permethrin (per METH rin)

U.S. Brand Names A200® Lice [OTC]; Acticin®; Elimite®; Nix® [OTC]; Rid® Spray [OTC]

Canadian Brand Names Kwellada-P™; Nix®

Pharmacologic Category Antiparasitic Agent, Topical; Scabicidal Agent

Use Single-application treatment of infestation with *Pediculus humanus capitis* (head louse) and its nits or *Sarcoptes scabiei* (scabies); indicated for prophylactic use during epidemics of lice

Pregnancy Risk Factor B

Dosage Topical:

Head lice: Children >2 months and Adults: After hair has been washed with shampoo, rinsed with water, and towel dried, apply a sufficient volume of topical liquid (lotion or cream rinse) to saturate the hair and scalp. Leave on hair for 10 minutes before rinsing off with water; remove remaining nits; may repeat in 1 week if lice or nits still present.

Scabies: Apply cream from head to toe; leave on for 8-14 hours before washing off with water; for infants, also apply on the hairline, neck, scalp, temple, and forehead; may reapply in 1 week if live mites appear

Permethrin 5% cream was shown to be safe and effective when applied to an infant <1 month of age with neonatal scabies; time of application was limited to 6 hours before rinsing with soap and water

Additional Information Complete prescribing information for this medication should be consulted for additional detail.

Dosage Forms Excipient information presented when available (limited, particularly for generics); consult specific product labeling.

Cream, topical (Acticin®, Elimite®): 5% (60 g) [contains coconut oil]

Lotion, topical: 1% (59 mL)

Liquid, topical [creme rinse formulation] (Nix®): 1% (60 mL) [contains isopropyl alcohol 20%]

Solution, spray [for bedding and furniture]:

A200® Lice: 0.5% (180 mL)

Nix®: 0.25% (148 mL)

Rid®: 0.5% (150 mL)

Perphenazine (per FEN a zeen)

Canadian Brand Names Apo-Perphenazine®

Pharmacologic Category Antiemetic; Antipsychotic Agent, Typical, Phenothiazine

Additional Appendix Information

Antipsychotic Agents *on page 1644*

Use Treatment of schizophrenia; severe nausea and vomiting

Unlabeled/Investigational Use Ethanol withdrawal; behavioral symptoms associated with dementia (elderly); Tourette's syndrome; Huntington's chorea; spasmodic torticollis; Reye's syndrome; psychosis; psychosis/agitation related to Alzheimer's dementia

Pregnancy Risk Factor C

Medication Safety Issues

Sound-alike/look-alike issues:

Trilafon® may be confused with Tri-Levlen®

Dosage Oral: Adults:

Schizophrenia/psychoses:

Nonhospitalized: Initial: 4-8 mg 3 times/day; reduce dose as soon as possible to minimum effective dosage (maximum: 64 mg/day)

Hospitalized: 8-16 mg 2-4 times/day (maximum: 64 mg/day)

Nausea/vomiting: 8-16 mg/day in divided doses (maximum: 24 mg/day)

Elderly: Behavioral symptoms associated with dementia (unlabeled use): Initial: 2-4 mg 1-2 times/day; increase at 4- to 7-day intervals by 2-4 mg/day. Increase dose intervals (bid, tid, etc) as necessary to control behavior response or side effects. Maximum daily dose: 32 mg; gradual increase (titration) and bedtime administration may prevent some side effects or decrease their severity.

Hemodialysis: Not dialyzable (0% to 5%)

Dosing adjustment in hepatic impairment: Dosage reductions should be considered in patients with liver disease although no specific guidelines are available

Additional Information Complete prescribing information for this medication should be consulted for additional detail.

Dosage Forms Excipient information presented when available (limited, particularly for generics); consult specific product labeling.

Tablet: 2 mg, 4 mg, 8 mg, 16 mg

◆ **Perphenazine and Amitriptyline Hydrochloride** *see* Amitriptyline and Perphenazine *on page 93*

◆ **Persantine®** *see* Dipyridamole *on page 467*

◆ **Pertussis, Acellular (Adsorbed)** *see* Diphtheria and Tetanus Toxoids, Acellular Pertussis, Poliovirus and *Haemophilus* b Conjugate Vaccine *on page 462*

◆ **Pethidine Hydrochloride** *see* Meperidine *on page 943*

◆ **Pexeva®** *see* PARoxetine *on page 1146*

◆ **Pexicam® (Can)** *see* Piroxicam *on page 1201*

◆ **PFA** *see* Foscarnet *on page 667*

◆ **Pfizerpen®** *see* Penicillin G (Parenteral/Aqueous) *on page 1164*

◆ **Pfizerpen-AS® (Can)** *see* Penicillin G Procaine *on page 1166*

◆ **PGE_1** *see* Alprostadil *on page 70*

◆ **PGE_2** *see* Dinoprostone *on page 454*

◆ **PGI_2** *see* Epoprostenol *on page 534*

- ◆ **PGX** *see* Epoprostenol *on page 534*
- ◆ **Phanasin® [OTC]** *see* GuaiFENesin *on page 709*
- ◆ **Phanasin® Diabetic Choice [OTC]** *see* GuaiFENesin *on page 709*
- ◆ **Phanatuss® DM [OTC]** *see* Guaifenesin and Dextromethorphan *on page 710*
- ◆ **Phanatuss® HC [DSC]** *see* Hydrocodone and Guaifenesin *on page 741*
- ◆ **Pharmaflur® [DSC]** *see* Fluoride *on page 635*
- ◆ **Pharmaflur® 1.1 [DSC]** *see* Fluoride *on page 635*
- ◆ **Pharmorubicin® (Can)** *see* Epirubicin *on page 528*
- ◆ **Phenabid®** *see* Chlorpheniramine and Phenylephrine *on page 309*
- ◆ **Phenabid DM®** *see* Chlorpheniramine, Phenylephrine, and Dextromethorphan *on page 311*
- ◆ **Phenadoz™** *see* Promethazine *on page 1249*
- ◆ **Phenagesic [OTC]** *see* Acetaminophen and Phenyltoloxamine *on page 29*
- ◆ **PhenaVent™ [DSC]** *see* Guaifenesin and Phenylephrine *on page 712*
- ◆ **PhenaVent™ D [DSC]** *see* Guaifenesin and Phenylephrine *on page 712*
- ◆ **PhenaVent™ LA [DSC]** *see* Guaifenesin and Phenylephrine *on page 712*
- ◆ **PhenaVent™ Ped [DSC]** *see* Guaifenesin and Phenylephrine *on page 712*
- ◆ **Phenazo™ (Can)** *see* Phenazopyridine *on page 1177*

Phenazopyridine (fen az oh PEER i deen)

U.S. Brand Names AZO-Gesic® [OTC]; AZO-Standard® Maximum Strength [OTC]; AZO-Standard® [OTC]; Baridium® [OTC]; Prodium® [OTC]; Pyridium®; ReAzo [OTC]; Uristat® [OTC] [DSC]; UTI Relief® [OTC]

Canadian Brand Names Phenazo™

Index Terms Phenazopyridine Hydrochloride; Phenylazo Diamino Pyridine Hydrochloride

Pharmacologic Category Analgesic, Urinary

Use Symptomatic relief of urinary burning, itching, frequency and urgency in association with urinary tract infection or following urologic procedures

Pregnancy Risk Factor B

Medication Safety Issues

Sound-alike/look-alike issues:

Phenazopyridine may be confused with phenoxybenzamine

Pyridium® may be confused with Dyrenium®, Perdiem®, pyridoxine, pyrithione

Dosage Oral:

Children: 12 mg/kg/day in 3 divided doses administered after meals for 2 days

Adults: 100-200 mg 3 times/day after meals for 2 days when used concomitantly with an antibacterial agent

Dosing interval in renal impairment:

Cl_{cr} 50-80 mL/minute: Administer every 8-16 hours

Cl_{cr} <50 mL/minute: Avoid use

Additional Information Complete prescribing information for this medication should be consulted for additional detail.

Dosage Forms Excipient information presented when available (limited, particularly for generics); consult specific product labeling. [DSC] = Discontinued product

Tablet, as hydrochloride: 100 mg, 200 mg

AZO-Gesic®, Prodium®, ReAzo; Uristat® [DSC]: 95 mg

AZO-Standard®: 95 mg [gluten free]

AZO Standard® Maximum Strength: 97.5 mg [gluten free]

Baridium®, UTI Relief®: 97.2 mg

Pyridium®: 100 mg, 200 mg

- ◆ **Phenazopyridine Hydrochloride** *see* Phenazopyridine *on page 1177*
- ◆ **Phencarb GG** *see* Carbetapentane, Guaifenesin, and Phenylephrine *on page 255*

Phenelzine (FEN el zeen)

U.S. Brand Names Nardil®

Canadian Brand Names Nardil®

Index Terms Phenelzine Sulfate

Pharmacologic Category Antidepressant, Monoamine Oxidase Inhibitor

Additional Appendix Information

Antidepressant Agents *on page 1638*

Tyramine Content of Foods *on page 1850*

Use Symptomatic treatment of atypical, nonendogenous, or neurotic depression

Unlabeled/Investigational Use Selective mutism

Restrictions An FDA-approved medication guide concerning the use of antidepressants in children, adolescents, and young adults must be distributed when dispensing an outpatient prescription (new or refill) where this medication is to be used without direct supervision of a healthcare provider. Medication guides are available at http://www.fda.gov/cder/Offices/ODS/medication_guides.htm. Dispense to parents or guardians of children and adolescents receiving this medication.

Pregnancy Risk Factor C

Lactation Excretion in breast milk unknown/not recommended

Medication Safety Issues

Sound-alike/look-alike issues:

Phenelzine may be confused with phenytoin

Nardil® may be confused with Norinyl®

Contraindications Hypersensitivity to phenelzine or any component of the formulation; congestive heart failure; pheochromocytoma; abnormal liver function tests or history of hepatic disease; renal disease or severe renal impairment

Concurrent use of sympathomimetics (including amphetamines, cocaine, dopamine, epinephrine, methylphenidate, norepinephrine, or phenylephrine) and related compounds (methyldopa, levodopa, phenylalanine, tryptophan, or tyrosine), as well as ophthalmic $alpha_2$-agonists (apraclonidine, brimonidine); may result in hypertensive reactions

CNS depressants, cyclobenzaprine, dextromethorphan, ethanol, meperidine, bupropion, or buspirone; may result in delirium, excitation, hyperpyrexia, seizures, and coma.

At least 2 weeks should elapse between the discontinuation of serotoninergic agents (including SNRIs, SSRIs, and tricyclics) and other MAO inhibitors and the initiation of phenelzine. At least 5 weeks should elapse between the discontinuation of fluoxetine and the initiation of phenelzine. In all cases, a sufficient amount of time must be allowed for the clearance of the serotoninergic agent and any active metabolites prior to the initiation of phenelzine.

At least 2 weeks should elapse between the discontinuation of phenelzine and the initiation of the following agents: Serotoninergic agents (including SNRIs, SSRIs, fluoxetine, and tricyclics), bupropion, buspirone, and other antidepressants.

General anesthesia, spinal anesthesia (hypotension may be exaggerated). Use caution with local anesthetics containing sympathomimetic agents. Phenelzine should be discontinued ≥10 days prior to elective surgery.

Foods high in tyramine or dopamine content; foods and/or supplements containing tyrosine, phenylalanine, tryptophan, or caffeine; may result in hypertensive reactions

Warnings/Precautions [U.S. Boxed Warning]: Antidepressants increase the risk of suicidal thinking and behavior in children, adolescents, and young adults (18-24 years of age) with major depressive disorder (MDD) and other psychiatric disorders; consider risk prior to prescribing. Short-term studies did not show an increased risk in patients >24 years of age and showed a decreased risk in patients ≥65 years. Closely monitor for clinical worsening, suicidality, or unusual changes in behavior; the patient's family or caregiver should be instructed to closely observe the patient and communicate condition with healthcare provider. Such observation would generally include at least weekly face-to-face contact with patients or their family members or caregivers during the first 4 weeks of treatment, then every other week visits for the next 4 weeks, then at 12 weeks, and as clinically indicated beyond 12 weeks. Additional contact by telephone may be appropriate between face-to-face visits. Adults treated with antidepressants should be observed similarly for clinical worsening and suicidality, especially during the initial few months of a course of drug therapy, or at times of dose changes, either increases or decreases. A medication guide should be dispensed with each prescription. Phenelzine is not generally considered a first-line agent for the treatment of depression; phenelzine is typically used in patients who have failed to respond to other treatments. **Phenelzine is not FDA approved for the treatment of depression in children ≤16 years of age.**

The possibility of a suicide attempt is inherent in major depression and may persist until remission occurs. Monitor for worsening of depression or suicidality, especially during initiation of therapy (generally first 1-2 months) or with dose increases or decreases. Worsening depression and severe abrupt suicidality that are not part of the presenting symptoms may require discontinuation or modification of drug therapy. Use caution in high-risk patients during initiation of therapy. Prescriptions should be written for the smallest quantity consistent with good patient care. The patient's family or caregiver should be alerted to monitor patients for the emergence of suicidality and associated behaviors such as anxiety, agitation, panic attacks, insomnia, irritability, hostility, impulsivity, akathisia, hypomania, and mania; patients should be instructed to notify their healthcare provider if any of these symptoms or worsening depression occur.

May worsen psychosis in some patients or precipitate a shift to mania or hypomania in patients with bipolar disorder. Monotherapy in patients with bipolar disorder should be avoided. Patients presenting with depressive symptoms should be screened for bipolar disorder. Phenelzine is not FDA approved for the treatment of bipolar depression.

Sensitization to the effects of insulin may occur; monitor blood glucose closely in patients with diabetes. Use with caution in patients who have glaucoma, or hyperthyroidism. Hypertensive crisis may occur with tyramine-, tryptophan-, or dopamine-containing foods. Phentolamine is recommended for the treatment of hypertensive crisis. Do not use with other MAO inhibitors or antidepressants. Avoid products containing sympathomimetic stimulants or dextromethorphan. Concurrent use with antihypertensive agents may lead to exaggeration of hypotensive effects. May cause orthostatic hypotension; use with caution in patients with hypotension or patients who would not tolerate transient hypotensive episodes (cardiovascular or cerebrovascular disease); effects may be additive with other agents which cause orthostasis. Use with caution in patients at risk of seizures, or in patients receiving other drugs which may lower seizure threshold. Discontinue at least 48 hours prior to myelography. May increase the risks associated with electroconvulsive therapy. Consider discontinuing, when possible, prior to elective surgery.

Adverse Reactions Frequency not defined.

Cardiovascular: Edema, orthostatic hypotension

Central nervous system: Anxiety (acute), ataxia, coma, delirium, dizziness, drowsiness, fatigue, fever, headache, hyper-reflexia, mania, seizure, sleep disturbances, twitching

Dermatologic: Pruritus, rash

Endocrine & metabolic: Decreased sexual ability (anorgasmia, ejaculatory disturbances, impotence), hypermetabolic syndrome, hypernatremia

Gastrointestinal: Constipation, weight gain, xerostomia

Genitourinary: Urinary retention

Hematologic: Leukopenia

Hepatic: Hepatitis, jaundice, necrotizing hepatocellular necrosis (rare)

Neuromuscular & skeletal: Lupus-like syndrome, myoclonia, tremor, weakness

Ocular: Blurred vision, glaucoma

Miscellaneous: Diaphoresis, transient cardiac or respiratory depression (following ECT), withdrawal syndrome (nausea, vomiting, malaise)

Respiratory: Edema (glottis)

Drug Interactions

Avoid Concomitant Use

Avoid concomitant use of Phenelzine with any of the following: Alpha-/Beta-Agonists (Indirect-Acting); Alpha1-Agonists; Alpha2-Agonists (Ophthalmic); Amphetamines; Atomoxetine; BuPROPion; BusPIRone; Cyclobenzaprine; Dexmethylphenidate; Dextromethorphan; Linezolid; Maprotiline; Meperidine; Methyldopa; Methylphenidate; Mirtazapine; Propoxyphene; Selective Serotonin Reuptake Inhibitors; Serotonin 5-HT1D Receptor Agonists; Serotonin/Norepinephrine Reuptake Inhibitors; Sibutramine; Tetrabenazine; Tricyclic Antidepressants

Increased Effect/Toxicity

Phenelzine may increase the levels/effects of: Alcohol (Ethyl); Alpha-/Beta-Agonists (Direct-Acting); Alpha-/Beta-Agonists (Indirect-Acting); Alpha1-Agonists; Alpha2-Agonists (Ophthalmic); Amphetamines; Anticholinergics; Atomoxetine; Beta2-Agonists; BuPROPion; CNS Depressants; Dexmethylphenidate; Dextromethorphan; Linezolid; Lithium; Meperidine; Methyldopa; Methylphenidate; Mirtazapine; Rauwolfia Alkaloids; Selective Serotonin Reuptake Inhibitors; Serotonin 5-HT1D Receptor Agonists; Serotonin Modulators; Serotonin/Norepinephrine Reuptake Inhibitors; Succinylcholine; Tricyclic Antidepressants

The levels/effects of Phenelzine may be increased by: Altretamine; Anilidopiperidine Opioids; BusPIRone; COMT Inhibitors; Cyclobenzaprine; Levodopa; Maprotiline; Pramlintide; Propoxyphene; Sibutramine; Tetrabenazine; TraMADol

Decreased Effect

Phenelzine may decrease the levels/effects of: Acetylcholinesterase Inhibitors (Central)

The levels/effects of Phenelzine may be decreased by: Acetylcholinesterase Inhibitors (Central)

Ethanol/Nutrition/Herb Interactions

Ethanol: Avoid ethanol (based on CNS depressant effects and potential tyramine content)

Food: Concurrent ingestion of foods rich in tyramine may cause sudden and severe high blood pressure (hypertensive crisis). Avoid tyramine-containing foods with MAO-Is. Food's freshness is also an important concern; improperly stored or spoiled food can create an environment where tyramine concentrations may increase.

Herb/Nutraceuticals: Avoid supplements containing caffeine, tyrosine, tryptophan or phenylalanine. Ingestion of large quantities may increase the risk of severe side effects (eg, hypertensive reactions, serotonin syndrome).

Stability Protect from light.

Mechanism of Action Thought to act by increasing endogenous concentrations of norepinephrine, dopamine, and serotonin through inhibition of the enzyme (monoamine oxidase) responsible for the breakdown of these neurotransmitters

Pharmacodynamics/Kinetics

Onset of action: Therapeutic: 2-4 weeks; geriatric patients receiving an average of 55 mg/day developed a mean platelet MAO activity inhibition of about 85%.

Duration: May continue to have a therapeutic effect and interactions 2 weeks after discontinuing therapy

Absorption: Well absorbed

Metabolism: Oxidized via monoamine oxidase (primary pathway) and acetylation (minor pathway)

Half-life elimination: 11 hours

Excretion: Urine (primarily as metabolites and unchanged drug)

Dosage Oral:

Children: Selective mutism (unlabeled use): 30-60 mg/day

Adults: Depression: 15 mg 3 times/day; may increase to 60-90 mg/day during early phase of treatment, then reduce dose for maintenance therapy slowly after maximum benefit is obtained; takes 2-4 weeks for a significant response to occur

Elderly: Depression: Initial: 7.5 mg/day; increase by 7.5-15 mg/day every 3-4 days as tolerated; usual therapeutic dose: 15-60 mg/day in 3-4 divided doses

Monitoring Parameters Blood pressure, heart rate; diet, weight; mood (if depressive symptoms), suicidal ideation (especially during the initial months of therapy or when doses are increased or decreased)

Additional Information Pyridoxine deficiency has occurred; symptoms include numbness and edema of hands; may respond to supplementation.

Dosage Forms Excipient information presented when available (limited, particularly for generics); consult specific product labeling.

Tablet: 15 mg

◆ **Phenelzine Sulfate** *see* Phenelzine *on page* 1177

◆ **Phenergan®** *see* Promethazine *on page* 1249

◆ **Pheniramine and Naphazoline** *see* Naphazoline and Pheniramine *on page* 1040

PHENobarbital (fee noe BAR bi tal)

U.S. Brand Names Luminal® Sodium

Canadian Brand Names PMS-Phenobarbital

Index Terms Phenobarbital Sodium; Phenobarbitone; Phenylethylmalonylurea

Pharmacologic Category Anticonvulsant, Barbiturate; Barbiturate

Additional Appendix Information

Status Epilepticus *on page* 1831

Use Management of generalized tonic-clonic (grand mal) and partial seizures; sedative

Unlabeled/Investigational Use Febrile seizures in children; may also be used for prevention and treatment of neonatal hyperbilirubinemia and lowering of bilirubin in chronic cholestasis; neonatal seizures; management of sedative/hypnotic withdrawal

Restrictions C-IV

Pregnancy Risk Factor D

Pregnancy Considerations Crosses the placenta. Cardiac defect reported; hemorrhagic disease of newborn due to fetal vitamin K depletion may occur; may induce maternal folic acid deficiency; withdrawal symptoms observed in infant following delivery. Epilepsy itself, number of medications, genetic factors, or a combination of these probably influence the teratogenicity of anticonvulsant therapy. Benefit:risk ratio usually favors continued use during pregnancy and breast-feeding.

Lactation Enters breast milk/not recommended (AAP recommends use "with caution")

Medication Safety Issues

Sound-alike/look-alike issues:

PHENobarbital may be confused with PENTobarbital

Luminal® may be confused with Tuinal®

Contraindications Hypersensitivity to barbiturates or any component of the formulation; marked hepatic impairment; dyspnea or airway obstruction; porphyria; intra-arterial and SubQ administration

Warnings/Precautions Potential for drug dependency exists, abrupt cessation may precipitate withdrawal, including status epilepticus in epileptic patients. Do not administer to patients in acute pain. Use caution in elderly, debilitated, renally or hepatic dysfunction, and pediatric patients. May cause paradoxical responses, including agitation and hyperactivity, particularly in acute pain and pediatric patients. Use with caution in patients with depression or suicidal tendencies, or in patients with a history of drug abuse. Tolerance, psychological and physical dependence may occur with prolonged use. May cause CNS depression, which may impair physical or mental abilities. Effects with other sedative drugs or ethanol may be potentiated. May cause respiratory depression or hypotension, particularly when administered intravenously. Use with caution in hemodynamically unstable patients (hypovolemic shock, CHF) or patients with respiratory disease. Due to its long half-life and risk of dependence, phenobarbital is not recommended as a sedative in the elderly. Use has been associated with cognitive deficits in children. Use with caution in patients with hypoadrenalism.

Adverse Reactions Frequency not defined.

Cardiovascular: Bradycardia, hypotension, syncope

Central nervous system: Drowsiness, lethargy, CNS excitation or depression, impaired judgment, "hangover" effect, confusion, somnolence, agitation, hyperkinesia, ataxia, nervousness, headache, insomnia, nightmares, hallucinations, anxiety, dizziness

Dermatologic: Rash, exfoliative dermatitis, Stevens-Johnson syndrome

Gastrointestinal: Nausea, vomiting, constipation

Hematologic: Agranulocytosis, thrombocytopenia, megaloblastic anemia

Local: Pain at injection site, thrombophlebitis with I.V. use

Renal: Oliguria

Respiratory: Laryngospasm, respiratory depression, apnea (especially with rapid I.V. use), hypoventilation

Miscellaneous: Gangrene with inadvertent intra-arterial injection

Drug Interactions

Metabolism/Transport Effects Substrate of CYP2C9 (minor), 2C19 (major), 2E1 (minor); **Induces** CYP1A2 (strong), 2A6 (strong), 2B6 (strong), 2C8 (strong), 2C9 (strong), 3A4 (strong)

Avoid Concomitant Use

Avoid concomitant use of PHENobarbital with any of the following: Darunavir; Etravirine; Nilotinib; Ranolazine; Voriconazole

Increased Effect/Toxicity

PHENobarbital may increase the levels/effects of: Alcohol (Ethyl); CNS Depressants; Meperidine

The levels/effects of PHENobarbital may be increased by: Carbonic Anhydrase Inhibitors; Chloramphenicol; CYP2C19 Inhibitors (Moderate); CYP2C19 Inhibitors (Strong); Felbamate; Primidone; Rufinamide; Valproic Acid

Decreased Effect

PHENobarbital may decrease the levels/effects of: Acetaminophen; Aminocamptothecin; Bendamustine;

Beta-Blockers; Calcium Channel Blockers; Chloramphenicol; Contraceptive (Progestins); Corticosteroids (Systemic); CycloSPORINE; CYP1A2 Substrates; CYP2A6 Substrates; CYP2B6 Substrates; CYP2C8 Substrates (High risk); CYP2C9 Substrates (High risk); CYP3A4 Substrates; Darunavir; Disopyramide; Doxycycline; Etoposide; Etoposide Phosphate; Etravirine; Griseofulvin; Lacosamide; LamoTRIgine; Maraviroc; Methadone; Nilotinib; Oral Contraceptive (Estrogens); OXcarbazepine; Propafenone; QuiNIDine; Ranolazine; Rufinamide; Sorafenib; Teniposide; Theophylline Derivatives; Tipranavir; Tricyclic Antidepressants; Valproic Acid; Vitamin K Antagonists; Voriconazole

The levels/effects of PHENobarbital may be decreased by: Amphetamines; CYP2C19 Inducers (Strong); Folic Acid; Ketorolac; Leucovorin-Levoleucovorin; Mefloquine; Methylfolate; Pyridoxine; Rifamycin Derivatives; Tipranavir

Ethanol/Nutrition/Herb Interactions

Ethanol: Avoid ethanol (may increase CNS depression).

Food: May cause decrease in vitamin D and calcium.

Herb/Nutraceutical: Avoid evening primrose (seizure threshold decreased). Avoid valerian, St John's wort, kava kava, gotu kola (may increase CNS depression).

Stability Protect elixir from light. Not stable in aqueous solutions; use only clear solutions. Do not add to acidic solutions; precipitation may occur.

Mechanism of Action Long-acting barbiturate with sedative, hypnotic, and anticonvulsant properties. Barbiturates depress the sensory cortex, decrease motor activity, alter cerebellar function, and produce drowsiness, sedation, and hypnosis. In high doses, barbiturates exhibit anticonvulsant activity; barbiturates produce dose-dependent respiratory depression.

Pharmacodynamics/Kinetics

Onset of action: Oral: Hypnosis: 20-60 minutes; I.V.: ~5 minutes

Peak effect: I.V.: ~30 minutes

Duration: Oral: 6-10 hours; I.V.: 4-10 hours

Absorption: Oral: 70% to 90%

Protein binding: 20% to 45%; decreased in neonates

Metabolism: Hepatic via hydroxylation and glucuronide conjugation

Half-life elimination: Neonates: 45-500 hours; Infants: 20-133 hours; Children: 37-73 hours; Adults: 53-140 hours

Time to peak, serum: Oral: 1-6 hours

Excretion: Urine (20% to 50% as unchanged drug)

Dosage

Children:

Sedation: Oral: 2 mg/kg 3 times/day

Hypnotic: I.M., I.V.: 3-5 mg/kg at bedtime

Preoperative sedation: Oral, I.M., I.V.: 1-3 mg/kg 1-1.5 hours before procedure

Adults:

Sedation: Oral, I.M.: 30-120 mg/day in 2-3 divided doses

Hypnotic: Oral, I.M., I.V.: 100-320 mg at bedtime

Preoperative sedation: I.M.: 100-200 mg 1-1.5 hours before procedure

Anticonvulsant: Status epilepticus: **Loading dose:** I.V.:

Infants and Children: 10-20 mg/kg in a single or divided dose; in select patients may administer additional 5 mg/kg/dose every 15-30 minutes until seizure is controlled or a total dose of 40 mg/kg is reached

Adults: 300-800 mg initially followed by 120-240 mg/dose at 20-minute intervals until seizures are controlled or a total dose of 1-2 g

Anticonvulsant maintenance dose: Oral, I.V.:

Infants: 5-8 mg/kg/day in 1-2 divided doses

Children:

1-5 years: 6-8 mg/kg/day in 1-2 divided doses

5-12 years: 4-6 mg/kg/day in 1-2 divided doses

Children >12 years and Adults: 1-3 mg/kg/day in divided doses or 50-100 mg 2-3 times/day

Sedative/hypnotic withdrawal (unlabeled use): Initial daily requirement is determined by substituting phenobarbital 30 mg for every 100 mg pentobarbital used during tolerance testing; then daily requirement is decreased by 10% of initial dose

Dosing interval in renal impairment: Cl_{cr} <10 mL/minute: Administer every 12-16 hours

Hemodialysis: Moderately dialyzable (20% to 50%)

Dosing adjustment/comments in hepatic disease: Increased side effects may occur in severe liver disease; monitor plasma levels and adjust dose accordingly

Dietary Considerations Vitamin D: Loss in vitamin D due to malabsorption; increase intake of foods rich in vitamin D. Supplementation of vitamin D and/or calcium may be necessary. Sodium content of injection (65 mg, 1 mL): 6 mg (0.3 mEq).

Administration Avoid rapid I.V. administration >50 mg/minute; avoid intra-arterial and SubQ injection; parenteral solutions are highly alkaline; avoid extravasation

Monitoring Parameters Phenobarbital serum concentrations, mental status, CBC, LFTs, seizure activity

Reference Range

Therapeutic:

Infants and children: 15-30 mcg/mL (SI: 65-129 µmol/L)

Adults: 20-40 mcg/mL (SI: 86-172 µmol/L)

Toxic: >40 mcg/mL (SI: >172 µmol/L)

Toxic concentration: Slowness, ataxia, nystagmus: 35-80 mcg/mL (SI: 150-344 µmol/L)

Coma with reflexes: 65-117 mcg/mL (SI: 279-502 µmol/L)

Coma without reflexes: >100 mcg/mL (SI: >430 µmol/L)

Test Interactions Assay interference of LDH

Additional Information Injectable solutions contain propylene glycol.

Dosage Forms Excipient information presented when available (limited, particularly for generics); consult specific product labeling.

Elixir: 20 mg/5 mL (5 mL, 7.5 mL, 15 mL, 480 mL) [contains alcohol]

Injection, solution, as sodium: 65 mg/mL (1 mL); 130 mg/mL (1 mL) [contains alcohol and propylene glycol]

Luminal® Sodium: 60 mg/mL (1 mL); 130 mg/mL (1 mL) [contains alcohol 10% and propylene glycol]

Tablet: 15 mg, 30 mg, 60 mg, 100 mg

Extemporaneous Preparations An alcohol-free phenobarbital 10 mg/mL suspension can be prepared as follows: Levigate ten phenobarbital 60 mg tablets in a glass mortar into a fine powder. Mix 30 mL of Ora-Plus® and 30 mL of either Ora-Sweet® or Ora-Sweet® SF; stir vigorously. Add 15 mL of the Ora-Plus®/Ora-Sweet® (or Ora-Sweet® SF) mixture to the powder; triturate well. Transfer to a 2 ounce amber plastic bottle; qs to a final volume of 60 mL, making sure to rinse the mortar with the syrup mixture several times to ensure all drug is removed. Stable for up to 115 days at room temperature. Shake well prior to use.

May mix dose with chocolate syrup (1:1 volume) immediately before administration to mask the bitter aftertaste.

Cober M and Johnson CE, "Stability of an Extemporaneously Prepared Alcohol-Free Phenobarbital Suspension," *Am J Health Syst Pharm*, 2007, 64(6):644-6.

◆ **Phenobarbital, Belladonna, and Ergotamine Tartrate** *see* Belladonna, Phenobarbital, and Ergotamine *on page 178*

◆ **Phenobarbital, Hyoscyamine, Atropine, and Scopolamine** *see* Hyoscyamine, Atropine, Scopolamine, and Phenobarbital *on page 756*

◆ **Phenobarbital Sodium** *see* PHENobarbital *on page 1179*

◆ **Phenobarbitone** *see* PHENobarbital *on page 1179*

◆ **Phenoptin** *see* Saproterin *on page 1353*

Phenoxybenzamine (fen oks ee BEN za meen)

U.S. Brand Names Dibenzyline®

Canadian Brand Names Dibenzyline®

Index Terms Phenoxybenzamine Hydrochloride

Pharmacologic Category Alpha$_1$ Blocker; Antidote

Use Symptomatic management of pheochromocytoma

Unlabeled/Investigational Use Micturition problems associated with neurogenic bladder, functional outlet obstruction, and partial prostate obstruction; treatment of hypertensive crisis caused by sympathomimetic amines

Pregnancy Risk Factor C

Medication Safety Issues

Sound-alike/look-alike issues:

Phenoxybenzamine may be confused with phenazopyridine

Dosage Oral:

Children (unlabeled use): Initial: 0.25-1 mg/kg/day (maximum: 10 mg); increase slowly to blood pressure control

Adults:

Pheochromocytoma, hypertension: Initial: 10 mg twice daily; increase by 10 mg every other day until optimal blood pressure response is achieved; usual range: 20-40 mg 2-3 times/day. Doses up to 240 mg/day have been reported (Kinney, 2000).

Micturition disorders (unlabeled use): 10-20 mg 1-2 times/day

Additional Information Complete prescribing information for this medication should be consulted for additional detail.

Dosage Forms Excipient information presented when available (limited, particularly for generics); consult specific product labeling.

Capsule, as hydrochloride:

Dibenzyline®: 10 mg [contains benzyl alcohol]

◆ **Phenoxybenzamine Hydrochloride** *see* Phenoxybenzamine *on page 1181*

◆ **Phenoxymethyl Penicillin** *see* Penicillin V Potassium *on page 1167*

Phentermine (FEN ter meen)

U.S. Brand Names Adipex-P®; Ionamin®

Canadian Brand Names Ionamin®

Index Terms Phentermine Hydrochloride

Pharmacologic Category Anorexiant; Sympathomimetic

Use Short-term (few weeks) adjunct in exogenous obesity

Restrictions C-IV

Pharmacotherapy for weight loss is recommended only for obese patients with a body mass index ≥30 kg/m^2, or ≥27 kg/m^2 in the presence of other risk factors such as hypertension, diabetes, and/or dyslipidemia or a high waist circumference; therapy should be used in conjunction with a comprehensive weight management program. Rule out organic causes of obesity (eg, untreated hypothyroidism) prior to use.

Note: Phentermine is not approved for long-term use. The limited usefulness of medications in this class should be weighed against possible risks associated with their use. Consult weight loss guidelines for current pharmacotherapy recommendations.

Pregnancy Risk Factor C

Pregnancy Considerations Reproduction studies have not been conducted.

Medication Safety Issues

Sound-alike/look-alike issues:

Phentermine may be confused with phentolamine, phenytoin

Ionamin® may be confused with Imodium®

Contraindications Hypersensitivity or idiosyncrasy to phentermine or other sympathomimetic amines or any component of the formulation; advanced arteriosclerosis, cardiovascular disease, moderate-to-severe hypertension; pulmonary hypertension; hyperthyroidism, glaucoma, agitated states, patients with a history of drug abuse; use during or within 14 days following MAO inhibitor therapy

Warnings/Precautions Primary pulmonary hypertension (PPH), a rare and frequently fatal pulmonary disease, has been reported to occur in patients receiving a combination of phentermine and fenfluramine or dexfenfluramine. The possibility of an association between PPH and the use of phentermine alone cannot be ruled out. The use of phenteramine has been associated with the development of valvular heart disease. Avoid stimulants in patients with known serious structural cardiac abnormalities, cardiomyopathy, serious heart rhythm abnormalities, or other serious cardiac problems that could increase the risk of sudden death that these conditions alone carry. Caution should be used in patients with hypertension and other cardiovascular conditions that might be exacerbated by increases in blood pressure or heart rate.

Use caution with diabetes; antidiabetic agent requirements may be altered with anorexigens and concomitant dietary restrictions. Stimulants may unmask tics in individuals with coexisting Tourette's syndrome. Use caution with seizure disorders. Phentermine is pharmacologically related to the amphetamines, which have a high abuse potential; prolonged use may lead to dependency. Prescriptions should be written for the smallest quantity consistent with good patient care to minimize possibility of overdose. Amphetamines may impair the ability to engage in potentially hazardous activities.

Not recommended for use in patients who used other anorectic agents within the past year. Discontinue if satisfactory weight loss has not occurred within the first 4 weeks of treatment, or if tolerance develops. Safety and efficacy have not been established for use with other weight loss medications including over-the-counter or herbal products. Safety and efficacy have not been established in children ≤16 years of age.

Adverse Reactions Frequency not defined.

Cardiovascular: Hypertension, palpitation, primary pulmonary hypertension and/or regurgitant cardiac valvular disease, tachycardia

Central nervous system: Dizziness, dysphoria, euphoria, headache, insomnia, overstimulation, psychosis, restlessness

Dermatologic: Urticaria

Endocrine & metabolic: Changes in libido

Gastrointestinal: Constipation, diarrhea, unpleasant taste, xerostomia

Genitourinary: Impotence

Neuromuscular & skeletal: Tremor

Drug Interactions

Avoid Concomitant Use

Avoid concomitant use of Phentermine with any of the following: Iobenguane I 123; MAO Inhibitors

Increased Effect/Toxicity

Phentermine may increase the levels/effects of: Analgesics (Opioid); Sympathomimetics

The levels/effects of Phentermine may be increased by: Alkalinizing Agents; Antacids; Cannabinoids; Carbonic Anhydrase Inhibitors; MAO Inhibitors; Tricyclic Antidepressants

Decreased Effect

Phentermine may decrease the levels/effects of: Antihistamines; Ethosuximide; Iobenguane I 123; PHENObarbital; Phenytoin

The levels/effects of Phentermine may be decreased by: Ammonium Chloride; Antipsychotics; Gastrointestinal Acidifying Agents; Lithium; Methenamine

Mechanism of Action Phentermine is a sympathomimetic amine with pharmacologic properties similar to the amphetamines. The mechanism of action in reducing appetite appears to be secondary to CNS effects, including stimulation of the hypothalamus to release norepinephrine.

Pharmacodynamics/Kinetics

Duration: Resin produces more prolonged clinical effects

Absorption: Well absorbed; resin absorbed slower

Excretion: Primarily urine

Dosage Oral: Children >16 years and Adults: Obesity:

Phentermine hydrochloride: 18.75-37.5 mg/ day

Phentermine resin: 15-30 mg/day

Dietary Considerations Most effective when combined with a low calorie diet and behavior modification counseling.

Administration

Phentermine hydrochloride: Administer before breakfast or 1-2 hours after breakfast. Tablets may be divided in half and dose may be given in 2 divided doses. Avoid late evening administration.

Phentermine resin: Administer before breakfast or 10-14 hours before retiring. Swallow capsules whole.

Monitoring Parameters Weight, waist circumference; blood pressure

Reference Range

Adult classification of weight by BMI (kg/m^2):

- Underweight: <18.5
- Normal: 18.5-24.9
- Overweight: 25-29.9
- Obese, class I: 30-34.9
- Obese, class II: 35-39.9
- Extreme obesity (class III): ≥40

Waist circumference: In adults with a BMI of 25-34.9 kg/m^2, high-risk waist circumference is defined as:

- Men >102 cm (>40 in)
- Women >88 cm (>35 in)

Dosage Forms Excipient information presented when available (limited, particularly for generics); consult specific product labeling.

Capsule, as hydrochloride: 15 mg, 30 mg, 37.5 mg

Adipex-P®: 37.5 mg

Capsule, resin complex:

Ionamin®: 15 mg

Tablet, as hydrochloride: 37.5 mg

Adipex-P®: 37.5 mg

◆ **Phentermine Hydrochloride** *see* Phentermine *on page 1181*

Phentolamine (fen TOLE a meen)

U.S. Brand Names OraVerse™

Canadian Brand Names Regitine®; Rogitine®

Index Terms Phentolamine Mesylate; Regitine [DSC]

Pharmacologic Category Alpha$_1$ Blocker

Additional Appendix Information

Hypertension *on page 1820*

Use Diagnosis of pheochromocytoma and treatment of hypertension associated with pheochromocytoma or other forms of hypertension caused by excess sympathomimetic amines; as treatment of dermal necrosis after extravasation of drugs with alpha-adrenergic effects (norepinephrine, dopamine, epinephrine)

OraVerse™: Reversal of soft tissue anesthesia and the associated functional deficits resulting from a local dental anesthetic containing a vasoconstrictor

Unlabeled/Investigational Use Treatment of pralidoxime-induced hypertension

Pregnancy Risk Factor C

Lactation Excretion in breast milk unknown

Medication Safety Issues

Sound-alike/look-alike issues:

Phentolamine may be confused with phentermine, Ventolin®

Contraindications Hypersensitivity to phentolamine or any component of the formulation; renal impairment; coronary or cerebral arteriosclerosis; concurrent use with phosphodiesterase-5 (PDE-5) inhibitors including sildenafil (>25 mg), tadalafil, or vardenafil

OraVerse™: There are no contraindications listed in the manufacturer's labeling.

Warnings/Precautions Myocardial infarction, cerebrovascular spasm, and cerebrovascular occlusion have occurred following administration; use with caution in patients with gastritis or peptic ulcer, tachycardia, or a history of cardiac arrhythmias. Discontinue if symptoms of angina occur or worsen. OraVerse™: Efficacy has not been established in children <6 years of age or <15 kg (33 pounds).

Adverse Reactions Frequency not always defined.

Cardiovascular: Arrhythmia, flushing, hypertension (OraVerse™), hypotension, orthostatic hypotension, tachycardia (OraVerse™ ≤6%), bradycardia (OraVerse™ ≤4%)

Central nervous system: Dizziness, headache (OraVerse™ ≤6%)

Dermatologic: Pruritus (OraVerse™)

Gastrointestinal: Nausea, vomiting, diarrhea

Local: Injection site pain (OraVerse™ 4% to 6%)

Neuromuscular & skeletal: Paresthesia (OraVerse™), weakness

Respiratory: Nasal congestion

Postmarketing and/or case reports: Pulmonary hypertension

Drug Interactions

Avoid Concomitant Use

Avoid concomitant use of Phentolamine with any of the following: Alfuzosin; Silodosin; Tamsulosin

Increased Effect/Toxicity

Phentolamine may increase the levels/effects of: Alfuzosin; Amifostine; Calcium Channel Blockers; RiTUXimab; Silodosin; Tamsulosin

The levels/effects of Phentolamine may be increased by: Alfuzosin; Beta-Blockers; Diazoxide; Herbs (Hypotensive Properties); Phosphodiesterase 5 Inhibitors; Prostacyclin Analogues; Silodosin; Tamsulosin

Decreased Effect

The levels/effects of Phentolamine may be decreased by: Herbs (Hypertensive Properties); Methylphenidate; Yohimbine

Stability Reconstituted solution is stable for 48 hours at room temperature and 1 week when refrigerated.

OraVerse™: Store at 20°C to 25°C (68°F to 77°F); excursions permitted between 15°C to 30°C (59°F to 86°F).

Mechanism of Action Competitively blocks alpha-adrenergic receptors to produce brief antagonism of circulating epinephrine and norepinephrine to reduce hypertension caused by alpha effects of these catecholamines; also has a positive inotropic and chronotropic effect on the heart

OraVerse™: Causes vasodilation and increased blood flow in injection area via alpha-adrenergic blockade to accelerate reversal of soft tissue anesthetic

Pharmacodynamics/Kinetics
Onset of action: I.M.: 15-20 minutes; I.V.: Immediate
Peak effect: OraVerse™: 10-20 minutes
Duration: I.M.: 30-45 minutes; I.V.: 15-30 minutes
Metabolism: Hepatic
Half-life elimination: 19 minutes
Excretion: Urine (10% as unchanged drug)

Dosage
Treatment of alpha-adrenergic drug extravasation: SubQ:
Children: 0.1-0.2 mg/kg diluted in 10 mL 0.9% sodium chloride infiltrated into area of extravasation within 12 hours
Adults: Infiltrate area with small amount of solution made by diluting 5-10 mg in 10 mL 0.9% sodium chloride within 12 hours of extravasation; do not exceed 0.1-0.2 mg/kg or 5 mg total
If dose is effective, normal skin color should return to the blanched area within 1 hour
Diagnosis of pheochromocytoma: I.M., I.V.:
Children: 0.05-0.1 mg/kg/dose, maximum single dose: 5 mg
Adults: 5 mg
Surgery for pheochromocytoma: Hypertension: I.M., I.V.:
Children: 0.05-0.1 mg/kg/dose given 1-2 hours before procedure; repeat as needed every 2-4 hours until hypertension is controlled; maximum single dose: 5 mg
Adults: 5 mg given 1-2 hours before procedure and repeated as needed every 2-4 hours
Hypertensive crisis: Adults: 5-20 mg
Treatment of pralidoxime-induced hypertension (unlabeled use): I.V.:
Children: 1 mg
Adults and Elderly: 5 mg
Reversal of soft tissue (lip, tongue) anesthesia (OraVerse™): Infiltration or block technique:submucosal oral injection:
Children: 15-30 kg: 0.2 mg maximum dose
Children >30 kg and <12 years: 0.4 mg maximum dose
Adults: **Note:** Dose is based upon the number of cartridges of local anesthetic administered. Infiltration or block injection:
0.2 mg if one-half cartridge of anesthesia was administered
0.4 mg if 1 cartridge of anesthesia was administered
0.8 mg if 2 cartridges of anesthesia were administered

Administration
Vasoconstrictor (alpha-adrenergic agonist) extravasation: Infiltrate the area of extravasation with multiple small injections using only 27- or 30-gauge needles and changing the needle between each skin entry. Be careful not to cause so much swelling of the extremity or digit that a compartment syndrome occurs. If infiltration is severe, may also need to consult vascular surgeon.
Pheochromocytoma: Inject each 5 mg over 1 minute.

Monitoring Parameters Blood pressure, heart rate; area of infiltration; monitor patient for orthostasis; assist with ambulation

Test Interactions Increased LFTs rarely

Dosage Forms Excipient information presented when available (limited, particularly for generics); consult specific product labeling.
Injection, powder for reconstitution, as mesylate: 5 mg
Injection, solution, as mesylate [preservative free]:
OraVerse™: 0.4 mg/1.7 mL (1.7 mL) [contains edetate disodium; dental cartridge]

◆ **Phentolamine Mesylate** *see* Phentolamine *on page 1182*

◆ **Phenylalanine Mustard** *see* Melphalan *on page 936*

◆ **Phenylazo Diamino Pyridine Hydrochloride** *see* Phenazopyridine *on page 1177*

Phenylephrine (fen il EF rin)

U.S. Brand Names 4 Way® Fast Acting [OTC]; 4 Way® Menthol [OTC]; 4 Way® No Drip [OTC]; AK-Dilate®; Altafrin; Anu-Med [OTC]; Dimetapp® Toddler's [OTC]; Formulation R™ [OTC]; Little Noses® Decongestant [OTC]; LuSonal™; Medi-Phenyl [OTC]; Medicone® Suppositories [OTC]; Mydfrin®; Nasop12™; Neo-Synephrine® Extra Strength [OTC]; Neo-Synephrine® Injection; Neo-Synephrine® Mild [OTC]; Neo-Synephrine® Regular Strength [OTC]; Neofrin™; NāSop™ [DSC]; OcuNefrin™ [OTC]; Preparation H® [OTC]; Rectacaine [OTC]; Relief® [OTC] [DSC]; Rhinall [OTC]; Sudafed PE™ [OTC]; Triaminic® Infant Thin Strips® Decongestant [OTC] [DSC]; Triaminic® Thin Strips® Cold [OTC]; Tronolane® Suppository [OTC]; Tur-bi-kal® [OTC]; Vicks® Sinex® Nasal Spray [OTC]; Vicks® Sinex® UltraFine Mist [OTC]

Canadian Brand Names Dionephrine®; Mydfrin®; Neo-Synephrine®

Index Terms Phenylephrine Hydrochloride; Phenylephrine Tannate

Pharmacologic Category Alpha/Beta Agonist; Ophthalmic Agent, Antiglaucoma; Ophthalmic Agent, Mydriatic

Use Treatment of hypotension, vascular failure in shock; as a vasoconstrictor in regional analgesia; as a mydriatic in ophthalmic procedures and treatment of wide-angle glaucoma; supraventricular tachycardia

For OTC use as symptomatic relief of nasal and nasopharyngeal mucosal congestion, treatment of hemorrhoids, relief of redness of the eye due to irritation

Pregnancy Risk Factor C

Pregnancy Considerations Reproduction studies have not been conducted.

Lactation Excretion in breast milk unknown/not recommended

Medication Safety Issues
Sound-alike/look-alike issues:
Mydfrin® may be confused with Midrin®

High alert medication: The Institute for Safe Medication Practices (ISMP) includes this medication among its list of drugs which have a heightened risk of causing significant patient harm when used in error.

Contraindications Hypersensitivity to phenylephrine or any component of the formulation; hypertension; ventricular tachycardia
Oral: Use with or within 14 days of MAO inhibitor therapy
Nasop12™: Additional contraindications: Use in newborns; breast-feeding
Ophthalmic: Narrow-angle glaucoma

Warnings/Precautions Some products contain sulfites which may cause allergic reactions in susceptible individuals. Use with extreme caution in patients taking MAO inhibitors.

Intravenous: Use with caution in the elderly, patients with hyperthyroidism, bradycardia, partial heart block, myocardial disease, or severe CAD. Assure adequate circulatory volume to minimize need for vasoconstrictors. Avoid hypertension; monitor blood pressure closely and adjust infusion rate. Avoid extravasation; infuse into a large vein if possible. Avoid infusion into leg veins. Watch I.V. site closely. If extravasation occurs, infiltrate the area subcutaneously with diluted phentolamine (5-10 mg in 10-15 mL of saline) with a fine hypodermic needle. Phentolamine should be administered as soon as possible after extravasation is noted. **[U.S. Boxed Warning]: Should be administered by adequately trained individuals familiar with its use.**

Nasal, oral, rectal: Use caution with asthma, bowel obstruction/narrowing, hyperthyroidism, diabetes mellitus, cardiovascular disease, ischemic heart disease, increased intraocular pressure, prostatic hyperplasia or in the elderly. Rebound congestion may occur when nasal products are discontinued after chronic use. When used for self-medication (OTC), notify healthcare provider if symptoms do not improve within 7 days (oral, rectal) or 3 days (nasal), are accompanied by fever (oral), or if bleeding occurs (rectal). Not for OTC use in children <2 years of age.

Ophthalmic: When used for self-medication (OTC), notify healthcare provider in case of vision changes, continued redness, or if symptoms worsen or do not improve within 3 days.

Adverse Reactions Frequency not defined.

Cardiovascular: Arrhythmia (rare), decreased cardiac output, hypertension, pallor, precordial pain or discomfort, reflex bradycardia, severe peripheral and visceral vasoconstriction

Central nervous system: Anxiety, dizziness, excitability, giddiness, headache, insomnia, nervousness, restlessness

Endocrine & metabolic: Metabolic acidosis

Gastrointestinal: Gastric irritation, nausea

Local: I.V.: Extravasation which may lead to necrosis and sloughing of surrounding tissue, blanching of skin

Neuromuscular & skeletal: Paresthesia, pilomotor response, tremor, weakness

Renal: Decreased renal perfusion, reduced urine output

Respiratory: Respiratory distress

Miscellaneous: Hypersensitivity reactions (including rash, urticaria, leukopenia, agranulocytosis, thrombocytopenia)

Drug Interactions

Avoid Concomitant Use

Avoid concomitant use of Phenylephrine with any of the following: Iobenguane I 123; MAO Inhibitors

Increased Effect/Toxicity

Phenylephrine may increase the levels/effects of: Sympathomimetics

The levels/effects of Phenylephrine may be increased by: Cannabinoids; MAO Inhibitors; Tricyclic Antidepressants

Decreased Effect

Phenylephrine may decrease the levels/effects of: Iobenguane I 123

Ethanol/Nutrition/Herb Interactions Herb/Nutraceutical: Avoid ephedra, yohimbe (may cause CNS stimulation).

Stability

Solution for injection: Store vials at controlled room temperature of 15°C to 30°C (59°F to 86°F). Protect from light. Do not use solution if brown or contains a precipitate.

I.V. infusion: May dilute 10 mg in 500 mL NS or D_5W.

I.V. injection: Dilute with SWFI to a concentration of 1 mg/mL.

Ophthalmic solution:

0.12%: Store at controlled room temperature. Protect from light and excessive heat.

2.5% and 10%: Refer to product labeling. Some products are labeled to store at room temperature, others should be stored under refrigeration at 2°C to 8°C (36°F to 46°F). Do not use solution if brown or contains a precipitate.

Tablet, chewable: Store at controlled room temperature of 15°C to 30°C (59°F to 86°F). Protect from light.

Mechanism of Action Potent, direct-acting alpha-adrenergic stimulator with weak beta-adrenergic activity; causes vasoconstriction of the arterioles of the nasal mucosa and conjunctiva; activates the dilator muscle of the pupil to cause contraction; produces vasoconstriction of arterioles in the body; produces systemic arterial vasoconstriction

Pharmacodynamics/Kinetics

Onset of action: I.M., SubQ: 10-15 minutes; I.V.: Immediate; Ophthalmic: 10-15 minutes

Duration: I.M.: 0.5-2 hours; I.V.: 15-30 minutes; SubQ: 1 hour; Ophthalmic: Maximal mydriasis: 1 hour, recover time: 3-6 hours

Metabolism: Hepatic, via intestinal monoamine oxidase to phenolic conjugates

Excretion: Urine (90%)

Dosage

Hemorrhoids: Children ≥12 years and Adults: Rectal:

Cream/ointment: Apply to clean dry area, up to 4 times/day; may be used externally or inserted rectally using applicator.

Suppository: Insert 1 suppository rectally, up to 4 times/day

Hypotension/shock:

Children:

I.V. bolus: 5-20 mcg/kg/dose every 10-15 minutes as needed

I.V. infusion: 0.1-0.5 mcg/kg/minute

Adults:

I.V. bolus: 0.1-0.5 mg/dose every 10-15 minutes as needed (initial dose should not exceed 0.5 mg)

I.V. infusion: Initial dose: 100-180 mcg/minute; when blood pressure is stabilized, maintenance rate: 40-60 mcg/minute; rates up to 360 mcg/minute have been reported; dosing range: 0.4-9.1 mcg/kg/minute

Nasal decongestant:

Children:

2-6 years:

Intranasal: Instill 1 drop every 2-4 hours of 0.125% solution as needed. (**Note:** Therapy should not exceed 3 continuous days.)

Oral: Tannate salt (NāSop™ suspension): 1.87-3.75 mg every 12 hours

6-12 years:

Intranasal: Instill 1-2 sprays or instill 1-2 drops every 4 hours of 0.25% solution as needed. (**Note:** Therapy should not exceed 3 continuous days.)

Oral:

Hydrochloride salt: 10 mg every 4 hours

Tannate salt:

NāSop™ suspension: 3.75-7.5 mg every 12 hours

Nasop12™ chewable tablet: 1/2 to 1 tablet (5-10 mg) every 12 hours

Children >12 years and Adults:

Intranasal: Instill 1-2 sprays or instill 1-2 drops every 4 hours of 0.25% to 0.5% solution as needed; 1% solution may be used in adult in cases of extreme nasal congestion; do not use nasal solutions more than 3 days

Oral:

Hydrochloride salt: 10-20 mg every 4 hours

Tannate salt:

NāSop™ suspension: 7.5-15 mg every 12 hours

Nasop12™ chewable tablet: 1-2 tablets (10-20 mg) every 12 hours

Ocular procedures:

Infants <1 year: Instill 1 drop of 2.5% 15-30 minutes before procedures

Children and Adults: Instill 1 drop of 2.5% or 10% solution, may repeat in 10-60 minutes as needed

Ophthalmic irritation (OTC formulation for relief of eye redness): Adults: Instill 1-2 drops 0.12% solution into affected eye, up to 4 times/day; do not use for >72 hours

Paroxysmal supraventricular tachycardia: I.V.:

Children: 5-10 mcg/kg/dose over 20-30 seconds

Adults: 0.25-0.5 mg/dose over 20-30 seconds

Dietary Considerations NāSop™ contains phenylalanine 4 mg/tablet. LuSonal™ contains phenylalanine. Sudafed PE™ contains phenylalanine 1 mg/strip.

Administration

I.V.: May cause necrosis or sloughing tissue if extravasation occurs during I.V. administration or SubQ administration.

Extravasation management: Use phentolamine as antidote; mix 5 mg with 9 mL of NS. Inject a small amount of this dilution subcutaneously into extravasated area. Blanching should reverse immediately. Monitor site. If blanching should recur, additional injections of phentolamine may be needed.

Oral: Chewable tablet: Chew or crush well. May mix crushed tablet with food. Do not swallow whole.

Monitoring Parameters Blood pressure, pulse; excitability, irritability, anxiety

Additional Information Phenylephrine allows for close titration of blood pressure and should be used in patients with hypotension or shock due to peripheral vasodilation. Phenylephrine should not constitute sole therapy in patients with hypotension due to aortic dysfunction or hypovolemia. An important benefit of this drug is the short half-life, allowing rapid changes in dosage with prompt appropriate blood pressure responses. When administered intravenously, it should be used in intensive care settings or under very close monitoring.

Dosage Forms Excipient information presented when available (limited, particularly for generics); consult specific product labeling. [DSC] = Discontinued product

Cream, rectal, as hydrochloride:
- Formulation R™: 0.25% (54 g) [contains sodium benzoate]

Filmstrip, orally disintegrating, as hydrochloride:
- Sudafed PE™: 10 mg (5s, 10s) [contains phenylalanine 1 mg/strip; cherry menthol flavor]
- Triaminic® Infant Thin Strips® Decongestant: 1.25 mg [mixed berry flavor] [DSC]
- Triaminic® Thin Strips® Cold: 2.5 mg [raspberry flavor]

Injection, solution, as hydrochloride: 1% [10 mg/mL] (1 mL, 5 mL, 10 mL) [may contain sodium metabisulfite]
- Neo-Synephrine®: 1% (1 mL) [contains sodium metabisulfite]

Liquid, oral, as hydrochloride:
- LuSonal™: 7.5 mg/5 mL (480 mL) [contains phenylalanine; strawberry flavor]

Liquid, oral, as hydrochloride [drops]:
- Dimetapp® Toddler's: 1.25 mg/0.8 mL (15 mL) [alcohol free; contains sodium benzoate; grape flavor]

Ointment, rectal, as hydrochloride:
- Formulation R™, Preparation H®: 0.25% (30 g, 60 g) [contains benzoic acid]
- Rectacaine: 0.25% (30 g)

Solution, intranasal, as hydrochloride [drops]:
- Little Noses® Decongestant: 0.125% (15 mL) [contains benzalkonium chloride]
- Neo-Synephrine® Extra Strength: 1% (15 mL) [contains benzalkonium chloride]
- Neo-Synephrine® Regular Strength: 0.5% (15 mL) [contains benzalkonium chloride]
- Rhinall: 0.25% (30 mL) [contains benzalkonium chloride and sodium bisulfite]
- Tur-bi-kal®: 0.17% (30 mL) [contains benzalkonium chloride]

Solution, intranasal, as hydrochloride [spray]:
- 4 Way® Fast Acting: 1% (15 mL, 30 mL) [contains benzalkonium chloride]
- 4 Way® Menthol: 1% (15 mL) [contains benzalkonium chloride and menthol]
- 4 Way® No Drip: 1% (15 mL) [contains benzalkonium chloride]
- Neo-Synephrine® Extra Strength: 1% (15 mL) [contains benzalkonium chloride]
- Neo-Synephrine® Mild: 0.25% (15 mL) [contains benzalkonium chloride]
- Neo-Synephrine® Regular Strength: 0.5% (15 mL) [contains benzalkonium chloride]
- Rhinall: 0.25% (40 mL) [contains benzalkonium chloride and sodium bisulfite]
- Vicks® Sinex®, Vicks® Sinex® UltraFine Mist: 0.5% (15 mL) [contains benzalkonium chloride]

Solution, ophthalmic, as hydrochloride: 2.5% (2 mL, 3 mL, 5 mL, 15 mL) [may contain sodium bisulfite]
- AK-Dilate®: 2.5% (2 mL, 15 mL); 10% (5 mL) [contains benzyl alcohol]
- Altrafrin: 0.12% (15 mL) [OTC]; 2.5% (15 mL) [RX; contains benzalkonium chloride]; 10% (5 mL) [RX; contains benzalkonium chloride]
- Mydfrin®: 2.5% (3 mL, 5 mL) [contains sodium bisulfite]
- Neofrin™: 2.5% (15 mL); 10% (15 mL)
- OcuNefrin™: 0.12% (15 mL)
- Relief®: 0.12% (15 mL) [contains benzalkonium chloride] [DSC]

Suppository, rectal, as hydrochloride: 0.25% (12s)
- Anu-Med: 0.25% (12s)
- Formulation R™, Preparation H®: 0.25% (12s, 24s, 48s)
- Medicone®, Tronolane®: 0.25% (12s, 24s)
- Rectacaine: 0.25% (12s)

Suspension, oral, as tannate:
- NāSop™: 7.5 mg/5 mL (120 mL) [orange flavor] [DSC]

Tablet, chewable, as tannate:
- Nasop12™: 10 mg [grape flavor]

Tablet, as hydrochloride: 10 mg
- Medi-Phenyl: 5 mg
- Sudafed PE™: 10 mg

Tablet, orally dissolving, as hydrochloride:
- NāSop™: 10 mg [contains phenylalanine 4 mg/tablet; bubble gum flavor] [DSC]

◆ **Phenylephrine CM** *see* Chlorpheniramine, Phenylephrine, and Methscopolamine *on page 313*

◆ **Phenylephrine, Acetaminophen, and Dextromethorphan** *see* Acetaminophen, Dextromethorphan, and Phenylephrine *on page 32*

◆ **Phenylephrine and Chlorpheniramine** *see* Chlorpheniramine and Phenylephrine *on page 309*

◆ **Phenylephrine and Cyclopentolate** *see* Cyclopentolate and Phenylephrine *on page 376*

◆ **Phenylephrine and Diphenhydramine** *see* Diphenhydramine and Phenylephrine *on page 458*

◆ **Phenylephrine and Promethazine** *see* Promethazine and Phenylephrine *on page 1251*

Phenylephrine and Scopolamine

(fen il EF rin & skoe POL a meen)

U.S. Brand Names Murocoll-2®

Index Terms Scopolamine and Phenylephrine

Pharmacologic Category Anticholinergic/Adrenergic Agonist

Use Mydriasis, cycloplegia, and to break posterior synechiae in iritis

Pregnancy Risk Factor C

Medication Safety Issues

Sound-alike/look-alike issues:
- Murocoll-2® may be confused with Murocel®

Dosage Ophthalmic: Instill 1-2 drops into eye(s); repeat in 5 minutes

Additional Information Complete prescribing information for this medication should be consulted for additional detail.

Dosage Forms Excipient information presented when available (limited, particularly for generics); consult specific product labeling.

Solution, ophthalmic: Phenylephrine hydrochloride 10% and scopolamine hydrobromide 0.3% (5 mL) [contains benzalkonium chloride and sodium metabisulfite]

◆ **Phenylephrine, Chlorpheniramine, and Dextromethorphan** *see* Chlorpheniramine, Phenylephrine, and Dextromethorphan *on page 311*

- **Phenylephrine, Chlorpheniramine, and Dihydrocodeine** *see* Dihydrocodeine, Chlorpheniramine, and Phenylephrine *on page 448*
- **Phenylephrine, Chlorpheniramine, and Guaifenesin** *see* Chlorpheniramine, Phenylephrine, and Guaifenesin *on page 312*
- **Phenylephrine, Chlorpheniramine, and Phenyltoloxamine** *see* Chlorpheniramine, Phenylephrine, and Phenyltoloxamine *on page 314*
- **Phenylephrine, Chlorpheniramine, Codeine, and Potassium Iodide** *see* Chlorpheniramine, Phenylephrine, Codeine, and Potassium Iodide *on page 314*
- **Phenylephrine, Dextromethorphan, and Acetaminophen** *see* Acetaminophen, Dextromethorphan, and Phenylephrine *on page 32*
- **Phenylephrine, Ephedrine, Chlorpheniramine, and Carbetapentane** *see* Chlorpheniramine, Ephedrine, Phenylephrine, and Carbetapentane *on page 311*
- **Phenylephrine Hydrochloride** *see* Phenylephrine *on page 1183*
- **Phenylephrine Hydrochloride, Acetaminophen, and Diphenhydramine** *see* Acetaminophen, Diphenhydramine, and Phenylephrine *on page 33*
- **Phenylephrine Hydrochloride and Acetaminophen** *see* Acetaminophen and Phenylephrine *on page 29*
- **Phenylephrine Hydrochloride and Diphenhydramine Hydrochloride** *see* Diphenhydramine and Phenylephrine *on page 458*
- **Phenylephrine Hydrochloride and Guaifenesin** *see* Guaifenesin and Phenylephrine *on page 712*
- **Phenylephrine Hydrochloride, Carbetapentane Citrate, and Guaifenesin** *see* Carbetapentane, Guaifenesin, and Phenylephrine *on page 255*
- **Phenylephrine Hydrochloride, Chlorpheniramine maleate, Dextromethorphan Hydrobromide, and Guaifenesin** *see* Dextromethorphan, Chlorpheniramine, Phenylephrine, and Guaifenesin *on page 434*
- **Phenylephrine, Promethazine, and Codeine** *see* Promethazine, Phenylephrine, and Codeine *on page 1251*

Phenylephrine, Pyrilamine, and Guaifenesin

(fen il EF rin, peer IL a meen, & gwye FEN e sin)

U.S. Brand Names Ryna-12X®

Index Terms Guaifenesin, Pyrilamine Tannate, and Phenylephrine Tannate; Pyrilamine Tannate, Guaifenesin, and Phenylephrine Tannate

Pharmacologic Category Alpha/Beta Agonist; Decongestant; Expectorant; Histamine H_1 Antagonist; Histamine H_1 Antagonist, First Generation

Use Symptomatic relief of cough, nasal congestion, and discharge associated with the common cold, sinusitis, allergic rhinitis, and other respiratory tract conditions

Pregnancy Risk Factor C

Dosage Oral:

Relief of cough, congestion:

Children 2-6 years: 2.5-5 mL of the suspension every 12 hours

Children 6-11 years: 5-10 mL of the suspension **or** 1/2 to 1 tablet every 12 hours

Children ≥12 years and Adults: 1-2 tablets every 12 hours

Additional Information Complete prescribing information for this medication should be consulted for additional detail.

Dosage Forms Excipient information presented when available (limited, particularly for generics); consult specific product labeling.

Suspension:

Ryna-12X®: Phenylephrine tannate 5 mg, pyrilamine tannate 30 mg, and guaifenesin 100 mg per 5 mL (120 mL) [contains benzoic acid; grape flavor]

Tablet [scored]:

Ryna-12X®: Phenylephrine tannate 25 mg, pyrilamine tannate 60 mg, and guaifenesin 200 mg

- **Phenylephrine Tannate** *see* Phenylephrine *on page 1183*
- **Phenylephrine Tannate and Carbetapentane Tannate** *see* Carbetapentane and Phenylephrine *on page 255*
- **Phenylephrine Tannate and Diphenhydramine Tannate** *see* Diphenhydramine and Phenylephrine *on page 458*
- **Phenylephrine Tannate, Chlorpheniramine Tannate, and Methscopolamine Nitrate** *see* Chlorpheniramine, Phenylephrine, and Methscopolamine *on page 313*
- **Phenylethylmalonylurea** *see* PHENobarbital *on page 1179*
- **Phenylgesic [OTC]** *see* Acetaminophen and Phenyltoloxamine *on page 29*
- **Phenyl Salicylate, Methenamine, Methylene Blue, Benzoic Acid, and Hyoscyamine** *see* Methenamine, Phenyl Salicylate, Methylene Blue, Benzoic Acid, and Hyoscyamine *on page 962*
- **Phenyl Salicylate, Methenamine, Methylene Blue, Sodium Biphosphate, and Hyoscyamine** *see* Methenamine, Sodium Biphosphate, Phenyl Salicylate, Methylene Blue, and Hyoscyamine *on page 962*
- **Phenyltoloxamine, Chlorpheniramine, and Phenylephrine** *see* Chlorpheniramine, Phenylephrine, and Phenyltoloxamine *on page 314*
- **Phenyltoloxamine Citrate and Acetaminophen** *see* Acetaminophen and Phenyltoloxamine *on page 29*
- **Phenytek®** *see* Phenytoin *on page 1186*

Phenytoin (FEN i toyn)

U.S. Brand Names Dilantin®; Phenytek®

Canadian Brand Names Dilantin®

Index Terms Diphenylhydantoin; DPH; Phenytoin Sodium; Phenytoin Sodium, Extended; Phenytoin Sodium, Prompt

Pharmacologic Category Antiarrhythmic Agent, Class Ib; Anticonvulsant, Hydantoin

Additional Appendix Information

Anticonvulsant Drugs of Choice *on page 1637*

Status Epilepticus *on page 1831*

Use Management of generalized tonic-clonic (grand mal), complex partial seizures; prevention of seizures following head trauma/neurosurgery

Pregnancy Risk Factor D

Pregnancy Considerations Phenytoin crosses the placenta. Congenital malformations (including a pattern of malformations termed the "fetal hydantoin syndrome" or "fetal anticonvulsant syndrome") have been reported in infants. Isolated cases of malignancies (including neuroblastoma) and coagulation defects in the neonate following delivery have also been reported. Epilepsy itself, the number of medications, genetic factors, or a combination of these probably influence the teratogenicity of anticonvulsant therapy.

Total plasma concentrations of phenytoin are decreased by 56% in the mother during pregnancy; unbound plasma (free) concentrations are decreased by 31%. Because protein binding is decreased, monitoring of unbound plasma concentrations is recommended. Concentrations should be monitored through the 8th week postpartum. The use of folic acid throughout pregnancy and vitamin K during the last month of pregnancy is recommended.

A pregnancy registry is available for women exposed to antiepileptic drug (including phenytoin) at the Genetics and Teratology Unit Massachusetts General Hospital, 1-888-233-2334.

Lactation Enters breast milk/not recommended (AAP rates "compatible")

Medication Safety Issues

Sound-alike/look-alike issues:

Phenytoin may be confused with phenelzine, phentermine

Dilantin® may be confused with Dilaudid®, diltiazem, Dipentum®

High alert medication: The Institute for Safe Medication Practices (ISMP) includes this medication (I.V. formulation) among its list of drug classes which have a heightened risk of causing significant patient harm when used in error.

International issues:

Dilantin® may be confused with Dolantine® which is a brand name for pethidine in Belgium and Switzerland

Contraindications Hypersensitivity to phenytoin, other hydantoins, or any component of the formulation; pregnancy

Warnings/Precautions May increase frequency of petit mal seizures; I.V. form may cause hypotension, skin necrosis at I.V. site; avoid I.V. administration in small veins; use with caution in patients with porphyria; discontinue if rash or lymphadenopathy occurs; a spectrum of hematologic effects have been reported with use (eg, neutropenia, leukopenia, thrombocytopenia, pancytopenia, and anemias); use with caution in patients with hepatic dysfunction, sinus bradycardia, S-A block, or AV block; use with caution in elderly or debilitated patients, or in any condition associated with low serum albumin levels, which will increase the free fraction of phenytoin in the serum and, therefore, the pharmacologic response. Sedation, confusional states, or cerebellar dysfunction (loss of motor coordination) may occur at higher total serum concentrations, or at lower total serum concentrations when the free fraction of phenytoin is increased. Effects with other sedative drugs or ethanol may be potentiated. Abrupt withdrawal may precipitate status epilepticus. Severe reactions, including toxic epidermal necrolysis and Stevens-Johnson syndromes, although rarely reported, have resulted in fatalities; drug should be discontinued if there are any signs of rash. Patients of Asian descent with the variant *HLA-B*1502* may be at an increased risk of developing Stevens-Johnson syndrome and/or toxic epidermal necrolysis.

Adverse Reactions I.V. effects: Hypotension, bradycardia, cardiac arrhythmia, cardiovascular collapse (especially with rapid I.V. use), venous irritation and pain, thrombophlebitis

Effects not related to plasma phenytoin concentrations: Hypertrichosis, gingival hypertrophy, thickening of facial features, carbohydrate intolerance, folic acid deficiency, peripheral neuropathy, vitamin D deficiency, osteomalacia, systemic lupus erythematosus

Concentration-related effects: Nystagmus, blurred vision, diplopia, ataxia, slurred speech, dizziness, drowsiness, lethargy, coma, rash, fever, nausea, vomiting, gum tenderness, confusion, mood changes, folic acid depletion, osteomalacia, hyperglycemia

Related to elevated concentrations:

>20 mcg/mL: Far lateral nystagmus

>30 mcg/mL: 45° lateral gaze nystagmus and ataxia

>40 mcg/mL: Decreased mentation

>100 mcg/mL: Death

Cardiovascular: Hypotension, bradycardia, cardiac arrhythmia, cardiovascular collapse

Central nervous system: Psychiatric changes, slurred speech, dizziness, drowsiness, headache, insomnia

Dermatologic: Rash

Gastrointestinal: Constipation, nausea, vomiting, gingival hyperplasia, enlargement of lips

Hematologic: Leukopenia, thrombocytopenia, agranulocytosis

Hepatic: Hepatitis

Local: Thrombophlebitis

Neuromuscular & skeletal: Tremor, peripheral neuropathy, paresthesia

Ocular: Diplopia, nystagmus, blurred vision

Rarely seen effects: Blood dyscrasias, coarsening of facial features, dyskinesias, hepatitis, hypertrichosis, lymphadenopathy, lymphoma, pseudolymphoma, SLE-like syndrome, Stevens-Johnson syndrome, toxic epidermal necrolysis, venous irritation and pain

Drug Interactions

Metabolism/Transport Effects Substrate of CYP2C9 (major), 2C19 (major), 3A4 (minor); **Induces** CYP2B6 (strong), 2C8 (strong), 2C9 (strong), 2C19 (strong), 3A4 (strong)

Avoid Concomitant Use

Avoid concomitant use of Phenytoin with any of the following: Darunavir; Etravirine; Nilotinib; Ranolazine

Increased Effect/Toxicity

Phenytoin may increase the levels/effects of: Alcohol (Ethyl); Amprenavir; CNS Depressants; Fosamprenavir; Lithium; Vitamin K Antagonists

The levels/effects of Phenytoin may be increased by: Amiodarone; Antifungal Agents (Azole Derivatives, Systemic); Benzodiazepines; Calcium Channel Blockers; Capecitabine; CarBAMazepine; Carbonic Anhydrase Inhibitors; Chloramphenicol; Cimetidine; CYP2C19 Inhibitors (Moderate); CYP2C19 Inhibitors (Strong); CYP2C9 Inhibitors (Moderate); CYP2C9 Inhibitors (Strong); Dexmethylphenidate; Disulfiram; Efavirenz; Felbamate; Floxuridine; Fluconazole; Fluorouracil; Isoniazid; Methylphenidate; OXcarbazepine; Proton Pump Inhibitors; Rufinamide; Selective Serotonin Reuptake Inhibitors; Sulfonamide Derivatives; Tacrolimus; Ticlopidine; Topiramate; Trimethoprim; Vitamin K Antagonists

Decreased Effect

Phenytoin may decrease the levels/effects of: Acetaminophen; Aminocamptothecin; Amiodarone; Antifungal Agents (Azole Derivatives, Systemic); CarBAMazepine; Caspofungin; Chloramphenicol; Clozapine; Contraceptive (Progestins); CycloSPORINE; CYP2B6 Substrates; CYP2C19 Substrates; CYP2C8 Substrates (High risk); CYP2C9 Substrates (High risk); CYP3A4 Substrates; Darunavir; Disopyramide; Doxycycline; Efavirenz; Etoposide; Etoposide Phosphate; Etravirine; Felbamate; Flunarizine; HMG-CoA Reductase Inhibitors; Irinotecan; Lacosamide; LamoTRIgine; Levodopa; Loop Diuretics; Lopinavir; Maraviroc; Mebendazole; Meperidine; Methadone; Metyrapone; Mexiletine; Nilotinib; Oral Contraceptive (Estrogens); OXcarbazepine; Primidone; QUEtiapine; QuiNIDine; Ranolazine; Ritonavir; Rufinamide; Sirolimus; Sorafenib; Tacrolimus; Temsirolimus; Teniposide; Theophylline Derivatives; Thyroid Products; Tipranavir; Topiramate; Valproic Acid; Vecuronium; Zonisamide

The levels/effects of Phenytoin may be decreased by: Amphetamines; Amprenavir; Antacids; CarBAMazepine; Ciprofloxacin; Colesevelam; CYP2C19 Inducers (Strong); CYP2C9 Inducers (Highly Effective); Diazoxide; Folic Acid; Fosamprenavir; Ketorolac; Leucovorin-Levoleucovorin; Lopinavir; Mefloquine; Methylfolate; Pyridoxine; Rifamycin Derivatives; Ritonavir; Theophylline Derivatives; Tipranavir; Valproic Acid; Vigabatrin

Ethanol/Nutrition/Herb Interactions

Ethanol:

Acute use: Avoid or limit ethanol (inhibits metabolism of phenytoin). Watch for sedation.

Chronic use: Avoid or limit ethanol (stimulates metabolism of phenytoin).

Food: Phenytoin serum concentrations may be altered if taken with food. If taken with enteral nutrition, phenytoin serum concentrations may be decreased. Tube feedings decrease bioavailability; hold tube feedings 1-2 hours before and 1-2 hours after phenytoin administration. May decrease calcium, folic acid, and vitamin D levels.

Herb/Nutraceutical: Avoid evening primrose (seizure threshold decreased). Avoid valerian, St John's wort, kava kava, gotu kola (may increase CNS depression).

Stability

Capsule, tablet: Store below 30°C (86°F). Protect from light and moisture.

Oral suspension: Store at room temperature of 20°C to 25°C (68°F to 77°F); do not freeze. Protect from light.

Solution for injection: Store at room temperature of 15°C to 30°C (59°F to 86°F). Use only clear solutions free of precipitate and haziness; slightly yellow solutions may be used. Precipitation may occur if solution is refrigerated and may dissolve at room temperature.

Further dilution of the solution for I.V. infusion is controversial and no consensus exists as to the optimal concentration and length of stability. Stability is concentration and pH dependent. Based on limited clinical consensus, NS or LR are recommended diluents. Dilutions of 1-10 mg/mL have been used and should be administered as soon as possible after preparation (some recommend to discard if not used within 4 hours). Do not refrigerate.

Mechanism of Action Stabilizes neuronal membranes and decreases seizure activity by increasing efflux or decreasing influx of sodium ions across cell membranes in the motor cortex during generation of nerve impulses; prolongs effective refractory period and suppresses ventricular pacemaker automaticity, shortens action potential in the heart

Pharmacodynamics/Kinetics

Onset of action: I.V.: ~0.5-1 hour

Absorption: Oral: Slow

Distribution: V_d:

Neonates: Premature: 1-1.2 L/kg; Full-term: 0.8-0.9 L/kg

Infants: 0.7-0.8 L/kg

Children: 0.7 L/kg

Adults: 0.6-0.7 L/kg

Protein binding:

Neonates: ≥80% (≤20% free)

Infants: ≥85% (≤15% free)

Adults: 90% to 95%

Others: Decreased protein binding

Disease states resulting in a decrease in serum albumin concentration: Burns, hepatic cirrhosis, nephrotic syndrome, pregnancy, cystic fibrosis

Disease states resulting in an apparent decrease in affinity of phenytoin for serum albumin: Renal failure, jaundice (severe), other drugs (displacers), hyperbilirubinemia (total bilirubin >15 mg/dL), Cl_{cr} <25 mL/minute (unbound fraction is increased two- to threefold in uremia)

Metabolism: Follows dose-dependent capacity-limited (Michaelis-Menten) pharmacokinetics with increased V_{max} in infants >6 months of age and children versus adults; major metabolite (via oxidation), HPPA, undergoes enterohepatic recirculation

Bioavailability: Form dependent

Half-life elimination: Oral: 22 hours (range: 7-42 hours)

Time to peak, serum (form dependent): Oral: Extended-release capsule: 4-12 hours; Immediate release preparation: 2-3 hours

Excretion: Urine (<5% as unchanged drug); as glucuronides

Clearance: Highly variable, dependent upon intrinsic hepatic function and dose administered; increased clearance and decreased serum concentrations with febrile illness

Dosage

Status epilepticus: I.V.:

Infants and Children: Loading dose: 15-20 mg/kg in a single or divided dose; maintenance dose: Initial: 5 mg/kg/day in 2 divided doses; usual doses:

6 months to 3 years: 8-10 mg/kg/day

4-6 years: 7.5-9 mg/kg/day

7-9 years: 7-8 mg/kg/day

10-16 years: 6-7 mg/kg/day, some patients may require every 8 hours dosing

Adults: Loading dose: Manufacturer recommends 10-15 mg/kg, however, 15-20 mg/kg is generally recommended; maximum rate: 50 mg/minute

Anticonvulsant: Children and Adults: Oral:

Loading dose: 15-20 mg/kg; based on phenytoin serum concentrations and recent dosing history; administer oral loading dose in 3 divided doses given every 2-4 hours to decrease GI adverse effects and to ensure complete oral absorption; maintenance dose: same as I.V.

Neurosurgery (prophylactic): 100-200 mg at approximately 4-hour intervals during surgery and during the immediate postoperative period

Dosage adjustment in obesity: Adults: Loading dose: Use adjusted body weight (ABW) (Abernethy, 1985)

ABW = [(Actual body weight – IBW) x 1.33] + IBW

Maximum loading dose: 2000 mg (Erstad, 2004)

Maintenance doses should be based on ideal body weight, conventional daily doses with adjustments based upon therapeutic drug monitoring and clinical effectiveness. (Abernethy, 1985; Erstad, 2002; Erstad, 2004)

Dosing adjustment/comments in renal impairment or hepatic disease: Safe in usual doses in mild liver disease; clearance may be substantially reduced in cirrhosis and plasma level monitoring with dose adjustment advisable. Free phenytoin levels should be monitored closely.

Dietary Considerations

Folic acid: Phenytoin may decrease mucosal uptake of folic acid; to avoid folic acid deficiency and megaloblastic anemia, some clinicians recommend giving patients on anticonvulsants prophylactic doses of folic acid and cyanocobalamin. However, folate supplementation may increase seizures in some patients (dose dependent). Discuss with healthcare provider prior to using any supplements.

Calcium: Hypocalcemia has been reported in patients taking prolonged high-dose therapy with an anticonvulsant. Some clinicians have given an additional 4000 units/week of vitamin D (especially in those receiving poor nutrition and getting no sun exposure) to prevent hypocalcemia.

Vitamin D: Phenytoin interferes with vitamin D metabolism and osteomalacia may result; may need to supplement with vitamin D

Tube feedings: Tube feedings decrease phenytoin absorption. To avoid decreased serum levels with continuous NG feeds, hold feedings for 1-2 hours prior to and 1-2 hours after phenytoin administration, if possible. There is a variety of opinions on how to administer phenytoin with enteral feedings. Be **consistent** throughout therapy.

Sodium content of 1 g injection: 88 mg (3.8 mEq)

Administration

Oral: Suspension: Shake well prior to use. Absorption is impaired when phenytoin suspension is given concurrently to patients who are receiving continuous nasogastric feedings. A method to resolve this interaction is to divide the daily dose of phenytoin and withhold the administration of nutritional supplements for 1-2 hours before and after each phenytoin dose.

I.M.: Although approved for I.M. use, I.M. administration is not recommended due to erratic absorption and pain on injection. Fosphenytoin may be considered.

I.V.: Vesicant. Fosphenytoin may be considered for loading in patients who are in status epilepticus, hemodynamically unstable, or develop hypotension/bradycardia with I.V. administration of phenytoin. Phenytoin may be administered by IVP or IVPB administration. The maximum rate of I.V. administration is 50 mg/minute. Highly sensitive patients (eg, elderly, patients with preexisting cardiovascular conditions) should receive phenytoin more slowly (eg, 20 mg/minute). An in-line 0.22-5 micron filter is recommended for IVPB solutions due to the high potential for precipitation of the solution. Avoid extravasation. Following I.V. administration, NS should be injected through the same needle or I.V. catheter to prevent irritation.

pH: 10.0-12.3

SubQ: SubQ administration is not recommended because of the possibility of local tissue damage (due to high pH).

Monitoring Parameters Blood pressure, vital signs (with I.V. use); plasma phenytoin level, CBC, liver function. **Note:** If available, free phenytoin concentrations should be obtained in patients with renal impairment and/or hypoalbuminemia. If free phenytoin levels are unavailable, the adjusted total level is based upon equations in adult patients.

Reference Range Timing of serum samples: Because it is slowly absorbed, peak blood levels may occur 4-8 hours after ingestion of an oral dose. The serum half-life varies with the dosage and the drug follows Michaelis-Menten kinetics. The average adult half-life is about 24 hours. Steady-state concentrations are reached in 5-10 days.

Children and Adults: Toxicity is measured clinically, and some patients require levels outside the suggested therapeutic range

Therapeutic range:

Total phenytoin: 10-20 mcg/mL (children and adults), 8-15 mcg/mL (neonates)

Concentrations of 5-10 mcg/mL may be therapeutic for some patients but concentrations <5 mcg/mL are not likely to be effective

50% of patients show decreased frequency of seizures at concentrations >10 mcg/mL

86% of patients show decreased frequency of seizures at concentrations >15 mcg/mL

Add another anticonvulsant if satisfactory therapeutic response is not achieved with a phenytoin concentration of 20 mcg/mL

Free phenytoin: 1-2.5 mcg/mL

Total phenytoin:

Toxic: >30 mcg/mL (SI: <120-200 µmol/L)

Lethal: >100 mcg/mL (SI: >400 µmol/L)

When to draw levels: This is dependent on the disease state being treated and the clinical condition of the patient

Key points:

Slow absorption of extended capsules and prolonged half-life minimize fluctuations between peak and trough concentrations, timing of sampling not crucial

Trough concentrations are generally recommended for routine monitoring. Daily levels are not necessary and may result in incorrect dosage adjustments. If it is determined essential to monitor free phenytoin concentrations, concomitant monitoring of total phenytoin concentrations is not necessary and expensive.

After a loading dose: If rapid therapeutic levels are needed, initial levels may be drawn after 1 hour (I.V. loading dose) or within 24 hours (oral loading dose) to aid in determining maintenance dose or need to reload.

Rapid achievement: Draw within 2-3 days of therapy initiation to ensure that the patient's metabolism is not remarkably different from that which would be predicted by average literature-derived pharmacokinetic parameters; early levels should be used cautiously in design of new dosing regimens

Second concentration: Draw within 6-7 days with subsequent doses of phenytoin adjusted accordingly

If plasma concentrations have not changed over a 3- to 5-day period, monitoring interval may be increased to once weekly in the acute clinical setting

In stable patients requiring long-term therapy, generally monitor levels at 3- to 12-month intervals

Adjustment of serum concentration: See tables.

Note: Although it is ideal to obtain free phenytoin concentrations to assess serum concentrations in patients with hypoalbuminemia or renal failure (Cl_{cr} ≤10 mL/minute), it may not always be possible. If free phenytoin concentrations are unavailable, the following equations may be utilized in adult patients.

Adjustment of Serum Concentration in Adults With Low Serum Albumin

Measured Total Phenytoin Concentration (mcg/mL)	Patient's Serum Albumin (g/dL)			
	3.5	3	2.5	2
	Adjusted Total Phenytoin Concentration (mcg/mL)[1]			
5	6	7	8	10
10	13	14	17	20
15	19	21	25	30

[1]Adjusted concentration = measured total concentration divided by [(0.2 x albumin) + 0.1].

Adjustment of Serum Concentration in Adults With Renal Failure (Cl_{cr} ≤10 mL/min)

Measured Total Phenytoin Concentration (mcg/mL)	Patient's Serum Albumin (g/dL)				
	4	3.5	3	2.5	2
	Adjusted Total Phenytoin Concentration (mcg/mL)[1]				
5	10	11	13	14	17
10	20	22	25	29	33
15	30	33	38	43	50

[1]Adjusted concentration = measured total concentration divided by [(0.1 x albumin) + 0.1].

Dosage Forms Excipient information presented when available (limited, particularly for generics); consult specific product labeling.

Capsule, extended release, as sodium: 100 mg

Dilantin®: 30 mg [contains sodium benzoate], 100 mg

Phenytek®: 200 mg, 300 mg

Capsule, prompt release, as sodium: 100 mg

Injection, solution, as sodium: 50 mg/mL (2 mL, 5 mL) [contains alcohol and propylene glycol]

Suspension, oral: 100 mg/4 mL (4 mL); 125 mg/5 mL (240 mL)

Dilantin®: 125 mg/5 mL (240 mL) [contains alcohol <0.6%, sodium benzoate; orange vanilla flavor]

Tablet, chewable:

Dilantin®: 50 mg

◆ **Phenytoin Sodium** *see* Phenytoin *on page 1186*

◆ **Phenytoin Sodium, Extended** *see* Phenytoin *on page 1186*

◆ **Phenytoin Sodium, Prompt** *see* Phenytoin *on page 1186*

◆ **Phillips'® M-O [OTC]** *see* Magnesium Hydroxide and Mineral Oil *on page 916*

Physostigmine (fye zoe STIG meen)

Canadian Brand Names Eserine®; Isopto® Eserine

Index Terms Eserine Salicylate; Physostigmine Salicylate; Physostigmine Sulfate

Pharmacologic Category Acetylcholinesterase Inhibitor

Use Reverse toxic, life-threatening delirium caused by atropine, diphenhydramine, dimenhydrinate, *Atropa belladonna* (deadly nightshade), or jimson weed (*Datura* spp)

Pregnancy Risk Factor C

Lactation Excretion in breast milk unknown

Medication Safety Issues

Sound-alike/look-alike issues:

Physostigmine may be confused with Prostigmin®, pyridostigmine

Contraindications Hypersensitivity to physostigmine or any component of the formulation; GI or GU obstruction; asthma; gangrene; diabetes, cardiovascular disease; any vagotonic state; coadministration of choline esters and depolarizing neuromuscular-blocking agents

Warnings/Precautions Patient must have a normal QRS interval, as measured by ECG, in order to receive; use caution in poisoning with agents known to prolong intraventricular conduction. Concomitant administration of choline esters or depolarizing neuromuscular-blocking agents (ie, succinylcholine) are contraindicated. Use with caution in patients with epilepsy, asthma, diabetes, gangrene, cardiovascular disease, bradycardia. Discontinue if excessive salivation or emesis, frequent urination or diarrhea occur. Reduce dosage if excessive sweating or nausea occurs. Administer slowly over 5 minutes to prevent respiratory distress and seizures. Continuous infusions should never be used. Due to the possibility of hypersensitivity or overdose/cholinergic crisis, atropine should be readily available; not intended as a first-line agent for anticholinergic toxicity or Parkinson's disease. Asystole and seizures have been reported when physostigmine was administered to TCA poisoned patients. Physostigmine is not recommended in patients with known or suspected TCA intoxication. Products may contain benzyl alcohol. Products may contain sodium bisulfate.

Adverse Reactions Frequency not defined.

Cardiovascular: Asystole, bradycardia, palpitation

Central nervous system: Hallucinations, nervousness, restlessness, seizure

Gastrointestinal: Diarrhea, nausea, salivation, stomach pain

Genitourinary: Urinary frequency

Neuromuscular & skeletal: Twitching

Ocular: Lacrimation, miosis
Respiratory: Bronchospasm, dyspnea, pulmonary edema, respiratory paralysis
Miscellaneous: Diaphoresis

Drug Interactions

Avoid Concomitant Use There are no known interactions where it is recommended to avoid concomitant use.

Increased Effect/Toxicity

Physostigmine may increase the levels/effects of: Beta-Blockers; Cholinergic Agonists; Succinylcholine

The levels/effects of Physostigmine may be increased by: Corticosteroids (Systemic); Ginkgo Biloba

Decreased Effect

Physostigmine may decrease the levels/effects of: Neuromuscular-Blocking Agents (Nondepolarizing)

Ethanol/Nutrition/Herb Interactions Herb/Nutraceutical: Ginkgo biloba may enhance the adverse/toxic effect of physostigmine; monitor.

Stability Do not use solution if cloudy or dark brown.

Mechanism of Action Inhibits destruction of acetylcholine by acetylcholinesterase which facilitates transmission of impulses across myoneural junction and prolongs the central and peripheral effects of acetylcholine

Pharmacodynamics/Kinetics

Onset of action: ~5 minutes
Duration: 1-2 hours
Absorption: I.M.: Readily absorbed
Distribution: Crosses blood-brain barrier readily and reverses both central and peripheral anticholinergic effects
Metabolism: Hepatic and via hydrolysis by cholinesterases
Half-life elimination: 15-40 minutes

Dosage Reversal of toxic anticholinergic effects: **Note:** Administer slowly over 5 minutes to prevent respiratory distress and seizures. Continuous infusions of physostigmine should never be used.

Children: **Note:** Reserve for life-threatening situations only: I.V.: 0.01-0.03 mg/kg/dose; may repeat after 5-10 minutes to a maximum total dose of 2 mg or until response occurs or adverse cholinergic effects occur

Adults: I.M., I.V.: 0.5-2 mg to start, repeat every 20 minutes until response occurs or adverse effect occurs; repeat 1-4 mg every 30-60 minutes as life-threatening symptoms recur

Administration Injection: Infuse slowly I.V. over 5 minutes. Too rapid administration can cause bradycardia and hypersalivation leading to respiratory distress and seizures.

Monitoring Parameters ECG, vital signs

Test Interactions Increased aminotransferase [ALT/AST] (S), increased amylase (S)

Dosage Forms Excipient information presented when available (limited, particularly for generics); consult specific product labeling.

Injection, solution, as salicylate: 1 mg/mL (2 mL) [contains benzyl alcohol and sodium metabisulfite]

◆ **Physostigmine Salicylate** *see* Physostigmine *on page 1190*

◆ **Physostigmine Sulfate** *see* Physostigmine *on page 1190*

◆ **Phytomenadione** *see* Phytonadione *on page 1191*

Phytonadione (fye toe na DYE one)

U.S. Brand Names Mephyton®

Canadian Brand Names AquaMEPHYTON®; Konakion; Mephyton®

Index Terms Methylphytyl Napthoquinone; Phylloquinone; Phytomenadione; Vitamin K_1

Pharmacologic Category Vitamin, Fat Soluble

Use Prevention and treatment of hypoprothrombinemia caused by coumarin derivative-induced or other drug-induced vitamin K deficiency, hypoprothrombinemia caused by malabsorption or inability to synthesize vitamin K; hemorrhagic disease of the newborn

Unlabeled/Investigational Use Treatment of hypoprothrombinemia caused by anticoagulant rodenticides

Pregnancy Risk Factor C

Lactation Enters breast milk/use caution (AAP rates "compatible")

Medication Safety Issues

Sound-alike/look-alike issues:

Mephyton® may be confused with melphalan, methadone

Contraindications Hypersensitivity to phytonadione or any component of the formulation

Warnings/Precautions **[U.S. Boxed Warning]: Severe reactions resembling hypersensitivity (eg, anaphylaxis) reactions have occurred rarely during or immediately after I.V. administration.** Allergic reactions have also occurred with I.M. and SubQ injections; oral administration is the safest. In obstructive jaundice or with biliary fistulas concurrent administration of bile salts is necessary. Manufacturers recommend the SubQ route over other parenteral routes. SubQ is less predictable when compared to the oral route. The American College of Chest Physicians recommends the I.V. route in patients with serious or life-threatening bleeding secondary to warfarin. The I.V. route should be restricted to emergency situations where oral phytonadione cannot be used. Efficacy is delayed regardless of route of administration; patient management may require other treatments in the interim. Administer a dose that will quickly lower the INR into a safe range without causing resistance to warfarin. High phytonadione doses may lead to warfarin resistance for at least one week. Use caution in newborns especially premature infants; hemolysis, jaundice and hyperbilirubinemia have been reported with larger than recommended doses. Some dosage forms contain benzyl alcohol which has been associated with "gasping syndrome" in premature infants. In liver disease, if initial doses do not reverse coagulopathy then higher doses are unlikely to have any effect. Ineffective in hereditary hypoprothrombinemia. Use caution with renal dysfunction (including premature infants). Injectable products may contain aluminum; may result in toxic levels following prolonged administration.

Adverse Reactions Parenteral administration: Frequency not defined.

Cardiovascular: Cyanosis, flushing, hypotension
Central nervous system: Dizziness
Dermatologic: Scleroderma-like lesions
Endocrine & metabolic: Hyperbilirubinemia (newborn; greater than recommended doses)
Gastrointestinal: Abnormal taste
Local: Injection site reactions
Respiratory: Dyspnea
Miscellaneous: Anaphylactoid reactions, diaphoresis, hypersensitivity reactions

Drug Interactions

Avoid Concomitant Use There are no known interactions where it is recommended to avoid concomitant use.

Increased Effect/Toxicity There are no known significant interactions involving an increase in effect.

Decreased Effect

Phytonadione may decrease the levels/effects of: Vitamin K Antagonists

Stability

Injection: Store at 15°C to 30°C (59°F to 86°F). Dilute in preservative-free NS, D_5W, or D_5NS.

Note: Store Hospira product at 20°C to 25°C (68°F to 77°F).

Oral: Store tablets at 15°C to 30°C (59°F to 86°F). Protect from light.

Mechanism of Action Promotes liver synthesis of clotting factors (II, VII, IX, X); however, the exact mechanism as to this stimulation is unknown. Menadiol is a water soluble form of vitamin K; phytonadione has a more rapid and prolonged effect than menadione; menadiol sodium diphosphate (K_4) is half as potent as menadione (K_3).

Pharmacodynamics/Kinetics

Onset of action: Increased coagulation factors: Oral: 6-10 hours; I.V.: 1-2 hours

Peak effect: INR values return to normal: Oral: 24-48 hours; I.V.: 12-14 hours

Absorption: Oral: From intestines in presence of bile; SubQ: Variable

Metabolism: Rapidly hepatic

Excretion: Urine and feces

Dosage Note: According to the manufacturer, SubQ is the preferred parenteral route; I.M. route should be avoided due to the risk of hematoma formation; I.V. route should be restricted for emergency use only. The American College of Chest Physicians recommends the I.V. route in patients with serious or life-threatening bleeding secondary to use of vitamin K antagonists.

Adequate intake:

Children:

1-3 years: 30 mcg/day

4-8 years: 55 mcg/day

9-13 years: 60 mcg/day

14-18 years: 75 mcg/day

Adults: Males: 120 mcg/day; Females: 90 mcg/day

Hemorrhagic disease of the newborn:

Prophylaxis: I.M.: 0.5-1 mg within 1 hour of birth

Treatment: I.M., SubQ: 1 mg/dose/day; higher doses may be necessary if mother has been receiving oral anticoagulants

Hypoprothrombinemia due to drugs (other than coumarin derivatives) or factors limiting absorption or synthesis: Adults: Oral, SubQ, I.M., I.V.: Initial: 2.5-25 mg (rarely up to 50 mg)

Vitamin K deficiency (supratherapeutic INR) secondary to coumarin derivative (Ansell, 2008): Adults:

If INR above therapeutic range to <5 (no significant bleeding and rapid reversal unnecessary): Lower or hold next dose and monitor frequently; when INR approaches desired range, resume dosing with a lower dose.

If INR ≥5 and <9 (no significant bleeding): If no risk factors for bleeding exist, omit next 1 or 2 doses, monitor INR more frequently, and resume with an appropriately adjusted dose when INR in desired range.

Alternatively, if other risk factors for bleeding exist, omit next dose and administer vitamin K orally 1-2.5 mg; resume with an appropriately adjusted dose when INR in desired range.

If INR ≥5 and <9 (no significant bleeding and rapid reversal required for surgery): Administer vitamin K orally ≤5 mg and hold warfarin. Expect INR to be reduced within 24 hours; if INR still elevated, another 1-2 mg of vitamin K orally may be given.

If INR ≥9 (no significant bleeding): Hold warfarin, administer vitamin K orally 2.5-5 mg, expect INR to be reduced within 24-48 hours, monitor INR more frequently and give additional vitamin K at an appropriate dose if necessary. Resume warfarin at an appropriately adjusted dose when INR is in desired range.

If serious bleeding at any INR elevation: Hold warfarin, administer vitamin K 10 mg by slow I.V. infusion and supplement with FFP, PCC, or rFVIIa depending on the urgency of the situation; I.V. Vitamin K may be repeated every 12 hours.

If life-threatening bleeding: Hold warfarin, give FFP, PCC, or rFVIIa supplemented with vitamin K 10 mg slow I.V. infusion; repeat if necessary, depending on INR.

Notes:

If mild-moderate INR elevation without major bleeding occurs, administer vitamin K orally instead of subcutaneously.

Use of high doses of vitamin K (eg, 10-15 mg) may cause warfarin resistance for ≥1 week. During this period of resistance, heparin or low molecular weight heparin may be given until INR responds.

FFP=fresh frozen plasma; PCC=prothrombin complex concentrate; rFVIIa=recombinant factor VIIa

Administration

I.V. administration: Infuse slowly; rate of infusion should not exceed 1 mg/minute (3 mg/m^2/minute in children and infants). The injectable route should be used only if the oral route is not feasible or there is a greater urgency to reverse anticoagulation.

Oral: The parenteral preparation has been administered orally to neonates.

Monitoring Parameters PT, INR

Dosage Forms Excipient information presented when available (limited, particularly for generics); consult specific product labeling.

Injection, aqueous colloidal: 2 mg/mL (0.5 mL); 10 mg/mL (1 mL)

Tablet: 100 mcg [OTC]

Mephyton®: 5 mg

Extemporaneous Preparations A 1 mg/mL oral suspension was stable for only 3 days when refrigerated when compounded as follows:

Triturate six 5 mg tablets in a mortar, reduce to a fine powder, then add 5 mL each of water and methylcellulose 1% while mixing; then transfer to a graduate and qs to 30 mL with sorbitol

Shake well before using and keep in refrigerator

Nahata MC and Hipple TF, *Pediatric Drug Formulations*, 3rd ed, Cincinnati, OH: Harvey Whitney Books Co, 1997.

◆ **Pidorubicin** *see* Epirubicin *on page* 528

◆ **Pidorubicin Hydrochloride** *see* Epirubicin *on page* 528

Pilocarpine (pye loe KAR peen)

U.S. Brand Names Isopto® Carpine; Pilopine HS®; Salagen®

Canadian Brand Names Diocarpine; Isopto® Carpine; Pilopine HS®; Salagen®

Index Terms Pilocarpine Hydrochloride

Pharmacologic Category Cholinergic Agonist; Ophthalmic Agent, Antiglaucoma; Ophthalmic Agent, Miotic

Additional Appendix Information

Glaucoma Drug Therapy *on page* 1808

Use

Ophthalmic: Management of chronic simple glaucoma, chronic and acute angle-closure glaucoma

Oral: Symptomatic treatment of xerostomia caused by salivary gland hypofunction resulting from radiotherapy for cancer of the head and neck or Sjögren's syndrome

Unlabeled/Investigational Use Counter effects of cycloplegics

Pregnancy Risk Factor C

Medication Safety Issues

Sound-alike/look-alike issues:

Isopto® Carpine may be confused with Isopto® Carbachol

Salagen® may be confused with Salacid®, selegiline

International issues:
Salagen® may be confused with Poagen® which is a brand name for grass pollen extract in Portugal

Dosage Adults:

Ophthalmic:

Glaucoma:

Solution: Instill 1-2 drops up to 6 times/day; adjust the concentration and frequency as required to control elevated intraocular pressure

Gel: Instill 0.5" ribbon into lower conjunctival sac once daily at bedtime

To counteract the mydriatic effects of sympathomimetic agents (unlabeled use): Solution: Instill 1 drop of a 1% solution in the affected eye

Oral: Xerostomia:

Following head and neck cancer: 5 mg 3 times/day, titration up to 10 mg 3 times/day may be considered for patients who have not responded adequately; do not exceed 2 tablets/dose

Sjögren's syndrome: 5 mg 4 times/day

Dosage adjustment in hepatic impairment: Oral: Patients with moderate impairment: 5 mg 2 times/day regardless of indication; adjust dose based on response and tolerability. Do not use with severe impairment (Child-Pugh score 10-15).

Additional Information Complete prescribing information for this medication should be consulted for additional detail.

Dosage Forms Excipient information presented when available (limited, particularly for generics); consult specific product labeling.

Gel, ophthalmic, as hydrochloride (Pilopine HS®): 4% (4 g) [contains benzalkonium chloride]

Solution, ophthalmic, as hydrochloride: 0.5% (15 mL); 1% (2 mL, 15 mL); 2% (2 mL, 15 mL); 3% (15 mL); 4% (2 mL, 15 mL); 6% (15 mL) [may contain benzalkonium chloride]

Isopto® Carpine: 1% (15 mL); 2% (15 mL); 4% (15 mL) [contains benzalkonium chloride]

Tablet, as hydrochloride: 5 mg, 7.5 mg

Salagen®: 5 mg, 7.5 mg

◆ **Pilocarpine Hydrochloride** *see* Pilocarpine *on page 1192*

◆ **Pilopine HS®** *see* Pilocarpine *on page 1192*

◆ **Pimaricin** *see* Natamycin *on page 1045*

Pimecrolimus (pim e KROE li mus)

U.S. Brand Names Elidel®

Canadian Brand Names Elidel®

Pharmacologic Category Immunosuppressant Agent; Topical Skin Product

Use Short-term and intermittent long-term treatment of mild to moderate atopic dermatitis in patients not responsive to conventional therapy or when conventional therapy is not appropriate

Restrictions An FDA-approved medication guide must be distributed when dispensing an outpatient prescription (new or refill) where this medication is to be used without direct supervision of a healthcare provider. Medication guides are available at http://www.fda.gov/cder/Offices/ODS/medication_guides.htm.

Pregnancy Risk Factor C

Pregnancy Considerations There are no adequate and well-controlled studies in pregnant women; use only if clearly needed.

Lactation Excretion in breast milk unknown/not recommended

Contraindications Hypersensitivity to pimecrolimus or any component of the formulation

Warnings/Precautions [U.S. Boxed Warning]: Topical calcineurin inhibitors have been associated with rare cases of lymphoma and skin malignancy. Avoid use on malignant or premalignant skin conditions (eg, cutaneous T-cell lymphoma). Topical calcineurin agents are considered second-line therapies in the treatment of atopic dermatitis/eczema, and should be limited to use in patients who have failed treatment with other therapies. **[U.S. Boxed Warning]: They should be used for short-term and intermittent treatment using the minimum amount necessary for the control of symptoms should be used.** Application should be limited to involved areas. Diagnosis should be reconfirmed if sign/symptoms do not improve within 6 weeks of treatment. Safety of intermittent use for >1 year has not been established.

May cause local symptoms (eg, burning, soreness, stinging) during first few days of treatment; usually self-resolving. Should not be used in immunocompromised patients. Do not apply to areas of active bacterial or viral infection; infections at the treatment site should be cleared prior to therapy. Patients with atopic dermatitis are predisposed to skin infections, and pimecrolimus therapy has been associated with risk of developing eczema herpeticum, varicella zoster, and herpes simplex. Papilloma/warts have been observed with use; discontinue pimecrolimus until resolution if worsening or do not respond to conventional treatment. Pimecrolimus may be associated with development of lymphadenopathy; possible infectious causes should be investigated. Discontinue use in patients with unknown cause of lymphadenopathy or acute infectious mononucleosis. Not recommended for use in patients with skin disease which may increase the potential for systemic absorption (eg, Netherton's syndrome). Avoid artificial or natural sunlight exposure, even when Elidel® is not on the skin. Safety not established in patients with generalized erythroderma. **[U.S. Boxed Warning]: The use of Elidel® in children <2 years of age is not recommended,** particularly since the effect on immune system development is unknown.

Adverse Reactions

>10%:

Central nervous system: Headache (7% to 25%), fever (1% to 13%)

Local: Burning at application site (2% to 26%; tends to resolve/improve as lesions resolve)

Respiratory: Nasopharyngitis (8% to 27%), cough (2% to 16%), upper respiratory tract infection (4% to 19%), bronchitis (≤11%)

Miscellaneous: Influenza (3% to 13%)

1% to 10%:

Dermatologic: Skin infection (2% to 6%), folliculitis (1% to 6%), impetigo (2% to 4%), skin papilloma (warts) (≤3%), acne (≤2%), herpes simplex dermatitis (≤ 2%), molluscum contagiosum (≤2%), urticaria (≤1%)

Endocrine & metabolic: Dysmenorrhea (1% to 2%)

Gastrointestinal: Diarrhea (1% to 8%), gastroenteritis (≤7%), abdominal pain (≤4%), constipation (≤4%)

Local: Irritation at application site (≤6%), pruritus at application site (1% to 6%), erythema at application site (≤2%)

Ocular: Eye infection (≤1%)

Otic: Ear infection (1% to 6%), otitis media (1% to 3%)

Respiratory: Pharyngitis (1% to 8%), asthma (1% to 4%), asthma aggravated (≤4%), nasal congestion (1% to 3%), sinusitis (1% to 3%), epistaxis (≤3%), dyspnea (≤2%), pneumonia (≤2%), rhinorrhea (≤2%), wheezing (≤1%)

Miscellaneous: Viral infection (≤7%), tonsillitis (≤6%), hypersensitivity (3% to 5%), herpes simplex infection (≤4%), bacterial infection (1% to 2%)

<1% (Limited to important or life-threatening): Anaphylaxis, angioneurotic edema, eczema herpeticum, facial edema, flushing (ethanol-associated), lymphadenopathy, ocular irritation (following application near eyes), malignancy

(basal cell carcinoma, squamous cell carcinoma, malignant melanoma, lymphoma), skin discoloration

Drug Interactions

Metabolism/Transport Effects **Substrate** of CYP3A4 (minor)

Avoid Concomitant Use There are no known interactions where it is recommended to avoid concomitant use.

Increased Effect/Toxicity

The levels/effects of Pimecrolimus may be increased by: CYP3A4 Inhibitors (Moderate); CYP3A4 Inhibitors (Strong)

Decreased Effect There are no known significant interactions involving a decrease in effect.

Ethanol/Nutrition/Herb Interactions Ethanol: Avoid ethanol (topical pimecrolimus may increase the potential for experiencing facial flushing following the consumption of alcoholic beverages).

Stability Store at 15°C to 30°C (59°F to 86°F); do not freeze.

Mechanism of Action Penetrates inflamed epidermis to inhibit T cell activation by blocking transcription of proinflammatory cytokine genes such as interleukin-2, interferon gamma (Th1-type), interleukin-4, and interleukin-10 (Th2-type). Pimecrolimus binds to the intracellular protein FKBP-12, inhibiting calcineurin, which blocks cytokine transcription and inhibits T-cell activation. Prevents release of inflammatory cytokines and mediators from mast cells *in vitro* after stimulation by antigen/IgE.

Pharmacodynamics/Kinetics Absorption: Poor when applied to 13% to 62% body surface area in adults for up to a year; detectable blood levels were observed in a higher proportion of children, as compared to adults

Dosage Children ≥2 years and Adults: Topical: Apply thin layer to affected area twice daily; rub in gently and completely. **Note:** Limit application to involved areas. Continue as long as signs and symptoms persist; discontinue if resolution occurs; re-evaluate if symptoms persist >6 weeks.

Administration Do not use with occlusive dressings. Burning at the application site is most common in first few days; improves as atopic dermatitis improves. Limit application to areas of involvement. Continue as long as signs and symptoms persist; discontinue if resolution occurs; re-evaluate if symptoms persist >6 weeks.

Dosage Forms Excipient information presented when available (limited, particularly for generics); consult specific product labeling.

Cream, topical:

Elidel®: 1% (30 g, 60 g, 100 g)

Pimozide (PI moe zide)

U.S. Brand Names Orap®

Canadian Brand Names Apo-Pimozide®; Orap®

Pharmacologic Category Antipsychotic Agent, Typical

Additional Appendix Information

Antipsychotic Agents *on page 1644*

Use Suppression of severe motor and phonic tics in patients with Tourette's disorder who have failed to respond satisfactorily to standard treatment

Unlabeled/Investigational Use Psychosis; reported use in individuals with delusions focused on physical symptoms (ie, preoccupation with parasitic infestation); Huntington's chorea; psychosis/agitation related to Alzheimer's dementia

Pregnancy Risk Factor C

Dosage Oral: **Note:** An ECG should be performed baseline and periodically thereafter, especially during dosage adjustment:

Children ≤12 years: Tourette's disorder: Initial: 0.05 mg/kg preferably once at bedtime; may be increased every third day; usual range: 2-4 mg/day; do not exceed 10 mg/day (0.2 mg/kg/day)

Children >12 years and Adults: Tourette's disorder: Initial: 1-2 mg/day in divided doses, then increase dosage as needed every other day; range is usually 7-16 mg/day, maximum dose: 10 mg/day or 0.2 mg/kg/day are not generally recommended

Note: Sudden unexpected deaths have occurred in patients taking doses >10 mg. Therefore, dosages exceeding 10 mg/day are generally not recommended.

Dosing adjustment in hepatic impairment: Reduction of dose is necessary in patients with liver disease

Additional Information Complete prescribing information for this medication should be consulted for additional detail.

Dosage Forms Excipient information presented when available (limited, particularly for generics); consult specific product labeling.

Tablet: 1 mg, 2 mg

◆ **Pin-X® [OTC]** *see* Pyrantel Pamoate *on page 1270*

Pindolol (PIN doe lole)

Canadian Brand Names Apo-Pindol®; Gen-Pindolol; Novo-Pindol; Nu-Pindol; PMS-Pindolol; Visken®

Pharmacologic Category Beta Blocker With Intrinsic Sympathomimetic Activity

Additional Appendix Information

Beta-Blockers *on page 1648*

Use Treatment of hypertension, alone or in combination with other agents

Unlabeled/Investigational Use Potential augmenting agent for antidepressants; ventricular arrhythmias/tachycardia, antipsychotic-induced akathisia, situational anxiety; aggressive behavior associated with dementia

Pregnancy Risk Factor B

Pregnancy Considerations Adverse events were not observed in animal studies. Pindolol crosses the human placenta. Beta-blockers have been associated with bradycardia, hypotension, and IUGR; IUGR is probably related to maternal hypertension. Available evidence suggests beta-blockers are generally safe during pregnancy (JNC 7).

Lactation Enters breast milk/not recommended

Medication Safety Issues

Sound-alike/look-alike issues:

Pindolol may be confused with Parlodel®, Plendil®

Visken® may be confused with Visine®

Contraindications Bronchial asthma; cardiogenic shock; heart block (2nd or 3rd degree) except in patients with a functioning artificial pacemaker; overt cardiac failure; severe bradycardia

Warnings/Precautions Consider pre-existing conditions such as sick sinus syndrome before initiating. Use with caution in patients with inadequate myocardial function, undergoing anesthesia, bronchospastic disease, myasthenia gravis, peripheral vascular disease, renal impairment, psychiatric disease (may cause CNS depression) or impaired hepatic function. Use with caution in patients with diabetes mellitus; may potentiate hypoglycemia and/or mask signs and symptoms. Beta-blockers with intrinsic sympathomimetic activity (including pindolol) do not appear to be of benefit in HF. If use is warranted with compensated HF, use with caution and monitor for a worsening of the condition. If condition worsens, consider temporary discontinuation or dosage reduction of pindolol. Beta-blocker therapy should not be withdrawn abruptly (particularly in patients with CAD), but gradually tapered to avoid acute tachycardia, hypertension, and/or ischemia. Adequate alpha-blockade is required prior to use of any beta-blocker for patients with untreated pheochromocytoma. Use caution with history of severe anaphylaxis to allergens; patients taking beta-blockers may become more sensitive to repeated challenges. Treatment of anaphylaxis (eg, epinephrine) in patients taking beta-blockers may be ineffective or promote undesirable effects. Use with caution in patients receiving anesthetic agents which decrease myocardial function (eg, ether, cyclopropane and trichloroethylene). Use with caution in patients on concurrent verapamil or diltiazem; bradycardia or heart block may occur. Safety and efficacy have not been established in children.

Adverse Reactions

1% to 10%:

- Cardiovascular: Edema (6%), chest pain (3%), bradycardia (≤2%), heart block (≤2%), hypotension (≤2%), syncope (≤2%), tachycardia (≤2%), palpitation (≤1%)
- Central nervous system: Insomnia (10%), dizziness (9%), fatigue (8%), nervousness (7%), nightmares/vivid dreams (5%), anxiety (≤2%), lethargy (≤2%)
- Dermatologic: Hyperhidrosis (≤2%), pruritus (1%)
- Gastrointestinal: Nausea (5%), diarrhea (≤2%), vomiting (≤2%), weight gain (≤2%)
- Genitourinary: Impotence (≤2%)
- Hematologic: Claudication (≤2%)
- Hepatic: ALT increased (7%), AST increased (7%)
- Neuromuscular & skeletal: Muscle pain (10%), arthralgia (7%), weakness (4%), paresthesia (3%), muscle cramps (3%)
- Ocular: Burning eyes (≤2%), visual disturbances (≤2%), eye discomfort (≤2%)
- Renal: Polyuria (≤2%)
- Respiratory: Dyspnea (5%), wheezing (≤2%)
- Miscellaneous: Cold extremities (≤2%)

<1% (Limited to important or life-threatening): Alkaline phosphatase increased, hallucination, heart failure, lactic acid dehydrogenase increased, uric acid increased

Other adverse reactions (noted with other beta-adrenergic-blocking agents that should be considered potential adverse events with pindolol): Agranulocytosis, alopecia, catatonia, clouded sensorium, disorientation, emotional lability, fever, intensification of pre-existing AV block, ischemic colitis, laryngospasm, mental depression, mesenteric artery thrombosis, nonthrombocytopenic purpura, Peyronie's disease, rash (erythematous), respiratory distress, short-term memory loss, thrombocytopenic purpura

Drug Interactions

Metabolism/Transport Effects **Substrate** of CYP2D6 (major); **Inhibits** CYP2D6 (weak)

Avoid Concomitant Use

Avoid concomitant use of Pindolol with any of the following: Methacholine

Increased Effect/Toxicity

Pindolol may increase the levels/effects of: Alpha-/Beta-Agonists (Direct-Acting); Alpha1-Blockers; Alpha2-Agonists; Amifostine; Antipsychotic Agents (Phenothiazines); Cardiac Glycosides; Insulin; Lidocaine; Methacholine; Midodrine; RiTUXimab

The levels/effects of Pindolol may be increased by: Acetylcholinesterase Inhibitors; Aminoquinolines (Antimalarial); Amiodarone; Anilidopiperidine Opioids; Antipsychotic Agents (Phenothiazines); Calcium Channel Blockers (Nondihydropyridine); Diazoxide; Dipyridamole; Disopyramide; Herbs (Hypotensive Properties); Propafenone; Propoxyphene; Prostacyclin Analogues; QuiNIDine; Reserpine; Selective Serotonin Reuptake Inhibitors

Decreased Effect

Pindolol may decrease the levels/effects of: Beta2-Agonists; Theophylline Derivatives

The levels/effects of Pindolol may be decreased by: Barbiturates; Herbs (Hypertensive Properties); Methylphenidate; Nonsteroidal Anti-Inflammatory Agents; Rifamycin Derivatives; Yohimbine

Ethanol/Nutrition/Herb Interactions Herb/Nutraceutical: Avoid bayberry, blue cohosh, cayenne, ephedra, ginger, ginseng (American), kola, and licorice (may worsen hypertension). Avoid black cohosh, california poppy, coleus, golden seal, hawthorn, mistletoe, periwinkle, quinine, and shepherd's purse (may increase antihypertensive effect).

Stability Store below 30°C (86°F). Protect from light.

Mechanism of Action Blocks both $beta_1$- and $beta_2$-receptors and has mild intrinsic sympathomimetic activity; pindolol has negative inotropic and chronotropic effects and can significantly slow AV nodal conduction. Augmentive action of antidepressants thought to be mediated via a serotonin 1A autoreceptor antagonism.

Pharmacodynamics/Kinetics

- Absorption: Rapid, 50% to 95%
- Distribution: V_d: ~2 L/kg
- Protein binding: 40%
- Metabolism: Hepatic (60% to 65%) to conjugates
- Half-life elimination: 3-4 hours; prolonged with advanced age, and cirrhosis (range: 2.5-30 hours)
- Time to peak, serum: ~1 hour
- Excretion: Urine (35% to 40% as unchanged drug); feces (6% to 9%)

Dosage Oral:

Adults:

- Hypertension: Initial: 5 mg twice daily, increase as necessary by 10 mg/day every 3-4 weeks (maximum daily dose: 60 mg); usual dose range (JNC 7): 10-40 mg twice daily
- Antidepressant augmentation (unlabeled use): 2.5 mg 3 times/day

Elderly: Initial: 5 mg once daily, increase as necessary by 5 mg/day every 3-4 weeks

Dosing adjustment in renal impairment: Use with caution. Clearance significantly decreased in uremic patients. Dosage reduction may be necessary.

Dosage adjustment in hepatic impairment: Use with caution. Elimination half-life in cirrhotic patients may be 10 times as long compared to normal patients. Dosage reduction is necessary in severely impaired.

Dietary Considerations May be taken without regard to meals.

Monitoring Parameters Blood pressure, heart rate, respiratory function

Dosage Forms Excipient information presented when available (limited, particularly for generics); consult specific product labeling.

Tablet: 5 mg, 10 mg

◆ **Pink Bismuth** *see* Bismuth *on page 199*

Pioglitazone (pye oh GLI ta zone)

U.S. Brand Names Actos®

Canadian Brand Names Actos®; Apo-Pioglitazone; CO Pioglitazone; Gen-Pioglitazone; Novo-Pioglitazone; PMS-Pioglitazone; ratio-Pioglitazone; Sandoz-Pioglitazone; SPEF-Pioglitazone

Pharmacologic Category Antidiabetic Agent, Thiazolidinedione

Additional Appendix Information

Diabetes Mellitus Management, Adults *on page 1801*

Use

Type 2 diabetes mellitus (noninsulin dependent, NIDDM), monotherapy: Adjunct to diet and exercise, to improve glycemic control

Type 2 diabetes mellitus (noninsulin dependent, NIDDM), combination therapy with sulfonylurea, metformin, or insulin: When diet, exercise, and a single agent alone does not result in adequate glycemic control

Unlabeled/Investigational Use Polycystic ovary syndrome (PCOS)

Pregnancy Risk Factor C

Pregnancy Considerations Pioglitazone is classified as pregnancy category C due to adverse effects observed in animal studies. The use of pioglitazone in pregnant women is limited to very few case reports where pregnancy occurred during treatment for polycystic ovarian syndrome (PCOS); details concerning fetal outcomes are limited. Thiazolidinediones may cause ovulation in anovulatory premenopausal women, increasing the risk of pregnancy; adequate contraception in premenopausal women is recommended. Maternal hyperglycemia can be associated with adverse effects in the fetus, including macrosomia, neonatal hyperglycemia, and hyperbilirubinemia; the risk of congenital malformations is increased when the Hb A_{1c} is above the normal range. Diabetes can also be associated with adverse effects in the mother. Poorly-treated diabetes may cause end-organ damage that may in turn negatively affect obstetric outcomes. Physiologic glucose levels should be maintained prior to and during pregnancy to decrease the risk of adverse events in the mother and the fetus. Until additional safety and efficacy data are obtained, the use of oral agents is generally not recommended as routine management of GDM or type 2 diabetes mellitus during pregnancy. Insulin is the drug of choice for the control of diabetes mellitus during pregnancy.

Lactation Excretion in breast milk unknown/not recommended

Medication Safety Issues

Sound-alike/look-alike issues:

Actos® may be confused with Actidose®, Actonel®

Contraindications Hypersensitivity to pioglitazone or any component of the formulation; NYHA Class III/IV heart failure (initiation of therapy)

Warnings/Precautions [U.S. Boxed Warning]: Thiazolidinediones, including pioglitazone, may cause or exacerbate heart failure; closely monitor for signs and symptoms of heart failure (eg, rapid weight gain, dyspnea, edema), particularly after initiation or dose increases. Not recommended for use in any patient with symptomatic heart failure; initiation of therapy is contraindicated in patients with NYHA class III or IV heart failure. If used in patients with NYHA class II (systolic heart failure), initiate at lowest dosage and monitor closely. Use with caution in patients with edema; may increase plasma volume and/or cause fluid retention. Dose reduction or discontinuation is recommended if heart failure suspected. Dose-related weight gain observed with use; mechanism unknown but likely associated with fluid retention and fat accumulation.

Should not be used in diabetic ketoacidosis. Mechanism requires the presence of insulin; therefore use in type 1 diabetes is not recommended. Use with caution in premenopausal, anovulatory women - may result in a resumption of ovulation, increasing the risk of pregnancy. Use with caution in patients with anemia (may reduce hemoglobin and hematocrit). Increased incidence of bone fractures in females treated with pioglitazone; majority of fractures occurred in the lower limb and distal upper limb.

Use with caution in patients with elevated transaminases (AST or ALT); do not initiate in patients with active liver disease of ALT >2.5 times the upper limit of normal at baseline. During therapy, if ALT >3 times the upper limit of normal, reevaluate levels promptly and discontinue if elevation persists or if jaundice occurs at any time during use. Idiosyncratic hepatotoxicity has been reported with another thiazolidinedione agent (troglitazone); avoid use in patients who previously experienced jaundice during troglitazone therapy. Monitoring should include periodic determinations of liver function. Use caution with pre-existing macular edema or diabetic retinopathy. Postmarketing reports of new-onset or worsening diabetic macular edema with decreased visual acuity has been reported. Safety and efficacy have not been established in children.

Adverse Reactions

>10%:

Cardiovascular: Edema (5%; in combination trials with sulfonlyureas or insulin, the incidence of edema was as high as 15%)

Respiratory: Upper respiratory tract infection (13%)

1% to 10%:

Cardiovascular: Heart failure (requiring hospitalization; up to 6% in patients with prior macrovascular disease)

Central nervous system: Headache (9%), fatigue (4%)

Gastrointestinal: Tooth disorder (5%)

Hematologic: Anemia (≤2%)

Neuromuscular & skeletal: Myalgia (5%)

Respiratory: Sinusitis (6%), pharyngitis (5%)

<1% (Limited to important or life-threatening): Bladder cancer, blurred vision, CPK increased, dyspnea (associated with weight gain and/or edema), fractures (females; usually in distal upper limbs or distal lower limbs), hepatic failure (very rare), hepatitis, macular edema (new onset or worsening), transaminases increased, visual acuity decreased

Frequency not defined: HDL-cholesterol increased, hematocrit/hemoglobin decreased, hypoglycemia (in combination trials with sulfonylureas or insulin), serum triglycerides decreased, weight gain/loss

Drug Interactions

Metabolism/Transport Effects Substrate of CYP2C8 (major), 3A4 (minor); **Inhibits** CYP2C8 (moderate), 2C9 (weak), 2C19 (weak), 2D6 (moderate); **Induces** CYP3A4 (weak)

Avoid Concomitant Use

Avoid concomitant use of Pioglitazone with any of the following: Thioridazine

Increased Effect/Toxicity

Pioglitazone may increase the levels/effects of: CYP2C8 Substrates (High risk); CYP2D6 Substrates; Fesoterodine; Nebivolol; Tamoxifen; Thioridazine

The levels/effects of Pioglitazone may be increased by: CYP2C8 Inhibitors (Moderate); CYP2C8 Inhibitors (Strong); Gemfibrozil; Herbs (Hypoglycemic Properties); Insulin; Pegvisomant; Pregabalin; Trimethoprim

Decreased Effect

Pioglitazone may decrease the levels/effects of: Codeine; Maraviroc; TraMADol

The levels/effects of Pioglitazone may be decreased by: Bile Acid Sequestrants; Corticosteroids (Orally Inhaled); Corticosteroids (Systemic); CYP2C8 Inducers (Highly Effective); Luteinizing Hormone-Releasing Hormone Analogs; Rifampin; Somatropin

Ethanol/Nutrition/Herb Interactions

Ethanol: Caution with ethanol (may cause hypoglycemia).

Food: Peak concentrations are delayed when administered with food, but the extent of absorption is not affected. Pioglitazone may be taken without regard to meals.

Herb/Nutraceutical: Caution with alfalfa, aloe, bilberry, bitter melon, burdock, celery, damiana, fenugreek, garcinia, garlic, ginger, ginseng (American), gymnema, marshmallow, and stinging nettle (may cause hypoglycemia).

Mechanism of Action Thiazolidinedione antidiabetic agent that lowers blood glucose by improving target cell response to insulin, without increasing pancreatic insulin secretion. It has a mechanism of action that is dependent on the presence of insulin for activity. Pioglitazone is a potent and selective agonist for peroxisome proliferator-activated receptor-gamma (PPARgamma). Activation of nuclear PPARgamma receptors influences the production of a number of gene products involved in glucose and lipid metabolism. PPARgamma is abundant in the cells within the renal collecting tubules; fluid retention results from stimulation by thiazolidinediones which increases sodium reabsorption.

Pharmacodynamics/Kinetics

Onset of action: Delayed

Peak effect: Glucose control: Several weeks

Distribution: V_{ss} (apparent): 0.63 L/kg

Protein binding: 99.8%; primarily to albumin

Metabolism: Hepatic (99%) via CYP2C8 and 3A4 to both active and inactive metabolites

Half-life elimination: Parent drug: 3-7 hours; Total: 16-24 hours

Time to peak: ~2 hours; delayed with food

Excretion: Urine (15% to 30%) and feces as metabolites

Dosage Oral:

Adults:

Monotherapy: Initial: 15-30 mg once daily; if response is inadequate, the dosage may be increased in increments up to 45 mg once daily; maximum recommended dose: 45 mg once daily

Combination therapy: Maximum recommended dose: 45 mg/day

With sulfonylureas: Initial: 15-30 mg once daily; dose of sulfonylurea should be reduced if the patient reports hypoglycemia

With metformin: Initial: 15-30 mg once daily; it is unlikely that the dose of metformin will need to be reduced due to hypoglycemia

With insulin: Initial: 15-30 mg once daily; dose of insulin should be reduced by 10% to 25% if the patient reports hypoglycemia or if the plasma glucose falls to <100 mg/dL.

Dosage adjustment in patients with CHF (NYHA Class II) in mono- or combination therapy: Initial: 15 mg once daily; may be increased after several months of treatment, with close attention to heart failure symptoms

Elderly: No dosage adjustment is recommended in elderly patients.

Dosage adjustment in renal impairment: No dosage adjustment is required.

Dosage adjustment in hepatic impairment: Clearance is significantly lower in hepatic impairment (Child-Pugh Grade B/C). Therapy should not be initiated if the patient exhibits active liver disease or increased transaminases (>2.5 times ULN) at baseline. During treatment if ALT levels elevate >3 times ULN, the test should be repeated as soon as possible. If ALT levels remain >3 times ULN or if the patient is jaundiced, therapy should be discontinued.

Dietary Considerations Management of type 2 diabetes mellitus (noninsulin dependent, NIDDM) should include diet control. May be taken without regard to meals.

Administration May be administered without regard to meals

Monitoring Parameters Hemoglobin A_{1c}, serum glucose; signs and symptoms of heart failure; liver enzymes prior to initiation and periodically during treatment (per clinician judgment). If the ALT is increased to >2.5 times the upper limit of normal, liver function testing should be performed more frequently until the levels return to normal or pretreatment values. Patients with an elevation in ALT >3 times the upper limit of normal should be rechecked as soon as possible. If the ALT levels remain >3 times the upper limit of normal, therapy with pioglitazone should be discontinued. Routine ophthalmic exams are recommended; patients reporting visual deterioration should have a prompt referral to an ophthalmologist and consideration should be given to discontinuing pioglitazone.

Reference Range Recommendations for glycemic control in adults with diabetes:

Hb A_{1c}: <7%

Preprandial capillary plasma glucose: 70-130 mg/dL

Peak postprandial capillary blood glucose: <180 mg/dL

Blood pressure: <130/80 mm Hg

Dosage Forms Excipient information presented when available (limited, particularly for generics); consult specific product labeling.

Tablet:

Actos®: 15 mg, 30 mg, 45 mg

Pioglitazone and Glimepiride

(pye oh GLI ta zone & GLYE me pye ride)

U.S. Brand Names Duetact™

Index Terms Glimepiride and Pioglitazone; Glimepiride and Pioglitazone Hydrochloride

Pharmacologic Category Antidiabetic Agent, Sulfonylurea; Antidiabetic Agent, Thiazolidinedione; Hypoglycemic Agent, Oral

Use Management of type 2 diabetes mellitus (noninsulin dependent, NIDDM) as an adjunct to diet and exercise

Pregnancy Risk Factor C

Medication Safety Issues

High alert medication: The Institute for Safe Medication Practices (ISMP) includes this medication among its list of drugs which have a heightened risk of causing significant patient harm when used in error.

Dosage Oral: Type 2 diabetes mellitus:

Adults: Initial dose should be based on current dose of pioglitazone and/or sulfonylurea.

Patients inadequately controlled on **glimepiride** alone: Initial dose: 30 mg/2 mg or 30 mg/4 mg once daily

Patients inadequately controlled on **pioglitazone** alone: Initial dose: 30 mg/2 mg once daily

Patients with systolic dysfunction (eg, NYHA Class I and II): Initiate only after patient has been safely titrated to 30 mg of pioglitazone. Initial dose: 30 mg/2 mg or 30 mg/4 mg once daily.

Note: No exact dosing relationship exists between glimepiride and other sulfonlyureas. Dosing should be limited to less than or equal to the maximum initial dose of glimepiride (2 mg). When converting patients from other sulfonylureas with longer half lives (eg, chlorpropamide) to glimepiride, observe patient carefully for 1-2 weeks due to overlapping hypoglycemic effects.

Dosing adjustment: Dosage may be increased up to max dose and formulation strengths available; tablet should not be given more than once daily; see individual agents for frequency of adjustments. Dosage adjustments in patients with systolic dysfunction should be done carefully and patient monitored for symptoms of worsening heart failure.

Maximum dose: Pioglitazone 45 mg/glimepiride 8 mg daily

Elderly: Initial: Glimepiride 1 mg/day prior to initiating Duetact™; dose titration and maintenance dosing should be conservative to avoid hypoglycemia

Dosage adjustment in renal impairment: Cl_{cr} <22 mL/minute: Initial dose should be 1 mg of glimepiride and dosage increments should be based on fasting blood glucose levels

Dosage adjustment in hepatic impairment: Do not initiate treatment with active liver disease or ALT >2.5 times ULN. During treatment, if ALT levels elevate >3 times ULN, the test should be repeated as soon as possible. If ALT levels remain >3 times ULN or if the patient is jaundiced, Duetact™ should be discontinued.

Additional Information Complete prescribing information for this medication should be consulted for additional detail.

Dosage Forms Excipient information presented when available (limited, particularly for generics); consult specific product labeling.

Tablet:

Duetact™:

30 mg/2 mg: Pioglitazone 30 mg and glimepiride 2 mg

30 mg/4 mg: Pioglitazone 30 mg and glimepiride 4 mg

Pioglitazone and Metformin

(pye oh GLI ta zone & met FOR min)

U.S. Brand Names Actoplus Met™

Index Terms Metformin Hydrochloride and Pioglitazone Hydrochloride

Pharmacologic Category Antidiabetic Agent, Biguanide; Antidiabetic Agent, Thiazolidinedione

Use Management of type 2 diabetes mellitus (noninsulin dependent, NIDDM)

Pregnancy Risk Factor C

Dosage Oral: Type 2 diabetes mellitus:

Adults: Initial dose should be based on current dose of pioglitazone and/or metformin; daily dose should be divided and given with meals

Patients inadequately controlled on **metformin alone**: Initial dose: Pioglitazone 15-30 mg/day plus current dose of metformin

Patients inadequately controlled on **pioglitazone alone**: Initial dose: Metformin 1000-1700 mg/day plus current dose of pioglitazone

Note: When switching from combination pioglitazone and metformin as separate tablets: Use current dose.

Dosing adjustment: Doses may be increased as increments of pioglitazone 15 mg and/or metformin 500-850 mg, up to the maximum dose; doses should be titrated gradually. Guidelines for frequency of adjustment (adapted from rosiglitazone/metformin combination labeling):

After a change in the **metformin** dosage, titration can be done after 1-2 weeks

After a change in the **pioglitazone** dosage, titration can be done after 8-12 weeks

Maximum dose: Pioglitazone 45 mg/metformin 2550 mg daily

Elderly: The initial and maintenance dosing should be conservative, due to the potential for decreased renal function (monitor). Generally, elderly patients should not be titrated to the maximum; do not use in patients ≥80 years of age unless normal renal function has been established.

Dosage adjustment in renal impairment: Do not use with renal disease or renal dysfunction (serum creatinine ≥1.5 mg/dL in males or ≥1.4 mg/dL in females or abnormal clearance).

Dosage adjustment in hepatic impairment: Do not initiate treatment with active liver disease or ALT >2.5 times ULN. During treatment if ALT levels elevate >3 times ULN, the test should be repeated as soon as possible. If ALT levels remain >3 times ULN or if the patient is jaundiced, therapy should be discontinued.

Additional Information Complete prescribing information for this medication should be consulted for additional detail.

Dosage Forms Excipient information presented when available (limited, particularly for generics); consult specific product labeling.

Tablet:

Actoplus Met™:

15/500: Pioglitazone 15 mg and metformin hydrochloride 500 mg

15/850: Pioglitazone 15 mg and metformin hydrochloride 850 mg

Piperacillin (pi PER a sil in)

Canadian Brand Names Piperacillin for Injection, USP

Index Terms Piperacillin Sodium

Pharmacologic Category Antibiotic, Penicillin

Additional Appendix Information

Antimicrobial Drugs of Choice *on page 1752*

Community-Acquired Pneumonia in Adults *on page 1766*

Use Treatment of susceptible infections such as septicemia, acute and chronic respiratory tract infections, skin and soft tissue infections, and urinary tract infections due to susceptible strains of *Pseudomonas*, *Proteus*, and *Escherichia coli* and *Enterobacter*, active against some streptococci and some anaerobic bacteria; febrile neutropenia (as part of combination regimen)

Pregnancy Risk Factor B

Dosage

Usual dosage range:

Neonates: I.M., I.V.: 100 mg/kg every 12 hours

Infants and Children: I.M., I.V.: 200-300 mg/kg/day in divided doses every 4-6 hours

Adults: I.M., I.V.: 2-4 g/dose every 4-6 hours (maximum: 24 g/day)

Indication-specific dosing:

Children: I.M., I.V.:

Cystic fibrosis: 350-500 mg/kg/day in divided doses every 4-6 hours

Adults:

Burn wound sepsis: I.V.: 4 g every 4 hours with vancomycin and amikacin

Cholangitis, acute: I.V.: 4 g every 6 hours

Keratitis *(Pseudomonas)*: Ophthalmic: 6-12 mg/mL every 15-60 minutes around the clock for 24-72 hours, then slow reduction

Malignant otitis externa: I.V.: 4-6 g every 4-6 hours with tobramycin

Moderate infections: I.M., I.V.: 2-3 g/dose every 6-12 hours (maximum: 2 g I.M./site)

Prosthetic joint *(Pseudomonas)*: I.V.: 3 g every 6 hours with aminoglycoside

***Pseudomonas* infections:** I.V.: 4 g every 4 hours

Severe infections: I.M., I.V.: 3-4 g/dose every 4-6 hours (maximum: 24 g/24 hours)

Urinary tract infections: I.V.: 2-3 g/dose every 6-12 hours

Uncomplicated gonorrhea: I.M.: 2 g in a single dose accompanied by 1 g probenecid 30 minutes prior to injection

Dosing adjustment in renal impairment: Adults: I.V.:

Cl_{cr} 20-40 mL/minute: Administer 3-4 g every 8 hours

Cl_{cr} <20 mL/minute: Administer 3-4 g every 12 hours

Moderately dialyzable (20% to 50%)

Continuous arteriovenous or venovenous hemodiafiltration effects: Dose as for Cl_{cr} 10-50 mL/minute

Additional Information Complete prescribing information for this medication should be consulted for additional detail.

Dosage Forms Excipient information presented when available (limited, particularly for generics); consult specific product labeling.

Injection, powder for reconstitution: 2 g, 3 g, 4 g, 40 g

Piperacillin and Tazobactam Sodium

(pi PER a sil in & ta zoe BAK tam SOW dee um)

U.S. Brand Names Zosyn®

Canadian Brand Names Tazocin®

Index Terms Piperacillin Sodium and Tazobactam Sodium; Tazobactam and Piperacillin

Pharmacologic Category Antibiotic, Penicillin

Additional Appendix Information

Antimicrobial Drugs of Choice *on page 1752*

Community-Acquired Pneumonia in Adults *on page 1766*

Use Treatment of moderate-to-severe infections caused by susceptible organisms, including infections of the lower respiratory tract (community-acquired pneumonia, nosocomial pneumonia); urinary tract; uncomplicated and complicated skin and skin structures; gynecologic (endometritis, pelvic inflammatory disease); bone and joint infections; intra-abdominal infections (appendicitis with rupture/abscess, peritonitis); and septicemia. Tazobactam expands activity of piperacillin to include beta-lactamase producing strains of *S. aureus*, *H. influenzae*, *Bacteroides*, and other gram-negative bacteria.

Pregnancy Risk Factor B

Pregnancy Considerations Adverse events have not been observed in animal studies; therefore, piperacillin/tazobactam is classified as pregnancy category B. Piperacillin and tazobactam both cross the placenta and are found in the fetal serum, placenta, amniotic fluid, and fetal urine. When used during pregnancy, the clearance and volume of distribution of piperacillin/tazobactam are increased; half-life and AUC are decreased.

Lactation Enters breast milk/use caution

Medication Safety Issues

Sound-alike/look-alike issues:

Zosyn® may be confused with Zofran®, Zyvox®

Contraindications Hypersensitivity to penicillins, beta-lactamase inhibitors, or any component of the formulation

Warnings/Precautions Bleeding disorders have been observed, particularly in patients with renal impairment; discontinue if thrombocytopenia or bleeding occurs. Due to sodium load and to the adverse effects of high serum concentrations of penicillins, dosage modification is required in patients with impaired or underdeveloped renal function; use with caution in patients with seizures or in patients with history of beta-lactam allergy; associated with an increased incidence of rash and fever in cystic fibrosis patients. Prolonged use may result in fungal or bacterial superinfection, including *C. difficile*-associated diarrhea (CDAD) and pseudomembranous colitis; CDAD has been observed >2 months postantibiotic treatment. Safety and efficacy have not been established in children <2 months of age.

Adverse Reactions

>10%: Gastrointestinal: Diarrhea (7% to 11%)

>1% to 10%:

Cardiovascular: Hypertension (2%)

Central nervous system: Insomnia (7%), headache (8%), fever (2% to 5%), agitation (2%), pain (2%)

Dermatologic: Rash (4%), pruritus (3%)

Gastrointestinal: Constipation (1% to 8%), nausea (7%), vomiting (3% to 4%), dyspepsia (3%), stool changes (2%), abdominal pain (1% to 2%)

Hepatic: Transaminases increased

Local: Local reaction (3%), abscess (2%)

Respiratory: Pharyngitis (2%)

Miscellaneous: Moniliasis (2%), sepsis (2%), infection (2%)

≤1% (Limited to important and life-threatening): Agranulocytosis, anaphylaxis/anaphylactoid reaction, anemia, anxiety, arrhythmia, arthralgia, atrial fibrillation, back pain, bradycardia, bronchospasm, candidiasis, cardiac arrest, cardiac failure, circulatory failure, chest pain, cholestatic jaundice, confusion, convulsions, coughing, depression, diaphoresis, dizziness, dyspnea, dysuria, edema, epistaxis, erythema multiforme, flatulence, flushing, gastritis, genital pruritus, hallucination, hematuria, hemolytic anemia, hemorrhage, hepatitis, hiccough, hypoglycemia, hypotension, ileus, incontinence, inflammation, injection site reaction, interstitial nephritis, leukorrhea, malaise, mesenteric embolism, myalgia, myocardial infarction, oliguria, pancytopenia, phlebitis, photophobia, pseudomembranous colitis, pulmonary edema, pulmonary embolism, purpura, renal failure, rhinitis, rigors, Stevens-Johnson syndrome, syncope, tachycardia (supraventricular and ventricular), taste perversion, thirst, thrombocytopenia, thrombocytosis, thrombophlebitis, tinnitus, toxic epidermal necrolysis, tremor, ulcerative stomatitis, urinary retention, vaginitis, ventricular fibrillation, vertigo

Drug Interactions

Avoid Concomitant Use There are no known interactions where it is recommended to avoid concomitant use.

Increased Effect/Toxicity

Piperacillin and Tazobactam Sodium may increase the levels/effects of: Methotrexate

The levels/effects of Piperacillin and Tazobactam Sodium may be increased by: Uricosuric Agents

Decreased Effect

Piperacillin and Tazobactam Sodium may decrease the levels/effects of: Aminoglycosides; Typhoid Vaccine

The levels/effects of Piperacillin and Tazobactam Sodium may be decreased by: Fusidic Acid; Tetracycline Derivatives

Stability

Vials: Store at controlled room temperature of 20°C to 25°C (68°F to 77°F). Use single-dose vials immediately after reconstitution (discard unused portions after 24 hours at room temperature and 48 hours if refrigerated). Reconstitute with 5 mL of diluent per 1 g of piperacillin and then further dilute. After reconstitution, vials or solution are stable in NS or D_5W for 24 hours at room temperature and 48 hours (vials) or 7 days (solution) when refrigerated.

Premixed solution: Store frozen at -20°C (-4°F). Thawed solution is stable for 24 hours at room temperature or 14 days under refrigeration; do not refreeze.

Mechanism of Action Inhibits bacterial cell wall synthesis by binding to one or more of the penicillin binding proteins (PBPs); which in turn inhibits the final transpeptidation step of peptidoglycan synthesis in bacterial cell walls, thus inhibiting cell wall biosynthesis. Bacteria eventually lyse due to ongoing activity of cell wall autolytic enzymes (autolysins and murein hydrolases) while cell wall assembly is arrested. Tazobactam inhibits many beta-lactamases, including staphylococcal penicillinase and Richmond and Sykes types II, III, IV, and V, including extended spectrum enzymes; it has only limited activity against class I beta-lactamases other than class Ic types.

Pharmacodynamics/Kinetics Both AUC and peak concentrations are dose proportional; hepatic impairment does not affect kinetics

Distribution: Well into lungs, intestinal mucosa, skin, muscle, uterus, ovary, prostate, gallbladder, and bile; penetration into CSF is low in subject with noninflamed meninges

Protein binding: Piperacillin and tazobactam: ~30%

Metabolism:

Piperacillin: 6% to 9% to desethyl metabolite (weak activity)

Tazobactam: ~26% to inactive metabolite

Bioavailability:

Piperacillin: I.M.: 71%

Tazobactam: I.M.: 84%

Half-life elimination: Piperacillin and tazobactam: 0.7-1.2 hours

Time to peak, plasma: Immediately following infusion of 30 minutes

Excretion: Clearance of both piperacillin and tazobactam are directly proportional to renal function

Piperacillin: Urine (68% as unchanged drug); feces (10% to 20%)

Tazobactam: Urine (80% as unchanged drug; remainder as inactive metabolite)

Dosage

Usual dosage range:

Children: I.V.:

2-8 months: 80 mg of piperacillin component/kg every 8 hours

≥9 months and ≤40 kg: 100 mg of piperacillin component/kg every 8 hours

Adults: I.V.: 3.375 g every 6 hours **or** 4.5 g every 6-8 hours; maximum: 18 g/day

Indication-specific dosing: I.V.:

Children: **Note:** Dosing based on piperacillin component:

Appendicitis, peritonitis:

2-8 months: 80 mg/kg every 8 hours

≥9 months and ≤40 kg: 100 mg/kg every 8 hours

>40 kg: refer to Adult dosing

Cystic fibrosis, pseudomonal infections (unlabeled use): 350-450 mg/kg/day in divided doses

Adults:

Diverticulitis, intra-abdominal abscess, peritonitis: I.V.: 3.375 g every 6 hours; **Note:** Some clinicians use 4.5 g every 8 hours for empiric coverage since the % time>MIC is similar between the regimens for most pathogens; however, this regimen is NOT recommended for nosocomial pneumonia or *Pseudomonas* coverage.

Pneumonia (nosocomial): I.V.: 4.5 g every 6 hours for 7-14 days (when used empirically, combination with an aminoglycoside or antipseudomonal fluoroquinolone is recommended; consider discontinuation of additional agent if *P. aeruginosa* is not isolated)

Severe infections: I.V.: 3.375 g every 6 hours for 7-10 days; **Note:** Some clinicians use 4.5 g every 8 hours for empiric coverage since the %time>MIC is similar between the regimens for most pathogens; however, this regimen is NOT recommended for nosocomial pneumonia or *Pseudomonas* coverage.

Dosing interval in renal impairment:

Cl_{cr} 20-40 mL/minute: Administer 2.25 g every 6 hours (3.375 g every 6 hours for nosocomial pneumonia)

Cl_{cr} <20 mL/minute: Administer 2.25 g every 8 hours (2.25 g every 6 hours for nosocomial pneumonia)

Hemodialysis/CAPD: Administer 2.25 g every 12 hours (2.25 g every 8 hours for nosocomial pneumonia) with an additional dose of 0.75 g after each hemodialysis session

Continuous renal replacement therapy (CRRT): Drug clearance is highly dependent on the method of renal replacement, filter type, and flow rate. Appropriate dosing requires close monitoring of pharmacologic response, signs of adverse reactions due to drug accumulation, as well as drug levels in relation to target trough (if appropriate). The following are general recommendations only (based on dialysate flow/ultrafiltration rates of 1 L/hour) and should not supersede clinical judgment:

CVVH: 2.25 g every 6 hours

CVVHD/CVVHDF: 2.25-3.375 g every 6 hours

Note: Higher dose of 3.375 g should be considered when treating resistant pathogens (especially *Pseudomonas*); alternative recommendations suggest dosing of 4.5 g every 8 hours; regardless of regimen, there is some concern of tazobactam (TAZ) accumulation, given its lower clearance relative to piperacillin (PIP). Some clinicians advocate dosing with PIP to alternate with PIP/TAZ, particularly in CVVH-dependent patients, to lessen this concern.

Dietary Considerations

Infusion, premixed: 2.25 g contains sodium 5.58 mEq (128 mg); 3.375 g contains sodium 8.38 mEq (192 mg); 4.5 g contains sodium 11.17 mEq (256 mg)

Injection, powder for reconstitution: 2.25 g contains sodium 5.58 mEq (128 mg); 3.375 g contains sodium 8.38 mEq (192 mg); 4.5 g contains sodium 11.17 mEq (256 mg); 40.5 g contains sodium 100.4 mEq (2304 mg, bulk pharmacy vial)

Administration Administer by I.V. infusion over 30 minutes

Some penicillins (eg, carbenicillin, ticarcillin and piperacillin) have been shown to inactivate aminoglycosides *in vitro*. This has been observed to a greater extent with tobramycin and gentamicin, while amikacin has shown greater stability against inactivation. Concurrent use of these agents may pose a risk of reduced antibacterial efficacy *in vivo*, particularly in the setting of profound renal impairment. However, definitive clinical evidence is lacking. If combination penicillin/aminoglycoside therapy is desired in a patient with renal dysfunction, separation of doses (if feasible), and routine monitoring of aminoglycoside levels, CBC, and clinical response should be considered. **Note:** Reformulated Zosyn® containing EDTA has been shown to be compatible *in vitro* for Y-site infusion with amikacin and gentamicin, but not compatible with tobramycin.

Monitoring Parameters Creatinine, BUN, CBC with differential, PT, PTT; signs of bleeding; monitor for signs of anaphylaxis during first dose

Test Interactions Positive Coombs' [direct] test; false positive reaction for urine glucose using copper-reduction method (Clinitest®); may result in false positive results with the Platelia® *Aspergillus* enzyme immunoassay (EIA)

Some penicillin derivatives may accelerate the degradation of aminoglycosides *in vitro*, leading to a potential underestimation of aminoglycoside serum concentration. **Note:** Reformulated Zosyn® containing EDTA has been shown to be compatible *in vitro* for Y-site infusion with amikacin and gentamicin, but not compatible with tobramycin.

Dosage Forms Excipient information presented when available (limited, particularly for generics); consult specific product labeling.

Note: 8:1 ratio of piperacillin sodium/tazobactam sodium

Infusion [premixed iso-osmotic solution, frozen]:

2.25 g: Piperacillin 2 g and tazobactam 0.25 g (50 mL) [contains sodium 5.58 mEq (128 mg) and EDTA]

3.375 g: Piperacillin 3 g and tazobactam 0.375 g (50 mL) [contains sodium 8.38 mEq (192 mg) and EDTA]

4.5 g: Piperacillin 4 g and tazobactam 0.5 g (50 mL) [contains sodium 11.17 mEq (256 mg) and EDTA]

Injection, powder for reconstitution:

2.25 g: Piperacillin 2 g and tazobactam 0.25 g [contains sodium 5.58 mEq (128 mg) and EDTA]

3.375 g: Piperacillin 3 g and tazobactam 0.375 g [contains sodium 8.38 mEq (192 mg) and EDTA]

4.5 g: Piperacillin 4 g and tazobactam 0.5 g [contains sodium 11.17 mEq (256 mg) and EDTA]

40.5 g: Piperacillin 36 g and tazobactam 4.5 g [contains sodium 100.4 mEq (2304 mg) and EDTA; bulk pharmacy vial]

◆ **Piperacillin for Injection, USP (Can)** *see* Piperacillin *on page 1198*

◆ **Piperacillin Sodium** *see* Piperacillin *on page 1198*

◆ **Piperacillin Sodium and Tazobactam Sodium** *see* Piperacillin and Tazobactam Sodium *on page 1198*

◆ **Piperazine Estrone Sulfate** *see* Estropipate *on page 568*

◆ **Piperonyl Butoxide and Pyrethrins** *see* Pyrethrins and Piperonyl Butoxide *on page 1271*

Pirbuterol (peer BYOO ter ole)

U.S. Brand Names Maxair™ Autohaler™

Index Terms Pirbuterol Acetate

Pharmacologic Category $Beta_2$-Adrenergic Agonist

Additional Appendix Information

Bronchodilators *on page 1650*

Use Prevention and treatment of reversible bronchospasm including asthma

Pregnancy Risk Factor C

Lactation Excretion in breast milk unknown

Contraindications Hypersensitivity to pirbuterol, albuterol, or any component of the formulation

Warnings/Precautions Optimize anti-inflammatory treatment before initiating maintenance treatment with pirbuterol. Do not use as a component of chronic therapy without an anti-inflammatory agent. Only the mildest form of asthma (Step 1 and/or exercise-induced) would not require concurrent use based upon asthma guidelines. Patient must be instructed to seek medical attention in cases where acute symptoms are not relieved or a previous level of response is diminished. The need to increase frequency of use may indicate deterioration of asthma, and treatment must not be delayed.

Use caution in patients with cardiovascular disease (arrhythmia or hypertension or CHF), convulsive disorders, diabetes, glaucoma, hyperthyroidism, or hypokalemia. Beta-agonists may cause elevation in blood pressure, heart rate, and result in CNS stimulation/excitation. $Beta_2$-agonists may increase risk of arrhythmia, increase serum glucose, or decrease serum potassium.

Do not exceed recommended dose; serious adverse events including fatalities, have been associated with excessive use of inhaled sympathomimetics. Rarely, paradoxical bronchospasm may occur with use of inhaled bronchodilating agents; this should be distinguished from inadequate response. All patients should utilize a spacer device when using a metered-dose inhaler. Safety and efficacy have not been established in children <12 years of age.

Adverse Reactions

>10%:

Central nervous system: Nervousness, restlessness

Endocrine & metabolic: Serum glucose increased, serum potassium decreased

Neuromuscular & skeletal: Trembling

1% to 10%:

Cardiovascular: Tachycardia, palpitation

Central nervous system: Headache, dizziness, lightheadedness

Gastrointestinal: Taste changes, vomiting, nausea

<1% (Limited to important or life-threatening): Arrhythmias, chest pain, hypertension, hypokalemia, insomnia, paradoxical bronchospasm

Drug Interactions

Avoid Concomitant Use

Avoid concomitant use of Pirbuterol with any of the following: Iobenguane I 123

Increased Effect/Toxicity

Pirbuterol may increase the levels/effects of: Sympathomimetics

The levels/effects of Pirbuterol may be increased by: Atomoxetine; Cannabinoids; MAO Inhibitors; Tricyclic Antidepressants

Decreased Effect

Pirbuterol may decrease the levels/effects of: Iobenguane I 123

The levels/effects of Pirbuterol may be decreased by: Alpha-/Beta-Blockers; Beta-Blockers (Beta1 Selective); Beta-Blockers (Nonselective); Betahistine

Stability Store between 15°C and 30°C (59°F and 86°F).

Mechanism of Action Pirbuterol is a $beta_2$-adrenergic agonist with a similar structure to albuterol, specifically a pyridine ring has been substituted for the benzene ring in albuterol. The increased $beta_2$ selectivity of pirbuterol results from the substitution of a tertiary butyl group on the nitrogen of the side chain, which additionally imparts resistance of pirbuterol to degradation by monoamine oxidase and provides a lengthened duration of action in comparison to the less selective previous beta-agonist agents.

Pharmacodynamics/Kinetics

Onset of action: Peak effect: Therapeutic: Oral: 2-3 hours with peak serum concentration of 6.2-9.8 mcg/L; Inhalation: 0.5-1 hour

Half-life elimination: 2-3 hours

Metabolism: Hepatic

Excretion: Urine (10% as unchanged drug)

Dosage Children ≥12 years and Adults: 2 inhalations every 4-6 hours for prevention; two inhalations at an interval of at least 1-3 minutes, followed by a third inhalation in treatment of bronchospasm, not to exceed 12 inhalations/day

Administration Inhalation: Shake inhaler well before use.

Monitoring Parameters Respiratory rate; FEV_1, peak flow, and/or other pulmonary function tests; blood pressure, heart rate; CNS stimulation; serum glucose, serum potassium

Dosage Forms Excipient information presented when available (limited, particularly for generics); consult specific product labeling.

Aerosol for oral inhalation, as acetate:

Maxair™ Autohaler™: 200 mcg/actuation (14 g) [400 actuations; contains chlorofluorocarbons]

◆ **Pirbuterol Acetate** *see* Pirbuterol *on page 1200*

Piroxicam (peer OKS i kam)

U.S. Brand Names Feldene®

Canadian Brand Names Apo-Piroxicam®; Gen-Piroxicam; Novo-Pirocam; Nu-Pirox; Pexicam®

Pharmacologic Category Nonsteroidal Anti-inflammatory Drug (NSAID), Oral

Additional Appendix Information

Nonsteroidal Anti-inflammatory Agents *on page 1669*

Use Symptomatic treatment of acute and chronic rheumatoid arthritis and osteoarthritis

Unlabeled/Investigational Use Ankylosing spondylitis

Restrictions An FDA-approved medication guide must be distributed when dispensing an oral outpatient prescription (new or refill) where this medication is to be used without direct supervision of a healthcare provider. Medication guides are available at http://www.fda.gov/cder/Offices/ODS/medication_guides.htm.

Pregnancy Risk Factor C/D (3rd trimester)

Medication Safety Issues

International issues:

Flogene® [Brazil] may be confused with Florone® which is a brand name for diflorasone in the U.S.

Dosage Oral:

Children (unlabeled use): 0.2-0.3 mg/kg/day once daily; maximum dose: 15 mg/day

Adults: 10-20 mg/day once daily; although associated with increase in GI adverse effects, doses >20 mg/day have been used (ie, 30-40 mg/day)

Dosing adjustment in renal impairment: Not recommended in patients with advanced renal disease

Dosing adjustment in hepatic impairment: Reduction of dosage is necessary

Additional Information Complete prescribing information for this medication should be consulted for additional detail.

Dosage Forms Excipient information presented when available (limited, particularly for generics); consult specific product labeling.

Capsule: 10 mg, 20 mg

◆ ***p*-Isobutylhydratropic Acid** *see* Ibuprofen *on page 760*

◆ **Pit** *see* Oxytocin *on page 1126*

- ◆ **Pitocin®** *see* Oxytocin *on page 1126*
- ◆ **Pitrex (Can)** *see* Tolnaftate *on page 1487*
- ◆ **PLA** *see* Poly-L-Lactic Acid *on page 1210*
- ◆ **Plan B® [RX/OTC]** *see* Levonorgestrel *on page 879*
- ◆ **Plan B™ (Can)** *see* Levonorgestrel *on page 879*
- ◆ **Plantago Seed** *see* Psyllium *on page 1268*
- ◆ **Plantain Seed** *see* Psyllium *on page 1268*
- ◆ **Plaquenil®** *see* Hydroxychloroquine *on page 751*
- ◆ **Plaretase® 8000** *see* Pancrelipase *on page 1136*
- ◆ **Plasbumin®** *see* Albumin *on page 49*
- ◆ **Plasbumin®-5 (Can)** *see* Albumin *on page 49*
- ◆ **Plasbumin®-25 (Can)** *see* Albumin *on page 49*
- ◆ **Plavix®** *see* Clopidogrel *on page 356*
- ◆ **Plendil®** *see* Felodipine *on page 606*

Plerixafor (pler IX a fore)

U.S. Brand Names Mozobil™

Index Terms AMD3100; LM3100

Pharmacologic Category Hematopoietic Stem Cell Mobilizer

Use Mobilization of hematopoietic stem cells (HSC) for collection and subsequent autologous transplantation (in combination with G-CSF) in patients with non-Hodgkin's lymphoma (NHL) and multiple myeloma (MM)

Pregnancy Risk Factor D

Pregnancy Considerations Adverse effects (including fetal mortality, decreased fetal weights, and teratogenicity) have been reported in animal studies. May cause fetal harm if administered to pregnant women. There are no adequate and well-controlled studies in pregnant women. Women of childbearing potential should use effective contraceptive measures to avoid becoming pregnant during treatment.

Lactation Excretion in breast milk unknown/not recommended

Contraindications There are no contraindications listed within the manufacturer's labeling.

Warnings/Precautions Increases circulating leukocytes when used in conjunction with G-CSF; monitor WBC; use with caution in patients with neutrophil count >50,000/mm^3. Thrombocytopenia has been observed with use; monitor platelet count. Not intended for mobilization in patients with leukemia; may contaminate apheresis product by mobilizing leukemic cells. When used in combination with G-CSF, tumor cells released from marrow could be collected in leukapheresis product; potential effect of tumor cell reinfusion is unknown. Splenomegaly and splenic rupture have been reported (rarely) with G-CSF use; instruct patients to report left upper quadrant pain or scapular/shoulder tip pain; promptly evaluate in any patient who report these.

Primary route of elimination is urinary; dosage reduction is recommended in patients with moderate-severe renal impairment (Cl_{cr} ≤50 mL/minute). Medications that may reduce renal function or compete for active tubular secretion may increase serum concentrations of plerixafor. Use has not been studied in patients weighing >175% of ideal body weight. Safety and efficacy have not been established in children.

Adverse Reactions Adverse reactions reported with G-CSF combination therapy.

>10%:

Central nervous system: Fatigue (27%), headache (22%), dizziness (11%)

Gastrointestinal: Diarrhea (37%), nausea (34%)

Local: Injection site reactions (34%, including erythema, hematoma, hemorrhage, induration, inflammation, irritation, pain, paresthesia, pruritus, rash, swelling, urticaria)

Neuromuscular & skeletal: Arthralgia (13%)

5% to 10%:

Central nervous system: Insomnia (7%)

Gastrointestinal: Vomiting (10%), flatulence (7%)

<5% (Limited to important or life-threatening): Abdominal discomfort, abdominal distension, abdominal pain, constipation, diaphoresis, dyspepsia, dyspnea, erythema, hypesthesia (oral), hypoxia, leukocytes increased, malaise, musculoskeletal pain, orthostatic hypotension, periorbital swelling, syncope, thrombocytopenia, urticaria, vasovagal reaction, xerostomia

Drug Interactions

Avoid Concomitant Use There are no known interactions where it is recommended to avoid concomitant use.

Increased Effect/Toxicity There are no known significant interactions involving an increase in effect.

Decreased Effect There are no known significant interactions involving a decrease in effect.

Stability Store at 25°C (77°F); excursions permitted to 15°C to 30°C (59°F to 86°F). The manufacturer recommends discarding unused drug remaining in the vial after use.

Mechanism of Action Reversibly inhibits binding of stromal cell-derived factor-1-alpha (SDF-1α), expressed on bone marrow stromal cells, to the CXC chemokine receptor 4 (CXCR4), resulting in mobilization of hematopoietic stem and progenitor cells from bone marrow into peripheral blood. Plerixafor used in combination with G-CSF results in synergistic increase in CD34+ cell mobilization. Mobilized CD34+ cells are capable of engrafting with extended repopulating capacity.

Pharmacodynamics/Kinetics

Onset of action: Peak CD34+ mobilization: Plerixafor monotherapy: 6-9 hours after administration; Plerixafor + G-CSF: 10-14 hours

Duration: WBC counts return toward baseline at ~24 after administration

Absorption: SubQ: Rapid

Distribution: 0.3L/kg; primarily to extravascular fluid space

Protein binding: ≤58%

Metabolism: Not metabolized

Half-life elimination: Terminal: 3-6 hours

Time to peak, plasma: SubQ: 30-60 minutes

Excretion: Urine (~70%; as parent drug)

Dosage Note: Dosing is based on actual body weight. Begin plerixafor after patient has received G-CSF 10 mcg/kg once daily for 4 days; plerixafor, G-CSF and apheresis should be continued daily until sufficient cell collection up to a maximum of 4 days.

SubQ: Adults: HSC mobilization: 0.24 mg/kg once daily ~11 hours prior to apheresis for up to 4 consecutive days; maximum dose: 40 mg/day

Dosage adjustment in renal impairment:

Cl_{cr} >50 mL/minute: No adjustment required

Cl_{cr} ≤50 mL/minute: 0.16 mg/kg; maximum dose: 27 mg/day

Hemodialysis: Insufficient information for dosing recommendation

Administration Administer subcutaneously, ~11 hours prior to initiation of apheresis. In some clinical trials, plerixafor administration began in the evening prior to apheresis. (G-CSF was begun on day 1, plerixafor initiated in the evening on day 4 and apheresis in the morning on day 5; with G-CSF, plerixafor and apheresis then continued daily until sufficient cell collection for autologous transplant.)

Monitoring Parameters CBC with differential and platelets

Dosage Forms Excipient information presented when available (limited, particularly for generics); consult specific product labeling.
Injection, solution [preservative free]:
Mozobil™: 20 mg/mL (1.2 mL)

- **Pletal®** *see* Cilostazol *on page 325*
- **Plexion®** *see* Sulfur and Sulfacetamide *on page 1411*
- **Plexion SCT®** *see* Sulfur and Sulfacetamide *on page 1411*
- **Plexion TS® [DSC]** *see* Sulfur and Sulfacetamide *on page 1411*
- **Pliaglis™** *see* Lidocaine and Tetracaine *on page 888*
- **PMPA** *see* Tenofovir *on page 1438*
- **PMS-Alendronate (Can)** *see* Alendronate *on page 58*
- **PMS-Alendronate-FC (Can)** *see* Alendronate *on page 58*
- **PMS-Amantadine (Can)** *see* Amantadine *on page 78*
- **PMS-Amiodarone (Can)** *see* Amiodarone *on page 87*
- **PMS-Amitriptyline (Can)** *see* Amitriptyline *on page 90*
- **PMS-Amoxicillin (Can)** *see* Amoxicillin *on page 98*
- **PMS-Anagrelide (Can)** *see* Anagrelide *on page 115*
- **PMS-Atenolol (Can)** *see* Atenolol *on page 149*
- **PMS-Azithromycin (Can)** *see* Azithromycin *on page 166*
- **PMS-Baclofen (Can)** *see* Baclofen *on page 172*
- **PMS-Bethanechol (Can)** *see* Bethanechol *on page 192*
- **PMS-Bicalutamide (Can)** *see* Bicalutamide *on page 197*
- **PMS-Bisoprolol (Can)** *see* Bisoprolol *on page 200*
- **PMS-Brimonidine Tartrate (Can)** *see* Brimonidine *on page 212*
- **PMS-Bromocriptine (Can)** *see* Bromocriptine *on page 213*
- **PMS-Bupropion SR (Can)** *see* BuPROPion *on page 223*
- **PMS-Buspirone (Can)** *see* BusPIRone *on page 226*
- **PMS-Butorphanol (Can)** *see* Butorphanol *on page 231*
- **PMS-Captopril (Can)** *see* Captopril *on page 249*
- **PMS-Carbamazepine (Can)** *see* CarBAMazepine *on page 252*
- **PMS-Carvedilol (Can)** *see* Carvedilol *on page 264*
- **PMS-Cefaclor (Can)** *see* Cefaclor *on page 268*
- **PMS-Cetirizine (Can)** *see* Cetirizine *on page 295*
- **PMS-Chloral Hydrate (Can)** *see* Chloral Hydrate *on page 300*
- **PMS-Cholestyramine (Can)** *see* Cholestyramine Resin *on page 319*
- **PMS-Cimetidine (Can)** *see* Cimetidine *on page 326*
- **PMS-Ciprofloxacin (Can)** *see* Ciprofloxacin *on page 329*
- **PMS-Citalopram (Can)** *see* Citalopram *on page 337*
- **PMS-Clarithromycin (Can)** *see* Clarithromycin *on page 341*
- **PMS-Clindamycin (Can)** *see* Clindamycin *on page 344*
- **PMS-Clobetasol (Can)** *see* Clobetasol *on page 347*
- **PMS-Clonazepam (Can)** *see* ClonazePAM *on page 352*
- **PMS-Clozapine (Can)** *see* Clozapine *on page 359*
- **PMS-Deferoxamine (Can)** *see* Deferoxamine *on page 411*
- **PMS-Desipramine (Can)** *see* Desipramine *on page 418*
- **PMS-Desmopressin (Can)** *see* Desmopressin *on page 421*
- **PMS-Desonide (Can)** *see* Desonide *on page 424*
- **PMS-Dexamethasone (Can)** *see* Dexamethasone *on page 425*
- **PMS-Dicitrate (Can)** *see* Sodium Citrate and Citric Acid *on page 1383*
- **PMS-Diclofenac (Can)** *see* Diclofenac *on page 437*
- **PMS-Diclofenac SR (Can)** *see* Diclofenac *on page 437*
- **PMS-Diphenhydramine (Can)** *see* DiphenhydrAMINE *on page 456*
- **PMS-Dipivefrin (Can)** *see* Dipivefrin *on page 466*
- **PMS-Docusate Calcium (Can)** *see* Docusate *on page 473*
- **PMS-Docusate Sodium (Can)** *see* Docusate *on page 473*
- **PMS-Enalapril (Can)** *see* Enalapril *on page 515*
- **PMS-Erythromycin (Can)** *see* Erythromycin *on page 544*
- **PMS-Famciclovir (Can)** *see* Famciclovir *on page 602*
- **PMS-Fenofibrate Micro (Can)** *see* Fenofibrate *on page 607*
- **PMS-Fluconazole (Can)** *see* Fluconazole *on page 625*
- **PMS-Flunisolide (Can)** *see* Flunisolide *on page 632*
- **PMS-Fluorometholone (Can)** *see* Fluorometholone *on page 636*
- **PMS-Fluoxetine (Can)** *see* FLUoxetine *on page 638*
- **PMS-Fluphenazine Decanoate (Can)** *see* Fluphenazine *on page 641*
- **PMS-Fluvoxamine (Can)** *see* Fluvoxamine *on page 652*
- **PMS-Fosinopril (Can)** *see* Fosinopril *on page 670*
- **PMS-Furosemide (Can)** *see* Furosemide *on page 676*
- **PMS-Gabapentin (Can)** *see* Gabapentin *on page 678*
- **PMS-Gemfibrozil (Can)** *see* Gemfibrozil *on page 687*
- **PMS-Glimepiride (Can)** *see* Glimepiride *on page 696*
- **PMS-Glyburide (Can)** *see* GlyBURIDE *on page 701*
- **PMS-Haloperidol LA (Can)** *see* Haloperidol *on page 720*
- **PMS-Hydrochlorothiazide (Can)** *see* Hydrochlorothiazide *on page 737*
- **PMS-Hydromorphone (Can)** *see* HYDROmorphone *on page 747*
- **PMS-Hydroxyzine (Can)** *see* HydrOXYzine *on page 754*
- **PMS-Indapamide (Can)** *see* Indapamide *on page 781*
- **PMS-Ipratropium (Can)** *see* Ipratropium *on page 811*
- **PMS-ISMN (Can)** *see* Isosorbide Mononitrate *on page 824*
- **PMS-Isoniazid (Can)** *see* Isoniazid *on page 820*
- **PMS-Isosorbide (Can)** *see* Isosorbide Dinitrate *on page 823*
- **PMS-Lactulose (Can)** *see* Lactulose *on page 847*
- **PMS-Lamotrigine (Can)** *see* LamoTRIgine *on page 850*
- **PMS-Leflunomide (Can)** *see* Leflunomide *on page 859*
- **PMS-Levetiracetam (Can)** *see* Levetiracetam *on page 872*
- **PMS-Levobunolol (Can)** *see* Levobunolol *on page 873*
- **PMS-Lindane (Can)** *see* Lindane *on page 889*
- **PMS-Lisinopril (Can)** *see* Lisinopril *on page 894*
- **PMS-Lithium Carbonate (Can)** *see* Lithium *on page 897*
- **PMS-Lithium Citrate (Can)** *see* Lithium *on page 897*
- **PMS-Loperamine (Can)** *see* Loperamide *on page 900*
- **PMS-Lorazepam (Can)** *see* LORazepam *on page 905*
- **PMS-Lovastatin (Can)** *see* Lovastatin *on page 910*
- **PMS-Loxapine (Can)** *see* Loxapine *on page 912*

Pneumococcal Conjugate Vaccine (7-Valent)

(noo moe KOK al KON ju gate vak SEEN, seven vay lent)

U.S. Brand Names Prevnar®

Canadian Brand Names Prevnar®

Index Terms Diphtheria CRM_{197} Protein; PCV; PCV7; Pneumococcal 7-Valent Conjugate Vaccine

Pharmacologic Category Vaccine, Inactivated (Bacterial)

Additional Appendix Information

Immunization Recommendations *on page* 1708

Use

Immunization of infants and toddlers against *Streptococcus pneumoniae* infection caused by serotypes included in the vaccine

Immunization of infant and toddlers against otitis media caused by serotypes included in the vaccine

Advisory Committee on Immunization Practices (ACIP) recommends routine vaccination for the following:

All children 2-23 months

Children ≥2-59 months with cochlear implants

Children ages 24-59 months with: Sickle cell disease (including other sickle cell hemoglobinopathies, asplenia, splenic dysfunction), HIV infection, immunocompromising conditions (congenital immunodeficiencies excluding chronic granulomatous disease, renal failure, nephrotic syndrome, diseases associated with immunosuppressive or radiation therapy, solid organ transplant), chronic illnesses (cardiac disease, cerebrospinal fluid leaks, diabetes mellitus, pulmonary disease excluding asthma unless on high dose corticosteroids)

Consider use in all children 24-59 months with priority given to:

Children 24-35 months

Children 24-59 months who are of Alaska native, American Indian, or African-American descent

Children 24-59 months who attend group day care centers

Pregnancy Risk Factor C

Pregnancy Considerations Reproduction studies have not been conducted. This product is indicated for use in infants and toddlers.

Lactation Excretion in breast milk unknown/not recommended

Medication Safety Issues

Sound-alike/look-alike issues:

Prevnar® may be confused with PREVEN®

Contraindications Hypersensitivity to pneumococcal vaccine or any component of the formulation, including diphtheria toxoid

Warnings/Precautions Use caution in latex sensitivity. Children with impaired immune responsiveness may have a reduced response to active immunization. The decision to administer or delay vaccination because of current or recent febrile illness depends on the severity of symptoms and the etiology of the disease. Immunization should be delayed during the course of an acute severe febrile illness; may administer to patients with mild acute illness (with or without fever). Use caution in children with coagulation disorders (including thrombocytopenia) where intramuscular injections should not be used. Epinephrine 1:1000 should be readily available. Use of pneumococcal conjugate vaccine does not replace use of the 23-valent pneumococcal polysaccharide vaccine in children ≥24 months of age with sickle cell disease, asplenia, HIV infection, chronic illness or if immunocompromised. Not to be used to treat pneumococcal infections or to provide immunity against diphtheria. Febrile seizures have been reported (rare). Antipyretics should be administered at the time of vaccination to patients at risk for seizures to reduce the risk of postvaccination fever. In order to maximize vaccination rates, the ACIP recommends simultaneous administration of all age-appropriate vaccines (live or inactivated) for which a person is eligible at a single clinic visit, unless contraindications exist. Safety and efficacy have not been established in children <6 weeks or ≥10 years of age. Not for I.V. use.

Adverse Reactions All serious adverse reactions must be reported to the U.S. Department of Health and Human Services (DHHS) Vaccine Adverse Event Reporting System (VAERS) 1-800-822-7967.

>10%:

Central nervous system: Fever, irritability, drowsiness, restlessness

Dermatologic: Erythema

Gastrointestinal: Decreased appetite, vomiting, diarrhea

Local: Induration, tenderness, nodule

1% to 10%: Dermatologic: Rash

Postmarketing and/or case reports: Anaphylactic reaction, anaphylactoid reaction, angioneurotic edema, apnea, bronchospasm, crying, dyspnea, erythema multiforme, facial edema, febrile seizure, hypersensitivity reaction, injection site reaction (eg, dermatitis, lymphadenopathy, pruritus, urticaria), shock

Drug Interactions

Avoid Concomitant Use There are no known interactions where it is recommended to avoid concomitant use.

Increased Effect/Toxicity There are no known significant interactions involving an increase in effect.

Decreased Effect

The levels/effects of Pneumococcal Conjugate Vaccine (7-Valent) may be decreased by: Immunosuppressants

Stability Store refrigerated at 2°C to 8°C (36°F to 46°F); do not freeze.

Mechanism of Action Promotes active immunization against invasive disease caused by *S. pneumoniae* capsular serotypes 4, 6B, 9V, 14, 18C, 19F, and 23F, all which are individually conjugated to CRM197 protein

Dosage I.M.:

Infants: 2-6 months: 0.5 mL at approximately 2-month intervals for 3 consecutive doses, followed by a fourth dose of 0.5 mL at 12-15 months of age; first dose may be given as young as 6 weeks of age, but is typically given at 2 months of age. In case of a moderate shortage of vaccine, defer the fourth dose until shortage is resolved; in case of a severe shortage of vaccine, defer third and fourth doses until shortage is resolved.

Previously Unvaccinated Older Infants and Children:

7-11 months: 0.5 mL for a total of 3 doses; 2 doses at least 4 weeks apart, followed by a third dose after the 1-year birthday (12-15 months), separated from the second dose by at least 2 months. In case of a severe shortage of vaccine, defer the third dose until shortage is resolved.

12-23 months: 0.5 mL for a total of 2 doses, separated by at least 2 months. In case of a severe shortage of vaccine, defer the second dose until shortage is resolved.

24-59 months:

Healthy Children: 0.5 mL as a single dose. In case of a severe shortage of vaccine, defer dosing until shortage is resolved.

Children with sickle cell disease, asplenia, HIV infection, chronic illness or immunocompromising conditions: 0.5 mL for a total of 2 doses, separated by 2 months

Previously Vaccinated with PPSV (ACIP recommendations): Children 24-59 months of age at high risk for pneumococcal disease but have already received the PPSV may benefit from the immunologic response induced by PCV. Suggested dosing: Starting ≥2 months after last PPSV dose: One dose of PCV, followed by a second dose ≥2 months later.

Previously Vaccinated with PCV and with a lapse in vaccine administration (ACIP recommendations) :

7-11 months: Previously received 1 or 2 doses PCV: 0.5 mL dose at 7-11 months of age, followed by a second dose ≥2 months later at 12-15 months of age

12-23 months:

Previously received 1 dose before 12 months of age: 0.5 mL dose, followed by a second dose ≥2 months later

Previously received 2 doses before age 12 months: 0.5 mL dose ≥2 months after the most recent dose

24-59 months: Any incomplete schedule: 0.5 mL as a single dose; **Note:** Patients with chronic diseases or immunosuppressing conditions should receive 2 doses ≥2 months apart

Administration Shake well prior to use. Administer I.M. (deltoid muscle for toddlers and young children or lateral midthigh in infants). Do not inject I.V.; avoid intradermal route.

For patients at risk of hemorrhage following intramuscular injection, the ACIP recommends "it should be administered intramuscularly if, in the opinion of the physician familiar with the patients bleeding risk, the vaccine can be administered with reasonable safety by this route. If the patient receives antihemophilia or other similar therapy, intramuscular vaccination can be scheduled shortly after such therapy is administered. A fine needle (23 gauge or smaller) can be used for the vaccination and firm pressure applied to the site (without rubbing) for at least 2 minutes. The patient should be instructed concerning the risk of hematoma from the injection."

Administration with other vaccines:

PCV with other inactivated vaccines: May be given simultaneously or at any interval between doses.

PCV with live vaccines: May be given simultaneously or at any interval between doses

Vaccine administration with antibody-containing products: PCV and antibody-containing products may be given simultaneously at different sites or at any interval between doses. Examples of antibody containing products include I.M. and I.V. immune globulin, hepatitis B immune globulin, tetanus immune globulin, varicella zoster immune globulin, rabies immune globulin, whole blood, packed red cells, plasma, and platelet products.

Monitoring Parameters Monitor for syncope for ≥15 minutes following vaccination.

Additional Information Federal law requires that the date of administration, the vaccine manufacturer, lot number of vaccine, and the administering person's name, title and address be entered into the patient's permanent medical record.

Dosage Forms Excipient information presented when available (limited, particularly for generics); consult specific product labeling.

Injection, suspension:

Prevnar®: 2 mcg of each capsular saccharide for serotypes 4, 9V, 14, 18C, 19F, and 23F, and 4 mcg of serotype 6B [bound to diphtheria CRM_{197} protein ~20 mcg] per 0.5 mL (0.5 mL) [contains aluminum, natural rubber/natural latex in packaging, soy, and yeast]

Pneumococcal Polysaccharide Vaccine (Polyvalent)

(noo moe KOK al pol i SAK a ride vak SEEN, pol i VAY lent)

U.S. Brand Names Pneumovax® 23

Canadian Brand Names Pneumo 23™; Pneumovax® 23

Index Terms 23-Valent Pneumococcal Polysaccharide Vaccine; 23PS; PPSV; PPV23

Pharmacologic Category Vaccine, Inactivated (Bacterial)

Additional Appendix Information

Guidelines for the Prevention of Opportunistic Infections in HIV Infected Persons *on page 1740*

Immunization Recommendations *on page 1708*

Use Immunization against pneumococcal disease caused by serotypes included in the vaccine. Use is recommended for the following:

Immunocompetent individuals:

- Routine vaccination for persons ≥50 years of age
- Persons ≥2 years with the following chronic conditions: cardiovascular disease, pulmonary disease, diabetes mellitus, liver disease
- Persons ≥2 years with alcoholism, cerebrospinal fluid leaks, functional or anatomic asplenia
- Persons ≥2 years in special living environments or social settings
- Adults 19-64 years who smoke cigarettes

Immunocompromised individuals: Persons ≥2 years with HIV infection, leukemia, lymphoma, Hodgkin's disease, multiple myeloma, generalized malignancy, chronic renal failure, nephritic syndrome, chronic immunosuppressive therapy (including corticosteroids), persons who received an organ or bone marrow transplant

In addition, the Advisory Committee on Immunization Practices (ACIP) recommends routine vaccination for all immunocompetent persons ≥65 years of age and persons aged 2-64 years with cochlear implants. Routine vaccination is not recommended for Alaska Natives or American Indian persons unless they have underlying conditions which are indications for vaccination; in special situations, vaccination may be recommended when living in an area at increased risk of invasive pneumococcal disease.

Pregnancy Risk Factor C

Pregnancy Considerations Animal reproduction studies have not been conducted. Vaccination should be considered in pregnant women at high risk for infection.

Lactation Excretion in breast milk unknown/use caution

Contraindications Hypersensitivity to pneumococcal vaccine or any component of the formulation

Warnings/Precautions Use caution in patients with severe cardiovascular or pulmonary disease where a systemic reaction may pose a significant risk. May cause relapse in patients with stable idiopathic thrombocytopenia purpura. Epinephrine injection (1:1000) must be immediately available in the case of anaphylaxis.

Patients who will be receiving immunosuppressive therapy (including Hodgkin's disease, cancer chemotherapy, or transplantation) should be vaccinated at least 2 weeks prior to the initiation of therapy. Immune responses may be impaired for several months following intensive immunosuppressive therapy (up to 2 years in Hodgkin's disease patients). Patients who will undergo splenectomy should also be vaccinated 2 weeks prior to surgery, if possible. Patients with HIV should be vaccinated as soon as possible (following confirmation of the diagnosis). Safety and efficacy have not been established in children <2 years of age. In order to maximize vaccination rates, the ACIP recommends simultaneous administration of all age-appropriate vaccines (live or inactivated) for which a person is eligible at a single clinic visit, unless contraindications exist. If a person has not received any pneumococcal vaccine or if pneumococcal vaccination status is unknown, PPSV should be administered as indicated.

Adverse Reactions All serious adverse reactions must be reported to the U.S. Department of Health and Human Services (DHHS) Vaccine Adverse Event Reporting System (VAERS) 1-800-822-7967.

Frequency not defined.

Central nervous system: Chills, Guillain-Barré syndrome, fever ≤102°F*, fever >102°F, headache, malaise, pain, radiculoneuropathy, seizure (febrile)

Dermatologic: Angioneurotic edema, cellulitis, rash, urticaria

Gastrointestinal: Nausea, vomiting

Hematologic: Hemolytic anemia (in patients with other hematologic disorders), leukocytosis, thrombocytopenia (in patients with stabilized ITP)

Local: Injection site reaction* (erythema, induration, swelling, soreness, warmth); peripheral edema in injected extremity

Neuromuscular & skeletal: Arthralgia, arthritis, limb mobility decreased, myalgia, paresthesia, weakness

Miscellaneous: Anaphylactoid reaction, C-reactive protein increased, lymphadenitis, serum sickness

*Reactions most commonly reported in clinical trials.

Drug Interactions

Avoid Concomitant Use There are no known interactions where it is recommended to avoid concomitant use.

Increased Effect/Toxicity There are no known significant interactions involving an increase in effect.

Decreased Effect

The levels/effects of Pneumococcal Polysaccharide Vaccine (Polyvalent) may be decreased by: Immunosuppressants

Stability Store under refrigeration at 2°C to 8°C (36°F to 46°F).

Mechanism of Action Although there are more than 80 known pneumococcal capsular types, pneumococcal disease is mainly caused by only a few types of pneumococci. Pneumococcal vaccine contains capsular polysaccharides of 23 pneumococcal types of *Streptococcal pneumoniae* which represent at least 85% to 90% of pneumococcal disease isolates in the United States. The pneumococcal vaccine with 23 pneumococcal capsular polysaccharide types became available in 1983. The 23 capsular pneumococcal vaccine contains purified capsular polysaccharides of pneumococcal types 1, 2, 3, 4, 5, 6B, 7F, 8, 9N, 9V, 10A, 11A, 12F, 14, 15B, 17F, 18C, 19F, 19A, 20, 22F, 23F, and 33F. These are the main pneumococcal types associated with serious infections in the United States.

Dosage I.M., SubQ:

Children >2 years and Adults: 0.5 mL

Revaccination:

Immunocompetent individuals: Revaccination generally not recommended

Children ≥2 years and Adults at highest risk for infection: One revaccination ≥5 years after first dose of PPSV. May consider giving the revaccination dose ≥3 years after first dose of PPSV in children who will be ≤10 years of age at the time of revaccination. Patients at highest risk for infection include those with asplenia, sickle cell anemia, HIV infection, leukemia, lymphoma, Hodgkin's disease, multiple myeloma, generalized malignancy, chronic renal failure, nephrotic syndrome, conditions associated with immunosuppression, and patients on immunosuppressive therapy (including corticosteroids)

Adults ≥65 years: One revaccination if ≥5 years after first dose of PPSV and if <65 years of age of initial vaccination.

Previously vaccinated with PCV vaccine: Children ≥2 years and Adults (ACIP recommendations):

With sickle cell disease, asplenia, immunocompromised or HIV infection: 0.5 mL at ≥2 years of age and ≥2 months after last dose of PCV; one revaccination with PPSV should be given ≥5 years for children >10 years of age and after 3-5 years for children ≤10 years of age; revaccination should not be administered <3 years after the previous PPSV dose

With chronic illness: 0.5 mL at ≥2 years of age and ≥2 months after last dose of PCV; revaccination with PPSV is not recommended

Administration Do not inject I.V., avoid intradermal (may cause severe local reactions); administer SubQ or I.M. (deltoid muscle or lateral midthigh)

For patients at risk of hemorrhage following intramuscular injection, the ACIP recommends "it should be administered intramuscularly if, in the opinion of the physician familiar with the patients bleeding risk, the vaccine can be administered with reasonable safety by this route. If the patient receives antihemophilia or other similar therapy, intramuscular vaccination can be scheduled shortly after such therapy is administered. A fine needle (23 gauge or smaller) can be used for the vaccination and firm pressure applied to the site (without rubbing) for at least 2 minutes. The patient should be instructed concerning the risk of hematoma from the injection."

Administration with other vaccines:

PPSV with other inactivated vaccines: May be given simultaneously or at any interval between doses.

PPSV with live vaccines: May be given simultaneously or at any interval between doses

Vaccine administration with antibody-containing products: PPSV and antibody-containing products may be given simultaneously at different sites or at any interval between doses. Examples of antibody containing products include I.M. and I.V. immune globulin, hepatitis B immune globulin, tetanus immune globulin, varicella zoster immune globulin, rabies immune globulin, whole blood, packed red cells, plasma, and platelet products.

Monitoring Parameters Monitor for syncope for ≥15 minutes following vaccination.

Additional Information Federal law requires that the date of administration, the vaccine manufacturer, lot number of vaccine, and the administering person's name, title, and address be entered into the patient's permanent medical record.

Dosage Forms Excipient information presented when available (limited, particularly for generics); consult specific product labeling.

Injection, solution:

Pneumovax® 23: 25 mcg each of 23 capsular polysaccharide isolates/0.5 mL (0.5 mL, 2.5 mL)

- **Pneumotussin® [DSC]** *see* Hydrocodone and Guaifenesin *on page 741*
- **Pneumovax® 23** *see* Pneumococcal Polysaccharide Vaccine (Polyvalent) *on page 1206*
- **PNU-140690E** *see* Tipranavir *on page 1477*
- **Podactin Cream [OTC]** *see* Miconazole *on page 989*
- **Podactin Powder [OTC]** *see* Tolnaftate *on page 1487*
- **Podocon-25®** *see* Podophyllum Resin *on page 1207*
- **Podofilm® (Can)** *see* Podophyllum Resin *on page 1207*
- **Podophyllin** *see* Podophyllum Resin *on page 1207*

Podophyllum Resin (po DOF fil um REZ in)

U.S. Brand Names Podocon-25®

Canadian Brand Names Podofilm®

Index Terms Mandrake; May Apple; Podophyllin

Pharmacologic Category Keratolytic Agent

Use Topical treatment of benign growths including external genital and perianal warts, papillomas, fibroids; compound benzoin tincture generally is used as the medium for topical application

Pregnancy Risk Factor X

Dosage Topical:

Children and Adults: 10% to 25% solution in compound benzoin tincture; apply drug to dry surface, use 1 drop at a time allowing drying between drops until area is covered; total volume should be limited to <0.5 mL per treatment session

Condylomata acuminatum: 25% solution is applied daily; use a 10% solution when applied to or near mucous membranes

Verrucae: 25% solution is applied 3-5 times/day directly to the wart

Additional Information Complete prescribing information for this medication should be consulted for additional detail.

Dosage Forms Excipient information presented when available (limited, particularly for generics); consult specific product labeling.

Liquid, topical: 25% (15 mL) [in benzoin tincture]

- **Poliovirus, inactivated (IPV)** *see* Diphtheria and Tetanus Toxoids, Acellular Pertussis, and Poliovirus Vaccine *on page 462*
- **Poliovirus, Inactivated (IPV)** *see* Diphtheria and Tetanus Toxoids, Acellular Pertussis, Poliovirus and *Haemophilus* b Conjugate Vaccine *on page 462*

Poliovirus Vaccine (Inactivated)

(POE lee oh VYE rus vak SEEN, in ak ti VAY ted)

U.S. Brand Names IPOL®

Canadian Brand Names IPOL®

Index Terms Enhanced-potency Inactivated Poliovirus Vaccine; IPV; Salk Vaccine

Pharmacologic Category Vaccine

Additional Appendix Information

Immunization Recommendations *on page 1708*

Use Active immunization against poliomyelitis caused by poliovirus types 1, 2 and 3. Routine immunization of adults in the United States is generally not recommended. Adults with previous wild poliovirus disease, who have never been immunized, or those who are incompletely immunized may receive inactivated poliovirus vaccine if they fall into one of the following categories:

- Travelers to regions or countries where poliomyelitis is endemic or epidemic
- Healthcare workers in close contact with patients who may be excreting poliovirus
- Laboratory workers handling specimens that may contain poliovirus
- Members of communities or specific population groups with diseases caused by wild poliovirus
- Incompletely vaccinated or unvaccinated adults in a household or with other close contact with children receiving oral poliovirus (may be at increased risk of vaccine associated paralytic poliomyelitis)

Pregnancy Risk Factor C

Pregnancy Considerations Animal reproduction studies have not been conducted. Although adverse effects of IPV have not been documented in pregnant women or their fetuses, vaccination of pregnant women should be avoided on theoretical grounds. Pregnant women at increased risk for infection and requiring immediate protection against polio may be administered the vaccine.

Lactation Excretion into breast milk unknown/use caution

Contraindications Hypersensitivity to any component of the vaccine

Warnings/Precautions Patients with prior clinical poliomyelitis, incomplete immunization with oral poliovirus vaccine (OPV), HIV infection, severe combined immunodeficiency, hypogammaglobulinemia, agammaglobulinemia, or altered immunity (due to corticosteroids, alkylating agents, antimetabolites or radiation) may receive inactivated poliovirus vaccine (IPV). Immune response may be decreased in patients receiving immune globulin. Vaccination may be deferred with an acute febrile illness; minor illnesses with or without a low-grade fever are not reasons to postpone vaccination. Immediate treatment for anaphylactic/anaphylactoid reaction should be available during vaccine use.

The injection contains 2-phenoxyethanol, calf serum protein, formaldehyde, neomycin, streptomycin, and polymyxin B; the packaging contains natural latex rubber. Safety and efficacy have not been established in children <6 weeks of age.

Adverse Reactions All serious adverse reactions must be reported to the U.S. Department of Health and Human Services (DHHS) Vaccine Adverse Event Reporting System (VAERS) 1-800-822-7967.

Percentages noted with concomitant administration of DTP or DTaP vaccine and observed within 48 hours of injection.

>10%:

Central nervous system: Irritability (7% to 65%), tiredness (4% to 61%), fever ≥39°C (≤38%)

Gastrointestinal: Anorexia (1% to 17%)

Local: Injection Site: Tenderness (≤29%), pain (13%), swelling (≤11%)

1% to 10%:

Gastrointestinal: Vomiting (1% to 3%)

Local: Injection site: Erythema (≤3%), induration (1%)

Miscellaneous: Persistent crying (up to 1% reported within 72 hours)

Postmarketing and/or case reports: Guillain-Barré syndrome has been temporally related to another inactivated poliovirus vaccine

Drug Interactions

Avoid Concomitant Use There are no known interactions where it is recommended to avoid concomitant use.

Increased Effect/Toxicity There are no known significant interactions involving an increase in effect.

Decreased Effect

The levels/effects of Poliovirus Vaccine (Inactivated) may be decreased by: Immunosuppressants

Stability Store under refrigeration 2°C to 8°C (35°F to 46°F); do not freeze.

Dosage I.M., SubQ:

Children:

Primary immunization: Administer three 0.5 mL doses, preferably 8 or more weeks apart, at 2, 4, and 6-18 months of age. First dose may be given as early as 6 weeks of age. Do not administer more frequently than 4 weeks apart.

Booster dose: 0.5 mL at 4-6 years of age

Adults:

Previously unvaccinated: Two 0.5 mL doses administered at 1- to 2-month intervals, followed by a third dose 6-12 months later. If <3 months, but at least 2 months are available before protection is needed, 3 doses may be administered at least 1 month apart. If administration must be completed within 1-2 months, give 2 doses at least 1 month apart. If <1 month is available, give 1 dose.

Incompletely vaccinated: Adults with at least 1 previous dose of OPV, <3 doses of IPV, or a combination of OPV and IPV equaling <3 doses, administer at least one 0.5 mL dose of IPV. Additional doses to complete the series may be given if time permits.

Completely vaccinated: One 0.5 mL dose

Administration Do not administer I.V.; for I.M. or SubQ administration. Administer to midlateral aspect of the thigh in infants and small children. Administer in the deltoid area to adults or older children.

Additional Information Federal law requires that the date of administration, the vaccine manufacturer, lot number of vaccine, and the administering person's name, title, and address be entered into the patient's permanent medical record.

As the global eradication of poliomyelitis continues, the risk for importation of wild-type poliovirus into the United States decreases dramatically. To eliminate the risk for vaccine-associated paralytic poliomyelitis (VAPP), an all-IPV schedule is recommended for routine childhood vaccination in the United States. Oral poliovirus vaccine (OPV), is not commercially available in the United States, but has been stockpiled for use in the following special circumstances:

Mass vaccination campaigns to control outbreaks of paralytic polio

Unvaccinated children who will be traveling within 4 weeks to areas where polio is endemic or epidemic

Children of parents who do not accept the recommended number of vaccine injections; these children may receive OPV only for the third or fourth dose or both. In this situation, healthcare providers should administer OPV only after discussing the risk for VAPP with parents or caregivers.

Currently, the primary risk for paralytic polio in U.S. residents is through travel to countries where polio remains endemic or where polio outbreaks are occurring. Unvaccinated persons traveling to countries that use OPV should be aware of the risk caused by OPV and should consider polio vaccination prior to travel.

Dosage Forms Excipient information presented when available (limited, particularly for generics); consult specific product labeling.

Injection, suspension:

IPOL®: Type 1 poliovirus 40 D-antigen units, type 2 poliovirus 8 D-antigen units, and type 3 poliovirus 32 D-antigen units per 0.5 mL (0.5 mL, 5 mL) [contains 2-phenoxyethanol, formaldehyde, calf serum protein, neomycin (may have trace amounts), streptomycin (may have trace amounts), and polymyxin B (may have trace amounts)]

- **Polocaine®** *see* Mepivacaine *on page 945*
- **Polocaine® Dental** *see* Mepivacaine *on page 945*
- **Polocaine® MPF** *see* Mepivacaine *on page 945*
- **Polycitra®** *see* Citric Acid, Sodium Citrate, and Potassium Citrate *on page 339*
- **Polycitra®-K** *see* Potassium Citrate and Citric Acid *on page 1218*
- **Polycitra®-LC** *see* Citric Acid, Sodium Citrate, and Potassium Citrate *on page 339*
- **Poly-Dex™** *see* Neomycin, Polymyxin B, and Dexamethasone *on page 1052*

Polyethylene Glycol 3350

(pol i ETH i leen GLY kol 3350)

U.S. Brand Names GlycoLax®; MiraLax® [OTC]

Index Terms PEG

Pharmacologic Category Laxative, Osmotic

Additional Appendix Information

Laxatives, Classification and Properties *on page 1660*

Use Treatment of occasional constipation in adults

Unlabeled/Investigational Use Treatment of constipation in children

Pregnancy Risk Factor C

Medication Safety Issues

Sound-alike/look-alike issues:

MiraLax™ may be confused with Mirapex®

International issues:

MiraLax™ may be confused with Murelax® which is a brand name for oxazepam in Australia

Dosage Oral: Adults: Occasional constipation: 17 g of powder (~1 heaping tablespoon) dissolved in 8 oz of water, once daily; do not use for >2 weeks.

Additional Information Complete prescribing information for this medication should be consulted for additional detail.

Dosage Forms Excipient information presented when available (limited, particularly for generics); consult specific product labeling. [DSC] = Discontinued product

Powder, for oral solution: PEG 3350 17 g/packet (12s); PEG 3350 255 g (14 oz); PEG 3350 527 g (26 oz)

GlycoLax®: PEG 3350 17 g/packet (14s) [DSC]; PEG 3350 255 g (16 oz) [DSC]; PEG 3350 527 g (24 oz)

MiraLax®: PEG 3350 17 g/packet (12s) [DSC]; PEG 3350 255 g (14 oz); PEG 3350 527 g (26 oz) [DSC]

Polyethylene Glycol-Electrolyte Solution

(pol i ETH i leen GLY kol ee LEK troe lite soe LOO shun)

U.S. Brand Names Colyte®; GoLYTELY®; MoviPrep®; NuLYTELY®; TriLyte®

Canadian Brand Names Colyte™; Klean-Prep®; PegLyte®

Index Terms Electrolyte Lavage Solution

Pharmacologic Category Laxative, Osmotic

Use Bowel cleansing prior to GI examination

Unlabeled/Investigational Use Whole bowel irrigation (WBI) in the following toxic ingestions: Packets of illicit drugs (body packers, body stuffers), potentially toxic sustained-release or enteric-coated agents, substantial amounts of iron (AACT, 2004)

Pregnancy Risk Factor C

Pregnancy Considerations Reproduction studies have not been conducted in animals or in humans.

Lactation Excretion in breast milk unknown/use caution

Medication Safety Issues

Sound-alike/look-alike issues:

GoLYTELY® may be confused with NuLYTELY®
NuLYTELY® may be confused with GoLYTELY®
TriLyte® may be confused with TriLipix™

Contraindications Hypersensitivity to polyethylene glycol or any component of the formulation; ileus, gastrointestinal obstruction, gastric retention, bowel perforation, toxic colitis, toxic megacolon

Warnings/Precautions Seizures associated with electrolyte abnormalities (eg, hyponatremia, hypokalemia) have occurred. Use caution with concomitant administration of medications that alter electrolyte balance or in patients with underlying hyponatremia. Do not add flavorings, unless provided by the manufacturer, as additional ingredients before use; observe unconscious or semiconscious patients with impaired gag reflex or those who are otherwise prone to regurgitation or aspiration during administration; use with caution in patients with severe ulcerative colitis. Evaluate patients with symptoms of bowel obstruction (nausea, vomiting, abdominal pain or distension) prior to use.

MoviPrep®: May be safer to use in patients who cannot tolerate fluid load (eg, heart failure, renal insufficiency, ascites). Use cautiously in patients with G6PD deficiency. Contains phenylalanine.

Adverse Reactions

>10%:

Central nervous system: Malaise (18% to 27%)
Gastrointestinal: Abdominal distension (<60%), anal irritation (<52%), nausea (14% to 47%), abdominal pain (13% to 39%), vomiting (7% to 12%)
Neuromuscular & skeletal: Rigors (34%)
Miscellaneous: Thirst (<47%)

1% to 10%:

Central nervous system: Dizziness (7%), headache (2%)
Gastrointestinal: Dyspepsia (1% to 3%)

Frequency not defined, postmarketing, and/or case reports: Abdominal cramps, abdominal fullness, allergic reactions, anaphylaxis, aspiration, asystole, bloating, chest tightness, dehydration (children), dermatitis, dyspnea (acute), esophageal perforation, facial edema, flatulence, hypersensitivity reactions, hypokalemia (children), Mallory-Weiss tear, pulmonary edema, rash, rhinorrhea, seizure, throat tightness, upper GI bleeding, urticaria

Drug Interactions

Avoid Concomitant Use There are no known interactions where it is recommended to avoid concomitant use.

Increased Effect/Toxicity There are no known significant interactions involving an increase in effect.

Decreased Effect There are no known significant interactions involving a decrease in effect.

Stability

CoLyte®, GoLYTELY®, NuLYTELY®, TriLyte®: Store at controlled room temperature of 25°C (77°F) before reconstitution. Use within 48 hours of preparation; refrigerate reconstituted solution; tap water may be used for preparation of the solution; shake container vigorously several times to ensure dissolution of powder.

MoviPrep®: Store at controlled room temperature of 25°C (77°F) before reconstitution. Mix the contents of pouch A and pouch B (one each) in container provided. Add 1 L of lukewarm water; mix the solution until dissolved. Repeat mixing procedure if second liter is needed. Refrigerate reconstituted solution. Use within 24 hours of preparation.

Mechanism of Action Induces catharsis by strong electrolyte and osmotic effects

Pharmacodynamics/Kinetics Onset of effect: Oral: ~1-2 hours

Dosage

Oral:

Children ≥6 months: Bowel cleansing prior to GI exam (CoLyte®, GoLYTELY®, NuLYTELY®, TriLyte®): 25 mL/kg/hour (some studies have used up to 40 mL/kg/hour) for 4-10 hours (until rectal effluent is clear). Maximum total dose: 4 L. **Note:** The solution may be given via nasogastric tube to patients who are unwilling or unable to drink the solution. Patients <2 years should be monitored closely.

Adults: Bowel cleansing prior to GI exam:

CoLyte®, GoLYTELY®, NuLYTELY®, TriLyte®: 240 mL (8 oz) every 10 minutes, until 4 L are consumed or the rectal effluent is clear; rapid drinking of each portion is preferred to drinking small amounts continuously. Ideally, patients should fast for ~3-4 hours prior to administration; absolutely no solid food for at least 2 hours before the solution is given. **Note:** The solution may be given via nasogastric tube to patients who are unwilling or unable to drink the solution.

MoviPrep®: Administer 2 L total with an additional 1 L of clear fluid prior to colonoscopy as follows:

Split dose: Evening before colonoscopy: 240 mL (8 oz) every 15 minutes until 1 L is consumed. Then drink 16 oz of clear liquid. On the morning of the colonoscopy, repeat process with second liter over 1 hour and then drink 16 oz of clear liquid at least 1 hour before the procedure.

Full dose: Evening before colonoscopy (~6 PM): 240 mL (8 oz every 15 minutes) until 1 L is consumed; 90 minutes later (~7:30 PM), repeat dose. Then drink 32 oz of clear liquid.

Nasogastric tube (CoLyte®, GoLYTELY®, NuLYTELY®, TriLyte®):

Bowel cleansing prior to GI exam:

Children ≥6 months: 25 mL/kg/hour until rectal effluent is clear.

Adults: Bowel cleansing prior to GI exam: 20-30 mL/minute (1.2-1.8 L/hour); the first bowel movement should occur ~1 hour after the start of administration.

Toxic ingestion (unlabeled use; AACT, 2004):

Children ≥9 months to 6 years: 500 mL/hour until rectal effluent is clear

Children 6-12 years: 1000 mL/hour until rectal effluent is clear

Adolescents and Adults: 1500-2000 mL/hour until rectal effluent is clear

Note: May take several hours for the rectal effluent to become clear. Duration may be extended if evidence of continued presence of toxins in GI tract (eg, radiographic evidence or ongoing elimination of toxins)

Dietary Considerations

CoLyte®, GoLYTELY®, NuLYTELY®, TriLyte®: Ideally, the patient should fast for ~3-4 hours prior to administration, but in no case should solid food be given for at least 2 hours before the solution is given. Some products contain aspartame which is metabolized to phenylalanine.

MoviPrep®: Patient should not eat solid food from start of solution administration until after colonoscopy. Patient may have clear liquid soup/plain yogurt for dinner; finish at least 1 hour before start of colon prep.

Administration Oral: Rapid drinking of each portion is preferred to drinking small amounts continuously. Do not add flavorings, unless provided by the manufacturer, as additional ingredients before use. Chilled solution often more palatable. Oral medications should not be administered within 1 hour of start of therapy.

Monitoring Parameters Electrolytes, serum glucose, BUN, urine osmolality; children <2 years of age should be monitored for hypoglycemia, dehydration, hypokalemia

Dosage Forms Excipient information presented when available (limited, particularly for generics); consult specific product labeling.

Powder, for oral solution: PEG 3350 240 g, sodium sulfate 22.72 g, sodium bicarbonate 6.72 g, sodium chloride 5.84 g, and potassium chloride 2.98 g (4000 mL)

Colyte®: PEG 3350 240 g, sodium sulfate 22.72 g, sodium bicarbonate 6.72 g, sodium chloride 5.84 g, and potassium chloride 2.98 g (4000 mL) [available with citrus berry, lemon lime, cherry, orange, and pineapple flavor packets]

GoLYTELY®:

PEG 3350 236 g, sodium sulfate 22.74 g, sodium bicarbonate 6.74 g, sodium chloride 5.86 g, and potassium chloride 2.97 g (4000 mL) [regular and pineapple flavor]

PEG 3350 227.1 g, sodium sulfate 21.5 g, sodium bicarbonate 6.36 g, sodium chloride 5.53 g, and potassium chloride 2.82 g per packet (1s) [regular flavor; makes 1 gallon of solution after mixing]

MoviPrep®: Pouch A: PEG 3350 100g, sodium sulfate 7.5 g, sodium chloride 2.69 g, potassium chloride 1.015 g; Pouch B: Ascorbic acid 4.7 g, sodium ascorbate 5.9 g (1000 mL) [contains phenylalanine 2.33 mg/treatment; lemon flavor; packaged with 2 of Pouch A and 2 of Pouch B in carton and a disposable reconstitution container]

NuLYTELY®: PEG 3350 420 g, sodium bicarbonate 5.72 g, sodium chloride 11.2 g, and potassium chloride 1.48 (4000 mL) [cherry, lemon-lime, orange, and pineapple flavors]

TriLyte®: PEG 3350 420 g, sodium bicarbonate 5.72 g, sodium chloride 11.2 g, and potassium chloride 1.48 g (4000 mL) [supplied with flavor packets]

- **Polygam® S/D [DSC]** *see* Immune Globulin (Intravenous) *on page 777*
- **Poly Hist Forte®** *see* Chlorpheniramine, Pyrilamine, and Phenylephrine *on page 315*
- **Poly Hist PD** *see* Chlorpheniramine, Pyrilamine, and Phenylephrine *on page 315*
- **Poly-Iron 150 [OTC]** *see* Polysaccharide-Iron Complex *on page 1212*

Poly-L-Lactic Acid (POL i el LAK tik AS id)

U.S. Brand Names Sculptra®

Index Terms New-Fill®; PLA

Pharmacologic Category Cosmetic Agent, Implant

Use Restoration and/or correction of facial lipoatrophy in patients with HIV

Dosage Intradermal or SubQ: Adults: Lipoatrophy: ~0.05-0.2 mL per individual injection depending on technique used; ~20 injections may be needed per cheek. Treatment should be individualized. Separate treatments by ≥2 weeks. Typical course involves 3-6 treatments. Supplemental injections may be needed. Do not overfill contour deficiency. For patients with severe facial fat loss, the average treatment requires ~1 vial per cheek area per treatment.

Additional Information Complete prescribing information for this medication should be consulted for additional detail.

Dosage Forms Excipient information presented when available (limited, particularly for generics); consult specific product labeling.

Injection, powder for suspension:

Sculptra®: Poly-L-lactic acid USP

Polymyxin B (pol i MIKS in bee)

U.S. Brand Names Poly-Rx

Index Terms Polymyxin B Sulfate

Pharmacologic Category Antibiotic, Irrigation; Antibiotic, Miscellaneous

Additional Appendix Information

Prevention of Wound Infection and Sepsis in Surgical Patients *on page 1738*

Use Treatment of acute infections caused by susceptible strains of *Pseudomonas aeruginosa*; used occasionally for gut decontamination; parenteral use of polymyxin B has mainly been replaced by less toxic antibiotics, reserved for life-threatening infections caused by organisms resistant to the preferred drugs (eg, pseudomonal meningitis - intrathecal administration)

Pregnancy Risk Factor B (per expert opinion)

Pregnancy Considerations **[U.S. Boxed Warning]: Safety in pregnant women has not been established.**

Lactation Excretion in breast milk unknown/use caution

Medication Safety Issues

High alert medication: The Institute for Safe Medication Practices (ISMP) includes this medication (intrathecal administration) among its list of drug classes which have a heightened risk of causing significant patient harm when used in error.

Contraindications Hypersensitivity to polymyxin B or any component of the formulation; concurrent use of neuromuscular blockers

Warnings/Precautions **[U.S. Boxed Warning]: May cause neurotoxicity, nephrotoxicity, and/or neuromuscular blockade and respiratory paralysis;** usual risk factors include pre-existing renal impairment, concomitant neuro-/nephrotoxic medications, advanced age and dehydration. Use with caution in patients with impaired renal function (modify dosage); polymyxin B-induced nephrotoxicity may be manifested by albuminuria, cellular casts, and azotemia. Discontinue therapy with decreasing urinary output and increasing BUN; neurotoxic reactions are usually associated with high serum levels, often in patients with renal dysfunction. Avoid concurrent or sequential use of other nephrotoxic and neurotoxic drugs (eg, aminoglycosides). The drug's neurotoxicity can result in respiratory paralysis from neuromuscular blockade, especially when the drug is given soon after anesthesia or muscle relaxants. Polymyxin B sulfate is most toxic when given parenterally; avoid parenteral use whenever possible. Prolonged use may result in fungal or bacterial superinfection, including *C. difficile*-associated diarrhea (CDAD) and pseudomembranous colitis; CDAD has been observed >2 months postantibiotic treatment. **[U.S. Boxed Warnings]: Safety in pregnant women not established; intramuscular/intrathecal administration only to hospitalized patients.**

Adverse Reactions Frequency not defined (limited to important or life-threatening):

Central nervous system: Neurotoxicity (irritability, drowsiness, ataxia, perioral paresthesia, numbness of the extremities, and blurred vision); dizziness

Neuromuscular & skeletal: Neuromuscular blockade

Renal: Nephrotoxicity

Respiratory: Respiratory arrest

Drug Interactions

Avoid Concomitant Use There are no known interactions where it is recommended to avoid concomitant use.

Increased Effect/Toxicity

Polymyxin B may increase the levels/effects of: Colistimethate; Neuromuscular-Blocking Agents

The levels/effects of Polymyxin B may be increased by: Capreomycin

Decreased Effect There are no known significant interactions involving a decrease in effect.

Stability Prior to reconstitution, store at room temperature of 15°C to 30°C (59°F to 86°F). Protect from light. After reconstitution, store under refrigeration at 2°C to 8°C (36°F to 46°F). Discard any unused solution after 72 hours.

Mechanism of Action Binds to phospholipids, alters permeability, and damages the bacterial cytoplasmic membrane permitting leakage of intracellular constituents

Pharmacodynamics/Kinetics

Absorption: Well absorbed from peritoneum; minimal from GI tract (except in neonates) from mucous membranes or intact skin

Distribution: Minimal into CSF; does not cross placenta

Half-life elimination: 4.5-6 hours; prolonged with renal impairment

Time to peak, serum: I.M.: ~2 hours

Excretion: Urine (>60% primarily as unchanged drug)

Dosage

Otic (in combination with other drugs): 1-2 drops, 3-4 times/day; should be used sparingly to avoid accumulation of excess debris

Infants <2 years:

I.M.: Up to 40,000 units/kg/day divided every 6 hours (not routinely recommended due to pain at injection sites)

I.V.: Up to 40,000 units/kg/day divided every 12 hours

Intrathecal: 20,000 units/day for 3-4 days, then 25,000 units every other day for at least 2 weeks after CSF cultures are negative and CSF (glucose) has returned to within normal limits

Children ≥2 years and Adults:

I.M.: 25,000-30,000 units/kg/day divided every 4-6 hours (not routinely recommended due to pain at injection sites)

I.V.: 15,000-25,000 units/kg/day divided every 12 hours

Intrathecal: 50,000 units/day for 3-4 days, then every other day for at least 2 weeks after CSF cultures are negative and CSF (glucose) has returned to within normal limits

Total daily dose should not exceed 2,000,000 units/day

Bladder irrigation: Continuous irrigant or rinse in the urinary bladder for up to 10 days using 20 mg (equal to 200,000 units) added to 1 L of normal saline; usually no more than 1 L of irrigant is used per day unless urine flow rate is high; administration rate is adjusted to patient's urine output

Topical irrigation or topical solution: 500,000 units/L of normal saline; topical irrigation should not exceed 2 million units/day in adults

Gut sterilization: Oral: 15,000-25,000 units/kg/day in divided doses every 6 hours

Clostridium difficile enteritis: Oral: 25,000 units every 6 hours for 10 days

Ophthalmic: A concentration of 0.1% to 0.25% is administered as 1-3 drops every hour, then increasing the interval as response indicates to 1-2 drops 4-6 times/day

Dosing adjustment/interval in renal impairment:

Cl_{cr} 20-50 mL/minute: Administer 75% to 100% of the normal daily dose given in divided doses every 12 hours

Cl_{cr} 5-20 mL/minute: Administer 50% of normal daily dose given in divided doses every 12 hours

Cl_{cr} <5 mL/minute: Administer 15% of normal daily dose given in divided doses every 12 hours

Administration Dissolve 500,000 units in 300-500 mL D_5W for continuous I.V. drip; dissolve 500,000 units in 2 mL water for injection, saline, or 1% procaine solution for I.M. injection; dissolve 500,000 units in 10 mL physiologic solution for intrathecal administration

Extravasation management: Monitor I.V. site closely; extravasation may cause serious injury with possible necrosis and tissue sloughing. Rotate infusion site frequently.

Monitoring Parameters Neurologic symptoms and signs of superinfection; renal function (decreasing urine output and increasing BUN may require discontinuance of therapy)

Reference Range Serum concentrations >5 mcg/mL are toxic in adults

Additional Information 1 mg = 10,000 units

Dosage Forms Excipient information presented when available (limited, particularly for generics); consult specific product labeling.

Injection, powder for reconstitution: 500,000 units

Powder [for prescription compounding]:

Poly-Rx: 100 million units (13 g)

◆ **Polymyxin B and Bacitracin** *see* Bacitracin and Polymyxin B *on page* 171

◆ **Polymyxin B and Neomycin** *see* Neomycin and Polymyxin B *on page* 1051

◆ **Polymyxin B and Trimethoprim** *see* Trimethoprim and Polymyxin B *on page* 1520

◆ **Polymyxin B, Bacitracin, and Neomycin** *see* Bacitracin, Neomycin, and Polymyxin B *on page* 171

◆ **Polymyxin B, Bacitracin, Neomycin, and Hydrocortisone** *see* Bacitracin, Neomycin, Polymyxin B, and Hydrocortisone *on page* 172

◆ **Polymyxin B, Neomycin, and Dexamethasone** *see* Neomycin, Polymyxin B, and Dexamethasone *on page* 1052

◆ **Polymyxin B, Neomycin, and Gramicidin** *see* Neomycin, Polymyxin B, and Gramicidin *on page* 1052

◆ **Polymyxin B, Neomycin, and Hydrocortisone** *see* Neomycin, Polymyxin B, and Hydrocortisone *on page* 1052

◆ **Polymyxin B, Neomycin, and Prednisolone** *see* Neomycin, Polymyxin B, and Prednisolone *on page* 1053

◆ **Polymyxin B Sulfate** *see* Polymyxin B *on page* 1210

◆ **Poly-Pred®** *see* Neomycin, Polymyxin B, and Prednisolone *on page* 1053

◆ **Poly-Rx** *see* Polymyxin B *on page* 1210

Polysaccharide-Iron Complex
(pol i SAK a ride-EYE ern KOM pleks)

U.S. Brand Names Ferrex 150 [OTC]; Niferex® [OTC]; Nu-Iron® 150 [OTC]; Poly-Iron 150 [OTC]; ProFe [OTC]

Index Terms Iron-Polysaccharide Complex

Pharmacologic Category Iron Salt

Use Prevention and treatment of iron-deficiency anemias

Medication Safety Issues

Sound-alike/look-alike issues:

Niferex® may be confused with Nephrox®

Dosage

Dietary Reference Intake: Dose is RDA presented as elemental iron unless otherwise noted:

0-6 months: 0.27 mg/day (adequate intake)

7-12 months: 11 mg/day

1-3 years: 7 mg/day

4-8 years: 10 mg/day

9-13 years: 8 mg/day

14-18 years: Male: 11 mg/day; Female: 15 mg/day; Pregnant female: 27 mg/day; Lactating female: 10 mg/day

19-50 years: Male: 8 mg/day; Female: 18 mg/day; Pregnant female: 27 mg/day; Lactating female: 9 mg/day

≥50 years: 8 mg/day

Iron deficiency: Oral:

Children ≥6 years: Tablets/elixir: 50-100 mg/day; may be given in divided doses

Adults:

Elixir: 50-100 mg twice daily

Capsules: 150-300 mg/day

Additional Information Complete prescribing information for this medication should be consulted for additional detail.

Dosage Forms Excipient information presented when available (limited, particularly for generics); consult specific product labeling.

Capsule: Elemental iron 150 mg

Ferrex 150, Nu-Iron® 150: Elemental iron 150 mg

Niferex®: Elemental iron 60 mg

Poly-Iron 150: Elemental iron 150 mg [contains tartrazine]

ProFe: Elemental iron 180 mg

Elixir:

Niferex®: Elemental iron 100 mg/5 mL (240 mL) [contains alcohol 10%; dye free, sugar free]

◆ **Polysporin® [OTC]** *see* Bacitracin and Polymyxin B *on page* 171

◆ **Polytrim®** *see* Trimethoprim and Polymyxin B *on page* 1520

◆ **Polytrim™ (Can)** *see* Trimethoprim and Polymyxin B *on page* 1520

◆ **Poly Tussin DM** *see* Chlorpheniramine, Phenylephrine, and Dextromethorphan *on page* 311

◆ **Polyvinylpyrrolidone with Iodine** *see* Povidone-Iodine *on page* 1222

◆ **Ponstan® (Can)** *see* Mefenamic Acid *on page* 932

◆ **Ponstel®** *see* Mefenamic Acid *on page* 932

◆ **Pontocaine®** *see* Tetracaine *on page* 1451

◆ **Pontocaine® Niphanoid®** *see* Tetracaine *on page* 1451

Porfimer (POR fi mer)

U.S. Brand Names Photofrin®

Canadian Brand Names Photofrin®

Index Terms CL-184116; Dihematoporphyrin Ether; Porfimer Sodium

Pharmacologic Category Antineoplastic Agent, Miscellaneous

Use Palliation in patients with obstructing (partial or complete) esophageal cancer; treatment of microinvasive endobronchial nonsmall cell lung cancer (NSCLC); reduction of obstruction and palliation in patients with obstructing (partial or complete) NSCLC; ablation of high-grade dysplasia in Barrett's esophagus

Unlabeled/Investigational Use Treatment of gastric cancer (obstruction); treatment of actinic keratoses and low-risk basal and squamous cell skin cancers

Pregnancy Risk Factor C

Medication Safety Issues

High alert medication: The Institute for Safe Medication Practices (ISMP) includes this medication among its list of drug classes which have a heightened risk of causing significant patient harm when used in error.

Dosage I.V.: Adults: 2 mg/kg, followed by exposure to the appropriate laser light; repeat courses must be separated by at least 30 days (esophageal or endobronchial cancer) or 90 days (Barrett's esophagus; delay subsequent treatment for insufficient healing) for a maximum of 3 courses

Additional Information Complete prescribing information for this medication should be consulted for additional detail.

Dosage Forms Excipient information presented when available (limited, particularly for generics); consult specific product labeling.

Injection, powder for reconstitution, as sodium:

Photofrin®: 75 mg

◆ **Porfimer Sodium** *see* Porfimer *on page* 1212

◆ **Portia™** *see* Ethinyl Estradiol and Levonorgestrel *on page 577*

Posaconazole (poe sa KON a zole)

U.S. Brand Names Noxafil®

Canadian Brand Names Posanol™

Index Terms SCH 56592

Pharmacologic Category Antifungal Agent, Oral

Additional Appendix Information

Antifungal Agents *on page 1640*

Use Prophylaxis of invasive *Aspergillus* and *Candida* infections in severely-immunocompromised patients [eg, hematopoietic stem cell transplant (HSCT) recipients with graft-versus-host disease (GVHD) or those with prolonged neutropenia secondary to chemotherapy for hematologic malignancies]; treatment of oropharyngeal candidiasis (including patients refractory to itraconazole and/or fluconazole)

Unlabeled/Investigational Use Salvage therapy of refractory invasive fungal infections; mucormycosis

Pregnancy Risk Factor C

Pregnancy Considerations Posaconazole has been shown to be teratogenic in animal studies. There are no adequate and well-controlled studies in pregnant women. Use only if the benefit to the mother justifies potential risk to the fetus.

Lactation Excretion in breast milk unknown/not recommended

Medication Safety Issues

Sound-alike/look-alike issues:

Noxafil® may be confused with minoxidil

International issues:

Noxafil® may be confused with Noxidil® which is a brand name for minoxidil in Thailand

Contraindications Hypersensitivity to posaconazole or any component of the formulation; coadministration of cisapride, ergot alkaloids, pimozide, quinidine, or sirolimus

Warnings/Precautions Use caution in hepatic impairment; hepatic dysfunction has occurred, ranging from mild/moderate increases of ALT/AST, alkaline phosphatase, and/or clinical hepatitis to severe reactions (cholestasis, hepatic failure including death). Use caution in patients with an increased risk of arrhythmia (concurrent QT_c-prolonging drugs, hypokalemia). Correct electrolyte abnormalities (eg, potassium, magnesium, and calcium) before initiating therapy. Concurrent use may significantly increase cyclosporine levels and may result in rare serious adverse events (eg, nephrotoxicity, leukoencephalopathy, and death); dose reduction and close monitoring are recommended with initiation of posaconazole therapy.

Use caution in hypersensitivity with other azole antifungal agents; cross-reaction may occur, but has not been established. Consider alternative therapy or closely monitor for breakthrough fungal infections in patients receiving drugs that decrease absorption or increase the metabolism of posaconazole or in any patient unable to eat or tolerate an oral liquid nutritional supplement. Use caution in severe renal impairment or GI disturbances; monitor for breakthrough fungal infections. Safety and efficacy have not been established in children <13 years of age.

Adverse Reactions Note: A higher frequency of adverse reactions was observed in studies with refractory oropharyngeal candidiasis patients and percentages are included below.

>10%: Gastrointestinal: Diarrhea (3% to 11%)

1% to 10%:

Cardiovascular: QT_c prolongation (4%), hypertension (1%)

Central nervous system: Headache (1% to 8%), dizziness (1% to 3%), fatigue (1% to 3%), insomnia (1% to 3%), fever (up to 3%), somnolence (1%)

Dermatologic: Rash (1% to 4%), pruritus (1% to 2%)

Endocrine & metabolic: Hypokalemia (3%)

Gastrointestinal: Nausea (5% to 8%), vomiting (4% to 7%), abdominal pain (1% to 5%), flatulence (1% to 5%), anorexia (1% to 3%), mucositis (2%), dyspepsia (1% to 2%), xerostomia (1% to 2%), taste perversion (1%), constipation (up to 1%)

Hematologic: Neutropenia (2% to 8%), anemia (up to 3%), thrombocytopenia (up to 2%)

Hepatic: Bilirubin increased (2% to 3%), ALT increased (2% to 3%), AST increased (2% to 3%), GGT increased (2% to 3%), alkaline phosphatase increased (1% to 2%), hepatocellular damage (1%)

Neuromuscular & skeletal: Weakness (1% to 3%), myalgia (up to 2%), tremor (1%)

Ocular: Blurred vision (1%)

Renal: Serum creatinine increased (2%)

<1% (Limited to important or life-threatening): Adrenal insufficiency, allergic/hypersensitivity reactions, cholestasis, hemolytic uremic syndrome, hepatic failure, hepatitis, pulmonary embolus, thrombotic thrombocytopenic purpura, torsade de pointes

Drug Interactions

Metabolism/Transport Effects Inhibits CYP3A4 (strong)

Avoid Concomitant Use

Avoid concomitant use of Posaconazole with any of the following: Alfuzosin; Cisapride; Conivaptan; Dofetilide; Efavirenz; Ergot Derivatives; Nilotinib; Pimozide; QuiNIDine; Ranolazine; Rivaroxaban; Salmeterol; Silodosin

Increased Effect/Toxicity

Posaconazole may increase the levels/effects of: Alfentanil; Alfuzosin; Alosetron; Aprepitant; Benzodiazepines (metabolized by oxidation); Bosentan; BusPIRone; Busulfan; Calcium Channel Blockers; CarBAMazepine; Cardiac Glycosides; Ciclesonide; Cilostazol; Cinacalcet; Cisapride; Conivaptan; Corticosteroids (Orally Inhaled); Corticosteroids (Systemic); CycloSPORINE; CYP3A4 Substrates; Docetaxel; Dofetilide; Eletriptan; Eplerenone; Ergot Derivatives; Erlotinib; Eszopiclone; FentaNYL; Fesoterodine; Fosaprepitant; Gefitinib; HMG-CoA Reductase Inhibitors; Imatinib; Irinotecan; Ixabepilone; Losartan; Macrolide Antibiotics; Maraviroc; Methadone; Nilotinib; Phenytoin; Phosphodiesterase 5 Inhibitors; Pimecrolimus; Pimozide; Protease Inhibitors; QuiNIDine; Ramelteon; Ranolazine; Repaglinide; Rifamycin Derivatives; Rivaroxaban; Salmeterol; Silodosin; Sirolimus; Solifenacin; Sorafenib; Sunitinib; Tacrolimus; Temsirolimus; Tolterodine; VinCRIStine; Vitamin K Antagonists; Ziprasidone; Zolpidem

The levels/effects of Posaconazole may be increased by: Macrolide Antibiotics; Protease Inhibitors

Decreased Effect

Posaconazole may decrease the levels/effects of: Amphotericin B; Saccharomyces boulardii

The levels/effects of Posaconazole may be decreased by: Antacids; Didanosine; Efavirenz; Grapefruit Juice; H2-Antagonists; Phenytoin; Rifamycin Derivatives; Sucralfate

Ethanol/Nutrition/Herb Interactions Food: Bioavailability increased ~3-4 times when posaconazole administered with a meal or an oral liquid nutritional supplement. Grapefruit juice may decrease the levels/effects of posaconazole; concurrent use should be avoided.

Stability Store at controlled room temperature of 25°C (77°F); do not freeze.

Mechanism of Action Interferes with fungal cytochrome P450 (latosterol-14α-demethylase) activity, decreasing ergosterol synthesis (principal sterol in fungal cell membrane) and inhibiting fungal cell membrane formation.

Pharmacodynamics/Kinetics

Absorption: Food and/or liquid nutritional supplements increase absorption; fasting states do not provide sufficient absorption to ensure adequate plasma concentrations

Distribution: V_d: 465-1774 L

Protein binding: ≥97%; predominantly bound to albumin

Metabolism: Not significantly metabolized; ~15% to 17% undergoes non-CYP-mediated metabolism, primarily via hepatic glucuronidation into metabolites

Half-life elimination: 35 hours (range: 20-66 hours)

Time to peak, plasma: ~3-5 hours

Excretion: Feces 71% to 77% (~66% as unchanged drug); urine 13% to 14% (<0.2% as unchanged drug)

Dosage Oral: Children ≥13 years and Adults:

Aspergillosis, invasive:

Prophylaxis: 200 mg 3 times/day

Treatment of refractory infection (unlabeled use): 200 mg 4 times/day initially; after disease stabilization may decrease frequency to 400 mg twice daily in divided doses. **Note:** Duration of therapy should be a minimum of 6-12 weeks or throughout period of immunosuppression.

Candidal infections:

Prophylaxis: 200 mg 3 times/day

Treatment of oropharyngeal infection: Initial: 100 mg twice daily for 1 day; maintenance: 100 mg once daily for 13 days

Treatment of refractory oropharyngeal infection: 400 mg twice daily

Mucormycosis (unlabeled use): 800 mg/day in 2 or 4 divided doses

Dosage adjustment in renal impairment: No adjustment necessary; use caution in severe renal impairment and monitor for breakthrough fungal infections. Variability in posaconazole exposure observed with Cl_{cr}<20 mL/minute.

Dosage adjustment in hepatic impairment: No adjustment necessary; use with caution

Dietary Considerations Give with meals. If alternative antifungal therapy can not be given to patients without food intake or severe diarrhea/vomiting, close monitoring for breakthrough fungal infections must be performed. Adequate posaconazole absorption from GI tract and subsequent plasma concentrations are dependent on food for efficacy. Lower average plasma concentrations have been associated with an increased risk of treatment failure.

Administration Shake well before use. Must be administered with a full meal or an oral liquid nutritional supplement. Administer oral suspension using dosing spoon provided by the manufacturer; spoon should be rinsed clean with water after each use and before storage.

Monitoring Parameters Hepatic function (eg, AST/ALT, alkaline phosphatase and bilirubin) prior to initiation and during treatment; renal function; electrolyte disturbances (eg, calcium, magnesium, potassium); CBC

Dosage Forms Excipient information presented when available (limited, particularly for generics); consult specific product labeling.

Suspension, oral:

Noxafil®: 40 mg/mL (123 mL) [contains sodium benzoate; delivers 105 mL of suspension; cherry flavor; packaged with calibrated dosing spoon]

◆ **Posanol™ (Can)** *see* Posaconazole *on page 1213*

◆ **Post Peel Healing Balm [OTC]** *see* Hydrocortisone *on page 743*

Potassium Acetate (poe TASS ee um AS e tate)

Pharmacologic Category Electrolyte Supplement, Parenteral

Use Potassium deficiency; to avoid chloride when high concentration of potassium is needed, source of bicarbonate

Pregnancy Risk Factor C

Medication Safety Issues

Consider special storage requirements for intravenous potassium salts; I.V. potassium salts have been administered IVP in error, leading to fatal outcomes.

Contraindications Severe renal impairment; hyperkalemia

Warnings/Precautions Close monitoring of serum potassium concentrations is needed to avoid hyperkalemia. Use with caution in patients with renal impairment, cardiac disease, acid/base disorders, or potassium-altering conditions/disorders. Use with caution in digitalized patients or patients receiving concomitant medications or therapies that increase potassium (eg, ACEIs, potassium-sparing diuretics, potassium containing salt substitutes). Do **NOT** administer undiluted or I.V. push; inappropriate parenteral administration may be fatal. Always administer potassium further diluted; refer to appropriate dilution and administration rate recommendations. Pain and phlebitis may occur during parenteral infusion requiring a decrease in infusion rate or potassium concentration. Potassium acetate solution for injection contains aluminum; use caution with impaired renal function and in premature infants.

Adverse Reactions

1% to 10%:

Cardiovascular: Bradycardia

Endocrine & metabolic: Hyperkalemia

Neuromuscular & skeletal: Weakness

Respiratory: Dyspnea

Local: Local tissue necrosis with extravasation

<1% (Limited to important or life-threatening): Abdominal pain, alkalosis, chest pain, mental confusion, paralysis, paresthesia, phlebitis, throat pain

Drug Interactions

Avoid Concomitant Use There are no known interactions where it is recommended to avoid concomitant use.

Increased Effect/Toxicity

Potassium Acetate may increase the levels/effects of: ACE Inhibitors; Angiotensin II Receptor Blockers; Potassium-Sparing Diuretics

The levels/effects of Potassium Acetate may be increased by: Eplerenone

Decreased Effect There are no known significant interactions involving a decrease in effect.

Mechanism of Action Potassium is the major cation of intracellular fluid and is essential for the conduction of nerve impulses in heart, brain, and skeletal muscle; contraction of cardiac, skeletal and smooth muscles; maintenance of normal renal function, acid-base balance, carbohydrate metabolism, and gastric secretion

Pharmacodynamics/Kinetics

Distribution: Enters cells via active transport from extracellular fluid

Excretion: Primarily urine; skin and feces (small amounts); most intestinal potassium reabsorbed

Dosage I.V. doses should be incorporated into the patient's maintenance I.V. fluids, intermittent I.V. potassium administration should be reserved for severe depletion situations and requires ECG monitoring; doses listed as mEq of potassium

Children:

Treatment of hypokalemia: I.V.: 2-5 mEq/kg/day

I.V. intermittent infusion (must be diluted prior to administration): 0.5-1 mEq/kg/dose (maximum: 30 mEq/dose) to infuse at 0.3-0.5 mEq/kg/hour (maximum: 1 mEq/kg/hour)

Note: Use caution in premature neonates; potassium acetate for injection contains aluminum.

Adults:

Treatment of hypokalemia: I.V.: 40-100 mEq/day

I.V. intermittent infusion (must be diluted prior to administration): 5-10 mEq/dose (maximum: 40 mEq/dose) to infuse over 2-3 hours (maximum: 40 mEq over 1 hour)

Note: Continuous cardiac monitor recommended for rates >0.5 mEq/hour

Potassium dosage/rate of infusion guidelines:

Serum potassium >2.5 mEq/L: Maximum infusion rate: 10 mEq/hour; maximum concentration: 40 mEq/L; maximum 24-hour dose: 200 mEq

Serum potassium <2.5 mEq/L: Maximum infusion rate: 40 mEq/hour; maximum concentration: 80 mEq/L; maximum 24-hour dose: 400 mEq

Dosage adjustment in renal impairment: Use caution; potassium acetate injection contains aluminum

Administration Potassium must be diluted prior to parenteral administration; maximum recommended concentration (peripheral line): 80 mEq/L; maximum recommended concentration (central line): 150 mEq/L or 15 mEq/100 mL; in severely fluid-restricted patients (with central lines): 200 mEq/L or 20 mEq/100 mL has been used; maximum rate of infusion, see Dosage, I.V. intermittent infusion

Additional Information 1 mEq of acetate is equivalent to the alkalinizing effect of 1 mEq of bicarbonate.

Dosage Forms Excipient information presented when available (limited, particularly for generics); consult specific product labeling.

Injection, solution: 2 mEq/mL (20 mL, 50 mL, 100 mL) [contains aluminum]

Injection, solution [concentrate]: 4 mEq/mL (50 mL) [contains aluminum]

Potassium Acid Phosphate

(poe TASS ee um AS id FOS fate)

U.S. Brand Names K-Phos® Original

Pharmacologic Category Urinary Acidifying Agent

Use Acidifies urine and lowers urinary calcium concentration; reduces odor and rash caused by ammoniacal urine; increases the antibacterial activity of methenamine

Pregnancy Risk Factor C

Contraindications Severe renal impairment; hyperkalemia, hyperphosphatemia; infected magnesium ammonium phosphate stones

Warnings/Precautions Use with caution in patients receiving concomitant medications or therapies that increase potassium (eg, ACEI, potassium-sparing diuretics, potassium containing salt substitutes). Use caution in patients with renal insufficiency or severe tissue breakdown (eg, chemotherapy or hemodialysis). May cause GI upset (eg, nausea, vomiting, diarrhea, abdominal pain, discomfort) and lead to GI ulceration, bleeding, perforation and/or obstruction. Close monitoring of serum potassium concentrations is needed to avoid hyperkalemia.

Adverse Reactions

>10%: Gastrointestinal: Diarrhea, nausea, stomach pain, flatulence, vomiting

1% to 10%:

Cardiovascular: Bradycardia

Endocrine & metabolic: Hyperkalemia

Local: Local tissue necrosis with extravasation

Neuromuscular & skeletal: Weakness

Respiratory: Dyspnea

<1% (Limited to important or life-threatening): Arrhythmia, dyspnea, edema, hyperphosphatemia, hypocalcemia, mental confusion, paralysis, paresthesia, tetany

Drug Interactions

Avoid Concomitant Use There are no known interactions where it is recommended to avoid concomitant use.

Increased Effect/Toxicity

Potassium Acid Phosphate may increase the levels/effects of: ACE Inhibitors; Angiotensin II Receptor Blockers; Potassium-Sparing Diuretics

The levels/effects of Potassium Acid Phosphate may be increased by: Eplerenone

Decreased Effect There are no known significant interactions involving a decrease in effect.

Mechanism of Action The principal intracellular cation; involved in transmission of nerve impulses, muscle contractions, enzyme activity, and glucose utilization

Pharmacodynamics/Kinetics

Absorption: Well absorbed from upper GI tract

Distribution: Enters cells via active transport from extracellular fluid

Excretion: Primarily urine; skin and feces (small amounts); most intestinal potassium reabsorbed

Dosage Adults: Oral: 1000 mg dissolved in 6-8 oz of water 4 times/day with meals and at bedtime; for best results, soak tablets in water for 2-5 minutes, then stir and swallow

Dietary Considerations May be taken with meals.

Monitoring Parameters Serum potassium, sodium, phosphate, calcium; serum salicylates (if taking salicylates)

Test Interactions Decreased ammonia (B)

Dosage Forms Excipient information presented when available (limited, particularly for generics); consult specific product labeling.

Tablet [scored]: 500 mg [phosphorus 114 mg and potassium 144 mg (3.7 mEq) per tablet; sodium free]

Potassium Bicarbonate and Potassium Chloride

(poe TASS ee um bye KAR bun ate & poe TASS ee um KLOR ide)

U.S. Brand Names K-Lyte/Cl® [DSC]

Index Terms Potassium Bicarbonate and Potassium Chloride (Effervescent)

Pharmacologic Category Electrolyte Supplement, Oral

Use Treatment or prevention of hypokalemia

Pregnancy Risk Factor C

Dosage Oral:

Children: 1-4 mEq/kg/24 hours in divided doses as required to maintain normal serum potassium

Adults:

Prevention: 16-24 mEq/day in 2-4 divided doses

Treatment: 40-100 mEq/day in 2-4 divided doses

Additional Information Complete prescribing information for this medication should be consulted for additional detail.

Dosage Forms Excipient information presented when available (limited, particularly for generics); consult specific product labeling. [DSC] = Discontinued product

Tablet for solution, oral [effervescent]: Potassium chloride 25 mEq [potassium bicarbonate 0.5 g and potassium chloride 1.5 g]

K-Lyte/Cl®: Potassium chloride 25 mEq [potassium bicarbonate 0.5 g and potassium chloride 1.5 g; citrus or fruit punch flavor] [DSC]

◆ **Potassium Bicarbonate and Potassium Chloride (Effervescent)** *see* Potassium Bicarbonate and Potassium Chloride *on page 1215*

Potassium Bicarbonate and Potassium Citrate

(poe TASS ee um bye KAR bun ate & poe TASS ee um SIT rate)

U.S. Brand Names Effer-K™; K-Lyte®; K-Lyte® DS; Klor-Con®/EF

Index Terms Potassium Bicarbonate and Potassium Citrate (Effervescent)

Pharmacologic Category Electrolyte Supplement, Oral

Use Treatment or prevention of hypokalemia

Pregnancy Risk Factor C

Medication Safety Issues

Sound-alike/look-alike issues:

Klor-Con® may be confused with Klaron®, K-Lor®

Dosage Oral:

Children: 1-4 mEq/kg/24 hours in divided doses as required to maintain normal serum potassium

Adults:

Prevention: 16-24 mEq/day in 2-4 divided doses

Treatment: 40-100 mEq/day in 2-4 divided doses

Additional Information Complete prescribing information for this medication should be consulted for additional detail.

Dosage Forms Excipient information presented when available (limited, particularly for generics); consult specific product labeling.

Tablet, effervescent:

Effer-K™: Potassium 25 mEq [cherry berry, lemon citrus, orange, or unflavored]

Klor-Con®/EF: Potassium 25 mEq [sugar free; orange flavor]

K-Lyte®: Potassium 25 mEq [orange flavor]

K-Lyte® DS: Potassium 50 mEq [orange flavor]

◆ **Potassium Bicarbonate and Potassium Citrate (Effervescent)** *see* Potassium Bicarbonate and Potassium Citrate *on page* 1216

Potassium Chloride

(poe TASS ee um KLOR ide)

U.S. Brand Names K-Lor®; K-Tab®; Kaon-Cl-10®; Kay Ciel® [DSC]; Klor-Con®; Klor-Con® 10; Klor-Con® 8; Klor-Con® M; Klor-Con®/25; microK®; microK® 10

Canadian Brand Names Apo-K®; K-10®; K-Dur®; K-Lor®; K-Lyte®/Cl; Micro-K Extencaps®; Roychlor®; Slo-Pot; Slow-K®

Index Terms KCl

Pharmacologic Category Electrolyte Supplement, Oral; Electrolyte Supplement, Parenteral

Use Treatment or prevention of hypokalemia

Pregnancy Risk Factor C

Pregnancy Considerations Reproduction studies have not been conducted. Potassium supplementation (that does not cause maternal hyperkalemia) would not be expected to cause adverse fetal events.

Lactation Enters breast milk/compatible

Medication Safety Issues

Sound-alike/look-alike issues:

Kaon-Cl-10® may be confused with kaolin

KCl may be confused with HCl

K-Lor® may be confused with Klor-Con®

Klor-Con® may be confused with Klaron®, K-Lor®

microK® may be confused with Micronase®

High alert medication: The Institute for Safe Medication Practices (ISMP) includes this medication (I.V. formulation) among its list of drugs which have a heightened risk of causing significant patient harm when used in error.

Per JCAHO recommendations, concentrated electrolyte solutions should not be available in patient care areas.

Consider special storage requirements for intravenous potassium salts; I.V. potassium salts have been administered IVP in error, leading to fatal outcomes.

Contraindications Hypersensitivity to any component of the formulation; hyperkalemia. In addition, solid oral dosage forms are contraindicated in patients in whom there is a structural, pathological, and/or pharmacologic cause for delay or arrest in passage through the GI tract.

Warnings/Precautions Close monitoring of serum potassium concentrations is needed to avoid hyperkalemia. Use with caution in patients with renal impairment, cardiac disease, acid/base disorders, or potassium-altering conditions/disorders. Use with caution in digitalized patients or patients receiving concomitant medications or therapies that increase potassium (eg, ACEI, potassium-sparing diuretics, potassium containing salt substitutes). Do **NOT** administer undiluted or I.V. push; inappropriate parenteral administration may be fatal. Always administer potassium further diluted; refer to appropriate dilution and administration rate recommendations. Pain and phlebitis may occur during parenteral infusion requiring a decrease in infusion rate or potassium concentration. Avoid administering potassium diluted in dextrose solutions during initial therapy; potential for transient decreases in serum potassium due to intracellular shift of potassium from dextrose-stimulated insulin release. May cause GI upset (eg, nausea, vomiting, diarrhea, abdominal pain, discomfort) and lead to GI ulceration, bleeding, perforation and/or obstruction. Oral liquid preparations (not solid) should be used in patients with esophageal compression or delayed gastric emptying.

Adverse Reactions Frequency not defined.

Dermatologic: Rash

Endocrine & metabolic: Hyperkalemia

Gastrointestinal: Abdominal pain/discomfort, diarrhea, flatulence, GI bleeding (oral), GI obstruction (oral), GI perforation (oral), nausea, vomiting

Drug Interactions

Avoid Concomitant Use There are no known interactions where it is recommended to avoid concomitant use.

Increased Effect/Toxicity

Potassium Chloride may increase the levels/effects of: ACE Inhibitors; Angiotensin II Receptor Blockers; Potassium-Sparing Diuretics

The levels/effects of Potassium Chloride may be increased by: Anticholinergic Agents; Eplerenone

Decreased Effect There are no known significant interactions involving a decrease in effect.

Stability

Capsule: MicroK®: Store between 20°C to 25°C (68°F to 77°F).

Powder for oral solution: Klor-Con®: Store at room temperature of 15°C to 30°C (59°F to 86°F).

Solution for injection: Store at room temperature; do not freeze. Use only clear solutions. Use admixtures within 24 hours.

Tablet: K-Tab®: Store below 30°C (86°F).

Mechanism of Action Potassium is the major cation of intracellular fluid and is essential for the conduction of nerve impulses in heart, brain, and skeletal muscle; contraction of cardiac, skeletal and smooth muscles; maintenance of normal renal function, acid-base balance, carbohydrate metabolism, and gastric secretion

Pharmacodynamics/Kinetics

Absorption: Well absorbed from upper GI tract

Distribution: Enters cells via active transport from extracellular fluid

Excretion: Primarily urine; skin and feces (small amounts); most intestinal potassium reabsorbed

Dosage I.V. doses should be incorporated into the patient's maintenance I.V. fluids; intermittent I.V. potassium administration should be reserved for severe depletion situations in patients undergoing ECG monitoring. Doses expressed as mEq of potassium.

Normal daily requirements: Oral, I.V.:
Children: 1-2 mEq/kg/day
Adults: 40-80 mEq/day
Prevention of hypokalemia: Oral:
Children: 1-2 mEq/kg/day in 1-2 divided doses
Adults: 20-40 mEq/day in 1-2 divided doses
Treatment of hypokalemia: Children:
Oral: 1-2 mEq/kg initially, then as needed based on frequently obtained lab values. If deficits are severe or ongoing losses are great, I.V. route should be considered.
I.V. intermittent infusion: 0.5-1 mEq/kg/dose (maximum dose: 40 mEq). If infusion exceeds 0.5 mEq/kg/hour, physician should be at bedside and patient should have continuous ECG monitoring; repeat as needed based on frequently obtained lab values.
Treatment of hypokalemia: Adults:
Oral:
Asymptomatic, mild hypokalemia: Usual dosage range: 40-100 mEq/day divided in 2-5 doses; generally recommended to limit doses to 20-25 mEq/dose to avoid GI discomfort.
Mild-to-moderate hypokalemia: Some clinicians may administer up to 120-240 mEq/day divided in 3-4 doses; limit doses to 40-60 mEq/dose. If deficits are severe or ongoing losses are great, I.V. route should be considered.
I.V. intermittent infusion: Peripheral or central line: ≤10 mEq/hour; repeat as needed based on frequently obtained lab values; central line infusion and continuous ECG monitoring highly recommended for infusions >10 mEq/hour.
Potassium dosage/rate of infusion general guidelines (per product labeling): **Note:** High variability exists in dosing/infusion rate recommendations; therapy guided by patient condition and specific institutional guidelines.
Serum potassium >2.5 mEq/L: Maximum infusion rate: 10 mEq/hour; maximum concentration: 40 mEq/L; maximum 24-hour dose: 200 mEq
Serum potassium <2 mEq/L and symptomatic (excluding emergency treatment of cardiac arrest): Maximum infusion rate (central line only): 40 mEq/hour in presence of continuous ECG monitoring and frequent lab monitoring; In selected situations, patients may require up to 400 mEq/24 hours.

Dietary Considerations Administer with plenty of fluid to decrease stomach irritation and discomfort. Some dietary sources of potassium include leafy green vegetables (eg, spinach, cabbage), tomatoes, cucumbers, zucchini, fruits (eg, apples, oranges, and bananas), root vegetables (eg, carrots, radishes), beans, and peas.

Administration

Parenteral: Potassium must be diluted prior to parenteral administration. Do not administer I.V. push. In general, the dose, concentration of infusion and rate of administration may be dependant on patient condition and specific institution policy. Some clinicians recommend that the maximum concentration for peripheral infusion is 10 mEq/100 mL and maximum rate of administration for peripheral infusion is 10 mEq/hour. ECG monitoring is recommended for peripheral or central infusions >10 mEq/hour in adults. Concentrations and rates of infusion may be greater with central line administration. Some clinicians recommend that the maximum concentration for central infusion is 20-40 mEq/100 mL and maximum rate of administration for central infusion is 40 mEq/hour.
Oral: Oral dosage forms should be taken with meals and a full glass of water or other liquid.
Capsule: MicroK®: Swallow whole, do not chew. Capsules may also be opened and contents sprinkled on a spoonful of applesauce or pudding and should be swallowed immediately without chewing. No more than 20 mEq should be given as a single dose.
Powder: Klor-Con®: Dissolve in 4-5 ounces of water or other beverage prior to administration.
Tablet: K-Tab®, Kaon-Cl®, Klor-Con®: Swallow tablets whole; do not crush, chew or suck on tablet. No more than 20 mEq should be given as a single dose.
Klor-Con® M: Tablet may also be broken in half and each half swallowed separately; the whole tablet may be dissolved in ~4 ounces of water (allow ~2 minutes to dissolve, stir well and drink immediately)

Monitoring Parameters Serum potassium, glucose, chloride, pH, urine output (if indicated), cardiac monitor (if intermittent infusion or potassium infusion rates 0.5 mEq/kg/hour in children or >10 mEq/hour in adults)

Dosage Forms Excipient information presented when available (limited, particularly for generics); consult specific product labeling. [DSC] = Discontinued product
Capsule, extended release, microencapsulated: 8 mEq [600 mg]; 10 mEq [750 mg]
microK®: 8 mEq [600 mg]
microK® 10: 10 mEq [750 mg]
Infusion [premixed in D_5W]: 20 mEq (1000 mL); 30 mEq (1000 mL); 40 mEq (1000 mL)
Infusion [premixed in D_5W and LR]: 20 mEq (1000 mL); 30 mEq (1000 mL); 40 mEq (1000 mL)
Infusion [premixed in D_5W and sodium chloride 0.2%]: 5 mEq (250 mL); 10 mEq (500 mL, 1000 mL); 20 mEq (1000 mL); 30 mEq (1000 mL); 40 mEq (1000 mL)
Infusion [premixed in D_5W and sodium chloride 0.225%: 10 mEq (500 mL, 1000 mL); 20 mEq (1000 mL); 30 mEq (1000 mL); 40 mEq (1000 mL)
Infusion [premixed in D_5W and sodium chloride 0.3%]: 10 mEq (500 mL); 20 mEq (1000 mL)
Infusion [premixed in D_5W and sodium chloride 0.33%]: 10 mEq (500 mL); 20 mEq (1000 mL)
Infusion [premixed in D_5W and sodium chloride 0.45%]: 10 mEq (500 mL, 1000 mL); 20 mEq (1000 mL); 30 mEq (1000 mL); 40 mEq (1000 mL)
Infusion [premixed in D_5W and NS]: 20 mEq (1000 mL); 40 mEq (1000 mL)
Infusion [premixed in $D_{10}W$ and sodium chloride 0.2%]: 5 mEq (250 mL)
Infusion [premixed in sodium chloride 0.45%]: 20 mEq (1000 mL); 40 mEq (1000 mL)
Infusion [premixed in NS]: 20 mEq (1000 mL); 40 mEq (1000 mL)
Infusion [premixed in SWFI; highly concentrated]: 10 mEq (50 mL, 100 mL); 20 mEq (50 mL, 100 mL); 30 mEq (100 mL); 40 mEq (100 mL)
Injection, solution [concentrate]: 2 mEq/mL (5 mL, 10 mL, 15 mL, 20 mL, 30 mL, 250 mL, 500 mL)
Powder, for oral solution: 20 mEq/packet (30s, 100s, 1000s)
K-Lor™: 20 mEq/packet (30s, 100s) [fruit flavor]
Kay Ciel® 10%: 20 mEq/packet (30s, 100s) [sugar free] [DSC]
Klor-Con®: 20 mEq/packet (30s, 100s) [sugar free; fruit flavor]
Klor-Con®/25: 25 mEq/packet (30s, 100s) [sugar free; fruit flavor]
Solution, oral: 20 mEq/15 mL (15 mL, 30 mL, 480 mL, 3840 mL); 40 mEq/15 mL (15 mL, 480 mL)
Tablet, extended release: 8 mEq [600 mg]; 10 mEq [750 mg]; 20 mEq [1500 mg]
K-Tab®: 10 mEq [750 mg]
Kaon-Cl® 10: 10 mEq [750 mg]
Tablet, extended release, microencapsulated: 10 mEq, 20 mEq
Klor-Con® M10: 10 mEq [750 mg]
Klor-Con® M15: 15 mEq [1125 mg; scored]
Klor-Con® M20: 20 mEq [1500 mg; scored]

Tablet, extended release, wax matrix: 8 mEq, 10 mEq
Klor-Con® 8: 8 mEq [600 mg]
Clor-Con® 10: 10 mEq [750 mg]

Potassium Citrate and Citric Acid

(poe TASS ee um SIT rate & SI trik AS id)

U.S. Brand Names Cytra-K; Polycitra®-K

Index Terms Citric Acid and Potassium Citrate

Pharmacologic Category Alkalinizing Agent, Oral

Use Treatment of metabolic acidosis; alkalinizing agent in conditions where long-term maintenance of an alkaline urine is desirable

Pregnancy Risk Factor A

Dosage Urine alkalizing agent:

Children: Solution: 5-15 mL after meals and at bedtime; adjust dose based on urinary pH

Adults:

Powder: One packet dissolved in water after meals and at bedtime; adjust dose to urinary pH

Solution: 15-30 mL after meals and at bedtime; adjust dose based on urinary pH

Additional Information Complete prescribing information for this medication should be consulted for additional detail.

Dosage Forms Excipient information presented when available (limited, particularly for generics); consult specific product labeling.

Note: Equivalent to potassium 2 mEq/mL and bicarbonate 2 mEq/mL

Powder for solution, oral:

Cytra-K: Potassium citrate monohydrate 3300 mg and citric acid 1002 mg per packet (100s) [sugar free; fruit flavor]

Polycitra®-K: Potassium citrate monohydrate 3300 mg and citric acid 1002 mg per packet (100s) [sugar free]

Solution:

Cytra-K: Potassium citrate monohydrate 1100 mg and citric acid monohydrate 334 mg per 5 mL (480 mL) [alcohol free, sugar free; contains sodium benzoate; berry citrus flavor]

Polycitra®-K: Potassium citrate monohydrate 1100 mg and citric acid monohydrate 334 mg per 5 mL (480 mL) [alcohol free, sugar free]

◆ **Potassium Citrate, Citric Acid, and Sodium Citrate** *see* Citric Acid, Sodium Citrate, and Potassium Citrate *on page* 339

Potassium Gluconate

(poe TASS ee um GLOO coe nate)

Pharmacologic Category Electrolyte Supplement, Oral

Use Treatment or prevention of hypokalemia

Pregnancy Risk Factor A

Contraindications Severe renal impairment, untreated Addison's disease, heat cramps, hyperkalemia, severe tissue trauma; solid oral dosage forms are contraindicated in patients in whom there is a structural, pathological, and/or pharmacologic cause for delay or arrest in passage through the GI tract

Warnings/Precautions Use caution in patients with acid/base disorders, cardiovascular disease, potassium-altering conditions/disorders, or renal impairment. Use with caution in patients receiving concomitant medications or therapies that increase potassium (eg, ACEI, potassium-sparing diuretics, potassium containing salt substitutes). Close monitoring of serum potassium concentrations is needed to avoid hyperkalemia. May cause GI upset (eg, nausea, vomiting, diarrhea, abdominal pain, discomfort) and lead to GI ulceration, bleeding, perforation and/or obstruction. Oral liquid preparations (not solid) should be used in patients with esophageal compression or delayed gastric emptying.

Adverse Reactions

>10%: Gastrointestinal: Diarrhea, nausea, stomach pain, flatulence, vomiting (oral)

1% to 10%:

Cardiovascular: Bradycardia

Endocrine & metabolic: Hyperkalemia

Neuromuscular & skeletal: Weakness

Respiratory: Dyspnea

<1% (Limited to important or life-threatening): Mental confusion, paralysis, paresthesia, phlebitis

Drug Interactions

Avoid Concomitant Use There are no known interactions where it is recommended to avoid concomitant use.

Increased Effect/Toxicity

Potassium Gluconate may increase the levels/effects of: ACE Inhibitors; Angiotensin II Receptor Blockers; Potassium-Sparing Diuretics

The levels/effects of Potassium Gluconate may be increased by: Eplerenone

Decreased Effect There are no known significant interactions involving a decrease in effect.

Stability Store at room temperature.

Mechanism of Action Potassium is the major cation of intracellular fluid and is essential for the conduction of nerve impulses in heart, brain, and skeletal muscle; contraction of cardiac, skeletal and smooth muscles; maintenance of normal renal function, acid-base balance, carbohydrate metabolism, and gastric secretion

Pharmacodynamics/Kinetics

Absorption: Well absorbed from upper GI tract

Distribution: Enters cells via active transport from extracellular fluid

Excretion: Primarily urine; skin and feces (small amounts); most intestinal potassium reabsorbed

Dosage Oral (doses listed as mEq of potassium):

Normal daily requirement:

Children: 2-3 mEq/kg/day

Adults: 40-80 mEq/day

Prevention of hypokalemia during diuretic therapy:

Children: 1-2 mEq/kg/day in 1-2 divided doses

Adults: 16-24 mEq/day in 1-2 divided doses

Treatment of hypokalemia:

Children: 2-5 mEq/kg/day in 2-4 divided doses

Adults: 40-100 mEq/day in 2-4 divided doses

Monitoring Parameters Serum potassium, chloride, glucose, pH, urine output (if indicated)

Test Interactions Decreased ammonia (B)

Additional Information 9.4 g potassium gluconate is approximately equal to 40 mEq potassium (4.3 mEq potassium/g potassium gluconate).

Dosage Forms Excipient information presented when available (limited, particularly for generics); consult specific product labeling.

Caplet: 595 mg [equivalent to potassium 99 mg]

Capsule: 99 mg [strength expressed as base]

Tablet: 99 mg [strength expressed as base]; 550 mg [equivalent to potassium 90 mg]; 595 mg [equivalent to potassium 99 mg]

Tablet, timed release: 95 mg [strength expressed as base]

Potassium Iodide (poe TASS ee um EYE oh dide)

U.S. Brand Names Iosat™ [OTC]; SSKI®; ThyroSafe™ [OTC]; ThyroShield™ [OTC]

Index Terms KI

Pharmacologic Category Antithyroid Agent; Expectorant

Use Expectorant for the symptomatic treatment of chronic pulmonary diseases complicated by mucous; reduce thyroid vascularity prior to thyroidectomy and management of thyrotoxic crisis; block thyroidal uptake of radioactive isotopes of iodine in a radiation emergency or other exposure to radioactive iodine

Unlabeled/Investigational Use Lymphocutaneous and cutaneous sporotrichosis

Pregnancy Risk Factor D

Pregnancy Considerations Iodide crosses the placenta (may cause hypothyroidism and goiter in fetus/newborn). Use as an expectorant during pregnancy is contraindicated by the AAP. Use for protection against thyroid cancer secondary to radioactive iodine exposure is considered acceptable based upon risk/benefit, keeping in mind the dose and duration. Repeat dosing should be avoided if possible.

Lactation Enters breast milk/use caution (AAP rates "compatible")

Medication Safety Issues

Sound-alike/look-alike issues:

Potassium iodide products, including saturated solution of potassium iodide (SSKI®) may be confused with potassium iodide and iodine (Strong Iodide Solution or Lugol's solution)

Contraindications Hypersensitivity to iodine or any component of the formulation; hyperkalemia; pulmonary edema; impaired renal function; hyperthyroidism; iodine-induced goiter; dermatitis herpetiformis; hypocomplementemic vasculitis

Warnings/Precautions Prolonged use can lead to hypothyroidism; cystic fibrosis patients have an exaggerated response; can cause acne flare-ups, can cause dermatitis; use with caution in patients with a history of thyroid disease, Addison's disease, cardiac disease, myotonia congenita, tuberculosis, acute bronchitis; use with caution in patients receiving concomitant medications or therapies that increase potassium (eg, ACEI, potassium-sparing diuretics, potassium containing salt substitutes).

Adverse Reactions Frequency not defined.

Cardiovascular: Irregular heart beat

Central nervous system: Confusion, tiredness, fever

Dermatologic: Skin rash

Endocrine & metabolic: Goiter, salivary gland swelling/tenderness, thyroid adenoma, swelling of neck/throat, myxedema, lymph node swelling, hyper-/hypothyroidism

Gastrointestinal: Diarrhea, gastrointestinal bleeding, metallic taste, nausea, stomach pain, stomach upset, vomiting

Neuromuscular & skeletal: Numbness, tingling, weakness, joint pain

Miscellaneous: Chronic iodine poisoning (with prolonged treatment/high doses); iodism, hypersensitivity reactions (angioedema, cutaneous and mucosal hemorrhage, serum sickness-like symptoms)

Drug Interactions

Avoid Concomitant Use

Avoid concomitant use of Potassium Iodide with any of the following: Sodium Iodide I131

Increased Effect/Toxicity

Potassium Iodide may increase the levels/effects of: ACE Inhibitors; Angiotensin II Receptor Blockers; Lithium; Potassium-Sparing Diuretics

The levels/effects of Potassium Iodide may be increased by: Eplerenone

Decreased Effect

Potassium Iodide may decrease the levels/effects of: Sodium Iodide I131; Vitamin K Antagonists

Stability Store at controlled room temperature of 25°C (77°F); excursions permitted to 15°C to 30°C (59°F to 86°F). Protect from light; keep tightly closed.

SSKI®: If exposed to cold, crystallization may occur. Warm and shake to redissolve. If solution becomes brown/yellow, it should be discarded. May be mixed in water, fruit juice, or milk.

Preparation of oral solution:

Concentration of 16.25 mg/5 mL oral solution: Crush one 130 mg tablet into a fine powder. Add 20 mL of water and mix until powder is dissolved. Add an additional 20 mL of low-fat milk (white or chocolate), orange juice, flat soda, raspberry syrup or infant formula. Final concentration will be 16.25 mg/5 mL. Stable for 7 days under refrigeration.

Concentration of 8.125 mg/5 mL oral solution: Crush one 65 mg tablet into a fine powder. Add 20 mL of water and mix until powder is dissolved. Add an additional 20 mL of low-fat milk (white or chocolate), orange juice, flat soda, raspberry syrup, or infant formula. Final concentration will be 8.125 mg/5 mL. Stable for 7 days under refrigeration.

Mechanism of Action Reduces viscosity of mucus by increasing respiratory tract secretions; inhibits secretion of thyroid hormone, fosters colloid accumulation in thyroid follicles. Following radioactive iodine exposure, potassium iodide blocks uptake of radioiodine by the thyroid, reducing the risk of thyroid cancer.

Pharmacodynamics/Kinetics

Onset of action: Hyperthyroidism: 24-48 hours

Peak effect: 10-15 days after continuous therapy

Duration: Radioactive iodine exposure: ~24 hours

Dosage Oral:

Adults: RDA: 150 mcg (iodine)

Expectorant: Adults: SSKI®: 300-600 mg 3-4 times/day

Preoperative thyroidectomy: Children and Adults: 50-250 mg (1-5 drops SSKI®) 3 times/day; administer for 10 days before surgery

To reduce risk of thyroid cancer following nuclear accident (Iosat™, ThyroSafe™, ThyroShield™): Dosing should continue until risk of exposure has passed or other measures are implemented:

Children (see adult dose for children >68 kg):

Infants <1 month: 16.25 mg once daily

1 month to 3 years: 32.5 mg once daily

3-18 years: 65 mg once daily

Children >68 kg and Adults (including pregnant/lactating women): 130 mg once daily

Thyrotoxic crisis:

Infants <1 year: 150-250 mg (3-5 drops SSKI®) 3 times/day

Children and Adults: 300-500 mg (6-10 drops SSKI®) 3 times/day

Sporotrichosis (cutaneous, lymphocutaneous; unlabeled use): Adults: Oral: Initial: 5 drops (SSKI®) 3 times/day; increase to 40-50 drops (SSKI®) 3 times/day as tolerated for 3-6 months

Dietary Considerations SSKI®: Take with food to decrease gastric irritation.

Administration SSKI®: Dilute in a glassful of water, fruit juice, or milk. Take with food to decrease gastric irritation

Monitoring Parameters Thyroid function tests, signs/symptoms of hyperthyroidism; thyroid function should be monitored in pregnant women, neonates, and young infants if repeat doses are required following radioactive iodine exposure

Test Interactions May alter thyroid function tests.

Additional Information 10 drops of SSKI® = potassium iodide 500 mg

Dosage Forms Excipient information presented when available (limited, particularly for generics); consult specific product labeling.

Solution, oral:

SSKI®: 1 g/mL (30 mL, 240 mL) [contains sodium thiosulfate]

ThyroShield™: 65 mg/mL (30 mL) [black raspberry flavor]

Tablet:

Iosat™: 130 mg

ThyroSafe™: 65 mg [equivalent to iodine 50 mg]

Extemporaneous Preparations Preparation of oral solution:

Concentration of 16.25 mg/5 mL oral solution: Crush one 130 mg tablet into a fine powder. Add 20 mL of water and mix until powder is dissolved. Add an additional 20 mL of low-fat milk (white or chocolate), orange juice, flat soda, raspberry syrup or infant formula. Final concentration will be 16.25 mg/5 mL.

Concentration of 8.125 mg/5 mL oral solution: Crush one 65 mg tablet into a fine powder. Add 20 mL of water and mix until powder is dissolved. Add an additional 20 mL of low-fat milk (white or chocolate), orange juice, flat soda, raspberry syrup, or infant formula. Final concentration will be 8.125 mg/5 mL.

Potassium Iodide and Iodine

(poe TASS ee um EYE oh dide & EYE oh dine)

Index Terms Lugol's Solution; Strong Iodine Solution

Pharmacologic Category Antithyroid Agent

Use Reduce thyroid vascularity prior to thyroidectomy and management of thyrotoxic crisis; block thyroidal uptake of radioactive isotopes of iodine in a radiation emergency or other exposure to radioactive iodine

Pregnancy Risk Factor D (potassium iodide)

Pregnancy Considerations Iodide crosses the placenta (may cause hypothyroidism and goiter in fetus/newborn). Use for protection against thyroid cancer secondary to radioactive iodine exposure is considered acceptable based upon risk/benefit, keeping in mind the dose and duration. Repeat dosing should be avoided if possible.

Lactation Enters breast milk/use caution (AAP rates "compatible")

Medication Safety Issues

Sound-alike/look-alike issues:

Potassium iodide and iodine (Strong Iodide Solution or Lugol's solution) may be confused with potassium iodide products, including saturated solution of potassium iodide (SSKI®)

Contraindications Hypersensitivity to iodine or any component of the formulation; hyperkalemia; pulmonary edema; impaired renal function; hyperthyroidism; iodine-induced goiter; dermatitis herpetiformis; hypocomplementemic vasculitis

Warnings/Precautions Prolonged use can lead to hypothyroidism; cystic fibrosis patients have an exaggerated response; can cause acne flare-ups, can cause dermatitis; use with caution in patients with a history of thyroid disease, Addison's disease, cardiac disease, myotonia congenita, tuberculosis, acute bronchitis; use with caution in patients receiving concomitant medications or therapies that increase potassium (eg, ACEI, potassium-sparing diuretics, potassium containing salt substitutes).

Adverse Reactions Frequency not defined.

Cardiovascular: Irregular heart beat

Central nervous system: Confusion, tiredness, fever

Dermatologic: Skin rash

Endocrine & metabolic: Goiter, salivary gland swelling/tenderness, thyroid adenoma, swelling of neck/throat, myxedema, lymph node swelling, hyper-/hypothyroidism

Gastrointestinal: Diarrhea, gastrointestinal bleeding, metallic taste, nausea, stomach pain, stomach upset, vomiting

Neuromuscular & skeletal: Numbness, tingling, weakness, joint pain

Miscellaneous: Chronic iodine poisoning (with prolonged treatment/high doses); iodism, hypersensitivity reactions (angioedema, cutaneous and mucosal hemorrhage, serum sickness-like symptoms)

Drug Interactions

Avoid Concomitant Use

Avoid concomitant use of Potassium Iodide and Iodine with any of the following: Sodium Iodide I131

Increased Effect/Toxicity

Potassium Iodide and Iodine may increase the levels/effects of: ACE Inhibitors; Angiotensin II Receptor Blockers; Lithium; Potassium-Sparing Diuretics

The levels/effects of Potassium Iodide and Iodine may be increased by: Eplerenone

Decreased Effect

Potassium Iodide and Iodine may decrease the levels/effects of: Sodium Iodide I131; Vitamin K Antagonists

Stability Store at controlled room temperature of 25°C (77°F); excursions permitted to 15°C to 30°C (59°F to 86°F). Protect from light and keep container tightly closed.

Mechanism of Action Inhibits secretion of thyroid hormone, fosters colloid accumulation in thyroid follicles. Following radioactive iodine exposure, potassium iodide blocks uptake of radioiodine by the thyroid, reducing the risk of thyroid cancer.

Pharmacodynamics/Kinetics

Onset of action: Hyperthyroidism: 24-48 hours

Peak effect: 10-15 days after continuous therapy

Dosage RDA, Adults: 150 mcg (iodine)

Children and Adults: Oral:

Preoperative thyroidectomy: 0.1-0.3 mL (3-5 drops) of strong iodine (Lugol's solution) 3 times/day; administer for 10 days before surgery

Thyrotoxic crisis: 1 mL strong iodine (Lugol's solution) 3 times/day

Monitoring Parameters

Thyroid function tests, signs/symptoms of hyperthyroidism; thyroid function should be monitored in pregnant women, neonates, and young infants if repeat doses are required following radioactive iodine exposure

Test Interactions May alter thyroid function tests.

Dosage Forms Excipient information presented when available (limited, particularly for generics); consult specific product labeling.

Solution, oral: Potassium iodide 100 mg/mL and iodine 50 mg/mL (480 mL)

Solution, topical: Potassium iodide 100 mg/mL and iodine 50 mg/mL (8 mL)

◆ **Potassium Iodide, Chlorpheniramine, Phenylephrine, and Codeine** *see* Chlorpheniramine, Phenylephrine, Codeine, and Potassium Iodide *on page* 314

Potassium Phosphate (poe TASS ee um FOS fate)

U.S. Brand Names Neutra-Phos®-K [OTC] [DSC]

Index Terms Phosphate, Potassium

Pharmacologic Category Electrolyte Supplement, Oral; Electrolyte Supplement, Parenteral

Use Treatment and prevention of hypophosphatemia; **Note:** The concomitant amount of potassium must be calculated into the total electrolyte content. For each 1 mmol of phosphate, ~1.5 mEq of potassium will be administered. Therefore, if ordering 30 mmol of potassium phosphate, the patient will receive ~45 mEq of potassium.

Pregnancy Risk Factor C

Medication Safety Issues

Sound-alike/look-alike issues:

Neutra-Phos®-K may be confused with K-Phos Neutral®

High alert medication: The Institute for Safe Medication Practices (ISMP) includes this medication (I.V. formulation) among its list of drugs which have a heightened risk of causing significant patient harm when used in error.

Per JCAHO recommendations, concentrated electrolyte solutions should not be available in patient care areas.

Consider special storage requirements for intravenous potassium salts; I.V. potassium salts have been administered IVP in error, leading to fatal outcomes.

Safe Prescribing: Because inorganic phosphate exists as monobasic and dibasic anions, with the mixture of valences dependent on pH, ordering by mEq amounts is unreliable and may lead to large dosing errors. In addition, I.V. phosphate is available in the sodium and potassium salt; therefore, the content of these cations must be considered when ordering phosphate. The most reliable method of ordering I.V. phosphate is by millimoles, then specifying the potassium or sodium salt. For example, an order for 15 mmol of phosphate as potassium phosphate in one liter of normal saline. The dosing of phosphate should be 0.2-0.3 mmol/kg with a usual daily requirement of 30-60 mmol/day or 15 mmol of phosphate per liter of TPN or 15 mmol phosphate per 1000 calories of dextrose. Would also provide 22 mEq of potassium.

Contraindications Hyperphosphatemia, hyperkalemia, hypocalcemia, hypomagnesemia, renal failure

Warnings/Precautions Close monitoring of serum potassium concentrations is needed to avoid hyperkalemia. Use with caution in patients with renal insufficiency, cardiac disease, metabolic alkalosis. Use with caution in digitalized patients and patients receiving concomitant potassium-altering therapies. Oral formulations may cause GI upset. Admixture of phosphate and calcium in I.V. fluids can result in calcium phosphate precipitation. Use extreme caution when administering potassium phosphate parenterally. Parenteral potassium may cause pain and phlebitis, requiring a decrease in infusion rate or potassium concentration.

Adverse Reactions

>10%: Gastrointestinal: Diarrhea, nausea, stomach pain, flatulence, vomiting

1% to 10%:

Cardiovascular: Bradycardia

Endocrine & metabolic: Hyperkalemia

Neuromuscular & skeletal: Weakness

Respiratory: Dyspnea

<1% (Limited to important or life-threatening): Acute renal failure, arrhythmia, chest pain, decreased urine output, dyspnea, edema, mental confusion, paralysis, paresthesia, phlebitis, tetany (with large doses of phosphate)

Drug Interactions

Avoid Concomitant Use There are no known interactions where it is recommended to avoid concomitant use.

Increased Effect/Toxicity

Potassium Phosphate may increase the levels/effects of: ACE Inhibitors; Angiotensin II Receptor Blockers; Potassium-Sparing Diuretics

The levels/effects of Potassium Phosphate may be increased by: Bisphosphonate Derivatives; Eplerenone

Decreased Effect

The levels/effects of Potassium Phosphate may be decreased by: Antacids; Calcium Salts; Iron Salts; Magnesium Salts; Sucralfate

Ethanol/Nutrition/Herb Interactions Food: Avoid administering with oxalate (berries, nuts, chocolate, beans, celery, tomato) or phytate-containing foods (bran, whole wheat).

Stability Store at room temperature; do not freeze. Use only clear solutions. Up to 10-15 mEq of calcium may be added per liter before precipitate may occur.

Stability of parenteral admixture at room temperature (25°C) is 24 hours.

Phosphate salts may precipitate when mixed with calcium salts. Solubility is improved in amino acid parenteral nutrition solutions. Check with a pharmacist to determine compatibility.

Dosage

Oral:

Normal Requirements Elemental Phosphorus:

0-6 months: 240 mg

6-12 months: 360 mg

1-10 years: 800 mg

>10 years: 1200 mg

Pregnancy lactation: Additional 400 mg/day

Adults: 800 mg

Oral Maintenance:

Children <4 years: 1 capsule (250 mg phosphorus/8 mmol) 4 times/day; dilute as instructed

Children >4 years and Adults: 1-2 capsules (250-500 mg phosphorus/8-16 mmol) 4 times/day; dilute as instructed

I.V.: **Caution: The concomitant amount of potassium must be calculated into the total electrolyte content. For each 1 mmol of phosphate, ~1.5 mEq of potassium will be administered. Therefore, if ordering 30 mmol of potassium phosphate, the patient will receive ~45 mEq of potassium. With orders for I.V. phosphate, there is considerable confusion associated with the use of millimoles (mmol) versus milliequivalents (mEq) to express the phosphate requirement.** The most reliable method of ordering I.V. phosphate is by millimoles, then specifying the potassium or sodium salt (see Medication Safety Issues). Doses listed as mmol of phosphate.

Acute treatment of hypophosphatemia: It is recommended that repletion of severe hypophosphatemia be done I.V. because large doses of oral phosphate may cause diarrhea and intestinal absorption may be unreliable. Intermittent I.V. infusion should be reserved for severe depletion situations; requires continuous cardiac monitoring. Guidelines differ based on degree of illness, need/use of TPN, and severity of hypophosphatemia. If potassium >4.0 mEq/L consider phosphate replacement strategy without potassium (eg, sodium phosphates). Obese patients and/or severe renal impairment were excluded from phosphate supplement trials.

Children and Adults: **Note:** There are no prospective studies of parenteral phosphate replacement in children. The following weight-based guidelines for adult dosing may be cautiously employed in pediatric patients.

General replacement guidelines (Lentz, 1978):

Low dose: 0.08 mmol/kg over 6 hours; use if losses are recent and uncomplicated

Intermediate dose: 0.16-0.24 mmol/kg over 4-6 hours; use if serum phosphorus level 0.5-1 mg/dL (0.16-0.32 mmoles/L)

Note: The initial dose may be increased by 25% to 50% if the patient is symptomatic secondary to hypophosphatemia and lowered by 25% to 50% if the patient is hypercalcemic.

Patients receiving TPN; supplemental dose (Clark, 1995):

Low dose: 0.16 mmol/kg over 4-6 hours; use if serum phosphorus level 2.3-3 mg/dL (0.73-0.96 mmoles/L)

Intermediate dose: 0.32 mmol/kg over 4-6 hours; use if serum phosphorus level 1.6-2.2 mg/dL (0.51-0.72 mmoles/L)

High dose: 0.64 mmol/kg over 8-12 hours; use if serum phosphorus <1.5 mg/dL (<0.5 mmoles/L)

Critically-ill adult trauma patients receiving TPN (Brown, 2006):

Low dose: 0.32 mmol/kg over 4-6 hours; use if serum phosphorus level 2.3-3 mg/dL (0.73-0.96 mmoles/L)

Intermediate dose: 0.64 mmol/kg over 4-6 hours; use if serum phosphorus level 1.6-2.2 mg/dL (0.51-0.72 mmoles/L)

High dose: 1 mmol/kg over 8-12 hours; use if serum phosphorus <1.5 mg/dL (<0.5 mmoles/L)

Maintenance: I.V. solutions: Doses may be incorporated into the patient's maintenance I.V. fluids.

Children: 0.5-1.5 mmol/kg/24 hours I.V. or 2-3 mmol/kg/24 hours orally in divided doses

Adults: 15-30 mmol/24 hours I.V. or 50-150 mmol/24 hours orally in divided doses

Administration Injection must be diluted in appropriate I.V. solution and volume prior to administration and administered over a minimum of 4 hours

Monitoring Parameters Serum potassium, calcium, phosphate, sodium, cardiac monitor (when intermittent infusion or high-dose I.V. replacement needed)

Test Interactions Decreased ammonia (B)

Dosage Forms Excipient information presented when available (limited, particularly for generics); consult specific product labeling. [DSC] = Discontinued product

Injection, solution: Potassium 4.4 mEq and phosphorus 3 mmol per mL (5 mL, 15 mL, 50 mL) [equivalent to potassium 170 mg and elemental phosphorus 93 mg per mL]

Powder for oral solution:

Neutra-Phos®-K: Monobasic potassium phosphate and dibasic potassium phosphate per packet (100s) [equivalent to elemental potassium 556 mg (14.25 mEq) and phosphorus 250 mg (14.25 mEq) per packet; sodium and sugar free; fruit flavor] [DSC]

Potassium Phosphate and Sodium Phosphate

(poe TASS ee um FOS fate & SOW dee um FOS fate)

U.S. Brand Names K-Phos® MF; K-Phos® Neutral; K-Phos® No. 2; Neutra-Phos® [OTC] [DSC]; Phos-NaK; Phospha 250™ Neutral; Uro-KP-Neutral®

Index Terms Sodium Phosphate and Potassium Phosphate

Pharmacologic Category Electrolyte Supplement, Oral

Use Treatment of conditions associated with excessive renal phosphate loss or inadequate GI absorption of phosphate; to acidify the urine to lower calcium concentrations; to increase the antibacterial activity of methenamine; reduce odor and rash caused by ammonia in urine

Pregnancy Risk Factor C

Medication Safety Issues

Sound-alike/look-alike issues:

K-Phos® Neutral may be confused with Neutra-Phos-K®

Dosage Oral:

Children ≥4 years: Elemental phosphorus 250 mg 4 times/day after meals and at bedtime

Adults: Elemental phosphorus 250-500 mg 4 times/day after meals and at bedtime

Additional Information Complete prescribing information for this medication should be consulted for additional detail.

Dosage Forms Excipient information presented when available (limited, particularly for generics); consult specific product labeling. [DSC] = Discontinued product

Caplet:

Uro-KP-Neutral®: Dipotassium phosphate, disodium phosphate, and monobasic sodium phosphate [equivalent to elemental phosphorus 258 mg, sodium 262.4 mg (10.8 mEq), and potassium 49.4 mg (1.3 mEq)]

Powder, for oral solution:

Neutra-Phos®: Dibasic potassium phosphate, monobasic potassium phosphate, dibasic sodium phosphate, and monosodium phosphate per packet (100s) [equivalent to elemental phosphorus 250 mg (14.25 mEq), sodium 164 mg (7.1 mEq), and potassium 278 mg (7.1 mEq) per packet] [DSC]

Phos-NaK: Dibasic potassium phosphate, monobasic potassium phosphate, dibasic sodium phosphate, and monosodium phosphate per packet (100s) [sugar free; equivalent to elemental phosphorus 250 mg, sodium 160 mg (6.9 mEq), and potassium 280 mg (7.1 mEq) per packet; fruit flavor]

Tablet:

K-Phos® MF: Potassium acid phosphate 155 mg and sodium acid phosphate 350 mg [equivalent to elemental phosphorus 125.6 mg, sodium 67 mg (2.9 mEq), and potassium 44.5 mg (1.1 mEq)]

K-Phos® Neutral: Monobasic potassium phosphate 155 mg, dibasic sodium phosphate 852 mg, and monobasic sodium phosphate 130 mg [equivalent to elemental phosphorus 250 mg, sodium 298 mg (13 mEq), and potassium 45 mg (1.1 mEq)]

K-Phos® No. 2: Potassium acid phosphate 305 mg and sodium acid phosphate 700 mg [equivalent to elemental phosphorus 250 mg, sodium 134 mg (5.8 mEq), and potassium 88 mg (2.3 mEq)]

Phospha 250™ Neutral: Monobasic potassium phosphate 155 mg, dibasic sodium phosphate 852 mg, and monobasic sodium phosphate 130 mg [equivalent to elemental phosphorus 250 mg, sodium 298 mg (13 mEq), and potassium 45 mg (1.1 mEq)]

◆ **Povidine™ [OTC]** *see* Povidone-Iodine *on page* 1222

Povidone-Iodine (POE vi done EYE oh dyne)

U.S. Brand Names Betadine®; Operand® [OTC]; Povidine™ [OTC]; Summer's Eve® Medicated Douche [OTC]; Vagi-Gard® [OTC]

Canadian Brand Names Betadine®; Proviodine

Index Terms Polyvinylpyrrolidone with Iodine; PVP-I

Pharmacologic Category Antiseptic, Ophthalmic; Antiseptic, Topical; Antiseptic, Vaginal; Topical Skin Product

Use External antiseptic with broad microbicidal spectrum for the prevention or treatment of topical infections associated with surgery, burns, minor cuts/scrapes; relief of minor vaginal irritation

Pregnancy Risk Factor C (ophthalmic)

Medication Safety Issues

Sound-alike/look-alike issues:

Betadine® may be confused with Betagan®, betaine

International issues:

Alphadine®: Brand name for ranitidine in Greece

Oralon® [Japan] may be confused with Oralone® which is a brand name for triamcinolone in the U.S.

Dosage

Antiseptic: Apply topically to affected area as needed. Ophthalmic solution may be used to irrigate the eye or applied to area around the eye such as skin, eyelashes, or lid margins.

Surgical scrub: Topical: Apply solution to wet skin or hands, scrub for ~5 minutes, rinse; refer to product labeling for specific procedure-related instructions.

Vaginal irritation: Douche: Insert 0.3% solution vaginally once daily for 5-7 days

Additional Information Complete prescribing information for this medication should be consulted for additional detail.

Dosage Forms Excipient information presented when available (limited, particularly for generics); consult specific product labeling. [DSC] = Discontinued product

Gel, topical: 10% (120 g)

Operand®: 10% (120 g)

Liquid, topical [prep-swab ampul]: 10% (0.65 mL)

Ointment, topical: 10% (1 g)

Povidine™: 10% (30 g)
Pad [prep pads]: 10% (200s)
Betadine® SwabAids: 10% (100s)
Solution, ophthalmic:
Betadine®: 5% (30 mL)
Solution, perineal [concentrate]:
Operand®: 10% (240 mL)
Solution, topical: 10% (22 mL, 60 mL, 90 mL, 240 mL, 480 mL, 3840 mL)
Betadine®: 10% (15 mL, 120 mL, 240 mL, 480 mL, 960 mL, 3840 mL)
Operand®: 10% (60 mL, 120 mL, 240 mL, 480 mL, 960 mL, 3840 mL)
Povidine™: 10% (240 mL)
Solution, topical [cleanser]:
Betadine® Skin Cleanser: 7.5% (120 mL)
Solution, topical [paint sponge]: 10% (50s)
Solution, topical [paint]: 10% (60 mL, 90 mL, 120 mL)
Solution, topical [surgical scrub]: 7.5% (60 mL, 120 mL)
Betadine® Surgical Scrub: 7.5% (120 mL, 480 mL, 960 mL, 3840 mL)
Operand®: 7.5% (60 mL, 120 mL, 240 mL, 480 mL, 960 mL, 3840 mL)
Solution, topical [spray]: 10% (60 mL)
Betadine®: 5% (90 mL) [CFC free; contains dry natural rubber]
Operand®: 10% (59 mL)
Solution, topical [surgical scrub sponge]: 10% (50s)
Solution, vaginal [concentrate, douche]:
Operand®: 10% (240 mL)
Vagi-Gard®: 10% (180 mL, 240 mL)
Solution, vaginal [douche]:
Summer's Eve® Medicated Douche: 0.3% (135 mL) [contains sodium benzoate]
Solution [concentrate, whirlpool]:
Operand®: 10% (3840 mL)
Swabsticks: 10% (25s, 50s, 1000s)
Betadine®: 10% (50s, 200s)
Swabsticks [gel saturated]: 10% (50s)
Swabsticks, topical [surgical scrub]: 7.5% (25s, 50s, 1000s)

◆ **PPD** *see* Tuberculin Tests *on page 1527*

◆ **PPL** *see* Benzylpenicilloyl-polylysine *on page 186*

◆ **PPS** *see* Pentosan Polysulfate Sodium *on page 1171*

◆ **PPSV** *see* Pneumococcal Polysaccharide Vaccine (Polyvalent) *on page 1206*

◆ **PPV23** *see* Pneumococcal Polysaccharide Vaccine (Polyvalent) *on page 1206*

Pralidoxime (pra li DOKS eem)

U.S. Brand Names Protopam®

Canadian Brand Names Protopam®

Index Terms 2-PAM; 2-Pyridine Aldoxime Methochloride; Pralidoxime Chloride

Pharmacologic Category Antidote

Use Reverse muscle paralysis caused by toxic exposure to organophosphate anticholinesterase pesticides and chemicals; control of overdose of anticholinesterase medications used to treat myasthenia gravis (ambenonium, neostigmine, pyridostigmine)

Unlabeled/Investigational Use Treatment of nerve agent toxicity (chemical warfare) in combination with atropine

Pregnancy Risk Factor C

Lactation Excretion in breast milk unknown/not recommended

Medication Safety Issues

Sound-alike/look-alike issues:

Pralidoxime may be confused with pramoxine, pyridoxine

Protopam® may be confused with Proloprim®, protamine, Protropin®

Contraindications Hypersensitivity to pralidoxime or any component of the formulation; poisonings due to phosphorus, inorganic phosphates, or organic phosphates without anticholinesterase activity; poisonings due to pesticides of carbamate class (may increase toxicity of carbaryl)

Warnings/Precautions Use with caution in patients with myasthenia gravis; dosage modification required in patients with impaired renal function. Clinical symptoms consistent with highly-suspected organophosphorous poisoning should be treated with antidote immediately; administration should not be delayed for confirmatory laboratory tests. Treatment should always include proper evacuation and decontamination procedures; medical personnel should protect themselves from inadvertent contamination. Antidotal administration is intended only for initial management; definitive and more extensive medical care is required following administration. Individuals should not rely solely on antidote for treatment, as other supportive measures (eg, artificial respiration) may still be required.

Adverse Reactions Frequency not defined.

Cardiovascular: Hypertension, tachycardia
Central nervous system: Dizziness, drowsiness, headache
Dermatologic: Rash
Gastrointestinal: Nausea
Hepatic: ALT increased (transient), AST increased (transient)
Local: Pain at injection site after I.M. administration
Neuromuscular & skeletal: Muscle rigidity, weakness
Ocular: Accommodation impaired, blurred vision, diplopia
Renal: Renal function decreased
Respiratory: Hyperventilation, laryngospasm

Drug Interactions

Avoid Concomitant Use There are no known interactions where it is recommended to avoid concomitant use.

Increased Effect/Toxicity There are no known significant interactions involving an increase in effect.

Decreased Effect There are no known significant interactions involving a decrease in effect.

Stability Store at controlled room temperature of 20°C to 25°C (68°F to 77°F). For I.V. administration, dilute 1 g with 20 mL SWI. Solution should be further diluted and administered as 1-2 g in 100 mL NS. If not practical or in cases of fluid overload, may prepare as a 5% solution.

Mechanism of Action Reactivates cholinesterase that had been inactivated by phosphorylation due to exposure to organophosphate pesticides by displacing the enzyme from its receptor sites; removes the phosphoryl group from the active site of the inactivated enzyme

Pharmacodynamics/Kinetics

Protein binding: None
Metabolism: Hepatic
Half-life elimination: 74-77 minutes
Time to peak, serum: I.V.: 5-15 minutes
Excretion: Urine (80% to 90% as metabolites and unchanged drug)

Dosage

Organic phosphorus poisoning (use in conjunction with atropine; atropine effects should be established before pralidoxime is administered): I.V. (may be given I.M. or SubQ if I.V. is not feasible):

Children: 20-50 mg/kg/dose; repeat in 1-2 hours if muscle weakness has not been relieved, then at 8- to 12-hour intervals if cholinergic signs recur

Adults: Initial: 30 mg/kg over 20 minutes, maintenance: I.V. infusion: 4-8 mg/kg/hour

Treatment of acetylcholinesterase inhibitor toxicity: Adults: I.V.: Initial: 1-2 g followed by increments of 250 mg every 5 minutes until response is observed

Nerve agent toxicity management (unlabeled use): **Note:** Atropine is a component of the management of nerve agent toxicity; consult atropine monograph for specific route and dose. To be effective, pralidoxime must be administered within minutes to a few hours following exposure (depending on the nerve agent).

Infants and Children:

Prehospital ("in the field"): Mild-to-moderate symptoms: I.M.: 15 mg/kg; severe symptoms: 25 mg/kg

Hospital/emergency department: Mild-to-severe symptoms: I.V.: 15 mg/kg (up to 1 g)

Adults:

Prehospital ("in the field"): Mild-to-moderate symptoms: I.M.: 600 mg; severe symptoms: 1800 mg

Hospital/emergency department: Mild-to-severe symptoms: I.V.: 15 mg/kg (up to 1 g)

Frail patients, elderly:

Prehospital ("in the field"): Mild-to-moderate symptoms: I.M.: 10 mg/kg; severe symptoms: 25 mg/kg

Hospital/emergency department: Mild-to-severe symptoms: I.V.: 5-10 mg/kg

Elderly: Refer to adult dosing; dosing should be cautious, considering possibility of decreased hepatic, renal, or cardiac function

Dosing adjustment in renal impairment: Dose should be reduced

Administration I.V.: Infuse over 15-30 minutes at a rate not to exceed 200 mg/minute; may administer I.M. or SubQ if I.V. is not accessible. If a more concentrated 5% solution is used, infuse over at least 5 minutes.

Monitoring Parameters Heart rate, respiratory rate, blood pressure, continuous ECG; cardiac monitor and blood pressure monitor required for I.V. administration

Reference Range Minimum therapeutic concentration: 4 mcg/mL

Additional Information Pralidoxime is most effective when given immediately after poisoning. If the poison has been ingested, exposure may continue due to slow absorption from the lower bowel; relapses may occur after initial improvement and treatment may need continued for several days in these patients. In cases of dermal exposure to organophosphate poisoning, clothing should be removed and hair and skin washed with sodium bicarbonate or alcohol as soon as possible.

Dosage Forms Excipient information presented when available (limited, particularly for generics); consult specific product labeling.

Injection, powder for reconstitution, as chloride:

Protopam®: 1 g

Injection, solution: 300 mg/mL (2 mL) [contains benzyl alcohol; prefilled auto injector]

◆ **Pralidoxime and Atropine** *see* Atropine and Pralidoxime *on page 159*

◆ **Pralidoxime Chloride** *see* Pralidoxime *on page 1223*

Pramipexole (pra mi PEKS ole)

U.S. Brand Names Mirapex®

Canadian Brand Names Apo-Pramipexole; Mirapex®; Novo-Pramipexole; PMS-Pramipexole; SANDOZ-Pramipexole

Pharmacologic Category Anti-Parkinson's Agent, Dopamine Agonist

Additional Appendix Information

Antiparkinsonian Agents *on page 1643*

Use Treatment of the signs and symptoms of idiopathic Parkinson's disease; treatment of moderate-to-severe primary Restless Legs Syndrome (RLS)

Unlabeled/Investigational Use Treatment of depression

Pregnancy Risk Factor C

Pregnancy Considerations Early embryonic loss and postnatal growth inhibition were observed in animal studies. There are no adequate and well-controlled studies in pregnant women.

Lactation Excretion in breast milk unknown/not recommended

Medication Safety Issues

Sound-alike/look-alike issues:

Mirapex® may be confused with Mifeprex®, MiraLax™

Contraindications Hypersensitivity to pramipexole or any component of the formulation

Warnings/Precautions Caution should be taken in patients with renal insufficiency; dose adjustment necessary. Caution in patients with pre-existing dyskinesias; may be exacerbated. May cause orthostatic hypotension; Parkinson's disease patients appear to have an impaired capacity to respond to a postural challenge. Use with caution in patients at risk of hypotension or where transient hypotensive episodes would be poorly tolerated. Parkinson's patients being treated with dopaminergic agonists ordinarily require careful monitoring for signs and symptoms of postural hypotension, especially during dose escalation. May cause hallucinations.

Dopamine agonists have been associated with compulsive behaviors and/or loss of impulse control, which has manifested as pathological gambling, libido increases (hypersexuality), and/or binge eating. Causality has not been established, and controversy exists as to whether this phenomenon is related to the underlying disease, prior behaviors/addictions and/or drug therapy. Dose reduction or discontinuation of therapy has been reported to reverse these behaviors in some, but not all cases.

Dopaminergic agents have been associated with a syndrome resembling neuroleptic malignant syndrome on abrupt withdrawal or significant dosage reduction after long-term use. Ergot-derived dopamine agonists have also been associated with fibrotic complications (eg, retroperitoneal fibrosis, pleural thickening, and pulmonary infiltrates). Although pramipexole is not an ergot, there have been postmarketing reports of possible fibrotic complications with pramipexole; monitor closely for signs and symptoms of fibrosis.

Pramipexole has been associated with somnolence, particularly at higher dosages (>1.5 mg/day). In addition, patients have been reported to fall asleep during activities of daily living, including driving, while taking this medication. Whether these patients exhibited somnolence prior to these events is not clear. Patients should be advised of this issue and factors which may increase risk (sleep disorders, other sedating medications, or concomitant medications which increase pramipexole concentrations) and instructed to report daytime somnolence or sleepiness to the prescriber. Patients should use caution in performing activities which require alertness (driving or operating machinery), and to avoid other medications which may cause CNS depression, including ethanol.

Pathologic degenerative changes were observed in the retinas of albino rats during studies with this agent, but were not observed in the retinas of albino mice or in other species. The significance of these data for humans remains uncertain. Augmentation (earlier onset of symptoms in the evening/afternoon, increase and/or spread of symptoms to other extremities) or rebound (shifting of symptoms to early morning hours) may occur in some RLS patients. Safety and efficacy have not been established in children.

Adverse Reactions Parkinson's disease (PD) unless identified as RLS:

>10%:

Cardiovascular: Postural hypotension (dose related; PD 53%)

Central nervous system: Dizziness (PD 25%), headache (RLS 16%), somnolence (dose related; RLS 6%; PD 9% to 22%), insomnia (RLS 13%; PD 17% to 27%), hallucinations (PD 9% to 17%), abnormal dreams (RLS up to 8%)

Gastrointestinal: Nausea (dose related; RLS: 5% to 27%; PD 28%), constipation (dose related; RLS: 4%; PD 10% to 14%)

Neuromuscular & skeletal: Weakness (PD 10% to 14%), dyskinesia (PD 47%), EPS

1% to 10%:

Cardiovascular: Edema, syncope, tachycardia, chest pain

Central nervous system: Malaise, confusion (PD 4% to 10%), amnesia (dose related), dystonias, akathisia, thinking abnormalities, myoclonus, hyperesthesia, paranoia, fever

Endocrine & metabolic: Decreased libido

Gastrointestinal: Anorexia, diarrhea (RLS 3% to7%), dysphagia, weight loss, xerostomia (up to 7%)

Genitourinary: Urinary frequency (PD 6%), impotence, urinary incontinence

Neuromuscular & skeletal: Muscle twitching, leg cramps, arthritis, bursitis, myasthenia, gait abnormalities, hypertonia

Ocular: Vision abnormalities

Respiratory: Dyspnea, nasal congestion (RLS up to 6%), rhinitis

Miscellaneous: Influenza (RLS 3%)

<1% (Limited to important or life-threatening): Augmentation (RLS ~20% but similar to placebo), compulsive gambling, liver transaminases increased, rebound (RLS), rhabdomyolysis, tolerance (RLS)

Reported with dopamine agonists: Impulsive/compulsive behaviors (eg, pathological gambling, hypersexuality, binge eating)

Frequency not defined, dose related: Falling asleep during activities of daily living

Drug Interactions

Avoid Concomitant Use There are no known interactions where it is recommended to avoid concomitant use.

Increased Effect/Toxicity

Pramipexole may increase the levels/effects of: Alcohol (Ethyl); CNS Depressants

Decreased Effect

The levels/effects of Pramipexole may be decreased by: Antipsychotics (Atypical); Antipsychotics (Typical); Metoclopramide

Ethanol/Nutrition/Herb Interactions

Ethanol: Avoid ethanol (may increase CNS depression).

Food: Food intake does not affect the extent of drug absorption, although the time to maximal plasma concentration is delayed by 60 minutes when taken with a meal.

Herb/Nutraceutical: Avoid valerian, St John's wort, SAMe, kava kava (may increase risk of serotonin syndrome and/or excessive sedation).

Stability Store at 15°C to 30°C (59°F to 86°F). Protect from light.

Mechanism of Action Pramipexole is a nonergot dopamine agonist with specificity for the D_2 subfamily dopamine receptor, and has also been shown to bind to D_3 and D_4 receptors. By binding to these receptors, it is thought that pramipexole can stimulate dopamine activity on the nerves of the striatum and substantia nigra.

Pharmacodynamics/Kinetics

Absorption: Rapid

Distribution: V_d: 500 L

Protein binding: 15%

Bioavailability: >90%

Half-life elimination: ~8 hours; Elderly: 12-14 hours

Time to peak, serum: ~2 hours

Excretion: Urine (90% as unchanged drug)

Dosage Oral: Adults:

Parkinson's disease: Initial: 0.375 mg/day given in 3 divided doses, increase gradually by 0.125 mg/dose every 5-7 days; range: 1.5-4.5 mg/day

Restless legs syndrome: Initial: 0.125 mg once daily 2-3 hours before bedtime. Dose may be doubled every 4-7 days up to 0.5 mg/day. Maximum dose: 0.5 mg/day (manufacturer's recommendation).

Note: Most patients require <0.5 mg/day, but higher doses have been used (2 mg/day). If augmentation occurs, dose earlier in the day.

Dosage adjustment in renal impairment: Use caution; renally-eliminated

Parkinson's disease:

Cl_{cr} 35-59 mL/minute: Initial: 0.125 mg twice daily (maximum dose: 1.5 mg twice daily)

Cl_{cr} 15-34 mL/minute: Initial: 0.125 mg once daily (maximum dose: 1.5 mg once daily)

Cl_{cr} <15 mL/minute (or hemodialysis patients): Not adequately studied

Restless legs syndrome:

Cl_{cr} 20-60 mL/minute: Duration between titration should be increased to 14 days

Cl_{cr} <20 mL/minute: Not adequately studied

Dietary Considerations May be taken with food to decrease nausea.

Administration Doses should be titrated gradually in all patients to avoid the onset of intolerable side effects. The dosage should be increased to achieve a maximum therapeutic effect, balanced against the side effects of dyskinesia, hallucinations, somnolence, and dry mouth.

Monitoring Parameters Monitor for improvement in symptoms of Parkinson's disease (eg, mentation, behavior, daily living activities, motor examinations), blood pressure, body weight changes, and heart rate

Dosage Forms Excipient information presented when available (limited, particularly for generics); consult specific product labeling. [CAN] = Canadian product

Tablet, as dihydrochloride monohydrate: 0.25 mg [CAN; generic not available in U.S.], 0.5 mg [CAN; generic not available in U.S.], 1 mg [CAN; generic not available in U.S.], 1.5 mg [CAN; generic not available in U.S.]

Mirapex®: 0.125 mg, 0.25 mg, 0.5 mg, 0.75 mg, 1 mg, 1.5 mg

Pramlintide (PRAM lin tide)

U.S. Brand Names Symlin®

Index Terms Pramlintide Acetate

Pharmacologic Category Amylinomimetic; Antidiabetic Agent

Use

Adjunctive treatment with mealtime insulin in type 1 diabetes mellitus (insulin dependent, IDDM) patients who have failed to achieve desired glucose control despite optimal insulin therapy

Adjunctive treatment with mealtime insulin in type 2 diabetes mellitus (noninsulin dependent, NIDDM) patients who have failed to achieve desired glucose control despite optimal insulin therapy, with or without concurrent sulfonylurea and/or metformin

Restrictions An FDA-approved medication guide must be distributed when dispensing an outpatient prescription (new or refill) where this medication is to be used without direct supervision of a healthcare provider. Medication guides are available at http://www.fda.gov/cder/Offices/ODS/medication_guides.htm.

Pregnancy Risk Factor C

Pregnancy Considerations Due to adverse events observed in some animal studies, pramlintide is classified as pregnancy category C. Based on *in vitro* data, pramlintide has a low potential to cross the placenta. Maternal hyperglycemia can be associated with adverse effects in the fetus, including macrosomia, neonatal hyperglycemia, and hyperbilirubinemia; the risk of congenital malformations is increased when the Hb A_{1c} is above the normal range. Diabetes can also be associated with adverse effects in the mother. Poorly-treated diabetes may cause end-organ damage that may in turn negatively affect obstetric outcomes. Physiologic glucose levels should be maintained prior to and during pregnancy to decrease the risk of adverse events in the mother and the fetus. Until additional safety and efficacy data are obtained, the use of pramlintide is generally not recommended in the routine management of diabetes mellitus during pregnancy. Insulin is the drug of choice for the control of diabetes mellitus during pregnancy.

Lactation Excretion in breast milk unknown/use caution

Medication Safety Issues

High alert medication: The Institute for Safe Medication Practices (ISMP) includes this medication among its list of drug classes which have a heightened risk of causing significant patient harm when used in error.

Dosing: The concentration of this product is 600 micrograms (mcg)/mL. Manufacturer recommended dosing ranges from 15 mcg to 120 mcg, which corresponds to injectable volumes of 0.025 mL to 0.2 mL. Patients and healthcare providers should exercise caution when administering this product to avoid inadvertent calculation of the dose based on "units," which could result in a sixfold overdose.

Contraindications Hypersensitivity to pramlintide or any component of the formulation; confirmed diagnosis of gastroparesis; hypoglycemia unawareness

Warnings/Precautions [U.S. Boxed Warning]: Coadministration with insulin may induce severe hypoglycemia (usually within 3 hours following administration); coadministration with insulin therapy is an approved indication but does require an initial dosage reduction of insulin and frequent pre and post blood glucose monitoring to reduce risk of severe hypoglycemia. Concurrent use of other glucose-lowering agents may increase risk of hypoglycemia. Avoid use in patients with poor compliance with their insulin regimen and/or blood glucose monitoring. Do not use in patients with Hb A_{1c} levels >9% or recent, recurrent episodes of hypoglycemia; obtain detailed history of glucose control (eg, Hb A_{1c}, incidence of hypoglycemia, glucose monitoring, and medication compliance) and body weight before initiating therapy. Use caution in patients with visual or dexterity impairment. Use caution when driving or operating heavy machinery until effects on blood sugar are known. Use caution with certain antihypertensive agents (eg, beta-adrenergic blockers) or neuropathic conditions which may mask signs/symptoms of hypoglycemia. Use caution in patients with history of nausea; avoid use in patients with conditions or concurrent medications likely to impair gastric motility (eg, anticholinergics); do not use in patients requiring medication(s) to stimulate gastric emptying. Safety and efficacy in pediatric patients have not been established.

Adverse Reactions

>10%:

Central nervous system: Headache (5% to 13%)

Gastrointestinal: Nausea (28% to 48%), vomiting (7% to 11%), anorexia (≤17%)

Endocrine & metabolic: Severe hypoglycemia (type 1 diabetes ≤17%)

Miscellaneous: Inflicted injury (8% to 14%)

1% to 10%:

Central nervous system: Fatigue (3% to 7%), dizziness (2% to 6%)

Endocrine & metabolic: Severe hypoglycemia (type 2 diabetes ≤8%)

Gastrointestinal: Abdominal pain (2% to 8%)

Respiratory: Pharyngitis (3% to 5%), cough (2% to 6%)

Neuromuscular & skeletal: Arthralgia (2% to 7%)

Miscellaneous: Allergic reaction (≤6%)

Postmarketing and/or case reports: Injection site reactions

Drug Interactions

Avoid Concomitant Use There are no known interactions where it is recommended to avoid concomitant use.

Increased Effect/Toxicity

Pramlintide may increase the levels/effects of: Anticholinergics

Decreased Effect There are no known significant interactions involving a decrease in effect.

Ethanol/Nutrition/Herb Interactions

Ethanol: Use caution with ethanol (may increase hypoglycemia).

Herb/Nutraceutical: Use caution with garlic, chromium, gymnema (may increase hypoglycemia).

Stability Store unopened vials at 2°C to 8°C (36°F to 46°F); do not freeze. Opened vials may be kept refrigerated or at room temperature ≤30°C (≤86°F). Discard opened vial after 30 days. Protect from light.

Mechanism of Action Synthetic analog of human amylin cosecreted with insulin by pancreatic beta cells; reduces postprandial glucose increases via the following mechanisms: 1) prolongation of gastric emptying time, 2) reduction of postprandial glucagon secretion, and 3) reduction of caloric intake through centrally-mediated appetite suppression

Pharmacodynamics/Kinetics

Duration: 3 hours

Protein binding: ~60%

Metabolism: Primarily renal to des-lys[1] pramlintide (active metabolite)

Bioavailability: ~30% to 40%

Half-life elimination: ~48 minutes

Time to peak, plasma: 20 minutes

Excretion: Primarily urine

Dosage SubQ: Adults: **Note:** When initiating pramlintide, reduce current insulin dose (including rapidly- and mixed-acting preparations) by 50% to avoid hypoglycemia.

Type 1 diabetes mellitus (insulin dependent, IDDM): Initial: 15 mcg immediately prior to meals; titrate in 15 mcg increments every 3 days (if no significant nausea occurs) to target dose of 30-60 mcg (consider discontinuation if intolerant of 30 mcg dose)

Type 2 diabetes mellitus (noninsulin dependent, NIDDM): Initial: 60 mcg immediately prior to meals; after 3-7 days, increase to 120 mcg prior to meals if no significant nausea occurs (if nausea occurs at 120 mcg dose, reduce to 60 mcg)

If pramlintide is discontinued for any reason, restart therapy with same initial titration protocol.

Dosage adjustment in renal impairment: No dosage adjustment required; not evaluated in dialysis patients

Dietary Considerations Dietary modification based on ADA recommendations is a part of therapy; pramlintide to be administered prior to major meals consisting of ≥250 Kcal or ≥30 g carbohydrates

Administration Do not mix with other insulins; administer subcutaneously into abdominal or thigh areas at sites distinct from concomitant insulin injections (do not administer into arm due to variable absorption); rotate injection sites frequently. Allow solution to reach room temperature before administering; may reduce injection site reactions. For oral medications in which a rapid onset of action is desired, administer 1 hour before, or 2 hours after pramlintide, if possible. When using the pen-injector, do not transfer drug to a syringe; dosing errors could occur.

Monitoring Parameters Prior to initiating therapy: Hb A_{1c}, hypoglycemic history, body weight. During therapy: urine sugar and acetone, pre- and postprandial and bedtime serum glucose, electrolytes, Hb A_{1c}, lipid profile

Dosage Forms Excipient information presented when available (limited, particularly for generics); consult specific product labeling.

Injection, solution, as acetate:

Symlin®: 600 mcg/mL (5 mL); 1000 mcg/mL (1.5 mL) [60 pen-injector]; 1000 mcg/mL (2.7 mL) [120 pen-injector]

- **Pramlintide Acetate** *see* Pramlintide *on page 1225*
- **Pramosone®** *see* Pramoxine and Hydrocortisone *on page 1227*
- **Pramox® HC (Can)** *see* Pramoxine and Hydrocortisone *on page 1227*

Pramoxine and Hydrocortisone

(pra MOKS een & hye droe KOR ti sone)

U.S. Brand Names Analpram-HC®; Epifoam®; Pramosone®; ProctoFoam®-HC

Canadian Brand Names Pramox® HC; Proctofoam™-HC

Index Terms Hydrocortisone and Pramoxine; Pramoxine Hydrochloride and Hydrocortisone Acetate

Pharmacologic Category Anesthetic/Corticosteroid

Use Relief of inflammatory and pruritic manifestations of corticosteroid-responsive dermatoses

Pregnancy Risk Factor C

Medication Safety Issues

Sound-alike/look-alike issues:

Pramosone® may be confused with predniSONE

Zone-A Forte® may be confused with Zonalon®

Dosage Topical/rectal: Apply to affected areas 3-4 times/day

Additional Information Complete prescribing information for this medication should be consulted for additional detail.

Dosage Forms Excipient information presented when available (limited, particularly for generics); consult specific product labeling.

Cream, topical:

Analpram-HC®: Pramoxine hydrochloride 1% and hydrocortisone acetate 1% (4 g, 30 g); pramoxine hydrochloride 1% and hydrocortisone acetate 2.5% (4 g, 30 g)

Pramosone®: Pramoxine hydrochloride 1% and hydrocortisone acetate 1% (30 g, 60 g); pramoxine hydrochloride 1% and hydrocortisone acetate 2.5% (30 g, 60 g)

Foam, rectal (ProctoFoam®-HC): Pramoxine hydrochloride 1% and hydrocortisone acetate 1% (10 g)

Foam, topical (Epifoam®): Pramoxine hydrochloride 1% and hydrocortisone acetate 1% (10 g)

Lotion, topical:

Analpram-HC®: Pramoxine hydrochloride 1% and hydrocortisone acetate 2.5% (60 mL)

Pramosone®: Pramoxine hydrochloride 1% and hydrocortisone acetate 1% (60 mL, 120 mL, 240 mL); pramoxine hydrochloride 1% and hydrocortisone acetate 2.5% (60 mL, 120 mL)

Ointment, topical (Pramosone®): Pramoxine hydrochloride 1% and hydrocortisone acetate 1% (30 g); pramoxine hydrochloride 1% and hydrocortisone acetate 2.5% (30 g)

- **Pramoxine Hydrochloride and Hydrocortisone Acetate** *see* Pramoxine and Hydrocortisone *on page 1227*
- **PrandiMet™** *see* Repaglinide and Metformin *on page 1305*
- **Prandin®** *see* Repaglinide *on page 1303*
- **Prascion®** *see* Sulfur and Sulfacetamide *on page 1411*
- **Prascion® AV [DSC]** *see* Sulfur and Sulfacetamide *on page 1411*
- **Prascion® FC** *see* Sulfur and Sulfacetamide *on page 1411*
- **Prascion® RA** *see* Sulfur and Sulfacetamide *on page 1411*
- **Prascion® TS** *see* Sulfur and Sulfacetamide *on page 1411*
- **Pravachol®** *see* Pravastatin *on page 1227*
- **PravASA (Can)** *see* Aspirin and Pravastatin *on page 146*

Pravastatin (prav a STAT in)

U.S. Brand Names Pravachol®

Canadian Brand Names Apo-Pravastatin®; CO Pravastatin; DOM-Pravastatin; GEN-Pravastatin; Novo-Pravastatin; NU-Pravastatin; PHL-Pravastatin; PMS-Pravastatin; Pravachol®; RAN-Pravastatin; ratio-Pravastatin; Riva-Pravastatin; Sandoz-Pravastatin

Index Terms Pravastatin Sodium

Pharmacologic Category Antilipemic Agent, HMG-CoA Reductase Inhibitor

Additional Appendix Information

Hyperlipidemia Management *on page 1815*

Lipid-Lowering Agents *on page 1661*

Use Use with dietary therapy for the following:

Primary prevention of coronary events: In hypercholesterolemic patients without established coronary heart disease to reduce cardiovascular morbidity (myocardial infarction, coronary revascularization procedures) and mortality.

Secondary prevention of cardiovascular events in patients with established coronary heart disease: To slow the progression of coronary atherosclerosis; to reduce cardiovascular morbidity (myocardial infarction, coronary vascular procedures) and to reduce mortality; to reduce the risk of stroke and transient ischemic attacks

Hyperlipidemias: Reduce elevations in total cholesterol, LDL-C, apolipoprotein B, and triglycerides (elevations of 1 or more components are present in Fredrickson type IIa, IIb, III, and IV hyperlipidemias)

Heterozygous familial hypercholesterolemia (HeFH): In pediatric patients, 8-18 years of age, with HeFH having LDL-C ≥190 mg/dL **or** LDL ≥160 mg/dL with positive family history of premature cardiovascular disease (CVD) or 2 or more CVD risk factors in the pediatric patient

Pregnancy Risk Factor X

Pregnancy Considerations Cholesterol biosynthesis may be important in fetal development. Contraindicated in pregnancy. Administer to women of childbearing potential only when conception is highly unlikely and patients have been informed of potential hazards.

Lactation Enters breast milk/contraindicated

Medication Safety Issues

Sound-alike/look-alike issues:

Pravachol® may be confused with Prevacid®, Prinivil®, propranolol

Contraindications Hypersensitivity to pravastatin or any component of the formulation; active liver disease; unexplained persistent elevations of serum transaminases; pregnancy; breast-feeding

Warnings/Precautions Secondary causes of hyperlipidemia should be ruled out prior to therapy. Liver function must be monitored by periodic laboratory assessment. Rhabdomyolysis with acute renal failure has occurred.

Risk may be increased with concurrent use of other drugs which may cause rhabdomyolysis (including colchicine, gemfibrozil, fibric acid derivatives, or niacin at doses ≥1 g/day). Temporarily discontinue in any patient experiencing an acute or serious condition predisposing to renal failure secondary to rhabdomyolysis. Based upon current evidence, HMG-CoA reductase inhibitor therapy should be continued in the perioperative period unless risk outweighs cardioprotective benefit. Use with caution in patients with advanced age, these patients are predisposed to myopathy. Use caution in patients with previous liver disease or heavy ethanol use. Treatment in patients <8 years of age is not recommended.

Adverse Reactions As reported in short-term trials; safety and tolerability with long-term use were similar to placebo

1% to 10%:

Cardiovascular: Chest pain (4%)

Central nervous system: Headache (2% to 6%), fatigue (4%), dizziness (1% to 3%)

Dermatologic: Rash (4%)

Gastrointestinal: Nausea/vomiting (7%), diarrhea (6%), heartburn (3%)

Hepatic: Transaminases increased (>3x normal on two occasions - 1%)

Neuromuscular & skeletal: Myalgia (2%)

Respiratory: Cough (3%)

Miscellaneous: Influenza (2%)

<1% (Limited to important or life-threatening): Allergy, lens opacity, libido change, memory impairment, muscle weakness, neuropathy, paresthesia, taste disturbance, tremor, vertigo

Postmarketing and/or case reports: Anaphylaxis, angioedema, cholestatic jaundice, cirrhosis, cranial nerve dysfunction, dermatomyositis, erythema multiforme, ESR increase, fulminant hepatic necrosis, gynecomastia, hemolytic anemia, hepatitis, hepatoma, lupus erythematosus-like syndrome, myopathy, pancreatitis, peripheral nerve palsy, polymyalgia rheumatica, positive ANA, purpura, rhabdomyolysis, Stevens-Johnson syndrome, vasculitis

Additional class-related events or case reports (not necessarily reported with pravastatin therapy): Angioedema, cataracts, depression, dyspnea, eosinophilia, erectile dysfunction, facial paresis, hypersensitivity reaction, impaired extraocular muscle movement, impotence, leukopenia, malaise, memory loss, ophthalmoplegia, paresthesia, peripheral neuropathy, photosensitivity, psychic disturbance, skin discoloration, thrombocytopenia, thyroid dysfunction, toxic epidermal necrolysis, transaminases increased, vomiting

Drug Interactions

Metabolism/Transport Effects **Substrate** of CYP3A4 (minor); **Inhibits** CYP2C9 (weak), 2D6 (weak), 3A4 (weak)

Avoid Concomitant Use There are no known interactions where it is recommended to avoid concomitant use.

Increased Effect/Toxicity

Pravastatin may increase the levels/effects of: DAPTOmycin; Vitamin K Antagonists

The levels/effects of Pravastatin may be increased by: Antifungal Agents (Azole Derivatives, Systemic); Colchicine; CycloSPORINE; Eltrombopag; Fenofibrate; Fenofibric Acid; Gemfibrozil; Niacin; Niacinamide; P-Glycoprotein Inhibitors; Protease Inhibitors

Decreased Effect

The levels/effects of Pravastatin may be decreased by: P-Glycoprotein Inducers; Phenytoin; Rifamycin Derivatives

Ethanol/Nutrition/Herb Interactions

Ethanol: Consumption of large amounts of ethanol may increase the risk of liver damage with HMG-CoA reductase inhibitors.

Food: Red yeast rice contains an estimated 2.4 mg lovastatin per 600 mg rice.

Herb/Nutraceutical: St John's wort may decrease pravastatin levels.

Stability Store at 25°C (77°F); excursions permitted to 15°C to 30°C (59°F to 86°F). Protect from moisture and light.

Mechanism of Action Pravastatin is a competitive inhibitor of 3-hydroxy-3-methylglutaryl coenzyme A (HMG-CoA) reductase, which is the rate-limiting enzyme involved in *de novo* cholesterol synthesis.

Pharmacodynamics/Kinetics

Onset of action: Several days

Peak effect: 4 weeks

Absorption: Rapidly absorbed; average absorption 34%

Protein binding: 50%

Metabolism: Hepatic to at least two metabolites

Bioavailability: 17%

Half-life elimination: ~2-3 hours

Time to peak, serum: 1-1.5 hours

Excretion: Feces (70%); urine (≤20%, 8% as unchanged drug)

Dosage Oral: **Note:** Doses should be individualized according to the baseline LDL-cholesterol levels, the recommended goal of therapy, and patient response; adjustments should be made at intervals of 4 weeks or more; doses may need adjusted based on concomitant medications

Children: HeFH:

8-13 years: 20 mg/day

14-18 years: 40 mg/day

Dosage adjustment for pravastatin based on concomitant cyclosporine: Refer to adult dosing section

Adults: Hyperlipidemias, primary prevention of coronary events, secondary prevention of cardiovascular events: Initial: 40 mg once daily; titrate dosage to response; usual range: 10-80 mg; (maximum dose: 80 mg once daily)

Dosage adjustment for pravastatin based on concomitant cyclosporine: Initial: 10 mg/day, titrate with caution (maximum dose: 20 mg/day)

Elderly: No specific dosage recommendations. Clearance is reduced in the elderly, resulting in an increase in AUC between 25% to 50%. However, substantial accumulation is not expected.

Dosing adjustment in renal impairment: Initial: 10 mg/day

Dosing adjustment in hepatic impairment: Initial: 10 mg/day

Dietary Considerations May be taken without regard to meals. Before initiation of therapy, patients should be placed on a standard cholesterol-lowering diet for 6 weeks and the diet should be continued during drug therapy. Red yeast rice contains an estimated 2.4 mg lovastatin per 600 mg rice.

Administration May be taken without regard to meals.

Monitoring Parameters Obtain baseline LFTs and total cholesterol profile; creatine phosphokinase due to possibility of myopathy. Repeat LFTs prior to elevation of dose May be measured when clinically indicated and/or periodically thereafter.

Dosage Forms Excipient information presented when available (limited, particularly for generics); consult specific product labeling.

Tablet, as sodium: 10 mg, 20 mg, 40 mg, 80 mg

Pravachol®: 10 mg; 20 mg [DSC]; 40 mg, 80 mg

◆ **Pravastatin and Aspirin** *see* Aspirin and Pravastatin *on page 146*

◆ **Pravastatin Sodium** *see* Pravastatin *on page 1227*

◆ **Pravigard™ PAC [DSC]** *see* Aspirin and Pravastatin *on page 146*

Praziquantel (pray zi KWON tel)

U.S. Brand Names Biltricide®
Canadian Brand Names Biltricide®
Pharmacologic Category Anthelmintic
Use All stages of schistosomiasis caused by all *Schistosoma* species pathogenic to humans; clonorchiasis and opisthorchiasis
Unlabeled/Investigational Use Cysticercosis and many intestinal tapeworms
Pregnancy Risk Factor B
Lactation Enters breast milk
Contraindications Hypersensitivity to praziquantel or any component of the formulation; ocular cysticercosis
Warnings/Precautions Use caution in patients with severe hepatic disease; patients with cerebral cysticercosis require hospitalization. Use caution with concurrent administration of strong inducers of cytochrome P450; therapeutic levels of praziquantel may not be achieved.
Adverse Reactions
1% to 10%:
Central nervous system: Dizziness, drowsiness, headache, malaise, CSF reaction syndrome in patients being treated for neurocysticercosis
Gastrointestinal: Abdominal pain, loss of appetite, nausea, vomiting
Miscellaneous: Diaphoresis
<1% (Limited to important or life-threatening): Diarrhea, fever, itching, rash, urticaria
Drug Interactions
Metabolism/Transport Effects **Inhibits** CYP2D6 (weak)
Avoid Concomitant Use
Avoid concomitant use of Praziquantel with any of the following: Rifampin
Increased Effect/Toxicity
The levels/effects of Praziquantel may be increased by: Cimetidine; CYP3A4 Inhibitors (Moderate); CYP3A4 Inhibitors (Strong); Dasatinib; Ketoconazole
Decreased Effect
The levels/effects of Praziquantel may be decreased by: Aminoquinolines (Antimalarial); CYP3A4 Inducers (Strong); Deferasirox; Herbs (CYP3A4 Inducers); Rifampin
Mechanism of Action Increases the cell permeability to calcium in schistosomes, causing strong contractions and paralysis of worm musculature leading to detachment of suckers from the blood vessel walls and to dislodgment
Pharmacodynamics/Kinetics
Absorption: Oral: ~80%
Distribution: CSF concentration is 14% to 20% of plasma concentration; enters breast milk
Protein binding: ~80%
Metabolism: Extensive first-pass effect
Half-life elimination: Parent drug: 0.8-1.5 hours; Metabolites: 4.5 hours
Time to peak, serum: 1-3 hours
Excretion: Urine (99% as metabolites)
Dosage Children >4 years and Adults: Oral:
Schistosomiasis: 20 mg/kg/dose 2-3 times/day for 1 day at 4- to 6-hour intervals
Flukes (unlabeled use): 25 mg/kg/dose every 8 hours for 1-2 days
Cysticercosis (unlabeled use): 50 mg/kg/day divided every 8 hours for 14 days
Tapeworms (unlabeled use): 10-20 mg/kg as a single dose (25 mg/kg for *Hymenolepis nana*)
Clonorchiasis/opisthorchiasis: 3 doses of 25 mg/kg as a 1-day treatment
Dosage Forms Excipient information presented when available (limited, particularly for generics); consult specific product labeling.
Tablet [tri-scored]: 600 mg

Prazosin (PRAZ oh sin)

U.S. Brand Names Minipress®
Canadian Brand Names Apo-Prazo®; Minipress®; Novo-Prazin; Nu-Prazo
Index Terms Furazosin; Prazosin Hydrochloride
Pharmacologic Category $Alpha_1$ Blocker
Use Treatment of hypertension
Unlabeled/Investigational Use Post-traumatic stress disorder (PTSD); benign prostatic hyperplasia; Raynaud's syndrome
Pregnancy Risk Factor C
Medication Safety Issues
Sound-alike/look-alike issues:
Prazosin may be confused with predniSONE

International issues:
Prazac® [Denmark] may be confused with Prozac® which is a brand name for fluoxetine in the U.S.
Prazepam [multiple international markets] may be confused with prazosin.
Dosage Oral:
Children (unlabeled use): Initial: 0.05-0.1 mg/kg/day in 3 divided doses; maximum: 0.5 mg/kg/day
Adults:
Hypertension: Initial: 1 mg/dose 2-3 times/day; usual maintenance dose: 3-15 mg/day in divided doses 2-4 times/day; maximum daily dose: 20 mg
Hypertensive urgency: 10-20 mg once, may repeat in 30 minutes
PTSD (unlabeled use): Initial: 2 mg at bedtime; titrate as tolerated to 10-15 mg at bedtime
Raynaud's (unlabeled use): 0.5-3 mg twice daily
Benign prostatic hyperplasia (unlabeled use): 2 mg twice daily
Additional Information Complete prescribing information for this medication should be consulted for additional detail.
Dosage Forms Excipient information presented when available (limited, particularly for generics); consult specific product labeling.
Capsule, as hydrochloride: 1 mg, 2 mg, 5 mg

◆ **Prazosin Hydrochloride** *see* Prazosin *on page* 1229
◆ **Precedex®** *see* Dexmedetomidine *on page* 428
◆ **Precose®** *see* Acarbose *on page* 24
◆ **Pred Forte®** *see* PrednisoLONE *on page* 1230
◆ **Pred-G®** *see* Prednisolone and Gentamicin *on page* 1232
◆ **Pred Mild®** *see* PrednisoLONE *on page* 1230

Prednicarbate (pred ni KAR bate)

U.S. Brand Names Dermatop®
Canadian Brand Names Dermatop®
Pharmacologic Category Corticosteroid, Topical
Additional Appendix Information
Corticosteroids *on page* 1652
Use Relief of the inflammatory and pruritic manifestations of corticosteroid-responsive dermatoses (medium potency topical corticosteroid)
Pregnancy Risk Factor C
Medication Safety Issues
Sound-alike/look-alike issues:
Dermatop® may be confused with Dimetapp®
Dosage Adults: Topical: Apply a thin film to affected area twice daily. Therapy should be discontinued when control is achieved; if no improvement is seen, reassessment of diagnosis may be necessary.

Additional Information Complete prescribing information for this medication should be consulted for additional detail.

Dosage Forms Excipient information presented when available (limited, particularly for generics); consult specific product labeling.

Cream: 0.1% (15 g, 60 g)
 Dermatop®: 0.1% (15 g [DSC], 60 g)
Ointment: 0.1% (15 g, 60 g)
 Dermatop®: 0.1% (15 g [DSC], 60 g)

PrednisoLONE (pred NISS oh lone)

U.S. Brand Names Econopred® Plus [DSC]; Millipred™; Omnipred™; Orapred ODT™; Orapred®; Pediapred®; Pred Forte®; Pred Mild®; Prelone®

Canadian Brand Names Diopred®; Hydeltra T.B.A.®; Inflamase® Mild; Novo-Prednisolone; Ophtho-Tate®; Pediapred®; Pred Forte®; Pred Mild®; Sab-Prenase

Index Terms Deltahydrocortisone; Metacortandralone; Prednisolone Acetate; Prednisolone Acetate, Ophthalmic; Prednisolone Sodium Phosphate; Prednisolone Sodium Phosphate, Ophthalmic

Pharmacologic Category Corticosteroid, Ophthalmic; Corticosteroid, Systemic

Additional Appendix Information

Corticosteroids *on page 1652*

Use Treatment of palpebral and bulbar conjunctivitis; corneal injury from chemical, radiation, thermal burns, or foreign body penetration; endocrine disorders, rheumatic disorders, collagen diseases, dermatologic diseases, allergic states, ophthalmic diseases, respiratory diseases, hematologic disorders, neoplastic diseases, edematous states, and gastrointestinal diseases; resolution of acute exacerbations of multiple sclerosis; management of fulminating or disseminated tuberculosis and trichinosis; acute or chronic solid organ rejection

Pregnancy Risk Factor C

Pregnancy Considerations Ophthalmic prednisolone was shown to be teratogenic in animal studies and adverse events have been observed with corticosteroids in animal reproduction studies. Prednisolone crosses the placenta; prior to reaching the fetus, prednisolone is converted by placental enzymes to prednisone. As a result, the amount of prednisolone reaching the fetus is ~8-10 times lower than the maternal serum concentration (healthy women at term; similar results observed with preterm pregnancies complicated by HELLP syndrome). Some studies have shown an association between first trimester corticosteroid use and oral clefts; adverse events in the fetus/neonate have been noted in case reports following large doses of systemic corticosteroids during pregnancy. Women exposed to prednisolone during pregnancy for the treatment of an autoimmune disease may contact the OTIS Autoimmune Diseases Study at 877-311-8972.

Lactation Enters breast milk/use caution (AAP rates "compatible")

Medication Safety Issues

Sound-alike/look-alike issues:
 PrednisoLONE may be confused with predniSONE
 Pediapred® may be confused with Pediazole®

Contraindications Hypersensitivity to prednisolone or any component of the formulation; acute superficial herpes simplex keratitis; live or attenuated virus vaccines (with immunosuppressive doses of corticosteroids); systemic fungal infections; varicella

Warnings/Precautions May cause hypercorticism or suppression of hypothalamic-pituitary-adrenal (HPA) axis, particularly in younger children or in patients receiving high doses for prolonged periods. HPA axis suppression may lead to adrenal crisis. Withdrawal and discontinuation of a corticosteroid should be done slowly and carefully. Particular care is required when patients are transferred from systemic corticosteroids to inhaled products due to possible adrenal insufficiency or withdrawal from steroids, including an increase in allergic symptoms. Patients receiving >20 mg per day of prednisone (or equivalent) may be most susceptible. Fatalities have occurred due to adrenal insufficiency in asthmatic patients during and after transfer from systemic corticosteroids to aerosol steroids; aerosol steroids do **not** provide the systemic steroid needed to treat patients having trauma, surgery, or infections.

Acute myopathy has been reported with high dose corticosteroids, usually in patients with neuromuscular transmission disorders; may involve ocular and/or respiratory muscles; monitor creatine kinase; recovery may be delayed. Corticosteroid use may cause psychiatric disturbances, including depression, euphoria, insomnia, mood swings, and personality changes. Pre-existing psychiatric conditions may be exacerbated by corticosteroid use. Prolonged use of corticosteroids may also increase the incidence of secondary infection, mask acute infection (including fungal infections), prolong or exacerbate viral infections, or limit response to vaccines. Exposure to chickenpox should be avoided; corticosteroids should not be used to treat ocular herpes simplex. Corticosteroids should not be used for cerebral malaria or viral hepatitis. Close observation is required in patients with latent tuberculosis and/or TB reactivity; restrict use in active TB (only in conjunction with antituberculosis treatment). Prolonged use of corticosteroids may result in glaucoma; damage to the optic nerve (not indicated for treatment of optic neuritis), defects in visual acuity and fields of vision, and posterior subcapsular cataract formation may occur. Use following cataract surgery may delay healing or increase the incidence of bleb formation. Prolonged treatment with corticosteroids has been associated with the development of Kaposi's sarcoma (case reports); if noted, discontinuation of therapy should be considered.

Use with caution in patients with thyroid disease, hepatic impairment, renal impairment, cardiovascular disease, diabetes, glaucoma, cataracts, myasthenia gravis, patients at risk for osteoporosis, patients at risk for seizures, or GI diseases (diverticulitis, peptic ulcer, ulcerative colitis) due to perforation risk. Use caution following acute MI (corticosteroids have been associated with myocardial rupture). Because of the risk of adverse effects, systemic corticosteroids should be used cautiously in the elderly in the smallest possible effective dose for the shortest duration. Do not use occlusive dressings on weeping or exudative lesions and general caution with occlusive dressings should be observed; adverse effects may be increased. Discontinue if skin irritation or contact dermatitis should occur; do not use in patients with decreased skin circulation. Withdraw therapy with gradual tapering of dose. May affect growth velocity; growth should be routinely monitored in pediatric patients.

Adverse Reactions Frequency not defined.

Ophthalmic formulation:

Endocrine & metabolic: Hypercorticoidism (rare)

Ocular: Conjunctival hyperemia, conjunctivitis, corneal ulcers, delayed wound healing, glaucoma, intraocular pressure increased, keratitis, loss of accommodation, optic nerve damage, mydriasis, posterior subcapsular cataract formation, ptosis, secondary ocular infection

Oral formulation:

Cardiovascular: Cardiomyopathy, CHF, edema, facial edema, hypertension

Central nervous system: Convulsions, headache, insomnia, malaise, nervousness, pseudotumor cerebri, psychic disorders, vertigo

Dermatologic: Bruising, facial erythema, hirsutism, petechiae, skin test reaction suppression, thin fragile skin, urticaria

Endocrine & metabolic: Carbohydrate tolerance decreased, Cushing's syndrome, diabetes mellitus, growth suppression, hyperglycemia, hypernatremia, hypokalemia, hypokalemic alkalosis, menstrual irregularities, negative nitrogen balance, pituitary adrenal axis suppression

Gastrointestinal: Abdominal distention, increased appetite, indigestion, nausea, pancreatitis, peptic ulcer, ulcerative esophagitis, weight gain

Hepatic: LFTs increased (usually reversible)

Neuromuscular & skeletal: Arthralgia, aseptic necrosis (humeral/femoral heads), fractures, muscle mass decreased, muscle weakness, osteoporosis, steroid myopathy, tendon rupture, weakness

Ocular: Cataracts, exophthalmus, eyelid edema, glaucoma, intraocular pressure increased, irritation

Respiratory: Epistaxis

Miscellaneous: Diaphoresis increased, impaired wound healing

Drug Interactions

Metabolism/Transport Effects **Substrate** of CYP3A4 (minor); **Inhibits** CYP3A4 (weak)

Avoid Concomitant Use

Avoid concomitant use of PrednisoLONE with any of the following: Natalizumab; Vaccines (Live)

Increased Effect/Toxicity

PrednisoLONE may increase the levels/effects of: Acetylcholinesterase Inhibitors; Amphotericin B; CycloSPORINE; Loop Diuretics; Natalizumab; NSAID (COX-2 Inhibitor); NSAID (Nonselective); Thiazide Diuretics; Vaccines (Live); Warfarin

The levels/effects of PrednisoLONE may be increased by: Antifungal Agents (Azole Derivatives, Systemic); Aprepitant; Calcium Channel Blockers (Nondihydropyridine); CycloSPORINE; Estrogen Derivatives; Fluconazole; Fosaprepitant; Macrolide Antibiotics; Neuromuscular-Blocking Agents (Nondepolarizing); Quinolone Antibiotics; Salicylates; Trastuzumab

Decreased Effect

PrednisoLONE may decrease the levels/effects of: Antidiabetic Agents; Calcitriol; Corticorelin; Isoniazid; Salicylates; Vaccines (Inactivated)

The levels/effects of PrednisoLONE may be decreased by: Aminoglutethimide; Antacids; Barbiturates; Bile Acid Sequestrants; Echinacea; Primidone; Rifamycin Derivatives

Ethanol/Nutrition/Herb Interactions

Ethanol: Avoid ethanol (may increase gastric mucosal irritation).

Food: Prednisolone interferes with calcium absorption. Limit caffeine.

Herb/Nutraceutical: St John's wort may decrease prednisolone levels. Avoid cat's claw, echinacea (have immunostimulant properties).

Stability Store Orapred ODT™ at 20°C to 25°C (68°F to 77°F) in blister pack. Protect from moisture.

Mechanism of Action Decreases inflammation by suppression of migration of polymorphonuclear leukocytes and reversal of increased capillary permeability; suppresses the immune system by reducing activity and volume of the lymphatic system

Pharmacodynamics/Kinetics

Duration: 18-36 hours

Protein binding (concentration dependent): 65% to 91%; decreased in elderly

Metabolism: Primarily hepatic, but also metabolized in most tissues, to inactive compounds

Half-life elimination: 3.6 hours; End-stage renal disease: 3-5 hours

Excretion: Primarily urine (as glucuronides, sulfates, and unconjugated metabolites)

Dosage Dose depends upon condition being treated and response of patient; dosage for infants and children should be based on severity of the disease and response of the patient rather than on strict adherence to dosage indicated by age, weight, or body surface area. Oral dosage expressed in terms of prednisolone base. Consider alternate day therapy for long-term therapy. Discontinuation of long-term therapy requires gradual withdrawal by tapering the dose. Patients undergoing unusual stress while receiving corticosteroids, should receive increased doses prior to, during, and after the stressful situation.

Children: Oral:

Acute asthma: 1-2 mg/kg/day in divided doses 1-2 times/day for 3-5 days

Anti-inflammatory or immunosuppressive dose: 0.1-2 mg/kg/day in divided doses 1-4 times/day

Nephrotic syndrome:

Initial (first 3 episodes): 2 mg/kg/day **or** 60 mg/m^2/day (maximum: 80 mg/day) in divided doses 3-4 times/day until urine is protein free for 3 consecutive days (maximum: 28 days); followed by 1-1.5 mg/kg/dose **or** 40 mg/m^2/dose given every other day for 4 weeks

Maintenance (long-term maintenance dose for frequent relapses): 0.5-1 mg/kg/dose given every other day for 3-6 months

Adults: Oral:

Usual range: 5-60 mg/day

Multiple sclerosis: 200 mg/day for 1 week followed by 80 mg every other day for 1 month

Rheumatoid arthritis: Initial: 5-7.5 mg/day; adjust dose as necessary

Ophthalmic suspension/solution: Conjunctivitis, corneal injury: Children and Adults: Instill 1-2 drops into conjunctival sac every hour during day, every 2 hours at night until favorable response is obtained, then use 1 drop every 4 hours.

Elderly: Use lowest effective dose

Dosing adjustment in hyperthyroidism: Prednisolone dose may need to be increased to achieve adequate therapeutic effects

Hemodialysis: Slightly dialyzable (5% to 20%); administer dose posthemodialysis

Peritoneal dialysis: Supplemental dose is not necessary

Dietary Considerations Should be taken after meals or with food or milk to decrease GI effects; increase dietary intake of pyridoxine, vitamin C, vitamin D, folate, calcium, and phosphorus.

Administration Administer oral formulation with food or milk to decrease GI effects.

Orapred ODT™: Do not break or use partial tablet. Remove tablet from blister pack just prior to use. May swallow whole or allow to dissolve on tongue.

Monitoring Parameters Blood pressure; blood glucose, electrolytes; intraocular pressure (use >6 weeks); bone mineral density

Test Interactions Response to skin tests

Dosage Forms Excipient information presented when available (limited, particularly for generics); consult specific product labeling. [DSC] = Discontinued product

Solution, ophthalmic, as sodium phosphate: 1% (5 mL, 10 mL, 15 mL) [contains benzalkonium chloride]

Solution, oral, as base: Prednisolone 15 mg/5 mL (240 mL, 480 mL)

Solution, oral, as sodium phosphate: Prednisolone base 5 mg/5 mL (120 mL, 240 mL); prednisolone base 15 mg/5 mL (240 mL)

Millipred™: 13.4 mg/5 mL (237 mL) [equivalent to prednisolone base 10 mg/5 mL; dye free; grape flavor]

Orapred®: 20 mg/5 mL (20 mL, 240 mL) [equivalent to prednisolone base 15 mg/5 mL; dye free; contains alcohol 2%, sodium benzoate; grape flavor]

Pediapred®: 6.7 mg/5 mL (120 mL) [equivalent to prednisolone base 5 mg/5 mL; dye free; raspberry flavor]

Suspension, ophthalmic, as acetate: 1% (5 mL, 10 mL, 15 mL)

Econopred® Plus [DSC], Omnipred™: 1% (5 mL, 10 mL) [contains benzalkonium chloride]

Pred Forte®: 1% (1 mL, 5 mL, 10 mL, 15 mL) [contains benzalkonium chloride and sodium bisulfite]

Pred Mild®: 0.12% (5 mL, 10 mL) [contains benzalkonium chloride and sodium bisulfite]

Syrup, as base: 5 mg/5 mL (120 mL); 15 mg/5 mL (5 mL [DSC], 240 mL, 480 mL)

Prelone®: 15 mg/5 mL (240 mL, 480 mL) [contains alcohol 5%, benzoic acid; cherry flavor]

Tablet, as base: 5 mg

Tablet, orally disintegrating, as sodium phosphate [strength expressed as base]:

Orapred ODT™: 10 mg, 15 mg, 30 mg [grape flavor]

◆ **Prednisolone Acetate** *see* PrednisoLONE *on page 1230*

◆ **Prednisolone Acetate, Ophthalmic** *see* PrednisoLONE *on page 1230*

Prednisolone and Gentamicin

(pred NIS oh lone & jen ta MYE sin)

U.S. Brand Names Pred-G®

Index Terms Gentamicin and Prednisolone

Pharmacologic Category Antibiotic/Corticosteroid, Ophthalmic

Use Treatment of steroid responsive inflammatory conditions and superficial ocular infections due to microorganisms susceptible to gentamicin

Pregnancy Risk Factor C

Dosage Ophthalmic: Children and Adults:

Ointment: Apply 1/2 inch ribbon in the conjunctival sac 1-3 times/day

Suspension: 1 drop 2-4 times/day; during the initial 24-48 hours, the dosing frequency may be increased if necessary up to 1 drop every hour

Additional Information Complete prescribing information for this medication should be consulted for additional detail.

Dosage Forms Excipient information presented when available (limited, particularly for generics); consult specific product labeling.

Ointment, ophthalmic:

Pred-G®: Prednisolone acetate 0.6% and gentamicin sulfate 0.3% (3.5 g)

Suspension, ophthalmic:

Pred-G®: Prednisolone acetate 1% and gentamicin sulfate 0.3% (5 mL, 10 mL) [contains benzalkonium chloride]

◆ **Prednisolone and Sulfacetamide** *see* Sulfacetamide and Prednisolone *on page 1405*

◆ **Prednisolone, Neomycin, and Polymyxin B** *see* Neomycin, Polymyxin B, and Prednisolone *on page 1053*

◆ **Prednisolone Sodium Phosphate** *see* PrednisoLONE *on page 1230*

◆ **Prednisolone Sodium Phosphate, Ophthalmic** *see* PrednisoLONE *on page 1230*

PredniSONE (PRED ni sone)

U.S. Brand Names PredniSONE Intensol™; Sterapred®; Sterapred® DS

Canadian Brand Names Apo-Prednisone®; Novo-Prednisone; Winpred™

Index Terms Deltacortisone; Deltadehydrocortisone

Pharmacologic Category Corticosteroid, Systemic

Additional Appendix Information

Corticosteroids *on page 1652*

Use Treatment of a variety of diseases, including:

Allergic states (including adjunctive treatment of anaphylaxis)

Autoimmune disorders (including systemic lupus erythematosus [SLE])

Collagen diseases

Dermatologic conditions/diseases

Edematous states (including nephrotic syndrome)

Endocrine disorders

Gastrointestinal diseases

Hematologic disorders (including idiopathic thrombocytopenia purpura [ITP])

Multiple sclerosis exacerbations

Neoplastic diseases

Ophthalmic diseases

Respiratory diseases (including acute asthma exacerbation)

Rheumatic disorders (including rheumatoid arthritis)

Trichinosis with neurologic or myocardial involvement

Tuberculous meningitis

Unlabeled/Investigational Use Adjunctive therapy for *Pneumocystis jiroveci* (formerly *carinni*) pneumonia (PCP); autoimmune hepatitis; adjunctive therapy for pain management in immunocompetent patients with herpes zoster; tuberculosis (severe, paradoxical reactions)

Pregnancy Considerations Adverse events have been observed with corticosteroids in animal reproduction studies. Prednisone and prednisolone cross the human placenta. In the mother, prednisone is converted to the active metabolite prednisolone by the liver. Prior to reaching the fetus, prednisolone is converted by placental enzymes back to prednisone. As a result, the level of prednisone remaining in the maternal serum and reaching the fetus are similar, however, the amount of prednisolone reaching the fetus is ~8-10 times lower than the maternal serum concentration (healthy women at term). Some studies have shown an association between first trimester prednisone use and oral clefts; adverse events in the fetus/neonate have been noted in case reports following large doses of systemic corticosteroids during pregnancy. Pregnant women exposed to prednisone for antirejection therapy following a transplant may contact the National Transplantation Pregnancy Registry (NTPR) at 215-955-4820. Women exposed to prednisone during pregnancy for the treatment of an autoimmune disease (eg, rheumatoid arthritis) may contact the OTIS Autoimmune Diseases Study at 877-311-8972.

Lactation Enters breast milk/AAP rates "compatible"

Medication Safety Issues

Sound-alike/look-alike issues:

PredniSONE may be confused with methylPREDNISolone, Pramosone®, prazosin, prednisoLONE, Prilosec®, primidone, promethazine

Contraindications Hypersensitivity to any component of the formulation; systemic fungal infections; administration of live or live attenuated vaccines with immunosuppressive doses of prednisone

Warnings/Precautions May cause hypercorticism or suppression of hypothalamic-pituitary-adrenal (HPA) axis, particularly in younger children or in patients receiving high doses for prolonged periods. HPA axis suppression may lead to adrenal crisis. Withdrawal and discontinuation of a corticosteroid should be done slowly and carefully. Particular care is required when patients are transferred from systemic corticosteroids to inhaled products due to possible adrenal insufficiency or withdrawal from steroids, including an increase in allergic symptoms. Patients receiving >20 mg per day of prednisone (or equivalent) may be most susceptible. Fatalities have occurred due to adrenal insufficiency in asthmatic patients during and after transfer from systemic corticosteroids to aerosol steroids; aerosol steroids do **not** provide the systemic steroid needed to treat patients having trauma, surgery, or infections.

Acute myopathy has been reported with high dose corticosteroids, usually in patients with neuromuscular transmission disorders; may involve ocular and/or respiratory muscles; monitor creatine kinase; recovery may be delayed. Prolonged use of corticosteroids may increase the incidence of secondary infection, mask acute infection (including fungal infections), prolong or exacerbate viral infections, or limit response to vaccines. Exposure to chickenpox should be avoided. Corticosteroids should not be used to treat ocular herpes simplex or cerebral malaria. Close observation is required in patients with latent tuberculosis and/or TB reactivity; restrict use in active TB (only in conjunction with antituberculosis treatment). Prolonged treatment with corticosteroids has been associated with the development of Kaposi's sarcoma (case reports); if noted, discontinuation of therapy should be considered. Prolonged use may cause posterior subcapsular cataracts, glaucoma (with possible nerve damage) and may increase the risk for ocular infections. Corticosteroid use may cause psychiatric disturbances, including depression, euphoria, insomnia, mood swings, and personality changes. Pre-existing psychiatric conditions may be exacerbated by corticosteroid use.

Use with caution in patients with HF, diabetes, GI diseases (diverticulitis, peptic ulcer, ulcerative colitis; due to risk of perforation), hepatic impairment, myasthenia gravis, MI, patients with or who are at risk for osteoporosis, seizure disorders or thyroid disease. May affect growth velocity; growth should be routinely monitored in pediatric patients.

Prior to use, the dose and duration of treatment should be based on the risk versus benefit for each individual patient. In general, use the smallest effective dose for the shortest duration of time to minimize adverse events. A gradual tapering of dose may be required prior to discontinuing therapy.

Adverse Reactions

Frequency not defined.

Cardiovascular: Congestive heart failure (in susceptible patients), hypertension

Central nervous system: Emotional instability, headache, intracranial pressure increased (with papilledema), psychic derangements (including euphoria, insomnia, mood swings, personality changes, severe depression), seizure, vertigo

Dermatologic: Bruising, facial erythema, petechiae, thin fragile skin, urticaria, wound healing impaired

Endocrine & metabolic: Adrenocortical and pituitary unresponsiveness (in times of stress), carbohydrate intolerance, Cushing's syndrome, diabetes mellitus, fluid retention, growth suppression (in children), hypokalemic alkalosis, hypothyroidism enhanced, menstrual irregularities, negative nitrogen balance due to protein catabolism, potassium loss, sodium retention

Gastrointestinal: Abdominal distension, pancreatitis, peptic ulcer (with possible perforation and hemorrhage), ulcerative esophagitis

Hepatic: ALT increased, AST increased, alkaline phosphatase increased

Neuromuscular & skeletal: Aseptic necrosis of femoral and humeral heads, muscle mass loss, muscle weakness, osteoporosis, pathologic fracture of long bones, steroid myopathy, tendon rupture (particularly Achilles tendon), vertebral compression fractures

Ocular: Exophthalmos, glaucoma, intraocular pressure increased, posterior subcapsular cataracts

Miscellaneous: Allergic reactions, anaphylactic reactions, diaphoresis, hypersensitivity reactions, infections, Kaposi's sarcoma

Drug Interactions

Metabolism/Transport Effects Substrate of CYP3A4 (minor); **Induces** CYP2C19 (weak), 3A4 (weak)

Avoid Concomitant Use

Avoid concomitant use of PredniSONE with any of the following: Natalizumab; Vaccines (Live)

Increased Effect/Toxicity

PredniSONE may increase the levels/effects of: Acetylcholinesterase Inhibitors; Amphotericin B; CycloSPORINE; Loop Diuretics; Natalizumab; NSAID (COX-2 Inhibitor); NSAID (Nonselective); Thiazide Diuretics; Vaccines (Live); Warfarin

The levels/effects of PredniSONE may be increased by: Antifungal Agents (Azole Derivatives, Systemic); Aprepitant; Calcium Channel Blockers (Nondihydropyridine); CycloSPORINE; Estrogen Derivatives; Fluconazole; Fosaprepitant; Macrolide Antibiotics; Neuromuscular-Blocking Agents (Nondepolarizing); Quinolone Antibiotics; Salicylates; Trastuzumab

Decreased Effect

PredniSONE may decrease the levels/effects of: Antidiabetic Agents; Calcitriol; Corticorelin; Isoniazid; Maraviroc; Salicylates; Vaccines (Inactivated)

The levels/effects of PredniSONE may be decreased by: Aminoglutethimide; Antacids; Barbiturates; Bile Acid Sequestrants; Echinacea; Primidone; Rifamycin Derivatives; Somatropin

Ethanol/Nutrition/Herb Interactions

Ethanol: Avoid ethanol (may increase gastric mucosal irritation)

Food: Prednisone interferes with calcium absorption. Limit caffeine.

Herb/Nutraceutical: St John's wort may decrease prednisone levels. Avoid cat's claw, echinacea (have immunostimulant properties).

Mechanism of Action Decreases inflammation by suppression of migration of polymorphonuclear leukocytes and reversal of increased capillary permeability; suppresses the immune system by reducing activity and volume of the lymphatic system; suppresses adrenal function at high doses. Antitumor effects may be related to inhibition of glucose transport, phosphorylation, or induction of cell death in immature lymphocytes. Antiemetic effects are thought to occur due to blockade of cerebral innervation of the emetic center via inhibition of prostaglandin synthesis.

Pharmacodynamics/Kinetics

Absorption: 50% to 90% (may be altered in IBS or hyperthyroidism)

Protein binding (concentration dependent): 65% to 91%

Metabolism: Hepatically converted from prednisone (inactive) to prednisolone (active); may be impaired with hepatic dysfunction

Half-life elimination: Normal renal function: ~3.5 hours

Excretion: Urine (small portion)

Dosage Oral:

General dosing range: Children and Adults: Initial: 5-60 mg/day: **Note:** Dose depends upon condition being treated and response of patient; dosage for infants and children should be based on severity of the disease and response of the patient rather than on strict adherence to dosage indicated by age, weight, or body surface area. Consider alternate day therapy for long-term therapy. Discontinuation of long-term therapy requires gradual withdrawal by tapering the dose.

Prednisone taper (other regimens also available):

Day 1: 30 mg divided as 10 mg before breakfast, 5 mg at lunch, 5 mg at dinner, 10 mg at bedtime

Day 2: 5 mg at breakfast, 5 mg at lunch, 5 mg at dinner, 10 mg at bedtime
Day 3: 5 mg 4 times/day (with meals and at bedtime)
Day 4: 5 mg 3 times/day (breakfast, lunch, bedtime)
Day 5: 5 mg 2 times/day (breakfast, bedtime)
Day 6: 5 mg before breakfast

Indication-specific dosing:
Children:
Acute asthma (NIH guidelines, 2007):
0-11 years 1-2 mg/kg/day for 3-10 days (maximum: 60 mg/day)
≥12 years: Refer to Adults dosing
Autoimmune hepatitis (unlabeled use; Czaja 2002): Initial treatment: 2 mg/kg/day for 2 weeks (maximum: 60 mg/day), followed by a taper over 6-8 weeks to a dose of 0.1-0.2 mg/kg/day or 5 mg/day
Nephrotic syndrome (Pediatric Nephrology Panel recommendations [Hogg, 2000]): Initial: 2 mg/kg/day or 60 mg/m^2/day given every day in 1-3 divided doses (maximum: 80 mg/day) until urine is protein free or for 4-6 weeks; followed by maintenance dose: 2 mg/kg/dose or 40 mg/m^2/dose given every other day in the morning; gradually taper and discontinue after 4-6 weeks. **Note:** No definitive treatment guidelines exist. Dosing is dependant on institution protocols and individual response.
PCP pneumonia (AIDSinfo guidelines, 2008): 1 mg/kg twice daily for 5 days, *followed by* 0.5-1 mg/kg twice daily for 5 days, *followed by* 0.5 mg/kg once daily for 11-21 days
Adolescents and Adults:
PCP pneumonia (AIDSinfo guidelines, 2008): Note: Begin within 72 hours of PCP therapy: 40 mg twice daily for 5 days, *followed by* 40 mg once daily for 5 days, *followed by* 20 mg once daily for 11 days or until antimicrobial regimen is completed
Adults:
Acute asthma (NIH guidelines, 2007): 40-60 mg per day for 3-10 days; administer as single or 2divided doses
Anaphylaxis, adjunctive treatment (Lieberman 2005): 0.5 mg/kg
Antineoplastic: Usual range: 10 mg/day to 100 mg/m^2/day (depending on indication). **Note:** Details concerning dosing in combination regimens should also be consulted.
Autoimmune hepatitis (unlabeled use; Czaja 2002): Initial treatment: 60 mg/day for 1 week, *followed by* 40 mg/day for 1 week, *then* 30 mg/day for 2 weeks, *then* 20 mg/day. Half this dose should be given when used in combination with azathioprine
Herpes zoster (unlabeled use; Dworkin 2007): 60 mg/day for 7 days, *followed by* 30 mg/day for 7 days, *then* 15 mg/day for 7 days
Idiopathic thrombocytopenia purpura (American Society of Hematology 1997): 1-2 mg/kg/day
Rheumatoid arthritis (American College of Rheumatology 2002): ≤10 mg/day
Systemic lupus erythematosus (American College of Rheumatology 1999):
Mild SLE: ≤10 mg/day
Refractory or severe organ-threatening disease: 20-60 mg/day
Thyrotoxicosis (type II amiodarone induced; unlabeled use): 30-40 mg/day for 7-14 days, gradually taper over 3 months
Tuberculosis, severe, paradoxical reactions (unlabeled use, AIDS info guidelines 2008): 1 mg/kg/day, gradually reduce after 1-2 weeks
Elderly: Use the lowest effective dose

Dosing adjustment in hepatic impairment: Prednisone is inactive and must be metabolized by the liver to prednisolone. This conversion may be impaired in patients with liver disease, however, prednisolone levels are observed to be higher in patients with severe liver failure than in normal patients. Therefore, compensation for the inadequate conversion of prednisone to prednisolone occurs.
Dosing adjustment in hyperthyroidism: Prednisone dose may need to be increased to achieve adequate therapeutic effects
Hemodialysis: Supplemental dose is not necessary
Peritoneal dialysis: Supplemental dose is not necessary

Dietary Considerations Should be taken after meals or with food or milk; may require increased dietary intake of pyridoxine, vitamin C, vitamin D, folate, calcium, and phosphorus; may require decreased dietary intake of sodium

Administration Administer with food to decrease gastrointestinal upset

Monitoring Parameters Blood pressure, blood glucose, electrolytes

Following prolonged use: Bone mass density, growth in children, signs and symptoms of infection, cataract formation

Test Interactions Decreased response to skin tests

Additional Information Tapering of corticosteroids after a short course of therapy (<7-10 days) is generally not required unless the disease/inflammatory process is slow to respond. Tapering after prolonged exposure is dependent upon the individual patient, duration of corticosteroid treatments, and size of steroid dose. Recovery of the HPA axis may require several months. Subtle but important HPA axis suppression may be present for as long as several months after a course of as few as 10-14 days duration. Testing of HPA axis (cosyntropin) may be required, and signs/symptoms of adrenal insufficiency should be monitored in patients with a history of use.

Dosage Forms Excipient information presented when available (limited, particularly for generics); consult specific product labeling.
Solution, oral: 1 mg/mL (5 mL, 120 mL, 500 mL) [contains alcohol 5%, sodium benzoate; peppermint vanilla flavor]
Solution, oral [concentrate]:
PredniSONE Intensol™: 5 mg/mL (30 mL) [contains alcohol 30%]
Tablet: 1 mg, 2.5 mg, 5 mg, 10 mg, 20 mg, 50 mg
Sterapred®: 5 mg [supplied as 21 tablet 6-day unit-dose package or 48 tablet 12-day unit-dose package]
Sterapred® DS: 10 mg [supplied as 21 tablet 6-day unit-dose package or 48 tablet 12-day unit-dose package]

◆ **PredniSONE Intensol™** *see* PredniSONE *on page 1232*

Pregabalin (pre GAB a lin)

U.S. Brand Names Lyrica®
Canadian Brand Names Lyrica®
Index Terms CI-1008; S-(+)-3-isobutylgaba
Pharmacologic Category Analgesic, Miscellaneous; Anticonvulsant, Miscellaneous
Additional Appendix Information
Anticonvulsant Drugs of Choice *on page 1637*
Use Management of pain associated with diabetic peripheral neuropathy; management of postherpetic neuralgia; adjunctive therapy for partial-onset seizure disorder in adults; management of fibromyalgia
Restrictions C-V
Pregnancy Risk Factor C
Pregnancy Considerations Increased incidence of fetal abnormalities, particularly skeletal malformations, were observed in animal studies. Male-mediated teratogenicity has been observed in animal studies; implications in

humans are not defined. Impaired male and female fertility has been noted in animal studies. There are no adequate and well-controlled studies in pregnant women. Use only when potential benefit to the mother outweighs possible risk to the fetus.

Lactation Excretion in breast milk unknown/not recommended

Contraindications Hypersensitivity to pregabalin or any component of the formulation

Warnings/Precautions Angioedema has been reported; may be life threatening; use with caution in patients with a history of angioedema episodes. Concurrent use with other drugs known to cause angioedema (eg, ACE inhibitors) may increase risk. Hypersensitivity reactions, including skin redness, blistering, hives, rash, dyspnea and wheezing have been reported; discontinue treatment of hypersensitivity occurs. May cause CNS depression and/or dizziness, which may impair physical or mental abilities. Patients must be cautioned about performing tasks which require mental alertness (eg, operating machinery or driving). Effects with other sedative drugs or ethanol may be potentiated. Visual disturbances (blurred vision, decreased acuity and visual field changes) have been associated with pregabalin therapy; patients should be instructed to notify their physician if these effects are noted.

Pregabalin has been associated with increases in CPK and rare cases of rhabdomyolysis. Patients should be instructed to notify their prescriber if unexplained muscle pain, tenderness, or weakness, particularly if fever and/or malaise are associated with these symptoms. Use may be associated with weight gain and peripheral edema; use caution in patients with congestive heart failure, hypertension, or diabetes. Effect on weight gain/edema may be additive to thiazolidinedione antidiabetic agent; particularly in patients with prior cardiovascular disease. May decrease platelet count or prolong PR interval.

Has been noted to be tumorigenic (increased incidence of hemangiosarcoma) in animal studies; significance of these findings in humans is unknown. Pregabalin has been associated with discontinuation symptoms following abrupt cessation, and increases in seizure frequency (when used as an antiepileptic) may occur. Should not be discontinued abruptly; dosage tapering over at least 1 week is recommended. Use caution in renal impairment; dosage adjustment required. Safety and efficacy have not been established in pediatric patients.

Adverse Reactions Note: Frequency of adverse effects may be influenced by dose or concurrent therapy. In add-on trials in epilepsy, frequency of CNS and adverse effects were higher than those reported in pain management trials. Range noted below is inclusive of all trials.

>10%:

- Cardiovascular: Peripheral edema (up to 16%)
- Central nervous system: Dizziness (8% to 45%), somnolence (4% to 28%), ataxia (up to 20%), headache (up to 14%)
- Gastrointestinal: Weight gain (up to 16%), xerostomia (1% to 15%)
- Neuromuscular & skeletal: Tremor (up to 11%)
- Ocular: Blurred vision (1% to 12%), diplopia (up to 12%)
- Miscellaneous: Infection (up to 14%), accidental injury (2% to 11%)

1% to 10%:

- Cardiovascular: Chest pain (up to 4%), edema (up to 6%)
- Central nervous system: Neuropathy (up to 9%), thinking abnormal (up to 9%), fatigue (up to 8%), confusion (up to 7%), euphoria (up to 7%), speech disorder (up to 7%), attention disturbance (up to 6%), incoordination (up to 6%), amnesia (up to 6%), pain (up to 5%), memory impaired (up to 4%), vertigo (up to 4%), feeling abnormal (up to 3%), hypoesthesia (up to 3%), anxiety (up to 2%), depression (up to 2%), disorientation (up to 2%), lethargy (up to 2%), fever (≥1%), depersonalization (≥1%), hypertonia (≥1%), stupor (≥1%), nervousness (up to 1%)
- Dermatologic: Facial edema (up to 3%), bruising (≥1%), pruritus (≥1%)
- Endocrine & metabolic: Fluid retention (up to 3%), hypoglycemia (up to 3%), libido decreased (≥1%)
- Gastrointestinal: Constipation (up to 10%), appetite increased (up to 7%), flatulence (up to 3%), vomiting (up to 3%), abdominal distension (up to 2%), abdominal pain (≥1%), gastroenteritis (≥1%)
- Genitourinary: Incontinence (up to 2%), anorgasmia (≥1%), impotence (≥1%), urinary frequency (≥1%)
- Hematologic: Thrombocytopenia (3%)
- Neuromuscular & skeletal: Balance disorder (up to 9%), abnormal gait (up to 8%), weakness (up to 7%), arthralgia (up to 6%), twitching (up to 5%), back pain (up to 4%), muscle spasm (up to 4%), myoclonus (up to 4%), paresthesia (>2%), CPK increased (2%), leg cramps (≥1%), myalgia (≥1%), myasthenia (up to 1%)
- Ocular: Visual abnormalities (up to 5%), visual field defect (≥2%), eye disorder (up to 2%), nystagmus (>2%), conjunctivitis (≥1%)
- Otic: Otitis media (≥1%), tinnitus (≥1%)
- Respiratory: Sinusitis (up to 7%), dyspnea (up to 3%), bronchitis (up to 3%), pharyngolaryngeal pain (up to 3%)
- Miscellaneous: Flu-like syndrome (up to 2%), allergic reaction (≥1%)

<1% (Limited to important or life-threatening): Abscess, acute renal failure, addiction (rare), agitation, albuminuria, anaphylactoid reaction, anemia, angioedema, aphasia, aphthous stomatitis, apnea, ascites, atelectasis, blepharitis, blindness, bronchiolitis, cellulitis, cerebellar syndrome, cervicitis, chills, cholecystitis, cholelithiasis, chondrodystrophy, circumoral paresthesia, cogwheel rigidity, colitis, coma, corneal ulcer, crystalluria (urate), delirium, delusions, diarrhea, dysarthria, dysautonomia, dyskinesia, dysphagia, dystonia, dysuria, encephalopathy, eosinophilia, esophageal ulcer, esophagitis, exfoliative dermatitis, extraocular palsy, extrapyramidal syndrome, gastritis, GI hemorrhage, glomerulitis, glucose tolerance decreased, granuloma, Guillain-Barré syndrome, hallucinations, heart failure, hematuria, hostility, hyper-/hypokinesia; hypersensitivity (including skin redness, blistering, hives, rash, dyspnea, and wheezing); hypotension, hypotonia, intracranial hypertension, laryngismus, leukopenia, leukorrhea, leukocytosis, lymphadenopathy, manic reaction, melena, myelofibrosis, nausea, nephritis, neuralgia, ocular hemorrhage, oliguria, optic atrophy, pancreatitis, papilledema, paranoid reaction, pelvic pain, periodontal abscess, peripheral neuritis, polycythemia, postural hypotension, prothrombin decreased, psychotic depression, ptosis, pulmonary edema, pulmonary fibrosis, purpura, pyelonephritis, rectal hemorrhage, renal calculus, retinal edema, retinal vascular disorder, retroperitoneal fibrosis, rhabdomyolysis, schizophrenic reaction, shock, skin necrosis, skin ulcer, spasm (generalized), ST depression, Stevens-Johnson syndrome, subcutaneous nodule, suicide, suicide attempt, syncope, thrombocythemia, thrombophlebitis, tongue edema, torticollis, trismus, uveitis, ventricular fibrillation

Drug Interactions

Avoid Concomitant Use There are no known interactions where it is recommended to avoid concomitant use.

Increased Effect/Toxicity

Pregabalin may increase the levels/effects of: Alcohol (Ethyl); Antidiabetic Agents (Thiazolidinedione); CNS Depressants

Decreased Effect

The levels/effects of Pregabalin may be decreased by: Ketorolac; Mefloquine

Ethanol/Nutrition/Herb Interactions

Ethanol: Avoid ethanol (may increase CNS depression).

Herb/Nutraceutical: Avoid valerian, St John's wort, kava kava, gotu kola (may increase CNS depression).

Stability Store at 15°C to 30°C (59°F to 86°F).

Mechanism of Action Binds to alpha$_2$-delta subunit of voltage-gated calcium channels within the CNS, inhibiting excitatory neurotransmitter release. Although structurally related to GABA, it does not bind to GABA or benzodiazepine receptors. Exerts antinociceptive and anticonvulsant activity. Decreases symptoms of painful peripheral neuropathies and, as adjunctive therapy in partial seizures, decreases the frequency of seizures.

Pharmacodynamics/Kinetics

Onset of action: Pain management: Effects may be noted as early as the first week of therapy.

Distribution: V_d: 0.5 L/kg

Protein binding: 0%

Metabolism: Negligible

Bioavailability: >90%

Half-life elimination: 6.3 hours

Time to peak, plasma: 1.5 hours (3 hours with food)

Excretion: Urine (90% as unchanged drug; minor metabolites)

Dosage Oral: Adults:

Fibromyalgia: Initial: 150 mg/day in divided doses (75 mg 2 times/day); may be increased to 300 mg/day (150 mg 2 times/day) within 1 week based on tolerability and effect; may be further increased to 450 mg/day (225 mg 2 times/day). Maximum dose: 450 mg/day (dosages up to 600 mg/day were evaluated with no significant additional benefit and an increase in adverse effects)

Neuropathic pain (diabetes-associated): Initial: 150 mg/day in divided doses (50 mg 3 times/day); may be increased within 1 week based on tolerability and effect; maximum dose: 300 mg/day (dosages up to 600 mg/day were evaluated with no significant additional benefit and an increase in adverse effects)

Postherpetic neuralgia: Initial: 150 mg/day in divided doses (75 mg 2 times/day or 50 mg 3 times/day); may be increased to 300 mg/day within 1 week based on tolerability and effect; further titration (to 600 mg/day) after 2-4 weeks may be considered in patients who do not experience sufficient relief of pain provided they are able to tolerate pregabalin. Maximum dose: 600 mg/day

Partial-onset seizures (adjunctive therapy): Initial: 150 mg per day in divided doses (75 mg 2 times/day or 50 mg 3 times/day); may be increased based on tolerability and effect (optimal titration schedule has not been defined). Maximum dose: 600 mg/day

Discontinuing therapy: Pregabalin should not be abruptly discontinued; taper dosage over at least 1 week

Dosage adjustment in renal impairment: In renally-impaired patients, dosage adjustment depends on renal function and daily dosage.

Pregabalin Renal Impairment Dosing

Cl_{cr} (mL/minute)	Total Pregabalin Daily Dose (mg/day)				Dosing Frequency
≥60	150	300	450	600	2-3 divided doses
30-60	75	150	225	300	2-3 divided doses
15-30	25-50	75	100-150	150	1-2 divided doses
<15	25	25-50	50-75	75	Single daily dose

Posthemodialysis supplementary dosage (as a single additional dose):
25 mg/day schedule: Single supplementary dose of 25 mg **or** 50 mg
25-50 mg/day schedule: Single supplementary dose of 50 mg **or** 75 mg
50-75 mg/day schedule: Single supplementary dose of 75 mg **or** 100 mg
75 mg/day schedule: Single supplementary dose of 100 mg **or** 150 mg

Dietary Considerations May be taken with or without food.

Administration May be administered with or without food.

Monitoring Parameters Measures of efficacy (pain intensity/seizure frequency); degree of sedation; symptoms of myopathy or ocular disturbance; weight gain/edema; CPK; skin integrity (in patients with diabetes).

Dosage Forms Excipient information presented when available (limited, particularly for generics); consult specific product labeling.

Capsule:

Lyrica®: 25 mg, 50 mg, 75 mg, 100 mg, 150 mg, 200 mg, 225 mg, 300 mg

- **Pregnenedione** *see* Progesterone *on page 1247*
- **Pregnyl®** *see* Chorionic Gonadotropin (Human) *on page 320*
- **Prelone®** *see* PrednisoLONE *on page 1230*
- **Premarin®** *see* Estrogens (Conjugated/Equine) *on page 563*
- **Premjact® [OTC]** *see* Lidocaine *on page 884*
- **Premphase®** *see* Estrogens (Conjugated/Equine) and Medroxyprogesterone *on page 566*
- **Premplus® (Can)** *see* Estrogens (Conjugated/Equine) and Medroxyprogesterone *on page 566*
- **Prempro™** *see* Estrogens (Conjugated/Equine) and Medroxyprogesterone *on page 566*
- **Preparation H® [OTC]** *see* Phenylephrine *on page 1183*
- **Preparation H® Hydrocortisone [OTC]** *see* Hydrocortisone *on page 743*
- **Pre-Pen® [DSC]** *see* Benzylpenicilloyl-polylysine *on page 186*
- **Prepidil®** *see* Dinoprostone *on page 454*
- **Preservative-Free Cosopt® (Can)** *see* Dorzolamide and Timolol *on page 482*
- **Pressyn® (Can)** *see* Vasopressin *on page 1552*
- **Pressyn® AR (Can)** *see* Vasopressin *on page 1552*
- **Pretz® [OTC]** *see* Sodium Chloride *on page 1381*
- **Pretz-D® [OTC]** *see* EPHEDrine *on page 524*
- **Prevacid®** *see* Lansoprazole *on page 853*
- **Prevacid® NapraPAC™** *see* Lansoprazole and Naproxen *on page 855*
- **Prevacid® SoluTab™** *see* Lansoprazole *on page 853*
- **Prevalite®** *see* Cholestyramine Resin *on page 319*
- **Prevex® B (Can)** *see* Betamethasone *on page 188*
- **Prevex® HC (Can)** *see* Hydrocortisone *on page 743*
- **PreviDent®** *see* Fluoride *on page 635*
- **PreviDent® 5000 Plus™** *see* Fluoride *on page 635*
- **Previfem®** *see* Ethinyl Estradiol and Norgestimate *on page 584*

Primaquine (PRIM a kween)

Index Terms Primaquine Phosphate; Prymaccone

Pharmacologic Category Aminoquinoline (Antimalarial)

Additional Appendix Information

Malaria Treatment *on page* 1770

Use Prevention of relapse of *P. vivax* malaria

Unlabeled/Investigational Use Prevention of relapse of *P. ovale* malaria; treatment of *Pneumocystis jiroveci* pneumonia (PCP); prevention of chloroquine-resistant malaria

Lactation Excretion in breast milk unknown

Medication Safety Issues

Sound-alike/look-alike issues:

Primaquine may be confused with primidone

Contraindications Use in acutely-ill patients who have a tendency to develop granulocytopenia (eg, rheumatoid arthritis, SLE); concurrent use with other medications causing hemolytic anemia or myeloid bone marrow suppression; concurrent use with or recent use of quinacrine

Warnings/Precautions Use with caution in patients with G6PD deficiency (hemolytic anemia may occur), NADH methemoglobin reductase deficiency (methemoglobinemia may occur); do not exceed recommended dosage and duration. Moderate-to-severe hemolytic reactions may occur in individuals with G6PD deficiency and personal or familial history of favism. Geographic regions with a high prevalence of G6PD deficiency (eg, Africa, southern Europe, Mediterranean region, Middle East, southeast Asia, Oceania) are associated with a higher incidence of hemolytic anemia. Promptly discontinue with signs of hemolytic anemia (darkening of urine, marked fall in hemoglobin or erythrocyte count). The CDC recommends screening for G6PD deficiency prior to therapy initiation. Anemia, methemoglobinemia, and leukopenia have been associated with primaquine use; monitor during treatment. **[U.S. Boxed Warning]: Should be prescribed only by physicians familiar with its use.**

Adverse Reactions Frequency not defined.

Cardiovascular: Arrhythmias (rare)

Central nervous system: Headache

Dermatologic: Pruritus

Gastrointestinal: Abdominal cramps, dyspepsia, nausea, vomiting

Hematologic: Agranulocytosis, anemia, hemolytic anemia (in patients with G6PD deficiency), leukopenia, leukocytosis, methemoglobinemia (in NADH-methemoglobin reductase-deficient individuals)

Ocular: Interference with visual accommodation

Drug Interactions

Metabolism/Transport Effects Substrate of CYP3A4 (major); **Inhibits** CYP1A2 (strong), 2D6 (weak), 3A4 (weak); **Induces** CYP1A2 (weak)

Avoid Concomitant Use

Avoid concomitant use of Primaquine with any of the following: Mefloquine

Increased Effect/Toxicity

Primaquine may increase the levels/effects of: Antipsychotic Agents (Phenothiazines); Bendamustine; Beta-Blockers; Cardiac Glycosides; CYP1A2 Substrates; Mefloquine

The levels/effects of Primaquine may be increased by: Mefloquine

Decreased Effect

Primaquine may decrease the levels/effects of: Anthelmintics

The levels/effects of Primaquine may be decreased by: CYP3A4 Inducers (Strong); Deferasirox; Herbs (CYP3A4 Inducers)

Ethanol/Nutrition/Herb Interactions Ethanol: Avoid ethanol (due to GI irritation).

Mechanism of Action Eliminates the primary tissue exoerythrocytic forms of *P. falciparum*; disrupts mitochondria and binds to DNA

Pharmacodynamics/Kinetics

Absorption: Well absorbed

Metabolism: Hepatic to carboxyprimaquine (active)

Half-life elimination: 3.7-9.6 hours

Time to peak, serum: 1-2 hours

Excretion: Urine (small amounts as unchanged drug)

Dosage Oral: Dosage expressed as mg of base (15 mg base = 26.3 mg primaquine phosphate). **Note:** The CDC recommends screening for G6PD deficiency prior to initiating treatment with primaquine.

Relapse prevention of *P. vivax* malaria: CDC recommendations: Uncomplicated malaria (*P. vivax* and *P. ovale*):

Children: 0.5 mg/kg once daily for 14 days (maximum dose: 30 mg/day); alternative regimen (recommended for mild G6PD deficiency): 45 mg once weekly for 8 weeks

Adults: 30 mg once daily for 14 days; alternative regimen (recommended for mild G6PD deficiency): 45 mg once weekly for 8 weeks

Prevention of chloroquine-resistant malaria (unlabeled use; CDC guidelines): Initiate 1-2 days prior to travel and continue for 7 days after departure from malaria-endemic area:

Children: 0.5 mg/kg once daily

Adults: 30 mg once daily

Pneumocystis jiroveci pneumonia treatment (unlabeled use): CDC recommendation (as alternative):

Children: 0.3 mg/kg once daily for 21 days (in combination with clindamycin)

Adults: 30 mg once daily for 21 days (in combination with clindamycin)

Administration Take with meals to decrease adverse GI effects. Drug has a bitter taste.

Monitoring Parameters Periodic CBC, visual color check of urine, glucose, electrolytes; if hemolysis suspected, monitor CBC, haptoglobin, peripheral smear, urinalysis dipstick for occult blood, G6PD deficiency screening (prior to initiating treatment; CDC recommendation)

Dosage Forms Excipient information presented when available (limited, particularly for generics); consult specific product labeling.

Tablet, as phosphate: 26.3 mg [15 mg base]

Primidone (PRI mi done)

U.S. Brand Names Mysoline®

Canadian Brand Names Apo-Primidone®

Index Terms Desoxyphenobarbital; Primaclone

Pharmacologic Category Anticonvulsant, Miscellaneous; Barbiturate

Use Management of grand mal, psychomotor, and focal seizures

Unlabeled/Investigational Use Benign familial tremor (essential tremor)

Pregnancy Risk Factor D

Pregnancy Considerations Crosses the placenta. Dysmorphic facial features; hemorrhagic disease of newborn due to fetal vitamin K depletion, maternal folic acid deficiency may occur. Epilepsy itself, number of medications, genetic factors, or a combination of these probably influence the teratogenicity of anticonvulsant therapy. Benefit:risk ratio usually favors continued use during pregnancy.

Lactation Enters breast milk/not recommended (AAP recommends use "with caution")

Medication Safety Issues

Sound-alike/look-alike issues:

Primidone may be confused with predniSONE, primaquine

Contraindications Hypersensitivity to primidone, phenobarbital, or any component of the formulation; porphyria; pregnancy

Warnings/Precautions Use with caution in patients with renal or hepatic impairment, pulmonary insufficiency; abrupt withdrawal may precipitate status epilepticus. Potential for drug dependency exists. Do not administer to patients in acute pain. Use caution in elderly, debilitated, or pediatric patients - may cause paradoxical responses. May cause CNS depression, which may impair physical or mental abilities. Patients must cautioned about performing tasks which require mental alertness (eg, operating machinery or driving). Effects with other sedative drugs or ethanol may be potentiated. Use with caution in patients with depression or suicidal tendencies, or in patients with a history of drug abuse. Tolerance or psychological and physical dependence may occur with prolonged use. Primidone's metabolite, phenobarbital, has been associated with cognitive deficits in children. Use with caution in patients with hypoadrenalism.

Adverse Reactions Frequency not defined.

Central nervous system: Drowsiness, vertigo, ataxia, lethargy, behavior change, fatigue, hyperirritability

Dermatologic: Rash

Gastrointestinal: Nausea, vomiting, anorexia

Genitourinary: Impotence

Hematologic: Agranulocytopenia, agranulocytosis, anemia

Ocular: Diplopia, nystagmus

Drug Interactions

Metabolism/Transport Effects Metabolized to phenobarbital; **Induces** CYP1A2 (strong), 2B6 (strong), 2C8 (strong), 2C9 (strong), 3A4 (strong)

Avoid Concomitant Use

Avoid concomitant use of Primidone with any of the following: Nilotinib; Nisoldipine; Ranolazine

Increased Effect/Toxicity

Primidone may increase the levels/effects of: Alcohol (Ethyl); Barbiturates; CNS Depressants

The levels/effects of Primidone may be increased by: Carbonic Anhydrase Inhibitors; Felbamate; Valproic Acid

Decreased Effect

Primidone may decrease the levels/effects of: Bendamustine; Corticosteroids (Systemic); CYP1A2 Substrates; CYP2B6 Substrates; CYP2C8 Substrates (High risk); CYP2C9 Substrates (High risk); CYP3A4 Substrates; LamoTRIgine; Maraviroc; Nilotinib; Nisoldipine; QuiNIDine; Ranolazine; Rufinamide; Sorafenib; Valproic Acid

The levels/effects of Primidone may be decreased by: Carbonic Anhydrase Inhibitors; Folic Acid; Ketorolac; Leucovorin-Levoleucovorin; Mefloquine; Methylfolate; Phenytoin

Ethanol/Nutrition/Herb Interactions

Ethanol: Avoid ethanol (may increase CNS depression).

Food: Protein-deficient diets increase duration of action of primidone.

Herb/Nutraceutical: Avoid valerian, St John's wort, kava kava, gotu kola (may increase CNS depression).

Stability Protect from light.

Mechanism of Action Decreases neuron excitability, raises seizure threshold similar to phenobarbital; primidone has two active metabolites, phenobarbital and phenylethylmalonamide (PEMA); PEMA may enhance the activity of phenobarbital

Pharmacodynamics/Kinetics

Absorption: 60% to 80%

Distribution: Adults: V_d: 0.6 L/kg

Protein binding: 30%

Metabolism: Hepatic to phenobarbital (active) by oxidation and to phenylethylmalonamide (PEMA; active) by scission of the heterocyclic ring

Half-life elimination (age dependent): Primidone: Mean 5-15 hours (variable); PEMA: 16 hours (variable)

Time to peak, serum: ~3 hours (variable)

Excretion: Urine (40% as unchanged drug; the remainder is unconjugated PEMA, phenobarbital and its metabolites)

Dosage Oral:

Children <8 years: Initial: 50-125 mg/day given at bedtime; increase by 50-125 mg/day increments every 3-7 days; usual dose: 10-25 mg/kg/day in divided doses 3-4 times/day

Children ≥8 years and Adults: Initial: 125-250 mg/day at bedtime; increase by 125-250 mg/day every 3-7 days; usual dose: 750-1500 mg/day in divided doses 3-4 times/day with maximum dosage of 2 g/day

Adults: Essential tremor (unlabeled use): 750 mg early in divided doses

Dosing interval in renal impairment:

Cl_{cr} 50-80 mL/minute: Administer every 8 hours

Cl_{cr} 10-50 mL/minute: Administer every 8-12 hours

Cl_{cr} <10 mL/minute: Administer every 12-24 hours

Hemodialysis: Moderately dialyzable (20% to 50%); administer dose postdialysis or administer supplemental 30% dose

Dietary Considerations Folic acid: Low erythrocyte and CSF folate concentrations. Megaloblastic anemia has been reported. To avoid folic acid deficiency and megaloblastic anemia, some clinicians recommend giving patients on anticonvulsants prophylactic doses of folic acid and cyanocobalamin.

Monitoring Parameters Serum primidone and phenobarbital concentration, CBC, neurological status. Due to CNS effects, monitor closely when initiating drug in elderly. Monitor CBC at 6-month intervals to compare with baseline obtained at start of therapy. Since elderly metabolize phenobarbital at a slower rate than younger adults, it is suggested to measure both primidone and phenobarbital levels together.

Reference Range Therapeutic: Children <5 years: 7-1[illegible] mcg/mL (SI: 32-46 µmol/L); Adults: 5-12 mcg/mL (SI: 23-55 µmol/L); toxic effects rarely present with levels <1[illegible] mcg/mL (SI: 46 µmol/L) if phenobarbital concentrations are low. Dosage of primidone is adjusted with reference mostly to the phenobarbital level; Toxic: >15 mcg/mL (SI: >6[illegible] µmol/L)

Dosage Forms Excipient information presented when available (limited, particularly for generics); consult specific product labeling.

Tablet: 50 mg, 250 mg [generic tablet may contain sodium benzoate]

Dosage forms available in Canada: Tablet: 125 mg, 250 mg. **Note:** 50 mg tablet is **not** available in Canada.

- **Primsol®** *see* Trimethoprim *on page 1519*
- **Prinivil®** *see* Lisinopril *on page 894*
- **Prinzide®** *see* Lisinopril and Hydrochlorothiazide *on page 896*
- **Priorix™ (Can)** *see* Measles, Mumps, and Rubella Vaccines (Combined) *on page 923*
- **Priscoline® [DSC]** *see* Tolazoline *on page 1485*
- **PrismaSol** *see* Electrolyte Solution, Renal Replacement *on page 510*
- **Pristinamycin** *see* Quinupristin and Dalfopristin *on page 1284*
- **Pristiq™** *see* Desvenlafaxine *on page 424*
- **Privigen™** *see* Immune Globulin (Intravenous) *on page 777*
- **Privine® [OTC]** *see* Naphazoline *on page 1040*
- **ProAir™ HFA** *see* Albuterol *on page 51*
- **ProAmatine®** *see* Midodrine *on page 993*
- **PRO-Amiodarone (Can)** *see* Amiodarone *on page 87*

Probenecid (proe BEN e sid)

Canadian Brand Names Benuryl™

Index Terms Benemid [DSC]

Pharmacologic Category Uricosuric Agent

Additional Appendix Information

Treatment of Sexually Transmitted Infections *on page 1773*

Use Prevention of hyperuricemia associated with gout or gouty arthritis; prolongation and elevation of beta-lactam plasma levels

Lactation Excretion in breast milk unknown

Medication Safety Issues

Sound-alike/look-alike issues:

Probenecid may be confused with Procanbid®

Contraindications Hypersensitivity to probenecid or any component of the formulation; high-dose aspirin therapy; blood dyscrasias; uric acid kidney stones; children <2 years of age

Warnings/Precautions Use with caution in patients with peptic ulcer. Salicylates may diminish the therapeutic effect of probenecid. This effect may be more pronounced with high, chronic doses, however, the manufacturer recommends the use of an alternative analgesic even in place of small doses of aspirin. Use of probenecid with penicillin in patients with renal insufficiency is not recommended. Probenecid monotherapy may not be effective in patients with a creatinine clearance <30 mL/minute. May cause exacerbation of acute gouty attack

Adverse Reactions Frequency not defined.

Cardiovascular: Flushing

Central nervous system: Dizziness, fever, headache

Dermatologic: Alopecia, dermatitis, pruritus, rash

Gastrointestinal: Anorexia, nausea, sore gums, vomiting

Genitourinary: Hematuria, polyuria

Hematologic: Anemia, aplastic anemia, hemolytic anemia, leukopenia

Hepatic: Hepatic necrosis

Neuromuscular & skeletal: Costovertebral pain, gouty arthritis (acute)

Renal: Nephrotic syndrome, renal colic

Miscellaneous: Anaphylaxis, hypersensitivity

Drug Interactions

Metabolism/Transport Effects Inhibits CYP2C19 (weak)

Avoid Concomitant Use

Avoid concomitant use of Probenecid with any of the following: Ketorolac

Increased Effect/Toxicity

Probenecid may increase the levels/effects of: Carbapenems; Cephalosporins; Dapsone; Doripenem; Gemifloxacin; Ketoprofen; Ketorolac; LORazepam; Methotrexate; Mycophenolate; Nonsteroidal Anti-Inflammatory Agents; Penicillins; Quinolone Antibiotics; Sodium Benzoate; Sodium Phenylacetate; Theophylline Derivatives; Zidovudine

Decreased Effect

The levels/effects of Probenecid may be decreased by: Salicylates

Mechanism of Action Competitively inhibits the reabsorption of uric acid at the proximal convoluted tubule, thereby promoting its excretion and reducing serum uric acid levels; increases plasma levels of weak organic acids (penicillins, cephalosporins, or other beta-lactam antibiotics) by competitively inhibiting their renal tubular secretion

Pharmacodynamics/Kinetics

Onset of action: Effect on penicillin levels: 2 hours

Absorption: Rapid and complete

Metabolism: Hepatic

Half-life elimination (dose dependent): Normal renal function: 6-12 hours

Time to peak, serum: 2-4 hours

Excretion: Urine

Dosage Oral:

Children:

<2 years: Contraindicated

2-14 years: Prolong penicillin serum levels: Initial: 25 mg/kg, then 40 mg/kg/day given 4 times/day (maximum: 500 mg/dose)

Gonorrhea: >45 kg: Refer to adult guidelines

Adults:

Hyperuricemia with gout: 250 mg twice daily for one week; increase to 250-500 mg/day; may increase by 500 mg/month, if needed, to maximum of 2-3 g/day (dosages may be increased by 500 mg every 6 months if serum urate concentrations are controlled)

Prolong penicillin serum levels: 500 mg 4 times/day

Gonorrhea: CDC guidelines (alternative regimen): Probenecid 1 g orally with cefoxitin 2 g I.M.

Pelvic inflammatory disease: CDC guidelines: Cefoxitin 2 g I.M. plus probenecid 1 g orally as a single dose

Neurosyphilis: CDC guidelines (alternative regimen): Procaine penicillin 2.4 million units/day I.M. plus probenecid 500 mg 4 times/day; both administered for 10-14 days

Dosing adjustment in renal impairment: Cl_{cr} <30 mL/minute: Avoid use

Dietary Considerations Drug may cause GI upset; take with food if GI upset. Drink plenty of fluids.

Administration Administer with food or antacids to minimize GI effects

Monitoring Parameters Uric acid, renal function, CBC

Test Interactions False-positive glucosuria with Clinitest®, a falsely high determination of theophylline has occurred and the renal excretion of phenolsulfonphthalein 17-ketosteroids and bromsulfophthalein (BSP) may be inhibited

Additional Information Avoid fluctuation in uric acid (increase or decrease); may precipitate gout attack. Use of sodium bicarbonate or potassium citrate is suggested until serum uric acid normalizes and tophaceous deposits disappear.

Dosage Forms Excipient information presented when available (limited, particularly for generics); consult specific product labeling.

Tablet: 500 mg

◆ **Probenecid and Colchicine** *see* Colchicine and Probenecid *on page 365*

◆ **Pro-Bicalutamide (Can)** *see* Bicalutamide *on page 197*

◆ **PRO-Bisoprolol (Can)** *see* Bisoprolol *on page 200*

Procainamide (pro KANE a mide)

U.S. Brand Names Procanbid® [DSC]

Canadian Brand Names Apo-Procainamide®; Procainamide Hydrochloride Injection, USP; Procan® SR; Pronestyl®-SR

Index Terms PCA (error-prone abbreviation); Procainamide Hydrochloride; Procaine Amide Hydrochloride

Pharmacologic Category Antiarrhythmic Agent, Class Ia

Use Treatment of ventricular tachycardia (VT), premature ventricular contractions, paroxysmal atrial tachycardia (PSVT), and atrial fibrillation (AF); prevent recurrence of ventricular tachycardia, paroxysmal supraventricular tachycardia, atrial fibrillation or flutter

Unlabeled/Investigational Use

ACLS guidelines:

Stable monomorphic VT (EF >40%, no CHF)

Stable wide complex tachycardia, likely VT (EF >40%, no CHF, patient stable)

Atrial fibrillation or flutter, including pre-excitation syndrome (EF >40%, no CHF)

AV reentrant, narrow complex tachycardia (eg, reentrant SVT) [preserved ventricular function]

PALS guidelines: Tachycardia with pulses and poor perfusion (possible VT)

Pregnancy Risk Factor C

Lactation Enters breast milk/use caution (AAP rates "compatible")

Medication Safety Issues

Sound-alike/look-alike issues:

Procanbid® may be confused with probenecid

Pronestyl® may be confused with Ponstel®

High alert medication: The Institute for Safe Medication Practices (ISMP) includes this medication among its list of drugs which have a heightened risk of causing significant patient harm when used in error.

PCA is an error-prone abbreviation (mistaken as patient controlled analgesia)

Contraindications Hypersensitivity to procaine, other ester-type local anesthetics, or any component of the formulation; complete heart block (except in patients with a functioning artificial pacemaker); second-degree AV block (without a functional pacemaker); various types of hemiblock (without a functional pacemaker); SLE; torsade de pointes; concurrent cisapride use; QT prolongation

Warnings/Precautions Monitor and adjust dose to prevent QT_c prolongation. Watch for proarrhythmic effects. May precipitate or exacerbate HF. Correct electrolyte disturbances, especially hypokalemia or hypomagnesemia, prior to use and throughout therapy. Reduce dosage in renal impairment. May increase ventricular response rate in patients with atrial fibrillation or flutter; control AV conduction before initiating. Correct hypokalemia before initiating therapy; hypokalemia may worsen toxicity. Use caution in digoxin-induced toxicity (can further depress AV conduction). Reduce dose if first-degree heart block occurs. Use caution with concurrent use of other antiarrhythmics. Avoid use in myasthenia gravis (may worsen condition). Hypersensitivity reactions can occur. Some tablets contain tartrazine; injection may contain bisulfite.

[U.S. Boxed Warning]: Potentially fatal blood dyscrasias have occurred with therapeutic doses; close monitoring is recommended during the first 3 months of therapy.

[U.S. Boxed Warning]: Long-term administration leads to the development of a positive antinuclear antibody (ANA) test in 50% of patients which may result in a drug-induced lupus erythematosus-like syndrome (in 20% to 30% of patients); discontinue procainamide with SLE symptoms and choose an alternative agent.

[U.S. Boxed Warning] In the Cardiac Arrhythmia Suppression Trial (CAST), recent (>6 days but <2 years ago) myocardial infarction patients with asymptomatic, non-life-threatening ventricular arrhythmias did not benefit and may have been harmed by attempts to suppress the arrhythmia with flecainide or encainide. An increased mortality or nonfatal cardiac arrest rate (7.7%) was seen in the active treatment group compared with patients in the placebo group (3%). The applicability of the CAST results to other populations is unknown. Antiarrhythmic agents should be reserved for patients with life-threatening ventricular arrhythmias.

Adverse Reactions

>1%:

Cardiovascular: Hypotension (I.V., up to 5%)

Dermatologic: Rash

Gastrointestinal: Diarrhea (3% to 4%), nausea, vomiting, taste disorder, GI complaints (3% to 4%)

<1% (Limited to important or life-threatening): Agranulocytosis, angioneurotic edema, aplastic anemia, arrhythmia (proarrhythmic effect, new or worsened), bone marrow suppression, cerebellar ataxia, cholestasis, demyelinating polyradiculoneuropathy, depressed myocardial contractility, depression, disorientation, drug fever, granulomatous hepatitis, hallucinations, hemolytic anemia, hepatic failure, hypoplastic anemia, leukopenia, mania, myasthenia gravis (worsened), myocarditis, myopathy, neuromuscular blockade, neutropenia, pancreatitis, pancytopenia, paradoxical increase in ventricular rate in atrial fibrillation/flutter, pericarditis, peripheral neuropathy, pleural effusion, positive ANA, positive Coombs' test, pruritus, pseudo-obstruction, psychosis, pulmonary embolism, QT prolongation (excessive), rash, respiratory failure due to myopathy, second-degree heart block, SLE-like syndrome, thrombocytopenia (0.5%), torsade de pointes, tremor, urticaria, vasculitis, ventricular arrhythmia

Drug Interactions

Metabolism/Transport Effects Substrate of CYP2D6 (major)

Avoid Concomitant Use

Avoid concomitant use of Procainamide with any of the following: Nilotinib; Tetrabenazine; Thioridazine; Ziprasidone

Increased Effect/Toxicity

Procainamide may increase the levels/effects of: Amiodarone; Neuromuscular-Blocking Agents; QTc-Prolonging Agents; Tetrabenazine; Thioridazine; Ziprasidone

The levels/effects of Procainamide may be increased by: Alfuzosin; Cimetidine; Ciprofloxacin; CYP2D6 Inhibitors (Moderate); CYP2D6 Inhibitors (Strong); Darunavir; Gadobutrol; Nilotinib; Trimethoprim

Decreased Effect

The levels/effects of Procainamide may be decreased by: Amiodarone

Ethanol/Nutrition/Herb Interactions

Ethanol: Avoid ethanol (acute ethanol administration reduces procainamide serum concentrations).

Herb/Nutraceutical: Avoid ephedra (may worsen arrhythmia).

Stability Procainamide may be stored at room temperature up to 27°C; however, refrigeration retards oxidation, which causes color formation. The solution is initially colorless but may turn slightly yellow on standing. Injection of air into the vial causes the solution to darken. Solutions darker than a light amber should be discarded.

Minimum volume: 1 g/250 mL NS/D_5W.

Stability of admixture at room temperature in D_5W or NS: 24 hours.

Some information indicates that procainamide may be subject to greater decomposition in D_5W unless the admixture is refrigerated or the pH is adjusted. Procainamide is believed to form an association complex with dextrose - the bioavailability of procainamide in this complex is not known and the complex formation is reversible.

Mechanism of Action Decreases myocardial excitability and conduction velocity and may depress myocardial contractility, by increasing the electrical stimulation threshold of ventricle, His-Purkinje system and through direct cardiac effects

Pharmacodynamics/Kinetics

Onset of action: I.M. 10-30 minutes

Distribution: V_d: Children: 2.2 L/kg; Adults: 2 L/kg; Congestive heart failure or shock: Decreased V_d

Protein binding: 15% to 20%

Metabolism: Hepatic via acetylation to produce N-acetyl procainamide (NAPA) (active metabolite)

Bioavailability: Oral: 75% to 95%

Half-life elimination:

Procainamide (hepatic acetylator, phenotype, cardiac and renal function dependent):

Children: 1.7 hours; Adults: 2.5-4.7 hours; Anephric: 11 hours

NAPA (dependent upon renal function):

Children: 6 hours; Adults: 6-8 hours; Anephric: 42 hours

Time to peak, serum: Capsule: 45 minutes to 2.5 hours; I.M.: 15-60 minutes

Excretion: Urine (25% as NAPA)

Dosage Must be titrated to patient's response

Children:

Oral: 15-50 mg/kg/24 hours divided every 3-6 hours

I.M.: 50 mg/kg/24 hours divided into doses of 1/8 to 1/4 every 3-6 hours in divided doses until oral therapy is possible

I.V. (infusion requires use of an infusion pump):

Load: 3-6 mg/kg/dose over 5 minutes not to exceed 100 mg/dose; may repeat every 5-10 minutes to maximum of 15 mg/kg/load

Maintenance as continuous I.V. infusion: 20-80 mcg/kg/minute; maximum: 2 g/24 hours

Possible VT (pulses and poor perfusion) [PALS 2005 Guidelines]: I.V.; I.O.: 15 mg/kg over 30-60 minutes

Adults:

Oral: Usual dose: 50 mg/kg/24 hours: maximum: 5 g/24 hours (**Note:** Twice-daily dosing approved for Procanbid®.)

Immediate release formulation: 250-500 mg/dose every 3-6 hours

Extended release formulation: 500 mg to 1 g every 6 hours; Procanbid®: 1000-2500 mg every 12 hours

I.M.: 0.5-1 g every 4-8 hours until oral therapy is possible

I.V. (infusion requires use of an infusion pump):

Loading dose: 15-18 mg/kg administered as slow infusion over 25-30 minutes **or** 100-200 mg/dose repeated every 5 minutes as needed to a total dose of 1 g. Reduce loading dose to 12 mg/kg in severe renal or cardiac impairment.

Maintenance dose: 1-4 mg/minute by continuous infusion. Maintenance infusions should be reduced by one-third in patients with moderate renal or cardiac impairment and by two-thirds in patients with severe renal or cardiac impairment.

ACLS guidelines: Infuse 20 mg/minute until arrhythmia is controlled, hypotension occurs, QRS complex widens by 50% of its original width, or total of 17 mg/kg is given.

Dosing interval in renal impairment:

Oral:

Cl_{cr} 10-50 mL/minute: Administer every 6-12 hours.

Cl_{cr} <10 mL/minute: Administer every 8-24 hours.

I.V.:

Loading dose: Reduce dose to 12 mg/kg in severe renal impairment.

Maintenance infusion: Reduce dose by one-third in patients with mild renal impairment. Reduce dose by two-thirds in patients with severe renal impairment.

Dialysis:

Procainamide: Moderately hemodialyzable (20% to 50%): 200 mg supplemental dose posthemodialysis is recommended.

N-acetylprocainamide: Not dialyzable (0% to 5%)

Procainamide/N-acetylprocainamide: Not peritoneal dialyzable (0% to 5%)

Procainamide/N-acetylprocainamide: Replace by blood level during continuous arteriovenous or venovenous hemofiltration

Dosing adjustment in hepatic impairment: Reduce dose by 50%.

Dietary Considerations Should be taken with water on an empty stomach.

Administration

Oral: Do **not** crush or chew extended release drug products.

Must dilute prior to I.V. administration; maximum rate: 50 mg/minute; administer around-the-clock rather than 4 times/day to promote less variation in peak and trough serum levels.

Infusion rate: **2 g/250 mL** (I.V. infusion requires use of an infusion pump):

1 mg/minute: 7.5 mL/hour

2 mg/minute: 15 mL/hour

3 mg/minute: 22.5 mL/hour

4 mg/minute: 30 mL/hour

5 mg/minute: 37.5 mL/hour

6 mg/minute: 45 mL/hour

Monitoring Parameters ECG, blood pressure, CBC with differential, platelet count; cardiac monitor and blood pressure monitor required during I.V. administration; blood levels in patients with renal failure or receiving constant infusion >3 mg/minute for longer than 24 hours

Reference Range

Timing of serum samples: Draw trough just before next oral dose; draw 6-12 hours after I.V. infusion has started; half-life is 2.5-5 hours

Therapeutic levels: Procainamide: 4-10 mcg/mL; NAPA 15-25 mcg/mL; Combined: 10-30 mcg/mL

Toxic concentration: Procainamide: >10-12 mcg/mL

Dosage Forms Excipient information presented when available (limited, particularly for generics); consult specific product labeling. [DSC] = Discontinued product

Capsule, as hydrochloride: 250 mg, 500 mg [DSC]

Injection, solution, as hydrochloride: 100 mg/mL (10 mL); 500 mg/mL (2 mL) [contains sodium metabisulfite]

Tablet, extended release, as hydrochloride: 750 mg [DSC]

Procanbid®: 500 mg, 1000 mg [DSC]

Extemporaneous Preparations Note: Several formulations have been described, some being more complex; for all formulations, the pH must be 4-6 to prevent degradation; some preparations require adjustment of pH; shake well before use

A suspension of 50 mg/mL can be made with the capsules, distilled water, and a 2:1 simple syrup/cherry syrup mixture; stability 2 weeks under refrigeration (ASHP, 1987)

Concentrations of 5, 50, and 100 mg/mL oral liquid preparations (made with the capsules, sterile water for irrigation and cherry syrup) stored at 4°C to 6°C (pH 6) were stable for at least 6 months (Metras, 1992).

A sucrose-based syrup (procainamide 50 mg/mL) made with capsules, distilled water, simple syrup, parabens, and cherry flavoring had a calculated stability of 456 days at 25°C and measured stability of 42 days at 40°C (pH ~5) while a maltitol-based syrup (procainamide 50 mg/mL) made with capsules, distilled water, Lycasin® (a syrup vehicle with 75% w/w maltitol), parabens, sodium bisulfate, saccharin, sodium acetate, pineapple and apricot flavoring, FD & C yellow number 6 (pH adjusted to 5 with glacial acetic acid) had a calculated stability of 97 days at 25°C and a measured stability of 94 days at 40°C. The maltitol-based syrup was more stable than the sucrose-based syrup when temperature was >37°C, but the sucrose-based syrup was more stable at temperatures <37°C (Alexander, 1993).

Alexander KS, Pudipeddi M, and Parker GA, "Stability of Procainamide Hydrochloride Syrups Compounded From Capsules," *Am J Hosp Pharm*, 1993, 50(4):693-8.

Handbook in Extemporaneous Formulations, Bethesda, MD: American Society of Hospital Pharmacists, 1987.

Metras JI, Swenson CF, and MacDermott MP, "Stability of Procainamide Hydrochloride in an Extemporaneously Compounded Oral Liquid," *Am J Hosp Pharm*, 1992, 49 (7):1720-4.

Swenson CF, "Importance of Following Instructions When Compounding," *Am J Hosp Pharm*, 1993, 50 (2):261.

◆ **Procainamide Hydrochloride** *see* Procainamide *on page 1240*

◆ **Procainamide Hydrochloride Injection, USP (Can)** *see* Procainamide *on page 1240*

Procaine (PROE kane)

U.S. Brand Names Novocain®

Index Terms Procaine Hydrochloride

Pharmacologic Category Local Anesthetic

Use Produces spinal anesthesia

Pregnancy Risk Factor C

Pregnancy Considerations Reproduction studies have not been conducted. Local anesthetics cross the placenta; effects to the fetus depend on procedure and type of administration.

Lactation Excretion in breast milk unknown/use caution

Medication Safety Issues

High alert medication: The Institute for Safe Medication Practices (ISMP) includes this medication (epidural administration) among its list of drug classes which have a heightened risk of causing significant patient harm when used in error.

Contraindications Hypersensitivity to procaine, PABA, parabens, other ester local anesthetics, or any component of the formulation; septicemia; infection at the injection site; cerebrospinal system infections (eg, meningitis, syphilis)

Warnings/Precautions Careful and constant monitoring of the patient's state of consciousness should be done following each local anesthetic injection; at such times, restlessness, anxiety, tinnitus, dizziness, blurred vision, tremors, depression, or drowsiness may be early warning signs of CNS toxicity. Treatment is primarily symptomatic and supportive. Intravascular injections should be avoided. Local anesthetics have been associated with rare occurrences of sudden respiratory arrest, seizures, and cardiac arrest. Patients with cardiac diseases, hyperthyroidism, or other endocrine diseases may be more susceptible to toxic effects of local anesthetics. Preparations may contain metabisulfite. Resuscitative equipment should be readily available during use. Use caution with heart block; large doses should be avoided. Use caution in the elderly, children, debilitated, acutely ill, patients with increased intra-abdominal pressure or obstetrical analgesia; reduced dose may be needed.

Adverse Reactions Frequency not defined.

Cardiovascular: Bradycardia, cardiac arrest, edema, hyper-/hypotension

Central nervous system: Dizziness, drowsiness, nervousness, seizure, tremor

Dermatologic: Cutaneous lesions (onset may be delayed), urticaria

Ocular: Blurred vision

Respiratory: Respiratory arrest

Miscellaneous: Allergic reactions

Drug Interactions

Avoid Concomitant Use

Avoid concomitant use of Procaine with any of the following: Sulfonamide Derivatives

Increased Effect/Toxicity There are no known significant interactions involving an increase in effect.

Decreased Effect

Procaine may decrease the levels/effects of: Sulfonamide Derivatives

Mechanism of Action Blocks both the initiation and conduction of nerve impulses by decreasing the neuronal membrane's permeability to sodium ions, which results in inhibition of depolarization with resultant blockade of conduction

Pharmacodynamics/Kinetics

Onset of action: 2-5 minutes

Duration (patient, type of block, concentration, and method of anesthesia dependent); 0.5-1.5 hours

Metabolism: Rapidly hydrolyzed by plasma enzymes to PABA and diethylaminoethanol (80% conjugated before elimination)

Half-life elimination: 7.7 minutes

Excretion: Urine (as metabolites and some unchanged drug)

Dosage Dose varies with procedure, desired depth, and duration of anesthesia, desired muscle relaxation, vascularity of tissues, physical condition, and age of patient

Adults: Spinal analgesia: Extent of anesthesia:

Perineum: Total dose: 50 mg; Procaine 10%: 0.5 mL with 0.5 mL diluent

Perineum and lower extremities: Total dose: 100 mg; Procaine 10%: 1 mL with 1 mL diluent

Up to costal margin: Total dose: 200 mg; Procaine 10%: 2 mL with 1 mL diluent

Dosage Forms Excipient information presented when available (limited, particularly for generics); consult specific product labeling.

Injection, solution, as hydrochloride:

Novocain®: 10% (2 mL) [contains sodium bisulfite]

◆ **Procaine Amide Hydrochloride** *see* Procainamide *on page 1240*

◆ **Procaine Benzylpenicillin** *see* Penicillin G Procaine *on page 1166*

◆ **Procaine Hydrochloride** *see* Procaine *on page 1242*

◆ **Procaine Penicillin G** *see* Penicillin G Procaine *on page 1166*

◆ **Pro-Calcitonin (Can)** *see* Calcitonin *on page 234*

◆ **Procanbid® [DSC]** *see* Procainamide *on page 1240*

◆ **Procan® SR (Can)** *see* Procainamide *on page 1240*

Procarbazine (proe KAR ba zeen)

U.S. Brand Names Matulane®

Canadian Brand Names Matulane®; Natulan®

Index Terms Benzmethyzin; N-Methylhydrazine; NSC-77213; Procarbazine Hydrochloride

Pharmacologic Category Antineoplastic Agent, Alkylating Agent

Additional Appendix Information

Tyramine Content of Foods *on page 1850*

Use Treatment of Hodgkin's disease

Unlabeled/Investigational Use Treatment of non-Hodgkin's lymphoma, brain tumors, melanoma, lung cancer, multiple myeloma

Pregnancy Risk Factor D

Pregnancy Considerations Animal studies have demonstrated teratogenic effects. There are no adequate and well-controlled studies in pregnant women. There are, however, case reports of fetal malformations in the offspring of pregnant women exposed to procarbazine as part of a combination chemotherapy regimen. Women of childbearing potential should avoid becoming pregnant during treatment.

Lactation Excretion in breast milk unknown/not recommended

Medication Safety Issues

Sound-alike/look-alike issues:

Procarbazine may be confused with dacarbazine

Matulane® may be confused with Modane®

High alert medication: The Institute for Safe Medication Practices (ISMP) includes this medication among its list of drugs which have a heightened risk of causing significant patient harm when used in error.

Contraindications Hypersensitivity to procarbazine or any component of the formulation; pre-existing bone marrow aplasia; ethanol ingestion; pregnancy

Warnings/Precautions Hazardous agent - use appropriate precautions for handling and disposal. Use with caution in patients with pre-existing renal or hepatic impairment. Procarbazine possesses MAO inhibitor activity and has potential for severe drug and food interactions; follow MAO-I diet. Avoid ethanol consumption, may cause disulfiram-like reaction. May cause hemolysis and/or presence of Heinz inclusion bodies in erythrocytes. Bone marrow depression may occur 2-8 weeks after treatment initiation. Allow ≥1 month interval between radiation therapy or myelosuppressive chemotherapy and initiation of treatment. Withhold treatment for CNS toxicity, leukopenia (WBC <4000/mm^3), thrombocytopenia (platelets <100,000/mm^3), hypersensitivity, stomatitis, diarrhea or hemorrhage. Procarbazine is a carcinogen which may cause acute leukemia. May cause infertility. **[U.S. Boxed Warning]: Should be administered under the supervision of an experienced cancer chemotherapy physician.**

Adverse Reactions Most frequencies not defined.

Cardiovascular: Edema, flushing, hypotension, syncope, tachycardia

Central nervous system: Apprehension, ataxia, chills, coma, confusion, depression, dizziness, drowsiness, fatigue, fever, hallucination, headache, insomnia, lethargy, nervousness, nightmares, pain, seizure, slurred speech

Dermatologic: Alopecia, dermatitis, hyperpigmentation, petechiae, pruritus, purpura, rash, urticaria

Endocrine & metabolic: Gynecomastia (in prepubertal and early pubertal males)

Hematologic: Eosinophilia; hemolysis (in patients with G6PD deficiency); hemolytic anemia; myelosuppression (leukopenia, anemia, thrombocytopenia); pancytopenia

Gastrointestinal: Abdominal pain, anorexia, constipation, diarrhea, dysphagia, hematemesis, melena; nausea and vomiting ([60% to 90%], increasing the dose in a stepwise fashion over several days may minimize); stomatitis, xerostomia

Genitourinary: Azoospermia (reported with combination chemotherapy), hematuria, nocturia, polyuria, reproductive dysfunction (>10%)

Hepatic: Hepatic dysfunction, jaundice

Neuromuscular & skeletal: Arthralgia, falling, foot drop, myalgia, neuropathy, paresthesia, reflex diminished, tremor, unsteadiness, weakness

Ocular: Diplopia, inability to focus, nystagmus, papilledema, photophobia, retinal hemorrhage

Otic: Hearing loss

Respiratory: Cough, epistaxis, hemoptysis, hoarseness, pleural effusion, pneumonitis, pulmonary toxicity (<1%)

Miscellaneous: Allergic reaction, diaphoresis, herpes, infection, secondary malignancies (2% to 15%; reported with combination therapy)

Drug Interactions

Avoid Concomitant Use

Avoid concomitant use of Procarbazine with any of the following: Alpha-/Beta-Agonists (Indirect-Acting); Alpha1-Agonists; Alpha2-Agonists (Ophthalmic); Amphetamines; Atomoxetine; BuPROPion; BusPIRone; Cyclobenzaprine; Dexmethylphenidate; Dextromethorphan; Linezolid; Maprotiline; Meperidine; Methyldopa; Methylphenidate; Mirtazapine; Natalizumab; Propoxyphene; Selective Serotonin Reuptake Inhibitors; Serotonin 5-HT1D Receptor Agonists; Serotonin/Norepinephrine Reuptake Inhibitors; Sibutramine; Tetrabenazine; Tricyclic Antidepressants; Vaccines (Live)

Increased Effect/Toxicity

Procarbazine may increase the levels/effects of: Alpha-/Beta-Agonists (Direct-Acting); Alpha-/Beta-Agonists (Indirect-Acting); Alpha1-Agonists; Alpha2-Agonists (Ophthalmic); Amphetamines; Atomoxetine; Beta2-Agonists; BuPROPion; Dexmethylphenidate; Dextromethorphan; Linezolid; Lithium; Meperidine; Methyldopa; Methylphenidate; Mirtazapine; Natalizumab; Rauwolfia Alkaloids; Selective Serotonin Reuptake Inhibitors; Serotonin 5-HT1D Receptor Agonists; Serotonin Modulators; Serotonin/Norepinephrine Reuptake Inhibitors; Tricyclic Antidepressants; Vaccines (Live); Vitamin K Antagonists

The levels/effects of Procarbazine may be increased by: Altretamine; Anilidopiperidine Opioids; BusPIRone; COMT Inhibitors; Cyclobenzaprine; Levodopa; Maprotiline; Propoxyphene; Sibutramine; Tetrabenazine; TraMADol; Trastuzumab

Decreased Effect

Procarbazine may decrease the levels/effects of: Cardiac Glycosides; Vaccines (Inactivated); Vitamin K Antagonists

The levels/effects of Procarbazine may be decreased by: Echinacea

Ethanol/Nutrition/Herb Interactions

Ethanol: May enhance the adverse/toxic effects of procarbazine; concurrent use not recommended.

Food: Concurrent ingestion of foods rich in tyramine may cause sudden and severe high blood pressure (hypertensive crisis). Avoid tyramine-containing foods with MAO-Is. Food's freshness is also an important concern; improperly stored or spoiled food can create an environment where tyramine concentrations may increase.

Herb/Nutraceuticals: Avoid supplements containing caffeine, tyrosine, tryptophan, or phenylalanine. Ingestion of large quantities may increase the risk of severe side effects (eg, hypertensive reactions, serotonin syndrome).

Stability Protect from light.

Mechanism of Action Mechanism of action is not clear, methylating of nucleic acids; inhibits DNA, RNA, and protein synthesis; may damage DNA directly and suppresses mitosis; metabolic activation required by host

Pharmacodynamics/Kinetics

Absorption: Rapid and complete

Distribution: Crosses blood-brain barrier; equilibrates between plasma and CSF

Metabolism: Hepatic and renal

Half-life elimination: 1 hour

Time to peak, plasma: 1 hour

Excretion: Urine and respiratory tract (<5% as unchanged drug, 70% as metabolites)

Dosage Refer to individual protocols. Manufacturer states that the dose is based on patient's ideal weight if the patient is obese or has abnormal fluid retention. Other studies suggest that ideal body weight may not be necessary. Oral (may be given as a single daily dose or in 2-3 divided doses):

Children:

BMT aplastic anemia conditioning regimen: 12.5 mg/kg/day every other day for 4 doses

Hodgkin's disease: MOPP/IC-MOPP regimens: 100 mg/m^2/day for 14 days and repeated every 4 weeks

Neuroblastoma and medulloblastoma: Doses as high as 100-200 mg/m^2/day once daily have been used

Adults: Initial: 2-4 mg/kg/day in single or divided doses for 7 days then increase dose to 4-6 mg/kg/day until response is obtained or leukocyte count decreased <4000/mm^3 or the platelet count decreased <100,000/mm^3; maintenance: 1-2 mg/kg/day

Dosing in renal impairment: The FDA-approved labeling does not contain dosing adjustment guidelines; use with caution; may result in increased toxicity.

Dosing in hepatic impairment: The FDA-approved labeling does not contain dosing adjustment guidelines; use with caution; may result in increased toxicity. The following guidelines have been used by some clinicians:

Floyd, 2006:

Transaminases 1.6-6 times ULN: Administer 75% of dose

Transaminases >6 times ULN: Use clinical judgment

Serum bilirubin >5 mg/dL or transaminases >3 times ULN: Avoid use

King, 2001: Serum bilirubin >5 mg/dL or transaminases >180 units/L: Avoid use

Dietary Considerations Avoid tyramine-containing foods/beverages. Some examples include aged or matured cheese, air-dried or cured meats (including sausages and salamis), fava or broad bean pods, tap/draft beers, Marmite concentrate, sauerkraut, soy sauce and other soybean condiments.

Administration May be given as a single daily dose or in 2-3 divided doses.

Monitoring Parameters CBC with differential, platelet and reticulocyte count, urinalysis, liver function test, renal function test.

Dosage Forms Excipient information presented when available (limited, particularly for generics); consult specific product labeling.

Capsule, as hydrochloride:

Matulane®: 50 mg

◆ **Procarbazine Hydrochloride** *see* Procarbazine *on page 1242*

◆ **Procardia®** *see* NIFEdipine *on page 1064*

◆ **Procardia XL®** *see* NIFEdipine *on page 1064*

◆ **Pro-Cefadroxil (Can)** *see* Cefadroxil *on page 269*

◆ **Pro-Cefuroxime (Can)** *see* Cefuroxime *on page 288*

◆ **Procetofene** *see* Fenofibrate *on page 607*

◆ **Prochieve®** *see* Progesterone *on page 1247*

Prochlorperazine (proe klor PER a zeen)

U.S. Brand Names Compro™

Canadian Brand Names Apo-Prochlorperazine®; Nu-Prochlor; Stemetil®

Index Terms Chlormeprazine; Compazine; Prochlorperazine Edisylate; Prochlorperazine Maleate

Pharmacologic Category Antiemetic; Antipsychotic Agent, Typical, Phenothiazine

Use Management of nausea and vomiting; psychotic disorders including schizophrenia; anxiety

Unlabeled/Investigational Use Behavioral syndromes in dementia; psychosis/agitation related to Alzheimer's dementia

Pregnancy Considerations Crosses the placenta. Isolated reports of congenital anomalies, however, some included exposures to other drugs. Jaundice, extrapyramidal signs, hyper-/hyporeflexes have been noted in newborns. Available evidence with use of occasional low doses suggests safe use during pregnancy.

Lactation Excretion in breast milk unknown/use caution

Medication Safety Issues

Sound-alike/look-alike issues:

Prochlorperazine may be confused with chlorproMAZINE

Compazine® may be confused with Copaxone®, Coumadin®

CPZ (occasional abbreviation for Compazine®) is an error-prone abbreviation (mistaken as chlorpromazine)

Contraindications Hypersensitivity to prochlorperazine or any component of the formulation (cross-reactivity between phenothiazines may occur); severe CNS depression; coma; pediatric surgery; Reye's syndrome; should not be used in children <2 years of age or <9 kg

Warnings/Precautions Elderly patients with dementia-related psychosis treated with antipsychotics are at an increased risk of death compared to placebo. An increased incidence of cerebrovascular adverse events (including fatalities) has been reported in elderly patients with dementia-related psychosis. Prochlorperazine is not approved for this indication.

May be sedating; use with caution in disorders where CNS depression is a feature. May obscure intestinal obstruction or brain tumor. May impair physical or mental abilities. Effects with other sedative drugs or ethanol may be potentiated. Use with caution in Parkinson's disease; hemodynamic instability; bone marrow suppression; predisposition to seizures; subcortical brain damage; and in severe cardiac, hepatic, renal or respiratory disease. Caution in breast cancer or other prolactin-dependent tumors. May alter temperature regulation or mask toxicity of other drugs. Use caution with exposure to heat. May alter cardiac conduction. May cause orthostatic hypotension. Hypotension may occur following administration, particularly when parenteral form is used or in high dosages. Antipsychotic use has been associated with esophageal dysmotility and aspiration; use with caution in patients at risk of pneumonia (ie, Alzheimer's disease). May be associated with pigmentary retinopathy.

Phenothiazines may cause anticholinergic effects; therefore, they should be used with caution in patients with decreased gastrointestinal motility, urinary retention, BPH, xerostomia, or visual problems. Conditions which also may be exacerbated by cholinergic blockade include narrow-angle glaucoma (screening is recommended) and worsening of myasthenia gravis. May cause extrapyramidal symptoms (EPS), including pseudoparkinsonism, acute dystonic reactions, akathisia, and tardive dyskinesia (risk of these reactions is high relative to other neuroleptics). Risk of dystonia (and possibly other EPS) may be greater with increased doses, use of conventional antipsychotics, males, and younger patients. Use caution in the elderly. Children with acute illness or dehydration are more susceptible to neuromuscular reactions; use cautiously.

May be associated with neuroleptic malignant syndrome (NMS).

Adverse Reactions Reported with prochlorperazine or other phenothiazines. Frequency not defined.

Cardiovascular: Cardiac arrest, hypotension, peripheral edema, Q-wave distortions, T-wave distortions

Central nervous system: Agitation, catatonia, cerebral edema, cough reflex suppressed, dizziness, drowsiness, fever (mild - I.M.), headache, hyperactivity, hyperpyrexia, impairment of temperature regulation, insomnia, neuroleptic malignant syndrome (NMS), paradoxical excitement, restlessness, seizure

Dermatologic: Angioedema, contact dermatitis, discoloration of skin (blue-gray), epithelial keratopathy, erythema, eczema, exfoliative dermatitis (injectable), itching, photosensitivity, rash, skin pigmentation, urticaria

Endocrine & metabolic: Amenorrhea, breast enlargement, galactorrhea, gynecomastia, glucosuria, hyperglycemia, hypoglycemia, lactation, libido (changes in), menstrual irregularity, SIADH

Gastrointestinal: Appetite increased, atonic colon, constipation, ileus, nausea, weight gain, xerostomia

Genitourinary: Ejaculating dysfunction, ejaculatory disturbances, impotence, incontinence, polyuria, priapism, urinary retention, urination difficulty

Hematologic: Agranulocytosis, aplastic anemia, eosinophilia, hemolytic anemia, leukopenia, pancytopenia, thrombocytopenic purpura

Hepatic: Biliary stasis, cholestatic jaundice, hepatotoxicity

Neuromuscular & skeletal: Dystonias (torticollis, opisthotonos, carpopedal spasm, trismus, oculogyric crisis, protusion of tongue); extrapyramidal symptoms (pseudoparkinsonism, akathisia, dystonias, tardive dyskinesia); SLE-like syndrome, tremor

Ocular: blurred vision, cornea and lens changes, lenticular/corneal deposits, miosis, mydriasis, pigmentary retinopathy

Respiratory: Asthma, laryngeal edema, nasal congestion

Miscellaneous: Allergic reactions, diaphoresis

Drug Interactions

Avoid Concomitant Use There are no known interactions where it is recommended to avoid concomitant use.

Increased Effect/Toxicity

Prochlorperazine may increase the levels/effects of: Alcohol (Ethyl); Analgesics (Opioid); Anticholinergics; Beta-Blockers; CNS Depressants

The levels/effects of Prochlorperazine may be increased by: Acetylcholinesterase Inhibitors (Central); Antimalarial Agents; Beta-Blockers; Lithium formulations; Pramlintide; Tetrabenazine

Decreased Effect

Prochlorperazine may decrease the levels/effects of: Amphetamines; Anti-Parkinson's Agents (Dopamine Agonist)

The levels/effects of Prochlorperazine may be decreased by: Antacids; Lithium formulations

Ethanol/Nutrition/Herb Interactions

Ethanol: Avoid ethanol (may increase CNS depression).

Food: Limit caffeine.

Herb/Nutraceutical: Avoid dong quai, St John's wort (may also cause photosensitization). Avoid kava kava, gotu kola, valerian, St John's wort (may increase CNS depression).

Stability

Injection: Store at <30°C (<86°F); do not freeze. Protect from light. Clear or slightly yellow solutions may be used. I.V. infusion: Injection may be diluted in 50-100 mL NS or D_5W.

Suppository, tablet: Store at 15°C to 30°C (59°F to 86°F). Protect from light.

Mechanism of Action Prochlorperazine is a piperazine phenothiazine antipsychotic which blocks postsynaptic mesolimbic dopaminergic D_1 and D_2 receptors in the brain, including the chemoreceptor trigger zone; exhibits a strong alpha-adrenergic and anticholinergic blocking effect and depresses the release of hypothalamic and hypophyseal hormones; believed to depress the reticular activating system, thus affecting basal metabolism, body temperature, wakefulness, vasomotor tone and emesis

Pharmacodynamics/Kinetics

Onset of action: Oral: 30-40 minutes; I.M.: 10-20 minutes; Rectal: ~60 minutes

Peak antiemetic effect: I.V.: 30-60 minutes

Duration: Rectal: 12 hours; Oral: 3-4 hours; I.M., I.V.: Adults: 4-6 hours; I.M.: Children: 12 hours

Distribution: V_d: 1400-1548 L; crosses placenta; enters breast milk

Metabolism: Primarily hepatic; N-desmethyl prochlorperazine (major active metabolite)

Bioavailability: Oral: 12.5%

Half-life elimination: Oral: 3-5 hours; I.V.: ~7 hours

Dosage

Antiemetic: Children (therapy >1 day usually not required): **Note:** Not recommended for use in children <9 kg or <2 years:

Oral, rectal: >9 kg: 0.4 mg/kg/24 hours in 3-4 divided doses; **or**

9-13 kg: 2.5 mg every 12-24 hours as needed; maximum: 7.5 mg/day

13.1-17 kg: 2.5 mg every 8-12 hours as needed; maximum: 10 mg/day

17.1-37 kg: 2.5 mg every 8 hours or 5 mg every 12 hours as needed; maximum: 15 mg/day

I.M.: 0.13 mg/kg/dose; change to oral as soon as possible

Antiemetic: Adults:

Oral (tablet): 5-10 mg 3-4 times/day; usual maximum: 40 mg/day; larger doses may rarely be required

I.M. (deep): 5-10 mg every 3-4 hours; usual maximum: 40 mg/day

I.V.: 2.5-10 mg; maximum 10 mg/dose or 40 mg/day; may repeat dose every 3-4 hours as needed

Rectal: 25 mg twice daily

Surgical nausea/vomiting: Adults: **Note:** Should not exceed 40 mg/day

I.M.: 5-10 mg 1-2 hours before induction or to control symptoms during or after surgery; may repeat once if necessary

I.V. (administer slow IVP <5 mg/minute): 5-10 mg 15-30 minutes before induction or to control symptoms during or after surgery; may repeat once if necessary

Rectal (unlabeled use): 25 mg

Antipsychotic:

Children 2-12 years (not recommended in children <9 kg or <2 years):

Oral, rectal: 2.5 mg 2-3 times/day; do not give more than 10 mg the first day; increase dosage as needed to maximum daily dose of 20 mg for 2-5 years and 25 mg for 6-12 years

I.M.: 0.13 mg/kg/dose; change to oral as soon as possible

Adults:

Oral: 5-10 mg 3-4 times/day; titrate dose slowly every 2-3 days; doses up to 150 mg/day may be required in some patients for treatment of severe disturbances

I.M.: Initial: 10-20 mg; if necessary repeat initial dose every 1-4 hours to gain control; more than 3-4 doses are rarely needed. If parenteral administration is still required; give 10-20 mg every 4-6 hours; change to oral as soon as possible.

Nonpsychotic anxiety: Oral (tablet): Adults: Usual dose: 15-20 mg/day in divided doses; do not give doses >20 mg/day or for longer than 12 weeks

Elderly: Behavioral symptoms associated with dementia (unlabeled use): Initial: 2.5-5 mg 1-2 times/day; increase dose at 4- to 7-day intervals by 2.5-5 mg/day; increase dosing intervals (twice daily, 3 times/day, etc) as necessary to control response or side effects; maximum daily dose should probably not exceed 75 mg in elderly; gradual increases (titration) may prevent some side effects or decrease their severity

Dietary Considerations Increase dietary intake of riboflavin; should be administered with food or water. Rectal suppositories may contain coconut and palm oil.

Administration May be administered orally, I.M., or I.V.

I.M.: Inject by deep IM into outer quadrant of buttocks.

I.V.: Doses should be given as a short (~30 minute) infusion to avoid orthostatic hypotension; administer at ≤5 mg/minute

Monitoring Parameters Vital signs; lipid profile, fasting blood glucose/Hgb A_{1c}; BMI; mental status, abnormal involuntary movement scale (AIMS); periodic ophthalmic exams (if chronically used); extrapyramidal symptoms (EPS)

Test Interactions False-positives for phenylketonuria, pregnancy, urinary amylase, uroporphyrins, urobilinogen

Additional Information Not recommended as an antipsychotic due to inferior efficacy compared to other phenothiazines.

Dosage Forms Excipient information presented when available (limited, particularly for generics); consult specific product labeling.

Injection, solution, as edisylate: 5 mg/mL (2 mL, 10 mL) [contains benzyl alcohol]

Suppository, rectal: 25 mg (12s) [may contain coconut and palm oil]

Compro™: 25 mg (12s) [contains coconut and palm oils]

Tablet, as maleate: 5 mg, 10 mg [strength expressed as base]

◆ **Prochlorperazine Edisylate** *see* Prochlorperazine *on page 1244*

◆ **Prochlorperazine Maleate** *see* Prochlorperazine *on page 1244*

◆ **Pro-Clonazepam (Can)** *see* ClonazePAM *on page 352*

◆ **Procrit®** *see* Epoetin Alfa *on page 531*

◆ **Proctocort®** *see* Hydrocortisone *on page 743*

◆ **ProctoCream® HC** *see* Hydrocortisone *on page 743*

◆ **Proctofene** *see* Fenofibrate *on page 607*

◆ **ProctoFoam®-HC** *see* Pramoxine and Hydrocortisone *on page 1227*

◆ **Proctofoam™-HC (Can)** *see* Pramoxine and Hydrocortisone *on page 1227*

◆ **Procto-Kit™** *see* Hydrocortisone *on page 743*

◆ **Procto-Pak™** *see* Hydrocortisone *on page 743*

◆ **Proctosert** *see* Hydrocortisone *on page 743*

◆ **Proctosol-HC®** *see* Hydrocortisone *on page 743*

◆ **Proctozone-HC™** *see* Hydrocortisone *on page 743*

Procyclidine (proe SYE kli deen)

U.S. Brand Names Kemadrin® [DSC]

Canadian Brand Names PMS-Procyclidine

Index Terms Procyclidine Hydrochloride

Pharmacologic Category Anti-Parkinson's Agent, Anticholinergic; Anticholinergic Agent

Additional Appendix Information

Antiparkinsonian Agents *on page 1643*

Use Relieves symptoms of parkinsonian syndrome and drug-induced extrapyramidal symptoms

Pregnancy Risk Factor C

Lactation Excretion in breast milk unknown/not recommended

Medication Safety Issues

Sound-alike/look-alike issues:

Kemadrin® may be confused with Coumadin®

Contraindications Hypersensitivity to procyclidine or any component of the formulation; angle-closure glaucoma; myasthenia gravis; safe use in children not established

Warnings/Precautions Use with caution in hot weather or during exercise. Elderly patients frequently develop increased sensitivity and require strict dosage regulation - side effects may be more severe in elderly patients with atherosclerotic changes. Use with caution in patients with tachycardia, cardiac arrhythmias, hypertension, hypotension, prostatic hyperplasia (especially in the elderly) or any tendency toward urinary retention, liver or kidney disorders and obstructive disease of the GI or GU tract. When given in large doses or to susceptible patients, may cause weakness and inability to move particular muscle groups. May be associated with confusion or hallucinations (generally at higher dosages); intensification of symptoms or toxic psychosis may occur in patients with mental disorders. May cause CNS depression, which may impair physical or mental abilities; patients must be cautioned about performing tasks which require mental alertness (eg, operating machinery or driving). Safety and efficacy have not been established in children.

Adverse Reactions Frequency not defined.

Cardiovascular: Palpitation, tachycardia

Central nervous system: Ataxia, confusion, drowsiness, fatigue, giddiness, headache, lightheadedness, loss of memory

Dermatologic: Dry skin, photosensitivity, rash

Gastrointestinal: Constipation, dry throat, epigastric distress, nausea, vomiting, xerostomia

Genitourinary: Difficult urination

Neuromuscular & skeletal: Weakness

Ocular: Blurred vision, increased intraocular pain, mydriasis

Respiratory: Dry nose

Miscellaneous: Diaphoresis decreased

Drug Interactions

Avoid Concomitant Use There are no known interactions where it is recommended to avoid concomitant use.

Increased Effect/Toxicity

Procyclidine may increase the levels/effects of: Anticholinergics; Cannabinoids; Potassium Chloride

The levels/effects of Procyclidine may be increased by: Pramlintide

Decreased Effect

Procyclidine may decrease the levels/effects of: Acetylcholinesterase Inhibitors (Central); Secretin

The levels/effects of Procyclidine may be decreased by: Acetylcholinesterase Inhibitors (Central)

Ethanol/Nutrition/Herb Interactions Ethanol: Avoid ethanol.

Mechanism of Action Thought to act by blocking excess acetylcholine at cerebral synapses; many of its effects are due to its pharmacologic similarities with atropine; it exerts an antispasmodic effect on smooth muscle, is a potent mydriatic; inhibits salivation

Pharmacodynamics/Kinetics

Onset of action: 30-40 minutes

Duration: 4-6 hours

Dosage Adults: Oral: 2.5 mg 3 times/day after meals; if tolerated, gradually increase dose, maximum of 20 mg/day if necessary

Dosing adjustment in hepatic impairment: Decrease dose to a twice daily dosing regimen

Dietary Considerations Should be taken after meals to minimize stomach upset.

Administration Should be administered after meals to minimize stomach upset.

Monitoring Parameters Symptoms of EPS or Parkinson's disease, pulse, anticholinergic effects (ie, CNS, bowel and bladder function)

Dosage Forms Excipient information presented when available (limited, particularly for generics); consult specific product labeling. [DSC] = Discontinued product

Tablet, as hydrochloride:

Kemadrin®: 5 mg [scored] [DSC]

- **Procyclidine Hydrochloride** *see* Procyclidine *on page 1246*
- **Procytox® (Can)** *see* Cyclophosphamide *on page 376*
- **Pro-Diclo-Rapide (Can)** *see* Diclofenac *on page 437*
- **Prodium® [OTC]** *see* Phenazopyridine *on page 1177*
- **Pro-Enalapril (Can)** *see* Enalapril *on page 515*
- **Profasi® HP (Can)** *see* Chorionic Gonadotropin (Human) *on page 320*
- **ProFe [OTC]** *see* Polysaccharide-Iron Complex *on page 1212*
- **Profen II® [DSC]** *see* Guaifenesin and Pseudoephedrine *on page 713*
- **Profen II DM®** *see* Guaifenesin, Pseudoephedrine, and Dextromethorphan *on page 715*
- **Profen Forte™ DM** *see* Guaifenesin, Pseudoephedrine, and Dextromethorphan *on page 715*
- **Pro-Feno-Super (Can)** *see* Fenofibrate *on page 607*
- **Profilnine® SD** *see* Factor IX Complex (Human) *on page 601*
- **Proflavanol C™ (Can)** *see* Ascorbic Acid *on page 139*
- **Pro-Fluconazole (Can)** *see* Fluconazole *on page 625*
- **PRO-Fluoxetine (Can)** *see* FLUoxetine *on page 638*

Progesterone (proe JES ter one)

U.S. Brand Names Crinone®; Endometrin®; First™-Progesterone VGS; Prochieve®; Prometrium®

Canadian Brand Names Crinone®; Prometrium®

Index Terms Pregnenedione; Progestin

Pharmacologic Category Progestin

Use

Oral: Prevention of endometrial hyperplasia in nonhysterectomized, postmenopausal women who are receiving conjugated estrogen tablets; secondary amenorrhea

I.M.: Amenorrhea; abnormal uterine bleeding due to hormonal imbalance

Intravaginal gel: Part of assisted reproductive technology (ART) for infertile women with progesterone deficiency; secondary amenorrhea

Vaginal tablet: Part of ART for infertile women with progesterone deficiency

Pregnancy Risk Factor B (Prometrium®, per manufacturer); none established for vaginal gel, vaginal tablet, or injection

Pregnancy Considerations There is an increased risk of minor birth defects in children whose mothers take progesterones during the first 4 months of pregnancy. Hypospadias has been reported in male and mild masculinization of the external genitalia has been reported in female babies exposed during the first trimester. Cleft lip, cleft palate, congenital heart disease, patent ductus arteriosus, ventricular septal defect, intrauterine death, and spontaneous abortion have been noted in case reports following use of oral progesterone during pregnancy. High doses of progesterone would be expected to impair fertility. According to the American College of Obstetricians and Gynecologists, additional studies are needed to evaluate the use of progesterone to reduce the risk of preterm birth. If needed, use should be restricted to women with history of previous spontaneous abortion at <37 weeks. The vaginal gel and tablet are indicated for use in ART. The oral capsules are contraindicated for use during pregnancy.

Lactation Enters breast milk/use caution (AAP rates "compatible")

Contraindications Hypersensitivity to progesterone or any component of the formulation; undiagnosed abnormal vaginal bleeding; history of or current thrombophlebitis or venous thromboembolic disorders (including DVT, PE); active or recent (within 1 year) arterial thromboembolic disease (eg, stroke, MI); known or suspected carcinoma of the breast or genital organs; hepatic dysfunction or disease; missed abortion or ectopic pregnancy; diagnostic test for pregnancy; capsules are also contraindicated for use during pregnancy

Warnings/Precautions [U.S. Boxed Warning]: Progestins used in combination with estrogen should not be used to prevent coronary heart disease. Use caution with cardiovascular disease or dysfunction. Progestins used in combination with estrogen may increase the risks of hypertension, myocardial infarction (MI), stroke, pulmonary emboli (PE), and deep vein thrombosis; incidence of these effects was shown to be significantly increased in postmenopausal women using CEE in combination with MPA. Similar risk should be assumed with other progestins.

[U.S. Boxed Warning]: The risk of dementia may be increased in postmenopausal women; increased incidence was observed in women ≥65 years of age taking CEE alone or in combination with MPA.

Discontinue pending examination in cases of sudden partial or complete vision loss, sudden onset of proptosis, diplopia, or migraine; discontinue permanently if papilledema or retinal vascular lesions are observed on examination. Use with caution in patients with diseases that may be exacerbated by fluid retention, including asthma, epilepsy, migraine, diabetes or renal dysfunction. Use caution with history of depression. Patients should be warned that progesterone might cause transient dizziness or drowsiness during initial therapy. Whenever possible, progestins in combination with estrogens should be discontinued at least 4-6 weeks prior to surgeries associated with an increased risk of thromboembolism or during periods of prolonged immobilization. Progestins used in combination with estrogen should be used for shortest duration possible consistent with treatment goals. Conduct periodic risk:benefit assessments.

Products may contain palm oil, peanut oil, sesame oil, or benzyl alcohol. Not for use prior to menarche.

Adverse Reactions

Injection (I.M.):

Cardiovascular: Cerebral edema, cerebral thrombosis, edema

Central nervous system: Depression, fever, insomnia, somnolence

Dermatologic: Acne, allergic rash (rare), alopecia, hirsutism, pruritus, rash, urticaria

Endocrine & metabolic: Amenorrhea, breakthrough bleeding, breast tenderness, galactorrhea, menstrual flow changes, spotting

Gastrointestinal: Nausea, weight gain/loss

Genitourinary: Cervical erosion changes, cervical secretion changes

Hepatic: Cholestatic jaundice

Local: Injection site: Irritation, pain, redness

Ocular: Optic neuritis, retinal thrombosis

Respiratory: Pulmonary embolism

Miscellaneous: Anaphylactoid reactions

Oral capsule (percentages reported when used in combination with or cycled with conjugated estrogens):

>10%:

Central nervous system: Headache (10% to 31%), dizziness (15% to 24%), depression (19%)

Endocrine & metabolic: Breast tenderness (27%), breast pain (6% to 16%)

Gastrointestinal: Abdominal pain (6% to 12%), abdominal bloating (10% to 20%)

Genitourinary: Urinary problems (11%)

Neuromuscular & skeletal: Joint pain (20%), musculoskeletal pain (6% to 12%)

Miscellaneous: Viral infection (7% to 12%)

5% to 10%:

Cardiovascular: Chest pain (7%)

Central nervous system: Fatigue (8% to 9%), emotional lability (6%), irritability (5% to 8%), worry (8%)

Gastrointestinal: Nausea/vomiting (8%), diarrhea (8%)

Respiratory: Upper respiratory tract infection (5%), cough (8%)

Miscellaneous: Night sweats (7%)

<5% (Limited to important or life-threatening): Acne, aggression, alopecia, ALT increased, anaphylactic reaction, angina pectoris, anxiety, arthralgia, arthritis, AST increased, blurred vision, breast cancer, cholecystectomy, cholestasis, cholestatic hepatitis, circulatory collapse, confusion, consciousness depressed/loss, constipation, convulsion, depersonalization, diplopia, disorientation, dyspepsia, dysphagia, edema, endometrial carcinoma, facial edema, fungal vaginitis, gastroenteritis, GGT increased, hemorrhagic rectum, hepatic enzymes increased, hepatic failure, hepatic necrosis, hepatitis, hernia, hiatus, hyperglycemia, hypersensitivity, hypertension, hypertonia, hypotension, insomnia, jaundice, leg cramps, leukorrhea, lymphadenopathy, muscle cramps, ovarian cyst, palpitation, pancreatitis (acute), paresthesia, personality disorder, pruritus, sedation, somnolence, speech disorder, stupor, suicidal ideation, syncope, tachycardia, TIA, tinnitus, tongue swelling, urticaria, uterine fibroid, vaginal dryness, vaginitis, verruca, vertigo, vision abnormal, visual disturbance, xerostomia

Vaginal gel (percentages reported with ART); also refer to oral capsule reactions listing for additional effects noted with progesterone:

>10%:

Central nervous system: Somnolence (27%), headache (13% to 17%), nervousness (16%), depression (11%)

Endocrine & metabolic: Breast enlargement (40%), breast pain (13%), libido decreased (11%)

Gastrointestinal: Constipation (27%), nausea (7% to 22%), cramps (15%), abdominal pain (12%)

Genitourinary: Perineal pain (17%), nocturia (13%)

5% to 10%:

Central nervous system: Pain (8%), dizziness (5%)

Gastrointestinal: Diarrhea (8%), bloating (7%), vomiting (5%)

Genitourinary: Vaginal discharge (7%), dyspareunia (6%), genital moniliasis (5%), genital pruritus (5%)

Neuromuscular & skeletal: Arthralgia (8%)

Vaginal tablet (percentages reported with ART); also refer to oral capsule reactions listing for additional effects noted with progesterone:

>10%:

Gastrointestinal: Abdominal pain (12%)

Miscellaneous: Post-oocyte retrieval pain (25% to 28%)

1% to 10%:

Central nervous system: Headache (3% to 4%), fatigue (2% to 3%)

Endocrine & metabolic: Ovarian hyperstimulation syndrome (7%)

Gastrointestinal: Nausea (7% to 8%), abdominal distension (4%), constipation (2% to 3%), vomiting (2% to 3%)

Genitourinary: Uterine spasm (3% to 4%), vaginal bleeding (3%), urinary tract infection (1% to 2%)

<1%: Burning, discomfort, itching, peripheral edema, urticaria, vaginal irritation

Drug Interactions

Metabolism/Transport Effects Substrate of CYP1A2 (minor), 2A6 (minor), 2C9 (minor), 2C19 (major), 2D6 (minor), 3A4 (major); **Inhibits** CYP2C9 (weak), 2C19 (weak), 3A4 (weak)

Avoid Concomitant Use

Avoid concomitant use of Progesterone with any of the following: Dabigatran Etexilate; Rivaroxaban; Silodosin; Topotecan

Increased Effect/Toxicity

Progesterone may increase the levels/effects of: Dabigatran Etexilate; P-Glycoprotein Substrates; Rivaroxaban; Silodosin; Topotecan

The levels/effects of Progesterone may be increased by: Herbs (Progestogenic Properties)

Decreased Effect

The levels/effects of Progesterone may be decreased by: Aminoglutethimide; CYP2C19 Inducers (Strong); CYP3A4 Inducers (Strong); Deferasirox; Herbs (CYP3A4 Inducers)

Ethanol/Nutrition/Herb Interactions

Food: Food increases oral bioavailability.

Herb/Nutraceutical: St John's wort may decrease progesterone levels. Herbs with progestogenic properties may enhance the adverse/toxic effects of progestin; example herbs include bloodroot, chasteberry, damiana, oregano, yucca.

Stability Store at controlled room temperature.

Mechanism of Action Natural steroid hormone that induces secretory changes in the endometrium, promotes mammary gland development, relaxes uterine smooth muscle, blocks follicular maturation and ovulation, and maintains pregnancy. When used as part of an ART program in the luteal phase, progesterone supports embryo implantation.

Pharmacodynamics/Kinetics

Absorption: Vaginal gel: Prolonged

Absorption half-life: 25-50 hours

Protein binding: Albumin (50% to 54%) and cortisol-binding protein (43% to 48%)

Metabolism: Hepatic to metabolites

Half-life elimination: Vaginal gel: 5-20 minutes

Time to peak: Oral: Within 3 hours; I.M.: ~8 hours; Vaginal tablet: ~17-24 hours

Excretion: Urine, bile, feces

Dosage Adults:

I.M.: Females:

Amenorrhea: 5-10 mg/day for 6-8 consecutive days

Functional uterine bleeding: 5-10 mg/day for 6 doses

Oral: Females:

Prevention of endometrial hyperplasia (in postmenopausal women with a uterus who are receiving daily conjugated estrogen tablets): 200 mg as a single daily dose every evening for 12 days sequentially per 28-day cycle

Amenorrhea: 400 mg every evening for 10 days

Intravaginal gel: Females:

ART in women who require progesterone supplementation: 90 mg (8% gel) once daily; if pregnancy occurs, may continue treatment for up to 10-12 weeks

ART in women with partial or complete ovarian failure: 90 mg (8% gel) intravaginally twice daily; if pregnancy occurs, may continue up to 10-12 weeks

Secondary amenorrhea: 45 mg (4% gel) intravaginally every other day for up to 6 doses; women who fail to respond may be increased to 90 mg (8% gel) every other day for up to 6 doses

Intravaginal tablet: Females: ART: 100 mg 2-3 times daily starting at oocyte retrieval and continuing for up to 10 weeks.

Administration

I.M.: Administer deep I.M. only

Intravaginal:

Vaginal gel: (A small amount of gel will remain in the applicator following insertion): Administer into the vagina directly from sealed applicator. Remove applicator from wrapper; holding applicator by thickest end, shake down to move contents to thin end; while holding applicator by flat section of thick end, twist off tab; gently insert into vagina and squeeze thick end of applicator.

For use at altitudes above 2500 feet: Remove applicator from wrapper; hold applicator on both sides of bubble in the thick end; using a lancet, make a single puncture in the bubble to relieve air pressure; holding applicator by thickest end, shake down to move contents to thin end; while holding applicator by flat section of thick end, twist off tab; gently insert into vagina and squeeze thick end of applicator.

Vaginal tablet: Insert tablet in vagina using disposable applicator provided.

Monitoring Parameters Routine physical examination that includes blood pressure and Papanicolaou smear, breast exam, mammogram. Adequate diagnostic measures, including endometrial sampling, if indicated, should be performed to rule out malignancy in all cases of undiagnosed abnormal vaginal bleeding. Signs and symptoms of thromboembolic disorders, vision changes

Test Interactions Thyroid function, metyrapone, liver function, coagulation tests, endocrine function tests

Dosage Forms Excipient information presented when available (limited, particularly for generics); consult specific product labeling.

Capsule:

Prometrium®: 100 mg, 200 mg [contains peanut oil]

Gel, vaginal:

Crinone®: 8% (1.45 g) [90 mg/dose; contains palm oil; 6 or 18 prefilled applicators]

Prochieve®: 4% (1.45 g) [45 mg/dose; contains palm oil; 6 prefilled applicators]; 8% (1.45 g) [90 mg/dose; contains palm oil; 6 or 18 prefilled applicators]

Injection, oil: 50 mg/mL (10 mL) [contains benzyl alcohol 10%, sesame oil]

Powder, for prescription compounding [micronized]: Progesterone USP (10 g, 25 g, 100 g, 1000 g)

Powder, for prescription compounding [wettable]: Progesterone USP (10 g, 25 g, 100 g, 1000 g)

First™-Progesterone VGS 25: Progesterone USP (0.75 g) [makes 30 progesterone 25 mg vaginal suppositories; kit contains fatty acid base, suppository mold, stirrer, filling tool, guide plate, mold cover with dispensing tool]

First™-Progesterone VGS 50: Progesterone USP (1.5 g) [makes 30 progesterone 50 mg vaginal suppositories; kit contains fatty acid base, suppository mold, stirrer, filling tool, guide plate, mold cover with dispensing tool]

First™-Progesterone VGS 100: Progesterone USP (3 g) [makes 30 progesterone 100 mg vaginal suppositories; kit contains fatty acid base, suppository mold, stirrer, filling tool, guide plate, mold cover with dispensing tool]

First™-Progesterone VGS 200: Progesterone USP (6 g) [makes 30 progesterone 200 mg vaginal suppositories; kit contains fatty acid base, suppository mold, stirrer, filling tool, guide plate, mold cover with dispensing tool]

First™-Progesterone VGS 400: Progesterone USP (12 g) [makes 30 progesterone 400 mg vaginal suppositories; kit contains fatty acid base, suppository mold, stirrer, filling tool, guide plate, mold cover with dispensing tool]

Tablet, vaginal:

Endometrin®: 100 mg (21s) [packaged with applicators]

- ◆ **Progestin** *see* Progesterone *on page 1247*
- ◆ **Proglycem®** *see* Diazoxide *on page 436*
- ◆ **Prograf®** *see* Tacrolimus *on page 1419*
- ◆ **Proguanil and Atovaquone** *see* Atovaquone and Proguanil *on page 154*
- ◆ **Proguanil Hydrochloride and Atovaquone** *see* Atovaquone and Proguanil *on page 154*
- ◆ **Pro-Hydroxyquine (Can)** *see* Hydroxychloroquine *on page 751*
- ◆ **Pro-Indapamide (Can)** *see* Indapamide *on page 781*
- ◆ **Pro-ISMN (Can)** *see* Isosorbide Mononitrate *on page 824*
- ◆ **Proleukin®** *see* Aldesleukin *on page 53*
- ◆ **Pro-Levocarb (Can)** *see* Carbidopa and Levodopa *on page 256*
- ◆ **Prolex®-D [DSC]** *see* Guaifenesin and Phenylephrine *on page 712*
- ◆ **Prolex®-PD [DSC]** *see* Guaifenesin and Phenylephrine *on page 712*
- ◆ **Pro-Lisinopril (Can)** *see* Lisinopril *on page 894*
- ◆ **PRO-Lovastatin (Can)** *see* Lovastatin *on page 910*
- ◆ **Promacet** *see* Butalbital and Acetaminophen *on page 230*
- ◆ **Promacta®** *see* Eltrombopag *on page 512*

Promethazine (proe METH a zeen)

U.S. Brand Names Phenadoz™; Phenergan®; Promethegan™

Canadian Brand Names Bioniche Promethazine; Histantil; Phenergan®; PMS-Promethazine

Index Terms Promethazine Hydrochloride

Pharmacologic Category Antiemetic; Histamine H_1 Antagonist; Histamine H_1 Antagonist, First Generation

Use Symptomatic treatment of various allergic conditions; antiemetic; motion sickness; sedative; postoperative pain (adjunctive therapy); anesthetic (adjunctive therapy); anaphylactic reactions (adjunctive therapy)

Pregnancy Risk Factor C

Pregnancy Considerations Teratogenic effects were not observed in animal studies. Crosses the placenta. Possible respiratory depression if drug is administered near time of delivery; behavioral changes, EEG alterations, impaired platelet aggregation reported with use during labor.

Lactation Excretion in breast milk unknown/use caution

Medication Safety Issues

Sound-alike/look-alike issues:

Promethazine may be confused with chlorproMAZINE, predniSONE, promazine

Phenergan® may be confused with Phenaphen®, Phrenilin®, Theragran®

High alert medication: The Institute for Safe Medication Practices (ISMP) includes this medication (I.V. formulation) among its list of drugs which have a heightened risk of causing significant patient harm when used in error.

Administration issues:

To prevent or minimize tissue damage during I.V. administration, the Institute for Safe Medication Practices (ISMP) has the following recommendations:

Limit concentration available to the 25 mg/mL product

Consider limiting initial doses to 6.25-12.5 mg

Further dilute the 25 mg/mL strength into 10-20 mL NS

Administer through a large bore vein (not hand or wrist)

Administer via running I.V. line at port furthest from patient's vein

Consider administering over 10-15 minutes
Instruct patients to report immediately signs of pain or burning

Contraindications Hypersensitivity to promethazine or any component of the formulation (cross-reactivity between phenothiazines may occur); coma; treatment of lower respiratory tract symptoms, including asthma; children <2 years of age

Warnings/Precautions [U.S. Boxed Warning]: Respiratory fatalities have been reported in children <2 years of age. In children ≥2 years, use the lowest possible dose; other drugs with respiratory depressant effects should be avoided. Not for SubQ or intra-arterial administration. Injection may contain sodium metabisulfite. I.M. is the preferred route of parenteral administration. I.V. use has been associated with severe tissue damage; discontinue immediately if burning or pain occurs with administration. May be sedating; use with caution in disorders where CNS depression is a feature. May impair physical or mental abilities; patients must be cautioned about performing tasks which require mental alertness. Use with caution in Parkinson's disease; hemodynamic instability; bone marrow suppression; subcortical brain damage; and in severe cardiac, hepatic, renal, or respiratory disease. Avoid use in Reye's syndrome. May lower seizure threshold; use caution in persons with seizure disorders or in persons using narcotics or local anesthetics which may also affect seizure threshold. May alter temperature regulation or mask toxicity of other drugs due to antiemetic effects. May alter cardiac conduction (life-threatening arrhythmias have occurred with therapeutic doses of phenothiazines). May cause orthostatic hypotension; use with caution in patients at risk of hypotension or where transient hypotensive episodes would be poorly tolerated (cardiovascular disease or cerebrovascular disease).

Phenothiazines may cause anticholinergic effects; therefore, they should be used with caution in patients with decreased gastrointestinal motility, urinary retention, BPH, xerostomia, or visual problems. Conditions which also may be exacerbated by cholinergic blockade include narrow-angle glaucoma (screening is recommended) and worsening of myasthenia gravis. May cause extrapyramidal symptoms, including pseudoparkinsonism, acute dystonic reactions, akathisia, and tardive dyskinesia. May be associated with neuroleptic malignant syndrome (NMS).

Adverse Reactions

Cardiovascular: Bradycardia, hypertension, nonspecific QT changes, postural hypotension, tachycardia
Central nervous system: Akathisia, catatonic states, confusion, delirium, disorientation, dizziness, drowsiness, dystonias, euphoria, excitation, extrapyramidal symptoms, fatigue, hallucinations, hysteria, insomnia, lassitude, nervousness, neuroleptic malignant syndrome, nightmares, pseudoparkinsonism, sedation, seizure, somnolence, tardive dyskinesia
Dermatologic: Angioneurotic edema, dermatitis, photosensitivity, skin pigmentation (slate gray), urticaria
Endocrine & metabolic: Amenorrhea, breast engorgement, gynecomastia, hyper-/hypoglycemia, lactation
Gastrointestinal: Constipation, nausea, vomiting, xerostomia
Genitourinary: Ejaculatory disorder, impotence, urinary retention
Hematologic: Agranulocytosis, aplastic anemia, eosinophilia, hemolytic anemia, leukopenia, thrombocytopenia, thrombocytopenic purpura
Hepatic: Jaundice
Local: Venous thrombosis; injection site reactions (burning, erythema, pain, edema)
Neuromuscular & skeletal: Incoordination, tremor
Ocular: Blurred vision, corneal and lenticular changes, diplopia, epithelial keratopathy, pigmentary retinopathy
Otic: Tinnitus
Respiratory: Apnea, asthma, nasal congestion, respiratory depression

Drug Interactions

Metabolism/Transport Effects Substrate (major) of CYP2B6, 2D6; **Inhibits** CYP2D6 (weak)

Avoid Concomitant Use

Avoid concomitant use of Promethazine with any of the following: Sibutramine

Increased Effect/Toxicity

Promethazine may increase the levels/effects of: Anticholinergics; Serotonin Modulators

The levels/effects of Promethazine may be increased by: CYP2B6 Inhibitors (Moderate); CYP2B6 Inhibitors (Strong); CYP2D6 Inhibitors (Moderate); CYP2D6 Inhibitors (Strong); Darunavir; Pramlintide; Sibutramine

Decreased Effect

Promethazine may decrease the levels/effects of: Acetylcholinesterase Inhibitors (Central)

The levels/effects of Promethazine may be decreased by: Acetylcholinesterase Inhibitors (Central); CYP2B6 Inducers (Strong)

Ethanol/Nutrition/Herb Interactions

Ethanol: Avoid ethanol (may increase CNS depression).
Herb/Nutraceutical: Avoid valerian, St John's wort, kava kava, gotu kola (may increase CNS depression).

Stability

Injection: Prior to dilution, store at room temperature. Protect from light. Solutions in NS or D_5W are stable for 24 hours at room temperature.
Suppositories: Store refrigerated at 2°C to 8°C (36°F to 46°F).
Tablets: Store at room temperature. Protect from light.

Mechanism of Action Blocks postsynaptic mesolimbic dopaminergic receptors in the brain; exhibits a strong alpha-adrenergic blocking effect and depresses the release of hypothalamic and hypophyseal hormones; competes with histamine for the H_1-receptor; reduces stimuli to the brainstem reticular system

Pharmacodynamics/Kinetics

Onset of action: I.M.: ~20 minutes; I.V.: 3-5 minutes
Peak effect: C_{max}: 9.04 ng/mL (suppository); 19.3 ng/mL (syrup)
Duration: 2-6 hours
Absorption:
I.M.: Bioavailability may be greater than with oral or rectal administration
Oral: Rapid and complete; large first pass effect limits systemic bioavailability
Distribution: V_d: 171 L
Protein binding: 93%
Metabolism: Hepatic; primarily oxidation; forms metabolites
Half-life elimination: 9-16 hours
Time to maximum serum concentration: 4.4 hours (syrup); 6.7-8.6 hours (suppositories)
Excretion: Primarily urine and feces (as inactive metabolites)

Dosage

Children ≥2 years:
Allergic conditions: Oral, rectal: 0.1 mg/kg/dose (maximum: 12.5 mg) every 6 hours during the day and 0.5 mg/kg/dose (maximum: 25 mg) at bedtime as needed
Antiemetic: Oral, I.M., I.V., rectal: 0.25-1 mg/kg 4-6 times/day as needed (maximum: 25 mg/dose)
Motion sickness: Oral, rectal: 0.5 mg/kg/dose 30 minutes to 1 hour before departure, then every 12 hours as needed (maximum dose: 25 mg twice daily)
Sedation: Oral, I.M., I.V., rectal: 0.5-1 mg/kg/dose every 6 hours as needed (maximum: 50 mg/dose)

Adults:

Allergic conditions (including allergic reactions to blood or plasma):

Oral, rectal: 25 mg at bedtime **or** 12.5 mg before meals and at bedtime (range: 6.25-12.5 mg 3 times/day)

I.M., I.V.: 25 mg, may repeat in 2 hours when necessary; switch to oral route as soon as feasible

Antiemetic: Oral, I.M., I.V., rectal: 12.5-25 mg every 4-6 hours as needed

Motion sickness: Oral, rectal: 25 mg 30-60 minutes before departure, then every 12 hours as needed

Sedation: Oral, I.M., I.V., rectal: 12.5-50 mg/dose

Dietary Considerations Increase dietary intake of riboflavin.

Administration Formulations available for oral, rectal, I.M./I.V.; not for SubQ or intra-arterial administration. Administer I.M. into deep muscle (preferred route of administration). I.V. administration is **not** the preferred route; severe tissue damage may occur. Solution for injection should be administered in a maximum concentration of 25 mg/mL (more dilute solutions are recommended). Administer via running I.V. line at port furthest from patient's vein, or through a large bore vein (not hand or wrist). Consider administering over 10-15 minutes (maximum: 25 mg/minute). Discontinue immediately if burning or pain occurs with administration.

Monitoring Parameters Relief of symptoms, mental status

Test Interactions Alters the flare response in intradermal allergen tests; hCG-based pregnancy tests may result in false-negatives or false-positives; increased serum glucose may be seen with glucose tolerance tests

Dosage Forms Excipient information presented when available (limited, particularly for generics); consult specific product labeling. [DSC] = Discontinued product

Injection, solution, as hydrochloride: 25 mg/mL (1 mL); 50 mg/mL (1 mL)

Phenergan®: 25 mg/mL (1 mL); 50 mg/mL (1 mL) [contains sodium metabisulfite]

Suppository, rectal, as hydrochloride: 12.5 mg, 25 mg, 50 mg

Phenadoz™: 12.5 mg, 25 mg

Phenergan®: 25 mg, 50 mg [DSC]

Promethegan™: 12.5 mg, 25 mg, 50 mg

Syrup, as hydrochloride: 6.25 mg/5 mL (120 mL, 480 mL) [contains alcohol]

Tablet, as hydrochloride: 12.5 mg, 25 mg, 50 mg

Phenergan®: 25 mg [DSC]

Promethazine and Codeine

(proe METH a zeen & KOE deen)

Index Terms Codeine and Promethazine

Pharmacologic Category Alpha/Beta Agonist; Analgesic, Opioid; Histamine H_1 Antagonist; Histamine H_1 Antagonist, First Generation

Use Temporary relief of coughs and upper respiratory symptoms associated with allergy or the common cold

Restrictions C-V

Pregnancy Risk Factor C

Dosage Oral:

Children <16 years: **Note:** Use of promethazine/codeine combination is contraindicated in children <16 years of age

Children ≥16 years and Adults: 5 mL every 4-6 hours (maximum: 30 mL/24 hours)

Additional Information Complete prescribing information for this medication should be consulted for additional detail.

Dosage Forms Excipient information presented when available (limited, particularly for generics); consult specific product labeling.

Syrup: Promethazine hydrochloride 6.25 mg and codeine phosphate 10 mg per 5 mL (120 mL, 473 mL) [contains alcohol]

Promethazine and Dextromethorphan

(proe METH a zeen & deks troe meth OR fan)

Index Terms Dextromethorphan and Promethazine

Pharmacologic Category Antitussive; Histamine H_1 Antagonist; Histamine H_1 Antagonist, First Generation

Use Temporary relief of coughs and upper respiratory symptoms associated with allergy or the common cold

Pregnancy Risk Factor C

Dosage Oral:

Children:

<2 years: Use of promethazine is contraindicated

2-6 years: 1.25-2.5 mL every 4-6 hours up to 10 mL in 24 hours

6-12 years: 2.5-5 mL every 4-6 hours up to 20 mL in 24 hours

Adults: 5 mL every 4-6 hours up to 30 mL in 24 hours

Additional Information Complete prescribing information for this medication should be consulted for additional detail.

Dosage Forms Excipient information presented when available (limited, particularly for generics); consult specific product labeling.

Syrup: Promethazine hydrochloride 6.25 mg and dextromethorphan hydrobromide 15 mg per 5 mL (120 mL, 480 mL) [contains alcohol 7%]

◆ **Promethazine and Meperidine** *see* Meperidine and Promethazine *on page 944*

Promethazine and Phenylephrine

(proe METH a zeen & fen il EF rin)

Index Terms Phenylephrine and Promethazine

Pharmacologic Category Alpha/Beta Agonist; Histamine H_1 Antagonist; Histamine H_1 Antagonist, First Generation

Use Temporary relief of upper respiratory symptoms associated with allergy or the common cold

Pregnancy Risk Factor C

Dosage Oral:

Children:

<2 years: Use of promethazine is contraindicated

2-6 years: 1.25-2.5 mL every 4-6 hours, not to exceed 7.5 mL in 24 hours

6-12 years: 2.5-5 mL every 4-6 hours, not to exceed 30 mL in 24 hours

Children >12 years and Adults: 5 mL every 4-6 hours, not to exceed 30 mL in 24 hours

Additional Information Complete prescribing information for this medication should be consulted for additional detail.

Dosage Forms Excipient information presented when available (limited, particularly for generics); consult specific product labeling.

Syrup: Promethazine hydrochloride 6.25 mg and phenylephrine hydrochloride 5 mg per 5 mL (473 mL) [contains alcohol]

◆ **Promethazine Hydrochloride** *see* Promethazine *on page 1249*

Promethazine, Phenylephrine, and Codeine

(proe METH a zeen, fen il EF rin, & KOE deen)

Index Terms Codeine, Promethazine, and Phenylephrine; Phenylephrine, Promethazine, and Codeine

Pharmacologic Category Alpha/Beta Agonist; Analgesic, Opioid; Antitussive; Histamine H_1 Agonist; Histamine H_1 Antagonist, First Generation

Use Temporary relief of coughs and upper respiratory symptoms including nasal congestion associated with allergy or the common cold

Restrictions C-V

Pregnancy Risk Factor C

Dosage Oral:

Children <16 years: **Note:** Use of promethazine/codeine combination is contraindicated in children <16 years of age

Children ≥16 years and Adults: 5 mL every 4-6 hours, not to exceed 30 mL/24 hours

Additional Information Complete prescribing information for this medication should be consulted for additional detail.

Dosage Forms Excipient information presented when available (limited, particularly for generics); consult specific product labeling.

Syrup: Promethazine hydrochloride 6.25 mg, phenylephrine hydrochloride 5 mg, and codeine phosphate 10 mg per 5 mL (480 mL) [contains alcohol and sodium benzoate]

◆ **Promethegan™** *see* Promethazine *on page* 1249

◆ **Prometrium®** *see* Progesterone *on page* 1247

◆ **PRO-Mirtazapine (Can)** *see* Mirtazapine *on page* 1002

◆ **Promit® [DSC]** *see* Dextran 1 *on page* 431

◆ **Pro-Naproxen EC (Can)** *see* Naproxen *on page* 1041

◆ **Pronestyl®-SR (Can)** *see* Procainamide *on page* 1240

◆ **Pronto® Complete Lice Removal System [OTC]** *see* Pyrethrins and Piperonyl Butoxide *on page* 1271

◆ **Pronto® Lice Control (Can)** *see* Pyrethrins and Piperonyl Butoxide *on page* 1271

◆ **Pronto® Plus Hair and Scalp Masque [OTC] [DSC]** *see* Pyrethrins and Piperonyl Butoxide *on page* 1271

◆ **Pronto® Plus Lice Killing Mousse Plus Vitamin E [OTC]** *see* Pyrethrins and Piperonyl Butoxide *on page* 1271

◆ **Pronto® Plus Lice Killing Mousse Shampoo Plus Natural Extracts and Oils [OTC]** *see* Pyrethrins and Piperonyl Butoxide *on page* 1271

◆ **Pronto® Plus Warm Oil Treatment and Conditioner [OTC]** *see* Pyrethrins and Piperonyl Butoxide *on page* 1271

◆ **Propaderm® (Can)** *see* Beclomethasone *on page* 176

Propafenone (pro PAF en one)

U.S. Brand Names Rythmol®; Rythmol® SR

Canadian Brand Names Apo-Propafenone®; PMS-Propafenone; Rythmol® Gen-Propafenone

Index Terms Propafenone Hydrochloride

Pharmacologic Category Antiarrhythmic Agent, Class Ic

Use Treatment of life-threatening ventricular arrhythmias

Rythmol® SR: Maintenance of normal sinus rhythm in patients with symptomatic atrial fibrillation

Unlabeled/Investigational Use Supraventricular tachycardias, including those patients with Wolff-Parkinson-White syndrome

Pregnancy Risk Factor C

Pregnancy Considerations There are no adequate and well-controlled studies in pregnant women; use only if potential benefit to the mother justifies potential risk to the fetus.

Lactation Enters breast milk/use caution

Contraindications Hypersensitivity to propafenone or any component of the formulation; sinoatrial, AV, and intraventricular disorders of impulse generation and/or conduction (except in patients with a functioning artificial pacemaker); sinus bradycardia; cardiogenic shock; uncompensated cardiac failure; hypotension; bronchospastic disorders; uncorrected electrolyte abnormalities; concurrent use of ritonavir (see Drug Interactions)

Warnings/Precautions Monitor for proarrhythmic events. May prolong QT_c interval; use caution with other QT_c-prolonging drugs. **[U.S. Boxed Warning]: In the Cardiac Arrhythmia Suppression Trial (CAST), recent (>6 days but <2 years ago) myocardial infarction patients with asymptomatic, non-life-threatening ventricular arrhythmias did not benefit and may have been harmed by attempts to suppress the arrhythmia with flecainide or encainide. An increased mortality or nonfatal cardiac arrest rate (7.7%) was seen in the active treatment group compared with patients in the placebo group (3%). The applicability of the CAST results to other populations is unknown. Antiarrhythmic agents should be reserved for patients with life-threatening ventricular arrhythmias.** Can cause or unmask a variety of conduction disturbances. May alter pacing and sensing thresholds of artificial pacemakers. Patients with bronchospastic disease should generally not receive this drug. Monitor for worsening HF if patient has underlying condition. Correct electrolyte disturbances, especially hypokalemia or hypomagnesemia, prior to use and throughout therapy. Administer cautiously in significant hepatic dysfunction. Use with caution in patients with myasthenia gravis; may exacerbate condition. Safety and efficacy have not been established in children.

Adverse Reactions

1% to 10%:

Cardiovascular: New or worsened arrhythmia (proarrhythmic effect) (2% to 10%), angina (2% to 5%), CHF (1% to 4%), ventricular tachycardia (1% to 3%), palpitation (1% to 3%), AV block (first-degree) (1% to 3%), syncope (1% to 2%), increased QRS interval (1% to 2%), chest pain (1% to 2%), PVCs (1% to 2%), bradycardia (1% to 2%), edema (0% to 1%), bundle branch block (0% to 1%), atrial fibrillation (1%), hypotension (0% to 1%), intraventricular conduction delay (0% to 1%)

Central nervous system: Dizziness (4% to 15%), fatigue (2% to 6%), headache (2% to 5%), ataxia (0% to 2%), insomnia (0% to 2%), anxiety (1% to 2%), drowsiness (1%)

Dermatologic: Rash (1% to 3%)

Gastrointestinal: Nausea/vomiting (2% to 11%), unusual taste (3% to 23%), constipation (2% to 7%), dyspepsia (1% to 3%), diarrhea (1% to 3%), xerostomia (1% to 2%), anorexia (1% to 2%), abdominal pain (1% to 2%), flatulence (0% to 1%)

Neuromuscular & skeletal: Tremor (0% to 1%), arthralgia (0% to 1%), weakness (1% to 2%)

Ocular: Blurred vision (1% to 6%)

Respiratory: Dyspnea (2% to 5%)

Miscellaneous: Diaphoresis (1%)

<1% (Limited to important or life-threatening): Agranulocytosis, alopecia, amnesia, anemia, apnea, AV block (second or third degree), AV dissociation, cardiac arrest, cholestasis (0.1%), coma, confusion, CHF, depression, granulocytopenia, hepatitis (0.03%), hyperglycemia, impotence, increased bleeding time, leukopenia, lupus erythematosus, mania, memory loss, nephrotic syndrome, paresthesia, peripheral neuropathy, pruritus, psychosis, purpura, renal failure, seizure (0.3%), SIADH, sinus node dysfunction, thrombocytopenia, tinnitus, vertigo

Drug Interactions

Metabolism/Transport Effects Substrate of CYP1A2 (minor), 2D6 (major), 3A4 (minor); **Inhibits** CYP1A2 (weak), 2D6 (weak)

Avoid Concomitant Use

Avoid concomitant use of Propafenone with any of the following: Nilotinib; Ritonavir; Tetrabenazine; Thioridazine; Tipranavir; Ziprasidone

Increased Effect/Toxicity

Propafenone may increase the levels/effects of: Beta-Blockers; Cardiac Glycosides; QTc-Prolonging Agents; Tetrabenazine; Thioridazine; Vitamin K Antagonists; Ziprasidone

The levels/effects of Propafenone may be increased by: Alfuzosin; Cimetidine; Ciprofloxacin; CYP2D6 Inhibitors (Moderate); CYP2D6 Inhibitors (Strong); Darunavir; Gadobutrol; Nilotinib; Ritonavir; Selective Serotonin Reuptake Inhibitors; Tipranavir

Decreased Effect

The levels/effects of Propafenone may be decreased by: Barbiturates; Rifamycin Derivatives

Ethanol/Nutrition/Herb Interactions

Food: Propafenone serum concentrations may be increased if taken with food.

Herb/Nutraceutical: St John's wort may decrease propafenone levels. Avoid ephedra (may worsen arrhythmia).

Stability Store at 25°C (77°F); excursions permitted to 15°C to 30°C (59°F to 86°F).

Mechanism of Action Propafenone is a class 1c antiarrhythmic agent which possesses local anesthetic properties, blocks the fast inward sodium current, and slows the rate of increase of the action potential. Prolongs conduction and refractoriness in all areas of the myocardium, with a slightly more pronounced effect on intraventricular conduction; it prolongs effective refractory period, reduces spontaneous automaticity and exhibits some beta-blockade activity.

Pharmacodynamics/Kinetics

Absorption: Well absorbed

Metabolism: Hepatic; two genetically determined metabolism groups exist: fast or slow metabolizers; 10% of Caucasians are slow metabolizers; exhibits nonlinear pharmacokinetics; when dose is increased from 300-900 mg/day, serum concentrations increase tenfold; this nonlinearity is thought to be due to saturable first-pass effect

Bioavailability: 150 mg: 3.4%; 300 mg: 10.6%

Half-life elimination: Single dose (100-300 mg): 2-8 hours; Chronic dosing: 10-32 hours

Time to peak: 150 mg dose: 2 hours, 300 mg dose: 3 hours

Dosage Oral: Adults: **Note:** Patients who exhibit significant widening of QRS complex or second- or third-degree AV block may need dose reduction.

Ventricular arrhythmias:

Immediate release tablet: Initial: 150 mg every 8 hours, increase at 3- to 4-day intervals up to 300 mg every 8 hours.

Extended release capsule: Initial: 225 mg every 12 hours; dosage increase may be made at a minimum of 5-day intervals; may increase to 325 mg every 12 hours; if further increase is necessary, may increase to 425 mg every 12 hours

Paroxysmal atrial fibrillation (unlabeled dose): Immediate release tablet: Outpatient: "Pill-in-the-pocket" dose: 450 mg (weight <70 kg); 600 mg (weight ≥70 kg). May not repeat in ≤24 hours. **Note:** An initial inpatient conversion trial should have been successful before sending patient home on this approach. Patient must be taking an AV nodal-blocking agent (eg, beta-blocker, nondihydropyridine calcium channel blocker) prior to initiation of antiarrhythmic.

Dosing adjustment in hepatic impairment: Reduction is necessary; however, specific guidelines are not available.

Dietary Considerations

Capsule: May be taken without regard to food. Rythmol® SR capsules contain soy lecithin.

Tablet: Should be taken at the same time in relation to meals each day, either always with meals or always between meals.

Administration Capsules should be swallowed whole; do not crush or chew.

Monitoring Parameters ECG, blood pressure, pulse (particularly at initiation of therapy)

Dosage Forms Excipient information presented when available (limited, particularly for generics); consult specific product labeling.

Capsule, extended release, as hydrochloride (Rythmol® SR): 225 mg, 325 mg, 425 mg [contains soy lecithin]

Tablet, as hydrochloride (Rythmol®): 150 mg, 225 mg, 300 mg

◆ **Propafenone Hydrochloride** *see* Propafenone *on page 1252*

Propantheline (proe PAN the leen)

Index Terms Propantheline Bromide

Pharmacologic Category Anticholinergic Agent

Use Adjunctive treatment of peptic ulcer, irritable bowel syndrome, pancreatitis, ureteral and urinary bladder spasm; reduce duodenal motility during diagnostic radiologic procedures

Pregnancy Risk Factor C

Dosage Oral:

Antisecretory:

Children: 1-2 mg/kg/day in 3-4 divided doses

Adults: 15 mg 3 times/day before meals or food and 30 mg at bedtime

Elderly: 7.5 mg 3 times/day before meals and at bedtime

Antispasmodic:

Children: 2-3 mg/kg/day in divided doses every 4-6 hours and at bedtime

Adults: 15 mg 3 times/day before meals or food and 30 mg at bedtime

Additional Information Complete prescribing information for this medication should be consulted for additional detail.

Dosage Forms Excipient information presented when available (limited, particularly for generics); consult specific product labeling.

Tablet, as bromide: 15 mg [contains lactose 23.2 mg]

◆ **Propantheline Bromide** *see* Propantheline *on page 1253*

Proparacaine (proe PAR a kane)

U.S. Brand Names Alcaine®; Ophthetic®; Parcaine™

Canadian Brand Names Alcaine®; Diocaine®

Index Terms Proparacaine Hydrochloride; Proxymetacaine

Pharmacologic Category Local Anesthetic, Ophthalmic

Use Anesthesia for tonometry, gonioscopy; suture removal from cornea; removal of corneal foreign body; cataract extraction, glaucoma surgery; short operative procedure involving the cornea and conjunctiva

Pregnancy Risk Factor C

Medication Safety Issues

Sound-alike/look-alike issues:

Proparacaine may be confused with propoxyphene

Dosage Children and Adults:

Ophthalmic surgery: Instill 1 drop of 0.5% solution in eye every 5-10 minutes for 5-7 doses

Tonometry, gonioscopy, suture removal: Instill 1-2 drops of 0.5% solution in eye just prior to procedure

Additional Information Complete prescribing information for this medication should be consulted for additional detail.

Dosage Forms Excipient information presented when available (limited, particularly for generics); consult specific product labeling.

Solution, ophthalmic, as hydrochloride: 0.5% (15 mL) [contains benzalkonium chloride]

Alcaine®: 0.5% (15 mL) [contains benzalkonium chloride]

Ophthetic®: 0.5% (15 mL) [contains benzalkonium chloride]

Parcaine™: 0.5% (15 mL) [contains benzalkonium chloride]

Proparacaine and Fluorescein

(proe PAR a kane & FLURE e seen)

U.S. Brand Names Flucaine®; Fluoracaine® [DSC]

Index Terms Fluorescein and Proparacaine

Pharmacologic Category Diagnostic Agent; Local Anesthetic

Use Anesthesia for tonometry, gonioscopy; suture removal from cornea; removal of corneal foreign body; cataract extraction, glaucoma surgery

Pregnancy Risk Factor C

Dosage

Ophthalmic surgery: Children and Adults: Instill 1 drop in each eye every 5-10 minutes for 5-7 doses

Tonometry, gonioscopy, suture removal: Adults: Instill 1-2 drops in each eye just prior to procedure

Additional Information Complete prescribing information for this medication should be consulted for additional detail.

Dosage Forms Excipient information presented when available (limited, particularly for generics); consult specific product labeling. [DSC] = Discontinued product

Solution, ophthalmic: Proparacaine hydrochloride 0.5% and fluorescein sodium 0.25% (5 mL)

Flucaine®, Fluoracaine® [DSC]: Proparacaine hydrochloride 0.5% and fluorescein sodium 0.25% (5 mL)

◆ **Proparacaine Hydrochloride** *see* Proparacaine *on page 1253*

◆ **Propecia®** *see* Finasteride *on page 622*

◆ **Propine®** *see* Dipivefrin *on page 466*

◆ **Proplex® T [DSC]** *see* Factor IX Complex (Human) *on page 601*

Propofol (PROE po fole)

U.S. Brand Names Diprivan®

Canadian Brand Names Diprivan®

Pharmacologic Category General Anesthetic

Additional Appendix Information

Status Epilepticus *on page 1831*

Use Induction of anesthesia for inpatient or outpatient surgery in patients ≥3 years of age; maintenance of anesthesia for inpatient or outpatient surgery in patients >2 months of age; in adults, for induction and maintenance of monitored anesthesia care sedation during procedures; sedation in intubated, mechanically-ventilated ICU patients

Unlabeled/Investigational Use Postoperative antiemetic; refractory delirium tremens (case reports); moderate sedation (conscious sedation)

Pregnancy Risk Factor B

Pregnancy Considerations Propofol should only be used in pregnancy if clearly needed. Propofol is not recommended for obstetrics, including cesarean section deliveries. Propofol crosses the placenta and may be associated with neonatal CNS and respiratory depression.

Lactation Enters breast milk/not recommended

Medication Safety Issues

Sound-alike/look-alike issues:

Diprivan® may be confused with Diflucan®, Ditropan®

Propofol may be confused with fospropofol

High alert medication: The Institute for Safe Medication Practices (ISMP) includes this medication among its list of drugs which have a heightened risk of causing significant patient harm when used in error.

Contraindications Hypersensitivity to propofol or any component of the formulation; hypersensitivity to eggs, egg products, soybeans, or soy products

Warnings/Precautions May rarely cause hypersensitivity, anaphylaxis, anaphylactoid reactions, angioedema, bronchospasm, and erythema; medications for the treatment of hypersensitivity reactions should be available for immediate use. The major cardiovascular effect of propofol is hypotension especially if patient is hypovolemic or if bolus dosing is used; use with caution in patients who are hemodynamically unstable, hypovolemic, or have abnormally low vascular tone (eg, sepsis). Use requires careful patient monitoring, should only be used by experienced personnel who are not actively engaged in the procedure or surgery. If used in a nonintubated and/or nonmechanically-ventilated patient, qualified personnel and appropriate equipment for rapid institution of respiratory and/or cardiovascular support must be immediately available. Use to induce moderate (conscious) sedation in patients warrants monitoring equivalent to that seen with deep anesthesia.

Use a lower induction dose, a slower maintenance rate of administration, and avoid rapidly administered boluses in the elderly, debilitated, or ASA-PS (American Society of Anesthesiologists - Physical Status) 3/4 patients to reduce the incidence of unwanted cardiorespiratory depressive events. Use caution in patients with severe cardiac disease (ejection fraction <50%) or respiratory disease; may have more profound adverse cardiovascular responses to propofol. Use caution in patients with a history of epilepsy or seizures; seizure may occur during recovery phase. Use caution in patients with increased intracranial pressure or impaired cerebral circulation; substantial decreases in mean arterial pressure and subsequent decreases in cerebral perfusion pressure may occur; consider continuous infusion or administer as a slow bolus.

Propofol-related infusion syndrome is a serious side effect with a high mortality rate characterized by dysrhythmia (eg, bradycardia or tachycardia), heart failure, hyperkalemia, lipemia, metabolic acidosis, and/or rhabdomyolysis or myoglobinuria with subsequent renal failure. Risk factors include poor oxygen delivery, sepsis, serious cerebral injury, and the administration of high doses of propofol (usually doses >83 mcg/kg/minute or >5 mg/kg/hour for >48 hours), but has also been reported following large dose, short term infusions during surgical anesthesia. The onset of the syndrome is rapid, occurring within 4 days of initiation. Alternate sedative therapy should be considered for patients with escalating doses of vasopressors or inotropes, when cardiac failure occurs during high-dose propofol infusion, when metabolic acidosis is observed, or in whom lengthy and/or high-dose sedation is needed.

Because propofol is formulated within a 10% fat emulsion, hypertriglyceridemia is an expected side effect. Patients who develop hypertriglyceridemia (eg, >500 mg/dL) are at risk of developing pancreatitis. An alternative sedative agent should be employed if significant hypertriglyceridemia occurs. Use with caution in patients with preexisting pancreatitis; use of propofol may exacerbate this condition. Use caution in patients with preexisting hyperlipidemia as evidenced by increased serum triglyceride levels or serum turbidity. Transient local pain may occur during I.V. injection; perioperative myoclonia has occurred. Propofol should only be used in pregnancy if clearly needed. Not recommended for use in obstetrics, including cesarean section deliveries. Safety and efficacy in pediatric intensive care unit patients have not been established. Concurrent use of fentanyl and propofol in pediatric patients may result in bradycardia.

Concomitant use may lead to increased sedative or anesthetic effects of propofol, more pronounced decreases in systolic, diastolic, and mean arterial pressures and cardiac output. Lower doses of propofol may be needed. In addition, fentanyl may cause serious bradycardia when used with propofol in pediatric patients. Alfentanil use with propofol has precipitated seizure activity in patients without any history of epilepsy. Discontinue opioids and paralytic agents prior to weaning. Avoid abrupt discontinuation prior to weaning or daily wake up assessments. Abrupt discontinuation can result in rapid awakening, anxiety, agitation, and resistance to mechanical ventilation; wean the infusion rate so the patient awakens slowly. Propofol lacks analgesic properties; pain management requires specific use of analgesic agents, at effective dosages, propofol must be titrated separately from the analgesic agent.

Propofol vials and prefilled syringes have the potential to support the growth of various microorganisms despite product additives intended to suppress microbial growth. To limit the potential for contamination, recommendations in product labeling for handling and administering propofol should be strictly adhered to. Some formulations may contain edetate disodium which may lead to decreased zinc levels in patients with prolonged therapy (>5 days) or a predisposition to zinc deficiency (eg, burns, diarrhea, or sepsis). A holiday from propofol infusion should take place after 5 days of therapy to allow for evaluation and necessary replacement of zinc. Some formulations may contain sulfites. Some products may contain benzyl alcohol; benzyl alcohol has been associated with the "gasping syndrome" in neonates and low-birth-weight infants.

Adverse Reactions

>10%:

Cardiovascular: Hypotension (children 17%; adults 3% to 26%)

Central nervous system: Movement (children 17%; adults 3% to 10%)

Local: Injection site burning, stinging, or pain (children 10%; adults 18%)

Respiratory: Apnea lasting 30-60 seconds (children 10%; adults 24%), apnea lasting >60 seconds (children 5%; adults 12%)

1% to 10%:

Cardiovascular: Hypertension (children 8%), arrhythmia (1% to 3%), bradycardia (1% to 3%), cardiac output decreased (1% to 3%; concurrent opioid use increases incidence), tachycardia (1% to 3%)

Dermatologic: Pruritus (1% to 3%), rash (children 5%; adults 1% to 3%)

Endocrine & metabolic: Hypertriglyceridemia (3% to 10%)

Respiratory: Respiratory acidosis during weaning (3% to 10%)

<1% (Limited to important or life-threatening): Agitation, amblyopia, anaphylaxis, anaphylactoid reaction, anticholinergic syndrome, asystole, atrial arrhythmia, bigeminy, cardiac arrest, chills, cough, dizziness, delirium, discoloration (green [urine, hair, or nailbeds]), extremity pain, fever, flushing, hemorrhage, hypersalivation, hypertonia, hypomagnesemia, hypoxia, infusion site reactions (including pain, swelling, blisters and/or tissue necrosis following accidental extravasation); laryngospasm, leukocytosis, lung function decreased, myalgia, myoclonia (rarely including convulsions and opisthotonos), nausea, pancreatitis, paresthesia, phlebitis, postoperative unconsciousness with or without increase in muscle tone, premature atrial contractions, premature ventricular contractions, pulmonary edema, propofol-related infusion syndrome (see Note), rhabdomyolysis, somnolence, syncope, thrombosis, urine cloudy, vision abnormality, wheezing

Note: Propofol-related infusion syndrome (PRIS) is a serious side effect with a high mortality rate characterized by dysrhythmia (eg, bradycardia or tachycardia), heart failure, hyperkalemia, lipemia, metabolic acidosis, and/or rhabdomyolysis or myoglobinuria with subsequent renal failure.

Drug Interactions

Metabolism/Transport Effects **Substrate** of CYP1A2 (minor), 2A6 (minor), 2B6 (major), 2C9 (major), 2C19 (minor), 2D6 (minor), 2E1 (minor), 3A4 (minor); **Inhibits** CYP1A2 (moderate), 2C9 (weak), 2C19 (moderate), 2D6 (weak), 2E1 (weak), 3A4 (strong)

Avoid Concomitant Use There are no known interactions where it is recommended to avoid concomitant use.

Increased Effect/Toxicity

Propofol may increase the levels/effects of: Ropivacaine

The levels/effects of Propofol may be increased by: Alfentanil; CYP2B6 Inhibitors (Moderate); CYP2B6 Inhibitors (Strong)

Decreased Effect There are no known significant interactions involving a decrease in effect.

Ethanol/Nutrition/Herb Interactions Food: Edetate disodium, an ingredient of propofol emulsion, may lead to decreased zinc levels in patients on prolonged therapy (>5 days) or those predisposed to deficiency (burns, diarrhea, and/or major sepsis).

Stability Store between 4°C to 22°C (40°F to 72°F); refrigeration is not required. Do not freeze. Protect from light. If transferred to a syringe or other container prior to administration, use within 6 hours. If used directly from vial/ prefilled syringe, use within 12 hours. Shake well before use. Do not use if there is evidence of separation of phases of emulsion.

Does not need to be diluted; however, propofol may be further diluted in 5% dextrose in water to a concentration of ≥2 mg/mL and is stable for 8 hours at room temperature.

Mechanism of Action Propofol is a sterically hindered, alkyl-phenolic compound with intravenous general anesthetic properties. The drug is unrelated to any of the currently used barbiturate, opioid, benzodiazepine, arylcyclohexylamine, or imidazole intravenous anesthetic agents.

Pharmacodynamics/Kinetics

Onset of action: Anesthetic: Bolus infusion (dose dependent): 9-51 seconds (average 30 seconds)

Duration (dose and rate dependent): 3-10 minutes

Distribution: V_d: 2-10 L/kg; after a 10-day infusion, V_d approaches 60 L/kg; decreased in the elderly

Protein binding: 97% to 99%

Metabolism: Hepatic to water-soluble sulfate and glucuronide conjugates (~50%)

Half-life elimination: Biphasic: Initial: 40 minutes; Terminal: 4-7 hours (after 10-day infusion, may be up to 1-3 days)

Excretion: Urine (~88% as metabolites, 40% as glucuronide metabolite); feces (<2%)

Dosage Dosage must be individualized based on total body weight and titrated to the desired clinical effect; wait at least 3-5 minutes between dosage adjustments to clinically assess drug effects; smaller doses are required when used with narcotics; the following are general dosing guidelines:

General anesthesia:

Induction: I.V.:

Children (healthy) 3-16 years, ASA-PS 1 or 2: 2.5-3.5 mg/kg over 20-30 seconds; use a lower dose for children ASA-PS 3 or 4

Adults (healthy), ASA-PS 1 or 2, <55 years: 2-2.5 mg/kg (~40 mg every 10 seconds until onset of induction)

Elderly, debilitated, or ASA-PS 3 or 4: 1-1.5 mg/kg (~20 mg every 10 seconds until onset of induction); **do not use rapid bolus dose (single or repeated)**

Cardiac anesthesia: 0.5-1.5 mg/kg (~20 mg every 10 seconds until onset of induction)

Neurosurgical patients: 1-2 mg/kg (~20 mg every 10 seconds until onset of induction)

Maintenance: I.V. infusion:

Children (healthy) 2 months to 16 years, ASA-PS 1 or 2: Initial: 200-300 mcg/kg/minute; after 30 minutes, if clinical signs of light anesthesia are absent, decrease the infusion rate; usual infusion rate: 125-150 mcg/kg/minute (range: 125-300 mcg/kg/minute); children ≤5 years may require larger infusion rates compared to older children

Adults (healthy), ASA-PS 1 or 2, <55 years: Initial: 100-200 mcg/kg/minute for 10-15 minutes; decrease by 30% to 50% during first 30 minutes of maintenance; usual infusion rate: 50-100 mcg/kg/minute to optimize recovery time

Elderly, debilitated, ASA-PS 3 or 4: 50-100 mcg/kg/minute

Cardiac anesthesia:

Low-dose propofol with primary opioid: 50-100 mcg/kg/minute (see manufacturer's labeling)

Primary propofol with secondary opioid: 100-150 mcg/kg/minute

Neurosurgical patients: 100-200 mcg/kg/minute

Maintenance: I.V. intermittent bolus: Adults (healthy), ASA-PS 1 or 2, <55 years: 25-50 mg increments as needed

Monitored anesthesia care sedation:

Initiation:

Adults (healthy), ASA-PS 1 or 2, <55 years: Slow I.V. infusion: 100-150 mcg/kg/minute for 3-5 minutes **or** slow injection: 0.5 mg/kg over 3-5 minutes

Elderly, debilitated, neurosurgical, or ASA-PS 3 or 4 patients: Use 80% of healthy adult dose; **do not use rapid bolus doses (single or repeated)**

Maintenance:

Adults (healthy), ASA-PS 1 or 2, <55 years: I.V. infusion using variable rates (preferred over intermittent boluses): 25-75 mcg/kg/minute **or** incremental bolus doses: 10 mg or 20 mg

Elderly, debilitated, neurosurgical, or ASA-PS 3 or 4 patients: Use 80% of healthy adult dose; **do not use rapid bolus doses (single or repeated)**

ICU sedation in intubated mechanically-ventilated patients: Avoid rapid bolus injection; individualize dose and titrate to response. Continuous infusion: Initial: 5 mcg/kg/minute; increase by 5-10 mcg/kg/minute every 5-10 minutes until desired sedation level is achieved; usual maintenance (Jacobi, 2002): 5-80 mcg/kg/minute; use 80% of healthy adult dose in elderly, debilitated, and ASA-PS 3 or 4 patients; reduce dose after adequate sedation established and adjust to response (eg, evaluate frequently to use minimum dose for sedation). Daily interruption with retitration is recommended to minimize prolonged sedative effects (Jacobi, 2002).

Refractory status epilepticus (unlabeled use): Adults: 1-2 mg/kg bolus, then 1.5-10 mg/kg/hour (intubation required)

Dietary Considerations Propofol is formulated in an oil-in-water emulsion. If on parenteral nutrition, may need to adjust the amount of lipid infused. Propofol emulsion contains 1.1 kcal/mL. Soybean fat emulsion is used as a vehicle for propofol. Formulations also contain egg phosphatide and glycerol.

Administration Strict aseptic technique must be maintained in handling although a preservative has been added. Do not use if contamination is suspected. Do not administer through the same I.V. catheter with blood or plasma. Tubing and any unused portions of propofol vials should be discarded after 12 hours.

To reduce pain associated with injection, use larger veins of forearm or antecubital fossa; lidocaine I.V. (1 mL of a 1% solution) may also be used prior to administration or it may be added to propofol immediately before administration in a quantity not to exceed 20 mg lidocaine per 200 mg propofol. Do not use filter <5 micron for administration.

Monitoring Parameters Cardiac monitor, blood pressure, oxygen saturation (during monitored anesthesia care sedation), arterial blood gas (with prolonged infusions). With prolonged infusions (eg, ICU sedation), monitor for metabolic acidosis, hyperkalemia, rhabdomyolysis or elevated CPK, hepatomegaly, and progression of cardiac and renal failure.

ICU sedation: Assess and adjust sedation according to scoring system; assess CNS function daily. Serum triglyceride levels should be obtained prior to initiation of therapy and every 3-7 days thereafter, especially if receiving for >48 hours with doses exceeding 50 mcg/kg/minute (Devlin, 2005); use intravenous port opposite propofol infusion or temporarily suspend infusion and flush port prior to blood draw.

Diprivan®: Monitor zinc levels in patients predisposed to deficiency (burns, diarrhea, major sepsis) or after 5 days of treatment.

Dosage Forms Excipient information presented when available (limited, particularly for generics); consult specific product labeling.

Injection, emulsion: 10 mg/mL (20 mL, 50 mL, 100 mL) [products may contain egg lecithin, and soybean oil; may contain benzyl alcohol, sodium benzoate, or sodium metabisulfite]

Diprivan®: 10 mg/mL (20 mL, 50 mL, 100 mL) [contains egg lecithin, soybean oil, and disodium edetate]

Propoxyphene (proe POKS i feen)

U.S. Brand Names Darvon-N®; Darvon®

Canadian Brand Names 642® Tablet; Darvon-N®

Index Terms Dextropropoxyphene; Propoxyphene Hydrochloride; Propoxyphene Napsylate

Pharmacologic Category Analgesic, Opioid

Additional Appendix Information

Narcotic / Opioid Analgesics *on page 1663*

Use Management of mild to moderate pain

Restrictions C-IV

Pregnancy Risk Factor C/D (prolonged use)

Pregnancy Considerations Withdrawal symptoms have been reported in the neonate following propoxyphene use during pregnancy. Teratogenic effects have also been noted in case reports. Opioid analgesics are considered pregnancy risk factor D if used for prolonged periods or in large doses near term.

Lactation Enters breast milk/use caution (AAP rates "compatible")

Medication Safety Issues

Sound-alike/look-alike issues:

Propoxyphene may be confused with proparacaine

Darvon® may be confused with Devrom®, Diovan®

Darvon-N® may be confused with Darvocet-N®

High alert medication: The Institute for Safe Medication Practices (ISMP) includes this medication among its list of drug classes which have a heightened risk of causing significant patient harm when used in error.

Contraindications Hypersensitivity to propoxyphene or any component of the formulation

Warnings/Precautions **[U.S. Boxed Warning]: When given in excessive doses, either alone or in combination with other CNS depressants (including alcohol), propoxyphene is a major cause of drug-related deaths; recommended dosage must not be exceeded and alcohol intake should be limited.** Avoid use in severely depressed or suicidal patients. Should not be prescribed in patients who are addiction prone or suicidal. Use caution in patients taking CNS depressant medications or antidepressants, and in patients who use alcohol in excess. Use with caution in patients with CNS depression coma, head trauma, thyroid dysfunction, adrenal insufficiency, morbid obesity, and prostatic hyperplasia/urinary stricture. Use with caution in patients with biliary tract dysfunction; acute pancreatitis may cause constriction of sphincter of Oddi. May cause hypotension; use with caution in patients with hypovolemia, cardiovascular disease (including acute MI), or drugs which may exaggerate hypotensive effects (including phenothiazines or general anesthetics). May obscure diagnosis or clinical course of patients with acute abdominal conditions.

May cause CNS depression, which may impair physical or mental abilities; patients must be cautioned about performing tasks which require mental alertness (eg, operating machinery or driving). Effects may be potentiated when used with other sedative drugs or ethanol. Use caution in patients dependent on opiates, substitution may result in acute opiate withdrawal symptoms. Tolerance or drug dependence may result from extended use. Propoxyphene should be used with caution in patients with renal or hepatic dysfunction, debilitated patients or in the elderly; consider dosing adjustment.

An opioid-containing analgesic regimen should be tailored to each patient's needs and based upon the type of pain being treated (acute versus chronic), the route of administration, degree of tolerance for opioids (naive versus chronic user), age, weight, and medical condition. The optimal analgesic dose varies widely among patients; doses should be titrated to pain relief/prevention. Safety and efficacy have not been established in children.

Adverse Reactions Frequency not defined.

Cardiovascular: Bundle branch block, hypotension

Central nervous system: Confusion, dizziness, dysphoria, drowsiness, fatigue, hallucinations, headache, increased intracranial pressure, lightheadedness, malaise, mental depression, nervousness, paradoxical CNS stimulation, paradoxical excitement and insomnia, restlessness, sedation, vertigo

Dermatologic: Rash, urticaria

Endocrine & metabolic: Decreased urinary 17-OHCS, hypoglycemia

Gastrointestinal: Abdominal pain, anorexia, biliary spasm, constipation, nausea, paralytic ileus, stomach cramps, vomiting, xerostomia

Genitourinary: Decreased urination, ureteral spasms

Hepatic: LFTs increased, jaundice

Neuromuscular & skeletal: Weakness

Ocular: Visual disturbances

Respiratory: Dyspnea

Miscellaneous: Histamine release, hypersensitivity reaction psychologic and physical dependence with prolonged use

Drug Interactions

Metabolism/Transport Effects **Inhibits** CYP2C9 (weak), 2D6 (weak), 3A4 (weak)

Avoid Concomitant Use

Avoid concomitant use of Propoxyphene with any of the following: MAO Inhibitors

Increased Effect/Toxicity

Propoxyphene may increase the levels/effects of: Alcohol (Ethyl); Alvimopan; Beta-Blockers; CarBAMazepine; CNS Depressants; Desmopressin; MAO Inhibitors; Selective Serotonin Reuptake Inhibitors; Tricyclic Antidepressants; Vitamin K Antagonists

The levels/effects of Propoxyphene may be increased by: Amphetamines; Antipsychotic Agents (Phenothiazines); Succinylcholine

Decreased Effect

Propoxyphene may decrease the levels/effects of: Pegvisomant

The levels/effects of Propoxyphene may be decreased by: Ammonium Chloride

Ethanol/Nutrition/Herb Interactions

Ethanol: Avoid or limit ethanol (may increase CNS depression). Watch for sedation.

Food: May decrease rate of absorption, but may slightly increase bioavailability.

Stability Store at controlled room temperature of 15°C to 30°C (59°F to 86°F).

Mechanism of Action Propoxyphene is a weak narcotic analgesic which acts through binding to opiate receptors to inhibit ascending pain pathways. Propoxyphene, as with other narcotic (opiate) analgesics, blocks pain perception in the cerebral cortex by binding to specific receptor molecules (opiate receptors) within the neuronal membranes of synapses. This binding results in a decreased synaptic chemical transmission throughout the CNS thus inhibiting the flow of pain sensations into the higher centers. Mu and kappa are the two subtypes of the opiate receptor which propoxyphene binds to cause analgesia.

Pharmacodynamics/Kinetics

Onset of action: 0.5-1 hour

Duration: 4-6 hours

Metabolism: Hepatic to active metabolite (norpropoxyphene) and inactive metabolites; first-pass effect

Half-life elimination: Adults: Parent drug: 6-12 hours; Norpropoxyphene: 30-36 hours

Excretion: Urine (primarily as metabolites)

Dosage Oral:

Children: Doses for children are not well established; doses of the hydrochloride of 2-3 mg/kg/d divided every 6 hours have been used

Adults:

Hydrochloride: 65 mg every 3-4 hours as needed for pain; maximum: 390 mg/day

Napsylate: 100 mg every 4 hours as needed for pain; maximum: 600 mg/day

Elderly:

Hydrochloride: 65 mg every 4-6 hours as needed for pain

Napsylate: 100 mg every 4-6 hours as needed for pain

Dosing adjustment in renal impairment: Serum concentrations of propoxyphene may be increased or elimination may be delayed. Avoid use in Cl_{cr} <10 mL/minute. Specific dosing recommendations not available for less severe impairment.

Not dialyzable (0% to 5%)

Dosing adjustment in hepatic impairment: Serum concentrations of propoxyphene may be increased or elimination may be delayed; specific dosing recommendations not available.

Dietary Considerations May administer with food if gastrointestinal distress occurs.

Administration Should be administered with glass of water on an empty stomach. Food may decrease rate of absorption, but may slightly increase bioavailability.

Monitoring Parameters Pain relief, respiratory and mental status, blood pressure

Reference Range

Therapeutic: Ranges published vary between laboratories and may not correlate with clinical effect

Therapeutic concentration: 0.1-0.4 mcg/mL (SI: 0.3-1.2 µmol/L)

Toxic: >0.5 mcg/mL (SI: >1.5 µmol/L)

Test Interactions False-positive methadone test

Additional Information 100 mg of napsylate = 65 mg of hydrochloride

Propoxyphene hydrochloride: Darvon®

Propoxyphene napsylate: Darvon-N®

Dosage Forms Excipient information presented when available (limited, particularly for generics); consult specific product labeling.

Capsule, as hydrochloride: 65 mg

Darvon®: 65 mg

Tablet, as napsylate:

Darvon-N®: 100 mg

Propoxyphene and Acetaminophen

(proe POKS i feen & a seet a MIN oh fen)

U.S. Brand Names Balacet 325™; Darvocet A500®; Darvocet-N® 100; Darvocet-N® 50

Canadian Brand Names Darvocet-N® 100; Darvocet-N® 50

Index Terms Acetaminophen and Propoxyphene; Propoxyphene Hydrochloride and Acetaminophen; Propoxyphene Napsylate and Acetaminophen

Pharmacologic Category Analgesic Combination (Opioid)

Use Management of mild to moderate pain

Restrictions C-IV

Pregnancy Risk Factor C

Medication Safety Issues

Sound-alike/look-alike issues:

Darvocet-N® may be confused with Darvon-N®

High alert medication: The Institute for Safe Medication Practices (ISMP) includes this medication among its list of drug classes which have a heightened risk of causing significant patient harm when used in error.

Duplicate therapy issues: This product contains acetaminophen, which may be a component of other combination products. Do not exceed the maximum recommended daily dose of acetaminophen.

Dosage Oral: Adults:

Darvocet A500®, Darvocet-N® 100: 1 tablet every 4 hours as needed; maximum: 600 mg propoxyphene napsylate/day

Darvocet-N® 50: 1-2 tablets every 4 hours as needed; maximum: 600 mg propoxyphene napsylate/day

Propoxyphene hydrochloride 65 mg and acetaminophen 650 mg: 1 tablet every 4 hours as needed; maximum: 390 mg/day propoxyphene hydrochloride, 4 g/day acetaminophen)

Note: Formulations contain significant amounts of acetaminophen; intake should be limited to <4 g acetaminophen/day (less in patients with hepatic impairment/ethanol abuse)

Elderly: Refer to adult dosing

Dosing adjustment in renal/hepatic impairment: Serum concentrations of propoxyphene may be increased or elimination may be delayed; specific dosing recommendations not available.

Additional Information Complete prescribing information for this medication should be consulted for additional detail.

Dosage Forms Excipient information presented when available (limited, particularly for generics); consult specific product labeling.

Tablet, 50/325:

Darvocet-N® 50: Propoxyphene napsylate 50 mg and acetaminophen 325 mg

Tablet, 65/650: Propoxyphene hydrochloride 65 mg and acetaminophen 650 mg

Tablet, 100/325:

Balacet 325™: Propoxyphene napsylate 100 mg and acetaminophen 325 mg

Tablet, 100/500: Propoxyphene hydrochloride 100 mg and acetaminophen 500 mg

Darvocet A500®: Propoxyphene napsylate 100 mg and acetaminophen 500 mg

Tablet, 100/650: Propoxyphene napsylate 100 mg and acetaminophen 650 mg

Darvocet-N® 100: Propoxyphene napsylate 100 mg and acetaminophen 650 mg

Propoxyphene, Aspirin, and Caffeine

(proe POKS i feen, AS pir in, & KAF een)

U.S. Brand Names Darvon® Compound [DSC]

Index Terms Aspirin, Caffeine, and Propoxyphene; Caffeine, Propoxyphene, and Aspirin; Propoxyphene Hydrochloride, Aspirin, and Caffeine

Pharmacologic Category Analgesic Combination (Opioid)

Use Treatment of mild-to-moderate pain

Restrictions C-IV

Pregnancy Risk Factor C

Medication Safety Issues

Sound-alike/look-alike issues:

Darvon® may be confused with Devrom®, Diovan®

High alert medication: The Institute for Safe Medication Practices (ISMP) includes this medication among its list of drug classes which have a heightened risk of causing significant patient harm when used in error.

Dosage Oral: Adults: Pain: One capsule (providing propoxyphene 65 mg) every 4 hours as needed; maximum propoxyphene 390 mg/day. This will also provide aspirin 389 mg and caffeine 32.4 mg per capsule.

Elderly: Refer to adult dosing; consider increasing dosing interval

Dosage adjustment in renal impairment: Serum concentrations of propoxyphene may be increased or elimination may be delayed; specific dosing recommendations not available. Avoid use with Cl_{cr} <10 mL/minute.

Dosage adjustment in hepatic impairment: Serum concentrations or propoxyphene may be increased or elimination may be delayed; specific dosing recommendations not available.

Additional Information Complete prescribing information for this medication should be consulted for additional detail.

Dosage Forms Excipient information presented when available (limited, particularly for generics); consult specific product labeling. [DSC] = Discontinued product

Capsule (Darvon® Compound 65): Propoxyphene hydrochloride 65 mg, aspirin 389 mg, and caffeine 32.4 mg [DSC]

◆ **Propoxyphene Hydrochloride** *see* Propoxyphene *on page 1256*

◆ **Propoxyphene Hydrochloride and Acetaminophen** *see* Propoxyphene and Acetaminophen *on page 1258*

◆ **Propoxyphene Hydrochloride, Aspirin, and Caffeine** *see* Propoxyphene, Aspirin, and Caffeine *on page 1258*

◆ **Propoxyphene Napsylate** *see* Propoxyphene *on page 1256*

◆ **Propoxyphene Napsylate and Acetaminophen** *see* Propoxyphene and Acetaminophen *on page 1258*

Propranolol (proe PRAN oh lole)

U.S. Brand Names Inderal® [DSC]; Inderal® LA; InnoPran XL™

Canadian Brand Names Apo-Propranolol®; Dom-Propranolol; Inderal®; Inderal®-LA; Novo-Pranol; Nu-Propranolol; PMS-Propranolol; Propranolol Hydrochloride Injection, USP

Index Terms Propranolol Hydrochloride

Pharmacologic Category Antiarrhythmic Agent, Class II; Beta-Adrenergic Blocker, Nonselective

Additional Appendix Information

Beta-Blockers *on page 1648*

Use Management of hypertension; angina pectoris; pheochromocytoma; essential tremor; supraventricular arrhythmias (such as atrial fibrillation and flutter, AV nodal re-entrant tachycardias), ventricular tachycardias (catecholamine-induced arrhythmias, digoxin toxicity); prevention of myocardial infarction; migraine headache prophylaxis; symptomatic treatment of hypertrophic subaortic stenosis (hypertrophic obstructive cardiomyopathy)

Unlabeled/Investigational Use Tremor due to Parkinson's disease; ethanol withdrawal; aggressive behavior (not recommended for dementia-associated aggression), anxiety, schizophrenia; antipsychotic-induced akathisia; primary and secondary prophylaxis of variceal hemorrhage; acute panic; thyrotoxicosis; tetralogy of Fallot (TOF) hypercyanotic spells

Pregnancy Risk Factor C (manufacturer); D (2nd and 3rd trimesters - expert analysis)

Pregnancy Considerations Embryotoxicity has been observed in some animal studies. Propranolol crosses the placenta. Beta-blockers have been associated with bradycardia, hypotension, and IUGR. IUGR is probably related to maternal hypertension. Available evidence suggests beta-blockers are generally safe during pregnancy (JNC 7). Neonatal hypoglycemia, respiratory depression and congenital abnormalities have been reported following maternal use of beta-blockers.

Lactation Enters breast milk/use caution (AAP rates "compatible")

Medication Safety Issues

Sound-alike/look-alike issues:

Propranolol may be confused with Pravachol®, Propulsid®

Inderal® may be confused with Adderall®, Enduron®, Enduronyl®, Imdur®, Imuran®, Inderide®, Isordil®, Toradol®

Inderal® 40 may be confused with Enduronyl® Forte

High alert medication: The Institute for Safe Medication Practices (ISMP) includes this medication among its list of drugs which have a heightened risk of causing significant patient harm when used in error.

Significant differences exist between oral and I.V. dosing. Use caution when converting from one route of administration to another.

International issues:

Inderal® may be confused with Indiaral® which is a brand name for loperamide in France

Contraindications Hypersensitivity to propranolol, beta-blockers, or any component of the formulation; uncompensated congestive heart failure (unless the failure is due to tachyarrhythmias being treated with propranolol), cardiogenic shock, severe sinus bradycardia or heart block (2nd or 3rd degree), severe hyperactive airway disease (asthma or COPD)

Warnings/Precautions Consider pre-existing conditions such as sick sinus syndrome before initiating. Administer cautiously in compensated heart failure and monitor for a worsening of the condition (efficacy of propranolol in HF has not been demonstrated). Beta-blocker therapy should not be withdrawn abruptly (particularly in patients with CAD), but gradually tapered to avoid acute tachycardia, hypertension, and/or ischemia. Use caution in patient with peripheral vascular disease (PVD). Use caution with concurrent use of beta-blockers and either verapamil or diltiazem; bradycardia or heart block can occur. Avoid concurrent I.V. use of both agents.

Use cautiously in patients with diabetes because it can mask prominent hypoglycemic symptoms. Use caution in hyperthyroidism since beta-blockade may mask signs of thyrotoxicosis. May alter thyroid-function tests. Use with caution in myasthenia gravis or psychiatric disease (may cause CNS depression). Use cautiously in renal and hepatic dysfunction; dosage adjustment required in hepatic impairment. Use care with anesthetic agents which decrease myocardial function. In general, patients with bronchospastic disease should not receive beta-blockers; if used at all, should be used cautiously with close monitoring. Adequate alpha-blockade is required prior to use of any beta-blocker for patients with untreated pheochromocytoma. Use caution with history of severe anaphylaxis to allergens; patients taking beta-blockers may become more sensitive to repeated challenges. Treatment of anaphylaxis (eg, epinephrine) in patients taking beta-blockers may be ineffective or promote undesirable effects. Safety and efficacy in children have not been established.

Adverse Reactions Frequency not defined.

Cardiovascular: Angina, arterial insufficiency, AV conduction disturbance increased, bradycardia, cardiogenic shock, CHF, hypotension, impaired myocardial contractility, mesenteric arterial thrombosis (rare), Raynaud's syndrome, syncope

Central nervous system: Amnesia, catatonia, cognitive dysfunction, confusion, depression, dizziness, emotional lability, fatigue, hallucinations, hypersomnolence, insomnia, lethargy, lightheadedness, psychosis, vertigo, vivid dreams

Dermatologic: Alopecia, contact dermatitis, cutaneous ulcers, eczematous eruptions, erythema multiforme, exfoliative dermatitis, hyperkeratosis, nail changes, oculomucocutaneous reactions, pruritus, psoriasiform eruptions, rash, Stevens-Johnson syndrome, toxic epidermal necrolysis, ulcers, ulcerative lichenoid, urticaria

Endocrine & metabolic: Hyper-/hypoglycemia, hyperkalemia, hyperlipidemia

Gastrointestinal: Anorexia, cramping, constipation, diarrhea, ischemic colitis, nausea, stomach discomfort, vomiting

Genitourinary: Impotence, interstitial nephritis (rare), oliguria (rare), Peyronie's disease, proteinuria (rare)

Hematologic: Agranulocytosis, nonthrombocytopenic purpura, thrombocytopenia, thrombocytopenic purpura

Hepatic: Alkaline phosphatase increased, transaminases increased

Neuromuscular & skeletal: Arthropathy, carpal tunnel syndrome (rare), myotonus, paresthesia, polyarthritis, weakness

Ocular: Hyperemia of the conjunctiva, mydriasis, visual acuity decreased, visual disturbances, xerophthalmia

Renal: BUN increased

Respiratory: Bronchospasm, dyspnea, laryngospasm, pharyngitis, pulmonary edema, respiratory distress, wheezing

Miscellaneous: Anaphylactic/anaphylactoid allergic reaction, cold extremities, lupus-like syndrome (rare)

Drug Interactions

Metabolism/Transport Effects Substrate of CYP1A2 (major), 2C19 (minor), 2D6 (major), 3A4 (minor); **Inhibits** CYP1A2 (weak), 2D6 (weak)

Avoid Concomitant Use

Avoid concomitant use of Propranolol with any of the following: Dabigatran Etexilate; Methacholine; Rivaroxaban; Topotecan

Increased Effect/Toxicity

Propranolol may increase the levels/effects of: Alpha-/Beta-Agonists (Direct-Acting); Alpha1-Blockers; Alpha2-Agonists; Amifostine; Antipsychotic Agents (Phenothiazines); Cardiac Glycosides; Dabigatran Etexilate; Insulin; Lidocaine; Methacholine; Midodrine; P-Glycoprotein Substrates; RiTUXimab; Rivaroxaban; Serotonin 5-HT1D Receptor Agonists; Topotecan

The levels/effects of Propranolol may be increased by: Acetylcholinesterase Inhibitors; Alcohol (Ethyl); Aminoquinolines (Antimalarial); Amiodarone; Anilidopiperidine Opioids; Antipsychotic Agents (Phenothiazines); Calcium Channel Blockers (Nondihydropyridine); CYP1A2 Inhibitors (Moderate); CYP1A2 Inhibitors (Strong); CYP2D6 Inhibitors (Moderate); CYP2D6 Inhibitors (Strong); Darunavir; Diazoxide; Dipyridamole; Disopyramide; Fluvoxamine; Herbs (Hypotensive Properties); Propafenone; Propoxyphene; Prostacyclin Analogues; QuiNIDine; Reserpine; Selective Serotonin Reuptake Inhibitors; Zileuton

Decreased Effect

Propranolol may decrease the levels/effects of: Beta2-Agonists; Theophylline Derivatives

The levels/effects of Propranolol may be decreased by: Alcohol (Ethyl); Barbiturates; CYP1A2 Inducers (Strong); Herbs (Hypertensive Properties); Methylphenidate; Nonsteroidal Anti-Inflammatory Agents; Rifamycin Derivatives; Yohimbine

Ethanol/Nutrition/Herb Interactions

Ethanol: Ethanol may increase or decrease plasma levels of propranolol. Reports are variable and have shown both enhanced as well as inhibited hepatic metabolism (of propranolol). Caution advised with consumption of alcohol and monitor for heart rate and/or blood pressure changes.

Food: Propranolol serum levels may be increased if taken with food. Protein-rich foods may increase bioavailability; a change in diet from high carbohydrate/low protein to low carbohydrate/high protein may result in increased oral clearance.

Cigarette: Smoking may decrease plasma levels of propranolol by increasing metabolism.

Herb/Nutraceutical: Avoid dong quai if using for hypertension (has estrogenic activity). Avoid bayberry, blue cohosh, cayenne, ephedra, ginger, ginseng (american), gotu kola, licorice, yohimbe (may worsen hypertension). Avoid black cohosh, california poppy, coleus, garlic, golden seal, hawthorn, mistletoe, periwinkle, quinine, shepherd's purse (have antihypertensive activity, may cause hypotension).

Stability

Injection: Store at 20°C to 25°C (68°F to 77°F); protect from freezing or excessive heat. Once diluted, propranolol is stable for 24 hours at room temperature in D_5W or NS. Protect from light. Solution has a maximum stability at pH of 3 and decomposes rapidly in alkaline pH.

Capsule, tablet: Store at 20°C to 25°C (68°F to 77°F); protect from freezing or excessive heat. Protect from light and moisture.

Mechanism of Action Nonselective beta-adrenergic blocker (class II antiarrhythmic); competitively blocks response to $beta_1$- and $beta_2$-adrenergic stimulation which results in decreases in heart rate, myocardial contractility, blood pressure, and myocardial oxygen demand. Nonselective beta-adrenergic blockers (propranolol, nadolol) reduce portal pressure by producing splanchnic vasoconstriction ($beta_2$ effect) thereby reducing portal blood flow.

Pharmacodynamics/Kinetics

Onset of action: Beta-blockade: Oral: 1-2 hours

Duration: Immediate release: 6-12 hours; Extended-release formulations: ~24-27 hours

Distribution: V_d: 4 L/kg in adults; crosses placenta; small amounts enter breast milk

Protein binding: Newborns: 68%; Adults: 90%

Metabolism: Hepatic to active and inactive compounds; extensive first-pass effect

Bioavailability: 30% to 40%

Half-life elimination: Neonates and Infants: Possible increased half-life; Children: 3.9-6.4 hours; Adults: Immediate release formulation: 3-6 hours; Extended-release formulations: 8-10 hours

Time to peak: Immediate release: 1-4 hours; Extended-release formulations: ~6-14 hours

Excretion: Urine (96% to 99%)

Dosage

Akathisia (unlabeled use): Oral: Adults: 30-120 mg/day in 2-3 divided doses

Essential tremor: Oral: Adults: 40 mg twice daily initially; maintenance doses: Usually 120-320 mg/day

Hypertension:

- Oral:
  - Children (unlabeled use): Initial: 0.5-1 mg/kg/day in divided doses every 6-12 hours; increase gradually every 5-7 days; maximum: 16 mg/kg/24 hours
  - Adults: Initial: 40 mg twice daily; increase dosage every 3-7 days; usual dose: 120-240 mg divided in 2-3 doses/day; maximum daily dose: 640 mg; usual dosage range (JNC 7): 40-160 mg/day in 2 divided doses
    - Extended release formulations:
      - Inderal® LA: Initial: 80 mg once daily; usual maintenance: 120-160 mg once daily; maximum daily dose: 640 mg; usual dosage range (JNC 7): 60-180 mg/day once daily
      - InnoPran XL™: Initial: 80 mg once daily at bedtime; if initial response is inadequate, may be increased at 2-3 week intervals to a maximum dose of 120 mg

Hypertrophic subaortic stenosis: Oral: Adults: 20-40 mg 3-4 times/day

- Inderal® LA: 80-160 mg once daily

Migraine headache prophylaxis: Oral:

- Children (unlabeled use): Initial: 2-4 mg/kg/day **or**
  - ≤35 kg: 10-20 mg 3 times/day
  - >35 kg: 20-40 mg 3 times/day
- Adults: Initial: 80 mg/day divided every 6-8 hours; increase by 20-40 mg/dose every 3-4 weeks to a maximum of 160-240 mg/day given in divided doses every 6-8 hours; if satisfactory response not achieved within 6 weeks of starting therapy, drug should be withdrawn gradually over several weeks
  - Inderal® LA: Initial: 80 mg once daily; effective dose range: 160-240 mg once daily

Post-MI mortality reduction: Oral: Adults: Initial: 40 mg 3 times/day; usual dosage range: 180-240 mg/day in 3-4 divided doses

Pheochromocytoma: Oral: Adults: 30-60 mg/day in divided doses

Stable angina: Oral: Adults: 80-320 mg/day in doses divided 2-4 times/day

- Inderal® LA: Initial: 80 mg once daily; maximum dose: 320 mg once daily

Tachyarrhythmias:

- Oral:
  - Children (unlabeled use): Initial: 0.5-1 mg/kg/day in divided doses every 6-8 hours; titrate dosage upward every 3-7 days; usual dose: 2-6 mg/kg/day; higher

doses may be needed; do not exceed 16 mg/kg/day or 60 mg/day

Adults: 10-30 mg/dose every 6-8 hours

Elderly: Initial: 10 mg twice daily; increase dosage every 3-7 days; usual dosage range: 10-320 mg given in 2 divided doses

I.V.:

Children (unlabeled use): 0.01-0.1 mg/kg/dose slow IVP over 10 minutes; maximum dose: 1 mg for infants; 3 mg for children

Adults: 1-3 mg/dose slow IVP; repeat every 2-5 minutes up to a total of 5 mg; titrate initial dose to desired response

or

0.1 mg/kg divided into 3 equal doses given at 2-3 minute intervals. May repeat total dose in 2 minutes if necessary (ACLS guidelines, 2005)

Note: Once response achieved or maximum dose administered, additional doses should not be given for at least 4 hours.

Elderly: Use caution; initiate at lower end of the dosing range.

Hypercyanotic spells (TOF) (unlabeled use): Children:

Oral: Palliation: Initial: 1 mg/kg/day every 6 hours; if ineffective, may increase dose after 1 week by 1 mg/kg/day to a maximum of 5 mg/kg/day; if patient becomes refractory, may increase slowly to a maximum of 10-15 mg/kg/day. Allow 24 hours between dosing changes.

I.V.: 0.01-0.2 mg/kg/dose infused over 10 minutes; maximum dose: 5 mg

Thyrotoxicosis (unlabeled use):

Oral:

Children: 2 mg/kg/day, divided every 6-8 hours, titrate to effective dose

Adolescents and Adults: Oral: 10-40 mg/dose every 6 hours

I.V.: Adults: 1-3 mg/dose slow IVP as a single dose

Variceal hemorrhage prophylaxis (unlabeled use; Garcia-Tsao, 2007): Oral: Adults:

Primary prophylaxis: Initial: 20 mg twice daily; adjust to maximal tolerated dose. **Note:** Risk factors for hemorrhage include Child-Pugh class B/C or variceal red wale markings on endoscopy.

Secondary prophylaxis: Initial: 20 mg twice daily; adjust to maximal tolerated dose

Dosing adjustment in renal impairment:

Not dialyzable (0% to 5%); supplemental dose is not necessary.

Peritoneal dialysis effects: Supplemental dose is not necessary.

Dosing adjustment in hepatic disease: Marked slowing of heart rate may occur in chronic liver disease with conventional doses; low initial dose and regular heart rate monitoring

Dietary Considerations Tablets (immediate release) should be taken on an empty stomach; capsules (extended release) may be taken with or without food, but should always be taken consistently (with food or on an empty stomach)

Administration I.V. dose is much smaller than oral dose. When administered acutely for cardiac treatment, monitor ECG and blood pressure. May administer by rapid infusion (I.V. push) at a rate of 1 mg/minute or by slow infusion over ~30 minutes. Necessary monitoring for surgical patients who are unable to take oral beta-blockers (prolonged ileus) has not been defined. Some institutions require monitoring of baseline and postinfusion heart rate and blood pressure when a patient's response to beta-blockade has not been characterized (ie, the patient's initial dose or following a change in dose). Consult individual institutional policies and procedures. Do not crush long-acting oral forms.

Monitoring Parameters Acute cardiac treatment: Monitor ECG, heart rate, and blood pressure with I.V. administration; heart rate and blood pressure with oral administration

Reference Range Therapeutic: 50-100 ng/mL (SI: 190-390 nmol/L) at end of dose interval

Dosage Forms Excipient information presented when available (limited, particularly for generics); consult specific product labeling. [DSC] = Discontinued product

Capsule, extended release, as hydrochloride: 60 mg, 80 mg, 120 mg, 160 mg

InnoPran XL™: 80 mg, 120 mg

Capsule, sustained release, as hydrochloride:

Inderal® LA: 60 mg, 80 mg, 120 mg, 160 mg

Injection, solution, as hydrochloride: 1 mg/mL (1 mL)

Inderal®: 1 mg/mL (1 mL) [DSC]

Solution, oral, as hydrochloride: 4 mg/mL (500 mL); 8 mg/mL (500 mL) [strawberry-mint flavor; contains alcohol 0.6%]

Tablet, as hydrochloride: 10 mg, 20 mg, 40 mg, 60 mg, 80 mg

Propranolol and Hydrochlorothiazide

(proe PRAN oh lole & hye droe klor oh THYE a zide)

U.S. Brand Names Inderide®

Index Terms Hydrochlorothiazide and Propranolol

Pharmacologic Category Beta Blocker, Nonselective; Diuretic, Thiazide

Use Management of hypertension

Pregnancy Risk Factor C

Medication Safety Issues

Sound-alike/look-alike issues:

Inderide® may be confused with Inderal®

Dosage Oral: Adults: Hypertension: Dose is individualized; typical dosages of **hydrochlorothiazide**: 12.5-50 mg/day; initial dose of **propranolol**: 80 mg/day

Daily dose of tablet form should be divided into 2 daily doses; may be used to maximum dosage of up to 160 mg of propranolol; higher dosages would result in higher than optimal thiazide dosages.

Additional Information Complete prescribing information for this medication should be consulted for additional detail.

Dosage Forms Excipient information presented when available (limited, particularly for generics); consult specific product labeling.

Tablet: Propranolol hydrochloride 40 mg and hydrochlorothiazide 25 mg; propranolol hydrochloride 80 mg and hydrochlorothiazide 25 mg

Inderide®: 40/25: Propranolol hydrochloride 40 mg and hydrochlorothiazide 25 mg

◆ **Propranolol Hydrochloride** *see* Propranolol *on page 1259*

◆ **Propranolol Hydrochloride Injection, USP (Can)** *see* Propranolol *on page 1259*

◆ **Proprinal [OTC]** *see* Ibuprofen *on page 760*

◆ **Proprinal® Cold and Sinus [OTC]** *see* Pseudoephedrine and Ibuprofen *on page 1267*

◆ **Propulsid®** *see* Cisapride *on page 334*

◆ **Propylene Glycol Diacetate, Acetic Acid, and Hydrocortisone** *see* Acetic Acid, Propylene Glycol Diacetate, and Hydrocortisone *on page 35*

◆ **2-Propylpentanoic Acid** *see* Valproic Acid and Derivatives *on page 1538*

Propylthiouracil (proe pil thye oh YOOR a sil)

Canadian Brand Names Propyl-Thyracil®

Index Terms PTU (error-prone abbreviation)

Pharmacologic Category Antithyroid Agent; Thioamide

Use Palliative treatment of hyperthyroidism as an adjunct to ameliorate hyperthyroidism in preparation for surgical treatment or radioactive iodine therapy; management of thyrotoxic crisis

Pregnancy Risk Factor D

Pregnancy Considerations Propylthiouracil crosses the placenta and because adverse events may occur in the fetus following maternal use, it is classified as pregnancy category D. The rate of congenital defects does not appear to be increased with maternal propylthiouracil use; however, fetal thyroid function may be transiently suppressed. Untreated hyperthyroidism may also cause adverse events in the mother (eg, heart failure, miscarriage, preeclampsia, thyroid storm), fetus (eg, goiter, growth restriction, hypo/hyperthyroidism, still birth) and neonate (eg, hyper-/hypothyroidism, neuropsychologic damage). The thioamides are treatment of choice for hyperthyroidism during pregnancy. In order to prevent adverse events to the fetus, the lowest effective dose should be used in order to achieve maternal levels of T_4 in the high euthyroid or low hyperthyroid range. Thyroid function should be monitored closely.

Lactation Enters breast milk/contraindicated (per manufacturer) (AAP rates "compatible")

Medication Safety Issues

Sound-alike/look-alike issues:

Propylthiouracil may be confused with Purinethol®

PTU is an error-prone abbreviation (mistaken as mercaptopurine [Purinethol®; 6-MP])

Contraindications Hypersensitivity to propylthiouracil or any component of the formulation; breast-feeding (per manufacturer; however, expert analysis and the AAP state this drug may be used in nursing mothers)

Warnings/Precautions Has been associated (rarely) with significant bone marrow depression. The most severe manifestation is agranulocytosis. Aplastic anemia, thrombocytopenia, and leukopenia may also occur. Use with caution in patients receiving other drugs known to cause myelosuppression particularly agranulocytosis. Discontinue if significant bone marrow suppression occurs, particularly agranulocytosis or aplastic anemia.

Rare, severe hepatic reactions (hepatic necrosis, hepatitis) may occur. Symptoms suggestive of hepatic dysfunction should prompt evaluation. Discontinue in the presence of hepatitis (transaminase >3x upper limit of normal). In addition, other rare hypersensitivity reactions have been reported, including the development of ANCA-positive vasculitis, drug fever, interstitial pneumonitis, exfoliative dermatitis, glomerulonephritis, leukocytoclastic vasculitis, and a lupus-like syndrome; prompt discontinuation is warranted in patients who develop symptoms consistent with a form of autoimmunity or other hypersensitivity during therapy.

May cause hypoprothrombinemia and bleeding; use with particular caution in patients >40 years of age. Thyroid hyperplasia or carcinoma may occur with prolonged usage (>1 year). Safety and efficacy have not been established in children <6 years of age.

Adverse Reactions Frequency not defined.

Cardiovascular: ANCA-positive vasculitis, cutaneous vasculitis, edema, leukocytoclastic vasculitis

Central nervous system: Dizziness, drowsiness, drug fever, fever, headache, neuritis, vertigo

Dermatologic: Alopecia, erythema nodosum, exfoliative dermatitis, pruritus, skin rash, urticaria

Endocrine & metabolic: Goiter, swollen salivary glands, weight gain

Gastrointestinal: Constipation, loss of taste perception, nausea, stomach pain, vomiting

Hematologic: Agranulocytosis, aplastic anemia, bleeding, leukopenia, thrombocytopenia

Hepatic: Cholestatic jaundice, hepatitis

Neuromuscular & skeletal: Arthralgia, paresthesia

Renal: Acute renal failure, glomerulonephritis, nephritis

Respiratory: Alveolar hemorrhage, interstitial pneumonitis

Miscellaneous: SLE-like syndrome

Drug Interactions

Avoid Concomitant Use

Avoid concomitant use of Propylthiouracil with any of the following: Sodium Iodide I131

Increased Effect/Toxicity There are no known significant interactions involving an increase in effect.

Decreased Effect

Propylthiouracil may decrease the levels/effects of: Sodium Iodide I131; Vitamin K Antagonists

Ethanol/Nutrition/Herb Interactions Food: Propylthiouracil serum levels may be altered if taken with food.

Mechanism of Action Inhibits the synthesis of thyroid hormones by blocking the oxidation of iodine in the thyroid gland; blocks synthesis of thyroxine and triiodothyronine

Pharmacodynamics/Kinetics

Onset of action: Therapeutic: 24-36 hours

Peak effect: Remission: 4 months of continued therapy

Duration: 2-3 hours

Distribution: Concentrated in the thyroid gland

Protein binding: 75% to 80%

Metabolism: Hepatic

Bioavailability: 80% to 95%

Half-life elimination: 1.5-5 hours; End-stage renal disease: 8.5 hours

Time to peak, serum: ~1 hour

Excretion: Urine (35%)

Dosage Oral: Administer in 3 equally divided doses at approximately 8-hour intervals. Adjust dosage to maintain T_3, T_4, and TSH levels in normal range; elevated T_3 may be sole indicator of inadequate treatment. Elevated TSH indicates excessive antithyroid treatment.

Children: Initial: 5-7 mg/kg/day **or** 150-200 mg/m^2/day in divided doses every 8 hours

or

6-10 years: 50-150 mg/day

>10 years: 150-300 mg/day

Maintenance: Determined by patient response **or** 1/3 to 2/3 of the initial dose in divided doses every 8-12 hours. This usually begins after 2 months on an effective initial dose.

Adults: Initial: 300-400 mg/day in divided doses every 6-8 hours. In patients with severe hyperthyroidism, very large goiters, or both, the initial dosage is usually 400 mg/day; an occasional patient will require 600-900 mg/day; maintenance: 100-150 mg/day in divided doses every 8-12 hours

Thyrotoxic crisis (recommendations vary widely and have not been evaluated in comparative trials): Dosages of 200-300 mg every 4-6 hours have been recommended for short-term initial therapy (until initial response), followed by gradual reduction to a maintenance dosage (100-150 mg/day in divided doses).

Elderly: Use lower dose recommendations; Initial: 150-300 mg/day

Withdrawal of therapy: Therapy should be withdrawn gradually with evaluation of the patient every 4-6 weeks for the first 3 months then every 3 months for the first year after discontinuation of therapy to detect any reoccurrence of a hyperthyroid state.

Dosing adjustment in renal impairment: Adjustment is not necessary

Dietary Considerations Administer at the same time in relation to meals each day, either always with meals or always between meals.

Monitoring Parameters CBC with differential, prothrombin time, liver function tests, thyroid function tests (TSH, T_3, T_4); periodic blood counts are recommended chronic therapy

Reference Range Normal laboratory values:
Total T_4: 5-12 mcg/dL
Serum T_3: 90-185 ng/dL
Free thyroxine index (FT_4 I): 6-10.5
TSH: 0.5-4.0 microunits/mL

Additional Information Preferred over methimazole in thyroid storm due to inhibition of peripheral conversion as well as synthesis of thyroid hormone.

Dosage Forms Excipient information presented when available (limited, particularly for generics); consult specific product labeling.
Tablet: 50 mg

Extemporaneous Preparations A 5 mg/mL oral suspension was stable for 10 days when refrigerated when compounded as follows:
Triturate six 50 mg tablets in a mortar, reduce to a fine powder, add 30 mL of carboxymethylcellulose 1.5%, transfer to a graduate and qs to 60 mL
Shake well before using and keep in refrigerator; protect from light
Nahata MC and Hipple TF, *Pediatric Drug Formulations*, 3rd ed, Cincinnati, OH: Harvey Whitney Books Co, 1997.

◆ **Propyl-Thyracil® (Can)** *see* Propylthiouracil *on page 1261*
◆ **2-Propylvaleric Acid** *see* Valproic Acid and Derivatives *on page 1538*
◆ **ProQuad®** *see* Measles, Mumps, Rubella, and Varicella Virus Vaccine *on page 923*
◆ **Proquin® XR** *see* Ciprofloxacin *on page 329*
◆ **PRO-Risperidone (Can)** *see* Risperidone *on page 1323*
◆ **Proscar®** *see* Finasteride *on page 622*
◆ **Prosed®/DS** *see* Methenamine, Phenyl Salicylate, Methylene Blue, Benzoic Acid, and Hyoscyamine *on page 962*
◆ **ProSom® [DSC]** *see* Estazolam *on page 553*
◆ **PRO-Sotalol (Can)** *see* Sotalol *on page 1394*
◆ **Prostacyclin** *see* Epoprostenol *on page 534*
◆ **Prostacyclin PGI_2** *see* Iloprost *on page 767*
◆ **Prostaglandin E_1** *see* Alprostadil *on page 70*
◆ **Prostaglandin E_2** *see* Dinoprostone *on page 454*
◆ **Prostaglandin F_2** *see* Carboprost Tromethamine *on page 260*
◆ **Prostigmin®** *see* Neostigmine *on page 1053*
◆ **Prostin E_2®** *see* Dinoprostone *on page 454*
◆ **Prostin® VR (Can)** *see* Alprostadil *on page 70*
◆ **Prostin VR Pediatric®** *see* Alprostadil *on page 70*

Protamine Sulfate (PROE ta meen SUL fate)

Pharmacologic Category Antidote

Use Treatment of heparin overdosage; neutralize heparin during surgery or dialysis procedures

Unlabeled/Investigational Use Treatment of low molecular weight heparin (LMWH) overdose

Pregnancy Risk Factor C

Lactation Excretion in breast milk unknown

Medication Safety Issues
Sound-alike/look-alike issues:
Protamine may be confused with ProAmatine®, Protonix®, Protopam®, Protropin®

Contraindications Hypersensitivity to protamine or any component of the formulation

Warnings/Precautions May not be totally effective in some patients following cardiac surgery despite adequate doses; may cause hypersensitivity reaction in patients with a history of allergy to fish (have epinephrine 1:1000 available) and in patients sensitized to protamine (via protamine-containing insulins); too rapid administration can cause severe hypotensive and anaphylactoid-like reactions. Heparin rebound associated with anticoagulation and bleeding has been reported to occur occasionally; symptoms typically occur 8-9 hours after protamine administration, but may occur as long as 18 hours later.

Adverse Reactions Frequency not defined.
Cardiovascular: Sudden fall in blood pressure, bradycardia, flushing, hypotension
Central nervous system: Lassitude
Gastrointestinal: Nausea, vomiting
Hematologic: Hemorrhage
Respiratory: Dyspnea, pulmonary hypertension
Miscellaneous: Hypersensitivity reactions

Drug Interactions
Avoid Concomitant Use There are no known interactions where it is recommended to avoid concomitant use.
Increased Effect/Toxicity There are no known significant interactions involving an increase in effect.
Decreased Effect There are no known significant interactions involving a decrease in effect.

Stability Refrigerate; do not freeze. Stable for at least 2 weeks at room temperature. Preservative-free formulation does not require refrigeration. Reconstitute vial with 5 mL sterile water. If using protamine in neonates, reconstitute with preservative-free sterile water for injection; resulting solution equals 10 mg/mL.

Mechanism of Action Combines with strongly acidic heparin to form a stable complex (salt) neutralizing the anticoagulant activity of both drugs

Pharmacodynamics/Kinetics Onset of action: I.V.: Heparin neutralization: ~5 minutes

Dosage
Heparin neutralization: I.V.: Protamine dosage is determined by the dosage of heparin; 1 mg of protamine neutralizes 90 USP units of heparin (lung) and 115 USP units of heparin (intestinal); maximum dose: 50 mg
Heparin overdosage, following intravenous administration: I.V.: Since blood heparin concentrations decrease rapidly **after** administration, adjust the protamine dosage depending upon the duration of time since heparin administration as follows: See table.

Time Elapsed	Dose of Protamine (mg) to Neutralize 100 units of Heparin
Immediate	1-1.5
30-60 min	0.5-0.75
>2 h	0.25-0.375

Heparin overdosage, following SubQ injection: I.V.: 1-1.5 mg protamine per 100 units heparin; this may be done by a portion of the dose (eg, 25-50 mg) given slowly I.V. followed by the remaining portion as a continuous infusion over 8-16 hours (the expected absorption time of the SubQ heparin dose)
LMWH overdose (unlabeled use): **Note:** Antifactor Xa activity never completely neutralized (maximum: ~60% to 75%)
Enoxaparin: 1 mg protamine for each mg of enoxaparin; if PTT prolonged 2-4 hours after first dose, consider additional dose of 0.5 mg for each mg of enoxaparin.
Dalteparin or tinzaparin: 1 mg protamine for each 100 anti-Xa int. units of dalteparin or tinzaparin; if PTT prolonged 2-4 hours after first dose, consider additional dose of 0.5 mg for each 100 anti-Xa int. units of dalteparin or tinzaparin.
Note: Excessive protamine doses may worsen bleeding potential.

Administration For I.V. use only; **incompatible** with cephalosporins and penicillins; administer slow IVP (50 mg over 10 minutes); rapid I.V. infusion causes hypotension; resulting solution equals 10 mg/mL; inject without further dilution over 1-3 minutes; maximum of 50 mg in any 10-minute period

Monitoring Parameters Coagulation test, aPTT or ACT, cardiac monitor and blood pressure monitor required during administration

Dosage Forms Excipient information presented when available (limited, particularly for generics); consult specific product labeling.

Injection, solution, as sulfate [preservative free]: 10 mg/mL (5 mL, 25 mL)

◆ **Protein C** *see* Protein C Concentrate (Human) *on page 1264*

◆ **Protein C (Activated), Human, Recombinant** *see* Drotrecogin Alfa *on page 496*

◆ **Protein-Bound Paclitaxel** *see* Paclitaxel (Protein Bound) *on page 1129*

Protein C Concentrate (Human)

(PROE teen cee KON suhn trate HYU man)

U.S. Brand Names Ceprotin

Index Terms Protein C

Pharmacologic Category Anticoagulant

Use Replacement therapy for severe congenital protein C deficiency for the prevention and/or treatment of venous thromboembolism and purpura fulminans

Pregnancy Risk Factor C

Medication Safety Issues

Sound-alike/look-alike issues:

Ceprotin may be confused with aprotinin, Cipro®

Protein C concentrate (human) may be confused with activated protein C (human, recombinant) which refers to drotrecogin alfa

Dosage Patient variables (including age, clinical condition, and plasma levels of protein C) will influence dosing and duration of therapy. Individualize dosing based on protein C activity and patient pharmacokinetic profile. Dosing is dependent on the severity of protein C deficiency, age of patient, clinical condition, and patient's level of protein C. The frequency, duration, and dose should be individualized.

I.V.: Children and Adults: Severe congenital protein C deficiency:

Acute episode/short-term prophylaxis: Initial dose: 100-120 int. units/kg (for determination of recovery and half-life)

Subsequent 3 doses: 60-80 int. units/kg every 6 hours (adjust to maintain peak protein C activity of 100%)

Maintenance dose: 45-60 int. units/kg every 6 or 12 hours (adjust to maintain recommended maintenance trough protein C activity levels >25%)

Long-term prophylaxis: Maintenance dose: 45-60 int. units/kg every 12 hours (recommended maintenance trough protein C activity levels >25%)

Note: Maintain target peak protein C activity of 100% during acute episodes and short-term prophylaxis. Maintain trough levels of protein C activity >25%. Higher peak levels of protein C may be necessary in prophylactic therapy of patients at increased risk for thrombosis (eg, infection, trauma, surgical intervention).

Additional Information Complete prescribing information for this medication should be consulted for additional detail.

Dosage Forms

Injection, powder for reconstitution:

Ceprotin: ~500 int. units [actual potency printed on vial label; contains human albumin and sodium; may contain trace amounts of mouse protein or heparin; packaged with diluent]; ~1000 int. units [actual potency printed on vial label; contains human albumin and sodium; may contain trace amounts of mouse protein or heparin; packaged with diluent]

◆ **Prothrombin Complex Concentrate** *see* Factor IX Complex (Human) *on page 601*

◆ **Protonix®** *see* Pantoprazole *on page 1140*

◆ **Protopam®** *see* Pralidoxime *on page 1223*

◆ **Protopic®** *see* Tacrolimus *on page 1419*

Protriptyline (proe TRIP ti leen)

U.S. Brand Names Vivactil®

Index Terms Protriptyline Hydrochloride

Pharmacologic Category Antidepressant, Tricyclic (Secondary Amine)

Additional Appendix Information

Antidepressant Agents *on page 1638*

Use Treatment of depression

Restrictions An FDA-approved medication guide concerning the use of antidepressants in children, adolescents, and young adults must be distributed when dispensing an outpatient prescription (new or refill) where this medication is to be used without direct supervision of a healthcare provider. Medication guides are available at http://www.fda.gov/cder/Offices/ODS/medication_guides.htm. Dispense to parents or guardians of children and adolescents receiving this medication.

Pregnancy Risk Factor C

Medication Safety Issues

Sound-alike/look-alike issues:

Vivactil® may be confused with Vyvanse™

Dosage Oral:

Adolescents: 15-20 mg/day

Adults: 15-60 mg/day in 3-4 divided doses

Elderly: Initial: 5-10 mg/day; increase every 3-7 days by 5-10 mg; usual dose: 15-20 mg/day

Additional Information Complete prescribing information for this medication should be consulted for additional detail.

Dosage Forms Excipient information presented when available (limited, particularly for generics); consult specific product labeling.

Tablet, as hydrochloride: 5 mg, 10 mg

Vivactil®: 5 mg, 10 mg

◆ **Protriptyline Hydrochloride** *see* Protriptyline *on page 1264*

◆ **Proventil® [DSC]** *see* Albuterol *on page 51*

◆ **Proventil® HFA** *see* Albuterol *on page 51*

◆ **Provera®** *see* MedroxyPROGESTERone *on page 930*

◆ **Provera-Pak (Can)** *see* MedroxyPROGESTERone *on page 930*

◆ **PRO-Verapamil SR (Can)** *see* Verapamil *on page 1557*

◆ **Provigil®** *see* Modafinil *on page 1009*

◆ **Proviodine (Can)** *see* Povidone-Iodine *on page 1222*

◆ **Provisc®** *see* Hyaluronate and Derivatives *on page 734*

◆ **Provocholine®** *see* Methacholine *on page 956*

◆ **Proxymetacaine** *see* Proparacaine *on page 1253*

◆ **Prozac®** *see* FLUoxetine *on page 638*

◆ **Prozac® Weekly™** *see* FLUoxetine *on page 638*

◆ **PRP-OMP** *see* *Haemophilus* b Conjugate Vaccine *on page 718*

◆ **PRP-T** *see* *Haemophilus* b Conjugate Vaccine *on page 718*

◆ **Prudoxin™** *see* Doxepin *on page 484*

◆ **Prussian Blue** *see* Ferric Hexacyanoferrate *on page 615*

◆ **Prymaccone** *see* Primaquine *on page 1237*

◆ **23PS** *see* Pneumococcal Polysaccharide Vaccine (Polyvalent) *on page 1206*

◆ **PS-341** *see* Bortezomib *on page 204*

◆ **Pseudacarb™** *see* Carbetapentane and Pseudoephedrine *on page 255*

Pseudoephedrine (soo doe e FED rin)

U.S. Brand Names Genaphed® [OTC]; Kidkare Decongestant [OTC]; Nasofed™; Oranyl [OTC]; Silfedrine Children's [OTC]; Sudafed® 12 Hour [OTC]; Sudafed® 24 Hour [OTC]; Sudafed® Children's [OTC]; Sudafed® Maximum Strength Nasal Decongestant [OTC]; Sudo-Tab® [OTC]; SudoGest [OTC]; Unifed [OTC]

Canadian Brand Names Balminil Decongestant; Benylin® D for Infants; Contac® Cold 12 Hour Relief Non Drowsy; Drixoral® ND; Eltor®; PMS-Pseudoephedrine; Pseudofrin; Robidrine®; Sudafed® Decongestant

Index Terms *d*-Isoephedrine Hydrochloride; Pseudoephedrine Hydrochloride; Pseudoephedrine Sulfate

Pharmacologic Category Alpha/Beta Agonist

Use Temporary symptomatic relief of nasal congestion due to common cold, upper respiratory allergies, and sinusitis; also promotes nasal or sinus drainage

Pregnancy Risk Factor C

Pregnancy Considerations Use during the 1st trimester may be associated with a possible risk of gastroschisis, small intestinal atresia, and hemifacial microsomia due pseudoephedrine's vasoconstrictive effects. However, additional studies are needed to define the magnitude of risk.

Lactation Enters breast milk/use caution (AAP rates "compatible")

Medication Safety Issues

Sound-alike/look-alike issues:

Dimetapp® may be confused with Dermatop®, Dimetabs®, Dimetane®

Sudafed® may be confused with Sufenta®

Contraindications Hypersensitivity to pseudoephedrine or any component of the formulation; with or within 14 days of MAO inhibitor therapy; newborns; breast-feeding

Warnings/Precautions Use with caution in the elderly; may be more sensitive to adverse effects; administer with caution to patients with hypertension, hyperthyroidism, diabetes mellitus, cardiovascular disease, ischemic heart disease, increased intraocular pressure, prostatic hyperplasia, or renal impairment. When used for self-medication (OTC), notify healthcare provider if symptoms do not improve within 7 days or are accompanied by fever. Discontinue and contact healthcare provider if nervousness, dizziness, or sleeplessness occur. Not for OTC use in children <2 years of age. Some products may contain phenylalanine.

Adverse Reactions Frequency not defined.

Cardiovascular: Arrhythmia, hypotension, palpitation, tachycardia

Central nervous system: Chills, confusion, coordination impaired, dizziness, drowsiness, excitability, fatigue, hallucination, headache, insomnia, nervousness, neuritis, restlessness, seizure, transient stimulation, vertigo

Dermatologic: Photosensitivity, rash, urticaria

Gastrointestinal: Anorexia, constipation, diarrhea, dry throat, nausea, vomiting, xerostomia

Genitourinary: Difficult urination, dysuria, polyuria, urinary retention

Hematologic: Agranulocytosis, hemolytic anemia, thrombocytopenia

Neuromuscular & skeletal: Tremor, weakness

Ocular: Blurred vision, diplopia

Otic: Tinnitus

Respiratory: Chest/throat tightness, dry nose, dyspnea, nasal congestion, thickening of bronchial secretions, wheezing

Miscellaneous: Anaphylaxis, diaphoresis

Drug Interactions

Avoid Concomitant Use

Avoid concomitant use of Pseudoephedrine with any of the following: Iobenguane I 123; MAO Inhibitors

Increased Effect/Toxicity

Pseudoephedrine may increase the levels/effects of: Bromocriptine; Sympathomimetics

The levels/effects of Pseudoephedrine may be increased by: Antacids; Cannabinoids; Carbonic Anhydrase Inhibitors; MAO Inhibitors; Serotonin/Norepinephrine Reuptake Inhibitors

Decreased Effect

Pseudoephedrine may decrease the levels/effects of: Iobenguane I 123

Ethanol/Nutrition/Herb Interactions

Food: Onset of effect may be delayed if pseudoephedrine is taken with food.

Herb/Nutraceutical: Avoid ephedra, yohimbe (may cause hypertension).

Mechanism of Action Directly stimulates alpha-adrenergic receptors of respiratory mucosa causing vasoconstriction; directly stimulates beta-adrenergic receptors causing bronchial relaxation, increased heart rate and contractility

Pharmacodynamics/Kinetics

Onset of action: Decongestant: Oral: 15-30 minutes

Duration: Immediate release tablet: 4-6 hours; Extended release: ≤12 hours

Absorption: Rapid

Metabolism: Partially hepatic

Half-life elimination: 9-16 hours

Excretion: Urine (70% to 90% as unchanged drug, 1% to 6% as active norpseudoephedrine); dependent on urine pH and flow rate; alkaline urine decreases renal elimination of pseudoephedrine

Dosage Oral:

Hydrochloride salt: General dosing guidelines:

Children:

<2 years: 4 mg/kg/day in divided doses every 6 hours

2-5 years: 15 mg every 4-6 hours; maximum: 60 mg/24 hours

6-12 years: 30 mg every 4-6 hours; maximum: 120 mg/24 hours

Adults: 30-60 mg every 4-6 hours, sustained release: 120 mg every 12 hours; maximum: 240 mg/24 hours

Tannate salt: Nasofed™ oral suspension:

Children 2-5 years: 1.25-2.5 mL (12.5-25 mg) every 12 hours

Children 6-11 years: 2.5-5 mL (25-50 mg) every 12 hours

Children ≥12 years & Adults: 5-10 mL (50-100 mg) every 12 hours

Dosing adjustment in renal impairment: Consider reducing dose

Dietary Considerations Should be taken with water or milk to decrease GI distress. Nasofed™ oral suspension contains phenylalanine 7 mg/5 mL; Sudafed® Children's chewable tablet contains phenylalanine 0.78 mg/tablet.

Administration Do not crush extended release drug product, swallow whole.

Test Interactions Interferes with urine detection of amphetamine (false-positive)

Dosage Forms Excipient information presented when available (limited, particularly for generics); consult specific product labeling.

Caplet, extended release, as hydrochloride:

Sudafed® 12 Hour: 120 mg

Liquid, as hydrochloride: 30 mg/5 mL (120 mL)

Silfedrine Children's: 15 mg/5 mL (120 mL, 480 mL) [alcohol and sugar free; grape flavor]

Sudafed® Children's: 15 mg/5 mL (120 mL) [alcohol and sugar free; contains sodium benzoate; grape flavor]
Unifed: 30 mg/5 mL (120 mL, 480 mL, 3840 mL)
Liquid, oral, as hydrochloride [drops]:
Kidkare Decongestant: 7.5 mg/0.8 mL (30 mL) [alcohol free; contains benzoic acid and sodium benzoate; cherry flavor]
Suspension, oral, as tannate:
Nasofed™: 50 mg/5 mL (118 mL) [contains phenylalanine 7 mg/5 mL, propylene glycol; strawberry flavor]
Syrup, as hydrochloride: 30 mg/5 mL (118 mL, 473 mL)
Tablet, as hydrochloride: 30 mg, 60 mg
Genaphed®, Oranyl, Sudafed®, Sudo-Tab®: 30 mg
SudoGest: 30 mg, 60 mg
Tablet, chewable, as hydrochloride:
Sudafed® Children's: 15 mg [sugar free; contains phenylalanine 0.78 mg/tablet; orange flavor]
Tablet, extended release, as hydrochloride:
Sudafed® 24 Hour: 240 mg

- ◆ **Pseudoephedrine, Acetaminophen, and Chlorpheniramine** *see* Acetaminophen, Chlorpheniramine, and Pseudoephedrine *on page 31*
- ◆ **Pseudoephedrine, Acetaminophen, and Dextromethorphan** *see* Acetaminophen, Dextromethorphan, and Pseudoephedrine *on page 33*
- ◆ **Pseudoephedrine and Acetaminophen** *see* Acetaminophen and Pseudoephedrine *on page 30*
- ◆ **Pseudoephedrine and Brompheniramine** *see* Brompheniramine and Pseudoephedrine *on page 214*
- ◆ **Pseudoephedrine and Carbetapentane** *see* Carbetapentane and Pseudoephedrine *on page 255*
- ◆ **Pseudoephedrine and Carbinoxamine** *see* Carbinoxamine and Pseudoephedrine *on page 258*
- ◆ **Pseudoephedrine and Chlorpheniramine** *see* Chlorpheniramine and Pseudoephedrine *on page 310*

Pseudoephedrine and Codeine

(soo doe e FED rin & KOE deen)

U.S. Brand Names Notuss®-DC; Nucofed® [DSC]

Index Terms Codeine and Pseudoephedrine; Codeine Phosphate and Pseudoephedrine Hydrochloride; Pseudoephedrine Hydrochloride and Codeine Phosphate

Pharmacologic Category Antitussive/Decongestant

Use Temporary symptomatic relief of congestion and cough due to upper respiratory infections including common cold, bronchitis, sinusitis, and influenza

Restrictions Capsule: C-III; Liquid: C-V

Pregnancy Risk Factor C

Dosage Oral: Relief of congestion and cough:
Children 6-11 years: 2.5-5 mL every 4-6 hours as needed (maximum: 20 mL/24 hours)
Children ≥12 years and Adults: One capsule every 6 hours as needed (maximum: 4 capsules/24 hours) **or** 5-10 mL every 4-6 hours as needed (maximum: 40 mL/24 hours)

Additional Information Complete prescribing information for this medication should be consulted for additional detail.

Dosage Forms Excipient information presented when available (limited, particularly for generics); consult specific product labeling. [DSC] = Discontinued product
Capsule:
Nucofed®: Pseudoephedrine hydrochloride 60 mg and codeine phosphate 20 mg [DSC]
Liquid, oral:
Notuss®-DC: Pseudoephedrine hydrochloride 30 mg and codeine phosphate 10 mg per 5 mL (473 mL) [dye free, ethanol free, gluten free, sugar free; contains propylene glycol; bubblegum flavor]

- ◆ **Pseudoephedrine and Desloratadine** *see* Desloratadine and Pseudoephedrine *on page 421*
- ◆ **Pseudoephedrine and Dexbrompheniramine** *see* Dexbrompheniramine and Pseudoephedrine *on page 428*

Pseudoephedrine and Dextromethorphan

(soo doe e FED rin & deks troe meth OR fan)

U.S. Brand Names Pedia Relief Cough and Cold [OTC]; Pedia Relief Infants [OTC]; PediaCare® Infants' Decongestant & Cough [OTC] [DSC]; Sudafed® Children's Cold & Cough [OTC]; SudoGest Children's [OTC]

Canadian Brand Names Balminil DM D; Benylin® DM-D; Koffex DM-D; Novahistex® DM Decongestant; Novahistine® DM Decongestant; Robitussin® Childrens Cough & Cold

Index Terms Dextromethorphan and Pseudoephedrine

Pharmacologic Category Antitussive/Decongestant

Use Temporary symptomatic relief of nasal congestion and cough due to common cold, hay fever, upper respiratory allergies

Dosage Relief of nasal congestion and cough: Oral:
General dosing guidelines base on pseudoephedrine component:
Children 2-6 years: 15 mg every 4-6 hours (maximum: 60 mg/24 hours)
Children 6-12 years: 30 mg every 4-6 hours (maximum: 120 mg/24 hours)
Children ≥12 years and Adults: 60 mg every 4-6 hours (maximum: 240 mg/24 hours)

Product-specific dosing:
Children 2-6 years (Sudafed® Children's Cold & Cough): 5 mL every 4 hours (maximum: 20 mL/24 hours)
Children 6-12 years (Sudafed® Children's Cold & Cough): 10 mL every 4 hours (maximum: 40 mL/24 hours)
Children ≥12 years and Adults (Sudafed® Children's Cold & Cough): 20 mL every 4 hours (maximum: 80 mL/24 hours)

Additional Information Complete prescribing information for this medication should be consulted for additional detail.

Dosage Forms Excipient information presented when available (limited, particularly for generics); consult specific product labeling. [DSC] = Discontinued product
Liquid:
Sudafed® Children's Cold & Cough: Pseudoephedrine hydrochloride 15 mg and dextromethorphan hydrobromide 5 mg per 5 mL (120 mL) [alcohol free, sugar free; contains sodium benzoate; cherry berry flavor]
Liquid, oral [drops]:
PediaCare® Infants' Decongestant & Cough: Pseudoephedrine hydrochloride 7.5 mg and dextromethorphan hydrobromide 2.5 mg per 0.8 mL (15 mL) [alcohol free; contains sodium benzoate; cherry flavor] [DSC]
Pedia Relief Infants: Pseudoephedrine hydrochloride 7.5 mg and dextromethorphan hydrobromide 2.5 mg per 0.8 mL (15 mL) [cherry flavor]
Syrup:
Pedia Relief Cough and Cold: Pseudoephedrine hydrochloride 15 mg and dextromethorphan hydrobromide 7.5 mg per 5 mL (120 mL) [cherry flavor]
SudoGest Children's: Pseudoephedrine hydrochloride 15 mg and dextromethorphan hydrobromide 5 mg per 5 mL (120 mL)

- ◆ **Pseudoephedrine and Diphenhydramine** *see* Diphenhydramine and Pseudoephedrine *on page 459*
- ◆ **Pseudoephedrine and Fexofenadine** *see* Fexofenadine and Pseudoephedrine *on page 619*

◆ **Pseudoephedrine and Guaifenesin** *see* Guaifenesin and Pseudoephedrine *on page 713*

Pseudoephedrine and Ibuprofen

(soo doe e FED rin & eye byoo PROE fen)

U.S. Brand Names Advil® Cold & Sinus [OTC]; Advil® Cold, Children's [OTC] [DSC]; Proprinal® Cold and Sinus [OTC]

Canadian Brand Names Advil® Cold & Sinus; Children's Advil® Cold; Sudafed® Sinus Advance

Index Terms Ibuprofen and Pseudoephedrine

Pharmacologic Category Decongestant/Analgesic

Use For temporary relief of cold, sinus and flu symptoms (including nasal congestion, sinus pressure, headache, minor body aches and pains, and fever)

Pregnancy Risk Factor Ibuprofen: B/D (3rd trimester)

Dosage OTC labeling: Oral: Children ≥12 years and Adults: Ibuprofen 200 mg and pseudoephedrine 30 mg per dose: One dose every 4-6 hours as needed; may increase to 2 doses if necessary (maximum: 6 doses/24 hours). Contact healthcare provider if symptoms have not improved within 7 days when treating cold symptoms or within 3 days when treating fever.

Additional Information Complete prescribing information for this medication should be consulted for additional detail.

Dosage Forms Excipient information presented when available (limited, particularly for generics); consult specific product labeling. [DSC] = Discontinued product

Caplet:

Advil® Cold and Sinus, Proprinal® Cold and Sinus: Pseudoephedrine hydrochloride 30 mg and ibuprofen 200 mg

Capsule, liquid filled:

Advil® Cold and Sinus: Pseudoephedrine hydrochloride 30 mg and ibuprofen 200 mg [solubilized ibuprofen as free acid and potassium salt; contains potassium 20 mg/capsule and coconut oil]

Suspension:

Advil® Cold, Children's: Pseudoephedrine hydrochloride 15 mg and ibuprofen 100 mg per 5 mL (120 mL) [alcohol free; contains sodium 3 mg/5 mL and sodium benzoate; grape flavor] [DSC]

◆ **Pseudoephedrine and Loratadine** *see* Loratadine and Pseudoephedrine *on page 905*

Pseudoephedrine and Methscopolamine

(soo doe e FED rin & meth skoe POL a meen)

U.S. Brand Names AlleRx™-D; Amdry-D; Extendryl PSE

Index Terms Methscopolamine and Pseudoephedrine; Pseudoephedrine hydrochloride and Methscopolamine Nitrate

Pharmacologic Category Decongestant/Anticholingeric Combination

Use Relief of symptoms of allergic rhinitis, vasomotor rhinitis, sinusitis, and the common cold

Pregnancy Risk Factor C

Dosage Oral: Children ≥12 years and Adults (Allerx™-D, Amdry-D): One tablet every 12 hours (maximum: 2 tablets/24 hours)

Additional Information Complete prescribing information for this medication should be consulted for additional detail.

Dosage Forms Excipient information presented when available (limited, particularly for generics); consult specific product labeling.

Tablet: Pseudoephedrine hydrochloride 120 mg and methscopolamine nitrate 2.5 mg

Allerx™-D, Amdry-D: Pseudoephedrine hydrochloride 120 mg and methscopolamine nitrate 2.5 mg

Tablet, extended release:

Extendryl PSE: Pseudoephedrine hydrochloride 120 mg and methscopolamine nitrate 2.5 mg

◆ **Pseudoephedrine and Naproxen** *see* Naproxen and Pseudoephedrine *on page 1043*

◆ **Pseudoephedrine and Triprolidine** *see* Triprolidine and Pseudoephedrine *on page 1522*

◆ **Pseudoephedrine, Chlorpheniramine, and Acetaminophen** *see* Acetaminophen, Chlorpheniramine, and Pseudoephedrine *on page 31*

◆ **Pseudoephedrine, Chlorpheniramine, and Codeine** *see* Chlorpheniramine, Pseudoephedrine, and Codeine *on page 314*

◆ **Pseudoephedrine, Chlorpheniramine, and Dextromethorphan** *see* Chlorpheniramine, Pseudoephedrine, and Dextromethorphan *on page 315*

◆ **Pseudoephedrine, Codeine, and Triprolidine** *see* Triprolidine, Pseudoephedrine, and Codeine *on page 1523*

◆ **Pseudoephedrine, Dextromethorphan, and Acetaminophen** *see* Acetaminophen, Dextromethorphan, and Pseudoephedrine *on page 33*

◆ **Pseudoephedrine, Dextromethorphan, and Guaifenesin** *see* Guaifenesin, Pseudoephedrine, and Dextromethorphan *on page 715*

◆ **Pseudoephedrine, Guaifenesin, and Codeine** *see* Guaifenesin, Pseudoephedrine, and Codeine *on page 715*

◆ **Pseudoephedrine Hydrochloride** *see* Pseudoephedrine *on page 1265*

◆ **Pseudoephedrine Hydrochloride and Acrivastine** *see* Acrivastine and Pseudoephedrine *on page 40*

◆ **Pseudoephedrine Hydrochloride and Codeine Phosphate** *see* Pseudoephedrine and Codeine *on page 1266*

◆ **Pseudoephedrine Hydrochloride and Hydrocodone Bitartrate** *see* Hydrocodone and Pseudoephedrine *on page 742*

◆ **Pseudoephedrine hydrochloride and Methscopolamine Nitrate** *see* Pseudoephedrine and Methscopolamine *on page 1267*

◆ **Pseudoephedrine Hydrochloride, Guaifenesin, and Dihydrocodeine Bitartrate** *see* Dihydrocodeine, Pseudoephedrine, and Guaifenesin *on page 448*

◆ **Pseudoephedrine, Hydrocodone, and Carbinoxamine** *see* Hydrocodone, Carbinoxamine, and Pseudoephedrine *on page 743*

◆ **Pseudoephedrine, Hydrocodone, and Guaifenesin** *see* Hydrocodone, Pseudoephedrine, and Guaifenesin *on page 743*

◆ **Pseudoephedrine Sulfate** *see* Pseudoephedrine *on page 1265*

◆ **Pseudoephedrine Tannate and Dexchlorpheniramine Tannate** *see* Dexchlorpheniramine and Pseudoephedrine *on page 428*

◆ **Pseudoephedrine, Triprolidine, and Codeine** *see* Triprolidine, Pseudoephedrine, and Codeine *on page 1523*

◆ **Pseudofrin (Can)** *see* Pseudoephedrine *on page 1265*

◆ **Pseudo GG TR** *see* Guaifenesin and Pseudoephedrine *on page 713*

◆ **Pseudo Max** *see* Guaifenesin and Pseudoephedrine *on page 713*

◆ **Pseudo Max DMX** *see* Guaifenesin, Pseudoephedrine, and Dextromethorphan *on page 715*

◆ **Pseudomonic Acid A** *see* Mupirocin *on page 1024*

- ◆ **Pseudovent™ [DSC]** *see* Guaifenesin and Pseudoephedrine *on page 713*
- ◆ **Pseudovent™ 400 [DSC]** *see* Guaifenesin and Pseudoephedrine *on page 713*
- ◆ **Pseudovent™ DM [DSC]** *see* Guaifenesin, Pseudoephedrine, and Dextromethorphan *on page 715*
- ◆ **Pseudovent™-Ped [DSC]** *see* Guaifenesin and Pseudoephedrine *on page 713*
- ◆ **Psoriatec™** *see* Anthralin *on page 118*

Psyllium (SIL i yum)

U.S. Brand Names Bulk-K [OTC]; Fiberall®; Fibro-Lax [OTC]; Fibro-XL [OTC]; Genfiber™ [OTC]; Hydrocil® Instant [OTC]; Konsyl-D™ [OTC]; Konsyl® Easy Mix™ [OTC]; Konsyl® Orange [OTC]; Konsyl® Original [OTC]; Konsyl® [OTC]; Metamucil® Plus Calcium [OTC]; Metamucil® Smooth Texture [OTC]; Metamucil® [OTC]; Natural Fiber Therapy Smooth Texture [OTC]; Natural Fiber Therapy [OTC]; Reguloid [OTC]

Canadian Brand Names Metamucil®

Index Terms Plantago Seed; Plantain Seed; Psyllium Husk; Psyllium Hydrophilic Mucilloid

Pharmacologic Category Antidiarrheal; Laxative, Bulk-Producing

Additional Appendix Information

Laxatives, Classification and Properties *on page 1660*

Use OTC labeling: Dietary fiber supplement; treatment of occasional constipation; reduce risk of coronary heart disease (CHD)

Unlabeled/Investigational Use Treatment of diarrhea, chronic constipation, irritable bowel syndrome, inflammatory bowel disease, colon cancer, or diabetes

Medication Safety Issues

Sound-alike/look-alike issues:

Fiberall® may be confused with Feverall®
Hydrocil® may be confused with Hydrocet®
Modane® may be confused with Matulane®, Moban®

Contraindications Hypersensitivity to psyllium or any component of the formulation; fecal impaction; GI obstruction

Warnings/Precautions Use with caution in patients with esophageal strictures, ulcers, stenosis, intestinal adhesions, or difficulty swallowing. Use with caution in the elderly; may have insufficient fluid intake which may predispose them to fecal impaction and bowel obstruction. Products must be taken with at least 8 ounces of fluid in order to prevent choking. To reduce the risk of CHD, the soluble fiber from psyllium should be used in conjunction with a diet low in saturated fat and cholesterol. Some products may contain calcium, potassium, sodium, soy lecithin, or phenylalanine.

When used for self-medication (OTC), do not use in the presence of abdominal pain, nausea or vomiting. Notify healthcare provider in case of sudden changes of bowel habits which last >2 weeks or in case of rectal bleeding. Not for self-treatment of constipation lasting >1 week

Adverse Reactions Frequency not defined.

Gastrointestinal: Abdominal cramps, constipation, diarrhea, esophageal or bowel obstruction

Respiratory: Bronchospasm

Miscellaneous: Anaphylaxis upon inhalation in susceptible individuals, rhinoconjunctivitis

Drug Interactions

Avoid Concomitant Use There are no known interactions where it is recommended to avoid concomitant use.

Increased Effect/Toxicity There are no known significant interactions involving an increase in effect.

Decreased Effect There are no known significant interactions involving a decrease in effect.

Mechanism of Action Psyllium is a soluble fiber. It absorbs water in the intestine to form a viscous liquid which promotes peristalsis and reduces transit time.

Pharmacodynamics/Kinetics

Onset of action: Relief of constipation: 12-72 hours

Absorption: None; small amounts of grain extracts present in the preparation have been reportedly absorbed following colonic hydrolysis

Dosage Oral: General dosing guidelines; consult specific product labeling.

Adequate intake for total fiber: Note: The definition of "fiber" varies; however, the soluble fiber in psyllium is only one type of fiber which makes up the daily recommended intake of total fiber.

Children 1-3 years: 19 g/day
Children 4-8 years: 25 g/day
Children 9-13 years: Male: 31 g/day; Female: 26 g/day
Children 14-18 years: Male: 38 g/day; Female: 26 g/day
Adults 19-50 years: Male: 38 g/day; Female: 25 g/day
Adults ≥51 years: Male: 30 g/day; Female: 21 g/day
Pregnancy: 28 g/day
Lactation: 29 g/day

Constipation:

Children 6-11 years: Psyllium: 1.25-15 g per day in divided doses

Children ≥12 years and Adults: Psyllium: 2.5-30 g per day in divided doses

Reduce risk of CHD: Children ≥12 years and Adults: Soluble fiber ≥7 g (psyllium seed husk ≥10.2 g) per day

Dietary Considerations Products should be taken with at least 8 ounces of fluids. Some products contain dextrose, sucrose, calcium, potassium, phenylalanine, as well as additional ingredients. Check individual product information for caloric and nutritional value.

When used to reduce the risk of CHD, the amount of **soluble fiber** from psyllium should be ≥7 g/day and it should be used in conjunction with a diet low in saturated fat and cholesterol.

Fiberall® contains phenylalanine.

Metamucil® Smooth Texture orange flavor, sugar free formulation contains phenylalanine 25 mg per teaspoonful. Metamucil® Smooth Texture berry burst flavor contains phenylalanine 16 mg per teaspoonful. Metamucil® Smooth Texture pink lemonade flavor, sugar free formulation contains phenylalanine 19 mg per teaspoonful. Metamucil® wafers contain soy lecithin. Konsyl® Orange sugar free contains calcium 6 mg, phenylalanine 21 mg, potassium 31 mg, and sodium 3 mg per teaspoon.

Administration Inhalation of psyllium dust may cause sensitivity to psyllium (eg, runny nose, watery eyes, wheezing). Drink at least 8 ounces of liquid with each dose. Powder must be mixed in a glass of water or juice. Capsules should be swallowed one at a time. When more than one dose is required, they should be divided throughout the day. Separate dose by at least 2 hours from other drug therapies.

Dosage Forms Excipient information presented when available (limited, particularly for generics); consult specific product labeling.

Capsule:

Fibro XL: 0.675 g [sugar free; provides dietary fiber 3.8 g and soluble fiber 3 g per 7 capsules]

Genfiber™: 0.52 g [provides dietary fiber 3 g and soluble fiber 2 g per 6 capsules]

Konsyl®: 0.52 g [sugar free; contains calcium 8 mg, potassium <11 mg and sodium 1 mg per capsule; provides dietary fiber 3 g and soluble fiber 2 g per 5 capsules]

Metamucil®: 0.52 g [contains potassium 5 mg/capsule; provides dietary fiber 3 g and soluble fiber 2.1 g per 6 capsules]

Metamucil® Plus Calcium: 0.52 g [contains calcium 60 mg and potassium 6 mg per capsule; provides dietary fiber 3 g and soluble fiber 2.1 g per 5 capsules]
Reguloid: 0.52 g [provides dietary fiber 3 g and soluble fiber 2 g per 6 capsules]

Powder:
Bulk-K: 4.7 g/teaspoon (392 g) [provides dietary fiber 3.8 g and soluble fiber 3 g per teaspoon]
Fiberall®: 0.05 g/tablespoon (454 g) [sugar free; contains phenylalanine; psyllium is in combination with other fiber sources providing total dietary fiber 3.5 g and soluble fiber 2 g per tablespoon; also contains vitamins and minerals; orange flavor]
Fibro-Lax: 4.7 g/teaspoon (140 g, 392 g) [provides dietary fiber 3.8 g and soluble fiber 3 g per teaspoon]
Genfiber®:
3.4 g/teaspoon (397 g, 595 g) [contains sodium ≤5 mg teaspoon; provides dietary fiber 3 g and soluble fiber 2 g per teaspoon; natural flavor]
3.4 g/tablespoon (397 g) [contains sodium ≤5 mg tablespoon; provides dietary fiber 3 g and soluble fiber 2 g per tablespoon; orange flavor]
Hydrocil® Instant:
3.5 g/packet (30s, 500s) [sugar free; provides dietary fiber 3 g and soluble fiber 2.4 g per packet]
3.5 g/teaspoon (300 g) [sugar free; provides dietary fiber 3 g and soluble fiber 2.4 g per teaspoon]
Konsyl®: Original:
6 g/packet (30s, 100s, 500s) [sugar free; contains calcium 10 mg, sodium 5 mg, and potassium 55 mg per packet; provides dietary fiber 5 g and soluble fiber 3 g per packet]
6 g/teaspoon (300 g, 450 g) [sugar free; contains calcium 10 mg, sodium 5 mg, and potassium 55 mg per teaspoon; provides dietary fiber 5 g and soluble fiber 3 g per teaspoon]
Konsyl-D™:
3.4 g/packet (100s, 500s) [contains calcium 6 mg, dextrose 3.1 g, potassium 31 mg and sodium 3 mg per packet; provides dietary fiber 3 g and soluble fiber 2 g per packet]
3.4 g/teaspoon (325 g, 397 g, 500 g) [contains calcium 6 mg, dextrose 3.1 g, potassium 31 mg, and sodium 3 mg per teaspoon; provides dietary fiber 3 g and soluble fiber 2 g per teaspoon]
Konsyl® Easy Mix:
6 g/packet (500s) [sugar free; contains calcium 10 mg, potassium 55 mg, and sodium 5 mg per packet; provides dietary fiber 5 g and soluble fiber 3 g per packet]
6 g/teaspoon (250 g) [sugar free; contains calcium 10 mg, potassium 55 mg, and sodium 5 mg per teaspoon; provides dietary fiber 5 g and soluble fiber 3 g per teaspoon]
Konsyl® Orange:
3.4 g/packet (30s) [contains calcium 6 mg, potassium 31 mg, sodium 3 mg, and sucrose 8g per packet; provides dietary fiber 3 g and soluble fiber 2 g per packet; orange flavor]
3.4 g/tablespoon (538 g) [contains calcium 6 mg, potassium 31 mg, sodium 3 mg, and sucrose 8g per tablespoon; provides dietary fiber 3 g and soluble fiber 2 g per tablespoon; orange flavor]
3.4 g/teaspoon (425 g) [sugar free; contains calcium 6 mg, phenylalanine 21 mg, potassium 31 mg, and sodium 3 mg per teaspoon; provides dietary fiber 3 g and soluble fiber 2 g per teaspoon; orange flavor]
Metamucil®:
3.4 g/teaspoon (390 g, 570 g, 870 g) [contains sodium 5 mg and potassium 30 mg per teaspoon; provides dietary fiber 3 g and soluble fiber ~2 g per teaspoon; unflavored]
3.4g/tablespoon (570 g, 870 g, 1254 g) [contains sodium 5 mg and potassium 30 mg per tablespoon; provides dietary fiber 3 g and soluble fiber ~2 g per tablespoon; orange flavor]
Metamucil® Smooth Texture:
3.3 g/teaspoon (288 g, 432 g, 684 g) [sugar free; contains phenylalanine 19 mg, potassium 35 mg, and sodium 5 mg per teaspoon; provides dietary fiber 3 g and soluble fiber ~2 g per teaspoon; pink lemonade flavor]
3.4 g/packet (30s) [contains sodium 5 mg and potassium 30 mg per packet; provides dietary fiber 3 g and soluble fiber ~2 g per packet; orange flavor]
3.4 g/packet (30s) [sugar free; contains phenylalanine 16 mg, sodium 5 mg, and potassium 30 mg per packet; provides dietary fiber 3 g and soluble fiber ~2 g per packet; berry burst flavor]
3.4 g/packet (30s) [sugar free; contains phenylalanine 25 mg, sodium 5 mg, and potassium 30 mg per packet; provides dietary fiber 3 g and soluble fiber ~2 g per packet; orange flavor]
3.4 g/tablespoon (609 g, 912 g, 1368g 1446 g) [contains sodium 5 mg and potassium 30 mg per dose tablespoon; provides dietary fiber 3 g and soluble fiber ~2 g per tablespoon; orange flavor]
3.4 g/teaspoon (300 g, 450 g, 690 g) [sugar free; contains sodium 5 mg and potassium 30 mg per dose teaspoon; provides dietary fiber 3 g and soluble fiber ~2 g per teaspoon; unflavored]
3.4 g/teaspoon (173 g, 300 g, 450 g, 660 g, 1020 g) [sugar free; contains phenylalanine 25 mg, sodium 5 mg, and potassium 30 mg per teaspoon; provides dietary fiber 3 g and soluble fiber ~2 g per teaspoon; orange flavor]
3.4 g/teaspoon (283 g, 425 g, 660 g) [sugar free; contains potassium 30 mg, sodium 5 mg and phenylalanine 16 mg per teaspoon; provides dietary fiber 3 g and soluble fiber ~2 g per teaspoon; berry burst flavor]
Natural Fiber Therapy: 3.4 g/tablespoon (369 g, 539 g) [natural and orange flavors]
Natural Fiber Therapy Smooth Texture: 3.4 g/teaspoon (300 g) [sugar free; orange flavor]
Reguloid®:
3.4 g/teaspoon (284 g, 426 g) [sugar free; contains phenylalanine 30 mg and sodium 6 mg per teaspoon; provides dietary fiber 3 g and soluble fiber 3 g per teaspoon; orange flavor]
3.4 g/teaspoon (284 g, 426 g) [sugar free; contains phenylalanine 6 mg and sodium 2 mg per teaspoon; provides dietary fiber 3 g and soluble fiber 2 g per teaspoon; regular flavor]
3.4 g/tablespoon (369 g, 540 g) [contains sodium 9 mg per tablespoon; provides dietary fiber 3 g and soluble fiber 2 g per tablespoon; orange flavor]
3.4 g/tablespoon (369 g, 540 g) [contains sodium 4 mg per tablespoon; provides dietary fiber 2 g and soluble fiber 2 g per tablespoon; regular flavor]

Wafers:
Metamucil®: 3.4 g/2 wafers (24s) [contains soya lecithin, wheat, sodium 20 mg, and potassium 60 mg per 2 wafers; provides dietary fiber 6 g and soluble fiber 3 g per 2 wafers; apple and cinnamon spice flavors]

◆ **Psyllium Husk** *see* Psyllium *on page 1268*

◆ **Psyllium Hydrophilic Mucilloid** *see* Psyllium *on page 1268*

◆ **P-Tann D** *see* Chlorpheniramine and Phenylephrine *on page 309*

◆ **Pteroylglutamic Acid** *see* Folic Acid *on page 655*

◆ **PTU (error-prone abbreviation)** *see* Propylthiouracil *on page 1261*

◆ **Pulmicort® (Can)** *see* Budesonide *on page 215*

- ◆ **Pulmicort Flexhaler™** *see* Budesonide *on page 215*
- ◆ **Pulmicort Respules®** *see* Budesonide *on page 215*
- ◆ **Pulmophylline (Can)** *see* Theophylline *on page 1455*
- ◆ **Pulmozyme®** *see* Dornase Alfa *on page 481*
- ◆ **Puregon® (Can)** *see* Follitropin Beta *on page 658*
- ◆ **Purified Chick Embryo Cell** *see* Rabies Vaccine *on page 1287*
- ◆ **Purinethol®** *see* Mercaptopurine *on page 946*
- ◆ **PVP-I** *see* Povidone-Iodine *on page 1222*
- ◆ **Pylera™** *see* Bismuth, Metronidazole, and Tetracycline *on page 199*

Pyrantel Pamoate (pi RAN tel PAM oh ate)

U.S. Brand Names Pin-X® [OTC]; Reese's® Pinworm Medicine [OTC]

Canadian Brand Names Combantrin™

Pharmacologic Category Anthelmintic

Use Treatment of pinworms (*Enterobius vermicularis*) and roundworms (*Ascaris lumbricoides*)

Unlabeled/Investigational Use Treatment of whipworms (*Trichuris trichiura*) and hookworms (*Ancylostoma duodenale*)

Pregnancy Risk Factor C

Contraindications Hypersensitivity to pyrantel pamoate or any component of the formulation

Warnings/Precautions Use with caution in patients with liver impairment, anemia, malnutrition, or pregnancy. Since pinworm infections are easily spread to others, treat all family members in close contact with the patient.

Adverse Reactions Frequency not defined.

Central nervous system: Dizziness, drowsiness, insomnia, headache

Dermatologic: Rash

Gastrointestinal: Abdominal cramps, anorexia, diarrhea, nausea, vomiting, tenesmus

Hepatic: Liver enzymes increased

Neuromuscular & skeletal: Weakness

Drug Interactions

Avoid Concomitant Use There are no known interactions where it is recommended to avoid concomitant use.

Increased Effect/Toxicity There are no known significant interactions involving an increase in effect.

Decreased Effect

The levels/effects of Pyrantel Pamoate may be decreased by: Aminoquinolines (Antimalarial)

Stability Protect from light.

Mechanism of Action Causes the release of acetylcholine and inhibits cholinesterase; acts as a depolarizing neuromuscular blocker, paralyzing the helminths

Pharmacodynamics/Kinetics

Absorption: Oral: Poor

Metabolism: Partially hepatic

Time to peak, serum: 1-3 hours

Excretion: Feces (50% as unchanged drug); urine (7% as unchanged drug)

Dosage Children and Adults (purgation is not required prior to use): Oral: **Note:** Dose is expressed as pyrantel base:

Roundworm, pinworm, or trichostrongyliasis: 11 mg/kg administered as a single dose; maximum dose: 1 g. (**Note:** For pinworm infection, dosage should be repeated in 2 weeks and all family members should be treated).

Hookworm (unlabeled use): 11 mg/kg administered once daily for 3 days

Administration May be mixed with milk or fruit juice

Monitoring Parameters Stool for presence of eggs, worms, and occult blood, serum AST and ALT

Dosage Forms Excipient information presented when available (limited, particularly for generics); consult specific product labeling.

Caplet, as pamoate:

Reese's® Pinworm Medicine: 180 mg [equivalent to pyrantel base 62.5 mg/tablet]

Suspension, oral as pamoate:

Pin-X®: 144 mg/mL (30 mL, 60 mL) [equivalent to pyrantel base 50 mg/mL; sugar free; contains sodium benzoate; caramel flavor]

Reese's® Pinworm Medicine: 144 mg/mL (30 mL) [equivalent to pyrantel base 50 mg/mL]

Tablet, chewable, as pamoate:

Pin-X®: 720.5 mg [equivalent to pyrantel base 250 mg/tablet; contains aspartame; orange flavor]

Pyrazinamide (peer a ZIN a mide)

Canadian Brand Names Tebrazid™

Index Terms Pyrazinoic Acid Amide

Pharmacologic Category Antitubercular Agent

Additional Appendix Information

Antimicrobial Drugs of Choice *on page 1752*

Guidelines for the Prevention of Opportunistic Infections in HIV Infected Persons *on page 1740*

Tuberculosis *on page 1776*

Use Adjunctive treatment of tuberculosis in combination with other antituberculosis agents

Pregnancy Risk Factor C

Lactation Enters breast milk/use caution

Contraindications Hypersensitivity to pyrazinamide or any component of the formulation; acute gout; severe hepatic damage

Warnings/Precautions Use with caution in patients with a history of alcoholism, renal failure, chronic gout, diabetes mellitus, or porphyria. Dose-related hepatotoxicity ranging from transient ALT/AST elevations to jaundice, hepatitis and/or liver atrophy (rare) has occurred. Use with caution in patients receiving concurrent medications associated with hepatotoxicity (particularly with rifampin).

Adverse Reactions

1% to 10%:

Central nervous system: Malaise

Gastrointestinal: Anorexia, nausea, vomiting

Neuromuscular & skeletal: Arthralgia, myalgia

<1% (Limited to important or life-threatening): Acne, angioedema (rare), anticoagulant effect, dysuria, fever, gout, hepatotoxicity, interstitial nephritis, itching, photosensitivity, porphyria, rash, sideroblastic anemia, thrombocytopenia, urticaria

Drug Interactions

Avoid Concomitant Use There are no known interactions where it is recommended to avoid concomitant use.

Increased Effect/Toxicity

Pyrazinamide may increase the levels/effects of: Rifampin

Decreased Effect

Pyrazinamide may decrease the levels/effects of: CycloSPORINE

Mechanism of Action Converted to pyrazinoic acid in susceptible strains of *Mycobacterium* which lowers the pH of the environment; exact mechanism of action has not been elucidated

Pharmacodynamics/Kinetics Bacteriostatic or bactericidal depending on drug's concentration at infection site

Absorption: Well absorbed

Distribution: Widely into body tissues and fluids including liver, lung, and CSF

Relative diffusion from blood into CSF: Adequate with or without inflammation (exceeds usual MICs)

CSF:blood level ratio: Inflamed meninges: 100%

Protein binding: 50%

Metabolism: Hepatic

Half-life elimination: 9-10 hours

Time to peak, serum: Within 2 hours

Excretion: Urine (4% as unchanged drug)

Dosage Oral: Treatment of tuberculosis:

Note: Used as part of a multidrug regimen. Treatment regimens consist of an initial 2-month phase, followed by a continuation phase of 4 or 7 additional months; frequency of dosing may differ depending on phase of therapy.

Children:

Daily therapy: 15-30 mg/kg/day (maximum: 2 g/day)

Twice weekly directly observed therapy (DOT): 50 mg/kg/dose (maximum: 4 g/dose)

Adults (dosing is based on lean body weight):

Daily therapy: 15-30 mg/kg/day

40-55 kg: 1000 mg

56-75 kg: 1500 mg

76-90 kg: 2000 mg (maximum dose regardless of weight)

Twice weekly directly observed therapy (DOT): 50 mg/kg

40-55 kg: 2000 mg

56-75 kg: 3000 mg

76-90 kg: 4000 mg (maximum dose regardless of weight)

Three times/week DOT: 25-30 mg/kg (maximum: 2.5 g)

40-55 kg: 1500 mg

56-75 kg: 2500 mg

76-90 kg: 3000 mg (maximum dose regardless of weight)

Elderly: Start with a lower daily dose (15 mg/kg) and increase as tolerated.

Dosing adjustment in renal impairment: Cl_{cr} <50 mL/minute: Avoid use or reduce dose to 12-20 mg/kg/day

Avoid use in hemo- and peritoneal dialysis as well as continuous arteriovenous or venovenous hemofiltration.

Dosing adjustment in hepatic impairment: Reduce dose

Monitoring Parameters Periodic liver function tests, serum uric acid, sputum culture, chest x-ray 2-3 months into treatment and at completion

Test Interactions Reacts with Acetest® and Ketostix® to produce pinkish-brown color

Dosage Forms Excipient information presented when available (limited, particularly for generics); consult specific product labeling.

Tablet: 500 mg

Extemporaneous Preparations Pyrazinamide suspension can be compounded with simple syrup or 0.5% methylcellulose with simple syrup at a concentration of 100 mg/mL; the suspension is stable for 2 months at 4°C or 25°C when stored in glass or plastic bottles

To prepare pyrazinamide suspension in 0.5% methylcellulose with simple syrup: Crush 200 pyrazinamide 500 mg tablets and mix with a suspension containing 500 mL of 1% methylcellulose and 500 mL simple syrup. Add to this a suspension containing 140 crushed pyrazinamide tablets in 350 mL of 1% methylcellulose and 350 mL of simple syrup to make 1.7 L of suspension containing pyrazinamide 100 mg/mL in 0.5% methylcellulose with simple syrup.

Nahata MC, Morosco RS, and Peritre SP, "Stability of Pyrazinamide in Two Suspensions," *Am J Health Syst Pharm*, 1995, 52:1558-60.

◆ **Pyrazinoic Acid Amide** *see* Pyrazinamide *on page 1270*

Pyrethrins and Piperonyl Butoxide

(pye RE thrins & pi PER oh nil byo TOKS ide)

U.S. Brand Names A-200® Lice Treatment Kit [OTC]; A-200® Maximum Strength [OTC]; Licide® [OTC]; Pronto® Complete Lice Removal System [OTC]; Pronto® Plus Hair and Scalp Masque [OTC] [DSC]; Pronto® Plus Lice Killing Mousse Plus Vitamin E [OTC]; Pronto® Plus Lice Killing Mousse Shampoo Plus Natural Extracts and Oils [OTC]; Pronto® Plus Warm Oil Treatment and Conditioner [OTC]; RID® Maximum Strength [OTC]; Tisit® Blue Gel [OTC]; Tisit® [OTC]

Canadian Brand Names Pronto® Lice Control; R & C™ II; R & C™ Shampoo/Conditioner; RID® Mousse

Index Terms Piperonyl Butoxide and Pyrethrins

Pharmacologic Category Antiparasitic Agent, Topical; Pediculocide; Shampoo, Pediculocide

Use Treatment of *Pediculus humanus* infestations (head lice, body lice, pubic lice, and their eggs)

Pregnancy Risk Factor C

Dosage Application of pyrethrins:

Topical products:

Apply enough solution to completely wet infested area, including hair

Allow to remain on area for 10 minutes

Wash and rinse with large amounts of warm water.

Use fine-toothed comb to remove lice and eggs from hair

Shampoo hair to restore body and luster

Treatment may be repeated if necessary once in a 24-hour period

Repeat treatment in 7-10 days to kill newly hatched lice

Note: Keep out of eyes when rinsing hair; protect eyes with a wash cloth or towel

Solution for furniture, bedding: Spray on entire area to be treated; allow to dry before use. Intended for use on items which cannot be laundered or dry cleaned. **Not for use on humans or animals.**

Additional Information Complete prescribing information for this medication should be consulted for additional detail.

Dosage Forms Excipient information presented when available (limited, particularly for generics); consult specific product labeling. [DSC] = Discontinued product

Cream, topical:

Pronto® Plus Hair and Scalp Masque: Pyrethrins 0.33% and piperonyl butoxide 4% (60 g) [green cream shampoo; contains coconut and sesame oil; apple herb scent; packaged with nit removal comb] [DSC]

Foam, topical [mousse]:

RID® Maximum Strength: Pyrethrins 0.33% and piperonyl butoxide 4% (156 g) [packaged with nit removal comb] [DSC]

Gel, topical:

Tisit® Blue Gel: Pyrethrins 0.33% and piperonyl butoxide 3% (30 g)

Kit:

A-200® Lice Treatment Kit:

Shampoo: Pyrethrins 0.33% and piperonyl butoxide 4% (120 mL)

Solution [spray; for bedding; not for human or animal use]: Permethrin 0.5% (180 mL)

[packaged with nit removal comb]

Pronto® Complete Lice Removal System:

Shampoo: Pyrethrins 0.33% and piperonyl butoxide 4% (60 mL)

Solution, topical: Benzalkonium chloride 0.1% (60 mL) [lice egg remover antiseptic]

[packaged with household furniture spray and nit removal comb]

Liquid, topical:

Tisit®: Pyrethrins 0.33% and piperonyl butoxide 2% (60 mL, 120 mL) [packaged with nit removal comb]

Oil, topical:

Pronto® Plus Warm Oil Treatment and Conditioner: Pyrethrins 0.33% and piperonyl butoxide 4% (36 mL) [fruity herbal scent; packaged with nit removal comb]

Shampoo: Pyrethrins 0.33% and piperonyl butoxide 4% (60 mL, 120 mL)

A-200® Maximum Strength: Pyrethrins 0.33% and piperonyl butoxide 4% (60 mL, 120 mL) [contains benzyl alcohol; packaged with nit removal comb]

Licide®: Pyrethrins 0.33% and piperonyl butoxide 4% (120 mL) [packaged with nit removal comb; also available in a kit containing shampoo, household spray, and nit removal comb]

Pronto® Plus Lice Killing Mousse Shampoo Plus Natural Extracts and Oils: Pyrethrins 0.33% and piperonyl butoxide 4% (60 mL) [packaged with nit removal comb]

Pronto® Plus Lice Killing Mousse Shampoo Plus Vitamin E: Pyrethrins 0.33% and piperonyl butoxide 4% (120 mL) [blue mousse shampoo; contains vitamin E; packaged with nit removal comb]

RID® Maximum Strength: Pyrethrins 0.33% and piperonyl butoxide 4% (60 mL, 120 mL, 180 mL, 240 mL) [packaged with nit removal comb; also available in a kit containing shampoo, gel, and furniture spray]

Tisit®: Pyrethrins 0.33% and piperonyl butoxide 3% (60 mL, 120 mL) [also available in a kit containing shampoo, nit removal comb, and furniture spray]

Solution [spray; for furniture, garments, bedding; not for human or animal use]:

Tisit®: Pyrethrins 0.4% and piperonyl butoxide 2% (150 mL)

◆ **Pyri-500 [OTC]** *see* Pyridoxine *on page* 1273

◆ **2-Pyridine Aldoxime Methochloride** *see* Pralidoxime *on page* 1223

◆ **Pyridium®** *see* Phenazopyridine *on page* 1177

Pyridostigmine (peer id oh STIG meen)

U.S. Brand Names Mestinon®; Mestinon® Timespan®; Regonol®

Canadian Brand Names Mestinon®; Mestinon®-SR

Index Terms Pyridostigmine Bromide

Pharmacologic Category Acetylcholinesterase Inhibitor

Use Symptomatic treatment of myasthenia gravis; antidote for nondepolarizing neuromuscular blockers

Military use: Pretreatment for Soman nerve gas exposure

Pregnancy Risk Factor B

Pregnancy Considerations Safety has not been established for use during pregnancy. The potential benefit to the mother should outweigh the potential risk to the fetus. When pyridostigmine is needed in myasthenic mothers, giving dose parenterally 1 hour before completion of the second stage of labor may facilitate delivery and protect the neonate during the immediate postnatal state.

Lactation Enters breast milk/compatible

Medication Safety Issues

Sound-alike/look-alike issues:

Pyridostigmine may be confused with physostigmine

Mestinon® may be confused with Metatensin®

Regonol® may be confused with Reglan®, Renagel®

Contraindications Hypersensitivity to pyridostigmine, bromides, or any component of the formulation; GI or GU obstruction

Warnings/Precautions Use with caution in patients with epilepsy, asthma, bradycardia, hyperthyroidism, cardiac arrhythmias, or peptic ulcer; adequate facilities should be available for cardiopulmonary resuscitation when testing and adjusting dose for myasthenia gravis; have atropine and epinephrine ready to treat hypersensitivity reactions; overdosage may result in cholinergic crisis, this must be distinguished from myasthenic crisis; anticholinesterase insensitivity can develop for brief or prolonged periods. Regonol® injection contains 1% benzyl alcohol as the preservative (not intended for use in newborns). **[U.S. Boxed Warning]: Regonol® injection must be administered by trained personnel.**

Adverse Reactions Frequency not defined.

Cardiovascular: Arrhythmias (especially bradycardia), AV block, cardiac arrest, decreased carbon monoxide, flushing, hypotension, nodal rhythm, nonspecific ECG changes, syncope, tachycardia

Central nervous system: Convulsions, dizziness, drowsiness, dysphonia, headache, loss of consciousness

Dermatologic: Skin rash, thrombophlebitis (I.V.), urticaria

Gastrointestinal: Abdominal pain, diarrhea, dysphagia, flatulence, hyperperistalsis, nausea, salivation, stomach cramps, vomiting

Genitourinary: Urinary urgency

Neuromuscular & skeletal: Arthralgia, dysarthria, fasciculations, muscle cramps, myalgia, spasms, weakness

Ocular: Amblyopia, lacrimation, small pupils

Respiratory: Bronchial secretions increased, bronchiolar constriction, bronchospasm, dyspnea, laryngospasm, respiratory arrest, respiratory depression, respiratory muscle paralysis

Miscellaneous: Allergic reactions, anaphylaxis, diaphoresis increased

Drug Interactions

Avoid Concomitant Use There are no known interactions where it is recommended to avoid concomitant use.

Increased Effect/Toxicity

Pyridostigmine may increase the levels/effects of: Beta-Blockers; Cholinergic Agonists; Succinylcholine

The levels/effects of Pyridostigmine may be increased by: Corticosteroids (Systemic); Ginkgo Biloba

Decreased Effect

Pyridostigmine may decrease the levels/effects of: Neuromuscular-Blocking Agents (Nondepolarizing)

The levels/effects of Pyridostigmine may be decreased by: Methocarbamol

Stability

Injection: Protect from light.

Tablet:

30 mg: Store under refrigeration at 2°C to 8°C (36°F to 46°F). Protect from light. Stable at room temperature for up to 3 months.

Mestinon®: Store at 25°C (77°F). Protect from moisture.

Mechanism of Action Inhibits destruction of acetylcholine by acetylcholinesterase which facilitates transmission of impulses across myoneural junction

Pharmacodynamics/Kinetics

Onset of action: Oral, I.M.: 15-30 minutes; I.V. injection: 2-5 minutes

Duration: Oral: Up to 6-8 hours (due to slow absorption); I.V.: 2-3 hours

Absorption: Oral: Very poor

Distribution: 19 ± 12 L

Metabolism: Hepatic

Bioavailability: 10% to 20%

Half-life elimination: 1-2 hours; Renal failure: ≤6 hours

Excretion: Urine (80% to 90% as unchanged drug)

Dosage

Myasthenia gravis:

Oral:

Children: 7 mg/kg/24 hours divided into 5-6 doses

Adults: Highly individualized dosing ranges: 60-1500 mg/day, usually 600 mg/day divided into 5-6 doses, spaced to provide maximum relief

Sustained release formulation: Highly individualized dosing ranges: 180-540 mg once or twice daily (doses separated by at least 6 hours); **Note:** Most clinicians reserve sustained release dosage form for bedtime dose only.

I.M., slow I.V. push:
Children: 0.05-0.15 mg/kg/dose
Adults: To supplement oral dosage pre- and post-operatively during labor and postpartum, during myasthenic crisis, or when oral therapy is impractical: ~1/30th of oral dose; observe patient closely for cholinergic reactions
or
I.V. infusion: Initial: 2 mg/hour with gradual titration in increments of 0.5-1 mg/hour, up to a maximum rate of 4 mg/hour

Pretreatment for Soman nerve gas exposure (military use): Oral: Adults: 30 mg every 8 hours beginning several hours prior to exposure; discontinue at first sign of nerve agent exposure, then begin atropine and pralidoxime

Reversal of nondepolarizing muscle relaxants: **Note:** Atropine sulfate (0.6-1.2 mg) I.V. immediately prior to pyridostigmine to minimize side effects: I.V.:
Children: Dosing range: 0.1-0.25 mg/kg/dose*
Adults: 0.1-0.25 mg/kg/dose; 10-20 mg is usually sufficient*
*Full recovery usually occurs ≤15 minutes, but ≥30 minutes may be required

Dosage adjustment in renal dysfunction: Lower dosages may be required due to prolonged elimination; no specific recommendations have been published

Administration Do **not** crush sustained release tablet.

Monitoring Parameters Observe for cholinergic reactions, particularly when administered I.V.

Test Interactions Increased aminotransferase [ALT/AST] (S), increased amylase (S)

Dosage Forms Excipient information presented when available (limited, particularly for generics); consult specific product labeling.
Injection, solution, as bromide:
Regonol®: 5 mg/mL (2 mL) [contains benzyl alcohol]
Syrup, as bromide:
Mestinon®: 60 mg/5 mL (480 mL) [raspberry flavor; contains alcohol 5%, sodium benzoate]
Tablet, as bromide: 60 mg
Mestinon®: 60 mg
Tablet, sustained release, as bromide:
Mestinon® Timespan®: 180 mg

◆ **Pyridostigmine Bromide** *see* Pyridostigmine *on page 1272*

Pyridoxine (peer i DOKS een)

U.S. Brand Names Aminoxin [OTC]; Pyri-500 [OTC]

Index Terms Pyridoxine Hydrochloride; Vitamin B_6

Pharmacologic Category Vitamin, Water Soluble

Additional Appendix Information
Guidelines for the Prevention of Opportunistic Infections in HIV Infected Persons *on page 1740*

Use Prevention and treatment of vitamin B_6 deficiency, pyridoxine-dependent seizures in infants

Unlabeled/Investigational Use Treatment and prophylaxis of neurological toxicities (ie, seizures, coma) associated with isoniazid, hydrazine, and Gyromitrin-containing mushroom (false morel) overdose/toxicity

Pregnancy Risk Factor A/C (dose exceeding RDA recommendation)

Pregnancy Considerations Crosses the placenta; available evidence suggests safe use during pregnancy

Lactation Enters breast milk/compatible

Medication Safety Issues
Sound-alike/look-alike issues:
Pyridoxine may be confused with paroxetine, pralidoxime, Pyridium®

Contraindications Hypersensitivity to pyridoxine or any component of the formulation

Warnings/Precautions Severe, permanent peripheral neuropathies have been reported; neurotoxicity is more common with long-term administration of large doses (>2 g/day). Dependence and withdrawal may occur with doses >200 mg/day. Single vitamin deficiency is rare; evaluate for other deficiencies. Some parenteral products contain aluminum; use caution in patients with impaired renal function and neonates. High doses may be required to reverse neurological toxicity secondary to isoniazid toxicity. Emergency departments should ensure an adequate supply in the event of an acute isoniazid overdose.

Adverse Reactions Frequency not defined.
Central nervous system: Headache, seizure (following very large I.V. doses)
Endocrine & metabolic: Acidosis
Gastrointestinal: Nausea
Hepatic: Increased AST
Neuromuscular & skeletal: Neuropathy, paresthesia
Miscellaneous: Allergic reactions

Drug Interactions

Avoid Concomitant Use There are no known interactions where it is recommended to avoid concomitant use.

Increased Effect/Toxicity There are no known significant interactions involving an increase in effect.

Decreased Effect
Pyridoxine may decrease the levels/effects of: Altretamine; Barbiturates; Levodopa; Phenytoin

Stability Protect from light.

Mechanism of Action Precursor to pyridoxal, which functions in the metabolism of proteins, carbohydrates, and fats; pyridoxal also aids in the release of liver and muscle-stored glycogen and in the synthesis of GABA (within the central nervous system) and heme

Pharmacodynamics/Kinetics
Absorption: Enteral, parenteral: Well absorbed
Metabolism: Via 4-pyridoxic acid (active form) and other metabolites
Half-life elimination: 15-20 days
Excretion: Urine

Dosage
Recommended daily allowance (RDA):
Children:
1-3 years: 0.9 mg
4-6 years: 1.3 mg
7-10 years: 1.6 mg
Adults:
Male: 1.7-2.0 mg
Female: 1.4-1.6 mg
Pyridoxine-dependent Infants:
Oral: 2-100 mg/day
I.M., I.V., SubQ: 10-100 mg
Dietary deficiency: Oral:
Children: 5-25 mg/24 hours for 3 weeks, then 1.5-2.5 mg/day in multiple vitamin product
Adults: 10-20 mg/day for 3 weeks
Drug-induced neuritis (eg, isoniazid, hydralazine, penicillamine, cycloserine): Oral:
Children:
Treatment: 10-50 mg/24 hours
Prophylaxis: 1-2 mg/kg/24 hours
Adults:
Treatment: 100-200 mg/24 hours
Prophylaxis: 25-100 mg/24 hours
Treatment of seizures and/or coma from acute isoniazid toxicity (unlabeled use): I.V.: Children and Adults:
Acute ingestion of known amount: A total dose of pyridoxine equal to the amount of isoniazid ingested should be given (ie, if 9 g of isoniazid were ingested, give a total dose of 9 g pyridoxine). Administer at a rate

of 1 g/minute if actively seizing; administer over 30 minutes if not actively seizing.

Acute ingestion of unknown amount: 5 g given at a rate of 1 g/minute; repeat doses (every 5-10 minutes) may be needed for persistent seizure activity or CNS toxicity

Treatment of acute hydrazine toxicity (unlabeled use; Nagappan, 2000): I.V.: Adults: A total dose of 25 mg/kg should be given over 15-30 minutes

Treatment of seizures from acute Gyromitrin-containing mushroom toxicity (unlabeled use; Diaz, 2005): I.V.: Children and Adults: 25 mg/kg over 15-30 minutes; repeat dose as needed to control seizures

Administration Burning may occur at the injection site after I.M. or SubQ administration; seizures have occurred following I.V. administration of very large doses. In patients with active seizures, administer dose at a rate of 1 g/minute; for patients without active seizures, administer dose over 15-30 minutes. If the parenteral formulation is not available, anecdotal reports suggest that pyridoxine tablets may be crushed and made into a slurry and given at the same dose. However, oral administration is not recommended for acutely poisoned patients with seizure activity.

Monitoring Parameters For treatment of isoniazid, hydrazine, or Gyromitrin-containing mushroom toxicity, anion gap, arterial blood gases, electrolytes, neurological exam, seizure activity

Reference Range Over 50 ng/mL (SI: 243 nmol/L) (varies considerably with method). A broad range is ~25-80 ng/mL (SI: 122-389 nmol/L). HPLC method for pyridoxal phosphate has normal range of 3.5-18 ng/mL (SI: 17-88 nmol/L).

Test Interactions Urobilinogen

Dosage Forms Excipient information presented when available (limited, particularly for generics); consult specific product labeling.

Capsule, as hydrochloride: 50 mg, 250 mg

Aminoxin: 20 mg

Injection, solution, as hydrochloride: 100 mg/mL (1 mL)

Liquid, oral, as hydrochloride: 200 mg/5 mL (120 mL)

Tablet, as hydrochloride: 25 mg, 50 mg, 100 mg, 250 mg, 500 mg

Tablet, sustained release, as hydrochloride:

Pyri-500: 500 mg

Extemporaneous Preparations A 1 mg/mL oral solution was stable for 30 days when refrigerated when compounded as follows:

Withdraw 100 mg (1 mL of a 100 mg/mL injection) from a vial with a needle and syringe, add to 99 mL of simple syrup in an amber bottle

Keep in refrigerator

Nahata MC and Hipple TF, *Pediatric Drug Formulations*, 3rd ed, Cincinnati, OH: Harvey Whitney Books Co, 1997.

◆ **Pyridoxine, Folic Acid, and Cyanocobalamin** *see* Folic Acid, Cyanocobalamin, and Pyridoxine *on page 655*

◆ **Pyridoxine Hydrochloride** *see* Pyridoxine *on page 1273*

◆ **Pyrilamine Tannate, Guaifenesin, and Phenylephrine Tannate** *see* Phenylephrine, Pyrilamine, and Guaifenesin *on page 1186*

Pyrimethamine (peer i METH a meen)

U.S. Brand Names Daraprim®

Canadian Brand Names Daraprim®

Pharmacologic Category Antimalarial Agent

Additional Appendix Information

Guidelines for the Prevention of Opportunistic Infections in HIV Infected Persons *on page 1740*

Malaria Treatment *on page 1770*

Use Prophylaxis of malaria due to susceptible strains of plasmodia; used in conjunction with quinine and sulfadiazine for the treatment of uncomplicated attacks of chloroquine-resistant *P. falciparum* malaria; used in conjunction with fast-acting schizonticide to initiate transmission control and suppression cure; synergistic combination with sulfonamide in treatment of toxoplasmosis

Pregnancy Risk Factor C

Pregnancy Considerations There are no adequate or well-controlled studies in pregnant women. Teratogenicity has been reported in animal studies. If administered during pregnancy (ie, for toxoplasmosis), supplementation of folate is strongly recommended. Pregnancy should be avoided during therapy.

Lactation Enters breast milk/not recommended (AAP rates "compatible")

Medication Safety Issues

Sound-alike/look-alike issues:

Daraprim® may be confused with Dantrium®, Daranide®

Contraindications Hypersensitivity to pyrimethamine or any component of the formulation; chloroguanide; resistant malaria; megaloblastic anemia secondary to folate deficiency

Warnings/Precautions When used for more than 3-4 days, it may be advisable to administer leucovorin to prevent hematologic complications; monitor CBC and platelet counts every 2 weeks; use with caution in patients with impaired renal or hepatic function or with possible G6PD. Use caution in patients with seizure disorders or possible folate deficiency (eg, malabsorption syndrome, pregnancy, alcoholism).

Adverse Reactions Frequency not defined.

Cardiovascular: Arrhythmias (large doses)

Central nervous system: Depression, fever, insomnia, lightheadedness, malaise, seizure

Dermatologic: Abnormal skin pigmentation, dermatitis, erythema multiforme, rash, Stevens-Johnson syndrome, toxic epidermal necrolysis

Gastrointestinal: Anorexia, abdominal cramps, atrophic glossitis, diarrhea, vomiting, xerostomia,

Hematologic: Megaloblastic anemia, leukopenia, pancytopenia, thrombocytopenia, pulmonary eosinophilia

Genitourinary: Hematuria

Miscellaneous: Anaphylaxis

Drug Interactions

Metabolism/Transport Effects Inhibits CYP2C9 (moderate), 2D6 (moderate)

Avoid Concomitant Use There are no known interactions where it is recommended to avoid concomitant use.

Increased Effect/Toxicity

Pyrimethamine may increase the levels/effects of: Antipsychotic Agents (Phenothiazines); CYP2C9 Substrates (High risk); CYP2D6 Substrates; Fesoterodine; Nebivolol; Tamoxifen

Decreased Effect

Pyrimethamine may decrease the levels/effects of: Codeine; TraMADol

The levels/effects of Pyrimethamine may be decreased by: Methylfolate

Stability Store at 15°C to 25°C (59°F to 77°F). Protect from light.

Mechanism of Action Inhibits parasitic dihydrofolate reductase, resulting in inhibition of vital tetrahydrofolic acid synthesis

Pharmacodynamics/Kinetics

Onset of action: ~1 hour

Absorption: Well absorbed

Distribution: Widely, mainly in blood cells, kidneys, lungs, liver, and spleen; crosses into CSF; crosses placenta; enters breast milk

Protein binding: 80% to 87%

Metabolism: Hepatic
Half-life elimination: 80-95 hours
Time to peak, serum: 1.5-8 hours
Excretion: Urine (20% to 30% as unchanged drug)

Dosage

Malaria chemoprophylaxis (for areas where chloroquine-resistant *P. falciparum* exists): Begin prophylaxis 2 weeks before entering endemic area:
- Children: 0.5 mg/kg once weekly; not to exceed 25 mg/dose
- **or**
- Children:
  - <4 years: 6.25 mg once weekly
  - 4-10 years: 12.5 mg once weekly
- Children >10 years and Adults: 25 mg once weekly
- Dosage should be continued for all age groups for at least 6-10 weeks after leaving endemic areas

Chloroquine-resistant *P. falciparum* malaria (when used in conjunction with quinine and sulfadiazine):
- Children:
  - <10 kg: 6.25 mg/day once daily for 3 days
  - 10-20 kg: 12.5 mg/day once daily for 3 days
  - 20-40 kg: 25 mg/day once daily for 3 days
- Adults: 25 mg twice daily for 3 days

Toxoplasmosis:
- Infants (congenital toxoplasmosis): Oral: 1 mg/kg once daily for 6 months with sulfadiazine then every other month with sulfa, alternating with spiramycin.
- Children: Loading dose: 2 mg/kg/day divided into 2 equal daily doses for 1-3 days (maximum: 100 mg/day) followed by 1 mg/kg/day divided into 2 doses for 4 weeks; maximum: 25 mg/day
  - With sulfadiazine or trisulfapyrimidines: 2 mg/kg/day divided every 12 hours for 3 days, followed by 1 mg/kg/day once daily or divided twice daily for 4 weeks given with trisulfapyrimidines or sulfadiazine
- Adults: 50-75 mg/day together with 1-4 g of a sulfonamide for 1-3 weeks depending on patient's tolerance and response, then reduce dose by 50% and continue for 4-5 weeks **or** 25-50 mg/day for 3-4 weeks

Prophylaxis for first episode of *Toxoplasma gondii*:
- Children ≥1 month of age: 1 mg/kg/day once daily with dapsone, plus oral folinic acid 5 mg every 3 days
- Adolescents and Adults: 50 mg once weekly with dapsone, plus oral folinic acid 25 mg once weekly

Prophylaxis to prevent recurrence of *Toxoplasma gondii*:
- Children ≥1 month of age: 1 mg/kg/day once daily given with sulfadiazine or clindamycin, plus oral folinic acid 5 mg every 3 days
- Adolescents and Adults: 25-50 mg once daily in combination with sulfadiazine or clindamycin, plus oral folinic acid 10-25 mg daily; atovaquone plus oral folinic acid has also been used in combination with pyrimethamine.

Administration Administer with meals to minimize GI distress.

Monitoring Parameters CBC, including platelet counts

Additional Information Leucovorin may be administered in a dosage of 3-9 mg/day for 3 days or 5 mg every 3 days or as required to reverse symptoms of or to prevent hematologic problems due to folic acid deficiency

Dosage Forms Excipient information presented when available (limited, particularly for generics); consult specific product labeling.
Tablet: 25 mg

Extemporaneous Preparations Pyrimethamine tablets may be crushed to prepare oral suspensions of the drug in water, cherry syrup or sucrose-containing solutions at a concentration of 1 mg/mL; stable at room temperature for 5-7 days

AHFS Drug Information, McEvoy G, ed, Bethesda, MD: American Society of Health-System Pharmacists, 1996.

- ◆ **Pyrimethamine and Sulfadoxine** *see* Sulfadoxine and Pyrimethamine *on page 1407*
- ◆ **QDALL® [DSC]** *see* Chlorpheniramine and Pseudoephedrine *on page 310*
- ◆ **Quadrivalent Human Papillomavirus Vaccine** *see* Papillomavirus (Types 6, 11, 16, 18) Vaccine (Human, Recombinant) *on page 1142*
- ◆ **Quad Tann®** *see* Chlorpheniramine, Ephedrine, Phenylephrine, and Carbetapentane *on page 311*
- ◆ **Quad Tann® Pediatric** *see* Chlorpheniramine, Ephedrine, Phenylephrine, and Carbetapentane *on page 311*
- ◆ **Qualaquin™** *see* QuiNINE *on page 1282*
- ◆ **Quartuss™** *see* Dextromethorphan, Chlorpheniramine, Phenylephrine, and Guaifenesin *on page 434*
- ◆ **Quasense™** *see* Ethinyl Estradiol and Levonorgestrel *on page 577*
- ◆ **Quaternium-18 Bentonite** *see* Bentoquatam *on page 183*

Quazepam (KWAZ e pam)

U.S. Brand Names Doral®
Canadian Brand Names Doral®
Pharmacologic Category Benzodiazepine
Additional Appendix Information
Benzodiazepines *on page 1646*
Use Treatment of insomnia
Restrictions C-IV
Pregnancy Risk Factor X
Medication Safety Issues
Sound-alike/look-alike issues:
Quazepam may be confused with oxazepam

Dosage Adults: Oral: Initial: 15 mg at bedtime; in some patients, the dose may be reduced to 7.5 mg after a few nights
Elderly: Dosing should be cautious; begin at lower end of dosing range (ie, 7.5 mg)
Dosing adjustment in hepatic impairment: Dose reduction may be necessary

Additional Information Complete prescribing information for this medication should be consulted for additional detail.

Dosage Forms Excipient information presented when available (limited, particularly for generics); consult specific product labeling.
Tablet:
Doral®: 15 mg

- ◆ **Quelicin®** *see* Succinylcholine *on page 1402*
- ◆ **Questran®** *see* Cholestyramine Resin *on page 319*
- ◆ **Questran® Light** *see* Cholestyramine Resin *on page 319*
- ◆ **Questran® Light Sugar Free (Can)** *see* Cholestyramine Resin *on page 319*

QUEtiapine (kwe TYE a peen)

U.S. Brand Names Seroquel®; Seroquel® XR
Canadian Brand Names Apo-Quetiapine; CO-Quetiapine; Gen-Quetiapine; Novo-Quetiapine; PMS-Quetiapine; ratio-Quetiapine; Riva-Quetiapine; Sandoz-Quetiapine; Seroquel®; Seroquel® XR
Index Terms Quetiapine Fumarate
Pharmacologic Category Antipsychotic Agent, Atypical
Additional Appendix Information
Antipsychotic Agents *on page 1644*
Use Treatment of schizophrenia; treatment of acute manic episodes associated with bipolar I disorder (as monotherapy or in combination with lithium or divalproex);

maintenance treatment of bipolar I disorder (in combination with lithium or divalproex); treatment of depressive episodes associated with bipolar disorder

Unlabeled/Investigational Use Autism, psychosis (children); psychosis/agitation related to Alzheimer's dementia

Restrictions An FDA-approved medication guide concerning the use of antidepressants in children, adolescents, and young adults must be distributed when dispensing an outpatient prescription (new or refill) where this medication is to be used without direct supervision of a healthcare provider. Medication guides are available at http://www.fda.gov/cder/drug/antidepressants/MG_template.pdf. Dispense to parents or guardians of children and adolescents receiving this medication.

Pregnancy Risk Factor C

Pregnancy Considerations Healthcare providers are encouraged to enroll women 18-45 years of age exposed to quetiapine during pregnancy in the Atypical Antipsychotics Pregnancy Registry (1-866-961-2388).

Lactation Enters breast milk/use caution

Medication Safety Issues

Sound-alike/look-alike issues:

QUEtiapine may be confused with OLANZapine

Seroquel® may be confused with Serentil®, Serzone®, Sinequan®

Contraindications

U.S. labeling: There are no contraindications listed in manufacturers labeling.

Canadian labeling: Hypersensitivity to quetiapine or any component of the formulation

Warnings/Precautions [U.S. Boxed Warning]: Antidepressants increase the risk of suicidal thinking and behavior in children, adolescents, and young adults (18-24 years of age) with major depressive disorder (MDD) and other psychiatric disorders; consider risk prior to prescribing. Short-term studies did not show an increased risk in patients >24 years of age and showed a decreased risk in patients ≥65 years. Closely monitor all patients for clinical worsening, suicidality, or unusual changes in behavior; particularly during the initial 1-2 months of therapy or during periods of dosage adjustments (increased or decreases); the patient's family or caregiver should be instructed to closely observe the patient and communicate condition with healthcare provider. A medication guide concerning the use of antidepressants should be dispensed with each prescription. **Quetiapine is not FDA approved for use in children.**

[U.S. Boxed Warning]: Elderly patients with dementia-related psychosis treated with antipsychotic drugs are at an increased risk of death compared to placebo. An increased incidence of cerebrovascular adverse events (including fatalities) has been reported in elderly patients with dementia-related psychosis. Quetiapine is not approved for this indication.

May be sedating, use with caution in disorders where CNS depression is a feature. Use with caution in Parkinson's disease. May induce orthostatic hypotension associated with dizziness, tachycardia, and, in some cases, syncope, especially during the initial dose titration period. Should be used with particular caution in patients with known cardiovascular disease (history of MI or ischemic heart disease, heart failure, or conduction abnormalities), cerebrovascular disease, or conditions that predispose to hypotension. Esophageal dysmotility and aspiration have been associated with antipsychotic use; use with caution in patients at risk of aspiration pneumonia (eg, Alzheimer's disease). Development of cataracts has been observed in animal studies, therefore, lens examinations should be made upon initiation of therapy and every 6 months thereafter. Leukopenia, neutropenia, and agranulocytosis (sometimes fatal) have been reported in clinical trials and postmarketing reports; presence of risk factors (eg, pre-existing low WBC or history of drug-induced leuko-/neutropenia) should prompt periodic blood count assessment and discontinuation at first signs of blood dyscrasias.

Due to anticholinergic effects, use with caution in patients with decreased gastrointestinal motility, urinary retention, BPH, xerostomia, visual problems, narrow-angle glaucoma (screening is recommended), and myasthenia gravis. Relative to other antipsychotics, quetiapine has a moderate potency of cholinergic blockade. May cause extrapyramidal symptoms (EPS), pseudoparkinsonism, and/or tardive dyskinesia. Risk of dystonia (and probably other EPS) may be greater with increased doses, use of conventional antipsychotics, males, and younger patients. Impaired core body temperature regulation may occur; caution with strenuous exercise, heat exposure, dehydration, and concomitant medication possessing anticholinergic effects. Neuroleptic malignant syndrome (NMS) is a potentially fatal symptom complex that has been reported in association with administration of antipsychotic drugs. Clinical manifestations of NMS are hyperpyrexia, muscle rigidity, altered mental status, and evidence of autonomic instability (irregular pulse or blood pressure, tachycardia, diaphoresis, and cardiac dysrhythmia). Management of NMS should include immediate discontinuation of antipsychotic drugs and other drugs not essential to concurrent therapy, intensive symptomatic treatment and medication monitoring, and treatment of any concomitant medical problems for which specific treatment are available.

Use caution in patients with a history of seizures. May cause decreases in total free thyroxine, elevations of liver enzymes, cholesterol levels, and/or triglyceride increases.

May cause hyperglycemia; in some cases may be extreme and associated with ketoacidosis, hyperosmolar coma, or death. Use with caution in patients with diabetes or other disorders of glucose regulation; monitor for worsening of glucose control. Significant weight gain has been observed with antipsychotic therapy; incidence varies with product. Monitor waist circumference and BMI. Patients using immediate release tablets may be switched to extended release tablets at the same total daily dose taken once daily. Dosage adjustments may be necessary based on response and tolerability. May cause withdrawal symptoms (rare) with abrupt cessation; gradually taper dose during discontinuation.

Adverse Reactions Actual frequency may be dependant upon dose and/or indication. Unless otherwise noted, frequency of adverse effects is reported for the immediate release oral formulation in adults.

>10%:

Central nervous system: Somnolence (18% to 34%; extended release ≤52%), sedation (30%), headache (17% to 21%), agitation (6% to 20%), dizziness (9% to 18%), extrapyramidal symptoms (8% to 12%)

Endocrine & metabolic: Triglycerides increased (14% to 23%), cholesterol increased (9% to 16%)

Gastrointestinal: Xerostomia (9% to 44%), weight gain (dose-related; 5% to 23%), appetite increased (5%; extended release <5% to 12%)

1% to 10%:

Cardiovascular: Orthostatic hypotension (4% to 7%), tachycardia (6%), syncope (extended release <5%), palpitation (≥1%), peripheral edema (≥1%)

Central nervous system: Fatigue (10%), pain (7%), lethargy (5%), akathisia (extended release <5%), dystonia (extended release <5%), tardive dyskinesia (extended release <5%), anxiety (4%), fever (2%)

Dermatologic: Rash (4%)

Endocrine & metabolic: Hyperglycemia (≥200 mg/dL post glucose challenge or fasting glucose ≥126 mg/dL, 4%)

Gastrointestinal: Constipation (8% to 10%), dyspepsia (dose-related; 5% to 7%), abdominal pain (dose-related; 4% to 7%), vomiting (5% to 6%), drooling (extended release <5%), dysphagia (extended release <5%), gastroenteritis (2%), anorexia (≥1%)

Hematologic: Leukopenia (≥1%)

Hepatic: Transaminases increased (1% to 6%), GGT increased (1%)

Neuromuscular & skeletal: Weakness (5% to 10%), tremor (8%), back pain (3% to 5%), dysarthria (≥1%), hypertonia (≥1%)

Ocular: Blurred vision (extended release <5%), amblyopia (2%)

Respiratory: Pharyngitis (4% to 6%), nasal congestion (5%), rhinitis (3%), cough (≥1%), dyspnea (≥1%)

Miscellaneous: Diaphoresis (≥1%), flu-like syndrome (≥1%)

<1% (Limited to important or life-threatening): Abnormal dreams, acute renal failure, agranulocytosis, alkaline phosphatase increased, amnesia, anaphylactic reaction, anaphylaxis, anemia, angina, asthma, bradycardia, bundle branch block, cardiomyopathy, cataract formation, cerebral ischemia, cerebrovascular accident, CHF, confusion, creatinine increased, dehydration, diabetes mellitus, dysuria, eosinophilia, epistaxis, exfoliative dermatitis, hallucinations, hypoglycemia, hyper-/hypothyroidism, hypersensitivity, hypokalemia, hyponatremia, involuntary movements, leukocytosis, lymphadenopathy, myocarditis, neuroleptic malignant syndrome, neutropenia, pancreatitis, pneumonia, priapism, QRS duration increased, QT prolongation, rectal bleeding, restless leg syndrome, rhabdomyolysis, seizure, SIADH, Stevens-Johnson syndrome, ST segment elevation, suicide attempt, thrombocytopenia, tinnitus, T-wave abnormal, T-wave inversion, urinary retention, vertigo

Drug Interactions

Metabolism/Transport Effects

Substrate of CYP2D6 (minor), 3A4 (major)

Avoid Concomitant Use

Avoid concomitant use of QUEtiapine with any of the following: Nilotinib; Thioridazine; Ziprasidone

Increased Effect/Toxicity

QUEtiapine may increase the levels/effects of: Alcohol (Ethyl); Anticholinergics; CNS Depressants; QTc-Prolonging Agents; Thioridazine; Ziprasidone

The levels/effects of QUEtiapine may be increased by: Acetylcholinesterase Inhibitors (Central); Alfuzosin; Ciprofloxacin; CYP3A4 Inhibitors (Moderate); CYP3A4 Inhibitors (Strong); Dasatinib; Gadobutrol; Lithium formulations; Nilotinib; Pramlintide; Tetrabenazine

Decreased Effect

QUEtiapine may decrease the levels/effects of: Amphetamines; Anti-Parkinson's Agents (Dopamine Agonist)

The levels/effects of QUEtiapine may be decreased by: CYP3A4 Inducers (Strong); Deferasirox; Herbs (CYP3A4 Inducers); Lithium formulations; Phenytoin

Ethanol/Nutrition/Herb Interactions

Ethanol: Avoid ethanol (may cause excessive impairment in cognition/motor function).

Food: In healthy volunteers, administration of quetiapine (immediate release) with food resulted in an increase in the peak serum concentration and AUC (each by ~15%) compared to the fasting state. Administration of the extended release with a high-fat meal (~800-1000 calories) resulted in an increase in peak serum concentration by 44% to 52% and AUC by 20% to 22% for the 50 mg and 300 mg tablets; administration with a light meal had no significant effect on the C_{max} or AUC.

Herb/Nutraceutical: St John's wort may decrease quetiapine levels. Avoid valerian, St John's wort, kava kava, gotu kola (may increase CNS depression).

Stability Store at controlled room temperature of 25°C (77°F).

Mechanism of Action Quetiapine is a dibenzothiazepine atypical antipsychotic. It has been proposed that this drug's antipsychotic activity is mediated through a combination of dopamine type 2 (D_2) and serotonin type 2 ($5\text{-}HT_2$) antagonism. It is an antagonist at multiple neurotransmitter receptors in the brain: serotonin $5\text{-}HT_{1A}$ and $5\text{-}HT_2$, dopamine D_1 and D_2, histamine H_1, and adrenergic alpha$_1$- and alpha$_2$- receptors; but appears to have no appreciable affinity at cholinergic muscarinic and benzodiazepine receptors.

Antagonism at receptors other than dopamine and $5\text{-}HT_2$ with similar receptor affinities may explain some of the other effects of quetiapine. The drug's antagonism of histamine H_1-receptors may explain the somnolence observed with it. The drug's antagonism of adrenergic alpha$_1$-receptors may explain the orthostatic hypotension observed with it.

Pharmacodynamics/Kinetics

Absorption: Rapidly absorbed following oral administration

Distribution: V_d: 6-14 L/kg; V_{dss}: ~2 days

Protein binding, plasma: 83%

Metabolism: Primarily hepatic; via CYP3A4; forms the metabolite N-desalkyl quetiapine (active) and two inactive metabolites

Bioavailability: 9% ± 4%; tablet is 100% bioavailable relative to solution

Half-life elimination:

Mean: Terminal: Quetiapine: ~6 hours; Extended release: ~7 hours

Metabolite: N-desalkyl quetiapine: 9-12 hours

Time to peak, plasma: Immediate release: 1.5 hours; Extended release: 6 hours

Excretion: Urine (73% as metabolites, <1% as unchanged drug); feces (20%)

Dosage Oral:

Children and Adolescents:

Autism (unlabeled use): 100-350 mg/day (1.6-5.2 mg/kg/day)

Psychosis and mania (unlabeled use): Initial: 25 mg twice daily; titrate as necessary to 450 mg/day

Adults:

Bipolar disorder:

Depression:

Immediate release tablet: Initial: 50 mg/day the first day; increase to 100 mg/day on day 2, further increasing by 100 mg/day each day until a target dose of 300 mg/day is reached by day 4. Further increases up to 600 mg/day by day 8 have been evaluated in clinical trials, but no additional anti-depressant efficacy was noted.

Extended release tablet: Initial: 50 mg/day the first day; increase to 100 mg on day 2, further increasing by 100 mg/day each day until a target dose of 300 mg/day is reached by day 4.

Mania:

Immediate release tablet: Initial: 50 mg twice daily on day 1, increase dose in increments of 100 mg/day to 200 mg twice daily on day 4; may increase to a target dose of 800 mg/day by day 6 at increments ≤200 mg/day. Usual dosage range: 400-800 mg/day.

Extended release tablet: Initial: 300 mg on day 1; increase to 600 mg on day 2 and adjust dose to 400-800 mg once daily on day 3, depending on response and tolerance.

Maintenance therapy: Immediate release tablet: 200-400 mg twice daily with lithium or divalproex; **Note:** Average time of stabilization was 15 weeks in clinical trials.

Schizophrenia/psychoses:

Immediate release tablet: Initial: 25 mg twice daily; increase in increments of 25-50 mg 2-3 times/day on the second and third day, if tolerated, to a target dose of 300-400 mg/day in 2-3 divided doses by day 4. Make further adjustments as needed at intervals of at least 2 days in adjustments of 25-50 mg twice daily. Usual maintenance range: 300-800 mg/day.

Extended release tablet: Initial: 300 mg once daily; increase in increments of up to 300 mg/day (in intervals of ≥1 day). For dosage requirements <200 mg during initial titration, the immediate release formulation should be used. Usual maintenance range: 400-800 mg/day.

Note: Dose reductions should be attempted periodically to establish lowest effective dose in patients with psychosis. Patients being restarted after 1 week of no drug need to be titrated as above.

Elderly: 40% lower mean oral clearance of quetiapine in adults >65 years of age; higher plasma levels expected and, therefore, dosage adjustment may be needed; elderly patients usually require 50-200 mg/day of immediate release tablets or 50 mg/day of extended release tablets with a slower titration schedule. Increase immediate release dose by 25-50 mg/day or extended release dose by 50 mg/day to effective dose, based on clinical response and tolerability. If initiated with immediate release tablets, patient may transition to extended release formulation (at equivalent total daily dose) when effective dose has been reached. See "Note" in adult dosing.

Psychosis/agitation related to Alzheimer's dementia (unlabeled use): Initial: 12.5-50 mg/day; if necessary, gradually increase as tolerated not to exceed 200-300 mg/day

Dosing comments in renal insufficiency: 25% lower mean oral clearance of quetiapine than normal subjects; however, plasma concentrations similar to normal subjects receiving the same dose; no dosage adjustment required

Dosing comments in hepatic insufficiency: 30% lower mean oral clearance of quetiapine than normal subjects; higher plasma levels expected in hepatically impaired subjects; dosage adjustment may be needed

Immediate release tablet: Initial: 25 mg/day, increase dose by 25-50 mg/day to effective dose, based on clinical response and tolerability to patient. If initiated with immediate-release formulation, patient may transition to extended-release formulation (at equivalent total daily dose) when effective dose has been reached.

Extended release tablet: Initial: 50 mg/day; increase dose by 50 mg/day to effective dose, based on clinical response and tolerability to patient.

Dietary Considerations

Immediate-release tablet: May be taken with or without food.

Extended release tablet: Take without food or with a light meal (≤300 calories).

Administration

Immediate release tablet: May be administered with or without food.

Extended release tablet: Administer without food or with a light meal (≤300 calories), preferably in the evening. Swallow tablet whole; do not break, crush, or chew.

Monitoring Parameters Vital signs; fasting lipid profile and fasting blood glucose/Hgb A_{1c} (prior to treatment, at 3 months, then annually); CBC frequently during first few months of therapy in patients with pre-existing low WBC or a history of drug-induced leukopenia/neutropenia; BMI, personal/family history of obesity, waist circumference; blood pressure; mental status, abnormal involuntary movement scale (AIMS). Weight should be assessed prior to treatment, at 4 weeks, 8 weeks, 12 weeks, and then at quarterly intervals. Consider titrating to a different antipsychotic agent for a weight gain ≥5% of the initial weight. Patients should have eyes checked for cataracts every 6 months while on this medication. Observe for new or worsening depression, anxiety, irritability, aggression, or other symptoms of unusual behavior, mood, or suicidal ideation (especially at the beginning of therapy or when doses are increased or decreased).

Dosage Forms Excipient information presented when available (limited, particularly for generics); consult specific product labeling.

Tablet:

Seroquel®: 25 mg, 50 mg, 100 mg, 200 mg, 300 mg, 400 mg

Tablet, extended release:

Seroquel® XR: 50 mg, 200 mg, 300 mg, 400 mg

◆ **Quetiapine Fumarate** *see* QUEtiapine *on page 1275*

◆ **Quibron® [DSC]** *see* Theophylline and Guaifenesin *on page 1457*

◆ **Quinalbarbitone Sodium** *see* Secobarbital *on page 1358*

Quinapril (KWIN a pril)

U.S. Brand Names Accupril®

Canadian Brand Names Accupril®; GD-Quinapril

Index Terms Quinapril Hydrochloride

Pharmacologic Category Angiotensin-Converting Enzyme (ACE) Inhibitor

Additional Appendix Information

Angiotensin Agents *on page 1632*

Heart Failure (Systolic) *on page 1809*

Use Treatment of hypertension; treatment of heart failure

Unlabeled/Investigational Use Treatment of left ventricular dysfunction after myocardial infarction; pediatric hypertension; to delay the progression of nephropathy and reduce risks of cardiovascular events in hypertensive patients with type 1 or 2 diabetes mellitus

Pregnancy Risk Factor C (1st trimester); D (2nd and 3rd trimesters)

Pregnancy Considerations Due to adverse events observed in some animal studies, quinapril is considered pregnancy category C during the first trimester. Based on human data, quinapril is considered pregnancy category D if used during the second and third trimesters (per the manufacturer; however, one study suggests that fetal injury may occur at anytime during pregnancy). Quinapril crosses the placenta. First trimester exposure to ACE inhibitors may cause major congenital malformations. An increased risk of cardiovascular and/or central nervous system malformations was observed in one study; however, an increased risk of teratogenic events was not observed in other studies. Second and third trimester use of an ACE inhibitor is associated with oligohydramnios. Oligohydramnios due to decreased fetal renal function may lead to fetal limb contractures, craniofacial deformation, and hypoplastic lung development. The use of ACE inhibitors during the second and third trimesters is also associated with anuria, hypotension, renal failure (reversible or irreversible), skull hypoplasia, and death in the fetus/neonate. Chronic maternal hypertension itself is also associated with adverse events in the fetus/infant. ACE inhibitors are not recommended during pregnancy to treat maternal hypertension or heart failure. Those who are planning a pregnancy should be considered for other medication options if an ACE inhibitor is currently prescribed or the ACE inhibitor should be discontinued as soon as possible once pregnancy is detected. The exposed fetus should be monitored for fetal growth, amniotic fluid volume, and organ formation. Infants exposed to an ACE inhibitor *in utero*, especially during the second and third trimester, should be monitored for hyperkalemia, hypotension, and oliguria.

[U.S. Boxed Warning]: Based on human data, ACE inhibitors can cause injury and death to the developing fetus when used in the second and third trimesters. ACE inhibitors should be discontinued as soon as possible once pregnancy is detected.

Lactation Enters breast milk/use caution

Medication Safety Issues

Sound-alike/look-alike issues:

Accupril® may be confused with Accolate®, Accutane®, AcipHex®, Monopril®

International issues:

Accupril® may be confused with Acepril® which is a brand name for lisinopril in Denmark, a brand name for enalapril in Hungary and Switzerland, and a brand name for captopril in Great Britain

Contraindications Hypersensitivity to quinapril or any component of the formulation; angioedema related to previous treatment with an ACE inhibitor

Warnings/Precautions Anaphylactic reactions may occur rarely with ACE inhibitors. At any time during treatment (especially following first dose) angioedema may occur rarely with ACE inhibitors; it may involve the head and neck (potentially compromising airway) or the intestine (presenting with abdominal pain). African-Americans and patients with idiopathic or hereditary angioedema may be at an increased risk. Prolonged frequent monitoring may be required especially if tongue, glottis, or larynx are involved as they are associated with airway obstruction. Patients with a history of airway surgery may have a higher risk of airway obstruction. Aggressive early and appropriate management is critical. Use in patients with previous angioedema associated with ACE inhibitor therapy is contraindicated. Severe anaphylactoid reactions may be seen during hemodialysis (eg, CVVHD) with high-flux dialysis membranes (eg, AN69), and rarely, during low density lipoprotein apheresis with dextran sulfate cellulose. Rare cases of anaphylactoid reactions have been reported in patients undergoing sensitization treatment with hymenoptera (bee, wasp) venom while receiving ACE inhibitors.

Symptomatic hypotension with or without syncope can occur with ACE inhibitors (usually with the first several doses); effects are most often observed in volume-depleted patients; close monitoring of patient is required especially with initial dosing and dosing increases; blood pressure must be lowered at a rate appropriate for the patient's clinical condition. Initiation of therapy in patients with ischemic heart disease or cerebrovascular disease warrants close observation due to the potential consequences posed by falling blood pressure (eg, MI, stroke). Use with caution in hypertrophic cardiomyopathy with outflow tract obstruction, severe aortic stenosis, or before, during, or immediately after major surgery. **[U.S. Boxed Warning]: Based on human data, ACEIs can cause injury and death to the developing fetus when used in the second and third trimesters. ACEIs should be discontinued as soon as possible once pregnancy is detected.**

Hyperkalemia may occur with ACE inhibitors; risk factors include renal dysfunction, diabetes mellitus, concomitant use of potassium-sparing diuretics, potassium supplements, and/or potassium-containing salts. Use cautiously, if at all, with these agents and monitor potassium closely. Cough may occur with ACE inhibitors. Other causes of cough should be considered (eg, pulmonary congestion in patients with heart failure) and excluded prior to discontinuation.

May be associated with deterioration of renal function and/or increases in serum creatinine, particularly in patients with low renal blood flow (eg, renal artery stenosis, heart failure) whose glomerular filtration rate (GFR) is dependent on efferent arteriolar vasoconstriction by angiotensin II; deterioration may result in oliguria, acute renal failure, and progressive azotemia. Small increases in serum creatinine may occur following initiation; consider discontinuation only in patients with progressive and/or significant deterioration in renal function. Use with caution in patients with unstented unilateral/bilateral renal artery stenosis. When unstented bilateral renal artery stenosis is present, use is generally avoided due to the elevated risk of deterioration in renal function unless possible benefits outweigh risks.

Rare toxicities associated with ACE inhibitors include cholestatic jaundice (which may progress to fulminant hepatic necrosis), agranulocytosis, neutropenia, or leukopenia with myeloid hypoplasia. Patients with collagen vascular diseases (especially with concomitant renal impairment) or renal impairment alone may be at increased risk for hematologic toxicity; periodically monitor CBC with differential in these patients. Safety and efficacy have not been established in children.

Adverse Reactions Note: Frequency ranges include data from hypertension and heart failure trials. Higher rates of adverse reactions have generally been noted in patients with CHF. However, the frequency of adverse effects associated with placebo is also increased in this population.

1% to 10%:

Cardiovascular: Hypotension (3%), chest pain (2%), first-dose hypotension (up to 3%)

Central nervous system: Dizziness (4% to 8%), headache (2% to 6%), fatigue (3%)

Dermatologic: Rash (1%)

Endocrine & metabolic: Hyperkalemia (2%)

Gastrointestinal: Vomiting/nausea (1% to 2%), diarrhea (1.7%)

Neuromuscular & skeletal: Myalgias (2% to 5%), back pain (1%)

Renal: BUN/serum creatinine increased (2%, transient elevations may occur with a higher frequency), worsening of renal function (in patients with bilateral renal artery stenosis or hypovolemia)

Respiratory: Upper respiratory symptoms, cough (2% to 4%; up to 13% in some studies), dyspnea (2%)

<1% (Limited to important or life-threatening): Acute renal failure, agranulocytosis, alopecia, amblyopia, anaphylactoid reaction, angina, angioedema, arrhythmia, arthralgia, depression, dermatopolymyositis, edema, eosinophilic pneumonitis, exfoliative dermatitis, hemolytic anemia, hepatitis, hyperkalemia, hypertensive crisis, impotence, insomnia, MI, orthostatic hypotension, pancreatitis, paresthesia, pemphigus, photosensitivity, pruritus, shock, somnolence, stroke, syncope, thrombocytopenia, vertigo

A syndrome which may include fever, myalgia, arthralgia, interstitial nephritis, vasculitis, rash, eosinophilia and positive ANA, and elevated ESR has been reported with ACE inhibitors. In addition, pancreatitis, hepatic necrosis, neutropenia, and/or agranulocytosis (particularly in patients with collagen-vascular disease or renal impairment) have been associated with many ACE inhibitors.

Drug Interactions

Avoid Concomitant Use There are no known interactions where it is recommended to avoid concomitant use.

Increased Effect/Toxicity

Quinapril may increase the levels/effects of: Allopurinol; Amifostine; AzaTHIOprine; CycloSPORINE; Ferric Gluconate; Gold Sodium Thiomalate; Lithium; RiTUXimab

The levels/effects of Quinapril may be increased by: Angiotensin II Receptor Blockers; Diazoxide; Eplerenone; Herbs (Hypotensive Properties); Loop Diuretics; Potassium Salts; Potassium-Sparing Diuretics; Prostacyclin Analogues; Sirolimus; Temsirolimus; Thiazide Diuretics; Trimethoprim

Decreased Effect

Quinapril may decrease the levels/effects of: Quinolone Antibiotics; Tetracycline Derivatives

The levels/effects of Quinapril may be decreased by: Antacids; Aprotinin; Herbs (Hypertensive Properties); Methylphenidate; Nonsteroidal Anti-Inflammatory Agents; Salicylates; Yohimbine

Ethanol/Nutrition/Herb Interactions Herb/Nutraceutical: Avoid bayberry, blue cohosh, cayenne, ephedra, ginger, ginseng (American), kola, licorice (may worsen hypertension). Avoid black cohosh, California poppy, coleus, golden seal, hawthorn, mistletoe, periwinkle, quinine, shepherd's purse (may have increased antihypertensive effect).

Stability Store at room temperature. To prepare solution for oral administration, mix prior to administration and use within 10 minutes.

Mechanism of Action Competitive inhibitor of angiotensin-converting enzyme (ACE); prevents conversion of angiotensin I to angiotensin II, a potent vasoconstrictor; results in lower levels of angiotensin II which causes an increase in plasma renin activity and a reduction in aldosterone secretion; a CNS mechanism may also be involved in hypotensive effect as angiotensin II increases adrenergic outflow from CNS; vasoactive kallikreins may be decreased in conversion to active hormones by ACE inhibitors, thus reducing blood pressure

Pharmacodynamics/Kinetics

Onset of action: 1 hour

Duration: 24 hours

Absorption: Quinapril: ≥60%

Protein binding: Quinapril: 97%; Quinaprilat: 97%

Metabolism: Rapidly hydrolyzed to quinaprilat, the active metabolite

Half-life elimination: Quinapril: 0.8 hours; Quinaprilat: 3 hours; increases as Cl_{cr} decreases

Time to peak, serum: Quinapril: 1 hour; Quinaprilat: ~2 hours

Excretion: Urine (50% to 60% primarily as quinaprilat)

Dosage Oral:

Children (unlabeled use): Hypertension: Initial 5-10 mg once daily; maximum: 80 mg/day

Adults:

Hypertension: Initial: 10-20 mg once daily, adjust according to blood pressure response at peak and trough blood levels; initial dose may be reduced to 5 mg in patients receiving diuretic therapy if the diuretic is continued; usual dose range (JNC 7): 10-40 mg once daily

Heart failure: Initial: 5 mg once or twice daily, titrated at weekly intervals to 20-40 mg daily in 2 divided doses; target dose (heart failure): 20 mg twice daily (ACC/AHA 2005 Heart Failure Guidelines)

Elderly: Initial: 2.5-5 mg/day; increase dosage at increments of 2.5-5 mg at 1- to 2-week intervals.

Dosing adjustment in renal impairment: Lower initial doses should be used; after initial dose (if tolerated), administer initial dose twice daily; may be increased at weekly intervals to optimal response:

Hypertension: Initial:

Cl_{cr} >60 mL/minute: Administer 10 mg/day

Cl_{cr} 30-60 mL/minute: Administer 5 mg/day

Cl_{cr} 10-30 mL/minute: Administer 2.5 mg/day

Heart failure: Initial:

Cl_{cr} >30 mL/minute: Administer 5 mg/day

Cl_{cr} 10-30 mL/minute: Administer 2.5 mg/day

Dosing comments in hepatic impairment: In patients with alcoholic cirrhosis, hydrolysis of quinapril to quinaprilat is impaired; however, the subsequent elimination of quinaprilat is unaltered.

Monitoring Parameters Blood pressure; serum creatinine and potassium; if patient has collagen vascular disease and/or renal impairment, periodically monitor CBC with differential

Dosage Forms Excipient information presented when available (limited, particularly for generics); consult specific product labeling.

Tablet: 5 mg, 10 mg, 20 mg, 40 mg

Accupril®: 5 mg, 10 mg, 20 mg, 40 mg

Quinapril and Hydrochlorothiazide

(KWIN a pril & hye droe klor oh THYE a zide)

U.S. Brand Names Accuretic®; Quinaretic

Canadian Brand Names Accuretic®

Index Terms Hydrochlorothiazide and Quinapril

Pharmacologic Category Angiotensin-Converting Enzyme (ACE) Inhibitor; Diuretic, Thiazide

Use Treatment of hypertension (not for initial therapy)

Pregnancy Risk Factor C (1st trimester); D (2nd and 3rd trimesters)

Dosage Oral:

Children: Safety and efficacy have not been established.

Adults: Initial:

Patients who have failed quinapril monotherapy:

Quinapril 10 mg/hydrochlorothiazide 12.5 mg **or**

Quinapril 20 mg/hydrochlorothiazide 12.5 mg once daily

Patients with adequate blood pressure control on hydrochlorothiazide 25 mg/day, but significant potassium loss:

Quinapril 10 mg/hydrochlorothiazide 12.5 mg **or**

Quinapril 20 mg/hydrochlorothiazide 12.5 mg once daily

Note: Clinical trials of quinapril/hydrochlorothiazide combinations used quinapril doses of 2.5-40 mg/day and hydrochlorothiazide doses of 6.25-25 mg/day.

Elderly: If previous response to individual components is unknown, initial dose selection should be cautious, at the low end of adult dosage range; titration should occur at 1- to 2-week intervals.

Dosage adjustment in renal impairment: Cl_{cr} <30 mL/minute/1.73 m^2 or serum creatinine ≤3 mg/dL: Use is not recommended.

Additional Information Complete prescribing information for this medication should be consulted for additional detail.

Dosage Forms Excipient information presented when available (limited, particularly for generics); consult specific product labeling.

Tablet:

10/12.5: Quinapril 10 mg and hydrochlorothiazide 12.5 mg

20/12.5: Quinapril 20 mg and hydrochlorothiazide 12.5 mg

20/25: Quinapril 20 mg and hydrochlorothiazide 25 mg

Accuretic® 10/12.5, Quinaretic 10/12.5: Quinapril 10 mg and hydrochlorothiazide 12.5 mg

Accuretic® 20/12.5, Quinaretic 20/12.5: Quinapril 20 mg and hydrochlorothiazide 12.5 mg

Accuretic® 20/25, Quinaretic 20/25: Quinapril 20 mg and hydrochlorothiazide 25 mg

◆ **Quinapril Hydrochloride** *see* Quinapril *on page* 1278

◆ **Quinaretic** *see* Quinapril and Hydrochlorothiazide *on page* 1280

◆ **Quinate® (Can)** *see* QuiNIDine *on page* 1280

QuiNIDine (KWIN i deen)

Canadian Brand Names Apo-Quinidine®; BioQuin® Durules™; Novo-Quinidin; Quinate®

Index Terms Quinidine Gluconate; Quinidine Polygalacturonate; Quinidine Sulfate

Pharmacologic Category Antiarrhythmic Agent, Class Ia

Additional Appendix Information

Malaria Treatment *on page 1770*

Use Prophylaxis after cardioversion of atrial fibrillation and/or flutter to maintain normal sinus rhythm; prevent recurrence of paroxysmal supraventricular tachycardia, paroxysmal AV junctional rhythm, paroxysmal ventricular tachycardia, paroxysmal atrial fibrillation, and atrial or ventricular premature contractions; has activity against *Plasmodium falciparum* malaria

Pregnancy Risk Factor C

Lactation Enters breast milk/compatible

Medication Safety Issues

Sound-alike/look-alike issues:

QuiNIDine may be confused with cloNIDine, quiNINE, Quinora®

High alert medication: The Institute for Safe Medication Practices (ISMP) includes this medication (I.V. formulation) among its list of drug classes which have a heightened risk of causing significant patient harm when used in error.

Contraindications Hypersensitivity to quinidine or any component of the formulation; thrombocytopenia; thrombocytopenic purpura; myasthenia gravis; heart block greater than first degree; idioventricular conduction delays (except in patients with a functioning artificial pacemaker); those adversely affected by anticholinergic activity; concurrent use of quinolone antibiotics which prolong QT interval, cisapride, amprenavir, or ritonavir

Warnings/Precautions Monitor and adjust dose to prevent QT_c prolongation. Watch for proarrhythmic effects. Correct hypokalemia before initiating therapy. Hypokalemia may worsen toxicity. **[U.S. Boxed Warning]: Antiarrhythmic drugs have not been shown to enhance survival in non-life-threatening ventricular arrhythmias and may increase mortality; the risk is greatest with structural heart disease. Quinidine may increase mortality in treatment of atrial fibrillation/flutter.** May precipitate or exacerbate HF. Reduce dosage in hepatic impairment. Use may cause digoxin-induced toxicity (adjust digoxin's dose). Use caution with concurrent use of other antiarrhythmics. Hypersensitivity reactions can occur. Can unmask sick sinus syndrome (causes bradycardia); use with caution in patients with heart block. Has been associated with severe hepatotoxic reactions, including granulomatous hepatitis. Hemolysis may occur in patients with G6PD (glucose-6-phosphate dehydrogenase) deficiency. Different salt products are not interchangeable.

Adverse Reactions

Frequency not defined: Hypotension, syncope

>10%:

Cardiovascular: QT_c prolongation (modest prolongation is common, however, excessive prolongation is rare and indicates toxicity)

Central nervous system: Lightheadedness (15%)

Gastrointestinal: Diarrhea (35%), upper GI distress, bitter taste, diarrhea, anorexia, nausea, vomiting, stomach cramping (22%)

1% to 10%:

Cardiovascular: Angina (6%), palpitation (7%), new or worsened arrhythmia (proarrhythmic effect)

Central nervous system: Syncope (1% to 8%), headache (7%), fatigue (7%), sleep disturbance (3%), tremor (2%), nervousness (2%), incoordination (1%)

Dermatologic: Rash (5%)

Neuromuscular & skeletal: Weakness (5%)

Ocular: Blurred vision

Otic: Tinnitus

Respiratory: Wheezing

<1% (Limited to important or life-threatening): Abnormal pigmentation, acute psychotic reactions, agranulocytosis, angioedema, arthralgia, bronchospasm, cerebral hypoperfusion (possibly resulting in ataxia, apprehension, and seizure), cholestasis, confusion, delirium, depression, drug-induced lupus-like syndrome, eczematous dermatitis, esophagitis, exacerbated bradycardia (in sick sinus syndrome), exfoliative rash, fever, flushing, granulomatous hepatitis, hallucinations, heart block, hemolytic anemia, hepatotoxic reaction (rare), hearing impaired, CPK increased, lichen planus, livedo reticularis, lymphadenopathy, melanin pigmentation of the hard palate, myalgia, mydriasis, nephropathy, optic neuritis, pancytopenia, paradoxical increase in ventricular rate during atrial fibrillation/flutter, photosensitivity, pneumonitis, pruritus, psoriaform rash, QT_c prolongation (excessive), respiratory depression, sicca syndrome, tachycardia, thrombocytopenia, thrombocytopenic purpura, torsade de pointes, urticaria, uveitis, vascular collapse, vasculitis, ventricular fibrillation, ventricular tachycardia, vertigo, visual field loss

Note: Cinchonism, a syndrome which may include tinnitus, high-frequency hearing loss, deafness, vertigo, blurred vision, diplopia, photophobia, headache, confusion, and delirium has been associated with quinidine use. Usually associated with chronic toxicity, this syndrome has also been described after brief exposure to a moderate dose in sensitive patients. Vomiting and diarrhea may also occur as isolated reactions to therapeutic quinidine levels.

Drug Interactions

Metabolism/Transport Effects Substrate of CYP2C9 (minor), 2E1 (minor), 3A4 (major); **Inhibits** CYP2C9 (weak), 2D6 (strong), 3A4 (strong)

Avoid Concomitant Use

Avoid concomitant use of QuiNIDine with any of the following: Alfuzosin; Antifungal Agents (Azole Derivatives, Systemic); Dabigatran Etexilate; Eplerenone; Mefloquine; Nilotinib; Nisoldipine; Protease Inhibitors; Ranolazine; Rivaroxaban; Salmeterol; Silodosin; Tamoxifen; Tetrabenazine; Thioridazine; Topotecan; Ziprasidone

Increased Effect/Toxicity

QuiNIDine may increase the levels/effects of: Alfuzosin; Alosetron; Amiodarone; Beta-Blockers; Cardiac Glycosides; Ciclesonide; CYP2D6 Substrates; CYP3A4 Substrates; Dabigatran Etexilate; Dextromethorphan; Eplerenone; FentaNYL; Fesoterodine; Haloperidol; Ixabepilone; Maraviroc; Mefloquine; Neuromuscular-Blocking Agents; Nilotinib; Nisoldipine; P-Glycoprotein Substrates; Pimecrolimus; QTc-Prolonging Agents; Ranolazine; Rivaroxaban; Salmeterol; Silodosin; Sorafenib; Tamoxifen; Tetrabenazine; Thioridazine; Topotecan; Tricyclic Antidepressants; Vitamin K Antagonists; Ziprasidone

The levels/effects of QuiNIDine may be increased by: Alfuzosin; Antacids; Antifungal Agents (Azole Derivatives, Systemic); Calcium Channel Blockers (Nondihydropyridine); Carbonic Anhydrase Inhibitors; Cimetidine; Ciprofloxacin; CYP3A4 Inhibitors (Moderate); CYP3A4 Inhibitors (Strong); Dasatinib; Fluconazole; Gadobutrol; Macrolide Antibiotics; Nilotinib; P-Glycoprotein Inhibitors; Protease Inhibitors; Selective Serotonin Reuptake Inhibitors; Tricyclic Antidepressants

Decreased Effect

QuiNIDine may decrease the levels/effects of: Codeine; Dihydrocodeine; Hydrocodone; TraMADol

The levels/effects of QuiNIDine may be decreased by: Amiodarone; Barbiturates; Calcium Channel Blockers (Dihydropyridine); CYP3A4 Inducers (Strong); Deferasirox; Herbs (CYP3A4 Inducers); Kaolin; P-Glycoprotein Inducers; Phenytoin; Potassium-Sparing Diuretics; Primidone; Rifamycin Derivatives

Ethanol/Nutrition/Herb Interactions

Food: Dietary salt intake may alter the rate and extent of quinidine absorption. A decrease in dietary salt may lead to an increase in quinidine serum concentrations. Avoid changes in dietary salt intake. Quinidine serum levels may be increased if taken with food. Food has a variable effect on absorption of sustained release formulation. The rate of absorption of quinidine may be decreased following the ingestion of grapefruit juice. In addition, CYP3A4 metabolism of quinidine may be reduced by grapefruit juice. Grapefruit juice should be avoided. Excessive intake of fruit juices or vitamin C may decrease urine pH and result in increased clearance of quinidine with decreased serum concentration. Alkaline foods may result in increased quinidine serum concentrations.

Herb/Nutraceutical: St John's wort may decrease quinidine levels. Avoid ephedra (may worsen arrhythmia).

Stability Do not use discolored parenteral solution.

Mechanism of Action Class Ia antiarrhythmic agent; depresses phase O of the action potential; decreases myocardial excitability and conduction velocity, and myocardial contractility by decreasing sodium influx during depolarization and potassium efflux in repolarization; also reduces calcium transport across cell membrane

Pharmacodynamics/Kinetics

Distribution: V_d: Adults: 2-3.5 L/kg, decreased with congestive heart failure, malaria; increased with cirrhosis; crosses placenta; enters breast milk

Protein binding:

Newborns: 60% to 70%; decreased protein binding with cyanotic congenital heart disease, cirrhosis, or acute myocardial infarction

Adults: 80% to 90%

Metabolism: Extensively hepatic (50% to 90%) to inactive compounds

Bioavailability: Sulfate: 80%; Gluconate: 70%

Half-life elimination, plasma: Children: 2.5-6.7 hours; Adults: 6-8 hours; prolonged with elderly, cirrhosis, and congestive heart failure

Excretion: Urine (15% to 25% as unchanged drug)

Dosage Dosage expressed in terms of the salt: 267 mg of quinidine gluconate = 200 mg of quinidine sulfate.

Children: Test dose for idiosyncratic reaction (sulfate, oral or gluconate, I.M.): 2 mg/kg or 60 mg/m^2

Oral (quinidine sulfate): 15-60 mg/kg/day in 4-5 divided doses or 6 mg/kg every 4-6 hours; usual 30 mg/kg/day or 900 mg/m^2/day given in 5 daily doses

I.V. **not** recommended (quinidine gluconate): 2-10 mg/kg/dose given at a rate ≤10 mg/minute every 3-6 hours as needed

Adults: Test dose: Oral, I.M.: 200 mg administered several hours before full dosage (to determine possibility of idiosyncratic reaction)

Oral (for malaria):

Sulfate: 100-600 mg/dose every 4-6 hours; begin at 200 mg/dose and titrate to desired effect (maximum daily dose: 3-4 g)

Gluconate: 324-972 mg every 8-12 hours

I.M.: 400 mg/dose every 2-6 hours; initial dose: 600 mg (gluconate)

I.V.: 200-400 mg/dose diluted and given at a rate ≤10 mg/minute; may require as much as 500-750 mg

Dosing adjustment in renal impairment: Cl_{cr} <10 mL/minute: Administer 75% of normal dose.

Hemodialysis: Slightly hemodialyzable (5% to 20%); 200 mg supplemental dose posthemodialysis is recommended.

Peritoneal dialysis: Not dialyzable (0% to 5%)

Dosing adjustment/comments in hepatic impairment: Larger loading dose may be indicated; reduce maintenance doses by 50% and monitor serum levels closely.

Dietary Considerations Administer with food or milk to decrease gastrointestinal irritation. Avoid changes in dietary salt intake.

Administration Administer around-the-clock to promote less variation in peak and trough serum levels

Oral: Do not crush, chew, or break sustained release dosage forms.

Parenteral: When injecting I.M., aspirate carefully to avoid injection into a vessel; maximum I.V. infusion rate: 10 mg/minute.

Monitoring Parameters Cardiac monitor required during I.V. administration; CBC, liver and renal function tests, should be routinely performed during long-term administration

Reference Range Therapeutic: 2-5 mcg/mL (SI: 6.2-15.4 μmol/L). Patient-dependent therapeutic response occurs at levels of 3-6 mcg/mL (SI: 9.2-18.5 μmol/L). Optimal therapeutic level is method dependent; >6 mcg/mL (SI: >18 μmol/L).

Dosage Forms Excipient information presented when available (limited, particularly for generics); consult specific product labeling.

Injection, solution, as gluconate: 80 mg/mL (10 mL) [equivalent to quinidine base 50 mg/mL]

Tablet, as sulfate: 200 mg, 300 mg

Tablet, extended release, as gluconate: 324 mg [equivalent to quinidine base 202 mg]

Tablet, extended release, as sulfate: 300 mg [equivalent to quinidine base 249 mg]

Extemporaneous Preparations A 10 mg/mL oral liquid preparation made from tablets and three different vehicles (cherry syrup, a 1:1 mixture of Ora-Sweet® and Ora-Plus®, or a 1:1 mixture of Ora-Sweet® SF and Ora-Plus®) was stable for 60 days when stored in amber plastic prescription bottles in the dark at room temperature (25°C) or under refrigeration (5°C). Grind six 200 mg tablets in a mortar into a fine powder; add 15 mL of the vehicle and mix well to form a uniform paste; mix while adding the vehicle in geometric proportions to **almost** 120 mL; transfer to a calibrated bottle and qsad to 120 mL; label "shake well" and "protect from light" (Allen 1998).

Allen LV and Erickson MA, "Stability of Bethanechol Chloride, Pyrazinamide, Quinidine Sulfate, Rifampin, and Tetracycline in Extemporaneously Compounded Oral Liquids," *Am J Health Syst Pharm*, 1998, 55 (17):1804-9.

◆ **Quinidine Gluconate** *see* QuiNIDine *on page* 1280

◆ **Quinidine Polygalacturonate** *see* QuiNIDine *on page* 1280

◆ **Quinidine Sulfate** *see* QuiNIDine *on page* 1280

QuiNINE (KWYE nine)

U.S. Brand Names Qualaquin™

Canadian Brand Names Apo-Quinine®; Novo-Quinine; Quinine-Odan™

Index Terms Quinine Sulfate

Pharmacologic Category Antimalarial Agent

Additional Appendix Information

Malaria Treatment *on page* 1770

Use In conjunction with other antimalarial agents, treatment of uncomplicated chloroquine-resistant *P. falciparum* malaria

Unlabeled/Investigational Use Treatment of *Babesia microti* infection in conjunction with clindamycin

Note: Prevention/treatment of nocturnal leg cramps (unapproved) removed following FDA-issued warning regarding severe adverse events (eg, cardiac arrhythmias, thrombocytopenia, and severe hypersensitivity reactions) and potentially serious drug interactions associated with quinine; use not justified in this condition.

Pregnancy Risk Factor C

Pregnancy Considerations Teratogenic effects have been reported in some animal studies. Quinine crosses the human placenta. Cord plasma to maternal plasma quinine ratios have been reported as 0.18-0.46 and should not be considered therapeutic to the infant. Teratogenic effects, optic nerve hypoplasia, and deafness have been reported in the infant following maternal use of very high doses; however, therapeutic doses used for malaria are generally considered safe. Quinine may also cause significant hypoglycemia when used during pregnancy. Malaria infection in pregnant women may be more severe than in nonpregnant women. The CDC recommends the use of quinine sulfate for the treatment of chloroquine-resistant *P. falciparum* malaria during pregnancy. Pregnant women should be advised not to travel to areas of *P. falciparum* resistance to chloroquine.

Lactation Enters breast milk/use caution (AAP rate "compatible")

Medication Safety Issues

Sound-alike/look-alike issues:

QuiNINE may be confused with quiNIDine

Contraindications Hypersensitivity to quinine or any component of the formulation; hypersensitivity to mefloquine or quinidine (cross sensitivity reported); prolonged QT interval; myasthenia gravis; optic neuritis; G6PD deficiency; history of black water fever; thrombotic thrombocytopenia purpura, hemolytic uremic syndrome, thrombocytopenia

Warnings/Precautions Use caution with medications or clinical conditions which may prolong the QT interval or cause cardiac arrhythmias. Use may cause significant hypoglycemia. Use caution with atrial fibrillation or flutter, renal or hepatic impairment. Quinine interacts with many medications due to its hepatic metabolism; use caution with other medications metabolized via the CYP3A4 isoenzyme system. Severe hypersensitivity reactions (eg, Stevens-Johnson syndrome, anaphylactic shock) have occurred; discontinue following any signs of sensitivity. Other events, including thrombocytopenia and hemolytic uremic syndrome, may also be attributed to hypersensitivity reactions. Because of the potential for severe and/or life-threatening side effects, as well as the absence of clinical effectiveness, quinine is no longer recommended for the treatment of nocturnal leg cramps.

Adverse Reactions

Frequency not defined.

Cardiovascular: Atrial fibrillation, atrioventricular block, bradycardia, cardiac arrest, chest pain, hypotension, irregular rhythm, nodal escape beats, palpitation, postural hypotension, QT prolongation, syncope, tachycardia, torsade de pointes, unifocal premature ventricular contractions, U waves, vasodilation, ventricular fibrillation, ventricular tachycardia

Central nervous system: Aphasia, ataxia, chills, coma, confusion, disorientation, dizziness, dystonic reaction, fever, flushing, headache, mental status altered, restlessness, seizure, suicide, vertigo

Dermatologic: Acral necrosis, allergic contact dermatitis, bullous dermatitis, bruising, cutaneous rash (urticaria, papular, scarlatinal), cutaneous vasculitis, diaphoresis, exfoliative dermatitis, erythema multiforme, petechiae, photosensitivity, pruritus, Stevens-Johnson syndrome, toxic epidermal necrolysis

Endocrine & metabolic: Hypoglycemia

Gastrointestinal: Abdominal pain, anorexia, diarrhea, esophagitis, gastric irritation, nausea, vomiting

Hematologic: Agranulocytosis, aplastic anemia, coagulopathy, disseminated intravascular coagulation, hemolytic anemia, hemolytic uremic syndrome, hemorrhage, hypoprothrombinemia, leukopenia, neutropenia, pancytopenia, thrombocytopenia, thrombotic thrombocytopenic purpura

Hepatic: Granulomatous hepatitis, hepatitis, jaundice, liver function test abnormalities

Neuromuscular & skeletal: Myalgia, tremor, weakness

Ocular: Blindness, blurred vision (with or without scotomata), color vision disturbance, diminished visual fields, diplopia, night blindness, optic neuritis, photophobia, pupillary dilation, vision loss (sudden)

Otic: Deafness, hearing impaired, tinnitus

Respiratory: Asthma, dyspnea, pulmonary edema

Renal: Acute interstitial nephritis, hemoglobinuria, renal failure, renal impairment

Miscellaneous: Black water fever, hypersensitivity syndrome, lupus anticoagulant, lupus-like syndrome

Drug Interactions

Metabolism/Transport Effects **Substrate** of CYP1A2 (minor), 2C19 (minor), 3A4 (major); **Inhibits** CYP2C8 (moderate), 2C9 (moderate), 2D6 (moderate), 3A4 (weak)

Avoid Concomitant Use

Avoid concomitant use of QuiNINE with any of the following: Mefloquine

Increased Effect/Toxicity

QuiNINE may increase the levels/effects of: Antihypertensives; Antipsychotic Agents (Phenothiazines); Cardiac Glycosides; CYP2C8 Substrates (High risk); CYP2C9 Substrates (High risk); CYP2D6 Substrates; Fesoterodine; Herbs (Hypotensive Properties); Mefloquine; Nebivolol; Tamoxifen

The levels/effects of QuiNINE may be increased by: CYP3A4 Inhibitors (Moderate); CYP3A4 Inhibitors (Strong); Dasatinib; Mefloquine

Decreased Effect

QuiNINE may decrease the levels/effects of: Codeine; TraMADol

The levels/effects of QuiNINE may be decreased by: CYP3A4 Inducers (Strong); Deferasirox; Herbs (CYP3A4 Inducers)

Ethanol/Nutrition/Herb Interactions Herb/Nutraceutical: St John's wort may decrease quinine levels. Black cohosh, California poppy, coleus, golden seal, hawthorn, mistletoe, periwinkle, and shepherd's purse may cause excessive decreases in blood pressure.

Stability Store at 25°C to 30°C (77°F to 86°F); do not refrigerate or freeze.

Mechanism of Action Depresses oxygen uptake and carbohydrate metabolism; intercalates into DNA, disrupting the parasite's replication and transcription; cardiovascular effects similar to quinidine

Pharmacodynamics/Kinetics

Absorption: Readily, mainly from upper small intestine

Distribution: 2.5-7.1 L/kg; varies with severity of infection

Intraerythrocytic levels are ~30% to 50% of the plasma concentration; distributes poorly to the CSF (~2% to 7% of plasma concentration)

Protein binding: 69% to 92% in healthy subjects; 78% to 95% with malaria

Metabolism: Primarily hepatic via CYP450 enzymes, including CYP3A4 and 2C19; forms metabolites; major metabolite, 3-hydroxyquinine, is less active than parent

Bioavailability: 76% to 88% in healthy subjects; increased with malaria

Half-life elimination:

Children: ~3 hours in healthy subjects; ~12 hours with malaria

Healthy adults: 10-13 hours

Time to peak, serum:

Children: 2 hours in healthy subjects; 4 hours with malaria

Adults: 1-3 hours in healthy subjects; 1.2-11 hours with malaria

Excretion: Urine (<20% as unchanged drug)

Dosage Note: Actual duration of treatment for malaria may be dependent upon the geographic region or pathogen.

Children: Oral:

Treatment of chloroquine-resistant malaria (CDC guidelines): 30 mg/kg/day in divided doses every 8 hours for 3-7 days with tetracycline, doxycycline, or clindamycin (consider risk versus benefit of using tetracycline or doxycycline in children <8 years of age)

Babesiosis (unlabeled use): 25 mg/kg/day divided every 8 hours for 7 days with clindamycin

Adults: Oral:

Treatment of chloroquine-resistant malaria: 648 mg every 8 hours for 7 days with tetracycline, doxycycline, or clindamycin

Babesiosis (unlabeled use): 650 mg every 8 hours for 7 days with clindamycin

Dosing interval/adjustment in renal impairment:

Cl_{cr} 10-50 mL/minute: Administer every 8-12 hours

Cl_{cr} <10 mL/minute: Administer every 24 hours

Severe chronic renal failure not on dialysis: Initial dose: 648 mg followed by 324 mg every 12 hours

Dialysis: Administer dose after dialysis

Peritoneal dialysis: Dose as for Cl_{cr} <10 mL/minute

Continuous arteriovenous or hemodialysis: Dose as for Cl_{cr} 10-50 mL/minute

Dosing adjustment in hepatic impairment:

Child-Pugh Class B: No dosing adjustment required; monitor closely

Child-Pugh Class C: Data not available

Dietary Considerations Take with food to decrease incidence of gastric upset.

Administration Avoid use of aluminum- or magnesium-containing antacids because of drug absorption problems. Swallow dose whole to avoid bitter taste. May be administered with food.

Monitoring Parameters Monitor CBC with platelet count, liver function tests, blood glucose, ophthalmologic examination

Reference Range Toxic: >10 mcg/mL

Test Interactions Positive Coombs' [direct]; false elevation of urinary steroids (when assayed by Zimmerman method) and catecholamines

Dosage Forms Excipient information presented when available (limited, particularly for generics); consult specific product labeling. [DSC] = Discontinued product

Capsule, as sulfate: 325 mg [DSC]

Qualaquin™: 324 mg

Tablet, as sulfate: 260 mg [DSC]

◆ **Quinine-Odan™ (Can)** *see* QuiNINE *on page 1282*

◆ **Quinine Sulfate** *see* QuiNINE *on page 1282*

◆ **Quinol** *see* Hydroquinone *on page 749*

◆ **Quintasa® (Can)** *see* Mesalamine *on page 949*

Quinupristin and Dalfopristin

(kwi NYOO pris tin & dal FOE pris tin)

U.S. Brand Names Synercid®

Canadian Brand Names Synercid®

Index Terms Pristinamycin; RP-59500

Pharmacologic Category Antibiotic, Streptogramin

Additional Appendix Information

Antibiotic Treatment of Adults With Infective Endocarditis *on page 1748*

Antimicrobial Drugs of Choice *on page 1752*

Use Treatment of serious or life-threatening infections associated with vancomycin-resistant *Enterococcus faecium* bacteremia; treatment of complicated skin and skin structure infections caused by methcillin-susceptible *Staphylococcus aureus* or *Streptococcus pyogenes*

Has been studied in the treatment of a variety of infections caused by *Enterococcus faecium* (not *E. fecalis*) including vancomycin-resistant strains. May also be effective in the treatment of serious infections caused by *Staphylococcus* species including those resistant to methicillin.

Pregnancy Risk Factor B

Pregnancy Considerations Because adverse effects were not observed in animal reproduction studies, quinupristin/dalfopristin is classified pregnancy category B. There are no adequate and well-controlled studies of quinupristin/dalfopristin in pregnant women.

Lactation Excretion in breast milk unknown/use caution

Contraindications Hypersensitivity to quinupristin, dalfopristin, pristinamycin, or virginiamycin, or any component of the formulation

Warnings/Precautions Use with caution in patients with hepatic or renal dysfunction. May cause pain and phlebitis when infused through a peripheral line (not relieved by hydrocortisone or diphenhydramine). Prolonged use may result in fungal or bacterial superinfection, including *C. difficile*-associated diarrhea (CDAD) and pseudomembranous colitis; CDAD has been observed >2 months postantibiotic treatment. May cause arthralgias, myalgias, and hyperbilirubinemia. May inhibit the metabolism of many drugs metabolized by CYP3A4. Concurrent therapy with cisapride (which may prolong QT_c interval and lead to arrhythmias) should be avoided. Safety and efficacy have not been established in children <16 years of age.

Adverse Reactions

>10%:

Hepatic: Hyperbilirubinemia (3% to 35%)

Local: Inflammation at infusion site (38% to 42%), local pain (40% to 44%), local edema (17% to 18%), infusion site reaction (12% to 13%)

Neuromuscular & skeletal: Arthralgia (up to 47%), myalgia (up to 47%)

1% to 10%:

Central nervous system: Pain (2% to 3%), headache (2%)

Dermatologic: Pruritus (2%), rash (3%)

Endocrine & metabolic: Hyperglycemia (1%)

Gastrointestinal: Nausea (3% to 5%), diarrhea (3%), vomiting (3% to 4%)

Hematologic: Anemia (3%)

Hepatic: GGT increased (2%), LDH increased (3%)

Local: Thrombophlebitis (2%)

Neuromuscular & skeletal: CPK increased (2%)

<1% (Limited to important or life-threatening): Allergic reaction, anaphylactoid reaction, angina, apnea, arrhythmia, cardiac arrest, coagulation disorder, dysautonomia, dyspnea, encephalopathy, gout, hematuria, hemolytic anemia, hepatitis, hyperkalemia, hypotension, maculopapular rash, mesenteric artery occlusion, myasthenia, neuropathy, pancreatitis, pancytopenia, paraplegia, paresthesia, pericarditis, pleural effusion, pseudomembranous colitis, respiratory distress, seizure, shock, stomatitis, syncope, thrombocytopenia, urticaria

Drug Interactions

Metabolism/Transport Effects Quinupristin: **Inhibits** CYP3A4 (weak)

Avoid Concomitant Use There are no known interactions where it is recommended to avoid concomitant use.

Increased Effect/Toxicity

Quinupristin and Dalfopristin may increase the levels/effects of: Calcium Channel Blockers; CycloSPORINE

Decreased Effect There are no known significant interactions involving a decrease in effect.

Stability Store unopened vials under refrigeration (2°C to 8°C/36°F to 46°F). Reconstitute single dose vial with 5 mL of 5% dextrose in water or sterile water for injection. Swirl gently to dissolve; do not shake (to limit foam formation). The reconstituted solution should be diluted within 30 minutes. Stability of the diluted solution prior to the infusion is established as 5 hours at room temperature or 54 hours if refrigerated at 2°C to 8°C. Reconstituted solution should be added to at least 250 mL of 5% dextrose in water for peripheral administration (increase to 500 mL or 750 mL if necessary to limit venous irritation). An infusion volume of 100 mL may be used for central line infusions. Do not freeze solution.

Mechanism of Action Quinupristin/dalfopristin inhibits bacterial protein synthesis by binding to different sites on the 50S bacterial ribosomal subunit thereby inhibiting protein synthesis

Pharmacodynamics/Kinetics

Distribution: Quinupristin: 0.45 L/kg; Dalfopristin: 0.24 L/kg

Protein binding: Moderate

Metabolism: To active metabolites via nonenzymatic reactions

Half-life elimination: Quinupristin: 0.85 hour; Dalfopristin: 0.7 hour (mean elimination half-lives, including metabolites: 3 and 1 hours, respectively)

Excretion: Feces (75% to 77% as unchanged drug and metabolites); urine (15% to 19%)

Dosage I.V.:

Children (limited information): Dosages similar to adult dosing have been used in the treatment of complicated skin/soft tissue infections and infections caused by vancomycin-resistant *Enterococcus faecium*

CNS shunt infection due to vancomycin-resistant *Enterococcus faecium*: 7.5 mg/kg/dose every 8 hours; concurrent intrathecal doses of 1-2 mg/day have been administered for up to 68 days

Adults:

Vancomycin-resistant *Enterococcus faecium*: 7.5 mg/kg every 8 hours

Complicated skin and skin structure infection: 7.5 mg/kg every 12 hours

Dosage adjustment in renal impairment: No adjustment required in renal failure, hemodialysis, or peritoneal dialysis

Dosage adjustment in hepatic impairment: Pharmacokinetic data suggest dosage adjustment may be necessary; however, specific recommendations have not been proposed

Elderly: No dosage adjustment is required

Administration Line should be flushed with 5% dextrose in water prior to and following administration. Infusion should be completed over 60 minutes (toxicity may be increased with shorter infusion). If severe venous irritation occurs following peripheral administration of quinupristin/dalfopristin diluted in 250 mL 5% dextrose in water, consideration should be given to increasing the infusion volume to 500 mL or 750 mL, changing the infusion site, or infusing by a peripherally-inserted central catheter (PICC) or a central venous catheter.

Dosage Forms Excipient information presented when available (limited, particularly for generics); consult specific product labeling.

Injection, powder for reconstitution:

Synercid®: 500 mg: Quinupristin 150 mg and dalfopristin 350 mg

◆ **Quixin®** *see* Levofloxacin *on page* 875

◆ **QVAR®** *see* Beclomethasone *on page* 176

◆ **R 14-15** *see* Erlotinib *on page* 541

◆ **R & C™ II (Can)** *see* Pyrethrins and Piperonyl Butoxide *on page* 1271

◆ **R & C™ Shampoo/Conditioner (Can)** *see* Pyrethrins and Piperonyl Butoxide *on page* 1271

◆ **RabAvert®** *see* Rabies Vaccine *on page* 1287

Rabeprazole (ra BEP ra zole)

U.S. Brand Names AcipHex®

Canadian Brand Names AcipHex®; Novo-Rabeprazole EC; Pariet®; PMS-Rabeprazole; Ran-Rabeprazole; Sandoz-Rabeprazole

Index Terms Pariprazole

Pharmacologic Category Proton Pump Inhibitor; Substituted Benzimidazole

Use Short-term (4-8 weeks) treatment and maintenance of erosive or ulcerative gastroesophageal reflux disease (GERD); symptomatic GERD; short-term (up to 4 weeks) treatment of duodenal ulcers; long-term treatment of pathological hypersecretory conditions, including Zollinger-Ellison syndrome; *H. pylori* eradication (in combination with amoxicillin and clarithromycin)

Canadian labeling: Additional uses (not in U.S. labeling): Treatment of nonerosive reflux disease (NERD); treatment of gastric ulcers

Unlabeled/Investigational Use Maintenance of duodenal ulcer

Pregnancy Risk Factor B

Pregnancy Considerations Not shown to be teratogenic in animal studies, however, adequate and well-controlled studies have not been done in humans; use during pregnancy only if clearly needed

Lactation Excretion in breast milk unknown/not recommended

Medication Safety Issues

Sound-alike/look-alike issues:

AcipHex® may be confused with Acephen®, Accupril®, Aricept®, pHisoHex®

Rabeprazole may be confused with aripiprazole,donepezil, lansoprazole, omeprazole, raloxifene

Contraindications Hypersensitivity to rabeprazole, substituted benzimidazoles (ie, esomeprazole, lansoprazole, omeprazole, pantoprazole), or any component of the formulation

Warnings/Precautions Use of proton pump inhibitors may increase the risk of gastrointestinal infections (eg, *Salmonella, Campylobacter*). Use caution in severe hepatic impairment. Relief of symptoms with rabeprazole does not preclude the presence of a gastric malignancy. Safety and efficacy have not been established in patients <12 years of age.

Adverse Reactions

1% to 10%:

Central nervous system: Pain (3%), headache (2% to 5%)

Gastrointestinal: Diarrhea (3%), flatulence (3%), constipation (2%), nausea (2%)

Respiratory: Pharyngitis (3%)

Miscellaneous: Infection (2%)

<1% (Limited to important or life-threatening): Abdomen enlarged, abdominal pain, abnormal stools, abnormal vision, agitation, agranulocytosis, albuminuria, allergic reaction, alopecia, amblyopia, anaphylaxis, anemia, angina pectoris, angioedema, anorexia, apnea, arrhythmia, arthralgia, arthritis, ascites, asthma, bloody diarrhea, bone pain, bradycardia, breast enlargement, bullous and other drug eruptions of skin, bundle branch block, bursitis, cataract, cellulitis, cerebral hemorrhage, chest pain substernal, cholangitis, cholecystitis, cholelithiasis, colitis, coma, constipation, contact dermatitis, convulsions, corneal opacity, CPK increased, cystitis, deafness, delirium, depression, diaphoresis, diabetes mellitus, diplopia, disorientation, dizziness, duodenitis, dysmenorrhea, dyspepsia, dysphagia, dyspnea, dysuria, edema, electrocardiogram abnormal, embolus, epistaxis, erythema multiforme, esophageal stenosis, esophagitis, extrapyramidal syndrome, eye hemorrhage, facial edema, fever, flatulence, fungal dermatitis, gastritis, gastroenteritis, gastrointestinal hemorrhage, gingivitis, glaucoma, glossitis, gout, gynecomastia, hematuria, hemolytic anemia, hepatic encephalopathy, hepatic cirrhosis, hepatic enzymes increased, hepatitis,

hepatoma, hernia, hyperammonemia, hypercholesteremia, hyperglycemia, hyperkinesia, hyperlipemia, hypertension, hyper-/hypothyroidism, hypertonia, hypokalemia, hyponatremia, hypoxia, impotence, injection site hemorrhage/pain/reaction, insomnia, interstitial nephritis, interstitial pneumonia, jaundice, kidney calculus, leukocytosis, leukopenia, leukorrhea, liver fatty deposit, lymphadenopathy, malaise, melena, menorrhagia, metrorrhagia, MI, migraine, myalgia, nausea, neck rigidity, nervousness, neuralgia, neuropathy, neutropenia, orchitis, palpitation, pancreatitis, pancytopenia, paresthesia, peripheral edema, photosensitivity, polycystic kidney, polyuria, proctitis, pruritus, PSA increased, psoriasis, pulmonary embolus, QT_c prolongation, rash, rectal hemorrhage, retinal degeneration, rhabdomyolysis, salivary gland enlargement, sinus bradycardia, skin discoloration, somnolence, Stevens-Johnson syndrome, stomatitis, strabismus, sudden death, supraventricular tachycardia, syncope, tachycardia, taste abnormal, thrombocytopenia, thrombophlebitis, thrombosis, thirst (rare) tinnitus, toxic epidermal necrolysis, tremor, TSH increased, ulcerative colitis, urinary incontinence, urticaria, vasodilation, ventricular arrhythmias, vertigo, vomiting, weakness, weight gain/loss, xerostomia

Drug Interactions

Metabolism/Transport Effects Substrate (major) of CYP2C19, 3A4; **Inhibits** CYP2C8 (moderate), 2C19 (moderate), 2DC (weak), 3A4 (weak)

Avoid Concomitant Use

Avoid concomitant use of Rabeprazole with any of the following: Erlotinib; Mesalamine; Nelfinavir

Increased Effect/Toxicity

Rabeprazole may increase the levels/effects of: CYP2C19 Substrates; CYP2C8 Substrates (High risk); Methotrexate; Saquinavir; Voriconazole

The levels/effects of Rabeprazole may be increased by: Fluconazole; Ketoconazole

Decreased Effect

Rabeprazole may decrease the levels/effects of: Atazanavir; Clopidogrel; Dabigatran Etexilate; Dasatinib; Erlotinib; Indinavir; Iron Salts; Itraconazole; Ketoconazole; Mesalamine; Mycophenolate; Nelfinavir

The levels/effects of Rabeprazole may be decreased by: CYP2C19 Inducers (Strong); CYP3A4 Inducers (Strong); Deferasirox; Herbs (CYP3A4 Inducers); Tipranavir

Ethanol/Nutrition/Herb Interactions

Ethanol: Avoid ethanol (may cause gastric mucosal irritation).

Food: High-fat meals may delay absorption, but C_{max} and AUC are not altered.

Herb/Nutraceutical: St John's wort may increase the metabolism and thus decrease the levels/effects of rabeprazole.

Stability Store at 25°C (77°F). Protect from moisture.

Mechanism of Action Potent proton pump inhibitor; suppresses gastric acid secretion by inhibiting the parietal cell H+/K+ ATP pump

Pharmacodynamics/Kinetics

Onset of action: Within 1 hour

Duration: 24 hours

Absorption: Oral: Well absorbed within 1 hour

Protein binding, serum: ~96%

Metabolism: Hepatic via CYP3A and 2C19 to inactive metabolites

Bioavailability: Oral: ~52%

Half-life elimination (dose dependent): 1-2 hours

Time to peak, plasma: 2-5 hours

Excretion: Urine (90% primarily as thioether carboxylic acid metabolites); remainder in feces

Dosage Oral:

Children ≥12 years: *U.S. labeling:* Short-term treatment of GERD: 20 mg once daily for ≤8 weeks

Adults >18 years and Elderly:

Erosive/ulcerative GERD: Treatment: 20 mg once daily for 4-8 weeks; if inadequate response, may repeat up to an additional 8 weeks; maintenance: 20 mg once daily

Canadian labeling: 20 mg once daily for 4 weeks; if inadequate response, may repeat for an additional 4 weeks (lack of symptom control after 4 weeks warrants further evaluation); maintenance: 10 mg once daily (maximum: 20 mg once daily)

Symptomatic GERD: Treatment: 20 mg once daily for 4 weeks; if inadequate response, may repeat for an additional 4 weeks

Canadian labeling: 10 mg once daily (maximum: 20 mg once daily) for 4 weeks; lack of symptom control after 4 weeks warrants further evaluation

Duodenal ulcer: 20 mg/day before breakfast for 4 weeks; additional therapy may be required for some patients

Gastric ulcers (*Canadian labeling*): 20 mg once daily up to 6 weeks; additional therapy may be required for some patients

H. pylori eradication: 20 mg twice daily for 7 days; to be administered with amoxicillin 1000 mg and clarithromycin 500 mg, also given twice daily for 7 days.

Hypersecretory conditions: 60 mg once daily; dose may need to be adjusted as necessary. Doses as high as 100 mg once daily and 60 mg twice daily have been used, and continued as long as necessary (up to 1 year in some patients).

NERD (*Canadian labeling*): Treatment: 10 mg (maximum: 20 mg once daily) for 4 weeks; lack of symptom control after 4 weeks warrants further evaluation

Dosage adjustment in renal impairment: No dosage adjustment required

Dosage adjustment in hepatic impairment:

Mild to moderate: Elimination decreased; no dosage adjustment required

Severe: Use caution

Dietary Considerations May be taken with or without food; best if taken before breakfast.

Administration May be administered with or without food; best if taken before breakfast. Do not crush, split, or chew tablet. May be administered with an antacid.

Dosage Forms Excipient information presented when available (limited, particularly for generics); consult specific product labeling. [CAN] = Canadian brand name

Tablet, delayed release, enteric coated, as sodium:

AcipHex®: 20 mg

Pariet® [CAN]: 10 mg, 20 mg

Rabies Immune Globulin (Human)

(RAY beez i MYUN GLOB yoo lin, HYU man)

U.S. Brand Names HyperRAB™ S/D; Imogam® Rabies-HT

Canadian Brand Names HyperRAB™ S/D; Imogam® Rabies Pasteurized

Index Terms RIG

Pharmacologic Category Immune Globulin

Additional Appendix Information

Immunization Recommendations *on page 1708*

Use Part of postexposure prophylaxis of persons with rabies exposure who lack a history of pre-exposure or postexposure prophylaxis with rabies vaccine or a recently documented neutralizing antibody response to previous rabies vaccination

Pregnancy Risk Factor C

Pregnancy Considerations Reproduction studies have not be conducted. Pregnancy is not a contraindication to postexposure prophylaxis.

Contraindications There are no contraindications listed within the FDA-approved manufacturer's labeling.

Warnings/Precautions Hypersensitivity and anaphylactic reactions can occur; immediate treatment (including epinephrine 1:1000) should be available. Use with caution in patients with isolated immunoglobulin A deficiency or a history of systemic hypersensitivity to human immunoglobulins. Use with caution in patients with thrombocytopenia or coagulation disorders; I.M. injections may be contraindicated. Product of human plasma; may potentially contain infectious agents which could transmit disease. Screening of donors, as well as testing and/or inactivation or removal of certain viruses, reduces the risk. Infections thought to be transmitted by this product should be reported to the manufacturer. Not for intravenous administration.

Adverse Reactions Frequency not defined.

Central nervous system: Fever (mild), headache, malaise

Dermatologic: Angioedema, rash, urticaria

Local: Soreness at injection site, tenderness, stiffness

Renal: Nephrotic syndrome

Miscellaneous: Anaphylaxis

Drug Interactions

Avoid Concomitant Use There are no known interactions where it is recommended to avoid concomitant use.

Increased Effect/Toxicity There are no known significant interactions involving an increase in effect.

Decreased Effect

Rabies Immune Globulin (Human) may decrease the levels/effects of: Vaccines (Live)

Stability Store between 2°C to 8°C (36°F to 46°F); do not freeze. Discard product exposed to freezing.

Mechanism of Action Rabies immune globulin is a solution of globulins dried from the plasma or serum of selected adult human donors who have been immunized with rabies vaccine and have developed high titers of rabies antibody. It generally contains 10% to 18% of protein of which not less than 80% is monomeric immunoglobulin G.

Dosage Children and Adults: Postexposure prophylaxis: Local wound infiltration: 20 units/kg in a single dose, RIG should always be administered as part of rabies vaccine regimen. If anatomically feasible, the full rabies immune globulin dose should be infiltrated around and into the wound(s); remaining volume should be administered I.M. at a site distant from the vaccine administration site. If rabies vaccine was initiated without rabies immune globulin, rabies immune globulin may be administered through the seventh day after the administration of the first dose of the vaccine. Administration of RIG is not recommended after the seventh day post vaccine since an antibody response to the vaccine is expected during this time period.

Note: Persons known to have an adequate titer or who have previously received postexposure prophylaxis with rabies vaccine should not receive RIG.

Administration Do not administer I.V.

Postexposure wound infiltration: If anatomically feasible, the full rabies immune globulin dose should be infiltrated around and into the wound(s); remaining volume should be administered I.M. in the deltoid muscle of the upper arm or lateral thigh muscle. The gluteal area should be avoided to reduce the risk of sciatic nerve damage. Do not administer rabies vaccine in the same syringe or at the same administration site as RIG.

Dosage Forms Excipient information presented when available (limited, particularly for generics); consult specific product labeling.

Injection, solution [preservative free]:

HyperRAB™ S/D: 150 int. units/mL (2 mL, 10 mL) [solvent/detergent treated]

Imogam® Rabies-HT: 150 int. units/mL (2 mL, 10 mL) [heat treated]

Rabies Vaccine (RAY beez vak SEEN)

U.S. Brand Names Imovax® Rabies; RabAvert®

Canadian Brand Names Imovax® Rabies; RabAvert®

Index Terms HDCV; Human Diploid Cell Cultures Rabies Vaccine; PCEC; Purified Chick Embryo Cell

Pharmacologic Category Vaccine, Inactivated (Viral)

Use Pre-exposure and postexposure vaccination against rabies

The Advisory Committee on Immunization Practices (ACIP) recommends a primary course of prophylactic immunization (pre-exposure vaccination) for the following:

- Persons with continuous risk of infection including rabies research laboratory and biologics production workers
- Persons with frequent risk of infection in areas where rabies is enzootic, including rabies diagnostic laboratory workers, cavers, veterinarians and their staff, animal control and wildlife workers; persons who frequently handle bats
- Persons with infrequent risk of infection, including veterinarians and animal control staff with terrestrial animals in areas where rabies infection is rare, veterinary students, travelers visiting areas where rabies is enzootic and immediate access to medical care and biologicals is limited

The ACIP recommends the use of postexposure vaccination for a particular person be assessed by the severity and likelihood versus the actual risk of acquiring rabies. Consideration should include the type of exposure, epidemiology of rabies in the area, species of the animal, circumstances of the incident, and the availability of the exposing animal for observation or rabies testing. Postexposure vaccination is used in both previously vaccinated and previously unvaccinated individuals.

Pregnancy Risk Factor C

Pregnancy Considerations Animal reproduction studies have not been conducted. Pregnancy is not a contraindication to postexposure prophylaxis. Pre-exposure prophylaxis during pregnancy may also be considered if risk of rabies is great.

Lactation Excretion in breast milk unknown

Contraindications

Pre-exposure prophylaxis: Hypersensitivity to rabies vaccine or any component of the formulation

Postexposure prophylaxis: There are no contraindications listed within the FDA-approved manufacturer's labeling.

Warnings/Precautions Rabies vaccine should not be used in persons with a confirmed diagnosis of rabies; use after the onset of symptoms may be detrimental. Postexposure vaccination may begin regardless of the length of time from documented or likely exposure, as long as clinical signs of rabies are not present. Immediate treatment (including epinephrine 1:1000) for anaphylactoid and/or hypersensitivity reactions should be available during vaccine use. Once postexposure prophylaxis has begun, administration should generally not be interrupted or discontinued due to local or mild adverse events. Continuation of vaccination following severe systemic reactions should consider the persons risk of developing rabies. Report serious reactions to the State Health Department or the manufacturer/distributor. An immune complex reaction is possible 2-21 days following booster doses of HDCV. Symptoms may include arthralgia, arthritis, angioedema, fever, generalized urticaria, malaise, nausea, and vomiting Immune response may be decreased in immunosuppressed patients. Imovax® Rabies contains albumin and neomycin. RabAvert® contains amphotericin B, bovine gelatin, chicken protein, chlortetracycline, and neomycin. For I. M. administration only.

Adverse Reactions All serious adverse reactions must be reported to the U.S. Department of Health and Human Services (DHHS) Vaccine Adverse Event Reporting System (VAERS) 1-800-822-7967.

>10%:

Central nervous system: Dizziness, headache, malaise

Gastrointestinal: Abdominal pain, nausea

Local: Erythema, itching, pain, swelling

Neuromuscular & skeletal: Myalgia

Miscellaneous: Lymphadenopathy

Uncommon, frequency not defined, postmarketing, and/or case reports:

Cardiovascular: Circulatory reactions, edema, palpitation

Central nervous system: Chills, fatigue, fever >38°C (100°F), Guillain-Barré syndrome, encephalitis, meningitis, multiple sclerosis, myelitis, neuroparalysis, vertigo

Dermatologic: Pruritus, urticaria, urticaria pigmentosa

Endocrine & metabolic: Hot flashes

Local: Limb swelling (extensive)

Neuromuscular & skeletal: Limb pain, monoarthritis, paralysis (transient), paresthesias (transient)

Otic: Retrobulbar neuritis, visual disturbances

Respiratory: Bronchospasm

Miscellaneous: Allergic reactions, anaphylaxis, hypersensitivity reactions, swollen lymph nodes

Drug Interactions

Avoid Concomitant Use There are no known interactions where it is recommended to avoid concomitant use.

Increased Effect/Toxicity There are no known significant interactions involving an increase in effect.

Decreased Effect

The levels/effects of Rabies Vaccine may be decreased by: Immunosuppressants

Stability Prior to reconstitution, store under refrigeration at 2°C to 8°C (36°F to 46°F); do not freeze. Protect from light. Reconstitute with provided diluent; gently swirl to dissolve. Use immediately after reconstitution.

Imovax®: Suspension will appear pink to red

RabAvert®: Suspension will appear clear to slightly opaque

Mechanism of Action Rabies vaccine is an inactivated virus vaccine which promotes immunity by inducing an active immune response. The production of specific antibodies requires about 7-10 days to develop. Rabies immune globulin or antirabies serum, equine (ARS) is given in conjunction with rabies vaccine to provide immune protection until an antibody response can occur.

Pharmacodynamics/Kinetics

Onset of action: I.M.: Rabies antibody: ~7-10 days

Peak effect: ~30-60 days

Duration: ≥1 year

Dosage

Pre-exposure vaccination: 1 mL I.M. on days 0, 7, and 21 to 28. **Note:** Prolonging the interval between doses does not interfere with immunity achieved after the concluding dose of the basic series.

Postexposure vaccination: All postexposure treatment should begin with immediate cleansing of the wound with soap and water

Persons not previously immunized as above: I.M.: 5 doses (1 mL each) on days 0, 3, 7, 14, 28. In addition, patients should also receive rabies immune globulin with the first dose (day 0)

Persons who have previously received postexposure prophylaxis with rabies vaccine, received a recommended I.M. pre-exposure series of rabies vaccine or have a previously documented rabies antibody titer considered adequate: I.M.: Two doses (1 mL each) on days 0 and 3; do not administer rabies immune globulin

Booster (for persons with continuous or frequent risk of infection): 1 mL I.M. based on antibody titers

Administration For I.M. administration only; this rabies vaccine product must not be administered intradermally; in adults and children, administer I.M. injections in the deltoid muscle, not the gluteal; for younger children, use the outer aspect of the thigh.

For patients at risk of hemorrhage following intramuscular injection, the ACIP recommends "it should be administered intramuscularly if, in the opinion of the physician familiar with the patients bleeding risk, the vaccine can be administered with reasonable safety by this route. If the patient receives antihemophilia or other similar therapy, intramuscular vaccination can be scheduled shortly after such therapy is administered. A fine needle (23 gauge or smaller) can be used for the vaccination and firm pressure applied to the site (without rubbing) for at least 2 minutes. The patient should be instructed concerning the risk of hematoma from the injection."

Administration with other vaccines:

Rabies vaccine with other inactivated vaccines: May be given simultaneously or at any interval between doses.

Rabies vaccine with live vaccines: May be given simultaneously or at any interval between doses.

Vaccine administration with antibody-containing products: Rabies vaccine may be given simultaneously at different sites or at any interval between doses. Examples of antibody containing products include I.M. and I.V. immune globulin, hepatitis B immune globulin, tetanus immune globulin, varicella zoster immune globulin, rabies immune globulin, whole blood, packed red cells, plasma, and platelet products.

Monitoring Parameters Monitor for syncope for ≥15 minutes following vaccination.

Antibody response to vaccination is not recommended for otherwise healthy persons who complete the pre-exposure or Postexposure regimen. Serologic testing to determine if the antibody titer is at an acceptable level is required for the following persons (booster vaccination recommended if titer is below the acceptable level):

Persons with continuous risk of infection: Serologic testing every 6 monthsPersons with frequent risk of infection: Serologic testing every 2 years

Monitoring of antibody response to vaccination is not recommended for otherwise healthy persons who complete the pre-exposure or Postexposure regimen.

Reference Range Adequate adaptive immune response: antibody titers of 0.5 int. units/mL [WHO] or complete virus neutralization at a 1:5 serum dilution by the rapid fluorescent focus inhibition test (RFFIT) [ACIP]

Additional Information Federal law requires that the date of administration, the vaccine manufacturer, lot number of vaccine, and the administering person's name, title, and address be entered into the patient's permanent medical record.

Dosage Forms Injection, powder for reconstitution [preservative free]:

Imovax® Rabies: ≥2.5 int. units [HDCV; grown in human diploid cell culture; contains albumin (human), neomycin (may have trace amounts)]

RabAvert®: ≥2.5 int. units [contains albumin (human), amphotericin B (may have trace amounts), bovine gelatin, chicken egg protein, chlortetracycline (may have trace amounts), neomycin (may have trace amounts); PCEC; grown in chicken fibroblast culture]

◆ **Racepinephrine** *see* EPINEPHrine *on page 525*

◆ **Radiogardase®** *see* Ferric Hexacyanoferrate *on page 615*

◆ **rAHF** *see* Antihemophilic Factor (Recombinant) *on page 121*

◆ **R-albuterol** *see* Levalbuterol *on page 870*

◆ **Ralivia™ ER (Can)** *see* TraMADol *on page 1497*

◆ **Ralix** *see* Chlorpheniramine, Phenylephrine, and Methscopolamine *on page 313*

Raloxifene (ral OKS i feen)

U.S. Brand Names Evista®

Canadian Brand Names Evista®

Index Terms Keoxifene Hydrochloride; NSC-706725; Raloxifene Hydrochloride

Pharmacologic Category Selective Estrogen Receptor Modulator (SERM)

Use Prevention and treatment of osteoporosis in postmenopausal women; risk reduction for invasive breast cancer in postmenopausal women with osteoporosis and in postmenopausal women with high risk for invasive breast cancer

Pregnancy Risk Factor X

Pregnancy Considerations Animal studies have demonstrated teratogenicity and fetal loss. There are no adequate and well-controlled studies in pregnant women. Raloxifene should not be used by pregnant women or by women planning to become pregnant in the immediate future.

Lactation Excretion in breast milk unknown/contraindicated

Medication Safety Issues

Sound-alike/look-alike issues:

Evista® may be confused with Avinza™

Contraindications History of or current venous thromboembolic disorders (including DVT, PE, and retinal vein thrombosis); pregnancy; breast-feeding

Warnings/Precautions Hazardous agent - use appropriate precautions for handling and disposal. **[U.S. Boxed Warning]: May increase the risk for DVT or PE;** use with caution in patients at high risk for venous thromboembolism; the risk for DVT and PE are higher in the first 4 months of treatment. Discontinue at least 72 hours prior to and during prolonged immobilization (postoperative recovery or prolonged bedrest). Use is contraindicated with a history of or current venous thromboembolic disorders. **[U.S. Boxed Warning]: The risk of death due to stroke may be increased in women with coronary heart disease or in women at risk for coronary events;** use with caution in patients with cardiovascular disease. Not be used for the prevention of cardiovascular disease. Use caution with moderate-to-severe renal dysfunction, hepatic impairment, unexplained uterine bleeding, and in women with a history of elevated triglycerides in response to treatment with oral estrogens (or estrogen/progestin). Safety with concomitant estrogen therapy has not been established. Safety and efficacy in premenopausal women or men have not been established. Not indicated for treatment of invasive breast cancer, to reduce the risk of recurrence of invasive breast cancer or to reduce the risk of noninvasive breast cancer. The efficacy (for breast cancer risk reduction) in women with inherited BRCA1 and BRCA1 mutations has not been established.

Adverse Reactions Note: Raloxifene has been associated with increased risk of thromboembolism (DVT, PE) and superficial thrombophlebitis; risk is similar to reported risk of HRT

>10%:

Cardiovascular: Peripheral edema (3% to 14%)

Endocrine & metabolic: Hot flashes (8% to 29%)

Neuromuscular & skeletal: Arthralgia (11% to 16%), leg cramps/muscle spasm (6% to 12%)

Miscellaneous: Flu syndrome (14% to 15%), infection (11% to 15%)

1% to 10%:

Cardiovascular: Chest pain (3% to 4%), syncope (2%), varicose vein (2%), venous thromboembolism (1% to 2%)

Central nervous system: Headache (9%), depression (6%), insomnia (6%), vertigo (4%), fever (3% to 4%), migraine (2%), hypoesthesia (≤2%)

Dermatologic: Rash (6%)

Endocrine & metabolic: Breast pain (4%)

Gastrointestinal: Nausea (8% to 9%), weight gain (9%), abdominal pain (7%), diarrhea (7%), dyspepsia (6%), vomiting (3% to 5%), flatulence (2% to 3%), cholelithiasis (≤3%), gastroenteritis (≤3%)

Genitourinary: Vaginal bleeding (6%), cystitis (3% to 5%), urinary tract infection (4%), vaginitis (4%), leukorrhea (3%), urinary tract disorder (3%), uterine disorder (3%), vaginal hemorrhage (3%), endometrial disorder (≤3%)

Neuromuscular & skeletal: Myalgia (8%), arthritis (4%), tendon disorder (4%), neuralgia (≤2%)

Ocular: Conjunctivitis (2%)

Respiratory: Bronchitis (10%), rhinitis (10%), sinusitis (8% to 10%), cough (6% to 9%), pharyngitis (5% to 8%), pneumonia (3%), laryngitis (≤2%)

Miscellaneous: Diaphoresis (3%)

<1% (Limited to important or life-threatening): Apolipoprotein A1 increased, apolipoprotein B decreased, death related to VTE, fibrinogen decreased, hypertriglyceridemia (in women with a history of increased triglycerides in response to oral estrogens), intermittent claudication, LDL cholesterol decreased, lipoprotein decreased, muscle spasm, retinal vein occlusion, stroke related to VTE, superficial thrombophlebitis, total serum cholesterol decreased

Drug Interactions

Avoid Concomitant Use There are no known interactions where it is recommended to avoid concomitant use.

Increased Effect/Toxicity There are no known significant interactions involving an increase in effect.

Decreased Effect

Raloxifene may decrease the levels/effects of: Levothyroxine

The levels/effects of Raloxifene may be decreased by: Bile Acid Sequestrants

Ethanol/Nutrition/Herb Interactions Ethanol: Avoid ethanol (may increase risk of osteoporosis).

Stability Store between 15°C to 30°C (59°F to 86°F).

Mechanism of Action A selective estrogen receptor modulator (SERM), meaning that it affects some of the same receptors that estrogen does, but not all, and in some instances, it antagonizes or blocks estrogen; it acts like estrogen to prevent bone loss and has the potential to block some estrogen effects in the breast and uterine tissues. Raloxifene decreases bone resorption, increasing bone mineral density and decreasing fracture incidence.

Pharmacodynamics/Kinetics

Onset of action: 8 weeks

Absorption: Rapid; ~60%

Distribution: 2348 L/kg

Protein binding: >95% to albumin and α-glycoprotein; does not bind to sex-hormone-binding globulin

Metabolism: Hepatic, extensive first-pass effect; metabolized to glucuronide conjugates

Bioavailability: ~2%

Half-life elimination: 28-33 hours

Excretion: Primarily feces; urine (<0.2% as unchanged drug; <6% as glucuronide conjugates)

Dosage Adults: Females: Oral:

Osteoporosis: 60 mg/day

Invasive breast cancer risk reduction: 60 mg/day

Dosage adjustment in hepatic impairment: Child-Pugh class A: Plasma concentrations were higher and correlated with total bilirubin. Safety and efficacy in hepatic insufficiency have not been established.

Dietary Considerations Supplemental calcium or vitamin D may be required if dietary intake is not adequate.

Administration May be administered any time of the day without regard to meals.

Monitoring Parameters Bone mineral density (BMD), CBC, lipid profile; adequate diagnostic measures, including endometrial sampling, if indicated, should be performed to rule out malignancy in all cases of undiagnosed abnormal vaginal bleeding

Additional Information The decrease in estrogen-related adverse effects with the selective estrogen-receptor modulators in general and raloxifene in particular should improve compliance and decrease the incidence of cardiovascular events and fractures while not increasing breast cancer.

Dosage Forms Excipient information presented when available (limited, particularly for generics); consult specific product labeling.

Tablet, as hydrochloride:

Evista®: 60 mg

◆ **Raloxifene Hydrochloride** *see* Raloxifene *on page 1289*

Raltegravir (ral TEG ra vir)

U.S. Brand Names Isentress™

Canadian Brand Names Isentress™

Index Terms MK-0518

Pharmacologic Category Antiretroviral Agent, Integrase Inhibitor

Additional Appendix Information

Antiretroviral Therapy for HIV Infection: Adults and Adolescents *on page 1758*

Perinatal HIV Guidelines *on page 1730*

Use Treatment of HIV-1 infection in combination with other antiretroviral agents in treatment-experienced patients with virus that shows multidrug resistance and active replication

Pregnancy Risk Factor C

Pregnancy Considerations Animal studies revealed treatment-related increases in rib formation at 3-4 times human doses; no other embryo-/fetotoxic or teratogenic effects noted. There are no adequate and well-controlled studies in pregnant women and available data is insufficient to recommend use in pregnancy. An antiretroviral registry has been established to monitor maternal and fetal outcomes in women receiving antiretroviral drugs. Physicians are encouraged to register patients at 1-800-258-4263 or www.APRegistry.com.

Lactation Excretion in breast milk unknown/contraindicated

Contraindications

U.S. labeling: There are no contraindications listed in the manufacturer's labeling.

Canadian labeling: Hypersensitivity to raltegravir or any other component of the formulation

Warnings/Precautions Patients may develop immune reconstitution syndrome resulting in the occurrence of an inflammatory response to an indolent or residual opportunistic infection; further evaluation and treatment may be required. Myopathy and rhabdomyolysis have been reported; use caution in patients with risk factors for CK elevations and/or skeletal muscle abnormalities. Use caution with medications known to induce (eg, rifampin) or inhibit (eg, atazanavir) UGT1A1 glucuronidation, as serum levels/therapeutic effects may be reduced or increased, respectively. Safety and efficacy have not been established in children <16 years of age.

Adverse Reactions

>10%: Endocrine & metabolic: Total cholesterol increased (grade 2: 16%; grade 3: 6%)

2% to 10%:

Cardiovascular: Hypertension (3%)

Central nervous system: Fatigue (8%), dizziness (4%), insomnia (4%)

Dermatologic: Rash (5%), pruritus (3% to 4%), folliculitis (2%)

Endocrine & metabolic: Glucose increased (≤250 mg/dL: 9%), LDL-cholesterol increased (grade 2: 9%; grade 3: 4%), hypertriglyceridemia (grade 3: 4%)

Gastrointestinal: Abdominal pain (5%), vomiting (4%), amylase increased (2.1-5 x ULN: 4%), gastroenteritis (3%), lipase increased (1.6-3 x ULN: 3%), anorexia (2%), constipation (2%)

Hepatic: Hyperbilirubinemia (9%; 2.6-5 x ULN: 3%), AST increased (2.6-5 x ULN: 9%), ALT increased (5.1-10 x ULN: 3%), alkaline phosphatase increased (2.6-5 x ULN: 2%)

Neuromuscular & skeletal: Arthralgia (3%), extremity pain (3%), creatine kinase increased (all grades: 2%)

Renal: Creatinine increased (1.4-1.8 x ULN: 3%)

Respiratory: Nasopharyngitis (6%), cough (5%), influenza (3%), sinusitis (3%)

Miscellaneous: Herpes zoster (4%), lymphadenopathy (3%), anogenital warts (2%)

Frequency <2% or not defined: Acneiform dermatitis, allodynia, anemia, anxiety, appetite increased, asthenia, back pain, cellulitis, central obesity, chest discomfort, chills, depression, diabetes mellitus, dreams abnormal, drug hypersensitivity, dry skin, dyspepsia, dyslipidemia, epistaxis, erectile dysfunction, erythema, facial wasting, flatulence, neutropenia, fever, gastritis, GERD, glossitis, gynecomastia, headache, hepatitis, hepatomegaly, herpes simplex, hyperhidrosis, hyperlactacidemia, irritability, lipodystrophy, macrocytic anemia, maculopapular rash, MI, muscle atrophy, muscle spasms, myalgia, myositis, nephropathy, nephrotic syndrome, neuropathy, night sweats, nocturia, palpitation, paresthesia, pollakiuria, prurigo, renal failure, renal tubular necrosis, skin infection, somnolence, Stevens-Johnson syndrome, vertigo, ventricular extrasystoles, visual disturbance, weight changes

Drug Interactions

Avoid Concomitant Use There are no known interactions where it is recommended to avoid concomitant use.

Increased Effect/Toxicity There are no known significant interactions involving an increase in effect.

Decreased Effect

The levels/effects of Raltegravir may be decreased by: Efavirenz; Rifampin; Tipranavir

Ethanol/Nutrition/Herb Interactions

Food: High-fat meal increased AUC by 19%, but raltegravir was administered without regard to meals in clinical trials.

Herb/Nutraceutical: St John's wort may decrease the levels/effects of raltegravir.

Stability Store at controlled room temperature of 20°C to 25°C (68°F to 77°F).

Mechanism of Action Incorporation of viral DNA into the host cell's genome is required to produce a self-replicating provirus and propagation of infectious virion particles. The viral cDNA strand produced by reverse transcriptase is subsequently processed and inserted into the human genome by the enzyme HIV-1 integrase (encoded by the pol gene of HIV). Raltegravir inhibits the catalytic activity of integrase, thus preventing integration of the proviral gene into human DNA.

Pharmacodynamics/Kinetics

Absorption: AUC increased 19% with high-fat meal

Protein binding: ~83%

Metabolism: Primarily hepatic glucuronidation mediated by UGT1A1

Half-life elimination: ~9 hours

Time to peak, plasma: ~3 hours

Excretion: Feces (51%, as unchanged drug); urine (32%; 9% as unchanged drug)

Dosage Oral: Adolescents ≥16 years and Adults: 400 mg twice daily

Dosage adjustment in renal impairment: No dosage adjustment required in severe impairment.

Dosage adjustment in hepatic impairment: No dosage adjustment required with mild-to-moderate impairment. No data available in severe impairment.

Dietary Considerations May be taken with or without food.

Monitoring Parameters Viral load, CD4 count, lipid profile

Dosage Forms Excipient information presented when available (limited, particularly for generics); consult specific product labeling.

Tablet:

Isentress™: 400 mg

Ramelteon (ra MEL tee on)

U.S. Brand Names Rozerem®

Index Terms TAK-375

Pharmacologic Category Hypnotic, Nonbenzodiazepine

Use Treatment of insomnia characterized by difficulty with sleep onset

Restrictions An FDA-approved patient medication guide is available and must be distributed when dispensing an outpatient prescription (new or refill) where this medication is to be used without direct supervision of a healthcare provider. Medication guides are available at http://www.fda.gov/cder/Offices/ODS/medication_guides.htm.

Pregnancy Risk Factor C

Pregnancy Considerations Animal studies have demonstrated teratogenic effects. May cause disturbances of reproductive hormonal regulation (eg, disruption of menses or decreased libido). There are no adequate and well-controlled studies in pregnant women.

Lactation Excretion in breast milk unknown/use caution

Medication Safety Issues

Sound-alike/look-alike issues:

Ramelteon may be confused with Remeron®

Rozerem® may be confused with Razadyne™, Remeron®

Contraindications History of angioedema with previous ramelteon therapy (do not rechallenge); concurrent use with fluvoxamine

Warnings/Precautions Symptomatic treatment of insomnia should be initiated only after careful evaluation of potential causes of sleep disturbance. Failure of sleep disturbance to resolve after a reasonable period of treatment may indicate psychiatric and/or medical illness. Because of the rapid onset of action, administer immediately prior to bedtime or after the patient has gone to bed and is having difficulty falling asleep. Hypnotics/sedatives have been associated with abnormal thinking and behavior changes including decreased inhibition, aggression, bizarre behavior, agitation, hallucinations, and depersonalization. These changes may occur unpredictably and may indicate previously unrecognized psychiatric disorders; evaluate appropriately. Postmarketing studies have indicated that the use of hypnotic/sedative agents (including ramelteon) for sleep has been associated with hypersensitivity reactions including anaphylaxis as well as angioedema. Do not rechallenge patients who have developed angioedema with ramelteon therapy. An increased risk for hazardous sleep-related activities such as sleep-driving; cooking and eating food, and making phone calls while asleep have also been noted. Use caution with pre-existing depression or other psychiatric conditions. Caution when using with other CNS depressants; avoid engaging in hazardous activities or activities requiring mental alertness. Not recommended for use in patients with severe sleep apnea or COPD. Use caution with moderate hepatic impairment; not recommended in patients with severe impairment. May cause disturbances of hormonal regulation. Use caution when administered concomitantly with strong CYP1A2 inhibitors. Safety and efficacy in pediatric patients have not been established.

Adverse Reactions 1% to 10%:

Central nervous system: Dizziness (4% to 5%), somnolence (3% to 5%), fatigue (3% to 4%), insomnia worsened (3%), depression (2%)

Endocrine & metabolic: Serum cortisol decreased (1%)

Gastrointestinal: Nausea (3%), taste perversion (2%)

Neuromuscular & skeletal: Myalgia (2%), arthralgia (2%)

Respiratory: Upper respiratory infection (3%)

Miscellaneous: Influenza (1%)

Postmarketing and/or case reports: Anaphylaxis, angioedema, complex sleep-related behavior (sleep-driving, cooking or eating food, making phone calls), prolactin levels increased, testosterone levels decreased

Drug Interactions

Metabolism/Transport Effects **Substrate** of CYP1A2 (major), CYP3A4 (minor), CYP2C family (minor)

Avoid Concomitant Use

Avoid concomitant use of Ramelteon with any of the following: Fluvoxamine

Increased Effect/Toxicity

Ramelteon may increase the levels/effects of: Alcohol (Ethyl); CNS Depressants

The levels/effects of Ramelteon may be increased by: Antifungal Agents (Azole Derivatives, Systemic); CYP1A2 Inhibitors (Moderate); CYP1A2 Inhibitors (Strong); Fluconazole; Fluvoxamine

Decreased Effect

The levels/effects of Ramelteon may be decreased by: Rifamycin Derivatives

Ethanol/Nutrition/Herb Interactions

Ethanol: Avoid ethanol (may increase CNS depression).

Food: Taking with high-fat meal delays T_{max} and increases AUC (~31%); do not take with high-fat meal.

Herb/Nutraceutical: Avoid valerian, St John's wort, kava kava, gotu kola (may increase CNS depression).

Stability Store at 25°C (77°F); excursions permitted to 15°C to 30°C (59°F to 86°F). Protect from moisture.

Mechanism of Action Potent, selective agonist of melatonin receptors MT_1 and MT_2 (with little affinity for MT_3) within the suprachiasmic nucleus of the hypothalamus, an area responsible for determination of circadian rhythms and synchronization of the sleep-wake cycle. Agonism of MT_1 is thought to preferentially induce sleepiness, while MT_2 receptor activation preferentially influences regulation of circadian rhythms. Ramelteon is eightfold more selective for MT_1 than MT_2 and exhibits nearly sixfold higher affinity for MT_1 than melatonin, presumably allowing for enhanced effects on sleep induction.

Pharmacodynamics/Kinetics

Onset of action: 30 minutes

Absorption: Rapid; high-fat meal delays T_{max} and increases AUC (~31%)

Distribution: 74 L

Protein binding: ~82%

Metabolism: Extensive first-pass effect; oxidative metabolism primarily through CYP1A2 and to a lesser extent through CYP2C and CYP3A4; forms active metabolite (M-II)

Bioavailability: Absolute: 1.8%

Half-life elimination: Ramelteon: 1-2.6 hours; M-II: 2-5 hours

Time to peak, plasma: Median: 0.5-1.5 hours

Excretion: Primarily as metabolites: Urine (84%); feces (4%)

Dosage

Oral: Adults: One 8 mg tablet within 30 minutes of bedtime

Dosage adjustment in renal impairment: No dosage adjustment required

Dosage adjustment in hepatic impairment: No adjustment required for mild-to-moderate impairment; use caution. Not recommended with severe impairment.

Dietary Considerations Taking with high-fat meal delays T_{max} and increases AUC (~31%); do not take with high-fat meal.

Administration Do not administer with a high-fat meal. Swallow tablet whole; do not break.

Dosage Forms Excipient information presented when available (limited, particularly for generics); consult specific product labeling.

Tablet:

Rozerem®: 8 mg

Ramipril (RA mi pril)

U.S. Brand Names Altace®

Canadian Brand Names Altace®; Apo-Ramipril®; CO Ramipril; GEN-Ramipril; Novo-Ramipril; RAN-Ramipril; ratio-Ramipril; Sandoz-Ramipril

Pharmacologic Category Angiotensin-Converting Enzyme (ACE) Inhibitor

Additional Appendix Information

Angiotensin Agents *on page 1632*

Heart Failure (Systolic) *on page 1809*

Use Treatment of hypertension, alone or in combination with thiazide diuretics; treatment of left ventricular dysfunction after MI; to reduce risk of MI, stroke, and death in patients at increased risk for these events

Unlabeled/Investigational Use Treatment of heart failure; to delay the progression of nephropathy and reduce risks of cardiovascular events in hypertensive patients with type 1 or 2 diabetes mellitus

Pregnancy Risk Factor C (1st trimester); D (2nd and 3rd trimesters)

Pregnancy Considerations Due to adverse events observed in some animal studies, ramipril is considered pregnancy category C during the first trimester. Based on human data, ramipril is considered pregnancy category D if used during the second and third trimesters (per the manufacturer; however, one study suggests that fetal injury may occur at anytime during pregnancy). Ramipril crosses the placenta. First trimester exposure to ACE inhibitors may cause major congenital malformations. An increased risk of cardiovascular and/or central nervous system malformations was observed in one study; however, an increased risk of teratogenic events was not observed in other studies. Second and third trimester use of an ACE inhibitor is associated with oligohydramnios. Oligohydramnios due to decreased fetal renal function may lead to fetal limb contractures, craniofacial deformation, and hypoplastic lung development. The use of ACE inhibitors during the second and third trimesters is also associated with anuria, hypotension, renal failure (reversible or irreversible), skull hypoplasia, and death in the fetus/neonate. Chronic maternal hypertension itself is also associated with adverse events in the fetus/infant. ACE inhibitors are not recommended during pregnancy to treat maternal hypertension or heart failure. Those who are planning a pregnancy should be considered for other medication options if an ACE inhibitor is currently prescribed or the ACE inhibitor should be discontinued as soon as possible once pregnancy is detected. The exposed fetus should be monitored for fetal growth, amniotic fluid volume, and organ formation. Infants exposed to an ACE inhibitor *in utero*, especially during the second and third trimester, should be monitored for hyperkalemia, hypotension, and oliguria.

[U.S. Boxed Warning]: Based on human data, ACE inhibitors can cause injury and death to the developing fetus when used in the second and third trimesters. ACE inhibitors should be discontinued as soon as possible once pregnancy is detected.

Lactation Excretion in breast milk unknown/not recommended

Medication Safety Issues

Sound-alike/look-alike issues:

Ramipril may be confused with enalapril, Monopril®

Altace® may be confused with alteplase, Amaryl®, Amerge®, Artane®

International issues:

Altace® may be confused with Altace® HCT which is a brand name for ramipril/hydrochlorothiazide combination product in Canada

Contraindications Hypersensitivity to ramipril or any component of the formulation; prior hypersensitivity (including angioedema) to ACE inhibitors

Warnings/Precautions Anaphylactic reactions may occur rarely with ACE inhibitors. At any time during treatment (especially following first dose) angioedema may occur rarely with ACE inhibitors; it may involve the head and neck (potentially compromising airway) or the intestine (presenting with abdominal pain). African-Americans and patients with idiopathic or hereditary angioedema may be at an increased risk. Prolonged frequent monitoring may be required especially if tongue, glottis, or larynx are involved as they are associated with airway obstruction. Patients with a history of airway surgery may have a higher risk of airway obstruction. Aggressive early and appropriate management is critical. Use in patients with previous angioedema associated with ACE inhibitor therapy is contraindicated. Severe anaphylactoid reactions may be seen during hemodialysis (eg, CVVHD) with high-flux dialysis membranes (eg, AN69), and rarely, during low density lipoprotein apheresis with dextran sulfate cellulose. Rare cases of anaphylactoid reactions have been reported in patients undergoing sensitization treatment with hymenoptera (bee, wasp) venom while receiving ACE inhibitors.

Symptomatic hypotension with or without syncope can occur with ACE inhibitors (usually with the first several doses); effects are most often observed in volume-depleted patients; close monitoring of patient is required especially with initial dosing and dosing increases; blood pressure must be lowered at a rate appropriate for the patient's clinical condition. Initiation of therapy in patients with ischemic heart disease or cerebrovascular disease warrants close observation due to the potential consequences posed by falling blood pressure (eg, MI, stroke). Use with caution in hypertrophic cardiomyopathy with outflow tract obstruction, severe aortic stenosis, or before, during, or immediately after major surgery. **[U.S. Boxed Warning]: Based on human data, ACEIs can cause injury and death to the developing fetus when used in the second and third trimesters. ACEIs should be discontinued as soon as possible once pregnancy is detected.**

Hyperkalemia may occur with ACE inhibitors; risk factors include renal dysfunction, diabetes mellitus, concomitant use of potassium-sparing diuretics, potassium supplements, and/or potassium containing salts. Use cautiously, if at all, with these agents and monitor potassium closely. Cough may occur with ACE inhibitors. Other causes of cough should be considered (eg, pulmonary congestion in patients with heart failure) and excluded prior to discontinuation.

May be associated with deterioration of renal function and/or increases in serum creatinine, particularly in patients with low renal blood flow (eg, renal artery stenosis, heart failure) whose glomerular filtration rate (GFR) is dependent on efferent arteriolar vasoconstriction by angiotensin II;

deterioration may result in oliguria, acute renal failure, and progressive azotemia. Small increases in serum creatinine may occur following initiation; consider discontinuation only in patients with progressive and/or significant deterioration in renal function. Use with caution in patients with unstented unilateral/bilateral renal artery stenosis. When unstented bilateral renal artery stenosis is present, use is generally avoided due to the elevated risk of deterioration in renal function unless possible benefits outweigh risks.

Rare toxicities associated with ACE inhibitors include cholestatic jaundice (which may progress to fulminant hepatic necrosis), agranulocytosis, neutropenia, or leukopenia with myeloid hypoplasia. Patients with collagen vascular diseases (especially with concomitant renal impairment) or renal impairment alone may be at increased risk for hematologic toxicity; periodically monitor CBC with differential in these patients. Safety and efficacy have not been established in children.

Adverse Reactions Note: Frequency ranges include data from hypertension and heart failure trials. Higher rates of adverse reactions have generally been noted in patients with CHF. However, the frequency of adverse effects associated with placebo is also increased in this population.

>10%: Respiratory: Cough (increased) (7% to 12%)

1% to 10%:

- Cardiovascular: Hypotension (11%), angina (up to 3%), postural hypotension (2%), syncope (up to 2%)
- Central nervous system: Headache (1% to 5%), dizziness (2% to 4%), fatigue (2%), vertigo (up to 2%)
- Endocrine & metabolic: Hyperkalemia (1% to 10%)
- Gastrointestinal: Nausea/vomiting (1% to 2%)
- Neuromuscular & skeletal: Chest pain (noncardiac) (1%)
- Renal: Renal dysfunction (1%), serum creatinine increased (1% to 2%), BUN increased (<1% to 3%); transient increases of creatinine and/or BUN may occur more frequently
- Respiratory: Cough (estimated 1% to 10%)

<1% (Limited to important or life-threatening): Agitation, agranulocytosis, amnesia, anaphylactoid reaction, angioedema, arrhythmia, bone marrow depression, convulsions, depression, dysphagia, dyspnea, edema, eosinophilia, erythema multiforme, hearing loss, hemolytic anemia, hepatitis, hypersensitivity reactions (urticaria, rash, fever), impotence, insomnia, myalgia, MI, neuropathy, onycholysis, pancreatitis, pancytopenia, paresthesia, pemphigoid, pemphigus, photosensitivity, proteinuria, somnolence, Stevens-Johnson syndrome, symptomatic hypotension, thrombocytopenia, toxic epidermal necrolysis

Worsening of renal function may occur in patients with bilateral renal artery stenosis or in hypovolemia. In addition, a syndrome which may include fever, myalgia, arthralgia, interstitial nephritis, vasculitis, rash, eosinophilia and positive ANA, and elevated ESR has been reported with ACE inhibitors. Risk of pancreatitis and/or agranulocytosis may be increased in patients with collagen vascular disease or renal impairment.

Drug Interactions

Avoid Concomitant Use There are no known interactions where it is recommended to avoid concomitant use.

Increased Effect/Toxicity

Ramipril may increase the levels/effects of: Allopurinol; Amifostine; AzaTHIOprine; CycloSPORINE; Ferric Gluconate; Gold Sodium Thiomalate; Lithium; RiTUXimab

The levels/effects of Ramipril may be increased by: Angiotensin II Receptor Blockers; Diazoxide; Eplerenone; Herbs (Hypotensive Properties); Loop Diuretics; Potassium Salts; Potassium-Sparing Diuretics; Prostacyclin Analogues; Sirolimus; Temsirolimus; Thiazide Diuretics; Trimethoprim

Decreased Effect

The levels/effects of Ramipril may be decreased by: Antacids; Aprotinin; Herbs (Hypertensive Properties); Methylphenidate; Nonsteroidal Anti-Inflammatory Agents; Salicylates; Yohimbine

Ethanol/Nutrition/Herb Interactions Herb/Nutraceutical: Avoid bayberry, blue cohosh, cayenne, ephedra, ginger, ginseng (American), kola, licorice (may worsen hypertension). Avoid black cohosh, California poppy, coleus, golden seal, hawthorn, mistletoe, periwinkle, quinine, shepherd's purse (may have increased antihypertensive effect).

Stability Store at controlled room temperature.

Mechanism of Action Ramipril is an ACE inhibitor which prevents the formation of angiotensin II from angiotensin I and exhibits pharmacologic effects that are similar to captopril. Ramipril must undergo enzymatic saponification by esterases in the liver to its biologically active metabolite, ramiprilat. The pharmacodynamic effects of ramipril result from the high-affinity, competitive, reversible binding of ramiprilat to angiotensin-converting enzyme, thus preventing the formation of the potent vasoconstrictor angiotensin II. This isomerized enzyme-inhibitor complex has a slow rate of dissociation, which results in high potency and a long duration of action; a CNS mechanism may also be involved in the hypotensive effect as angiotensin II increases adrenergic outflow from CNS; vasoactive kallikreins may be decreased in conversion to active hormones by ACE inhibitors, thus reducing blood pressure

Pharmacodynamics/Kinetics

Onset of action: 1-2 hours

Duration: 24 hours

Absorption: Well absorbed (50% to 60%)

Distribution: Plasma levels decline in a triphasic fashion; rapid decline is a distribution phase to peripheral compartment, plasma protein and tissue ACE (half-life: 2-4 hours); second phase is an apparent elimination phase representing the clearance of free ramiprilat (half-life: 9-18 hours); and final phase is the terminal elimination phase representing the equilibrium phase between tissue binding and dissociation

Protein binding:
- Ramipril: 73%
- Ramiprilat: 56%

Metabolism: Hepatic to the active form, ramiprilat

Bioavailability:
- Ramipril: 28%
- Ramiprilat: 44%

Half-life elimination: Ramiprilat: Effective: 13-17 hours; Terminal: >50 hours

Time to peak, serum:
- Ramipril: ~1 hour
- Ramiprilat: 2-4 hours

Excretion: Urine (60%) and feces (40%) as parent drug and metabolites

Dosage Adults: Oral:

Hypertension: 2.5-5 mg once daily, maximum: 20 mg/day

Reduction in risk of MI, stroke, and death from cardiovascular causes: Initial: 2.5 mg once daily for 1 week, then 5 mg once daily for the next 3 weeks, then increase as tolerated to 10 mg once daily (may be given as divided dose)

Heart failure postmyocardial infarction: Initial: 2.5 mg twice daily titrated upward, if possible, to 5 mg twice daily.

Heart failure (unlabeled use): Initial: 1.25-2.5 mg once daily; target dose: 10 mg once daily (ACC/AHA 2005 Heart Failure Guidelines)

Note: The dose of any concomitant diuretic should be reduced. If the diuretic cannot be discontinued, initiate therapy with 1.25 mg. After the initial dose, the patient should be monitored carefully until blood pressure has stabilized.

Dosing adjustment in renal impairment:

Cl_{cr} <40 mL/minute: Administer 25% of normal dose.

Renal failure and hypertension: Administer 1.25 mg once daily, titrated upward as possible.

Renal failure and heart failure: Administer 1.25 mg once daily, increasing to 1.25 mg twice daily up to 2.5 mg twice daily as tolerated.

Administration Capsule is usually swallowed whole, but may be may be mixed in water, apple juice, or applesauce.

Monitoring Parameters Blood pressure; serum creatinine and potassium; if patient has collagen vascular disease and/or renal impairment, periodically monitor CBC with differential

Test Interactions Increases BUN, creatinine, potassium, positive Coombs' [direct]; decreases cholesterol (S); may cause false-positive results in urine acetone determinations using sodium nitroprusside reagent

Dosage Forms Excipient information presented when available (limited, particularly for generics); consult specific product labeling.

Capsule: 1.25 mg, 2.5 mg, 5 mg, 10 mg

Altace®: 1.25 mg, 2.5 mg, 5 mg, 10 mg

Tablet:

Altace®: 1.25 mg, 2.5 mg, 5 mg, 10 mg

- ◆ **RAN™-Atenolol (Can)** *see* Atenolol *on page* 149
- ◆ **RAN™-Carvedilol (Can)** *see* Carvedilol *on page* 264
- ◆ **Ran-Cefprozil (Can)** *see* Cefprozil *on page* 281
- ◆ **RAN™-Ciprofloxacin (Can)** *see* Ciprofloxacin *on page* 329
- ◆ **RAN™-Citalopram (Can)** *see* Citalopram *on page* 337
- ◆ **Ranexa®** *see* Ranolazine *on page* 1297
- ◆ **RAN™-Fentanyl Transdermal System (Can)** *see* FentaNYL *on page* 610
- ◆ **RAN-Fosinopril (Can)** *see* Fosinopril *on page* 670

Ranibizumab (ra ni BIZ oo mab)

U.S. Brand Names Lucentis®

Canadian Brand Names Lucentis®

Index Terms rhuFabV2

Pharmacologic Category Monoclonal Antibody; Ophthalmic Agent; Vascular Endothelial Growth Factor (VEGF) Inhibitor

Use Treatment of neovascular (wet) age-related macular degeneration (AMD)

Pregnancy Risk Factor C

Pregnancy Considerations Reproduction studies have not been conducted. Use during pregnancy only if clearly needed.

Lactation Excretion in breast milk unknown/use caution

Contraindications Hypersensitivity to ranibizumab or any component of the formulation; ocular or periocular infection

Canadian labeling: Additional contraindications: Active intraocular inflammation

Warnings/Precautions Intravitreous injections may be associated with endophthalmitis and retinal detachments. Proper aseptic injection techniques should be used and patients should be instructed to report any signs of infection immediately. Intraocular pressure may increase following injection. Intravitreal injections of ranibizumab may induce temporary visual disturbances that impair the ability to drive or operate machinery. Affected patients should be advised to abstain from driving or using machinery until resolution of disturbances. Use for >24 months has not been evaluated.

Risk of thromboembolic events, particularly stroke, may be increased following intravitreal administration of VEGF inhibitors. Rare hypersensitivity reactions (including anaphylaxis) have been associated with another VEGF inhibitor, pegaptanib, occurring within several hours of use; monitor closely. Equipment and appropriate personnel should be available for monitoring and treatment of anaphylaxis. Safety and efficacy have not been established in children.

Additionally in Canadian labeling: Safety and efficacy of ranibizumab administered concurrently to both eyes or in recipients of previous intravitreal injections has not been established.

Adverse Reactions Note: Rates of ocular adverse reactions reported for control group when percentages overlapped with treatment group.

>10%:

Central nervous system: Headache (2% to 15%)

Neuromuscular & skeletal: Arthralgia (3% to 11%)

Ocular: Conjunctival hemorrhage (43% to 77%; control: 29% to 66%), eye pain (17% to 37%; control 11% to 33%), vitreous floaters (3% to 32%), intraocular pressure increased (8% to 24%), vitreous detachment (7% to 22%; control 13% to 18%), intraocular inflammation (5% to 18%; control 3% to 11%), eye irritation (4% to 19%; control 6% to 20%), visual disturbance (up to 14%), blepharitis (3% to 13%), retinal disorder (≤13%), retinal degeneration (1% to 11%)

Note: Cataract, foreign body sensation, lacrimation increased, pruritus, and subretinal fibrosis occurred in >10% of patients, but also occurred in similar percentages to the control; visual acuity blurred/decreased occurred more often in the control.

Respiratory: Nasopharyngitis (5% to 16%), upper respiratory tract infection (2% to 15%)

1% to 10%:

Cardiovascular: Arterial thromboembolic events (≤5%; stroke ≤3%), atrial fibrillation (≤5%)

Endocrine & metabolic: Hypercholesterolemia (1% to 8%), diabetes mellitus (≤5%)

Gastrointestinal: Nausea (2% to 9%), viral gastroenteritis ≤5%)

Hematologic: Anemia (3% to 8%; control up to 8%)

Ocular: Conjunctival hyperemia (≤9%), posterior capsule opacification (≤8%), injection site hemorrhage (≤5%), vitreous hemorrhage (≤4%)

Note: Ocular hyperemia, maculopathy, dry eye, and ocular discomfort occurred in 1% to 10% of patients, but also occurred in similar percentages to the control; retinal exudates occurred more often in the control.

Respiratory: Bronchitis (3% to 10%), cough (3% to 10%), sinusitis (2% to 8%), chronic obstructive pulmonary disease (COPD) (≤5%), dyspnea (≤5%)

Miscellaneous: Influenza (2% to 10%), ranibizumab antibodies (1% to 6%), herpes zoster (≤5%)

<1% (Limited to important or life-threatening): Endophthalmitis, iatrogenic traumatic cataracts, retinal tear, rhegmatogenous retinal detachments

Drug Interactions

Avoid Concomitant Use There are no known interactions where it is recommended to avoid concomitant use.

Increased Effect/Toxicity There are no known significant interactions involving an increase in effect.

Decreased Effect There are no known significant interactions involving a decrease in effect.

Stability Store in original carton under refrigeration at 2°C to 8°C (36°F to 46°F); protect from light. Do not freeze.

Mechanism of Action Ranibizumab is a recombinant humanized monoclonal antibody fragment which binds to and inhibits human vascular endothelial growth factor A (VEGF-A). Ranibizumab inhibits VEGF from binding to its receptors and thereby suppressing neovascularization and slowing vision loss.

Pharmacodynamics/Kinetics

Absorption: Low levels are detected in the serum following intravitreal injection

Half-life elimination: Vitreous: ~9 days

Dosage Intravitreal: Adults:

Age-related macular degeneration (AMD): 0.5 mg (0.05 mL) once a month. **Note:** Frequency may be reduced after the first 4 injections to once every 3 months if monthly injections are not feasible; however, this regimen has reportedly resulted in a ~5 letter (1 line) loss of visual acuity over 9 months, as compared to monthly dosing.

Canadian labeling: AMD: 0.5 mg (0.05 mL) once a month. Frequency may be reduced after the first 3 injections to once every 3 months if monthly injections are not feasible.

Dosage adjustment in renal impairment: Dose adjustment not expected

Dosage adjustment in hepatic impairment: Dose adjustment not expected

Administration For ophthalmic intravitreal injection only. Remove contents from vial using a 5 micron 19-gauge filter needle attached to a tuberculin syringe. Discard filter needle and replace with a sterile 30 gauge 1/2 inch needle for injection. Adequate anesthesia and a broad-spectrum antimicrobial agent should be administered prior to the procedure.

Monitoring Parameters Intraocular pressure (within 30 minutes and between 2-7 days following administration); retinal perfusion, endophthalmitis

Dosage Forms Excipient information presented when available (limited, particularly for generics); consult specific product labeling. [CAN] = Canadian product availability

Injection, solution [preservative free]:

Lucentis®: 10 mg/mL (0.2 mL)

Lucentis® [CAN]: 10 mg/mL (0.3 mL)

◆ **Raniclor™** *see* Cefaclor *on page 268*

Ranitidine (ra NI ti deen)

U.S. Brand Names Zantac 150™ [OTC]; Zantac 75® [OTC]; Zantac®; Zantac® EFFERdose®

Canadian Brand Names Acid Reducer; Acid Reducer Maximum Strength Non Prescription; Alti-Ranitidine; Apo-Ranitidine®; BCI-Ranitidine; CO Ranitidine; Dom-Ranitidine; Gen-Ranidine; Novo-Ranidine; Nu-Ranit; PMS-Ranitidine; Ranitidine Injection, USP; Ratio-Ranitidine; Rhoxal-Ranitidine; Riva-Ranitidine; Sandoz-Ranitidine; ScheinPharm Ranitidine; Zantac 75®; Zantac Maximum Strength Non-Prescription; Zantac®

Index Terms Ranitidine Hydrochloride

Pharmacologic Category Histamine H_2 Antagonist

Use

Zantac®: Short-term and maintenance therapy of duodenal ulcer, gastric ulcer, gastroesophageal reflux, active benign ulcer, erosive esophagitis, and pathological hypersecretory conditions; as part of a multidrug regimen for *H. pylori* eradication to reduce the risk of duodenal ulcer recurrence

Zantac 75® [OTC]: Relief of heartburn, acid indigestion, and sour stomach

Unlabeled/Investigational Use Recurrent postoperative ulcer, upper GI bleeding, prevention of acid-aspiration pneumonitis during surgery, and prevention of stress-induced ulcers

Pregnancy Risk Factor B

Pregnancy Considerations Ranitidine crosses the placenta, teratogenic effects to the fetus have not been reported in animal studies. Use with caution during pregnancy.

Lactation Enters breast milk/use caution

Medication Safety Issues

Sound-alike/look-alike issues:

Ranitidine may be confused with amantadine, rimantadine

Zantac® may be confused with Xanax®, Zarontin®, Zofran®, Zyrtec®

International issues:

Antagon®: Brand name for astemizole in Mexico; brand name for ganirelix in the U.S.

Contraindications Hypersensitivity to ranitidine or any component of the formulation

Warnings/Precautions Ranitidine has been associated with confusional states (rare). Use with caution in patients with hepatic impairment; use with caution in renal impairment, dosage modification required. Avoid use in patients with history of acute porphyria (may precipitate attacks); long-term therapy may be associated with vitamin B_{12} deficiency. Symptoms of GI distress may be associated with a variety of conditions; symptomatic response to H_2 antagonists does not rule out the potential for significant pathology (eg, malignancy). EFFERdose® formulation contains phenylalanine. Safety and efficacy of ranitidine have not been established for pediatric patients <1 month of age

Adverse Reactions Frequency not defined (limited to important or life-threatening):

Cardiovascular: Arrhythmias, vasculitis

Central nervous system: Dizziness, hallucinations, headache, mental confusion, somnolence, vertigo

Dermatologic: Erythema multiforme, rash

Gastrointestinal: Pancreatitis

Hematologic: Acquired hemolytic anemia, agranulocytosis, aplastic anemia, granulocytopenia, leukopenia, pancytopenia, thrombocytopenia

Hepatic: Hepatic failure

Respiratory: Pneumonia (causal relationship not established)

Miscellaneous: Anaphylaxis, hypersensitivity reactions

Drug Interactions

Metabolism/Transport Effects Substrate (minor) of CYP1A2, 2C19, 2D6; **Inhibits** CYP1A2 (weak), 2D6 (weak)

Avoid Concomitant Use

Avoid concomitant use of Ranitidine with any of the following: Erlotinib; Mesalamine

Increased Effect/Toxicity

Ranitidine may increase the levels/effects of: Saquinavir

The levels/effects of Ranitidine may be increased by: P-Glycoprotein Inhibitors

Decreased Effect

Ranitidine may decrease the levels/effects of: Antifungal Agents (Azole Derivatives, Systemic); Atazanavir; Cefpodoxime; Cefuroxime; Dasatinib; Erlotinib; Fosamprenavir; Indinavir; Iron Salts; Mesalamine; Nelfinavir

The levels/effects of Ranitidine may be decreased by: P-Glycoprotein Inducers

Ethanol/Nutrition/Herb Interactions

Ethanol: Avoid ethanol (may cause gastric mucosal irritation).

Food: Does not interfere with absorption of ranitidine.

Stability

Injection: Vials: Store between 4°C to 30°C (39°F to 86°F). Protect from light. Solution is a clear, colorless to yellow solution; slight darkening does not affect potency.

Premixed bag: Store between 2°C to 25°C (36°F to 77°F). Protect from light.

EFFERdose® formulations: Store between 2°C to 30°C (36°F to 86°F).

Syrup: Store between 4°C to 25°C (39°F to 77°F). Protect from light.

Tablet: Store in dry place, between 15°C to 30°C (59°F to 86°F). Protect from light.

Vials can be mixed with NS or D_5W; solutions are stable for 48 hours at room temperature.

Intermittent bolus injection: Dilute to maximum of 2.5 mg/mL.

Intermittent infusion: Dilute to maximum of 0.5 mg/mL.

Mechanism of Action Competitive inhibition of histamine at H_2-receptors of the gastric parietal cells, which inhibits gastric acid secretion, gastric volume, and hydrogen ion concentration are reduced. Does not affect pepsin secretion, pentagastrin-stimulated intrinsic factor secretion, or serum gastrin.

Pharmacodynamics/Kinetics

Absorption: Oral: 50%

Distribution: Normal renal function: V_d: 1.7 L/kg; Cl_{cr} 25-35 mL/minute: 1.76 L/kg minimally penetrates the blood-brain barrier; enters breast milk

Protein binding: 15%

Metabolism: Hepatic to N-oxide, S-oxide, and N-desmethyl metabolites

Bioavailability: Oral: 48%

Half-life elimination:

Oral: Normal renal function: 2.5-3 hours; Cl_{cr} 25-35 mL/minute: 4.8 hours

I.V.: Normal renal function: 2-2.5 hours

Time to peak, serum: Oral: 2-3 hours; I.M.: ≤15 minutes

Excretion: Urine: Oral: 30%, I.V.: 70% (as unchanged drug); feces (as metabolites)

Dosage

Children 1 month to 16 years:

Duodenal and gastric ulcer:

Oral:

Treatment: 2-4 mg/kg/day divided twice daily; maximum treatment dose: 300 mg/day

Maintenance: 2-4 mg/kg once daily; maximum maintenance dose: 150 mg/day

I.V.: 2-4 mg/kg/day divided every 6-8 hours; maximum: 200 mg/day

GERD and erosive esophagitis:

Oral: 5-10 mg/kg/day divided twice daily; maximum: GERD: 300 mg/day, erosive esophagitis: 600 mg/day

I.V. (unlabeled): 2-4 mg/kg/day divided every 6-8 hours; maximum: 200 mg/day **or as an alternative**

Continuous infusion: Initial: 1 mg/kg/dose for one dose followed by infusion of 0.08-0.17 mg/kg/hour or 2-4 mg/kg/day

Children ≥12 years: Prevention of heartburn: Oral: Zantac 75® [OTC]: 75 mg 30-60 minutes before eating food or drinking beverages which cause heartburn; maximum: 150 mg/24 hours; do not use for more than 14 days

Adults:

Duodenal ulcer: Oral: Treatment: 150 mg twice daily, or 300 mg once daily after the evening meal or at bedtime; maintenance: 150 mg once daily at bedtime

Helicobacter pylori eradication: 150 mg twice daily; requires combination therapy

Pathological hypersecretory conditions:

Oral: 150 mg twice daily; adjust dose or frequency as clinically indicated; doses of up to 6 g/day have been used

I.V.: Continuous infusion for Zollinger-Ellison: 1 mg/kg/hour; measure gastric acid output at 4 hours, if >10 mEq or if patient is symptomatic, increase dose in increments of 0.5 mg/kg/hour; doses of up to 2.5 mg/kg/hour have been used

Gastric ulcer, benign: Oral: 150 mg twice daily; maintenance: 150 mg once daily at bedtime

Erosive esophagitis: Oral: Treatment: 150 mg 4 times/day; maintenance: 150 mg twice daily

Prevention of heartburn: Oral: Zantac 75® [OTC]: 75 mg 30-60 minutes before eating food or drinking beverages which cause heartburn; maximum: 150 mg in 24 hours; do not use for more than 14 days

Patients not able to take oral medication:

I.M.: 50 mg every 6-8 hours

I.V.: Intermittent bolus or infusion: 50 mg every 6-8 hours

Continuous I.V. infusion: 6.25 mg/hour

Elderly: Ulcer healing rates and incidence of adverse effects are similar in the elderly, when compared to younger patients; dosing adjustments not necessary based on age alone

Dosing adjustment in renal impairment: Adults: Cl_{cr} <50 mL/minute:

Oral: 150 mg every 24 hours; adjust dose cautiously if needed

I.V.: 50 mg every 18-24 hours; adjust dose cautiously if needed

Hemodialysis: Adjust dosing schedule so that dose coincides with the end of hemodialysis

Dosing adjustment/comments in hepatic disease: Patients with hepatic impairment may have minor changes in ranitidine half-life, distribution, clearance, and bioavailability; dosing adjustments not necessary, monitor

Dietary Considerations Oral dosage forms may be taken with or without food.

Zantac® EFFERdose®: Effervescent tablet 25 mg contains sodium 1.33 mEq/tablet and phenylalanine 2.81 mg/tablet

Administration

Ranitidine injection may be administered I.M. or I.V.:

I.M.: Injection is administered undiluted

I.V.: Must be diluted; may be administered IVP or IVPB or continuous I.V. infusion

IVP: Ranitidine (usually 50 mg) should be diluted to a total of 20 mL with NS or D_5W and administered over at least 5 minutes

IVPB: Administer over 15-20 minutes

Continuous I.V. infusion: Administer at 6.25 mg/hour and titrate dosage based on gastric pH by continuous infusion over 24 hours

EFFERdose®: Should not be chewed, swallowed whole, or dissolved on tongue: 25 mg tablet: Dissolve in at least 5 mL (1 teaspoonful) of water; wait until completely dissolved before administering

Monitoring Parameters AST, ALT, serum creatinine; when used to prevent stress-related GI bleeding, measure the intragastric pH and try to maintain pH >4; signs and symptoms of peptic ulcer disease, occult blood with GI bleeding, monitor renal function to correct dose; monitor for side effects

Test Interactions False-positive urine protein using Multistix®, gastric acid secretion test, skin test allergen extracts, serum creatinine, urine protein test

Dosage Forms Excipient information presented when available (limited, particularly for generics); consult specific product labeling.

Capsule 150 mg, 300 mg

Infusion [premixed in NaCl 0.45%; preservative free]:

Zantac®: 50 mg (50 mL)

Injection, solution: 25 mg/mL (2 mL, 6 mL)

Zantac®: 25 mg/mL (2 mL, 6 mL, 40 mL) [contains phenol 0.5% as preservative]

Syrup: 15 mg/mL (5 mL, 10 mL, 473 mL)

Zantac®: 15 mg/mL (473 mL) [contains alcohol 7.5%; peppermint flavor]

Tablet: 75 mg [OTC], 150 mg, 300 mg

Zantac®: 150 mg, 300 mg

Zantac 75®: 75 mg

Zantac 150™: 150 mg

Tablet, for solution, oral [effervescent]:

Zantac® EFFERdose®: 25 mg [contains phenylalanine 2.81 mg/tablet, sodium 1.33 mEq/tablet, sodium benzoate]

◆ **Ranitidine Hydrochloride** *see* Ranitidine *on page* 1295

- ◆ **Ranitidine Injection, USP (Can)** *see* Ranitidine *on page 1295*
- ◆ **Ran-Lisinopril (Can)** *see* Lisinopril *on page 894*
- ◆ **RAN™-Lovastatin (Can)** *see* Lovastatin *on page 910*
- ◆ **RAN™-Metformin (Can)** *see* MetFORMIN *on page 954*

Ranolazine (ra NOE la zeen)

U.S. Brand Names Ranexa®

Pharmacologic Category Cardiovascular Agent, Miscellaneous

Use Treatment of chronic angina

Pregnancy Risk Factor C

Pregnancy Considerations Adverse effects were observed in animal studies. There are no adequate and well-controlled studies in pregnant women.

Lactation Excretion in breast milk unknown/not recommended

Medication Safety Issues

Sound-alike/look-alike issues:

Ranexa™ may be confused with Celexa®

Contraindications Clinically significant hepatic impairment; concurrent strong CYP3A inhibitors; concurrent inducers of CYP3A

Warnings/Precautions Ranolazine does not relieve acute angina attacks. Has been shown to prolong QT interval in a dose/plasma concentration-related manner. Hepatically-impaired patients may have a more significant increase in QT interval. Use with caution in patients with mild (Child-Pugh class A) or moderate (Child-Pugh class B) hepatic impairment; use is contraindicated with clinically significant hepatic impairment. Use caution in patients ≥75 years of age; they may experience more adverse events. Use caution and monitor blood pressure in patients with renal dysfunction; has not been evaluated in patients requiring dialysis.

Ranolazine is a substrate for and a moderate inhibitor of P-glycoprotein. Inhibitors of P-glycoprotein may increase serum concentrations of ranolazine. Ranolazine may increase serum concentrations of substrates for P-glycoprotein (eg, digoxin). Ranolazine is primarily metabolized by CYP3A; use is contraindicated with inducers and strong inhibitors of CYP3A. Ranolazine has potential to prolong the QT-interval; use caution when administered concomitantly with QT-prolonging drugs. Use caution when administering ranolazine to patients with a history of malignant neoplasms or adenomatous polyps. Safety and efficacy in children have not been established.

Adverse Reactions

>10%:

Central nervous system: Dizziness (5% to 13%; dose related)

Gastrointestinal: Constipation (5% to 8%; 19% in the elderly)

>0.5% to 10%:

Cardiovascular: Syncope (≤3%), bradycardia (≤2%), hypotension (≤2%), orthostatic hypotension (≤2%), palpitation (≤2%), peripheral edema (≤2%), QT_c prolongation (>500 msec: ≤1%)

Central nervous system: Headache (3% to 6%), vertigo (≤2%)

Gastrointestinal: Nausea (4% to 9%), abdominal pain (≤2%), vomiting (≤2%), xerostomia (≤2%)

Hematologic: Hematocrit decreased (1%)

Otic: Tinnitus (≤2%)

Respiratory: Dyspnea (≤2%)

≤0.5% (Limited to important or life-threatening): Angioedema, blood pressure increased, blurred vision, confusion, eosinophilia, hemoglobin A_{1c} decreased, hematuria, hypoesthesia, leukopenia, pancytopenia, paresthesia, pulmonary fibrosis, renal failure, serum creatinine increased, thrombocytopenia, T-wave amplitude decreased, T-wave changes (notched), torsade de pointes (case report [Morrow, 2007]), tremor, weakness

Drug Interactions

Metabolism/Transport Effects Substrate of CYP3A4 (major), 2D6 (minor), P-glycoprotein; **Inhibits** CYP3A4 (weak), 2D6 (moderate), P-glycoprotein

Avoid Concomitant Use

Avoid concomitant use of Ranolazine with any of the following: Antifungal Agents (Azole Derivatives, Systemic); Calcium Channel Blockers (Nondihydropyridine); CYP3A4 Inducers (Strong); CYP3A4 Inhibitors (Strong); Dabigatran Etexilate; Nilotinib; Rifampin; Rivaroxaban; Silodosin; Tetrabenazine; Thioridazine; Topotecan; Ziprasidone

Increased Effect/Toxicity

Ranolazine may increase the levels/effects of: CYP2D6 Substrates; Dabigatran Etexilate; Digoxin; Fesoterodine; Nebivolol; P-Glycoprotein Substrates; QTc-Prolonging Agents; Rivaroxaban; Silodosin; Simvastatin; Tamoxifen; Tetrabenazine; Thioridazine; Topotecan; Ziprasidone

The levels/effects of Ranolazine may be increased by: Alfuzosin; Antifungal Agents (Azole Derivatives, Systemic); Calcium Channel Blockers (Nondihydropyridine); Ciprofloxacin; CYP3A4 Inhibitors (Moderate); CYP3A4 Inhibitors (Strong); Dasatinib; Gadobutrol; Nilotinib; P-Glycoprotein Inhibitors

Decreased Effect

Ranolazine may decrease the levels/effects of: Codeine; TraMADol

The levels/effects of Ranolazine may be decreased by: CYP3A4 Inducers (Strong); Deferasirox; Herbs (CYP3A4 Inducers); P-Glycoprotein Inducers; Rifampin

Ethanol/Nutrition/Herb Interactions Food: Limit the use of grapefruit, grapefruit juice, or grapefruit-containing products; if use is significant and consistent, the dose of ranolazine should be limited to 500 mg twice daily.

Stability Store at 25°C (77°F); excursions permitted to 15°C to 30°C (59°F to 86°F).

Mechanism of Action Ranolazine exerts antianginal and anti-ischemic effects without changing hemodynamic parameters (heart rate or blood pressure). At therapeutic levels, ranolazine inhibits the late phase of the inward sodium channel (late I_{Na}) in ischemic cardiac myocytes during cardiac repolarization reducing intracellular sodium concentrations and thereby reducing calcium influx via Na^+-Ca^{2+} exchange. Decreased intracellular calcium reduces ventricular tension and myocardial oxygen consumption. It is thought that ranolazine produces myocardial relaxation and reduces anginal symptoms through this mechanism although this is uncertain. At higher concentrations, ranolazine inhibits the rapid delayed rectifier potassium current (I_{Kr}) thus prolonging the ventricular action potential duration and subsequent prolongation of the QT interval.

Pharmacodynamics/Kinetics

Absorption: Highly variable; ranolazine is a substrate of P-glycoprotein; concurrent use of P-glycoprotein inhibitors may increase absorption

Protein binding: ~62%

Metabolism: Hepatic via CYP3A (major) and 2D6 (minor); gut

Bioavailability: 35% to 55%

Half-life elimination: Terminal: 7 hours

Time to peak, plasma: 2-5 hours

Excretion: Primarily urine (75% mostly as metabolites); feces (25% mostly as metabolites); in feces and urine, <5% to 7% excreted unchanged

Dosage Oral: Chronic angina:

Adults: Initial: 500 mg twice daily; maximum recommended dose: 1000 mg twice daily

Elderly: Select dose cautiously, starting at the lower end of the dosing range

Dosage adjustment for ranolazine with concomitant medications:

Diltiazem, verapamil, and other moderate CYP3A inhibitors: Dose should not exceed 500 mg twice daily

P-glycoprotein inhibitors (eg, cyclosporine): Down-titrate ranolazine based on clinical response

Dosage adjustment in renal impairment: Dosage adjustment recommendations have not been established. However, plasma ranolazine levels increased ~50% in patients with varying degrees of renal dysfunction. Patients with severe renal dysfunction had an increase in mean diastolic blood pressure of 10-15 mm Hg. Monitor blood pressure closely in these patients. Ranolazine has not been evaluated in patients requiring dialysis.

Dosage adjustment in hepatic impairment: Use with caution in patients with mild (Child-Pugh class A) and moderate (Child-Pugh class B) hepatic impairment. Use is contraindicated with clinically significant hepatic impairment.

Dietary Considerations May be taken with or without food.

Administration May be taken with or without meals. Swallow tablet whole; do not crush, break, or chew.

Monitoring Parameters Baseline and follow up ECG to evaluate QT interval; blood pressure in patients with renal dysfunction; correct and maintain serum potassium in normal limits

Dosage Forms Excipient information presented when available (limited, particularly for generics); consult specific product labeling.

Tablet, extended release:

Ranexa®: 500 mg, 1000 mg

- ◆ **RAN-Ondansetron (Can)** *see* Ondansetron *on page 1102*
- ◆ **Ran-Pantoprazole (Can)** *see* Pantoprazole *on page 1140*
- ◆ **RAN-Pravastatin (Can)** *see* Pravastatin *on page 1227*
- ◆ **Ran-Rabeprazole (Can)** *see* Rabeprazole *on page 1285*
- ◆ **RAN-Ramipril (Can)** *see* Ramipril *on page 1292*
- ◆ **Ran-Risperidone (Can)** *see* Risperidone *on page 1323*
- ◆ **Ran-Tamsulosin (Can)** *see* Tamsulosin *on page 1426*
- ◆ **Rapaflo®** *see* Silodosin *on page 1370*
- ◆ **Rapamune®** *see* Sirolimus *on page 1372*
- ◆ **Raphon [OTC]** *see* EPINEPHrine *on page 525*
- ◆ **Raptiva®** *see* Efalizumab *on page 507*

Rasagiline (ra SA ji leen)

U.S. Brand Names Azilect®

Index Terms AGN 1135; Rasagiline Mesylate; TVP-1012

Pharmacologic Category Anti-Parkinson's Agent, MAO Type B Inhibitor

Additional Appendix Information

Antiparkinsonian Agents *on page 1643*

Use Initial monotherapy or as adjunct to levodopa in the treatment of idiopathic Parkinson's disease

Pregnancy Risk Factor C

Pregnancy Considerations Animal studies have documented decreased offspring survival and birth weight. An increased incidence of teratogenic effects, embryo-fetal deaths, and cardiovascular abnormalities were also noted with rasagiline in combination with levodopa/carbidopa. There are no adequate and well-controlled studies in pregnant women.

Lactation Excretion in breast milk unknown/use caution

Medication Safety Issues

Sound-alike/look-alike issues:

Azilect® may be confused with Aricept®

Contraindications Hypersensitivity to rasagiline or any component of the formulation; concomitant use of amphetamine, tramadol, propoxyphene, methadone, dextromethorphan, St John's wort, mirtazapine, cyclobenzaprine, or sympathomimetic amines (eg, pseudoephedrine, ephedrine); use of meperidine or other MAO inhibitor within 14 days of rasagiline; elective surgery requiring general anesthesia, local anesthesia containing sympathomimetic vasoconstrictors; patients with pheochromocytoma

Warnings/Precautions

Cardiovascular system: Hypertensive crisis may occur with tyramine, tryptophan, or dopamine-containing foods; avoid for at least 2 weeks following discontinuation of rasagiline. May cause orthostatic hypotension, particularly in combination with levodopa; use with caution in patients with hypotension or patients who would not tolerate transient hypotensive episodes (cardiovascular or cerebrovascular disease); orthostasis is usually most problematic during first 2 months of therapy and tends to abate thereafter. Due to the potential for hemodynamic instability, patients should not undergo elective surgery requiring general anesthesia and should avoid local anesthesia containing sympathomimetic vasoconstrictors within 14 days of discontinuing rasagiline. If surgery is required, benzodiazepines, mivacurium, fentanyl, morphine or codeine may be used cautiously.

Central nervous system: May cause hallucinations; signs of severe CNS toxicity (some fatal), including hyperpyrexia, hyperthermia, rigidity, altered mental status, seizure and coma have been reported with selective and nonselective MAO inhibitor use in combination with antidepressants. Do not use within 5 weeks of fluoxetine discontinuation; do not initiate tricyclic, SSRI or SNRI therapy within 2 weeks of discontinuing rasagiline. Addition to levodopa therapy may result in exacerbation of dyskinesias, requiring a reduction in levodopa dosage.

Dermatologic: Risk of melanoma may be increased with rasagiline, although increased risk has been associated with Parkinson's disease itself; patients should have regular and frequent skin examinations.

Organ dysfunction: Use caution in mild hepatic impairment; dose reduction recommended. Do not use with moderate to severe hepatic impairment.

Safety and efficacy in pediatric patients have not been established.

Adverse Reactions Unless otherwise noted, the following adverse reactions are as reported for monotherapy. Spectrum of adverse events was generally similar with adjunctive (levodopa) therapy, though the incidence tended to be higher.

>10%:

Central nervous system: Dyskinesia (18% adjunct therapy), headache (14%)

Gastrointestinal: Nausea (10% to 12% adjunct therapy)

1% to 10%:

Cardiovascular: Postural hypotension (6% to 9% adjunct therapy; dose dependent), bundle branch block angina, chest pain, syncope

Central nervous system: Depression (5%), hallucinations (4% to 5% adjunct therapy), fever (3%), malaise (2%), vertigo (2%), anxiety, dizziness

Dermatologic: Bruising (2%), alopecia, skin carcinoma, vesiculobullous rash

Endocrine & metabolic: Impotence, libido decreased

Gastrointestinal: Constipation (4% to 9% adjunct therapy), weight loss (2% to 9% adjunct therapy; dose dependent), dyspepsia (7%), xerostomia (2% to 6%

adjunct therapy; dose dependent), gastroenteritis (3%), anorexia, diarrhea, gastrointestinal hemorrhage, vomiting

Genitourinary: Hematuria, urinary incontinence

Hematologic: Leukopenia

Hepatic: Liver function tests increased

Neuromuscular & skeletal: Arthralgia (7%), neck pain (2%), arthritis (2%), paresthesia (2%), abnormal gait, hyperkinesias, hypertonia, neuropathy, tremor, weakness

Ocular: Conjunctivitis (3%)

Renal: Albuminuria

Respiratory: Rhinitis (3%), asthma, cough increased

Miscellaneous: Fall (5%), flu-like syndrome (5%), allergic reaction

<1% (Limited to important or life-threatening): Acute kidney failure, aphasia, apnea, atrial arrhythmia, bigeminy, blepharitis, blindness, bone necrosis, cerebral hemorrhage, cerebral ischemia, circumoral paresthesia, deafness, deep thrombophlebitis, delirium, diplopia, dysautonomia, dysesthesia, emphysema, esophageal ulcer, exfoliative dermatitis, facial paralysis, glaucoma, gynecomastia, heart failure, hematemesis, hemiplegia, hemorrhage (various locations), hostility, hypocalcemia, incoordination, interstitial pneumonia, intestinal obstruction, intestinal perforation, intestinal stenosis, jaundice, keratitis, kidney calculus, large intestine perforation, laryngismus, larynx edema, leukoderma, leukorrhea, lung fibrosis, macrocytic anemia, manic depressive reaction, mania, megacolon, menstrual abnormalities, MI, muscle atrophy, myelitis, neuralgia, neuritis, neurosis, nocturia, paranoid reaction, parosmia, personality disorder, pleural effusion, pneumothorax, polyuria, psychosis, psychotic depression, ptosis, purpura, retinal degeneration, retinal detachment, seizure, stomach ulcer, strabismus, stupor, thrombocythemia, thrombosis, tongue edema, urinary disorders, vaginal moniliasis, ventricular fibrillation, ventricular tachycardia, vestibular disorder, visual field defect

Drug Interactions

Metabolism/Transport Effects **Substrate** of CYP1A2 (major)

Avoid Concomitant Use

Avoid concomitant use of Rasagiline with any of the following: Alpha-/Beta-Agonists (Indirect-Acting); Alpha1-Agonists; Alpha2-Agonists (Ophthalmic); Amphetamines; Atomoxetine; BuPROPion; BusPIRone; Cyclobenzaprine; Dexmethylphenidate; Dextromethorphan; Linezolid; Maprotiline; Meperidine; Methyldopa; Methylphenidate; Mirtazapine; Propoxyphene; Selective Serotonin Reuptake Inhibitors; Serotonin 5-HT1D Receptor Agonists; Serotonin/Norepinephrine Reuptake Inhibitors; Sibutramine; Tetrabenazine; Tricyclic Antidepressants

Increased Effect/Toxicity

Rasagiline may increase the levels/effects of: Alpha-/Beta-Agonists (Direct-Acting); Alpha-/Beta-Agonists (Indirect-Acting); Alpha1-Agonists; Alpha2-Agonists (Ophthalmic); Amphetamines; Atomoxetine; Beta2-Agonists; BuPROPion; Dexmethylphenidate; Dextromethorphan; Linezolid; Lithium; Meperidine; Methyldopa; Methylphenidate; Mirtazapine; Rauwolfia Alkaloids; Selective Serotonin Reuptake Inhibitors; Serotonin 5-HT1D Receptor Agonists; Serotonin Modulators; Serotonin/Norepinephrine Reuptake Inhibitors; Tricyclic Antidepressants

The levels/effects of Rasagiline may be increased by: Altretamine; Anilidopiperidine Opioids; BusPIRone; COMT Inhibitors; Cyclobenzaprine; CYP1A2 Inhibitors (Moderate); CYP1A2 Inhibitors (Strong); Levodopa; Maprotiline; Propoxyphene; Sibutramine; Tetrabenazine; TraMADol

Decreased Effect

The levels/effects of Rasagiline may be decreased by: CYP1A2 Inducers (Strong)

Ethanol/Nutrition/Herb Interactions

Ethanol: Avoid ethanol. Avoid beverages containing tyramine (hearty red wine and beer).

Food: Concurrent ingestion of foods rich in tyramine may cause sudden and severe high blood pressure (hypertensive crisis). Avoid tyramine-containing foods with MAO-Is. Food's freshness is also an important concern; improperly stored or spoiled food can create an environment where tyramine concentrations may increase.

Herb/Nutraceutical: Avoid valerian, St John's wort, SAMe, kava kava (may increase risk of serotonin syndrome and/or excessive sedation); Avoid supplements containing caffeine, tyrosine, tryptophan, or phenylalanine. Ingestion of large quantities may increase the risk of severe side effects (eg, hypertensive reactions, serotonin syndrome).

Stability Store at 15°C to 30°C (59°F to 86°F).

Mechanism of Action Potent, irreversible and selective inhibitor of brain monoamine oxidase (MAO) type B, which plays a major role in the catabolism of dopamine. Inhibition of dopamine depletion in the striatal region of the brain reduces the symptomatic motor deficits of Parkinson's disease. There is also experimental evidence of rasagiline conferring neuroprotective effects (antioxidant, antiapoptotic), which may delay onset of symptoms and progression of neuronal deterioration.

Pharmacodynamics/Kinetics

Onset of action: Therapeutic: Within 1 hour

Duration: ~1 week (irreversible inhibition); may require ~14-40 days for complete restoration of (brain) MAO-B activity

Absorption: Rapid

Protein binding: 88% to 94%

Metabolism: Hepatic N-dealkylation and/or hydroxylation via CYP1A2 to multiple inactive metabolites (nonamphetamine derivatives)

Distribution: V_{dss}: 87 L

Bioavailability: 36%

Half-life elimination: ~1.3-3 hours (no correlation with biologic effect due to irreversible inhibition)

Time to peak, plasma: 30 minutes to 1 hour

Excretion: Urine (62%, >99% as metabolites); feces (7%)

Dosage Oral: Adults: Parkinson's disease:

Monotherapy: 1 mg once daily

Adjunctive therapy with levodopa: Initial: 0.5 mg once daily; may increase to 1 mg once daily based on response and tolerability

Note: When added to existing levodopa therapy, a dose reduction of levodopa may be required to avoid exacerbation of dyskinesias; typical dose reductions of ~9% to 13% were employed in clinical trials

Dose reduction with concomitant ciprofloxacin or other CYP1A2 inhibitors: 0.5 mg once daily

Dosage adjustment in renal impairment:

Mild impairment: No adjustment necessary

Moderate-to-severe impairment: No data available

Dosage adjustment in hepatic impairment:

Mild impairment (Child-Pugh ≤6): 0.5 mg once daily

Moderate-to-severe impairment: Not recommended

Dietary Considerations Avoid tyramine-containing foods/beverages. Some examples include aged or matured cheese, air-dried or cured meats (including sausages and salamis), fava or broad bean pods, tap/draft beers, Marmite concentrate, sauerkraut, soy sauce and other soybean condiments.

Monitoring Parameters Blood pressure; symptoms of parkinsonism; general mood and behavior (increased anxiety, or presence of mania or agitation); skin examination for presence of melanoma (higher incidence in Parkinson's patients- drug causation not established)

Additional Information When adding rasagiline to levodopa/carbidopa, the dose of the latter can usually be decreased. Studies are investigating the use of rasagiline in early Parkinson's disease to slow the progression of the disease.

Dosage Forms Excipient information presented when available (limited, particularly for generics); consult specific product labeling.

Tablet:
Azilect®: 0.5 mg, 1 mg

◆ **Rasagiline Mesylate** *see* Rasagiline *on page* 1298

Rasburicase (ras BYOOR i kayse)

U.S. Brand Names Elitek™

Canadian Brand Names Fasturtec®

Index Terms NSC-721631; Recombinant Urate Oxidase

Pharmacologic Category Enzyme; Enzyme, Urate-Oxidase (Recombinant)

Use Initial management of uric acid levels in pediatric patients with leukemia, lymphoma, and solid tumor malignancies receiving anticancer therapy expected to result in tumor lysis and elevation of plasma uric acid

Unlabeled/Investigational Use Prevention and treatment of malignancy-associated hyperuricemia in adults

Pregnancy Risk Factor C

Pregnancy Considerations Reproduction studies have not been conducted.

Lactation Excretion in breast milk unknown/not recommended

Contraindications Hypersensitivity, hemolytic or methemoglobinemia reactions to rasburicase or any component of the formulation; glucose-6-phosphatase dehydrogenase (G6PD) deficiency

Warnings/Precautions **[U.S. Boxed Warning]: Hypersensitivity reactions (including anaphylaxis), methemoglobinemia, and severe hemolysis have been reported;** reactions may occur at any time during treatment (including the initial dose); discontinue **immediately and permanently** in patients developing any of these reactions. Hemolysis may be associated with G6PD deficiency; patients at higher risk for G6PD deficiency should be screened prior to therapy. **[U.S. Boxed Warning]: Enzymatic degradation of uric acid in blood samples will occur if left at room temperature;** specific guidelines for the collection of plasma uric acid samples must be followed. Rasburicase is immunogenic and can elicit an antibody response; administration of more than one course is not recommended.

Adverse Reactions As reported in patients receiving rasburicase with antitumor therapy versus active-control:

>10%:
- Central nervous system: Fever (5% to 46%), headache (26%)
- Dermatologic: Rash (13%)
- Gastrointestinal: Vomiting (50%), nausea (27%), abdominal pain (20%), constipation (20%), mucositis (2% to 15%), diarrhea (≤1% to 20%)

1% to 10%:
- Hematologic: Neutropenia with fever (4%), neutropenia (2%)
- Respiratory: Respiratory distress (3%)
- Miscellaneous: Sepsis (3%)

<1% (Limited to important or life-threatening): Anaphylaxis, convulsions, hemolysis, methemoglobinemia, pulmonary edema

Drug Interactions

Avoid Concomitant Use There are no known interactions where it is recommended to avoid concomitant use.

Increased Effect/Toxicity There are no known significant interactions involving an increase in effect.

Decreased Effect There are no known significant interactions involving a decrease in effect.

Stability Prior to reconstitution, store with diluent at 2°C to 8°C (36°F to 46°F); do not freeze. Protect from light. Reconstitute each vial with 1 mL of the provided diluent. Mix by gently swirling; do **not** shake or vortex. Discard if discolored or containing particulate matter. Total dose should be further diluted in NS to a final volume of 50 mL. Reconstituted and final solution may be stored up to 24 hours at 2°C to 8°C (36°F to 46°F). Discard unused product.

Mechanism of Action Rasburicase is a recombinant urate-oxidase enzyme, which converts uric acid to allantoin (an inactive and soluble metabolite of uric acid); it does not inhibit the formation of uric acid.

Pharmacodynamics/Kinetics

Distribution: Pediatric patients: 110-127 mL/kg
Half-life elimination: Pediatric patients: 18 hours

Dosage I.V.:

Children: Management of uric acid levels: 0.15 mg/kg or 0.2 mg/kg once daily for 5 days (manufacturer-recommended duration); begin chemotherapy 4-24 hours after the first dose

Limited data suggest that a single prechemotherapy dose (versus multiple-day administration) may be sufficiently efficacious. Monitoring electrolytes, hydration status, and uric acid concentrations are necessary to identify the need for additional doses. Other clinical manifestations of tumor lysis syndrome (eg, hyperphosphatemia, hypocalcemia, and hyperkalemia) may occur.

Adults (unlabeled use): Management of malignancy-associated hyperuricemia: 0.2 mg/kg/day for 3-7 days, beginning the day before or day of chemotherapy **or** 0.15-0.2 mg/kg as a single dose, repeated if needed based on uric acid levels **or** 3-6 mg as a single dose, repeated (1.5-6 mg) if needed based on uric acid levels

Administration I.V. infusion over 30 minutes; do **not** administer as a bolus infusion. Do **not** filter during infusion. If not possible to administer through a separate line, I.V. line should be flushed with at least 15 mL saline prior to and following rasburicase infusion.

Monitoring Parameters Plasma uric acid levels, CBC

Test Interactions Specific handling procedures must be followed to prevent the degradation of uric acid in plasma samples. Blood must be collected in prechilled tubes containing heparin anticoagulant. Samples must then be **immediately** immersed in an ice water bath. Prepare samples by centrifugation in a precooled centrifuge (4°C). Samples must be kept in ice water bath and analyzed within 4 hours of collection.

Dosage Forms Excipient information presented when available (limited, particularly for generics); consult specific product labeling.

Injection, powder for reconstitution:
Elitek™: 1.5 mg [packaged with three 1 mL ampuls of diluent]; 7.5 mg [packaged with 5 mL of diluent]

◆ **Rasilez® (Can)** *see* Aliskiren *on page* 63
◆ **rATG** *see* Antithymocyte Globulin (Rabbit) *on page* 125
◆ **ratio-Aclavulanate (Can)** *see* Amoxicillin and Clavulanate Potassium *on page* 100
◆ **ratio-Acyclovir (Can)** *see* Acyclovir *on page* 40
◆ **ratio-Alendronate (Can)** *see* Alendronate *on page* 58
◆ **ratio-Amcinonide (Can)** *see* Amcinonide *on page* 81
◆ **Ratio-Amiodarone (Can)** *see* Amiodarone *on page* 87
◆ **Ratio-Amiodarone I.V. (Can)** *see* Amiodarone *on page* 87
◆ **ratio-Azithromycin (Can)** *see* Azithromycin *on page* 166
◆ **ratio-Bicalutamide (Can)** *see* Bicalutamide *on page* 197

- ◆ **ratio-Brimonidine (Can)** *see* Brimonidine *on page 212*
- ◆ **RATIO-Bupropion SR (Can)** *see* BuPROPion *on page 223*
- ◆ **ratio-Buspirone (Can)** *see* BusPIRone *on page 226*
- ◆ **ratio-Carvedilol (Can)** *see* Carvedilol *on page 264*
- ◆ **Ratio-Cefuroxime (Can)** *see* Cefuroxime *on page 288*
- ◆ **ratio-Ciprofloxacin (Can)** *see* Ciprofloxacin *on page 329*
- ◆ **ratio-Citalopram (Can)** *see* Citalopram *on page 337*
- ◆ **ratio-Clarithromycin (Can)** *see* Clarithromycin *on page 341*
- ◆ **ratio-Clindamycin (Can)** *see* Clindamycin *on page 344*
- ◆ **RATIO-Clobetasol (Can)** *see* Clobetasol *on page 347*
- ◆ **ratio-Cotridin (Can)** *see* Triprolidine, Pseudoephedrine, and Codeine *on page 1523*
- ◆ **ratio-Diltiazem CD (Can)** *see* Diltiazem *on page 450*
- ◆ **ratio-Emtec (Can)** *see* Acetaminophen and Codeine *on page 27*
- ◆ **ratio-Enalapril (Can)** *see* Enalapril *on page 515*
- ◆ **ratio-Famotidine (Can)** *see* Famotidine *on page 603*
- ◆ **ratio-Fenofibrate MC (Can)** *see* Fenofibrate *on page 607*
- ◆ **ratio-Fentanyl (Can)** *see* FentaNYL *on page 610*
- ◆ **ratio-Fluoxetine (Can)** *see* FLUoxetine *on page 638*
- ◆ **ratio-Fluticasone (Can)** *see* Fluticasone *on page 644*
- ◆ **RATIO-Gabapentin (Can)** *see* Gabapentin *on page 678*
- ◆ **ratio-Glimepiride (Can)** *see* Glimepiride *on page 696*
- ◆ **ratio-Glyburide (Can)** *see* GlyBURIDE *on page 701*
- ◆ **ratio-Inspra-Sal (Can)** *see* Albuterol *on page 51*
- ◆ **ratio-Ipra Sal UDV (Can)** *see* Ipratropium and Albuterol *on page 812*
- ◆ **ratio-Ketorolac (Can)** *see* Ketorolac *on page 841*
- ◆ **ratio-Lamotrigine (Can)** *see* LamoTRIgine *on page 850*
- ◆ **ratio-Lenoltec (Can)** *see* Acetaminophen and Codeine *on page 27*
- ◆ **ratio-Lisinopril (Can)** *see* Lisinopril *on page 894*
- ◆ **ratio-Lovastatin (Can)** *see* Lovastatin *on page 910*
- ◆ **RATIO-Metformin (Can)** *see* MetFORMIN *on page 954*
- ◆ **ratio-Methotrexate (Can)** *see* Methotrexate *on page 965*
- ◆ **RATIO-Methylphenidate (Can)** *see* Methylphenidate *on page 973*
- ◆ **ratio-Mirtazapine (Can)** *see* Mirtazapine *on page 1002*
- ◆ **ratio-Mometasone (Can)** *see* Mometasone *on page 1012*
- ◆ **Ratio-Morphine (Can)** *see* Morphine Sulfate *on page 1016*
- ◆ **Ratio-Morphine SR (Can)** *see* Morphine Sulfate *on page 1016*
- ◆ **ratio-Omeprazole (Can)** *see* Omeprazole *on page 1100*
- ◆ **RATIO-Ondansetron (Can)** *see* Ondansetron *on page 1102*
- ◆ **ratio-Orciprenaline® (Can)** *see* Metaproterenol *on page 952*
- ◆ **Ratio-Pantoprazole (Can)** *see* Pantoprazole *on page 1140*
- ◆ **ratio-Paroxetine (Can)** *see* PARoxetine *on page 1146*
- ◆ **ratio-Pentoxifylline (Can)** *see* Pentoxifylline *on page 1173*
- ◆ **ratio-Pioglitazone (Can)** *see* Pioglitazone *on page 1195*
- ◆ **ratio-Pravastatin (Can)** *see* Pravastatin *on page 1227*
- ◆ **ratio-Quetiapine (Can)** *see* QUEtiapine *on page 1275*
- ◆ **ratio-Ramipril (Can)** *see* Ramipril *on page 1292*
- ◆ **Ratio-Ranitidine (Can)** *see* Ranitidine *on page 1295*
- ◆ **Ratio-Risperidone (Can)** *see* Risperidone *on page 1323*
- ◆ **ratio-Salbutamol (Can)** *see* Albuterol *on page 51*
- ◆ **ratio-Sertraline (Can)** *see* Sertraline *on page 1362*
- ◆ **ratio-Simvastatin (Can)** *see* Simvastatin *on page 1370*
- ◆ **RATIO-Sotalol (Can)** *see* Sotalol *on page 1394*
- ◆ **ratio-Sumatriptan (Can)** *see* SUMAtriptan *on page 1414*
- ◆ **ratio-Tamsulosin (Can)** *see* Tamsulosin *on page 1426*
- ◆ **ratio-Temazepam (Can)** *see* Temazepam *on page 1432*
- ◆ **ratio-Theo-Bronc (Can)** *see* Theophylline *on page 1455*
- ◆ **ratio-Topiramate (Can)** *see* Topiramate *on page 1489*
- ◆ **ratio-Trazodone (Can)** *see* TraZODone *on page 1505*
- ◆ **ratio-Valproic (Can)** *see* Valproic Acid and Derivatives *on page 1538*
- ◆ **ratio-Valproic ECC (Can)** *see* Valproic Acid and Derivatives *on page 1538*
- ◆ **RATIO-Venlafaxine XR (Can)** *see* Venlafaxine *on page 1554*
- ◆ **Razadyne™** *see* Galantamine *on page 679*
- ◆ **Razadyne™ ER** *see* Galantamine *on page 679*
- ◆ **6R-BH4** *see* Sapropterin *on page 1353*
- ◆ **Reactine™ (Can)** *see* Cetirizine *on page 295*
- ◆ **Rea-Lo® [OTC]** *see* Urea *on page 1530*
- ◆ **ReAzo [OTC]** *see* Phenazopyridine *on page 1177*
- ◆ **Rebetol®** *see* Ribavirin *on page 1310*
- ◆ **Rebetron®** *see* Interferon Alfa-2b and Ribavirin *on page 804*
- ◆ **Rebif®** *see* Interferon Beta-1a *on page 806*
- ◆ **Reclast®** *see* Zoledronic Acid *on page 1587*
- ◆ **Reclipsen™** *see* Ethinyl Estradiol and Desogestrel *on page 575*
- ◆ **Recombinant α-L-Iduronidase (Glycosaminoglycan α-L-Iduronohydrolase)** *see* Laronidase *on page 857*
- ◆ **Recombinant Hirudin** *see* Lepirudin *on page 863*
- ◆ **Recombinant Human Deoxyribonuclease** *see* Dornase Alfa *on page 481*
- ◆ **Recombinant Human Insulin-Like Growth Factor-1** *see* Mecasermin *on page 926*
- ◆ **Recombinant Human Interleukin-11** *see* Oprelvekin *on page 1106*
- ◆ **Recombinant Human Luteinizing Hormone** *see* Lutropin Alfa *on page 912*
- ◆ **Recombinant Human Parathyroid Hormone (1-34)** *see* Teriparatide *on page 1444*
- ◆ **Recombinant Human Platelet-Derived Growth Factor B** *see* Becaplermin *on page 176*
- ◆ **Recombinant Human Thyrotropin** *see* Thyrotropin Alfa *on page 1465*
- ◆ **Recombinant Interleukin-11** *see* Oprelvekin *on page 1106*
- ◆ **Recombinant Plasminogen Activator** *see* Reteplase *on page 1306*
- ◆ **Recombinant Urate Oxidase** *see* Rasburicase *on page 1300*
- ◆ **Recombinate** *see* Antihemophilic Factor (Recombinant) *on page 121*
- ◆ **Recombivax HB®** *see* Hepatitis B Vaccine (Recombinant) *on page 728*
- ◆ **Rectacaine [OTC]** *see* Phenylephrine *on page 1183*
- ◆ **Red Cross™ Canker Sore [OTC]** *see* Benzocaine *on page 183*

Remifentanil (rem i FEN ta nil)

U.S. Brand Names Ultiva®

Canadian Brand Names Ultiva®

Index Terms GI87084B

Pharmacologic Category Analgesic, Opioid; Anilidopiperidine Opioid

Use Analgesic for use during the induction and maintenance of general anesthesia; for continued analgesia into the immediate postoperative period; analgesic component of monitored anesthesia

Unlabeled/Investigational Use Management of pain in mechanically-ventilated patients

Restrictions C-II

Pregnancy Risk Factor C

Pregnancy Considerations Remifentanil has been shown to cross the placenta. Neonatal respiratory depression and sedation may occur.

Lactation Excretion in breast milk unknown/use caution

Medication Safety Issues

Sound-alike/look-alike issues:

Remifentanil may be confused with alfentanil

High alert medication: The Institute for Safe Medication Practices (ISMP) includes this medication among its list of drug classes which have a heightened risk of causing significant patient harm when used in error.

Contraindications Not for intrathecal or epidural administration, due to the presence of glycine in the formulation; hypersensitivity to remifentanil, fentanyl, or fentanyl analogs, or any component of the formulation

Warnings/Precautions Remifentanil is not recommended as the sole agent in general anesthesia, because the loss of consciousness cannot be assured and due to the high incidence of apnea, hypotension, tachycardia and muscle rigidity; it should be administered by individuals specifically trained in the use of anesthetic agents and should not be used in diagnostic or therapeutic procedures outside the monitored anesthesia setting; resuscitative and intubation equipment should be readily available. May cause hypotension; use with caution in patients with hypovolemia, cardiovascular disease (including acute MI), or drugs which may exaggerate hypotensive effects (including phenothiazines or general anesthetics). Shares the toxic potentials of opiate agonists, and precautions of opiate agonist therapy should be observed. In patients <55 years of age, intraoperative awareness has been reported when used with propofol rates of ≤75 mcg/kg/minute.

Use with caution when administering to patients with bradycardia. Inject slowly over 3-5 minutes; rapid I.V. infusion may result in skeletal muscle and chest wall rigidity, impaired ventilation, or respiratory distress/arrest; nondepolarizing skeletal muscle relaxant may be required. Interruption of an infusion will result in offset of effects within 5-10 minutes; the discontinuation of remifentanil infusion should be preceded by the establishment of adequate postoperative analgesia orders, especially for patients in whom postoperative pain is anticipated. Use caution in the morbidly obese. Safety and efficacy for postoperative analgesic or monitored anesthesia care have not been established in children.

Adverse Reactions

>10%: Gastrointestinal: Nausea, vomiting

1% to 10%:

Cardiovascular: Bradycardia (dose dependent), hypertension, hypotension (dose dependent), tachycardia

Central nervous system: Agitation, dizziness, fever, headache

Dermatologic: Pruritus

Neuromuscular & skeletal: Muscle rigidity (dose dependent)

Ocular: Visual disturbances

Respiratory: Apnea, hypoxia, respiratory depression

Miscellaneous: Postoperative pain, shivering

<1% (Limited to important or life-threatening): Anaphylactic/anaphylactoid reactions, anemia, anxiety, arrhythmia, asystole, bronchospasm, confusion, constipation, CPK-MB increased, diarrhea, dysphagia, electrolyte disorders, hallucinations, heart block, pleural effusion, prolonged emergence from anesthesia, pulmonary edema, syncope, thrombocytopenia, xerostomia

Drug Interactions

Avoid Concomitant Use There are no known interactions where it is recommended to avoid concomitant use.

Increased Effect/Toxicity

Remifentanil may increase the levels/effects of: Alcohol (Ethyl); Alvimopan; Beta-Blockers; Calcium Channel Blockers (Nondihydropyridine); CNS Depressants; Desmopressin; MAO Inhibitors; Selective Serotonin Reuptake Inhibitors

The levels/effects of Remifentanil may be increased by: Amphetamines; Antipsychotic Agents (Phenothiazines); Succinylcholine

Decreased Effect

Remifentanil may decrease the levels/effects of: Pegvisomant

The levels/effects of Remifentanil may be decreased by: Ammonium Chloride

Stability Prior to reconstitution, store at 2°C to 25°C (36°F to 77°F). Prepare solution by adding 1 mL of diluent per

1 mg of remifentanil. Shake well. Further dilute to a final concentration of 20, 25, 50, or 250 mcg/mL. Stable for 24 hours at room temperature after reconstitution and further dilution to concentrations of 20-250 mcg/mL (4 hours if diluted with LR).

Mechanism of Action Binds with stereospecific mu-opioid receptors at many sites within the CNS, increases pain threshold, alters pain reception, inhibits ascending pain pathways

Pharmacodynamics/Kinetics

Onset of action: I.V.: 1-3 minutes

Distribution: V_d: 100 mL/kg; increased in children

Protein binding: ~70% (primarily $alpha_1$ acid glycoprotein)

Metabolism: Rapid via blood and tissue esterases

Half-life elimination (dose dependent): Terminal: 10-20 minutes; effective: 3-10 minutes

Excretion: Urine

Dosage I.V. continuous infusion: Dose should be based on ideal body weight (IBW) in obese patients (>30% over IBW).

Children Birth to 2 months: Maintenance of anesthesia with nitrous oxide (70%): 0.4 mcg/kg/minute (range: 0.4-1 mcg/kg/minute); supplemental bolus dose of 1 mcg/kg may be administered, smaller bolus dose may be required with potent inhalation agents, potent neuraxial anesthesia, significant comorbidities, significant fluid shifts, or without atropine pretreatment. Clearance in neonates is highly variable; dose should be carefully titrated.

Children 1-12 years: Maintenance of anesthesia with halothane, sevoflurane, or isoflurane: 0.25 mcg/kg/minute (range: 0.05-1.3 mcg/kg/minute); supplemental bolus dose of 1 mcg/kg may be administered every 2-5 minutes. Consider increasing concomitant anesthetics with infusion rate >1 mcg/kg/minute. Infusion rate can be titrated upward in increments up to 50% or titrated downward in decrements of 25% to 50%. May titrate every 2-5 minutes.

Adults:

Induction of anesthesia: 0.5-1 mcg/kg/minute; if endotracheal intubation is to occur in <8 minutes, an initial dose of 1 mcg/kg may be given over 30-60 seconds

Coronary bypass surgery: 1 mcg/kg/minute

Maintenance of anesthesia: **Note:** Supplemental bolus dose of 1 mcg/kg may be administered every 2-5 minutes. Consider increasing concomitant anesthetics with infusion rate >1 mcg/kg/minute. Infusion rate can be titrated upward in increments of 25% to 100% or downward in decrements of 25% to 50%. May titrate every 2-5 minutes.

With nitrous oxide (66%): 0.4 mcg/kg/minute (range: 0.1-2 mcg/kg/minute)

With isoflurane: 0.25 mcg/kg/minute (range: 0.05-2 mcg/kg/minute)

With propofol: 0.25 mcg/kg/minute (range: 0.05-2 mcg/kg/minute)

Coronary bypass surgery: 1 mcg/kg/minute (range: 0.125-4 mcg/kg/minute); supplemental dose: 0.5-1 mcg/kg

Continuation as an analgesic in immediate postoperative period: 0.1 mcg/kg/minute (range: 0.025-0.2 mcg/kg/minute). Infusion rate may be adjusted every 5 minutes in increments of 0.025 mcg/kg/minute. Bolus doses are not recommended. Infusion rates >0.2 mcg/kg/minute are associated with respiratory depression.

Coronary bypass surgery, continuation as an analgesic into the ICU: 1 mcg/kg/minute (range: 0.05-1 mcg/kg/minute)

Analgesic component of monitored anesthesia care: **Note:** Supplemental oxygen is recommended:

Single I.V. dose given 90 seconds prior to local anesthetic:

Remifentanil alone: 1 mcg/kg over 30-60 seconds

With midazolam: 0.5 mcg/kg over 30-60 seconds

Continuous infusion beginning 5 minutes prior to local anesthetic:

Remifentanil alone: 0.1 mcg/kg minute

With midazolam: 0.05 mcg/kg/minute

Continuous infusion given after local anesthetic:

Remifentanil alone: 0.05 mcg/kg/minute (range: 0.025-0.2 mcg/kg/minute)

With midazolam: 0.025 mcg/kg/minute (range: 0.025-0.2 mcg/kg/minute)

Note: Following local or anesthetic block, infusion rate should be decreased to 0.05 mcg/kg/minute; rate adjustments of 0.025 mcg/kg/minute may be done at 5-minute intervals

Critically-ill patients (unlabeled dose): Continuous infusion: 42-1050 mcg/hour (based on 70 kg patient) **or** 0.6-15 mcg/kg/hour

Elderly: Elderly patients have an increased sensitivity to effect of remifentanil, doses should be decreased by 1/2 and titrated

Administration An infusion device should be used to administer continuous infusions. During the maintenance of general anesthesia, I.V. boluses may be administered over 30-60 seconds. Injections should be given into I.V. tubing close to the venous cannula; tubing should be cleared after treatment to prevent residual effects when other fluids are administered through the same I.V. line.

Monitoring Parameters Respiratory and cardiovascular status, blood pressure, heart rate

Additional Information Ultra short-acting narcotic that is unique compared to other short-acting narcotics. This agent is not considered suitable as the sole agent for induction; remifentanil should be used in combination with other induction agents. Bolus doses are not recommended for sedation cases and in treatment of postoperative pain due to risk of respiratory depression and muscle rigidity. Due to remifentanil's short duration of action, when postoperative pain is anticipated, discontinuation of an infusion of remifentanil should be preceded by an adequate postoperative analgesic (ie, fentanyl, morphine).

Dosage Forms Excipient information presented when available (limited, particularly for generics); consult specific product labeling.

Injection, powder for reconstitution: 1 mg, 2 mg, 5 mg [contains glycine 15 mg]

- ◆ **Reminyl® [DSC]** *see* Galantamine *on page 679*
- ◆ **Reminyl® (Can)** *see* Galantamine *on page 679*
- ◆ **Reminyl® ER (Can)** *see* Galantamine *on page 679*
- ◆ **Remodulin®** *see* Treprostinil *on page 1506*
- ◆ **Renagel®** *see* Sevelamer *on page 1365*
- ◆ **Renal Replacement Solution** *see* Electrolyte Solution, Renal Replacement *on page 510*
- ◆ **Renedil® (Can)** *see* Felodipine *on page 606*
- ◆ **Renova®** *see* Tretinoin (Topical) *on page 1509*
- ◆ **Renvela®** *see* Sevelamer *on page 1365*
- ◆ **ReoPro®** *see* Abciximab *on page 21*
- ◆ **Reopro® (Can)** *see* Abciximab *on page 21*

Repaglinide (re PAG li nide)

U.S. Brand Names Prandin®

Canadian Brand Names GlucoNorm®; Prandin®

Pharmacologic Category Antidiabetic Agent, Meglitinide Derivative

Additional Appendix Information

Diabetes Mellitus Management, Adults *on page 1801*

Use Management of type 2 diabetes mellitus (noninsulin dependent, NIDDM) as an adjunct to diet and exercise;

may be used in combination with metformin or thiazolidinediones

Pregnancy Risk Factor C

Pregnancy Considerations Adverse events have been observed in some animal studies; therefore, repaglinide is classified as pregnancy category C. Information describing the effects of repaglinide on pregnancy outcomes is limited. Maternal hyperglycemia can be associated with adverse effects in the fetus, including macrosomia, neonatal hyperglycemia, and hyperbilirubinemia; the risk of congenital malformations is increased when the Hb A_{1c} is above the normal range. Diabetes can also be associated with adverse effects in the mother. Poorly-treated diabetes may cause end-organ damage that may in turn negatively affect obstetric outcomes. Physiologic glucose levels should be maintained prior to and during pregnancy to decrease the risk of adverse events in the mother and the fetus. Until additional safety and efficacy data are obtained, the use of oral agents is generally not recommended as routine management of GDM or type 2 diabetes mellitus during pregnancy. Insulin is the drug of choice for the control of diabetes mellitus during pregnancy.

Lactation Excretion in breast milk unknown/not recommended

Medication Safety Issues

Sound-alike/look-alike issues:

Prandin® may be confused with Avandia®

High alert medication: The Institute for Safe Medication Practices (ISMP) includes this medication among its list of drug classes which have a heightened risk of causing significant patient harm when used in error.

Contraindications Hypersensitivity to repaglinide or any component of the formulation; diabetic ketoacidosis, with or without coma (treat with insulin); type 1 diabetes (insulin dependent, IDDM)

Warnings/Precautions Use with caution in patients with moderate-to-severe hepatic impairment. Use caution in severe renal dysfunction, elderly, malnourished, or patients with adrenal/pituitary dysfunction; may be more susceptible to glucose-lowering effects. May cause hypoglycemia; appropriate patient selection, dosage, and patient education are important to avoid hypoglycemic episodes. It may be necessary to discontinue repaglinide and administer insulin if the patient is exposed to stress (fever, trauma, infection, surgery). Theoretically, repaglinide may increase cardiovascular events as observed in some studies using sulfonylureas, but there are no long-term studies assessing this concern. Not indicated for use in combination with NPH insulin as there have been case reports of myocardial ischemia; further evaluation required to assess the safety of this combination. Safety and efficacy have not been established in pediatric patients.

Adverse Reactions

>10%:

Central nervous system: Headache (9% to 11%)

Endocrine & metabolic: Hypoglycemia (16% to 31%)

Respiratory: Upper respiratory tract infection (10% to 16%)

1% to 10%:

Cardiovascular: Ischemia (4%), chest pain (2% to 3%)

Gastrointestinal: Diarrhea (4% to 5%), constipation (2% to 3%), tooth disorder (≤2%)

Genitourinary: Urinary tract infection (2% to 3%)

Neuromuscular & skeletal: Arthralgia (3% to 6%), back pain (5% to 6%)

Respiratory: Sinusitis (3% to 6%), bronchitis (2% to 6%)

Miscellaneous: Allergy (1% to 2%)

<1% (Limited to important or life-threatening): Alopecia, anaphylactoid reaction, arrhythmias, ECG abnormal, hemolytic anemia, hepatic dysfunction (severe), hepatitis, hypertension, jaundice, leukopenia, liver function tests increased, MI, palpitation, pancreatitis, Stevens-Johnson syndrome, thrombocytopenia

Drug Interactions

Metabolism/Transport Effects Substrate of CYP2C8 (major), 3A4 (major)

Avoid Concomitant Use There are no known interactions where it is recommended to avoid concomitant use.

Increased Effect/Toxicity

The levels/effects of Repaglinide may be increased by: Antifungal Agents (Azole Derivatives, Systemic); CycloSPORINE; CYP2C8 Inhibitors (Moderate); CYP2C8 Inhibitors (Strong); CYP3A4 Inhibitors (Moderate); CYP3A4 Inhibitors (Strong); Dasatinib; Eltrombopag; Gemfibrozil; Herbs (Hypoglycemic Properties); Macrolide Antibiotics; Pegvisomant; Trimethoprim

Decreased Effect

The levels/effects of Repaglinide may be decreased by: Corticosteroids (Orally Inhaled); Corticosteroids (Systemic); CYP2C8 Inducers (Highly Effective); CYP3A4 Inducers (Strong); Deferasirox; Herbs (CYP3A4 Inducers); Luteinizing Hormone-Releasing Hormone Analogs; Rifamycin Derivatives; Somatropin

Ethanol/Nutrition/Herb Interactions

Ethanol: Avoid ethanol (may cause hypoglycemia).

Food: When given with food, the AUC of repaglinide is decreased.

Herb/Nutraceutical: St John's wort may decrease repaglinide levels. Avoid gymnema, garlic (may cause hypoglycemia).

Stability Do not store above 25°C (77°F). Protect from moisture.

Mechanism of Action Nonsulfonylurea hypoglycemic agent of the meglitinide class (the nonsulfonylurea moiety of glyburide) used in the management of type 2 diabetes mellitus; stimulates insulin release from the pancreatic beta cells

Pharmacodynamics/Kinetics

Onset of action: Single dose: Increased insulin levels: ~15-60 minutes

Duration: 4-6 hours

Absorption: Rapid and complete

Distribution: V_d: 31 L

Protein binding, plasma: >98% to albumin

Metabolism: Hepatic via CYP3A4 and CYP2C8 isoenzymes and glucuronidation to inactive metabolites

Bioavailability: Mean absolute: ~56%

Half-life elimination: ~1 hour

Time to peak, plasma: ~1 hour

Excretion: Within 96 hours: Feces (~90%, <2% as parent drug); Urine (~8%)

Dosage Adults: Oral: Should be taken within 15 minutes of the meal, but time may vary from immediately preceding the meal to as long as 30 minutes before the meal

Initial: For patients not previously treated or whose Hb A_{1c} is <8%, the starting dose is 0.5 mg before each meal. For patients previously treated with blood glucose-lowering agents whose Hb A_{1c} is ≥8%, the initial dose is 1 or 2 mg before each meal.

Dose adjustment: Determine dosing adjustments by blood glucose response, usually fasting blood glucose. Double the preprandial dose up to 4 mg until satisfactory blood glucose response is achieved. At least 1 week should elapse to assess response after each dose adjustment.

Dose range: 0.5-4 mg taken with meals. Repaglinide may be dosed preprandial 2, 3, or 4 times/day in response to changes in the patient's meal pattern. Maximum recommended daily dose: 16 mg.

Patients receiving other oral hypoglycemic agents: When repaglinide is used to replace therapy with other oral hypoglycemic agents, it may be started the day after the final dose is given. Observe patients carefully for hypoglycemia because of potential overlapping of drug effects. When transferred from longer half-life sulfonylureas (eg, chlorpropamide), close monitoring may be indicated for up to ≥1 week.

Combination therapy: If repaglinide monotherapy does not result in adequate glycemic control, metformin or a thiazolidinedione may be added. Or, if metformin or thiazolidinedione therapy does not provide adequate control, repaglinide may be added. The starting dose and dose adjustments for combination therapy are the same as repaglinide monotherapy. Carefully adjust the dose of each drug to determine the minimal dose required to achieve the desired pharmacologic effect. Failure to do so could result in an increase in the incidence of hypoglycemic episodes. Use appropriate monitoring of FPG and Hb A_{1c} measurements to ensure that the patient is not subjected to excessive drug exposure or increased probability of secondary drug failure. If glucose is not achieved after a suitable trial of combination therapy, consider discontinuing these drugs and using insulin.

Dosing adjustment in renal impairment:

Cl_{cr} 40-80 mL/minute (mild to moderate renal dysfunction): Initial dosage adjustment does not appear to be necessary.

Cl_{cr} 20-40 mL/minute: Initiate 0.5 mg with meals; titrate carefully.

Cl_{cr} <20 mL/minute: Not studied.

Dosing adjustment in hepatic impairment: Use conservative initial and maintenance doses. Use longer intervals between dosage adjustments.

Dietary Considerations Administer repaglinide 15-30 minutes before meals. Dietary modification based on ADA recommendations is a part of therapy. May cause hypoglycemia. Must be able to recognize symptoms of hypoglycemia (palpitations, tachycardia, sweaty palms, diaphoresis, lightheadedness).

Administration Administer repaglinide 15-30 minutes before meals. Patients who are anorexic or NPO, may need to have their dose held to avoid hypoglycemia. Patients consuming extra meals should be instructed to add a dose for the extra meal.

Monitoring Parameters Monitor fasting blood glucose (periodically) and glycosylated hemoglobin (Hb A_{1c}) levels (every 3 months) with a goal of decreasing these levels towards the normal range. During dose adjustment, fasting glucose can be used to determine response.

Reference Range Recommendations for glycemic control in adults with diabetes:

Hb A_{1c}: <7%

Preprandial capillary plasma glucose: 70-130 mg/dL

Peak postprandial capillary blood glucose: <180 mg/dL

Blood pressure: <130/80 mm Hg

Dosage Forms Excipient information presented when available (limited, particularly for generics); consult specific product labeling.

Tablet:

Prandin®: 0.5 mg, 1 mg, 2 mg

Repaglinide and Metformin

(re PAG li nide & met FOR min)

U.S. Brand Names PrandiMet™

Index Terms Metformin and Repaglinide; Repaglinide and Metformin Hydrochloride

Pharmacologic Category Antidiabetic Agent, Biguanide; Antidiabetic Agent, Meglitinide Derivative; Hypoglycemic Agent, Oral

Additional Appendix Information

Diabetes Mellitus Management, Adults *on page 1801*

Use Management of type 2 diabetes mellitus (noninsulin dependent, NIDDM), as an adjunct to diet and exercise, in patients currently receiving or not adequately controlled on metformin and/or a meglitinide

Pregnancy Risk Factor C

Medication Safety Issues

Sound-alike/look-alike issues:

PrandiMet™ may be confused with Avandamet®, Prandin®

High alert medication: The Institute for Safe Medication Practices (ISMP) includes this medication among its list of drug classes which have a heightened risk of causing significant patient harm when used in error.

Dosage Oral: Adults: Type 2 diabetes mellitus:

Patients currently taking repaglinide and metformin: Initial doses should be based on (but not exceeding) the patient's current doses of repaglinide and metformin; daily doses should be divided and given 2-3 times daily with meals (maximum single dose: 4 mg/dose [repaglinide], 1000 mg/dose [metformin]; maximum daily dose: 10 mg/day [repaglinide], 2500 mg/day [metformin])

Patients inadequately controlled on metformin alone: Initial dose: repaglinide 1 mg/ metformin 500 mg twice daily with meals. Titrate slowly to reduce the risk of repaglinide-induced hypoglycemia.

Patients inadequately controlled on a meglitinide alone: Initial dose: metformin 500 mg twice daily plus repaglinide at a dose similar to (but not exceeding) the patient's current dose. Titrate slowly to reduce the risk of metformin-induced gastrointestinal adverse effects.

Dosing adjustment in renal impairment: Do not use in renal impairment; metformin use is contraindicated in patients with renal impairment (serum creatinine ≥1.5 mg/dL in males or ≥1.4 mg/dL in females)

Dosing adjustment in hepatic impairment: Avoid use in patients with impaired liver function

Additional Information Complete prescribing information for this medication should be consulted for additional detail.

Dosage Forms Excipient information presented when available (limited, particularly for generics); consult specific product labeling.

Tablet:

PrandiMet™:

1/500: Repaglinide 1 mg and metformin hydrochloride 500 mg

2/500: Repaglinide 2 mg and metformin hydrochloride 500 mg

- **Repaglinide and Metformin Hydrochloride** *see* Repaglinide and Metformin *on page 1305*
- **Repan®** *see* Butalbital, Acetaminophen, and Caffeine *on page 229*
- **Reprexain®** *see* Hydrocodone and Ibuprofen *on page 742*
- **Repronex®** *see* Menotropins *on page 941*
- **Requa® Activated Charcoal [OTC]** *see* Charcoal *on page 299*
- **Requip®** *see* Ropinirole *on page 1337*
- **Requip® XL™** *see* Ropinirole *on page 1337*
- **Rescon®** *see* Chlorpheniramine, Phenylephrine, and Methscopolamine *on page 313*
- **Rescon® MX** *see* Chlorpheniramine, Phenylephrine, and Methscopolamine *on page 313*
- **Rescon DM [OTC]** *see* Chlorpheniramine, Pseudoephedrine, and Dextromethorphan *on page 315*
- **Rescon GG [OTC]** *see* Guaifenesin and Phenylephrine *on page 712*
- **Rescon-Jr®** *see* Chlorpheniramine and Phenylephrine *on page 309*
- **Rescriptor®** *see* Delavirdine *on page 414*

- **Resectisol®** *see* Mannitol *on page* *919*

Reserpine (re SER peen)

Pharmacologic Category Central Monoamine-Depleting Agent; Rauwolfia Alkaloid

Additional Appendix Information

Hypertension *on page* *1820*

Use Management of mild-to-moderate hypertension; treatment of agitated psychotic states (schizophrenia)

Unlabeled/Investigational Use Management of tardive dyskinesia

Pregnancy Risk Factor C

Medication Safety Issues

Sound-alike/look-alike issues:

Reserpine may be confused with Risperdal®, risperidone

Dosage Note: When used for management of hypertension, full antihypertensive effects may take as long as 3 weeks.

Oral:

Children: Hypertension: 0.01-0.02 mg/kg/24 hours divided every 12 hours; maximum dose: 0.25 mg/day (not recommended in children)

Adults:

Hypertension:

Manufacturer's labeling: Initial: 0.5 mg/day for 1-2 weeks; maintenance: 0.1-0.25 mg/day

Note: Clinically, the need for a "loading" period (as recommended by the manufacturer) is not well supported, and alternative dosing is preferred.

Alternative dosing (unlabeled): Initial: 0.1 mg once daily; adjust as necessary based on response.

Usual dose range (JNC 7): 0.05-0.25 mg once daily; 0.1 mg every other day may be given to achieve 0.05 mg once daily

Schizophrenia (labeled use) or tardive dyskinesia (unlabeled use): Dosing recommendations vary; initial dose recommendations generally range from 0.05-0.25 mg (although manufacturer recommends 0.5 mg once daily initially in schizophrenia). May be increased in increments of 0.1-0.25 mg; maximum dose in tardive dyskinesia: 5 mg/day.

Elderly: Initial: 0.05 mg once daily, increasing by 0.05 mg every week as necessary

Dosing adjustment in renal impairment: Cl_{cr} <10 mL/minute: Avoid use

Dialysis: Not removed by hemo or peritoneal dialysis; supplemental dose is not necessary

Additional Information Complete prescribing information for this medication should be consulted for additional detail.

Dosage Forms Excipient information presented when available (limited, particularly for generics); consult specific product labeling.

Tablet: 0.1 mg, 0.25 mg

- **Resource® GlutaSolve® [OTC]** *see* Glutamine *on page* *700*
- **Respa®-1st** *see* Guaifenesin and Pseudoephedrine *on page* *713*
- **Respa-DM®** *see* Guaifenesin and Dextromethorphan *on page* *710*
- **Respahist®** *see* Brompheniramine and Pseudoephedrine *on page* *214*
- **Respaire®-60 SR [DSC]** *see* Guaifenesin and Pseudoephedrine *on page* *713*
- **Respaire®-120 SR [DSC]** *see* Guaifenesin and Pseudoephedrine *on page* *713*
- **Respa® PE [DSC]** *see* Guaifenesin and Phenylephrine *on page* *712*
- **Respi-Tann™** *see* Carbetapentane and Pseudoephedrine *on page* *255*
- **Restasis®** *see* CycloSPORINE *on page* *379*
- **Restoril®** *see* Temazepam *on page* *1432*
- **Restylane®** *see* Hyaluronate and Derivatives *on page* *734*

Retapamulin (re te PAM ue lin)

U.S. Brand Names Altabax™

Pharmacologic Category Antibiotic, Pleuromutilin; Antibiotic, Topical

Use Treatment of impetigo caused by susceptible strains of *S. pyogenes* or methicillin-susceptible *S. aureus*

Pregnancy Risk Factor B

Dosage Topical: Impetigo:

Children ≥9 months: Apply to affected area twice daily for 5 days. Total treatment area should not exceed 2% of total body surface area.

Adults: Apply to affected area twice daily for 5 days. Total treatment area should not exceed 100 cm^2 total body surface area.

Additional Information Complete prescribing information for this medication should be consulted for additional detail.

Dosage Forms

Ointment, topical:

Altabax™: 1% (5 g, 10 g, 15 g)

- **Retavase®** *see* Reteplase *on page* *1306*

Reteplase (RE ta plase)

U.S. Brand Names Retavase®

Canadian Brand Names Retavase®

Index Terms r-PA; Recombinant Plasminogen Activator

Pharmacologic Category Thrombolytic Agent

Use Management of ST-elevation myocardial infarction (STEMI); improvement of ventricular function; reduction of the incidence of CHF and the reduction of mortality following AMI

Recommended criteria for treatment: STEMI: Chest pain ≥20 minutes duration, onset of chest pain within 12 hours of treatment (or within prior 12-24 hours in patients with continuing ischemic symptoms), and ST-segment elevation >0.1 mV in at least two contiguous precordial leads or two adjacent limb leads on ECG or new or presumably new left bundle branch block (LBBB)

Pregnancy Risk Factor C

Lactation Excretion in breast milk unknown/use caution

Medication Safety Issues

High alert medication: The Institute for Safe Medication Practices (ISMP) includes this medication (I.V.) among its list of drugs which have a heightened risk of causing significant patient harm when used in error.

Contraindications Hypersensitivity to reteplase or any component of the formulation; active internal bleeding; history of cerebrovascular accident; recent intracranial or intraspinal surgery or trauma; intracranial neoplasm, arteriovenous malformations, or aneurysm; known bleeding diathesis; severe uncontrolled hypertension

Warnings/Precautions Concurrent heparin anticoagulation can contribute to bleeding; careful attention to all potential bleeding sites. I.M. injections and nonessential handling of the patient should be avoided. Venipunctures should be performed carefully and only when necessary. If arterial puncture is necessary, use an upper extremity vessel that can be manually compressed. If serious bleeding occurs then the infusion of anistreplase and heparin should be stopped.

For the following conditions the risk of bleeding is higher with use of reteplase and should be weighed against the benefits of therapy: recent major surgery (eg, CABG, obstetrical delivery, organ biopsy, previous puncture of noncompressible vessels), cerebrovascular disease, recent gastrointestinal or genitourinary bleeding, recent trauma including CPR, hypertension (systolic BP >180 mm Hg and/or diastolic BP >110 mm Hg), high likelihood of left heart thrombus (eg, mitral stenosis with atrial fibrillation), acute pericarditis, subacute bacterial endocarditis, hemostatic defects including ones caused by severe renal or hepatic dysfunction, significant hepatic dysfunction, pregnancy, diabetic hemorrhagic retinopathy or other hemorrhagic ophthalmic conditions, septic thrombophlebitis or occluded AV cannula at seriously infected site, advanced age (eg, >75 years), patients receiving oral anticoagulants, any other condition in which bleeding constitutes a significant hazard or would be particularly difficult to manage because of location.

Coronary thrombolysis may result in reperfusion arrhythmias. Follow standard MI management. Rare anaphylactic reactions can occur. Safety and efficacy in pediatric patients have not been established.

Adverse Reactions Bleeding is the most frequent adverse effect associated with reteplase. Heparin and aspirin have been administered concurrently with reteplase in clinical trials. The incidence of adverse events is a reflection of these combined therapies, and are comparable with comparison thrombolytics.

>10%: Local: Injection site bleeding (4.6% to 48.6%)

1% to 10%:

- Gastrointestinal: Bleeding (1.8% to 9.0%)
- Genitourinary: Bleeding (0.9% to 9.5%)
- Hematologic: Anemia (0.9% to 2.6%)

<1% (Limited to important or life-threatening): Allergic/anaphylactoid reactions, cholesterol embolization, intracranial hemorrhage (0.8%)

Other adverse effects noted are frequently associated with MI (and therefore may or may not be attributable to Retavase®) and include arrhythmia, arrest, cardiac reinfarction, cardiogenic shock, embolism, hypotension, pericarditis, pulmonary edema, tamponade, thrombosis

Drug Interactions

Avoid Concomitant Use There are no known interactions where it is recommended to avoid concomitant use.

Increased Effect/Toxicity

Reteplase may increase the levels/effects of: Anticoagulants; Drotrecogin Alfa

The levels/effects of Reteplase may be increased by: Antiplatelet Agents; Herbs (Anticoagulant/Antiplatelet Properties); Nonsteroidal Anti-Inflammatory Agents; Salicylates

Decreased Effect

The levels/effects of Reteplase may be decreased by: Aprotinin

Stability Dosage kits should be stored at 2°C to 25°C (36°F to 77°F) and remain sealed until use in order to protect from light. Reteplase should be reconstituted using the diluent, syringe, needle, and dispensing pin provided with each kit.

Mechanism of Action Reteplase is a nonglycosylated form of tPA produced by recombinant DNA technology using *E. coli*; it initiates local fibrinolysis by binding to fibrin in a thrombus (clot) and converts entrapped plasminogen to plasmin

Pharmacodynamics/Kinetics

Onset of action: Thrombolysis: 30-90 minutes

Half-life elimination: 13-16 minutes

Excretion: Feces and urine

Clearance: Plasma: 250-450 mL/minute

Dosage

Children: Not recommended

Adults: 10 units I.V. over 2 minutes, followed by a second dose 30 minutes later of 10 units I.V. over 2 minutes; withhold second dose if serious bleeding or anaphylaxis occurs

Note: All patients should receive 162-325 mg of chewable nonenteric coated aspirin as soon as possible and then daily. Administer concurrently with heparin 60 units/kg bolus (maximum: 4000 units) followed by continuous infusion of 12 units/kg/hour (maximum: 1000 units/hour) and adjust to aPTT target of 50-70 seconds (or 1.5-2 times the upper limit of control).

Administration Reteplase should be reconstituted using the diluent, syringe, needle and dispensing pin provided with each kit and the each reconstituted dose should be administered I.V. over 2 minutes; no other medication should be added to the injection solution

Monitoring Parameters Monitor for signs of bleeding (hematuria, GI bleeding, gingival bleeding)

Dosage Forms Excipient information presented when available (limited, particularly for generics); consult specific product labeling.

Injection, powder for reconstitution [preservative free]:

Retavase®: 10.4 units [equivalent to reteplase 18.1 mg; contains sucrose and polysorbate 80; packaged with sterile water for injection]

- ◆ **Retin-A®** *see* Tretinoin (Topical) *on page 1509*
- ◆ **Retin-A® Micro** *see* Tretinoin (Topical) *on page 1509*
- ◆ **Retinoic Acid** *see* Tretinoin (Topical) *on page 1509*
- ◆ **Retinova® (Can)** *see* Tretinoin (Topical) *on page 1509*
- ◆ **Retisert®** *see* Fluocinolone *on page 633*
- ◆ **Retrovir®** *see* Zidovudine *on page 1581*
- ◆ **Revatio®** *see* Sildenafil *on page 1368*
- ◆ **Revex® [DSC]** *see* Nalmefene *on page 1036*
- ◆ **ReVia®** *see* Naltrexone *on page 1039*
- ◆ **Revitalose C-1000® (Can)** *see* Ascorbic Acid *on page 139*
- ◆ **Revlimid®** *see* Lenalidomide *on page 861*
- ◆ **Revolade®** *see* Eltrombopag *on page 512*
- ◆ **Reyataz®** *see* Atazanavir *on page 146*
- ◆ **rFSH-alpha** *see* Follitropin Alfa *on page 656*
- ◆ **rFSH-beta** *see* Follitropin Beta *on page 658*
- ◆ **rFVIIa** *see* Factor VIIa (Recombinant) *on page 598*
- ◆ **R-Gene®** *see* Arginine *on page 133*
- ◆ **r-hCG** *see* Chorionic Gonadotropin (Recombinant) *on page 321*
- ◆ **rhDNase** *see* Dornase Alfa *on page 481*
- ◆ **Rheumatrex® Dose Pack®** *see* Methotrexate *on page 965*
- ◆ **rhFSH-alpha** *see* Follitropin Alfa *on page 656*
- ◆ **rhFSH-beta** *see* Follitropin Beta *on page 658*
- ◆ **rhGAA** *see* Alglucosidase Alfa *on page 62*
- ◆ **r-h α-GAL** *see* Agalsidase Beta *on page 47*
- ◆ **RhIG** *see* Rh_o(D) Immune Globulin *on page 1308*
- ◆ **rhIGF-1** *see* Mecasermin *on page 926*
- ◆ **rhIGF-1/rhIGFBP-3** *see* Mecasermin *on page 926*
- ◆ **rhIL-11** *see* Oprelvekin *on page 1106*
- ◆ **Rhinacon A** *see* Chlorpheniramine, Phenylephrine, and Phenyltoloxamine *on page 314*
- ◆ **Rhinalar® (Can)** *see* Flunisolide *on page 632*
- ◆ **Rhinall [OTC]** *see* Phenylephrine *on page 1183*
- ◆ **Rhinaris-CS Anti-Allergic Nasal Mist (Can)** *see* Cromolyn *on page 372*

◆ **Rhinocort® Aqua®** *see* Budesonide *on page 215*
◆ **Rhinocort® Aqua™ (Can)** *see* Budesonide *on page 215*
◆ **Rhinocort® Turbuhaler® (Can)** *see* Budesonide *on page 215*
◆ **RhinoFlex™** *see* Acetaminophen and Phenyltoloxamine *on page 29*
◆ **RhinoFlex 650** *see* Acetaminophen and Phenyltoloxamine *on page 29*
◆ **rhKGF** *see* Palifermin *on page 1129*
◆ **r-hLH** *see* Lutropin Alfa *on page 912*
◆ **Rho(D) Immune Globulin (Human)** *see* Rh_o(D) Immune Globulin *on page 1308*
◆ **Rho®-Clonazepam (Can)** *see* ClonazePAM *on page 352*
◆ **Rhodacine® (Can)** *see* Indomethacin *on page 783*

Rh_o(D) Immune Globulin

(ar aych oh (dee) i MYUN GLOB yoo lin)

U.S. Brand Names HyperRHO™ S/D Full Dose; HyperRHO™ S/D Mini Dose; MICRhoGAM®; RhoGAM®; Rhophylac®; WinRho® SDF

Canadian Brand Names WinRho® SDF

Index Terms RhIG; Rho(D) Immune Globulin (Human); RhoIGIV; RhoIVIM

Pharmacologic Category Immune Globulin

Use

Suppression of Rh isoimmunization: Use in the following situations when an Rh_o(D)-negative individual is exposed to Rh_o(D)-positive blood: During delivery of an Rh_o(D)-positive infant; abortion; amniocentesis; chorionic villus sampling; ruptured tubal pregnancy; abdominal trauma; hydatidiform mole; transplacental hemorrhage. Used when the mother is Rh_o(D) negative, the father of the child is either Rh_o(D) positive or Rh_o(D) unknown, the baby is either Rh_o(D) positive or Rh_o(D) unknown.

Transfusion: Suppression of Rh isoimmunization in Rh_o(D)-negative individuals transfused with Rh_o(D) antigen-positive RBCs or blood components containing Rh_o(D) antigen-positive RBCs

Treatment of idiopathic thrombocytopenic purpura (ITP): Used in the following nonsplenectomized Rh_o(D) positive individuals: Children with acute or chronic ITP, adults with chronic ITP, children and adults with ITP secondary to HIV infection

Pregnancy Risk Factor C

Pregnancy Considerations Animal studies have not been conducted. Available evidence suggests that Rh_o(D) immune globulin administration during pregnancy does not harm the fetus or affect future pregnancies.

Lactation Does not enter breast milk

Contraindications Hypersensitivity to immune globulins or any component of the formulation; prior sensitization to Rh_o(D)

Warnings/Precautions Rare but serious signs and symptoms (eg, back pain, shaking, chills, fever, discolored urine; onset within 4 hours of infusion) of intravascular hemolysis (IVH) have been reported in postmarketing experience in patients treated for ITP. Clinically-compromising anemia, acute renal insufficiency and disseminated intravascular coagulation (DIC) have also been reported. ITP patients should be advised of the signs and symptoms of IVH and instructed to report them immediately.

Product of human plasma; may potentially contain infectious agents which could transmit disease. Screening of donors, as well as testing and/or inactivation or removal of certain viruses, reduces the risk. Infections thought to be transmitted by this product should be reported to the manufacturer. Not for replacement therapy in immune globulin deficiency syndromes. Use caution with IgA deficiency, may contain trace amounts of IgA; patients who are IgA deficient may have the potential for developing IgA antibodies, anaphylactic reactions may occur. Administer I.M. injections with caution in patients with thrombocytopenia or coagulation disorders. Some products may contain maltose, which may result in falsely-elevated blood glucose readings. Use caution with renal dysfunction; may require an infusion rate reduction or discontinuation. Safety and efficacy have not been established for Rhophylac® in patients with anemia.

ITP: Do not administer I.M. or SubQ for the treatment of ITP; administer dose I.V. only. Safety and efficacy not established in Rh_o(D) negative, non-ITP thrombocytopenia, or splenectomized patients. When using WinRho® SDF, decrease dose with hemoglobin <10 g/dL; use with extreme caution if hemoglobin <8 g/dL. Safety and efficacy have not been established for Rhophylac® in patients with anemia.

Rh_o(D) suppression: For use in the mother; do not administer to the neonate.

Adverse Reactions Frequency not defined.

Cardiovascular: Hyper-/hypotension, pallor, tachycardia, vasodilation

Central nervous system: Chills, dizziness, fever, headache, malaise, somnolence

Dermatologic: Pruritus, rash

Gastrointestinal: Abdominal pain, diarrhea, nausea, vomiting

Hematologic: Haptoglobin decreased, hemoglobin decreased (patients with ITP), intravascular hemolysis (patients with ITP)

Hepatic: Bilirubin increased, LDH increased

Local: Injection site reaction: Discomfort, induration, mild pain, redness, swelling

Neuromuscular & skeletal: Arthralgia, back pain, hyperkinesia, myalgia, weakness

Renal: Acute renal insufficiency

Miscellaneous: Anaphylaxis, diaphoresis, infusion-related reactions, positive anti-C antibody test (transient), shivering

Postmarketing and/or case reports: Anemia (clinically-compromising), DIC, dyspnea, erythema, hemoglobinuria (transient in patients with ITP), injection site irritation, vertigo

Drug Interactions

Avoid Concomitant Use There are no known interactions where it is recommended to avoid concomitant use.

Increased Effect/Toxicity There are no known significant interactions involving an increase in effect.

Decreased Effect

Rho(D) Immune Globulin may decrease the levels/effects of: Vaccines (Live)

Stability Store at 2°C to 8°C (35°F to 46°F); do not freeze.

Rhophylac®: Protect from light.

Mechanism of Action

Rh suppression: Prevents isoimmunization by suppressing the immune response and antibody formation by Rh_o(D) negative individuals to Rh_o(D) positive red blood cells.

ITP: Not completely characterized; Rh_o(D) immune globulin is thought to form anti-D-coated red blood cell complexes which bind to macrophage Fc receptors within the spleen; blocking or saturating the spleens ability to clear antibody-coated cells, including platelets. In this manner, platelets are spared from destruction.

Pharmacodynamics/Kinetics

Onset of platelet increase: ITP: Platelets should rise within 1-2 days

Peak effect: In 7-14 days

Duration: Suppression of Rh isoimmunization: ~12 weeks; Treatment of ITP: 30 days (variable)

Distribution: V_d: I.M.: 8.59 L

Bioavailability: I.M.: Rhophylac®: 69%

Half-life elimination: 12-30 days
Time to peak, plasma: I.M.: 5-10 days; I.V. (WinRho® SDF): ≤2 hours

Dosage

ITP: Children and Adults:
Rhophylac®: I.V.: 50 mcg/kg
WinRho® SDF: I.V.:
Initial: 50 mcg/kg as a single injection, or can be given as a divided dose on separate days. If hemoglobin is <10 g/dL: Dose should be reduced to 25-40 mcg/kg.
Subsequent dosing: 25-60 mcg/kg can be used if required to elevate platelet count
Maintenance dosing if patient **did respond** to initial dosing: 25-60 mcg/kg based on platelet and hemoglobin levels
Maintenance dosing if patient **did not respond** to initial dosing:
Hemoglobin 8-10 g/dL: Redose between 25-40 mcg/kg
Hemoglobin >10 g/dL: Redose between 50-60 mcg/kg
Hemoglobin <8 g/dL: Use with caution

Rh_o (D) suppression: Adults: **Note:** One "full dose" (300 mcg) provides enough antibody to prevent Rh sensitization if the volume of RBC entering the circulation is ≤15 mL. When >15 mL is suspected, a fetal red cell count should be performed to determine the appropriate dose.
Pregnancy:
Antepartum prophylaxis: In general, dose is given at 28 weeks. If given early in pregnancy, administer every 12 weeks to ensure adequate levels of passively acquired anti-Rh
HyperRHO™ S/D Full Dose, RhoGAM®: I.M.: 300 mcg
Rhophylac®, WinRho® SDF: I.M., I.V.: 300 mcg
Postpartum prophylaxis: In general, dose is administered as soon as possible after delivery, preferably within 72 hours. Can be given up to 28 days following delivery
HyperRHO™ S/D Full Dose, RhoGAM®: I.M.: 300 mcg
Rhophylac®: I.M., I.V.: 300 mcg
WinRho® SDF: I.M., I.V.: 120 mcg
Threatened abortion, any time during pregnancy (with continuation of pregnancy):
HyperRHO™ S/D Full Dose, RhoGAM®: I.M.: 300 mcg; administer as soon as possible
Rhophylac®, WinRho® SDF: I.M., I.V.: 300 mcg; administer as soon as possible
Abortion, miscarriage, termination of ectopic pregnancy:
RhoGAM®: I.M.: ≥13 weeks gestation: 300 mcg.
HyperRHO™ S/D Mini Dose, MICRhoGAM®: <13 weeks gestation: I.M.: 50 mcg
Rhophylac®: I.M., I.V.: 300 mcg
WinRho® SDF: I.M., I.V.: After 34 weeks gestation: 120 mcg; administer immediately or within 72 hours
Amniocentesis, chorionic villus sampling:
HyperRHO™ S/D Full Dose, RhoGAM®: I.M.: At 15-18 weeks gestation or during the 3rd trimester: 300 mcg. If dose is given between 13-18 weeks, repeat at 26-28 weeks and within 72 hours of delivery.
Rhophylac®: I.M., I.V.: 300 mcg
WinRho® SDF: I.M., I.V.: Before 34 weeks gestation: 300 mcg; administer immediately, repeat dose every 12 weeks during pregnancy; After 34 weeks gestation: 120 mcg, administered immediately or within 72 hours
Excessive fetomaternal hemorrhage (>15 mL): Rhophylac®: I.M., I.V.: 300 mcg within 72 hours plus 20 mcg/mL fetal RBCs in excess of 15 mL if excess transplacental bleeding is quantified **or** 300 mcg/dose if bleeding cannot be quantified
Abdominal trauma, manipulation:
HyperRHO™ S/D Full Dose, RhoGAM®: I.M.: 2nd or 3rd trimester: 300 mcg. If dose is given between 13-18 weeks, repeat at 26-28 weeks and within 72 hours of delivery
Rhophylac®: I.M., I.V.: 300 mcg within 72 hours
WinRho® SDF: I.M./I.V.: After 34 weeks gestation: 120 mcg; administer immediately or within 72 hours

Transfusion:
Children and Adults: WinRho® SDF: Administer within 72 hours after exposure of incompatible blood transfusions or massive fetal hemorrhage.
I.V.: Calculate dose as follows; administer 600 mcg every 8 hours until the total dose is administered:
Exposure to Rh_o(D) positive whole blood: 9 mcg/mL blood
Exposure to Rh_o(D) positive red blood cells: 18 mcg/mL cells
I.M.: Calculate dose as follows; administer 1200 mcg every 12 hours until the total dose is administered:
Exposure to Rh_o(D) positive whole blood: 12 mcg/mL blood
Exposure to Rh_o(D) positive red blood cells: 24 mcg/mL cells
Adults:
HyperRHO™ S/D Full Dose, RhoGAM®: I.M.: Multiply the volume of Rh positive whole blood administered by the hematocrit of the donor unit to equal the volume of RBCs transfused. The volume of RBCs is then divided by 15 mL, providing the number of 300 mcg doses (vials/syringes) to administer. If the dose calculated results in a fraction, round up to the next higher whole 300 mcg dose (vial/syringe).
Rhophylac®: I.M., I.V.: 20 mcg/2 mL transfused blood or 20 mcg/mL erythrocyte concentrate

Dosage adjustment in renal impairment: I.V. infusion: Use caution; may require infusion rate reduction or discontinuation.

Administration The total volume can be administered in divided doses at different sites at one time or may be divided and given at intervals, provided the total dosage is given within 72 hours of the fetomaternal hemorrhage or transfusion.
I.M.: Administer into the deltoid muscle of the upper arm or anterolateral aspect of the upper thigh; avoid gluteal region due to risk of sciatic nerve injury. If large doses (>5 mL) are needed, administration in divided doses at different sites is recommended. **Note:** Do not administer I.M. Rho(D) immune globulin for ITP.
I.V.:
WinRho® SDF: Infuse over at least 3-5 minutes; do not administer with other medications
Rhophylac®: ITP: Infuse at 2 mL per 15-60 seconds
Note: If preparing dose using liquid formulation, withdraw the entire contents of the vial to ensure accurate calculation of the dosage requirement.

Monitoring Parameters Signs and symptoms of intravascular hemolysis (IVH), anemia, and renal insufficiency; observe patient for side effects for at least 20 minutes following administration; patients with suspected IVH should have CBC, haptoglobin, plasma hemoglobin, urine dipstick, BUN, serum creatinine, liver function tests, DIC-specific tests (D-dimer, fibrin degradation products [FDP] or fibrin split products [FSP]) for differential diagnosis. Clinical response may be determined by monitoring platelets, red blood cell (RBC) counts, hemoglobin, and reticulocyte levels.

Test Interactions Some infants born to women given Rh_o(D) antepartum have a weakly positive Coombs' test at birth. Fetal-maternal hemorrhage may cause false blood-typing result in the mother; when there is any doubt to the patients' Rh type, Rh_o(D) immune globulin should be administered. WinRho® SDF liquid contains maltose; may result in falsely elevated blood glucose levels with dehydrogenase pyrroloquinolinequinone or glucose-dye-oxidoreductase testing methods. WinRho® SDF contains trace amounts of anti-A, B, C and E; may alter Coombs' tests following administration.

Additional Information A "full dose" of Rh_o(D) immune globulin has previously been referred to as a 300 mcg dose. It is not the actual anti-D content. Although dosing has traditionally been expressed in mcg, potency is listed in int. units (1 mcg = 5 int. units). ITP patients requiring transfusions should be transfused with Rho-negative blood cells to avoid exacerbating hemolysis; platelet products may contain red blood cells; caution should be exercised if platelets are from Rh_o-positive donors.

Dosage Forms Excipient information presented when available (limited, particularly for generics); consult specific product labeling. [DSC] = Discontinued product

Injection, solution [preservative free]:
- HyperRHO™ S/D Full Dose: 300 mcg [for I.M. use only]
- HyperRHO™ S/D Mini Dose: 50 mcg [for I.M. use only]
- MICRhoGAM®: 50 mcg [for I.M. use only; contains polysorbate 80]
- RhoGAM®: 300 mcg [for I.M. use only; contains polysorbate 80]
- Rhophylac®: 300 mcg/2 mL (2 mL) [1500 int. units; for I.M. or I.V. use; contains human albumin]
- WinRho® SDF:
  - 120 mcg/~0.5 mL (~0.5 mL) [600 int. units; contains maltose and polysorbate 80; for I.M. or I.V. use] [DSC]
  - 300 mcg/~1.3 mL (~1.3 mL) [1500 int. units; contains maltose and polysorbate 80; for I.M. or I.V. use]
  - 500 mcg/~2.2 mL (~2.2 mL) [2500 int. units; contains maltose and polysorbate 80; for I.M. or I.V. use]
  - 1000 mcg/~4.4 mL (~4.4 mL) [5000 int. units; contains maltose and polysorbate 80; for I.M. or I.V. use]
  - 3000 mcg/~13 mL (~13 mL) [15,000 int. units; contains maltose and polysorbate 80; for I.M. or I.V. use]

◆ **Rhodis™ (Can)** *see* Ketoprofen *on page 839*

◆ **Rhodis-EC™ (Can)** *see* Ketoprofen *on page 839*

◆ **Rhodis SR™ (Can)** *see* Ketoprofen *on page 839*

◆ **RhoGAM®** *see* Rh_o(D) Immune Globulin *on page 1308*

◆ **RhoIGIV** *see* Rh_o(D) Immune Globulin *on page 1308*

◆ **RhoIVIM** *see* Rh_o(D) Immune Globulin *on page 1308*

◆ **Rho®-Loperamine (Can)** *see* Loperamide *on page 900*

◆ **Rho®-Nitro (Can)** *see* Nitroglycerin *on page 1073*

◆ **Rhophylac®** *see* Rh_o(D) Immune Globulin *on page 1308*

◆ **Rhotral (Can)** *see* Acebutolol *on page 25*

◆ **Rhotrimine® (Can)** *see* Trimipramine *on page 1521*

◆ **Rhoxal-acebutolol (Can)** *see* Acebutolol *on page 25*

◆ **Rhoxal-atenolol (Can)** *see* Atenolol *on page 149*

◆ **Rhoxal-cyclosporine (Can)** *see* CycloSPORINE *on page 379*

◆ **Rhoxal-diltiazem CD (Can)** *see* Diltiazem *on page 450*

◆ **Rhoxal-diltiazem SR (Can)** *see* Diltiazem *on page 450*

◆ **Rhoxal-diltiazem T (Can)** *see* Diltiazem *on page 450*

◆ **Rhoxal-Fluvoxamine (Can)** *see* Fluvoxamine *on page 652*

◆ **Rhoxal-glimepiride (Can)** *see* Glimepiride *on page 696*

◆ **Rhoxal-Loperamide (Can)** *see* Loperamide *on page 900*

◆ **RHOXAL-Metformin (Can)** *see* MetFORMIN *on page 954*

◆ **Rhoxal-minocycline (Can)** *see* Minocycline *on page 999*

◆ **Rhoxal-nabumetone (Can)** *see* Nabumetone *on page 1030*

◆ **Rhoxal-orphendrine (Can)** *see* Orphenadrine *on page 1108*

◆ **Rhoxal-pamidronate (Can)** *see* Pamidronate *on page 1134*

◆ **Rhoxal-paroxetine (Can)** *see* PARoxetine *on page 1146*

◆ **Rhoxal-Ranitidine (Can)** *see* Ranitidine *on page 1295*

◆ **Rhoxal-salbutamol (Can)** *see* Albuterol *on page 51*

◆ **Rhoxal-sertraline (Can)** *see* Sertraline *on page 1362*

◆ **RHOXAL-Sotalol (Can)** *see* Sotalol *on page 1394*

◆ **Rhoxal-sumatriptan (Can)** *see* SUMAtriptan *on page 1414*

◆ **Rhoxal-ticlopidine (Can)** *see* Ticlopidine *on page 1468*

◆ **Rhoxal-valproic (Can)** *see* Valproic Acid and Derivatives *on page 1538*

◆ **rhPTH(1-34)** *see* Teriparatide *on page 1444*

◆ **Rh-TSH** *see* Thyrotropin Alfa *on page 1465*

◆ **rHuEPO-α** *see* Epoetin Alfa *on page 531*

◆ **rhuFabV2** *see* Ranibizumab *on page 1294*

◆ **rhuGM-CSF** *see* Sargramostim *on page 1355*

◆ **rhu Keratinocyte Growth Factor** *see* Palifermin *on page 1129*

◆ **rHu-KGF** *see* Palifermin *on page 1129*

◆ **rhuMAb-E25** *see* Omalizumab *on page 1099*

◆ **rHuMAb-EGFr** *see* Panitumumab *on page 1138*

◆ **rhuMAb-VEGF** *see* Bevacizumab *on page 193*

◆ **RiaSTAP™** *see* Fibrinogen Concentrate (Human) *on page 619*

◆ **RibaPak™** *see* Ribavirin *on page 1310*

◆ **Ribasphere®** *see* Ribavirin *on page 1310*

Ribavirin (rye ba VYE rin)

U.S. Brand Names Copegus®; Rebetol®; RibaPak™; Ribasphere®; Virazole®

Canadian Brand Names Virazole®

Index Terms RTCA; Tribavirin

Pharmacologic Category Antiviral Agent

Use

Inhalation: Treatment of patients with respiratory syncytial virus (RSV) infections; specially indicated for treatment of severe lower respiratory tract RSV infections in patients with an underlying compromising condition (prematurity, bronchopulmonary dysplasia and other chronic lung conditions, congenital heart disease, immunodeficiency, immunosuppression), and recent transplant recipients

Oral capsule:
- In combination with interferon alfa-2b (Intron® A) injection for the treatment of chronic hepatitis C in patients with compensated liver disease who have relapsed after alpha interferon therapy or were previously untreated with alpha interferons
- In combination with peginterferon alfa-2b (PEG-Intron®) injection for the treatment of chronic hepatitis C in patients with compensated liver disease who were previously untreated with alpha interferons

Oral solution: In combination with interferon alfa 2b (Intron® A) injection for the treatment of chronic hepatitis C in patients with compensated liver disease who were previously untreated with alpha interferons or patients who have relapsed after alpha interferon therapy

Oral tablet: In combination with peginterferon alfa-2a (Pegasys®) injection for the treatment of chronic hepatitis C in patients with compensated liver disease who were previously untreated with alpha interferons (includes patients with histological evidence of cirrhosis [Child-Pugh class A] and patients with clinically-stable HIV disease)

Unlabeled/Investigational Use Used in other viral infections including influenza A and B and adenovirus

Restrictions An FDA-approved medication guide must be distributed when dispensing an outpatient prescription (new or refill) for treatment of hepatitis C where this medication is to be used without direct supervision of a healthcare provider. Medication guides are available at http://www.fda.gov/cder/Offices/ODS/medication_guides.htm.

Pregnancy Risk Factor X

Pregnancy Considerations **[U.S. Boxed Warning]: Significant teratogenic effects have been observed in all animal studies** at ~0.01 times the maximum recommended daily human dose. Use is contraindicated in pregnancy. Negative pregnancy test is required before initiation and monthly thereafter. Avoid pregnancy in female patients and female partners of male patients during therapy by using two effective forms of contraception; continue contraceptive measures for at least 6 months after completion of therapy. If patient or female partner becomes pregnant during treatment, she should be counseled about potential risks of exposure. If pregnancy occurs during use or within 6 months after treatment, report to the ribavirin pregnancy registry (800-593-2214).

Lactation Excretion in breast milk unknown/not recommended

Medication Safety Issues

Sound-alike/look-alike issues:

Ribavirin may be confused with riboflavin, rifampin, Robaxin®

Contraindications Hypersensitivity to ribavirin or any component of the formulation; women of childbearing age who will not use contraception reliably; pregnancy

Additional contraindications for oral formulation: Male partners of pregnant women; hemoglobinopathies (eg, thalassemia major, sickle cell anemia); patients with autoimmune hepatitis; ribavirin tablets are contraindicated in patients with hepatic decompensation (Child-Pugh class B and C)

Refer to individual monographs for Interferon Alfa-2b (Intron® A) and Peginterferon Alfa-2a (Pegasys®) for additional contraindication information.

Warnings/Precautions

Oral: **[U.S. Boxed Warning]: Significant teratogenic effects have been observed in all animal studies.** A negative pregnancy test is required before initiation and monthly thereafter. Avoid pregnancy in female patients and female partners of male patients, during therapy, and for at least 6 months after treatment; two forms of contraception should be used. Safety and efficacy have not been established in patients who have failed other alpha interferon therapy, received organ transplants, or been coinfected with hepatitis B or HIV (Copegus® may be used in HIV coinfected patients unless CD4+ cell count is <100 cells/microL). Oral products should not be used for HIV infection, adenovirus, RSV, or influenza infections. **[U.S. Boxed Warning]: Monotherapy not effective for chronic hepatitis C infection.** Severe psychiatric events have occurred including depression and suicidal behavior during combination therapy. Avoid use in patients with a psychiatric history; discontinue if severe psychiatric symptoms occur. Acute hypersensitivity reactions (eg, anaphylaxis, angioedema, bronchoconstriction, and urticaria) have been observed (rarely) with ribavirin and alfa interferon combination therapy. Severe cutaneous reactions, including Stevens-Johnson syndrome and exfoliative dermatitis have been reported (rarely) with ribavirin and alfa interferon combination therapy; discontinue with signs or symptoms of severe skin reactions. Use with caution in patients with renal impairment; avoid use in patients with Cl_{cr} <50 mL/minute. Elderly patients are more susceptible to adverse effects; use caution. **[U.S. Boxed Warning]: Hemolytic anemia is the primary toxicity of oral therapy; usually occurring within 1-2 weeks of therapy initiation;** observed in ~10% to 13% of patients when alfa interferons were combined with ribavirin. Assess cardiac disease before initiation. Anemia may worsen underlying cardiac disease; avoid use in patients with significant/unstable cardiac disease. If deterioration in cardiovascular status occurs, discontinue therapy. Patients with renal dysfunction and/or those >50 years of age should be carefully assessed for development of anemia. Use caution in pulmonary disease; pulmonary symptoms have been associated with administration. Discontinue therapy if evidence of hepatic decompensation (Child-Pugh score ≥6) is observed. Use caution in patients with sarcoidosis (exacerbation reported). Dental and periodontal disorders have been reported with ribavirin and interferon therapy; patients should be instructed to brush teeth twice daily and have regular dental exams. Safety and efficacy have not been established in patients <3 years of age.

Inhalation: **[U.S. Boxed Warning]: Use with caution in patients requiring assisted ventilation because precipitation of the drug in the respiratory equipment may interfere with safe and effective patient ventilation; sudden deterioration of respiratory function has been observed;** monitor carefully in patients with COPD and asthma for deterioration of respiratory function. Ribavirin is potentially mutagenic, tumor-promoting, and gonadotoxic. Although anemia has not been reported with inhalation therapy, consider monitoring for anemia 1-2 weeks post-treatment. Pregnant healthcare workers may consider unnecessary occupational exposure; ribavirin has been detected in healthcare workers' urine. Healthcare professionals or family members who are pregnant (or may become pregnant) should be counseled about potential risks of exposure and counseled about risk reduction strategies. Hazardous agent - use appropriate precautions for handling and disposal.

Adverse Reactions

Inhalation:

1% to 10%:

Central nervous system: Fatigue, headache, insomnia

Gastrointestinal: Nausea, anorexia

Hematologic: Anemia

<1%: Hypotension, cardiac arrest, digitalis toxicity, conjunctivitis, mild bronchospasm, worsening of respiratory function, apnea

Note: Incidence of adverse effects (approximate) in healthcare workers: Headache (51%); conjunctivitis (32%); rhinitis, nausea, rash, dizziness, pharyngitis, and lacrimation (10% to 20%); bronchospasm and/or chest pain (case reports in individuals with underlying airway disease)

Oral (all adverse reactions are documented while receiving combination therapy with alfa interferons; percentages as reported in adults); asterisked (*) percentages are those similar to interferon therapy alone:

>10%:

Central nervous system: Fatigue (60% to 70%)*, headache (43% to 66%)*, fever (32% to 46%)*, insomnia (26% to 41%), depression (20% to 36%)*, irritability (23% to 33%), dizziness (14% to 26%), impaired concentration (10% to 21%)*, emotional lability (7% to 12%)*

Dermatologic: Alopecia (27% to 36%), pruritus (13% to 29%), rash (5% to 28%), dry skin (10% to 24%), dermatitis (≤16%)

Endocrine and metabolic: Hyperuricemia (33% to 38%)

Gastrointestinal: Nausea (25% to 47%), anorexia (21% to 32%), weight decrease (10% to 29%), vomiting (9% to 25%)*, diarrhea (10% to 22%), dyspepsia (6% to 16%),

abdominal pain (8% to 13%), xerostomia (≤12%), RUQ pain (≤12%)
Hematologic: Leukopenia (6% to 45%), neutropenia (8% to 42%; grade 4: 2% to 11%; 40% with HIV coinfection), hemoglobin decreased (21% to 36%), anemia (11% to 17%), thrombocytopenia (<1% to 15%), lymphopenia (12% to 14%), hemolytic anemia (10% to 13%)
Hepatic: Bilirubin increase (10% to 32%)
Neuromuscular & skeletal: Myalgia (40% to 64%)*, rigors (25% to 48%), arthralgia (22% to 34%)*, musculoskeletal pain (19% to 28%)
Respiratory: Dyspnea (13% to 26%), cough (7% to 23%), pharyngitis (≤13%), sinusitis (≤12%)*
Miscellaneous: Flu-like syndrome (13% to 18%)*, viral infection (≤12%), diaphoresis (≤11%)

1% to 10%:
Cardiovascular: Chest pain (5% to 9%)*, flushing (≤4%)
Central nervous system: Pain (≤10%), mood alteration (≤6%; 9% with HIV coinfection), agitation (5% to 8%), nervousness (6%)*, memory impairment (≤6%), malaise (≤6%), suicidal ideation (adolescents: 2%; adults: 1%)
Dermatologic: Eczema (4% to 5%)
Endocrine & metabolic: Menstrual disorder (≤7%), hypothyroidism (≤5%)
Gastrointestinal: Taste perversion (4% to 9%), constipation (≤5%)
Hepatic: Hepatomegaly (≤4%), transaminases increased (1% to 3%), hepatic decompensation (2% with HIV coinfection)
Neuromuscular & skeletal: Weakness (9% to 10%), back pain (5%)
Ocular: Blurred vision (≤6%), conjunctivitis (≤5%)
Respiratory: Rhinitis (≤8%), exertional dyspnea (≤7%)
Miscellaneous: Fungal infection (≤6%), bacterial infection (3% to 5%)

<1% (Limited to important or life-threatening): Aggression, angina, anxiety, aplastic anemia, arrhythmia; autoimmune disorders (systemic lupus erythematosus, rheumatoid arthritis, sarcoidosis); cerebral hemorrhage, cholangitis, colitis, coma, corneal ulcer, dehydration, diabetes mellitus, drug abuse relapse/overdose, exfoliative dermatitis, fatty liver, hearing impairment/loss, gastrointestinal bleeding, gout, hallucination, hepatic dysfunction, hyper-/hypothyroidism, hypersensitivity (including anaphylaxis, angioedema, bronchoconstriction, and urticaria), myositis, pancreatitis, peptic ulcer, peripheral neuropathy, pneumonitis, psychosis, psychotic disorder, pulmonary dysfunction, pulmonary embolism, pulmonary infiltrates, pure red cell aplasia; skin reactions (erythema multiforme, exfoliative dermatitis, urticaria, vesiculobullous eruptions); sarcoidosis exacerbation, Stevens-Johnson syndrome, suicide, thrombotic thrombocytopenic purpura, thyroid function test abnormalities

Note: Incidence of anorexia, headache, fever, suicidal ideation, and vomiting are higher in children.

Drug Interactions

Avoid Concomitant Use There are no known interactions where it is recommended to avoid concomitant use.

Increased Effect/Toxicity

Ribavirin may increase the levels/effects of: Reverse Transcriptase Inhibitors (Nucleoside)

The levels/effects of Ribavirin may be increased by: Interferons (Alfa)

Decreased Effect

Ribavirin may decrease the levels/effects of: Influenza Virus Vaccine

Ethanol/Nutrition/Herb Interactions Food: Oral: High-fat meal increases the AUC and C_{max}.

Stability

Inhalation: Store vials in a dry place at 15°C to 30°C (59°F to 86°F). Do not use any water containing an antimicrobial agent to reconstitute drug. Reconstituted solution is stable for 24 hours at room temperature. Should not be mixed with other aerosolized medication.

Oral: Store at controlled room temperature of 25°C (77°F). Solution may also be refrigerated at 2°C to 8°C (36°F to 46°F).

Mechanism of Action Inhibits replication of RNA and DNA viruses; inhibits influenza virus RNA polymerase activity and inhibits the initiation and elongation of RNA fragments resulting in inhibition of viral protein synthesis

Pharmacodynamics/Kinetics

Absorption: Inhalation: Systemic; dependent upon respiratory factors and method of drug delivery; maximal absorption occurs with the use of aerosol generator via endotracheal tube; highest concentrations in respiratory tract and erythrocytes
Distribution: Oral capsule: Single dose: V_d 2825 L; distribution significantly prolonged in the erythrocyte (16-40 days), which can be used as a marker for intracellular metabolism
Protein binding: Oral: None
Metabolism: Hepatically and intracellularly (forms active metabolites); may be necessary for drug action
Bioavailability: Oral: 64%
Half-life elimination, plasma:
Children: Inhalation: 6.5-11 hours
Adults: Oral:
Capsule, single dose (Rebetol®, Ribasphere®): 24 hours in healthy adults, 44 hours with chronic hepatitis C infection (increases to ~298 hours at steady state)
Tablet, single dose (Copegus®): ~120-170 hours
Time to peak, serum: Inhalation: At end of inhalation period; Oral capsule: Multiple doses: 3 hours; Tablet: 2 hours
Excretion: Inhalation: Urine (40% as unchanged drug and metabolites); Oral capsule: Urine (61%), feces (12%)

Dosage

Aerosol inhalation: Infants and Children: Use with Viratek® small particle aerosol generator (SPAG-2) at a concentration of 20 mg/mL (6 g reconstituted with 300 mL of sterile water without preservatives). Continuous aerosol administration: 12-18 hours/day for 3 days, up to 7 days in length

Oral capsule or solution: Children ≥3 years: Chronic hepatitis C (in combination with interferon alfa-2b): Rebetol®: Oral: **Note:** Oral solution should be used in children 3-5 years of age, children ≤25 kg, or those unable to swallow capsules.
Capsule/solution: 15 mg/kg/day in 2 divided doses (morning and evening)
Capsule dosing recommendations:
25-36 kg: 400 mg/day (200 mg morning and evening)
37-49 kg: 600 mg/day (200 mg in the morning and 400 mg in the evening)
50-61 kg: 800 mg/day (400 mg in the morning and evening)
>61 kg: Refer to adult dosing
Note: Treatment duration may vary. Consult current guidelines and literature.

Oral capsule (Rebetol®, Ribasphere®): Adults:
Chronic hepatitis C (in combination with interferon alfa-2b):
≤75 kg: 400 mg in the morning, then 600 mg in the evening
>75 kg: 600 mg in the morning, then 600 mg in the evening
Chronic hepatitis C (in combination with peginterferon alfa-2b): 400 mg twice daily
Note: Treatment duration may vary. Consult current guidelines and literature.

Oral tablet (Copegus®, in combination with peginterferon alfa-2b): Adults: Chronic hepatitis C:
Monoinfection, genotype 1,4:
<75 kg: 1000 mg/day in 2 divided doses

≥75 kg: 1200 mg/day in 2 divided doses
Monoinfection, genotype 2,3: 800 mg/day in 2 divided doses
Coinfection with HIV: 800 mg/day in 2 divided doses
Note: Treatment duration may vary. Consult current guidelines and literature. Pretreatment platelets should be ≥90,000/mm^3 (75,000/mm^3 for cirrhosis or 70,000/mm^3 for coinfection with HIV), ANC ≥1500/mm^3, hemoglobin ≥12 g/dL for women and ≥13 g/dL for men (11 g/dL for HIV coinfected women and 12 g/dL for coinfected men), and TSH and T_4 within normal limits or controlled adequately. CD4+ cell count should be ≥200 cells/microL (or CD4+ count 100-200 cells/microL and HIV-1 RNA <5000 copies/mL) for coinfection with HIV.

Dosage adjustment for toxicity: Oral: Capsule, solution, tablet:
Patient **without** cardiac history:
Hemoglobin <10 g/dL:
Children: Decrease dose to 7.5 mg/kg/day
Adults: Decrease dose to 600 mg/day
Hemoglobin <8.5 g/dL: Children and Adults: Permanently discontinue treatment
Patient **with** cardiac history:
Hemoglobin has decreased ≥2 g/dL during any 4-week period of treatment:
Children: Decrease dose to 7.5 mg/kg/day
Adults: Decrease dose to 600 mg/day
Hemoglobin <12 g/dL after 4 weeks of reduced dose: Children and Adults: Permanently discontinue treatment

Dosage adjustment in renal impairment: Cl_{cr} <50 mL/minute: Oral route is not recommended
Dosage adjustment in renal impairment: Hepatic decompensation (Child-Pugh class B and C): Use of ribavirin tablets is contraindicated.

Dietary Considerations When used in combination with interferon alfa-2b, capsules and solution may be taken with or without food, but always in a consistent manner in regard to food intake (ie, always take with food or always take on an empty stomach). When used in combination with peginterferon alfa 2b, capsules should be taken with food. Tablets should be taken with food.

Administration
Inhalation: Ribavirin should be administered in well-ventilated rooms (at least 6 air changes/hour). In mechanically-ventilated patients, ribavirin can potentially be deposited in the ventilator delivery system depending on temperature, humidity, and electrostatic forces; this deposition can lead to malfunction or obstruction of the expiratory valve, resulting in inadvertently high positive end-expiratory pressures. The use of one-way valves in the inspiratory lines, a breathing circuit filter in the expiratory line, and frequent monitoring and filter replacement have been effective in preventing these problems. Solutions in SPAG-2 unit should be discarded at least every 24 hours and when the liquid level is low before adding newly reconstituted solution. Should not be mixed with other aerosolized medication.
Oral: Administer concurrently with interferon alfa injection. Capsule should not be opened, crushed, chewed, or broken. Capsules are not for use in children <5 years of age. Use oral solution for children 3-5 years, those ≤25 kg, or those who cannot swallow capsules.
Capsule, in combination with interferon alfa-2b: May be administered with or without food, but always in a consistent manner in regard to food intake.
Capsule, in combination with peginterferon alfa 2b: Administer with food.
Solution, in combination with interferon alfa-2b: May be administered with or without food, but always in a consistent manner in regard to food intake.
Tablet: Should be administered with food.

Monitoring Parameters
Inhalation: Respiratory function, hemoglobin, reticulocyte count, CBC with differential, I & O
Oral: Hemoglobin and hematocrit (pretreatment, 2- and 4 weeks after initiation), CBC with differential; pretreatment and monthly pregnancy test for women of childbearing age; LFTs, renal function, TSH, serum HCV RNA ; pretreatment ECG in patients with pre-existing cardiac disease; dental exams

Reference Range
Early viral response (EVR): >2 log decrease in HCV RNA after 12 weeks of treatment
End of treatment response (ETR): Absence of detectable HCV RNA at end of the recommended treatment period
Sustained treatment response (STR): Absence of HCV RNA in the serum 6 months following completion of full treatment course

Dosage Forms Excipient information presented when available (limited, particularly for generics); consult specific product labeling.
Capsule: 200 mg
Rebetol®, Ribasphere®: 200 mg
Combination package [dose pack]:
RibaPak™ 400/600 [each package contains]:
Tablet: 400 mg (7s)
Tablet: 600 mg (2s)
Powder for solution, for nebulization:
Virazole®: 6 g (1s) [reconstituted product contains ribavirin 20 mg/mL]
Solution, oral:
Rebetol®: 40 mg/mL (100 mL) [contains propylene glycol and sodium benzoate; bubble-gum flavor]
Tablet: 200 mg
Copegus®: 200 mg
Ribasphere®: 200 mg, 400 mg, 600 mg
Tablet [dose pack]:
RibaPak™: 400 mg (14s); 600 mg (14s)

◆ **Ribavirin and Interferon Alfa-2b Combination Pack** *see* Interferon Alfa-2b and Ribavirin *on page 804*

◆ **Ribo-100** *see* Riboflavin *on page 1313*

Riboflavin (RYE boe flay vin)

U.S. Brand Names Ribo-100
Index Terms Lactoflavin; Vitamin B_2; Vitamin G
Pharmacologic Category Vitamin, Water Soluble
Use Prevention of riboflavin deficiency and treatment of ariboflavinosis
Pregnancy Risk Factor A/C (dose exceeding RDA recommendation)
Medication Safety Issues
Sound-alike/look-alike issues:
Riboflavin may be confused with ribavirin
Dosage Oral:
Riboflavin deficiency:
Children: 2.5-10 mg/day in divided doses
Adults: 5-30 mg/day in divided doses
Recommended daily allowance:
Children: 0.4-1.8 mg
Adults: 1.2-1.7 mg
Additional Information Complete prescribing information for this medication should be consulted for additional detail.
Dosage Forms Excipient information presented when available (limited, particularly for generics); consult specific product labeling.
Tablet: 25 mg, 50 mg, 100 mg
Ribo-100: 100 mg

◆ **Rid-A-Pain Dental [OTC]** *see* Benzocaine *on page 183*

◆ **Ridaura®** *see* Auranofin *on page 160*

- ◆ **RID® Maximum Strength [OTC]** *see* Pyrethrins and Piperonyl Butoxide *on page 1271*
- ◆ **RID® Mousse (Can)** *see* Pyrethrins and Piperonyl Butoxide *on page 1271*
- ◆ **Rid® Spray [OTC]** *see* Permethrin *on page 1176*

Rifabutin (rif a BYOO tin)

U.S. Brand Names Mycobutin®

Canadian Brand Names Mycobutin®

Index Terms Ansamycin

Pharmacologic Category Antibiotic, Miscellaneous; Antitubercular Agent

Use Prevention of disseminated *Mycobacterium avium* complex (MAC) in patients with advanced HIV infection

Unlabeled/Investigational Use Utilized in multidrug regimens for treatment of MAC

Pregnancy Risk Factor B

Lactation Excretion in breast milk unknown

Medication Safety Issues

Sound-alike/look-alike issues:

Rifabutin may be confused with rifampin

Contraindications Hypersensitivity to rifabutin, any other rifamycins, or any component of the formulation; rifabutin is contraindicated in patients with a WBC <1000/mm^3 or a platelet count <50,000/mm^3

Warnings/Precautions Rifabutin as a single agent must not be administered to patients with active tuberculosis since its use may lead to the development of tuberculosis that is resistant to both rifabutin and rifampin. Rifabutin should be discontinued in patients with AST >500 units/L or if total bilirubin is >3 mg/dL. Use with caution in patients with liver impairment. Modification of dosage should be considered in patients with renal impairment. Prolonged use may result in fungal or bacterial superinfection, including *C. difficile*-associated diarrhea (CDAD) and pseudomembranous colitis; CDAD has been observed >2 months postantibiotic treatment.

Adverse Reactions

>10%:

Dermatologic: Rash (11%)

Genitourinary: Discoloration of urine (30%)

Hematologic: Neutropenia (25%), leukopenia (17%)

1% to 10%:

Central nervous system: Headache (3%)

Gastrointestinal: Abdominal pain (4%), vomiting/nausea (3%), diarrhea (3%), eructation (3%), anorexia (2%), flatulence (2%)

Hematologic: Anemia, thrombocytopenia (5%)

Hepatic: ALT increased (7% to 9%), AST increased (7% to 9%)

Neuromuscular & skeletal: Myalgia

<1% (Limited to important or life-threatening): Chest pain, dyspepsia, dyspnea, fever, insomnia, taste perversion, uveitis

Drug Interactions

Metabolism/Transport Effects Substrate of CYP3A4 (major); **Induces** CYP3A4 (strong)

Avoid Concomitant Use

Avoid concomitant use of Rifabutin with any of the following: Mycophenolate; Nilotinib; Ranolazine; Voriconazole

Increased Effect/Toxicity

Rifabutin may increase the levels/effects of: Clopidogrel; Isoniazid

The levels/effects of Rifabutin may be increased by: Antifungal Agents (Azole Derivatives, Systemic); Delavirdine; Fluconazole; Macrolide Antibiotics; Nevirapine; Protease Inhibitors; Voriconazole

Decreased Effect

Rifabutin may decrease the levels/effects of: Alfentanil; Amiodarone; Angiotensin II Receptor Blockers; Antiemetics (5HT3 Antagonists); Antifungal Agents (Azole Derivatives, Systemic); Aprepitant; Atovaquone; Barbiturates; Benzodiazepines (metabolized by oxidation); BusPIRone; Calcium Channel Blockers; Contraceptive (Progestins); Corticosteroids (Systemic); CycloSPORINE; CYP3A4 Substrates; Dapsone; Delavirdine; Disopyramide; Efavirenz; Etravirine; FentaNYL; Fluconazole; Gefitinib; HMG-CoA Reductase Inhibitors; Imatinib; Maraviroc; Morphine Sulfate; Mycophenolate; Nevirapine; Nilotinib; Oral Contraceptive (Estrogens); Phenytoin; Propafenone; Protease Inhibitors; QuiNIDine; Ramelteon; Ranolazine; Repaglinide; Sorafenib; Sunitinib; Tacrolimus; Tamoxifen; Temsirolimus; Terbinafine; Tocainide; Typhoid Vaccine; Vitamin K Antagonists; Voriconazole; Zaleplon; Zolpidem

The levels/effects of Rifabutin may be decreased by: CYP3A4 Inducers (Strong); Deferasirox; Efavirenz; Herbs (CYP3A4 Inducers); Nevirapine

Ethanol/Nutrition/Herb Interactions Food: High-fat meal may decrease the rate but not the extent of absorption.

Mechanism of Action Inhibits DNA-dependent RNA polymerase at the beta subunit which prevents chain initiation

Pharmacodynamics/Kinetics

Absorption: Readily, 53%

Distribution: V_d: 9.32 L/kg; distributes to body tissues including the lungs, liver, spleen, eyes, and kidneys

Protein binding: 85%

Metabolism: To active and inactive metabolites

Bioavailability: Absolute: HIV: 20%

Half-life elimination: Terminal: 45 hours (range: 16-69 hours)

Time to peak, serum: 2-4 hours

Excretion: Urine (10% as unchanged drug, 53% as metabolites); feces (10% as unchanged drug, 30% as metabolites)

Dosage Oral:

Children >1 year:

Prophylaxis: 5 mg/kg daily; higher dosages have been used in limited trials

Treatment (unlabeled use): Patients not receiving NNRTIs or protease inhibitors:

Initial phase (2 weeks to 2 months): 10-20 mg/kg daily (maximum: 300 mg).

Second phase: 10-20 mg/kg daily (maximum: 300 mg) or twice weekly

Adults:

Prophylaxis: 300 mg once daily (alone or in combination with azithromycin)

Treatment (unlabeled use):

Patients not receiving NNRTIs or protease inhibitors:

Initial phase: 5 mg/kg daily (maximum: 300 mg)

Second phase: 5 mg/kg daily or twice weekly

Dosage adjustment for concurrent nelfinavir, amprenavir, indinavir: Reduce rifabutin dose to 150 mg/day; no change in dose if administered twice weekly

Dosage adjustment for concurrent efavirenz (no concomitant protease inhibitor): Increase rifabutin dose to 450-600 mg daily, or 600 mg 3 times/week

Dosage adjustment in renal impairment: Cl_{cr} <30 mL/minute: Reduce dose by 50%

Dietary Considerations May be taken with meals or without food or mix with applesauce.

Administration Should be administered on an empty stomach, but may be taken with meals to minimize nausea or vomiting.

Monitoring Parameters Periodic liver function tests, CBC with differential, platelet count

Dosage Forms Excipient information presented when available (limited, particularly for generics); consult specific product labeling.

Capsule: 150 mg

◆ **Rifadin®** *see* Rifampin *on page 1315*

◆ **Rifampicin** *see* Rifampin *on page 1315*

Rifampin (rif AM pin)

U.S. Brand Names Rifadin®

Canadian Brand Names Rifadin®; Rofact™

Index Terms Rifampicin

Pharmacologic Category Antibiotic, Miscellaneous; Antitubercular Agent

Use Management of active tuberculosis in combination with other agents; elimination of meningococci from the nasopharynx in asymptomatic carriers

Unlabeled/Investigational Use Prophylaxis of *Haemophilus influenzae* type b infection; *Legionella* pneumonia; used in combination with other anti-infectives in the treatment of staphylococcal infections; treatment of *M. leprae* infections

Pregnancy Risk Factor C

Pregnancy Considerations Teratogenic effects have bee reported in animal studies. Rifampin crosses the human placenta. Due to the risk of tuberculosis to the fetus, treatment is recommended when the probability of maternal disease is moderate to high. Postnatal hemorrhages have been reported in the infant and mother with isoniazid administration during the last few weeks of pregnancy.

Lactation Enters breast milk/not recommended (AAP rates "compatible")

Medication Safety Issues

Sound-alike/look-alike issues:

Rifadin® may be confused with Rifater®, Ritalin®

Rifampin may be confused with ribavirin, rifabutin, Rifamate®, rifapentine, rifaximin

Contraindications Hypersensitivity to rifampin, any rifamycins, or any component of the formulation; concurrent use of amprenavir, saquinavir/ritonavir (possibly other protease inhibitors)

Warnings/Precautions Use with caution and modify dosage in patients with liver impairment; observe for hyperbilirubinemia; discontinue therapy if this in conjunction with clinical symptoms or any signs of significant hepatocellular damage develop. Use with caution in patients receiving concurrent medications associated with hepatotoxicity. Use with caution in patients with a history of alcoholism (even if ethanol consumption is discontinued during therapy). Since rifampin since rifampin has enzyme-inducing properties, porphyria exacerbation is possible; use with caution in patients with porphyria; do not use for meningococcal disease, only for short-term treatment of asymptomatic carrier states

Regimens of >600 mg once or twice weekly have been associated with a high incidence of adverse reactions including a flu-like syndrome, hypersensitivity, thrombocytopenia, leukopenia, and anemia. Urine, feces, saliva, sweat, tears, and CSF may be discolored to red/orange; remove soft contact lenses during therapy since permanent staining may occur. Do not administer I.V. form via I.M. or SubQ routes; restart infusion at another site if extravasation occurs. Prolonged use may result in fungal or bacterial superinfection, including *C. difficile*-associated diarrhea (CDAD) and pseudomembranous colitis; CDAD has been observed >2 months postantibiotic treatment. Monitor for compliance in patients on intermittent therapy.

Adverse Reactions

Frequency not defined:

Cardiovascular: Edema, flushing

Central nervous system: Ataxia, behavioral changes, concentration impaired, confusion, dizziness, drowsiness, fatigue, fever, headache, numbness, psychosis

Dermatologic: Pemphigoid reaction, pruritus, urticaria

Endocrine & metabolic: Adrenal insufficiency, menstrual disorders

Hematologic: Agranulocytosis (rare), DIC, eosinophilia, hemoglobin decreased, hemolysis, hemolytic anemia, leukopenia, thrombocytopenia (especially with high-dose therapy)

Hepatic: Hepatitis (rare), jaundice

Neuromuscular & skeletal: Myalgia, osteomalacia, weakness

Ocular: Exudative conjunctivitis, visual changes

Renal: Acute renal failure, BUN increased, hemoglobinuria, hematuria, interstitial nephritis, uric acid increased

Miscellaneous: Flu-like syndrome

1% to 10%:

Dermatologic: Rash (1% to 5%)

Gastrointestinal (1% to 2%): Anorexia, cramps, diarrhea, epigastric distress, flatulence, heartburn, nausea, pseudomembranous colitis, pancreatitis vomiting

Hepatic: LFTs increased (up to 14%)

Drug Interactions

Metabolism/Transport Effects **Induces** CYP1A2 (strong), 2A6 (strong), 2B6 (strong), 2C8 (strong), 2C9 (strong), 2C19 (strong), 3A4 (strong)

Avoid Concomitant Use

Avoid concomitant use of Rifampin with any of the following: Atazanavir; Etravirine; Mycophenolate; Nilotinib; Praziquantel; Ranolazine; Voriconazole

Increased Effect/Toxicity

Rifampin may increase the levels/effects of: Clopidogrel; Isoniazid

The levels/effects of Rifampin may be increased by: Antifungal Agents (Azole Derivatives, Systemic); Delavirdine; Eltrombopag; Fluconazole; Macrolide Antibiotics; P-Glycoprotein Inhibitors; Protease Inhibitors; Pyrazinamide; Voriconazole

Decreased Effect

Rifampin may decrease the levels/effects of: Alfentanil; Amiodarone; Angiotensin II Receptor Blockers; Antidiabetic Agents (Thiazolidinedione); Antiemetics (5HT3 Antagonists); Antifungal Agents (Azole Derivatives, Systemic); Aprepitant; Atazanavir; Atovaquone; Barbiturates; Bendamustine; Benzodiazepines (metabolized by oxidation); Beta-Blockers; BusPIRone; Calcium Channel Blockers; Caspofungin; Chloramphenicol; Contraceptive (Progestins); Corticosteroids (Systemic); CycloSPORINE; CYP1A2 Substrates; CYP2A6 Substrates; CYP2B6 Substrates; CYP2C19 Substrates; CYP2C8 Substrates (High risk); CYP2C9 Substrates (High risk); CYP3A4 Substrates; Dabigatran Etexilate; Dapsone; Delavirdine; Disopyramide; Efavirenz; Erlotinib; Etravirine; Exemestane; FentaNYL; Fexofenadine; Fluconazole; Fosaprepitant; Gefitinib; HMG-CoA Reductase Inhibitors; Imatinib; LamoTRIgine; Maraviroc; Methadone; Morphine Sulfate; Mycophenolate; Nevirapine; Nilotinib; Oral Contraceptive (Estrogens); P-Glycoprotein Substrates; Phenytoin; Praziquantel; Propafenone; Protease Inhibitors; QuiNIDine; Raltegravir; Ramelteon; Ranolazine; Repaglinide; Sirolimus; Sorafenib; Sulfonylureas; Sunitinib; Tacrolimus; Tamoxifen; Temsirolimus; Terbinafine; Thyroid Products; Tocainide; Typhoid Vaccine; Valproic Acid; Vitamin K Antagonists; Voriconazole; Zaleplon; Zidovudine; Zolpidem

The levels/effects of Rifampin may be decreased by: P-Glycoprotein Inducers

Ethanol/Nutrition/Herb Interactions

Ethanol: Avoid ethanol (may increase risk of hepatotoxicity).

Food: Food decreases the extent of absorption; rifampin concentrations may be decreased if taken with food.

Herb/Nutraceutical: St John's wort may decrease rifampin levels.

Stability Rifampin powder is reddish brown. Intact vials should be stored at room temperature and protected from excessive heat and light. Reconstitute powder for injection with SWFI. Prior to injection, dilute in appropriate volume of compatible diluent (eg, 100 mL D_5W). Reconstituted vials are stable for 24 hours at room temperature.

Stability of parenteral admixture at room temperature (25°C) is 4 hours for D_5W and 24 hours for NS.

Mechanism of Action Inhibits bacterial RNA synthesis by binding to the beta subunit of DNA-dependent RNA polymerase, blocking RNA transcription

Pharmacodynamics/Kinetics

Duration: ≤24 hours

Absorption: Oral: Well absorbed; food may delay or slightly reduce peak

Distribution: Highly lipophilic; crosses blood-brain barrier well

Relative diffusion from blood into CSF: Adequate with or without inflammation (exceeds usual MICs)

CSF:blood level ratio: Inflamed meninges: 25%

Protein binding: 80%

Metabolism: Hepatic; undergoes enterohepatic recirculation

Half-life elimination: 3-4 hours; prolonged with hepatic impairment; End-stage renal disease: 1.8-11 hours

Time to peak, serum: Oral: 2-4 hours

Excretion: Feces (60% to 65%) and urine (~30%) as unchanged drug

Dosage

Usual dosage ranges: Oral, I.V.:

Infants and Children: 10-20 mg/kg/day as a single dose or in 2 divided doses; maximum: 600 mg/day

Adults: 600 mg once or twice daily

Indication-specific dosing: Oral, I.V.:

***H. influenzae* prophylaxis (unlabeled use):**

Infants and Children: 20 mg/kg/day every 24 hours for 4 days, not to exceed 600 mg/dose

Adults: 600 mg every 24 hours for 4 days

Leprosy (unlabeled use): Adults:

Multibacillary: 600 mg once monthly for 24 months in combination with ofloxacin and minocycline

Paucibacillary: 600 mg once monthly for 6 months in combination with dapsone

Single lesion: 600 mg as a single dose in combination with ofloxacin 400 mg and minocycline 100 mg

Meningitis *(Pneumococcus* or *Staphylococcus)* (unlabeled use): Recommended only for organisms known to be rifampin-susceptible and highly penicillin- or cephalosporin-resistant. May be used in place of or in addition to vancomycin when dexamethasone therapy employed.

Infants and Children: 20 mg/kg/day as a single dose or in 2 divided doses; maximum: 600 mg/day

Adults: 600 mg once daily

Meningococcal meningitis prophylaxis (unlabeled use):

Infants <1 month: 10 mg/kg/day in divided doses every 12 hours for 2 days

Infants ≥1 month and Children: 20 mg/kg/day in divided doses every 12 hours for 2 days (maximum: 600 mg/dose)

Adults: 600 mg every 12 hours for 2 days

Nasal carriers of *Staphylococcus aureus* (unlabeled use):

Children: 15 mg/kg/day divided every 12 hours for 5-10 days in combination with other antibiotics

Adults: 600 mg/day for 5-10 days in combination with other antibiotics

Nontuberculous mycobacterium (*M. kansasii*) (unlabeled use): Adults: 10 mg/kg/day (maximum: 600 mg/day) for duration to include 12 months of culture-negative sputum; typically used in combination with ethambutol and isoniazid

Synergy for *Staphylococcus aureus* infections (unlabeled use): Adults: 300-600 mg twice daily with other antibiotics

Tuberculosis, active: Note: A four-drug regimen (isoniazid, rifampin, pyrazinamide, and ethambutol) is preferred for the initial, empiric treatment of TB. When the drug susceptibility results are available, the regimen should be altered as appropriate.

Infants and Children <12 years:

Daily therapy: 10-20 mg/kg/day usually as a single dose (maximum: 600 mg/day)

Twice weekly directly observed therapy (DOT): 10-20 mg/kg (maximum: 600 mg)

Adults:

Daily therapy: 10 mg/kg/day (maximum: 600 mg/day)

Twice weekly directly observed therapy (DOT): 10 mg/kg (maximum: 600 mg); 3 times/week: 10 mg/kg (maximum: 600 mg)

Tuberculosis, latent infection (LTBI): As an alternative to isoniazid:

Children: 10-20 mg/kg/day (maximum: 600 mg/day) for 6 months

Adults: 10 mg/kg/day (maximum: 600 mg/day) for 4 months. **Note:** Combination with pyrazinamide should not generally be offered (*MMWR*, Aug 8, 2003).

Dosing adjustment in hepatic impairment: Dose reductions may be necessary to reduce hepatotoxicity

Hemodialysis or peritoneal dialysis: Plasma rifampin concentrations are not significantly affected by hemodialysis or peritoneal dialysis.

Dietary Considerations Rifampin should be taken on an empty stomach.

Administration

I.V.: Administer I.V. preparation once daily by slow I.V. infusion over 30 minutes to 3 hours at a final concentration not to exceed 6 mg/mL.

Oral: Administer on an empty stomach (ie, 1 hour prior to, or 2 hours after meals or antacids) to increase total absorption. The compounded oral suspension must be shaken well before using. May mix contents of capsule with applesauce or jelly.

Monitoring Parameters Periodic (baseline and every 2-4 weeks during therapy) monitoring of liver function (AST, ALT, bilirubin), CBC; hepatic status and mental status, sputum culture, chest x-ray 2-3 months into treatment

Test Interactions Positive Coombs' reaction [direct], rifampin inhibits standard assay's ability to measure serum folate and B_{12}; transient increase in LFTs and decreased biliary excretion of contrast media

Dosage Forms Excipient information presented when available (limited, particularly for generics); consult specific product labeling.

Capsule: 150 mg, 300 mg

Injection, powder for reconstitution: 600 mg

Extemporaneous Preparations For pediatric and adult patients with difficulty swallowing or where lower doses are needed, the package insert lists an extemporaneous liquid suspension as follows:

Rifampin 1% w/v suspension (10 mg/mL) can be compounded using one of four syrups (Syrup NF, simple syrup, Syrpalta® syrup, or raspberry syrup)

Empty contents of four 300 mg capsules or eight 150 mg capsules onto a piece of weighing paper

If necessary, crush contents to produce a fine powder

Transfer powder blend to a 4 oz amber glass or plastic prescription bottle

Rinse paper and spatula with 20 mL of syrup and add the rinse to bottle; shake vigorously

Add 100 mL of syrup to the bottle and shake vigorously

This compounding procedure results in a 1% w/v suspension containing 10 mg rifampin/mL; stability studies indicate suspension is stable at room temperature (25°C ± 3°C) or in refrigerator (2°C to 8°C) for 4 weeks; shake well prior to administration

Rifapentine (rif a PEN teen)

U.S. Brand Names Priftin®

Canadian Brand Names Priftin®

Pharmacologic Category Antitubercular Agent

Use Treatment of pulmonary tuberculosis; rifapentine must always be used in conjunction with at least one other antituberculosis drug to which the isolate is susceptible; it may also be necessary to add a third agent (either streptomycin or ethambutol) until susceptibility is known.

Pregnancy Risk Factor C

Pregnancy Considerations Has been shown to be teratogenic in rats and rabbits. Rat offspring showed cleft palates, right aortic arch, and delayed ossification and increased number of ribs. Rabbits displayed ovarian agenesis, pes varus, arhinia, microphthalmia, and irregularities of the ossified facial tissues. Rat studies also show decreased fetal weight, increased number of stillborns, and decreased gestational survival. There are no adequate and well-controlled studies in pregnant women. Rifapentine should be used during pregnancy only if the potential benefits justifies the potential risk to the fetus.

Lactation Excretion in breast milk unknown/contraindicated

Medication Safety Issues

Sound-alike/look-alike issues:

Rifapentine may be confused with rifampin

Contraindications Hypersensitivity to rifapentine, rifampin, rifabutin, any rifamycin analog, or any component of the formulation

Warnings/Precautions Patients with abnormal liver tests and/or liver disease should only be given rifapentine when absolutely necessary and under strict medical supervision. Monitoring of liver function tests should be carried out prior to therapy and then every 2-4 weeks during therapy if signs of liver disease occur or worsen, rifapentine should be discontinued. All patients treated with rifapentine should have baseline measurements of liver function tests and enzymes, bilirubin, and a complete blood count. Patients should be seen monthly and specifically questioned regarding symptoms associated with adverse reactions. Routine laboratory monitoring in people with normal baseline measurements is generally not necessary. Use with caution in patients with porphyria; exacerbation is possible.

Rifapentine may produce a red-orange discoloration of body tissues/fluids including skin, teeth, tongue, urine, feces, saliva, sputum, tears, sweat, and cerebral spinal fluid. Contact lenses may become permanently stained. Prolonged use may result in fungal or bacterial superinfection, including *C. difficile*-associated diarrhea (CDAD) and pseudomembranous colitis; CDAD has been observed >2 months postantibiotic treatment. Experience in treating TB in HIV-infected patients is limited. Compliance with dosing regimen is absolutely necessary for successful drug therapy.

Adverse Reactions

>10%: Endocrine & metabolic: Hyperuricemia (most likely due to pyrazinamide from initiation phase combination therapy)

1% to 10%:

Cardiovascular: Hypertension

Central nervous system: Headache, dizziness

Dermatologic: Rash, pruritus, acne

Gastrointestinal: Anorexia, nausea, vomiting, dyspepsia, diarrhea

Genitourinary: Pyuria, proteinuria, hematuria, urinary casts

Hematologic: Neutropenia, lymphopenia, anemia, leukopenia, thrombocytosis

Hepatic: ALT increased, AST increased

Neuromuscular & skeletal: Arthralgia, pain

Respiratory: Hemoptysis

<1% (Limited to important or life-threatening): Aggressive reaction, arthrosis, gout, hepatitis, hyperkalemia, pancreatitis, purpura, thrombocytopenia

Drug Interactions

Metabolism/Transport Effects **Induces** CYP2C8 (strong), 2C9 (strong), 3A4 (strong)

Avoid Concomitant Use

Avoid concomitant use of Rifapentine with any of the following: Etravirine; Mycophenolate; Nilotinib; Ranolazine; Voriconazole

Increased Effect/Toxicity

Rifapentine may increase the levels/effects of: Clopidogrel; Isoniazid

The levels/effects of Rifapentine may be increased by: Antifungal Agents (Azole Derivatives, Systemic); Delavirdine; Fluconazole; Protease Inhibitors; Voriconazole

Decreased Effect

Rifapentine may decrease the levels/effects of: Alfentanil; Amiodarone; Angiotensin II Receptor Blockers; Antiemetics (5HT3 Antagonists); Antifungal Agents (Azole Derivatives, Systemic); Aprepitant; Atovaquone; Barbiturates; Benzodiazepines (metabolized by oxidation); Beta-Blockers; BusPIRone; Calcium Channel Blockers; Contraceptive (Progestins); Corticosteroids (Systemic); CycloSPORINE; CYP2C8 Substrates (High risk); CYP2C9 Substrates (High risk); CYP3A4 Substrates; Dapsone; Delavirdine; Disopyramide; Etravirine; FentaNYL; Fluconazole; Gefitinib; HMG-CoA Reductase Inhibitors; Imatinib; Maraviroc; Methadone; Morphine Sulfate; Mycophenolate; Nilotinib; Oral Contraceptive (Estrogens); Phenytoin; Propafenone; Protease Inhibitors; QuiNIDine; Ramelteon; Ranolazine; Repaglinide; Sorafenib; Sunitinib; Tacrolimus; Tamoxifen; Temsirolimus; Terbinafine; Tocainide; Vitamin K Antagonists; Voriconazole; Zaleplon; Zidovudine; Zolpidem

Ethanol/Nutrition/Herb Interactions Food: Food increases AUC and maximum serum concentration by 43% and 44% respectively as compared to fasting conditions.

Stability Store at room temperature (15°C to 30°C; 59°F to 86°F). Protect from excessive heat and humidity.

Mechanism of Action Inhibits DNA-dependent RNA polymerase in susceptible strains of *Mycobacterium tuberculosis* (but not in mammalian cells). Rifapentine is bactericidal against both intracellular and extracellular MTB organisms. MTB resistant to other rifamycins including rifampin are likely to be resistant to rifapentine. Cross-resistance does not appear between rifapentine and other nonrifamycin antimycobacterial agents.

Pharmacodynamics/Kinetics

Absorption: Food increases AUC and C_{max} by 43% and 44% respectively.

Distribution: V_d: ~70.2 L; rifapentine and metabolite accumulate in human monocyte-derived macrophages with intracellular/extracellular ratios of 24:1 and 7:1 respectively

Protein binding: Rifapentine and 25-desacetyl metabolite: 97.7% and 93.2%, primarily to albumin

Metabolism: Hepatic; hydrolyzed by an esterase and esterase enzyme to form the active metabolite 25-desacetyl rifapentine

Bioavailability: ~70%

Half-life elimination: Rifapentine: 14-17 hours; 25-desacetyl rifapentine: 13 hours
Time to peak, serum: 5-6 hours
Excretion: Urine (17% primarily as metabolites)

Dosage
Children: No dosing information available
Adults: **Rifapentine should not be used alone**; initial phase should include a 3- to 4-drug regimen
Intensive phase (initial 2 months) of short-term therapy: 600 mg (four 150 mg tablets) given twice weekly (with an interval of not less than 72 hours between doses); following the intensive phase, treatment should continue with rifapentine 600 mg once weekly for 4 months in combination with INH or appropriate agent for susceptible organisms
Dosing adjustment in renal or hepatic impairment: Unknown

Monitoring Parameters Patients with pre-existing hepatic problems should have liver function tests monitored every 2-4 weeks during therapy

Test Interactions Rifampin has been shown to inhibit standard microbiological assays for serum folate and vitamin B_{12}; this should be considered for rifapentine; therefore, alternative assay methods should be considered.

Additional Information Rifapentine has only been studied in patients with tuberculosis receiving a 6-month short-course intensive regimen approval. Outcomes have been based on 6-month follow-up treatment observed in clinical trial 008 as a surrogate for the 2-year follow-up generally accepted as evidence for efficacy in the treatment of pulmonary tuberculosis.

Dosage Forms Excipient information presented when available (limited, particularly for generics); consult specific product labeling.
Tablet: 150 mg

Rifaximin (rif AX i min)

U.S. Brand Names Xifaxan™

Pharmacologic Category Antibiotic, Miscellaneous

Use Treatment of travelers' diarrhea caused by noninvasive strains of *E. coli*

Pregnancy Risk Factor C

Pregnancy Considerations Adverse events have been observed in animal reproduction studies; therefore, the manufacturer classifies rifaximin as pregnancy category C. Due to the limited oral absorption of rifaximin (<0.4%), exposure to the fetus is expected to be extremely low.

Lactation Excretion in breast milk unknown/not recommended

Medication Safety Issues
Sound-alike/look-alike issues:
Rifaximin may be confused with rifampin

Contraindications Hypersensitivity to rifaximin, other rifamycin antibiotics, or any component of the formulation; diarrhea with fever or blood in the stool

Warnings/Precautions Efficacy has not been established for the treatment of diarrhea due to pathogens other than *E. coli*, including *C. jejuni*, *Shigella* and *Salmonella*. Consider alternative therapy if symptoms persist or worsen after 24-48 hours of treatment. Not for treatment of systemic infections; <1% is absorbed orally. Prolonged use may result in fungal or bacterial superinfection, including *C. difficile*-associated diarrhea (CDAD) and pseudomembranous colitis; CDAD has been observed >2 months postantibiotic treatment. Safety and efficacy have not been established in children <12 years of age.

Adverse Reactions Incidence of adverse effects reported as ≥2% occurred more in the placebo group than the rifaximin group except for headache.
2% to 10%: Central nervous system: Headache (10%; placebo 9%)
<2%, postmarketing, and/or case reports (limited to important or life-threatening): Abnormal dreams, allergic dermatitis, angioneurotic edema (includine tongue and facial edema with dysphagia), exfoliative dermatitis, fatigue, flushing, hypersensitivity reactions, insomnia, motion sickness, pruritus, rash, sunburn, tinnitus, urticaria

Drug Interactions
Metabolism/Transport Effects Induces CYP3A4 (minor)
Avoid Concomitant Use There are no known interactions where it is recommended to avoid concomitant use.
Increased Effect/Toxicity There are no known significant interactions involving an increase in effect.
Decreased Effect
Rifaximin may decrease the levels/effects of: Maraviroc; Typhoid Vaccine

Stability Store at controlled room temperature of 20°C to 25°C (68°F to 77°F).

Mechanism of Action Rifaximin inhibits bacterial RNA synthesis by binding to bacterial DNA-dependent RNA polymerase.

Pharmacodynamics/Kinetics
Absorption: Oral: <0.4%
Distribution: 80% to 90% in the gut
Half-life elimination: ~6 hours
Excretion: Feces (~97% as unchanged drug); urine (<1%)

Dosage Oral: Children ≥12 years and Adults: Travelers' diarrhea: 200 mg 3 times/day for 3 days

Dietary Considerations May be taken with or without food.

Administration May be administered with or without food.

Monitoring Parameters Temperature, blood in stool, change in symptoms

Dosage Forms Excipient information presented when available (limited, particularly for generics); consult specific product labeling.
Tablet: 200 mg

◆ **rIFN-A** *see* Interferon Alfa-2a *on page* *799*
◆ **rIFN beta-1a** *see* Interferon Beta-1a *on page* *806*
◆ **rIFN beta-1b** *see* Interferon Beta-1b *on page* *807*
◆ **RIG** *see* Rabies Immune Globulin (Human) *on page* *1286*
◆ **rIL-11** *see* Oprelvekin *on page* *1106*

Rilonacept (ri LON a sept)

U.S. Brand Names Arcalyst™

Pharmacologic Category Interleukin-1 Inhibitor

Use Orphan drug: Treatment of cryopyrin-associated periodic syndromes (CAPS) including familial cold autoinflammatory syndrome (FCAS) and Muckle-Wells syndrome (MWS)

Pregnancy Risk Factor C

Pregnancy Considerations Animal studies have demonstrated teratogenic effects and fetal loss. There are no adequate and well-controlled studies in pregnant women. Use during pregnancy only if potential benefit to the mother outweighs potential risk to the fetus.

Lactation Excretion in breast milk unknown/use caution

Contraindications There are no contraindications listed in the manufacturer's labeling.

Warnings/Precautions May cause rare hypersensitivity, anaphylaxis, or anaphylactoid reactions; medications for the treatment of hypersensitivity reactions should be available for immediate use. Caution should be exercised when considering use in patients with a history of new/recurrent infections, with conditions that predispose them to infections, or with latent or localized infections. Therapy should not be initiated in patients with active or chronic infections. Use may impair defenses against malignancies; impact on the development and course of malignancies is not fully defined. Use may increase total cholesterol, HDL, LDL, and triglycerides; periodic assessment of lipid profile should occur. Tumor necrosis factor (TNF)-blocking agents should not be used in combination with rilonacept; risk of serious infection is increased. Immunizations should be up to date including pneumococcal and influenza vaccines before initiating therapy. Live vaccines should not be given concurrently. Administration of inactivated (killed) vaccines while on therapy may not be effective. Use with caution in the elderly due to the potential higher risk for infections. Safety and efficacy has not been established in patients <12 years of age.

Adverse Reactions

>10%:

Local: Injection site reactions (48%; majority mild-moderate; typically lasting 1-2 days; characterized by erythema, bruising, dermatitis, inflammation, pain, pruritus, swelling, urticaria, vesicles, warmth, and hemorrhage)

Respiratory: Upper respiratory tract infection (26%)

Miscellaneous: Infection (48% during winter months; 18% during summer months), antibody formation to rilonacept (35%)

1% to 10%:

Central nervous system: Hypoesthesia (9%)

Respiratory: Cough (9%), sinusitis (9%)

<1% (Limited to important or life-threatening): HDL cholesterol increased, LDL cholesterol increased, neutropenia (transient), triglycerides increased, total cholesterol increased

Drug Interactions

Avoid Concomitant Use

Avoid concomitant use of Rilonacept with any of the following: Anti-TNF Agents; Natalizumab; Vaccines (Live)

Increased Effect/Toxicity

Rilonacept may increase the levels/effects of: Natalizumab; Vaccines (Live)

The levels/effects of Rilonacept may be increased by: Anti-TNF Agents; Trastuzumab

Decreased Effect

Rilonacept may decrease the levels/effects of: Vaccines (Inactivated)

The levels/effects of Rilonacept may be decreased by: Echinacea

Stability Store powder in refrigerator at 2°C to 8°C (36°F to 46°F); do not freeze. Do not shake. Protect from light. Reconstitute rilonacept 220 mg powder for injection with SWFI 2.3 mL; do not use bacteriostatic water containing benzyl alcohol or parabens. After reconstituting with SWFI, gently shake the vial for 1 minute, then allow solution to sit for 1 minute. Each reconstituted vial allows for withdrawal of 2 mL (160 mg) for SubQ administration. After reconstitution, may be stored at controlled room temperature. Protect from light. Use within 3 hours of reconstitution.

Mechanism of Action Cryopyrin-associated periodic syndromes (CAPS) refers to rare genetic syndromes caused by mutations in the nucleotide-binding domain, leucine rich family (NLR), pyrin domain containing 3 (NLRP-3) gene or the cold-induced autoinflammatory syndrome-1 (CIAS1) gene. Cryopyrin, a protein encoded by this gene, regulates interleukin-1 beta (IL-1β) activation. Deficiency of cryopyrin results in excessive inflammation. Rilonacept reduces inflammation by binding to IL-1β (some binding of IL-1α and IL-1 receptor antagonist) and preventing interaction with cell surface receptors.

Pharmacodynamics/Kinetics Onset of action: Steady state reached by 6 weeks

Dosage SubQ: Cryopyrin-associated periodic syndromes:

Children ≥12 years: Loading dose 4.4 mg/kg (maximum dose: 320 mg) given as 1-2 separate injections (maximum: 2 mL/injection) on the same day, followed by 2.2 mg/kg (maximum dose: 160 mg) once weekly. **Note:** Do not administer more frequently than once weekly.

Adults: Loading dose 320 mg given as 2 separate injections (160 mg each) on the same day at 2 different sites, followed a week later by 160 mg, then once weekly. **Note:** Do not administer more frequently than once weekly.

Administration SubQ: Rotate injection sites (thigh, abdomen, upper arm); injections should never be made at sites that are bruised, red, tender, or hard

Monitoring Parameters CBC with differential, lipid profile, C-reactive protein (CRP), serum amyloid A; signs of infection

Dosage Forms Excipient information presented when available (limited, particularly for generics); consult specific product labeling.

Injection, powder for reconstitution:

Arcalyst™: 220 mg

◆ **Rilutek®** *see* Riluzole *on page* 1319

Riluzole (RIL yoo zole)

U.S. Brand Names Rilutek®

Canadian Brand Names Rilutek®

Index Terms 2-Amino-6-Trifluoromethoxy-benzothiazole; RP-54274

Pharmacologic Category Glutamate Inhibitor

Use Treatment of amyotrophic lateral sclerosis (ALS); riluzole can extend survival or time to tracheostomy

Pregnancy Risk Factor C

Pregnancy Considerations Impaired fertility, decreased implantation, increased intrauterine death, and adverse effects on offspring growth and viability were observed in animal studies. There are no adequate or well-controlled studies in pregnant women.

Lactation Excretion in breast milk unknown/not recommended

Contraindications Severe hypersensitivity reactions to riluzole or any component of the formulation

Warnings/Precautions Among 4000 patients given riluzole for ALS, there were 3 cases of marked neutropenia (ANC <500/mm^3), all seen within the first 2 months of treatment. Use with caution in patients with concomitant renal insufficiency. Use with caution in patients with current evidence or history of abnormal liver function; do not administer if baseline liver function tests are elevated. May cause elevations in transaminases (usually transient); discontinue if jaundice develops. The elderly, female, or Japanese patients may have decreased clearance of riluzole; use with caution. May cause dizziness or somnolence; caution should be used performing tasks which require alertness (operating machinery or driving). Safety and efficacy have not been established in children.

Adverse Reactions

>10%:

Gastrointestinal: Nausea (12% to 21%)

Neuromuscular & skeletal: Weakness (15% to 20%)

Respiratory: Lung function decreased (10% to 16%)

1% to 10%:

Cardiovascular: Edema, hypertension, tachycardia

Central nervous system: Agitation, circumoral paresthesia, depression, dizziness, headache, insomnia, malaise, somnolence, tremor, vertigo

Dermatologic: Alopecia, eczema, pruritus

Gastrointestinal: Abdominal pain, anorexia, diarrhea, dyspepsia, flatulence, oral moniliasis, stomatitis, vomiting

Hepatic: Liver function tests increased

Neuromuscular & skeletal: Arthralgia, back pain
Respiratory: Cough increased, rhinitis, sinusitis
Miscellaneous: Aggravation reaction

<1% (Limited to important or life-threatening): Exfoliative dermatitis, neutropenia, postural hypertension, seizure

Drug Interactions

Metabolism/Transport Effects **Substrate** of CYP1A2 (major)

Avoid Concomitant Use There are no known interactions where it is recommended to avoid concomitant use.

Increased Effect/Toxicity There are no known significant interactions involving an increase in effect.

Decreased Effect

The levels/effects of Riluzole may be decreased by: CYP1A2 Inducers (Strong)

Ethanol/Nutrition/Herb Interactions

Ethanol: Avoid ethanol (due to CNS depression and possible risk of liver toxicity).

Food: A high-fat meal decreases absorption of riluzole (decreasing AUC by 20% and peak blood levels by 45%). Charbroiled food may increase riluzole elimination.

Stability Store at 20°C to 25°C (68°F to 77°F). Protect from bright light.

Mechanism of Action Mechanism of action is not known. Pharmacologic properties include inhibitory effect on glutamate release, inactivation of voltage-dependent sodium channels; and ability to interfere with intracellular events that follow transmitter binding at excitatory amino acid receptors

Pharmacodynamics/Kinetics

Absorption: 90%; high-fat meal decreases AUC by 20% and peak blood levels by 45%

Protein binding, plasma: 96%, primarily to albumin and lipoproteins

Metabolism: Extensively hepatic to six major and a number of minor metabolites via CYP1A2 dependent hydroxylation and glucuronidation

Bioavailability: Oral: Absolute: 60%

Half-life elimination: 12 hours

Excretion: Urine (90%; 85% as metabolites, 2% as unchanged drug) and feces (5%) within 7 days

Dosage Adults: Oral: 50 mg every 12 hours; no increased benefit can be expected from higher daily doses, but adverse events are increased

Dosage adjustment in smoking: Cigarette smoking is known to induce CYP1A2; patients who smoke cigarettes would be expected to eliminate riluzole faster. There is no information, however, on the effect of, or need for, dosage adjustment in these patients.

Dosage adjustment in special populations: Females and Japanese patients may possess a lower metabolic capacity to eliminate riluzole compared with male and Caucasian subjects, respectively

Dosage adjustment in renal impairment: Use with caution in patients with concomitant renal insufficiency

Dosage adjustment in hepatic impairment: Use with caution in patients with current evidence or history of abnormal liver function indicated by significant abnormalities in serum transaminase, bilirubin or GGT levels. Baseline elevations of several LFTs (especially elevated bilirubin) should preclude use of riluzole.

Dietary Considerations Take at least 1 hour before, or 2 hours after, a meal.

Administration Administer at the same time each day, 1 hour before or 2 hours after a meal.

Monitoring Parameters Monitor serum aminotransferases including ALT levels before and during therapy. Evaluate serum ALT levels every month during the first 3 months of therapy, every 3 months during the remainder of the first year and periodically thereafter. Evaluate ALT levels more frequently in patients who develop elevations. Maximum increases in serum ALT usually occurred within 3 months after the start of therapy and were usually transient when <5 times ULN (upper limits of normal).

In trials, if ALT levels were <5 times ULN, treatment continued and ALT levels usually returned to below 2 times ULN within 2-6 months. There is no experience with continued treatment of ALS patients once ALT values exceed 5 times ULN.

If a decision is made to continue treatment in patients when the ALT exceeds 5 times ULN, frequent monitoring (at least weekly) of complete liver function is recommended. Discontinue treatment if ALT exceeds 10 times ULN or if clinical jaundice develops. Monitor temperature, especially during first 2 months of therapy.

Dosage Forms Excipient information presented when available (limited, particularly for generics); consult specific product labeling.

Tablet: 50 mg

Rimantadine (ri MAN ta deen)

U.S. Brand Names Flumadine®

Canadian Brand Names Flumadine®

Index Terms Rimantadine Hydrochloride

Pharmacologic Category Antiviral Agent, Adamantane

Additional Appendix Information

Community-Acquired Pneumonia in Adults *on page 1766*

Guidelines for the Prevention of Opportunistic Infections in HIV Infected Persons *on page 1740*

Use Prophylaxis (adults and children >1 year of age) and treatment (adults) of influenza A viral infection (per manufacturer labeling; also refer to current ACIP guidelines for recommendations during current flu season)

Note: In certain circumstances, the ACIP recommends use of rimantadine in combination with oseltamivir for the treatment or prophylaxis of influenza A infection when resistance to oseltamivir is suspected.

Pregnancy Risk Factor C

Pregnancy Considerations Animal data suggest embryotoxicity, maternal toxicity, and offspring mortality at doses 7-11 times the recommended human dose. There are no adequate and well-controlled studies in pregnant women.

Lactation Excretion in breast milk unknown/ not recommended

Medication Safety Issues

Sound-alike/look-alike issues:

Rimantadine may be confused with amantadine, ranitidine, Rimactane®

Flumadine® may be confused with fludarabine, flunisolide, flutamide

Contraindications Hypersensitivity to drugs of the adamantine class, including rimantadine and amantadine, or any component of the formulation

Warnings/Precautions Use with caution in patients with renal and hepatic dysfunction; avoid use, if possible, in patients with recurrent and eczematoid dermatitis, uncontrolled psychosis, or severe psychoneurosis. An increase in seizure incidence may occur in patients with seizure disorders; discontinue drug if seizures occur; resistance may develop during treatment; viruses exhibit cross-resistance between amantadine and rimantadine. Due to increased resistance, the ACIP has recommended that rimantadine and amantadine no longer be used for the treatment or prophylaxis of influenza A in the United States until susceptibility has been re-established; consult current guidelines.

Adverse Reactions

1% to 10%:

Central nervous system: Dizziness (1% to 2%), insomnia (2% to 3%), concentration impaired (2%), anxiety (1%), fatigue (1%), headache (1%), nervousness (1% to 2%)

Gastrointestinal: Nausea (3%), anorexia (2%), vomiting (2%), xerostomia (2%), abdominal pain (1%)
Neuromuscular & skeletal: Weakness (1%)
<1% (Limited to important or life-threatening): Agitation, ataxia, bronchospasm, cardiac failure, confusion, convulsions, cough, depression, diarrhea, dyspepsia, dyspnea, euphoria, gait abnormality, hallucinations, heart block, hyperkinesias, hypertension, lactation, palpitation, pallor, parosmia, pedal edema, rash, somnolence, syncope, tachycardia, taste alteration, tinnitus, tremor

Drug Interactions

Avoid Concomitant Use There are no known interactions where it is recommended to avoid concomitant use.

Increased Effect/Toxicity There are no known significant interactions involving an increase in effect.

Decreased Effect

Rimantadine may decrease the levels/effects of: Influenza Virus Vaccine

Ethanol/Nutrition/Herb Interactions Food: Food does not affect rate or extent of absorption

Stability Store at 15°C to 30°C (59°F to 86°F).

Mechanism of Action Exerts its inhibitory effect on three antigenic subtypes of influenza A virus (H1N1, H2N2, H3N2) early in the viral replicative cycle, possibly inhibiting the uncoating process; it has no activity against influenza B virus and is two- to eightfold more active than amantadine

Pharmacodynamics/Kinetics

Onset of action: Antiviral activity: No data exist establishing a correlation between plasma concentration and antiviral effect
Absorption: Tablet and syrup formulations are equally absorbed
Metabolism: Extensively hepatic
Half-life elimination: 25.4 hours; prolonged in elderly
Time to peak: 6 hours
Excretion: Urine (<25% as unchanged drug)
Clearance: Hemodialysis does not contribute to clearance

Dosage Oral:

Prophylaxis:
Children 1-10 years: 5 mg/kg/day; maximum: 150 mg/day
Children >10 years and Adults: 100 mg twice daily
Elderly: 100 mg/day in nursing home patients or all elderly patients who may experience adverse effects using the adult dose

Treatment:
Adults: 100 mg twice daily
Elderly: 100 mg once daily in patients ≥65 years

Dosage adjustment in renal impairment:
Cl_{cr} >10 mL/minute: Dose adjustment not required
Cl_{cr} ≤10 mL/minute: 100 mg/day

Dosage adjustment in hepatic impairment: Severe dysfunction: 100 mg/day

Administration Initiation of rimantadine within 48 hours of the onset of influenza A illness halves the duration of illness and significantly reduces the duration of viral shedding and increased peripheral airways resistance; continue therapy for 5-7 days after symptoms begin

Monitoring Parameters Monitor for CNS or GI effects in elderly or patients with renal or hepatic impairment

Dosage Forms Excipient information presented when available (limited, particularly for generics); consult specific product labeling. [DSC] = Discontinued product

Syrup, as hydrochloride:
Flumadine®: 50 mg/5 mL (240 mL) [raspberry flavor] [DSC]
Tablet, as hydrochloride: 100 mg
Flumadine®: 100 mg

◆ **Rimantadine Hydrochloride** *see* Rimantadine *on page 1320*

Rimexolone (ri MEKS oh lone)

U.S. Brand Names Vexol®

Canadian Brand Names Vexol®

Pharmacologic Category Corticosteroid, Ophthalmic

Use Treatment of inflammation after ocular surgery and the treatment of anterior uveitis

Pregnancy Risk Factor C

Medication Safety Issues

Sound-alike/look-alike issues:
Vexol® may be confused with VoSol®

Dosage Adults: Ophthalmic: Instill 1 drop in conjunctival sac 2-4 times/day up to every 4 hours; may use every 1-2 hours during first 1-2 days

Additional Information Complete prescribing information for this medication should be consulted for additional detail.

Dosage Forms Excipient information presented when available (limited, particularly for generics); consult specific product labeling.

Suspension, ophthalmic: 1% (5 mL, 10 mL) [contains benzalkonium chloride]

◆ **Rinate™ Pediatric** *see* Chlorpheniramine and Phenylephrine *on page 309*

◆ **Riomet®** *see* MetFORMIN *on page 954*

◆ **Riopan Plus® [OTC] [DSC]** *see* Magaldrate and Simethicone *on page 914*

◆ **Riopan Plus® Double Strength [OTC] [DSC]** *see* Magaldrate and Simethicone *on page 914*

◆ **Riphenidate (Can)** *see* Methylphenidate *on page 973*

Risedronate (ris ED roe nate)

U.S. Brand Names Actonel®

Canadian Brand Names Actonel®

Index Terms Risedronate Sodium

Pharmacologic Category Bisphosphonate Derivative

Use Treatment of Paget's disease of the bone; treatment and prevention of glucocorticoid-induced osteoporosis; treatment and prevention of osteoporosis in postmenopausal women; treatment of osteoporosis in men

Pregnancy Risk Factor C

Pregnancy Considerations Teratogenic and nonteratogenic embryo/fetal effects have been reported in animal studies. There are no adequate and well-controlled studies in pregnant women. Bisphosphonates are incorporated into the bone matrix and gradually released over time. Theoretically, there may be a risk of fetal harm when pregnancy follows the completion of therapy. Based on limited case reports with pamidronate, serum calcium levels in the newborn may be altered if administered during pregnancy.

Lactation Excretion in breast milk unknown/not recommended

Medication Safety Issues

Sound-alike/look-alike issues:
Actonel® may be confused with Actos®

Contraindications Hypersensitivity to risedronate, bisphosphonates, or any component of the formulation; hypocalcemia; inability to stand or sit upright for at least 30 minutes

Warnings/Precautions Bisphosphonates may cause upper gastrointestinal disorders such as dysphagia, esophagitis, esophageal ulcer, and gastric ulcer; risk increases in patients unable to comply with dosing instructions. Use with caution in patients with dysphagia, esophageal disease, gastritis, duodenitis, or ulcers (may worsen underlying condition). Discontinue if new or worsening symptoms occur. Use caution in patients with renal impairment (not recommended in patients with a Cl_{cr} <30 mL/minute). Hypocalcemia must be corrected before therapy initiation with risedronate. Ensure adequate calcium and vitamin D intake, especially for patients with Paget's disease in whom the pretreatment rate of bone turnover may be greatly elevated.

Bisphosphonate therapy has been associated with osteonecrosis, primarily of the jaw; this has been observed mostly in cancer patients, but also in patients with postmenopausal osteoporosis and other diagnoses. Dental exams and preventative dentistry should be performed prior to placing patients with risk factors on chronic bisphosphonate therapy. Invasive dental procedures should be avoided during treatment.

Infrequently, severe (and occasionally debilitating) bone, joint, and/or muscle pain have been reported during bisphosphonate treatment. The onset of pain ranged from a single day to several months. Symptoms usually resolve upon discontinuation. Some patients experienced recurrence when rechallenged with same drug or another bisphosphonate; avoid use in patients with a history of these symptoms in association with bisphosphonate therapy.

When using for glucocorticoid-induced osteoporosis, evaluate sex steroid hormonal status prior to treatment initiation; consider appropriate hormone replacement if necessary. Safety and efficacy in pediatric patients have not been established.

Adverse Reactions Frequency may vary with dose and indication.

>10%:

- Cardiovascular: Hypertension (11%)
- Central nervous system: Headache (10% to 18%)
- Dermatologic: Rash (8% to 12%)
- Endocrine & metabolic: Serum PTH levels decreased (<30%)
- Gastrointestinal: Diarrhea (5% to 20%), constipation (7% to 13%), nausea (7% to 13%), abdominal pain (7% to 12%), dyspepsia (7% to 11%)
- Genitourinary: Urinary tract infection (11%)
- Neuromuscular & skeletal: Arthralgia (12% to 33%), back pain (18% to 28%)
- Miscellaneous: Infection (≤31%)

1% to 10%:

- Cardiovascular: Peripheral edema (8%), chest pain (5% to 7%), arrhythmia (2%)
- Central nervous system: Depression (7%), dizziness (7%), insomnia (5%)
- Endocrine & metabolic: Hypocalcemia (≤5%), hypophosphatemia (<3%)
- Gastrointestinal: Gastritis (3%), duodenitis (≤1%), glossitis (≤1%)
- Genitourinary: Prostatic hyperplasia (5%; benign), nephrolithiasis (3%)
- Neuromuscular & skeletal: Joint disorder (7%), myalgia (5% to 7%), neck pain (5%), weakness (5%), neuralgia (4%)
- Ocular: Cataract (7%), dry eyes (3%)
- Respiratory: Bronchitis (3% to 10%), pharyngitis (6%), rhinitis (6%), dyspnea (4%)
- Miscellaneous: Flu-like syndrome (10%), acute phase reaction (≤8%; includes fever, influenza-like illness)

<1% (Limited to important or life-threatening): Allergic reaction, angioedema, arthritis, bullous skin reaction, cough, dysphagia, esophagitis, esophageal ulcer, gastric ulcer, hypersensitivity reaction, iritis, joint pain, liver function test abnormality, musculoskeletal pain (rarely severe or incapacitating), osteonecrosis (primarily of the jaw), sinusitis, uveitis

Drug Interactions

Avoid Concomitant Use There are no known interactions where it is recommended to avoid concomitant use.

Increased Effect/Toxicity

Risedronate may increase the levels/effects of: Phosphate Supplements

The levels/effects of Risedronate may be increased by: Aminoglycosides; Nonsteroidal Anti-Inflammatory Agents

Decreased Effect

The levels/effects of Risedronate may be decreased by: Antacids; Calcium Salts; Iron Salts; Magnesium Salts

Ethanol/Nutrition/Herb Interactions

Ethanol: Avoid ethanol (may increase risk of osteoporosis).

Food: Food reduces absorption (similar to other bisphosphonates); mean oral bioavailability is decreased when given with food.

Stability Store at room temperature of 20°C to 25°C (68°F to 77°F).

Mechanism of Action A bisphosphonate which inhibits bone resorption via actions on osteoclasts or on osteoclast precursors; decreases the rate of bone resorption, leading to an indirect increase in bone mineral density. In Paget's disease, characterized by disordered resorption and formation of bone, inhibition of resorption leads to an indirect decrease in bone formation; but the newly-formed bone has a more normal architecture.

Pharmacodynamics/Kinetics

Onset of action: May require weeks
Absorption: Rapid
Distribution: V_d: 13.8 L/kg
Protein binding: ~24%
Metabolism: None
Bioavailability: Poor, ~0.54% to 0.75%
Half-life elimination: Initial: 1.5 hours; Terminal: 480-561 hours
Time to peak, serum: 1 hour
Excretion: Urine (up to 85%); feces (as unabsorbed drug)

Dosage Oral: Adults:

Paget's disease of bone: 30 mg once daily for 2 months

Retreatment may be considered (following post-treatment observation of at least 2 months) if relapse occurs, or if treatment fails to normalize serum alkaline phosphatase. For retreatment, the dose and duration of therapy are the same as for initial treatment. No data are available on more than one course of retreatment.

Osteoporosis (postmenopausal) prevention and treatment: 5 mg once daily **or** 35 mg once weekly **or** one 75 mg tablet taken on 2 consecutive days once a month (total of 2 tablets/month) **or** 150 mg once a month

Osteoporosis (male) treatment: 35 mg once weekly

Osteoporosis (glucocorticoid-induced) prevention and treatment: 5 mg once daily

Dosage adjustment in renal impairment:

Cl_{cr} ≥30 mL/minute: No adjustment required
Cl_{cr} <30 mL/minute: **Not** recommended for use

Dietary Considerations Take ≥30 minutes before the first food or drink of the day other than water. Supplemental calcium and/or vitamin D may be required if dietary intake is not adequate.

Administration It is imperative to administer risedronate at least 30 minutes before the patient takes any food, drink, or other medications orally to avoid interference with absorption. The patient should take risedronate on an empty stomach with a full glass (8 oz) of **plain water** (not mineral water) and avoid lying down for 30 minutes after swallowing tablet to help delivery to stomach. Tablet should be swallowed whole; do not crush or chew.

Monitoring Parameters Alkaline phosphatase should be periodically measured; serum calcium, phosphorus; monitor pain and fracture rate; bone mineral density

Evaluate sex steroid hormonal status prior to treatment initiation (when treating glucocorticoid-induced osteoporosis).

Reference Range Calcium (total): Adults: 9.0-11.0 mg/dL (2.05-2.54 mmol/L), may slightly decrease with aging; phosphorus: 2.5-4.5 mg/dL (0.81-1.45 mmol/L)

Test Interactions Bisphosphonates may interfere with diagnostic imaging agents such as technetium-99m-diphosphonate in bone scans.

Dosage Forms Excipient information presented when available (limited, particularly for generics); consult specific product labeling.

Tablet, as sodium:

Actonel®: 5 mg, 30 mg, 35 mg, 75 mg, 150 mg

Risedronate and Calcium

(ris ED roe nate & KAL see um)

U.S. Brand Names Actonel® and Calcium

Index Terms Calcium and Risedronate; Risedronate Sodium and Calcium Carbonate

Pharmacologic Category Bisphosphonate Derivative; Calcium Salt

Use Treatment and prevention of osteoporosis in postmenopausal women

Pregnancy Risk Factor C

Medication Safety Issues

Sound-alike/look-alike issues:

Actonel® may be confused with Actos®

Dosage

Oral: Adults: Osteoporosis in postmenopausal females:

Risedronate: 35 mg once weekly on day 1 of 7-day treatment cycle

Calcium carbonate: 1250 mg (elemental calcium 500 mg) once daily on days 2 through 7 of 7-day treatment cycle

Dosage adjustment in renal impairment: Cl_{cr} <30 mL/minute: Not recommended for use

Additional Information Complete prescribing information for this medication should be consulted for additional detail.

Dosage Forms Excipient information presented when available (limited, particularly for generics); consult specific product labeling.

Combination package [each package contains]:

Tablet (Actonel®): Risedronate 35 mg (4s)

Tablet: Calcium carbonate 1250 mg (24s) [equivalent to elemental calcium 500 mg]

◆ **Risedronate Sodium** *see* Risedronate *on page* 1321

◆ **Risedronate Sodium and Calcium Carbonate** *see* Risedronate and Calcium *on page* 1323

◆ **Risperdal®** *see* Risperidone *on page* 1323

◆ **Risperdal M-Tab** *see* Risperidone *on page* 1323

◆ **Risperdal® M-Tab®** *see* Risperidone *on page* 1323

◆ **Risperdal® Consta®** *see* Risperidone *on page* 1323

Risperidone (ris PER i done)

U.S. Brand Names Risperdal®; Risperdal® Consta®; Risperdal® M-Tab®

Canadian Brand Names Apo-Risperidone®; CO Risperidone; Dom-Risperidone; Gen-Risperidone; Novo-Risperidone; PHL-Risperidone; PMS-Risperidone ODT; PRO-Risperidone; Ran-Risperidone; Ratio-Risperidone; Risperdal®; Risperdal® Consta®; Risperdal® M-Tab®; Riva-Risperidone; Sandoz Risperidone

Index Terms Risperdal M-Tab

Pharmacologic Category Antimanic Agent; Antipsychotic Agent, Atypical

Use Treatment of schizophrenia; treatment of acute mania or mixed episodes associated with bipolar I disorder (as monotherapy in children or adults, or in combination with lithium or valproate in adults); treatment of irritability/aggression associated with autistic disorder

Unlabeled/Investigational Use Treatment of Tourette's disorder; treatment of pervasive developmental disorder; psychosis/agitation related to Alzheimer's dementia

Pregnancy Risk Factor C

Pregnancy Considerations Animal studies indicate an increase in fetal mortality. Reversible EPS symptoms were noted in neonates following use of risperidone during the last trimester. Agenesis of the corpus callosum has also been noted in one case report. There are no adequate and well-controlled studies in pregnant women. When using Risperdal® Consta®, patients should notify healthcare provider if they become or intend to become pregnant during therapy or within 12 weeks of last injection. Risperidone may cause hyperprolactinemia, which may decrease reproductive function in both males and females. Healthcare providers are encouraged to enroll women 18-45 years of age exposed to risperidone during pregnancy in the Atypical Antipsychotics Pregnancy Registry (1-866-961-2388).

Lactation Enters breast milk/not recommended

Medication Safety Issues

Sound-alike/look-alike issues:

Risperidone may be confused with reserpine

Risperdal® may be confused with lisinopril, reserpine

Contraindications Hypersensitivity to risperidone or any component of the formulation

Warnings/Precautions **[U.S. Boxed Warning]: Elderly patients with dementia-related psychosis treated with antipsychotic drugs are at an increased risk of death compared to placebo.** An increased incidence of cerebrovascular adverse events (including fatalities) has been reported in elderly patients with dementia-related psychosis. Risperidone is not approved for the treatment of dementia-related psychosis.

Low to moderately sedating, use with caution in disorders where CNS depression is a feature. Use with caution in Parkinson's disease. Caution in patients with predisposition to seizures; or severe cardiac disease. Use with caution in renal or hepatic dysfunction; dose reduction recommended. Esophageal dysmotility and aspiration have been associated with antipsychotic use; use with caution in patients at risk of aspiration pneumonia (ie, Alzheimer's disease). Elevates prolactin levels; effects seen in adults and children. Use with caution in breast cancer or other prolactin-dependent tumors. May alter temperature regulation. May mask toxicity of other drugs or conditions (eg intestinal obstruction, Reyes syndrome, brain tumor) due to antiemetic effects.

Use with caution in patients with cardiovascular diseases (eg, heart failure, history of myocardial infarction or ischemia, cerebrovascular disease, conduction abnormalities). May cause orthostatic hypotension; use with caution in patients at risk of this effect (eg, concurrent medication use which may predispose to hypotension/bradycardia or presence of hypovolemia) or in those who would not tolerate transient hypotensive episodes. May alter cardiac conduction (low risk relative to other neuroleptics); life-threatening arrhythmias have occurred with therapeutic doses of neuroleptics.

May cause anticholinergic effects (confusion, agitation, constipation, xerostomia, blurred vision, urinary retention); therefore, they should be used with caution in patients with decreased gastrointestinal motility, urinary retention, BPH, xerostomia, or visual problems. Conditions which also may be exacerbated by cholinergic blockade include narrow-angle glaucoma (screening is recommended) and worsening of myasthenia gravis. Relative to other neuroleptics, risperidone has a low potency of cholinergic blockade.

May cause extrapyramidal symptoms (EPS), including pseudoparkinsonism, acute dystonic reactions, akathisia, and tardive dyskinesia (risk of these reactions is low relative to other neuroleptics, and is dose dependent). Risk of dystonia (and probably other EPS) may be greater with increased doses, use of conventional antipsychotics, males, and younger patients. Risk of neuroleptic malignant syndrome (NMS) may be increased in patients with Parkinson's disease or Lewy body dementia; monitor for symptoms of confusion, obtundation, postural instability and extrapyramidal symptoms. May cause hyperglycemia; in some cases may be extreme and associated with ketoacidosis, hyperosmolar coma, or death. Use with caution in patients with diabetes or other disorders of glucose regulation; monitor for worsening of glucose control. Significant weight gain has been observed with antipsychotic therapy; incidence varies with product. Monitor waist circumference and BMI. Rare cases of priapism have been reported.

The possibility of a suicide attempt is inherent in psychotic illness or bipolar disorder; use caution in high-risk patients during initiation of therapy. Prescriptions should be written for the smallest quantity consistent with good patient care. Safety and efficacy have not been established in children <5 years of age (<18 years of age for I.M. injection). Long-term effects on growth or sexual maturation have not been evaluated. Vehicle used in injectable (polylactide-co-glycolide microspheres) has rarely been associated with retinal artery occlusion in patients with abnormal arteriovenous anastomosis.

Adverse Reactions The frequency of adverse effects is reported as absolute percentages and is not based upon net frequencies as compared to placebo. Actual frequency may be dependant upon dose and/or indication. Events are reported from placebo-controlled studies and not with combination therapy. Unless otherwise noted, frequency of adverse effects is reported for the oral formulation in adults.

>10%:

Central nervous system: Somnolence (children 12% to 67%; adults 5% to 14%; I.M. injection 5% to 6%), fatigue (children 18% to 42%; adults 1% to 3%), headache (I.M. injection 15% to 21%), fever (children 20%; adults 1% to 2%), dystonia (children 9% to 18%; adults 5% to 11%), anxiety (children ≤16%; adults 2% to 16%), dizziness (children 7% to 16%; adults 4% to 10%), Parkinsonism (children 2% to 16%; adults 12% to 20%)

Dermatologic: Rash (children ≤11%; adults 2% to 4%)

Gastrointestinal: Appetite increased (children 4% to 49%), vomiting (children 10% to 25%), salivation increased (children ≤22%; adults 1% to 3%), constipation (children 21%; adults 8% to 9%), abdominal pain (children 15% to 18%; adults 3% to 4%), nausea (children 8% to 16%; adults 4% to 9%), dyspepsia (children 5% to 16%; adults 4% to 10%), xerostomia (children 13%; adults ≤4%)

Genitourinary: Urinary incontinence (children 5% to 22%; adults <2%)

Neuromuscular & skeletal: Tremor (adults 6%; children 10% to 12%)

Respiratory: Rhinitis (children 13% to 36%; adults 7% to 11%), upper respiratory infection (children 34%; adults 2% to 3%), cough (children 34%; adults 3%)

1% to 10%:

Cardiovascular: Tachycardia (children ≤7%; adults 1% to 5%), chest pain (1% to 3%), creatine phosphokinase increased (≤2%), postural hypotension (≤2%), arrhythmia (≤1%), edema (≤1%), hypotension (≤1%), syncope (≤1%)

Central nervous system: Akathisia (children ≤10%; adults 5% to 9%), automatism (children 7%), confusion (children 5%)

Dermatologic: Seborrhea (up to 2%), acne (1%)

Endocrine & metabolic: Lactation nonpuerperal (children 2% to 5%; adults 1%), ejaculation failure (≤1%)

Gastrointestinal: Diarrhea (children 7% to 8%; adults ≤3%), anorexia (children 8%; adults ≤2%;), weight gain (children 5%; adults ≤1%), toothache (I.M. injection 1% to 3%)

Genitourinary: Urinary tract infection (≤3%)

Hematologic: Anemia (I.M. injection <2%; oral ≤1%)

Hepatic: Transaminases increased (I.M. injection ≥1%; oral 1%)

Neuromuscular & skeletal: Dyskinesia (children 7%; adults 1%), arthralgia (2% to 3%), back pain (2% to 3%), myalgia (≤2%), weakness (1%)

Ocular: Abnormal vision (children 4% to 7%; adults 1% to 3%), blurred vision (I.M. injection 2% to 3%)

Otic: Earache (1%)

Respiratory: Dyspnea (children 2% to 5%; adults 2%), epistaxis (≤2%)

≤1% (Limited to important or life-threatening): Agranulocytosis, allergic reaction, amenorrhea, amnesia, anaphylactic reaction, anemias (oral formulations), angina pectoris, angioedema, antidiuretic hormone disorder, aphasia, apnea, ascites, aspiration, asthma, atrial fibrillation, AV block, bronchospasm, cachexia, catatonic reaction, cerebrovascular accident, cerebrovascular disorder, cholecystitis, cholelithiasis, cholestatic hepatitis, cholinergic syndrome, coma, dehydration, delirium, depression, diabetes mellitus, diabetic ketoacidosis, diverticulitis, dysphagia, esophagitis, esophageal dysmotility, fecal incontinence, flu-like syndrome, gastroenteritis, hematemesis, hematuria, hemorrhage, hepatic failure, hepatocellular damage, hyper-/hypoglycemia, hyperphosphatemia, hypertriglyceridemia, hyperuricemia, hypokalemia, hyponatremia, hypoproteinemia, intestinal obstruction, jaundice, leukocytosis, leukopenia, leukorrhea, lymphadenopathy, mastitis, menstrual irregularities, migraine, myocardial infarction, myocarditis, palpitation, pancreatitis, Pelger-Huët anomaly, pituitary adenomas, pneumonia, precocious puberty, premature atrial contractions, priapism, pulmonary embolism, purpura, QT_c prolongation, RBC disorders, renal insufficiency, retinal artery occlusion (I.M. formulation), rigors, sarcoidosis, skin exfoliation, skin ulceration, ST depression, stomatitis, stridor, stroke, superficial phlebitis, synostosis, T wave inversions, thrombocytopenia, thrombophlebitis, thrombotic thrombocytopenic purpura, tinnitus, tongue discoloration, tongue edema, tongue paralysis, torticollis, transient ischemic attack, urinary retention, urticaria, ventricular extrasystoles, ventricular tachycardia, water intoxication, withdrawal syndrome, xerophthalmia

Drug Interactions

Metabolism/Transport Effects **Substrate** of CYP2D6 (major), 3A4 (minor); **Inhibits** CYP2D6 (weak), 3A4 (weak)

Avoid Concomitant Use

Avoid concomitant use of Risperidone with any of the following: Nilotinib; Thioridazine; Ziprasidone

Increased Effect/Toxicity

Risperidone may increase the levels/effects of: Alcohol (Ethyl); Anticholinergics; CNS Depressants; QTc-Prolonging Agents; Thioridazine; Ziprasidone

The levels/effects of Risperidone may be increased by: Acetylcholinesterase Inhibitors (Central); Alfuzosin; Ciprofloxacin; CYP2D6 Inhibitors (Moderate); CYP2D6 Inhibitors (Strong); Darunavir; Gadobutrol; Lithium formulations; Nilotinib; Pramlintide; Selective Serotonin Reuptake Inhibitors; Tetrabenazine; Valproic Acid; Verapamil

Decreased Effect

Risperidone may decrease the levels/effects of: Amphetamines; Anti-Parkinson's Agents (Dopamine Agonist)

The levels/effects of Risperidone may be decreased by: CarBAMazepine; Lithium formulations

Ethanol/Nutrition/Herb Interactions

Ethanol: Avoid ethanol (may increase CNS depression).

Herb/Nutraceutical: Avoid kava kava, gotu kola, valerian, St John's wort (may increase CNS depression).

Stability

Injection: Risperdal® Consta®: Store in refrigerator at 2°C to 8°C (36°F to 46°F) and protect from light. May be stored at room temperature of 25°C (77°F) for up to 7 days prior to administration. Bring to room temperature prior to reconstitution. Reconstitute with provided diluent only. Shake vigorously to mix; will form thick, milky suspension. Following reconstitution, store at room temperature and use within 6 hours. Suspension settles in ~2 minutes; shake vigorously to resuspend prior to administration.

Oral solution, tablet: Store at 15°C to 25°C (59°F to 77°F). Protect from light and moisture. Keep orally-disintegrating tablets sealed in foil pouch until ready to use. Do not freeze solution.

Mechanism of Action Risperidone is a benzisoxazole atypical antipsychotic with mixed serotonin-dopamine antagonist activity that binds to 5-HT_2-receptors in the CNS and in the periphery with a very high affinity; binds to dopamine-D_2 receptors with less affinity. The binding affinity to the dopamine-D_2 receptor is 20 times lower than the 5-HT_2 affinity. The addition of serotonin antagonism to dopamine antagonism (classic neuroleptic mechanism) is thought to improve negative symptoms of psychoses and reduce the incidence of extrapyramidal side effects. $Alpha_1$, $alpha_2$ adrenergic, and histaminergic receptors are also antagonized with high affinity. Risperidone has low to moderate affinity for 5-HT_{1C}, 5-HT_{1D}, and 5-HT_{1A} receptors, weak affinity for D_1 and no affinity for muscarinics or $beta_1$ and $beta_2$ receptors

Pharmacodynamics/Kinetics

Absorption:

- Oral: Rapid and well absorbed; food does not affect rate or extent
- Injection: <1% absorbed initially; main release occurs at ~3 weeks and is maintained from 4-6 weeks

Distribution: V_d: 1-2 L/kg

Protein binding, plasma: Risperidone 90%; 9-hydroxyrisperidone: 77%

Metabolism: Extensively hepatic via CYP2D6 to 9-hydroxyrisperidone (similar pharmacological activity as risperidone); *N*-dealkylation is a second minor pathway

Bioavailability: Oral: 70%; Tablet (relative to solution): 94%; orally-disintegrating tablets and oral solution are bioequivalent to tablets

Half-life elimination: Active moiety (risperidone and its active metabolite 9-hydroxyrisperidone)

- Oral: 20 hours (mean)
  - Extensive metabolizers: Risperidone: 3 hours; 9-hydroxyrisperidone: 21 hours
  - Poor metabolizers: Risperidone: 20 hours; 9-hydroxyrisperidone: 30 hours
- Injection: 3-6 days; related to microsphere erosion and subsequent absorption of risperidone

Time to peak, plasma: Oral: Risperidone: Within 1 hour; 9-hydroxyrisperidone: Extensive metabolizers: 3 hours; Poor metabolizers: 17 hours

Excretion: Urine (70%); feces (14%)

Dosage

Oral:

Children ≥5 years and Adolescents: Autism:

- <15 kg: Use with caution; specific dosing recommendations not available
- <20 kg: Initial: 0.25 mg/day; may increase dose to 0.5 mg/day after ≥4 days, maintain dose for ≥14 days. In patients not achieving sufficient clinical response, may increase dose by 0.25 mg/day in ≥2-week intervals. Therapeutic effect reached plateau at 1 mg/day in clinical trials. Following clinical response, consider gradually lowering dose. May be administered once daily or in divided doses twice daily.
- ≥20 kg: Initial: 0.5 mg/day; may increase dose to 1 mg/day after ≥4 days, maintain dose for ≥14 days. In patients not achieving sufficient clinical response, may increase dose by 0.5 mg/day in ≥2-week intervals. Therapeutic effect reached plateau at 2.5 mg/day (3 mg/day in children >45 kg) in clinical trials. Following clinical response, consider gradually lowering dose. May be administered once daily or in divided doses twice daily.

Children and Adolescents:

- Pervasive developmental disorder (unlabeled use): Initial: 0.25 mg twice daily; titrate up 0.25 mg/day every 5-7 days; optimal dose range: 0.75-3 mg/day
- Schizophrenia: Adolescents 13-17 years: Initial: 0.5 mg once daily; dose may be adjusted in increments of 0.5-1 mg/day at intervals ≥24 hours to a dose of 3 mg/day. Doses ranging from 1-6 mg/day have been evaluated, however, doses >3 mg/day do not confer additional benefit and are associated with increased adverse events.
- Bipolar disorder: Children and Adolescents 10-17 years: Initial: 0.5 mg once daily; dose may be adjusted in increments of 0.5-1 mg/day at intervals ≥24 hours to a dose of 2.5 mg/day. Doses ranging from 0.5-6 mg/day have been evaluated, however doses >2.5 mg/day do not confer additional benefit and are associated with increased adverse events.
- Tourette's disorder (unlabeled use): Initial: 0.5 mg; titrate to 2-4 mg/day

Adults:

Schizophrenia:

- Initial: 1 mg twice daily; may be increased by 1-2 mg/day at intervals ≥24 hours to a recommended dosage range of 4-8 mg/day; may be given as a single daily dose once maintenance dose is achieved; daily dosages >6 mg do not appear to confer any additional benefit, and the incidence of extrapyramidal symptoms is higher than with lower doses. Further dose adjustments should be made in increments/decrements of 1-2 mg/day on a weekly basis. Dose range studied in clinical trials: 4-16 mg/day.
- Maintenance: Recommended dosage range: 2-8 mg/day

Bipolar mania:

- Initial: 2-3 mg once daily; if needed, adjust dose by 1 mg/day in intervals ≥24 hours; dosing range: 1-6 mg/day
- Maintenance: No dosing recommendation available for treatment >3 weeks duration.

Elderly:

- Oral: A starting dose of 0.5 mg twice daily, and titration should progress slowly in increments of no more than 0.5 mg twice daily; increases to dosages >1.5 mg twice daily should occur at intervals of ≥1 week.
  - Psychosis/agitation related to Alzheimer's dementia (unlabeled use): Initial: 0.25-1 mg/day; if necessary, gradually increase as tolerated not to exceed 1.5-2 mg/day
- I.M. (Risperdal® Consta®): A lower initial dose of 12.5 mg may be appropriate.
- **Note:** Additional monitoring of renal function and orthostatic blood pressure may be warranted. If once-a-day dosing in the elderly or debilitated patient is considered, a twice daily regimen should be used to titrate to the target dose, and this dose should be maintained for 2-3 days prior to attempts to switch to a once-daily regimen.

I.M.: Adults: Schizophrenia (Risperdal® Consta®): 25 mg every 2 weeks; some patients may benefit from larger doses; maximum dose not to exceed 50 mg every 2 weeks. Dosage adjustments should not be made more frequently than every 4 weeks. A lower initial dose of 12.5 mg may be appropriate in some patients.

Note: Oral risperidone (or other antipsychotic) should be administered with the initial injection of Risperdal® Consta® and continued for 3 weeks (then discontinued) to maintain adequate therapeutic plasma concentrations prior to main release phase of risperidone from injection site. When switching from depot administration to a short-acting formulation, administer short-acting agent in place of the next regularly-scheduled depot injection.

Dosing adjustment in renal impairment:

Oral: Starting dose of 0.5 mg twice daily; titration should progress slowly in increments of no more than 0.5 mg twice daily; increases to dosages >1.5 mg twice daily should occur at intervals of ≥1 week. Clearance of the active moiety is decreased by 60% in patients with moderate-to-severe renal disease compared to healthy subjects.

I.M.: An initial dose of 12.5 mg may be considered

Dosing adjustment in hepatic impairment:

Oral: Starting dose of 0.5 mg twice daily; titration should progress slowly in increments of no more than 0.5 mg twice daily; increases to dosages >1.5 mg twice daily should occur at intervals of ≥1 week. The mean free fraction of risperidone in plasma was increased by 35% in patients with hepatic impairment compared to healthy subjects.

I.M.: An initial dose of 12.5 mg may be considered

Dietary Considerations May be taken with or without food. Risperdal® M-Tabs® contain phenylalanine.

Administration

Oral:

Oral solution can be mixed with water, coffee, orange juice, or low-fat milk, but is **not compatible** with cola or tea. May be administered with or without food.

In children or adolescents experiencing somnolence, half the daily dose may be administered twice daily **or** the once-daily dose may be administered at bedtime.

When reinitiating treatment after discontinuation, the initial titration schedule should be followed.

Risperdal® M-Tabs® should not be removed from blister pack until administered. Using dry hands, place immediately on tongue. Tablet will dissolve within seconds, and may be swallowed with or without liquid. Do not split or chew.

I.M.: Risperdal® Consta® should be administered into either the deltoid muscle or the upper outer quadrant of the gluteal area. Avoid inadvertent injection into vasculature. Injection should alternate between the two arms or buttocks. Do not combine two different dosage strengths into one single administration. Do not substitute any components of the dose-pack; administer with needle provided (1-inch needle for deltoid administration or 2-inch needle for gluteal administration).

Monitoring Parameters Vital signs; fasting lipid profile and fasting blood glucose/Hgb A_{1c} (prior to treatment, at 3 months, then annually); BMI, personal/family history of obesity, waist circumference; blood pressure; mental status, abnormal involuntary movement scale (AIMS), extrapyramidal symptoms; orthostatic blood pressure changes for 3-5 days after starting or increasing dose. Weight should be assessed prior to treatment, at 4 weeks, 8 weeks, 12 weeks, and then at quarterly intervals. Consider titrating to a different antipsychotic agent for a weight gain ≥5% of the initial weight.

Additional Information Risperdal® Consta® is an injectable formulation of risperidone using the extended release Medisorb® drug-delivery system; small polymeric microspheres degrade slowly, releasing the medication at a controlled rate.

Dosage Forms Excipient information presented when available (limited, particularly for generics); consult specific product labeling.

Injection, microspheres for reconstitution, extended release:

Risperdal® Consta®: 12.5 mg, 25 mg, 37.5 mg, 50 mg [contains polylactide-co-glycolide; supplied in a dose-pack containing vial with active ingredient in microsphere formulation, prefilled syringe with diluent, needle-free vial access device, and 2 safety needles (1- and 2-inch)]

Solution, oral: 1 mg/mL (30 mL)

Risperdal®: 1 mg/mL (30 mL) [contains benzoic acid]

Tablet: 0.25 mg, 0.5 mg, 1 mg, 2 mg, 3 mg, 4 mg

Risperdal®: 0.25 mg, 0.5 mg, 1 mg, 2 mg, 3 mg, 4 mg

Tablet, orally disintegrating: 0.5 mg, 1 mg, 2 mg, 3 mg, 4 mg

Risperdal® M-Tabs®: 0.5 mg [contains phenylalanine 0.14 mg]; 1 mg [contains phenylalanine 0.28 mg]; 2 mg [contains phenylalanine 0.42 mg]; 3 mg [contains phenylalanine 0.63 mg]; 4 mg [contains phenylalanine 0.84 mg]

◆ **Ritalin®** *see* Methylphenidate *on page 973*

◆ **Ritalin® LA** *see* Methylphenidate *on page 973*

◆ **Ritalin-SR®** *see* Methylphenidate *on page 973*

◆ **Ritalin® SR (Can)** *see* Methylphenidate *on page 973*

Ritonavir (ri TOE na veer)

U.S. Brand Names Norvir®

Canadian Brand Names Norvir®; Norvir® SEC

Pharmacologic Category Antiretroviral Agent, Protease Inhibitor

Additional Appendix Information

Antiretroviral Therapy for HIV Infection: Adults and Adolescents *on page 1758*

Management of Healthcare Worker Exposures to HBV, HCV, and HIV *on page 1719*

Perinatal HIV Guidelines *on page 1730*

Use Treatment of HIV infection; should always be used as part of a multidrug regimen (at least three antiretroviral agents); may be used as a pharmacokinetic "booster" for other protease inhibitors

Pregnancy Risk Factor B

Pregnancy Considerations No increased risk of overall birth defects has been observed following 1st trimester exposure according to data collected by the antiretroviral pregnancy registry. Early studies have shown lower plasma levels during pregnancy compared to postpartum. If needed during pregnancy, use in combination with another PI to boost levels of second PI. Pregnancy and protease inhibitors are both associated with an increased risk of hyperglycemia. Glucose levels should be closely monitored. The Perinatal HIV Guidelines Working Group considers ritonavir to be an alternative PI for use during pregnancy. Healthcare professionals are encouraged to contact the antiretroviral pregnancy registry to monitor outcomes of pregnant women exposed to antiretroviral medications (1-800-258-4263 or www.APRegistry.com).

Lactation Excretion in breast milk unknown/contraindicated

Medication Safety Issues

Sound-alike/look-alike issues:

Ritonavir may be confused with Retrovir®

Norvir® may be confused with Norvasc®

Contraindications Hypersensitivity to ritonavir or any component of the formulation; concurrent alfuzosin, amiodarone, cisapride, dihydroergotamine, ergonovine, ergotamine, flecainide, methylergonovine, midazolam, pimozide, propafenone, quinidine, triazolam, and voriconazole (when ritonavir ≥800 mg/day)

Warnings/Precautions [U.S. Boxed Warning]: Ritonavir may interact with many medications, resulting in potentially serious and/or life-threatening adverse events. Use with caution in patients taking strong CYP3A4 inhibitors, moderate or strong CYP3A4 inducers and major CYP3A4 substrates (see Drug Interactions); consider alternative agents that avoid or lessen the potential for CYP-mediated interactions. Not recommended for use with alfuzosin, amiodarone, cisapride, ergot derivatives, flecainide, lovastatin, midazolam, pimozide, propafenone quinidine, simvastatin, St John's wort, triazolam, or voriconazole. Pancreatitis has been observed; use with caution in patients with increased triglycerides; monitor serum lipase and amylase and for gastrointestinal symptoms. Increases in total cholesterol and triglycerides have been reported; screening should be done prior to therapy and periodically throughout treatment.

Protease inhibitors have been associated with a variety of hypersensitivity events (some severe), including rash, anaphylaxis (rare), angioedema, bronchospasm, erythema multiforme, and/or Stevens-Johnson syndrome (rare). It is generally recommended to discontinue treatment if severe rash or moderate symptoms accompanied by other systemic symptoms occur. Use with caution in patients with cardiomyopathy, ischemic heart disease, pre-existing conduction abnormalities, or structural heart disease; may be at increased risk of conduction abnormalities (eg, second- or third-degree AV block). Ritonavir has been associated with AV block due to prolongation of PR interval; use caution with drugs that prolong the PR interval. Use with caution in patients with hemophilia A or B; increased bleeding during protease inhibitor therapy has been reported. Changes in glucose tolerance, hyperglycemia, exacerbation of diabetes, DKA, and new-onset diabetes mellitus have been reported in patients receiving protease inhibitors. May be associated with fat redistribution (buffalo hump, increased abdominal girth, breast engorgement, facial atrophy, and dyslipidemia). Immune reconstitution syndrome may develop resulting in the occurrence of an inflammatory response to an indolent or residual opportunistic infection; further evaluation and treatment may be required. May cause hepatitis or exacerbate pre-existing hepatic dysfunction; use with caution in patients with hepatitis B or C and in hepatic disease. Safety and efficacy have not been established in children <1 month of age.

Adverse Reactions Percentages as reported for combined experiences in both treatment-naive and experienced adults:

>10%:

Endocrine & metabolic: Hypercholesterolemia (>240 mg/dL: 37% to 45%), triglycerides increased (>800 mg/dL: 17% to 34%; >1500 mg/dL: 1% to 13%)

Gastrointestinal: Nausea (26% to 30%), diarrhea (15% to 23%), vomiting (14% to 17%), taste perversion (7% to 11%)

Hepatic: GGT increased (5% to 20%)

Neuromuscular & skeletal: Weakness (10% to 15%), creatine phosphokinase increased (9% to 12%)

2% to 10%:

Cardiovascular: Vasodilation (2%)

Central nervous system: Fever (1% to 5%), dizziness (3% to 4%), insomnia (2% to 3%), somnolence (2% to 3%), depression (2%), anxiety (up to 2%)

Dermatologic: Rash (up to 4%)

Endocrine & metabolic: Uric acid increased (up to 4%)

Gastrointestinal: Abdominal pain (6% to 8%), anorexia (2% to 8%), dyspepsia (up to 6%), local throat irritation (2% to 3%)

Hepatic: Transaminases increased (6% to 10%)

Neuromuscular & skeletal: Paresthesia (3% to 7%), arthralgia (up to 2%), myalgia (2%)

Respiratory: Pharyngitis (≤1% to 3%)

Miscellaneous: Diaphoresis (2% to 3%)

<2% (Limited to important or life-threatening): Abnormal vision. acute myeloblastic leukemia, adrenal cortex insufficiency, adrenal suppression, anaphylaxis, allergic reaction, amnesia, anemia, angioedema, aphasia, asthma, atrioventricular block (first, second, or third degree), bleeding increased (in patients with hemophilia A or B), bronchospasm, cachexia, cerebral ischemia, cerebral venous thrombosis, chest pain, cholestatic jaundice, coma, Cushing's syndrome, dehydration, dementia, depersonalization, diabetes mellitus, dyspnea, edema, esophageal ulcer, gastroenteritis, gastrointestinal hemorrhage, hallucinations, hepatic coma, hepatitis, hepatomegaly, hepatosplenomegaly, hyper-/hypotension, hypercholesteremia, hypothermia, hypoventilation, ileus, interstitial pneumonia, kidney failure, larynx edema, leukopenia, lymphadenopathy, lymphocytosis, manic reaction, MI, myeloproliferative disorder, neuropathy, orthostatic hypotension,palpitation, pancreatitis, paralysis, postural hypotension, pseudomembranous colitis, rectal hemorrhage, redistribution of body fat,right bundle branch block, seizure, skin melanoma, Stevens-Johnson syndrome, subdural hematoma, syncope, tachycardia, thrombocytopenia, tongue edema, ulcerative colitis, urticaria, vasospasm

Drug Interactions

Metabolism/Transport Effects Substrate of CYP1A2 (minor), 2B6 (minor), 2D6 (major), 3A4 (major); **Inhibits** CYP2C8 (strong), 2C9 (weak), 2C19 (weak), 2D6 (strong), 2E1 (weak), 3A4 (strong); **Induces** CYP1A2 (weak), 2C8 (weak), 2C9 (weak), 3A4 (weak)

Avoid Concomitant Use

Avoid concomitant use of Ritonavir with any of the following: Alfuzosin; Amiodarone; Cisapride; Dabigatran Etexilate; Disulfiram; Eplerenone; Ergot Derivatives; Etravirine; Flecainide; Nilotinib; Nisoldipine; Pimozide; Propafenone; QuiNIDine; Ranolazine; Rivaroxaban; Salmeterol; Silodosin; St Johns Wort; Tamoxifen; Thioridazine; Topotecan; Voriconazole

Increased Effect/Toxicity

Ritonavir may increase the levels/effects of: Alfuzosin; Alosetron; Amiodarone; Antifungal Agents (Azole Derivatives, Systemic); Benzodiazepines (metabolized by oxidation); Calcium Channel Blockers (Dihydropyridine); Calcium Channel Blockers (Nondihydropyridine); CarBAMazepine; Ciclesonide; Cisapride; Clarithromycin; Corticosteroids (Orally Inhaled); CycloSPORINE; CYP2C8 Substrates (High risk); CYP2D6 Substrates; CYP3A4 Substrates; Dabigatran Etexilate; Digoxin; Dronabinol; Enfuvirtide; Eplerenone; Ergot Derivatives; FentaNYL; Fesoterodine; Flecainide; Fusidic Acid; HMG-CoA Reductase Inhibitors; Ixabepilone; Maraviroc; Meperidine; Methadone; Nebivolol; Nefazodone; Nilotinib; Nisoldipine; P-Glycoprotein Substrates; Phosphodiesterase 5 Inhibitors; Pimecrolimus; Pimozide; Propafenone; Protease Inhibitors; QuiNIDine; Ranolazine; Rifamycin Derivatives; Rivaroxaban; Salmeterol; Silodosin; Sirolimus; Sorafenib; Tacrolimus; Tamoxifen; Temsirolimus; Tenofovir; Tetrabenazine; Thioridazine; Topotecan; TraZODone; Tricyclic Antidepressants

The levels/effects of Ritonavir may be increased by: Antifungal Agents (Azole Derivatives, Systemic); Clarithromycin; CycloSPORINE; Delavirdine; Disulfiram; Efavirenz; Enfuvirtide; Fusidic Acid; P-Glycoprotein Inhibitors

Decreased Effect

Ritonavir may decrease the levels/effects of: Abacavir; Atovaquone; BuPROPion; Clarithromycin; Codeine; Delavirdine; Etravirine; LamoTRIgine; Meperidine; Oral Contraceptive (Estrogens); Phenytoin; Theophylline

Derivatives; TraMADol; Valproic Acid; Voriconazole; Warfarin; Zidovudine

The levels/effects of Ritonavir may be decreased by: Antacids; CarBAMazepine; CYP3A4 Inducers (Strong); Deferasirox; Efavirenz; Garlic; Nevirapine; Oral Contraceptive (Estrogens); P-Glycoprotein Inducers; Phenytoin; Rifamycin Derivatives; St Johns Wort; Tenofovir

Ethanol/Nutrition/Herb Interactions

Food: Food enhances absorption.

Herb/Nutraceutical: St John's wort may decrease ritonavir serum levels. Avoid use.

Stability

Capsule: Store under refrigeration at 2°C to 8°C (36°F to 46°F); may be left out at room temperature of <25°C (<77°F) if used within 30 days. Protect from light. Avoid exposure to excessive heat.

Solution: Store at room temperature at 20°C to 25°C (68°F to 77°F); do not refrigerate. Avoid exposure to excessive heat.

Mechanism of Action Ritonavir inhibits HIV protease and renders the enzyme incapable of processing the gag-pol polyprotein precursor which leads to production of noninfectious immature HIV particles

Pharmacodynamics/Kinetics

Absorption: Variable; increased with food

Distribution: High concentrations in serum and lymph nodes; V_d: 0.16-0.66 L/kg

Protein binding: 98% to 99%

Metabolism: Hepatic via CYP3A4 and 2D6; five metabolites, low concentration of an active metabolite (M-2) achieved in plasma (oxidative)

Half-life elimination: 3-5 hours

Time to peak, plasma: Oral solution: 2 hours (fasted); 4 hours (nonfasted)

Excretion: Urine (~11%; ~4% as unchanged drug); feces (~86%; ~34% as unchanged drug)

Dosage Treatment of HIV infection: Oral:

Children >1 month: 350-400 mg/m^2 twice daily (maximum dose: 600 mg twice daily). Initiate dose at 250 mg/m^2 twice daily; titrate dose upward every 2-3 days by 50 mg/m^2 twice daily.

Adults: 600 mg twice daily; dose escalation tends to avoid nausea that many patients experience upon initiation of full dosing. Escalate the dose as follows: 300 mg twice daily for 1 day, 400 mg twice daily for 2 days, 500 mg twice daily for 1 day, then 600 mg twice daily. Ritonavir may be better tolerated when used in combination with other antiretrovirals by initiating the drug alone and subsequently adding the second agent within 2 weeks.

Pharmacokinetic "booster" in combination with other protease inhibitors: 100-400 mg/day

Refer to individual monographs; specific dosage recommendations often require adjustment of both agents.

Note: Dosage adjustments for ritonavir when administered in combination therapy:

Amprenavir: Adjustments necessary for each agent:

Amprenavir 1200 mg with ritonavir 200 mg once daily

or

Amprenavir 600 mg with ritonavir 100 mg twice daily

Amprenavir plus efavirenz (3-drug regimen): Amprenavir 1200 mg twice daily plus ritonavir 200 mg twice daily plus efavirenz at standard dose

Indinavir: Adjustments necessary for both agents:

Indinavir 800 mg twice daily plus ritonavir 100-200 mg twice daily **or**

Indinavir 400 mg twice daily plus ritonavir 400 mg twice daily

Nelfinavir: Ritonavir 400 mg twice daily

Rifabutin: Decrease rifabutin dose to 150 mg every other day

Saquinavir: Ritonavir 400 mg twice daily

Dosing adjustment in renal impairment: None necessary

Dosing adjustment in hepatic impairment: No adjustment required in mild or moderate impairment; however, careful monitoring is required in moderate hepatic impairment (levels may be decreased); caution advised with severe impairment (no data available)

Dietary Considerations Should be taken with food. Oral solution contains 43% ethanol by volume.

Administration Administer with food. Liquid formulations usually have an unpleasant taste. Consider mixing it with chocolate milk or a liquid nutritional supplement. Whenever possible, administer oral solution with calibrated dosing syringe. Shake liquid well before use.

Monitoring Parameters Triglycerides, cholesterol, CBC, LFTs, CPK, uric acid, basic HIV monitoring, viral load, CD4 count, glucose, serum amylase and lipase

Additional Information Potential compliance problems, frequency of administration and adverse effects should be discussed with patients before initiating therapy to help prevent the emergence of resistance.

Dosage Forms Excipient information presented when available (limited, particularly for generics); consult specific product labeling.

Capsule, soft gelatin:

Norvir®: 100 mg [contains ethanol and polyoxyl 35 castor oil]

Solution:

Norvir®: 80 mg/mL (240 mL) [contains ethanol, polyoxyl 35 castor oil, and propylene glycol; peppermint and caramel flavor]

- **Ritonavir and Lopinavir** *see* Lopinavir and Ritonavir *on page 901*
- **Rituxan®** *see* RiTUXimab *on page 1328*

RiTUXimab (ri TUK si mab)

U.S. Brand Names Rituxan®

Canadian Brand Names Rituxan®

Index Terms Anti-CD20 Monoclonal Antibody; C2B8 Monoclonal Antibody; IDEC-C2B8; NSC-687451

Pharmacologic Category Antineoplastic Agent, Monoclonal Antibody; Monoclonal Antibody

Use Treatment of low-grade or follicular CD20-positive, B-cell non-Hodgkin's lymphoma (NHL); treatment of diffuse large B-cell CD20-positive NHL; treatment of moderately- to severely-active rheumatoid arthritis (RA) in combination with methotrexate

Unlabeled/Investigational Use Treatment of autoimmune hemolytic anemia (AIHA) in children; chronic immune thrombocytopenic purpura (ITP); chronic lymphocytic leukemia (CLL); small lymphocytic lymphoma (SLL); pemphigus vulgaris, Waldenström's macroglobulinemia (WM); treatment of systemic autoimmune diseases (other than rheumatoid arthritis); treatment of refractory chronic graft-versus-host disease (GVHD)

Restrictions An FDA-approved medication guide is available; distribute to each patient to whom this medication is dispensed.

Pregnancy Risk Factor C

Pregnancy Considerations Animal studies have demonstrated adverse effects including decreased (reversible) B-cells and immunosuppression. There are no adequate and well-controlled studies in pregnant women. IgG molecules are known to cross the placenta (rituximab is an engineered IgG molecule) and rituximab has been detected in the serum of infants exposed *in utero*. B-Cell lymphocytopenia lasting <6 months may occur in exposed infants. Use during pregnancy only if clearly needed.

Lactation Excretion in breast milk unknown/not recommended

Medication Safety Issues

Sound-alike/look-alike issues:

Rituxan® may be confused with Remicade®

RiTUXimab may be confused with inFLIXimab

High alert medication: The Institute for Safe Medication Practices (ISMP) includes this medication among its list of drug classes which have a heightened risk of causing significant patient harm when used in error.

The rituximab dose for rheumatoid arthritis is a flat dose (1000 mg) and is not based on body surface area (BSA).

Contraindications There are no contraindications listed in the manufacturer's labeling.

Warnings/Precautions [U.S. Boxed Warning]: Severe (occasionally fatal) infusion-related reactions have been reported, usually with the first infusion; fatalities have been reported within 24 hours of infusion; monitor closely and discontinue with grades 3 or 4 infusion reactions. Reactions usually occur within 30-120 minutes and may include hypotension, angioedema, bronchospasm, hypoxia, urticaria, and in more severe cases pulmonary infiltrates, acute respiratory distress syndrome, myocardial infarction, ventricular fibrillation, cardiogenic shock and/or anaphylaxis. Risk factors associated with fatal outcomes include chronic lymphocytic leukemia, female gender, mantle cell lymphoma, or pulmonary infiltrates. Closely monitor patients with a history of prior cardiopulmonary reactions or with pre-existing cardiac or pulmonary conditions and patients with high numbers of circulating malignant cells (>25,000/mm^3). Discontinue infusion for severe reactions; treatment is symptomatic. Medications for the treatment of hypersensitivity reactions (eg, bronchodilators, epinephrine, antihistamines, corticosteroids) should be available for immediate use. Discontinue infusion for serious or life-threatening cardiac arrhythmias; subsequent doses should include cardiac monitoring during and after the infusion. Mild-to-moderate infusion-related reactions (eg, chills, fever, rigors) occur frequently and are typically managed through slowing or interrupting the infusion. Infusion may be resumed at a 50% infusion rate reduction upon resolution of symptoms. Due to the potential for hypotension, consider withholding antihypertensives 12 hours prior to treatment.

[U.S. Boxed Warning]: Progressive multifocal leukoencephalopathy (PML) due to JC virus infection has been reported with rituximab use. Cases were reported in patients with hematologic malignancies receiving rituximab either with combination chemotherapy, or with hematopoietic stem cell transplant. Cases were also reported in patients receiving rituximab for autoimmune diseases who had received prior or concurrent immunosuppressant therapy. Onset may be delayed, although most cases were diagnosed within 12 months of the last rituximab dose. Evaluate any neurological change promptly; consider neurology consultation, brain MRI and lumbar puncture for suspected PML. Discontinue rituximab in patients who develop PML; consider reducing/discontinuing concurrent chemotherapy or immunosuppressants. Other serious and potentially fatal viral infections, either new or reactivated, associated with rituximab use include cytomegalovirus, herpes simplex virus, parvovirus B19, varicella zoster virus, West Nile virus, and hepatitis C. Viral infections may be delayed; occurring up to 1 year after discontinuation of rituximab. Rarely, reactivation of hepatitis B (with fulminant hepatitis and hepatic failure) has been reported in association with rituximab; screen high-risk patients prior to therapy initiation.

[U.S. Boxed Warning]: Tumor lysis syndrome leading to acute renal failure requiring dialysis may occur 12-24 hours following the first dose. Hyperkalemia, hypocalcemia, hyperuricemia, and/or hyperphosphatemia may occur. Consider prophylaxis (allopurinol, hydration) in patients at high risk (high numbers of circulating malignant cells ≥25,000/mm^3 or high tumor burden). May cause renal toxicity in patients with hematologic malignancies; consider discontinuation with increasing serum creatinine or oliguria. **[U.S. Boxed Warning]: Severe and sometimes fatal mucocutaneous reactions (lichenoid dermatitis, paraneoplastic pemphigus, Stevens-Johnson syndrome, toxic epidermal necrolysis and vesiculobullous dermatitis) have been reported,** occurring from 1-13 weeks following exposure. Discontinue in patients experiencing severe mucocutaneous skin reactions; the safety of re-exposure following mucocutaneous reactions has not been evaluated. Use caution with pre-existing cardiac or pulmonary disease, or prior cardiopulmonary events. Rheumatoid arthritis patients are at increased risk for cardiovascular events; monitor closely during and after each infusion. Elderly patients are at higher risk for cardiac (supraventricular arrhythmia) and pulmonary adverse events (pneumonia, pneumonitis). Bowel obstruction and perforation have been reported with an average onset of symptoms of ~6 days; complaints of abdominal pain should be evaluated, especially if early in the treatment course. Live vaccines should not be given concurrently with rituximab; there is no data available concerning secondary transmission of live vaccines with or following rituximab treatment. RA patients should be brought up to date with nonlive immunizations (following current guidelines) before initiating therapy; evaluate risks of therapy delay versus benefit (of nonlive vaccines) for NHL patients. Safety and efficacy of rituximab in combination with biologic agents or disease-modifying antirheumatic drugs (DMARD) other than methotrexate have not been established. Safety and efficacy of retreatment for RA have not been established. Not approved for use in children.

Adverse Reactions Note: Patients treated with rituximab for rheumatoid arthritis (RA) may experience fewer adverse reactions.

>10%:

Central nervous system: Fever (5% to 53%), chills (3% to 33%), headache (19%), pain (12%)

Dermatologic: Rash (15%; grades 3/4: 1%), pruritus (5% to 14%), angioedema (11%; grades 3/4: 1%)

Gastrointestinal: Nausea (8% to 23%), abdominal pain (2% to 14%)

Hematologic: Cytopenias (grades 3/4: ≤48%; may be prolonged), lymphopenia (48%; grades 3/4: 40%; median duration 14 days), leukopenia (14%; grades 3/4: 4%), neutropenia (14%; grades 3/4: 6%; median duration 13 days), thrombocytopenia (12%; grades 3/4: 2%)

Neuromuscular & skeletal: Weakness (2% to 26%)

Respiratory: Cough (13%), rhinitis (3% to 12%)

Miscellaneous: Infusion-related reactions (lymphoma: first dose 77%; decreases with subsequent infusions; may include angioedema, bronchospasm, chills, dizziness, fever, headache, hyper-/hypotension, myalgia, nausea, pruritus, rash, rigors, urticaria, and vomiting; reactions reported are lower [first infusion: 32%] in RA); infection (31%; grades 3/4: 4%; bacterial: 19%; viral 10%; fungal: 1%), night sweats (15%)

1% to 10%:

Cardiovascular: Hypotension (10%), peripheral edema (8%), hypertension (6% to 8%), flushing (5%), edema (<5%)

Central nervous system: Dizziness (10%), anxiety (2% to 5%), agitation (<5%), depression (<5%), hypoesthesia (<5%), insomnia (<5%), malaise (<5%), nervousness (<5%), neuritis (<5%), somnolence (<5%), vertigo (<5%), migraine (RA: 2%)

Dermatologic: Urticaria (2% to 8%)

Endocrine & metabolic: Hyperglycemia (9%), hypoglycemia (<5%), hypercholesterolemia (2%)
Gastrointestinal: Diarrhea (10%), vomiting (10%), dyspepsia (3%), anorexia (<5%), weight loss (<5%)
Hematologic: Anemia (8%; grades 3/4: 3%)
Local: Pain at the injection site (<5%)
Neuromuscular & skeletal: Back pain (10%), myalgia (10%), arthralgia (6% to 10%), paresthesia (2%), arthritis (<5%), hyperkinesia (<5%), hypertonia (<5%), neuropathy (<5%)
Ocular: Conjunctivitis (<5%), lacrimation disorder (<5%)
Respiratory: Throat irritation (2% to 9%), bronchospasm (8%), dyspnea (7%), upper respiratory tract infection (RA: 7%), sinusitis (6%)
Miscellaneous: LDH increased (7%)

Postmarketing and/or case reports: Acute renal failure, anaphylactoid reaction/anaphylaxis, angina, aplastic anemia, ARDS, arrhythmia, bowel obstruction, bronchiolitis obliterans, cardiac failure, cardiogenic shock, disease progression (Kaposi's sarcoma), fatal infusion-related reactions, fulminant hepatitis, gastrointestinal perforation, hemolytic anemia, hepatic failure, hepatitis, hepatitis B reactivation, hyperviscosity syndrome (in Waldenström's macroglobulinemia), hypogammaglobulinemia, hypoxia, interstitial pneumonitis, lichenoid dermatitis, lupus-like syndrome, marrow hypoplasia, MI, neutropenia (late-onset occurring >40 days after last dose), optic neuritis, pancytopenia (prolonged), paraneoplastic pemphigus (uncommon), pleuritis, pneumonia, pneumonitis, polyarticular arthritis, progressive multifocal leukoencephalopathy (PML), pure red cell aplasia, renal toxicity, serum sickness, Stevens-Johnson syndrome, supraventricular arrhythmia, systemic vasculitis, toxic epidermal necrolysis, tumor lysis syndrome, urticaria, uveitis, vasculitis with rash, ventricular fibrillation, ventricular tachycardia, vesiculobullous dermatitis, viral reactivation (includes JC virus, cytomegalovirus, herpes simplex virus, parvovirus B19, varicella zoster virus, West Nile virus, and hepatitis C)

Drug Interactions

Avoid Concomitant Use

Avoid concomitant use of RiTUXimab with any of the following: Natalizumab; Vaccines (Live)

Increased Effect/Toxicity

RiTUXimab may increase the levels/effects of: Natalizumab; Vaccines (Live)

The levels/effects of RiTUXimab may be increased by: Abciximab; Antihypertensives; Herbs (Hypoglycemic Properties); Trastuzumab

Decreased Effect

RiTUXimab may decrease the levels/effects of: Vaccines (Inactivated)

The levels/effects of RiTUXimab may be decreased by: Echinacea

Ethanol/Nutrition/Herb Interactions Herb/Nutraceutical: Avoid echinacea (may diminish the therapeutic effect of immunosuppressants). Avoid hypoglycemic herbs, including alfalfa, aloe, bilberry, bitter melon, burdock, celery, damiana, fenugreek, garcinia, garlic, ginger, ginseng (American), gymnema, marshmallow, and stinging nettle (may enhance the hypoglycemic effect of rituximab).

Stability Store vials under refrigeration at 2°C to 8°C (36°F to 46°F); do not freeze. Do not shake. Protect vials from direct sunlight.

Withdraw the necessary amount of rituximab and dilute to a final concentration of 1-4 mg/mL with 0.9% sodium chloride or 5% dextrose in water. Gently invert the bag to mix the solution; do not shake. Solutions for infusion are stable at 2°C to 8°C (36°F to 46°F) for 24 hours and at room temperature for an additional 24hours.

Mechanism of Action Rituximab is a monoclonal antibody directed against the CD20 antigen on B-lymphocytes. CD20 regulates cell cycle initiation; and, possibly, functions as a calcium channel. Rituximab binds to the antigen on the cell surface, activating complement-dependent B-cell cytotoxicity; and to human Fc receptors, mediating cell killing through an antibody-dependent cellular toxicity. B-cells are believed to play a role in the development and progression of rheumatoid arthritis. Signs and symptoms of RA are reduced by targeting B-cells and the progression of structural damage is delayed.

Pharmacodynamics/Kinetics

Duration: Detectable in serum 3-6 months after completion of treatment; B-cell recovery begins ~6 months following completion of treatment; median B-cell levels return to normal by 12 months following completion of treatment

Absorption: I.V.: Immediate and results in a rapid and sustained depletion of circulating and tissue-based B cells

Distribution: 4.3 L (following two 1000 mg doses for rheumatoid arthritis)

Half-life elimination:

Cancer: Proportional to dose; wide ranges reflect variable tumor burden and changes in CD20 positive B-cell populations with repeated doses:

>100 mg/m^2: 4.4 days (range 1.6-10.5 days)

375 mg/m^2:

Following first dose: Mean half-life: 3.2 days (range 1.3-6.4 days)

Following fourth dose: Mean half-life: 8.6 days (range 3.5-17 days)

RA: Mean terminal half-life: 19 days

Excretion: Uncertain; may undergo phagocytosis and catabolism in the reticuloendothelial system (RES)

Dosage Note: Pretreatment with acetaminophen and an antihistamine is recommended.

Children: AIHA, chronic ITP (unlabeled uses): I.V.: 375 mg/m^2 once weekly for 2-4 doses

Adults: I.V. infusion (refer to individual protocols):

NHL (relapsed/refractory, low-grade or follicular CD20-positive, B-cell): 375 mg/m^2 once weekly for 4 or 8 doses

Retreatment following disease progression: 375 mg/m^2 once weekly for 4 doses

NHL (diffuse large B-cell): 375 mg/m^2 given on day 1 of each chemotherapy cycle for up to 8 doses

NHL (follicular, CD20-positive, B-cell, previously untreated): 375 mg/m^2 given on day 1 of each chemotherapy cycle for up to 8 doses

NHL (nonprogressing, low-grade, CD20-positive, B-cell, after first line CVP): 375 mg/m^2 once weekly for 4 doses every 6 months for up to 4 cycles (initiate after 6-8 cycles of chemotherapy are completed)

Rheumatoid arthritis: 1000 mg on days 1 and 15 in combination with methotrexate

Note: Premedication with a corticosteroid (eg, methylprednisolone 100 mg I.V.) 30 minutes prior to each rituximab dose is recommended. In clinical trials, patients received oral corticosteroids on a tapering schedule from baseline through day 16.

CLL/SLL (unlabeled use): 100 mg day 1, then 375 mg/m^2 3 times/week for 11 doses

Refractory pemphigus vulgaris (unlabeled use): 375 mg/m^2 once weekly of weeks 1, 2, and 3 of a 4-week cycle, repeat for 1 additional cycle, then 1 dose per month for 4 months (total of 10 doses in 6 months)

Refractory chronic GVHD, Waldenström's macroglobulinemia (unlabeled uses): 375 mg/m^2 once weekly for 4 weeks

Combination therapy with ibritumomab: 250 mg/m^2 I.V. day 1; repeat in 7-9 days with ibritumomab (also see Ibritumomab monograph):

Administration Do **not** administer I.V. push or bolus.

Initial infusion: Start rate of 50 mg/hour; if there is no reaction, increase the rate by 50 mg/hour increments every 30 minutes, to a maximum rate of 400 mg/hour.

Subsequent infusions: If patient did not tolerate initial infusion follow initial infusion guidelines. If patient tolerated initial infusion, start at 100 mg/hour; if there is no reaction, increase the rate by 100 mg/hour increments every 30 minutes, to a maximum rate of 400 mg/hour.

Note: If a reaction occurs, slow or stop the infusion. If the reaction abates, restart infusion at 50% of the previous rate.

In patients with NHL who are receiving a corticosteroid as part of their combination chemotherapy regimen and after tolerance has been established at the recommended infusion rate in cycle 1, a rapid infusion rate has been used beginning with cycle 2. The daily corticosteroid, acetaminophen, and diphenhydramine are administered prior to treatment, then the rituximab dose is administered over 90 minutes, with 20% of the dose administered in the first 30 minutes and the remaining 80% is given over 60 minutes (Sehn, 2007).

Monitoring Parameters CBC with differential and platelets, peripheral CD20$^+$ cells; HAMA/HACA titers (high levels may increase the risk of allergic reactions); renal function, fluid balance; vital signs; monitor for infusion reactions, cardiac monitoring during and after infusion in rheumatoid arthritis patients and in patients with pre-existing cardiac disease or if arrhythmias develop during or after subsequent infusions

Screen for hepatitis B in high-risk patients prior to initiation of rituximab therapy (the NCCN NHL guidelines recommend screening **all** NHL patients prior to therapy). In addition, carriers and patients with evidence of recovery from prior hepatitis B infection should be monitored closely for clinical and laboratory signs of HBV infection during therapy and for up to a year following completion of treatment. High-risk patients should be screened for hepatitis C (per NCCN guidelines).

Complaints of abdominal pain, especially early in the course of treatment, should prompt a thorough diagnostic evaluation and appropriate treatment. Signs or symptoms of progressive multifocal leukoencephalopathy (focal neurologic deficits, which may present as hemiparesis, visual field deficits, cognitive impairment, aphasia, ataxia, and/or cranial nerve deficits). If PML is suspected, obtain brain MRI scan and lumbar puncture.

Dosage Forms Excipient information presented when available (limited, particularly for generics); consult specific product labeling.

Injection, solution [preservative free]:

Rituxan®: 10 mg/mL (10 mL, 50 mL) [contains polysorbate 80]

◆ **Riva-Alendronate (Can)** *see* Alendronate *on page 58*

◆ **RIVA-Amiodarone (Can)** *see* Amiodarone *on page 87*

◆ **Riva-Atenolol (Can)** *see* Atenolol *on page 149*

◆ **Riva-Buspirone (Can)** *see* BusPIRone *on page 226*

◆ **Riva-Ciprofloxacin (Can)** *see* Ciprofloxacin *on page 329*

◆ **Riva-Citalopram (Can)** *see* Citalopram *on page 337*

◆ **Riva-Clindamycin (Can)** *see* Clindamycin *on page 344*

◆ **Riva-Diclofenac (Can)** *see* Diclofenac *on page 437*

◆ **Riva-Diclofenac-K (Can)** *see* Diclofenac *on page 437*

◆ **Riva-Dicyclomine (Can)** *see* Dicyclomine *on page 441*

◆ **Riva-Enalapril (Can)** *see* Enalapril *on page 515*

◆ **Riva-Famotidine (Can)** *see* Famotidine *on page 603*

◆ **Riva-Fenofibrate Micro (Can)** *see* Fenofibrate *on page 607*

◆ **Riva-Fluconazole (Can)** *see* Fluconazole *on page 625*

◆ **Riva-Fluoxetine (Can)** *see* FLUoxetine *on page 638*

◆ **Riva-Fluvox (Can)** *see* Fluvoxamine *on page 652*

◆ **Riva-Fosinopril (Can)** *see* Fosinopril *on page 670*

◆ **RIVA-Gabapentin (Can)** *see* Gabapentin *on page 678*

◆ **Riva-Indapamide (Can)** *see* Indapamide *on page 781*

◆ **Riva-Lisinopril (Can)** *see* Lisinopril *on page 894*

◆ **Riva-Loperamide (Can)** *see* Loperamide *on page 900*

◆ **Riva-Lorazepam (Can)** *see* LORazepam *on page 905*

◆ **Riva-Lovastatin (Can)** *see* Lovastatin *on page 910*

◆ **RIVA-Metformin (Can)** *see* MetFORMIN *on page 954*

◆ **RIVA-Metoprolol (Can)** *see* Metoprolol *on page 982*

◆ **Riva-Mirtazapine (Can)** *see* Mirtazapine *on page 1002*

◆ **Riva-Naproxen (Can)** *see* Naproxen *on page 1041*

◆ **Rivanase AQ (Can)** *see* Beclomethasone *on page 176*

◆ **Riva-Norfloxacin (Can)** *see* Norfloxacin *on page 1080*

◆ **Riva-Oxazepam (Can)** *see* Oxazepam *on page 1116*

◆ **Riva-Oxybutynin (Can)** *see* Oxybutynin *on page 1119*

◆ **Riva-Pantoprazole (Can)** *see* Pantoprazole *on page 1140*

◆ **Riva-Pravastatin (Can)** *see* Pravastatin *on page 1227*

◆ **Riva-Quetiapine (Can)** *see* QUEtiapine *on page 1275*

◆ **Riva-Ranitidine (Can)** *see* Ranitidine *on page 1295*

◆ **Riva-Risperidone (Can)** *see* Risperidone *on page 1323*

◆ **Riva-Sertraline (Can)** *see* Sertraline *on page 1362*

◆ **Riva-Simvastatin (Can)** *see* Simvastatin *on page 1370*

◆ **Rivasol (Can)** *see* Zinc Sulfate *on page 1584*

◆ **Riva-Sotalol (Can)** *see* Sotalol *on page 1394*

Rivastigmine (ri va STIG meen)

U.S. Brand Names Exelon®

Canadian Brand Names Exelon®

Index Terms ENA 713; Rivastigmine Tartrate; SDZ ENA 713

Pharmacologic Category Acetylcholinesterase Inhibitor (Central)

Use Treatment of mild-to-moderate dementia associated with Alzheimer's disease or Parkinson's disease

Unlabeled/Investigational Use Severe dementia associated with Alzheimer's disease; Lewy body dementia

Pregnancy Risk Factor B

Pregnancy Considerations Teratogenic effects were not observed in animal studies. There are no adequate and well-controlled studies in pregnant women. Should be used only if the benefit outweighs the potential risk to the fetus.

Lactation Excretion in breast milk unknown/use caution

Contraindications Hypersensitivity to rivastigmine, other carbamate derivatives (eg, neostigmine, pyridostigmine, physostigmine), or any component of the formulation

Warnings/Precautions Significant nausea, vomiting, anorexia, and weight loss are associated with use; occurs more frequently in women and during the titration phase. Nausea and/or vomiting may be severe, particularly at doses higher than recommended. Monitor weight during therapy. Therapy should be initiated at lowest dose and titrated; if treatment is interrupted for more than several days, reinstate at the lowest daily dose. Cholinesterase inhibitors may have vagotonic effects which may cause bradycardia and/or heart block with or without a history of cardiac disease. Alzheimer's treatment guidelines consider bradycardia to be a relative contraindication for use of centrally-active cholinesterase inhibitors. Use caution in patients with a history of peptic ulcer disease or concurrent NSAID use. Use caution in patients undergoing anesthesia who will receive succinylcholine-type muscle relaxation, patients with sick-sinus syndrome, bradycardia or supraventricular conduction conditions, urinary obstruction, seizure disorders, or pulmonary conditions such as asthma or COPD. Use caution in patients with low body weight (<50 kg) due to increased risk of adverse reactions. Safety and efficacy in children have not been established.

Adverse Reactions **Note:** Many concentration-related effects are reported at a lower frequency by transdermal route.

>10%:

Central nervous system: Dizziness (2% to 21%), headache (3% to 17%)

Gastrointestinal: Nausea (7% to 47%), vomiting (6% to 31%), diarrhea (5% to 19%), anorexia (3% to 17%), abdominal pain (1% to 13%)

1% to 10%:

Cardiovascular: Syncope (3%), hypertension (3%)

Central nervous system: Fatigue (2% to 9%), insomnia (1% to 9%), confusion (8%), depression (4% to 6%), anxiety (2% to 5%), malaise (5%), somnolence (4% to 5%), hallucinations (4%), aggressiveness (3%), parkinsonism symptoms worsening (2% to 3%), vertigo (≤2%)

Gastrointestinal: Dyspepsia (9%), constipation (5%), flatulence (4%), weight loss (3% to 8%), eructation (2%), dehydration (2%)

Genitourinary: Urinary tract infection (1% to 7%)

Neuromuscular & skeletal: Weakness (2% to 6%), tremor (1%; up to 10% in Parkinson's patients)

Respiratory: Rhinitis (4%)

Miscellaneous: Diaphoresis (4%), flu-like syndrome (3%)

<1% (Limited to important or life-threatening symptoms; reactions may be at a similar frequency to placebo): Abnormal hepatic function, acute renal failure, albuminuria, allergy, anemia, angina, aphasia, apnea, apraxia, ataxia, atrial fibrillation, AV block, bradycardia, bronchospasm, bundle branch block, cachexia, cardiac arrest, cardiac failure, chest pain, cholecystitis, diplopia, diverticulitis, dysphagia, dyspnea, dysphonia, edema, esophagitis, extrasystoles, fecal incontinence, gastritis, gastroesophageal reflux, GGT increased, glaucoma, hematuria, hot flashes, hyper-/hypoglycemia, hypercholesterolemia, hyper-/hypokinesia, hypertonia, hypokalemia, hyponatremia, hypotension (including postural), hypothermia, hypothyroidism, intestinal obstruction, intracranial hemorrhage, mastitis, MI, migraine, neuralgia, palpitation, pancreatitis, paresthesia, periorbital or facial edema, peripheral ischemia, peripheral neuropathy, pneumonia, pruritus, psychiatric disorders (eg, delirium, depersonalization, psychosis, emotional lability, suicidal ideation or tendencies), rash, retinopathy, rigors, seizure, sick-sinus syndrome, sudden cardiac death, supraventricular tachycardia, thrombocytopenia, thrombophlebitis, thrombosis, transient ischemic attack, ulcerative stomatitis, urinary incontinence, urticaria, vasovagal syncope

Drug Interactions

Avoid Concomitant Use There are no known interactions where it is recommended to avoid concomitant use.

Increased Effect/Toxicity

Rivastigmine may increase the levels/effects of: Antipsychotics; Beta-Blockers; Cholinergic Agonists; Succinylcholine

The levels/effects of Rivastigmine may be increased by: Corticosteroids (Systemic); Ginkgo Biloba

Decreased Effect

Rivastigmine may decrease the levels/effects of: Anticholinergics; Neuromuscular-Blocking Agents (Nondepolarizing)

The levels/effects of Rivastigmine may be decreased by: Anticholinergics

Ethanol/Nutrition/Herb Interactions

Smoking: Nicotine increases the clearance of rivastigmine by 23%.

Ethanol: Avoid ethanol (due to risk of sedation; may increase GI irritation).

Food: Food delays absorption by 90 minutes, lowers C_{max} by 30% and increases AUC by 30%.

Herb/Nutraceutical: Avoid ginkgo biloba (may increase cholinergic effects).

Stability

Oral: Store at 15°C to 30°C (59°F to 86°F); do not freeze. Store solution in an upright position.

Transdermal patch: Store at 15°C to 30°C (59°F to 86°F). Patches should be kept in sealed pouch until use.

Mechanism of Action A deficiency of cortical acetylcholine is thought to account for some of the symptoms of Alzheimer's disease and the dementia of Parkinson's disease; rivastigmine increases acetylcholine in the central nervous system through reversible inhibition of its hydrolysis by cholinesterase

Pharmacodynamics/Kinetics

Duration: Anticholinesterase activity (CSF): ~10 hours (6 mg oral dose)

Absorption: Oral: Fasting: Rapid and complete within 1 hour

Distribution: V_d: 1.8-2.7 L/kg; penetrates blood-brain barrier (CSF levels are ~40% of plasma levels following oral administration)

Protein binding: 40%

Metabolism: Extensively via cholinesterase-mediated hydrolysis in the brain; metabolite undergoes N-demethylation and/or sulfate conjugation hepatically; CYP minimally involved; linear kinetics at 3 mg twice daily, but nonlinear at higher doses

Bioavailability: Oral: 36% to 40%

Half-life elimination: Oral: 1.5 hours; Transdermal patch: 3 hours (after removal)

Time to peak: Oral: 1 hour; Transdermal patch: 10-16 hours following first dose

Excretion: Urine (97% as metabolites); feces (0.4%)

Dosage Adults:

Oral: **Note:** Exelon® oral solution and capsules are bioequivalent.

Mild-to-moderate Alzheimer's dementia: Initial: 1.5 mg twice daily; may increase by 3 mg/day (1.5 mg/dose) every 2 weeks based on tolerability (maximum recommended dose: 6 mg twice daily)

Note: If GI adverse events occur, discontinue treatment for several doses then restart at the same or next lower dosage level; antiemetics have been used to control GI symptoms. If treatment is interrupted for longer than several days, restart the treatment at the lowest dose and titrate as previously described.

Mild-to-moderate Parkinson's-related dementia: Initial: 1.5 mg twice daily; may increase by 3 mg/day (1.5 mg/dose) every 4 weeks based on tolerability (maximum recommended dose: 6 mg twice daily)

Transdermal patch: Mild-to-moderate Alzheimer's- or Parkinson's-related dementia:

Initial: 4.6 mg/24 hours; if well tolerated, may be increased (after at least 4 weeks) to 9.5 mg/24 hours (recommended effective dose)

Maintenance: 9.5 mg/24 hours (maximum dose: 9.5 mg/24 hours)

Note: If intolerance is noted (nausea, vomiting), patch should be removed and treatment interrupted for several days and restarted at the same or lower dosage. If interrupted for more than several days, reinitiate at lowest dosage and increase to maintenance dose after 4 weeks.

Conversion from oral therapy: If oral daily dose <6 mg, switch to 4.6 mg/24 hours patch; if oral daily dose 6-12 mg, switch to 9.5 mg/24 hours patch. Apply patch on the next day following last oral dose.

Elderly: Following oral administration, clearance is significantly lower in patients >60 years of age, but dosage adjustments are not recommended. Age was not associated with exposure in patients treated transdermally. Titrate dose to individual's tolerance.

Dosage adjustment in renal impairment: Dosage adjustments are not recommended, however, titrate the dose to the individual's tolerance.

Dosage adjustment in hepatic impairment: Clearance is significantly reduced in mild to moderately impaired patients. Although dosage adjustments are not recommended, use lowest possible dose and titrate according to individual's tolerance. Consider intervals of >2 weeks between dosage adjustments.

Dietary Considerations Capsules should be taken with meals.

Administration

Oral: Should be administered with meals (breakfast or dinner). Capsule should be swallowed whole. Liquid form is available for patients who cannot swallow capsules (can be swallowed directly from syringe or mixed with water, soda, or cold fruit juice). Stir well and drink within 4 hours of mixing.

Topical: Apply transdermal patch to upper or lower back (alternatively, nay apply to upper arm or chest). Avoid reapplication to same spot of skin for 14 days (may rotate sections of back, for example). Do not apply to red, irritated, or broken skin. Avoid areas of recent application of lotion or powder. After removal, fold patch to press adhesive surfaces together, and discard. Avoid eye contact; wash hands after handling patch. Replace patch every 24 hours. Avoid exposing the patch to external sources of heat (eg, sauna, excessive light) for prolonged periods of time.

Monitoring Parameters Cognitive function at periodic intervals (MMSE), symptoms of GI intolerance, weight

Dosage Forms Excipient information presented when available (limited, particularly for generics); consult specific product labeling.

Capsule:

Exelon®: 1.5 mg, 3 mg, 4.5 mg, 6 mg

Solution, oral:

Exelon®: 2 mg/mL (120 mL) [contains sodium benzoate]

Transdermal system [once-daily patch]:

Exelon®: 4.6 mg/24 hours (30s) [5 cm^2; contains rivastigmine 9 mg]; 9.5 mg/24 hours (30s) [10 cm^2; contains rivastigmine 18 mg]

- ◆ **Rivastigmine Tartrate** *see* Rivastigmine *on page* 1331
- ◆ **Riva-Sumatriptan (Can)** *see* SUMAtriptan *on page* 1414
- ◆ **RIVA-Terbinafine (Can)** *see* Terbinafine *on page* 1441
- ◆ **RIVA-Valacyclovir (Can)** *see* Valacyclovir *on page* 1535
- ◆ **RIVA-Venlafaxine XR (Can)** *see* Venlafaxine *on page* 1554
- ◆ **Riva-Verapamil SR (Can)** *see* Verapamil *on page* 1557
- ◆ **Riva-Zide (Can)** *see* Hydrochlorothiazide and Triamterene *on page* 739
- ◆ **Rivotril® (Can)** *see* ClonazePAM *on page* 352

Rizatriptan (rye za TRIP tan)

U.S. Brand Names Maxalt-MLT®; Maxalt®

Canadian Brand Names Maxalt RPD™; Maxalt™

Index Terms MK462

Pharmacologic Category Antimigraine Agent; Serotonin 5-$HT_{1B,\ 1D}$ Receptor Agonist

Additional Appendix Information

Antimigraine Drugs: 5-HT_1 Receptor Agonists *on page* 1642

Use Acute treatment of migraine with or without aura

Pregnancy Risk Factor C

Pregnancy Considerations There are no adequate and well-controlled studies using rizatriptan in pregnant women. Use only if potential benefit to the mother outweighs the potential risk to the fetus. A pregnancy registry has been established to monitor outcomes of women exposed to rizatriptan during pregnancy (800-986-8999). In some animal studies, administration was associated with decreased weight gain, developmental toxicity and increased mortality in the offspring. Teratogenic effects were not observed.

Lactation Excretion in breast milk unknown/use caution

Contraindications Hypersensitivity to rizatriptan or any component of the formulation; documented ischemic heart disease or Prinzmetal's angina; uncontrolled hypertension; basilar or hemiplegic migraine; during or within 2 weeks of MAO inhibitors; during or within 24 hours of treatment with another 5-HT_1 agonist, or an ergot-containing or ergot-type medication (eg, methysergide, dihydroergotamine)

Warnings/Precautions Only indicated for treatment of acute migraine; if a patient does not respond to the first dose, the diagnosis of migraine should be reconsidered. Coronary artery vasospasm, transient ischemia, myocardial infarction, ventricular tachycardia/fibrillation, cardiac arrest, and death have been reported with 5-HT_1 agonist administration. Patients who experience sensations of chest pain/pressure/tightness or symptoms suggestive of angina following dosing should be evaluated for coronary artery disease or Prinzmetal's angina before receiving additional doses. Should not be given to patients who have risk factors for CAD (eg, hypertension, hypercholesterolemia, smoker, obesity, diabetes, strong family history of CAD, menopause, male >40 years of age) without adequate cardiac evaluation. Patients with suspected CAD should have cardiovascular evaluation to rule out CAD before considering use; if cardiovascular evaluation "is satisfactory", first dose should be given in the healthcare provider's office. Periodic evaluation of cardiovascular status should be done in all patients. Significant elevation in blood pressure, including hypertensive crisis, has also been reported on rare occasions in patients with and without a history of hypertension. Cerebral/subarachnoid hemorrhage, stroke, peripheral vascular ischemia, and colonic ischemia have been reported with 5-HT_1 agonist administration.

Use with caution in elderly or patients with hepatic or renal impairment (including dialysis patients). Symptoms of agitation, confusion, hallucinations, hyper-reflexia, myoclonus, shivering, and tachycardia may occur with concomitant proserotonergic drugs (eg, SSRIs/SNRIs or triptans) or agents which reduce rizatriptan's metabolism. Concurrent use of serotonin precursors (eg, tryptophan) is not recommended. Safety and efficacy have not been established in children <18 years of age. Maxalt-MLT® tablets contain phenylalanine.

Adverse Reactions

1% to 10%:

Cardiovascular: Systolic/diastolic blood pressure increases (5-10 mm Hg), chest pain (5%), palpitation

Central nervous system: Dizziness, drowsiness, fatigue (13% to 30%, dose related)

Dermatologic: Skin flushing

Endocrine & metabolic: Mild increase in growth hormone, hot flashes

Gastrointestinal: Abdominal pain, dry mouth (<5%), nausea

Respiratory: Dyspnea

<1% (Limited to important or life-threatening): Akinesia, angina, angioedema, arrhythmia, bradycardia, bradykinesia, decreased mental activity, myalgia, myocardial ischemia, MI, neck pain/stiffness, neurological/psychiatric abnormalities, pruritus, stroke, syncope, tachycardia, tinnitus, toxic epidermal necrolysis, wheezing

Drug Interactions

Avoid Concomitant Use

Avoid concomitant use of Rizatriptan with any of the following: Ergot Derivatives; MAO Inhibitors; Sibutramine

Increased Effect/Toxicity

Rizatriptan may increase the levels/effects of: Ergot Derivatives; Serotonin Modulators

The levels/effects of Rizatriptan may be increased by: Ergot Derivatives; MAO Inhibitors; Propranolol; Sibutramine

Decreased Effect There are no known significant interactions involving a decrease in effect.

Ethanol/Nutrition/Herb Interactions Food: Food delays absorption.

Stability Store in blister pack until administration.

Mechanism of Action Selective agonist for serotonin (5-HT_{1D} receptor) in cranial arteries to cause vasoconstriction and reduce sterile inflammation associated with antidromic neuronal transmission correlating with relief of migraine

Pharmacodynamics/Kinetics

Onset of action: ~30 minutes
Duration: 14-16 hours
Protein binding: 14%
Metabolism: Via monoamine oxidase-A; first-pass effect
Bioavailability: 40% to 50%
Half-life elimination: 2-3 hours
Time to peak: 1-1.5 hours
Excretion: Urine (82%, 8% to 16% as unchanged drug); feces (12%)

Dosage Note: In patients with risk factors for coronary artery disease, following adequate evaluation to establish the absence of coronary artery disease, the initial dose should be administered in a setting where response may be evaluated (physician's office or similarly staffed setting). ECG monitoring may be considered.

Oral: 5-10 mg, repeat after 2 hours if significant relief is not attained; maximum: 30 mg in a 24-hour period (use 5 mg dose in patients receiving propranolol with a maximum of 15 mg in 24 hours)

Note: For orally-disintegrating tablets (Maxalt-MLT®): Patient should be instructed to place tablet on tongue and allow to dissolve. Dissolved tablet will be swallowed with saliva.

Dietary Considerations Orally-disintegrating tablet contains phenylalanine (1.05 mg per 5 mg tablet, 2.10 mg per 10 mg tablet).

Monitoring Parameters Headache severity, signs/symptoms suggestive of angina; consider monitoring blood pressure, heart rate, and/or ECG with first dose in patients with likelihood of unrecognized coronary disease, such as patients with significant hypertension, hypercholesterolemia, obese patients, patients with diabetes, smokers with other risk factors or strong family history of coronary artery disease

Dosage Forms Excipient information presented when available (limited, particularly for generics); consult specific product labeling.

Tablet:
Maxalt®: 5 mg, 10 mg

Tablet, orally disintegrating:
Maxalt-MLT®: 5 mg [contains phenylalanine 1.05 mg/tablet; peppermint flavor]; 10 mg [contains phenylalanine 2.1 mg/tablet; peppermint flavor]

- ◆ **rLFN-α2** *see* Interferon Alfa-2b *on page* 801
- ◆ **R-modafinil** *see* Armodafinil *on page* 136
- ◆ **Ro 5488** *see* Tretinoin (Oral) *on page* 1508
- ◆ **Robafen® AC** *see* Guaifenesin and Codeine *on page* 710
- ◆ **Robafen DM [OTC]** *see* Guaifenesin and Dextromethorphan *on page* 710
- ◆ **Robafen DM Clear [OTC]** *see* Guaifenesin and Dextromethorphan *on page* 710
- ◆ **Robaxin®** *see* Methocarbamol *on page* 964
- ◆ **Robidrine® (Can)** *see* Pseudoephedrine *on page* 1265
- ◆ **Robinul®** *see* Glycopyrrolate *on page* 703
- ◆ **Robinul® Forte** *see* Glycopyrrolate *on page* 703
- ◆ **Robitussin® [OTC]** *see* GuaiFENesin *on page* 709
- ◆ **Robitussin® (Can)** *see* GuaiFENesin *on page* 709
- ◆ **Robitussin® Childrens Cough & Cold (Can)** *see* Pseudoephedrine and Dextromethorphan *on page* 1266
- ◆ **Robitussin® Children's Cough & Cold Long-Acting [OTC]** *see* Dextromethorphan and Chlorpheniramine *on page* 433
- ◆ **Robitussin® Cough and Allergy [OTC] [DSC]** *see* Chlorpheniramine, Phenylephrine, and Dextromethorphan *on page* 311
- ◆ **Robitussin® Cough and Cold [OTC]** *see* Guaifenesin, Pseudoephedrine, and Dextromethorphan *on page* 715
- ◆ **Robitussin® Cough and Cold CF [OTC]** *see* Guaifenesin, Pseudoephedrine, and Dextromethorphan *on page* 715
- ◆ **Robitussin® Cough and Cold Infant CF [OTC]** *see* Guaifenesin, Pseudoephedrine, and Dextromethorphan *on page* 715
- ◆ **Robitussin® Cough and Cold Nighttime [OTC]** *see* Chlorpheniramine, Phenylephrine, and Dextromethorphan *on page* 311
- ◆ **Robitussin® Cough and Congestion [OTC]** *see* Guaifenesin and Dextromethorphan *on page* 710
- ◆ **Robitussin® Cough & Cold® (Can)** *see* Guaifenesin, Pseudoephedrine, and Dextromethorphan *on page* 715
- ◆ **Robitussin® Cough & Cold Long-Acting [OTC]** *see* Dextromethorphan and Chlorpheniramine *on page* 433
- ◆ **Robitussin® DM [OTC]** *see* Guaifenesin and Dextromethorphan *on page* 710
- ◆ **Robitussin® DM (Can)** *see* Guaifenesin and Dextromethorphan *on page* 710
- ◆ **Robitussin® DM Infant [OTC] [DSC]** *see* Guaifenesin and Dextromethorphan *on page* 710
- ◆ **Robitussin® Night Time Cough & Cold [OTC]** *see* Diphenhydramine and Phenylephrine *on page* 458
- ◆ **Robitussin® Pediatric Cough and Cold Nighttime [OTC]** *see* Chlorpheniramine, Phenylephrine, and Dextromethorphan *on page* 311
- ◆ **Robitussin® Sugar Free Cough [OTC]** *see* Guaifenesin and Dextromethorphan *on page* 710
- ◆ **Rocaltrol®** *see* Calcitriol *on page* 235
- ◆ **Rocephin®** *see* CefTRIAXone *on page* 285

Rocuronium (roe kyoor OH nee um)

U.S. Brand Names Zemuron®

Canadian Brand Names Zemuron®

Index Terms ORG 946; Rocuronium Bromide

Pharmacologic Category Neuromuscular Blocker Agent, Nondepolarizing

Use Adjunct to general anesthesia to facilitate both rapid sequence and routine endotracheal intubation and to relax skeletal muscles during surgery; to facilitate mechanical ventilation in ICU patients

Pregnancy Risk Factor C

Pregnancy Considerations Teratogenic effects were not observed in animal studies. Rocuronium crosses the placenta; umbilical venous plasma levels are ~18% of the maternal concentration. The manufacturer does not recommend use for rapid sequence induction during cesarean section.

Lactation Excretion in breast milk unknown/use caution

Medication Safety Issues

Sound-alike/look-alike issues:

Zemuron® may be confused with Remeron®

High alert medication: The Institute for Safe Medication Practices (ISMP) includes this medication among its list of drugs which have a heightened risk of causing significant patient harm when used in error.

Contraindications Hypersensitivity to rocuronium or any component of the formulation

Warnings/Precautions Use with caution in patients with cardiovascular disease, pulmonary disease, hepatic impairment; ventilation must be supported during neuromuscular blockade; certain clinical conditions may result in potentiation or antagonism of neuromuscular blockade:

Potentiation: Electrolyte abnormalities, severe hyponatremia, severe hypocalcemia, severe hypokalemia, hypermagnesemia, neuromuscular diseases, acidosis, acute intermittent porphyria, renal failure, hepatic failure

Antagonism: Alkalosis, hypercalcemia, demyelinating lesions, peripheral neuropathies, diabetes mellitus

Increased sensitivity in patients with myasthenia gravis, Eaton-Lambert syndrome; resistance in burn patients (>30% of body) for period of 5-70 days postinjury; resistance in patients with muscle trauma, denervation, immobilization, infection. Cross-sensitivity with other neuromuscular-blocking agents may occur; use extreme caution in patients with previous anaphylactic reactions. Use caution in the elderly. Should be administered by adequately trained individuals familiar with its use. Use appropriate anesthesia, pain control, and sedation Immediate treatment (including epinephrine 1:1000) for anaphylactoid and/or hypersensitivity reactions should be available during use. Safety and efficacy have not been established in children <3 months of age

Adverse Reactions

>1%: Cardiovascular: Transient hypotension (<1% to 2%) and hypertension (<1% to 2%)

<1% (Limited to important or life-threatening): Abnormal ECG, acute quadriplegic myopathy syndrome (prolonged use), anaphylaxis, arrhythmia, bronchospasm, edema, hiccups, injection site pruritus, myositis ossificans (prolonged use), nausea, rash, rhonchi, shock, tachycardia, vomiting, wheezing

Drug Interactions

Avoid Concomitant Use There are no known interactions where it is recommended to avoid concomitant use.

Increased Effect/Toxicity

Rocuronium may increase the levels/effects of: Botulinum Toxin Type A; Botulinum Toxin Type B; Cardiac Glycosides; Corticosteroids (Systemic)

The levels/effects of Rocuronium may be increased by: Aminoglycosides; Calcium Channel Blockers; Capreomycin; Colistimethate; Inhalational Anesthetics; Ketorolac; Lincosamide Antibiotics; Lithium; Loop Diuretics; Magnesium Salts; Polymyxin B; Procainamide; QuiNIDine; Tetracycline Derivatives; Vancomycin

Decreased Effect

The levels/effects of Rocuronium may be decreased by: Acetylcholinesterase Inhibitors; Loop Diuretics

Stability Store under refrigeration (2°C to 8°C), do not freeze. When stored at room temperature, it is stable for 60 days; once opened, use within 30 days. Dilutions up to 5 mg/mL in 0.9% sodium chloride, dextrose 5% in water, 5% dextrose in sodium chloride 0.9%, or lactated Ringer's are stable for up to 24 hours at room temperature.

Mechanism of Action Blocks acetylcholine from binding to receptors on motor endplate inhibiting depolarization

Pharmacodynamics/Kinetics

Onset of action: Good intubation conditions in 1-2 minutes; maximum neuromuscular blockade within 4 minutes

Duration: ~30 minutes (with standard doses, increases with higher doses)

Distribution: V_d: ~0.25 L/kg

Protein binding: ~30%

Metabolism: Minimally hepatic; 17-desacetylrocuronium (5% to 10% activity of parent drug)

Half-life elimination: 60-70 minutes

Excretion: Feces (50%); urine (30%)

Dosage Administer I.V.; dose to effect; doses will vary due to interpatient variability; use ideal body weight for obese patients

Children ≥3 months:

Initial: 0.6 mg/kg under halothane anesthesia produce excellent to good intubating conditions within 1 minute and will provide a median time of 41 minutes of clinical relaxation in children 3 months to 1 year of age, and 27 minutes in children 1-12 years

Maintenance: 0.075-0.125 mg/kg administered upon return of T_1 to 25% of control provides clinical relaxation for 7-10 minutes

Adults:

Tracheal intubation: I.V.:

Initial: 0.6 mg/kg is expected to provide approximately 31 minutes of clinical relaxation under opioid/nitrous oxide/oxygen anesthesia with neuromuscular block sufficient for intubation attained in 1-2 minutes; lower doses (0.45 mg/kg) may be used to provide 22 minutes of clinical relaxation with median time to neuromuscular block of 1-3 minutes; maximum blockade is achieved in <4 minutes

Maximum: 0.9-1.2 mg/kg may be given during surgery under opioid/nitrous oxide/oxygen anesthesia without adverse cardiovascular effects and is expected to provide 58-67 minutes of clinical relaxation; neuromuscular blockade sufficient for intubation is achieved in <2 minutes with maximum blockade in <3 minutes

Maintenance: 0.1, 0.15, and 0.2 mg/kg administered at 25% recovery of control T_1 (defined as 3 twitches of train-of-four) provides a median of 12, 17, and 24 minutes of clinical duration under anesthesia

Rapid sequence intubation: 0.6-1.2 mg/kg in appropriately premedicated and anesthetized patients with excellent or good intubating conditions within 2 minutes

Continuous infusion: Initial: 0.01-0.012 mg/kg/minute only after early evidence of spontaneous recovery of neuromuscular function is evident; infusion rates have ranged from 4-16 mcg/kg/minute

ICU: 10 mcg/kg/minute; adjust dose to maintain appropriate degree of neuromuscular blockade (eg, 1 or 2 twitches on train-of-four)

Dosing adjustment in hepatic impairment: Reductions are necessary in patients with liver disease

Administration Administer I.V. only; may be administered undiluted as a bolus injection or via a continuous infusion using an infusion pump

Monitoring Parameters Peripheral nerve stimulator measuring twitch response, heart rate, blood pressure, assisted ventilation status

Additional Information Rocuronium is classified as an intermediate-duration neuromuscular-blocking agent. Do not mix in the same syringe with barbiturates. Rocuronium does not relieve pain or produce sedation.

Dosage Forms Excipient information presented when available (limited, particularly for generics); consult specific product labeling.

Injection, solution, as bromide: 10 mg/mL (5 mL, 10 mL)

Zemuron®: 10 mg/mL (5 mL, 10 mL)

- ◆ **Rocuronium Bromide** *see* Rocuronium *on page 1334*
- ◆ **Rofact™ (Can)** *see* Rifampin *on page 1315*
- ◆ **Roferon®-A [DSC]** *see* Interferon Alfa-2a *on page 799*
- ◆ **Roferon®-A (Can)** *see* Interferon Alfa-2a *on page 799*
- ◆ **Rogaine® (Can)** *see* Minoxidil *on page 1001*
- ◆ **Rogaine® Extra Strength for Men [OTC]** *see* Minoxidil *on page 1001*
- ◆ **Rogaine® for Men [OTC]** *see* Minoxidil *on page 1001*
- ◆ **Rogaine® for Women [OTC]** *see* Minoxidil *on page 1001*
- ◆ **Rogitine® (Can)** *see* Phentolamine *on page 1182*
- ◆ **Rolaids® [OTC]** *see* Calcium Carbonate and Magnesium Hydroxide *on page 239*
- ◆ **Rolaids® Extra Strength [OTC]** *see* Calcium Carbonate and Magnesium Hydroxide *on page 239*
- ◆ **Rolaids® Softchews [OTC]** *see* Calcium Carbonate *on page 238*
- ◆ **Romazicon®** *see* Flumazenil *on page 631*
- ◆ **Romilar® AC** *see* Guaifenesin and Codeine *on page 710*

Romiplostim (roe mi PLOE stim)

U.S. Brand Names Nplate™

Index Terms AMG 531

Pharmacologic Category Colony Stimulating Factor; Thrombopoietic Agent

Use Treatment of thrombocytopenia in patients with chronic immune (idiopathic) thrombocytopenia purpura (ITP) who have had insufficient response to corticosteroids, immune globulin, or splenectomy

Restrictions Approved for use only under a risk management and restricted distribution program, Nplate™ NEXUS (Network of Experts Understanding and Supporting Nplate™ and Patients) program (1-877-675-2831 or www.nplate.com). Prescribers and patients must be registered with the program.

An FDA-approved medication guide is available; distribute to each patient to whom this medication is dispensed.

Pregnancy Risk Factor C

Pregnancy Considerations Adverse effects were observed in animal studies. There are no adequate and well-controlled studies in pregnant women. Use during pregnancy only if the potential benefit to the mother outweighs the potential risk to the fetus. The Nplate™ pregnancy registry has been established to monitor outcomes of women exposed to romiplostim during pregnancy (1-877-675-2831).

Lactation Excretion in breast milk unknown/ not recommended.

Contraindications There are no contraindications listed within the manufacturer's labeling.

Warnings/Precautions May increase the risk for bone marrow reticulin formation or progression. Collagen fibrosis with cytopenias was not observed in clinical trials, although patients receiving romiplostim may be at risk for marrow fibrosis with cytopenias. Onset of new or worsening cellular abnormalities or cytopenias may warrant therapy discontinuation and subsequent bone marrow biopsy. Thromboembolism may occur with treatment; use with caution in patients with a history of cerebrovascular disease. Stimulation of cell surface thrombopoietin (TPO) receptors may increase the risk for hematologic malignancies; may increase the risk for progression of underlying myelodysplastic syndrome (MDS).

Inadequate platelet response may be due to neutralizing antibodies (to romiplostim or TPO) or bone marrow fibrosis. Indicated only when the degree of thrombocytopenia and clinical conditions increase the risk for bleeding; use the lowest dose necessary to achieve and maintain platelet count platelet count ≥50,000/mm^3. Do not use to normalize platelet counts. Discontinue if platelet count does not respond to a level to avoid clinically important bleeding after 4 weeks at the maximum recommended dose. May be used in combination with other therapies for ITP, including corticosteroids, danazol, azathioprine, immune globulin, or Rho(D) immune globulin. Reduce dose of or discontinue ITP medications when platelet count ≥50,000/mm^3.

Upon discontinuation of therapy, thrombocytopenia may worsen. Severity may be greater than pretreatment level. Risk of bleeding is increased, particularly in patients receiving anticoagulants or antiplatelet agents; monitor closely. Rebound thrombocytopenia generally resolves within 14 days.

Use with caution in patients with hepatic and renal impairment (has not been studied). Safety and efficacy have not been established in children.

Adverse Reactions

>10%:

Central nervous system: Headache (35%), fatigue (33%), dizziness (17%), insomnia (16%)

Gastrointestinal: Diarrhea (17%), nausea (13%), abdominal pain (11%)

Neuromuscular & skeletal: Arthralgia (26%), myalgia (14%), back pain (13%), limb pain (13%)

Respiratory: Epistaxis (32%), upper respiratory tract infection (17%)

1% to 10%:

Gastrointestinal: Dyspepsia (7%)

Hematologic: Rebound thrombocytopenia (7%), bone marrow reticulin formation/deposition (4%)

Neuromuscular & skeletal: Shoulder pain (8%), paresthesia (6%)

Miscellaneous: Antibody formation (romiplostim 10%; TPO 5%)

<1% (Limited to important or life-threatening): Thromboembolism

Drug Interactions

Avoid Concomitant Use There are no known interactions where it is recommended to avoid concomitant use.

Increased Effect/Toxicity There are no known significant interactions involving an increase in effect.

Decreased Effect There are no known significant interactions involving a decrease in effect.

Stability Store intact vials refrigerated at 2°C to 8°C (36°F to 46°F); do not freeze. Protect from light. Reconstitute with preservative free SWFI to a final concentration of 500 mcg/mL. Gently invert vial and swirl; do not shake. Reconstituted solution may be stored at room temperature of 25°C (77°F) or refrigerated at 2°C to 8°C (36°F to 46°F) for up to 24 hours. Protect reconstituted solution from light.

Mechanism of Action Thrombopoietin (TPO) peptide mimetic which increases platelet counts in ITP by binding to and activating the human TPO receptor.

Pharmacodynamics/Kinetics

Onset of action: Platelet count increase: SubQ: 4-9 days; Peak platelet count increase: Days 12-16

Duration: Platelet counts return to baseline by day 28

Absorption: SubQ: Slow

Half-life elimination: Median: 3.5 days (range: 1-34 days)

Time to peak, plasma: SubQ: Median: 14 hours (range: 7-50 hours)

Dosage Note: Initial dose is based on actual body weight. Discontinue if platelet count does not respond to a level that avoids clinically important bleeding after 4 weeks at the maximum recommended dose.

SubQ: Adults: ITP: Initial: 1 mcg/kg once weekly; adjust dose by 1 mcg/kg/week to achieve platelet count ≥50,000/mm^3 and to reduce the risk of bleeding; Maximum: 10 mcg/kg (median dose needed to achieve response in clinical trials: 2 mcg/kg)

Dosage adjustment recommendations:

Platelet count <50,000/mm^3: Increase dose by 1 mcg/kg

Platelet count >200,000/mm^3 for 2 consecutive weeks: Reduce dose by 1 mcg/kg

Platelet count >400,000/mm^3: Withhold dose; assess platelet count weekly; when platelet count <200,000/mm^3, resume with the dose reduced by 1 mcg/kg

Dietary Considerations Nplate™ 250 mcg vial contains sucrose 15 mg and 500 mcg vial contains sucrose 25 mg.

Administration Administer SubQ. Administration volume may be small; use appropriate syringe (with graduations to 0.01 mL) for administration.

Monitoring Parameters CBC with differential and platelets (baseline, during treatment [weekly until platelet response stable for 4 weeks then monthly] and weekly for at least 2 weeks following completion of treatment)

Evaluate for neutralizing antibodies in patients with inadequate response (blood samples may be submitted to Amgen for assay [1-800-772-6436]).

Reference Range Target platelet count of 50,000-200,000/mm^3; platelet life span: 8-11 days

Dosage Forms Excipient information presented when available (limited, particularly for generics); consult specific product labeling.

Injection, powder for reconstitution:

Nplate™: 250 mcg [contains sucrose 15 mg/vial]; 500 mcg [contains sucrose 25 mg/vial]

- **Romycin®** *see* Erythromycin *on page 544*
- **Rondec®** *see* Chlorpheniramine and Phenylephrine *on page 309*
- **Rondec®-DM** *see* Chlorpheniramine, Phenylephrine, and Dextromethorphan *on page 311*

Ropinirole (roe PIN i role)

U.S. Brand Names Requip®; Requip® XL™

Canadian Brand Names Requip®

Index Terms Ropinirole Hydrochloride

Pharmacologic Category Anti-Parkinson's Agent, Dopamine Agonist

Additional Appendix Information

Antiparkinsonian Agents *on page 1643*

Use Treatment of idiopathic Parkinson's disease; in patients with early Parkinson's disease who were not receiving concomitant levodopa therapy as well as in patients with advanced disease on concomitant levodopa; treatment of moderate-to-severe primary Restless Legs Syndrome (RLS)

Pregnancy Risk Factor C

Pregnancy Considerations Teratogenic effects have been observed in animal studies. There are no adequate and well-controlled studies in pregnant women; use only if potential benefit outweighs the risk to the fetus.

Lactation Excretion in breast milk unknown/not recommended

Medication Safety Issues

Sound-alike/look-alike issues:

Requip® may be confused with Reglan®

Ropinirole may be confused with ropivacaine

Contraindications Hypersensitivity to ropinirole or any component of the formulation

Warnings/Precautions Syncope, sometimes associated with bradycardia, was observed in association with ropinirole in both early Parkinson's disease (without levodopa) patients and advanced Parkinson's disease (with levodopa) patients. Dopamine agonists appear to impair the systemic regulation of blood pressure resulting in postural hypotension, especially during dose escalation. Parkinson's disease patients appear to have an impaired capacity to respond to a postural challenge; use with caution in patients at risk of hypotension (ie, those receiving antihypertensive drugs) or where transient hypotensive episodes would be poorly tolerated (cardiovascular disease or cerebrovascular disease). Parkinson's patients being treated with dopaminergic agonists ordinarily require careful monitoring for signs and symptoms of postural hypotension, especially during dose escalation, and should be informed of this risk. May cause hallucinations; risk may be increased in the elderly. Use with caution in patients with pre-existing dyskinesia, severe hepatic or renal dysfunction. Avoid use in patients with a major psychotic disorder; may exacerbate psychosis.

Patients treated with ropinirole have reported falling asleep while engaging in activities of daily living; this has been reported to occur without significant warning signs. Monitor for daytime somnolence or pre-existing sleep disorder; caution with concomitant sedating medication; discontinue if significant daytime sleepiness or episodes of falling asleep occur. Patients must be cautioned about performing tasks which require mental alertness (eg, operating machinery or driving). Use with caution in patients receiving other CNS depressants or psychoactive agents. Effects with other sedative drugs or ethanol may be potentiated.

Dopamine agonists have been associated with compulsive behaviors and/or loss of impulse control, which has manifested as pathological gambling, libido increases (hypersexuality), and/or binge eating. Causality has not been established, and controversy exists as to whether this phenomenon is related to the underlying disease, prior behaviors/addictions and/or drug therapy. Dose reduction or discontinuation of therapy has been reported to reverse these behaviors in some, but not all cases.

Some patients treated for RLS may experience worsening of symptoms in the early morning hours (rebound) or an increase and/or spread of daytime symptoms (augmentation); clinical management of these phenomena has not been evaluated in controlled clinical trials. Pathologic degenerative changes were observed in the retinas of albino rats during studies with this agent, but were not observed in the retinas of albino mice or in other species. The significance of these data for humans remains uncertain.

Other dopaminergic agents have been associated with a syndrome resembling neuroleptic malignant syndrome on withdrawal or significant dosage reduction after long-term use. Risk of fibrotic complications (eg, pleural effusion/fibrosis, interstitial lung disease) and melanoma has been reported in patients receiving ropinirole; drug causation has not been established. Safety and efficacy have not been established in children.

Adverse Reactions

Data inclusive of trials in early Parkinson's disease (without levodopa) and Restless Legs Syndrome:

>10%:

Cardiovascular: Syncope (1% to 12%)

Central nervous system: Somnolence (11% to 40%), dizziness (6% to 40%), fatigue (8% to 11%)

Gastrointestinal: Nausea (immediate release: 40% to 60%; extended release: 19%), vomiting (11% to 12%)

Miscellaneous: Viral infection (11%)

1% to 10%:

Cardiovascular: Dependent/leg edema (2% to 7%), orthostasis (1% to 6%), hypertension (5%), chest pain (4%), flushing (3%), palpitation (3%), peripheral

ischemia (2% to 3%), atrial fibrillation (2%), extrasystoles (2%), hypotension (2%), tachycardia (2%)
Central nervous system: Pain (3% to 8%), headache (extended release: 6%), confusion (5%), hallucinations (up to 5%; dose related), hypoesthesia (4%), amnesia (3%), malaise (3%), yawning (3%), concentration impaired (2%), vertigo (2%)
Dermatologic: Hyperhidrosis (3%)
Gastrointestinal: Constipation (≥5%), dyspepsia (4% to 10%), abdominal pain (3% to 7%), xerostomia (3% to 5%), diarrhea (5%), anorexia (4%), flatulence (3%)
Genitourinary: Urinary tract infection (5%), impotence (3%)
Hepatic: Alkaline phosphatase increased (3%)
Neuromuscular & skeletal: Weakness (6%), arthralgia (4%), muscle cramps (3%), paresthesia (3%), hyperkinesia (2%)
Ocular: Abnormal vision (6%), xerophthalmia (2%)
Respiratory: Pharyngitis (6% to 9%), rhinitis (4%), sinusitis (4%), bronchitis (3%), dyspnea (3%), influenza (3%), cough (3%), nasal congestion (2%)
Miscellaneous: Diaphoresis increased (3% to 6%)

Advanced Parkinson's disease (with levodopa):
>10%:
Central nervous system: Dizziness (immediate release: 26%; extended-release: 8%), somnolence (immediate release: 20%, extended release: 7%), headache (17%)
Gastrointestinal: Nausea (immediate release: 30%; extended-release: 11%)
Neuromuscular & skeletal: Dyskinesias (immediate release: 34%; extended-release: 13%; dose related)
1% to 10%:
Cardiovascular: Hypotension (2% to 5%; including orthostatic), peripheral edema (4%), syncope (3%), hypertension (3%; dose related)
Central nervous system: Hallucinations (7% to 10%; dose related), confusion (9%), anxiety (2% to 6%), amnesia (5%), nervousness (5%), pain (5%), vertigo (4%), abnormal dreaming (3%), paresis (3%), aggravated parkinsonism, insomnia
Gastrointestinal: Abdominal pain (6% to 9%), vomiting (7%), constipation (4% to 6%), diarrhea (3% to 5%), xerostomia (2% to 5%), dysphagia (2%), flatulence (2%), salivation increased (2%), weight loss (2%)
Genitourinary: Urinary tract infection (6%), pyuria (2%), urinary incontinence (2%)
Hematologic: Anemia (2%)
Neuromuscular & skeletal: Falls (2% to 10%; dose related), arthralgia (7%), tremor (6%), hypokinesia (5%), paresthesia (5%), arthritis (3%), back pain (3%)
Ocular: Diplopia (2%)
Respiratory: Upper respiratory tract infection (9%), dyspnea (3%)
Miscellaneous: Injury, diaphoresis increased (7%), viral infection, increased drug level (7%)

Other adverse effects (all phase 2/3 trials for Parkinson's disease and Restless Leg Syndrome):
≥1%: Asthma, BUN increased, depression, gastroenteritis, gastrointestinal reflux, irritability, migraine, muscle spasm, myalgia, neck pain, neuralgia, osteoarthritis, pharyngolaryngeal pain, rash, rigors, sleep disorder, tendonitis
<1% (Limited to important or life-threatening): Abnormal coordination, acidosis, agitation, aneurysm, angina, aphasia, behavioral disorders, bradycardia, bundle branch block, cardiac arrest, cardiac failure, cardiac valvulopathy, cardiomegaly, cellulitis, cholecystitis, cholelithiasis, choreoathetosis, colitis, coma, conjunctival hemorrhage, dehydration, diabetes mellitus, diverticulitis, Dupuytren's contracture, dysphonia, electrolyte disturbances, eosinophilia, extrapyramidal symptoms, gangrene, gastrointestinal hemorrhage, gastrointestinal ulceration, glaucoma, goiter, gynecomastia, hematuria, hemiparesis, hemiplegia, hepatitis (ischemic), hyperbilirubinemia, hypercholesterolemia, hyper-/hypothyroidism, hyper-/hypotonia, hypoglycemia, hyponatremia, hyperphosphatemia, hyperuricemia; impulsive/compulsive behaviors (eg, pathological gambling, hypersexuality, binge eating); infections (bacterial, viral or fungal); interstitial lung disease, intestinal obstruction, leukocytosis, leukopenia, limb embolism, liver enzymes increased, lymphadenopathy, lymphedema, lymphocytosis, lymphopenia, menstrual abnormalities, mitral insufficiency, MI, neoplasms (various), pancreatitis, paralysis, peripheral neuropathy, photosensitivity, pleural effusion, pleural fibrosis, proteinuria, psychiatric disorders, pulmonary edema, pulmonary embolism, renal calculus, renal failure (acute), seizure, sepsis, SIADH, skin disorders, stomatitis, stupor, subarachnoid hemorrhage, suicide attempt, SVT, thrombocytopenia, thrombosis, tinnitus, tongue edema, torticollis, urticaria, vagina/uterine hemorrhage, ventricular tachycardia, visual disturbances

Drug Interactions

Metabolism/Transport Effects Substrate of CYP1A2 (major), 3A4 (minor); **Inhibits** CYP1A2 (weak)

Avoid Concomitant Use There are no known interactions where it is recommended to avoid concomitant use.

Increased Effect/Toxicity
The levels/effects of Ropinirole may be increased by: Ciprofloxacin; CYP1A2 Inhibitors (Moderate); CYP1A2 Inhibitors (Strong); Estrogen Derivatives

Decreased Effect
The levels/effects of Ropinirole may be decreased by: Antipsychotics (Atypical); Antipsychotics (Typical); CYP1A2 Inducers (Strong); Metoclopramide

Ethanol/Nutrition/Herb Interactions
Ethanol: Avoid ethanol (may increase CNS depression).
Herb/Nutraceutical: Avoid kava kava, gotu kola, valerian, St John's wort (may increase CNS depression).

Stability Store at controlled room temperature of 20°C to 25°C (68°F to 77°F). Protect from light.

Mechanism of Action Ropinirole has a high relative *in vitro* specificity and full intrinsic activity at the D_2 and D_3 dopamine receptor subtypes, binding with higher affinity to D_3 than to D_2 or D_4 receptor subtypes; relevance of D_3 receptor binding in Parkinson's disease is unknown. Ropinirole has moderate *in vitro* affinity for opioid receptors. Ropinirole and its metabolites have negligible *in vitro* affinity for dopamine D_1, 5-HT_1, 5-HT_2, benzodiazepine, GABA, muscarinic, alpha$_1$-, alpha$_2$-, and beta-adrenoreceptors. Although precise mechanism of action of ropinirole is unknown, it is believed to be due to stimulation of postsynaptic dopamine D_2-type receptors within the caudate putamen in the brain. Ropinirole caused decreases in systolic and diastolic blood pressure at doses >0.25 mg. The mechanism of ropinirole-induced postural hypotension is believed to be due to D_2-mediated blunting of the noradrenergic response to standing and subsequent decrease in peripheral vascular resistance.

Pharmacodynamics/Kinetics
Absorption: Not affected by food
Distribution: V_d: 525 L
Protein binding: 40%
Metabolism: Extensively hepatic via CYP1A2 to inactive metabolites; first-pass effect
Bioavailability: Absolute: 45% to 55%
Half-life elimination: ~6 hours
Time to peak: Immediate release: ~1-2 hours; Extended release: 6-10 hours; T_{max} increased by 2.5-3 hours when drug taken with food
Excretion: Urine (<10% as unchanged drug, 60% as metabolites)
Clearance: Reduced by 15% to 30% in patients >65 years of age

Dosage Oral: Adults:

Parkinson's disease:

Immediate release tablet: The dosage should be increased to achieve a maximum therapeutic effect, balanced against the principal side effects of nausea, dizziness, somnolence and dyskinesia. Recommended starting dose is 0.25 mg 3 times/day; based on individual patient response, the dosage should be titrated with weekly increments as described below:

- Week 1: 0.25 mg 3 times/day; total daily dose: 0.75 mg
- Week 2: 0.5 mg 3 times/day; total daily dose: 1.5 mg
- Week 3: 0.75 mg 3 times/day; total daily dose: 2.25 mg
- Week 4: 1 mg 3 times/day; total daily dose: 3 mg

Note: After week 4, if necessary, daily dosage may be increased by 1.5 mg/day on a weekly basis up to a dose of 9 mg/day, and then by up to 3 mg/day weekly to a total of 24 mg/day

Parkinson's disease discontinuation taper: Ropinirole should be gradually tapered over 7 days as follows: reduce frequency of administration from 3 times daily to twice daily for 4 days, then reduce to once daily for remaining 3 days.

Extended release tablet: Initial: 2 mg once daily for 1-2 weeks, followed by increases of 2 mg/day at weekly or longer intervals based on therapeutic response and tolerability (maximum: 24 mg/day); **Note:** When discontinuing gradually taper over 7 days.

Restless legs syndrome: Immediate release tablets: Initial: 0.25 mg once daily 1-3 hours before bedtime. Dose may be increased after 2 days to 0.5 mg daily, and after 7 days to 1 mg daily. Dose may be further titrated upward in 0.5 mg increments every week until reaching a daily dose of 3 mg during week 6. If symptoms persist or reappear, the daily dose may be increased to a maximum of 4 mg beginning week 7.

Note: Doses up to 4 mg per day may be discontinued without tapering.

Converting from ropinirole immediate release tablets to ropinirole extended-release tablets: Choose a once daily extended-release dose that most closely matches current immediate-release daily dose.

Dosage adjustment in renal impairment: No adjustment needed in patients with moderate renal impairment (Cl_{cr} 30-50 mL/minute); has not been studied in patients with severe impairment.

Removal by hemodialysis is unlikely.

Dosage adjustment in hepatic impairment: Titrate with caution; has not been studied.

Dietary Considerations May be taken with or without food; taking with food may reduce nausea.

Administration May be administered with or without food; taking with food may reduce nausea. Swallow extended-release tablet whole; do not crush, split, or chew.

Monitoring Parameters

Blood pressure (orthostatic); daytime alertness

Additional Information If therapy with a drug known to be a potent inhibitor of CYP1A2 is stopped or started during treatment with ropinirole, adjustment of ropinirole dose may be required. Ropinirole binds to melanin-containing tissues (ie, eyes, skin) in pigmented rats. After a single dose, long-term retention of drug was demonstrated, with a half-life in the eye of 20 days; not known if ropinirole accumulates in these tissues over time.

Dosage Forms Excipient information presented when available (limited, particularly for generics); consult specific product labeling. [DSC] = Discontinued product

Combination package:

Requip® [starter kit; contents per each administration card]: Tablet: 0.25 mg (2s), 0.5 mg (5s), 1 mg (7s) [DSC]

Tablet: 0.25 mg, 0.5 mg, 1 mg, 2 mg, 3 mg, 4 mg, 5 mg

Requip®: 0.25 mg, 0.5 mg, 1 mg, 2 mg, 3 mg, 4 mg, 5 mg

Tablet, extended-release:

Requip® XL™: 2 mg, 4 mg, 8 mg

◆ **Ropinirole Hydrochloride** *see* Ropinirole *on page 1337*

Ropivacaine (roe PIV a kane)

U.S. Brand Names Naropin®

Canadian Brand Names Naropin®

Index Terms Ropivacaine Hydrochloride

Pharmacologic Category Local Anesthetic

Use Local anesthetic for use in surgery, postoperative pain management, and obstetrical procedures when local or regional anesthesia is needed

Pregnancy Risk Factor B

Pregnancy Considerations Teratogenic events were not observed in animal studies. When used for epidural block during labor and delivery, systemically absorbed ropivacaine may cross the placenta, resulting in varying degrees of fetal or neonatal effects (eg, CNS or cardiovascular depression). Fetal or neonatal adverse events include fetal bradycardia (12%), neonatal jaundice (8%), low Apgar scores (3%), fetal distress (2%), neonatal respiratory disorder (3%). Maternal hypotension may also result from systemic absorption. In cases of hypotension, position pregnant woman in left lateral decubitus position to prevent aortocaval compression by the gravid uterus. Epidural anesthesia may prolong the second stage of labor.

Lactation Excretion in breast milk unknown/use caution

Medication Safety Issues

Sound-alike/look-alike issues:

Ropivacaine may be confused with bupivacaine, ropinirole

High alert medication: The Institute for Safe Medication Practices (ISMP) includes this medication (epidural administration) among its list of drug classes which have a heightened risk of causing significant patient harm when used in error.

Contraindications Hypersensitivity to ropivacaine, amide-type local anesthetics (eg, bupivacaine, mepivacaine, lidocaine), or any component of the formulation

Warnings/Precautions Careful and constant monitoring of the patient's state of consciousness should be done following each local anesthetic injection; at such times, restlessness, anxiety, tinnitus, dizziness, blurred vision, tremors, depression, or drowsiness may be early warning signs of CNS toxicity. Treatment is primarily symptomatic and supportive. Intravascular injections should be avoided. Local anesthetics have been associated with rare occurrences of sudden respiratory arrest, seizures, and cardiac arrest. When administering this agent, have ready access to drugs and equipment for resuscitation. Use with caution in patients with liver disease, cardiovascular disease, neurological or psychiatric disorders, and in the elderly or debilitated; these patients may be at greater risk for toxicity. Cardiovascular adverse events (bradycardia, hypotension) may be age-related (more common in patients >61 years of age). Use caution in patients on type III antiarrhythmics (eg, amiodarone); consider ECG monitoring since cardiac effects may be additive. Use cautiously in hypotension, hypovolemia, or heart block. Ropivacaine is not recommended for use in emergency situations where rapid administration is necessary. Safety and efficacy have not been established in pediatric patients.

Adverse Reactions

>10%:

Cardiovascular: Hypotension (dose-related and age-related: 32% to 69%), bradycardia (6% to 20%)

Gastrointestinal: Nausea (11% to 29%), vomiting (7% to 14%)
Neuromuscular & skeletal: Back pain (7% to 16%)
1% to 10%:
Cardiovascular: Hypertension, tachycardia, chest pain (1% to 5%)
Central nervous system: Fever (3% to 9%), headache (5% to 8%), dizziness (3%), chills (2% to 3%), anxiety (1%), lightheadedness
Dermatologic: Pruritus (1% to 5%)
Endocrine & metabolic: Hypokalemia
Genitourinary: Urinary retention (1% to 5%), urinary tract infection (1% to 5%)
Hematologic: Anemia (6%)
Neuromuscular & skeletal: Paresthesia (2% to 6%), hypoesthesia, rigors, circumoral paresthesia
Renal: Oliguria
Respiratory: Dyspnea
Miscellaneous: Shivering
<1% (Limited to important or life-threatening): Accidental I.V. injection (0.2%), angioedema, allergic reaction, apnea (usually associated with epidural block in head/neck region), bronchospasm, cardiac arrest, cardiovascular collapse, dyskinesia, hallucination, hyperthermia, laryngeal edema, myocardial depression, MI, rash, seizure, syncope, tinnitus, urticaria, ventricular arrhythmia

Drug Interactions

Metabolism/Transport Effects Substrate of CYP1A2 (major), 2B6 (minor), 2D6 (minor), 3A4 (minor; may be major in cases of 1A2 inhibition/deficiency)

Avoid Concomitant Use There are no known interactions where it is recommended to avoid concomitant use.

Increased Effect/Toxicity

The levels/effects of Ropivacaine may be increased by: Ciprofloxacin; CYP1A2 Inhibitors (Moderate); CYP1A2 Inhibitors (Strong); Fluvoxamine; Fospropofol; Propofol

Decreased Effect There are no known significant interactions involving a decrease in effect.

Stability Store at 20°C to 25°C (68°F to 77°F). Infusions should be discarded after 24 hours.

Mechanism of Action Blocks both the initiation and conduction of nerve impulses by decreasing the neuronal membrane's permeability to sodium ions, which results in inhibition of depolarization with resultant blockade of conduction

Pharmacodynamics/Kinetics

Onset of action: Anesthesia (route dependent): 3-15 minutes
Duration (dose and route dependent): 3-15 hours
Metabolism: Hepatic, via CYP1A2 to metabolites
Half-life elimination: Epidural: 5-7 hours
Excretion: Urine (86% as metabolites)

Dosage Dose varies with procedure, onset and depth of anesthesia desired, vascularity of tissues, duration of anesthesia, and condition of patient: Adults:

Surgical anesthesia:
Lumbar epidural: 15-30 mL of 0.5% to 1% solution
Lumbar epidural block for cesarean section:
20-30 mL dose of 0.5% solution
15-20 mL dose of 0.75% solution
Thoracic epidural block: 5-15 mL dose of 0.5% to 0.75% solution
Major nerve block:
35-50 mL dose of 0.5% solution (175-250 mg)
10-40 mL dose of 0.75% solution (75-300 mg)
Field block: 1-40 mL dose of 0.5% solution (5-200 mg)
Labor pain management: Lumbar epidural: Initial: 10-20 mL 0.2% solution; continuous infusion dose: 6-14 mL/hour of 0.2% solution with incremental injections of 10-15 mL/hour of 0.2% solution
Postoperative pain management:
Lumbar or thoracic epidural: Continuous infusion dose: 6-14 mL/hour of 0.2% solution
Infiltration/minor nerve block:
1-100 mL dose of 0.2% solution
1-40 mL dose of 0.5% solution

Administration Administered via local infiltration, epidural block and epidural infusion, or intermittent bolus

Monitoring Parameters Heart rate, blood pressure, ECG monitoring (if used with antiarrhythmics)

Dosage Forms Excipient information presented when available (limited, particularly for generics); consult specific product labeling.

Infusion, as hydrochloride:
Naropin®: 2 mg/mL (100 mL, 200 mL)
Injection, solution, as hydrochloride [preservative free]:
Naropin®: 2 mg/mL (10 mL, 20 mL); 5 mg/mL (20 mL, 30 mL); 7.5 mg/mL (20 mL); 10 mg/mL (10 mL, 20 mL)

◆ **Ropivacaine Hydrochloride** *see* Ropivacaine *on page 1339*

◆ **Rosac®** *see* Sulfur and Sulfacetamide *on page 1411*

◆ **Rosanil®** *see* Sulfur and Sulfacetamide *on page 1411*

Rosiglitazone (roh si GLI ta zone)

U.S. Brand Names Avandia®

Canadian Brand Names Avandia®

Pharmacologic Category Antidiabetic Agent, Thiazolidinedione

Additional Appendix Information

Diabetes Mellitus Management, Adults *on page 1801*

Use Type 2 diabetes mellitus (noninsulin dependent, NIDDM):

Monotherapy: Improve glycemic control as an adjunct to diet and exercise
Note: Canadian labeling approves use as monotherapy only when metformin is contraindicated or not tolerated.
Combination therapy: **Note:** Use when diet, exercise, and a single agent do not result in adequate glycemic control.
U.S. labeling: In combination with a sulfonylurea, metformin, or sulfonylurea plus metformin
Canadian labeling: In combination with metformin; in combination with a sulfonylurea only when metformin use is contraindicated or not tolerated

Unlabeled/Investigational Use Polycystic ovary syndrome (PCOS)

Restrictions An FDA-approved medication guide must be distributed when dispensing an outpatient prescription (new or refill) where this medication is to be used without direct supervision of a healthcare provider. Medication guides are available at http://www.fda.gov/cder/Offices/ODS/medication_guides.htm.

Pregnancy Risk Factor C

Pregnancy Considerations Rosiglitazone is classified as pregnancy category C due to adverse effects observed in initial animal studies. Rosiglitazone has been found to cross the placenta during the first trimester of pregnancy. Inadvertent use early in pregnancy has not shown adverse fetal effects although in the majority of cases, the medication was stopped as soon as pregnancy was detected. Thiazolidinediones may cause ovulation in anovulatory premenopausal women, increasing the risk of pregnancy; adequate contraception in premenopausal women is recommended. Maternal hyperglycemia can be associated with adverse effects in the fetus, including macrosomia, neonatal hyperglycemia, and hyperbilirubinemia; the risk of congenital malformations is increased when the Hb A_{1c} is above the normal range. Diabetes can also be associated with adverse effects in the mother. Poorly-treated diabetes may cause end-organ damage that may in turn negatively affect obstetric outcomes.

Physiologic glucose levels should be maintained prior to and during pregnancy to decrease the risk of adverse events in the mother and the fetus. Until additional safety and efficacy data are obtained, the use of oral agents is generally not recommended as routine management of GDM or type 2 diabetes mellitus during pregnancy. Insulin is the drug of choice for the control of diabetes mellitus during pregnancy.

Lactation Excretion in breast milk unknown/not recommended

Medication Safety Issues

Sound-alike/look-alike issues:

Avandia® may be confused with Avalide®, Coumadin®, Prandin®

International issues:

Avandia® may be confused with Avanza® which is a brand name for mirtazapine in Australia

Contraindications

U.S. labeling: NYHA Class III/IV heart failure (initiation of therapy)

Canadian labeling: Hypersensitivity to rosiglitazone or any component of the formulation; any stage of heart failure (eg, NYHA Class I, II, III, IV); serious hepatic impairment; pregnancy

Warnings/Precautions [U.S. Boxed Warning]: Thiazolidinediones, including rosiglitazone, may cause or exacerbate congestive heart failure; closely monitor for signs/symptoms of congestive heart failure (eg, rapid weight gain, dyspnea, edema), particularly after initiation or dose increases. Not recommended for use in any patient with symptomatic heart failure. In the U.S., initiation of therapy is contraindicated in patients with NYHA class III or IV heart failure; in Canada use is contraindicated in patients with any stage of heart failure (NYHA Class I, II, III, IV). Use with caution in patients with edema; may increase plasma volume and/or cause fluid retention, leading to heart failure. Dose-related weight gain observed with use; mechanism unknown but likely associated with fluid retention and fat accumulation. Use may also be associated with an increased risk of angina and MI. Use caution in patients at risk for cardiovascular events and monitor closely. Discontinue if any deterioration in cardiac status occurs.

Should not be used in diabetic ketoacidosis. Mechanism requires the presence of insulin; therefore, use in type 1 diabetes (insulin dependent, IDDM) is not recommended. Combination therapy with other hypoglycemic agents may increase risk for hypoglycemic events; dose reduction with the concomitant agent may be warranted. Concomitant use with nitrates is not recommended due to increased risk of myocardial ischemia. Avoid use with insulin due to an increased risk of edema, congestive heart failure, and myocardial ischemic events.

Use with caution in patients with elevated transaminases (AST or ALT); do not initiate in patients with active liver disease or ALT >2.5 times ULN at baseline; evaluate patients with ALT ≤2.5 times ULN at baseline or during therapy for cause of enzyme elevation; during therapy, if ALT >3 times ULN, reevaluate levels promptly and discontinue if elevation persists or if jaundice occurs at any time during use. Idiosyncratic hepatotoxicity has been reported with another thiazolidinedione agent (troglitazone); avoid use in patients who previously experienced jaundice during troglitazone therapy. Monitoring should include periodic determinations of liver function. Increased incidence of bone fractures in females treated with rosiglitazone observed during analysis of long-term trial; majority of fractures occurred in the upper arm, hand, and foot (differing from the hip or spine fractures usually associated with postmenopausal osteoporosis). May decrease hemoglobin/hematocrit and/or WBC count (slight); effects may be related to increased plasma volume and/or dose related; use with caution in patients with anemia.

Rosiglitazone has been associated with new onset and/or worsening of macular edema in patients with diabetes. Rosiglitazone should be used with caution in patients with a pre-existing macular edema or diabetic retinopathy. Discontinuation of rosiglitazone should be considered in any patient who reports visual deterioration. In addition, ophthalmological consultation should be initiated in these patients. Use with caution in premenopausal, anovulatory women; may result in resumption of ovulation, increasing the risk of pregnancy. Safety and efficacy in pediatric patients have not been established.

Additional Canadian warnings (not included in U.S. labeling): If glycemic control is inadequate, rosiglitazone may be added to metformin or a sulfonylurea (if metformin use is contraindicated or not tolerated); use of triple therapy (rosiglitazone in combination with both metformin and a sulfonylurea) is not indicated due to increased risks of heart failure and fluid retention.

Adverse Reactions Note: The rate of certain adverse reactions (eg, anemia, edema, hypoglycemia) may be higher with some combination therapies.

>10%: Endocrine & metabolic: HDL-cholesterol increased, LDL-cholesterol increased, total cholesterol increased, weight gain

1% to 10%:

Cardiovascular: Edema (5%), hypertension (4%); heart failure/CHF (up to 2% to 3% in patients receiving insulin; incidence likely higher in patients with pre-existing HF; myocardial ischemia (3%; incidence likely higher in patients with preexisting CAD)

Central nervous system: Headache (6%)

Endocrine & metabolic: Hypoglycemia (1% to 3%; combination therapy with insulin: 12% to 14%)

Gastrointestinal: Diarrhea (3%)

Hematologic: Anemia (2%)

Neuromuscular & skeletal: Fractures (up to 9%; incidence greater in females; usually upper arm, hand, or foot), arthralgia (5%), back pain (4% to 5%)

Respiratory: Upper respiratory tract infection (4% to 10%), nasopharyngitis (6%)

Miscellaneous: Injury (8%)

<1% (Limited to important or life-threatening): Anaphylaxis, angina, angioedema, bilirubin increased, blurred vision, cardiac arrest, dyspnea, coronary artery disease, coronary thrombosis, hematocrit decreased, hemoglobin decreased, hepatic failure, hepatitis, HDL-cholesterol decreased, jaundice (reversible), macular edema, MI, pleural effusion, pruritus, pulmonary edema, rash, Stevens-Johnson syndrome, thrombocytopenia, transaminases increased, urticaria, visual acuity decreased, weight gain (rapid, excessive; usually due to fluid accumulation), WBC count decreased

Note: Rare cases of hepatocellular injury have been reported in men in their 60s within 2-3 weeks after initiation of rosiglitazone therapy. LFTs in these patients revealed severe hepatocellular injury which responded with rapid improvement of liver function and resolution of symptoms upon discontinuation of rosiglitazone. Patients were also receiving other potentially hepatotoxic medications (Al-Salman, 2000; Freid, 2000).

Drug Interactions

Metabolism/Transport Effects Substrate of CYP2C8 (major), 2C9 (minor); **Inhibits** CYP2C8 (moderate), 2C9 (weak), 2C19 (weak), 2D6 (weak)

Avoid Concomitant Use There are no known interactions where it is recommended to avoid concomitant use.

Increased Effect/Toxicity

Rosiglitazone may increase the levels/effects of: CYP2C8 Substrates (High risk)

The levels/effects of Rosiglitazone may be increased by: CYP2C8 Inhibitors (Moderate); CYP2C8 Inhibitors (Strong); Gemfibrozil; Herbs (Hypoglycemic Properties); Insulin; Pegvisomant; Pregabalin; Trimethoprim; Vasodilators (Organic Nitrates)

Decreased Effect

The levels/effects of Rosiglitazone may be decreased by: Bile Acid Sequestrants; Corticosteroids (Orally Inhaled); Corticosteroids (Systemic); CYP2C8 Inducers (Highly Effective); Luteinizing Hormone-Releasing Hormone Analogs; Rifampin; Somatropin

Ethanol/Nutrition/Herb Interactions

Ethanol: Avoid ethanol (may cause hypoglycemia).

Food: Peak concentrations are lower by 28% and delayed when administered with food, but these effects are not believed to be clinically significant.

Herb/Nutraceutical: Avoid alfalfa, aloe, bilberry, bitter melon, burdock, celery, damiana, fenugreek, garcinia, garlic, ginger, ginseng (American), gymnema, marshmallow, stinging nettle (may cause hypoglycemia).

Stability Store at 15°C to 30°C (59°F to 86°F). Protect from light.

Mechanism of Action Thiazolidinedione antidiabetic agent that lowers blood glucose by improving target cell response to insulin, without increasing pancreatic insulin secretion. It has a mechanism of action that is dependent on the presence of insulin for activity. Rosiglitazone is an agonist for peroxisome proliferator-activated receptor-gamma (PPARgamma). Activation of nuclear PPAR-gamma receptors influences the production of a number of gene products involved in glucose and lipid metabolism. Thiazolidinedione antidiabetic agent that lowers blood glucose by improving target cell response to insulin, without increasing pancreatic insulin secretion. It has a mechanism of action that is dependent on the presence of insulin for activity. PPARgamma is abundant in the cells within the renal collecting tubules; fluid retention results from stimulation by thiazolidinediones which increases sodium reabsorption.

Pharmacodynamics/Kinetics

Onset of action: Delayed; Maximum effect: Up to 12 weeks

Distribution: V_{dss} (apparent): 17.6 L

Protein binding: 99.8%; primarily albumin

Metabolism: Hepatic (99%) via CYP2C8; minor metabolism via CYP2C9

Bioavailability: 99%

Half-life elimination: 3-4 hours

Time to peak, plasma: 1 hour; delayed with food

Excretion: Urine (64%) and feces (23%) as metabolites

Dosage Oral:

Adults: **Note:** All patients should be initiated at the lowest recommended dose.

Monotherapy: Initial: 4 mg daily as a single daily dose or in divided doses twice daily. If response is inadequate after 8-12 weeks of treatment, the dosage may be increased to 8 mg daily as a single daily dose or in divided doses twice daily. In clinical trials, the 4 mg twice-daily regimen resulted in the greatest reduction in fasting plasma glucose and Hb A_{1c}.

Combination therapy: When adding rosiglitazone to existing therapy, continue current dose(s) of previous agents:

U.S. labeling: With sulfonylureas or metformin (or sulfonylurea plus metformin): Initial: 4 mg daily as a single daily dose or in divided doses twice daily. If response is inadequate after 8-12 weeks of treatment, the dosage may be increased to 8 mg daily as a single daily dose or in divided doses twice daily. Reduce dose of sulfonylurea if hypoglycemia occurs. It is unlikely that the dose of metformin will need to be reduced due to hypoglycemia.

Canadian labeling:

With metformin: Initial: 4 mg daily as a single daily dose or in divided doses twice daily. If response is inadequate after 8-12 weeks of treatment, the dosage may be increased to 8 mg daily as a single daily dose or in divided doses twice daily.

With a sulfonylurea: 4 mg daily as a single daily dose or in divided doses twice daily. Dose should not exceed 4 mg daily when using in combination with a sulfonylurea. Reduce dose of sulfonylurea if hypoglycemia occurs.

Elderly: No dosage adjustment is recommended

Dosage adjustment in renal impairment: No dosage adjustment is required

Dosage comment in hepatic impairment: Clearance is significantly lower in hepatic impairment. Therapy should not be initiated if the patient exhibits active liver disease or increased transaminases (ALT >2.5 times the upper limit of normal) at baseline.

Dietary Considerations Management of type 2 diabetes mellitus (noninsulin dependent, NIDDM) should include diet control. May be taken without regard to meals.

Monitoring Parameters Hemoglobin A_{1c}, fasting serum glucose; signs and symptoms of fluid retention or heart failure; liver enzymes (prior to initiation of therapy, then periodically thereafter); ophthalmic exams. Evaluate patients with ALT ≤2.5 times ULN at baseline or during therapy for cause of enzyme elevation. Patients with an elevation in ALT >3 times ULN should be rechecked as soon as possible. If the ALT levels remain >3 times ULN, therapy with rosiglitazone should be discontinued.

Reference Range Recommendations for glycemic control in adults with diabetes:

Hb A_{1c}: <7%

Preprandial capillary plasma glucose: 70-130 mg/dL

Peak postprandial capillary blood glucose: <180 mg/dL

Dosage Forms Excipient information presented when available (limited, particularly for generics); consult specific product labeling.

Tablet:

Avandia®: 2 mg, 4 mg, 8 mg

Rosiglitazone and Glimepiride

(roh si GLI ta zone & GLYE me pye ride)

U.S. Brand Names Avandaryl®

Index Terms Glimepiride and Rosiglitazone Maleate

Pharmacologic Category Antidiabetic Agent, Sulfonylurea; Antidiabetic Agent, Thiazolidinedione

Use Management of type 2 diabetes mellitus (noninsulin dependent, NIDDM) as an adjunct to diet and exercise

Restrictions An FDA-approved medication guide must be distributed when dispensing an outpatient prescription (new or refill) where this medication is to be used without direct supervision of a healthcare provider. Medication guides are available at http://www.fda.gov/cder/Offices/ODS/medication_guides.htm.

Pregnancy Risk Factor C

Medication Safety Issues

High alert medication: The Institute for Safe Medication Practices (ISMP) includes this medication among its list of drugs which have a heightened risk of causing significant patient harm when used in error.

Dosage Oral: Adults: Type 2 diabetes mellitus:

Initial: Rosiglitazone 4 mg and glimepiride 1 mg once daily **or** rosiglitazone 4 mg and glimepiride 2 mg once daily (for patients previously treated with sulfonylurea or thiazolidinedione monotherapy)

Patients switching from combination rosiglitazone and glimepiride as separate tablets: Use current dose

Titration:

Dose adjustment in patients previously on sulfonylurea monotherapy: May take 2 weeks to observe decreased blood glucose and 2-3 months to see full effects of rosiglitazone component. If not adequately controlled after 8-12 weeks, increase daily dose of rosiglitazone component.

Dose adjustment in patients previously on thiazolidinedione monotherapy: If not adequately controlled after 1-2 weeks, increase daily dose of glimepiride component in ≤2 mg increments in 1-2 week intervals.

Maximum dose:

U.S. labeling: Rosiglitazone 8 mg and glimepiride 4 mg once daily

Canadian labeling: Rosiglitazone 4 mg and glimepiride 4 mg once daily

Elderly: Rosiglitazone 4 mg and glimepiride 1 mg once daily; carefully titrate dose.

Dosage adjustment in renal impairment: Rosiglitazone 4 mg and glimepiride 1 mg once daily; carefully titrate dose.

Dosage adjustment in hepatic impairment: Rosiglitazone 4 mg and glimepiride 1 mg once daily; carefully titrate dose.

ALT ≤2.5 times ULN: Use with caution

ALT >2.5 times ULN: Do not initiate therapy

ALT >3 times ULN or jaundice: Discontinue

Additional Information Complete prescribing information for this medication should be consulted for additional detail.

Dosage Forms Excipient information presented when available (limited, particularly for generics); consult specific product labeling.

Tablet:

Avandaryl® 4 mg/1 mg: Rosiglitazone maleate 4 mg and glimepiride 1 mg

Avandaryl® 4 mg/2 mg: Rosiglitazone maleate 4 mg and glimepiride 2 mg

Avandaryl® 4 mg/4 mg: Rosiglitazone maleate 4 mg and glimepiride 4 mg

Avandaryl® 8 mg/2 mg: Rosiglitazone maleate 8 mg and glimepiride 2 mg

Avandaryl® 8 mg/4 mg: Rosiglitazone maleate 8 mg and glimepiride 4 mg

Rosiglitazone and Metformin

(roh si GLI ta zone & met FOR min)

U.S. Brand Names Avandamet®

Canadian Brand Names Avandamet®

Index Terms Metformin and Rosiglitazone; Metformin Hydrochloride and Rosiglitazone Maleate; Rosiglitazone Maleate and Metformin Hydrochloride

Pharmacologic Category Antidiabetic Agent, Biguanide; Antidiabetic Agent, Thiazolidinedione

Use Management of type 2 diabetes mellitus (noninsulin dependent, NIDDM) as an adjunct to diet and exercise in patients where dual rosiglitazone and metformin therapy is appropriate

Restrictions An FDA-approved medication guide must be distributed when dispensing an outpatient prescription (new or refill) where this medication is to be used without direct supervision of a healthcare provider. Medication guides are available at http://www.fda.gov/cder/Offices/ODS/medication_guides.htm.

Pregnancy Risk Factor C

Medication Safety Issues

Sound-alike/look-alike issues:

Avandamet® may be confused with Anzemet®

Dosage Oral:

Adults: Type 2 diabetes mellitus: Daily dose should be divided and given with meals:

First-line therapy (drug-naive patients): Initial: Rosiglitazone 2 mg and metformin 500 mg once or twice daily; may increase by 2 mg/500 mg per day after 4 weeks to a maximum of 8 mg/2000 mg per day.

Second-line therapy:

Patients inadequately controlled on **metformin alone**: Initial dose: Rosiglitazone 4 mg/day plus current dose of metformin

Patients inadequately controlled on **rosiglitazone alone**: Initial dose: Metformin 1000 mg/day plus current dose of rosiglitazone

Note: When switching from combination rosiglitazone and metformin as separate tablets: Use current dose

Dose adjustment: Doses may be increased as increments of rosiglitazone 4 mg and/or metformin 500 mg, up to the maximum dose; doses should be titrated gradually.

After a change in the metformin dosage, titration can be done after 1-2 weeks

After a change in the rosiglitazone dosage, titration can be done after 8-12 weeks

Maximum dose: Rosiglitazone 8 mg/metformin 2000 mg daily

Elderly: The initial and maintenance dosing should be conservative, due to the potential for decreased renal function (monitor). Generally, elderly patients should not be titrated to the maximum; do not use in patients ≥80 years unless normal renal function has been established.

Dosage adjustment in renal impairment: Do not use with renal disease or renal dysfunction (serum creatinine ≥1.5 mg/dL in males or ≥1.4 mg/dL in females or abnormal clearance)

Dosage adjustment in hepatic impairment: Do not initiate therapy with active liver disease or ALT >2.5 times the upper limit of normal

Additional Information Complete prescribing information for this medication should be consulted for additional detail.

Dosage Forms Excipient information presented when available (limited, particularly for generics); consult specific product labeling.

Tablet:

Avandamet®: 2/500: Rosiglitazone 2 mg and metformin hydrochloride 500 mg

Avandamet®: 4/500: Rosiglitazone 4 mg and metformin hydrochloride 500 mg

Avandamet®: 2/1000: Rosiglitazone 2 mg and metformin hydrochloride 1000 mg

Avandamet®: 4/1000: Rosiglitazone 4 mg and metformin hydrochloride 1000 mg

◆ **Rosiglitazone Maleate and Metformin Hydrochloride** *see* Rosiglitazone and Metformin *on page* 1343

◆ **Rosula®** *see* Sulfur and Sulfacetamide *on page* 1411

◆ **Rosula® Clarifying** *see* Sulfur and Sulfacetamide *on page* 1411

◆ **Rosula® NS** *see* Sulfacetamide *on page* 1405

Rosuvastatin (roe soo va STAT in)

U.S. Brand Names Crestor®

Canadian Brand Names Crestor®

Index Terms Rosuvastatin Calcium

Pharmacologic Category Antilipemic Agent, HMG-CoA Reductase Inhibitor

Additional Appendix Information

Hyperlipidemia Management *on page* 1815

Lipid-Lowering Agents *on page* 1661

Use Used with dietary therapy for hyperlipidemias to reduce elevations in total cholesterol (TC), LDL-C, apolipoprotein B, nonHDL-C, and triglycerides (TG) in patients with primary hypercholesterolemia (elevations of 1 or more components are present in Fredrickson type IIa, IIb, and IV hyperlipidemias); treatment of primary dysbetalipoproteinemia (Fredrickson type III hyperlipidemia); treatment of homozygous familial hypercholesterolemia (FH); to slow progression of atherosclerosis as an adjunct to diet to lower TC and LDL-C

Pregnancy Risk Factor X

Pregnancy Considerations Cholesterol biosynthesis may be important in fetal development. Contraindicated in pregnancy. Administer to women of childbearing potential only when conception is highly unlikely and patients have been informed of potential hazards.

Lactation Excretion in breast milk unknown/contraindicated

Contraindications Hypersensitivity to rosuvastatin or any component of the formulation; active liver disease; unexplained persistent elevations of serum transaminases (>3 times ULN); pregnancy; breast-feeding

Warnings/Precautions Secondary causes of hyperlipidemia should be ruled out prior to therapy. Liver function must be monitored by periodic laboratory assessment. Use with caution in patients who consume large amounts of ethanol or have a history of liver disease. Rhabdomyolysis with acute renal failure has occurred. Discontinue in any patient in which CPK levels are markedly elevated (>10 times ULN) or if myopathy is suspected/diagnosed. An increased incidence of rosuvastatin-associated myopathy has been reported during concomitant therapy with fibric acid derivatives, niacin, cyclosporine, and lopinavir/ritonavir, and in certain subgroups of the Asian population. Monitor closely if used with other drugs associated with myopathy (eg, colchicine). Risk is also elevated at higher dosages of rosuvastatin. Patients should be instructed to report unexplained muscle pain, tenderness, or weakness, particularly if associated with fever and/or malaise. Use caution in patients predisposed to myopathy (eg, renal failure, advanced age, inadequately treated hypothyroidism). Temporarily withhold in patients experiencing an acute or serious condition predisposing to renal failure secondary to rhabdomyolysis (sepsis, hypotension, major surgery, trauma, severe metabolic or endocrine or electrolyte disorders, uncontrolled seizures). Based upon current evidence, HMG-CoA reductase inhibitor therapy should be continued in the perioperative period unless risk outweighs cardioprotective benefit. Safety and efficacy have not been established in children (limited experience with homozygous FH in patients >8 years of age).

Adverse Reactions

>10%: Neuromuscular & skeletal: Myalgia (3% to 13%)

2% to 10%:

- Central nervous system: Headache (6%), dizziness (4%)
- Gastrointestinal: Nausea (3%), abdominal pain (2%), constipation (2%)
- Hepatic: ALT increased (2%; >3 times ULN)
- Neuromuscular & skeletal: Arthralgia (10%), CPK increased (3%), weakness (3%)

<2%, postmarketing, and/or case reports: Alkaline phosphatase increased, AST increased, bilirubin increased, GGT increased, hematuria (microscopic), hepatitis, hyperglycemia; hypersensitivity reactions (including angioedema, pruritis, rash, urticaria); memory deficits, myoglobinuria, myositis, myopathy, pancreatitis, proteinuria (dose related), renal failure, rhabdomyolysis, thyroid function test abnormalities

Adverse reactions reported with other HMG-CoA reductase inhibitors include a hypersensitivity syndrome (symptoms may include anaphylaxis, angioedema, arthralgia, erythema multiforme, eosinophilia, hemolytic anemia, lupus syndrome, photosensitivity, polymyalgia rheumatica, positive ANA, purpura, Stevens-Johnson syndrome, toxic epidermal necrolysis, urticaria, vasculitis)

Drug Interactions

Metabolism/Transport Effects Substrate (minor) of CYP2C9, 3A4

Avoid Concomitant Use There are no known interactions where it is recommended to avoid concomitant use.

Increased Effect/Toxicity

Rosuvastatin may increase the levels/effects of: DAPTOmycin; Vitamin K Antagonists

The levels/effects of Rosuvastatin may be increased by: Amiodarone; Colchicine; CycloSPORINE; Eltrombopag; Fenofibrate; Fenofibric Acid; Gemfibrozil; Niacin; Niacinamide; Protease Inhibitors

Decreased Effect There are no known significant interactions involving a decrease in effect.

Ethanol/Nutrition/Herb Interactions

Ethanol: Avoid excessive ethanol consumption (due to potential hepatic effects).

Food: Red yeast rice contains an estimated 2.4 mg lovastatin per 600 mg rice.

Stability Store between 20°C and 25°C (68°F to 77°F). Protect from moisture.

Mechanism of Action Inhibitor of 3-hydroxy-3-methylglutaryl coenzyme A (HMG-CoA) reductase, the rate-limiting enzyme in cholesterol synthesis (reduces the production of mevalonic acid from HMG-CoA); this then results in a compensatory increase in the expression of LDL receptors on hepatocyte membranes and a stimulation of LDL catabolism

Pharmacodynamics/Kinetics

Onset of action: Within 1 week; maximal at 4 weeks

Distribution: V_d: 134 L

Protein binding: 88%

Metabolism: Hepatic (10%), via CYP2C9 (1 active metabolite identified)

Bioavailability: 20% (high first-pass extraction by liver)

Asian patients have been noted to have increased bioavailability.

Half-life elimination: 19 hours

Time to peak, plasma: 3-5 hours

Excretion: Feces (90%), primarily as unchanged drug

Dosage Adults: Oral:

Hyperlipidemia, mixed dyslipidemia, hypertriglyceridemia, primary dysbetalipoproteinemia, slowing progression of atherosclerosis:

Initial dose:

General dosing: 10 mg once daily; 20 mg once daily may be used in patients with severe hyperlipidemia (LDL >190 mg/dL) and aggressive lipid targets

Conservative dosing: Patients requiring less aggressive treatment or predisposed to myopathy (including patients of Asian descent): 5 mg once daily

Titration: After 2 weeks, may be increased by 5-10 mg once daily; dosing range: 5-40 mg/day (maximum dose: 40 mg once daily)

Note: The 40 mg dose should be reserved for patients who have not achieved goal cholesterol levels on a dose of 20 mg/day, including patients switched from another HMG-CoA reductase inhibitor.

Homozygous familial hypercholesterolemia (FH): Initial: 20 mg once daily (maximum dose: 40 mg/day)

Dosage adjustment with concomitant medications:

Cyclosporine: Rosuvastatin dose should not exceed 5 mg/day

Gemfibrozil or lopinavir/ritonavir: Rosuvastatin dose should not exceed 10 mg/day

Dosage adjustment for hematuria and/or persistent, unexplained proteinuria while on 40 mg/day: Reduce dose and evaluate causes

Dosage adjustment in renal impairment:

Mild-to-moderate impairment: No dosage adjustment required.

Cl_{cr} <30 mL/minute/1.73 m^2: Initial: 5 mg/day; do not exceed 10 mg once daily

Dietary Considerations May be taken with or without food. Red yeast rice contains an estimated 2.4 mg lovastatin per 600 mg rice.

Administration May be administered with or without food.

Monitoring Parameters Total cholesterol, LDL, and HDL cholesterol within 2-4 weeks of treatment initiation or dose change; liver function tests should be determined at baseline (prior to initiation), 3 months following initiation, 3 months after any increase in dose, and periodically thereafter (eg, semiannually); baseline CPK (recheck CPK in any patient with symptoms suggestive of myopathy)

Dosage Forms Excipient information presented when available (limited, particularly for generics); consult specific product labeling.

Tablet:

Crestor®: 5 mg, 10 mg, 20 mg, 40 mg

◆ **Rosuvastatin Calcium** *see* Rosuvastatin *on page 1343*

◆ **Rotarix®** *see* Rotavirus Vaccine *on page 1345*

◆ **RotaTeq®** *see* Rotavirus Vaccine *on page 1345*

Rotavirus Vaccine (ROE ta vye rus vak SEEN)

U.S. Brand Names Rotarix®; RotaTeq®

Index Terms Human Rotavirus Vaccine, Attenuated (HRV); Pentavalent Human-Bovine Reassortant Rotavirus Vaccine (PRV); Rotavirus Vaccine, Pentavalent; RV1 (Rotarix®); RV5 (RotaTeq®)

Pharmacologic Category Vaccine, Live (Viral)

Use Prevention of rotavirus gastroenteritis in infants and children

The Advisory Committee on Immunization Practices (ACIP) recommends routine vaccination of all infants.

Pregnancy Risk Factor C

Pregnancy Considerations

Reproduction studies have not been conducted. Not indicated for use in women of reproductive age. Infants living in households with pregnant women may be vaccinated.

Contraindications Hypersensitivity to rotavirus vaccine or any component of the formulation

In addition, Rotarix® is contraindicated with a history of an uncorrected congenital malformation of the GI tract.

Warnings/Precautions Information is not available for use in postexposure prophylaxis. May consider deferring administration in patients with moderate or severe acute illness (with or without fever); may administer to patients with mild acute illness (with or without fever). Use caution with history of GI disorders, acute GI illness, chronic diarrhea, failure to thrive, congenital abdominal disorders, abdominal surgery, and intussusception. Vaccine may be used with controlled gastroesophageal reflux disease. Consider delaying administration to infants with acute diarrhea or vomiting. Rotarix® is contraindicated with a history of an uncorrected congenital malformation of the GI tract. Virus from live virus vaccines may be transmitted to nonvaccinated contacts; use caution in presence immunocompromised family members. Safety and efficacy have not been established for use in immunocompromised infants (including blood dyscrasias, leukemia, lymphoma, malignant neoplasms affecting bone marrow or lymphatic system), infants on immunosuppressants (including high-dose corticosteroids; may be administered with topical corticosteroids or inhaled steroids), primary and acquired immunodeficiencies (including HIV), or infants receiving blood products or immunoglobulins within 42 days. Intussusception was observed with a previous licensed rotavirus vaccine; an increased risk in intussusception was not observed in clinical trials with current vaccines, however, cases have been noted in postmarketing reports. Immediate treatment (including epinephrine 1:1000) for anaphylactoid and/or hypersensitivity reactions should be available during vaccine use. Some packaging may contain natural latex/natural rubber. Not intended for use in adults. Safety and efficacy of RotaTeq® have not been established in infants <6 weeks or >32 weeks of age. Safety and efficacy of Rotarix® have not been established in infants <6 weeks or >24 weeks of age. In order to maximize vaccination rates, the ACIP recommends simultaneous administration of all age-appropriate vaccines (live or inactivated) for which a person is eligible at a single clinic visit, unless contraindications exist.

Adverse Reactions All serious adverse reactions must be reported to the U.S. Department of Health and Human Services (DHHS) Vaccine Adverse Event Reporting System (VAERS) 1-800-822-7967 or www.-vaers.hhs.gov.

Note: Ranges reported; actual percentage may vary between products.

>10%:

Central nervous system: Fever ≥38.1°C (17% to 20%; equal to placebo), irritability (3% to 11%)

Gastrointestinal: Diarrhea (4% to 24%), vomiting (3% to 15%)

Otic: Otitis media (15%)

1% to 10%:

Gastrointestinal: Flatulence (2%)

Respiratory: Nasopharyngitis (7%), bronchospasm (1%)

<1% (Limited to important or life-threatening): Hematochezia, idiopathic thrombocytopenic purpura, intussusception, Kawasaki disease, seizure, urticaria

Drug Interactions

Avoid Concomitant Use

Avoid concomitant use of Rotavirus Vaccine with any of the following: Immunosuppressants

Increased Effect/Toxicity

The levels/effects of Rotavirus Vaccine may be increased by: Immunosuppressants

Decreased Effect

Rotavirus Vaccine may decrease the levels/effects of: Tuberculin Tests

The levels/effects of Rotavirus Vaccine may be decreased by: Immune Globulins

Stability

Rotarix®: Prior to reconstitution, store powder under refrigeration at 2°C to 8°C (36°F to 46°F); diluent may be stored at room temperature 20°C to 25°C (68°F to 77°F). Protect from light; discard if frozen. Reconstitute only with provided diluent and transfer adapter. Shake vigorously to form suspension. Following reconstitution, may be refrigerated or stored at room temperature for up to 24 hours. Discard if frozen.

RotaTeq®: Store and transport under refrigeration at 2°C to 8°C (36°F to 46°F). Use as soon as possible once removed from refrigerator. Protect from light.

Mechanism of Action A live vaccine; replicates in the small intestine and promotes active immunity to rotavirus gastroenteritis. Rotarix® is specifically indicated for prevention of rotavirus gastroenteritis caused by serotypes G1, G3, G4 and G9 and RotaTeq® is specifically indicated for prevention of rotavirus gastroenteritis caused by serotypes G1, G2, G3, and G4. However, vaccines may provide immunity to other serotypes.

Pharmacodynamics/Kinetics Note: There is no established relationship between antibody response and protection against gastroenteritis.

Seroconversion:

Rotarix®: Antirotavirus IgA antibodies were noted 1-2 months following competition of the 2-dose series in 77% to 87% of infants.

RotaTeq®: A threefold increase in antirotavirus IgA was noted following completion of the 3-dose regimen in 93% to 100% of infants.

Duration: Following administration of rotavirus vaccine, efficacy of protecting against any grade of rotavirus gastroenteritis through two seasons was 70% to 79%

Dosage Oral: **Manufacturer's labeling:**

Infants 6-24 weeks of age: Rotarix®: A total of two 1mL doses, the first dose given at 6-14 weeks of age. The first and second dose should be separated by ≥4 weeks. The 2-dose series should be completed by 24 weeks of age.

Infants 6-32 weeks: RotaTeq®: A total of three 2 mL doses given at 2-, 4-, and 6 months of age; the first given at 6-14 weeks of age, followed by subsequent doses at 4- to 10-week intervals. Routine administration of the first dose at >12 weeks of age is not recommended (insufficient data). Administer all doses by 32 weeks of age. Infants who have had rotavirus gastroenteritis before getting the full course of vaccine should still initiate or complete the 3-dose schedule; initial infection provides only partial immunity.

ACIP recommendations: The first dose can be given at 6-14 weeks of age. The series should not be started in infants ≥15 weeks. The final dose in the series should be administered by 8 months 0 days of age. A total of three doses, administered at 2-, 4-, and 6 months of age, however, if Rotarix® is used at ages 2- and 4 months, a dose at 6 months is not indicated. The ACIP Provisional Recommendations for vaccination recommend completing the vaccine series with the same product whenever possible. If continuing with same product will cause vaccination to be deferred, or if product used previously is unknown, vaccination should be completed with the product available. If RotaTeq® was used in any previous doses, or if the specific product used was unknown, a total of three doses should be given

Dietary Considerations Do not mix or dilute vaccine. May be administered before or after food, milk, or breast milk.

Administration

Rotarix®: Using oral applicator, administer contents into infant's inner cheek. If most of dose is spit out or regurgitated, may administer a replacement dose at the same visit. Dispose of applicator and vaccine vial in biologic waste container.

RotaTeq®: Gently squeeze dose from ready-to-use dosing tube into infant's inner cheek. If infant spits or regurgitates vaccine, a replacement dose is not recommended. In general, vaccine administration should be deferred for 42 days following an antibody-containing product. However, if deferral causes first dose of vaccine to be scheduled at ≥13 weeks of age, a shorter deferral interval should be used. After use, dispose of the empty tube and cap in a biologic waste container.

Administration with other vaccines:

Rotavirus vaccine with inactivated vaccines: May be given simultaneously or at any interval between doses

Rotavirus vaccine with other live vaccines:

Intranasal: If not given simultaneously, wait at least 4 weeks between administration

Injectable: May be given simultaneously or at any interval between doses of live injectable vaccines

Vaccine administration with antibody-containing products: Do not give rotavirus vaccine simultaneously. Defer rotavirus vaccine for 6 weeks after receipt of antibody containing product unless deferral will cause first dose of rotavirus vaccine to be given ≥13 weeks of age. Examples of antibody-containing products include I.M. and I.V. immune globulin, hepatitis B immune globulin, tetanus immune globulin, varicella zoster immune globulin, rabies immune globulin, whole blood, packed red cells, plasma, and platelet products.

Test Interactions Tuberculin tests: Rotavirus vaccine may diminish the diagnostic effect of tuberculin tests.

Additional Information Federal law requires that the date of administration, the vaccine manufacturer, lot number of vaccine, and the administering person's name, title and address be entered into the patient's permanent medical record.

Dosage Forms Excipient information presented when available (limited, particularly for generics); consult specific product labeling.

Powder, for suspension, oral [preservative free; human derived]:

Rotarix®: G1P[8] ≥10^6 infectious units per 1 mL [oral applicator contains natural latex/natural rubber]

Suspension, oral [preservative free; bovine and human derived]:

RotaTeq®: G1 ≥2.2 10^6 infectious units, G2 ≥2.8 10^6 infectious units, G3 ≥2.2 10^6 infectious units, G4 ≥2 10^6 infectious units, and P1 [8] ≥2.3 10^6 infectious units per 2 mL (2 mL)

◆ **Rotavirus Vaccine, Pentavalent** *see* Rotavirus Vaccine *on page 1345*

Rotigotine (roe TIG oh teen)

U.S. Brand Names Neupro® [DSC]

Index Terms N-0923

Pharmacologic Category Anti-Parkinson's Agent, Dopamine Agonist

Additional Appendix Information

Antiparkinsonian Agents *on page 1643*

Use Treatment of the signs and symptoms of early-stage idiopathic Parkinson's disease

Pregnancy Risk Factor C

Pregnancy Considerations Fetal death and adverse effects on embryo-fetal development were observed in some, but not all animal studies. There are no adequate and well-controlled studies in pregnant women.

Lactation Excretion in breast milk unknown/not recommended

Medication Safety Issues

Sound-alike/look-alike issues:

Neupro® may be confused with Neupogen®

Transdermal patch contains metal (eg, aluminum); remove patch prior to MRI.

Contraindications Hypersensitivity to rotigotine or any component of the formulation

Warnings/Precautions Use commonly associated with somnolence. In addition, patients falling asleep during activities of daily living, including driving, have also been reported and may occur without significant warning signs. Monitor for daytime somnolence or pre-existing sleep disorder. Patients must be cautioned about performing tasks which require mental alertness (eg, operating machinery or driving). Use with caution in patients receiving other CNS depressants or psychoactive agents; discontinue if significant daytime sleepiness or episodes of falling asleep occur. Effects with other sedative drugs or ethanol may be potentiated.

Dopamine agonists may cause orthostatic hypotension and syncope; Parkinson's disease patients appear to have an impaired capacity to respond to a postural challenge. Use with caution in patients at risk of hypotension (such as those receiving antihypertensive drugs) or where transient hypotensive episodes would be poorly tolerated (cardiovascular disease or cerebrovascular disease). Parkinson's patients being treated with dopaminergic agonists ordinarily require careful monitoring for signs and symptoms of postural hypotension, especially during dose escalation, and should be informed of this risk. Therapy has also been associated with inconsistent increases in blood pressure, increased heart rate (average increase of 2-4 bpm), and fluid retention.

Dopamine agonists have been associated with compulsive behaviors and/or loss of impulse control, which has manifested as pathological gambling, libido increases (hypersexuality), and/or binge eating. Causality has not been established, and controversy exists as to whether this phenomenon is related to the underlying disease, prior behaviors/addictions and/or drug therapy. Dose reduction or discontinuation of therapy has been reported to reverse these behaviors in some, but not all cases.

Use with caution in patients with pre-existing dyskinesia; therapy may exacerbate. Therapy may also cause hallucinations. Risk for melanoma development is increased in Parkinson's disease patients; drug causation or factors contributing to risk have not been established. Other dopaminergic agents have been associated with a syndrome resembling neuroleptic malignant syndrome on withdrawal and/or significant dosage reduction. Taper treatment when discontinuing therapy; do not stop abruptly. Rare cases of pleural, retroperitoneal fibrosis and/or cardiac valvulopathy have been reported in patients treated with ergot-derived dopamine agonists, generally with prolonged use. The potential of rotigotine, a nonergot-derived dopamine agonist, to cause similar fibrotic complications is unknown.

Patch contains aluminum; remove patch prior to magnetic resonance imaging or cardioversion to avoid skin burns. Patch also contains sodium metabisulfite which may cause allergic reaction in susceptible individuals. Patients should be instructed to rotate application sites to reduce incidence of application site reactions. Reactions increasing in severity, spreading outside of application site or persistent reactions (lasting longer than several days) prompt assessment and any generalized skin reaction require discontinuation of therapy. Patients should be instructed to avoid patch exposure to heat sources; heat application may result in several fold increases in drug absorption. Safety and effectiveness have not been established in children <18 years of age.

Adverse Reactions

>10%:

Central nervous system: Somnolence (13% to 25%), dizziness (18%), headache (14%), insomnia (6% to 14%)

Gastrointestinal: Nausea (34% to 48%), vomiting (10% to 20%)

Local: Application site reactions (21% to 37%)

1% to 10%:

Cardiovascular: Sinus tachycardia (9%), peripheral edema (7%), orthostatic hypotension (5% to 7%), hypertension (3%), syncope

Central nervous system: Fatigue (8%), abnormal dreams (2% to 5%), hallucination (≤3%), vertigo (3%), ataxia, confusion, fever, hypoesthesia, malaise

Dermatologic: Erythematous rash (2% to 6%), contact dermatitis, pruritus, purpura

Endocrine & metabolic: Hypoglycemia (7%)

Gastrointestinal: Constipation (dose related; 5%), dyspepsia (4%), anorexia (dose related; 3%), xerostomia (3%), weight gain (3%), weight loss (≤2%)

Genitourinary: Urinary tract infection (3%), urinary incontinence

Hematologic: Hemoglobin decreased

Hepatic: Albumin decreased, GGT increased

Neuromuscular & skeletal: Back pain (6%), arthralgia (4%), myalgia (≤2%), abnormal gait, hypertonia, leg pain, neuralgia, paresthesia

Ocular: Vision changes (dose related; 3%)

Respiratory: Sinusitis (3%)

Miscellaneous: Accident (5%), diaphoresis increased (4%)

<1% (Limited to important or life-threatening): Allergic reaction, appetite increased, atrial fibrillation, AV block, BUN increased, bundle branch block, flushing, heart failure, hot flashes, hyperesthesia, impotence, paranoia, psychosis, photopsia, rigors, saliva increased, seizure, sexual urgency, thrombocytopenia, tinnitus, ventricular arrhythmia, ventricular tachycardia

Reported with dopamine agonists: Impulsive/compulsive behaviors (eg, pathological gambling, hypersexuality, binge eating)

Drug Interactions

Avoid Concomitant Use There are no known interactions where it is recommended to avoid concomitant use.

Increased Effect/Toxicity

Rotigotine may increase the levels/effects of: Alcohol (Ethyl); CNS Depressants

Decreased Effect

The levels/effects of Rotigotine may be decreased by: Antipsychotics (Atypical); Antipsychotics (Typical); Metoclopramide

Ethanol/Nutrition/Herb Interactions Ethanol: Avoid ethanol (may increase CNS depression).

Stability Store at 15°C to 30°C (59°F to 86°F). Store in original pouch until application.

Mechanism of Action Rotigotine is a nonergot dopamine agonist with specificity for D_3-, D_2-, and D_1-dopamine receptors. Although the precise mechanism of action of rotigotine is unknown, it is believed to be due to stimulation of postsynaptic dopamine D_2-type auto receptors within the substantia nigra in the brain, leading to improved dopaminergic transmission in the motor areas of the basal ganglia, notably the caudate nucleus/putamen regions.

Pharmacodynamics/Kinetics

Distribution: V_d: 84 L/kg

Protein binding: ~90%

Metabolism: Extensive conjugation and N-dealkylation

Half-life elimination: After removal of patch: ~5-7 hours

Time to peak, plasma: 15-18 hours; can occur 4-27 hours post application

Excretion: Urine (~71% as metabolites, <1% as unchanged drug); feces (~11%)

Dosage Topical: Transdermal: Adults: Initial: Apply 2 mg/24 hours patch once daily; may increase by 2 mg/24 hours weekly, based on clinical response and tolerability (maximum: 6 mg/24 hours)

Dosage reductions or discontinuation: Decrease by 2 mg/24 hours every other day

Note: In clinical trials, the lowest effective dose was 4 mg/24 hours and doses >6 mg/24 hours did not provide any additional therapeutic benefit and increased incidence of adverse effects

Dosage adjustment in renal impairment: Severe impairment (Cl_{cr} 15-29 mL/minute): No dosage adjustment required

Dosage adjustment in hepatic impairment:

Moderate hepatic impairment (Child-Pugh class B): No dosage adjustment required

Severe hepatic impairment: Not studied

Administration Inspect patches for formation of crystals. Do not use if crystallization is present. Apply to clean, dry, hairless area of skin on the front of the abdomen, thigh, hip, flank, shoulder, or upper arm at approximately the same time daily. Remove from pouch immediately before use and press patch firmly in place on skin for 20-30 seconds. Application sites should be rotated on a daily basis. Do not apply to same application site for more than once every 14 days or apply patch to oily, irritated or damaged skin. Avoid exposing patch to external heat sources (eg, heating pad, electric blanket, heat lamp, hot tub). If applied to hairy area, shave ≥3 days prior to applying patch. If patch detaches, immediately apply a new one to a new site.

Monitoring Parameters Blood pressure (orthostatic); daytime alertness; periodic skin evaluations (melanoma development)

Dosage Forms Excipient information presented when available (limited, particularly for generics); consult specific product labeling. [DSC] = Discontinued product

Transdermal system [once-daily patch]:

Neupro®:

2 mg/24 hours (7s, 30s) [10 cm^2, total rotigotine 4.5 mg; contains sodium metabisulfite] [DSC]

4 mg/24 hours (7s, 30s) [20 cm^2, total rotigotine 9 mg; contains sodium metabisulfite] [DSC]

6 mg/24 hours (7s, 30s) [30 cm^2, total rotigotine 13.5 mg; contains sodium metabisulfite] [DSC]

- **Rowasa®** *see* Mesalamine *on page 949*
- **Roxanol™** *see* Morphine Sulfate *on page 1016*
- **Roxicet™** *see* Oxycodone and Acetaminophen *on page 1122*
- **Roxicet™ 5/500** *see* Oxycodone and Acetaminophen *on page 1122*
- **Roxicodone®** *see* OxyCODONE *on page 1120*
- **Roychlor® (Can)** *see* Potassium Chloride *on page 1216*
- **Rozerem®** *see* Ramelteon *on page 1291*
- **RP-6976** *see* Docetaxel *on page 471*
- **RP-54274** *see* Riluzole *on page 1319*
- **RP-59500** *see* Quinupristin and Dalfopristin *on page 1284*
- **r-PA** *see* Reteplase *on page 1306*
- **rPDGF-BB** *see* Becaplermin *on page 176*
- **(R,R)-Formoterol L-Tartrate** *see* Arformoterol *on page 131*
- **RS-25259** *see* Palonosetron *on page 1132*
- **RS-25259-197** *see* Palonosetron *on page 1132*
- **R-Tanna** *see* Chlorpheniramine and Phenylephrine *on page 309*
- **R-Tanna Pediatric** *see* Chlorpheniramine and Phenylephrine *on page 309*
- **RTCA** *see* Ribavirin *on page 1310*
- **RU 0211** *see* Lubiprostone *on page 912*
- **RU-486** *see* Mifepristone *on page 994*
- **RU-23908** *see* Nilutamide *on page 1068*
- **RU-38486** *see* Mifepristone *on page 994*
- **Rubella, Measles and Mumps Vaccines, Combined** *see* Measles, Mumps, and Rubella Vaccines (Combined) *on page 923*
- **Rubella, Varicella, Measles, and Mumps Vaccine** *see* Measles, Mumps, Rubella, and Varicella Virus Vaccine *on page 923*

Rubella Virus Vaccine (Live)

(rue BEL a VYE rus vak SEEN, live)

U.S. Brand Names Meruvax® II

Index Terms German Measles Vaccine

Pharmacologic Category Vaccine

Additional Appendix Information

Immunization Recommendations *on page 1708*

Use Selective active immunization against rubella

Note: Trivalent measles - mumps - rubella (MMR) vaccine is the preferred immunizing agent for most children and many adults.

Pregnancy Risk Factor C

Pregnancy Considerations Animal reproduction studies have not been conducted. Women who are pregnant when vaccinated or who become pregnant within 28 days of vaccination should be counseled on the theoretical risks to the fetus. The risk of rubella-associated malformations in these women is so small as to be negligible. MMR is the vaccine of choice if recipients are likely to be susceptible to measles or mumps as well as to rubella. Evidence of rubella immunity should be determined in women of childbearing potential.

Lactation Enters breast milk/use caution

Medication Safety Issues

Sound-alike/look-alike issues:

Meruvax® II may be confused with Attenuvax®

Contraindications Hypersensitivity to rubella vaccine or any component of the vaccine; history of anaphylactic reactions to neomycin; individuals with blood dyscrasias, leukemia, lymphomas, or other malignant neoplasms affecting the bone marrow or lymphatic systems; concurrent immunosuppressive therapy (not including steroid replacement); primary and acquired immunodeficiency states; family history of congenital or hereditary immunodeficiency; active/untreated tuberculosis; current febrile illness; pregnancy

Warnings/Precautions Immediate treatment for anaphylactic/anaphylactoid reaction should be available during vaccine use. Use with caution in patients with thrombocytopenia and those who develop thrombocytopenia after first dose; thrombocytopenia may worsen. Defer vaccine following blood, plasma, or immune globulin (human) administration. The manufacturer contraindicates use with febrile infections; however, the ACIP notes that patients with minor illnesses with or without fever (diarrhea, mild upper respiratory tract infection, otitis media) may receive vaccines. Leukemia patients who are in remission and who have not received chemotherapy for at least 3 months may be vaccinated; patients with HIV infection, who are asymptomatic and not severely immunosuppressed may be vaccinated. Therapy to treat tuberculosis should be started prior to administering vaccine to patients with untreated, active tuberculosis. Contains gelatin, human albumin, neomycin, sorbitol and sucrose. A history of contact dermatitis to neomycin is not a contraindication to use, however, do not use with previous anaphylactic reaction to neomycin. Vaccination is recommended for individuals in certain high-risk groups (students entering institutions of higher learning, healthcare workers, travelers to endemic areas, etc). Safety and efficacy have not been established in children <12 months of age.

Adverse Reactions All serious adverse reactions must be reported to the U.S. Department of Health and Human Services (DHHS) Vaccine Adverse Event Reporting System (VAERS) 1-800-822-7967.

Frequency not defined.

Cardiovascular: Syncope, vasculitis

Central nervous system: Dizziness, encephalitis, fever, Guillain-Barré syndrome, headache, irritability, malaise, polyneuritis, polyneuropathy

Dermatologic: Angioneurotic edema, erythema multiforme, pruritus, purpura, rash, Stevens-Johnson syndrome, urticaria

Gastrointestinal: Diarrhea, nausea, sore throat, vomiting

Hematologic: Leukocytosis, thrombocytopenia

Local: Injection site reactions which include burning, induration, pain, redness, stinging, wheal and flare

Neuromuscular & skeletal: Arthralgia/arthritis (variable; highest rates in women, 12% to 26% versus children, up to 3%), myalgia, paresthesia

Ocular: Conjunctivitis, optic neuritis, papillitis, retrobulbar neuritis

Otic: Nerve deafness, otitis media

Respiratory: Bronchial spasm, cough, rhinitis

Miscellaneous: Anaphylactoid reactions, anaphylaxis, regional lymphadenopathy

Drug Interactions

Avoid Concomitant Use

Avoid concomitant use of Rubella Virus Vaccine (Live) with any of the following: Immunosuppressants

Increased Effect/Toxicity

The levels/effects of Rubella Virus Vaccine (Live) may be increased by: Immunosuppressants

Decreased Effect

Rubella Virus Vaccine (Live) may decrease the levels/ effects of: Tuberculin Tests

The levels/effects of Rubella Virus Vaccine (Live) may be decreased by: Immune Globulins

Stability Vaccine is to be shipped at 10°C (50°F). May use dry ice. Protect from light at all times. Prior to reconstitution, store at 2°C to 8°C (36°F to 46°F) or colder. Discard reconstituted vaccine after 8 hours.

Mechanism of Action Rubella vaccine is a live attenuated vaccine that contains the Wistar Institute RA 27/3 strain, which is adapted to and propagated in human diploid cell culture. Promotes active immunity by inducing rubella hemagglutination-inhibiting antibodies.

Pharmacodynamics/Kinetics Onset of action: Antibodies to vaccine: 2-4 weeks

Dosage Children ≥12 months and Adults: SubQ: 0.5 mL

Primary immunization is recommended at 12-15 months; revaccination with MMR-II at 4-6 years of age is recommended prior to elementary school. Previously unvaccinated children of susceptible pregnant women should be vaccinated.

Adults without documentation of immunity: Vaccination is recommended for students entering colleges and other institutions of higher education, for military personal, for healthcare workers, for international travelers who visit endemic areas, and to women of childbearing potential. Do not administer to women who may become pregnant within 4 weeks of receiving vaccine; administer following completion or termination of pregnancy

Administration SubQ injection only in outer aspect of upper arm; avoid injection into blood vessel. **Not for I.V. administration.**

Test Interactions May depress tuberculin skin test sensitivity

Additional Information Live virus vaccine. Federal law requires that the date of administration, the vaccine manufacturer, lot number of vaccine, and the administering person's name, title, and address be entered into the patient's permanent record.

Acceptable presumptive evidence of immunity includes one of the following:

1. Documentation of adequate vaccination
2. Laboratory evidence of immunity
3. Documentation of physician-diagnosed disease

Dosage Forms Excipient information presented when available (limited, particularly for generics); consult specific product labeling.

Injection, powder for reconstitution [preservative free]:

Meruvax® II: ≥1000 $TCID_{50}$ (Wistar RA 27/3 Strain) [contains gelatin, human albumin, sorbitol, sucrose, and neomycin]

- ◆ **Rubeola Vaccine** *see* Measles Virus Vaccine (Live) *on page 924*
- ◆ **Rubex® [DSC]** *see* DOXOrubicin *on page 486*
- ◆ **Rubidomycin Hydrochloride** *see* DAUNOrubicin Hydrochloride *on page 407*
- ◆ **RUF 331** *see* Rufinamide *on page 1349*

Rufinamide (roo FIN a mide)

U.S. Brand Names Banzel™

Index Terms CGP 33101; E 2080; RUF 331; Xilep

Pharmacologic Category Anticonvulsant, Triazole Derivative

Use Adjunctive therapy in the treatment of generalized seizures of Lennox-Gastaut syndrome

Restrictions An FDA-approved patient medication guide is available and must be distributed when dispensing an outpatient prescription (new or refill) where this medication is to be used without direct supervision of a healthcare provider. Medication guides are available at http://www.fda.gov/cder/Offices/ODS/medication_guides.htm.

Pregnancy Risk Factor C

Dosage Oral: Lennox-Gastaut (adjunctive):

Children ≥4 years: Initial: 10 mg/kg/day in 2 equally divided doses; increase dose by ~10 mg/kg/day every other day to a target dose of 45 mg/kg/day or 3200 mg/day (whichever is lower) in 2 equally divided doses

Adults: Initial: 400-800 mg/day in 2 equally divided doses; increase dose by 400-800 mg/day every 2 days until maximum daily dose: 3200 mg/day in 2 equally divided doses

Dosage adjustment in renal impairment: Cl_{cr} <30 mL/minute: No dosage adjustment needed

Hemodialysis: No specific guidelines available; consider dosage adjustment for loss of drug

Dosage adjustment in hepatic impairment:

Mild-to-moderate impairment: Use caution

Severe impairment: Use in severe impairment has not been studied and is not recommended

Additional Information Complete prescribing information for this medication should be consulted for additional detail.

Dosage Forms Excipient information presented when available (limited, particularly for generics); consult specific product labeling.

Tablet:

Banzel™: 200 mg, 400 mg

- ◆ **Ru-Hist Forte** *see* Chlorpheniramine, Pyrilamine, and Phenylephrine *on page 315*
- ◆ **Rulox [OTC]** *see* Aluminum Hydroxide and Magnesium Hydroxide *on page 76*
- ◆ **Rulox No. 1 [DSC]** *see* Aluminum Hydroxide and Magnesium Hydroxide *on page 76*
- ◆ **Ru-Tuss DM** *see* Guaifenesin, Pseudoephedrine, and Dextromethorphan *on page 715*
- ◆ **Rutuss Jr** *see* Guaifenesin and Pseudoephedrine *on page 713*
- ◆ **RV1 (Rotarix®)** *see* Rotavirus Vaccine *on page 1345*
- ◆ **RV5 (RotaTeq®)** *see* Rotavirus Vaccine *on page 1345*
- ◆ **Rylosol (Can)** *see* Sotalol *on page 1394*
- ◆ **Ryna-12X®** *see* Phenylephrine, Pyrilamine, and Guaifenesin *on page 1186*
- ◆ **Rynatan®** *see* Chlorpheniramine and Phenylephrine *on page 309*
- ◆ **Rynatan® Pediatric** *see* Chlorpheniramine and Phenylephrine *on page 309*
- ◆ **Rynatuss®** *see* Chlorpheniramine, Ephedrine, Phenylephrine, and Carbetapentane *on page 311*
- ◆ **Rythmodan® (Can)** *see* Disopyramide *on page 468*
- ◆ **Rythmodan®-LA (Can)** *see* Disopyramide *on page 468*
- ◆ **Rythmol®** *see* Propafenone *on page 1252*
- ◆ **Rythmol® Gen-Propafenone (Can)** *see* Propafenone *on page 1252*
- ◆ **Rythmol® SR** *see* Propafenone *on page 1252*

- **S2® [OTC]** *see* EPINEPHrine *on page 525*
- **S-(+)-3-isobutylgaba** *see* Pregabalin *on page 1234*
- **S-4661** *see* Doripenem *on page 480*
- **Sab-Diclofenac (Can)** *see* Diclofenac *on page 437*
- **SAB-Dimenhydrinate (Can)** *see* DimenhyDRINATE *on page 453*
- **SAB-Gentamicin (Can)** *see* Gentamicin *on page 692*
- **Sab-Naproxen (Can)** *see* Naproxen *on page 1041*
- **Sab-Prenase (Can)** *see* PrednisoLONE *on page 1230*
- **SAB-Trifluridine (Can)** *see* Trifluridine *on page 1517*

Sacrosidase (sak ROE si dase)

U.S. Brand Names Sucraid®

Canadian Brand Names Sucraid®

Pharmacologic Category Enzyme, Gastrointestinal

Use Orphan drug: Oral replacement therapy in sucrase deficiency, as seen in congenital sucrase-isomaltase deficiency (CSID)

Restrictions Sucraid® is not available in retail pharmacies or via mail-order pharmacies. To obtain the product, please refer to http://www.sucraid.net/ or call 1-866-740-2743.

Pregnancy Risk Factor C

Dosage Oral:

Infants ≥5 months and Children <15 kg: 8500 int. units (1 mL) per meal or snack

Children >15 kg and Adults: 17,000 int. units (2 mL) per meal or snack

Doses should be diluted with 2-4 oz of water, milk, or formula with each meal or snack. Approximately one-half of the dose may be taken before, and the remainder of a dose taken at the completion of each meal or snack.

Additional Information Complete prescribing information for this medication should be consulted for additional detail.

Dosage Forms Excipient information presented when available (limited, particularly for generics); consult specific product labeling.

Solution, oral:

Sucraid®: 8500 int. units per mL (118 mL)

- **Safe Tussin® DM [OTC]** *see* Guaifenesin and Dextromethorphan *on page 710*
- **SAHA** *see* Vorinostat *on page 1569*
- **Saizen®** *see* Somatropin *on page 1388*
- **Salagen®** *see* Pilocarpine *on page 1192*
- **Salazopyrin® (Can)** *see* Sulfasalazine *on page 1409*
- **Salazopyrin En-Tabs® (Can)** *see* Sulfasalazine *on page 1409*
- **Salbu-2 (Can)** *see* Albuterol *on page 51*
- **Salbu-4 (Can)** *see* Albuterol *on page 51*
- **Salbutamol** *see* Albuterol *on page 51*
- **Salbutamol and Ipratropium** *see* Ipratropium and Albuterol *on page 812*
- **Salbutamol Sulphate** *see* Albuterol *on page 51*
- **Salflex® (Can)** *see* Salsalate *on page 1352*
- **Salicylazosulfapyridine** *see* Sulfasalazine *on page 1409*
- **Salicylsalicylic Acid** *see* Salsalate *on page 1352*
- **Saline Mist [OTC]** *see* Sodium Chloride *on page 1381*
- **SalineX® [OTC] [DSC]** *see* Sodium Chloride *on page 1381*
- **Salk Vaccine** *see* Poliovirus Vaccine (Inactivated) *on page 1207*

Salmeterol (sal ME te role)

U.S. Brand Names Serevent® Diskus®

Canadian Brand Names Serevent® Diskhaler® Disk; Serevent® Diskus®

Index Terms Salmeterol Xinafoate

Pharmacologic Category Beta2-Adrenergic Agonist, Long-Acting; Beta$_2$-Adrenergic Agonist

Additional Appendix Information

Bronchodilators *on page 1650*

Use Maintenance treatment of asthma; prevention of bronchospasm with reversible obstructive airway disease, including patients with symptoms of nocturnal asthma; prevention of exercise-induced bronchospasm; maintenance treatment of bronchospasm associated with COPD

Restrictions An FDA-approved medication guide must be distributed when dispensing an outpatient prescription (new or refill) where this medication is to be used without direct supervision of a healthcare provider. Medication guides are available at http://www.fda.gov/cder/Offices/ODS/medication_guides.htm.

Pregnancy Risk Factor C

Pregnancy Considerations Animal studies have demonstrated (dose-dependent) teratogenicity. There are no adequate and well-controlled studies in pregnant women. Beta-agonists may interfere with uterine contractility if administered during labor. Use only if clearly needed.

Lactation Enters breast milk/use caution

Medication Safety Issues

Sound-alike/look-alike issues:

Salmeterol may be confused with Salbutamol, Solu-Medrol®

Serevent® may be confused with Atrovent®, Combivent®, Serentil®, sertraline, Sinemet®, Spiriva®, Zoloft®

Contraindications Hypersensitivity to salmeterol or any component of the formulation

Warnings/Precautions

Asthma treatment: [U.S. Boxed Warning]: Long-acting beta$_2$-agonists (LABAs) may increase the risk of asthma-related deaths. Salmeterol should only be used as adjuvant therapy in patients not adequately controlled on inhaled corticosteroids or whose disease requires two maintenance therapies. In a large, randomized clinical trial (SMART, 2006), salmeterol was associated with a small, but statistically significant increase in asthma-related deaths (when added to usual asthma therapy); risk may be greater in African-American patients versus Caucasians. Do **not** use for acute asthmatic symptoms. Short-acting beta$_2$-agonist (eg, albuterol) should be used for acute symptoms and symptoms occurring between treatments. Do **not** initiate in patients with significantly worsening or acutely deteriorating asthma; reports of severe (sometimes fatal) respiratory events have been reported when salmeterol has been initiated in this situation. Salmeterol is not a substitute for inhaled or oral corticosteroids; should not be used as monotherapy for the treatment of asthma. Corticosteroids should not be stopped or reduced when salmeterol is initiated. During the initiation of salmeterol watch for signs of worsening asthma. Patients must be instructed to use short-acting beta$_2$-agonists (eg, albuterol) for acute asthmatic or COPD symptoms and to seek medical attention in cases where acute symptoms are not relieved or a previous level of response is diminished. The need to increase frequency of use of short-acting beta$_2$-agonist may indicate deterioration of asthma, and treatment must not be delayed. Because LABAs may disguise poorly controlled persistent asthma, frequent or chronic use of LABAs for exercise-induced bronchospasm is discouraged by the NIH Asthma Guidelines (NIH, 2007).

Salmeterol should not be used more than twice daily; do not use with other long-acting beta$_2$-agonists.

Concurrent diseases: Use caution in patients with cardiovascular disease (eg, arrhythmia, hypertension, or HF), seizure disorders, diabetes, glaucoma, hyperthyroidism, hepatic impairment, or hypokalemia. Beta-agonists may cause elevation in blood pressure, heart rate, CNS stimulation/excitation, increased risk of arrhythmia, increase serum glucose, or decrease serum potassium.

Adverse events: Immediate hypersensitivity reactions (urticaria, angioedema, rash, bronchospasm) have been reported. There have been reports of laryngeal spasm, irritation, swelling (stridor, choking) with use. Salmeterol should not be used more than twice daily; do not exceed recommended dose; do not use with other long-acting beta$_2$-agonists; serious adverse events have been associated with excessive use of inhaled sympathomimetics. Rarely, paradoxical bronchospasm may occur with use of inhaled bronchodilating agents; this should be distinguished from inadequate response. Powder for oral inhalation contains lactose; very rare anaphylactic reactions have been reported in patients with severe milk protein allergy.

Safety and efficacy have not been established in children <4 years of age.

Adverse Reactions

>10%:

- Central nervous system: Headache (13% to 17%)
- Neuromuscular & skeletal: Pain (1% to 12%)

1% to 10%:

- Cardiovascular: Hypertension (4%), edema (1% to 3%), pallor
- Central nervous system: Dizziness (4%), sleep disturbance (1% to 3%), fever (1% to 3%), anxiety (1% to 3%), migraine (1% to 3%)
- Dermatologic: Rash (1% to 4%), contact dermatitis (1% to 3%), eczema (1% to 3%), urticaria (3%), photodermatitis (1% to 2%)
- Endocrine & metabolic: Hyperglycemia (1% to 3%)
- Gastrointestinal: Throat irritation (7%), nausea (1% to 3%), dyspepsia (1% to 3%), dental pain (1% to 3%), gastrointestinal infection (1% to 3%), oropharyngeal candidiasis (1% to 3%), xerostomia (1% to 3%)
- Neuromuscular & skeletal: Muscular cramps/spasm (3%), articular rheumatism (1% to 3%), arthralgia (1% to 3%), joint pain (1% to 3%), muscular stiffness (1% to 3%), paresthesia (1% to 3%), rigidity (1% to 3%)
- Ocular: Keratitis/conjunctivitis (1% to 3%)
- Respiratory: Nasal congestion (4% to 9%), tracheitis/bronchitis (7%), pharyngitis (≤6%), cough (5%), influenza (5%), viral respiratory tract infection (5%), sinusitis (4% to 5%), rhinitis (4% to 5%), asthma (3% to 4%)

<1% (Limited to important or life-threatening): Abdominal pain, agitation, aggression, anaphylactic reaction (Diskus®: severe milk allergy), angioedema, aphonia, arrhythmia, atrial fibrillation, bronchospasm and immediate bronchospasm, cataracts, chest congestion, chest tightness, choking, contusions, Cushing syndrome, Cushingoid features, depression, dysmenorrhea, dyspnea, earache, ecchymoses, edema (facial, oropharyngeal), eosinophilic conditions, glaucoma, growth velocity reduction in children/adolescents, hypercorticism, hypersensitivity reaction (immediate and delayed), hypokalemia, hypothyroidism, intraocular pressure increased, laryngeal spasm/irritation, irregular menstruation, myositis, osteoporosis, pallor, paradoxical tracheitis, paranasal sinus pain, PID, restlessness, stridor, supraventricular tachycardia, syncope, tremor, vaginal candidiasis, vaginitis, vulvovaginitis, rare cases of vasculitis (Churg-Strauss syndrome), ventricular tachycardia, weight gain

Drug Interactions

Metabolism/Transport Effects Substrate of CYP3A4 (major)

Avoid Concomitant Use

Avoid concomitant use of Salmeterol with any of the following: CYP3A4 Inhibitors (Strong); Iobenguane I 123

Increased Effect/Toxicity

Salmeterol may increase the levels/effects of: Sympathomimetics

The levels/effects of Salmeterol may be increased by: Atomoxetine; Cannabinoids; CYP3A4 Inhibitors (Moderate); CYP3A4 Inhibitors (Strong); MAO Inhibitors; Tricyclic Antidepressants

Decreased Effect

Salmeterol may decrease the levels/effects of: Iobenguane I 123

The levels/effects of Salmeterol may be decreased by: Alpha-/Beta-Blockers; Beta-Blockers (Beta1 Selective); Beta-Blockers (Nonselective); Betahistine

Stability Inhalation powder: Store at controlled room temperature 20°C to 25°C (68°F to 77°F) in a dry place away from direct heat or sunlight. Stable for 6 weeks after removal from foil pouch.

Mechanism of Action Relaxes bronchial smooth muscle by selective action on beta$_2$-receptors with little effect on heart rate; salmeterol acts locally in the lung.

Pharmacodynamics/Kinetics

Onset of action: Asthma: 30-48 minutes, COPD: 2 hours

Peak effect: Asthma: 3 hours, COPD: 2-5 hours

Duration: 12 hours

Absorption: Systemic: Inhalation: Undetectable to poor

Protein binding: 96%

Metabolism: Hepatic; hydroxylated via CYP3A4

Half-life elimination: 5.5 hours

Time to peak, serum: ~20 minutes

Excretion: Feces (60%), urine (25%)

Dosage Inhalation, powder (50 mcg/inhalation):

Asthma, maintenance and prevention: Children ≥4 years and Adults: One inhalation twice daily (~12 hours apart); maximum: 1 inhalation twice daily. **Note:** For long-term asthma control, long acting beta$_2$-agonists (LABAs) should be used in combination with inhaled corticosteroids and not as monotherapy.

Exercise-induced asthma, prevention: Children ≥4 years and Adults: One inhalation at least 30 minutes prior to exercise; additional doses should not be used for 12 hours; should not be used in individuals already receiving salmeterol twice daily. **Note:** Because LABAs may disguise poorly controlled persistent asthma, frequent or chronic use of LABAs for exercise-induced bronchospasm is discouraged by the NIH Asthma Guidelines (NIH, 2007).

COPD maintenance: Adults: One inhalation twice daily (~12 hours apart); maximum: 1 inhalation twice daily

Dosage adjustment in hepatic impairment: No dosage adjustment required; manufacturer suggests close monitoring of patients with hepatic impairment.

Dietary Considerations Powder for oral inhalation contains lactose; very rare anaphylactic reactions have been reported in patients with severe milk protein allergy.

Administration Inhalation: **Not** to be used for the relief of acute attacks. Not for use with a spacer device. Administer with Diskus® in a level, horizontal position. Do not wash mouthpiece; Diskus® should be kept dry.

Monitoring Parameters FEV$_1$, peak flow, and/or other pulmonary function tests; blood pressure, heart rate; CNS stimulation. Monitor for increased use of short-acting beta$_2$-agonist inhalers; may be marker of a deteriorating asthma condition.

Dosage Forms Excipient information presented when available (limited, particularly for generics); consult specific product labeling. [CAN] = Canadian brand name

Powder for oral inhalation:
Serevent® Diskus®: Salmeterol xinafoate 50 mcg (28s, 60s) [delivers 50 mcg/inhalation; contains lactose]
Serevent® Diskhaler® Disk [CAN]: Salmeterol xinafoate 50 mcg (60s) [delivers 50 mcg/inhalation; contains lactose] [not available in U.S]

Salsalate (SAL sa late)

U.S. Brand Names Amigesic® [DSC]
Canadian Brand Names Amigesic®; Salflex®
Index Terms Disalicylic Acid; Salicylsalicylic Acid
Pharmacologic Category Salicylate
Use Treatment of minor pain or fever; arthritis
Pregnancy Risk Factor C/D (3rd trimester)
Medication Safety Issues
Sound-alike/look-alike issues:
Salsalate may be confused with sucralfate, sulfasalazine
Dosage Adults: Oral: 3 g/day in 2-3 divided doses
Dosing comments in renal impairment: In patients with end-stage renal disease undergoing hemodialysis: 750 mg twice daily with an additional 500 mg after dialysis
Additional Information Complete prescribing information for this medication should be consulted for additional detail.
Dosage Forms Excipient information presented when available (limited, particularly for generics); consult specific product labeling. [DSC] = Discontinued product
Tablet: 500 mg, 750 mg
Amigesic®: 500 mg [DSC], 750 mg [DSC]

- ◆ **Sandoz-Rabeprazole (Can)** *see* Rabeprazole *on page* 1285
- ◆ **Sandoz-Ramipril (Can)** *see* Ramipril *on page* 1292
- ◆ **Sandoz-Ranitidine (Can)** *see* Ranitidine *on page* 1295
- ◆ **Sandoz Risperidone (Can)** *see* Risperidone *on page* 1323
- ◆ **Sandoz-Sertraline (Can)** *see* Sertraline *on page* 1362
- ◆ **Sandoz-Simvastatin (Can)** *see* Simvastatin *on page* 1370
- ◆ **SANDOZ-Sotalol (Can)** *see* Sotalol *on page* 1394
- ◆ **Sandoz-Sumatriptan (Can)** *see* SUMAtriptan *on page* 1414
- ◆ **Sandoz-Tamsulosin (Can)** *see* Tamsulosin *on page* 1426
- ◆ **SANDOZ-Terbinafine (Can)** *see* Terbinafine *on page* 1441
- ◆ **Sandoz-Ticlopidine (Can)** *see* Ticlopidine *on page* 1468
- ◆ **Sandoz-Timolol (Can)** *see* Timolol *on page* 1472
- ◆ **Sandoz-Tobramycin (Can)** *see* Tobramycin *on page* 1481
- ◆ **Sandoz-Topiramate (Can)** *see* Topiramate *on page* 1489
- ◆ **Sandoz-Trifluridine (Can)** *see* Trifluridine *on page* 1517
- ◆ **Sandoz-Valproic (Can)** *see* Valproic Acid and Derivatives *on page* 1538
- ◆ **SANDOZ-Venlafaxine XR (Can)** *see* Venlafaxine *on page* 1554
- ◆ **Sans Acne® (Can)** *see* Erythromycin *on page* 544
- ◆ **Santyl®** *see* Collagenase *on page* 367

Sapropterin (sap roe TER in)

U.S. Brand Names Kuvan™

Index Terms 6R-BH4; Phenoptin; Sapropterin Dihydrochloride

Pharmacologic Category Enzyme Cofactor

Use Adjunct to dietary management in the treatment of tetrahydrobiopterin (BH4) responsive phenylketonuria (PKU)

Pregnancy Risk Factor C

Medication Safety Issues

Sound-alike/look-alike issues:

Sapropterin may be confused with cyproterone

Dosage Oral: PKU: Children ≥4 years and Adults: Initial: 10 mg/kg once daily; adjust after 1 month based on blood phenylalanine levels (if phenylalanine levels do not decrease from baseline, increase dose to 20 mg/kg once daily); discontinue if phenylalanine levels do not decrease after 1 month of treatment at 20 mg/kg/day (nonresponder). Maintenance range: 5-20 mg/kg once daily

Additional Information Complete prescribing information for this medication should be consulted for additional detail.

Dosage Forms Excipient information presented when available (limited, particularly for generics); consult specific product labeling.

Tablet, as dihydrochloride:

Kuvan™: 100 mg

- ◆ **Sapropterin Dihydrochloride** *see* Sapropterin *on page* 1353

Saquinavir (sa KWIN a veer)

U.S. Brand Names Invirase®

Canadian Brand Names Invirase®

Index Terms Saquinavir Mesylate

Pharmacologic Category Antiretroviral Agent, Protease Inhibitor

Additional Appendix Information

Antiretroviral Therapy for HIV Infection: Adults and Adolescents *on page* 1758

Management of Healthcare Worker Exposures to HBV, HCV, and HIV *on page* 1719

Perinatal HIV Guidelines *on page* 1730

Use Treatment of HIV infection; used in combination with at least two other antiretroviral agents

Pregnancy Risk Factor B

Pregnancy Considerations Adverse events were not observed in animal studies and saquinavir crosses the human placenta in minimal amounts. Based on limited data, Invirase® 1000 mg (capsules and tablets) administered twice daily with ritonavir 100 mg twice daily provide adequate levels in pregnant women. The Perinatal HIV Guidelines Working Group considers Invirase® capsules and ritonavir to be an alternative combination for use during pregnancy. Pregnancy and protease inhibitors are both associated with an increased risk of hyperglycemia. Glucose levels should be closely monitored. Health professionals are encouraged to contact the antiretroviral pregnancy registry to monitor outcomes of pregnant women exposed to antiretroviral medications (1-800-258-4263 or www.APRegistry.com).

Lactation Excretion in breast milk unknown/contraindicated

Medication Safety Issues

Sound-alike/look-alike issues:

Saquinavir may be confused with Sinequan®

Contraindications Hypersensitivity to saquinavir or any component of the formulation; severe hepatic impairment; coadministration with amiodarone, cisapride, flecainide, midazolam, pimozide, propafenone, quinidine, rifampin, triazolam, or ergot derivatives

Warnings/Precautions Use caution in patients with hepatic insufficiency. May exacerbate pre-existing hepatic dysfunction; use with caution in patients with hepatitis B or C and in cirrhosis. May be associated with fat redistribution (buffalo hump, increased abdominal girth, breast engorgement, facial atrophy). Use caution in hemophilia. May increase cholesterol and/or triglycerides. Changes in glucose tolerance, hyperglycemia, exacerbation of diabetes, DKA, and new-onset diabetes mellitus have been reported in patients receiving protease inhibitors.

Use with caution in patients taking strong CYP3A4 inhibitors, moderate or strong CYP3A4 inducers and major CYP3A4 substrates (see Drug Interactions); consider alternative agents that avoid or lessen the potential for CYP-mediated interactions. St. John's Wort, lovastatin, and simvastatin should not be used concurrently with saquinavir/ritonavir. A listing of medications that should not be used is available with each bottle and patients should be provided with this information. Patients may develop immune reconstitution syndrome resulting in the occurrence of an inflammatory response to an indolent or residual opportunistic infection; further evaluation and treatment may be required. Invirase® may be used only if combined with ritonavir. Safety and efficacy have not been established in children ≤16 years of age.

Adverse Reactions

Incidence data shown for saquinavir soft gel capsule formulation (no longer available) in combination with ritonavir.

10%: Gastrointestinal: Nausea (11%)

1% to 10%:

Cardiovascular: Chest pain

Central nervous system: Fatigue (6%), fever (3%), anxiety, depression, headache, insomnia, pain

Dermatologic: Pruritus (3%), rash (3%), dry lips/skin (2%), eczema (2%), verruca

Endocrine & metabolic: Lipodystrophy (5%), hyperglycemia (3%), hypoglycemia, hyperkalemia, libido disorder, serum amylase increased

Gastrointestinal: Diarrhea (8%), vomiting (7%), abdominal pain (6%), constipation (2%), abdominal discomfort, appetite decreased, buccal mucosa ulceration, dyspepsia, flatulence, taste alteration

Hepatic: AST increased, ALT increased, bilirubin increased

Neuromuscular & skeletal: Back pain (2%), CPK increased, paresthesia, weakness

Renal: Creatinine kinase increased

Respiratory: Pneumonia (5%), bronchitis (3%), sinusitis (3%)

Miscellaneous: Influenza (3%)

Incidence not currently defined (limited to significant reactions; reported for hard or soft gel capsule with/without ritonavir)

Cardiovascular: Cyanosis, heart valve disorder (including murmur), hyper-/hypotension, peripheral vasoconstriction, syncope, thrombophlebitis

Central nervous system: Agitation, amnesia, ataxia, confusion, hallucination, hyper-/hyporeflexia, myelopolyradiculoneuritis, neuropathies, poliomyelitis, progressive multifocal encephalopathy, psychosis, seizures, somnolence, speech disorder, suicide attempt

Dermatologic: Alopecia, bullous eruption, dermatitis, erythema, maculopapular rash, photosensitivity, Stevens-Johnson syndrome, skin ulceration, urticaria

Endocrine & metabolic: Dehydration, diabetes, electrolyte changes, TSH increased

Gastrointestinal: Ascites, colic, dysphagia, esophagitis, bloody stools, gastritis, intestinal obstruction, hemorrhage (rectal), pancreatitis, stomatitis

Genitourinary: impotence, prostate enlarged, hematuria, UTI

Hematologic; Acute myeloblastic leukemia, anemia (including hemolytic), leukopenia, neutropenia, pancytopenia, splenomegaly, thrombocytopenia

Hepatic: Alkaline phosphatase increased, GGT increased, hepatitis, hepatomegaly, hepatosplenomegaly, jaundice, liver disease exacerbation

Neuromuscular & skeletal: Arthritis, LDH increased

Ocular: Blepharitis, visual disturbance

Otic: Otitis, hearing decreased, tinnitus

Renal: Nephrolithiasis, renal calculus

Respiratory: Dyspnea, hemoptysis, pharyngitis, upper respiratory tract infection

Miscellaneous: Infections (bacterial, fungal, viral)

Drug Interactions

Metabolism/Transport Effects **Substrate** of CYP2D6 (minor), 3A4 (major); **Inhibits** CYP2C9 (weak), 2C19 (weak), 2D6 (weak), 3A4 (moderate)

Avoid Concomitant Use

Avoid concomitant use of Saquinavir with any of the following: Alfuzosin; Amiodarone; Cisapride; Dabigatran Etexilate; Darunavir; Eplerenone; Ergot Derivatives; Nilotinib; Nisoldipine; Pimozide; QuiNIDine; Ranolazine; Rivaroxaban; Salmeterol; Silodosin; St Johns Wort; Topotecan

Increased Effect/Toxicity

Saquinavir may increase the levels/effects of: Alfuzosin; Alosetron; Amiodarone; Antifungal Agents (Azole Derivatives, Systemic); Benzodiazepines (metabolized by oxidation); Calcium Channel Blockers (Dihydropyridine); Calcium Channel Blockers (Nondihydropyridine); CarBAMazepine; Ciclesonide; Cisapride; Clarithromycin; Corticosteroids (Orally Inhaled); CycloSPORINE; CYP3A4 Substrates; Dabigatran Etexilate; Digoxin; Enfuvirtide; Eplerenone; Ergot Derivatives; Etravirine; FentaNYL; Fesoterodine; Fusidic Acid; HMG-CoA Reductase Inhibitors; Ixabepilone; Maraviroc; Meperidine; Methadone; Nefazodone; Nilotinib; Nisoldipine; P-Glycoprotein Substrates; Phosphodiesterase 5 Inhibitors; Pimecrolimus; Pimozide; Protease Inhibitors; QuiNIDine; Ranolazine; Rifamycin Derivatives; Rivaroxaban; Salmeterol; Silodosin; Sirolimus; Sorafenib; Tacrolimus; Temsirolimus; Topotecan; TraZODone; Tricyclic Antidepressants

The levels/effects of Saquinavir may be increased by: Antifungal Agents (Azole Derivatives, Systemic); Clarithromycin; CycloSPORINE; Delavirdine; Efavirenz; Enfuvirtide; Etravirine; Fusidic Acid; H2-Antagonists; P-Glycoprotein Inhibitors; Proton Pump Inhibitors

Decreased Effect

Saquinavir may decrease the levels/effects of: Abacavir; Clarithromycin; Darunavir; Delavirdine; Etravirine; Meperidine; Oral Contraceptive (Estrogens); Theophylline Derivatives; Valproic Acid; Zidovudine

The levels/effects of Saquinavir may be decreased by: Antacids; CarBAMazepine; CYP3A4 Inducers (Strong); Deferasirox; Efavirenz; Garlic; Nevirapine; Oral Contraceptive (Estrogens); P-Glycoprotein Inducers; Rifamycin Derivatives; St Johns Wort

Ethanol/Nutrition/Herb Interactions

Food: A high-fat meal maximizes bioavailability. Saquinavir levels may increase if taken with grapefruit juice.

Herb/Nutraceutical: Saquinavir serum concentrations may be decreased by St John's wort; avoid concurrent use. Garlic capsules may decrease saquinavir serum concentrations; avoid use if saquinavir is the only protease inhibitor.

Stability Invirase®: Store at room temperature.

Mechanism of Action As an inhibitor of HIV protease, saquinavir prevents the cleavage of viral polyprotein precursors which are needed to generate functional viral proteins required for the maturation of an infectious HIV virion.

Pharmacodynamics/Kinetics

Absorption: Poor; increased with high fat meal; Fortovase® has improved absorption over Invirase®

Distribution: V_d: 700 L; does not distribute into CSF

Protein binding, plasma: ~98%

Metabolism: Extensively hepatic via CYP3A4; extensive first-pass effect

Bioavailability: Invirase®: ~4%

Excretion: Feces (81% to 88%), urine (1% to 3%) within 5 days

Dosage

Oral:

Children >16 years and Adults (Invirase®): 1000 mg (five 200 mg capsules or two 500 mg tablets) twice daily given in combination with ritonavir 100 mg twice daily. This combination should be given together and within 2 hours after a full meal in combination with a nucleoside analog. **Note:** Saquinavir (Invirase®) should not be used in "unboosted regimens."

Dosage adjustments when administered in combination therapy: Lopinavir and ritonavir (Kaletra™): Invirase® 1000 mg twice daily

Elderly: Clinical studies did not include sufficient numbers of patients ≥65 years of age; use caution due to increased frequency of organ dysfunction

Dietary Considerations Administer within 2 hours of a meal. Invirase® capsules contain lactose 63.3 mg/capsule (not expected to induce symptoms of intolerance).

Administration Take saquinavir within 2 hours after a full meal. When used with ritonavir, saquinavir and ritonavir should be administered at the same time.

Monitoring Parameters Monitor viral load, CD4 count, triglycerides, cholesterol, glucose

Dosage Forms Excipient information presented when available (limited, particularly for generics); consult specific product labeling.

Capsule:

Invirase®: 200 mg [contains lactose 63.3 mg/capsule]

Tablet:

Invirase®: 500 mg

◆ **Saquinavir Mesylate** *see* Saquinavir *on page 1353*

◆ **Sarafem®** *see* FLUoxetine *on page 638*

Sargramostim (sar GRAM oh stim)

U.S. Brand Names Leukine®

Canadian Brand Names Leukine®

Index Terms GM-CSF; Granulocyte-Macrophage Colony Stimulating Factor; NSC-613795; rhuGM-CSF

Pharmacologic Category Colony Stimulating Factor

Use

Acute myelogenous leukemia (AML) following induction chemotherapy in older adults (≥55 years of age) to shorten time to neutrophil recovery and to reduce the incidence of severe and life-threatening infections and infections resulting in death

Bone marrow transplant (allogeneic or autologous) failure or engraftment delay

Myeloid reconstitution after allogeneic bone marrow transplantation

Myeloid reconstitution after autologous bone marrow transplantation: Non-Hodgkin's lymphoma (NHL), acute lymphoblastic leukemia (ALL), Hodgkin's lymphoma

Peripheral stem cell transplantation: Mobilization and myeloid reconstitution following autologous peripheral stem cell transplantation

Pregnancy Risk Factor C

Pregnancy Considerations Clinical effects to the fetus: Animal reproduction studies have not been conducted. It is not known whether sargramostim can cause fetal harm when administered to a pregnant woman or can affect reproductive capability. Sargramostim should be given to a pregnant woman only if clearly needed.

Lactation Excretion in breast milk unknown/use caution

Medication Safety Issues

Sound-alike/look-alike issues:

Leukine® may be confused with Leukeran®, leucovorin

Contraindications Hypersensitivity to sargramostim, yeast-derived products, or any component of the formulation; concurrent (24 hours preceding/following) myelosuppressive chemotherapy or radiation therapy; patients with excessive (≥10%) leukemic myeloid blasts in bone marrow or peripheral blood

Warnings/Precautions Simultaneous administration, or administration 24 hours preceding/following cytotoxic chemotherapy or radiotherapy is not recommended. Use with caution in patients with pre-existing cardiac problems or HF; supraventricular arrhythmias have been reported in patients with history of arrhythmias. Edema, capillary leak syndrome, pleural and/or pericardial effusion have been reported; use with caution in patients with pre-existing fluid retention; may worsen. Use with caution in patients with hepatic or renal impairment; monitor hepatic and/or renal function in patients with history of hepatic or renal dysfunction. Elevations in bilirubin, transaminases, and serum creatinine have been observed with use. Dyspnea may occur; monitor respiratory symptoms during and following infusion; use with caution in patients with hypoxia or pulmonary infiltrates.

With rapid increase in blood counts (ANC >20,000/mm^3, WBC >50,000/mm^3, or platelets >500,000/mm^3); decrease dose by 50% or discontinue drug (counts will fall to normal within 3-7 days after discontinuing drug). May potentially act as a growth factor for any tumor type, particularly myeloid malignancies; caution should be exercised when using in any malignancy with myeloid characteristics; tumors of nonhematopoietic origin may have surface receptors for sargramostim. Discontinue use if disease progression occurs during treatment.

There is a "first-dose effect" (refer to Adverse Reactions for details) which is seen (rarely) with the first dose of a cycle and does not usually occur with subsequent doses within that cycle. Anaphylaxis or other serious allergic reactions have been reported; discontinue immediately if occur. Solution contains benzyl alcohol; do not use in premature infants or neonates.

Adverse Reactions

>10%:

Cardiovascular: Hypertension (34%), pericardial effusion (4% to 25%), edema (13% to 25%), chest pain (15%), peripheral edema (11%), tachycardia (11%)

Central nervous system: Fever (81%), malaise (57%), headache (26%), chills (25%), anxiety (11%), insomnia (11%)

Dermatologic: Rash (44%), pruritus (23%)

Endocrine & metabolic: Hyperglycemia (25%), hypercholesterolemia (17%), hypomagnesemia (15%)

Gastrointestinal: Diarrhea (≤89%), nausea (58% to 70%), vomiting (46% to 70%), abdominal pain (38%), weight loss (37%), anorexia (13%), hematemesis (13%), dysphagia (11%), gastrointestinal hemorrhage (11%)

Genitourinary: Urinary tract disorder (14%)

Hepatic: Hyperbilirubinemia (30%)

Neuromuscular & skeletal: Weakness (66%), bone pain (21%), arthralgia (11% to 21%) myalgia (18%)

Ocular: Eye hemorrhage (11%)

Renal: BUN increased (23%), serum creatinine increased (15%)

Respiratory: Pharyngitis (23%), epistaxis (17%), dyspnea (15%)

1% to 10%: Respiratory: Pleural effusion (1%)

<1% (Limited to important or life-threatening): Allergic reaction, anaphylaxis, arrhythmia, capillary leak syndrome, constipation, dizziness, eosinophilia; first-dose effect (syndrome with respiratory distress, hypoxia, flushing, hypotension, syncope, and/or tachycardia occurring with the first dose of a treatment cycle); injection site reaction, lethargy, leukocytosis, liver function abnormalities (transient), pain, pericarditis, prothrombin time prolonged, rigors, sore throat, supraventricular arrhythmia (transient), thrombocytosis, thrombophlebitis, thrombosis

Drug Interactions

Avoid Concomitant Use There are no known interactions where it is recommended to avoid concomitant use.

Increased Effect/Toxicity There are no known significant interactions involving an increase in effect.

Decreased Effect There are no known significant interactions involving a decrease in effect.

Stability Store at 2°C to 8°C (36°F to 46°F); do not freeze. Do not shake.

Solution for injection: May be stored for up to 20 days at 2°C to 8°C (36°F to 46°F) once the vial has been entered. Discard remaining solution after 20 days.

Powder for injection: May be reconstituted with preservative free SWFI or bacteriostatic water for injection (with benzyl alcohol 0.9%). Preparations made with SWFI should be administered as soon as possible, and discarded within 6 hours of reconstitution. Preparations made with bacteriostatic water may be stored for up to 20 days at 2°C to 8°C (36°F to 46°F). Gently swirl to reconstitute; do not shake.

Sargramostim may also be further diluted in 25-50 mL NS to a concentration ≥10 mcg/mL for I.V. infusion administration; preparations diluted with NS are stable for 48 hours at room temperature and refrigeration.

If the final concentration of sargramostim is <10 mcg/mL, 1 mg of human albumin/1 mL of NS (eg, 1 mL of 5% human albumin/50 mL of NS) should be added.

Mechanism of Action Stimulates proliferation, differentiation and functional activity of neutrophils, eosinophils, monocytes, and macrophages, as indicated.

Pharmacodynamics/Kinetics

Onset of action: Increase in WBC: 7-14 days

Duration: WBCs return to baseline within 1 week of discontinuing drug

Half-life elimination: I.V.: 60 minutes; SubQ: 2.7 hours

Time to peak, serum: SubQ: 1-3 hours

Dosage

Children (unlabeled use) and Adults: I.V. infusion over ≥2 hours or SubQ: **Rounding the dose to the nearest vial size enhances patient convenience and reduces costs without clinical detriment**

Myeloid reconstitution after allogeneic or autologous bone marrow transplant: I.V.: 250 mcg/m^2/day (over 2 hours), begin 2-4 hours after the marrow infusion and ≥24 hours after chemotherapy or radiotherapy, when the post marrow infusion ANC is <500 cells/mm^3, and continue until ANC >1500 cells/mm^3 for 3 consecutive days

If a severe adverse reaction occurs, reduce dose by 50% or temporarily discontinue the dose until the reaction abates

If blast cells appear or progression of the underlying disease occurs, discontinue treatment

If ANC >20,000 cells/mm^3, interrupt treatment or reduce the dose by 50%

Neutrophil recovery following chemotherapy in AML: I.V.: 250 mcg/m^2/day (over 4 hours) starting approximately on day 11 or 4 days following the completion of induction chemotherapy, if day 10 bone marrow is hypoplastic with <5% blasts

If a second cycle of chemotherapy is necessary, administer ~4 days after the completion of chemotherapy if the bone marrow is hypoplastic with <5% blasts

Continue sargramostim until ANC is >1500 cells/mm^3 for 3 consecutive days or a maximum of 42 days

Discontinue sargramostim immediately if leukemic regrowth occurs

If a severe adverse reaction occurs, reduce the dose by 50% or temporarily discontinue the dose until the reaction abates

If ANC >20,000 cells/mm^3, interrupt treatment or reduce the dose by 50%

Mobilization of peripheral blood progenitor cells: I.V., SubQ: 250 mcg/m^2/day I.V. over 24 hours or SubQ once daily

Continue the same dose through the period of PBPC collection

The optimal schedule for PBPC collection has not been established (usually begun by day 5 and performed daily until protocol specified targets are achieved)

If WBC >50,000 cells/mm^3, reduce the dose by 50%

If adequate numbers of progenitor cells are not collected, consider other mobilization therapy

Postperipheral blood progenitor cell transplantation: I.V., SubQ: 250 mcg/m^2/day I.V. over 24 hours or SubQ once daily beginning immediately following infusion of progenitor cells and continuing until ANC is >1500 cells/mm^3 for 3 consecutive days is attained

BMT failure or engraftment delay: I.V.: 250 mcg/m^2/day over 2 hours for 14 days

May be repeated after 7 days off therapy if engraftment has not occurred

If engraftment still has not occurred, a third course of 500 mcg/m^2/day for 14 days may be tried after another 7 days off therapy; if there is still no improvement, it is unlikely that further dose escalation will be beneficial

If a severe adverse reaction occurs, reduce the dose by 50% or temporarily discontinue the dose until the reaction abates

If blast cells appear or disease progression occurs, discontinue treatment

If ANC >20,000 cells/mm^3, interrupt treatment or reduce the dose by 50%

Administration Can premedicate with analgesics and antipyretics (eg, acetaminophen) to control adverse events (eg, fever, chills, myalgia, etc); control bone pain with non-narcotic analgesics. Sargramostim is administered as a subcutaneous injection or intravenous infusion; intravenous infusion should be over 2-24 hours; continuous infusions may be more effective than short infusion or bolus injection. An in-line membrane filter should **NOT** be used for intravenous administration. When administering GM-CSF subcutaneously, rotate injection sites.

Monitoring Parameters Vital signs, hydration status, weight, CBC with differential twice weekly during therapy, renal/liver function tests at least biweekly during therapy (in patients displaying renal or hepatic dysfunction prior to initiation of treatment), pulmonary function

Reference Range Excessive leukocytosis: ANC >20,000/mm^3 or WBC >50,000 cells/mm^3

Test Interactions May interfere with bone imaging studies; increased hematopoietic activity of the bone marrow may appear as transient positive bone imaging changes

Additional Information Reimbursement Hotline (Leukine®): 1-800-321-4669

Dosage Forms Excipient information presented when available (limited, particularly for generics); consult specific product labeling.

Injection, powder for reconstitution:

Leukine®: 250 mcg [contains sucrose 10 mg/mL]

Injection, solution:

Leukine®: 500 mcg/mL (1 mL) [contains benzyl alcohol and sucrose 10 mg/mL]

◆ **Sarna® HC (Can)** *see* Hydrocortisone *on page* 743

◆ **Sarnol®-HC [OTC]** *see* Hydrocortisone *on page* 743

◆ **Savella™** *see* Milnacipran *on page* 997

◆ **SB-265805** *see* Gemifloxacin *on page* 688

◆ **SB-497115** *see* Eltrombopag *on page* 512

◆ **SB-497115-GR** *see* Eltrombopag *on page* 512

◆ **SC 33428** *see* IDArubicin *on page* 765

◆ **Scandonest® 3% Plain** *see* Mepivacaine *on page* 945

◆ **SCH 13521** *see* Flutamide *on page* 643

◆ **SCH 56592** *see* Posaconazole *on page* 1213

◆ **ScheinPharm Ranitidine (Can)** *see* Ranitidine *on page* 1295

◆ **SCIG** *see* Immune Globulin (Subcutaneous) *on page* 779

◆ **S-Citalopram** *see* Escitalopram *on page* 547

◆ **Scleromate®** *see* Morrhuate Sodium *on page* 1020

◆ **Sclerosol®** *see* Talc (Sterile) *on page* 1424

◆ **Scopace™** *see* Scopolamine Derivatives *on page* 1356

◆ **Scopolamine and Phenylephrine** *see* Phenylephrine and Scopolamine *on page* 1185

◆ **Scopolamine Base** *see* Scopolamine Derivatives *on page* 1356

◆ **Scopolamine Butylbromide** *see* Scopolamine Derivatives *on page* 1356

Scopolamine Derivatives

(skoe POL a meen dah RIV ah tives)

U.S. Brand Names Isopto® Hyoscine; Scopace™; Transderm Scōp®

Canadian Brand Names Buscopan®; Transderm-V®

Index Terms Hyoscine Butylbromide; Hyoscine Hydrobromide; Scopolamine Base; Scopolamine Butylbromide; Scopolamine Hydrobromide

Pharmacologic Category Anticholinergic Agent

Additional Appendix Information

Cycloplegic Mydriatics *on page 1655*

Use

Scopolamine base:

Transdermal: Prevention of nausea/vomiting associated with motion sickness and recovery from anesthesia and surgery

Scopolamine hydrobromide:

Injection: Preoperative medication to produce amnesia, sedation, tranquilization, antiemetic effects, and decrease salivary and respiratory secretions

Ophthalmic: Produce cycloplegia and mydriasis; treatment of iridocyclitis

Oral: Symptomatic treatment of postencephalitic parkinsonism and paralysis agitans; in spastic states; inhibits excessive motility and hypertonus of the gastrointestinal tract in such conditions as the irritable colon syndrome, mild dysentery, diverticulitis, pylorospasm, and cardiospasm

Scopolamine butylbromide [not available in the U.S.]:

Oral/injection: Treatment of smooth muscle spasm of the genitourinary or gastrointestinal tract; injection may also be used to prior to radiological/diagnostic procedures to prevent spasm

Pregnancy Risk Factor C

Pregnancy Considerations Teratogenic effects were not observed in animal studies; embryotoxic events were observed in some studies. Scopolamine crosses the placenta; may cause respiratory depression and/or neonatal hemorrhage when used during pregnancy. Transdermal scopolamine has been used as an adjunct to epidural anesthesia for cesarean delivery without adverse CNS effects on the newborn. Except when used prior to cesarean section, use during pregnancy only if the benefit to the mother outweighs the potential risk to the fetus.

Lactation Enters breast milk/use caution (AAP rates "compatible")

Medication Safety Issues

Transdermal patch may contain conducting metal (eg, aluminum); remove patch prior to MRI.

Contraindications Hypersensitivity to scopolamine, other belladonna alkaloids, or any component of the formulation; narrow-angle glaucoma; acute hemorrhage; paralytic ileus; tachycardia secondary to cardiac insufficiency; myasthenia gravis

Tablet formulations are contraindicated in patients with prostatic hyperplasia, pyloric obstruction, or patients with an idiosyncrasy to anticholinergic drugs.

Injectable formulations are contraindicated in patients with chronic lung disease (repeated administration).

Warnings/Precautions Use with caution in patients with coronary artery disease, tachyarrhythmias, heart failure, or hypertension; evaluate tachycardia prior to administration. Use with caution with hepatic or renal impairment; adverse CNS effects occur more often in these patients. Use with caution in infants and children since they may be more susceptible to adverse effects of scopolamine. Use injectable, ophthalmic, and transdermal products with caution in patients with prostatic hyperplasia (nonobstructive) or urinary retention; oral products are contraindicated. Discontinue if patient reports unusual visual disturbances or pain within the eye. Use caution in hiatal hernia, reflux esophagitis, and ulcerative colitis. Use with caution in patients with a history of seizure or psychosis; may exacerbate these conditions. Patients with idiosyncratic reaction to anticholinergics, including scopolamine, may experience disorientation, delirium and/or marked somnolence; may be accompanied by dilated pupils, rapid pulse and xerostomia. May cause CNS depression, which may impair physical or mental abilities; patients must be cautioned about performing tasks which require mental alertness (eg, operating machinery or driving).

Transdermal patch may contain conducting metal (eg, aluminum); remove patch prior to MRI. Ophthalmic products may contain benzalkonium chloride which may be absorbed by contact lenses; remove contacts prior to administration and wait 15 minutes before reinserting. Scopolamine (hyoscine) hydrobromide should not be interchanged with scopolamine butylbromide formulations; dosages are not equivalent. Safety and efficacy have not been established for the use of transdermal and oral scopolamine in children.

Adverse Reactions Frequency not defined.

Ophthalmic: Note: Systemic adverse effects have been reported following ophthalmic administration.

Central nervous system: Drowsiness, somnolence, visual hallucination

Dermatologic: Eczematoid dermatitis

Ocular: Blurred vision, edema, exudate, follicular conjunctivitis, increased intraocular pressure, local irritation, photophobia, vascular congestion

Respiratory: Congestion

Systemic:

Cardiovascular: Flushing, orthostatic hypotension, palpitation, tachycardia, ventricular fibrillation

Central nervous system: Acute toxic psychosis (rare), agitation (rare), ataxia, confusion, delusion (rare), disorientation, dizziness, drowsiness, fatigue, hallucination (rare), headache, loss of memory, paranoid behavior (rare), restlessness

Dermatologic: Dry skin, erythema, increased sensitivity to light, rash

Endocrine & metabolic: Decreased flow of breast milk, thirst

Gastrointestinal: Bloated feeling, constipation, dry throat, dysphagia, nausea, vomiting, xerostomia

Genitourinary: Dysuria, urinary retention

Local: Irritation at injection site

Neuromuscular & skeletal: Tremor, weakness

Ocular: Accommodation impaired, blurred vision, cycloplegia, dryness, glaucoma (narrow-angle), increased intraocular pain, itching, photophobia, pupil dilation

Respiratory: Dry nose

Miscellaneous: Diaphoresis (decreased), heat intolerance

Drug Interactions

Avoid Concomitant Use There are no known interactions where it is recommended to avoid concomitant use.

Increased Effect/Toxicity

Scopolamine Derivatives may increase the levels/effects of: Alcohol (Ethyl); Anticholinergics; Cannabinoids; CNS Depressants; Potassium Chloride

The levels/effects of Scopolamine Derivatives may be increased by: Pramlintide

Decreased Effect

Scopolamine Derivatives may decrease the levels/effects of: Acetylcholinesterase Inhibitors (Central); Secretin

The levels/effects of Scopolamine Derivatives may be decreased by: Acetylcholinesterase Inhibitors (Central)

Ethanol/Nutrition/Herb Interactions Ethanol: Avoid ethanol (may increase CNS depression).

Stability

Injection: Store at room temperature of 15°C to 30°C (58°F to 86°F). Protect from light.

Hydrobromide injection: Avoid acid solutions, hydrolysis occurs at pH <3.

Butylbromide injection: Stable in D_5W, NS, $D_{10}W$, and LR for up to 8 hours.

Ophthalmic solution: Store at 8°C to 27°C (46°F to 80°F). Protect from light.

Tablet: Store at room temperature of 15°C to 30°C (58°F to 86°F).

Transdermal system: Store at 20°C to 25°C (68°F to 77°F).

Mechanism of Action Blocks the action of acetylcholine at parasympathetic sites in smooth muscle, secretory glands and the CNS; increases cardiac output, dries secretions, antagonizes histamine and serotonin; dilates pupils

Pharmacodynamics/Kinetics

Onset of action: Oral, I.M.: 0.5-1 hour; I.V.: 10 minutes

Peak effect: 20-60 minutes; may take 3-7 days for full recovery; transdermal: 24 hours

Duration: Oral, I.M.: 4-6 hours; I.V.: 2 hours

Absorption: Tertiary salts (hydrobromide) are well absorbed; quaternary salts (butylbromide) are poorly absorbed (local concentrations in the GI tract following oral dosing may be high)

Metabolism: Hepatic

Half-life elimination: 4.8 hours

Excretion: Urine (<10%, as parent drug and metabolites)

Dosage Note: Scopolamine (hyoscine) hydrobromide should not be interchanged with scopolamine butylbromide formulations. Dosages are not equivalent.

Scopolamine base: Transdermal patch: Adults:

Preoperative: Apply 1 patch to hairless area behind ear the night before surgery or 1 hour prior to cesarean section (apply no sooner than 1 hour before surgery to minimize newborn exposure); remove 24 hours after surgery

Motion sickness: Apply 1 patch behind the ear at least 4 hours prior to exposure and every 3 days as needed; effective if applied as soon as 2-3 hours before anticipated need, best if 12 hours before

Scopolamine hydrobromide:

Antiemetic: SubQ:

Children: 0.006 mg/kg

Adults: 0.6-1 mg

Preoperative: I.M., I.V., SubQ:

Children 6 months to 3 years: 0.1-0.15 mg

Children 3-6 years: 0.2-0.3 mg

Adults: 0.3-0.65 mg

Sedation, tranquilization: I.M., I.V., SubQ: Adults: 0.6 mg 3-4 times/day

Refraction: Ophthalmic:

Children: Instill 1 drop of 0.25% to eye(s) twice daily for 2 days before procedure

Adults: Instill 1-2 drops of 0.25% to eye(s) 1 hour before procedure

Iridocyclitis: Ophthalmic:

Children: Instill 1 drop of 0.25% to eye(s) up to 3 times/day

Adults: Instill 1-2 drops of 0.25% to eye(s) up to 4 times/day

Parkinsonism, spasticity, motion sickness: Adults: Oral: 0.4-0.8 mg. May repeat every 8-12 hours as needed; the dosage may be cautiously increased in parkinsonism and spastic states. For motion sickness, administration at least 1 hour before exposure is recommended.

Scopolamine butylbromide:

Gastrointestinal/genitourinary spasm (Buscopan® [CAN]; not available in the U.S.): Adults:

Oral: 10-20 mg daily (1-2 tablets); maximum: 6 tablets/day

I.M., I.V., SubQ: 10-20 mg; maximum: 100 mg/day. Intramuscular injections should be administered 10-15 minutes prior to radiological/diagnostic procedures

Administration

I.V.:

Hydrobromide: Dilute with an equal volume of sterile water and administer by direct I.V.; inject over 2-3 minutes

Butylbromide: No dilution is necessary prior to injection; inject at a rate of 1 mL/minute

Ophthalmic: Remove contact lenses prior to administration; wait 15 minutes before reinserting if using products containing benzalkonium chloride. Wash hands following administration.

Transdermal: Topical patch is programmed to deliver 1 mg over 3 days. Once applied, do not remove the patch for 3 full days. Apply to hairless area of skin behind the ear. Wash hands before and after applying the disc to avoid drug contact with eyes.

Monitoring Parameters Body temperature, heart rate, urinary output, intraocular pressure

Test Interactions Interferes with gastric secretion test

Dosage Forms Excipient information presented when available (limited, particularly for generics); consult specific product labeling. [CAN] = Canadian brand name

Injection, solution, as hydrobromide: 0.4 mg/mL (1 mL)

Injection, solution, as hyoscine-N-butylbromide:

Buscopan® [CAN]: 20 mg/mL [not available in U.S.]

Solution, ophthalmic, as hydrobromide:

Isopto® Hyoscine: 0.25% (5 mL) [contains benzalkonium chloride]

Tablet, as hyoscine-N-butylbromide:

Buscopan® [CAN]: 10 mg [not available in U.S.]

Tablet, soluble, as hydrobromide:

Scopace™: 0.4 mg

Transdermal system:

Transderm Scōp®: 1.5 mg (4s, 10s, 24s) [releases ~1 mg over 72 hours]

- **Scopolamine Hydrobromide** *see* Scopolamine Derivatives *on page 1356*
- **Scopolamine, Hyoscyamine, Atropine, and Phenobarbital** *see* Hyoscyamine, Atropine, Scopolamine, and Phenobarbital *on page 756*
- **Scot-Tussin® DM Maximum Strength [OTC]** *see* Dextromethorphan and Chlorpheniramine *on page 433*
- **Scot-Tussin® Expectorant [OTC]** *see* GuaiFENesin *on page 709*
- **Scot-Tussin® Senior [OTC]** *see* Guaifenesin and Dextromethorphan *on page 710*
- **Sculptra®** *see* Poly-L-Lactic Acid *on page 1210*
- **SD/01** *see* Pegfilgrastim *on page 1152*
- **SDX-105** *see* Bendamustine *on page 181*
- **SDZ ENA 713** *see* Rivastigmine *on page 1331*
- **Seasonale®** *see* Ethinyl Estradiol and Levonorgestrel *on page 577*
- **Seasonique™** *see* Ethinyl Estradiol and Levonorgestrel *on page 577*
- **Seb-Prev™** *see* Sulfacetamide *on page 1405*

Secobarbital (see koe BAR bi tal)

U.S. Brand Names Seconal®

Index Terms Quinalbarbitone Sodium; Secobarbital Sodium

Pharmacologic Category Barbiturate

Use Preanesthetic agent; short-term treatment of insomnia

Restrictions C-II

Pregnancy Risk Factor D

Medication Safety Issues

Sound-alike/look-alike issues:

Seconal® may be confused with Sectral®

Dosage Oral:

Children:

Preoperative sedation: 2-6 mg/kg (maximum dose: 100 mg/dose) 1-2 hours before procedure

Sedation: 6 mg/kg/day divided every 8 hours

Adults:
Hypnotic: Usual: 100 mg/dose at bedtime; range: 100-200 mg/dose
Preoperative sedation: 100-300 mg 1-2 hours before procedure

Additional Information Complete prescribing information for this medication should be consulted for additional detail.

Dosage Forms Excipient information presented when available (limited, particularly for generics); consult specific product labeling.
Capsule, as sodium: 100 mg

- **Secobarbital Sodium** *see* Secobarbital *on page 1358*
- **Seconal®** *see* Secobarbital *on page 1358*
- **Sectral®** *see* Acebutolol *on page 25*
- **Secura® Antifungal [OTC]** *see* Miconazole *on page 989*
- **Sedapap®** *see* Butalbital and Acetaminophen *on page 230*
- **Selax® (Can)** *see* Docusate *on page 473*
- **Select™ 1/35 (Can)** *see* Ethinyl Estradiol and Norethindrone *on page 581*

Selegiline (se LE ji leen)

U.S. Brand Names Eldepryl®; Emsam®; Zelapar™

Canadian Brand Names Apo-Selegiline®; Gen-Selegiline; Novo-Selegiline; Nu-Selegiline

Index Terms Deprenyl; L-Deprenyl; Selegiline Hydrochloride

Pharmacologic Category Anti-Parkinson's Agent, MAO Type B Inhibitor; Antidepressant, Monoamine Oxidase Inhibitor

Additional Appendix Information

Antidepressant Agents *on page 1638*
Antiparkinsonian Agents *on page 1643*
Tyramine Content of Foods *on page 1850*

Use Adjunct in the management of parkinsonian patients in which levodopa/carbidopa therapy is deteriorating (oral products); treatment of major depressive disorder (transdermal product)

Unlabeled/Investigational Use Early Parkinson's disease; attention-deficit/hyperactivity disorder (ADHD); negative symptoms of schizophrenia; extrapyramidal symptoms

Restrictions An FDA-approved medication guide concerning the use of antidepressants in children, adolescents, and young adults must be distributed when dispensing a transdermal selegiline outpatient prescription (new or refill) where this medication is to be used without direct supervision of a healthcare provider. Medication guides are available at http://www.fda.gov/cder/Offices/ODS/medication_guides.htm. Dispense to parents or guardians of children and adolescents receiving this medication.

Pregnancy Risk Factor C

Pregnancy Considerations Teratogenic and adverse behavioral events were noted in animal studies. There are no adequate and well-controlled studies in pregnant women.

Lactation Excretion in breast milk unknown/use caution

Medication Safety Issues
Sound-alike/look-alike issues:
Selegiline may be confused with Salagen®, Serentil®, sertraline, Serzone®, Stelazine®
Eldepryl® may be confused with Elavil®, enalapril
Zelapar™ may be confused with zaleplon, Zemplar®

Contraindications Hypersensitivity to selegiline or any component of the formulation; concomitant use of meperidine
Orally disintegrating tablet: Additional contraindications: Concomitant use of dextromethorphan, methadone, propoxyphene, tramadol, oral selegiline, other MAO inhibitors
Transdermal: Additional contraindications: Pheochromocytoma; concomitant use of bupropion, selective or dual serotonin reuptake inhibitors (including SSRIs and SNRIs), tricyclic antidepressants, buspirone, tramadol, propoxyphene, methadone, dextromethorphan, St. John's wort, mirtazapine, cyclobenzaprine, oral selegiline and other MAO inhibitors; carbamazepine, and oxcarbazepine; elective surgery requiring general anesthesia, local anesthesia containing sympathomimetic vasoconstrictors; sympathomimetics (and related compounds); foods high in tyramine content; supplements containing tyrosine, phenylalanine, tryptophan, or caffeine

Warnings/Precautions
Oral: MAO-B selective inhibition should not pose a problem with tyramine-containing products as long as the typical oral doses are employed, however, rare reactions have been reported. Increased risk of nonselective MAO inhibition occurs with oral capsule/tablet doses >10 mg/day or orally disintegrating tablet doses >2.5 mg/day. Use of oral selegiline with tricyclic antidepressants and SSRIs has also been associated with rare reactions and should generally be avoided. Addition to levodopa therapy may result in exacerbation of levodopa adverse effects, requiring a reduction in levodopa dosage.

Transdermal: Nonselective MAO inhibition occurs with transdermal delivery and is necessary for antidepressant efficacy. Hypertensive crisis as a result of ingesting tyramine-rich foods is always a concern with nonselective MAO inhibition. Although transdermal delivery minimizes inhibition of MAO-A in the gut, there is limited data with higher transdermal doses; dietary restrictions are recommended with doses >6 mg/24 hours.

Transdermal: **[U.S. Boxed Warning]: Antidepressants increase the risk of suicidal thinking and behavior in children, adolescents, and young adults (18-24 years of age) with major depressive disorder (MDD) and other psychiatric disorders;** consider risk prior to prescribing. Short-term studies did not show an increased risk in patients >24 years of age and showed a decreased risk in patients ≥65 years. Closely monitor patients for worsening of depression, suicidality and/or associated behaviors, particularly during the initial 1-2 months of therapy or during periods of dosage adjustments (increases or decreases); the patient's family or caregiver should be instructed to closely observe the patient and communicate condition with healthcare provider. A medication guide concerning the use of antidepressants should be dispensed with each prescription. **Transdermal selegiline is not FDA approved for use in children <12 years of age.**

Transdermal: The possibility of a suicide attempt is inherit in major depression and may persist until remission occurs. Patients treated with antidepressants (for any indication) should be observed for clinical worsening and suicidality, especially during the initial few months of a course of drug therapy, or at times of dose changes, either increases or decreases. Use caution in high-risk patients. Worsening depression and severe abrupt suicidality that are not part of the presenting symptoms may require discontinuation or modification of drug therapy. Use caution in high-risk patients during initiation of therapy. The patient's family or caregiver should be alerted to monitor patients for the emergence of suicidality and associated behaviors (such as agitation, irritability, hostility, and hypomania) and call healthcare provider.

Transdermal selegiline may worsen psychosis in some patients or precipitate a shift to mania or hypomania in patients with bipolar disorder. Monotherapy in patients with bipolar disorder should be avoided. Patients presenting with depressive symptoms should be screened for bipolar disorder. **Selegiline is not FDA approved for the treatment of bipolar depression.**

Adverse Reactions Unless otherwise noted, the percentage of adverse events is reported for the transdermal patch (**Note:** ODT = orally disintegrating tablet, Oral = capsule/tablet)

>10%:

Central nervous system: Headache (18%; ODT 7%; oral 2%), insomnia (12%; ODT 7%), dizziness (ODT 11%; oral 7%)

Gastrointestinal: Nausea (ODT 11%; oral 10%)

Local: Application site reaction (24%)

1% to 10%:

Cardiovascular: Hypotension (including postural 3% to 10%), chest pain (≥1%; ODT 2%), hypertension (≥1%), peripheral edema (≥1%)

Central nervous system: Pain (ODT 8%), hallucinations (ODT 4%; oral 3%), confusion (ODT 4%; oral 3%), headache (ODT 7%; oral 2%), ataxia (ODT 3%), somnolence (ODT 3%), agitation (≥1%), amnesia (≥1%), paresthesia (≥1%), thinking abnormal (≥1%), depression (<1%; ODT 2%)

Dermatologic: Rash (4%), ecchymosis (ODT 2%), bruising (≥1%), pruritus (≥1%), acne (≥1%)

Endocrine & metabolic: Weight loss (5%), hypokalemia (ODT 2%), sexual side effects (≤1%)

Gastrointestinal: Diarrhea (9%; ODT 2%), xerostomia (8%; ODT 4%), stomatitis (ODT 5%), abdominal pain (oral 4%), dyspepsia (4%; ODT 5%), constipation (≥1%; ODT 4%), flatulence (≥1%; ODT 2%), anorexia (≥1%), gastroenteritis (≥1%), taste perversion (≥1%; ODT 2%), vomiting (≥1%; ODT 3%), tooth disorder (ODT 2%), dysphagia (ODT 2%)

Genitourinary: Dysmenorrhea (≥1%), metrorrhagia (≥1%), UTI (≥1%), urinary frequency (≥1%)

Neuromuscular & skeletal: Dyskinesia (ODT 6%), back pain (ODT 5%), ataxia (<1%; ODT 3%), leg cramps (ODT 3%), myalgia (≥1%; ODT 3%), neck pain (≥1%), tremor (<1%; ODT 3%)

Otic: Tinnitus (≥1%)

Respiratory: Rhinitis (ODT 7%), pharyngitis (3%; ODT 4%), sinusitis (3%), cough (≥1%), bronchitis (≥1%), dyspnea (<1%; ODT 3%)

Miscellaneous: Diaphoresis (≥1%)

Oral and/or transdermal patch: <1% or frequency not defined (limited to important or life-threatening): Abnormal liver function tests, alkaline phosphatase increased, appetite increased, arrhythmia, asthma, ataxia, atrial fibrillation, bacterial infection, behavior/mood changes, bilirubinemia, bradycardia, bradykinesia, breast neoplasm (female), breast pain, chorea, circumoral paresthesia, colitis, dehydration, delusions, dental caries, depersonalization, depression, emotional lability, epistaxis, eructation, euphoria, face edema, fever, fungal infection, gastritis, generalized spasm, glossitis, heat stroke, hematuria (female), hernia, hostility, hypercholesterolemia, hyperesthesia, hyperglycemia, hyperkinesias, hypertonia, hypoglycemic reaction, hyponatremia, kidney calculus (female), lactate dehydrogenase increased, laryngismus, leukocytosis, leukopenia, libido increased, loss of balance, lymphadenopathy, maculopapular rash, manic reaction, melena, migraine, moniliasis, myasthenia, myocardial infarct, myoclonus, neoplasia, neurosis, osteoporosis, otitis external, palpitation, paranoid reaction, parasitic infection, parosmia, pelvic pain, periodontal abscess, peripheral vascular disorder, pneumonia, polyuria (female), prostatic hyperplasia, rectal hemorrhage, salivation increased, skin hypertrophy, skin benign neoplasm, suicide attempt, syncope, tachycardia, tenosynovitis, tongue edema, twitching, urinary retention, urinary urgency (male and female), urination impaired (male), urticaria, vaginal hemorrhage, vaginal moniliasis, vaginitis, vasodilatation, vertigo, vesiculobullous rash, viral infection, visual field defect

Drug Interactions

Metabolism/Transport Effects **Substrate** of CYP1A2 (minor), 2A6 (minor), 2B6 (major), 2C8 (minor), 2C19 (minor), 2D6 (minor), 3A4 (minor); **Inhibits** CYP1A2 (weak), 2A6 (weak), 2C9 (weak), 2C19 (weak), 2D6 (weak), 2E1 (weak), 3A4 (weak)

Avoid Concomitant Use

Avoid concomitant use of Selegiline with any of the following: Alpha-/Beta-Agonists (Indirect-Acting); Alpha1-Agonists; Alpha2-Agonists (Ophthalmic); Amphetamines; Atomoxetine; BuPROPion; BusPIRone; Cyclobenzaprine; Dexmethylphenidate; Dextromethorphan; Linezolid; Maprotiline; Meperidine; Methyldopa; Methylphenidate; Mirtazapine; Propoxyphene; Selective Serotonin Reuptake Inhibitors; Serotonin 5-HT1D Receptor Agonists; Serotonin/Norepinephrine Reuptake Inhibitors; Sibutramine; Tetrabenazine; Tricyclic Antidepressants

Increased Effect/Toxicity

Selegiline may increase the levels/effects of: Alpha-/Beta-Agonists (Direct-Acting); Alpha-/Beta-Agonists (Indirect-Acting); Alpha1-Agonists; Alpha2-Agonists (Ophthalmic); Amphetamines; Atomoxetine; Beta2-Agonists; BuPROPion; Dexmethylphenidate; Dextromethorphan; Linezolid; Lithium; Meperidine; Methyldopa; Methylphenidate; Mirtazapine; Rauwolfia Alkaloids; Selective Serotonin Reuptake Inhibitors; Serotonin 5-HT1D Receptor Agonists; Serotonin Modulators; Serotonin/Norepinephrine Reuptake Inhibitors; Tricyclic Antidepressants

The levels/effects of Selegiline may be increased by: Altretamine; Anilidopiperidine Opioids; BusPIRone; COMT Inhibitors; Cyclobenzaprine; CYP2B6 Inhibitors (Moderate); CYP2B6 Inhibitors (Strong); Levodopa; Maprotiline; Oral Contraceptive (Estrogens); Oral Contraceptive (Progestins); Propoxyphene; Sibutramine; Tetrabenazine; TraMADol

Decreased Effect

The levels/effects of Selegiline may be decreased by: CYP2B6 Inducers (Strong)

Ethanol/Nutrition/Herb Interactions

Ethanol: Avoid ethanol (based on CNS depressant effects and potential tyramine content)

Food: Concurrent ingestion of foods rich in tyramine may cause sudden and severe high blood pressure (hypertensive crisis). Avoid tyramine-containing foods with MAO-Is. Food's freshness is also an important concern; improperly stored or spoiled food can create an environment where tyramine concentrations may increase.

Herb/Nutraceuticals: Avoid valerian, St John's wort, SAMe, kava kava. Avoid supplements containing caffeine, tryptophan, or phenylalanine. Ingestion of large quantities may increase the risk of severe side effects (eg, hypertensive reactions, serotonin syndrome).

Stability

Capsule, tablet: Store at controlled room temperature 15°C to 30°C (59°F to 86°F).

Orally-disintegrating tablet: Store at controlled room temperature 15°C to 30°C (59°F to 86°F). Use within 3 months of opening pouch and immediately after opening individual blister.

Transdermal: Store at 20°C to 25°C (68°F to 77°F).

Mechanism of Action Potent, irreversible inhibitor of monoamine oxidase (MAO). Plasma concentrations achieved via administration of oral dosage forms in recommended doses confer selective inhibition of MAO type B, which plays a major role in the metabolism of dopamine; selegiline may also increase dopaminergic activity by interfering with dopamine reuptake at the synapse. When administered transdermally in recommended doses, selegiline achieves higher blood levels and effectively inhibits both MAO-A and MAO-B, which blocks catabolism of other centrally-active biogenic amine neurotransmitters.

Pharmacodynamics/Kinetics

Onset of action: Therapeutic: Oral: Within 1 hour

Duration: Oral: 24-72 hours

Absorption:

Orally disintegrating tablet: Rapid; greater bioavailability than capsule/tablet

Transdermal: 25% to 30% (of total selegiline content) over 24 hours

Protein binding: ~90%

Metabolism: Hepatic, primarily via CYP2B6 to active (N-desmethylselegiline, amphetamine, methamphetamine) and inactive metabolites

Half-life elimination: Oral: 10 hours; Transdermal: 18-25 hours

Excretion: Urine (primarily metabolites); feces

Dosage

Capsule/tablet:

Children and Adolescents: ADHD (unlabeled use): 5-15 mg/day

Adults: Parkinson's disease: 5 mg twice daily with breakfast and lunch or 10 mg in the morning

Elderly: Parkinson's disease: Initial: 5 mg in the morning, may increase to a total of 10 mg/day

Orally disintegrating tablet (Zelapar™): Adults: Parkinson's disease: Initial 1.25 mg daily for at least 6 weeks; may increase to 2.5 mg daily based on clinical response (maximum: 2.5 mg daily)

Transdermal (Emsam®): Depression:

Adults: Initial: 6 mg/24 hours once daily; may titrate based on clinical response in increments of 3 mg/day every 2 weeks up to a maximum of 12 mg/24 hours

Elderly: 6 mg/24 hours

Dosage adjustment in renal impairment: No adjustment necessary.

Dosage adjustment in hepatic impairment: No adjustment necessary in mild-moderate hepatic impairment.

Dietary Considerations Avoid tyramine-containing foods/beverages. Some examples include aged or matured cheese, air-dried or cured meats (including sausages and salamis), fava or broad bean pods, tap/draft beers, Marmite concentrate, sauerkraut, soy sauce and other soybean condiments.

Emsam® 9 mg/24 hours or 12 mg/24 hours: Avoid tyramine-rich foods or beverages beginning the first day of treatment or for 2 weeks after discontinuation or dose reduction to 6 mg/24 hours.

Zelapar™: Phenylalanine 1.25 mg per 1.25 mg tablet; do not take with food or liquid

Administration

Oral: Orally disintegrating tablet (Zelapar™): Take in morning before breakfast; place on top of tongue and allow to dissolve. Avoid food or liquid 5 minutes before and after administration.

Topical: Transdermal (Emsam®): Apply to clean, dry, intact skin to the upper torso (below the neck and above the waist), upper thigh, or outer surface of the upper arm. Avoid exposure of application site to external heat source, which may increase the amount of drug absorbed. Apply at the same time each day and rotate application sites. Wash hands with soap and water after handling. Avoid touching the sticky side of the patch.

Monitoring Parameters Blood pressure; symptoms of parkinsonism; general mood and behavior (increased anxiety, presence of mania or agitation); suicidal ideation (especially at the beginning of therapy or when doses are increased or decreased)

Additional Information When adding selegiline to levodopa/carbidopa, the dose of the latter can usually be decreased.

Dosage Forms Excipient information presented when available (limited, particularly for generics); consult specific product labeling.

Capsule, oral, as hydrochloride: 5 mg

Eldepryl®: 5 mg

Tablet, oral, as hydrochloride: 5 mg

Tablet, orally-disintegrating:

Zelapar™: 1.25 mg [contains phenylalanine 1.25 mg/tablet]

Transdermal system, topical [once-daily patch]:

Emsam®: 6 mg/24 hours (30s) [20 cm^2, total selegiline 20 mg]; 9 mg/24 hours (30s) [30 cm^2, total selegiline 30 mg]; 12 mg/24 hours (30s) [40 cm^2, total selegiline 40 mg]

◆ **Selegiline Hydrochloride** *see* Selegiline *on page* 1359

◆ **Selenicaps [OTC]** *see* Selenium *on page* 1361

◆ **Selenimin [OTC]** *see* Selenium *on page* 1361

Selenium (se LEE nee um)

U.S. Brand Names Selenicaps [OTC]; Selenimin [OTC]

Pharmacologic Category Trace Element, Parenteral

Use Trace metal supplement

Pregnancy Risk Factor C

Dosage I.V. in TPN solutions:

Children: 3 mcg/kg/day

Adults:

Metabolically stable: 20-40 mcg/day

Deficiency from prolonged TPN support: 100 mcg/day for 24 and 31 days

Additional Information Complete prescribing information for this medication should be consulted for additional detail.

Dosage Forms Excipient information presented when available (limited, particularly for generics); consult specific product labeling.

Capsule: 200 mcg

Selenicaps: 200 mcg [sugar, gluten free]

Injection, solution: 40 mcg/mL (10 mL)

Tablet: 50 mcg, 100 mcg, 200 mcg

Selenimin: 50 mcg, 125 mcg, 200 mcg

Tablet, timed release: 200 mcg

Selenium Sulfide (se LEE nee um SUL fide)

U.S. Brand Names Dandrex [OTC]; Head & Shoulders® Intensive Treatment [OTC]; Selseb®; Selsun blue® 2-in-1 Treatment [OTC]; Selsun blue® Daily Treatment [OTC]; Selsun blue® Medicated Treatment [OTC]; Selsun blue® Moisturizing Treatment [OTC]; Tersi

Canadian Brand Names Versel®

Pharmacologic Category Topical Skin Product

Use Treatment of itching and flaking of the scalp associated with dandruff, to control scalp seborrheic dermatitis; treatment of tinea versicolor

Pregnancy Risk Factor C

Dosage Topical: Adults:

Dandruff, seborrhea: Massage 5-10 mL of shampoo into wet scalp, leave on scalp 2-3 minutes, rinse thoroughly; rub foam into affected skin twice daily

Tinea versicolor: Apply the 2.5% lotion to affected area and lather with small amounts of water; leave on skin for 10 minutes, then rinse thoroughly; apply every day for 7 days; rub foam into affected skin twice daily

Additional Information Complete prescribing information for this medication should be consulted for additional detail.

Dosage Forms Excipient information presented when available (limited, particularly for generics); consult specific product labeling.

Aerosol, topical [foam]:
Tersi: 2.25% (70 g)
Lotion, topical: 2.5% (120 mL)
Shampoo, topical: 1% (210 mL)
Dandrex: 1% (240 mL)
Head & Shoulders® Intensive Treatment: 1% (420 mL)
Selseb®: 2.25% (180 mL)
Selsun blue® Daily Treatment: 1% (207 mL, 325 mL)
Selsun blue® Medicated Treatment: 1% (120 mL, 207 mL, 325 mL) [contains menthol]
Selsun blue® Moisturizing Treatment: 1% (207 mL, 325 mL) [contains aloe and moisturizers]
Selsun blue® 2-in-1 Treatment: 1% (207 mL, 325 mL) [contains conditioner]

◆ **Selfemra™** *see* FLUoxetine *on page 638*

◆ **Selseb®** *see* Selenium Sulfide *on page 1361*

◆ **Selsun blue® 2-in-1 Treatment [OTC]** *see* Selenium Sulfide *on page 1361*

◆ **Selsun blue® Daily Treatment [OTC]** *see* Selenium Sulfide *on page 1361*

◆ **Selsun blue® Medicated Treatment [OTC]** *see* Selenium Sulfide *on page 1361*

◆ **Selsun blue® Moisturizing Treatment [OTC]** *see* Selenium Sulfide *on page 1361*

◆ **Selzentry™** *see* Maraviroc *on page 921*

◆ **Semprex®-D** *see* Acrivastine and Pseudoephedrine *on page 40*

◆ **Senna and Docusate** *see* Docusate and Senna *on page 474*

◆ **Senna-S** *see* Docusate and Senna *on page 474*

◆ **Senokot-S® [OTC]** *see* Docusate and Senna *on page 474*

◆ **SenoSol™-SS [OTC]** *see* Docusate and Senna *on page 474*

◆ **Sensipar®** *see* Cinacalcet *on page 328*

◆ **Sensorcaine®** *see* Bupivacaine *on page 220*

◆ **Sensorcaine®-MPF** *see* Bupivacaine *on page 220*

◆ **Sensorcaine®-MPF Spinal** *see* Bupivacaine *on page 220*

◆ **Sepasoothe®** *see* Benzocaine *on page 183*

◆ **Septra®** *see* Sulfamethoxazole and Trimethoprim *on page 1407*

◆ **Septra® DS** *see* Sulfamethoxazole and Trimethoprim *on page 1407*

◆ **Septra® Injection (Can)** *see* Sulfamethoxazole and Trimethoprim *on page 1407*

◆ **Serax®** *see* Oxazepam *on page 1116*

◆ **Serevent® Diskhaler® Disk (Can)** *see* Salmeterol *on page 1350*

◆ **Serevent® Diskus®** *see* Salmeterol *on page 1350*

Sermorelin Acetate (ser moe REL in AS e tate)

U.S. Brand Names Geref® Diagnostic [DSC]

Pharmacologic Category Diagnostic Agent; Growth Hormone

Use Geref® Diagnostic: For evaluation of the ability of the pituitary gland to secrete growth hormone (GH)

Pregnancy Risk Factor C

Dosage

Children and Adults: Diagnostic: I.V.: 1 mcg/kg as a single dose in the morning following an overnight fast

Note: Response to diagnostic test may be decreased in patients >40 years

Additional Information Complete prescribing information for this medication should be consulted for additional detail.

Dosage Forms Excipient information presented when available (limited, particularly for generics); consult specific product labeling. [DSC] = Discontinued product

Injection, powder for reconstitution, as acetate: 50 mcg [packaged with diluent] [DSC]

◆ **Seromycin®** *see* CycloSERINE *on page 378*

◆ **Serophene®** *see* ClomiPHENE *on page 349*

◆ **Seroquel®** *see* QUEtiapine *on page 1275*

◆ **Seroquel® XR** *see* QUEtiapine *on page 1275*

◆ **Serostim®** *see* Somatropin *on page 1388*

Sertaconazole (ser ta KOE na zole)

U.S. Brand Names Ertaczo®

Index Terms Sertaconazole Nitrate

Pharmacologic Category Antifungal Agent, Topical

Use Topical treatment of tinea pedis (athlete's foot)

Pregnancy Risk Factor C

Dosage Topical: Children ≥12 years and Adults: Apply between toes and to surrounding healthy skin twice daily for 4 weeks

Additional Information Complete prescribing information for this medication should be consulted for additional detail.

Dosage Forms Excipient information presented when available (limited, particularly for generics); consult specific product labeling.

Cream, topical, as nitrate:
Ertaczo®: 2% (30 g, 60 g)

◆ **Sertaconazole Nitrate** *see* Sertaconazole *on page 1362*

Sertraline (SER tra leen)

U.S. Brand Names Zoloft®

Canadian Brand Names Apo-Sertraline®; CO Sertraline; Dom-Sertraline; Gen-Sertraline; GMD-Sertraline; Novo-Sertraline; Nu-Sertraline; PHL-Sertraline; PMS-Sertraline; ratio-Sertraline; Rhoxal-sertraline; Riva-Sertraline; Sandoz-Sertraline; Zoloft®

Index Terms Sertraline Hydrochloride

Pharmacologic Category Antidepressant, Selective Serotonin Reuptake Inhibitor

Additional Appendix Information

Antidepressant Agents *on page 1638*

Selective Serotonin Reuptake Inhibitors (SSRIs) Pharmacokinetics *on page 1670*

Use Treatment of major depression; obsessive-compulsive disorder (OCD); panic disorder; post-traumatic stress disorder (PTSD); premenstrual dysphoric disorder (PMDD); social anxiety disorder

Unlabeled/Investigational Use Eating disorders; generalized anxiety disorder (GAD); impulse control disorders; treatment of mild dementia-associated agitation in nonpsychotic patients

Restrictions An FDA-approved medication guide concerning the use of antidepressants in children, adolescents, and young adults must be distributed when dispensing an outpatient prescription (new or refill) where this medication is to be used without direct supervision of a healthcare provider. Medication guides are available at http://www.fda.gov/cder/Offices/ODS/medication_guides.htm. Dispense to parents or guardians of children and adolescents receiving this medication.

Pregnancy Risk Factor C

Pregnancy Considerations Due to adverse effects observed in animal studies, sertraline is classified as pregnancy category C. Sertraline crosses the human placenta. Nonteratogenic effects in the newborn following SSRI exposure late in the third trimester include respiratory distress, cyanosis, apnea, seizures, temperature instability, feeding difficulty, vomiting, hypoglycemia, hypo- or hypertonia, hyper-reflexia, jitteriness, irritability, constant crying, and tremor. An increased risk of low birth weight, lower APGAR scores, and blunted behavioral response to pain for a prolonged period after delivery has also been reported. Exposure to SSRIs after the twentieth week of gestation has been associated with persistent pulmonary hypertension of the newborn (PPHN). Adverse effects may be due to toxic effects of the SSRI or drug discontinuation. The long-term effects of *in utero* SSRI exposure on infant development and behavior are not known.

Due to pregnancy-induced physiologic changes, women who are pregnant may require increased doses of sertraline to achieve euthymia. Women treated for major depression and who are euthymic prior to pregnancy are more likely to experience a relapse when medication is discontinued as compared to pregnant women who continue taking antidepressant medications. The ACOG recommends that therapy with SSRIs or SNRIs during pregnancy be individualized; treatment of depression during pregnancy should incorporate the clinical expertise of the mental health clinician, obstetrician, primary healthcare provider, and pediatrician (ACOG, 2007). If treatment during pregnancy is required, consider tapering therapy during the third trimester in order to prevent withdrawal symptoms in the infant. If this is done and the woman is considered to be at risk from her major depressive disorder, the medication can be restarted following delivery, although the dose should be readjusted to that required before pregnancy.

Lactation Enters breast milk/use caution (AAP rates "of concern")

Medication Safety Issues

Sound-alike/look-alike issues:

Sertraline may be confused with selegiline, Serentil®, Serevent®

Zoloft® may be confused with Zocor®

Contraindications Hypersensitivity to sertraline or any component of the formulation; use of MAO inhibitors within 14 days; concurrent use of pimozide; concurrent use of sertraline oral concentrate with disulfiram

Warnings/Precautions [U.S. Boxed Warning]: Antidepressants increase the risk of suicidal thinking and behavior in children, adolescents, and young adults (18-24 years of age) with major depressive disorder (MDD) and other psychiatric disorders; consider risk prior to prescribing. Short-term studies did not show an increased risk in patients >24 years of age and showed a decreased risk in patients ≥65 years. Closely monitor patients for clinical worsening, suicidality, or unusual changes in behavior, particularly during the initial 1-2 months of therapy or during periods of dosage adjustments (increases or decreases); the patient's family or caregiver should be instructed to closely observe the patient and communicate condition with healthcare provider. A medication guide concerning the use of antidepressants should be dispensed with each prescription. **Sertraline is not FDA approved for use in children with major depressive disorder (MDD). However, it is approved for the treatment of obsessive-compulsive disorder (OCD) in children ≥6 years of age.**

The possibility of a suicide attempt is inherent in major depression and may persist until remission occurs. Use caution in high-risk patients. Worsening depression and severe abrupt suicidality that are not part of the presenting symptoms may require discontinuation or modification of drug therapy. The patient's family or caregiver should be alerted to monitor patients for the emergence of suicidality and associated behaviors (such as agitation, irritability, hostility, impulsivity, and hypomania) and call healthcare provider.

May worsen psychosis in some patients or precipitate a shift to mania or hypomania in patients with bipolar disorder. Patients presenting with depressive symptoms should be screened for bipolar disorder. Monotherapy in patients with bipolar disorder should be avoided. **Sertraline is not FDA approved for the treatment of bipolar depression.**

The potential for severe reaction exists when used with MAO inhibitors, SSRIs/SNRIs or triptans; serotonin syndrome (hyperthermia, muscular rigidity, mental status changes/agitation, autonomic instability) may occur; concomitant use with MAO inhibitors is contraindicated. Has a very low potential to impair cognitive or motor performance. However, caution patients regarding activities requiring alertness until response to sertraline is known. Does not appear to potentiate the effects of alcohol, however, ethanol use is not advised.

Use caution in patients with a previous seizure disorder or condition predisposing to seizures such as brain damage, alcoholism, or concurrent therapy with other drugs which lower the seizure threshold. May increase the risks associated with electroconvulsive therapy. Use with caution in patients with hepatic or renal dysfunction and in elderly patients. May cause hyponatremia/SIADH (elderly at increased risk); volume depletion (diuretics may increase risk). Use with caution in patients with renal insufficiency or other concurrent illness (due to limited experience). Sertraline acts as a mild uricosuric; use with caution in patients at risk of uric acid nephropathy. Use caution with concomitant use of NSAIDs, ASA, or other drugs that affect coagulation; the risk of bleeding may be potentiated. Use with caution in patients where weight loss is undesirable. May cause or exacerbate sexual dysfunction.

Use oral concentrate formulation with caution in patients with latex sensitivity; dropper dispenser contains dry natural rubber. Monitor growth in pediatric patients. Discontinuation symptoms (eg, dysphoric mood, irritability, agitation, confusion, anxiety, insomnia, hypomania) may occur upon abrupt discontinuation. Taper dose when discontinuing therapy.

Adverse Reactions

>10%:

Central nervous system: Dizziness, fatigue, headache, insomnia, somnolence

Endocrine & metabolic: Libido decreased

Gastrointestinal: Anorexia, diarrhea, nausea, xerostomia

Genitourinary: Ejaculatory disturbances

Neuromuscular & skeletal: Tremors

Miscellaneous: Diaphoresis

1% to 10%:

Cardiovascular: Chest pain, palpitation

Central nervous system: Agitation, anxiety, hypoesthesia, malaise, nervousness, pain

Dermatologic: Rash

Endocrine & metabolic: Impotence

Gastrointestinal: Appetite increased, constipation, dyspepsia, flatulence, vomiting, weight gain

Neuromuscular & skeletal: Back pain, hypertonia, myalgia, paresthesia, weakness

Ocular: Visual difficulty, abnormal vision

Otic: Tinnitus

Respiratory: Rhinitis

Miscellaneous: Yawning

<1% (Limited to important or life-threatening): Abdominal pain, acute renal failure, agranulocytosis, allergic reaction, anaphylactoid reaction, angioedema, aplastic

anemia, atrial arrhythmia, AV block, bilirubin increased, blindness, bradycardia, cataract, dystonia, extrapyramidal symptoms, galactorrhea, gum hyperplasia, gynecomastia, hallucinations, hepatic failure, hepatitis, hepatomegaly, hyperglycemia, hyperprolactinemia, hypothyroidism, jaundice, leukopenia, lupus-like syndrome, micturition disorders, neuroleptic malignant syndrome, oculogyric crisis, serotonin syndrome, SIADH, Stevens-Johnson syndrome (and other severe dermatologic reactions), optic neuritis, pancreatitis (rare), photosensitivity, priapism, psychosis, PT/INR increased, pulmonary hypertension, QT_c prolongation, serum sickness, thrombocytopenia, torsade de pointes, transaminases increased, vasculitis, ventricular tachycardia

Additional adverse reactions reported in pediatric patients (frequency >2%): Aggressiveness, epistaxis, hyperkinesia, purpura, sinusitis, urinary incontinence

Drug Interactions

Metabolism/Transport Effects Substrate of CYP2B6 (minor), 2C9 (minor), 2C19 (major), 2D6 (major), 3A4 (minor); **Inhibits** CYP1A2 (weak), 2B6 (moderate), 2C8 (weak), 2C9 (weak), 2C19 (moderate), 2D6 (moderate), 3A4 (moderate)

Avoid Concomitant Use

Avoid concomitant use of Sertraline with any of the following: Disulfiram; Iobenguane I 123; MAO Inhibitors; Pimozide; Sibutramine; Thioridazine

Increased Effect/Toxicity

Sertraline may increase the levels/effects of: Alcohol (Ethyl); Alpha-/Beta-Blockers; Anticoagulants; Antidepressants (Serotonin Reuptake Inhibitor/Antagonist); Antiplatelet Agents; Aspirin; Beta-Blockers; BusPIRone; CarBAMazepine; Clozapine; CNS Depressants; CYP2B6 Substrates; CYP2C19 Substrates; CYP2D6 Substrates; CYP3A4 Substrates; Desmopressin; Dextromethorphan; Drotrecogin Alfa; Eplerenone; Fesoterodine; Galantamine; Haloperidol; Ibritumomab; Lithium; Maraviroc; Methadone; NSAID (COX-2 Inhibitor); NSAID (Nonselective); Phenytoin; Pimecrolimus; Pimozide; Propafenone; Ranolazine; Risperidone; Salicylates; Salmeterol; Serotonin Modulators; Tamoxifen; Thioridazine; Thrombolytic Agents; Tositumomab and Iodine I 131 Tositumomab; TraMADol; Tricyclic Antidepressants; Vitamin K Antagonists

The levels/effects of Sertraline may be increased by: Analgesics (Opioid); BusPIRone; Cimetidine; CYP2D6 Inhibitors (Moderate); CYP2D6 Inhibitors (Strong); Dasatinib; Disulfiram; Herbs (Anticoagulant/Antiplatelet Properties); Macrolide Antibiotics; MAO Inhibitors; Metoclopramide; Omega-3-Acid Ethyl Esters; Pentosan Polysulfate Sodium; Prostacyclin Analogues; Sibutramine; TraMADol; Tryptophan

Decreased Effect

Sertraline may decrease the levels/effects of: Iobenguane I 123

The levels/effects of Sertraline may be decreased by: CarBAMazepine; Cyproheptadine; Darunavir; Efavirenz

Ethanol/Nutrition/Herb Interactions

Ethanol: Avoid ethanol (may increase CNS depression).

Food: Sertraline average peak serum levels may be increased if taken with food.

Herb/Nutraceutical: Avoid valerian, St John's wort, kava kava, gotu kola (may increase CNS depression).

Stability Tablets and oral solution should be stored at controlled room temperature of 15°C to 30°C (59°F to 86°F).

Mechanism of Action Antidepressant with selective inhibitory effects on presynaptic serotonin (5-HT) reuptake and only very weak effects on norepinephrine and dopamine neuronal uptake. *In vitro* studies demonstrate no significant affinity for adrenergic, cholinergic, GABA, dopaminergic, histaminergic, serotonergic, or benzodiazepine receptors.

Pharmacodynamics/Kinetics

Onset of action: Depression: The onset of action is within a week, however, individual response varies greatly and full response may not be seen until 8-12 weeks after initiation of treatment.

Absorption: Slow

Protein binding: 98%

Metabolism: Hepatic; may involve CYP2C19 and CYP2D6; extensive first pass metabolism; forms metabolite N-desmethylsertraline

Bioavailability: Bioavailability of tablets and solution are equivalent

Half-life elimination: Sertraline: 26 hours; N-desmethylsertraline: 66 hours (range: 62-104 hours)

Time to peak, plasma: Sertraline: 4.5-8.4 hours

Excretion: Urine and feces

Dosage Oral:

Children and Adolescents: Obsessive-compulsive disorder:

6-12 years: Initial: 25 mg once daily

13-17 years: Initial: 50 mg once daily

Note: May increase daily dose, at intervals of not less than 1 week, to a maximum of 200 mg/day. If somnolence is noted, give at bedtime.

Adults:

Depression/obsessive-compulsive disorder: Oral: Initial: 50 mg/day (see "Note" above)

Panic disorder, post-traumatic stress disorder, social anxiety disorder: Initial: 25 mg once daily; increase to 50 mg once daily after 1 week (see "Note" above)

Premenstrual dysphoric disorder: 50 mg/day either daily throughout menstrual cycle **or** limited to the luteal phase of menstrual cycle, depending on physician assessment. Patients not responding to 50 mg/day may benefit from dose increases (50 mg increments per menstrual cycle) up to 150 mg/day when dosing throughout menstrual cycle **or** up to 100 mg day when dosing during luteal phase only. If a 100 mg/day dose has been established with luteal phase dosing, a 50 mg/day titration step for 3 days should be utilized at the beginning of each luteal phase dosing period.

Elderly: Depression/obsessive-compulsive disorder: Start treatment with 25 mg/day in the morning and increase by 25 mg/day increments every 2-3 days if tolerated to 50-100 mg/day; additional increases may be necessary; maximum dose: 200 mg/day. **Note:** Patients with Alzheimer's dementia-related depression may require a lower starting dosage of 12.5 mg/day, with titration intervals of 1-2 weeks, up to 150-200 mg/day maximum.

Dosage adjustment/comment in renal impairment: Multiple-dose pharmacokinetics are unaffected by renal impairment.

Hemodialysis: Not removed by hemodialysis

Dosage adjustment/comment in hepatic impairment: Sertraline is extensively metabolized by the liver; caution should be used in patients with hepatic impairment; a lower dose or less frequent dosing should be used.

Administration Oral concentrate: Must be diluted before use. Immediately before administration, use the dropper provided to measure the required amount of concentrate; mix with 4 ounces (1/2 cup) of water, ginger ale, lemon/lime soda, lemonade, or orange juice **only**. Do not mix with any other liquids than these. The dose should be taken immediately after mixing; do not mix in advance. A slight haze may appear after mixing; this is normal. **Note:** Use with caution in patients with latex sensitivity; dropper dispenser contains dry natural rubber.

Monitoring Parameters Monitor nutritional intake and weight; mental status for depression, suicidal ideation (especially at the beginning of therapy or when doses are increased or decreased), anxiety, social functioning, mania, panic attacks; akathisia; growth in pediatric patients

Additional Information Buspirone (15-60 mg/day) may be useful in treatment of sexual dysfunction during treatment with a selective serotonin reuptake inhibitor. May exacerbate tics in Tourette's syndrome.

Dosage Forms Excipient information presented when available (limited, particularly for generics); consult specific product labeling.

Solution, oral [concentrate]: 20 mg/mL (60 mL)

Zoloft®: 20 mg/mL (60 mL) [contains ethanol 12%; natural rubber/natural latex in packaging]

Tablet: 25 mg, 50 mg, 100 mg

Zoloft®: 25 mg, 50 mg, 100 mg

◆ **Sertraline Hydrochloride** *see* Sertraline *on page 1362*

◆ **Serzone** *see* Nefazodone *on page 1047*

Sevelamer (se VEL a mer)

U.S. Brand Names Renagel®; Renvela®

Canadian Brand Names Renagel®

Index Terms Sevelamer Carbonate; Sevelamer Hydrochloride

Pharmacologic Category Phosphate Binder

Use Reduction or control of serum phosphorous in patients with chronic kidney disease on hemodialysis

Pregnancy Risk Factor C

Pregnancy Considerations Animal studies have shown reduced or irregular ossification of fetal bones. Because sevelamer may cause a reduction in the absorption of some vitamins, it should be used with caution in pregnant women.

Lactation Excretion in breast milk unknown/use caution (not absorbed systemically but may alter maternal nutrition)

Medication Safety Issues

Sound-alike/look-alike issues:

Renagel® may be confused with Reglan®, Regonol®, Renal Caps, Renvela®

Renvela® may be confused with Reglan®, Regonol®, Renagel®, Renal Caps

Sevelamer may be confused with Savella™

International issues:

Renagel® may be confused with Remegel® which is a brand name for calcium carbonate in Ireland, Italy, and Great Britain

Contraindications Hypophosphatemia; bowel obstruction

Warnings/Precautions Use with caution in patients with gastrointestinal disorders including dysphagia, swallowing disorders, severe gastrointestinal motility disorders (including constipation), or major gastrointestinal surgery. May cause reductions in vitamin D, E, K, and folic acid absorption. May bind to some drugs in the gastrointestinal tract and decrease their absorption; when changes in absorption of oral medications may have significant clinical consequences (such as antiarrhythmic and antiseizure medications), these medications should be taken at least 1 hour before or 3 hours after a dose of sevelamer. Tablets should not be taken apart or chewed; broken or crushed tablets will rapidly expand in water/saliva and may be a choking hazard.

Adverse Reactions Note: A decreased incidence of gastrointestinal adverse events was observed in a clinical trial of sevelamer carbonate compared to sevelamer hydrochloride.

>10%:

Dermatologic: Pruritus (13%)

Gastrointestinal: Vomiting (22%), nausea (7% to 20%), diarrhea (4% to 19%), dyspepsia (5% to 16%)

Neuromuscular & skeletal: Limb pain (13%), arthralgia (12%)

Respiratory: Nasopharyngitis (14%), bronchitis (11%)

1% to 10%:

Cardiovascular: Hypertension (10%)

Central nervous system: Headache (9%), pyrexia (5%)

Endocrine & metabolic: Hypercalcemia (5% to 7%)

Gastrointestinal: Abdominal pain (9%), flatulence (4% to 8%), constipation (2% to 8%)

Neuromuscular & skeletal: Back pain (4%)

Respiratory: Dyspnea (10%), cough (7%), upper respiratory tract infection (5%)

Miscellaneous: Peritonitis (peritoneal dialysis: 8%)

Postmarketing and/or case reports: Fecal impaction, ileus (rare), intestinal obstruction (rare), intestinal perforation (rare), rash

Drug Interactions

Avoid Concomitant Use There are no known interactions where it is recommended to avoid concomitant use.

Increased Effect/Toxicity There are no known significant interactions involving an increase in effect.

Decreased Effect

Sevelamer may decrease the levels/effects of: Mycophenolate; Quinolone Antibiotics

Stability Store at controlled room temperature of 25°C (77°F); excursions permitted to 15°C to 30°C (59°F to 86°F). Protect from moisture.

Mechanism of Action Sevelamer (a polymeric compound) binds phosphate within the intestinal lumen, limiting absorption and decreasing serum phosphate concentrations without altering calcium, aluminum, or bicarbonate concentrations. Increased serum bicarbonate levels have been observed with the use of sevelamer carbonate, compared to sevelamer hydrochloride.

Pharmacodynamics/Kinetics

Absorption: Not systemically absorbed

Excretion: Feces

Dosage Oral: **Note:** The dosing of sevelamer carbonate and sevelamer hydrochloride are expected to be similar, when switching from one product to another, the same dose (on a mg per mg basis) should be utilized.

Children (unlabeled use): Sevelamer hydrochloride: Doses of 121-163 mg/kg/day divided 3 times/day given with meals have been used in small studies. Doses should be rounded to nearest tablet size.

Maintenance dose adjustment based on serum phosphorous concentration (based on age).

Adults: Patients not taking a phosphate binder: 800-1600 mg 3 times/day with meals; the initial dose may be based on serum phosphorous levels:

>5.5 mg/dL to <7.5 mg/dL: 800 mg 3 times/day

≥7.5 mg/dL to <9.0 mg/dL: 1200-1600 mg 3 times/day

≥9.0 mg/dL: 1600 mg 3 times/day

Maintenance dose adjustment based on serum phosphorous concentration (goal range of 3.5-5.5 mg/dL; maximum dose studied was equivalent to 13 g/day [sevelamer hydrochloride] or 14 g/day [sevelamer carbonate]):

>5.5 mg/dL: Increase by 1 tablet per meal at 2-week intervals

3.5-5.5 mg/dL: Maintain current dose

<3.5 mg/dL: Decrease by 1 tablet per meal

Dosage adjustment when switching between phosphate binder products: 667 mg of calcium acetate is equivalent to 800 mg sevelamer (carbonate or hydrochloride)

Dietary Considerations Take with meals. Reduced levels of folic acid, and vitamins D, E, and K may occur; most hemodialysis patients in clinical trials received vitamin supplementation.

Administration Must be administered with meals. Tablets should be swallowed whole; do not crush, chew, or break.

Monitoring Parameters Serum chemistries, including phosphorus, calcium, bicarbonate, chloride

Dosage Forms Excipient information presented when available (limited, particularly for generics); consult specific product labeling.

Tablet, as carbonate:
Renvela®: 800 mg

Tablet, as hydrochloride:
Renagel®: 400 mg, 800 mg

- **Sevelamer Carbonate** *see* Sevelamer *on page 1365*
- **Sevelamer Hydrochloride** *see* Sevelamer *on page 1365*

Sevoflurane (see voe FLOO rane)

U.S. Brand Names Sojourn™; Ultane®
Canadian Brand Names Sevorane® AF
Pharmacologic Category General Anesthetic, Inhalation
Use Induction and maintenance of general anesthesia
Pregnancy Risk Factor B
Medication Safety Issues

Sound-alike/look-alike issues:
Ultane® may be confused with Ultram®

High alert medication: The Institute for Safe Medication Practices (ISMP) includes this medication among its list of drug classes which have a heightened risk of causing significant patient harm when used in error.

Dosage Minimum alveolar concentration (MAC), the concentration that abolishes movement in response to a noxious stimulus (surgical incision) in 50% of patients, is 2.6% (25 years of age) for sevoflurane. Surgical levels of anesthesia are generally achieved with concentrations from 0.5% to 3%; the concentration at which amnesia and loss of awareness occur is 0.6%.

Minimum alveolar concentrations (MAC) values for surgical levels of anesthesia:

0 to 1 month old full-term neonates: Sevoflurane in oxygen: 3.3%
1 to <6 months: Sevoflurane in oxygen: 3%
6 months to <3 years:
Sevoflurane in oxygen: 2.8%
Sevoflurane in 60% N_2O/40% oxygen: 2%
3-12 years: Sevoflurane in oxygen: 2.5%
25 years:
Sevoflurane in oxygen: 2.6%
Sevoflurane in 65% N_2O/35% oxygen: 1.4%
40 years:
Sevoflurane in oxygen: 2.1%
Sevoflurane in 65% N_2O/35% oxygen: 1.1%
60 years:
Sevoflurane in oxygen: 1.7%
Sevoflurane in 65% N_2O/35% oxygen: 0.9%
80 years:
Sevoflurane in oxygen: 1.4%
Sevoflurane in 65% N_2O/35% oxygen: 0.7%

Dosage adjustment in renal impairment: Use with caution in renal insufficiency.

Dosage adjustment in hepatic impairment: Use with caution in patients with underlying hepatic conditions.

Additional Information Complete prescribing information for this medication should be consulted for additional detail.

Dosage Forms Excipient information presented when available (limited, particularly for generics); consult specific product labeling.

Liquid for inhalation: 100% (250 mL)
Sojourn™, Ultane®: 100% (250 mL)

- **Sevorane® AF (Can)** *see* Sevoflurane *on page 1366*
- **Shingles Vaccine** *see* Zoster Vaccine *on page 1593*
- **Shohl's Solution (Modified)** *see* Sodium Citrate and Citric Acid *on page 1383*

Sibutramine (si BYOO tra meen)

U.S. Brand Names Meridia®
Canadian Brand Names Meridia®
Index Terms Sibutramine Hydrochloride Monohydrate
Pharmacologic Category Anorexiant; Sympathomimetic
Additional Appendix Information

Obesity Treatment Guidelines for Adults *on page 1829*

Use Management of obesity
Restrictions C-IV

Pharmacotherapy for weight loss is recommended only for obese patients with a body mass index ≥30 kg/m^2, or ≥27 kg/m^2 in the presence of other risk factors such as hypertension, diabetes, and/or dyslipidemia or a high waist circumference; therapy should be used in conjunction with a comprehensive weight management program. Rule out organic causes of obesity (eg, untreated hypothyroidism) prior to use.

Pregnancy Risk Factor C

Pregnancy Considerations Teratogenic effects were not observed in animal studies except at doses also causing maternal toxicity. There are no adequate and well-controlled studies in pregnant women. Use in pregnancy is not recommended.

Lactation Excretion in breast milk unknown/not recommended

Medication Safety Issues

Sound-alike/look-alike issues:
Meridia® may be confused with Aredia®

Contraindications Hypersensitivity to sibutramine or any component of the formulation; during or within 2 weeks of MAO inhibitors or concomitant centrally-acting appetite suppressants; anorexia nervosa, bulimia nervosa; poorly-controlled or uncontrolled hypertension, coronary artery disease, CHF arrhythmia; stroke

Warnings/Precautions The use of some anorexigens has been associated with the development of valvular heart disease. Avoid use in patients with known serious structural cardiac abnormalities, cardiomyopathy, serious heart rhythm abnormalities, or other serious cardiac problems that could increase the risk of sudden death that these conditions alone carry.

May cause increase in blood pressure or pulse rate. For patients experiencing a sustained increase in blood pressure or pulse, dose reduction or discontinuation should be considered. Caution should be used in patients with hypertension and other cardiovascular conditions that might be exacerbated by increases in blood pressure or heart rate. Should not be used in patients with coronary artery disease, HF, arrhythmia, or stroke.

Primary pulmonary hypertension (PPH), a rare and frequently fatal disease of the lungs, has been found to occur with increased frequency in patients receiving some anorexigens. Although not reported in clinical trials, it is possible that sibutramine may share this potential, and patients should be monitored closely.

Use with caution in mild-moderate renal impairment or hepatic dysfunction, seizure disorder, gallstones, narrow-angle glaucoma, and elderly patients; not for use in patients with severe renal or hepatic impairment. Use caution with diabetes; antidiabetic agent requirements may be altered with anorexigens and concomitant dietary restrictions. Avoid concurrent use with other serotonergic agents, due to the risk of developing serotonin syndrome. Rare cases of bleeding have been reported; use caution in patients with bleeding disorders. Stimulants may unmask tics in individuals with coexisting Tourette's syndrome. Rare reports of depression, suicide and suicidal ideation have been documented; use caution and monitor closely in patients with history of psychiatric symptoms. May impair the ability to engage in potentially hazardous activities. Safety and efficacy have not been established in children <16 years of age.

Adverse Reactions

>10%:

Central nervous system: Headache (30%), insomnia (11%)

Gastrointestinal: Xerostomia (17%), anorexia (13%), constipation (12%)

1% to 10%:

Cardiovascular: Tachycardia (3%), vasodilation (2%), hypertension (2%), palpitation (2%), chest pain (2%)

Central nervous system: Dizziness (7%), nervousness (5%), anxiety (5%), depression (4%), somnolence (2%), CNS stimulation (2%), emotional lability (1%)

Dermatologic: Rash (4%)

Endocrine & metabolic: Dysmenorrhea (4%)

Gastrointestinal: Appetite increased (9%), nausea (6%), abdominal pain (5%), dyspepsia (5%), gastritis (2%), taste perversion (2%)

Genitourinary: Vaginal *Monilia* (1%)

Hepatic: Abnormal LFTs (2%)

Neuromuscular & skeletal: Back pain (8%), weakness (6%), arthralgia (6%), neck pain (2%), myalgia (2%), paresthesia (2%), tenosynovitis (1%), joint disorder (1%)

Otic: Ear disorder (2%)

Respiratory: Pharyngitis (10%), rhinitis (10%), sinusitis (5%), cough (4%)

Miscellaneous: Flu-like syndrome (8%), diaphoresis (3%), allergic reactions (2), thirst (2%)

<1%: Bruising

Frequency not defined:

Cardiovascular: Peripheral edema

Central nervous system: Thinking abnormal, agitation, fever

Dermatologic: Pruritus

Endocrine & metabolic: Menstrual disorders/irregularities

Gastrointestinal: Diarrhea, flatulence, gastroenteritis, tooth disorder

Neuromuscular & skeletal: Arthritis, hypertonia, leg cramps

Ocular: Amblyopia

Respiratory: Bronchitis, dyspnea

Postmarketing and/or case reports (frequency not defined; limited to important or life-threatening): Amnesia, anaphylactic shock, anaphylactoid reaction, anemia, angina, angioedema, arrhythmia, arthrosis, atrial fibrillation, blurred vision, cardiac arrest, cerebrovascular accident, CHF, cholecystitis, cholelithiasis, GI hemorrhage, goiter, hematuria, hyper-/hypoglycemia, hyper-/hypothyroidism, hypersensitivity reaction, impotence, interstitial nephritis, intestinal obstruction, intraocular pressure increased, leukopenia, lymphadenopathy, mania, mouth/stomach ulcer, mydriasis, photosensitivity, seizure, serotonin syndrome, stroke, suicidal ideation, syncope, thrombocytopenia, tongue edema, torsade de pointes, Tourette's syndrome, urinary retention, urticaria, transient ischemic attack, vascular headache, ventricular arrhythmia, vertigo

Drug Interactions

Metabolism/Transport Effects Substrate of CYP3A4 (major)

Avoid Concomitant Use

Avoid concomitant use of Sibutramine with any of the following: Ergot Derivatives; Iobenguane I 123; Serotonin Modulators

Increased Effect/Toxicity

Sibutramine may increase the levels/effects of: Ergot Derivatives; Serotonin Modulators; Sympathomimetics

The levels/effects of Sibutramine may be increased by: Cannabinoids; CYP3A4 Inhibitors (Moderate); CYP3A4 Inhibitors (Strong); Dasatinib

Decreased Effect

Sibutramine may decrease the levels/effects of: Iobenguane I 123

Ethanol/Nutrition/Herb Interactions

Ethanol: Avoid excess ethanol ingestion.

Herb/Nutraceutical: St John's wort and SAMe may decrease sibutramine levels.

Stability Store at room temperature of 15°C to 30°C (59°F to 86°F).

Mechanism of Action Sibutramine and its two primary metabolites block the neuronal uptake of norepinephrine, serotonin, and (to a lesser extent) dopamine. There is no monoamine-releasing (or depleting) activity.

Pharmacodynamics/Kinetics

Absorption: 77%; rapid

Protein binding, plasma: Parent drug and metabolites: >94%

Metabolism: Hepatic; undergoes first-pass metabolism via CYP3A4; forms two primary metabolites (M_1 and M_2; active)

Half-life elimination: Sibutramine: 1 hour; Metabolites: M_1: 14 hours; M_2: 16 hours

Time to peak: Sibutramine: 1.2 hours; Metabolites (M_1 and M_2): 3-4 hours

Excretion: Primarily urine (77% as inactive metabolites); feces

Dosage Children ≥16 years and Adults:

Initial: 10 mg once daily; after 4 weeks may titrate up to 15 mg once daily as needed and tolerated (may be used for up to 2 years, per manufacturer labeling)

Maintenance: 5-15 mg once daily

Dosage adjustment in renal/hepatic impairment: Should not be used in patients with severe renal or hepatic impairment

Dietary Considerations Sibutramine, as an appetite suppressant, is the most effective when combined with a low calorie diet and behavior modification counseling.

Administration May take with or without food.

Monitoring Parameters Weight, waist circumference, blood pressure, heart rate. Do initial blood pressure and heart rate evaluation and then monitor regularly during therapy. If patient has sustained increases in either blood pressure or pulse rate, consider discontinuing or reducing the dose of the drug.

Reference Range

Adult classification of weight by BMI (kg/m^2):

Underweight: <18.5

Normal: 18.5-24.9

Overweight: 25-29.9

Obese, class I: 30-34.9

Obese, class II: 35-39.9

Extreme obesity (class III): ≥40

Waist circumference: In adults with a BMI of 25-34.9 kg/m^2, high-risk waist circumference is defined as:

Men >102 cm (>40 in)

Women >88 cm (>35 in)

Additional Information Physicians should carefully evaluate patients for history of drug abuse and follow such patients closely, observing them for signs of misuse or abuse (eg, development of tolerance, excessive increases of doses, drug seeking behavior).

Dosage Forms Excipient information presented when available (limited, particularly for generics); consult specific product labeling.

Capsule, as hydrochloride:

Meridia®: 5 mg, 10 mg, 15 mg

◆ **Sibutramine Hydrochloride Monohydrate** *see* Sibutramine *on page 1366*

◆ **Silace [OTC]** *see* Docusate *on page 473*

◆ **Siladryl® Allergy [OTC]** *see* DiphenhydrAMINE *on page 456*

Sildenafil (sil DEN a fil)

U.S. Brand Names Revatio®; Viagra®

Canadian Brand Names Viagra®

Index Terms UK92480

Pharmacologic Category Phosphodiesterase-5 Enzyme Inhibitor

Use

Revatio®: Treatment of pulmonary arterial hypertension (WHO Group I)

Viagra®: Treatment of erectile dysfunction (ED)

Unlabeled/Investigational Use Pulmonary arterial hypertension in children

Pregnancy Risk Factor B

Pregnancy Considerations Teratogenic effects were not observed in animal studies. There are no adequate and well-controlled studies in pregnant women. Less than 0.001% appears in the semen.

Lactation Excretion in breast milk unknown/use caution

Medication Safety Issues

Sound-alike/look-alike issues:

Revatio® may be confused with ReVia®

Sildenafil may be confused with silodosin, tadalafil, vardenafil

Viagra® may be confused with Allegra®, Vaniqa™

Contraindications Hypersensitivity to sildenafil or any component of the formulation; concurrent use (regularly/intermittently) of organic nitrates in any form (eg, nitroglycerin, isosorbide dinitrate)

Warnings/Precautions Decreases in blood pressure may occur due to vasodilator effects; use with caution in patients with left ventricular outflow obstruction (aortic stenosis or hypertrophic obstructive cardiomyopathy); may be more sensitive to hypotensive actions. Concurrent use with alpha-adrenergic antagonist therapy or substantial ethanol consumption may cause symptomatic hypotension; patients should be hemodynamically stable prior to initiating therapy at the lowest possible dose. Use with caution in patients with hypotension (<90/50 mm Hg); uncontrolled hypertension (>170/110 mm Hg); life-threatening arrhythmias, stroke or MI within the last 6 months; cardiac failure or coronary artery disease causing unstable angina; safety and efficacy have not been studied in these patients. There is a degree of cardiac risk associated with sexual activity; therefore, physicians should consider the cardiovascular status of their patients prior to initiating any treatment for erectile dysfunction.

Sildenafil should be used with caution in patients with anatomical deformation of the penis (angulation, cavernosal fibrosis, or Peyronie's disease) and in patients who have conditions which may predispose them to priapism (sickle cell anemia, multiple myeloma, leukemia). All patients should be instructed to seek medical attention if erection persists >4 hours.

Vision loss may occur rarely and be a sign of nonarteritic anterior ischemic optic neuropathy (NAION). Risk may be increased with history of vision loss. Other risk factors for NAION include low cup-to-disc ratio ("crowded disc"), coronary artery disease, diabetes, hypertension, hyperlipidemia, smoking, and age >50 years. May cause dose-related impairment of color discrimination. Use caution in patients with retinitis pigmentosa; a minority have genetic disorders of retinal phosphodiesterases (no safety information available). Sudden decrease or loss of hearing has been reported rarely; hearing changes may be accompanied by tinnitus and dizziness. A direct relationship between therapy and vision or hearing loss has not been determined.

The potential underlying causes of erectile dysfunction should be evaluated prior to treatment. The safety and efficacy of sildenafil with other treatments for erectile dysfunction have not been established; use is not recommended. Efficacy with concurrent bosentan therapy has not been evaluated; use with caution. Use with caution in patients taking strong CYP3A4 inhibitors or alpha-blockers. Concomitant use with all forms of nitrates is contraindicated. If nitrate administration is medically necessary, it is not known when nitrates can be safely administered following the use of sildenafil (per manufacturer); the ACC/AHA 2007 guidelines supports administration of nitrates only if 24 hours have elapsed.

Use caution in patients with bleeding disorders or with active peptic ulcer disease; safety and efficacy have not been established. Use with caution in the elderly, or patients with renal or hepatic dysfunction; dose adjustment may be needed.

Adverse Reactions Based upon normal doses for either indication. (Adverse effects such as flushing, diarrhea, myalgia, and visual disturbances may be increased with doses >100 mg/24 hours.)

>10%:

Central nervous system: Headache (16% to 46%)

Gastrointestinal: Dyspepsia (7% to 17%; dose related)

2% to 10%:

Cardiovascular: Flushing (10%)

Central nervous system: Insomnia (≤7%), pyrexia (6%), dizziness (2%)

Dermatologic: Erythema (6%), rash (2%)

Gastrointestinal: Diarrhea (3% to 9%), gastritis (≤3%)

Genitourinary: Urinary tract infection (3%)

Hepatic: LFTs increased

Neuromuscular & skeletal: Myalgia (≤7%), paresthesia (≤3%)

Ocular: Abnormal vision (color changes, blurred vision, or increased sensitivity to light 3% to 11%; dose related)

Respiratory: Epistaxis (9% to 13%), dyspnea exacerbated (≤7%), nasal congestion (4%), rhinitis (4%), sinusitis (3%)

<2% (Limited to important or life-threatening): Allergic reaction, amnesia (transient global), anemia, angina pectoris, anorgasmia, asthma, AV block, cardiac arrest, cardiomyopathy, cataract, cerebral thrombosis, cerebrovascular hemorrhage, colitis, cystitis, depression, dysphagia, edema, exfoliative dermatitis, eye hemorrhage, gout, hearing decreased, hearing loss, heart failure, hematuria, hemorrhage, hyper-/hypoglycemia, hypernatremia, hyper-/hypotension, hyperuricemia, intracerebral hemorrhage, intraocular pressure increased, leukopenia, migraine, myocardial ischemia, MI, myasthenia, mydriasis, neuralgia, nonarteritic ischemic optic neuropathy (NAION), palpitation, postural hypotension, priapism, pulmonary hemorrhage, rectal hemorrhage, retinal vascular disease or bleeding, seizure, shock, stomatitis, subarachnoid hemorrhage, syncope, tachycardia, tendon rupture, TIA, urinary incontinence, ventricular arrhythmia, vertigo, visual field loss, vitreous detachment/traction, vomiting

Drug Interactions

Metabolism/Transport Effects Substrate of CYP2C9 (minor), 3A4 (major); **Inhibits** CYP1A2 (weak), 2C9 (weak), 2C19 (weak), 2D6 (weak), 2E1 (weak), 3A4 (weak)

Avoid Concomitant Use

Avoid concomitant use of Sildenafil with any of the following: Vasodilators (Organic Nitrates)

Increased Effect/Toxicity

Sildenafil may increase the levels/effects of: Alpha1-Blockers; Bosentan; HMG-CoA Reductase Inhibitors; Vasodilators (Organic Nitrates)

The levels/effects of Sildenafil may be increased by: Antifungal Agents (Azole Derivatives, Systemic); CYP3A4 Inhibitors (Moderate); CYP3A4 Inhibitors (Strong); Dasatinib; Macrolide Antibiotics; Protease Inhibitors; Sapropterin

Decreased Effect

The levels/effects of Sildenafil may be decreased by: Bosentan; Etravirine

Ethanol/Nutrition/Herb Interactions

Food: Amount and rate of absorption of sildenafil is reduced when taken with a high-fat meal. Serum concentrations/toxicity may be increased with grapefruit juice; avoid concurrent use.

Herb/Nutraceutical: St John's wort may decrease sildenafil levels.

Stability Store tablets at controlled room temperature of 25°C (77°F); excursions permitted to 15°C to 30°C (59°F to 86°F).

Mechanism of Action

Erectile dysfunction: Does not directly cause penile erections, but affects the response to sexual stimulation. The physiologic mechanism of erection of the penis involves release of nitric oxide (NO) in the corpus cavernosum during sexual stimulation. NO then activates the enzyme guanylate cyclase, which results in increased levels of cyclic guanosine monophosphate (cGMP), producing smooth muscle relaxation and inflow of blood to the corpus cavernosum. Sildenafil enhances the effect of NO by inhibiting phosphodiesterase type 5 (PDE-5), which is responsible for degradation of cGMP in the corpus cavernosum; when sexual stimulation causes local release of NO, inhibition of PDE-5 by sildenafil causes increased levels of cGMP in the corpus cavernosum, resulting in smooth muscle relaxation and inflow of blood to the corpus cavernosum; at recommended doses, it has no effect in the absence of sexual stimulation.

Pulmonary arterial hypertension (PAH): Inhibits phosphodiesterase type 5 (PDE-5) in smooth muscle of pulmonary vasculature where PDE-5 is responsible for the degradation of cyclic guanosine monophosphate (cGMP). Increased cGMP concentration results in pulmonary vasculature relaxation; vasodilation in the pulmonary bed and the systemic circulation (to a lesser degree) may occur.

Pharmacodynamics/Kinetics

Onset of action: ~60 minutes

Duration: 2-4 hours

Absorption: Rapid; slower with a high-fat meal

Distribution: V_{dss}: 105 L

Protein binding, plasma: ~96%

Metabolism: Hepatic via CYP3A4 (major) and CYP2C9 (minor route); forms metabolite (active)

Bioavailability: 40%

Half-life elimination: 4 hours

Time to peak: 30-120 minutes; delayed by 60 minutes with a high-fat meal

Excretion: Feces (80%); urine (13%)

Dosage Oral:

Children ≥1 month: Pulmonary arterial hypertension (unlabeled use): 0.25-2 mg/kg/dose every 4-6 hours. Most reports used 0.5 mg/kg/dose and titrated up to 2 mg/kg/dose

Adults:

Erectile dysfunction (Viagra®): Usual dose: 50 mg once daily 1 hour (range: 30 minutes to 4 hours) before sexual activity; dosing range: 25-100 mg once daily

Pulmonary arterial hypertension (Revatio®): Pulmonary arterial hypertension (Revatio®): 20 mg 3 times/day, taken 4-6 hours apart

Elderly >65 years: Use with caution

Revatio®: Refer to adult dosing.

Viagra®: Starting dose of 25 mg should be considered.

Dosage considerations for patients stable on alpha-blockers: Viagra®: Initial 25 mg

Dosage adjustment for concomitant use of potent CYP34A inhibitors:

Revatio®:

Erythromycin, saquinavir: No dosage adjustment

Itraconazole, ketoconazole, ritonavir: Not recommended

Viagra®:

Erythromycin, itraconazole, ketoconazole, saquinavir: Starting dose of 25 mg should be considered

Ritonavir: Maximum: 25 mg every 48 hours

Dosage adjustment in renal impairment:

Revatio®: Dose adjustment not necessary

Viagra®: Cl_{cr} <30 mL/minute: Starting dose of 25 mg should be considered

Dosage adjustment in hepatic impairment:

Revatio®: Child-Pugh class A and B: Dose adjustment not necessary

Viagra®: Child-Pugh class A and B: Starting dose of 25 mg should be considered; not studied in severe impairment (Child-Pugh class C)

Administration

Revatio®: Administer tablets at least 4-6 hours apart

Viagra®: Administer orally 30 minutes to 4 hours before sexual activity

Additional Information Sildenafil is ~10 times more selective for PDE-5 as compared to PDE6. This enzyme is found in the retina and is involved in phototransduction. At higher plasma levels, interference with PDE6 is believed to be the basis for changes in color vision noted in some patients.

Dosage Forms Excipient information presented when available (limited, particularly for generics); consult specific product labeling.

Tablet:

Revatio®: 20 mg

Viagra®: 25 mg, 50 mg, 100 mg

Extemporaneous Preparations A stable suspension of sildenafil citrate (2.5 mg/mL) may be prepared as follows: Triturate thirty (30) sildenafil 25 mg tablets (Viagra®) to a fine powder in a mortar and pestle. Create a uniform paste by stirring in a small volume of suspending agent (1:1 mixture of methylcellulose 1% and simple syrup NF or a 1:1 mixture of Ora-Sweet® and Ora-Plus®). Continue adding vehicle to the paste in a geometric manner, with mixing, until near the desired volume. Transfer suspension to a graduated cylinder and QS to 300 mL with vehicle. Final suspension should be transferred to amber plastic bottles, labeled with "shake well" and dated for 90-day expiration at room temperature (25°C) or under refrigeration (4°C).

Nahata MC, Morosco RS, and Brady MT, "Extemporaneous Sildenafil Citrate Oral Suspensions for the Treatment of Pulmonary Hypertension in Children," *Am J Health-Syst Pharm*, 2006, 63:254-7.

◆ **Silexin [OTC]** *see* Guaifenesin and Dextromethorphan *on page 710*

◆ **Silfedrine Children's [OTC]** *see* Pseudoephedrine *on page 1265*

Silodosin (SI lo doe sin)

U.S. Brand Names Rapaflo®
Index Terms KMD 3213
Pharmacologic Category Alpha$_1$ Blocker
Use Treatment of signs and symptoms of benign prostatic hyperplasia (BPH)
Pregnancy Risk Factor B
Medication Safety Issues
Sound-alike/look-alike issues:
Rapaflo® may be confused with Rapamune®, Raptiva®
Silodosin may be confused with sildenafil
Dosage Oral: Adults: BPH: 8 mg once daily with a meal
Dosage adjustment in renal impairment:
Cl_{cr} >50 mL/minute: No adjustment needed
Cl_{cr} 30-50 mL/minute: 4 mg once daily
Cl_{cr} <30 mL/minute: Use is contraindicated
Dosage adjustment in hepatic impairment:
Mild-to-moderate impairment (Child-Pugh classes A and B): No adjustment needed
Severe impairment (Child-Pugh class C): Use is contraindicated
Additional Information Complete prescribing information for this medication should be consulted for additional detail.
Dosage Forms Excipient information presented when available (limited, particularly for generics); consult specific product labeling.
Capsule:
Rapaflo®: 4 mg, 8 mg

◆ **Silphen® [OTC]** *see* DiphenhydrAMINE *on page 456*

◆ **Sil-Tex** *see* Guaifenesin and Phenylephrine *on page 712*

◆ **Siltussin DAS [OTC]** *see* GuaiFENesin *on page 709*

◆ **Siltussin DM [OTC]** *see* Guaifenesin and Dextromethorphan *on page 710*

◆ **Siltussin DM DAS [OTC]** *see* Guaifenesin and Dextromethorphan *on page 710*

◆ **Siltussin SA [OTC]** *see* GuaiFENesin *on page 709*

◆ **Silvadene®** *see* Silver Sulfadiazine *on page 1370*

Silver Nitrate (SIL ver NYE trate)

Index Terms $AgNO_3$
Pharmacologic Category Antibiotic, Topical; Cauterizing Agent, Topical; Topical Skin Product, Antibacterial
Use Cauterization of wounds and sluggish ulcers, removal of granulation tissue and warts; aseptic prophylaxis of burns
Pregnancy Risk Factor C
Dosage Children and Adults:
Sticks: Apply to mucous membranes and other moist skin surfaces only on area to be treated 2-3 times/week for 2-3 weeks
Topical solution: Apply a cotton applicator dipped in solution on the affected area 2-3 times/week for 2-3 weeks
Additional Information Complete prescribing information for this medication should be consulted for additional detail.
Dosage Forms Excipient information presented when available (limited, particularly for generics); consult specific product labeling.
Applicator sticks, topical: Silver nitrate 75% and potassium nitrate 25% (6", 12", 18")
Solution, topical: 0.5% (960 mL); 10% (30 mL); 25% (30 mL); 50% (30 mL)

Silver Sulfadiazine (SIL ver sul fa DYE a zeen)

U.S. Brand Names Silvadene®; SSD®; SSD® AF; Thermazene®
Canadian Brand Names Flamazine®
Pharmacologic Category Antibiotic, Topical
Additional Appendix Information
Sulfonamide Derivatives *on page 1671*
Use Prevention and treatment of infection in second and third degree burns
Pregnancy Risk Factor B
Dosage Children and Adults: Topical: Apply once or twice daily with a sterile-gloved hand; apply to a thickness of 1/16"; burned area should be covered with cream at all times
Additional Information Complete prescribing information for this medication should be consulted for additional detail.
Dosage Forms Excipient information presented when available (limited, particularly for generics); consult specific product labeling.
Cream, topical: 1% (25 g, 50 g, 85 g, 400 g)
Silvadene®, Thermazene®: 1% (20 g, 50 g, 85 g, 400 g, 1000 g)
SSD®: 1% (25 g, 50 g, 85 g, 400 g)
SSD® AF: 1% (50 g, 400 g)

◆ **Simcor®** *see* Niacin and Simvastatin *on page 1060*

◆ **Simethicone, Aluminum Hydroxide, and Magnesium Hydroxide** *see* Aluminum Hydroxide, Magnesium Hydroxide, and Simethicone *on page 76*

◆ **Simethicone and Loperamide Hydrochloride** *see* Loperamide and Simethicone *on page 901*

◆ **Simethicone and Magaldrate** *see* Magaldrate and Simethicone *on page 914*

◆ **Simply Saline® [OTC]** *see* Sodium Chloride *on page 1381*

◆ **Simply Saline® Baby [OTC]** *see* Sodium Chloride *on page 1381*

◆ **Simply Saline® Nasal Moist® [OTC]** *see* Sodium Chloride *on page 1381*

◆ **Simply Sleep® [OTC]** *see* DiphenhydrAMINE *on page 456*

◆ **Simply Sleep® (Can)** *see* DiphenhydrAMINE *on page 456*

◆ **Simuc [DSC]** *see* Guaifenesin and Phenylephrine *on page 712*

◆ **Simuc-DM** *see* Guaifenesin and Dextromethorphan *on page 710*

◆ **Simulect®** *see* Basiliximab *on page 174*

Simvastatin (sim va STAT in)

U.S. Brand Names Zocor®
Canadian Brand Names Apo-Simvastatin®; CO Simvastatin; Dom-Simvastatin; Gen-Simvastatin; Novo-Simvastatin; Nu-Simvastatin; PHL-Simvastatin; PMS-Simvastatin; ratio-Simvastatin; Riva-Simvastatin; Sandoz-Simvastatin; Taro-Simvastatin; Zocor®
Pharmacologic Category Antilipemic Agent, HMG-CoA Reductase Inhibitor
Additional Appendix Information
Hyperlipidemia Management *on page 1815*
Lipid-Lowering Agents *on page 1661*
Use Used with dietary therapy for the following:
Secondary prevention of cardiovascular events in hypercholesterolemic patients with established coronary heart

disease (CHD) or at high risk for CHD: To reduce cardiovascular morbidity (myocardial infarction, coronary revascularization procedures) and mortality; to reduce the risk of stroke and transient ischemic attacks

Hyperlipidemias: To reduce elevations in total cholesterol, LDL-C, apolipoprotein B, and triglycerides, and increase HDL-C in patients with primary hypercholesterolemia (elevations of 1 or more components are present in Fredrickson type IIa, IIb, III, and IV hyperlipidemias); treatment of homozygous familial hypercholesterolemia

Heterozygous familial hypercholesterolemia (HeFH): In adolescent patients (10-17 years of age, females >1 year postmenarche) with HeFH having LDL-C ≥190 mg/dL **or** LDL ≥160 mg/dL with positive family history of premature cardiovascular disease (CVD), or 2 or more CVD risk factors in the adolescent patient

Pregnancy Risk Factor X

Pregnancy Considerations Cholesterol biosynthesis may be important in fetal development. Contraindicated in pregnancy. Administer to women of childbearing potential only when conception is highly unlikely and patients have been informed of potential hazards. If pregnancy occurs during treatment, discontinue simvastatin immediately.

Lactation Excretion in breast milk unknown/contraindicated

Medication Safety Issues

Sound-alike/look-alike issues:

Zocor® may be confused with Cozaar®, Yocon®, Zoloft®

International issues:

Cardin® [Poland] may be confused with Cardene® which is a brand name for nicardipine in the U.S.

Cardin® [Poland] may be confused with Cardem® which is a brand name for celiprolol in Spain

Contraindications Hypersensitivity to simvastatin or any component of the formulation; active liver disease; unexplained persistent elevations of serum transaminases; pregnancy; breast-feeding

Warnings/Precautions Secondary causes of hyperlipidemia should be ruled out prior to therapy. Liver function must be monitored by laboratory assessment. Rhabdomyolysis with acute renal failure has occurred. Risk is dose-related and is increased with concurrent use of lipid-lowering agents which may cause rhabdomyolysis (gemfibrozil, fibric acid derivatives, or niacin at doses ≥1 g/day), during concurrent use with danazol or strong CYP3A4 inhibitors (including amiodarone, clarithromycin, cyclosporine, erythromycin, telithromycin, itraconazole, ketoconazole, nefazodone, grapefruit juice in large quantities, verapamil, or protease inhibitors such as indinavir, nelfinavir, or ritonavir). Monitor closely if used with other drugs associated with myopathy (eg, colchicine). Weigh the risk versus benefit when combining any of these drugs with simvastatin. Do not initiate simvastatin-containing treatment in a patient with pre-existing therapy of cyclosporine or danazol, unless the patient has previously demonstrated tolerance to ≥5 mg/day simvastatin. Temporarily discontinue in any patient experiencing an acute or serious major medical or surgical condition which may increase the risk of rhabdomyolysis. Discontinue temporarily for elective surgical procedures. Based upon current evidence, HMG-CoA reductase inhibitor therapy should be continued in the perioperative period unless risk outweighs cardioprotective benefit. Use caution in patients with renal insufficiency. Use with caution in patients with advanced age, these patients are predisposed to myopathy. Use with caution in patients who consume large amounts of ethanol or have a history of liver disease. Use is contraindicated with active liver disease and with unexplained transaminase elevations. Safety and efficacy have not been established in patients <10 years of age or in premenarcheal girls.

Adverse Reactions

1% to 10%:

Gastrointestinal: Constipation (2%), flatulence (1% to 2%), dyspepsia (1%)

Hepatic: Transaminases increased (>3x ULN; 1%)

Neuromuscular & skeletal: CPK elevation (>3x normal on one or more occasions; 5%)

Respiratory: Upper respiratory infection (2%)

<1% (Limited to important or life-threatening): Abdominal pain, depression, dermatomyositis, diarrhea, dizziness, fatigue, headache, hypotension, insomnia, lichen planus, muscle pain, muscle tenderness, muscle weakness, myopathy, nausea, photosensitivity, pruritus, thrombocytopenia, vertigo, weakness

Additional class-related events or case reports (not necessarily reported with simvastatin therapy): Alopecia, alkaline phosphatase increased, alteration in taste, alopecia, anaphylaxis, angioedema, anorexia, anxiety, arthralgia, arthritis, bilirubin increased, cataracts, chills, cholestatic jaundice, cirrhosis, decreased libido, depression, dermatomyositis, dryness of skin/mucous membranes, dyspnea, eosinophilia, erectile dysfunction/impotence, erythema multiforme, facial paresis, fatty liver, fever, flushing, fulminant hepatic necrosis, gynecomastia, hemolytic anemia, hepatic failure, hepatitis, hepatoma, hyperbilirubinemia, hypersensitivity reaction, impaired extraocular muscle movement, increased alkaline phosphatase, increased CPK (>10x normal), increased ESR, increased GGT, leukopenia, malaise, memory loss, myopathy, nail changes, nodules, ophthalmoplegia, pancreatitis, paresthesia, peripheral nerve palsy, peripheral neuropathy, photosensitivity, polymyalgia rheumatica, positive ANA, pruritus, psychic disturbance, purpura, rash, renal failure (secondary to rhabdomyolysis), rhabdomyolysis, skin discoloration, Stevens-Johnson syndrome, systemic lupus erythematosus-like syndrome, thrombocytopenia, thyroid dysfunction, toxic epidermal necrolysis, transaminases increased, tremor, urticaria, vasculitis, vertigo, vomiting

Drug Interactions

Metabolism/Transport Effects Substrate of CYP3A4 (major); **Inhibits** CYP2C8 (weak), 2C9 (weak), 2D6 (weak)

Avoid Concomitant Use There are no known interactions where it is recommended to avoid concomitant use.

Increased Effect/Toxicity

Simvastatin may increase the levels/effects of: DAPTOmycin; Vitamin K Antagonists

The levels/effects of Simvastatin may be increased by: Amiodarone; Antifungal Agents (Azole Derivatives, Systemic); Calcium Channel Blockers (Nondihydropyridine); Colchicine; CycloSPORINE; CYP3A4 Inhibitors (Moderate); CYP3A4 Inhibitors (Strong); Danazol; Dasatinib; Eltrombopag; Fenofibrate; Fenofibric Acid; Fluconazole; Gemfibrozil; Grapefruit Juice; Imatinib; Macrolide Antibiotics; Nefazodone; Niacin; Niacinamide; Protease Inhibitors; Ranolazine; Sildenafil

Decreased Effect

The levels/effects of Simvastatin may be decreased by: Bosentan; CYP3A4 Inducers (Strong); Deferasirox; Etravirine; Phenytoin; Rifamycin Derivatives; St Johns Wort

Ethanol/Nutrition/Herb Interactions

Ethanol: Avoid excessive ethanol consumption (due to potential hepatic effects).

Food: Simvastatin serum concentration may be increased when taken with grapefruit juice; avoid concurrent intake of large quantities (>1 quart/day). Red yeast rice contains an estimated 2.4 mg lovastatin per 600 mg rice.

Herb/Nutraceutical: St John's wort may decrease simvastatin levels.

Stability Tablets should be stored in tightly-closed containers at temperatures between 5°C to 30°C (41°F to 86°F).

Mechanism of Action Simvastatin is a methylated derivative of lovastatin that acts by competitively inhibiting 3-hydroxy-3-methylglutaryl-coenzyme A (HMG-CoA) reductase, the enzyme that catalyzes the rate-limiting step in cholesterol biosynthesis

Pharmacodynamics/Kinetics

Onset of action: >3 days

Peak effect: 2 weeks

Absorption: 85%

Protein binding:~95%

Metabolism: Hepatic via CYP3A4; extensive first-pass effect

Bioavailability: <5%

Half-life elimination: Unknown

Time to peak: 1.3-2.4 hours

Excretion: Feces (60%); urine (13%)

Dosage Oral: **Note:** Doses should be individualized according to the baseline LDL-cholesterol levels, the recommended goal of therapy, and the patient's response; adjustments should be made at intervals of 4 weeks or more; doses may need adjusted based on concomitant medications

Children 10-17 years (females >1 year postmenarche):

HeFH: 10 mg once daily in the evening; range: 10-40 mg/day (maximum: 40 mg/day)

Dosage adjustment for simvastatin with concomitant amiodarone, cyclosporine, danazol, gemfibrozil, or verapamil: Refer to drug-specific dosing in adult dosing section

Adults:

Homozygous familial hypercholesterolemia: 40 mg once daily in the evening **or** 80 mg/day (given as 20 mg, 20 mg, and 40 mg evening dose)

Prevention of cardiovascular events, hyperlipidemias: 20-40 mg once daily in the evening; range: 5-80 mg/day

Patients requiring only moderate reduction of LDL-cholesterol may be started at 10 mg once daily

Patients requiring reduction of >45% in low-density lipoprotein (LDL) cholesterol may be started at 40 mg once daily in the evening

Patients with CHD or at high risk for CHD: Dosing should be started at 40 mg once daily in the evening; simvastatin should be started simultaneously with diet therapy.

Dosage adjustment with concomitant medications:

Cyclosporine or danazol: Initial: 5 mg simvastatin, should **not** exceed 10 mg/day

Gemfibrozil: Simvastatin dose should **not** exceed 10 mg/day

Amiodarone or verapamil: Simvastatin dose should **not** exceed 20 mg/day

Dosing adjustment/comments in renal impairment: Because simvastatin does not undergo significant renal excretion, modification of dose should not be necessary in patients with mild to moderate renal insufficiency.

Severe renal impairment: Cl_{cr} <10 mL/minute: Initial: 5 mg/day with close monitoring.

Dietary Considerations Red yeast rice contains an estimated 2.4 mg lovastatin per 600 mg rice.

Administration May be taken without regard to meals. Administer in the evening for maximal efficacy.

Monitoring Parameters Creatine phosphokinase levels due to possibility of myopathy; serum cholesterol (total and fractionated)

Obtain liver function tests prior to initiation, dose, and thereafter when clinically indicated. Patients titrated to the 80 mg dose should be tested prior to initiation and 3 months after initiating the 80 mg dose. Thereafter, periodic monitoring (ie, semiannually) is recommended for the first year of treatment. Patients with elevated transaminase levels should have a second (confirmatory) test and frequent monitoring until values normalize. Discontinue if increase in ALT/AST is persistently >3 times ULN.

Dosage Forms Excipient information presented when available (limited, particularly for generics); consult specific product labeling.

Tablet: 5 mg, 10 mg, 20 mg, 40 mg, 80 mg

Zocor®: 5 mg, 10 mg, 20 mg, 40 mg, 80 mg

- ◆ **Simvastatin and Ezetimibe** *see* Ezetimibe and Simvastatin *on page* *598*
- ◆ **Simvastatin and Niacin** *see* Niacin and Simvastatin *on page* *1060*
- ◆ **Sina-12X** *see* Guaifenesin and Phenylephrine *on page* *712*
- ◆ **Sinemet®** *see* Carbidopa and Levodopa *on page* *256*
- ◆ **Sinemet® CR** *see* Carbidopa and Levodopa *on page* *256*
- ◆ **Sinequan® [DSC]** *see* Doxepin *on page* *484*
- ◆ **Sinequan® (Can)** *see* Doxepin *on page* *484*
- ◆ **Singulair®** *see* Montelukast *on page* *1014*
- ◆ **Sinutab® Non Drowsy (Can)** *see* Acetaminophen and Pseudoephedrine *on page* *30*
- ◆ **Sinutab® Non-Drying [OTC]** *see* Guaifenesin and Pseudoephedrine *on page* *713*
- ◆ **Sinutab® Sinus [OTC]** *see* Acetaminophen and Phenylephrine *on page* *29*
- ◆ **Sinutab® Sinus & Allergy (Can)** *see* Acetaminophen, Chlorpheniramine, and Pseudoephedrine *on page* *31*
- ◆ **Sinutab® Sinus Allergy Maximum Strength [OTC]** *see* Acetaminophen, Chlorpheniramine, and Pseudoephedrine *on page* *31*
- ◆ **SINUvent® PE** *see* Guaifenesin and Phenylephrine *on page* *712*
- ◆ **Sirdalud®** *see* TiZANidine *on page* *1480*

Sirolimus (sir OH li mus)

U.S. Brand Names Rapamune®

Canadian Brand Names Rapamune®

Pharmacologic Category Immunosuppressant Agent; mTOR Kinase Inhibitor

Use Prophylaxis of organ rejection in patients receiving renal transplants, in combination with corticosteroids and cyclosporine (cyclosporine may be withdrawn in low-to-moderate immunological risk patients after 2-4 months, in conjunction with an increase in sirolimus dosage; in high-risk patients, use in combination with cyclosporine and corticosteroids is recommended for the first year)

Unlabeled/Investigational Use Prophylaxis of organ rejection in heart transplant recipients; immunosuppression in peripheral stem cell/bone marrow transplantation

Pregnancy Risk Factor C

Pregnancy Considerations Embryotoxicity and fetotoxicity may occur, as evidenced by increased mortality, reduced fetal weights and delayed ossification in animal studies. There are no adequate and well-controlled studies in pregnant women. Effective contraception must be initiated before therapy with sirolimus and continued for 12 weeks after discontinuation.

The National Transplantation Pregnancy Registry (NTPR, Temple University) is a registry for pregnant women taking immunosuppressants following any solid organ transplant. The NTPR encourages reporting of all immunosuppressant exposures during pregnancy in transplant recipients at 877-955-6877.

Lactation Excretion in breast milk unknown/not recommended

Medication Safety Issues

Sound-alike/look-alike issues:

Rapamune® may be confused with Rapaflo®

Sirolimus may be confused with tacrolimus, temsirolimus

Contraindications Hypersensitivity to sirolimus or any component of the formulation

Warnings/Precautions [U.S. Boxed Warning]: Immunosuppressive agents, including sirolimus, increase the risk of infection and may be associated with the development of lymphoma. Immune suppression may also increase the risk of opportunistic infections and sepsis. Prophylactic treatment for *Pneumocystis jirovec* pneumonia (PCP) should be administered for 1 year post-transplant; prophylaxis for cytomegalovirus (CMV) should be taken for 3 months in patients at risk for CMV.

[U.S. Boxed Warning]: Sirolimus is not recommended for *de novo* use in liver or lung transplant patients. Studies indicate an association with an increase risk of hepatic artery thrombosis, graft failure, and increased mortality when used in combination with cyclosporine and/or tacrolimus for liver transplantation. Cases of bronchial anastomotic dehiscence have been reported in lung transplant patients when sirolimus was used as part of an immunosuppressive regimen; most of these reactions were fatal.

In renal transplant patients, *de novo* use without cyclosporine has been associated with higher rates of acute rejection. May increase serum creatinine and decrease GFR. Use caution when used concurrently with medications which may alter renal function. May delay recovery of renal function in patients with delayed allograft function. Monitor renal function closely when combined with cyclosporine; consider dosage adjustment or discontinue in patients with increasing serum creatinine. Increased urinary protein excretion has been observed when converting renal transplant patients from calcineurin inhibitors to sirolimus during maintenance therapy. A higher level of proteinuria prior to sirolimus conversion correlates with a higher degree of proteinuria after conversion. In some patients, proteinuria may reach nephrotic levels.

Use caution with hepatic impairment; a reduction in the maintenance dose is recommended. Has been associated with an increased risk of fluid accumulation and lymphocele; peripheral edema, lymphedema, and pleural and pericardial effusions (including significant effusions and tamponade) were reported; use with caution in patients in whom fluid accumulation may be poorly tolerated, such as in cardiovascular disease (heart failure or hypertension) and pulmonary disease. Cases of interstitial lung disease (eg, pneumonitis, bronchiolitis obliterans organizing pneumonia, pulmonary fibrosis) have been observed; risk may be increased with higher trough levels. Avoid concurrent use of strong CYP3A4 inhibitors or strong inducers of either CYP3A4 or P-glycoprotein. Concurrent use with a calcineurin inhibitor (cyclosporine, tacrolimus) may increase the risk of calcineurin inhibitor-induced hemolytic uremic syndrome/thrombotic thrombocytopenic purpura/thrombotic microangiopathy (HUS/TTP/TMA).

Hypersensitivity reactions, including anaphylactic/anaphylactoid reactions, angioedema, exfoliative dermatitis, and hypersensitivity vasculitis have been reported. Concurrent use with other drugs known to cause angioedema (eg, ACE inhibitors) may increase risk. Immunosuppressant therapy is associated with an increased risk of skin cancer; limit sun and ultraviolet light exposure; use appropriate sun protection. May increase serum lipids (cholesterol and triglycerides); use with caution in patients with hyperlipidemia. May be associated with wound dehiscence and impaired healing; use caution in the perioperative period. Patients with a body mass index (BMI) >30 kg/m^2 are at increased risk for abnormal wound healing. Safety and efficacy of combination therapy with cyclosporine high-risk patients has not been studied beyond 12 months of treatment; adjustment of immunosuppressive therapy beyond 12 months should be considered based on clinical judgement. Not labeled for use in children <13 years of age, or in adolescent patients <18 years of age considered at high immunological risk.

Adverse Reactions Incidence of many adverse effects is dose related.

>20%:

Cardiovascular: Peripheral edema (54% to 64%), hypertension (39% to 49%), edema (16% to 24%), chest pain (16% to 24%)

Central nervous system: Fever (23% to 34%), headache (23% to 34%), pain (24% to 33%), insomnia (13% to 22%)

Dermatologic: Acne (20% to 31%), rash (10% to 20%)

Endocrine & metabolic: Hypertriglyceridemia (38% to 57%), hypercholesterolemia (38% to 46%), hypophosphatemia (15% to 23%), hypokalemia (11% to 21%)

Gastrointestinal: Diarrhea (25% to 42%), constipation (28% to 38%), abdominal pain (28% to 36%), nausea (25% to 36%), vomiting (19% to 25%), dyspepsia (17% to 25%), weight gain (8% to 21%)

Genitourinary: Urinary tract infection (20% to 33%)

Hematologic: Anemia (23% to 37%), thrombocytopenia (13% to 30%)

Neuromuscular & skeletal: Weakness (22% to 40%), arthralgia (25% to 31%), tremor (21% to 31%), back pain (16% to 26%)

Renal: Serum creatinine increased (35% to 40%)

Respiratory: Dyspnea (22% to 30%), upper respiratory infection (20% to 26%), pharyngitis (16% to 21%)

3% to 20%:

Cardiovascular: Atrial fibrillation, CHF, DVT, facial edema, hypervolemia, hypotension, palpitation, peripheral vascular disorder, postural hypotension, syncope, tachycardia, thrombosis, vasodilation, venous thromboembolism

Central nervous system: Chills, malaise, anxiety, confusion, depression, dizziness, emotional lability, hypoesthesia, hypotonia, neuropathy, somnolence

Dermatologic: Dermatitis (fungal), hirsutism, pruritus, skin hypertrophy, dermal ulcer, ecchymosis, cellulitis, skin carcinoma (up to 3%; includes basal cell carcinoma, squamous cell carcinoma, melanoma), wound healing abnormal

Endocrine & metabolic: Cushing's syndrome, diabetes mellitus, glycosuria, acidosis, dehydration, hypercalcemia, hyperglycemia, hyperphosphatemia, hypocalcemia, hypoglycemia, hypomagnesemia, hyponatremia, hyperkalemia (12% to 17%)

Gastrointestinal: Enlarged abdomen, anorexia, dysphagia, eructation, esophagitis, flatulence, gastritis, gastroenteritis, gingivitis, gingival hyperplasia, ileus, mouth ulceration, oral moniliasis, stomatitis, weight loss

Genitourinary: Pelvic pain, scrotal edema, testis disorder, impotence

Hematologic: Leukocytosis, polycythemia, TTP, hemolytic-uremic syndrome, hemorrhage, leukopenia (9% to 15%)

Hepatic: Abnormal liver function tests, alkaline phosphatase increased, ascites, LDH increased, transaminases increased

Local: Thrombophlebitis

Neuromuscular & skeletal: Arthrosis, bone necrosis, CPK increased, leg cramps, myalgia, osteoporosis, tetany, hypertonia, paresthesia

Ocular: Abnormal vision, cataract, conjunctivitis

Otic: Ear pain, deafness, otitis media, tinnitus

Renal: Albuminuria, bladder pain, BUN increased, dysuria, hematuria, hydronephrosis, kidney pain, tubular necrosis, nocturia, oliguria, pyelonephritis, pyuria, nephropathy (toxic), urinary frequency, urinary incontinence, urinary retention

Respiratory: Asthma, atelectasis, bronchitis, cough, epistaxis, hypoxia, lung edema, pleural effusion, pneumonia, pulmonary embolism, rhinitis, sinusitis

Miscellaneous: Abscess, diaphoresis, flu-like syndrome, herpesvirus infection, hernia, infection (including opportunistic), lymphadenopathy, lymphocele, lymphoproliferative disease/lymphoma (1% to 3%), peritonitis, sepsis

Infrequent, postmarketing, and/or case reports: Anaphylactoid reaction, anaphylaxis, anastomotic disruption, angioedema, azoospermia, cytomegalovirus, Epstein-Barr virus, exfoliative dermatitis, fascial dehiscence, hepatic necrosis, hepatotoxicity, hypersensitivity reaction, hypersensitivity vasculitis; interstitial lung disease (dose–related; includes pneumonitis, pulmonary fibrosis, and bronchiolitis obliterans organizing pneumonia [BOOP] with no identified infectious etiology); joint disorders, lymphedema, nephrotic syndrome, neutropenia, pancreatitis, pancytopenia, pericardial effusion, *Pneumocystis* pneumonia, proteinuria, pulmonary hemorrhage, tamponade, tuberculosis, wound dehiscence

Note: Hepatic artery thrombosis and graft failure have been reported in liver transplant patients (not an approved use); bronchial anastomotic dehiscence has been reported in lung transplant patients (not an approved use); and calcineurin inhibitor-induced hemolytic uremic syndrome/thrombotic thrombocytopenic purpura/thrombotic microangiopathy (HUS/TTP/TMA) has been reported with concurrent cyclosporine and/or tacrolimus.

Drug Interactions

Metabolism/Transport Effects Substrate of CYP3A4 (major), P-glycoprotein; **Inhibits** CYP3A4 (weak)

Avoid Concomitant Use

Avoid concomitant use of Sirolimus with any of the following: Natalizumab; Vaccines (Live)

Increased Effect/Toxicity

Sirolimus may increase the levels/effects of: ACE Inhibitors; CycloSPORINE; Natalizumab; Tacrolimus; Vaccines (Live)

The levels/effects of Sirolimus may be increased by: Antifungal Agents (Azole Derivatives, Systemic); CycloSPORINE; CYP3A4 Inhibitors (Moderate); CYP3A4 Inhibitors (Strong); Dasatinib; Herbs (Hypoglycemic Properties); Macrolide Antibiotics; P-Glycoprotein Inhibitors; Protease Inhibitors; Trastuzumab

Decreased Effect

Sirolimus may decrease the levels/effects of: Vaccines (Inactivated)

The levels/effects of Sirolimus may be decreased by: CYP3A4 Inducers (Strong); Deferasirox; Echinacea; Herbs (CYP3A4 Inducers); P-Glycoprotein Inducers; Phenytoin; Rifampin

Ethanol/Nutrition/Herb Interactions

Food: Avoid grapefruit juice; may decrease clearance of sirolimus. Ingestion with high-fat meals decreases peak concentrations but increases AUC by 23% to 35%. Sirolimus should be taken consistently either with or without food to minimize variability.

Herb/Nutraceutical: St John's wort may decrease sirolimus levels; avoid concurrent use. Avoid cat's claw, echinacea (have immunostimulant properties; consider therapy modifications). Herbs with hypoglycemic properties may increase the risk of sirolimus-induced hypoglycemia; includes alfalfa, aloe, bilberry, bitter melon, burdock, celery, damiana, fenugreek, garcinia, garlic, ginger, ginseng (American), gymnema, marshmallow, stinging nettle.

Stability

Oral solution: Store under refrigeration, 2°C to 8°C (36°F to 46°F). Protect from light. A slight haze may develop in refrigerated solutions, but the quality of the product is not affected. After opening, solution should be used in 1 month. If necessary, may be stored at temperatures up to 25°C (77°F) for ≤15 days after opening. Product may be stored in amber syringe for a maximum of 24 hours (at room temperature or refrigerated). Solution should be used immediately following dilution.

Tablet: Store at room temperature of 20°C to 25°C (68°F to 77°F). Protect from light.

Mechanism of Action Sirolimus inhibits T-lymphocyte activation and proliferation in response to antigenic and cytokine stimulation and inhibits antibody production. Its mechanism differs from other immunosuppressants. Sirolimus binds to FKBP-12, an intracellular protein, to form an immunosuppressive complex which inhibits the regulatory kinase, mTOR (mammalian target of rapamycin). This inhibition suppresses cytokine mediated T-cell proliferation, halting progression from the G1 to the S phase of the cell cycle. It inhibits acute rejection of allografts and prolongs graft survival.

Pharmacodynamics/Kinetics

Absorption: Rapid

Distribution: 12 L/kg (range: 4-20 L/kg)

Protein binding: 92%, primarily to albumin

Metabolism: Extensively hepatic via CYP3A4; to 7 major metabolites

Bioavailability: Oral solution: 14%; Oral tablet: 18%

Half-life elimination: Mean: 62 hours (range: 46-78 hours); extended in hepatic impairment (Child-Pugh class A or B) to 113 hours

Time to peak: 1-2 hours

Excretion: Feces (91% due to P-glycoprotein-mediated efflux into gut lumen); urine (2%)

Dosage Oral:

Combination therapy with cyclosporine: Doses should be taken 4 hours after cyclosporine, and should be taken consistently either with or without food.

Low- to moderate-risk renal transplant patients: Children ≥13 years and Adults: Dosing by body weight:

<40 kg: Loading dose: 3 mg/m^2 on day 1, followed by maintenance dosing of 1 mg/m^2 once daily

≥40 kg: Loading dose: 6 mg on day 1; maintenance: 2 mg once daily

High-risk renal transplant patients: Adults: Loading dose: Up to 15 mg on day 1; maintenance: 5 mg/day; obtain trough concentration between days 5-7 and adjust accordingly. Continue concurrent cyclosporine/sirolimus therapy for 1 year following transplantation. Further adjustment of the regimen must be based on clinical status.

Dosage adjustment: Sirolimus dosages should be adjusted to maintain trough concentrations within desired range based on risk and concomitant therapy. Maximum daily dose: 40 mg. Dosage should be adjusted at intervals of 7-14 days to account for the long half-life of sirolimus. In general, dose proportionality may be assumed. New sirolimus dose **equals** current dose **multiplied by** (target concentration/current concentration). **Note:** If large dose increase is required, consider loading dose calculated as:

Loading dose **equals** (new maintenance dose **minus** current maintenance dose) **multiplied by** 3

Maximum dose in 1 day: 40 mg; if required dose is >40 mg (due to loading dose), divide over 2 days. Serum concentrations should not be used as the sole basis for dosage adjustment (monitor clinical signs/symptoms, tissue biopsy, and laboratory parameters).

Maintenance therapy after withdrawal of cyclosporine: Cyclosporine withdrawal is not recommended in high immunological risk patients. Following 2-4 months of combined therapy, withdrawal of cyclosporine may be considered in low-to-moderate risk patients. Cyclosporine should be discontinued over 4-8 weeks, and a necessary increase in the dosage of sirolimus (up to fourfold) should be anticipated due to removal of metabolic inhibition by cyclosporine and to maintain adequate immunosuppressive effects. Dose-adjusted trough target concentrations are typically 16-24 ng/mL for the first year post-transplant and 12-20 ng/mL thereafter (measured by chromatographic methodology).

Dosage adjustment in renal impairment: No dosage adjustment (in loading or maintenance dose) is necessary in renal impairment. However, adjustment of regimen (including discontinuation of therapy) should be considered when used concurrently with cyclosporine and elevated or increasing serum creatinine is noted.

Dosage adjustment in hepatic impairment:

Loading dose: No adjustment required

Maintenance dose:

Mild-to-moderate hepatic impairment: reduce maintenance dose by ~33%

Severe hepatic impairment: reduce maintenance dose by ~50%

Dietary Considerations Take consistently, with or without food, to minimize variability of absorption.

Administration Initial dose should be administered as soon as possible after transplant. Sirolimus should be taken 4 hours after oral cyclosporine (Neoral® or Gengraf®).

Solution: Mix with at least 2 ounces of water or orange juice. No other liquids should be used for dilution. Patient should drink diluted solution immediately. The cup should then be refilled with an additional 4 ounces of water or orange juice, stirred vigorously, and the patient should drink the contents at once.

Tablet: Do not crush, split, or chew.

Monitoring Parameters Monitor LFTs and CBC during treatment. Monitor sirolimus levels in all patients (especially in pediatric patients, patients ≥13 years of age weighing <40 kg, patients with hepatic impairment, or on concurrent potent inhibitors or inducers of CYP3A4, and/or if cyclosporine dosing is markedly reduced or discontinued), and when changing dosage forms of sirolimus. Also monitor serum cholesterol and triglycerides, blood pressure, serum creatinine, and urinary protein. Serum drug concentrations should be determined 3-4 days after loading doses and 7-14 days after dosage adjustments; however, these concentrations should not be used as the sole basis for dosage adjustment, especially during withdrawal of cyclosporine (monitor clinical signs/symptoms, tissue biopsy, and laboratory parameters). **Note:** Specific ranges will vary with assay methodology (chromatographic or immunoassay) and are not interchangeable.

Reference Range Note: Differences in sensitivity and specificity exist between methods of detection (eg, immunoassay vs HPLC); on average, chromatographic methods yield values ~20% lower than (whole blood) immunoassay determinations. Target range may vary based on assay conditions.

Serum trough concentrations (based on HPLC methods):

Concomitant cyclosporine: 4-12 ng/mL

After cyclosporine withdrawal: 16-24 ng/mL for the first year after transplant; after 1 year: 12-20 ng/mL

Note: Trough concentrations vary based on clinical context and use of additional immunosuppressants. The following represents typical ranges.

When combined with tacrolimus and mycophenolate mofetil (MMF) without steroids: 6-8 ng/mL

As a substitute for tacrolimus (starting 4-8 weeks post-transplant), in combination with MMF and steroids: 8-12 ng/mL

Following conversion from tacrolimus to sirolimus >6 months post-transplant due to chronic allograft nephropathy: 4-6 ng/mL

Additional Information

Sirolimus tablets and oral solution are not bioequivalent, due to differences in absorption. Clinical equivalence was seen using 2 mg tablet and 2 mg solution. It is not known if higher doses are also clinically equivalent. Monitor sirolimus levels if cages in dosage forms are made.

Sirolimus solution may cause irritation if administered undiluted.

High-risk renal transplant patients are defined (per the manufacturer's labeling) as African-American transplant recipients and/or repeat renal transplant recipients who lost a previous allograft based on an immunologic process and/or patients with high PRA (panel-reactive antibodies; peak PRA level >80%). Individual transplant centers may have differences in their definitions. For example, some centers would consider a PRA >50% to be at higher risk of rejection.

Dosage Forms Excipient information presented when available (limited, particularly for generics); consult specific product labeling.

Solution, oral:

Rapamune®: 1 mg/mL (60 mL) [contains ethanol 1.5% to 2.5%; packaged with oral syringes and a carrying case]

Tablet:

Rapamune®: 1 mg, 2 mg

SitaGLIPtin (sit a GLIP tin)

U.S. Brand Names Januvia™

Index Terms MK-0431; Sitagliptin Phosphate

Pharmacologic Category Antidiabetic Agent, Dipeptidyl Peptidase IV (DPP-IV) Inhibitor

Use

U.S. labeling: Management of type 2 diabetes mellitus (noninsulin dependent, NIDDM) as an adjunct to diet and exercise as monotherapy or in combination therapy with other antidiabetic agents

Canadian labeling: Management of NIDDM in combination with metformin therapy, diet, and exercise. **Note:** Use as monotherapy is not approved in Canadian labeling.

Pregnancy Risk Factor B

Pregnancy Considerations Adverse events have not been observed in animal reproduction studies; therefore, sitagliptan is classified as pregnancy category B. There are no adequate and well controlled studies in pregnant women. Maternal hyperglycemia can be associated with adverse effects in the fetus, including macrosomia, neonatal hyperglycemia, and hyperbilirubinemia; the risk of congenital malformations is increased when the Hb A_{1c} is above the normal range. Diabetes can also be associated with adverse effects in the mother. Poorly-treated diabetes may cause end-organ damage that may in turn negatively affect obstetric outcomes. Physiologic glucose levels should be maintained prior to and during pregnancy to decrease the risk of adverse events in the mother and the fetus. Until additional safety and efficacy data are obtained, the use of oral agents is generally not recommended as routine management of GDM or type 2 diabetes mellitus during pregnancy. Insulin is the drug of choice for the control of diabetes mellitus during pregnancy. Health professionals are encouraged to report any prenatal exposure to sitagliptin by contacting Merck's pregnancy registry (1-800-986-8999).

Lactation Excretion in breast milk unknown/use caution

Medication Safety Issues

Sound-alike/look-alike issues:

Januvia™ may be confused with Jantoven™

SitaGLIPtin may be confused with SUMAtriptan

Contraindications Serious hypersensitivity (eg, anaphylaxis, angioedema) or any component of the formulation; type 1 diabetes mellitus (insulin dependent, IDDM), diabetic ketoacidosis

Warnings/Precautions Use caution when used in conjunction with sulfonylureas; risk of hypoglycemia is increased. Monitor blood glucose closely; dosage adjustments of the sulfonylurea may be necessary. Use with caution in patients with moderate-to-severe renal dysfunction and end-stage renal disease (ESRD) requiring hemodialysis or peritoneal dialysis; dosing adjustment required. Rare hypersensitivity reactions, including anaphylaxis, angioedema, and/or severe dermatologic reactions such as Stevens-Johnson syndrome, have been reported in postmarketing surveillance; discontinue if signs/symptoms of hypersensitivity reactions occur. Safety and efficacy have not been established in children <18 years of age.

Adverse Reactions

1% to 10%:

Gastrointestinal: Diarrhea (3%), abdominal pain (2%), nausea (1%)

Respiratory: Nasopharyngitis (5%)

Postmarketing and/or case reports: Anaphylaxis, angioedema, exfoliative dermatitis, hypoglycemia (risk increased in conjunction with sulfonylureas), hypersensitivity, liver enzymes increased, rash, serum creatinine increased, Stevens-Johnson syndrome, urticaria, white blood cells increased

Drug Interactions

Metabolism/Transport Effects Substrate (minor) of CYP2C8, 3A4

Avoid Concomitant Use There are no known interactions where it is recommended to avoid concomitant use.

Increased Effect/Toxicity There are no known significant interactions involving an increase in effect.

Decreased Effect There are no known significant interactions involving a decrease in effect.

Stability Store at 20°C to 25°C (68°F to 77°F).

Mechanism of Action Sitagliptin inhibits dipeptidyl peptidase IV (DPP-IV) enzyme resulting in prolonged active incretin levels. Incretin hormones (eg, glucagon-like peptide-1 [GLP-1] and glucose-dependent insulinotropic polypeptide [GIP]) regulate glucose homeostasis by increasing insulin synthesis and release from pancreatic beta cells and decreasing glucagon secretion from pancreatic alpha cells. Decreased glucagon secretion results in decreased hepatic glucose production. Under normal physiologic circumstances, incretin hormones are released by the intestine throughout the day and levels are increased in response to a meal; incretin hormones are rapidly inactivated by the DPP-IV enzyme.

Pharmacodynamics/Kinetics

Absorption: Rapid

Distribution: ~198 L

Protein binding: 38%

Metabolism: Not extensively metabolized; minor metabolism via CYP3A4 and 2C8 to metabolites (inactive) suggested by *in vitro* studies

Bioavailability: ~87%

Half-life elimination: 12 hours

Time to peak, plasma: 1-4 hours

Excretion: Urine 87% (79% as unchanged drug, 16% as metabolites); feces 13%

Dosage Oral: Adults: Type 2 diabetes: 100 mg once daily

Concomitant use with sulfonylureas: Reduced dose of sulfonylurea may be needed

Dosage adjustment in renal impairment:

Cl_{cr} ≥50 mL/minute: No adjustment required

Cl_{cr} ≥30 to <50 mL/minute: 50 mg once daily

S_{cr}: Males: >1.7 to ≤3.0 mg/dL; Females: >1.5 to ≤2.5 mg/dL: 50 mg once daily

Cl_{cr}<30 mL/minute: 25 mg once daily

S_{cr}: Males: >3.0 mg/dL; Females: >2.5 mg/dL: 25 mg once daily

ESRD requiring hemodialysis or peritoneal dialysis: 25 mg once daily; administered without regard to timing of hemodialysis

Dosage adjustment in hepatic impairment:

Mild-to-moderate impairment (Child-Pugh score 7-9): No dosage adjustment required

Severe impairment (Child-Pugh score >9): Not studied

Dietary Considerations May be taken with or without food.

Administration May be administered with or without food.

Monitoring Parameters Hgb A_{1C} and serum glucose; renal function prior to initiation and periodically during treatment.

Reference Range Recommendations for glycemic control in adults with diabetes:

Hb A_{1c}: <7%

Preprandial capillary plasma glucose: 70-130 mg/dL

Peak postprandial capillary blood glucose: <180 mg/dL

Blood pressure: <130/80 mm Hg

Dosage Forms Excipient information presented when available (limited, particularly for generics); consult specific product labeling.

Tablet:

Januvia™: 25 mg, 50 mg, 100 mg

Sitagliptin and Metformin

(sit a GLIP tin & met FOR min)

U.S. Brand Names Janumet™

Index Terms Metformin and Sitagliptin; Sitagliptin Phosphate and Metformin Hydrochloride

Pharmacologic Category Antidiabetic Agent, Biguanide; Antidiabetic Agent, Dipeptidyl Peptidase IV (DPP-IV) Inhibitor; Hypoglycemic Agent, Oral

Additional Appendix Information

Diabetes Mellitus Management, Adults *on page 1801*

Use Management of type 2 diabetes mellitus (noninsulin dependent, NIDDM) in patients not adequately controlled on metformin or sitagliptin monotherapy and as an adjunct to diet and exercise

Pregnancy Risk Factor B

Medication Safety Issues

Sound-alike/look-alike issues:

Janumet™ may be confused with Jantoven™

Dosage Oral: Type 2 diabetes mellitus:

Adults: Initial doses should be based on current dose of sitagliptin and metformin; daily doses should be divided and given twice daily with meals. Maximum: Sitagliptin 100 mg/metformin 2000 mg daily

Patients inadequately controlled on metformin alone: Initial dose: Sitagliptin 100 mg/day plus current dose of metformin. **Note:** Per manufacturer labeling, patients currently receiving metformin 850 mg twice daily should receive an initial dose of sitagliptin 50 mg and metformin 1000 mg twice daily

Patients inadequately controlled on sitagliptin alone: Initial dose: Metformin 1000 mg/day plus sitagliptin 100 mg/day. **Note:** Patients currently receiving a renally adjusted dose of sitagliptin should not be switched to combination product.

Dosing adjustment: Metformin component may be gradually increased up to the maximum dose. Maximum dose: Sitagliptin 100 mg/metformin 2000 mg daily

Elderly: The initial and maintenance dosing should be conservative, due to the potential for decreased renal function (monitor). Do not use in patients ≥80 years of age unless normal renal function has been established.

Dosage adjustment in renal impairment: Do not use with renal disease or renal dysfunction (serum creatinine ≥1.5 mg/dL in males or ≥1.4 mg/dL in females or abnormal clearance).

Dosage adjustment in hepatic impairment: Avoid metformin; liver disease is a risk factor for the development of lactic acidosis during metformin therapy.

Additional Information Complete prescribing information for this medication should be consulted for additional detail.

Dosage Forms Excipient information presented when available (limited, particularly for generics); consult specific product labeling.

Tablet:

Janumet™:

50/500: Sitagliptin 50 mg and metformin hydrochloride 500 mg

50/1000: Sitagliptin 50 mg and metformin hydrochloride 1000 mg

◆ **Sitagliptin Phosphate** *see* SitaGLIPtin *on page 1375*
◆ **Sitagliptin Phosphate and Metformin Hydrochloride** *see* Sitagliptin and Metformin *on page 1376*
◆ **Skeeter Stik [OTC]** *see* Benzocaine *on page 183*
◆ **Skelaxin®** *see* Metaxalone *on page 954*
◆ **Skelid®** *see* Tiludronate *on page 1470*
◆ **SKF 104864** *see* Topotecan *on page 1491*
◆ **SKF 104864-A** *see* Topotecan *on page 1491*
◆ **Sleep-ettes D [OTC]** *see* DiphenhydrAMINE *on page 456*
◆ **Sleepinal® [OTC]** *see* DiphenhydrAMINE *on page 456*
◆ **S-leucovorin** *see* LEVOleucovorin *on page 878*
◆ **6S-leucovorin** *see* LEVOleucovorin *on page 878*
◆ **Slo-Niacin® [OTC]** *see* Niacin *on page 1057*
◆ **Slo-Pot (Can)** *see* Potassium Chloride *on page 1216*
◆ **Slow FE® [OTC]** *see* Ferrous Sulfate *on page 617*
◆ **Slow-K® (Can)** *see* Potassium Chloride *on page 1216*
◆ **Slow-Mag® [OTC]** *see* Magnesium Chloride *on page 914*

Smallpox Vaccine (SMAL poks vak SEEN)

U.S. Brand Names ACAM2000™

Index Terms Dried Smallpox Vaccine; Live Smallpox Vaccine; Vaccinia Vaccine

Pharmacologic Category Vaccine

Use Active immunization against vaccinia virus, the causative agent of smallpox in persons determined to be at risk for smallpox infection. The ACIP recommends vaccination of laboratory workers at risk of exposure from cultures or contaminated animals which may be a source of vaccinia or related Orthopoxviruses capable of causing infections in humans (monkeypox, cowpox, or variola). The ACIP also recommends that consideration be given for vaccination in healthcare workers having contact with clinical specimens, contaminated material, or patients receiving vaccinia or recombinant vaccinia viruses. ACIP recommends revaccination every 10 years. The Armed Forces recommend vaccination of certain personnel categories. Recommendations for use in response to bioterrorism are regularly updated by the CDC, and may be found at www.cdc.gov.

Restrictions The smallpox vaccine is not available for general public use. All supplies are currently owned by the federal government for inclusion in the Strategic National Stockpile. In October 2002, the FDA approved the licensing of the stockpile of smallpox vaccine. This approval allows the vaccine to be distributed and administered in the event of a smallpox attack. The bulk of current supplies have been designated for use by the U.S. military. Additionally, laboratory workers who may be at risk of exposure may require vaccination. Bioterrorism experts have proposed immunization of first responders (including police, fire, and emergency workers), but these plans may not be implemented until additional stocks of vaccine are licensed.

ACAM2000™ is subject to a Risk Minimization Action Plan (RiskMAP) which includes mandatory adverse event reporting, risk management evaluation, and education for both healthcare providers administering the vaccine and patients. Patients who receive the vaccine must be given an FDA-approved medication guide which is available at http://www.fda.gov/cber/label/acam2000pi.pdf.

Pregnancy Risk Factor D

Pregnancy Considerations [U.S. Boxed Warning]: Pregnant women should not be vaccinated in nonemergency situations. Animal reproduction studies have not been conducted. Vaccinia vaccine has not been associated with the development of congenital malformations. On rare occasions, vaccination has been reported to cause fetal infection. Fetal vaccina infection is associated with stillbirth or neonatal mortality. Pregnancy should be avoided for at least 28 days following vaccination. Healthcare providers may enroll pregnant women who were inadvertently vaccinated during pregnancy (or within 42 days prior to conception) in the CDC pregnancy registry by calling 404-639-8253 or 877-554-4625. Military cases should be reported to the Department of Defense.

Lactation Excretion in breast milk unknown/not recommended

Contraindications There are no absolute contraindications regarding vaccination of individuals with a high-risk exposure to smallpox. The decision to vaccinate in an emergency situation must be based on a careful analysis of potential benefits and possible risks.

For non-emergent use: Hypersensitivity to the vaccine or any component of the formulation; patients with a history of eczema or patients whose household contacts have acute or chronic exfoliative skin conditions (atopic dermatitis, eczema, burns, impetigo, Varicella zoster, or wounds); history of Darier disease (or if household contact has active disease); immunosuppressed patients and their household contacts, including patients with congenital or acquired immune deficiencies (including HIV, agammaglobulinemia, leukemia, lymphoma, neoplastic disease of the bone marrow or lymphatic system), patients receiving radiation, immunosuppressive drugs, or systemic corticosteroids ≥20 mg/day or ≥2 mg/kg body weight of prednisone for >2 weeks; patients using ocular steroid medications; moderate to severe intercurrent illness; cardiac disease, including previous MI, angina, CHF, cardiomyopathy, chest pain, or shortness of breath requiring medical therapy; pregnancy or suspected pregnancy (including household contacts of pregnant women); breast-feeding.

Warnings/Precautions [U.S. Boxed Warning]: Acute myopericarditis and/or pericarditis, encephalitis, encephalomyelitis, and encephalopathy have been observed following vaccination. [U.S. Boxed Warning]: Progressive vaccinia, ocular vaccinia, general vaccinia, and severe vaccinial skin infections have been observed following vaccination. [U.S. Boxed Warning]: Severe skin and systemic reactions, including Stevens-Johnson syndrome, have also occurred. [U.S. Boxed Warning]: Immunocompromised patients or those with eczema, cardiovascular disease, or risk factors for cardiovascular disease may be at an increased risk for severe adverse reactions and

should not be vaccinated in nonemergency situations. [U.S. Boxed Warning]: Pregnant women should not be vaccinated in nonemergency situations due to the risk of *in utero* transmission.

For vaccination by scarification (multiple punctures into superficial layers of the skin) only. **Not for I.M., I.V., or SubQ injection.** Some dosage forms may contain chlortetracycline, dihydrostreptomycin, neomycin, polymyxin B, and/or human albumin. Virus may be cultured from vaccination sites until scab separates from lesion. Individuals should be instructed to avoid contact with patients at high risk of transmission/adverse effects, including pregnant or breastfeeding women and patients with eczema or immunodeficiency during this time. Patients should be advised not to donate blood or organs for 21-30 days; contacts who have inadvertently contracted vaccinia should avoid donating blood for 14 days. Appropriate precautions should be used for the handling and disposal of vaccine and all supplies. **[U.S. Boxed Warning]: Not for use in infants <12 months of age (in emergency situations)** or in pediatric patients <18 years of age (in nonemergency situations). Safety and efficacy has not been established in patients ≥65 years of age.

Adverse Reactions All serious adverse reactions must be reported to the U.S. Department of Health and Human Services (DHHS) Vaccine Adverse Event Reporting System (VAERS) 1-800-822-7967. In addition, clinicians may enroll patients with adverse reactions in the CDC Registry at 877-554-4625. Serious adverse reactions to ACAM2000™ may also be reported to the manufacturer, Acambis Inc, at 866-440-9440.

>10%:

- Central nervous system: Fever (up to 70%; may be ≥102°F in up to 20% of children; frequency in adults may be lower), fatigue (48% to 56%), headache (35% to 51%), malaise (28% to 37%)
- Dermatologic: Erythema (22% to 24%); rash (6% to 11% erythematous, folliculitis, papulovesicular, urticarial, nonspecific)
- Gastrointestinal: Nausea (10% to 19%), diarrhea (12% to 16%)
- Local: Injection site: Pruritus (82% to 92%), erythema (61% to 74%), pain (37% to 67%), edema (28% to 48%)
- Neuromuscular & skeletal: Myalgia (27% to 46%), rigors (21% to 23%)
- Miscellaneous: Lymph node pain (19% to 57%), feeling hot (20% to 32%), exercise tolerance decreased (8% to 11%), lymphadenopathy (6% to 8%)

1% to 10%:

- Gastrointestinal: Constipation (6%), vomiting (3% to 5%)
- Neuromuscular & skeletal: Arthralgia, back pain
- Respiratory: Dyspnea (3% to 4%)

Frequency not defined: Abdominal pain, blindness, Bell's palsy, cardiomyopathy (nonischemic/dilated), contact dermatitis, corneal scarring, death, dizziness, eczema vaccinatum, encephalitis, encephalomyelitis, encephalopathy, erythema multiforme, generalized vaccinia, Guillain-Barré syndrome, hypersensitivity reactions; inadvertent inoculation at other sites (including autoinoculation to eyelid, face, genitalia, lips, mouth, nose, rectum); ischemic heart disease, keratitis, meningitis, myocarditis, myopericarditis (asymptomatic or symptomatic), ocular vaccinia, paresthesia, pericarditis, photophobia, progressive vaccinia, secondary pyogenic infection, seizure, Stevens-Johnson syndrome, vaccinial skin infection, vertigo

Drug Interactions

Avoid Concomitant Use

Avoid concomitant use of Smallpox Vaccine with any of the following: Immunosuppressants

Increased Effect/Toxicity

Smallpox Vaccine may increase the levels/effects of: Varicella Virus Vaccine

The levels/effects of Smallpox Vaccine may be increased by: Immunosuppressants

Decreased Effect

Smallpox Vaccine may decrease the levels/effects of: Tuberculin Tests

The levels/effects of Smallpox Vaccine may be decreased by: Immune Globulins

Stability Store at -15°C to -25°C (5°F to -13°F); prior to reconstitution, may be stored at 2°C to 8°C (36°F to 46°F) for up to 18 months. Bring to room temperature prior to reconstitution. Using the syringe provided, inject 0.3 mL of provided diluent into the vaccine vial. Swirl gently until the solution becomes a slightly hazy, colorless to straw-colored liquid free from particulate matter; avoid contact between the solution and the rubber stopper. Following reconstitution, stable for 6 to 8 hours at room temperature of 20°C to 25°C (68°F to 77°F) or for up to 30 days when refrigerated at 2°C to 8°C (36°F to 46°F). The provided diluent should be stored at room temperature of 15°C to 30°C (59°F to 86°F).

Mechanism of Action Vaccinia virus is similar to the variola (smallpox) virus. By inducing a localized infection with vaccinia virus, immunity to both vaccinia and smallpox is achieved. Vaccination results in viral replication, production of neutralizing antibodies, immunity, and cellular hypersensitivity.

Pharmacodynamics/Kinetics Onset of action: Neutralizing antibodies appear 10-13 days after vaccination.

Dosage Not for I.M., I.V., or SubQ injection: Vaccination by scarification (multiple-puncture technique) only: **Note:** A trace of blood should appear at vaccination site after 15-20 seconds; if no trace of blood is visible, an additional 3 insertions should be made using the same needle, without reinserting the needle into the vaccine bottle.

Children ≥12 months (in emergency conditions only) and Adults (ACAM2000™):

Primary vaccination and revaccination: Use a single drop of vaccine suspension and 15 needle punctures (using the same bifurcated needle) into the superficial skin

Note: According to the manufacturer, revaccination is recommended every 3 years for patients at a continued high risk for smallpox infection. This recommendation differs from the current ACIP recommendations for routine nonemergency smallpox revaccination. Additional information can be obtained from the Department of Defense and the CDC.

Dosage adjustment in renal impairment: No dosage adjustment required

Administration Vaccination should only be performed by healthcare providers trained in the safe and efficacious administration of the smallpox vaccine via the percutaneous route. Using a bifurcated needle, 1 drop of vaccine is introduced into the superficial layers of the skin using a multiple-puncture technique. The skin over the insertion of the deltoid muscle or the posterior aspect of the arm over the triceps are the preferred sites for vaccination.

A single-use bifurcated needle should be dipped carefully into the reconstituted vaccine (following removal of rubber stopper). Visually confirm that the needle picks up a drop of vaccine solution. Deposit the drop of vaccine onto clean, dry skin at the vaccination site. If alcohol is used to clean the skin, allow site to dry completely prior to administration to prevent the inactivation of the vaccine by the alcohol. Holding the bifurcated needle perpendicular to the skin, punctures are to be made rapidly within a diameter of about 5 mm into the superficial skin of the vaccination site.

The puncture strokes should be vigorous enough to allow a trace of blood to appear after approximately 15-20 seconds. Wipe off any remaining vaccine with dry sterile gauze. Dispose of all materials in a biohazard waste container. All materials must be burned, boiled, or autoclaved. If no evidence of vaccine take is apparent after 7 days, the individual may be vaccinated again.

To prevent transmission of the virus, avoid scratching the vaccination site and cover with gauze; cover gauze with a semipermeable barrier or clothing. Ointment or salves should not be applied to the vaccination site. Good handwashing prevents inadvertent inoculation. Vaccinees should change bandages away from others and launder their own linens separately to prevent transmission.

Monitoring Parameters Monitor vaccination site; inspect after 6-8 days. Evidence of a major reaction (vesicular or pustular lesion or an area of palpable induration surrounding a central lesion) confirms success of vaccination. An equivocal reaction (all responses other than a major reaction) requires revaccination in patients undergoing primary vaccination only (preferably with another vial or vaccine lot, if available). Consult CDC or state or local health department if response to a second vaccination from a different vial or lot is equivocal.

Test Interactions Rapid plasma regain (RPR) test: Smallpox vaccine may induce false-positive RPR test for syphilis; confirm positive RPR test using a more specific test (eg, FTA assay).

Tuberculin skin (PPD) and blood tests: Smallpox vaccine may diminish the diagnostic utility of tuberculin skin (PPD) and blood tests; avoid skin test for ≥1 month after vaccine to prevent false-negative results.

Additional Information Initial reaction of the vaccine includes formation of a papule (2-5 days following vaccination). The papule forms a vesicle on day 5 or day 6, which becomes pustular, with surrounding erythema and induration. The maximal area of erythema usually occurs between day 8 and day 10, and crusting of the lesion normally occurs between day 14 and day 21. Formation of a major cutaneous reaction in patients undergoing primary vaccination by day 6-8 is indicative of successful acquisition of protective immunity. In patients previously vaccinated, the major cutaneous reaction typically seen by day 6-8 may be modified and/or reduced; a lack of cutaneous response does not indicate vaccination failure and revaccination is not required in these patients. At the peak of the reaction, systemic symptoms (fever, malaise) and lymphadenopathy may occur. All materials used in vaccination must be burned, boiled, or autoclaved. Vaccination can decrease the rate of severe or fatal smallpox if administered during the first 4 days of exposure.

If vaccination failure occurs, revaccination should be attempted using a different vial or vaccine lot. If the second vaccination (from a different vial or lot) also fails, contact the Centers for Disease Control and Prevention (CDC) at 404-639-3670 and/or the state or local health department prior to administering any additional vaccine.

Dosage Forms Excipient information presented when available (limited, particularly for generics); consult specific product labeling. [DSC] = Discontinued product

Injection, powder for reconstitution [purified monkey cell source]:

- ACAM2000™: 1-5 x 10^8 plaque-forming units per mL [contains polymyxin B, neomycin (trace amounts) and human albumin; packed with diluent, tuberculin syringes for reconstitution, and 100 bifurcated needles for administration]

◆ **SMZ-TMP** *see* Sulfamethoxazole and Trimethoprim *on page 1407*

◆ **(+)-(*S*)-*N*-Methyl-γ-(1-naphthyloxy)-2-thiophenepropylamine Hydrochloride** *see* DULoxetine *on page 498*

◆ **Sodium 2-Mercaptoethane Sulfonate** *see* Mesna *on page 951*

◆ **Sodium 4-Hydroxybutyrate** *see* Sodium Oxybate *on page 1384*

◆ **Sodium *L*-Triiodothyronine** *see* Liothyronine *on page 892*

Sodium Acetate (SOW dee um AS e tate)

Pharmacologic Category Electrolyte Supplement, Parenteral

Use Sodium source in large volume I.V. fluids to prevent or correct hyponatremia in patients with restricted intake; used to counter acidosis through conversion to bicarbonate

Pregnancy Risk Factor C

Contraindications Alkalosis, hypocalcemia, low sodium diets, edema, cirrhosis

Warnings/Precautions Avoid extravasation, use with caution in patients with edema, heart failure, severe hepatic failure or renal impairment. Use with caution in patients with acid/base alterations; contains acetate, monitor closely during acid/base correction. Close monitoring of serum sodium concentrations is needed to avoid hypernatremia. Solution for injection contains aluminum; use with caution in patients with impaired renal function and in premature infants.

Adverse Reactions 1% to 10%:

Cardiovascular: Thrombosis, hypervolemia

Dermatologic: Chemical cellulitis at injection site (extravasation)

Endocrine & metabolic: Hypernatremia, dilution of serum electrolytes, overhydration, hypokalemia, metabolic alkalosis, hypocalcemia

Gastrointestinal: Gastric distension, flatulence

Local: Phlebitis

Respiratory: Pulmonary edema

Miscellaneous: Congestive conditions

Drug Interactions

Avoid Concomitant Use There are no known interactions where it is recommended to avoid concomitant use.

Increased Effect/Toxicity There are no known significant interactions involving an increase in effect.

Decreased Effect There are no known significant interactions involving a decrease in effect.

Stability Protect from light, heat, and freezing.

Dosage Sodium acetate is metabolized to bicarbonate on an equimolar basis outside the liver; administer in large volume I.V. fluids as a sodium source. Refer to Sodium Bicarbonate monograph.

Maintenance electrolyte requirements of sodium in parenteral nutrition solutions:

- Daily requirements: 3-4 mEq/kg/24 hours or 25-40 mEq/1000 kcal/24 hours
- Maximum: 100-150 mEq/24 hours

Dietary Considerations Sodium and acetate content of 1 g: 7.3 mEq

Administration Must be diluted prior to I.V. administration; infusion hypertonic solutions (>154 mEq/L) via a central line; maximum rate of administration: 1 mEq/kg/hour

Dosage Forms Excipient information presented when available (limited, particularly for generics); consult specific product labeling. [DSC] = Discontinued product

Injection, solution [concentrate]: 2 mEq/mL (20 mL, 50 mL, 100 mL; 250 mL [DSC]); 4 mEq/mL (50 mL, 100 mL)

◆ **Sodium Acid Carbonate** *see* Sodium Bicarbonate *on page 1380*

◆ **Sodium Acid Phosphate and Methenamine** *see* Methenamine and Sodium Acid Phosphate *on page 962*

◆ **Sodium Aurothiomalate** *see* Gold Sodium Thiomalate *on page 704*

◆ **Sodium Benzoate and Caffeine** *see* Caffeine *on page 232*

◆ **Sodium Benzoate and Sodium Phenylacetate** *see* Sodium Phenylacetate and Sodium Benzoate *on page 1384*

Sodium Bicarbonate (SOW dee um bye KAR bun ate)

U.S. Brand Names Brioschi® [OTC]; Neut®

Index Terms Baking Soda; $NaHCO_3$; Sodium Acid Carbonate; Sodium Hydrogen Carbonate

Pharmacologic Category Alkalinizing Agent; Antacid; Electrolyte Supplement, Oral; Electrolyte Supplement, Parenteral

Use Management of metabolic acidosis; gastric hyperacidity; as an alkalinization agent for the urine; treatment of hyperkalemia; management of overdose of certain drugs, including tricyclic antidepressants and aspirin

Unlabeled/Investigational Use Prevention of contrast-induced nephropathy (CIN)

Pregnancy Risk Factor C

Lactation Enters breast milk/compatible

Contraindications Alkalosis, hypernatremia, severe pulmonary edema, hypocalcemia, unknown abdominal pain

Warnings/Precautions Rapid administration in neonates and children <2 years of age has led to hypernatremia, decreased CSF pressure and intracranial hemorrhage. **Use of I.V. $NaHCO_3$ should be reserved for documented metabolic acidosis and for hyperkalemia-induced cardiac arrest.** Routine use in cardiac arrest is not recommended. Avoid extravasation, tissue necrosis can occur due to the hypertonicity of $NaHCO_3$. May cause sodium retention especially if renal function is impaired; not to be used in treatment of peptic ulcer; use with caution in patients with HF, edema, cirrhosis, or renal failure. Not the antacid of choice for the elderly because of sodium content and potential for systemic alkalosis.

Adverse Reactions Frequency not defined.

Cardiovascular: Cerebral hemorrhage, CHF (aggravated), edema

Central nervous system: Tetany

Gastrointestinal: Belching, flatulence (with oral), gastric distension

Endocrine & metabolic: Hypernatremia, hyperosmolality, hypocalcemia, hypokalemia, increased affinity of hemoglobin for oxygen-reduced pH in myocardial tissue necrosis when extravasated, intracranial acidosis, metabolic alkalosis, milk-alkali syndrome (especially with renal dysfunction)

Respiratory: Pulmonary edema

Drug Interactions

Avoid Concomitant Use

Avoid concomitant use of Sodium Bicarbonate with any of the following: Mesalamine

Increased Effect/Toxicity

Sodium Bicarbonate may increase the levels/effects of: Alpha-/Beta-Agonists; Amphetamines; Memantine; QuiNIDine; Tocainide

Decreased Effect

Sodium Bicarbonate may decrease the levels/effects of: ACE Inhibitors; Anticonvulsants (Hydantoin); Antifungal Agents (Azole Derivatives, Systemic); Antipsychotic Agents (Phenothiazines); Atazanavir; Bisacodyl; Cefpodoxime; Cefuroxime; Corticosteroids (Oral); CycloSPORINE; Dabigatran Etexilate; Dasatinib; Delavirdine; Erlotinib; Iron Salts; Isoniazid; Lithium; Mesalamine; Methenamine; Penicillamine; Phosphate Supplements; Protease Inhibitors; Tetracycline Derivatives; Trientine

Ethanol/Nutrition/Herb Interactions Herb/Nutraceutical: Concurrent doses with iron may decrease iron absorption.

Stability Store injection at room temperature; do not freeze. Protect from heat. Use only clear solutions.

Prevention of contrast-induced nephropathy (unlabeled use): Remove 154 mL from 1000 mL bag of D_5W; replace with 154 mL of 8.4% sodium bicarbonate; resultant concentration is 154 mEq/L (Merten, 2004); more practically, institutions may remove 150 mL from 1000 mL bag of D_5W and replace with 150 mL of 8.4% sodium bicarbonate; resultant concentration is 150 mEq/L

Mechanism of Action Dissociates to provide bicarbonate ion which neutralizes hydrogen ion concentration and raises blood and urinary pH

Pharmacodynamics/Kinetics

Onset of action: Oral: Rapid; I.V.: 15 minutes

Duration: Oral: 8-10 minutes; I.V.: 1-2 hours

Absorption: Oral: Well absorbed

Excretion: Urine (<1%)

Dosage

Cardiac arrest: **Routine use of $NaHCO_3$ is not recommended.** May be considered in the setting of prolonged cardiac arrest only after adequate alveolar ventilation has been established and effective cardiac compressions. **Note:** In some cardiac arrest situations (eg, metabolic acidosis, hyperkalemia, or tricyclic antidepressant overdose), sodium bicarbonate may be beneficial.

Infants and Children: I.V.: 0.5-1 mEq/kg/dose repeated every 10 minutes or as indicated by arterial blood gases; rate of infusion should not exceed 10 mEq/minute; neonates and children <2 years of age should receive 4.2% (0.5 mEq/mL) solution

Adults: I.V.: Initial: 1 mEq/kg/dose one time; maintenance: 0.5 mEq/kg/dose every 10 minutes or as indicated by arterial blood gases

Metabolic acidosis: Infants, Children, and Adults: Dosage should be based on the following formula if blood gases and pH measurements are available:

HCO_3^- (mEq) = 0.3 x weight (kg) x base deficit (mEq/L)

Administer 1/2 dose initially, then remaining 1/2 dose over the next 24 hours; monitor pH, serum HCO_3^-, and clinical status

Note: If acid-base status is not available: Dose for older Children and Adults: 2-5 mEq/kg I.V. infusion over 4-8 hours; subsequent doses should be based on patient's acid-base status

Chronic renal failure: Oral: Initiate when plasma HCO_3^- <15 mEq/L

Children: 1-3 mEq/kg/day

Adults: Start with 20-36 mEq/day in divided doses, titrate to bicarbonate level of 18-20 mEq/L

Hyperkalemia: Adults: I.V.: 50 mEq over 5 minutes (as appropriate, consider methods of enhancing potassium removal/excretion)

Renal tubular acidosis: Oral:

Distal:

Children: 2-3 mEq/kg/day

Adults: 0.5-2 mEq/kg/day in 4-5 divided doses

Proximal: Children and Adults: Initial: 5-10 mEq/kg/day; maintenance: Increase as required to maintain serum bicarbonate in the normal range

Urine alkalinization: Oral:

Children: 1-10 mEq (84-840 mg)/kg/day in divided doses every 4-6 hours; dose should be titrated to desired urinary pH

Adults: Initial: 48 mEq (4 g), then 12-24 mEq (1-2 g) every 4 hours; dose should be titrated to desired urinary pH; doses up to 16 g/day (200 mEq) in patients <60 years and 8 g (100 mEq) in patients >60 years

Antacid: Adults: Oral: 325 mg to 2 g 1-4 times/day

Prevention of contrast-induced nephropathy (unlabeled use): Adults: I.V. infusion: 154 mEq/L sodium bicarbonate in D_5W solution: 3 mL/kg/hour for 1 hour immediately before contrast injection, then 1mL/kg/hour during contrast exposure and for 6 hours after procedure

To prepare solution, remove 154 mL from 1000 mL bag of D_5W; replace with 154 mL of 8.4% sodium bicarbonate; resultant concentration is 154 mEq/L (Merten, 2004); more practically, institutions may remove 150 mL from 1000 mL bag of D_5W and replace with 150 mL of 8.4% sodium bicarbonate; resultant concentration is 150 mEq/L

Dietary Considerations Oral product should be administered 1-3 hours after meals.

Sodium content:

Injection: 50 mL, 8.4% = 1150 mg = 50 mEq; each mL of 8.4% $NaHCO_3$ contains 23 mg sodium; 1 mEq $NaHCO_3$ = 84 mg

Granules: 2.69 g packet or capful = 770 mg sodium

Powder: 30 mEq sodium per 1/2 teaspoon

Administration For I.V. administration to infants, use the 0.5 mEq/mL solution or dilute the 1 mEq/mL solution 1:1 with **sterile water**; for direct I.V. infusion in emergencies, administer slowly (maximum rate in infants: 10 mEq/minute); for infusion, dilute to a maximum concentration of 0.5 mEq/mL in dextrose solution and infuse over 2 hours (maximum rate of administration: 1 mEq/kg/hour)

Dosage Forms Excipient information presented when available (limited, particularly for generics); consult specific product labeling.

Granules, for solution, oral [effervescent]:

Brioschi®: 2.69 g/packet (12s) [contains sodium 770 mg/packet; lemon flavor]; 2.69 g/capful (120 g, 240 g) [contains sodium 770 mg/capful; lemon flavor]

Infusion [premixed in water for injection]: 5% (500 mL) [5.95 mEq/10 mL]

Injection, solution:

4.2% (10 mL) [5 mEq/10 mL]

7.5% (50 mL) [8.92 mEq/10 mL]

8.4% (10 mL, 50 mL, 250 mL, 500 mL) [10 mEq/10 mL]

Neut®: 4% (5 mL) [2.4 mEq/5 mL; contains edetate disodium]

Powder: Sodium bicarbonate USP (120 g, 480 g) [contains sodium 30 mEq per 1/2 teaspoon]

Tablet: 325 mg [3.8 mEq]; 650 mg [7.6 mEq]

◆ **Sodium Biphosphate, Methenamine, Methylene Blue, Phenyl Salicylate, and Hyoscyamine** *see* Methenamine, Sodium Biphosphate, Phenyl Salicylate, Methylene Blue, and Hyoscyamine *on page 962*

Sodium Chloride (SOW dee um KLOR ide)

U.S. Brand Names 4-Way® Saline Moisturizing Mist [OTC]; Altachlore [OTC]; Altamist [OTC]; Ayr® Allergy Sinus [OTC]; Ayr® Baby Saline [OTC]; Ayr® Saline No-Drip [OTC]; Ayr® Saline [OTC]; Breathe Free® [OTC]; Deep Sea [OTC]; Entsol® [OTC]; Humist® for Kids [OTC]; Humist® [OTC]; Hyper-Sal™; Little Noses® Saline [OTC]; Little Noses® Stuffy Nose Kit [OTC] ; Muro 128® [OTC]; Mycinaire™ [OTC] [DSC]; Na-Zone® [OTC]; Nasal Moist® Saline [OTC]; Nasal Spray [OTC]; NāSal™ [OTC]; Ocean® for Kids [OTC]; Ocean® [OTC]; Pretz® [OTC]; Saline Mist [OTC]; SalineX® [OTC] [DSC]; Simply Saline® Baby [OTC]; Simply Saline® Nasal Moist® [OTC] ; Simply Saline® [OTC]; Syrex; Wound Wash Saline™ [OTC]

Index Terms NaCl; Normal Saline; Salt

Pharmacologic Category Electrolyte Supplement, Parenteral; Genitourinary Irrigant; Irrigant; Lubricant, Ocular; Sodium Salt

Use

Parenteral: Restores sodium ion in patients with restricted oral intake (especially hyponatremia states or low salt syndrome). In general, parenteral saline uses:

Bacteriostatic sodium chloride: Dilution or dissolving drugs for I.M., I.V., or SubQ injections

Concentrated sodium chloride: Additive for parenteral fluid therapy

Hypertonic sodium chloride: For severe hyponatremia and hypochloremia

Hypotonic sodium chloride: Hydrating solution

Normal saline: Restores water/sodium losses

Pharmaceutical aid/diluent for infusion of compatible drug additives

Ophthalmic: Reduces corneal edema

Inhalation: Restores moisture to pulmonary system; loosens and thins congestion caused by colds or allergies; diluent for bronchodilator solutions that require dilution before inhalation

Intranasal: Restores moisture to nasal membranes

Irrigation: Wound cleansing, irrigation, and flushing

Unlabeled/Investigational Use Traumatic brain injury (hypertonic sodium chloride)

Pregnancy Risk Factor C

Medication Safety Issues

Per JCAHO recommendations, concentrated electrolyte solutions (eg, NaCl >0.9%) should not be available in patient care areas.

High alert medication: The Institute for Safe Medication Practices (ISMP) includes this medication (I.V. formulation >0.9% concentration) among its list of drugs which have a heightened risk of causing significant patient harm when used in error.

Contraindications Hypersensitivity to sodium chloride or any component of the formulation; hypertonic uterus, hypernatremia, fluid retention

Warnings/Precautions Use with caution in patients with HF, renal insufficiency, liver cirrhosis, hypertension, edema; sodium toxicity is almost exclusively related to how fast a sodium deficit is corrected; both rate and magnitude are extremely important; do not use bacteriostatic sodium chloride in newborns since benzyl alcohol preservatives have been associated with toxicity. Wound Wash Saline™ is for single-patient use only.

Irrigants: For external use only; not for parenteral use. Do not use during electrosurgical procedures. Irrigating fluids may be absorbed into systemic circulation; monitor for fluid or solute overload.

Adverse Reactions Frequency not defined.

Cardiovascular: Congestive conditions

Endocrine & metabolic: Extravasation, hypervolemia, hypernatremia, dilution of serum electrolytes, overhydration, hypokalemia

Local: Thrombosis, phlebitis, extravasation

Respiratory: Pulmonary edema

Drug Interactions

Avoid Concomitant Use There are no known interactions where it is recommended to avoid concomitant use.

Increased Effect/Toxicity There are no known significant interactions involving an increase in effect.

Decreased Effect

Sodium Chloride may decrease the levels/effects of: Lithium

Stability Store injection at room temperature; do not freeze. Protect from heat. Use only clear solutions.

Mechanism of Action Principal extracellular cation; functions in fluid and electrolyte balance, osmotic pressure control, and water distribution

Pharmacodynamics/Kinetics

Absorption: Oral, I.V.: Rapid

Distribution: Widely distributed

Excretion: Primarily urine; also sweat, tears, saliva

Dosage

Children: I.V.: Hypertonic solutions (>0.9%) should only be used for the initial treatment of acute serious symptomatic hyponatremia; maintenance: 3-4 mEq/kg/day; maximum: 100-150 mEq/day; dosage varies widely depending on clinical condition

Replacement: Determined by laboratory determinations mEq

Sodium deficiency (mEq/kg) = [% dehydration (L/kg)/ 100 x 70 (mEq/L)] + [0.6 (L/kg) x (140 - serum sodium) (mEq/L)]

Children ≥2 years and Adults:

Intranasal: 2-3 sprays in each nostril as needed

Irrigation: Spray affected area

Children and Adults: Inhalation: Bronchodilator diluent: 1-3 sprays (1-3 mL) to dilute bronchodilator solution in nebulizer prior to administration

Adults:

GU irrigant: 1-3 L/day by intermittent irrigation

Replacement I.V.: Determined by laboratory determinations mEq

Sodium deficiency (mEq/kg) = [% dehydration (L/kg)/100 x 70 (mEq/L)] + [0.6 (L/kg) x (140 - serum sodium) (mEq/L)]

To correct acute, serious hyponatremia: mEq sodium = [desired sodium (mEq/L) - actual sodium (mEq/L)] x [0.6 x wt (kg)]; for acute correction use 125 mEq/L as the desired serum sodium; acutely correct serum sodium in 5 mEq/L/dose increments; more gradual correction in increments of 10 mEq/L/day is indicated in the asymptomatic patient

Chloride maintenance electrolyte requirement in parenteral nutrition: 2-4 mEq/kg/24 hours or 25-40 mEq/1000 kcals/24 hours; maximum: 100-150 mEq/24 hours

Sodium maintenance electrolyte requirement in parenteral nutrition: 3-4 mEq/kg/24 hours or 25-40 mEq/1000 kcals/24 hours; maximum: 100-150 mEq/24 hours.

Approximate Deficits of Water and Electrolytes in Moderately Severe Dehydration[1]

Condition	Water (mL/kg)	Sodium (mEq/kg)
Fasting and thirsting	100-120	5-7
Diarrhea		
isonatremic	100-120	8-10
hypernatremic	100-120	2-4
hyponatremic	100-120	10-12
Pyloric stenosis	100-120	8-10
Diabetic acidosis	100-120	9-10

[1]A **negative** deficit indicates total body **excess** prior to treatment.

Adapted from Behrman RE, Kleigman RM, Nelson WE, et al, eds, *Nelson Textbook of Pediatrics*, 14th ed, WB Saunders Co, 1992.

Ophthalmic:

Ointment: Apply once daily or more often

Solution: Instill 1-2 drops into affected eye(s) every 3-4 hours

Administration Irrigation solution: Do not warm >66°C (150°F); not for I.V. use. Wound Wash Saline™: Before use, expel a short stream into air to clear nozzle.

Monitoring Parameters Serum sodium, potassium, chloride, and bicarbonate levels; I & O, weight

Reference Range Serum/plasma sodium levels:

Neonates:

Full-term: 133-142 mEq/L

Premature: 132-140 mEq/L

Children ≥2 months to Adults: 135-145 mEq/L

Dosage Forms Excipient information presented when available (limited, particularly for generics); consult specific product labeling. [DSC] = Discontinued product

Aerosol, intranasal [spray; preservative free]:

Entsol®: 3% (100 mL) [chlorofluorocarbon free]

Gel, intranasal:

Ayr® Saline: <0.5% (14 g) [contains soybean oil and aloe]

Entsol®: 3% (20 g) [contains benzalkonium chloride; with aloe and vitamin E]

Simply Saline® Nasal Moist®: 0.65% (30 g) [contains aloe]

Gel, intranasal [spray]:

Ayr® Saline No-Drip: <0.5% (22 mL) [contains benzalkonium chloride, benzyl alcohol, and soybean oil]

Injection, solution: 0.45% (25 mL, 50 mL, 100 mL, 250 mL, 500 mL, 1000 mL); 0.9% (25 mL, 50 mL, 100 mL, 150 mL, 250 mL, 500 mL, 1000 mL, 1 g); 3% (500 mL); 5% (500 mL)

Injection, solution [preservative free]: 0.9% (2 mL, 3 mL, 5 mL, 10 mL, 20 mL, 50 mL, 100 mL)

Injection, solution [I.V. flush]: 0.9% (10 mL)

Injection, solution [I.V. flush; preservative free]: 0.9% (1 mL, 2 mL, 2.5 mL, 3 mL, 5 mL, 10 mL)

Syrex: 0.9% (2.5 mL, 3 mL, 5 mL, 10 mL)

Injection, solution [bacteriostatic]: 0.9% (10 mL, 20 mL, 30 mL)

Injection, solution [concentrate]: 14.6% (40 mL); 23.4% (100 mL, 250 mL)

Injection, solution [concentrate; preservative free]: 14.6% (20 mL, 40 mL); 23.4% (30 mL, 100 mL, 200 mL)

Ointment, ophthalmic: 5% (3.5 g)

Altachlore: 5% (3.5 g)

Ointment, ophthalmic [preservative free]:

Muro 128®: 5% (3.5 g)

Powder for solution, intranasal [preservative free]:

Entsol®: 3% (10.5 g)

Solution for blood processing [not for injection]: 0.9% (3000 mL)

Solution for inhalation [preservative free]: 0.9% (3 mL, 5 mL, 15 mL); 3% (15 mL)

Solution for inhalation [hypertonic; preservative free]: 10% (15 mL)

Solution for inhalation [hypotonic; preservative free]: 0.45% (5 mL)

Solution for injection [I.V. flush; preservative free]: 0.9% (2.5 mL, 5 mL, 10 mL)

Solution for irrigation: 0.45% (2000 mL); 0.9% (250 mL, 500 mL, 1000 mL, 1500 mL, 2000 mL, 3000 mL, 4000 mL, 5000 mL)

Solution for irrigation [preservative free]: 0.45% (1500 mL [DSC]; 2000 mL); 0.9% (250 mL, 500 mL, 1000 mL, 1500 mL, 2000 mL, 3000 mL)

Solution for irrigation [slush solution]: 0.9% (1000 mL)

Solution for nebulization [preservative free]:

Hyper-Sal™: 7% (4 mL)

Solution, intranasal [preservative free]:

Simply Saline®: 3% (44 mL)

Solution, intranasal [drops]:

Ayr® Saline: 0.65% (50 mL) [alcohol free; contains benzalkonium chloride]

NāSal™: 0.65% (15 mL) [alcohol free; contains benzalkonium chloride]

SalineX®: 0.4% (15 mL) [contains benzalkonium chloride] [DSC]

Solution, intranasal [drops, mist, spray]

Humist®: 0.65% (45 mL) [ethanol free]

Humist® for Kids: 0.65% (30 mL) [ethanol free; bubblegum flavor]

Ocean®: 0.65% (45 mL, 473 mL) [gluten free; contains benzalkonium chloride and benzyl alcohol]

Ocean® for Kids: 0.65% (37.5 mL) [alcohol free; contains benzalkonium chloride]

Solution, intranasal [drops, spray]:
Ayr® Baby Saline: 0.65% (30 mL) [ethanol free; contains benzalkonium chloride]
Little Noses® Saline: 0.65% (30 mL) [contains benzalkonium chloride]
Little Noses® Stuffy Nose Kit: 0.65% (15 mL) [contains benzalkonium chloride]
Solution, intranasal [drops, spray, stream]:
Saline Mist: 0.65% (45 mL) [contains benzalkonium chloride] [DSC]
Solution, intranasal [irrigation]:
Pretz®: 0.75% (237 mL, 960 mL) [contains benzalkonium chloride and sodium benzoate; with yerba santa]
Solution, intranasal [mist]:
Ayr® Allergy Sinus: 2.65% (50 mL)
Ayr® Saline: 0.65% (50 mL) [ethanol free; contains benzalkonium chloride]
Entsol®: 3% (30 mL) [contains benzalkonium chloride]
Mycinaire™: 0.65% (30 mL) [contains benzalkonium chloride] [DSC]
Saline Mist: 0.65% (45 mL) [contains benzalkonium chloride]
SalineX®: 0.4% (50 mL) [contains benzalkonium chloride] [DSC]
4-Way® Moisturizing Mist: 0.74% (29.6 mL) [ethanol free; contains benzalkonium chloride and menthol]
Solution, intranasal [mist, preservative free]:
Simply Saline®: 0.9% (44 mL, 90 mL)
Simply Saline® Baby: 0.9% (45 mL)
Solution, intranasal [nasal wash; preservative free]:
Entsol®: 3% (240 mL)
Solution, intranasal [spray]:
Altamist: 0.65% (60 mL) [contains benzalkonium chloride]
Breathe Free®: 0.65% (44.3 mL) [contains benzalkonium chloride]
Deep Sea: 0.65% (45 mL) [contains benzalkonium chloride and benzyl alcohol]
Na-Zone®: 0.65% (60 mL) [contains benzalkonium chloride]
Nasal Moist® Saline: 0.65% (45 mL)
Nasal Spray: 0.65% (45 mL) [contains benzalkonium chloride and benzyl alcohol]
NāSal™: 0.65% (30 mL) [ethanol free; contains benzalkonium chloride and thimerosal]
Solution, intranasal [spray, isotonic, buffered]:
Pretz®: 0.75% (50 mL) [contains benzalkonium chloride and sodium benzoate; with yerba santa]
Solution, ophthalmic: 5% (15 mL)
Solution, ophthalmic [drops]: 5% (15 mL)
Altachlore: 5% (15 mL, 30 mL)
Muro 128®: 2% (15 mL); 5% (15 mL, 30 mL)
Solution, topical [preservative free]:
Wound Wash Saline™: 0.9% (90 mL, 210 mL)
Swab, intranasal:
Ayr® Saline: <0.5% (20) [contains aloe and soybean oil]
Tablet for solution, topical: 1000 mg

Sodium Chondroitin Sulfate and Sodium Hyaluronate

(SOW de um kon DROY tin SUL fate & SOW de um hye al yoor ON ate)

U.S. Brand Names DisCoVisc®; Viscoat®

Index Terms Chondroitin Sulfate and Sodium Hyaluronate; Sodium Hyaluronate and Chondroitin Sulfate

Pharmacologic Category Ophthalmic Agent, Viscoelastic

Use Ophthalmic surgical aid in the anterior segment during cataract extraction and intraocular lens implantation

Pregnancy Risk Factor C

Dosage Ophthalmic: Adults: Carefully introduce (using a 27-gauge cannula) into anterior chamber during surgery

Additional Information Complete prescribing information for this medication should be consulted for additional detail.

Dosage Forms Excipient information presented when available (limited, particularly for generics); consult specific product labeling.

Injection, solution, intraocular:
DisCoVisc®: Sodium chondroitin sulfate ≤4% and sodium hyaluronate ≤1.7% (0.5 mL, 1 mL) [provided in a kit which also contains 27-gauge cannula and cannula locking ring]
Viscoat®: Sodium chondroitin sulfate ≤4% and sodium hyaluronate ≤3% (0.5 mL, 0.75 mL) [packaging contains latex; packaged with 27-gauge cannula and cannula locking ring]

Sodium Citrate and Citric Acid

(SOW dee um SIT rate & SI trik AS id)

U.S. Brand Names Bicitra®; Cytra-2; Oracit®; Shohl's Solution (Modified)

Canadian Brand Names PMS-Dicitrate

Index Terms Modified Shohl's Solution

Pharmacologic Category Alkalinizing Agent, Oral

Use Treatment of metabolic acidosis; alkalinizing agent in conditions where long-term maintenance of an alkaline urine is desirable

Pregnancy Risk Factor Not established

Dosage Oral: Systemic alkalization:
Infants and Children: 2-3 mEq/kg/day in divided doses 3-4 times/day **or** 5-15 mL with water after meals and at bedtime
Adults: 10-30 mL with water after meals and at bedtime

Additional Information Complete prescribing information for this medication should be consulted for additional detail.

Dosage Forms Excipient information presented when available (limited, particularly for generics); consult specific product labeling. **Note:** Contains sodium 1 mEq/mL and is equivalent to bicarbonate 1 mEq/mL

Solution, oral: Sodium citrate 500 mg and citric acid 334 mg per 5 mL (480 mL)
Bicitra®: Sodium citrate 500 mg and citric acid 334 mg per 5 mL (480 mL) [sugar free; grape flavor]
Cytra-2: Sodium citrate 500 mg and citric acid 334 mg per 5 mL (480 mL) [alcohol free, dye free, sugar free; contains propylene glycol and sodium benzoate; grape flavor]
Oracit®: Sodium citrate 490 mg and citric acid 640 mg per 5 mL (15 mL, 30 mL, 500 mL, 3840 mL)
Shohl's Solution (Modified): Sodium citrate 500 mg and citric acid 300 mg per 5 mL (480 mL) [contains alcohol]

- ◆ **Sodium Citrate, Citric Acid, and Potassium Citrate** *see* Citric Acid, Sodium Citrate, and Potassium Citrate *on page* 339
- ◆ **Sodium Diuril®** *see* Chlorothiazide *on page* 308
- ◆ **Sodium Edecrin®** *see* Ethacrynic Acid *on page* 573
- ◆ **Sodium Edetate** *see* Edetate Disodium *on page* 505
- ◆ **Sodium Etidronate** *see* Etidronate Disodium *on page* 586
- ◆ **Sodium Ferric Gluconate** *see* Ferric Gluconate *on page* 615
- ◆ **Sodium Fluorescein** *see* Fluorescein *on page* 634
- ◆ **Sodium Fluoride** *see* Fluoride *on page* 635
- ◆ **Sodium Hyaluronate** *see* Hyaluronate and Derivatives *on page* 734
- ◆ **Sodium Hyaluronate and Chondroitin Sulfate** *see* Sodium Chondroitin Sulfate and Sodium Hyaluronate *on page* 1383

◆ **Sodium Hydrogen Carbonate** *see* Sodium Bicarbonate *on page 1380*

Sodium Hypochlorite Solution
(SOW dee um hye poe KLOR ite soe LOO shun)

U.S. Brand Names Dakin's Solution; Di-Dak-Sol

Index Terms Modified Dakin's Solution

Pharmacologic Category Disinfectant, Antibacterial (Topical)

Use Treatment of athlete's foot (0.5%); wound irrigation (0.5%); disinfection of utensils and equipment (5%)

Pregnancy Risk Factor C

Dosage Topical irrigation

Additional Information Complete prescribing information for this medication should be consulted for additional detail.

Dosage Forms Excipient information presented when available (limited, particularly for generics); consult specific product labeling.

Solution, topical:

Dakin's: 0.125% (480 mL); 0.25% (480 mL); 0.5% (480 mL, 3840 mL)

Di-Dak-Sol: 0.0125% (480 mL)

◆ **Sodium Hyposulfate** *see* Sodium Thiosulfate *on page 1386*

◆ **Sodium Nafcillin** *see* Nafcillin *on page 1033*

◆ **Sodium Nitroferricyanide** *see* Nitroprusside *on page 1075*

◆ **Sodium Nitroprusside** *see* Nitroprusside *on page 1075*

Sodium Oxybate (SOW dee um ox i BATE)

U.S. Brand Names Xyrem®

Canadian Brand Names Xyrem®

Index Terms 4-Hydroxybutyrate; Gamma Hydroxybutyric Acid; GHB; Sodium 4-Hydroxybutyrate

Pharmacologic Category Central Nervous System Depressant

Use Treatment of cataplexy and daytime sleepiness in patients with narcolepsy

Restrictions C-I (illicit use); C-III (medical use)

Sodium oxybate oral solution will be available only to prescribers enrolled in the Xyrem® Patient Success Program® and dispensed to the patient through the designated centralized pharmacy (1-866-997-3688). Prior to dispensing the first prescription, prescribers will be sent educational materials to be reviewed with the patient and enrollment forms for the postmarketing surveillance program. Patients must be seen at least every 3 months; prescriptions can be written for a maximum of 3 months (the first prescription may only be written for a 1-month supply).

An FDA-approved medication guide must be distributed when dispensing an outpatient prescription (new or refill) where this medication is to be used without direct supervision of a healthcare provider. Medication guides are available at http://www.fda.gov/cder/Offices/ODS/medication_guides.htm.

Pregnancy Risk Factor B

Dosage Oral:

Children ≥16 years and Adults: Narcolepsy: Initial: 4.5 g/day, in 2 equal doses; first dose to be given at bedtime after the patient is in bed, and second dose to be given 2.5-4 hours later. Dose may be increased or adjusted in 2-week intervals; average dose: 6-9 g/day (maximum: 9 g/day)

Elderly: Safety and efficacy have not been studied in patients >65 years.

Dosage adjustment in renal impairment: Adjustment not necessary; consider sodium content

Dosage adjustment in hepatic impairment: Decrease starting dose to half and titrate doses carefully in patients with liver dysfunction. Elimination half-life significantly longer in patients with Child's class C liver dysfunction.

Additional Information Complete prescribing information for this medication should be consulted for additional detail.

Dosage Forms Excipient information presented when available (limited, particularly for generics); consult specific product labeling.

Solution, oral:

Xyrem®: 500 mg/mL (180 mL) [contains sodium 91 mg/mL; supplied in a kit containing bottle adapter, two dosing cups, and oral syringe (as measuring device)]

◆ **Sodium PAS** *see* Aminosalicylic Acid *on page 86*

Sodium Phenylacetate and Sodium Benzoate
(SOW dee um fen il AS e tate & SOW dee um BENZ oh ate)

U.S. Brand Names Ammonul®

Index Terms NAPA and NABZ; Sodium Benzoate and Sodium Phenylacetate

Pharmacologic Category Antidote; Urea Cycle Disorder (UCD) Treatment Agent

Use Adjunct to treatment of acute hyperammonemia and encephalopathy in patients with urea cycle disorders involving partial or complete deficiencies of carbamyl-phosphate synthetase (CPS), ornithine transcarbamoylase (OTC), argininosuccinate lysase (ASL), or argininosuccinate synthetase (ASS); for use with hemodialysis in acute neonatal hyperammonemic coma, moderate-to-severe hyperammonemic encephalopathy and hyperammonemia which fails to respond to initial therapy

Pregnancy Risk Factor C

Dosage Administer as a loading dose over 90-120 minutes, followed by an equivalent maintenance infusion given over 24 hours. Dosage based on weight and specific enzyme deficiency; therapy should continue until ammonia levels are in normal range. Repeat loading doses are not recommended due to the prolonged plasma levels.

Children ≤20 kg:

CPS and OTC deficiency: Ammonul® 2.5 mL/kg and arginine 10% 2 mL/kg (provides sodium phenylacetate 250 mg/kg, sodium benzoate 250 mg/kg, and arginine hydrochloride 200 mg/kg).

ASS and ASL deficiency: Ammonul® 2.5 mL/kg and arginine 10% 6 mL/kg (provides sodium phenylacetate 250 mg/kg, sodium benzoate 250 mg/kg, and arginine hydrochloride 600 mg/kg)

Note: Pending a specific diagnosis in infants, the bolus and maintenance dose of arginine should be 6 mL/kg. If ASS or ASL are excluded as diagnostic possibilities, reduce dose of arginine to 2 mL/kg/day.

Children >20 kg and Adults:

CPS and OTC deficiency: Ammonul® 55 mL/m^2 and arginine 10% 2 mL/kg (provides sodium phenylacetate 5.5 g/m^2, sodium benzoate 5.5 g/m^2, and arginine hydrochloride 200 mg/kg)

ASS and ASL deficiency: Ammonul® 55 mL/m^2 and arginine 10% 6 mL/kg (provides sodium phenylacetate 5.5 g/m^2, sodium benzoate 5.5 g/m^2, and arginine hydrochloride 600 mg/kg)

Dosage adjustment in renal impairment: Use with caution; monitor closely

Dialysis: Ammonia clearance is ~10 times greater with hemodialysis than by peritoneal dialysis or hemofiltration. Exchange transfusion is ineffective.

Dosage adjustment in hepatic impairment: Use with caution

Additional Information Complete prescribing information for this medication should be consulted for additional detail.

Dosage Forms Excipient information presented when available (limited, particularly for generics); consult specific product labeling.

Injection, solution [concentrate]:

Ammonul®: Sodium phenylacetate 100 mg and sodium benzoate 100 mg per 1 mL (50 mL)

Sodium Phenylbutyrate

(SOW dee um fen il BYOO ti rate)

U.S. Brand Names Buphenyl®

Index Terms Ammonapse

Pharmacologic Category Urea Cycle Disorder (UCD) Treatment Agent

Use Adjunctive therapy in the chronic management of patients with urea cycle disorder involving deficiencies of carbamoylphosphate synthetase, ornithine transcarbamylase, or argininosuccinic acid synthetase

Pregnancy Risk Factor C

Dosage Oral: Management of urea cycle disorders:

Children <20 kg: Powder: 450-600 mg/kg/day, administered in equally divided amounts with each meal or feeding, 3-6 times daily (maximum dose: 20 g/day)

Children ≥20 kg and Adults: Powder or tablet: 9.9-13 g/m^2/day, administered in equally divided amounts with each meal or feeding, 3-6 times daily (maximum dose: 20 g/day)

Additional Information Complete prescribing information for this medication should be consulted for additional detail.

Dosage Forms Excipient information presented when available (limited, particularly for generics); consult specific product labeling.

Powder, for oral solution:

Buphenyl®: 3 g/level teaspoon (250 g) [contains sodium 125 mg/g; packaged with measuring devices]

Tablet:

Buphenyl®: 500 mg [contains sodium 124 mg/g]

◆ **Sodium Phosphate and Potassium Phosphate** *see* Potassium Phosphate and Sodium Phosphate *on page 1222*

Sodium Polystyrene Sulfonate

(SOW dee um pol ee STYE reen SUL fon ate)

U.S. Brand Names Kayexalate®; Kionex®; SPS®

Canadian Brand Names Kayexalate®; PMS-Sodium Polystyrene Sulfonate

Pharmacologic Category Antidote

Use Treatment of hyperkalemia

Pregnancy Risk Factor C

Lactation Excretion in breast milk unknown/use caution

Medication Safety Issues

Sound-alike/look-alike issues:

Kayexalate® may be confused with Kaopectate®

Always prescribe either one-time doses or as a specific number of doses (eg, 15 g q6h x 2 doses). Scheduled doses with no dosage limit could be given for days leading to dangerous hypokalemia.

International issues:

Kionex™ may be confused with Kinex® which is a brand name for biperiden in Mexico

Contraindications Hypersensitivity to sodium polystyrene sulfonate or any component of the formulation; hypernatremia, hypokalemia, obstructive bowel disease

Warnings/Precautions Use with caution in patients with severe HF, hypertension, edema, or renal failure; avoid using the commercially available liquid product in neonates due to the preservative content; large oral doses may cause fecal impaction (especially in elderly); enema will reduce the serum potassium faster than oral administration, but the oral route will result in a greater reduction over several hours.

Adverse Reactions Frequency not defined.

Endocrine & metabolic: Hypernatremia, hypokalemia, hypocalcemia, hypomagnesemia

Gastrointestinal: Anorexia, colonic necrosis (rare), constipation, fecal impaction, intestinal obstruction (due to concretions in association with aluminum hydroxide), nausea, vomiting

Drug Interactions

Avoid Concomitant Use There are no known interactions where it is recommended to avoid concomitant use.

Increased Effect/Toxicity

Sodium Polystyrene Sulfonate may increase the levels/effects of: Antacids

Decreased Effect There are no known significant interactions involving a decrease in effect.

Stability Store prepared suspensions at 15°C to 30°C (59°F to 86°F). Store repackaged product in refrigerator and use within 14 days. Freshly prepared suspensions should be used within 24 hours. Do not heat resin suspension.

Mechanism of Action Removes potassium by exchanging sodium ions for potassium ions in the intestine before the resin is passed from the body

Pharmacodynamics/Kinetics

Onset of action: 2-24 hours

Absorption: None

Excretion: Completely feces (primarily as potassium polystyrene sulfonate)

Dosage

Children:

Oral: 1 g/kg/dose every 6 hours

Rectal: 1 g/kg/dose every 2-6 hours (In small children and infants, employ lower doses by using the practical exchange ratio of 1 mEq K^+/g of resin as the basis for calculation)

Adults: Hyperkalemia:

Oral: 15 g 1-4 times/day

Rectal: 30-50 g every 6 hours

Dietary Considerations Do **not** mix in orange juice. Powder for suspension contains sodium 100 mg/g (4.1 mEq/g). SPS® suspension contains sodium 1500 mg/60 mL (65 mEq/60 mL).

Administration

Oral: Administer orally (or NG) as a suspension using the commercially available suspension or the powder for suspension. **Do not mix in orange juice.** Chilling the oral mixture will increase palatability. Shake suspension well prior to administration.

Powder for suspension: For each 1 g of the powdered resin, add 3–4 mL of water or syrup (amount of fluid usually ranges from 20–100 mL)

Rectal: Enema route is less effective than oral administration. Administer cleansing enema first. Retain enema in colon for at least 30-60 minutes and for several hours, if possible. Enema should be followed by irrigation with normal saline to prevent necrosis.

Monitoring Parameters Exchange capacity is 1 mEq/g *in vivo*, and *in vitro* capacity is 3.1 mEq/g, therefore, a wide range of exchange capacity exists such that close monitoring of serum electrolytes (potassium, sodium, calcium, magnesium) is necessary; ECG

Reference Range Serum potassium: Adults: 3.5-5.2 mEq/L

Additional Information 1 g of resin binds approximately 1 mEq of potassium

Dosage Forms Excipient information presented when available (limited, particularly for generics); consult specific product labeling.

Powder for suspension, oral/rectal:

Kayexalate®: 15 g/4 level teaspoons (480 g) [contains sodium 100 mg (4.1 mEq)/g]

Kionex®: 15 g/4 level teaspoons (454 g) [contains sodium 100 mg (4.1 mEq)/g]

Suspension, oral/rectal: 15 g/60 mL (60 mL, 120 mL, 200 mL, 500 mL)

SPS®: 15 g/60 mL (60 mL, 120 mL, 480 mL) [contains alcohol 0.3%, sodium 1500 mg (65 mEq)/60 mL, propylene glycol, and sorbitol; cherry flavor]

◆ **Sodium Sulfacetamide** *see* Sulfacetamide *on page 1405*

◆ **Sodium Sulfacetamide and Sulfur** *see* Sulfur and Sulfacetamide *on page 1411*

Sodium Tetradecyl (SOW dee um tetra DEK il)

U.S. Brand Names Sotradecol®

Canadian Brand Names Trombovar®

Index Terms Sodium Tetradecyl Sulfate

Pharmacologic Category Sclerosing Agent

Use Treatment of small, uncomplicated varicose veins of the lower extremities

Pregnancy Risk Factor C

Dosage I.V.: Test dose: 0.5 mL given several hours prior to administration of larger dose; 0.5-2 mL (preferred maximum: 1 mL) in each vein, maximum: 10 mL per treatment session; 3% solution reserved for large varices

Additional Information Complete prescribing information for this medication should be consulted for additional detail.

Dosage Forms Excipient information presented when available (limited, particularly for generics); consult specific product labeling.

Injection, as sulfate:

Sotradecol®: 1% (2 mL) [contains benzyl alcohol]; 3% (2 mL) [contains benzyl alcohol]

◆ **Sodium Tetradecyl Sulfate** *see* Sodium Tetradecyl *on page 1386*

Sodium Thiosulfate (SOW dee um thye oh SUL fate)

U.S. Brand Names Versiclear™

Index Terms Disodium Thiosulfate Pentahydrate; Pentahydrate; Sodium Hyposulfate; Sodium Thiosulphate; Thiosulfuric Acid Disodium Salt

Pharmacologic Category Antidote

Use

Parenteral: Used alone or with sodium nitrite or amyl nitrite in cyanide poisoning; reduce the risk of nephrotoxicity associated with cisplatin therapy; treatment of cyanide poisoning due to nitroprusside

Topical: Treatment of tinea versicolor

Unlabeled/Investigational Use Management of I.V. extravasation

Pregnancy Risk Factor C

Pregnancy Considerations Safety has not been established in pregnant women. Use only when potential benefit to the mother outweighs the possible risk to the fetus.

Contraindications Hypersensitivity to sodium thiosulfate or any component of the formulation

Warnings/Precautions Safety in pregnancy has not been established; discontinue topical use if irritation or sensitivity occurs; rapid I.V. infusion has caused transient hypotension and ECG changes in dogs; can increase risk of thiocyanate intoxication; use caution with renal impairment. Fire victims may present with both cyanide and carbon monoxide poisoning. Collection of pretreatment blood cyanide concentrations does not preclude administration and should not delay administration in the emergency management of highly suspected or confirmed cyanide toxicity. Patients receiving treatment for acute cyanide toxicity must be monitored for return of symptoms for 24-48 hours.

Adverse Reactions Frequency not defined

Cardiovascular: Hypotension (infusion rate-dependent)

Dermatologic: Contact dermatitis, local irritation

Gastrointestinal: Nausea, vomiting

Miscellaneous: Hypersensitivity reactions

Drug Interactions

Avoid Concomitant Use There are no known interactions where it is recommended to avoid concomitant use.

Increased Effect/Toxicity There are no known significant interactions involving an increase in effect.

Decreased Effect There are no known significant interactions involving a decrease in effect.

Mechanism of Action

Cyanide toxicity: Accelerates the clearance of cyanide via the rhodanase-catalyzed detoxification of cyanide to thiocyanate (much less toxic than cyanide). The accelerated action of rhodanase is a result of the exogenous sulfur provided by sodium thiosulfate.

Cisplatin toxicity: Complexes with cisplatin to form a compound that is nontoxic to either normal or cancerous cells

Pharmacodynamics/Kinetics

Absorption: Oral: Poor

Distribution: Extracellular fluid

Half-life elimination: 0.65 hour

Excretion: Urine (28.5% as unchanged drug)

Dosage

Cyanide poisoning: I.V.: **Note:** Death from cyanide poisoning may occur rapidly, do not delay antidote administration in the event of highly suspected or confirmed cyanide poisoning; usually given in conjunction with amyl nitrite and sodium nitrite

Children: 7 g/m^2 (maximum dose: 12.5 g) given over 10 minutes; may repeat at 1/2 the original dose if symptoms return

Adults: 12.5 g given over 10 minutes; may repeat at 1/2 the original dose if symptoms return

Cisplatin rescue should be given before or during cisplatin administration: I.V. infusion (in sterile water): 12 g/m^2 over 6 hours or 9 g/m^2 I.V. push followed by 1.2 g/m^2 continuous infusion for 6 hours

Tinea versicolor: Children and Adults: Topical: 20% to 25% solution: Apply a thin layer to affected areas twice daily

Drug extravasation (unlabeled use): Children and Adults: SubQ: 1/6 M (~4%) solution: Inject into the affected area; various volumes have also been suggested for direct injection into existing I.V. line; however, the optimal volume and efficacy of such practices have not been thoroughly evaluated. **Note:** Use only for large cisplatin infiltrates (>20 mL) and cisplatin concentrations >0.5 mg/mL.

Administration

I.V.: Inject slowly, over at least 10 minutes; rapid administration may cause hypotension.

Topical: Do not apply to or near eyes.

Monitoring Parameters Monitor for signs of thiocyanate toxicity; monitor for hypotension and hypersensitivity reactions

Dosage Forms Excipient information presented when available (limited, particularly for generics); consult specific product labeling.

Injection, solution [preservative free]: 100 mg/mL (10 mL); 250 mg/mL (50 mL)

Lotion: Sodium thiosulfate 25% and salicylic acid 1% (120 mL) [contains isopropyl alcohol 10%]

- ◆ **Sodium Thiosulphate** *see* Sodium Thiosulfate *on page 1386*
- ◆ **Soflax™ (Can)** *see* Docusate *on page 473*
- ◆ **Sojourn™** *see* Sevoflurane *on page 1366*
- ◆ **Solage** *see* Mequinol and Tretinoin *on page 946*
- ◆ **Solagé®** *see* Mequinol and Tretinoin *on page 946*
- ◆ **Solaquin® [OTC]** *see* Hydroquinone *on page 749*
- ◆ **Solaquin® (Can)** *see* Hydroquinone *on page 749*
- ◆ **Solaquin Forte®** *see* Hydroquinone *on page 749*
- ◆ **Solaraze®** *see* Diclofenac *on page 437*
- ◆ **Solarcaine® Aloe Extra Burn Relief [OTC]** *see* Lidocaine *on page 884*
- ◆ **Solia™** *see* Ethinyl Estradiol and Desogestrel *on page 575*

Solifenacin (sol i FEN a sin)

U.S. Brand Names VESIcare®

Index Terms Solifenacin Succinate; YM905

Pharmacologic Category Anticholinergic Agent

Use Treatment of overactive bladder with symptoms of urinary frequency, urgency, or urge incontinence

Pregnancy Risk Factor C

Pregnancy Considerations Decreased fetal weight, increased incidence of cleft palate, and delayed physical development were observed in some animal studies. There are no adequate or well-controlled studies in pregnant women. Use during pregnancy only if the benefit to the mother outweighs the potential risk to the fetus.

Lactation Excretion in breast milk unknown/not recommended

Medication Safety Issues

Sound-alike/look-alike issues:

VESIcare® may be confused with Visicol®

Contraindications Hypersensitivity to solifenacin or any component of the formulation; urinary retention; gastric retention; uncontrolled narrow-angle glaucoma.

Warnings/Precautions May cause drowsiness and/or blurred vision, which may impair physical or mental abilities; patients must be cautioned about performing tasks which require mental alertness (eg, operating machinery or driving). Heat prostration may occur in the presence of increased environmental temperature; use caution in hot weather and/or exercise. Use with caution in patients with bladder outflow obstruction, gastrointestinal obstructive disorders, and decreased gastrointestinal motility. Use with caution in patients with a known history of QT prolongation or other risk factors for QT prolongation (eg, concomitant use of medications known to prolong QT interval and/or electrolyte abnormalities); the risk for QT prolongation is dose-related. Use with caution in patients with controlled (treated) narrow-angle glaucoma; use is contraindicated with uncontrolled narrow-angle glaucoma. Dosage adjustment is required for patients with severe renal impairment (Cl_{cr} <30 mL/minute) or moderate (Child-Pugh class B) hepatic impairment; use is not recommended with severe hepatic impairment (Child-Pugh class C). Patients on potent CYP3A4 inhibitors require the lower dose of solifenacin. Safety and efficacy in pediatric patients have not been established.

Adverse Reactions

>10%: Gastrointestinal: Xerostomia (11% to 28%; dose-related), constipation (5% to 13%; dose-related)

1% to 10%:

Cardiovascular: Edema (≤1%), hypertension (≤1%)

Central nervous system: Headache (3% to 6%), fatigue (1% to 2%), depression (≤1%)

Gastrointestinal: Dyspepsia (1% to 4%), nausea (2% to 3%), upper abdominal pain (1% to 2%)

Genitourinary: Urinary tract infection (3% to 5%), urinary retention (≤1%)

Ocular: Blurred vision (4% to 5%), dry eyes (≤2%)

Respiratory: Cough (≤1%)

Miscellaneous: Influenza (≤2%)

<1% (Limited to important or life-threatening): Angioneurotic edema, confusion, fecal impaction, gastrointestinal obstruction, hallucination, hypersensitivity, pruritus, QT_c prolongation, rash, torsade de pointes, urticaria

Drug Interactions

Metabolism/Transport Effects **Substrate** of CYP3A4 (major)

Avoid Concomitant Use There are no known interactions where it is recommended to avoid concomitant use.

Increased Effect/Toxicity

Solifenacin may increase the levels/effects of: Anticholinergics; Cannabinoids; Potassium Chloride

The levels/effects of Solifenacin may be increased by: Antifungal Agents (Azole Derivatives, Systemic); CYP3A4 Inhibitors (Moderate); CYP3A4 Inhibitors (Strong); Dasatinib; Pramlintide

Decreased Effect

Solifenacin may decrease the levels/effects of: Acetylcholinesterase Inhibitors (Central); Secretin

The levels/effects of Solifenacin may be decreased by: Acetylcholinesterase Inhibitors (Central); CYP3A4 Inducers (Strong); Deferasirox; Herbs (CYP3A4 Inducers)

Ethanol/Nutrition/Herb Interactions

Food: Grapefruit juice may increase the serum level effects of solifenacin.

Herb/Nutraceutical: St John's wort (*Hypericum*) may decrease the levels/effects of solifenacin.

Stability Store at controlled room temperature of 25°C (77°F).

Mechanism of Action Inhibits muscarinic receptors resulting in decreased urinary bladder contraction, increased residual urine volume, and decreased detrusor muscle pressure.

Pharmacodynamics/Kinetics

Distribution: V_d: 600 L

Protein binding: ~98% bound primarily to alpha$_1$-acid glycoprotein

Metabolism: Extensively hepatic; via N-oxidation and 4 R-hydroxylation, forms one active and three inactive metabolites; primary pathway for elimination is via CYP3A4

Bioavailability: ~90%

Half-life elimination: 45-68 hours following chronic dosing

Time to peak, plasma: 3-8 hours

Excretion: Urine 69% (<15% as unchanged drug); feces 23%

Dosage Oral: Adults: 5 mg/day; if tolerated, may increase to 10 mg/day

Dosage adjustment with concomitant CYP3A4 inhibitors: Maximum solifenacin dose: 5 mg/day

Dosage adjustment in renal impairment: Use with caution in reduced renal function

Cl_{cr} <30 mL/minute: Maximum dose: 5 mg/day

Dosage adjustment in hepatic impairment: Use with caution in reduced hepatic function

Moderate (Child-Pugh class B): Maximum dose: 5 mg/day

Severe (Child-Pugh class C): Use is not recommended

Dietary Considerations May be taken with or without food.

Administration Swallow tablet whole; administer with liquids; may be taken without regard to food.

Monitoring Parameters Anticholinergic effects (eg, fixed and dilated pupils, blurred vision, tremors, or dry skin); creatinine clearance (prior to treatment for dosing adjustment); liver function

Dosage Forms Excipient information presented when available (limited, particularly for generics); consult specific product labeling.

Tablet, as succinate:

VESIcare®: 5 mg, 10 mg

- **Solifenacin Succinate** *see* Solifenacin *on page* *1387*
- **Soliris™** *see* Eculizumab *on page* *502*
- **Solodyn™** *see* Minocycline *on page* *999*
- **Soltamox™ [DSC]** *see* Tamoxifen *on page* *1424*
- **Soluble Fluorescein** *see* Fluorescein *on page* *634*
- **Solu-Cortef®** *see* Hydrocortisone *on page* *743*
- **Solu-Medrol®** *see* MethylPREDNISolone *on page* *976*
- **Soma®** *see* Carisoprodol *on page* *261*
- **Soma® Compound** *see* Carisoprodol and Aspirin *on page* *261*
- **Soma® Compound w/Codeine [DSC]** *see* Carisoprodol, Aspirin, and Codeine *on page* *262*
- **Somatrem** *see* Somatropin *on page* *1388*

Somatropin (soe ma TROE pin)

U.S. Brand Names Genotropin Miniquick®; Genotropin®; Humatrope®; Norditropin®; Norditropin® NordiFlex®; Nutropin AQ®; Nutropin®; Omnitrope™; Saizen®; Serostim®; Tev-Tropin®; Zorbtive®

Canadian Brand Names Humatrope®; Nutropine®; Nutropin® AQ; Saizen®; Serostim®

Index Terms hGH; Human Growth Hormone; Somatrem

Pharmacologic Category Growth Hormone

Use

Children:

Treatment of growth failure due to inadequate endogenous growth hormone secretion (Genotropin®, Humatrope®, Norditropin®, Nutropin®, Nutropin AQ®, Omnitrope™, Saizen®, Tev-Tropin®)

Treatment of short stature associated with Turner syndrome (Genotropin®, Humatrope®, Norditropin®, Nutropin®, Nutropin AQ®)

Treatment of Prader-Willi syndrome (Genotropin®)

Treatment of growth failure associated with chronic renal insufficiency (CRI) up until the time of renal transplantation (Nutropin®, Nutropin AQ®)

Treatment of growth failure in children born small for gestational age who fail to manifest catch-up growth by 2 years of age (Genotropin®) or by 2-4 years of age (Norditropin®)

Treatment of idiopathic short stature (nongrowth hormone-deficient short stature) defined by height standard deviation score (SDS) less than or equal to -2.25 and growth rate not likely to attain normal adult height (Genotropin®, Humatrope®, Nutropin®, Nutropin AQ®)

Treatment of short stature or growth failure associated with short stature homeobox gene (SHOX) deficiency (Humatrope®)

Treatment of short stature associated with Noonan syndrome (Norditropin®)

Adults:

HIV patients with wasting or cachexia with concomitant antiviral therapy (Serostim®)

Replacement of endogenous growth hormone in patients with adult growth hormone deficiency who meet both of the following criteria (Genotropin®, Humatrope®, Norditropin®, Nutropin®, Nutropin AQ®, Omnitrope™, Saizen®):

Biochemical diagnosis of adult growth hormone deficiency by means of a subnormal response to a standard growth hormone stimulation test (peak growth hormone ≤5 mcg/L). Confirmatory testing may not be required in patients with congenital/genetic growth hormone deficiency or multiple pituitary hormone deficiencies due to organic diseases.

and

Adult-onset: Patients who have adult growth hormone deficiency whether alone or with multiple hormone deficiencies (hypopituitarism) as a result of pituitary disease, hypothalamic disease, surgery, radiation therapy, or trauma

or

Childhood-onset: Patients who were growth hormone deficient during childhood, confirmed as an adult before replacement therapy is initiated

Treatment of short-bowel syndrome (Zorbtive®)

Unlabeled/Investigational Use Investigational: Congestive heart failure; pediatric HIV patients with wasting/cachexia (Serostim®); HIV-associated adipose redistribution syndrome (HARS) (Serostim®)

Pregnancy Risk Factor B/C (depending upon manufacturer)

Pregnancy Considerations Reproduction studies have not been conducted with all agents. Teratogenic effects were not observed in animal studies. During normal pregnancy, maternal production of endogenous growth hormone decreases as placental growth hormone production increases. Data with somatropin use during pregnancy is limited.

Lactation Excretion in breast milk unknown/use caution

Medication Safety Issues

Sound-alike/look-alike issues:

Somatrem may be confused with somatropin

Somatropin may be confused with somatrem, sumatriptan

International issues:

Genotropin® may be confused with Genatropine® which is a brand name for atropine in France

Contraindications Hypersensitivity to growth hormone or any component of the formulation; growth promotion in pediatric patients with closed epiphyses; progression of any underlying intracranial lesion or actively growing intracranial tumor; acute critical illness due to complications following open heart or abdominal surgery; multiple accidental trauma or acute respiratory failure; evidence of active malignancy; active proliferative or severe nonproliferative diabetic retinopathy; use in patients with Prader-Willi syndrome **without** growth hormone deficiency (except Genotropin®) or in patients with Prader-Willi syndrome **with** growth hormone deficiency who are severely obese or have severe respiratory impairment

Warnings/Precautions Initiation of somatropin is contraindicated with acute critical illness due to complications following open heart or abdominal surgery, multiple accidental trauma, or acute respiratory failure; mortality may be increased. The safety of continuing somatropin in patients who develop these illnesses during therapy has not been established; use with caution. Use in contraindicated with active malignancy; monitor patients with preexisting tumors or growth failure secondary to an intracranial lesion for recurrence or progression of underlying disease.

Somatropin may decrease insulin sensitivity; use with caution in patients with diabetes or with risk factors for impaired glucose tolerance. Untreated/undiagnosed hypothyroidism may decrease response to therapy. Intracranial hypertension (IH) with headache, nausea, papilledema, visual changes, and/or vomiting has been reported with growth hormone product, funduscopic examinations are recommended. Patients with Turner syndrome, chronic renal failure and Prader-Willi syndrome may be at increased risk for IH. Progression of scoliosis may occur in children experiencing rapid growth. Patients with growth hormone deficiency may develop slipped capital epiphyses more frequently, evaluate any child with new onset of a limp or with complaints of hip or knee pain. Patients with Turner syndrome are at increased risk for otitis media and other ear/hearing disorders, cardiovascular disorders (including stroke, aortic aneurysm, hypertension), and thyroid disease, monitor carefully. Concurrent glucocorticoid therapy may inhibit growth promotion effects; may require dosage adjustment or replacement glucocorticoid therapy in patients with ACTH deficiency. Fluid retention may occur frequently in adults during use; manifestations of fluid retention (eg, edema, arthralgia, myalgia, nerve compression syndromes/paresthesias) are generally transient and dose dependent. Products may contain benzyl alcohol or m-cresol. When administering to newborns, reconstitute with sterile water or saline for injection. Not for I.V. injection.

Fatalities have been reported in pediatric patients with Prader-Willi syndrome following the use of growth hormone. The reported fatalities occurred in patients with one or more risk factors, including severe obesity, sleep apnea, respiratory impairment, or unidentified respiratory infection; male patients with one or more of these factors may be at greater risk. Treatment interruption is recommended in patients who show signs of upper airway obstruction, including the onset of, or increased, snoring. In addition, evaluation of and/or monitoring for sleep apnea and respiratory infections are recommended.

Patients with HIV infection should be maintained on antiretroviral therapy to prevent the potential increase in viral replication.

Safety and efficacy have not been established for the treatment of Noonan syndrome in children with significant cardiac disease.

Adverse Reactions

Growth hormone deficiency: Adverse reactions reported with growth hormone deficiency vary greatly by age. Generally, percentages are less in pediatric patients than adults, and many of the reactions reported in adults are dose related. Percentages reported also vary by product. Below is a listing by age group; events reported more commonly overall are noted with an asterisk (*).

Children: Antibodies development, arthralgia, edema, eosinophilia, glycosuria, Hb A_{1c} increased, headache, hematoma, hematuria, hyperglycemia (mild), hypertriglyceridemia, hypoglycemia, hypothyroidism, injection site reaction, leg pain, lipoatrophy, muscle pain, psoriasis exacerbation, rash, seizure, weakness

Adults: Arthralgia*, back pain, bronchitis, carpal tunnel syndrome, chest pain, depression, diaphoresis, dizziness, edema*, fatigue, flu-like syndrome*, glucose intolerance, glucosuria, headache*, hyperglycemia (mild), hypertension, hypoesthesia, hypothyroidism, infection, insomnia, leg edema, muscle pain, myalgia*, nausea, pain in extremities, paresthesia*, peripheral edema*, rhinitis, skeletal pain*, stiffness in extremities, upper respiratory tract infection, weakness

Additional/postmarketing reactions observed with growth hormone deficiency: Gynecomastia, increased growth of pre-existing nevi, pancreatitis

HARS: Serostim®: Limited to >10%: Edema (peripheral) (19% to 45%), arthralgia (28% to 37%), pain (extremity) (5% to 19%), hypoesthesia (9% to 15%), headache (4% to 14%), blood glucose increased (4% to 14%), paresthesia (11% to 13%), myalgia (3% to 13%)

Idiopathic short stature: Percentages reported using Humatrope® versus placebo: Myalgia (24%), scoliosis (19%), otitis media (16%), arthralgia (11%), arthrosis (11 %), hyperlipidemia (8%), gynecomastia (5%), hip pain (3%), hypertension (3%). Additional adverse reactions listed as reported using other products from ISS NCGS Cohort (frequencies <1%): Aggressiveness, benign intracranial hypertension, diabetes, edema, hair loss, headache, injection site reaction

Prader-Willi syndrome: Genotropin® (frequency not defined): Aggressiveness, arthralgia, edema, hair loss, headache, benign intracranial hypertension, myalgia; fatalities associated with use in this population have been reported

Turner syndrome: Percentages reported using Humatrope® compared to untreated patients. Additional adverse reactions reported from other products, frequency not specified: Surgical procedures (45%), otitis media (43%), ear disorders (18%), hypothyroidism (14%), nevi increased (11%), peripheral edema (7%), joint pain, respiratory illness, urinary tract infection

HIV patients with wasting or cachexia: Serostim® (limited to ≥5%): Musculoskeletal disorders (arthralgia, arthrosis, myalgia: 78%), peripheral edema (26%), headache (13%), nausea (9%), paresthesia (8%), edema (6%), gynecomastia (6%), hypoesthesia (5%)

Short-bowel syndrome: Zorbtive® (limited to >10%): Peripheral edema (69% to 81%), facial edema (44% to 50%), arthralgia (31% to 44%), nausea (13% to 31%), injection site pain (up to 31%), flatulence (25%), injection site reaction (19% to 25%), abdominal pain (13% to 25%), vomiting (19%), pain (6% to 19%), chest pain (up to 19%), dehydration (up to 19%), infection (up to 19%), rhinitis (up to 19%), hearing symptoms (13%), dizziness (6% to 13%), rash (6% to 13%), diaphoresis (up to 13%), generalized edema (up to 13%), malaise (up to 13%), moniliasis (up to 13%), myalgia (up to 13%)

SHOX deficiency: Humatrope®: Arthralgia (11%), gynecomastia (8%), excessive cutaneous nevi (7%), scoliosis (4%)

Small for gestational age: Genotropin® (frequency not defined): Mild, transient hyperglycemia; benign intracranial hypertension (rare); central precocious puberty; jaw prominence (rare); aggravation of pre-existing scoliosis (rare); injection site reactions; progression of pigmented nevi

Drug Interactions

Avoid Concomitant Use There are no known interactions where it is recommended to avoid concomitant use.

Increased Effect/Toxicity There are no known significant interactions involving an increase in effect.

Decreased Effect

Somatropin may decrease the levels/effects of: Antidiabetic Agents; Cortisone; PredniSONE

The levels/effects of Somatropin may be decreased by: Estrogen Derivatives

Stability

Genotropin®: Store at 2°C to 8°C (36°F to 46°F); do not freeze. Protect from light. Reconstitute with diluent provided. Following reconstitution of 5.8 mg and 13.8 mg cartridge, store under refrigeration and use within 21 days.

Genotropin® Miniquick®: Store in refrigerator prior to dispensing, but may be stored ≤25°C (77°F) for up to 3 months after dispensing. Reconstitute with diluent provided. Consult the instructions provided with the reconstitution device. Once reconstituted, solution must be refrigerated and used within 24 hours. Discard unused portion.

Humatrope®:

Vial: Before and after reconstitution, store at 2°C to 8°C (36°F to 46°F); do not freeze. When reconstituted with provided diluent or bacteriostatic water for injection, use within 14 days. When reconstituted with sterile water for injection, use within 24 hours and discard unused portion. Reconstitute 5.5 mg vial with 1.5-5 mL diluent provided; swirl gently, do not shake.

Cartridge: Before and after reconstitution, store at 2°C to 8°C (36°F to 46°F); do not freeze. Consult HumatroPen™ User Guide for complete instructions for reconstitution. **Do not use diluent provided with vials.** Following reconstitution with provided diluent, stable for

28 days under refrigeration. Dilute with solution provided with cartridges **ONLY**; do not use diluent provided with vials.

Norditropin®: Store at 2°C to 8°C (36°F to 46°F); do not freeze. Avoid direct light.

Cartridge: When refrigerated, must be used within 4 weeks once inserted into pen. Orange cartridges (5 mg/1.5 mL) may also be stored up to 3 weeks at ≤25°C (77°F).

Prefilled pen: When refrigerated, must be used within 4 weeks once inserted into pen. Orange and blue cartridges may also be stored up to 3 weeks at ≤25°C (77°F).

Nutropin®: Before and after reconstitution, store at 2°C to 8°C (36°F to 46°F); do not freeze.

Vial: Reconstitute with bacteriostatic water for injection. Swirl gently, do not shake. Use reconstituted vials within 14 days. When reconstituted with sterile water for injection, use immediately and discard unused portion.

AQ formulation: Use within 28 days following initial use.

Omnitrope™:

Powder for injection: Prior to reconstitution, store under refrigeration at 2°C to 8°C (36°F to 46°F); do not freeze. Protect from light. Reconstitute with provided diluent. Swirl gently; do not shake. Following reconstitution with the provided diluents, the 5.8 mg vial may be stored under refrigeration for up to 3 weeks. Store vial in carton to protect from light.

Solution: Prior to use, store under refrigeration at 2°C to 8°C (36°F to 46°F). Once the cartridge is loaded into the pen delivery system, store under refrigeration for up to 21 days after first use.

Saizen®: Prior to reconstitution, store at room temperature 15°C to 30°C (59°F to 86°F). Following reconstitution with bacteriostatic water for injection, reconstituted solution should be refrigerated and used within 14 days. When reconstituted with sterile water for injection, use immediately and discard unused portion. The Saizen® easy click cartridge, when reconstituted with the provided bacteriostatic water, should be stored under refrigeration and used within 21 days.

5 mg vial: Reconstitute with 1-3 mL bacteriostatic water for injection or sterile water for injection; Gently swirl; do not shake.

8.8 mg vial: Reconstitute with 2-3 mL bacteriostatic water for injection or sterile water for injection. Gently swirl; do not shake.

Serostim®: Prior to reconstitution, store at room temperature 15°C to 30°C (59°F to 86°F). Reconstitute with sterile water for injection. When reconstituted with sterile water for injection, use immediately and discard unused portion.

Tev-Tropin®: Prior to reconstitution, store at 2°C to 8°C (36°F to 46°F). Reconstitute with 1-5 mL of diluent provided. Gently swirl; do not shake. May use preservative free NS for use in newborns. Following reconstitution with bacteriostatic NS, solution should be refrigerated and used within 14 days. Some cloudiness may occur; do not use if cloudiness persists after warming to room temperature.

Zorbtive®: Store unopened vials and diluent at room temperature of 15°C to 30°C (59°F to 86°F). Store reconstituted vial under refrigeration at 2°C to 8°C (36°F to 46°F) for up to 14 days; do not freeze.

8.8 mg vial: Reconstitute with 1-2 mL bacteriostatic water for injection. Swirl gently.

Mechanism of Action Somatropin is a purified polypeptide hormones of recombinant DNA origin; somatropin contains the identical sequence of amino acids found in human growth hormone; human growth hormone stimulates growth of linear bone, skeletal muscle, and organs; stimulates erythropoietin which increases red blood cell mass; exerts both insulin-like and diabetogenic effects; enhances the transmucosal transport of water, electrolytes, and nutrients across the gut

Pharmacodynamics/Kinetics

Duration: Maintains supraphysiologic levels for 18-20 hours

Absorption: I.M., SubQ: Well absorbed

Distribution: ~1 L/kg

Metabolism: Hepatic and renal (~90%)

Bioavailability: SubQ: ~70% to 90%

Half-life elimination: Preparation and route of administration dependent; SubQ: ~2-4 hours

Excretion: Urine

Dosage

Children (individualize dose):

Chronic renal insufficiency (CRI): Nutropin®, Nutropin® AQ: SubQ: Weekly dosage: 0.35 mg/kg divided into daily injections; continue until the time of renal transplantation

Dosage recommendations in patients treated for CRI who require dialysis:

Hemodialysis: Administer dose at night prior to bedtime or at least 3-4 hours after hemodialysis to prevent hematoma formation from heparin

CCPD: Administer dose in the morning following dialysis

CAPD: Administer dose in the evening at the time of overnight exchange

Growth hormone deficiency:

Genotropin®, Omnitrope™: SubQ: Weekly dosage: 0.16-0.24 mg/kg divided into 6-7 daily doses

Humatrope®: I.M., SubQ: Weekly dosage: 0.18 mg/kg; maximum replacement dose: 0.3 mg/kg/week; dosing should be divided into equal doses given 3 times/week on alternating days, 6 times/week, or daily

Norditropin®: SubQ: 0.024-0.034 mg/kg/day, 6-7 times/week

Nutropin®, Nutropin® AQ: SubQ: Weekly dosage: 0.3 mg/kg divided into daily doses; pubertal patients: ≤0.7 mg/kg/week divided daily

Tev-Tropin®: SubQ: Up to 0.1 mg/kg administered 3 times/week

Saizen®: I.M., SubQ: 0.18 mg/kg/week in divided doses administered daily **or** as 0.06 mg/kg/dose administered 3 times/week **or** as 0.03 mg/kg/dose administered 6 times/week

Note: Therapy should be discontinued when patient has reached satisfactory adult height, when epiphyses have fused, or when the patient ceases to respond. Growth of 5 cm/year or more is expected, if growth rate does not exceed 2.5 cm in a 6-month period, double the dose for the next 6 months; if there is still no satisfactory response, discontinue therapy

HIV patients with wasting or cachexia (unlabeled use): Serostim®: SubQ: Limited data; doses of 0.04 mg/kg/day were reported in five children, 6-17 years of age; doses of 0.07 mg/kg/day were reported in six children, 8-14 years of age

Idiopathic short stature:

Genotropin®: SubQ: Weekly dosage: 0.47 mg/kg divided into equal doses 6-7 times per week

Humatrope®: SubQ: Weekly dosage: 0.37 mg/kg divided into equal doses 6-7 times per week

Nutropin®, Nutropin AQ®: SubQ: Weekly dosage: Up to 0.3 mg/kg divided into daily doses

Noonan syndrome: Norditropin®: SubQ: Up to 0.066 mg/kg/day

Prader-Willi syndrome: Genotropin®: SubQ: Weekly dosage: 0.24 mg/kg divided into 6-7 doses

SHOX deficiency: Humatrope®: SubQ: 0.35 mg/kg/week divided into equal daily doses

Small for gestational age:

Genotropin®: SubQ: Weekly dosage: 0.48 mg/kg divided into 6-7 doses

Norditropin®: SubQ: Up to 0.067 mg/kg/day

Alternate dosing (small for gestational age): In older/early pubertal children or children with very short stature, consider initiating therapy at higher doses (0.067 mg/kg/day) and then consider reducing the dose (0.033 mg/kg/day) if substantial catch-up growth observed. In younger children (<4 years) with less severe short stature, consider initiating therapy with lower doses (0.033 mg/kg/day) and then titrating the dose upwards as needed.

Turner syndrome:

Genotropin®: SubQ: Weekly dosage: 0.33 mg/kg divided into 6-7 doses

Humatrope®, Nutropin®, Nutropin® AQ: SubQ: Weekly dosage: ≤0.375 mg/kg divided into equal doses 3-7 times per week

Norditropin®: Up to 0.067 mg/kg/day

Adults:

Growth hormone deficiency: Adjust dose based on individual requirements: To minimize adverse events in older or overweight patients, reduced dosages may be necessary. During therapy, dosage should be decreased if required by the occurrence of side effects or excessive IGF-I levels.

Norditropin®: SubQ: Initial dose ≤0.004 mg/kg/day; after 6 weeks of therapy, may increase dose up to 0.016 mg/kg/day

Nutropin®, Nutropin® AQ: SubQ: ≤0.006 mg/kg/day; dose may be increased up to a maximum of 0.025 mg/kg/day in patients <35 years of age, or up to a maximum of 0.0125 mg/kg/day in patients ≥35 years of age

Humatrope®: SubQ: ≤0.006 mg/kg/day; dose may be increased up to a maximum of 0.0125 mg/kg/day

Genotropin®, Omnitrope™: SubQ: Weekly dosage: ≤0.04 mg/kg divided into 6-7 daily doses; dose may be increased at 4- to 8-week intervals to a maximum of 0.08 mg/kg/week

Saizen®: SubQ: ≤0.005 mg/kg/day; dose may be increased to not more than 0.01 mg/kg/day after 4 weeks

Alternate dosing (growth hormone deficiency): SubQ: Initial: 0.2 mg/day (range: 0.15-0.3 mg/day); may increase every 1-2 months by 0.1-0.2 mg/day

Dosage adjustment with estrogen supplementation (growth hormone deficiency): Larger doses of somatropin may be needed for women taking oral estrogen replacement products; dosing not affected by topical products

HARS (unlabeled use): Serostim®: SubQ: Induction: 4 mg once daily at bedtime for 12 weeks; Maintenance: 2 mg or 4 mg every other day at bedtime for 12-24 weeks. **Note:** Every-other-day dosing during induction has also been studied. Although a greater response was seen with daily dosing, it was associated with an increased incidence of adverse events.

HIV patients with wasting or cachexia: Serostim®: SubQ: 0.1 mg/kg once daily at bedtime (maximum: 6 mg/day). Alternately, patients at risk for side effects may be started at 0.1 mg/kg every other day. Patients who continue to lose weight after 12 weeks should be re-evaluated for opportunistic infections or other clinical events; rotate injection sites to avoid lipodystrophy Adjust dose if needed to manage side effects.

Daily dose based on body weight:

<35 kg: 0.1 mg/kg

35-45 kg: 4 mg

45-55 kg: 5 mg

>55 kg: 6 mg

Short-bowel syndrome (Zorbtive®): SubQ: 0.1 mg/kg once daily for 4 weeks (maximum: 8 mg/day)

Fluid retention (moderate) or arthralgias: Treat symptomatically or reduce dose by 50%

Severe toxicity: Discontinue therapy for up to 5 days; when symptoms resolve, restart at 50% of dose. If severe toxicity recurs or does not disappear within 5 days after discontinuation, permanently discontinue treatment.

Elderly: Patients ≥65 years of age may be more sensitive to the action of growth hormone and more prone to adverse effects; in general, dosing should be cautious, beginning at low end of dosing range

Dosage adjustment in renal impairment Reports indicate patients with chronic renal failure tend to have decreased clearance; specific dosing suggestions not available

Dosage adjustment in hepatic impairment: Clearance may be reduced in patients with severe hepatic dysfunction; specific dosing suggestions not available

Dietary Considerations

Prader-Willi syndrome: All patients should have effective weight control (use is contraindicated in severely-obese patients).

Short-bowel syndrome: Intravenous parenteral nutrition requirements may need reassessment as gastrointestinal absorption improves.

Administration Do not shake; administer SubQ or I.M. (not all products are approved for I.M. administration). Rotate administration sites to avoid tissue atrophy. When administering to newborns, reconstitute with sterile water for injection.

Norditropin® cartridge must be administered using the corresponding color-coded NordiPen® injection pen.

Omnitrope™: Solution in the cartridges must be administered using the Omnitrope™ pen; when installing a new cartridge, prime pen prior to first use.

Humatrope®: When administering for growth hormone deficiency, SubQ route is preferred

Tev-Tropin®: SubQ injections of solutions >1 mL not recommended.

Monitoring Parameters Growth curve, periodic thyroid function tests, bone age (annually), periodical urine testing for glucose, somatomedin C (IGF-I) levels; funduscopic examinations at initiation of therapy and periodically during treatment; serum phosphorus, alkaline phosphatase and parathyroid hormone. If growth deceleration is observed in children treated for growth hormone deficiency, and not due to other causes, evaluate for presence of antibody formation. Strict blood glucose monitoring in patients with diabetes. Progression or recurrence of pre-existing tumors or malignant transformation of skin lesions.

CRI: Progression of renal osteodystrophy

Prader-Willi syndrome: Monitor for sleep apnea, respiratory infections, snoring (onset of or increased)

Turner syndrome: Ear disorders including otitis media; cardiovascular disorders

Noonan syndrome: Prior to use, verify short stature syndrome.

Dosage Forms Excipient information presented when available (limited, particularly for generics); consult specific product labeling.

Injection, powder for reconstitution [rDNA origin]:

Genotropin®: 5.8 mg [~15 int. units/mL; delivers 5 mg/mL; contains m-cresol]; 13.8 mg [~36 int. units/mL; delivers 12 mg/mL; contains m-cresol]

Genotropin Miniquick® [preservative free]: 0.2 mg, 0.4 mg, 0.6 mg, 0.8 mg, 1 mg, 1.2 mg, 1.4 mg, 1.6 mg, 1.8 mg, 2 mg [each strength delivers 0.25 mL]

Humatrope®: 5 mg [15 int. units], 6 mg [18 int. units], 12 mg [36 int. units], 24 mg [72 int. units]

Nutropin®: 5 mg [~15 int. units; packaged with diluent containing benzyl alcohol]; 10 mg [~30 int. units; packaged with diluent containing benzyl alcohol]

Omnitrope™: 5.8 mg [~17.4 int. units; packaged with diluent containing benzyl alcohol]

Saizen®: 5 mg [~15 int. units; contains sucrose 34.2 mg; packaged with diluent containing benzyl alcohol]; 8.8 mg [~26.4 int. units; contains sucrose 60.2 mg; packaged with diluent containing benzyl alcohol]
Serostim®: 4 mg [~12 int. units; contains sucrose 27.3 mg; packaged with diluent containing benzyl alcohol; 5 mg [~15 int. units; contains sucrose 34.2 mg]; 6 mg [~18 int. units; contains sucrose 41 mg]; 8.8 mg [~26.4 int. units; contains sucrose 60.19 mg; packaged with diluent containing benzyl alcohol]
Tev-Tropin®: 5 mg [15 int. units/mL; packaged with diluent containing benzyl alcohol]
Zorbtive®: 8.8 mg [~26.4 int. units; contains sucrose 60.19 mg; packaged with diluent containing benzyl alcohol]

Injection, solution [rDNA origin]:
Norditropin®: 5 mg/1.5 mL (1.5 mL); 15 mg/1.5 mL (1.5 mL)
Norditropin® NordiFlex®: 5 mg/1.5 mL (1.5 mL); 10 mg/1.5 mL (1.5 mL); 15 mg/1.5 mL (1.5 mL)
Nutropin AQ®: 5 mg/mL (2 mL) [~15 int. units/mL]
Omnitrope™: 5 mg/1.5 mL (1.5 mL); 10 mg/1.5 mL (1.5 mL)

- **Somatuline® Autogel® (Can)** *see* Lanreotide *on page 853*
- **Somatuline® Depot** *see* Lanreotide *on page 853*
- **Somavert®** *see* Pegvisomant *on page 1159*
- **Sominex® [OTC]** *see* DiphenhydrAMINE *on page 456*
- **Sominex® Maximum Strength [OTC]** *see* DiphenhydrAMINE *on page 456*
- **Somnote®** *see* Chloral Hydrate *on page 300*
- **Som Pam (Can)** *see* Flurazepam *on page 643*
- **Sonata®** *see* Zaleplon *on page 1576*

Sorafenib (sor AF e nib)

U.S. Brand Names Nexavar®

Canadian Brand Names Nexavar®

Index Terms BAY 43-9006; NSC-724772; Sorafenib Tosylate

Pharmacologic Category Antineoplastic Agent, Tyrosine Kinase Inhibitor; Vascular Endothelial Growth Factor (VEGF) Inhibitor

Use Treatment of advanced renal cell cancer (RCC), unresectable hepatocellular cancer (HCC)

Unlabeled/Investigational Use Treatment of advanced thyroid cancer

Pregnancy Risk Factor D

Pregnancy Considerations Animal studies have demonstrated teratogenicity and fetal loss. There are no adequate and well-controlled studies in pregnant women. Because sorafenib inhibits angiogenesis, a critical component of fetal development, adverse effects on pregnancy would be expected. Women of childbearing potential should be advised to avoid pregnancy. Men and women should use effective birth control during treatment and for at least 2 weeks after treatment is discontinued.

Lactation Excretion in breast milk unknown/not recommended

Medication Safety Issues

Sound-alike/look-alike issues:
Nexavar® may be confused with Nexium®
Sorafenib may be confused with sunitinib

High alert medication: The Institute for Safe Medication Practices (ISMP) includes this medication among its list of drug classes which have a heightened risk of causing significant patient harm when used in error.

Contraindications Hypersensitivity to sorafenib or any component of the formulation

Warnings/Precautions Hazardous agent - use appropriate precautions for handling and disposal. May cause hypertension, especially in the first 6 weeks of treatment; monitor; use caution in patients with underlying or poorly-controlled hypertension. May cause cardiac ischemia or infarction; consider discontinuing (temporarily or permanently) in patients who develop these; use in patients with unstable coronary artery disease or recent myocardial infarction has not been studied. Use with caution in patients with cardiovascular disease. Serious bleeding events may occur; monitor PT/INR in patients on warfarin therapy. May complicate wound healing; temporarily withhold treatment for patients undergoing major surgical procedures. Gastrointestinal perforation has been reported (rare); monitor patients for signs/symptoms (abdominal pain, constipation, or vomiting); discontinue treatment if gastrointestinal perforation occurs. Avoid concurrent use (if possible) with strong CYP3A4 inducers (eg, carbamazepine, dexamethasone, phenobarbital, phenytoin, rifampin, St. John's wort); may decrease sorafenib levels/effects. Use caution when administering sorafenib with compounds that are metabolized predominantly via UGT1A1 (eg, irinotecan). Hand-foot skin reaction and rash are the most common adverse events; usually managed with topical treatment, treatment delays, and/or dose reductions. Sorafenib levels may be lower in HCC patients with mild-to-moderate hepatic impairment (Child-Pugh classes A and B); has not been studied in patients with severe hepatic impairment or in patients on dialysis. Use with extreme caution in patients with HCC with elevated bilirubin levels. The optimal dose in non-HCC patients with hepatic impairment has not been established. Safety and efficacy have not been established in children.

Adverse Reactions

>10%:
Cardiovascular: Hypertension (9% to 17%; grade 3: 3% to 4%; grade 4: <1%; onset: ~3 weeks)
Central nervous system: Fatigue (37% to 46%), sensory neuropathy (≤13%), pain (11%)
Dermatologic: Rash/desquamation (19% to 40%; grade 3: ≤1%), hand-foot syndrome (21% to 30%; grade 3: 6% to 8%), alopecia (14% to 27%), pruritus (14% to 19%), dry skin (10% to 11%), erythema
Endocrine & metabolic: Hypoalbuminemia (≤59%), hypophosphatemia (35% to 45%; grade 3: 11% to 13%; grade 4: <1%)
Gastrointestinal: Diarrhea (43% to 55%; grade 3: 2% to 10%; grade 4: <1%), lipase increased (40% to 41% [usually transient]), amylase increased (30% to 34% [usually transient]), abdominal pain (11% to 31%), weight loss (10% to 30%), anorexia (16% to 29%), nausea (23% to 24%), vomiting (15% to 16%), constipation (14% to 15%)
Hematologic: Lymphopenia (23% to 47%; grades 3/4: ≤13%), thrombocytopenia (12% to 46%; grades 3/4: 1% to 4%), INR increased (≤42%), neutropenia (≤18%; grades 3/4: ≤5%), hemorrhage (15% to 18%; grade 3: 2% to 3%; grade 4: ≤2%), leukopenia
Hepatic: Liver dysfunction (≤11%; grade 3: 2%; grade 4: 1%)
Neuromuscular & skeletal: Muscle pain, weakness
Respiratory: Dyspnea (≤14%), cough (≤13%)

1% to 10%:
Cardiovascular: Cardiac ischemia/infarction (≤3%), flushing
Central nervous system: Headache (≤10%), depression, fever
Dermatologic: Acne, exfoliative dermatitis
Gastrointestinal: Appetite decreased, dyspepsia, dysphagia, esophageal varices bleeding (2%), glossodynia, mucositis, stomatitis, xerostomia

Genitourinary: Erectile dysfunction
Hematologic: Anemia
Hepatic: Transaminases increased (transient)
Neuromuscular & skeletal: Joint pain (≤10%), arthralgia, myalgia
Respiratory: Hoarseness
Miscellaneous: Influenza-like symptoms

<1% (Limited to important or life-threatening): Acute renal failure, alkaline phosphatase increased, arrhythmia, bilirubin increased, bone pain, cardiac failure, cerebral hemorrhage, CHF, dehydration, eczema, epistaxis, erythema multiforme, folliculitis, gastritis, gastrointestinal hemorrhage, gastrointestinal perforation, gastrointestinal reflux, gynecomastia, hypersensitivity (skin reaction, urticaria), hypertensive crisis, hyponatremia, hypothyroidism, infection, jaundice, MI, mouth pain, myocardial ischemia, pancreatitis, pleural effusion, preeclampsia-like syndrome (reversible hypertension and proteinuria), renal failure, respiratory hemorrhage, reversible posterior leukoencephalopathy syndrome (RPLS), rhinorrhea, skin cancer (squamous cell/keratoacanthomas), thromboembolism, tinnitus, transient ischemic attack, tumor pain, voice alteration

Drug Interactions

Metabolism/Transport Effects Substrate of CYP3A4 (minor); **Inhibits** CYP2B6 (moderate), 2C8 (strong), 2C9 (moderate)

Avoid Concomitant Use

Avoid concomitant use of Sorafenib with any of the following: Natalizumab; Vaccines (Live)

Increased Effect/Toxicity

Sorafenib may increase the levels/effects of: CYP2B6 Substrates; CYP2C8 Substrates (High risk); CYP2C9 Substrates (High risk); DOXOrubicin; Fluorouracil; Irinotecan; Natalizumab; Vaccines (Live); Vitamin K Antagonists; Warfarin

The levels/effects of Sorafenib may be increased by: CYP3A4 Inhibitors (Strong); Trastuzumab

Decreased Effect

Sorafenib may decrease the levels/effects of: Cardiac Glycosides; Dacarbazine; Fluorouracil; Vaccines (Inactivated); Vitamin K Antagonists

The levels/effects of Sorafenib may be decreased by: CYP3A4 Inducers (Strong); Echinacea; Herbs (CYP3A4 Inducers)

Ethanol/Nutrition/Herb Interactions

Food: Bioavailability is decreased 29% with a high-fat meal (bioavailability is similar to fasting state when administered with a moderate-fat meal).
Herb/Nutraceutical: Avoid St John's wort (may decrease the levels/effects of sorafenib).

Stability Store at room temperature of 25°C (77°F); excursions permitted to 15°C and 30°C (59°F and 86°F). Protect from moisture.

Mechanism of Action Multikinase inhibitor; inhibits tumor growth and angiogenesis by inhibiting intracellular Raf kinases (CRAF, BRAF, and mutant BRAF), and cell surface kinase receptors (VEGFR-2, VEGFR-3, PDGFR-beta, cKIT, and FLT-3)

Pharmacodynamics/Kinetics

Protein binding: 99.5%
Metabolism: Hepatic, via CYP3A4 (primarily oxidated to the pyridine N-oxide; active, minor) and UGT1A9 (glucuronidation)
Bioavailability: 38% to 49%; reduced when administered with a high-fat meal
Half-life elimination: 25-48 hours
Time to peak, plasma: ~3 hours
Excretion: Feces (77%, 51% as unchanged drug); urine (19%, as metabolites)

Dosage Oral: Adults:

Advanced renal cell carcinoma: 400 mg twice daily
Hepatocellular cancer: 400 mg twice daily
Thyroid cancer (unlabeled use): 400 mg twice daily (Gupta-Abramson, 2008)

Dosage adjustment for concomitant CYP3A4 inducers: Avoid the concomitant use of a strong CYP3A4 inducer (eg, carbamazepine, dexamethasone, phenobarbital, phenytoin, rifampin, St. John's wort) with sorafenib. If a strong CYP3A4 inducer is required, the sorafenib dose may need to be increased, with careful monitoring. When the strong CYP3A4 inducer is discontinued, reduce sorafenib to the indicated dose.

Dosage adjustment for toxicity: Temporary interruption and/or dosage reduction may be necessary for management of adverse drug reactions. The dose may be reduced to 400 mg once daily and then further reduced to 400 mg every other day.

Dose modification for severe/persistent hypertension (despite antihypertensive therapy) or cardiac ischemia/infarction: Consider temporarily or permanently discontinuing treatment.

Dose modification for hemorrhage requiring medical intervention or gastrointestinal perforation: Consider permanently discontinuing treatment.

Dose modification for skin toxicity:

- Grade 1 (numbness, dysesthesia, paresthesia, tingling, painless swelling, erythema or discomfort of the hands or feet which do not disrupt normal activities): Continue sorafenib and consider symptomatic treatment with topical therapy.
- Grade 2 (painful erythema and swelling of the hands or feet and/or discomfort affecting normal activities):
  - 1st occurrence: Continue sorafenib and consider symptomatic treatment with topical therapy. **Note:** If no improvement within 7 days, see dosing for 2nd or 3rd occurrence.
  - 2nd or 3rd occurrence: Hold treatment until resolves to grade 0-1; resume treatment with dose reduced by one dose level (400 mg daily or 400 mg every other day)
  - 4th occurrence: Discontinue treatment
- Grade 3 (moist desquamation, ulceration, blistering, or severe pain of the hands or feet or severe discomfort that prevents working or performing daily activities):
  - 1st or 2nd occurrence: Hold treatment until resolves to grade 0-1; resume treatment with dose reduced by one dose level (400 mg daily or 400 mg every other day)
  - 3rd occurrence: Discontinue treatment

Dosage adjustment in renal impairment: No adjustment is required for mild, moderate, or severe renal impairment (not dependant on dialysis); has not been studied in dialysis patients.

Dosage adjustment in hepatic impairment: No adjustment required for mild (Child-Pugh class A) to moderate (Child-Pugh class B) hepatic impairment; not studied in severe hepatic impairment (Child-Pugh class C). Use with extreme caution in patients with HCC with elevated bilirubin levels.

Dietary Considerations Take without food (1 hour before or 2 hours after eating).

Administration Administer with water on an empty stomach (1 hour before or 2 hours after eating). Swallow tablet whole.

Monitoring Parameters CBC with differential, electrolytes, phosphorus, lipase and amylase levels; blood pressure (baseline, weekly for the first 6 weeks, then periodic)

Dosage Forms Excipient information presented when available (limited, particularly for generics); consult specific product labeling.

Tablet, as tosylate:
Nexavar®: 200 mg

◆ **Sorafenib Tosylate** *see* Sorafenib *on page 1392*

Sorbitol (SOR bi tole)

Pharmacologic Category Genitourinary Irrigant; Laxative, Osmotic

Additional Appendix Information

Laxatives, Classification and Properties *on page 1660*

Use Genitourinary irrigant in transurethral prostatic resection or other transurethral resection or other transurethral surgical procedures; diuretic; humectant; sweetening agent; hyperosmotic laxative; facilitate the passage of sodium polystyrene sulfonate through the intestinal tract

Pregnancy Risk Factor C

Dosage Hyperosmotic laxative (as single dose, at infrequent intervals):

Children 2-11 years:

Oral: 2 mL/kg (as 70% solution)

Rectal enema: 30-60 mL as 25% to 30% solution

Children >12 years and Adults:

Oral: 30-150 mL (as 70% solution)

Rectal enema: 120 mL as 25% to 30% solution

Adjunct to sodium polystyrene sulfonate: 15 mL as 70% solution orally until diarrhea occurs (10-20 mL/2 hours) or 20-100 mL as an oral vehicle for the sodium polystyrene sulfonate resin

When administered with charcoal:

Oral:

Children: 4.3 mL/kg of 35% sorbitol with 1 g/kg of activated charcoal

Adults: 4.3 mL/kg of 70% sorbitol with 1 g/kg of activated charcoal every 4 hours until first stool containing charcoal is passed

Topical: 3% to 3.3% as transurethral surgical procedure irrigation

Additional Information Complete prescribing information for this medication should be consulted for additional detail.

Dosage Forms Excipient information presented when available (limited, particularly for generics); consult specific product labeling.

Solution, genitourinary irrigation: 3% (3000 mL, 5000 mL); 3.3% (2000 mL, 4000 mL)

Solution, oral: 70% (30 mL, 480 mL, 3840 mL)

◆ **Soriatane® [DSC]** *see* Acitretin *on page 38*

◆ **Soriatane® (Can)** *see* Acitretin *on page 38*

◆ **Soriatane® CK Convenience Kit™** *see* Acitretin *on page 38*

◆ **Sorine®** *see* Sotalol *on page 1394*

Sotalol (SOE ta lole)

U.S. Brand Names Betapace AF®; Betapace®; Sorine®

Canadian Brand Names Apo-Sotalol®; Betapace AF®; CO Sotalol; DOM-Sotalol; Gen-Sotalol; Lin-Sotalol; MED-Sotalol; Novo-Sotalol; Nu-Sotalol; PHL-Sotalol; PMS-Sotalol; PRO-Sotalol; RATIO-Sotalol; RHOXAL-Sotalol; Riva-Sotalol; Rylosol; SANDOZ-Sotalol

Index Terms Sotalol Hydrochloride

Pharmacologic Category Antiarrhythmic Agent, Class II; Antiarrhythmic Agent, Class III; Beta-Adrenergic Blocker, Nonselective

Additional Appendix Information

Beta-Blockers *on page 1648*

Use Treatment of documented ventricular arrhythmias (ie, sustained ventricular tachycardia), that in the judgment of the physician are life-threatening; maintenance of normal sinus rhythm in patients with symptomatic atrial fibrillation and atrial flutter who are currently in sinus rhythm. Manufacturer states substitutions should not be made for Betapace AF® since Betapace AF® is distributed with a patient package insert specific for atrial fibrillation/flutter.

Pregnancy Risk Factor B

Pregnancy Considerations There are no adequate and well-controlled studies in pregnant women. Beta-blockers have been associated with bradycardia, hypotension, and IUGR; IUGR is probably related to maternal hypertension. Sotalol has been shown to cross the placenta, and is found in amniotic fluid; therefore, sotalol should be used during pregnancy only if the potential benefit outweighs the potential risk. Cases of neonatal hypoglycemia have been reported following maternal use of beta-blockers at parturition or during breast-feeding. Monitor breast-fed infant for symptoms of beta-blockade.

Lactation Enters breast milk/use caution (AAP rates "compatible")

Medication Safety Issues

Sound-alike/look-alike issues:

Sotalol may be confused with Stadol®

Betapace® may be confused with Betapace AF®

Betapace AF® may be confused with Betapace®

Contraindications Hypersensitivity to sotalol or any component of the formulation; bronchial asthma; sinus bradycardia; second- and third-degree AV block (unless a functioning pacemaker is present); congenital or acquired long QT syndromes; cardiogenic shock; uncontrolled congestive heart failure. Betapace AF® is contraindicated in patients with significantly reduced renal filtration (Cl_{cr} <40 mL/minute).

Warnings/Precautions [U.S. Boxed Warning] Manufacturer recommends initiation (or reinitiation) and doses increased in a hospital setting with continuous monitoring and staff familiar with the recognition and treatment of life-threatening arrhythmias. Some experts will initiate therapy on an outpatient basis in a patient without heart disease or bradycardia, who has a baseline uncorrected QT interval <450 msec, and normal serum potassium and magnesium levels; close EKG monitoring during this time is necessary. ACC/AHA guidelines for management of atrial fibrillation also recommend that for outpatient initiation the patient not have risk factors predisposing to drug-induced ventricular proarrhythmia (Fuster, 2001). Dosage should be adjusted gradually with 3 days between dosing increments to achieve steady-state concentrations, and to allow time to monitor QT intervals. Creatinine clearance must be calculated prior to dosing. Use cautiously in the renally-impaired (dosage adjustment required).

Watch for proarrhythmic effects; monitor and adjust dose to prevent QTc prolongation. Concurrent use with other QT_c-prolonging drugs (including Class I and Class III antiarrhythmics) is generally not recommended; withhold for 3 half-lives. Correct electrolyte imbalances before initiating (especially hypokalemia and hypomagnesemia). Consider pre-existing conditions such as sick sinus syndrome before initiating. Conduction abnormalities can occur particularly sinus bradycardia. Use cautiously within the first 2 weeks post-MI (experience limited). Administer cautiously in compensated heart failure and monitor for a worsening of the condition. Use caution in patients with PVD (can aggravate arterial insufficiency). Beta-blocker therapy should not be withdrawn abruptly (particularly in patients with CAD), but gradually tapered to avoid acute tachycardia, hypertension, and/or ischemia. Use caution with concurrent use of beta-blockers and either verapamil or diltiazem; bradycardia or heart block can occur. Use cautiously in diabetics because it can mask prominent hypoglycemic symptoms. Use with caution in patients with bronchospastic disease, myasthenia gravis, peripheral vascular disease, or psychiatric disease. Use care with anesthetic agents which decrease myocardial function. Adequate alpha-blockade is required prior to use of any beta-blocker for patients with untreated pheochromocytoma. Use caution with history of severe anaphylaxis to allergens; patients taking beta-blockers may become more sensitive to repeated challenges. Treatment of anaphylaxis (eg, epinephrine) in patients taking beta-blockers may be ineffective or promote undesirable effects. Safety and efficacy have not been established in children.

[U.S. Boxed Warning]: Betapace® should not be substituted for Betapace® AF; Betapace® AF is distributed with an educational insert specifically for patients with atrial fibrillation/flutter.

Adverse Reactions

>10%:

Cardiovascular: Bradycardia (16%), chest pain (16%), palpitation (14%)

Central nervous system: Fatigue (20%), dizziness (20%), lightheadedness (12%)

Neuromuscular & skeletal: Weakness (13%)

Respiratory: Dyspnea (21%)

1% to 10%:

Cardiovascular: Edema (8%), abnormal ECG (7%), hypotension (6%), proarrhythmia (5%), syncope (5%), CHF (5%), peripheral vascular disorders (3%)

Central nervous system: Headache (8%), sleep problems (8%), mental confusion (6%), anxiety (4%), depression (4%)

Dermatologic: Itching/rash (5%)

Endocrine & metabolic: Sexual ability decreased (3%)

Gastrointestinal: Nausea/vomiting (10%), diarrhea (7%), stomach discomfort (3% to 6%), flatulence (2%)

Genitourinary: Impotence (2%)

Hematologic: Bleeding (2%)

Neuromuscular & skeletal: Extremity pain (7%), paresthesia (4%), back pain (3%)

Ocular: Visual problems (5%)

Respiratory: Upper respiratory problems (5% to 8%), asthma (2%)

<1% (Limited to important or life-threatening): Alopecia, bronchiolitis obliterans with organized pneumonia (BOOP), cold extremities, diaphoresis, eosinophilia, leukocytoclastic vasculitis, leukopenia, paralysis, phlebitis, photosensitivity reaction, pruritus, pulmonary edema, Raynaud's phenomenon, red crusted skin, retroperitoneal fibrosis, serum transaminases increased, skin necrosis after extravasation, thrombocytopenia, vertigo

Drug Interactions

Avoid Concomitant Use

Avoid concomitant use of Sotalol with any of the following: Methacholine; Nilotinib; Tetrabenazine; Ziprasidone

Increased Effect/Toxicity

Sotalol may increase the levels/effects of: Alpha-/Beta-Agonists (Direct-Acting); Alpha1-Blockers; Alpha2-Agonists; Amifostine; Antipsychotic Agents (Phenothiazines); Cardiac Glycosides; Insulin; Lidocaine; Methacholine; Midodrine; QTc-Prolonging Agents; RiTUXimab; Tetrabenazine; Ziprasidone

The levels/effects of Sotalol may be increased by: Acetylcholinesterase Inhibitors; Aminoquinolines (Antimalarial); Amiodarone; Anilidopiperidine Opioids; Antipsychotic Agents (Phenothiazines); Calcium Channel Blockers (Nondihydropyridine); Ciprofloxacin; Diazoxide; Dipyridamole; Disopyramide; Gadobutrol; Herbs (Hypotensive Properties); Nilotinib; Propafenone; Propoxyphene; Prostacyclin Analogues; QuiNIDine; Reserpine; Selective Serotonin Reuptake Inhibitors

Decreased Effect

Sotalol may decrease the levels/effects of: Beta2-Agonists; Theophylline Derivatives

The levels/effects of Sotalol may be decreased by: Barbiturates; Herbs (Hypertensive Properties); Methylphenidate; Nonsteroidal Anti-Inflammatory Agents; Rifamycin Derivatives; Yohimbine

Ethanol/Nutrition/Herb Interactions

Food: Sotalol peak serum concentrations may be decreased if taken with food.

Herb/Nutraceutical: Avoid ephedra (may worsen arrhythmia).

Stability Store at 25°C (77°F); excursions permitted to 15°C to 30°C (59°F to 86°F).

Mechanism of Action

Beta-blocker which contains both beta-adrenoreceptor-blocking (Vaughan Williams Class II) and cardiac action potential duration prolongation (Vaughan Williams Class III) properties

Class II effects: Increased sinus cycle length, slowed heart rate, decreased AV nodal conduction, and increased AV nodal refractoriness

Class III effects: Prolongation of the atrial and ventricular monophasic action potentials, and effective refractory prolongation of atrial muscle, ventricular muscle, and atrioventricular accessory pathways in both the antegrade and retrograde directions

Sotalol is a racemic mixture of *d-* and *l*-sotalol; both isomers have similar Class III antiarrhythmic effects while the *l*-isomer is responsible for virtually all of the beta-blocking activity

Sotalol has both $beta_1$- and $beta_2$-receptor blocking activity

The beta-blocking effect of sotalol is a noncardioselective [half maximal at about 80 mg/day and maximal at doses of 320-640 mg/day]. Significant beta-blockade occurs at oral doses as low as 25 mg/day.

The Class III effects are seen only at oral doses ≥160 mg/day

Pharmacodynamics/Kinetics

Onset of action: Rapid, 1-2 hours

Peak effect: 2.5-4 hours

Duration: 8-16 hours

Absorption: Decreased 20% to 30% by meals compared to fasting

Distribution: Low lipid solubility; enters milk of laboratory animals and is reported to be present in human milk

Protein binding: None

Metabolism: None

Bioavailability: 90% to 100%

Half-life elimination: 12 hours; Children: 9.5 hours; terminal half-life decreases with age <2 years (may by ≥1 week in neonates)

Excretion: Urine (as unchanged drug)

Dosage Sotalol should be initiated and doses increased in a hospital with facilities for cardiac rhythm monitoring and assessment. Proarrhythmic events can occur after initiation of therapy and with each upward dosage adjustment.

Children: Oral: The safety and efficacy of sotalol in children have not been established

Note: Dosing per manufacturer, based on pediatric pharmacokinetic data; wait at least 36 hours between dosage adjustments to allow monitoring of QT intervals

≤2 years: Dosage should be adjusted (decreased) by plotting of the child's age on a logarithmic scale; see graph on next page or refer to manufacturer's package labeling.

>2 years: Initial: 90 mg/m^2/day in 3 divided doses; may be incrementally increased to a maximum of 180 mg/m^2/day

Adults: Oral:

Ventricular arrhythmias (Betapace®, Sorine®):

Initial: 80 mg twice daily

Dose may be increased gradually to 240-320 mg/day; allow 3 days between dosing increments in order to attain steady-state plasma concentrations and to allow monitoring of QT intervals

Most patients respond to a total daily dose of 160-320 mg/day in 2-3 divided doses.

Sotalol Age Factor Nomogram for Patients ≤2 Years of Age

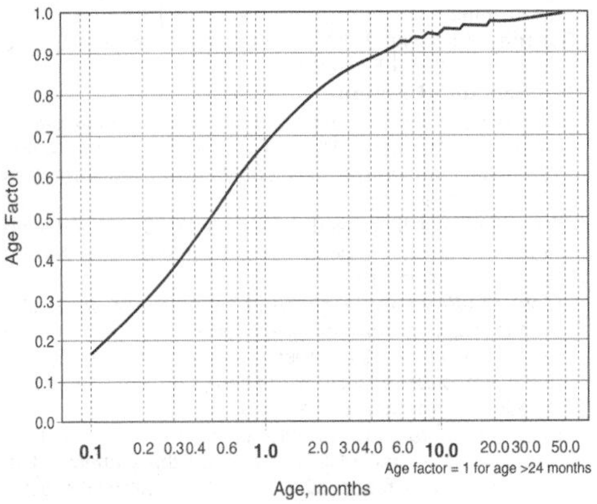

Adapted from U.S. Food and Drug Administration.
http://www.fda.gov/cder/foi/label/2001/2115s3lbl.PDF

Some patients, with life-threatening refractory ventricular arrhythmias, may require doses as high as 480-640 mg/day; however, these doses should only be prescribed when the potential benefit outweighs the increased of adverse events.

Atrial fibrillation or atrial flutter (Betapace AF®): Initial: 80 mg twice daily

If the initial dose does not reduce the frequency of relapses of atrial fibrillation/flutter and is tolerated without excessive QT prolongation (not >520 msec) after 3 days, the dose may be increased to 120 mg twice daily. This may be further increased to 160 mg twice daily if response is inadequate and QT prolongation is not excessive.

Elderly: Age does not significantly alter the pharmacokinetics of sotalol, but impaired renal function in elderly patients can increase the terminal half-life, resulting in increased drug accumulation

Dosage adjustment in renal impairment: Adults: Impaired renal function can increase the terminal half-life, resulting in increased drug accumulation. Sotalol (Betapace AF®) is contraindicated per the manufacturer for treatment of atrial fibrillation/flutter in patients with a Cl_{cr} <40 mL/minute.

Ventricular arrhythmias (Betapace®, Sorine®):

Cl_{cr} >60 mL/minute: Administer every 12 hours

Cl_{cr} 30-60 mL/minute: Administer every 24 hours

Cl_{cr} 10-30 mL/minute: Administer every 36-48 hours

Cl_{cr} <10 mL/minute: Individualize dose

Atrial fibrillation/flutter (Betapace AF®):

Cl_{cr} >60 mL/minute: Administer every 12 hours

Cl_{cr} 40-60 mL/minute: Administer every 24 hours

Cl_{cr} <40 mL/minute: Use is contraindicated

Dialysis: Hemodialysis would be expected to reduce sotalol plasma concentrations because sotalol is not bound to plasma proteins and does not undergo extensive metabolism; administer dose postdialysis or administer supplemental 80 mg dose; peritoneal dialysis does not remove sotalol; supplemental dose is not necessary

Dietary Considerations Administer on an empty stomach.

Administration Food may decrease adsorption

Monitoring Parameters Serum magnesium, potassium, ECG

Additional Information Pharmacokinetics in children are more relevant for BSA than age.

Dosage Forms Excipient information presented when available (limited, particularly for generics); consult specific product labeling.

Tablet, as hydrochloride: 80 mg, 80 mg [artrial fibrillation], 120 mg, 120 mg [artrial fibrillation], 160 mg, 160 mg, [artrial fibrillation], 240 mg

Betapace®: 80 mg, 120 mg, 160 mg, 240 mg

Betapace AF®: 80 mg, 120 mg, 160 mg [artrial fibrillation]

Sorine®: 80 mg, 120 mg, 160 mg, 240 mg

Extemporaneous Preparations To make a 5 mg/mL oral solution, using a 6-ounce amber plastic prescription bottle, add five sotalol 120 mg tablets to 120 mL of simple syrup containing 0.1% sodium benzoate (tablets do not need to be crushed). Shake well. Allow tablets to hydrate for ~2 hours; shake intermittently until tablets completely disintegrate. Store at Store at room temperature; shake well before use. Stable for 3 months. (Refer to manufacturer's current labeling.)

◆ **Sotalol Hydrochloride** *see* Sotalol *on page 1394*

◆ **Sotradecol®** *see* Sodium Tetradecyl *on page 1386*

◆ **Sotret®** *see* Isotretinoin *on page 825*

◆ **SPA** *see* Albumin *on page 49*

◆ **Spacol [DSC]** *see* Hyoscyamine *on page 756*

◆ **Spacol T/S [DSC]** *see* Hyoscyamine *on page 756*

◆ **Spastrin® [DSC]** *see* Belladonna, Phenobarbital, and Ergotamine *on page 178*

◆ **SPD417** *see* CarBAMazepine *on page 252*

◆ **Spectazole® [DSC]** *see* Econazole *on page 502*

Spectinomycin (spek ti noe MYE sin)

U.S. Brand Names Trobicin® [DSC]

Index Terms Spectinomycin Hydrochloride

Pharmacologic Category Antibiotic, Miscellaneous

Additional Appendix Information

Treatment of Sexually Transmitted Infections *on page 1773*

Use Treatment of uncomplicated gonorrhea

Pregnancy Risk Factor B

Lactation Enters breast milk/effect on infant unknown

Medication Safety Issues

Sound-alike/look-alike issues:

Trobicin® may be confused with tobramycin

Contraindications Hypersensitivity to spectinomycin or any component of the formulation

Warnings/Precautions Since spectinomycin is ineffective in the treatment of syphilis and may mask symptoms, all patients should be tested for syphilis at the time of gonorrheal diagnosis and 3 months later. Prolonged use may result in fungal or bacterial superinfection, including *C. difficile*-associated diarrhea (CDAD) and pseudomembranous colitis; CDAD has been observed >2 months postantibiotic treatment. Safety and efficacy have not been established in children.

Adverse Reactions <1% (Limited to important or life-threatening): Abdominal cramps, chills, dizziness, headache, nausea, vomiting

Drug Interactions

Avoid Concomitant Use There are no known interactions where it is recommended to avoid concomitant use.

Increased Effect/Toxicity There are no known significant interactions involving an increase in effect.

Decreased Effect

Spectinomycin may decrease the levels/effects of: Typhoid Vaccine

Stability Reconstitute with supplied diluent only. Use reconstituted solutions within 24 hours.

Mechanism of Action A bacteriostatic antibiotic that selectively binds to the 30s subunits of ribosomes, and thereby inhibiting bacterial protein synthesis

Pharmacodynamics/Kinetics

Duration: Up to 8 hours

Absorption: I.M.: Rapid and almost complete

Distribution: Concentrates in urine; does not distribute well into the saliva

Half-life elimination: 1.7 hours

Time to peak: ~1 hour

Excretion: Urine (70% to 100% as unchanged drug)

Dosage I.M.:

Children:

<45 kg: 40 mg/kg/dose 1 time (ceftriaxone preferred)

≥45 kg: Refer to adult dosing.

Children >8 years who are allergic to PCNS/cephalosporins may be treated with oral tetracycline

Adults:

Uncomplicated urethral, cervical, pharyngeal, or rectal gonorrhea: 2 g deep I.M. or 4 g where antibiotic resistance is prevalent 1 time; 4 g (10 mL) dose should be given as two 5 mL injections, followed by adequate chlamydial treatment (doxycycline 100 mg twice daily for 7 days)

Disseminated gonococcal infection: 2 g every 12 hours

Dosing adjustment in renal impairment: None necessary

Hemodialysis: 50% removed by hemodialysis

Administration For I.M. use only

Dosage Forms Excipient information presented when available (limited, particularly for generics); consult specific product labeling.

Injection, powder for reconstitution, as hydrochloride:

Trobicin®: 2 g [diluent contains benzyl alcohol] [DSC]

- **Spectinomycin Hydrochloride** *see* Spectinomycin *on page 1396*
- **Spectracef®** *see* Cefditoren *on page 272*
- **SPEF-Pioglitazone (Can)** *see* Pioglitazone *on page 1195*
- **SPI 0211** *see* Lubiprostone *on page 912*
- **Spiriva® (Can)** *see* Tiotropium *on page 1476*
- **Spiriva® HandiHaler®** *see* Tiotropium *on page 1476*

Spironolactone (speer on oh LAK tone)

U.S. Brand Names Aldactone®

Canadian Brand Names Aldactone®; Novo-Spiroton

Pharmacologic Category Diuretic, Potassium-Sparing; Selective Aldosterone Blocker

Additional Appendix Information

Heart Failure (Systolic) *on page 1809*

Use Management of edema associated with excessive aldosterone excretion; hypertension; congestive heart failure; primary hyperaldosteronism; hypokalemia; cirrhosis of liver accompanied by edema or ascites

Unlabeled/Investigational Use Female acne (adjunctive therapy); hirsutism; hypertension (pediatric); diuretic (pediatric)

Pregnancy Risk Factor C/D in pregnancy-induced hypertension (per expert analysis)

Pregnancy Considerations Teratogenic effects were not observed in animal studies; however, doses used were less than or equal to equivalent doses in humans. The antiandrogen effects of spironolactone have been shown to cause feminization of the male fetus in animal studies. Two case reports did not demonstrate this effect in humans however, the authors caution that adequate data is lacking. Diuretics are generally avoided in pregnancy due to the theoretical risk that decreased plasma volume may cause placental insufficiency. Diuretics should not be used during pregnancy in the presence of reduced placental perfusion (eg, pre-eclampsia, intrauterine growth restriction).

Lactation Enters breast milk/not recommended (AAP rates "compatible")

Medication Safety Issues

Sound-alike/look-alike issues:

Aldactone® may be confused with Aldactazide®

International issues:

Aldactone®: Brand name for potassium canrenoate in Austria, Czech Republic, Germany, and Hungary

Contraindications Hypersensitivity to spironolactone or any component of the formulation; anuria; acute renal insufficiency; significant impairment of renal excretory function; hyperkalemia; pregnancy (pregnancy-induced hypertension - per expert analysis)

Warnings/Precautions Avoid potassium supplements, potassium-containing salt substitutes, a diet rich in potassium, or other drugs that can cause hyperkalemia. Excess amounts can lead to profound diuresis with fluid and electrolyte loss; close medical supervision and dose evaluation are required. Watch for and correct electrolyte disturbances; adjust dose to avoid dehydration. In cirrhosis, avoid electrolyte and acid/base imbalances that might lead to hepatic encephalopathy. Gynecomastia is related to dose and duration of therapy. Discontinue use prior to adrenal vein catheterization. When evaluating a heart failure patient for spironolactone treatment, creatinine should be ≤2.5 mg/dL in men or ≤2 mg/dL in women and potassium <5 mEq/L. **[U.S. Boxed Warning]: Shown to be a tumorigen in chronic toxicity animal studies. Avoid unnecessary use.**

Adverse Reactions Incidence of adverse events is not always reported (mean daily dose 26 mg).

Cardiovascular: Edema (2%, placebo 2%)

Central nervous system: Disorders (23%, placebo 21%) which may include drowsiness, lethargy, headache, mental confusion, drug fever, ataxia, fatigue

Dermatologic: Maculopapular, erythematous cutaneous eruptions, urticaria, hirsutism, eosinophilia

Endocrine & metabolic: Gynecomastia (men 9%; placebo 1%), breast pain (men 2%; placebo 0.1%), serious hyperkalemia (2%, placebo 1%), hyponatremia, dehydration, hyperchloremic metabolic acidosis (in decompensated hepatic cirrhosis), impotence, menstrual irregularities, amenorrhea, postmenopausal bleeding

Gastrointestinal: Disorders (29%, placebo 29%) which may include anorexia, nausea, cramping, diarrhea, gastric bleeding, ulceration, gastritis, vomiting

Hematologic: Agranulocytosis

Hepatic: Cholestatic/hepatocellular toxicity

Renal: Increased BUN concentration

Miscellaneous: Deepening of the voice, anaphylactic reaction, breast cancer

Drug Interactions

Avoid Concomitant Use There are no known interactions where it is recommended to avoid concomitant use.

Increased Effect/Toxicity

Spironolactone may increase the levels/effects of: ACE Inhibitors; Amifostine; Ammonium Chloride; RiTUXimab

The levels/effects of Spironolactone may be increased by: Angiotensin II Receptor Blockers; Diazoxide;

Drospirenone; Eplerenone; Herbs (Hypotensive Properties); Potassium Salts; Prostacyclin Analogues

Decreased Effect

Spironolactone may decrease the levels/effects of: Cardiac Glycosides; Mitotane; QuiNIDine

The levels/effects of Spironolactone may be decreased by: Herbs (Hypertensive Properties); Methylphenidate; Yohimbine

Ethanol/Nutrition/Herb Interactions

Food: Food increases absorption.

Herb/Nutraceutical: Avoid natural licorice (due to mineralocorticoid activity)

Stability Protect from light.

Mechanism of Action Competes with aldosterone for receptor sites in the distal renal tubules, increasing sodium chloride and water excretion while conserving potassium and hydrogen ions; may block the effect of aldosterone on arteriolar smooth muscle as well

Pharmacodynamics/Kinetics

Duration: 2-3 days

Protein binding: 91% to 98%

Metabolism: Hepatic to multiple metabolites, including canrenone (active)

Half-life elimination: 78-84 minutes

Time to peak, serum: 1-3 hours (primarily as the active metabolite)

Excretion: Urine and feces

Dosage To reduce delay in onset of effect, a loading dose of 2 or 3 times the daily dose may be administered on the first day of therapy. Oral:

Children:

Diuretic, hypertension (unlabeled use): Children 1-17 years: Initial: 1 mg/kg/day divided every 12-24 hours (maximum dose: 3.3 mg/kg/day, up to 100 mg/day)

Diagnosis of primary aldosteronism (unlabeled use): 125-375 mg/m^2/day in divided doses

Adults:

Edema, hypokalemia: 25-200 mg/day in 1-2 divided doses

Hypertension (JNC 7): 25-50 mg/day in 1-2 divided doses

Diagnosis of primary aldosteronism: 100-400 mg/day in 1-2 divided doses

Acne in women (unlabeled use): 25-200 mg once daily

Hirsutism in women (unlabeled use): 50-200 mg/day in 1-2 divided doses

CHF, severe (with ACE inhibitor and a loop diuretic ± digoxin): 12.5-25 mg/day; maximum daily dose: 50 mg (higher doses may occasionallly be used). In the RALES trial, 25 mg every other day was the lowest maintenance dose possible.

Note: If potassium >5.4 mEq/L, consider dosage reduction.

Elderly: Initial: 25-50 mg/day in 1-2 divided doses, increasing by 25-50 mg every 5 days as needed.

Dosing interval in renal impairment:

Cl_{cr} 10-50 mL/minute: Administer every 12-24 hours.

Cl_{cr} <10 mL/minute: Avoid use.

Dietary Considerations Should be taken with food to decrease gastrointestinal irritation and to increase absorption. Excessive potassium intake (eg, salt substitutes, low-salt foods, bananas, nuts) should be avoided.

Monitoring Parameters Blood pressure, serum electrolytes (potassium, sodium), renal function, I & O ratios and daily weight throughout therapy

CHF: Potassium levels and renal function should be checked in 3 days and 1 week after initiation, then every 2-4 weeks for 3-12 months, then every 3-6 months.

Test Interactions May cause false elevation in serum digoxin concentrations measured by RIA

Additional Information Maximum diuretic effect may be delayed 2-3 days and maximum hypertensive effects may be delayed 2-3 weeks.

Dosage Forms Excipient information presented when available (limited, particularly for generics); consult specific product labeling.

Tablet: 25 mg, 50 mg, 100 mg

Aldactone®: 25 mg

Aldactone®: 50 mg, 100 mg [scored]

Extemporaneous Preparations A 25 mg/mL oral suspension can be prepared by crushing one hundred twenty (120) 25 mg tablets in a mortar (reducing to a fine powder), and then mixing in 20 mL of vehicle (a 1:1 combination of Ora-Sweet® or Ora-Sweet® SF and Ora-Plus®) to create a uniform paste. Continue to add vehicle in geometric amounts (while mixing) until near-final volume is achieved. Transfer to a graduate and add sufficient quantity to make 120 mL. Label "shake well" and "refrigerate." Refrigerated stability is 60 days.

Allen LV Jr and Erickson MA III, "Stability of Ketoconazole, Metolazone, Metronidazole, Procainamide Hydrochloride, and Spironolactone in Extemporaneously Compounded Oral Liquids," *Am J Health Syst Pharm*, 1996, 53:2073-8.

Nahata MC, Morosco RS, and Hipple TF, 4th ed, *Pediatric Drug Formulations*, Cincinnati, OH: Harvey Whitney Books Co, 2000.

- **Spironolactone and Hydrochlorothiazide** *see* Hydrochlorothiazide and Spironolactone *on page 739*
- **SPM 927** *see* Lacosamide *on page 847*
- **Sporanox®** *see* Itraconazole *on page 829*
- **SPP100** *see* Aliskiren *on page 63*
- **Sprintec®** *see* Ethinyl Estradiol and Norgestimate *on page 584*
- **Sprycel®** *see* Dasatinib *on page 404*
- **SPS®** *see* Sodium Polystyrene Sulfonate *on page 1385*
- **Sronyx™** *see* Ethinyl Estradiol and Levonorgestrel *on page 577*
- **SSD®** *see* Silver Sulfadiazine *on page 1370*
- **SSD® AF** *see* Silver Sulfadiazine *on page 1370*
- **SSKI®** *see* Potassium Iodide *on page 1218*
- **Stadol® [DSC]** *see* Butorphanol *on page 231*
- **Staflex** *see* Acetaminophen and Phenyltoloxamine *on page 29*
- **Stagesic™** *see* Hydrocodone and Acetaminophen *on page 740*
- **Stalevo®** *see* Levodopa, Carbidopa, and Entacapone *on page 875*
- **StanGard®** *see* Fluoride *on page 635*
- **StanGard® Perio** *see* Fluoride *on page 635*
- **Stannous Fluoride** *see* Fluoride *on page 635*
- **Starlix®** *see* Nateglinide *on page 1045*
- **Statex® (Can)** *see* Morphine Sulfate *on page 1016*
- **Statuss™ DM** *see* Chlorpheniramine, Phenylephrine, and Dextromethorphan *on page 311*

Stavudine (STAV yoo deen)

U.S. Brand Names Zerit®

Canadian Brand Names Zerit®

Index Terms d4T

Pharmacologic Category Antiretroviral Agent, Reverse Transcriptase Inhibitor (Nucleoside)

Additional Appendix Information

Antiretroviral Therapy for HIV Infection: Adults and Adolescents *on page 1758*

Management of Healthcare Worker Exposures to HBV, HCV, and HIV *on page 1719*

Perinatal HIV Guidelines *on page 1730*

Use Treatment of HIV infection in combination with other antiretroviral agents

Pregnancy Risk Factor C

Pregnancy Considerations No increased risk of overall birth defects has been observed following 1st trimester exposure according to data collected by the antiretroviral pregnancy registry. Cases of fatal and nonfatal lactic acidosis, with or without pancreatitis, have been reported in pregnant women. It is not known if pregnancy itself potentiates this known side effect; however, pregnant women may be at increased risk of lactic acidosis and liver damage. Combination treatment with didanosine may also contribute to the risk of lactic acidosis, and should be considered only if benefit outweighs risk. Hepatic enzymes and electrolytes should be monitored frequently during the 3rd trimester of pregnancy. Pharmacokinetics of stavudine are not significantly altered during pregnancy; dose adjustments are not needed. There are no adequate and well-controlled studies in pregnant women; however, the Perinatal HIV Guidelines Working Group considers stavudine to be an alternative NRTI in dual nucleoside combination regimens; use with didanosine only if no alternatives are available, do not use with zidovudine. Health professionals are encouraged to contact the antiretroviral pregnancy registry to monitor outcomes of pregnant women exposed to antiretroviral medications (1-800-258-4263 or www.APRegistry.com).

Lactation Excretion in breast milk unknown/contraindicated

Medication Safety Issues

Sound-alike/look-alike issues:

Zerit® may be confused with Ziac®

Contraindications Hypersensitivity to stavudine or any component of the formulation

Warnings/Precautions Use with caution in patients who demonstrate previous hypersensitivity to zidovudine, didanosine, zalcitabine, pre-existing bone marrow suppression, renal insufficiency (dosage adjustment recommended), or peripheral neuropathy. Peripheral neuropathy may be the dose-limiting side effect; if neuropathy recurs after interruption and reinitiation of therapy (at a reduced dose), consider permanent discontinuation. Zidovudine should not be used in combination with stavudine. **[U.S. Boxed Warning]: Lactic acidosis and severe hepatomegaly with steatosis have been reported with stavudine use, including fatal cases;** combination therapy with didanosine may increase risk; use with caution in patients with risk factors for liver disease (although acidosis has occurred in patients without known risk factors, risk may be increased with female gender, obesity, pregnancy, or prolonged exposure). Suspend treatment in any patient who develops clinical or laboratory findings suggestive of lactic acidosis or hepatotoxicity. Severe motor weakness (resembling Guillain-Barré syndrome) has been reported (including fatal cases, usually in association with lactic acidosis); manufacturer recommends discontinuation if motor weakness develops (with or without lactic acidosis). May cause redistribution of fat (eg, buffalo hump, peripheral wasting with increased abdominal girth, cushingoid appearance). Patients may develop immune reconstitution syndrome resulting in the occurrence of an inflammatory response to an indolent or residual opportunistic infection; further evaluation and treatment may be required. **[U.S. Boxed Warning]: Pancreatitis (including some fatal cases) has occurred during combination therapy (didanosine with or without hydroxyurea).** Risk increased when used in combination regimen with didanosine (with or without hydroxyurea). Suspend therapy with agents toxic to the pancreas (including stavudine, didanosine, or hydroxyurea) in patients with suspected pancreatitis. Use with caution in combination with interferon alfa with or without ribavirin in HIV/HBV coinfected patients; monitor closely for hepatic decompensation, anemia, or neutropenia; dose reduction or discontinuation of interferon and/or ribavirin may be required if toxicity evident.

Adverse Reactions Adverse reactions reported below represent experience with combination therapy with other nucleoside analogues and protease inhibitors.

>10%:

- Central nervous system: Headache (25% to 46%)
- Dermatologic: Rash (18% to 30%)
- Gastrointestinal: Nausea (43% to 53%; less than comparator group), vomiting (18% to 30%; less than comparator group), diarrhea (34% to 45%)
- Hepatic: Hyperbilirubinemia (65% to 68%; grade 3/4: 7% to 16%), AST increased (42% to 53%; grade 3/4: 5% to 7%), ALT increased (40% to 50%; grade 3/4: 6% to 8%), GGT increased (15% to 28%; grade 3/4: 2% to 5%)
- Neuromuscular & skeletal: Peripheral neuropathy (8% to 21%)
- Miscellaneous: Amylase increased (21% to 31%; grade 3/4: 4% to 8%), lipase increased (~27%; grade 3/4: 5% to 6%)

Postmarketing and/or case reports: Abdominal pain, allergic reaction, anemia, anorexia, chills, diabetes mellitus, fever, hepatic failure, hepatitis, hepatomegaly (with steatosis; some fatal), hyperglycemia, hyperlactatemia (symptomatic), insomnia, lactic acidosis (some fatal), leukopenia, macrocytosis, motor weakness (severe), myalgia, pancreatitis, redistribution/accumulation of body fat, thrombocytopenia

Drug Interactions

Avoid Concomitant Use There are no known interactions where it is recommended to avoid concomitant use.

Increased Effect/Toxicity

Stavudine may increase the levels/effects of: Didanosine

The levels/effects of Stavudine may be increased by: Ribavirin

Decreased Effect

The levels/effects of Stavudine may be decreased by: DOXOrubicin; DOXOrubicin (Liposomal); Zidovudine

Stability Capsules and powder for reconstitution may be stored at controlled room temerature of 25°C (77°F). Reconstitute powder for oral suspension with 202 mL of purified water as specified on the bottle. Shake vigorously until suspended. Final suspension will be 1 mg/mL (200 mL). Reconstituted oral solution should be stored in refrigerator at 2°C to 8°C (36°F to 46°F) and is stable for 30 days.

Mechanism of Action Stavudine is a thymidine analog which interferes with HIV viral DNA dependent DNA polymerase resulting in inhibition of viral replication; nucleoside reverse transcriptase inhibitor

Pharmacodynamics/Kinetics

Distribution: V_d: 46 L

Bioavailability: 86.4%

Metabolism: Undergoes intracellular phosphorylation to an active metabolite

Half-life elimination: 1.2-1.6 hours

Time to peak, serum: 1 hour

Excretion: Urine (42% as unchanged drug)

Dosage Oral:

Newborns (Birth to 13 days): 0.5 mg/kg every 12 hours

Children:

- >14 days and <30 kg: 1 mg/kg every 12 hours
- ≥30 kg: Refer to adult dosing

Adults:

- ≥60 kg: 40 mg every 12 hours
- <60 kg: 30 mg every 12 hours

Dosing adjustment for toxicity: If symptoms of peripheral neuropathy occur, discontinue until symptoms resolve. Treatment may then be resumed at 50% the recommended dose. If symptoms recur at lower dose, permanent discontinuation should be considered.

Dosing adjustment in renal impairment:

Children: Specific recommendations not available. Reduction in dose or increase in dosing interval should be considered.

Adults:

Cl_{cr} >50 mL/minute:

≥60 kg: 40 mg every 12 hours

<60 kg: 30 mg every 12 hours

Cl_{cr} 26-50 mL/minute:

≥60 kg: 20 mg every 12 hours

<60 kg: 15 mg every 12 hours

Cl_{cr} 10-25 mL/minute, hemodialysis (administer dose after hemodialysis on day of dialysis):

≥60 kg: 20 mg every 24 hours

<60 kg: 15 mg every 24 hours

Elderly: Older patients should be closely monitored for signs and symptoms of peripheral neuropathy; dosage should be carefully adjusted to renal function

Dietary Considerations May be taken without regard to meals. Oral solution contains sucrose 50 mg/mL.

Administration May be administered without regard to meals. Oral solution should be shaken vigorously prior to use.

Monitoring Parameters Monitor liver function tests and renal function tests; signs and symptoms of peripheral neuropathy; monitor viral load and CD4 count

Additional Information Potential compliance problems, frequency of administration and adverse effects should be discussed with patients before initiating therapy to help prevent the emergence of resistance.

Dosage Forms Excipient information presented when available (limited, particularly for generics); consult specific product labeling.

Capsule: 15 mg, 20 mg, 30 mg, 40 mg

Zerit®: 15 mg, 20 mg, 30 mg, 40 mg

Powder for solution, oral:

Zerit®: 1 mg/mL (200 mL) [dye free; contains sucrose 50 mg/mL; fruit flavor]

- **Stavzor™** *see* Valproic Acid and Derivatives *on page 1538*
- **Stemetil® (Can)** *see* Prochlorperazine *on page 1244*
- **Sterapred®** *see* PredniSONE *on page 1232*
- **Sterapred® DS** *see* PredniSONE *on page 1232*
- **Sterile Talc** *see* Talc (Sterile) *on page 1424*
- **Sterile Talc Powder™** *see* Talc (Sterile) *on page 1424*
- **STI-571** *see* Imatinib *on page 768*
- **Stieprox® (Can)** *see* Ciclopirox *on page 324*
- **Stimate®** *see* Desmopressin *on page 421*
- **Sting-Kill [OTC]** *see* Benzocaine *on page 183*
- **St. Joseph® Adult Aspirin [OTC]** *see* Aspirin *on page 142*
- **Stop®** *see* Fluoride *on page 635*
- **Strattera®** *see* Atomoxetine *on page 150*

Streptomycin (strep toe MYE sin)

Index Terms Streptomycin Sulfate

Pharmacologic Category Antibiotic, Aminoglycoside; Antitubercular Agent

Use Part of combination therapy of active tuberculosis; used in combination with other agents for treatment of streptococcal or enterococcal endocarditis, mycobacterial infections, plague, tularemia, and brucellosis

Pregnancy Risk Factor D

Pregnancy Considerations Streptomycin crosses the placenta. Many case reports of hearing impairment in children exposed *in utero* have been published. Impairment has ranged from mild hearing loss to bilateral deafness. Because of several reports of total irreversible bilateral congenital deafness in children whose mothers received streptomycin during pregnancy, the manufacturer classifies streptomycin as pregnancy risk factor D.

Lactation Enters breast milk/not recommended (AAP rates "compatible")

Medication Safety Issues

Sound-alike/look-alike issues:

Streptomycin may be confused with streptozocin

Contraindications Hypersensitivity to streptomycin or any component of the formulation; pregnancy

Warnings/Precautions [U.S. Boxed Warning]: May cause neurotoxicity, nephrotoxicity, and/or neuromuscular blockade and respiratory paralysis; usual risk factors include pre-existing renal impairment, concomitant neuro-/nephrotoxic medications, advanced age and dehydration. The drug's neurotoxicity can result in respiratory paralysis from neuromuscular blockade, especially when the drug is given soon after anesthesia or muscle relaxants. Use with caution in patients with pre-existing vertigo, tinnitus, hearing loss, neuromuscular disorders, or renal impairment; modify dosage in patients with renal impairment; ototoxicity is directly proportional to the amount of drug given and the duration of treatment; tinnitus or vertigo are indications of vestibular injury and impending bilateral irreversible damage; renal damage is usually reversible. **[U.S. Boxed Warning]: Parenteral form should be used only where appropriate audiometric and laboratory testing facilities are available.** Prolonged use may result in fungal or bacterial superinfection, including *C. difficile*-associated diarrhea (CDAD) and pseudomembranous colitis; CDAD has been observed >2 months postantibiotic treatment.

Adverse Reactions Frequency not defined.

Cardiovascular: Hypotension

Central nervous system: Neurotoxicity, drowsiness, headache, drug fever, paresthesia

Dermatologic: Skin rash

Gastrointestinal: Nausea, vomiting

Hematologic: Eosinophilia, anemia

Neuromuscular & skeletal: Arthralgia, weakness, tremor

Otic: Ototoxicity (auditory), ototoxicity (vestibular)

Renal: Nephrotoxicity

Respiratory: Difficulty in breathing

Drug Interactions

Avoid Concomitant Use

Avoid concomitant use of Streptomycin with any of the following: Gallium Nitrate

Increased Effect/Toxicity

Streptomycin may increase the levels/effects of: Bisphosphonate Derivatives; Botulinum Toxin Type A; Botulinum Toxin Type B; CARBOplatin; Colistimethate; CycloSPORINE; Gallium Nitrate; Neuromuscular-Blocking Agents

The levels/effects of Streptomycin may be increased by: Amphotericin B; Capreomycin; CISplatin; Loop Diuretics; Nonsteroidal Anti-Inflammatory Agents; Vancomycin

Decreased Effect

Streptomycin may decrease the levels/effects of: Typhoid Vaccine

The levels/effects of Streptomycin may be decreased by: Penicillins

Stability Depending upon manufacturer, reconstituted solution remains stable for 2-4 weeks when refrigerated. Exposure to light causes darkening of solution without apparent loss of potency.

Mechanism of Action Inhibits bacterial protein synthesis by binding directly to the 30S ribosomal subunits causing faulty peptide sequence to form in the protein chain

Pharmacodynamics/Kinetics

Absorption:

Oral: Poorly absorbed

I.M.: Well absorbed

Distribution: To extracellular fluid including serum, abscesses, ascitic, pericardial, pleural, synovial, lymphatic, and peritoneal fluids; poorly distributed into CSF

Protein binding: 34%

Half-life elimination: Newborns: 4-10 hours; Adults: 2-4.7 hours, prolonged with renal impairment

Time to peak: I.M.: Within 1 hour

Excretion: Urine (90% as unchanged drug); feces, saliva, sweat, and tears (<1%)

Dosage Note: For I.M. administration; I.V. use is not recommended

Usual dosage range:

Children: 20-40 mg/kg/day (maximum: 1 g)

Adults: 15-30 mg/kg/day or 1-2 g/day

Indication-specific dosing:

Children: **Tuberculosis:** I.M.:

Daily therapy: 20-40 mg/kg/day (maximum: 1 g/day)

Directly observed therapy (DOT): Twice weekly: 25-30 mg/kg (maximum: 1.5 g)

Directly observed therapy DOT: 3 times/week: 25-30 mg/kg (maximum: 1.5 g)

Adults: I.M.:

Brucellosis: 1 g/day for 14-21 days (with doxycycline, 100 mg twice daily for 6 weeks)

Endocarditis:

Enterococcal: 1 g every 12 hours for 2 weeks, 500 mg every 12 hours for 4 weeks in combination with penicillin

Streptococcal: 1 g every 12 hours for 1 week, 500 mg every 12 hours for 1 week

***Mycobacterium avium* complex:** Adjunct therapy (with macrolide, rifamycin, and ethambutol): 15 mg/kg 3 times/week for first 2-3 months for severe disease

Plague: 15 mg/kg (or 1 g) every 12 hours until the patient is afebrile for at least 3 days

Tuberculosis:

Daily therapy: 15 mg/kg/day (maximum: 1 g)

Directly observed therapy (DOT): Twice weekly: 25-30 mg/kg (maximum: 1.5 g)

Directly observed therapy DOT: 3 times/week: 25-30 mg/kg (maximum: 1.5 g)

Tularemia: 10-15 mg/kg every 12 hours (maximum: 2 g/day) for 7-10 days or until patient is afebrile for 5-7 days

Elderly: I.M.: 10 mg/kg/day, not to exceed 750 mg/day; dosing interval should be adjusted for renal function; some authors suggest not to give more than 5 days/week or give as 20-25 mg/kg/dose twice weekly

Dosing interval in renal impairment:

Cl_{cr} 10-50 mL/minute: Administer every 24-72 hours

Cl_{cr} <10 mL/minute: Administer every 72-96 hours

Removed by hemo- and peritoneal dialysis: Administer dose postdialysis

Administration Inject deep I.M. into large muscle mass; I.V. administration is not recommended; has been administered intravenously over 30-60 minutes.

Monitoring Parameters Hearing (audiogram), BUN, creatinine; serum concentration of the drug should be monitored in all patients; eighth cranial nerve damage is usually preceded by high-pitched tinnitus, roaring noises, sense of fullness in ears, or impaired hearing and may persist for weeks after drug is discontinued

Reference Range Therapeutic: Peak: 20-30 mcg/mL; Trough: <5 mcg/mL; Toxic: Peak: >50 mcg/mL; Trough: >10 mcg/mL

Test Interactions False-positive urine glucose with Benedict's solution or Clinitest®; penicillin may decrease aminoglycoside serum concentrations *in vitro*

Dosage Forms Excipient information presented when available (limited, particularly for generics); consult specific product labeling.

Injection, powder for reconstitution: 1 g

- **Streptomycin Sulfate** *see* Streptomycin *on page 1400*
- **Striant®** *see* Testosterone *on page 1445*
- **Strifon Forte® (Can)** *see* Chlorzoxazone *on page 318*
- **Stromectol®** *see* Ivermectin *on page 831*
- **Strong Iodine Solution** *see* Potassium Iodide and Iodine *on page 1220*
- **Strontium-89 Chloride** *see* Strontium-89 *on page 1401*

Strontium-89 (STRON shee um atey nine)

U.S. Brand Names Metastron®

Canadian Brand Names Metastron®

Index Terms Strontium-89 Chloride

Pharmacologic Category Radiopharmaceutical

Use Relief of bone pain in patients with skeletal metastases

Pregnancy Risk Factor D

Dosage Adults: I.V.: 148 megabecquerel (4 millicurie) administered by slow I.V. injection over 1-2 minutes or 1.5-2.2 megabecquerel (40-60 microcurie)/kg; repeated doses are generally not recommended at intervals <90 days; measure the patient dose by a suitable radioactivity calibration system immediately prior to administration

Additional Information Complete prescribing information for this medication should be consulted for additional detail.

Dosage Forms Excipient information presented when available (limited, particularly for generics); consult specific product labeling.

Injection, solution, as chloride [preservative free]:

Metastron®: 10.9-22.6 mg/mL (4 mL) [148 megabecquerel, 4 millicurie per vial]

- **SU11248** *see* Sunitinib *on page 1416*
- **Suberoylanilide Hydroxamic Acid** *see* Vorinostat *on page 1569*
- **Sublimaze®** *see* FentaNYL *on page 610*
- **Suboxone®** *see* Buprenorphine and Naloxone *on page 223*
- **Subutex®** *see* Buprenorphine *on page 221*

Succimer (SUKS si mer)

U.S. Brand Names Chemet®

Canadian Brand Names Chemet®

Index Terms DMSA

Pharmacologic Category Antidote

Use Treatment of lead poisoning in children with serum lead levels >45 mcg/dL

Unlabeled/Investigational Use

Treatment of lead poisoning in symptomatic adults

Pregnancy Risk Factor C

Pregnancy Considerations Adverse events were observed in animal reproduction studies. Following maternal occupational exposure, lead crosses the placenta in amounts related to maternal plasma levels. Possible outcomes of maternal lead exposure >10 mcg/dL includes spontaneous abortion, postnatal developmental delay, and reduced birth weight. Chelation therapy during pregnancy is for maternal benefit only and should be limited to the treatment of severe, symptomatic lead poisoning.

Lactation Excretion in breast milk unknown/not recommended

Contraindications Hypersensitivity to succimer or any component of the formulation

Warnings/Precautions Remove sources of lead exposure prior to treatment. Consult experts before using chelation drug therapy for lead removal. Succimer should not be used to treat encephalopathy associated with lead toxicity. Caution in patients with renal or hepatic impairment; adequate hydration should be maintained during therapy. Succimer is dialyzable, however, the lead chelates are not. Rebounding serum lead levels may occur after treatment.

Adverse Reactions Note: Percentages as reported in pediatric patients unless otherwise noted.

>10%: Gastrointestinal: Appetite decreased, diarrhea, hemorrhoid symptoms, metallic taste, loose stools, nausea, vomiting

1% to 10%:

Cardiovascular: Arrhythmia (adults 2%)

Central nervous system: Chills, dizziness, drowsiness, fatigue, fever, headache, sleepiness

Dermatologic: Rash (including papular rash, herpetic rash and mucocutaneous eruptions); pruritus

Endocrine & metabolic: Cholesterol increased

Gastrointestinal: Abdominal cramps, mucosal irritation, sore throat

Genitourinary: Proteinuria (adults), urine output decreased (adults), voiding difficulty (adults)

Hepatic: Alkaline phosphatase increased, ALT increased, AST increased

Neuromuscular & skeletal: Back pain, flank pain, leg pain (adults), neuropathy, paresthesia, rib pain

Ocular: Cloudy film in eye, watery eyes

Otic: Otitis media, plugged ears

Respiratory: Cough, nasal congestion, rhinorrhea

Miscellaneous: Flu-like syndrome, moniliasis

<1% (Limited to important or life-threatening): Allergic reactions (especially with retreatment), eosinophilia, neutropenia (causal relationship not established)

Drug Interactions

Avoid Concomitant Use There are no known interactions where it is recommended to avoid concomitant use.

Increased Effect/Toxicity There are no known significant interactions involving an increase in effect.

Decreased Effect There are no known significant interactions involving a decrease in effect.

Stability Store between 15°C to 25°C (59°F to 77°F); avoid excessive heat.

Mechanism of Action Succimer is an analog of dimercaprol. It forms water soluble chelates with heavy metals which are subsequently excreted renally. Succimer binds heavy metals; however, the chemical form of these chelates is not known.

Pharmacodynamics/Kinetics

Absorption: Rapid but incomplete

Protein binding: Highly bound to albumin

Metabolism: Rapidly and extensively to mixed succimer cysteine disulfides

Half-life elimination: 2 days

Time to peak, serum: ~1-2 hours

Excretion: Urine (~25%) with peak urinary excretion between 2-4 hours (90% as mixed succimer-cysteine disulfide conjugates, 10% as unchanged drug); feces (as unabsorbed drug)

Dosage Note: For the treatment of high blood lead levels in children, the CDC recommends chelation treatment when blood lead levels are >45 mcg/dL (CDC, 2002). Children with blood lead levels >70 mcg/dL or symptomatic lead poisoning should be treated with parenteral agents (AAP, 2005). In adults, available guidelines recommend chelation therapy with blood lead levels >50 mcg/dL and significant symptoms; chelation therapy may also be indicated with blood lead levels ≥100 mcg/dL and/or symptoms. (Kosnett, 2007).

Children: Oral: 10 mg/kg/dose (or 350 mg/m^2/dose) every 8 hours for 5 days followed by 10 mg/kg/dose (or 350 mg/m^2/dose) every 12 hours for 14 days. Maximum: 500 mg/dose. For children <5 years of age, dose should be based on mg/m^2; dosing by mg/kg may be suboptimal.

Adults (mild symptoms or blood lead levels 70-100 mg/dL; unlabeled use): 10 mg/kg/dose (or 350 mg/m^2/dose) every 8 hours for 5 days, followed by 10 mg/kg/dose (or 350 mg/m^2/dose) every 12 hours for 14 days; Maximum: 500 mg/dose

Note: Treatment courses may be repeated, but 2-week intervals between courses is generally recommended.

Dosing adjustment in renal/hepatic impairment: Administer with caution and monitor closely

Administration Capsule can be separated and contents sprinkled on a small amount of soft food, or the contents placed on a spoon and administered followed by fruit drink.

Monitoring Parameters Blood lead levels (baseline and 7-21 days after completing chelation therapy); serum aminotransferase, CBC with differential, platelets (baseline, and weekly during treatment); hemoglobin or hematocrit, iron status, free erythrocyte protoporphyrin or zinc protoporphyrin; neurodevelopmental changes

Test Interactions False-positive ketones (U) using nitroprusside methods, falsely decreased serum CPK; falsely decreased uric acid measurement

Dosage Forms Excipient information presented when available (limited, particularly for generics); consult specific product labeling.

Capsule:

Chemet®:100 mg

Succinylcholine (suks in il KOE leen)

U.S. Brand Names Anectine®; Quelicin®

Canadian Brand Names Quelicin®

Index Terms Succinylcholine Chloride; Suxamethonium Chloride

Pharmacologic Category Neuromuscular Blocker Agent, Depolarizing

Additional Appendix Information

Neuromuscular-Blocking Agents *on page 1665*

Use Adjunct to general anesthesia to facilitate both rapid sequence and routine endotracheal intubation and to relax skeletal muscles during surgery; to reduce the intensity of muscle contractions of pharmacologically- or electrically-induced convulsions; does not relieve pain or produce sedation

Pregnancy Risk Factor C

Pregnancy Considerations Reproduction studies have not been conducted. Small amounts cross the placenta. Sensitivity to succinylcholine may be increased due to a ~24% decrease in plasma cholinesterase activity during pregnancy and several days postpartum.

Lactation Excretion in breast milk unknown/use caution

Medication Safety Issues

High alert medication: The Institute for Safe Medication Practices (ISMP) includes this medication among its list of drugs which have a heightened risk of causing significant patient harm when used in error.

Contraindications Hypersensitivity to succinylcholine or any component of the formulation; personal or familial history of malignant hyperthermia; myopathies associated with elevated serum creatine phosphokinase (CPK) values; acute phase of injury following major burns, multiple trauma, extensive denervation of skeletal muscle or upper motor neuron injury

Warnings/Precautions [U.S. Boxed Warning]: Use caution in children and adolescents. Acute rhabdomyolysis with hyperkalemia, ventricular arrhythmias and cardiac arrest have been reported (rarely) in children with undiagnosed skeletal muscle myopathy. Use in children should be reserved for emergency intubation or where immediate airway control is necessary.

Use with caution in patients with pre-existing hyperkalemia, extensive or severe burns; severe hyperkalemia may develop in patients with chronic abdominal infections, burn injuries, children with skeletal muscle myopathy, subarachnoid hemorrhage, or conditions which cause degeneration of the nervous system. Alkalosis, hypercalcemia, demyelinating lesions, peripheral neuropathies, denervation, infection, muscle trauma, and diabetes mellitus may result in antagonism of neuromuscular blockade. Electrolyte abnormalities, severe hyponatremia, severe hypocalcemia, severe hypokalemia, hypermagnesemia, neuromuscular diseases, acidosis, acute intermittent porphyria, Eaton-Lambert syndrome, myasthenia gravis, renal failure, and hepatic failure may result in potentiation of neuromuscular blockade. May increase vagal tone.

Succinylcholine is metabolized by plasma cholinesterase; use with caution (if at all) in patients suspected of being homozygous for the atypical plasma cholinesterase gene.

Use with caution in patients with extensive or severe burns; risk of hyperkalemia is increased following injury. May increase intraocular pressure; use caution with narrow angle glaucoma or penetrating eye injuries. Risk of bradycardia may be increased with second dose and may occur more in children. Use may be associated with acute onset of malignant hyperthermia; risk may be increased with concomitant administration of volatile anesthetics. Use with caution in the elderly; effects and duration are more variable.

Maintenance of an adequate airway and respiratory support is critical. Should be administered by adequately trained individuals familiar with its use.

Adverse Reactions

Frequency not defined.

Cardiovascular: Arrhythmias, bradycardia (higher with second dose, more frequent in children), cardiac arrest, hyper-/hypotension, tachycardia

Dermatologic: Rash

Endocrine & metabolic: Hyperkalemia

Gastrointestinal: Salivation (excessive)

Neuromuscular & skeletal: Jaw rigidity, muscle fasciculation, postoperative muscle pain, rhabdomyolysis (with possible myoglobinuric acute renal failure)

Ocular: Intraocular pressure increased

Renal: Acute renal failure (secondary to rhabdomyolysis)

Respiratory: Apnea, respiratory depression (prolonged)

Miscellaneous: Anaphylaxis, malignant hyperthermia

Postmarketing and/or case reports: Acute quadriplegic myopathy syndrome (prolonged use), myositis ossificans (prolonged use)

Drug Interactions

Avoid Concomitant Use There are no known interactions where it is recommended to avoid concomitant use.

Increased Effect/Toxicity

Succinylcholine may increase the levels/effects of: Analgesics (Opioid); Botulinum Toxin Type A; Botulinum Toxin Type B; Cardiac Glycosides

The levels/effects of Succinylcholine may be increased by: Acetylcholinesterase Inhibitors; Aminoglycosides; Capreomycin; Colistimethate; Cyclophosphamide; Echothiophate Iodide; Lincosamide Antibiotics; Lithium; Loop Diuretics; Magnesium Salts; Phenelzine; Polymyxin B; Procainamide; QuiNIDine; Tetracycline Derivatives; Vancomycin

Decreased Effect

The levels/effects of Succinylcholine may be decreased by: Loop Diuretics

Stability Refrigerate at 2°C to 8°C (36°F to 46°F); however, stable for ≤3 months unrefrigerated (25°C). May dilute to a final concentration of 1-2 mg/mL. Do not mix with alkaline solutions (pH > 8.5). Stability of parenteral admixture (1-2 mg/mL) at refrigeration temperature (4°C) is 24 hours in D_5W or NS.

Mechanism of Action Acts similar to acetylcholine, produces depolarization of the motor endplate at the myoneural junction which causes sustained flaccid skeletal muscle paralysis produced by state of accommodation that developes in adjacent excitable muscle membranes

Pharmacodynamics/Kinetics

Onset of action: I.M.: 2-3 minutes; I.V.: Complete muscular relaxation: 30-60 seconds

Duration: I.M.: 10-30 minutes; I.V.: 4-6 minutes with single administration

Metabolism: Rapidly hydrolyzed by plasma pseudocholinesterase

Excretion: Urine

Dosage I.M., I.V.: Dose to effect; doses will vary due to interpatient variability; use ideal body weight for obese patients

I.M.: Children and Adults: Up to 3-4 mg/kg, total dose should not exceed 150 mg

I.V.:

Children: **Note:** Because of the risk of malignant hyperthermia, use of continuous infusions is not recommended in infants and children

Smaller Children: Intermittent: Initial: 2 mg/kg/dose one time; maintenance: 0.3-0.6 mg/kg/ dose every 5-10 minutes as needed

Older Children and Adolescents: Intermittent: Initial: 1 mg/kg/dose one time; maintenance: 0.3-0.6 mg/kg every 5-10 minutes as needed

Adults: Initial:

Short surgical procedures: 0.6 mg/kg (range 0.3-1.1 mg/kg)

Long surgical procedures:

Continuous infusion: 2.5-4.3 mg/minute; adjust dose based on response

Intermittent: Initial: 0.3-1.1 mg/kg; maintenance: 0.04-0.07 mg/kg/dose as required

Note: Initial dose of succinylcholine must be increased when nondepolarizing agent pretreatment used because of the antagonism between succinylcholine and nondepolarizing neuromuscular-blocking agents.

Dose adjustment with reduced plasma cholinesterase activity: Administer a test dose of 5-10 mg to evaluate sensitivity, or cautiously administer 1 mg/mL by slow I.V. infusion to produce neuromuscular blockade

Dosing adjustment in hepatic impairment: Dose should be decreased in patients with severe liver disease

Administration May be administered by rapid I.V. injection without further dilution. I.M. injections should be made deeply, preferably high into deltoid muscle; use only when I.V. access is not available.

Monitoring Parameters Monitor cardiac, blood pressure, and oxygenation during administration; temperature, serum potassium and calcium, assisted ventilator status; neuromuscular function with a peripheral nerve stimulator

Dosage Forms Excipient information presented when available (limited, particularly for generics); consult specific product labeling.

Injection, solution, as chloride:

Anectine®: 20 mg/mL (10 mL)

Quelicin®: 20 mg/mL (10 mL)

Injection, solution, as chloride [preservative free]:

Quelicin®: 100 mg/mL (10 mL)

◆ **Succinylcholine Chloride** *see* Succinylcholine *on page 1402*

◆ **Suclor™** *see* Chlorpheniramine and Pseudoephedrine *on page 310*

◆ **Sucraid®** *see* Sacrosidase *on page 1350*

Sucralfate (soo KRAL fate)

U.S. Brand Names Carafate®

Canadian Brand Names Novo-Sucralate; Nu-Sucralate; PMS-Sucralate; Sulcrate®; Sulcrate® Suspension Plus

Index Terms Aluminum Sucrose Sulfate, Basic

Pharmacologic Category Gastrointestinal Agent, Miscellaneous

Use Short-term (≤8 weeks) management of duodenal ulcers; maintenance therapy for duodenal ulcers

Unlabeled/Investigational Use Gastric ulcers; suspension may be used topically for treatment of stomatitis due to cancer chemotherapy and other causes of esophageal and gastric erosions; GERD, esophagitis; treatment of NSAID mucosal damage; prevention of stress ulcers; postsclerotherapy for esophageal variceal bleeding

Pregnancy Risk Factor B

Medication Safety Issues

Sound-alike/look-alike issues:

Sucralfate may be confused with salsalate

Carafate® may be confused with Cafergot®

Dosage Oral:

Children (unlabeled use): Doses of 40-80 mg/kg/day divided every 6 hours have been used

Stomatitis (unlabeled use): 5-10 mL (1 g/10 mL suspension), swish and spit or swish and swallow 4 times/day

Adults:

Stress ulcer (unlabeled use):

Prophylaxis: 1 g 4 times/day

Treatment: 1 g every 4 hours

Duodenal ulcer:

Treatment: 1 g 4 times/day on an empty stomach and at bedtime for 4-8 weeks, or alternatively 2 g twice daily; treatment is recommended for 4-8 weeks in adults

Maintenance: Prophylaxis: 1 g twice daily

Stomatitis (unlabeled use): 10 mL (1 g/10 mL suspension), swish and spit or swish and swallow 4 times/day

Dosage comment in renal impairment: Aluminum salt is minimally absorbed (<5%), however, may accumulate in renal failure

Additional Information Complete prescribing information for this medication should be consulted for additional detail.

Dosage Forms Excipient information presented when available (limited, particularly for generics); consult specific product labeling.

Suspension, oral: 1 g/10 mL (10 mL)

Carafate®: 1 g/10 mL (420 mL)

Tablet: 1 g

Carafate®: 1 g

◆ **Sucrets® [OTC]** *see* Dyclonine *on page 501*

◆ **Sudafed® 12 Hour [OTC]** *see* Pseudoephedrine *on page 1265*

◆ **Sudafed® 24 Hour [OTC]** *see* Pseudoephedrine *on page 1265*

◆ **Sudafed® Children's [OTC]** *see* Pseudoephedrine *on page 1265*

◆ **Sudafed® Children's Cold & Cough [OTC]** *see* Pseudoephedrine and Dextromethorphan *on page 1266*

◆ **Sudafed® Cold & Cough Extra Strength (Can)** *see* Acetaminophen, Dextromethorphan, and Pseudoephedrine *on page 33*

◆ **Sudafed® Decongestant (Can)** *see* Pseudoephedrine *on page 1265*

◆ **Sudafed® Head Cold and Sinus Extra Strength (Can)** *see* Acetaminophen and Pseudoephedrine *on page 30*

◆ **Sudafed® Maximum Strength Nasal Decongestant [OTC]** *see* Pseudoephedrine *on page 1265*

◆ **Sudafed® Maximum Strength Sinus Nighttime [OTC] [DSC]** *see* Triprolidine and Pseudoephedrine *on page 1522*

◆ **Sudafed® Multi-Symptom Sinus and Cold [OTC]** *see* Acetaminophen and Pseudoephedrine *on page 30*

◆ **Sudafed PE™ [OTC]** *see* Phenylephrine *on page 1183*

◆ **Sudafed PE® Nighttime Cold [OTC]** *see* Acetaminophen, Diphenhydramine, and Phenylephrine *on page 33*

◆ **Sudafed PE® Severe Cold [OTC]** *see* Acetaminophen, Diphenhydramine, and Phenylephrine *on page 33*

◆ **Sudafed PE® Sinus & Allergy [OTC]** *see* Chlorpheniramine and Phenylephrine *on page 309*

◆ **Sudafed PE® Sinus Headache [OTC]** *see* Acetaminophen and Phenylephrine *on page 29*

◆ **Sudafed® Sinus Advance (Can)** *see* Pseudoephedrine and Ibuprofen *on page 1267*

◆ **Sudafed® Sinus & Allergy [OTC]** *see* Chlorpheniramine and Pseudoephedrine *on page 310*

◆ **SudaHist®** *see* Chlorpheniramine and Pseudoephedrine *on page 310*

◆ **Sudal® 12** *see* Chlorpheniramine and Pseudoephedrine *on page 310*

◆ **SudaTex-DM** *see* Guaifenesin, Pseudoephedrine, and Dextromethorphan *on page 715*

◆ **SudaTex-G** *see* Guaifenesin and Pseudoephedrine *on page 713*

◆ **SudoGest [OTC]** *see* Pseudoephedrine *on page 1265*

◆ **SudoGest Children's [OTC]** *see* Pseudoephedrine and Dextromethorphan *on page 1266*

◆ **Sudo-Tab® [OTC]** *see* Pseudoephedrine *on page 1265*

◆ **Sufenta®** *see* SUFentanil *on page 1404*

SUFentanil (soo FEN ta nil)

U.S. Brand Names Sufenta®

Canadian Brand Names Sufentanil Citrate Injection, USP; Sufenta®

Index Terms Sufentanil Citrate

Pharmacologic Category Analgesic, Opioid; Anilidopiperidine Opioid; General Anesthetic

Use Analgesic supplement in maintenance of balanced general anesthesia; primary anesthetic for induction and maintenance of anesthesia in patients undergoing major surgical procedures; epidural anesthetic in conjunction with bupivacaine in labor and delivery

Restrictions C-II

Pregnancy Risk Factor C/D (prolonged use or high doses at term)

Medication Safety Issues

Sound-alike/look-alike issues:

SUFentanil may be confused with alfentanil, fentaNYL

Sufenta® may be confused with Alfenta®, Sudafed®, Survanta®

High alert medication: The Institute for Safe Medication Practices (ISMP) includes this medication among its list of drugs which have a heightened risk of causing significant patient harm when used in error.

Dosage

I.V.:

Children 2-12 years: Induction: 10-25 mcg/kg (10-15 mcg/kg most common dose) with 100% O_2; Maintenance: Up to 1-2 mcg/kg total dose

Adults: Dose should be based on body weight. **Note:** In obese patients (eg, >20% above ideal body weight), use lean body weight to determine dosage.

Surgical analgesia (surgery 1-2 hours long): Total dose:1-2 mcg/kg; ≥75% of dose administered prior to intubation; administered with N_2O/O_2; Maintenance: 5-20 mcg as needed. Total dose should not exceed 1 mcg/kg/hour of expected surgical time.

Epidural: Adults: Analgesia: Labor and delivery: 10-15 mcg with 10 mL bupivacaine 0.125% with/without epinephrine. May repeat at ≥1-hour interval for 2 additional doses.

Additional Information Complete prescribing information for this medication should be consulted for additional detail.

Dosage Forms Excipient information presented when available (limited, particularly for generics); consult specific product labeling.

Injection, solution [preservative free]: 50 mcg/mL (1 mL, 2 mL, 5 mL)

Sufenta®: 50 mcg/mL (1 mL, 2 mL, 5 mL)

◆ **Sufentanil Citrate** *see* SUFentanil *on page 1404*

◆ **Sufentanil Citrate Injection, USP (Can)** *see* SUFentanil *on page 1404*

◆ **Sular®** *see* Nisoldipine *on page 1070*

◆ **Sulbactam and Ampicillin** *see* Ampicillin and Sulbactam *on page 111*

Sulconazole (sul KON a zole)

U.S. Brand Names Exelderm®

Canadian Brand Names Exelderm®

Index Terms Sulconazole Nitrate

Pharmacologic Category Antifungal Agent, Topical

Use Treatment of superficial fungal infections of the skin, including tinea cruris (jock itch), tinea corporis (ringworm), tinea versicolor, and possibly tinea pedis (athlete's foot, cream only)

Pregnancy Risk Factor C

Dosage Adults: Topical: Apply a small amount to the affected area and gently massage once or twice daily for 3 weeks (tinea cruris, tinea corporis, tinea versicolor) to 4 weeks (tinea pedis).

Additional Information Complete prescribing information for this medication should be consulted for additional detail.

Dosage Forms Excipient information presented when available (limited, particularly for generics); consult specific product labeling.

Cream, as nitrate:

Exelderm®: 1% (15 g, 30 g, 60 g)

Solution, topical, as nitrate:

Exelderm®: 1% (30 mL)

◆ **Sulconazole Nitrate** *see* Sulconazole *on page 1405*

◆ **Sulcrate® (Can)** *see* Sucralfate *on page 1404*

◆ **Sulcrate® Suspension Plus (Can)** *see* Sucralfate *on page 1404*

Sulfacetamide (sul fa SEE ta mide)

U.S. Brand Names Bleph®-10; Carmol® Scalp Treatment; Klaron®; Mexar™ [DSC]; Ovace®; Ovace® Plus; Rosula® NS; Seb-Prev™

Canadian Brand Names Cetamide™; Diosulf™

Index Terms Sodium Sulfacetamide; Sulfacetamide Sodium

Pharmacologic Category Acne Products; Antibiotic, Ophthalmic; Antibiotic, Sulfonamide Derivative; Topical Skin Product, Acne

Additional Appendix Information

Sulfonamide Derivatives *on page 1671*

Use

Ophthalmic: Treatment and prophylaxis of conjunctivitis due to susceptible organisms; corneal ulcers; adjunctive treatment with systemic sulfonamides for therapy of trachoma

Dermatologic: Scaling dermatosis (seborrheic); bacterial infections of the skin; acne vulgaris

Pregnancy Risk Factor C

Medication Safety Issues

Sound-alike/look-alike issues:

Bleph®-10 may be confused with Blephamide®

Klaron® may be confused with Klor-Con®

Dosage

Children >2 months and Adults: Ophthalmic:

Ointment: Apply to lower conjunctival sac 1-4 times/day and at bedtime

Solution: Instill 1-2 drops several times daily up to every 2-3 hours in lower conjunctival sac during waking hours and less frequently at night; increase dosing interval as condition responds. Usual duration of treatment: 7-10 days

Trachoma: Instill 2 drops into the conjunctival sac every 2 hours; must be used in conjunction with systemic therapy

Children >12 years and Adults: Topical:

Acne: Apply thin film to affected area twice daily

Seborrheic dermatitis: Apply at bedtime and allow to remain overnight; in severe cases, may apply twice daily. Duration of therapy is usually 8-10 applications; dosing interval may be increased as eruption subsides. Applications once or twice weekly, or every other week may be used to prevent eruptions.

Secondary cutaneous bacterial infections: Apply 2-4 times/day until infection clears

Additional Information Complete prescribing information for this medication should be consulted for additional detail.

Dosage Forms Excipient information presented when available (limited, particularly for generics); consult specific product labeling. [DSC] = Discontinued product

Aerosal, topical, as sodium [foam]:

Ovace®: 10% (50 g [DSC], 100 g)

Cream, topical, as sodium:

Ovace®: 10% (30 g, 60 g) [DSC]

Seb-Prev™: 10% (30 g, 60 g)

Gel, topical, as sodium:

Ovace® [DSC], Seb-Prev™: 10% (30 g, 60 g)

Lotion, topical, as sodium: 10% (120 mL)

Carmol® Scalp Treatment: 10% (85 g) [contains urea 10%]

Klaron®: 10% (120 mL) [contains sodium metabisulfite]

Lotion, topical, as sodium [wash]:

Ovace®: 10% (180 mL, 360 mL)

Lotion, topical, as sodium [emulsion-based wash]:

Ovace® Plus: 10% (180 mL, 360 mL)

Ointment, ophthalmic, as sodium: 10% (3.5 g) [DSC]

Pad, topical, as sodium:

Rosula® NS: 10% (30s) [contains urea 10%]

Soap, topical, as sodium [wash]:

Mexar™: 10% (170 mL) [DSC]

Seb-Prev™: 10% (170 mL, 340 mL)

Solution, ophthalmic, as sodium [drops]: 10% (15 mL)

Bleph®-10: 10% (5 mL) [contains benzalkonium chloride]

Suspension, topical, as sodium: 10% (118 mL)

Sulfacetamide and Prednisolone
(sul fa SEE ta mide & pred NIS oh lone)

U.S. Brand Names Blephamide®

Canadian Brand Names Blephamide®; Dioptimyd®

Index Terms Prednisolone and Sulfacetamide

Pharmacologic Category Antibiotic/Corticosteroid, Ophthalmic

Use Steroid-responsive inflammatory ocular conditions in which a corticosteroid is indicated and where infection is present or there is a risk of infection

Pregnancy Risk Factor C

Medication Safety Issues

Sound-alike/look-alike issues:

Blephamide® may be confused with Bleph®-10

Dosage Ophthalmic:Children ≥6 years and Adults:

Ointment: Apply ~1/2 inch ribbon to lower conjunctival sac 3-4 times/day and 1-2 times at night

Solution: Instill 2 drops every 4 hours

Suspension: Instill 2 drops every 4 hours during the day and at bedtime

Additional Information Complete prescribing information for this medication should be consulted for additional detail.

Dosage Forms Excipient information presented when available (limited, particularly for generics); consult specific product labeling.

Ointment, ophthalmic:

Blephamide®: Sulfacetamide sodium 10% and prednisolone acetate 0.2% (3.5 g)

Solution, ophthalmic [drops]: Sulfacetamide sodium 10% and prednisolone sodium phosphate 0.25% (5 mL, 10 mL)

Suspension, ophthalmic [drops]:

Blephamide®: Sulfacetamide sodium 10% and prednisolone acetate 0.2% (5 mL, 10 mL) [contains benzalkonium chloride]

- **Sulfacetamide and Sulfur** *see* Sulfur and Sulfacetamide *on page 1411*
- **Sulfacetamide Sodium** *see* Sulfacetamide *on page 1405*
- **Sulfacet-R®** *see* Sulfur and Sulfacetamide *on page 1411*

SulfADIAZINE (sul fa DYE a zeen)

Pharmacologic Category Antibiotic, Sulfonamide Derivative

Additional Appendix Information

Guidelines for the Prevention of Opportunistic Infections in HIV Infected Persons *on page 1740*

Sulfonamide Derivatives *on page 1671*

Use Treatment of urinary tract infections and nocardiosis; adjunctive treatment in toxoplasmosis; uncomplicated attack of malaria

Unlabeled/Investigational Use Rheumatic fever prophylaxis

Pregnancy Risk Factor B/D (at term)

Lactation Enters breast milk/contraindicated

Medication Safety Issues

Sound-alike/look-alike issues:

SulfaDIAZINE may be confused with sulfasalazine, sulfiSOXAZOLE

Contraindications Hypersensitivity to any sulfa drug or any component of the formulation; porphyria; children <2 months of age unless indicated for the treatment of congenital toxoplasmosis; sunscreens containing PABA; pregnancy (at term)

Warnings/Precautions Fatalities associated with severe reactions including Stevens-Johnson syndrome, toxic epidermal necrolysis, hepatic necrosis, agranulocytosis, aplastic anemia and other blood dyscrasias; discontinue use at first sign of rash. Use with caution in patients with impaired hepatic function or impaired renal function, G6PD deficiency; dosage modification required in patients with renal impairment; fluid intake should be maintained ≥1500 mL/day, or administer sodium bicarbonate to keep urine alkaline; more likely to cause crystalluria because it is less soluble than other sulfonamides. Chemical similarities are present among sulfonamides, sulfonylureas, carbonic anhydrase inhibitors, thiazides, and loop diuretics (except ethacrynic acid). Use in patients with sulfonamide allergy is specifically contraindicated in product labeling, however, a risk of cross-reaction exists in patients with allergy to any of these compounds; avoid use when previous reaction has been severe. Prolonged use may result in fungal or bacterial superinfection, including *C. difficile*-associated diarrhea (CDAD) and pseudomembranous colitis; CDAD has been observed >2 months postantibiotic treatment.

Adverse Reactions Frequency not defined.

Central nervous system: Dizziness, fever, headache

Dermatologic: Lyell's syndrome, Stevens-Johnson syndrome, itching, rash, photosensitivity

Endocrine & metabolic: Thyroid function disturbance

Gastrointestinal: Anorexia, diarrhea, nausea, vomiting

Genitourinary: Crystalluria

Hematologic: Aplastic anemia, granulocytopenia, hemolytic anemia, leukopenia, thrombocytopenia

Hepatic: Hepatitis, jaundice

Renal: Hematuria, acute nephropathy, interstitial nephritis

Miscellaneous: Serum sickness-like reactions

Drug Interactions

Metabolism/Transport Effects Substrate of CYP2C9 (major), 2E1 (minor), 3A4 (minor); **Inhibits** CYP2C9 (strong)

Avoid Concomitant Use

Avoid concomitant use of SulfADIAZINE with any of the following: Procaine

Increased Effect/Toxicity

SulfADIAZINE may increase the levels/effects of: CycloSPORINE; CYP2C9 Substrates (High risk); Methotrexate; Phenytoin; Sulfonylureas; Vitamin K Antagonists

The levels/effects of SulfADIAZINE may be increased by: CYP2C9 Inhibitors (Moderate); CYP2C9 Inhibitors (Strong)

Decreased Effect

SulfADIAZINE may decrease the levels/effects of: CycloSPORINE; Typhoid Vaccine

The levels/effects of SulfADIAZINE may be decreased by: CYP2C9 Inducers (Highly Effective); Procaine

Ethanol/Nutrition/Herb Interactions

Food: Avoid large quantities of vitamin C or acidifying agents (cranberry juice) to prevent crystalluria.

Herb/Nutraceutical: Avoid dong quai, St John's wort (may also cause photosensitization).

Stability Tablets may be crushed to prepare oral suspension of the drug in water or with a sucrose-containing solution. Aqueous suspension with concentrations of 100 mg/mL should be stored in the refrigerator and used within 7 days.

Mechanism of Action Interferes with bacterial growth by inhibiting bacterial folic acid synthesis through competitive antagonism of PABA

Pharmacodynamics/Kinetics

Absorption: Well absorbed

Distribution: Throughout body tissues and fluids including pleural, peritoneal, synovial, and ocular fluids; throughout total body water; readily diffused into CSF; enters breast milk

Metabolism: Via N-acetylation

Half-life elimination: 10 hours

Time to peak: Within 3-6 hours

Excretion: Urine (43% to 60% as unchanged drug, 15% to 40% as metabolites)

Dosage Oral:

Asymptomatic meningococcal carriers:

Infants 1-12 months: 500 mg once daily for 2 days

Children 1-12 years: 500 mg twice daily for 2 days

Adults: 1 g twice daily for 2 days

Congenital toxoplasmosis:

Newborns and Children <2 months: 100 mg/kg/day divided every 6 hours in conjunction with pyrimethamine 1 mg/kg/day once daily and supplemental folinic acid 5 mg every 3 days for 6 months

Children >2 months: 25-50 mg/kg/dose 4 times/day

Nocardiosis: 4-8 g/day for a minimum of 6 weeks
Toxoplasmosis:
Children >2 months: Loading dose: 75 mg/kg; maintenance dose: 120-150 mg/kg/day, maximum dose: 6 g/day; divided every 4-6 hours in conjunction with pyrimethamine 2 mg/kg/day divided every 12 hours for 3 days followed by 1 mg/kg/day once daily with supplemental folinic acid
Adults: 2-6 g/day in divided doses every 6 hours in conjunction with pyrimethamine 50-75 mg/day and with supplemental folinic acid
Prevention of recurrent attacks of rheumatic fever (unlabeled use):
>30 kg: 1 g/day
<30 kg: 0.5 g/day

Dietary Considerations Supplemental folinic acid should be administered to reverse symptoms or prevent problems due to folic acid deficiency.

Administration Tablets may be crushed to prepare oral suspension of the drug in water or with a sucrose-containing solution. Aqueous suspension with concentrations of 100 mg/mL should be stored in the refrigerator and used within 7 days. Administer around-the-clock to promote less variation in peak and trough serum levels.

Dosage Forms Excipient information presented when available (limited, particularly for generics); consult specific product labeling.
Tablet: 500 mg

Sulfadoxine and Pyrimethamine
(sul fa DOKS een & peer i METH a meen)

U.S. Brand Names Fansidar®

Index Terms Pyrimethamine and Sulfadoxine

Pharmacologic Category Antimalarial Agent

Use Treatment of *Plasmodium falciparum* malaria in patients in whom chloroquine resistance is suspected; malaria prophylaxis for travelers to areas where chloroquine-resistant malaria is endemic

Pregnancy Risk Factor C/D (at term)

Dosage Children and Adults: Oral:
Treatment of acute attack of malaria: A single dose of the following number of Fansidar® tablets is used in sequence with quinine or alone:
2-11 months: 1/4 tablet
1-3 years: 1/2 tablet
4-8 years: 1 tablet
9-14 years: 2 tablets
>14 years: 3 tablets
Malaria prophylaxis: A single dose should be carried for self-treatment in the event of febrile illness when medical attention is not immediately available:
2-11 months: 1/4 tablet
1-3 years: 1/2 tablet
4-8 years: 1 tablet
9-14 years: 2 tablets
>14 years and Adults: 3 tablets

Additional Information Complete prescribing information for this medication should be consulted for additional detail.

Dosage Forms Excipient information presented when available (limited, particularly for generics); consult specific product labeling.
Tablet: Sulfadoxine 500 mg and pyrimethamine 25 mg

Sulfamethoxazole and Trimethoprim
(sul fa meth OKS a zole & trye METH oh prim)

U.S. Brand Names Bactrim™; Bactrim™ DS; Septra®; Septra® DS; Sulfatrim®

Canadian Brand Names Apo-Sulfatrim®; Apo-Sulfatrim® DS; Apo-Sulfatrim® Pediatric; Novo-Trimel; Novo-Trimel D.S.; Nu-Cotrimox; Septra® Injection

Index Terms Co-Trimoxazole; SMZ-TMP; Sulfatrim; TMP-SMZ; Trimethoprim and Sulfamethoxazole

Pharmacologic Category Antibiotic, Miscellaneous; Antibiotic, Sulfonamide Derivative

Additional Appendix Information
Animal and Human Bites *on page 1747*
Antimicrobial Drugs of Choice *on page 1752*
Desensitization Protocols *on page 1691*
Guidelines for the Prevention of Opportunistic Infections in HIV Infected Persons *on page 1740*

Use
Oral treatment of urinary tract infections due to *E. coli*, *Klebsiella* and *Enterobacter* sp, *M. morganii*, *P. mirabilis* and *P. vulgaris*; acute otitis media in children; acute exacerbations of chronic bronchitis in adults due to susceptible strains of *H. influenzae* or *S. pneumoniae*; treatment and prophylaxis of *Pneumocystis jiroveci* pneumonitis (PCP); traveler's diarrhea due to enterotoxigenic *E. coli*; treatment of enteritis caused by *Shigella flexneri* or *Shigella sonnei*
I.V. treatment or severe or complicated infections when oral therapy is not feasible, for documented PCP, empiric treatment of PCP in immune compromised patients; treatment of documented or suspected shigellosis, typhoid fever, *Nocardia asteroides* infection, or other infections caused by susceptible bacteria

Unlabeled/Investigational Use Cholera and *Salmonella*-type infections and nocardiosis; chronic prostatitis; as prophylaxis in neutropenic patients with *P. jiroveci* infections, in leukemia patients, and in patients following renal transplantation, to decrease incidence of PCP; treatment of *Cyclospora* infection, typhoid fever, *Nocardia asteroides* infection; prophylaxis against urinary tract infection

Pregnancy Risk Factor C/D (at term - expert analysis)

Pregnancy Considerations Do not use at term to avoid kernicterus in the newborn; use during pregnancy only if risks outweigh the benefits since folic acid metabolism may be affected.

Lactation Enters breast milk/contraindicated (AAP rates "compatible with restrictions")

Medication Safety Issues
Sound-alike/look-alike issues:
Bactrim™ may be confused with bacitracin, Bactine®, Bactroban®
Co-trimoxazole may be confused with clotrimazole
Septra® may be confused with Ceptaz®, Sectral®
Septra® DS may be confused with Semprex®-D

Contraindications Hypersensitivity to any sulfa drug, trimethoprim, or any component of the formulation; megaloblastic anemia due to folate deficiency; infants <2 months of age; marked hepatic damage or severe renal disease (if patient not monitored); pregnancy (at term); breast-feeding

Warnings/Precautions Use with caution in patients with G6PD deficiency, impaired renal or hepatic function or potential folate deficiency (malnourished, chronic anticonvulsant therapy, or elderly); maintain adequate hydration to prevent crystalluria; adjust dosage in patients with renal impairment. Injection vehicle contains benzyl alcohol and sodium metabisulfite.

Chemical similarities are present among sulfonamides, sulfonylureas, carbonic anhydrase inhibitors, thiazides, and loop diuretics (except ethacrynic acid). Use in patients with sulfonamide allergy is specifically contraindicated in product labeling, however, a risk of cross-reaction exists in patients with allergy to any of these compounds; avoid use when previous reaction has been severe.

Fatalities associated with severe reactions including Stevens-Johnson syndrome, toxic epidermal necrolysis, hepatic necrosis, agranulocytosis, aplastic anemia and other blood dyscrasias; discontinue use at first sign of rash or serious adverse reactions. Elderly patients appear at greater risk for more severe adverse reactions. May cause hypoglycemia, particularly in malnourished, or patients with renal or hepatic impairment. Use with caution in patients with porphyria or thyroid dysfunction. Slow acetylators may be more prone to adverse reactions. Caution in patients with allergies or asthma. May cause hyperkalemia (associated with high doses of trimethoprim). Incidence of adverse effects appears to be increased in patients with AIDS. Prolonged use may result in fungal or bacterial superinfection, including *C. difficile*-associated diarrhea (CDAD) and pseudomembranous colitis; CDAD has been observed >2 months postantibiotic treatment.

Adverse Reactions The most common adverse reactions include gastrointestinal upset (nausea, vomiting, anorexia) and dermatologic reactions (rash or urticaria). Rare, life-threatening reactions have been associated with co-trimoxazole, including severe dermatologic reactions, blood dyscrasias, and hepatotoxic reactions. Most other reactions listed are rare, however, frequency cannot be accurately estimated.

Cardiovascular: Allergic myocarditis

Central nervous system: Apathy, aseptic meningitis, ataxia, chills, depression, fatigue, fever, hallucinations, headache, insomnia, kernicterus (in neonates), nervousness, peripheral neuritis, seizure, vertigo

Dermatologic: Photosensitivity, pruritus, rash, skin eruptions, urticaria; rare reactions include erythema multiforme, exfoliative dermatitis, Henoch-Schönlein purpura, Stevens-Johnson syndrome, and toxic epidermal necrolysis

Endocrine & metabolic: Hyperkalemia (generally at high dosages), hypoglycemia (rare), hyponatremia

Gastrointestinal: Abdominal pain, anorexia, diarrhea, glottis, nausea, pancreatitis, pseudomembranous colitis, stomatitis, vomiting

Hematologic: Agranulocytosis, aplastic anemia, eosinophilia, hemolysis (with G6PD deficiency), hemolytic anemia, hypoprothrombinemia, leukopenia, megaloblastic anemia, methemoglobinemia, neutropenia, thrombocytopenia

Hepatic: Hepatotoxicity (including hepatitis, cholestasis, and hepatic necrosis), hyperbilirubinemia, transaminases increased

Neuromuscular & skeletal: Arthralgia, myalgia, rhabdomyolysis, weakness

Otic: Tinnitus

Renal: BUN increased, crystalluria, diuresis (rare), interstitial nephritis, nephrotoxicity (in association with cyclosporine), renal failure, serum creatinine increased, toxic nephrosis (with anuria and oliguria)

Respiratory: Cough, dyspnea, pulmonary infiltrates

Miscellaneous: Allergic reaction, anaphylaxis, angioedema, periarteritis nodosa (rare), serum sickness, systemic lupus erythematosus (rare)

Drug Interactions

Metabolism/Transport Effects

Sulfamethoxazole: **Substrate** of CYP2C9 (major), 3A4 (minor); **Inhibits** CYP2C9 (moderate)

Trimethoprim: **Substrate** (major) of CYP2C9, 3A4; **Inhibits** CYP2C8 (moderate), 2C9 (moderate)

Avoid Concomitant Use

Avoid concomitant use of Sulfamethoxazole and Trimethoprim with any of the following: Dofetilide; Procaine

Increased Effect/Toxicity

Sulfamethoxazole and Trimethoprim may increase the levels/effects of: ACE Inhibitors; Amantadine; Angiotensin II Receptor Blockers; Antidiabetic Agents (Thiazolidinedione); AzaTHIOprine; CycloSPORINE; CYP2C8 Substrates (High risk); CYP2C9 Substrates (High risk); Dapsone; Dofetilide; LamiVUDine; Memantine; Methotrexate; Phenytoin; Procainamide; Repaglinide; Sulfonylureas; Vitamin K Antagonists

The levels/effects of Sulfamethoxazole and Trimethoprim may be increased by: Amantadine; CYP2C9 Inhibitors (Moderate); CYP2C9 Inhibitors (Strong); Dapsone; Memantine

Decreased Effect

Sulfamethoxazole and Trimethoprim may decrease the levels/effects of: CycloSPORINE; Typhoid Vaccine

The levels/effects of Sulfamethoxazole and Trimethoprim may be decreased by: CYP2C9 Inducers (Highly Effective); CYP3A4 Inducers (Strong); Deferasirox; Herbs (CYP3A4 Inducers); Leucovorin-Levoleucovorin; Procaine

Ethanol/Nutrition/Herb Interactions Herb/Nutraceutical: Avoid dong quai; St John's wort (may diminish effects and also cause photosensitization).

Stability

Injection: Store at room temperature; do not refrigerate. Less soluble in more alkaline pH. Protect from light. Solution must be diluted prior to administration. Following dilution, store at room temperature; do not refrigerate. Manufacturer recommended dilutions and stability of parenteral admixture at room temperature (25°C):

5 mL/125 mL D_5W; stable for 6 hours.

5 mL/100 mL D_5W; stable for 4 hours.

5 mL/75 mL D_5W; stable for 2 hours.

Studies have also confirmed limited stability in NS; detailed references should be consulted.

Suspension, tablet: Store at controlled room temperature of 15°C to 25°C (59°F to 77°F). Protect from light.

Mechanism of Action Sulfamethoxazole interferes with bacterial folic acid synthesis and growth via inhibition of dihydrofolic acid formation from para-aminobenzoic acid; trimethoprim inhibits dihydrofolic acid reduction to tetrahydrofolate resulting in sequential inhibition of enzymes of the folic acid pathway

Pharmacodynamics/Kinetics

Absorption: Oral: Almost completely, 90% to 100%

Protein binding: SMX: 68%, TMP: 45%

Metabolism: SMX: N-acetylated and glucuronidated; TMP: Metabolized to oxide and hydroxylated metabolites

Half-life elimination: SMX: 9 hours, TMP: 6-17 hours; both are prolonged in renal failure

Time to peak, serum: Within 1-4 hours

Excretion: Both are excreted in urine as metabolites and unchanged drug

Effects of aging on the pharmacokinetics of both agents has been variable; increase in half-life and decreases in clearance have been associated with reduced creatinine clearance

Dosage Dosage recommendations are based on the trimethoprim component. Double-strength tablets are equivalent to sulfamethoxazole 800 mg and trimethoprim 160 mg.

Usual dosage ranges:

Children >2 months:

Mild-to-moderate infections: Oral: 8-12 mg TMP/kg/day in divided doses every 12 hours

Serious infection:

Oral: 20 mg TMP/kg/day in divided doses every 6 hours

I.V.: 8-12 mg TMP/kg/day in divided doses every 6 hours

Adults:

Oral: One double strength tablet (sulfamethoxazole 800 mg; trimethoprim 160 mg) every 12-24 hours

I.V.: 8-20 mg TMP/kg/day divided every 6-12 hours

Indication-specifc dosing:
Children >2 months:
Acute otitis media: Oral: 8 mg TMP/kg/day in divided doses every 12 hours for 10 days. **Note:** Recommended by the American Academy of Pediatrics as an alternative agent in penicillin-allergic patients at a dose of 6-10 mg TMP/kg/day (AOM guidelines, 2004).
Urinary tract infection:
Treatment:
Oral: 6-12 mg TMP/kg/day in divided doses every 12 hours
I.V.: 8-10 mg TMP/kg/day in divided doses every 6, 8, or 12 hours for up to 14 days with serious infections
Prophylaxis: Oral: 2 mg TMP/kg/dose daily or 5 mg TMP/kg/dose twice weekly
Pneumocystis jiroveci:
Treatment: Oral, I.V.: 15-20 mg TMP/kg/day in divided doses every 6-8 hours
Prophylaxis: Oral, 150 mg TMP/m^2/day in divided doses every 12 hours for 3 days/week; dose should not exceed trimethoprim 320 mg and sulfamethoxazole 1600 mg daily
Alternative prophylaxis dosing schedules include:
150 mg TMP/m^2/day as a single daily dose 3 times/week on consecutive days
or
150 mg TMP/m^2/day in divided doses every 12 hours administered 7 days/week
or
150 mg TMP/m^2/day in divided doses every 12 hours administered 3 times/week on alternate days
Shigellosis:
Oral: 8 mg TMP/kg/day in divided doses every 12 hours for 5 days
I.V.: 8-10 mg TMP/kg/day in divided doses every 6, 8, or 12 hours for up to 5 days
***Cyclospora* (unlabeled use):** Oral, I.V.: 5 mg TMP/kg twice daily for 7-10 days
Adults:
Urinary tract infection:
Oral: One double-strength tablet every 12 hours
Duration of therapy: Uncomplicated: 3-5 days; Complicated: 7-10 days
Pyelonephritis: 14 days
Prostatitis: Acute: 2 weeks; Chronic: 2-3 months
I.V.: 8-10 mg TMP/kg/day in divided doses every 6, 8, or 12 hours for up to 14 days with severe infections
Chronic bronchitis (acute): Oral: One double-strength tablet every 12 hours for 10-14 days
Meningitis (bacterial): I.V.: 10-20 mg TMP/kg/day in divided doses every 6-12 hours
Shigellosis:
Oral: One double strength tablet every 12 hours for 5 days
I.V.: 8-10 mg TMP/kg/day in divided doses every 6, 8, or 12 hours for up to 5 days
Travelers' diarrhea: Oral: One double strength tablet every 12 hours for 5 days
Sepsis: I.V.: 20 TMP/kg/day divided every 6 hours
***Pneumocystis jiroveci*:**
Prophylaxis: Oral: 1 double strength tablet daily or 3 times/week
Treatment: Oral, I.V.: 15-20 mg TMP/kg/day in 3-4 divided doses
Cyclospora (unlabeled use): Oral, I.V.: 160 mg TMP twice daily for 7-10 days. **Note:** AIDS patients: Oral: 1 double strength tablet 2-4 times/day for 10 days, then 1 double strength tablet 3 times/week for 10 weeks (Verdier, 2000 and Pape, 1994).
Nocardia (unlabeled use): Oral, I.V.:
Cutaneous infections: 5-10 mg TMP/kg/day in 2-4 divided doses
Severe infections (pulmonary/cerebral): 15 mg TMP/kg/day in 2-4 divided doses for 3-4 weeks, then 10 mg TMP/kg/day in 2-4 divided doses. Treatment duration is controversial; an average of 7 months has been reported.
Note: Therapy for severe infection may be initiated I.V. and converted to oral therapy (frequently converted to approximate dosages of oral solid dosage forms: 2 DS tablets every 8-12 hours). Although not widely available, sulfonamide levels should be considered in patients with questionable absorption, at risk for dose-related toxicity, or those with poor therapeutic response.

Dosing adjustment in renal impairment: Oral, I.V.:
Cl_{cr} 15-30 mL/minute: Administer 50% of recommended dose
Cl_{cr} <15 mL/minute: Use is not recommended

Dietary Considerations Should be taken with 8 oz of water.

Administration
I.V.: Infuse over 60-90 minutes, must dilute well before giving; may be given less diluted in a central line; not for I.M. injection
Oral: May be taken with or without food. Administer with at least 8 ounces of water.

Monitoring Parameters Perform culture and sensitivity testing prior to initiating therapy; CBC, serum potassium, creatinine, BUN

Test Interactions Increased creatinine (Jaffé alkaline picrate reaction); increased serum methotrexate by dihydrofolate reductase method

Dosage Forms Excipient information presented when available (limited, particularly for generics); consult specific product labeling. **Note:** The 5:1 ratio (SMX:TMP) remains constant in all dosage forms.
Injection, solution: Sulfamethoxazole 80 mg and trimethoprim 16 mg per mL (5 mL, 10 mL, 30 mL)
Suspension, oral: Sulfamethoxazole 200 mg and trimethoprim 40 mg per 5 mL (480 mL)
Sulfatrim®: Sulfamethoxazole 200 mg and trimethoprim 40 mg per 5 mL (100 mL, 480 mL) [contains alcohol ≤0.5% propylene glycol; cherry flavor]
Tablet: Sulfamethoxazole 400 mg and trimethoprim 80 mg
Bactrim™: Sulfamethoxazole 400 mg and trimethoprim 80 mg
Septra®: Sulfamethoxazole 400 mg and trimethoprim 80 mg
Tablet, double strength: Sulfamethoxazole 800 mg and trimethoprim 160 mg
Bactrim™ DS: Sulfamethoxazole 800 mg and trimethoprim 160 mg
Septra® DS: Sulfamethoxazole 800 mg and trimethoprim 160 mg

◆ **Sulfamylon®** *see* Mafenide *on page 913*

Sulfasalazine (sul fa SAL a zeen)

U.S. Brand Names Azulfidine®; Azulfidine® EN-tabs®; Sulfazine; Sulfazine EC

Canadian Brand Names Alti-Sulfasalazine; Salazopyrin En-Tabs®; Salazopyrin®

Index Terms Salicylazosulfapyridine

Pharmacologic Category 5-Aminosalicylic Acid Derivative

Additional Appendix Information
Sulfonamide Derivatives *on page 1671*

Use Management of ulcerative colitis; enteric coated tablets are also used for rheumatoid arthritis (including juvenile rheumatoid arthritis) in patients who inadequately respond to analgesics and NSAIDs

Unlabeled/Investigational Use Ankylosing spondylitis, collagenous colitis, Crohn's disease, psoriasis, psoriatic arthritis, juvenile chronic arthritis

Pregnancy Risk Factor B/D (at term)

Lactation Enters breast milk/use caution (AAP recommends use "with caution")

Medication Safety Issues

Sound-alike/look-alike issues:

Sulfasalazine may be confused with salsalate, sulfaDIAZINE, sulfiSOXAZOLE

Azulfidine® may be confused with Augmentin®, azaTHIOprine

Contraindications Hypersensitivity to sulfasalazine, sulfa drugs, salicylates, or any component of the formulation; porphyria; GI or GU obstruction; pregnancy (at term)

Warnings/Precautions Use with caution in patients with renal impairment; impaired hepatic function or urinary obstruction, blood dyscrasias, severe allergies or asthma, or G6PD deficiency; may cause folate deficiency (consider providing 1 mg/day folate supplement). Deaths from irreversible neuromuscular, central nervous system, fibrosing alveolitis, agranulocytosis, aplastic anemia, and other blood dyscrasias have been reported. In males, oligospermia (rare) has been reported. Chemical similarities are present among sulfonamides, sulfonylureas, carbonic anhydrase inhibitors, thiazides, and loop diuretics (except ethacrynic acid). Use in patients with sulfonamide allergy is specifically contraindicated in product labeling, however, a risk of cross-reaction exists in patients with allergy to any of these compounds; avoid use when previous reaction has been severe. Safety and efficacy have not been established in children <2 years of age.

Adverse Reactions

>10%:

Central nervous system: Headache (33%)

Dermatologic: Photosensitivity

Gastrointestinal: Anorexia, nausea, vomiting, diarrhea (33%), gastric distress

Genitourinary: Reversible oligospermia (33%)

<3% (Limited to important or life-threatening): Alopecia, anaphylaxis, aplastic anemia, ataxia, crystalluria, depression, epidermal necrolysis, exfoliative dermatitis, granulocytopenia, hallucinations, Heinz body anemia, hemolytic anemia, hepatitis, interstitial nephritis, jaundice, leukopenia, Lyell's syndrome, myelodysplastic syndrome, nephropathy (acute), neutropenic enterocolitis, pancreatitis, peripheral neuropathy, photosensitization, pruritus, rhabdomyolysis, seizure, serum sickness-like reactions, skin discoloration, Stevens-Johnson syndrome, thrombocytopenia, thyroid function disturbance, urine discoloration, urticaria, vasculitis, vertigo

Additional events reported with sulfonamides and/or 5-ASA derivatives: Cholestatic jaundice, eosinophilia pneumonitis, erythema multiforme, fibrosing alveolitis, hepatic necrosis, Kawasaki-like syndrome, SLE-like syndrome, pericarditis, seizure, transverse myelitis

Drug Interactions

Avoid Concomitant Use There are no known interactions where it is recommended to avoid concomitant use.

Increased Effect/Toxicity

Sulfasalazine may increase the levels/effects of: Thiopurine Analogs; Varicella Virus-Containing Vaccines

Decreased Effect

Sulfasalazine may decrease the levels/effects of: Cardiac Glycosides; Methylfolate

Ethanol/Nutrition/Herb Interactions

Food: May impair folate absorption.

Herb/Nutraceutical: Avoid dong quai, St John's wort (may also cause photosensitization)

Stability Protect from light.

Mechanism of Action Acts locally in the colon to decrease the inflammatory response and systemically interferes with secretion by inhibiting prostaglandin synthesis

Pharmacodynamics/Kinetics

Absorption: 10% to 15% as unchanged drug from small intestine

Distribution: Small amounts enter feces and breast milk

Metabolism: Via colonic intestinal flora to sulfapyridine and 5-aminosalicylic acid (5-ASA); following absorption, sulfapyridine undergoes N-acetylation and ring hydroxylation while 5-ASA undergoes N-acetylation

Half-life elimination: 5.7-10 hours

Excretion: Primarily urine (as unchanged drug, components, and acetylated metabolites)

Dosage Oral:

Children ≥2 years: Ulcerative colitis: Initial: 40-60 mg/kg/day in 3-6 divided doses; maintenance dose: 20-30 mg/kg/day in 4 divided doses

Children ≥6 years: Juvenile rheumatoid arthritis: Enteric coated tablet: 30-50 mg/kg/day in 2 divided doses; Initial: Begin with 1/4 to 1/3 of expected maintenance dose; increase weekly; maximum: 2 g/day typically

Adults:

Ulcerative colitis: Initial: 1 g 3-4 times/day, 2 g/day maintenance in divided doses; may initiate therapy with 0.5-1 g/day

Rheumatoid arthritis: Enteric coated tablet: Initial: 0.5-1 g/day; increase weekly to maintenance dose of 2 g/day in 2 divided doses; maximum: 3 g/day (if response to 2 g/day is inadequate after 12 weeks of treatment)

Dosing interval in renal impairment:

Cl_{cr} 10-30 mL/minute: Administer twice daily

Cl_{cr} <10 mL/minute: Administer once daily

Dosing adjustment in hepatic impairment: Avoid use

Dietary Considerations Since sulfasalazine impairs folate absorption, consider providing 1 mg/day folate supplement.

Administration GI intolerance is common during the first few days of therapy (administer with meals).

Dosage Forms Excipient information presented when available (limited, particularly for generics); consult specific product labeling.

Tablet: 500 mg

Azulfidine®, Sulfazine: 500 mg

Tablet, delayed release, enteric coated: 500 mg

Azulfidine® EN-tabs®, Sulfazine EC: 500 mg

◆ **Sulfatol®** *see* Sulfur and Sulfacetamide *on page* 1411

◆ **Sulfatol®-M** *see* Sulfur and Sulfacetamide *on page* 1411

◆ **Sulfatrim** *see* Sulfamethoxazole and Trimethoprim *on page* 1407

◆ **Sulfatrim®** *see* Sulfamethoxazole and Trimethoprim *on page* 1407

◆ **Sulfazine** *see* Sulfasalazine *on page* 1409

◆ **Sulfazine EC** *see* Sulfasalazine *on page* 1409

SulfiSOXAZOLE (sul fi SOKS a zole)

U.S. Brand Names Gantrisin®

Canadian Brand Names Novo-Soxazole; Sulfizole®

Index Terms Sulfisoxazole Acetyl; Sulphafurazole

Pharmacologic Category Antibiotic, Sulfonamide Derivative

Additional Appendix Information

Antimicrobial Drugs of Choice *on page* 1752

Sulfonamide Derivatives *on page* 1671

Use Treatment of urinary tract infections, otitis media, *Chlamydia*; nocardiosis

Pregnancy Risk Factor B/D (near term)

Lactation Enters breast milk/compatible

Medication Safety Issues

Sound-alike/look-alike issues:

SulfiSOXAZOLE may be confused with sulfaDIAZINE, sulfamethoxazole, sulfasalazine

Gantrisin® may be confused with Gastrosed™

Contraindications Hypersensitivity to sulfisoxazole, any sulfa drug, or any component of the formulation; porphyria; infants <2 months of age (sulfas compete with bilirubin for protein binding sites); patients with urinary obstruction; sunscreens containing PABA; pregnancy (at term)

Warnings/Precautions Fatalities associated with severe reactions including Stevens-Johnson syndrome, toxic epidermal necrolysis, hepatic necrosis, agranulocytosis, aplastic anemia and other blood dyscrasias; discontinue use at first sign of rash. Use with caution in patients with G6PD deficiency (hemolysis may occur), hepatic or renal impairment; dosage modification required in patients with renal impairment; risk of crystalluria should be considered in patients with impaired renal function. Chemical similarities are present among sulfonamides, sulfonylureas, carbonic anhydrase inhibitors, thiazides, and loop diuretics (except ethacrynic acid). Use in patients with sulfonamide allergy is specifically contraindicated in product labeling, however, a risk of cross-reaction exists in patients with allergy to any of these compounds; avoid use when previous reaction has been severe. Prolonged use may result in fungal or bacterial superinfection, including *C. difficile*-associated diarrhea (CDAD) and pseudomembranous colitis; CDAD has been observed >2 months postantibiotic treatment.

Adverse Reactions Frequency not defined.

Cardiovascular: Vasculitis

Central nervous system: Dizziness, fever, headache

Dermatologic: Itching, Lyell's syndrome, rash, photosensitivity, Stevens-Johnson syndrome

Endocrine & metabolic: Thyroid function disturbance

Gastrointestinal: Anorexia, diarrhea, nausea, vomiting

Genitourinary: Crystalluria, hematuria

Hematologic: Aplastic anemia, granulocytopenia, hemolytic anemia, leukopenia, thrombocytopenia

Hepatic: Hepatitis, jaundice

Renal: Interstitial nephritis

Miscellaneous: Serum sickness-like reactions

Drug Interactions

Metabolism/Transport Effects Substrate of CYP2C9 (major); **Inhibits** CYP2C9 (strong)

Avoid Concomitant Use

Avoid concomitant use of SulfiSOXAZOLE with any of the following: Procaine

Increased Effect/Toxicity

SulfiSOXAZOLE may increase the levels/effects of: CycloSPORINE; CYP2C9 Substrates (High risk); Methotrexate; Phenytoin; Sulfonylureas; Vitamin K Antagonists

The levels/effects of SulfiSOXAZOLE may be increased by: CYP2C9 Inhibitors (Moderate); CYP2C9 Inhibitors (Strong)

Decreased Effect

SulfiSOXAZOLE may decrease the levels/effects of: CycloSPORINE; Typhoid Vaccine

The levels/effects of SulfiSOXAZOLE may be decreased by: CYP2C9 Inducers (Highly Effective); Procaine

Ethanol/Nutrition/Herb Interactions

Food: Interferes with folate absorption.

Herb/Nutraceutical: Avoid dong quai, St John's wort (may also cause photosensitization).

Stability Protect from light.

Mechanism of Action Interferes with bacterial growth by inhibiting bacterial folic acid synthesis through competitive antagonism of PABA

Pharmacodynamics/Kinetics

Absorption: Sulfisoxazole acetyl is hydrolyzed in GI tract to sulfisoxazole which is readily absorbed

Distribution: Crosses placenta; enters breast milk

CSF:blood level ratio: Normal meninges: 50% to 80%; Inflamed meninges: 80+%

Protein binding: 85% to 88%

Metabolism: Hepatic via acetylation and glucuronide conjugation to inactive compounds

Half-life elimination: 4-7 hours; prolonged with renal impairment

Time to peak, serum: 2-3 hours

Excretion: Urine (95%, 40% to 60% as unchanged drug) within 24 hours

Dosage Oral: Not for use in patients <2 months of age:

Children >2 months: Initial: 75 mg/kg, followed by 120-150 mg/kg/day in divided doses every 4-6 hours; not to exceed 6 g/day

Adults: Initial: 2-4 g, then 4-8 g/day in divided doses every 4-6 hours

Dosing interval in renal impairment:

Cl_{cr} 10-50 mL/minute: Administer every 8-12 hours

Cl_{cr} <10 mL/minute: Administer every 12-24 hours

Hemodialysis: >50% removed by hemodialysis

Dietary Considerations Should be taken with a glass of water on an empty stomach.

Administration Administer around-the-clock to promote less variation in peak and trough serum levels.

Monitoring Parameters CBC, urinalysis, renal function tests, temperature

Test Interactions False-positive protein in urine; false-positive urine glucose with Clinitest®

Dosage Forms Excipient information presented when available (limited, particularly for generics); consult specific product labeling.

Suspension, oral [pediatric]

Gantrisin®: 500 mg/5 mL (480 mL) [contains alcohol 0.3%; raspberry flavor]

◆ **Sulfisoxazole Acetyl** *see* SulfiSOXAZOLE *on page 1410*

◆ **Sulfisoxazole and Erythromycin** *see* Erythromycin and Sulfisoxazole *on page 547*

◆ **Sulfizole® (Can)** *see* SulfiSOXAZOLE *on page 1410*

Sulfur and Sulfacetamide

(SUL fur & sul fa SEE ta mide)

U.S. Brand Names AVAR™ [DSC]; AVAR™-e; AVAR™-e Green [DSC]; Clarifoam™ EF; Clenia™; Plexion SCT®; Plexion TS® [DSC]; Plexion®; Prascion®; Prascion® AV [DSC]; Prascion® FC; Prascion® RA; Prascion® TS; Rosac®; Rosanil®; Rosula®; Rosula® Clarifying; Sulfacet-R®; Sulfatol®; Sulfatol®-M; Suphera™

Canadian Brand Names Sulfacet-R®

Index Terms Sodium Sulfacetamide and Sulfur; Sulfacetamide and Sulfur; Sulfur and Sulfacetamide Sodium

Pharmacologic Category Acne Products; Antibiotic, Sulfonamide Derivative; Antiseborrheic Agent, Topical; Topical Skin Product, Acne

Use Aid in the treatment of acne vulgaris, acne rosacea, and seborrheic dermatitis

Pregnancy Risk Factor C

Dosage Topical: Children ≥12 years and Adults: Apply in a thin film 1-3 times/day. Cleansing products should be used 1-2 times/day.

Dosage adjustment in renal impairment: Use is contraindicated.

Additional Information Complete prescribing information for this medication should be consulted for additional detail.

Dosage Forms Excipient information presented when available (limited, particularly for generics); consult specific product labeling. [DSC] = Discontinued product

Aerosol, topical [foam]:
- Clarifoam™ EF: Sulfur 5% and sulfacetamide sodium 10% (60 g)

Cleanser, topical:
- AVAR™: Sulfur 5% and sulfacetamide sodium 10% (228 g)
- Plexion®: Sulfur 5% and sulfacetamide sodium 10% (170 g, 340 g)
- Prascion®: Sulfur 5% and sulfacetamide sodium 10% (170 g, 340 g)
- Prascion® AV: Sulfur 5% and sulfacetamide sodium 10% (227 g) [DSC]
- Rosanil®: Sulfur 5% and sulfacetamide sodium 10% (170 g, 390 g)
- Rosula®: Sulfur 5% and sulfacetamide sodium 10% (355 mL) [contains urea 10%]

Cleanser, topoical [emulsion-based]:
- Sulfatol®: Sulfur 5% and sulfacetamide sodium 10% (355 mL) [contains urea 10%]

Cream, topical:
- AVAR™-e: Sulfur 5% and sulfacetamide sodium 10% (45 g) [contains benzyl alcohol]
- AVAR™-e Green: Sulfur 5% and sulfacetamide sodium 10% (45 g) [contains benzyl alcohol; color corrective cream]
- Clenia™: Sulfur 5% and sulfacetamide sodium 10% (28 g)
- Plexion SCT®: Sulfur 5% and sulfacetamide sodium 10% (120 g) [contains benzyl alcohol]
- Prascion® RA: Sulfur 5% and sulfacetamide sodium 10% (45 g) [contains benzyl alcohol and sunscreen]
- Rosac®: Sulfur 5% and sulfacetamide sodium 10% (45 g) [contains benzyl alcohol and sunscreen]
- Suphera™: Sulfur 5% and sulfacetamide sodium 10% (113 g)

Gel, topical:
- AVAR™: Sulfur 5% and sulfacetamide sodium 10% (45 g) [contains benzyl alcohol]
- Rosula®: Sulfur 5% and sulfacetamide sodium 10% (45 mL) [contains urea 10% and benzyl alcohol]

Gel, topical [emulsion-based]:
- Sulfatol®: Sulfur 5% and sulfacetamide sodium 10% (45 mL) [contains urea 10%]

Lotion, topical: Sulfur 5% and sulfacetamide sodium 10% (25 g, 30 g, 45 g, 60 g)
- Sulfacet-R®: Sulfur 5% and sulfacetamide sodium 10% (25 g) [contains sodium metabisulfite; tint formulation]
- Sulfatol-M®: Sulfur 5% and sulfacetamide sodium 10% (25 g) [contains sodium metabisulfite; tint formulation]
- Sulfatol-M®: Sulfur 5% and sulfacetamide sodium 10% (25 g) [contains sodium metabisulfite; tint-free formulation]

Pad, topical [cleansing cloth]:
- Plexion®: Sulfur 5% and sulfacetamide sodium 10% (30s, 60s) [contains aloe vera]
- Prascion® FC: Sulfur 5% and sulfacetamide sodium 10% (30s, 60s)

Suspension, topical: Sulfur 5% and sulfacetamide sodium 10% (30 g)
- Plexion® TS: Sulfur 5% and sulfacetamide sodium 10% (30 g) [contains benzyl alcohol] [DSC]
- Prascion® TS: Sulfur 5% and sulfacetamide sodium 10% (30 g)

Wash, topical: Sulfur 5% and sulfacetamide sodium 10% (170 g, 340 g)
- Clenia™: Sulfur 5% and sulfacetamide sodium 10% (170 g, 340 g)
- Rosac®: Sulfur 1% and sulfacetamide sodium 10% (170 g)

Wash, topical [emulsion-based]:
- Rosula® Clarifying: Sulfur 4% and sulfacetamide sodium 10% (473 mL) [contains urea 10%]

◆ **Sulfur and Sulfacetamide Sodium** *see* Sulfur and Sulfacetamide *on page 1411*

Sulindac (SUL in dak)

U.S. Brand Names Clinoril®

Canadian Brand Names Apo-Sulin®; Novo-Sundac; Nu-Sundac

Pharmacologic Category Nonsteroidal Anti-inflammatory Drug (NSAID), Oral

Additional Appendix Information

Nonsteroidal Anti-inflammatory Agents *on page 1669*

Use Management of inflammatory diseases including osteoarthritis, rheumatoid arthritis, acute gouty arthritis, ankylosing spondylitis, acute painful shoulder (bursitis/tendonitis)

Restrictions An FDA-approved medication guide must be distributed when dispensing an oral outpatient prescription (new or refill) where this medication is to be used without direct supervision of a healthcare provider. Medication guides are available at http://www.fda.gov/cder/Offices/ODS/medication_guides.htm.

Pregnancy Risk Factor C/D (3rd trimester)

Pregnancy Considerations Animal studies have not documented teratogenic effects. However, known effects of NSAIDs suggest the potential for premature ductus arteriosus closure, particularly in late pregnancy.

Lactation Excretion in breast milk unknown/not recommended

Medication Safety Issues

Sound-alike/look-alike issues:

Clinoril® may be confused with Cleocin®, Clozaril®, Oruvail®

Contraindications Hypersensitivity or allergic-type reactions to sulindac, aspirin, other NSAIDs, or any component of the formulation; perioperative pain in the setting of coronary artery bypass graft (CABG) surgery

Warnings/Precautions [U.S. Boxed Warning]: NSAIDs are associated with an increased risk of adverse cardiovascular thrombotic events, including MI, stroke, and new onset or worsening of pre-existing hypertension. Use caution with fluid retention, heart failure, or hypertension. Concurrent administration of ibuprofen, and potentially other nonselective NSAIDs, may interfere with aspirin's cardioprotective effect. NSAID use may compromise existing renal function; dose-dependent decreases in prostaglandin synthesis may result from NSAID use, reducing renal blood flow which may cause renal decompensation. Patients with impaired renal function, dehydration, heart failure, liver dysfunction, those taking diuretics, and ACE inhibitors, and the elderly are at greater risk of renal toxicity. Rehydrate patient before starting therapy; monitor renal function closely. Not recommended for use in patients with advanced renal disease. Long-term NSAID use may result in renal papillary necrosis. Use caution in patients with renal lithiasis; sulindac metabolites have been reported as components of renal stones. Use hydration in patients with a history of renal stones. Use with caution in patients with decreased hepatic function. May require dosage adjustment in hepatic dysfunction; sulfide and sulfone metabolites may accumulate. **[U.S. Boxed Warning]: Use is contraindicated for treatment of perioperative pain in the setting of coronary artery bypass graft (CABG) surgery.** Risk of MI and stroke may be increased with use following CABG surgery.

[U.S. Boxed Warning]: NSAIDs may increase risk of gastrointestinal irritation, inflammation, ulceration,

bleeding, and perforation. Use the lowest effective dose for the shortest duration of time, consistent with individual patient goals, to reduce risk of cardiovascular or GI adverse events. Pancreatitis has been reported; discontinue with suspected pancreatitis.

Platelet adhesion and aggregation may be decreased, may prolong bleeding time; patients with coagulation disorders or who are receiving anticoagulants should be monitored closely. Anemia may occur; patients on long-term NSAID therapy should be monitored for anemia. NSAIDs may cause serious skin adverse events including exfoliative dermatitis, Stevens-Johnson syndrome (SJS) and toxic epidermal necrolysis (TEN); discontinue use at first sign of skin rash or hypersensitivity. Anaphylactoid reactions may occur. Do not use in patients who experience bronchospasm, asthma, rhinitis, or urticaria with NSAID or aspirin therapy. Use caution in other forms of asthma. May increase the risk of aseptic meningitis, especially in patients with systemic lupus erythematosus (SLE) and mixed connective tissue disorders. Safety and efficacy have not been established in children.

Withhold for at least 4-6 half-lives prior to surgical or dental procedures.

Adverse Reactions

1% to 10%:

Cardiovascular: Edema (1% to 3%)

Central nervous system: Dizziness (3% to 9%), headache (3% to 9%), nervousness (1% to 3%)

Dermatologic: Rash (3% to 9%), pruritus (1% to 3%)

Gastrointestinal: GI pain (10%), constipation (3% to 9%), diarrhea (3% to 9%), dyspepsia (3% to 9%), nausea (3% to 9%), abdominal cramps (1% to 3%), anorexia (1% to 3%), flatulence (1% to 3%), vomiting (1% to 3%)

Otic: Tinnitus (1% to 3%)

<1% (Limited to important or life-threatening): Agranulocytosis, ageusia, alopecia, anaphylaxis, angioneurotic edema, aplastic anemia, arrhythmia, aseptic meningitis, bitter taste, blurred vision, bone marrow depression, bronchial spasm, bruising, CHF, cholestasis, colitis, conjunctivitis, crystalluria, depression, dry mucous membranes, dyspnea, dysuria, epistaxis, erythema multiforme, exfoliative dermatitis, fever, gastritis, GI bleeding, GI perforation, glossitis, gynecomastia, hearing decreased, hematuria, hemolytic anemia, hepatitis, hepatic failure, hyperglycemia, hyperkalemia, hypersensitivity reaction, hypersensitivity syndrome (includes chills, diaphoresis, fever, flushing), hypersensitivity vasculitis, hypertension, insomnia, intestinal stricture, interstitial nephritis, jaundice, leukopenia, liver function abnormal, metallic taste, necrotizing fascitis, nephrotic syndrome, neuritis, neutropenia, palpitation, pancreatitis, paresthesia, peptic ulcer, photosensitivity, proteinuria, psychosis, purpura, renal calculi, renal failure, renal impairment, retinal disturbances, seizure, somnolence, Stevens-Johnson syndrome, stomatitis, syncope, thrombocytopenia, toxic epidermal necrolysis, urine discoloration, vaginal bleeding, vertigo, visual disturbance, weakness

Drug Interactions

Avoid Concomitant Use

Avoid concomitant use of Sulindac with any of the following: Ketorolac

Increased Effect/Toxicity

Sulindac may increase the levels/effects of: Aminoglycosides; Anticoagulants; Antiplatelet Agents; Bisphosphonate Derivatives; CycloSPORINE; Desmopressin; Methotrexate; Nonsteroidal Anti-Inflammatory Agents; Pemetrexed; Quinolone Antibiotics; Salicylates; Thrombolytic Agents; Vancomycin; Vitamin K Antagonists

The levels/effects of Sulindac may be increased by: Antidepressants (Tricyclic, Tertiary Amine); Corticosteroids (Systemic); Dimethyl Sulfoxide; Herbs (Anticoagulant/Antiplatelet Properties); Ketorolac; Probenecid; Selective Serotonin Reuptake Inhibitors; Serotonin/Norepinephrine Reuptake Inhibitors; Treprostinil

Decreased Effect

Sulindac may decrease the levels/effects of: ACE Inhibitors; Angiotensin II Receptor Blockers; Antiplatelet Agents; Beta-Blockers; Eplerenone; HydrALAZINE; Loop Diuretics; Salicylates; Thiazide Diuretics

The levels/effects of Sulindac may be decreased by: Bile Acid Sequestrants; Salicylates

Ethanol/Nutrition/Herb Interactions

Ethanol: Avoid ethanol (may enhance gastric mucosal irritation).

Herb/Nutraceutical: Avoid alfalfa, anise, bilberry, bladderwrack, bromelain, cat's claw, celery, chamomile, coleus, cordyceps, dong quai, evening primrose, fenugreek, feverfew, garlic, ginger, ginkgo biloba, ginseng (American, Panax, Siberian), grapeseed, green tea, guggul, horse chestnut seed, horseradish, licorice, prickly ash, red clover, reishi, SAMe (S-adenosylmethionine), sweet clover, turmeric, white willow (all have additional antiplatelet activity).

Stability Store at room temperature of 15°C to 30°C (59°F to 86°F).

Mechanism of Action Reversibly inhibits cyclooxygenase-1 and 2 (COX-1 and 2) enzymes, which result in decreased formation of prostaglandin precursors; has antipyretic, analgesic, and anti-inflammatory properties

Pharmacodynamics/Kinetics

Absorption: 90%

Protein binding: Sulindac, sulfone, and sulfide metabolites: 93% to 98% primarily to albumin

Distribution: Crosses blood-brain barrier (brain concentrations <4% of plasma concentrations) and placental barriers

Metabolism: Hepatic; prodrug metabolized to sulfide metabolite (active) for therapeutic effects and to sulfone metabolites (inactive); parent and inactive sulfone metabolite undergo extensive enterohepatic recirculation

Half-life elimination: Parent drug: ~8 hours; Active metabolite: ~16 hours

Excretion: Urine (~50%, primarily as inactive metabolites, <1% as active metabolite); feces (~25%, primarily as metabolites)

Dosage Oral:

Children: Dose not established

Adults: **Note:** Maximum daily dose: 400 mg

Osteoarthritis, rheumatoid arthritis, ankylosing spondylitis: 150 mg twice daily

Acute painful shoulder (bursitis/tendonitis): 200 mg twice daily; usual treatment: 7-14 days

Acute gouty arthritis: 200 mg twice daily; usual treatment: 7 days

Dosing adjustment in renal impairment: Not recommended with advanced renal impairment; if required, decrease dose and monitor closely

Dosing adjustment in hepatic impairment: Dose reduction is necessary; discontinue if abnormal liver function tests occur

Dietary Considerations Drug may cause GI upset, bleeding, ulceration, perforation; take with food or milk to minimize GI upset.

Administration Should be administered with food or milk.

Monitoring Parameters Liver enzymes, BUN, serum creatinine, CBC, blood pressure; signs and symptoms of GI bleeding; ophthalmic exam (if ocular complaints develop during treatment)

Test Interactions Increased chloride (S), increased sodium (S), increased bleeding time

Dosage Forms Excipient information presented when available (limited, particularly for generics); consult specific product labeling.

Tablet: 150 mg, 200 mg
Clinoril®: 200 mg

Extemporaneous Preparations A suspension of sulindac can be prepared by triturating 1000 mg sulindac (5 x 200 mg tablets) with 50 mg of kelco and 400 mg of Veegum® until a powder mixture is formed; then add 30 mL of sorbitol 35% (prepared from 70% sorbitol) to form a slurry; finally add a sufficient quantity of 35% sorbitol to make a final volume of 100 mL; the final suspension is 10 mg/mL and is stable for 7 days

◆ **Sulphafurazole** *see* SulfiSOXAZOLE *on page 1410*

SUMAtriptan (soo ma TRIP tan)

U.S. Brand Names Imitrex®

Canadian Brand Names Apo-Sumatriptan®; CO Sumatriptan; Dom-Sumatriptan; Gen-Sumatriptan; Imitrex®; Imitrex® DF; Imitrex® Nasal Spray; Novo-Sumatriptan; PHL-Sumatriptan; PMS-Sumatriptan; ratio-Sumatriptan; Rhoxal-sumatriptan; Riva-Sumatriptan; Sandoz-Sumatriptan; Sumatryx

Index Terms Sumatriptan Succinate

Pharmacologic Category Antimigraine Agent; Serotonin $5\text{-HT}_{1B,\ 1D}$ Receptor Agonist

Additional Appendix Information

Antimigraine Drugs: 5-HT_1 Receptor Agonists *on page 1642*

Sulfonamide Derivatives *on page 1671*

Use

Oral, SubQ: Acute treatment of migraine with or without aura

SubQ: Acute treatment of cluster headache episodes

Pregnancy Risk Factor C

Pregnancy Considerations There are no adequate and well-controlled studies using sumatriptan in pregnant women. Use only if potential benefit to the mother outweighs the potential risk to the fetus. A pregnancy registry has been established to monitor outcomes of women exposed to sumatriptan during pregnancy (800-336-2176). Preliminary data from the registry do not suggest a greater risk of birth defects than the general population and so far a specific pattern of malformations has not been identified. However, sample sizes are small and studies are ongoing. In some (but not all) animal studies, administration was associated with embryolethality, fetal malformations and pup mortality.

Lactation Enters breast milk/use caution (AAP rates "compatible")

Medication Safety Issues

Sound-alike/look-alike issues:

SUMAtriptan may be confused with sitaGLIPtin, somatropin, zolmitriptan

International issues:

Imitrex® may be confused with Nitrex® which is a brand name for isosorbide mononitrate in Italy

Contraindications Hypersensitivity to sumatriptan or any component of the formulation; patients with ischemic heart disease or signs or symptoms of ischemic heart disease (including Prinzmetal's angina, angina pectoris, myocardial infarction, silent myocardial ischemia); cerebrovascular syndromes (including strokes, transient ischemic attacks); peripheral vascular syndromes (including ischemic bowel disease); uncontrolled hypertension; use within 24 hours of ergotamine derivatives; use within 24 hours of another 5-HT_1 agonist; concurrent administration or within 2 weeks of discontinuing an MAO inhibitor, specifically MAO type A inhibitors; management of hemiplegic or basilar migraine; prophylactic treatment of migraine; severe hepatic impairment; not for I.V. administration

Warnings/Precautions Sumatriptan is indicated only in patients ≥18 years of age with a clear diagnosis of migraine or cluster headache. Cardiac events (coronary artery vasospasm, transient ischemia, myocardial infarction, ventricular tachycardia/fibrillation, cardiac arrest and death), cerebral/subarachnoid hemorrhage, and stroke have been reported with 5-HT_1 agonist administration. Do not give to patients with risk factors for CAD until a cardiovascular evaluation has been performed; if evaluation is satisfactory, the healthcare provider should administer the first dose and cardiovascular status should be periodically evaluated.

Significant elevation in blood pressure, including hypertensive crisis, has also been reported on rare occasions in patients with and without a history of hypertension. Vasospasm-related reactions have been reported other than coronary artery vasospasm. Peripheral vascular ischemia and colonic ischemia with abdominal pain and bloody diarrhea have occurred. Use with caution in patients with a history of seizure disorder or in patients with a lowered seizure threshold. Use with caution in patients with hepatic impairment. Symptoms of agitation, confusion, hallucinations, hyper-reflexia, myoclonus, shivering, and tachycardia (serotonin syndrome) may occur with concomitant proserotonergic drugs (ie, SSRIs/SNRIs or triptans) or agents which reduce sumatriptan's metabolism. Concurrent use of serotonin precursors (eg, tryptophan) is not recommended. Safety and efficacy in pediatric patients have not been established.

Adverse Reactions

Injection:

>10%:

Central nervous system: Dizziness (12%), warm/hot sensation (11%)

Local: Pain at injection site (59%)

Neuromuscular & skeletal: Paresthesia (14%)

1% to 10%:

Cardiovascular: Chest pain/tightness/heaviness/pressure (2% to 3%), hyper-/hypotension (1%)

Central nervous system: Burning (7%), feeling of heaviness (7%), flushing (7%), pressure sensation (7%), feeling of tightness (5%), drowsiness (3%), malaise/fatigue (1%), feeling strange (2%), headache (2%), tight feeling in head (2%), cold sensation (1%), anxiety (1%)

Gastrointestinal: Abdominal discomfort (1%), dysphagia (1%)

Neuromuscular & skeletal: Neck, throat, and jaw pain/tightness/pressure (2% to 5%), mouth/tongue discomfort (5%), weakness (5%), myalgia (2%); muscle cramps (1%), numbness (5%)

Ocular: Vision alterations (1%)

Respiratory: Throat discomfort (3%), nasal disorder/discomfort (2%)

Miscellaneous: Diaphoresis (2%)

Nasal spray:

>10%: Gastrointestinal: Bad taste (13% to 24%), nausea (11% to 13%), vomiting (11% to 13%)

1% to 10%:

Central nervous system: Dizziness (1% to 2%)

Respiratory: Nasal disorder/discomfort (2% to 4%), throat discomfort (1% to 2%)

Tablet:

1% to 10%:

Cardiovascular: Chest pain/tightness/heaviness/pressure (1% to 2%), hyper-/hypotension (1%), palpitation (1%), syncope (1%)

Central nervous system: Burning (1%), dizziness (>1%), drowsiness (>1%), malaise/fatigue (2% to 3%), headache (>1%), nonspecified pain (1% to 2%, placebo 1%), vertigo (<1% to 2%), migraine (>1%), sleepiness (>1%)

Gastrointestinal: Diarrhea (1%), nausea (>1%), vomiting (>1%), hyposalivation (>1%)

Genitourinary: Hematuria (1%)

Hematologic: Hemolytic anemia (1%)
Neuromuscular & skeletal: Neck, throat, and jaw pain/tightness/pressure (2% to 3%), paresthesia (3% to 5%), myalgia (1%), numbness (1%)
Otic: Ear hemorrhage (1%), hearing loss (1%), sensitivity to noise (1%), tinnitus (1%)
Respiratory: Allergic rhinitis (1%), dyspnea (1%), nasal inflammation (1%), nose/throat hemorrhage (1%), sinusitis (1%), upper respiratory inflammation (1%)
Miscellaneous: Hypersensitivity reactions (1%), nonspecified pressure/tightness/heaviness (1% to 3%, placebo 2%); warm/cold sensation (2% to 3%, placebo 2%)

Route unspecified: <1%: Postmarketing and uncontrolled studies (limited to important or life-threatening): Abdominal aortic aneurysm, abdominal discomfort, abnormal menstrual cycle, abnormal/elevated liver function tests, accommodation disorders, acute renal failure, agitation, anaphylactoid reaction, anaphylaxis, anemia, angioneurotic edema, arrhythmia, atrial fibrillation, bronchospasm, cerebral ischemia, cerebrovascular accident, convulsions, deafness, death, decreased appetite, dental pain, diarrhea, dyspeptic symptoms, dysphagia, dystonic reaction, ECG changes, fluid disturbances (including retention), flushing, gastrointestinal pain, hallucinations, heart block, hematuria, hemolytic anemia, hiccups, hypersensitivity reactions, intestinal obstruction, intracranial pressure increased, ischemic colitis, joint ache, muscle stiffness, nose/throat hemorrhage, numbness of tongue, optic neuropathy (ischemic), pancytopenia, paresthesia, phlebitis, photosensitivity, Prinzmetal's angina, pruritus, psychomotor disorders, pulmonary embolism, rash, Raynaud syndrome, sensation changes, shock, subarachnoid hemorrhage, swallowing disorders, syncope, thrombocytopenia, thrombophlebitis, thrombosis, transient myocardial ischemia, TSH increased, vasculitis, vision loss, xerostomia

Drug Interactions

Avoid Concomitant Use

Avoid concomitant use of SUMAtriptan with any of the following: Ergot Derivatives; MAO Inhibitors; Sibutramine

Increased Effect/Toxicity

SUMAtriptan may increase the levels/effects of: Ergot Derivatives; Serotonin Modulators

The levels/effects of SUMAtriptan may be increased by: Ergot Derivatives; MAO Inhibitors; Sibutramine

Decreased Effect There are no known significant interactions involving a decrease in effect.

Stability Store at 2°C to 20°C (36°F to 86°F). Protect from light.

Mechanism of Action Selective agonist for serotonin (5-HT_{1D} receptor) in cranial arteries to cause vasoconstriction and reduces sterile inflammation associated with antidromic neuronal transmission correlating with relief of migraine

Pharmacodynamics/Kinetics

Onset of action: ~30 minutes
Distribution: V_d: 2.4 L/kg
Protein binding: 14% to 21%
Metabolism: Hepatic, primarily via MAO-A isoenzyme
Bioavailability: SubQ: 97% ± 16% of that following I.V. injection; Oral: 15%
Half-life elimination: Injection, tablet: 2.5 hours; Nasal spray: 2 hours
Time to peak, serum: 5-20 minutes
Excretion:
Injection: Urine (38% as indole acetic acid metabolite, 22% as unchanged drug)
Nasal spray: Urine (42% as indole acetic acid metabolite, 3% as unchanged drug)
Tablet: Urine (60% as indole acetic acid metabolite, 3% as unchanged drug); feces (40%)

Dosage Adults:
Oral: A single dose of 25 mg, 50 mg, or 100 mg (taken with fluids). If a satisfactory response has not been obtained at 2 hours, a second dose may be administered. Results from clinical trials show that initial doses of 50 mg and 100 mg are more effective than doses of 25 mg, and that 100 mg doses do not provide a greater effect than 50 mg and may have increased incidence of side effects. Although doses of up to 300 mg/day have been studied, the total daily dose should not exceed 200 mg. The safety of treating an average of >4 headaches in a 30-day period have not been established.
Intranasal: A single dose of 5 mg, 10 mg, or 20 mg administered in one nostril. A 10 mg dose may be achieved by administering a single 5 mg dose in each nostril. If headache returns, the dose may be repeated once after 2 hours, not to exceed a total daily dose of 40 mg. The safety of treating an average of >4 headaches in a 30-day period has not been established.
SubQ: Up to 6 mg; if side effects are dose-limiting, lower doses may be used. A second injection may be administered at least 1 hour after the initial dose, but not more than 2 injections in a 24-hour period.

Dosage adjustment in renal impairment: Dosage adjustment not necessary

Dosage adjustment in hepatic impairment: Bioavailability of oral sumatriptan is increased with liver disease. If treatment is needed, do not exceed single doses of 50 mg. The nasal spray has not been studied in patients with hepatic impairment, however, because the spray does not undergo first-pass metabolism, levels would not be expected to alter. Use of all dosage forms is contraindicated with severe hepatic impairment.

Administration

Oral: Should be taken with fluids as soon as symptoms appear
Injection solution: For SubQ administration; do not administer I.V.; may cause coronary vasospasm. An autoinjection device (STATdose System®) is available for use with the 4 mg and 6 mg cartridges.

Dosage Forms Excipient information presented when available (limited, particularly for generics); consult specific product labeling. **Note:** Strength expressed as sumatriptan base

Injection, solution, as succinate: 8 mg/mL (0.5 mL); 12 mg/mL (0.5 mL)
Imitrex®: 8 mg/mL (0.5 mL); 12 mg/mL (0.5 mL)
Solution, intranasal [spray]: 5 mg/0.1 mL (6s); 20 mg/0.1 mL (6s)
Imitrex®: 5 mg/0.1 mL (6s); 20 mg/0.1 mL (6s)
Tablet, as succinate: 25 mg, 50 mg, 100 mg
Imitrex®: 25 mg, 50 mg, 100 mg

Sumatriptan and Naproxen

(soo ma TRIP tan & na PROKS en)

U.S. Brand Names Treximet™

Index Terms Naproxen and Sumatriptan; Naproxen Sodium and Sumatriptan; Naproxen Sodium and Sumatriptan Succinate; Sumatriptan Succinate and Naproxen; Sumatriptan Succinate and Naproxen Sodium

Pharmacologic Category Antimigraine Agent; Nonsteroidal Anti-inflammatory Drug (NSAID), Oral; Serotonin 5-$HT_{1B,\ 1D}$ Receptor Agonist

Use Acute treatment of migraine with or without aura

Restrictions

An FDA-approved medication guide must be distributed when dispensing an oral outpatient prescription (new or refill) where this medication is to be used without direct supervision of a healthcare provider. Medication guides are available at http://www.fda.gov/cder/Offices/ODS/medication_guides.htm.

Pregnancy Risk Factor C

Medication Safety Issues

Sound-alike/look-alike issues:

Naproxen may be confused with Natacyn®, Nebcin®, neomycin, niacin

SUMAtriptan may be confused with somatropin, zolmitriptan

Treximet™ may be confused with Trexall™

Dosage Oral: Adults: 1 tablet (sumatriptan 85 mg and naproxen 500 mg). If a satisfactory response has not been obtained at 2 hours, a second dose may be administered (maximum: 2 tablets/24 hours). **Note:** The safety of treating an average of >5 migraine headaches in a 30-day period has not been established.

Dosage adjustment in renal impairment:

Cl_{cr} ≥30 mL/minute Dosage adjustment not necessary

Cl_{cr} <30 mL/minute: Use not recommended

Dosage adjustment in hepatic impairment: Mild-to-severe impairment: Use is contraindicated by the manufacturer

Additional Information Complete prescribing information for this medication should be consulted for additional detail.

Dosage Forms Excipient information presented when available (limited, particularly for generics); consult specific product labeling.

Tablet:

Treximet™ 85/500: Sumatriptan 85 mg and naproxen sodium 500 mg [contains sodium 61.2 mg/tablet (~2.7 mEq/tablet)]

- **Sumatriptan Succinate** *see* SUMAtriptan *on page 1414*
- **Sumatriptan Succinate and Naproxen** *see* Sumatriptan and Naproxen *on page 1415*
- **Sumatriptan Succinate and Naproxen Sodium** *see* Sumatriptan and Naproxen *on page 1415*
- **Sumatryx (Can)** *see* SUMAtriptan *on page 1414*
- **Summer's Eve® Medicated Douche [OTC]** *see* Povidone-Iodine *on page 1222*
- **Summer's Eve® SpecialCare™ Medicated Anti-Itch Cream [OTC] [DSC]** *see* Hydrocortisone *on page 743*

Sunitinib (su NIT e nib)

U.S. Brand Names Sutent®

Canadian Brand Names Sutent®

Index Terms NSC-736511; SU11248; Sunitinib Malate

Pharmacologic Category Antineoplastic Agent, Tyrosine Kinase Inhibitor; Vascular Endothelial Growth Factor (VEGF) Inhibitor

Use Treatment of gastrointestinal stromal tumor (GIST) intolerance to or disease progression on imatinib; treatment of advanced renal cell cancer (RCC)

Pregnancy Risk Factor D

Pregnancy Considerations Animal studies have demonstrated teratogenicity and fetal loss. There are no adequate and well-controlled studies in pregnant women. Because sunitinib inhibits angiogenesis, a critical component of fetal development, adverse effects on pregnancy would be expected. Women of childbearing potential should be advised to avoid pregnancy.

Lactation Excretion in breast milk unknown/not recommended

Medication Safety Issues

Sound-alike/look-alike issues:

Sunitinib may be confused with sorafenib

High alert medication: The Institute for Safe Medication Practices (ISMP) includes this medication among its list of drug classes which have a heightened risk of causing significant patient harm when used in error.

Contraindications There are no contraindications listed within the FDA-approved manufacturer's labeling.

Canadian labeling: Hypersensitivity to sunitinib or any component of the formulation; pregnancy

Warnings/Precautions May cause a decrease in left ventricular ejection fraction (LVEF), including grade 3 reductions; monitor with baseline and periodic LVEF evaluations. Mean onset of symptomatic HF is 22 days from treatment initiation. Interrupt therapy or decrease dose with LVEF <50% or >20% reduction from baseline. Discontinue with clinical signs and symptoms of heart failure (HF). QT_c prolongation and torsade de pointes have been observed; a baseline and periodic ECG should be obtained; correct electrolyte abnormalities prior to treatment and monitor and correct potassium, calcium and magnesium levels during therapy; use caution in patients with a history of QT_c prolongation, with medications known to prolong the QT_c interval, or patients with pre-existing (relevant) cardiac disease, bradycardia, or electrolyte imbalance. Use caution with cardiac dysfunction; patients with MI, bypass grafts, HF, vascular diseases (including CVA and TIA), and PE were excluded from clinical trials. May cause hypertension; monitor and control with antihypertensives if needed; interrupt therapy until hypertension is controlled for severe hypertension. Use caution and closely monitor in patients with underlying or poorly-controlled hypertension. Use with caution in patients concurrently taking strong CYP3A4 inhibitors (may increase sunitinib levels; eg, ketoconazole) or inducers (may decrease sunitinib levels; eg, rifampin); dosage adjustments of sunitinib may be required.

Hemorrhagic events have been reported including epistaxis, rectal, gingival, upper GI, genital, wound bleeding, tumor-related, and hemoptysis/pulmonary hemorrhage. Microangiopathic hemolytic anemia (MAHA) has been reported when sunitinib has been used in combination with bevacizumab. Serious and fatal gastrointestinal complications, including gastrointestinal perforation, have occurred (rarely). Hypothyroidism may occur; the risk for hypothyroidism appears to increase with therapy duration; hyperthyroidism, sometimes followed by hypothyroidism has also been reported; monitor thyroid function at baseline and if symptomatic. Adrenal function abnormalities have been reported; monitor for adrenal insufficiency for patients with trauma, severe infection, or undergoing surgery. May cause skin and/or hair depigmentation or discoloration. Reversible posterior leukoencephalopathy syndrome (RPLS) has been reported (rarely); symptoms include confusion, headache, hypertension, lethargy, seizure, blindness and/or other vision, or neurologic disturbances; interrupt treatment and begin hypertension management. Has not been studied in patients with severe hepatic impairment (Child-Pugh class C). Safety and effectiveness in children have not been established.

Adverse Reactions

>10%:

Cardiovascular: Hypertension (15% to 30%; grades 3/4: 4% to 10%), LVEF decreased (11% to 21%; grades 3/4: 1%), heart failure (≤15%), peripheral edema (11%)

Central nervous system: Fatigue (42% to 58%), fever (17% to 18%), headache (13% to 18%), chills (11%), insomnia (11%)

Dermatologic: Hyperpigmentation (19% to 33%), skin discoloration (19% to 30%), rash (14% to 27%), hand-foot syndrome (12% to 21%), dry skin (17% to 18%), hair color changes (7% to 16%)

Endocrine & metabolic: Hyperuricemia (15% to 41%), hypophosphatemia (9% to 36%), hypocalcemia (35%), hypoglycemia (19%), hypoalbuminemia (18%), hyperglycemia (15%), hyponatremia (6% to 14%), hypokalemia (12%), hyperkalemia (6% to 11%), hypernatremia (10% to 11%)

Gastrointestinal: Diarrhea (40% to 58%), lipase increased (25% to 52%), nausea (31% to 49%), taste perversion (21% to 44%), mucositis/stomatitis (29% to 43%), anorexia (31% to 38%), constipation (16% to 34%), abdominal pain (22% to 33%), dyspepsia (28%), vomiting (24% to 28%), amylase increased (5% to 17%), weight loss (12%), xerostomia (12%), GERD/ reflux (11%)

Hematologic: Leukopenia (up to 78%; grades 3/4: 5%), neutropenia (53% to 72%; grades 3/4: 10% to 12%), anemia (26% to 72%; grades 3/4: 3% to 7%), thrombocytopenia (38% to 65%; grades 3/4: 5% to 8%), lymphopenia (38% to 59%; grades 3/4: up to 59%), hemorrhage/bleeding (18% to 30%)

Hepatic: AST increased (39% to 52%), ALT increased (39% to 46%), alkaline phosphatase increased (24% to 42%), hyperbilirubinemia (10% to 19%)

Neuromuscular & skeletal: Creatine kinase increased (41%), weakness (21% to 22%), back pain (11% to 19%), arthralgia (12% to 18%), limb pain (14% to 17%), myalgia (14%)

Renal: Creatinine increased (12% to 66%)

Respiratory: Dyspnea (10% to 28%), cough (8% to 17%)

1% to 10%:

Cardiovascular: Venous thrombotic events (2% to 3%), DVT (1% to 3%), myocardial ischemia (1%)

Central nervous system: Depression (8%), dizziness (7%)

Dermatologic: Skin blistering (7%), alopecia (5%)

Endocrine & metabolic: Dehydration (8%), hypothyroidism (3% to 7%)

Gastrointestinal: Flatulence (10%), glossodynia (10%), oral pain (6% to 10%), appetite disturbance (9%), pancreatitis (1%)

Neuromuscular & skeletal: Peripheral neuropathy (10%)

Ocular: Periorbital edema (7%), lacrimation increased (6%)

Respiratory: Pulmonary embolism (1%)

<1% (Limited to important or life-threatening): Acute renal failure, adrenal dysfunction, atrial flutter, febrile neutropenia, gastrointestinal perforation, hepatic failure, hyperthyroidism, infection, microangiopathic hemolytic anemia (when used in combination with bevacizumab), MI, myopathy, nephrotic syndrome, neutropenic infection, preeclampsia-like syndrome (proteinuria and reversible hypertension), proteinuria, pulmonary hemorrhage, QT_c prolongation, reversible posterior leukoencephalopathy syndrome (RPLS), rhabdomyolysis, seizure, thrombotic microangiopathy, torsade de pointes, ventricular arrhythmia

Drug Interactions

Metabolism/Transport Effects Substrate of CYP3A4 (major)

Avoid Concomitant Use

Avoid concomitant use of Sunitinib with any of the following: Bevacizumab; Natalizumab; Nilotinib; Tetrabenazine; Thioridazine; Vaccines (Live); Ziprasidone

Increased Effect/Toxicity

Sunitinib may increase the levels/effects of: Bevacizumab; Natalizumab; QTc-Prolonging Agents; Tetrabenazine; Thioridazine; Vaccines (Live); Vitamin K Antagonists; Ziprasidone

The levels/effects of Sunitinib may be increased by: Alfuzosin; Antifungal Agents (Azole Derivatives, Systemic); Ciprofloxacin; CYP3A4 Inhibitors (Moderate); CYP3A4 Inhibitors (Strong); Dasatinib; Gadobutrol; Nilotinib; Trastuzumab

Decreased Effect

Sunitinib may decrease the levels/effects of: Cardiac Glycosides; Vaccines (Inactivated); Vitamin K Antagonists

The levels/effects of Sunitinib may be decreased by: CYP3A4 Inducers (Strong); Deferasirox; Echinacea; Herbs (CYP3A4 Inducers); Rifamycin Derivatives

Ethanol/Nutrition/Herb Interactions

Food: Grapefruit juice may increase the levels/effects of sunitinib. Food has no effect on the bioavailability of sunitinib.

Herb/Nutraceutical: Avoid St John's wort (may increase metabolism and decrease sunitinib concentrations).

Stability Store at room temperature of 25°C (77°F); excursions permitted to 15°C and 30°C (59°F and 86°F).

Mechanism of Action Exhibits antitumor and antiangiogenic properties by inhibiting multiple receptor tyrosine kinases, including platelet-derived growth factors (PDGFRα and PDGFRβ), vascular endothelial growth factors (VEGFR1, VEGFR2, and VEGFR3), FMS-like tyrosine kinase-3 (FLT3), colony-stimulating factor type 1 (CSF-1R), and glial cell-line-derived neurotrophic factor receptor (RET).

Pharmacodynamics/Kinetics

Distribution: V_d/F: 2230 L

Protein binding: Sunitinib: 95%; SU12662: 90%

Metabolism: Hepatic; primarily metabolized by CYP3A4 to the N-desethyl metabolite SU12662 (active)

Half-life elimination: Sunitinib: 40-60 hours; SU12662: 80-110 hours

Time to peak, plasma: 6-12 hours

Excretion: Feces (61%); urine (16%)

Dosage Oral: Adults: Gastrointestinal stromal tumor, renal cell cancer: 50 mg once daily for 4 weeks of a 6-week treatment cycle (4 weeks on, 2 weeks off). **Note:** Dosage modifications should be done in increments of 12.5 mg; individualize based on safety and tolerability.

Dosage adjustment with concurrent CYP3A4 inhibitor: Dose reductions are more likely to be needed when sunitinib is administered concomitantly with strong CYP3A4 inhibitors (eg, clarithromycin, erythromycin, itraconazole, ketoconazole, nefazodone, protease inhibitors, telithromycin, voriconazole); dose reductions to a minimum of 37.5 mg/day should be considered with strong CYP3A4 inhibitors.

Dosage adjustment with concurrent CYP3A4 inducer: May require increased doses; dosage increases to a maximum of 87.5 mg/day with careful monitoring should be considered with strong CYP3A4 inducers (eg, carbamazepine, dexamethasone, phenobarbital, phenytoin, rifampin, St. John's wort).

Dosage adjustment for toxicity:

Cardiac toxicity:

Ejection fraction <50% and >20% below baseline without evidence of CHF: Interrupt treatment and/or reduce dose

LV dysfunction with CHF clinical manifestations: Discontinue treatment

Severe hypertension: Temporarily interrupt treatment until hypertension is controlled

Hepatic failure, nephrotic syndrome, or pancreatitis: Discontinue treatment

RPLS or thrombotic microangiopathy: Temporarily withhold treatment; after resolution, may resume with discretion.

Dosage adjustment in renal impairment: Not studied in patients with serum creatinine >2 x ULN; pharmacokinetics were unaltered in patients with Cl_{cr} ≥42 mL/minute.

Dosage adjustment in hepatic impairment: No adjustment is necessary with mild-to-moderate (Child-Pugh Class A or B) hepatic impairment; not studied in patients with severe (Child-Pugh Class C) hepatic impairment. Studies excluded patients with ALT/AST >2.5 x ULN, or if due to liver metastases, ALT/AST >5 x ULN.

Dietary Considerations May be taken with or without food. Avoid grapefruit juice.

Administration May be taken with or without food.

Monitoring Parameters LVEF, baseline (and periodic with cardiac risk factors), ECG (12-lead; baseline and periodic), blood pressure, adrenal function, CBC with differential and platelets (prior to each treatment cycle), serum chemistries including magnesium, phosphate, and potassium (prior to each treatment cycle), thyroid function (baseline; then if symptomatic), urinalysis (for proteinuria development or worsening)

Dosage Forms Excipient information presented when available (limited, particularly for generics); consult specific product labeling.

Capsule:

Sutent®: 12.5 mg, 25 mg, 50 mg

Extemporaneous Preparations

Sunitinib 10 mg/mL oral suspension: In a mortar, mix the contents of three 50-mg sunitinib capsules with a 1:1 mixture of Ora-Sweet® and Ora-Plus® to a final volume of 15 mL, yielding a final sunitinib concentration of 10 mg/mL; transfer to amber plastic bottle. This suspension maintains an average concentration of 96% to 106% (of the original concentration) at room temperature or refrigerated for up to 60 days in plastic amber prescription bottles. Note: Shake well before use.

Navid F, Christensen R, Minkin P, et al, "Stability of Sunitinib in Oral Suspension," *Ann Pharmacother*, 2008, 42(7):962-6.

- **Sunitinib Malate** *see* Sunitinib *on page 1416*
- **Supartz™** *see* Hyaluronate and Derivatives *on page 734*
- **Supeudol® (Can)** *see* OxyCODONE *on page 1120*
- **Suphera™** *see* Sulfur and Sulfacetamide *on page 1411*
- **Suplasyn® (Can)** *see* Hyaluronate and Derivatives *on page 734*
- **Supprelin® LA** *see* Histrelin *on page 732*
- **Suprax®** *see* Cefixime *on page 275*
- **Surfak® [OTC]** *see* Docusate *on page 473*
- **Surmontil®** *see* Trimipramine *on page 1521*
- **Survanta®** *see* Beractant *on page 187*
- **Sustiva®** *see* Efavirenz *on page 508*
- **SuTan** *see* Dexchlorpheniramine and Pseudoephedrine *on page 428*
- **Sutent®** *see* Sunitinib *on page 1416*
- **Su-Tuss DM** *see* Guaifenesin and Dextromethorphan *on page 710*
- **Su-Tuss®-HD [DSC]** *see* Hydrocodone, Pseudoephedrine, and Guaifenesin *on page 743*
- **Suxamethonium Chloride** *see* Succinylcholine *on page 1402*
- **Sween Cream® [OTC]** *see* Vitamin A and Vitamin D *on page 1565*
- **Symax SL** *see* Hyoscyamine *on page 756*
- **Symax SR** *see* Hyoscyamine *on page 756*
- **Symbicort®** *see* Budesonide and Formoterol *on page 218*
- **Symbyax®** *see* Olanzapine and Fluoxetine *on page 1095*
- **Symlin®** *see* Pramlintide *on page 1225*
- **Symmetrel®** *see* Amantadine *on page 78*
- **Sympt-X [OTC]** *see* Glutamine *on page 700*
- **Sympt-X G.I. [OTC]** *see* Glutamine *on page 700*
- **SymTan™ [DSC]** *see* Hydrocodone and Pseudoephedrine *on page 742*
- **Synacthen** *see* Cosyntropin *on page 372*
- **Synagis®** *see* Palivizumab *on page 1132*
- **Synalar® [DSC]** *see* Fluocinolone *on page 633*
- **Synalar® (Can)** *see* Fluocinolone *on page 633*
- **Synalgos®-DC** *see* Dihydrocodeine, Aspirin, and Caffeine *on page 448*
- **Synarel®** *see* Nafarelin *on page 1032*
- **Syn-Diltiazem® (Can)** *see* Diltiazem *on page 450*
- **Synera™** *see* Lidocaine and Tetracaine *on page 888*
- **Synercid®** *see* Quinupristin and Dalfopristin *on page 1284*
- **Synphasic® (Can)** *see* Ethinyl Estradiol and Norethindrone *on page 581*
- **Syntest D.S. [DSC]** *see* Estrogens (Esterified) and Methyltestosterone *on page 568*
- **Syntest H.S. [DSC]** *see* Estrogens (Esterified) and Methyltestosterone *on page 568*
- **Synthroid®** *see* Levothyroxine *on page 881*
- **Syntocinon® (Can)** *see* Oxytocin *on page 1126*
- **Synvisc®** *see* Hyaluronate and Derivatives *on page 734*
- **Syprine®** *see* Trientine *on page 1515*
- **Syrex** *see* Sodium Chloride *on page 1381*
- **SyringeAvitene™** *see* Collagen Hemostat *on page 367*
- **Syrup of Ipecac** *see* Ipecac Syrup *on page 811*
- **T_3 Sodium (error-prone abbreviation)** *see* Liothyronine *on page 892*
- **T_3/T_4 Liotrix** *see* Liotrix *on page 892*
- **T_4** *see* Levothyroxine *on page 881*
- **T-20** *see* Enfuvirtide *on page 518*
- **642® Tablet (Can)** *see* Propoxyphene *on page 1256*
- **Tabloid®** *see* Thioguanine *on page 1459*
- **Taclonex®** *see* Calcipotriene and Betamethasone *on page 234*
- **Taclonex Scalp®** *see* Calcipotriene and Betamethasone *on page 234*

Tacrine (TAK reen)

U.S. Brand Names Cognex®

Index Terms Tacrine Hydrochloride; Tetrahydroaminoacrine; THA

Pharmacologic Category Acetylcholinesterase Inhibitor (Central)

Use Treatment of mild-to-moderate dementia of the Alzheimer's type

Unlabeled/Investigational Use Lewy body dementia

Pregnancy Risk Factor C

Lactation Excretion in breast milk unknown/not recommended

Medication Safety Issues

Sound-alike/look-alike issues:

Cognex® may be confused with Corgard®

International issues:

Cognex® may be confused with Codex® which is a brand name for *Saccharomyces boulardii* in Italy

Contraindications Hypersensitivity to tacrine, acridine derivatives, or any component of the formulation; patients previously treated with tacrine who developed jaundice

Warnings/Precautions The use of tacrine has been associated with elevations in serum transaminases; serum transaminases (specifically ALT) must be monitored throughout therapy; use extreme caution in patients with current evidence of a history of abnormal liver function tests. Cholinesterase inhibitors may have vagotonic effects which may cause bradycardia and/or heart block with or without a history of cardiac disease. Alzheimer's treatment guidelines consider bradycardia to be a relative contraindication for use of centrally-active cholinesterase inhibitors. Use caution in patients with urinary tract obstruction (bladder outlet obstruction or prostatic hyperplasia), asthma, and sick-sinus syndrome, bradycardia, or conduction abnormalities (tacrine may cause bradycardia and/or heart block). Also, patients with cardiovascular disease, asthma, or peptic ulcer should use cautiously. Use with caution in patients with a history of seizures. May cause nausea, vomiting, or loose stools. Abrupt discontinuation or dosage decrease may worsen cognitive function. May be associated with neutropenia. May exaggerate neuromuscular blockade effects of depolarizing neuromuscular-blocking agents like succinylcholine. Safety and efficacy have not been established in children.

Adverse Reactions

>10%:

- Central nervous system: Dizziness, headache
- Gastrointestinal: Diarrhea, nausea, vomiting
- Miscellaneous: Transaminases increased

1% to 10%:

- Cardiovascular: Flushing
- Central nervous system: Ataxia, confusion, depression, fatigue, insomnia, somnolence
- Dermatologic: Rash
- Gastrointestinal: Abdominal pain, anorexia, constipation, dyspepsia, flatulence, weight loss
- Neuromuscular & skeletal: Myalgia, tremor
- Respiratory: Rhinitis

Drug Interactions

Metabolism/Transport Effects **Substrate** of CYP1A2 (major); **Inhibits** CYP1A2 (weak)

Avoid Concomitant Use There are no known interactions where it is recommended to avoid concomitant use.

Increased Effect/Toxicity

Tacrine may increase the levels/effects of: Antipsychotics; Beta-Blockers; Cholinergic Agonists; Succinylcholine; Theophylline Derivatives

The levels/effects of Tacrine may be increased by: Corticosteroids (Systemic); CYP1A2 Inhibitors (Moderate); CYP1A2 Inhibitors (Strong); Fluvoxamine; Ginkgo Biloba

Decreased Effect

Tacrine may decrease the levels/effects of: Anticholinergics; Neuromuscular-Blocking Agents (Nondepolarizing)

The levels/effects of Tacrine may be decreased by: Anticholinergics

Ethanol/Nutrition/Herb Interactions Food: Food decreases bioavailability.

Mechanism of Action Centrally-acting cholinesterase inhibitor. It elevates acetylcholine in cerebral cortex by slowing the degradation of acetylcholine.

Pharmacodynamics/Kinetics

- Absorption: Oral: Rapid
- Distribution: V_d: Mean: 349 L; reduced by food
- Protein binding, plasma: 55%
- Metabolism: Extensively by CYP450 to multiple metabolites; first pass effect
- Bioavailability: Absolute: 17%
- Half-life elimination, serum: 2-4 hours; Steady-state: 24-36 hours
- Time to peak, plasma: 1-2 hours

Dosage Adults: Initial: 10 mg 4 times/day; may increase by 40 mg/day adjusted every 6 weeks; maximum: 160 mg/day; best administered separate from meal times.

Dose adjustment based upon transaminase elevations:

- ALT ≤3 times ULN*: Continue titration
- ALT >3 to ≤5 times ULN*: Decrease dose by 40 mg/day, resume when ALT returns to normal
- ALT >5 times ULN*: Stop treatment, may rechallenge upon return of ALT to normal

*ULN = upper limit of normal

Patients with clinical jaundice confirmed by elevated total bilirubin (>3 mg/dL) should not be rechallenged with tacrine

Dietary Considerations Give with food if GI side effects are intolerable.

Monitoring Parameters ALT levels and other liver enzymes weekly for at least the first 18 weeks, then monitor once every 3 months

Reference Range In clinical trials, serum concentrations >20 ng/mL were associated with a much higher risk of development of symptomatic adverse effects

Dosage Forms Excipient information presented when available (limited, particularly for generics); consult specific product labeling.

Capsule, as hydrochloride: 10 mg, 20 mg, 30 mg, 40 mg

◆ **Tacrine Hydrochloride** *see* Tacrine *on page 1418*

Tacrolimus (ta KROE li mus)

U.S. Brand Names Prograf®; Protopic®

Canadian Brand Names Advagraf™; Prograf®; Protopic®

Index Terms FK506

Pharmacologic Category Immunosuppressant Agent; Topical Skin Product

Use

- Oral/injection: Potent immunosuppressive drug used in heart, kidney, or liver transplant recipients
- Topical: Moderate-to-severe atopic dermatitis in patients not responsive to conventional therapy or when conventional therapy is not appropriate

Unlabeled/Investigational Use Potent immunosuppressive drug used in lung, small bowel transplant recipients; immunosuppressive drug for peripheral stem cell/bone marrow transplantation

Restrictions An FDA-approved medication guide must be distributed when dispensing the outpatient prescription (new or refill) for tacrolimus ointment where this medication is to be used without direct supervision of a healthcare provider. Medication guides are available at http://www.fda.gov/cder/Offices/ODS/medication_guides.htm.

Pregnancy Risk Factor C

Pregnancy Considerations Tacrolimus crosses the placenta and reaches concentrations four times greater than maternal plasma concentrations. Neonatal hyperkalemia and renal dysfunction have been reported.

The National Transplantation Pregnancy Registry (NTPR, Temple University) is a registry for pregnant women taking immunosuppressants following any solid organ transplant. The NTPR encourages reporting of all immunosuppressant exposures during pregnancy in transplant recipients at 877-955-6877.

Lactation Enters breast milk/contraindicated

Medication Safety Issues

Sound-alike/look-alike issues:

- Prograf® may be confused with Gengraf®, Prozac®
- Tacrolimus may be confused with sirolimus, temsirolimus

Contraindications Hypersensitivity to tacrolimus or any component of the formulation

Warnings/Precautions

Oral/injection: Insulin-dependent post-transplant diabetes mellitus (PTDM) has been reported (1% to 20%); risk increases in African-American and Hispanic kidney transplant patients. **[U.S. Boxed Warning]: Increased susceptibility to infection and the possible development of lymphoma may result from immunosuppression with tacrolimus.** Nephrotoxicity and neurotoxicity have been reported, especially with higher doses; to avoid excess nephrotoxicity do not administer simultaneously with cyclosporine; monitoring of serum concentrations (trough for oral therapy) is essential to prevent organ rejection and reduce drug-related toxicity. Tonic clonic seizures may have been triggered by tacrolimus. A period of 24 hours should elapse between discontinuation of cyclosporine and the initiation of tacrolimus. Use caution in renal or hepatic dysfunction, dosing adjustments may be required. Delay initiation if postoperative oliguria occurs. Use may be associated with the development of hypertension (common). Myocardial hypertrophy has been reported (rare). Each mL of injection contains polyoxyl 60 hydrogenated castor oil (HCO-60) (200 mg) and dehydrated alcohol USP 80% v/v. Anaphylaxis has been reported with the injection, use should be reserved for those patients not able to take oral medications. **[U.S. Boxed Warning]: Should be administered under the supervision of a physician experienced in immunosuppressive therapy in a facility appropriate for monitoring and managing therapy.**

Topical: [U.S. Boxed Warning]: Topical calcineurin inhibitors have been associated with rare cases of malignancy (including skin and lymphoma), therefore it should be limited to short-term and intermittent treatment using the minimum amount necessary for the control of symptoms and only on involved areas. Use in children <2 years of age is not recommended, children ages 2-15 should only use the 0.03% ointment. Avoid use on malignant or premalignant skin conditions (eg cutaneous T-cell lymphoma). Should not be used in immunocompromised patients. Do not apply to areas of active bacterial or viral infection; infections at the treatment site should be cleared prior to therapy. Topical calcineurin agents are considered second-line therapies in the treatment of atopic dermatitis/eczema, and should be limited to use in patients who have failed treatment with other therapies. Patients with atopic dermatitis are predisposed to skin infections, and tacrolimus therapy has been associated with risk of developing eczema herpeticum, varicella zoster, and herpes simplex. If atopic dermatitis is not improved in <6 weeks, re-evaluate to confirm diagnosis. May be associated with development of lymphadenopathy; possible infectious causes should be investigated. Discontinue use in patients with unknown cause of lymphadenopathy or acute infectious mononucleosis. Acute renal failure has been observed (rarely) with topical use. Not recommended for use in patients with skin disease which may increase systemic absorption (eg, Netherton's syndrome). Minimize sunlight exposure during treatment. Safety not established in patients with generalized erythroderma. Safety of intermittent use for >1 year has not been established, particularly since the effect on immune system development is unknown.

Adverse Reactions

Oral, I.V.:

≥15%:

Cardiovascular: Chest pain, hypertension, pericardial effusion (heart transplant)

Central nervous system: Dizziness, headache, insomnia, tremor (headache and tremor are associated with high whole blood concentrations and may respond to decreased dosage)

Dermatologic: Pruritus, rash

Endocrine & metabolic: Diabetes mellitus, hyperglycemia, hyper-/hypokalemia, hyperlipemia, hypomagnesemia, hypophosphatemia

Gastrointestinal: Abdominal pain, constipation, diarrhea, dyspepsia, nausea, vomiting

Genitourinary: Urinary tract infection

Hematologic: Anemia, leukocytosis, leukopenia, thrombocytopenia

Hepatic: Ascites

Neuromuscular & skeletal: Arthralgia, back pain, paresthesia, tremor, weakness

Renal: Abnormal kidney function, BUN increased, creatinine increased, oliguria, urinary tract infection

Respiratory: Atelectasis, bronchitis, dyspnea, increased cough, pleural effusion

Miscellaneous: CMV infection, infection

<15%:

Cardiovascular: Abnormal ECG (QRS or ST segment abnormal), angina pectoris, cardiopulmonary failure, deep thrombophlebitis, heart rate decreased, hemorrhage, hemorrhagic stroke, hypervolemia, hypotension, generalized edema, peripheral vascular disorder, phlebitis, postural hypotension, tachycardia, thrombosis, vasodilation

Central nervous system: Abnormal dreams, abnormal thinking, agitation, amnesia, anxiety, chills, confusion, depression, dizziness, elevated mood, emotional lability, encephalopathy, hallucinations, nervousness, paralysis, psychosis, quadriparesis, seizure, somnolence

Dermatologic: Acne, alopecia, cellulitis, exfoliative dermatitis, fungal dermatitis, hirsutism, increased diaphoresis, photosensitivity reaction, skin discoloration, skin disorder, skin ulcer

Endocrine & metabolic: Acidosis, alkalosis, Cushing's syndrome, decreased bicarbonate, decreased serum iron, diabetes mellitus, hypercalcemia, hypercholesterolemia, hyperphosphatemia, hypoproteinemia, increased alkaline phosphatase

Gastrointestinal: Anorexia, appetite increased, cramps, duodenitis, dysphagia, enlarged abdomen, esophagitis (including ulcerative), flatulence, gastritis, gastroesophagitis, GI perforation/hemorrhage, ileus, oral moniliasis, pancreatic pseudocyst, rectal disorder, stomatitis, weight gain

Genitourinary: Bladder spasm, cystitis, dysuria, nocturia, oliguria, urge incontinence, urinary frequency, urinary incontinence, urinary retention, vaginitis

Hematologic: Bruising, coagulation disorder, decreased prothrombin, hypochromic anemia, polycythemia

Hepatic: Abnormal liver function tests, ALT increased, AST increased, bilirubinemia, cholangitis, cholestatic jaundice, GGT increased, hepatitis (including granulomatous), jaundice, liver damage, increase LDH

Neuromuscular & skeletal: Hypertonia, incoordination, joint disorder, leg cramps, myalgia, myasthenia, myoclonus, nerve compression, neuropathy, osteoporosis

Ocular: Abnormal vision, amblyopia

Otic: Ear pain, otitis media, tinnitus

Renal: Albuminuria, renal tubular necrosis, toxic nephropathy

Respiratory: Asthma, lung disorder, pharyngitis, pneumonia, pneumothorax, pulmonary edema, respiratory disorder, rhinitis, sinusitis, voice alteration

Miscellaneous: Abscess, abnormal healing, allergic reaction, crying, flu-like syndrome, generalized spasm, hernia, herpes simplex, peritonitis, sepsis, writing impaired

Topical:

>10%:

Central nervous system: Headache (5% to 20%), fever (1% to 21%)

Dermatologic: Skin burning (43% to 58%; tends to improve as lesions resolve), pruritus (41% to 46%), erythema (12% to 28%)

Respiratory: Increased cough (18% children)

Miscellaneous: Flu-like syndrome (23% to 28%), allergic reaction (4% to 12%)

Oral, I.V., topical: Postmarketing and/or case reports (limited to important or life-threatening): Acute renal failure, alopecia, anaphylaxis, anaphylactoid reaction, angioedema, ARDS, arrhythmia, atrial fibrillation, atrial flutter, bile duct stenosis, blindness, cardiac arrest, cerebral infarction, cerebrovascular accident, deafness, delirium, depression, DIC, hemiparesis, hemolytic-uremic syndrome, hemorrhagic cystitis, hepatic necrosis, hepatotoxicity, hyperglycemia, leukoencephalopathy, lymphoproliferative disorder (related to EBV), myocardial hypertrophy (associated with ventricular dysfunction; reversible upon discontinuation), MI, neutropenia, pancreatitis (hemorrhagic and necrotizing), pancytopenia, paresthesia, photosensitivity reaction (topical), quadriplegia, QT_c prolongation, respiratory failure, seizure, skin discoloration (topical), Stevens-Johnson syndrome, syncope, toxic epidermal necrolysis, thrombocytopenic purpura, torsade de pointes, TTP, veno-occlusive hepatic disease, venous thrombosis, ventricular fibrillation

Note: Calcineurin inhibitor-induced hemolytic uremic syndrome/thrombotic thrombocytopenic purpura/thrombotic microangiopathy (HUS/TTP/TMA) have been reported (with concurrent sirolimus).

Drug Interactions

Metabolism/Transport Effects **Substrate** of CYP3A4 (major); **Inhibits** CYP3A4 (weak)

Avoid Concomitant Use

Avoid concomitant use of Tacrolimus with any of the following: Dabigatran Etexilate; Grapefruit Juice; Natalizumab; Rivaroxaban; Silodosin; Topotecan; Vaccines (Live)

Increased Effect/Toxicity

Tacrolimus may increase the levels/effects of: Alcohol (Ethyl); Dabigatran Etexilate; Natalizumab; P-Glycoprotein Substrates; Phenytoin; Rivaroxaban; Silodosin; Topotecan; Vaccines (Live)

The levels/effects of Tacrolimus may be increased by: Antidepressants (Serotonin Reuptake Inhibitor/Antagonist); Antifungal Agents (Azole Derivatives, Systemic); Calcium Channel Blockers (Dihydropyridine); Calcium Channel Blockers (Nondihydropyridine); CYP3A4 Inhibitors (Moderate); CYP3A4 Inhibitors (Strong); Dasatinib; Fluconazole; Grapefruit Juice; Macrolide Antibiotics; MetroNIDAZOLE; P-Glycoprotein Inhibitors; Protease Inhibitors; Sirolimus; Temsirolimus; Trastuzumab

Decreased Effect

Tacrolimus may decrease the levels/effects of: Vaccines (Inactivated)

The levels/effects of Tacrolimus may be decreased by: Caspofungin; Cinacalcet; CYP3A4 Inducers (Strong); Deferasirox; Echinacea; P-Glycoprotein Inducers; Phenytoin; Rifamycin Derivatives; St Johns Wort

Ethanol/Nutrition/Herb Interactions

Ethanol: Localized flushing (redness, warm sensation) may occur at application site of topical tacrolimus following ethanol consumption.

Food: Decreases rate and extent of absorption. High-fat meals have most pronounced effect (35% decrease in AUC, 77% decrease in C_{max}). Grapefruit juice, CYP3A4 inhibitor, may increase serum level and/or toxicity of tacrolimus; avoid concurrent use.

Herb/Nutraceutical: St John's wort: May reduce tacrolimus serum concentrations (avoid concurrent use).

Stability

Injection: Prior to dilution, store at 5°C to 25°C (41°F to 77°F). Following dilution, stable for 24 hours in D_5W or NS in glass or polyolefin containers. Dilute with 5% dextrose injection or 0.9% sodium chloride injection to a final concentration between 0.004 mg/mL and 0.02 mg/mL.

Capsules and ointment: Store at room temperature of 15°C to 30°C (59°F to 86°F).

Mechanism of Action Suppresses cellular immunity (inhibits T-lymphocyte activation), possibly by binding to an intracellular protein, FKBP-12

Pharmacodynamics/Kinetics

Absorption: Better in resected patients with a closed stoma; unlike cyclosporine, clamping of the T-tube in liver transplant patients does not alter trough concentrations or AUC

Oral: Incomplete and variable; food within 15 minutes of administration decreases absorption (27%)

Topical: Serum concentrations range from undetectable to 20 ng/mL (<5 ng/mL in majority of adult patients studied)

Protein binding: 99%

Metabolism: Extensively hepatic via CYP3A4 to eight possible metabolites (major metabolite, 31-demethyl tacrolimus, shows same activity as tacrolimus *in vitro*)

Bioavailability: Oral: Adults: 7% to 28%, Children: 10% to 52%; Topical: <0.5%; Absolute: Unknown

Half-life elimination: Variable, 21-61 hours in healthy volunteers

Time to peak: 0.5-4 hours

Excretion: Feces (~92%); feces/urine (<1% as unchanged drug)

Dosage

Oral:

Children: **Note:** Patients without pre-existing renal or hepatic dysfunction have required (and tolerated) higher doses than adults to achieve similar blood concentrations. It is recommended that therapy be initiated at high end of the recommended adult I.V. and oral dosing ranges; dosage adjustments may be required. If switching from I.V. to oral, the oral dose should be started 8-12 hours after stopping the infusion. Adjunctive therapy with corticosteroids is recommended early post-transplant.

Liver transplant: Initial dose: 0.15-0.20 mg/kg/day in 2 divided doses, given every 12 hours; begin oral dose no sooner than 6 hours post-transplant

Adults: **Note:** If switching from I.V. to oral, the oral dose should be started 8-12 hours after stopping the infusion. Adjunctive therapy with corticosteroids is recommended early post-transplant.

Heart transplant: Initial dose: 0.075 mg/kg/day in 2 divided doses, given every 12 hours; begin oral dose no sooner than 6 hours post-transplant

Kidney transplant: Initial dose: 0.2 mg/kg/day in 2 divided doses, given every 12 hours; initial dose may be given within 24 hours of transplant, but should be delayed until renal function has recovered; African-American patients may require larger doses to maintain trough concentration

Liver transplant: Initial dose: 0.1-0.15 mg/kg/day in 2 divided doses, given every 12 hours; begin oral dose no sooner than 6 hours post-transplant

I.V.: Children and Adults: **Note:** I.V. route should only be used in patients not able to take oral medications and continued only until oral medication can be tolerated; anaphylaxis has been reported. Begin no sooner than 6 hours post-transplant; adjunctive therapy with corticosteroids is recommended.

Heart transplant: Initial dose: 0.01 mg/kg/day as a continuous infusion

Kidney, liver transplant: Initial dose: 0.03-0.05 mg/kg/day as a continuous infusion

Prevention of graft-vs-host disease: 0.03 mg/kg/day as continuous infusion

Topical: Children ≥2 years and Adults: Atopic dermatitis (moderate to severe): Apply minimum amount of 0.03% or 0.1% ointment to affected area twice daily; rub in gently and completely. Discontinue use when symptoms have cleared. If no improvement within 6 weeks, patients should be re-examined to confirm diagnosis.

Dosing adjustment in renal impairment: Evidence suggests that lower doses should be used; patients should receive doses at the lowest value of the recommended I.V. and oral dosing ranges; further reductions in dose below these ranges may be required.

Tacrolimus therapy should usually be delayed up to 48 hours or longer in patients with postoperative oliguria.

Hemodialysis: Not removed by hemodialysis; supplemental dose is not necessary.

Peritoneal dialysis: Significant drug removal is unlikely based on physiochemical characteristics.

Dosing adjustment in hepatic impairment: Use of tacrolimus in liver transplant recipients experiencing post-transplant hepatic impairment may be associated with increased risk of developing renal insufficiency related to high whole blood levels of tacrolimus. The presence of moderate-to-severe hepatic dysfunction (serum bilirubin >2 mg/dL; Child-Pugh score ≥10) appears to affect the metabolism of tacrolimus. The half-life of the drug was prolonged and the clearance reduced after I.V. administration. The bioavailability of tacrolimus was also increased after oral administration. The higher plasma concentrations as determined by ELISA, in patients with severe hepatic dysfunction are probably due to the accumulation of metabolites of lower activity. These patients should be monitored closely and dosage adjustments should be considered. Some evidence indicates that lower doses could be used in these patients.

Dietary Considerations Capsule: Take on an empty stomach; be consistent with timing and composition of meals if GI intolerance occurs (per manufacturer).

Administration

I.V.: Administer by I.V. continuous infusion only. Do not use PVC tubing when administering dilute solutions. Usually intended to be administered as a continuous infusion over 24 hours.

Oral: If dosed once daily (not common), administer in the morning. If dosed twice daily, doses should be 12 hours apart. If the morning and evening doses differ, the larger dose (differences are never >0.5-1 mg) should be given in the morning. If dosed 3 times/day, separate doses by 8 hours.

Topical: Do not use with occlusive dressings. Burning at the application site is most common in first few days; improves as atopic dermatitis improves. Limit application to involved areas. Continue as long as signs and symptoms persist; discontinue if resolution occurs; re-evaluate if symptoms persist >6 weeks.

Monitoring Parameters Renal function, hepatic function, serum electrolytes (especially potassium), glucose and blood pressure, measure 3 times/week for first few weeks, then gradually decrease frequency as patient stabilizes. Whole blood concentrations should be used for monitoring (trough for oral therapy). Signs/symptoms of anaphylactic reactions during infusion should also be monitored. Patients should be monitored during the first 30 minutes of the infusion, and frequently thereafter.

Reference Range

Heart: Typical whole blood trough concentrations:
- One week to 3 months: 8-20 ng/mL
- Months 3-18: 6-18 ng/mL

Kidney transplant: Whole blood trough concentrations:
- Months 1-3: 7-20 ng/mL
- Months 4-12: 5-15 ng/mL

Liver transplant: Whole blood trough concentrations:
- Months 1-12: 5-20 ng/mL

Additional Information Additional dosing considerations:

Switch from I.V. to oral therapy: Threefold increase in dose

Pediatric patients: About 2 times higher dose compared to adults

Liver dysfunction: Decrease I.V. dose; decrease oral dose

Renal dysfunction: Does not affect kinetics; decrease dose to decrease levels if renal dysfunction is related to the drug

Dosage Forms Excipient information presented when available (limited, particularly for generics); consult specific product labeling.

Capsule (Prograf®): 0.5 mg, 1 mg, 5 mg

Injection, solution (Prograf®): 5 mg/mL (1 mL) [contains dehydrated alcohol 80% and polyoxyl 60 hydrogenated castor oil]

Ointment, topical (Protopic®): 0.03% (30 g, 60 g, 100 g); 0.1% (30 g, 60 g, 100 g)

Extemporaneous Preparations Tacrolimus 0.5 mg/mL oral suspension: Mix the contents of six 5-mg tacrolimus capsules with equal amounts of Ora-Plus® and Simple Syrup, N.F., to make a final volume of 60 mL. The suspension is stable for 56 days at room temperature in glass or plastic amber prescription bottles.

Esquivel C, So S, McDiarmid S, Andrews W, and Colombani PM, "Suggested Guidelines for the Use of Tacrolimus in Pediatric Liver Transplant Patients," *Transplantation*, 1996, 61(5):847-8.

Foster JA, Jacobson PA, Johnson CE, et al, "Stability of Tacrolimus in an Extemporaneously Compounded Oral Liquid (Abstract of Meeting Presentation)," *American Society of Health-System Pharmacists Annual Meeting*, 1996, 53:P-52(E).

Tacrolimus 1 mg/mL oral suspension: Mix the contents of six 5-mg capsules in approximately 5 mL of sterile water; add capsule contents to an empty amber bottle first, then add sterile water and agitate bottle until drug disperses and a slurry is formed. Add equal parts of Ora-Plus® (suspending agent) and Ora-Sweet® (sweetening agent) to a total volume of 30 mL. The suspension is stable for 4 months at room temperature in plastic amber prescription bottles.

Elefante A, Muindi J, West K, et al, "Long-Term Stability of a Patient-Convenient 1 mg/mL Suspension of Tacrolimus for Accurate Maintenance of Stable Therapeutic Levels," *Bone Marrow Transplant*, 2006, 37 (8):781-4.

Tadalafil (tah DA la fil)

U.S. Brand Names Cialis®

Canadian Brand Names Cialis®

Index Terms GF196960

Pharmacologic Category Phosphodiesterase-5 Enzyme Inhibitor

Use Treatment of erectile dysfunction (ED)

Pregnancy Risk Factor B

Pregnancy Considerations Teratogenic events were not reported in animal reproduction studies. Postnatal development and pup survival was decreased at some doses. Tadalafil is not indicated for use in women. Less than 0.0005% is found in the semen of healthy males.

Lactation Excretion in breast milk unknown

Medication Safety Issues

Sound-alike/look-alike issues:

Tadalafil may be confused with sildenafil, vardenafil

Contraindications Concurrent use (regularly/intermittently) of organic nitrates in any form (eg, nitroglycerin, isosorbide dinitrate)

Warnings/Precautions There is a degree of cardiac risk associated with sexual activity; therefore, physicians should consider the cardiovascular status of their patients prior to initiating any treatment for erectile dysfunction. Use with caution in patients with hypotension (<90/50 mm Hg), uncontrolled hypertension (>170/100 mm Hg), NYHA class II-IV heart failure within the last 6 months, uncontrolled arrhythmias, stroke within the last 6 months, MI within the last 3 months; safety and efficacy have not been studied in these patients. Use caution in patients with left ventricular outflow obstruction (eg, aortic stenosis). Concurrent use with alpha-adrenergic antagonist therapy or substantial alcohol consumption may cause symptomatic hypotension; patients should be hemodynamically stable prior to initiating tadalafil therapy at the lowest possible dose. Use caution in patients receiving strong CYP3A4 inhibitors, the elderly, or those with hepatic impairment or renal impairment; dosage adjustment/limitation is needed. Use caution in patients with bleeding disorders or peptic ulcer disease.

Agents for the treatment of erectile dysfunction should be used with caution in patients with anatomical deformation of the penis (angulation, cavernosal fibrosis, or Peyronie's disease), or in patients who have conditions which may predispose them to priapism (sickle cell anemia, multiple myeloma, leukemia). All patients should be instructed to seek immediate medical attention if erection persists >4 hours. The safety and efficacy of tadalafil with other treatments for erectile dysfunction have not been studied and are, therefore, not recommended as combination therapy.

Rare cases of nonarteritic anterior ischemic optic neuropathy (NAION) have been reported; risk may be increased with history of vision loss. Other risk factors for NAION include heart disease, diabetes, hypertension, smoking, age >50 years, or history of certain eye problems. Sudden decrease or loss of hearing has been reported rarely; hearing changes may be accompanied by tinnitus and dizziness. A direct relationship between therapy and vision or hearing loss has not been determined.

Patients with genetic retinal disorders (eg, retinitis pigmentosa) were not evaluated in clinical trials; use is not recommended. Safety and efficacy in children ≤18 years of age have not been established.

Adverse Reactions Similar adverse events are reported with once-daily dosing, but are generally lower than with doses used as needed.

>10%: Central nervous system: Headache (3% to 15%)

2% to 10%:

- Cardiovascular: Flushing (1% to 3%), hypertension (1% to 3%)
- Gastrointestinal: Dyspepsia (3% to 10%)
- Neuromuscular & skeletal: Back pain (3% to 6%), CPK increased (2%), myalgia (1% to 4%), limb pain (1% to 3%)
- Respiratory: Upper respiratory tract infection (3% to 4%), cough (2% to 4%), nasal congestion (2% to 4%)

<2% (Limited to important or life-threatening): Abdominal pain (upper), amnesia (transient global), angina pectoris, arthralgia, blurred vision, chest pain, color perception change, color vision decreased, conjunctival hyperemia, conjunctivitis, diaphoresis, diarrhea, dizziness, dysphagia, dyspnea, epistaxis, esophagitis, exfoliative dermatitis, eye pain, eyelid swelling, facial edema, fatigue, gastritis, gastroesophageal reflux, hearing decreased, hearing loss, hepatic enzymes increased, hyper-/hypotension, hypoesthesia, GGTP increased, insomnia, lacrimation, migraine, MI, nausea, neck pain, nonarteritic ischemic optic neuropathy, pain, palpitation, paresthesia, pharyngitis, photophobia, postural hypotension, priapism (reported with drugs in this class), pruritus, rash, retinal artery occlusion, retinal vein occlusion, seizure, somnolence, Stevens-Johnson syndrome, stroke, sudden cardiac death, syncope, tachycardia, tinnitus, urinary tract infection, urticaria, vertigo, visual changes (color vision), visual field loss, vomiting, weakness, xerostomia

Drug Interactions

Metabolism/Transport Effects **Substrate of** CYP3A4 (major)

Avoid Concomitant Use

Avoid concomitant use of Tadalafil with any of the following: Vasodilators (Organic Nitrates)

Increased Effect/Toxicity

Tadalafil may increase the levels/effects of: Alpha1-Blockers; Vasodilators (Organic Nitrates)

The levels/effects of Tadalafil may be increased by: Antifungal Agents (Azole Derivatives, Systemic); CYP3A4 Inhibitors (Moderate); CYP3A4 Inhibitors (Strong); Dasatinib; Macrolide Antibiotics; Protease Inhibitors; Sapropterin

Decreased Effect

The levels/effects of Tadalafil may be decreased by: Etravirine

Ethanol/Nutrition/Herb Interactions

Ethanol: Substantial consumption of ethanol may increase the risk of hypotension and orthostasis. Lower ethanol consumption has not been associated with significant changes in blood pressure or increase in orthostatic symptoms.

Food: Rate and extent of absorption are not affected by food. Grapefruit juice may increase serum levels/toxicity of tadalafil. When used on an as-needed basis, do not give more than a single 10 mg dose of tadalafil more frequently than every 72 hours in patients who regularly consume grapefruit juice. When used on a once-daily basis, the dose of tadalafil should not exceed 2.5 mg/day in patients who regularly consume grapefruit juice.

Herb/Nutraceutical: St John's wort: Use caution with concomitant use.

Stability Store at controlled room temperature of 25°C (77°F); excursions permitted to 15°C to 30°C (59°F to 86°F).

Mechanism of Action Does not directly cause penile erections, but affects the response to sexual stimulation. The physiologic mechanism of erection of the penis involves release of nitric oxide (NO) in the corpus cavernosum during sexual stimulation. NO then activates the enzyme guanylate cyclase, which results in increased levels of cyclic guanosine monophosphate (cGMP), producing smooth muscle relaxation and inflow of blood to the corpus cavernosum. Tadalafil enhances the effect of NO by inhibiting phosphodiesterase type 5 (PDE-5), which is responsible for degradation of cGMP in the corpus cavernosum; when sexual stimulation causes local release of NO, inhibition of PDE-5 by tadalafil causes increased levels of cGMP in the corpus cavernosum, resulting in smooth muscle relaxation and inflow of blood to the corpus cavernosum. At recommended doses, it has no effect in the absence of sexual stimulation.

Pharmacodynamics/Kinetics

Onset of action: Within 1 hour

Duration: Up to 36 hours

Distribution: V_d: 63 L

Protein binding: 94%

Metabolism: Hepatic, via CYP3A4 to metabolites (inactive)

Half-life elimination: 17.5 hours

Time to peak, plasma: ~2 hours (range: 30 minutes to 6 hours)

Excretion: Feces (61%, as metabolites); urine (36%, as metabolites)

Dosage Oral: Erectile dysfunction:

Adults:

As-needed dosing: 10 mg at least 30 minutes prior to anticipated sexual activity (dosing range: 5-20 mg); to be given as one single dose and not given more than once daily. **Note:** Erectile function may be improved for up to 36 hours following a single dose; adjust dose.

Once-daily dosing: 2.5 mg once daily (dosing range: 2.5-5 mg/day) to be given at approximately the same time daily without regard to timing of sexual activity

Elderly: No dose adjustment for patients >65 years of age; use with caution in patients with concomitant medications or renal/hepatic impairment

Dosing adjustment with concomitant medications:

Alpha$_1$-blockers: If stabilized on either alpha-blockers or tadalafil therapy, initiate new therapy with the other agent at the lowest possible dose.

CYP3A4 inhibitors: Dose reduction of tadalafil is recommended with strong CYP3A4 inhibitors. When used on an as-needed basis, the dose of tadalafil should not exceed 10 mg, and tadalafil should not be taken more frequently than once every 72 hours. When used on a once-daily basis, the dose of tadalafil should not exceed 2.5 mg. Examples of such inhibitors include amprenavir, atazanavir, clarithromycin, conivaptan, delavirdine, diclofenac, fosamprenavir, imatinib, indinavir, isoniazid, itraconazole, ketoconazole, miconazole, nefazodone, nelfinavir, nicardipine, propofol, quinidine, ritonavir, and telithromycin.

Dosage adjustment in renal impairment:

As-needed use:

Cl_{cr} 51-80 mL/minute: Dosage adjustment not required

Cl_{cr} 31-50 mL/minute: Initial dose 5 mg once daily; maximum dose 10 mg not to be given more frequently than every 48 hours

Cl_{cr} <30 mL/minute and on hemodialysis: Maximum dose 5 mg not to be given more frequently than every 72 hours

Once-daily use:

Cl_{cr} 51-80 mL/minute: Dosage adjustment not required

Cl_{cr} 31-50 mL/minute: Dose adjustment not needed

Cl_{cr} <30 mL/minute and on hemodialysis: Use not recommended

Dosage adjustment in hepatic impairment:

As-needed use:

Mild-to-moderate hepatic impairment (Child-Pugh class A or B): Use with caution; dose should not exceed 10 mg once daily

Severe hepatic impairment (Child-Pugh class C): Use is not recommended

Once-daily use:

Mild-to-moderate hepatic impairment (Child-Pugh class A or B): Use with caution

Severe hepatic impairment: Use is not recommended

Dietary Considerations May be taken with or without food.

Administration May be administered with or without food, prior to anticipated sexual activity. When used on an as-needed basis, should be taken at least 30 minutes prior to sexual activity. When used on a once-daily basis, should be taken at the same time each day, without regard to timing of sexual activity.

Monitoring Parameters Monitor for response and adverse effects.

Dosage Forms Excipient information presented when available (limited, particularly for generics); consult specific product labeling.

Tablet:

Cialis®: 2.5 mg, 5 mg, 10 mg, 20 mg

- ◆ **Tagamet® HB (Can)** *see* Cimetidine *on page 326*
- ◆ **Tagamet® HB 200 [OTC]** *see* Cimetidine *on page 326*
- ◆ **TAK-375** *see* Ramelteon *on page 1291*
- ◆ **Talc** *see* Talc (Sterile) *on page 1424*
- ◆ **Talc for Pleurodesis** *see* Talc (Sterile) *on page 1424*

Talc (Sterile) (talk STARE il)

U.S. Brand Names Sclerosol®; Sterile Talc Powder™

Index Terms Intrapleural Talc; Sterile Talc; Talc; Talc for Pleurodesis

Pharmacologic Category Sclerosing Agent

Use Prevention of recurrence of malignant pleural effusion in symptomatic patients

Pregnancy Risk Factor B

Dosage Adults: Pleural effusion:

Intrapleural aerosol: 4-8 g (1-2 cans) as a single dose

Intrapleural instillation: 5 g

Additional Information Complete prescribing information for this medication should be consulted for additional detail.

Dosage Forms Excipient information presented when available (limited, particularly for generics); consult specific product labeling.

Aerosol, intrapleural [powder]:

Sclerosol®: 4 g g [contains chlorofluorocarbon]

Powder, intrapleural:

Sterile Talc Powder™: Talc USP (5 g)

- ◆ **Talwin®** *see* Pentazocine *on page 1169*
- ◆ **Talwin® Nx** *see* Pentazocine *on page 1169*
- ◆ **Tambocor™** *see* Flecainide *on page 623*
- ◆ **Tamiflu®** *see* Oseltamivir *on page 1109*
- ◆ **Tamofen® (Can)** *see* Tamoxifen *on page 1424*

Tamoxifen (ta MOKS i fen)

U.S. Brand Names Soltamox™ [DSC]

Canadian Brand Names Apo-Tamox®; Gen-Tamoxifen; Nolvadex®; Nolvadex®-D; Novo-Tamoxifen; Tamofen®

Index Terms ICI-46474; Tamoxifen Citrate

Pharmacologic Category Antineoplastic Agent, Estrogen Receptor Antagonist; Selective Estrogen Receptor Modulator (SERM)

Use Treatment of metastatic (female and male) breast cancer; adjuvant treatment of breast cancer; reduce risk of invasive breast cancer in women with ductal carcinoma *in situ* (DCIS); reduce the incidence of breast cancer in women at high risk

Unlabeled/Investigational Use Treatment of mastalgia, gynecomastia, melanoma and desmoid tumors; induction of ovulation; treatment of precocious puberty in females, secondary to McCune-Albright syndrome

Restrictions An FDA-approved medication guide must be distributed when dispensing the outpatient prescription (new or refill) to females for breast cancer prevention or treatment of ductal carcinoma *in situ* where this medication is to be used without direct supervision of a healthcare provider. Medication guides are available at http://www.fda.gov/cder/Offices/ODS/medication_guides.htm.

Pregnancy Risk Factor D

Pregnancy Considerations Animal studies have demonstrated fetal adverse effects and fetal loss. There are no adequate and well-controlled studies in pregnant women. There have been reports of vaginal bleeding, birth defects and fetal loss in pregnant women. Tamoxifen use during pregnancy may have a potential long term risk to the fetus of a DES-like syndrome. For sexually-active women of childbearing age, initiate during menstruation (negative β-hCG immediately prior to initiation in women with irregular cycles). Tamoxifen may induce ovulation. Barrier or nonhormonal contraceptives are recommended. Pregnancy should be avoided during treatment and for 2 months after treatment has been discontinued.

Lactation Excretion in breast milk unknown/not recommended

Medication Safety Issues

Sound-alike/look-alike issues:

Tamoxifen may be confused with pentoxifylline, Tambocor™

Contraindications Hypersensitivity to tamoxifen or any component of the formulation; concurrent warfarin therapy or history of deep vein thrombosis or pulmonary embolism (when tamoxifen is used for cancer risk reduction)

Warnings/Precautions Hazardous agent - use appropriate precautions for handling and disposal. **[U.S. Boxed Warning]: Serious and life-threatening events (including stroke, pulmonary emboli, and uterine malignancy) have occurred at an incidence greater than placebo during use for cancer risk reduction;**these events are rare, but require consideration in risk:benefit evaluation. An increased incidence of thromboembolic events, including DVT and pulmonary embolism, has been associated with use for breast cancer; risk is increased with concomitant chemotherapy; use with caution in individuals with a history of thromboembolic events. Thrombocytopenia and/or leukopenia may occur; neutropenia and pancytopenia have been reported rarely. Although the relationship to tamoxifen therapy is uncertain, rare hemorrhagic episodes have occurred in patients with significant thrombocytopenia. Use with caution in patients with hyperlipidemias; infrequent postmarketing cases of hyperlipemias have been reported. Decreased visual acuity, retinal vein thrombosis, retinopathy, corneal changes, color perception changes, and increased incidence of cataracts (and the need for cataract surgery), have been reported. Hypercalcemia has occurred in patients with bone metastasis, usually within a few weeks of therapy initiation; institute appropriate hypercalcemia management; discontinue if severe. Local disease flare and increased bone and tumor pain may occur in patients with metastatic breast cancer; may be associated with (good) tumor response.

Tamoxifen use may be associated with changes in bone mineral density (BMD) and the effects may be dependant upon menstrual status. In postmenopausal women, tamoxifen use is associated with a protective effect on bone mineral density (BMD), preventing loss of BMD which lasts over the 5 year treatment period. In premenopausal women, a decline (from baseline) in BMD mineral density has been observed in women who continued to menstruate; may be associated with an increased risk of fractures. Liver abnormalities such as cholestasis, fatty liver, hepatitis, and hepatic necrosis have occurred. Hepatocellular carcinomas have been reported in some studies; relationship to treatment is unclear. Endometrial hyperplasia, polyps, endometriosis, uterine fibroids, and ovarian cysts have occurred. May increase risk of uterine or endometrial cancer; monitor. Amenorrhea and menstrual irregularities have been reported with tamoxifen use.

Adverse Reactions

>10%:

- Cardiovascular: Flushing (33% to 41%), hypertension (11%), peripheral edema (11%)
- Central nervous system: Pain (3% to 16%), mood changes (12% to 18%), depression (2% to 12%)
- Dermatologic: Skin changes (6% to 19%), rash (13%)
- Endocrine & metabolic: Hot flashes (3% to 80%), fluid retention (32%), altered menses (13% to 25%), amenorrhea (16%)
- Gastrointestinal: Nausea (5% to 26%), weight loss (23%)
- Genitourinary: Vaginal bleeding (2% to 23%), vaginal discharge (13% to 55%)
- Neuromuscular & skeletal: Weakness (19%), arthritis (14%), arthralgia (11%)
- Respiratory: Pharyngitis (14%)

1% to 10%:

- Cardiovascular: Chest pain (5%), venous thrombotic events (5%), edema (4%), cardiovascular ischemia (3%), cerebrovascular ischemia (3%), angina (2%), deep venous thrombus (≤2%), MI (1%)
- Central nervous system: Insomnia (9%), dizziness (8%), headache (8%), anxiety (6%), fatigue (4%)
- Dermatologic: Alopecia (<1% to 5%)
- Endocrine & metabolic: Oligomenorrhea (9%), breast pain (6%), menstrual disorder (6%), breast neoplasm (5%), hypercholesterolemia (4%)
- Gastrointestinal: Abdominal pain (9%), weight gain (9%), constipation (4% to 8%), diarrhea (7%), dyspepsia (6%), throat irritation (oral solution 5%), abdominal cramps (1%), anorexia (1%)
- Genitourinary: Urinary tract infection (10%), leukorrhea (9%), vaginal hemorrhage (6%), vaginitis (5%), ovarian cyst (3%)
- Hematologic: Thrombocytopenia (≤10%), anemia (5%)
- Hepatic: AST increased (5%), serum bilirubin increased (2%)
- Neuromuscular & skeletal: Back pain (10%), bone pain (6% to 10%), osteoporosis (7%), fracture (7%), arthrosis (5%), myalgia (5%), paresthesia (5%), musculoskeletal pain (3%)
- Ocular: Cataract (7%)
- Renal: Serum creatinine increased (≤2%)
- Respiratory: Cough (4% to 9%), dyspnea (8%), bronchitis (5%), sinusitis (5%)
- Miscellaneous: Infection/sepsis (≤9%), diaphoresis (6%), flu-like syndrome (6%), allergic reaction (3%)

<1or frequency not defined (limited to important or life-threatening): Angioedema, bullous pemphigoid, cholestasis, corneal changes, endometrial cancer, endometrial hyperplasia, endometrial polyps, endometriosis, erythema multiforme, fatty liver, hepatic necrosis, hepatitis, hypercalcemia, hyperlipidemia, hypersensitivity reactions, hypertriglyceridemia, impotence (males), interstitial pneumonitis, lightheadedness, loss of libido (males), pancreatitis, phlebitis, pruritus vulvae, pulmonary embolism, retinal vein thrombosis, retinopathy, second primary tumors, Stevens-Johnson syndrome, stroke, superficial phlebitis, taste disturbances; tumor pain and local disease flare (including increase in lesion size and erythema) during treatment of metastatic breast cancer (generally resolves with continuation); uterine fibroids, vaginal dryness, visual color perception changes

Drug Interactions

Metabolism/Transport Effects **Substrate** of CYP2A6 (minor), 2B6 (minor), 2C9 (major), 2D6 (major), 2E1 (minor), 3A4 (major); **Inhibits** CYP2B6 (weak), 2C8 (moderate), 2C9 (weak), 3A4 (weak), p-glycoprotein

Avoid Concomitant Use

Avoid concomitant use of Tamoxifen with any of the following: CYP2D6 Inhibitors (Strong); Dabigatran Etexilate; Rivaroxaban; Silodosin; Topotecan; Vitamin K Antagonists

Increased Effect/Toxicity

Tamoxifen may increase the levels/effects of: CYP2C8 Substrates (High risk); Dabigatran Etexilate; P-Glycoprotein Substrates; Rivaroxaban; Silodosin; Topotecan; Vitamin K Antagonists

The levels/effects of Tamoxifen may be increased by: CYP2C9 Inhibitors (Moderate); CYP2C9 Inhibitors (Strong); CYP2D6 Inhibitors (Moderate); CYP2D6 Inhibitors (Strong); CYP3A4 Inhibitors (Moderate); CYP3A4 Inhibitors (Strong); Darunavir; Dasatinib

Decreased Effect

Tamoxifen may decrease the levels/effects of: Anastrozole; Letrozole

The levels/effects of Tamoxifen may be decreased by: Aminoglutethimide; CYP2C9 Inducers (Highly Effective); CYP3A4 Inducers (Strong); Deferasirox; Herbs (CYP3A4 Inducers); Rifamycin Derivatives

Ethanol/Nutrition/Herb Interactions Herb/Nutraceutical: Avoid black cohosh, dong quai in estrogen-dependent tumors. Avoid St John's wort (may decrease levels/effects of tamoxifen).

Stability

Solution: Store at room temperature at or below 25°C (77°F); do not refrigerate or freeze. Protect from light. Use within 3 months of opening.

Tablet: Store at room temperature of 20°C to 25°C (68°F to 77°F). Protect from light.

Mechanism of Action Competitively binds to estrogen receptors on tumors and other tissue targets, producing a nuclear complex that decreases DNA synthesis and inhibits estrogen effects; nonsteroidal agent with potent antiestrogenic properties which compete with estrogen for binding sites in breast and other tissues; cells accumulate in the G_0 and G_1 phases; therefore, tamoxifen is cytostatic rather than cytocidal.

Pharmacodynamics/Kinetics

Absorption: Well absorbed; tablet and oral solution are bioequivalent

Distribution: High concentrations found in uterus, endometrial and breast tissue

Protein binding: 99%

Metabolism: Hepatic (via CYP3A4) to major metabolites, N-desmethyl tamoxifen (major) and 4-hydroxytamoxifen (minor), and a tamoxifen derivative (minor); undergoes enterohepatic recirculation

Half-life elimination: Distribution: 7-14 hours; Elimination: 5-7 days; Metabolites: 14 days

Time to peak, serum: 5 hours

Excretion: Feces (26% to 51%); urine (9% to 13%)

Dosage Oral (refer to individual protocols):

Children: Female: Precocious puberty and McCune-Albright syndrome (unlabeled use): A dose of 20 mg/day has been reported in patients 2-10 years of age; safety and efficacy have not been established for treatment of longer than 1 year duration

Adults:

Breast cancer treatment:

Metastatic (males and females) or adjuvant therapy (females): 20-40 mg/day; daily doses >20 mg should be given in 2 divided doses (morning and evening); doses >20 mg/day are not more effective in adjuvant therapy

DCIS (females): 20 mg once daily for 5 years

Breast cancer risk reduction (pre- and postmenopausal high-risk females): 20 mg/day for 5 years

Induction of ovulation (unlabeled use): 5-40 mg twice daily for 4 days

Administration Administer once or twice daily. Doses >20 mg/day should be given in divided doses.

Monitoring Parameters CBC with platelets, serum calcium, LFTs; triglycerides and cholesterol (in patients with pre-existing hyperlipemias); abnormal vaginal bleeding; breast and gynecologic exams (baseline and routine), mammogram (baseline and routine)

Test Interactions T_4 elevations (which may be explained by increases in thyroid-binding globulin) have been reported; not accompanied by clinical hyperthyroidism

Additional Information Oral clonidine is being studied for the treatment of tamoxifen-induced "hot flashes." The tumor flare reaction may indicate a good therapeutic response, and is often considered a good prognostic factor.

Dosage Forms Excipient information presented when available (limited, particularly for generics); consult specific product labeling. [DSC] = Discontinued product

Solution, oral:

Soltamox™: 10 mg/5 mL (150 mL) [sugar free; licorice flavor] [DSC]

Tablet: 10 mg, 20 mg

◆ **Tamoxifen Citrate** *see* Tamoxifen *on page 1424*

Tamsulosin (tam SOO loe sin)

U.S. Brand Names Flomax®

Canadian Brand Names Flomax®; Flomax® CR; Gen-Tamsulosin; Novo-Tamsulosin; Ran-Tamsulosin; ratio-Tamsulosin; Sandoz-Tamsulosin

Index Terms Tamsulosin Hydrochloride

Pharmacologic Category Alpha$_1$ Blocker

Use Treatment of signs and symptoms of benign prostatic hyperplasia (BPH)

Unlabeled/Investigational Use Symptomatic treatment of bladder outlet obstruction or dysfunction

Pregnancy Risk Factor B

Pregnancy Considerations Teratogenic effects were not observed in animal studies, however, tamsulosin is not approved for use in women.

Medication Safety Issues

Sound-alike/look-alike issues:

Flomax® may be confused with Flonase®, Flovent®, Foltx®, Fosamax®, Volmax®

Tamsulosin may be confused with tacrolimus, tamoxifen, terazosin

International issues:

Flomax®: Brand name for morniflumate in Italy

Flomax® may be confused with Flomox® which is a brand name for cefcapene in Japan

Contraindications Hypersensitivity to tamsulosin or any component of the formulation

Warnings/Precautions Not intended for use as an antihypertensive drug. May cause significant orthostatic hypotension and syncope, especially with first dose; anticipate a similar effect if therapy is interrupted for a few days, if dosage is rapidly increased, or if another antihypertensive drug (particularly vasodilators) or a PDE-5 inhibitor (eg, sildenafil, tadalafil, vardenafil) is introduced. "First-dose" orthostatic hypotension may occur 4-8 hours after dosing; may be dose related. Patients should be cautioned about performing hazardous tasks when starting new therapy or adjusting dosage upward. Discontinue if symptoms of angina occur or worsen. Rule out prostatic carcinoma before beginning therapy with tamsulosin. Intraoperative floppy iris syndrome has been observed in cataract surgery patients who were on or were previously treated with alpha$_1$-blockers; causality has not been established and there appears to be no benefit in discontinuing alpha-blocker therapy prior to surgery. Priapism has been associated with use (rarely). Rarely, patients with a sulfa allergy have also developed an allergic reaction to tamsulosin; avoid use when previous reaction has been severe. Not indicated for use in women or children.

Adverse Reactions

>10%:

Cardiovascular: Orthostatic hypotension (6 % to 19%)

Central nervous system: Headache (19% to 21%), dizziness (15% to 17%)

Genitourinary: Abnormal ejaculation (8% to 18%)

Respiratory: Rhinitis (13% to 18%)

Miscellaneous: Infection (9% to 11%)

1% to 10%:

Cardiovascular: Chest pain (4%)

Central nervous system: Somnolence (3% to 4%), insomnia (1% to 2%), vertigo (≤1%)

Endocrine & metabolic: Libido decreased (1% to 2%)

Gastrointestinal: Diarrhea (4% to 6%), nausea (3% to 4%), tooth disorder (1% to 2%)

Neuromuscular & skeletal: Weakness (8% to 9%), back pain (7% to 8%)

Ocular: Blurred vision (≤2%)

Respiratory: Pharyngitis (5% to 6%), cough (3% to 5%), sinusitis (2% to 4%)

<1% (Limited to important or life-threatening): Allergic reactions (angioedema, pruritus, rash, urticaria, respiratory symptoms); constipation, hypotension, intraoperative floppy iris syndrome, orthostasis (symptomatic), palpitation, priapism, skin desquamation, syncope, transaminases increased, vomiting

Drug Interactions

Metabolism/Transport Effects Substrate (major) of CYP2D6, 3A4

Avoid Concomitant Use

Avoid concomitant use of Tamsulosin with any of the following: Alfuzosin; Alpha1-Blockers; Silodosin

Increased Effect/Toxicity

Tamsulosin may increase the levels/effects of: Alfuzosin; Alpha1-Blockers; Calcium Channel Blockers; Silodosin

The levels/effects of Tamsulosin may be increased by: Alfuzosin; Alpha1-Blockers; Beta-Blockers; CYP2D6

Inhibitors (Moderate); CYP2D6 Inhibitors (Strong); CYP3A4 Inhibitors (Moderate); CYP3A4 Inhibitors (Strong); Darunavir; Dasatinib; Phosphodiesterase 5 Inhibitors; Silodosin

Decreased Effect

The levels/effects of Tamsulosin may be decreased by: CYP3A4 Inducers (Strong); Deferasirox; Herbs (CYP3A4 Inducers)

Ethanol/Nutrition/Herb Interactions

Food: Fasting increases bioavailability by 30% and peak concentration 40% to 70%.

Herb/Nutraceutical: St John's wort: May decrease the levels/effects of tamsulosin. Avoid herbs with hypotensive properties (black cohosh, California poppy, coleus, golden seal, hawthorn, mistletoe, periwinkle, quinine, Shepherd's purse); may enhance the hypotensive effect of tamsulosin. Avoid saw palmetto (due to limited experience with this combination).

Stability Store at room temperature of 25°C (77°F); excursions permitted to 15°C to 30°C (59°F to 86°F).

Mechanism of Action Tamsulosin is an antagonist of $alpha_{1A}$-adrenoreceptors in the prostate. Smooth muscle tone in the prostate is mediated by $alpha_{1A}$-adrenoreceptors; blocking them leads to relaxation of smooth muscle in the bladder neck and prostate causing an improvement of urine flow and decreased symptoms of BPH. Approximately 75% of the $alpha_1$-receptors in the prostate are of the $alpha_{1A}$ subtype.

Pharmacodynamics/Kinetics

Absorption: >90%

Protein binding: 94% to 99%, primarily to $alpha_1$ acid glycoprotein (AAG)

Metabolism: Hepatic via CYP3A4 and 2D6; metabolites undergo extensive conjugation to glucuronide or sulfate

Bioavailability: Fasting: 30% increase

Distribution: V_d: 16 L

Steady-state: By the fifth day of once-daily dosing

Half-life elimination: Healthy volunteers: 9-13 hours; Target population: 14-15 hours

Time to peak: Fasting: 4-5 hours; With food: 6-7 hours

Excretion: Urine (76%, <10% as unchanged drug); feces (21%)

Dosage Oral: Adults:

BPH: 0.4 mg once daily ~30 minutes after the same meal each day; dose may be increased after 2-4 weeks to 0.8 mg once daily in patients who fail to respond. If therapy is interrupted for several days, restart with 0.4 mg once daily.

Bladder outlet obstruction (unlabeled use): 0.4 mg once daily ~30 minutes after the same meal each day

Dosage adjustment in renal impairment:

Cl_{cr} ≥10 mL/minute: No adjustment needed

Cl_{cr} <10 mL/minute: Not studied

Dosage adjustment in hepatic impairment:

Mild-to-moderate impairment: No adjustment needed

Severe impairment: Not studied

Dietary Considerations Take once daily, 30 minutes after the same meal each day.

Administration Administer 30 minutes after the same meal each day. Capsules should be swallowed whole; do not crush, chew, or open.

Dosage Forms Excipient information presented when available (limited, particularly for generics); consult specific product labeling.

Capsule, as hydrochloride:

Flomax®: 0.4 mg

- ◆ **Tamsulosin Hydrochloride** *see* Tamsulosin *on page 1426*
- ◆ **Tanac® [OTC]** *see* Benzocaine *on page 183*
- ◆ **TanaCof-XR** *see* Brompheniramine *on page 214*
- ◆ **Tanafed DMX™** *see* Chlorpheniramine, Pseudoephedrine, and Dextromethorphan *on page 315*
- ◆ **Tannate PD-DM** *see* Chlorpheniramine, Pseudoephedrine, and Dextromethorphan *on page 315*
- ◆ **Tannate Pediatric** *see* Chlorpheniramine and Phenylephrine *on page 309*
- ◆ **Tanta-Orciprenaline® (Can)** *see* Metaproterenol *on page 952*
- ◆ **TAP-144** *see* Leuprolide *on page 868*
- ◆ **Tapazole®** *see* Methimazole *on page 963*
- ◆ **Tarceva®** *see* Erlotinib *on page 541*
- ◆ **Targretin®** *see* Bexarotene *on page 195*
- ◆ **Tarka®** *see* Trandolapril and Verapamil *on page 1500*
- ◆ **Taro-Amcinonide (Can)** *see* Amcinonide *on page 81*
- ◆ **Taro-Carbamazepine Chewable (Can)** *see* CarBAMazepine *on page 252*
- ◆ **Taro-Ciprofloxacin (Can)** *see* Ciprofloxacin *on page 329*
- ◆ **Taro-Clindamycin (Can)** *see* Clindamycin *on page 344*
- ◆ **Taro-Clobetasol (Can)** *see* Clobetasol *on page 347*
- ◆ **Taro-Desoximetasone (Can)** *see* Desoximetasone *on page 424*
- ◆ **Taro-Enalapril (Can)** *see* Enalapril *on page 515*
- ◆ **Taro-Fluconazole (Can)** *see* Fluconazole *on page 625*
- ◆ **Taro-Mometasone (Can)** *see* Mometasone *on page 1012*
- ◆ **Taro-Simvastatin (Can)** *see* Simvastatin *on page 1370*
- ◆ **Taro-Sone® (Can)** *see* Betamethasone *on page 188*
- ◆ **Taro-Warfarin (Can)** *see* Warfarin *on page 1570*
- ◆ **Tasigna®** *see* Nilotinib *on page 1066*
- ◆ **Tasmar®** *see* Tolcapone *on page 1485*
- ◆ **Tavist® Allergy [OTC]** *see* Clemastine *on page 343*
- ◆ **Tavist® ND ALLERGY [OTC]** *see* Loratadine *on page 904*
- ◆ **Taxol®** *see* Paclitaxel *on page 1127*
- ◆ **Taxotere®** *see* Docetaxel *on page 471*

Tazarotene (taz AR oh teen)

U.S. Brand Names Avage™; Tazorac®

Canadian Brand Names Tazorac®

Pharmacologic Category Acne Products; Keratolytic Agent; Topical Skin Product, Acne

Use Topical treatment of facial acne vulgaris; topical treatment of stable plaque psoriasis of up to 20% body surface area involvement; mitigation (palliation) of facial skin wrinkling, facial mottled hyper-/hypopigmentation, and benign facial lentigines

Pregnancy Risk Factor X

Pregnancy Considerations May cause fetal harm if administered to a pregnant woman. A negative pregnancy test should be obtained 2 weeks prior to treatment; treatment should begin during a normal menstrual period.

Lactation Excretion in breast milk unknown/use caution

Contraindications Hypersensitivity to tazarotene, other retinoids or vitamin A derivatives (isotretinoin, tretinoin, etretinate), or any component of the formulation; use in women of childbearing potential who are unable to comply with birth control requirements; pregnancy (negative pregnancy test required)

Warnings/Precautions Women of childbearing potential must use adequate contraceptive measures because of potential teratogenicity. Treatment can increase skin sensitivity to weather extremes of wind or cold. Also, concomitant topical medications (eg, medicated or abrasive soaps, cleansers, or cosmetics with a strong drying effect) should be used with caution due to increased skin irritation. May cause photosensitivity; exposure to sunlight should be avoided unless deemed medically necessary, and in such cases, exposure should be minimized (including use of sunscreens/protective clothing) during use of tazarotene. Risk may be increased by concurrent therapy with known photosensitizers (thiazides, tetracyclines, fluoroquinolones, phenothiazines, sulfonamides). For external use only; avoid contact with eyes, eyelids, and mouth. Not for use on eczematous, broken, or sunburned skin; not for treatment of lentigo maligna. Avoid application over extensive areas; specifically, safety and efficacy of gel applied over >20% of BSA have not been established. Safety and efficacy in children <12 years of age have not been established.

Adverse Reactions Percentage of incidence varies with formulation and/or strength:

>10%: Dermatologic: Burning/stinging, desquamation, dry skin, erythema, pruritus, skin pain, worsening of psoriasis

1% to 10%: Dermatologic: Contact dermatitis, discoloration, fissuring, hypertriglyceridemia, inflammation, irritation, localized bleeding, rash

Frequency not defined:

Dermatologic: Photosensitization

Neuromuscular & skeletal: Peripheral neuropathy

Drug Interactions

Avoid Concomitant Use There are no known interactions where it is recommended to avoid concomitant use.

Increased Effect/Toxicity There are no known significant interactions involving an increase in effect.

Decreased Effect There are no known significant interactions involving a decrease in effect.

Stability Store at room temperature of 25°C (77°F), away from heat and direct light; do not freeze.

Mechanism of Action Synthetic, acetylenic retinoid which modulates differentiation and proliferation of epithelial tissue and exerts some degree of anti-inflammatory and immunological activity

Pharmacodynamics/Kinetics

Duration: Therapeutic: Psoriasis: Effects have been observed for up to 3 months after a 3-month course of topical treatment

Absorption: Minimal following cutaneous application (≤6% of dose)

Distribution: Retained in skin for prolonged periods after topical application.

Protein binding: >99%

Metabolism: Prodrug, rapidly metabolized via esterases to an active metabolite (tazarotenic acid) following topical application and systemic absorption; tazarotenic acid undergoes further hepatic metabolism

Half-life elimination: 18 hours

Excretion: Urine and feces (as metabolites)

Dosage Topical: **Note:** In patients experiencing excessive pruritus, burning, skin redness, or peeling, discontinue until integrity of the skin is restored, or reduce dosing to an interval the patient is able to tolerate.

Children ≥12 years and Adults:

Acne: Tazorac® cream/gel 0.1%: Cleanse the face gently. After the skin is dry, apply a thin film of tazarotene (2 mg/cm^2) once daily, in the evening, to the skin where the acne lesions appear; use enough to cover the entire affected area

Psoriasis: Tazorac® gel 0.05% or 0.1%: Apply once daily, in the evening, to psoriatic lesions using enough (2 mg/cm^2) to cover only the lesion with a thin film to no more than 20% of body surface area. If a bath or shower is taken prior to application, dry the skin before applying. Unaffected skin may be more susceptible to irritation, avoid application to these areas.

Children ≥17 years and Adults: Palliation of fine facial wrinkles, facial mottled hyper/hypopigmentation, benign facial lentigines: Avage™: Apply a pea-sized amount once daily to clean dry face at bedtime; lightly cover entire face including eyelids if desired. Emollients or moisturizers may be applied before or after; if applied before tazarotene, ensure cream or lotion has absorbed into the skin and has dried completely.

Adults: Psoriasis: Tazorac® cream 0.05% or 0.1%: Apply once daily, in the evening, to psoriatic lesions using enough (2 mg/cm^2) to cover only the lesion with a thin film to no more than 20% of body surface area. If a bath or shower is taken prior to application, dry the skin before applying. Unaffected skin may be more susceptible to irritation, avoid application to these areas.

Administration Do not apply to eczematous or sunburned skin; apply thin film to affected areas; avoid eyes and mouth

Monitoring Parameters Disease severity in plaque psoriasis during therapy (reduction in erythema, scaling, induration); routine blood chemistries (including transaminases) are suggested during long-term topical therapy; pregnancy test prior to treatment of female patients

Dosage Forms Excipient information presented when available (limited, particularly for generics); consult specific product labeling.

Cream:

Avage™: 0.1% (30 g) [contains benzyl alcohol]

Tazorac®: 0.05% (30 g, 60 g); 0.1% (30 g, 60 g) [contains benzyl alcohol]

Gel (Tazorac®): 0.05% (30 g, 100 g); 0.1% (30 g, 100 g) [contains benzyl alcohol]

◆ **Tazicef®** *see* Ceftazidime *on page 282*

◆ **Tazobactam and Piperacillin** *see* Piperacillin and Tazobactam Sodium *on page 1198*

◆ **Tazocin® (Can)** *see* Piperacillin and Tazobactam Sodium *on page 1198*

◆ **Tazorac®** *see* Tazarotene *on page 1427*

◆ **Taztia XT™** *see* Diltiazem *on page 450*

◆ **TB Skin Test** *see* Tuberculin Tests *on page 1527*

◆ **3TC** *see* LamiVUDine *on page 848*

◆ **3TC® (Can)** *see* LamiVUDine *on page 848*

◆ **3TC, Abacavir, and Zidovudine** *see* Abacavir, Lamivudine, and Zidovudine *on page 19*

◆ **T-Cell Growth Factor** *see* Aldesleukin *on page 53*

◆ **TCGF** *see* Aldesleukin *on page 53*

◆ **TCN** *see* Tetracycline *on page 1451*

◆ **Td** *see* Diphtheria and Tetanus Toxoid *on page 460*

◆ **Td Adsorbed (Can)** *see* Diphtheria and Tetanus Toxoid *on page 460*

◆ **Tdap** *see* Diphtheria and Tetanus Toxoids, and Acellular Pertussis Vaccine *on page 463*

◆ **TDF** *see* Tenofovir *on page 1438*

◆ **Tebrazid™ (Can)** *see* Pyrazinamide *on page 1270*

◆ **Tecta™ (Can)** *see* Pantoprazole *on page 1140*

Tegaserod (teg a SER od)

U.S. Brand Names Zelnorm®

Canadian Brand Names Zelnorm® [DSC]

Index Terms HTF919; Tegaserod Maleate

Pharmacologic Category Serotonin 5-HT_4 Receptor Agonist

Use Emergency treatment of irritable bowel syndrome with constipation (IBS-C) and chronic idiopathic constipation (CIC) in women (<55 years of age) in which no alternative therapy exists

Restrictions Available in U.S. under an emergency investigational new drug (IND) process. Emergency situations are defined as immediately life-threatening or requiring hospitalization. Physicians with patients who may qualify can contact the FDA's Division of Drug Information via email (druginfo@fda.hhs.gov), by calling (301-796-3400), or at http://www.fda.gov/cder. The FDA may either deny the request or authorize shipment of Zelnorm® by Novartis. Additional information can be found at http://www.zelnorm.com or http://www.fda.gov/cder/drug/infopage/zelnorm/default.htm

Pregnancy Risk Factor B

Pregnancy Considerations Safety and efficacy have not been established in pregnant women. Use during pregnancy only if clearly needed.

Lactation Excretion in breast milk unknown/not recommended

Contraindications Per product labeling: Hypersensitivity to tegaserod or any component of the formulation; severe renal impairment; moderate or severe hepatic impairment; history of bowel obstruction, symptomatic gallbladder disease, suspected sphincter of Oddi dysfunction, or abdominal adhesions. Treatment should not be started in patients with diarrhea or in those who experience diarrhea frequently.

Exclusion criteria under the emergency-IND process: Unstable angina, history of MI or stroke, hypertension, hyperlipidemia, diabetes, age ≥55 years, smoking, obesity, depression, anxiety, or suicidal ideation.

Warnings/Precautions Serious cardiovascular events (eg, MI, stroke, unstable angina) may occur; patients should seek emergency care following any sign and symptom suggestive of a serious cardiac event. Use under the emergency IND process will not be permitted in patients with unstable angina, a history of MI or stroke, cigarette smoking, hypertension, hyperlipidemia, obesity, or diabetes. In addition, use will not be permitted in patients with depression, anxiety, or with any signs of suicidal ideation or behavior. Use has been associated with rare intestinal ischemic events. Discontinue immediately with new or sudden worsening abdominal pain or rectal bleeding. Diarrhea may occur after the start of treatment, most cases reported as a single episode within the first week of therapy, and may resolve with continued dosing. However, serious consequences of diarrhea (hypovolemia, syncope) have been reported. Patients should be warned to contact healthcare provider immediately if they develop severe diarrhea, or diarrhea with severe cramping, abdominal pain, or dizziness. Use caution with mild hepatic impairment; not recommended with moderate or severe impairment. Potential benefits should be weighed against potential risks in patients eligible for emergency-IND use. Safety and efficacy have not been established in males with IBS or patients <18 years of age. Use in elderly women (≥55 years of age) is contraindicated.

Adverse Reactions

>10%:

Central nervous system: Headache (15%)

Gastrointestinal: Abdominal pain (12%)

1% to 10%:

Central nervous system: Dizziness (4%), migraine (2%)

Gastrointestinal: Diarrhea (9%; severe <1%), nausea (8%), flatulence (6%)

Neuromuscular & skeletal: Back pain (5%), arthropathy (2%), leg pain (1%)

<1% (Limited to important or life-threatening): Albuminuria, alopecia, ALT increased, angina pectoris, arrhythmia, AST increased, bile duct stone, cramps, cholecystitis (with increased transaminases), gangrenous bowel, hepatitis, hypersensitivity reaction, hypokalemia (secondary to diarrhea), hypotension, ischemic colitis, mesenteric ischemia, MI, pruritus, rectal bleeding, renal pain, severe diarrhea (complicated by hypovolemia, hypotension, syncope), sphincter of Oddi spasm (suspected), stroke, syncope, tenesmus, unstable angina, vertigo

Drug Interactions

Avoid Concomitant Use There are no known interactions where it is recommended to avoid concomitant use.

Increased Effect/Toxicity There are no known significant interactions involving an increase in effect.

Decreased Effect There are no known significant interactions involving a decrease in effect.

Ethanol/Nutrition/Herb Interactions Food: Bioavailability is decreased by 40% to 65% and C_{max} is decreased by 20% to 40% when taken with food. T_{max} is prolonged from 1 hour up to 2 hours when taken following a meal, but decreased to 0.7 hours when taken 30 minutes before a meal.

Stability Store at controlled room temperature of 15°C to 30°C (59°F to 86°F). Protect from moisture.

Mechanism of Action Tegaserod is a partial neuronal 5-HT_4 receptor agonist. Its action at the receptor site leads to stimulation of the peristaltic reflex and intestinal secretion, and moderation of visceral sensitivity.

Pharmacodynamics/Kinetics

Distribution: V_d: 368 ± 223 L

Protein binding: 98% primarily to α_1-acid glycoprotein

Metabolism: GI: Hydrolysis in the stomach; Hepatic: Oxidation, conjugation, and glucuronidation; metabolite (negligible activity); significant first-pass effect

Bioavailability: Fasting: 10%

Half-life elimination: I.V.: 11 ± 5 hours

Time to peak: 1 hour

Excretion: Feces (~66% as unchanged drug); urine (~33% as metabolites)

Dosage Oral:

Adults (<55 years of age): Females:

IBS with constipation: 6 mg twice daily, before meals, for 4-6 weeks; may consider continuing treatment for an additional 4-6 weeks in patients who respond initially

Chronic idiopathic constipation: 6 mg twice daily, before meals; the need for continued therapy should be reassessed periodically

Elderly: Use in women ≥55 years of age is contraindicated.

Dosage adjustment in renal impairment: C_{max} and AUC of the inactive metabolite are increased with renal impairment.

Mild-to-moderate impairment: No dosage adjustment recommended

Severe impairment: Use is contraindicated

Dosage adjustment in hepatic impairment: C_{max} and AUC of tegaserod are increased with hepatic impairment.

Mild impairment: No dosage adjustment recommended; however, use caution

Moderate-to-severe impairment: Use is contraindicated

Dietary Considerations Take on an empty stomach, 30 minutes before meals.

Administration Administer 30 minutes before meals.

Dosage Forms Excipient information presented when available (limited, particularly for generics); consult specific product labeling.

Tablet:

Zelnorm®: 2 mg, 6 mg

◆ **Tegaserod Maleate** *see* Tegaserod *on page* 1428

◆ **Tegretol®** *see* CarBAMazepine *on page* 252

◆ **Tegretol®-XR** *see* CarBAMazepine *on page* 252

◆ **Tekturna®** *see* Aliskiren *on page* 63

◆ **Tekturna HCT®** *see* Aliskiren and Hydrochlorothiazide *on page* 64

Telithromycin (tel ith roe MYE sin)

U.S. Brand Names Ketek®

Canadian Brand Names Ketek®

Index Terms HMR 3647

Pharmacologic Category Antibiotic, Ketolide

Use Treatment of community-acquired pneumonia (mild-to-moderate) caused by susceptible strains of *Streptococcus pneumoniae* (including multidrug-resistant isolates), *Haemophilus influenzae*, *Chlamydophila pneumoniae*, *Moraxella catarrhalis*, and *Mycoplasma pneumoniae*

Restrictions An FDA-approved Medication Guide is available and must be dispensed with every prescription. Copies may be found at: http://www.fda.gov/cder/foi/label/2007/021144s012medg.pdf

Pregnancy Risk Factor C

Pregnancy Considerations Because adverse effects were observed in some animal studies, telithromycin is classified pregnancy category C. There are no adequate and well-controlled studies of telithromycin in pregnant women.

Lactation Excretion in breast milk unknown/use caution

Contraindications Hypersensitivity to telithromycin, macrolide antibiotics, or any component of the formulation; myasthenia gravis; history of hepatitis and/or jaundice associated with telithromycin or other macrolide antibiotic use; concurrent use of cisapride or pimozide

Warnings/Precautions Acute hepatic failure and severe liver injury, including hepatitis and hepatic necrosis (leading to some fatalities) have been reported, in some cases after only a few doses; if signs/symptoms of hepatitis or liver damage occur, discontinue therapy and initiate liver function tests. **[U.S. Boxed Warning]: Life-threatening (including fatal) respiratory failure has occurred in patients with myasthenia gravis;** use in these patients is contraindicated. May prolong QT_c interval, leading to a risk of ventricular arrhythmias; closely-related antibiotics have been associated with malignant ventricular arrhythmias and torsade de pointes. Avoid in patients with prolongation of QTc interval due to congenital causes, history of long QT syndrome, uncorrected electrolyte disturbances (hypokalemia or hypomagnesemia), significant bradycardia (<50 bpm), or concurrent therapy with QT_c-prolonging drugs (eg, class Ia and class III antiarrhythmics). Avoid use in patients with a prior history of confirmed cardiogenic syncope or ventricular arrhythmias while receiving macrolide antibiotics or other QT_c-prolonging drugs. May cause severe visual disturbances (eg, changes in accommodation ability, diplopia, blurred vision). May cause loss of consciousness (possibly vagal-related); caution patients that these events may interfere with ability to operate machinery or drive, and to use caution until effects are known. Use caution in renal impairment; severe impairment (Cl_{cr} <30 mL/minute) requires dosage adjustment. Pseudomembranous colitis has been reported. Safety and efficacy not established in pediatric patients <13 years of age per Canadian approved labeling and <18 years of age per U.S. approved labeling.

Adverse Reactions

>10%: Gastrointestinal: Diarrhea (10% to 11%)

2% to 10%:

- Central nervous system: Headache (2% to 6%), dizziness (3% to 4%)
- Gastrointestinal: Nausea (7% to 8%), vomiting (2% to 3%), loose stools (2%), dysgeusia (2%)

≥0.2% to <2%:

- Central nervous system: Fatigue, insomnia, somnolence, vertigo
- Dermatologic: Rash
- Gastrointestinal: Abdominal distension, abdominal pain, anorexia, constipation, dyspepsia, flatulence, gastritis, gastroenteritis, GI upset, glossitis, stomatitis, watery stools, xerostomia
- Genitourinary: Vaginal candidiasis, vaginitis
- Hematologic: Platelets increased
- Hepatic: Transaminases increased
- Ocular: Blurred vision, accommodation delayed, diplopia
- Miscellaneous: Candidiasis, diaphoresis increased

<0.2% (Limited to important or life-threatening): Acute repiratory failure, alkaline phosphatase increased, allergic reaction, anaphylaxis, angioedema, anxiety, arrhythmia, bilirubin increased, bradycardia, edema (facial), eosinophilia, erythema multiforme, flushing, hepatitis, hepatitis, hepatocellular injury (including necrosis), hypotension, jaundice, liver failure, loss of consciousness (may be vagal-related), muscle cramps, myasthenia gravis exacerbation (rare), palpitation, pancreatitis, paresthesia, pruritus, pseudomembranous colitis, QT_c prolongation, syncope, torsade de pointes

Drug Interactions

Metabolism/Transport Effects Substrate of CYP1A2 (minor), 3A4 (major); **Inhibits** CYP2D6 (weak), 3A4 (strong)

Avoid Concomitant Use

Avoid concomitant use of Telithromycin with any of the following: Alfuzosin; Cisapride; Disopyramide; Nilotinib; Pimozide; Ranolazine; Rivaroxaban; Salmeterol; Silodosin; Tetrabenazine; Thioridazine; Ziprasidone

Increased Effect/Toxicity

Telithromycin may increase the levels/effects of: Alfentanil; Alfuzosin; Alosetron; Antifungal Agents (Azole Derivatives, Systemic); Benzodiazepines (metabolized by oxidation); BusPIRone; Calcium Channel Blockers; CarBAMazepine; Cardiac Glycosides; Ciclesonide; Cilostazol; Cisapride; Clozapine; Colchicine; Corticosteroids (Systemic); CycloSPORINE; CYP3A4 Substrates; Disopyramide; Eletriptan; Eplerenone; Ergot Derivatives; FentaNYL; Fesoterodine; HMG-CoA Reductase Inhibitors; Ixabepilone; Maraviroc; Nilotinib; Phosphodiesterase 5 Inhibitors; Pimecrolimus; Pimozide; QTc-Prolonging Agents; QuiNIDine; Ranolazine; Repaglinide; Rifamycin Derivatives; Rivaroxaban; Salmeterol; Selective Serotonin Reuptake Inhibitors; Silodosin; Sirolimus; Sorafenib; Tacrolimus; Temsirolimus; Tetrabenazine; Thioridazine; Vitamin K Antagonists; Ziprasidone; Zopiclone

The levels/effects of Telithromycin may be increased by: Alfuzosin; Antifungal Agents (Azole Derivatives, Systemic); Ciprofloxacin; CYP3A4 Inhibitors (Moderate); CYP3A4 Inhibitors (Strong); Dasatinib; Gadobutrol; Nilotinib

Decreased Effect

Telithromycin may decrease the levels/effects of: Clopidogrel; Typhoid Vaccine

The levels/effects of Telithromycin may be decreased by: CYP3A4 Inducers (Strong); Deferasirox; Etravirine; Herbs (CYP3A4 Inducers)

Ethanol/Nutrition/Herb Interactions Herb/nutraceutical: St John's wort: May decrease the levels/effects of telithromycin.

Stability Store at 15°C to 30°C (59°F to 86°F).

Mechanism of Action Inhibits bacterial protein synthesis by binding to two sites on the 50S ribosomal subunit. Telithromycin has also been demonstrated to alter secretion of IL-1alpha and TNF-alpha; the clinical significance of this immunomodulatory effect has not been evaluated.

Pharmacodynamics/Kinetics

Absorption: Rapid

Distribution: 2.9 L/kg

Protein binding: 60% to 70%; primarily to albumin

Metabolism: Hepatic, via CYP3A4 (50%) and non-CYP-mediated pathways

Bioavailability: 57% (significant first-pass metabolism)

Half-life elimination: 10 hours

Time to peak, plasma: 1 hour

Excretion: Urine (13% unchanged drug, remainder as metabolites); feces (7%)

Dosage Oral:

Children ≥13 years and Adults: Tonsillitis/pharyngitis (unlabeled use; Canadian indication): 800 mg once daily for 5 days

Adults:

Community-acquired pneumonia: 800 mg once daily for 7-10 days

Dosage adjustment in renal impairment:

U.S. product labeling: Cl_{cr} <30 mL/minute, including dialysis: 600 mg once daily; when renal impairment is accompanied by hepatic impairment, reduce dosage to 400 mg once daily

Canadian product labeling: Cl_{cr} <30 mL/minute: Reduce dose to 400 mg once daily

Hemodialysis: Administer following dialysis

Dosage adjustment in hepatic impairment: No adjustment recommended, unless concurrent severe renal impairment is present

Dietary Considerations May be taken with or without food.

Administration May be administered with or without food.

Monitoring Parameters Liver function tests; signs/symptoms of liver failure (eg, jaundice, fatigue, malaise, anorexia, nausea, bilirubinemia, acholic stools, liver tenderness, hepatomegaly); visual acuity

Dosage Forms Excipient information presented when available (limited, particularly for generics); consult specific product labeling.

Tablet:

Ketek®: 300 mg [not available in Canada], 400 mg

Telmisartan (tel mi SAR tan)

U.S. Brand Names Micardis®

Canadian Brand Names Micardis®

Pharmacologic Category Angiotensin II Receptor Blocker

Additional Appendix Information

Angiotensin Agents *on page 1632*

Use Treatment of hypertension; may be used alone or in combination with other antihypertensive agents

Pregnancy Risk Factor C (1st trimester); D (2nd and 3rd trimesters)

Pregnancy Considerations Medications which act on the renin-angiotensin system are reported to have the following fetal/neonatal effects: Hypotension, neonatal skull hypoplasia, anuria, renal failure, and death; oligohydramnios is also reported. These effects are reported to occur with exposure during the second and third trimesters. There are no adequate and well-controlled studies in pregnant women. **[U.S. Boxed Warning]: Based on human data, drugs that act on the angiotensin system can cause injury and death to the developing fetus when used in the second and third trimesters. Angiotensin receptor blockers should be discontinued as soon as possible once pregnancy is detected.**

Lactation Enters breast milk/not recommended

Contraindications Hypersensitivity to telmisartan or any component of the formulation

Warnings/Precautions [U.S. Boxed Warning]: Based on human data, drugs that act on the angiotensin system can cause injury and death to the developing fetus when used in the second and third trimesters. Angiotensin receptor blockers should be discontinued as soon as possible once pregnancy is detected. May cause hyperkalemia; avoid potassium supplementation unless specifically required by healthcare provider. Avoid use or use a smaller dose in patients who are volume depleted; correct depletion first. May be associated with deterioration of renal function and/or increases in serum creatinine, particularly in patients with low renal blood flow (eg, renal artery stenosis, heart failure) whose glomerular filtration rate (GFR) is dependent on efferent arteriolar vasoconstriction by angiotensin II. Use with caution in unstented unilateral/bilateral renal artery stenosis. When unstented bilateral renal artery stenosis is present, use is generally avoided due to the elevated risk of deterioration in renal function unless possible benefits outweigh risks. Use with caution with pre-existing renal insufficiency; significant aortic/mitral stenosis. Use with caution in patients who have biliary obstructive disorders or hepatic dysfunction. Safety and efficacy have not been established in children.

Adverse Reactions May be associated with worsening of renal function in patients dependent on renin-angiotensin-aldosterone system.

1% to 10%:

Cardiovascular: Hypertension (1%), chest pain (1%), peripheral edema (1%)

Central nervous system: Headache (1%), dizziness (1%), pain (1%), fatigue (1%)

Gastrointestinal: Diarrhea (3%), dyspepsia (1%), nausea (1%), abdominal pain (1%)

Genitourinary: Urinary tract infection (1%)

Neuromuscular & skeletal: Back pain (3%), myalgia (1%)

Respiratory: Upper respiratory infection (7%), sinusitis (3%), pharyngitis (1%), cough (2%)

Miscellaneous: Flu-like syndrome (1%)

<1% (Limited to important or life-threatening): Abnormal vision, allergic reaction, anemia, angina, angioedema, angioneurotic edema, atrial fibrillation, bradycardia, creatinine kinase increased, CHF, cramps, depression, dyspnea, edema, eosinophilia, epistaxis, erectile dysfunction, erythema, facial edema, gout, hepatic dysfunction, hyperkalemia, hypersensitivity, hypotension, impotence, increased serum creatinine and BUN, insomnia, MI, migraine, muscle cramps, orthostatic hypotension (more frequent in dialysis patients), paresthesia, pruritus, rhabdomyolysis, rash, renal dysfunction, renal failure, somnolence, syncope, thrombocytopenia, tinnitus, uric acid increased, urticaria, vertigo, weakness

Drug Interactions

Metabolism/Transport Effects Inhibits CYP2C19 (weak)

Avoid Concomitant Use There are no known interactions where it is recommended to avoid concomitant use.

Increased Effect/Toxicity

Telmisartan may increase the levels/effects of: ACE Inhibitors; Amifostine; Cardiac Glycosides; Lithium; Potassium-Sparing Diuretics; RiTUXimab

The levels/effects of Telmisartan may be increased by: Diazoxide; Eplerenone; Herbs (Hypotensive Properties); Potassium Salts; Prostacyclin Analogues; Trimethoprim

Decreased Effect

The levels/effects of Telmisartan may be decreased by: Herbs (Hypertensive Properties); Methylphenidate; Nonsteroidal Anti-Inflammatory Agents; Yohimbine

Ethanol/Nutrition/Herb Interactions Herb/Nutraceutical: Avoid dong quai if using for hypertension (has estrogenic activity). Avoid ephedra, yohimbe, ginseng (may worsen hypertension). Avoid garlic (may have increased antihypertensive effect).

Mechanism of Action Angiotensin II acts as a vasoconstrictor. In addition to causing direct vasoconstriction, angiotensin II also stimulates the release of aldosterone. Once aldosterone is released, sodium as well as water are reabsorbed. The end result is an elevation in blood pressure. Telmisartan is a nonpeptide AT1 angiotensin II receptor antagonist. This binding prevents angiotensin II from binding to the receptor thereby blocking the vasoconstriction and the aldosterone secreting effects of angiotensin II.

Pharmacodynamics/Kinetics Orally active, not a prodrug
Onset of action: 1-2 hours
Peak effect: 0.5-1 hours
Duration: Up to 24 hours
Protein binding: >99.5%
Metabolism: Hepatic via conjugation to inactive metabolites; not metabolized via CYP
Bioavailability (dose dependent): 42% to 58%
Half-life elimination: Terminal: 24 hours
Excretion: Feces (97%)
Clearance: Total body: 800 mL/minute

Dosage Adults: Oral: Initial: 40 mg once daily; usual maintenance dose range: 20-80 mg/day. Patients with volume depletion should be initiated on the lower dosage with close supervision.

Dosage adjustment in renal impairment: No adjustment required; hemodialysis patients are more susceptible to orthostatic hypotension

Dosage adjustment in hepatic impairment: Supervise patients closely.

Dietary Considerations May be taken without regard to food.

Monitoring Parameters Supine blood pressure, electrolytes, serum creatinine, BUN, urinalysis, symptomatic hypotension, and tachycardia

Dosage Forms Excipient information presented when available (limited, particularly for generics); consult specific product labeling.
Tablet: 20 mg, 40 mg, 80 mg

Telmisartan and Hydrochlorothiazide
(tel mi SAR tan & hye droe klor oh THYE a zide)

U.S. Brand Names Micardis® HCT

Canadian Brand Names Micardis® Plus

Index Terms Hydrochlorothiazide and Telmisartan

Pharmacologic Category Angiotensin II Receptor Blocker; Diuretic, Thiazide

Use Treatment of hypertension; combination product should not be used for initial therapy

Pregnancy Risk Factor C (1st trimester); D (2nd and 3rd trimesters)

Dosage Adults: Oral: Replacement therapy: Combination product can be substituted for individual titrated agents. Initiation of combination therapy when monotherapy has failed to achieve desired effects:

Patients currently on telmisartan: Initial dose if blood pressure is not currently controlled on monotherapy of 80 mg telmisartan: Telmisartan 80 mg/hydrochlorothiazide 12.5 mg once daily; may titrate up to telmisartan 160 mg/hydrochlorothiazide 25 mg if needed

Patients currently on hydrochlorothiazide: Initial dose if blood pressure is not currently controlled on monotherapy of 25 mg once daily: Telmisartan 80 mg/hydrochlorothiazide 12.5 mg once daily or telmisartan 80 mg/hydrochlorothiazide 25 mg once daily; may titrate up to telmisartan 160 mg/hydrochlorothiazide 25 mg if blood pressure remains uncontrolled after 2-4 weeks of therapy. Patients who develop hypokalemia may be switched to telmisartan 80 mg/hydrochlorothiazide 12.5 mg.

Dosage adjustment in renal impairment:
Cl_{cr} >30 mL/minute: Usual recommended dose
Cl_{cr} ≤30 mL/minute: Not recommended

Dosage adjustment in hepatic impairment: Dosing should be started at telmisartan 40 mg/hydrochlorothiazide 12.5 mg; do **not** use in patients with severe hepatic impairment

Elderly: No dosing adjustment needed based on age; monitor renal and hepatic function

Additional Information Complete prescribing information for this medication should be consulted for additional detail.

Dosage Forms Excipient information presented when available (limited, particularly for generics); consult specific product labeling. [CAN]: Canadian brand name
Tablet:
Micardis® HCT [available in U.S.]:
40/12.5: Telmisartan 40 mg and hydrochlorothiazide 12.5 mg
80/12.5: Telmisartan 80 mg and hydrochlorothiazide 12.5 mg
80/25: Telmisartan 80 mg and hydrochlorothiazide 25 mg
Micardis® Plus [CAN]: 80/25: Telmisartan 80 mg and hydrochlorothiazide 25 mg [Not available in U.S.]

◆ **Telzir® (Can)** *see* Fosamprenavir *on page 664*

Temazepam (te MAZ e pam)

U.S. Brand Names Restoril®

Canadian Brand Names Apo-Temazepam®; CO Temazepam; Dom-Temazepam; Gen-Temazepam; Novo-Temazepam; Nu-Temazepam; PHL-Temazepam; PMS-Temazepam; ratio-Temazepam; Restoril®

Pharmacologic Category Hypnotic, Benzodiazepine

Additional Appendix Information
Benzodiazepines *on page 1646*

Use Short-term treatment of insomnia

Unlabeled/Investigational Use Treatment of anxiety; adjunct in the treatment of depression; management of panic attacks

Restrictions C-IV

An FDA-approved patient medication guide is available and must be distributed when dispensing an outpatient prescription (new or refill) where this medication is to be used without direct supervision of a healthcare provider. Medication guides are available at http://www.fda.gov/cder/Offices/ODS/medication_guides.htm.

Pregnancy Risk Factor X

Medication Safety Issues
Sound-alike/look-alike issues:
Temazepam may be confused with flurazepam, LORazepam
Restoril® may be confused with Vistaril®, Zestril®

Dosage Oral:
Adults: 15-30 mg at bedtime
Elderly or debilitated patients: 15 mg

Additional Information Complete prescribing information for this medication should be consulted for additional detail.

Dosage Forms Excipient information presented when available (limited, particularly for generics); consult specific product labeling.
Capsule: 7.5 mg, 15 mg, 22.5 mg, 30 mg
Restoril®: 7.5 mg, 15 mg, 22.5 mg, 30 mg

◆ **Temodal® (Can)** *see* Temozolomide *on page 1432*
◆ **Temodar®** *see* Temozolomide *on page 1432*
◆ **Temovate®** *see* Clobetasol *on page 347*
◆ **Temovate E®** *see* Clobetasol *on page 347*

Temozolomide (te moe ZOE loe mide)

U.S. Brand Names Temodar®

Canadian Brand Names Temodal®; Temodar®

Index Terms NSC-362856; TMZ

Pharmacologic Category Antineoplastic Agent, Alkylating Agent (Triazene)

Use Treatment of adult patients with refractory anaplastic astrocytoma; newly-diagnosed glioblastoma multiforme

Unlabeled/Investigational Use Metastatic melanoma

Pregnancy Risk Factor D

Pregnancy Considerations May cause fetal harm when administered to pregnant women. Animal studies, at doses less than used in humans, resulted in numerous birth defects. Testicular toxicity was demonstrated in animal studies using smaller doses than recommended for cancer treatment. There are no adequate and well-controlled studies in pregnant women. Male and female patients should avoid pregnancy while receiving drug.

Lactation Excretion in breast milk unknown/not recommended

Medication Safety Issues

High alert medication: The Institute for Safe Medication Practices (ISMP) includes this medication among its list of drugs which have a heightened risk of causing significant patient harm when used in error.

Contraindications Hypersensitivity to temozolomide or any component of the formulation; hypersensitivity to dacarbazine (since both drugs are metabolized to MTIC); pregnancy

Warnings/Precautions Hazardous agent - use appropriate precautions for handling and disposal. Pneumocystis *jiroveci* pneumonia (PCP) may occur; risk is increased in those receiving steroids or longer dosing regimens; PCP prophylaxis is required in patients receiving radiotherapy in combination with the 42-day temozolomide regimen. Myelosuppression may occur; an increased incidence has been reported in geriatric and female patients. Rare cases of myelodysplastic syndrome and secondary malignancies, including acute myeloid leukemia have been reported. Use caution in patients with severe hepatic or renal impairment.

Adverse Reactions Note: With CNS malignancies, it is difficult to distinguish between CNS adverse events caused by temozolomide versus the effects of progressive disease.

>10%:

- Cardiovascular: Peripheral edema (11%)
- Central nervous system: Fatigue (34% to 61%), headache (23% to 41%), seizure (6% to 23%), hemiparesis (18%), fever (13%), dizziness (5% to 12%), coordination abnormality (11%)
- Dermatologic: Alopecia (55%), rash (8% to 13%)
- Gastrointestinal: Nausea (49% to 53%; grades 3/4: 1% to 10%), vomiting (29% to 42%; grades 3/4: 2% to 6%), constipation (22% to 33%), anorexia (9% to 27%), diarrhea (10% to 16%)
- Hematologic: Lymphopenia (grades 3/4: 55%), thrombocytopenia (grades 3/4: adults: 4% to 19%; children: 25%), neutropenia (grades 3/4: adults: 8% to 14%; children: 20%), leukopenia (grades 3/4: 11%)
- Neuromuscular & skeletal: Weakness (7% to 13%)
- Miscellaneous: Viral infection (11%)

1% to 10%:

- Central nervous system: Amnesia (10%), insomnia (4% to 10%), somnolence (9%), ataxia (8%), paresis (8%), anxiety (7%), memory impairment (7%), depression (6%), confusion (5%)
- Dermatologic: Pruritus (5% to 8%), dry skin (5%), radiation injury (2% maintenance phase after radiotherapy), erythema (1%)
- Endocrine & metabolic: Hypercorticism (8%), breast pain (females 6%)
- Gastrointestinal: Stomatitis (9%), abdominal pain (5% to 9%), dysphagia (7%), taste perversion (5%), weight gain (5%)
- Genitourinary: Incontinence (8%), urinary tract infection (8%), urinary frequency (6%)
- Hematologic: Anemia (grades 3/4: 4%)
- Neuromuscular & skeletal: Paresthesia (9%), back pain (8%), abnormal gait (6%), arthralgia (6%), myalgia (5%)
- Ocular: Blurred vision (5% to 8%), diplopia (5%), vision abnormality (visual deficit/vision changes 5%)
- Respiratory: Pharyngitis (8%), upper respiratory tract infection (8%), cough (5% to 8%), sinusitis (6%), dyspnea (5%)
- Miscellaneous: Allergic reaction (up to 3%)

Postmarketing and/or case reports: Anaphylaxis, aplastic anemia, erythema multiforme, myelodysplastic syndrome, opportunistic infection (eg, PCP), pancytopenia, secondary malignancies (including myeloid leukemia)

Drug Interactions

Avoid Concomitant Use

Avoid concomitant use of Temozolomide with any of the following: Natalizumab; Vaccines (Live)

Increased Effect/Toxicity

Temozolomide may increase the levels/effects of: Natalizumab; Vaccines (Live)

The levels/effects of Temozolomide may be increased by: Trastuzumab

Decreased Effect

Temozolomide may decrease the levels/effects of: Vaccines (Inactivated)

The levels/effects of Temozolomide may be decreased by: Echinacea

Ethanol/Nutrition/Herb Interactions Food: Food reduces rate and extent of absorption.

Stability Store at room temperature of 15°C to 30°C (59°F to 86°F).

Mechanism of Action Like dacarbazine, temozolomide is converted to the active alkylating metabolite MTIC [(methyl-triazene-1-yl)-imidazole-4-carboxamide]. Unlike dacarbazine, however, this conversion is spontaneous, nonenzymatic, and occurs under physiologic conditions in all tissues to which the drug distributes.

Pharmacodynamics/Kinetics

- Absorption: Rapid and complete
- Distribution: V_d: Parent drug: 0.4 L/kg; penetrates blood-brain barrier; CSF levels are ~35% to 39% of plasma levels
- Protein binding: 15%
- Metabolism: Prodrug, hydrolyzed to the active form, MTIC; MTIC is eventually eliminated as CO_2 and 5-aminoimidazole-4-carboxamide (AIC), a natural constituent in urine
- Bioavailability: 100%
- Half-life elimination: Mean: Parent drug: 1.8 hours
- Time to peak: Empty stomach: 1 hour
- Excretion: Urine (~38%; parent drug 6%); feces 0.8%

Dosage Oral (refer to individual protocols): Adults:

Anaplastic astrocytoma (refractory): Initial dose: 150 mg/m^2/day for 5 days; repeat every 28 days. Subsequent doses of 100-200 mg/m^2/day for 5 days per treatment cycle; based upon hematologic tolerance.

- ANC <1000/mm^3 or platelets <50,000/mm^3 on day 22 or day 29 (day 1 of next cycle): Postpone therapy until ANC >1500/mm^3 and platelets >100,000/mm^3; reduce dose by 50 mg/m^2/day for subsequent cycle
- ANC 1000-1500/mm^3 or platelets 50,000-100,000/mm^3 on day 22 or day 29 (day 1 of next cycle): Postpone therapy until ANC >1500/mm^3 and platelets >100,000/mm^3; maintain initial dose
- ANC >1500/mm^3 and platelets >100,000/mm^3 on day 22 or day 29 (day 1 of next cycle): Increase dose to or maintain dose at 200 mg/m^2/day for 5 days for subsequent cycle

Glioblastoma multiforme (high-grade glioma):

Concomitant phase: 75 mg/m^2/day for 42 days with radiotherapy (60Gy administered in 30 fractions). **Note:** PCP prophylaxis is required during concomitant phase and should continue in patients who develop lymphocytopenia until recovery (common toxicity criteria [CTC] ≤1). Obtain weekly CBC.

ANC ≥1500/mm^3, platelet count ≥100,000/mm^3, and nonhematologic CTC ≤grade 1 (excludes alopecia, nausea/vomiting): Temodar® 75 mg/m^2/day may be continued throughout the 42-day concomitant period up to 49 days

Dosage modification:

ANC ≥500/mm^3 but <1500/mm^3 **or** platelet count ≥10,000/mm^3 but <100,000/mm^3 **or** nonhematologic CTC grade 2 (excludes alopecia, nausea/vomiting): Interrupt therapy

ANC <500/mm^3 **or** platelet count <10,000/mm^3 **or** nonhematologic CTC grade 3/4 (excludes alopecia, nausea/vomiting): Discontinue therapy

Maintenance phase (consists of 6 treatment cycles): Begin 4 weeks after concomitant phase completion. **Note:** Each subsequent cycle is 28 days (consisting of 5 days of drug treatment followed by 23 days without treatment). Draw CBC within 48 hours of day 22; hold next cycle and do weekly CBC until ANC >1500/mm^3 and platelet count >100,000/mm^3; dosing modification should be based on lowest blood counts and worst nonhematologic toxicity during the previous cycle.

Cycle 1: 150 mg/m^2/day for 5 days; repeat every 28 days

Dosage modification for next cycle:

ANC <1000/mm^3, platelet count <50,000/mm^3, or nonhematologic CTC grade 3 (excludes for alopecia, nausea/vomiting) during previous cycle: Decrease dose by 50 mg/m^2/day for 5 days, unless dose has already been lowered to 100 mg/m^2/day, then discontinue therapy.

If dose reduction <100 mg/m^2/day is required or nonhematologic CTC grade 4 (excludes for alopecia, nausea/vomiting), or if the same grade 3 nonhematologic toxicity occurs after dose reduction: Discontinue therapy

Cycle 2: 200 mg/m^2/day for 5 days every 28 days, unless prior toxicity, then refer to Dosage Modifications under "Cycle 1" and give adjusted dose for 5 days

Cycles 3-6: Continue with previous cycle's dose for 5 days every 28 days unless toxicity has occurred then, refer to Dosage Modifications under "Cycle 1" and give adjusted dose for 5 days

Metastatic melanoma (unlabeled use): 200 mg/m^2/day for 5 days every 28 days (for up to 12 cycles). For subsequent cycles reduce dose to 75% of the original dose for grade 3/4 hematologic toxicity and reduce the dose to 50% of the original dose for grade 3/4 nonhematologic toxicity.

Elderly: Refer to adult dosing. **Note:** Patients ≥70 years of age had a higher incidence of grade 4 neutropenia and thrombocytopenia in the first cycle of therapy than patients <70 years of age.

Dosage adjustment in renal impairment: No guidelines exist. Caution should be used when administered to patients with severe renal impairment (Cl_{cr} <36 mL/minute). Temozolomide has not been studied in dialysis patients.

Dosage adjustment in hepatic impairment: Caution should be used when administering to patients with severe hepatic impairment.

Dietary Considerations The incidence of nausea/vomiting is decreased when the drug is taken on an empty stomach.

Administration Capsules should not be opened or chewed but swallowed whole with a glass of water. May be administered on an empty stomach to reduce nausea and vomiting. Bedtime administration may be advised.

Monitoring Parameters CBC with differential and platelets (prior to each cycle; weekly during glioma concomitant phase treatment; at or within 48 hours of day 22 and weekly until ANC >1500/mm^3 for glioma maintenance and astrocytoma treatment)

Dosage Forms Excipient information presented when available (limited, particularly for generics); consult specific product labeling.

Capsule:

Temodar®: 5 mg, 20 mg, 100 mg, 140 mg, 180 mg, 250 mg

Extemporaneous Preparations Temozolomide 10 mg/mL oral suspension: In a glass mortar, mix the contents of ten 100-mg capsules and 500 mg of povidine K-30 powder; add 25 mg anhydrous citric acid dissolved in 1.5 mL purified water; mix to form a paste; add 50 mL Ora-Plus® (add a small amount at first, mix, add balance); mix; transfer to amber plastic bottle; add enough Ora-Sweet® or Ora-Sweet® SF to bring a total volume of 100 mL by rinsing the mortar with small amounts of Ora-Sweet®; repeat rinsing 3 more times. The suspension is stable for 7 days at room temperature or 60 days refrigerated in plastic amber prescription bottles. **Note:** Use appropriate handling precautions during preparation.

Trissel LA, Yanping Z, and Koontz SE. "Temozolomide Stability in Extemporaneously Compounded Oral Suspension," *Int J Pharm Compounding*, 2006, 10 (5):396-9.

◆ **Tempra® (Can)** *see* Acetaminophen *on page 25*

Temsirolimus (tem sir OH li mus)

U.S. Brand Names Torisel®

Canadian Brand Names Torisel®

Index Terms CCI-779; NSC-683864

Pharmacologic Category Antineoplastic Agent, mTOR Kinase Inhibitor

Use Treatment of advanced renal cell cancer (RCC)

Pregnancy Risk Factor D

Pregnancy Considerations Embryotoxicity and fetotoxicity may occur, as evidenced by increased mortality, reduced fetal weights, and delayed ossification in animal studies. There are no adequate and well-controlled studies in pregnant women. Women of childbearing potential should be advised to avoid pregnancy. Men and women should use effective birth control during temsirolimus treatment, and continue for 3 months after temsirolimus discontinuation.

Lactation Excretion in breast milk unknown/not recommended

Medication Safety Issues

Sound-alike/look-alike issues:

Temsirolimus may be confused with sirolimus, tacrolimus

High alert medication: The Institute for Safe Medication Practices (ISMP) includes this medication among its list of drug classes which have a heightened risk of causing significant patient harm when used in error.

Temsirolimus, for the treatment of advanced renal cell cancer, is a flat dose (25 mg) and is not based on body surface area (BSA).

Contraindications There are no contraindications listed within the FDA-approved manufacturer's labeling.

Canadian labeling: Additional contraindications (not in U.S. labeling): History of anaphylaxis after exposure to temsirolimus, sirolimus, or any component of the formulation

Warnings/Precautions Hazardous agent - use appropriate precautions for handling and disposal.

Hypersensitivity/infusion reactions (eg, anaphylaxis, apnea, dyspnea, flushing, loss of consciousness, hypotension, and/or chest pain) have been reported. Infusion reaction may occur with initial or subsequent infusions.

Premedicate with an antihistamine (H_1 antagonist) prior to infusion; monitor during infusion; interrupt infusion for severe reaction. With discretion, treatment may be resumed at a slower infusion rate; administer an H_1 antagonist (if not given as premedication) and/or an H_2 antagonist 30 minutes prior to resuming infusion. Use with caution in patients with hypersensitivity to polysorbate 80. Angioneurotic edema has been reported; concurrent use with other drugs known to cause angioedema (eg, ACE inhibitors) may increase risk.

Use with caution in patients taking strong CYP3A4 inhibitors and moderate or strong CYP3A4 inducers (see Drug Interactions); consider alternative agents that avoid or lessen the potential for CYP-mediated interactions. Patients should not be immunized with live, viral vaccines during or shortly after treatment and should avoid close contact with recently vaccinated (live vaccine) individuals. Patients who are receiving anticoagulant therapy or those with CNS tumors/metastases may be at increased risk for developing intracerebral bleeding.

Increases in serum glucose are common; may alter insulin and/or oral hypoglycemic therapy requirements in patients with diabetes; monitor. Serum cholesterol and triglyceride elevations are also common; may require initiation or dose increases of antihyperlipidemic agents. Treatment may result in immunosuppression, may increase risk of opportunistic infections and/or sepsis. Interstitial lung disease (ILD), sometimes fatal, has been reported; symptoms include dyspnea, cough, hypoxia, and/or fever, although asymptomatic cases may present; promptly evaluate worsening respiratory symptoms. Cases of bowel perforation (fatal) have occurred; promptly evaluate any new or worsening abdominal pain or bloody stools. Temsirolimus may be associated with impaired wound healing; use caution in the perioperative period. Cases of acute renal failure with rapid progression have been reported, including cases unresponsive to dialysis.

Has not been studied in patients with hepatic impairment; use caution; temsirolimus is predominantly cleared by the liver. Safety and efficacy in children have not been established.

Adverse Reactions

>10%:

- Cardiovascular: Edema (35%), peripheral edema (27%), chest pain (16%)
- Central nervous system: Pain (28%), fever (24%), headache (15%), insomnia (12%)
- Dermatologic: Rash (47%), pruritus (19%), nail disorder/thinning (14%), dry skin (11%)
- Endocrine & metabolic: Hyperglycemia (26% to 89%; grades 3/4: 16%), hypercholesterolemia (24% to 87%; grades 3/4: 2%), hyperlipidemia (27% to 83%; grades 3/4: 44%), hypophosphatemia (49%; grades 3/4: 18%), hypokalemia (21%; grades 3/4: 5%)
- Gastrointestinal: Mucositis (41%), nausea (37%), anorexia (32%), diarrhea (27%), abdominal pain (21%), constipation (20%), stomatitis (20%), taste disturbance (20%), vomiting (19%), weight loss (19%)
- Genitourinary: Urinary tract infection (15%)
- Hematologic: Anemia (45% to 94%; grades 3/4: 20%), lymphopenia (53%; grades 3/4: 16%), thrombocytopenia (14% to 40%; grades 3/4: 1%; dose-limiting toxicity), leukopenia (6% to 32%; grades 3/4: 1%), neutropenia (7% to 19%; grades 3/4: 3% to 5%)
- Hepatic: Alkaline phosphatase increased (68%; grades 3/4: 3%), AST increased (8% to 38%; grades 3/4: 1% to 2%)
- Neuromuscular & skeletal: Weakness (51%), back pain (20%), arthralgia (18%)
- Renal: Creatinine increased (14% to 57%; grades 3/4: 3%)
- Respiratory: Dyspnea (28%), cough (26%), epistaxis (12%), pharyngitis (12%)
- Miscellaneous: Infection (20% to 27%; includes abscess, bronchitis, cellulitis, herpes simplex, herpes zoster)

1% to 10%:

- Cardiovascular: Hypertension (7%), venous thromboembolism (2%, includes DVT and PE), thrombophlebitis (1%)
- Central nervous system: Chills (8%), depression (4%)
- Dermatologic: Acne (10%), wound healing impaired (1%)
- Gastrointestinal: Bowel perforation (fatal: 1%)
- Hepatic: Hyperbilirubinemia (8%)
- Neuromuscular & skeletal: Myalgia (8%)
- Ocular: Conjunctivitis (7%)
- Respiratory: Rhinitis (10%), pneumonia (8%), upper respiratory tract infection (7%), interstitial lung disease (2%)
- Miscellaneous: Allergic/hypersensitivity/infusion reaction (9%; includes anaphylaxis, apnea, chest pain, dyspnea, flushing, hypotension, loss of consciousness)

<1% (Limited to important or life-threatening): Acute renal failure, angioneurotic edema, pneumonitis

Drug Interactions

Metabolism/Transport Effects **Substrate** of CYP3A4 (major); **Inhibits** CYP3A4 (weak), 2D6 (weak)

Avoid Concomitant Use

Avoid concomitant use of Temsirolimus with any of the following: Natalizumab; Vaccines (Live)

Increased Effect/Toxicity

Temsirolimus may increase the levels/effects of: ACE Inhibitors; CycloSPORINE; Natalizumab; Tacrolimus; Vaccines (Live)

The levels/effects of Temsirolimus may be increased by: Antifungal Agents (Azole Derivatives, Systemic); CYP3A4 Inhibitors (Moderate); CYP3A4 Inhibitors (Strong); Dasatinib; Herbs (Hypoglycemic Properties); Macrolide Antibiotics; P-Glycoprotein Inhibitors; Protease Inhibitors; Trastuzumab

Decreased Effect

Temsirolimus may decrease the levels/effects of: Vaccines (Inactivated)

The levels/effects of Temsirolimus may be decreased by: CarBAMazepine; CYP3A4 Inducers (Strong); Deferasirox; Echinacea; Herbs (CYP3A4 Inducers); P-Glycoprotein Inducers; Phenytoin; Rifamycin Derivatives

Ethanol/Nutrition/Herb Interactions Herb/Nutraceutical: St John's wort may decrease sirolimus (the active metabolite of temsirolimus) levels; avoid concurrent use. Herbs with hypoglycemic properties may increase the risk of temsirolimus-induced hypoglycemia; includes alfalfa, aloe, bilberry, bitter melon, burdock, celery, damiana, fenugreek, garcinia, garlic, ginger, ginseng (American), gymnema, marshmallow, stinging nettle. Avoid grapefruit and grapefruit juice (may increase the levels/effects of sirolimus).

Stability Store intact vials under refrigeration at 2°C to 8°C (36°F to 46°F). Protect from light during storage, preparation, and handling. Vials should be diluted with 1.8 mL of provided diluent to a concentration of 10 mg/mL (vial contains overfill). Mix by inverting vial. Diluted solution in the vial (10 mg/mL) is stable for 24 hours at room temperature. After allowing air bubbles to subside, further dilute in 250 mL of NS in a non-DEHP/non-PVC container (glass, polyolefin or polypropylene). Avoid excessive shaking (may result in foaming). Solutions diluted for infusion (in normal saline) must be infused within 6 hours of preparation. Use appropriate precautions for handling and disposal.

Mechanism of Action Temsirolimus and its active metabolite, sirolimus, are targeted inhibitors of mTOR (mammalian target of rapamycin) kinase activity. Temsirolimus (and sirolimus) bind to FKBP-12, an intracellular protein, to form a complex which inhibits mTOR signaling, halting the cell cycle at the G1 phase in tumor cells. In renal cell carcinoma, mTOR inhibition also exhibits anti-angiogenesis activity by reducing levels of HIF-1 and HIF-2 alpha (hypoxia inducible factors) and vascular endothelial growth factor (VEGF).

Pharmacodynamics/Kinetics

Distribution: V_{dss}: 172 L

Metabolism: Hepatic; via CYP3A4 to sirolimus (primary active metabolite) and 4 minor metabolites

Half-life elimination: Temsirolimus: ~17 hours; Sirolimus: ~55 hours

Time to peak, plasma: Temsirolimus: At end of infusion; Sirolimus: 0.5-2 hours after temsirolimus infusion

Excretion: Feces (78%); urine (<5%)

Dosage Note: For infusion reaction prophylaxis, premedicate with an H_1 antagonist (eg, diphenhydramine 25-50 mg I.V.) 30 minutes prior to infusion.

I.V.: Adults: RCC: 25 mg weekly

Dosage adjustment for concomitant CYP3A4 inhibitors/inducers:

CYP3A4 inhibitors: Dose reductions are likely to be needed when temsirolimus is administered concomitantly with a strong CYP3A4 inhibitor (an alternate medication for CYP3A4 enzyme inhibitors should be investigated first); in the event that temsirolimus must be administered concomitantly with a potent enzyme inhibitor, consider reducing temsirolimus to 12.5 mg/week with careful monitoring. (When a strong CYP3A4 inhibitor is discontinued; allow ~1 week to elapse prior to adjusting the temsirolimus upward to the dose used prior to initiation of the CYP3A4 inhibitor.)

CYP3A4 inducers: Concomitant administration with CYP3A4 inducers may require increased temsirolimus doses (alternatives to the enzyme-inducing agent should be utilized first); consider adjusting temsirolimus dose to 50 mg/week, with careful monitoring. (If the strong CYP3A4 enzyme inducer is discontinued, reduce the temsirolimus to the dose used prior to initiation of the CYP3A4 inducer.)

Dosage adjustment for toxicity :

Hematologic toxicity: ANC <1000/mm^3 or platelets <75,000/mm^3: Withhold treatment until resolves and reinitiate treatment with a 5 mg/week dose reduction; minimum dose: 15 mg/week if adjustment for toxicity is needed.

Nonhematologic toxicity: Any toxicity ≥grade 3: Withhold treatment until resolves to ≤grade 2; reinitiate treatment with a 5 mg/week dose reduction; minimum dose: 15 mg/week if adjustment for toxicity is needed.

Dosage adjustment in renal impairment: Not studied in renal dysfunction, however, due to the minimal renal elimination (<5%), dosage adjustment for renal dysfunction is not recommended.

Hemodialysis: Has not been studied in hemodialysis patients.

Dosage adjustment in hepatic impairment (DOH) The FDA-approved labeling does not contain hepatic dosing adjustment guidelines. Patients with AST >3 times ULN (>5 times ULN in the presence of liver metastases) and total bilirubin >1.5 times ULN were excluded from clinical trials. Temsirolimus is primarily cleared hepatically.

Administration Infuse over 30-60 minute via an infusion pump (preferred). Use non-DEHP containing administration tubing. Administer through an inline polyethersulfone filter ≤5 micron. Premedicate with an H_1 antagonist (eg, diphenhydramine 25-50 mg I.V.) 30 minutes prior to infusion. Monitor during infusion; interrupt infusion for hypersensitivity/infusion reaction; monitor for 30-60 minutes; may reinitiate at a reduced infusion rate (over 60 minutes) with discretion, 30 minutes after administration of a histamine H_1 antagonist and/or a histamine H_2 antagonist (eg, famotidine or ranitidine).

Monitoring Parameters CBC with differential and platelets (weekly), serum chemistries including glucose (baseline and every other week), serum cholesterol and triglycerides (baseline and periodic), liver and renal function tests

Monitor for infusion reactions; infection; symptoms of ILD (or radiographic changes)

Dosage Forms Excipient information presented when available (limited, particularly for generics); consult specific product labeling.

Injection, solution [concentrate]:

Torisel®: 25 mg/mL [contains dehydrated ethanol, propylene glycol; diluent contains dehydrated ethanol, polyethylene glycol, polysorbate 80]

Tenecteplase (ten EK te plase)

U.S. Brand Names TNKase®

Canadian Brand Names TNKase®

Pharmacologic Category Thrombolytic Agent

Use Thrombolytic agent used in the management of ST-elevation myocardial infarction (STEMI) for the lysis of thrombi in the coronary vasculature to restore perfusion and reduce mortality.

Recommended criteria for treatment: STEMI: Chest pain ≥20 minutes duration, onset of chest pain within 12 hours of treatment (or within prior 12-24 hours in patients with continuing ischemic symptoms), and S-T segment elevation >0.1 mV in at least two contiguous precordial leads or two adjacent limb leads on ECG or new or presumably new left bundle branch block (LBBB)

Unlabeled/Investigational Use Acute MI - combination regimen of tenecteplase (unlabeled dose), abciximab, and heparin (unlabeled dose)

Pregnancy Risk Factor C

Pregnancy Considerations Administer to pregnant women only if the potential benefits justify the risk to the fetus.

Lactation Use caution

Medication Safety Issues

Sound-alike/look-alike issues:

TNKase® may be confused with t-PA

TNK (occasional abbreviation for TNKase®) is an error-prone abbreviation (mistaken as TPA)

High alert medication: The Institute for Safe Medication Practices (ISMP) includes this medication (I.V.) among its list of drugs which have a heightened risk of causing significant patient harm when used in error.

Contraindications Hypersensitivity to tenecteplase or any component of the formulation; active internal bleeding; history of stroke; intracranial/intraspinal surgery or trauma within 2 months; intracranial neoplasm; arteriovenous malformation or aneurysm; bleeding diathesis; severe uncontrolled hypertension

Warnings/Precautions Stop antiplatelet agents and heparin if serious bleeding occurs. Avoid I.M. injections and nonessential handling of the patient for a few hours after administration. Monitor for bleeding complications. Venipunctures should be performed carefully and only when necessary. If arterial puncture is necessary, then use an upper extremity that can be easily compressed manually. For the following conditions, the risk of bleeding is higher with use of tenecteplase and should be weighed against the benefits: Recent major surgery, cerebrovascular disease, recent GI or GU bleed, recent trauma, uncontrolled hypertension (systolic BP ≥180 mm Hg and/or diastolic BP ≥110 mm Hg), suspected left heart thrombus, acute pericarditis, subacute bacterial endocarditis, hemostatic defects, severe hepatic dysfunction, pregnancy, hemorrhagic diabetic retinopathy or other hemorrhagic ophthalmic conditions, septic thrombophlebitis or occluded arteriovenous cannula at seriously infected site, advanced age (see Usual Dosing, Elderly), anticoagulants, recent administration of GP IIb/IIIa inhibitors. Coronary thrombolysis may result in reperfusion arrhythmias. Caution with readministration of tenecteplase. Safety and efficacy have not been established in pediatric patients. Cholesterol embolism has rarely been reported.

Adverse Reactions As with all drugs which may affect hemostasis, bleeding is the major adverse effect associated with tenecteplase. Hemorrhage may occur at virtually any site. Risk is dependent on multiple variables, including the dosage administered, concurrent use of multiple agents which alter hemostasis, and patient predisposition. Rapid lysis of coronary artery thrombi by thrombolytic agents may be associated with reperfusion-related arterial and/or ventricular arrhythmia.

>10%:
- Local: Hematoma (12% minor)
- Hematologic: Bleeding (22% minor: ASSENT-2 trial)

1% to 10%:
- Central nervous system: Stroke (2%)
- Gastrointestinal: GI hemorrhage (1% major, 2% minor), epistaxis (2% minor)
- Genitourinary: GU bleeding (4% minor)
- Hematologic: Bleeding (5% major; ASSENT-2 trial)
- Local: Bleeding at catheter puncture site (4% minor), hematoma (2% major)
- Respiratory: Pharyngeal (3% minor)

The incidence of stroke and bleeding increase with age above 65 years.

<1% (Limited to important or life-threatening): Anaphylaxis, angioedema, bleeding at catheter puncture site (<1% major), cholesterol embolism (clinical features may include livedo reticularis, "purple toe" syndrome, acute renal failure, gangrenous digits, hypertension, pancreatitis, MI, cerebral infarction, spinal cord infarction, retinal artery occlusion, bowel infarction, rhabdomyolysis), GU bleeding (<1% major), intracranial hemorrhage (0.9%), laryngeal edema, rash, respiratory tract bleeding, retroperitoneal bleeding, urticaria

Additional cardiovascular events associated with use in MI: Arrhythmias, AV block, cardiac arrest, cardiac tamponade, cardiogenic shock, electromechanical dissociation, embolism, fever, heart failure, hypotension, mitral regurgitation, myocardial reinfarction, myocardial rupture, nausea, pericardial effusion, pericarditis, pulmonary edema, recurrent myocardial ischemia, thrombosis, vomiting

Drug Interactions

Avoid Concomitant Use There are no known interactions where it is recommended to avoid concomitant use.

Increased Effect/Toxicity

Tenecteplase may increase the levels/effects of: Anticoagulants; Drotrecogin Alfa

The levels/effects of Tenecteplase may be increased by: Antiplatelet Agents; Herbs (Anticoagulant/Antiplatelet Properties); Nonsteroidal Anti-Inflammatory Agents; Salicylates

Decreased Effect

The levels/effects of Tenecteplase may be decreased by: Aprotinin

Stability Store at room temperature not to exceed 30°C (86°F) or under refrigeration 2°C to 8°C (36°F to 46°F). Tenecteplase should be reconstituted using the supplied 10 mL syringe with TwinPak™ Dual Cannula Device and 10 mL sterile water for injection. If reconstituted and not used immediately, store in refrigerator and use within 8 hours.

Mechanism of Action Initiates fibrinolysis by binding to fibrin and converting plasminogen to plasmin.

Pharmacodynamics/Kinetics

Distribution: V_d is weight related and approximates plasma volume

Metabolism: Primarily hepatic

Half-life elimination: 90-130 minutes

Excretion: Clearance: Plasma: 99-119 mL/minute

Dosage I.V.:

Adult: Recommended total dose should not exceed 50 mg and is based on patient's weight; administer as a bolus over 5 seconds

If patient's weight:
- <60 kg, dose: 30 mg
- ≥60 to <70 kg, dose: 35 mg
- ≥70 to <80 kg, dose: 40 mg
- ≥80 to <90 kg, dose: 45 mg
- ≥90 kg, dose: 50 mg

Note: All patients should receive 162-325 mg of chewable nonenteric coated aspirin as soon as possible and then daily. Administer concurrently with heparin 60 units/kg bolus (maximum: 4000 units) followed by continuous infusion of 12 units/kg/hour (maximum: 1000 units/hour) and adjust to aPTT target of 50-70 seconds (or 1.5-2 times the upper limit of control).

Elderly: Although dosage adjustments are not recommended, the elderly have a higher incidence of morbidity and mortality with the use of tenecteplase. The 30-day mortality in the ASSENT-2 trial was 2.5% for patients <65 years, 8.5% for patients 65-74 years, and 16.2% for patients ≥75 years. The intracranial hemorrhage rate was 0.4% for patients <65, 1.6 % for patients 65-74 years, and 1.7 % for patients ≥75 years. The risks and benefits of use should be weighted carefully in the elderly.

Combination regimen (unlabeled): Half-dose tenecteplase (15-25 mg based on weight) and abciximab 0.25 mg/kg bolus then 0.125 mcg/kg/minute (maximum: 10 mcg/minute) for 12 hours with heparin dosing as follows: Concurrent bolus of 40 units/kg (maximum: 3000 units), then 7 units/kg/hour (maximum: 800 units/hour) as continuous infusion. Adjust to aPTT target of 50-70 seconds.

Note: The 2004 ACC/AHA guidelines for the management of patients with STEMI suggests that abciximab and half-dose reteplase or tenecteplase may be considered for prevention of reinfarction in patients with anterior MI, who are <75 years of age and have no risk factors for bleeding. However, more recently the American College of Chest Physicians recommends against the combination of half-dose reteplase or tenecteplase and standard-dose abciximab (with low dose unfractionated heparin) in any patient with STEMI due to the lack of mortality benefit and the risk of major bleeding (Goodman, 2008).

Dosage adjustment in renal impairment: No formal recommendations for renal impairment

Dosage adjustment in hepatic impairment: Severe hepatic failure is a relative contraindication. Recommendations were not made for mild to moderate hepatic impairment.

Administration Tenecteplase should be reconstituted using the supplied 10 mL syringe with TwinPak™ dual cannula device and 10 mL sterile water for injection. Do not shake when reconstituting. Slight foaming is normal and will dissipate if left standing for several minutes. The reconstituted solution is 5 mg/mL. Any unused solution should be discarded. Tenecteplase is **incompatible** with dextrose solutions. Dextrose-containing lines must be flushed with a saline solution before and after administration. Administer as a single I.V. bolus over 5 seconds. Avoid I.M. injections and nonessential handling of patient.

Monitoring Parameters CBC, aPTT, signs and symptoms of bleeding, ECG monitoring

Dosage Forms Excipient information presented when available (limited, particularly for generics); consult specific product labeling.

Injection, powder for reconstitution [recombinant]:

TNKase®: 50 mg

◆ **Tenex®** *see* GuanFACINE *on page 717*

Teniposide (ten i POE side)

U.S. Brand Names Vumon®

Canadian Brand Names Vumon®

Index Terms EPT; VM-26

Pharmacologic Category Antineoplastic Agent, Miscellaneous

Use Treatment of acute lymphocytic leukemia, small cell lung cancer

Pregnancy Risk Factor D

Medication Safety Issues

Sound-alike/look-alike issues:

Teniposide may be confused with etoposide

High alert medication: The Institute for Safe Medication Practices (ISMP) includes this medication among its list of drugs which have a heightened risk of causing significant patient harm when used in error.

Dosage I.V.:

Children: 130 mg/m^2/week, increasing to 150 mg/m^2 after 3 weeks and up to 180 mg/m^2 after 6 weeks

Acute lymphoblastic leukemia (ALL): 165 mg/m^2 twice weekly for 8-9 doses **or** 250 mg/m^2 weekly for 4-8 weeks

Adults: 50-180 mg/m^2 once or twice weekly for 4-6 weeks or 20-60 mg/m^2/day for 5 days

Small cell lung cancer: 80-90 mg/m^2/day for 5 days every 4-6 weeks

Dosage adjustment in renal/hepatic impairment: Data is insufficient, but dose adjustments may be necessary in patient with significant renal or hepatic impairment

Dosage adjustment in Down syndrome patients: Reduce initial dosing; administer the first course at half the usual dose. Patients with both Down syndrome and leukemia may be especially sensitive to myelosuppressive chemotherapy.

Additional Information Complete prescribing information for this medication should be consulted for additional detail.

Dosage Forms Excipient information presented when available (limited, particularly for generics); consult specific product labeling.

Injection, solution: 10 mg/mL (5 mL) [contains benzyl alcohol, dehydrated ethanol 42.7%, and polyoxyethylated castor oil]

Tenofovir (te NOE fo veer)

U.S. Brand Names Viread®

Canadian Brand Names Viread®

Index Terms PMPA; TDF; Tenofovir Disoproxil Fumarate

Pharmacologic Category Antiretroviral Agent, Reverse Transcriptase Inhibitor (Nucleotide)

Additional Appendix Information

Antiretroviral Therapy for HIV Infection: Adults and Adolescents *on page 1758*

Management of Healthcare Worker Exposures to HBV, HCV, and HIV *on page 1719*

Perinatal HIV Guidelines *on page 1730*

Use Management of HIV infections in combination with at least two other antiretroviral agents; treatment of chronic hepatitis B virus (HBV)

Pregnancy Risk Factor B

Pregnancy Considerations Animal studies have shown decreased fetal growth and reduced fetal bone porosity. Clinical studies in children have shown bone demineralization with chronic use. Tenofovir crosses the human placenta; limited data indicate decreased maternal bioavailability during the 3rd trimester. Due to the potential for bone effects, use in pregnancy only if clearly needed. Cases of lactic acidosis/hepatic steatosis syndrome have been reported in pregnant women receiving nucleoside analogues. It is not known if pregnancy itself potentiates this known side effect; however, pregnant women may be at increased risk of lactic acidosis and liver damage. Hepatic enzymes and electrolytes should be monitored frequently during the 3rd trimester of pregnancy in women receiving nucleoside analogues. Health professionals are encouraged to contact the Antiretroviral Pregnancy Registry to monitor outcomes of pregnant women exposed to antiretroviral medications (1-800-258-4263 or www.APRegistry.com).

Lactation Excretion in breast milk unknown/contraindicated

Contraindications There are no contraindications listed within the FDA-approved labeling.

Warnings/Precautions [U.S Boxed Warning]: Lactic acidosis and severe hepatomegaly with steatosis have been reported with tenofovir and other nucleoside analogues, including fatal cases; use with caution in patients with risk factors for liver disease (risk may be increased in obese patients or prolonged exposure) and suspend treatment in any patient who develops clinical or laboratory findings suggestive of lactic acidosis (transaminase elevation may/may not accompany hepatomegaly and steatosis). May cause redistribution of fat (eg, buffalo hump, peripheral wasting with increased abdominal girth, cushingoid appearance). Immune reconstitution syndrome may develop resulting in the occurrence of an inflammatory response to an indolent or residual opportunistic infection; further evaluation and treatment may be required. Use caution in hepatic impairment; no dosage adjustment is required; limited studies indicate the pharmacokinetics of tenofovir are not altered in hepatic dysfunction.

May cause osteomalacia; increased biochemical markers of bone metabolism, serum parathyroid hormone levels, and 1,25 vitamin D levels have been noted with tenofovir use. A 5% to 7% loss of bone mineral density (BMD) has been reported in some patients. BMD monitoring should be considered in patients with a history of bone fracture or risk factors for osteopenia.

Use caution in renal impairment. Calculate creatinine clearance prior to initiation of therapy and monitor renal function (including recalculation of creatinine clearance and serum phosphorus) during therapy. Dosage adjustment required in patients with Cl_{cr} <50 mL/minute. May cause acute renal failure or Fanconi syndrome; use caution with other nephrotoxic agents (especially those which compete for active tubular secretion), patients with low body weight, or concurrent medications which increase tenofovir levels. Use caution in the elderly: dosage adjustment based on renal function may be required.

[U.S. Boxed Warning]: If treating HBV, acute exacerbation of hepatitis B may occur upon discontinuation. Monitor liver function closely for several months after discontinuing treatment; reinitiation of antihepatitis B therapy may be required. Treatment of HBV in patients with unrecognized/untreated HIV may lead to HIV resistance; patients should be tested for presence of HIV infection prior to initiating therapy. Do not use as monotherapy in treatment of HIV. Treatment of HIV in patients with unrecognized/untreated HBV may lead to rapid HBV resistance. Patients should be tested for presence of chronic hepatitis B prior to initiation of therapy. Use with caution in patients taking strong CYP3A4 inhibitors, moderate or strong CYP3A4 inducers and major CYP3A4 substrates (see Drug Interactions); consider alternative agents that avoid or lessen the potential for CYP-mediated interactions. Do not use concurrently with adefovir or tenofovir combination products. Safety and efficacy have not been established in pediatric patients.

Adverse Reactions Percentages listed were from clinical trials with tenofovir addition to prior antiretroviral therapy. Only adverse events from treatment naïve patient studies which varied significantly were noted (eg, rash event). Frequencies listed are treatment-emergent adverse effects noted at higher frequency than in the placebo group. Patients treated for chronic hepatitis B had similar reactions and frequencies.

>10%:

Cardiovascular: Chest pain (3%)

Central nervous system: Pain (7% to 12%)

Gastrointestinal: Diarrhea (9% to 16%), nausea (8% to 11%)

Neuromuscular & skeletal: Weakness (7% to 11%)

1% to 10%:

Central nervous system: Depression (4% to 9%; treatment naïve 11%), fatigue (9%), headache (5% to 8%; treatment naïve 14%), fever (2% to 4%; treatment naïve 8%), dizziness (1% to 8%), anxiety (treatment naïve 6%), insomnia (3% to 5%)

Dermatologic: Rash event (maculopapular, pustular, or vesiculobullous rash, pruritus or urticaria 5% to 7%; treatment naïve 18%)

Endocrine & metabolic: Triglycerides increased (grades 3/4: 4% to 11%), hyperglycemia (grades 3/4: 2%)

Gastrointestinal: Vomiting (4% to 7%), abdominal pain (4% to 7%), serum amylase increased (grades 3/4: 4%; treatment naïve 9%), dyspepsia (3% to 4%), flatulence (3% to 4%), anorexia (3% to 4%), weight loss (2% to 4%)

Genitourinary: Hematuria (grades 3/4: 7%)

Hematologic: Neutropenia (1% to 2%; grade 3/4: 3%)

Hepatic: Transaminases increased (2% to 10%), alkaline phosphatase increased (grades 3/4: 1%)

Neuromuscular & skeletal: Creatine kinase (grade 3/4: 7% to 12%), back pain (3% to 4%; treatment naïve 9%), neuropathy (peripheral 3% to 5%), myalgia (3% to 4%)

Renal: Glycosuria (≤3%)

Respiratory: Respiratory tract infection (upper; 8%), sinusitis (8%), pharyngitis (5%), pneumonia (2% to 3%; treatment naïve 5%)

Miscellaneous: Diaphoresis (3%)

Postmarketing and/or case reports: Acute tubular necrosis, allergic reaction, bone mineral density decreased, dyspnea, Fanconi syndrome, hepatic steatosis, hepatitis, hypokalemia, hypophosphatemia, immune reconstitution syndrome, interstitial nephritis, lactic acidosis, muscle weakness, nephrogenic diabetes insipidus, nephrotoxicity, osteomalacia, pancreatitis, proteinuria, proximal renal tubulopathy, renal failure, renal myopathy, rhabdomyolysis, serum creatinine increased

Drug Interactions

Metabolism/Transport Effects Inhibits CYP1A2 (weak)

Avoid Concomitant Use There are no known interactions where it is recommended to avoid concomitant use.

Increased Effect/Toxicity

Tenofovir may increase the levels/effects of: Adefovir; Didanosine

The levels/effects of Tenofovir may be increased by: Acyclovir-Valacyclovir; Atazanavir; Ganciclovir-Valganciclovir; Lopinavir; Protease Inhibitors

Decreased Effect

Tenofovir may decrease the levels/effects of: Atazanavir; Didanosine; Protease Inhibitors

The levels/effects of Tenofovir may be decreased by: Adefovir

Ethanol/Nutrition/Herb Interactions Food: Fatty meals may increase the bioavailability of tenofovir. Tenofovir may be taken with or without food.

Stability Store at 25°C (77°F); excursions permitted to 15°C to 30°C (59°F to 86°F).

Mechanism of Action Tenofovir disoproxil fumarate (TDF) is an analog of adenosine 5'-monophosphate; it interferes with the HIV viral RNA dependent DNA polymerase resulting in inhibition of viral replication. TDF is first converted intracellularly by hydrolysis to tenofovir and subsequently phosphorylated to the active tenofovir diphosphate; nucleotide reverse transcriptase inhibitor. Tenofovir inhibits replication of HBV by inhibiting HBV polymerase.

Pharmacodynamics/Kinetics

Distribution: 1.2-1.3 L/kg

Protein binding: ≤7% to serum proteins

Metabolism: Tenofovir disoproxil fumarate (TDF) is converted intracellularly by hydrolysis (by non-CYP enzymes) to tenofovir, then phosphorylated to the active tenofovir diphosphate

Bioavailability: ~25% (fasting); increases ~40% with high-fat meal

Half-life elimination: ~17 hours

Time to peak, serum: Fasting: 36-84 minutes; With food: 96-144 minutes

Excretion: Urine (70% to 80%) via filtration and active secretion, primarily as unchanged tenofovir

Dosage Oral: Adults: HIV infection, hepatitis B infection: 300 mg once daily

Note: Concurrent use with adefovir and/or tenofovir combination products should be avoided.

Dosage adjustment in renal impairment:

Cl_{cr} ≥50 mL/minute: No adjustment necessary

Cl_{cr} 30-49 mL/minute: 300 mg every 48 hours

Cl_{cr} 10-29 mL/minute: 300 mg every 72-96 hours

Cl_{cr} <10 mL/minute without hemodialysis: No recommendation available.

Hemodialysis: 300 mg every 7 days or after a total of ~12 hours of dialysis (usually once weekly assuming 3 dialysis sessions lasting about 4 hours each)

Dosage adjustment in hepatic impairment: No dosage adjustment required.

Dietary Considerations May be taken with or without food. Consider calcium and vitamin D supplementation in patients with history of bone fracture or osteopenia.

Administration May be administered with or without food.

Monitoring Parameters

Patients with HIV: CBC with differential, reticulocyte count, serum creatine kinase, CD4 count, HIV RNA plasma levels, renal and hepatic function tests, bone density (long-term), serum phosphorus; testing for HBV is recommended prior to the initiation of antiretroviral therapy

Patients with HBV: HIV status (prior to initiation of therapy); bone density (long-term), serum phosphorus; serum creatinine (prior to initiation and during therapy; every 3 months in patients with medical conditions which predispose to renal insufficiency and in all patients treated for >1 year; more frequent monitoring required if preexisting renal insufficiency detected [Lok, 2007]); viral load; LFTs for several months following discontinuation of tenofovir.

Patients with HIV and HBV coinfection should be monitored for several months following tenofovir discontinuation.

Additional Information Approval was based on two clinical trials involving patients who were previously treated with antiretrovirals with continued evidence of HIV replication despite therapy. The risk:benefit ratio for untreated patients has not been established (studies currently ongoing), however, patients who received tenofovir showed significant decreases in HIV replication as compared to continuation of standard therapy.

A high rate of early virologic nonresponse was observed when abacavir, lamivudine, and tenofovir were used as the initial regimen in treatment-naive patients. A high rate of early virologic nonresponse was also observed when didanosine, lamivudine, and tenofovir were used as the initial regimen in treatment-naive patients. Use of either of these combinations is not recommended; patients currently on either of these regimens should be closely monitored for modification of therapy. Early virologic failure was also observed with tenofovir and didanosine delayed release capsules, plus either efavirenz or nevirapine; use caution in treatment-naive patients with high baseline viral loads.

Dosage Forms Excipient information presented when available (limited, particularly for generics); consult specific product labeling.

Tablet, as disoproxil fumarate:

Viread®: 300 mg [equivalent to 245 mg tenofovir disoproxil]

◆ **Tenofovir and Emtricitabine** *see* Emtricitabine and Tenofovir *on page 515*

◆ **Tenofovir Disoproxil Fumarate** *see* Tenofovir *on page 1438*

◆ **Tenofovir Disoproxil Fumarate, Efavirenz, and Emtricitabine** *see* Efavirenz, Emtricitabine, and Tenofovir *on page 509*

◆ **Tenolin (Can)** *see* Atenolol *on page 149*

◆ **Tenoretic®** *see* Atenolol and Chlorthalidone *on page 150*

◆ **Tenormin®** *see* Atenolol *on page 149*

◆ **Tensilon® (Can)** *see* Edrophonium *on page 505*

◆ **Tenuate® (Can)** *see* Diethylpropion *on page 443*

◆ **Tenuate® Dospan® (Can)** *see* Diethylpropion *on page 443*

◆ **Terazol® (Can)** *see* Terconazole *on page 1443*

◆ **Terazol® 3** *see* Terconazole *on page 1443*

◆ **Terazol® 7** *see* Terconazole *on page 1443*

Terazosin (ter AY zoe sin)

Canadian Brand Names Alti-Terazosin; Apo-Terazosin®; Hytrin®; Novo-Terazosin; Nu-Terazosin; PMS-Terazosin

Pharmacologic Category Alpha$_1$ Blocker

Use Management of mild to moderate hypertension; alone or in combination with other agents such as diuretics or beta-blockers; benign prostate hyperplasia (BPH)

Unlabeled/Investigational Use Pediatric hypertension

Pregnancy Risk Factor C

Lactation Excretion in breast milk unknown

Contraindications Hypersensitivity to quinazolines (doxazosin, prazosin, terazosin) or any component of the formulation; concurrent use with phosphodiesterase-5 (PDE-5) inhibitors including sildenafil (>25 mg), tadalafil, or vardenafil

Warnings/Precautions Can cause significant orthostatic hypotension and syncope, especially with first dose; anticipate a similar effect if therapy is interrupted for a few days, if dosage is rapidly increased, or if another antihypertensive drug (particularly vasodilators) or a PDE-5 inhibitor is introduced. Discontinue if symptoms of angina occur or worsen. Patients should be cautioned about performing hazardous tasks when starting new therapy or adjusting dosage upward. Prostate cancer should be ruled out before starting for BPH. Use with caution in hepatic impairment. Intraoperative floppy iris syndrome has been observed in cataract surgery patients who were on or were previously treated with alpha$_1$-blockers. Causality has not been established and there appears to be no benefit in discontinuing alpha-blocker therapy prior to surgery. Safety and efficacy in children have not been established.

Adverse Reactions Asthenia, postural hypotension, dizziness, somnolence, nasal congestion/rhinitis, and impotence were the only events noted in clinical trials to occur at a frequency significantly greater than placebo ($p < 0.05$).

>10%:

- Central nervous system: Dizziness, headache
- Neuromuscular & skeletal: Muscle weakness

1% to 10%:

- Cardiovascular: Edema, palpitation, chest pain, peripheral edema (3%), orthostatic hypotension (3% to 4%), tachycardia
- Central nervous system: Fatigue, nervousness, drowsiness
- Gastrointestinal: Dry mouth
- Genitourinary: Urinary incontinence
- Ocular: Blurred vision
- Respiratory: Dyspnea, nasal congestion

<1% (Limited to important or life-threatening): Allergic reactions, anaphylaxis, atrial fibrillation, priapism, sexual dysfunction, syncope (0.8%), thrombocytopenia

Drug Interactions

Avoid Concomitant Use

Avoid concomitant use of Terazosin with any of the following: Alfuzosin; Silodosin; Tamsulosin

Increased Effect/Toxicity

Terazosin may increase the levels/effects of: Alfuzosin; Amifostine; Calcium Channel Blockers; RiTUXimab; Silodosin; Tamsulosin

The levels/effects of Terazosin may be increased by: Alfuzosin; Beta-Blockers; Diazoxide; Herbs (Hypotensive Properties); Phosphodiesterase 5 Inhibitors; Prostacyclin Analogues; Silodosin; Tamsulosin

Decreased Effect

The levels/effects of Terazosin may be decreased by: Herbs (Hypertensive Properties); Methylphenidate; Yohimbine

Ethanol/Nutrition/Herb Interactions Herb/Nutraceutical: Avoid dong quai if using for hypertension (has estrogenic activity). Avoid ephedra, yohimbe, ginseng (may worsen hypertension). Avoid saw palmetto. Avoid garlic (may have increased antihypertensive effect).

Mechanism of Action Alpha$_1$-specific blocking agent with minimal alpha$_2$ effects; this allows peripheral postsynaptic blockade, with the resultant decrease in arterial tone, while preserving the negative feedback loop which is mediated by the peripheral presynaptic alpha$_2$-receptors; terazosin relaxes the smooth muscle of the bladder neck, thus reducing bladder outlet obstruction

Pharmacodynamics/Kinetics

- Onset of action: 1-2 hours
- Absorption: Rapid
- Protein binding: 90% to 95%
- Metabolism: Extensively hepatic
- Half-life elimination: 9.2-12 hours
- Time to peak, serum: ~1 hour
- Excretion: Feces (60%); urine (40%)

Dosage Oral:

Hypertension:

Children (unlabeled use): Initial: 1 mg once daily; gradually increase dose as necessary, up to maximum of 20 mg/day

Adults: Initial: 1 mg at bedtime; slowly increase dose to achieve desired blood pressure, up to 20 mg/day; usual dose range (JNC 7): 1-20 mg once daily

Dosage reduction may be needed when adding a diuretic or other antihypertensive agent; if drug is discontinued for greater than several days, consider beginning with initial dose and retitrate as needed; dosage may be given on a twice daily regimen if response is diminished at 24 hours and hypotensive is observed at 2-4 hours following a dose

Benign prostatic hyperplasia: Adults: Initial: 1 mg at bedtime, increasing as needed; most patients require 10 mg day; if no response after 4-6 weeks of 10 mg/day, may increase to 20 mg/day

Dietary Considerations May be taken without regard to meals at the same time each day.

Monitoring Parameters Standing and sitting/supine blood pressure, especially following the initial dose at 2-4 hours following the dose and thereafter at the trough point to ensure adequate control throughout the dosing interval; urinary symptoms

Dosage Forms Excipient information presented when available (limited, particularly for generics); consult specific product labeling.

Capsule: 1 mg, 2 mg, 5 mg, 10 mg

Terbinafine (TER bin a feen)

U.S. Brand Names Lamisil AT® [OTC]; Lamisil®

Canadian Brand Names Apo-Terbinafine®; CO Terbinafine; Gen-Terbinafine; Lamisil®; Novo-Terbinafine; PHL-Terbinafine; PMS-Terbinafine; RIVA-Terbinafine; SANDOZ-Terbinafine; Terbinafine-250

Index Terms Terbinafine Hydrochloride

Pharmacologic Category Antifungal Agent, Oral; Antifungal Agent, Topical

Use Active against most strains of *Trichophyton mentagrophytes*, *Trichophyton rubrum*; may be effective for infections of *Microsporum gypseum* and *M. nanum*, *Trichophyton verrucosum*, *Epidermophyton floccosum*, *Candida albicans*, and *Scopulariopsis brevicaulis*

Oral: Onychomycosis of the toenail or fingernail due to susceptible dermatophytes; treatment of tinea capitis

Topical: Antifungal for the treatment of tinea pedis (athlete's foot), tinea cruris (jock itch), and tinea corporis (ringworm) [OTC/prescription formulations]; tinea versicolor [prescription formulations]

Pregnancy Risk Factor B

Pregnancy Considerations Adverse events were not observed in animal studies. There are no adequate and well-controlled studies in pregnant women. Avoid use in pregnancy since treatment of onychomycosis is postponable.

Lactation Enters breast milk/not recommended

Medication Safety Issues

Sound-alike/look-alike issues:

Terbinafine may be confused with terbutaline

Lamisil® may be confused with Lamictal®, Lomotil®

International issues:

Lamisil® may be confused with Lemesil® which is a brand name for nimesulide in Greece and Romania

Contraindications History of or allergic reaction to oral terbinafine

Warnings/Precautions While rare, the following complications have been reported with oral use and may require discontinuation of therapy: Changes in the ocular lens and retina, pancytopenia, neutropenia, Stevens-Johnson syndrome, toxic epidermal necrolysis. Precipitation or exacerbation of cutaneous or systemic lupus erythematosus has been observed; discontinue if signs and/or symptoms develop. Rare cases of hepatic failure, including fatal cases, have been reported following oral treatment of onychomycosis. Not recommended for use in patients with active or chronic liver disease. Discontinue if symptoms or signs of hepatobiliary dysfunction or cholestatic hepatitis develop. If irritation/sensitivity develops with topical use, discontinue therapy. Oral products are not recommended for use with pre-existing liver or renal disease (Cl_{cr} ≤50 mL/minute). Use caution in patients sensitive to allylamine antifungals (eg, naftifine, butenafine); cross sensitivity to terbinafine may exist.

Adverse Reactions

Oral: Adverse events listed for tablets unless otherwise specified. Oral granules were studied in patients 4-12 years of age.

>10%: Central nervous system: Headache (13%; granules 7%)

1% to 10%:

Central nervous system: Fever (granules 7%)

Dermatologic: Rash (6%; granules 2%), pruritus (3%; granules 1%), urticaria (1%)

Gastrointestinal: Diarrhea (6%; granules 3%), vomiting (granules 5%), dyspepsia (4%), nausea (3%; granules 2%), taste disturbance (3%), abdominal pain (2%; granules 2% to 4%), toothache (granules 1%)

Hepatic: Liver enzyme abnormalities (3%)

Respiratory: Nasopharyngitis (granules 10%), cough (granules 6%), nasal congestion (granules 2%), pharyngeal pain (granules 2%), rhinorrhea (granules 2%)

<1%, postmarketing, and/or case reports: Acute pancreatitis, anemia, angioedema, agranulocytosis, allergic reactions, alopecia, anaphylaxis, appetite decreased, arthralgia, dizziness, fatigue, generalized exanthematous pustulosis (acute), hepatic failure, malaise, myalgia, neutropenia (severe), ocular lens and retina changes, precipitation/exacerbation of cutaneous and systemic lupus erythematosus, pancytopenia, psoriasiform eruption, psoriasis exacerbation, rhabdomyolysis, Stevens-Johnson syndrome, thrombocytopenia, toxic epidermal necrolysis, visual field acuity decreased, visual field defects, vomiting

Topical: 1% to 10%:

Dermatologic: Burning, contact dermatitis, dryness, exfoliation, irritation, pruritus, rash

Local: Irritation, stinging

Drug Interactions

Metabolism/Transport Effects Substrate (minor) of 1A2, 2C9, 2C19, 3A4; **Inhibits** CYP2D6 (strong); **Induces** CYP3A4 (weak)

Avoid Concomitant Use

Avoid concomitant use of Terbinafine with any of the following: Tamoxifen; Thioridazine

Increased Effect/Toxicity

Terbinafine may increase the levels/effects of: CYP2D6 Substrates; Fesoterodine; Nebivolol; Tamoxifen; Tetrabenazine; Thioridazine; Tricyclic Antidepressants

Decreased Effect

Terbinafine may decrease the levels/effects of: Codeine; CycloSPORINE; Maraviroc; *Saccharomyces boulardii;* TraMADol

The levels/effects of Terbinafine may be decreased by: Rifamycin Derivatives

Stability

Cream: Store at 5°C to 30°C (41°F to 86°F).

Granules: Store at controlled room temperature if 15°C to 30°C (59°F to 86°F).

Solution: Store at 5°C to 25°C (41°F to 77°F); do not refrigerate.

Tablet: Store below 25°C (77°F). Protect from light.

Mechanism of Action Synthetic allylamine derivative which inhibits squalene epoxidase, a key enzyme in sterol biosynthesis in fungi. This results in a deficiency in ergosterol within the fungal cell wall and results in fungal cell death.

Pharmacodynamics/Kinetics

Absorption: Topical: Limited (<5%); Oral: >70% (children and adults)

Distribution: V_d: 1000 L; distributed to sebum and skin predominantly

Protein binding: Plasma: >99% (children and adults)

Metabolism: Hepatic; no active metabolites; first-pass effect; little effect on CYP

Bioavailability: Oral: 40% (children 36% to 64%)

Half-life elimination:

Topical: 14-35 hours

Oral: Terminal half-life: 200-400 hours; very slow release of drug from skin and adipose tissues occurs; effective half-life: ~36 hours (children 27-31 hours)

Time to peak, plasma: 1-2 hours (children and adults)

Excretion: Urine (70% to 75%; children 70%)

Dosage

Oral:

Granules: Tinea capitis: Children ≥4 years:

<25 kg: 125 mg once daily for 6 weeks

25-35 kg: 187.5 mg once daily for 6 weeks

>35 kg: 250 mg once daily for 6 weeks

Tablet: Onychomycosis:

Children (unlabeled use):

10-20 kg: 62.5 mg once daily for 6 weeks (fingernails) **or** 12 weeks (toenails)

20-40 kg: 125 mg once daily for 6 weeks (fingernails) **or** 12 weeks (toenails)

>40 kg: 250 mg once daily for 6 weeks (fingernails) **or** 12 weeks (toenails)

Adults:

Superficial mycoses: Fingernail: 250 mg/day for up to 6 weeks; toenail: 250 mg/day for 12 weeks; doses may be given in 2 divided doses

Systemic mycosis (unlabeled use): 250-500 mg/day for up to 16 months

Topical:

Cream, gel, solution: Children ≥12 years and Adults:

Athlete's foot (tinea pedis): Apply to affected area twice daily for at least 1 week, not to exceed 4 weeks [OTC/prescription formulations]

Ringworm (tinea corporis) and jock itch (tinea cruris): Apply cream to affected area once or twice daily for at least 1 week, not to exceed 4 weeks; apply gel or solution once daily for 7 days [OTC formulations]

Cream, solution: Adults: Tinea versicolor: Apply to affected area twice daily for 1 week [prescription formulation]

Dosing adjustment in renal impairment: Cl_{cr} <50 mL/minute: Clearance decreased by ~50%; oral administration is not recommended

Dosing adjustment in hepatic impairment: Clearance is decreased by ~50% with hepatic cirrhosis; oral administration is not recommended

Administration Tablets may be administered without regard to meals. Granules should be sprinkled on a spoonful of nonacidic food (eg, mashed potatoes); swallow granules without chewing.

Monitoring Parameters AST/ALT prior to initiation, repeat if used >6 weeks; CBC

Additional Information Due to potential toxicity, the manufacturer recommends confirmation of diagnosis testing of nail specimens prior to treatment of onychomycosis. Patients should not be considered therapeutic failures until they have been symptom-free for 2-4 weeks off following a course of treatment; GI complaints usually subside with continued administration.

A meta-analysis of efficacy studies for toenail infections revealed that weighted average mycological cure rates for continuous therapy were 36.7% (griseofulvin), 54.7% (itraconazole), and 77% (terbinafine). Cure rate for 4-month pulse therapy for itraconazole and terbinafine were 73.3% and 80%. Additionally, the final outcome measure of final costs per cured infections for continuous therapy was significantly lower for terbinafine.

Dosage Forms Excipient information presented when available (limited, particularly for generics); consult specific product labeling.

Cream, topical, as hydrochloride: 1% (12 g, 24 g)

Lamisil AT®: 1% (12 g, 15 g, 24 g, 30 g, 36 g) [contains benzyl alcohol]

Gel, topical:

Lamisil AT®: 1% (6 g, 12 g) [contains benzyl alcohol]

Granules, oral:

Lamisil® 125 mg/packet (42s); 187.5 mg/packet (42s)

Solution, topical, as hydrochloride [spray]:

Lamisil AT®: 1% (30 mL) [contains ethanol]

Tablet, oral: 250 mg

Lamisil®: 250 mg

◆ **Terbinafine-250 (Can)** *see* Terbinafine *on page 1441*

◆ **Terbinafine Hydrochloride** *see* Terbinafine *on page 1441*

Terbutaline (ter BYOO ta leen)

Canadian Brand Names Bricanyl®

Index Terms Brethaire [DSC]; Bricanyl [DSC]

Pharmacologic Category $Beta_2$-Adrenergic Agonist

Additional Appendix Information

Bronchodilators *on page 1650*

Use Bronchodilator in reversible airway obstruction and bronchial asthma

Unlabeled/Investigational Use Tocolytic agent (management of preterm labor)

Pregnancy Risk Factor B

Lactation Enters breast milk/compatible

Medication Safety Issues

Sound-alike/look-alike issues:

Terbutaline may be confused with terbinafine, TOLBUTamide

Contraindications Hypersensitivity to terbutaline or any component of the formulation; cardiac arrhythmias associated with tachycardia; tachycardia caused by digitalis intoxication

Warnings/Precautions When used for tocolysis, there is some risk of maternal pulmonary edema, which has been associated with the following risk factors, excessive hydration, multiple gestation, occult sepsis and underlying cardiac disease. To reduce risk, limit fluid intake to 2.5-3 L/day, limit sodium intake, maintain maternal pulse to <130 beats/minute.

Use caution in patients with cardiovascular disease (arrhythmia or hypertension or HF), convulsive disorders, diabetes, glaucoma, hyperthyroidism, or hypokalemia. Beta-agonists may cause elevation in blood pressure, heart rate, and result in CNS stimulation/excitation. $Beta_2$-agonists may increase risk of arrhythmia, increase serum glucose, or decrease serum potassium.

When used as a bronchodilator, optimize anti-inflammatory treatment before initiating maintenance treatment with terbutaline. Do not use as a component of chronic therapy without an anti-inflammatory agent. Only the mildest form of asthma (Step 1 and/or exercise-induced) would not require concurrent use based upon asthma guidelines. Patient must be instructed to seek medical attention in cases where acute symptoms are not relieved or a previous level of response is diminished. The need to increase frequency of use may indicate deterioration of asthma, and treatment must not be delayed.

Immediate hypersensitivity reactions (urticaria, angioedema, rash, bronchospasm) have been reported. Do not exceed recommended dose; serious adverse events including fatalities, have been associated with excessive use of inhaled sympathomimetics. Rarely, paradoxical bronchospasm may occur with use of inhaled bronchodilating agents; this should be distinguished from inadequate response.

Adverse Reactions

>10%:
- Central nervous system: Nervousness, restlessness
- Endocrine & metabolic: Serum glucose increased, serum potassium decreased
- Neuromuscular & skeletal: Trembling

1% to 10%:
- Cardiovascular: Tachycardia, hypertension, pounding heartbeat
- Central nervous system: Dizziness, lightheadedness, drowsiness, headache, insomnia
- Gastrointestinal: Dry mouth, nausea, vomiting, bad taste in mouth
- Neuromuscular & skeletal: Muscle cramps, weakness
- Miscellaneous: Diaphoresis

<1% (Limited to important or life-threatening): Arrhythmia, chest pain, hypokalemia, paradoxical bronchospasm

Drug Interactions

Avoid Concomitant Use

Avoid concomitant use of Terbutaline with any of the following: Iobenguane I 123

Increased Effect/Toxicity

Terbutaline may increase the levels/effects of: Sympathomimetics

The levels/effects of Terbutaline may be increased by: Atomoxetine; Cannabinoids; MAO Inhibitors; Tricyclic Antidepressants

Decreased Effect

Terbutaline may decrease the levels/effects of: Iobenguane I 123

The levels/effects of Terbutaline may be decreased by: Alpha-/Beta-Blockers; Beta-Blockers (Beta1 Selective); Beta-Blockers (Nonselective); Betahistine

Ethanol/Nutrition/Herb Interactions Herb/Nutraceutical: Avoid ephedra, yohimbe (may cause CNS stimulation).

Stability Store injection at room temperature; do not freeze. Protect from heat and light. Use only clear solutions. Store powder for inhalation (Bricanyl® Turbuhaler [CAN]) at room temperature between 15°C and 30°C (58°F and 86°F).

Mechanism of Action Relaxes bronchial smooth muscle by action on $beta_2$-receptors with less effect on heart rate

Pharmacodynamics/Kinetics

Onset of action: Oral: 30-45 minutes; SubQ: 6-15 minutes
Protein binding: 25%
Metabolism: Hepatic to inactive sulfate conjugates
Bioavailability: SubQ doses are more bioavailable than oral
Half-life elimination: 11-16 hours
Excretion: Urine

Dosage

Children <12 years: Bronchoconstriction:
- Oral: Initial: 0.05 mg/kg/dose 3 times/day, increased gradually as required; maximum: 0.15 mg/kg/dose 3-4 times/day or a total of 5 mg/24 hours
- SubQ: 0.005-0.01 mg/kg/dose to a maximum of 0.3 mg/dose; may repeat in 15-20 minutes

Children ≥6 years and Adults: Bronchospasm (acute): Inhalation (Bricanyl® [CAN] MDI: 500 mcg/puff, *not labeled for use in the U.S.*): One puff as needed; may repeat with 1 inhalation (after 5 minutes); more than 6 inhalations should not be necessary in any 24 hour period. **Note:** If a previously effective dosage regimen fails to provide the usual relief, or the effects of a dose last for >3 hours, medical advice should be sought immediately; this is a sign of seriously worsening asthma that requires reassessment of therapy.

Children >12 years and Adults: Bronchoconstriction:
- Oral:
  - 12-15 years: 2.5 mg every 6 hours 3 times/day; not to exceed 7.5 mg in 24 hours
  - >15 years: 5 mg/dose every 6 hours 3 times/day; if side effects occur, reduce dose to 2.5 mg every 6 hours; not to exceed 15 mg in 24 hours
- SubQ: 0.25 mg/dose; may repeat in 15-30 minutes (maximum: 0.5 mg/4-hour period)

Adults: Premature labor (tocolysis; unlabeled use):
- Acute: I.V. 2.5-10 mcg/minute; increased gradually every 10-20 minutes; effective maximum dosages from 17.5-30 mcg/minute have been used with caution. Duration of infusion is at least 12 hours.
- Maintenance: Oral: 2.5-10 mg every 4-6 hours for as long as necessary to prolong pregnancy depending on patient tolerance

Dosing adjustment/comments in renal impairment:
- Cl_{cr} 10-50 mL/minute: Administer at 50% of normal dose
- Cl_{cr} <10 mL/minute: Avoid use

Administration

I.V.: Use infusion pump.
Oral: Administer around-the-clock to promote less variation in peak and trough serum levels

Monitoring Parameters Serum potassium, glucose; heart rate, blood pressure, respiratory rate; monitor for signs and symptoms of pulmonary edema (when used as a tocolytic); monitor FEV_1, peak flow, and/or other pulmonary function tests (when used as bronchodilator)

Dosage Forms Excipient information presented when available (limited, particularly for generics); consult specific product labeling. [CAN] = Canadian brand name

Injection, solution, as sulfate: 1 mg/mL (1 mL)
Powder for oral inhalation:
- Bricanyl® Turbuhaler [CAN]: 500 mcg/actuation [50 or 200 metered actuations] [not available in U.S.]

Tablet, as sulfate: 2.5 mg, 5 mg

Extemporaneous Preparations A 1 mg/mL suspension made from terbutaline tablets in simple syrup NF is stable 30 days when refrigerated

Horner RK and Johnson CE, "Stability of An Extemporaneously Compounded Terbutaline Sulfate Oral Liquid," *Am J Hosp Pharm*, 1991, 48(2):293-5.

Terconazole (ter KONE a zole)

U.S. Brand Names Terazol® 3; Terazol® 7; Zazole™

Canadian Brand Names Terazol®

Index Terms Triaconazole

Pharmacologic Category Antifungal Agent, Vaginal

Additional Appendix Information

Treatment of Sexually Transmitted Infections *on page 1773*

Use Local treatment of vulvovaginal candidiasis

Pregnancy Risk Factor C

Lactation Excretion in breast milk unknown/not recommended

Medication Safety Issues

Sound-alike/look-alike issues:
- Terconazole may be confused with tioconazole

International issues:
- Terazol® may be confused with Theradol® which is a brand name for tramadol in the Netherlands

Contraindications Hypersensitivity to terconazole or any component of the formulation

Warnings/Precautions Should be discontinued if sensitization or irritation occurs. Microbiological studies (KOH smear and/or cultures) should be repeated in patients not responding to terconazole in order to confirm the diagnosis and rule out other pathogens. Petrolatum-based vaginal products may damage rubber or latex condoms or diaphragms; separate use by 3 days. Safety and efficacy have not been established in children.

Adverse Reactions

1% to 10%:

Central nervous system: Fever, chills

Gastrointestinal: Abdominal pain

Genitourinary: Vulvar/vaginal burning, dysmenorrhea

<1% (Limited to important or life-threatening): Burning or itching of penis of sexual partner, flu-like syndrome, polyuria; vulvar itching, soreness, edema, or discharge

Drug Interactions

Avoid Concomitant Use There are no known interactions where it is recommended to avoid concomitant use.

Increased Effect/Toxicity There are no known significant interactions involving an increase in effect.

Decreased Effect There are no known significant interactions involving a decrease in effect.

Stability Store at room temperature of 13°C to 30°C (59°F to 86°F).

Mechanism of Action Triazole ketal antifungal agent; involves inhibition of fungal cytochrome P450. Specifically, terconazole inhibits cytochrome P450-dependent 14-alpha-demethylase which results in accumulation of membrane disturbing 14-alpha-demethylsterols and ergosterol depletion.

Pharmacodynamics/Kinetics Absorption: Extent of systemic absorption after vaginal administration may be dependent on presence of a uterus; 5% to 8% in women who had a hysterectomy versus 12% to 16% in nonhysterectomy women

Dosage Adults: Female:

Terazol® 3, Zazole™ 0.8% vaginal cream: Insert 1 applicatorful intravaginally at bedtime for 3 consecutive days

Terazol® 7, Zazole™ 0.4% vaginal cream: Insert 1 applicatorful intravaginally at bedtime for 7 consecutive days

Terazol® 3 vaginal suppository: Insert 1 suppository intravaginally at bedtime for 3 consecutive days

Additional Information Watch for local irritation; assist patient in administration, if necessary; assess patient's ability to self-administer, may be difficult in patients with arthritis or limited range of motion

Dosage Forms Excipient information presented when available (limited, particularly for generics); consult specific product labeling.

Cream, vaginal: 0.4% (45 g); 0.8% (20 g)

Terazol® 7: 0.4% (45 g) [packaged with measured-dose applicator]

Terazol® 3: 0.8% (20 g) [packaged with measured-dose applicator]

Zazole™: 0.4% (45 g) [packaged with measured-dose applicator]; 0.8% (20 g) [packaged with measured-dose applicator]

Suppository, vaginal:

Terazol® 3: 80 mg (3s) [may contain coconut and/or palm kernel oil]

◆ **Terfluzine (Can)** *see* Trifluoperazine *on page 1516*

Teriparatide (ter i PAR a tide)

U.S. Brand Names Forteo®

Canadian Brand Names Forteo®

Index Terms Parathyroid Hormone (1-34); Recombinant Human Parathyroid Hormone (1-34); rhPTH(1-34)

Pharmacologic Category Parathyroid Hormone Analog

Use Treatment of osteoporosis in postmenopausal women at high risk of fracture; treatment of primary or hypogonadal osteoporosis in men at high risk of fracture

Restrictions An FDA-approved medication guide must be distributed when dispensing an outpatient prescription (new or refill) where this medication is to be used without direct supervision of a healthcare provider. Medication guides are available at http://www.fda.gov/cder/Offices/ODS/medication_guides.htm.

Pregnancy Risk Factor C

Pregnancy Considerations Adverse events were observed in animal studies; the effect on human fetal development has not been studied. Teriparatide is not indicated for use in pregnant or premenopausal women.

Lactation Excretion in breast milk unknown/not recommended

Contraindications Hypersensitivity to teriparatide or any component of the formulation

Warnings/Precautions [U.S. Boxed Warning]: In animal studies, teriparatide has been associated with an increase in osteosarcoma; risk was dependent on both dose and duration. Avoid use in patients with an increased risk of osteosarcoma (including Paget's disease, prior radiation, unexplained elevation of alkaline phosphatase, or in patients with open epiphyses). Do not use in patients with a history of skeletal metastases, hyperparathyroidism, or pre-existing hypercalcemia. Not for use in patients with metabolic bone disease other than osteoporosis. Use caution in patients with active or recent urolithiasis. Use caution in patients at risk of orthostasis (including concurrent antihypertensive therapy), or in patients who may not tolerate transient hypotension (cardiovascular or cerebrovascular disease). Use caution in patients with cardiac, renal or hepatic impairment (limited data available concerning safety and efficacy). Use of teriparatide for longer than 2 years is not recommended. Not approved for use in pediatric patients.

Adverse Reactions

>10%: Endocrine & metabolic: Hypercalcemia (transient increases noted 4-6 hours postdose [women 11%; men 6%])

1% to 10%:

Cardiovascular: Chest pain (3%), syncope (3%)

Central nervous system: Dizziness (8%), depression (4%), vertigo (4%)

Dermatologic: Rash (5%)

Endocrine & metabolic: Hyperuricemia (3%)

Gastrointestinal: Nausea (9%), dyspepsia (5%), vomiting (3%), tooth disorder (2%)

Neuromuscular & skeletal: Arthralgia (10%), weakness (9%), leg cramps (3%), muscle spasm

Respiratory: Rhinitis (10%), pharyngitis (6%), dyspnea (4%), pneumonia (4%)

Miscellaneous: Antibodies to teriparatide (3% of women in long-term treatment; hypersensitivity reactions or decreased efficacy were not associated in preclinical trials)

Postmarketing and/or case reports: Acute dyspnea, allergic reactions, edema (facial/oral), hypercalcemia >11 mg/dL; injection site reactions (bleeding, bruising, erythema, pain, pruritus, swelling); urticaria

Drug Interactions

Avoid Concomitant Use There are no known interactions where it is recommended to avoid concomitant use.

Increased Effect/Toxicity There are no known significant interactions involving an increase in effect.

Decreased Effect There are no known significant interactions involving a decrease in effect.

Ethanol/Nutrition/Herb Interactions

Ethanol: Excessive intake may increase risk of osteoporosis.

Herb/Nutraceutical: Ensure adequate calcium and vitamin D intake.

Stability Store at 2°C to 8°C (36°F to 46°F); do not freeze. Protect from light. Discard pen 28 days after first injection.

Do not use if solution is cloudy, colored or contains solid particles.

Mechanism of Action Teriparatide is a recombinant formulation of endogenous parathyroid hormone (PTH), containing a 34-amino-acid sequence which is identical to the N-terminal portion of this hormone. The pharmacologic activity of teriparatide is similar to the physiologic activity of PTH, stimulating osteoblast function, increasing gastrointestinal calcium absorption, increasing renal tubular reabsorption of calcium. Treatment with teriparatide increases bone mineral density, bone mass, and strength. In postmenopausal women, it has been shown to decrease osteoporosis-related fractures.

Pharmacodynamics/Kinetics

Distribution: V_d: 0.12 L/kg

Metabolism: Hepatic (nonspecific proteolysis)

Bioavailability: 95%

Half-life elimination: Serum: I.V.: 5 minutes; SubQ: 1 hour

Time to peak, serum: 30 minutes

Excretion: Urine (as metabolites)

Dosage SubQ: Adults: 20 mcg once daily; **Note:** Initial administration should occur under circumstances in which the patient may sit or lie down, in the event of orthostasis.

Dosage adjustment in renal impairment: No dosage adjustment required. Bioavailability and half-life increase with Cl_{cr} <30 mL/minute.

Administration Administer by subcutaneous injection into the thigh or abdominal wall. Initial administration should occur under circumstances in which the patient may sit or lie down, in the event of orthostasis.

Monitoring Parameters Serum calcium, serum phosphorus, uric acid; blood pressure; bone mineral density

Test Interactions Transiently increases serum calcium; maximal effect 4-6 hours postdose; generally returns to baseline ~16 hours postdose

Additional Information Teriparatide was formerly marketed as a diagnostic agent (Perithar™); that agent was withdrawn from the market in 1997. Teriparatide (Forteo®) is manufactured through recombinant DNA technology using a strain of *E. coli*.

Dosage Forms Excipient information presented when available (limited, particularly for generics); consult specific product labeling.

Injection, solution:

Forteo®: 250 mcg/mL (3 mL) [prefilled syringe, delivers teriparatide 20 mcg/dose]

◆ **Tersi** *see* Selenium Sulfide *on page* 1361

◆ **Teslac® [DSC]** *see* Testolactone *on page* 1445

◆ **Teslac® (Can)** *see* Testolactone *on page* 1445

◆ **TESPA** *see* Thiotepa *on page* 1462

◆ **Tessalon®** *see* Benzonatate *on page* 185

◆ **Testim®** *see* Testosterone *on page* 1445

Testolactone (tes toe LAK tone)

U.S. Brand Names Teslac® [DSC]

Canadian Brand Names Teslac®

Pharmacologic Category Androgen

Use Palliative treatment of advanced or disseminated breast carcinoma

Restrictions C-III

Pregnancy Risk Factor C

Medication Safety Issues

Sound-alike/look-alike issues:

Testolactone may be confused with testosterone

Dosage Adults: Females: Oral: 250 mg 4 times/day for at least 3 months; desired response may take as long as 3 months

Additional Information Complete prescribing information for this medication should be consulted for additional detail.

Dosage Forms Excipient information presented when available (limited, particularly for generics); consult specific product labeling. [DSC] = Discontinued product

Tablet:

Teslac®: 50 mg [DSC]

◆ **Testopel®** *see* Testosterone *on page* 1445

Testosterone (tes TOS ter one)

U.S. Brand Names Androderm®; AndroGel®; Delatestryl®; Depo®-Testosterone; First®-Testosterone; First®-Testosterone MC; Striant®; Testim®; Testopel®

Canadian Brand Names Andriol®; Androderm®; AndroGel®; Andropository; Delatestryl®; Depotest® 100; Everone® 200; Virilon® IM

Index Terms Testosterone Cypionate; Testosterone Enanthate

Pharmacologic Category Androgen

Use

Injection: Androgen replacement therapy in the treatment of delayed male puberty; male hypogonadism (primary or hypogonadotropic); inoperable metastatic female breast cancer (enanthate only)

Pellet: Androgen replacement therapy in the treatment of delayed male puberty; male hypogonadism (primary or hypogonadotropic)

Topical (buccal system, gel, transdermal system): Male hypogonadism (primary or hypogonadotropic)

Capsule (not available in U.S.): Androgen replacement therapy in the treatment of delayed male puberty; male hypogonadism (primary or hypogonadotropic); replacement therapy in impotence or for male climacteric symptoms due to androgen deficiency

Unlabeled/Investigational Use Androgen deficiency in men with AIDS wasting; postmenopausal women with decreased sexual desire (in combination with estrogen therapy)

Restrictions C-III

Pregnancy Risk Factor X

Pregnancy Considerations Testosterone may cause adverse effects, including masculinization of the female fetus, if used during pregnancy. Females who are or may become pregnant should also avoid skin-to-skin contact to areas where testosterone has been applied topically on another person.

Lactation Enters breast milk/contraindicated

Medication Safety Issues

Sound-alike/look-alike issues:

Testosterone may be confused with testolactone

Testoderm® may be confused with Estraderm®

Transdermal patch may contain conducting metal (eg, aluminum); remove patch prior to MRI.

Contraindications Hypersensitivity to testosterone or any component of the formulation; males with carcinoma of the breast or prostate; pregnancy or women who may become pregnant; breast-feeding

Depo®-Testosterone: Also contraindicated in serious hepatic, renal, or cardiac disease

Andriol®: Also contraindicated in hepatic, renal, or cardiac disease; hypercalcemia; nephrosis or nephritic phase of nephritis; prepubertal males; patients who are easily sexually stimulated

Warnings/Precautions When used to treat delayed male puberty, perform radiographic examination of the hand and wrist every 6 months to determine the rate of bone maturation. May cause hypercalcemia in patients with prolonged immobilization or cancer. May accelerate bone maturation without producing compensating gain in linear growth. Has both androgenic and anabolic activity, the anabolic action may enhance hypoglycemia. May alter serum cholesterol; use caution with history of MI or coronary artery disease. Use caution in elderly patients or patients with other demographic factors which may increase the risk of prostatic carcinoma; careful monitoring is required. Urethral obstruction may develop in patients with BPH; treatment should be discontinued if this should occur (use lower dose if restarted). Withhold treatment pending urological evaluation if PSA >3 ng/mL. May cause fluid retention; use caution in patients with cardiovascular disease or other edematous conditions. May cause gynecomastia. Large doses may suppress spermatogenesis.

Prolonged use of high doses of androgens has been associated with serious hepatic effects (peliosis hepatis, hepatic neoplasms, cholestatic hepatitis, jaundice). May potentiate sleep apnea in some male patients (obesity or chronic lung disease). Testosterone may be transferred to another person following skin-to-skin contact with the application site; virilization of female sexual partners has been reported with male use of the topical gel. Transdermal patch may contain conducting metal (eg, aluminum); remove patch prior to MRI. Gels and buccal system have not been evaluated in males <18 years of age; safety and efficacy of injection have not been established in males <12 years of age. Some testosterone products may be chemically synthesized from soy. Some products may contain benzyl alcohol.

Adverse Reactions Frequency rarely defined.

Cardiovascular: Deep venous thrombosis, edema, hypertension, vasodilation

Central nervous system: Aggressive behavior, amnesia, anxiety, dizziness, emotional lability, excitation, headache, malaise, mental depression, nervousness, seizure, sleep apnea, sleeplessness

Dermatologic: Acne, alopecia, dry skin, hair discoloration, hirsutism (increase in pubic hair growth), pruritus, rash, seborrhea

Endocrine & metabolic: Breast soreness, gonadotropin secretion decreased, growth acceleration, gynecomastia, hot flashes, hypercalcemia, hyperchloremia, hypercholesterolemia, hyper-/hypokalemia, hyperlipidemia, hypernatremia, hypoglycemia, inorganic phosphate retention, libido changes, menstrual problems (including amenorrhea), virilism, water retention

Gastrointestinal: GI bleeding, GI irritation, nausea, taste disorder, vomiting, weight gain

Following buccal administration (most common): Bitter taste, gum edema, gum or mouth irritation, gum pain, gum tenderness, taste perversion

Genitourinary: Bladder irritability, epididymitis, impotence, oligospermia, priapism, prostatic carcinoma, prostatic hyperplasia, PSA increased, testicular atrophy, urination impaired

Hepatic: Bilirubin increased, cholestatic hepatitis, cholestatic jaundice, hepatic dysfunction, hepatic necrosis, hepatocellular neoplasms, liver function test changes, peliosis hepatis

Hematologic: Anemia, bleeding, hematocrit/hemoglobin increased, leukopenia, polycythemia, suppression of clotting factors

Local: Application site reaction (gel), injection site pain

Transdermal system: Pruritus at application site (37%), burn-like blisters under system (12%), erythema at application site (7%), vesicles at application site (6%), allergic contact dermatitis to system (4%), burning at application site (3%), induration at application site (3%)

Neuromuscular & skeletal: Paresthesia, weakness

Ocular: Lacrimation increased

Renal: Creatinine increased

Respiratory: Dyspnea

Miscellaneous: Anaphylactoid reactions, diaphoresis, hypersensitivity reactions, smell disorder

Postmarketing and/or case reports: Injection: Cough, coughing fits, respiratory distress

Drug Interactions

Metabolism/Transport Effects Substrate (minor) of CYP2B6, 2C9, 2C19, 3A4; **Inhibits** CYP3A4 (weak)

Avoid Concomitant Use There are no known interactions where it is recommended to avoid concomitant use.

Increased Effect/Toxicity

Testosterone may increase the levels/effects of: CycloSPORINE; Vitamin K Antagonists

Decreased Effect There are no known significant interactions involving a decrease in effect.

Ethanol/Nutrition/Herb Interactions Herb/Nutraceutical: St John's wort may decrease testosterone levels.

Stability

Androderm®: Store at room temperature. Do not store outside of pouch. Excessive heat may cause system to burst.

AndroGel®, Delatestryl®, Striant®, Testim®: Store at room temperature.

Depo® Testosterone: Store at room temperature. Protect from light.

Testopel®: Store in a cool location.

Mechanism of Action Principal endogenous androgen responsible for promoting the growth and development of the male sex organs and maintaining secondary sex characteristics in androgen-deficient males

Pharmacodynamics/Kinetics

Duration (route and ester dependent): I.M.: Cypionate and enanthate esters have longest duration, ≤2-4 weeks; gel: 24-48 hours

Absorption: Transdermal gel: ~10% of applied dose

Protein binding: 98%; bound to sex hormone-binding globulin (40%) and albumin

Metabolism: Hepatic; forms metabolites, including dihydrotestosterone (DHT) and estradiol (both active)

Half-life elimination: 10-100 minutes

Excretion: Urine (90%); feces (6%)

Dosage

Adolescents and Adults: Male:

I.M.:

Hypogonadism: Testosterone enanthate or testosterone cypionate: 50-400 mg every 2-4 weeks (FDA-approved dosing range); 75-100 mg/week or 150-200 mg every 2 weeks (per practice guidelines)

Delayed puberty: Testosterone enanthate: 50-200 mg every 2-4 weeks for a limited duration

Pellet (for subcutaneous implantation): Delayed male puberty, male hypogonadism: 150-450 mg every 3-6 months

Oral: Delayed puberty, hypogonadism, or hypogonadotropic hypogonadism: Capsule (Andriol®; not available in U.S.): Initial: 120-160 mg/day in 2 divided doses for 2-3 weeks; adjust according to individual response; usual maintenance dose: 40-120 mg/day (in divided doses)

Adults:

I.M.: Females: Inoperable metastatic breast cancer: Testosterone enanthate: 200-400 mg every 2-4 weeks

Topical: Primary male hypogonadism **or** hypogonadotropic hypogonadism:

Buccal: 30 mg twice daily (every 12 hours) applied to the gum region above the incisor tooth

Transdermal system: Androderm®: Initial: Apply 5 mg/day once nightly to clean, dry area on the back, abdomen, upper arms, or thighs (do **not** apply to scrotum); dosing range: 2.5-7.5 mg/day; in nonvirilized patients, dose may be initiated at 2.5 mg/day

Gel: AndroGel®, Testim®: 5 g (to deliver 50 mg of testosterone with 5 mg systemically absorbed) applied once daily (preferably in the morning) to clean, dry, intact skin of the shoulder and upper arms. AndroGel® may also be applied to the abdomen. Dosage may be increased to a maximum of 10 g (100 mg). **Do not apply testosterone gel to the genitals.**

Dose adjustment based on testosterone levels:

Less than normal range: Increase dose from 5 g to 7.5 g to 10 g

Greater than normal range: Decrease dose. Discontinue if consistently above normal at 5 g/day

Dosing adjustment/comments in hepatic disease: Reduce dose

Dietary Considerations Testosterone USP may be synthesized from soy. Food and beverages have not been found to interfere with buccal system; ensure system is in place following eating, drinking, or brushing teeth.

Administration

I.M.: Warm to room temperature; shaking vial will help redissolve crystals that have formed after storage. Administer by deep I.M. injection into the upper outer quadrant of the gluteus maximus.

Oral, buccal application (Striant®): One mucoadhesive for buccal application (buccal system) should be applied to a comfortable area above the incisor tooth. Apply flat side of system to gum. Rotate to alternate sides of mouth with each application. Hold buccal system firmly in place for 30 seconds to ensure adhesion. The buccal system should adhere to gum for 12 hours. If the buccal system falls out, replace with a new system. If the system falls out within 4 hours of next dose, the new buccal system should remain in place until the time of the following scheduled dose. System will soften and mold to shape of gum as it absorbs moisture from mouth. Do not chew or swallow the buccal system. The buccal system will not dissolve; gently remove by sliding downwards from gum; avoid scratching gum.

Oral, capsule (Andriol®; not available in the U.S.): Should be administered with meals. Should be swallowed whole; do not crush or chew.

Transdermal patch (Androderm®): Apply patch to clean, dry area of skin on the arm, back, or upper buttocks. Following patch removal, mild skin irritation may be treated with OTC hydrocortisone cream. A small amount of triamcinolone acetonide 0.1% cream may be applied under the system to decrease irritation; do not use ointment. Patch should be applied nightly. Rotate administration sites, allowing 7 days between applying to the same site.

Topical gel: AndroGel®, Testim®: Apply (preferably in the morning) to clean, dry, intact skin of the shoulder and upper arms (AndroGel® may also be applied to the abdomen). Apply at the same time each day. Upon opening the packet(s), the entire contents should be squeezed into the palm of the hand and immediately applied to the application site(s). Alternatively, a portion may be squeezed onto palm of hand and applied, repeating the process until entire packet has been applied. Application sites should be allowed to dry for a few minutes prior to dressing. Hands should be washed with soap and water after application. **Do not apply testosterone gel to the genitals**. For optimal absorption, after application wait at least 5-6 hours prior to showering or swimming; however waiting at least 1 hour should have minimal affect on absorption if done infrequently. Alcohol-based gels are flammable; avoid fire or smoking until gel has dried. Testosterone may be transferred to another person following skin-to-skin contact with the application site. Thoroughly wash hands after application and cover application site with clothing (ie shirt) once gel has dried, or clean application site thoroughly with soap and water prior to contact in order to minimize transfer.

AndroGel® multidose pump: Prime pump 3 times (and discard this portion of product) prior to initial use.

Monitoring Parameters Periodic liver function tests, PSA and prostate exam (prior to therapy, at 3 months, then as based on current guidelines), cholesterol, hemoglobin and hematocrit (prior to therapy, at 3 months, then annually); radiologic examination of wrist and hand every 6 months (when using in prepubertal children). Withhold initial treatment with hematocrit >50%, hyperviscosity, untreated obstructive sleep apnea, or uncontrolled severe heart failure. Monitor urine and serum calcium and signs of virilization in women treated for breast cancer.

PSA: Withhold initial treatment if PSA >3 ng/mL, or with palpable prostate nodule or induration without further urological evaluation. Do not treat with severe untreated BPH with IPSS symptom score >19.

Serum testosterone: Monitor 3 months after initiating treatment, then annually.

Injection: Measure midway between injections

AndroGel®: Morning serum testosterone levels 14 days after start of therapy

Androderm®: Morning serum testosterone levels following application the previous evening

Striant®: Application area of gums; total serum testosterone 4-12 weeks after initiating treatment, prior to morning dose

Reference Range Testosterone, urine: Male: 100-1500 ng/24 hours; Female: 100-500 ng/24 hours

Test Interactions May cause a decrease in thyroid function tests

Dosage Forms Excipient information presented when available (limited, particularly for generics); consult specific product labeling. [CAN] = Canadian brand name

Capsule, gelatin, as undecanoate:

Andriol™ [CAN]: 40 mg (10s) [not available in U.S.]

Gel, topical:

AndroGel®:

1.25 g/actuation (75 g) [1% metered-dose pump; delivers 5 g/4 actuations; provides sixty 1.25 g actuations; contains ethanol 67%; may be chemically synthesized from soy]

2.5 g (30s) [1% unit dose packets; contains ethanol 67%; may be chemically synthesized from soy]

5 g (30s) [1% unit dose packets; contains ethanol; may be chemically synthesized from soy]

Testim®: 5 g (30s) [1% unit-dose tube; contains ethanol 74%; may be chemically synthesized from soy]

Implant, subcutaneous:

Testopel®: 75 mg (10s, 100s)

Injection, in oil, as cypionate: 100 mg/mL (10 mL); 200 mg/mL (1 mL, 10 mL)

Depo®-Testosterone: 100 mg/mL (10 mL); 200 mg/mL (1 mL, 10 mL) [contains benzyl alcohol, benzyl benzoate, and cottonseed oil]

Injection, in oil, as enanthate: 200 mg/mL (5 mL)

Delatestryl®: 200 mg/mL (1 mL, 5 mL) [contains sesame oil]

Kit [for prescription compounding; testosterone 2%]:

First®-Testosterone:

Injection, in oil: Testosterone propionate 100 mg/mL (12 mL) [contains sesame oil and benzyl alcohol]

Ointment: White petrolatum (48 g)

First®-Testosterone MC:

Injection, in oil: Testosterone propionate 100 mg/mL (12 mL) [contains sesame oil and benzyl alcohol]

Cream: Moisturizing cream (48 g)

Mucoadhesive, for buccal application [buccal system]:

Striant®: 30 mg (10s) [may be chemically synthesized from soy]

Transdermal system, topical:

Androderm®: 2.5 mg/day (60s) [contains ethanol]; 5 mg/day (30s) [contains ethanol]

◆ **Testosterone Cypionate** *see* Testosterone *on page 1445*

- **Testosterone Enanthate** *see* Testosterone *on page 1445*
- **Testred®** *see* MethylTESTOSTERone *on page 979*
- **Tetanus and Diphtheria Toxoid** *see* Diphtheria and Tetanus Toxoid *on page 460*

Tetanus Immune Globulin (Human)

(TET a nus i MYUN GLOB yoo lin HYU man)

U.S. Brand Names HyperTET™ S/D

Canadian Brand Names HyperTET™ S/D

Index Terms TIG

Pharmacologic Category Immune Globulin

Use Prophylaxis against tetanus following injury in patients where immunization status is not known or uncertain

The Advisory Committee on Immunization Practices (ACIP) recommends passive immunization with TIG for the following:

- Persons with a wound that is not clean or minor and in whom contraindications to a tetanus-toxoid containing vaccine exist and they have not completed a primary series of tetanus toxoid immunization.
- Persons who are wounded in bombings or similar mass casualty events who have penetrating injuries or nonintact skin exposure and who cannot confirm receipt of a tetanus booster within the previous 5 years. In case of shortage, use should be reserved for persons ≥60 years of age.

Pregnancy Risk Factor C

Pregnancy Considerations Animal reproduction studies have not been conducted. Tetanus immune globulin and a tetanus toxoid containing vaccine are recommended by the ACIP as part of the standard wound management to prevent tetanus in pregnant women.

Warnings/Precautions Hypersensitivity and anaphylactic reactions can occur; immediate treatment (including epinephrine 1:1000) should be available. Use caution in patients with isolated immunoglobulin A deficiency or a history of systemic hypersensitivity to human immunoglobulins. Use with caution in patients with thrombocytopenia or coagulation disorders; I.M. injections may be contraindicated. Product of human plasma; may potentially contain infectious agents which could transmit disease. Screening of donors, as well as testing and/or inactivation or removal of certain viruses, reduces the risk. Infections thought to be transmitted by this product should be reported to the manufacturer. Skin testing should not be performed as local irritation can occur and be misinterpreted as a positive reaction. Not for intravenous administration.

Adverse Reactions Frequency not defined.

Central nervous system: Temperature increased

Dermatologic: Angioneurotic edema (rare)

Local: Injection site: pain, soreness, tenderness

Renal: Nephritic syndrome (rare)

Miscellaneous: Anaphylactic shock (rare)

Drug Interactions

Avoid Concomitant Use There are no known interactions where it is recommended to avoid concomitant use.

Increased Effect/Toxicity There are no known significant interactions involving an increase in effect.

Decreased Effect

Tetanus Immune Globulin (Human) may decrease the levels/effects of: Vaccines (Live)

Stability Store at 2°C to 8°C (26°F to 46°F). Do not use if frozen.

Mechanism of Action Passive immunity toward tetanus

Pharmacodynamics/Kinetics Absorption: Well absorbed

Dosage I.M.:

Prophylaxis of tetanus:

Children <7 years: 4 units/kg; some recommend administering 250 units to small children

Children ≥7 years and Adults: 250 units

Treatment of tetanus: Children and Adults: 500-6000 units. Infiltration of part of the dose around the wound is recommended.

Tetanus Prophylaxis in Wound Management

Number of Prior Tetanus Toxoid Doses	Clean, Minor Wounds		All Other Wounds	
	Td[1]	TIG[2]	Td[1]	TIG[2]
Unknown or <3	Yes	No	Yes	Yes
≥3[3]	No[4]	No	No[5]	No

[1]Adult tetanus and diphtheria toxoids; use pediatric preparations (DT or DTP) if the patient is <7 years old.

[2]Tetanus immune globulin.

[3]If only three doses of fluid tetanus toxoid have been received, a fourth dose of toxoid, preferably an adsorbed toxoid, should be given.

[4]Yes, if >10 years since last dose.

[5]Yes, if >5 years since last dose.

Adapted from Centers for Disease Control, "Diphtheria, Tetanus, and Pertussis: Recommendations for Vaccine Use and Other Preventive Measures: Recommendations of the Immunization Practices Advisory Committee (ACIP)," *MMWR* 1991:40(RR-10).

Administration Do not administer I.V.; I.M. use only. Administer in the anterolateral aspects of the upper thigh or the deltoid muscle of the upper arm. Avoid gluteal region due to risk of injury to sciatic nerve; if gluteal region is used, administer only in the upper outer quadrant. If tetanus vaccine and tetanus immune globulin are administered simultaneously, separate sites should be used for each injection. When used for the treatment of tetanus, infiltration of part of the dose around the wound is recommended.

Vaccine administration with antibody-containing products*:

Antibody-containing products and inactivated vaccines: May be given simultaneously at different sites or at any interval between doses.

Antibody-containing products and live vaccines: Do not give simultaneously.

*Examples of antibody-containing products include I.M. and I.V. immune globulin, hepatitis B immune globulin, tetanus immune globulin, varicella zoster immune globulin, rabies immune globulin, whole blood, packed red cells, plasma, and platelet products.

Additional Information Tetanus immune globulin (TIG) must not contain <50 units/mL. Protein makes up 10% to 18% of TIG preparations. The great majority of this (≥90%) is IgG. TIG has almost no color or odor and it is a sterile, nonpyrogenic, concentrated preparation of immunoglobulins that has been derived from the plasma of adults hyperimmunized with tetanus toxoid. The pooled material from which the immunoglobulin is derived may be from fewer than 1000 donors. This plasma has been shown to be free of hepatitis B surface antigen.

Dosage Forms Excipient information presented when available (limited, particularly for generics); consult specific product labeling.

Injection, solution [preservative free]:

HyperTET™ S/D: 250 units/mL (1 mL) [prefilled syringe]

- **Tetanus Toxoid** *see* Diphtheria and Tetanus Toxoids, Acellular Pertussis, Poliovirus and *Haemophilus* b Conjugate Vaccine *on page 462*

Tetanus Toxoid (Adsorbed)

(TET a nus TOKS oyd, ad SORBED)

Pharmacologic Category Vaccine, Inactivated (Bacterial)

Additional Appendix Information

Immunization Recommendations *on page 1708*

Use Active immunization against tetanus when combination antigen preparations are not indicated. **Note:** Tetanus and diphtheria toxoids for adult use (Td) is the preferred immunizing agent for most adults and for children after their seventh birthday. Young children should receive trivalent DTaP (diphtheria/tetanus/acellular pertussis), as part of their childhood immunization program, unless pertussis is contraindicated, then DT is warranted.

Pregnancy Risk Factor C

Pregnancy Considerations Animal studies have not been conducted. The ACIP recommends vaccination in previously unvaccinated women or in women with an incomplete vaccination series, whose child may be born in unhygienic conditions. Tetanus immune globulin and a tetanus toxoid-containing vaccine are recommended by the ACIP as part of the standard wound management to prevent tetanus in pregnant women. Vaccination using Td is preferred.

Lactation Excretion in breast milk unknown/use caution

Medication Safety Issues

Sound-alike/look-alike issues:

Tetanus toxoid products may be confused with influenza virus vaccine and tuberculin products. Medication errors have occurred when tetanus toxoid products have been inadvertently administered instead of tuberculin skin tests (PPD) and influenza virus vaccine. These products are refrigerated and often stored in close proximity to each other.

Contraindications Hypersensitivity to tetanus toxoid or any component of the formulation

Warnings/Precautions Avoid injection into a blood vessel; allergic reactions may occur; epinephrine 1:1000 must be available. Patients who are immunocompromised may have reduced response; may be used in patients with HIV infection. May defer elective immunization during febrile illness or acute infection; defer elective immunization during outbreaks of poliomyelitis. In patients with a history of severe local reaction (Arthus-type) or temperature of >39.4°C (>103°F) following previous dose, do not give further routine or emergency doses of tetanus and diphtheria toxoids for 10 years. Use caution in patients on anticoagulants, with thrombocytopenia, or bleeding disorders (bleeding may occur following intramuscular injection). Use with caution if Guillain-Barré syndrome occurred within 6 weeks of prior tetanus toxoid. Contains thimerosal; vial stopper may contain natural latex rubber. This product is not indicated for use in children <7 years of age. In order to maximize vaccination rates, the ACIP recommends simultaneous administration of all age-appropriate vaccines (live or inactivated) for which a person is eligible at a single clinic visit, unless contraindications exist.

Adverse Reactions All serious adverse reactions must be reported to the U.S. Department of Health and Human Services (DHHS) Vaccine Adverse Event Reporting System (VAERS) 1-800-822-7967.

Frequency not defined.

Cardiovascular: Hypotension

Central nervous system: Brachial neuritis, fever, malaise, pain

Gastrointestinal: Nausea

Local: Edema, induration (with or without tenderness), rash, redness, urticaria, warmth

Neuromuscular: Arthralgia, Guillain-Barré syndrome

Miscellaneous: Anaphylactic reaction, Arthus-type hypersensitivity reaction

Drug Interactions

Avoid Concomitant Use There are no known interactions where it is recommended to avoid concomitant use.

Increased Effect/Toxicity There are no known significant interactions involving an increase in effect.

Decreased Effect

The levels/effects of Tetanus Toxoid (Adsorbed) may be decreased by: Immunosuppressants

Stability Store at 2°C to 8°C (26°F to 46°F); do not freeze.

Mechanism of Action Tetanus toxoid preparations contain the toxin produced by virulent tetanus bacilli (detoxified growth products of *Clostridium tetani*). The toxin has been modified by treatment with formaldehyde so that it has lost toxicity but still retains ability to act as antigen and produce active immunity; the aluminum salt, a mineral adjuvant, delays the rate of absorption and prolongs and enhances its properties; duration ~10 years.

Pharmacodynamics/Kinetics Duration: Primary immunization: ~10 years

Dosage Children ≥7 years and Adults: I.M.:

Primary immunization: 0.5 mL; repeat 0.5 mL at 4-8 weeks after first dose and at 6-12 months after second dose

Routine booster dose: Recommended every 10 years

Note: In most patients, Td is the recommended product for primary immunization, booster doses, and tetanus immunization in wound management (refer to Diphtheria and Tetanus Toxoid monograph on page 460)

Administration Inject intramuscularly in the area of the vastus lateralis (midthigh laterally) or deltoid. Do not inject into gluteal area. Shake well prior to withdrawing dose; do not use if product does not form a suspension.

For patients at risk of hemorrhage following intramuscular injection, the ACIP recommends "it should be administered intramuscularly if, in the opinion of the physician familiar with the patients bleeding risk, the vaccine can be administered with reasonable safety by this route. If the patient receives antihemophilia or other similar therapy, intramuscular vaccination can be scheduled shortly after such therapy is administered. A fine needle (23 gauge or smaller) can be used for the vaccination and firm pressure applied to the site (without rubbing) for at least 2 minutes. The patient should be instructed concerning the risk of hematoma from the injection."

Administration with other vaccines:

Tetanus toxoid vaccine with other inactivated vaccines: May be given simultaneously or at any interval between doses.

Tetanus toxoid vaccine with live vaccines: May be given simultaneously or at any interval between doses

Vaccine administration with antibody-containing products: Tetanus toxoid vaccine may be be given simultaneously at different sites or at any interval between doses. Examples of antibody-containing products include I.M. and I.V. immune globulin, hepatitis B immune globulin, tetanus immune globulin, varicella zoster immune globulin, rabies immune globulin, whole blood, packed red cells, plasma, and platelet products.

Additional Information Federal law requires that the date of administration, the vaccine manufacturer, lot number of vaccine, and the administering person's name, title and address be entered into the patient's permanent medical record.

Dosage Forms Excipient information presented when available (limited, particularly for generics); consult specific product labeling.

Injection, suspension: Tetanus 5 Lf units per 0.5 mL (0.5 mL) [contains trace amounts of thimerosal]

Tetanus Toxoid (Fluid)

(TET a nus TOKS oyd FLOO id)

Index Terms Tetanus Toxoid Plain

Pharmacologic Category Toxoid

Additional Appendix Information

Immunization Recommendations *on page 1708*

Use Indicated as booster dose in the active immunization against tetanus in the rare adult or child who is allergic to the aluminum adjuvant (a product containing adsorbed tetanus toxoid is preferred); not indicated for primary immunization

Unlabeled/Investigational Use Anergy testing (no longer recommended)

Pregnancy Risk Factor C

Pregnancy Considerations Reproduction studies have not been conducted and effects to the fetus are not known. Deferring immunization until the 2nd trimester may be considered.

Medication Safety Issues

Sound-alike/look-alike issues:

Tetanus toxoid products may be confused with influenza virus vaccine and tuberculin products. Medication errors have occurred when tetanus toxoid products have been inadvertently administered instead of tuberculin skin tests (PPD) and influenza virus vaccine. These products are refrigerated and often stored in close proximity to each other.

Contraindications Hypersensitivity to tetanus toxoid or any component of the formulation

Warnings/Precautions Immediate treatment (including epinephrine 1:1000) for anaphylactoid and/or hypersensitivity reactions should be available during use. Patients who are immunocompromised may have reduced response; may be used in patients with HIV infection. May defer elective immunization during febrile illness or acute infection; defer elective immunization during outbreaks of poliomyelitis. In patients with a history of severe local reaction (Arthus-type) following previous dose, do not give further routine or emergency doses of tetanus and diphtheria toxoids for 10 years. Use caution in patients on anticoagulants, with thrombocytopenia, or bleeding disorders (bleeding may occur following intramuscular injection). Contains thimerosal; vial stopper contains natural latex rubber. Safety and efficacy in children <6 weeks of age have not been established; this product is not indicated for use in children <7 years of age.

Adverse Reactions All serious adverse reactions must be reported to the U.S. Department of Health and Human Services (DHHS) Vaccine Adverse Event Reporting System (VAERS) 1-800-822-7967.

Frequency not defined.

Cardiovascular: Hypotension

Central nervous system: Brachial neuritis, fever, Guillain-Barré syndrome, malaise

Dermatologic: Rash, urticaria

Gastrointestinal: Nausea

Local: Edema, induration (with or without tenderness), redness, warmth

Neuromuscular & skeletal: Arthralgia

Miscellaneous: Anaphylaxis, Arthus-type hypersensitivity reactions (severe local reaction developing 2-8 hours following injection)

Drug Interactions

Avoid Concomitant Use There are no known interactions where it is recommended to avoid concomitant use.

Increased Effect/Toxicity There are no known significant interactions involving an increase in effect.

Decreased Effect

The levels/effects of Tetanus Toxoid (Fluid) may be decreased by: Immunosuppressants

Stability Refrigerate 2°C to 8°C (35°F to 46°F); do not freeze.

Mechanism of Action Tetanus toxoid preparations contain the toxin produced by virulent tetanus bacilli (detoxified growth products of *Clostridium tetani*). The toxin has been modified by treatment with formaldehyde so that is has lost toxicity but still retains ability to act as antigen and produce active immunity.

Dosage

Primary immunization: Not indicated for this use.

Booster doses: I.M., SubQ: 0.5 mL every 10 years

Anergy testing (unlabeled use; no longer recommended for this indication): Intradermal: 0.1 mL; doses that have been used range from 0.1 mL of a 1:10 dilution to 0.1 mL of the undiluted product

Administration

I.M. Shake well prior to use. Administer I.M. in lateral aspect of midthigh or deltoid muscle of upper arm

For patients at risk of hemorrhage following intramuscular injection, the ACIP recommends "it should be administered intramuscularly if, in the opinion of the physician familiar with the patients bleeding risk, the vaccine can be administered with reasonable safety by this route. If the patient receives antihemophilia or other similar therapy, intramuscular vaccination can be scheduled shortly after such therapy is administered. A fine needle (23 gauge or smaller) can be used for the vaccination and firm pressure applied to the site (without rubbing) for at least 2 minutes. The patient should be instructed concerning the risk of hematoma from the injection."

SubQ: Shake well prior to use. Administer in area of the lateral aspect of midthigh or deltoid. SubQ route may be preferred in patients with thrombocytopenia or coagulation disorders.

Additional Information Federal law requires that the date of administration, the vaccine manufacturer, lot number of vaccine, and the administering person's name, title and address be entered into the patient's permanent medical record.

Dosage Forms Excipient information presented when available (limited, particularly for generics); consult specific product labeling. [DSC] = Discontinued product

Injection, solution: Tetanus 4 Lf units per 0.5 mL (7.5 mL) [contains thimerosal; vial stopper contains dry natural latex rubber] [DSC]

◆ **Tetanus Toxoid Plain** *see* Tetanus Toxoid (Fluid) *on page 1450*

◆ **Tetanus Toxoid, Reduced Diphtheria Toxoid, and Acellular Pertussis, Adsorbed** *see* Diphtheria and Tetanus Toxoids, and Acellular Pertussis Vaccine *on page 463*

Tetrabenazine (tet ra BEN a zeen)

U.S. Brand Names Xenazine®

Canadian Brand Names Nitoman™

Pharmacologic Category Central Monoamine-Depleting Agent

Use Treatment of chorea associated with Huntington's disease

Canadian labeling: Treatment of hyperkinetic movement disorders, including Huntington's chorea, hemiballismus, senile chorea, Tourette syndrome, and tardive dyskinesia

Restrictions An FDA-approved patient medication guide is available and must be distributed when dispensing an outpatient prescription (new or refill) where this medication is to be used without direct supervision of a healthcare provider.

Pregnancy Risk Factor C

Dosage Oral: Dose should be individualized; titrate slowly

Chorea associated with Huntington's disease: Adults:

Initial: 12.5 mg once daily, may increase to 12.5 mg twice daily after 1 week

Maintenance: May be increased by 12.5 mg/day at weekly intervals; doses >37.5 mg/day should be divided into 3 doses (maximum single dose 25 mg)

Patients requiring doses >50 mg/day: Genotype for CYP2D6:

Extensive/intermediate metabolizers: Maximum: 100 mg/day; 37.5 mg/dose

Poor metabolizers: Maximum: 50 mg/day; 25 mg/dose

Concomitant use with strong CYP2D6 inhibitors (eg, fluoxetine, paroxetine, quinidine): Dose of tetrabenazine should be reduced by 50% in patients receiving strong CYP2D6 inhibitors, follow dosing for poor CYP2D6 metabolizers. Use caution when adding a CYP2D6 inhibitor to patients already taking tetrabenazine.

Note: If treatment is interrupted for >5 days, retitration is recommended. If treatment is interrupted for <5 days resume at previous maintenance dose.

Canadian labeling: Hyperkinetic movement disorders:

Adults: Initial: 12.5 mg twice daily (may be given 3 times/day); may be increased by 12.5 mg/day every 3-5 days; should be titrated slowly to maximal tolerated and effective dose (dose is individualized)

Usual maximum tolerated dosage: 25 mg 3 times/day; maximum recommended dose: 200 mg/day

Note: If there is no improvement at the maximum tolerated dose after 7 days, improvement is unlikely; discontinuation should be considered.

Elderly and/or debilitated patients: Consider initiation at lower doses; must be titrated slowly to individualize dosage

Dosage adjustment for toxicity: For toxicity/adverse reaction, including akathisia, restlessness, parkinsonism, insomnia, depression, suicidality, anxiety, sedation (intolerable): Suspend upward dosage titration and reduce dose; consider discontinuing if adverse reaction does not resolve (may be discontinued without tapering.

Dosage adjustment in hepatic impairment: Use is contraindicated

Additional Information Complete prescribing information for this medication should be consulted for additional detail.

Dosage Forms Excipient information presented when available (limited, particularly for generics); consult specific product labeling. [CAN] = Canadian product

Tablet:

Nitoman™ [CAN]: 25 mg [not available in the U.S.]

Xenazine®: 12.5 mg, 25 mg

Tetracaine (TET ra kane)

U.S. Brand Names Pontocaine®; Pontocaine® Niphanoid®

Canadian Brand Names Ametop™; Pontocaine®

Index Terms Amethocaine Hydrochloride; Tetracaine Hydrochloride

Pharmacologic Category Local Anesthetic

Use Spinal anesthesia; local anesthesia in the eye for various diagnostic and examination purposes; topically applied to nose and throat for various diagnostic procedures

Pregnancy Risk Factor C

Dosage Adults:

Ophthalmic: Short-term anesthesia of the eye: 0.5% solution: Instill 1-2 drops; prolonged use (especially for at-home self-medication) is not recommended

Injection: Spinal anesthesia: **Note:** Dosage varies with the anesthetic procedure, the degree of anesthesia required, and the individual patient response; it is administered by subarachnoid injection for spinal anesthesia.

Perineal anesthesia: 5 mg

Perineal and lower extremities: 10 mg

Anesthesia extending up to costal margin: 15 mg; doses up to 20 mg may be given, but are reserved for exceptional cases

Low spinal anesthesia (saddle block): 2-5 mg

Topical mucous membranes (rhinolaryngology): Used as a 0.25% or 0.5% solution by direct application or nebulization; total dose should not exceed 20 mg

Additional Information Complete prescribing information for this medication should be consulted for additional detail.

Dosage Forms Excipient information presented when available (limited, particularly for generics); consult specific product labeling.

Injection, powder for reconstitution, as hydrochloride [preservative free]:

Pontocaine® Niphanoid®: 20 mg

Injection, solution, as hydrochloride [preservative free]: 1% [10 mg/mL] (2 mL)

Pontocaine®): 1% [10 mg/mL] (2 mL) [contains sodium bisulfite]

Solution, ophthalmic, as hydrochloride: 0.5% [5 mg/mL] (2 mL, 15 mL)

Solution, topical, as hydrochloride (Pontocaine®): 2% [20 mg/mL] (30 mL, 118 mL) [for rhinolaryngology]

◆ **Tetracaine and Lidocaine** *see* Lidocaine and Tetracaine *on page 888*

◆ **Tetracaine, Benzocaine, and Butamben** *see* Benzocaine, Butamben, and Tetracaine *on page 185*

◆ **Tetracaine Hydrochloride** *see* Tetracaine *on page 1451*

◆ **Tetracosactide** *see* Cosyntropin *on page 372*

Tetracycline (tet ra SYE kleen)

Canadian Brand Names Apo-Tetra®; Nu-Tetra

Index Terms Achromycin; TCN; Tetracycline Hydrochloride

Pharmacologic Category Antibiotic, Tetracycline Derivative

Additional Appendix Information

Antimicrobial Drugs of Choice *on page 1752*

Helicobacter pylori Treatment *on page 1813*

Malaria Treatment *on page 1770*

Treatment of Sexually Transmitted Infections *on page 1773*

Use Treatment of susceptible bacterial infections of both gram-positive and gram-negative organisms; also infections due to *Mycoplasma*, *Chlamydia*, and *Rickettsia*; indicated for acne, exacerbations of chronic bronchitis, and treatment of gonorrhea and syphilis in patients who are allergic to penicillin; as part of a multidrug regimen for *H. pylori* eradication to reduce the risk of duodenal ulcer recurrence

Pregnancy Risk Factor D

Pregnancy Considerations Tetracyclines cross the placenta, enter fetal circulation, and may cause permanent discoloration of teeth if used during the second or third trimester. Maternal hepatic toxicity has been associated with the use of tetracycline during pregnancy, especially in patients with azotemia or pyelonephritis. Because use during pregnancy may cause fetal harm, tetracycline is classified as pregnancy category D.

Lactation Enters breast milk/not recommended (AAP rates "compatible")

Medication Safety Issues

Sound-alike/look-alike issues:

Tetracycline may be confused with tetradecyl sulfate

Achromycin may be confused with actinomycin, Adriamycin PFS®

Contraindications Hypersensitivity to tetracycline or any component of the formulation; do not administer to children ≤8 years of age; pregnancy

Warnings/Precautions Use with caution in patients with renal or hepatic impairment (eg, elderly); dosage modification required in patients with renal impairment since it may increase BUN as an antianabolic agent. Hepatotoxicity has been reported rarely; risk may be increased in patients with pre-existing hepatic or renal impairment. Pseudotumor cerebri has been reported with tetracycline use (usually resolves with discontinuation); outdated drug can cause nephropathy; use protective measure to avoid photosensitivity. Prolonged use may result in fungal or bacterial superinfection, including *C. difficile*-associated diarrhea (CDAD) and pseudomembranous colitis; CDAD has been observed >2 months postantibiotic treatment. May cause tissue hyperpigmentation, enamel hypoplasia, or permanent tooth discoloration; use of tetracyclines should be avoided during tooth development (children ≤8 years of age) unless other drugs are not likely to be effective or are contraindicated. However, recommended in treatment of anthrax exposure. Do not use during pregnancy. In addition to affecting tooth development, tetracycline use has been associated with retardation of skeletal development and reduced bone growth.

Adverse Reactions Frequency not defined.

Cardiovascular: Pericarditis

Central nervous system: Intracranial pressure increased, bulging fontanels in infants, pseudotumor cerebri, paresthesia

Dermatologic: Photosensitivity, pruritus, pigmentation of nails, exfoliative dermatitis

Endocrine & metabolic: Diabetes insipidus syndrome

Gastrointestinal: Discoloration of teeth and enamel hypoplasia (young children), nausea, diarrhea, vomiting, esophagitis, anorexia, abdominal cramps, antibiotic-associated pseudomembranous colitis, staphylococcal enterocolitis, pancreatitis

Hematologic: Thrombophlebitis

Hepatic: Hepatotoxicity

Renal: Acute renal failure, azotemia, renal damage

Miscellaneous: Superinfection, anaphylaxis, hypersensitivity reactions, candidal superinfection

Drug Interactions

Metabolism/Transport Effects **Substrate** of CYP3A4 (major); **Inhibits** CYP3A4 (moderate)

Avoid Concomitant Use

Avoid concomitant use of Tetracycline with any of the following: Retinoic Acid Derivatives

Increased Effect/Toxicity

Tetracycline may increase the levels/effects of: CYP3A4 Substrates; Eplerenone; FentaNYL; Maraviroc; Neuromuscular-Blocking Agents; Pimecrolimus; Ranolazine; Retinoic Acid Derivatives; Salmeterol; Vitamin K Antagonists

Decreased Effect

Tetracycline may decrease the levels/effects of: Atovaquone; Penicillins; Typhoid Vaccine

The levels/effects of Tetracycline may be decreased by: Antacids; Bile Acid Sequestrants; Bismuth; Bismuth Subsalicylate; CYP3A4 Inducers (Strong); Deferasirox; Herbs (CYP3A4 Inducers); Iron Salts; Magnesium Salts; Quinapril; Zinc Salts

Ethanol/Nutrition/Herb Interactions

Food: Tetracycline serum concentrations may be decreased if taken with dairy products.

Herb/Nutraceutical: Avoid dong quai, St John's wort (may also cause photosensitization)

Stability Outdated tetracyclines have caused a Fanconi-like syndrome. Protect oral dosage forms from light.

Mechanism of Action Inhibits bacterial protein synthesis by binding with the 30S and possibly the 50S ribosomal subunit(s) of susceptible bacteria; may also cause alterations in the cytoplasmic membrane

Pharmacodynamics/Kinetics

Absorption: Oral: 75%

Distribution: Small amount appears in bile

Relative diffusion from blood into CSF: Good only with inflammation (exceeds usual MICs)

CSF:blood level ratio: Inflamed meninges: 25%

Protein binding: ~65%

Half-life elimination: Normal renal function: 8-11 hours; End-stage renal disease: 57-108 hours

Time to peak, serum: Oral: 2-4 hours

Excretion: Urine (60% as unchanged drug); feces (as active form)

Dosage

Usual dosage range:

Children >8 years: Oral: 25-50 mg/kg/day in divided doses every 6 hours

Adults: Oral: 250-500 mg/dose every 6 hours

Indication-specific dosing:

Adults: Oral:

Acne: 250-500 twice daily

Chronic bronchitis, acute exacerbation: 500 mg 4 times/day

Erlichiosis: 500 mg 4 times/day for 7-14 days

Peptic ulcer disease: Eradication of *Helicobacter pylori*: 500 mg 2-4 times/day depending on regimen; requires combination therapy with at least one other antibiotic and an acid-suppressing agent (proton pump inhibitor or H_2 blocker)

Periodontitis: 250 mg every 6 hours until improvement (usually 10 days)

Vibrio cholerae: 500 mg 4 times/day for 3 days

Dosing interval in renal impairment:

Cl_{cr} 50-80 mL/minute: Administer every 8-12 hours

Cl_{cr} 10-50 mL/minute: Administer every 12-24 hours

Cl_{cr} <10 mL/minute: Administer every 24 hours

Dialysis: Slightly dialyzable (5% to 20%) via hemo- and peritoneal dialysis or via continuous arteriovenous or venovenous hemofiltration; no supplemental dosage necessary

Dosing adjustment in hepatic impairment: Use caution; no dosing adjustment required

Administration Should be administered on an empty stomach (ie, 1 hour prior to, or 2 hours after meals) to increase total absorption. Administer at least 1-2 hours prior to, or 4 hours after antacid because aluminum and magnesium cations may chelate with tetracycline and reduce its total absorption.

Monitoring Parameters Renal, hepatic, and hematologic function test, temperature, WBC, cultures and sensitivity, appetite, mental status

Test Interactions False-negative urine glucose with Clinistix®

Dosage Forms Excipient information presented when available (limited, particularly for generics); consult specific product labeling.

Capsule, as hydrochloride: 250 mg, 500 mg

◆ **Tetracycline Hydrochloride** *see* Tetracycline *on page 1451*

◆ **Tetracycline, Metronidazole, and Bismuth Subcitrate Potassium** *see* Bismuth, Metronidazole, and Tetracycline *on page 199*

◆ **Tetracycline, Metronidazole, and Bismuth Subsalicylate** *see* Bismuth, Metronidazole, and Tetracycline *on page 199*
◆ **Tetrahydroaminoacrine** *see* Tacrine *on page 1418*
◆ **Tetrahydrocannabinol** *see* Dronabinol *on page 494*
◆ **2,2,2-tetramine** *see* Trientine *on page 1515*
◆ **Tetra Tannate Pediatric** *see* Chlorpheniramine, Ephedrine, Phenylephrine, and Carbetapentane *on page 311*
◆ **Teveten®** *see* Eprosartan *on page 536*
◆ **Teveten® HCT** *see* Eprosartan and Hydrochlorothiazide *on page 537*
◆ **Teveten® Plus (Can)** *see* Eprosartan and Hydrochlorothiazide *on page 537*
◆ **Tev-Tropin®** *see* Somatropin *on page 1388*
◆ **Texacort®** *see* Hydrocortisone *on page 743*
◆ **TG** *see* Thioguanine *on page 1459*
◆ **6-TG (error-prone abbreviation)** *see* Thioguanine *on page 1459*
◆ **THA** *see* Tacrine *on page 1418*

Thalidomide (tha LI doe mide)

U.S. Brand Names Thalomid®

Canadian Brand Names Thalomid®

Index Terms NSC-66847

Pharmacologic Category Angiogenesis Inhibitor; Immunomodulator, Systemic; Tumor Necrosis Factor (TNF) Blocking Agent

Use Treatment of multiple myeloma; treatment and maintenance of cutaneous manifestations of erythema nodosum leprosum (ENL)

Unlabeled/Investigational Use Treatment of Crohn's disease; graft-versus-host reactions after bone marrow transplantation; AIDS-related aphthous stomatitis; Behçet's syndrome; Waldenström's macroglobulinemia; Langerhans cell histiocytosis; may be effective in rheumatoid arthritis, discoid lupus erythematosus, and erythema multiforme

Restrictions Thalidomide is approved for marketing only under a special distribution program. This program, called the "System for Thalidomide Education and Prescribing Safety" (STEPS® 1-888-423-5436), has been approved by the FDA. Prescribers and pharmacists must be registered with the program. No more than a 4-week supply should be dispensed. Blister packs should be dispensed intact (do not repackage capsules). Prescriptions must be filled within 7 days. Subsequent prescriptions may be filled only if fewer than 7 days of therapy remain on the previous prescription. A new prescription is required for further dispensing (a telephone prescription may not be accepted.)

Pregnancy Risk Factor X

Pregnancy Considerations **[U.S. Boxed Warning]: Thalidomide is a known teratogen; effective contraception must be used for at least 4 weeks before initiating therapy, during therapy, and for 4 weeks following discontinuation of thalidomide for women of childbearing potential.** Embryotoxic with limb defects noted from the 27th to 40th gestational day of exposure; all cases of phocomelia occur from the 27th to 42nd gestational day; fetal cardiac, gastrointestinal, bone, external ear, eye, and genitourinary tract abnormalities have also been described. Mortality at or shortly after birth has also been reported. Either abstinence or two forms of effective contraception must be used for at least 4 weeks before initiating therapy, during therapy, and for 4 weeks following discontinuation of thalidomide. A negative pregnancy test (sensitivity of at least 50 mIU/mL) within 24 hours prior to beginning therapy, weekly during the first 4 weeks, and every 4 weeks (every 2 weeks for women with irregular menstrual cycles) thereafter is required for women of childbearing potential. Males (even those vasectomized) must use a latex condom during any sexual contact with women of childbearing age. Risk to the fetus from semen of male patients is unknown. Thalidomide must be immediately discontinued and the patient referred to a reproductive toxicity specialist if pregnancy occurs during treatment. Any suspected fetal exposure to thalidomide must be reported to the FDA via the MedWatch program (1-800-FDA-1088) and to Celgene Corporation (1-888-423-5436).

Lactation Excretion in breast milk unknown/not recommended

Medication Safety Issues

Sound-alike/look-alike issues:

Thalidomide may be confused with flutamide

High alert medication: The Institute for Safe Medication Practices (ISMP) includes this medication among its list of drugs which have a heightened risk of causing significant patient harm when used in error.

International issues:

Thalomid® may be confused with Thilomide® which is a brand name for lodoxamide in Greece and Turkey

Contraindications Hypersensitivity to thalidomide or any component of the formulation; neuropathy (peripheral); patient unable to comply with STEPS® program (including males); women of childbearing potential unless alternative therapies are inappropriate and adequate precautions are taken to avoid pregnancy; pregnancy

Warnings/Precautions Hazardous agent - use appropriate precautions for handling and disposal. **[U.S. Boxed Warning]: Thalidomide is a known teratogen; effective contraception must be used for at least 4 weeks before initiating therapy, during therapy, and for 4 weeks following discontinuation of thalidomide for women of childbearing potential.** Use caution with drugs which may decrease the efficacy of hormonal contraceptives.

[U.S. Boxed Warning]: Thrombotic events have been reported, generally in patients with other risk factors for thrombosis (neoplastic disease, inflammatory disease, or concurrent therapy with combination chemotherapy. Use in combination with dexamethasone is associated with increased risk for deep vein thrombosis (DVT) and pulmonary embolism (PE), monitor for signs and symptoms of thromboembolism; patients at risk may benefit from prophylactic anticoagulation or aspirin.

May cause sedation; patients must be warned to use caution when performing tasks which require alertness. Use caution in patients with renal or hepatic impairment, neurological disorders, or constipation. Thalidomide has been associated with the development of peripheral neuropathy, which may be irreversible; use caution with other medications which may cause peripheral neuropathy. Consider immediate discontinuation (if clinically appropriate) in patients who develop neuropathy. May cause seizures; use caution in patients with a history of seizures, concurrent therapy with drugs which alter seizure threshold, or conditions which predispose to seizures. May cause neutropenia; discontinue therapy if absolute neutrophil count decreases to $<750/mm^3$. Use caution in patients with HIV infection; has been associated with increased viral loads. May cause orthostasis and/or bradycardia; use with caution in patients with cardiovascular disease or in patients who would not tolerate transient hypotensive episodes. Hypersensitivity, Stevens-Johnson syndrome (SJS) and toxic epidermal necrolysis (TEN) have been reported; withhold therapy and evaluate with skin rashes; permanently discontinue if rash is exfoliative, purpuric, bullous or if SJS or TEN is suspected. Safety and efficacy have not been established in children <12 years of age.

Adverse Reactions

>10%:

Cardiovascular: Edema (57%), thrombosis/embolism (23%; grade 3: 13%, grade 4: 9%), hypotension (16%)

Central nervous system: Fatigue (79%; grade 3: 3%, grade 4: 1%), somnolence (36% to 38%), dizziness (4% to 20%), sensory neuropathy (54%), confusion (28%), anxiety/agitation (9% to 26%), fever (19% to 23%), motor neuropathy (22%), headache (13% to 19%)

Dermatologic: Rash (21% to 31%), rash/desquamation (30%; grade 3: 4%), dry skin (21%), maculopapular rash (4% to 19%), acne (3% to 11%)

Endocrine & metabolic: Hypocalcemia (72%)

Gastrointestinal: Constipation (3% to 55%), anorexia (3% to 28%), nausea (4% to 24%), weight loss (23%), weight gain (22%), diarrhea (4% to 19%), oral moniliasis (4% to 11%)

Hematologic: Leukopenia (17% to 35%), neutropenia (31%), anemia (6% to 13%), lymphadenopathy (6% to 13%)

Hepatic: AST increased (3% to 25%), bilirubin increased (14%)

Neuromuscular & skeletal: Muscle weakness (40%), tremor (4% to 26%), weakness (6% to 22%), myalgia (17%), paresthesia (6% to 16%), arthralgia (13%)

Renal: Hematuria (11%)

Respiratory: Dyspnea (42%)

Miscellaneous: Diaphoresis (13%)

1% to 10%:

Cardiovascular: Facial edema (4%), peripheral edema (3% to 8%)

Central nervous system: Insomnia (9%), nervousness (3% to 9%), malaise (8%), vertigo (8%), pain (3% to 8%)

Dermatologic: Dermatitis (fungal 4% to 9%), pruritus (3% to 8%), nail disorder (3% to 4%)

Endocrine & metabolic: Hyperlipemia (6% to 9%)

Gastrointestinal: Xerostomia (8% to 9%), flatulence (8%), tooth pain (4%)

Genitourinary: Impotence (3% to 8%)

Hepatic: LFTs abnormal (9%)

Neuromuscular & skeletal: Neuropathy (8%), back pain (4% to 6%), neck pain (4%), neck rigidity (4%)

Renal: Albuminuria (3% to 8%)

Respiratory: Pharyngitis (4% to 8%), rhinitis (4%), sinusitis (4% to 8%)

Miscellaneous: Infection (6% to 8%)

Postmarketing and/or case reports (limited to important or life-threatening): Acute renal failure, alkaline phosphatase increased, ALT increased, amenorrhea, aphthous stomatitis, arrhythmia, atrial fibrillation, bile duct obstruction, bradycardia, BUN increased, carpal tunnel, CML, creatinine clearance decreased, creatinine increased, deafness, depression, diplopia, dysesthesia, ECG abnormalities, electrolyte imbalances, enuresis, eosinophilia, epistaxis, erythema multiforme, erythema nodosum, erythroleukemia, exfoliative dermatitis, febrile neutropenia, foot drop, galactorrhea, granulocytopenia, gynecomastia, hepatomegaly, Hodgkin's disease, hypercalcemia, hyper-/hypokalemia, hypersensitivity, hypertension, hyper-/hypothyroidism, hyperuricemia, hypomagnesemia, hyponatremia, hypoproteinemia, intestinal obstruction, intestinal perforation, interstitial pneumonitis, LDH increased, lethargy, leukocytosis, lymphedema, lymphopenia, mental status changes, metrorrhagia, migraine, myxedema, nystagmus, oliguria, orthostatic hypotension, pancytopenia, paresthesia, petechiae, peripheral neuritis, photosensitivity, pleural effusion, prothrombin time changes, psychosis, pulmonary embolus, pulmonary hypertension, purpura, Raynaud's syndrome, seizure, status epilepticus, Stevens-Johnson syndrome, stomach ulcer, stupor, suicide attempt, syncope, tachycardia, thrombocytopenia, toxic epidermal necrolysis, tumor lysis syndrome

Drug Interactions

Avoid Concomitant Use

Avoid concomitant use of Thalidomide with any of the following: Anakinra; Natalizumab; Rilonacept; Vaccines (Live)

Increased Effect/Toxicity

Thalidomide may increase the levels/effects of: Abatacept; Alcohol (Ethyl); Anakinra; CNS Depressants; Natalizumab; Pamidronate; Rilonacept; Vaccines (Live); Zoledronic Acid

The levels/effects of Thalidomide may be increased by: Dexamethasone; Trastuzumab

Decreased Effect

Thalidomide may decrease the levels/effects of: Vaccines (Inactivated)

The levels/effects of Thalidomide may be decreased by: Echinacea

Ethanol/Nutrition/Herb Interactions

Ethanol: Avoid ethanol (may increase sedation).

Herb/Nutraceutical: Avoid cat's claw and echinacea (have immunostimulant properties; consider therapy modifications).

Stability Store at 15°C to 30°C (50°F to 86°F). Protect from light. Keep in original package.

Mechanism of Action Has immunomodulatory and antiangiogenic characteristics. Immunologic effects may vary based on conditions; may suppress excessive tumor necrosis factor-alpha production in patients with ENL, yet may increase plasma tumor necrosis factor-alpha levels in HIV-positive patients. In multiple myeloma, thalidomide is associated with an increase in natural killer cells and increased levels of interleukin-2 and interferon gamma. Other proposed mechanisms of action include suppression of angiogenesis, prevention of free-radical-mediated DNA damage, increased cell mediated cytotoxic effects, and altered expression of cellular.

Pharmacodynamics/Kinetics

Distribution: V_d: 120 L

Protein binding: 55% to 66%

Metabolism: Nonenzymatic hydrolysis in plasma; forms multiple metabolites

Half-life elimination: 5-7 hours

Time to peak, plasma: 3-6 hours

Excretion: Urine (<1% as unchanged drug)

Dosage Oral:

Multiple myeloma: 200 mg once daily (with dexamethasone 40 mg daily on days 1-4, 9-12, and 17-20 of a 28-day treatment cycle)

Cutaneous ENL:

Initial: 100-300 mg/day taken once daily at bedtime with water (at least 1 hour after evening meal)

Patients weighing <50 kg: Initiate at lower end of the dosing range

Severe cutaneous reaction or patients previously requiring high dose may be initiated at 400 mg/day; doses may be divided, but taken 1 hour after meals

Maintenance: Dosing should continue until active reaction subsides (usually at least 2 weeks), then tapered in 50 mg decrements every 2-4 weeks

Patients who flare during tapering or with a history or requiring prolonged maintenance should be maintained on the minimum dosage necessary to control the reaction. Efforts to taper should be repeated every 3-6 months, in increments of 50 mg every 2-4 weeks.

Behçet's syndrome (unlabeled use): 100-400 mg/day

Graft-vs-host reactions (unlabeled use): 100-1600 mg/day; usual initial dose: 200 mg 4 times/day for use up to 700 days

AIDS-related aphthous stomatitis (unlabeled use): 200 mg twice daily for 5 days, then 200 mg/day for up to 8 weeks

Discoid lupus erythematosus (unlabeled use): 100-400 mg/day; maintenance dose: 25-50 mg

Dietary Considerations Should be taken at least 1 hour after the evening meal.

Administration Oral: Administer with water, preferably at bedtime once daily on an empty stomach, at least 1 hour after the evening meal. Doses >400 mg/day may be given in 2-3 divided doses. Avoid extensive handling of capsules; capsules should remain in blister pack until ingestion. If exposed to the powder content from broken capsules or body fluids from patients receiving thalidomide, the exposed area should be washed with soap and water.

Monitoring Parameters CBC with differential, platelets; signs of neuropathy monthly for the first 3 months, then periodically during treatment; consider monitoring of sensory nerve application potential amplitudes (at baseline and every 6 months) to detect asymptomatic neuropathy. In HIV-seropositive patients: viral load after 1 and 3 months, then every 3 months. Pregnancy testing (sensitivity of at least 50 mIU/mL) is required within 24 hours prior to initiation of therapy, weekly during the first 4 weeks, then every 4 weeks in women with regular menstrual cycles or every 2 weeks in women with irregular menstrual cycles.

Reference Range Therapeutic plasma thalidomide levels in graft-vs-host reactions are 5-8 mcg/mL, although it has been suggested that lower plasma levels (0.5-1.5 mcg/mL) may be therapeutic; peak serum thalidomide level after a 200 mg dose: 1.2 mcg/mL

Dosage Forms Excipient information presented when available (limited, particularly for generics); consult specific product labeling.

Capsule:

Thalomid®: 50 mg, 100 mg, 200 mg

◆ **Thalitone®** *see* Chlorthalidone *on page 318*

◆ **Thalomid®** *see* Thalidomide *on page 1453*

◆ **THAM®** *see* Tromethamine *on page 1524*

◆ **THC** *see* Dronabinol *on page 494*

◆ **Theo-24®** *see* Theophylline *on page 1455*

◆ **TheoCap™** *see* Theophylline *on page 1455*

◆ **Theochron™** *see* Theophylline *on page 1455*

◆ **Theochron® SR (Can)** *see* Theophylline *on page 1455*

Theophylline (thee OFF i lin)

U.S. Brand Names Elixophyllin®; Theo-24®; TheoCap™; Theochron™; Uniphyl®

Canadian Brand Names Apo-Theo LA®; Novo-Theophyl SR; PMS-Theophylline; Pulmophylline; ratio-Theo-Bronc; Theochron® SR; Uniphyl® SRT

Index Terms Theophylline Anhydrous

Pharmacologic Category Theophylline Derivative

Additional Appendix Information

Asthma *on page 1793*

Use Treatment of symptoms and reversible airway obstruction due to chronic asthma, or other chronic lung diseases; apnea of prematurity

Note: The National Heart, Lung, and Blood Institute Guidelines (2007) do not recommend oral theophylline as a long-term control medication for asthma in children ≤4years of age; use may be considered as an alternative (but not preferred) agent in older children and adults. The guidelines do not recommend theophylline I.V. for the treatment of exacerbations of asthma.

Pregnancy Risk Factor C

Pregnancy Considerations Adverse events were observed in animal reproduction studies. Theophylline crosses the placenta; adverse effects may be seen in the newborn. Use is generally safe when used at the recommended doses (serum concentrations 5-12 mcg/mL) however maternal adverse events may be increased and efficacy may be decreased in pregnant women. Theophylline metabolism may change during pregnancy; the half-life is similar to that observed in otherwise healthy, nonsmoking adults with asthma during the first and second trimesters (~8.7 hours), but may increase to 13 hours (range 8-18 hours) during the third trimester. The volume of distribution is also increased during the third trimester. Monitor serum levels. The recommendations for the use of theophylline in pregnant women with asthma are similar to those used in nonpregnant adults (National Heart, Lung, and Blood Institute Guidelines, 2004).

Lactation Enters breast milk/compatible (AAP rates "compatible")

Contraindications Hypersensitivity to theophylline or any component of the formulation; premixed injection may contain corn-derived dextrose and its use is contraindicated in patients with allergy to corn-related products

Warnings/Precautions If a patient develops signs and symptoms of theophylline toxicity (eg, persistent, repetitive vomiting), a serum theophylline level should be measured and subsequent doses held. Due to potential saturation of theophylline clearance at serum levels in or (in some patients) less than the therapeutic range, dosage adjustment should be made in small increments (maximum: 25%). Due to wider interpatient variability, theophylline serum level measurements must be used to optimize therapy and prevent serious toxicity. Use with caution in patients with peptic ulcer, hyperthyroidism, seizure disorders, and patients with tachyarrhythmias (eg, sinus tachycardia, atrial fibrillation); use may exacerbate these conditions. Theophylline clearance may be decreased in patients with acute pulmonary edema, congestive heart failure, cor-pulmonale, fever, hepatic disease, acute hepatitis, cirrhosis, hypothyroidism, sepsis with multiorgan failure, and shock; clearance may also be decreased in neonates, infants <3 months of age with decreased renal function, children <1 year of age, the elderly >60 years of age, and patients following cessation of smoking.

Adverse Reactions Frequency not defined. Adverse events observed at therapeutic serum levels:

Cardiovascular: Flutter, tachycardia

Central nervous system: Headache, hyperactivity (children), insomnia, restlessness, seizures

Endocrine & metabolic: Hypercalcemia (with concomitant hyperthyroid disease)

Gastrointestinal: Nausea, reflux or ulcer aggravation, vomiting

Genitourinary: Difficulty urinating (elderly males with prostatism)

Neuromuscular & skeletal: Tremor

Renal: Diuresis (transient)

Drug Interactions

Metabolism/Transport Effects **Substrate** of CYP1A2 (major), 2C9 (minor), 2D6 (minor), 2E1 (major), 3A4 (major); **Inhibits** CYP1A2 (weak)

Avoid Concomitant Use

Avoid concomitant use of Theophylline with any of the following: Iobenguane I 123

Increased Effect/Toxicity

Theophylline may increase the levels/effects of: Sympathomimetics

The levels/effects of Theophylline may be increased by: Allopurinol; Cannabinoids; Cimetidine; CYP1A2 Inhibitors (Moderate); CYP1A2 Inhibitors (Strong); CYP2E1 Inhibitors (Moderate); CYP3A4 Inhibitors (Moderate); CYP3A4 Inhibitors (Strong); Dasatinib; Disulfiram; Fluvoxamine; Interferons; Isoniazid; Macrolide Antibiotics; Mexiletine; Pentoxifylline; Quinolone Antibiotics; Tacrine; Thiabendazole; Ticlopidine; Zileuton

Decreased Effect

Theophylline may decrease the levels/effects of: Adenosine; Benzodiazepines; Iobenguane I 123; Lithium; Phenytoin; Regadenoson; Zafirlukast

The levels/effects of Theophylline may be decreased by: Aminoglutethimide; Barbiturates; Beta-Blockers (Beta1 Selective); Beta-Blockers (Nonselective); CarBAMazepine; CYP1A2 Inducers (Strong); CYP3A4 Inducers (Strong); Deferasirox; Herbs (CYP3A4 Inducers); Moricizine; Phenytoin; Protease Inhibitors; Thyroid Products

Ethanol/Nutrition/Herb Interactions Food: Food does not appreciably affect the absorption of liquid, fast-release products, and most sustained release products; however, food may induce a sudden release (dose-dumping) of once-daily sustained release products resulting in an increase in serum drug levels and potential toxicity. Avoid excessive amounts of caffeine. Avoid extremes of dietary protein and carbohydrate intake. Changes in diet may affect the elimination of theophylline; charbroiled foods may increase elimination, reducing half-life by 50%.

Stability Elixir, tablet, premixed infusion: Store at controlled room temperature of 25°C (77°F).

Mechanism of Action Causes bronchodilatation, diuresis, CNS and cardiac stimulation, and gastric acid secretion by blocking phosphodiesterase which increases tissue concentrations of cyclic adenine monophosphate (cAMP) which in turn promotes catecholamine stimulation of lipolysis, glycogenolysis, and gluconeogenesis and induces release of epinephrine from adrenal medulla cells

Pharmacodynamics/Kinetics

Absorption: Oral: Dosage form dependent

Distribution: 0.45 L/kg based on ideal body weight; distributes poorly into body fat; V_d may increase in premature neonates, patients with hepatic cirrhosis, acidemia (uncorrected), the elderly

Metabolism: Children >1 year and Adults: Hepatic; involves CYP1A2, 2E1 and 3A4; forms active metabolites (caffeine and 3-methylxanthine)

Protein binding: 40%, primarily to albumin

Half-life elimination: Highly variable and dependent upon age, liver function, cardiac function, lung disease, and smoking history

- Premature infants, postnatal age 3-15 days: 30 hours (range: 17-43 hours)
- Premature infants, postnatal age 25-57 days: 20 hours (range: 9.4-30.6 hours)
- Children 6-17 years: 3.7 hours (range: 1.5-5.9 hours)
- Adults 16-60 years with asthma, nonsmoking, otherwise healthy: 8.7 hours (range: 6.1-12.8 hours)

Time to peak, serum:

- Oral: Liquid: 1 hour; Tablet, enteric-coated: 5 hours; Tablet, uncoated: 2 hours
- I.V.: Within 30 minutes

Excretion: Urine

- Neonates: 50% as unchanged theophylline
- Children >3 months and Adults: ~10% as unchanged theophylline

Dosage Note: Doses should be individualized based on peak serum concentrations and should be based on ideal body weight.

Acute symptoms: Loading dose: Children and Adults: Oral, I.V.:

If no theophylline received within the previous 24 hours: 4.6 mg/kg loading dose (~5.8 mg/kg hydrous aminophylline) I.V. or 5 mg/kg orally. Loading dose intended to achieve a serum level of approximately 10 mcg/mL; loading doses should be given intravenously (preferred) or with a rapidly absorbed oral product (not an extended-release product). **Note:** On the average, for every 1 mg/kg theophylline given, blood levels will rise 2 mcg/mL.

If theophylline has been administered in the previous 24 hours: A loading dose is not recommended without obtaining a serum theophylline concentration. The loading dose should be calculated as follows:

Dose = (desired serum theophylline concentration - measured serum theophylline concentration) (V_d)

Acute symptoms: Maintenance dose: Children and Adults: I.V.: **Note:** To achieve a target concentration of 10 mcg/mL unless otherwise noted. Lower initial doses may be required in patients with reduced theophylline clearance. Dosage should be adjusted according to serum level measurements during the first 12- to 24-hour period.

- Neonates ≤24 days: 1 mg/kg every 12 hours to achieve a target concentration of 7.5 mcg/mL for apnea of prematurity
- Neonates >24 days: 1.5 mg/kg every 12 hours to achieve a target concentration of 7.5 mcg/mL for apnea of prematurity
- Infants 6-52 weeks: mg/kg/hour = (0.008) (age in weeks) + 0.21
- Children 1-9 years: 0.8 mg/kg/hour
- Children 9-12 years: 0.7 mg/kg/hour
- Adolescents 12-16 years (cigarette or marijuana smokers): 0.7 mg/kg/hour
- Adolescents 12-16 years (nonsmokers): 0.5 mg/kg/hour; maximum 900 mg/day unless serum levels indicate need for larger dose
- Adults 16-60 years (otherwise healthy, nonsmokers): 0.4 mg/kg/hour; maximum 900 mg/day unless serum levels indicate need for larger dose
- Adults >60 years: 0.3 mg/kg/hour; maximum 400 mg/day unless serum levels indicate need for larger dose
- Cardiac decompensation, cor pulmonale, hepatic dysfunction, sepsis with multiorgan failure, shock: 0.2 mg/kg/hour; maximum 400 mg/day unless serum levels indicate need for larger dose

Treatment of chronic conditions: Oral:

Infants <1 year: **Note:** Doses should be adjusted to maintain the peak steady state serum concentrations. The time to reach steady state will vary based on age and the presence of risk factors which may affect theophylline clearance. Theophylline serum levels obtained prior to reaching steady state should not be used to increase the maintenance dose even if the serum concentration is <10 mcg/mL. Peak steady state theophylline serum concentrations should be 5-10 mcg/mL in neonates and 10-15 mcg/mL in older infants.

- Premature Neonates <24 days postnatal age: 1 mg/kg/dose every 12 hours
- Premature Neonates ≥24 days postnatal age: 1.5 mg/kg/dose every 12 hours
- Full-term Infants and Infants <26 weeks: Total daily dose (mg)= [(0.2 x age in weeks) +5] x (weight in kg); divide dose into 3 equal amounts and administer at 8-hour intervals
- Full-term Infants and Infants ≥26 weeks and <52 weeks: Total daily dose (mg) = [(0.2 x age in weeks) +5] x (weight in kg); divide dose into 4 equal amounts and administer at 6-hour intervals

Children 1-15 years and <45 kg **without** risk factors for impaired theophylline clearance: 12-14 mg/kg/day in divided doses, every 4-6 hours for 3 days (maximum dose: 300 mg/day), then increase to 16 mg/kg/day in divided doses every 4-6 hours for 3 days (maximum dose: 400 mg/day); maintenance dose: 20 mg/kg/day in divided doses every 4-6 hours (maximum dose: 600 mg/day)

Increase dose only if tolerated. Consider lowering dose or using a slower titration if caffeine-like adverse events occur. Smaller doses given more frequently may be used in patients with a more rapid metabolism to prevent breakthrough symptoms which could occur due to low trough concentration prior to the next dose. Reliably absorbed slow release formulations can be used to decrease serum fluctuations and permit longer dosing intervals.

Adults 16-60 years **without** risk factors for impaired theophylline clearance: 300 mg/day in divided doses every 6-8 hours for 3 days, then increase to 400 mg/day in divided doses every 6-8 hours for 3 days; maintenance dose: 600 mg/day in divided doses every 6-8 hours

Increase dose only if tolerated. Consider lowering dose or using a slower titration if caffeine-like adverse events occur. Smaller doses given more frequently may be used in patients with a more rapid metabolism to prevent breakthrough symptoms which could occur due to low trough concentration prior to the next dose. Reliably absorbed slow release formulations can be used to decrease serum fluctuations and permit longer dosing intervals.

Dose adjustment in patients **with** risk factors for impaired theophylline clearance and patients in whom monitoring serum theophylline levels is not feasible:

Children 1-15 years: Do not exceed a dose of 16 mg/kg/day or 400 mg/day

Children ≥16 and Adults: Do not exceed a dose of 400 mg/day

Dose adjustment in the elderly (>60 years): Do not exceed a dose of 400 mg/day

Dosage adjustment after serum theophylline measurement:

Within normal limits: 10-19.9 mcg/mL: Maintain dosage if tolerated. Recheck serum theophylline concentration at 24-hour intervals (for acute I.V. dosing) or at 6- to 12-month intervals (for oral dosing). Finer adjustments in dosage may be needed for some patients. If levels ≥15 mcg/mL, consider 10% dose reduction to improve safety margin.

Too high:

20-24.9 mcg/mL: Decrease doses by about 25%. Recheck serum theophylline concentrations (see "Note").

25-30 mcg/mL: Skip next dose (oral) or stop infusion for 12 hours (children) or 24 hours (adults) and decrease subsequent doses by about 25%. Recheck serum theophylline concentrations (see **"Note"**).

>30 mcg/mL: Stop dosing and treat overdose; if resumed, decrease subsequent doses by 50%. Recheck serum theophylline concentrations (see "Note").

Too low: <9.9 mcg/mL: If tolerated, but symptoms remain, increase dose by about 25%. Recheck serum theophylline concentrations (see **"Note"**).

Note: Recheck serum theophylline levels after 3 days when using oral dosing, or after 12 hours (children) or 24 hours (adults) when dosing intravenously. Patients maintained with oral therapy may be reassessed at 6- to 12-month intervals.

Dietary Considerations Should be taken with water 1 hour before or 2 hours after meals. Premixed injection may contain corn-derived dextrose and its use is contraindicated in patients with allergy to corn-related products.

Administration Oral: Long-acting preparations should be taken with a full glass of water, swallowed whole, or cut in half if scored. Do **not** crush. Extended release capsule forms may be opened and the contents sprinkled on soft foods; do **not** chew beads.

Monitoring Parameters Monitor heart rate, CNS effects (insomnia, irritability); respiratory rate (COPD patients often have resting controlled respiratory rates in low 20s); arterial or capillary blood gases (if applicable)

Theophylline levels: Serum theophylline levels should be monitored prior to making dose increases; in the presence of signs or symptoms of toxicity; or when a new illness, worsening of a present illness, or medication changes occur that may change theophylline clearance

I.V. loading dose: Measure serum concentrations 30 minutes after the end of an I.V. loading dose

I.V. infusion: Measure serum concentrations one half-life after starting a continuous infusion, then every 12-24 hours

Reference Range Therapeutic levels:

Asthma: 5-15 mcg/mL (peak level)

Toxic concentration: >20 mcg/mL

Test Interactions Plasma glucose, uric acid, free fatty acids, total cholesterol, HDL, HDL/LDL ratio, and urinary free cortisol excretion may be increased by theophylline. Theophylline may decrease triiodothyronine.

Dosage Forms Excipient information presented when available (limited, particularly for generics); consult specific product labeling.

Capsule, extended release:

TheoCap™: 125 mg, 200 mg [12 hour]

Theo-24®: 100 mg, 200 mg, 300 mg, 400 mg [24 hours]

Elixir:

Elixophyllin®: 80 mg/15 mL (473 mL) [contains alcohol 20%; mixed fruit flavor]

Infusion [premixed in D_5W]: 200 mg (50 mL, 100 mL); 400 mg (250 mL, 500 mL); 800 mg (250 mL, 500 mL, 1000 mL)

Tablet, controlled release:

Uniphyl®: 400 mg, 600 mg [24 hours]

Tablet, extended release: 100 mg, 200 mg, 300 mg, 400 mg, 450 mg, 600 mg

Theochron™: 100 mg, 200 mg, 300 mg, 450 mg [12-24 hours]

Theophylline and Guaifenesin

(thee OFF i lin & gwye FEN e sin)

U.S. Brand Names Elixophyllin-GG®; Quibron® [DSC]

Index Terms Guaifenesin and Theophylline

Pharmacologic Category Theophylline Derivative

Use Symptomatic treatment of bronchospasm associated with bronchial asthma, chronic bronchitis, and pulmonary emphysema

Pregnancy Risk Factor C

Dosage Adults: Oral: 16 mg/kg/day or 400 mg theophylline/day, in divided doses, every 6-8 hours

Additional Information Complete prescribing information for this medication should be consulted for additional detail.

Dosage Forms Excipient information presented when available (limited, particularly for generics); consult specific product labeling. [DSC] = Discontinued product

Capsule:

Quibron®: Theophylline 150 mg and guaifenesin 90 mg [DSC]

Liquid:

Elixophyllin-GG®: Theophylline 100 mg and guaifenesin 100 mg per 15 mL (240 mL, 480 mL) [alcohol free, dye free, sugar free; cherry-berry flavor]

◆ **Theophylline Anhydrous** *see* Theophylline *on page 1455*

◆ **TheraCys®** *see* BCG Vaccine *on page 176*

◆ **Thera-Flur-N® [DSC]** *see* Fluoride *on page 635*

◆ **Thermazene®** *see* Silver Sulfadiazine *on page 1370*

Thiabendazole (thye a BEN da zole)

U.S. Brand Names Mintezol®

Index Terms Tiabendazole

Pharmacologic Category Anthelmintic

Use Treatment of strongyloidiasis, cutaneous larva migrans, visceral larva migrans, dracunculiasis, trichinosis, and mixed helminthic infections

Unlabeled/Investigational Use Cutaneous larva migrans (topical application)

Pregnancy Risk Factor C

Pregnancy Considerations Cleft palate and skeletal defects were observed in some animal studies. There are no adequate and well-controlled studies in pregnant women.

Lactation Excretion in breast milk unknown/not recommended

Contraindications Hypersensitivity to thiabendazole or any component of the formulation; not for use as prophylactic treatment of enterobiasis (pinworm) infestation

Warnings/Precautions Erythema multiforme and Stevens-Johnson syndrome have been reported (including fatalities); discontinue at first sign of reaction. Use with caution in patients with renal or hepatic impairment, malnutrition or anemia, or dehydration. Causes sedation; caution must be used in performing tasks which require alertness. Not suitable treatment for mixed infections with *Ascaris*. Ophthalmic changes may occur and persist >1 year. Safety and efficacy are limited in children <14 kg (30 lb).

Adverse Reactions Frequency not defined.

Central nervous system: Chills, delirium, dizziness, drowsiness, hallucinations, headache, seizure

Dermatologic: Angioedema, pruritus, rash, Stevens-Johnson syndrome

Endocrine & metabolic: Hyperglycemia

Gastrointestinal: Abdominal pain, anorexia, diarrhea, drying of mucous membranes, nausea, vomiting

Genitourinary: Crystalluria, enuresis, hematuria, malodor of urine

Hematologic: Leukopenia

Hepatic: Cholestasis, hepatic failure, hepatotoxicity, jaundice

Neuromuscular & skeletal: Incoordination, numbness

Ocular: Abnormal sensation in eyes, blurred vision, dry eyes, Sicca syndrome, vision decreased, xanthopsia

Otic: Tinnitus

Renal: Nephrotoxicity

Miscellaneous: Anaphylaxis, hypersensitivity reactions, lymphadenopathy

Drug Interactions

Metabolism/Transport Effects **Substrate** of CYP1A2 (minor); **Inhibits** CYP1A2 (strong)

Avoid Concomitant Use There are no known interactions where it is recommended to avoid concomitant use.

Increased Effect/Toxicity

Thiabendazole may increase the levels/effects of: Bendamustine; CYP1A2 Substrates; Theophylline Derivatives

Decreased Effect

The levels/effects of Thiabendazole may be decreased by: Aminoquinolines (Antimalarial)

Mechanism of Action Inhibits helminth-specific mitochondrial fumarate reductase

Pharmacodynamics/Kinetics

Absorption: Rapid and well absorbed

Metabolism: Rapidly hepatic; metabolized to 5-hydroxy form

Half-life elimination: 1.2 hours

Time to peak, plasma: Oral suspension: Within 1-2 hours

Excretion: Urine (90%) and feces (5%) primarily as conjugated metabolites

Dosage Purgation is not required prior to use; drinking of fruit juice aids in expulsion of worms by removing the mucous to which the intestinal tapeworms attach themselves.

Children and Adults:

Oral: 50 mg/kg/day divided every 12 hours (if >68 kg: 1.5 g/dose); maximum dose: 3 g/day

Treatment duration:

Strongyloidiasis, ascariasis, uncinariasis: For 2 consecutive days

Cutaneous larva migrans: For 2 consecutive days; if active lesions are still present 2 days after completion, a second course of treatment is recommended.

Visceral larva migrans: For 7 consecutive days

Trichinosis: For 2-4 consecutive days; optimal dosage not established

Dracunculosis: 50-75 mg/kg/day divided every 12 hours for 3 days

Topical (unlabeled): Cutaneous larva migrans: Apply directly to larval tracks 2-3 times/day for up to 2 weeks; application frequencies may range from 2-6 times/day. **Note:** Not available as a topical formulation; oral suspension (10% to 15%) has been used topically, as well as a number of extemporaneous formulations.

Dosing comments in renal/hepatic impairment: Use with caution

Monitoring Parameters Periodic renal and hepatic function tests

Dosage Forms Excipient information presented when available (limited, particularly for generics); consult specific product labeling. [DSC] = Discontinued product

Suspension, oral: 500 mg/5 mL (120 mL) [DSC]

Tablet, chewable: 500 mg [orange flavor]

Extemporaneous Preparations Topical application of thiabendazole has been recommended for the treatment of cutaneous larva migrans (*Redbook*, 2003; *Med Letter*, 2002). In some cases, the commercially-available 10% oral suspension has been used for topical application. Alternatively, a number of extemporaneous preparations have used crushed tablets to prepare distinct formulations. These include a 10% ointment (in white petrolatum), a 15% topical lotion (suspended with compound tragacanth powder 250 mg/40 mL), a 15% cream (in either hydrophilic or fat-based creams), and topical solutions (2% to 4% in DMSO). The stability of these formulations has not been established, and there are no comparative studies evaluating different formulations. All preparations have been applied between 2-6 times daily for up to 2 weeks.

◆ **Thiamazole** *see* Methimazole *on page 963*

◆ **Thiamin** *see* Thiamine *on page 1458*

Thiamine (THYE a min)

Canadian Brand Names Betaxin®

Index Terms Aneurine Hydrochloride; Thiamin; Thiamine Hydrochloride; Thiaminium Chloride Hydrochloride; Vitamin B_1

Pharmacologic Category Vitamin, Water Soluble

Use Treatment of thiamine deficiency including beriberi, Wernicke's encephalopathy, Korsakoff's syndrome, neuritis associated with pregnancy, or in alcoholic patients; dietary supplement

Pregnancy Risk Factor A/C (dose exceeding RDA recommendation)

Medication Safety Issues

Sound-alike/look-alike issues:

Thiamine may be confused with Tenormin®, Thorazine®

International issues:

Doxal® [Brazil] may be confused with Doxil® which is a brand name for doxorubicin in the U.S.

Doxal® [Brazil]: Brand name for doxycycline in Austria; brand name for pyridoxine in Brazil; brand name for doxepin in Finland

Dosage

Adequate Intake:

0-6 months: 0.2 mg/day

7-12 months: 0.3 mg/day

Recommended daily intake:

1-3 years: 0.5 mg

4-8 years: 0.6 mg

9-13 years: 0.9 mg

14-18 years: Female: 1 mg; Male: 1.2 mg

≥19 years: Female: 1.1 mg; Male: 1.2 mg

Pregnancy, lactation: 1.4 mg

Parenteral nutrition supplementation:

Infants: 1.2 mg/day

Adults: 6 mg/day; may be increased to 25-50 mg/day with history of alcohol abuse

Thiamine deficiency (beriberi):

Children: 10-25 mg/dose I.M. or I.V. daily (if critically ill), or 10-50 mg/dose orally every day for 2 weeks, then 5-10 mg/dose orally daily for 1 month

Adults: 5-30 mg/dose I.M. or I.V. 3 times/day (if critically ill); then orally 5-30 mg/day in single or divided doses 3 times/day for 1 month

Alcohol withdrawal syndrome: Adults: 100 mg/day I.M. or I.V. for several days, followed by 50-100 mg/day orally

Wernicke's encephalopathy: Adults: Treatment: Initial: 100 mg I.V., then 50-100 mg/day I.M. or I.V. until consuming a regular, balanced diet. Larger doses may be needed in patients with alcohol abuse.

Additional Information Complete prescribing information for this medication should be consulted for additional detail.

Dosage Forms Excipient information presented when available (limited, particularly for generics); consult specific product labeling.

Injection, solution, as hydrochloride: 100 mg/mL (2 mL)

Tablet, as hydrochloride: 50 mg, 100 mg, 250 mg, 500 mg

◆ **Thiamine Hydrochloride** *see* Thiamine *on page 1458*

◆ **Thiaminium Chloride Hydrochloride** *see* Thiamine *on page 1458*

Thioguanine (thye oh GWAH neen)

U.S. Brand Names Tabloid®

Canadian Brand Names Lanvis®

Index Terms 2-Amino-6-Mercaptopurine; 6-TG (error-prone abbreviation); 6-Thioguanine (error-prone abbreviation); NSC-752; TG; Tioguanine

Pharmacologic Category Antineoplastic Agent, Antimetabolite (Purine Antagonist)

Use Treatment of acute myelogenous (nonlymphocytic) leukemia; treatment of chronic myelogenous leukemia and granulocytic leukemia

Restrictions The I.V. formulation is not available in U.S.

Pregnancy Risk Factor D

Lactation Excretion in breast milk unknown

Medication Safety Issues

High alert medication: The Institute for Safe Medication Practices (ISMP) includes this medication among its list of drugs which have a heightened risk of causing significant patient harm when used in error.

6-thioguanine and 6-TG are error-prone abbreviations (associated with six-fold overdoses of thioguanine)

Contraindications Hypersensitivity to thioguanine or any component of the formulation; pregnancy

Warnings/Precautions Hazardous agent - use appropriate precautions for handling and disposal. Use with caution and reduce dose in patients with renal or hepatic impairment. Not recommended for long-term continuous therapy due to potential for hepatotoxicity (hepatic veno-occlusive disease). Discontinue in patients with evidence of hepatotoxicity. Thioguanine is potentially carcinogenic and teratogenic; myelosuppression may be delayed. Caution with history of previous therapy resistance with either thioguanine or mercaptopurine (there is usually complete cross resistance between these two). Patients with genetic deficiency of thiopurine methyltransferase (TPMT) or who are receiving drugs which inhibit this enzyme (mesalazine, olsalazine, sulfasalazine) may be highly sensitive to myelosuppressive effects.

Adverse Reactions

>10%: Hematologic: Myelosuppressive:

WBC: Moderate

Platelets: Moderate

Onset: 7-10 days

Nadir: 14 days

Recovery: 21 days

1% to 10%:

Dermatologic: Skin rash

Endocrine & metabolic: Hyperuricemia

Gastrointestinal: Mild nausea or vomiting, anorexia, stomatitis, diarrhea

Neuromuscular & skeletal: Unsteady gait

<1% (Limited to important or life-threatening): Ascites, esophageal varices, hepatic necrosis, hepatitis, jaundice, LFTs increased, neurotoxicity, photosensitivity, portal hypertension, splenomegaly, thrombocytopenia, veno-occlusive hepatic disease

Drug Interactions

Avoid Concomitant Use

Avoid concomitant use of Thioguanine with any of the following: Natalizumab; Vaccines (Live)

Increased Effect/Toxicity

Thioguanine may increase the levels/effects of: Natalizumab; Vaccines (Live)

The levels/effects of Thioguanine may be increased by: 5-ASA Derivatives; Trastuzumab

Decreased Effect

Thioguanine may decrease the levels/effects of: Vaccines (Inactivated)

The levels/effects of Thioguanine may be decreased by: Echinacea

Ethanol/Nutrition/Herb Interactions Food: Enhanced absorption if administered between meals.

Stability Store tablet at room temperature.

Mechanism of Action Purine analog that is incorporated into DNA and RNA resulting in the blockage of synthesis and metabolism of purine nucleotides

Pharmacodynamics/Kinetics

Absorption: 30% (highly variable)

Distribution: Crosses placenta

Metabolism: Hepatic; rapidly and extensively via TPMT to 2-amino-6-methylthioguanine (active) and inactive compounds

Half-life elimination: Terminal: 11 hours

Time to peak, serum: Within 8 hours

Excretion: Urine

Dosage Total daily dose can be given at one time.

Oral (refer to individual protocols):

Infants and Children <3 years: Combination drug therapy for acute nonlymphocytic leukemia: 3.3 mg/kg/day in divided doses twice daily for 4 days

Children and Adults: 2-3 mg/kg/day calculated to nearest 20 mg or 75-200 mg/m^2/day in 1-2 divided doses for 5-7 days or until remission is attained

Dosing comments in renal or hepatic impairment: Reduce dose

Monitoring Parameters CBC with differential and platelet count; liver function tests (weekly when beginning therapy then monthly, more frequently in patients with liver disease or concurrent hepatotoxic drugs); hemoglobin, hematocrit, serum uric acid; some laboratories offer testing for TPMT deficiency

Hepatotoxicity may present with signs of portal hypertension (splenomegaly, esophageal varices, thrombocytopenia) or veno-occlusive disease (fluid retention, ascites, hepatomegaly with tenderness, or hyperbilirubinemia)

Dosage Forms Excipient information presented when available (limited, particularly for generics); consult specific product labeling.

Tablet [scored]:

Tabloid®: 40 mg

Extemporaneous Preparations A 20 mg/mL oral suspension can be prepared by crushing fifteen 40 mg tablets in a mortar, and then adding 10 mL of methylcellulose 1% (in small amounts). Transfer to a graduate, then add a sufficient quantity of syrup to make 30 mL of suspension. Label "shake well." Room temperature stability is 60 days.

Dressman JB and Poust RI, "Stability of Allopurinol and Five Antineoplastics in Suspension," *Am J Hosp Pharm*, 1983, 40:616-8.

Nahata MC, Morosco RS, and Hipple TF, 4th ed, *Pediatric Drug Formulations*, Cincinnati, OH: Harvey Whitney Books Co, 2000.

◆ **6-Thioguanine (error-prone abbreviation)** *see* Thioguanine *on page 1459*

Thiopental (thye oh PEN tal)

U.S. Brand Names Pentothal®

Canadian Brand Names Pentothal®

Index Terms Thiopental Sodium

Pharmacologic Category Anticonvulsant, Barbiturate; Barbiturate; General Anesthetic

Use Induction of anesthesia; adjunct for intubation in head injury patients; control of convulsive states; treatment of elevated intracranial pressure

Restrictions C-III

Pregnancy Risk Factor C

Medication Safety Issues

High alert medication: The Institute for Safe Medication Practices (ISMP) includes this medication among its list of drugs which have a heightened risk of causing significant patient harm when used in error.

Contraindications Hypersensitivity to thiopental, barbiturates, or any component of the formulation; status asthmaticus; severe cardiovascular disease; porphyria (variegate or acute intermittent); should not be administered by intra-arterial injection

Warnings/Precautions Laryngospasm or bronchospasms may occur; use with extreme caution in patients with reactive airway diseases (asthma or COPD). Use with caution when the hypnotic may be prolonged or potentiated (excessive premedication, Addison's disease, hepatic or renal dysfunction, myxedema, increased blood urea, severe anemia, or myasthenia gravis). Potential for drug dependency exists, abrupt cessation may precipitate withdrawal, including status epilepticus in epileptic patients. Do not administer to patients in acute pain. Use caution in patients with unstable aneurysms, cardiovascular disease, renal impairment, or hepatic disease. Use caution in elderly, debilitated, or pediatric patients. May cause paradoxical responses, including agitation and hyperactivity, particularly in acute pain and pediatric patients. Effects with other sedative drugs or ethanol may be potentiated. May cause respiratory depression or hypotension. Use with caution in hemodynamically unstable patients (hypotension or shock) or patients with respiratory disease. Repeated dosing or continuous infusions may cause cumulative effects. Extravasation or intra-arterial injection causes necrosis due to pH of 10.6, ensure patient has intravenous access.

Adverse Reactions Frequency not defined.

Cardiovascular: Bradycardia, hypotension, syncope

Central nervous system: Drowsiness, lethargy, CNS excitation or depression, impaired judgment, "hangover" effect, confusion, somnolence, agitation, hyperkinesia, ataxia, nervousness, headache, insomnia, nightmares, hallucinations, anxiety, dizziness, shivering

Dermatologic: Rash, exfoliative dermatitis, Stevens-Johnson syndrome

Gastrointestinal: Nausea, vomiting, constipation

Hematologic: Agranulocytosis, thrombocytopenia, megaloblastic anemia, immune hemolytic anemia (rare)

Local: Pain at injection site, thrombophlebitis with I.V. use

Renal: Oliguria

Respiratory: Laryngospasm, respiratory depression, apnea (especially with rapid I.V. use), hypoventilation, sneezing, cough, bronchospasm

Miscellaneous: Gangrene with inadvertent intra-arterial injection, anaphylaxis, anaphylactic reactions

Drug Interactions

Avoid Concomitant Use There are no known interactions where it is recommended to avoid concomitant use.

Increased Effect/Toxicity

Thiopental may increase the levels/effects of: Alcohol (Ethyl); CNS Depressants; Meperidine

The levels/effects of Thiopental may be increased by: Carbonic Anhydrase Inhibitors; Chloramphenicol; Felbamate; Primidone; Valproic Acid

Decreased Effect

Thiopental may decrease the levels/effects of: Acetaminophen; Beta-Blockers; Calcium Channel Blockers; Chloramphenicol; Contraceptive (Progestins); Corticosteroids (Systemic); CycloSPORINE; Disopyramide; Doxycycline; Etoposide; Etoposide Phosphate; LamoTRIgine; Methadone; Oral Contraceptive (Estrogens); Propafenone; QuiNIDine; Teniposide; Theophylline Derivatives; Tricyclic Antidepressants; Valproic Acid; Vitamin K Antagonists

The levels/effects of Thiopental may be decreased by: Ketorolac; Mefloquine; Pyridoxine; Rifamycin Derivatives

Stability Reconstituted solutions remain stable for 3 days at room temperature and 7 days when refrigerated.

Mechanism of Action Short-acting barbiturate with sedative, hypnotic, and anticonvulsant properties. Barbiturates depress the sensory cortex, decrease motor activity, alter cerebellar function, and produce drowsiness, sedation, and hypnosis. In high doses, barbiturates exhibit anticonvulsant activity; barbiturates produce dose-dependent respiratory depression.

Pharmacodynamics/Kinetics

Onset of action: Anesthetic: I.V.: 30-60 seconds

Duration: 5-30 minutes

Distribution: V_d: ~1.6 L/kg

Protein binding: 72% to 86%

Metabolism: Hepatic, primarily to inactive metabolites but pentobarbital is also formed

Half-life elimination: 3-11.5 hours; decreased in children

Dosage I.V.:

Induction anesthesia:

Infants: 5-8 mg/kg

Children 1-12 years: 5-6 mg/kg

Adults: 3-5 mg/kg

Maintenance anesthesia:

Children: 1 mg/kg as needed

Adults: 25-100 mg as needed

Increased intracranial pressure: Children and Adults: 1.5-5 mg/kg/dose; repeat as needed to control intracranial pressure

Seizures:

Children: 2-3 mg/kg/dose; repeat as needed

Adults: 75-250 mg/dose; repeat as needed

Dosing adjustment in renal impairment: Cl_{cr} <10 mL/minute: Administer at 75% of normal dose

Note: Accumulation may occur with chronic dosing due to lipid solubility; prolonged recovery may result from redistribution of thiopental from fat stores

Dietary Considerations Sodium content of 1 g (injection): 86.8 mg (3.8 mEq)

Administration Administer slowly over 20-30 seconds. Rapid I.V. injection may cause hypotension or decreased cardiac output; avoid extravasation, necrosis may occur. Check I.V. catheter placement prior to administration.

Monitoring Parameters Respiratory rate, heart rate, blood pressure

Reference Range Therapeutic: Hypnotic: 1-5 mcg/mL (SI: 4.1-20.7 µmol/L); Coma: 30-100 mcg/mL (SI: 124-413 µmol/L); Anesthesia: 7-130 mcg/mL (SI: 29-536 µmol/L); Toxic: >10 mcg/mL (SI: >41 µmol/L)

Additional Information Thiopental switches from linear to nonlinear pharmacokinetics following prolonged continuous infusions.

Dosage Forms Excipient information presented when available (limited, particularly for generics); consult specific product labeling.

Injection, powder for reconstitution, as sodium: 250 mg, 400 mg, 500 mg, 1 g

◆ **Thiopental Sodium** *see* Thiopental *on page 1460*

◆ **Thiophosphoramide** *see* Thiotepa *on page 1462*

Thioridazine (thye oh RID a zeen)

Canadian Brand Names Mellaril®

Index Terms Thioridazine Hydrochloride

Pharmacologic Category Antipsychotic Agent, Typical, Phenothiazine

Additional Appendix Information

Antipsychotic Agents *on page 1644*

Use Management of schizophrenic patients who fail to respond adequately to treatment with other antipsychotic drugs, either because of insufficient effectiveness or the inability to achieve an effective dose due to intolerable adverse effects from those medications

Unlabeled/Investigational Use Behavior problems (children); severe psychoses (children); schizophrenia/psychoses (children); depressive disorders/dementia (children and adults); behavioral symptoms associated with dementia (elderly); psychosis/agitation related to Alzheimer's dementia

Pregnancy Risk Factor C

Lactation Excretion in breast milk unknown/not recommended

Medication Safety Issues

Sound-alike/look-alike issues:

Thioridazine may be confused with thiothixene, Thorazine®

Mellaril® may be confused with Elavil®, Mebaral®

Contraindications Hypersensitivity to thioridazine or any component of the formulation (cross-reactivity between phenothiazines may occur); severe CNS depression; circulatory collapse; severe hypotension; bone marrow suppression; blood dyscrasias; coma; in combination with other drugs that are known to prolong the QT_c interval; in patients with congenital long QT syndrome or a history of cardiac arrhythmias; concurrent use with medications that inhibit the metabolism of thioridazine (fluoxetine, paroxetine, fluvoxamine, propranolol, pindolol); patients known to have genetic defect leading to reduced levels of activity of CYP2D6

Warnings/Precautions [U.S. Boxed Warning]: Thioridazine has dose-related effects on ventricular repolarization leading to QT_c prolongation, a potentially life-threatening effect. Therefore, it should be reserved for patients with schizophrenia who have failed to respond to adequate levels of other antipsychotic drugs. May cause orthostatic hypotension; use with caution in patients at risk of this effect or those who would tolerate transient hypotensive episodes (cerebrovascular disease, cardiovascular disease, or other medications which may predispose).

Highly sedating, use with caution in disorders where CNS depression is a feature. Use with caution in Parkinson's disease. Use caution in patients with hemodynamic instability; predisposition to seizures; subcortical brain damage; severe cardiac, hepatic, renal, or respiratory disease. Esophageal dysmotility and aspiration have been associated with antipsychotic use; use with caution in patients at risk of pneumonia (ie, Alzheimer's disease). Caution in breast cancer or other prolactin-dependent tumors (may elevate prolactin levels). May alter temperature regulation or mask toxicity of other drugs due to antiemetic effects. Check blood counts periodically and discontinue at first signs of blood dyscrasias; use is contraindicated in patients with bone marrow suppression.

Elderly patients with dementia-related psychosis treated with antipsychotics are at an increased risk of death compared to placebo. An increased incidence of cerebrovascular adverse events (including fatalities) has been reported in elderly patients with dementia-related psychosis. Thioridazine is not approved for this indication. Phenothiazines may cause anticholinergic effects (confusion, agitation, constipation, xerostomia, blurred vision, urinary retention); therefore, they should be used with caution in patients with decreased gastrointestinal motility, urinary retention, BPH, xerostomia, or visual problems. Conditions which also may be exacerbated by cholinergic blockade include narrow-angle glaucoma (screening is recommended) and worsening of myasthenia gravis. Relative to other neuroleptics, thioridazine has a high potency of cholinergic blockade.

May cause extrapyramidal symptoms (EPS), including pseudoparkinsonism, acute dystonic reactions, akathisia, and tardive dyskinesia (risk of these reactions is low relative to other neuroleptics). Risk of dystonia (and possibly other EPS) may be greater with increased doses, use of conventional antipsychotics, males, and younger patients. Use caution in the elderly. May be associated with neuroleptic malignant syndrome (NMS). Doses exceeding recommended doses may cause pigmentary retinopathy.

Adverse Reactions Frequency not defined.

Cardiovascular: Hypotension, orthostatic hypotension, peripheral edema, ECG changes

Central nervous system: EPS (pseudoparkinsonism, akathisia, dystonias, tardive dyskinesia), dizziness, drowsiness, neuroleptic malignant syndrome (NMS), impairment of temperature regulation, lowering of seizure threshold

Dermatologic: Increased sensitivity to sun, rash, discoloration of skin (blue-gray)

Endocrine & metabolic: Changes in menstrual cycle, libido (changes in), breast pain, galactorrhea, amenorrhea

Gastrointestinal: Constipation, weight gain, nausea, vomiting, stomach pain, xerostomia, diarrhea

Genitourinary: Difficulty in urination, ejaculatory disturbances, urinary retention, priapism

Hematologic: Agranulocytosis, leukopenia

Hepatic: Cholestatic jaundice, hepatotoxicity

Neuromuscular & skeletal: Tremor, seizure

Ocular: Pigmentary retinopathy, blurred vision, cornea and lens changes

Respiratory: Nasal congestion

Drug Interactions

Metabolism/Transport Effects Substrate of CYP2C19 (minor), 2D6 (major); **Inhibits** CYP1A2 (weak), 2C9 (weak), 2D6 (moderate), 2E1 (weak)

Avoid Concomitant Use

Avoid concomitant use of Thioridazine with any of the following: CYP2D6 Inhibitors; Fluvoxamine; Nilotinib; QTc-Prolonging Agents; Ziprasidone

Increased Effect/Toxicity

Thioridazine may increase the levels/effects of: Alcohol (Ethyl); Analgesics (Opioid); Anticholinergics; Beta-Blockers; CNS Depressants; CYP2D6 Substrates; Fesoterodine; Tamoxifen; Ziprasidone

The levels/effects of Thioridazine may be increased by: Acetylcholinesterase Inhibitors (Central); Alfuzosin; Antimalarial Agents; Beta-Blockers; Ciprofloxacin; CYP2D6 Inhibitors; Darunavir; Fluvoxamine; Gadobutrol; Lithium formulations; Nilotinib; Pramlintide; QTc-Prolonging Agents; Tetrabenazine

Decreased Effect

Thioridazine may decrease the levels/effects of: Amphetamines; Anti-Parkinson's Agents (Dopamine Agonist); TraMADol

The levels/effects of Thioridazine may be decreased by: Antacids; Lithium formulations

Ethanol/Nutrition/Herb Interactions

Ethanol: Avoid ethanol (may increase CNS depression).

Herb/Nutraceutical: Avoid kava kava, valerian, St John's wort, gotu kola (may increase CNS depression). Avoid dong quai, St John's wort (may also cause photosensitization).

Stability Protect from light.

Mechanism of Action Thioridazine is a piperidine phenothiazine which blocks postsynaptic mesolimbic dopaminergic receptors in the brain; exhibits a strong alpha-adrenergic blocking effect and depresses the release of hypothalamic and hypophyseal hormones

Pharmacodynamics/Kinetics

Duration: 4-5 days

Half-life elimination: 21-25 hours

Time to peak, serum: ~1 hour

Dosage Oral:

Children >2-12 years (unlabeled use): Range: 0.5-3 mg/kg/day in 2-3 divided doses; usual: 1 mg/kg/day; maximum: 3 mg/kg/day

- Behavior problems (unlabeled use): Initial: 10 mg 2-3 times/day, increase gradually
- Severe psychoses (unlabeled use): Initial: 25 mg 2-3 times/day, increase gradually

Children >12 years (unlabeled use) and Adults:

- Schizophrenia/psychoses: Initial: 50-100 mg 3 times/day with gradual increments as needed and tolerated; maximum: 800 mg/day in 2-4 divided doses
- Depressive disorders/dementia (unlabeled use): Initial: 25 mg 3 times/day; maintenance dose: 20-200 mg/day

Elderly: Behavioral symptoms associated with dementia (unlabeled use): Oral: Initial: 10-25 mg 1-2 times/day; increase at 4- to 7-day intervals by 10-25 mg/day; increase dose intervals (once daily, twice daily, etc) as necessary to control response or side effects. Maximum daily dose: 400 mg; gradual increases (titration) may prevent some side effects or decrease their severity.

Hemodialysis: Not dialyzable (0% to 5%)

Administration Do not take antacid within 2 hours of taking drug.

Monitoring Parameters Baseline and periodic ECG; vital signs; serum potassium, lipid profile, fasting blood glucose and Hgb A_{1c}; BMI; mental status, abnormal involuntary movement scale (AIMS); periodic eye exam; do not initiate if QT_c >450 msec

Reference Range Toxic: >1 mg/mL; lethal: 2-8 mg/dL

Test Interactions False-positives for phenylketonuria, urinary amylase, uroporphyrins, urobilinogen

Dosage Forms Excipient information presented when available (limited, particularly for generics); consult specific product labeling. [DSC] = Discontinued product

Tablet, as hydrochloride: 10 mg, 15 mg [DSC], 25 mg, 50 mg, 100 mg, 150 mg [DSC], 200 mg [DSC]

◆ **Thioridazine Hydrochloride** *see* Thioridazine *on page 1461*

◆ **Thiosulfuric Acid Disodium Salt** *see* Sodium Thiosulfate *on page 1386*

Thiotepa (thye oh TEP a)

Index Terms TESPA; Thiophosphoramide; Triethylenethiophosphoramide; TSPA

Pharmacologic Category Antineoplastic Agent, Alkylating Agent

Use Treatment of superficial tumors of the bladder; palliative treatment of adenocarcinoma of breast or ovary; lymphomas and sarcomas; controlling intracavitary effusions caused by metastatic tumors; I.T. use: CNS leukemia/lymphoma, CNS metastases

Pregnancy Risk Factor D

Pregnancy Considerations Animal studies have demonstrated teratogenicity and fetal loss. There are no adequate and well-controlled studies in pregnant women. May cause harm if administered during pregnancy. Effective contraception is recommended for men and women of childbearing potential.

Lactation Enters breast milk/not recommended

Medication Safety Issues

High alert medication: The Institute for Safe Medication Practices (ISMP) includes this medication among its list of drugs which have a heightened risk of causing significant patient harm when used in error.

Contraindications Hypersensitivity to thiotepa or any component of the formulation; pregnancy

Warnings/Precautions Hazardous agent - use appropriate precautions for handling and disposal. Myelosuppression is common. Potentially mutagenic, carcinogenic, and teratogenic. Reduce dosage and use extreme caution in patients with hepatic, renal, or bone marrow damage. Use should be limited to cases where benefit outweighs risk.

Adverse Reactions

>10%:

- Hematopoietic: Myelosuppression (dose related and cumulative): Anemia and pancytopenia may become fatal; careful hematologic monitoring is required; intravesical administration may cause bone marrow suppression as well.
- Hematologic: Myelosuppression (WBC: moderate; platelets: severe; onset: 7-10 days, nadir: 14 days, recovery: 28 days)
- Local: Injection site pain

1% to 10%:

- Central nervous system: Dizziness, fatigue, fever, headache
- Dermatologic: Alopecia, depigmentation (with topical treatment), hyperpigmentation (with high-dose therapy), pruritus, rash, urticaria
- Endocrine & metabolic: Amenorrhea, hyperuricemia
- Gastrointestinal: Anorexia, nausea and vomiting rarely occur
  - Emetic potential: Low (<10%)
- Genitourinary: Dysuria, hemorrhagic cystitis (intravesicular administration: rare), urinary retention
- Neuromuscular & skeletal: Weakness
- Ocular: Conjunctivitis
- Renal: Hematuria
- Miscellaneous: Tightness of the throat, allergic reactions

<1% (Limited to important or life-threatening): Carcinogenesis: Like other alkylating agents, this drug is carcinogenic.

BMT:

Central nervous system: Confusion, inappropriate behavior, somnolence

Dermatologic: Hyperpigmentation

Gastrointestinal: Mucositis, mild nausea and vomiting

Hepatic: Serum transaminitis, hyperbilirubinemia

Drug Interactions

Metabolism/Transport Effects Inhibits CYP2B6 (strong)

Avoid Concomitant Use

Avoid concomitant use of Thiotepa with any of the following: Natalizumab; Vaccines (Live)

Increased Effect/Toxicity

Thiotepa may increase the levels/effects of: CYP2B6 Substrates; Natalizumab; Vaccines (Live)

The levels/effects of Thiotepa may be increased by: Trastuzumab

Decreased Effect

Thiotepa may decrease the levels/effects of: Vaccines (Inactivated)

The levels/effects of Thiotepa may be decreased by: Echinacea

Ethanol/Nutrition/Herb Interactions

Ethanol: Avoid ethanol (due to GI irritation).

Herb/Nutraceutical: Avoid black cohosh, dong quai in estrogen-dependent tumors.

Stability Store intact vials under refrigeration (2°C to 8°C). Protect from light. Reconstitute each vial to 10 mg/mL. Reconstituted solutions (10 mg/mL) are stable for up to 28 days under refrigeration (4°C to 8°C) or 7 days at room temperature (25°C). Filter through a 0.22 micron filter prior to administration.

Solutions for infusion should be diluted to a concentration ≥5 mg/mL in 5% dextrose or 1, 3, or 5 mg/mL in 0.9% sodium chloride injection:

Diluted in D_5W (≥5 mg/mL): Stable for 14 days under refrigeration (4°C) or 3 days at room temperature (23°C).

Diluted in NS:

1, 3, or 5 mg/mL concentration: Stable for 48 hours under refrigeration (4°C to 8°C) or 24 hours at room temperature (25°C).

≤0.5 mg/mL concentration: Stable for <1 hour.

Intrathecal: Dilute in 1-5 mL NS or Elliott's B solution.

Intravesicular: Dilute in 30-60 mL SWFI or NS.

Mechanism of Action Alkylating agent that reacts with DNA phosphate groups to produce cross-linking of DNA strands leading to inhibition of DNA, RNA, and protein synthesis; mechanism of action has not been explored as thoroughly as the other alkylating agents, it is presumed that the aziridine rings open and react as nitrogen mustard; reactivity is enhanced at a lower pH

Pharmacodynamics/Kinetics

Absorption: Intracavitary instillation: Unreliable (10% to 100%) through bladder mucosa; I.M.: variable

Metabolism: Extensively hepatic; major metabolite (active): TEPA

Half-life elimination: Terminal (dose-dependent clearance): 109 minutes

Excretion: Urine (as metabolites and unchanged drug)

Dosage Refer to individual protocols.

Children: Sarcomas: I.V.: 25-65 mg/m^2 as a single dose every 21 days

Adults:

I.M., I.V., SubQ: 30-60 mg/m^2 once weekly

I.V.: 0.3-0.4 mg/kg by rapid I.V. administration every 1-4 weeks, **or** 0.2 mg/kg or 6-8 mg/m^2/day for 4-5 days every 2-4 weeks

High-dose therapy for bone marrow transplant: I.V.: 500 mg/m^2, up to 900 mg/m^2

I.M.: 15-30 mg in various schedules have been given

Intracavitary: 0.6-0.8 mg/kg or 30-60 mg weekly

Intrapericardial: 15-30 mg

Intrathecal: 10-15 mg or 5-11.5 mg/m^2

Dosing comments/adjustment in renal impairment: Use with extreme caution, reduced dose may be warranted.

Administration

I.V.: Administer either as a short (10-60 minute) infusion or 1-2 minute push; a 1 mg/mL solution is considered isotonic; not a vesicant

Intravesical lavage: Instill directly into the bladder and retain for at least 2 hours; patient should be repositioned every 15-30 minutes for maximal exposure

Monitoring Parameters CBC with differential and platelet count (monitor for at least 3 weeks after treatment); uric acid, urinalysis

Additional Information A 1 mg/mL solution is considered isotonic.

Dosage Forms Excipient information presented when available (limited, particularly for generics); consult specific product labeling.

Injection, powder for reconstitution: 15 mg, 30 mg

Thiothixene (thye oh THIKS een)

U.S. Brand Names Navane®

Canadian Brand Names Navane®

Index Terms Tiotixene

Pharmacologic Category Antipsychotic Agent, Typical

Additional Appendix Information

Antipsychotic Agents *on page 1644*

Use Management of schizophrenia

Unlabeled/Investigational Use Psychotic disorders (children); rapid tranquilization of the agitated patient (children); nonpsychotic patient, dementia behavior (elderly); psychosis/agitation related to Alzheimer's dementia

Pregnancy Risk Factor C

Lactation Excretion in breast milk unknown/not recommended

Medication Safety Issues

Sound-alike/look-alike issues:

Thiothixene may be confused with thioridazine

Navane® may be confused with Norvasc®, Nubain®

Contraindications Hypersensitivity to thiothixene or any component of the formulation; severe CNS depression; circulatory collapse; blood dyscrasias; coma

Warnings/Precautions [U.S. Boxed Warning]: Elderly patients with dementia-related psychosis treated with antipsychotics are at an increased risk of death compared to placebo. An increased incidence of cerebrovascular adverse events (including fatalities) has been reported in elderly patients with dementia-related psychosis. Thiothixene is not approved for this indication. May alter cardiac conduction; life-threatening arrhythmias have occurred with therapeutic doses of antipsychotics. Avoid use in patients with underlying QT prolongation, in those taking medicines that prolong the QT interval, or cause polymorphic ventricular tachycardia; monitor ECG closely for dose-related QT effects. Myelosuppression (eg, leukopenia, agranulocytosis) has been observed with antipsychotic use; check blood counts periodically and discontinue at first signs of blood dyscrasias; use is contraindicated in patients with bone marrow suppression. Antipsychotic use has been associated with esophageal dysmotility and aspiration; use with caution in patients at risk of pneumonia (ie, Alzheimer's disease). May cause extrapyramidal symptoms (EPS), including pseudoparkinsonism, acute dystonic reactions, akathisia, and tardive dyskinesia (risk of these reactions is high relative to other neuroleptics). Risk of dystonia (and possibly other EPS) may be greater with increased doses, use of conventional antispychotics, males, and younger patients. Use may be associated with NMS; monitor for mental status changes, fever, muscle rigidity, and/or autonomic instability (risk may be increased in patients with Parkinson's disease or Lewy body dementia). May cause orthostatic hypotension; use with caution in patients at risk of this effect or in those who would not tolerate transient hypotensive episodes (cerebrovascular disease, cardiovascular disease, hypovolemia, or concurrent medication use which may predispose to hypotension/bradycardia). May be associated with pigmentary retinopathy. May be sedating, use with caution in disorders where CNS depression is a feature; patients must be cautioned about performing tasks which require mental alertness (eg, operating machinery or driving). Impaired core body temperature regulation may occur; caution with strenuous exercise, heat exposure, dehydration, and concomitant medication possessing anticholinergic effects.

May be sedating, use with caution in disorders where CNS depression is a feature; patients must be cautioned about performing tasks which require mental alertness (eg, operating machinery or driving). May cause anticholinergic effects (constipation, xerostomia, blurred vision, urinary retention); use with caution in patients with decreased gastrointestinal motility, paralytic ileus, urinary retention, BPH, xerostomia, or visual problems. Relative to other neuroleptics, thiothixene has a low potency of cholinergic blockade. May mask toxicity of other drugs or conditions (eg, intestinal obstruction, Reye's syndrome, brain tumor) due to antiemetic effects.

Use with caution in patients with severe cardiovascular disease, narrow-angle glaucoma, hepatic impairment, myasthenia gravis, Parkinson's disease, breast cancer or other prolactin-dependent tumors, renal impairment, respiratory disease, or seizure disorder. Safety and efficacy have not been established in children <12 years of age.

Adverse Reactions Frequency not defined.

Cardiovascular: Hypotension, nonspecific ECG changes, syncope, tachycardia

Central nervous system: Agitation, dizziness, drowsiness, extrapyramidal symptoms (akathisia, dystonias, lightheadedness, pseudoparkinsonism, tardive dyskinesia), insomnia restlessness

Dermatologic: Discoloration of skin (blue-gray), photosensitivity, pruritus, rash, urticaria

Endocrine & metabolic: Amenorrhea, breast pain, libido (changes in), changes in menstrual cycle, galactorrhea, gynecomastia, hyper-/hypoglycemia, hyperprolactinemia, lactation

Gastrointestinal: Constipation, nausea, salivation increased, stomach pain, vomiting, weight gain, xerostomia

Genitourinary: Difficulty in urination, ejaculatory disturbances, impotence

Hematologic: Leukocytes, leukopenia

Neuromuscular & skeletal: Tremors

Ocular: Blurred vision, pigmentary retinopathy

Respiratory: Nasal congestion

Miscellaneous: Diaphoresis

Drug Interactions

Metabolism/Transport Effects **Substrate** of CYP1A2 (major); **Inhibits** CYP2D6 (weak)

Avoid Concomitant Use

Avoid concomitant use of Thiothixene with any of the following: Nilotinib; Thioridazine; Ziprasidone

Increased Effect/Toxicity

Thiothixene may increase the levels/effects of: Alcohol (Ethyl); Anticholinergics; CNS Depressants; QTc-Prolonging Agents; Thioridazine; Ziprasidone

The levels/effects of Thiothixene may be increased by: Acetylcholinesterase Inhibitors (Central); Alfuzosin; Ciprofloxacin; CYP1A2 Inhibitors (Moderate); CYP1A2 Inhibitors (Strong); Gadobutrol; Lithium formulations; Nilotinib; Pramlintide; Tetrabenazine

Decreased Effect

Thiothixene may decrease the levels/effects of: Amphetamines; Anti-Parkinson's Agents (Dopamine Agonist)

The levels/effects of Thiothixene may be decreased by: CYP1A2 Inducers (Strong); Lithium formulations

Ethanol/Nutrition/Herb Interactions

Ethanol: Avoid ethanol (may increase CNS depression).

Herb/Nutraceutical: Avoid kava kava, valerian, St John's wort, gotu kola (may increase CNS depression).

Mechanism of Action Thiothixene is a thioxanthene antipsychotic which elicits antipsychotic activity by postsynaptic blockade of CNS dopamine receptors resulting in inhibition of dopamine-mediated effects; also has alpha-adrenergic blocking activity

Pharmacodynamics/Kinetics

Metabolism: Extensively hepatic

Half-life elimination: >24 hours with chronic use

Dosage Oral:

Children <12 years (unlabeled use): Schizophrenia/psychoses: 0.25 mg/kg/24 hours in divided doses (dose not well established; use not recommended)

Children >12 years (unlabeled use) and Adults:

Mild-to-moderate psychosis: 2 mg 3 times/day, up to 20-30 mg/day; more severe psychosis: Initial: 5 mg 2 times/day, may increase gradually, if necessary; maximum: 60 mg/day

Rapid tranquilization of the agitated patient (administered every 30-60 minutes): 5-10 mg; average total dose for tranquilization: 15-30 mg

Elderly: Nonpsychotic patient, dementia behavior (unlabeled use): Initial: 1-2 mg 1-2 times/day; increase dose at 4- to 7-day intervals by 1-2 mg/day. Increase dosing intervals (bid, tid, etc) as necessary to control response or side effects; maximum daily dose: 30 mg. Gradual increases in dose may prevent some side effects or decrease their severity.

Hemodialysis: Not dialyzable (0% to 5%)

Monitoring Parameters Vital signs; lipid profile, fasting blood glucose/Hgb A_{1c}; BMI; mental status, abnormal involuntary movement scale (AIMS), extrapyramidal symptoms (EPS)

Test Interactions May cause false-positive pregnancy test

Dosage Forms Excipient information presented when available (limited, particularly for generics); consult specific product labeling. [DSC] = Discontinued product

Capsule: 1 mg, 2 mg, 5 mg, 10 mg

Navane®: 1 mg [DSC], 2 mg, 5 mg, 10 mg, 20 mg

- **Thonzonium, Neomycin, Colistin, and Hydrocortisone** *see* Neomycin, Colistin, Hydrocortisone, and Thonzonium *on page* 1051
- **Thorets [OTC]** *see* Benzocaine *on page* 183
- **Thrive™ [OTC]** *see* Nicotine *on page* 1062
- **Thrombate III®** *see* Antithrombin III *on page* 124
- **Thymocyte Stimulating Factor** *see* Aldesleukin *on page* 53
- **Thymoglobulin®** *see* Antithymocyte Globulin (Rabbit) *on page* 125
- **Thyrogen®** *see* Thyrotropin Alfa *on page* 1465

Thyroid, Desiccated (THYE roid DES i kay tid)

U.S. Brand Names Armour® Thyroid; Nature-Throid™; Westhroid™

Index Terms Desiccated Thyroid; Thyroid Extract; Thyroid USP

Pharmacologic Category Thyroid Product

Use Replacement or supplemental therapy in hypothyroidism; pituitary TSH suppressants (thyroid nodules, thyroiditis, multinodular goiter, thyroid cancer), thyrotoxicosis, diagnostic suppression tests

Pregnancy Risk Factor A

Dosage Oral:

Children: See table.

Recommended Pediatric Dosage for Congenital Hypothyroidism

Age	Daily Dose (mg)	Daily Dose/kg (mg)
0-6 mo	15-30	4.8-6
6-12 mo	30-45	3.6-4.8
1-5 y	45-60	3-3.6
6-12 y	60-90	2.4-3
>12 y	>90	1.2-1.8

Adults: Initial: 15-30 mg; increase with 15 mg increments every 2-4 weeks; use 15 mg in patients with cardiovascular disease or myxedema. Maintenance dose: Usually 60-120 mg/day; monitor TSH and clinical symptoms.

Thyroid cancer: Requires larger amounts than replacement therapy

Additional Information Complete prescribing information for this medication should be consulted for additional detail.

Dosage Forms Excipient information presented when available (limited, particularly for generics); consult specific product labeling.

Tablet: 30 mg, 32.5 mg, 60 mg, 65 mg, 120 mg, 130 mg, 180 mg

Armour® Thyroid: 15 mg, 30 mg, 60 mg, 90 mg, 120 mg, 180 mg, 240 mg, 300 mg

Nature-Throid™: 16.25 mg, 32.5 mg, 65 mg, 130 mg, 195 mg

Westhroid™: 32.5 mg, 65 mg, 130 mg

◆ **Thyroid Extract** *see* Thyroid, Desiccated *on page 1464*

◆ **Thyroid USP** *see* Thyroid, Desiccated *on page 1464*

◆ **Thyrolar®** *see* Liotrix *on page 892*

◆ **ThyroSafe™ [OTC]** *see* Potassium Iodide *on page 1218*

◆ **ThyroShield™ [OTC]** *see* Potassium Iodide *on page 1218*

Thyrotropin Alfa (thye roe TROH pin AL fa)

U.S. Brand Names Thyrogen®

Canadian Brand Names Thyrogen®

Index Terms Human Thyroid Stimulating Hormone; Recombinant Human Thyrotropin; Rh-TSH; Thyrotropin Alpha; TSH

Pharmacologic Category Diagnostic Agent

Use As an adjunctive diagnostic tool for serum thyroglobulin (Tg) testing; adjunctive treatment for radioiodine ablation of thyroid tissue remnants after total or near-total thyroidectomy in patients with well-differentiated thyroid cancer without evidence of metastatic disease

Potential clinical uses include: Patients with an undetectable Tg on thyroid hormone suppressive therapy to exclude the diagnosis of residual or recurrent thyroid cancer, patients requiring serum Tg testing and radioiodine imaging who are unwilling to undergo thyroid hormone withdrawal testing and whose treating physician believes that use of a less sensitive test is justified, patients who are either unable to mount an adequate endogenous TSH response to thyroid hormone withdrawal or in whom withdrawal is medically contraindicated, and patients without evidence of metastatic disease to ablate thyroid remnants (in combination with radioiodine [I^{131}]) following near-total thyroidectomy.

Pregnancy Risk Factor C

Medication Safety Issues

Sound-alike/look-alike issues:

Thyrogen® may be confused with Thyrolar®

Dosage I.M.: Children >16 years and Adults: Radioiodine imaging or ablation: 0.9 mg, followed 24 hours later by a second 0.9 mg dose

For radioiodine imaging or remnant ablation, radioiodine administration should be given 24 hours following the second thyrotropin injection. Diagnostic scanning should be performed 48 hours after radioiodine administration (72 hours after the second thyrotropin injection). Post-therapy scanning may be delayed (additional days) to allow decline of background activity.

For serum Tg testing, serum Tg should be obtained 72 hours after final injection of thyrotropin.

Additional Information Complete prescribing information for this medication should be consulted for additional detail.

Dosage Forms Excipient information presented when available (limited, particularly for generics); consult specific product labeling.

Injection, powder for reconstitution:

Thyrogen®: 1.1 mg

◆ **Thyrotropin Alpha** *see* Thyrotropin Alfa *on page 1465*

◆ **Tiabendazole** *see* Thiabendazole *on page 1457*

TiaGABine (tye AG a been)

U.S. Brand Names Gabitril®

Canadian Brand Names Gabitril®

Index Terms Tiagabine Hydrochloride

Pharmacologic Category Anticonvulsant, Miscellaneous

Use Adjunctive therapy in adults and children ≥12 years of age in the treatment of partial seizures

Pregnancy Risk Factor C

Lactation Enters breast milk/not recommended

Medication Safety Issues

Sound-alike/look-alike issues:

TiaGABine may be confused with tiZANidine

Contraindications Hypersensitivity to tiagabine or any component of the formulation

Warnings/Precautions New-onset seizures and status epilepticus have been associated with tiagabine use when taken for unlabeled indications. Often these seizures have occurred shortly after the initiation of treatment or shortly after a dosage increase. Seizures have also occurred with very low doses or after several months of therapy. In most cases, patients were using concomitant medications (eg, antidepressants, antipsychotics, stimulants, narcotics). In these instances, the discontinuation of tiagabine, followed by an evaluation for an underlying seizure disorder, is suggested. Use for unapproved indications, however, has not been proven to be safe or effective and is not recommended. When tiagabine is used as an adjunct in partial seizures (an FDA-approved indication), it should not be abruptly discontinued because of the possibility of increasing seizure frequency, unless safety concerns require a more rapid withdrawal. Rarely, nonconvulsive status epilepticus has been reported following abrupt discontinuation or dosage reduction.

Use with caution in patients with hepatic impairment. Experience in patients not receiving enzyme-inducing drugs has been limited; caution should be used in treating any patient who is not receiving one of these medications (decreased dose and slower titration may be required). Weakness, sedation, and confusion may occur with tiagabine use. Patients must be cautioned about performing tasks which require mental alertness (eg, operating machinery or driving). Effects with other sedative drugs or ethanol may be potentiated. May cause serious rash, including Stevens-Johnson syndrome. Safety and efficacy have not been established in children <12 years of age.

Adverse Reactions

>10%:

Central nervous system: Concentration decreased, dizziness, nervousness, somnolence

Gastrointestinal: Nausea

Neuromuscular & skeletal: Weakness, tremor

1% to 10%:

Cardiovascular: Chest pain, edema, hypertension, palpitation, peripheral edema, syncope, tachycardia, vasodilation

Central nervous system: Agitation, ataxia, chills, confusion, difficulty with memory, confusion, depersonalization, depression, euphoria, hallucination, hostility, insomnia, malaise, migraine, paranoid reaction, personality disorder, speech disorder

Dermatologic: Alopecia, bruising, dry skin, pruritus, rash

Gastrointestinal: Abdominal pain, diarrhea, gingivitis, increased appetite, mouth ulceration, stomatitis, vomiting, weight gain/loss

Neuromuscular & skeletal: Abnormal gait, arthralgia, dysarthria, hyper-/hypokinesia, hyper-/hypotonia, myasthenia, myalgia, myoclonus, neck pain, paresthesia, reflexes decreased, stupor, twitching, vertigo

Ocular: Abnormal vision, amblyopia, nystagmus

Otic: Ear pain, hearing impairment, otitis media, tinnitus

Respiratory: Bronchitis, cough, dyspnea, epistaxis, pneumonia

Miscellaneous: Allergic reaction, cyst, diaphoresis, flu-like syndrome, lymphadenopathy

<1% (Limited to important or life-threatening): Abortion, abscess, anemia, angina, apnea, asthma, blepharitis, blindness, cellulitis, cerebral ischemia, cholelithiasis, CNS neoplasm, coma, deafness, dehydration, dysphagia, dystonia, electrocardiogram abnormal, encephalopathy, hemorrhage, erythrocytes abnormal, leukopenia, fecal incontinence, herpes simplex/zoster, glossitis, goiter, hematuria, hemoptysis, hepatomegaly, hypercholesteremia, hyper-/hypoglycemia, hyperlipemia, hypokalemia, hyponatremia, hypotension, hypothyroidism, impotence, kidney failure, liver function tests abnormal, MI, neoplasm, peripheral vascular disorder, paralysis, photophobia, psychosis, petechia, photosensitivity, seizure (when used for unlabeled uses), sepsis, spasm, suicide attempt, thrombocytopenia, thrombophlebitis, urinary retention, urinary urgency, urticaria, visual field defect

Drug Interactions

Metabolism/Transport Effects Substrate of 3A4 (major)

Avoid Concomitant Use There are no known interactions where it is recommended to avoid concomitant use.

Increased Effect/Toxicity

TiaGABine may increase the levels/effects of: Alcohol (Ethyl); CNS Depressants

The levels/effects of TiaGABine may be increased by: CYP3A4 Inhibitors (Moderate); CYP3A4 Inhibitors (Strong); Dasatinib

Decreased Effect

The levels/effects of TiaGABine may be decreased by: CYP3A4 Inducers (Strong); Deferasirox; Herbs (CYP3A4 Inducers); Ketorolac; Mefloquine

Ethanol/Nutrition/Herb Interactions

Ethanol: Avoid ethanol (may increase CNS depression).

Food: Food reduces the rate but not the extent of absorption.

Herb/Nutraceutical: St John's wort may decrease tiagabine levels. Avoid valerian, St John's wort, kava kava, gotu kola (may increase CNS depression).

Mechanism of Action The exact mechanism by which tiagabine exerts antiseizure activity is not definitively known; however, *in vitro* experiments demonstrate that it enhances the activity of gamma aminobutyric acid (GABA), the major neuroinhibitory transmitter in the nervous system; it is thought that binding to the GABA uptake carrier inhibits the uptake of GABA into presynaptic neurons, allowing an increased amount of GABA to be available to postsynaptic neurons; based on *in vitro* studies, tiagabine does not inhibit the uptake of dopamine, norepinephrine, serotonin, glutamate, or choline

Pharmacodynamics/Kinetics

Absorption: Rapid (45 minutes); prolonged with food

Protein binding: 96%, primarily to albumin and α_1-acid glycoprotein

Metabolism: Hepatic via CYP (primarily 3A4)

Bioavailability: Oral: Absolute: 90%

Half-life elimination: 2-5 hours when administered with enzyme inducers; 7-9 hours when administered without enzyme inducers

Time to peak, plasma: 45 minutes

Excretion: Feces (63%); urine (25%); 2% as unchanged drug; primarily as metabolites

Dosage Oral (administer with food):

Patients receiving enzyme-inducing AED regimens:

Children 12-18 years: 4 mg once daily for 1 week; may increase to 8 mg daily in 2 divided doses for 1 week; then may increase by 4-8 mg weekly to response or up to 32 mg daily in 2-4 divided doses

Adults: 4 mg once daily for 1 week; may increase by 4-8 mg weekly to response or up to 56 mg daily in 2-4 divided doses; usual maintenance: 32-56 mg/day

Patients **not** receiving enzyme-inducing AED regimens: The estimated plasma concentrations of tiagabine in patients not taking enzyme-inducing medications is twice that of patients receiving enzyme-inducing AEDs. Lower doses are required; slower titration may be necessary.

Dietary Considerations Take with food.

Monitoring Parameters A reduction in seizure frequency is indicative of therapeutic response to tiagabine in patients with partial seizures; complete blood counts, renal function tests, liver function tests, and routine blood chemistry should be monitored periodically during therapy

Reference Range Maximal plasma level after a 24 mg/dose: 552 ng/mL

Additional Information Animal studies suggest that tiagabine may bind to retina and uvea; however, no treatment-related ophthalmoscopic changes were seen long-term; periodic monitoring may be considered.

Dosage Forms Excipient information presented when available (limited, particularly for generics); consult specific product labeling.

Tablet, as hydrochloride:

Gabitril®: 2 mg, 4 mg, 12 mg, 16 mg

◆ **Tiagabine Hydrochloride** *see* TiaGABine *on page 1465*

◆ **Tiamol® (Can)** *see* Fluocinonide *on page 634*

◆ **Tiazac®** *see* Diltiazem *on page 450*

◆ **Tiazac® XC (Can)** *see* Diltiazem *on page 450*

Ticarcillin and Clavulanate Potassium

(tye kar SIL in & klav yoo LAN ate poe TASS ee um)

U.S. Brand Names Timentin®

Canadian Brand Names Timentin®

Index Terms Ticarcillin and Clavulanic Acid

Pharmacologic Category Antibiotic, Penicillin

Additional Appendix Information

Antimicrobial Drugs of Choice *on page 1752*

Use Treatment of lower respiratory tract, urinary tract, skin and skin structures, bone and joint, gynecologic (endometritis) and intra-abdominal (peritonitis) infections, and septicemia caused by susceptible organisms. Clavulanate expands activity of ticarcillin to include beta-lactamase producing strains of *S. aureus*, *H. influenzae*, *Bacteroides* species, and some other gram-negative bacilli

Pregnancy Risk Factor B

Pregnancy Considerations Adverse events were not observed in animal reproduction studies; therefore, ticarcillin/clavulanate is classified as pregnancy category B. Ticarcillin and clavulanate cross the placenta. Human experience with the penicillins during pregnancy has shown no evidence of adverse effects to the fetus. Ticarcillin/clavulanate is approved for the treatment of postpartum gynecologic infections, including endometritis, caused by susceptible organisms.

Lactation Enters breast milk/use caution

Contraindications Hypersensitivity to ticarcillin, clavulanate, any penicillin, or any component of the formulation

Warnings/Precautions Use with caution and modify dosage in patients with renal impairment; serious and occasionally severe or fatal hypersensitivity (anaphylactoid) reactions have been reported in patients on penicillin therapy (especially with a history of beta-lactam hypersensitivity and/or a history of sensitivity to multiple allergens); use with caution in patients with seizures and in patients with HF due to high sodium load. Particularly in patients with renal impairment, bleeding disorders have been observed; discontinue if thrombocytopenia or bleeding occurs. Prolonged use may result in fungal or bacterial superinfection, including *C. difficile*-associated diarrhea (CDAD) and pseudomembranous colitis; CDAD has been observed >2 months postantibiotic treatment. Safety and efficacy have not been established in children <3 months of age.

Adverse Reactions Frequency not defined.

Central nervous system: Confusion, drowsiness, fever, headache, Jarisch-Herxheimer reaction, seizure

Dermatologic: Erythema multiforme, pruritus, rash, Stevens-Johnson syndrome, toxic epidermal necrolysis, urticaria

Endocrine & metabolic: Electrolyte imbalance

Gastrointestinal: *Clostridium difficile* colitis, diarrhea, nausea, vomiting

Hematologic: Bleeding, eosinophilia, hemolytic anemia, leukopenia, neutropenia, positive Coombs' reaction, prothrombin time prolonged, thrombocytopenia

Hepatic: Hepatotoxicity, jaundice

Local: Injection site reaction (pain, burning, induration); thrombophlebitis

Neuromuscular & skeletal: Myoclonus

Renal: BUN increased, interstitial nephritis (acute), serum creatinine increased

Miscellaneous: Anaphylaxis, hypersensitivity reactions

Drug Interactions

Avoid Concomitant Use There are no known interactions where it is recommended to avoid concomitant use.

Increased Effect/Toxicity

Ticarcillin and Clavulanate Potassium may increase the levels/effects of: Methotrexate

The levels/effects of Ticarcillin and Clavulanate Potassium may be increased by: Uricosuric Agents

Decreased Effect

Ticarcillin and Clavulanate Potassium may decrease the levels/effects of: Aminoglycosides; Typhoid Vaccine

The levels/effects of Ticarcillin and Clavulanate Potassium may be decreased by: Fusidic Acid; Tetracycline Derivatives

Stability

Vials: Store intact vials at <24°C (<75°F). Reconstituted solution is stable for 6 hours at room temperature and 72 hours when refrigerated. I.V. infusion in NS or LR is stable for 24 hours at room temperature, 7 days when refrigerated, or 30 days when frozen. I.V. infusion in D_5W solution is stable for 24 hours at room temperature, 3 days when refrigerated, or 7 days when frozen. After freezing, thawed solution is stable for 8 hours at room temperature. Darkening of drug indicates loss of potency of clavulanate potassium.

Premixed solution: Store frozen at ≤-20°C (-4°F). Thawed solution is stable for 24 hours at room temperature or 7 days under refrigeration; do not refreeze.

Mechanism of Action Inhibits bacterial cell wall synthesis by binding to one or more of the penicillin binding proteins (PBPs); which in turn inhibits the final transpeptidation step of peptidoglycan synthesis in bacterial cell walls, thus inhibiting cell wall biosynthesis. Bacteria eventually lyse due to ongoing activity of cell wall autolytic enzymes (autolysins and murein hydrolases) while cell wall assembly is arrested.

Pharmacodynamics/Kinetics

Absorption: Ticarcillin: Not absorbed orally

Protein binding: Ticarcillin: ~45%; Clavulanic acid: ~25%

Metabolism: Clavulanic acid: Hepatic

Half-life elimination: Ticarcillin: 1.1 hours;Clavulanic acid: 1.1 hours

Excretion: Ticarcillin: Urine (60% to 70%); Clavulanic acid: Urine (35% to 45% as unchanged drug)

Clearance: Clavulanic acid does not affect clearance of ticarcillin

Dosage Note: Timentin® (ticarcillin/clavulanate) is a combination product; each 3.1 g dosage form contains 3 g ticarcillin disodium and 0.1 g clavulanic acid.

Usual dosage range:

Children and Adults <60 kg: I.V.: 200-300 mg of ticarcillin component/kg/day in divided doses every 4-6 hours

Children ≥60 kg and Adults: I.V.: 3.1 g (ticarcillin 3 g plus clavulanic acid 0.1 g) every 4-6 hours (maximum: 24 g of ticarcillin component/day)

Indication-specific dosing:

Children: I.V.:

Bite wounds (animal): 200 mg of ticarcillin component/kg/day in divided doses

Neutropenic fever: 75 mg of ticarcillin component/kg every 6 hours (maximum: 3.1 g/dose)

Pneumonia (nosocomial): 300 mg of ticarcillin component/kg/day in 4 divided doses (maximum: 18-24 g of ticarcillin component/day)

Children ≥60 kg and Adults: I.V.:

Amnionitis, cholangitis, diverticulitis, endometritis, epididymo-orchitis, mastoiditis, orbital cellulitis, peritonitis, pneumonia (aspiration): 3.1 g every 6 hours

Liver abscess, parafascial space infections, septic thrombophlebitis: 3.1 g every 4 hours

***Pseudomonas* infections:** 3.1 g every 4 hours

Urinary tract infections: 3.1 g every 6-8 hours

Dosing adjustment in renal impairment: Loading dose: I.V.: 3.1 g one dose, followed by maintenance dose based on creatinine clearance:

Cl_{cr} 30-60 mL/minute: Administer 2 g of ticarcillin component every 4 hours or 3.1 g every 8 hours

Cl_{cr} 10-30 mL/minute: Administer 2 g of ticarcillin component every 8 hours or 3.1 g every 12 hours

Cl_{cr} <10 mL/minute: Administer 2 g of ticarcillin component every 12 hours

Cl_{cr} <10 mL/minute with concomitant hepatic dysfunction: 2 g of ticarcillin component every 24 hours

Moderately dialyzable (20% to 50%)

Continuous ambulatory peritoneal dialysis: 3.1 g every 12 hours

Hemodialysis: 2 g of ticarcillin component every 12 hours; supplemented with 3.1 g after each dialysis

Continuous renal replacement therapy (CRRT): Drug clearance is highly dependent on the method of renal replacement, filter type, and flow rate. Appropriate dosing requires close monitoring of pharmacologic response, signs of adverse reactions due to drug accumulation, as well as drug levels in relation to target trough (if appropriate). The following are general recommendations only (based on dialysate flow/ultrafiltration rates of 1 L/hour) and should not supersede clinical judgment:

CVVH: 2 g every 6-8 hours

CVVHD/CVVHDF: 3.1 g every 6 hours

Note: Do not administer in intervals exceeding every 8 hours. Clavulanate component is hepatically eliminated; extending the dosing interval beyond 8 hours may result in loss of beta-lactamase inhibition.

Dosing adjustment in hepatic dysfunction: With concomitant renal dysfunction (Cl_{cr} <10 mL/minute): 2 g of ticarcillin component every 24 hours

Dietary Considerations Sodium content of 1 g: 4.51 mEq; potassium content of 1 g: 0.15 mEq

Administration Infuse over 30 minutes.

Some penicillins (eg, carbenicillin, ticarcillin and piperacillin) have been shown to inactivate aminoglycosides *in vitro*. This has been observed to a greater extent with tobramycin and gentamicin, while amikacin has shown greater stability against inactivation. Concurrent use of these agents may pose a risk of reduced antibacterial efficacy *in vivo*, particularly in the setting of profound renal impairment. However, definitive clinical evidence is lacking. If combination penicillin/aminoglycoside therapy is desired in a patient with renal dysfunction, separation of doses (if feasible), and routine monitoring of aminoglycoside levels, CBC, and clinical response should be considered.

Monitoring Parameters Observe for signs and symptoms of anaphylaxis during first dose.

Test Interactions Positive Coombs' test, false-positive urinary proteins

Some penicillin derivatives may accelerate the degradation of aminoglycosides *in vitro*, leading to a potential underestimation of aminoglycoside serum concentration.

Dosage Forms Excipient information presented when available (limited, particularly for generics); consult specific product labeling.

Infusion [premixed, frozen]: Ticarcillin 3 g and clavulanic acid 0.1 g (100 mL) [contains sodium 4.51 mEq and potassium 0.15 mEq per g]

Injection, powder for reconstitution: Ticarcillin 3 g and clavulanic acid 0.1 g (3.1 g, 31 g) [contains sodium 4.51 mEq and potassium 0.15 mEq per g]

◆ **Ticarcillin and Clavulanic Acid** *see* Ticarcillin and Clavulanate Potassium *on page 1466*

◆ **TICE® BCG** *see* BCG Vaccine *on page 176*

◆ **Ticlid® [DSC]** *see* Ticlopidine *on page 1468*

◆ **Ticlid® (Can)** *see* Ticlopidine *on page 1468*

Ticlopidine (tye KLOE pi deen)

U.S. Brand Names Ticlid® [DSC]

Canadian Brand Names Alti-Ticlopidine; Apo-Ticlopidine®; Gen-Ticlopidine; Novo-Ticlopidine; Nu-Ticlopidine; Rhoxal-ticlopidine; Sandoz-Ticlopidine; Ticlid®

Index Terms Ticlopidine Hydrochloride

Pharmacologic Category Antiplatelet Agent

Use Platelet aggregation inhibitor that reduces the risk of thrombotic stroke in patients who have had a stroke or stroke precursors. **Note:** Due to its association with life-threatening hematologic disorders, ticlopidine should be reserved for patients who are intolerant to aspirin, or who have failed aspirin therapy. Adjunctive therapy (with aspirin) following successful coronary stent implantation to reduce the incidence of subacute stent thrombosis.

Unlabeled/Investigational Use Protection of aortocoronary bypass grafts, diabetic microangiopathy, ischemic heart disease, prevention of postoperative DVT, reduction of graft loss following renal transplant

Pregnancy Risk Factor B

Lactation Excretion in breast milk unknown

Contraindications Hypersensitivity to ticlopidine or any component of the formulation; active pathological bleeding such as peptic ulcer disease (PUD) or intracranial hemorrhage; severe liver dysfunction; hematopoietic disorders (neutropenia, thrombocytopenia, a past history of TTP or aplastic anemia)

Warnings/Precautions Use with caution in patients who may be at risk of increased bleeding (eg, PUD, trauma, or surgery). Consider discontinuing 10-14 days before elective surgery (except in patients with cardiac stents that have not completed their full course of dual antiplatelet therapy; patient-specific situations need to be discussed with cardiologist; AHA/ACC/SCAI/ACS/ADA Science Advisory provides recommendations). Use caution in concurrent treatment with anticoagulants (eg, heparin, warfarin) or other antiplatelet drugs; bleeding risk is increased. Use with caution in patients with mild-to-moderate hepatic impairment; use is contraindicated with severe hepatic impairment. Use with caution in patients with moderate-to-severe renal impairment (experience is limited); bleeding times may be significantly prolonged and the risk of hematologic adverse effects (eg, neutropenia) may be increased. **[U.S. Boxed Warning]: May cause life-threatening hematologic reactions, including neutropenia, agranulocytosis, thrombotic thrombocytopenia purpura (TTP), and aplastic anemia.** Routine monitoring is required (see Monitoring Parameters). Monitor for signs and symptoms of neutropenia including WBC count. Discontinue if the absolute neutrophil count falls to <1200/mm^3 or if the platelet count falls to <80,000/mm^3. Safety and efficacy have not been established in children.

Adverse Reactions As with all drugs which may affect hemostasis, bleeding is associated with ticlopidine. Hemorrhage may occur at virtually any site. Risk is dependent on multiple variables, including the use of multiple agents which alter hemostasis and patient susceptibility.

>10%:

Endocrine & metabolic: Total cholesterol increased (increases of ~8% to 10% within 1 month of therapy), triglycerides increased

Gastrointestinal: Diarrhea (13%)

1% to 10%:

Central nervous system: Dizziness (1%)

Dermatologic: Rash (5%), purpura (2%), pruritus (1%)

Gastrointestinal: Nausea (7%), dyspepsia (7%), gastrointestinal pain (4%), vomiting (2%), flatulence (2%), anorexia (1%)

Hematologic: Neutropenia (2%)

Hepatic: Alkaline phosphatase increased (>2 x upper limit of normal; 8%), abnormal liver function test (1%)

<1% (Limited to important or life-threatening): Agranulocytosis, anaphylaxis, angioedema, aplastic anemia, arthropathy, bilirubin increased, bone marrow suppression, bronchiolitis obliterans-organized pneumonia, chronic diarrhea, conjunctival bleeding, eosinophilia, erythema multiforme, erythema nodosum, exfoliative dermatitis, gastrointestinal bleeding, hematuria, hemolytic anemia, hepatic necrosis, hepatitis, hyponatremia, intracranial bleeding (rare), jaundice, maculopapular rash, menorrhagia, myositis, nephrotic syndrome, pancytopenia, peptic ulcer, peripheral neuropathy, pneumonitis (allergic), positive ANA, renal failure, sepsis, serum creatinine increased, serum sickness, Stevens-Johnson syndrome,

systemic lupus erythematosus, thrombocytopenia (immune), thrombocytosis, thrombotic thrombocytopenic purpura, urticaria, vasculitis

Drug Interactions

Metabolism/Transport Effects Substrate of CYP3A4 (major); **Inhibits** CYP1A2 (weak), 2C9 (weak), 2C19 (strong), 2D6 (moderate), 2E1 (weak), 3A4 (weak)

Avoid Concomitant Use

Avoid concomitant use of Ticlopidine with any of the following: Thioridazine

Increased Effect/Toxicity

Ticlopidine may increase the levels/effects of: Anticoagulants; Antiplatelet Agents; CYP2C19 Substrates; CYP2D6 Substrates; Drotrecogin Alfa; Fesoterodine; Ibritumomab; Nebivolol; Phenytoin; Salicylates; Tamoxifen; Theophylline Derivatives; Thioridazine; Thrombolytic Agents; Tositumomab and Iodine I 131 Tositumomab

The levels/effects of Ticlopidine may be increased by: Dasatinib; Herbs (Anticoagulant/Antiplatelet Properties); Nonsteroidal Anti-Inflammatory Agents; Omega-3-Acid Ethyl Esters; Pentosan Polysulfate Sodium; Prostacyclin Analogues

Decreased Effect

Ticlopidine may decrease the levels/effects of: Codeine; TraMADol

The levels/effects of Ticlopidine may be decreased by: CYP3A4 Inducers (Strong); Deferasirox; Herbs (CYP3A4 Inducers); Nonsteroidal Anti-Inflammatory Agents

Ethanol/Nutrition/Herb Interactions

Food: Ticlopidine bioavailability may be increased (20%) if taken with food. High-fat meals increase absorption, antacids decrease absorption.

Herb/Nutraceutical: Avoid alfalfa, anise, bilberry, bladderwrack, bromelain, cat's claw, chamomile, coleus, cordyceps, dong quai, evening primrose oil, fenugreek, feverfew, garlic, ginger, ginkgo biloba, ginseng (American), ginseng (Panax), ginseng (Siberian), grape seed, green tea, guggul, horse chestnut seed, horseradish, licorice, prickly ash, red clover, reishi, SAMe (S-adenosylmethionine), sweet clover, turmeric, white willow (all have additional antiplatelet activity).

Mechanism of Action Ticlopidine requires *in vivo* biotransformation to an unidentified active metabolite. This active metabolite irreversibly blocks the P2Y12 component of ADP receptors, which prevents activation of the GPIIb/IIIa receptor complex, thereby reducing platelet aggregation. Platelets blocked by ticlopidine are affected for the remainder of their lifespan.

Pharmacodynamics/Kinetics

Onset of action: ~6 hours

Peak effect: 3-5 days; serum levels do not correlate with clinical antiplatelet activity

Absorption: Well absorbed

Protein binding: Parent drug: 98%; <15% bound to alpha$_1$-acid glycoprotein

Metabolism: Extensively hepatic; has at least 1 active metabolite

Half-life elimination: 13 hours

Time to peak, serum: ~2 hours

Excretion: Urine (60%); feces (23%)

Dosage Oral: Adults:

Stroke prevention: 250 mg twice daily

Coronary artery stenting (initiate after successful implantation): 250 mg twice daily (in combination with antiplatelet doses of aspirin) for up to 30 days

Unstable angina, non-ST-segment elevation myocardial infarction (UA/NSTEMI) undergoing percutaneous coronary intervention (PCI) in patients unable to receive clopidogrel (unlabeled dosing): Initial: 500 mg loading dose given at least 6 hours prior to PCI, followed by 250 mg twice daily (in combination with aspirin 75-325 mg once daily). Duration of therapy dependent upon type of stent implanted during PCI.

Note: *Coronary artery stents:* Duration of ticlopidine (clopidogrel preferred) in combination with aspirin: According to the ACC/AHA/SCAI guidelines, ideally 12 months following drug-eluting stent (DES) placement in patients not at high risk for bleeding; at a minimum, 1, 3, and 6 months for bare metal (BMS), sirolimus-eluting, and paclitaxel-eluting stents, respectively, for uninterrupted therapy (Smith, 2005). The 2008 *Chest* guidelines recommend for patients who undergo PCI and receive a BMS (with ongoing ACS) or a DES (with or without ongoing ACS) that ticlopidine (clopidogrel preferred) be continued for at least 12 months. In patients receiving a BMS without ongoing ACS, ticlopidine (or clopidogrel) may be continued for at least 1 month. In patients receiving a DES, therapy with ticlopidine (or clopidogrel) beyond 12 months may be considered in patients without bleeding or tolerability issues (Becker, 2008). Premature interruption of therapy may result in stent thrombosis with subsequent fatal and nonfatal myocardial infarction.

Dosage adjument in renal impairment: No adjustment is necessary

Dosage adjustment in hepatic impairment: No specific guidelines for patients with hepatic impairment; use with caution. Use is contraindicated with severe renal impairment.

Dietary Considerations Should be taken with food to reduce stomach upset.

Administration Administer with food.

Monitoring Parameters Signs of bleeding; CBC with differential every 2 weeks starting the second week through the third month of treatment; more frequent monitoring is recommended for patients whose absolute neutrophil counts have been consistently declining or are 30% less than baseline values. The peak incidence of TTP occurs between 3-4 weeks, the peak incidence of neutropenia occurs at approximately 4-6 weeks, and the incidence of aplastic anemia peaks after 4-8 weeks of therapy. Few cases have been reported after 3 months of treatment. Liver function tests (alkaline phosphatase and transaminases) should be performed in the first 4 months of therapy if liver dysfunction is suspected.

Dosage Forms Excipient information presented when available (limited, particularly for generics); consult specific product labeling. [DSC] = Discontinued product

Tablet, as hydrochloride: 250 mg

Ticlid®: 250 mg [DSC]

◆ **Ticlopidine Hydrochloride** *see* Ticlopidine *on page 1468*

◆ **TIG** *see* Tetanus Immune Globulin (Human) *on page 1448*

◆ **Tigan®** *see* Trimethobenzamide *on page 1518*

Tigecycline (tye ge SYE kleen)

U.S. Brand Names Tygacil®

Index Terms GAR-936

Pharmacologic Category Antibiotic, Glycylcycline

Use Treatment of complicated skin and skin structure infections caused by susceptible organisms, including methicillin-resistant *Staphylococcus aureus* and vancomycin-sensitive *Enterococcus faecalis*; treatment of complicated intra-abdominal infections

Pregnancy Risk Factor D

Pregnancy Considerations Because adverse effects were observed in animals and because of the potential for permanent tooth discoloration, tigecycline is classified pregnancy category D. Tigecycline frequently causes nausea and vomiting and, therefore, may not be ideal for use in a patient with pregnancy-related nausea.

Lactation Excretion in breast milk unknown/use caution

Contraindications Hypersensitivity to tigecycline or any component of the formulation

Warnings/Precautions Due to structural similarity with tetracyclines, use caution in patients with prior hypersensitivity and/or severe adverse reactions associated with tetracycline use. Due to structural similarities with tetracyclines, may be associated with photosensitivity, pseudotumor cerebri, pancreatitis, and antianabolic effects (including increased BUN, azotemia, acidosis, and hyperphosphatemia) observed with this class. May cause fetal harm if used during pregnancy; patients should be advised of potential risks associated with use. Permanent discoloration of the teeth may occur if used during tooth development (fetal stage through children up to 8 years of age). Use caution in hepatic impairment; dosage adjustment may be required with severe impairment.

Prolonged use may result in fungal or bacterial superinfection, including *C. difficile*-associated diarrhea (CDAD) and pseudomembranous colitis; CDAD has been observed >2 months postantibiotic treatment. Use with caution if using as monotherapy for patients with intestinal perforation (in the small sample of available cases, septic shock occurred more frequently than patients treated with imipenem/cilastatin comparator). Safety and efficacy in children <18 years of age have not been established.

Adverse Reactions Note: Frequencies relative to placebo are not available; some frequencies are lower than those experienced with comparator drugs.

>10%: Gastrointestinal: Nausea (25% to 30%; severe in 1%), vomiting (20%; severe in 1%), diarrhea (13%)

2% to 10%:

Cardiovascular: Hypertension (5%), peripheral edema (3%), hypotension (2%), phlebitis (2%)

Central nervous system: Fever (7%), headache (6%), dizziness (4%), pain (4%), insomnia (2%)

Dermatologic: Pruritus (3%), rash (2%)

Endocrine & metabolic: Hypoproteinemia (5%), hyperglycemia (2%), hypokalemia (2%)

Gastrointestinal: Abdominal pain (7%), constipation (3%), dyspepsia (3%)

Hematologic: Thrombocythemia (6%), anemia (4%), leukocytosis (4%)

Hepatic: ALT increased (6%), AST increased (4%), alkaline phosphatase increased (4%), amylase increased (3%), bilirubin increased (2%), LDH increased (4%)

Local: Reaction to procedure (9%)

Neuromuscular & skeletal: Weakness (3%)

Renal: BUN increased (2%)

Respiratory: Cough increased (4%), dyspnea (3%), pulmonary physical finding (2%)

Miscellaneous: Abnormal healing (4%), infection (8%), abscess (3%), diaphoresis increased (2%)

<2% (Limited to important or life-threatening): Abnormal stools, allergic reaction, anorexia, aPTT prolonged, back pain, bradycardia, chills, creatinine increased, dry mouth, eosinophilia, hypocalcemia, hypoglycemia, hyponatremia, injection site edema, injection site inflammation, injection site pain, injection site phlebitis, injection site reaction, INR increased, jaundice, leukorrhea, pancreatitis (acute), PT prolonged, septic shock, tachycardia, taste perversion, thrombocytopenia, thrombophlebitis, vaginal moniliasis, vaginitis, vasodilatation

Drug Interactions

Avoid Concomitant Use There are no known interactions where it is recommended to avoid concomitant use.

Increased Effect/Toxicity

Tigecycline may increase the levels/effects of: Warfarin

Decreased Effect There are no known significant interactions involving a decrease in effect.

Stability Store at 15°C to 30°C (59°F to 86°F) prior to reconstitution. Add 5.3 mL NS or D_5W to each 50 mg vial. Swirl gently to dissolve. Resulting solution is 10 mg/mL. Reconstituted solution must be further diluted to allow I.V. administration. Transfer to 100 mL I.V. bag for infusion (final concentration should not exceed 1 mg/mL). Once reconstituted, may be stored at room temperature for up to 24 hours (up to 6 hours in the vial and after further dilution, in the I.V. bag). Alternatively, may be refrigerated for up to 45 hours following immediate transfer of the reconstituted solution into the I.V. bag. Reconstituted solution is red-orange.

Mechanism of Action Binds to the 30S ribosomal subunit of susceptible bacteria, inhibiting protein synthesis.

Pharmacodynamics/Kinetics Note: Systemic clearance is reduced by 55% and half-life increased by 43% in moderate hepatic impairment.

Distribution: V_d: 7-9 L/kg; extensive tissue distribution

Protein binding: 71% to 89%

Metabolism: Hepatic, via glucuronidation, N-acetylation, and epimerization to several metabolites, each <10% of the dose

Half-life elimination: Single dose: 27 hours; following multiple doses: 42 hours

Excretion: Urine (33%; with 22% as unchanged drug); feces (59%; primarily as unchanged drug)

Dosage I.V.: Adults:

Initial: 100 mg as a single dose

Maintenance dose: 50 mg every 12 hours

Recommended duration of therapy: Intra-abdominal infections or complicated skin/skin structure infections: 5-14 days.

Dosage adjustment in renal impairment: No dosage adjustment required in renal impairment or after hemodialysis.

Dosage adjustment in hepatic impairment:

Mild-to-moderate hepatic disease: No dosage adjustment required

Severe hepatic impairment (Child-Pugh class C): Initial dose of 100 mg should be followed with 25 mg every 12 hours

Administration Infuse over 30-60 minutes through dedicated line or via Y-site

Additional Information Generally considered bacteriostatic. Tigecycline is a derivative of minocycline (9-t-butylglycylamido minocycline), but is not classified as a tetracycline. It has demonstrated activity against a variety of gram-positive and -negative bacterial pathogens.

Dosage Forms Excipient information presented when available (limited, particularly for generics); consult specific product labeling.

Injection, powder for reconstitution:

Tygacil®: 50 mg [contains lactose 100 mg]

◆ **Tikosyn®** *see* Dofetilide *on page 474*

◆ **Tilade® [DSC]** *see* Nedocromil *on page 1047*

◆ **Tilade® (Can)** *see* Nedocromil *on page 1047*

◆ **Tilia™ Fe** *see* Ethinyl Estradiol and Norethindrone *on page 581*

Tiludronate (tye LOO droe nate)

U.S. Brand Names Skelid®

Index Terms Tiludronate Disodium

Pharmacologic Category Bisphosphonate Derivative

Use Treatment of Paget's disease of the bone (osteitis deformans) in patients who have a level of serum alkaline phosphatase (SAP) at least twice the upper limit of normal, or who are symptomatic, or who are at risk for future complications of their disease

Pregnancy Risk Factor C

Pregnancy Considerations Teratogenic and nonteratogenic embryo/fetal effects have been reported in animal studies. There are no adequate and well-controlled studies in pregnant women. Bisphosphonates are incorporated into the bone matrix and gradually released over time. Theoretically, there may be a risk of fetal harm when pregnancy follows the completion of therapy. Based on limited case reports with pamidronate, serum calcium levels in the newborn may be altered if bisphosphonates are administered during pregnancy.

Lactation Excretion in breast milk unknown/use caution

Medication Safety Issues

International issues:

Skelid® may be confused with Skaelud® which is a brand name for pyrithione zinc in Denmark

Contraindications Hypersensitivity to tiludronate, bisphosphonates, or any component of the formulation

Warnings/Precautions Not recommended in patients with severe renal impairment (Cl_{cr} <30 mL/minute). Use with caution in patients with active upper GI problems (eg, dysphagia, symptomatic esophageal diseases, gastritis, duodenitis, ulcers).

Bisphosphonate therapy has been associated with osteonecrosis, primarily of the jaw; this has been observed mostly in cancer patients, but also in patients with postmenopausal osteoporosis and other diagnoses. Dental exams and preventative dentistry should be performed prior to placing patients with risk factors on chronic bisphosphonate therapy. Invasive dental procedures should be avoided during treatment.

Infrequently, severe (and occasionally debilitating) bone, joint, and/or muscle pain have been reported during bisphosphonate treatment. The onset of pain ranged from a single day to several months. Symptoms usually resolve upon discontinuation. Some patients experienced recurrence when rechallenged with same drug or another bisphosphonate; avoid use in patients with a history of these symptoms in association with bisphosphonate therapy. Safety and efficacy have not been established in children.

Adverse Reactions

1% to 10%:

Cardiovascular: Chest pain (3%), edema (3%), flushing, hypertension, syncope

Central nervous system: Anxiety, fatigue, insomnia, nervousness, somnolence, vertigo

Dermatologic: Rash (3%), skin disorder (3%), pruritus

Endocrine & metabolic: Hyperparathyroidism (3%)

Gastrointestinal: Nausea (9%), diarrhea (9%), dyspepsia (5%), vomiting (4%), flatulence (3%), tooth disorder (3%), abdominal pain, anorexia, constipation, gastritis, xerostomia

Genitourinary: Urinary tract infection

Neuromuscular & skeletal: Arthrosis (3%), paresthesia (4%), fractures, muscle spasm, weakness

Ocular: Cataract (3%), conjunctivitis (3%), glaucoma (3%)

Respiratory: Rhinitis (5%), sinusitis (5%), pharyngitis (3%), bronchitis

Miscellaneous: Accidental injury (4%), infection (3%), diaphoresis

<1% (Limited to important or life-threatening): Musculoskeletal pain (sometimes severe and/or incapacitating), osteonecrosis (primarily of the jaw), Stevens-Johnson syndrome

Drug Interactions

Avoid Concomitant Use There are no known interactions where it is recommended to avoid concomitant use.

Increased Effect/Toxicity

Tiludronate may increase the levels/effects of: Phosphate Supplements

The levels/effects of Tiludronate may be increased by: Aminoglycosides; Indomethacin; Nonsteroidal Anti-Inflammatory Agents

Decreased Effect

The levels/effects of Tiludronate may be decreased by: Antacids; Aspirin; Calcium Salts; Iron Salts; Magnesium Salts

Ethanol/Nutrition/Herb Interactions Food: In single-dose studies, the bioavailability of tiludronate was reduced by 90% when an oral dose was administered with, or 2 hours after, a standard breakfast compared to the same dose administered after an overnight fast and 4 hours before a standard breakfast.

Stability Store at 25°C (77°F); excursions permitted to 15°C to 30°C (59°F to 86°F). Do not remove tablets from foil strips until they are to be used.

Mechanism of Action Inhibition of normal and abnormal bone resorption. Inhibits osteoclasts through at least two mechanisms: disruption of the cytoskeletal ring structure, possibly by inhibition of protein-tyrosine-phosphatase, thus leading to the detachment of osteoclasts from the bone surface area and the inhibition of the osteoclast proton pump.

Pharmacodynamics/Kinetics

Onset of action: Delayed, may require several weeks

Absorption: Rapid

Distribution: Widely to bone and soft tissue

Protein binding: ~90%, primarily to albumin

Metabolism: Little, if any

Bioavailability: ~6% (range: 2% to 11%); reduced by 90% when given with food

Half-life elimination: Healthy volunteers: Single dose: 50 hours; Cl_{cr} 11-18 mL/minute: 205 hours; Pagetic patients: Repeated dosing: 150 hours

Time to peak, plasma: Within 2 hours

Excretion: Urine (~60%, as tiludronic acid within 13 days)

Dosage Oral: Adults: 400 mg (2 tablets of tiludronic acid) daily for a period of 3 months; allow an interval of 3 months to assess response

Dosing adjustment in renal impairment: Cl_{cr} <30 mL/minute: **Not recommended**

Dosing adjustment in hepatic impairment: Adjustment is not necessary

Dietary Considerations Do not take within 2 hours of food. Ensure adequate intake of vitamin D and calcium supplements during treatment.

Administration Administer as a single oral dose, take with 6-8 oz of plain water. Should not be taken with beverages containing minerals (eg, mineral water), food, or with other medications (may reduce absorption). Do not take within 2 hours of food. Take calcium or mineral supplements at least 2 hours before or after tiludronate. Take aluminum- or magnesium-containing antacids at least 2 hours after taking tiludronate. Do not take tiludronate within 2 hours of indomethacin.

Test Interactions Bisphosphonates may interfere with diagnostic imaging agents such as technetium-99m-diphosphonate in bone scans.

Dosage Forms Excipient information presented when available (limited, particularly for generics); consult specific product labeling.

Tablet, tiludronic acid:

Skelid®: 200 mg [equivalent to 240 mg tiludronate disodium]

◆ **Tiludronate Disodium** *see* Tiludronate *on page* 1470

◆ **Tim-AK (Can)** *see* Timolol *on page* 1472

◆ **Time-C [OTC]** *see* Ascorbic Acid *on page* 139

◆ **Time-C-Bio [OTC]** *see* Ascorbic Acid *on page* 139

◆ **Timentin®** *see* Ticarcillin and Clavulanate Potassium *on page* 1466

Timolol (TIM oh lol)

U.S. Brand Names Betimol®; Istalol®; Timolol GFS; Timoptic-XE®; Timoptic®; Timoptic® in OcuDose®

Canadian Brand Names Alti-Timolol; Apo-Timol®; Apo-Timop®; Gen-Timolol; Nu-Timolol; Phoxal-timolol; PMS-Timolol; Sandoz-Timolol; Tim-AK; Timoptic-XE®; Timoptic®

Index Terms Timolol Hemihydrate; Timolol Maleate

Pharmacologic Category Beta-Adrenergic Blocker, Nonselective; Ophthalmic Agent, Antiglaucoma

Additional Appendix Information

Beta-Blockers *on page 1648*

Glaucoma Drug Therapy *on page 1808*

Use

Ophthalmic: Treatment of elevated intraocular pressure such as glaucoma or ocular hypertension

Oral: Treatment of hypertension and angina; to reduce mortality following myocardial infarction; prophylaxis of migraine

Pregnancy Risk Factor C (manufacturer); D (2nd and 3rd trimesters - expert analysis)

Pregnancy Considerations Timolol was shown to cross the placenta in an *in vitro* perfusion study. Beta-blockers have been associated with bradycardia, hypotension, hypoglycemia, and intrauterine growth rate (IUGR); IUGR is probably related to maternal hypertension. Available evidence suggests beta-blockers are generally safe during pregnancy (JNC 7). Cases of neonatal hypoglycemia have been reported following maternal use of beta-blockers at parturition or during breast-feeding. Bradycardia and arrhythmia have been reported in an infant following ophthalmic administration of timolol during pregnancy.

Lactation Enters breast milk/use caution (AAP rates "compatible")

Medication Safety Issues

Sound-alike/look-alike issues:

Timolol may be confused with atenolol, Tylenol®

Timoptic® may be confused with Betoptic® S, Talacen®, Viroptic®

Bottle cap color change:

Timoptic®: Both the 0.25% and 0.5% strengths are now packaged in bottles with yellow caps; previously, the color of the cap on the product corresponded to different strengths.

International issues:

Betimol® may be confused with Betanol® which is a brand name for metipranolol in Monaco

Contraindications Hypersensitivity to timolol or any component of the formulation; sinus bradycardia; sinus node dysfunction; heart block greater than first degree (except in patients with a functioning artificial pacemaker); cardiogenic shock; uncompensated cardiac failure; bronchospastic disease; pregnancy (2nd and 3rd trimesters)

Warnings/Precautions Consider pre-existing conditions such as sick sinus syndrome before initiating. Administer cautiously in compensated heart failure and monitor for a worsening of the condition. **[U.S. Boxed Warning]: Beta-blocker therapy should not be withdrawn abruptly (particularly in patients with CAD), but gradually tapered to avoid acute tachycardia, hypertension, and/or ischemia.** Use caution with concurrent use of beta-blockers and either verapamil or diltiazem; bradycardia or heart block can occur. Beta-blockers can aggravate symptoms in patients with PVD. Patients with bronchospastic disease should generally not receive beta-blockers - monitor closely if used in patients with potential risk of bronchospasm. Use cautiously in patients with diabetes because it can mask prominent hypoglycemic symptoms. Use cautiously in severe renal impairment: marked hypotension can occur in patients maintained on hemodialysis. Use care with anesthetic agents which decrease myocardial function. Can worsen myasthenia gravis. Use with caution in patients with a history of psychiatric illness; may cause or exacerbate CNS depression. Similar reactions found with systemic administration may occur with topical administration. Adequate alpha-blockade is required prior to use of any beta-blocker for patients with untreated pheochromocytoma. Use caution with history of severe anaphylaxis to allergens; patients taking beta-blockers may become more sensitive to repeated challenges. Treatment of anaphylaxis (eg, epinephrine) in patients taking beta-blockers may be ineffective or promote undesirable effects.

Ophthalmic: Systemic absorption and adverse effects may occur, including bradycardia and/or hypotension. Should not be used alone in angle-closure glaucoma (has no effect on pupillary constriction). Multidose vials have been associated with development of bacterial keratitis; avoid contamination. Some product do contain benzalkonium chloride which may be absorbed by soft contact lenses; do not administer while wearing soft contact lenses.

Adverse Reactions

Ophthalmic:

>10%: Ocular: Burning, stinging

1% to 10%:

Cardiovascular: Hypertension

Central nervous system: Headache

Ocular: Blepharitis, blurred vision, cataract, conjunctival injection, conjunctivitis, foreign body sensation, hyperemia, itching, tearing, visual acuity decreased

Miscellaneous: Infection

Systemic:

1% to 10%:

Cardiovascular: Bradycardia

Central nervous system: Fatigue, dizziness

Respiratory: Dyspnea

Frequency not defined (reported with any dosage form):

Cardiovascular: Angina pectoris, arrhythmia, bradycardia, cardiac failure, cardiac arrest, cerebral vascular accident, cerebral ischemia, edema, hypotension, heart block, palpitation, Raynaud's phenomenon

Central nervous system: Anxiety, confusion, depression, disorientation, dizziness, hallucinations, insomnia, memory loss, nervousness, nightmares, somnolence

Dermatologic: Alopecia, angioedema, pseudopemphigoid, psoriasiform rash, psoriasis exacerbation, rash, urticaria

Endocrine & metabolic: Hypoglycemia masked, libido decreased

Gastrointestinal: Anorexia, diarrhea, dyspepsia, nausea, xerostomia

Genitourinary: Impotence, retoperitoneal fibrosis

Hematologic: Claudication

Neuromuscular & skeletal: Myasthenia gravis exacerbation, paresthesia

Ocular: Corneal sensitivity decreased, cystoid macular edema, diplopia, dry eyes, keratitis, ocular discharge, ocular pain, ptosis, refractive changes, visual disturbances

Otic: Tinnitus

Respiratory: Bronchospasm, cough, dyspnea, nasal congestion, pulmonary edema, respiratory failure

Miscellaneous: Allergic reactions, cold hands/feet, Peyronie's disease, systemic lupus erythematosus

Drug Interactions

Metabolism/Transport Effects Substrate of CYP2D6 (major); **Inhibits** CYP2D6 (weak)

Avoid Concomitant Use

Avoid concomitant use of Timolol with any of the following: Methacholine

Increased Effect/Toxicity

Timolol may increase the levels/effects of: Alpha-/Beta-Agonists (Direct-Acting); Alpha1-Blockers; Alpha2-Agonists; Amifostine; Antipsychotic Agents (Phenothiazines); Cardiac Glycosides; Insulin; Lidocaine; Methacholine; Midodrine; RiTUXimab

The levels/effects of Timolol may be increased by: Acetylcholinesterase Inhibitors; Aminoquinolines (Antimalarial); Amiodarone; Anilidopiperidine Opioids; Antipsychotic Agents (Phenothiazines); Calcium Channel Blockers (Nondihydropyridine); CYP2D6 Inhibitors (Moderate); CYP2D6 Inhibitors (Strong); Darunavir; Diazoxide; Dipyridamole; Disopyramide; Herbs (Hypotensive Properties); Propafenone; Propoxyphene; Prostacyclin Analogues; QuiNIDine; Reserpine; Selective Serotonin Reuptake Inhibitors

Decreased Effect

Timolol may decrease the levels/effects of: Beta2-Agonists; Theophylline Derivatives

The levels/effects of Timolol may be decreased by: Barbiturates; Herbs (Hypertensive Properties); Methylphenidate; Nonsteroidal Anti-Inflammatory Agents; Rifamycin Derivatives; Yohimbine

Stability Ophthalmic drops: Store at room temperature; do not freeze. Protect from light.

Timolol GFS: Store at 2°C to 25°C (36°F to 77°F). Protect from light.

Timoptic® in OcuDose®: Store in the protective foil wrap and use within 1 month after opening foil package.

Mechanism of Action Blocks both $beta_1$- and $beta_2$-adrenergic receptors, reduces intraocular pressure by reducing aqueous humor production or possibly outflow; reduces blood pressure by blocking adrenergic receptors and decreasing sympathetic outflow, produces a negative chronotropic and inotropic activity through an unknown mechanism

Pharmacodynamics/Kinetics

Onset of action:

Hypotensive: Oral: 15-45 minutes

Peak effect: 0.5-2.5 hours

Intraocular pressure reduction: Ophthalmic: 30 minutes

Peak effect: 1-2 hours

Duration: ~4 hours; Ophthalmic: Intraocular: 24 hours

Protein binding: 60%

Metabolism: Extensively hepatic; extensive first-pass effect

Half-life elimination: 2-2.7 hours; prolonged with renal impairment

Excretion: Urine (15% to 20% as unchanged drug)

Dosage

Ophthalmic:

Children and Adults:

Solution: Initial: Instill 1 drop (0.25% solution) into affected eye(s) twice daily; increase to 0.5% solution if response not adequate; decrease to 1 drop/day if controlled; do not exceed 1 drop twice daily of 0.5% solution

Gel-forming solution (Timolol GFS, Timoptic-XE®): Instill 1 drop (either 0.25% or 0.5% solution) once daily

Adults: Solution (Istalol®): Instill 1 drop (0.5% solution) once daily in the morning

Oral: Adults:

Hypertension: Initial: 10 mg twice daily, increase gradually every 7 days, usual dosage: 20-40 mg/day in 2 divided doses; maximum: 60 mg/day

Prevention of myocardial infarction: 10 mg twice daily initiated within 1-4 weeks after infarction

Migraine headache: Initial: 10 mg twice daily, increase to maximum of 30 mg/day

Dietary Considerations Oral product should be administered with food at the same time each day.

Administration Ophthalmic: Administer other topically-applied ophthalmic medications at least 10 minutes before Timoptic-XE®; wash hands before use; invert closed bottle and shake once before use; remove cap carefully so that tip does not touch anything; hold bottle between thumb and index finger; use index finger of other hand to pull down the lower eyelid to form a pocket for the eye drop and tilt head back; place the dispenser tip close to the eye and gently squeeze the bottle to administer 1 drop; remove pressure after a single drop has been released; **do not allow the dispenser tip to touch the eye**; replace cap and store bottle in an upright position in a clean area; do **not** enlarge hole of dispenser; do **not** wash tip with water, soap, or any other cleaner. Some ophthalmic solutions contain benzalkonium chloride; wait at least 10 minutes after instilling solution before inserting soft contact lenses.

Monitoring Parameters Blood pressure, apical and radial pulses, fluid I & O, daily weight, respirations, mental status, and circulation in extremities before and during therapy; monitor for systemic effect of beta-blockade even when administering ophthalmic product

Dosage Forms Excipient information presented when available (limited, particularly for generics); consult specific product labeling. [DSC] = Discontinued product

Note: Unless otherwise specified, strength expressed as base.

Gel-forming solution, ophthalmic, as maleate:

Timolol GFS: 0.25% (2.5 mL, 5 mL); 0.5% (2.5 mL, 5 mL)

Timoptic-XE®: 0.25% (5 mL); 0.5% (5 mL)

Solution, ophthalmic, as hemihydrate:

Betimol®: 0.25% (5 mL, 10 mL [DSC], 15 mL [DSC]); 0.5% (5 mL, 10 mL, 15 mL) [contains benzalkonium chloride]

Solution, ophthalmic, as maleate: 0.25% (5 mL, 10 mL, 15 mL); 0.5% (5 mL, 10 mL, 15 mL)

Istalol®: 0.5% (10 mL) [contains benzalkonium chloride and potassium sorbate]

Timoptic®: 0.25% (5 mL); 0.5% (5 mL, 10 mL) [contains benzalkonium chloride]

Solution, ophthalmic, as maleate [preservative free]:

Timoptic® in OcuDose®: 0.25% (0.2 mL); 0.5% (0.2 mL)

Tablet, as maleate: 5 mg, 10 mg, 20 mg [strength expressed as salt]

- ◆ **Timolol and Brimonidine** *see* Brimonidine and Timolol *on page 212*
- ◆ **Timolol and Dorzolamide** *see* Dorzolamide and Timolol *on page 482*
- ◆ **Timolol GFS** *see* Timolol *on page 1472*
- ◆ **Timolol Hemihydrate** *see* Timolol *on page 1472*
- ◆ **Timolol Maleate** *see* Timolol *on page 1472*
- ◆ **Timoptic®** *see* Timolol *on page 1472*
- ◆ **Timoptic® in OcuDose®** *see* Timolol *on page 1472*
- ◆ **Timoptic-XE®** *see* Timolol *on page 1472*
- ◆ **Tinactin® Antifungal [OTC]** *see* Tolnaftate *on page 1487*
- ◆ **Tinactin® Antifungal Deodorant [OTC]** *see* Tolnaftate *on page 1487*
- ◆ **Tinactin® Antifungal Jock Itch [OTC]** *see* Tolnaftate *on page 1487*
- ◆ **Tinaderm [OTC]** *see* Tolnaftate *on page 1487*
- ◆ **Ting® Cream [OTC]** *see* Tolnaftate *on page 1487*
- ◆ **Ting® Spray Liquid [OTC]** *see* Tolnaftate *on page 1487*

Tinzaparin (tin ZA pa rin)

U.S. Brand Names Innohep®

Canadian Brand Names Innohep®

Index Terms Tinzaparin Sodium

Pharmacologic Category Low Molecular Weight Heparin

Additional Appendix Information

Anticoagulants, Injectable *on page 1636*

Use Treatment of acute symptomatic deep vein thrombosis, with or without pulmonary embolism, in conjunction with warfarin sodium

Pregnancy Risk Factor B

Pregnancy Considerations Teratogenic events were not observed in animal studies. Tinzaparin does not cross the human placenta. A pharmacokinetic study in pregnant women found no dose adjustment was needed during pregnancy. Pregnancy may increase the risk of thromboembolism; risk may be further increased with certain pre-existing conditions. As with all anticoagulants, bleeding is the major adverse effect of tinzaparin. Vaginal bleeding was reported in ~10% of pregnant patients during tinzaparin therapy. Contains benzyl alcohol; use with caution in pregnant women.

Lactation Excretion in breast milk unknown/use caution

Medication Safety Issues

High alert medication: The Institute for Safe Medication Practices (ISMP) includes this medication among its list of drug classes which have a heightened risk of causing significant patient harm when used in error.

2009 National Patient Safety Goals: The Joint Commission on Accreditation of Healthcare Organizations requires healthcare organizations that provide anticoagulant therapy to have a process in place to reduce the risk of anticoagulant-associated patient harm. Patients receiving anticoagulants should receive individualized care through a defined process that includes standardized ordering, dispensing, administration, monitoring and education. This does not apply to routine short-term use of anticoagulants for prevention of venous thromboembolism when the expectation is that the patient's laboratory values will remain within or close to normal values (NPSG.03.05.01).

Contraindications Hypersensitivity to tinzaparin sodium, heparin, or any component of the formulation; active major bleeding; heparin-induced thrombocytopenia (current or history of)

Warnings/Precautions [U.S. Boxed Warning]: Patients with recent or anticipated neuraxial anesthesia (epidural or spinal anesthesia) are at risk of spinal or epidural hematoma and subsequent paralysis. Consider risk versus benefit prior to neuraxial anesthesia; risk is increased by concomitant agents that may alter hemostasis, as well as traumatic or repeated epidural or spinal puncture, and indwelling epidural catheters. Patient should be observed closely for signs and symptoms of neurological impairment. Not to be used interchangeably (unit for unit) with heparin or any other low molecular weight heparins.

Monitor patient closely for signs or symptoms of bleeding. Certain patients are at increased risk of bleeding. Risk factors include bacterial endocarditis; congenital or acquired bleeding disorders; active ulcerative or angiodysplastic GI diseases; severe uncontrolled hypertension; history of hemorrhagic stroke; use shortly after brain, spinal, or ophthalmologic surgery; patients treated concomitantly with platelet inhibitors; recent GI bleeding; thrombocytopenia or platelet defects; severe liver disease; hypertensive or diabetic retinopathy; or in patients undergoing invasive procedures. Monitor platelet count closely. Rare cases of thrombocytopenia have occurred. Manufacturer recommends discontinuation of therapy if platelets are <100,000/mm^3. Rare cases of thrombocytopenia with thrombosis have occurred.

Reduced tinzaparin clearance was observed in patients with moderate-to-severe renal impairment; use with caution or avoid use in patients with renal insufficiency. The 2008 *Chest* guidelines recommend that patients with Cl_{cr} <30 mL/minute be treated with unfractionated heparin instead of LMWH (Hirsh, 2008). Use with caution in the elderly (delayed elimination may occur). Use in patients ≥70 years of age with renal insufficiency (Cl_{cr} ≤30 mL/minute or ≥75 years of age and Cl_{cr} ≤60 mL/minute) has been associated with an increased risk of death compared to use of unfractionated heparin; consider alternative treatments in these patients. Safety and efficacy in pediatric patients have not been established.

Heparin can cause hyperkalemia by suppressing aldosterone production; similar reactions could occur with LMWHs. Monitor for hyperkalemia which most commonly occurs in patients with risk factors for the development of hyperkalemia (eg, renal dysfunction, concomitant use of potassium-sparing diuretics or potassium supplements, hematoma in body tissues). For subcutaneous use only; do not administer intramuscularly or intravenously. Clinical experience is limited in patients with BMI >40 kg/m^2. Derived from porcine intestinal mucosa. Contains benzyl alcohol and sodium metabisulfite

Adverse Reactions As with all anticoagulants, bleeding is the major adverse effect of tinzaparin. Hemorrhage may occur at virtually any site. Risk is dependent on multiple variables.

>10%:
- Hepatic: ALT increased (13%)
- Local: Injection site hematoma (16%)

1% to 10%:
- Cardiovascular: Angina pectoris, chest pain (2%), hyper-/hypotension, tachycardia
- Central nervous system: Confusion, dizziness, fever (2%), headache (2%), insomnia, pain (2%)
- Dermatologic: Bullous eruption, pruritus, rash (1%), skin disorder
- Gastrointestinal: Constipation (1%), dyspepsia, flatulence, nausea (2%), nonspecified gastrointestinal disorder, vomiting (1%)
- Genitourinary: Dysuria, urinary retention, urinary tract infection (4%)
- Hematologic: Anemia, hematoma, hemorrhage (2%), thrombocytopenia (1%)
- Hepatic: AST increased (9%)
- Local: Thrombophlebitis (deep)
- Neuromuscular & skeletal: Back pain (2%)
- Renal: Hematuria (1%)
- Respiratory: Dyspnea (1%), epistaxis (2%), pneumonia, pulmonary embolism (2%), respiratory disorder
- Miscellaneous: Impaired healing, infection, unclassified reactions

<1% (Limited to important or life-threatening): Abscess, acute febrile reaction, agranulocytosis, allergic purpura, allergic reaction, angioedema, anaphylactoid reaction, anorectal bleeding, cardiac arrhythmia, cellulitis, cerebral hemorrhage, cholestatic hepatitis, coronary thrombosis, dependent edema, epidermal necrolysis, erythematous gastrointestinal hemorrhage, granulocytopenia, hemarthrosis, hematemesis, hemoptysis, injection site bleeding, intracranial hemorrhage, ischemic necrosis, melena, MI, necrosis, neoplasm, ocular hemorrhage, pancytopenia, peripheral ischemia, priapism, purpura, rash, retroperitoneal/intra-abdominal bleeding, severe thrombocytopenia, skin necrosis, spinal epidural hematoma, Stevens-Johnson syndrome, thromboembolism, urticaria, vaginal hemorrhage, wound hematoma

Drug Interactions

Avoid Concomitant Use There are no known interactions where it is recommended to avoid concomitant use.

Increased Effect/Toxicity

Tinzaparin may increase the levels/effects of: Anticoagulants; Drotrecogin Alfa; Ibritumomab; Tositumomab and Iodine I 131 Tositumomab

The levels/effects of Tinzaparin may be increased by: Antiplatelet Agents; Dasatinib; Herbs (Anticoagulant/Antiplatelet Properties); Nonsteroidal Anti-Inflammatory Agents; Pentosan Polysulfate Sodium; Prostacyclin Analogues; Salicylates; Thrombolytic Agents

Decreased Effect There are no known significant interactions involving a decrease in effect.

Stability Store at 15°C to 30°C (59°F to 86°F).

Mechanism of Action Standard heparin consists of components with molecular weights ranging from 4000-30,000 daltons with a mean of 16,000 daltons. Heparin acts as an anticoagulant by enhancing the inhibition rate of clotting proteases by antithrombin III, impairing normal hemostasis and inhibition of factor Xa. Low molecular weight heparins have a small effect on the activated partial thromboplastin time and strongly inhibit factor Xa. The primary inhibitory activity of tinzaparin is through antithrombin. Tinzaparin is derived from porcine heparin that undergoes controlled enzymatic depolymerization. The average molecular weight of tinzaparin ranges between 5500 and 7500 daltons which is distributed as <2000 daltons (<10%), 2000-8000 daltons (60% to 72%), and >8000 daltons (22% to 36%). The anti-Xa activity is approximately 100 int. units/mg.

Pharmacodynamics/Kinetics

Onset of action: 2-3 hours

Distribution: 3-5 L

Half-life elimination: 3-4 hours

Metabolism: Partially metabolized by desulphation and depolymerization

Bioavailability: 87%

Time to peak: 4-5 hours

Excretion: Urine

Dosage SubQ:

Adults: DVT with or without pulmonary embolism (PE): 175 anti-Xa int. units/kg of body weight once daily. The 2008 *Chest* guidelines recommend starting warfarin on the first treatment day and continuing tinzaparin until INR is between 2 and 3 (usually 5-7 days). Administer tinzaparin for at least 5 days and until INR ≥2 for at least 24 hours (Hirsh, 2008).

Note: To calculate the volume of solution to administer per dose: Volume to be administered (mL) = patient weight (kg) x 0.00875 mL/kg (may be rounded off to the nearest 0.05 mL)

Elderly: No significant differences in safety or response were seen when used in patients ≥65 years of age. However, increased sensitivity to tinzaparin in elderly patients may be possible due to a decline in renal function. Increased all-cause mortality noted in patients ≥70 years of age with Cl_{cr} ≤30 mL/minute or ≥75 years of age and Cl_{cr} ≤60 mL/minute; consider alternative treatments in these patients.

Dosing adjustment in obesity: Weight based dosing (175 anti-Xa int. units/kg of body weight once daily) provided in product labeling for patients up to 162 kg. Limited clinical experience in patients with a BMI >40 kg/m^2.

Dosage adjustment in renal impairment:

Cl_{cr} ≤50 mL/minute: Use with caution; clearance is decreased

Cl_{cr} <30 mL/minute: Per manufacturer's labeling, use with caution. The 2008 *Chest* guidelines recommend avoiding use (in patients requiring therapeutic anticoagulation); if used, consider monitoring anti-Xa levels (Hirsh, 2008).

Dosage adjustment in hepatic impairment: No specific dosage adjustment has been recommended.

Administration Patient should be lying down or sitting. Administer by deep SubQ injection, alternating between the left and right anterolateral and left and right posterolateral abdominal wall. Vary site daily. The entire needle should be introduced into the skin fold formed by the thumb and forefinger. Hold the skin fold until injection is complete. To minimize bruising, do not rub the injection site.

Monitoring Parameters CBC including platelet count and hematocrit or hemoglobin, and stool for occult blood; the monitoring of PT and/or aPTT is not of clinical value. Patients receiving both warfarin and tinzaparin should have their INR drawn just prior to the next scheduled dose of tinzaparin.

According to 2008 *Chest* guidelines, routine monitoring of anti-Xa levels is generally not recommended; however, anti-Xa levels may be beneficial in certain patients (eg, obese patients, patients with severe renal insufficiency receiving therapeutic doses, and possibly pregnant women receiving therapeutic doses; Hirsh, 2008)

Dosage Forms Excipient information presented when available (limited, particularly for generics); consult specific product labeling.

Injection, solution, as sodium:

Innohep®: 20,000 anti-Xa int. units/mL (2 mL) [contains benzyl alcohol and sodium metabisulfite]

◆ **Tinzaparin Sodium** *see* Tinzaparin *on page* 1473

Tioconazole (tye oh KONE a zole)

U.S. Brand Names 1-Day™ [OTC]; Vagistat®-1 [OTC]

Pharmacologic Category Antifungal Agent, Vaginal

Use Local treatment of vulvovaginal candidiasis

Pregnancy Risk Factor C

Lactation Excretion in breast milk unknown/not recommended

Medication Safety Issues

Sound-alike/look-alike issues:

Tioconazole may be confused with terconazole

Contraindications Hypersensitivity to tioconazole or any component of the formulation

Warnings/Precautions If irritation or sensitization occurs, discontinue use. Petrolatum-based vaginal products may damage rubber or latex condoms or diaphragms. Separate use by 3 days. Safety and efficacy have not been established in children.

Drug Interactions

Metabolism/Transport Effects Inhibits CYP1A2 (weak), 2A6 (weak), 2C9 (weak), 2C19 (weak), 2D6 (weak), 2E1 (weak)

Avoid Concomitant Use There are no known interactions where it is recommended to avoid concomitant use.

Increased Effect/Toxicity There are no known significant interactions involving an increase in effect.

Decreased Effect There are no known significant interactions involving a decrease in effect.

Stability Store at room temperature.

Mechanism of Action A 1-substituted imidazole derivative with a broad antifungal spectrum against a wide variety of dermatophytes and yeasts, including *Trichophyton mentagrophytes*, *T. rubrum*, *T. erinacei*, *T. tonsurans*, *Microsporum canis*, *Microsporum gypseum*, and *Candida albicans*. Both agents appear to be similarly effective against *Epidermophyton floccosum*.

Pharmacodynamics/Kinetics

Onset of action: Some improvement: Within 24 hours; Complete relief: Within 7 days

Absorption: Intravaginal: Systemic (small amounts)

Distribution: Vaginal fluid: 24-72 hours

Excretion: Urine and feces

Dosage Adults: Vaginal: Insert 1 applicatorful in vagina, just prior to bedtime, as a single dose

Administration Insert high into vagina

Dosage Forms Excipient information presented when available (limited, particularly for generics); consult specific product labeling.

Ointment, vaginal: 6.5% (4.6 g) [with applicator]

◆ **Tioguanine** *see* Thioguanine *on page 1459*

◆ **Tiotixene** *see* Thiothixene *on page 1463*

Tiotropium (ty oh TRO pee um)

U.S. Brand Names Spiriva® HandiHaler®

Canadian Brand Names Spiriva®

Index Terms Tiotropium Bromide Monohydrate

Pharmacologic Category Anticholinergic Agent

Use Maintenance treatment of bronchospasm associated with COPD (bronchitis and emphysema)

Pregnancy Risk Factor C

Pregnancy Considerations Adverse events (fetal loss, decreased birth weights, delayed sexual maturation) were observed in some animal studies. There are no adequate and well-controlled studies in pregnant women. Use only when expected benefit to mother outweighs potential risk to the fetus.

Lactation Excretion in breast milk unknown/use caution

Medication Safety Issues

Sound-alike/look-alike issues:

Spiriva® may be confused with Inspra™, Serevent®

Spiriva® capsules for inhalation are for administration via HandiHaler® device and are **not** for oral use

Contraindications Hypersensitivity to tiotropium, atropine or its derivatives, including ipratropium, or any component of the formulation (contains lactose)

Warnings/Precautions Rarely, paradoxical bronchospasm may occur with use of inhaled bronchodilating agents; this should be distinguished from inadequate response. Not indicated for the initial (rescue) treatment of acute episodes of bronchospasm; use with caution in patients with myasthenia gravis, narrow-angle glaucoma, prostatic hyperplasia, or bladder neck obstruction; avoid inadvertent instillation of powder into the eyes. Immediate hypersensitivity reactions may occur. The contents of Spiriva® capsules are for inhalation only via the HandiHaler® device. There have been reports of incorrect administration (swallowing of the capsules). Safety and efficacy have not been established in pediatric patients.

Adverse Reactions

>10%:

Gastrointestinal: Xerostomia (16%)

Respiratory: Upper respiratory tract infection (41% vs 37% with placebo), sinusitis (11% vs 9% with placebo)

1% to 10%:

Cardiovascular: Angina (1% to 7%), edema (dependent, 5%)

Central nervous system: Depression (1% to 3%), dysphonia (1% to 3%)

Dermatologic: Rash (4%)

Endocrine & metabolic: Hypercholesterolemia (1% to 3%), hyperglycemia (1% to 3%)

Gastrointestinal: Dyspepsia (6%), abdominal pain (5%), constipation (4%), vomiting (4%), reflux, ulcerative stomatitis

Genitourinary: Urinary tract infection (7%)

Neuromuscular & skeletal: Myalgia (4%), arthritis (≥3%), leg pain (1% to 3%), paresthesia (1% to 3%), skeletal pain (1% to 3%)

Ocular: Cataract (1% to 3%)

Respiratory: Pharyngitis (9%), rhinitis (6%), epistaxis (4%), cough (≥3%), laryngitis (1% to 3%)

Miscellaneous: Infection (4%), moniliasis (4%), flu-like syndrome (≥3%), allergic reaction (1% to 3%), herpes zoster (1% to 3%)

<1%, postmarketing, and/or case reports (limited to important or life-threatening): Angioedema; application site irritation (glossitis, mouth ulceration, pharyngolaryngeal pain); atrial fibrillation, blurred vision, candidiasis (oral), dizziness, dysphagia, glaucoma, hoarseness, hypersensitivity reactions, ileus (paralytic), intestinal obstruction, intraocular pressure increased, palpitation, paradoxical bronchospasm, pruritus, pupil dilation (if powder comes in contact with eyes), stroke, supraventricular tachycardia, tachycardia, throat irritation, urinary difficulty, urinary retention, urticaria

Drug Interactions

Metabolism/Transport Effects Substrate (minor) of CYP2D6, 3A4

Avoid Concomitant Use There are no known interactions where it is recommended to avoid concomitant use.

Increased Effect/Toxicity

Tiotropium may increase the levels/effects of: Anticholinergics; Cannabinoids; Potassium Chloride

The levels/effects of Tiotropium may be increased by: Pramlintide

Decreased Effect

Tiotropium may decrease the levels/effects of: Acetylcholinesterase Inhibitors (Central); Secretin

The levels/effects of Tiotropium may be decreased by: Acetylcholinesterase Inhibitors (Central)

Stability Store at 25°C (77°F); excursions permitted to 15°C to 30°C (59°F to 86°F). Do not store capsules in HandiHaler® device. Capsules should be stored in the blister pack and only removed immediately before use. Once protective foil is peeled back and/or removed the capsule should be used immediately; if capsule is not used immediately it should be discarded.

Mechanism of Action Blocks the action of acetylcholine at parasympathetic sites in bronchial smooth muscle causing bronchodilation

Pharmacodynamics/Kinetics

Absorption: Poorly absorbed from GI tract, systemic absorption may occur from lung

Distribution: V_d: 32 L/kg

Protein binding: 72%

Metabolism: Hepatic (minimal), via CYP2D6 and CYP3A4

Bioavailability: Following inhalation, 19.5%; oral solution: 2% to 3%

Half-life elimination: 5-6 days

Time to peak, plasma: 5 minutes (following inhalation)

Excretion: Urine (14% of an inhaled dose); feces (primarily nonabsorbed drug)

Dosage Oral inhalation: Adults: Contents of 1 capsule (18 mcg) inhaled once daily using HandiHaler® device

Dosage adjustment in renal impairment: Plasma concentrations increase in renal impairment. Use caution in moderate-severe impairment; no specific dosage adjustment recommended.

Administration Administer once daily at the same time each day. Remove capsule from foil blister immediately before use. Capsule should not be swallowed. Place capsule in the capsule-chamber in the base of the HandiHaler® Inhaler. Must only use the HandiHaler® Inhaler. Close mouthpiece until a click is heard, leaving dustcap open. Exhale fully. Do not exhale into inhaler. Tilt head slightly back and inhale (rapidly, steadily and deeply); the capsule vibration may be heard within the device. Hold breath as long as possible. If any powder remains in capsule, exhale and inhale again. Repeat until capsule is empty. Throw away empty capsule; do not leave in inhaler. Do not use a spacer with the HandiHaler® Inhaler. Do not use HandiHaler® device for other medications. Always keep capsules and inhaler dry.

Delivery of dose: Instruct patient to place mouthpiece gently between teeth, closing lips around inhaler. Instruct patient to inhale deeply and hold breath held for 5-10 seconds. The amount of drug delivered is small, and the individual will not sense the medication as it is inhaled.

Remove mouthpiece prior to exhalation. Patient should not breathe out through the mouthpiece.

Monitoring Parameters FEV_1, peak flow (or other pulmonary function studies)

Dosage Forms Excipient information presented when available (limited, particularly for generics); consult specific product labeling.

Powder for oral inhalation [capsule]:

Spiriva® HandiHaler®: 18 mcg/capsule (5s, 30s, 90s) [contains lactose]

◆ **Tiotropium Bromide Monohydrate** *see* Tiotropium *on page 1476*

Tipranavir (tip RA na veer)

U.S. Brand Names Aptivus®

Canadian Brand Names Aptivus®

Index Terms PNU-140690E; TPV

Pharmacologic Category Antiretroviral Agent, Protease Inhibitor

Additional Appendix Information

Antiretroviral Therapy for HIV Infection: Adults and Adolescents *on page 1758*

Perinatal HIV Guidelines *on page 1730*

Use Treatment of HIV-1 infections in combination with ritonavir and other antiretroviral agents; limited to highly treatment-experienced or multiprotease inhibitor-resistant patients.

Pregnancy Risk Factor C

Pregnancy Considerations It is not known if tipranavir crosses the human placenta. Pregnancy and protease inhibitors are both associated with an increased risk of hyperglycemia. Glucose levels should be closely monitored. Women receiving estrogen (as hormonal contraception or replacement therapy) have an increased incidence of rash. Alternative forms of contraception may be needed. Health professionals are encouraged to contact the antiretroviral pregnancy registry to monitor outcomes of pregnant women exposed to antiretroviral medications (1-800-258-4263 or www.APRegistry.com).

Lactation Excretion in breast milk unknown/contraindicated

Contraindications Concurrent therapy of tipranavir/ritonavir with amiodarone, cisapride, ergot derivatives (eg, dihydroergotamine, ergonovine, ergotamine, methylergonovine), flecainide, lovastatin, midazolam, pimozide, propafenone, quinidine, rifampin, simvastatin, St John's wort, and triazolam; moderate-to-severe hepatic impairment (Child-Pugh class B and C)

Warnings/Precautions Coadministration with ritonavir is required. **[U.S. Boxed Warning]: In combination with ritonavir, may cause hepatitis (including fatalities) and/or exacerbate pre-existing hepatic dysfunction (causal relationship not established); patients with chronic hepatitis B or C are at increased risk.** Monitor patients closely; discontinue use if signs or symptoms of toxicity occur or if asymptomatic AST/ALT elevations >10 times upper limit of normal or AST/ALT elevations >5-10 times upper limit of normal concurrently with total bilirubin >2.5 times the upper limit of normal occur. Use with caution in patients with mild hepatic impairment; contraindicated in moderate-to-severe impairment. May be associated with fat redistribution (buffalo hump, increased abdominal girth, breast engorgement, facial atrophy). Use caution in hemophilia. May increase cholesterol and/or triglycerides; hypertriglyceridemia may increase risk of pancreatitis. May cause hyperglycemia. Use with caution in patients with sulfonamide allergy. Protease inhibitors have been associated with a variety of hypersensitivity events (some severe), including rash, anaphylaxis (rare), angioedema, bronchospasm, erythema multiforme, and/or Stevens-Johnson syndrome (rare). It is generally recommended to discontinue treatment if severe rash or moderate symptoms accompanied by other systemic symptoms occur. Immune reconstitution syndrome, including inflammatory responses to indolent infections, has been associated with antiretroviral therapy; additional evaluation and treatment may be required.

[U.S. Boxed Warning]: Tipranavir has been associated with rare reports of fatal and nonfatal intracranial hemorrhage; causal relationship not established. Events often occurred in patients with medical conditions (eg, CNS lesions, head trauma, recent neurosurgery, coagulopathy, alcohol abuse) or concurrent therapy which may have influenced these events. Tipranavir may inhibit platelet aggregation. Use with caution in patients who may be at risk for increased bleeding (trauma, surgery or other medical conditions) or in patients receiving concurrent medications which may increase the risk of bleeding, including antiplatelet agents and anticoagulants.

Use with caution in patients taking strong CYP3A4 inhibitors and moderate CYP3A4 inducers. Concomitant use with selected major CYP3A4 substrates and strong CYP3A4 inducers is contraindicated (see Drug Interactions); consider alternative agents that avoid or lessen the potential for CYP-mediated interactions. Coadministration with anticoagulants or antiplatelet agents may increase the risk of bleeding. Women receiving estrogen (as hormonal contraception or replacement therapy) have an increased incidence of rash. Alternative forms of contraception may be needed. Oral solution formulation contains vitamin E; additional vitamin E supplements should be avoided. Safety and efficacy have not been established in children <2 years of age.

Adverse Reactions

>10%:

Dermatologic: Rash (children 21%; adults 3% to 10%)

Endocrine & metabolic: Hypercholesterolemia (>300 mg/dL: 22%), hypertriglyceridemia (>400 mg/dL: 61%)

Gastrointestinal: Diarrhea (15%)

Hepatic: Transaminases increased (>2.5 x ULN: 26% to 32%; grade 3/4: 10% to 20%)

Neuromuscular & skeletal: CPK increased (grade 3/4: children 11%)

2% to 10%:

Central nervous system: Fever (6% to 8%), fatigue (6%), headache (5%)

Endocrine & metabolic: Dehydration (2%)

Gastrointestinal: Nausea (5% to 9%), amylase increased (grade 3: 6% to 8%), vomiting (6%), abdominal pain (4%), diarrhea (children 4%), weight loss (3%)

Hematologic: Bleeding (children 8%), WBC decreased (grades 3: 5%), anemia (3%), neutropenia (2%)

Hepatic: ALT increased (2%, grades 3/4: 10%), AST increased (grades 3/4: 6%), GGT increased (2%)

Neuromuscular & skeletal: Myalgia (2%)

Respiratory: Cough (children 6%), dyspnea (2%), epistaxis (children 4%)

<2% (Limited to important or life-threatening): Abdominal distension, anorexia, appetite decreased, diabetes mellitus, dizziness, dyspepsia, exanthem, facial wasting, flatulence, flu-like syndrome, gastroesophageal reflux, hepatic failure, hepatic steatosis, hepatitis, hyperbilirubinemia, hyperglycemia, hypersensitivity, immune reconstitution syndrome, insomnia, intracranial hemorrhage, lipase increased, lipoatrophy, lipodystrophy (acquired), lipohypertrophy, malaise, mitochondrial toxicity, muscle cramp, neuropathy (peripheral), pancreatitis, pruritus, renal insufficiency, sleep disorder, somnolence, thrombocytopenia

Drug Interactions

Metabolism/Transport Effects Substrate of CYP3A4 (major; minimal metabolism when coadministered with ritonavir)

Avoid Concomitant Use

Avoid concomitant use of Tipranavir with any of the following: Amiodarone; Cisapride; Ergot Derivatives; Etravirine; Flecainide; Pimozide; Propafenone; QuiNIDine; St Johns Wort

Increased Effect/Toxicity

Tipranavir may increase the levels/effects of: Amiodarone; Antifungal Agents (Azole Derivatives, Systemic); Benzodiazepines (metabolized by oxidation); Calcium Channel Blockers (Dihydropyridine); Calcium Channel Blockers (Nondihydropyridine); CarBAMazepine; Cisapride; Clarithromycin; Corticosteroids (Orally Inhaled); CycloSPORINE; Digoxin; Enfuvirtide; Eplerenone; Ergot Derivatives; FentaNYL; Flecainide; Fusidic Acid; HMG-CoA Reductase Inhibitors; Meperidine; Methadone; Nefazodone; Phosphodiesterase 5 Inhibitors; Pimozide; Propafenone; Protease Inhibitors; QuiNIDine; Rifamycin Derivatives; Sirolimus; Tacrolimus; Temsirolimus; Tenofovir; TraZODone; Tricyclic Antidepressants

The levels/effects of Tipranavir may be increased by: Antifungal Agents (Azole Derivatives, Systemic); Clarithromycin; CycloSPORINE; Delavirdine; Disulfiram; Efavirenz; Enfuvirtide; Estrogen Derivatives; Fusidic Acid; MetroNIDAZOLE

Decreased Effect

Tipranavir may decrease the levels/effects of: Abacavir; Clarithromycin; Dabigatran Etexilate; Delavirdine; Didanosine; Estrogen Derivatives; Etravirine; Meperidine; P-Glycoprotein Substrates; PHENobarbital; Phenytoin; Proton Pump Inhibitors; Raltegravir; Theophylline Derivatives; Valproic Acid; Zidovudine

The levels/effects of Tipranavir may be decreased by: Antacids; CarBAMazepine; CYP3A4 Inducers (Strong); Deferasirox; Efavirenz; Garlic; Nevirapine; PHENobarbital; Phenytoin; Rifamycin Derivatives; St Johns Wort; Tenofovir

Ethanol/Nutrition/Herb Interactions

Ethanol: Capsules contain dehydrated alcohol 7% w/w (0.1g per capsule)

Food: Bioavailability is increased with a high-fat meal.

Herb/Nutraceutical: St Johns wort may decrease the levels/effects of tipranavir/ritonavir; concurrent use is contraindicated. Vitamin E (high dose) may increase the risk of bleeding.

Stability

Capsule: Prior to opening bottle, store under refrigeration at 2°C to 8°C (36°F to 46°F). After bottle is opened, may be stored at controlled room temperature of 25°C (77°F) for up to 60 days.

Oral solution: Store at 15°C to 30°C (59°F to 86°F). After bottle is open, use within 60 days. Do not refrigerator or freeze oral solution.

Mechanism of Action Tipranavir is a nonpeptide inhibitor of HIV-1 protease. It binds to the protease activity site and inhibits the activity of the enzyme. HIV protease is required for the cleavage of viral polyprotein precursors into individual functional proteins found in infectious HIV. Inhibition prevents cleavage of these polyproteins, resulting in the formation of immature, noninfectious viral particles.

Pharmacodynamics/Kinetics

Absorption: Incomplete (percentage not established)

Distribution: V_d: 7.7-10 L

Protein binding: >99% (albumin, alpha$_1$-acid glycoprotein)

Metabolism: Hepatic, via CYP3A4 (minimal when coadministered with ritonavir)

Bioavailability: Not established; increased with high-fat meal

Half-life elimination: Children 2-<6 years of age: ~8 hours, 6-<12 years of age: ~7 hours, 12-18 years: ~5 hours; Adults: 6 hours

Time to peak, plasma: 3 hours

Excretion: Feces (82%); urine (4%); primarily as unchanged drug (when coadministered with ritonavir)

Dosage Oral:

Children ≥2 years: 14 mg/kg or 375 mg/m^2 (maximum: 500 mg/dose) twice daily. **Note:** Coadministration with ritonavir (6 mg/kg or 150 mg/m^2 [maximum 200 mg/dose] twice daily) is required.

If intolerance or toxicity develops and virus is not resistant to multiple protease inhibitors: May decrease dose to 12 mg/kg or 290 mg/m^2 twice daily. **Note:** Coadministration with ritonavir (5 mg/kg or 115 mg/m^2 twice daily) is required.

Adults: 500 mg twice daily with a high-fat meal. **Note:** Coadministration with ritonavir (200 mg twice daily) is required.

Dosage adjustment in renal impairment: No adjustment required

Dosage adjustment in hepatic impairment:

Mild impairment (Child-Pugh class A): No adjustment required

Moderate-to-severe impairment (Child-Pugh class B-C): Concurrent use is contraindicated

Dietary Considerations Contains dehydrated ethanol 7% w/w (0.1 g per capsule). Oral solution formulation contains vitamin E; additional vitamin E supplements should be avoided.

Administration Should be administered with a high-fat meal (bioavailability is increased); coadministration with ritonavir is required

Monitoring Parameters Viral load, CD4, serum glucose, liver function tests, bilirubin

Dosage Forms Excipient information presented when available (limited, particularly for generics); consult specific product labeling.

Capsule, soft gelatin:

Aptivus®: 250 mg [contains dehydrated ethanol 7% per capsule]

Solution:

Aptivus®: 100 mg/mL (95 mL) [contains vitamin E, propylene glycol; buttermint-butter toffee flavor]

Tirofiban (tye roe FYE ban)

U.S. Brand Names Aggrastat®

Canadian Brand Names Aggrastat®

Index Terms MK383; Tirofiban Hydrochloride

Pharmacologic Category Antiplatelet Agent, Glycoprotein IIb/IIIa Inhibitor

Additional Appendix Information

Glycoprotein Antagonists *on page 1656*

Use In combination with heparin, is indicated for the treatment of acute coronary syndrome, including patients who are to be managed medically and those undergoing PTCA or atherectomy. In this setting, it has been shown to decrease the rate of a combined endpoint of death, new myocardial infarction or refractory ischemia/repeat cardiac procedure.

Pregnancy Risk Factor B

Lactation Excretion in breast milk unknown/contraindicated

Medication Safety Issues

Sound-alike/look-alike issues:

Aggrastat® may be confused with Aggrenox®, argatroban

High alert medication: The Institute for Safe Medication Practices (ISMP) includes this medication among its list

of drugs which have a heightened risk of causing significant patient harm when used in error.

Contraindications Hypersensitivity to tirofiban or any component of the formulation; active internal bleeding or a history of bleeding diathesis within the previous 30 days; history of intracranial hemorrhage, intracranial neoplasm, arteriovenous malformation, or aneurysm; history of thrombocytopenia following prior exposure; history of CVA within 30 days or any history of hemorrhagic stroke; major surgical procedure or severe physical trauma within the previous month; history, symptoms, or findings suggestive of aortic dissection; severe hypertension (systolic BP >180 mm Hg and/or diastolic BP >110 mm Hg); concomitant use of another parenteral GP IIb/IIIa inhibitor; acute pericarditis

Warnings/Precautions Bleeding is the most common complication encountered during this therapy; most major bleeding occurs at the arterial access site for cardiac catheterization. Caution in patients with platelets <150,000/mm^3; patients with hemorrhagic retinopathy; chronic dialysis patients; when used in combination with other drugs impacting on coagulation. To minimize bleeding complications, care must be taken in sheath insertion/removal. Sheath hemostasis should be achieved at least 4 hours before hospital discharge. Other trauma and vascular punctures should be minimized. Avoid obtaining vascular access through a noncompressible site (eg, subclavian or jugular vein). Patients with severe renal insufficiency require dosage reduction. Safety and efficacy have not been established in children.

Adverse Reactions Bleeding is the major drug-related adverse effect. Patients received background treatment with aspirin and heparin. Major bleeding was reported in 1.4% to 2.2%; minor bleeding in 10.5% to 12%; transfusion was required in 4% to 4.3%.

>1% (nonbleeding adverse events):

Cardiovascular: Bradycardia (4%), coronary artery dissection (5%), edema (2%)

Central nervous system: Dizziness (3%), fever (>1%), headache (>1%), vasovagal reaction (2%)

Gastrointestinal: Nausea (>1%)

Genitourinary: Pelvic pain (6%)

Hematologic: Thrombocytopenia: <90,000/mm^3 (1.5%), <50,000/mm^3 (0.3%)

Neuromuscular & skeletal: Leg pain (3%)

Miscellaneous: Diaphoresis (2%)

<1% (Limited to important or life-threatening): Acutely decreased platelets in association with fever, anaphylaxis, GI bleeding (0.1% to 0.2%), GU bleeding (up to 0.1%), hemopericardium, intracranial bleeding (up to 0.1%), pulmonary alveolar hemorrhage, rash, retroperitoneal bleeding (up to 0.6%), severe (<10,000/mm^3) thrombocytopenia (rare), spinal-epidural hematoma

Drug Interactions

Avoid Concomitant Use There are no known interactions where it is recommended to avoid concomitant use.

Increased Effect/Toxicity

Tirofiban may increase the levels/effects of: Anticoagulants; Antiplatelet Agents; Drotrecogin Alfa; Ibritumomab; Salicylates; Thrombolytic Agents; Tositumomab and Iodine I 131 Tositumomab

The levels/effects of Tirofiban may be increased by: Dasatinib; Herbs (Anticoagulant/Antiplatelet Properties); Nonsteroidal Anti-Inflammatory Agents; Omega-3-Acid Ethyl Esters; Pentosan Polysulfate Sodium; Prostacyclin Analogues

Decreased Effect

The levels/effects of Tirofiban may be decreased by: Nonsteroidal Anti-Inflammatory Agents

Stability Store at 25°C (77°F); do not freeze. Protect from light during storage.

Mechanism of Action A reversible antagonist of fibrinogen binding to the GP IIb/IIIa receptor, the major platelet surface receptor involved in platelet aggregation. When administered intravenously, it inhibits *ex vivo* platelet aggregation in a dose- and concentration-dependent manner. When given according to the recommended regimen, >90% inhibition is attained by the end of the 30-minute infusion. Platelet aggregation inhibition is reversible following cessation of the infusion.

Pharmacodynamics/Kinetics

Distribution: 35% unbound

Metabolism: Minimally hepatic

Half-life elimination: 2 hours

Excretion: Urine (65%) and feces (25%) primarily as unchanged drug

Clearance: Elderly: Reduced by 19% to 26%

Dosage Adults: I.V.: Initial rate of 0.4 mcg/kg/minute for 30 minutes and then continued at 0.1 mcg/kg/minute; dosing should be continued through angiography and for 12-24 hours after angioplasty or atherectomy. See table.

Tirofiban Dosing (Using 50 mcg/mL Concentration)

Patient Weight (kg)	Patients With Normal Renal Function		Patients With Renal Dysfunction	
	30-Min Loading Infusion Rate (mL/h)	Maintenance Infusion Rate (mL/h)	30-Min Loading Infusion Rate (mL/h)	Maintenance Infusion Rate (mL/h)
30-37	16	4	8	2
38-45	20	5	10	3
46-54	24	6	12	3
55-62	28	7	14	4
63-70	32	8	16	4
71-79	36	9	18	5
80-87	40	10	20	5
88-95	44	11	22	6
96-104	48	12	24	6
105-112	52	13	26	7
113-120	56	14	28	7
121-128	60	15	30	8
128-137	64	16	32	8
138-145	68	17	34	9
146-153	72	18	36	9

Dosing adjustment in severe renal impairment: Cl_{cr} <30 mL/minute: Reduce dose to 50% of normal rate.

Administration Intended for intravenous delivery using sterile equipment and technique. Do not add other drugs or remove solution directly from the bag with a syringe. Do not use plastic containers in series connections; such use can result in air embolism by drawing air from the first container if it is empty of solution. Discard unused solution 24 hours following the start of infusion. May be administered through the same catheter as heparin. Tirofiban injection must be diluted to a concentration of 50 mcg/mL (premixed solution does not require dilution). Infuse over 30 minutes.

Monitoring Parameters Platelet count. Hemoglobin and hematocrit should be monitored prior to treatment, within 6 hours following loading infusion, and at least daily thereafter during therapy. Platelet count may need to be monitored earlier in patients who received prior glycoprotein IIb/IIa antagonists. Persistent reductions of platelet counts <90,000/mm^3 may require interruption or discontinuation of infusion. Because tirofiban requires concurrent heparin therapy, aPTT levels should also be followed. Monitor vital signs and laboratory results prior to, during, and after therapy. Assess infusion insertion site during and after therapy (every 15 minutes or as institutional policy).

Observe and teach patient bleeding precautions (avoid invasive procedures and activities that could result in injury). Monitor closely for signs of unusual or excessive bleeding (eg, CNS changes, blood in urine, stool, or vomitus, unusual bruising or bleeding). Breast-feeding is contraindicated.

Dosage Forms Excipient information presented when available (limited, particularly for generics); consult specific product labeling. [DSC] = Discontuned product

Infusion [premixed in sodium chloride]:

Aggrastat®: 50 mcg/mL (100 mL, 250 mL)

Injection, solution:

Aggrastat®: 250 mcg/mL (50 mL) [DSC]

◆ **Tirofiban Hydrochloride** *see* Tirofiban *on page 1478*

◆ **Tisit® [OTC]** *see* Pyrethrins and Piperonyl Butoxide *on page 1271*

◆ **Tisit® Blue Gel [OTC]** *see* Pyrethrins and Piperonyl Butoxide *on page 1271*

◆ **Titralac™ [OTC]** *see* Calcium Carbonate *on page 238*

◆ **Ti-U-Lac® H (Can)** *see* Urea and Hydrocortisone *on page 1531*

TiZANidine (tye ZAN i deen)

U.S. Brand Names Zanaflex Capsules™; Zanaflex®

Canadian Brand Names Apo-Tizanidine®; Gen-Tizanidine; Zanaflex®

Index Terms Sirdalud®

Pharmacologic Category $Alpha_2$-Adrenergic Agonist

Use Skeletal muscle relaxant used for treatment of muscle spasticity

Unlabeled/Investigational Use Tension headaches, low back pain, and trigeminal neuralgia

Pregnancy Risk Factor C

Lactation Excretion in breast milk unknown/not recommended

Medication Safety Issues

Sound-alike/look-alike issues:

TiZANidine may be confused with tiaGABine

Zanaflex® capsules and Zanaflex® tablets (or generic tizanidine tablets) are not interchangeable

Contraindications Hypersensitivity to tizanidine or any component of the formulation; concomitant therapy with ciprofloxacin or fluvoxamine (potent CYP1A2 inhibitors)

Warnings/Precautions Significant hypotension (possibly with bradycardia or orthostatic hypotension) and sedation may occur; use caution in patients with cardiac disease or those at risk for severe hypotensive or sedative effects. Avoid concomitant administration with CYP1A2 inhibitors; increased tizanidine levels/effects (severe hypotension and sedation) may occur. These effects may also be increased with concomitant administration with other CNS depressants and/or antihypertensives; use caution. Elderly patients are at risk due to decreased clearance, particulary in elderly patients with renal insufficiency (Cl_{cr} <25 mL/minute) compared to healthy elderly subjects; this may lead to an increased risk of adverse effects and/or a longer duration of effects. Use caution in any patient with renal impairment; reduced initial doses recommended in patient with Cl_{cr} <25 mL/minute. Use with extreme caution or avoid in hepatic impairment due to extensive hepatic metabolism and potential hepatotoxicity; AST/ALT elevations (≥2 times baseline) and rarely hepatic failure have occurred; monitoring recommended.

Use has been associated with visual hallucinations or delusions, generally in first 6 weeks of therapy; use caution in patients with psychiatric disorders. Withdrawal resulting in rebound hypertension, tachycardia, and hypertonia may occur upon discontinuation; doses should be decreased slowly, particularly in patients receiving high doses for prolonged periods. Pharmacokinetics and bioequivalence between capsules and tablets altered by nonfasting vs fasting conditions. Limited data exists for chronic use of single doses >8 mg and multiple doses >24 mg/day. Safety and efficacy have not been established in children.

Adverse Reactions Frequency percentages below reported during multiple-dose studies, unless specified otherwise.

>10%:

Cardiovascular: Hypotension (single-dose study with doses ≥8 mg: 16% to 33%)

Central nervous system: Somnolence (48%), dizziness (16%)

Gastrointestinal: Xerostomia (49%)

Neuromuscular & skeletal: Weakness (41%)

1% to 10%:

Cardiovascular: Bradycardia (single-dose study with doses ≥8 mg: 2% to 10%)

Central nervous system: Nervousness (3%), speech disorder (3%), visual hallucinations/delusions (3%; generally occurring in first 6 weeks of therapy), anxiety (1%), depression (1%), fever (1%)

Dermatologic: Rash (1%), skin ulcer (1%)

Gastrointestinal: Constipation (4%), vomiting (3%), abdominal pain (1%), diarrhea (1%), dyspepsia (1%)

Genitourinary: UTI (10%), urinary frequency (3%)

Hepatic: Liver enzymes increased (3% to 5%)

Neuromuscular & skeletal: Dyskinesia (3%), back pain (1%), myasthenia (1%), paresthesia (1%)

Ocular: Blurred vision (3%)

Respiratory: Pharyngitis (3%), rhinitis (3%)

Miscellaneous: Infection (6%), flu-like syndrome (3%), diaphoresis (1%)

<1%, frequency not defined, and postmarketing experience (limited to important or life-threatening): Adrenal insufficiency, allergic reaction, anemia, angina, arrhythmia, carcinoma, cholelithiasis, deafness, dementia, dyslipidemia, gastrointestinal hemorrhage, glaucoma, heart failure, hepatomegaly, hemiplegia, hepatic failure, hepatitis, hepatoma, hyperglycemia, hypokalemia, hyponatremia, hypoproteinemia, hypothyroidism, jaundice, leukopenia, leukocytosis, MI, optic neuritis, palpitation, postural hypotension, psychotic-like symptoms, pulmonary embolus, respiratory acidosis, retinal hemorrhage, sepsis, suicide attempt, syncope, thrombocythemia, thrombocytopenia, ventricular extrasystoles, ventricular tachycardia

Drug Interactions

Metabolism/Transport Effects Substrate of CYP1A2 (major)

Avoid Concomitant Use

Avoid concomitant use of TiZANidine with any of the following: Ciprofloxacin; Fluvoxamine; Iobenguane I 123

Increased Effect/Toxicity

TiZANidine may increase the levels/effects of: Alcohol (Ethyl); Amifostine; CNS Depressants; RiTUXimab

The levels/effects of TiZANidine may be increased by: Beta-Blockers; Ciprofloxacin; CYP1A2 Inhibitors (Moderate); CYP1A2 Inhibitors (Strong); Diazoxide; Fluvoxamine; Herbs (Hypotensive Properties); Oral Contraceptive (Estrogens); Prostacyclin Analogues

Decreased Effect

TiZANidine may decrease the levels/effects of: Iobenguane I 123

The levels/effects of TiZANidine may be decreased by: Antidepressants (Alpha2-Antagonist); Herbs (Hypertensive Properties); Methylphenidate; Serotonin/Norepinephrine Reuptake Inhibitors; Tricyclic Antidepressants; Yohimbine

Ethanol/Nutrition/Herb Interactions

Ethanol: Avoid ethanol (may increase CNS depression).

Food: The tablet and capsule dosage forms are not bioequivalent when administered with food. Food increases both the time to peak concentration and the extent of absorption for both the tablet and capsule. However, maximal concentrations of tizanidine achieved when administered with food were increased by 30% for the tablet, but decreased by 20% for the capsule. Under fed conditions, the capsule is approximately 80% bioavailable relative to the tablet.

Herb/Nutraceutical: Avoid valerian, St John's wort, kava kava, gotu kola (may increase CNS depression). Avoid black cohosh, California poppy, coleus, golden seal, hawthorn, mistletoe, periwinkle, quinine, shepherd's purse (may increase hypotensive effects).

Mechanism of Action An $alpha_2$-adrenergic agonist agent which decreases excitatory input to alpha motor neurons; an imidazole derivative chemically-related to clonidine, which acts as a centrally acting muscle relaxant with $alpha_2$-adrenergic agonist properties; acts on the level of the spinal cord

Pharmacodynamics/Kinetics

Duration: 3-6 hours

Absorption: Tablets and capsules are bioequivalent under fasting conditions, but not under nonfasting conditions.

Tablets administered with food: Peak plasma concentration is increased by ~30%; time to peak increased by 25 minutes; extent of absorption increased by ~30%.

Capsules administered with food: Peak plasma concentration decreased by 20%; time to peak increased by 2-3 hours; extent of absorption increased by ~10%.

Capsules opened and sprinkled on applesauce are not bioequivalent to administration of intact capsules under fasting conditions. Peak plasma concentration and AUC are increased by 15% to 20%.

Protein binding: ~30%

Metabolism: Extensively hepatic

Bioavailability: ~40% (extensive first-pass metabolism)

Half-life elimination: 2.5 hours

Time to peak, serum:

Fasting state: Capsule, tablet: 1 hour

Fed state: Capsule: 3-4 hours, Tablet: 1.5 hours

Excretion: Urine (60%); feces (20%)

Dosage

Adults: 2-4 mg 3 times/day

Usual initial dose: 4 mg, may increase by 2-4 mg as needed for satisfactory reduction of muscle tone every 6-8 hours to a maximum of 3 doses in any 24-hour period

Maximum: 36 mg/day

Elderly: No specific dosing guidelines exist; clearance is decreased; dose cautiously

Dosing adjustment in renal impairment: Cl_{cr} <25 mL/minute: Use with caution; clearance reduced >50%. During initial dose titration, use reduced doses. If higher doses necessary, increase dose instead of increasing dosing frequency.

Dosing adjustment in hepatic impairment: Avoid use in hepatic impairment; if used, lowest possible dose should be used initially with close monitoring for adverse effects (eg, hypotension).

Dietary Considerations Administration with food compared to administration in the fasting state results in clinically-significant differences in absorption and other pharmacokinetic parameters. Patients should be consistent and should not switch administration of the tablets or the capsules between the fasting and nonfasting state. In addition, switching between the capsules and the tablets in the fed state will also result in significant differences. Opening capsule contents to sprinkle on applesauce compared to swallowing intact capsules whole will also result in significant absorption differences. Patients should be consistent with regards to administration.

Administration Capsules may be opened and contents sprinkled on food; however, extent of absorption is increased up to 20% relative to administration of the capsule under fasted conditions.

Monitoring Parameters Monitor liver function (aminotransferases) at baseline, 1, 3, 6 months and periodically thereafter; blood pressure; renal function

Dosage Forms Excipient information presented when available (limited, particularly for generics); consult specific product labeling.

Capsule:

Zanaflex Capsules™: 2 mg, 4 mg, 6 mg

Tablet: 2 mg, 4 mg

Zanaflex®: 2 mg [DSC], 4 mg [scored]

- **TMC-114** *see* Darunavir *on page 402*
- **TMC125** *see* Etravirine *on page 594*
- **TMP** *see* Trimethoprim *on page 1519*
- **TMP-SMZ** *see* Sulfamethoxazole and Trimethoprim *on page 1407*
- **TMZ** *see* Temozolomide *on page 1432*
- **TNKase®** *see* Tenecteplase *on page 1436*
- **TOBI®** *see* Tobramycin *on page 1481*
- **TobraDex®** *see* Tobramycin and Dexamethasone *on page 1484*
- **Tobradex® (Can)** *see* Tobramycin and Dexamethasone *on page 1484*

Tobramycin (toe bra MYE sin)

U.S. Brand Names AKTob®; TOBI®; Tobrex®

Canadian Brand Names PMS-Tobramycin; Sandoz-Tobramycin; TOBI®; Tobramycin Injection, USP; Tobrex®

Index Terms Tobramycin Sulfate

Pharmacologic Category Antibiotic, Aminoglycoside; Antibiotic, Ophthalmic

Additional Appendix Information

Aminoglycoside Dosing and Monitoring *on page 1630*

Antimicrobial Drugs of Choice *on page 1752*

Prevention of Wound Infection and Sepsis in Surgical Patients *on page 1738*

Use Treatment of documented or suspected infections caused by susceptible gram-negative bacilli including *Pseudomonas aeruginosa*; topically used to treat superficial ophthalmic infections caused by susceptible bacteria. Tobramycin solution for inhalation is indicated for the management of cystic fibrosis patients (>6 years of age) with *Pseudomonas aeruginosa*.

Pregnancy Risk Factor D (injection, inhalation); B (ophthalmic)

Pregnancy Considerations Tobramycin crosses the placenta and produces detectable serum levels in the fetus. Because of several reports of total irreversible bilateral congenital deafness in children whose mothers received streptomycin during pregnancy, the manufacturer classifies systemic tobramycin as pregnancy risk factor D. There have been no reports of fetal toxicity in humans from tobramycin. No adequate and well-controlled studies have been conducted in pregnant women and it is not known whether tobramycin can cause fetal harm. Although the manufacturer considers tobramycin pregnancy risk factor D, tobramycin-specific clinical data would suggest a pregnancy risk factor C.

Due to pregnancy induced physiologic changes, some pharmacokinetic parameters of tobramycin may be altered. Pregnant women have an average-to-larger volume of distribution which may result in lower serum peak levels than for the same dose in nonpregnant women. Serum half-life is also shorter.

Lactation Enters breast milk/not recommended

Medication Safety Issues

Sound-alike/look-alike issues:

Tobramycin may be confused with Trobicin®, vancomycin

AKTob® may be confused with AK-Trol®

Nebcin® may be confused with Inapsine®, Naprosyn®, Nubain®

Tobrex® may be confused with TobraDex®

High alert medication: The Institute for Safe Medication Practices (ISMP) includes this medication (intrathecal administration) among its list of drug classes which have a heightened risk of causing significant patient harm when used in error.

Contraindications Hypersensitivity to tobramycin, other aminoglycosides, or any component of the formulation; pregnancy (injection/inhalation)

Warnings/Precautions [U.S. Boxed Warning]: Aminoglycosides may cause neurotoxicity and/or nephrotoxicity; usual risk factors include pre-existing renal impairment, concomitant neuro-/nephrotoxic medications, advanced age and dehydration. Ototoxicity may be directly proportional to the amount of drug given and the duration of treatment; tinnitus or vertigo are indications of vestibular injury and impending hearing loss; renal damage is usually reversible. May cause neuromuscular blockade and respiratory paralysis; especially when given soon after anesthesia or muscle relaxants.

Not intended for long-term therapy due to toxic hazards associated with extended administration; use caution in pre-existing renal insufficiency, vestibular or cochlear impairment, myasthenia gravis, hypocalcemia, conditions which depress neuromuscular transmission. Dosage modification required in patients with impaired renal function. Prolonged use may result in fungal or bacterial superinfection, including *C. difficile*-associated diarrhea (CDAD) and pseudomembranous colitis; CDAD has been observed >2 months postantibiotic treatment. Solution may contain sodium metabisulfate; use caution in patients with sulfite allergy.

Adverse Reactions

Injection: Frequency not defined:

Central nervous system: Confusion, disorientation, dizziness, fever, headache, lethargy, vertigo

Dermatologic: Exfoliative dermatitis, itching, rash, urticaria

Endocrine & metabolic: Serum calcium, magnesium, potassium, and/or sodium decreased

Gastrointestinal: Diarrhea, nausea, vomiting

Hematologic: Anemia, eosinophilia, granulocytopenia, leukocytosis, leukopenia, thrombocytopenia

Hepatic: ALT increased, AST increased, bilirubin increased, LDH increased

Local: Pain at the injection site

Otic: Hearing loss, tinnitus, ototoxicity (auditory), ototoxicity (vestibular), roaring in the ears

Renal: BUN increased, cylindruria, serum creatinine increased, oliguria, proteinuria

Inhalation:

>10%:

Gastrointestinal: Sputum discoloration (21%)

Respiratory: Voice alteration (13%)

1% to 10%:

Central nervous system: Malaise (6%)

Otic: Tinnitus (3%)

Postmarketing and/or case reports: Hearing loss

Ophthalmic: <1% (Limited to important or life-threatening): Ocular: Conjunctival erythema, lid itching, lid swelling

Drug Interactions

Avoid Concomitant Use

Avoid concomitant use of Tobramycin with any of the following: Gallium Nitrate

Increased Effect/Toxicity

Tobramycin may increase the levels/effects of: Bisphosphonate Derivatives; Botulinum Toxin Type A; Botulinum Toxin Type B; CARBOplatin; Colistimethate; CycloSPORINE; Gallium Nitrate; Neuromuscular-Blocking Agents

The levels/effects of Tobramycin may be increased by: Amphotericin B; Capreomycin; CISplatin; Loop Diuretics; Nonsteroidal Anti-Inflammatory Agents; Vancomycin

Decreased Effect

Tobramycin may decrease the levels/effects of: Typhoid Vaccine

The levels/effects of Tobramycin may be decreased by: Penicillins

Stability

Injection: Stable at room temperature both as the clear, colorless solution and as the dry powder. Reconstituted solutions remain stable for 24 hours at room temperature and 96 hours when refrigerated. Dilute in 50-100 mL NS, D_5W for I.V. infusion.

Separate administration of extended-spectrum penicillins (eg, carbenicillin, ticarcillin, piperacillin) from tobramycin in patients with severe renal impairment; tobramycin's efficacy may be reduced if given concurrently.

Ophthalmic solution: Store at 8°C to 27°C (46°F to 80°F).

Solution, for inhalation (TOBI®): Store under refrigeration at 2°C to 8°C (36°F to 46°F). May be stored in foil pouch at room temperature of 25°C (77°F) for up to 28 days. Avoid intense light. Solution may darken over time; however, do not use if cloudy or contains particles.

Mechanism of Action Interferes with bacterial protein synthesis by binding to 30S and 50S ribosomal subunits resulting in a defective bacterial cell membrane

Pharmacodynamics/Kinetics

Absorption:

Oral: Poorly absorbed

I.M.: Rapid and complete

Inhalation: Peak serum concentrations are ~1 mcg/mL following a 300 mg dose

Distribution: V_d: 0.2-0.3 L/kg; Pediatrics: 0.2-0.7 L/kg; to extracellular fluid including serum, abscesses, ascitic, pericardial, pleural, synovial, lymphatic, and peritoneal fluids; poor penetration into CSF, eye, bone, prostate

Inhalation: Tobramycin remains concentrated primarily in the airways

Protein binding: <30%

Half-life elimination:

Neonates: ≤1200 g: 11 hours; >1200 g: 2-9 hours

Adults: 2-3 hours; directly dependent upon glomerular filtration rate

Adults with impaired renal function: 5-70 hours

Time to peak, serum: I.M.: 30-60 minutes; I.V.: ~30 minutes

Excretion: Normal renal function: Urine (~90% to 95%) within 24 hours

Dosage Note: Dosage individualization is **critical** because of the low therapeutic index.

Use of ideal body weight (IBW) for determining the mg/kg/dose appears to be more accurate than dosing on the basis of total body weight (TBW). In morbid obesity, dosage requirement may best be estimated using a dosing weight of IBW + 0.4 (TBW - IBW).

Initial and periodic plasma drug levels (eg, peak and trough with conventional dosing) should be determined, particularly in critically-ill patients with serious infections or in disease states known to significantly alter aminoglycoside pharmacokinetics (eg, cystic fibrosis, burns, or major surgery).

Usual dosage range:

Infants and Children <5 years: I.M., I.V.: 2.5 mg/kg/dose every 8 hours

Children ≥5 years: I.M., I.V.: 2-2.5 mg/kg/dose every 8 hours

Note: Higher individual doses and/or more frequent intervals (eg, every 6 hours) may be required in selected clinical situations (cystic fibrosis) or serum levels document the need.

Children and Adults:

Inhalation:

Aerosolized tobramycin injection (unlabeled use): 80 mg 2 times/day. **Note:** Injectable formulation may contain preservatives, which may increase risk of bronchospasm.

TOBI®: Children ≥6 years and Adults: 300 mg every 12 hours (do not administer doses <6 hours apart); administer in repeated cycles of 28 days on drug followed by 28 days off drug.

Intrathecal: 4-8 mg/day

Ophthalmic: Children ≥2 months and Adults:

Ointment: Instill 1/2" (1.25 cm) 2-3 times/day every 3-4 hours

Solution: Instill 1-2 drops every 2-4 hours, up to 2 drops every hour for severe infections

Topical: Apply 3-4 times/day to affected area

Adults: I.M., I.V.:

Conventional: 1-2.5 mg/kg/dose every 8-12 hours; to ensure adequate peak concentrations early in therapy, higher initial dosage may be considered in selected patients when extracellular water is increased (edema, septic shock, postsurgical, and/or trauma)

Once-daily: 4-7 mg/kg/dose once daily; some clinicians recommend this approach for all patients with normal renal function; this dose is at least as efficacious with similar, if not less, toxicity than conventional dosing.

Indication-specific dosing:

Neonates:

Meningitis: I.M., I.V.:

0-7 days: <2000 g: 2.5 mg/kg every 18-24 hours; >2000 g: 2.5 mg/kg every 12 hours

8-28 days: <2000 g: 2.5 mg/kg every 8-12 hours; >2000 g: 2.5 mg/kg every 8 hours

Children:

Cystic fibrosis:

I.M., I.V.: 2.5-3.3 mg/kg every 6-8 hours; **Note:** Some patients may require larger or more frequent doses if serum levels document the need (eg, cystic fibrosis or febrile granulocytopenic patients).

Inhalation: See adult dosing.

Adults:

I.M., I.V.:

Brucellosis: 240 mg (I.M.) daily or 5 mg/kg (I.V.) daily for 7 days; either regimen recommended in combination with doxycycline

Cholangitis: 4-6 mg/kg once daily with ampicillin

Diverticulitis, complicated: 1.5-2 mg/kg every 8 hours (with ampicillin and metronidazole)

Infective endocarditis or synergy (for gram-positive infections): I.M., I.V.: 1 mg/kg every 8 hours (with ampicillin)

Meningitis *(Enterococcus or Pseudomonas aeruginosa)*: I.V.: Loading dose: 2 mg/kg, then 1.7 mg/kg/dose every 8 hours (administered with another bacteriocidal drug)

Pelvic inflammatory disease: Loading dose: 2 mg/kg, then 1.5 mg/kg every 8 hours **or** 4.5 mg/kg once daily

Plague *(Yersinia pestis)*: Treatment: 5 mg/kg/day, followed by postexposure prophylaxis with doxycycline

Pneumonia, hospital- or ventilator-associated: 7 mg/kg/day (with antipseudomonal beta-lactam or carbapenem)

Prophylaxis against endocarditis (dental, oral, upper respiratory procedures, GI/GU procedures): 1.5 mg/kg with ampicillin (50 mg/kg) 30 minutes prior to procedure. **Note:** AHA guidelines now recommend prophylaxis only in patients undergoing invasive procedures and in whom underlying cardiac conditions may predispose to a higher risk of adverse outcomes should infection occur. As of April 2007, routine prophylaxis no longer recommended by the AHA.

Tularemia: 5 mg/kg/day divided every 8 hours for 1-2 weeks

Urinary tract infection: 1.5 mg/kg/dose every 8 hours

Inhalation:

Cystic fibrosis:

Aerosolized tobramycin injection (unlabeled use): 80 mg 2 times/day; **Note:** Injectable formulation may contain preservatives, which may increase risk of bronchospasm.

TOBI®: 300 mg every 12 hours (do not administer doses <6 hours apart); administer in repeated cycles of 28 days on drug followed by 28 days off drug.

Dosing interval in renal impairment: I.M., I.V.:

Conventional dosing:

Cl_{cr} ≥60 mL/minute: Administer every 8 hours

Cl_{cr} 40-60 mL/minute: Administer every 12 hours

Cl_{cr} 20-40 mL/minute: Administer every 24 hours

Cl_{cr} 10-20 mL/minute: Administer every 48 hours

Cl_{cr} <10 mL/minute: Administer every 72 hours

High-dose therapy: Interval may be extended (eg, every 48 hours) in patients with moderate renal impairment (Cl_{cr} 30-59 mL/minute) and/or adjusted based on serum level determinations.

Hemodialysis: Dialyzable; 30% removal of aminoglycosides occurs during 4 hours of HD - administer dose after dialysis and follow levels

Continuous arteriovenous or venovenous hemofiltration: Dose as for Cl_{cr} of 10-40 mL/minute and follow levels

Administration in CAPD fluid:

Gram-negative infection: 4-8 mg/L (4-8 mcg/mL) of CAPD fluid

Gram-positive infection (ie, synergy): 3-4 mg/L (3-4 mcg/mL) of CAPD fluid

Administration IVPB/I.M.: Dose as for Cl_{cr} <10 mL/minute and follow levels

Dosing adjustment/comments in hepatic disease: Monitor plasma concentrations

Dietary Considerations May require supplementation of calcium, magnesium, potassium.

Administration

I.V.: Infuse over 30-60 minutes. Flush with saline before and after administration.

Inhalation (TOBI®): To be inhaled over ~15 minutes using a handheld nebulizer (PARI-LC PLUS™). If multiple different nebulizer treatments are required, administer bronchodilator first, followed by chest physiotherapy, any other nebulized medications, and then TOBI® last. Do not mix with other nebulizer medications.

Ophthalmic: Contact lenses should not be worn during treatment of ophthalmic infections.

Ointment: Do not touch tip of tube to eye. Instill ointment into pocket between eyeball and lower lid; patient should look downward before closing eye.

Solution: Allow 5 minutes between application of "multiple-drop" therapy.

Suspension: Shake well before using; tilt head back, instill suspension in conjunctival sac and close eye(s). Do not touch dropper to eye. Apply light finger pressure on lacrimal sac for 1 minute following instillation.

Some penicillins (eg, carbenicillin, ticarcillin and piperacillin) have been shown to inactivate aminoglycosides *in vitro*. This has been observed to a greater extent with tobramycin and gentamicin, while amikacin has shown greater stability against inactivation. Concurrent use of these agents may pose a risk of reduced antibacterial efficacy *in vivo*, particularly in the setting of profound renal impairment. However, definitive clinical evidence is lacking. If combination penicillin/aminoglycoside therapy is desired in a patient with renal dysfunction, separation of doses (if feasible), and routine monitoring of aminoglycoside levels, CBC, and clinical response should be considered.

Monitoring Parameters Urinalysis, urine output, BUN, serum creatinine, peak and trough plasma tobramycin levels; be alert to ototoxicity; hearing should be tested before and during treatment

Some penicillin derivatives may accelerate the degradation of aminoglycosides *in vitro*. This may be clinically-significant for certain penicillin (ticarcillin, piperacillin, carbenicillin) and aminoglycoside (gentamicin, tobramycin) combination therapy in patients with significant renal impairment. Close monitoring of aminoglycoside levels is warranted.

Reference Range

Timing of serum samples: Draw peak 30 minutes after 30-minute infusion has been completed or 1 hour following I.M. injection or beginning of infusion; draw trough immediately before next dose

Therapeutic levels:

Peak:

Serious infections: 6-8 mcg/mL (SI: 12-17 µmol/L)

Life-threatening infections: 8-10 mcg/mL (SI: 17-21 µmol/L)

Urinary tract infections: 4-6 mcg/mL (SI: 7-12 µmol/L)

Synergy against gram-positive organisms: 3-5 mcg/mL

Trough:

Serious infections: 0.5-1 mcg/mL

Life-threatening infections: 1-2 mcg/mL

The American Thoracic Society (ATS) recommends trough levels of <1 mcg/mL for patients with hospital-acquired pneumonia.

Monitor serum creatinine and urine output; obtain drug levels after the third dose unless otherwise directed

Inhalation: Serum levels are ~1 mcg/mL one hour following a 300 mg dose in patients with normal renal function.

Test Interactions Some penicillin derivatives may accelerate the degradation of aminoglycosides *in vitro*, leading to a potential underestimation of aminoglycoside serum concentration.

Additional Information Once-daily dosing: Higher peak serum drug concentration to MIC ratios, demonstrated aminoglycoside postantibiotic effect, decreased renal cortex drug uptake, and improved cost-time efficiency are supportive reasons for the use of once daily dosing regimens for aminoglycosides. Current research indicates these regimens to be as effective for non-life-threatening infections, with no higher incidence of nephrotoxicity, than those requiring multiple daily doses. Doses are determined by calculating the entire day's dose via usual multiple dose calculation techniques and administering this quantity as a single dose. Doses are then adjusted to maintain mean serum concentrations above the MIC(s) of the causative organism(s). (Example: 2.5-5 mg/kg as a single dose; expected Cp_{max}: 10-20 mcg/mL and Cp_{min}: <1 mcg/mL). Further research is needed for universal recommendation in all patient populations and gram-negative disease; exceptions may include those with known high clearance (eg, children, patients with cystic fibrosis, or burns who may require shorter dosage intervals) and patients with renal function impairment for whom longer than conventional dosage intervals are usually required.

Dosage Forms Excipient information presented when available (limited, particularly for generics); consult specific product labeling.

Infusion [premixed in NS]: 60 mg (50 mL); 80 mg (100 mL)

Injection, powder for reconstitution: 1.2 g

Injection, solution: 10 mg/mL (2 mL, 8 mL); 40 mg/mL (2 mL, 30 mL, 50 mL) [may contain sodium metabisulfite]

Ointment, ophthalmic (Tobrex®): 0.3% (3.5 g)

Solution for nebulization [preservative free] (TOBI®): 60 mg/mL (5 mL)

Solution, ophthalmic (AKTob®, Tobrex®): 0.3% (5 mL) [contains benzalkonium chloride]

Tobramycin and Dexamethasone

(toe bra MYE sin & deks a METH a sone)

U.S. Brand Names TobraDex®

Canadian Brand Names Tobradex®

Index Terms Dexamethasone and Tobramycin

Pharmacologic Category Antibiotic/Corticosteroid, Ophthalmic

Use Treatment of external ocular infection caused by susceptible gram-negative bacteria and steroid responsive inflammatory conditions of the palpebral and bulbar conjunctiva, lid, cornea, and anterior segment of the globe

Pregnancy Risk Factor C

Medication Safety Issues

Sound-alike/look-alike issues:

TobraDex® may be confused with Tobrex®

Dosage Children and Adults: Ophthalmic: Instill 1-2 drops of solution every 4 hours; apply ointment 2-3 times/day; for severe infections apply ointment every 3-4 hours, or solution 2 drops every 30-60 minutes initially, then reduce to less frequent intervals

Additional Information Complete prescribing information for this medication should be consulted for additional detail.

Dosage Forms Excipient information presented when available (limited, particularly for generics); consult specific product labeling.

Ointment, ophthalmic: Tobramycin 0.3% and dexamethasone 0.1% (3.5 g)

Suspension, ophthalmic: Tobramycin 0.3% and dexamethasone 0.1% (2.5 mL, 5 mL, 10 mL) [contains benzalkonium chloride]

◆ **Tobramycin and Loteprednol Etabonate** *see* Loteprednol and Tobramycin *on page 910*

◆ **Tobramycin Injection, USP (Can)** *see* Tobramycin *on page 1481*

◆ **Tobramycin Sulfate** *see* Tobramycin *on page 1481*

◆ **Tobrex®** *see* Tobramycin *on page 1481*

◆ **Today® [OTC]** *see* Nonoxynol 9 *on page 1077*

◆ **Tofranil®** *see* Imipramine *on page 774*

◆ **Tofranil-PM®** *see* Imipramine *on page 774*

TOLAZamide (tole AZ a mide)

Canadian Brand Names Tolinase®

Pharmacologic Category Antidiabetic Agent, Sulfonylurea

Additional Appendix Information

Diabetes Mellitus Management, Adults *on page 1801*

Sulfonamide Derivatives *on page 1671*

Use Adjunct to diet for the management of mild to moderately severe, stable, type 2 diabetes mellitus (noninsulin dependent, NIDDM)

Pregnancy Risk Factor C

Medication Safety Issues

Sound-alike/look-alike issues:

TOLAZamide may be confused with tolazoline, TOLBUTamide

Tolinase® may be confused with Orinase®

High alert medication: The Institute for Safe Medication Practices (ISMP) includes this medication among its list of drugs which have a heightened risk of causing significant patient harm when used in error.

Dosage Oral: Adults: Doses >500 mg/day should be given in 2 divided doses:

Initial: 100-250 mg/day with breakfast or the first main meal of the day

Fasting blood sugar <200 mg/dL: 100 mg/day

Fasting blood sugar >200 mg/dL: 250 mg/day

Patient is malnourished, underweight, elderly, or not eating properly: 100 mg/day

Adjust dose in increments of 100-250 mg/day at weekly intervals to response; maximum daily dose: 1 g (doses >1 g/day are not likely to improve control)

Conversion from insulin to tolazamide:

<20 units day = 100 mg/day

21-<40 units/day = 250 mg/day

≥40 units/day = 250 mg/day and 50% of insulin dose

Dosing adjustment in renal impairment: Conservative initial and maintenance doses are recommended because tolazamide is metabolized to active metabolites, which are eliminated in the urine

Dosing comments in hepatic impairment: Conservative initial and maintenance doses and careful monitoring of blood glucose are recommended

Additional Information Complete prescribing information for this medication should be consulted for additional detail.

Dosage Forms Excipient information presented when available (limited, particularly for generics); consult specific product labeling.

Tablet: 250 mg, 500 mg

Tolazoline (tole AZ oh leen)

U.S. Brand Names Priscoline® [DSC]

Index Terms Benzazoline Hydrochloride; Tolazoline Hydrochloride

Pharmacologic Category Vasodilator

Use Treatment of persistent pulmonary vasoconstriction and hypertension of the newborn (persistent fetal circulation), peripheral vasospastic disorders

Pregnancy Risk Factor C

Medication Safety Issues

Sound-alike/look-alike issues:

Tolazoline may be confused with TOLAZamide

Priscoline® may be confused with Apresoline®

Dosage

Neonates: Initial: I.V.: 1-2 mg/kg over 10-15 minutes via scalp vein or upper extremity; maintenance: 1-2 mg/kg/hour; use lower maintenance doses in patients with decreased renal function. Also used in neonates for acute vasospasm "cath toes" at 0.25 mg/kg/hour (no load); maximum dose: 6-8 mg/kg/hour.

Dosing interval in renal impairment in newborns: Urine output <0.9 mL/kg/hour: Decrease dose to 0.08 mg/kg/hour for every 1 mg/kg of loading dose

Adults: Peripheral vasospastic disorder: I.M., I.V., SubQ: 10-50 mg 4 times/day

Additional Information Complete prescribing information for this medication should be consulted for additional detail.

Dosage Forms Excipient information presented when available (limited, particularly for generics); consult specific product labeling. [DSC] = Discontinued product

Injection, solution, as hydrochloride [DSC]: 25 mg/mL (4 mL)

◆ **Tolazoline Hydrochloride** *see* Tolazoline *on page 1485*

TOLBUTamide (tole BYOO ta mide)

Canadian Brand Names Apo-Tolbutamide®

Index Terms Tolbutamide Sodium

Pharmacologic Category Antidiabetic Agent, Sulfonylurea

Additional Appendix Information

Diabetes Mellitus Management, Adults *on page 1801*

Sulfonamide Derivatives *on page 1671*

Use Adjunct to diet for the management of type 2 diabetes mellitus (noninsulin dependent, NIDDM)

Pregnancy Risk Factor C

Medication Safety Issues

Sound-alike/look-alike issues:

TOLBUTamide may be confused with terbutaline, TOLAZamide

Orinase® may be confused with Orabase®, Ornex®, Tolinase®

High alert medication: The Institute for Safe Medication Practices (ISMP) includes this medication among its list of drugs which have a heightened risk of causing significant patient harm when used in error.

Dosage Oral: **Note:** Divided doses may improve gastrointestinal tolerance.

Adults: Initial: 1-2 g/day as a single dose in the morning or in divided doses throughout the day. Maintenance dose: 0.25-3 g/day; however, a maintenance dose >2 g/day is seldom required.

Elderly: Initial: 250 mg 1-3 times/day; usual: 500-2000 mg; maximum: 3 g/day

Dosing adjustment in renal impairment: Adjustment is not necessary

Hemodialysis: Not dialyzable (0% to 5%)

Dosing adjustment in hepatic impairment: Reduction of dose may be necessary in patients with impaired liver function

Additional Information Complete prescribing information for this medication should be consulted for additional detail.

Dosage Forms Excipient information presented when available (limited, particularly for generics); consult specific product labeling.

Tablet: 500 mg

◆ **Tolbutamide Sodium** *see* TOLBUTamide *on page 1485*

Tolcapone (TOLE ka pone)

U.S. Brand Names Tasmar®

Pharmacologic Category Anti-Parkinson's Agent, COMT Inhibitor

Additional Appendix Information

Antiparkinsonian Agents *on page 1643*

Use Adjunct to levodopa and carbidopa for the treatment of signs and symptoms of idiopathic Parkinson's disease in patients with motor fluctuations not responsive to other therapies

Restrictions A patient signed consent form acknowledging the risks of hepatic injury should be obtained by the treating physician.

Pregnancy Risk Factor C

Pregnancy Considerations Tolcapone may be teratogenic based on animal studies. There are no adequate and well-controlled studies in pregnant women. Use only if benefit outweighs risk.

Lactation Excretion in breast milk unknown/not recommended

Contraindications Hypersensitivity to tolcapone or any component of the formulation; history of liver disease or tolcapone-induced hepatocellular injury; nontraumatic rhabdomyolysis or hyperpyrexia and confusion

Warnings/Precautions [U.S. Boxed Warning]: Due to reports of fatal liver injury associated with use of this drug, the manufacturer is advising that tolcapone be reserved for patients who are experiencing inadequate symptom control or who are not appropriate candidates for other available treatments. Patients must provide written consent acknowledging the risks of hepatic injury. Liver disease should be excluded prior to initiation; laboratory monitoring is recommended. Discontinue if signs and/or symptoms of hepatic injury are noted (eg, transaminases >2 times upper limit of normal) or if clinical improvement is not evident after 3 weeks of therapy. Use with caution in patients with pre-existing dyskinesias; exacerbation of pre-existing dyskinesia and severe rhabdomyolysis has been reported. Levodopa dosage reduction may be required, particularly in patients with levodopa dosages >600 mg daily or with moderate-to-severe dyskinesia prior to initiation.

May cause orthostatic hypotension and syncope; Parkinson's disease patients appear to have an impaired capacity to respond to a postural challenge; use with caution in patients at risk of hypotension (such as those receiving antihypertensive drugs) or where transient hypotensive episodes would be poorly tolerated (cardiovascular disease or cerebrovascular disease). Parkinson's patients being treated with dopaminergic agonists ordinarily require careful monitoring for signs and symptoms of postural hypotension, especially during dose escalation, and should be informed of this risk. May cause hallucinations, which may improve with reduction in levodopa therapy. Use with caution in patients with lower gastrointestinal disease or an increased risk of dehydration; tolcapone has been associated with delayed development of diarrhea (onset after 2-12 weeks).

Tolcapone, in conjunction with other drug therapy that alters brain biogenic amine concentrations (eg, MAO inhibitors, SSRIs), has been associated with a syndrome resembling neuroleptic malignant syndrome (hyperpyrexia and confusion - some fatal) on abrupt withdrawal or dosage reduction. Concomitant use of tolcapone and nonselective MAO inhibitors should be avoided. Selegiline is a selective MAO type B inhibitor (when given orally at ≤10 mg/day) and can be taken with tolcapone. Dopaminergic agents from the ergot class have also been associated with fibrotic complications, such as retroperitoneal fibrosis, pulmonary infiltrates or effusion and pleural thickening. It is unknown whether non-ergot, pro-dopaminergic agents like tolcapone confer this risk. Use caution in patients with hepatic impairment or severe renal impairment. Safety and efficacy in pediatric patients have not been established.

Adverse Reactions

>10%:

Cardiovascular: Orthostatic hypotension (17%)

Central nervous system: Sleep disorder (24% to 25%), excessive dreaming (16% to 21%), somnolence (14% to 32%), hallucinations (8% to 24%) dizziness (6% to 13%), headache (10% to 11%), confusion (10% to 11%)

Gastrointestinal: Nausea (28% to 50%), anorexia (19% to 23%), diarrhea (16% to 34%; approximately 3% to 4% severe)

Neuromuscular & skeletal: Dyskinesia (42% to 51%), dystonia (19% to 22%), muscle cramps (17% to 18%)

1% to 10%:

Cardiovascular: Syncope (4% to 5%), chest pain (1% to 3%), hypotension (2%), palpitation

Central nervous system: Fatigue (3% to 7%), loss of balance (2% to 3%), agitation (1%), euphoria (1%), hyperactivity (1%), malaise (1%), panic reaction (1%), irritability (1%), mental deficiency (1%), fever (1%), depression, hypoesthesia, tremor, speech disorder, vertigo, emotional lability, hyperkinesia

Dermatologic: Alopecia (1%), bleeding (1%), tumor (1%), rash

Gastrointestinal: Vomiting (8% to 10%), constipation (6% to 8%), xerostomia (5% to 6%), abdominal pain (5% to 6%), dyspepsia (3% to 4%), flatulence (2% to 4%), tooth disorder

Genitourinary: UTI (5%), hematuria (4% to 5%), urine discoloration (2% to 3%), urination disorder (1% to 2%), uterine tumor (1%), incontinence, impotence

Hepatic: Transaminases increased (1% to 3%; 3 times ULN, usually with first 6 months of therapy)

Neuromuscular & skeletal: Paresthesia (1% to 3%), hyper-/hypokinesia (1% to 3%), arthritis (1% to 2%), neck pain (2%), stiffness (2%), myalgia, rhabdomyolysis

Ocular: Cataract (1%), eye inflammation (1%)

Otic: Tinnitus

Respiratory: Upper respiratory infection (5% to 7%), dyspnea (3%), sinus congestion (1% to 2%), bronchitis, pharyngitis

Miscellaneous: Diaphoresis (4% to 7%), influenza (3% to 4%), burning (1% to 2%), flank pain, injury, infection

<1% (Limited to important or life-threatening): Abnormal stools, abscess, allergic reaction, amnesia, anemia, antisocial reaction, apathy, apnea, arteriosclerosis, arthrosis, asthma, bladder calculus, breast neoplasm, carcinoma, cardiovascular disorder, cellulitis, cerebral ischemia, cerebrovascular accident, chills, cholecystitis, cholelithiasis, choreoathetosis, colitis, cough increased, death, dehydration, delirium, delusions, diabetes mellitus, diplopia, duodenal ulcer, dysphagia, dysuria, ear pain, eczema, edema, encephalopathy, epistaxis, erythema multiforme, esophagitis, extrapyramidal syndrome, eye hemorrhage, eye pain, facial edema, furunculosis, gastroenteritis, gastrointestinal carcinoma, gastrointestinal hemorrhage, glaucoma, hemiplegia, hernia, herpes simplex, herpes zoster, hiccup, hostility, hypercholesteremia, hyperventilation, hypoxia, infection (bacterial), infection (fungal), joint disorder, kidney calculus, lacrimation disorder, laryngitis, leukemia, libido changes, lung edema, manic reaction, meningitis, mouth ulceration, myoclonus, neoplasm, nervousness, neuralgia, neuropathy, nocturia, oliguria, otitis media, ovarian carcinoma, pain, paranoid reaction, parosmia, pericardial effusion, polyuria, prostatic carcinoma, prostatic disorder, pruritus, psychosis, rectal disorder, rhinitis, salivation increased, seborrhea, skin discoloration, skin disorder, stomach atony, surgical procedure, tenosynovitis, thinking abnormal, thirst, thrombocytopenia, thrombosis, tongue disorder, twitching, urinary retention, urinary tract disorder, urticaria, uterine atony, uterine disorder, uterine hemorrhage, vaginitis, viral infection

Drug Interactions

Metabolism/Transport Effects Inhibits CYP2C9 (weak)

Avoid Concomitant Use There are no known interactions where it is recommended to avoid concomitant use.

Increased Effect/Toxicity

Tolcapone may increase the levels/effects of: Alcohol (Ethyl); CNS Depressants; COMT Substrates; MAO Inhibitors

Decreased Effect There are no known significant interactions involving a decrease in effect.

Ethanol/Nutrition/Herb Interactions

Ethanol: Avoid ethanol (may increase CNS depression).

Food: Tolcapone, taken with food within 1 hour before or 2 hours after the dose, decreases bioavailability by 10% to 20%.

Avoid valerian, St John's wort, kava kava, gotu kola (may increase CNS depression).

Stability Store at 20°C to 25°C (68°F to 77°F).

Mechanism of Action Tolcapone is a selective and reversible inhibitor of catechol-o-methyltransferase

(COMT). In the presence of a decarboxylase inhibitor (eg, carbidopa), COMT is the major degradation pathway for levodopa. Inhibition of COMT leads to more sustained plasma levels of levodopa and enhanced central dopaminergic activity.

Pharmacodynamics/Kinetics

Absorption: Rapid

Distribution: 9 L

Protein binding: >99.0%

Metabolism: Hepatic, via glucuronidation, to inactive metabolite (>99%)

Bioavailability: 65%

Half-life elimination: 2-3 hours

Time to peak: ~2 hours

Excretion: Urine (60% as metabolites, 0.5% as unchanged drug); feces (40%)

Dosage Note: If clinical improvement is not observed after 3 weeks of therapy (regardless of dose), tolcapone treatment should be discontinued.

Oral: Adults: Initial: 100 mg 3 times/day; may increase as tolerated to 200 mg 3 times/day. **Note:** Levodopa dose may need to be decreased upon initiation of tolcapone (average reduction in clinical trials was 30%). As many as 70% of patients receiving levodopa doses >600 mg daily required levodopa dosage reduction in clinical trials. Patients with moderate-to-severe dyskinesia prior to initiation are also more likely to require dosage reduction.

Dosage adjustment in renal impairment: No adjustment necessary for mild-moderate impairment. Use caution with severe impairment; no safety information available in patients with Cl_{cr}<25 mL/minute.

Dosage adjustment in hepatic impairment: Do not use. Discontinue immediately if signs/symptoms of hepatic impairment develop.

Dietary Considerations May be taken without regard to food.

Administration May be administered with or without food. In clinical studies, the first dose of the day was administered with carbidopa/levodopa, and the subsequent doses were administered 6 hours and 12 hours later.

Monitoring Parameters Blood pressure, symptoms of Parkinson's disease, liver enzymes at baseline and then every 2-4 weeks for the first 6 months of therapy; thereafter, periodic monitoring should be conducted as deemed clinically relevant. If the dose is increased to 200 mg 3 times/day, reinitiate LFT monitoring every 2-4 weeks for 6 months, and then resume periodic monitoring. Discontinue therapy if the ALT or AST exceeds 2 times ULN or if the clinical signs and symptoms suggest the onset of liver failure.

Dosage Forms Excipient information presented when available (limited, particularly for generics); consult specific product labeling.

Tablet:

Tasmar®: 100 mg, 200 mg

◆ **Tolectin** *see* Tolmetin *on page 1487*

◆ **Tolinase® (Can)** *see* TOLAZamide *on page 1484*

Tolmetin (TOLE met in)

Index Terms Tolectin; Tolmetin Sodium

Pharmacologic Category Nonsteroidal Anti-inflammatory Drug (NSAID), Oral

Additional Appendix Information

Nonsteroidal Anti-inflammatory Agents *on page 1669*

Use Treatment of rheumatoid arthritis and osteoarthritis, juvenile rheumatoid arthritis

Restrictions An FDA-approved medication guide must be distributed when dispensing an oral outpatient prescription (new or refill) where this medication is to be used without direct supervision of a healthcare provider. Medication guides are available at http://www.fda.gov/cder/Offices/ODS/medication_guides.htm.

Pregnancy Risk Factor C/D (3rd trimester)

Dosage Oral:

Children ≥2 years:

JRA: Initial: 20 mg/kg/day in 3-4 divided doses, then 15-30 mg/kg/day in 3-4 divided doses (maximum dose: 30 mg/kg/day)

Analgesic (unlabeled use): 5-7 mg/kg/dose every 6-8 hours

Adults: RA, osteoarthritis: 400 mg 3 times/day; usual dose: 600 mg to 1.8 g/day; maximum: 1.8 g/day

Additional Information Complete prescribing information for this medication should be consulted for additional detail.

Dosage Forms Excipient information presented when available (limited, particularly for generics); consult specific product labeling.

Capsule: 400 mg

Tablet: 200 mg, 600 mg

◆ **Tolmetin Sodium** *see* Tolmetin *on page 1487*

Tolnaftate (tole NAF tate)

U.S. Brand Names Blis-To-Sol® [OTC]; FungiGuard [OTC]; Mycocide® NS [OTC]; Podactin Powder [OTC]; Tinactin® Antifungal Deodorant [OTC]; Tinactin® Antifungal Jock Itch [OTC]; Tinactin® Antifungal [OTC]; Tinaderm [OTC]; Ting® Cream [OTC]; Ting® Spray Liquid [OTC]

Canadian Brand Names Pitrex

Pharmacologic Category Antifungal Agent, Topical

Use Treatment of tinea pedis, tinea cruris, tinea corporis

Pregnancy Risk Factor C

Medication Safety Issues

Sound-alike/look-alike issues:

Tolnaftate may be confused with Tornalate®

Tinactin® may be confused with Talacen®

Dosage Children ≥2 years and Adults: Topical: Wash and dry affected area; spray aerosol or apply 1-3 drops of solution or a small amount of cream, or powder and rub into the affected areas 2 times/day

Note: May use for up to 4 weeks for tinea pedis or tinea corporis, and up to 2 weeks for tinea cruris

Additional Information Complete prescribing information for this medication should be consulted for additional detail.

Dosage Forms Excipient information presented when available (limited, particularly for generics); consult specific product labeling. [DSC] = Discontinued product

Aerosol, topical [spray]:

Tinactin® Antifungal: 1% (150 g) [contains ethanol 29% v/v]

Ting®: 1% (128 g) [contains ethanol 41% v/v]

Aerosol, topical [powder, spray]:

Tinactin® Antifungal Deodorant: 1% (133 g) [contains ethanol 11% v/v, talc]

Tinactin® Antifungal: 1% (133 g) [contains ethanol 11% v/v, talc]

Tinactin® Antifungal Jock Itch: 1% (133 g) [contains ethanol 11%, talc]

Cream, topical: 1% (15 g, 30 g)

FungiGuard, Tinactin® Antifungal Jock Itch, Ting®: 1% (15 g)

Tinactin® Antifungal: 1% (15 g, 30 g)

Liquid, topical:

Blis-To-Sol®: 1% (30 mL, 55 mL)

FungiGuard: 1% (30 mL) [contains vitamin E and aloe]

Liquid, topical [spray]:
Tinactin® Antifungal: 1% (59 mL) [contains ethanol 70% v/v]
Powder, topical: 1% (45 g)
Podactin: 1% (45 g)
Tinactin® Antifungal: 1% (108 g)
Solution, topical: 1% (10 mL)
Mycocide® NS: 1% (30 mL)
Tinaderm: 1% (10 mL)

Tolterodine (tole TER oh deen)

U.S. Brand Names Detrol®; Detrol® LA

Canadian Brand Names Detrol®; Detrol® LA; Unidet®

Index Terms Tolterodine Tartrate

Pharmacologic Category Anticholinergic Agent

Use Treatment of patients with an overactive bladder with symptoms of urinary frequency, urgency, or urge incontinence

Pregnancy Risk Factor C

Pregnancy Considerations Teratogenic effects were observed in some animal studies. There are no adequate and well-controlled studies in pregnant women. Use during pregnancy only if the potential benefit to the mother outweighs the possible risk to the fetus.

Lactation Excretion in breast milk unknown/not recommended

Medication Safety Issues

Sound-alike/look-alike issues:
Tolterodine may be confused with fesoterodine
Detrol® may be confused with Ditropan®

International issues:
Detrol® may be confused with Desurol® which is a brand name for oxolinic acid in the Czech Republic

Contraindications Hypersensitivity to tolterodine or any component of the formulation; urinary retention; gastric retention; uncontrolled narrow-angle glaucoma

Warnings/Precautions May cause drowsiness and/or blurred vision, which may impair physical or mental abilities; patients must be cautioned about performing tasks which require mental alertness (eg, operating machinery or driving). Use with caution in patients with bladder flow obstruction, may increase the risk of urinary retention. Use with caution in patients with gastrointestinal obstructive disorders (ie, pyloric stenosis), may increase the risk of gastric retention. Use with caution in patients with myasthenia gravis and controlled (treated) narrow-angle glaucoma; metabolized in the liver and excreted in the urine and feces, dosage adjustment is required for patients with renal or hepatic impairment. Tolterodine has been associated with QT_c prolongation at high (supratherapeutic) doses. The manufacturer recommends caution in patients with congenital prolonged QT or in patients receiving concurrent therapy with QT_c-prolonging drugs (class Ia or III antiarrhythmics). However, the mean change in QT_c even at supratherapeutic dosages was less than 15 msec. Individuals who are CYP2D6 poor metabolizers or in the presence of inhibitors of CYP2D6 and CYP3A4 may be more likely to exhibit prolongation. Dosage adjustment is recommended in patients receiving CYP3A4 inhibitors (a lower dose of tolterodine is recommended). Safety and efficacy in pediatric patients have not been established.

Adverse Reactions As reported with immediate release tablet, unless otherwise specified

>10%: Gastrointestinal: Dry mouth (35%; extended release capsules 23%)

1% to 10%:
Cardiovascular: Chest pain (2%)
Central nervous system: Headache (7%; extended release capsules 6%), somnolence (3%; extended release capsules 3%), fatigue (4%; extended release capsules 2%), dizziness (5%; extended release capsules 2%), anxiety (extended release capsules 1%)
Dermatologic: Dry skin (1%)
Gastrointestinal: Abdominal pain (5%; extended release capsules 4%), constipation (7%; extended release capsules 6%), dyspepsia (4%; extended release capsules 3%), diarrhea (4%), weight gain (1%)
Genitourinary: Dysuria (2%; extended release capsules 1%)
Neuromuscular & skeletal: Arthralgia (2%)
Ocular: Abnormal vision (2%; extended release capsules 1%), dry eyes (3%; extended release capsules 3%)
Respiratory: Bronchitis (2%), sinusitis (extended release capsules 2%)
Miscellaneous: Flu-like syndrome (3%), infection (1%)

<1% (Limited to important or life-threatening): Anaphylactoid reactions, angioedema, confusion, dementia aggravated, disorientation, hallucinations, memory impairment, palpitation, peripheral edema, QT_c prolongation, tachycardia

Drug Interactions

Metabolism/Transport Effects Substrate of CYP2C9 (minor), 2C19 (minor), 2D6 (major), 3A4 (major)

Avoid Concomitant Use There are no known interactions where it is recommended to avoid concomitant use.

Increased Effect/Toxicity

Tolterodine may increase the levels/effects of: Anticholinergics; Cannabinoids; Potassium Chloride; Warfarin

The levels/effects of Tolterodine may be increased by: Antifungal Agents (Azole Derivatives, Systemic); CYP2D6 Inhibitors (Moderate); CYP2D6 Inhibitors (Strong); CYP3A4 Inhibitors (Moderate); CYP3A4 Inhibitors (Strong); Darunavir; Dasatinib; Fluconazole; Pramlintide; VinBLAStine

Decreased Effect

Tolterodine may decrease the levels/effects of: Acetylcholinesterase Inhibitors (Central); Secretin

The levels/effects of Tolterodine may be decreased by: Acetylcholinesterase Inhibitors (Central); CYP3A4 Inducers (Strong); Deferasirox; Herbs (CYP3A4 Inducers)

Ethanol/Nutrition/Herb Interactions

Food: Increases bioavailability (~53% increase) of tolterodine tablets (dose adjustment not necessary); does not affect the pharmacokinetics of tolterodine extended release capsules. As a CYP3A4 inhibitor, grapefruit juice may increase the serum level and/or toxicity of tolterodine, but unlikely secondary to high oral bioavailability.

Herb/Nutraceutical: St John's wort (*Hypericum*) appears to induce CYP3A enzymes.

Stability Store at 25°C (77°F); excursions permitted to 15°C to 30°C (59°F to 86°F). Protect from light.

Mechanism of Action Tolterodine is a competitive antagonist of muscarinic receptors. In animal models, tolterodine demonstrates selectivity for urinary bladder receptors over salivary receptors. Urinary bladder contraction is mediated by muscarinic receptors. Tolterodine increases residual urine volume and decreases detrusor muscle pressure.

Pharmacodynamics/Kinetics

Absorption: Immediate release tablet: Rapid; ≥77%

Distribution: I.V.: V_d: 113 ± 27 L

Protein binding: >96% (primarily to $alpha_1$-acid glycoprotein)

Metabolism: Extensively hepatic, primarily via CYP2D6 (some metabolites share activity) and 3A4 usually (minor pathway). In patients with a genetic deficiency of CYP2D6, metabolism via 3A4 predominates.

Bioavailability: Immediate release tablet: Increased 53% with food

Half-life elimination:

Immediate release tablet: Extensive metabolizers: ~2 hours; Poor metabolizers: ~10 hours

Extended release capsule: Extensive metabolizers: ~7 hours; Poor metabolizers: ~18 hours

Time to peak: Immediate release tablet: 1-2 hours; Extended release tablet: 2-6 hours

Excretion: Urine (77%); feces (17%); primarily as metabolites (<1% unchanged drug) of which the active 5-hydroxymethyl metabolite accounts for 5% to 14% (<1% in poor metabolizers); as unchanged drug (<1%; <2.5% in poor metabolizers)

Dosage

Oral: Adults: Treatment of overactive bladder:

Immediate release tablet: 2 mg twice daily; the dose may be lowered to 1 mg twice daily based on individual response and tolerability

Dosing adjustment in patients concurrently taking CYP3A4 inhibitors: 1 mg twice daily

Extended release capsule: 4 mg once a day; dose may be lowered to 2 mg daily based on individual response and tolerability

Dosing adjustment in patients concurrently taking CYP3A4 inhibitors: 2 mg daily

Elderly: Safety and efficacy in patients >64 years was found to be similar to that in younger patients; no dosage adjustment is needed based on age

Dosing adjustment in renal impairment: Use with caution (studies conducted in patients with Cl_{cr} 10-30 mL/minute):

Immediate release tablet: 1 mg twice daily

Extended release capsule: 2 mg daily

Dosing adjustment in hepatic impairment:

Immediate release tablet: 1 mg twice daily

Extended release capsule: 2 mg daily

Administration Extended release capsule: Swallow whole; do not crush, chew, or open

Monitoring Parameters Renal function (BUN, creatinine); hepatic function

Dosage Forms Excipient information presented when available (limited, particularly for generics); consult specific product labeling.

Capsule, extended release, as tartrate (Detrol® LA): 2 mg, 4 mg

Tablet, as tartrate (Detrol®): 1 mg, 2 mg

- **Tolterodine Tartrate** *see* Tolterodine *on page* 1488
- **Tomoxetine** *see* Atomoxetine *on page* 150
- **Topamax®** *see* Topiramate *on page* 1489
- **Topicaine® [OTC]** *see* Lidocaine *on page* 884
- **Topicort®** *see* Desoximetasone *on page* 424
- **Topicort®-LP** *see* Desoximetasone *on page* 424
- **Topilene® (Can)** *see* Betamethasone *on page* 188

Topiramate (toe PYRE a mate)

U.S. Brand Names Topamax®

Canadian Brand Names Apo-Topiramate; Co-Topiramate; Dom-Topiramate; Gen-Topiramate; Novo-Topiramate; PHL-Topiramate; PMS-Topiramate; ratio-Topiramate; Sandoz-Topiramate; Topamax®

Pharmacologic Category Anticonvulsant, Miscellaneous

Additional Appendix Information

Anticonvulsant Drugs of Choice *on page* 1637

Use Monotherapy or adjunctive therapy for partial onset seizures and primary generalized tonic-clonic seizures; adjunctive treatment of seizures associated with Lennox-Gastaut syndrome; prophylaxis of migraine headache

Unlabeled/Investigational Use Infantile spasms, neuropathic pain, cluster headache

Pregnancy Risk Factor C

Pregnancy Considerations Topiramate was found to be teratogenic in animal studies; however, there is limited information in pregnant women; use only if benefit to the mother outweighs the risk to the fetus. Based on limited data, topiramate was found to cross the placenta. Postmarketing experience includes reports of hypospadias following *in vitro* exposure to topiramate.

Lactation Enters breast milk/not recommended

Medication Safety Issues

Sound-alike/look-alike issues:

Topamax® may be confused with Tegretol®, Tegretol®-XR, Toprol-XL®

Contraindications Hypersensitivity to topiramate or any component of the formulation

Warnings/Precautions Use with caution in patients with hepatic, respiratory, or renal impairment. Topiramate may decrease serum bicarbonate concentrations (up to 67% of patients); treatment-emergent metabolic acidosis is less common. Risk may be increased in patients with a predisposing condition (organ dysfunction, ketogenic diet, or concurrent treatment with other drugs which may cause acidosis). Metabolic acidosis may occur at dosages as low as 50 mg/day. Monitor serum bicarbonate as well as potential complications of chronic acidosis (nephrolithiasis, osteomalacia, and reduced growth rates in children). Kidney stones have been reported in both children and adults; the risk of kidney stones is about 2-4 times that of the untreated population; the risk of this event may be reduced by increasing fluid intake.

Cognitive dysfunction, psychiatric disturbances (mood disorders), and sedation (somnolence or fatigue) may occur with topiramate use; incidence may be related to rapid titration and higher doses. Topiramate may also cause paresthesia, dizziness, and ataxia. Topiramate has been associated with acute myopia and secondary angle-closure glaucoma in adults and children, typically within 1 month of initiation; discontinue in patients with acute onset of decreased visual acuity or ocular pain. Hyperammonemia with or without encephalopathy may occur with concomitant valproate administration; use with caution in patients with inborn errors of metabolism or decreased hepatic mitochondrial activity. Topiramate may be associated (rarely) with severe oligohydrosis and hyperthermia, most frequently in children; use caution and monitor closely during strenuous exercise, during exposure to high environmental temperature, or in patients receiving drugs with anticholinergic activity.

Avoid abrupt withdrawal of topiramate therapy, it should be withdrawn/tapered slowly to minimize the potential of increased seizure frequency. Doses were also gradually withdrawn in migraine prophylaxis studies. Effects with other sedative drugs or ethanol may be potentiated. Safety and efficacy have not been established in children <2 years of age for adjunctive treatment of seizures and <10 years of age for monotherapy treatment of seizures. Safety and efficacy have not been established in children for migraine prophylaxis.

Adverse Reactions Adverse events are reported for placebo-controlled trials of adjunctive therapy in adult and pediatric patients. Unless otherwise noted, the percentages refer to incidence in epilepsy trials. Note: A wide range of dosages were studied; incidence of adverse events was frequently lower in the pediatric population studied.

>10%:

Central nervous system: Dizziness (4% to 32%), ataxia (6% to 16%), somnolence (15% to 29%), psychomotor slowing (3% to 21%), nervousness (9% to 19%), memory difficulties (2% to 14%), speech problems (2% to 13%), fatigue (9% to 30%), difficulty concentrating (5% to 14%), depression (9% to 13%), confusion (4% to 14%)

Endocrine & metabolic: Serum bicarbonate decreased (dose-related: 7% to 67%; marked reductions [to <17 mEq/L] 1% to 11%)

Gastrointestinal: Nausea (6% to 12%; migraine trial: 14%), weight loss (8% to 13%), anorexia (4% to 24%)

Neuromuscular & skeletal: Paresthesia (1% to 19%; migraine trial: 35% to 51%)

Ocular: Nystagmus (10% to 11%), abnormal vision (<1% to 13%)

Respiratory: Upper respiratory infection (migraine trial: 12% to 13%)

Miscellaneous: Injury (6% to 14%)

1% to 10%:

Cardiovascular: Chest pain (2% to 4%), edema (1% to 2%), bradycardia (1%), pallor (up to 1%), hypertension (1% to 2%)

Central nervous system: Abnormal coordination (4%), hypoesthesia (1% to 2%; migraine trial: 8%), convulsions (1%), depersonalization (1% to 2%), apathy (1% to 3%), cognitive problems (3%), emotional lability (3%), agitation (3%), aggressive reactions (2% to 9%), tremor (3% to 9%), stupor (1% to 2%), mood problems (4% to 9%), anxiety (2% to 10%), insomnia (4% to 8%), neurosis (1%), vertigo (1% to 2%)

Dermatologic: Pruritus (migraine trial: 2% to 4%), skin disorder (1% to 3%), alopecia (2%), dermatitis (up to 2%), hypertrichosis (up to 2%), rash erythematous (up to 2%), eczema (up to 1%), seborrhea (up to 1%), skin discoloration (up to 1%)

Endocrine & metabolic: Hot flashes (1% to 2%); metabolic acidosis (hyperchloremia, nonanion gap), dehydration, breast pain (up to 4%), menstrual irregularities (1% to 2%), hypoglycemia (1%), libido decreased (<1% to 2%)

Gastrointestinal: Dyspepsia (2% to 7%), abdominal pain (5% to 7%), constipation (3% to 5%), xerostomia (2% to 4%), fecal incontinence (1%), gingivitis (1%), diarrhea (2%; migraine trial: 11%), vomiting (1% to 3%), gastroenteritis (1% to 3%), appetite increased (1%), GI disorder (1%), (2% to 4%; migraine trial: 12% to 15%), dysphagia (1%), flatulence (1%), GERD (1%), glossitis (1%), gum hyperplasia (1%), weight increase (1%)

Genitourinary: Impotence, dysuria/incontinence (<1% to 4%), prostatic disorder (2%), UTI (2% to 3%), premature ejaculation (migraine trial: 3%), cystitis (2%)

Hematologic: Leukopenia (1% to 2%), purpura (8%), hematoma (1%), prothrombin time increased (1%), thrombocytopenia (1%)

Neuromuscular & skeletal: Myalgia (2%), weakness (3% to 6%), back pain (1% to 5%), leg pain (2% to 4%), rigors (1%), hypertonia, arthralgia (1% to 7%), gait abnormal (2% to 8%), involuntary muscle contractions (2%; migraine trial: 4%), skeletal pain (1%), hyperkinesia (up to 5%), hyporeflexia (up to 2%)

Ocular: Conjunctivitis (1%), diplopia (2% to 10%), myopia (up to 1%)

Otic: Hearing decreased (1% to 2%), tinnitus (1% to 2%), otitis media (migraine trial: 1% to 2%)

Renal: Nephrolithiasis, renal calculus (1% to 2%), hematuria (<1% to 2%)

Respiratory: Pharyngitis (3% to 6%), sinusitis (4% to 6%; migraine trial: 8% to 10%), epistaxis (1% to 4%), rhinitis (4% to 7%), dyspnea (1% to 2%), pneumonia (5%), coughing (migraine trial: 2% to 3%), bronchitis (migraine trial: 3%)

Miscellaneous: Flu-like syndrome (3% to 7%), allergy (2% to 3%), body odor (up to 1%), fever (migraine trial: 1% to 2%), viral infection (migraine trial: 3% to 4%), infection (<1% to 2%), diaphoresis (≤1%), thirst (2%)

<1% (Limited to important or life-threatening): Accommodation abnormality, anemia, angina, apraxia, AV block, bone marrow depression, deep vein thrombosis, dehydration, delirium, diabetes mellitus, dyskinesia, electrolyte imbalance, encephalopathy (with valproate therapy), eosinophilia, erythema multiforme, euphoria, eye pain, granulocytopenia, hepatic failure, hepatitis, hyperammonemia (with valproate therapy), hyperthermia (severe), hypokalemia, hypotension, liver enzymes increased, lymphadenopathy, lymphopenia, manic reaction, migraine aggravated, neuropathy, oligohydrosis, pancreatitis, pancytopenia, paranoid reaction, pemphigus, photosensitivity, psychosis, pulmonary embolism, rash, renal tubular acidosis, Stevens-Johnson syndrome, suicidal behavior, syncope, syndrome of acute myopia/secondary angle-closure glaucoma, tongue edema, toxic epidermal necrolysis

Drug Interactions

Metabolism/Transport Effects **Inhibits** CYP2C19 (weak); **Induces** CYP3A4 (weak)

Avoid Concomitant Use There are no known interactions where it is recommended to avoid concomitant use.

Increased Effect/Toxicity

Topiramate may increase the levels/effects of: Alcohol (Ethyl); CNS Depressants; Phenytoin; Valproic Acid

Decreased Effect

Topiramate may decrease the levels/effects of: Maraviroc; Oral Contraceptive (Estrogens)

The levels/effects of Topiramate may be decreased by: CarBAMazepine; Ketorolac; Mefloquine; Phenytoin

Ethanol/Nutrition/Herb Interactions

Ethanol: Avoid ethanol (may increase CNS depression).

Food: Ketogenic diet may increase the possibility of acidosis and/or kidney stones.

Herb/Nutraceutical: Avoid evening primrose (seizure threshold decreased).

Stability Store at room temperature of 15°C to 30°C (59°F to 86°F). Protect from moisture.

Mechanism of Action Anticonvulsant activity may be due to a combination of potential mechanisms: Blocks neuronal voltage-dependent sodium channels, enhances GABA(A) activity, antagonizes AMPA/kainate glutamate receptors, and weakly inhibits carbonic anhydrase.

Pharmacodynamics/Kinetics

Absorption: Good, rapid; unaffected by food

Protein binding: 15% to 41% (inversely related to plasma concentrations)

Metabolism: Hepatic via P450 enzymes

Bioavailability: 80%

Half-life elimination: Mean: Adults: Normal renal function: 21 hours; shorter in pediatric patients; clearance is 50% higher in pediatric patients; Elderly: ~24 hours

Time to peak, serum: ~1-4 hours

Excretion: Urine (~70% to 80% as unchanged drug)

Dialyzable: ~30%

Dosage Oral: **Note:** Do not abruptly discontinue therapy; taper dosage gradually to prevent rebound effects. (In clinical trials, adult doses were withdrawn by decreasing in weekly intervals of 50-100 mg/day gradually over 2-8 weeks for seizure treatment, and by decreasing in weekly intervals by 25-50 mg/day for migraine prophylaxis.)

Epilepsy, monotherapy: Children ≥10 years and Adults: Partial onset seizure and primary generalized tonic-clonic seizure: Initial: 25 mg twice daily; may increase weekly by 50 mg/day up to 100 mg twice daily (week 4 dose); thereafter, may further increase weekly by 100 mg/day up to the recommended maximum of 200 mg twice daily.

Epilepsy, adjunctive therapy:

Children 2-16 years:

Partial onset seizure or seizure associated with Lennox-Gastaut syndrome: Initial dose titration should begin at 25 mg (or less, based on a range of 1-3 mg/kg/day)

nightly for the first week; dosage may be increased in increments of 1-3 mg/kg/day (administered in 2 divided doses) at 1- or 2-week intervals to a total daily dose of 5-9 mg/kg/day

Primary generalized tonic-clonic seizure: Use initial dose listed above, but use slower initial titration rate; titrate to recommended maintenance dose by the end of 8 weeks

Adolescents ≥17 years and Adults:

Partial onset seizures: Initial: 25-50 mg/day (given in 2 divided doses) for 1 week; increase at weekly intervals by 25-50 mg/day until response; usual maintenance dose: 100-200 mg twice daily. Doses >1600 mg/day have not been studied.

Primary generalized tonic-clonic seizures: Use initial dose as listed above for partial onset seizures, but use slower initial titration rate; titrate upwards to recommended dose by the end of 8 weeks; usual maintenance dose: 200 mg twice daily. Doses >1600 mg/day have not been studied.

Adults:

Migraine prophylaxis: Initial: 25 mg/day (in the evening), titrated at weekly intervals in 25 mg increments, up to the recommended total daily dose of 100 mg/day given in 2 divided doses

Cluster headache (unlabeled use): Initial: 25 mg/day, titrated at weekly intervals in 25 mg increments, up to 200 mg/day

Neuropathic pain (unlabeled use): Initial: 25 mg/day, titrated at weekly intervals in 25-50 mg increments to target dose of 400 mg daily in 2 divided doses. Reported dosage range studied: 25-800 mg/day

Dosing adjustment in renal impairment: Cl_{cr} <70 mL/minute: Administer 50% dose and titrate more slowly

Hemodialysis: Supplemental dose may be needed during hemodialysis

Dosing adjustment in hepatic impairment: Clearance may be reduced

Administration Oral: May be administered without regard to meals

Capsule sprinkles: May be swallowed whole or opened to sprinkle the contents on soft food (drug/food mixture should not be chewed).

Tablet: Because of bitter taste, tablets should not be broken.

Monitoring Parameters Seizure frequency, hydration status; electrolytes (recommended monitoring includes serum bicarbonate at baseline and periodically during treatment), serum creatinine; monitor for symptoms of acute acidosis and complications of long-term acidosis (nephrolithiasis, osteomalacia, and reduced growth rates in children); ammonia level in patients with unexplained lethargy, vomiting, or mental status changes; intraocular pressure, symptoms of secondary angle closure glaucoma

Additional Information May be associated with weight loss in some patients

Dosage Forms Excipient information presented when available (limited, particularly for generics); consult specific product labeling.

Capsule, sprinkle:

Topamax®: 15 mg, 25 mg

Tablet:

Topamax®: 25 mg, 50 mg, 100 mg, 200 mg

◆ **Topisone® (Can)** *see* Betamethasone *on page 188*

◆ **Toposar®** *see* Etoposide *on page 591*

Topotecan (toe poe TEE kan)

U.S. Brand Names Hycamtin®

Canadian Brand Names Hycamtin®

Index Terms Hycamptamine; NSC-609699; SKF 104864; SKF 104864-A; Topotecan Hydrochloride

Pharmacologic Category Antineoplastic Agent, Camptothecin; Antineoplastic Agent, Natural Source (Plant) Derivative

Use Treatment of ovarian cancer and small cell lung cancer; cervical cancer (in combination with cisplatin)

Unlabeled/Investigational Use Investigational: Treatment of nonsmall cell lung cancer, myelodysplastic syndrome, sarcoma (pediatrics), neuroblastoma (pediatrics), refractory solid tumors (pediatrics)

Pregnancy Risk Factor D

Pregnancy Considerations Animal studies found reduced fetal body weight, eye, brain, skull, and vertebrae malformations. May cause fetal harm in pregnant women. Use during pregnancy is contraindicated.

Lactation Excretion in breast milk unknown/contraindicated

Medication Safety Issues

Sound-alike/look-alike issues:

Hycamtin® may be confused with Hycomine®, Mycamine®

High alert medication: The Institute for Safe Medication Practices (ISMP) includes this medication among its list of drugs which have a heightened risk of causing significant patient harm when used in error.

Contraindications Hypersensitivity to topotecan or any component of the formulation; severe bone marrow depression; pregnancy; breast-feeding

Warnings/Precautions Hazardous agent - use appropriate precautions for handling and disposal. The dose-limiting toxicity is bone marrow suppression (primarily neutropenia; may also cause thrombocytopenia and anemia); monitor bone marrow function. Neutropenia is not cumulative overtime. **[U.S. Boxed Warning]: Should only administer to patients with adequate bone marrow reserves, baseline neutrophils at least 1500 cells/mm^3** and platelet counts at least 100,000/mm^3. In a clinical study comparing I.V. to oral topotecan, G-CSF support was administered in a higher percentage of patients receiving oral topotecan. Topotecan-induced neutropenia may lead to neutropenic colitis; should be considered in patients presenting with neutropenia, fever and abdominal pain. Diarrhea has been reported with oral topotecan; may be severe; incidence may be higher in the elderly; educate patients on proper management. Use caution in renal impairment; may require dose adjustment. **[U.S. Boxed Warning]: Should be administered under the supervision of an experienced cancer chemotherapy physician.** Safety and efficacy in children have not been established.

Adverse Reactions

>10%:

Central nervous system: Fatigue (11% to 29%), fever (5% to 28%), pain (23%), headache (18%)

Dermatologic: Alopecia (10% to 49%), rash (16%)

Gastrointestinal: Nausea (27% to 64%), vomiting (19% to 45%), diarrhea (14% to 32%; Oral: grade 3: 4%; grade 4: ≤1%; onset: 9 days), constipation (29%), abdominal pain (22%), anorexia (7% to 19%), stomatitis (18%)

Hematologic: Neutropenia (83% to 97%; grade 4: 32% to 80%; nadir 8-11 days; duration: 7 days; recovery <21 days), leukopenia (86% to 97%; grade 4: 15% to 32%), anemia (89% to 98%; grade 4: 7% to 10%), thrombocytopenia (69% to 81%; grade 4: 6% to 29%; duration: 3 days), neutropenic fever/sepsis (2% to 28%)

Neuromuscular & skeletal: Weakness (3% to 25%)

Respiratory: Dyspnea (22%), cough (15%)

1% to 10%:

Hepatic: Transient increases in liver enzymes (8%)

Neuromuscular & skeletal: Paresthesia (7%)

Miscellaneous: Sepsis (grades 3/4: 5%)

<1% (Limited to important or life-threatening): Abdominal pain, allergic reactions, anaphylactoid reactions,

angioedema, bleeding (severe, associated with thrombocytopenia), dermatitis (severe), injection site reactions (mild erythema, bruising), neutropenic colitis, pancytopenia, pruritus (severe)

Drug Interactions

Avoid Concomitant Use

Avoid concomitant use of Topotecan with any of the following: Natalizumab; P-Glycoprotein Inhibitors; Vaccines (Live)

Increased Effect/Toxicity

Topotecan may increase the levels/effects of: Natalizumab; Vaccines (Live)

The levels/effects of Topotecan may be increased by: BCRP/ABCG2 Inhibitors; Filgrastim; P-Glycoprotein Inhibitors; Platinum Derivatives; Trastuzumab

Decreased Effect

Topotecan may decrease the levels/effects of: Vaccines (Inactivated)

The levels/effects of Topotecan may be decreased by: Echinacea

Ethanol/Nutrition/Herb Interactions Ethanol: Avoid ethanol (due to GI irritation).

Stability

I.V.: Store intact vials of lyophilized powder for injection at room temperature of 20°C to 25°C (68°F to 77°F); protect from light. Reconstitute with 4 mL SWFI. This solution is stable for up to 28 days at room temperature of 20°C to 25°C (68°F to 77°F). Topotecan should be further diluted in 50-100 mL D_5W or NS. This solution is stable for 24 hours at room temperature or up to 7 days under refrigeration.

Oral: Store at 15°C to 30°C (59°F to 86°F). Protect from light

Mechanism of Action Binds to topoisomerase I and stabilizes the cleavable complex so that religation of the cleaved DNA strand cannot occur. This results in the accumulation of cleavable complexes and single-strand DNA breaks. Topotecan acts in S phase of the cell cycle.

Pharmacodynamics/Kinetics

Absorption: Oral: Rapid

Distribution: V_{dss} of the lactone is high (mean: 87.3 L/mm^2; range: 25.6-186 L/mm^2), suggesting wide distribution and/or tissue sequestering

Protein binding: ~35%

Metabolism: Undergoes a rapid, pH-dependent hydrolysis of the lactone ring to yield a relatively inactive hydroxy acid in plasma; metabolized in the liver to N-demethylated metabolite

Bioavailability: Oral: ~40%

Half-life elimination: I.V.: 2-3 hours; renal impairment: 5 hours; Oral: 3-6 hours

Time to peak, plasma: Oral 1-2 hours; delayed with high-fat meal (1.5-4 hours)

Excretion:

I.V.: Urine (51%; 3% as N-desmethyl topotecan); feces (18%; 2% as N-desmethyl topotecan)

Oral: Urine (20%; 2% as N-desmethyl topotecan); feces (33%; <2% as N-desmethyl topotecan)

Dosage Adults (refer to individual protocols): **Note:** Baseline neutrophil count should be >1500/mm^3; retreatment neutrophil count should be >1000/mm^3; baseline and retreatment platelet count should be >100,000/mm^3; (also, for oral topotecan, retreatment hemoglobin should be ≥9 g/dL):

Small cell lung cancer:

IVPB: 1.5 mg/m^2/day for 5 days; repeated every 21 days

Oral: 2.3 mg/m^2/day for 5 days; repeated every 21 days (round dose to the nearest 0.25 mg); if patient vomits after dose is administered, do not give a replacement dose.

Metastatic ovarian cancer:

IVPB: 1.5 mg/m^2/day for 5 days; repeated every 21 days

I.V. continuous infusion (unlabeled dose) 0.2-0.7 mg/m^2/day for 7-21 days

Cervical cancer: IVPB: 0.75 mg/m^2/day for 3 days (followed by cisplatin 50 mg/m^2 on day 1 only, [with hydration]); repeated every 21 days

Dosage adjustment for toxicity:

I.V.:

Ovarian and small cell lung cancer: Dosage adjustment for hematological effects: Severe neutropenia or platelet count <25,000/mm^3: Reduce dose to 1.25 mg/m^2/day for subsequent cycles (may consider G-CSF support [beginning on day 6] prior to instituting dose reduction for neutropenia)

Cervical cancer: Severe febrile neutropenia (ANC <1000/mm^3 with temperature of 38°C) or platelet count <10,000/mm^3: Reduce topotecan to 0.6 mg/m^2/day for subsequent cycles (may consider C-CSF support [beginning on day 4] prior to instituting dose reduction for neutropenic fever.

For neutropenic fever despite G-CSF use, reduce dose to 0.45 mg/m^2/day for subsequent cycles). **Note:** Cisplatin may also require dose adjustment.

Oral:

Small cell lung cancer: Severe neutropenia (neutrophils <500/mm^3 associated with fever or infection or lasting >7 days) or prolonged neutropenia (neutrophils ≥500/mm^3 to ≤1000/mm^3 lasting beyond day 21) or platelets <25,000/mm^3 or grades 3/4 diarrhea: Reduce dose to 1.9 mg/m^2/day for subsequent cycles (may consider same dosage reduction for grade 2 diarrhea if clinically indicated).

Dosing adjustment in renal impairment:

The FDA-approved labeling recommends the following dosage adjustment:

I.V.:

Cl_{cr} 20-39 mL/minute: Reduce to 0.75 mg/m^2/dose

Cl_{cr} <20 mL/minute: Insufficient data available for dosing recommendation

Note: For topotecan in combination with cisplatin for cervical cancer, do not initiate treatment in patients with serum creatinine >1.5 mg/dL; consider discontinuing treatment in patients with serum creatinine >1.5 mg/dL in subsequent cycles.

Oral:

Cl_{cr} 30-49 mL/minute: Reduce dose to 1.8 mg/m^2/day

Cl_{cr} <30 mL/minute: Insufficient data available for dosing recommendation

The following guidelines have been used by some clinicians:

Aronoff, 2007: *I.V.:*

Children:

Cl_{cr} 30-50 mL/minute: Administer 75% of dose

Cl_{cr} 10-29 mL/minute: Administer 50% of dose or reduce by 0.75 mg/m^2/dose

Cl_{cr} <10 mL/minute: Administer 25% of dose

Hemodialysis: 0.75 mg/m^2

Continuous renal replacement therapy (CRRT): Administer 50% of dose or reduce by 0.75 mg/m^2/dose

Adults:

Cl_{cr} >50 mL/minute: Administer 75% of dose

Cl_{cr} 10-50 mL/minute: Administer 50% of dose

Cl_{cr} <10 mL/minute: Administer 25% of dose

Hemodialysis: Avoid use

Continuous ambulatory peritoneal dialysis (CAPD): Avoid use

Continuous renal replacement therapy (CRRT): 0.75 mg/m^2

Kintzel, 1995:

Cl_{cr} 46-60 mL/minute: Administer 80% of dose

Cl_{cr} 31-45 mL/minute: Administer 75% of dose

Cl_{cr} <30 mL/minute: Administer 70% of dose

Dosing adjustment in hepatic impairment: The FDA-approved labeling recommends the following:

I.V.: Bilirubin 1.5-10 mg/dL: No adjustment necessary

Oral: Bilirubin >1.5 mg/dL: No adjustment necessary

Dietary Considerations May be taken with or without food.

Administration

I.V.: Administer IVPB over 30 minutes or by 24-hour continuous infusion. For combination chemotherapy with cisplatin, administer pretreatment hydration.

Oral: Administer with or without food. Swallow whole; do not crush, chew, or divide capsule. If vomiting occurs after dose, do not take replacement dose.

Monitoring Parameters CBC with differential and platelet count, renal function tests, bilirubin

Test Interactions None known

Dosage Forms Excipient information presented when available (limited, particularly for generics); consult specific product labeling.

Capsule:

Hycamtin®: 0.25 mg, 1 mg

Injection, powder for reconstitution:

Hycamtin®: 4 mg

◆ **Topotecan Hydrochloride** *see* Topotecan *on page 1491*

◆ **Toprol-XL®** *see* Metoprolol *on page 982*

◆ **Topsyn® (Can)** *see* Fluocinonide *on page 634*

◆ **Toradol® (Can)** *see* Ketorolac *on page 841*

◆ **Toradol® IM (Can)** *see* Ketorolac *on page 841*

Toremifene (tore EM i feen)

U.S. Brand Names Fareston®

Canadian Brand Names Fareston®

Index Terms FC1157a; Toremifene Citrate

Pharmacologic Category Antineoplastic Agent, Estrogen Receptor Antagonist; Selective Estrogen Receptor Modulator (SERM)

Use Treatment of postmenopausal metastatic breast cancer (estrogen receptor positive or estrogen receptor status unknown)

Pregnancy Risk Factor D

Pregnancy Considerations Animal studies have demonstrated embryotoxicity and fetal adverse effects. There are no adequate and well-controlled studies in pregnant women. May cause fetal harm if administered during pregnancy.

Lactation Excretion in breast milk unknown/not recommended

Contraindications Hypersensitivity to toremifene or any component of the formulation

Warnings/Precautions Hazardous agent - use appropriate precautions for handling and disposal. Hypercalcemia and tumor flare have been reported during the first weeks of treatment in some breast cancer patients with bone metastases. Tumor flare is a syndrome of diffuse musculoskeletal pain and erythema with increased size of tumor lesions that later regress. It is often accompanied by hypercalcemia. Tumor flare does not imply treatment failure or represent tumor progression. Institute appropriate measures if hypercalcemia occurs, and if severe, discontinue treatment. Drugs that decrease renal calcium excretion (eg, thiazide diuretics) may increase the risk of hypercalcemia in patients receiving toremifene. Leukopenia and thrombocytopenia have been reported rarely. Endometrial hyperplasia has been reported; endometrial cancer has been reported, although a role of toremifene in endometrial cancer development has not been established. Use with caution in patients with hepatic failure. Avoid use in patients with thromboembolic disease.

Adverse Reactions

>10%:

Endocrine & metabolic: Hot flashes (35%)

Gastrointestinal: Nausea (14%)

Genitourinary: Vaginal discharge (13%)

Hepatic: Alkaline phosphatase increased (8% to 19%), AST increased (5% to 19%)

Miscellaneous: Diaphoresis (20%)

1% to 10%:

Cardiovascular: Edema (5%), arrhythmia (≤2%), CVA/TIA (≤2%), thrombosis (≤2%), cardiac failure (≤1%), MI (≤1%)

Central nervous system: Dizziness (9%)

Endocrine & metabolic: Hypercalcemia (≤3%)

Gastrointestinal: Vomiting (4%)

Genitourinary: Vaginal bleeding (2%)

Hepatic: Bilirubin increased (1% to 2%)

Local: Thrombophlebitis (≤2%)

Ocular: Cataracts (≤10%), xerophthalmia (≤9%), visual field abnormal (≤4%), corneal keratopathy (≤2%), glaucoma (≤2%), vision abnormal/diplopia (≤2%)

Respiratory: Pulmonary embolism (≤2%)

<1% (Limited to important or life-threatening): Alopecia, angina, anorexia, arthritis, ataxia, constipation, corneal opacity (reversible), corneal verticulata, deep vein thrombosis, depression, dermatitis, dyspnea, endometrial cancer, endometrial hyperplasia, fatigue, hepatitis (toxic), incoordination, ischemic attack, jaundice, lethargy, leukopenia, paresis, pruritus, QT prolongation, retinopathy, rigors, skin discoloration, thrombocytopenia, thrombophlebitis, tremor, tumor flare, vaginal dryness, vertigo, weakness

Drug Interactions

Metabolism/Transport Effects Substrate of CYP1A2 (minor), 3A4 (major)

Avoid Concomitant Use There are no known interactions where it is recommended to avoid concomitant use.

Increased Effect/Toxicity There are no known significant interactions involving an increase in effect.

Decreased Effect

The levels/effects of Toremifene may be decreased by: CYP3A4 Inducers (Strong); Deferasirox; Herbs (CYP3A4 Inducers)

Ethanol/Nutrition/Herb Interactions Herb/Nutraceutical: Avoid St John's wort (may decrease toremifene levels).

Stability Store at 25°C (77°F); excursions permitted to 15°C to 30°C (59°F to 86°F). Protect from heat and light.

Mechanism of Action Nonsteroidal, triphenylethylene derivative with potent antiestrogenic properties (also has estrogenic effects). Competitively binds to estrogen receptors on tumors and other tissue targets, producing a nuclear complex that decreases DNA synthesis and inhibits estrogen effects. Competes with estrogen for binding sites in breast and other tissues; cells accumulate in the G_0 and G_1 phases; therefore, toremifene is cytostatic rather than cytocidal.

Pharmacodynamics/Kinetics

Absorption: Well absorbed

Distribution: V_d: 580 L (range: 457-958 L)

Protein binding, plasma: >99.5%, primarily to albumin

Metabolism: Extensively hepatic, principally by CYP3A4 to N-demethyltoremifene, which is also antiestrogenic but with weak *in vivo* antitumor potency

Half-life elimination: ~5 days

Time to peak, serum: ~3 hours (range: 2-6 hours)

Excretion: Primarily feces; urine (10%) during a 1-week period

Dosage Adults: Oral: 60 mg once daily, generally continued until disease progression is observed

Dosage adjustment in renal impairment: No dosage adjustment necessary

Dosage adjustment in hepatic impairment: Toremifene is extensively metabolized in the liver and dosage adjustments may be indicated in patients with liver disease; however, no specific guidelines have been developed

Administration Administer orally, as a single daily dose.

Monitoring Parameters Obtain periodic complete blood counts, calcium levels, and liver function tests. Closely monitor patients with bone metastases for hypercalcemia during the first few weeks of treatment. Leukopenia and thrombocytopenia have been reported rarely; monitor leukocyte and platelet counts during treatment.

Dosage Forms Excipient information presented when available (limited, particularly for generics); consult specific product labeling.

Tablet:

Fareston®: 60 mg

◆ **Toremifene Citrate** *see* Toremifene *on page 1493*

◆ **Torisel®** *see* Temsirolimus *on page 1434*

Torsemide (TORE se mide)

U.S. Brand Names Demadex®

Pharmacologic Category Diuretic, Loop

Additional Appendix Information

Heart Failure (Systolic) *on page 1809*

Sulfonamide Derivatives *on page 1671*

Use Management of edema associated with congestive heart failure and hepatic or renal disease; used alone or in combination with antihypertensives in treatment of hypertension; I.V. form is indicated when rapid onset is desired

Pregnancy Risk Factor B

Pregnancy Considerations A decrease in fetal weight, an increase in fetal resorption, and delayed fetal ossification has occurred in animal studies.

Lactation Excretion in breast milk unknown/use caution

Medication Safety Issues

Sound-alike/look-alike issues:

Torsemide may be confused with furosemide

Demadex® may be confused with Denorex®

Contraindications Hypersensitivity to torsemide, any component of the formulation, or any sulfonylureas; anuria

Warnings/Precautions Loop diuretics are potent diuretics; excess amounts can lead to profound diuresis with fluid and electrolyte loss; close medical supervision and dose evaluation are required. Watch for and correct electrolyte disturbances; adjust dose to avoid dehydration. In cirrhosis, avoid electrolyte and acid/base imbalances that might lead to hepatic encephalopathy. Coadministration of antihypertensives may increase the risk of hypotension.

Monitor fluid status and renal function in an attempt to prevent oliguria, azotemia, and reversible increases in BUN and creatinine; close medical supervision of aggressive diuresis required. Rapid I.V. administration (associated with other loop diuretics), renal impairment, excessive doses, and concurrent use of other ototoxins is associated with ototoxicity; has been seen with oral torsemide.

Chemical similarities are present among sulfonamides, sulfonylureas, carbonic anhydrase inhibitors, thiazides, and loop diuretics (except ethacrynic acid). Use in patients with sulfonylurea allergy is specifically contraindicated in product labeling, however, a risk of cross-reaction exists in patients with allergy to any of these compounds; avoid use when previous reaction has been severe. Discontinue if signs of hypersensitivity are noted.

Adverse Reactions

1% to 10%:

Cardiovascular: Edema (1.1%), ECG abnormality (2%), chest pain (1.2%)

Central nervous system: Headache (7.3%), dizziness (3.2%), insomnia (1.2%), nervousness (1%)

Endocrine & metabolic: Hyperglycemia, hyperuricemia, hypokalemia

Gastrointestinal: Diarrhea (2%), constipation (1.8%), nausea (1.8%), dyspepsia (1.6%), sore throat (1.6%)

Genitourinary: Excessive urination (6.7%)

Neuromuscular & skeletal: Weakness (2%), arthralgia (1.8%), myalgia (1.6%)

Respiratory: Rhinitis (2.8%), cough increase (2%)

<1% (Limited to important or life-threatening): Angioedema, atrial fibrillation, GI hemorrhage, hypernatremia hypotension, hypovolemia, rash, rectal bleeding, shunt thrombosis, syncope, ventricular tachycardia

Drug Interactions

Metabolism/Transport Effects Substrate of CYP2C8 (minor), 2C9 (major); **Inhibits** CYP2C19 (weak)

Avoid Concomitant Use There are no known interactions where it is recommended to avoid concomitant use.

Increased Effect/Toxicity

Torsemide may increase the levels/effects of: ACE Inhibitors; Allopurinol; Amifostine; Aminoglycosides; Dofetilide; Neuromuscular-Blocking Agents; RiTUXimab

The levels/effects of Torsemide may be increased by: Corticosteroids (Orally Inhaled); Corticosteroids (Systemic); CYP2C9 Inhibitors (Moderate); CYP2C9 Inhibitors (Strong); Diazoxide; Eltrombopag; Herbs (Hypotensive Properties); Prostacyclin Analogues

Decreased Effect

Torsemide may decrease the levels/effects of: Neuromuscular-Blocking Agents

The levels/effects of Torsemide may be decreased by: Bile Acid Sequestrants; CYP2C9 Inducers (Highly Effective); Herbs (Hypertensive Properties); Methylphenidate; Nonsteroidal Anti-Inflammatory Agents; Phenytoin; Yohimbine

Ethanol/Nutrition/Herb Interactions Herb/Nutraceutical: Avoid dong quai if using for hypertension (has estrogenic activity). Avoid ephedra, yohimbe, ginseng (may worsen hypertension). Avoid garlic (may have increased antihypertensive effect).

Stability If torsemide is to be administered via continuous infusion, stability has been demonstrated through 24 hours at room temperature in plastic containers for the following fluids and concentrations:

200 mg torsemide (10 mg/mL) added to 250 mL D_5W, 250 mL NS or 500 mL 0.45% sodium chloride.

50 mg torsemide (10 mg/mL) added to 500 mL D_5W, 250 mL NS or 500 mL 0.45% sodium chloride.

Mechanism of Action Inhibits reabsorption of sodium and chloride in the ascending loop of Henle and distal renal tubule, interfering with the chloride-binding cotransport system, thus causing increased excretion of water, sodium, chloride, magnesium, and calcium; does not alter GFR, renal plasma flow, or acid-base balance

Pharmacodynamics/Kinetics

Onset of action: Diuresis: 30-60 minutes

Peak effect: 1-4 hours

Duration: ~6 hours

Absorption: Oral: Rapid

Protein binding, plasma: ~97% to 99%

Metabolism: Hepatic (80%) via CYP

Bioavailability: 80% to 90%

Half-life elimination: 2-4; Cirrhosis: 7-8 hours

Excretion: Urine (20% as unchanged drug)

Dosage Adults: Oral, I.V.:

Congestive heart failure: 10-20 mg once daily; may increase gradually for chronic treatment by doubling dose until the diuretic response is apparent (for acute treatment, I.V. dose may be repeated every 2 hours with double the dose as needed). **Note:** ACC/AHA 2005 guidelines for chronic heart failure recommend a maximum daily oral dose of 200 mg; maximum single I.V. dose of 100-200 mg

Continuous I.V. infusion: 20 mg I.V. load then 5-20 mg/hour

Chronic renal failure: 20 mg once daily; increase as described above

Hepatic cirrhosis: 5-10 mg once daily with an aldosterone antagonist or a potassium-sparing diuretic; increase as described above

Hypertension: 2.5-5 mg once daily; increase to 10 mg after 4-6 weeks if an adequate hypotensive response is not apparent; if still not effective, an additional antihypertensive agent may be added

Administration I.V. injections should be administered over ≥2 minutes; the oral form may be administered regardless of meal times; patients may be switched from the I.V. form to the oral and vice-versa with no change in dose; no dosage adjustment is needed in the elderly or patients with hepatic impairment

To administer as a continuous infusion: 50 mg or 200 mg torsemide should be diluted in 250 mL or 500 mL of compatible solution in plastic containers

Monitoring Parameters Renal function, electrolytes, and fluid status (weight and I & O), blood pressure

Additional Information 10-20 mg torsemide is approximately equivalent to furosemide 40 mg or bumetanide 1 mg.

Dosage Forms Excipient information presented when available (limited, particularly for generics); consult specific product labeling. [DSC] = Discontinued product

Injection, solution:

Demadex®: 10 mg/mL (2 mL [DSC], 5 mL [DSC])

Tablet: 5 mg, 10 mg, 20 mg, 100 mg

Demadex®: 5 mg, 10 mg, 20 mg, 100 mg [scored]

◆ **Tositumomab I-131** *see* Tositumomab and Iodine I 131 Tositumomab *on page 1495*

Tositumomab and Iodine I 131 Tositumomab

(toe si TYOO mo mab & EYE oh dyne eye one THUR tee one toe si TYOO mo mab)

U.S. Brand Names Bexxar®

Index Terms 131 I Anti-B1 Antibody; 131 I-Anti-B1 Monoclonal Antibody; Anti-CD20-Murine Monoclonal Antibody I-131; B1; B1 Antibody; Iodine I 131 Tositumomab and Tositumomab; Tositumomab I-131

Pharmacologic Category Antineoplastic Agent, Monoclonal Antibody; Radiopharmaceutical

Use Treatment of relapsed or refractory CD20 positive, low-grade, follicular, or transformed non-Hodgkin's lymphoma

Pregnancy Risk Factor X

Medication Safety Issues

High alert medication: The Institute for Safe Medication Practices (ISMP) includes this medication among its list of drugs which have a heightened risk of causing significant patient harm when used in error.

Dosage I.V.: Adults: Dosing consists of four components administered in 2 steps. Thyroid protective agents (SSKI, Lugol's solution or potassium iodide), acetaminophen and diphenhydramine should be given prior to or with treatment.

Step 1: Dosimetric step (Day 0):

Tositumomab 450 mg in NS 50 mL administered over 60 minutes

Iodine I 131 tositumomab (containing I-131 5.0 mCi and tositumomab 35mg) in NS 30 mL administered over 20 minutes

Note: Whole body dosimetry and biodistribution should be determined on Day 0; days 2, 3, or 4; and day 6 or 7 prior to administration of Step 2. If biodistribution is not acceptable, do not administer the therapeutic step. On day 6 or 7, calculate the patient specific activity of iodine I 131 tositumomab to deliver 75 cGy TBD or 65 cGy TBD (in mCi).

Step 2: Therapeutic step (Day 7):

Tositumomab 450 mg in NS 50 mL administered over 60 minutes

Iodine I 131 tositumomab:

Platelets ≥150,000/mm^3: Iodine I 131 calculated to deliver 75 cGy total body irradiation and tositumomab 35 mg over 20 minutes

Platelets ≥100,000/mm^3 and <150,000/mm^3: Iodine I 131 calculated to deliver 65 cGy total body irradiation and tositumomab 35 mg over 20 minutes

Additional Information Complete prescribing information for this medication should be consulted for additional detail.

Dosage Forms Excipient information presented when available (limited, particularly for generics); consult specific product labeling.

Note: Not all components are shipped from the same facility. When ordering, ensure that all will arrive on the same day.

Kit [dosimetric package]: Tositumomab 225 mg/16.1 mL [2 vials], tositumomab 35 mg/2.5 mL [1 vial], and iodine I 131 tositumomab 0.1 mg/mL and 0.61mCi/mL (20 mL) [1 vial]

Kit [therapeutic package]: Tositumomab 225 mg/16.1 mL [2 vials], tositumomab 35 mg/2.5 mL [1 vial], and iodine I 131 tositumomab 1.1 mg/mL and 5.6 mCi/mL (20 mL) [1 or 2 vials]

Total Parenteral Nutrition

(TOE tal par EN ter al noo TRISH un)

Index Terms Hyperal; Hyperalimentation; Parenteral Nutrition; PN; TPN

Pharmacologic Category Caloric Agent; Intravenous Nutritional Therapy

Use Infusion of nutrient solutions into the bloodstream to support nutritional needs during a time when patient is unable to absorb nutrients via the gastrointestinal tract, cannot take adequate nutrition orally or enterally, or have had (or are expected to have) inadequate oral intake for 7-14 days

Medication Safety Issues

High alert medication: The Institute for Safe Medication Practices (ISMP) includes this medication among its list of drugs which have a heightened risk of causing significant patient harm when used in error.

Dosage PN is a highly-individualized therapy. The following general guidelines may be used in the estimation of needs. Electrolytes, vitamins, and trace minerals should be added to TPN mixtures based on patients individualized needs.

Neonates: I.V.: **Note:** When indicated for premature neonates, start on day 1 of life if possible.

Total calories:

Term: 85-105 kcal/kg/day

Preterm (stable): 90-120 kcal/kg/day

Fluid:

<1.5 kg: 130-150 mL/kg/day

1.5-2 kg: 110-130 mL/kg/day

2-10 kg: 100 mL/kg/day

Carbohydrate (dextrose): 40% to 50 % of caloric intake; advance as tolerated

Term: Initial: 6-8 mg/kg/minute; goal: 10-14 mg/kg/minute

Premature: Initial: 6 mg/kg/minute; goal: 10-13 mg/kg/minute

Protein (amino acids):
Term: Initial: 2.5 g/kg/day; goal: 3 g/kg/day
Extremely (<1000 g) and very (<1500 g) low-birth-weight (stable): Initial: 1-1.5 g/kg/day; goal: 3.5-3.85 g/kg/day to promote utero growth rates.
Sepsis, hypoxia: Initial: 1 g/kg/day; goal: 3-3.85 g/kg/day

Fat:
Term: Initial: 0.5-1 g/kg/day (maximum: 3 g/kg/day); administer over 24 hours
Preterm: Initial: 0.25-0.5 g/kg/day (maximum: 3 g/kg/day or 1 g/kg/day if on phototherapy); administer over 24 hours
Note: Monitor triglycerides while receiving intralipids. If triglycerides >200 mg/dL, stop infusion and restart at 0.5-1g/kg/day

Heparin: 1 unit/mL of parenteral nutrition fluids should be added to enhance clearance of lipid emulsions

Children: I.V.: **Note:** Give within 5-7 days if unable to meet needs orally or with enteral nutrition:

Total calories:
<6 months: 85-105 kcal/kg/day
6-12 months: 80-100 kcal/kg/day
1-7 years: 75-90 kcal/kg/day
7-12 years: 50-75 kcal/kg/day
12-18 years: 30-50 kcal/kg/day

Fluid:
2-10 kg: 100 mL/kg
>10-20 kg: 1000 mL for 10 kg plus 50 mL/kg for each kg >10
>20 kg: 1500 mL for 10 kg plus 20 mL/kg for each kg >20

Carbohydrate (dextrose): 40% to 50% of caloric intake
<1 year: Initial: 6-8 mg/kg/minute; goal: 10-14 mg/kg/minute
1-10 years: Initial: 10% to 12.5%; daily increase: 5% increments (maximum: 15 mg/kg/minute)
>10 years: Initial: 10% to 15%; daily increase: 5% increments (maximum: 8.5 mg/kg/minute)

Protein (amino acids):
1-12 months: Initial: 2-3 g/kg/day; daily increase: 1 g/kg/day (maximum: 3 g/kg/day)
1-10 years: Initial: 1-2 g/kg/day; daily increase: 1 g/kg/day (maximum: 2-2.5 g/kg/day)
>10 years: Initial: 0.8-1.5 g/kg/day; daily increase: 1 g/kg/day (maximum: 1.5-2 g/kg/day)

Fat: Initial: 1 g/kg/day; daily increase: 1 g/kg/day (maximum: 3 g/kg/day); **Note:** Monitor triglycerides while receiving intralipids.

Adults: I.V.:

Total calories: Calculate using Harris-Benedict equation or based on stress level as indicated below:

Harris-Benedict Equation (BEE):
Females: 655.1 + [(9.56 x W) + (1.85 x H) - (4.68 x A)]
Males: 66.47 + [(13.75 x W) + (5 x H) - (6.76 x A)]
Then multiply BEE x (activity factor) x (stress factor)
W = weight in kg; H = height in cm; A = age in years
Activity factor = 1.2 sedentary, 1.3 normal activity, 1.4 active, 1.5 very active
Stress factor = 1.5 for trauma, stressed, or surgical patients and underweight (to promote weight gain); 2.0 for severe burn patients

Stress level:
Normal/mild stress level: 20-25 kcal/kg/day
Moderate stress level: 25-30 kcal/kg/day
Severe stress level: 30-40 kcal/kg/day
Pregnant women in second or third trimester: Add an additional 300 kcal/day

Fluid: mL/day = 30-40 mL/kg

Carbohydrate (dextrose):
5 g/kg/day or 3.5 mg/kg/minute (maximum rate: 4-7 mg/kg/minute)
Minimum recommended amount: 400 calories/day or 100 g/day

Protein (amino acids):
Maintenance: 0.8-1 g/kg/day
Normal/mild stress level: 1-1.2 g/kg/day
Moderate stress level: 1.2-1.5 g/kg/day
Severe stress level: 1.5-2 g/kg/day
Burn patients (severe): Increase protein until significant wound healing achieved
Solid organ transplant: Perioperative: 1.5-2 g/kg/day
Renal failure:
Acute (severely malnourished or hypercatabolic): 1.5-1.8 g/kg/day
Chronic, with dialysis: 1.2-1.3 g/kg/day
Chronic, without dialysis: 0.6-0.8 g/kg/day
Continuous hemofiltration: ≥1 g/kg/day
Hepatic failure:
Acute management when other treatments have failed:
With encephalopathy: 0.6-1 g/kg/day
Without encephalopathy: 1-1.5 g/kg/day
Chronic encephalopathy: Use branch chain amino acid enriched diets only if unresponsive to pharmacotherapy
Pregnant women in second or third trimester: Add an additional 10-14 g/day

Fat:
Initial: 20% to 40 % of total calories (maximum: 60% of total calories or 2.5 g/kg/day); **Note:** Monitor triglycerides while receiving intralipids.
Safe for use in pregnancy
I.V. lipids are safe in adults with pancreatitis if triglyceride levels <400 mg/dL

Additional Information Complete prescribing information for this medication should be consulted for additional detail.

Dosage Forms Excipient information presented when available (limited, particularly for generics); consult specific product labeling. TPN is usually compounded from optimal combinations of macronutrients (water, protein, dextrose, and lipids) and micronutrients (electrolytes, trace elements, and vitamins) to meet the specific nutritional requirements of a patient. Individual hospitals may have designated standard TPN formulas. There are a few commercially-available amino acids with electrolytes solutions; however, these products may not meet an individual's specific nutrition requirements.
See Fat Emulsion on page 605 monographs for additional information.

◆ **Totect™** *see* Dexrazoxane *on page* 430
◆ **Touro® CC** *see* Guaifenesin, Pseudoephedrine, and Dextromethorphan *on page* 715
◆ **Touro® CC-LD** *see* Guaifenesin, Pseudoephedrine, and Dextromethorphan *on page* 715
◆ **Touro® Allergy** *see* Brompheniramine and Pseudoephedrine *on page* 214
◆ **Touro® DM** *see* Guaifenesin and Dextromethorphan *on page* 710
◆ **Touro® HC [DSC]** *see* Hydrocodone and Guaifenesin *on page* 741
◆ **Touro LA®** *see* Guaifenesin and Pseudoephedrine *on page* 713
◆ **Toviaz™** *see* Fesoterodine *on page* 617
◆ **tPA** *see* Alteplase *on page* 72
◆ **TPN** *see* Total Parenteral Nutrition *on page* 1495
◆ **TPV** *see* Tipranavir *on page* 1477
◆ **tRA** *see* Tretinoin (Oral) *on page* 1508
◆ **Tracleer®** *see* Bosentan *on page* 206

◆ **Tramacet (Can)** *see* Acetaminophen and Tramadol *on page 30*

TraMADol (TRA ma dole)

U.S. Brand Names Ultram®; Ultram® ER

Canadian Brand Names Ralivia™ ER; Tridural™; Zytram® XL

Index Terms Tramadol Hydrochloride

Pharmacologic Category Analgesic, Opioid

Use Relief of moderate to moderately-severe pain

Pregnancy Risk Factor C

Pregnancy Considerations Adverse events were observed in animal studies. Tramadol has been shown to cross the human placenta when administered during labor. Postmarketing reports following tramadol use during pregnancy include neonatal seizures, withdrawal syndrome, fetal death, and stillbirth. Not recommended for use during labor and delivery.

Lactation Enters breast milk/not recommended

Medication Safety Issues

Sound-alike/look-alike issues:

TraMADol may be confused with Toradol®, Trandate®, traZODone, Voltaren®

Ultram® may be confused with Ultane®, Ultracet®, Voltaren®

International issues:

Theradol® [Netherlands] may be confused with Foradil® which is a brand name for formoterol in the U.S.

Theradol® [Netherlands] may be confused with Terazol® which is a brand name for terconazole in the U.S.

Theradol® [Netherlands] may be confused with Toradol® which is a brand name for ketorolac in the U.S.

Contraindications Hypersensitivity to tramadol, opioids, or any component of the formulation; opioid-dependent patients; acute intoxication with alcohol, hypnotics, centrally-acting analgesics, opioids, or psychotropic drugs

Note: Based on Canadian product labeling:

Tramadol is contraindicated during or within 14 days following MAO inhibitor therapy

Extended release formulations (Ralivia™ ER [CAN], Tridural™[CAN], and Zytram® XL [CAN]): Additional contraindications: Severe (Cl_{cr} <30 mL/minute) renal dysfunction, severe (Child-Pugh Class C) hepatic dysfunction

Warnings/Precautions Rare but serious anaphylactoid reactions (including fatalities) often following initial dosing have been reported. Pruritus, hives, bronchospasm, angioedema, toxic epidermal necrolysis (TEN) and Stevens-Johnson syndrome also have been reported with use. Previous anaphylactoid reactions to opioids may increase risks for similar reactions to tramadol. Caution patients to swallow tablets whole. Rapid release and absorption of tramadol from tablets that are broken, crushed, or chewed may lead to a potentially lethal overdose. May cause CNS depression, which may impair physical or mental abilities; patients must be cautioned about performing tasks which require mental alertness (eg, operating machinery or driving). May cause CNS depression and/or respiratory depression, particularly when combined with other CNS depressants. Use with caution and reduce dosage when administered to patients receiving other CNS depressants. An increased risk of seizures may occur in patients receiving serotonin reuptake inhibitors (SSRIs or anorectics), tricyclic antidepressants, other cyclic compounds (including cyclobenzaprine, promethazine), neuroleptics, or drugs which may lower seizure threshold. Patients with a history of seizures, or with a risk of seizures (head trauma, metabolic disorders, CNS infection, or malignancy, or during ethanol/drug withdrawal) are also at increased risk. Avoid use with serotonergic agents such as TCAs, MAO inhibitors (contraindicated in Canadian product labeling), triptans, venlafaxine, trazodone, lithium, sibutramine, meperidine, dextromethorphan, St John's wort, SNRIs and SSRIs; concomitant use has been associated with the development of serotonin syndrome.

Elderly (particularly >75 years of age), debilitated patients and patients with chronic respiratory disorders may be at greater risk of adverse events. Use with caution in patients with increased intracranial pressure or head injury. Avoid use in patients who are suicidal or addiction prone. Use caution in heavy alcohol users. Use caution in treatment of acute abdominal conditions; may mask pain. Use tramadol with caution and reduce dosage in patients with liver disease or renal dysfunction. Tolerance or drug dependence may result from extended use (withdrawal symptoms have been reported); abrupt discontinuation should be avoided. Tapering of dose at the time of discontinuation limits the risk of withdrawal symptoms. Safety and efficacy in pediatric patients have not been established.

Adverse Reactions

>10%:

Cardiovascular: Flushing (8% to 16%)

Central nervous system: Dizziness (16% to 33%), headache (12% to 32%), insomnia (7% to 11%), somnolence (7% to 25%)

Dermatologic: Pruritus (6% to 12%)

Gastrointestinal: Constipation (10% to 46%), nausea (15% to 40%), vomiting (5% to 17%), dyspepsia (1% to 13%)

Neuromuscular & skeletal: Weakness (4% to 12%)

1% to 10%:

Cardiovascular: Chest pain (1% to <5%), postural hypotension (2% to 5%), vasodilation (1% to <5%)

Central nervous system: Anxiety (1% to <5%), confusion (1% to <5%), coordination impaired (1% to <5%), depression (1% to <5%), euphoria (1% to <5%), hypoesthesia (1% to <5%), lethargy (1% to <5%), nervousness (1% to <5%), pain (1% to <5%), pyrexia (1% to <5%), restlessness (1% to <5%), malaise (<1% to <5%)

Dermatologic: Dermatitis (1% to <5%), rash (1% to <5%)

Endocrine & metabolic: Hot flashes (2% to 9%), menopausal symptoms (1% to <5%)

Gastrointestinal: Diarrhea (5% to 10%), xerostomia (5% to 10%), anorexia (1% to <6%), abdominal pain (1% to <5%), appetite decreased (1% to <5%), weight loss (1% to <5%), flatulence (<1% to <5%)

Genitourinary: Urinary tract infection (1% to <5%), urinary frequency (<1% to <5%), urinary retention (<1% to <5%)

Neuromuscular & skeletal: Arthralgia (1% to <5%), back pain (1% to <5%), hypertonia (1% to <5%), rigors (1% to <5%), paresthesia (1% to <5%), tremor (1% to <5%), creatinine phosphokinase increased (1% to <5%)

Ocular: Blurred vision (1% to <5%), miosis (1% to <5%)

Respiratory: Bronchitis (1% to <5%), congestion (nasal/sinus) (1% to <5%), cough (1% to <5%), dyspnea (1% to <5%), nasopharyngitis (1% to <5%), rhinorrhea (1% to <5%), sinusitis (1% to <5%), sneezing (1% to <5%), sore throat (1% to <5%), upper respiratory infection (1% to <5%)

Miscellaneous: Diaphoresis (2% to 9%), flu-like syndrome (1% to < 5%), shivering (<1% to <5%)

<1% (Limited to important or life-threatening): Abnormal ECG, abnormal gait, agitation, allergic reaction, amnesia, anaphylactoid reactions, anaphylaxis, angioedema, appendicitis, ALT increased, AST increased, bronchospasm, cataracts, cellulitis, cholecystitis, cholelithiasis, clamminess, cognitive dysfunction, concentration difficulty, creatinine increased, deafness, disorientation, dreams abnormal, dysuria, ear infection, edema, gastroenteritis, gastrointestinal bleeding, hallucination,

hematuria, hemoglobin decreased, hepatitis, hyperglycemia, hyper-/hypotension, irritability, joint stiffness, libido decreased, liver enzymes increased, liver failure, menstrual disorder, MI, migraine, muscle cramps, muscle spasms, muscle twitching, myalgia, myocardial ischemia, night sweats, palpitation, pancreatitis, peripheral edema, peripheral ischemia, pneumonia, proteinuria, pulmonary edema, pulmonary embolism, sedation, seizure, serotonin syndrome, sleep disorder, speech disorder, Stevens-Johnson syndrome, stomatitis, suicidal tendency, syncope, taste perversion, tachycardia, tinnitus, toxic epidermal necrolysis, urticaria, vertigo, vesicles

A withdrawal syndrome may occur with abrupt discontinuation; includes anxiety, diarrhea, hallucinations (rare), nausea, pain, piloerection, rigors, sweating, and tremor. Uncommon discontinuation symptoms may include severe anxiety, panic attacks, or paresthesia.

Drug Interactions

Metabolism/Transport Effects Substrate of CYP2D6 (major), 3A4 (major)

Avoid Concomitant Use

Avoid concomitant use of TraMADol with any of the following: Sibutramine

Increased Effect/Toxicity

TraMADol may increase the levels/effects of: Alcohol (Ethyl); CNS Depressants; MAO Inhibitors; Selective Serotonin Reuptake Inhibitors; Serotonin Modulators

The levels/effects of TraMADol may be increased by: CYP3A4 Inhibitors (Moderate); CYP3A4 Inhibitors (Strong); Dasatinib; Selective Serotonin Reuptake Inhibitors; Sibutramine; Tricyclic Antidepressants

Decreased Effect

The levels/effects of TraMADol may be decreased by: CYP2D6 Inhibitors (Moderate); CYP2D6 Inhibitors (Strong); CYP3A4 Inducers (Strong); Deferasirox; Herbs (CYP3A4 Inducers)

Ethanol/Nutrition/Herb Interactions

Ethanol: Avoid ethanol (may increase CNS depression).

Food:

Immediate release: Does not affect the rate or extent of absorption.

Extended release: Reduced C_{max} and AUC and T_{max} occurred 3 hours earlier when taken with a high-fat meal.

Herb/Nutraceutical: Avoid valerian, St John's wort, kava kava, gotu kola (may increase CNS depression).

Stability Store at controlled room temperature of 25°C (77°F).

Mechanism of Action Tramadol and active metabolite (M1) binds to μ-opiate receptors in the CNS causing inhibition of ascending pain pathways, altering the perception of and response to pain; also inhibits the reuptake of norepinephrine and serotonin, which also modifies the ascending pain pathway

Pharmacodynamics/Kinetics

Onset of action: Immediate release: ~1 hour

Duration: 9 hours

Absorption: Immediate release formulation: Rapid and complete; Extended release formulation: Delayed

Distribution: V_d: 2.5-3 L/kg

Protein binding, plasma: 20%

Metabolism: Extensively hepatic via demethylation, glucuronidation, and sulfation; has pharmacologically active metabolite formed by CYP2D6 (M1; O-desmethyl tramadol)

Bioavailability: Immediate release: 75%; Extended release: Ultram® ER: 85% to 90% (as compared to immediate release), Zytram® XL, Tridural™: 70%

Half-life elimination: Tramadol: ~6-8 hours; Active metabolite: 7-9 hours; prolonged in elderly, hepatic or renal impairment; Zytram® XL: ~16 hours; Ralivia™ ER, Tridural™: ~5-9 hours

Time to peak: Immediate release: ~2 hours; Extended release: Ultram® ER: ~12 hours, Tridural™: ~4 hours

Excretion: Urine (30% as unchanged drug; 60% as metabolites)

Dosage Moderate-to-severe chronic pain: Oral:

Adults:

Immediate release formulation: 50-100 mg every 4-6 hours (not to exceed 400 mg/day)

For patients not requiring rapid onset of effect, tolerability may be improved by starting dose at 25 mg/day and titrating dose by 25 mg every 3 days, until reaching 25 mg 4 times/day. The total daily dose may then be increased by 50 mg every 3 days as tolerated, to reach dose of 50 mg 4 times/day. After titration, 50-100 mg may be given every 4-6 hours as needed up to a maximum 400 mg/day.

Extended release formulations:

Ultram® ER: Patients not currently on immediate-release: 100 mg once daily; titrate every 5 days (maximum: 300 mg/day); Patients currently on immediate-release: Calculate 24-hour immediate release total and initiate total daily dose (round dose to the next lowest 100 mg increment); titrate (maximum: 300 mg/day)

Ralivia™ ER (Canadian labeling, not available in U.S.): 100 mg once daily; titrate every 5 days as needed based on clinical response and severity of pain (maximum: 300 mg/day)

Tridural™ (Canadian labeling, not available in U.S.): 100 mg once daily; titrate by 100 mg/day every 2 days as needed based on clinical response and severity of pain (maximum: 300 mg/day)

Zytram® XL (Canadian labeling, not available in U.S.): 150 mg once daily; if pain relief is not achieved may titrate by increasing dosage incrementally, with sufficient time to evaluate effect of increased dosage; generally not more often than every 7 days (maximum: 400 mg/day)

Elderly >75 years:

Immediate release: 50 mg every 6 hours (not to exceed 300 mg/day); see dosing adjustments for renal and hepatic impairment.

Extended release formulation: Use with great caution. See adult dosing.

Dosing adjustment in renal impairment:

Immediate release: Cl_{cr} <30 mL/minute: Administer 50-100 mg dose every 12 hours (maximum: 200 mg/day)

Extended release: Should not be used in patients with Cl_{cr} <30 mL/minute

Dosing adjustment in hepatic impairment:

Immediate release: Cirrhosis: Recommended dose: 50 mg every 12 hours

Extended release: Should not be used in patients with severe (Child-Pugh Class C) hepatic dysfunction

Dietary Considerations May be taken with or without food. Extended release formulation: Be consistent; always give with food or always give on an empty stomach.

Administration Extended release tablet: Swallow whole; do not crush, chew, or split

Monitoring Parameters Pain relief, respiratory rate, blood pressure, and pulse; signs of tolerance or abuse

Reference Range 100-300 ng/mL; however, serum level monitoring is not required

Dosage Forms Excipient information presented when available (limited, particularly for generics); consult specific product labeling. [CAN] = Canadian brand name

Tablet, as hydrochloride: 50 mg

Ultram®: 50 mg

Tablet, extended release, as hydrochloride:

Ultram® ER: 100 mg, 200 mg, 300 mg

Ralivia™ ER [CAN]: 100 mg, 200 mg, 300 mg [not available in the U.S.]

Tridural™ [CAN]: 100 mg, 200 mg, 300 mg [not available in the U.S.]

Zytram® XL [CAN]: 150 mg, 200 mg, 300 mg, 400 mg [not available in the U.S.]

◆ **Tramadol Hydrochloride** *see* TraMADol *on page 1497*

◆ **Tramadol Hydrochloride and Acetaminophen** *see* Acetaminophen and Tramadol *on page 30*

◆ **Trandate®** *see* Labetalol *on page 845*

Trandolapril (tran DOE la pril)

U.S. Brand Names Mavik®

Canadian Brand Names Mavik™

Pharmacologic Category Angiotensin-Converting Enzyme (ACE) Inhibitor

Additional Appendix Information

Angiotensin Agents *on page 1632*

Heart Failure (Systolic) *on page 1809*

Use Treatment of hypertension alone or in combination with other antihypertensive agents; treatment of heart failure or left ventricular dysfunction after myocardial infarction

Unlabeled/Investigational Use As a class, ACE inhibitors are recommended in the treatment of heart failure; to delay the progression of nephropathy and reduce risks of cardiovascular events in hypertensive patients with type 1 or 2 diabetes mellitus

Pregnancy Risk Factor C (1st trimester); D (2nd and 3rd trimesters)

Pregnancy Considerations Due to adverse events observed in some animal studies, trandolapril is considered pregnancy category C during the first trimester. Based on human data, trandolapril is considered pregnancy category D if used during the second and third trimesters (per the manufacturer; however, one study suggests that fetal injury may occur at anytime during pregnancy). First trimester exposure to ACE inhibitors may cause major congenital malformations. An increased risk of cardiovascular and/or central nervous system malformations was observed in one study; however, an increased risk of teratogenic events was not observed in other studies. Second and third trimester use of an ACE inhibitor is associated with oligohydramnios. Oligohydramnios due to decreased fetal renal function may lead to fetal limb contractures, craniofacial deformation, and hypoplastic lung development. The use of ACE inhibitors during the second and third trimesters is also associated with anuria, hypotension, renal failure (reversible or irreversible), skull hypoplasia, and death in the fetus/neonate. Chronic maternal hypertension itself is also associated with adverse events in the fetus/infant. ACE inhibitors are not recommended during pregnancy to treat maternal hypertension or heart failure. Those who are planning a pregnancy should be considered for other medication options if an ACE inhibitor is currently prescribed or the ACE inhibitor should be discontinued as soon as possible once pregnancy is detected. The exposed fetus should be monitored for fetal growth, amniotic fluid volume, and organ formation. Infants exposed to an ACE inhibitor *in utero*, especially during the second and third trimester, should be monitored for hyperkalemia, hypotension, and oliguria.

[U.S. Boxed Warning]: Based on human data, ACE inhibitors can cause injury and death to the developing fetus when used in the second and third trimesters. ACE inhibitors should be discontinued as soon as possible once pregnancy is detected.

Lactation Excretion in breast milk unknown/not recommended

Contraindications Hypersensitivity to trandolapril or any component of the formulation; history of angioedema related to previous treatment with an ACE inhibitor

Warnings/Precautions Anaphylactic reactions may occur rarely with ACE inhibitors. At any time during treatment (especially following first dose) angioedema may occur rarely with ACE inhibitors; it may involve the head and neck (potentially compromising the airway) or the intestine (presenting with abdominal pain). African-Americans and patients with idiopathic or hereditary angioedema may be at an increased risk. Prolonged frequent monitoring may be required especially if tongue, glottis, or larynx are involved as they are associated with airway obstruction. Patients with a history of airway surgery may have a higher risk of airway obstruction. Aggressive early and appropriate management is critical. Use in patients with previous angioedema associated with ACE inhibitor therapy is contraindicated. Severe anaphylactoid reactions may be seen during hemodialysis (eg, CVVHD) with high-flux dialysis membranes (eg, AN69). Rare cases of anaphylactoid reactions have been reported in patients undergoing sensitization treatment with hymenoptera (bee, wasp) venom while receiving ACE inhibitors.

Symptomatic hypotension with or without syncope can occur with ACE inhibitors (usually with the first several doses); effects are most often observed in volume-depleted patients; correct volume depletion prior to initiation; close monitoring of patient is required especially with initial dosing and dosing increases; blood pressure must be lowered at a rate appropriate for the patient's clinical condition. Initiation of therapy in patients with ischemic heart disease or cerebrovascular disease warrants close observation due to the potential consequences posed by falling blood pressure (eg, MI, stroke). Use with caution in hypertrophic cardiomyopathy with outflow tract obstruction, severe aortic stenosis, or before, during, or immediately after major surgery. **[U.S. Boxed Warning]: Based on human data, ACEIs can cause injury and death to the developing fetus when used in the second and third trimesters. ACEIs should be discontinued as soon as possible once pregnancy is detected.**

Hyperkalemia may occur with ACE inhibitors; risk factors include renal dysfunction, diabetes mellitus, concomitant use of potassium-sparing diuretics, potassium supplements, and/or potassium-containing salts. Use cautiously, if at all, with these agents and monitor potassium closely. Cough may occur with ACE inhibitors. Other causes of cough should be considered (eg, pulmonary congestion in patients with heart failure) and excluded prior to discontinuation.

Dosage adjustment needed in severe renal dysfunction (Cl_{cr}<30 mL/minute) or hepatic cirrhosis. May be associated with deterioration of renal function and/or increases in serum creatinine, particularly in patients with low renal blood flow (eg, renal artery stenosis, heart failure) whose glomerular filtration rate (GFR) is dependent on efferent arteriolar vasoconstriction by angiotensin II; deterioration may result in oliguria, acute renal failure, and progressive azotemia. Small increases in serum creatinine may occur following initiation; consider discontinuation only in patients with progressive and/or significant deterioration in renal function. Use with caution in patients with unstented unilateral/bilateral renal artery stenosis. When unstented bilateral renal artery stenosis is present, use is generally avoided due to the elevated risk of deterioration in renal function unless possible benefits outweigh risks.

Rare toxicities associated with ACE inhibitors include cholestatic jaundice (which may progress to fulminant hepatic necrosis), agranulocytosis, neutropenia, or leukopenia with myeloid hypoplasia. Patients with collagen vascular diseases (especially with concomitant renal impairment) or renal impairment alone may be at increased risk for hematologic toxicity; periodically monitor CBC with differential in these patients. Safety and efficacy have not been established in children.

Adverse Reactions Note: Frequency ranges include data from hypertension and heart failure trials. Higher rates of adverse reactions have generally been noted in patients with CHF. However, the frequency of adverse effects associated with placebo is also increased in this population.

>1%:

Cardiovascular: Hypotension (<1% to 11%), bradycardia (<1% to 4.7%), intermittent claudication (3.8%), stroke (3.3%), syncope (5.9%)

Central nervous system: Dizziness (1.3% to 23%), asthenia (3.3%)

Endocrine & metabolic: Elevated uric acid (15%), hyperkalemia (5.3%), hypocalcemia (4.7%)

Gastrointestinal: Dyspepsia (6.4%), gastritis (4.2%)

Neuromuscular & skeletal: Myalgia (4.7%)

Renal: Elevated BUN (9%), elevated serum creatinine (1.1% to 4.7%)

Respiratory: Cough (1.9% to 35%)

<1% (Limited to important or life-threatening): Angina, angioedema, anxiety, AV block (first-degree), dyspnea, gout, impotence, increased ALT, increased serum creatinine, insomnia, laryngeal edema, muscle pain, neutropenia, pancreatitis, paresthesia, pruritus, rash, symptomatic hypotension, thrombocytopenia, vertigo. Worsening of renal function may occur in patients with bilateral renal artery stenosis or in hypovolemic patients. In addition, a syndrome which may include fever, myalgia, arthralgia, interstitial nephritis, vasculitis, rash, eosinophilia and positive ANA, and elevated ESR has been reported with ACE inhibitors.

Drug Interactions

Avoid Concomitant Use There are no known interactions where it is recommended to avoid concomitant use.

Increased Effect/Toxicity

Trandolapril may increase the levels/effects of: Allopurinol; Amifostine; AzaTHIOprine; CycloSPORINE; Ferric Gluconate; Gold Sodium Thiomalate; Lithium; RiTUXimab

The levels/effects of Trandolapril may be increased by: Angiotensin II Receptor Blockers; Diazoxide; Eplerenone; Herbs (Hypotensive Properties); Loop Diuretics; Potassium Salts; Potassium-Sparing Diuretics; Prostacyclin Analogues; Sirolimus; Temsirolimus; Thiazide Diuretics; Trimethoprim

Decreased Effect

The levels/effects of Trandolapril may be decreased by: Antacids; Aprotinin; Herbs (Hypertensive Properties); Methylphenidate; Nonsteroidal Anti-Inflammatory Agents; Salicylates; Yohimbine

Ethanol/Nutrition/Herb Interactions Herb/Nutraceutical: Avoid bayberry, blue cohosh, cayenne, ephedra, ginger, ginseng (American), kola, licorice (may worsen hypertension). Avoid black cohosh, California poppy, coleus, golden seal, hawthorn, mistletoe, periwinkle, quinine, shepherd's purse (may have increased antihypertensive effect).

Mechanism of Action Trandolapril is an ACE inhibitor which prevents the formation of angiotensin II from angiotensin I. Trandolapril must undergo enzymatic hydrolysis, mainly in liver, to its biologically active metabolite, trandolaprilat. A CNS mechanism may also be involved in the hypotensive effect as angiotensin II increases adrenergic outflow from the CNS. Vasoactive kallikrein's may be decreased in conversion to active hormones by ACE inhibitors, thus reducing blood pressure.

Pharmacodynamics/Kinetics

Onset of action: 1-2 hours

Peak effect: Reduction in blood pressure: 6 hours

Duration: Prolonged; 72 hours after single dose

Absorption: Rapid

Distribution:

Trandolapril: ~18L

Trandolaprilat (active metabolite) is very lipophilic in comparison to other ACE inhibitors

Protein binding: 80%

Metabolism: Hepatically hydrolyzed to active metabolite, trandolaprilat

Bioavailability:

Trandolapril: 10%

Trandolaprilat: 70%

Half-life elimination:

Trandolapril: 6 hours; Trandolaprilat: Effective: 10 hours, Terminal: 24 hours

Time to peak: Parent: 1 hour; Active metabolite trandolaprilat: 4-10 hours

Excretion: Urine (33%); feces (66%)

Clearance: Reduce dose in renal failure; creatinine clearances ≤30 mL/minute result in accumulation of active metabolite

Dosage Adults: Oral:

Hypertension: Initial dose in patients not receiving a diuretic: 1 mg/day (2 mg/day in black patients). Adjust dosage according to the blood pressure response. Make dosage adjustments at intervals of ≥1 week. Most patients have required dosages of 2-4 mg/day. There is a little experience with doses >8 mg/day. Patients inadequately treated with once daily dosing at 4 mg may be treated with twice daily dosing. If blood pressure is not adequately controlled with trandolapril monotherapy, a diuretic may be added.

Usual dose range (JNC 7): 1-4 mg once daily

Heart failure postmyocardial infarction or left ventricular dysfunction postmyocardial infarction: Initial: 1 mg/day; titrate patients (as tolerated) towards the target dose of 4 mg/day. If a 4 mg dose is not tolerated, patients can continue therapy with the greatest tolerated dose.

Dosing adjustment in renal impairment: Cl_{cr} ≤30 mL/minute: Recommended starting dose: 0.5 mg/day.

Dosing adjustment in hepatic impairment: Cirrhosis: Recommended starting dose: 0.5 mg/day.

Monitoring Parameters Blood pressure; serum creatinine and potassium; if patient has collagen vascular disease and/or renal impairment, periodically monitor CBC with differential

Dosage Forms Excipient information presented when available (limited, particularly for generics); consult specific product labeling.

Tablet: 1 mg, 2 mg, 4 mg

Mavik®: 1 mg, 2 mg, 4 mg

Trandolapril and Verapamil

(tran DOE la pril & ver AP a mil)

U.S. Brand Names Tarka®

Canadian Brand Names Tarka®

Index Terms Verapamil and Trandolapril

Pharmacologic Category Angiotensin-Converting Enzyme (ACE) Inhibitor; Calcium Channel Blocker

Use Treatment of hypertension; however, not indicated for initial treatment of hypertension

Pregnancy Risk Factor C/D (2nd and 3rd trimesters)

Dosage Dose is individualized

Additional Information Complete prescribing information for this medication should be consulted for additional detail.

Dosage Forms Excipient information presented when available (limited, particularly for generics); consult specific product labeling.

Tablet, variable release:

1/240: Trandolapril 1 mg [immediate release] and verapamil hydrochloride 240 mg [sustained release]

2/180: Trandolapril 2 mg [immediate release] and verapamil hydrochloride 180 mg [sustained release]

2/240: Trandolapril 2 mg [immediate release] and verapamil hydrochloride 240 mg [sustained release]

4/240: Trandolapril 4 mg [immediate release] and verapamil hydrochloride 240 mg [sustained release]

Tranexamic Acid (tran eks AM ik AS id)

U.S. Brand Names Cyklokapron®

Canadian Brand Names Cyklokapron®; Tranexamic Acid Injection BP

Pharmacologic Category Antihemophilic Agent

Use Short-term use (2-8 days) in hemophilia patients during and following tooth extraction to reduce or prevent hemorrhage

Unlabeled/Investigational Use Has been used as an alternative to aminocaproic acid for subarachnoid hemorrhage

Pregnancy Risk Factor B

Medication Safety Issues

Sound-alike/look-alike issues:

Cyklokapron® may be confused with cycloSPORINE

Dosage Children and Adults: I.V.: 10 mg/kg immediately before surgery, then 25 mg/kg/dose orally 3-4 times/day for 2-8 days

Alternatively:

Oral: 25 mg/kg 3-4 times/day beginning 1 day prior to surgery

I.V.: 10 mg/kg 3-4 times/day in patients who are unable to take oral

Dosing adjustment/interval in renal impairment:

Cl_{cr} 50-80 mL/minute: Administer 50% of normal dose or 10 mg/kg twice daily I.V. or 15 mg/kg twice daily orally

Cl_{cr} 10-50 mL/minute: Administer 25% of normal dose or 10 mg/kg/day I.V. or 15 mg/kg/day orally

Cl_{cr} <10 mL/minute: Administer 10% of normal dose or 10 mg/kg/dose every 48 hours I.V. or 15 mg/kg/dose every 48 hours orally

Additional Information Complete prescribing information for this medication should be consulted for additional detail.

Dosage Forms Excipient information presented when available (limited, particularly for generics); consult specific product labeling.

Injection, solution: 100 mg/mL (10 mL)

Tablet: 500 mg [Not marketed in U.S.; available from manufacturer for select cases]

◆ **Tranexamic Acid Injection BP (Can)** *see* Tranexamic Acid *on page* 1501

◆ **Transamine Sulphate** *see* Tranylcypromine *on page* 1501

◆ **Transderm-V® (Can)** *see* Scopolamine Derivatives *on page* 1356

◆ **Transderm-Nitro® (Can)** *see* Nitroglycerin *on page* 1073

◆ **Transderm Scōp®** *see* Scopolamine Derivatives *on page* 1356

◆ ***trans*-Retinoic Acid** *see* Tretinoin (Oral) *on page* 1508

◆ ***trans*-Retinoic Acid** *see* Tretinoin (Topical) *on page* 1509

◆ **Tranxene® SD™** *see* Clorazepate *on page* 358

◆ **Tranxene® SD™-Half Strength** *see* Clorazepate *on page* 358

◆ **Tranxene T-Tab®** *see* Clorazepate *on page* 358

◆ **Tranxene® T-Tab®** *see* Clorazepate *on page* 358

Tranylcypromine (tran il SIP roe meen)

U.S. Brand Names Parnate®

Canadian Brand Names Parnate®

Index Terms Transamine Sulphate; Tranylcypromine Sulfate

Pharmacologic Category Antidepressant, Monoamine Oxidase Inhibitor

Additional Appendix Information

Antidepressant Agents *on page* 1638

Tyramine Content of Foods *on page* 1850

Use Treatment of major depressive episode without melancholia

Unlabeled/Investigational Use Post-traumatic stress disorder

Restrictions An FDA-approved medication guide concerning the use of antidepressants in children, adolescents, and young adults must be distributed when dispensing an outpatient prescription (new or refill) where this medication is to be used without direct supervision of a healthcare provider. Medication guides are available at http://www.fda.gov/cder/Offices/ODS/medication_guides.htm. Dispense to parents or guardians of children and adolescents receiving this medication.

Pregnancy Risk Factor C

Lactation Enters breast milk/not recommended

Contraindications Hypersensitivity to tranylcypromine, other MAO inhibitors, dibenzazepine derivatives, or any component of the formulation; cardiovascular disease; cerebrovascular defect; headache history; hepatic disease; hypertension; pheochromocytoma; renal disease; concurrent use of antihistamines, antiparkinson drugs, antihypertensives, bupropion, buspirone, CNS depressants, dexfenfluramine, dextromethorphan, diuretics, ethanol, meperidine, and SSRIs; general anesthesia (discontinue 10 days prior to elective surgery); local vasoconstrictors; spinal anesthesia (hypotension may be exaggerated); sympathomimetics (and related compounds); foods high in tyramine content; supplements containing tyrosine, phenylalanine, tryptophan, or caffeine

Warnings/Precautions Risk of suicide: [U.S. Boxed Warning]: Antidepressants increase the risk of suicidal thinking and behavior in children, adolescents, and young adults (18-24 years of age) with major depressive disorder (MDD) and other psychiatric disorders; consider risk prior to prescribing. Short-term studies did not show an increased risk in patients >24 years of age and showed a decreased risk inpatients >65 years. Closely monitor for clinical worsening, suicidality, or unusual changes in behavior such as anxiety, agitation, panic attacks, insomnia, irritability, hostility, impulsivity, akathisia, hypomania, and mania. The patient's family or caregiver should be instructed to closely observe the patient and communicate condition with healthcare provider. Such observation would generally include at least weekly face-to-face contact with patients or their family members or caregivers during the first 4 weeks of treatment, then every other week visits for the next 4 weeks, then at 12 weeks, and as clinically indicated beyond 12 weeks. Additional contact by telephone may be appropriate between face-to-face visits. A medication guide should be dispensed with each prescription. **Tranylcypromine is not FDA approved for treatment of children and adolescents.**

All patients treated with antidepressants should be observed similarly for clinical worsening and suicidality, especially during the initial few months of a course of drug therapy, or at times of dose changes, either increases or decreases. The possibility of a suicide attempt is inherent in major depression and may persist until remission occurs. Worsening depression and severe abrupt suicidality that are not part of the presenting symptoms may require discontinuation or modification of drug therapy. Use caution in high-risk patients during initiation of therapy. Prescriptions should be written for the smallest quantity consistent with good patient care.

Hypertensive crisis may occur with foods/supplements high in tyramine, tryptophan, phenylalanine, or tyrosine content; treatment with phentolamine is recommended for hypertensive crisis. Use with caution in patients who have glaucoma, hyperthyroidism, diabetes or hypotension. May cause orthostatic hypotension (especially at dosages >30 mg/day). Use with caution in patients at risk of seizures, or in patients receiving other drugs which may lower seizure threshold. Discontinue at least 48 hours prior to myelography. May increase the risks associated with electroconvulsive therapy. Consider discontinuing, when possible, prior to elective surgery. Use with caution in patients with renal impairment. Do not use with other MAO inhibitors or antidepressants. Avoid products containing sympathomimetic stimulants or dextromethorphan. Concurrent use with antihypertensive agents may lead to exaggeration of hypotensive effects. May worsen psychosis in some patients or precipitate a shift to mania or hypomania in patients with bipolar disorder. **Tranylcypromine is not FDA approved for the treatment of bipolar depression.**

Elderly patients: Interactions with tyramine or tryptophan-containing foods and orthostasis have limited tranylcypromine's use.

Adverse Reactions Frequency not defined.

Cardiovascular: Edema, orthostatic hypotension, palpitation, tachycardia

Central nervous system: Agitation, akinesia, anxiety, ataxia, chills, confusion, disorientation, dizziness, drowsiness, fatigue, headache, hyper-reflexia, insomnia, mania, memory loss, restlessness, sleep disturbances, twitching

Dermatologic: Alopecia, cystic acne (flare), pruritus, rash, urticaria, scleroderma (localized)

Endocrine & metabolic: Hypernatremia, hypermetabolic syndrome; sexual dysfunction (anorgasmia, ejaculatory disturbances, impotence); SIADH

Gastrointestinal: Abdominal pain, anorexia, constipation, diarrhea, nausea, vomiting, weight gain, xerostomia

Genitourinary: Incontinence, urinary retention

Hematologic: Agranulocytosis, anemia, leukopenia, thrombocytopenia

Hepatic: Hepatitis

Neuromuscular & skeletal: Akinesis, muscle spasm, myoclonus, numbness, paresthesia, tremor, weakness

Ocular: Blurred vision, glaucoma

Otic: Tinnitus

Miscellaneous: Diaphoresis

Drug Interactions

Metabolism/Transport Effects Inhibits CYP1A2 (moderate), 2A6 (strong), 2C8 (weak), 2C9 (weak), 2C19 (moderate), 2D6 (moderate), 2E1 (weak), 3A4 (weak)

Avoid Concomitant Use

Avoid concomitant use of Tranylcypromine with any of the following: Alpha-/Beta-Agonists (Indirect-Acting); Alpha1-Agonists; Alpha2-Agonists (Ophthalmic); Amphetamines; Atomoxetine; BuPROPion; BusPIRone; Cyclobenzaprine; Dexmethylphenidate; Dextromethorphan; Linezolid; Maprotiline; Meperidine; Methyldopa; Methylphenidate; Mirtazapine; Propoxyphene; Selective Serotonin Reuptake Inhibitors; Serotonin 5-HT1D Receptor Agonists; Serotonin/Norepinephrine Reuptake Inhibitors; Sibutramine; Tetrabenazine; Thioridazine; Tricyclic Antidepressants

Increased Effect/Toxicity

Tranylcypromine may increase the levels/effects of: Alcohol (Ethyl); Alpha-/Beta-Agonists (Direct-Acting); Alpha-/Beta-Agonists (Indirect-Acting); Alpha1-Agonists; Alpha2-Agonists (Ophthalmic); Amphetamines; Anticholinergics; Atomoxetine; Beta2-Agonists; BuPROPion; CNS Depressants; CYP1A2 Substrates; CYP2A6 Substrates; CYP2C19 Substrates; CYP2D6 Substrates; Dexmethylphenidate; Dextromethorphan; Fesoterodine; Linezolid; Lithium; Meperidine; Methyldopa; Methylphenidate; Mirtazapine; Nebivolol; Rauwolfia Alkaloids; Selective Serotonin Reuptake Inhibitors; Serotonin 5-HT1D Receptor Agonists; Serotonin Modulators; Serotonin/Norepinephrine Reuptake Inhibitors; Tamoxifen; Thioridazine; Tricyclic Antidepressants

The levels/effects of Tranylcypromine may be increased by: Altretamine; Anilidopiperidine Opioids; BusPIRone; COMT Inhibitors; Cyclobenzaprine; Levodopa; Maprotiline; Pramlintide; Propoxyphene; Sibutramine; Tetrabenazine; TraMADol

Decreased Effect

Tranylcypromine may decrease the levels/effects of: Acetylcholinesterase Inhibitors (Central); Codeine

The levels/effects of Tranylcypromine may be decreased by: Acetylcholinesterase Inhibitors (Central)

Ethanol/Nutrition/Herb Interactions

Ethanol: Avoid ethanol (based on CNS depressant effects and potential tyramine content)

Food: Concurrent ingestion of foods rich in tyramine may cause sudden and severe high blood pressure (hypertensive crisis). Avoid tyramine-containing foods with MAO-Is. Food's freshness is also an important concern; improperly stored or spoiled food can create an environment where tyramine concentrations may increase.

Herb/Nutraceuticals: Avoid valerian, St John's wort, SAMe. Avoid supplements containing caffeine, gingko, yohimbime, ephedra, tyrosine, tryptophan or phenylalanine. Ingestion of large quantities may increase the risk of severe side effects (eg, hypertensive reactions, serotonin syndrome).

Mechanism of Action Tranylcypromine is a nonhydrazine monoamine oxidase inhibitor. It increases endogenous concentrations of epinephrine, norepinephrine, dopamine, and serotonin through inhibition of the enzyme (monoamine oxidase) responsible for the breakdown of these neurotransmitters.

Pharmacodynamics/Kinetics

Onset of action: Therapeutic: 2 days to 3 weeks continued dosing

Half-life elimination: 90-190 minutes

Time to peak, serum: ~2 hours

Excretion: Urine

Dosage Adults: Oral: 10 mg twice daily, increase by 10 mg increments at 1- to 3-week intervals; maximum: 60 mg/day; usual effective dose: 30 mg/day

Dietary Considerations Avoid foods containing tryptophan and caffeine. Avoid tyramine-containing foods/beverages. Some examples include aged or matured cheese, air-dried or cured meats (including sausages and salamis), fava or broad bean pods, tap/draft beers, Marmite concentrate, sauerkraut, soy sauce and other soybean condiments.

Monitoring Parameters Blood pressure, mental status, suicidal ideation (especially at the beginning of therapy or when doses are increased or decreased)

Additional Information Tranylcypromine has a more rapid onset of therapeutic effect than other MAO inhibitors, but causes more severe hypertensive reactions.

Dosage Forms Excipient information presented when available (limited, particularly for generics); consult specific product labeling.

Tablet: 10 mg

◆ **Tranylcypromine Sulfate** *see* Tranylcypromine *on page 1501*

Trastuzumab (tras TU zoo mab)

U.S. Brand Names Herceptin®

Canadian Brand Names Herceptin®

Index Terms NSC-688097

Pharmacologic Category Antineoplastic Agent, Monoclonal Antibody; Monoclonal Antibody

Use Adjuvant treatment of HER-2 overexpressing breast cancer; treatment of HER-2 overexpressing metastatic breast cancer

Pregnancy Risk Factor D

Pregnancy Considerations Reproductive studies in cynomolgus monkeys showed no evidence of impaired fertility or fetal harm. Trastuzumab inhibits HER2 protein, which has a role in embryonic development. Anhydramnios and oligohydramnios (reversible in some cases) have been reported with use during the second and third trimester of pregnancy. There are no adequate and well-controlled studies in pregnant women. Effective contraception is recommended during and for 6 months after treatment for women of childbearing potential. If used during pregnancy, monitor for oligohydramnios. Women exposed to trastuzumab during pregnancy are encouraged to enroll in the Cancer and Childbirth Registry (1-800-690-6720).

The National Comprehensive Cancer Network (NCCN) breast cancer guidelines (v2.2008) recommend administering trastuzumab in the postpartum period (if trastuzumab is indicated).

Lactation Excretion in breast milk unknown/not recommended

Medication Safety Issues

High alert medication: The Institute for Safe Medication Practices (ISMP) includes this medication among its list of drug classes which have a heightened risk of causing significant patient harm when used in error.

Contraindications There are no contraindications listed within the manufacturer's labeling.

Warnings/Precautions Hazardous agent - use appropriate precautions for handling and disposal. **[U.S. Boxed Warning]: Trastuzumab is associated with symptomatic and asymptomatic reductions in left ventricular ejection fraction (LVEF) and severe heart failure (HF) and may result in mural thrombus formation and stroke, and even cardiac death; discontinue for cardiomyopathy.** Evaluate LVEF in all patients prior to and during treatments. Extreme caution should be used in patients with pre-existing cardiac disease or dysfunction. Concomitant administration of anthracyclines and prior exposure to anthracyclines or radiation therapy significantly increases the risk of cardiomyopathy; other potential risk factors include advanced age, high or low body mass index, smoking, diabetes, and hyper/hypothyroidism. Discontinuation should be strongly considered in patients who develop a clinically significant reduction in LVEF during therapy; treatment with HF medications (eg, ACE inhibitors, beta-blockers) should be initiated. Cardiomyopathy due to trastuzumab is generally reversible over a period of 1-3 months after discontinuation. (When LVEF returns to baseline, reinitiation may be considered if indicated.) Trastuzumab is also associated with arrhythmias and hypertension.

[U.S. Boxed Warning]: Serious adverse events, including hypersensitivity reaction (anaphylaxis), infusion reactions (including fatalities), and pulmonary events (including acute respiratory distress syndrome [ARDS]) have been associated with trastuzumab. Discontinue for anaphylaxis, angioedema, ARDS or interstitial pneumonitis. Most of these events occur with the first infusion; pulmonary events may occur during or within 24 hours of the first infusion; delayed reactions have occurred. Interrupt infusion for dyspnea or significant hypotension. Retreatment of patients who experienced severe hypersensitivity reactions has been attempted (with premedication). Some patients tolerated retreatment, while others experienced a second severe reaction. When used in combination with myelosuppressive chemotherapy, trastuzumab may increase the incidence of neutropenia (moderate-to-severe) and febrile neutropenia. May cause serious pulmonary toxicity (dyspnea, hypoxia, interstitial pneumonitis, pulmonary infiltrates, pleural effusion, non-cardiogenic pulmonary edema, pulmonary insufficiency, acute respiratory distress syndrome, and/or pulmonary fibrosis); use caution in patients with pre-existing pulmonary disease or patients with extensive pulmonary tumor involvement. Safety and efficacy in children have not been established.

Adverse Reactions Note: Percentages reported with single-agent therapy.

>10%:

Cardiovascular: LVEF decreased (4% to 22%)

Central nervous system: Pain (47%), fever (6% to 36%), chills (5% to 32%), headache (10% to 26%), insomnia (14%), dizziness (4% to 13%)

Dermatologic: Rash (4% to 18%)

Gastrointestinal: Nausea (6% to 33%), diarrhea (7% to 25%), vomiting (4% to 23%), abdominal pain (2% to 22%), anorexia (14%)

Neuromuscular & skeletal: Weakness (4% to 42%), back pain (5% to 22%)

Respiratory: Cough (5% to 26%), dyspnea (3% to 22%), rhinitis (2% to 14%), pharyngitis (12%)

Miscellaneous: Infusion reaction (21% to 40%, chills and fever most common; severe: 1%), infection (20%)

1% to 10%:

Cardiovascular: Peripheral edema (5% to 10%), edema (8%), CHF (2% to 7%; severe: <1%), tachycardia (5%), hypertension (4%), arrhythmia (3%), palpitation (3%)

Central nervous system: Depression (6%)

Dermatologic: Acne (2%), nail disorder (2%), pruritus (2%)

Gastrointestinal: Constipation (2%), dyspepsia (2%)

Genitourinary: Urinary tract infection (3% to 5%)

Hematologic: Anemia (4%), leukopenia (3%)

Neuromuscular & skeletal: Paresthesia (2% to 9%), bone pain (3% to 7%), arthralgia (6% to 8%), myalgia (4%), muscle spasm (3%), peripheral neuritis (2%), neuropathy (1%)

Respiratory: Sinusitis (2% to 9%), nasopharyngitis (8%), upper respiratory infection (3%), epistaxis (2%), pharyngolaryngeal pain (2%)

Miscellaneous: Flu-like syndrome (2% to 10%), accidental injury (6%), influenza (4%), allergic reaction (3%), herpes simplex (2%)

<1% (Limited to important or life-threatening): Acute respiratory distress syndrome (ARDS), amblyopia, anaphylaxis, anaphylactoid reaction, angioedema, apnea, ascites, asthma, ataxia, bone necrosis, bronchospasm, cardiac arrest, cardiomyopathy, cellulitis, coagulopathy, colitis, confusion, deafness, esophageal ulcer, gastroenteritis, glomerulonephritis (membraneous, focal and fibrillary), glomerulopathy, glomerulosclerosis, hematemesis, hemorrhage, hemorrhagic cystitis, hepatic failure, hepatitis, herpes zoster, hydrocephalus, hydronephrosis, hypercalcemia, hypersensitivity, hypotension, hypothyroidism, hypoxia, ileus, intestinal obstruction, interstitial pneumonitis, laryngitis, leukemia (acute), lymphangitis, mania, mural thrombosis, myopathy, nephrotic syndrome, neutropenia, pancreatitis, pancytopenia, paroxysmal nocturnal dyspnea, pathological

fracture, pericardial effusion, pleural effusion, pneumonitis, pneumothorax, pulmonary edema (noncardiogenic), pulmonary fibrosis, pulmonary hypertension, pulmonary infiltrate, pyelonephritis, radiation injury, renal failure, respiratory distress, respiratory failure, seizure, sepsis, shock, skin ulcers, stroke, syncope, stomatitis, thyroiditis (autoimmune), vascular thrombosis, ventricular dysfunction, volume overload

Drug Interactions

Avoid Concomitant Use There are no known interactions where it is recommended to avoid concomitant use.

Increased Effect/Toxicity

Trastuzumab may increase the levels/effects of: Antineoplastic Agents (Anthracycline); Immunosuppressants

The levels/effects of Trastuzumab may be increased by: Abciximab; Paclitaxel

Decreased Effect

Trastuzumab may decrease the levels/effects of: Paclitaxel

Stability Prior to reconstitution, store intact vials under refrigeration at 2°C to 8°C (36°F to 46°F). Reconstitute each vial with 20 mL of bacteriostatic sterile water for injection (SWFI) to a concentration of 21 mg/mL. Swirl gently; do not shake. Allow vial to rest for ~5 minutes. Following reconstitution with bacteriostatic SWFI, the solution in the vial is stable refrigerated for 28 days from the date of reconstitution; do not freeze. If the patient has a known hypersensitivity to benzyl alcohol, trastuzumab may be reconstituted with sterile water for injection without preservatives, which must be used immediately.

Determine the appropriate volume for the trastuzumab dose and further dilute in 250 mL NS prior to administration. Avoid rapid expulsion from syringe; gently invert bag to mix. The solution for infusion is stable for 24 hours refrigerated; do not freeze.

Mechanism of Action Trastuzumab is a monoclonal antibody which binds to the extracellular domain of the human epidermal growth factor receptor 2 protein (HER-2); it mediates antibody-dependent cellular cytotoxicity by inhibiting proliferation of cells which overexpress HER-2 protein.

Pharmacodynamics/Kinetics

Distribution: V_d: 44 mL/kg; not likely to cross the (intact) blood brain barrier (due to the large molecule size)

Half-life elimination: Weekly dosing: Mean: 6 days (range: 1-32 days); every 3 week regimen: Mean: 16 days (range: 11-23 days)

Dosage Details concerning dosing in combination regimens should also be consulted. Adults: I.V. infusion:

Adjuvant treatment of breast cancer:

With concurrent paclitaxel or docetaxel:

Initial loading dose: 4 mg/kg infused over 90 minutes

Maintenance dose: 2 mg/kg infused over 30 minutes weekly for total of 12 weeks, followed 1 week later (when concurrent chemotherapy completed) by 6 mg/kg infused over 30-60 minutes every 3 weeks for total therapy duration of 52 weeks

With concurrent docetaxel/carboplatin:

Initial loading dose: 4 mg/kg infused over 90 minutes

Maintenance dose: 2 mg/kg infused over 30 minutes weekly for total of 18 weeks, followed 1 week later (when concurrent chemotherapy completed) by 6 mg/kg infused over 30-60 minutes every 3 weeks for total therapy duration of 52 weeks

Following completion of anthracycline-based chemotherapy:

Initial loading dose: 8 mg/kg infused over 90 minutes

Maintenance dose: 6 mg/kg infused over 30 minutes every 3 weeks for total therapy duration of 52 weeks

Metastatic breast cancer (either as a single agent or in combination with paclitaxel):

Initial loading dose: 4 mg/kg infused over 90 minutes

Maintenance dose: 2 mg/kg infused over 30 minutes weekly until disease progression

Dosage adjustment for toxicity:

Cardiotoxicity: LVEF ≥16% decrease from baseline within normal limits or LVEF below normal limits and ≥10% decrease from baseline: Withhold treatment for 4 weeks and repeat LVEF every 4 weeks. May resume trastuzumab treatment if LVEF returns to normal limits within 4-8 weeks and remains at ≤15% decrease from baseline value. Discontinue permanently for persistent (>8 weeks) LVEF decline or for >3 incidents of treatment interruptions for cardiomyopathy.

Infusion-related events:

Mild-moderate infusion reactions: Decrease infusion rate

Dyspnea, clinically significant hypotension: Interrupt infusion

Severe or life-threatening infusion reactions: Consider permanent discontinuation

Dosing adjustment in renal impairment: Data suggest that the disposition of trastuzumab is not altered based on age or serum creatinine (up to 2 mg/dL); however, no formal interaction studies have been performed

Dosing adjustment in hepatic impairment: No data is currently available

Administration Administered by I.V. infusion; loading doses are infused over 90 minutes; maintenance doses may be infused over 30 minutes if tolerated. Do not administer with D_5W. Do not administer I.V. push or by rapid bolus. Treatment with acetaminophen, diphenhydramine, and/or meperidine is usually effective for managing infusion-related events.

Monitoring Parameters HER2 expression assessment (pretherapy); monitor vital signs during infusion; signs and symptoms of cardiac dysfunction; LVEF (baseline, every 3 months during treatment, upon therapy completion and every 6 months for at least 2 years; if treatment is withheld for significant LVEF dysfunction, monitor LVEF at 4-week intervals)

Dosage Forms Excipient information presented when available (limited, particularly for generics); consult specific product labeling.

Injection, powder for reconstitution:

Herceptin®: 440 mg [packaged with bacteriostatic water for injection; diluent contains benzyl alcohol]

◆ **Trasylol®** *see* Aprotinin *on page* 131

◆ **Travatan®** *see* Travoprost *on page* 1504

◆ **Travatan® Z** *see* Travoprost *on page* 1504

Travoprost (TRA voe prost)

U.S. Brand Names Travatan®; Travatan® Z

Canadian Brand Names Travatan®; Travatan® Z

Pharmacologic Category Ophthalmic Agent, Antiglaucoma; Prostaglandin, Ophthalmic

Additional Appendix Information

Glaucoma Drug Therapy *on page* 1808

Use Reduction of elevated intraocular pressure in patients with open-angle glaucoma or ocular hypertension who are intolerant of the other IOP-lowering medications or insufficiently responsive (failed to achieve target IOP determined after multiple measurements over time) to another IOP-lowering medication

Pregnancy Risk Factor C

Medication Safety Issues

Sound-alike/look-alike issues:

Travatan® may be confused with Xalatan®

Dosage Ophthalmic: Adults: Glaucoma (open angle) or ocular hypertension: Instill 1 drop into affected eye(s) once daily in the evening; do not exceed once-daily dosing (may decrease IOP-lowering effect). If used with other topical ophthalmic agents, separate administration by at least 5 minutes.

Additional Information Complete prescribing information for this medication should be consulted for additional detail.

Dosage Forms Excipient information presented when available (limited, particularly for generics); consult specific product labeling.

Solution, ophthalmic:

Travatan®: 0.004% (2.5 mL, 5 mL) [contains benzalkonium chloride]

Travatan® Z: 0.004% (2.5 mL, 5 mL)

TraZODone (TRAZ oh done)

Canadian Brand Names Alti-Trazodone; Apo-Trazodone D®; Apo-Trazodone®; Desyrel®; Gen-Trazodone; Novo-Trazodone; Nu-Trazodone; PMS-Trazodone; ratio-Trazodone; Trazorel®

Index Terms Trazodone Hydrochloride

Pharmacologic Category Antidepressant, Serotonin Reuptake Inhibitor/Antagonist

Additional Appendix Information

Antidepressant Agents *on page 1638*

Use Treatment of depression

Unlabeled/Investigational Use Potential augmenting agent for antidepressants, hypnotic

Restrictions An FDA-approved medication guide concerning the use of antidepressants in children, adolescents, and young adults must be distributed when dispensing an outpatient prescription (new or refill) where this medication is to be used without direct supervision of a healthcare provider. Medication guides are available at http://www.fda.gov/cder/Offices/ODS/medication_guides.htm. Dispense to parents or guardians of children and adolescents receiving this medication.

Pregnancy Risk Factor C

Pregnancy Considerations Trazodone is classified as pregnancy category C due to adverse effects observed in animal studies. When trazodone is taken during pregnancy, an increased risk of major malformations has not been observed in the small number of pregnancies studied. The long-term effects on neurobehavior have not been evaluated.

Women treated for major depression and who are euthymic prior to pregnancy are more likely to experience a relapse when medication is discontinued as compared to pregnant women who continue taking antidepressant medications. Therapy during pregnancy should be individualized; treatment of depression during pregnancy should incorporate the clinical expertise of the mental health clinician, obstetrician, primary healthcare provider, and pediatrician. If treatment during pregnancy is required, consider tapering therapy during the third trimester to prevent potential withdrawal symptoms in the infant. If this is done and the woman is considered to be at risk of relapse from her major depressive disorder, the medication can be restarted following delivery.

Lactation Enters breast milk/use caution (AAP rates "of concern")

Medication Safety Issues

Sound-alike/look-alike issues:

Desyrel® may be confused with Demerol®, Delsym®, Zestril®

TraZODone may be confused with traMADol

International issues:

Desyrel® may be confused with Deseril® which is a brand name for methysergide in multiple international markets

Contraindications Hypersensitivity to trazodone or any component of the formulation

Warnings/Precautions **[U.S. Boxed Warning]: Antidepressants increase the risk of suicidal thinking and behavior in children, adolescents, and young adults (18-24 years of age) with major depressive disorder (MDD) and other psychiatric disorders;** consider risk prior to prescribing. Short-term studies did not show an increased risk in patients >24 years of age and showed a decreased risk in patients ≥65 years. Closely monitor for clinical worsening, suicidality, or unusual changes in behavior; the patient's family or caregiver should be instructed to closely observe the patient and communicate condition with healthcare provider. A medication guide should be dispensed with each prescription. **Trazodone is not FDA approved for use in children.**

The possibility of a suicide attempt is inherent in major depression and may persist until remission occurs. Monitor for worsening of depression or suicidality, especially during initiation of therapy (generally first 1-2 months) or with dose increases or decreases. Use caution in high-risk patients. Worsening depression and severe abrupt suicidality that are not part of the presenting symptoms may require discontinuation or modification of drug therapy. The patient's family or caregiver should be alerted to monitor patients for the emergence of suicidality and associated behaviors (such as agitation, irritability, hostility, impulsivity, and hypomania) and call healthcare provider.

May worsen psychosis in some patients or precipitate a shift to mania or hypomania in patients with bipolar disorder. Patients presenting with depressive symptoms should be screened for bipolar disorder. Monotherapy in patients with bipolar disorder should be avoided. **Trazodone is not FDA approved for the treatment of bipolar depression.**

Priapism, including cases resulting in permanent dysfunction, has occurred with the use of trazodone. Not recommended for use in a patient during the acute recovery phase of MI. Trazodone should be initiated with caution in patients who are receiving concurrent or recent therapy with a MAO inhibitor.

The risks of sedation and/or postural hypotension are high relative to other antidepressants. Trazodone frequently causes sedation, which may result in impaired performance of tasks requiring alertness (eg, operating machinery or driving). Sedative effects may be additive with other CNS depressants and ethanol. Use with caution in patients with a history of cardiovascular disease (including previous MI, stroke, tachycardia, or conduction abnormalities). The risk of conduction abnormalities with this agent is low relative to other antidepressants.

Consider discontinuing, when possible, prior to elective surgery. Therapy should not be abruptly discontinued in patients receiving high doses for prolonged periods. Use caution in patients with a previous seizure disorder or condition predisposing to seizures such as brain damage, alcoholism, or concurrent therapy with other drugs which lower the seizure threshold. Use with caution in patients with hepatic or renal dysfunction and in elderly patients.

Adverse Reactions

>10%:

Central nervous system: Dizziness, headache, sedation

Gastrointestinal: Nausea, xerostomia

Ocular: Blurred vision

1% to 10%:

Cardiovascular: Syncope, hyper-/hypotension, edema

Central nervous system: Confusion, decreased concentration, fatigue, incoordination

Gastrointestinal: Diarrhea, constipation, weight gain/loss

Neuromuscular & skeletal: Tremor, myalgia

Respiratory: Nasal congestion

<1% (Limited to important or life-threatening): Agitation, allergic reactions, alopecia, anxiety, bradycardia, extrapyramidal symptoms, hepatitis, priapism, rash, seizure, speech impairment, tachycardia, urinary retention

Drug Interactions

Metabolism/Transport Effects Substrate of CYP2D6 (minor), 3A4 (major); **Inhibits** CYP2D6 (moderate), 3A4 (weak)

Avoid Concomitant Use

Avoid concomitant use of TraZODone with any of the following: Sibutramine

Increased Effect/Toxicity

TraZODone may increase the levels/effects of: Alcohol (Ethyl); CNS Depressants; CYP2D6 Substrates; Fesoterodine; Nebivolol; Serotonin Modulators; Tamoxifen

The levels/effects of TraZODone may be increased by: BusPIRone; CYP3A4 Inhibitors (Moderate); CYP3A4 Inhibitors (Strong); Dasatinib; Protease Inhibitors; Selective Serotonin Reuptake Inhibitors; Sibutramine; Venlafaxine

Decreased Effect

TraZODone may decrease the levels/effects of: Codeine; Dabigatran Etexilate; P-Glycoprotein Substrates; TraMADol

The levels/effects of TraZODone may be decreased by: CYP3A4 Inducers (Strong); Deferasirox; Herbs (CYP3A4 Inducers)

Ethanol/Nutrition/Herb Interactions

Ethanol: Avoid ethanol (may increase CNS depression).

Food: Time to peak serum levels may be increased if trazodone is taken with food.

Herb/Nutraceutical: Avoid valerian, St John's wort, SAMe, kava kava (may increase risk of serotonin syndrome and/or excessive sedation).

Mechanism of Action Inhibits reuptake of serotonin, causes adrenoreceptor subsensitivity, and induces significant changes in 5-HT presynaptic receptor adrenoreceptors. Trazodone also significantly blocks histamine (H_1) and alpha$_1$-adrenergic receptors.

Pharmacodynamics/Kinetics

Onset of action: Therapeutic (antidepressant): 1-3 weeks; sleep aid: 1-3 hours

Protein binding: 85% to 95%

Metabolism: Hepatic via CYP3A4 to an active metabolite (mCPP)

Half-life elimination: 7-8 hours, two compartment kinetics

Time to peak, serum: 30-100 minutes; delayed with food (up to 2.5 hours)

Excretion: Primarily urine; secondarily feces

Dosage Oral: Therapeutic effects may take up to 6 weeks to occur; therapy is normally maintained for 6-12 months after optimum response is reached to prevent recurrence of depression

Children 6-12 years: Depression (unlabeled use): Initial: 1.5-2 mg/kg/day in divided doses; increase gradually every 3-4 days as needed; maximum: 6 mg/kg/day in 3 divided doses

Adolescents: Depression (unlabeled use): Initial: 25-50 mg/day; increase to 100-150 mg/day in divided doses

Adults:

Depression: Initial: 150 mg/day in 3 divided doses (may increase by 50 mg/day every 3-7 days); maximum: 600 mg/day

Sedation/hypnotic (unlabeled use): 25-50 mg at bedtime (often in combination with daytime SSRIs); may increase up to 200 mg at bedtime

Elderly: 25-50 mg at bedtime with 25-50 mg/day dose increase every 3 days for inpatients and weekly for outpatients, if tolerated; usual dose: 75-150 mg/day

Administration Dosing after meals may decrease lightheadedness and postural hypotension

Monitoring Parameters Suicidal ideation (especially at the beginning of therapy or when doses are increased or decreased)

Reference Range

Plasma levels do not always correlate with clinical effectiveness

Therapeutic: 0.5-2.5 mcg/mL

Potentially toxic: >2.5 mcg/mL

Toxic: >4 mcg/mL

Dosage Forms Excipient information presented when available (limited, particularly for generics); consult specific product labeling.

Tablet, as hydrochloride: 50 mg, 100 mg, 150 mg, 300 mg

◆ **Trazodone Hydrochloride** *see* TraZODone *on page 1505*

◆ **Trazorel® (Can)** *see* TraZODone *on page 1505*

◆ **Treanda®** *see* Bendamustine *on page 181*

◆ **Trecator®** *see* Ethionamide *on page 585*

◆ **Trelstar® (Can)** *see* Triptorelin *on page 1523*

◆ **Trelstar® Depot** *see* Triptorelin *on page 1523*

◆ **Trelstar® LA** *see* Triptorelin *on page 1523*

◆ **Trental®** *see* Pentoxifylline *on page 1173*

Treprostinil (tre PROST in il)

U.S. Brand Names Remodulin®

Canadian Brand Names Remodulin®

Index Terms Treprostinil Sodium

Pharmacologic Category Prostacyclin; Prostaglandin; Vasodilator

Use Treatment of pulmonary arterial hypertension (PAH) in patients with NYHA Class II-IV symptoms to decrease exercise-associated symptoms; to diminish clinical deterioration when transitioning from epoprostenol (I.V.)

Pregnancy Risk Factor B

Pregnancy Considerations Some skeletal malformations and maternal toxicity noted in animal studies. There are no adequate and well-controlled studies in pregnant women. Use with caution and only if clearly needed.

Lactation Excretion in breast milk unknown/use caution

Contraindications There are no contraindications listed in the FDA-approved labeling.

Warnings/Precautions Abrupt withdrawal/large dosage reductions may worsen symptoms of PAH. Chronic continuous I.V. infusion of treprostinil via a chronic indwelling central venous catheter has been associated with serious blood stream infections. This method of administration should be reserved for patients who are intolerant of the SubQ route or in whom the benefit outweighs the potential risks. Treprostinil should only be used by clinicians experienced in the treatment of PAH. Prior to initiation, patients should be carefully evaluated for ability to administer treprostinil and care for the infusion system. Initiation must occur in a setting where adequate personnel and equipment necessary for hemodynamic monitoring and emergency treatment is available. Use with caution in patients with hepatic impairment; dose reduction is recommended for the initial dose in patients with mild-to-moderate hepatic insufficiency; has not been studied in severe hepatic impairment. Use caution in renal impairment. Use with caution in patients ≥65 years of age. Safety and efficacy have not been established in patients ≤16 years of age.

Adverse Reactions

>10%:

Cardiovascular: Vasodilation (11%)

Central nervous system: Headache (27%)

Dermatologic: Rash (14%)

Gastrointestinal: Diarrhea (25%), nausea (22%)
Local: Infusion site pain (SubQ 85%, may improve after several months of therapy); infusion site reaction (SubQ 83%)
Neuromuscular & Skeletal: Jaw pain (13%)

1% to 10%:
Cardiovascular: Edema (9%), hypotension (4%)
Central nervous system: Dizziness (9%)
Dermatologic: Pruritus (8%)

Postmarketing and/or case reports: Anxiety, arm swelling, bone pain, cellulitis, central venous catheter-related line infections, central venous catheter-related sepsis, hematoma, pain, paresthesia, restlessness, thrombocytopenia, thrombophlebitis

Drug Interactions

Avoid Concomitant Use There are no known interactions where it is recommended to avoid concomitant use.

Increased Effect/Toxicity

Treprostinil may increase the levels/effects of: Anticoagulants; Antihypertensives; Antiplatelet Agents; Nonsteroidal Anti-Inflammatory Agents; Salicylates

Decreased Effect There are no known significant interactions involving a decrease in effect.

Stability Store vials at 15°C to 30°C (59°F to 86°F). Contents of a vial should not be used past 30 days after initial needle access into the vial. For SubQ infusion, product should not be diluted prior to use. Contents of a single-reservoir syringe of treprostinil can be administered up to 72 hours at 37°C. For I.V. infusion, dilute in SWFI, NS, or Flolan® sterile diluent to a final volume of either 50 mL or 100 mL (dependent on system reservoir and calculated dose). Stability for up to 48 hours has been shown for concentrations as low as 4000 ng/mL. Solutions diluted for infusion may be used for up to 48 hours at 37°C.

Mechanism of Action Treprostinil is a direct vasodilator of both pulmonary and systemic arterial vascular beds; also inhibits platelet aggregation.

Pharmacodynamics/Kinetics

Absorption: SubQ: Rapidly and completely
Distribution: 14 L/70 kg lean body weight
Protein binding: 91%
Metabolism: Hepatic (enzymes unknown); forms 5 metabolites (HU1-HU5)
Bioavailability: SubQ: 100%
Half-life elimination: Terminal: ~2-4 hours
Excretion: Urine (79%; 4% as unchanged drug, 64% as metabolites); feces (13%)

Dosage Note: Prior to initiation, patients should be carefully evaluated for ability to administer treprostinil and care for the infusion system outside of inpatient setting. Immediate access to back up pump, infusion sets, and medication is essential to prevent treatment interruptions.

Adults: PAH: SubQ (preferred) or I.V. infusion:

Initial: New to prostacyclin therapy: 1.25 ng/kg/minute continuous; if dose cannot be tolerated due to systemic effects, reduce to 0.625 ng/kg/minute. Increase at rate not >1.25 ng/kg/minute per week for first 4 weeks, and not >2.5 ng/kg/minute per week for remainder of therapy. Limited experience with doses >40 ng/kg/minute. **Note:** Dose must be carefully and individually titrated (symptom improvement with minimal adverse effects). Avoid abrupt withdrawal. If infusion is restarted within a few hours of discontinuation, the same dose rate may be used. Interruptions for longer periods may require retitration.

Transitioning from epoprostenol (see table): SubQ (preferred) or I.V. infusion: **Note:** Transition should occur in a hospital setting to follow response (eg, walking distance, sign/symptoms of disease progression). May take 24-48 hours to transition. Transition is accomplished by initiating the infusion of treprostinil, and increasing it while simultaneously reducing the dose of intravenous epoprostenol. During transition, increases in PAH symptoms should be first treated with an increase in treprostinil dose. Occurrence of prostacyclin associated side effects should be treated by decreasing the dose of epoprostenol.

Transitioning From I.V. Epoprostenol to SubQ (Preferred) or I.V. Treprostinil

Step	Epoprostenol Dose	Treprostinil Dose
1	Maintain current dose	Initiate at 10% initial epoprostenol dose
2	Decrease to 80% initial dose	Increase to 30% initial epoprostenol dose
3	Decrease to 60% initial dose	Increase to 50% initial epoprostenol dose
4	Decrease to 40% initial dose	Increase to 70% initial epoprostenol dose
5	Decrease to 20% initial dose	Increase to 90% initial epoprostenol dose
6	Decrease to 5% initial dose	Increase to 110% initial epoprostenol dose
7	Discontinue epoprostenol	Maintain current dose plus additional 5% to 10% as needed

Elderly: Limited experience in patients ≥65 years; refer to adult dosing; use caution

Dosage adjustment in renal impairment: No specific dosage adjustment recommended; use with caution.

Dosage adjustment in hepatic impairment:

Mild-to-moderate: Initial: 0.625 ng/kg/minute; increase with caution.

Severe: Has not been studied in patients with severe hepatic impairment.

Dietary Considerations Sodium chloride content of solution for injection:

1 mg/mL, 2.5 mg/mL, and 5 mg/mL each contain sodium chloride 5.3 mg/mL

10 mg/mL contains sodium chloride 4 mg/mL

Administration Prior to initiation, patients should be carefully evaluated for ability to administer treprostinil and care for the infusion system outside of inpatient setting. Avoid abrupt withdrawal (including interruptions in delivery) or rapid large dosage reductions. Immediate access to back up pump, infusion sets, and medication is essential to prevent treatment interruptions.

I.V. infusion: I.V. use is recommended when SubQ infusion is not tolerated or when the benefit outweighs the potential risks of an indwelling central venous catheter. Solution must be diluted in SWFI or NS prior to use and administered by continuous infusion using a central indwelling catheter and infusion pump. Peripheral infusion may be used temporarily until central line is established.

SubQ infusion (preferred): Administer undiluted via continuous SubQ infusion using an appropriately-designed infusion pump. Infusion site reactions may be helped by moving the infusion site every 3 days, local application of topical hot and cold packs, topical or oral analgesics. Injection site pain and erythema may improve after several months of therapy.

Monitoring Parameters BP, dyspnea, fatigue, activity tolerance, symptoms of excessive dose (eg, headache, nausea, vomiting)

Dosage Forms Excipient information presented when available (limited, particularly for generics); consult specific product labeling.

Injection, solution: 1 mg/mL (20 mL) [contains sodium chloride 5.3 mg/mL]; 2.5 mg/mL (20 mL) [contains sodium chloride 5.3 mg/mL]; 5 mg/mL (20 mL) [contains sodium chloride 5.3 mg/mL]; 10 mg/mL (20 mL) [contains sodium chloride 4 mg/mL]

Tretinoin (Oral) (TRET i noyn, oral)

U.S. Brand Names Vesanoid®

Canadian Brand Names Vesanoid®

Index Terms *trans*-Retinoic Acid; All-*trans*-Retinoic Acid; ATRA; NSC-122758; Ro 5488; tRA

Pharmacologic Category Antineoplastic Agent, Miscellaneous; Retinoic Acid Derivative

Use Induction of remission in patients with acute promyelocytic leukemia (APL), French American British (FAB) classification M3 (including the M3 variant)

Pregnancy Risk Factor D

Pregnancy Considerations **[U.S. Boxed Warning]: High risk of teratogenicity; not to be used in women of childbearing potential** unless the woman is capable of complying with effective contraceptive measures. Repeat pregnancy testing and contraception counseling monthly throughout the period of treatment. Major fetal abnormalities and spontaneous abortions have been reported with other retinoids. Effective contraception must be used during treatment and for 1 month following discontinuation of therapy.

Lactation Enters breast milk/not recommended

Medication Safety Issues

Sound-alike/look-alike issues:

Tretinoin may be confused with isotretinoin, trientine

High alert medication: The Institute for Safe Medication Practices (ISMP) includes this medication among its list of drugs which have a heightened risk of causing significant patient harm when used in error.

Contraindications Sensitivity to parabens, vitamin A, other retinoids, or any component of the formulation; pregnancy

Warnings/Precautions Hazardous agent - use appropriate precautions for handling and disposal. **[U.S. Boxed Warning]: Patients with acute promyelocytic leukemia (APL) are at high risk and can have severe adverse reactions to tretinoin.**

[U.S. Boxed Warning]: About 25% of patients with APL and treated with tretinoin, have experienced retinoic acid-APL (RA-APL) syndrome, characterized by fever, dyspnea, acute respiratory distress, weight gain, radiographic pulmonary infiltrates and pleural or pericardial effusions, edema, and hepatic, renal, and/or multiorgan failure. This syndrome has occasionally been accompanied by impaired myocardial contractility and episodic hypotension. It has been observed with or without concomitant leukocytosis. Endotracheal intubation and mechanical ventilation have been required in some cases due to progressive hypoxemia, and several patients have expired with multiorgan failure. The syndrome usually occurs during the first month of treatment, with some cases reported following the first dose.

Management of the syndrome has not been defined, but high-dose steroids given at the first suspicion of RA-APL syndrome appear to reduce morbidity and mortality. At the first signs suggestive of the syndrome, immediately initiate high-dose steroids (dexamethasone 10 mg I.V.) every 12 hours for 3 days or until resolution of symptoms, regardless of the leukocyte count. The majority of patients do not require termination of tretinoin therapy during treatment of the RA-APL syndrome.

[U.S. Boxed Warning]: During treatment, ~40% of patients will develop rapidly evolving leukocytosis; may be associated with a higher risk of life-threatening complications.

If signs and symptoms of the RA-APL syndrome are present together with leukocytosis, initiate treatment with high-dose steroids immediately. Consider adding full-dose chemotherapy (including an anthracycline, if not contraindicated) to the tretinoin therapy on day 1 or 2 for patients presenting with a WBC count of >5 x 10^9/L or immediately, for patients presenting with a WBC count of <5 x 10^9/L, if the WBC count reaches ≥6 x 10^9/L by day 5, or ≥10 x 10^9/L by day 10 or ≥15 x 10^9/L by day 28.

[U.S. Boxed Warning]: High risk of teratogenicity; not to be used in women of childbearing potential unless the woman is capable of complying with effective contraceptive measures. Repeat pregnancy testing and contraception counseling monthly throughout the period of treatment.

Retinoids have been associated with pseudotumor cerebri (benign intracranial hypertension), especially in children. Concurrent use of other drugs associated with this effect (eg, tetracyclines) may increase risk. Early signs and symptoms include papilledema, headache, nausea, vomiting and visual disturbances.

Up to 60% of patients experienced hypercholesterolemia or hypertriglyceridemia, which were reversible upon completion of treatment. Elevated liver function test results occur in 50% to 60% of patients during treatment. Carefully monitor liver function test results during treatment and give consideration to a temporary withdrawal of tretinoin if test results reach >5 times the upper limit of normal. **[U.S. Boxed Warning]: Should be administered under the supervision of an experienced cancer chemotherapy physician.** Safety and efficacy have not been established in children <1 year of age.

Adverse Reactions Virtually all patients experience some drug-related toxicity, especially headache, fever, weakness and fatigue. These adverse effects are seldom permanent or irreversible nor do they usually require therapy interruption.

>10%:

Cardiovascular: Peripheral edema (52%), chest discomfort (32%), edema (29%), arrhythmias (23%), flushing (23%), hypotension (14%), hypertension (11%)

Central nervous system: Headache (86%), fever (83%), malaise (66%), pain (37%), dizziness (20%), anxiety (17%), insomnia (14%), depression (14%), confusion (11%)

Dermatologic: Skin/mucous membrane dryness (77%), rash (54%), pruritus (20%), alopecia (14%)

Endocrine & metabolic: Hypercholesterolemia and/or hypertriglyceridemia (60%)

Gastrointestinal: Nausea/vomiting (57%), liver function tests increased (50% to 60%), GI hemorrhage (34%), abdominal pain (31%), mucositis (26%), diarrhea (23%), weight gain (23%), constipation (17%), dyspepsia (14%), abdominal distention (11%), weight loss (17%), xerostomia, anorexia (17%)

Hematologic: Hemorrhage (60%), leukocytosis (40%), disseminated intravascular coagulation (DIC) (26%)

Local: Phlebitis (11%), injection site reactions (17%)

Neuromuscular & skeletal: Bone pain (77%), paresthesia (17%), myalgia (14%)

Ocular: Visual disturbances (17%)

Otic: Earache/ear fullness (23%)

Renal: Renal insufficiency (11%)

Respiratory: Upper respiratory tract disorders (63%), dyspnea (60%), respiratory insufficiency (26%), pleural effusion (20%), pneumonia (14%), rales (14%), expiratory wheezing (14%), dry nose

Miscellaneous: Shivering (63%), infections (58%), retinoic acid-acute promyelocytic leukemia syndrome (25%), diaphoresis increased (20%)

1% to 10%:

Cardiovascular: Cerebral hemorrhage (9%), pallor (6%), cardiac failure (6%), cardiac arrest (3%), MI (3%), enlarged heart (3%), heart murmur (3%), stroke (3%), myocarditis (3%), pericarditis (3%), pulmonary hypertension (3%), secondary cardiomyopathy (3%), ischemia

Central nervous system: Intracranial hypertension (9%), agitation (9%), hallucination (6%), agnosia (3%), aphasia (3%), cerebellar edema (3%), cerebral hemorrhage (9%), seizure (3%), coma (3%), CNS depression (3%), dysarthria (3%), encephalopathy (3%), hypotaxia (3%), light reflex absent (3%), spinal cord disorder (3%), unconsciousness (3%), dementia (3%), forgetfulness (3%), somnolence (3%), slow speech (3%), hypothermia (3%)

Dermatologic: Cellulitis (8%), photosensitivity

Endocrine & metabolic: Acidosis (3%)

Gastrointestinal: Hepatosplenomegaly (9%), ulcer (3%)

Genitourinary: Dysuria (9%), acute renal failure (3%), micturition frequency (3%), renal tubular necrosis (3%), enlarged prostate (3%)

Hepatic: Ascites (3%), hepatitis (3%)

Neuromuscular & skeletal: Tremor (3%), leg weakness (3%), abnormal gait (3%), bone inflammation (3%), asterixis, dysarthria, facial paralysis, flank pain, hemiplegia, hyporeflexia

Ocular: Visual acuity change (6%), visual field deficit (3%), dry eyes

Otic: Hearing loss

Renal: Acute renal failure, renal tubular necrosis

Respiratory: Lower respiratory tract disorders (9%), pulmonary infiltration (6%), bronchial asthma (3%), pulmonary/larynx edema

Miscellaneous: Face edema

<1% (Limited to important or life-threatening): Arterial thrombosis, basophilia, cataracts, conjunctivitis, erythema nodosum, hypercalcemia, hyperuricemia, inflammatory bowel syndrome, irreversible hearing loss, pancreatitis, pseudomotor cerebri, renal infarct, Sweet's syndrome, vasculitis, venous thrombosis

Drug Interactions

Metabolism/Transport Effects **Substrate** (minor) of CYP2A6 (minor), 2B6 (minor), 2C8 (major), 2C9 (minor); **Inhibits** CYP2C9 (weak); **Induces** CYP2E1 (weak)

Avoid Concomitant Use

Avoid concomitant use of Tretinoin (Oral) with any of the following: Natalizumab; Tetracycline Derivatives; Vaccines (Live)

Increased Effect/Toxicity

Tretinoin (Oral) may increase the levels/effects of: Natalizumab; Vaccines (Live)

The levels/effects of Tretinoin (Oral) may be increased by: CYP2C8 Inhibitors (Moderate); CYP2C8 Inhibitors (Strong); Tetracycline Derivatives; Trastuzumab

Decreased Effect

Tretinoin (Oral) may decrease the levels/effects of: Oral Contraceptive (Estrogens); Oral Contraceptive (Progestins); Vaccines (Inactivated)

The levels/effects of Tretinoin (Oral) may be decreased by: CYP2C8 Inducers (Highly Effective); Echinacea

Ethanol/Nutrition/Herb Interactions

Ethanol: Avoid ethanol (may increase CNS depression).

Food: Absorption of retinoids has been shown to be enhanced when taken with food.

Herb/Nutraceutical: St John's wort may decrease tretinoin levels. Avoid dong quai, St John's wort (may also cause photosensitization). Avoid additional vitamin A supplementation. May lead to vitamin A toxicity.

Stability Store capsule at 15°C to 30°C (59°F to 86°F);. Protect from light.

Mechanism of Action Tretinoin appears to bind one or more nuclear receptors and inhibits clonal proliferation and/or granulocyte differentiation

Pharmacodynamics/Kinetics

Protein binding: >95%

Metabolism: Hepatic via CYP; primary metabolite: 4-oxo-all-*trans*-retinoic acid

Half-life elimination: Terminal: Parent drug: 0.5-2 hours

Time to peak, serum: 1-2 hours

Excretion: Urine (63%); feces (30%)

Dosage Oral: Children and Adults:

Remission induction: 45 mg/m^2/day in 2-3 divided doses for up to 30 days after complete remission (maximum duration of treatment: 90 days)

Remission maintenance: 45-200 mg/m^2/day in 2-3 divided doses for up to 12 months.

Dietary Considerations To enhance absorption, some clinicians recommend giving with a fatty meal. Capsule contains soybean oil.

Administration Administer with meals; do not crush capsules

Monitoring Parameters Monitor the patient's hematologic profile, coagulation profile, liver function test results and triglyceride and cholesterol levels frequently

Dosage Forms Excipient information presented when available (limited, particularly for generics); consult specific product labeling.

Capsule: 10 mg

Vesanoid®: 10 mg [contains soybean oil and parabens]

Tretinoin (Topical) (TRET i noyn, TOP i kal)

U.S. Brand Names Atralin™; Avita®; Renova®; Retin-A®; Retin-A® Micro; Tretin-X™

Canadian Brand Names Rejuva-A®; Retin-A®; Retin-A® Micro; Retinova®

Index Terms *trans*-Retinoic Acid; Retinoic Acid; Vitamin A Acid

Pharmacologic Category Acne Products; Retinoic Acid Derivative; Topical Skin Product, Acne

Use Treatment of acne vulgaris; photodamaged skin; palliation of fine wrinkles, mottled hyperpigmentation, and tactile roughness of facial skin as part of a comprehensive skin care and sun avoidance program

Unlabeled/Investigational Use Some skin cancers

Pregnancy Risk Factor C

Pregnancy Considerations Oral tretinoin is teratogenic and fetotoxic in rats at doses 1000 and 500 times the topical human dose, respectively. Tretinoin does not appear to be teratogenic when used topically since it is rapidly metabolized by the skin; however, there are rare reports of fetal defects. Use for acne only if benefit to mother outweighs potential risk to fetus. During pregnancy, do not use for palliation of fine wrinkles, mottled hyperpigmentation, and tactile roughness of facial skin.

Lactation Enters breast milk/compatible

Medication Safety Issues

Sound-alike/look-alike issues:

Tretinoin may be confused with isotretinoin, trientine

International issues:

Renova® may be confused with Remov® which is a brand name for nimesulide in Italy

Contraindications Hypersensitivity to tretinoin or any component of the formulation; sunburn

Warnings/Precautions Use with caution in patients with eczema; avoid excessive exposure to sunlight and sunlamps; avoid contact with abraded skin, sunburned skin, mucous membranes, eyes, mouth, angles of the nose. Treatment can increase skin sensitivity to weather extremes of wind or cold. Also, concomitant topical medications (eg, medicated or abrasive soaps, cleansers, or cosmetics with a strong drying effect) should be used with caution due to increased skin irritation. Palliation of fine wrinkles, mottled hyperpigmentation, and tactile roughness of facial skin: Do not use the 0.05% cream for longer than 48 weeks or the 0.02% cream for longer than 52 weeks. Not for use on moderate- to heavily-pigmented skin. Gel is flammable; do not expose to high temperatures or flame. Safety and efficacy have not been established in children <12 years of age.

Adverse Reactions

>10%: Dermatologic: Excessive dryness, erythema, scaling of the skin, pruritus

1% to 10%:

Dermatologic: Hyperpigmentation or hypopigmentation, photosensitivity, initial acne flare-up

Local: Edema, blistering, stinging

Drug Interactions

Metabolism/Transport Effects **Substrate** of CYP2A6 (minor), 2B6 (minor), 2C8 (major), 2C9 (minor); **Inhibits** CYP2C9 (weak); **Induces** CYP2E1 (weak)

Avoid Concomitant Use There are no known interactions where it is recommended to avoid concomitant use.

Increased Effect/Toxicity There are no known significant interactions involving an increase in effect.

Decreased Effect There are no known significant interactions involving a decrease in effect.

Ethanol/Nutrition/Herb Interactions

Food: Avoid excessive intake of vitamin A (cod liver oil, halibut fish oil).

Herb/Nutraceutical: Avoid dong quai, St John's wort (may also cause photosensitization). Avoid excessive amounts of vitamin A supplements.

Stability Store at 25°C (77°F). Gel is flammable; keep away from heat and flame.

Mechanism of Action Keratinocytes in the sebaceous follicle become less adherent which allows for easy removal; inhibits microcomedone formation and eliminates lesions already present

Pharmacodynamics/Kinetics

Absorption: Minimal

Metabolism: Hepatic for the small amount absorbed

Excretion: Urine and feces

Dosage Topical:

Children >12 years and Adults: Acne vulgaris: Begin therapy with a weaker formulation of tretinoin (0.025% cream, 0.04% microsphere gel, or 0.01% gel) and increase the concentration as tolerated; apply once daily to acne lesions before retiring or on alternate days; if stinging or irritation develop, decrease frequency of application

Adults ≥18: Palliation of fine wrinkles, mottled hyperpigmentation, and tactile roughness of facial skin: Pea-sized amount of the 0.02% or 0.05% cream applied to entire face once daily in the evening

Elderly: Use of the 0.02% cream in patients 65-71 years of age showed similar improvement in fine wrinkles as seen in patients <65 years. Safety and efficacy of the 0.02% cream have not been established in patients >71 years of age. Safety and efficacy of the 0.05% cream have not been established in patients >50 years of age.

Administration Palliation of fine wrinkles, mottled hyperpigmentation, and tactile roughness of facial skin: Cream: Prior to application, gently wash face with a mild soap. Pat dry. Wait 20-30 minutes to apply cream. Avoid eyes, ears, nostrils, and mouth.

Dosage Forms Excipient information presented when available (limited, particularly for generics); consult specific product labeling. [DSC] = Discontinued product

Cream, topical: 0.025% (20 g, 45 g); 0.05% (20 g, 45 g); 0.1% (20 g, 45 g)

Avita®: 0.025% (20 g, 45 g)

Renova®: 0.02% (40 g, 60 g) [contains benzyl alcohol]

Retin-A®: 0.025% (20 g, 45 g); 0.05% (20 g, 45 g); 0.1% (20 g, 45 g)

Tretin-X™: 0.025% (35 g); 0.05% (35 g); 0.1% (35 g)

Gel, topical: 0.01% (15 g, 45 g); 0.025% (15 g, 45 g)

Atralin™: 0.05% (45 g) [contains benzyl alcohol and fish collagen]

Avita®: 0.025% (20 g, 45 g) [contains ethanol 83%]

Retin-A®: 0.01% (15 g, 45 g); 0.025% (15 g, 45 g) [contains ethanol 90%]

Tretin-X™: 0.025% (35 g); 0.01% (35 g) [contains ethanol 90%]

Gel, topical [microsphere gel]:

Retin-A® Micro: 0.04% (20 g, 45 g, 50 g); 0.1% (20 g, 45 g, 50 g) [contains benzyl alcohol]

◆ **Trexall™** *see* Methotrexate *on page 965*

◆ **Treximet™** *see* Sumatriptan and Naproxen *on page 1415*

◆ **Triaconazole** *see* Terconazole *on page 1443*

◆ **Triaderm (Can)** *see* Triamcinolone *on page 1510*

◆ **Triall™** *see* Chlorpheniramine, Phenylephrine, and Methscopolamine *on page 313*

Triamcinolone (trye am SIN oh lone)

U.S. Brand Names Aristospan®; Azmacort®; Kenalog-10®; Kenalog-40®; Kenalog®; Nasacort® AQ; Tri-Nasal® [DSC]; Triderm®; Triesence™; Trivaris™; Zytopic™

Canadian Brand Names Aristospan®; Kenalog®; Kenalog® in Orabase; Nasacort® AQ; Oracort; Triaderm; Trinasal®

Index Terms Triamcinolone Acetonide, Aerosol; Triamcinolone Acetonide, Parenteral; Triamcinolone Diacetate, Oral; Triamcinolone Diacetate, Parenteral; Triamcinolone Hexacetonide; Triamcinolone, Oral

Pharmacologic Category Corticosteroid, Inhalant (Oral); Corticosteroid, Nasal; Corticosteroid, Ophthalmic; Corticosteroid, Systemic; Corticosteroid, Topical

Additional Appendix Information

Corticosteroids *on page 1652*

Use

Intra-articular (soft tissue): Acute gouty arthritis, acute/subacute bursitis, acute tenosynovitis, epicondylitis, rheumatoid arthritis, synovitis of osteoarthritis

Intralesional: Alopecia areata, discoid lupus erythematosus, keloids, granuloma annulare lesions (localized hypertrophic, infiltrated, or inflammatory), lichen planus plaques, lichen simplex chronicus plaques, psoriatic plaques, necrobiosis lipoidica diabeticorum, cystic tumors of aponeurosis or tendon (ganglia)

Nasal inhalation: Management of seasonal and perennial allergic rhinitis

Ophthalmic: Intravitreal: treatment of sympathetic ophthalmia, temporal arteritis, uveitis, ocular inflammatory conditions unresponsive to topical corticosteroids

Triesence™: Visualization during vitrectomy

Oral inhalation: Control of bronchial asthma and related bronchospastic conditions

Oral topical: Adjunctive treatment and temporary relief of symptoms associated with oral inflammatory lesions and ulcerative lesions resulting from trauma

Systemic: Adrenocortical insufficiency, dermatologic diseases, endocrine disorders, gastrointestinal diseases, hematologic and neoplastic disorders, nervous system disorders, nephrotic syndrome, rheumatic disorders, allergic states, respiratory diseases, systemic lupus erythematosus (SLE), and other diseases requiring anti-inflammatory or immunosuppressive effects

Topical: Inflammatory dermatoses responsive to steroids

Pregnancy Risk Factor C/D (ophthalmic suspension)

Pregnancy Considerations Triamcinolone was shown to be teratogenic following inhalation in animal studies and adverse events have been observed with corticosteroids in animal reproduction studies. Some studies have shown an association between first trimester corticosteroid use and oral clefts; adverse events in the fetus/neonate have been noted in case reports following large doses of systemic corticosteroids during pregnancy.

Lactation Excretion in breast milk unknown/use caution

Medication Safety Issues

Sound-alike/look-alike issues:

Kenalog® may be confused with Ketalar®

Nasacort® may be confused with NasalCrom®

TAC (occasional abbreviation for triamcinolone) is an error-prone abbreviation (mistaken as tetracaine-adrenaline-cocaine)

Contraindications Hypersensitivity to triamcinolone or any component of the formulation; systemic fungal infections; primary treatment of status asthmaticus or other acute episodes of asthma; fungal, viral, or bacterial infections of the mouth or throat (oral topical formulation); cerebral malaria; idiopathic thrombocytopenic purpura (I.M. injection)

Warnings/Precautions May cause hypercorticism or suppression of hypothalamic-pituitary-adrenal (HPA) axis, particularly in younger children or in patients receiving high doses for prolonged periods. HPA axis suppression may lead to adrenal crisis. Withdrawal and discontinuation of a corticosteroid should be done slowly and carefully. Particular care is required when patients are transferred from systemic corticosteroids to inhaled products due to possible adrenal insufficiency or withdrawal from steroids, including an increase in allergic symptoms. Patients receiving >20 mg per day of prednisone (or equivalent) may be most susceptible. Fatalities have occurred due to adrenal insufficiency in asthmatic patients during and after transfer from systemic corticosteroids to aerosol steroids; aerosol steroids do not provide the systemic steroid needed to treat patients having trauma, surgery, or infections.

May cause hypercorticism or suppression of hypothalamic-pituitary-adrenal (HPA) axis, particularly in younger children or in patients receiving high doses for prolonged periods. HPA axis suppression may lead to adrenal crisis. Withdrawal and discontinuation of a corticosteroid should be done slowly and carefully. Particular care is required when patients are transferred from systemic corticosteroids to inhaled products due to possible adrenal insufficiency or withdrawal from steroids, including an increase in allergic symptoms. Patients receiving >20 mg per day of prednisone (or equivalent) may be most susceptible. Fatalities have occurred due to adrenal insufficiency in asthmatic patients during and after transfer from systemic corticosteroids to aerosol steroids; aerosol steroids do not provide the systemic steroid needed to treat patients having trauma, surgery, or infections.

Bronchospasm may occur with wheezing after inhalation; if this occurs stop steroid and treat with a fast-acting bronchodilator (eg, albuterol). Supplemental steroids (oral or parenteral) may be needed during stress or severe asthma attacks. Not to be used in status asthmaticus or for the relief of acute bronchospasm. Acute myopathy has been reported with high dose corticosteroids, usually in patients with neuromuscular transmission disorders; may involve ocular and/or respiratory muscles; monitor creatine kinase; recovery may be delayed. Corticosteroid use may cause psychiatric disturbances, including depression, euphoria, insomnia, mood swings, and personality changes. Pre-existing psychiatric conditions may be exacerbated by corticosteroid use. Prolonged use of corticosteroids may also increase the incidence of secondary infection, mask acute infection (including fungal infections), prolong or exacerbate viral infections, or limit response to vaccines. Exposure to chickenpox should be avoided; corticosteroids should not be used to treat ocular herpes simplex. Corticosteroids should not be used for cerebral malaria or viral hepatitis. Close observation is required in patients with latent tuberculosis and/or TB reactivity; restrict use in active TB (only in conjunction with antituberculosis treatment). Use with caution in patients with threadworm infection; may cause serious hyperinfection. Prolonged treatment with corticosteroids has been associated with the development of Kaposi's sarcoma (case reports); if noted, discontinuation of therapy should be considered.

Use with caution in patients with thyroid disease, hepatic impairment, renal impairment, cardiovascular disease, diabetes, glaucoma, cataracts, myasthenia gravis, patients at risk for osteoporosis, patients at risk for seizures, or GI diseases (diverticulitis, peptic ulcer, ulcerative colitis) due to perforation risk. Use caution following acute MI (corticosteroids have been associated with myocardial rupture). Because of the risk of adverse effects, systemic corticosteroids should be used cautiously in the elderly in the smallest possible effective dose for the shortest duration. Azmacort® (metered dose inhaler) comes with its own spacer device attached and may be easier to use in older patients. Avoid nasal corticosteroid use in patients with recent nasal septal ulcers, nasal surgery or nasal trauma until healing has occurred. Do not use occlusive dressings on weeping or exudative lesions and general caution with occlusive dressings should be observed; discontinue if skin irritation or contact dermatitis should occur; do not use in patients with decreased skin circulation; avoid the use of high potency steroids on the face. Patients should not be immunized with live, viral vaccines while receiving immunosuppressive doses of corticosteroids. The ability to respond to dead viral vaccines is unknown. Some injection suspension formulations contain benzyl alcohol.

Intravitreal injection (Triesence™, Trivaris™) has been associated with endophthalmitis and visual disturbances. Blindness has been reported following injection into nasal turbinates and intralesional injections into the head. Safety of intraturbinal, subconjunctival, subtenons, retrobulbar, or intravitreal injection has not been demonstrated. Some formulations should not be administered intravitreally.

Orally-inhaled and intranasal corticosteroids may cause a reduction in growth velocity in pediatric patients (~1 centimeter per year [range 0.3-1.8 cm per year] and related to dose and duration of exposure). To minimize the systemic effects of orally-inhaled and intranasal corticosteroids, each patient should be titrated to the lowest effective dose. Growth should be routinely monitored in pediatric patients. Withdraw systemic therapy with gradual tapering of dose. There have been reports of systemic corticosteroid withdrawal symptoms (eg, joint/muscle pain, lassitude, depression) when withdrawing oral inhalation therapy. Injection suspension contains benzyl alcohol; benzyl alcohol has been associated with the "gasping syndrome" in neonates and low-birth-weight infants.

Oral topical: Discontinue if local irritation or sensitization should develop. If significant regeneration or repair of oral tissues has not occurred in seven days, re-evaluation of the etiology of the oral lesion is advised.

Adverse Reactions

Inhalation (nasal, oral):

>10%:

Central nervous system: Headache (2% to 51%)

Respiratory: Pharyngitis (5% to 25%)

1% to 10%:
- Cardiovascular: Facial edema (1% to 3%)
- Central nervous system: Pain (1% to 3%)
- Dermatologic: Photosensitivity (1% to 3%), rash (1% to 3%)
- Endocrine & metabolic: Dysmenorrhea (≥2%)
- Gastrointestinal: Taste perversion (5% to 8%), dyspepsia (3% to 5%), abdominal pain (1% to 5%), nausea (2% to 3%), diarrhea (1% to 3%), oral moniliasis (1% to 3%), toothache (1% to 3%), vomiting (1% to 3%), weight gain (1% to 3%), xerostomia (1% to 3%)
- Genitourinary: Cystitis (1% to 3%), urinary tract infection (1% to 3%), vaginal moniliasis (1% to 3%)
- Local: Nasal burning (≥2%; transient), nasal stinging (≥2%; transient)
- Neuromuscular & skeletal: Back pain (2% to 8%), bursitis (1% to 3%), myalgia (1% to 3%), tenosynovitis (1% to 3%)
- Ocular: Conjunctivitis (1% to 4%)
- Otic: Otitis media (≥2%)
- Respiratory: Sinusitis (2% to 9%), cough (≤8%), epistaxis (≤5%), bronchitis (children 3%), chest congestion (1% to 3%), asthma (≥2%), rhinitis (≥2%)
- Miscellaneous: Flu-like syndrome (2% to 9%), voice alteration (1% to 3%), allergic reaction (≥2%), infection (≥2%)

<1% (Limited to important or life-threatening): Anaphylaxis, blood cortisol decreased, bone mineral density loss (rare; prolonged use), cataracts, dizziness, dry throat, dyspnea, fatigue, glaucoma, growth suppression, hoarseness, hypersensitivity, insomnia, intraocular pressure increased, nasal septum perforation, oral candidiasis, osteoporosis (rare; prolonged use), pruritus, sneezing, throat irritation, urticaria (rare), wheezing, wound healing impaired

Injection:

Frequency not defined; reactions reported with corticosteroid therapy in general:
- Cardiovascular: Arrhythmia, bradycardia, cardiac arrest, cardiac enlargement, CHF, circulatory collapse, edema, hypertension, hypertrophic cardiomyopathy (premature infants), myocardial rupture (following recent MI), syncope, tachycardia, thromboembolism, vasculitis
- Central nervous system: Arachnoiditis (I.T.), depression, emotional instability, euphoria, headache, insomnia, intracranial pressure increased, malaise, meningitis (I.T.), mood changes, neuritis, neuropathy, personality change, pseudotumor cerebri (with discontinuation), seizure, vertigo
- Dermatologic: Abscess (sterile), acne, allergic dermatitis, angioedema, atrophy (cutaneous/subcutaneous), bruising, dry skin, erythema, hair thinning, hirsutism, hyper-/hypopigmentation, hypertrichosis, impaired wound healing, lupus erythematosus-like lesions, petechiae, purpura, rash, skin test suppression, striae, thin skin
- Endocrine & metabolic: Carbohydrate intolerance, Cushingoid state, diabetes mellitus, fluid retention, glucose intolerance, growth suppression (children), hypokalemia, hypokalemic alkalosis, menstrual irregularities, negative nitrogen balance, sodium retention, sperm motility altered
- Gastrointestinal: Abdominal distention, appetite increased, GI hemorrhage, GI perforation, nausea, pancreatitis, peptic ulcer, ulcerative esophagitis, weight gain
- Hepatic: Hepatomegaly, liver function tests increased
- Local: Thrombophlebitis
- Neuromuscular & skeletal: Aseptic necrosis of femoral and humeral heads, calcinosis, Charcot-like arthropathy, fractures, joint tissue damage, muscle mass loss, myopathy, osteoporosis, parasthesia, tendon rupture, vertebral compression fractures, weakness
- Ocular: Cataracts, exophthalmos, glaucoma, ocular pressure increased, papilledema
- Renal: Glycosuria
- Respiratory: Pulmonary edema
- Miscellaneous: Abnormal fat deposits, anaphylactoid reaction, anaphylaxis, diaphoresis, hiccups, infection, moon face

Ophthalmic:

>10%: Ocular: Cataract progression (20% to 60%), intraocular pressure increased (20% to 60%)

1% to 10%: Ocular: ≤2%: Blurred vision, conjunctival hemorrhage, discomfort (transient), endophthalmitis, glaucoma, hypopyon, inflammation, optic disc vascular disorder, retinal detachment, vitreous floaters, visual acuity decreased

<1%, postmarketing, and/or case reports: Exophthalmos

Topical:

Frequency not defined:
- Dermatologic: Acneiform eruptions, allergic contact dermatitis, dryness, folliculitis,, hypertrichosis, hypopigmentation, itching, miliaria, perioral dermatitis, skin atrophy, skin infection (secondary), skin maceration, striae
- Local: Burning, irritation

Drug Interactions

Avoid Concomitant Use

Avoid concomitant use of Triamcinolone with any of the following: Natalizumab; Vaccines (Live)

Increased Effect/Toxicity

Triamcinolone may increase the levels/effects of: Acetylcholinesterase Inhibitors; Amphotericin B; CycloSPORINE; Loop Diuretics; Natalizumab; NSAID (COX-2 Inhibitor); NSAID (Nonselective); Thiazide Diuretics; Vaccines (Live); Warfarin

The levels/effects of Triamcinolone may be increased by: Antifungal Agents (Azole Derivatives, Systemic); Aprepitant; Calcium Channel Blockers (Nondihydropyridine); CycloSPORINE; Estrogen Derivatives; Fluconazole; Fosaprepitant; Macrolide Antibiotics; Neuromuscular-Blocking Agents (Nondepolarizing); Quinolone Antibiotics; Salicylates; Trastuzumab

Decreased Effect

Triamcinolone may decrease the levels/effects of: Antidiabetic Agents; Calcitriol; Corticorelin; Isoniazid; Salicylates; Vaccines (Inactivated)

The levels/effects of Triamcinolone may be decreased by: Aminoglutethimide; Barbiturates; Echinacea; Primidone; Rifamycin Derivatives

Ethanol/Nutrition/Herb Interactions

Ethanol: Avoid ethanol (may enhance gastric mucosal irritation).

Food: Triamcinolone interferes with calcium absorption.

Herb/Nutraceutical: Avoid cat's claw, echinacea (have immunostimulant properties).

Stability

Injection, suspension:

Acetonide injectable suspension:

Kenalog®: Store at 20°C to 25°C (68°F to 77°F); avoid freezing. Protect from light.

Triesence™ : Store at 4°C to 25°C (39°F to 77°F); do not freeze. Protect from light.

Trivaris™: Store at 2°C to 8°C (36°F to 46°F); avoid freezing. Protect from light.

Hexacetonide injectable suspension: Avoid diluents containing parabens, phenol, or other preservatives (may cause flocculation). Diluted suspension stable up to 1 week. Suspension for intralesional use may be diluted with D_5NS, $D_{10}NS$ or SWFI to a 1:1, 1:2, or 1:4 concentration. Solutions for intra-articular use, may be diluted with lidocaine 1% or 2%.

Inhalation, oral: Store at controlled room temperature of 20°C to 25°C (68°F to 77°F); avoid excessive heat. Do not puncture.

Intranasal: Store at controlled room temperature of 20°C to 25°C (68°F to 77°F); do not freeze.

Topical:

Ointment: Store at room temperature.

Spray: Store at room temperature; avoid excessive heat.

Mechanism of Action Decreases inflammation by suppression of migration of polymorphonuclear leukocytes and reversal of increased capillary permeability; suppresses the immune system by reducing activity and volume of the lymphatic system; suppresses adrenal function at high doses

Pharmacodynamics/Kinetics

Duration: Oral: 8-12 hours

Absorption: Topical: Systemic

Distribution: V_d: 99.5 L

Protein binding: ~68%

Time to peak: I.M.: 8-10 hours

Half-life elimination: Biologic: 18-36 hours; Intravitreal: Nonvitrectomized patients: 13-24 days, Vitrectomized patients: ~3 days (based upon 1 patient)

Excretion: Urine (~40%); feces (~60%)

Dosage The lowest possible dose should be used to control the condition; when dose reduction is possible, the dose should be reduced gradually. Parenteral dose is usually 1/3 to 1/2 the oral dose given every 12 hours. In life-threatening situations, parenteral doses larger than the oral dose may be needed.

Injection:

Acetonide:

Intra-articular, intrabursal, tendon sheaths: Adults: Initial: Smaller joints: 2.5-5 mg, larger joints: 5-15 mg; may require up to 10 mg for small joints and up to 40 mg for large joints; maximum dose/treatment (several joints at one time): 20-80 mg

Intradermal: Adults: Initial: 1 mg

I.M.: Range: 2.5-100 mg/day

Children: Initial: 0.11-1.6 mg/kg/day in 3-4 divided doses

Children 6-12 years: Initial: 40 mg

Children >12 years and Adults: Initial: 60 mg

Hay fever/pollen asthma: 40-100 mg as a single injection/season

Multiple sclerosis (acute exacerbation): 160 mg daily for 1 week, followed by 64 mg every other day for 1 month

Hexacetonide: Adults:

Intralesional, sublesional: Up to 0.5 mg/square inch of affected skin; range: 2-48 mg

Intra-articular: Large joints: 10-20 mg; small joints: 2-6 mg

Triamcinolone Dosing

	Acetonide	Hexacetonide
Intrasynovial	5-40 mg	
Intralesional	1-30 mg (usually 1 mg per injection site); 10 mg/mL suspension usually used	Up to 0.5 mg/sq inch affected area
Sublesional	1-30 mg	
Systemic I.M.	2.5-60 mg/dose (usual adult dose: 60 mg; may repeat with 20-100 mg dose when symptoms recur)	
Intra-articular	2.5-40 mg	2-20 mg average
large joints	5-15 mg	10-20 mg
small joints	2.5-5 mg	2-6 mg
Tendon sheaths	2.5-10 mg	
Intradermal	1 mg/site	

Intranasal: Perennial allergic rhinitis, seasonal allergic rhinitis:

Nasal spray:

Children 2-5 years: 110 mcg/day as 1 spray in each nostril once daily (maximum: 110 mcg/day)

Children 6-11 years: Initial: 110 mcg/day as 1 spray in each nostril once daily; may increase to 220 mcg/day as 2 sprays in each nostril if response not adequate; once symptoms controlled may reduce to 110 mcg/day

Children ≥12 years and Adults: 220 mcg/day as 2 sprays in each nostril once daily; once symptoms controlled reduce to 110 mcg/day

Nasal inhaler:

Children 6-11 years: Initial: 220 mcg/day as 2 sprays in each nostril once daily

Children ≥12 years and Adults: Initial: 220 mcg/day as 2 sprays in each nostril once daily; may increase dose to 440 mcg/day (given once daily or divided and given 2 or 4 times/day)

Ophthalmic injection: Intravitreal: Children and Adults

Ocular disease: Initial: 4 mg as a single dose; additional doses may be given as needed over the course of treatment

Visualization during vitrectomy (Triesence™): 1-4 mg

Oral inhalation: Asthma:

Children 6-12 years: 75-150 mcg 3-4 times/day **or** 150-300 mcg twice daily; maximum dose: 900 mcg/day

Children >12 years and Adults: 150 mcg 3-4 times/day **or** 300 mcg twice daily; maximum dose: 1200 mcg/day

NIH Asthma Guidelines (NIH, 2007) (administer in divided doses twice daily):

Children: 5-11 years:

"Low" dose: 300-600 mcg/day

"Medium" dose: >600-900 mcg/day

"High" dose: >900 mcg/day

Children ≥12 years and Adults:

"Low" dose: 300-750 mcg/day

"Medium" dose: >750-1500 mcg/day

"High" dose: >1500 mcg/day

Oral topical: Oral inflammatory lesions/ulcers: Press a small dab (about 1/4 inch) to the lesion until a thin film develops. A larger quantity may be required for coverage of some lesions. For optimal results use only enough to coat the lesion with a thin film; do not rub in.

Topical:

Cream, Ointment:

0.025%: Apply thin film to affected areas 2-4 times/day

0.1% or 0.5%: Apply thin film to affected areas 2-3 times/day

Spray: Apply to affected area 3-4 times/day

Dietary Considerations May be taken with food to decrease GI distress. Ensure adequate intake of calcium and vitamins (or consider supplementation) in patients on medium-to-high doses of systemic corticosteroids.

Administration

Injection: Shake well prior to use. Avoid injecting into a previously infected joint; do not inject into unstable joints

I.M.: Inject deep in large muscle mass, avoid deltoid.

SubQ: Avoid subcutaneous administration.

Trivaris™: Can be administered intravitreally also; **not for I.V. use**. Bring to room temperature prior to administration. A 27 gauge 1/2-inch needle is recommended for intravitreal administration.

Nasal spray, inhalation: Shake well prior to use. Gently blow nose to clear nostrils.

Nasacort® AQ: Prime prior to first use, by shaking contents well and releasing 5 sprays into the air. If product is not used for more than 2 weeks, reprime with 1 spray.

Ophthalmic injection (intravitreal): Triescence™: Not for I.V. use. Shake vial well prior to use. Administer under controlled aseptic conditions (eg, sterile gloves, sterile drape, sterile eyelid speculum). Adequate anesthesia and a broad-spectrum bactericidal agent should be administered prior to injection. Inject immediately after withdrawing from vial. If administration is required in the second eye, a new vial should be used. Do not use if agglomerated (clumpy or granular appearance).

Oral inhalation: Shake well prior to use. Rinse mouth and throat after using inhaler to prevent candidiasis. Use spacer device provided with Azmacort®. To prime inhaler prior to first use, shake inhaler, then press cannister to release 2 puffs. Inhaler will need to reprimed if not used for longer than 3 days.

Oral topical: Apply small dab to lesion until a thin film develops; do not rub in. Apply at bedtime or after meals if applications are needed throughout the day.

Topical:

Ointment: Apply a thin film sparingly. Do not use on open skin or wounds. Do not occlude area unless directed; if using occluding dressing, monitor for infection.

Spray: Avoid eyes and do not inhale if spraying near face. Occlusive dressing may be used if instructed; monitor for infection.

Monitoring Parameters Ophthalmic injection (intravitreal): Following injection monitor for increased intraocular pressure and endophthalmitis; check for perfusion of optic nerve head immediately after injection, tonometry within 30 minutes, biomicroscopy between 2-7 days after injection.

Additional Information 16 mg triamcinolone is equivalent to 100 mg cortisone (no mineralocorticoid activity).

Effects of inhaled/intranasal steroids on growth have been observed in the absence of laboratory evidence of HPA axis suppression, suggesting that growth velocity is a more sensitive indicator of systemic corticosteroid exposure in pediatric patients than some commonly used tests of HPA axis function. The long-term effects of this reduction in growth velocity associated with orally-inhaled and intranasal corticosteroids, including the impact on final adult height, are unknown. The potential for "catch up" growth following discontinuation of treatment with inhaled corticosteroids has not been adequately studied.

Product Availability Trivaris™: FDA approved June 2008; availability currently undetermined

Dosage Forms Excipient information presented when available (limited, particularly for generics); consult specific product labeling. [DSC] = Discontinued product

Aerosol for oral inhalation, as acetonide:

Azmacort®: 75 mcg per actuation (20 g) [contains chlorofluorocarbon; 240 actuations]

Aerosol, topical, as acetonide:

Kenalog®: 0.2 mg/2-second spray (63 g) [contains dehydrated ethanol 10.3%]

Cream, as acetonide: 0.025% (15 g, 80 g, 454 g); 0.1% (15 g, 80 g, 454 g, 2270 g); 0.5% (15 g)

Triderm®: 0.1% (30 g, 85 g)

Zytopic™: 0.1% (85 g)

Injection, suspension, as acetonide:

Kenalog-10®: 10 mg/mL (5 mL) [contains benzyl alcohol, polysorbate 80; not for I.V. or I.M. use]

Kenalog-40®: 40 mg/mL (1 mL, 5 mL, 10 mL) [contains benzyl alcohol, polysorbate 80; not for I.V. or intradermal use]

Triesence™: 40 mg/mL (1 mL) [contains polysorbate 80; not for I.V. use]

Trivaris™: 80 mg/mL (0.1 mL) [preservative free; not for I.V. use; (for intra-articular, intramuscular, intravitreal use)]

Injection, suspension, as hexacetonide:

Aristospan®: 5 mg/mL (5 mL); 20 mg/mL (1 mL, 5 mL) [contains benzyl alcohol, polysorbate 80; not for I.V. use]

Lotion, as acetonide: 0.025% (60 mL); 0.1% (60 mL)

Ointment, topical, as acetonide: 0.025% (15 g, 80 g, 454 g); 0.05% (430 g); 0.1% (15 g, 80 g, 454 g); 0.5% (15 g)

Paste, oral, topical, as acetonide: 0.1% (5 g)

Powder, for prescription compounding, as acetonide [micronized]: Triamcinolone acetonide USP (5 g)

Solution, intranasal, as acetonide [spray]:

Tri-Nasal®: 50 mcg/inhalation (15 mL) [120 actuations] [DSC]

Suspension, intranasal, as acetonide [spray]:

Nasacort® AQ: 55 mcg/inhalation (16.5 g) [120 actuations]

- **Triamcinolone Acetonide, Aerosol** *see* Triamcinolone *on page 1510*
- **Triamcinolone Acetonide, Parenteral** *see* Triamcinolone *on page 1510*
- **Triamcinolone and Nystatin** *see* Nystatin and Triamcinolone *on page 1087*
- **Triamcinolone Diacetate, Oral** *see* Triamcinolone *on page 1510*
- **Triamcinolone Diacetate, Parenteral** *see* Triamcinolone *on page 1510*
- **Triamcinolone Hexacetonide** *see* Triamcinolone *on page 1510*
- **Triamcinolone, Oral** *see* Triamcinolone *on page 1510*
- **Triaminic® Cold & Allergy (Can)** *see* Chlorpheniramine and Pseudoephedrine *on page 310*
- **Triaminic® Cold and Allergy [OTC]** *see* Chlorpheniramine and Phenylephrine *on page 309*
- **Triaminic® Infant Thin Strips® Decongestant [OTC] [DSC]** *see* Phenylephrine *on page 1183*
- **Triaminic® Thin Strips® Cold [OTC]** *see* Phenylephrine *on page 1183*
- **Triaminic® Thin Strips™ Cough and Runny Nose [OTC]** *see* DiphenhydrAMINE *on page 456*

Triamterene (trye AM ter een)

U.S. Brand Names Dyrenium®

Pharmacologic Category Diuretic, Potassium-Sparing

Use Alone or in combination with other diuretics in treatment of edema and hypertension; decreases potassium excretion caused by kaliuretic diuretics

Pregnancy Risk Factor B (manufacturer); D (expert analysis)

Medication Safety Issues
Sound-alike/look-alike issues:
Triamterene may be confused with trimipramine
Dyrenium® may be confused with Pyridium®

Dosage Oral:
Children (unlabeled use): Hypertension: Initial: 1-2 mg/kg/day in 2 divided doses; maximum: 3-4 mg/kg/day, up to 300 mg/day
Adults: Hypertension, edema: 100-300 mg/day in 1-2 divided doses; maximum dose: 300 mg/day; usual dosage range (JNC 7): 50-100 mg/day
Dosing comments in renal impairment: Cl_{cr} <10 mL/minute: Avoid use.
Dosing adjustment in hepatic impairment: Dose reduction is recommended in patients with cirrhosis.

Additional Information Complete prescribing information for this medication should be consulted for additional detail.

Dosage Forms Excipient information presented when available (limited, particularly for generics); consult specific product labeling.
Capsule: 50 mg, 100 mg [contains benzyl alcohol]

- ◆ **Triamterene and Hydrochlorothiazide** *see* Hydrochlorothiazide and Triamterene *on page* 739
- ◆ **Triatec-8 (Can)** *see* Acetaminophen and Codeine *on page* 27
- ◆ **Triatec-8 Strong (Can)** *see* Acetaminophen and Codeine *on page* 27
- ◆ **Triatec-30 (Can)** *see* Acetaminophen and Codeine *on page* 27

Triazolam (trye AY zoe lam)

U.S. Brand Names Halcion®
Canadian Brand Names Apo-Triazo®; Gen-Triazolam; Halcion®
Pharmacologic Category Hypnotic, Benzodiazepine
Additional Appendix Information
Benzodiazepines *on page* 1646
Use Short-term treatment of insomnia
Restrictions C-IV

An FDA-approved patient medication guide is available and must be distributed when dispensing an outpatient prescription (new or refill) where this medication is to be used without direct supervision of a healthcare provider. Medication guides are available at http://www.fda.gov/cder/Offices/ODS/medication_guides.htm.

Pregnancy Risk Factor X

Medication Safety Issues
Sound-alike/look-alike issues:
Triazolam may be confused with alPRAZolam
Halcion® may be confused with halcinonide, Haldol®

Dosage Oral (onset of action is rapid, patient should be in bed when taking medication):
Children <18 years: Dosage not established
Adults:
Insomnia (short-term): 0.125-0.25 mg at bedtime (maximum dose: 0.5 mg/day)
Preprocedure sedation (dental): 0.25 mg taken the evening before oral surgery; or 0.25 mg 1 hour before procedure
Elderly: Insomnia (short-term use): Initial: 0.125 mg at bedtime; maximum dose: 0.25 mg/day
Dosing adjustment/comments in hepatic impairment: Reduce dose or avoid use in cirrhosis

Additional Information Complete prescribing information for this medication should be consulted for additional detail.

Dosage Forms Excipient information presented when available (limited, particularly for generics); consult specific product labeling. [DSC] = Discontinued product
Tablet: 0.125 mg, 0.25 mg
Halcion®: 0.125 mg [DSC], 0.25 mg

- ◆ **Tribavirin** *see* Ribavirin *on page* 1310
- ◆ **Tricardio B** *see* Folic Acid, Cyanocobalamin, and Pyridoxine *on page* 655
- ◆ **Trichloroacetaldehyde Monohydrate** *see* Chloral Hydrate *on page* 300
- ◆ **Trichloromonofluoromethane and Dichlorodifluoromethane** *see* Dichlorodifluoromethane and Trichloromonofluoromethane *on page* 437
- ◆ **Tricitrates** *see* Citric Acid, Sodium Citrate, and Potassium Citrate *on page* 339
- ◆ **TriCor®** *see* Fenofibrate *on page* 607
- ◆ **Tricosal** *see* Choline Magnesium Trisalicylate *on page* 319
- ◆ **Tri-Cyclen® (Can)** *see* Ethinyl Estradiol and Norgestimate *on page* 584
- ◆ **Tri-Cyclen® Lo (Can)** *see* Ethinyl Estradiol and Norgestimate *on page* 584
- ◆ **Triderm®** *see* Triamcinolone *on page* 1510
- ◆ **Tridural™ (Can)** *see* TraMADol *on page* 1497
- ◆ **Trien** *see* Trientine *on page* 1515

Trientine (TRYE en teen)

U.S. Brand Names Syprine®
Canadian Brand Names Syprine®
Index Terms 2,2,2-tetramine; Trien; Trientine Hydrochloride; Triethylene Tetramine Dihydrochloride
Pharmacologic Category Chelating Agent
Use Treatment of Wilson's disease in patients intolerant to penicillamine
Pregnancy Risk Factor C
Lactation Excretion in breast milk unknown/use caution

Medication Safety Issues
Sound-alike/look-alike issues:
Trientine may be confused with Trental®, tretinoin

Contraindications Hypersensitivity to trientine or any component of the formulation

Warnings/Precautions May cause iron-deficiency anemia, copper deficiency and subsequent iron overload and/or sideroblastic anemia. Monitor patients for neurologic worsening with initiation of therapy; can rarely occur. Monitor for development of hypersensitivity reactions.

Adverse Reactions Frequency not defined.
Central nervous system: Dystonia, malaise
Dermatologic: Rash, thickening and fissuring of skin
Endocrine & metabolic: Iron deficiency
Gastrointestinal: Abdominal pain, anorexia, aphthoid ulcer, colitis, epigastric pain, gastritis, heartburn, loss of taste
Hematologic: Aplastic anemia (rare), anemia, sideroblastic anemia (reversible)
Hepatic: Iron overload
Local: Tenderness
Neuromuscular & skeletal: Muscle cramps, muscle pain, muscular spasm, myasthenia gravis, rhabdomyolysis, weakness
Miscellaneous: Fixed drug eruption, lupus-like reactions

Drug Interactions
Avoid Concomitant Use There are no known interactions where it is recommended to avoid concomitant use.
Increased Effect/Toxicity There are no known significant interactions involving an increase in effect.
Decreased Effect
Trientine may decrease the levels/effects of: Calcium Salts; Iron Salts; Magnesium Salts; Zinc Salts

The levels/effects of Trientine may be decreased by: Antacids; Calcium Salts; Carbonic Anhydrase Inhibitor Diuretics; Iron Salts; Magnesium Salts; Zinc Salts

Stability Store at 2°C to 8°C (36°F to 46°F).

Mechanism of Action Trientine hydrochloride is an oral chelating agent structurally dissimilar from penicillamine and other available chelating agents; an effective oral chelator of copper used to induce adequate cupriuresis

Pharmacodynamics/Kinetics

Absorption: Poor

Metabolism: To acetyltrien (chelating activity significantly less than parent)

Excretion: Urine (1% as parent; 8% as metabolite)

Dosage Oral (administer on an empty stomach):

Children <12 years: 500-750 mg/day in divided doses 2-4 times/day; maximum: 1.5 g/day. The practice guideline suggests 20 mg/kg/day rounded off to the nearest 250 mg, given in 2-3 divided doses (Roberts, 2003).

Children ≥12 years and Adults: 750-1250 mg/day in divided doses 2-4 times/day; maximum dose: 2 g/day. The practice guideline suggests typical doses of 750-1500 mg/day in 2-3 divided doses with maintenance therapy of 750-1000 mg/day (Roberts, 2003)

Dietary Considerations Should be taken 1 hour before or 2 hours after meals and at least 1 hour apart from any drug, food, or milk.

Administration Do not chew capsule, swallow whole followed by a full glass of water; notify healthcare provider of any fever or skin changes; any skin exposed to the contents of a capsule should be promptly washed with water

Monitoring Parameters Periodic 24-hour urinary copper assessment (every 6-12 months); free serum copper level

Reference Range Urinary copper excretion: 200-500 mcg (3-8 micromoles)/day

Dosage Forms Excipient information presented when available (limited, particularly for generics); consult specific product labeling.

Capsule, as hydrochloride: 250 mg

- **Trientine Hydrochloride** *see* Trientine *on page 1515*
- **Triesence™** *see* Triamcinolone *on page 1510*

Triethanolamine Polypeptide Oleate-Condensate

(trye eth a NOLE a meen pol i PEP tide OH lee ate-KON den sate)

U.S. Brand Names Cerumenex® [DSC]

Canadian Brand Names Cerumenex®

Pharmacologic Category Otic Agent, Cerumenolytic

Use Removal of ear wax (cerumen)

Pregnancy Risk Factor C

Dosage Children and Adults: Otic: Fill ear canal, insert cotton plug; allow to remain 15-30 minutes; flush ear with lukewarm water as a single treatment; if a second application is needed for unusually hard impactions, repeat the procedure

Additional Information Complete prescribing information for this medication should be consulted for additional detail.

Dosage Forms Excipient information presented when available (limited, particularly for generics); consult specific product labeling. [DSC] = Discontinued product

Solution, otic: 10% (6 mL, 12 mL) [DSC]

- **Triethylene Tetramine Dihydrochloride** *see* Trientine *on page 1515*
- **Triethylenethiophosphoramide** *see* Thiotepa *on page 1462*

Trifluoperazine (trye floo oh PER a zeen)

Canadian Brand Names Apo-Trifluoperazine®; Novo-Trifluzine; PMS-Trifluoperazine; Terfluzine

Index Terms Trifluoperazine Hydrochloride

Pharmacologic Category Antipsychotic Agent, Typical, Phenothiazine

Additional Appendix Information

Antipsychotic Agents *on page 1644*

Use Treatment of schizophrenia

Unlabeled/Investigational Use Management of psychotic disorders; behavioral symptoms associated with dementia behavior (elderly); psychosis/agitation related to Alzheimer's dementia

Pregnancy Risk Factor C

Lactation Enters breast milk/not recommended (AAP rates "of concern")

Medication Safety Issues

Sound-alike/look-alike issues:

Trifluoperazine may be confused with triflupromazine, trihexyphenidyl

Stelazine® may be confused with selegiline

Contraindications Hypersensitivity to trifluoperazine or any component of the formulation (cross-reactivity between phenothiazines may occur); severe CNS depression; bone marrow suppression; blood dyscrasias; severe hepatic disease; coma

Warnings/Precautions Elderly patients with dementia-related psychosis treated with antipsychotics are at an increased risk of death compared to placebo. An increased incidence of cerebrovascular adverse events (including fatalities) has been reported in elderly patients with dementia-related psychosis. Trifluoperazine is not approved for this indication.

May be sedating, use with caution in disorders where CNS depression is a feature. Use with caution in Parkinson's disease. Caution in patients with hemodynamic instability; predisposition to seizures; subcortical brain damage; hepatic impairment; severe cardiac, renal, or respiratory disease. Esophageal dysmotility and aspiration have been associated with antipsychotic use - use with caution in patients at risk of pneumonia (ie, Alzheimer's disease). Caution in breast cancer or other prolactin-dependent tumors (may elevate prolactin levels). May alter temperature regulation or mask toxicity of other drugs due to antiemetic effects. May alter cardiac conduction - life-threatening arrhythmias have occurred with therapeutic doses of phenothiazines. May cause orthostatic hypotension - use with caution in patients at risk of this effect or those who would tolerate transient hypotensive episodes (cerebrovascular disease, cardiovascular disease or other medications which may predispose). Check blood counts periodically and discontinue at first signs of blood dyscrasias; use is contraindicated in patients with bone marrow suppression. Safety in children <6 years of age has not been established.

Due to anticholinergic effects, should be used with caution in patients with decreased gastrointestinal motility, urinary retention, BPH, xerostomia, visual problems, narrow-angle glaucoma (screening is recommended) and myasthenia gravis. Relative to other antipsychotics, trifluoperazine has a low potency of cholinergic blockade.

May cause extrapyramidal symptoms (EPS), including pseudoparkinsonism, acute dystonic reactions, akathisia, and tardive dyskinesia (risk of these reactions is high relative to other neuroleptics). Risk of dystonia (and possibly other EPS) may be greater with increased doses, use of conventional antipsychotics, males, and younger patients. Use caution in the elderly. May be associated with neuroleptic malignant syndrome (NMS) or pigmentary retinopathy.

Adverse Reactions Frequency not defined.

Cardiovascular: Hypotension, orthostatic hypotension, cardiac arrest

Central nervous system: Extrapyramidal symptoms (pseudoparkinsonism, akathisia, dystonias, tardive dyskinesia), dizziness, headache, neuroleptic malignant syndrome (NMS), impairment of temperature regulation, lowering of seizure threshold

Dermatologic: Increased sensitivity to sun, rash, discoloration of skin (blue-gray), photosensitivity

Endocrine & metabolic: Changes in menstrual cycle, libido (changes in), breast pain, hyperglycemia, hypoglycemia, gynecomastia, lactation, galactorrhea

Gastrointestinal: Constipation, weight gain, nausea, vomiting, stomach pain, xerostomia

Genitourinary: Difficulty in urination, ejaculatory disturbances, urinary retention, priapism

Hematologic: Agranulocytosis, leukopenia, pancytopenia, thrombocytopenic purpura, eosinophilia, hemolytic anemia, aplastic anemia

Hepatic: Cholestatic jaundice, hepatotoxicity

Neuromuscular & skeletal: Tremor

Ocular: Pigmentary retinopathy, cornea and lens changes

Respiratory: Nasal congestion

Drug Interactions

Metabolism/Transport Effects Substrate of CYP1A2 (major)

Avoid Concomitant Use There are no known interactions where it is recommended to avoid concomitant use.

Increased Effect/Toxicity

Trifluoperazine may increase the levels/effects of: Alcohol (Ethyl); Analgesics (Opioid); Anticholinergics; Beta-Blockers; CNS Depressants

The levels/effects of Trifluoperazine may be increased by: Acetylcholinesterase Inhibitors (Central); Antimalarial Agents; Beta-Blockers; CYP1A2 Inhibitors (Moderate); CYP1A2 Inhibitors (Strong); Lithium formulations; Pramlintide; Tetrabenazine

Decreased Effect

Trifluoperazine may decrease the levels/effects of: Amphetamines; Anti-Parkinson's Agents (Dopamine Agonist)

The levels/effects of Trifluoperazine may be decreased by: Antacids; CYP1A2 Inducers (Strong); Lithium formulations

Ethanol/Nutrition/Herb Interactions

Ethanol: Avoid ethanol (may increase CNS depression).

Herb/Nutraceutical: Avoid kava kava, gotu kola, valerian, St John's wort (may increase CNS depression). Avoid dong quai, St John's wort (may also cause photosensitization).

Mechanism of Action Trifluoperazine is a piperazine phenothiazine antipsychotic which blocks postsynaptic mesolimbic dopaminergic receptors in the brain; exhibits alpha-adrenergic blocking effect and depresses the release of hypothalamic and hypophyseal hormones

Pharmacodynamics/Kinetics

Metabolism: Extensively hepatic

Half-life elimination: >24 hours with chronic use

Dosage Oral:

Children 6-12 years: Schizophrenia/psychoses: Hospitalized or well-supervised patients: Initial: 1 mg 1-2 times/day, gradually increase until symptoms are controlled or adverse effects become troublesome; maximum: 15 mg/day

Adults:

Schizophrenia/psychoses:

Outpatients: 1-2 mg twice daily

Hospitalized or well-supervised patients: Initial: 2-5 mg twice daily with optimum response in the 15-20 mg/day range; do not exceed 40 mg/day

Nonpsychotic anxiety: 1-2 mg twice daily; maximum: 6 mg/day; therapy for anxiety should not exceed 12 weeks; do not exceed 6 mg/day for longer than 12 weeks when treating anxiety; agitation, jitteriness, or insomnia may be confused with original neurotic or psychotic symptoms

Elderly:

Schizophrenia/psychoses:

Refer to adult dosing. Dose selection should start at the low end of the dosage range and titration must be gradual.

Behavioral symptoms associated with dementia behavior (unlabeled use): Initial: 0.5-1 mg 1-2 times/day; increase dose at 4- to 7-day intervals by 0.5-1 mg/day; increase dosing intervals (bid, tid, etc) as necessary to control response or side effects. Maximum daily dose: 40 mg. Gradual increases (titration) may prevent some side effects or decrease their severity.

Hemodialysis: Not dialyzable (0% to 5%)

Dietary Considerations May be taken with food to decrease GI distress.

Monitoring Parameters Vital signs; lipid profile, fasting blood glucose/Hgb A_{1c}; BMI; mental status, abnormal involuntary movement scale (AIMS)

Reference Range Therapeutic response and blood levels have not been established

Test Interactions False-positive for phenylketonuria

Additional Information Do not exceed 6 mg/day for longer than 12 weeks when treating anxiety. Agitation, jitteriness, or insomnia may be confused with original neurotic or psychotic symptoms.

Dosage Forms Excipient information presented when available (limited, particularly for generics); consult specific product labeling.

Tablet: 1 mg, 2 mg, 5 mg, 10 mg

◆ **Trifluoperazine Hydrochloride** *see* Trifluoperazine *on page 1516*

◆ **Trifluorothymidine** *see* Trifluridine *on page 1517*

Trifluridine (trye FLURE i deen)

U.S. Brand Names Viroptic®

Canadian Brand Names SAB-Trifluridine; Sandoz-Trifluridine; Viroptic®

Index Terms F_3T; Trifluorothymidine

Pharmacologic Category Antiviral Agent, Ophthalmic

Use Treatment of primary keratoconjunctivitis and recurrent epithelial keratitis caused by herpes simplex virus types I and II

Pregnancy Risk Factor C

Medication Safety Issues

Sound-alike/look-alike issues:

Viroptic® may be confused with Timoptic®

Dosage Adults: Instill 1 drop into affected eye every 2 hours while awake, to a maximum of 9 drops/day, until re-epithelialization of corneal ulcer occurs; then use 1 drop every 4 hours for another 7 days; do **not** exceed 21 days of treatment; if improvement has not taken place in 7-14 days, consider another form of therapy

Additional Information Complete prescribing information for this medication should be consulted for additional detail.

Dosage Forms Excipient information presented when available (limited, particularly for generics); consult specific product labeling.

Solution, ophthalmic: 1% (7.5 mL)

Viroptic®: 1% (7.5 mL)

◆ **Triglide™** *see* Fenofibrate *on page 607*

Trihexyphenidyl (trye heks ee FEN i dil)

Canadian Brand Names Apo-Trihex®

Index Terms Artane; Benzhexol Hydrochloride; Trihexyphenidyl Hydrochloride

Pharmacologic Category Anti-Parkinson's Agent, Anticholinergic; Anticholinergic Agent

Additional Appendix Information

Antiparkinsonian Agents *on page 1643*

Use Adjunctive treatment of Parkinson's disease; treatment of drug-induced extrapyramidal symptoms

Pregnancy Risk Factor C

Lactation Excretion in breast milk unknown/use caution

Medication Safety Issues

Sound-alike/look-alike issues:

Trihexyphenidyl may be confused with trifluoperazine

Artane may be confused with Altace®, Anturane®, Aramine®

Contraindications Hypersensitivity to trihexyphenidyl or any component of the formulation; narrow-angle glaucoma; pyloric or duodenal obstruction; stenosing peptic ulcers; bladder neck obstructions; achalasia; myasthenia gravis

Warnings/Precautions Use with caution in hot weather or during exercise, especially when administered concomitantly with other atropine-like drugs to chronically-ill patients, alcoholics, patients with CNS disease, or persons doing manual labor in a hot environment. Elderly patients require strict dosage regulation. Use with caution in patients with tachycardia, cardiac arrhythmias, hypertension, hypotension, glaucoma, prostatic hyperplasia or any tendency toward urinary retention, liver or kidney disorders, and obstructive disease of the GI or GU tract. May exacerbate mental symptoms when used to treat extrapyramidal symptoms. When given in large doses or to susceptible patients, may cause weakness. Does not improve symptoms of tardive dyskinesias.

Adverse Reactions Frequency not defined.

Cardiovascular: Tachycardia

Central nervous system: Confusion, agitation, euphoria, drowsiness, headache, dizziness, nervousness, delusions, hallucinations, paranoia

Dermatologic: Dry skin, increased sensitivity to light, rash

Gastrointestinal: Constipation, xerostomia, dry throat, ileus, nausea, vomiting, parotitis

Genitourinary: Urinary retention

Neuromuscular & skeletal: Weakness

Ocular: Blurred vision, mydriasis, increase in intraocular pressure, glaucoma, blindness (long-term use in narrow-angle glaucoma)

Respiratory: Dry nose

Miscellaneous: Diaphoresis (decreased)

Drug Interactions

Avoid Concomitant Use There are no known interactions where it is recommended to avoid concomitant use.

Increased Effect/Toxicity

Trihexyphenidyl may increase the levels/effects of: Anticholinergics; Cannabinoids; Potassium Chloride

The levels/effects of Trihexyphenidyl may be increased by: Pramlintide

Decreased Effect

Trihexyphenidyl may decrease the levels/effects of: Acetylcholinesterase Inhibitors (Central); Secretin

The levels/effects of Trihexyphenidyl may be decreased by: Acetylcholinesterase Inhibitors (Central)

Ethanol/Nutrition/Herb Interactions Ethanol: Avoid ethanol (may increase CNS depression).

Mechanism of Action Exerts a direct inhibitory effect on the parasympathetic nervous system. It also has a relaxing effect on smooth musculature; exerted both directly on the muscle itself and indirectly through parasympathetic nervous system (inhibitory effect)

Pharmacodynamics/Kinetics

Onset of action: Peak effect: ~1 hour

Half-life elimination: 3.3-4.1 hours

Time to peak, serum: 1-1.5 hours

Excretion: Primarily urine

Dosage Adults: Oral: Initial: 1-2 mg/day, increase by 2 mg increments at intervals of 3-5 days; usual dose: 5-15 mg/day in 3-4 divided doses

Administration Tolerated best if given in 3 daily doses and with food. High doses may be divided into 4 doses, at meal times and at bedtime. Patients may be switched to sustained-action capsules when stabilized on conventional dosage forms.

Monitoring Parameters IOP monitoring and gonioscopic evaluations should be performed periodically

Additional Information Incidence and severity of side effects are dose related. Patients may be switched to sustained-action capsules when stabilized on conventional dosage forms.

Dosage Forms Excipient information presented when available (limited, particularly for generics); consult specific product labeling.

Elixir, as hydrochloride: 2 mg/5 mL (480 mL)

Tablet, as hydrochloride: 2 mg, 5 mg

- **Trihexyphenidyl Hydrochloride** *see* Trihexyphenidyl *on page 1518*
- **TriHIBit®** *see* Diphtheria and Tetanus Toxoids, Acellular Pertussis, and *Haemophilus influenzae* b Conjugate Vaccine *on page 462*
- **Tri-Hist** *see* Chlorpheniramine, Pyrilamine, and Phenylephrine *on page 315*
- **Trikacide (Can)** *see* MetroNIDAZOLE *on page 984*
- **Trikof-D® [DSC]** *see* Guaifenesin, Pseudoephedrine, and Dextromethorphan *on page 715*
- **Trileptal®** *see* OXcarbazepine *on page 1116*
- **TriLipix™** *see* Fenofibric Acid *on page 609*
- **Tri-Luma™** *see* Fluocinolone, Hydroquinone, and Tretinoin *on page 633*
- **TriLyte®** *see* Polyethylene Glycol-Electrolyte Solution *on page 1209*

Trimethobenzamide (trye meth oh BEN za mide)

U.S. Brand Names Tigan®

Canadian Brand Names Tigan®

Index Terms Trimethobenzamide Hydrochloride

Pharmacologic Category Anticholinergic Agent; Antiemetic

Use Treatment of postoperative nausea and vomiting; treatment of nausea associated with gastroenteritis

Pregnancy Considerations Teratogenic effects were not observed in animal studies. Safety and efficacy have not been established in pregnant patients. Trimethobenzamide has been used to treat nausea and vomiting of pregnancy.

Lactation Excretion in breast milk unknown

Medication Safety Issues

Sound-alike/look-alike issues:

Tigan® may be confused with Tiazac®, Ticar®, Ticlid®

Trimethobenzamide may be confused with metoclopramide, trimethoprim

Contraindications Hypersensitivity to trimethobenzamide or any component of the formulation; injection contraindicated in children

Warnings/Precautions May mask emesis due to Reye's syndrome or mimic CNS effects of Reye's syndrome in patients with emesis of other etiologies. Antiemetic effects may mask toxicity of other drugs or conditions (eg, intestinal obstruction). May cause drowsiness; patient should avoid tasks requiring alertness (eg, driving, operating machinery). May cause extrapyramidal symptoms (EPS) which may be confused with CNS symptoms of primary disease responsible for emesis. Risk of CNS adverse effects (eg, coma, EPS, seizure) may be increased in patients with acute febrile illness, dehydration, electrolyte imbalance, encephalitis, or gastroenteritis; use caution. Allergic-type skin reactions have been reported with use; discontinue with signs of sensitization. Trimethobenzamide clearance is predominantly renal; dosage reductions may be recommended in patient with renal impairment. Use capsule formulation with caution in children; antiemetics are not recommended for uncomplicated vomiting in children, limit antiemetic use to prolonged vomiting of known etiology. Use of injection is contraindicated in children.

Adverse Reactions Frequency not defined.

Cardiovascular: Hypotension (I.V. administration)

Central nervous system: Coma, depression, disorientation, dizziness, drowsiness, EPS, headache, Parkinson-like symptoms, seizure

Dermatologic: Allergic-type skin reactions

Gastrointestinal: Diarrhea

Hematologic: Blood dyscrasias

Hepatic: Jaundice

Local: Injection site burning, pain, redness, stinging, or swelling

Neuromuscular & skeletal: Muscle cramps, opisthotonos

Ocular: Blurred vision

Miscellaneous: Hypersensitivity reactions

Drug Interactions

Avoid Concomitant Use There are no known interactions where it is recommended to avoid concomitant use.

Increased Effect/Toxicity

Trimethobenzamide may increase the levels/effects of: Anticholinergics; Cannabinoids; Potassium Chloride

The levels/effects of Trimethobenzamide may be increased by: Pramlintide

Decreased Effect

Trimethobenzamide may decrease the levels/effects of: Acetylcholinesterase Inhibitors (Central); Secretin

The levels/effects of Trimethobenzamide may be decreased by: Acetylcholinesterase Inhibitors (Central)

Ethanol/Nutrition/Herb Interactions Ethanol: Concomitant use should be avoided (sedative effects may be additive).

Stability Store capsules and injection solution at room temperature of 25°C (77°F); excursions permitted to 15°C to 30°C (59°F to 86°F).

Mechanism of Action Acts centrally to inhibit the medullary chemoreceptor trigger zone by blocking emetic impulses to the vomiting center

Pharmacodynamics/Kinetics

Onset of action: Antiemetic: Oral: 10-40 minutes; I.M.: 15-35 minutes

Duration: 3-4 hours

Metabolism: Via oxidation, forms metabolite trimethobenzamide N-oxide

Bioavailability: Oral: 60% to 100%

Half-life elimination: 7-9 hours

Time to peak: Oral: ~45 minutes; I.M.: ~30 minutes

Excretion: Urine (30% to 50%, as unchanged drug)

Dosage

Children >40 kg: Oral: 300 mg 3-4 times/day

Adults:

Oral: 300 mg 3-4 times/day

I.M.: 200 mg 3-4 times/day

Postoperative nausea and vomiting (PONV): I.M.: 200 mg, followed 1 hour later by a second 200 mg dose

Elderly: Refer to adult dosing. Consider dosage reduction or increasing dosing interval in elderly patients with renal impairment (specific adjustment guidelines are not provided in the manufacturer's labeling).

Dosage adjustment in renal impairment: Cl_{cr} ≤70 mL/minute: Consider dosage reduction or increasing dosing interval (specific adjustment guidelines are not provided in the manufacturer's labeling)

Administration

Injection: Administer I.M. only; not for I.V. administration. Inject deep into upper outer quadrant of gluteal muscle.

Capsule: Administer capsule orally without regard to meals.

Monitoring Parameters Renal function (at baseline)

Dosage Forms Excipient information presented when available (limited, particularly for generics); consult specific product labeling.

Capsule, as hydrochloride: 300 mg

Tigan®: 300 mg

Injection, solution, as hydrochloride: 100 mg/mL (2 mL)

Tigan®: 100 mg/mL (20 mL)

Injection, solution, as hydrochloride [preservative free]:

Tigan®: 100 mg/mL (2 mL)

◆ **Trimethobenzamide Hydrochloride** *see* Trimethobenzamide *on page 1518*

Trimethoprim (trye METH oh prim)

U.S. Brand Names Primsol®

Canadian Brand Names Apo-Trimethoprim®

Index Terms TMP

Pharmacologic Category Antibiotic, Miscellaneous

Use Treatment of urinary tract infections due to susceptible strains of *E. coli*, *P. mirabilis*, *K. pneumoniae*, *Enterobacter* sp and coagulase-negative *Staphylococcus* including *S. saprophyticus*; acute otitis media in children; acute exacerbations of chronic bronchitis in adults; in combination with other agents for treatment of toxoplasmosis, *Pneumocystis carinii*; treatment of superficial ocular infections involving the conjunctiva and cornea

Pregnancy Risk Factor C

Pregnancy Considerations There are no well-controlled studies on the use of trimethoprim during pregnancy. Because trimethoprim may interfere with folic acid metabolism, consider using only if the potential benefit to the mother outweighs the possible risk to the fetus.

Lactation Enters breast milk/use caution (AAP rates "compatible")

Medication Safety Issues

Sound-alike/look-alike issues:

Trimethoprim may be confused with trimethaphan

Proloprim® may be confused with Prolixin®, Protropin®

Contraindications Hypersensitivity to trimethoprim or any component of the formulation; megaloblastic anemia due to folate deficiency

Warnings/Precautions Use with caution in patients with impaired renal or hepatic function or with possible folate deficiency. Prolonged use may result in fungal or bacterial superinfection, including *C. difficile*-associated diarrhea (CDAD) and pseudomembranous colitis; CDAD has been observed >2 months postantibiotic treatment.

Adverse Reactions Frequency not defined.

Central nervous system: Aseptic meningitis (rare), fever

Dermatologic: Maculopapular rash (3% to 7% at 200 mg/day; incidence higher with larger daily doses), erythema multiforme (rare), exfoliative dermatitis (rare), pruritus (common), phototoxic skin eruptions, Stevens-Johnson syndrome (rare), toxic epidermal necrolysis (rare)

Endocrine & metabolic: Hyperkalemia, hyponatremia

Gastrointestinal: Epigastric distress, glossitis, nausea, vomiting

Hematologic: Leukopenia, megaloblastic anemia, methemoglobinemia, neutropenia, thrombocytopenia
Hepatic: Liver enzyme elevation, cholestatic jaundice (rare)
Renal: BUN and creatinine increased
Miscellaneous: Anaphylaxis, hypersensitivity reactions

Drug Interactions

Metabolism/Transport Effects Substrate (major) of CYP2C9, 3A4; **Inhibits** CYP2C8 (moderate), 2C9 (moderate)

Avoid Concomitant Use

Avoid concomitant use of Trimethoprim with any of the following: Dofetilide

Increased Effect/Toxicity

Trimethoprim may increase the levels/effects of: ACE Inhibitors; Amantadine; Angiotensin II Receptor Blockers; Antidiabetic Agents (Thiazolidinedione); AzaTHIOprine; CYP2C8 Substrates (High risk); CYP2C9 Substrates (High risk); Dapsone; Dofetilide; LamiVUDine; Memantine; Methotrexate; Phenytoin; Procainamide; Repaglinide

The levels/effects of Trimethoprim may be increased by: Amantadine; CYP2C9 Inhibitors (Moderate); CYP2C9 Inhibitors (Strong); Dapsone; Memantine

Decreased Effect

Trimethoprim may decrease the levels/effects of: Typhoid Vaccine

The levels/effects of Trimethoprim may be decreased by: CYP2C9 Inducers (Highly Effective); CYP3A4 Inducers (Strong); Deferasirox; Herbs (CYP3A4 Inducers); Leucovorin-Levoleucovorin

Stability Protect the 200 mg tablet from light.

Mechanism of Action Inhibits folic acid reduction to tetrahydrofolate, and thereby inhibits microbial growth

Pharmacodynamics/Kinetics

Absorption: Readily and extensive
Distribution: Widely into body tissues and fluids (middle ear, prostate, bile, aqueous humor, CSF); crosses placenta; enters breast milk
Protein binding: 42% to 46%
Metabolism: Partially hepatic
Half-life elimination: 8-14 hours; prolonged with renal impairment
Time to peak, serum: 1-4 hours
Excretion: Urine (60% to 80%) as unchanged drug

Dosage Oral:

Children: 4 mg/kg/day in divided doses every 12 hours
Adults: 100 mg every 12 hours or 200 mg every 24 hours for 10 days; longer treatment periods may be necessary for prostatitis (ie, 4-16 weeks); in the treatment of *Pneumocystis carinii* pneumonia; dose may be as high as 15-20 mg/kg/day in 3-4 divided doses

Dosing interval in renal impairment:

Cl_{cr} 15-30 mL/minute: Administer 100 mg every 18 hours or 50 mg every 12 hours
Cl_{cr} <15 mL/minute: Administer 100 mg every 24 hours or avoid use

Hemodialysis: Moderately dialyzable (20% to 50%)

Dietary Considerations May cause folic acid deficiency, supplements may be needed. Should be taken with milk or food.

Administration Administer with milk or food.

Reference Range Therapeutic: Peak: 5-15 mg/L; Trough: 2-8 mg/L

Dosage Forms Excipient information presented when available (limited, particularly for generics); consult specific product labeling.

Solution, oral:
Primsol®: 50 mg (base)/5 mL (473 mL) [dye free, ethanol free; contains propylene glycol, sodium benzoate; bubble gum flavor]

Tablet: 100 mg

Trimethoprim and Polymyxin B

(trye METH oh prim & pol i MIKS in bee)

U.S. Brand Names Polytrim®

Canadian Brand Names PMS-Polytrimethoprim; Polytrim™

Index Terms Polymyxin B and Trimethoprim

Pharmacologic Category Antibiotic, Ophthalmic

Use Treatment of surface ocular bacterial conjunctivitis and blepharoconjunctivitis

Pregnancy Risk Factor C

Dosage Instill 1-2 drops in eye(s) every 4-6 hours

Elderly: No overall differences observed between elderly and other adults

Additional Information Complete prescribing information for this medication should be consulted for additional detail.

Dosage Forms Excipient information presented when available (limited, particularly for generics); consult specific product labeling.

Solution, ophthalmic: Trimethoprim 1 mg and polymyxin B sulfate 10,000 units per mL (10 mL) [contains benzalkonium chloride]

◆ **Trimethoprim and Sulfamethoxazole** *see* Sulfamethoxazole and Trimethoprim *on page 1407*

Trimetrexate

(tri me TREKS ate)

U.S. Brand Names NeuTrexin® [DSC]

Index Terms NSC-352122; Trimetrexate Glucuronate

Pharmacologic Category Antineoplastic Agent, Miscellaneous

Use Alternative therapy for the treatment of moderate-to-severe *Pneumocystis jiroveci* pneumonia (PCP) in immunocompromised patients, including patients with acquired immunodeficiency syndrome (AIDS), who are intolerant of, or are refractory to, sulfamethoxazole/trimethoprim therapy or for whom sulfamethoxazole/trimethoprim and pentamidine are contraindicated

Unlabeled/Investigational Use Treatment of nonsmall cell lung cancer, metastatic colorectal cancer, metastatic head and neck cancer, pancreatic adenocarcinoma, cutaneous T-cell lymphoma

Pregnancy Risk Factor D

Medication Safety Issues

High alert medication: The Institute for Safe Medication Practices (ISMP) includes this medication among its list of drugs which have a heightened risk of causing significant patient harm when used in error.

Dosage Note: Concurrent leucovorin 20 mg/m^2 every 6 hours must be administered daily (oral or I.V.) during treatment and for 72 hours past the last dose of trimetrexate.

Adults: I.V.:

Pneumocystis jiroveci pneumonia (PCP): 45 mg/m^2 once daily for 21 days; **alternative dosing based on weight:**
<50 kg:Trimetrexate 1.5 mg/kg/day; leucovorin 0.6 mg/kg 4 times/day
50-80 kg: Trimetrexate 1.2 mg/kg/day; leucovorin 0.5 mg/kg/4 times/day
>80 kg: Trimetrexate 1 mg/kg/day; leucovorin 0.5 mg/kg/4 times/day
Note: Oral doses of leucovorin should be rounded up to the next higher 25 mg increment.

Antineoplastic (unlabeled use): 6-16 mg/m^2 once daily for 5 days every 21-28 days **or** 150-200 mg/m^2 every 2 weeks

Dosage adjustment in hepatic impairment: Although it may be necessary to reduce the dose in patients with liver dysfunction, no specific dosage recommendations exist for treatment initiation with hepatic impairment.

Dosage Adjustment in Hematologic Toxicity

Toxicity Grade	Neutrophils (Polys/Bands)	Platelets	Dosage Recommendations	
			Trimetrexate	Leucovorin
1	>1000/mm^3	>75,000/mm^3	45 mg/m^2 once daily	20 mg/m^2 every 6 h
2	750-1000/mm^3	50,000-75,000/mm^3	45 mg/m^2 once daily	40 mg/m^2 every 6 h
3	500-749/mm^3	25,000-49,999/mm^3	22 mg/m^2 once daily	40 mg/m^2 every 6 h
4	<500/mm^3	<25,000/mm^3	Day 1-9: Discontinue Day 10-21: Interrupt up to 96 hours (see **Note**)	40 mg/m^2 every 6 h

Note:

If Grade 4 hematologic toxicity occurs prior to day 10: Trimetrexate should be discontinued and leucovorin administered for an additional 72 hours.

If Grade 4 hematologic toxicity occurs at day 10 or later: Trimetrexate may be held up to 96 hours to allow counts to recover.

If counts recover to Grade 3 within 96 hours, trimetrexate should be administered at a dose of 22 mg/m^2 and leucovorin 40 mg/m^2 every 6 hours.

When counts recover to Grade 2 toxicity, trimetrexate may be increased to 45 mg/m^2. Continue leucovorin at 40 mg/m^2 for duration of treatment.

Discontinue trimetrexate if counts do not improve to less than or equal to Grade 3 toxicity within 96 hours. Continue leucovorin at 40 mg/m^2 every 6 hours for 72 hours following last dose.

Hepatic toxicity (during treatment): Hold drug therapy if transaminase levels or alkaline phosphatase levels increase to >5 times the upper limit of normal.

Renal toxicity (during treatment): Hold drug therapy if serum creatinine levels increase to >2.5 mg/dL and elevation is considered secondary to trimetrexate.

Other toxicities: Hold drug therapy in patients experiencing severe mucosal toxicity that interferes with oral intake. Treatment should be discontinued for fever that cannot be controlled with antipyretics (oral temperature ≥40.5°C/105°F).

In addition: If trimetrexate treatment is interrupted for toxicity, leucovorin therapy must continue for 72 hours past the last administered dose of trimetrexate.

Additional Information Complete prescribing information for this medication should be consulted for additional detail.

Dosage Forms Excipient information presented when available (limited, particularly for generics); consult specific product labeling. [DSC] = Discontinued product

Injection, powder for reconstitution [preservative free]:

NeuTrexin®: 25 mg, 200 mg [DSC]

◆ **Trimetrexate Glucuronate** *see* Trimetrexate *on page 1520*

Trimipramine (trye MI pra meen)

U.S. Brand Names Surmontil®

Canadian Brand Names Apo-Trimip®; Nu-Trimipramine; Rhotrimine®; Surmontil®

Index Terms Trimipramine Maleate

Pharmacologic Category Antidepressant, Tricyclic (Tertiary Amine)

Additional Appendix Information

Antidepressant Agents *on page 1638*

Use Treatment of depression

Restrictions An FDA-approved medication guide concerning the use of antidepressants in children, adolescents, and young adults must be distributed when dispensing an outpatient prescription (new or refill) where this medication is to be used without direct supervision of a healthcare provider. Medication guides are available at http://www.fda.gov/cder/Offices/ODS/medication_guides.htm. Dispense to parents or guardians of children and adolescents receiving this medication.

Pregnancy Risk Factor C

Lactation Enters breast milk/contraindicated

Medication Safety Issues

Sound-alike/look-alike issues:

Trimipramine may be confused with triamterene, trimeprazine

Contraindications Hypersensitivity to trimipramine, any component of the formulation, or other dibenzodiazepines; use of MAO inhibitors within 14 days; use in a patient during the acute recovery phase of MI

Warnings/Precautions [U.S. Boxed Warning]: Antidepressants increase the risk of suicidal thinking and behavior in children, adolescents, and young adults (18-24 years of age) with major depressive disorder (MDD) and other psychiatric disorders; consider risk prior to prescribing. Short-term studies did not show an increased risk in patients >24 years of age and showed a decreased risk in patients ≥65 years. Closely monitor for clinical worsening, suicidality, or unusual changes in behavior; the patient's family or caregiver should be instructed to closely observe the patient and communicate condition with healthcare provider. A medication guide should be dispensed with each prescription. **Trimipramine is not FDA approved for use in children.**

The possibility of a suicide attempt is inherent in major depression and may persist until remission occurs. Monitor for worsening of depression or suicidality, especially during initiation of therapy (generally first 1-2 months) or with dose increases or decreases. Use caution in high-risk patients. Worsening depression and severe abrupt suicidality that are not part of the presenting symptoms may require discontinuation or modification of drug therapy. The patient's family or caregiver should be alerted to monitor patients for the emergence of suicidality and associated behaviors (such as agitation, irritability, hostility, impulsivity, and hypomania) and call healthcare provider.

May worsen psychosis in some patients or precipitate a shift to mania or hypomania in patients with bipolar disorder. Patients presenting with depressive symptoms should be screened for bipolar disorder. Monotherapy in patients with bipolar disorder should be avoided. **Trimipramine is not FDA approved for the treatment of bipolar depression.**

The degree of sedation, anticholinergic effects, orthostasis, and conduction abnormalities are high relative to other antidepressants. Trimipramine often causes drowsiness/sedation, resulting in impaired performance of tasks requiring alertness (eg, operating machinery or driving). Sedative effects may be additive with other CNS depressants and/or ethanol. Use with caution in patients with a history of cardiovascular disease (including previous MI, stroke, tachycardia, or conduction abnormalities). Use with caution in patients with urinary retention, benign prostatic hyperplasia, narrow-angle glaucoma, xerostomia, visual problems, constipation, or a history of bowel obstruction.

May alter glucose control - use with caution in patients with diabetes. Consider discontinuing, when possible, prior to elective surgery. Therapy should not be abruptly discontinued in patients receiving high doses for prolonged periods. May lower seizure threshold - use caution in patients with a previous seizure disorder or condition predisposing to seizures such as brain damage, alcoholism, or concurrent therapy with other drugs which lower the seizure threshold. May increase the risks associated with electroconvulsive therapy. Use with caution in hyperthyroid patients or those receiving thyroid supplementation. Use with caution in patients with hepatic or renal dysfunction and in elderly patients.

Adverse Reactions Frequency not defined.

Cardiovascular: Arrhythmias, hyper-/hypotension, tachycardia, palpitation, heart block, stroke, MI

Central nervous system: Headache, exacerbation of psychosis, confusion, delirium, hallucinations, nervousness, restlessness, delusions, agitation, insomnia, nightmares, anxiety, seizure, drowsiness

Dermatologic: Photosensitivity, rash, petechiae, itching

Endocrine & metabolic: Sexual dysfunction, breast enlargement, galactorrhea, SIADH

Gastrointestinal: Xerostomia, constipation, increased appetite, nausea, unpleasant taste, weight gain, diarrhea, heartburn, vomiting, anorexia, trouble with gums, decreased lower esophageal sphincter tone may cause GE reflux

Genitourinary: Difficult urination, urinary retention, testicular edema

Hematologic: Agranulocytosis, eosinophilia, purpura, thrombocytopenia

Hepatic: Cholestatic jaundice, increased liver enzymes

Neuromuscular & skeletal: Tremors, numbness, tingling, paresthesia, incoordination, ataxia, peripheral neuropathy, extrapyramidal symptoms

Ocular: Blurred vision, eye pain, disturbances in accommodation, mydriasis, increased intraocular pressure

Otic: Tinnitus

Miscellaneous: Allergic reactions

Drug Interactions

Metabolism/Transport Effects Substrate (major) of CYP2C19, 2D6, 3A4

Avoid Concomitant Use

Avoid concomitant use of Trimipramine with any of the following: Iobenguane I 123; MAO Inhibitors; Nilotinib; Sibutramine; Tetrabenazine; Thioridazine; Ziprasidone

Increased Effect/Toxicity

Trimipramine may increase the levels/effects of: Alcohol (Ethyl); Alpha-/Beta-Agonists (Direct-Acting); Alpha1-Agonists; Amphetamines; Anticholinergics; Aspirin; Beta2-Agonists; CNS Depressants; Desmopressin; NSAID (COX-2 Inhibitor); NSAID (Nonselective); QTc-Prolonging Agents; QuiNIDine; Serotonin Modulators; Sulfonylureas; Tetrabenazine; Thioridazine; TraMADol; Vitamin K Antagonists; Yohimbine; Ziprasidone

The levels/effects of Trimipramine may be increased by: Alfuzosin; Altretamine; BuPROPion; Cimetidine; Cinacalcet; Ciprofloxacin; CYP2C19 Inhibitors (Moderate); CYP2C19 Inhibitors (Strong); CYP2D6 Inhibitors (Moderate); CYP2D6 Inhibitors (Strong); CYP3A4 Inhibitors (Moderate); CYP3A4 Inhibitors (Strong); Darunavir; Dasatinib; Dexmethylphenidate; DULoxetine; Gadobutrol; Lithium; MAO Inhibitors; Methylphenidate; Nilotinib; Pramlintide; Propoxyphene; Protease Inhibitors; QuiNIDine; Selective Serotonin Reuptake Inhibitors; Sibutramine; Terbinafine; Valproic Acid

Decreased Effect

Trimipramine may decrease the levels/effects of: Acetylcholinesterase Inhibitors (Central); Alpha2-Agonists; Iobenguane I 123

The levels/effects of Trimipramine may be decreased by: Acetylcholinesterase Inhibitors (Central); Barbiturates; CarBAMazepine; CYP2C19 Inducers (Strong); CYP3A4 Inducers (Strong); Deferasirox; St Johns Wort

Ethanol/Nutrition/Herb Interactions

Ethanol: Avoid ethanol (may increase CNS depression).

Food: Grapefruit juice may inhibit the metabolism of some TCAs and clinical toxicity may result.

Herb/Nutraceutical: Avoid valerian, St John's wort, SAMe, kava kava (may increase risk of serotonin syndrome and/or excessive sedation).

Stability Solutions stable at a pH of 4-5. Turns yellowish or reddish on exposure to light. Slight discoloration does not affect potency; marked discoloration is associated with loss of potency. Capsules stable for 3 years following date of manufacture.

Mechanism of Action Increases the synaptic concentration of serotonin and/or norepinephrine in the central nervous system by inhibition of their reuptake by the presynaptic neuronal membrane

Pharmacodynamics/Kinetics

Distribution: V_d: 17-48 L/kg

Protein binding: 95%; free drug: 3% to 7%

Metabolism: Hepatic; significant first-pass effect

Bioavailability: 18% to 63%

Half-life elimination: 16-40 hours

Excretion: Urine

Dosage Oral:

Adults: 50-150 mg/day as a single bedtime dose up to a maximum of 200 mg/day outpatient and 300 mg/day inpatient

Elderly: Adequate studies have not been done in the elderly. In general, dosing should be cautious, starting at the lower end of dosing range.

Monitoring Parameters Blood pressure and pulse rate prior to and during initial therapy; evaluate mental status, suicidal ideation (especially at the beginning of therapy or when doses are increased or decreased); monitor weight; ECG in older adults

Additional Information May cause alterations in bleeding time.

Dosage Forms Excipient information presented when available (limited, particularly for generics); consult specific product labeling.

Capsule: 25 mg, 50 mg, 100 mg

- **Trimipramine Maleate** *see* Trimipramine *on page 1521*
- **Tri-Nasal® [DSC]** *see* Triamcinolone *on page 1510*
- **Trinasal® (Can)** *see* Triamcinolone *on page 1510*
- **TriNessa®** *see* Ethinyl Estradiol and Norgestimate *on page 584*
- **Trinipatch® 0.2 (Can)** *see* Nitroglycerin *on page 1073*
- **Trinipatch® 0.4 (Can)** *see* Nitroglycerin *on page 1073*
- **Trinipatch® 0.6 (Can)** *see* Nitroglycerin *on page 1073*
- **Tri-Norinyl®** *see* Ethinyl Estradiol and Norethindrone *on page 581*
- **Triostat®** *see* Liothyronine *on page 892*
- **Tripedia®** *see* Diphtheria and Tetanus Toxoids, and Acellular Pertussis Vaccine *on page 463*
- **Triphasil®** *see* Ethinyl Estradiol and Levonorgestrel *on page 577*
- **Triple Antibiotic** *see* Bacitracin, Neomycin, and Polymyxin B *on page 171*
- **Triplex™ AD** *see* Chlorpheniramine, Pyrilamine, and Phenylephrine *on page 315*
- **Tri-Previfem®** *see* Ethinyl Estradiol and Norgestimate *on page 584*

Triprolidine and Pseudoephedrine

(trye PROE li deen & soo doe e FED rin)

U.S. Brand Names Allerfrim [OTC]; Aprodine® [OTC]; Genac® [OTC]; Silafed® [OTC]; Sudafed® Maximum Strength Sinus Nighttime [OTC] [DSC]; Tri-Sudo® [OTC] [DSC]; Zymine®-D

Canadian Brand Names Actifed®

Index Terms Pseudoephedrine and Triprolidine

Pharmacologic Category Alpha/Beta Agonist; Histamine H_1 Antagonist; Histamine H_1 Antagonist, First Generation

Use Temporary relief of nasal congestion, decongest sinus openings, running nose, sneezing, itching of nose or throat and itchy, watery eyes due to common cold, hay fever, or other upper respiratory allergies

Pregnancy Risk Factor C

Medication Safety Issues

Sound-alike/look-alike issues:

Aprodine® may be confused with Aphrodyne®

Dosage Oral:

Liquid (Zymine®-D):

Children:

2-4 years: 1.25 mL every 4-6 hours (maximum pseudoephedrine: 60 mg/24 hours)

4-6 years: 2.5 mL every 4-6 hours (maximum pseudoephedrine: 60 mg/24 hours)

6-12 years: 2.5-5 mL every 4-6 hours (maximum pseudoephedrine: 120 mg/24 hours)

Children ≥12 years and Adults: 5-10 mL every 4-6 hours (maximum pseudoephedrine: 240 mg/24 hours)

Syrup (Allerfrim, Aprodine®):

Children 6-12 years: 5 mL every 4-6 hours; do not exceed 4 doses in 24 hours

Children >12 years and Adults: 10 mL every 4-6 hours; do not exceed 4 doses in 24 hours

Tablet (Aprodine®):

Children 6-12 years: 1/2 tablet every 4-6 hours; do not exceed 4 doses in 24 hours

Children >12 years and Adults: One tablet every 4-6 hours; do not exceed 4 doses in 24 hours

Additional Information Complete prescribing information for this medication should be consulted for additional detail.

Dosage Forms Excipient information presented when available (limited, particularly for generics); consult specific product labeling. [DSC] = Discontinued product

Liquid:

Zymine®-D: Triprolidine hydrochloride 1.25 mg and pseudoephedrine hydrochloride 45 mg per 5 mL (480 mL)

Syrup: Triprolidine hydrochloride 1.25 mg and pseudoephedrine hydrochloride 30 mg per 5 mL (120 mL) [DSC]

Allerfrim: Triprolidine hydrochloride 1.25 mg and pseudoephedrine hydrochloride 30 mg per 5 mL (120 mL, 480 mL) [contains sodium benzoate]

Aprodine®: Triprolidine hydrochloride 1.25 mg and pseudoephedrine hydrochloride 30 mg per 5 mL (120 mL)

Silafed®: Triprolidine hydrochloride 1.25 mg and pseudoephedrine hydrochloride 30 mg per 5 mL (120 mL, 240 mL)

Tablet:

Allerfrim, Aprodine®, Genac®, Sudafed® Maximum Strength Sinus Nighttime, Tri-Sudo® [DSC]: Triprolidine hydrochloride 2.5 mg and pseudoephedrine hydrochloride 60 mg

◆ **Triprolidine, Codeine, and Pseudoephedrine** *see* Triprolidine, Pseudoephedrine, and Codeine *on page 1523*

Triprolidine, Pseudoephedrine, and Codeine (trye PROE li deen, soo doe e FED rin, & KOE deen)

Canadian Brand Names CoActifed®; Covan®; ratio-Cotridin

Index Terms Codeine, Pseudoephedrine, and Triprolidine; Codeine, Triprolidine, and Pseudoephedrine; Pseudoephedrine, Codeine, and Triprolidine; Pseudoephedrine, Triprolidine, and Codeine; Triprolidine, Codeine, and Pseudoephedrine

Pharmacologic Category Alpha/Beta Agonist; Analgesic, Opioid; Antitussive; Histamine H_1 Antagonist; Histamine H_1 Antagonist, First Generation

Use Symptomatic relief of upper respiratory symptoms and cough

Restrictions C-V (CDSA-I)

Pregnancy Risk Factor C

Medication Safety Issues

Sound-alike/look-alike issues:

Triacin-C® may be confused with triacetin

Dosage Oral:

Children:

2-6 years: 2.5 mL 4 times/day

7-12 years: 5 mL 4 times/day **or** 1/2 tablet 4 times/day

Children >12 years and Adults: 10 mL 4 times/day **or** 1 tablet 4 times/day

Additional Information Complete prescribing information for this medication should be consulted for additional detail.

Dosage Forms Excipient information presented when available (limited, particularly for generics); consult specific product labeling. [CAN] = Canadian brand name

Syrup:

CoActifed® [CAN], ratio-Cotridin [CAN]: Triprolidine hydrochloride 2 mg, pseudoephedrine hydrochloride 30 mg, and codeine phosphate 10 mg per 5 mL (100 mL, 2000 mL) [not available in U.S.]

CoVan® [CAN]: Triprolidine hydrochloride 2 mg, pseudoephedrine hydrochloride 30 mg, and codeine phosphate 10 mg per 5 mL (500 mL) [not available in U.S.]

Tablet:

CoActifed® [CAN]: Triprolidine hydrochloride 4 mg, pseudoephedrine hydrochloride 60 mg, and codeine phosphate 20 mg (50s) [not available in U.S.]

◆ **TripTone® [OTC]** *see* DimenhyDRINATE *on page 453*

◆ **Triptoraline** *see* Triptorelin *on page 1523*

Triptorelin (trip toe REL in)

U.S. Brand Names Trelstar® Depot; Trelstar® LA

Canadian Brand Names Trelstar® ; Trelstar® Depot; Trelstar® LA

Index Terms AY-25650; CL-118,532; D-Trp(6)-LHRH; Triptoraline; Triptorelin Pamoate; Tryptoreline

Pharmacologic Category Gonadotropin Releasing Hormone Agonist

Use Palliative treatment of advanced prostate cancer as an alternative to orchiectomy or estrogen administration

Unlabeled/Investigational Use Treatment of endometriosis, growth hormone deficiency, hyperandrogenism, *in vitro* fertilization, ovarian carcinoma, pancreatic carcinoma, precocious puberty, uterine leiomyomata

Pregnancy Risk Factor X

Pregnancy Considerations Contraindicated in women who are or may become pregnant.

Lactation Excretion in breast milk unknown/contraindicated

Contraindications Hypersensitivity to triptorelin or any component of the formulation, other LHRH agonists or LHRH; pregnancy

Warnings/Precautions Hazardous agent - use appropriate precautions for handling and disposal. Transient increases in testosterone can lead to worsening symptoms (bone pain, hematuria, bladder outlet obstruction) of prostate cancer during the first few weeks of therapy. Cases of spinal cord compression have been reported with LHRH agonists. Closely observe patients with metastatic vertebral lesions or lower urinary tract obstruction. Hypersensitivity reactions including angioedema and anaphylaxis have rarely occurred. Rare cases of pituitary apoplexy (frequently secondary to pituitary adenoma) have been observed with leuprolide administration (onset from 1 hour to usually <2 weeks); may present as sudden headache, vomiting, visual or mental status changes, and infrequently cardiovascular collapse; immediate medical attention required. Safety and efficacy has not established in pediatric population.

Adverse Reactions As reported with Trelstar® Depot and Trelstar® LA; frequency of effect may vary by product:

>10%:

Central nervous system: Headache (30% to 50%)

Endocrine & metabolic: Hot flashes (95% to 100%), glucose increased

Hematologic: Hemoglobin decreased, RBC count decreased

Hepatic: Alkaline phosphatase increased, ALT increased, AST increased

Neuromuscular & skeletal: Skeletal pain (12% to 13%)

Renal: BUN increased

1% to 10%:

Cardiovascular: Leg edema (6%), hypertension (4%), chest pain (2%), peripheral edema (1%)

Central nervous system: Dizziness (1% to 3%), pain (2% to 3%), emotional lability (1%), fatigue (2%), insomnia (2%)

Dermatologic: Rash (2%), pruritus (1%)

Endocrine & metabolic: Alkaline phosphatase increased (2%), breast pain (2%), gynecomastia (2%), libido decreased (2%), tumor flare (8%)

Gastrointestinal: Nausea (3%), anorexia (2%), constipation (2%), dyspepsia (2%), vomiting (2%), abdominal pain (1%), diarrhea (1%)

Genitourinary: Dysuria (5%), impotence (2% to 7%), urinary retention (1%), urinary tract infection (1%)

Hematologic: Anemia (1%)

Local: Injection site pain (4%)

Neuromuscular & skeletal: Leg pain (2% to 5%), back pain (3%), arthralgia (2%), leg cramps (2%), myalgia (1%), weakness (1%)

Ocular: Conjunctivitis (1%), eye pain (1%)

Respiratory: Cough (2%), dyspnea (1%), pharyngitis (1%)

Postmarketing and/or case reports (limited to important or life-threatening): Anaphylaxis, angioedema, hypersensitivity reactions, pituitary apoplexy, renal dysfunction, spinal cord compression

Drug Interactions

Avoid Concomitant Use There are no known interactions where it is recommended to avoid concomitant use.

Increased Effect/Toxicity There are no known significant interactions involving an increase in effect.

Decreased Effect

Triptorelin may decrease the levels/effects of: Antidiabetic Agents

Stability

Trelstar® Depot: Store at 15°C to 30°C (59°F to 86°F).

Trelstar® LA: Store at 20°C to 25°C (68°F to 77°F).

Reconstitution: Reconstitute with 2 mL sterile water for injection. Shake well to obtain a uniform suspension.

Debioclip™: Follow manufacturer's instructions for mixing prior to use.

Mechanism of Action Causes suppression of ovarian and testicular steroidogenesis due to decreased levels of LH and FSH with subsequent decrease in testosterone (male) and estrogen (female) levels. After chronic and continuous administration, usually 2-4 weeks after initiation, a sustained decrease in LH and FSH secretion occurs.

Pharmacodynamics/Kinetics

Absorption: Oral: Not active

Distribution: V_d: 30-33 L

Protein binding: None

Metabolism: Unknown; unlikely to involve CYP; no known metabolites

Half-life elimination: 2.8 ± 1.2 hours

Moderate to severe renal impairment: 6.5-7.7 hours

Hepatic impairment: 7.6 hours

Time to peak: 1-3 hours

Excretion: Urine (42% as intact peptide); hepatic

Dosage I.M.: Adults: Prostate cancer:

Trelstar® Depot: 3.75 mg once every 28 days

Trelstar® LA: 11.25 mg once every 84 days

Dosage adjustment in renal/hepatic impairment: Although this drug is excreted renally, no guidelines for adjustments are available.

Administration Administer by I.M. injection into the buttock; alternate injection sites.

Monitoring Parameters Serum testosterone levels, prostate-specific antigen

Test Interactions Pituitary-gonadal function may be suppressed with chronic administration and for up to 8 weeks after triptorelin therapy has been discontinued.

Dosage Forms Excipient information presented when available (limited, particularly for generics); consult specific product labeling.

Injection, powder for reconstitution:

Trelstar® Depot: 3.75 mg [contains polylactide-co-glycolide; polysorbate 80]

Trelstar® LA: 11.25 mg [contains polylactide-co-glycolide; polysorbate 80]

- **Triptorelin Pamoate** *see* Triptorelin *on page 1523*
- **Triquilar® (Can)** *see* Ethinyl Estradiol and Levonorgestrel *on page 577*
- **Tris Buffer** *see* Tromethamine *on page 1524*
- **Trisenox®** *see* Arsenic Trioxide *on page 137*
- **Tris(hydroxymethyl)aminomethane** *see* Tromethamine *on page 1524*
- **Tri-Sprintec®** *see* Ethinyl Estradiol and Norgestimate *on page 584*
- **Tri-Sudo® [OTC] [DSC]** *see* Triprolidine and Pseudoephedrine *on page 1522*
- **Trital DM** *see* Chlorpheniramine, Phenylephrine, and Dextromethorphan *on page 311*
- **Trivagizole-3® (Can)** *see* Clotrimazole *on page 359*
- **Trivalent Inactivated Influenza Vaccine (TIV)** *see* Influenza Virus Vaccine *on page 788*
- **Trivaris™** *see* Triamcinolone *on page 1510*
- **Tri-Vent™ DM [DSC]** *see* Guaifenesin, Pseudoephedrine, and Dextromethorphan *on page 715*
- **Tri-Vent™ DPC [DSC]** *see* Chlorpheniramine, Phenylephrine, and Dextromethorphan *on page 311*
- **Tri-Vent™ HC [DSC]** *see* Hydrocodone, Carbinoxamine, and Pseudoephedrine *on page 743*
- **Trivora®** *see* Ethinyl Estradiol and Levonorgestrel *on page 577*
- **Trizivir®** *see* Abacavir, Lamivudine, and Zidovudine *on page 19*
- **Trobicin® [DSC]** *see* Spectinomycin *on page 1396*
- **Trocaine® [OTC]** *see* Benzocaine *on page 183*
- **Trombovar® (Can)** *see* Sodium Tetradecyl *on page 1386*

Tromethamine (troe METH a meen)

U.S. Brand Names THAM®

Index Terms Tris Buffer; Tris(hydroxymethyl) aminomethane

Pharmacologic Category Alkalinizing Agent, Parenteral

Use Correction of metabolic acidosis associated with cardiac bypass surgery or cardiac arrest; to correct excess acidity of stored blood that is preserved with acid citrate dextrose (ACD); indicated in infants needing alkalinization after receiving maximum sodium bicarbonate (8-10 mEq/kg/24 hours)

Pregnancy Risk Factor C

Pregnancy Considerations Animal studies have not been conducted. There are no adequate and well-controlled studies in pregnant women. Use only if potential benefit outweighs possible risk to the fetus.

Lactation Excretion in breast milk unknown/use caution

Medication Safety Issues

Sound-alike/look-alike issues:

Tromethamine may be confused with TrophAmine®

Contraindications Hypersensitivity to tromethamine or any component of the formulation; uremia or anuria; chronic respiratory acidosis (neonates); salicylate intoxication (neonates)

Warnings/Precautions Reduce dose and monitor pH carefully in renal impairment; drug should not be given for a period of longer than 24 hours unless for a life-threatening situation. May cause respiratory depression; monitor closely especially if patient not intubated. May cause hypoglycemia with extremely large doses. Avoid extravasation; may cause tissue necrosis.

Adverse Reactions Frequency not defined.

Cardiovascular: Hypervolemia, venospasm

Endocrine & metabolic: Hyperkalemia, hypoglycemia (usually doses >500 mg/kg administered over <1 hour)

Hepatic: Hepatic necrosis (resulted during delivery via umbilical venous catheter)

Local: Necrosis with extravasation, phlebitis, tissue irritation

Respiratory: Apnea, pulmonary edema, respiratory depression

Drug Interactions

Avoid Concomitant Use There are no known interactions where it is recommended to avoid concomitant use.

Increased Effect/Toxicity

Tromethamine may increase the levels/effects of: Amphetamines

Decreased Effect There are no known significant interactions involving a decrease in effect.

Stability Store at 20°C to 25°C (68°F to 77°F); protect from freezing

Mechanism of Action Acts as a proton acceptor, which combines with hydrogen ions, liberating bicarbonate buffer, to correct acidosis. It buffers both metabolic and respiratory acids, limiting carbon dioxide generation. Also an osmotic diuretic.

Pharmacodynamics/Kinetics

Distribution: Distributes quickly into extracellular space; at steady state distributes into a volume slightly greater than total body water; penetrates slowly intracellularly

Half-life elimination: 5.6 hours

Excretion: Urine (>75%) within 8 hours

Dosage

Neonates and Infants: Metabolic acidosis associated with RDS: Initial: Approximately 1 mL/kg for each pH unit below 7.4; additional doses determined by changes in PaO_2, pH, and pCO_2; **Note:** Although THAM® solution does not raise pCO_2 when treating metabolic acidosis with concurrent respiratory acidosis, bicarbonate may be preferred because the osmotic effects of THAM® are greater.

Adults: Dose depends on buffer base deficit; when deficit is known: tromethamine (mL of 0.3 M solution) = body weight (kg) x base deficit (mEq/L) x 1.1

Metabolic acidosis with cardiac arrest:

I.V.: 3.6-10.8 g (111-333 mL); additional amounts may be required to control acidosis after arrest reversed

Open chest: Intraventricular: 2-6 g (62-185 mL). **Note:** Do not inject into cardiac muscle

Acidosis associated with cardiac bypass surgery: Average dose: 9 mL/kg (2.7 mEq/kg); 500 mL is adequate for most adults; maximum dose: 500 mg/kg in ≤1 hour

Excess acidity of acid citrate dextrose (ACD) blood in coronary artery surgery: 15-77 mL of 0.3 molar solution added to each 500 mL of blood

Dosing comments in renal impairment: Use with caution; monitor for toxicity

Administration Maximum concentration: 0.3 molar; infuse slowly over at least 1 hour; to avoid glucose or potassium changes, should not exceed 16.5 mL/kg in 1 hour

Monitoring Parameters Serum electrolytes (especially potassium, blood glucose); renal function, arterial blood gases, ECG monitoring, fluid status, ventilation rate

Check infusion site frequently during administration.

Reference Range Blood pH (physiologic): 7.38-7.42

Additional Information 1 mM = 120 mg = 3.3 mL = 1 mEq of THAM®

Dosage Forms Excipient information presented when available (limited, particularly for generics); consult specific product labeling.

Injection, solution:

THAM®: 18 g [0.3 molar] (500 mL)

- **Tronolane® Suppository [OTC]** *see* Phenylephrine *on page 1183*
- **Tropicacyl®** *see* Tropicamide *on page 1525*

Tropicamide (troe PIK a mide)

U.S. Brand Names Mydral™; Mydriacyl®; Tropicacyl®

Canadian Brand Names Diotrope®; Mydriacyl®

Index Terms Bistropamide

Pharmacologic Category Ophthalmic Agent, Mydriatic

Additional Appendix Information

Cycloplegic Mydriatics *on page 1655*

Use Short-acting mydriatic used in diagnostic procedures; as well as preoperatively and postoperatively; treatment of some cases of acute iritis, iridocyclitis, and keratitis

Pregnancy Risk Factor C

Dosage Ophthalmic: Children and Adults (individuals with heavily pigmented eyes may require larger doses):

Cycloplegia: Instill 1-2 drops (1%); may repeat in 5 minutes

Exam must be performed within 30 minutes after the repeat dose; if the patient is not examined within 20-30 minutes, instill an additional drop

Mydriasis: Instill 1-2 drops (0.5%) 15-20 minutes before exam; may repeat every 30 minutes as needed

Additional Information Complete prescribing information for this medication should be consulted for additional detail.

Dosage Forms Excipient information presented when available (limited, particularly for generics); consult specific product labeling.

Solution, ophthalmic [drops]: 0.5% (15 mL); 1% (2 mL, 3 mL, 15 mL)

Mydriacyl®: 1% (3 mL, 15 mL) [contains benzalkonium chloride]

Mydral™, Tropicacyl®: 0.5% (15 mL); 1% (15 mL) [contains benzalkonium chloride]

- **Trosec (Can)** *see* Trospium *on page 1525*

Trospium (TROSE pee um)

U.S. Brand Names Sanctura®; Sanctura® XR

Canadian Brand Names Trosec

Index Terms Trospium Chloride

Pharmacologic Category Anticholinergic Agent

Use Treatment of overactive bladder with symptoms of urgency, incontinence, and urinary frequency

Pregnancy Risk Factor C

Pregnancy Considerations Adverse events were observed in animal studies. There are no adequate or well-controlled studies in pregnant women; use only if clearly needed.

Lactation Excretion in breast milk unknown/use caution

Contraindications Hypersensitivity to trospium or any component of the formulation; urinary retention; gastric retention; uncontrolled narrow-angle glaucoma

Warnings/Precautions May cause drowsiness and/or blurred vision, which may impair physical or mental abilities; patients must be cautioned about performing tasks which require mental alertness (eg, operating machinery or driving). May occur in the presence of increased environmental temperature; use caution in hot weather and/or exercise. Use with caution in patients with bladder flow obstruction, may increase the risk of urinary retention. Use with caution in patients with gastrointestinal obstructive disorders (eg, pyloric stenosis); may increase the risk of gastric retention. Use caution in patients with decreased GI motility (eg, myasthenia gravis, ulcerative colitis). Avoid use of extended release formulation in severe renal impairment (Cl_{cr} <30 mL/minute). Use immediate release formulation with caution in renal dysfunction; dosage adjustment is required. Active tubular secretion (ATS) is a route of elimination; use caution with other medications that are eliminated by ATS (eg, procainamide, pancuronium, vancomycin, morphine). Use with extreme caution in patients with controlled (treated) narrow-angle glaucoma. Use caution in patients with moderate-to-severe hepatic dysfunction. Use caution in Alzheimer's patients. Use caution in the elderly (≥65 years of age); increased anticholinergic side effects are seen. Safety and efficacy in pediatric patients have not been established.

Adverse Reactions

>10%: Gastrointestinal: Xerostomia (9% to 22%)

1% to 10%:

Cardiovascular: Tachycardia

Central nervous system: Headache (4% to 7%), fatigue (2%)

Dermatologic: Dry skin

Gastrointestinal: Constipation (9% to 10%), abdominal pain (1% to 3%), dyspepsia (1% to 2%), flatulence (1% to 2%), nausea (1%), abdominal distention (<2%), taste abnormal, vomiting

Genitourinary: Urinary retention (≤1%), urinary tract infection (1% to 7%)

Ocular: Dry eyes (1% to 2%), blurred vision (1%)

Respiratory: Nasopharyngitis (3%), nasal dryness (1%)

Miscellaneous: Influenza (2%)

<1% (Limited to important or life-threatening): Anaphylaxis, angioneurotic edema, back pain, chest pain, delirium, feces hard, gastritis, hallucinations, hypertensive crisis, palpitation, rash, rhabdomyolysis, somnolence, Stevens-Johnson syndrome, supraventricular tachycardia, syncope, T-wave inversion

Drug Interactions

Avoid Concomitant Use There are no known interactions where it is recommended to avoid concomitant use.

Increased Effect/Toxicity

Trospium may increase the levels/effects of: Anticholinergics; Cannabinoids; Potassium Chloride

The levels/effects of Trospium may be increased by: Pramlintide

Decreased Effect

Trospium may decrease the levels/effects of: Acetylcholinesterase Inhibitors (Central); Secretin

The levels/effects of Trospium may be decreased by: Acetylcholinesterase Inhibitors (Central)

Ethanol/Nutrition/Herb Interactions

Ethanol: Avoid use since ethanol may enhance the sedative effects of trospium. Ethanol should not be ingested within 2 hours of the administration of the trospium extended release formulation.

Food: Administration with a fatty meal reduces the absorption and bioavailability of trospium.

Stability Store at 20°C to 25°C (68°F to 77°F).

Mechanism of Action Trospium antagonizes the effects of acetylcholine on muscarinic receptors in cholinergically innervated organs. It reduces the smooth muscle tone of the bladder.

Pharmacodynamics/Kinetics

Absorption: <10%; decreased with food

Distribution: V_d: 395 - >600 L, primarily in plasma

Protein binding: 48% to 85% *in vitro*

Metabolism: Hypothesized to be via esterase hydrolysis and conjugation; forms metabolites

Bioavailability: Immediate release formulation: ~10% (range: 4% to 16%)

Half-life elimination: Immediate release formulation: 20 hours

Severe renal insufficiency (Cl_{cr} <30 mL/minute): ~33 hours; extended release formulation: ~35 hours

Time to peak, plasma: 5-6 hours

Excretion: Feces (85%); urine (~6%; mostly as unchanged drug) primarily via active tubular secretion

Dosage Oral:

Adults: Immediate release formulation: 20 mg twice daily; extended release formulation: 60 mg once daily

Elderly ≥75 years: Immediate release formulation: Consider initial dose of 20 mg once daily (based on tolerability) at bedtime

Dosage adjustment in renal impairment: Cl_{cr} ≤30 mL/minute: Immediate release formulation: 20 mg once daily at bedtime; Extended release formulation: Use not recommended

Dietary Considerations Give 1 hour prior to meals or on an empty stomach.

Administration Administer tablets at bedtime on an empty stomach. Administer extended release capsules in the morning with a full glass of water 1 hour before eating.

Dosage Forms Excipient information presented when available (limited, particularly for generics); consult specific product labeling.

Capsule, extended release, as chloride:

Sanctura® XR: 60 mg

Tablet, as chloride:

Sanctura®: 20 mg

◆ **Trospium Chloride** *see* Trospium *on page* 1525

◆ **Trusopt®** *see* Dorzolamide *on page* 482

◆ **Truvada®** *see* Emtricitabine and Tenofovir *on page* 515

Trypsin, Balsam Peru, and Castor Oil

(TRIP sin, BAL sam pe RUE, & KAS tor oyl)

U.S. Brand Names Allanderm-T™; Granulex®; Optase™; Xenaderm™

Index Terms Balsam Peru, Trypsin, and Castor Oil; Castor Oil, Trypsin, and Balsam Peru

Pharmacologic Category Protectant, Topical

Use Treatment of decubitus ulcers, varicose ulcers, debridement of eschar, dehiscent wounds and sunburn; promote wound healing; reduce odor from necrotic wounds

Medication Safety Issues

Sound-alike/look-alike issues:

Granulex® may be confused with Regranex®

Dosage Topical: Apply a minimum of twice daily or as often as necessary

Additional Information Complete prescribing information for this medication should be consulted for additional detail.

Dosage Forms Excipient information presented when available (limited, particularly for generics); consult specific product labeling.

Aerosol, topical: Trypsin 0.12 mg, balsam Peru 87 mg, and castor oil 788 mg per gram (120 g)

Granulex®: Trypsin 0.12 mg, balsam Peru 87 mg, and castor oil 788 mg per gram (60 g, 120 g)

Gel, topical:

Optase™: Trypsin 0.12 mg, balsam Peru 87 mg, and castor oil 788 mg per gram (95 g)

Ointment, topical:

Allanderm-T™, Xenaderm™: Trypsin 90 USP units, balsam Peru 87 mg, and castor oil 788 mg per gram (30 g, 60 g)

◆ **Tryptoreline** *see* Triptorelin *on page 1523*

◆ **TSH** *see* Thyrotropin Alfa *on page 1465*

◆ **TSPA** *see* Thiotepa *on page 1462*

◆ **TST** *see* Tuberculin Tests *on page 1527*

◆ **Tuberculin Purified Protein Derivative** *see* Tuberculin Tests *on page 1527*

◆ **Tuberculin Skin Test** *see* Tuberculin Tests *on page 1527*

Tuberculin Tests (too BER kyoo lin tests)

U.S. Brand Names Aplisol®; Tubersol®

Index Terms Mantoux; PPD; TB Skin Test; TST; Tuberculin Purified Protein Derivative; Tuberculin Skin Test

Pharmacologic Category Diagnostic Agent

Use Skin test in diagnosis of tuberculosis

Pregnancy Risk Factor C

Pregnancy Considerations Reproduction studies have not been conducted. Pregnancy is not a contraindication to testing.

Medication Safety Issues

Sound-alike/look-alike issues:

Aplisol® may be confused with Anusol®, A.P.L.®, Aplitest®, Atropisol®

Administration issues:

Tuberculin products may be confused with tetanus toxoid products and influenza virus vaccine. Medication errors have occurred when tuberculin skin tests (PPD) have been inadvertently administered instead of tetanus toxoid products and influenza virus vaccine. These products are refrigerated and often stored in close proximity to each other.

Contraindications Hypersensitivity to tuberculin purified protein derivative (PPD) or any component of the formulation; previous severe reaction to tuberculin PPD skin test (TST)

Warnings/Precautions Patients with a previous severe reaction to TST (vesiculation, ulceration, necrosis) at the injection site should not receive tuberculin PPD again. Do not administer to persons with documented tuberculosis or a clear history of treatment for tuberculosis; persons with extensive burns or eczema. Skin testing may be deferred with major viral infections or live-virus vaccination within 1 month. Tuberculous or other bacterial infections, viral infection, live virus vaccination, malignancy, immunosuppressive agents, and conditions which impair immune response may cause a decreased response to test. Very young children (<6 weeks of age) may also have an absent or delayed response. For intradermal administration only; do not administer I.V., I.M., or SubQ. Epinephrine (1:1000) should be available to treat possible allergic reactions.

Adverse Reactions Suspected adverse reactions should be reported to the Food and Drug Administration (FDA) MedWatch Program at 1-800-332-1088

Frequency not defined:

Dermatologic: Rash

Local: Injection site reactions: Bleeding, bruising, discomfort, erythematous reaction, hematoma, necrosis, pain, pruritus, redness, scarring, ulceration, vesiculation

Miscellaneous: Anaphylaxis

Drug Interactions

Avoid Concomitant Use There are no known interactions where it is recommended to avoid concomitant use.

Increased Effect/Toxicity There are no known significant interactions involving an increase in effect.

Decreased Effect

The levels/effects of Tuberculin Tests may be decreased by: Vaccines (Live)

Stability Aplisol®, Tubersol®: Store under refrigeration at 2°C to 8°C (36°F to 46°F); do not freeze. Protect from light. Opened vials should be discarded after 30 days.

Mechanism of Action Tuberculosis results in individuals becoming sensitized to certain antigenic components of the *M. tuberculosis* organism. Culture extracts called tuberculins are contained in tuberculin skin test preparations. Upon intracutaneous injection of these culture extracts, a classic delayed (cellular) hypersensitivity reaction occurs. This reaction is characteristic of a delayed course (peak occurs >24 hours after injection, induration of the skin secondary to cell infiltration, and occasional vesiculation and necrosis). Delayed hypersensitivity reactions to tuberculin may indicate infection with a variety of nontuberculosis mycobacteria, or vaccination with the live attenuated mycobacterial strain of *M. bovis* vaccine, BCG, in addition to previous natural infection with *M. tuberculosis*.

Pharmacodynamics/Kinetics

Onset of action: Delayed hypersensitivity reactions: 5-6 hours

Peak effect: 48-72 hours

Duration: Reactions subside over a few days

Dosage Children and Adults: Intradermal: 0.1 mL

TST interpretation: Criteria for positive TST read at 48-72 hours (see Note below for healthcare workers):

Induration ≥5 mm: Persons with HIV infection (or risk factors for HIV infection, but unknown status), recent close contact to person with known active TB, persons with chest x-ray consistent with healed TB, persons who are immunosuppressed

Induration ≥10 mm: Persons with clinical conditions which increase risk of TB infection, recent immigrants, I.V. drug users, residents and employees of high-risk settings, children <4 years of age

Induration ≥15 mm: Persons who do not meet any of the above criteria (no risk factors for TB)

Note: A two-step test is recommended when testing will be performed at regular intervals (eg, for healthcare workers). If the first test is negative, a second TST should be administered 1-3 weeks after the first test was read.

TST interpretation (CDC guidelines) in a healthcare setting:

Baseline test: ≥10 mm is positive (either first or second step)

Serial testing without known exposure: Increase of ≥10 mm is positive

Known exposure:

≥5 mm is positive in patients with baseline of 0 mm

≥10 mm is positive in patients with negative baseline or previous screening result of ≥0mm

Read test at 48-72 hours following placement. Test results with 0 mm induration or measured induration less than the defined cutoff point are considered to signify absence of infection with *M. tuberculosis*. Test results should be documented in millimeters even if classified as negative. Erythema and redness of skin are not indicative of a positive test result.

Administration For intradermal administration only. Administer to upper third of forearm (palm up) ≥2 inches from elbow, wrist, or other injection site. If neither arm can be used, may administer to back of shoulder. Administer using inch 1/4 to 1/2 inch 27-gauge needle or finer tuberculin syringe. Should form wheal (6-10 mm in diameter) as liquid is injected which will remain ~10 minutes. Avoid pressure or bandage at injection site. Document date and time of injection, person placing TST, location of injection site and lot number of solution.

Monitoring Parameters Monitor for immediate hypersensitivity reactions for ~15 minutes following injection.

Test Interactions False-positive reactions may occur with BCG vaccination or previous mycobacteria (nonTB) infection (previous BCG vaccination is not a contraindication to testing). False-negative reactions may occur with impaired cell mediated immunity.

Additional Information Situations where risk of tuberculosis infection may be increased are with contacts of recently-diagnosed persons with active disease, contact with immigrants from countries where tuberculosis is still common, or reactivation with impaired immunity (HIV infection, diabetes, renal failure, immunosuppressant use, pulmonary silicosis). Healthcare workers, staff of correctional facilities, and travelers at high risk of exposure should have routine testing. Patients with HIV infection should be tested as soon as possible following diagnosis.

The date of administration, the product manufacturer, and lot number of product must be entered into the patient's permanent medical record. Results should be recorded in millimeters (even if 0), not "negative" or "positive".

Dosage Forms Excipient information presented when available (limited, particularly for generics); consult specific product labeling.

Injection, solution:

Aplisol®, Tubersol®: 5 TU/0.1 mL (1 mL, 5 mL) [contains polysorbate 80]

◆ **Tubersol®** *see* Tuberculin Tests *on page 1527*

◆ **Tucks® Anti-Itch [OTC]** *see* Hydrocortisone *on page 743*

◆ **Tums® [OTC]** *see* Calcium Carbonate *on page 238*

◆ **Tums® E-X [OTC]** *see* Calcium Carbonate *on page 238*

◆ **Tums® Extra Strength Sugar Free [OTC]** *see* Calcium Carbonate *on page 238*

◆ **Tums® Smoothies™ [OTC]** *see* Calcium Carbonate *on page 238*

◆ **Tums® Ultra [OTC]** *see* Calcium Carbonate *on page 238*

◆ **Tur-bi-kal® [OTC]** *see* Phenylephrine *on page 1183*

◆ **Tusnel-DM Pediatric®** *see* Guaifenesin, Pseudoephedrine, and Dextromethorphan *on page 715*

◆ **Tusnel Liquid®** *see* Guaifenesin, Pseudoephedrine, and Dextromethorphan *on page 715*

◆ **Tusnel Pediatric®** *see* Guaifenesin, Pseudoephedrine, and Dextromethorphan *on page 715*

◆ **TussiCaps™** *see* Hydrocodone and Chlorpheniramine *on page 741*

◆ **Tussigon®** *see* Hydrocodone and Homatropine *on page 742*

◆ **Tussionex®** *see* Hydrocodone and Chlorpheniramine *on page 741*

◆ **Tussi-Organidin® DM NR** *see* Guaifenesin and Dextromethorphan *on page 710*

◆ **Tussi-Organidin® DM-S NR** *see* Guaifenesin and Dextromethorphan *on page 710*

◆ **Tussi-Organidin® NR** *see* Guaifenesin and Codeine *on page 710*

◆ **Tussi-Organidin® S-NR** *see* Guaifenesin and Codeine *on page 710*

◆ **Tusso-C™** *see* Guaifenesin and Codeine *on page 710*

◆ **Tusso-DF® [DSC]** *see* Hydrocodone and Guaifenesin *on page 741*

◆ **Tussplex™ DM** *see* Chlorpheniramine, Phenylephrine, and Dextromethorphan *on page 311*

◆ **TVP-1012** *see* Rasagiline *on page 1298*

◆ **Twelve Resin-K** *see* Cyanocobalamin *on page 374*

◆ **Twilite® [OTC]** *see* DiphenhydrAMINE *on page 456*

◆ **Twinject®** *see* EPINEPHrine *on page 525*

◆ **Twinrix®** *see* Hepatitis A and Hepatitis B Recombinant Vaccine *on page 725*

◆ **Ty21a Vaccine** *see* Typhoid Vaccine *on page 1529*

◆ **Tycolene [OTC]** *see* Acetaminophen *on page 25*

◆ **Tycolene Maximum Strength [OTC]** *see* Acetaminophen *on page 25*

◆ **Tygacil®** *see* Tigecycline *on page 1469*

◆ **Tykerb®** *see* Lapatinib *on page 856*

◆ **Tylenol® [OTC]** *see* Acetaminophen *on page 25*

◆ **Tylenol® (Can)** *see* Acetaminophen *on page 25*

◆ **Tylenol® 8 Hour [OTC]** *see* Acetaminophen *on page 25*

◆ **Tylenol® Allergy Multi-Symptom Nighttime [OTC]** *see* Acetaminophen, Diphenhydramine, and Phenylephrine *on page 33*

◆ **Tylenol® Allergy Sinus (Can)** *see* Acetaminophen, Chlorpheniramine, and Pseudoephedrine *on page 31*

◆ **Tylenol® Arthritis Pain [OTC]** *see* Acetaminophen *on page 25*

◆ **Tylenol® Children's [OTC]** *see* Acetaminophen *on page 25*

◆ **Tylenol® Children's with Flavor Creator [OTC]** *see* Acetaminophen *on page 25*

◆ **Tylenol® Children's Plus Cold Nighttime [OTC] [DSC]** *see* Acetaminophen, Chlorpheniramine, and Pseudoephedrine *on page 31*

◆ **Tylenol® Cold Day Non-Drowsy [OTC]** *see* Acetaminophen, Dextromethorphan, and Pseudoephedrine *on page 33*

◆ **Tylenol® Cold Daytime (Can)** *see* Acetaminophen, Dextromethorphan, and Pseudoephedrine *on page 33*

◆ **Tylenol® Cold Daytime, Children's [OTC]** *see* Acetaminophen and Pseudoephedrine *on page 30*

◆ **Tylenol® Cold Head Congestion Daytime [OTC]** *see* Acetaminophen, Dextromethorphan, and Phenylephrine *on page 32*

◆ **Tylenol® Cold, Infants [OTC] [DSC]** *see* Acetaminophen and Pseudoephedrine *on page 30*

◆ **Tylenol® Cold Multi-Symptom Daytime [OTC]** *see* Acetaminophen, Dextromethorphan, and Phenylephrine *on page 32*

◆ **Tylenol® Decongestant (Can)** *see* Acetaminophen and Pseudoephedrine *on page 30*

◆ **Tylenol Elixir with Codeine (Can)** *see* Acetaminophen and Codeine *on page 27*

◆ **Tylenol® Extra Strength [OTC]** *see* Acetaminophen *on page 25*

◆ **Tylenol® Flu Non-Drowsy Maximum Strength [OTC]** *see* Acetaminophen, Dextromethorphan, and Pseudoephedrine *on page 33*

◆ **Tylenol® Infants [OTC]** *see* Acetaminophen *on page 25*

◆ **Tylenol® Junior [OTC]** *see* Acetaminophen *on page 25*

◆ **Tylenol No. 1 (Can)** *see* Acetaminophen and Codeine *on page 27*

◆ **Tylenol No. 1 Forte (Can)** *see* Acetaminophen and Codeine *on page 27*

◆ **Tylenol No. 2 with Codeine (Can)** *see* Acetaminophen and Codeine *on page 27*

Typhoid Vaccine (TYE foid vak SEEN)

U.S. Brand Names Typhim Vi®; Vivotif®

Canadian Brand Names Typherix®; Typhim Vi®; Vivotif®

Index Terms Ty21a Vaccine; Typhoid Vaccine Live Oral Ty21a; Vi Vaccine

Pharmacologic Category Vaccine

Additional Appendix Information

Immunization Recommendations *on page 1708*

Use Active immunization against typhoid fever caused by *Salmonella typhi*

Not for routine vaccination. In the United States and Canada, use should be limited to:

- Travelers to areas with a prolonged risk of exposure to *S. typhi*
- Persons with intimate exposure to a *S. typhi* carrier
- Laboratory technicians with exposure to *S. typhi*
- Travelers with achlorhydria or hypochlorhydria (Canadian recommendation)

Pregnancy Risk Factor C

Pregnancy Considerations Reproduction studies have not been conducted. The manufacturer of the Typhim Vi® injection suggests delaying vaccination until the 2nd or 3rd trimester if possible. Untreated typhoid fever may lead to miscarriage or vertical intrauterine transmission causing neonatal typhoid (rare).

Lactation Excretion in breast milk unknown/use caution

Contraindications Hypersensitivity to any component of the vaccine. In addition, the oral vaccine is contraindicated with congenital or acquired immunodeficient state, acute febrile illness, acute GI illness

Warnings/Precautions Not all recipients of typhoid vaccine will be fully protected against typhoid fever. Travelers should take all necessary precautions to avoid contact or ingestion of potentially contaminated food or water sources. Should not be used to treat typhoid fever.

Injection: Administer at least 2 weeks prior to expected exposure. Vaccination may be deferred during acute infection or febrile illness. Immune response may be decreased in those receiving immunosuppressive therapy or are otherwise immunocompromised. Use caution with coagulation disorders (including thrombocytopenia) where intramuscular injections should not be used. Epinephrine 1:1000 should be readily available. Safety and efficacy have not been established in children <2 years of age.

Oral: Full immunization schedule should be completed at least 1 week prior to expected exposure. The complete immunization schedule must be followed to achieve optimum immune response. Vaccination may be deferred with persistent diarrhea or vomiting. Safety and efficacy have not been established in children <6 years of age.

Adverse Reactions In the U.S., all serious adverse reactions must be reported to the Department of Health and Human Services (DHHS) Vaccine Adverse Event Reporting System (VAERS) 1-800-822-7967. In Canada, adverse reactions are reported to the Canadian Adverse Events following Immunization Surveillance System (CAEFISS) via the Adverse Event Following Immunization Report Form available at http://www.phac-aspc.gc.ca/im/aefi-form_e.html.

Oral:

1% to 10%:

Central nervous system: Headache (5%), fever (3%)

Dermatologic: Rash (1%)

Gastrointestinal: Abdominal pain (6%), diarrhea (3%), nausea (6%), vomiting (2%)

Postmarketing and/or case reports: Anaphylactic reaction, demyelinating disease, myalgia, pain, RA, urticaria, sepsis, weakness

Injection (incidence may vary based on age and/or product used):

>10%:

Central nervous system: Headache (16% to 20%), fever (undefined; 2% to 32%), malaise (4% to 24%)

Local: Injection site: Tenderness (97% to 98%), pain (27% to 41%), soreness (up to 16%), induration (5% to 15%)

Neuromuscular & skeletal: General aches (1% to 13%)

1% to 10%:

Central nervous system: Fever ≥100°F (2%), >102°F (2%)

Dermatologic: Pruritus (up to 8%)

Gastrointestinal: Nausea (up to 8%), vomiting (2%)

Local: Injection site: Erythema (up to 5%), swelling (up to 4%)

Neuromuscular & skeletal: Myalgia (3% to 7%)

Postmarketing and/or case reports: Abdominal pain, allergic reactions, anaphylaxis, arthralgia, cervical pain, diarrhea, dizziness, flu-like syndrome, Guillain-Barré syndrome, hypotension, injection site inflammation (including angioedema and urticaria), loss of consciousness, lymphadenopathy, malaise, perforated jejunum, rash, serum sickness, tremor, urticaria, vasodilation, weakness

Drug Interactions

Avoid Concomitant Use

Avoid concomitant use of Typhoid Vaccine with any of the following: Immunosuppressants

Increased Effect/Toxicity

The levels/effects of Typhoid Vaccine may be increased by: Immunosuppressants; Mefloquine

Decreased Effect

Typhoid Vaccine may decrease the levels/effects of: Tuberculin Tests

The levels/effects of Typhoid Vaccine may be decreased by: Antibiotics; Immune Globulins

Ethanol/Nutrition/Herb Interactions Ethanol: Avoid alcohol within 2 hours of taking the capsule; may disrupt the enteric coating

Stability

Typherix®: Store between 2°C to 8°C (35°F to 46°F); do not freeze. Discard if vaccine has been frozen. Protect from light.

Typhim Vi®: Store between 2°C to 8°C (35°F to 46°F); do not freeze.

Vivotif®: Store between 2°C to 8°C (35°F to 46°F).

Mechanism of Action Virulent strains of *Salmonella typhi* cause disease by penetrating the intestinal mucosa and entering the systemic circulation via the lymphatic vasculature. One possible mechanism of conferring immunity may be the provocation of a local immune response in the intestinal tract induced by oral ingesting of a live strain with subsequent aborted infection. The ability of *Salmonella typhi* to produce clinical disease (and to elicit an immune response) is dependent on the bacteria having a complete lipopolysaccharide. The live attenuate Ty21a strain lacks the enzyme UDP-4-galactose epimerase so that lipopolysaccharide is only synthesized under conditions that induce bacterial autolysis. Thus, the strain remains avirulent despite the production of sufficient lipopolysaccharide to evoke a protective immune response. Despite low levels of lipopolysaccharide synthesis, cells lyse before gaining a virulent phenotype due to the intracellular accumulation of metabolic intermediates.

Pharmacodynamics/Kinetics

Onset of action: Immunity to *Salmonella typhi*: Oral: ~1 week

Duration: Immunity: Oral: ~4-7 years; Parenteral: Typhim Vi®: >17-21 months, Typherix®: ~3 years

Dosage Immunization:

Oral: Children ≥6 years and Adults:

Primary immunization: One capsule on alternate days (day 1, 3, 5, and 7) for a total of 4 doses; all doses should be complete at least 1 week prior to potential exposure

Booster immunization: Repeat full course of primary immunization every 5 years

I.M.: Children ≥2 years and Adults: 0.5 mL given at least 2 weeks prior to expected exposure

Reimmunization:

Typhim Vi®: 0.5 mL; optimal schedule has not been established; a single dose every 2 years is currently recommended for repeated or continued exposure

Typherix®: 0.5 mL every 3 years

Administration Injection: Typhim Vi® and Typherix® may be given I.M. and are indicated for children ≥2 years of age; administer as a single 0.5 mL (25 mcg) injection in deltoid muscle. **Do not administer Typhim Vi® or Typherix® intravascularly. Note:** For patients at risk of hemorrhage following intramuscular injection, the ACIP recommends "it should be administered intramuscularly if, in the opinion of the physician familiar with the patients bleeding risk, the vaccine can be administered with reasonable safety by this route. If the patient receives antihemophilia or other similar therapy, intramuscular vaccination can be scheduled shortly after such therapy is administered. A fine needle (23 gauge or smaller) can be used for the vaccination and firm pressure applied to the site (without rubbing) for at least 2 minutes. The patient should be instructed concerning the risk of hematoma from the injection."

Oral: Swallow capsule whole soon after placing into mouth; do not chew or open capsule. Capsule should be taken with a cold or lukewarm beverage (≤37°C/98.6°F). Take one hour prior to a meal. Avoid alcohol within 2 hours of administration.

Additional Information Federal law requires that the date of administration, the vaccine manufacturer, lot number of vaccine, and the administering person's name, title, and address be entered into the patient's permanent medical record.

Dosage Forms Excipient information presented when available (limited, particularly for generics); consult specific product labeling. [CAN] = Canadian brand name

Capsule, enteric coated:

Vivotif®: Viable *S. typhi* Ty21a 2-6.8 x 10^9 colony-forming units and nonviable *S. typhi* Ty21a 5-50 x 10^9 bacterial cells [contains lactose 100-180 mg/capsule and sucrose 26-130 mg/capsule]

Injection, solution:

Typherix® [CAN]: Vi capsular polysaccharide 25 mcg/0.5 mL (0.5 mL) [derived from *S. typhi* Ty2 strain] [not available in U.S.]

Typhim Vi®: Purified Vi capsular polysaccharide 25 mcg/0.5 mL (0.5 mL, 10 mL) [derived from *S. typhi* Ty2 strain]

- **Typhoid Vaccine Live Oral Ty21a** *see* Typhoid Vaccine *on page 1529*
- **Tysabri®** *see* Natalizumab *on page 1044*
- **506U78** *see* Nelarabine *on page 1047*
- **U-90152S** *see* Delavirdine *on page 414*
- **UCB-P071** *see* Cetirizine *on page 295*
- **UK** *see* Urokinase *on page 1533*
- **UK-88,525** *see* Darifenacin *on page 401*
- **UK-427,857** *see* Maraviroc *on page 921*
- **UK92480** *see* Sildenafil *on page 1368*
- **UK109496** *see* Voriconazole *on page 1567*
- **Ulcidine (Can)** *see* Famotidine *on page 603*
- **Ultane®** *see* Sevoflurane *on page 1366*
- **Ultiva®** *see* Remifentanil *on page 1302*
- **Ultracaps MT [DSC]** *see* Pancrelipase *on page 1136*
- **Ultracet®** *see* Acetaminophen and Tramadol *on page 30*
- **Ultram®** *see* TraMADol *on page 1497*
- **Ultram® ER** *see* TraMADol *on page 1497*
- **Ultra Mide® [OTC]** *see* Urea *on page 1530*
- **UltraMide 25™ (Can)** *see* Urea *on page 1530*
- **Ultramop™ (Can)** *see* Methoxsalen *on page 968*
- **Ultraprin [OTC]** *see* Ibuprofen *on page 760*
- **Ultraquin™ (Can)** *see* Hydroquinone *on page 749*
- **Ultrase®** *see* Pancrelipase *on page 1136*
- **Ultrase® MT** *see* Pancrelipase *on page 1136*
- **Ultravate®** *see* Halobetasol *on page 719*
- **Umecta®** *see* Urea *on page 1530*
- **Unasyn®** *see* Ampicillin and Sulbactam *on page 111*
- **Unburn®** *see* Lidocaine *on page 884*
- **Unidet® (Can)** *see* Tolterodine *on page 1488*
- **Unifed [OTC]** *see* Pseudoephedrine *on page 1265*
- **Unipen® (Can)** *see* Nafcillin *on page 1033*
- **Uniphyl®** *see* Theophylline *on page 1455*
- **Uniphyl® SRT (Can)** *see* Theophylline *on page 1455*
- **Uniretic®** *see* Moexipril and Hydrochlorothiazide *on page 1011*
- **Unisom® Maximum Strength SleepGels® [OTC]** *see* DiphenhydrAMINE *on page 456*
- **Unithroid®** *see* Levothyroxine *on page 881*
- **Univasc®** *see* Moexipril *on page 1010*
- **Unna's Boot** *see* Zinc Gelatin *on page 1584*
- **Unna's Paste** *see* Zinc Gelatin *on page 1584*
- **Urasal® (Can)** *see* Methenamine *on page 961*

Urea (yoor EE a)

U.S. Brand Names Aquacare® [OTC]; Aquaphilic® With Carbamide [OTC]; Carmol® 10 [OTC]; Carmol® 20 [OTC]; Carmol® 40; Carmol® Deep Cleaning; Cerovel™; DPM™ [OTC]; Gormel® [OTC]; Hydro 40™; Kerafoam™; Keralac™; Keralac™ Nailstik; Kerol™; Kerol™ Redi-Cloths;

Kerol™ ZX; Lanaphilic® [OTC]; Nutraplus® [OTC]; Rea-Lo® [OTC]; Ultra Mide® [OTC]; Umecta® ; Ureacin® [OTC]; Vanamide™

Canadian Brand Names UltraMide 25™; Uremol®; Urisec®

Index Terms Carbamide

Pharmacologic Category Diuretic, Osmotic; Keratolytic Agent; Topical Skin Product

Use Keratolytic agent to soften nails or skin; OTC: Moisturizer for dry, rough skin

Pregnancy Risk Factor C

Dosage Topical: Adults: Hyperkeratotic conditions, dry skin: Apply 1-3 times/day

Additional Information Complete prescribing information for this medication should be consulted for additional detail.

Dosage Forms Excipient information presented when available (limited, particularly for generics); consult specific product labeling. [DSC] = Discontinued product

Aerosol, topical [foam]:
- Hydro 40™: 40% (70 g)
- Kerafoam™: 30% (60 g)

Cloth, topical:
- Kerol™ Redi-Cloths: 42% (30s) [contains lactic acid, vitamin E and zinc]

Cream, topical: 40% (30 g, 85 g, 199 g)
- Aquacare®: 10% (75 g)
- Carmol® 20: 20% (90 g)
- Carmol® 40: 40% (30 g, 90 g, 210 g)
- Cerovel™: 40% (133 g) [DSC]
- DPM™: 20% (118 g) [contains menthol and peppermint oil]
- Gormel®: 20% (75 g, 120 g, 454 g, 2270 g)
- Keralac™: 50% (142 g, 255 g) [contains lactic acid, vitamin E, and zinc]
- Nutraplus®: 10% (90 g, 454 g)
- Rea-Lo®: 30% (60 g, 240 g)
- Ureacin®-20: 20% (120 g)
- Vanamide™: 40% (85 g, 199 g)

Emulsion, topical:
- Kerol™: 50% (283.5 g) [contains lactic acid, vitamin E, and zinc]
- Umecta®: 40% (120 mL, 480 mL)

Gel: 40% (15 mL)
- Carmol® 40: 40% (15 mL)
- Cerovel™: 40% (25 mL)
- Keralac™: 50% (18 mL) [contains lactic acid and zinc]

Lotion, topical: 40% (240 mL)
- Aquacare®: 10% (240 mL)
- Carmol® 10: 10% (180 mL)
- Carmol® 40: 40% (240 mL)
- Cerovel™: 40% (325 mL)
- Keralac™: 35% (207 mL, 325 mL) [contains lactic acid, vitamin E, and zinc]
- Nutraplus®: 10% (240 mL, 480 mL)
- Ultra Mide®: 25% (120 mL, 240 mL)
- Ureacin®-10: 10% (240 mL)

Ointment, topical:
- Aquaphilic® with Carbamide: 10% (180 g, 480 g); 20% (480 g)
- Keralac™: 50% (90 g)
- Lanaphilic®: 10% (454 g); 20% (454 g)

Shampoo, topical:
- Carmol® Deep Cleaning: 10% (240 mL)

Solution, topical:
- Keralac™ Nailstick: 50% (2.4 mL)
- Kerol™ ZX: 50% (12 mL) [contains lactic acid, vitamin E, and zinc]

Suspension, topical: 50% (284 g)
- Kerol™: 50% (284 g) [contains lactic acid, salicylic acid and vitamin E]
- Umecta®: 40% (18 mL) [nail film with applicator], (300 mL)

Urea and Hydrocortisone
(yoor EE a & hye droe KOR ti sone)

U.S. Brand Names Carmol-HC®

Canadian Brand Names Ti-U-Lac® H; Uremol® HC

Index Terms Hydrocortisone and Urea

Pharmacologic Category Corticosteroid, Topical

Use Inflammation of corticosteroid-responsive dermatoses

Pregnancy Risk Factor C

Dosage Apply thin film and rub in well 1-4 times/day. Therapy should be discontinued when control is achieved; if no improvement is seen, reassessment of diagnosis may be necessary.

Additional Information Complete prescribing information for this medication should be consulted for additional detail.

Dosage Forms Excipient information presented when available (limited, particularly for generics); consult specific product labeling.

Cream: Urea 10% and hydrocortisone acetate 1% (30 g) [in water soluble vanishing cream base]

- ◆ **Urea, Chlorophyllin, and Papain** *see* Chlorophyllin, Papain, and Urea *on page* 306
- ◆ **Ureacin® [OTC]** *see* Urea *on page* 1530
- ◆ **Urea Peroxide** *see* Carbamide Peroxide *on page* 254
- ◆ **Urecholine®** *see* Bethanechol *on page* 192
- ◆ **Urelle®** *see* Methenamine, Sodium Biphosphate, Phenyl Salicylate, Methylene Blue, and Hyoscyamine *on page* 962
- ◆ **Uremol® (Can)** *see* Urea *on page* 1530
- ◆ **Uremol® HC (Can)** *see* Urea and Hydrocortisone *on page* 1531
- ◆ **Urex™** *see* Methenamine *on page* 961
- ◆ **Urimar-T** *see* Methenamine, Sodium Biphosphate, Phenyl Salicylate, Methylene Blue, and Hyoscyamine *on page* 962
- ◆ **Urisec® (Can)** *see* Urea *on page* 1530
- ◆ **Urispas®** *see* Flavoxate *on page* 623
- ◆ **Uristat® [OTC] [DSC]** *see* Phenazopyridine *on page* 1177

Urofollitropin (yoor oh fol li TROE pin)

U.S. Brand Names Bravelle®

Canadian Brand Names Bravelle®; Fertinorm® H.P.

Index Terms Follicle-Stimulating Hormone, Human; FSH; hFSH

Pharmacologic Category Gonadotropin; Ovulation Stimulator

Use Ovulation induction in patients who previously received pituitary suppression; development of multiple follicles with Assisted Reproductive Technologies (ART)

Pregnancy Risk Factor X

Pregnancy Considerations Ectopic pregnancy, congenital abnormalities, spontaneous abortion, and multiple births have been reported. The incidence of congenital abnormality may be slightly higher after ART than with spontaneous conception; higher incidence may be related to parenteral characteristics (maternal age, sperm characteristics).

Lactation Excretion in breast milk unknown/not recommended

Contraindications Hypersensitivity to follitropins or any component of the formulation; high levels of FSH indicating primary ovarian failure; uncontrolled thyroid or adrenal dysfunction; the presence of any cause of infertility other than anovulation; presence of an organic intracranial lesion (eg, pituitary tumor); abnormal vaginal bleeding of undetermined origin; ovarian cysts or enlargement not due to polycystic ovary syndrome; pregnancy

Warnings/Precautions These medications should only be used by physicians who are thoroughly familiar with infertility problems and their management. To minimize risks, use only at the lowest effective dose. Monitor ovarian response with serum estradiol and vaginal ultrasound on a regular basis.

Ovarian enlargement which may be accompanied by abdominal distention or abdominal pain, occurs in ~20% of those treated with urofollitropin and hCG, and generally regresses without treatment within 2-3 weeks. If ovaries are abnormally enlarged on the last day of treatment, withhold hCG to reduce the risk of ovarian hyperstimulation syndrome (OHSS). OHSS is characterized by severe ovarian enlargement, abdominal pain/distention, nausea, vomiting, diarrhea, dyspnea, and oliguria, and may be accompanied by ascites, pleural effusion, hypovolemia, electrolyte imbalance, hemoperitoneum, and thromboembolic events. If hyperstimulation occurs, stop treatment and hospitalize patient. This syndrome develops rapidly within 24 hours to several days and generally occurs during the 7-10 days immediately following treatment. Hemoconcentration associated with fluid loss into the abdominal cavity has occurred and should be assessed by fluid intake and output, weight, hematocrit, serum and urinary electrolytes, urine specific gravity, BUN and creatinine, and abdominal girth. Determinations should be performed daily or more often if the need arises. Treatment is primarily symptomatic and consists of bedrest, fluid and electrolyte replacement, and analgesics. The ascitic, pleural and pericardial fluids should not be removed unless needed to relieve symptoms of cardiopulmonary distress.

Serious pulmonary conditions (atelectasis, acute respiratory distress syndrome, and exacerbation of asthma) have been reported. Thromboembolic events, both in association with and separate from ovarian hyperstimulation syndrome, have been reported.

Multiple births may result from the use of these medications; advise patient of the potential risk of multiple births before starting the treatment. Safety and efficacy have not been established in children or the elderly. May contain lactose.

Adverse Reactions Percentage may vary by indication, route of administration.

>10%:

- Central nervous system: Headache
- Endocrine & metabolic: Ovarian enlargement, ovarian hyperstimulation syndrome
- Gastrointestinal: Abdominal cramps

1% to 10%:

- Cardiovascular: Hypertension
- Central nervous system: Depression, emotional lability, fever, pain
- Dermatologic: Acne, exfoliative dermatitis, rash
- Endocrine & metabolic: Breast tenderness, hot flashes, ovarian disorder (pain, cyst)
- Gastrointestinal: Abdomen enlarged, abdominal pain, constipation, diarrhea, dehydration, nausea, vomiting, weight gain
- Genitourinary: Cervical disorder, urinary tract infection, pelvic pain/cramps, uterine spasms, vaginal discharge, vaginal hemorrhage, vaginal spotting
- Local: Injection site reaction
- Neuromuscular & skeletal: Neck pain
- Respiratory: Respiratory disorder, sinusitis
- Miscellaneous: Infection, postretrieval pain

Postmarketing, case reports, or events reported with gonadotropins: Acute respiratory distress syndrome, adnexal torsion, anaphylactic reactions, arterial occlusion, atelectasis, cerebral vascular occlusion, deep vein thrombosis, hemoperitoneum, hypersensitivity reactions, ovarian neoplasms, pulmonary embolism

Drug Interactions

Avoid Concomitant Use There are no known interactions where it is recommended to avoid concomitant use.

Increased Effect/Toxicity There are no known significant interactions involving an increase in effect.

Decreased Effect There are no known significant interactions involving a decrease in effect.

Stability Lyophilized powder may be stored in the refrigerator or at room temperature of 3°C to 25°C (37°F to 77°F). Protect from light. Dissolve contents of vial in sterile saline 1 mL; gently swirl (do not shake). Do not use if solution is not clear or contains particles. If more than 1 vial is required for a single dose, up to 6 vials can be reconstituted with sterile saline 1 mL and administered as a single injection. This is done by first reconstituting 1 vial with sterile saline as previously described, withdrawing the entire contents of the reconstituted vial, and (using this as the diluent for the second vial) injecting into the second vial, etc. Use immediately after reconstitution.

Mechanism of Action Urofollitropin is a preparation of highly purified follicle-stimulating hormone (FSH) extracted from the urine of postmenopausal women. Follitropins stimulate ovarian follicular growth in women who do not have primary ovarian failure. FSH is required for normal follicular growth, maturation, gonadal steroid production, and spermatogenesis.

Pharmacodynamics/Kinetics

Half-life elimination

- I.M.: 37 hours, 15 hours following multiple doses
- SubQ: 32 hours, 21 hours following multiple doses

Time to peak, plasma:

- I.M.: 17 hours, 11 hours following multiple doses
- SubQ: 21 hours, 10 hours following multiple doses

Dosage Note: Dose should be individualized. Use the lowest dose consistent with the expectation of good results. Over the course of treatment, doses may vary depending on individual patient response.

Adults: Females:

Ovulation induction: I.M., SubQ: Initial: 150 int. units daily for the first 5 days of treatment. Dose adjustments ≤75-150 int. units can be made every ≥2 days; maximum daily dose: 450 int. units; treatment >12 days is not recommended. If response to follitropin is appropriate, hCG is given 1 day following the last dose. Withhold hCG if serum estradiol is >2000 pg/mL, if the ovaries are abnormally enlarged, or if abdominal pain occurs.

ART: SubQ: 225 int. units daily for the first 5 days; dose may be adjusted based on patient response, but adjustments should not be made more frequently than once every 2 days; maximum adjustment: 75-150 int. units; maximum daily dose: 450 int. units; maximum duration of treatment: 12 days. When a sufficient number of follicles of adequate size are present, the final maturation of the follicles is induced by administering hCG. Withhold hCG in cases where the ovaries are abnormally enlarged on the last day of therapy.

Administration Administer I.M. or SubQ; gently massage site after administration.

I.M.: Administer in upper quadrant of buttock near hip

SubQ: Administer on lower abdomen; thigh is not recommended unless abdomen cannot be used

Monitoring Parameters Monitor sufficient follicular maturation. This may be directly estimated by sonographic visualization of the ovaries and endometrial lining or measuring serum estradiol levels. The combination of both ultrasonography and measurement of estradiol levels is useful for monitoring for the growth and development of follicles and timing hCG administration.

The clinical evaluation of estrogenic activity (changes in vaginal cytology and changes in appearance and volume of cervical mucus) provides an indirect estimate of the estrogenic effect upon the target organs and, therefore, it should only be used adjunctively with more direct estimates of follicular development (ultrasonography and serum estradiol determinations).

The clinical confirmation of ovulation is obtained by direct and indirect indices of progesterone production. The indices most generally used are: rise in basal body temperature, increase in serum progesterone, and menstruation following the shift in basal body temperature.

Monitor for signs and symptoms of OHSS for at least 2 weeks following hCG administration.

Dosage Forms Excipient information presented when available (limited, particularly for generics); consult specific product labeling.

Injection, powder for reconstitution [human origin]:

Bravelle®: 75 int. units [contains lactose; packaged with diluent]

Urokinase (ur oh KYE nase)

U.S. Brand Names Kinlytic™

Index Terms Abbokinase; UK

Pharmacologic Category Thrombolytic Agent

Use Thrombolytic agent for the lysis of acute massive pulmonary emboli or pulmonary emboli with unstable hemodynamics

Unlabeled/Investigational Use Thrombolytic agent used in treatment of recent severe or massive deep vein thrombosis, and occluded I.V. or dialysis cannulas; peripheral arterial occlusive disease

Pregnancy Risk Factor B

Pregnancy Considerations Urokinase was not found to be teratogenic in animal studies; it is not known if it crosses the human placenta. Placental separation and hemorrhage have been reported in one patient treated at 3 months gestation. Use during pregnancy only if clearly needed.

Lactation Excretion in breast milk unknown/use caution

Medication Safety Issues

High alert medication: The Institute for Safe Medication Practices (ISMP) includes this medication among its list of drugs which have a heightened risk of causing significant patient harm when used in error.

Contraindications Hypersensitivity to urokinase or any component of the formulation; active internal bleeding; recent (within 2 months) CVA, intracranial surgery or intraspinal surgery; recent trauma (including cardiopulmonary resuscitation); intracranial neoplasm, arteriovenous malformation, or aneurysm; known bleeding diathesis; severe uncontrolled arterial hypertension

Warnings/Precautions The risk of bleeding is increased with use; fatal hemorrhage has been reported. Concurrent heparin anticoagulation can contribute to bleeding; careful attention to all potential bleeding sites. I.M. injections and nonessential handling of the patient should be avoided. Venipunctures should be performed carefully and only when necessary. If arterial puncture is necessary, use an upper extremity vessel that can be manually compressed. If serious bleeding occurs, then the infusion of urokinase and heparin should be stopped.

For the following conditions, the risk of bleeding is higher with use of thrombolytics and should be weighed against the benefits of therapy: recent (within 10 days) major surgery, obstetrical delivery, organ biopsy, or previous puncture of noncompressible vessels; pregnancy, cerebrovascular disease, recent (within 10 days) gastrointestinal bleeding, high likelihood of left heart thrombus (in the setting of mitral stenosis with atrial fibrillation), subacute bacterial endocarditis, hemostatic defects including those caused by severe renal or hepatic dysfunction, diabetic hemorrhagic retinopathy, and/or any other condition in which bleeding constitutes a significant hazard or would be particularly difficult to manage because of location. Use is contraindicated in recent trauma, including CPR. Use with caution in patients receiving oral anticoagulants or platelet inhibitors; increased risk of bleeding. Cholesterol embolization has been reported rarely with the use of thrombolytics, usually associated with invasive vascular procedures and/or anticoagulant therapy. Hypersensitivity reactions, including fatal anaphylaxis (rare), bronchospasm, orolingual edema and urticaria have been reported. Infusion reactions (eg, chills, rigor, hypoxia, hyper-/hypotension, tachycardia) may also occur. Reactions usually occur within the first hour of infusion. Safety and efficacy in pediatric patients have not been established.

Adverse Reactions As with all drugs which may affect hemostasis, bleeding is the major adverse effect associated with urokinase. Hemorrhage may occur at virtually any site. Risk is dependent on multiple variables, including the dosage administered, concurrent use of multiple agents which alter hemostasis, and patient predisposition.

>10%: Local: Injection site: Bleeding (5% decrease in hematocrit reported in 37% patients; most bleeding occurring at external incisions or injection sites, but also reported in other areas)

<1% (Limited to important or life-threatening): Allergic reaction (includes anaphylaxis, bronchospasm, orolingual edema, urticaria, skin rash, pruritus), cardiac arrest, cerebral vascular accident, chest pain, cholesterol embolism, diaphoresis, hemiplegia, intracranial hemorrhage, retroperitoneal hemorrhage, MI, pulmonary edema, recurrent pulmonary embolism, reperfusion ventricular arrhythmia, stroke, substernal pain, thrombocytopenia, vascular embolization (cerebral and distal); infusion reactions (most occurring within 1 hour) including acidosis, back pain, chills, cyanosis, dyspnea, fever, hyper-/hypotension, hypoxia, nausea, rigors, tachycardia, vomiting

Drug Interactions

Avoid Concomitant Use There are no known interactions where it is recommended to avoid concomitant use.

Increased Effect/Toxicity

Urokinase may increase the levels/effects of: Anticoagulants; Drotrecogin Alfa

The levels/effects of Urokinase may be increased by: Antiplatelet Agents; Herbs (Anticoagulant/Antiplatelet Properties); Nonsteroidal Anti-Inflammatory Agents; Salicylates

Decreased Effect

The levels/effects of Urokinase may be decreased by: Aprotinin

Stability Prior to reconstitution, store in refrigerator at 2°C to 8°C (36°F to 46°F). Reconstitute vial with 5 mL preservative free sterile water for injection by gently rolling and tilting; do not shake. Contains no preservatives; should not be reconstituted until immediately before using. Discard unused portion. Solution will look pale and straw colored. May filter through ≤0.45 micron filter. Prior to infusion, solution should be further diluted in D_5W or NS; the manufacturer recommends a total infusion volume of 195 mL.

Mechanism of Action Promotes thrombolysis by directly activating plasminogen to plasmin, which degrades fibrin, fibrinogen, and other procoagulant plasma proteins

Pharmacodynamics/Kinetics

Onset of action: I.V.: Fibrinolysis occurs rapidly

Duration: ≥4 hours

Distribution: 11.5 L

Half-life elimination: 6.4-18.8 minutes

Excretion: Urine and feces (small amounts)

Dosage

Children and Adults: Deep vein thrombosis (unlabeled use): I.V.: Loading: 4400 units/kg over 10 minutes, then 4400 units/kg/hour for 12 hours

Adults:

Acute pulmonary embolism: I.V.: Loading: 4400 int. units/kg over 10 minutes; maintenance: 4400 int. units/kg/hour for 12 hours. To prevent recurrent thrombosis, anticoagulation treatment is recommended after the completion of urokinase infusion; if heparin is used, do not administer heparin loading dose. Do not start anticoagulation until aPTT has decreased to less than twice the normal control value.

Acute peripheral arterial occlusion of leg (unlabeled use; Ouriel, 1998): I.V.: 4000 int. units/minute for 4 hours, followed by 2000 int. units/minute for up to a total duration of therapy of 48 hours. **Note:** Systemic heparinization should not be given concurrently.

Occluded I.V. catheters (unlabeled use):

5000 units in each lumen over 1-2 minutes, leave in lumen for 1-4 hours, then aspirate; may repeat with 10,000 units in each lumen if 5000 units fails to clear the catheter; **do not infuse into the patient**; volume to instill into catheter is equal to the volume of the catheter

I.V. infusion: 200 units/kg/hour in each lumen for 12-48 hours at a rate of at least 20 mL/hour

Dialysis patients: 5000 units is administered in each lumen over 1-2 minutes; leave urokinase in lumen for 1-2 days, then aspirate

Administration Solution may be filtered with ≤0.45 micron filter during I.V. therapy. Administer using an infusion pump. When prepared to a total volume of 195 mL, the loading dose should be administered at 90 mL/hour over 10 minutes. The maintenance dose should be administered at 15 mL/hour over 12 hours. I.V. tubing should be flushed with NS or D_5W to ensure total dose is administered.

Monitoring Parameters Blood pressure (avoid using lower extremities for BP), pulse; CBC, platelet count, aPTT, urinalysis

Product Availability

Kinlytic™: ImaRx Therapeutics retired the trade name Abbokinase® for urokinase and is currently marketing urokinase under the trade name Kinlytic™

Dosage Forms Excipient information presented when available (limited, particularly for generics); consult specific product labeling.

Injection, powder for reconstitution:

Kinlytic™: 250,000 int. units [contains albumin (human)]

- ◆ **Uro-KP-Neutral®** *see* Potassium Phosphate and Sodium Phosphate *on page* 1222
- ◆ **Urolene Blue® [DSC]** *see* Methylene Blue *on page* 971
- ◆ **Uro-Mag® [OTC]** *see* Magnesium Oxide *on page* 916
- ◆ **Uromax® (Can)** *see* Oxybutynin *on page* 1119
- ◆ **Uromitexan (Can)** *see* Mesna *on page* 951
- ◆ **Uroqid-Acid® No. 2** *see* Methenamine and Sodium Acid Phosphate *on page* 962
- ◆ **Uroxatral®** *see* Alfuzosin *on page* 61
- ◆ **Urso® (Can)** *see* Ursodiol *on page* 1534
- ◆ **Urso 250™** *see* Ursodiol *on page* 1534
- ◆ **Ursodeoxycholic Acid** *see* Ursodiol *on page* 1534

Ursodiol (ur soe DYE ol)

U.S. Brand Names Actigall®; Urso 250™; Urso Forte™

Canadian Brand Names DOM-Ursodiol C; PHL-Ursodiol C; PMS-Ursodiol C; Urso®; Urso® DS

Index Terms Ursodeoxycholic Acid

Pharmacologic Category Gallstone Dissolution Agent

Use Actigall®: Gallbladder stone dissolution; prevention of gallstones in obese patients experiencing rapid weight loss; Urso®: Primary biliary cirrhosis

Unlabeled/Investigational Use Liver transplantation

Pregnancy Risk Factor B

Dosage Adults: Oral:

Gallstone dissolution: 8-10 mg/kg/day in 2-3 divided doses; use beyond 24 months is not established; obtain ultrasound images at 6-month intervals for the first year of therapy; 30% of patients have stone recurrence after dissolution

Gallstone prevention: 300 mg twice daily

Primary biliary cirrhosis: 13-15 mg/kg/day in 2-4 divided doses (with food)

Additional Information Complete prescribing information for this medication should be consulted for additional detail.

Dosage Forms Excipient information presented when available (limited, particularly for generics); consult specific product labeling.

Capsule (Actigall®): 300 mg

Tablet:

Urso 250™: 250 mg

Urso Forte™: 500 mg

- ◆ **Urso® DS (Can)** *see* Ursodiol *on page* 1534
- ◆ **Urso Forte™** *see* Ursodiol *on page* 1534
- ◆ **Uta®** *see* Methenamine, Sodium Biphosphate, Phenyl Salicylate, Methylene Blue, and Hyoscyamine *on page* 962
- ◆ **Utira™-C** *see* Methenamine, Sodium Biphosphate, Phenyl Salicylate, Methylene Blue, and Hyoscyamine *on page* 962
- ◆ **UTI Relief® [OTC]** *see* Phenazopyridine *on page* 1177
- ◆ **Utradol™ (Can)** *see* Etodolac *on page* 587
- ◆ **Uvadex®** *see* Methoxsalen *on page* 968

Vaccinia Immune Globulin (Intravenous)

(vax IN ee a i MYUN GLOB yoo lin IN tra VEE nus)

U.S. Brand Names CNJ-016™

Index Terms VIGIV

Pharmacologic Category Immune Globulin

Use Treatment of infectious complications of smallpox (vaccinia virus) vaccination, such as eczema vaccinatum, progressive vaccinia, and severe generalized vaccinia; treatment of vaccinia infections in individuals with concurrent skin conditions or accidental virus exposure to eyes (except vaccinia keratitis), mouth, or other areas where viral infection would pose significant risk

Pregnancy Risk Factor C

Pregnancy Considerations Immune globulins cross the placenta in increased amounts after 30 weeks gestation. There are no adequate and well-controlled studies in pregnant women; use only if benefits outweigh the risks.

Lactation Excretion in breast milk unknown/use caution

Contraindications Hypersensitivity to immune globulin or any component of the formulation; isolated vaccinia keratitis; selective IgA deficiency

Warnings/Precautions Hypersensitivity and anaphylactic reactions can occur; immediate treatment (including epinephrine 1:1000) should be available. Contains trace amounts of IgA; use caution in IgA-deficient patients. Aseptic meningitis syndrome (AMS) has been reported with intravenous immune globulin administration (rare); may occur with high doses (≥2 g/kg). Intravenous immune globulin has been associated with antiglobulin hemolysis; monitor for signs of hemolytic anemia. Monitor for transfusion-related acute lung injury (TRALI); noncardiogenic pulmonary edema has been reported with intravenous immune globulin use. Acute renal dysfunction (increased serum creatinine, oliguria, acute renal failure) can rarely occur; usually within 7 days of use (more likely with products stabilized with sucrose). Use with caution in the elderly, patients with renal disease, diabetes mellitus, volume depletion, sepsis, paraproteinemia, and nephrotoxic medications due to risk of renal dysfunction. In patients at risk of renal dysfunction, the rate of infusion and concentration of solution should be minimized. discontinue if renal function deteriorates. Patients should not be volume depleted prior to therapy. Thrombotic events have been reported with administration of intravenous immune globulin; use with caution in patients with cardiovascular risk factors. Product of human plasma; may potentially contain infectious agents which could transmit disease. Screening of donors, as well as testing and/or inactivation or removal of certain viruses, reduces the risk. Infections thought to be transmitted by this product should be reported to the manufacturer. Some products may contain maltose, which may result in falsely-elevated blood glucose readings. Use with caution in the elderly; safety and efficacy have not been established. Safety and efficacy have not been established in children. For intravenous administration only.

Adverse Reactions Note: Actual frequency varies by dose, rate of infusion, and specific product used

Cardiovascular: Flushing

Central nervous system: Cold or hot feeling, dizziness, fatigue, headache, pain, pallor, pyrexia

Dermatologic: Erythema, urticaria

Gastrointestinal: Abdominal pain, appetite decreased, nausea, vomiting

Local: Injection site reaction

Neuromuscular & skeletal: Arthralgia, back pain, paraesthesia, muscle cramp, rigors, tremor, weakness

Miscellaneous: Diaphoresis

Postmarketing and/or case reports (as reported with other IVIG products): Apnea, acute respiratory distress syndrome, bronchospasm, bullous dermatitis, cardiac arrest, coma, Coombs' test positive, cyanosis, dyspnea, epidermolysis, erythema multiforme, hemolysis, hepatic dysfunction, hypoxemia, hypotension, leukopenia, loss of consciousness, lung injury (transfusion associated), pancytopenia, pulmonary edema, seizure, Stevens-Johnson syndrome, syncope, thromboembolism, vascular collapse

Drug Interactions

Avoid Concomitant Use There are no known interactions where it is recommended to avoid concomitant use.

Increased Effect/Toxicity There are no known significant interactions involving an increase in effect.

Decreased Effect

Vaccinia Immune Globulin (Intravenous) may decrease the levels/effects of: Vaccines (Live)

Stability Store between 2°C and 8°C (35.6°F to 46.4°F).

CNJ-016™ (Cangene product): If frozen, use within 60 days of thawing at 2°C and 8°C. Infusion should begin within 4 hours after entering vial.

DynPort product: Use within 6 hours of piercing vial stopper; complete infusion within 12 hours of spiking vial.

Mechanism of Action Antibodies obtained from pooled human plasma of individuals immunized with the smallpox vaccine provide passive immunity

Pharmacodynamics/Kinetics

Distribution: V_d: CNJ-016™ (Cangene product): 6630 L

Half-life elimination:

CNJ-016™ (Cangene product): 30 days (range 13-67 days)

DynPort product: 22 days

Dosage I.V.:

Adults:

CNJ-016™ (Cangene product): 6000 units/kg; 9000 units/kg may be considered if patient does not respond to initial dose.

DynPort product: Total dose: 2 mL/kg (100 mg/kg); higher doses (200-500 mg/kg) may be considered if patient does not respond to initial recommended dose (sucrose-related renal impairment is worsened at doses ≥400 mg/kg)

Elderly: Safety and efficacy have not been established

Dosage adjustment in renal impairment: Use caution. Doses ≥400 mg/kg of the DynPort product are not recommended.

Dietary Considerations DynPort solution for injection contains sodium 0.02-0.03 mEq/mL.

Administration Do not shake; avoid foaming. For intravenous use only. Predilution is not recommended. If dedicated line is not available, flush with NS prior to administration of VIGIV. Do not exceed recommended rates of infusion.

CNJ-016™ (Cangene product): Patients ≥50 kg: Infuse at ≤2 mL/minute; Patients <50 kg: Infuse at 0.04 mL/kg/minute. Maximum assessed rate of infusion: 4 mL/minute. Decrease rate of infusion if minor adverse reactions develop in patients with risk factors for thrombosis/thromboembolism and/or renal insufficiency.

DynPort product: Infuse at 1 mL/kg/hour for 30 minutes, then 2 mL/kg/hour for 30 minutes, then 3 mL/kg/hour until complete. Administer through 0.22 micron filtered set; use of infusion pump is recommended.

Monitoring Parameters During infusion, monitor patient for signs of infusion-related reactions, including (but not limited to) flushing, fever, chills, respiratory distress, blood pressure or heart rate changes.

Test Interactions CNJ-016™ contains maltose. Falsely-elevated blood glucose levels may occur when glucose monitoring devices and test strips utilizing the glucose dehydrogenase pyrroloquinolinequinone (GDH-PQQ) based methods are used. Glucose monitoring devices and test strips which utilize the glucose-specific method are recommended.

Dosage Forms Excipient information presented when available (limited, particularly for generics); consult specific product labeling.

Injection, solution [preservative free; solvent-detergent treated]:

CNJ-016™ (Cangene product): ≥50,000 units/15 mL (15 mL) [contains maltose 10% and polysorbate 80 0.03%]

DynPort product: 50 mg/mL (50 mL) [contains sucrose 50 mg/mL, human albumin 10 mg/mL, sodium 0.02-0.03 mEq/mL]

◆ **Vaccinia Vaccine** *see* Smallpox Vaccine *on page* 1377

◆ **Vagifem®** *see* Estradiol *on page* 554

◆ **Vagi-Gard® [OTC]** *see* Povidone-Iodine *on page* 1222

◆ **Vagistat®-1 [OTC]** *see* Tioconazole *on page* 1475

Valacyclovir (val ay SYE kloe veer)

U.S. Brand Names Valtrex®

Canadian Brand Names APO-Valacyclovir; PMS-Valacyclovir; RIVA-Valacyclovir; Valtrex®

Index Terms Valacyclovir Hydrochloride

Pharmacologic Category Antiviral Agent, Oral

Additional Appendix Information

Guidelines for the Prevention of Opportunistic Infections in HIV Infected Persons *on page* 1740

Treatment of Sexually Transmitted Infections *on page* 1773

Use Treatment of herpes zoster (shingles) in immunocompetent patients; treatment of first-episode and recurrent genital herpes; suppression of recurrent genital herpes and reduction of heterosexual transmission of genital herpes in immunocompetent patients; suppression of genital herpes in HIV-infected individuals; treatment of herpes labialis (cold sores); chickenpox in immunocompetent children

Unlabeled/Investigational Use Prophylaxis of cancer-related HSV, VZV, and CMV infections; treatment of cancer-related HSV, VZV infection

Pregnancy Risk Factor B

Pregnancy Considerations Teratogenic events were not observed in animal studies. Data from a pregnancy registry has shown no increased rate of birth defects than that of the general population; however, the registry is small and use during pregnancy is only warranted if the potential benefit to the mother justifies the risk of the fetus.

Lactation Enters breast milk/use caution

Medication Safety Issues

Sound-alike/look-alike issues:

Valtrex® may be confused with Valcyte™, Zovirax®

Valacyclovir may be confused with acyclovir, valganciclovir, vancomycin

Contraindications Hypersensitivity to valacyclovir, acyclovir, or any component of the formulation

Warnings/Precautions Thrombotic thrombocytopenic purpura/hemolytic uremic syndrome has occurred in immunocompromised patients (at doses of 8 g/day). Safety and efficacy have not been established for treatment/suppression of recurrent genital herpes or disseminated herpes in patients with profound immunosuppression (eg, advanced HIV with CD4 <100 cells/mm^3). Use caution in patients with renal impairment, the elderly, and/or those receiving nephrotoxic agents. Acute renal failure and CNS effects have been observed in patients with renal dysfunction; dose adjustment may be required. Decreased precipitation in renal tubules may occur leading to urinary precipitation; adequately hydrate patient. For cold sores, treatment should begin at with earliest symptom (tingling, itching, burning). For genital herpes, treatment should begin as soon as possible after the first signs and symptoms (within 72 hours of onset of first diagnosis or within 24 hours of onset of recurrent episodes). For herpes zoster, treatment should begin within 72 hours of onset of rash. For chickenpox, treatment should begin with earliest sign or symptom. Use with caution in the elderly; CNS effects have been reported. Safety and efficacy have not been established in patients <2 years of age.

Adverse Reactions

>10%:

Central nervous system: Headache (13% to 38%)

Gastrointestinal: Nausea (5% to 15%), abdominal pain (1% to 11%)

Hematologic: Neutropenia (≤18%)

Hepatic: ALT increased (≤14%), AST increased (2% to 16%)

Respiratory: Nasopharyngitis (≤16%)

1% to 10%:

Central nervous system: Fatigue (≤8%), depression (≤7%), fever (children 4%), dizziness (2% to 4%)

Dermatologic: Rash (≤8%)

Endocrine: Dysmenorrhea (≤1% to 8%), dehydration (children 2%)

Gastrointestinal: Vomiting (<1% to 6%), diarrhea (children 5%; adults <1%)

Hematologic: Thrombocytopenia (≤3%)

Hepatic: Alkaline phosphatase increased (≤4%)

Neuromuscular & skeletal: Arthralgia (<1 to 6%)

Respiratory: Rhinorrhea (children 2%)

Miscellaneous: Herpes simplex (children 2%)

<1% (Limited to important or life-threatening): Acute hypersensitivity reactions (angioedema, anaphylaxis, dyspnea, pruritus, rash, urticaria); aggression, agitation, alopecia, anemia, aplastic anemia, ataxia, creatinine increased, coma, confusion, consciousness decreased, diarrhea, dysarthria, encephalopathy, facial edema, erythema multiforme, hallucinations (auditory and visual), hemolytic uremic syndrome (HUS), hepatitis, hypertension, leukocytoclastic vasculitis, leukopenia, mania, photosensitivity reaction, psychosis, rash, renal failure, renal pain, seizure, tachycardia, thrombotic thrombocytopenic purpura (TTP), thrombocytopenia, tremor, urinary precipitation, visual disturbances

Drug Interactions

Avoid Concomitant Use

Avoid concomitant use of Valacyclovir with any of the following: Zoster Vaccine

Increased Effect/Toxicity

Valacyclovir may increase the levels/effects of: Mycophenolate; Tenofovir; Zidovudine

The levels/effects of Valacyclovir may be increased by: Mycophenolate

Decreased Effect

Valacyclovir may decrease the levels/effects of: Zoster Vaccine

Stability Store at 15°C to 25°C (59°F to 77°F).

Mechanism of Action Valacyclovir is rapidly and nearly completely converted to acyclovir by intestinal and hepatic metabolism. Acyclovir is converted to acyclovir monophosphate by virus-specific thymidine kinase then further converted to acyclovir triphosphate by other cellular enzymes. Acyclovir triphosphate inhibits DNA synthesis and viral replication by competing with deoxyguanosine triphosphate for viral DNA polymerase and being incorporated into viral DNA.

Pharmacodynamics/Kinetics

Absorption: Rapid

Distribution: Acyclovir is widely distributed throughout the body including brain, kidney, lungs, liver, spleen, muscle, uterus, vagina, and CSF

Protein binding: ~14% to 18%

Metabolism: Hepatic; valacyclovir is rapidly and nearly completely converted to acyclovir and L-valine by first-pass effect; acyclovir is hepatically metabolized to a very small extent by aldehyde oxidase and by alcohol and aldehyde dehydrogenase (inactive metabolites)

Bioavailability: ~55% once converted to acyclovir

Half-life elimination: Normal renal function: Adults: Acyclovir: 2.5-3.3 hours, Valacyclovir: ~30 minutes; End-stage renal disease: Acyclovir: 14-20 hours; During hemodialysis: 4 hours

Excretion: Urine, primarily as acyclovir (89%); **Note:** Following oral administration of radiolabeled valacyclovir, 46% of the label is eliminated in the feces (corresponding to nonabsorbed drug), while 47% of the radiolabel is eliminated in the urine.

Dosage Oral:

Children 2 to <18 years: Chickenpox: 20 mg/kg/dose 3 times/day for 5 days (maximum: 1 g 3 times/day)

Children ≥12 and Adults: Herpes labialis (cold sores): 2 g twice daily for 1 day (separate doses by ~12 hours)

Adults:

CMV prophylaxis in allogeneic HSCT recipients (unlabeled use): 2 g 4 times/day

Herpes zoster (shingles): 1 g 3 times/day for 7 days

HSV, VZV in cancer patients (unlabeled use): Prophylaxis: 500 mg 2-3 times/day; Treatment: 1 g 3 times/day

Genital herpes:

Initial episode: 1 g twice daily for 10 days

Recurrent episode: 500 mg twice daily for 3 days

Reduction of transmission: 500 mg once daily (source partner)

Suppressive therapy:
Immunocompetent patients: 1000 mg once daily (500 mg once daily in patients with <9 recurrences per year)
HIV-infected patients (CD4 ≥100 cells/mm^3): 500 mg twice daily

Dosing adjustment in renal impairment:
Herpes zoster: Adults:
Cl_{cr} 30-49 mL/minute: 1 g every 12 hours
Cl_{cr} 10-29 mL/minute: 1 g every 24 hours
Cl_{cr} <10 mL/minute: 500 mg every 24 hours
Genital herpes: Adults:
Initial episode:
Cl_{cr} 10-29 mL/minute: 1 g every 24 hours
Cl_{cr} <10 mL/minute: 500 mg every 24 hours
Recurrent episode: Cl_{cr} <29 mL/minute: 500 mg every 24 hours
Suppressive therapy: Cl_{cr} <29 mL/minute:
For usual dose of 1 g every 24 hours, decrease dose to 500 mg every 24 hours
For usual dose of 500 mg every 24 hours, decrease dose to 500 mg every 48 hours
HIV-infected patients: 500 mg every 24 hours
Herpes labialis: Adolescents and Adults:
Cl_{cr} 30-49 mL/minute: 1 g every 12 hours for 2 doses
Cl_{cr} 10-29 mL/minute: 500 mg every 12 hours for 2 doses
Cl_{cr} <10 mL/minute: 500 mg as a single dose
Hemodialysis: Dialyzable (~33% removed during 4-hour session); administer dose postdialysis
Chronic ambulatory peritoneal dialysis/continuous arteriovenous hemofiltration dialysis: Pharmacokinetic parameters are similar to those in patients with ESRD; supplemental dose not needed following dialysis

Dosing adjustment in hepatic impairment: No adjustment required.

Dietary Considerations May be taken with or without food.

Administration If GI upset occurs, administer with meals.

Monitoring Parameters Urinalysis, BUN, serum creatinine, liver enzymes, and CBC

Dosage Forms Excipient information presented when available (limited, particularly for generics); consult specific product labeling.
Caplet:
Valtrex®: 500 mg, 1000 mg

Extemporaneous Preparations
To prepare a valacyclovir 25 mg/mL oral suspension, crush five valacyclovir 500 mg caplets (10 caplets for 50 mg/mL suspension) into a fine powder in a mortar. Gradually add 5 mL aliquots of Suspension Structured Vehicle USP-NF (SSV) to powder and triturate until a paste is formed. Continue adding 5 mL aliquots of SSV to the mortar until a suspension is formed (minimum 20 mL SSV and maximum 40 mL SSV). Transfer to 100 mL bottle. Add the cherry flavor (amount recommended on package) to the mortar and dissolve in ~5 mL of SSV. Add to bottle once dissolved. Rinse the mortar at least 3 times with ~5 mL of SSV, transferring contents between additions of SSV. Continue to add the SSV to bring final volume to 100 mL. The preparation is stable for 28 days under refrigeration; shake well before using. (Refer to manufacturer's current labeling.)

◆ **Valacyclovir Hydrochloride** *see* Valacyclovir *on page 1535*

◆ **Valcyte™** *see* Valganciclovir *on page 1537*

◆ **23-Valent Pneumococcal Polysaccharide Vaccine** *see* Pneumococcal Polysaccharide Vaccine (Polyvalent) *on page 1206*

Valganciclovir (val gan SYE kloh veer)

U.S. Brand Names Valcyte™
Canadian Brand Names Valcyte™
Index Terms Valganciclovir Hydrochloride
Pharmacologic Category Antiviral Agent
Use Treatment of cytomegalovirus (CMV) retinitis in patients with acquired immunodeficiency syndrome (AIDS); prevention of CMV disease in high-risk patients (donor CMV positive/recipient CMV negative) undergoing kidney, heart, or kidney/pancreas transplantation
Pregnancy Risk Factor C
Pregnancy Considerations Valganciclovir is converted to ganciclovir and shares its reproductive toxicity. **[U.S. Boxed Warning]: Ganciclovir may adversely affect spermatogenesis and fertility;** due to its mutagenic potential, contraceptive precautions for female and male patients need to be followed during and for at least 90 days after therapy with this drug.
Lactation Excretion in breast milk unknown/contraindicated
Medication Safety Issues
Sound-alike/look-alike issues:
Valcyte™ may be confused with Valium®, Valtrex®
Valganciclovir may be confused with valacyclovir
Contraindications Hypersensitivity to valganciclovir, ganciclovir, acyclovir, or any component of the formulation; absolute neutrophil count <500/mm^3; platelet count <25,000/mm^3; hemoglobin <8 g/dL
Warnings/Precautions Hazardous agent - use appropriate precautions for handling and disposal. **[U.S. Boxed Warning]: May cause dose- or therapy-limiting granulocytopenia, anemia, and/or thrombocytopenia;** use caution in patients with impaired renal function (dose adjustment required). **[U.S. Boxed Warning]: Ganciclovir may adversely affect spermatogenesis and fertility;** due to its mutagenic potential, contraceptive precautions for female and male patients need to be followed during and for at least 90 days after therapy with the drug. Due to differences in bioavailability, valganciclovir tablets cannot be substituted for ganciclovir capsules on a one-to-one basis. Not indicated for use in liver transplant patients (higher incidence of tissue-invasive CMV relative to oral ganciclovir was observed in trials). Safety and efficacy not established in pediatric patients.
Adverse Reactions
>10%:
Central nervous system: Fever (31%), headache (9% to 22%), insomnia (16%)
Gastrointestinal: Diarrhea (16% to 41%), nausea (8% to 30%), vomiting (21%), abdominal pain (15%)
Hematologic: Granulocytopenia (11% to 27%), anemia (8% to 26%)
Ocular: Retinal detachment (15%)
1% to 10%:
Central nervous system: Peripheral neuropathy (9%), paresthesia (8%), seizure (<5%), psychosis, hallucinations (<5%), confusion (<5%), agitation (<5%)
Hematologic: Thrombocytopenia (8%), pancytopenia (<5%), bone marrow depression (<5%), aplastic anemia (<5%), bleeding (potentially life-threatening due to thrombocytopenia <5%)
Renal: Renal function decreased (<5%)
Miscellaneous: Local and systemic infection, including sepsis (<5%); allergic reaction (<5%)
<1% (Limited to important or life-threatening): Valganciclovir is expected to share the toxicities which may occur at a low incidence or due to idiosyncratic reactions which have been associated with ganciclovir
Drug Interactions
Avoid Concomitant Use There are no known interactions where it is recommended to avoid concomitant use.

Increased Effect/Toxicity

Valganciclovir may increase the levels/effects of: Mycophenolate; Reverse Transcriptase Inhibitors (Nucleoside); Tenofovir

The levels/effects of Valganciclovir may be increased by: Mycophenolate

Decreased Effect There are no known significant interactions involving a decrease in effect.

Ethanol/Nutrition/Herb Interactions Food: Coadministration with a high-fat meal increased AUC by 30%.

Stability Store at 25°C (77°F); excursions permitted to 15°C to 30°C (59°F to 86°F).

Mechanism of Action Valganciclovir is rapidly converted to ganciclovir in the body. The bioavailability of ganciclovir from valganciclovir is increased 10-fold compared to oral ganciclovir. A dose of 900 mg achieved systemic exposure of ganciclovir comparable to that achieved with the recommended doses of intravenous ganciclovir of 5 mg/kg. Ganciclovir is phosphorylated to a substrate which competitively inhibits the binding of deoxyguanosine triphosphate to DNA polymerase resulting in inhibition of viral DNA synthesis.

Pharmacodynamics/Kinetics

Absorption: Well absorbed; high-fat meal increases AUC by 30%

Distribution: Ganciclovir: V_d: 15.26 L/1.73 m^2; widely to all tissue including CSF and ocular tissue

Protein binding: 1% to 2%

Metabolism: Converted to ganciclovir by intestinal mucosal cells and hepatocytes

Bioavailability: With food: 60%

Half-life elimination: Ganciclovir: 4.08 hours; prolonged with renal impairment; Severe renal impairment: Up to 68 hours

Excretion: Urine (primarily as ganciclovir)

Dosage Oral: Adults:

CMV retinitis:

Induction: 900 mg twice daily for 21 days (with food)

Maintenance: Following induction treatment, or for patients with inactive CMV retinitis who require maintenance therapy: Recommended dose: 900 mg once daily (with food)

Prevention of CMV disease following transplantation: 900 mg once daily (with food) beginning within 10 days of transplantation; continue therapy until 100 days post-transplantation

Dosage adjustment in renal impairment:

Induction dose:

Cl_{cr} 40-59 mL/minute: 450 mg twice daily

Cl_{cr} 25-39 mL/minute: 450 mg once daily

Cl_{cr} 10-24 mL/minute: 450 mg every 2 days

Maintenance dose:

Cl_{cr} 40-59 mL/minute: 450 mg once daily

Cl_{cr} 25-39 mL/minute: 450 mg every 2 days

Cl_{cr} 10-24 mL/minute: 450 mg twice weekly

Note: Valganciclovir is not recommended in patients receiving hemodialysis. For patients on hemodialysis (Cl_{cr} <10 mL/minute), it is recommended that ganciclovir be used (dose adjusted as specified for ganciclovir).

Dietary Considerations Should be taken with meals.

Administration Avoid direct contact with broken or crushed tablets. Consideration should be given to handling and disposal according to guidelines issued for antineoplastic drugs. However, there is no consensus on the need for these precautions.

Monitoring Parameters Retinal exam (at least every 4-6 weeks), CBC, platelet counts, serum creatinine

Dosage Forms Excipient information presented when available (limited, particularly for generics); consult specific product labeling.

Tablet, as hydrochloride: 450 mg [valganciclovir hydrochloride 496.3 mg equivalent to valganciclovir 450 mg]

- **Valganciclovir Hydrochloride** *see* Valganciclovir *on page 1537*
- **Valisone® Scalp Lotion (Can)** *see* Betamethasone *on page 188*
- **Valium®** *see* Diazepam *on page 434*
- **Valorin [OTC]** *see* Acetaminophen *on page 25*
- **Valorin Extra [OTC]** *see* Acetaminophen *on page 25*
- **Valproate Semisodium** *see* Valproic Acid and Derivatives *on page 1538*
- **Valproate Sodium** *see* Valproic Acid and Derivatives *on page 1538*
- **Valproic Acid** *see* Valproic Acid and Derivatives *on page 1538*

Valproic Acid and Derivatives

(val PROE ik AS id & dah RIV ah tives)

U.S. Brand Names Depacon®; Depakene®; Depakote®; Depakote® ER; Depakote® Sprinkle; Stavzor™

Canadian Brand Names Alti-Divalproex; Apo-Divalproex®; Apo-Valproic®; Depakene®; Dom-Divalproex; Epival® I.V.; Gen-Divalproex; Novo-Divalproex; Nu-Divalproex; PHL-Divalproex; PHL-Valproic Acid; PHL-Valproic Acid E.C.; PMS-Valproic Acid; PMS-Valproic Acid E.C.; ratio-Valproic; ratio-Valproic ECC; Rhoxal-valproic; Sandoz-Valproic

Index Terms 2-Propylpentanoic Acid; 2-Propylvaleric Acid; Dipropylacetic Acid; Divalproex Sodium; DPA; Valproate Semisodium; Valproate Sodium; Valproic Acid

Pharmacologic Category Anticonvulsant, Miscellaneous; Antimanic Agent; Histone Deacetylase Inhibitor

Additional Appendix Information

Anticonvulsant Drugs of Choice *on page 1637*

Use

Depacon®, Depakene®, Depakote®, Depakote® ER, Depakote® Sprinkle, Stavzor™: Monotherapy and adjunctive therapy in the treatment of patients with complex partial seizures; monotherapy and adjunctive therapy of simple and complex absence seizures; adjunctive therapy in patients with multiple seizure types that include absence seizures

Depakote®, Depakote® ER, Stavzor™: Mania associated with bipolar disorder; migraine prophylaxis

Unlabeled/Investigational Use Status epilepticus

Pregnancy Risk Factor D

Pregnancy Considerations [U.S. Boxed Warning]: May cause teratogenic effects such as neural tube defects (eg, spina bifida). Teratogenic effects have been reported in animals and humans. Valproic acid crosses the placenta. Neural tube, cardiac, facial (characteristic pattern of dysmorphic facial features), skeletal, multiple other defects reported. Epilepsy itself, number of medications, genetic factors, or a combination of these probably influence the teratogenicity of anticonvulsant therapy. Information from the North American Antiepileptic Drug Pregnancy Registry notes a fourfold increase in congenital malformations with exposure to valproic acid monotherapy during the 1st trimester of pregnancy when compared to monotherapy with other antiepileptic drugs (AED). The risk of neural tube defects is ~1% to 2% (general population risk estimated to be 0.14% to 0.2%). The effect of folic acid supplementation to decrease this risk is unknown, however, folic acid supplementation is recommended for all women contemplating pregnancy. An information sheet describing the teratogenic potential is available from the manufacturer.

Nonteratogenic effects have also been reported. Afibrinogenemia leading to fatal hemorrhage and hepatotoxicity have been noted in case reports of infants following *in utero* exposure to valproic acid. Use in women of childbearing potential requires that benefits of use in mother be weighed against the potential risk to fetus, especially when used for conditions not associated with permanent injury or risk of death (eg, migraine). Health professionals and patients are encouraged to contact the North American Antiepileptic Drug Pregnancy registry to monitor outcomes of pregnant women exposed to valproic acid and other AEDs (1-888-233-2334).

Lactation Enters breast milk/not recommended (AAP considers "compatible")

Medication Safety Issues

Sound-alike/look-alike issues:

Depakene® may be confused with Depakote®

Depakote® may be confused with Depakene®, Depakote® ER, Senokot®

Depakote® ER may be confused with Depakote®

Contraindications Hypersensitivity to valproic acid, derivatives, or any component of the formulation; hepatic disease or significant impairment; urea cycle disorders

Warnings/Precautions

[U.S. Boxed Warning]: Hepatic failure resulting in fatalities has occurred in patients; children <2 years of age are at considerable risk. Other risk factors include organic brain disease, mental retardation with severe seizure disorders, congenital metabolic disorders, and patients on multiple anticonvulsants. Hepatotoxicity has usually been reported within 6 months of therapy initiation. Monitor patients closely for appearance of malaise, weakness, facial edema, anorexia, jaundice, and vomiting; discontinue immediately with signs/symptom of significant or suspected impairment. Liver function tests should be performed at baseline and at regular intervals after initiation of therapy, especially within the first 6 months. Hepatic dysfunction may progress despite discontinuing treatment. Should only be used as monotherapy in children <2 years of age and patients at high risk for hepatotoxicity. Contraindicated with severe impairment.

[U.S. Boxed Warning]: Cases of life-threatening pancreatitis, occurring at the start of therapy or following years of use, have been reported in adults and children. Some cases have been hemorrhagic with rapid progression of initial symptoms to death. Promptly evaluate symptoms of abdominal pain, nausea, vomiting, and/or anorexia; should generally be discontinued if pancreatitis is diagnosed.

[U.S. Boxed Warning]: May cause teratogenic effects such as neural tube defects (eg, spina bifida). Use in women of childbearing potential requires that benefits of use in mother be weighed against the potential risk to fetus, especially when used for conditions not associated with permanent injury or risk of death (eg, migraine).

May cause severe thrombocytopenia, inhibition of platelet aggregation, and bleeding. Tremors may indicate overdosage; use with caution in patients receiving other anticonvulsants. Hypersensitivity reactions affecting multiple organs have been reported in association with valproic acid use; may include dermatologic and/or hematologic changes (eosinophilia, neutropenia, thrombocytopenia) or symptoms of organ dysfunction.

Hyperammonemia and/or encephalopathy, sometimes fatal, have been reported following the initiation of valproic acid therapy and may be present with normal transaminase levels. Ammonia levels should be measured in patients who develop unexplained lethargy and vomiting, changes in mental status, or in patients who present with hypothermia (unintentional drop in core body temperature to <35°C/95°F). Discontinue therapy if ammonia levels are increased and evaluate for possible urea cycle disorder (UCD); contraindicated in patients with UCD. Evaluation of UCD should be considered for the following patients prior to the start of therapy: History of unexplained encephalopathy or coma; encephalopathy associated with protein load; pregnancy or postpartum encephalopathy; unexplained mental retardation; history of elevated plasma ammonia or glutamine; history of cyclical vomiting and lethargy; episodic extreme irritability, ataxia; low BUN or protein avoidance; family history of UCD or unexplained infant deaths (particularly male); or signs or symptoms of UCD (hyperammonemia, encephalopathy, respiratory alkalosis). Hypothermia has been reported with valproic acid therapy; may or may not be associated with hyperammonemia; may also occur with concomitant topiramate therapy.

In vitro studies have suggested valproic acid stimulates the replication of HIV and CMV viruses under experimental conditions. The clinical consequence of this is unknown, but should be considered when monitoring affected patients.

FDA reports demonstrate a statistically significant increased risk of suicidality; relative risk appears to be higher in patients with epilepsy compared to patients treated for psychiatric or other considerations. Use of Depacon® injection is not recommended for post-traumatic seizure prophylaxis following acute head trauma. Anticonvulsants should not be discontinued abruptly because of the possibility of increasing seizure frequency; valproic acid should be withdrawn gradually to minimize the potential of increased seizure frequency, unless safety concerns require a more rapid withdrawal. Concomitant use with carbapenem antibiotics may reduce valproic acid levels to subtherapeutic levels; monitor levels frequently and consider alternate therapy if levels drop significantly or lack of seizure control occurs. Concomitant use with clonazepam may induce absence status. Patients treated for bipolar disorder should be monitored closely for clinical worsening or suicidality; prescriptions should be written for the smallest quantity consistent with good patient care.

CNS depression may occur with valproic acid use. Patients must be cautioned about performing tasks which require mental alertness (operating machinery or driving). Effects with other sedative drugs or ethanol may be potentiated. Use with caution in the elderly.

Adverse Reactions

>10%:

Central nervous system: Headache (≤31%), somnolence (≤30%), dizziness (12% to 25%), insomnia (>1% to 15%), nervousness (>1% to 11%), pain (1% to 11%)

Dermatologic: Alopecia (>1% to 24%)

Gastrointestinal: Nausea (15% to 48%), vomiting (7% to 27%), diarrhea (7% to 23%), abdominal pain (7% to 23%), dyspepsia (7% to 23%), anorexia (>1% to 12%)

Hematologic: Thrombocytopenia (1% to 24%; dose related)

Neuromuscular & skeletal: Tremor (≤57%), weakness (6% to 27%)

Ocular: Diplopia (>1% to 16%), amblyopia/blurred vision (≤12%)

Miscellaneous: Infection (≤20%), flu-like syndrome (12%)

1% to 10%:

Cardiovascular: Peripheral edema (>1% to 8%), chest pain (>1% to <5%), edema (>1% to <5%), facial edema (>1% to <5%), hypertension (>1% to <5%), hypotension (>1% to <5%), palpitation (>1% to <5%), postural hypotension (>1% to <5%), tachycardia (>1% to <5%), vasodilation(>1% to <5%), arrhythmia

Central nervous system: Ataxia (>1% to 8%), amnesia (>1% to 7%), emotional lability (>1% to 6%), fever (>1% to 6%), abnormal thinking (≤6%), depression (>1% to 5%), abnormal dreams (>1% to <5%), agitation (>1% to <5%), anxiety (>1% to <5%), catatonia (>1% to <5%), chills (>1% to <5%), confusion (>1% to <5%), coordination abnormal (>1% to <5%), hallucination (>1% to <5%), malaise (>1% to <5%), personality disorder (>1% to <5%), speech disorder (>1% to <5%), tardive dyskinesia (>1% to <5%), vertigo (>1% to <5%), euphoria (1%), hypoesthesia (1%)

Dermatologic: Rash (>1% to 6%), bruising (>1% to 5%), discoid lupus erythematosus (>1% to <5%), dry skin (>1% to <5%), furunculosis (>1% to <5%), petechia (>1% to <5%), pruritus (>1% to <5), seborrhea (>1% to <5%)

Endocrine & metabolic: Amenorrhea (>1% to <5%), dysmenorrhea (>1% to <5%), metrorrhagia (>1% to <5%), hypoproteinemia

Gastrointestinal: Weight gain (4% to 9%), weight loss (6%), appetite increased (≤6%), constipation (>1% to 5%), xerostomia (>1% to 5%), eructation (>1% to <5%), fecal incontinence (>1% to <5%), flatulence (>1% to <5%), gastroenteritis (>1% to <5%), glossitis (>1% to <5%), hematemesis (>1% to <5%), pancreatitis (>1% to <5%), periodontal abscess (>1% to <5%), stomatitis (>1% to <5%), taste perversion (>1% to <5%), dysphagia, gum hemorrhage, mouth ulceration

Genitourinary: Cystitis (>1% to 5%), dysuria (>1% to 5%), urinary frequency (>1% to <5%), urinary incontinence (>1% to <5%), vaginal hemorrhage (>1% to 5%), vaginitis (>1% to <5%)

Hepatic: ALT increased (>1% to <5%), AST increased (>1% to <5%)

Local: Injection site pain (3%), injection site reaction (2%), injection site inflammation (1%)

Neuromuscular & skeletal: Back pain (≤8%), abnormal gait (>1% to <5%), arthralgia (>1% to <5%), arthrosis (>1% to <5%), dysarthria (>1% to <5%), hypertonia (>1% to <5%), hypokinesia (>1% to <5%), leg cramps (>1% to <5%), myalgia (>1% to <5%), myasthenia (>1% to <5%), neck pain (>1% to <5%), neck rigidity (>1% to <5%), paresthesia (>1% to <5%), reflex increased (>1% to <5%), twitching (>1% to <5%)

Ocular: Nystagmus (1% to 8%), dry eyes (>1% to 5%), eye pain (>1% to 5%), abnormal vision (>1% to <5%), conjunctivitis (>1% to <5%)

Otic: Tinnitus (1% to 7%), ear pain (>1% to 5%), deafness (>1% to <5%), otitis media (>1% to <5%)

Respiratory: Pharyngitis (2% to 8%), bronchitis (5%), rhinitis (>1% to 5%), dyspnea (1% to 5%), cough (>1% to <5%), epistaxis (>1% to <5%), pneumonia (>1% to <5%), sinusitis (>1% to <5%)

Miscellaneous: Diaphoresis (1%), hiccups

<1% (Limited to important and/or life-threatening): Aggression, agranulocytosis, allergic reaction, anaphylaxis, anemia, aplastic anemia, asterixis, behavioral deterioration, bilirubin increased, bleeding time altered, bone marrow suppression, bone pain, bradycardia, breast enlargement, cutaneous vasculitis, carnitine decreased, cerebral atrophy (reversible), coma (rare), dementia, encephalopathy (rare), enuresis, eosinophilia, erythema multiforme, Fanconi-like syndrome (rare, in children), galactorrhea, hematoma formation, hemorrhage, hepatic failure, hepatotoxicity, hostility, hyperactivity, hyperammonemia, hyperammonemic encephalopathy (in patients with UCD), hyperglycinemia, hypersensitivity reactions (severe, with multiorgan dysfunction), hypofibrinogenemia, hyponatremia, hypothermia, inappropriate ADH secretion, intermittent porphyria, LDH increased, leukopenia, lupus, lymphocytosis, macrocytosis, menstrual irregularities, pancytopenia parkinsonism, parotid gland swelling, photosensitivity, platelet aggregation inhibited, polycystic ovary disease (rare), psychosis, seeing "spots before the eyes," Stevens-Johnson syndrome, suicidal behavior/ideation, thyroid function tests abnormal, toxic epidermal necrolysis (rare), urinary tract infection

Drug Interactions

Metabolism/Transport Effects For valproic acid: **Substrate** (minor) of CYP2A6, 2B6, 2C9, 2C19, 2E1; **Inhibits** CYP2C9 (weak), 2C19 (weak), 2D6 (weak), 3A4 (weak); **Induces** CYP2A6 (weak)

Avoid Concomitant Use There are no known interactions where it is recommended to avoid concomitant use.

Increased Effect/Toxicity

Valproic Acid and Derivatives may increase the levels/effects of: Barbiturates; Ethosuximide; LamoTRIgine; LORazepam; Primidone; Risperidone; Rufinamide; Tricyclic Antidepressants; Vorinostat; Zidovudine

The levels/effects of Valproic Acid and Derivatives may be increased by: ChlorproMAZINE; Felbamate; Salicylates; Topiramate

Decreased Effect

Valproic Acid and Derivatives may decrease the levels/effects of: Aminocamptothecin; CarBAMazepine; OXcarbazepine; Phenytoin

The levels/effects of Valproic Acid and Derivatives may be decreased by: Barbiturates; CarBAMazepine; Carbapenems; Ethosuximide; Methylfolate; Phenytoin; Primidone; Protease Inhibitors; Rifampin

Ethanol/Nutrition/Herb Interactions

Ethanol: Avoid ethanol (may increase CNS depression).

Food: Food may delay but does not affect the extent of absorption. Valproic acid serum concentrations may be decreased if taken with food. Milk has no effect on absorption.

Herb/Nutraceutical: Avoid evening primrose (seizure threshold decreased).

Stability

Depakote® tablet, Depakene® solution: Store below 30°C (86°F).

Depakote® Sprinkles: Store below 25°C (77°F).

Depakote® ER, Stavzor™: Store at controlled room temperature of 25°C (77°F).

Depakene® capsule: Store at controlled room temperature of 15°C to 25°C (59°F to 77°F).

Depacon®: Store vial at room temperature of 15°C to 30°C (59°F to 86°F). Injection should be diluted in 50 mL of a compatible diluent. Stable in D_5W, NS, and LR for at least 24 hours when stored in glass or PVC.

Mechanism of Action Causes increased availability of gamma-aminobutyric acid (GABA), an inhibitory neurotransmitter, to brain neurons or may enhance the action of GABA or mimic its action at postsynaptic receptor sites

Pharmacodynamics/Kinetics

Distribution: Total valproate: 11 L/1.73 m^2; free valproate 92 L/1.73 m^2

Protein binding (dose dependent): 80% to 90%; decreased in the elderly and with hepatic or renal dysfunction

Metabolism: Extensively hepatic via glucuronide conjugation and mitochondrial beta-oxidation. The relationship between dose and total valproate concentration is nonlinear; concentration does not increase proportionally with the dose, but increases to a lesser extent due to saturable plasma protein binding. The kinetics of unbound drug are linear.

Bioavailability: Depakote® ER: ~90% relative to I.V. dose and ~89% relative to delayed release formulation

Half-life elimination (increased in neonates and with liver disease): Children >2 months: 7-13 hours; Adults: 9-16 hours

Time to peak, serum: Depakote® tablet: ~4 hours; Depakote® ER: 4-17 hours; Stavzor™: 2 hours

Excretion: Urine (30% to 50% as glucuronide conjugate, 3% as unchanged drug)

Dosage

Seizure disorders: **Note:** Administer doses >250 mg/day in divided doses.

Oral:

Simple and complex absence seizures: Children and Adults: Initial: 15 mg/kg/day; increase by 5-10 mg/kg/day at weekly intervals until therapeutic levels are achieved; maximum: 60 mg/kg/day. Larger maintenance doses may be required in younger children.

Complex partial seizures: Children ≥10 years and Adults: Initial: 10-15 mg/kg/day; increase by 5-10 mg/kg/day at weekly intervals until therapeutic levels are achieved; maximum: 60 mg/kg/day. Larger maintenance doses may be required in younger children.

Note: Regular release and delayed release formulations are usually given in 2-4 divided doses/day; extended release formulation (Depakote® ER) is usually given once daily. Conversion to Depakote® ER from a stable dose of Depakote® may require an increase in the total daily dose between 8% and 20% to maintain similar serum concentrations. Depakote® ER is not recommended for use in children <10 years of age.

I.V.: Administer as a 60-minute infusion (≤20 mg/minute) with the same frequency as oral products; switch patient to oral products as soon as possible. Rapid infusions ≤45 mg/kg over 5-10 minutes (1.5-6 mg/kg/minute) were generally well tolerated in a clinical trial.

Rectal (unlabeled): Dilute syrup 1:1 with water for use as a retention enema; loading dose: 17-20 mg/kg one time; maintenance: 10-15 mg/kg/dose every 8 hours

Status epilepticus (unlabeled use): Adults:

Loading dose: I.V.: 15-45 mg/kg administered at ≤6 mg/kg/minute.

Maintenance dose: I.V. infusion: 1-4 mg/kg/hour; titrate dose as needed based upon patient response and evaluation of drug-drug interactions

Mania: Adults: Oral:

Depakote® tablet, Stavzor™: Initial: 750 mg/day in divided doses; dose should be adjusted as rapidly as possible to desired clinical effect; maximum recommended dosage: 60 mg/kg/day

Depakote® ER: Initial: 25 mg/kg/day given once daily; dose should be adjusted as rapidly as possible to desired clinical effect; maximum recommended dose: 60 mg/kg/day.

Migraine prophylaxis:

Children ≥12 years (Stavzor™): 250 mg twice daily; adjust dose based on patient response, up to 1000 mg/day

Children ≥16 years and Adults: Oral:

Depakote® tablet: 250 mg twice daily; adjust dose based on patient response, up to 1000 mg/day

Depakote® ER: 500 mg once daily for 7 days, then increase to 1000 mg once daily; adjust dose based on patient response; usual dosage range 500-1000 mg/day

Elderly: Elimination is decreased in the elderly. Studies of elderly patients with dementia show a high incidence of somnolence. In some patients, this was associated with weight loss. Starting doses should be lower and increases should be slow, with careful monitoring of nutritional intake and dehydration. Safety and efficacy for use in patients >65 years have not been studied for migraine prophylaxis.

Dosing adjustment in renal impairment: A 27% reduction in clearance of unbound valproate is seen in patients with Cl_{cr} <10 mL/minute. Hemodialysis reduces valproate concentrations by 20%, therefore no dose adjustment is needed in patients with renal failure. Protein binding is reduced, monitoring only total valproate concentrations may be misleading.

Dosing adjustment/comments in hepatic impairment: Reduce dose. Clearance is decreased with liver impairment. Hepatic disease is also associated with decreased albumin concentrations and 2- to 2.6-fold increase in the unbound fraction. Free concentrations of valproate may be elevated while total concentrations appear normal. Use is contraindicated in severe impairment.

Dietary Considerations Valproic acid may cause GI upset; take with large amount of water or food to decrease GI upset. May need to split doses to avoid GI upset.

Depakote® Sprinkle capsule contents may be mixed with semisolid food (eg, applesauce or pudding) in patients having difficulty swallowing; particles should be swallowed and not chewed.

Valproate sodium oral solution will generate valproic acid in carbonated beverages and may cause mouth and throat irritation; do not mix valproate sodium oral solution with carbonated beverages.

Administration

Depakote® ER: Swallow whole; do not crush or chew. Patients who need dose adjustments smaller than 500 mg/day for migraine prophylaxis should be changed to Depakote® delayed release tablets.

Depakote® Sprinkle capsules may be swallowed whole or open capsule and sprinkle on small amount (1 teaspoonful) of soft food and use immediately (do not store or chew).

Depacon®: Following dilution to final concentration, administer over 60 minutes at a rate ≤20 mg/minute. Alternatively, single doses up to 45 mg/kg have been administered as a rapid infusion over 5-10 minutes (1.5-6 mg/kg/minute).

Depakene® capsule, Stavzor™: Swallow whole; do not chew.

Monitoring Parameters Liver enzymes (at baseline and during therapy), CBC with platelets (baseline and periodic intervals), PT/PTT (especially prior to surgery), serum ammonia (with symptoms of lethargy, mental status change), serum valproate levels

Reference Range

Therapeutic:

Epilepsy: 50-100 mcg/mL (SI: 350-690 μmol/L)

Mania: 85-125 mcg/mL (SI: 350-860 μmol/L)

Toxic: Some laboratories may report >200 mcg/mL (SI: >1390 μmol/L) as a toxic threshold, although clinical toxicity can occur at lower concentrations. Probability of thrombocytopenia increases with total valproate levels ≥110 mcg/mL in females or ≥135 mcg/mL in males.

Seizure control: May improve at levels >100 mcg/mL (SI: 690 μmol/L), but toxicity may occur at levels of 100-150 mcg/mL (SI: 690-1040 μmol/L)

Mania: Clinical response seen with trough levels between 85-125 mcg/mL; risk of toxicity increases at levels >125 mcg/mL

Test Interactions False-positive result for urine ketones; accuracy of thyroid function tests

Additional Information Extended release tablets have 10% to 20% less fluctuation in serum concentration than delayed release tablets. Extended release tablets are not bioequivalent to delayed release tablets.

Dosage Forms Excipient information presented when available (limited, particularly for generics); consult specific product labeling. **Note:** Strength expressed as valproic acid

Capsule, softgel, as valproic acid: 250 mg

Depakene®: 250 mg

Capsule, softgel, delayed release, as valproic acid:

Stavzor™: 125 mg, 250 mg, 500 mg

Capsule, sprinkles, as divalproex sodium:

Depakote® Sprinkle: 125 mg

Injection, solution, as valproate sodium: 100 mg/mL (5 mL)

Depacon®: 100 mg/mL (5 mL) [contains edetate disodium]

Syrup, as valproic acid: 250 mg/5 mL (5 mL, 10 mL, 480 mL)

Depakene®: 250 mg/5 mL (480 mL)

Tablet, delayed release, as divalproex sodium: 125 mg, 250 mg, 500 mg

Depakote®: 125 mg, 250 mg, 500 mg

Tablet, delayed release, enteric coated, as divalproex sodium: 125 mg, 250 mg, 500 mg

Tablet, extended release, as divalproex sodium:

Depakote® ER: 250 mg, 500 mg

Valrubicin (val ROO bi sin)

U.S. Brand Names Valstar® [DSC]

Canadian Brand Names Valstar®; Valtaxin®

Index Terms *N*-trifluoroacetyladriamycin-14-valerate; AD3L

Pharmacologic Category Antineoplastic Agent, Anthracycline

Use Intravesical therapy of BCG-refractory carcinoma *in situ* of the urinary bladder

Pregnancy Risk Factor C

Pregnancy Considerations There are no adequate and well-controlled studies in pregnant women. All patients of reproductive age should use an effective method of contraception during the treatment period.

Lactation Excretion in breast milk unknown/not recommended

Medication Safety Issues

Sound-alike/look-alike issues:

Valstar® may be confused with valsartan

High alert medication: The Institute for Safe Medication Practices (ISMP) includes this medication among its list of drugs which have a heightened risk of causing significant patient harm when used in error.

Contraindications Hypersensitivity to anthracyclines, Cremophor® EL, or any component of the formulation; concurrent urinary tract infection or small bladder capacity (unable to tolerate a 75 mL instillation)

Warnings/Precautions Hazardous agent - use appropriate precautions for handling and disposal. Do not administer if mucosal integrity of bladder has been compromised or bladder perforation is present. Irritable bladder symptoms may occur during instillation and retention. Use caution in patients with severe irritable bladder symptoms. Red-tinged urine is typical for the first 24 hours after instillation. Prolonged symptoms or discoloration should prompt contact with the physician. Valrubicin should be used cautiously (if at all) in patients having a history of hypersensitivity reactions to other medications prepared with Cremophor® EL.

Adverse Reactions

>10%: Genitourinary: Frequency (61%), dysuria (56%), urgency (57%), bladder spasm (31%), hematuria (29%), bladder pain (28%), urinary incontinence (22%), cystitis (15%), urinary tract infection (15%)

1% to 10%:

Cardiovascular: Chest pain (2%), vasodilation (2%), peripheral edema (1%)

Central nervous system: Headache (4%), malaise (4%), dizziness (3%), fever (2%)

Dermatologic: Rash (3%)

Endocrine & metabolic: Hyperglycemia (1%)

Gastrointestinal: Abdominal pain (5%), nausea (5%), diarrhea (3%), vomiting (2%), flatulence (1%)

Genitourinary: Nocturia (7%), burning symptoms (5%), urinary retention (4%), urethral pain (3%), pelvic pain (1%), hematuria (microscopic) (3%)

Hematologic: Anemia (2%)

Neuromuscular & skeletal: Weakness (4%), back pain (3%), myalgia (1%)

Respiratory: Pneumonia (1%)

<1% (Limited to important or life-threatening): Pruritus, skin irritation, taste disturbance, tenesmus, urethritis, urine flow decreased

Drug Interactions

Avoid Concomitant Use

Avoid concomitant use of Valrubicin with any of the following: Natalizumab; Vaccines (Live)

Increased Effect/Toxicity

Valrubicin may increase the levels/effects of: Natalizumab; Vaccines (Live)

The levels/effects of Valrubicin may be increased by: Bevacizumab; Taxane Derivatives; Trastuzumab

Decreased Effect

Valrubicin may decrease the levels/effects of: Cardiac Glycosides; Vaccines (Inactivated)

The levels/effects of Valrubicin may be decreased by: Cardiac Glycosides; Echinacea

Stability Store unopened vials under refrigeration at 2°C to 8°C (36°F to 48°F). Stable for 12 hours when diluted in 0.9% sodium chloride. Allow vial to warm to room temperature without heating. Dilute 800 mg (20 mL) with 55 mL NS.

Mechanism of Action Blocks function of DNA topoisomerase II; inhibits DNA synthesis, causes extensive chromosomal damage, and arrests cell development; unlike other anthracyclines, does not appear to intercalate DNA

Pharmacodynamics/Kinetics

Absorption: Well absorbed into bladder tissue, negligible systemic absorption. Trauma to mucosa may increase absorption, and perforation greatly increases absorption with significant systemic myelotoxicity.

Metabolism: Negligible after intravesical instillation and 2-hour retention

Excretion: Urine when expelled from urinary bladder (98.6% as intact drug; 0.4% as *N*-trifluoroacetyladriamycin)

Dosage Adults: Intravesical: 800 mg once weekly for 6 weeks

Dosing adjustment in renal impairment: No specific adjustment recommended

Dosing adjustment in hepatic impairment: No specific adjustment recommended

Administration Intravesicular bladder lavage, usually in 75 mL of 0.9% sodium chloride injection. Retain in the bladder for 2 hours, then void. Due to the Cremophor® EL diluent, valrubicin should be administered through non-PVC tubing.

Monitoring Parameters Cystoscopy, biopsy, and urine cytology every 3 months for recurrence or progression

Dosage Forms Excipient information presented when available (limited, particularly for generics); consult specific product labeling. [DSC] = Discontinued product

Injection, solution [DSC]: 40 mg/mL (5 mL) [contains Cremophor® EL 50% (polyoxyethyleneglycol triricinoleate) and dehydrated alcohol 50%]

Valsartan (val SAR tan)

U.S. Brand Names Diovan®

Canadian Brand Names Diovan®

Pharmacologic Category Angiotensin II Receptor Blocker

Additional Appendix Information

Angiotensin Agents *on page 1632*

Heart Failure (Systolic) *on page 1809*

Use Alone or in combination with other antihypertensive agents in the treatment of essential hypertension; reduction of cardiovascular mortality in patients with left ventricular dysfunction postmyocardial infarction; treatment of heart failure (NYHA Class II-IV)

Pregnancy Risk Factor D

Pregnancy Considerations Medications which act on the renin-angiotensin system are reported to have the following fetal/neonatal effects: Hypotension, neonatal skull hypoplasia, anuria, renal failure, and death; oligohydramnios is also reported. These effects are reported to occur with exposure during the second and third trimesters. **[U.S. Boxed Warning]: Based on human data, drugs that act on the angiotensin system can cause injury and death to the developing fetus when used in the second and third trimesters. Angiotensin receptor blockers should be discontinued as soon as possible once pregnancy is detected.**

Lactation Excretion in breast milk unknown/not recommended

Medication Safety Issues

Sound-alike/look-alike issues:

Valsartan may be confused with losartan, Valstar™

Diovan® may be confused with Darvon®, Dioval®, Zyban®

Contraindications

U.S. labeling: There are no contraindications listed in manufacturer's labeling.

Canadian labeling: Hypersensitivity to valsartan or any component of the formulation

Warnings/Precautions **[U.S. Boxed Warning]: Based on human data, drugs that act on the angiotensin system can cause injury and death to the developing fetus when used in the second and third trimesters. Angiotensin receptor blockers should be discontinued as soon as possible once pregnancy is detected.** May cause hyperkalemia; avoid potassium supplementation unless specifically required by healthcare provider. During the initiation of therapy, hypotension may occur, particularly in patients with heart failure or post-MI patients. Use extreme caution with concurrent administration of potassium-sparing diuretics or potassium supplements, in patients with mild-to-moderate hepatic dysfunction (adjust dose), in those who may be sodium/water depleted (eg, on high-dose diuretics), and in the elderly; correct depletion first.

Use caution with unstented unilateral/bilateral renal artery stenosis. When unstented bilateral renal artery stenosis is present, use is generally avoided due to the elevated risk of deterioration in renal function unless possible benefits outweigh risks. Use with caution with preexisting renal insufficiency; significant aortic/mitral stenosis. May be associated with deterioration of renal function and/or increases in serum creatinine, particularly in patients with low renal blood flow (eg, renal artery stenosis, heart failure) whose glomerular filtration rate (GFR) is dependent on efferent arteriolar vasoconstriction by angiotensin II. Use caution in patients with severe renal impairment or significant hepatic dysfunction. Monitor renal function closely in patients with severe heart failure; changes in renal function should be anticipated and dosage adjustments of valsartan or concomitant medications may be needed. In Canada, use is not approved in patients <18 years of age.

Adverse Reactions

>10%:

Central nervous system: Dizziness (heart failure trials 17%)

Renal: BUN increased >50% (heart failure trials 17%)

1% to 10%:

Cardiovascular: Hypotension (heart failure trials 7%; MI trial 1%), postural hypotension (heart failure trials 2%), syncope (up to >1%)

Central nervous system: Dizziness (hypertension trial 2% to 8%), fatigue (heart failure trials 3%; hypertension trial 2%), postural dizziness (heart failure trials 2%), headache (heart failure trials >1%), vertigo (up to >1%)

Endocrine & metabolic: Serum potassium increased by >20% (4% to 10%), hyperkalemia (heart failure trials 2%)

Gastrointestinal: Diarrhea (heart failure trials 5%), abdominal pain (2%), nausea (heart failure trials >1%), upper abdominal pain (heart failure trials >1%)

Hematologic: Neutropenia (2%)

Neuromuscular & skeletal: Arthralgia (heart failure trials 3%), back pain (up to 3%)

Ocular: Blurred vision (heart failure trials >1%)

Renal: Creatinine doubled (MI trial 4%), creatinine increased >50% (heart failure trials 4%), renal dysfunction (up to >1%)

Respiratory: Cough (1% to 3%)

Miscellaneous: Viral infection (3%)

All indications: <1% (Limited to important or life-threatening): Allergic reactions, alopecia, anaphylaxis, anemia, angioedema, anorexia, anxiety, chest pain, constipation, dyspepsia, dyspnea, flatulence, hematocrit/hemoglobin decreased, hepatitis, impotence, insomnia, liver function tests increased, microcytic anemia, muscle cramps, myalgia, palpitation, paresthesia, photosensitivity, pruritus, rash, rhabdomyolysis, somnolence, taste disorder, thrombocytopenia, vomiting, weakness, xerostomia

Drug Interactions

Metabolism/Transport Effects **Inhibits** CYP2C9 (weak)

Avoid Concomitant Use There are no known interactions where it is recommended to avoid concomitant use.

Increased Effect/Toxicity

Valsartan may increase the levels/effects of: ACE Inhibitors; Amifostine; Lithium; Potassium-Sparing Diuretics; RiTUXimab

The levels/effects of Valsartan may be increased by: Diazoxide; Eltrombopag; Eplerenone; Herbs (Hypotensive Properties); Potassium Salts; Prostacyclin Analogues; Trimethoprim

Decreased Effect

The levels/effects of Valsartan may be decreased by: Herbs (Hypertensive Properties); Methylphenidate; Nonsteroidal Anti-Inflammatory Agents; Yohimbine

Ethanol/Nutrition/Herb Interactions

Food: Decreases rate and extent of absorption by 50% and 40%, respectively.

Herb/Nutraceutical: Avoid bayberry, blue cohosh, cayenne, ephedra, ginger, ginseng (American), kola, licorice (may worsen hypertension). Avoid black cohosh, California poppy, coleus, golden seal, hawthorn, mistletoe, periwinkle, quinine, shepherd's purse (may have increased antihypertensive effect).

Stability Store at 25°C (77°F); excursions between 15°C to 30°C (59°F to 86°F) permitted. Protect from moisture.

Mechanism of Action Valsartan produces direct antagonism of the angiotensin II (AT2) receptors, unlike the ACE inhibitors. It displaces angiotensin II from the AT1 receptor and produces its blood pressure-lowering effects by antagonizing AT1-induced vasoconstriction, aldosterone release, catecholamine release, arginine vasopressin release, water intake, and hypertrophic responses. This action results in more efficient blockade of the cardiovascular effects of angiotensin II and fewer side effects than the ACE inhibitors.

Pharmacodynamics/Kinetics

Onset of antihypertensive effect: 2 weeks (maximal: 4 weeks)

Distribution: V_d: 17 L (adults)

Protein binding: 95%, primarily albumin

Metabolism: To inactive metabolite

Bioavailability: Tablet: 25% (range 10% to 35%); suspension: ~40% (~1.6 times more than tablet)

Half-life elimination: ~6 hours

Time to peak, serum: 2-4 hours

Excretion: Feces (83%) and urine (13%) as unchanged drug

Dosage Oral:
Hypertension:
Children 6-16 years: Initial: 1.3 mg/kg once daily (maximum: 40 mg/day); dose may be increased to achieve desired effect; doses >2.7 mg/kg (maximum: 160 mg) have not been studied
Adults: Initial: 80 mg or 160 mg once daily (in patients who are not volume depleted); dose may be increased to achieve desired effect; maximum recommended dose: 320 mg/day
Heart failure: Adults: Initial: 40 mg twice daily; titrate dose to 80-160 mg twice daily, as tolerated; maximum daily dose: 320 mg
Left ventricular dysfunction after MI: Adults: Initial: 20 mg twice daily; titrate dose to target of 160 mg twice daily as tolerated; may initiate ≥12 hours following MI

Dosing adjustment in renal impairment:
Children: Use is not recommended if Cl_{cr} <30 mL/minute.
Adults: No dosage adjustment necessary if Cl_{cr} >10 mL/minute.
Dialysis: Not significantly removed
Dosing adjustment in hepatic impairment In mild-to-moderate liver disease no adjustment is needed. Use caution in patients with liver disease. Patients with mild to moderate chronic disease have twice the exposure as healthy volunteers.

Dietary Considerations Avoid salt substitutes which contain potassium. May be taken with or without food.

Administration Administer with or without food.

Monitoring Parameters Baseline and periodic electrolyte panels, renal function, BP; in CHF, serum potassium during dose escalation and periodically thereafter

Additional Information Valsartan may have an advantage over losartan due to minimal metabolism requirements and consequent use in mild-to-moderate hepatic impairment.

Dosage Forms Excipient information presented when available (limited, particularly for generics); consult specific product labeling.
Tablet:
Diovan®: 40 mg, 80 mg, 160 mg, 320 mg

Extemporaneous Preparations To prepare valsartan suspension, add 80 mL of Ora-Plus® to an 8-ounce amber glass bottle containing eight (8) valsartan 80 mg tablets. Shake well ≥2 minutes. Allow the suspension to stand for a minimum of 1 hour then shake for 1 minute. Then add 80 mL of Ora-Sweet SF® to the bottle and shake for at least 10 seconds. Resulting 160 mL suspension will contain valsartan 4 mg/mL. Store for either up to 30 days at room temperature (below 30°C/86°F) or up to 75 days under refrigeration (2-8°C/35-46°F) in the glass bottle. Shake well before use.
Product information, December, 2007; Novartis Pharmaceuticals Corp.

◆ **Valsartan and Amlodipine** *see* Amlodipine and Valsartan *on page 96*

Valsartan and Hydrochlorothiazide
(val SAR tan & hye droe klor oh THYE a zide)

U.S. Brand Names Diovan HCT®
Canadian Brand Names Diovan HCT®
Index Terms Hydrochlorothiazide and Valsartan
Pharmacologic Category Angiotensin II Receptor Blocker; Diuretic, Thiazide
Use Treatment of hypertension
Pregnancy Risk Factor D
Medication Safety Issues
Sound-alike/look-alike issues:
Diovan® may be confused with Darvon®, Dioval®, Zyban®

Dosage Oral: Dose is individualized; combination product may be used as initial therapy or substituted for individual components in patients currently maintained on both agents separately or in patients not adequately controlled with monotherapy (using one of the agents or an agent within same antihypertensive class).
Adults: Hypertension:
Initial therapy: Valsartan 160 mg and hydrochlorothiazide 12.5 mg once daily; dose may be titrated after 1-2 weeks of therapy. Maximum recommended daily doses: Valsartan 320 mg; hydrochlorothiazide 25 mg.
Add-on/replacement therapy: Valsartan 80-160 mg and hydrochlorthiazide 12.5-25 mg once daily; dose may be titrated after 3-4 weeks of therapy. Maximum recommended daily dose: Valsartan 320 mg; hydrochlorothiazide 25 mg.
Dosage adjustment in renal impairment:
Cl_{cr} >30 mL/minute: No adjustment needed
CL_{cr} ≤30 mL/minute: Use of combination not recommended. Contraindicated in patients with anuria.
Dosage adjustment in hepatic impairment: Use with caution; initiate at lower dose and titrate slowly

Additional Information Complete prescribing information for this medication should be consulted for additional detail.

Dosage Forms Excipient information presented when available (limited, particularly for generics); consult specific product labeling.
Tablet:
Diovan HCT® 80 mg/12.5 mg: Valsartan 80 mg and hydrochlorothiazide 12.5 mg
Diovan HCT® 160 mg/12.5 mg: Valsartan 160 mg and hydrochlorothiazide 12.5 mg
Diovan HCT® 160 mg/25 mg: Valsartan 160 mg and hydrochlorothiazide 25 mg
Diovan HCT® 320 mg/12.5 mg: Valsartan 320 mg and hydrochlorothiazide 12.5 mg
Diovan HCT® 320 mg/25 mg: Valsartan 320 mg and hydrochlorothiazide 25 mg

◆ **Valstar® [DSC]** *see* Valrubicin *on page 1542*
◆ **Valstar® (Can)** *see* Valrubicin *on page 1542*
◆ **Valtaxin® (Can)** *see* Valrubicin *on page 1542*
◆ **Valtrex®** *see* Valacyclovir *on page 1535*
◆ **Vanamide™** *see* Urea *on page 1530*
◆ **Vanceril® AEM (Can)** *see* Beclomethasone *on page 176*
◆ **Vancocin®** *see* Vancomycin *on page 1544*

Vancomycin (van koe MYE sin)

U.S. Brand Names Vancocin®
Canadian Brand Names Vancocin®
Index Terms Vancomycin Hydrochloride
Pharmacologic Category Antibiotic, Miscellaneous
Use Treatment of patients with infections caused by staphylococcal species and streptococcal species; used orally for staphylococcal enterocolitis or for antibiotic-associated pseudomembranous colitis produced by *C. difficile*
Unlabeled/Investigational Use Bacterial endophthalmitis
Pregnancy Risk Factor B (oral); C (injection)
Pregnancy Considerations Adverse effects have not been observed in animal studies and there are no controlled studies in pregnant women; however, oral vancomycin is not systemically absorbed. Therefore, I.V. vancomycin has been classified pregnancy category C and oral vancomycin has been classified pregnancy category B. Vancomycin crosses the placenta. *In vivo* studies and human case reports have documented placental transfer of vancomycin in the second and third

trimesters of pregnancy resulting in therapeutic fetal concentrations. Vancomycin has not caused adverse fetal effects, including hearing loss or nephrotoxicity, when administered during pregnancy. A case report has been published of a vancomycin dose rapidly administered over 3 minutes leading to maternal hypotension and fetal bradycardia.

The pharmacokinetics of vancomycin may be altered during pregnancy and pregnant patients may need a higher dose of vancomycin. Maternal half-life is unchanged, but the volume of distribution and the total plasma clearance are increased. Individualization of therapy through serum concentration monitoring may be warranted. Vancomycin is recommended for use in pregnant women for prevention of early-onset group B streptococcal (GBS) disease in newborns.

Lactation Enters breast milk/not recommended

Medication Safety Issues

Sound-alike/look-alike issues:

I.V. vancomycin may be confused with Invanz®

Vancomycin may be confused with clindamycin, gentamicin, tobramycin, valacyclovir, vecuronium, Vibramycin®

High alert medication: The Institute for Safe Medication Practices (ISMP) includes this medication (intrathecal administration) among its list of drug classes which have a heightened risk of causing significant patient harm when used in error.

Contraindications Hypersensitivity to vancomycin or any component of the formulation; avoid in patients with previous severe hearing loss

Warnings/Precautions May cause nephrotoxicity; usual risk factors include pre-existing renal impairment, concomitant nephrotoxic medications, advanced age, and dehydration. Discontinue treatment if signs of nephrotoxicity occur; renal damage is usually reversible. May cause neurotoxicity; usual risk factors include pre-existing renal impairment, concomitant neuro-/nephrotoxic medications, advanced age, and dehydration. Ototoxicity is proportional to the amount of drug given and the duration of treatment. Tinnitus or vertigo may be indications of vestibular injury and impending bilateral irreversible damage. Discontinue treatment if signs of ototoxicity occur. Prolonged therapy (>1 week) or total doses exceeding 25 g may increase the risk of neutropenia; prompt reversal of neutropenia is expected after discontinuation of therapy. Prolonged use may result in fungal or bacterial superinfection, including *C. difficile*-associated diarrhea (CDAD) and pseudomembranous colitis; CDAD has been observed >2 months postantibiotic treatment. Use with caution in patients with renal impairment or those receiving other nephrotoxic or ototoxic drugs; dosage modification required in patients with impaired renal function (especially elderly). Rapid I.V. administration may result in hypotension, flushing, erythema, urticaria, and/or pruritus; rate of infusion should be ≥60 minutes. Oral vancomycin is only indicated for the treatment of pseudomembranous colitis due to *C. difficile* and enterocolitis due to *S. aureus* and is not effective for systemic infections; parenteral vancomycin is not effective for the treatment of colitis due to *C. difficile* and enterocolitis due to *S. aureus*.

Adverse Reactions

Oral:

>10%: Gastrointestinal: Bitter taste, nausea, vomiting, stomatitis

1% to 10%:

Central nervous system: Chills, drug fever

Hematologic: Eosinophilia

<1% (Limited to important or life-threatening): Interstitial nephritis, ototoxicity, renal failure, skin rash, thrombocytopenia, vasculitis

Parenteral:

>10%:

Cardiovascular: Hypotension accompanied by flushing

Dermatologic: Erythematous rash on face and upper body (red neck or red man syndrome)

1% to 10%:

Central nervous system: Chills, drug fever

Hematologic: Eosinophilia, reversible neutropenia

<1% (Limited to important or life-threatening): Ototoxicity, renal failure, thrombocytopenia, vasculitis

Drug Interactions

Avoid Concomitant Use

Avoid concomitant use of Vancomycin with any of the following: Gallium Nitrate

Increased Effect/Toxicity

Vancomycin may increase the levels/effects of: Aminoglycosides; Colistimethate; Gallium Nitrate; Neuromuscular-Blocking Agents

The levels/effects of Vancomycin may be increased by: Nonsteroidal Anti-Inflammatory Agents

Decreased Effect

Vancomycin may decrease the levels/effects of: Typhoid Vaccine

Stability Reconstituted 500 mg and 1 g vials are stable at either room temperature or under refrigeration for 14 days. **Note:** Vials contain no bacteriostatic agent. Solutions diluted for administration in either D_5W or NS are stable under refrigeration for 14 days or at room temperature for 7 days. Reconstitute vials with 20 mL of SWFI for each 1 g of vancomycin (10 mL/500 mg vial; 20 mL/1 g vial; 100 mL/5 g vial; 200 mL/10 g vial). The reconstituted solution must be further diluted with at least 100 mL of a compatible diluent per 500 mg of vancomycin prior to parenteral administration.

Intrathecal: Vancomycin is available as a powder for injection and may be diluted to 1-5 mg/mL concentration in preservative free 0.9% sodium chloride for administration into the CSF.

Mechanism of Action Inhibits bacterial cell wall synthesis by blocking glycopeptide polymerization through binding tightly to D-alanyl-D-alanine portion of cell wall precursor

Pharmacodynamics/Kinetics

Absorption: Oral: Poor; I.M.: Erratic; Intraperitoneal: ~38%

Distribution: Widely in body tissue and fluids, except for CSF

Relative diffusion from blood into CSF: Good only with inflammation (exceeds usual MICs)

CSF:blood level ratio: Normal meninges: Nil; Inflamed meninges: 20% to 30%

Protein binding: 10% to 50%

Half-life elimination: Biphasic: Terminal:

Newborns: 6-10 hours

Infants and Children 3 months to 4 years: 4 hours

Children >3 years: 2.2-3 hours

Adults: 5-11 hours; significantly prolonged with renal impairment

End-stage renal disease: 200-250 hours

Time to peak, serum: I.V.: 45-65 minutes

Excretion: I.V.: Urine (80% to 90% as unchanged drug); Oral: Primarily feces

Dosage

Usual dosage range:

Infants >1 month and Children: I.V.: 10-15 mg/kg every 6 hours

Adults:

I.V.: 2-3 g/day (20-45 mg/kg/day) in divided doses every 6-12 hours; maximum 3 g/day; **Note:** Dose requires adjustment in renal impairment

Oral: 500-1000 mg/day in divided doses every 6 hours

Indication-specific dosing:

Infants >1 month and Children:

Colitis (*C. difficile*), enterocolitis (*S. aureus*): Oral: 40 mg/kg/day in 3-4 divided doses added to fluids for 7-10 days (maximum: 2000 mg/day)

Meningitis/CNS infection:

I.V.: 15 mg/kg every 6 hours

Intrathecal: 5-20 mg/day

Prophylaxis against infective endocarditis: I.V.:

Dental, oral, or upper respiratory tract surgery: 20 mg/kg 1 hour prior to the procedure. **Note:** American Heart Association (AHA) guidelines now recommend prophylaxis only in patients undergoing invasive procedures and in whom underlying cardiac conditions may predispose to a higher risk of adverse outcomes should infection occur.

GI/GU procedure: 20 mg/kg plus gentamicin 2 mg/kg 1 hour prior to surgery. **Note:** As of April 2007, routine prophylaxis no longer recommended by the AHA.

Susceptible gram-positive infections: I.V.: 10 mg/kg every 6 hours

Adults:

Catheter-related infections: Antibiotic lock technique: 2 mg/mL in SWFI/NS or D_5W; instill 3-5 mL into catheter port as a flush solution instead of heparin lock (**Note:** Do not mix with any other solutions.)

Colitis (*C. difficile*), enterocolitis (*S. aureus*): Oral: 500-2000 mg/day in 3-4 divided doses for 7-10 days (usual dose: 125-250 mg every 6 hours)

Endophthalmitis (unlabeled use): Intravitreal: Usual dose: 1 mg/0.1 mL NS instilled into vitreum; may repeat administration if necessary in 3-4 days, usually in combination with ceftazidime or an aminoglycoside

Note: Some clinicians have recommended using a lower dose of 0.2 mg/0.1 mL, based on concerns for retinotoxicity.

Hospital-acquired pneumonia (HAP): I.V.: 15 mg/kg/dose every 12 hours (American Thoracic Society [ATS] 2005 guidelines)

Meningitis *(Pneumococcus* or *Staphylococcus)*:

I.V.: 30-45 mg/kg/day in divided doses every 8-12 hours **or** 500-750 mg every 6 hours (with third-generation cephalosporin for PCN-resistant *Streptococcus pneumoniae*); maximum dose: 2-3 g/day

Intrathecal: Up to 20 mg/day

Prophylaxis against infective endocarditis: I.V.:

Dental, oral, or upper respiratory tract surgery: 1 g 1 hour before surgery. **Note:** AHA guidelines now recommend prophylaxis only in patients undergoing invasive procedures and in whom underlying cardiac conditions may predispose to a higher risk of adverse outcomes should infection occur

GI/GU procedure: 1 g plus 1.5 mg/kg gentamicin 1 hour prior to surgery. **Note:** As of April 2007, routine prophylaxis no longer recommended by the AHA.

Susceptible gram-positive infections: I.V.: 15-20 mg/kg/dose (usual: 750-1500 mg) every 12 hours

Dosing interval in renal impairment (vancomycin levels should be monitored in patients with any renal impairment):

Cl_{cr} >50 mL/minute: Start with 15-20 mg/kg/dose (usual: 750-1500 mg) every 12 hours

Cl_{cr} 20-49 mL/minute: Start with 15-20 mg/kg/dose (usual: 750-1500 mg) every 24 hours

Cl_{cr} <20 mL/minute: Will need longer intervals; determine by serum concentration monitoring

Dialysis: Variable, depending on method; poorly dialyzable by conventional hemodialysis (0% to 5%). Use of high-flux membranes and continuous renal replacement therapy (CRRT) increases vancomycin clearance, and generally requires replacement dosing.

Hemodialysis (HD): Following loading dose of 15-20 mg/kg, give 500 mg to 1 g after each dialysis session, depending on factors such as HD membrane type and flow rate; monitor levels closely.

Continuous ambulatory peritoneal dialysis (CAPD):

Administration via CAPD fluid: 15-30 mg/L (15-30 mcg/mL) of CAPD fluid

Systemic: 1 g loading dose, followed by 500 mg to 1 g every 48-72 hours with close monitoring of levels

Continuous renal replacement therapy (CRRT): Removal of vancomycin is highly dependent on the method of replacement, filter type, and flow rate. Appropriate dosing requires close monitoring of levels in relation to target trough. The following are general recommendations only (based on Trotman, et al, 2005), and require consideration of the aforementioned parameters.

CVVH: Following loading dose of 15-20 mg/kg, give 1 g every 48 hours

CVVHD or CVVHDF: Following loading dose of 15-20 mg/kg, give 1 g every 24 hours

Trotman RL, Williamson JC, Shoemaker DM, et al, "Antibiotic Dosing in Critically Ill Adult Patients Receiving Continuous Renal Replacement Therapy," *Clin Infect Dis*, 2005, 41:1159-66.

Dietary Considerations May be taken with food.

Administration Administer vancomycin by I.V. intermittent infusion over at least 60 minutes at a final concentration not to exceed 5 mg/mL. If a maculopapular rash appears on the face, neck, trunk, and/or upper extremities (red man syndrome), slow the infusion rate to over 1½ to 2 hours and increase the dilution volume. Hypotension, shock, and cardiac arrest (rare) have also been reported with too rapid of infusion. Reactions are often treated with antihistamines and steroids.

Vancomycin is available as a powder for injection and may be diluted to 1-5 mg/mL concentration in preservative free 0.9% sodium chloride for administration into the CSF.

May be administered by intravitreal injection (unlabeled use).

Oral: May be administered with food. If patient cannot swallow capsules, the powder for injection may be reconstituted and diluted for oral administration.

Not for I.M. administration.

Extravasation treatment: Monitor I.V. site closely; extravasation will cause serious injury with possible necrosis and tissue sloughing. Rotate infusion site frequently.

Monitoring Parameters Periodic renal function tests, urinalysis, serum vancomycin concentrations, WBC, audiogram

Reference Range

Timing of serum samples: Draw peak 1 hour after 1-hour infusion has completed; draw trough just before next dose

Therapeutic levels: Peak: 25-40 mcg/mL; Trough: 5-12 mcg/mL

Toxic: >80 mcg/mL (SI: >54 µmol/L)

The ATS guidelines recommend trough levels of 15-20 mcg/mL for hospital-acquired pneumonia. The Infectious Disease Society of America (ISDA) meningitis guidelines recommend trough levels of 15-20 mcg/mL.

Additional Information Because of its long half-life, vancomycin should be dosed on an every 12-hour basis. Monitoring of peak and trough serum levels is advisable. "Red man syndrome", characterized by skin rash and hypotension, is not an allergic reaction but rather is associated with too rapid infusion of the drug. To alleviate or prevent the reaction, infuse vancomycin at a rate of ≥30 minutes for each 500 mg of drug being administered (eg, 1 g over ≥60 minutes); 1.5 g over ≥90 minutes.

Dosage Forms Excipient information presented when available (limited, particularly for generics); consult specific product labeling.
Capsule (Vancocin®): 125 mg, 250 mg
Infusion [premixed in iso-osmotic dextrose] (Vancocin®): 500 mg (100 mL); 1 g (200 mL)
Injection, powder for reconstitution: 500 mg, 1 g, 5 g, 10 g

- **Vancomycin Hydrochloride** *see* Vancomycin *on page 1544*
- **Vandazole™** *see* MetroNIDAZOLE *on page 984*
- **Vaniqa™** *see* Eflornithine *on page 510*
- **Vanos™** *see* Fluocinonide *on page 634*
- **Vanoxide-HC®** *see* Benzoyl Peroxide and Hydrocortisone *on page 185*
- **Vanquish® Extra Strength Pain Reliever [OTC]** *see* Acetaminophen, Aspirin, and Caffeine *on page 31*
- **Vantas™** *see* Histrelin *on page 732*
- **Vantin®** *see* Cefpodoxime *on page 280*
- **Vaprisol®** *see* Conivaptan *on page 368*
- **VAQTA®** *see* Hepatitis A Vaccine *on page 726*

Vardenafil (var DEN a fil)

U.S. Brand Names Levitra®
Canadian Brand Names Levitra®
Index Terms Vardenafil Hydrochloride
Pharmacologic Category Phosphodiesterase-5 Enzyme Inhibitor
Use Treatment of erectile dysfunction (ED)
Pregnancy Risk Factor B
Pregnancy Considerations Teratogenic effects were not observed in animal studies; however, vardenafil is not indicated for use in women. No effects on sperm motility or morphology were observed in healthy males.
Lactation Excretion in breast milk unknown/not indicated for use in women.
Medication Safety Issues
Sound-alike/look-alike issues:
Vardenafil may be confused with sildenafil, tadalafil
Levitra® may be confused with Kaletra®, Lexiva®
Contraindications Hypersensitivity to vardenafil or any component of the formulation; concurrent (regular or intermittent) use of organic nitrates in any form (eg, nitroglycerin, isosorbide dinitrate)
Warnings/Precautions There is a degree of cardiac risk associated with sexual activity; therefore, physicians may wish to consider the patient's cardiovascular status prior to initiating any treatment for erectile dysfunction. Use caution in patients with anatomical deformation of the penis (angulation, cavernosal fibrosis, or Peyronie's disease) and in patients who have conditions which may predispose them to priapism (sickle cell anemia, multiple myeloma, leukemia). Instruct patients to seek immediate medical attention if erection persists >4 hours.

Use is not recommended in patients with hypotension (<90/50 mm Hg); uncontrolled hypertension (>170/100 mm Hg); unstable angina or angina during intercourse; life-threatening arrhythmias, stroke or MI within the last 6 months; cardiac failure or coronary artery disease causing unstable angina. Safety and efficacy have not been studied in these patients. Use caution in patients with left ventricular outflow obstruction (eg, aortic stenosis). Use caution with alpha-blockers, effective CYP3A4 inhibitors, the elderly, or those with hepatic impairment (Child-Pugh class B); dosage adjustment is needed.

Rare cases of nonarteritic ischemic optic neuropathy (NAION) have been reported; risk may be increased with history of vision loss. Other risk factors for NAION include heart disease, diabetes, hypertension, smoking, age >50 years, or history of certain eye problems. Sudden decrease or loss of hearing has been reported rarely; hearing changes may be accompanied by tinnitus and dizziness.

Safety and efficacy have not been studied in patients with the following conditions, therefore, use in these patients is not recommended at this time: Congenital QT prolongation, patients taking medications known to prolong the QT interval (avoid use in patients taking Class Ia or III antiarrhythmics); severe hepatic impairment (Child-Pugh class C); end-stage renal disease requiring dialysis; retinitis pigmentosa or other degenerative retinal disorders. The safety and efficacy of vardenafil with other treatments for erectile dysfunction have not been studied and are not recommended as combination therapy. Concomitant use with all forms of nitrates is contraindicated. If nitrate administration is medically necessary, it is not known when nitrates can be safely administered following the use of vardenafil; the ACC/AHA 2007 guidelines support administration of nitrates only if 24 hours have elapsed. Safety and efficacy have not been established in children. Potential underlying causes of erectile dysfunction should be evaluated prior to treatment.

Adverse Reactions
>10%:
Cardiovascular: Flushing (11%)
Central nervous system: Headache (15%)
2% to 10%:
Central nervous system: Dizziness (2%)
Gastrointestinal: Dyspepsia (4%), nausea (2%)
Neuromuscular & skeletal: CPK increased (2%)
Respiratory: Rhinitis (9%), sinusitis (3%)
Miscellaneous: Flu-like syndrome (3%)
<2% (Limited to important or life-threatening): Abnormal ejaculation, amnesia (transient global), anaphylactic reaction, angina, arthralgia, dyspnea, hearing decreased, hearing loss, hyper-/hypotension, insomnia, liver function tests abnormal, MI, myalgia, nonarteritic ischemic optic neuropathy (NAION), pain, photophobia, photosensitivity, postural hypotension, priapism, pruritus, rash, somnolence, syncope, tachycardia, tinnitus, vertigo, vision abnormal, visual acuity reduced, visual field defects, vision loss (temporary or permanent)

Drug Interactions
Metabolism/Transport Effects **Substrate** of CYP2C (minor), 3A5 (minor), 3A4 (major)
Avoid Concomitant Use
Avoid concomitant use of Vardenafil with any of the following: Vasodilators (Organic Nitrates)
Increased Effect/Toxicity
Vardenafil may increase the levels/effects of: Alpha1-Blockers; Vasodilators (Organic Nitrates)

The levels/effects of Vardenafil may be increased by: Antifungal Agents (Azole Derivatives, Systemic); CYP3A4 Inhibitors (Moderate); CYP3A4 Inhibitors (Strong); Dasatinib; Macrolide Antibiotics; Protease Inhibitors; Sapropterin
Decreased Effect
The levels/effects of Vardenafil may be decreased by: Etravirine

Ethanol/Nutrition/Herb Interactions Food: High-fat meals decrease maximum serum concentration 18% to 50%. Serum concentrations/toxicity may be increased with grapefruit juice; avoid concurrent use.
Stability Store at controlled room temperature of 25°C (77°F); excursions permitted to 15°C to 25°C (59°F to 86°F).
Mechanism of Action Does not directly cause penile erections, but affects the response to sexual stimulation. The physiologic mechanism of erection of the penis involves release of nitric oxide (NO) in the corpus

cavernosum during sexual stimulation. NO then activates the enzyme guanylate cyclase, which results in increased levels of cyclic guanosine monophosphate (cGMP), producing smooth muscle relaxation and inflow of blood to the corpus cavernosum. Vardenafil enhances the effect of NO by inhibiting phosphodiesterase type 5 (PDE-5), which is responsible for degradation of cGMP in the corpus cavernosum; when sexual stimulation causes local release of NO, inhibition of PDE-5 by vardenafil causes increased levels of cGMP in the corpus cavernosum, resulting in smooth muscle relaxation and inflow of blood to the corpus cavernosum; at recommended doses, it has no effect in the absence of sexual stimulation.

Pharmacodynamics/Kinetics

Onset of action: ~60 minutes

Absorption: Rapid

Distribution: V_d: 208 L

Protein binding: ~95% (parent drug and metabolite)

Metabolism: Hepatic via CYP3A4 (major), CYP2C and 3A5 (minor); forms metabolite (active)

Bioavailability: ~15%; Elderly (≥65 years): AUC increased by 52%; Hepatic impairment (moderate, Child-Pugh class B): AUC increased by 160%

Half-life elimination: Terminal: Vardenafil and metabolite: 4-5 hours

Time to peak, plasma: 0.5-2 hours

Excretion: Feces (91% to 95% as metabolites); urine (2% to 6%)

Dosage Oral: Adults: Erectile dysfunction: 10 mg 60 minutes prior to sexual activity; dosing range: 5-20 mg; to be given as one single dose and not given more than once daily

Elderly ≥65 years: Initial: 5 mg 60 minutes prior to sexual activity; to be given as one single dose and not given more than once daily

Dosing adjustment with concomitant medications:

Alpha-blocker (dose should be stable at time of vardenafil initiation): Initial vardenafil dose: 5 mg/24 hours; if an alpha-blocker is added to vardenafil therapy, it should be initiated at the smallest possible dose, and titrated carefully.

Atazanavir: Maximum vardenafil dose: 2.5 mg/24 hours

Clarithromycin: Maximum vardenafil dose: 2.5 mg/24 hours

Erythromycin: Maximum vardenafil dose: 5 mg/24 hours

Indinavir: Maximum vardenafil dose: 2.5 mg/24 hours

Itraconazole:

200 mg/day: Maximum vardenafil dose: 5 mg/24 hours

400 mg/day: Maximum vardenafil dose: 2.5 mg/24 hours

Ketoconazole:

200 mg/day: Maximum vardenafil dose: 5 mg/24 hours

400 mg/day: Maximum vardenafil dose: 2.5 mg/24 hours

Ritonavir: Maximum vardenafil dose: 2.5 mg/72 hours

Saquinavir: Maximum vardenafil dose: 2.5 mg/24 hours

Dosage adjustment in renal impairment: Dose adjustment not needed for mild, moderate, or severe impairment; use has not been studied in patients on renal dialysis

Dosage adjustment in hepatic impairment:

Child-Pugh class A: No adjustment required

Child-Pugh class B: Initial: 5 mg 60 minutes prior to sexual activity (maximum dose: 10 mg); to be given as one single dose and not given more than once daily

Child-Pugh class C: Has not been studied; use is not recommended by the manufacturer

Dietary Considerations May take with or without food.

Administration May be administered with or without food, 60 minutes prior to sexual activity.

Monitoring Parameters Monitor for response and adverse reactions.

Dosage Forms Excipient information presented when available (limited, particularly for generics); consult specific product labeling.

Tablet:

Levitra®: 2.5 mg, 5 mg, 10 mg, 20 mg

◆ **Vardenafil Hydrochloride** *see* Vardenafil *on page* 1547

Varenicline (var e NI kleen)

U.S. Brand Names Chantix®

Canadian Brand Names Champix®

Index Terms Varenicline Tartrate

Pharmacologic Category Partial Nicotine Agonist; Smoking Cessation Aid

Use Treatment to aid in smoking cessation

Restrictions An FDA-approved medication guide must be distributed when dispensing an outpatient prescription (new or refill) where this medication is to be used without direct supervision of a healthcare provider. Medication guides are available at http://www.fda.gov/cder/Offices/ODS/medication_guides.htm.

Pregnancy Risk Factor C

Pregnancy Considerations Teratogenic effects were not observed in animal studies, however, decreased fertility, decreased fetal weight, and increased auditory startle response were observed in the offspring. There are no adequate or well-controlled studies in pregnant women. Use only if benefit outweighs the potential risk to fetus.

Lactation Excretion in breast milk unknown/not recommended

Contraindications There are no contraindications listed within the manufacturer's labeling.

Warnings/Precautions Dose-dependent nausea may occur; both transient and persistent nausea has been reported. Dosage reduction may be considered for intolerable nausea. Neuropsychiatric symptoms, including suicidal thoughts and erratic/aggressive behavior, have been reported with use and following withdrawal of varenicline. Smoking cessation (with or without treatment) is associated with nicotine withdrawal symptoms and the exacerbation of underlying psychiatric illness; however, behavioral changes were also reported in patients who continued to smoke. Monitor patients for behavioral changes and psychiatric symptoms (eg, agitation, depression, suicidal behavior, suicidal ideation); inform patients to discontinue treatment and contact their healthcare provider immediately if they experience any behavioral and/or mood changes. Patients with pre-existing psychiatric illness (eg, bipolar disorder, major severe depression, schizophrenia) were not studied in clinical trials; safety and efficacy has not been established in these populations. Due to rare neuropsychiatric events, caution is warranted if treatment is initiated; worsening of psychiatric illness has been reported. May cause sedation, which may impair physical or mental abilities; patients must be cautioned about performing tasks which require mental alertness (eg, operating machinery or driving).

Use caution in renal dysfunction; dosage adjustment required. Safety and efficacy of varenicline with other smoking cessation therapies have not been established; increased adverse events when used concurrently with nicotine replacement therapy. The manufacturer does not recommend use in patients <18 years of age.

Adverse Reactions

>10%:

Central nervous system: Insomnia (18% to 19%), headache (15% to 19%), abnormal dreams (9% to 13%)

Gastrointestinal: Nausea (16% to 40%; dose related)

1% to 10%:

Central nervous system: Sleep disorder (≤5%), somnolence (3%), nightmares (1% to 2%), lethargy (1% to 2%), malaise (≤7%)

Dermatologic: Rash (≤3%)

Gastrointestinal: Flatulence (6% to 9%), abdominal pain (≤7%), constipation (5% to 8%), abnormal taste (5% to 8%), xerostomia (≤6%), dyspepsia (5%), vomiting (1% to 5%), appetite increased (3% to 4%), anorexia (≤2%), gastroesophageal reflux (1%)

Respiratory: Dyspnea (≤2%), rhinorrhea (≤1%)

<1% (Limited to important or life-threatening): Acute coronary syndrome, acute renal failure, aggression, agitation, amnesia, anemia, angina, anxiety, arrhythmia, asthma, atrial fibrillation, attention disturbance, behavioral changes, blindness (transient), blurred vision, bradycardia, bradyphrenia, cardiac flutter, cataract, cerebrovascular accident, chest pain, chills, conjunctivitis, coronary artery disease, cor pulmonale, deafness, depression, dermatitis, diabetes mellitus, diarrhea, disorientation, dissociation, dizziness, dysarthria, dysphagia, ECG abnormal, eczema, edema, emotional disorder, enterocolitis, epistaxis, erectile dysfunction, eructation, erythema, esophagitis, euphoria, facial palsy, fever, flu-like syndrome, flushing, gall bladder disorder, gastritis, gastric ulcer, gastrointestinal hemorrhage, gingivitis, hallucinations, hyperhidrosis, hyper-/hypokalemia, hyperlipidemia, hypersensitivity, hyper-/hypotension, hypoglycemia, intestinal obstruction, irritability, leukocytosis, libido decreased, liver function test abnormal, lymphadenopathy, mental impairment, MI, migraine, mood swings, mouth ulceration, muscle enzyme increased, musculoskeletal pain, multiple sclerosis, myositis, nephrolithiasis, night blindness, nocturia, nystagmus, ocular vascular disorder, osteoporosis, palpitation, pancreatitis, parosmia, peripheral ischemia, photophobia, photosensitivity, pleurisy, polyuria, psoriasis, psychomotor impairment, psychotic disorder, pulmonary embolism, restless leg syndrome, restlessness, seizure, sexual dysfunction, splenomegaly, suicidal behavior, suicidal ideation, suicide, syncope, tachycardia, thinking abnormal, thrombocytopenia, thrombosis, thyroid disorder, tinnitus, transient ischemic attack, tremor, urinary retention, urticaria, ventricular extrasystoles, vertigo, visual field defect, vitreous floaters, weight gain, xerophthalmia

Drug Interactions

Avoid Concomitant Use There are no known interactions where it is recommended to avoid concomitant use.

Increased Effect/Toxicity There are no known significant interactions involving an increase in effect.

Decreased Effect There are no known significant interactions involving a decrease in effect.

Stability Store at controlled room temperature of 25°C (77°F).

Mechanism of Action Partial neuronal alpha$_4$ β_2 nicotinic receptor agonist; prevents nicotine stimulation of mesolimbic dopamine system associated with nicotine addiction. Also binds to 5 HT_3 receptor (significance not determined) with moderate affinity. Varenicline stimulates dopamine activity but to a much smaller degree than nicotine does, resulting in decreased craving and withdrawal symptoms.

Pharmacodynamics/Kinetics

Absorption: Well absorbed; unaffected by food

Protein binding: ≤20%

Metabolism: Minimal (<10% of clearance is through metabolism)

Half-life elimination: ~24 hours

Time to peak, plasma: ~3-4 hours

Excretion: Primarily urine (92% as unchanged drug)

Dosage Oral: Adults:

Initial:

Days 1-3: 0.5 mg once daily

Days 4-7: 0.5 mg twice daily

Maintenance (≥ Day 8): 1 mg twice daily

Note: Start 1 week before target quit date. Patients who cannot tolerate adverse events may require temporary reduction in dose. If patient successfully quits smoking during the 12 weeks, may continue for another 12 weeks to help maintain success. If not successful in first 12 weeks, then stop medication and reassess factors contributing to failure.

Dosage adjustment for toxicity: Lower dose for a period of time, then increase again

Dosage adjustment in renal impairment:

Cl_{cr} ≥30 mL/minute: No adjustment required

Cl_{cr} <30 mL/minute: Initial: 0.5 mg once daily; maximum dose: 0.5 mg twice daily

Hemodialysis: Maximum dose: 0.5 mg once daily

Dosage adjustment in hepatic impairment: No adjustment required

Dietary Considerations Should be given with food and a full glass of water to decrease gastric upset.

Administration Administer with food and glass of water.

Monitoring Parameters Monitor for behavioral changes and psychiatric symptoms (eg, agitation, depression, suicidal behavior, suicidal ideation)

Additional Information In all studies, patients received an educational booklet on smoking cessation and received up to 10 minutes of counseling at each weekly visit. Dosing started 1 week before target quit date. Successful cessation of smoking may alter pharmacokinetic properties of other medications (eg, theophylline, warfarin, insulin).

Dosage Forms Excipient information presented when available (limited, particularly for generics); consult specific product labeling.

Tablet:

Chantix®: 0.5 mg, 1 mg

Combination package, oral [dose-pack]:

Chantix®:

Tablet, oral: 0.5 mg (11) [white tablets]

Tablet, oral: 1 mg (42) [light blue tablets]

◆ **Varenicline Tartrate** *see* Varenicline *on page 1548*

◆ **Varicella, Measles, Mumps, and Rubella Vaccine** *see* Measles, Mumps, Rubella, and Varicella Virus Vaccine *on page 923*

Varicella Virus Vaccine

(var i SEL a VYE rus vak SEEN)

U.S. Brand Names Varivax®

Canadian Brand Names Varilrix®; Varivax® III

Index Terms Chickenpox Vaccine; Varicella-Zoster Virus (VZV) Vaccine (Varicella); VZV Vaccine (Varicella)

Pharmacologic Category Vaccine

Additional Appendix Information

Immunization Recommendations *on page 1708*

Use Immunization against varicella in children ≥12 months of age and adults

The ACIP recommends vaccination for all children, adolescents, and adults who do not have evidence of immunity. Vaccination is especially important for:

- Persons with close contact to those at high risk for severe disease
- Persons living or working in environments where transmission is likely (teachers, child-care workers, residents and staff of institutional settings)
- Persons in environments where transmission has been reported
- Nonpregnant women of childbearing age
- Adolescents and adults in households with children
- International travelers

Postexposure prophylaxis: Vaccination within 3 days (possibly 5 days) after exposure to rash is effective in preventing illness or modifying severity of disease

Pregnancy Risk Factor C

Pregnancy Considerations Animal reproduction studies have not been conducted. Varivax® should not be administered to pregnant females and pregnancy should be avoided for 3 months (per manufacturer labeling; 1 month per ACIP) following vaccination. A pregnancy registry has been established for pregnant women exposed to varicella virus vaccine (800-986-8999). Varicella disease during the 1st or 2nd trimesters may result in congenital varicella syndrome. The onset of maternal varicella infection from 5 days prior to 2 days after delivery may cause varicella infection in the newborn. All women should be assessed for immunity during a prenatal visit; those without evidence of immunity should be vaccinated upon completion or termination of pregnancy.

Lactation Excretion in breast milk unknown/use caution

Medication Safety Issues

Sound-alike/look-alike issues:

Varicella virus vaccine has been given in error (instead of the indicated varicella immune globulin) to pregnant women exposed to varicella.

Both varicella vaccine and zoster vaccine are live, attenuated strains of varicella-zoster virus. Their indications, dosing, and composition are distinct. Varicella is indicated in children to prevent chickenpox, while zoster vaccine is indicated in older individuals to prevent reactivation of the virus which causes shingles. Zoster vaccine is **not** a substitute for varicella vaccine and should not be used in children.

Contraindications Hypersensitivity to any component of the vaccine; individuals with blood dyscrasias, leukemia, lymphomas, or other malignant neoplasms affecting the bone marrow or lymphatic systems; those receiving immunosuppressive therapy; primary and acquired immunodeficiency states; family history of congenital or hereditary immunodeficiency; active, untreated tuberculosis; current febrile illness (per manufacturer labeling); pregnancy

Warnings/Precautions Immediate treatment for anaphylactoid reaction should be available during vaccine use. Defer vaccination for at least 5 months following blood or plasma transfusions, immune globulin (IgG), or VZIG (avoid IgG or IVIG use for 2 months following vaccination); salicylates should be avoided for 6 weeks after vaccination. Vaccinated individuals should not have close association with susceptible high-risk individuals (newborns, pregnant women, immunocompromised persons) following vaccination. May administer to patients with mild acute illness (with or without low grade fever per CDC guidelines). Children with HIV infection with age-specific CD4+ T-lymphocyte percentages ≥15% may receive live attenuated varicella vaccine. Vaccination may be considered for adolescents and adults with CD4+ T-lymphocyte counts ≥200 cells/µL. Products may contain gelatin, neomycin, or albumin.

Adverse Reactions All serious adverse reactions must be reported to the U.S. Department of Health and Human Services (DHHS) Vaccine Adverse Event Reporting System (VAERS) 1-800-822-7967.

>10%:

Central nervous system: Fever (10% to 15%)

Local: Injection site reaction (19% to 33%)

1% to 10%:

Central nervous system: Chills, fatigue, headache, irritability, malaise, nervousness, sleep disturbance

Dermatologic: Generalized varicella-like rash (1% to 6%), contact rash, dermatitis, diaper rash, dry skin, eczema, heat rash, itching

Gastrointestinal: Abdominal pain, appetite decreased, cold/canker sore, constipation, diarrhea, nausea, vomiting

Hematologic: Lymphadenopathy

Local: Varicella-like rash at the injection site (1% to 3%)

Neuromuscular & skeletal: Arthralgia, myalgia, stiff neck

Otic: Otitis

Respiratory: Cough, lower/upper respiratory illness

Miscellaneous: Allergic reactions, teething

<1%: Febrile seizure, pneumonitis

<1% (Limited to important or life-threatening): Anaphylaxis, aseptic meningitis, ataxia, Bell's palsy, cellulitis, cerebellar ataxia (acute), cerebrovascular accident, disseminated varicella infection, dizziness, encephalitis, erythema multiforme, Guillain-Barré syndrome, hemiparesis (acute), Henoch-Schönlein purpura, hepatitis, herpes zoster, impetigo, nonfebrile seizure, paresthesia, pharyngitis, pneumonia, secondary skin infection, Stevens-Johnson syndrome, thrombocytopenia, transverse myelitis, urticaria

Drug Interactions

Avoid Concomitant Use

Avoid concomitant use of Varicella Virus Vaccine with any of the following: Immunosuppressants

Increased Effect/Toxicity

The levels/effects of Varicella Virus Vaccine may be increased by: 5-ASA Derivatives; Immunosuppressants; Salicylates; Smallpox Vaccine

Decreased Effect

Varicella Virus Vaccine may decrease the levels/effects of: Tuberculin Tests

The levels/effects of Varicella Virus Vaccine may be decreased by: Immune Globulins

Stability Store powder in freezer at -15°C (5°F) or colder; protect from light. Store diluent separately at room temperature or in refrigerator. Powder may be stored under refrigeration for up to 72 continuous hours prior to reconstitution; if not used within 72 hours, vaccine should be discarded. Use 0.7 mL of the provided diluent to reconstitute vaccine. Gently agitate to mix thoroughly. (Total volume of reconstituted vaccine will be ~0.5 mL.) Following reconstitution, discard reconstituted vaccine if not used within 30 minutes.

Canadian formulations: **Note:** Varicella vaccine has been reformulated to produce a refrigerator-stable preparation. Previously, the product required storage in a freezer prior to reconstitution. The new Canadian formulation may be stored in a freezer, but if transferred to a refrigerator, may not be refrozen. Individual product labeling should be consulted to confirm proper conditions.

Mechanism of Action As a live, attenuated vaccine, varicella virus vaccine offers active immunity to disease caused by the varicella-zoster virus

Pharmacodynamics/Kinetics

Onset of action: Seroconversion: ~4-6 weeks

Duration: Antibody titers detectable at 10 years postvaccination

Dosage SubQ:

Children 12 months to 12 years: 0.5 mL; a second dose may be administered ≥3 months later

Note: The ACIP recommends the routine childhood vaccination be 2 doses, with the first dose administered at 12-15 months of age. School age children should receive the second dose at 4-6 years of age, but it may be administered earlier provided ≥3 months have elapsed after the first dose. All children and adolescents who received only 1 dose of vaccine should receive a second dose.

Children ≥13 years to Adults: 2 doses of 0.5 mL separated by 4-8 weeks

Administration Do not administer I.V. Inject immediately after reconstitution. Inject SubQ into the outer aspect of the upper arm, if possible.

Monitoring Parameters Rash, fever

Additional Information Federal law requires that the date of administration, the vaccine manufacturer, lot number of vaccine, and the administering person's name, title, and address be entered into the patient's permanent medical record.

Evidence of immunity to varicella includes any of the following:

Documentation of age appropriate vaccination with varicella vaccine.

Laboratory evidence of immunity or laboratory confirmation of disease.

Birth in the United States prior to 1980 (except for health care personnel, pregnant women and the immunocompromised).

Diagnosis or verification of varicella disease by healthcare provider.

Diagnosis or verification of herpes zoster by healthcare provider.

Persons who lack evidence of immunity should be vaccinated.

Dosage Forms Excipient information presented when available (limited, particularly for generics); consult specific product labeling. [CAN] = Canadian brand name

Injection, powder for reconstitution [preservative free]:

Varivax®: 1350 plaque-forming units (PFU) [contains gelatin and trace amounts of neomycin; packaged with diluent]

Varivax® III [CAN]: 1350 plaque-forming units (PFU) [contains gelatin and trace amounts of neomycin; packaged with diluent; not available in U.S.]

Injection, powder for reconstitution (Valrilix® [CAN]): $10^{3.3}$ plaque-forming units (PFU) [contains albumin and gelatin; packaged with diluent; not available in U.S.]

Varicella-Zoster Immune Globulin (Human)

(var i SEL a- ZOS ter i MYUN GLOB yoo lin HYU man)

Canadian Brand Names VariZIG™

Index Terms VZIG

Pharmacologic Category Immune Globulin

Use In pregnant women, for the prevention or reduction in severity of maternal infection within 4 days of exposure to the varicella zoster virus.

Unlabeled/Investigational Use In the United States, the Centers for Disease Control and Prevention (CDC) recommends varicella-zoster immune globulin (VZIG) for the passive immunization of patients who are at a greater risk of complications following significant exposure to varicella and do not have evidence of immunity. Guidelines restrict administration to those patients meeting the following criteria:

- Immunocompromised patients without evidence of immunity, including those with neoplastic disease (eg, leukemia or lymphoma); primary or acquired immunodeficiency; immunosuppressive therapy (including steroid therapy equivalent to prednisone ≥2 mg/kg or 20 mg/day)
- Newborn of mother who had onset of varicella (chickenpox) within 5 days before delivery or within 48 hours after delivery
- Premature infants (≥28 weeks gestation) whose mother has no evidence of immunity
- Premature infants (<28 weeks gestation or ≤1000 g) regardless of maternal history
- Pregnant women without evidence of immunity

Significant exposure includes:

Continuous household contact

Face-to-face indoor contact (>5 minutes or >1 hour depending on reference)

Hospital contact (in same 2-4 bedroom or adjacent beds in a large ward or prolonged face-to-face contact with an infectious staff member or patient)

Restrictions Varicella-zoster immune globulin (VZIG) was discontinued in the United States in 2005. It is currently available as VariZIG™ under an Investigational New Drug Application Expanded Access protocol. Inventory for anticipated patients may be obtained by contacting FFF Enterprises at 800-843-7477 and faxing a release form. The release form can be accessed from the CDC (available at http://www.fda.gov/cber/infosheets/mphvzig020806.htm). VariZIG™ may also be prepositioned at qualified sites.

Pregnancy Considerations Animal reproduction studies have not been conducted. Clinical use of other immunoglobulins suggest that there are no adverse effects on the fetus. Pregnant women who do not have evidence of immunity to varicella may be at increased risk of infection following exposure. VZIG is used to prevent maternal complications, not fetal infection.

Lactation Excretion in breast milk unknown/use caution

Medication Safety Issues

Sound-alike/look-alike issues:

Varicella virus vaccine has been given in error (instead of the indicated varicella immune globulin) to pregnant women exposed to varicella.

Contraindications Severe reaction associated with past human immune globulin administration; hypersensitivity to any component of the formulation; patients with evidence of immunity; IgA deficiency

Note: U.S. CDC guidelines: Healthy and immunocompromised patients (except bone marrow transplant recipients [BMT]) with positive history of varicella infection are considered immune. BMT patients who had varicella infection *prior to* transplant are **not** considered immune; however, the expanded access protocol does not include use for this indication. BMT patients who develop varicella infection *after* transplant **are** considered immune. Patients who are fully vaccinated, but later became immunocompromised should be monitored closely; treatment with VZIG is not indicated, but other therapy may be needed if disease occurs.

Adverse Reactions

>10%:

Central nervous system: Headache (7% to 11%)

Local: Injection site pain (17% to 47%)

1% to 10%:

Central nervous system: Dizziness (up to 5%), fever (up to 5%), pain (up to 5%), chills (up to 2%), fatigue (up to 2%), flushing (up to 2%), insomnia (up to 2%)

Dermatologic: Rash (up to 4%), dermatitis (up to 2%), erythematous rash (up to 2%)

Gastrointestinal: Nausea (2% to 5%), dysgeusia (up to 2%)

Local: Injection site bruising, itching, or tenderness (up to 2%)

Neuromuscular & skeletal: Neck pain (up to 5%), myalgia (up to 2%)

Drug Interactions

Avoid Concomitant Use There are no known interactions where it is recommended to avoid concomitant use.

Increased Effect/Toxicity There are no known significant interactions involving an increase in effect.

Decreased Effect

Varicella-Zoster Immune Globulin (Human) may decrease the levels/effects of: Vaccines (Live)

Stability Prior to reconstitution, store at 2°C to 8°C (36°F to 48°F); do not freeze. Following reconstitution, may store at 2°C to 8°C (36°F to 48°F) for up to 12 hours. Reconstitute only with provided diluent. Inject diluent slowly and at an angle onto the inside glass wall of the vial. Gently invert vial and swirl to dissolve; do not shake. For I.V. administration, reconstitute with 2.5 mL/vial (provides 50 int. units/mL). For I.M. administration, reconstitute with 1.25 mL/vial (provides 100 int. units/mL).

Mechanism of Action Antibodies obtained from pooled human plasma of individuals with high titers of varicella-zoster provide passive immunity.

Pharmacodynamics/Kinetics
Duration: ≥6 weeks
Metabolism: Metabolized in the reticuloendothelial system
Bioavailability: 100%
Half-life elimination: I.V.: 18-24 days; I.M.: 24-30 days
Time to peak, plasma: I.V.: <3 hours; I.M.: 2-7 days

Dosage I.M., I.V.:
Children: Passive immunization (unlabeled use): Refer to adult dosing.
Adults: Prevention or reduction of maternal infection (approved use), passive immunization (unlabeled use): 125 int. units/10 kg (minimum dose: 125 int. units; maximum dose: 625 int. units). Administer within 96 hours of exposure.

Administration For I.M. or I.V. administration. Bring to room temperature prior to use. Should be given as soon as possible following exposure; efficacy has not been established for use >96 hours following exposure. For I.M. injection, administer into deltoid muscle or anterolateral aspect of upper thigh; avoid gluteal region. For I.V. administration, inject over 3-5 minutes.

Monitoring Parameters Observe for adverse effects for 20 minutes following administration. The CDC also recommends monitoring for signs and symptoms of varicella infection for 28 days after VZIG administration.

Test Interactions May cause false-positive test for immunity to VZV for 3 months following administration. May cause a false-positive Coomb's test.

Dosage Forms Excipient information presented when available (limited, particularly for generics); consult specific product labeling. [CAN = Canadian brand name]
Injection, powder for reconstitution [preservative free]:
VariZIG™ [CAN]: 125 int. units [package with diluent] [available in the U.S under expanded access protocol]

- ◆ **Varicella-Zoster Virus (VZV) Vaccine (Varicella)** *see* Varicella Virus Vaccine *on page 1549*
- ◆ **Varicella-Zoster (VZV) Vaccine (Zoster)** *see* Zoster Vaccine *on page 1593*
- ◆ **Varilrix® (Can)** *see* Varicella Virus Vaccine *on page 1549*
- ◆ **Varivax®** *see* Varicella Virus Vaccine *on page 1549*
- ◆ **Varivax® III (Can)** *see* Varicella Virus Vaccine *on page 1549*
- ◆ **VariZIG™ (Can)** *see* Varicella-Zoster Immune Globulin (Human) *on page 1551*
- ◆ **Vaseretic®** *see* Enalapril and Hydrochlorothiazide *on page 518*
- ◆ **Vasocon® (Can)** *see* Naphazoline *on page 1040*
- ◆ **Vasodilan® [DSC]** *see* Isoxsuprine *on page 827*

Vasopressin (vay soe PRES in)

Canadian Brand Names Pressyn®; Pressyn® AR

Index Terms 8-Arginine Vasopressin; ADH; Antidiuretic Hormone

Pharmacologic Category Antidiuretic Hormone Analog; Hormone, Posterior Pituitary

Use Treatment of diabetes insipidus; differential diagnosis of diabetes insipidus

Unlabeled/Investigational Use Adjunct in the treatment of GI hemorrhage and esophageal varices; pulseless arrest (ventricular tachycardia [VT]/ventricular fibrillation [VF], asystole/pulseless electrical activity [PEA]); vasodilatory shock (septic shock)

Pregnancy Risk Factor C

Pregnancy Considerations Animal reproduction studies have not been conducted. Vasopressin and desmopressin have been used safely during pregnancy based on case reports.

Lactation Enters breast milk/use caution

Medication Safety Issues
Sound-alike/look-alike issues:
Pitressin® may be confused with Pitocin®

Contraindications Hypersensitivity to vasopressin or any component of the formulation

Warnings/Precautions Use with caution in patients with seizure disorders, migraine, asthma, vascular disease, renal disease, cardiac disease; chronic nephritis with nitrogen retention, goiter with cardiac complications, or arteriosclerosis. I.V. infiltration may lead to severe vasoconstriction and localized tissue necrosis, gangrene of extremities, tongue, and ischemic colitis. May cause water toxication; early signs include drowsiness, listlessness, and headache, these should be recognized to prevent coma and seizures. Elderly patients should be cautioned not to increase their fluid intake beyond that sufficient to satisfy their thirst in order to avoid water intoxication and hyponatremia; under experimental conditions, the elderly have shown to have a decreased responsiveness to vasopressin with respect to its effects on water homeostasis.

Adverse Reactions Frequency not defined.
Cardiovascular: Arrhythmia, asystole (>0.04 units/minute), blood pressure increased, cardiac output decreased (>0.04 units/minute), chest pain, MI, vasoconstriction (with higher doses), venous thrombosis
Central nervous system: Pounding in head, fever, vertigo
Dermatologic: Ischemic skin lesions, circumoral pallor, urticaria
Gastrointestinal: Abdominal cramps, flatulence, mesenteric ischemia, nausea, vomiting
Genitourinary: Uterine contraction
Neuromuscular & skeletal: Tremor
Respiratory: Bronchial constriction
Miscellaneous: Diaphoresis

Drug Interactions
Avoid Concomitant Use There are no known interactions where it is recommended to avoid concomitant use.
Increased Effect/Toxicity There are no known significant interactions involving an increase in effect.
Decreased Effect There are no known significant interactions involving a decrease in effect.

Ethanol/Nutrition/Herb Interactions Ethanol: Avoid ethanol (due to effects on ADH).

Stability Store injection at room temperature; do not freeze. Protect from heat. Use only clear solutions.

Mechanism of Action Increases cyclic adenosine monophosphate (cAMP) which increases water permeability at the renal tubule resulting in decreased urine volume and increased osmolality; causes peristalsis by directly stimulating the smooth muscle in the GI tract; direct vasoconstrictor without inotropic or chronotropic effects

Pharmacodynamics/Kinetics
Onset of action: Nasal: 1 hour
Duration: Nasal: 3-8 hours; I.M., SubQ: 2-8 hours
Metabolism: Nasal/Parenteral: Hepatic, renal
Half-life elimination: Nasal: 15 minutes; Parenteral: 10-20 minutes
Excretion: Nasal: Urine; SubQ: Urine (5% as unchanged drug) after 4 hours

Dosage
Diabetes insipidus: **Note:** Highly variable dosage; titrated based on serum and urine sodium and osmolality in addition to fluid balance and urine output; vasopressin

rarely used for this indication; other therapies are available.

I.M., SubQ:

Children: 2.5-10 units 2-4 times/day as needed

Adults: 5-10 units 2-3 times/day as needed

Continuous I.V. infusion (unlabeled route): Children and Adults: 0.0005 unit/kg/hour; double dosage as needed every 30 minutes to a maximum of 0.01 unit/kg/hour

GI/variceal hemorrhage (unlabeled use): Continuous I.V. infusion: Dilute in NS or D_5W to 0.1-1 unit/mL. **Note:** Other therapies may be preferred.

GI hemorrhage (unlabeled use): Children: Initial I.V. bolus: 0.3 unit/kg (maximum: 20 units) may be given. Continuous I.V. infusion: 0.001-0.01 units/kg/minute; titrate dose as needed; maximum: 0.01 unit/kg/minute; if bleeding controlled for 12-24 hours, then taper off over 24-36 hours

Variceal hemorrhage (unlabeled use) [AASLD guidelines, 2007]: Adults: Initial: 0.2-0.4 units/minute, may titrate dose as needed to a maximum dose of 0.8 units/minute; maximum duration: 24 hours at highest effective dose continuously (to reduce incidence of adverse effects). Patient should also receive I.V. nitroglycerin concurrently to prevent myocardial ischemic complications; monitor closely for signs/symptoms of ischemia (myocardial, peripheral, bowel)

Pulseless arrest (unlabeled use) [ACLS, 2005]: Adults: I.V., I.O.: 40 units; may give 1 dose to replace first or second dose of epinephrine. I.V./I.O. drug administration is preferred, but if no access, may give endotracheally. ACLS guidelines do not recommend a specific endotracheal dose; however, may be given endotracheally using the same I.V. dose (Wenzel, 1997). Mix with 5-10 mL of water or normal saline, and administer down the endotracheal tube.

Vasodilatory shock/septic shock (unlabeled use): Adults: I.V.: 0.01-0.04 units/minute for the treatment of septic shock. Doses >0.04 units/minute may have more cardiovascular side effects. Most case reports have used 0.04 units/minute continuous infusion as a fixed dose.

Dosing adjustment in hepatic impairment: Some patients respond to much lower doses with cirrhosis

Administration

I.V.: Use extreme caution to avoid extravasation because of risk of necrosis and gangrene. In treatment of varices, infusions are often supplemented with nitroglycerin infusions to minimize cardiac effects.

GI hemorrhage: Administration requires the use of an infusion pump.

Infusion rates: 100 units in 500 mL D_5W rate

0.1 unit/minute: 30 mL/hour

0.2 unit/minute: 60 mL/hour

0.3 unit/minute: 90 mL/hour

0.4 unit/minute: 120 mL/hour

0.5 unit/minute: 150 mL/hour

0.6 unit/minute: 180 mL/hour

Vasodilatory shock: Administration through a central catheter is recommended.

Intranasal (topical administration on nasal mucosa): Administer injectable vasopressin on cotton plugs, as nasal spray, or by dropper. Should not be inhaled.

Endotracheal: If no I.V. /I.O. access may give endotracheally. ACLS guidelines do not recommend a specific endotracheal dose; however, may be given endotracheally using the same I.V. dose (Wenzel, 1997). Mix with 5-10 mL of water or normal saline, and administer down the endotracheal tube.

Monitoring Parameters Serum and urine sodium, urine specific gravity, urine and serum osmolality; urine output, fluid input and output, blood pressure, heart rate

Reference Range Plasma: 0-2 pg/mL (SI: 0-2 ng/L) if osmolality <285 mOsm/L; 2-12 pg/mL (SI: 2-12 ng/L) if osmolality >290 mOsm/L

Additional Information Vasopressin increases factor VIII levels and may be useful in hemophiliacs.

Dosage Forms Excipient information presented when available (limited, particularly for generics); consult specific product labeling.

Injection, solution: 20 units/mL (0.5 mL, 1 mL, 10 mL)

- **Vasotec®** *see* Enalapril *on page 515*
- **Vasotec® I.V. (Can)** *see* Enalapril *on page 515*
- **Vaxigrip® (Can)** *see* Influenza Virus Vaccine *on page 788*
- **VCF™ [OTC]** *see* Nonoxynol 9 *on page 1077*
- **Vectibix®** *see* Panitumumab *on page 1138*

Vecuronium (vek ue ROE nee um)

U.S. Brand Names Norcuron® [DSC]

Canadian Brand Names Norcuron®

Index Terms ORG NC 45

Pharmacologic Category Neuromuscular Blocker Agent, Nondepolarizing

Additional Appendix Information

Neuromuscular-Blocking Agents *on page 1665*

Use Adjunct to general anesthesia to facilitate endotracheal intubation and to relax skeletal muscles during surgery; to facilitate mechanical ventilation in ICU patients; does not relieve pain or produce sedation

Pregnancy Risk Factor C

Pregnancy Considerations Use in cesarean section has been reported. Umbilical venous concentrations were 11% of maternal.

Lactation Excretion in breast milk unknown/use caution

Medication Safety Issues

Sound-alike/look-alike issues:

Vecuronium may be confused with vancomycin

Norcuron® may be confused with Narcan®

High alert medication: The Institute for Safe Medication Practices (ISMP) includes this medication among its list of drugs which have a heightened risk of causing significant patient harm when used in error.

Contraindications Hypersensitivity to vecuronium or any component of the formulation

Warnings/Precautions Ventilation must be supported during neuromuscular blockade; certain clinical conditions may result in potentiation or antagonism of neuromuscular blockade:

Potentiation: Electrolyte abnormalities, severe hyponatremia, severe hypocalcemia, severe hypokalemia, hypermagnesemia, neuromuscular diseases, acidosis, acute intermittent porphyria, renal failure, hepatic failure

Antagonism: Alkalosis, hypercalcemia, demyelinating lesions, peripheral neuropathies, diabetes mellitus

Increased sensitivity in patients with myasthenia gravis, Eaton-Lambert syndrome; resistance in burn patients (>30% of body) for period of 5-70 days postinjury; resistance in patients with muscle trauma, denervation, immobilization, infection; use with caution in patients with hepatic or renal impairment; does not counteract bradycardia produced by anesthetics/vagal stimulation. Cross-sensitivity with other neuromuscular-blocking agents may occur; use extreme caution in patients with previous anaphylactic reactions. Use caution in the elderly. **[U.S. Boxed Warning]: Should be administered by adequately trained individuals familiar with its use.**

Adverse Reactions <1% (Limited to important or life-threatening): Bradycardia, circulatory collapse, edema, flushing, hypersensitivity reaction, hypotension, itching, rash, tachycardia, acute quadriplegic myopathy syndrome (prolonged use), myositis ossificans (prolonged use)

Drug Interactions

Avoid Concomitant Use There are no known interactions where it is recommended to avoid concomitant use.

Increased Effect/Toxicity

Vecuronium may increase the levels/effects of: Botulinum Toxin Type A; Botulinum Toxin Type B; Cardiac Glycosides; Corticosteroids (Systemic)

The levels/effects of Vecuronium may be increased by: Aminoglycosides; Calcium Channel Blockers; Capreomycin; Colistimethate; Inhalational Anesthetics; Ketorolac; Lincosamide Antibiotics; Lithium; Loop Diuretics; Magnesium Salts; Polymyxin B; Procainamide; QuiNIDine; Tetracycline Derivatives; Vancomycin

Decreased Effect

The levels/effects of Vecuronium may be decreased by: Acetylcholinesterase Inhibitors; CarBAMazepine; Loop Diuretics; Phenytoin

Stability Store intact vials of powder for injection at room temperature 15°C to 30°C (59°F to 86°F). Vials reconstituted with bacteriostatic water for injection (BWFI) may be stored for 5 days under refrigeration or at room temperature. Vials reconstituted with other compatible diluents (nonbacteriostatic) should be stored under refrigeration and used within 24 hours. Reconstitute with compatible solution for injection to final concentration of 1 mg/mL.

Mechanism of Action Blocks acetylcholine from binding to receptors on motor endplate inhibiting depolarization

Pharmacodynamics/Kinetics

Onset of action:

Good intubation conditions: Within 2.5-3 minutes

Maximum neuromuscular blockade: Within 3-5 minutes

Duration: 20-40 minutes

Metabolism: Active metabolite: 3-desacetyl vecuronium (1/2 the activity of parent drug)

Half-life elimination: 51-80 minutes

Excretion: Primarily feces (40% to 75%); urine (30% as unchanged drug and metabolites)

Dosage Administer I.V.; dose to effect; doses will vary due to interpatient variability; use ideal body weight for obese patients

Surgery:

Infants >7 weeks to 1 year: Initial: 0.08-0.1 mg/kg/dose; maintenance: 0.05-0.1 mg/kg every 60 minutes as needed

Children >1 year and Adults: Initial: 0.08-0.1 mg/kg or 0.04-0.06 mg/kg after initial dose of succinylcholine for intubation; maintenance: 0.01-0.015 mg/kg 25-40 minutes after initial dose, then 0.01-0.015 mg/kg every 12-15 minutes (higher doses will allow less frequent maintenance doses); may be administered as a continuous infusion at 0.8-2 mcg/kg/minute

Pretreatment/priming: Adults: 10% of intubating dose given 3-5 minutes before initial dose

ICU: Adults: 0.05-0.1 mg/kg bolus followed by 0.8-1.7 mcg/kg/minute once initial recovery from bolus observed or 0.1-0.2 mg/kg/dose every 1 hour

Note: Children (1-10 years) may require slightly higher initial doses and slightly more frequent supplementation; infants >7 weeks to 1 year may be more sensitive to vecuronium and have a longer recovery time

Dosing adjustment in renal impairment: Prolongation of blockade

Dosing adjustment in hepatic impairment: Dose reductions are necessary in patients with cirrhosis or cholestasis

Administration Concentration of 1 mg/mL may be administered by rapid I.V. injection. May further dilute reconstituted vial to 0.1-0.2 mg/mL in a compatible solution for I.V. infusion. Concentration of 1 mg/mL may be used for I.V. infusion in fluid-restricted patients.

Monitoring Parameters Blood pressure, heart rate

Additional Information Vecuronium is classified as an intermediate-duration neuromuscular-blocking agent. It produces minimal, if any, histamine release; does not relieve pain or produce sedation. It may produce cumulative effect on duration of blockade.

Dosage Forms Excipient information presented when available (limited, particularly for generics); consult specific product labeling.

Injection, powder for reconstitution, as bromide: 10 mg, 20 mg [may be supplied with diluent containing benzyl alcohol]

◆ **Velban** *see* VinBLAStine *on page 1560*

◆ **Velcade®** *see* Bortezomib *on page 204*

◆ **Velivet™** *see* Ethinyl Estradiol and Desogestrel *on page 575*

Venlafaxine (ven la FAX een)

U.S. Brand Names Effexor XR®; Effexor®

Canadian Brand Names Co-Venlafaxine XR; Effexor® XR; GEN-Venlafaxine XR; Novo-Venlafaxine XR; PMS-Venlafaxine XR; RATIO-Venlafaxine XR; RIVA-Venlafaxine XR; SANDOZ-Venlafaxine XR

Pharmacologic Category Antidepressant, Serotonin/Norepinephrine Reuptake Inhibitor

Additional Appendix Information

Antidepressant Agents *on page 1638*

Use Treatment of major depressive disorder, generalized anxiety disorder (GAD), social anxiety disorder (social phobia), panic disorder

Unlabeled/Investigational Use Obsessive-compulsive disorder (OCD); hot flashes; neuropathic pain; attention-deficit/hyperactivity disorder (ADHD)

Restrictions An FDA-approved medication guide concerning the use of antidepressants in children, adolescents, and young adults must be distributed when dispensing an outpatient prescription (new or refill) where this medication is to be used without direct supervision of a healthcare provider. Medication guides are available at http://www.fda.gov/cder/Offices/ODS/medication_guides.htm. Dispense to parents or guardians of children and adolescents receiving this medication.

Pregnancy Risk Factor C

Pregnancy Considerations Venlafaxine is classified as pregnancy category C due to adverse effects observed in animal studies. Venlafaxine and its active metabolite ODV cross the human placenta. Neonatal seizures and neonatal abstinence syndrome have been noted in case reports following maternal use of venlafaxine during pregnancy. Nonteratogenic effects in the newborn following SSRI/SNRI exposure late in the third trimester include respiratory distress, cyanosis, apnea, seizures, temperature instability, feeding difficulty, vomiting, hypoglycemia, hyper- or hypotonia, hyper-reflexia, jitteriness, irritability, constant crying, and tremor. The long-term effects on neurobehavior have not been studied.

Due to pregnancy-induced physiologic changes, some pharmacokinetic parameters of venlafaxine may be altered. Women should be monitored for decreased efficacy. Women treated for major depression and who are euthymic prior to pregnancy are more likely to experience a relapse when medication is discontinued as compared to pregnant women who continue taking antidepressant medications. The ACOG recommends that therapy with SSRIs or SNRIs during pregnancy be individualized; treatment of depression during pregnancy should incorporate the clinical expertise of the mental health clinician, obstetrician, primary healthcare provider, and pediatrician. If treatment during pregnancy is required, consider tapering therapy during the third trimester in order to prevent withdrawal symptoms in the infant. If this is done and the woman is considered to be at risk of relapse from her major depressive disorder, the medication can be restarted following delivery, although the dose should be readjusted to that required before pregnancy.

Lactation Enters breast milk/not recommended

Contraindications Hypersensitivity to venlafaxine or any component of the formulation; use of MAO inhibitors within 14 days; should not initiate MAO inhibitor within 7 days of discontinuing venlafaxine

Warnings/Precautions [U.S. Boxed Warning]: Antidepressants increase the risk of suicidal thinking and behavior in children, adolescents, and young adults (18-24 years of age) with major depressive disorder (MDD) and other psychiatric disorders; consider risk prior to prescribing. Short-term studies did not show an increased risk in patients >24 years of age and showed a decreased risk in patients ≥65 years. Closely monitor for clinical worsening, suicidality, or unusual changes in behavior; the patient's family or caregiver should be instructed to closely observe the patient and communicate condition with healthcare provider. Reduced growth rate has been observed with venlafaxine therapy in children. A medication guide should be dispensed with each prescription. **Venlafaxine is not FDA approved for use in children.**

The possibility of a suicide attempt is inherent in major depression and may persist until remission occurs. Monitor for worsening of depression or suicidality, especially during initiation of therapy (generally first 1-2 months) or with dose increases or decreases. Use caution in high-risk patients. Worsening depression and severe abrupt suicidality that are not part of the presenting symptoms may require discontinuation or modification of drug therapy. The patient's family or caregiver should be alerted to monitor patients for the emergence of suicidality and associated behaviors (such as agitation, irritability, hostility, impulsivity, and hypomania) and call healthcare provider.

May worsen psychosis in some patients or precipitate a shift to mania or hypomania in patients with bipolar disorder. Patients presenting with depressive symptoms should be screened for bipolar disorder. Monotherapy in patients with bipolar disorder should be avoided. **Venlafaxine is not FDA approved for the treatment of bipolar depression.**

The potential for severe reactions exists when used with MAO inhibitors, SSRIs/SNRIs or triptans (myoclonus, diaphoresis, hyperthermia, NMS features, seizures, and death). May cause sustained increase in blood pressure or tachycardia; dose related and increases are generally modest (12-15 mm Hg diastolic). Control pre-existing hypertension prior to initiation of venlafaxine. Use caution in patients with recent history of MI, unstable heart disease, or hyperthyroidism; may cause increase in anxiety, nervousness, insomnia; may cause weight loss (use with caution in patients where weight loss is undesirable); may cause increases in serum cholesterol. Use caution with hepatic or renal impairment; dosage adjustments recommended. May cause hyponatremia/SIADH (elderly at increased risk); volume depletion (diuretics may increase risk).

May impair platelet aggregation resulting in increased risk of bleeding events, particularly if used concomitantly with aspirin or NSAIDs. Bleeding related to SSRI or SNRI use has been reported to range from relatively minor bruising and epistaxis to life-threatening hemorrhage. Interstitial lung disease and eosinophilic pneumonia have been rarely reported; may present as progressive dyspnea, cough, and/or chest pain. Prompt evaluation and possible discontinuation of therapy may be necessary. Venlafaxine may increase the risks associated with electroconvulsive therapy. Use cautiously in patients with a history of seizures. The risks of cognitive or motor impairment, as well as the potential for anticholinergic effects are very low. May cause or exacerbate sexual dysfunction.

Abrupt discontinuation or dosage reduction after extended (≥6 weeks) therapy may lead to agitation, dysphoria, nervousness, anxiety, and other symptoms. When discontinuing therapy, dosage should be tapered gradually over at least a 2-week period. If intolerable symptoms occur following a decrease in dosage or upon discontinuation of therapy, then resuming the previous dose with a more gradual taper should be considered. Use caution in patients with increased intraocular pressure or at risk of acute narrow-angle glaucoma.

Adverse Reactions

>10%:

Central nervous system: Headache (25% to 38%), insomnia (15% to 24%), somnolence (12% to 23%), nervousness (6% to 21%), dizziness (11% to 20%)

Gastrointestinal: Nausea (21% to 58%), xerostomia (12% to 22%), anorexia (8% to 20%), constipation (8% to 15%)

Genitourinary: Abnormal ejaculation/orgasm (2% to 19%)

Neuromuscular & skeletal: Weakness (8% to 19%)

Miscellaneous: Diaphoresis (10% to 14%)

1% to 10%:

Cardiovascular: Hypertension (dose related; 3% in patients receiving <100 mg/day, up to 13% in patients receiving >300 mg/day), vasodilation (3% to 4%), palpitation (3%), tachycardia (2%), chest pain (2%), postural hypotension (1%), edema

Central nervous system: Abnormal dreams (3% to 7%), anxiety (5% to 6%), yawning (3% to 5%), agitation (2% to 4%), chills (3%), confusion (2%), abnormal thinking (2%), depersonalization (1%), depression (1% to 3%), fever, migraine, amnesia, hypoesthesia, trismus, vertigo

Dermatologic: Rash (3%), pruritus (1%), bruising

Endocrine & metabolic: Libido decreased (3% to 9%), hypercholesterolemia (5%), triglycerides increased

Gastrointestinal: Diarrhea (6% to 8%), dyspepsia (7%), vomiting (3% to 6%), abdominal pain (6%), flatulence (3% to 4%), taste perversion (2%), weight loss (1% to 4%), appetite increased, weight gain

Genitourinary: Impotence (4% to 10%), urinary frequency (3%), urination impaired (2%), urinary retention (1%), prostatic disorder

Neuromuscular & skeletal: Tremor (4% to 10%), hypertonia (3%), paresthesia (2% to 3%), twitching (1% to 3%), neck pain, arthralgia

Ocular: Abnormal or blurred vision (4% to 6%), mydriasis (2%)

Otic: Tinnitus (2%)

Respiratory: Pharyngitis (7%), sinusitis (2%), cough increased, dyspnea

Miscellaneous: Infection (6%), flu-like syndrome (6%), trauma (2%)

<1% (Limited to important or life-threatening): Agranulocytosis, anaphylaxis, anemia, aplastic anemia, aneurysm, angina pectoris, anuria, appendicitis, arrhythmia (including atrial and ventricular tachycardia, fibrillation, and torsade de pointes), arteritis, asthma, ataxia, atelectasis, atrioventricular block, bacteremia, balance/coordination impaired, basophilia, bigeminy, biliary pain, bilirubinemia, bleeding time increased, bradycardia, bradykinesia, BUN increased, bundle branch block, carcinoma, cardiovascular disorder (mitral valve and circulatory disturbance), cataract, catatonia, cellulitis, cerebral ischemia, cholelithiasis, congestive heart failure, coronary artery disease, creatinine increased, crystalluria, cyanosis, deafness, DVT, dehydration, delusions, dementia, diabetes mellitus, dystonia, ECG abnormalities (including QT prolongation), embolus, eosinophilia, erythema

multiforme, exfoliative dermatitis, extrapyramidal symptoms, extrasystoles, facial paralysis, fasciitis, fatty liver, gastrointestinal ulcer, glaucoma, glycosuria, granuloma, Guillain-Barré syndrome, heart arrest, hematemesis, hematoma, hemorrhage (eye, GI, mucocutaneous, rectal), hepatic necrosis, hepatic failure, hepatitis, homicidal ideation, hostility, hyperacusis, hypercalcinuria, hyperchlorhydria, hyper-/hypoglycemia, hyper-/hypokalemia, hyper-/hypophosphatemia, hyper-/hypothyroidism, hyperuricemia, hypocholesteremia, hyponatremia, hypoproteinemia, hypotension, interstitial lung disease (including eosinophilic pneumonia), intestinal obstruction, jaundice, kidney function abnormal, larynx edema, leukocytosis, leukoderma, leukopenia, liver enzymes increased, loss of consciousness, lymphadenopathy, lymphocytosis, maculopapular rash, menstrual abnormalities, miliaria, moniliasis, multiple myeloma, myasthenia, myocardial infarct, myoclonus, myopathy, neck rigidity, neuroleptic malignant-like syndrome, neuropathy, neutropenia, osteoporosis, pancreatitis, pancytopenia, peripheral vascular disorder, pleurisy, pneumonia, pyelonephritis, pyuria, renal failure, rhabdomyolysis, rheumatoid arthritis, seizure, serotonin syndrome, SIADH, skin atrophy, Stevens-Johnson syndrome, suicidal ideation (reported at a frequency up to 2% in children/adolescents with major depressive disorder), suicide attempt, syncope, tendon rupture, thrombocythemia, thrombocytopenia, tongue edema, toxic epidermal necrolysis, withdrawal syndrome

Drug Interactions

Metabolism/Transport Effects Substrate of CYP2C9 (minor), 2C19 (minor), 2D6 (major), 3A4 (major); **Inhibits** CYP2B6 (weak), 2D6 (weak), 3A4 (weak)

Avoid Concomitant Use

Avoid concomitant use of Venlafaxine with any of the following: Iobenguane I 123; MAO Inhibitors; Sibutramine

Increased Effect/Toxicity

Venlafaxine may increase the levels/effects of: Alcohol (Ethyl); Alpha-/Beta-Agonists; Aspirin; CNS Depressants; NSAID (Nonselective); Serotonin Modulators; TraZODone

The levels/effects of Venlafaxine may be increased by: CYP2D6 Inhibitors (Moderate); CYP2D6 Inhibitors (Strong); CYP3A4 Inhibitors (Moderate); CYP3A4 Inhibitors (Strong); Darunavir; Dasatinib; MAO Inhibitors; Metoclopramide; Sibutramine; Voriconazole

Decreased Effect

Venlafaxine may decrease the levels/effects of: Alpha2-Agonists; Indinavir; Iobenguane I 123

The levels/effects of Venlafaxine may be decreased by: CYP3A4 Inducers (Strong); Deferasirox; Herbs (CYP3A4 Inducers)

Ethanol/Nutrition/Herb Interactions

Ethanol: Avoid ethanol (may increase CNS effects).

Herb/Nutraceutical: Avoid valerian, St John's wort, SAMe, kava kava, tryptophan (may increase risk of serotonin syndrome and/or excessive sedation).

Stability Store at controlled room temperature of 20°C to 25°C (68°F to 77°F).

Mechanism of Action Venlafaxine and its active metabolite, o-desmethylvenlafaxine (ODV), are potent inhibitors of neuronal serotonin and norepinephrine reuptake and weak inhibitors of dopamine reuptake. Venlafaxine and ODV have no significant activity for muscarinic cholinergic, H_1-histaminergic, or alpha$_2$-adrenergic receptors. Venlafaxine and ODV do not possess MAO-inhibitory activity.

Pharmacodynamics/Kinetics

Absorption: Oral: 92% to 100%; food has no significant effect on the absorption of venlafaxine or formation of the active metabolite O-desmethylvenlafaxine (ODV)

Distribution: At steady state: Venlafaxine 7.5 ± 3.7 L/kg, ODV 5.7 ± 1.8 L/Kg

Protein binding: Bound to human plasma protein: Venlafaxine 27%, ODV 30%

Metabolism: Hepatic via CYP2D6 to active metabolite, O-desmethylvenlafaxine (ODV); other metabolites include N-desmethylvenlafaxine and N,O-didesmethylvenlafaxine

Bioavailability: Absolute: ~45%

Half-life elimination: Venlafaxine: 3-7 hours; ODV: 9-13 hours; Steady-state, plasma: Venlafaxine/ODV: Within 3 days of multiple-dose therapy; prolonged with cirrhosis (Adults: Venlafaxine: ~30%, ODV: ~60%) and with dialysis (Adults: Venlafaxine: ~180%, ODV: ~142%)

Time to peak:

Immediate release: Venlafaxine: 2 hours, ODV: 3 hours

Extended release: Venlafaxine: 5.5 hours, ODV: 9 hours

Excretion: Urine (~87%, 5% as unchanged drug, 29% as unconjugated ODV, 26% as conjugated ODV, 27% as minor inactive metabolites) within 48 hours

Clearance at steady state: Venlafaxine: 1.3 ± 0.6 L/hour/kg, ODV: 0.4 ± 0.2 L/hour/kg

Clearance decreased with:

Cirrhosis: Adults: Venlafaxine: ~50%, ODV: ~30%

Severe cirrhosis: Adults: Venlafaxine: ~90%

Renal impairment (Cl_{cr} 10-70 mL/minute): Adults: Venlafaxine: ~24%

Dialysis: Adults: Venlafaxine: ~57%, ODV: ~56%; due to large volume of distribution, a significant amount of drug is not likely to be removed.

Dosage Oral:

Children and Adolescents:

Attention-deficit/hyperactivity disorder (unlabeled use): Initial: 12.5 mg/day

Children <40 kg: Increase by 12.5 mg/week to maximum of 50 mg/day in 2 divided doses

Children ≥40 kg: Increase by 25 mg/week to maximum of 75 mg/day in 3 divided doses.

Mean dose: 60 mg or 1.4 mg/kg administered in 2-3 divided doses

Adults:

Depression:

Immediate-release tablets: 75 mg/day, administered in 2 or 3 divided doses, taken with food; dose may be increased in 75 mg/day increments at intervals of at least 4 days, up to 225-375 mg/day

Extended-release capsules or tablets: 75 mg once daily taken with food; for some new patients, it may be desirable to start at 37.5 mg/day for 4-7 days before increasing to 75 mg once daily; dose may be increased by up to 75 mg/day increments every 4 days as tolerated, up to a recommended maximum of 225 mg/day

Generalized anxiety disorder: Extended-release capsules: 75 mg once daily taken with food; for some new patients, it may be desirable to start at 37.5 mg/day for 4-7 days before increasing to 75 mg once daily; dose may be increased by up to 75 mg/day increments every 4 days as tolerated, up to a maximum of 225 mg/day

Panic disorder: Extended-release capsules: 37.5 mg once daily for 1 week; may increase to 75 mg daily, with subsequent weekly increases of 75 mg/day up to a maximum of 225 mg/day.

Social anxiety disorder:

Extended-release capsules: 75 mg once daily taken with food; for some new patients, it may be desirable to start at 37.5 mg/day for 4-7 days before increasing to 75 mg once daily; dose may be increased by up to 75 mg/day increments every 4 days as tolerated, up to a maximum of 225 mg/day

Extended release tablets: 75 mg once daily taken with food (maximum: 75 mg/day); no evidence that doses >75 mg/day offer any additional benefit

Obsessive-compulsive disorder (unlabeled use): Titrate to usual dosage range of 150-300 mg/day; however, doses up to 375 mg daily have been used; response may be seen in 4 weeks

Neuropathic pain (unlabeled use): Dosages evaluated varied considerably based on etiology of chronic pain, but efficacy has been shown for many conditions in the range of 75-225 mg/day; onset of relief may occur in 1-2 weeks, or take up to 6 weeks for full benefit.

Hot flashes (unlabeled use): Doses of 37.5-75 mg/day have demonstrated significant improvement of vasomotor symptoms after 4-8 weeks of treatment; in one study, doses >75 mg/day offered no additional benefit; however, higher doses (225 mg/day) may be beneficial in patients with perimenopausal depression.

Attention-deficit disorder (unlabeled use): Initial: Doses vary between 18.75 to 75 mg/day; may increase after 4 weeks to 150 mg/day; if tolerated, doses up to 225 mg/day have been used

Note: When discontinuing this medication after more than 1 week of treatment, it is generally recommended that the dose be tapered. If venlafaxine is used for 6 weeks or longer, the dose should be tapered over 2 weeks when discontinuing its use.

Elderly: Alzheimer's dementia-related depression:

Immediate-release tablets: Initial: 25 mg/day; may increase at weekly intervals to maximum of 375 mg/day in divided doses

Extended-release capsules: Initial: 37.5 mg/day; may increase at weekly intervals to maximum of 225 mg/day

Dosing adjustment in renal impairment: Cl_{cr} 10-70 mL/minute: Decrease dose by 25%; decrease total daily dose by 50% if dialysis patients; dialysis patients should receive dosing after completion of dialysis

Dosing adjustment in moderate hepatic impairment: Reduce total daily dosage by 50%

Dietary Considerations Should be taken with food.

Administration Administer with food.

Extended release formulations: Swallow capsule or tablet whole; do not crush or chew. Contents of capsule may be sprinkled on a spoonful of applesauce and swallowed immediately without chewing; followed with a glass of water to ensure complete swallowing of the pellets.

Monitoring Parameters Blood pressure should be regularly monitored, especially in patients with a high baseline blood pressure; may cause mean increase in heart rate of 4-9 beats/minute; cholesterol; mental status for depression, suicidal ideation (especially at the beginning of therapy or when doses are increased or decreased), anxiety, social functioning, mania, panic attacks; height and weight should be monitored in children

Reference Range Peak serum level of 163 ng/mL (325 ng/mL of ODV metabolite) obtained after a 150 mg oral dose

Test Interactions Increased thyroid, uric acid, glucose, potassium, AST, cholesterol (S)

Dosage Forms Excipient information presented when available (limited, particularly for generics); consult specific product labeling.

Capsule, extended release:

Effexor XR®: 37.5 mg, 75 mg, 150 mg

Tablet: 25 mg, 37.5 mg, 50 mg, 75 mg, 100 mg

Effexor®: 25 mg, 37.5 mg, 50 mg, 75 mg, 100 mg

Tablet, extended release: 37.5 mg, 75 mg, 150 mg, 225 mg

- ◆ **Venofer®** *see* Iron Sucrose *on page* 819
- ◆ **Ventavis®** *see* Iloprost *on page* 767
- ◆ **Ventolin® (Can)** *see* Albuterol *on page* 51
- ◆ **Ventolin® Diskus (Can)** *see* Albuterol *on page* 51
- ◆ **Ventolin® HFA** *see* Albuterol *on page* 51
- ◆ **Ventolin® I.V. Infusion (Can)** *see* Albuterol *on page* 51
- ◆ **Ventrodisk (Can)** *see* Albuterol *on page* 51
- ◆ **VePesid® [DSC]** *see* Etoposide *on page* 591
- ◆ **VePesid® (Can)** *see* Etoposide *on page* 591
- ◆ **Veracolate [OTC]** *see* Bisacodyl *on page* 198
- ◆ **Veramyst™** *see* Fluticasone *on page* 644

Verapamil (ver AP a mil)

U.S. Brand Names Calan®; Calan® SR; Covera-HS®; Isoptin® SR; Verelan®; Verelan® PM

Canadian Brand Names Apo-Verap®; Apo-Verap® SR; Calan®; Chronovera®; Covera-HS®; Covera®; Dom-Verapamil SR; Gen-Verapamil; Gen-Verapamil SR; Isoptin® SR; Med-Verapamil; Novo-Veramil SR; Nu-Verap; PHL-Verapamil; PMS-Verapamil SR; PRO-Verapamil SR; Riva-Verapamil SR; Verapamil Hydrochloride Injection, USP; Verelan SRC

Index Terms Iproveratril Hydrochloride; Verapamil Hydrochloride

Pharmacologic Category Antiarrhythmic Agent, Class IV; Calcium Channel Blocker

Additional Appendix Information

Calcium Channel Blockers *on page* 1651

Hypertension *on page* 1820

Use Orally for treatment of angina pectoris (vasospastic, chronic stable, unstable) and hypertension; I.V. for supraventricular tachyarrhythmias (PSVT, atrial fibrillation, atrial flutter)

Unlabeled/Investigational Use Migraine; hypertrophic cardiomyopathy; bipolar disorder (manic manifestations)

Pregnancy Risk Factor C

Pregnancy Considerations Use in pregnancy only when clearly needed and when the benefits outweigh the potential risk to the fetus. Crosses the placenta. One report of suspected heart block when used to control fetal supraventricular tachycardia. May exhibit tocolytic effects.

Lactation Enters breast milk (small amounts)/not recommended

Medication Safety Issues

Sound-alike/look-alike issues:

Calan® may be confused with Colace®

Covera-HS® may be confused with Provera®

Isoptin® may be confused with Isopto® Tears

Verelan® may be confused with Virilon®, Voltaren®

High alert medication: The Institute for Safe Medication Practices (ISMP) includes this medication (I.V. formulation) among its list of drug classes which have a heightened risk of causing significant patient harm when used in error.

Significant differences exist between oral and I.V. dosing. Use caution when converting from one route of administration to another.

International issues:

Calan®: Brand name for vinpocetine in Japan

Contraindications Hypersensitivity to verapamil or any component of the formulation; severe left ventricular dysfunction; hypotension (systolic pressure <90 mm Hg) or cardiogenic shock; sick sinus syndrome (except in patients with a functioning artificial pacemaker); second- or third-degree AV block (except in patients with a functioning artificial pacemaker); atrial flutter or fibrillation and an accessory bypass tract (WPW, Lown-Ganong-Levine syndrome)

Warnings/Precautions Increased angina and/or MI has occurred with initiation or dosage titration of calcium channel blockers. The most common side effect is peripheral edema; occurs within 2-3 weeks of starting therapy. Avoid use in heart failure; can exacerbate condition. Symptomatic hypotension with or without syncope can rarely occur; blood pressure must be lowered at a rate appropriate for the patient's clinical condition. Rare increases in liver function tests can be observed. Can cause first-degree AV block or sinus bradycardia. Other conduction abnormalities are rare. Use caution when using verapamil together with a beta-blocker. Avoid use of I.V. verapamil with an I.V. beta-blocker; can result in asystole. Use I.V. with caution in patients with hypertrophic subaortic stenosis (IHSS). Use I.V. with caution in patients with attenuated neuromuscular transmission (Duchenne's muscular dystrophy, myasthenia gravis). Adjust the dose in severe renal dysfunction; may require lower startingdoes in hepatic dysfunction. Verapamil significantly increases digoxin serum concentrations (adjust digoxin's dose). May prolong recovery from nondepolarizing neuromuscular-blocking agents.

Adverse Reactions

>10%: Gastrointestinal: Gingival hyperplasia (up to 19%), constipation (12% up to 42% in clinical trials)

1% to 10%:

Cardiovascular: Bradycardia (1.2 to 1.4%); first-, second-, or third-degree AV block (1.2%); CHF (1.8%); hypotension (2.5% to 3%); peripheral edema (1.9%), symptomatic hypotension (1.5% I.V.); severe tachycardia (1%)

Central nervous system: Dizziness (1.2% to 3.3%), fatigue (1.7%), headache (1.2% to 2.2%)

Dermatologic: Rash (1.2%)

Gastrointestinal: Nausea (0.9% to 2.7%)

Respiratory: Dyspnea (1.4%)

<1% (Limited to important or life-threatening): Alopecia, angina, arthralgia, asystole, atrioventricular dissociation, bronchial/laryngeal spasm, cerebrovascular accident, chest pain, claudication, confusion, diarrhea, dry mouth, ecchymosis, electrical mechanical dissociation (EMD), emotional depression, eosinophilia, equilibrium disorders, erythema multiforme, exanthema, exfoliative dermatitis, galactorrhea/hyperprolactinemia, GI obstruction, gingival hyperplasia, gynecomastia, hair color change, impotence, muscle cramps, MI, myoclonus, paresthesia, Parkinsonian syndrome, psychotic symptoms, purpura (vasculitis), rash, respiratory failure, rotary nystagmus, shakiness, shock, somnolence, Stevens-Johnson syndrome, syncope, urticaria, ventricular fibrillation, vertigo

Drug Interactions

Metabolism/Transport Effects Substrate of CYP1A2 (minor), 2B6 (minor), 2C9 (minor), 2C18 (minor), 2E1 (minor), 3A4 (major); **Inhibits** CYP1A2 (weak), 2C9 (weak), 2D6 (weak), 3A4 (moderate)

Avoid Concomitant Use

Avoid concomitant use of Verapamil with any of the following: Dabigatran Etexilate; Dofetilide; Ranolazine; Rivaroxaban; Topotecan

Increased Effect/Toxicity

Verapamil may increase the levels/effects of: Alcohol (Ethyl); Amifostine; Amiodarone; Benzodiazepines (metabolized by oxidation); Beta-Blockers; BusPIRone; Calcium Channel Blockers (Dihydropyridine); CarBAMazepine; Cardiac Glycosides; Colchicine; Corticosteroids (Systemic); CycloSPORINE; CYP3A4 Substrates; Dabigatran Etexilate; Dofetilide; Eletriptan; Eplerenone; Fexofenadine; HMG-CoA Reductase Inhibitors; Lithium; Magnesium Salts; Maraviroc; Midodrine; Neuromuscular-Blocking Agents (Nondepolarizing); Nitroprusside; P-Glycoprotein Substrates; Phenytoin; Pimecrolimus; QuiNIDine; Ranolazine; Risperidone; RiTUXimab; Rivaroxaban; Salicylates; Salmeterol; Tacrolimus; Topotecan

The levels/effects of Verapamil may be increased by: Alpha1-Blockers; Anilidopiperidine Opioids; Antifungal Agents (Azole Derivatives, Systemic); Cimetidine; Colchicine; CycloSPORINE; CYP3A4 Inhibitors (Moderate); CYP3A4 Inhibitors (Strong); Dasatinib; Diazoxide; Fluconazole; Grapefruit Juice; Herbs (Hypotensive Properties); Macrolide Antibiotics; Magnesium Salts; P-Glycoprotein Inhibitors; Prostacyclin Analogues; Protease Inhibitors; Quinupristin

Decreased Effect

Verapamil may decrease the levels/effects of: Clopidogrel

The levels/effects of Verapamil may be decreased by: Barbiturates; Calcium Salts; CarBAMazepine; CYP3A4 Inducers (Strong); Deferasirox; Herbs (CYP3A4 Inducers); Herbs (Hypertensive Properties); Methylphenidate; Nafcillin; P-Glycoprotein Inducers; Rifamycin Derivatives; Yohimbine

Ethanol/Nutrition/Herb Interactions

Ethanol: Avoid or limit ethanol (may increase ethanol levels).

Food: Grapefruit juice may increase the serum concentration of verapamil; avoid concurrent use.

Herb/Nutraceutical: St John's wort may decrease levels. Avoid dong quai if using for hypertension (has estrogenic activity). Avoid ephedra, yohimbe, ginseng (may worsen arrhythmia or hypertension). Avoid garlic (may have increased antihypertensive effect).

Stability Store injection at room temperature; do not freeze. Protect from heat. Use only clear solutions. Physically compatible in solutions of pH of 3-6, but may precipitate in solutions having a pH ≥6. Protect I.V. solution from light.

Mechanism of Action Inhibits calcium ion from entering the "slow channels" or select voltage-sensitive areas of vascular smooth muscle and myocardium during depolarization; produces a relaxation of coronary vascular smooth muscle and coronary vasodilation; increases myocardial oxygen delivery in patients with vasospastic angina; slows automaticity and conduction of AV node.

Pharmacodynamics/Kinetics

Onset of action: Peak effect: Oral: Immediate release: 1-2 hours; I.V.: 1-5 minutes

Duration: Oral: Immediate release tablets: 6-8 hours; I.V.: 10-20 minutes

Protein binding: 90%

Metabolism: Hepatic via multiple CYP isoenzymes; extensive first-pass effect

Bioavailability: Oral: 20% to 35%

Half-life elimination: Infants: 4.4-6.9 hours; Adults: Single dose: 2-8 hours, Multiple doses: 4.5-12 hours; prolonged with hepatic cirrhosis

Excretion: Urine (70%, 3% to 4% as unchanged drug); feces (16%)

Dosage

Children: SVT:

I.V.:

<1 year: 0.1-0.2 mg/kg over 2 minutes; repeat every 30 minutes as needed

1-15 years: 0.1-0.3 mg/kg over 2 minutes; maximum: 5 mg/dose, may repeat dose in 15 minutes if adequate response not achieved; maximum for second dose: 10 mg/dose

Oral (dose not well established):

1-5 years: 4-8 mg/kg/day in 3 divided doses **or** 40-80 mg every 8 hours

>5 years: 80 mg every 6-8 hours

Adults:

SVT: I.V.: 2.5-5 mg (over 2 minutes); second dose of 5-10 mg (~0.15 mg/kg) may be given 15-30 minutes after the initial dose if patient tolerates, but does not respond to initial dose; maximum total dose: 20 mg

Angina: Oral: Initial dose: 80-120 mg 3 times/day (elderly or small stature: 40 mg 3 times/day); range: 240-480 mg/day in 3-4 divided doses

Hypertension: Oral:
Immediate release: 80 mg 3 times/day; usual dose range (JNC 7): 80-320 mg/day in 2 divided doses
Sustained release: 240 mg/day; usual dose range (JNC 7): 120-360 mg/day in 1-2 divided doses; 120 mg/day in the elderly or small patients (no evidence of additional benefit in doses >360 mg/day).
Extended release:
Covera-HS®: Usual dose range (JNC 7): 120-360 mg once daily (once-daily dosing is recommended at bedtime)
Verelan® PM: Usual dose range: 200-400 mg once daily at bedtime

Dosing adjustment in renal impairment: Cl_{cr} <10 mL/minute: Administer at 50% to 75% of normal dose.
Dialysis: Not dialyzable (0% to 5%) via hemo- or peritoneal dialysis; supplemental dose is not necessary.

Dosing adjustment/comments in hepatic disease: Reduce dose in cirrhosis, reduce dose to 20% to 50% of normal and monitor ECG.

Dietary Considerations Calan® SR and Isoptin® SR products may be taken with food or milk, other formulations may be administered without regard to meals; sprinkling contents of Verelan® or Verelan® PM capsule onto applesauce does not affect oral absorption.

Administration
Oral: Do not crush or chew sustained or extended release products.
Calan® SR, Isoptin® SR: Administer with food.
Verelan®, Verelan® PM: Capsules may be opened and the contents sprinkled on 1 tablespoonful of applesauce, then swallowed without chewing.
I.V.: Rate of infusion: Over 2 minutes.

Monitoring Parameters Monitor blood pressure closely

Reference Range Therapeutic: 50-200 ng/mL (SI: 100-410 nmol/L) for parent; under normal conditions, norverapamil concentration is the same as parent drug. Toxic: >90 mcg/mL

Dosage Forms Excipient information presented when available (limited, particularly for generics); consult specific product labeling.
Caplet, sustained release, as hydrochloride: 120 mg, 180 mg, 240 mg
Calan® SR: 120 mg
Calan® SR: 180 mg, 240 mg [scored]
Capsule, extended release, oral, as hydrochloride: 120 mg, 180 mg, 240 mg
Capsule, extended release, controlled onset, as hydrochloride: 100 mg, 200 mg, 300 mg
Verelan® PM: 100 mg, 200 mg, 300 mg
Capsule, sustained release, as hydrochloride: 120 mg, 180 mg, 240 mg, 360 mg
Verelan®: 120 mg, 180 mg, 240 mg, 360 mg
Injection, solution, as hydrochloride: 2.5 mg/mL (2 mL, 4 mL)
Tablet, as hydrochloride: 40 mg, 80 mg, 120 mg
Calan®: 40 mg
Calan®: 80 mg, 120 mg [scored]
Tablet, extended release, as hydrochloride: 120 mg, 180 mg, 240 mg
Tablet, extended release, controlled onset, as hydrochloride:
Covera-HS®: 180 mg, 240 mg
Tablet, sustained release, as hydrochloride: 120 mg, 180 mg, 240 mg
Isoptin® SR: 120 mg
Isoptin® SR: 180 mg, 240 mg [scored]

Extemporaneous Preparations To prepare a verapamil 50 mg/mL liquid, crush 75 verapamil hydrochloride 80 mg tablets into a fine powder. Add ~40 mL of either Ora-Sweet® and Ora-Plus® (1:1 preparation), or Ora-Sweet® SF and Ora-Plus® (1:1 preparation), or cherry syrup. Mix to a uniform paste. Continue to add the vehicle to bring the final volume to 120 mL. The preparation is stable for 60 days; shake well before using and protect from light.

Allen LV and Erickson III MA, "Stability of Labetalol Hydrochloride, Metoprolol Tartrate, Verapamil Hydrochloride, and Spironolactone With Hydrochlorothiazide in Extemporaneously Compounded Oral Liquids," *Am J Health Syst Pharm*, 1996, 53:304-9.

- ◆ **Verapamil and Trandolapril** *see* Trandolapril and Verapamil *on page 1500*
- ◆ **Verapamil Hydrochloride** *see* Verapamil *on page 1557*
- ◆ **Verapamil Hydrochloride Injection, USP (Can)** *see* Verapamil *on page 1557*
- ◆ **Verdeso™** *see* Desonide *on page 424*
- ◆ **Verelan®** *see* Verapamil *on page 1557*
- ◆ **Verelan® PM** *see* Verapamil *on page 1557*
- ◆ **Verelan SRC (Can)** *see* Verapamil *on page 1557*
- ◆ **Vermox® [DSC]** *see* Mebendazole *on page 925*
- ◆ **Vermox® (Can)** *see* Mebendazole *on page 925*
- ◆ **Versed** *see* Midazolam *on page 990*
- ◆ **Versel® (Can)** *see* Selenium Sulfide *on page 1361*
- ◆ **Versiclear™** *see* Sodium Thiosulfate *on page 1386*
- ◆ **Vesanoid®** *see* Tretinoin (Oral) *on page 1508*
- ◆ **VESIcare®** *see* Solifenacin *on page 1387*
- ◆ **Vexol®** *see* Rimexolone *on page 1321*
- ◆ **VFEND®** *see* Voriconazole *on page 1567*
- ◆ **Viadur® [DSC]** *see* Leuprolide *on page 868*
- ◆ **Viadur® (Can)** *see* Leuprolide *on page 868*
- ◆ **Viagra®** *see* Sildenafil *on page 1368*
- ◆ **Vibramycin®** *see* Doxycycline *on page 491*
- ◆ **Vibra-Tabs®** *see* Doxycycline *on page 491*
- ◆ **Vicks® 44E [OTC]** *see* Guaifenesin and Dextromethorphan *on page 710*
- ◆ **Vicks® Casero™ Chest Congestion Relief [OTC]** *see* GuaiFENesin *on page 709*
- ◆ **Vicks® DayQuil® Cold/Flu Multi-Symptom Relief [OTC]** *see* Acetaminophen, Dextromethorphan, and Phenylephrine *on page 32*
- ◆ **Vicks® Pediatric Formula 44E [OTC]** *see* Guaifenesin and Dextromethorphan *on page 710*
- ◆ **Vicks® Sinex® Nasal Spray [OTC]** *see* Phenylephrine *on page 1183*
- ◆ **Vicks® Sinex® UltraFine Mist [OTC]** *see* Phenylephrine *on page 1183*
- ◆ **Vicks® Vitamin C [OTC]** *see* Ascorbic Acid *on page 139*
- ◆ **Vicodin®** *see* Hydrocodone and Acetaminophen *on page 740*
- ◆ **Vicodin® ES** *see* Hydrocodone and Acetaminophen *on page 740*
- ◆ **Vicodin® HP** *see* Hydrocodone and Acetaminophen *on page 740*
- ◆ **Vicoprofen®** *see* Hydrocodone and Ibuprofen *on page 742*
- ◆ **Vidaza®** *see* AzaCITIDine *on page 161*
- ◆ **Videx®** *see* Didanosine *on page 441*
- ◆ **Videx® EC** *see* Didanosine *on page 441*
- ◆ **Vigamox™** *see* Moxifloxacin *on page 1021*
- ◆ **VIGIV** *see* Vaccinia Immune Globulin (Intravenous) *on page 1534*
- ◆ **Vimpat®** *see* Lacosamide *on page 847*

VinBLAStine (vin BLAS teen)

Index Terms NSC-49842; Velban; Vinblastine Sulfate; Vincaleukoblastine; VLB

Pharmacologic Category Antineoplastic Agent, Natural Source (Plant) Derivative; Antineoplastic Agent, Vinca Alkaloid

Use Treatment of Hodgkin's and non-Hodgkin's lymphoma; testicular cancer; breast cancer; mycosis fungoides; Kaposi's sarcoma; histiocytosis (Letterer-Siwe disease); choriocarcinoma

Unlabeled/Investigational Use Treatment of bladder cancer, melanoma, nonsmall cell lung cancer (NSCLC), ovarian cancer, prostate cancer, renal cancer, soft tissue sarcoma (desmoid tumors)

Pregnancy Risk Factor D

Pregnancy Considerations Animal studies have demonstrated resorption and teratogenic effects. There are no adequate and well-controlled studies in pregnant women. Women of childbearing potential should avoid becoming pregnant during vinblastine treatment. Aspermia has been reported in males who have received treatment with vinblastine.

Lactation Excretion in breast milk unknown/not recommended

Medication Safety Issues

Sound-alike/look-alike issues:

VinBLAStine may be confused with vinCRIStine, vinorelbine

High alert medication: The Institute for Safe Medication Practices (ISMP) includes this medication among its list of drug classes which have a heightened risk of causing significant patient harm when used in error.

Note: Must be dispensed in overwrap which bears the statement **"Do not remove covering until the moment of injection. Fatal if given intrathecally. For I.V. use only."** Syringes should be labeled: **"Fatal if given intrathecally. For I.V. use only."**

Contraindications Significant granulocytopenia; presence of bacterial infection; I.T. administration is contraindicated (may result in death)

Warnings/Precautions Hazardous agent - use appropriate precautions for handling and disposal. **[U.S. Boxed Warning]: For I.V. use only. Intrathecal administration may result in death.** Must be dispensed in overwrap which bears the statement **"Do not remove covering until the moment of injection. Fatal if given intrathecally. For I.V. use only." [U.S. Boxed Warning]: Vinblastine is a moderate vesicant; avoid extravasation. Individuals administering should be experienced in vinblastine administration;** assure proper needle or catheter placement prior to administration. Leukopenia is common; granulocytopenia may be severe with higher doses. Leukopenia may be more pronounced in cachectic patients and patients with skin ulceration. Thrombocytopenia and anemia may occur rarely.

Use with caution in patients with hepatic impairment; toxicity may be increased; may require dosage modification. Neurotoxicity is rare at clinical doses; may occur with high doses (symptoms are similar to vincristine toxicity, including peripheral neuropathy, loss of deep tendon reflexes, headache, weakness, urinary retention, and GI symptoms). May rarely cause disabling neurotoxicity (usually reversible). Itraconazole may decrease the metabolism of vinblastine via CYP3A4 inhibition and may increase the effects of vinblastine via P-glycoprotein effects; severe myelosuppression and neurotoxicity may occur. Acute shortness of breath and severe bronchospasm have been reported, most often in association with concurrent administration of mitomycin; may occur within minutes to several hours following vinblastine administration or up to 14 days following mitomycin administration; use caution in patients with pre-existing pulmonary disease. Use with caution in patients with ischemic heart disease. **[U.S. Boxed Warning]: Should be administered under the supervision of an experienced cancer chemotherapy physician.**

Adverse Reactions Frequency not defined.

Common:

Cardiovascular: Hypertension

Central nervous system: Malaise

Dermatologic: Alopecia

Gastrointestinal: Constipation

Hematologic: Myelosuppression, leukopenia/granulocytopenia (nadir: 5-10 days; recovery: 7-14 days; dose-limiting toxicity)

Neuromuscular & skeletal: Bone pain, jaw pain, tumor pain

Less common:

Cardiovascular: Angina, cerebrovascular accident, coronary ischemia, ECG abnormalities, MI, Raynaud's phenomenon

Central nervous system: Depression, dizziness, headache, neurotoxicity (duration: >24 hours), seizure, vertigo

Dermatologic: Dermatitis, photosensitivity (rare), rash, skin blistering

Endocrine & metabolic: Aspermia, hyperuricemia, SIADH

Gastrointestinal: Abdominal pain, anorexia, diarrhea, gastrointestinal bleeding, hemorrhagic enterocolitis, ileus, metallic taste, nausea (mild), paralytic ileus, rectal bleeding, stomatitis, vomiting (mild)

Genitourinary: Urinary retention

Hematologic: Anemia, thrombocytopenia (recovery within a few days)

Local: Cellulitis (with extravasation), irritation, phlebitis (with extravasation), radiation recall

Neuromuscular & skeletal: Deep tendon reflex loss, myalgia, paresthesia, peripheral neuritis, weakness

Ocular: Nystagmus

Otic: Auditory damage, deafness, vestibular damage

Respiratory: Bronchospasm, dyspnea, pharyngitis

Drug Interactions

Metabolism/Transport Effects Substrate of CYP2D6 (minor), 3A4 (major); **Inhibits** CYP2D6 (weak), 3A4 (weak)

Avoid Concomitant Use

Avoid concomitant use of VinBLAStine with any of the following: Natalizumab; Vaccines (Live)

Increased Effect/Toxicity

VinBLAStine may increase the levels/effects of: Mitomycin; Natalizumab; Tolterodine; Vaccines (Live)

The levels/effects of VinBLAStine may be increased by: CYP3A4 Inhibitors (Moderate); CYP3A4 Inhibitors (Strong); Dasatinib; Itraconazole; Lopinavir; P-Glycoprotein Inhibitors; Trastuzumab

Decreased Effect

VinBLAStine may decrease the levels/effects of: Dabigatran Etexilate; P-Glycoprotein Substrates; Vaccines (Inactivated)

The levels/effects of VinBLAStine may be decreased by: CYP3A4 Inducers (Strong); Deferasirox; Echinacea; Herbs (CYP3A4 Inducers); P-Glycoprotein Inducers

Ethanol/Nutrition/Herb Interactions Herb/Nutraceutical: Avoid St John's wort (may decrease vinblastine levels). Avoid black cohosh, dong quai in estrogen-dependent tumors.

Stability Note: Must be dispensed in overwrap which bears the statement "Do not remove covering until the moment of injection. Fatal if given intrathecally. For I.V. use only." Syringes should be labeled: "Fatal if given intrathecally. For I.V. use only."

Store intact vials under refrigeration at 2°C to 8°C (36°F to 46°F). Protect from light. Reconstitute lyophilized powder to a concentration of 1 mg/mL with NS or bacteriostatic NS. For infusion, may dilute in 50 mL NS or D_5W; dilution in larger volumes (≥100 mL) of I.V. fluids is not recommended. Use appropriate precautions for handling and disposal. Solutions reconstituted in bacteriostatic NS are stable for 28 days under refrigeration.

Mechanism of Action Vinblastine binds to tubulin and inhibits microtubule formation, therefore, arresting the cell at metaphase by disrupting the formation of the mitotic spindle; it is specific for the M and S phases. Vinblastine may also interfere with nucleic acid and protein synthesis by blocking glutamic acid utilization.

Pharmacodynamics/Kinetics

Distribution: V_d: 27.3 L/kg; binds extensively to tissues; does not penetrate CNS or other fatty tissues; distributes to liver

Protein binding: 99%

Metabolism: Hepatic to active metabolite

Half-life elimination: Biphasic: Initial: 4 minutes; Terminal: 25 hours

Excretion: Feces (95%); urine (<1% as unchanged drug)

Dosage Details concerning dosing in combination regimens should also be consulted. **Note:** Frequency and duration of therapy may vary by indication, concomitant combination chemotherapy and hematologic response. **For I.V. use only.**

Children: I.V.:

Hodgkin's disease: Initial dose: 6 mg/m^2; do not administer more frequently than every 7 days

Letterer-Siwe disease: Initial dose: 6.5 mg/m^2; do not administer more frequently than every 7 days

Testicular cancer: Initial dose: 3 mg/m^2; do not administer more frequently than every 7 days

Adults: I.V.: Initial: 3.7 mg/m^2; adjust dose every 7 days (based on white blood cell response) up to 5.5 mg/m^2 (second dose); 7.4 mg/m^2 (third dose); 9.25 mg/m^2 (fourth dose); and 11.1 mg/m^2 (fifth dose); do not administer more frequently than every 7 days.

Usual range: 5.5-7.4 mg/m^2 every 7 days; Maximum dose: 18.5 mg/m^2; dosage adjustment goal is to reduce white blood cell count to ~3000/mm^3

Indication-specific dosing:

Hodgkin's disease: Usual dose: 6 mg/m^2 every 2 weeks (as part of a combination chemotherapy regimen) (Horning, 2002; Bartlett, 1995)

Testicular cancer: Usual dose: 0.11 mg/kg daily for 2 days every 3 weeks (as part of a combination chemotherapy regimen) (Loehrer, 1998) **or** 6 mg/m^2/day for 2 days every 3-4 weeks (as part of a combination chemotherapy regimen) (Clemm, 1986)

Bladder cancer (unlabeled use): Usual dose: 3 mg/m^2 every 7 days for 3 out of 4 weeks (as part of combination chemotherapy) (Sternberg, 2001) **or** 3 mg/m^2 days 2, 15, and 22 of a 28-day treatment cycle (as part of a combination chemotherapy regimen) (von der Maase, 2000)

Melanoma (unlabeled used): 2 mg/m^2 days 1-4 and 22-25 of a 6-week treatment cycle (as part of a combination chemotherapy regimen) (Eton, 2002)

Nonsmall cell lung cancer (unlabeled use): 4 mg/m^2 days 1, 8, 15, 22, and 29, then every 2 weeks (as part of combination chemotherapy) (Arriagada, 2004)

Ovarian cancer (unlabeled use): 0.11 mg/kg daily for 2 days every 3 weeks (as part of a combination chemotherapy regimen) (Loehrer, 1998)

Prostate cancer (unlabeled use): 4 mg/m^2 every week for 6 weeks of an 8-week treatment cycle (as part of combination chemotherapy) (Hudes, 1999)

Dosing adjustment in renal impairment: According to FDA-approved labeling, no adjustment is necessary in patients with renal impairment.

Dosing adjustment in hepatic impairment:

The FDA-approved labeling recommends the following guidelines: Serum bilirubin >3 mg/dL: Administer 50% of dose

The following guidelines have been used by some clinicians:

Serum bilirubin >3.1 or transaminases >3 times ULN: Avoid use (Floyd, 2006) **or**

Serum bilirubin 1.5-3 mg/dL or AST 60-180 units: Administer 50% of dose

Serum bilirubin 3-5 mg/dL: Administer 25% of dose

Serum bilirubin >5 mg/dL or AST >180 units: Avoid use

Administration FATAL IF GIVEN INTRATHECALLY. For I.V. administration only, usually as a slow (2-3 minutes) push, or a bolus (5-15 minutes) infusion; the manufacturer recommends an undiluted 1-minute infusion to prevent venous irritation/extravasation. Prolonged administration times and/or increased administration volumes may the risk of vein irritation and extravasation. Assure proper needle or catheter placement prior to administration.

Monitoring Parameters CBC with differential and platelet count, serum uric acid, hepatic function tests

Dosage Forms Excipient information presented when available (limited, particularly for generics); consult specific product labeling.

Injection, powder for reconstitution, as sulfate: 10 mg

Injection, solution, as sulfate: 1 mg/mL (10 mL) [contains benzyl alcohol]

◆ **Vinblastine Sulfate** *see* VinBLAStine *on page 1560*

◆ **Vincaleukoblastine** *see* VinBLAStine *on page 1560*

◆ **Vincasar PFS®** *see* VinCRIStine *on page 1561*

◆ **Vincasar® PFS® (Can)** *see* VinCRIStine *on page 1561*

VinCRIStine (vin KRIS teen)

U.S. Brand Names Vincasar PFS®

Canadian Brand Names Vincasar® PFS®

Index Terms Leurocristine Sulfate; NSC-67574; Oncovin; Vincristine Sulfate

Pharmacologic Category Antineoplastic Agent, Natural Source (Plant) Derivative; Antineoplastic Agent, Vinca Alkaloid

Use Treatment of leukemias, Hodgkin's disease, non-Hodgkin's lymphomas, Wilms' tumor, neuroblastoma, rhabdomyosarcoma

Pregnancy Risk Factor D

Lactation Enters breast milk/not recommended

Medication Safety Issues

Sound-alike/look-alike issues:

VinCRIStine may be confused with vinBLAStine

Oncovin® may be confused with Ancobon®

High alert medication: The Institute for Safe Medication Practices (ISMP) includes this medication among its list of drugs which have a heightened risk of causing significant patient harm when used in error.

To prevent fatal inadvertent intrathecal injection, it is recommended that all doses be dispensed in a small minibag. If dispensing vincristine in a syringe, vincristine must be packaged in the manufacturer-provided overwrap which bears the statement **"Do not remove covering until the moment of injection. For intravenous use only. Fatal if given intrathecally."**

Contraindications Hypersensitivity to vincristine or any component of the formulation; **for I.V. use only, fatal if given intrathecally**; patients with demyelinating form of Charcot-Marie-Tooth syndrome; pregnancy

Warnings/Precautions Hazardous agent - use appropriate precautions for handling and disposal. **[U.S. Boxed Warning]: Vincristine is a vesicant; avoid extravasation. (Individuals administering should be experienced in vincristine administration.)**

Dosage modification required in patients with impaired hepatic function or who have pre-existing neuromuscular disease. Use with caution in the elderly. Avoid eye contamination. Observe closely for shortness of breath, bronchospasm, especially in patients treated with mitomycin C. Alterations in mental status such as depression, confusion, or insomnia; constipation, paralytic ileus, and urinary tract disturbances may occur. All patients should be on a prophylactic bowel management regimen.

[U.S. Boxed Warning]: Intrathecal administration of vincristine has uniformly caused severe neurologic damage and/or death; vincristine should never be administered by this route. For I.V. use only. Neurologic effects of vincristine may be additive with those of other neurotoxic agents and spinal cord irradiation.

Adverse Reactions

>10%: Dermatologic: Alopecia (20% to 70%)

1% to 10%:

Cardiovascular: Orthostatic hypotension or hypertension, hyper-/hypotension

Central nervous system: CNS depression, confusion, cranial nerve paralysis, fever, headache, insomnia, motor difficulties, seizure

Intrathecal administration of vincristine has uniformly caused death; vincristine should never be administered by this route. Neurologic effects of vincristine may be additive with those of other neurotoxic agents and spinal cord irradiation.

Dermatologic: Rash

Endocrine & metabolic: Hyperuricemia

Gastrointestinal: Abdominal cramps, anorexia, bloating, constipation (and possible paralytic ileus secondary to neurologic toxicity), diarrhea, metallic taste, nausea (mild), oral ulceration, vomiting, weight loss

Genitourinary: Bladder atony (related to neurotoxicity), dysuria, polyuria, urinary retention

Hematologic: Leukopenia (mild), thrombocytopenia, myelosuppression (onset: 7 days; nadir: 10 days; recovery: 21 days)

Local: Phlebitis, tissue irritation and necrosis if infiltrated

Neuromuscular & skeletal: Cramping, jaw pain, leg pain, myalgia, numbness, weakness

Peripheral neuropathy: Frequently the dose-limiting toxicity of vincristine. Most frequent in patients >40 years of age; occurs usually after an average of 3 weekly doses, but may occur after just one dose. Manifested as loss of the deep tendon reflexes in the lower extremities, numbness, tingling, pain, paresthesia of the fingers and toes (stocking glove sensation), and "foot drop" or "wrist drop."

Ocular: Optic atrophy, photophobia

<1% (Limited to important or life-threatening): SIADH (rare), stomatitis

Drug Interactions

Metabolism/Transport Effects Substrate of CYP3A4 (major); **Inhibits** CYP3A4 (weak)

Avoid Concomitant Use

Avoid concomitant use of VinCRIStine with any of the following: Natalizumab; Vaccines (Live)

Increased Effect/Toxicity

VinCRIStine may increase the levels/effects of: Mitomycin; Natalizumab; Vaccines (Live); Vitamin K Antagonists

The levels/effects of VinCRIStine may be increased by: Antifungal Agents (Azole Derivatives, Systemic); CYP3A4 Inhibitors (Moderate); CYP3A4 Inhibitors (Strong); Dasatinib; Lopinavir; NIFEdipine; P-Glycoprotein Inhibitors; Trastuzumab

Decreased Effect

VinCRIStine may decrease the levels/effects of: Cardiac Glycosides; Vaccines (Inactivated); Vitamin K Antagonists

The levels/effects of VinCRIStine may be decreased by: CYP3A4 Inducers (Strong); Deferasirox; Echinacea; Herbs (CYP3A4 Inducers); P-Glycoprotein Inducers

Ethanol/Nutrition/Herb Interactions Herb/Nutraceutical: St John's wort may decrease vincristine levels.

Stability

Undiluted vials: Store under refrigeration. May be stable for up to 30 days at room temperature.

I.V. solution: **Note:** The World Health Organization (WHO) recommends dispensing vincristine in a minibag, rather than a syringe.

Diluted in 20-50 mL NS or D_5W, stable for 7 days under refrigeration, or 2 days at room temperature. In ambulatory pumps, solution is stable for 7-10 days at room temperature.

Mechanism of Action Binds to tubulin and inhibits microtubule formation, therefore, arresting the cell at metaphase by disrupting the formation of the mitotic spindle; it is specific for the M and S phases. Vincristine may also interfere with nucleic acid and protein synthesis by blocking glutamic acid utilization.

Pharmacodynamics/Kinetics

Absorption: Oral: Poor

Distribution: V_d: 163-165 L/m^2; poor penetration into CSF; rapidly removed from bloodstream and tightly bound to tissues; penetrates blood-brain barrier poorly

Protein binding: 75%

Metabolism: Extensively hepatic

Half-life elimination: Terminal: 24 hours

Excretion: Feces (~80%); urine (<1% as unchanged drug)

Dosage Note: Doses are often capped at 2 mg; however, this may reduce the efficacy of the therapy and may not be advisable. Refer to individual protocols; orders for single doses >2.5 mg or >5 mg/treatment cycle should be verified with the specific treatment regimen and/or an experienced oncologist prior to dispensing. I.V.:

Children ≤10 kg or BSA <1 m^2: Initial therapy: 0.05 mg/kg once weekly then titrate dose

Children >10 kg or BSA ≥1 m^2: 1-2 mg/m^2, may repeat once weekly for 3-6 weeks; maximum single dose: 2 mg

Neuroblastoma: I.V. continuous infusion with doxorubicin: 1 mg/m^2/day for 72 hours

Adults: 0.4-1.4 mg/m^2, may repeat every week **or**

0.4-0.5 mg/day continuous infusion for 4 days every 4 weeks **or**

0.25-0.5 mg/m^2/day for 5 days every 4 weeks

Dosing adjustment in renal impairment: No adjustment is necessary in patients with renal impairment.

Dosing adjustment in hepatic impairment:

The FDA-approved labeling recommends the following guidelines: Serum bilirubin >3 mg/dL: Administer 50% of normal dose

The following guidelines have been used by some clinicians:

Serum bilirubin 1.5-3 mg/dL or AST 60-180 units: Administer 50% of dose

Serum bilirubin 3-5 mg/dL: Administer 25% of dose

Serum bilirubin >5 mg/dL or AST >180 units: Avoid use

Floyd, 2006: Serum bilirubin 1.5-3 mg/dL or transaminases 2-3 times ULN or alkaline phosphatase elevated: Administer 50% of dose

Administration FATAL IF GIVEN INTRATHECALLY.

I.V.: Usually administered as short (10-15 minutes) infusion (preferred) or as slow (1-2 minutes) push; 24-hour continuous infusions are occasionally used

Intralesional injection has been reported for Kaposi's sarcoma.

Monitoring Parameters Serum electrolytes (sodium), hepatic function tests, neurologic examination, CBC, serum uric acid

Dosage Forms Excipient information presented when available (limited, particularly for generics); consult specific product labeling.

Injection, solution, as sulfate [preservative free]:
Vincasar PFS®: 1 mg/mL (1 mL, 2 mL)

◆ **Vincristine Sulfate** *see* VinCRIStine *on page 1561*

Vinorelbine (vi NOR el been)

U.S. Brand Names Navelbine®

Canadian Brand Names Navelbine®; Vinorelbine Injection, USP; Vinorelbine Tartrate for Injection

Index Terms Dihydroxydeoxynorvinkaleukoblastine; Vinorelbine Tartrate

Pharmacologic Category Antineoplastic Agent, Natural Source (Plant) Derivative; Antineoplastic Agent, Vinca Alkaloid

Use Treatment of nonsmall cell lung cancer (NSCLC)

Unlabeled/Investigational Use Treatment of breast cancer, cervical cancer, and ovarian cancer

Pregnancy Risk Factor D

Pregnancy Considerations Animal studies have demonstrated embryotoxicity, fetotoxicity, decreased fetal weight, and delayed ossification. There are no adequate and well-controlled studies in pregnant women. Women of child-bearing potential should avoid becoming pregnant during vinorelbine treatment.

Lactation Excretion in breast milk unknown/not recommended

Medication Safety Issues

Sound-alike/look-alike issues:
Vinorelbine may be confused with vinBLAStine

High alert medication: The Institute for Safe Medication Practices (ISMP) includes this medication among its list of drug classes which have a heightened risk of causing significant patient harm when used in error.

Vinorelbine is intended **for I. V. use only**: Inadvertent intrathecal administration of other vinca alkaloids has resulted in death. Syringes containing vinorelbine should be labeled **"For I.V. use only. Fatal if given intrathecally."**

Contraindications Pretreatment granulocyte counts <1000/mm^3

Warnings/Precautions Hazardous agent - use appropriate precautions for handling and disposal. **[U.S. Boxed Warning]: For I.V. use only; do not administer intrathecally;** intrathecal administration may result in death. **[U.S. Boxed Warning]: Avoid extravasation;** infiltration may cause irritation, thrombophlebitis and/or local tissue necrosis. **[U.S. Boxed Warning]: Severe granulocytopenia may occur with treatment;** granulocytopenia is a dose-limiting toxicity; granulocyte counts should be ≥1000/mm3 prior to treatment initiation; monitor closely for infections and/or fever; may require dosage adjustment. The incidence of granulocytopenia is significantly higher when given in combination with cisplatin when compared to single-agent vinorelbine. Use with caution in patients with compromised marrow reserve due to prior chemotherapy therapy or prior radiation therapy.

Fatal cases of interstitial pulmonary changes and ARDS have been reported (with single-agent therapy); promptly evaluate changes in baseline pulmonary symptoms or any new onset pulmonary symptoms. Acute shortness of breath and severe bronchospasm have been reported rarely; usually associated with the concurrent administration of mitomycin.

Dosage modification required in patients with impaired hepatic function and neurotoxicity; use with caution. May cause new onset or worsening of pre-existing neuropathy; use with caution in patients with neuropathy. May cause severe constipation (grade 3-4), paralytic ileus, intestinal obstruction, necrosis, and/or perforation. May have radiosensitizing effects with prior or concurrent radiation therapy; radiation recall reactions may occur in patients who have received prior radiation therapy. Avoid eye contamination (exposure may cause severe irritation). **[U.S. Boxed Warning]: Should be administered under the supervision of an experienced cancer chemotherapy physician.**

Adverse Reactions Note: Reported with single-agent therapy.

>10%:
- Central nervous system: Fatigue (27%)
- Dermatologic: Alopecia (12% to 30%)
- Gastrointestinal: Nausea (31% to 44%; grade 3: 1% to 2%), constipation (35%; grade 3: 3%), vomiting (20% to 31%; grade 3: 1% to 2%), diarrhea (12% to 17%)
- Hematologic: Leukopenia (83% to 92%; grade 4: 6% to 15%), granulocytopenia (90%; grade 4: 36%; nadir: 7-10 days; recovery 14-21 days; dose-limiting), neutropenia (85%; grade 4: 28%), anemia (83%; grades 3/4: 9%)
- Hepatic: AST increased (67%; grade 3: 5%; grade 4: 1%), total bilirubin increased (5% to 13%; grade 3: 4%; grade 4: 3%)
- Local: Injection site reaction (22% to 28%; includes erythema, vein discoloration), injection site pain (16%)
- Neuromuscular & skeletal: Weakness (36%), peripheral neuropathy (25%; grade 3: 1%; grade 4: <1%)
- Renal: Creatinine increased (13%)

1% to 10%:
- Cardiovascular: Chest pain (5%)
- Dermatologic: Rash (<5%)
- Gastrointestinal: Paralytic ileus (1%)
- Hematologic: Neutropenic fever/sepsis (8%; grade 4: 4%), thrombocytopenia (3% to 5%; grades 3/4: 1%)
- Local: Phlebitis (7% to 10%)
- Neuromuscular & skeletal: Loss of deep tendon reflexes (<5%), myalgia (<5%), arthralgia (<5%), jaw pain (<5%)
- Otic: Ototoxicity (≤1%)
- Respiratory: Dyspnea (7%)

<1% (Limited to important or life-threatening): Abdominal pain, allergic reactions, anaphylaxis, angioedema, back pain, DVT, dysphagia, esophagitis, flushing, gait instability, headache, hemorrhagic cystitis, hyper-/hypotension, hyponatremia, intestinal necrosis, intestinal obstruction, intestinal perforation, interstitial pulmonary changes, local rash, local urticaria, MI (rare), mucositis, muscle weakness, pancreatitis, paralytic ileus, pneumonia, pruritus, pulmonary edema, pulmonary embolus, radiation recall (dermatitis, esophagitis), skin blistering, syndrome of inappropriate ADH secretion, tachycardia, thromboembolic events, tumor pain, urticaria, vasodilation

Drug Interactions

Metabolism/Transport Effects Substrate of CYP2D6 (minor), 3A4 (major); **Inhibits** CYP2D6 (weak), 3A4 (weak)

Avoid Concomitant Use

Avoid concomitant use of Vinorelbine with any of the following: Natalizumab; Vaccines (Live)

Increased Effect/Toxicity

Vinorelbine may increase the levels/effects of: Mitomycin; Natalizumab; Vaccines (Live)

The levels/effects of Vinorelbine may be increased by: CISplatin; CYP3A4 Inhibitors (Moderate); CYP3A4

Inhibitors (Strong); Dasatinib; Paclitaxel; Paclitaxel (Protein Bound); Trastuzumab

Decreased Effect

Vinorelbine may decrease the levels/effects of: Vaccines (Inactivated)

The levels/effects of Vinorelbine may be decreased by: CYP3A4 Inducers (Strong); Deferasirox; Echinacea; Herbs (CYP3A4 Inducers)

Ethanol/Nutrition/Herb Interactions Herb/Nutraceutical: Avoid St John's wort (may decrease vinorelbine levels).

Stability Store intact vials under refrigeration at 2°C to 8°C (36°F to 46°F); do not freeze. Protect from light. Intact vials are stable at room temperature of 25°C (77°F) for up to 72 hours. Dilute in D_5W or NS to a final concentration of 1.5-3 mg/mL (for syringe) or 0.5-2 mg/mL (for I.V. bag). Dilutions in D_5W or NS are stable for 24 hours at room temperature.

Mechanism of Action Semisynthetic vinca alkaloid which binds to tubulin and inhibits microtubule formation, therefore, arresting the cell at metaphase by disrupting the formation of the mitotic spindle; it is specific for the M and S phases. Vinorelbine may also interfere with nucleic acid and protein synthesis by blocking glutamic acid utilization.

Pharmacodynamics/Kinetics

Absorption: Unreliable; must be given I.V.

Distribution: V_d: 25-40 L/kg; binds extensively to human platelets and lymphocytes (80% to 91%)

Protein binding: 80% to 91%

Metabolism: Extensively hepatic, via CYP3A4, to two metabolites, deacetylvinorelbine (active) and vinorelbine N-oxide

Bioavailability: Oral (not approved in the U. S.): 26% to 45%

Half-life elimination: Triphasic: Terminal: 28-44 hours

Excretion: Feces (46%); urine (18%, 10% to 12% as unchanged drug)

Clearance: Plasma: Mean: 0.97-1.26 L/hour/kg

Dosage Details concerning dosing in combination regimens should also be consulted.

I.V.: Adults:

NSCLC:

Single-agent therapy: 30 mg/m^2/dose every 7 days

Combination therapy with cisplatin: 25-30 mg/m^2/dose every 7 days (in combination with cisplatin)

Breast cancer (unlabeled use): 25 mg/m^2/dose every 7 days

Cervical cancer (unlabeled use): 30 mg/m^2/dose days 1 and 8 of a 21-day treatment cycle

Ovarian cancer (unlabeled use): 25 mg/m^2/dose every 7 days **or** 30 mg/m^2/dose days 1 and 8 of a 21-day treatment cycle

Dosage adjustment in hematological toxicity: Granulocyte counts should be ≥1000 cells/mm^3 prior to the administration of vinorelbine. Adjustments in the dosage of vinorelbine should be based on granulocyte counts obtained on the day of treatment as follows:

Granulocytes ≥1500 cells/mm^3 on day of treatment: Administer 100% of starting dose

Granulocytes 1000-1499 cells/mm^3 on day of treatment: Administer 50% of starting dose

Granulocytes <1000 cells/mm^3 on day of treatment: Do not administer. Repeat granulocyte count in one week; if 3 consecutive doses are held because granulocyte count is <1000 cells/mm^3, discontinue vinorelbine.

For patients who, during treatment, have experienced fever and/or sepsis while granulocytopenic or had 2 consecutive weekly doses held due to granulocytopenia, subsequent doses of vinorelbine should be:

75% of starting dose for granulocytes ≥1500 cells/mm^3

37.5% of starting dose for granulocytes 1000-1499 cells/mm^3

Dosage adjustment for neurotoxicity: Neurotoxicity ≥grade 2: Discontinue treatment

Dosage adjustment in renal impairment: No adjustment is necessary.

Dosing adjustment in hepatic impairment: The FDA-approved labeling guidelines are as follows: Vinorelbine should be administered with caution in patients with hepatic insufficiency. In patients who develop hyperbilirubinemia during treatment with vinorelbine, the dose should be adjusted for total bilirubin as follows:

Serum bilirubin ≤2 mg/dL: Administer 100% of dose

Serum bilirubin 2.1-3 mg/dL: Administer 50% of dose

Serum bilirubin >3 mg/dL: Administer 25% of dose

Dosing adjustment in patients with concurrent hematologic toxicity and hepatic impairment: Administer the lower of the doses determined from the adjustment recommendations.

Administration FATAL IF GIVEN INTRATHECALLY. Administer as a direct intravenous push or rapid bolus, over 6-10 minutes (up to 30 minutes). Longer infusions may increase the risk of pain and phlebitis. Intravenous doses should be followed by at least 75-125 mL of saline or D_5W to reduce the incidence of phlebitis and inflammation. Assure proper needle or catheter position prior to administration.

Monitoring Parameters CBC with differential and platelet count, hepatic function tests; monitor for new-onset pulmonary symptoms (or worsening from baseline); monitor for neuropathy

Dosage Forms Excipient information presented when available (limited, particularly for generics); consult specific product labeling.

Injection, solution [preservative free]: 10 mg/mL (1 mL, 5 mL)

Navelbine®: 10 mg/mL (1 mL, 5 mL)

◆ **Vinorelbine Injection, USP (Can)** *see* Vinorelbine *on page* 1563

◆ **Vinorelbine Tartrate** *see* Vinorelbine *on page* 1563

◆ **Vinorelbine Tartrate for Injection (Can)** *see* Vinorelbine *on page* 1563

◆ **Viokase®** *see* Pancrelipase *on page* 1136

◆ **Viosterol** *see* Ergocalciferol *on page* 538

◆ **Viracept®** *see* Nelfinavir *on page* 1049

◆ **Viramune®** *see* Nevirapine *on page* 1055

◆ **Virazole®** *see* Ribavirin *on page* 1310

◆ **Viread®** *see* Tenofovir *on page* 1438

◆ **Virilon®** *see* MethylTESTOSTERone *on page* 979

◆ **Virilon® IM (Can)** *see* Testosterone *on page* 1445

◆ **Viroptic®** *see* Trifluridine *on page* 1517

◆ **Viscoat®** *see* Sodium Chondroitin Sulfate and Sodium Hyaluronate *on page* 1383

◆ **Visine-A® [OTC]** *see* Naphazoline and Pheniramine *on page* 1040

◆ **Visine® Advanced Allergy (Can)** *see* Naphazoline and Pheniramine *on page* 1040

◆ **Visken® (Can)** *see* Pindolol *on page* 1194

◆ **Vistaril®** *see* HydrOXYzine *on page* 754

◆ **Vistide®** *see* Cidofovir *on page* 324

◆ **Vistra 650** *see* Acetaminophen and Phenyltoloxamine *on page* 29

◆ **Vita-C® [OTC]** *see* Ascorbic Acid *on page* 139

◆ **Vitamin C** *see* Ascorbic Acid *on page* 139

◆ **Vitamin D_2** *see* Ergocalciferol *on page* 538

◆ **Vitamin D_3 and Alendronate** *see* Alendronate and Cholecalciferol *on page* 60

◆ **Vitamin D and Calcium Carbonate** *see* Calcium and Vitamin D *on page 238*

Vitamin A (VYE ta min aye)

U.S. Brand Names Aquasol A®; Palmitate-A® [OTC]
Index Terms Oleovitamin A
Pharmacologic Category Vitamin, Fat Soluble
Use Treatment and prevention of vitamin A deficiency; parenteral (I.M.) route is indicated when oral administration is not feasible or when absorption is insufficient (malabsorption syndrome)
Pregnancy Risk Factor A/X (dose exceeding RDA recommendation)
Medication Safety Issues
Sound-alike/look-alike issues:
Aquasol® may be confused with Anusol®
Dosage
RDA:
<1 year: 375 mcg
1-3 years: 400 mcg
4-6 years: 500 mcg*
7-10 years: 700 mcg*
>10 years: 800-1000 mcg*
Male: 1000 mcg
Female: 800 mcg
* mcg retinol equivalent (0.3 mcg retinol = 1 unit vitamin A)
Vitamin A supplementation in measles (recommendation of the World Health Organization): Children: Oral: Administer as a single dose; repeat the next day and at 4 weeks for children with ophthalmologic evidence of vitamin A deficiency:
6 months to 1 year: 100,000 units
>1 year: 200,000 units
Note: Use of vitamin A in measles is recommended only for patients 6 months to 2 years of age hospitalized with measles and its complications **or** patients >6 months of age who have any of the following risk factors and who are not already receiving vitamin A: immunodeficiency, ophthalmologic evidence of vitamin A deficiency including night blindness, Bitot's spots or evidence of xerophthalmia, impaired intestinal absorption, moderate-to-severe malnutrition including that associated with eating disorders, or recent immigration from areas where high mortality rates from measles have been observed
Note: Monitor patients closely; dosages >25,000 units/kg have been associated with toxicity
Severe deficiency with xerophthalmia: Oral:
Children 1-8 years: 5000-10,000 units/kg/day for 5 days or until recovery occurs
Children >8 years and Adults: 500,000 units/day for 3 days, then 50,000 units/day for 14 days, then 10,000-20,000 units/day for 2 months
Deficiency (without corneal changes): Oral:
Infants <1 year: 100,000 units every 4-6 months
Children 1-8 years: 200,000 units every 4-6 months
Children >8 years and Adults: 100,000 units/day for 3 days then 50,000 units/day for 14 days
Deficiency: I.M.: **Note:** I.M. route is indicated when oral administration is not feasible or when absorption is insufficient (malabsorption syndrome):
Infants: 7500-15,000 units/day for 10 days
Children 1-8 years: 17,500-35,000 units/day for 10 days
Children >8 years and Adults: 100,000 units/day for 3 days, followed by 50,000 units/day for 2 weeks
Note: Follow-up therapy with an oral therapeutic multivitamin (containing additional vitamin A) is recommended:
Low Birth Weight Infants: Additional vitamin A is recommended, however, no dosage amount has been established
Children ≤8 years: 5000-10,000 units/day
Children >8 years and Adults: 10,000-20,000 units/day
Malabsorption syndrome (prophylaxis): Children >8 years and Adults: Oral: 10,000-50,000 units/day of water miscible product
Dietary supplement: Oral:
Infants up to 6 months: 1500 units/day
Children:
6 months to 3 years: 1500-2000 units/day
4-6 years: 2500 units/day
7-10 years: 3300-3500 units/day
Children >10 years and Adults: 4000-5000 units/day
Additional Information Complete prescribing information for this medication should be consulted for additional detail.
Dosage Forms Excipient information presented when available (limited, particularly for generics); consult specific product labeling.
Capsule [softgel]: 10,000 units; 25,000 units
Injection, solution (Aquasol A®): 50,000 units/mL (2 mL) [contains polysorbate 80]
Tablet (Palmitate-A®): 5000 units, 15,000 units

◆ **Vitamin A Acid** *see* Tretinoin (Topical) *on page 1509*

Vitamin A and Vitamin D
(VYE ta min aye & VYE ta min dee)

U.S. Brand Names A and D® Original [OTC]; Baza® Clear [OTC]; Sween Cream® [OTC]
Index Terms Cod Liver Oil
Pharmacologic Category Topical Skin Product
Use Temporary relief of discomfort due to chapped skin, diaper rash, minor burns, abrasions, as well as irritations associated with ostomy skin care
Pregnancy Risk Factor B
Dosage Topical: Apply locally with gentle massage as needed
Additional Information Complete prescribing information for this medication should be consulted for additional detail.
Dosage Forms Excipient information presented when available (limited, particularly for generics); consult specific product labeling.
Capsule, softgel: Vitamin A 1250 int. units and vitamin D 135 int. units; vitamin A 1250 int. units and vitamin D 130 int. units; vitamin A 5,000 int. units and vitamin D 400 int. units; vitamin A 10,000 int. units and vitamin D 400 int. units; vitamin A 10,000 int. units and vitamin D 5000 int. units; vitamin A 25,000 int. units and vitamin D 1000 int. units
Cream:
Sween Cream®: 2 g, 85 g, 184 g, 339 g [original]
Sween Cream®: 57 g, 142 g [fresh scent]
Sween Cream®: 57 g [fragrance free]
Ointment: 0.9 g, 5 g, 60 g, 120 g, 454 g [in lanolin-petrolatum base]
A and D® Original: 45 g, 120 g, 454 g
Baza® Clear: 50 g, 150 g, 240 g
Tablet: Vitamin A 10,000 int. units and vitamin D 400 int. units

◆ **Vitamin B_1** *see* Thiamine *on page 1458*
◆ **Vitamin B_2** *see* Riboflavin *on page 1313*
◆ **Vitamin B_3** *see* Niacin *on page 1057*
◆ **Vitamin B_3** *see* Niacinamide *on page 1059*
◆ **Vitamin B_6** *see* Pyridoxine *on page 1273*
◆ **Vitamin B_{12}** *see* Cyanocobalamin *on page 374*
◆ **Vitamin B_{12a}** *see* Hydroxocobalamin *on page 750*

Vitamin E (VYE ta min ee)

U.S. Brand Names Alph-E [OTC]; Alph-E-Mixed [OTC]; Aquasol E® [OTC]; Aquavit-E [OTC]; d-Alpha-Gems™ [OTC]; E-Gems Elite® [OTC]; E-Gems Plus® [OTC]; E-Gems® [OTC]; Ester-E™ [OTC]; Gamma E-Gems® [OTC]; Gamma-E Plus [OTC]; High Gamma Vitamin E Complete™ [OTC]; Key-E® Kaps [OTC]; Key-E® [OTC]

Index Terms *d*-Alpha Tocopherol; *dl*-Alpha Tocopherol

Pharmacologic Category Vitamin, Fat Soluble

Use Dietary supplement

Unlabeled/Investigational Use To reduce the risk of bronchopulmonary dysplasia or retrolental fibroplasia in infants exposed to high concentrations of oxygen; prevention and treatment of tardive dyskinesia; prevention and treatment of hemolytic anemia secondary to vitamin E deficiency

Pregnancy Risk Factor A/C (dose exceeding RDA recommendation)

Medication Safety Issues

Sound-alike/look-alike issues:

Aquasol E® may be confused with Anusol®

Dosage Vitamin E may be expressed as alpha-tocopherol equivalents (ATE), which refer to the biologically-active (R) stereoisomer content. Oral:

Recommended daily allowance (RDA):

Infants (adequate intake; RDA not established):

≤6 months: 4 mg

7-12 months: 6 mg

Children:

1-3 years: 6 mg; upper limit of intake should not exceed 200 mg/day

4-8 years: 7 mg; upper limit of intake should not exceed 300 mg/day

9-13 years: 11 mg; upper limit of intake should not exceed 600 mg/day

14-18 years: 15 mg; upper limit of intake should not exceed 800 mg/day

Adults: 15 mg; upper limit of intake should not exceed 1000 mg/day

Pregnant female:

≤18 years: 15 mg; upper level of intake should not exceed 800 mg/day

19-50 years: 15 mg; upper level of intake should not exceed 1000 mg/day

Lactating female:

≤18 years: 19 mg; upper level of intake should not exceed 800 mg/day

19-50 years: 19 mg; upper level of intake should not exceed 1000 mg/day

Vitamin E deficiency:

Children (with malabsorption syndrome): 1 unit/kg/day of water miscible vitamin E (to raise plasma tocopherol concentrations to the normal range within 2 months and to maintain normal plasma concentrations)

Adults: 60-75 units/day

Prevention of vitamin E deficiency: Adults: 30 units/day

Cystic fibrosis, beta-thalassemia, sickle cell anemia may require higher daily maintenance doses:

Children:

Cystic fibrosis: 100-400 units/day

Beta-thalassemia: 750 units/day

Adults:

Sickle cell: 450 units/day

Tardive dyskinesia (unlabeled use): 1600 units/day

Additional Information Complete prescribing information for this medication should be consulted for additional detail.

Dosage Forms Excipient information presented when available (limited, particularly for generics); consult specific product labeling.

Capsule: 400 int. units, 1000 int. units

Key-E® Kaps: 200 int. units, 400 int. units

Capsule, softgel: 200 int. units, 400 int. units, 600 int. units, 1000 int. units

Alph-E: 200 int. units, 400 int. units

Alph-E-Mixed: 200 int. units [contains mixed tocopherols]; 400 int. units [contains mixed tocopherols], 1000 int. units [sugar free; contains mixed tocopherols]

Aqua Gem E®: 200 units, 400 units

d-Alpha-Gems™: 400 int. units [derived from soybean oil]

E-Gems®: 30 int. units, 100 int. units, 200 int. units, 400 int. units, 600 int. units, 800 int. units, 1000 int. units, 1200 int. units [derived from soybean oil]

E-Gems Plus®: 200 int. units, 400 int. units, 800 int. units [contains mixed tocopherols]

E-Gems Elite®: 400 int. units [contains mixed tocopherols]

Ester-E™: 400 int. units

Gamma E-Gems®: 90 int. units [also contains mixed tocopherols]

Gamma-E Plus: 200 int. units [contains soybean oil]

High Gamma Vitamin E Complete™: 200 int. units [contains soybean oil, mixed tocopherols]

Cream: 50 int. units/g (60 g), 100 int. units/g (60 g), 1000 int. units/120 g (120 g), 30,000 int. units/57 g (57 g)

Key-E®: 30 int. units/g (60 g, 120 g, 600 g)

Lip balm (E-Gem® Lip Care): 1000 int. units/tube [contains vitamin A and aloe]

Oil, oral/topical: 100 int. units/0.25 mL (60 mL, 75 mL); 1150 units/0.25 mL (30 mL, 60 mL, 120 mL); 28,000 int. units/30 mL (30 mL)

Alph-E: 28,000 int. units/30 mL (30 mL) [topical]

E-Gems®: 100 units/10 drops (15 mL, 60 mL)

Ointment, topical (Key-E®): 30 units/g (60 g, 120 g, 480 g)

Powder (Key-E®): 700 int. units per 1/4 teaspoon (15 g, 75 g, 1000 g) [derived from soybean oil]

Solution, oral drops: 15 int. units/0.3 mL (30 mL)

Aquasol E®: 15 int. units/0.3 mL (12 mL, 30 mL) [latex free]

Aquavit-E: 15 int. units/0.3 mL (30 mL) [butterscotch flavor]

Suppository, rectal/vaginal (Key-E®): 30 int. units (12s, 24s) [contains coconut oil]

Tablet: 100 int. units, 200 int. units, 400 int. units, 500 int. units

Key-E®: 200 int. units, 400 int. units

◆ **Vitamin G** *see* Riboflavin *on page* 1313

◆ **Vitamin K_1** *see* Phytonadione *on page* 1191

◆ **Vitelle™ Irospan® [OTC] [DSC]** *see* Ferrous Sulfate and Ascorbic Acid *on page* 617

◆ **Vitrasert®** *see* Ganciclovir *on page* 681

◆ **Vitrax®** *see* Hyaluronate and Derivatives *on page* 734

◆ **Vitussin [DSC]** *see* Hydrocodone and Guaifenesin *on page* 741

◆ **Vi Vaccine** *see* Typhoid Vaccine *on page* 1529

◆ **Vivactil®** *see* Protriptyline *on page* 1264

◆ **Vivaglobin®** *see* Immune Globulin (Subcutaneous) *on page* 779

◆ **Vivarin® [OTC]** *see* Caffeine *on page* 232

◆ **Vivelle® [DSC]** *see* Estradiol *on page* 554

◆ **Vivelle-Dot®** *see* Estradiol *on page* 554

◆ **Vivitrol™** *see* Naltrexone *on page* 1039

◆ **Vivotif®** *see* Typhoid Vaccine *on page* 1529

◆ **VLB** *see* VinBLAStine *on page* 1560

◆ **VM-26** *see* Teniposide *on page* 1438

◆ **Volibris™ (Can)** *see* Ambrisentan *on page* 80

◆ **Voltaren®** *see* Diclofenac *on page* 437

◆ **Voltaren® Gel** *see* Diclofenac *on page* 437

◆ **Voltaren Ophtha® (Can)** *see* Diclofenac *on page 437*

◆ **Voltaren Ophthalmic®** *see* Diclofenac *on page 437*

◆ **Voltaren Rapide® (Can)** *see* Diclofenac *on page 437*

◆ **Voltaren®-XR** *see* Diclofenac *on page 437*

◆ **Voluven®** *see* Hetastarch *on page 731*

Voriconazole (vor i KOE na zole)

U.S. Brand Names VFEND®

Canadian Brand Names VFEND®

Index Terms UK109496

Pharmacologic Category Antifungal Agent, Oral; Antifungal Agent, Parenteral

Additional Appendix Information

Antifungal Agents *on page 1640*

Use Treatment of invasive aspergillosis; treatment of esophageal candidiasis; treatment of candidemia (in non-neutropenic patients); treatment of disseminated *Candida* infections of the skin and viscera; treatment of serious fungal infections caused by *Scedosporium apiospermum* and *Fusarium* spp (including *Fusarium solani*) in patients intolerant of, or refractory to, other therapy

Unlabeled/Investigational Use

Fungal infection prophylaxis in intermediate or high risk neutropenic cancer patients with myelodysplastic syndrome (MDS) or acute myelogenous leukemia (AML), neutropenic allogeneic hematopoietic stem cell recipients, and patients with significant graft-versus-host disease; empiric antifungal therapy (second-line) for persistent neutropenic fever

Pregnancy Risk Factor D

Pregnancy Considerations Voriconazole can cause fetal harm when administered to a pregnant woman. Voriconazole was teratogenic and embryotoxic in animal studies, and lowered plasma estradiol in animal models. Women of childbearing potential should use effective contraception during treatment. Should be used in pregnant woman only if benefit to mother justifies potential risk to the fetus.

Lactation Excretion in breast milk unknown/not recommended

Contraindications Hypersensitivity to voriconazole or any component of the formulation (cross-reaction with other azole antifungal agents may occur but has not been established, use caution); coadministration of CYP3A4 substrates which may lead to QT_c prolongation (cisapride, pimozide, or quinidine); coadministration with barbiturates (long acting), carbamazepine, efavirenz (with standard [eg, not adjusted] voriconazole and efavirenz doses), ergot derivatives, rifampin, rifabutin, ritonavir (≥800 mg/day), sirolimus, St John's wort

Warnings/Precautions Visual changes, including blurred vision, changes in visual acuity, color perception, and photophobia, are commonly associated with treatment. Patients should be warned to avoid tasks which depend on vision, including operating machinery or driving. Changes are reversible on discontinuation following brief exposure/treatment regimens (≤28 days).

Serious hepatic reactions (including hepatitis, cholestasis, and fulminant hepatic failure) have occurred during treatment, primarily in patients with serious concomitant medical conditions. However, hepatotoxicity has occurred in patients with no identifiable risk factors. Use caution in patients with pre-existing hepatic impairment (dose adjustment or discontinuation may be required).

Voriconazole tablets contain lactose; avoid administration in hereditary galactose intolerance, Lapp lactase deficiency, or glucose-galactose malabsorption. Suspension contains sucrose; use caution with fructose intolerance, sucrose-isomaltase deficiency, or glucose-galactose malabsorption. Avoid/limit use of intravenous formulation in patients with renal impairment; intravenous formulation contains excipient sulfobutyl ether beta-cyclodextrin (SBECD), which may accumulate in renal insufficiency. Acute renal failure has been observed in severely ill patients; use with caution in patients receiving concomitant nephrotoxic medications. Anaphylactoid-type infusion-related reactions may occur with intravenous dosing. Consider discontinuation of infusion if reaction is severe.

Use caution in patients taking strong cytochrome P450 inducers, CYP2C9 inhibitors, and major 3A4 substrates (see Drug Interactions); consider alternative agents that avoid or lessen the potential for CYP-mediated interactions. QT interval prolongation has been associated with voriconazole use; rare cases of arrhythmia (including torsade de pointes), cardiac arrest, and sudden death have been reported, usually in seriously ill patients with comorbidities and/or risk factors (eg, prior cardiotoxic chemotherapy, cardiomyopathy, electrolyte imbalance, or concomitant QT_c-prolonging drugs). Use with caution in these patient populations; correct electrolyte abnormalities (eg, hypokalemia, hypomagnesemia, hypocalcemia) prior to initiating therapy. Do not infuse concomitantly with blood products or short-term concentrated electrolyte solutions, even if the two infusions are running in separate intravenous lines (or cannulas). Rarely, serious cutaneous reactions (including Stevens-Johnson syndrome) have been reported with treatment. Consider discontinuing in patients developing a rash. Avoid strong, direct exposure to sunlight; may cause photosensitivity, especially with long-term use. Monitor pancreatic function in patients (children and adults) at risk for acute pancreatitis (eg, recent chemotherapy or hematopoietic stem cell transplantation); there have been postmarketing reports of pancreatitis in children. Safety and efficacy have not been established in children <12 years of age.

Adverse Reactions

>10%:

Central nervous system: Hallucinations (4% to 12%; auditory and/or visual and likely serum concentration-dependent)

Ocular: Visual changes (dose related; photophobia, color changes, increased or decreased visual acuity, or blurred vision occur in ~21%)

Renal: Creatinine increased (1% to 21%)

2% to 10%:

Cardiovascular: Tachycardia (≤2%)

Central nervous system: Fever (≤6%), chills (≤4%), headache (≤3%)

Dermatologic: Rash (≤7%)

Endocrine & metabolic: Hypokalemia (≤2%)

Gastrointestinal: Nausea (1% to 5%), vomiting (1% to 4%)

Hepatic: Alkaline phosphatase increased (4% to 5%), AST increased (2% to 4%), ALT increased (2% to 3%), cholestatic jaundice (1% to 2%)

Ocular: Photophobia (2% to 3%)

<2% (Limited to important or life-threatening): Acute tubular necrosis, adrenal cortical insufficiency, agranulocytosis, allergic reaction, anaphylactoid reaction, anemia (aplastic, hemolytic, macrocytic, megaloblastic, or microcytic), angioedema, anuria, ascites, atrial arrhythmia, atrial fibrillation, AV block, bigeminy, bleeding time increased, bone marrow depression, bone necrosis, bradycardia, brain edema, bundle branch block, BUN increased, cardiac arrest, cardiomegaly, cardiomyopathy, cerebral hemorrhage/ischemia, cerebrovascular accident, chest pain, CHF, cholecystitis, cholelithiasis, chromatopsia, color blindness, coma, confusion, cyanosis, delirium, dementia, depersonalization, depression, diabetes insipidus, diarrhea, DIC, discoid lupus erythematosus, duodenal ulcer perforation, DVT, dyspnea, edema, encephalopathy, endocarditis, eosinophilia,

erythema multiforme, exfoliative dermatitis, extrapyramidal symptoms, fixed drug eruption, fulminant hepatic failure, GI hemorrhage, GGT/LDH increased, glucose tolerance decreased, Guillain-Barré syndrome, hematemesis, hepatic coma, hepatic failure, hepatitis, hepatomegaly, hydronephrosis, hyper-/hypocalcemia, hyper-/hypoglycemia, hyper-/hypomagnesemia, hyper-/hyponatremia, hyper-/hypotension, hyper-/hypothyroidism, hyperbilirubinemia, hypercholesterolemia, hyperkalemia, hyperuricemia, hypophosphatemia, hypoxia, intestinal perforation, intracranial hypertension, jaundice, leukopenia, lung edema, lymphadenopathy, lymphangitis, maculopapular rash, MI, multiorgan failure, myasthenia, myopathy, nephritis, nephrosis, neuropathy, night blindness, nodal arrhythmia, oculogyric crisis, optic atrophy, optic neuritis, osteomalacia, osteoporosis, palpitation, pancreatitis, pancytopenia, papilledema, paresthesia, peripheral edema, peritonitis, petechia, photosensitivity, pleural effusion, postural hypotension, pruritus, pseudomembraneous colitis, psychosis, pulmonary embolus, purpura, QT interval prolongation, renal dysfunction, renal failure (acute), respiratory distress syndrome, retinal hemorrhage, seizure, sepsis, spleen enlarged, Stevens-Johnson syndrome, suicidal ideation, supraventricular extrasystoles, supraventricular tachycardia, syncope, thrombocytopenia, thrombophlebitis, thrombotic thrombocytopenic purpura, tongue edema, torsade de pointes, toxic epidermal necrolysis, uremia, urinary retention, urticaria, uveitis, vasodilation, ventricular arrhythmia, ventricular fibrillation, ventricular tachycardia, visual field defect

Drug Interactions

Metabolism/Transport Effects **Substrate** of CYP2C9 (major), 2C19 (major), 3A4 (minor); **Inhibits** CYP2C9 (weak), 2C19 (weak), 3A4 (moderate)

Avoid Concomitant Use

Avoid concomitant use of Voriconazole with any of the following: Alfuzosin; Barbiturates; CarBAMazepine; Cisapride; Conivaptan; Darunavir; Dofetilide; Ergot Derivatives; Lopinavir; Nilotinib; Pimozide; QuiNIDine; Ranolazine; Rifamycin Derivatives; Ritonavir; Rivaroxaban; Salmeterol; Silodosin; St Johns Wort; Tetrabenazine; Thioridazine

Increased Effect/Toxicity

Voriconazole may increase the levels/effects of: Alfentanil; Alfuzosin; Alosetron; Aprepitant; Benzodiazepines (metabolized by oxidation); Bosentan; BusPIRone; Busulfan; Calcium Channel Blockers; CarBAMazepine; Cardiac Glycosides; Ciclesonide; Cilostazol; Cinacalcet; Cisapride; Conivaptan; Corticosteroids (Orally Inhaled); Corticosteroids (Systemic); CycloSPORINE; CYP3A4 Substrates; Diclofenac; Docetaxel; Dofetilide; Eletriptan; Eplerenone; Ergot Derivatives; Erlotinib; Eszopiclone; FentaNYL; Fesoterodine; Fosaprepitant; Gefitinib; HMG-CoA Reductase Inhibitors; Imatinib; Irinotecan; Ixabepilone; Losartan; Macrolide Antibiotics; Maraviroc; Methadone; Nilotinib; Oral Contraceptive (Estrogens); Oral Contraceptive (Progestins); Phenytoin; Phosphodiesterase 5 Inhibitors; Pimecrolimus; Pimozide; Protease Inhibitors; QTc-Prolonging Agents; QuiNIDine; Ramelteon; Ranolazine; Repaglinide; Reverse Transcriptase Inhibitors (Non-Nucleoside); Rifamycin Derivatives; Rivaroxaban; Salmeterol; Silodosin; Sirolimus; Solifenacin; Sorafenib; Sunitinib; Tacrolimus; Temsirolimus; Tetrabenazine; Thioridazine; Tolterodine; Venlafaxine; VinCRIStine; Vitamin K Antagonists; Ziprasidone; Zolpidem

The levels/effects of Voriconazole may be increased by: Alfuzosin; Ciprofloxacin; CYP2C9 Inhibitors (Moderate); CYP2C9 Inhibitors (Strong); Gadobutrol; Macrolide Antibiotics; Nilotinib; Oral Contraceptive (Estrogens); Oral Contraceptive (Progestins); Protease Inhibitors; Proton Pump Inhibitors

Decreased Effect

Voriconazole may decrease the levels/effects of: Amphotericin B; Saccharomyces boulardii

The levels/effects of Voriconazole may be decreased by: Antacids; Barbiturates; CarBAMazepine; CYP2C19 Inducers (Strong); CYP2C9 Inducers (Highly Effective); Darunavir; Didanosine; Grapefruit Juice; Lopinavir; Phenytoin; Reverse Transcriptase Inhibitors (Non-Nucleoside); Rifamycin Derivatives; Ritonavir; St Johns Wort; Sucralfate

Ethanol/Nutrition/Herb Interactions

Food: May decrease voriconazole absorption. Voriconazole should be taken 1 hour before or 1 hour after a meal. Avoid grapefruit juice (may decrease voriconazole levels).

Herb/Nutraceutical: St John's wort may decrease voriconazole levels; concurrent use with voriconazole is contraindicated.

Stability

Powder for injection: Store at 15°C to 30°C (59°F to 86°F). Reconstitute 200 mg vial with 19 mL of sterile water for injection (use of automated syringe is not recommended). Resultant solution (20 mL) has a concentration of 10 mg/mL. Prior to infusion, must dilute to 0.5-5 mg/mL with NS, LR, D_5WLR, $D_5W^{1/2}$NS, D_5W, D_5W with KCl 20 mEq, $^{1/2}$ NS, or D_5WNS. Do not dilute with 4.2% sodium bicarbonate infusion. Reconstituted solutions are stable for up to 24 hours under refrigeration at 2°C to 8°C (36°F to 46°F).

Powder for oral suspension: Store at 2°C to 8°C (36°F to 46°F). Add 46 mL of water to the bottle to make 40 mg/mL suspension. Reconstituted oral suspension may be stored at 15°C to 30°C (59°F to 86°F). Discard after 14 days.

Tablets: Store at 15°C to 30°C (59°F to 86°F).

Mechanism of Action Interferes with fungal cytochrome P450 activity (selectively inhibits 14-alpha-lanosterol demethylation), decreasing ergosterol synthesis (principal sterol in fungal cell membrane) and inhibiting fungal cell membrane formation.

Pharmacodynamics/Kinetics

Absorption: Well absorbed after oral administration; administration of crushed tablets is considered bioequivalent to whole tablets

Distribution: V_d: 4.6 L/kg

Protein binding: 58%

Metabolism: Hepatic, via CYP2C19 (major pathway) and CYP2C9 and CYP3A4 (less significant); saturable (may demonstrate nonlinearity)

Bioavailability: 96%

Half-life elimination: Variable, dose-dependent

Time to peak: Oral: 1-2 hours; 0.5 hours (crushed tablet)

Excretion: Urine (as inactive metabolites; <2% as unchanged drug)

Dosage

Usual dosage ranges:

Children <12 years: Dosage not established

Children ≥12 years and Adults:

Oral: 100-300 mg every 12 hours

I.V.: 6 mg/kg every 12 hours for 2 doses; followed by maintenance dose of 4 mg/kg every 12 hours

Indication-specific dosing: Children ≥12 years and Adults:

Aspergillosis, invasive, including disseminated and extrapulmonary infection: Duration of therapy should be a minimum of 6-12 weeks or throughout period of immunosuppression:

I.V.: Initial: Loading dose: 6 mg/kg every 12 hours for 2 doses; followed by maintenance dose of 4 mg/kg every 12 hours

Oral: May consider oral therapy in place of I.V. with dosing of 4 mg/kg (rounded up to convenient tablet dosage form) every 12 hours; however, I.V. administration is preferred in serious infections since comparative efficacy with the oral formulation has not been established.

Scedosporiosis, fusariosis: I.V.: Initial: Loading dose: 6 mg/kg every 12 hours for 2 doses; followed by maintenance dose of 4 mg/kg every 12 hours

Candidemia and other deep tissue *Candida* infections: I.V.: Initial: Loading dose 6 mg/kg every 12 hours for 2 doses; followed by maintenance dose of 3-4 mg/kg every 12 hours

Endophthalmitis, fungal: I.V.: 6 mg/kg every 12 hours for 2 doses, then 200 mg orally twice daily

Esophageal candidiasis: Oral:

Patients <40 kg: 100 mg every 12 hours; maximum: 300 mg/day

Patients ≥40 kg: 200 mg every 12 hours; maximum: 600 mg/day

Note: Treatment should continue for a minimum of 14 days, and for at least 7 days following resolution of symptoms.

Conversion to oral dosing:

Patients <40 kg: 100 mg every 12 hours; increase to 150 mg every 12 hours in patients who fail to respond adequately

Patients ≥40 kg: 200 mg every 12 hours; increase to 300 mg every 12 hours in patients who fail to respond adequately

Dosage adjustment in patients unable to tolerate treatment:

I.V.: Dose may be reduced to 3 mg/kg every 12 hours

Oral: Dose may be reduced in 50 mg decrements to a minimum dosage of 200 mg every 12 hours in patients weighing ≥40 kg (100 mg every 12 hours in patients <40 kg)

Dosage adjustment in patients receiving concomitant CYP450 enzyme inducers or substrates:

Cyclosporine: Reduce cyclosporine dose by 1/2 and monitor closely.

Efavirenz: Oral: Increase maintenance dose of voriconazole to 400 mg every 12 hours and reduce efavirenz dose to 300 mg once daily

Phenytoin:

I.V.: Increase maintenance dosage to 5 mg/kg every 12 hours

Oral: Increase dose to 400 mg every 12 hours in patients ≥40 kg (200 mg every 12 hours in patients <40 kg)

Dosage adjustment in renal impairment: In patients with Cl_{cr} <50 mL/minute, accumulation of the intravenous vehicle (SBECD) occurs. After initial I.V. loading dose, oral voriconazole should be administered to these patients, unless an assessment of the benefit:risk to the patient justifies the use of I.V. voriconazole. Monitor serum creatinine and change to oral voriconazole therapy when possible.

Hemodialysis: Oral dosage adjustment not required; I.V. dosing not recommended since SBECD vehicle is cleared at half the rate of voriconazole and may accumulate

Dosage adjustment in hepatic impairment:

Mild-to-moderate hepatic dysfunction (Child-Pugh class A and B): Following standard loading dose, reduce maintenance dosage by 50%

Severe hepatic impairment: Should only be used if benefit outweighs risk; monitor closely for toxicity

Dietary Considerations Oral: Should be taken 1 hour before or 1 hour after a meal. Voriconazole tablets contain lactose; avoid administration in hereditary galactose intolerance, Lapp lactase deficiency, or glucose-galactose malabsorption. Suspension contains sucrose; use caution with fructose intolerance, sucrose-isomaltase deficiency, or glucose-galactose malabsorption.

Administration

Oral: Administer 1 hour before or 1 hour after a meal.

I.V.: Infuse over 1-2 hours (rate not to exceed 3 mg/kg/hour). Do not infuse concomitantly into same line or cannula with other drug infusions, including TPN.

Monitoring Parameters Hepatic function at initiation and during course of treatment; renal function; serum electrolytes (particularly calcium, magnesium and potassium) prior to therapy initiation; visual function (visual acuity, visual field and color perception) if treatment course continues >28 days; may consider obtaining voriconazole trough level in patients failing therapy or exhibiting signs of toxicity; pancreatic function (in patients at risk for acute pancreatitis)

Dosage Forms Excipient information presented when available (limited, particularly for generics); consult specific product labeling.

Injection, powder for reconstitution: 200 mg [contains SBECD 3200 mg]

Powder for oral suspension: 200 mg/5 mL (70 mL) [contains sodium benzoate and sucrose; orange flavor]

Tablet: 50 mg, 200 mg [contains lactose]

Vorinostat (vor IN oh stat)

U.S. Brand Names Zolinza™

Index Terms NSC-701852; SAHA; Suberoylanilide Hydroxamic Acid

Pharmacologic Category Antineoplastic Agent, Histone Deacetylase Inhibitor

Use Treatment of progressive, persistent, or recurrent cutaneous T-cell lymphoma (CTCL)

Pregnancy Risk Factor D

Pregnancy Considerations Animal studies have demonstrated adverse fetal effects, including fetal loss, decreased fetal weight, and skeletal malformation. There are no adequate and well-controlled studies in pregnant women. Inform patient of potential hazard if used during pregnancy or if pregnancy occurs during treatment.

Lactation Excretion in breast milk unknown/not recommended

Medication Safety Issues

High alert medication: The Institute for Safe Medication Practices (ISMP) includes this medication among its list of drug classes which have a heightened risk of causing significant patient harm when used in error.

Contraindications There are no contraindications listed within the manufacturer's labeling.

Warnings/Precautions Hazardous agent - use appropriate precautions for handling and disposal. Pulmonary embolism and deep vein thrombosis (DVT) have been reported; monitor. Use caution in patients with a history of thrombotic events. Dose-related thrombocytopenia and/or anemia may occur; may require dosage adjustments. QT_c prolongation has been observed; a baseline and periodic 12-lead ECG should be obtained. Correct electrolyte abnormalities prior to treatment and monitor and correct potassium, calcium, and magnesium levels during therapy. Use caution in patients with a history of QT_c prolongation or with medications known to prolong the QT interval. May cause hyperglycemia; monitor and use with caution in diabetics; may require diet and/or therapy modifications. Nausea, vomiting, and diarrhea may occur; antiemetics and antidiarrheals may be required; replace fluids and electrolytes to avoid dehydration. Safety and efficacy in children have not been established.

Adverse Reactions

>10%:

Cardiovascular: Peripheral edema (13%)

Central nervous system: Fatigue (46% to 73%), chills (12% to 16%), dizziness (15%), headache (12%), fever (11%)
Dermatologic: Alopecia (18% to 19%), pruritus (12%)
Endocrine & metabolic: Hyperglycemia (8% to 69%; grade 3: 5%), dehydration (16%)
Gastrointestinal: Diarrhea (49% to 52%), nausea (41% to 49%), taste perversion (24% to 46%), xerostomia (11% to 35%), weight loss (20% to 27%), anorexia (22% to 24%), vomiting (12% to 24%), appetite decreased (14% to 22%), constipation (11% to 15%)
Hematologic: Thrombocytopenia (22% to 54%; grades 3/4: 5% to 19%), anemia (2% to 14%; grades 3/4: 1% to 3%)
Neuromuscular & skeletal: Muscle spasm (16% to 20%)
Renal: Proteinuria (51%), creatinine increased (15% to 47%)
Respiratory: Dyspnea (34%), cough (11%), upper respiratory infection (11%)

1% to 10%:
Cardiovascular: QT_c prolongation (3% to 6%)
Dermatologic: Squamous cell carcinoma (4%)
Respiratory: Pulmonary embolism (5%)

<1% (Limited to important or life-threatening): Angioneurotic edema, blurred vision, chest pain, cholecystitis, creatine phosphokinase (CPK) increased, DVT, enterococcal infection, exfoliative dermatitis, gastrointestinal hemorrhage, hemoptysis, hypertension, hypocalcemia, hypokalemia, hyponatremia, hypophosphatemia, infection, lethargy, leukopenia, MI, neutropenia, pneumonia, renal failure, sepsis, spinal cord injury, streptococcal bacteremia, stroke (ischemic), syncope, T-cell lymphoma, transaminases increased, tumor hemorrhage, ureteric obstruction, ureteropelvic junction obstruction, urinary retention, vasculitis, weakness

Drug Interactions

Avoid Concomitant Use

Avoid concomitant use of Vorinostat with any of the following: Nilotinib; Tetrabenazine; Thioridazine; Ziprasidone

Increased Effect/Toxicity

Vorinostat may increase the levels/effects of: QTc-Prolonging Agents; Tetrabenazine; Thioridazine; Vitamin K Antagonists; Ziprasidone

The levels/effects of Vorinostat may be increased by: Alfuzosin; Ciprofloxacin; Gadobutrol; Nilotinib; Valproic Acid

Decreased Effect There are no known significant interactions involving a decrease in effect.

Stability Store at 20°C to 25°C (68°F to 77°F); excursions permitted to 15°C to 30°C (59°F to 86°F).

Mechanism of Action Inhibition of histone deacetylase enzymes, HDAC1, HDAC2, HDAC3, and HDAC6, which catalyze acetyl group removal from protein lysine residues (including histones and transcription factors). Inhibition of histone deacetylase results in accumulation of acetyl groups, leading to alterations in chromatin structure and transcription factor activation causing termination of cell growth leading to cell death.

Pharmacodynamics/Kinetics

Protein binding: ~71%
Metabolism: Glucuronidated and hydrolyzed (followed by beta-oxidation) to inactive metabolites
Bioavailability: Fasting: ~43%
Half-life elimination: ~2 hours
Time to peak, plasma: With high-fat meal: ~4 hours (range: 2-10 hours)
Excretion: Urine: 52% (<1% as unchanged drug, ~52% as inactive metabolites)

Dosage Oral: Adults: Cutaneous T-cell lymphoma: 400 mg once daily

Dosage adjustment for intolerance: Reduce dose to 300 mg once daily; may further reduce to 300 mg daily for 5 consecutive days per week

In clinical trials, treatment was withheld for grade 4 anemia or thrombocytopenia or other grade 3 or 4 drug related toxicity, until resolved to ≤ grade 1. Therapy was reinitiated with dose modification (Olsen, 2007).

Dosage adjustment in renal impairment: Not studied, however, based on the minimal renal elimination, adjustment may not be required.

Dosage adjustment in hepatic impairment: Not studied; use caution based on predominant hepatic metabolism.

Dietary Considerations Take with food.

Administration Administer with food. Do not open, crush, or chew capsules.

Monitoring Parameters Baseline, then periodic 12-lead ECG; baseline, then every other week serum electrolytes (including calcium, magnesium and potassium), CBC with differential and platelets, serum creatinine and blood glucose for 2 months, then monthly

Dosage Forms Excipient information presented when available (limited, particularly for generics); consult specific product labeling.

Capsule:
Zolinza™: 100 mg

◆ **VoSol® HC** *see* Acetic Acid, Propylene Glycol Diacetate, and Hydrocortisone *on page 35*

◆ **VoSpire ER®** *see* Albuterol *on page 51*

◆ **VP-16** *see* Etoposide *on page 591*

◆ **VP-16-213** *see* Etoposide *on page 591*

◆ **Vumon®** *see* Teniposide *on page 1438*

◆ **Vusion®** *see* Miconazole and Zinc Oxide *on page 990*

◆ **vWF:RCof** *see* Antihemophilic Factor/von Willebrand Factor Complex (Human) *on page 122*

◆ **Vytone®** *see* Iodoquinol and Hydrocortisone *on page 810*

◆ **Vytorin®** *see* Ezetimibe and Simvastatin *on page 598*

◆ **Vyvanse™** *see* Lisdexamfetamine *on page 893*

◆ **VZIG** *see* Varicella-Zoster Immune Globulin (Human) *on page 1551*

◆ **VZV Vaccine (Varicella)** *see* Varicella Virus Vaccine *on page 1549*

◆ **VZV Vaccine (Zoster)** *see* Zoster Vaccine *on page 1593*

Warfarin (WAR far in)

U.S. Brand Names Coumadin®; Jantoven®

Canadian Brand Names Apo-Warfarin®; Coumadin®; Gen-Warfarin; Novo-Warfarin; Taro-Warfarin

Index Terms Warfarin Sodium

Pharmacologic Category Anticoagulant, Coumarin Derivative; Vitamin K Antagonist

Use Prophylaxis and treatment of thromboembolic disorders (eg, venous, pulmonary) and embolic complications arising from atrial fibrillation or cardiac valve replacement; adjunct to reduce risk of systemic embolism (eg, recurrent MI, stroke) after myocardial infarction

Unlabeled/Investigational Use Prevention of recurrent transient ischemic attacks

Restrictions An FDA-approved medication guide must be distributed when dispensing an outpatient prescription (new or refill) where this medication is to be used without direct supervision of a healthcare provider. Medication guides are available at http://www.fda.gov/cder/Offices/ODS/medication_guides.htm.

Pregnancy Risk Factor X

Pregnancy Considerations Oral anticoagulants cross the placenta and produce fetal abnormalities. May also cause fatal fetal hemorrhage. Warfarin should not be used during pregnancy because of significant risks. Adjusted-dose heparin can be given safely throughout pregnancy in patients with venous thromboembolism.

Lactation Does not enter breast milk, only metabolites are excreted (AAP rates "compatible")

Medication Safety Issues

Sound-alike/look-alike issues:

Coumadin® may be confused with Avandia®, Cardura®, Compazine®, Kemadrin®

Jantoven™ may be confused with Janumet™, Januvia™

High alert medication: The Institute for Safe Medication Practices (ISMP) includes this medication among its list of drugs which have a heightened risk of causing significant patient harm when used in error.

2009 National Patient Safety Goals: The Joint Commission on Accreditation of Healthcare Organizations requires healthcare organizations that provide anticoagulant therapy to have a process in place to reduce the risk of anticoagulant-associated patient harm. Patients receiving anticoagulants should receive individualized care through a defined process that includes standardized ordering, dispensing, administration, monitoring and education. This does not apply to routine short-term use of anticoagulants for prevention of venous thromboembolism when the expectation is that the patient's laboratory values will remain within or close to normal values (NPSG.03.05.01).

Contraindications Hypersensitivity to warfarin or any component of the formulation; hemorrhagic tendencies (eg, patients bleeding from the GI, respiratory, or GU tract; aneurysm; cerebrovascular hemorrhage; following spinal puncture and other diagnostic or therapeutic procedures with potential for significant bleeding; history of bleeding diathesis); recent or potential surgery of the eye or CNS; major regional lumbar block anesthesia or surgery resulting in large, open surfaces; blood dyscrasias; severe uncontrolled or malignant hypertension; pericarditis or pericardial effusion; subacute bacterial endocarditis; history of warfarin-induced necrosis; an unreliable, noncompliant patient; alcoholism; patient who has a history of falls or is a significant fall risk; unsupervised senile or psychotic patient; eclampsia/pre-eclampsia, threatened abortion, pregnancy

Warnings/Precautions Use care in the selection of patients appropriate for this treatment. Ensure patient cooperation especially from the alcoholic, illicit drug user, demented, or psychotic patient; ability to comply with routine laboratory monitoring is essential. Use with caution in trauma, acute infection, moderate-severe renal insufficiency, prolonged dietary insufficiencies, moderate-severe hypertension, polycythemia vera, vasculitis, open wound, active TB, any disruption in normal GI flora, history of PUD, anaphylactic disorders, indwelling catheters, severe diabetes, thyroid disease, and menstruating and postpartum women. Use with caution in protein C deficiency. Use with caution in patients with heparin-induced thrombocytopenia and DVT. Warfarin monotherapy is contraindicated in the initial treatment of active HIT. Reduced liver function, regardless of etiology, may impair synthesis of coagulation factors leading to increased warfarin sensitivity.

[U.S. Boxed Warning]: May cause major or fatal bleeding. Risk factors for bleeding include high intensity anticoagulation (INR >4), age (>65 years), variable INRs, history of GI bleeding, hypertension, cerebrovascular disease, serious heart disease, anemia, malignancy, trauma, renal insufficiency, drug-drug interactions, long duration of therapy, or known genetic deficiency in CYP2C9 activity. Patient must be instructed to report bleeding, accidents, or falls. Unrecognized bleeding sites (eg, colon cancer) may be uncovered by anticoagulation. Patient must also report any new or discontinued medications, herbal or alternative products used, or significant changes in smoking or dietary habits. Necrosis or gangrene of the skin and other tissue can occur, usually in conjunction with protein C or S deficiency. "Purple toes syndrome," due to cholesterol microembolization, may rarely occur. Women may be at risk of developing ovarian hemorrhage at the time of ovulation. The elderly may be more sensitive to anticoagulant therapy. Safety and efficacy have not been established in children; monitor closely.

Presence of the CYP2C9*2 or *3 allele and/or polymorphism of the vitamin K oxidoreductase (VKORC1) gene may increase the risk of bleeding. Lower doses may be required in these patients; genetic testing may help determine appropriate dosing.

Adverse Reactions Bleeding is the major adverse effect of warfarin. Hemorrhage may occur at virtually any site. Risk is dependent on multiple variables, including the intensity of anticoagulation and patient susceptibility.

Cardiovascular: Angina, chest pain, edema, hemorrhagic shock, hypotension, pallor, syncope, vasculitis

Central nervous system: Coma, dizziness, fatigue, fever, headache, lethargy, malaise, pain, stroke

Dermatologic: Alopecia, bullous eruptions, dermatitis, rash, pruritus, urticaria

Gastrointestinal: Abdominal cramps, abdominal pain, anorexia, diarrhea, flatulence, gastrointestinal bleeding, mouth ulcers, nausea, taste disturbance, vomiting

Genitourinary: Hematuria, priapism

Hematologic: Agranulocytosis, anemia, leukopenia, retroperitoneal hematoma, unrecognized bleeding sites (eg, colon cancer) may be uncovered by anticoagulation

Hepatic: Cholestatic jaundice, hepatic injury, hepatitis, transaminases increased

Neuromuscular & skeletal: Joint pain, muscle pain, osteoporosis (potential association with long-term use), paralysis, paresthesia, weakness

Respiratory: Dyspnea, tracheobronchial calcification

Miscellaneous: Anaphylactic reaction, cold intolerance, hypersensitivity/allergic reactions, skin necrosis, gangrene, "purple toes" syndrome

Drug Interactions

Metabolism/Transport Effects Substrate of CYP1A2 (minor), 2C9 (major), 2C19 (minor), 3A4 (minor); **Inhibits** CYP2C9 (moderate), 2C19 (weak)

Avoid Concomitant Use

Avoid concomitant use of Warfarin with any of the following: Tamoxifen

Increased Effect/Toxicity

Warfarin may increase the levels/effects of: Anticoagulants; CYP2C9 Substrates (High risk); Drotrecogin Alfa; Phenytoin

The levels/effects of Warfarin may be increased by: Acetaminophen; Allopurinol; Amiodarone; Androgens; Antineoplastic Agents; Antiplatelet Agents; Atazanavir; Capecitabine; Cephalosporins; Cimetidine; Clopidogrel; Corticosteroids (Systemic); Cranberry; CYP2C9 Inhibitors (Moderate); CYP2C9 Inhibitors (Strong); Dasatinib; Disulfiram; Efavirenz; Etoposide; Fenofibrate; Fenofibric Acid; Fenugreek; Fibric Acid Derivatives; Fluconazole; Fluorouracil; Gefitinib; Ginkgo Biloba; Glucagon; Herbs (Anticoagulant/Antiplatelet Properties); HMG-CoA Reductase Inhibitors; Ifosfamide; Imatinib; Itraconazole; Ivermectin; Ketoconazole; Leflunomide; Macrolide Antibiotics; MetroNIDAZOLE; Miconazole; NSAID (COX-2 Inhibitor); NSAID (Nonselective); Omega-3-Acid Ethyl Esters; Orlistat; Pentosan Polysulfate Sodium; Phenytoin; Posaconazole; Propafenone; Propoxyphene; Prostacyclin Analogues; Proton Pump Inhibitors; QuiNIDine; Quinolone Antibiotics; Salicylates; Selective Serotonin Reuptake Inhibitors; Sitaxsentan; Sorafenib;

Sulfinpyrazone [Off Market]; Sulfonamide Derivatives; Tamoxifen; Tetracycline Derivatives; Thrombolytic Agents; Thyroid Products; Tigecycline; Tolterodine; Tricyclic Antidepressants; Vitamin A; Vitamin E; Voriconazole; Vorinostat; Zafirlukast; Zileuton

Decreased Effect

The levels/effects of Warfarin may be decreased by: Aminoglutethimide; Antineoplastic Agents; Antithyroid Agents; Aprepitant; AzaTHIOprine; Barbiturates; Bile Acid Sequestrants; Bosentan; CarBAMazepine; Coenzyme Q-10; Contraceptive (Progestins); CYP2C9 Inducers (Highly Effective); Darunavir; Dicloxacillin; Fosaprepitant; Ginseng (American); Glutethimide; Griseofulvin; Lopinavir; Mercaptopurine; Nafcillin; Oral Contraceptive (Estrogens); Phytonadione; Rifamycin Derivatives; Ritonavir; St Johns Wort

Ethanol/Nutrition/Herb Interactions

Ethanol: Avoid ethanol. Acute ethanol ingestion (binge drinking) decreases the metabolism of warfarin and increases PT/INR. Chronic daily ethanol use increases the metabolism of warfarin and decreases PT/INR.

Food: The anticoagulant effects of warfarin may be decreased if taken with foods rich in vitamin K. Vitamin E may increase warfarin effect. Cranberry juice may increase warfarin effect.

Herb/Nutraceutical: Cranberry, fenugreek, ginkgo biloba, glucosamine, may enhance bleeding or increase warfarin's effect. Ginseng (American), coenzyme Q_{10}, and St John's wort may decrease warfarin levels and effects. Avoid alfalfa, anise, bilberry, bladderwrack, bromelain, cat's claw, celery, chamomile, coleus, cordyceps, dong quai, evening primrose oil, fenugreek, feverfew, garlic, ginger, ginkgo biloba, ginseng (American), ginseng (Panax), ginseng (Siberian), grapeseed, green tea, guggul, horse chestnut seed, horseradish, licorice, omega-3-acids, prickly ash, red clover, reishi, SAMe (s-adenosylmethionine), sweet clover, turmeric, and white willow (all have additional antiplatelet activity).

Stability

Injection: Prior to reconstitution, store at 15°C to 30°C (59°F to 86°F). Following reconstitution with 2.7 mL of sterile water (yields 2 mg/mL solution), stable for 4 hours at 15°C to 30°C (59°F to 86°F). Protect from light.

Tablet: Store at 15°C to 30°C (59°F to 86°F). Protect from light.

Mechanism of Action Hepatic synthesis of coagulation factors II, VII, IX, and X, as well as proteins C and S, requires the presence of vitamin K. These clotting factors are biologically activated by the addition of carboxyl groups to key glutamic acid residues within the proteins' structure. In the process, "active" vitamin K is oxidatively converted to an "inactive" form, which is then subsequently reactivated by vitamin K epoxide reductase complex 1 (VKORC1). Warfarin competitively inhibits the subunit 1 of the multi-unit VKOR complex, thus depleting functional vitamin K reserves and hence reduces synthesis of active clotting factors.

Pharmacodynamics/Kinetics

Onset of action: Anticoagulation: Oral: 24-72 hours

Peak effect: Full therapeutic effect: 5-7 days; INR may increase in 36-72 hours

Duration: 2-5 days

Absorption: Oral: Rapid, complete

Distribution: 0.14 L/kg

Protein binding: 99%

Metabolism: Hepatic, primarily via CYP2C9; minor pathways include CYP2C8, 2C18, 2C19, 1A2, and 3A4

Genomic variants: Approximately 37% reduced clearance of S-warfarin in patients heterozygous for 2C9 (*1/*2 or *1/*3), and ~70% reduced in patients homozygous for reduced function alleles (*2/*2, *2/*3, or *3/*3)

Half-life elimination: 20-60 hours; Mean: 40 hours; highly variable among individuals

Time to peak, plasma: Oral: ~4 hours

Excretion: Urine (92%, primarily as metabolites)

Dosage Note: New labeling identifies genetic factors which may increase patient sensitivity to warfarin. Specifically, genetic variations in the proteins CYP2C9 and VKORC1, responsible for warfarin's primary metabolism and pharmacodynamic activity, respectively, have been identified as predisposing factors associated with decreased dose requirement and increased bleeding risk. A genotyping test is available, and may provide important guidance on initiation of anticoagulant therapy.

Oral:

Infants and Children (unlabeled use): Initial loading dose (if baseline INR is 1-1.3): 0.2 mg/kg (maximum: 10 mg/dose); adjust dose based on INR (reported ranges to maintain INR of 2-3: 0.09-0.33 mg/kg/day). Infants <12 months of age may require doses at or near the high end of this range; consistent anticoagulation may be difficult to maintain in children <5 years of age.

Adults: Initial dosing must be individualized. Consider the patient (hepatic function, cardiac function, age, nutritional status, concurrent therapy, risk of bleeding) in addition to prior dose response (if available) and the clinical situation. Start 2-5 mg daily for 2 days **or** 5-10 mg daily for 1-2 days (Ansell, 2008). Adjust dose according to INR results; usual maintenance dose ranges from 2-10 mg daily (individual patients may require loading and maintenance doses outside these general guidelines).

Note: Lower starting doses may be required for patients with hepatic impairment, poor nutrition, CHF, elderly, high risk of bleeding, or patients who are debilitated, or those with reduced function genomic variants of the catabolic enzymes CYP2C9 (*2 or *3 alleles) or VKORC1 (-1639 polymorphism). Higher initial doses may be reasonable in selected patients (ie, receiving enzyme-inducing agents and with low risk of bleeding).

I.V.: Adults: 2-5 mg/day administered as a slow bolus injection

Dosing adjustment in renal disease: No adjustment required, however, patients with renal failure have an increased risk of bleeding complications. Monitor closely.

Dosing adjustment in hepatic disease: Monitor effect at usual doses; the response to oral anticoagulants may be markedly enhanced in obstructive jaundice (due to reduced vitamin K absorption) and also in hepatitis and cirrhosis (due to decreased production of vitamin K-dependent clotting factors); INR should be closely monitored

Dietary Considerations Foods high in vitamin K (eg, beef liver, pork liver, green tea, and leafy green vegetables) inhibit anticoagulant effect. Do not change dietary habits once stabilized on warfarin therapy. A balanced diet with a consistent intake of vitamin K is essential. Avoid large amounts of alfalfa, asparagus, broccoli, Brussels sprouts, cabbage, cauliflower, green teas, kale, lettuce, spinach, turnip greens, and watercress; decreased efficacy of warfarin. It is recommended that the diet contain a CONSISTENT vitamin K content of 70-140 mcg/day. Check with healthcare provider before changing diet.

Administration

Oral: Administer with or without food. Take at the same time each day.

I.V.: Administer as a slow bolus injection over 1-2 minutes; avoid all I.M. injections

Monitoring Parameters Prothrombin time, hematocrit, INR; consider genotyping of CYP2C9 and VKORC1 prior to initiation of therapy, if available

Reference Range

INR = patient prothrombin time/mean normal prothrombin time

ISI = international sensitivity index

INR should be increased by 2-3.5 times depending upon indication. An INR >4 does not generally add additional therapeutic benefit and is associated with increased risk of bleeding.

Adult INR ranges based upon indication: See table.

Warfarin levels are not used for monitoring degree of anticoagulation. They may be useful if a patient with unexplained coagulopathy is using the drug surreptitiously or if it is unclear whether clinical resistance is due to true drug resistance or lack of drug intake.

Normal prothrombin time (PT): 10.9-12.9 seconds. Healthy premature newborns have prolonged coagulation test screening results (eg, PT, aPTT, TT) which return to normal adult values at approximately 6 months of age. Healthy prematures, however, do not develop spontaneous hemorrhage or thrombotic complications because of a balance between procoagulants and inhibitors.

Additional Information Prospective genotyping is available, and may provide important guidance on initiation of anticoagulant therapy. Commercial testing with PGxPredict™:WARFARIN is now available from PGxHealth™ (Division of Clinical Data, Inc, New Haven, CT). The test genotypes patients for presence of the CYP2C9*2 or *3 alleles and the VKORC1 -1639G>A polymorphism. The results of the test allow patients to be phenotyped as extensive, intermediate, or poor metabolizers (CYP2C9) and as low, intermediate, or high warfarin sensitivity (VKORC1). Ordering information is available at 888-592-7327 or warfarininfo@pgxhealth.com.

Dosage Forms Excipient information presented when available (limited, particularly for generics); consult specific product labeling.

Injection, powder for reconstitution, as sodium:

- Coumadin®: 5 mg

Tablet, as sodium: 1 mg, 2 mg, 2.5 mg, 3 mg, 4 mg, 5 mg, 6 mg, 7.5 mg, 10 mg

- Coumadin®: 1 mg, 2 mg, 2.5 mg, 3 mg, 4 mg, 5 mg, 6 mg, 7.5 mg [scored]
- Coumadin®: 10 mg [scored; dye free]
- Jantoven®: 1 mg, 2 mg, 2.5 mg, 3 mg, 4 mg, 5 mg, 6 mg, 7.5 mg [scored]
- Jantoven®: 10 mg [scored; dye free]

Adult Target INR Ranges Based Upon Indication

Indication	Targeted INR	Targeted INR Range
Cardiac		
Acute myocardial infarction (high risk)[1]	2.5	2-3[2,3]
Atrial fibrillation or atrial flutter	2.5	2-3
Valvular		
Bileaflet or Medtronic Hall tilting disk mechanical aortic valve in normal sinus rhythm and normal LA size	2.5	2-3
Bileaflet or tilting disk mechanical mitral valve	3	2.5-3.5
Caged ball or caged disk mechanical valve	3	2.5-3.5
Mechanical prosthetic valve with systemic embolism despite adequate anticoagulation	3 **or** 3.5[4]	2.5-3.5[4] **or** 3-4[4]
Mechanical valve and risk factors for thromboembolism (eg, AF, MI[5], LA enlargement, hypercoagulable state, low EF) or history of atherosclerotic vascular disease	3	2.5-3.5[6]
Bioprosthetic mitral valve	2.5	2-3[7]
Bioprosthetic mitral or aortic valve with prior history of systemic embolism	2.5	2-3[7]
Bioprosthetic mitral or aortic valve with evidence of LA thrombus at surgery	2.5	2-3[8]
Bioprosthetic mitral or aortic valve with risk factors for thromboembolism (eg, AF, hypercoagulable state or low EF)	2.5	2-3[9]
Prosthetic mitral valve thrombosis (resolved)	4	3.5-4.5[3]
Prosthetic aortic valve thrombosis (resolved)	3.5	3-4[3]
Rheumatic mitral valve disease and normal sinus rhythm (LA diameter >5.5 cm), AF, previous systemic embolism, or LA thrombus	2.5	2-3
Thromboembolism Treatment		
Venous thromboembolism	2.5	2-3[10,11]
Thromboprophylaxis		
Chronic thromboembolic pulmonary hypertension (CTPH)	2.5	2-3
Lupus inhibitor (no other risk factors)	2.5	2-3
Lupus inhibitor and recurrent thromboembolism	3	2.5-3.5
Major trauma patients with impaired mobility undergoing rehabilitation	2.5	2-3
Spinal cord injury (acute) undergoing rehabilitation	2.5	2-3
Total hip or knee replacement (elective) or hip fracture surgery	2.5	2-3[12]
Other Indications		
Cerebral venous sinus thrombosis	2.5	2-3[13]
Ischemic stroke due to AF	2.5	2-3

[1] High-risk includes large anterior MI, significant heart failure, intracardiac thrombus, atrial fibrillation, history of thromboembolism.

[2] Maintain anticoagulation for 3 months.

[3] Combine with aspirin 81 mg/day.

[4] Combine with aspirin 81 mg/day, if not previously receiving, **and/or** if previous target INR was 2.5, then new target INR should be 3 (2.5-3.5). If previous target INR was 3, then new target INR should be 3.5 (3-4).

[5] MI refers to anterior-apical ST-segment elevation myocardial infarction.

[6] Combine with aspirin 81 mg/day unless patient is at high risk of bleeding (eg, history of GI bleed, age >80 years).

[7] Maintain anticoagulation for 3 months after valve insertion then switch to aspirin 81 mg/day if no other indications for warfarin exist or clinically reassess need for warfarin in patients with prior history of systemic embolism.

[8] Maintain anticoagulation with warfarin until thrombus resolution.

[9] If patient has history of atherosclerotic vascular disease, combine with aspirin 81 mg/day unless patient is at high risk of bleeding (eg, history of GI bleed, age >80 years).

[10] Treat for 3 months in patients with VTE due to transient reversible risk factor. Treat for a minimum of 3 months in patients with unprovoked VTE and evaluate for long term therapy. Other risk groups (eg, cancer) may require >3 months of therapy.

[11] In patients with unprovoked VTE who prefer less frequent INR monitoring, low-intensity therapy (INR range: 1.5-1.9) with less frequent monitoring is recommended over stopping treatment.

[12] Continue for at least 10 days and up to 35 days after surgery.

[13] Continue for up to 12 months.

◆ **Warfarin Sodium** *see* Warfarin *on page* 1570

◆ **4 Way® Fast Acting [OTC]** *see* Phenylephrine *on page* 1183

Yellow Fever Vaccine (YEL oh FEE ver vak SEEN)

U.S. Brand Names YF-VAX®

Canadian Brand Names YF-VAX®

Pharmacologic Category Vaccine, Live (Viral)

Additional Appendix Information

Immunization Recommendations *on page 1708*

Use Induction of active immunity against yellow fever virus, primarily among persons traveling or living in areas where yellow fever infection exists and laboratory workers who may be exposed to the virus; vaccination may also be required for some international travelers

Pregnancy Risk Factor C

Pregnancy Considerations Animal reproduction studies have not been conducted. Adverse events were not observed in the mother or fetus following vaccination during the third trimester of pregnancy in Nigerian women; however maternal seroconversion was reduced. Inadvertent exposure early in the first trimester of pregnancy in Brazilian women did not show decreased maternal seroconversion; no major congenital abnormalities were noted. Vaccine should be administered if travel to an endemic area is unavoidable and the infant should be monitored after birth. Tests to verify maternal immune response may be considered. If a pregnant woman is to be vaccinated only to satisfy an international requirement (as opposed to decreasing risk of infection), efforts should be made to obtain a waiver letter.

Lactation Excretion in breast milk unknown/contraindicated

Contraindications Hypersensitivity to egg or chick embryo protein, or any component of the formulation; children <9 months of age (per manufacturer); children <6 months of age (CDC guidelines); acute or febrile disease; immunosuppressed patients; breast-feeding women

Warnings/Precautions Do not use in immunodeficient persons (including patients <24 months after hematopoietic stem cell transplant) or patients receiving immunosuppressants (eg, steroids, radiation). Patients who are immunosuppressed have a theoretical risk of encephalitis with yellow fever vaccine administration; consider delaying travel or obtaining a waiver letter. Patients on low-dose or short-term corticosteroids, or with asymptomatic HIV infection are not considered immunosuppressed and may be offered the vaccine. If vaccination is only to satisfy an international requirement (as opposed to decreasing risk of infection), efforts should be made to obtain a waiver letter. Immediate treatment (including epinephrine 1:1000) for anaphylactoid and/or hypersensitivity reactions should be available during vaccine use.

Chicken embryos are used in the manufacture of this vaccine. Use is contraindicated in patients with immediate-type hypersensitivity reactions to eggs; in general, persons who are able to eat eggs or egg products may receive the vaccine. The vial stopper contains latex; product may contain gelatin. Immunization should be delayed during the course of an acute or febrile illness. The presence of a low-grade fever is generally not a reason to postpone vaccination. Use with caution in the elderly; the risk of adverse events is increased in patients ≥65 years of age. Avoid use in pregnant women unless travel to high-risk areas is unavoidable. The manufacturer contraindicates use in infants <9 months of age due to risk of encephalitis. The CDC allows for use in infants 6-8 months of age when possible exposure with the yellow fever virus is unavoidable and the risk of infection exists. Infants <6 months of age should never be vaccinated.

Adverse Reactions All serious adverse reactions must be reported to the U.S. Department of Health and Human Services (DHHS) Vaccine Adverse Event Reporting System (VAERS) 1-800-822-7967.

Frequency not defined (adverse reactions may be increased in patients <9 months or ≥65 years of age)

Central nervous system: Fever (incidence of these reactions have been reported to be as low as <5% and as high as 10% to 30% depending on the study), focal neurological defects, headache, seizure

Local: Injection site reactions (edema, hypersensitivity, mass, pain)

Neuromuscular & skeletal: Myalgia, weakness

Miscellaneous: Guillain-Barré syndrome, hypersensitivity (immediate), vaccine-associated neurotropic disease (rare), viscerotropic disease (rare; may be associated with multiorgan failure)

Drug Interactions

Avoid Concomitant Use

Avoid concomitant use of Yellow Fever Vaccine with any of the following: Immunosuppressants

Increased Effect/Toxicity

The levels/effects of Yellow Fever Vaccine may be increased by: Immunosuppressants

Decreased Effect

Yellow Fever Vaccine may decrease the levels/effects of: Tuberculin Tests

Stability Store at 2°C to 8°C (35°F to 46°F); do not freeze. Reconstitute only with diluent provided. Inject diluent slowly into vial and allow to stand for 1-2 minutes. Gently swirl until a uniform suspension forms; swirl well before withdrawing dose. Avoid vigorous shaking to prevent foaming of suspension. Vaccine must be used within 60 minutes of reconstitution. Keep suspension refrigerated until used.

Pharmacodynamics/Kinetics

Onset of action: Seroconversion: 10-14 days

Duration: ≥30 years

Dosage SubQ:

Children ≥6 months (unlabeled use [CDC guidelines]): One dose (0.5 mL) ≥10 days before travel; Booster: Every 10 years for those at continued risk of exposure

Children ≥9 months (per manufacturer) and Adults: One dose (0.5 mL) ≥10 days before travel; Booster: Every 10 years for those at continued risk of exposure

Administration For SubQ injection only. Do not administer I.M. or I.V.

Monitoring Parameters Monitor for adverse effects 10-30 days after vaccination.

Additional Information Federal law requires that the date of administration, the vaccine manufacturer, lot number of vaccine, and the administering person's name, title, and address be entered into the patient's permanent medical record. A hypersensitivity screening test and desensitization procedure is available for persons with suspected or known severe egg sensitivity. Consult manufacturer's labeling for details. Some countries require a valid international Certification of Vaccination showing receipt of vaccine. The WHO requires revaccination every 10 years to maintain traveler's vaccination certificate.

The following CDC agencies may be contacted if serologic testing is needed or for advice when administering yellow fever vaccine to pregnant women, children <9 months, or patients with altered immune status:

Division of Vector-Borne Infectious Diseases: 970-221-6400

Division of Global Migration and Quarantine: 404-498-1600

Dosage Forms Excipient information presented when available (limited, particularly for generics); consult specific product labeling.

Injection, powder for reconstitution [17D-204 strain]:

YF-VAX®: ≥4.74 Log_{10} plaque-forming units (PFU) per 0.5 mL dose [single-dose or 5-dose vial; produced in chicken embryos; contains gelatin; packaged with diluent; vial stopper contains latex]

◆ **YF-VAX®** *see* Yellow Fever Vaccine *on page 1574*
◆ **YM087** *see* Conivaptan *on page 368*
◆ **YM905** *see* Solifenacin *on page 1387*
◆ **YM-08310** *see* Amifostine *on page 82*
◆ **Yodoxin®** *see* Iodoquinol *on page 810*
◆ **Z4942** *see* Ifosfamide *on page 766*
◆ **Zaditen® (Can)** *see* Ketotifen *on page 844*
◆ **Zaditor® [OTC]** *see* Ketotifen *on page 844*
◆ **Zaditor® (Can)** *see* Ketotifen *on page 844*

Zafirlukast (za FIR loo kast)

U.S. Brand Names Accolate®

Canadian Brand Names Accolate®

Index Terms ICI-204,219

Pharmacologic Category Leukotriene-Receptor Antagonist

Additional Appendix Information

Asthma *on page 1793*

Use Prophylaxis and chronic treatment of asthma in adults and children ≥5 years of age

Pregnancy Risk Factor B

Pregnancy Considerations There are no adequate and well-controlled trials in pregnant women. Teratogenic effects not observed in animal studies; fetal defects were observed when administered in maternally toxic doses.

Lactation Enters breast milk/contraindicated

Medication Safety Issues

Sound-alike/look-alike issues:

Accolate® may be confused with Accupril®, Accutane®, Aclovate®

Contraindications Hypersensitivity to zafirlukast or any component of the formulation

Warnings/Precautions Zafirlukast is not FDA approved for use in the reversal of bronchospasm in acute asthma attacks, including status asthmaticus. Therapy with zafirlukast can be continued during acute exacerbations of asthma.

Hepatic adverse events (including hepatitis, hyperbilirubinemia, and hepatic failure) have been reported; female patients may be at greater risk. Discontinue immediately if liver dysfunction is suspected. Periodic testing of liver function may be considered (early detection is generally believed to improve the likelihood of recovery). If hepatic dysfunction is suspected (due to clinical signs/symptoms), liver function tests should be measured immediately. Do not resume or restart if hepatic function studies are consistent with dysfunction. Use caution in patients with alcoholic cirrhosis; clearance is reduced.

Rare cases of eosinophilic vasculitis (Churg-Strauss) have been reported in patients receiving zafirlukast (usually, but not always, associated with reduction in concurrent steroid dosage). No causal relationship established. Monitor for eosinophilic vasculitis, rash, pulmonary symptoms, cardiac symptoms, or neuropathy.

An increased proportion of zafirlukast patients >55 years of age reported infections as compared to placebo-treated patients. These infections were mostly mild or moderate in intensity and predominantly affected the respiratory tract. Infections occurred equally in both sexes, were dose-proportional to total milligrams of zafirlukast exposure, and were associated with coadministration of inhaled corticosteroids. Safety and efficacy have not been established in patients <5 years of age.

Adverse Reactions

>10%: Central nervous system: Headache (13%)

1% to 10%:

- Central nervous system: Dizziness (2%), pain (2%), fever (2%)
- Gastrointestinal: Nausea (3%), diarrhea (3%), abdominal pain (2%), vomiting (2%), dyspepsia (1%)
- Hepatic: ALT increased (2%)
- Neuromuscular & skeletal: Back pain (2%), myalgia (2%), weakness (2%)
- Miscellaneous: Infection (4%)

<1% (Limited to important or life-threatening): Agranulocytosis, angioedema, arthralgia, behavior/mood changes, bleeding, bruising, edema, eosinophilia (systemic), eosinophilic pneumonia, hepatic failure, hepatitis, hyperbilirubinemia, hypersensitivity reactions, insomnia, malaise, pruritus, rash, suicidality, suicide, urticaria, vasculitis with clinical features of Churg-Strauss syndrome (rare)

Drug Interactions

Metabolism/Transport Effects Substrate of CYP2C9 (major); **Inhibits** CYP1A2 (weak), 2C8 (weak), 2C9 (moderate), 2C19 (weak), 2D6 (weak), 3A4 (weak)

Avoid Concomitant Use There are no known interactions where it is recommended to avoid concomitant use.

Increased Effect/Toxicity

Zafirlukast may increase the levels/effects of: CYP2C9 Substrates (High risk); Vitamin K Antagonists

The levels/effects of Zafirlukast may be increased by: CYP2C9 Inhibitors (Moderate); CYP2C9 Inhibitors (Strong)

Decreased Effect

The levels/effects of Zafirlukast may be decreased by: CYP2C9 Inducers (Highly Effective); Erythromycin; Theophylline Derivatives

Ethanol/Nutrition/Herb Interactions Food: Decreases bioavailability of zafirlukast by 40%.

Stability Store tablets at controlled room temperature (20°C to 25°C; 68°F to 77°F). Protect from light and moisture; dispense in original airtight container.

Mechanism of Action Zafirlukast is a selectively and competitive leukotriene-receptor antagonist (LTRA) of leukotriene D4 and E4 (LTD4 and LTE4), components of slow-reacting substance of anaphylaxis (SRSA). Cysteinyl leukotriene production and receptor occupation have been correlated with the pathophysiology of asthma, including airway edema, smooth muscle constriction, and altered cellular activity associated with the inflammatory process, which contribute to the signs and symptoms of asthma.

Pharmacodynamics/Kinetics

Protein binding: >99%, primarily to albumin
Metabolism: Extensively hepatic via CYP2C9
Bioavailability: Reduced 40% with food
Half-life elimination: 10 hours
Time to peak, serum: 3 hours
Excretion: Urine (10%); feces

Dosage Oral:

Children <5 years: Safety and effectiveness have not been established
Children 5-11 years: 10 mg twice daily
Children ≥12 years and Adults: 20 mg twice daily
Elderly: The mean dose (mg/kg) normalized AUC and C_{max} increase and plasma clearance decreases with increasing age. In patients >65 years of age, there is a two- to threefold greater C_{max} and AUC compared to younger adults.

Dosing adjustment in renal impairment: Dosage adjustment not required.

Dosing adjustment in hepatic impairment: In patients with hepatic impairment (ie, biopsy-proven cirrhosis), there is a 50% to 60% greater C_{max} and AUC compared to normal subjects.

Dietary Considerations Should be taken on an empty stomach (1 hour before or 2 hours after meals).

Administration Administer at least 1 hour before or 2 hours after a meal.

Monitoring Parameters Monitor for improvements in air flow; monitor closely for sign/symptoms of hepatic injury; periodic monitoring of LFTs may be considered (not proved to prevent serious injury, but early detection may enhance recovery)

Dosage Forms Excipient information presented when available (limited, particularly for generics); consult specific product labeling.

Tablet: 10 mg, 20 mg

Zaleplon (ZAL e plon)

U.S. Brand Names Sonata®

Pharmacologic Category Hypnotic, Nonbenzodiazepine

Use Short-term (7-10 days) treatment of insomnia (has been demonstrated to be effective for up to 5 weeks in controlled trial)

Restrictions C-IV

An FDA-approved patient medication guide is available and must be distributed when dispensing an outpatient prescription (new or refill) where this medication is to be used without direct supervision of a healthcare provider. Medication guides are available at http://www.fda.gov/cder/Offices/ODS/medication_guides.htm.

Pregnancy Risk Factor C

Pregnancy Considerations Not recommended for use during pregnancy

Lactation Enters breast milk/not recommended

Contraindications Hypersensitivity to zaleplon or any component of the formulation

Warnings/Precautions Symptomatic treatment of insomnia should be initiated only after careful evaluation of potential causes of sleep disturbance. Failure of sleep disturbance to resolve after 7-10 days may indicate psychiatric and/or medical illness.

Use with caution in patients with depression, particularly if suicidal risk may be present. Use with caution in patients with a history of drug dependence. Abrupt discontinuance may lead to withdrawal symptoms. Hypnotics/sedatives have been associated with abnormal thinking and behavior changes including decreased inhibition, aggression, bizarre behavior, agitation, hallucinations, and depersonalization. These changes may occur unpredictably and may indicate previously unrecognized psychiatric disorders; evaluate appropriately. May impair physical and mental capabilities. Patients must be cautioned about performing tasks which require mental alertness (operating machinery or driving). Amnesia can occur. Use with caution in patients receiving other CNS depressants or psychoactive medications. Effects with other sedative drugs or ethanol may be potentiated. Postmarketing studies have indicated that the use of hypnotic/sedative agents for sleep has been associated with hypersensitivity reactions including anaphylaxis as well as angioedema. An increased risk for hazardous sleep-related activities such as sleep-driving;

cooking and eating food, and making phone calls while asleep have also been noted.

Use with caution in the elderly, those with compromised respiratory function, or hepatic impairment (dosage adjustment recommended in mild-to-moderate hepatic impairment; avoid use in severe impairment). Because of the rapid onset of action, zaleplon should be administered immediately prior to bedtime or after the patient has gone to bed and is having difficulty falling asleep. Capsules contain tartrazine (FDC yellow #5); avoid in patients with sensitivity (caution in patients with asthma). Safety and efficacy have not been established in children.

Adverse Reactions

>10 %: Central nervous system: Headache (30% to 42%)

1% to 10%:

Cardiovascular: Chest pain (≥1%), peripheral edema (≤1%)

Central nervous system: Dizziness (7% to 9%), somnolence (5% to 6%), amnesia (2% to 4%), depersonalization (<1% to 2%), hypoesthesia (<1% to 2%), malaise (<1% to 2%), abnormal thinking (≥1%), anxiety (≥1%), depression (≥1%), fever (≥1%), migraine (≥1%), nervousness (≥1%), confusion (≤1%), hallucination (≤1%), vertigo (≤1%)

Dermatologic: Pruritus (≥1%), rash (≥1%), photosensitivity reaction (≤1%)

Endocrine & metabolic: Dysmenorrhea (3% to 4%)

Gastrointestinal: Nausea (6% to 8%), abdominal pain (6%), anorexia (<1% to 2%), constipation (≥1%), dyspepsia (≥1%), taste perversion (≥1%), xerostomia (≥1%), colitis (up to 1%)

Neuromuscular & skeletal: Weakness (5% to 7%), paresthesia (3%), tremor (2%), arthralgia (≥1%), arthritis (≥1%), back pain (≥1%), myalgia (≥1%), hypertonia (1%)

Ocular: Eye pain (3% to 4%), abnormal vision (<1% to 2%), conjunctivitis (≥1%)

Otic: Hyperacusis (1% to 2%), ear pain (≤1%)

Respiratory: Bronchitis (≥1%), epistaxis (≤1%)

Miscellaneous: Parosmia (<1% to 2%)

<1% (Limited to important or life-threatening): Alopecia, ALT increased, anaphylaxis, angioedema, anemia, angina, AST increased, ataxia, bigeminy, bilirubinemia, bleeding gums, bundle branch block, cardiospasm, cerebral ischemia, cholelithiasis, circumoral paresthesia, CNS stimulation; complex sleep-related behavior (sleep-driving, cooking or eating food, making phone calls); cyanosis, delusions, diabetes mellitus, duodenal ulcer, dysarthria, dystonia, dysuria, ecchymosis, eosinophilia, facial paralysis, gastroenteritis, glaucoma, goiter, hematuria, hyper-/hypoglycemia, hyper-/hypotension, hyperuricemia, hypothyroidism, impotence, incontinence, intestinal obstruction, ketosis, lactose intolerance, leukocytosis, lymphocytosis, liver function tests (abnormal), lymphadenopathy, myasthenia, myositis, osteoporosis, palpitation, peptic ulcer, pericardial effusion, photophobia, ptosis, pulmonary embolus, purpura, rash, rectal bleeding, sinus bradycardia, substernal chest pain, syncope, thrombophlebitis, tongue edema, ulcerative stomatitis, urinary retention, ventricular tachycardia, vasodilation, ventricular extrasystoles

Drug Interactions

Metabolism/Transport Effects **Substrate** of CYP3A4 (minor)

Avoid Concomitant Use There are no known interactions where it is recommended to avoid concomitant use.

Increased Effect/Toxicity

Zaleplon may increase the levels/effects of: Alcohol (Ethyl); CNS Depressants

The levels/effects of Zaleplon may be increased by: Cimetidine

Decreased Effect

The levels/effects of Zaleplon may be decreased by: Flumazenil; Rifamycin Derivatives

Ethanol/Nutrition/Herb Interactions

Ethanol: Avoid ethanol (may increase CNS depression).

Food: High fat meal prolonged absorption; delayed t_{max} by 2 hours, and reduced C_{max} by 35%.

Herb/Nutraceutical: St John's wort may decrease zaleplon levels. Avoid valerian, St John's wort, kava kava, gotu kola (may increase CNS depression).

Stability Store at controlled room temperature of 20°C to 25°C (68°F to 77°F). Protect from light.

Mechanism of Action Zaleplon is unrelated to benzodiazepines, barbiturates, or other hypnotics. However, it interacts with the benzodiazepine GABA receptor complex. Nonclinical studies have shown that it binds selectively to the brain omega-1 receptor situated on the alpha subunit of the GABA-A receptor complex.

Pharmacodynamics/Kinetics

Onset of action: Rapid

Duration: 6-8 hours

Absorption: Rapid and almost complete; high-fat meal delays absorption

Distribution: V_d: ~1.4 L/kg

Protein binding: ~45% to 75%

Metabolism: Extensive, primarily via aldehyde oxidase to form 5-oxo-zaleplon and, to a lesser extent, by CYP3A4 to desethylzaleplon; all metabolites are pharmacologically inactive

Bioavailability: ~30%

Half-life elimination: 1 hour

Time to peak, serum: 1 hour

Excretion: Urine (~70% primarily metabolites, <1% as unchanged drug); feces (~17%)

Clearance: Plasma: Oral: 3 L/hour/kg

Dosage Oral:

Adults: 10 mg at bedtime (range: 5-20 mg); has been used for up to 5 weeks of treatment in controlled trial setting

Elderly: 5 mg at bedtime; recommended maximum: 10 mg/day

Dosage adjustment in renal impairment: No adjustment for mild-to-moderate renal impairment; use in severe renal impairment has not been adequately studied

Dosage adjustment in hepatic impairment: Mild-to-moderate impairment: 5 mg; not recommended for use in patients with severe hepatic impairment

Dietary Considerations Avoid taking with or after a heavy, high-fat meal; reduces absorption.

Administration Immediately before bedtime or when the patient is in bed and cannot fall asleep

Additional Information Prescription quantities should not exceed a 1-month supply.

Dosage Forms Excipient information presented when available (limited, particularly for generics); consult specific product labeling.

Capsule: 5 mg, 10 mg

Sonata®: 5 mg, 10 mg [contains tartrazine]

◆ **Zamicet®** *see* Hydrocodone and Acetaminophen *on page 740*

◆ **Zanaflex®** *see* TiZANidine *on page 1480*

◆ **Zanaflex Capsules™** *see* TiZANidine *on page 1480*

Zanamivir (za NA mi veer)

U.S. Brand Names Relenza®

Canadian Brand Names Relenza®

Pharmacologic Category Antiviral Agent; Neuraminidase Inhibitor

Use Treatment of uncomplicated acute illness due to influenza virus A and B in patients who have been symptomatic for no more than 2 days; prophylaxis against influenza virus A and B

The Advisory Committee on Immunization Practices (ACIP) recommends that **treatment** be considered for the following:

- Persons hospitalized with laboratory confirmed influenza (may also have benefit if started >48 hours after onset of illness).
- Persons with laboratory confirmed influenza pneumonia.
- Persons with laboratory confirmed influenza and bacterial infections.
- Persons with laboratory confirmed influenza and who are at higher risk for influenza complications.
- Persons presenting for care within 48 hours of laboratory confirmed influenza onset and who want to decrease duration and/or severity of their symptoms or decrease the risk of transmission to those at high risk for complications.

The ACIP recommends that **prophylaxis** be considered for the following:

- Persons at high risk for influenza infection during the first 2 weeks following vaccination (eg, children <9 years and not previously vaccinated) if the virus is circulating in the community.
- Persons at high risk for influenza infection, but the vaccination is contraindicated.
- Unvaccinated family members or healthcare providers with prolonged exposure to or close contact with high-risk persons, unvaccinated persons, or infants <6 months of age.
- Persons at high risk for influenza infection, their family members and close contacts, and healthcare workers when the circulating strain of influenza is not matched with the vaccine.
- Persons with immune deficiency or those who may not respond to vaccination.
- Unvaccinated staff and persons during response to an outbreak in a closed institutional setting that has patients at high risk for infection (eg, extended care facilities).

Pregnancy Risk Factor C

Pregnancy Considerations Zanamivir has been shown to cross the placenta in animal models, however, no evidence of fetal malformations has been demonstrated. There are no adequate and well-controlled studies in pregnant women.

Lactation Excretion in breast milk unknown/use caution

Contraindications Hypersensitivity to zanamivir or any component of the formulation

Warnings/Precautions Allergic-like reactions, including anaphylaxis, oropharyngeal edema, and serious skin rashes have been reported. Rare occurrences of neuropsychiatric events (including confusion, delirium, hallucinations, and/or self-injury) have been reported from postmarketing surveillance; direct causation is difficult to establish (influenza infection may also be associated with behavioral and neurologic changes). Patients must be instructed in the use of the delivery system. No data are available to support the use of this drug in patients who begin use for treatment after 48 hours of symptoms. Effectiveness has not been established in patients with significant underlying medical conditions or for prophylaxis of influenza in nursing home patients. Not recommended for use in patients with underlying respiratory disease, such as asthma or COPD, due to lack of efficacy and risk of serious adverse effects. Bronchospasm, decreased lung function, and other serious adverse reactions, including those with fatal outcomes, have been reported in patients with and without airway disease; discontinue with bronchospasm or signs of decreased lung function. For a patient with an underlying airway disease where a medical decision has been made to use zanamivir, a fast-acting bronchodilator should be made available, and used prior to each dose. Not a substitute for annual flu vaccination; has not been shown to reduce risk of transmission of influenza to others. Consider primary or concomitant bacterial infections. Powder for oral inhalation contains lactose. Safety and efficacy of repeated courses or use with severe renal impairment have not been established. Indicated for children ≥5 years of age (for influenza prophylaxis) and children ≥7 years of age (for influenza treatment); children ages 5-6 years may have inadequate inhalation (via Diskhaler®) for the treatment of influenza.

Adverse Reactions Most adverse reactions occurred at a frequency which was less than or equal to the control (lactose vehicle).

>10%:

Central nervous system: Headache (prophylaxis 13% to 24%; treatment 2%)

Gastrointestinal: Throat/tonsil discomfort/pain (prophylaxis 8% to 19%)

Respiratory: Nasal signs and symptoms (prophylaxis 12% to 20%; treatment 2%), cough (prophylaxis 7% to 17%; treatment ≤2%)

Miscellaneous: Viral infection (prophylaxis 3% to 13%)

1% to 10%:

Central nervous system: Fever/chills (prophylaxis 5% to 9%; treatment <1.5%), fatigue (prophylaxis 5% to 8%; treatment <1.5%), malaise (prophylaxis 5% to 8%; treatment <1.5%), dizziness (treatment 1% to 2%)

Dermatologic: Urticaria (treatment <1.5%)

Gastrointestinal: Anorexia/appetite decreased (prophylaxis 2% to 4%), appetite increased (prophylaxis 2% to 4%), nausea (prophylaxis 1% to 2%; treatment ≤3%), diarrhea (prophylaxis 2%; treatment 2% to 3%), vomiting (prophylaxis 1% to 2%; treatment 1% to 2%), abdominal pain (treatment <1.5%)

Neuromuscular & skeletal: Muscle pain (prophylaxis 3% to 8%), musculoskeletal pain (prophylaxis 6%), arthralgia/articular rheumatism (prophylaxis 2%), arthralgia (treatment <1.5%), myalgia (treatment <1.5%)

Respiratory: Infection (ear/nose/throat; prophylaxis 2%; treatment 1% to 5%), sinusitis (treatment 3%), bronchitis (treatment 2%), nasal inflammation (prophylaxis 1%)

<1% (Limited to important or life-threatening): Abnormal behavior, agitation, allergic or allergic-like reaction (including oropharyngeal edema), anxiety, arrhythmia, asthma, bronchospasm, confusion, consciousness altered, delirium, delusions, dyspnea, facial edema, hallucination, hemorrhage (ear/nose/throat), nightmares, rash (including serious cutaneous reactions), seizure, syncope

Drug Interactions

Avoid Concomitant Use There are no known interactions where it is recommended to avoid concomitant use.

Increased Effect/Toxicity There are no known significant interactions involving an increase in effect.

Decreased Effect

Zanamivir may decrease the levels/effects of: Influenza Virus Vaccine

Stability Store at controlled room temperature (25°C) 77°F. Do not puncture blister until taking a dose using the Diskhaler®.

Mechanism of Action Zanamivir inhibits influenza virus neuraminidase enzymes, potentially altering virus particle aggregation and release.

Pharmacodynamics/Kinetics

Absorption: Inhalation: ~4% to 17%

Protein binding, plasma: <10%

Metabolism: None

Half-life elimination, serum: 2.5-5.1 hours

Excretion: Urine (as unchanged drug); feces (unabsorbed drug)

Dosage Oral inhalation:

Children ≥5 years and Adults: Prophylaxis (household setting): Two inhalations (10 mg) once daily for 10 days. Begin within 1½ days following onset of signs or symptoms of index case.

Children ≥7 years and Adults: Treatment: Two inhalations (10 mg total) twice daily for 5 days. Doses on first day should be separated by at least 2 hours; on subsequent days, doses should be spaced by ~12 hours. Begin within 2 days of signs or symptoms.

Adolescents and Adults: Prophylaxis (community outbreak): Two inhalations (10 mg) once daily for 28 days. Begin within 5 days of outbreak.

Administration Inhalation: Must be used with Diskhaler® delivery device. Patients who are scheduled to use an inhaled bronchodilator should use their bronchodilator prior to zanamivir. With the exception of the initial dose when used for treatment, administer at the same time each day.

Additional Information Majority of patients included in clinical trials were infected with influenza A, however, a number of patients with influenza B infections were also enrolled. Patients with lower temperature or less severe symptoms appeared to derive less benefit from therapy. No consistent treatment benefit was demonstrated in patients with chronic underlying medical conditions.

Dosage Forms Excipient information presented when available (limited, particularly for generics); consult specific product labeling.

Powder for oral inhalation: 5 mg/blister (20s) [4 blisters per Rotadisk® foil pack, 5 Rotadisk® per package; packaged with Diskhaler® inhalation device; contains lactose]

◆ **Zantac®** *see* Ranitidine *on page 1295*

◆ **Zantac 75® [OTC]** *see* Ranitidine *on page 1295*

◆ **Zantac 75® (Can)** *see* Ranitidine *on page 1295*

◆ **Zantac 150™ [OTC]** *see* Ranitidine *on page 1295*

◆ **Zantac® EFFERdose®** *see* Ranitidine *on page 1295*

◆ **Zantac Maximum Strength Non-Prescription (Can)** *see* Ranitidine *on page 1295*

◆ **Zarontin®** *see* Ethosuximide *on page 586*

◆ **Zaroxolyn®** *see* Metolazone *on page 981*

◆ **Zavesca®** *see* Miglustat *on page 996*

◆ **Zazole™** *see* Terconazole *on page 1443*

◆ **Z-Cof™ 12DM** *see* Guaifenesin, Pseudoephedrine, and Dextromethorphan *on page 715*

◆ **Z-Cof LA™** *see* Guaifenesin and Dextromethorphan *on page 710*

◆ **ZD1033** *see* Anastrozole *on page 116*

◆ **ZD1839** *see* Gefitinib *on page 683*

◆ **ZDV** *see* Zidovudine *on page 1581*

◆ **ZDV, Abacavir, and Lamivudine** *see* Abacavir, Lamivudine, and Zidovudine *on page 19*

◆ **Zeasorb®-AF [OTC]** *see* Miconazole *on page 989*

◆ **Zebeta®** *see* Bisoprolol *on page 200*

◆ **Zebutal™** *see* Butalbital, Acetaminophen, and Caffeine *on page 229*

◆ **Zegerid®** *see* Omeprazole and Sodium Bicarbonate *on page 1102*

◆ **Zelapar™** *see* Selegiline *on page 1359*

◆ **Zeldox** *see* Ziprasidone *on page 1585*

◆ **Zeldox® (Can)** *see* Ziprasidone *on page 1585*

◆ **Zelnorm®** *see* Tegaserod *on page 1428*

◆ **Zelnorm® [DSC] (Can)** *see* Tegaserod *on page 1428*

◆ **Zemplar®** *see* Paricalcitol *on page 1144*

◆ **Zemuron®** *see* Rocuronium *on page 1334*

◆ **Zenapax®** *see* Daclizumab *on page 389*

◆ **Zenchent™** *see* Ethinyl Estradiol and Norethindrone *on page 581*

◆ **Zeneca 182,780** *see* Fulvestrant *on page 675*

◆ **Zerit®** *see* Stavudine *on page 1398*

◆ **Zestoretic®** *see* Lisinopril and Hydrochlorothiazide *on page 896*

◆ **Zestril®** *see* Lisinopril *on page 894*

◆ **Zetia®** *see* Ezetimibe *on page 597*

◆ **Zevalin®** *see* Ibritumomab *on page 758*

◆ **Zgesic** *see* Acetaminophen and Phenyltoloxamine *on page 29*

◆ **Ziac®** *see* Bisoprolol and Hydrochlorothiazide *on page 201*

◆ **Ziagen®** *see* Abacavir *on page 18*

◆ **Ziana™** *see* Clindamycin and Tretinoin *on page 347*

Ziconotide (zi KOE no tide)

U.S. Brand Names Prialt®

Pharmacologic Category Analgesic, Nonopioid; Calcium Channel Blocker, N-Type

Use Management of severe chronic pain in patients requiring intrathecal (I.T.) therapy and who are intolerant or refractory to other therapies

Pregnancy Risk Factor C

Pregnancy Considerations Teratogenic effects were not observed in animal studies, but increased postimplantation pup loss was reported. Maternal toxicity was also noted. There are no adequate and well-controlled studies in pregnant women.

Lactation Excretion in breast milk unknown/not recommended

Medication Safety Issues

High alert medication: The Institute for Safe Medication Practices (ISMP) includes this medication among its list of drugs which have a heightened risk of causing significant patient harm when used in error.

Contraindications Hypersensitivity to ziconotide or any component of the formulation; history of psychosis; I.V. administration

I.T. administration is contraindicated in patients with infection at the injection site, uncontrolled bleeding, or spinal canal obstruction that impairs CSF circulation

Warnings/Precautions [U.S Boxed Warning]: Severe psychiatric symptoms and neurological impairment have been reported; interrupt or discontinue therapy if cognitive impairment, hallucinations, mood changes, or changes in consciousness occur. May cause or worsen depression and/or risk of suicide. Cognitive impairment may appear gradually during treatment and is generally reversible after discontinuation (may take up to 2 weeks for cognitive effects to reverse). Use caution in the elderly; may experience a higher incidence of confusion. Patients should be instructed to use caution in performing tasks which require alertness (eg, operating machinery or driving). May have additive effects with opiates or other CNS-depressant medications; may potentiate opioid-induced decreased GI motility; does not interact with opioid receptors or potentiate opiate-induced respiratory depression. Will not prevent or relieve symptoms associated with opiate withdrawal and opiates should not be abruptly discontinued. Unlike opioids, ziconotide therapy can be interrupted abruptly or discontinued without evidence of withdrawal.

Meningitis may occur with use of I.T. pumps; monitor for signs and symptoms of meningitis; treatment of meningitis may require removal of system and discontinuation of intrathecal therapy. Elevated serum creatine kinase can occur, particularly during the first 2 months of therapy;

consider dose reduction or discontinuing if combined with new neuromuscular symptoms (myalgias, myasthenia, muscle cramps, weakness) or reduction in physical activity. Safety and efficacy have not been established with renal or hepatic dysfunction, or in pediatric patients. Should not be used in combination with intrathecal opiates.

Adverse Reactions

>10%:

Central nervous system: Dizziness (46%), confusion (15% to 33%), memory impairment (7% to 22%), somnolence (17%), ataxia (14%), speech disorder (14%), headache (13%), aphasia (12%), hallucination (12%; including auditory and visual)

Gastrointestinal: Nausea (40%), diarrhea (18%), vomiting (16%)

Neuromuscular & skeletal: Creatine kinase increased (40%; ≥3 times ULN: 11%), weakness (18%), gait disturbances (14%)

Ocular: Blurred vision (12%)

2% to 10%:

Cardiovascular: Hypotension, peripheral edema, postural hypotension

Central nervous system: Abnormal thinking (8%), amnesia (8%), anxiety (8%), vertigo (7%), insomnia (6%), fever (5%), paranoid reaction (3%), delirium (2%), hostility (2%), stupor (2%), agitation, attention disturbance, balance impaired, burning sensation, coordination abnormal, depression, disorientation, fatigue, fever, hypoesthesia, irritability, lethargy, mental impairment, mood disorder, nervousness, pain, sedation

Dermatologic: Pruritus (7%)

Gastrointestinal: Anorexia (6%), taste perversion (5%), abdominal pain, appetite decreased, constipation, xerostomia

Genitourinary: Urinary retention (9%), dysuria, urinary hesitance

Neuromuscular & skeletal: Dysarthria (7%), paresthesia (7%), rigors (7%), tremor (7%), muscle spasm (6%), limb pain (5%), areflexia, muscle cramp, muscle weakness, myalgia

Ocular: Nystagmus (8%), diplopia, visual disturbance

Respiratory: Sinusitis (5%)

Miscellaneous: Diaphoresis (5%)

<2% (Limited to important or life-threatening): Acute renal failure, aspiration pneumonia (<1%), atrial fibrillation, cerebral vascular accident, ECG abnormalities, incoherence, loss of consciousness, mania, meningitis, myoclonus, psychosis (1%), psychotic disorder, respiratory distress, rhabdomyolysis, seizure (clonic and grand mal), sepsis, suicidal ideation, suicide attempt (<1%)

Drug Interactions

Avoid Concomitant Use There are no known interactions where it is recommended to avoid concomitant use.

Increased Effect/Toxicity

Ziconotide may increase the levels/effects of: Alcohol (Ethyl); CNS Depressants

Decreased Effect There are no known significant interactions involving a decrease in effect.

Ethanol/Nutrition/Herb Interactions Ethanol: Avoid ethanol (may increase CNS adverse effects).

Stability Prior to use, store vials at 2°C to 8°C (36°F to 46°F). Once diluted, may be stored at 2°C to 8°C (36°F to 46°F) for 24 hours; refrigerate during transit. Do not freeze. Protect from light.

Preservative free NS should be used when dilution is needed.

CADD-Micro® ambulatory infusion pump: Initial fill: Dilute to final concentration of 5 mcg/mL.

Medtronic SynchroMed® EL or SynchroMed® II infusion system: Prior to initial fill, rinse internal pump surfaces with 2 mL ziconotide (25 mcg/mL), repeat twice. Only the 25 mcg/mL concentration (undiluted) should be used for initial pump fill. When using the Medtronic SynchroMed® EL or SynchroMed® II Infusion System, solutions expire as follows:

25 mcg/mL: Undiluted:

Initial fill: Use within 14 days.

Refill: Use within 84 days.

100 mcg/mL:

Undiluted: Refill: Use within 84 days.

Diluted: Refill: Use within 40 days.

Mechanism of Action Ziconotide selectively binds to N-type voltage-sensitive calcium channels located on the nociceptive afferent nerves of the dorsal horn in the spinal cord. This binding is thought to block N-type calcium channels, leading to a blockade of excitatory neurotransmitter release and reducing sensitivity to painful stimuli.

Pharmacodynamics/Kinetics

Distribution: I.T.: V_d: ~140 mL

Protein binding: ~50%

Metabolism: Metabolized via endopeptidases and exopeptidases present on multiple organs including kidney, liver, lung; degraded to peptide fragments and free amino acids

Half-life elimination: I.V.: 1-1.6 hours (plasma); I.T.: 2.9-6.5 hours (CSF)

Excretion: I.V.: Urine (<1%)

Dosage I.T.:

Adults: Chronic pain: Initial dose: ≤2.4 mcg/day (0.1 mcg/hour)

Dose may be titrated by ≤2.4 mcg/day (0.1 mcg/hour) at intervals ≤2-3 times/week to a maximum dose of 19.2 mcg/day (0.8 mcg/hour) by day 21; average dose at day 21: 6.9 mcg/day (0.29 mcg/hour). A faster titration should be used only if the urgent need for analgesia outweighs the possible risk to patient safety.

Dosage adjustment for toxicity:

Cognitive impairment: Reduce dose or discontinue. Effects are generally reversible within 3-15 days of discontinuation.

Reduced level of consciousness: Discontinue until event resolves.

CK elevation with neuromuscular symptoms: Consider dose reduction or discontinuation.

Elderly: Refer to adult dosing; use with caution.

Administration Not for I.V. administration. For I.T. administration only using Medtronic SynchroMed® EL, SynchroMed® II Infusion System, or CADD-Micro® ambulatory infusion pump.

Medtronic SynchroMed® EL or SynchroMed® II Infusion Systems:

Naive pump priming (first time use with ziconotide): Use 2 mL of undiluted ziconotide 25 mcg/mL solution to rinse the internal surfaces of the pump; repeat twice for a total of 3 rinses

Initial pump fill: Use only undiluted 25 mcg/mL solution and fill pump after priming. Following the initial fill only, adsorption on internal device surfaces will occur, requiring the use of the undiluted solution and refill within 14 days.

Pump refills: Contents should be emptied prior to refill. Subsequent pump refills should occur at least every 40 days if using diluted solution or at least every 84 days if using undiluted solution.

CADD-Micro® ambulatory infusion pump: Refer to manufacturers' manual for initial fill and refill instructions

Monitoring Parameters Monitor for psychiatric or neurological impairment; signs and symptoms of meningitis or other infection; serum CPK (every other week for first month then monthly); pain relief

Dosage Forms Excipient information presented when available (limited, particularly for generics); consult specific product labeling.

Injection, solution, as acetate [preservative free]:
Prialt®: 25 mcg/mL (20 mL); 100 mcg/mL (1 mL, 5 mL)

Zidovudine (zye DOE vyoo deen)

U.S. Brand Names Retrovir®

Canadian Brand Names Apo-Zidovudine®; AZT™; Retrovir®

Index Terms Azidothymidine; AZT (error-prone abbreviation); Compound S; ZDV

Pharmacologic Category Antiretroviral Agent, Reverse Transcriptase Inhibitor (Nucleoside)

Additional Appendix Information

Management of Healthcare Worker Exposures to HBV, HCV, and HIV *on page 1719*

Perinatal HIV Guidelines *on page 1730*

Use Treatment of HIV infection in combination with at least two other antiretroviral agents; prevention of maternal/fetal HIV transmission as monotherapy

Unlabeled/Investigational Use Postexposure prophylaxis for HIV exposure as part of a multidrug regimen

Pregnancy Risk Factor C

Pregnancy Considerations Zidovudine crosses the placenta. No increased risk of overall birth defects has been observed following 1st trimester exposure according to data collected by the antiretroviral pregnancy registry. The use of zidovudine reduces the maternal-fetal transmission of HIV by ~70% and should be considered for antenatal and intrapartum therapy whenever possible. The Perinatal HIV Guidelines Working Group considers zidovudine the preferred NRTI for use in combination regimens during pregnancy. In HIV-infected mothers not previously on antiretroviral therapy, treatment may be delayed until after 10-12 weeks gestation. Cases of lactic acidosis/hepatic steatosis syndrome have been reported in pregnant women receiving nucleoside analogues. It is not known if pregnancy itself potentiates this known side effect; however, pregnant women may be at increased risk of lactic acidosis and liver damage. Hepatic enzymes and electrolytes should be monitored frequently during the 3rd trimester of pregnancy in women receiving nucleoside analogues. Women in labor with an unknown HIV status should have a rapid HIV test. If the test is positive, begin I.V. zidovudine therapy. (If a postpartum confirmatory test is negative, zidovudine therapy in the infant can be stopped). Health professionals are encouraged to contact the antiretroviral pregnancy registry to monitor outcomes of pregnant women exposed to antiretroviral medications (1-800-258-4263 or www.APRegistry.com).

Lactation Enters breast milk/contraindicated

Medication Safety Issues

Sound-alike/look-alike issues:

Azidothymidine may be confused with azaTHIOprine, aztreonam

Retrovir® may be confused with acyclovir, ritonavir

AZT is an error-prone abbreviation (mistaken as azathioprine, aztreonam)

Contraindications Life-threatening hypersensitivity to zidovudine or any component of the formulation

Warnings/Precautions **[U.S. Boxed Warning]: Often associated with hematologic toxicity including granulocytopenia, severe anemia requiring transfusions, or (rarely) pancytopenia.** Use with caution in patients with bone marrow compromise (granulocytes <1000 cells/mm^3 or hemoglobin <9.5 mg/dL); dosage adjustment may be required in patients who develop anemia or neutropenia. **[U.S. Boxed Warning]: Lactic acidosis and severe hepatomegaly with steatosis have been reported, including fatal cases;** use with caution in patients with risk factors for liver disease (risk may be increased in obese patients or prolonged exposure) and suspend treatment with zidovudine in any patient who develops clinical or laboratory findings suggestive of lactic acidosis (transaminase elevation may/may not accompany hepatomegaly and steatosis). Use caution in combination with interferon alfa with or without ribavirin in HIV/HBV coinfected patients; monitor closely for hepatic decompensation, anemia, or neutropenia; dose reduction or discontinuation of interferon and/or ribavirin may be required if toxicity evident. **[U.S. Boxed Warning]: Prolonged use has been associated with symptomatic myopathy and myositis.** May cause redistribution of fat (eg, buffalo hump, peripheral wasting with increased abdominal girth, cushingoid appearance). Immune reconstitution syndrome may develop resulting in the occurrence of an inflammatory response to an indolent or residual opportunistic infection; further evaluation and treatment may be required. Reduce dose in patients with severe renal impairment.

Adverse Reactions As reported in adult patients with asymptomatic HIV infection. Frequency and severity may increase with advanced disease.

>10%:

Central nervous system: Headache (63%), malaise (53%)

Gastrointestinal: Nausea (51%), anorexia (20%), vomiting (17%)

1% to 10%:

Gastrointestinal: Constipation (6%)

Hematologic: Granulocytopenia (2%; onset 6-8 weeks), anemia (1%; onset 2-4 weeks)

Hepatic: Transaminases increased (1% to 3%)

Neuromuscular & skeletal: Weakness (9%)

Frequency not defined:

Cardiovascular: Cardiomyopathy, chest pain, syncope, vasculitis

Central nervous system: Anxiety, chills, confusion, depression, dizziness, fatigue, insomnia, loss of mental acuity, mania, seizure, somnolence, vertigo

Dermatologic: Pruritus, rash, skin/nail pigmentation changes, Stevens-Johnson syndrome, toxic epidermal necrolysis, urticaria

Endocrine & metabolic: Body fat redistribution, gynecomastia

Gastrointestinal: Abdominal cramps, abdominal pain, dyspepsia, dysphagia, flatulence, mouth ulcer, oral mucosa pigmentation, pancreatitis, taste perversion

Genitourinary: Urinary frequency, urinary hesitancy

Hematologic: Aplastic anemia, hemolytic anemia, leukopenia, lymphadenopathy, pancytopenia with marrow hypoplasia, pure red cell aplasia

Hepatic: Hepatitis, hepatomegaly with steatosis, hyperbilirubinemia, jaundice, lactic acidosis

Neuromuscular & skeletal: Arthralgia, back pain, CPK increased, LDH increased, musculoskeletal pain, myalgia, neuropathy, muscle spasm, myopathy, myositis, paresthesia, rhabdomyolysis, tremor

Ocular: Amblyopia, macular edema, photophobia

Otic: Hearing loss

Respiratory: Cough, dyspnea, rhinitis, sinusitis

Miscellaneous: Allergic reactions, anaphylaxis, angioedema, diaphoresis, flu-like syndrome, immune reconstitution syndrome

Drug Interactions

Metabolism/Transport Effects **Substrate** (minor) of CYP2A6, 2C9, 2C19, 3A4

Avoid Concomitant Use There are no known interactions where it is recommended to avoid concomitant use.

Increased Effect/Toxicity

The levels/effects of Zidovudine may be increased by: Acyclovir-Valacyclovir; DOXOrubicin; DOXOrubicin (Liposomal); Fluconazole; Ganciclovir-Valganciclovir;

Interferons; Methadone; Probenecid; Ribavirin; Valproic Acid

Decreased Effect

Zidovudine may decrease the levels/effects of: Stavudine

The levels/effects of Zidovudine may be decreased by: DOXOrubicin; DOXOrubicin (Liposomal); Protease Inhibitors; Rifamycin Derivatives

Stability Store undiluted vials at 15°C to 25°C (59°F to 77°F). Protect from light. Solution for injection should be diluted with D_5W to a concentration ≤4 mg/mL. The solution is physically and chemically stable for 24 hours at room temperature and 48 hours if refrigerated. Attempt to administer diluted solution within 8 hours if stored at room temperature or 24 hours if refrigerated to minimize potential for microbially-contaminated solutions.

Mechanism of Action Zidovudine is a thymidine analog which interferes with the HIV viral RNA-dependent DNA polymerase resulting in inhibition of viral replication; nucleoside reverse transcriptase inhibitor

Pharmacodynamics/Kinetics

Distribution: Significant penetration into the CSF; crosses placenta

V_d: 1-2.2 L/kg

Relative diffusion from blood into CSF: Adequate with or without inflammation (exceeds usual MICs)

CSF:blood level ratio: Normal meninges: ~60%

Protein binding: 25% to 38%

Metabolism: Hepatic via glucuronidation to inactive metabolites; extensive first-pass effect

Bioavailability: 54% to 74%

Half-life elimination: Terminal: 0.5-3 hours

Time to peak, serum: 30-90 minutes

Excretion:

Oral: Urine (72% to 74% as metabolites, 14% to 18% as unchanged drug)

I.V.: Urine (45% to 60% as metabolites, 18% to 29% as unchanged drug)

Dosage

Prevention of maternal-fetal HIV transmission: **Note:** Consider use of zidovudine in combination with nevirapine (and possibly lamivudine) in select situations (eg, infants born to mothers with suboptimal viral suppression at delivery, infants born to mothers with only intrapartum therapy or no therapy, or infants born to mothers with known antiretroviral drug-resistant virus) (AIDSinfo guidelines, July 2008).

Neonatal: **Note:** Dosing should begin 6-12 hours after birth and continue for the first 6 weeks of life.

Oral:

Full-term infants: 2 mg/kg/dose every 6 hours

Infants ≥30 weeks and <35 weeks gestation at birth: 2 mg/kg/dose every 12 hours; at 2 weeks of age, advance to 2 mg/kg/dose every 8 hours

Infants <30 weeks gestation at birth: 2 mg/kg/dose every 12 hours; at 4 weeks of age, advance to 2 mg/kg/dose every 8 hours

I.V.: Infants unable to receive oral dosing:

Full term: 1.5 mg/kg/dose every 6 hours

Infants ≥30 weeks and <35 weeks gestation at birth: 1.5 mg/kg/dose every 12 hours; at 2 weeks of age, advance to 1.5 mg/kg/dose every 8 hours

Infants <30 weeks gestation at birth: 1.5 mg/kg/dose every 12 hours; at 4 weeks of age, advance to 1.5 mg/kg/dose every 8 hours

Maternal: Oral (per AIDSinfo guidelines): 100 mg 5 times/day **or** 200 mg 3 times/day **or** 300 mg twice daily. Begin at 14-34 weeks gestation and continue until start of labor.

During labor and delivery, administer zidovudine I.V. at 2 mg/kg as loading dose followed by a continuous I.V. infusion of 1 mg/kg/hour until the umbilical cord is clamped

Treatment of HIV infection:

Children 6 weeks to 12 years:

Oral: Dose should be calculated by body weight (in kg) or body surface area and should not exceed the recommended adult dose. **Note:** Doses calculated by body weight may not be the same as those calculated by body surface area.

Dosing based on body surface area: 160 mg/m^2/dose every 8 hours **or** 240 mg/m^2 every 12 hours (maximum: 200 mg every 8 hours); some Working Group members use a dose of 180 mg/m^2 to 240 mg/m^2 every 12 hours when using in drug combinations with other antiretroviral compounds, but data on this dosing in children is limited.

Dosing based on weight:

4 to <9 kg: 12 mg/kg/dose twice daily **or** 8 mg/kg/dose 3 times a day

≥9 to <30 kg: 9 mg/kg/dose twice daily **or** 6 mg/kg/dose 3 times a day

≥30 kg: 300 mg twice daily **or** 200 mg 3 times a day

I.V. continuous infusion: 20 mg/m^2/hour

I.V. intermittent infusion: 120 mg/m^2/dose every 6 hours

Adults:

Oral: 300 mg twice daily or 200 mg 3 times/day

I.V.: 1 mg/kg/dose administered every 4 hours around-the-clock (5-6 doses/day)

Prevention of HIV following needlesticks (unlabeled use):

Oral: Adults: 200 mg 3 times/day plus lamivudine 150 mg twice daily; a protease inhibitor (eg, indinavir) may be added for high risk exposures; begin therapy within 2 hours of exposure if possible

Patients should receive I.V. therapy only until oral therapy can be administered

Dosing adjustment for hematologic toxicity: Consider dose interruption for significant anemia (hemoglobin <7.5 g/dL or >25% reduction from baseline) and/or neutropenia (granulocyte count <750 cells/mm^3 or >50% reduction from baseline) until evidence of recovery. Anemia associated with chronic zidovudine may warrant dose reduction.

Dosing adjustment in renal impairment: Cl_{cr} <15 mL/minute including hemo-/peritoneal dialysis: 100 mg (oral) or 1 mg/kg (I.V.) every 6-8 hours

Continuous arteriovenous or venovenous hemodiafiltration effects: Administer 100 mg every 8 hours

Dosing adjustment in hepatic impairment: Insufficient data to make dosing recommendation

Dietary Considerations May be taken without regard to food.

Administration

Oral: Administer around-the-clock to promote less variation in peak and trough serum levels; may be administered without regard to food

I.M.: Do not administer I.M.

I.V.: Avoid rapid infusion or bolus injection

Neonates: Infuse over 30 minutes

Adults: Infuse loading dose over 1 hour, followed by continuous infusion

Monitoring Parameters Monitor CBC and platelet count at least every 2 weeks, liver function tests, MCV, serum creatinine kinase, viral load, and CD4 count; observe for appearance of opportunistic infections

Additional Information Potential compliance problems, frequency of administration, and adverse effects should be discussed with patients before initiating therapy to help prevent the emergence of resistance.

Dosage Forms Excipient information presented when available (limited, particularly for generics); consult specific product labeling.

Capsule:

Retrovir®: 100 mg

Injection, solution [preservative free]:
Retrovir®: 10 mg/mL (20 mL)
Syrup:
Retrovir®: 50 mg/5 mL (240 mL) [contains sodium benzoate; strawberry flavor]
Tablet: 300 mg
Retrovir®: 300 mg

- **Zidovudine, Abacavir, and Lamivudine** *see* Abacavir, Lamivudine, and Zidovudine *on page 19*

Zidovudine and Lamivudine
(zye DOE vyoo deen & la MI vyoo deen)

U.S. Brand Names Combivir®
Canadian Brand Names Combivir®
Index Terms AZT + 3TC (error-prone abbreviation); Lamivudine and Zidovudine
Pharmacologic Category Antiretroviral Agent, Reverse Transcriptase Inhibitor (Nucleoside)
Additional Appendix Information
Antiretroviral Therapy for HIV Infection: Adults and Adolescents *on page 1758*
Management of Healthcare Worker Exposures to HBV, HCV, and HIV *on page 1719*
Use Treatment of HIV infection when therapy is warranted based on clinical and/or immunological evidence of disease progression
Pregnancy Risk Factor C
Medication Safety Issues
Sound-alike/look-alike issues:
Combivir® may be confused with Combivent®, Epivir®

AZT is an error-prone abbreviation (mistaken as azaTHIOprine, aztreonam)
Dosage Children ≥12 years and Adults: Oral: One tablet twice daily
Note: Because this is a fixed-dose combination product, avoid use in patients requiring dosage reduction including children <12 years of age, renally-impaired patients with a creatinine clearance ≤50 mL/minute, hepatic impairment, or those patients experiencing dose-limiting adverse effects.
Additional Information Complete prescribing information for this medication should be consulted for additional detail.
Dosage Forms Excipient information presented when available (limited, particularly for generics); consult specific product labeling.
Tablet:
Combivir®: Zidovudine 300 mg and lamivudine 150 mg

- **Zilactin® (Can)** *see* Lidocaine *on page 884*
- **Zilactin-L® [OTC]** *see* Lidocaine *on page 884*
- **Zilactin®-B [OTC]** *see* Benzocaine *on page 183*
- **Zilactin-B® (Can)** *see* Benzocaine *on page 183*
- **Zilactin Baby® (Can)** *see* Benzocaine *on page 183*
- **Zilactin Toothache and Gum Pain® [OTC]** *see* Benzocaine *on page 183*

Zileuton (zye LOO ton)

U.S. Brand Names Zyflo CR™; Zyflo® [DSC]
Pharmacologic Category 5-Lipoxygenase Inhibitor
Additional Appendix Information
Asthma *on page 1793*
Use Prophylaxis and chronic treatment of asthma in children ≥12 years of age and adults
Pregnancy Risk Factor C
Pregnancy Considerations In developmental studies, reduced body weight and increased skeletal variations were observed in rats. There are no adequate and well-controlled studies in pregnant women.
Lactation Excretion in breast milk unknown/not recommended
Contraindications Hypersensitivity to zileuton or any component of the formulation; active liver disease or transaminase elevations greater than or equal to three times the upper limit of normal (≥3 times ULN)
Warnings/Precautions Not FDA approved for the reversal of bronchospasm in acute asthma attacks, including status asthmaticus; therapy may be continued during acute asthma exacerbations. Hepatic adverse effects have been reported (elevated transaminase levels); females >65 years and patients with pre-existing elevated transaminases may be at greater risk. Serum ALT should be monitored. Discontinue zileuton and follow transaminases until normal if patients develop clinical signs/symptoms of liver dysfunction or with transaminase levels >5 times ULN (use caution with history of liver disease and/or in those patients who consume substantial quantities of ethanol). Safety and efficacy have not been established in children <12 years of age.
Adverse Reactions
>10%: Central nervous system: Headache (23% to 25%)
1% to 10%:
Central nervous system: Pain (8%)
Dermatologic: Rash
Gastrointestinal: Dyspepsia (8%), nausea (6%), abdominal pain (5%), diarrhea, vomiting
Hematologic: Leukopenia (1% to 3%)
Hepatic: ALT increased (2% to 3%)
Neuromuscular & skeletal: Asthenia (4%), myalgia (3%)
Respiratory: Pharyngitis, sinusitis, upper respiratory tract infection
Miscellaneous: Hypersensitivity reactions

Frequency not defined:
Cardiovascular: Chest pain
Central nervous system: Dizziness, fever, insomnia, malaise, nervousness, somnolence
Dermatologic: Pruritus
Gastrointestinal: Constipation, flatulence
Genitourinary: Urinary tract infection, vaginitis
Neuromuscular & skeletal: Arthralgia, hypertonia, neck pain/rigidity
Ocular: Conjunctivitis
Miscellaneous: Lymphadenopathy
Postmarketing and/or case reports: Behavior/mood changes, hepatitis, hyperbilirubinemia, jaundice, liver failure, suicidality, suicide, urticaria
Drug Interactions
Metabolism/Transport Effects Substrate (minor) of CYP1A2, 2C9, 3A4; **Inhibits** CYP1A2 (moderate)
Avoid Concomitant Use There are no known interactions where it is recommended to avoid concomitant use.
Increased Effect/Toxicity
Zileuton may increase the levels/effects of: Propranolol; Theophylline; Warfarin
Decreased Effect There are no known significant interactions involving a decrease in effect.
Ethanol/Nutrition/Herb Interactions
Ethanol: Avoid ethanol (may increase CNS depression; may increase risk of hepatic toxicity).
Food:
Zyflo CR™: Improved absorption when administered with food.
Zyflo®: Absorption not improved when taken with food.
Herb/Nutraceutical: St John's wort may decrease zileuton levels.
Stability Store tablets at 15°C to 30°C (59°F to 86°F). Protect from light.
Mechanism of Action Specific 5-lipoxygenase inhibitor which inhibits leukotriene formation. Leukotrienes augment

neutrophil and eosinophil migration, neutrophil and monocyte aggregation, leukocyte adhesion, increased capillary permeability, and smooth muscle contraction (which contribute to inflammation, edema, mucous secretion, and bronchoconstriction in the airway of the asthmatic.)

Pharmacodynamics/Kinetics
- Absorption: Rapid
- Distribution: 1.2 L/kg
- Protein binding: 93%
- Metabolism: Hepatic and gastrointestinal; zileuton and N-dehydroxylated metabolite can be metabolized by CYP1A2, 2C9, and 3A4
- Bioavailability: Unknown
- Half-life elimination: ~3 hours
- Time to peak, serum: 1.7 hours
- Excretion: Urine (~95% primarily as metabolites); feces (~2%)

Dosage Oral:
- Children <12 years: Safety and effectiveness have not been established
- Children ≥12 years and Adults:
  - Zyflo®: 600 mg 4 times/day
  - Zyflo CR™: 1200 mg twice daily.

Dosing adjustment in renal impairment: Adjustment not required in renal failure or with hemodialysis

Dosing adjustment in hepatic impairment: Contraindicated with hepatic dysfunction

Dietary Considerations Zyflo®: May be taken with or without food; Zyflo CR™: Take with food.

Administration Zyflo®: Administer without regard to meals (eg, with or without food). Zyflo CR™: Do not crush, cut, or chew tablet; administer with food.

Monitoring Parameters Evaluate hepatic transaminases at initiation of, and during therapy. Monitor serum ALT before treatment begins, once-a-month for the first 3 months, every 2-3 months for the remainder of the first year, and periodically thereafter for patients receiving long-term zileuton therapy. If symptoms of liver dysfunction (right upper quadrant pain, nausea, fatigue, lethargy, pruritus, jaundice, or "flu-like" symptoms) develop or transaminase elevations >5 times ULN occur, discontinue therapy and follow transaminase levels until normal.

Dosage Forms Excipient information presented when available (limited, particularly for generics); consult specific product labeling. [DSC] = Discontinued product
- Tablet:
  - Zyflo®: 600 mg [DSC]
- Tablet, extended release:
  - Zyflo CR™: 600 mg

◆ **Zinacef®** *see* Cefuroxime *on page* 288

◆ **Zincate®** *see* Zinc Sulfate *on page* 1584

Zinc Chloride (zink KLOR ide)

Pharmacologic Category Trace Element

Use Cofactor for replacement therapy to different enzymes; helps maintain normal growth rates, normal skin hydration, and senses of taste and smell

Pregnancy Risk Factor C

Dosage Clinical response may not occur for up to 6-8 weeks
- Supplemental to I.V. solutions:
  - Premature Infants <1500 g, up to 3 kg: 300 mcg/kg/day
  - Infants (full term) and Children ≤5 years: 100 mcg/kg/day
  - Adults:
    - Stable with fluid loss from small bowel: 12.2 mg zinc/L TPN or 17.1 mg zinc/kg (added to 1000 mL I.V. fluids) of stool or ileostomy output
    - Metabolically stable: 2.5-4 mg/day; add 2 mg/day for acute catabolic states

Additional Information Complete prescribing information for this medication should be consulted for additional detail.

Dosage Forms Excipient information presented when available (limited, particularly for generics); consult specific product labeling.
- Injection, solution [preservative free]: 1 mg/mL (10 mL, 50 mL)

Zinc Gelatin (zink JEL ah tin)

U.S. Brand Names Gelucast®

Index Terms Dome Paste Bandage; Unna's Boot; Unna's Paste; Zinc Gelatin Boot

Pharmacologic Category Topical Skin Product

Use As a protectant and to support varicosities and similar lesions of the lower limbs

Dosage Topical: Apply externally as an occlusive boot

Additional Information Complete prescribing information for this medication should be consulted for additional detail.

Dosage Forms Excipient information presented when available (limited, particularly for generics); consult specific product labeling.
- Bandage: 3" x 10 yards; 4" x 10 yards

◆ **Zinc Gelatin Boot** *see* Zinc Gelatin *on page* 1584

◆ **Zincofax® (Can)** *see* Zinc Oxide *on page* 1584

Zinc Oxide (zink OKS ide)

U.S. Brand Names Ammens® Medicated Deodorant [OTC]; Balmex® [OTC]; Boudreaux's® Butt Paste [OTC]; Critic-Aid Skin Care® [OTC]; Desitin® Creamy [OTC]; Desitin® [OTC]

Canadian Brand Names Zincofax®

Index Terms Base Ointment; Lassar's Zinc Paste

Pharmacologic Category Topical Skin Product

Use Protective coating for mild skin irritations and abrasions; soothing and protective ointment to promote healing of chapped skin, diaper rash

Dosage Infants, Children, and Adults: Topical: Apply as required for affected areas several times daily

Additional Information Complete prescribing information for this medication should be consulted for additional detail.

Dosage Forms Excipient information presented when available (limited, particularly for generics); consult specific product labeling.
- Cream:
  - Balmex®: 11.3% (60 g, 120 g, 480 g) [contains aloe and vitamin E]
- Ointment, topical: 20% (30 g, 60 g, 454 g); 40% (120 g)
  - Desitin®: 40% (30 g, 60 g, 90 g, 120 g, 270 g, 480 g) [contains cod liver oil and lanolin]
  - Desitin® Creamy: 10% (60 g, 120 g)
- Paste, topical:
  - Boudreaux's® Butt Paste: 16% (30 g, 60 g, 120 g, 480 g) [contains castor oil, boric acid, mineral oil, and Peruvian balsam]
  - Critic-Aid Skin Care®: 20% (71 g, 170 g)
- Powder, topical (Ammens® Medicated Deodorant): 9.1% (187.5 g, 330 g) [original and shower fresh scent]

◆ **Zinc Oxide and Miconazole Nitrate** *see* Miconazole and Zinc Oxide *on page* 990

Zinc Sulfate (zink SUL fate)

U.S. Brand Names Orazinc® [OTC]; Zincate®

Canadian Brand Names Anuzinc; Rivasol

Index Terms $ZnSO_4$ (error-prone abbreviation)

Pharmacologic Category Trace Element

Use Zinc supplement (oral and parenteral); may improve wound healing in those who are deficient

Pregnancy Risk Factor C

Medication Safety Issues

Sound-alike/look-alike issues:

$ZnSO_4$ is an error-prone abbreviation (mistaken as morphine sulfate)

Dosage

RDA: Oral:

Birth to 6 months: 3 mg elemental zinc/day

6-12 months: 5 mg elemental zinc/day

1-10 years: 10 mg elemental zinc/day

≥11 years: 15 mg elemental zinc/day

Zinc deficiency: Oral:

Infants and Children: 0.5-1 mg elemental zinc/kg/day divided 1-3 times/day; somewhat larger quantities may be needed if there is impaired intestinal absorption or an excessive loss of zinc

Adults: 110-220 mg zinc sulfate (25-50 mg elemental zinc)/dose 3 times/day

Parenteral TPN: I.V.:

Infants (premature, birth weight <1500 g up to 3 kg): 300 mcg/kg/day

Infants (full term) and Children ≤5 years: 100 mcg/kg/day

Adults:

Acute metabolic states: 4.5-6 mg/day

Metabolically stable: 2.5-4 mg/day

Stable with fluid loss from the small bowel: 12.2 mg zinc/L of TPN solution, or an additional 17.1 mg zinc (added to 1000 mL I.V. fluids) per kg of stool or ileostomy output

Additional Information Complete prescribing information for this medication should be consulted for additional detail.

Dosage Forms Excipient information presented when available (limited, particularly for generics); consult specific product labeling.

Capsule (Orazinc®, Zincate®): 220 mg [elemental zinc 50 mg]

Injection, solution [preservative free]: 1 mg elemental zinc/mL (10 mL); 5 mg elemental zinc/mL (5 mL)

Tablet (Orazinc®): 110 mg [elemental zinc 25 mg]

◆ **Zinecard®** *see* Dexrazoxane *on page 430*

◆ **Zingo™** *see* Lidocaine *on page 884*

◆ **Ziox™** *see* Chlorophyllin, Papain, and Urea *on page 306*

◆ **Ziox 405™** *see* Chlorophyllin, Papain, and Urea *on page 306*

Ziprasidone (zi PRAS i done)

U.S. Brand Names Geodon®

Canadian Brand Names Zeldox®

Index Terms Zeldox; Ziprasidone Hydrochloride; Ziprasidone Mesylate

Pharmacologic Category Antipsychotic Agent, Atypical

Additional Appendix Information

Antipsychotic Agents *on page 1644*

Use Treatment of schizophrenia; treatment of acute manic or mixed episodes associated with bipolar disorder with or without psychosis; acute agitation in patients with schizophrenia

Unlabeled/Investigational Use Tourette's syndrome; psychosis/agitation related to Alzheimer's dementia

Pregnancy Risk Factor C

Pregnancy Considerations Developmental toxicity demonstrated in animals. There are no adequate and well-controlled studies in pregnant women. Use only if potential benefit justifies risk to the fetus. Healthcare providers are encouraged to enroll women 18-45 years of age exposed to ziprasidone during pregnancy in the Atypical Antipsychotics Pregnancy Registry (1-866-961-2388).

Lactation Excretion in breast milk unknown/not recommended

Contraindications Hypersensitivity to ziprasidone or any component of the formulation; history (or current) prolonged QT; congenital long QT syndrome; recent myocardial infarction; history of arrhythmias; uncompensated heart failure; concurrent use of other QT_c-prolonging agents including amiodarone, arsenic trioxide, bretylium, chlorpromazine, cisapride, class Ia antiarrhythmics (quinidine, procainamide), dofetilide, dolasetron, droperidol, ibutilide, levomethadyl, mefloquine, mesoridazine, pentamidine, pimozide, probucol, some quinolone antibiotics (moxifloxacin), sotalol, tacrolimus, and thioridazine

Warnings/Precautions [U.S. Boxed Warning]: Elderly patients with dementia-related behavioral disorders treated with atypical antipsychotics are at an increased risk of death compared to placebo. An increased incidence of cerebrovascular adverse events (including fatalities) has been reported in elderly patients with dementia-related psychosis. Ziprasidone is not approved for this indication.

May result in QT_c prolongation (dose related), which has been associated with the development of malignant ventricular arrhythmias (torsade de pointes) and sudden death. Note contraindications related to this effect. Observed prolongation was greater than with other atypical antipsychotic agents (risperidone, olanzapine, quetiapine), but less than with thioridazine. Avoid hypokalemia, hypomagnesemia. Use caution in patients with bradycardia. Discontinue in patients found to have persistent QT_c intervals >500 msec. Patients with symptoms of dizziness, palpitations, or syncope should receive further cardiac evaluation. May cause orthostatic hypotension.

May cause extrapyramidal symptoms (EPS). Risk of dystonia (and probably other EPS) may be greater with increased doses, use of conventional antipsychotics, males, and younger patients. Impaired core body temperature regulation may occur; caution with strenuous exercise, heat exposure, dehydration, and concomitant medication possessing anticholinergic effects; not reported in premarketing trials of ziprasidone. Antipsychotic use may also be associated with neuroleptic malignant syndrome (NMS). Use with caution in patients at risk of seizures.

Atypical antipsychotics have been associated with development of hyperglycemia. There is limited documentation with ziprasidone and specific risk associated with this agent is not known. Use caution in patients with diabetes or other disorders of glucose regulation; monitor for worsening of glucose control.

Cognitive and/or motor impairment (sedation) is common with ziprasidone. Use with caution in disorders where CNS depression is a feature. Use with caution in Parkinson's disease. Antipsychotic use has been associated with esophageal dysmotility and aspiration; use with caution in patients at risk of pneumonia (ie, Alzheimer's disease). Caution in breast cancer or other prolactin-dependent tumors; elevates prolactin levels. Use caution in renal or hepatic impairment. Ziprasidone has been associated with a fairly high incidence of rash (5%). Significant weight gain has been observed with antipsychotic therapy; incidence varies with product. Monitor waist circumference and BMI. Safety and efficacy have not been established in pediatric patients.

The possibility of a suicide attempt is inherent in psychotic illness or bipolar disorder; use caution in high-risk patients during initiation of therapy. Prescriptions should be written for the smallest quantity consistent with good patient care.

Adverse Reactions Note: Although minor QT_c prolongation (mean: 10 msec at 160 mg/day) may occur more frequently (incidence not specified), clinically-relevant prolongation (>500 msec) was rare (0.06%) and less than placebo (0.23%).

>10%:

Central nervous system: Extrapyramidal symptoms (2% to 31%), somnolence (8% to 31%), headache (3% to 18%), dizziness (3% to 16%)

Gastrointestinal: Nausea (4% to 12%)

1% to 10%:

Cardiovascular: Chest pain (5%), postural hypotension (5%), hypertension (2% to 3%), bradycardia (2%), tachycardia (2%), vasodilation (1%), facial edema, orthostatic hypotension

Central nervous system: Akathisia (2% to 10%), anxiety (2% to 5%), insomnia (3%), agitation (2%), speech disorder (2%), personality disorder (2%), psychosis (1%), akinesia, amnesia, ataxia, chills, confusion, coordination abnormal, delirium, dystonia, fever, hostility, hypothermia, oculogyric crisis, vertigo

Dermatologic: Rash (4%), fungal dermatitis (2%)

Endocrine & metabolic: Dysmenorrhea (2%)

Gastrointestinal: Weight gain (10%), constipation (2% to 9%), dyspepsia (1% to 8%), diarrhea (3% to 5%), vomiting (3% to 5%), salivation increased (4%), xerostomia (1% to 5%), tongue edema (3%), abdominal pain (2%), anorexia (2%), dysphagia (2%), rectal hemorrhage (2%), tooth disorder (1%), buccoglossal syndrome

Genitourinary: Priapism (1%)

Local: Injection site pain (7% to 9%)

Neuromuscular & skeletal: Weakness (2% to 6%), hypoesthesia (2%), myalgia (2%), paresthesia (2%), back pain (1%), cogwheel rigidity (1%), hypertonia (1%), abnormal gait, choreoathetosis, dysarthria, dyskinesia, hyper-/hypokinesia, hypotonia, neuropathy, tremor, twitching

Ocular: Vision abnormal (3% to 6%), diplopia

Respiratory: Infection (8%), rhinitis (1% to 4%), cough (3%), pharyngitis (3%), dyspnea (2%)

Miscellaneous: Diaphoresis (2%), furunculosis (2%), flu-like syndrome (1%), photosensitivity reaction, withdrawal syndrome

<1% (Limited to important or life-threatening): Akinesia, allergic reaction, angina, atrial fibrillation, ataxia, AV block (first degree), bundle branch block, cerebral infarction, cholestatic jaundice, choreoathetosis, delirium, dysarthria, dysphagia, eosinophilia, exfoliative dermatitis, galactorrhea, gout, gynecomastia, hemorrhage, hepatitis, jaundice, myocarditis, neuroleptic malignant syndrome, neuropathy, opisthotonos, photophobia, pneumonia, pulmonary embolism, QT_c prolongation >500 msec (0.06%), seizure (0.4%), sexual dysfunction (male and female), stroke, syncope (0.6%), tardive dyskinesia, tenosynovitis, thrombocytopenia, thyroiditis, torsade de pointes, torticollis, urinary retention

Drug Interactions

Metabolism/Transport Effects Substrate (minor) of CYP1A2, 3A4; **Inhibits** CYP2D6 (weak), 3A4 (weak)

Avoid Concomitant Use

Avoid concomitant use of Ziprasidone with any of the following: Nilotinib; QTc-Prolonging Agents; Thioridazine

Increased Effect/Toxicity

Ziprasidone may increase the levels/effects of: Alcohol (Ethyl); CNS Depressants; Thioridazine

The levels/effects of Ziprasidone may be increased by: Acetylcholinesterase Inhibitors (Central); Alfuzosin; Antifungal Agents (Azole Derivatives, Systemic); Ciprofloxacin; Gadobutrol; Lithium formulations; Nilotinib; QTc-Prolonging Agents; Tetrabenazine

Decreased Effect

Ziprasidone may decrease the levels/effects of: Amphetamines; Anti-Parkinson's Agents (Dopamine Agonist)

The levels/effects of Ziprasidone may be decreased by: CarBAMazepine; Lithium formulations

Ethanol/Nutrition/Herb Interactions

Ethanol: Avoid ethanol (may increase CNS depression).

Food: Administration with food increases serum levels twofold. Grapefruit juice may increase serum concentration of ziprasidone.

Herb/Nutraceutical: St John's wort may decrease serum levels of ziprasidone, due to a potential effect on CYP3A4. This has not been specifically studied. Avoid kava kava, chamomile (may increase CNS depression).

Stability

Capsule: Store at controlled room temperature of 15°C to 30°C (59°F to 86°F).

Vials for injection: Store at controlled room temperature of 15°C to 30°C (59°F to 86°F). Protect from light. Each vial should be reconstituted with 1.2 mL SWI. Shake vigorously. Will form a pale, pink solution containing 20 mg/mL ziprasidone. Following reconstitution, injection may be stored at room temperature up to 24 hours or up to 7 days if refrigerated. Protect from light.

Mechanism of Action Ziprasidone is a benzylisothiazolylpiperazine antipsychotic. The exact mechanism of action is unknown. However, *in vitro* radioligand studies show that ziprasidone has high affinity for D_2, D_3, 5-HT_{2A}, 5-HT_{1A}, 5-HT_{2C}, 5-HT_{1D}, and alpha$_1$-adrenergic; moderate affinity for histamine H_1 receptors; and no appreciable affinity for alpha$_2$-adrenergic receptors, beta-adrenergic, 5-HT_3, 5-HT_4, cholinergic, mu, sigma, or benzodiazepine receptors. Ziprasidone functions as an antagonist at the D_2, 5-HT_{2A}, and 5-HT_{1D} receptors and as an agonist at the 5-HT_{1A} receptor. Ziprasidone moderately inhibits the reuptake of serotonin and norepinephrine.

Pharmacodynamics/Kinetics

Absorption: Well absorbed

Distribution: V_d: 1.5 L/kg

Protein binding: 99%, primarily to albumin and alpha$_1$-acid glycoprotein

Metabolism: Extensively hepatic, primarily via aldehyde oxidase; less than 1/3 of total metabolism via CYP3A4 and CYP1A2 (minor)

Bioavailability: Oral (with food): 60% (up to twofold increase with food); I.M.: 100%

Half-life elimination: Oral: 7 hours; I.M.: 2-5 hours

Time to peak: Oral: 6-8 hours; I.M.: ≤60 minutes

Excretion: Feces (66%) and urine (20%) as metabolites; little as unchanged drug (1% urine, 4% feces)

Clearance: 7.5 mL/minute/kg

Dosage

Children and Adolescents: Tourette's syndrome (unlabeled use): Oral: 5-40 mg/day

Adults:

Bipolar mania: Oral: Initial: 40 mg twice daily (with food)

Adjustment: May increase to 60 or 80 mg twice daily on second day of treatment; average dose 40-80 mg twice daily

Schizophrenia: Oral: Initial: 20 mg twice daily (with food)

Adjustment: Increases (if indicated) should be made no more frequently than every 2 days; ordinarily patients should be observed for improvement over several weeks before adjusting the dose

Maintenance: Range 20-100 mg twice daily; however, dosages >80 mg twice daily are generally not recommended

Acute agitation (schizophrenia): I.M.: 10 mg every 2 hours **or** 20 mg every 4 hours; maximum: 40 mg/day;

oral therapy should replace I.M. administration as soon as possible

Elderly: No dosage adjustment is recommended; consider initiating at a low end of the dosage range, with slower titration

Dosage adjustment in renal impairment:

Oral: No dosage adjustment is recommended

I.M.: Cyclodextrin, an excipient in the I.M. formulation, is cleared by renal filtration; use with caution.

Ziprasidone is not removed by hemodialysis.

Dosage adjustment in hepatic impairment: No dosage adjustment is recommended

Administration

Oral: Administer with food.

Injection: For I.M. administration only.

Monitoring Parameters Vital signs; serum potassium and magnesium; fasting lipid profile and fasting blood glucose/ Hgb A_{1c} (prior to treatment, at 3 months, then annually); BMI, personal/family history of obesity, waist circumference; blood pressure; mental status, abnormal involuntary movement scale (AIMS), extrapyramidal symptoms. Weight should be assessed prior to treatment, at 4 weeks, 8 weeks, 12 weeks, and then at quarterly intervals. Consider titrating to a different antipsychotic agent for a weight gain ≥5% of the initial weight. The value of routine ECG screening or monitoring has not been established.

Test Interactions Increased cholesterol, triglycerides, eosinophils

Additional Information The increased potential to prolong QT_c, as compared to other available antipsychotic agents, should be considered in the evaluation of available alternatives.

Dosage Forms Excipient information presented when available (limited, particularly for generics); consult specific product labeling.

Capsule, as hydrochloride: 20 mg, 40 mg, 60 mg, 80 mg

Injection, powder for reconstitution, as mesylate: 20 mg

- ◆ **Ziprasidone Hydrochloride** *see* Ziprasidone *on page 1585*
- ◆ **Ziprasidone Mesylate** *see* Ziprasidone *on page 1585*
- ◆ **Zithromax®** *see* Azithromycin *on page 166*
- ◆ **Zithromax® TRI-PAK™** *see* Azithromycin *on page 166*
- ◆ **Zithromax® Z-PAK®** *see* Azithromycin *on page 166*
- ◆ **ZM-182,780** *see* Fulvestrant *on page 675*
- ◆ **Zmax®** *see* Azithromycin *on page 166*
- ◆ **$ZnSO_4$ (error-prone abbreviation)** *see* Zinc Sulfate *on page 1584*
- ◆ **Zocor®** *see* Simvastatin *on page 1370*
- ◆ **Zofran®** *see* Ondansetron *on page 1102*
- ◆ **Zofran® ODT** *see* Ondansetron *on page 1102*
- ◆ **Zoladex®** *see* Goserelin *on page 705*
- ◆ **Zoladex® LA (Can)** *see* Goserelin *on page 705*
- ◆ **Zoledronate** *see* Zoledronic Acid *on page 1587*

Zoledronic Acid (zoe le DRON ik AS id)

U.S. Brand Names Reclast®; Zometa®

Canadian Brand Names Aclasta®; Zometa®

Index Terms CGP-42446; NSC-721517; Zoledronate

Pharmacologic Category Antidote; Bisphosphonate Derivative

Use Treatment of hypercalcemia of malignancy (albumin-corrected serum calcium ≥12 mg/dL), multiple myeloma, bone metastases of solid tumors, Paget's disease of bone; osteoporosis (to reduce the incidence of fractures in postmenopausal women with osteoporosis or to reduce the incidence of new clinical fractures in patients with low-trauma hip fracture)

Unlabeled/Investigational Use Prevention of bone loss associated with aromatase inhibitor therapy in postmenopausal women with breast cancer; prevention of bone loss associated with androgen deprivation therapy in prostate cancer

Pregnancy Risk Factor D

Pregnancy Considerations Animal studies resulted in embryotoxicity and losses. Zoledronic acid should not be used during pregnancy; may cause fetal harm if administered to a pregnant woman. Bisphosphonates are incorporated into the bone matrix and gradually released over time. Theoretically, there may be a risk of fetal harm when pregnancy follows the completion of therapy. Based on limited case reports with pamidronate, serum calcium levels in the newborn may be altered if administered during pregnancy.

Lactation Excretion in breast milk unknown/not recommended

Medication Safety Issues

Sound-alike/look-alike issues:

Zometa® may be confused with Zofran®, Zoladex®

Contraindications Hypersensitivity to zoledronic acid, other bisphosphonates, or any component of the formulation; hypocalcemia (Reclast®)

Note: In Canada, Aclasta® is also contraindicated with uncorrected hypocalcemia at the time of infusion and in pregnancy and breast-feeding.

Warnings/Precautions Bisphosphonate therapy has been associated with osteonecrosis, primarily of the jaw; this has been observed mostly in cancer patients, but also in patients with postmenopausal osteoporosis and other diagnoses. Dental exams and preventative dentistry should be performed prior to placing patients with risk factors on chronic bisphosphonate therapy. Invasive dental procedures should be avoided during treatment.

Infrequently, severe (and occasionally debilitating) bone, joint, and/or muscle pain have been reported during bisphosphonate treatment. The onset of pain ranged from a single day to several months. Symptoms usually resolve upon discontinuation. Some patients experienced recurrence when rechallenged with same drug or another bisphosphonate; avoid use in patients with a history of these symptoms in association with bisphosphonate therapy.

May cause hypocalcemia in patients with Paget's disease, in whom the pretreatment rate of bone turnover may be greatly elevated. Hypocalcemia must be corrected before initiation of therapy in patients with Paget's disease and osteoporosis. Ensure adequate calcium and vitamin D intake during therapy. Use caution in patients with disturbances of calcium and mineral metabolism (eg, hypoparathyroidism, thyroid surgery, malabsorption syndromes).

Reclast®: Use is not recommended in patients with severe renal impairment (Cl_{cr} <35 mL/minute). When used in the treatment of Paget's disease significant renal deterioration has not been observed with the usual 5 mg dose administered over at least 15 minutes.

Zometa®: Use caution in renal dysfunction; dosage adjustment required. In cancer patients, renal toxicity has been reported with doses >4 mg or infusions administered over 15 minutes. Risk factors for renal deterioration include pre-existing renal insufficiency and repeated doses of zoledronic acid and other bisphosphonates. Dehydration and the use of other nephrotoxic drugs which may contribute to renal deterioration should be identified and managed. Use is not recommended in patients with severe renal impairment (serum creatinine >3 mg/dL) and bone metastases (limited data); use in patients with hypercalcemia of malignancy and severe renal impairment should only be done if the benefits outweigh the risks. Renal function should be assessed prior to treatment; if decreased after treatment, additional treatments should be withheld until renal function returns to within 10% of baseline. Diuretics should not be used before correcting hypovolemia. Renal deterioration, resulting in renal failure and dialysis has occurred in patients treated with zoledronic acid after single and multiple infusions at recommended doses of 4 mg over 15 minutes.

Aclasta® [CAN; not available in U.S.]: Use is not recommended in patients with severe renal impairment (Cl_{cr} <30 mL/minute).

Adequate hydration is required during treatment (urine output ~2 L/day); avoid overhydration, especially in patients with heart failure. Dehydration and concurrent use of other nephrotoxic drugs may increase the risk for renal impairment. Use caution in patients with aspirin-sensitive asthma (may cause bronchoconstriction), hepatic dysfunction, and the elderly. Women of childbearing age should be advised against becoming pregnant. Not approved for use in children.

Adverse Reactions Note: An acute reaction (eg, arthralgia, fever, flu-like symptoms, myalgia) may occur within the first 3 days following infusion in up to 44% of patients; usually resolves within 3-4 days of onset, although may take up to 14 days to resolve. The incidence may be decreased with acetaminophen (prior to infusion and for 72 hours postinfusion).

Zometa®:

>10%:

Cardiovascular: Leg edema (5% to 21%), hypotension (11%)

Central nervous system: Fatigue (39%), fever (32% to 44%), headache (5% to 19%), dizziness (18%), insomnia (15% to 16%), anxiety (11% to 14%), depression (14%), agitation (13%), confusion (7% to 13%), hypoesthesia (12%)

Dermatologic: Alopecia (12%), dermatitis (11%)

Endocrine & metabolic: Dehydration (5% to 14%), hypophosphatemia (12% to 13%), hypokalemia (12%), hypomagnesemia (11%)

Gastrointestinal: Nausea (29% to 46%), constipation (27% to 31%), vomiting (14% to 32%), diarrhea (17% to 24%), anorexia (9% to 22%), abdominal pain (14% to 16%), weight loss (16%), appetite decreased (13%)

Genitourinary: Urinary tract infection (12% to 14%)

Hematologic: Anemia (22% to 33%), neutropenia (12%)

Neuromuscular & skeletal: Bone pain (55%), weakness (5% to 24%), myalgia (23%), arthralgia (5% to 21%), back pain (15%), paresthesia (15%), limb pain (14%), skeletal pain (12%), rigors (11%)

Renal: Renal deterioration (8% to 17%; up to 40% in patients with abnormal baseline creatinine)

Respiratory: Dyspnea (22% to 27%), cough (12% to 22%)

Miscellaneous: Cancer progression (16%), moniliasis (12%)

1% to 10%:

Cardiovascular: Chest pain (5% to 10%)

Central nervous system: Somnolence (5% to 10%)

Endocrine & metabolic: Hypocalcemia (5% to 10%; grades 3/4: ≤1%), hypermagnesemia (2%)

Gastrointestinal: Dysphagia (5% to 10%), dyspepsia (10%), mucositis (5% to 10%), stomatitis (8%), sore throat (8%)

Hematologic: Thrombocytopenia (5% to 10%), pancytopenia (5% to 10%), granulocytopenia (5% to 10%)

Renal: Serum creatinine increased (grades 3/4: 2%)

Respiratory: Pleural effusion, upper respiratory tract infection (10%)

Miscellaneous: Metastases (5% to 10%), nonspecific infection (5% to 10%)

Reclast®:

>10%:

Cardiovascular: Hypertension (7% to 13%)

Central nervous system: Fever (9% to 18%), headache (4% to 12%)

Neuromuscular & skeletal: Arthralgia (9% to 24%), myalgia (5% to 12%), limb pain (6% to 11%)

Miscellaneous: Flu-like syndrome (1% to 11%)

1% to 10%:

Cardiovascular: Peripheral edema (3% to 6%), atrial fibrillation (2% to 3%)

Central nervous system: Dizziness (2% to 9%), fatigue (2% to 8%), chills (2% to 5%), lethargy (5%), pain (2% to 5%), malaise (1% to 2%), hyperthermia (≤2%)

Dermatologic: Rash (3%)

Endocrine & metabolic: Hypocalcemia (≤3%)

Gastrointestinal: Nausea (5% to 9%), constipation (6%), diarrhea (5% to 6%), dyspepsia (2% to 5%), vomiting (2% to 5%), abdominal pain (1% to 5%), abdominal distension (2%), anorexia (1% to 2%)

Neuromuscular & skeletal: Bone pain (3% to 9%), rigors (8%), shoulder pain (≤7%), weakness (2% to 5%), back pain (4%), muscle spasm (2% to 4%), musculoskeletal pain (≤3%), muscle stiffness (2%), paresthesia (2%)

Renal: Serum creatinine increased (2%)

Respiratory: Dyspnea (5%)

Zometa® and/or Reclast®: <1% (Limited to important or life-threatening): Allergic reaction, anaphylactic reaction/shock, angioneurotic edema, arrhythmia, blurred vision, bradycardia, bronchoconstriction, conjunctivitis, diaphoresis, episcleritis; flu-like syndrome (fever, chills, flushing, bone pain, arthralgia, myalgia); hematuria, hyperesthesia, hyperkalemia, hypernatremia, hypersensitivity, hypertension; injection site reaction (eg, itching, pain, redness); iritis, joint and/or muscle pain (sometimes severe and/or incapacitating), muscle cramps, osteonecrosis (primarily of the jaws), proteinuria, pruritus, rash, renal failure, renal impairment, taste perversion, tremor, urticaria, uveitis, weight gain, xerostomia

Drug Interactions

Avoid Concomitant Use There are no known interactions where it is recommended to avoid concomitant use.

Increased Effect/Toxicity

Zoledronic Acid may increase the levels/effects of: Phosphate Supplements

The levels/effects of Zoledronic Acid may be increased by: Aminoglycosides; Nonsteroidal Anti-Inflammatory Agents; Thalidomide

Decreased Effect There are no known significant interactions involving a decrease in effect.

Stability

Aclasta® [CAN]: Store at room temperature of 15°C to 30°C (59°F to 86°F).

Reclast®: Store at room temperature of 25°C (77°F); excursions permitted to 15°C to 30°C (59°F to 86°F). After opening, stable for 24 hours at 2°C to 8°C (36°F to 46°F).

Zometa®: Store vials at 25°C (77°F); excursions permitted to 15°C to 30°C (59°F to 86°F). Dilute solution for injection in 100 mL NS or D_5W prior to administration. Solutions for infusion may be stored for 24 hours at 15°C to 30°C (59°F to 86°F). Infusion of solution must be completed within 24 hours.

Mechanism of Action A bisphosphonate which inhibits bone resorption via actions on osteoclasts or on osteoclast precursors; inhibits osteoclastic activity and skeletal calcium release induced by tumors. Decreases serum calcium and phosphorus, and increases their elimination. In osteoporosis, zoledronic acid inhibits osteoclast-mediated resorption, therefore reducing bone turnover.

Pharmacodynamics/Kinetics

Distribution: Binds to bone

Protein binding: 28% to 53%
Half-life elimination: Triphasic; Terminal: 146 hours
Excretion: Urine (39% ± 16% as unchanged drug) within 24 hours; feces (<3%)

Dosage I.V.: Adults: **Note:** Patients treated for multiple myeloma, osteoporosis, and Paget's disease should receive a daily calcium supplement and multivitamin containing vitamin D (if dietary intake is inadequate).

Hypercalcemia of malignancy (albumin-corrected serum calcium ≥12 mg/dL) (Zometa®): 4 mg (maximum) given as a single dose. Wait at least 7 days before considering retreatment. Dosage adjustment may be needed in patients with decreased renal function following treatment.

Multiple myeloma or metastatic bone lesions from solid tumors (Zometa®): 4 mg every 3-4 weeks

Osteoporosis (Reclast®, Aclasta® [CAN]): 5 mg infused over at least 15 minutes every 12 months

Paget's disease (Reclast®, Aclasta® [CAN]): 5 mg infused over at least 15 minutes. **Note:** Data concerning retreatment is not available, but may be considered.

Prevention of aromatase inhibitor-induced bone loss in breast cancer (unlabeled use): 4 mg every 6 months

Prevention of androgen deprivation-induced bone loss in nonmetastatic prostate cancer (unlabeled use): 4 mg every 3-12 months

Dosage adjustment in renal impairment (at treatment initiation):

Reclast®: Cl_{cr} <35 mL/minute: Not recommended
Zometa®: Multiple myeloma and bone metastases:
- Cl_{cr} >60 mL/minute: 4 mg
- Cl_{cr} 50-60 mL/minute: 3.5 mg
- Cl_{cr} 40-49 mL/minute: 3.3 mg
- Cl_{cr} 30-39 mL/minute: 3 mg
- Cl_{cr} <30 mL/minute: Not recommended

Zometa®: Hypercalcemia of malignancy:
- Mild-to-moderate impairment: No adjustment necessary
- Severe impairment (serum creatinine >4.5 mg/dL): Evaluate risk versus benefit

Aclasta® [CAN]:
- Cl_{cr} ≥30 mL/minute: No adjustment recommended
- Cl_{cr} <30 mL/minute: Use is not recommended

Dosage adjustment for renal toxicity (during treatment):

Hypercalcemia of malignancy: Evidence of renal deterioration: Evaluate risk versus benefit.

Multiple myeloma and bone metastases: Evidence of renal deterioration: Withhold dose until renal function returns to within 10% of baseline: renal deterioration defined as follows:
- Normal baseline creatinine: Increase of 0.5 mg/dL
- Abnormal baseline creatinine: Increase of 1 mg/dL

Reinitiate dose at the same dose administered prior to treatment interruption.

Dosage adjustment in hepatic impairment: Specific guidelines are not available.

Dietary Considerations

Multiple myeloma or metastatic bone lesions from solid tumors: Take daily calcium supplement (500 mg) and daily multivitamin (with 400 int. units vitamin D).

Osteoporosis: Ensure adequate calcium and vitamin D supplementation. Postmenopausal women generally require calcium 1200 mg/day and vitamin D 800-1000 int. units/day.

Paget's disease: Take calcium 1500 mg/day and vitamin D 800 units/day, particularly during the first 2 weeks after administration.

Administration Infuse over 15-30 minutes; do not infuse over <15 minutes. Infuse in a line separate from other medications. Patients should be appropriately hydrated prior to treatment.

Reclast®: If refrigerated, allow to reach room temperature prior to administration. Acetaminophen or ibuprofen after administration may reduce the incidence of acute reaction (eg, arthralgia, fever, flu-like symptoms, myalgia).

Monitoring Parameters Prior to initiation of therapy, dental exam and preventative dentistry for patients at risk for osteonecrosis

Aclasta® [CAN]: Serum creatinine, calcium and vitamin D levels

Reclast®: Alkaline phosphatase, serum creatinine (prior to each dose and periodically thereafter in high risk patients), calcium and mineral (phosphorus and magnesium) levels

Zometa®: Serum creatinine prior to each dose; serum electrolytes, phosphate, magnesium, and hemoglobin/hematocrit should be evaluated regularly. Monitor serum calcium to assess response and avoid overtreatment.

Test Interactions Bisphosphonates may interfere with diagnostic imaging agents such as technetium-99m-diphosphonate in bone scans.

Dosage Forms Excipient information presented when available (limited, particularly for generics); consult specific product labeling. [CAN] = Canadian brand name

Infusion, solution [premixed]:
- Aclasta® [CAN]: 5 mg (100 mL) [not available in U.S.]
- Reclast®: 5 mg (100 mL)

Injection, solution:
- Zometa®: 4 mg/5 mL (5 mL) [as monohydrate 4.264 mg]

◆ **Zolinza™** *see* Vorinostat *on page* 1569

Zolmitriptan (zohl mi TRIP tan)

U.S. Brand Names Zomig-ZMT®; Zomig®

Canadian Brand Names Zomig®; Zomig® Nasal Spray; Zomig® Rapimelt

Index Terms 311C90

Pharmacologic Category Antimigraine Agent; Serotonin 5-$HT_{1B,\ 1D}$ Receptor Agonist

Use Acute treatment of migraine with or without aura

Pregnancy Risk Factor C

Pregnancy Considerations There are no adequate and well-controlled studies using zolmitriptan in pregnant women. Use only if potential benefit to the mother outweighs the potential risk to the fetus. In animal studies, administration was associated with embryolethality, fetal abnormalities, and pup mortality.

Lactation Excretion in breast milk unknown/use caution

Medication Safety Issues

Sound-alike/look-alike issues:
- Zolmitriptan may be confused with SUMAtriptan

Contraindications Hypersensitivity to zolmitriptan or any component of the formulation; ischemic heart disease or vasospastic coronary artery disease, including Prinzmetal's angina; signs or symptoms of ischemic heart disease; uncontrolled hypertension; symptomatic Wolff-Parkinson-White syndrome or arrhythmias associated with other cardiac accessory conduction pathway disorders; use with ergotamine derivatives (within 24 hours of); use within 24 hours of another 5-HT_1 agonist; concurrent administration or within 2 weeks of discontinuing an MAO inhibitor; management of hemiplegic or basilar migraine

Nasal spray: Additional contraindications with nasal spray: Cerebrovascular syndromes (eg, stroke, TIA); peripheral vascular disease (including ischemic bowel disease)

Warnings/Precautions Zolmitriptan is indicated only in patient populations with a clear diagnosis of migraine. Not for prophylactic treatment of migraine headaches. Cardiac events (coronary artery vasospasm, transient ischemia, myocardial infarction, ventricular tachycardia/fibrillation, cardiac arrest, and death) have been reported with 5-HT_1 agonist administration. Should not be given to patients who have risk factors for CAD (eg, hypertension, hypercholesterolemia, smoker, obesity, diabetes, strong family history of CAD, menopause, male >40 years of age) without adequate cardiac evaluation. Patients with suspected CAD should have cardiovascular evaluation to rule out CAD before considering zolmitriptan's use; if cardiovascular evaluation negative, first dose would be safest if given in the healthcare provider's office. Periodic evaluation of those without cardiovascular disease, but with continued risk factors, should be done. Significant elevation in blood pressure, including hypertensive crisis, has also been reported on rare occasions in patients with and without a history of hypertension. Vasospasm-related reactions have been reported other than coronary artery vasospasm. Peripheral vascular ischemia and colonic ischemia with abdominal pain and bloody diarrhea have occurred. Cerebral/subarachnoid hemorrhage and stroke have been reported with 5-HT_1 agonist administration; nasal spray contraindicated in patients with cerebrovascular syndromes. Rarely, partial vision loss and blindness (transient and permanent) have been reported with 5-HT_1 agonists. Use with caution in patients with hepatic impairment. Zomig-ZMT™ tablets contain phenylalanine. Symptoms of agitation, confusion, hallucinations, hyperreflexia, myoclonus, shivering, and tachycardia (serotonin syndrome) may occur with concomitant proserotonergic drugs (eg, SSRIs/SNRIs or triptans) or agents which reduce zolmitriptan's metabolism. Concurrent use of serotonin precursors (eg, tryptophan) is not recommended. Safety and efficacy not established in patients <18 years of age (oral) and <12 years of age (nasal).

Adverse Reactions Percentages noted from oral preparations.

1% to 10%:

- Cardiovascular: Chest pain (2% to 4%), palpitation (up to 2%)
- Central nervous system: Dizziness (6% to 10%), somnolence (5% to 8%), pain (2% to 3%), vertigo (≤2%)
- Gastrointestinal: Nausea (4% to 9%), xerostomia (3% to 5%), dyspepsia (1% to 3%), dysphagia (≤2%)
- Neuromuscular & skeletal: Paresthesia (5% to 9%), weakness (3% to 9%), warm/cold sensation (5% to 7%), hypoesthesia (1% to 2%), myalgia (1% to 2%), myasthenia (up to 2%)
- Miscellaneous: Neck/throat/jaw pain (4% to 10%), diaphoresis (up to 3%), allergic reaction (up to 1%)

<1% (Limited to important or life-threatening): Anaphylactoid reaction, anaphylaxis, angina, apnea, arrhythmia, ataxia, bronchospasm, cerebral ischemia, coronary artery vasospasm, cyanosis, eosinophilia, esophagitis, gastrointestinal infarction/necrosis, hallucinations, headache, hematemesis, hypertension, hypertensive crisis, ischemic colitis, melena, miscarriage, MI, myocardial ischemia, pancreatitis, photosensitivity, QT prolongation, rash, serotonin syndrome, splenic infarction, syncope, tetany, thrombocytopenia, tinnitus, ulcer, urticaria

Events related to other serotonin 5-HT_{1D} receptor agonists: Cardiac arrest, cerebral hemorrhage, peripheral vascular ischemia, stroke, subarachnoid hemorrhage, ventricular fibrillation

Drug Interactions

Metabolism/Transport Effects Substrate of CYP1A2 (minor)

Avoid Concomitant Use

Avoid concomitant use of Zolmitriptan with any of the following: Ergot Derivatives; MAO Inhibitors; Sibutramine

Increased Effect/Toxicity

Zolmitriptan may increase the levels/effects of: Ergot Derivatives; Serotonin Modulators

The levels/effects of Zolmitriptan may be increased by: Cimetidine; Ergot Derivatives; MAO Inhibitors; Sibutramine

Decreased Effect There are no known significant interactions involving a decrease in effect.

Ethanol/Nutrition/Herb Interactions Ethanol: Limit use (may have additive CNS toxicity).

Stability Store at 20°C to 25°C (68°F to 77°F). Protect from light and moisture.

Mechanism of Action Selective agonist for serotonin (5-HT_{1B} and 5-HT_{1D} receptors) in cranial arteries to cause vasoconstriction and reduce sterile inflammation associated with antidromic neuronal transmission correlating with relief of migraine

Pharmacodynamics/Kinetics

Onset of action: 0.5-1 hour

Absorption: Well absorbed

Distribution: V_d: 7 L/kg

Protein binding: 25%

Metabolism: Converted to an active N-desmethyl metabolite (2-6 times more potent than zolmitriptan)

Bioavailability: 40%

Half-life elimination: 2.8-3.7 hours

Time to peak, serum: Tablet: 1.5 hours; Orally-disintegrating tablet and nasal spray: 3 hours

Excretion: Urine (~60% to 65% total dose); feces (30% to 40%)

Dosage Oral:

Children: Safety and efficacy have not been established

Adults: Migraine:

- Tablet: Initial: ≤2.5 mg at the onset of migraine headache; may break 2.5 mg tablet in half
- Orally-disintegrating tablet: Initial: 2.5 mg at the onset of migraine headache
- Nasal spray: Initial: 1 spray (5 mg) at the onset of migraine headache
- **Note:** Use the lowest possible dose to minimize adverse events. If the headache returns, the dose may be repeated after 2 hours; do not exceed 10 mg within a 24-hour period. Controlled trials have not established the effectiveness of a second dose if the initial one was ineffective.

Elderly: No dosage adjustment needed but elderly patients are more likely to have underlying cardiovascular disease and should have careful evaluation of cardiovascular system before prescribing.

Dosage adjustment in renal impairment: No dosage adjustment recommended. There is a 25% reduction in zolmitriptan's clearance in patients with severe renal impairment (Cl_{cr} 5-25 mL/minute).

Dosage adjustment in hepatic impairment: Administer with caution in patients with liver disease, generally using doses <2.5 mg (doses <5 mg can only be achieved using oral tablets). Patients with moderate-to-severe hepatic impairment may have decreased clearance of zolmitriptan, and significant elevation in blood pressure was observed in some patients.

Administration Administer as soon as migraine headache starts.

Tablet: May be broken.

Orally-disintegrating tablet: Must be taken whole; do not break, crush or chew. Place on tongue and allow to dissolve. Administration with liquid is not required.

Nasal spray: Blow nose gently prior to use. After removing protective cap, instill device into nostril. Block opposite nostril; breathe in gently through nose while pressing plunger of spray device. One dose (5 mg) is equal to 1 spray in 1 nostril.

Additional Information Not recommended if the patient has risk factors for heart disease (high blood pressure, high cholesterol, obesity, diabetes, smoking, strong family history of heart disease, postmenopausal woman, or a male >40 years of age).

This agent is intended to relieve migraine, but not to prevent or reduce the number of attacks. Use only to treat an actual migraine attack.

Dosage Forms Excipient information presented when available (limited, particularly for generics); consult specific product labeling.

Solution, intranasal [spray]:

Zomig®: 5 mg/0.1 mL (0.1 mL)

Tablet:

Zomig®: 2.5 mg, 5 mg

Tablet, orally disintegrating:

Zomig-ZMT®: 2.5 mg [contains phenylalanine 2.81 mg/tablet; orange flavor]; 5 mg [contains phenylalanine 5.62 mg/tablet; orange flavor]

◆ **Zoloft®** *see* Sertraline *on page* 1362

Zolpidem (zole PI dem)

U.S. Brand Names Ambien CR®; Ambien®; Zolpimist®

Index Terms Zolpidem Tartrate

Pharmacologic Category Hypnotic, Nonbenzodiazepine

Use

Ambien®: Short-term treatment of insomnia (with difficulty of sleep onset)

Ambien CR®: Treatment of insomnia (with difficulty of sleep onset and/or sleep maintenance)

Restrictions C-IV

An FDA-approved patient medication guide is available and must be distributed when dispensing an outpatient prescription (new or refill) where this medication is to be used without direct supervision of a healthcare provider. The guide provides information about the appropriate use of zolpidem, and discusses concerns relating to "sleep-driving" and other activities of which the patient may have no recollection.

Pregnancy Risk Factor C

Pregnancy Considerations Teratogenic effects were not observed in animal studies. Children born of mothers taking sedative/hypnotics may be at risk for withdrawal; neonatal flaccidity has been reported in infants following maternal use of sedative/hypnotics during pregnancy.

Lactation Enters breast milk/not recommended (AAP rates "compatible")

Medication Safety Issues

Sound-alike/look-alike issues:

Ambien® may be confused with Ambi 10®

Contraindications Hypersensitivity to zolpidem or any component of the formulation

Warnings/Precautions Should be used only after evaluation of potential causes of sleep disturbance. Failure of sleep disturbance to resolve after 7-10 days may indicate psychiatric or medical illness. Hypnotics/sedatives have been associated with abnormal thinking and behavior changes including decreased inhibition, aggression, bizarre behavior, agitation, hallucinations, and depersonalization. These changes may occur unpredictably and may indicate previously unrecognized psychiatric disorders; evaluate appropriately. Sedative/hypnotics may produce withdrawal symptoms following abrupt discontinuation. Use with caution in patients with depression; worsening of depression, including suicide or suicidal ideation has been reported with the use of hypnotics. Intentional overdose may be an issue in this population. The minimum dose that will effectively treat the individual patient should be used. Prescriptions should be written for the smallest quantity consistent with good patient care. Causes CNS depression, which may impair physical and mental capabilities. Zolpidem should only be administered when the patient is able to stay in bed a full night (7-8 hours) before being active again. Effects with other sedative drugs or ethanol may be potentiated.

Use caution in patients with myasthenia gravis. Use caution in the elderly; dose adjustment recommended. Closely monitor elderly or debilitated patients for impaired cognitive or motor performance. Avoid use in patients with sleep apnea or a history of sedative-hypnotic abuse. Postmarketing studies have indicated that the use of hypnotic/sedative agents for sleep has been associated with hypersensitivity reactions including anaphylaxis as well as angioedema. An increased risk for hazardous sleep-related activities such as sleep-driving; cooking and eating food, and making phone calls while asleep have also been noted; amnesia may also occur. Discontinue treatment in patients who report a sleep-driving episode.

Use caution with respiratory disease. Use caution with hepatic impairment; dose adjustment required. Because of the rapid onset of action, administer immediately prior to bedtime or after the patient has gone to bed and is having difficulty falling asleep. Safety and efficacy have not been established in pediatric patients.

Adverse Reactions Actual frequency may be dosage form, dose, and/or age dependent

>10%: Central nervous system: Dizziness, headache, somnolence

1% to 10%:

Cardiovascular: Blood pressure increased, chest discomfort/pain, palpitation

Central nervous system: Abnormal dreams, anxiety, apathy, amnesia, ataxia, attention disturbance, body temperature increased, confusion, depersonalization, depression, disinhibition, disorientation, drowsiness, drugged feeling, euphoria, fatigue, fever, hallucinations, hypoesthesia, insomnia, memory disorder, lethargy, lightheadedness, mood swings, sleep disorder, stress

Dermatologic: Rash, urticaria, wrinkling

Endocrine & metabolic: Menorrhagia

Gastrointestinal: Abdominal discomfort, abdominal pain, abdominal tenderness, appetite disorder, constipation, diarrhea, dyspepsia, flatulence, gastroenteritis, gastroesophageal reflux, hiccup, nausea, vomiting, xerostomia

Genitourinary: Urinary tract infection

Neuromuscular & skeletal: Arthralgia, back pain, balance disorder, myalgia, neck pain, paresthesia, psychomotor retardation, tremor, weakness

Ocular: Asthenopia, blurred vision, depth perception altered, diplopia, red eye, visual disturbance

Otic: Labyrinthitis, tinnitus, vertigo

Renal: Dysuria

Respiratory: Pharyngitis, sinusitis, throat irritation, upper respiratory tract infection

Miscellaneous: Allergy, binge eating, flu-like syndrome

<1% (Limited to important or life-threatening): Agitation, anaphylaxis, angioedema, anorexia, arthritis, bronchitis, cerebrovascular disorder, cognition decreased, complex sleep-related behavior (sleep-driving, cooking or eating food, making phone calls), concentrating difficulty, constipation, cough, cystitis, diaphoresis, dysarthria, dysphagia, dyspnea, edema, emotional lability, eye irritation, falling, hepatic function abnormalities, hyperglycemia, hyper-/hypotension, illusion, leg cramps, menstrual disorder, nervousness, pallor, postural hypotension, pruritus, rhinitis, scleritis, somnambulism (sleepwalking), speech disorder, stupor, syncope, tachycardia, taste perversion, thirst, urinary incontinence, vaginitis

Drug Interactions

Metabolism/Transport Effects Substrate of CYP1A2 (minor), 2C9 (minor), 2C19 (minor), 2D6 (minor), 3A4 (major)

Avoid Concomitant Use There are no known interactions where it is recommended to avoid concomitant use.

Increased Effect/Toxicity

Zolpidem may increase the levels/effects of: Alcohol (Ethyl); CNS Depressants

The levels/effects of Zolpidem may be increased by: Antifungal Agents (Azole Derivatives, Systemic); CYP3A4 Inhibitors (Moderate); CYP3A4 Inhibitors (Strong); Dasatinib

Decreased Effect

The levels/effects of Zolpidem may be decreased by: CYP3A4 Inducers (Strong); Deferasirox; Flumazenil; Herbs (CYP3A4 Inducers); Rifamycin Derivatives

Ethanol/Nutrition/Herb Interactions

Ethanol: May enhance the adverse/toxic effects of zolpidem; avoid use.

Food: Maximum plasma concentration and bioavailability are decreased with food; time to peak plasma concentration is increased; half-life remains unchanged. Grapefruit juice may decrease the metabolism of zolpidem.

Herb/Nutraceutical: St John's wort may decrease the levels/effects of zolpidem; avoid concomitant use. In addition, concomitant use of valerian, kava kava, and gotu kola should be avoided due to the risk of increased CNS depression.

Stability Store Ambien® at controlled room temperature of 20°C to 25°C (68°F to 77°F). Store Ambien CR® at controlled room temperature of 15°C to 25°C (59°F to 77°F).

Mechanism of Action Zolpidem, an imidazopyridine hypnotic that is structurally dissimilar to benzodiazepines, enhances the activity of the inhibitory neurotransmitter, γ-aminobutyric acid (GABA), via selective agonism at the benzodiazepine-1 (BZ_1) receptor; the result is increased chloride conductance, neuronal hyperpolarization, inhibition of the action potential, and a decrease in neuronal excitability leading to sedative and hypotic effects. Because of its selectivity for the BZ_1 receptor site over the BZ_2 receptor site, zolpidem exhibits minimal anxiolytic, myorelaxant, and anticonvulsant properties (effects largely attributed to agonism at the BZ_2 receptor site).

Pharmacodynamics/Kinetics

Onset of action: 30 minutes

Duration: 6-8 hours

Absorption: Rapid

Distribution: V_d: 0.54 L/kg

Protein binding: ~93%

Metabolism: Hepatic methylation and hydroxylation via CYP3A4 (~60%), CYP2C9 (~22%), CYP1A2 (~14%), CYP2D6 (~3%), and CYP2C19 (~3%) to three inactive metabolites

Bioavailability: 70%

Half-life elimination: ~2.5 hours (range 1.4-4.5 hours); Cirrhosis: Up to 9.9 hours; Elderly: prolonged up to 32%

Time to peak, plasma: 1.6 hours; 2.2 hours with food

Excretion: Urine (48% to 67%, primarily as metabolites); feces (29% to 42%, primarily as metabolites)

Dosage Oral:

Adults:

Ambien®: 10 mg immediately before bedtime; maximum dose: 10 mg

Ambien CR®: 12.5 mg immediately before bedtime

Elderly:

Ambien®: 5 mg immediately before bedtime

Ambien CR®: 6.25 mg immediately before bedtime

Dosing adjustment in renal impairment: Dose adjustment not required; monitor closely

Hemodialysis: Not dialyzable

Dosing adjustment in hepatic impairment:

Ambien®: 5 mg

Ambien CR®: 6.25 mg

Dietary Considerations For faster sleep onset, do not administer with (or immediately after) a meal.

Administration Ingest immediately before bedtime due to rapid onset of action. Ambien CR® tablets should be swallowed whole; do not divide, crush, or chew.

Monitoring Parameters Daytime alertness; respiratory rate; behavior profile

Reference Range 80-150 ng/mL

Additional Information Causes fewer disturbances in sleep stages as compared to benzodiazepines. Time spent in sleep stages 3 and 4 are maintained; zolpidem decreases sleep latency; should not be prescribed in quantities exceeding a 1-month supply.

Product Availability Zolpimist® oral spray: FDA approved December, 2008; availability currently undetermined

Zolpimist® is an oral spray of zolpidem indicated for the short-term treatment of insomnia characterized by difficulties with sleep initiation.

Dosage Forms Excipient information presented when available (limited, particularly for generics); consult specific product labeling.

Tablet, as tartrate: 5 mg, 10 mg

Ambien®: 5 mg, 10 mg

Tablet, extended release, as tartrate:

Ambien CR®: 6.25 mg, 12.5 mg

- ◆ **Zolpidem Tartrate** *see* Zolpidem *on page* 1591
- ◆ **Zolpimist®** *see* Zolpidem *on page* 1591
- ◆ **Zometa®** *see* Zoledronic Acid *on page* 1587
- ◆ **Zomig®** *see* Zolmitriptan *on page* 1589
- ◆ **Zomig® Nasal Spray (Can)** *see* Zolmitriptan *on page* 1589
- ◆ **Zomig® Rapimelt (Can)** *see* Zolmitriptan *on page* 1589
- ◆ **Zomig-ZMT®** *see* Zolmitriptan *on page* 1589
- ◆ **Zomorph® (Can)** *see* Morphine Sulfate *on page* 1016
- ◆ **Zonalon®** *see* Doxepin *on page* 484
- ◆ **Zonegran®** *see* Zonisamide *on page* 1592

Zonisamide (zoe NIS a mide)

U.S. Brand Names Zonegran®

Canadian Brand Names Zonegran®

Pharmacologic Category Anticonvulsant, Miscellaneous

Additional Appendix Information

Anticonvulsant Drugs of Choice *on page* 1637

Use Adjunct treatment of partial seizures in children >16 years of age and adults with epilepsy

Unlabeled/Investigational Use Bipolar disorder

Pregnancy Risk Factor C

Pregnancy Considerations Fetal abnormalities and death have been reported in animals, however, there are no studies in pregnant women. Based on limited case reports, it appears zonisamide crosses the placenta. Use during pregnancy only if the potential benefits outweigh the potential risks.

Lactation Excretion in breast milk unknown/contraindicated

Medication Safety Issues

Sound-alike/look-alike issues:

Zonisamide may be confused with lacosamide

Contraindications Hypersensitivity to zonisamide, sulfonamides, or any component of the formulation

Warnings/Precautions Rare, but potentially fatal sulfonamide reactions have occurred following the use of zonisamide. These reactions include Stevens-Johnson syndrome and toxic epidermal necrolysis, usually appearing within 2-16 weeks of drug initiation. Discontinue zonisamide if rash develops. Chemical similarities are present among sulfonamides, sulfonylureas, carbonic anhydrase inhibitors, thiazides, and loop diuretics (except ethacrynic acid). Use in patients with sulfonamide allergy is specifically contraindicated in product labeling, however, a risk of cross-reaction exists in patients with allergy to any of these compounds; avoid use when previous reaction has been severe.

Decreased sweating (oligohydrosis) and hyperthermia requiring hospitalization have been reported in children. Discontinue zonisamide in patients who develop acute renal failure or a significant sustained increase in creatinine/BUN concentration. Kidney stones have been reported. Use cautiously in patients with renal or hepatic dysfunction. Significant CNS effects include psychiatric symptoms, psychomotor slowing, and fatigue or somnolence. Fatigue and somnolence occur within the first month of treatment, most commonly at doses of 300-500 mg/day. Effects with other sedative drugs or ethanol may be potentiated. Abrupt withdrawal may precipitate seizures; discontinue or reduce doses gradually. Safety and efficacy in children <16 years of age has not been established.

Adverse Reactions Adjunctive therapy: Frequencies noted in patients receiving other anticonvulsants:

>10%:

Central nervous system: Somnolence (17%), dizziness (13%)

Gastrointestinal: Anorexia (13%)

1% to 10%:

Central nervous system: Headache (10%), agitation/irritability (9%), fatigue (8%), tiredness (7%), ataxia (6%), confusion (6%), concentration decreased (6%), memory impairment (6%), depression (6%), insomnia (6%), speech disorders (5%), mental slowing (4%), anxiety (3%), nervousness (2%), schizophrenic/schizophreniform behavior (2%), difficulty in verbal expression (2%), status epilepticus (1%), convulsion (1%), hyperesthesia (1%), incoordination (1%)

Dermatologic: Rash (3%), bruising (2%), pruritus (1%)

Gastrointestinal: Nausea (9%), abdominal pain (6%), diarrhea (5%), dyspepsia (3%), weight loss (3%), constipation (2%), dry mouth (2%), taste perversion (2%), vomiting (1%)

Neuromuscular & skeletal: Paresthesia (4%), abnormal gait (1%), tremor (1%), weakness (1%)

Ocular: Diplopia (6%), nystagmus (4%), amblyopia (1%)

Otic: Tinnitus (1%)

Respiratory: Rhinitis (2%), pharyngitis (1%), increased cough (1%)

Miscellaneous: Flu-like syndrome (4%) accidental injury (1%)

<1% (Limited to important or life threatening symptoms): Agranulocytosis, allergic reaction, alopecia, aplastic anemia, apnea, atrial fibrillation, bladder calculus, cholangitis, cholecystitis, cholestatic jaundice, colitis, deafness, duodenitis, dysarthria, dyskinesia, dyspnea, dystonia, encephalopathy, esophagitis, facial paralysis, gingival hyperplasia, glaucoma, gum hemorrhage, gynecomastia, heart failure, hematemesis, hemoptysis, hirsutism, hyperthermia, impotence, leukopenia, lupus erythematosus, menorrhagia, movement disorder, myoclonus, nephrolithiasis, neuropathy, oculogyric crisis, oligohydrosis, peripheral neuritis, pulmonary embolus, rash, rectal hemorrhage, Stevens-Johnson syndrome, stroke, suicidal behavior/ideation, syncope, thrombocytopenia, toxic epidermal necrolysis, urinary retention, urticaria

Drug Interactions

Metabolism/Transport Effects Substrate of CYP2C19 (minor), 3A4 (major)

Avoid Concomitant Use There are no known interactions where it is recommended to avoid concomitant use.

Increased Effect/Toxicity

Zonisamide may increase the levels/effects of: Alcohol (Ethyl); CNS Depressants

The levels/effects of Zonisamide may be increased by: CYP3A4 Inhibitors (Moderate); CYP3A4 Inhibitors (Strong); Dasatinib

Decreased Effect

The levels/effects of Zonisamide may be decreased by: CYP3A4 Inducers (Strong); Deferasirox; Herbs (CYP3A4 Inducers); Ketorolac; Mefloquine; Phenytoin

Ethanol/Nutrition/Herb Interactions

Ethanol: Avoid ethanol (may increase CNS depression).

Food: Food delays time to maximum concentration, but does not affect bioavailability.

Stability Store at controlled room temperature 25°C (77°F). Protect from moisture and light.

Mechanism of Action The exact mechanism of action is not known. May stabilize neuronal membranes and suppress neuronal hypersynchronization through action at sodium and calcium channels. Does not affect GABA activity.

Pharmacodynamics/Kinetics

Distribution: V_d: 1.45 L/kg

Protein binding: 40%

Metabolism: Hepatic via CYP3A4; forms N-acetyl zonisamide and 2-sulfamoylacetyl phenol (SMAP)

Half-life elimination: 63 hours

Time to peak: 2-6 hours

Excretion: Urine (62%, 35% as unchanged drug, 65% as metabolites); feces (3%)

Dosage Oral:

Children >16 years and Adults:

Adjunctive treatment of partial seizures: Initial: 100 mg/day; dose may be increased to 200 mg/day after 2 weeks. Further dosage increases to 300 mg/day and 400 mg/day can then be made with a minimum of 2 weeks between adjustments, in order to reach steady state at each dosage level. Doses of up to 600 mg/day have been studied, however, there is no evidence of increased response with doses above 400 mg/day.

Mania (unlabeled use): Initial: 100-200 mg/day; maximum: 600 mg/day (Kanba, 1994)

Elderly: Data from clinical trials is insufficient for patients >65 years; begin dosing at the low end of the dosing range.

Dosage adjustment in renal/hepatic impairment: Slower titration and frequent monitoring are indicated in patients with renal or hepatic disease. There is insufficient experience regarding dosing/toxicity in patients with estimated GFR <50 mL/minute. Marked renal impairment (Cl_{cr} <20 mL/minute) was associated with a 35% increase in AUC.

Dietary Considerations May be taken with or without food.

Administration Capsules should be swallowed whole. Dose may be administered once or twice daily. Doses of 300 mg/day and higher are associated with increased side effects. Steady-state levels are reached in 14 days.

Monitoring Parameters Monitor BUN and serum creatinine

Dosage Forms Excipient information presented when available (limited, particularly for generics); consult specific product labeling.

Capsule: 25 mg, 50 mg, 100 mg

Zonegran®: 25 mg, 100 mg

- **Zorbtive®** *see* Somatropin *on page 1388*
- **ZORprin®** *see* Aspirin *on page 142*
- **Zostavax®** *see* Zoster Vaccine *on page 1593*

Zoster Vaccine (ZOS ter vak SEEN)

U.S. Brand Names Zostavax®

Index Terms Shingles Vaccine; Varicella-Zoster (VZV) Vaccine (Zoster); VZV Vaccine (Zoster)

Pharmacologic Category Vaccine, Live (Viral)

Use Prevention of herpes zoster (shingles) in patients ≥60 years of age

The Advisory Committee on Immunization Practices (ACIP) recommends routine vaccination of all patients ≥60 years of age, including:

- Patients who report a previous episode of zoster.
- Patients with chronic medical conditions (eg, chronic renal failure, diabetes mellitus, rheumatoid arthritis, chronic pulmonary disease) unless those conditions are contraindications.
- Residents of nursing homes and other long-term care facilities ≥60 years of age, without contraindications.

Pregnancy Risk Factor C

Pregnancy Considerations Animal reproduction studies have not been conducted. Use during pregnancy is contraindicated. Although women of childbearing potential are unlikely to receive the vaccine, women should avoid becoming pregnant for 4 weeks after vaccination. Risk to the fetus following exposure to wild-type varicella zoster virus is small and risk following exposure from the attenuated vaccine is probably even less. Inadvertent exposure to the vaccine during pregnancy should be reported to Merck's National Service Center (800-986-8999).

Lactation Excretion in breast milk unknown/use caution

Medication Safety Issues

Both varicella vaccine and zoster vaccine are live, attenuated strains of varicella-zoster virus. Their indications, dosing, and composition are distinct. Varicella vaccine is indicated for the prevention of chickenpox, while zoster vaccine is indicated in older individuals to prevent reactivation of the virus which causes shingles. Zoster vaccine is **not** a substitute for varicella vaccine and should not be used in children.

Contraindications Hypersensitivity to any component of the vaccine; individuals with leukemia, lymphomas, or other malignant neoplasms affecting the bone marrow or lymphatic systems; primary and acquired immunodeficiency states including AIDS or clinical manifestations of HIV; those receiving immunosuppressive therapy (including high-dose corticosteroids); pregnancy

In addition, ACIP recommends that the following immunocompromised patients should not receive zoster vaccine:

Patients undergoing hematopoietic stem cell transplant (limited data; assess risk/benefit, if needed, administer ≥24 months after transplantation);

Patients receiving recombinant human immune modulators, particularly antitumor necrosis factor agents (eg, adalimumab, infliximab, etanercept). Safety and efficacy of concurrent administration is unknown and not recommended. Defer vaccination for ≥1 month after discontinuation.

Patients with unspecified cellular immunodeficiency (exception, patients with impaired humoral immunity may receive vaccine).

Warnings/Precautions Zoster vaccine is not a substitute for varicella vaccine and should not be used in children. Not for use in the treatment of active zoster outbreak or in the treatment of postherpetic neuropathy (PHN). Avoid administration in patients with acute febrile illness; consider deferral of vaccination; may administer to patients with mild acute illness (with or without fever). Defer treatment in patients with active untreated tuberculosis. May be used in patients with a history of zoster infection.

Medications active against the herpesvirus family (eg, acyclovir, famciclovir, valacyclovir) may interfere with the zoster vaccine. In patients where immunosuppressant therapy is anticipated, zoster vaccine should be given at least 14 days to 1 month prior to beginning therapy when possible Use is contraindicated in severely immunocompromised patients (eg, patients receiving chemo-/radiation therapy or other immunosuppressive therapy [including high-dose corticosteroids]); may have a reduced response to vaccination. Patients receiving corticosteroids in low-to-moderate doses, topical (inhaled, nasal, skin), local injection (intra-articular, bursal, tendon) may receive vaccine. Vaccinated individuals do not need to take precautions against spreading varicella following vaccination; transmission of virus is rare unless rash develops. In case of rash, standard contact precautions should be followed.

Immediate treatment for anaphylactoid reaction should be available during vaccine use. Contains gelatin and neomycin; do not use in patients with a history of anaphylactic/anaphylactoid reaction. Contact dermatitis to neomycin is not a contraindication to the vaccine. Not for use in patients <60 years of age. The ACIP does not recommend zoster vaccination in patients of any age who have received the varicella vaccine.

Adverse Reactions All serious adverse reactions must be reported to the U.S. Department of Health and Human Services (DHHS) Vaccine Adverse Event Reporting System (VAERS) 1-800-822-7967.

>10%: Local: Injection site reaction (48%; includes erythema, tenderness, swelling, hematoma, pruritus, and/or warmth)

1% to 10% (**Note:** Rates similar to placebo):

Central nervous system: Fever (2%), headache (1%)
Dermatologic: Skin disorder (1%)
Gastrointestinal: Diarrhea (2%)
Neuromuscular & skeletal: Weakness (1%)
Respiratory: Respiratory tract infection (2%), rhinitis (1%)
Miscellaneous: Flu-like syndrome (2%)

<1%, postmarketing, and/or case reports following varicella vaccine have included (not reported specifically following zoster vaccine): Anaphylaxis, ataxia, Bell's palsy, cellulitis, cerebrovascular accident, dizziness, encephalitis, erythema multiforme, Guillain-Barré syndrome, Henoch-Schönlein purpura, herpes zoster, impetigo, nonfebrile seizure, paresthesia, pharyngitis, pyrexia, rash (noninjection site), secondary skin infection, Stevens-Johnson syndrome, thrombocytopenia, transverse myelitis

Drug Interactions

Avoid Concomitant Use

Avoid concomitant use of Zoster Vaccine with any of the following: Acyclovir-Valacyclovir; Famciclovir; Immunosuppressants

Increased Effect/Toxicity

The levels/effects of Zoster Vaccine may be increased by: Immunosuppressants

Decreased Effect

Zoster Vaccine may decrease the levels/effects of: Tuberculin Tests

The levels/effects of Zoster Vaccine may be decreased by: Acyclovir-Valacyclovir; Famciclovir; Immune Globulins

Stability During shipment, should be maintained at -15°C (5°F) or colder. Store powder in freezer at -15°C (5°F). Protect from light. Store diluent separately at room temperature or in refrigerator. Withdraw entire contents of the vial containing the provided diluent to reconstitute vaccine. Gently agitate to mix thoroughly. Withdraw entire contents of reconstituted vaccine vial for administration. Discard if reconstituted vaccine is not used within 30 minutes. Do not freeze reconstituted vaccine.

Mechanism of Action As a live, attenuated vaccine (Oka/Merck strain of varicella-zoster virus), zoster virus vaccine stimulates active immunity to disease caused by the varicella-zoster virus. Administration has been demonstrated to protect against the development of herpes zoster, with the highest efficacy in patients 60-69 years of age. It may also reduce the severity of complications, including postherpetic neuralgia, in patients who develop zoster following vaccination.

Pharmacodynamics/Kinetics

Onset of action: Seroconversion: ~6 weeks

Duration: Not established; protection has been demonstrated for at least 4 years

Dosage SubQ: Adults ≥60 years: 0.65 mL administered as a single dose; there is no data to support readministration of the vaccine

Dosage adjustment in renal impairment: No adjustment required

Administration Do not administer I.V.; inject immediately after reconstitution. Inject SubQ into the deltoid region of the upper arm, if possible. In persons anticipating immunosuppression, give at least 14 days to 1 month prior to starting immunosuppressant.

Administration with chronic use of acyclovir, famciclovir, or valacyclovir: Discontinue ≥24 hours before administration of zoster vaccine. Do not use for ≥14 days after vaccination.

Administration with other vaccines:

Zoster vaccine with inactivated vaccines: May be given simultaneously or at any interval between doses

Zoster vaccine with other live vaccines:

Intranasal or injectable: If not given simultaneously, wait at least 4 weeks between administration

Oral: May be given simultaneously or at any interval between doses of live or inactivated injectable vaccines

Vaccine administration with antibody-containing products: Zoster vaccine may be given with blood or antibody-containing products. Examples of antibody-containing products include I.M. and I.V. immune globulin, hepatitis B immune globulin, tetanus immune globulin, varicella zoster immune globulin, rabies immune globulin, whole blood, packed red cells, plasma, and platelet products

Monitoring Parameters Fever, rash

Additional Information Federal law requires that the date of administration, the vaccine manufacturer, lot number of vaccine, and the administering person's name, title, and address be entered into the patient's permanent medical record.

The varicella-zoster virus (VZV) is capable of causing two distinct manifestations of infection. Primary infection results in chickenpox (varicella). These infections tend to occur in young children or younger adults. Reactivation of latent infection (painful vesicular cutaneous eruption usually in a dermatomal pattern) occurs in older patients or in immunosuppressed populations. This is commonly referred to as shingles (herpes zoster). Although the vaccines are directed against the same causative organism, healthcare workers should be aware of differences in indications, dosing, populations, and composition of the vaccine. Neither vaccine is intended for administration during active outbreaks.

Dosage Forms Excipient information presented when available (limited, particularly for generics); consult specific product labeling.

Injection, powder for reconstitution [preservative free]

Zostavax®: 19,400 plaque-forming units (PFU) [contains gelatin, sucrose, and trace amounts of neomycin]

- ◆ **Zosyn®** *see* Piperacillin and Tazobactam Sodium *on page 1198*
- ◆ **Zovia®** *see* Ethinyl Estradiol and Ethynodiol Diacetate *on page 576*
- ◆ **Zovirax®** *see* Acyclovir *on page 40*
- ◆ **Ztuss™ Tablet [DSC]** *see* Hydrocodone, Pseudoephedrine, and Guaifenesin *on page 743*
- ◆ **Ztuss™ ZT [DSC]** *see* Hydrocodone and Guaifenesin *on page 741*
- ◆ **Zyban®** *see* BuPROPion *on page 223*
- ◆ **Zydone®** *see* Hydrocodone and Acetaminophen *on page 740*
- ◆ **Zyflo® [DSC]** *see* Zileuton *on page 1583*
- ◆ **Zyflo CR™** *see* Zileuton *on page 1583*
- ◆ **Zylet™** *see* Loteprednol and Tobramycin *on page 910*
- ◆ **Zyloprim®** *see* Allopurinol *on page 65*
- ◆ **Zymar®** *see* Gatifloxacin *on page 683*
- ◆ **Zym-Fluconazole (Can)** *see* Fluconazole *on page 625*
- ◆ **Zymine®-D** *see* Triprolidine and Pseudoephedrine *on page 1522*
- ◆ **Zyprexa®** *see* OLANZapine *on page 1093*
- ◆ **Zyprexa Zydis** *see* OLANZapine *on page 1093*
- ◆ **Zyprexa® Zydis®** *see* OLANZapine *on page 1093*
- ◆ **Zyrtec® [OTC]** *see* Cetirizine *on page 295*
- ◆ **Zyrtec® Allergy [OTC]** *see* Cetirizine *on page 295*
- ◆ **Zyrtec®, Children's Allergy [OTC]** *see* Cetirizine *on page 295*
- ◆ **Zyrtec®, Children's Hives Relief [OTC]** *see* Cetirizine *on page 295*
- ◆ **Zytopic™** *see* Triamcinolone *on page 1510*
- ◆ **Zytram® XL (Can)** *see* TraMADol *on page 1497*
- ◆ **Zyvox®** *see* Linezolid *on page 890*
- ◆ **Zyvoxam® (Can)** *see* Linezolid *on page 890*

APPENDIX TABLE OF CONTENTS

ABBREVIATIONS, ACRONYMS, AND SYMBOLS

Abbreviations Which May Be Used in This Reference

Abbreviation	Meaning
5-HT	5-hydroxytryptamine
AAP	American Academy of Pediatrics
ABG	arterial blood gases
ABW	adjusted body weight
AACT	American Academy of Clinical Toxicology
ACC	American College of Cardiology
ACE	angiotensin converting enzyme
ACLS	advanced cardiac life support
ACOG	American College of Obstetricians and Gynecologists
ACTH	adrenocorticotrophic hormone
ADH	alcohol dehydrogenase
ADHD	attention-deficit/hyperactivity disorder
ADLs	activities of daily living
AED	antiepileptic drug
AHA	American Heart Association
AIDS	acquired immune deficiency syndrome
AIMS	Abnormal Involuntary Movement Scale
ALS	amyotrophic lateral sclerosis
ALT	alanine aminotransferase
AMA	American Medical Association
ANC	absolute neutrophil count
ARB	angiotensin receptor blocker
ARDS	acute respiratory distress syndrome
AST	aspartate aminotransferase
AUC	area under the curve
BDI	Beck Depression Inventory
BEC	blood ethanol concentration
BLS	basic life support
BMI	body mass index
BP	blood pressure
BPH	benign prostatic hyperplasia
BPRS	Brief Psychiatric Rating Scale
BSA	body surface area
BUN	blood urea nitrogen
CABG	coronary artery bypass graft
CAD	coronary artery disease
CAN	Canadian
CAPD	continuous ambulatory peritoneal dialysis
CAS	chemical abstract service
CBC	complete blood count
CBT	cognitive behavioral therapy
Cl_{cr}	creatinine clearance
CDC	Centers for Disease Control and Prevention
CF	cystic fibrosis
CGI	Clinical Global Impression
CHD	coronary heart disease

Abbreviations Which May Be Used in This Reference *(continued)*

Abbreviation	Meaning
CHF	congestive heart failure; chronic heart failure
CIE	chemotherapy-induced emesis
C-II	schedule two controlled substance
C-III	schedule three controlled substance
C-IV	schedule four controlled substance
C-V	schedule five controlled substance
CIV	continuous I.V. infusion
C_{max}	maximum plasma concentration
C_{min}	minimum plasma concentration
CMV	cytomegalovirus
CNS	central nervous system or coagulase negative staphylococcus
COLD	chronic obstructive lung disease
COPD	chronic obstructive pulmonary disease
COX	cyclooxygenase
CPK	creatine phosphokinase
CRF	chronic renal failure
CRP	C-reactive protein
CRRT	continuous renal replacement therapy
CSF	cerebrospinal fluid
CT	computed tomography
CVVH	continuous venovenous hemofiltration
CVVHD	continuous venovenous hemodialysis
CVVHDF	continuous venovenous hemodiafiltration
CYP	cytochrome
D_5W	dextrose 5% in water
DBP	diastolic blood pressure
DEHP	di(3-ethylhexyl)phthalate
DIC	disseminated intravascular coagulation
DM	diabetes mellitus
DMARD	disease modifying antirheumatic drug
DSC	discontinued
DSM-IV	Diagnostic and Statistical Manual
DVT	deep vein thrombosis
EBV	Epstein-Barr virus
ECG	electrocardiogram
ECMO	extracorporeal membrane oxygenation
ECT	electroconvulsive therapy
ED	emergency department
EEG	electroencephalogram
EF	ejection fraction
EG	ethylene glycol
EGA	estimated gestational age
	enzyme immunoassay
	enzyme-linked immunosorbent assay
	extrapyramidal side effects
	erythrocyte sedimentation rate
	end stage renal disease
	alcohol
	Food and Drug Administration
	failure to thrive

Abbreviations Which May Be Used in This Reference *(continued)*

Abbreviation	Meaning
GABA	gamma-aminobutyric acid
GAD	generalized anxiety disorder
GERD	gastroesophageal reflux disease
GFR	glomerular filtration rate
GGT	gamma-glutamyltransferase
GI	gastrointestinal
GU	genitourinary
GVHD	graft versus host disease
HAM-A	Hamilton Anxiety Scale
HAM-D	Hamilton Depression Scale
HDL	high density lipoprotein
HF	heart failure
HFSA	Heart Failure Society of America
HIV	human immunodeficiency virus
HMG-CoA	3-hydroxy-3-methylglutaryl-coenzyme A
HOCM	hypertrophic obstructive cardiomyopathy
HPA	hypothalamic-pituitary-adrenal
HSV	herpes simplex virus
HTN	hypertension
HUS	hemolytic uremic syndrome
IBD	inflammatory bowel disease
IBS	irritable bowel syndrome
IBW	ideal body weight
ICD	implantable cardioverter defibrillator
ICH	intracranial hemorrhage
ICP	intracranial pressure
IDDM	insulin dependent diabetes mellitus
IDSA	Infectious Diseases Society of America
IHSS	idiopathic hypertrophic subaortic stenosis
I.M.	intramuscular
INR	international normalized ration
Int. unit	international unit
IOP	intraocular pressure
IUGR	intrauterine growth retardation
I.V.	intravenous
JIA	juvenile idiopathic arthritis
JNC	Joint National Committee
KIU	kallikrein inhibitor unit
LAMM	L-α-acetyl methadol
LDH	lactate dehydrogenase
LDL	low density lipoprotein
LFT	liver function test
LGA	large for gestational age
LR	lactated ringers
LVEF	left ventricular ejection fraction
LVH	left ventricular hypertrophy
MADRS	Montgomery Asbery Depression Rating Scale
MAOIs	monamine oxidase inhibitors
MDD	major depressive disorder
MDRD	modification of diet in renal disease

Abbreviations Which May Be Used in This Reference *(continued)*

Abbreviation	Meaning
mEq	milliequivalent
mg	milligram
MI	myocardial infarction
mL	milliliter
mm	millimeter
mM	millimolar
mm Hg	millimeters of mercury
MMSE	mini mental status examination
M/P	milk to plasma ratio
MPS I	mucopolysaccharidosis I
MRHD	maximum recommended human dose
MRI	magnetic resonance imaging
MUGA	multiple gated acquisition scan
NAS	neonatal abstinence syndrome
NF	National Formulary
NFD	Nephrogenic fibrosing dermopathy
ng	nanogram
NIDDM	Noninsulin dependent diabetes mellitus
NKA	no known allergies
NKDA	No known drug allergies
NMDA	n-methyl-d-aspartic acid
NMS	neuroleptic malignant syndrome
NNRTI	non-nucleoside reverse transcriptase inhibitor
NRTI	nucleoside reverse transcriptase inhibitor
NS	normal saline
NSAID	nonsteroidal anti-inflammatory drug
NSF	nephrogenic systemic fibrosis
NSTEMI	Non-ST-elevation myocardial infarction
OA	osteoarthritis
OCD	obsessive-compulsive disorder
OHSS	ovarian hyperstimulation syndrome
OTC	over-the-counter
PAT	paroxysmal atrial tachycardia
PD	Parkinson's disease; peritoneal dialysis
PDA	patent ductus arteriosus
PDE-5	phosphodiesterase-5
PE	pulmonary embolus
PEG tube	percutaneous endoscopic gastrostomy tube
PHN	post-herpetic neuralgia
PID	pelvic inflammatory disease
PMDD	premenstrual dysphoric disorder
[illegible]	postoperative nausea and vomiting
[illegible]	peripheral parenteral nutrition
[illegible]	premature rupture of membranes
[illegible]	paroxysmal supraventricular tachycardia
[illegible]	prothrombin time
[illegible]	post-traumatic stress disorder
[illegible]	partial thromboplastin time
[illegible]	peptic ulcer disease
[illegible]	peripheral vascular disease

Abbreviations Which May Be Used in This Reference *(continued)*

Abbreviation	Meaning
QT_c	corrected QT interval
QT_c-F	corrected QT interval by Fredricia's formula
RA	rheumatoid arthritis
REM	rapid eye movement
RPLS	reversible posterior leukoencephalopathy syndrome
SA	sinoatrial
SAD	seasonal affective disorder
SAH	subarachnoid hemorrhage
SBE	subacute bacterial endocarditis
SBP	systolic blood pressure
S_{Cr}	serum creatinine
SERM	selective estrogen receptor modulator
SGA	small for gestational age
SGOT	serum glutamic oxaloacetic aminotransferase
SGPT	serum glutamic pyruvate transaminase
SI	International System of Units or Systeme international d'Unites
SIADH	syndrome of inappropriate antidiuretic hormone secretion
SLE	systemic lupus erythematosus
SNRI	serotonin norepinephrine reuptake inhibitor
SSKI	saturated solution of potassium iodide
SSRIs	selective serotonin reuptake inhibitors
STD	sexually transmitted disease
STEM I	ST-elevation myocardial infarction
SubQ	subcutaneous
supp	suppository
SVT	supraventricular tachycardia
SWFI	sterile water for injection
syr	syrup
$T_{1/2}$	half-life
tab	tablet
TB	tuberculosis
TC	total cholesterol
TCA	tricyclic antidepressant
TD	tardive dyskinesia
TG	triglyceride
TIA	transient ischemic attack
TMA	thrombotic microangiopathy
T_{max}	time to maximum observed concentration, plasma
TNF	Tumor necrosis factor
TPN	total parenteral nutrition
tr, tinct	tincture
tsp	teaspoonful
UC	ulcerative colitis
ULN	upper limits of normal
URI	upper respiratory infection
USAN	United States Adopted Names
USP	United States Pharmacopeia
UTI	urinary tract infection
UV	ultraviolet
V_d	volume of distribution

Abbreviations Which May Be Used in This Reference *(continued)*

Abbreviation	Meaning
VEGF	vascular endothelial growth factor
VF	ventricular fibrillation
VT	ventricular tachycardia
VTE	venous thromboembolism
vWD	von Willebrand disease
VZV	varicella zoster virus
YBOC	Yale Brown Obsessive-Compulsive Scale
YMRS	Young Mania Rating Scale

Common Weights, Measures, or Apothecary Abbreviations

Abbreviation	Meaning
<[1]	less than
>[1]	greater than
≤	less than or equal to
≥	greater than or equal to
ac	before meals or food
ad	to, up to
ad lib	at pleasure
AM	morning
AMA	against medical advice
amp	ampul
amt	amount
aq	water
aq. dest.	distilled water
ASAP	as soon as possible
a.u.[1]	each ear
bid	twice daily
bm	bowel movement
C	Celsius, centigrade
cal	calorie
cap	capsule
cc[1]	cubic centimeter
cm	centimeter
comp	compound
cont	continue
d	day
d/c[1]	discharge
dil	dilute
disp	dispense
div	divide
dtd	give of such a dose
Dx	diagnosis
elix, el	elixir
emp	as directed
et	and
ex aq	in water
F	Fahrenheit
f, ft	make, let be made

Common Weights, Measures, or Apothecary Abbreviations *(continued)*

Abbreviation	Meaning
g	gram
gr	grain
gtt	a drop
h	hour
hs[1]	at bedtime
kcal	kilocalorie
kg	kilogram
L	liter
liq	a liquor, solution
M	molar
mcg	microgram
m. dict	as directed
mEq	milliequivalent
mg	milligram
microL	microliter
mL	milliliter
mm	millimeter
mM	millimolar
mm Hg	millimeters of mercury
ng	nanogram
no.	number
noc	in the night
non rep	do not repeat, no refills
NPO	nothing by mouth
NV	nausea and vomiting
O, Oct	a pint
o.d.[1]	right eye
o.l.	left eye
o.s.[1]	left eye
o.u.[1]	each eye
pc, post cib	after meals
PM	afternoon or evening
P.O.	by mouth
P.R.	rectally
prn	as needed
pulv	a powder
q	every
qad	every other day
qd[1,2]	every day, daily
qh	every hour
qid	four times a day
qod[1,2]	every other day
qs	a sufficient quantity
qs ad	a sufficient quantity to make
Rx	take, a recipe
SL	sublingual
stat	at once, immediately
SubQ	subcutaneous
supp	suppository
syr	syrup

Common Weights, Measures, or Apothecary Abbreviations *(continued)*

Abbreviation	Meaning
tab	tablet
tal	such
tid	three times a day
tr, tinct	tincture
trit	triturate
tsp	teaspoon
u.d.	as directed
ung	ointment
v.o.	verbal order
w.a.	while awake
x3	3 times
x4	4 times

[1]ISMP error-prone abbreviation.

[2]JCAHO Do Not Use list.

Additional abbreviations used and defined within a specific monograph or text piece may only apply to that text.

References

The Institute for Safe Medication Practices (ISMP) list of Error-Prone Abbreviations, Symbols, and Dose Designations. Available at: http://www.ismp.org/Tools/errorproneabbreviations.pdf.

The Joint Commission Official "Do Not Use" list. Available at: http://www.jointcommission.org/PatientSafety/DoNotUseList/.

APACHE II SCORING SYSTEM

The APACHE II score is the sum of the total acute physiology score (APS), age points, and chronic health points. Determination of these scores/points are outlined in the following tables. For an online scoring calculator, see http://www.sfar.org/scores2/scores2.html.

APACHE II Score	Points
APS points	
+ Age points	
+ Chronic health points	
Total APACHE II Score	

Glasgow Coma Scale

(circle appropriate response)

Eyes open	**Verbal – nonintubated**
4 - Spontaneously	5 - Oriented and controversed
3 - To verbal	4 - Disoriented and talks
2 - To painful stimuli	3 - Inappropriate words
1 - No response	2 - Incomprehensible sounds
	1 - No response
Motor response	
6 - To verbal command	**Verbal – intubated**
5 - Localizes to pain	5 - Seems able to talk
4 - Withdraws to pain	3 - Questionable ability to talk
3 - Decorticate	1 - Generally unresponsive
2 - Decerebrate	
1 - No response	

Age Points

Assign points to age as follows:	Points
≤44	0
45-54	2
55-64	3
65-74	5
≥75	6

Chronic Health Points

Liver Cardiovascular Pulmonary Kidney Immune	If the patient has a history of severe organ system insufficiency or is immunocompromised assign points as follows: a. for nonoperative or emergency postoperative patients - 5 points or b. for elective postoperative patients - 2 points **DEFINITIONS** Organ insufficiency or immunocompromised state must have been evident prior to this hospital admission and conform to the following criteria. **Liver:** Biopsy proven cirrhosis and documented portal hypertension; episodes of past upper GI bleeding attributed to portal hypertension; or prior episodes of hepatic failure/encephalopathy/coma **Cardiovascular:** New York Heart Association Class IV **Respiratory:** Chronic restrictive, obstructive, or vascular disease resulting in severe exercise restriction, ie, unable to climb stairs or perform household duties; or documented chronic hypoxia, hypercapnia, secondary polycythemia, severe pulmonary hypertension (>40 mm Hg), or respirator dependency **Renal:** Receiving chronic dialysis **Immunocompromised:** The patient has received therapy that suppresses resistance to infection, eg, immunosuppression, chemotherapy, radiation, long term or recent high dose steroids, or has a disease that is sufficiently advanced to suppress resistance to infection, eg, leukemia, lymphoma, AIDS **Chronic Health Points =**

Reference: Knaus WA, Draper EA, Wagner DP, et al, "APACHE II: A Severity of Disease Classification System," *Crit Care Med*, 1985, 13(10):818-29.

Total Acute Physiology Score (APS) (Choose the worst value in the past 24 hours)

	Physiologic Variable	High Abnormal Range								Low Abnormal Range
		+4	+3	+2	+1	0	+1	+2	+3	+4
1	Temperature rectal (°C)[1]	≥41	39-40.9		38.5-38.9	36-38.4	34-35.9	32-33.9	30-31.9	≤29.9
2	Mean arterial pressure (mm Hg)	≥160	130-159	110-129		70-109		50-69		≤49
3	Heart rate (ventricular response)	≥180	140-179	110-139		70-109		55-69	40-54	≤39
4	Respiratory rate (nonventilated or ventilated)	≥50	35-49		25-34	12-24	10-11	6-9		≤5
5	Oxygenation: A-aDO_2 or PaO_2 (mm Hg) a) FiO_2 ≥0.5: record A-aDO_2	≥500	350-499	200-349		<200				
	b) FiO_2 <0.5: record only PaO_2					PO_2 >70	PO_2 61-70		PO_2 55-60	PO_2 <55
6*	Arterial pH	≥7.7	7.6-7.69		7.5-7.59	7.33-7.49		7.25-7.32	7.15-7.24	<7.15
7	Serum sodium (mmol/L)	≥180	160-179	155-159	150-154	130-149		120-129	111-119	≤110
8	Serum potassium (mmol/L)	≥7	6-6.9		5.5-5.9	3.5-5.4	3-3.4	2.5-2.9		<2.5
9	Serum creatinine (mg/100 mL) double point score for acute renal failure	≥3.5	2-3.4	1.5-1.9		0.6-1.4		<0.6		
10	Hematocrit (%)	≥60		50-59.9	46-49.9	30-45.9		20-29.9		<20
11	White blood count (total/mm^3) (in 1000s)	≥40		20-39.9	15-19.9	3-14.9		1-2.9		<1
12	Glasgow coma score (GCS): Score = 15 minus actual GCS [see Glasgow Coma Scale table]									
A	Total acute physiology score (APS): Sum of the 12 individual variable points									
*	Serum HCO_3 (venous-mmol/L) Not preferred, use if no ABGs	≥52	41-51.9		32-40.9	22-31.9		18-21.9	15-17.9	<15

[1]Temperature may also be obtained by the following methods: Swan-Ganz core, bladder, tympanic membrane.

APOTHECARY / METRIC EQUIVALENTS

Approximate Liquid Measures

Basic equivalent: 1 fluid ounce = 30 mL

Examples:

1 gallon ... 3800 mL	1 gallon ... 128 fluid ounces
1 quart ... 960 mL	1 quart ... 32 fluid ounces
1 pint ... 480 mL	1 pint ... 16 fluid ounces
8 fluid oz ... 240 mL	15 minims ... 1 mL
4 fluid oz ... 120 mL	10 minims ... 0.6 mL

Approximate Household Equivalents

1 teaspoonful ... 5 mL	1 tablespoonful ... 15 mL

Weights

Basic equivalents:

1 oz ... 30 g	15 gr ... 1 g

Examples:

4 oz ... 120 g	1 gr ... 60 mg
2 oz ... 60 g	1/100 gr ... 600 mcg
10 gr ... 600 mg	1/150 gr ... 400 mcg
7 1/2 gr ... 500 mg	1/200 gr ... 300 mcg
16 oz ... 1 lb	

Metric Conversions

Basic equivalents:

1 g ... 1000 mg	1 mg ... 1000 mcg

Examples:

5 g ... 5000 mg	5 mg ... 5000 mcg
0.5 g ... 500 mg	0.5 mg ... 500 mcg
0.05 g ... 50 mg	0.05 mg ... 50 mcg

Exact Equivalents

1 g	=	15.43 gr	0.1 mg	=	1/600 gr
1 mL	=	16.23 minims	0.12 mg	=	1/500 gr
1 minim	=	0.06 mL	0.15 mg	=	1/400 gr
1 gr	=	64.8 mg	0.2 mg	=	1/300 gr
1 pint (pt)	=	473.2 mL	0.3 mg	=	1/200 gr
1 oz	=	28.35 g	0.4 mg	=	1/150 gr
1 lb	=	453.6 g	0.5 mg	=	1/120 gr
1 kg	=	2.2 lb	0.6 mg	=	1/100 gr
1 qt	=	946.4 mL	0.8 mg	=	1/80 gr
			1 mg	=	1/65 gr

Solids[1]

1/4 grain	=	15 mg
1/2 grain	=	30 mg
1 grain	=	60 mg
1 1/2 grains	=	90 mg
5 grains	=	300 mg
10 grains	=	600 mg

[1]Use exact equivalents for compounding and calculations requiring a high degree of accuracy.

AVERAGE WEIGHTS AND SURFACE AREAS

Average Height, Weight, and Surface Area by Age and Gender

Age	Girls			Boys		
	Height (cm)	Weight (kg)	BSA (m^2)	Height (cm)	Weight (kg)	BSA (m^2)
Birth	49.5	3.4	0.22	50	3.6	0.22
3 mo	59	5.6	0.3	61	6	0.32
6 mo	65	7.2	0.36	67	7.9	0.38
9 mo	70	8.3	0.4	72	9.3	0.43
12 mo	74.5	9.5	0.44	75.5	10.3	0.46
15 mo	77	10.3	0.47	79	11.1	0.49
18 mo	80	11	0.49	82	11.7	0.52
21 mo	83	11.6	0.52	85	12.2	0.54
2 y	86	12	0.54	87.5	12.6	0.55
2.5 y	91	13	0.57	92	13.5	0.59
3 y	94.5	13.8	0.6	96	14.3	0.62
3.5 y	97	15	0.64	98	15	0.64
4 y	101	16	0.67	102	16	0.67
4.5 y	104	17	0.7	105	17	0.7
5 y	107.5	18	0.73	109	18.5	0.75
6 y	115	20	0.80	115	21	0.82
7 y	121.5	23	0.88	122	23	0.88
8 y	127.5	25.5	0.95	127.5	26	0.96
9 y	133	29	1.04	133.5	28.5	1.03
10 y	138	33	1.12	138.5	32	1.1
11 y	144	37	1.22	143.5	36	1.2
12 y	151	41.5	1.32	149	40.5	1.29
13 y	157	46	1.42	156	45.5	1.4
14 y	160.5	49.5	1.49	163.5	51	1.52
15 y	162	52	1.53	170	56	1.63
16 y	162.5	54	1.56	173.5	61	1.71
17 y	163	55	1.58	175	64.5	1.77
Adult[1]	163.5	58	1.62	177	83.5	2.03

Data extracted from the CDC growth charts based on the 50th percentile height and weight for a given age.[2]

Body surfaced area calculation[3]: $\sqrt{[(Ht \times Wt) / 3600]}$

[1]McDowell MA, Fryar CD, Hirsch R, et al, "Anthropometric Reference Data for Children and Adults: U.S. Population, 1999-2002," *Adv Data*, 2005, (361):1-5.

[2]Centers for Disease Control and Prevention, "2000 CDC Growth Charts: United States," Available at: http://www.cdc.gov/growthcharts/. Accessed November 16, 2007.

[3]Mosteller RD, "Simplified Calculation of Body-Surface Area," *N Engl J Med*, 1987, 317(17):1098.

BODY MASS INDEX (BMI)

BMI = weight (kg) / [height (m)]^2

See "Obesity Treatment Guidelines for Adults" in Therapy Recommendations section.

BODY SURFACE AREA OF ADULTS AND CHILDREN

Calculating Body Surface Area in Children

In a child of average size, find weight and corresponding surface area on the boxed scale to the left; or, use the nomogram to the right. Lay a straightedge on the correct height and weight points for the child, then read the intersecting point on the surface area scale. (**Note:** 2.2 lb = 1 kg)

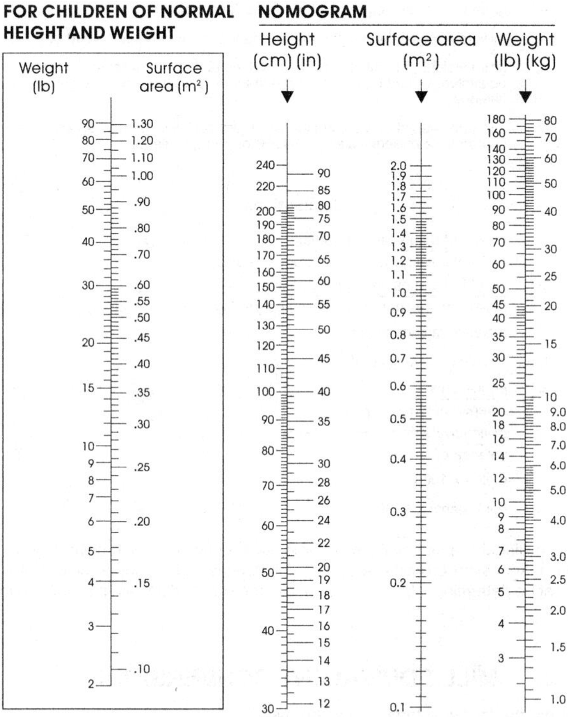

BODY SURFACE AREA FORMULA
(Adult and Pediatric)

$$\text{BSA (m}^2\text{)} = \sqrt{\frac{\text{ht (in)} \times \text{wt (lb)}}{3131}} \quad \text{or, in metric: BSA (m}^2\text{)} = \sqrt{\frac{\text{ht (cm)} \times \text{wt (kg)}}{3600}}$$

References

Lam TK and Leung DT, "More on Simplified Calculation of Body Surface Area," *N Engl J Med*, 1988, 318(17):1130 (letter).
Mosteller RD, "Simplified Calculation of Body Surface Area," *N Engl J Med*, 1987, 317(17):1098 (letter).

IDEAL BODY WEIGHT CALCULATION

Adults (18 years and older) (IBW is in kg)

IBW (male) = 50 + (2.3 x height in inches over 5 feet)

IBW (female) = 45.5 + (2.3 x height in inches over 5 feet)

Children (IBW is in kg; height is in cm)

a. 1-18 years

IBW = (height)^2 x 1.65) / 1000

b. 5 feet and taller
IBW (male) = 39 + (2.27 x height in inches over 5 feet)
IBW (female) = 42.2 + (2.27 x height in inches over 5 feet)

MILLIEQUIVALENT AND MILLIMOLE CALCULATIONS AND CONVERSIONS

DEFINITIONS AND CALCULATIONS

Definitions

mole	=	gram molecular weight of a substance (aka molar weight)
millimole (mM)	=	milligram molecular weight of a substance (a millimole is 1/1000 of a mole)
equivalent weight	=	gram weight of a substance which will combine with or replace 1 gram (1 mole) of hydrogen; an equivalent weight can be determined by dividing the molar weight of a substance by its ionic valence
milliequivalent (mEq)	=	milligram weight of a substance which will combine with or replace 1 milligram (1 millimole) of hydrogen (a milliequivalent is 1/1000 of an equivalent)

Calculations

$$\text{moles} = \frac{\text{weight of a substance (grams)}}{\text{molecular weight of that substance (grams)}}$$

$$\text{millimoles} = \frac{\text{weight of a substance (milligrams)}}{\text{molecular weight of that substance (milligrams)}}$$

$$\text{equivalents} = \text{moles x valence of ion}$$

$$\text{milliequivalents} = \text{millimoles x valence of ion}$$

$$\text{moles} = \frac{\text{equivalents}}{\text{valence of ion}}$$

$$\text{millimoles} = \frac{\text{milliequivalents}}{\text{valence of ion}}$$

$$\text{millimoles} = \text{moles x 1000}$$

$$\text{milliequivalents} = \text{equivalents x 1000}$$

Note: Use of equivalents and milliequivalents is valid only for those substances which have fixed ionic valences (eg, sodium, potassium, calcium, chlorine, magnesium bromine, etc). For substances with variable ionic valences (eg, phosphorous), a reliable equivalent value cannot be determined. In these instances, one should calculate millimoles (which are fixed and reliable) rather than milliequivalents.

MILLIEQUIVALENT CONVERSIONS

To convert mg/100 mL to mEq/L the following formula may be used:

$$\frac{\text{(mg/100 mL) x 10 x valence}}{\text{atomic weight}} = \text{mEq/L}$$

To convert mEq/L to mg/100 mL the following formula may be used:

$$\frac{\text{(mEq/L) x atomic weight}}{\text{10 x valence}} = \text{mg/100 mL}$$

To convert mEq/L to volume of percent of a gas the following formula may be used:

$$\frac{\text{(mEq/L) x 22.4}}{10} = \text{volume percent}$$

Valences and Atomic Weights of Selected Ions

Substance	Electrolyte	Valence	Molecular Wt
Calcium	Ca^{++}	2	40
Chloride	Cl^{-}	1	35.5
Magnesium	Mg^{++}	2	24
Phosphate	HPO_4^{--} (80%)	1.8	96[1]
pH = 7.4	$H_2PO_4^{-}$ (20%)	1.8	96[1]
Potassium	K^{+}	1	39
Sodium	Na^{+}	1	23
Sulfate	SO_4^{--}	2	96[1]

[1]The molecular weight of phosphorus only is 31, and sulfur only is 32.

Approximate Milliequivalents — Weights of Selected Ions

Salt	mEq/g Salt	mg Salt/mEq
Calcium carbonate [$CaCO_3$]	20	50
Calcium chloride [$CaCl_2 \cdot 2H_2O$]	14	74
Calcium gluceptate [$Ca(C_7H_{13}O_8)_2$]	4	245
Calcium gluconate [$Ca(C_6H_{11}O_7)_2 \cdot H_2O$]	5	224
Calcium lactate [$Ca(C_3H_5O_3)_2 \cdot 5H_2O$]	7	154
Magnesium gluconate [$Mg(C_6H_{11}O_7)_2 \cdot H_2O$]	5	216
Magnesium oxide [MgO]	50	20
Magnesium sulfate [$MgSO_4$]	17	60
Magnesium sulfate [$MgSO_4 \cdot 7H_2O$]	8	123
Potassium acetate [$K(C_2H_3O_2)$]	10	98
Potassium chloride [KCl]	13	75
Potassium citrate [$K_3(C_6H_5O_7) \cdot H_2O$]	9	108
Potassium iodide [KI]	6	166
Sodium acetate [$Na(C_2H_3O_2)$]	12	82
Sodium acetate [$Na(C_2H_3O_2) \cdot 3H_2O$]	7	136
Sodium bicarbonate [$NaHCO_3$]	12	84
Sodium chloride [NaCl]	17	58
Sodium citrate [$Na_3(C_6H_5O_7) \cdot 2H_2O$]	10	98
Sodium iodine [NaI]	7	150
Sodium lactate [$Na(C_3H_5O_3)$]	9	112
Zinc sulfate [$ZnSO_4 \cdot 7H_2O$]	7	144

CORRECTED SODIUM

Corrected Na^+ = measured Na^+ + [1.5 x (glucose – 150 divided by 100)]

Note: Do not correct for glucose <150.

WATER DEFICIT

Water deficit = 0.6 x body weight [1 – (140 divided by Na^+)]

Note: Body weight is estimated weight in kg when fully hydrated; **Na^+** is serum or plasma sodium. Use corrected Na^+ if necessary. Consult medical references for recommendations for replacement of deficit.

TOTAL SERUM CALCIUM CORRECTED FOR ALBUMIN LEVEL

[(Normal albumin – patient's albumin) x 0.8] + patient's measured total calcium

ACID-BASE ASSESSMENT

Henderson-Hasselbalch Equation

$pH = 6.1 + \log (HCO_3^- / (0.03)(pCO_2))$

Alveolar Gas Equation

PIO_2	=	FiO_2 x (total atmospheric pressure – vapor pressure of H_2O at 37°C)
	=	FiO_2 x (760 mm Hg – 47 mm Hg)
PAO_2	=	$PIO_2 - PACO_2 / R$

Alveolar/arterial oxygen gradient = $PAO_2 - PaO_2$

Normal ranges:

Children	15-20 mm Hg
Adults	20-25 mm Hg

where:

PIO_2	=	Oxygen partial pressure of inspired gas (mm Hg) (150 mm Hg in room air at sea level)
FiO_2	=	Fractional pressure of oxygen in inspired gas (0.21 in room air)

PAO_2	=	Alveolar oxygen partial pressure
$PACO_2$	=	Alveolar carbon dioxide partial pressure
PaO_2	=	Arterial oxygen partial pressure
R	=	Respiratory exchange quotient (typically 0.8, increases with high carbohydrate diet, decreases with high fat diet)

Acid-Base Disorders

Acute metabolic acidosis:
$PaCO_2$ expected = 1.5 (HCO_3^-) + 8 ± 2 **or**
Expected decrease in $PaCO_2$ = 1.3 (1-1.5) x decrease in HCO_3^-

Acute metabolic alkalosis:
Expected increase in $PaCO_2$ = 0.6 (0.5-1) x increase in HCO_3^-

Acute respiratory acidosis (<6 h duration):
For every $PaCO_2$ increase of 10 mm Hg, HCO_3 increases by 1 mEq/L

Chronic respiratory acidosis (>6 h duration):
For every $PaCO_2$ increase of 10 mm Hg, HCO_3 increases by 4 mEq/L

Acute respiratory alkalosis (<6 h duration):
For every $PaCO_2$ decrease of 10 mm Hg, HCO_3 decreases by 2 mEq/L

Chronic respiratory alkalosis (>6 h duration):
For every $PaCO_2$ decrease of 10 mm Hg, HCO_3 increases by 5 mEq/L

ACID-BASE EQUATION

H^+ (in mEq/L) = (24 x $PaCO_2$) divided by HCO_3^-

Aa GRADIENT

Aa gradient [(713)(FiO_2 – ($PaCO_2$ divided by 0.8))] – PaO_2

Aa gradient	=	alveolar-arterial oxygen gradient
FiO_2	=	inspired oxygen (expressed as a fraction)
$PaCO_2$	=	arterial partial pressure carbon dioxide (mm Hg)
PaO_2	=	arterial partial pressure oxygen (mm Hg)

OSMOLALITY

Definition: The summed concentrations of all osmotically active solute particles.

Predicted serum osmolality =
2 Na^+ + glucose (mg/dL) / 18 + BUN (mg/dL) / 2.8

The normal range of serum osmolality is 285-295 mOsm/L.

Differential diagnosis of increased serum osmolal gap (>10 mOsm/L)

Medications and toxins
Alcohols (ethanol, methanol, isopropanol, glycerol, ethylene glycol)
Mannitol

Calculated Osm

Osmolal gap = measured Osm – calculated Osm

0 to +10: Normal
>10: Abnormal
<0: Probable lab or calculation error

BICARBONATE DEFICIT

HCO_3^- deficit = (0.4 x wt in kg) x (HCO_3^- desired – HCO_3^- measured)

Note: In clinical practice, the calculated quantity may differ markedly from the actual amount of bicarbonate needed or that which may be safely administered.

ANION GAP

Definition: The difference in concentration between unmeasured cation and anion equivalents in serum.

Anion gap = Na^+ – (Cl^- + HCO_3^-)
(The normal anion gap is 10-14 mEq/L)

Differential Diagnosis of Increased Anion Gap Acidosis

Organic anions
- Lactate (sepsis, hypovolemia, seizures, large tumor burden)
- Pyruvate
- Uremia
- Ketoacidosis (β-hydroxybutyrate and acetoacetate)
- Amino acids and their metabolites
- Other organic acids

Inorganic anions
- Hyperphosphatemia
- Sulfates
- Nitrates

Differential Diagnosis of Decreased Anion Gap

Organic cations
- Hypergammaglobulinemia

Inorganic cations
- Hyperkalemia
- Hypercalcemia
- Hypermagnesemia

Medications and toxins
- Lithium

Hypoalbuminemia

RETICULOCYTE INDEX

(% retic divided by 2) x (patient's Hct divided by normal Hct) **or**
(% retic divided by 2) x (patient's Hgb divided by normal Hgb)

Normal index: 1.0
Good marrow response: 2.0-6.0

POUNDS / KILOGRAMS CONVERSION

1 pound = 0.45359 kilograms
1 kilogram = 2.2 pounds

lb	kg	lb	kg	lb	kg
1	0.45	70	31.75	140	63.50
5	2.27	75	34.02	145	65.77
10	4.54	80	36.29	150	68.04
15	6.80	85	38.56	155	70.31
20	9.07	90	40.82	160	72.58
25	11.34	95	43.09	165	74.84
30	13.61	100	45.36	170	77.11
35	15.88	105	47.63	175	79.38
40	18.14	110	49.90	180	81.65
45	20.41	115	52.16	185	83.92
50	22.68	120	54.43	190	86.18
55	24.95	125	56.70	195	88.45
60	27.22	130	58.91	200	90.72
65	29.48	135	61.24		

TEMPERATURE CONVERSION

Celsius to Fahrenheit = (°C x 9/5) + 32 = °F
Fahrenheit to Celsius = (°F - 32) x 5/9 = °C

°C	°F	°C	°F	°C	°F
100.0	212.0	39.0	102.2	36.8	98.2
50.0	122.0	38.8	101.8	36.6	97.9
41.0	105.8	38.6	101.5	36.4	97.5
40.8	105.4	38.4	101.1	36.2	97.2
40.6	105.1	38.2	100.8	36.0	96.8
40.4	104.7	38.0	100.4	35.8	96.4
40.2	104.4	37.8	100.1	35.6	96.1
40.0	104.0	37.6	99.7	35.4	95.7
39.8	103.6	37.4	99.3	35.2	95.4
39.6	103.3	37.2	99.0	35.0	95.0
39.4	102.9	37.0	98.6	0	32.0
39.2	102.6				

REFERENCE VALUES FOR CHILDREN

		Normal Values
CHEMISTRY		
Albumin	0-1 y	2-4 g/dL
	1 y to adult	3.5-5.5 g/dL
Ammonia	Newborns	90-150 mcg/dL
	Children	40-120 mcg/dL
	Adults	18-54 mcg/dL
Amylase	Newborns	0-60 units/L
	Adults	30-110 units/L
Bilirubin, conjugated, direct	Newborns	<1.5 mg/dL
	1 mo to adult	0-0.5 mg/dL
Bilirubin, total	0-3 d	2-10 mg/dL
	1 mo to adult	0-1.5 mg/dL
Bilirubin, unconjugated, indirect		0.6-10.5 mg/dL
Calcium	Newborns	7-12 mg/dL
	0-2 y	8.8-11.2 mg/dL
	2 y to adult	9-11 mg/dL
Calcium, ionized, whole blood		4.4-5.4 mg/dL
Carbon dioxide, total		23-33 mEq/L
Chloride		95-105 mEq/L
Cholesterol	Newborns	45-170 mg/dL
	0-1 y	65-175 mg/dL
	1-20 y	120-230 mg/dL
Creatinine	0-1 y	≤0.6 mg/dL
	1 y to adult	0.5-1.5 mg/dL
Glucose	Newborns	30-90 mg/dL
	0-2 y	60-105 mg/dL
	Children to Adults	70-110 mg/dL
Iron		
	Newborns	110-270 mcg/dL
	Infants	30-70 mcg/dL
	Children	55-120 mcg/dL
	Adults	70-180 mcg/dL
Iron binding	Newborns	59-175 mcg/dL
	Infants	100-400 mcg/dL
	Adults	250-400 mcg/dL
Lactic acid, lactate		2-20 mg/dL
Lead, whole blood		<10 mcg/dL
Lipase		
	Children	20-140 units/L
	Adults	0-190 units/L
Magnesium		1.5-2.5 mEq/L
Osmolality, serum		275-296 mOsm/kg
Osmolality, urine		50-1400 mOsm/kg

Chemistry		Normal Values
Phosphorus	Newborns	4.2-9 mg/dL
	6 wk to 19 mo	3.8-6.7 mg/dL
	19 mo to 3 y	2.9-5.9 mg/dL
	3-15 y	3.6-5.6 mg/dL
	>15 y	2.5-5 mg/dL
Potassium, plasma	Newborns	4.5-7.2 mEq/L
	2 d to 3 mo	4-6.2 mEq/L
	3 mo to 1 y	3.7-5.6 mEq/L
	1-16 y	3.5-5 mEq/L
Protein, total	0-2 y	4.2-7.4 g/dL
	>2 y	6-8 g/dL
Sodium		136-145 mEq/L
Triglycerides	Infants	0-171 mg/dL
	Children	20-130 mg/dL
	Adults	30-200 mg/dL
Urea nitrogen, blood	0-2 y	4-15 mg/dL
	2 y to Adult	5-20 mg/dL
Uric acid	Male	3-7 mg/dL
	Female	2-6 mg/dL
ENZYMES		
Alanine aminotransferase (ALT)	0-2 mo	8-78 units/L
	>2 mo	8-36 units/L
Alkaline phosphatase (ALKP)	Newborns	60-130 units/L
	0-16 y	85-400 units/L
	>16 y	30-115 units/L
Aspartate aminotransferase (AST)	Infants	18-74 units/L
	Children	15-46 units/L
	Adults	5-35 units/L
Creatine kinase (CK)	Infants	20-200 units/L
	Children	10-90 units/L
	Adult male	0-206 units/L
	Adult female	0-175 units/L
Lactate dehydrogenase (LDH)	Newborns	290-501 units/L
	1 mo to 2 y	110-144 units/L
	>16 y	60-170 units/L

Blood Gases

	Arterial	Capillary	Venous
pH	7.35-7.45	7.35-7.45	7.32-7.42
pCO_2 (mm Hg)	35-45	35-45	38-52
pO_2 (mm Hg)	70-100	60-80	24-48
HCO_3 (mEq/L)	19-25	19-25	19-25
TCO_2 (mEq/L)	19-29	19-29	23-33
O_2 saturation (%)	90-95	90-95	40-70
Base excess (mEq/L)	-5 to +5	-5 to +5	-5 to +5

Thyroid Function Tests

T_4 (thyroxine)	1-7 d	10.1-20.9 mcg/dL
	8-14 d	9.8-16.6 mcg/dL
	1 mo to 1 y	5.5-16 mcg/dL
	>1 y	4-12 mcg/dL
FTI	1-3 d	9.3-26.6
	1-4 wk	7.6-20.8
	1-4 mo	7.4-17.9
	4-12 mo	5.1-14.5
	1-6 y	5.7-13.3
	>6 y	4.8-14
T_3 by RIA	Newborns	100-470 ng/dL
	1-5 y	100-260 ng/dL
	5-10 y	90-240 ng/dL
	10 y to Adult	70-210 ng/dL
T_3 uptake		35%-45%
TSH	Cord	3-22 μIU/mL
	1-3 d	<40 μIU/mL
	3-7 d	<25 μIU/mL
	>7 d	0-10 μIU/mL

REFERENCE VALUES FOR ADULTS

CHEMISTRY

Test	Values	Remarks
Serum / Plasma		
Acetone	Negative	
Albumin	3.2-5 g/dL	
Alcohol, ethyl	Negative	
Aldolase	1.2-7.6 IU/L	
Ammonia	20-70 mcg/dL	Specimen to be placed on ice as soon as collected.
Amylase	30-110 units/L	
Bilirubin, direct	0-0.3 mg/dL	
Bilirubin, total	0.1-1.2 mg/dL	
Calcium	8.6-10.3 mg/dL	
Calcium, ionized	2.24-2.46 mEq/L	
Chloride	95-108 mEq/L	
Cholesterol, total	≤200 mg/dL	Fasted blood required – normal value affected by dietary habits. This reference range is for a general adult population.
HDL cholesterol	40-60 mg/dL	Fasted blood required – normal value affected by dietary habits.
LDL cholesterol	<160 mg/dL	If triglyceride is >400 mg/dL, LDL cannot be calculated accurately (Friedewald equation). Target LDL-C depends on patient's risk factors.
CO_2	23-30 mEq/L	
Creatine kinase (CK) isoenzymes		
CK-BB	0%	
CK-MB (cardiac)	0%-3.9%	
CK-MM (muscle)	96%-100%	
CK-MB levels must be both ≥4% and 10 IU/L to meet diagnostic criteria for CK-MB positive result consistent with myocardial injury.		
Creatine phosphokinase (CPK)	8-150 IU/L	
Creatinine	0.5-1.4 mg/dL	
Ferritin	13-300 ng/mL	
Folate	3.6-20 ng/dL	
GGT (gamma-glutamyltranspeptidase)		
male	11-63 IU/L	
female	8-35 IU/L	
GLDH	To be determined	
Glucose (preprandial)	<115 mg/dL	Goals different for diabetics.
Glucose, fasting	60-110 mg/dL	Goals different for diabetics.
Glucose, nonfasting (2-h postprandial)	<120 mg/dL	Goals different for diabetics.
Hemoglobin A_{1c}	<8	
Hemoglobin, plasma free	<2.5 mg/100 mL	
Hemoglobin, total glycosolated (Hb A_1)	4%-8%	
Iron	65-150 mcg/dL	
Iron binding capacity, total (TIBC)	250-420 mcg/dL	
Lactic acid	0.7-2.1 mEq/L	Specimen to be kept on ice and sent to lab as soon as possible.
Lactate dehydrogenase (LDH)	56-194 IU/L	
Lactate dehydrogenase (LDH) isoenzymes		
LD_1	20%-34%	
LD_2	29%-41%	
LD_3	15%-25%	

CHEMISTRY *(continued)*

Test	Values	Remarks
LD_4	1%-12%	
LD_5	1%-15%	
Flipped LD_1/LD_2 ratios (>1 may be consistent with myocardial injury) particularly when considered in combination with a recent CK-MB positive result.		
Lipase	23-208 units/L	
Magnesium	1.6-2.5 mg/dL	Increased by slight hemolysis.
Osmolality	289-308 mOsm/kg	
Phosphatase, alkaline		
adults 25-60 y	33-131 IU/L	
adults ≥61 y	51-153 IU/L	
infancy-adolescence	Values range up to 3-5 times higher than adults	
Phosphate, inorganic	2.8-4.2 mg/dL	
Potassium	3.5-5.2 mEq/L	Increased by slight hemolysis.
Prealbumin	>15 mg/dL	
Protein, total	6.5-7.9 g/dL	
AST	<35 IU/L (20-48)	
ALT (10-35)	<35 IU/L	
Sodium	134-149 mEq/L	
Thyroid stimulating hormone (TSH)		
adults ≤20 y	0.7-6.4 mIU/L	
21-54 y	0.4-4.2 mIU/L	
55-87 y	0.5-8.9 mIU/L	
Transferrin	>200 mg/dL	
Triglycerides	45-155 mg/dL	Fasted blood required.
Troponin I	<1.5 ng/mL	
Urea nitrogen (BUN)	7-20 mg/dL	
Uric acid		
male	2-8 mg/dL	
female	2-7.5 mg/dL	
Cerebrospinal Fluid		
Glucose	50-70 mg/dL	
Protein	15-45 mg/dL	CSF obtained by lumbar puncture.
Note: Bloody specimen gives erroneously high value due to contamination with blood proteins		
Urine (24-hour specimen is required for all these tests unless specified)		
Amylase	32-641 units/L	The value is in units/L and **not** calculated for total volume.
Amylase, fluid (random samples)		Interpretation of value left for physician, depends on the nature of fluid.
Calcium	Depends upon dietary intake	
Creatine		
male	150 mg/24 h	Higher value on children and during pregnancy.
female	250 mg/24 h	
Creatinine	1000-2000 mg/24 h	
Creatinine clearance (endogenous)		
male	85-125 mL/min	A blood sample must accompany urine specimen.
female	75-115 mL/min	
Glucose	1 g/24 h	
5-hydroxyindoleacetic acid	2-8 mg/24 h	
Iron	0.15 mg/24 h	Acid washed container required.
Magnesium	146-209 mg/24 h	

CHEMISTRY *(continued)*

Test	Values	Remarks
Osmolality	500-800 mOsm/kg	With normal fluid intake.
Oxalate	10-40 mg/24 h	
Phosphate	400-1300 mg/24 h	
Potassium	25-120 mEq/24 h	Varies with diet; the interpretation of urine electrolytes and osmolality should be left for the physician.
Sodium	40-220 mEq/24 h	
Porphobilinogen, qualitative	Negative	
Porphyrins, qualitative	Negative	
Proteins	0.05-0.1 g/24 h	
Salicylate	Negative	
Urea clearance	60-95 mL/min	A blood sample must accompany specimen.
Urea N	10-40 g/24 h	Dependent on protein intake.
Uric acid	250-750 mg/24 h	Dependent on diet and therapy.
Urobilinogen	0.5-3.5 mg/24 h	For qualitative determination on random urine, send sample to urinalysis section in Hematology Lab.
Xylose absorption test		
children	16%-33% of ingested xylose	
Feces		
Fat, 3-day collection	<5 g/d	Value depends on fat intake of 100 g/d for 3 days preceding and during collection.
Gastric Acidity		
Acidity, total, 12 h	10-60 mEq/L	Titrated at pH 7.

Blood Gases

	Arterial	Capillary	Venous
pH	7.35-7.45	7.35-7.45	7.32-7.42
pCO_2 (mm Hg)	35-45	35-45	38-52
pO_2 (mm Hg)	70-100	60-80	24-48
HCO_3 (mEq/L)	19-25	19-25	19-25
TCO_2 (mEq/L)	19-29	19-29	23-33
O_2 saturation (%)	90-95	90-95	40-70
Base excess (mEq/L)	-5 to +5	-5 to +5	-5 to +5

HEMATOLOGY

Complete Blood Count

Age	Hgb (g/dL)	Hct (%)	RBC (mill/mm^3)	RDW
0-3 d	15.0-20.0	45-61	4.0-5.9	<18
1-2 wk	12.5-18.5	39-57	3.6-5.5	<17
1-6 mo	10.0-13.0	29-42	3.1-4.3	<16.5
7 mo to 2 y	10.5-13.0	33-38	3.7-4.9	<16
2-5 y	11.5-13.0	34-39	3.9-5.0	<15
5-8 y	11.5-14.5	35-42	4.0-4.9	<15
13-18 y	12.0-15.2	36-47	4.5-5.1	<14.5
Adult male	13.5-16.5	41-50	4.5-5.5	<14.5
Adult female	12.0-15.0	36-44	4.0-4.9	<14.5

Age	MCV (fL)	MCH (pg)	MCHC (%)	Plts (x 10^3/mm^3)
0-3 d	95-115	31-37	29-37	250-450
1-2 wk	86-110	28-36	28-38	250-450
1-6 mo	74-96	25-35	30-36	300-700
7 mo to 2 y	70-84	23-30	31-37	250-600
2-5 y	75-87	24-30	31-37	250-550
5-8 y	77-95	25-33	31-37	250-550
13-18 y	78-96	25-35	31-37	150-450
Adult male	80-100	26-34	31-37	150-450
Adult female	80-100	26-34	31-37	150-450

WBC and Differential

Age	WBC (x 10^3/mm^3)	Segs	Bands	Lymphs	Monos
0-3 d	9.0-35.0	32-62	10-18	19-29	5-7
1-2 wk	5.0-20.0	14-34	6-14	36-45	6-10
1-6 mo	6.0-17.5	13-33	4-12	41-71	4-7
7 mo to 2 y	6.0-17.0	15-35	5-11	45-76	3-6
2-5 y	5.5-15.5	23-45	5-11	35-65	3-6
5-8 y	5.0-14.5	32-54	5-11	28-48	3-6
13-18 y	4.5-13.0	34-64	5-11	25-45	3-6
Adults	4.5-11.0	35-66	5-11	24-44	3-6

Age	Eosinophils	Basophils	Atypical Lymphs	No. of NRBCs
0-3 d	0-2	0-1	0-8	0-2
1-2 wk	0-2	0-1	0-8	0
1-6 mo	0-3	0-1	0-8	0
7 mo to 2 y	0-3	0-1	0-8	0
2-5 y	0-3	0-1	0-8	0
5-8 y	0-3	0-1	0-8	0
13-18 y	0-3	0-1	0-8	0
Adults	0-3	0-1	0-8	0

Segs = segmented neutrophils.

Bands = band neutrophils.

Lymphs = lymphocytes.

Monos = monocytes.

Erythrocyte Sedimentation Rates and Reticulocyte Counts

Sedimentation rate, Westergren	Children	0-20 mm/h
	Adult male	0-15 mm/h
	Adult female	0-20 mm/h
Sedimentation rate, Wintrobe	Children	0-13 mm/h
	Adult male	0-10 mm/h
	Adult female	0-15 mm/h
Reticulocyte count	Newborns	2%-6%
	1-6 mo	0%-2.8%
	Adults	0.5%-1.5%

LIVER DISEASE

Pugh's Modification of Child's Classification for Severity

Parameter	Points for Increasing Abnormality 1	2	3
Encephalopathy	None	1 or 2	3 or 4
Ascites	Absent	Slight	Moderate
Bilirubin (mg/dL)	<2.9	2.9-5.8	>5.8
Albumin (g/dL)	>3.5	2.8-3.5	<2.8
Prothrombin time (seconds over control)	1-4	4-6	>6

Scores:

Mild hepatic impairment = <6 points.

Moderate hepatic impairment = 6-10 points.

Severe hepatic impairment = >10 points.

Considerations for Drug Dose Adjustment

Extent of Change in Drug Dose	Conditions or Requirements to Be Satisfied
No or minor change	Mild liver disease
	Extensive elimination of drug by kidneys and no renal dysfunction
	Elimination by pathways of metabolism spared by liver disease
	Drug is enzyme-limited and given acutely
	Drug is flow/enzyme-sensitive and only given acutely by I.V. route
	No alteration in drug sensitivity
Decrease in dose up to 25%	Elimination by the liver does not exceed 40% of the dose; no renal dysfunction
	Drug is flow-limited and given by I.V. route, with no large change in protein binding
	Drug is flow/enzyme-limited and given acutely by oral route
	Drug has a large therapeutic ratio
>25% decrease in dose	Drug metabolism is affected by liver disease; drug administered chronically
	Drug has a narrow therapeutic range; protein binding altered significantly
	Drug is flow-limited and given orally
	Drug is eliminated by kidneys and renal function severely affected
	Altered sensitivity to drug due to liver disease

Reference

Arns PA, Wedlund PJ, and Branch RA, "Adjustment of Medications in Liver Failure," *The Pharmacologic Approach to the Critically Ill Patient*, 2nd ed, Chernow B, ed, Baltimore, MD: Williams & Wilkins, 1988, 85-111.

CREATININE CLEARANCE ESTIMATING METHODS IN PATIENTS WITH STABLE RENAL FUNCTION

These formulas provide an acceptable estimate of the patient's creatinine clearance **except** in the following instances.

- Patient's serum creatinine is changing rapidly (either increasing or decreasing).
- Patient is markedly emaciated.

In above situations, certain assumptions have to be made.

- In a patient with rapidly rising serum creatinine (ie, >0.5-0.7 mg/dL/day), it is best to assume that the patient's creatinine clearance is probably <10 mL/minute.
- In an emaciated patient, although their actual creatinine clearance is less than their calculated creatinine clearance (because of decreased creatinine production), it is not possible to easily predict how much less.

INFANTS

Estimation of creatinine clearance using serum creatinine and body length (to be used when an adequate timed specimen cannot be obtained). **Note:** This formula may not provide an accurate estimation of creatinine clearance for infants younger than 6 months of age and for patients with severe starvation or muscle wasting.

$$Cl_{cr} = K \times L/S_{cr}$$

where:

Cl_{cr} = creatinine clearance in mL/minute/1.73 m^2
K = constant of proportionality that is age specific

Age	K
Low birth weight ≤1 y	0.33
Full-term ≤1 y	0.45
2-12 y	0.55
13-21 y female	0.55
13-21 y male	0.70

L = length in cm
S_{cr} = serum creatinine concentration in mg/dL

Reference

Schwartz GJ, Brion LP, and Spitzer A, "The Use of Plasma Creatinine Concentration for Estimating Glomerular Filtration Rate in Infants, Children and Adolescents," *Pediatr Clin North Am*, 1987, 34(3):571-90.

CHILDREN (1-18 years)

Method 1: (Traub SL and Johnson CE, *Am J Hosp Pharm*, 1980, 37(2):195-201)

$$Cl_{cr} = 0.48 \times (\text{height}) / S_{cr}$$

where:

Cl_{cr} = creatinine clearance in mL/min/1.73 m^2
S_{cr} = serum creatinine in mg/dL
Height = height in cm

Method 2: Nomogram (Traub SL and Johnson CE, *Am J Hosp Pharm*, 1980, 37(2):195-201)

The nomogram below is for rapid evaluation of endogenous creatinine clearance (Cl_{cr}) in pediatric patients (aged 1-18 years).

To predict Cl_{cr}, connect the child's Scr (serum creatinine) and Ht (height) with a ruler and read the Cl_{cr} where the ruler intersects the center line.

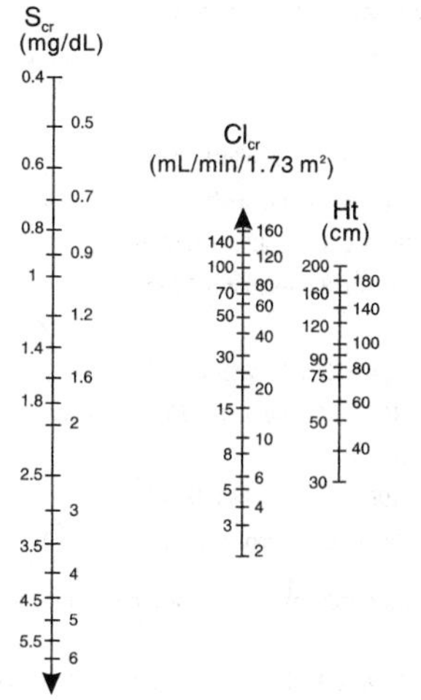

ADULTS (18 years and older)

Method 1: (Cockroft DW and Gault MH, *Nephron*, 1976, 16:31-41)

Estimated creatinine clearance (Cl_{cr}) (mL/min):

Male = (140 – age) x BW (kg) / 72 x S_{cr}
Female = male x 0.85

Note: Use of actual body weight (BW) in obese patients (and possibly patients with ascites) may significantly overestimate creatinine clearance. Some clinicians prefer to use an adjusted ideal body weight (IBW) in such cases [eg, IBW + 0.4(ABW-IBW)], especially when calculating dosages for aminoglycoside antibiotics.

Method 2: (Jelliffe RW, *Ann Intern Med*, 1973, 79:604)

Estimated creatinine clearance (Cl_{cr}) (mL/min/1.73 m^2):

Male = 98 – 0.8 (age – 20) / S_{cr}
Female = male x 0.90

RENAL FUNCTION TESTS

Endogenous Creatinine Clearance vs Age (timed collection)

Creatinine clearance (mL/min/1.73 m^2) = (Cr_uV/Cr_sT) (1.73/A)

where:

Cr_u	=	urine creatinine concentration (mg/dL)
V	=	total urine collected during sampling period (mL)
Cr_s	=	serum creatinine concentration (mg/dL)
T	=	duration of sampling period (min) (24 h = 1440 min)
A	=	body surface area (m^2)

Age-specific normal values

5-7 d	50.6 ± 5.8 mL/min/1.73 m^2
1-2 mo	64.6 ± 5.8 mL/min/1.73 m^2
5-8 mo	87.7 ± 11.9 mL/min/1.73 m^2
9-12 mo	86.9 ± 8.4 mL/min/1.73 m^2
≥18 mo	
male	124 ± 26 mL/min/1.73 m^2
female	109 ± 13.5 mL/min/1.73 m^2
Adults	
male	105 ± 14 mL/min/1.73 m^2
female	95 ± 18 mL/min/1.73 m^2

Note: In patients with renal failure (creatinine clearance <25 mL/min), creatinine clearance may be elevated over GFR because of tubular secretion of creatinine.

Calculation of Creatinine Clearance From a 24-Hour Urine Collection

Equation 1:

$$Cl_{cr} = \frac{U \times V}{P}$$

where:

Cl_{cr}	=	creatinine clearance
U	=	urine concentration of creatinine
V	=	total urine volume in the collection
P	=	plasma creatinine concentration

Equation 2:

$$Cl_{cr} = \frac{\text{(total urine volume [mL])} \times \text{(urine Cr concentration [mg/dL])}}{\text{(serum creatinine [mg/dL])} \times \text{(time of urine collection [minutes])}}$$

Occasionally, a patient will have a 12- or 24-hour urine collection done for direct calculation of creatinine clearance. Although a urine collection for 24 hours is best, it is difficult to do since many urine collections occur for a much shorter period. A 24-hour urine collection is the desired duration of urine collection because the urine excretion of creatinine is diurnal and thus the measured creatinine clearance will vary throughout the day as the creatinine in the urine varies. When the urine collection is less than 24 hours, the total excreted creatinine will be affected by the time of the day during which the collection is performed. A 24-hour urine collection is sufficient to be able to accurately average the diurnal creatinine excretion variations. If a patient has 24 hours of urine collected for creatinine clearance, equation 1 can be used for calculating the creatinine clearance. To use equation 1 to calculate the creatinine clearance, it will be necessary to know the duration of urine collection, the urine collection volume, the urine creatinine concentration, and the serum creatinine value that reflects the urine collection period. In most cases, a serum creatinine concentration is drawn anytime during the day, but it is best to have the value drawn halfway through the collection period.

Amylase:Creatinine Clearance Ratio

$$\frac{Amylase_u \times creatinine_p}{Amylase_p \times creatinine_u} \times 100$$

u = urine; p = plasma

Serum BUN:Serum Creatinine Ratio

Serum BUN (mg/dL:serum creatinine (mg/dL))

Normal BUN:creatinine ratio is 10-15

BUN:creatinine ratio >20 suggests prerenal azotemia (also seen with high urea-generation states such as GI bleeding)

BUN:creatinine ratio <5 may be seen with disorders affecting urea biosynthesis such as urea cycle enzyme deficiencies and with hepatitis.

Fractional Sodium Excretion

Fractional sodium secretion (FENa) = $Na_u Cr_s / Na_s Cr_u$ x 100%

where:

Na_u	=	urine sodium (mEq/L)
Na_s	=	serum sodium (mEq/L)
Cr_u	=	urine creatinine (mg/dL)
Cr_s	=	serum creatinine (mg/dL)

FENa <1% suggests prerenal failure
FENa >2% suggest intrinsic renal failure (for newborns, normal FENa is approximately 2.5%)

Note: Disease states associated with a falsely elevated FENa include severe volume depletion (>10%), early acute tubular necrosis, and volume depletion in chronic renal disease. Disorders associated with a lowered FENa include acute glomerulonephritis, hemoglobinuric or myoglobinuric renal failure, nonoliguric acute tubular necrosis, and acute urinary tract obstruction. In addition, FENa may be <1% in patients with acute renal failure **and** a second condition predisposing to sodium retention (eg, burns, congestive heart failure, nephrotic syndrome).

Urine Calcium:Urine Creatinine Ratio (spot sample)

Urine calcium (mg/dL): urine creatinine (mg/dL)

Normal values <0.21 (mean values 0.08 males, 0.06 females)

Premature infants show wide variability of calcium:creatinine ratio, and tend to have lower thresholds for calcium loss than older children. Prematures without nephrolithiasis had mean Ca:Cr ratio of 0.75 ± 0.76. Infants with nephrolithiasis had mean Ca:Cr ratio of 1.32 ± 1.03 (Jacinto JS, Modanlou HD, Crade M, et al, "Renal Calcification Incidence in Very Low Birth Weight Infants," *Pediatrics*, 1988, 81:31.)

Urine Protein:Urine Creatinine Ratio (spot sample)

P_u / Cr_u	Total Protein Excretion ($mg/m^2/d$)
0.1	80
1	800
10	8000

where:

P_u = urine protein concentration (mg/dL)
Cr_u = urine creatinine concentration (mg/dL)

AMINOGLYCOSIDE DOSING AND MONITORING

All aminoglycoside therapy should be individualized for specific patients in specific clinical situation. The following are guidelines for initiating therapy.

1. Loading dose based on estimated ideal body weight (IBW). **All patients require a loading dose independent of renal function.**

Agent	Dose
Gentamicin	2 mg/kg
Tobramycin	2 mg/kg
Amikacin	7.5 mg/kg

Significantly higher loading doses may be required in severely ill intensive care unit patients.

2. Initial maintenance doses as a percent of loading dose according to desired dosing interval and creatinine clearance (Cl_{cr}):
   Male Cl_{cr} (mL/min) = (140 – age) x IBW / 72 x serum creatinine
   Female = 0.85 x Cl_{cr} males

Cl_{cr} (mL/min)	Dosing Interval (h)		
	8	12	24
90	84%	—	—
80	80%	—	—
70	76%	88%	—
60	—	84%	—
50	—	79%	—
40	—	72%	92%
30	—	—	86%
25	—	—	81%
20	—	—	75%

Patients >65 years of age should not receive initial aminoglycoside maintenance dosing more often than every 12 hours.

3. Serum concentration monitoring
   - Serum concentration monitoring is necessary for **safe** and **effective** therapy, particularly in patients with serious infections and those with risk factors for toxicity.
   - Peak serum concentrations should be drawn 30 minutes after the completion of a 30-minute infusion. Trough serum concentrations should be drawn within 30 minutes prior to the administered dose.
   - Serum concentrations should be drawn after 5 half-lives, usually around the third dose or thereafter.
4. Desired measured serum concentrations

	Peak (mcg/mL)	Trough (mcg/mL)
Gentamicin	6-10	0.5-2.0
Tobramycin	6-10	0.5-2.0
Amikacin	20-30	<5

5. For patients receiving hemodialysis:
   - administer the **same** loading dose
   - administer 2/3 of the loading dose after each dialysis
   - **serum concentrations must be monitored**
   - watch for ototoxicity from accumulation of drug
6. For individual clinical situations the prescribing physician should feel free to consult Infectious Disease, the Pharmacology Service, or the Pharmacy.

"Once Daily" Aminoglycosides

High dose, "once daily" aminoglycoside therapy for treatment of gram-negative bacterial infections has been studied and remains controversial. The pharmacodynamics of aminoglycosides reveal dose-dependent killing which suggests an efficacy advantage of "high" peak serum concentrations. It is also suggested that allowing troughs to fall to unmeasurable levels decreases the risk of nephrotoxicity without detriment to efficacy. Because of a theoretical saturation of tubular cell uptake of aminoglycosides, decreasing the number of times the drug is administered in a particular time period may play a role in minimizing the risk of nephrotoxicity. Ototoxicity has not been sufficiently formally evaluated through audiometry or vestibular testing comparing "once daily" to standard therapy. Over 100 letters, commentaries, studies and reviews have been published on the topic of "once daily" aminoglycosides with varying dosing regimens, monitoring parameters, inclusion and exclusion criteria, and results (most of which have been favorable for the "once daily" regimens). The caveats of this simplified method of dosing are several, including assurance that creatinine clearances be calculated, that all patients are not candidates and should not be considered for this regimen, and that "once daily" is a semantic misnomer.

Because of the controversial nature of this method, it is beyond the scope of this book to present significant detail and dosing regimen recommendations. Considerable experience with two methods warrants mention. The Hartford Hospital has experience with over 2000 patients utilizing a 7 mg/kg dose, a dosing scheme for various creatinine clearance estimates, and a serum concentration monitoring nomogram.[1] Providence Medical Center utilizes a 5 mg/kg dosing regimen but only in patients with excellent renal function; serum concentrations are monitored 4-6 hours prior to the dose administered.[2] Two excellent reviews discuss the majority of studies and controversies regarding these dosing techniques.[3,4] An editorial accompanies one of the reviews and is worth examination.[5]

"Once daily" dosing may be a safe and effective method of providing aminoglycoside therapy to a large number of patients who require these efficacious yet toxic agents. As with any method of aminoglycoside administration, dosing must be individualized and the caveats of the method considered.

Footnotes

1. Nicolau DP, Freeman CD, Belliveau PP, et al, "Experience With a Once-Daily Aminoglycoside Program Administered to 2,184 Patients," *Antimicrob Agents Chemother*, 1995, 39(3):650-5.
2. Gilbert DN, "Once-Daily Aminoglycoside Therapy," *Antimicrob Agents Chemother*, 1991, 35(3):399-405.
3. Preston SL and Briceland LL, "Single Daily Dosing of Aminoglycosides," *Pharmacotherapy*, 1995, 15(3):297-316.
4. Bates RD and Nahata MC, "Once-Daily Administration of Aminoglycosides," *Ann Pharmacother*, 1994, 28(6):757-66.
5. Rotschafer JC and Rybak MJ, "Single Daily Dosing of Aminoglycosides: A Commentary," *Ann Pharmacother*, 1994, 28(6):797-801.

Aminoglycoside Penetration Into Various Tissues

Site	Extent of Distribution
Eye	Poor
CNS	Poor (<25%)
Pleural	Excellent
Bronchial secretions	Poor
Sputum	Fair (10%-50%)
Pulmonary tissue	Excellent
Ascitic fluid	Variable (43%-132%)
Peritoneal fluid	Poor
Bile	Variable (25%-90%)
Bile with obstruction	Poor
Synovial fluid	Excellent
Bone	Poor
Prostate	Poor
Urine	Excellent
Renal tissue	Excellent

Adapted from Neu HC, "Pharmacology of Aminoglycosides," *The Aminoglycosides*, Whelton E and Neu HC, eds, New York, NY: Marcel Dekker, Inc, 1981.

ANGIOTENSIN AGENTS

Comparison of Indications and Adult Dosages

Drug	Hypertension	CHF	Renal Dysfunction	Dialyzable	Strengths (mg)
ACE Inhibitors					
Benazepril (Lotensin®)	10-40 mg/day	Not FDA approved	Cl_{cr} <30 mL/min: 5 mg/day initially Maximum: 40 mg/day	Yes	Tablets 5, 10, 20, 40
Captopril (Capoten®)	25-100 mg/day bid-tid	6.25-100 mg tid Maximum: 450 mg/day	Cl_{cr} 10-50 mL/min: 75% of usual dose Cl_{cr} <10 mL/min: 50% of usual dose	Yes	Tablets 12.5, 25, 50, 100
Enalapril (Vasotec®)	2.5-40 mg/day qd-bid	2.5-20 mg bid Maximum: 20 mg bid	Cl_{cr} 30-80 mL/min: 5 mg/day initially Cl_{cr} <30 mL/min: 2.5 mg/day initially	Yes	Tablets 2.5, 5, 10, 20
Enalaprilat[1]	0.625 mg, 1.25 mg, 2.5 mg q6h Maximum: 5 mg q6h	Not FDA approved	Cl_{cr} <30 mL/min: 0.625 mg q6h	Yes	1.25 mg/mL (1 mL, 2 mL vials)
Fosinopril (Monopril®)	10-40 mg/day	10-40 mg/day	No dosage reduction necessary	Not well dialyzed	Tablets 10, 20, 40
Lisinopril (Prinivil®, Zestril®)	10-40 mg/day Maximum: 40 mg/day	5-40 mg/day	Cl_{cr} 10-30 mL/min: 5 mg/day initially Cl_{cr} <10 mL/min: 2.5 mg/day initially	Yes	Tablets 2.5, 5, 10, 20, 30, 40
Moexipril (Univasc®)	7.5-30 mg/day qd-bid Maximum: 30 mg/day	LV dysfunction (post-MI): 7.5-30 mg/day	Cl_{cr} <40 mL/min: 3.75 mg/day initially Maximum: 15 mg/day	Unknown	Tablets 7.5, 15
Perindopril (Aceon®)	4-8 mg/day	4-8 mg/day Maximum: 16 mg/day	Cl_{cr} 30-60 mL/min: 2 mg/day Cl_{cr} 15-29 mL/min: 2 mg qod Cl_{cr} <15 mL/min: 2 mg on dialysis days	Yes	Tablets 2, 4, 8
Quinapril (Accupril®)	10-40 mg/day qd-bid	5-20 mg bid	Cl_{cr} 30-60 mL/min: 5 mg/day initially Cl_{cr} <10-30 mL/min: 2.5 mg/day initially	Not well dialyzed	Tablets 5, 10, 20, 40
Ramipril (Altace®)	2.5-20 mg/day qd-bid	2.5-10 mg/day	Cl_{cr} <40 mL/min: 25% of normal dose	Unknown	Capsules 1.25, 2.5, 5, 10
Trandolapril (Mavik®)	1-4 mg/day Maximum: 8 mg/day qd-bid	LV dysfunction (post-MI): 1-4 mg/day	Cl_{cr} <30 mL/min: 0.5 mg/day initially	No	Tablets 1, 2, 4
Angiotensin II Receptor Blockers					
Candesartan (Atacand®)	8-32 mg/day	Target: 32 mg once daily	No dosage adjustment necessary	No	Tablets 4, 8, 16, 32
Eprosartan (Teveten®)	400-800 mg/day qd-bid	Not FDA approved	No dosage adjustment necessary	Unknown	Tablets 400, 600
Irbesartan (Avapro®)	150-300 mg/day	Not FDA approved	No dosage reduction necessary	No	Tablets 75, 150, 300
Losartan (Cozaar®)	25-100 mg qd or bid	Not FDA approved	No dosage adjustment necessary	No	Tablets 25, 50, 100
Olmesartan (Benicar®)	20-40 mg/day	Not FDA approved	No dosage adjustment necessary	Unknown	Tablets 5, 20, 40
Telmisartan (Micardis®)	20-80 mg/day	Not FDA approved	No dosage reduction necessary	No	Tablets 20, 40, 80
Valsartan (Diovan®)	80-320 mg/day	Target: 160 mg bid	Decrease dose only if Cl_{cr} <10 mL/minute	No	Tablets 40, 80, 160, 320

Comparison of Indications and Adult Dosages *continued*

Drug	Hypertension	CHF	Renal Dysfunction	Dialyzable	Strengths (mg)
Renin Inhibitors					
Aliskiren (Tekturna®)	150-300 mg once daily	Not FDA approved	No dosage adjustment necessary in mild-to-moderate impairment; not adequately studied in severe impairment	Unknown	Tablets 150, 300

Dosage is based on 70 kg adult with normal hepatic and renal function.

[1]Enalaprilat is the only available ACE inhibitor in a parenteral formulation.

ACE Inhibitors: Comparative Pharmacokinetics

Drug	Prodrug	Absorption (%)	Serum $t_{1/2}$ (h) Normal Renal Function	Serum Protein Binding (%)	Elimination	Onset of BP Lowering Action (h)	Peak BP Lowering Effects (h)	Duration of BP Lowering Effects (h)
Benazepril	Yes	37		~97	Renal (32%), biliary (~12%)	1	2-4	24
Benazeprilat			10-11 (effective)	~95%				
Captopril	No	60-75 (fasting)	1.9 (elimination)	25-30	Renal	0.25-0.5	1-1.5	~6
Enalapril	Yes	55-75	2	50-60	Renal (60%-80%), fecal	1	4-6	12-24
Enalaprilat			11 (effective)					
Fosinopril		36			Renal (~50%), biliary (~50%)	1		24
Fosinoprilat			12 (effective)	>99				
Moexipril	Yes		1	90	Fecal (53%), renal (8%)		1-2	>24
Moexiprilat			2-10	50				
Perindopril	Yes		1.5-3	60	Renal		3-7	
Perindoprilat			3-10 (effective)	10-20				
Quinapril	Yes	>60	0.8	97	Renal (~60%) as metabolite, fecal	1	2-4	24
Quinaprilat			2					
Ramipril	Yes	50-60	1-2	73	Renal (60%), fecal (40%)	1-2	3-6	24
Ramiprilat			13-17 (effective)	56				
Trandolapril	Yes		6	80	Renal (33%), fecal (66%)	1-2	6	≥24
Trandolaprilat			10	65-94				

Angiotensin II Receptor Blockers and Renin Inhibitors: Comparative Pharmacokinetics

Drug	Prodrug	Time to Peak	Bioavailability	Food "Area-Under-the-Curve"	Elimination Half-Life	Elimination Altered in Renal Dysfunction	Precautions in Severe Renal Dysfunction	Elimination Altered in Hepatic Dysfunction	Precautions in Hepatic Dysfunction	Protein Binding
Angiotensin II Receptor Blockers										
Candesartan (Atacand®)	Yes[1]	3-4 h	15%	No effect	9 h	Yes[2]	Yes	No	Yes	>99%
Eprosartan (Teveten®)	No	1-2 h	13%	No effect	5-9 h	No	Yes	No	Yes	98%
Irbesartan (Avapro®)	No	1.5-2 h	60%-80%	No effect	11-15 h	No	Yes	No	No	90%
Losartan (Cozaar®)	Yes[3]	1 h / 3-4 h[3]	33%	9%-10%	1.5-2 h / 6-9 h[3]	No	Yes	Yes	Yes	~99%
Olmesartan (Benicar®)	Yes	1-2 h	26%	No effect	13 h	Yes	Yes	Yes	No	99%
Telmisartan (Micardis®)	No	0.5-1 h	42%-58%	9.6%-20%	24 h	No	Yes	Yes	Yes	>99.5%
Valsartan (Diovan®)	No	2-4 h	25%	9%-40%	6 h	No	Yes	Yes	Yes	95%
Renin Inhibitors										
Aliskiren (Tekturna®)	No	1-3 h	~3%	85% (high-fat meal)	16-32 h	Yes[4]	Yes	No	No	?

[1]Candesartan cilexetil: Active metabolite candesartan.

[2]Dosage adjustments are not necessary.

[3]Losartan: Active metabolite E-3174.

[4]No initial dosage adjustment in mild-to-moderate impairment.

ANTICOAGULANTS, INJECTABLE

Name	Use	Limitation	Dose (SubQ unless otherwise noted)	Average MW (in daltons)
		Low Molecular Weight Heparins		
Dalteparin (Fragmin®)	Prophylaxis	Abdominal surgery[1] Abdominal surgery[2]	2500 units/d 5000 units/d	4000-6000
		Hip surgery[1]	5000 units/d postoperatively	
	Treatment	DVT[3]	100 units/kg bid 200 units/kg qd	4000-6000
		Unstable[4] angina Non-Q-wave MI	120 units/kg (max: 10,000 units) q12h for 5-8 d	
Enoxaparin (Lovenox®)	Prophylaxis	Hip or knee replacement	30 mg twice daily[5]	3500-5500
		High-risk hip replacement or abdominal surgery	40 mg once daily	
	Treatment	DVT or PE	1 mg/kg q12h	
		Acute coronary	1 mg/kg q12h	
Tinzaparin (Innohep®)	Treatment	DVT or PE	175 anti-Xa int. units/kg/day	5500-7500
		Heparin		
Heparin (Hep-Lock®)	Prophylaxis	Risk of thromboembolic disease	5000 units q8-12h	3000-30,000
	Treatment	Thrombosis or embolization	80 units/kg IVP then 20,000-40,000 units daily as continuous I.V. infusion	
	Treatment[3]	Unstable angina[3]	80 units/kg IVP then 20,000-40,000 units daily as continuous I.V. infusion	
		Heparinoid		
Danaparoid	Prophylaxis	Hip replacement	750 units bid	6500
	Treatment[3]		2000 units q12h	
		Selective Anti-Xa Inhibitor		
Fondaparinux[6] (Arixtra®)	Prophylaxis	Hip fracture Hip or knee replacement	2.5 mg once daily	1728
		Coumarin Derivatives		
Warfarin (Coumadin®)	Prophylaxis	NS	Variable	NS
	Treatment		2-5 mg/d	

NS = not stated.

[1]Patients with low risk of DVT.

[2]Patients with high risk of DVT.

[3]Not FDA approved.

[4]Patients >60 years of age may require a lower dose of heparin.

[5]Patients weighing <100 lb or ≥65 years of age may receive 0.5 mg/kg/dose every 12 hours.

[6]Synthetic pentasaccharide.

ANTICONVULSANT DRUGS OF CHOICE

Seizure Type	First Line Therapy	Alternatives
Partial (including secondary generalization)	Carbamazepine, lamotrigine, levetiracetam, or oxcarbazepine	Gabapentin, lacosamide, phenytoin, pregabalin, topiramate, valproate, or zonisamide
Generalized tonic-clonic	Lamotrigine or valproate	Carbamazepine, levetiracetam, oxcarbazepine, phenytoin, topiramate, or zonisamide
Childhood absence epilepsy	Ethosuximide (only if no generalized seizures), lamotrigine, or valproate	Clonazepam, levetiracetam, or zonisamide
Atypical absence, myoclonic, or atonic	Lamotrigine, levetiracetam, or valproate	Clonazepam, felbamate, topiramate, or zonisamide

Note: Table includes non-FDA approved indications.

References

"Drugs for Epilepsy," *Treat Guidel Med Lett*, 2008, 6(70):37-46.

Glauser T, Ben-Menachem E, Bourgeois B, et al, "ILAE Treatment Guidelines: Evidence-Based Analysis of Antiepileptic Drug Efficacy and Effectiveness as Initial Monotherapy for Epileptic Seizures and Syndromes," *Epilepsia*, 2006, 47(7):1094-120.

ANTIDEPRESSANT AGENTS

Comparison of Usual Dosage, Mechanism of Action, and Adverse Effects

Drug	Initial Dose	Usual Dosage (mg/d)	Dosage Forms	Adverse Effects						Comments
				ACH	Drowsiness	Orthostatic Hypotension	Conduction Abnormalities	GI Distress	Weight Gain	
Tricyclic Antidepressants and Related Compounds[1]										
Amitriptyline	25-75 mg qhs	100-300	T, I	4+	4+	3+	3+	1	4+	Also used in chronic pain, migraine, and as a hypnotic; contraindicated with cisapride
Amoxapine	50 mg bid	100-400	T	2+	2+	2+	2+	0	2+	May cause extrapyramidal symptom (EPS)
Clomipramine[2] (Anafranil®)	25-75 mg qhs	100-250	C	4+	4+	2+	3+	1+	4+	Approved for OCD
Desipramine (Norpramin®)	25-75 mg qhs	100-300	T	1+	2+	2+	2+	0	1+	Blood levels useful for therapeutic monitoring
Doxepin (Sinequan®, Zonalon®)	25-75 mg qhs	100-300	C, L	3+	4+	2+	2+	0	4+	
Imipramine (Tofranil®, Tofranil-PM®)	25-75 mg qhs	100-300	T, C	3+	3+	4+	3+	1+	4+	Blood levels useful for therapeutic monitoring
Maprotiline	25-75 mg qhs	100-225	T	2+	3+	2+	2+	0	2+	
Nortriptyline (Pamelor®)	25-50 mg qhs	50-150	C, L	2+	2+	1+	2+	0	1+	Blood levels useful for therapeutic monitoring
Protriptyline (Vivactil®)	15 mg qAM	15-60	T	2+	1+	2+	3+	1+	1+	
Trimipramine (Surmontil®)	25-75 mg qhs	100-300	C	4+	4+	3+	3+	0	4+	
Selective Serotonin Reuptake Inhibitors[3]										
Citalopram (Celexa™)	20 mg qAM	20-60	T	0	0	0	0	3+[4]	1+	
Escitalopram (Lexapro™)	10 mg qAM	10-20	T	0	0	0	0	3+	1+	S-enantiomer of citalopram
Fluoxetine (Prozac®, Prozac® Weekly™, Sarafem™)	10-20 mg qAM	20-80	C, L, T	0	0	0	0	3+[4]	1+	CYP2B6 and 2D6 inhibitor
Fluvoxamine[2]	50 mg qhs	100-300	T	0	0	0	0	3+[4]	1+	Contraindicated with pimozide, thioridazine, mesoridazine, CYP1A2, 2B6, 2C19, and 3A4 inhibitors
Paroxetine (Paxil®, Paxil® CR™)	10-20 mg qAM	20-50	T, L	1+	1+	0	0	3+[4]	2+	CYP2B6 and 2D6 inhibitor
Sertraline (Zoloft®)	25-50 mg qAM	50-200	T	0	0	0	0	3+[4]	1+	CYP2B6 and 2C19 inhibitor
Dopamine-Reuptake Blocking Compounds										
Bupropion (Wellbutrin®, Wellbutrin SR®, Wellbutrin XL™, Zyban®)	100 mg bid-tid IR[5] 150 mg qAM-bid SR[6]	300-450[7]	T	0	0	0	1+/0	1+	0	Contraindicated with seizures, bulimia, and anorexia; low incidence of sexual dysfunction IR: A 6-h interval between doses preferred SR: An 8-h interval between doses preferred

Comparison of Usual Dosage, Mechanism of Action, and Adverse Effects *continued*

Drug	Initial Dose	Usual Dosage (mg/d)	Dosage Forms	Adverse Effects						Comments
				ACH	Drowsiness	Orthostatic Hypotension	Conduction Abnormalities	GI Distress	Weight Gain	
Serotonin / Norepinephrine Reuptake Inhibitors[8]										
Duloxetine (Cymbalta®)	40-60 mg/d	40-60	C	1+	1+	0	1+	3+	0	Useful for stress incontinence and chronic pain
Desvenlafaxine (Pristiq™)	50 mg/d	50-100	T/SR	0	1+	1+	0	3+[4]	0	
Venlafaxine (Effexor®, Effexor® XR)	25 mg bid-tid IR 37.5 mg qd XR	75-375	T	1+	1+	0	1+	3+[4]	0	High-dose is useful to treat refractory depression; frequency of hypertension increases with dosage >225 mg/d
$5\text{-}HT_2$ Receptor Antagonist Properties										
Nefazodone	100 mg bid	300-600	T	1+	1+	2+	1+	1+	0	Contraindicated with carbamazepine, pimozide, astemizole, cisapride, and terfenadine; caution with triazolam and alprazolam; low incidence of sexual dysfunction
Trazodone (Desyrel®)	50 mg tid	150-600	T	0	4+	3+	1+	1+	2+	
Noradrenergic Antagonist										
Mirtazapine (Remeron®, Remeron® SolTab®)	15 mg qhs	15-45	T	1+	3+	1+	1+	0	3+	Dose >15 mg/d less sedating, low incidence of sexual dysfunction
Monoamine Oxidase Inhibitors										
Isocarboxazid (Marplan®)	10 mg tid	10-30	T	2+	2+	2+	1+	1+	2+	Diet must be low in tyramine; contraindicated with sympathomimetics and other antidepressants
Phenelzine (Nardil®)	15 mg tid	15-90	T	2+	2+	2+	0	1+	3+	
Tranylcypromine (Parnate®)	10 mg bid	10-60	T	2+	1+	2+	1+	1+	2+	
Selegiline (EmSam®)	6 mg/d	6-12	Transdermal	2+	1+	2+	0	1+	0	Low tyramine diet not required for 6 mg/d dosage

ACH = anticholinergic effects (dry mouth, blurred vision, urinary retention, constipation); 0 - 4+ = absent or rare - relatively common. T = tablet, L = liquid, I = injectable, C = capsule; IR = immediate release, SR = sustained release.

[1]**Important note:** A 1-week supply taken all at once in a patient receiving the maximum dose can be fatal.

[2]Not approved by FDA for depression. Approved for OCD.

[3]Flat dose response curve, headache, nausea, and sexual dysfunction are common side effects for SSRIs.

[4]Nausea is usually mild and transient.

[5]IR: 100 mg bid, may be increased to 100 mg tid no sooner than 3 days after beginning therapy.

[6]SR: 150 mg qAM, may be increased to 150 mg bid as early as day 4 of dosing.

[7]To minimize seizure risk, do not exceed IR 150 mg/dose or SR 200 mg/dose.

[8]Do not use with sibutramine; relatively safe in overdose.

ANTIFUNGAL AGENTS

Activities of Various Agents Against Specific Fungi

Organisms	Amphotericin B[1]	Caspofungin	Fluconazole	Flucytosine
Aspergillus spp	FA	FA	N	?
Blastomyces dermatitidis	FA	?	A	N
Candida albicans	FA	FA	FA	FA
Candida glabrata	A	A	?	A
Candida krusei	FA	A	?	A
Candida tropicalis	FA	A	?	A
Coccidioides immitis	FA	?	A	N
Cryptococcus spp	FA	N	FA	FA
Dermatophytes	A	?	A	?
Fusarium spp	A	N	N	N
Histoplasma capsulatum	FA	A?	A	N
Penicillium spp	A	?	?	A
Pseudoallescheria boydii	?	A	N	N
Sporothrix schenckii	A	?	?	?
Zygomycetes (Mucor, Rhizopus)	A	N	N	N

Organisms	Griseofulvin	Itraconazole	Ketoconazole	Micafungin
Aspergillus spp	N	FA	N	A
Blastomyces dermatitidis	N	FA	FA	?
Candida albicans	N	FA	FA	FA
Candida glabrata	N	?	?	FA
Candida krusei	N	A	?	A
Candida tropicalis	N	?	?	A
Coccidioides immitis	N	A	FA	?
Cryptococcus spp	N	A	A	N
Dermatophytes	FA	A	A	?
Fusarium spp	N	N	N	?
Histoplasma capsulatum	N	FA	FA	?
Penicillium spp	N	?	N	?
Pseudoallescheria boydii	N	N	N	?
Sporothrix schenckii	N	?	N	?
Zygomycetes (Mucor, Rhizopus)	N	N	N	N

Organisms	Miconazole	Nystatin	Terbinafine	Voriconazole
Aspergillus spp	N	A	N	FA
Blastomyces dermatitidis	N	A	N	A
Candida albicans	FA	FA	A	A
Candida glabrata	?	A	?	A
Candida krusei	?	A	?	A
Candida tropicalis	?	A	?	A
Coccidioides immitis	A	N	N	A
Cryptococcus spp	A	N	N	A
Dermatophytes	N	N	FA	?
Fusarium spp	N	N	N	FA
Histoplasma capsulatum	N	N	N	A
Penicillium spp	N	N	N	?
Pseudoallescheria boydii	N	N	N	FA
Sporothrix schenckii	?	N	N	?
Zygomycetes (Mucor, Rhizopus)	N	N	N	N?

Organisms	Anidulafungin	Posaconazole
Aspergillus spp	A	FA
Blastomyces dermatitidis	N	A
Candida albicans	FA	FA
Candida glabrata	FA	A
Candida krusei	A	A
Candida tropicalis	FA	A
Coccidioides immitis	?	A
Cryptococcus spp	N	A
Dermatophytes	N?	A
Fusarium spp	N	A
Histoplasma capsulatum	?	A
Penicillium spp	A	A
Pseudoallescheria boydii	?	A
Sporothrix schenckii	?	A
Zygomycetes (Mucor, Rhizopus)	N?	A

FA = FDA approved indication. A = active. ? = unknown or questionable. N = not active.

[1]Various lipid products have differing indications, but all have activity against the same organisms.

References

Espinel-Ingroff A, "Comparison of *In Vitro* Activities of the New Triazole SCH56592 and the Echinocandins MK-0991 (L-743,872) and LY303366 Against Opportunistic Filamentous and Dimorphic Fungi and Yeasts," *J Clin Microbiol*, 1998, 36(10):2950-6.

Sabatelli F, Patel R, Mann PA, et al, "*In Vitro* Activities of Posaconazole, Fluconazole, Itraconazole, Voriconazole, and Amphotericin B Against a Large Collection of Clinically Important Molds and Yeasts," *Antimicrob Agents Chemother*, 2006, 50(6):2009-15.

Torres HA, Hachem RY, Chemaly RF, et al, "Posaconazole: A Broad-Spectrum Triazole Antifungal," *Lancet Infect Dis*, 2005, 5(12):775-85.

Vazquez JA, "Anidulafungin: A New Echinocandin With a Novel Profile," *Clin Ther*, 2005, 27(6):657-73.

Zhanel GG, Karlowsky JA, Harding GA, et al, "*In Vitro* Activity of a New Semisynthetic Echinocandin, LY-303366, Against Systemic Isolates of *Candida* Species, *Cryptococcus neoformans*, *Blastomyces dermatitidis*, and *Aspergillus* Species," *Antimicrob Agents Chemother*, 1997, 41(4):863-5.

ANTIMIGRAINE DRUGS: 5-HT$_1$ RECEPTOR AGONISTS

Pharmacokinetic Differences

Pharmacokinetic Parameter	Almotriptan (Axert™)	Eletriptan (Relpax®)	Frovatriptan (Frova®)	Naratriptan (Amerge®)	Rizatriptan (Maxalt®, Maxalt-MLT®)		Sumatriptan (Imitrex®)			Zolmitriptan (Zomig®, Zomig-ZMT™)	
	Oral (6.25 mg)	Tablets	Oral	Oral	Tablets	Disintegrating Tablets	SubQ (6 mg)	Oral (100 mg)	Nasal (20 mg)	Oral (5 mg)	Oral (10 mg)
Onset	<60 min	<2 h	<2 h	30 min	~30 min	~30 min	10 min	30-60 min	<60 min	0.5-1 h	
Duration	Short	Short	Long	Long	Short	Short	Short	Short	Short	Short	
Time to peak serum concentration (h)	1-3	1.5-2	2-4	2-4	1-1.5	1.6-2.5	5-20	1.5-2.5	1	1.5	2-3.5
Average bioavailability (%)	70	50	20-30	70	45	—	97	15	17	40-46	46-49
Volume of distribution (L)	180-200	138	210-280	170	110-140	110-140	170	170	NA	—	402
Half-life (h)	3-4	4	26	6	2-3	2-3	2	2-2.5[1]	2	2.8-3.4	2.5-3.7
Fraction excreted unchanged in urine (%)	40	—	32	50	14	14	22	3	3	8	8

[1]With extended dosing, the half-life extends to 7 hours.

ANTIPARKINSONIAN AGENTS

Drugs Used for the Treatment of Parkinsonian Symptoms[1]

Drug	Mechanism	Initial Dose	Titration Schedule	Usual Daily Dosage	Recommended Dosing Schedule
Dopaminergic Agents					
Amantadine (Symmetrel®)	NMDA receptor antagonist and inhibits neuronal reuptake of dopamine	100 mg every other day	100 mg/dose every week, up to 300 mg 3 times/d	100-200 mg	Twice daily
Apomorphine (Apokyn™)	D_2 receptors (caudate-putamen)	1-2 mg	Complex; based on tolerance and response to test dose(s)	Variable; <20 mg	Individualized; 3-5 times/d prn
Bromocriptine (Parlodel®)	Moderate affinity for D_2 and D_3 dopamine receptors	1.25 mg twice daily	2.5 mg/d every 2-4 wk	2.5-100 mg	3 times/d
Cabergoline (Dostinex®)[2]	Selective to D_2 dopamine receptors	0.5 mg once daily	0.25-0.5 mg/d every 4 wk	0.5-5 mg	Once daily
Carbidopa/levodopa (Sinemet® CR)	Converts to dopamine; binds to all CNS dopamine receptors	10-25/100 mg 2-4 times/d	0.5-1 tablet (10 or 25/100 mg) every 1-2 d	50/200 to 200/2000 mg (3-8 tablets)	3 times/d or twice daily (for controlled release)
Entacapone (Comtan®)	COMT enzyme inhibitor	200 mg 3 times/d	Titrate down the doses of carbidopa/levodopa as required	600-1600 mg	3 times/d; up to 8 times/d
Levodopa/carbidopa/entacapone (Stalevo™)	Converts to dopamine; binds to all CNS dopamine receptors; COMT enzyme inhibitor	1 tablet 3-4 times/d (to replace previous dosing with individual agents)	As tolerated based on response and presence of dyskinesias	3-8 tablets per day	3-4 times/d
Pramipexole (Mirapex®)	High affinity for D_2 and D_3 dopamine receptors	0.125 mg 3 times/d	0.125 mg/dose every 5-7 d	1.5-4.5 mg	3 times/d
Rasagiline (Azilect®)	Inhibits MAO-B	0.5-1 mg once daily	≤1 mg daily	0.5-1 mg	Once daily
Ropinirole (Requip®)	High affinity for D_2 and D_3 dopamine receptors	0.25 mg 3 times/d	0.25 mg/dose weekly for 4 wk, then 1.5 mg/d every week up to 9 mg/d; 3 mg/d up to a max of 24 mg/d	0.75-24 mg	3 times/d
Rotigotine (Neupro® [DSC])	D_1, D_2, D_3 dopamine receptor agonist	2 mg/24 hours transdermal patch	Increase by 2 mg/24 hours weekly; maximum 6 mg/24 hours	2 mg/24 hours, 4 mg/24 hours, or 6 mg/24 hours	Once daily patch
Selegiline (Eldepryl®)	Inhibits MAO-B	5-10 mg twice daily	Titrate down the doses of carbidopa/levodopa as required	5-10 mg	Twice daily
Tolcapone (Tasmar®)	COMT enzyme inhibitor	100 mg 3 times/d	Titrate down the doses of carbidopa/levodopa as required	300-600 mg	3 times/d
Anticholinergic Agents					
Benztropine (Cogentin®)	Blocks cholinergic receptors, also has antihistamine effects	0.5-2 mg/d in 1-4 divided doses	0.5 mg/dose every 5-6 d	2-6 mg	1-2 times/d
Diphenhydramine (Benadryl®)	Blocks cholinergic receptors	12.5-25 mg 3-4 times/d	As tolerated	25-300 mg	3-4 times/d
Procyclidine (Kemadrin®)	Blocks cholinergic receptors	2.5 mg 3 times/d	Gradually as tolerated	7.5-20 mg	3 times/d
Trihexyphenidyl (Artane)	Blocks cholinergic receptors; also some direct effects	1-2 mg/d	2 mg/d at intervals of 3-5 d	5-15 mg	3-4 times/d

[1]The medications listed in the table represent treatment options for both idiopathic Parkinson's disease, as well as Parkinsonian symptoms resulting from other drug therapy.

[2]Cabergoline is not FDA approved for the treatment of Parkinson's disease.

ANTIPSYCHOTIC AGENTS

Antipsychotic Agent	Dosage Forms	I.M./P.O. Potency	Equiv. Dosages (approx) (mg)	Usual Adult Daily Maint. Dose (mg)	Sedation (Incidence)	Extrapyramidal Side Effects	Anticholinergic Side Effects	Orthostatic Hypotension	Comments
Aripiprazole (Abilify™)	Soln, tab		4	10-30	Low	Very low	Very low	Very low	Low weight gain; activating
Chlorpromazine (Thorazine® [DSC])	Conc, inj, supp, syr, tab	4:1	100	200-1000	High	Moderate	Moderate	Moderate / high	
Clozapine (Clozaril®)	Tab		100	75-900	High	Very low	High	High	~1% incidence of agranulocytosis; weekly-biweekly CBC required; potential for weight gain, lipid abnormalities, and diabetes
Fluphenazine (Permitil®, Prolixin®, Prolixin Decanoate®, Prolixin Enanthate®)	Conc, elix, inj, tab	2:1	2	0.5-20	Low	High	Low	Low	
Haloperidol (Haldol®, Haldol® Decanoate)	Conc, inj, tab	2:1	2	0.5-20	Low	High	Low	Low	
Loxapine (Loxitane®, Loxitane® C, Loxitane® I.M.)	Cap, conc, inj		10	25-250	Moderate	Moderate	Low	Low	
Molindone (Moban®)	Conc, tab		15	15-225	Low	Moderate	Low	Low	May cause less weight gain
Olanzapine (Zyprexa®, Zyprexa® Zydis®)	Inj, tab, tab (oral-disintegrating)		4	5-20	Moderate / high	Low	Moderate	Moderate	Potential for weight gain, lipid abnormalities, diabetes
Paliperidone (Invega™)	Tab (extended release)			3-12	Low / moderate	Low	Very low	Moderate	Active metabolite of risperidone
Perphenazine (Trilafon®)	Conc, inj, tab		10	16-64	Low	Moderate	Low	Low	
Pimozide (Orap™)	Tab		2	1-10	Moderate	High	Moderate	Low	Contraindicated with CYP3A inhibitors
Quetiapine (Seroquel®)	Tab		125	50-800	Moderate / high	Very low	Moderate	Moderate	Moderate weight gain; potential for lipid abnormalities; diabetes
Risperidone (Risperdal®)	Inj, soln, tab, tab (oral-disintegrating)		1	0.5-6	Low / moderate	Low	Very low	Moderate	Low to moderate weight gain; potential for diabetes
Thioridazine (Mellaril®)	Conc, tab		100	200-800	High	Low	High	Moderate / high	May cause irreversible retinitis pigmentosa at doses >800 mg/d; prolongs QTc; use only in treatment of refractory illness
Thiothixene (Navane®)	Cap, conc, powder for inj	4:1	4	5-40	Low	High	Low	Low / moderate	

Antipsychotic Agent	Dosage Forms	I.M./P.O. Potency	Equiv. Dosages (approx) (mg)	Usual Adult Daily Maint. Dose (mg)	Sedation (Incidence)	Extrapyramidal Side Effects	Anticholinergic Side Effects	Orthostatic Hypotension	Comments
Trifluoperazine (Stelazine® [DSC])	Conc, inj, tab		5	2-40	Low	High	Low	Low	
Ziprasidone (Geodon®)	Cap, powder for inj	2:1	40	40-160	Low / moderate	Low	Very low	Low / moderate	Low weight gain; contraindicated with QTc-prolonging agents

BENZODIAZEPINES

Agent	FDA-Approved Indication	Dosage Forms	Relative Potency	Peak Blood Levels (oral) (h)	Protein Binding (%)	Volume of Distribution (L/kg)	Major Active Metabolite	Onset	Metabolism	Half-Life (parent) (h)	Half-Life[1] (metabolite) (h)	Elimination	Usual Initial Dose	Adult Oral Dosage Range
Anxiolytic														
Alprazolam (Alprazolam Intensol®, Niravam™; Xanax XR®; Xanax®)	Anxiety, anxiety associated with depression, panic disorder treatment	Sol, tab	0.5	IR: 1-2 XR: 9	80	0.9-1.2	No	Intermediate	Hepatic via CYP3A4	12-15	—	Urine	0.25-0.5 tid	0.75-4 mg/d
Chlordiazepoxide (Librium®)	Anxiety, EtOH withdrawal, adjunct to anesthesia (I.V.)	Cap, powd for inj	10	2-4	90-98	0.3	Yes	Intermediate	Hepatic via CYP3A4	5-30	24-96	Urine	5-25 mg tid-qid	15-100 mg/d
Diazepam (Diastat® Rectal Delivery System, Diazepam Intensol®, Valium®)	Anxiety, EtOH withdrawal, adjunct to anesthesia (I.V.), anxiety/amnesiac during cardioversion (I.V.), anxiety/amnesia in endoscopic procedures, convulsions/status epilepticus (I.V.), adjunct in epilepsy (rectal gel), skeletal muscle spasms	Gel, inj, sol, tab	5	0.5-2	98	1.1	Yes	Rapid	Hepatic via 2C19 and 3A4	20-80	50-100	Urine	2-10 mg bid-qid	4-40 mg/d
Lorazepam (Ativan®)[2]	Anxiety, anxiety associated with depression, adjunct to anesthesia (I.V.), convulsions/status epilepticus (I.V.)	Inj, sol, tab	1	1-6	88-92	1.3	No	Intermediate	Hepatic	10-20	—	Urine and feces (minimal)	0.5-2 mg tid-qid	2-4 mg/d
Oxazepam (Serax®)	Anxiety, anxiety associated with depression, EtOH withdrawal	Cap, tab	15-30	2-4	86-99	0.6-2	No	Slow	Hepatic via glucoronide conjugation	5-20	—	Urine as unchanged (50%) and glucoronide	10-30 mg tid-qid	30-120 mg/d
Sedative / Hypnotic														
Estazolam (ProSom™)	Insomnia	Tab	0.3	2	93	—	No	Slow	Hepatic via CYP3A4	10-24	—	Urine	1 mg qhs	1-2 mg
Flurazepam (Dalmane®)	Insomnia	Cap	5	0.5-2	97	—	Yes	Rapid	Hepatic via CYP3A4	Not signifi-cant	40-114	Urine	15 mg qhs	15-60 mg
Quazepam (Doral®)	Insomnia	Tab	5	2	95	5	Yes	Intermediate	Hepatic via CYP3A4	25-41	28-114	Urine	15 mg qhs	7.5-15 mg
Temazepam (Restoril®)	Insomnia	Cap	5	2-3	96	1.4	No	Slow	Hepatic via CYP2B6, 2C8/9, 2C19, 3A4	10-40	—	Urine as inactive metabolites	15-30 mg qhs	15-30 mg
Triazolam (Halcion®)	Insomnia	Tab	0.1	1	89-94	0.8-1.3	No	Intermediate	Hepatic via CYP3A4	2.3	—	Urine as unchanged drug and metabolites	0.125-0.25 qhs	0.125-0.25 mg

Agent	FDA-Approved Indication	Dosage Forms	Relative Potency	Peak Blood Levels (oral) (h)	Protein Binding (%)	Volume of Distribution (L/kg)	Major Active Metabolite	Onset	Metabolism	Half-Life (parent) (h)	Half-Life[1] (metabolite) (h)	Elimination	Usual Initial Dose	Adult Oral Dosage Range
Miscellaneous														
Clonazepam (Klonopin™)	Adjunct in Lennox-Gastuat syndrome, akinetic seizures, myoclonic seizures, adjunct in absence seizures, panic disorder treatment	Tab	0.25-0.5	1-2	86	1.8-4	No	Intermediate	Hepatic via glucoronide and sulfate conjugation	18-50	—	Urine as glucoronide or sulfate conjugate	0.5 mg tid	1.5-20 mg/d
Clorazepate (Tranxene®)	Anxiety, EtOH withdrawal, adjunct in partial seizures	Cap, tab	7.5	1-2	80-95	—	Yes	Rapid	Decarboxylated in acidic stomach prior to absorption and hepatic via CYP3A4	Not significant	50-100	Urine	7.5-15 mg bid-qid	15-60 mg
Midazolam	Adjunct to anesthesia, anxiety/amnesiac during cardioversion, anxiety/amnesia in endoscopic procedures	Inj	NA	0.4-0.7[3]	95	0.8-6.6	No	Rapid	Hepatic via CYP3A4	2-5 h	—	Urine as glucoronide or feces (2% to 10%)	NA	NA

IR = immediate release; XR = extended release; NA = not available.

Rapid = 15 minutes or less; intermediate = 15-30 minutes; slow = 30-60 minutes.

[1]Significant metabolite.

[2]Reliable bioavailability when given I.M.

[3]I.V. only.

BETA-BLOCKERS

Agent	Adrenergic Receptor Blocking Activity	Lipid Solubility	Protein Bound (%)	Half-Life (h)	Bioavailability (%)	Primary (Secondary) Route of Elimination	Indications	Usual Dosage
Acebutolol (Sectral®)	$beta_1$	Low	15-25	3-4	40 7-fold[1]	Hepatic (renal)	Hypertension, arrhythmias	P.O.: 400-1200 mg/d
Atenolol (Tenormin®)	$beta_1$	Low	<5-10	6-9[2]	50-60 4-fold[1]	Renal (hepatic)	Hypertension, angina pectoris, acute MI	P.O.: 50-200 mg/d I.V.: 5 mg x 2 doses
Betaxolol (Kerlone®)	$beta_1$	Low	50-55	14-22	84-94	Hepatic (renal)	Hypertension	P.O.: 10-20 mg/d
Bisoprolol (Zebeta®)	$beta_1$	Low	26-33	9-12	80	Renal (hepatic)	Hypertension, heart failure	P.O.: 2.5-5 mg
Carteolol (Cartrol®)	$beta_1$ $beta_2$	Low	20-30	6	80-85	Renal	Hypertension	P.O.: 2.5-10 mg/d
Carvedilol (Coreg®)	$beta_1$ $beta_2$ $alpha_1$	ND	98	7-10	25-35	Bile into feces	Hypertension, heart failure (mild to severe)	P.O.: 6.25 mg twice daily
Esmolol (Brevibloc®)	$beta_1$	Low	55	0.15	NA 5-fold[1]	Red blood cell	Supraventricular tachycardia, sinus tachycardia, atrial fibrillation/flutter, hypertension	I.V. infusion: 25-300 mcg/kg/min
Labetalol (Trandate®)	$alpha_1$ $beta_1$ $beta_2$	Moderate	50	5.5-8	18-30 10-fold[1]	Renal (hepatic)	Hypertension	P.O.: 200-2400 mg/d I.V.: 20-80 mg at 10-min intervals up to a maximum of 300 mg **or** continuous infusion of 2 mg/min
Metoprolol (Lopressor®, Toprol-XL®)	$beta_1$	Moderate	10-12	3-7	50 10-fold[1] (Toprol XL®: 77)	Hepatic/renal	Hypertension, angina pectoris, acute MI, heart failure (mild to moderate; XL formulation only)	P.O.: 100-450 mg/d I.V.: Post-MI 15 mg Angina: 15 mg then 2-5 mg/hour Arrhythmias: 0.2 mg/kg
Nadolol (Corgard®)	$beta_1$ $beta_2$	Low	25-30	20-24	30 5- to 8-fold[1]	Renal	Hypertension, angina pectoris	P.O.: 40-320 mg/d
Penbutolol (Levatol®)	$beta_1$ $beta_2$	High	80-98	5	~100	Hepatic (renal)	Hypertension	P.O.: 20-80 mg/d
Pindolol	$beta_1$ $beta_2$	Moderate	57	3-4[2]	90 4-fold[1]	Hepatic (renal)	Hypertension	P.O.: 20-60 mg/d
Propranolol (Inderal®, various)	$beta_1$ $beta_2$	High	90	3-5[2]	30 20-fold[1]	Hepatic	Hypertension, angina pectoris, arrhythmias, prophylaxis (post-MI)	P.O.: 40-480 mg/d I.V.: Reflex tachycardia 1-10 mg
Propranolol long-acting (Inderal-LA®)	$beta_1$ $beta_2$	High	90	9-18	20- to 30-fold[1]	Hepatic	Hypertrophic subaortic stenosis, prophylaxis (post-MI)	P.O.: 180-240 mg/d

Agent	Adrenergic Receptor Blocking Activity	Lipid Solubility	Protein Bound (%)	Half-Life (h)	Bioavailability (%)	Primary (Secondary) Route of Elimination	Indications	Usual Dosage
Sotalol (Betapace®, Betapace AF®, Sorine®)	$beta_1$ $beta_2$	Low	0	12	90-100	Renal	Ventricular arrhythmias/ tachyarrhythmias	P.O.: 160-320 mg/d
Timolol (Blocadren®)	$beta_1$ $beta_2$	Low to moderate	<10	4	75 7-fold[1]	Hepatic (renal)	Hypertension, prophylaxis (post-MI)	P.O.: 20-60 mg/d P.O.: 20 mg/d

Dosage is based on 70 kg adult with normal hepatic and renal function.

Note: All $beta_1$-selective agents will inhibit $beta_2$ receptors at higher doses.

[1]Interpatient variations in plasma levels.

[2]Half-life increased to 16-27 hours in creatinine clearance of 15-35 mL/minute and >27 hours in creatinine clearance <15 mL/minute.

BRONCHODILATORS

Comparison of Inhaled Sympathomimetic Bronchodilators

Drug	Adrenergic Receptor	Onset (min)	Duration Activity (h)
Albuterol (Proventil®)	$Beta_1$ < $Beta_2$	<5	3-8
Arformoterol (Brovana™)	$Beta_1$ < $Beta_2$	7-20	
Epinephrine (various)	Alpha and $Beta_1$ and $Beta_2$	1-5	1-3
Formoterol (Foradil®)	$Beta_1$ < $Beta_2$	3-5	12
Isoproterenol (Isuprel®)	$Beta_1$ and $Beta_2$	2-5	0.5-2
Levalbuterol (Xopenex®)	$Beta_1$ < $Beta_2$	10-17	5-6
Metaproterenol (Alupent®)	$Beta_1$ < $Beta_2$	5-30	2-6
Pirbuterol (Maxair™)	$Beta_1$ < $Beta_2$	<5	5
Salmeterol (Serevent®)	$Beta_1$ < $Beta_2$	5-14	12
Terbutaline	$Beta_1$ < $Beta_2$	5-30	3-6

CALCIUM CHANNEL BLOCKERS

Comparative Pharmacokinetics

Agent	Bioavailability (%)	Protein Binding (%)	Onset of BP Effect (min)	Duration of BP Effect (h)	Half-Life (h)	Volume of Distribution	Route of Metabolism	Route of Excretion
Dihydropyridines								
Amlodipine (Norvasc®)	64-90	93-98	30-50	24	30-50	21 L/kg	Hepatic; inactive metabolites	Urine; 10% as parent
Clevidipine (Cleviprex™)		>99.5	2-4	5-15 min	1-15 min	0.17 L/kg	Blood and extravascular tissue esterases	Urine(63% to 74%; as metabolites); feces (7% to 22%)
Felodipine (Plendil®)	20	>99	2-5 h	24	11-16	10 L/kg	Hepatic; CYP3A4 substrate (major); inactive metabolites; extensive first pass	Urine (70%; as metabolites); feces 10%
Isradipine (DynaCirc® [DSC]) (immediate release)	15-24	95	20	>12	8	3 L/kg	Hepatic; CYP3A4 substrate (major); inactive metabolites; extensive first pass	Urine as metabolites
Nicardipine (Cardene®) (immediate release)	35	>95	30	≤8	2-4		Hepatic; CYP3A4 substrate (major); saturable first pass	Urine (60%; as metabolites); feces 35%
Nifedipine (Procardia®) (immediate release)	40-77	92-98	Within 20		2-5		Hepatic; CYP3A4 substrate (major); inactive metabolites	Urine as metabolites
Nimodipine (Nimotop®)	13	>95	ND	4-6	1-2		Hepatic; CYP3A4 substrate (major); metabolites inactive or less active than parent; extensive first pass	Urine (50%; as metabolites); feces 32%
Nisoldipine (Sular®)	5	>99	ND	6-12	7-12		Hepatic; CYP3A4 substrate (major); 1 active metabolite (10% of parent); extensive first pass	Urine as metabolites
Phenylalkylamines								
Verapamil (Calan®) (immediate release)	20-35	90	30	6-8	4.5-12		Hepatic; CYP3A4 substrate (major); 1 active metabolite (20% of parent); extensive first pass	Urine (70%; 3%-4% as unchanged drug); feces 16%
Benzothiazepines								
Diltiazem (Cardizem®) (immediate release)	~40	70-80	30-60	6-8	3-4.5	3-13 L/kg	Hepatic; CYP3A4 substrate (major); 1 major metabolite (20%-50% of parent); extensive first pass	Urine as metabolites

CORTICOSTEROIDS

Corticosteroids, Systemic Equivalencies

Glucocorticoid	Approximate Equivalent Dose (mg)	Routes of Administration	Relative Anti-inflammatory Potency	Relative Mineralocorticoid Potency	Protein Binding (%)	Half-life Plasma (min)	Half-life Biologic (h)
Short-Acting							
Cortisone	25	P.O., I.M.	0.8	2	90	30	8-12
Hydrocortisone	20	I.M., I.V.	1	2	90	80-118	8-12
Intermediate-Acting							
Methylprednisolone[1]	4	P.O., I.M., I.V.	5	0	—	78-188	18-36
Prednisolone	5	P.O., I.M., I.V., intra-articular, intradermal, soft tissue injection	4	1	90-95	115-212	18-36
Prednisone	5	P.O.	4	1	70	60	18-36
Triamcinolone[1]	4	P.O., I.M., intra-articular, intradermal, intrasynovial, soft tissue injection	5	0	—	200+	18-36
Long-Acting							
Betamethasone	0.6-0.75	P.O., I.M., intra-articular, intradermal, intrasynovial, soft tissue injection	25	0	64	300+	36-54
Dexamethasone	0.75	P.O., I.M., I.V., intra-articular, intradermal, soft tissue injection	25-30	0	—	110-210	36-54
Mineralocorticoids							
Fludrocortisone	—	P.O.	10	125	42	210+	18-36

[1]May contain propylene glycol as an excipient in injectable forms.

GUIDELINES FOR SELECTION AND USE OF TOPICAL CORTICOSTEROIDS

The quantity prescribed and the frequency of refills should be monitored to reduce the risk of adrenal suppression. In general, short courses of high-potency agents are preferable to prolonged use of low potency. After control is achieved, control should be maintained with a low potency preparation.

1. Low-to-medium potency agents are usually effective for treating thin, acute, inflammatory skin lesions; whereas, high or super-potent agents are often required for treating chronic, hyperkeratotic, or lichenified lesions.
2. Since the stratum corneum is thin on the face and intertriginous areas, low-potency agents are preferred but a higher potency agent may be used for 2 weeks.
3. Because the palms and soles have a thick stratum corneum, high or super-potent agents are frequently required.
4. Low potency agents are preferred for infants and the elderly. Infants have a high body surface area to weight ratio; elderly patients have thin, fragile skin.
5. The vehicle in which the topical corticosteroid is formulated influences the absorption and potency of the drug. Ointment bases are preferred for thick, lichenified lesions; they enhance penetration of the drug. Creams are preferred for acute and subacute dermatoses; they may be used on moist skin areas or intertriginous areas. Solutions, gels, and sprays are preferred for the scalp or for areas where a nonoil-based vehicle is needed.
6. In general, super-potent agents should not be used for longer than 2-3 weeks unless the lesion is limited to a small body area. Medium-to-high potency agents usually cause only rare adverse effects when treatment is limited to 3 months or less, and use on the face and intertriginous areas are avoided. If long-term treatment is needed, intermittent vs continued treatment is recommended.
7. Most preparations are applied once or twice daily. More frequent application may be necessary for the palms or soles because the preparation is easily removed by normal activity and penetration is poor due to a thick stratum corneum. Every-other-day or weekend-only application may be effective for treating some chronic conditions.

Corticosteroids, Topical

Steroid		Vehicle
	Very High Potency	
0.05%	Betamethasone dipropionate, augmented	Lotion, ointment
0.05%	Clobetasol propionate	Cream, foam, gel, lotion, ointment, shampoo, spray
0.05%	Diflorasone diacetate	Ointment
0.05%	Halobetasol propionate	Cream, ointment
	High Potency	
0.1%	Amcinonide	Cream, ointment, lotion
0.05%	Betamethasone dipropionate, augmented	Cream
0.05%	Betamethasone dipropionate	Cream, ointment
0.1%	Betamethasone valerate	Ointment
0.05%	Desoximetasone	Gel
0.25%	Desoximetasone	Cream, ointment
0.05%	Diflorasone diacetate	Cream, ointment
0.05%	Fluocinonide	Cream, ointment, gel
0.1%	Halcinonide	Cream, ointment
0.5%	Triamcinolone acetonide	Cream
	Intermediate Potency	
0.05%	Betamethasone dipropionate	Lotion
0.1%	Betamethasone valerate	Cream
0.1%	Clocortolone pivalate	Cream
0.05%	Desoximetasone	Cream
0.025%	Fluocinolone acetonide	Cream, ointment
0.05%	Flurandrenolide	Cream, ointment, lotion, tape
0.005%	Fluticasone propionate	Ointment
0.05%	Fluticasone propionate	Cream
0.1%	Hydrocortisone butyrate[1]	Ointment, solution
0.2%	Hydrocortisone valerate[1]	Cream, ointment
0.1%	Mometasone furoate[1]	Cream, ointment, lotion
0.1%	Prednicarbate	Cream, ointment
0.025%	Triamcinolone acetonide	Cream, ointment, lotion
0.1%	Triamcinolone acetonide	Cream, ointment, lotion

Corticosteroids, Topical *(continued)*

Steroid		Vehicle
Low Potency		
0.05%	Alclometasone dipropionate[1]	Cream, ointment
0.05%	Desonide	Cream
0.01%	Fluocinolone acetonide	Cream, solution
0.5%	Hydrocortisone[1]	Cream, ointment, lotion
0.5%	Hydrocortisone acetate[1]	Cream, ointment
1%	Hydrocortisone acetate[1]	Cream, ointment
1%	Hydrocortisone[1]	Cream, ointment, lotion, solution
2.5%	Hydrocortisone[1]	Cream, ointment, lotion

[1]Not fluorinated.

CYCLOPLEGIC MYDRIATICS

Agent	Peak Mydriasis	Peak Cycloplegia	Time to Recovery
Atropine	30-40 min	1-3 h	>14 d
Cyclopentolate	25-75 min	25-75 min	24 h
Homatropine	30-90 min	30-90 min	6 h - 4 d
Scopolamine	20-30 min	30 min - 1 h	5-7 d
Tropicamide	20-40 min	20-35 min	1-6 h

GLYCOPROTEIN ANTAGONISTS

Comparison of Glycoprotein IIb / IIIa Receptor Antagonists

	Abciximab (ReoPro®)	Tirofiban (Aggrastat®)	Eptifibatide (Integrilin®)
Type	Monoclonal antibody	Nonpeptide	Peptide
Mechanism of action	Steric hindrance and conformational changes	Mimics native protein sequence in receptor	Mimics native protein sequence in receptor
Biologic half-life	12-24 h	4-8 h	4-8 h
Reversible with platelet infusions	Yes	No (effect dissipates within 4-8 h)	No (effect dissipates within 4-8 h)
Speed of reversibility (return of platelet function)	Slow (>48 h)	Fast (2 h)	Fast (2 h)
Vitronectin activity	Yes	No	No
FDA-approved labeling			
Percutaneous coronary intervention (PCI)	Yes	No	Yes
Coronary stents	Yes	No	No
Unstable angina pre-PCI	When PCI planned	When PCI planned	When PCI planned
Unstable angina, medical stabilization	No	Yes	Yes
FDA-approved dosing for percutaneous coronary intervention	0.25 mg/kg bolus followed by 0.125 mcg/kg/min infusion (max: 10 mcg/min) x 12 h	Not approved for use in planned PCI	180 mcg/kg bolus immediately before the initiation of PCI, followed by 2 mcg/kg/min infusion until discharge or 18-24 hours. Repeat bolus 10 minutes after initial bolus.
FDA-approved dosing for unstable angina stabilization	0.25 mg/kg bolus followed by 10 mcg/min infusion x 18-24 h, concluding 1 h post-PCI	0.4 mcg/kg/min x 30 min followed by 0.1 mcg/kg/min infusion through angiography or 12-24 h after subsequent PCI	180 mcg/kg/bolus followed by 2 mcg/kg/min infusion until discharge, CABG procedure or up to 72 h
How supplied – volume of injectable (total drug contents/vial)	5 mL vial (10 mg)	50 mL vial (12.5 mg) 100 mL premixed solution (5 mg) 250 mL premixed solution (12.5 mg)	10 mL vial (20 mg) 100 mL vial (75 mg) 100 mL vial (200 mg)
Storage requirements	Refrigerate, do not freeze and do not shake	Can store at room temperature, do not freeze, protect from light during storage	Refrigerate and protect from light until administered

HEMODYNAMIC SUPPORT, INTRAVENOUS

Drug	Dose	Hemodynamic Effects				
		HR	MAP	PAOP	CI	SVR
Dopamine	1-3 mcg/kg/min	↑	0	↓	0/↑	0/↓
	3-10 mcg/kg/min	↑	↑	0	↑	0
	>10-20 mcg/kg/min	↑↑	↑↑	0	↑	↑
Epinephrine	0.01-0.05 mcg/kg/min	↑	↑	0/↓	↑↑	0/↓
	>0.05 mcg/kg/min	↑↑	↑↑	↑	↑↑	↑↑
Norepinephrine	0.02-3 mcg/kg/min	0/↑	↑↑↑	↑↑	0/↓/↑	↑↑↑
Phenylephrine	0.5-9 mcg/kg/min	0/↓	↑	↑	0/↓/↑	↑↑↑
Vasopressin	0.04 units/min	0/↓	↑↑	↑	0/↓	↑↑
Dobutamine	2-10 mcg/kg/min	0/↑	↑	↓	↑	0/↓
	>10-20 mcg/kg/min	↑↑	↓/↑	↓	↑	↓
Milrinone	0.375-0.75 mcg/kg/min	↑↑	0/↓/↑	↓	↑	↓↓
Nesiritide	2 mcg/kg bolus	0	↓	↓	0/↑	↓
	0.01-0.03 mcg/kg/min					
Nitroglycerin	0.1-2 mcg/kg/min	0/↑	0/↓	↓	0/↑	↓
Nitroprusside	0.25-3 mcg/kg/min	0/↑	0/↓	↓	↑	↓

HR = heart rate; MAP = mean arterial pressure; PAOP = pulmonary artery occlusion pressure; CI = cardiac index; SVR = systemic vascular resistance.

↑ = increase; ↓ = decrease; 0 = no change.

Drug	Dose	Receptor Activity				
		α_1	α_2	β_1	β_2	DA_1
Dobutamine	2-10 mcg/kg/min	+	0	+++	++	0
	>10-20 mcg/kg/min	++	0	++++	+++	0
Dopamine	1-3 mcg/kg/min	0	0	+	0	++++
	3-10 mcg/kg/min	0/+	0	++++	++	++++
	>10-20 mcg/kg/min	+++	0	++++	+	0
Epinephrine	0.01-0.05 mcg/kg/min	++	++	++++	+++	0
	>0.05 mcg/kg/min	++++	++++	+++	+	0
Norepinephrine	0.02-3 mcg/kg/min	++++	++	++	0	0
Phenylephrine	0.5-9 mcg/kg/min	++++	+	0	0	0
Vasopressin	0.04 units/min	0	0	0	0	0

Activity ranges from no activity (0) or maximal activity (++++).

DA = dopaminergic.

Reference

Sypniewski ES, "Hypovolemic and Cardigenic Shock," *Pharmacotherapy: A Pathophysiologic Approach*, 3rd ed, Dipiro JT, Talbert RL, Hayes PE, et al, eds, Stamford, CT: McGraw-Hill, 1997, 522-3.

INTRAVENOUS IMMUNE GLOBULIN

Brand Name	FDA-Approved Indications	Labeled Contraindications	IgA Content	Half-Life	pH	Osmolarity / Osmolality	Recommended Infusion Rates	Additional Comments
Carimune® NF	Primary immunodeficiency; ITP	IgA deficiency with IgA antibody; severe systemic reaction to human immune globulins	720 mcg/mL	3 weeks	6.4-6.8	3% solution in NS: 498 mOsmol/kg 6% solution in NS: 690 mOsmol/kg 9% solution in NS: 882 mOsmol/kg 12% solution in NS: 1074 mOsmol/kg 3% solution in D_5W: 444 mOsmol/kg 6% solution in D_5W: 636 mOsmol/kg 9% solution in D_5W: 828 mOsmol/kg 12% solution in D_5W: 1020 mOsmol/kg 3% solution in SWFI: 192 mOsmol/kg 6% solution in SWFI: 384 mOsmol/kg 9% solution in SWFI: 576 mOsmol/kg 12% solution in SWFI: 768 mOsmol/kg	Initial (3% solution): 0.5-1 mL/min Maximum (3% solution): 2 mg/kg/min	Contains sucrose
Flebogamma®	Primary immunodeficiency	IgA deficiency with IgA antibody; anaphylactic reactions to blood or blood derived products	<50 mcg/mL	30-45 days	5-6	240-350 mOsmol/L	Initial (5% solution): 0.01 mL/kg/min (0.5 mg/kg/min) Maximum (5% solution): 0.1 mL/kg/min (5 mg/kg/min) Maximum in patients with renal dysfunction (5% solution): 0.06 mL/kg/min (3 mg/kg/min)	Contains sorbitol
Gammagard Liquid	Primary immunodeficiency	IgA deficiency, history of anaphylaxis with immune globulin	37 mcg/mL	35 days	4.6-5.1	240-300 mOsmol/kg	Initial (10% solution): 0.5 mL/kg/h (0.8 mg/kg/min) Maximum (10% solution): 5 mL/kg/h (8.9 mg/kg/min); <2 mL/kg/h (3.3 mg/kg/min) in patients at risk for renal impairment or thrombosis	
Gammagard S/D	Primary immunodeficiency, ITP, CLL, Kawasaki syndrome	IgA deficiency	≤1 mcg/mL	~23-53 days	6.4-7.2		Initial (5% solution): 0.5 mL/kg/h Maximum (5% solution): 4 mL/kg/h Maximum concentration for infusion: 10%	Contains glucose
Gamunex®	Primary immunodeficiency, ITP, chronic inflammatory demyelinating polyneuropathy (CIDP)	IgA deficiency with IgA antibody; history of anaphylaxis with immune globulin	46 mcg/mL	35 days	4-4.5	258 mOsmol/kg	Initial (10% solution): 0.01 mL/kg/min Maximum (10% solution): 0.08 mL/kg/min Maximum concentration for infusion: 10%	

Brand Name	FDA-Approved Indications	Labeled Contraindications	IgA Content	Half-Life	pH	Osmolarity / Osmolality	Recommended Infusion Rates	Additional Comments
Octagam®	Primary immunodeficiency	IgA deficiency with IgA antibody	≤200 mcg/mL	Immunodeficiency: 40 days	5.1-6.0	310-380 mOsmol/kg	Initial: 30 mg/kg/h (0.01 mL/kg/min) Maximum: <200 mg/kg/h (<0.07 mL/kg/min) Maximum concentration for infusion: 5%	Contains maltose
Privigen™	Primary immunodeficiency, ITP	IgA deficiency; history of anaphylaxis with immune globulin; hyperprolinemia	≤25 mcg/mL	~37 days	4.6-5	240-440 mOsmol/kg	Initial: 0.5 mg/kg/min (0.005 mL/kg/min) Maximum primary immunodeficiency: 8 mg/kg/min (0.08 mL/kg/min; ITP: 4 mg/kg/min (0.04 mL/kg/min) Maximum concentration for solution: 10%	L-proline

Carimune® NF prescribing information, ZLB Behring LLC, Kankakee, IL, January 2005.

Flebogamma® 5% prescribing information, Grifols Biologicals, Inc, Los Angeles, CA, September 2004.

Gammagard Liquid prescribing information, Baxter Healthcare Corporation, Westlake Village, CA, April 2005.

Gammagard S/D prescribing information, Baxter Healthcare Corporation, Westlake Village, CA, March 2007.

Gamunex® prescribing information, Talecris Biotherapeutics, Inc, Research Triangle Park, NC, September 2008.

Octagam® prescribing information, Octapharma USA, Inc, Centreville, VA, March 2007.

Privigen™ prescribing information, CSL Behring, King of Prussia, PA, July 2007

LAXATIVES, CLASSIFICATION AND PROPERTIES

Laxative	Onset of Action	Site of Action	Mechanism of Action
Saline			
Magnesium citrate Magnesium hydroxide (Phillips'® Milk of Magnesia)	30 min to 3 h	Small and large intestine	Attract/retain water in intestinal lumen increasing intraluminal pressure; cholecystokinin release
Sodium phosphates (Fleet® Enema)	2-15 min	Colon	
Irritant / Stimulant			
Senna (Senokot®)	6-10 h	Colon	Direct action on intestinal mucosa; stimulate myenteric plexus; alter water and electrolyte secretion
Bisacodyl (Dulcolax®) tablets, suppositories	15 min to 1 h	Colon	
Castor oil	2-6 h	Small intestine	
Bulk-Producing			
Methylcellulose (Citrucel®) Psyllium (Metamucil®)	12-24 h (up to 72 h)	Small and large intestine	Holds water in stool; mechanical distention; malt soup extract reduces fecal pH
Lubricant			
Mineral oil	6-8 h	Colon	Lubricates intestine; retards colonic absorption of fecal water; softens stool
Surfactants / Stool Softener			
Docusate sodium (Colace®) Docusate calcium (Surfak®)	24-72 h	Small and large intestine	Detergent activity; facilitates admixture of fat and water to soften stool
Miscellaneous and Combination Laxatives			
Glycerin suppository	15-30 min	Colon	Local irritation; hyperosmotic action
Lactulose	24-48 h	Colon	Delivers osmotically active molecules to colon
Lubiprostone (Amitiza®)	24-48 h	Apical membrane of the GI epithelium	Activates intestinal chloride channels increasing intestinal fluid
Docusate/senna (Peri-Colace®)	8-12 h	Small and large intestine	Senna – mild irritant; docusate – stool softener
Polyethylene glycol 3350 (GlycoLax™, MiraLax™)	48 h	Small and large intestine	Nonabsorbable solution which acts as an osmotic agent
Sorbitol 70%	24-48 h	Colon	Delivers osmotically active molecules to colon

LIPID-LOWERING AGENTS

Effects on Lipoproteins

Drug	Total Cholesterol (%)	LDLC (%)	HDLC (%)	TG (%)
Bile-acid resins	↓20-25	↓20-35	→	↑5-20
Fibric acid derivatives	↓10	↓10 (↑)	↑10-20	↓40-55
HMG-CoA RI (statins)	↓15-60	↓20-40	↑2-15	↓7-25
Nicotinic acid	↓25	↓20	↑20	↓40
Probucol	↓10-15	↓<10	↓30	→
Ezetimibe	↓12-13	↓16-18	↑1-4	↓5-6

Lipid-Lowering Agents

Drug	Dose / Day	Effect on LDL (%)	Effect on HDL (%)	Effect on TG (%)
HMG-CoA Reductase Inhibitors				
Atorvastatin	10 mg 20 mg 40 mg 80 mg	-39 -43 -50 -60	+6 +9 +6 +5	-19 -26 -29 -37
Fluvastatin	20 mg 40 mg 80 mg	-22 -25 -36	+3 +4 +6	-12 -14 -18
Lovastatin	10 mg 20 mg 40 mg 80 mg	-21 -27 -31 -40	+5 +6 +5 +9.5	-10 -8 -8 -19
Pravastatin	10 mg 20 mg 40 mg 80 mg	-22 -32 -34 -37	+7 +2 +12 +3	-15 -11 -24 -19
Rosuvastatin	5 mg 10 mg 20 mg 40 mg	-45 -52 -55 -63	+13 +14 +8 +10	-35 -10 -23 -28
Simvastatin	5 mg 10 mg 20 mg 40 mg 80 mg	-26 -30 -38 -41 -47	+10 +12 +8 +13 +16	-12 -15 -19 -28 -33
Bile Acid Sequestrants				
Cholestyramine	4-24 g	-15 to -30	+3 to +5	+0 to +20
Colestipol	7-30 g	-15 to -30	+3 to +5	+0 to +20
Colesevelam	6 tablets 7 tablets	-15 -18	+3 +3	+10 +9
Fibric Acid Derivatives				
Fenofibrate	67-200 mg	-20 to -25	+1 to +20	-30 to -50
Gemfibrozil	600 mg twice daily	-5 to -10[1]	+10 to +20	-40 to -60
Niacin	1.5-6 g	-21 to -27	+10 to +35	-10 to -50
2-Azetidinone				
Ezetimibe	10 mg	-18	+1	-8
Omega-3-Acid Ethyl Esters	4 g	+44.5	+9.1	-44.9

Lipid-Lowering Agents *(continued)*

Drug	Dose / Day	Effect on LDL (%)	Effect on HDL (%)	Effect on TG (%)
Combination Products				
Ezetimibe and fenofibrate	10/160 mg	-20	+19	-44
Ezetimibe and simvastatin	10/10 mg 10/20 mg 10/40 mg 10/80 mg	-45 -52 -55 -60	+8 +10 +6 +6	-23 -24 -23 -31
Niacin and lovastatin	1000/20 mg 1000/40 mg 1500/40 mg 2000/40 mg	-30 -36 -37 -42	+20 +20 +27 +30	-32 -39 -44 -44
Niacin and simvastatin	1000/20 mg 1000/40 mg 2000/20 mg 2000/40 mg	-12 -7 -14 -5	+21 +15 +29 +24	-27 -23 -38 -32

[1]May increase LDL in some patients.

Recommended Liver Function Monitoring for HMG-CoA Reductase Inhibitors

Agent	Initial and After Elevation in Dose	6 Weeks[1]	12 Weeks[1]	Periodically
Atorvastatin (Lipitor®)	x		x	x
Fluvastatin (Lescol®)	x		x	x
Lovastatin (Mevacor®)	x	x	x	x
Pravastatin (Pravachol®)	x			x
Simvastatin (Zocor®)	x			x

[1]After initiation of therapy or any elevation in dose.

NARCOTIC / OPIOID ANALGESICS

Opioid Analgesics – Initial Oral Dosing Commonly Used for Severe Pain

Drug	Equianalgesic Dose (mg)		Initial Oral Dose	
	Oral[1]	Parenteral[2]	Children (mg/kg)	Adults (mg)
Buprenorphine	—	0.4	—	—
Butorphanol	—	2	—	—
Hydromorphone	7.5	1.5	0.06	4-8
Levorphanol	Acute: 4 Chronic: 1	Acute: 2 Chronic: 1	0.04	2-4
Meperidine	300	75	Not recommended	
Methadone	10	5	0.2	5-10
Morphine	30	10	0.3	15-30
Nalbuphine	—	10	—	—
Pentazocine	50	30	—	—
Oxycodone	20	—	0.3	10-20
Oxymorphone	—	1	—	—

From "Principles of Analgesic Use in the Treatment of Acute Pain and Cancer Pain," *Am Pain Soc*, Fifth Ed.

[1]Elderly: Starting dose should be lower for this population group.

[2]Standard parenteral doses for acute pain in adults; can be used to doses for I.V. infusions and repeated small I.V. boluses. Single I.V. boluses, use half the I.M. dose. Children >6 months: I.V. dose = parenteral equianalgesic dose x weight (kg)/100.

Comparative Pharmacology

Drug	Analgesic	Antitussive	Constipation	Respiratory Depression	Sedation	Emesis
Phenanthrenes						
Codeine	+	+++	+	+	+	+
Hydrocodone	++	+++				
Hydromorphone	++	++	+	++	+	+
Levorphanol	++	++		++	++	+
Morphine	++	++	++	++	++	++
Oxycodone	++	+++	++	++	++	++
Oxymorphone	++	+	+++	+++		+++
Phenylpiperidines						
Meperidine	++		+	++	+	
Diphenylheptanes						
Methadone	++	++	+	++	+	+
Propoxyphene	+			+	+	+
Agonist / Antagonist						
Pentazocine	++		+	++	++ or stimulation	++

Adapted from Catalano RB, "The Medical Approach to Management of Pain Caused by Cancer," *Semin Oncol*, 1975, 2(4):379-92.

NEUROMUSCULAR-BLOCKING AGENTS

Suggested Dosing Guidelines for the Use of Neuromuscular-Blocking Agents in the Intensive Care Unit

Agent	Intermittent Injection	Continuous Infusion
Intermediate Duration		
Atracurium	0.4-0.5 mg/kg every 25-35 minutes	0.4-1 mg/kg/h
Cisatracurium (Nimbex®)	0.15-0.2 mg/kg every 40-60 minutes	0.03-0.6 mg/kg/h
Rocuronium (Zemuron®)	0.6 mg/kg every 30 minutes	0.6 mg/kg/h
Vecuronium	0.1 mg/kg every 35-45 minutes	0.05-0.1 mg/kg/h
Long Duration		
Pancuronium	0.1 mg/kg every 90-100 minutes	0.05-0.1 mg/kg/h

Pharmacokinetic and Pharmacodynamic Properties of Neuromuscular Blocking Agents

Agent	Clearance (mL/kg/min)	V_{dss} (L/kg)	Half-life (min)	ED95[1] (mg/kg)	Initial Adult Dose[2,3] (mg/kg)	Onset (min)	Clinical Duration of Action of Initial Dose (min)	Administration as an Intraoperative Infusion (mcg/kg/min)
Ultra-Short Duration								
Succinylcholine	Unknown	Unknown	Unknown	0.2	1-1.5	0.5-1	4-6	10-100
Intermediate Duration								
Atracurium	5-7	0.2	20	0.2	0.4-0.5	2-3	60-70 (dose dependent)	4-12
Cisatracurium	4.6	0.15	22-29	0.05	0.15-0.2	2-3	25-93	1-3
Rocuronium	4	0.17-0.29	60-70	0.3	0.6-1.2	1-1.5	~30	4-16
Vecuronium	4.5	0.16-0.27	51-80	0.05	0.08-0.1	2-3	20-40	0.8-2
Long Duration								
Pancuronium	1-2	0.18-0.26	107-169	0.07	0.08-0.1	3-5	60-100	n/a

[1]ED95: Effective dose causing 95% blockade.

[2]Initial dose (intubation dose) is usually 2 x ED95 with the exception of cisatracurium where the recommended initial dose is 3-4 x ED95.

[3]Prior administration of succinylcholine generally enhances the magnitude and duration of nondepolarizing NMB agents; initial doses should be lower.

NICOTINE PRODUCTS

Dosage Form	Brand Name	Dosing	Recommended Treatment Duration	Strengths Available
Lozenge	Commit™ (OTC)	Patients who smoke their first cigarette within 30 minutes of waking should use the 4 mg strength; otherwise the 2 mg strength is recommended. 1-6 wk: One lozenge q1-2h 7-9 wk: One lozenge q2-4h 10-12 wk: One lozenge q4-8h	~12 wk	2 mg, 4 mg
Chewing gum	Nicorette® (OTC)	Chew 1 piece q1-2h for 6 wk, then decrease to 1 piece q2-4h for 3 wk, then 1 piece q4-8h for 3 wk, then discontinue.	~12 wk	2 mg, 4 mg
Transdermal	Nicoderm CQ® (OTC)	One 21 mg/d patch qd for 6 wk, then one 14 mg/d patch qd for 2 wk, then one 7 mg/d patch qd for 2 wk, then discontinue. Low-dose regimen[1]: One 14 mg/d patch qd for 6 wk, then one 7 mg/d patch qd for 2 wk, then discontinue.	~10 wk	Patch: 21 mg/d 14 mg/d 7 mg/d
	Nicotrol®	One 15 mg patch qd, worn for 16 h/d and removed for 8 h/d for a total of 6 wk, then discontinue.	~6 wk	Patch: 15 mg/16 h 10 mg/16 h 5 mg/16 h
Nasal spray	Nicotrol® NS	One dose is 2 sprays (1 spray in each nostril). Initial dose: 1-2 sprays q1h, should not exceed 10 sprays (5 doses)/h or 80 sprays (40 doses)/d.	~12 wk	10 mL spray 0.5/mg spray (200 actuations)
Inhaler	Nicotrol®	Inhaler releases 4 mg nicotine (the equivalent of 2 cigarettes smoked) for 20 min of active inhaler puffing. Usual dose: 6-16 cartridges/d for up to 12 wk, then reduce dose gradually over ensuing 12 wk, then discontinue.	~18-24 wk	10 mg/cartridge: releases 4 mg/ cartridge

[1]Transdermal low-dose regimens are intended for patients <100 lb, smoke <10 cigarettes/day, and/or have a history of cardiovascular disease.

NITRATES

Nitrates[1]	Dosage Form	Onset (min)	Duration
Nitroglycerin	I.V.	1-2	3-5 min
	Sublingual	1-3	30-60 min
	Translingual spray	2	30-60 min
	Oral, sustained release	40	4-8 h
	Topical ointment	20-60	2-12 h
	Transdermal	40-60	18-24 h
Isosorbide dinitrate	Sublingual and chewable	2-5	1-2 h
	Oral	20-40	4-6 h
	Oral, sustained release	Slow	8-12 h
Isosorbide mononitrate	Oral	60-120	5-12 h

[1]Hemodynamic and antianginal tolerance often develops within 24-48 hours of continuous nitrate administration.

Adapted from Corwin S and Reiffel JA, "Nitrate Therapy for Angina Pectoris," *Arch Intern Med*, 1985, 145:538-43 and Franciosa JA, "Nitroglycerin and Nitrates in Congestive Heart Failure," *Heart and Lung*, 1980, 9(5):873-82.

NONSTEROIDAL ANTI-INFLAMMATORY AGENTS

Comparative Dosages and Pharmacokinetics

Drug	Maximum Recommended Daily Dose (mg)	Time to Peak Levels[1] (h)	Half-life (h)
Acetic Acids			
Diclofenac potassium immediate release (Cataflam®)	200	1	1-2
Diclofenac sodium delayed release (Voltaren®)	225	2-3	1-2
Etodolac	1200	1-2	7.3
Indomethacin (Indocin®)	200	1-2	4.5
Indomethacin sustained release (Indocin® SR)	150	2-4	4.5-6
Ketorolac (Toradol®)	I.M.: 120[2] P.O.: 40	0.5-1	3.8-8.6
Sulindac (Clinoril®)	400	2-4	7.8 (16.4)[3]
Tolmetin (Tolectin®)	2000	0.5-1	1-1.5
Fenamates (Anthranilic Acids)			
Meclofenamate	400	0.5-1	2 (3.3)[4]
Mefenamic acid (Ponstel®)	1000	2-4	2-4
Propionic Acids			
Fenoprofen (Nalfon®)	3200	1-2	2-3
Flurbiprofen	300	1.5	5.7
Ibuprofen (various)	3200	1-2	1.8-2.5
Ketoprofen	300	0.5-2	2-4
Naproxen (Naprosyn®)	1500	2-4	12-15
Naproxen sodium (Anaprox®, others)	1375	1-2	12-13
Oxaprozin (Daypro®)	1800	3-5	42-50
Nonacidic Agent			
Nabumetone	2000	3-6	24
Salicylic Acid Derivative			
Diflunisal	1500	2-3	8-12
Salsalate	3000	2-3	7-8
COX-2 Inhibitor			
Celecoxib (Celebrex®)	400	3	11
Oxicam			
Meloxicam (Mobic®)	15	4-5	15-20
Piroxicam (Feldene®)	20	3-5	30-86

Dosage is based on 70 kg adult with normal hepatic and renal function.

[1]Food decreases the rate of absorption and may delay the time to peak levels.

[2]150 mg on the first day.

[3]Half-life of active sulfide metabolite.

[4]Half-life with multiple doses.

SELECTIVE SEROTONIN REUPTAKE INHIBITORS (SSRIS) PHARMACOKINETICS

SSRI	Half-Life (h)	Metabolite Half-Life	Peak Plasma Level (h)	% Protein Bound	Bioavailability (%)	Initial Dose
Citalopram (Celexa™)	35	S-desmethyl-citalopram: 59 hours	4	80	80	20 mg qAM
Escitalopram (Lexapro™)	27-32	S-desmethyl-citalopram: 59 hours	5	56	80	10 mg qAM
Fluoxetine (Prozac®, Prozac® Weekly™, Sarafem™)	Initial: 24-72 Chronic: 96-144	Norfluoxetine: 4-16 days	6-8	95	72	10-20 mg qAM
Fluvoxamine	16	N/A	3	80	53	50 mg qhs
Paroxetine (Paxil®, Paxil® CR™)	21	N/A	5	95	>90	10-20 mg qAM
Sertraline (Zoloft®)	26	N-desmethyl-sertraline: 62-104 hours	5-8	98	88	25-50 qAM

SULFONAMIDE DERIVATIVES

The following table lists commonly prescribed drugs which are either sulfonamide derivatives or are structurally similar to sulfonamides. Please note that the list may not be all inclusive. **Note:** The degree of cross-reaction between antibiotic sulfonamides (arylamine sulfonamides) and nonantibiotic sulfonamides is controversial.

Commonly Prescribed Drugs

Classification	Specific Drugs
Antimicrobial Agents	Mafenide acetate (Sulfamylon®) Silver sulfadiazine (Silvadene®) Sodium sulfacetamide Sulfadiazine Sulfamethoxazole (ie, Bactrim™ and co-trimoxazole) Sulfisoxazole (Gantrisin®)
Diuretics, Carbonic Anhydrase Inhibitors	Acetazolamide (Diamox®) Dichlorphenamide (Daranide®) Methazolamide
Diuretics, Loop	Bumetanide (Bumex®) Furosemide (Lasix®) Torsemide (Demadex®)
Diuretics, Thiazide	Chlorothiazide (Diuril®) Chlorthalidone (Thalitone®) Hydrochlorothiazide (various and combinations, eg, Dyazide®, Maxzide®) Indapamide Methyclothiazide Metolazone (Zaroxolyn®)
Hypoglycemic Agents, Oral	Chlorpropamide (Diabinese®) Glimepiride (Amaryl®) Glipizide (Glucotrol®) Glyburide (DiaBeta®, Glynase®, Micronase®) Tolazamide Tolbutamide
Other Agents	Celecoxib (Celebrex®) Dapsone Sulfasalazine (Azulfidine®) Sumatriptan (Imitrex®) Zonisamide (Zonegran®)

THIAZOLIDINEDIONES

Lipid Effects

Parameter	Pioglitazone (Actos®)	Rosiglitazone (Avandia®)
LDL	↑ up to 7%	↑ up to 18.6%
HDL	↑ up to 13%	↑ up to 18.5%
Total cholesterol	No significant change	↑
Total cholesterol/HDL ratio	↓	↓
LDL/HDL ratio	Slightly ↓	No change
Triglycerides	↓ up to 26%	Variable effects

Thiazolidinedione Pharmacokinetics

Parameter	Pioglitazone (Actos®)	Rosiglitazone (Avandia®)
Absorption	Food slightly delays but does not alter the extent of absorption	Absolute bioavailability is 99% Food ↓ C_{max} and delays T_{max}, but not change in AUC
T_{max}	2 h	1 h
Distribution	0.63 ± 0.41 L/kg	17.6 L
Plasma protein binding	>99% to serum albumin	99.8% to serum albumin
Metabolism	Extensive liver metabolism by hydroxylation and oxidation. Some metabolites are pharmacologically active. CYP2C8 and CYP3A4 metabolism	Extensive liver metabolism via N-demethylation and hydroxylation with no unchanged drug excreted in the urine CYP2C8 and some CYP2C9 metabolism
Excretion	Urine (15% to 30%) and feces	Urine (64%) and feces (23%)
Half-life	Pioglitazone: 3-7 h Pioglitazone and metabolites: 16-24 h	3.15-3.59 h
Effect of hemodialysis	Not removed	Not removed

CYTOCHROME P450 ENZYMES: SUBSTRATES, INHIBITORS, AND INDUCERS

INTRODUCTION

Most drugs are eliminated from the body, at least in part, by being chemically altered to less lipid-soluble products (ie, metabolized), and thus are more likely to be excreted via the kidneys or the bile. Phase I metabolism includes drug hydrolysis, oxidation, and reduction, and results in drugs that are more polar in their chemical structure, while Phase II metabolism involves the attachment of an additional molecule onto the drug (or partially metabolized drug) in order to create an inactive and/or more water soluble compound. Phase II processes include (primarily) glucuronidation, sulfation, glutathione conjugation, acetylation, and methylation.

Virtually any of the Phase I and II enzymes can be inhibited by some xenobiotic or drug. Some of the Phase I and II enzymes can be induced. Inhibition of the activity of metabolic enzymes will result in increased concentrations of the substrate (drug), whereas induction of the activity of metabolic enzymes will result in decreased concentrations of the substrate. For example, the well-documented enzyme-inducing effects of PHENobarbital may include a combination of Phase I and II enzymes. Phase II glucuronidation may be increased via induced UDP-glucuronosyltransferase (UGT) activity, whereas Phase I oxidation may be increased via induced cytochrome P450 (CYP) activity. However, for most drugs, the primary route of metabolism (and the primary focus of drug-drug interaction) is Phase I oxidation, and specifically, metabolism.

CYP enzymes may be responsible for the metabolism (at least partial metabolism) of approximately 75% of all drugs, with the CYP3A subfamily responsible for nearly half of this activity. Found throughout plant, animal, and bacterial species, CYP enzymes represent a superfamily of xenobiotic metabolizing proteins. There have been several hundred CYP enzymes identified in nature, each of which has been assigned to a family (1, 2, 3, etc), subfamily (A, B, C, etc), and given a specific enzyme number (1, 2, 3, etc) according to the similarity in amino acid sequence that it shares with other enzymes. Of these many enzymes, only a few are found in humans, and even fewer appear to be involved in the metabolism of xenobiotics (eg, drugs). The key human enzyme subfamilies include CYP1A, CYP2A, CYP2B, CYP2C, CYP2D, CYP2E, and CYP3A.

CYP enzymes are found in the endoplasmic reticulum of cells in a variety of human tissues (eg, skin, kidneys, brain, lungs), but their predominant sites of concentration and activity are the liver and intestine. Though the abundance of CYP enzymes throughout the body is relatively equally distributed among the various subfamilies, the relative contribution to drug metabolism is (in decreasing order of magnitude) CYP3A4 (nearly 50%), CYP2D6 (nearly 25%), CYP2C8/9 (nearly 15%), then CYP1A2, CYP2C19, CYP2A6, and CYP2E1. Owing to their potential for numerous drug-drug interactions, those drugs that are identified in preclinical studies as substrates of CYP3A enzymes are often given a lower priority for continued research and development in favor of drugs that appear to be less affected by (or less likely to affect) this enzyme subfamily.

Each enzyme subfamily possesses unique selectivity toward potential substrates. For example, CYP1A2 preferentially binds medium-sized, planar, lipophilic molecules, while CYP2D6 preferentially binds molecules that possess a basic nitrogen atom. Some CYP subfamilies exhibit polymorphism (ie, multiple allelic variants that manifest differing catalytic properties). The best described polymorphisms involve CYP2C9, CYP2C19, and CYP2D6. Individuals possessing "wild type" gene alleles exhibit normal functioning CYP capacity. Others, however, possess allelic variants that leave the person with a subnormal level of catalytic potential (so called "poor metabolizers"). Poor metabolizers would be more likely to experience toxicity from drugs metabolized by the affected enzymes (or less effects if the enzyme is responsible for converting a prodrug to it's active form as in the case of codeine). The percentage of people classified as poor metabolizers varies by enzyme and population group. As an example, approximately 7% of Caucasians and only about 1% of Orientals appear to be CYP2D6 poor metabolizers.

CYP enzymes can be both inhibited and induced by other drugs, leading to increased or decreased serum concentrations (along with the associated effects), respectively. Induction occurs when a drug causes an increase in the amount of smooth endoplasmic reticulum, secondary to increasing the amount of the affected CYP enzymes in the tissues. This "revving up" of the CYP enzyme system may take several days to reach peak activity, and likewise, may take several days, even months, to return to normal following discontinuation of the inducing agent.

CYP inhibition occurs via several potential mechanisms. Most commonly, a CYP inhibitor competitively (and reversibly) binds to the active site on the enzyme, thus preventing the substrate from binding to the same site, and preventing the substrate from being metabolized. The affinity of an inhibitor for an enzyme may be expressed by an inhibition constant (Ki) or IC50 (defined as the concentration of the inhibitor required to cause 50% inhibition under a given set of conditions). In addition to reversible competition for an enzyme site, drugs may inhibit enzyme activity by binding to sites on the enzyme other than that to which the substrate would bind, and thereby cause a change in the functionality or physical structure of the enzyme. A drug may also bind to the enzyme in an irreversible (ie, "suicide") fashion. In such a case, it is not the concentration of drug at the enzyme site that is important (constantly binding and releasing), but the number of molecules available for binding (once bound, always bound).

Although an inhibitor or inducer may be known to affect a variety of CYP subfamilies, it may only inhibit one or two in a clinically important fashion. Likewise, although a substrate is known to be at least partially metabolized by a variety of CYP enzymes, only one or two enzymes may contribute significantly enough to its overall metabolism to warrant concern when used with potential inducers or inhibitors. Therefore, when attempting to predict the level of risk of using two drugs that may affect each other via altered CYP function, it is important to identify the relative effectiveness of the inhibiting/inducing drug on the CYP subfamilies that significantly contribute to the metabolism of the substrate. The contribution of a specific CYP pathway to substrate metabolism should be considered not only in light of other known CYP pathways, but also other nonoxidative pathways for substrate metabolism (eg, glucuronidation) and transporter proteins (eg, P-glycoprotein) that may affect the presentation of a substrate to a metabolic pathway.

HOW TO USE THE TABLES

The following CYP SUBSTRATES, INHIBITORS, and INDUCERS tables provide a clinically relevant perspective on drugs that are affected by, or affect, cytochrome P450 (CYP) enzymes. Not all human, drug-metabolizing CYP enzymes are specifically (or separately) included in the tables. Some enzymes have been excluded because they do not appear to significantly contribute to the metabolism of marketed drugs (eg, CYP2C18). In the case of CYP3A4, the industry routinely uses this single enzyme designation to represent all enzymes in the CYP3A subfamily. CYP3A7 is present in fetal livers. It is effectively absent from adult livers. CYP3A4 (adult) and CYP3A7 (fetal) appear to share similar properties in their respective hosts. The impact of CYP3A7 in fetal and neonatal drug interactions has not been investigated.

The **CYP Substrates table** contains a list of drugs reported to be metabolized, at least in part, by one or more CYP enzymes. An enzyme that appears to play a clinically significant (major) role in a drug's metabolism is indicated by "•", and an enzyme whose role appears to be clinically insignificant (minor) is indicated by "o". A clinically significant designation is the result of a two-phase review. The first phase considered the contribution of each CYP enzyme to the overall metabolism of the drug. The enzyme pathway was considered potentially clinically relevant if it was responsible for at least 30% of the metabolism of the drug. If so, the drug was subjected to a second phase. The second phase considered the clinical relevance of a substrate's concentration being increased twofold, or decreased by one-half (such as might be observed if combined with an effective CYP inhibitor or inducer, respectively). If either of these changes was considered to present a clinically significant concern, the CYP pathway for the drug was designated "major." If neither change would appear to present a clinically significant concern, or if the CYP enzyme was responsible for a smaller portion of the overall metabolism (ie, <30%), the pathway was designated "minor."

The **CYP Inhibitors table** contains a list of drugs that are reported to inhibit one or more CYP enzymes. Enzymes that are strongly inhibited by a drug are indicated by "•". Enzymes that are moderately inhibited are indicated by "□". Enzymes that are weakly inhibited are indicated by "o". The designations are the result of a review of published clinical reports, available Ki data, and assessments published by other experts in the field. As it pertains to Ki values set in a ratio with achievable serum drug concentrations ([I]) under normal dosing conditions, the following parameters were employed: [I]/Ki ≥1 = strong; [I]/Ki 0.1-1 = moderate; [I]/Ki <0.1 = weak.

The **CYP Inducers table** contains a list of drugs that are reported to induce one or more CYP enzymes. Enzymes that appear to be effectively induced by a drug are indicated by "•", and enzymes that do not appear to be effectively induced are indicated by "o". The designations are the result of a review of published clinical reports and assessments published by experts in the field.

In general, clinically significant interactions are more likely to occur between substrates and either inhibitors or inducers of the same enzyme(s), all of which have been indicated by "•". However, these assessments possess a degree of subjectivity, at times based on limited indications regarding the significance of CYP effects of particular agents. An attempt has been made to balance a conservative, clinically-sensitive presentation of the data with a desire to avoid the numbing effect of a "beware of everything" approach. Even so, other potential interactions (ie, those involving enzymes indicated by "o") may warrant consideration in some cases. It is important to note that information related to CYP metabolism of drugs is expanding at a rapid pace, and thus, the contents of this table should only be considered to represent a "snapshot" of the information available at the time of publication.

Selected Readings

Bjornsson TD, Callaghan JT, Einolf HJ, et al, "The Conduct of *in vitro* and *in vivo* Drug-Drug Interaction Studies: A PhRMA Perspective," *J Clin Pharmacol*, 2003, 43(5):443-69.

Drug-Drug Interactions, Rodrigues AD, ed, New York, NY: Marcel Dekker, Inc, 2002.

Levy RH, Thummel KE, Trager WF, et al, eds, *Metabolic Drug Interactions*, Philadelphia, PA: Lippincott Williams & Wilkins, 2000.

Michalets EL, "Update: Clinically Significant Cytochrome P-450 Drug Interactions," *Pharmacotherapy*, 1998, 18(1):84-112.

Thummel KE and Wilkinson GR, " *In vitro* and *in vivo* Drug Interactions Involving Human CYP3A," *Annu Rev Pharmacol Toxicol*, 1998, 38:389-430.

Zhang Y and Benet LZ, "The Gut as a Barrier to Drug Absorption: Combined Role of Cytochrome P450 3A and P-Glycoprotein," *Clin Pharmacokinet*, 2001, 40(3):159-68.

Selected Websites

http://www.gentest.com
http://www.imm.ki.se/CYPalleles
http://medicine.iupui.edu/flockhart
http://www.mhc.com/Cytochromes

CYP Substrates

● = major substrate; ○ = minor substrate

Drug	1A2	2A6	2B6	2C8	2C9	2C19	2D6	2E1	3A4
Acenocoumarol	●				●	○			
Acetaminophen	○	○			○		○	○	○
Albendazole	○								○
Alfentanil									●
Alfuzosin									●
Aliskiren									○
Almotriptan							○		○
Alosetron	●				○				○
ALPRAZolam									●
Ambrisentan						●			●
Aminophylline	●							○	○
Amiodarone	○			●		○	○		●
Amitriptyline	○		○		○	○	●		○
AmLODIPine									●
Amoxapine							●		
Amprenavir					○				●
Anagrelide	○								
Apomorphine	○					○			○
Aprepitant	○					○			●
Arformoterol						○	○		
Argatroban									○
Aripiprazole							●		●
Armodafinil									●
Aspirin					○				
Atazanavir									●
Atomoxetine						○	●		
Atorvastatin									●
Azelastine	○					○	○		○
Azithromycin									○
Benzphetamine			○						●
Benztropine							○		
Benzydamine	○					○	○		○
Betaxolol	●						●		
Bexarotene									○
Bezafibrate									○
Bisoprolol							○		●
Bortezomib	○				○	●	○		●
Bosentan					●				●
Brinzolamide									○
Bromazepam									●
Bromocriptine									●
Budesonide									●
Bupivacaine	○					○	○		○
Buprenorphine									●
BuPROPion	○	○	●		○		○	○	○
BusPIRone							○		●

CYP Substrates *(continued)*

Drug	1A2	2A6	2B6	2C8	2C9	2C19	2D6	2E1	3A4
Busulfan									●
Caffeine	●				○		○	○	○
Candesartan					○				
Capsaicin								○	
Captopril							●		
CarBAMazepine				○					●
Carisoprodol						●			
Carteolol							○		
Carvedilol	○				●		●	○	○
Celecoxib					●				○
Cetirizine									○
Cevimeline							○		○
ChlordiazePOXIDE									●
Chloroquine							●		●
Chlorpheniramine							○		●
ChlorproMAZINE	○						●		○
ChlorproPAMIDE					○				
Chlorzoxazone	○	○					○	●	○
Ciclesonide							○		●
Cilostazol	○					○	○		●
Cisapride	○	○	○		○	○			●
Citalopram						●	○		●
Clarithromycin									●
Clobazam						●			●
ClomiPRAMINE	●					●	●		○
ClonazePAM									●
Clopidogrel	○								○
Clorazepate									●
Clozapine	●	○			○	○	○		○
Cocaine									●
Codeine[1]							●		○
Colchicine									●
Conivaptan									●
Cyclobenzaprine	●						○		○
Cyclophosphamide[2]		○	●		○	○			●
CycloSPORINE									●
Dacarbazine	●							●	
Dantrolene									●
Dapsone				○	●	○		○	●
Darifenacin							○		●
Darunavir									●
Dasatinib									●
Delavirdine							○		●
Desipramine	○						●		
Desogestrel						●			
Desvenlafaxine									○
Dexamethasone									○
Dexmedetomidine		●							
Dextromethorphan			○		○	○	●	○	○
Diazepam	○		○		○	●			●

CYP Substrates *(continued)*

Drug	1A2	2A6	2B6	2C8	2C9	2C19	2D6	2E1	3A4
Diclofenac	○		○	○	○	○	○		○
Digoxin									○
Dihydrocodeine[1]							○		
Dihydroergotamine									●
Diltiazem					○		○		●
Disopyramide									●
Disulfiram	○	○	○				○	○	○
Docetaxel									●
Dofetilide									○
Dolasetron					○				○
Domperidone									○
Donepezil							○		○
Dorzolamide					○				○
Doxepin	●						●		●
DOXOrubicin							●		●
Drospirenone									○
DULoxetine	●						●		
Dutasteride									○
Efavirenz			●						●
Eletriptan									●
Enalapril									○
Enflurane								●	
Eplerenone									●
Ergoloid mesylates									●
Ergonovine									●
Ergotamine									●
Erlotinib	○								●
Erythromycin			○						●
Escitalopram						●			●
Esomeprazole						●			●
Estazolam									○
Estradiol	●	○	○		○	○	○	○	●
Estrogens, conjugated A/synthetic	●	○	○		○	○	○	○	●
Estrogens, conjugated equine	●	○	○		○	○	○	○	●
Estrogens, conjugated esterified	●		○		○			○	●
Estropipate	●		○		○			○	●
Eszopiclone								○	●
Ethinyl estradiol					○				●
Ethosuximide									●
Etonogestrel									○
Etoposide	○							○	●
Exemestane									●
Felbamate								○	●
Felodipine									●
Fenofibrate									○
FentaNYL									●
Fexofenadine									○
Finasteride									○
Flecainide	○						●		
Flunisolide									●

CYP Substrates *(continued)*

Drug	1A2	2A6	2B6	2C8	2C9	2C19	2D6	2E1	3A4
FLUoxetine	○		○		●	○	●	○	○
Fluphenazine							●		
Flurazepam									●
Flurbiprofen					○				
Flutamide	●								●
Fluticasone									●
Fluvastatin				○	●		○		○
Fluvoxamine	●						●		
Formoterol		○			○	○	○		
Fosamprenavir (as amprenavir)					○				●
Fosaprepitant	○					○			●
Fosphenytoin (as phenytoin)					●	●			○
Frovatriptan	○								
Fulvestrant									○
Galantamine							○		○
Gefitinib									●
Gemfibrozil									○
Glimepiride					●				
GlipiZIDE					●				
Granisetron									○
Guanabenz	●								
Haloperidol	○						●		●
Halothane		○	○		○		○	●	○
HYDROcodone[1]							●		
Hydrocortisone									○
Ibuprofen					○	○			
Ifosfamide[3]		●	○	○	○	●			●
Imatinib	○				○	○	○		●
Imipramine	○		○			●	●		○
Imiquimod	○								○
Indinavir							○		●
Indomethacin					○	○			
Irbesartan					○				
Irinotecan			●						●
Isoflurane								●	
Isoniazid								●	
Isosorbide									●
Isosorbide dinitrate									●
Isosorbide mononitrate									●
Isradipine									●
Itraconazole									●
Ivermectin									○
Ixabepilone									●
Ketamine			●		●				●
Ketoconazole									●
Lansoprazole					○	●			●
Lapatinib				○					●
Letrozole		○							○
Levobupivacaine	○								○
Levonorgestrel									●

CYP Substrates *(continued)*

Drug	1A2	2A6	2B6	2C8	2C9	2C19	2D6	2E1	3A4
Lidocaine	○	○	○		○		●		●
Lomustine							●		
Loperamide			○						
Lopinavir									●
Loratadine							○		○
Losartan					●				●
Lovastatin									●
Maprotiline							●		
Maraviroc									●
MedroxyPROGESTERone									●
Mefenamic acid					○				
Mefloquine									●
Meloxicam					○				○
Meperidine			○			○			○
Mephobarbital			○		○	●			
Mestranol[4]					●				●
Methadone					○	○	○		●
Methamphetamine							●		
Methoxsalen		○							
Methsuximide						●			
Methylergonovine									●
MethylPREDNISolone									●
Metoclopramide	○						○		
Metoprolol						○	●		
Mexiletine	●						●		
Micafungin									○
Miconazole									●
Midazolam			○						●
Mifepristone									○
Mirtazapine	●				○		●		●
Moclobemide						●	●		
Modafinil									●
Mometasone									○
Montelukast					●				●
Moricizine									●
Morphine sulfate							○		
Naproxen	○				○				
Nateglinide					●				●
Nebivolol							●		
Nefazodone							●		●
Nelfinavir					○	●	○		●
Nevirapine			○				○		●
NiCARdipine	○				○		○	○	●
Nicotine	○	○	○		○	○	○	○	○
NIFEdipine							○		●
Nilotinib									●
Nilutamide						●			
NiMODipine									●
Nisoldipine									●
Norelgestromin									○

CYP Substrates *(continued)*

Drug	1A2	2A6	2B6	2C8	2C9	2C19	2D6	2E1	3A4
Norethindrone									●
Norgestrel									●
Nortriptyline	○					○	●		○
OLANZapine	●						○		
Omeprazole		○			○	●	○		●
Ondansetron	○				○		○	○	●
Orphenadrine	○		○				○		○
Oxybutynin									○
OxyCODONE[1]							●		
Paclitaxel				●	●				●
Palonosetron	○						○		○
Pantoprazole					○	●	○		○
Paricalcitol									●
PARoxetine							●		
Pentamidine						●			
Perphenazine	○				○	○	●		○
PHENobarbital					○	●		○	
Phenytoin					●	●			○
Pimecrolimus									○
Pimozide	●								●
Pindolol							●		
Pioglitazone				●					○
Piroxicam					○				
Pravastatin									○
PrednisoLONE									○
PredniSONE									○
Primaquine									●
Procainamide							●		
Progesterone	○	○			○	●	○		●
Proguanil	○					○			○
Promethazine			●				●		
Propafenone	○						●		○
Propofol	○	○	●		●	○	○	○	○
Propranolol	●					○	●		○
Protriptyline							●		
Quazepam						●			●
QUEtiapine							○		●
QuiNIDine					○			○	●
QuiNINE	○					○			●
Rabeprazole						●			●
Ramelteon	●								○
Ranitidine	○					○	○		
Ranolazine							○		●
Rasagiline	●								
Repaglinide				●					●
Rifabutin									●
Riluzole	●								
Risperidone							●		○
Ritonavir	○		○				●		●
Ropinirole	●								○

CYP Substrates *(continued)*

Drug	1A2	2A6	2B6	2C8	2C9	2C19	2D6	2E1	3A4
Ropivacaine	●		○				○		○
Rosiglitazone				●	○				
Rosuvastatin					○				○
Salmeterol									●
Saquinavir							○		●
Selegiline	○	○	●	○		○	○		○
Sertraline			○		○	●	●		○
Sevoflurane		○	○					●	○
Sibutramine									●
Sildenafil					○				●
Simvastatin									●
Sirolimus									●
SitaGLIPtin				○					○
Sitaxsentan					○				○
Solifenacin									●
Sorafenib									○
Spiramycin									●
SUFentanil									●
SulfaDIAZINE					●			○	○
Sulfamethoxazole					●				○
SulfiSOXAZOLE					●				
Sunitinib									●
Tacrine	●								
Tacrolimus									●
Tadalafil									●
Tamoxifen		○	○		●		●	○	●
Tamsulosin							●		●
Telithromycin	○								●
Temazepam			○		○	○			○
Temsirolimus									●
Teniposide									●
Terbinafine	○				○	○			○
Testosterone			○		○	○			○
Tetracycline									●
Theophylline	●				○		○	●	●
Thiabendazole	○								
Thioridazine						○	●		
Thiothixene	●								
TiaGABine									●
Ticlopidine									●
Timolol							●		
Tinidazole			○						●
Tiotropium							○		○
Tipranavir									●
TiZANidine	●								
TOLBUTamide					●	○			
Tolcapone					○				
Tolterodine					○	○	●		●
Toremifene	○								●
Torsemide				○	●				

CYP Substrates *(continued)*

Drug	1A2	2A6	2B6	2C8	2C9	2C19	2D6	2E1	3A4
TraMADol[1]							●		●
TraZODone							○		●
Tretinoin		○	○	●	○				
Triazolam									●
Trifluoperazine	●								
Trimethoprim					●				●
Trimipramine						●	●		●
Valproic acid		○	○		○	○		○	
Vardenafil									●
Venlafaxine					○	○	●		●
Verapamil	○		○		○			○	●
VinBLAStine							○		●
VinCRIStine									●
Vinorelbine							○		●
Voriconazole					●	●			○
Warfarin	○				●	○			○
Yohimbine							○		
Zafirlukast					●				
Zaleplon									○
Zidovudine		○			○	○			○
Zileuton	○				○				○
Ziprasidone	○								○
Zolmitriptan	○								
Zolpidem	○				○	○	○		●
Zonisamide						○			●
Zopiclone					●				●
Zuclopenthixol							●		

[1]This opioid analgesic is bioactivated *in vivo* via CYP2D6. Inhibiting this enzyme would decrease the effects of the analgesic. The active metabolite might also affect, or be affected by, CYP enzymes.

[2]Cyclophosphamide is bioactivated *in vivo* to acrolein via CYP2B6 and 3A4. Inhibiting these enzymes would decrease the effects of cyclophosphamide.

[3]Ifosfamide is bioactivated *in vivo* to acrolein via CYP3A4. Inhibiting this enzyme would decrease the effects of ifosfamide.

[4]Mestranol is bioactivated *in vivo* to ethinyl estradiol via CYP2C8/9. See Ethinyl Estradiol for additional CYP information.

CYP Inhibitors

● = strong inhibitor; □ = moderate inhibitor; o = weak inhibitor

Drug	1A2	2A6	2B6	2C8	2C9	2C19	2D6	2E1	3A4
Acebutolol							o		
Acetaminophen									o
AcetaZOLAMIDE									o
Albendazole	o								
Alosetron	o							o	
Amiodarone	o	□	o		□	o	□		□
Amitriptyline	o				o	o	o	o	
AmLODIPine	□	o	o	o	o		o		o
Amphetamine							o		
Amprenavir						o			●
Anastrozole	o			o	o				o
Apomorphine	o					o			
Aprepitant					o	o			□
Armodafinil						□			
Atazanavir	o			●	o				●
Atorvastatin									o
Azelastine			o		o	o	o		o
Azithromycin									o
Betamethasone									o
Betaxolol							o		
Bortezomib	o				o	□	o		o
Bromazepam								o	
Bromocriptine	o								o
Buprenorphine	o	o				o	o		
BuPROPion							o		
Caffeine	o								□
Candesartan				o	o				
Celecoxib				□			o		
Chloramphenicol					o				o
Chloroquine							□		
Chlorpheniramine							o		
ChlorproMAZINE							●	o	
Chlorzoxazone								o	o
Cholecalciferol					o	o	o		
Cimetidine	□				o	□	□	o	□
Cinacalcet							●		
Ciprofloxacin	●								o
Cisapride							o		o
Citalopram	o		o			o	o		
Clarithromycin	o								●
Clemastine							o		o
ClomiPRAMINE							□		
Clopidogrel					o				
Clotrimazole	o	o	o	o	o	o	o	o	□
Clozapine	o				o	o	□	o	o
Cocaine							●		o

CYP Inhibitors *(continued)*

Drug	1A2	2A6	2B6	2C8	2C9	2C19	2D6	2E1	3A4
Codeine							○		
Conivaptan									●
Cyclophosphamide									○
CycloSPORINE					○				□
Danazol									○
Darifenacin							□		○
Dasatinib									○
Delavirdine	○				●	●	●		●
Desipramine		□	□				□	○	□
Desvenlafaxine									○
Dexmedetomidine	○				○		●		○
Dextromethorphan							○		
Diazepam						○			○
Diclofenac	□				○			○	○
Dihydroergotamine									○
Diltiazem					○		○		□
DiphenhydrAMINE							□		
Disulfiram	○	○	○		○		○	●	○
Docetaxel									○
Dolasetron							○		
DOXOrubicin			□				○		○
Doxycycline									□
Drospirenone	○				○	○			○
DULoxetine							□		
Econazole								○	
Efavirenz					□	□			□
Entacapone	○	○			○	○	○	○	○
Eprosartan					○				
Ergotamine									○
Erythromycin	○								□
Escitalopram							○		
Esomeprazole						□			
Estradiol	○			○					
Estrogens, conjugated A/synthetic	○								
Estrogens, conjugated equine	○			○					
Ethinyl estradiol	○		○	○		○			○
Ethotoin						○			
Etoposide					○				○
Felbamate						○			
Felodipine				□	○		○		○
Fenofibrate		○		○	○	○			
FentaNYL									○
Fexofenadine							○		
Flavocoxid	○				○	○	○		○
Flecainide							○		
Fluconazole	○				●	●			□
FLUoxetine	□		○		○	□	●		○
Fluphenazine	○				○		○	○	
Flurazepam								○	
Flurbiprofen					●				

CYP Inhibitors *(continued)*

Drug	1A2	2A6	2B6	2C8	2C9	2C19	2D6	2E1	3A4
Flutamide	○								
Fluvastatin	○			○	□		○		○
Fluvoxamine	●		○		○	●	○		○
Fosamprenavir (as amprenavir)						○			●
Fosaprepitant					○	○			□
Gefitinib						○	○		
Gemfibrozil	□			●	●	●			
GlyBURIDE				○					○
Haloperidol							□		□
HydrALAZINE									○
HydrOXYzine							○		
Ibuprofen					●				
Ifosfamide									○
Imatinib					○		□		●
Imipramine	○					○	□	○	
Indinavir					○	○	○		●
Indomethacin					●	○			
Interferon alfa-2a	○								
Interferon alfa-2b	○								
Interferon gamma-1b	○							○	
Irbesartan				□	□		○		○
Isoflurane			○						
Isoniazid	○	□			○	●	□	□	●
Isradipine									○
Itraconazole									●
Ketoconazole	●	□	○	○	●	□	□		●
Ketoprofen					○				
Lansoprazole					○	□	○		○
Leflunomide					○				
Letrozole		●				○			
Lidocaine	●						□		□
Lomustine							○		○
Loratadine				○		□	○		
Losartan	○			□	□	○			○
Lovastatin					○		○		○
Mefenamic acid					●				
Mefloquine							○		○
Meloxicam					○				
Mephobarbital						○			
Mestranol	○		○			○			○
Methadone							□		○
Methimazole	○	○	○		○	○	□	○	○
Methotrimeprazine							○		
Methoxsalen	●	●			○	○	○	○	○
Methsuximide						○			
Methylnaltrexone							○		
Methylphenidate							○		
MethylPREDNISolone				○					○
Metoclopramide							○		
Metoprolol							○		

CYP Inhibitors *(continued)*

Drug	1A2	2A6	2B6	2C8	2C9	2C19	2D6	2E1	3A4
MetroNIDAZOLE					○				□
Metyrapone		○							
Mexiletine	●								
Micafungin									○
Miconazole	□	●	○		●	●	●	□	●
Midazolam				○	○				○
Mifepristone							○		○
Mirtazapine	○								○
Mitoxantrone									○
Moclobemide	○					○	○		
Modafinil	○	○			○	●		○	○
Montelukast				○	○				
Nateglinide					○				
Nefazodone	○		○	○			○		●
Nelfinavir	○		○		○	○	○		●
Nevirapine	○						○		○
NiCARdipine					●	□	□		●
Nicotine		○						○	
NIFEdipine	□				○		○		○
Nilutamide						○			
Nisoldipine	○								○
Nizatidine									○
Norfloxacin	●								□
Nortriptyline							○	○	
Ofloxacin	●								
OLANZapine	○				○	○	○		○
Omeprazole	○				□	●	○		○
Ondansetron	○				○		○		
Orphenadrine	○	○	○		○	○	○	○	○
OXcarbazepine						○			
Oxprenolol							○		
Oxybutynin				○			○		○
Pantoprazole					○				
PARoxetine	○		□		○	○	●		○
Peginterferon alfa-2a	○								
Peginterferon alfa-2b	○								
Pentamidine				○	○	○	○		○
Pentoxifylline	○								
Perphenazine	○						○		
Pilocarpine		○						○	○
Pimozide						○	○	○	○
Pindolol							○		
Pioglitazone				□	○	○	□		
Piroxicam					●				
Posaconazole									●
Pravastatin					○		○		○
Praziquantel							○		
PrednisoLONE									○
Primaquine	●						○		○
Probenecid						○			

CYP Inhibitors *(continued)*

Drug	1A2	2A6	2B6	2C8	2C9	2C19	2D6	2E1	3A4
Progesterone					○	○			○
Promethazine							○		
Propafenone	○						○		
Propofol	□				○	□	○	○	●
Propoxyphene					○		○		○
Propranolol	○						○		
Pyrimethamine					□		□		
QuiNIDine					○		●		●
QuiNINE				□	□		□		○
Quinupristin									○
Rabeprazole				□		□	○		○
Ranitidine	○						○		
Ranolazine							□		○
Risperidone							○		○
Ritonavir				●	○	○	●	○	●
Ropinirole	○								
Rosiglitazone				□	○	○	○		
Saquinavir					○	○	○		□
Selegiline	○	○			○	○	○	○	○
Sertraline	○		□	○	○	□	□		□
Sildenafil	○				○	○	○	○	○
Simvastatin				○	○		○		
Sirolimus									○
Sitaxsentan					●	●			□
Sorafenib			□	●	□				
Sulconazole	○	○			○	○	○	○	○
SulfaDIAZINE					●				
Sulfamethoxazole					□				
SulfiSOXAZOLE					●				
Tacrine	○								
Tacrolimus									○
Tamoxifen			○	□	○				○
Telithromycin							○		●
Telmisartan						○			
Temsirolimus							○		○
Teniposide					○				○
Tenofovir	○								
Terbinafine							●		
Testosterone									○
Tetracycline									□
Theophylline	○								
Thiabendazole	●								
Thioridazine	○				○		□	○	
Thiotepa			●						
Thiothixene							○		
Ticlopidine	○				○	●	□	○	○
Timolol							○		
Tioconazole	○	○			○	○	○	○	
Tocainide	○								
TOLBUTamide				○	●				

CYP Inhibitors *(continued)*

Drug	1A2	2A6	2B6	2C8	2C9	2C19	2D6	2E1	3A4
Tolcapone					○				
Topiramate						○			
Torsemide						○			
Tranylcypromine	□	●		○	○	□	□	○	○
TraZODone							□		○
Tretinoin					○				
Triazolam				○	○				
Trimethoprim				□	□				
Triprolidine							○		
Valproic acid					○	○	○		○
Valsartan					○				
Venlafaxine			○				○		○
Verapamil	○				○		○		□
VinBLAStine							○		○
VinCRIStine									○
Vinorelbine							○		○
Voriconazole					○	○			□
Warfarin					□	○			
Yohimbine							○		
Zafirlukast	○			○	□	○	○		○
Zileuton	□								
Ziprasidone							○		○

CYP Inducers

• = effectively induced; o = not effectively induced

Drug	1A2	2A6	2B6	2C8	2C9	2C19	2D6	2E1	3A4
Aminoglutethimide	•					•			•
Amobarbital		•							
Aprepitant					o				o
Armodafinil	o								o
Bexarotene									o
Bosentan					•				•
Calcitriol									o
CarBAMazepine	•		•	•	•	•			•
Colchicine				o	o			o	o
Cyclophosphamide			o	o	o				
Dexamethasone		o	o	o	o				•
Dicloxacillin									o
Efavirenz (in liver only)			o						•
Estradiol									o
Estrogens, conjugated A/synthetic									o
Estrogens, conjugated equine									o
Felbamate									o
Fosaprepitant					o				o
Fosphenytoin (as phenytoin)			•	•	•	•			•
Griseofulvin	o			o	o				o
Hydrocortisone									o
Ifosfamide				o	o				
Insulin preparations	o								
Isoniazid (after D/C)								o	
Lansoprazole	o								
MedroxyPROGESTERone									o
Mephobarbital		o							
Metyrapone									o
Modafinil	o		o						o
Moricizine	o								o
Nafcillin									•
Nevirapine			•						•
Norethindrone						o			
Omeprazole	o								
OXcarbazepine									•
Paclitaxel									o
Pantoprazole	o								o
PENTobarbital		•							•
PHENobarbital	•	•	•	•	•				•
Phenytoin			•	•	•	•			•
Pioglitazone									o
PredniSONE						o			o
Primaquine	o								
Primidone[1]	•		•	•	•				•
Rifabutin									•
Rifampin	•	•	•	•	•	•			•

CYP Inducers *(continued)*

Drug	1A2	2A6	2B6	2C8	2C9	2C19	2D6	2E1	3A4
Rifapentine				●	●				●
Rifaximin									○
Ritonavir (long-term)	○			○	○				○
Secobarbital		●		●	●				
Terbinafine									○
Topiramate									○
Tretinoin								○	
Valproic acid		○							

[1]Primidone is partially metabolized to PHENobarbital. See PHENobarbital for additional CYP information.

DESENSITIZATION PROTOCOLS

PENICILLIN DESENSITIZATION PROTOCOL: MUST BE DONE BY PHYSICIAN!

Acute penicillin desensitization should only be performed in an intensive care setting. Any remedial risk factor should be corrected. All β-adrenergic antagonists such as propranolol or even timolol ophthalmic drops should be discontinued. Asthmatic patients should be under optimal control. An intravenous line should be established, baseline electrocardiogram (ECG) and spirometry should be performed, and continuous ECG monitoring should be instituted. Premedication with antihistamines or steroids is not recommended, as these drugs have not proven effective in suppressing severe reactions but may mask early signs of reactivity that would otherwise result in a modification of the protocol.

Protocols have been developed for penicillin desensitization using both the oral and parenteral route. As of 1987 there were 93 reported cases of oral desensitization, 74 of which were done by Sullivan and his collaborators. Of these 74 patients, 32% experienced a transient allergic reaction either during desensitization (one-third) or during penicillin treatment after desensitization (two-thirds). These reactions were usually mild and self-limited in nature. Only one IgE-mediated reaction (wheezing and bronchospasm) required discontinuation of the procedure before desensitization could be completed. It has been argued that oral desensitization may be safer than parenteral desensitization, but most patients can also be safely desensitized by parenteral route.

During desensitization any dose that causes mild systemic reactions such as pruritus, fleeting urticaria, rhinitis, or mild wheezing should be repeated until the patient tolerates the dose without systemic symptoms or signs. More serious reactions such as hypotension, laryngeal edema, or asthma require appropriate treatment, and if desensitization is continued, the dose should be decreased by at least 10-fold and withheld until the patient is stable.

Once desensitized, the patient's treatment with penicillin must not lapse or the risk of an allergic reaction increases. If the patient requires a β-lactam antibiotic in the future and still remains skin test-positive to penicillin reagents, desensitization would be required again.

Several patients have been maintained on long-term, low-dose penicillin therapy (usually bid-tid) to sustain a chronic state of desensitization. Such individuals usually require chronic desensitization because of continuous occupationally related exposure to β-lactam drugs.

Order for placement/availability at the bedside in the event of a hypersensitivity reaction during scratch/skin testing and desensitization:

Hydrocortisone: 100 mg IVP
Diphenhydramine: 50 mg IVP
Epinephrine: 1:1000 SubQ

Several investigators have demonstrated that penicillin can be administered to history positive, skin test positive patients if initially small but gradually increasing doses are given. However, patients with a history of exfoliative dermatitis secondary to penicillin should not be re-exposed to the drug, even by desensitization.

Desensitization is a potentially dangerous procedure and should be only performed in an area where immediate access to emergency drugs and equipment can be assured.

Begin between 8-10 AM in the morning.

Follow desensitization as indicated for penicillin G or ampicillin.

AMPICILLIN

Oral Desensitization Protocol

1. Begin 0.03 mg of ampicillin
2. Double the dose administered every 30 minutes until complete
3. Example of oral dosing regimen:

Dose #	Ampicillin (mg)
1	0.03
2	0.06
3	0.12
4	0.23
5	0.47
6	0.94
7	1.87
8	3.75
9	7.5
10	15
11	30
12	60
13	125
14	250
15	500

PENICILLIN G

Parenteral Desensitization Protocol: Typical Schedule

Injection No.	Benzylpenicillin Concentration (units/mL)	Volume and Route (mL)[1]
1[2]	100	0.1 I.D.
2	↓	0.2 SubQ
3		0.4 SubQ
4		0.8 SubQ
5[2]	1000	0.1 I.D.
6	↓	0.3 SubQ
7		0.6 SubQ
8[2]	10,000	0.1 I.D.
9	↓	0.2 SubQ
10		0.4 SubQ
11		0.8 SubQ
12[2]	100,000	0.1 I.D.
13	↓	0.3 SubQ
14		0.6 SubQ
15[2]	1,000,000	0.1 I.D.
16	↓	0.2 SubQ
17		0.2 I.M.
18		0.4 I.M.
19	Continuous I.V. infusion (1,000,000 units/h)	

[1]Administer progressive doses at intervals of not less than 20 minutes.

[2]Observe and record skin wheal and flare response to intradermal dose.

Abbreviations: I.D. = intradermal, SubQ = subcutaneous, I.M. = intramuscular, I.V. = intravenous.

PENICILLIN

Oral Desensitization Protocol

Step[1]	Phenoxymethyl Penicillin (units/mL)	Amount (mL)	Dose (units)	Cumulative Dosage (units)
1	1000	0.1	100	100
2	1000	0.2	200	300
3	1000	0.4	400	700
4	1000	0.8	800	1500
5	1000	1.6	1600	3100
6	1000	3.2	3200	6300
7	1000	6.4	6400	12,700
8	10,000	1.2	12,000	24,700
9	10,000	2.4	24,000	48,700
10	10,000	4.8	48,000	96,700
11	80,000	1	80,000	176,700
12	80,000	2	160,000	336,700
13	80,000	4	320,000	656,700
14	80,000	8	640,000	1,296,700
		Observe patient for 30 minutes		
Change to benzylpenicillin G I.V.				
15	500,000	0.25	125,000	
16	500,000	0.50	250,000	
17	500,000	1	500,000	
18	500,000	2.25	1,125,000	

[1]Interval between steps, 15 min

ALLOPURINOL

Successful Desensitization for Treatment of a Fixed Drug Eruption

	Oral Dose of Allopurinol
Days 1-3	50 mcg/day
Days 4-6	100 mcg/day
Days 7-9	200 mcg/day
Days 10-12	500 mcg/day
Days 13-15	1 mg/day
Days 16-18	5 mg/day
Days 19-21	10 mg/day
Days 22-24	25 mg/day
Days 25-27	50 mg/day
Day 28	100 mg/day
Prednisone 10 mg/day through desensitization and 1 month after reaching dose of 100 mg allopurinol	

Modified from *J Allergy Clin Immunol*, 1996, 97:1171-2.

AMPHOTERICIN B

Challenge and Desensitization Protocol

1. Procedure supervised by physician
2. Epinephrine, 1:1000 wt/vol, multidose vial at bedside
3. Premixed albutenol solution at bedside for nebulization
4. Endotracheal intubation supplies at bedside with anesthesiologist on standby
5. Continuous cardiac telemetry with electronic monitoring of blood pressure
6. Continuous pulse oximetry
7. Premedication with methylprednisolone, 60 mg, I.V. and diphenhydramine, 25 mg I.V.
8. Amphotericin B (Fungizone®)[1] administration schedule
    a. 10^{-6}, infused over 10 minutes
    b. 10^{-5}, infused over 10 minutes
    c. 10^{-4}, infused over 10 minutes
    d. 10^{-3}, infused over 10 minutes
    e. 10^{-2}, infused over 10 minutes
    f. 10^{-1} (1 mg), infused over 30 minutes
    g. 30 mg in 250 mL 5% dextrose, infused over 4 hours

[1]Mixtures were prepared in 10 mL 5% dextrose by hospital intensive care unit pharmacy, unless otherwise noted.
From Kemp SF and Lockey RF, "Amphotericin B: Emergency Challenge in a Neutropenic, Asthmatic Patient With Fungal Sepsis," *J Allergy Clin Immunol*, 1995, 96(3):425-7.

BACTRIM™

Oral Desensitization Protocol

(Adapted from Gluckstein D and Ruskin J, "Rapid Oral Desensitization to Trimethoprim-Sulfamethoxazole (TMP-SMZ): Use in Prophylaxis for *Pneumocystis carinii* Pneumonia in Patients With AIDS Who Were Previously Intolerant to TMP-SMZ," *Clin Infect Dis*, 1995, 20:849-53.)

Please read the directions carefully before starting the protocol!

1. There must be a clear cut need for a sulfa drug or a sulfa drug combination product such as Bactrim™. The decision to use sulfa must be made prior to skin testing.
2. Informed consent from the patient or an appropriate relative must have been obtained.
3. A trained individual, physician, nurse, or aide, **must be with the patient** at all times.
4. A physician **must** be on the floor at all times.
5. Injectable epinephrine 0.3 mL 1:1000, diphenhydramine (Benadryl®) 50 mg, corticosteroids and oral ibuprofen 400 mg solution should be drawn up and available at the bedside.
6. Appropriate resuscitative equipment must be available.
7. All dilution of oral Bactrim™ should be made up prior to beginning procedure.
8. Patient should drink 180 mL of water after each Bactrim™ dose.

Dilution for Bactrim™ Desensitization

Final Concentration	Bottle #	Procedure
Oral Bactrim™ 40/200 mg/5 mL	A	Conventional oral Bactrim™ suspension 5 mL = 40/200 mg
Oral Bactrim™ 0.4/2 mg/mL	B	1. Add 5 mL conventional oral Bactrim™ suspension or A (concentration = 40/200 mg/5 mL) to 95 mL of sterile water 2. Shake well. This will give 100 mL of 40/200 mg Bactrim™; each mL = 0.4/2 mg Bactrim™. 3. Dispense 20 mL for use
Oral Bactrim™ 0.004/0.02 mg/mL	C	1. Add 1 mL of the 0.4/2 mg/mL Bactrim™ or B to 99 mL of sterile water 2. Shake well. This will give 100 mL of 0.4/2 mg Bactrim™; each mL = 0.004/0.02 mg Bactrim™. 3. Dispense 20 mL for use

Adverse Reactions and Response During the Protocol

Types of Reactions	Alteration of Protocol
Mild reactions (rash, fever, nausea)	I.V. diphenhydramine (Benadryl®) 50 mg and oral ibuprofen suspension 400 mg
Urticaria, dyspnea, severe vomiting, or hypotension	**STOP** the protocol IMMEDIATELY

- If patient tolerates up to Bactrim™ DS, he/she is desensitized.
- Assuming that there were no complications, the procedure will take up to 6 hours.

Sample Bactrim™ Desensitization Flow Sheet

Patient Name ____________________ Age _____ Gender ______________ Hospital # ______________________________

Diagnosis ____________________ Physician ________________________ Pager ________ History of sulfa reaction ______________________

# Hour	Actual Time	Suggested Dose	Form	Suggested Volume	Actual Dose	Form	Actual Volume	Reaction / Notes	Initial
0		Bactrim™ 0.004/0.02 mg (use **0.004/0.02 mg/mL** bottle or bottle C)	Susp (C)	1 mL					
1		Bactrim™ 0.04/0.2 mg (use 0.004/0.02 mg/mL bottle or bottle C)	Susp (C)	10 mL					
2		Bactrim™ 0.4/2 mg (use **0.4/2 mg/mL bottle** or bottle B)	Susp (B)	1 mL					
3		Bactrim™ 4/20 mg (use 0.4/2 mg/mL bottle or bottle B)	Susp (B)	10 mL					
4		Bactrim™ 40/200 mg (use **40/200 mg/5 mL unit dose** Bactrim™ or A)	Susp (A)	5 mL					
5		Bactrim™ 80/400 mg (use 40/200 mg/5 mL unit dose Bactrim™ or A)	Susp (A)	10 mL					
6		Bactrim™ DS tablet	Tablet	1 DS pill					

Note: Drink 180 mL of water after each Bactrim™ dose.

ALTERNATIVE BACTRIM™ PROTOCOL

Adapted from Leoung GS, Stanford JF, Giordano MF, et al, "Trimethoprim-Sulfamethoxazole (TMP-SMZ) Dose Escalation Versus Direct Rechallenge for *Pneumocystis carinii* Pneumonia, Prophylaxis in Human Immunodeficiency Virus-Infected Patients With Previous Adverse Reaction to TMP-SMZ," *J Infect Dis*, 2001, 184(8):992-7.

Trimethoprim-Sulfamethoxazole (TMP-SMZ) Dose-Escalation Regimen in Human Immunodeficiency Virus-Infected Patients With Previous Mild-to-Moderate Treatment-Limiting Rash and/or Fever

Dosing Level	Portion of Single-Strength TMP-SMZ (%)	Amount (Frequency) of Pediatric Suspension (mL)	Total TMP Dose (mg)	Total SMZ Dose (mg)
1	12.5	1.25 qd	10	50
2	25	1.25 bid	20	100
3	37.5	1.25 tid	30	150
4	50	2.5 bid	40	200
5	75	2.5 tid	60	300
6	100	1 single-strength tablet	80	400

Note: Each dosing level is a daily dose. For successful completion of the reintroduction phase, patients must have taken each dose level at least once. Patients were permitted to repeat dose levels once; dose levels were completed in increasing increments, and the level 6 dose was taken no later than day 13 of the reintroduction phase. Patients were permitted to withhold study drug for 2 days during the reintroduction phase (withholding study drug for >2 days during reintroduction resulted in permanent discontinuation). Patients were required to take an antihistamine during dose escalation.

VANCOMYCIN DESENSITIZATION PROTOCOL

(Adapted from Wong JT, Ripple RE, MacLean JA, et al, "Vancomycin Hypersensitivity: Synergism with Narcotics and Desensitization by a Rapid Continuous Intravenous Protocol," *J Allergy Clin Immunol*, 1994, 94(2 Pt 1):189-94.)

Please read the directions carefully before starting the protocol!

1. Vancomycin desensitization is indicated only for cases with a definitive need for vancomycin and persistent allergic reaction despite slowing of infusion rate and the addition of Benadryl® or cases with reported vancomycin anaphylactic reactions.
2. Informed consent from the patient or an appropriate relative must have been obtained.
3. A trained individual, physician, nurse, or aide, **must be with the patient** at all times.
4. A physician **must** be on the floor at all times.
5. Injectable epinephrine 0.3 mL 1:1000, diphenhydramine (Benadryl®) 50 mg, corticosteroids and oral ibuprofen 400 mg solution should be drawn up and available at the bedside.
6. Appropriate resuscitative equipment must be available.
7. All dilution of I.V. vancomycin should be made up prior to beginning procedure.
8. All patients are pretreated with 25-50 mg Benadryl®.
9. Infusion rates are to be tightly regulated with **syringe pump**.

Dilution for Vancomycin Desensitization

Final Concentration	Bottle #	Procedure
10 mg/mL	A	1. Dilute 1 g of vancomycin in 10 mL of sterile water 2. Shake well until the drug is completely dissolved 3. Add 2 mL of solution to 18 mL of 0.9% normal saline 4. Mix well 5. This will give 20 mL of 10 mg/mL concentration of vancomycin or (Bottle A) 6. Dispense 10-15 mL in a syringe for syringe pump. Label the syringe as "SYR A: conc = 10 mg/mL" with patient's name, ID, room number, date, and dispensor's initial/ pharmacist's initial.
1 mg/mL	B	1. Add 2 mL of bottle A vancomycin (10 mg/mL) to 18 mL of 0.9% normal saline 2. Mix well 3. This will give 20 mL of 1 mg/mL concentration vancomycin or (Bottle B) 4. Dispense 10-15 mL in a syringe for syringe pump. Label the syringe as "SYR B: conc = 1 mg/mL" with patient's name, ID, room number, date, and dispensor's initial/ pharmacist's initial.
0.1 mg/mL	C	1. Add 2 mL of Bottle B vancomycin (1 mg/mL) to 18 mL of 0.9% normal saline 2. Mix well 3. This will give 20 mL of 0.1 mg/mL concentration vancomycin or (Bottle C) 4. Dispense 10-15 mL in a syringe for syringe pump. Label the syringe as "SYR C: conc = 0.1 mg/mL" with patient's name, ID, room number, date, and dispensor's initial/ pharmacist's initial.
0.01 mg/mL	D	1. Add 2 mL of Bottle C vancomycin (0.1 mg/mL) to 18 mL of 0.9% normal saline 2. Mix well 3. This will give 20 mL of 0.01 mg/mL concentration vancomycin or (Bottle D) 4. Dispense 10-15 mL in a syringe for syringe pump. Label the syringe as "SYR D: conc = 0.01 mg/mL" with patient's name, ID, room number, date, and dispensor's initial/ pharmacist's initial.

Dilution for Vancomycin Desensitization *(continued)*

Final Concentration	Bottle #	Procedure
0.001 mg/mL	E	1. Add 2 mL of Bottle D vancomycin (0.01 mg/mL) to 18 mL of 0.9% normal saline 2. Mix well 3. This will give 20 mL of 0.001 mg/mL concentration vancomycin or (Bottle E) 4. Dispense 10-15 mL in a syringe for syringe pump. Label the syringe as "SYR E: conc = 0.001 mg/mL" with patient's name, ID, room number, date, and dispensor's initial/ pharmacist's initial.
0.0001 mg/mL	F	1. Add 2 mL of Bottle E vancomycin (0.001 mg/mL) to 18 mL of 0.9% normal saline 2. Mix well 3. This will give 20 mL of 0.0001 mg/mL concentration vancomycin or (Bottle F) 4. Dispense 10-15 mL in a syringe for syringe pump. Label the syringe as "SYR F: conc = 0.0001 mg/mL" with patient's name, ID, room number, date, and dispensor's initial/ pharmacist's initial.

Sample Vancomycin Desensitization Flow Sheet

Patient Name ______________________ Age __________ Gender ______________ Hospital # ______________________

Diagnosis ______________ Physician ________________ Pager __________ History of vancomycin reaction ______________

Time (h/min)	Actual Time	Vancomycin Concentration (mg/mL)	Syr #	Fluid Infusion Rate (mL/min)	VIR (mg/min)	Actual Concentration (mg/mL)	Syr #	Infusion Rate (mL/min)	Reaction / Notes	Initial
0:00		0.0001	F	1	0.0001					
0:10		0.001	E	0.33	0.00033					
0:20		0.001	E	1.0	0.001					
0:30		0.01	D	0.33	0.0033					
0:40		0.01	D	1.0	0.010					
0:50		0.1	C	0.33	0.033					
1:00		0.1	C	0.33	0.033					
1:10		1.0	B	0.33	0.33					
1:20		1.0	B	1	1					
1:30		10.0	A	0.22	2.2 [1]					
1:30		10.0	A	0.44	4.4 [1]					

[1]After a VIR of 2.2-4.4 mg/min is achieved, full dose of vancomycin can be administered at the VIR for the first day. The rate can be gradually advanced over the next few days as tolerated.

Patients in whom a VIR of 2.2-4.4 mg/min can **not** be achieved, continue to receive vancomycin at the highest tolerated infusion rate for the first day. The rate is to be gradually advanced over the next few days as tolerated.

ALTERNATIVE VANCOMYCIN PROTOCOL

Adapted from Wazny LD and Daghigh B, "Desensitization Protocols for Vancomycin Hypersensitivity," *Ann Pharmacother*, 2001, 35(11):1458-64.

Rapid Vancomycin Desensitization Protocol (Lerner and Dwyer)

Premedication

Diphenhydramine 50 mg I.V. and hydrocortisone 100 mg I.V. 15 minutes prior to initiation of protocol, then q6h throughout protocol.

Infusion No.	Dilution	Vancomycin Dose (mg)	Concentration (mg/mL)
1	1:10,000	0.02	0.0002
2	1:1000	0.20	0.002
3	1:100	2	0.02
4	1:10	20	0.2
5	Standard	500	2

Preparation

1. Prepare a standard bag of 500 mg vancomycin in 250 mL NS or D_5W; label as infusion no. 5, vancomycin 2 mg/mL.
2. Draw up 10 mL of the standard vancomycin 2 mg/mL preparation and place in 100 mL bag of NS or D_5W; label as infusion no. 4, vancomycin 0.2 mg/mL.
3. Draw up 10 mL of the 0.2 mg/mL solution and place in a 100 mL bag of NS or D_5W; label as infusion no. 3, vancomycin 0.02 mg/mL.
4. Draw up 10 mL of the 0.02 mg/mL solution and place in a 100 mL bag of NS or D_5W; label as infusion no. 2, vancomycin 0.002 mg/mL.
5. Draw up 10 mL of the 0.002 mg/mL solution and place in a 100 mL bag of NS or D_5W; label as infusion no. 1, vancomycin 0.0002 mg/mL.

Infusion Rate Directions

Initiate infusion rate at 0.5 mL/min (30 mL/h) and increase by 0.5 mL/min (30 mL/h) as tolerated every 5 minutes to a maximum rate of 5 mL/min (300 mL/h). If pruritus, hypotension, rash, or difficulty breathing occurs, stop infusion and reinfuse the previously tolerated infusion at the highest tolerated rate. This step may be repeated up to three times for any given concentration.

Upon completion of infusion no. 5, immediately administer the required dose of vancomycin in the usual dilution of NS or D_5W over 2 hours. Decrease rate if patient becomes symptomatic or, alternatively, increase rate if patient tolerates dose. Administer diphenhydramine 50 mg P.O. 60 minutes prior to each dose.

CEFTRIAXONE DESENSITIZATION PROTOCOL

Dose	Concentration (mg/mL)	Volume (mL)	Dose (mg)
Subcutaneous Route: 15-minute intervals between all doses			
1	0.2	0.5	0.1
2	0.2	1	0.2
3	2	0.25	0.5
4	2	0.5	1
5	2	1	2
6	16	0.25	4
7	16	0.5	8
8	16	1	16
Intravenous Route: Infuse over 20-30 minutes; 15 minutes between doses			
9	20	1.5 mL qs to 50 mL	30 mg/50 mL
10	20	3 mL qs to 50 mL	60 mg/50 mL
11	20	6 mL qs to 50 mL	120 mg/50 mL
12	20	12.5 mL qs to 50 mL	250 mg/50 mL
13	–	–	1 g/50 mL

Pharmacy Admixture Instructions

1. Mix ceftriaxone 1 g/50 mL NS (concentration 20 mg/mL); label **Bag A**.
2. Remove 1 mL from Bag A and add 99 mL NS (concentration 0.2 mg/mL); label **Bag B**.
3. Use **Bag B** to make doses 1 and 2.
4. Remove 1 mL from Bag A and add 9 mL NS (concentration 2 mg/mL); label **Bag C**.
5. Use Bag C to make doses 3, 4, and 5.
6. Remove 1 mL from Bag A and add 0.25 mL NS (concentration 16 mg/mL); label **Bag D**.
7. Use Bag D to make doses 6 and 7.
8. Repeat step 6 to make dose 8 (step 6 only makes 1.25 mL; therefore need to repeat to make dose 8).
9. Take a 50 mL bag of NS and remove overfill plus 1.5 mL; add 1.5 mL from Bag A to NS bag (30 mg/50 mL); this is dose 9.
10. Take a 50 mL bag of NS and remove overfill plus 3 mL; add 3 mL from Bag A to NS bag (60 mg/50 mL); this is dose 10.
11. Take a 50 mL bag of NS and remove overfill plus 6 mL; add 6 mL from Bag A to NS bag (120 mg/50 mL); this is dose 11.
12. Take a 50 mL bag of NS and remove overfill plus 12.5 mL; add 12.5 mL from Bag A to NS bag (250 mg/50 mL); this is dose 12.
13. Dispense 1 g/50 mL for dose 13.

CIPROFLOXACIN

Modified from *J Allergy Clin Immunol*, 1996, 97:1426-7.

Premedicated with diphenhydramine hydrochloride, ranitidine, and prednisone 1 hour before the desensitization.

The individual doses were administered at 15-minute intervals. Because the patient was intubated in the intensive care unit, vital signs were continually monitored. The patient's skin was inspected for development of urticaria, and his chest was auscultated for wheezing every 10 minutes. No rash, hypotension, or wheezing developed during desensitization. The procedure took 4 hours, and once finished, the patient had received an equivalent to his first scheduled dose (400 mg twice daily). The second dose was given 4 hours later, followed by routine administration of 400 mg every 12 hours, with a small dose (25 mg intravenously) between therapeutic doses to maintain a drug level in the blood. The patient subsequently received 4 weeks of ciprofloxacin treatment without difficulty.

Desensitization Regimen for Ciprofloxacin

Ciprofloxacin Concentration (mg/mL)	Volume Given (mL)	Absolute Amount (mg)	Cumulative Total Dose (mg)
0.1	0.1	0.01	0.01
0.1	0.2	0.02	0.03
0.1	0.4	0.04	0.07
0.1	0.8	0.08	0.15
1	0.16	0.16	0.31
1	0.32	0.32	0.63
1	0.64	0.64	1.27
2	0.6	1.2	2.47
2	1.2	2.4	4.87
2	2.4	4.8	9.67
2	5	10	19.67
2	10	20	39.67
2	20	40	79.67
2	40	80	159.67
2	120	240	399.67

Drug volumes <1 mL were mixed with normal saline solution to a final volume of 3 mL and then slowly infused; the other doses were administered over 10 minutes, except the last dose (240 mg in 120 mL), which was given with an infusion pump over 20 minutes.

IMIPENEM DESENSITIZATION PROTOCOL

Adapted from Saxon A, Adelman DC, Patel A, et al, "Imipenem Cross-Reactivity With Penicillin in Humans," *J Allergy Clin Immunol*, 1988, 82(2):213-7.

Indication: Need for imipenem in the setting of anaphylactic potential to penicillin. Cross-reactivity between imipenem and penicillin is high.

Subcutaneous Route: 15-minute intervals between all doses				
Dose	Solution No.	Concentration (mg/mL)	SubQ Injections q15min	
			Volume (mL)	Dosage (mg)
1	3	0.05	0.5	0.025
2		0.05	1	0.05
3	2	0.5	0.2	0.1
4		0.5	0.4	0.2
5		0.5	0.8	0.4
6	1	5	0.12	0.6
7		5	0.25	1.25
8		5	0.5	2.5
9		5	1	5
——— Wait 30 minutes ———				
Intravenous Route: Infuse over 20-30 minutes; 15 minutes between doses				
Dose	**Solution No.**	**I.V. Imipenem Dose (using 50 mL NSS)**	**Concentration (mg/mL)**	**Total Dosage (mg)**
10	1	2 mL in 50 mL NSS	10 mg/50 mL	10
11		4 mL in 50 mL NSS	20 mg/50 mL	20
12		8 mL in 50 mL NSS	40 mg/50 mL	40
13		12 mL in 50 mL NSS	60 mg/50 mL	60
	Add 10 mL NSS to 500 mg vial Primaxin®			
14		2.5 mL in 50 mL NSS	125 mg/50 mL	125
15		5 mL in 50 mL NSS	250 mg/50 mL	250

INSULIN

Lilly's appropriate diluting fluid, sterile saline, or distilled water, to which 1 mL of the patient's blood or the addition of 1 mL of 1% serum albumin (making a 0.1% solution) for each 10 mL of stock diluent, is a satisfactory diluent. The albumin in the blood or serum albumin solution is necessary to retain the integrity of the higher dilutions by preventing adsorption to glass or plastic. Dilution is stable 30 days under refrigeration or room temperature, but should be used within 24 hours due to a lack of preservative.

1. Make a 1:1 dilution of single species (beef, pork, or human) insulin (50 units/mL).
2. Add 0.5 mL of the above dilution to 4.5 mL of diluent (5 units/mL).
3. Add 0.5 mL of the 5 units/mL dilution to 4.5 mL of diluent (0.5 unit/mL).
4. Add 0.5 mL of the 0.5 unit/mL dilution to 4.5 mL of diluent (0.05 unit/mL).
5. Add 0.5 mL of the 0.05 unit/mL dilution to 4.5 mL of diluent (0.005 unit/mL).

The 5 vials containing 50, 5, 0.5, 0.05, and 0.005 unit/mL are ready for skin testing or desensitization procedures.

One may start desensitization by giving 0.02 mL of 0.05 unit/mL concentration (1/1000 unit) intradermally. If no reaction occurs, administer 0.04 and 0.08 mL of the same concentration at 30-minute intervals.

The procedure continues proceeding to the next greater concentration (0.5 unit/mL) and giving 0.02, 0.04, and 0.08 mL at 30-minute intervals.

In the same manner proceed through the 5 units/mL and 50 units/mL concentrations with the exception that these injections should be given subcutaneously.

Note: If a reaction is noted, back up 2 steps and try to proceed forward again.

If the patient reacts to the initial injection, it will be necessary to utilize the lower concentration (0.005 unit/mL) to initiate the procedure.

It is essential that manifestations of allergic reactions not be obscured. Therefore, antihistamines or steroids should not be used during desensitization except to treat severe allergic reactions. The use of these agents may obscure mild to moderate reactions to the lower doses and result in more severe reactions as doses increase, leading to failure of the desensitization program.

NELFINAVIR DESENSITIZATION PROTOCOL

Adapted from Abraham PE, Sorensen SJ, Baker WH, et al, "Nelfinavir Desensitization," *Ann Pharmacother*, 2001, 35(5):553-6.

Step	Time (min)	Nelfinavir Dose (mg)	
		q30min	Total
1	0	0.5	0.5
2	30	1	1.5
3	60	2	3.5
4	90	5	8.5
5	120	10	18.5
6	150	20	38.5
7	180	40	78.5
8	210	80	158.5
9	240	160	318.5
10	270	250	568.5
11	300	500	1068.5
12	330	750	1818.5
Observe patient in ICU for 2 hours before discharge			

RIFAMPIN and ETHAMBUTOL

Oral Desensitization in Mycobacterial Disease

Time from Start (h:min)	Rifampin (mg)	Ethambutol (mg)
0	0.1	0.1
00:45	0.5	0.5
01:30	1	1
02:15	2	2
03:00	4	4
03:45	8	8
04:30	16	16
05:15	32	32
06:00	50	50
06:45	100	100
07:30	150	200
11:00	300	400
Next day		
6:30 AM	300 mg twice daily	400 mg 3 times/day

From *Am J Respir Crit Care Med*, 1994, 149:815-7.

SKIN TESTS

PENICILLIN ALLERGY

The recommended battery of major and minor determinants used in penicillin skin testing will disclose those individuals with circulating IgE antibodies. This procedure is therefore useful to identify patients at risk for immediate or accelerated reactions. Skin tests are of no value in predicting the occurrence of non-IgE-mediated hypersensitivity reactions to penicillin such as delayed exanthem, drug fever, hemolytic anemia, interstitial nephritis, or exfoliative dermatitis. Based on large scale trials, skin testing solutions have been standardized.

Antihistamines, tricyclic antidepressants, and adrenergic drugs, all of which may inhibit skin test results, should be discontinued at least 24 hours prior to skin testing. Antihistamines with long half-lives (hydroxyzine, terfenadine, astemizole, etc) may attenuate skin test results up to a week, or longer after discontinuation.

When properly performed with due consideration for preliminary scratch tests and appropriate dilutions, skin testing with penicillin reagents can almost always be safely accomplished. Systemic reactions accompany about 1% of positive skin tests; these are usually mild but can be serious. **Therefore skin tests should be done in the presence of a physician and with immediate access to medications and equipment needed to treat anaphylaxis**.

History of Penicillin Allergy

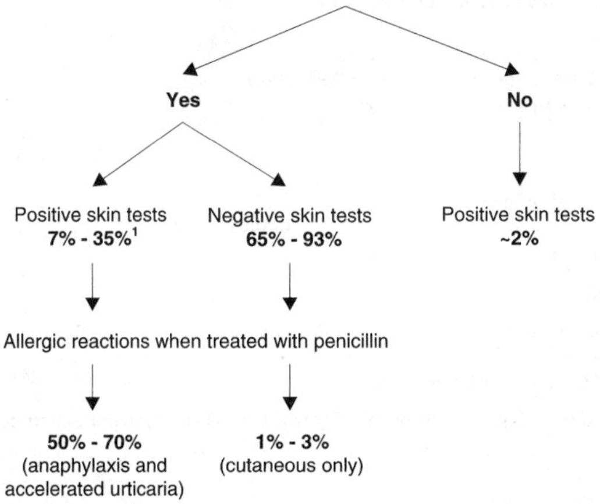

[1]One study found 65% positive.

Prevalence of positive and negative skin tests and subsequent allergic reactions in patients treated with penicilin (based on studies using both penicilloyl-polylysine and minor determinant mixture as skin test reagents).

Penicillin Skin Testing Protocol

Skin tests evaluate the patient for the presence of penicillin IgE – sensitive mast cells which are responsible for anaphylaxis and other immediate hypersensitivity reactions. Local or systemic allergic reactions rarely occur due to skin testing, therefore, a tourniquet, I.V., and epinephrine should be at the bedside. The breakdown products of penicillin provide the antigen which is responsible for the allergy. Testing is performed with benzylpenicilloyl-polylysine (Pre-Pen®), the major determinant, penicillin G which provides the minor determinants and the actual penicillin which will be administered.

Controls are important if the patient is extremely ill or is taking antihistamines, codeine, or morphine. Normal saline is the negative control. Morphine sulfate, a mast cell degranulator, can be used as a positive control, if the patient is not on morphine or codeine. Histamine is the preferred positive control, however, is not manufactured in a pharmaceutical formulation anymore. A false-positive or false-negative will make further skin testing invalid.

Control Solutions

Normal saline = negative control
Morphine sulfate (10 mg/100 mL 0.9% NaCl, 0.1 mg/mL) = positive control

Test Solutions

Order the necessary solutions as 0.5 mL in a tuberculin syringe. **Note:** May need to order 2 syringes of each – one for scratch testing and one for intradermal skin testing.

I. **Pre-Pen®: Benzylpenicilloyl-polylysine (0.25 mL ampul) = MAJOR DETERMINANT**

A. Undiluted Pre-Pen®

B. 1:100 concentration
To make: Dilute 0.1 mL of Pre-Pen® in 10 mL of 0.9% NaCl

C. 1:10,000 concentration
(Only necessary in patients with a history of anaphylaxis)
To make: Dilute 1 mL of the 1:100 solution in 100 mL of 0.9% NaCl

II. **Penicillin G sodium/potassium = MINOR DETERMINANT**

A. 5000 units/mL concentration

B. 5 units/mL concentration
(Only necessary in patients with a history of anaphylaxis)
To make: Dilute 0.1 mL of a 5000 units/mL solution in 100 mL of 0.9% NaCl

III. **Penicillin product to be administered — if not penicillin G**

A. **Ampicillin** 2.5 mg/mL concentration

To make: Dilute 250 mg in 100 mL of 0.9% NaCl

B. **Nafcillin** 2.5 mg/mL concentration
To make: Dilute 250 mg in 100 mL of 0.9% NaCl

Order for placement/availability at the bedside in the event of a hypersensitivity reaction during scratch/skin testing and desensitization:

Hydrocortisone: 100 mg IVP
Diphenhydramine: 50 mg IVP
Epinephrine: 1:1000 SubQ

Scratch / Skin Testing Protocol: Must Be Done by Physician!

1. Begin with the control solutions (ie, normal saline and morphine).
2. Administer **scratch tests** in the following order (beginning with the most dilute solution):

Pre-Pen®	Syringes: C,B,A
Penicillin G	Syringes: E,D
Ampicillin/Nafcillin	Syringe: F

The inner volar surface of the forearm is usually used.
A nonbleeding scratch of 3-5 mm in length is made in the epidermis with a 20-gauge needle.
If bleeding occurs, another site should be selected and another scratch made using less pressure.
A small drop of the test solution is then applied and rubbed gently into the scratch using an applicator, toothpick, or the side of the needle.
The scratch test site should be observed for the appearance of a wheal, erythema, and pruritus.
A positive reaction is signified by the appearance within 15 minutes of a pale wheal (usually with pseudopods) ranging from 5-15 mm or more in diameter.
As soon as a positive response is elicited, or 15 minutes has elapsed, the solution should be wiped off the scratch.
If the scratch test is negative or equivocal (ie, a wheal of <5 mm in diameter with little or no erythema or itching appears), an intradermal test may be performed.
If significant reaction, treat and proceed to desensitization.

3. Administer **intradermal tests** in the following order (beginning with the most dilute solution):

Pre-Pen®	Syringes: C,B,A
Penicillin G	Syringes: E,D
Ampicillin/Nafcillin	Syringe: F

Intradermal tests are usually performed on a sterilized area of the upper outer arm at a sufficient distance below the deltoid muscle to permit proximal application of a tourniquet if a severe reaction occurs.
Using a tuberculin syringe with a 3/8- 5/8 inch 26- to 30-gauge needle, an amount of each test solution sufficient to raise the smallest perceptible bleb (usually 0.01-0.02 mL) is injected immediately under the surface of the skin.
A separate needle and syringe must be used for each solution.
Each test and control site should be at least 15 cm apart.
Positive reactions are manifested as a wheal at the test site with a diameter at least 5 mm larger than the saline control, often accompanied by itching and a marked increase in the size of the bleb.
Skin responses to penicillin testing will develop within 15 minutes.
If no significant reaction, may challenge patient with reduced dosage of the penicillin to be administered.
Physician should be at the bedside during this challenge dose!
If significant reaction, treat and begin desensitization.

Delayed Hypersensitivity (Anergy)

Delayed cutaneous hypersensitivity (DCH) is a cell-mediated immunological response which has been used diagnostically to assess previous infection (eg, purified protein derivative (PPD) and coccidioidin) or as an indicator of the status of the immune system by using mumps, *Candida*, tetanus toxoid, or trichophyton to test for anergy. Anergy is a defect in cell-mediated immunity that is characterized by an impaired response, or lack of a response to DCH testing with injected antigens. Anergy has been associated with several disease states, malnutrition, and immunosuppressive therapy, and has been correlated with increased risk of infection, morbidity, and mortality.

Many of the skin test antigens have not been approved by the FDA as tests for anergy, and so the directions for use and interpretation of reactions to these products may differ from that of the product labeling. There is also disagreement in the published literature as to the selection and interpretation of these tests for anergy assessment, leading to different recommendations for use of these products.

General Guidelines

Read these guidelines before using any skin test.

Administration

1. Use a separate sterile TB syringe for each antigen. Immediately after the antigen is drawn up, make the injection intradermally in the flexor surface of the forearm.
2. A small bleb 6-10 mm in diameter will form if the injection is made at the correct depth. If a bleb does not form or if the antigen solution leaks from the site, the injection must be repeated.
3. When applying more than one skin test, make the injections at least 5 cm apart.
4. Do any serologic blood tests before testing or wait 48-96 hours.

Reading

1. Read all tests at 24, 48, and 72 hours. Reactions occurring before 24 hours are indicative of an immediate rather than a delayed hypersensitivity.
2. Measure the diameter of the induration in two directions (at right angles) with a ruler and record each diameter in millimeters. Ballpoint pen method of measurement is the most accurate.
3. Test results should be recorded by the nurse in the Physician's Progress Notes section of the chart, and should include the millimeters of induration present, and a picture of the arm showing the location of the test(s).

Factors Causing False-Negative Reactions

1. Improper administration, interpretation, or use of outdated antigen
2. Test is applied too soon after exposure to the antigen (DCH takes 2-20 weeks to develop)
3. Concurrent viral illnesses (eg, rubeola, influenza, mumps, and probably others) or recent administration of live attenuated virus vaccines (eg, measles)
4. Anergy may be associated with:
   a. Immune suppressing chronic illnesses such as diabetes, uremia, sarcoidosis, metastatic carcinomas, Hodgkin's, acute lymphocytic leukemia, hypothyroidism, chronic hepatitis, and cirrhosis.
   b. Some antineoplastic agents, radiation therapy, and corticosteroids. If possible, discontinue steroids at least 48 hours prior to DCH skin testing.
   c. Congenital immune deficiencies.
   d. Malnutrition, shock, severe burns, and trauma.
   e. Severe disseminated infections (miliary or cavitary TB, cocci granuloma, and other disseminated mycotic infections, gram-negative bacillary septicemia).
   f. Leukocytosis (>15,000 cells/mm^3).

Factors Causing False-Positive Reactions

1. Improper interpretation
2. Patient sensitivity to minor ingredients in the antigen solutions such as the phenol or thimerosal preservatives
3. Cross-reactions between similar antigens

Candida 1:1000
Dose = 0.1 mL intradermally (30% of children <18 months of age and 50% >18 months of age respond)
Can be used as a control antigen

Coccidioidin 1:1000
Dose = 0.1 mL intradermally (apply with PPD **and** a control antigen)
Mercury derivative used as a preservative for Spherulin®.

Multitest CMI (*Candida*, diphtheria toxoid, tetanus toxoid, *Streptococcus*, old tuberculin, *Trichophyton, Proteus* antigen, and negative control)
Press loaded unit into the skin with sufficient pressure to puncture the skin and allow adequate penetration of all points.

Mumps 40 cfu/mL
Dose = 0.1 mL intradermally (contraindicated in patients allergic to eggs, egg products, or thimerosal)

Dosage as Part of Disease Diagnosis

Tuberculin Testing
Purified Protein Derivative (PPD)

Preparation	Dilution	Units/0.1 mL
First strength	1:10,000	1
Intermediate strength	1:2000	5
Second strength	1:100	250

The usual initial dose is 0.1 mL of the intermediate strength. The first strength should be used in the individuals suspected of being highly sensitive. The second strength is used only for individuals who fail to respond to a previous injection of the first or intermediate strengths.

A positive reaction is ≥10 mm induration except in HIV-infected individuals where a positive reaction is ≥5 mm of induration.

Adverse Reactions

In patients who are highly sensitive, or when higher than recommended doses are used, exaggerated local reactions may occur, including erythema, pain, blisters, necrosis, and scarring. Although systemic reactions are rare, a few cases of lymph node enlargement, fever, malaise, and fatigue have been reported.

To prevent severe local reactions, never use second test strengths as the initial agent. Use diluted first strengths in patients with known or suspected hypersensitivity to the antigen.

Have epinephrine and antihistamines on hand to treat severe allergic reactions that may occur.

Treatment of Adverse Reactions

Severe reactions to intradermal skin tests are rare and treatment consists of symptomatic care.

Skin Testing

All skin tests are given intradermally into the flexor surface of one arm.

Purified protein derivative (PPD) is used most often in the diagnosis of tuberculosis. *Candida, Trichophyton*, and mumps skin tests are used most often as controls for anergy.

Dose: The usual skin test dose is as follows:

Antigen		Standard Dose	Concentration
PPD	1 TU	0.1 mL	1 TU – highly sensitive patients
	5 TU	0.1 mL	5 TU – standard dose
	250 TU	0.1 mL	250 TU – anergic patients in whom TB is suspected
Candida		0.02 mL	
Mumps		0.1 mL	
Trichophyton		0.02 mL	

Interpretation:

Skin Test	Reading Time	Positive Reaction
PPD	48-72 h	**≥5 mm considered positive for:** • close contacts to an infectious case • persons with abnormal chest x-ray indicating old healed TB • persons with known or suspected HIV infection **≥10 mm considered positive for:** • other medical risk factors • foreign born from high prevalence areas • medically underserved, low income populations • alcoholics and intravenous drug users • residents of long-term care facilities (including correctional facilities and nursing homes) • staff in settings where disease would pose a hazard to large number of susceptible persons **≥15 mm considered positive for:** • persons without risk factors for TB
Candida	24-72 h	≥5 mm induration
Mumps	24-36 h	≥5 mm
Trichophyton	24-72 h	≥5 mm induration

Recommended Interpretation of Skin Test Reactions

Reaction	Local Reaction	
	After Intradermal Injections of Antigens	After Dinitrochlorobenzene
1+	Erythema >10 mm and/or induration >1-5 mm	Erythema and/or induration covering <½ area of dose site
2+	Induration 6-10 mm	Induration covering >½ area of dose site
3+	Induration 11-20 mm	Vesiculation and induration at dose site or spontaneous flare at days 7-14 at the site
4+	Induration >20 mm	Bulla or ulceration at dose site or spontaneous flare at days 7-14 at the site

IMMUNIZATION RECOMMENDATIONS

Recommended Immunization Schedule for Ages 0-6 Years United States, 2009

Vaccine ▼ / Age ▶	Birth	1 mo	2 mo	4 mo	6 mo	12 mo	15 mo	18 mo	19-23 mo	2-3 y	4-6 y
Hepatitis B[1]	HepB	HepB		See footnote 1	HepB						
Rotavirus[2]			RV	RV	RV[2]						
Diphtheria, tetanus, pertussis[3]			DTaP	DTaP	DTaP	See footnote 3	DTaP				DTaP
Haemophilus influenzae type b[4]			Hib	Hib	Hib[4]	Hib					
Pneumococcal[5]			PCV	PCV	PCV	PCV				PPSV	
Inactivated poliovirus			IPV	IPV	IPV						IPV
Influenza[6]					Influenza (yearly)						
Measles, mumps, rubella[7]						MMR		See footnote 7			MMR
Varicella[8]						Varicella		See footnote 8			Varicella
Hepatitis A[9]						HepA (2 doses)				HepA series	
Meningococcal[10]										MCV	

☐ Range of recommended ages ■ Certain high-risk groups

Note: For those who fall behind or start late, see also the Catch-up Immunization Schedule table.

This schedule indicates the recommended ages for routine administration of currently licensed vaccines, as of December 17, 2008, for children aged 0-6 years. Any dose not administered at the recommended age should be administered at a subsequent visit, when indicated and feasible. Licensed combination vaccines may be used whenever any component of the combination is indicated and other components are not contraindicated and if approved by the Food and Drug Administration for that dose of the series. Providers should consult the relevant Advisory Committee on Immunization Practices statement for detailed recommendations, including **high-risk conditions: http://www.cdc.gov/vaccines/pubs/acip-list.htm**. Clinically significant adverse events that follow immunization should be reported to the Vaccine Adverse Event Reporting System (VAERS). Guidance about how to obtain and complete a VAERS form is available at **http://www.vaers.hhs.gov** or by telephone, 800-822-7967.

Footnotes to Recommended Immunization Schedule for Ages 0-6 Years

[1]**Hepatitis B vaccine (HepB).** *(Minimum age: birth)*

At birth:

- Administer monovalent HepB to all newborns before hospital discharge.
- If mother is hepatitis surface antigen (HB_sAg)-positive, administer HepB and 0.5 mL of hepatitis B immune globulin (HBIG) within 12 hours of birth.
- If mother's HB_sAg status is unknown, administer HepB within 12 hours of birth. Determine mother's HB_sAg status as soon as possible and, if HB_sAg-positive, administer HBIG (no later than age 1 week).

After the birth dose:

- The HepB series should be completed with either monovalent HepB or a combination vaccine containing HepB. The second dose should be administered at age 1 or 2 months. The final dose should be administered no earlier than age 24 weeks.
- Infants born to HB_sAg-positive mothers should be tested for HB_sAg and antibody to HB_sAg (anti-HBs) after completion of at least 3 doses of HepB series, at age 9-18 months (generally at the next well-child visit).

4-month dose:

- Administration of 4 doses of HepB to infants is permissible when combination vaccines containing HepB are administered after the birth dose.

[2]**Rotavirus vaccine (RV).** *(Minimum age: 6 weeks)*

- Administer the first dose at age 6-14 weeks (maximum age: 14 weeks 6 days). Vaccination should not be initiated for infants aged 15 weeks or older (ie, 15 weeks 0 days or older).
- Administer the final dose in the series by age 8 months 0 days.
- If Rotarix® is administered at ages 2 and 4 months, a dose at 6 months is not indicated.

[3]**Diphtheria and tetanus toxoids and acellular pertussis vaccine (DTaP).** *(Minimum age: 6 weeks)*

- The fourth dose may be administered as early as age 12 months, provided at least 6 months have elapsed since the third dose.
- Administer the final dose in the series at age 4-6 years.

[4] ***Haemophilus influenzae*** **type b conjugate vaccine (Hib).** *(Minimum age: 6 weeks)*

- If PRP-OMP (PedvaxHIB® or ComVax® [HepB-Hib]) is administered at ages 2 and 4 months, a dose at age 6 months is not indicated.
- TriHiBit® (DTaP/Hib) should not be used for doses at ages 2, 4, or 6 months but can be used as the final dose in children aged ≥12 months.

[5]**Pneumococcal vaccine.** *(Minimum age: 6 weeks for pneumococcal conjugate vaccine [PCV]; 2 years for pneumococcal polysaccharide vaccine [PPSV])*

- PCV is recommended for all children aged <5 years. Administer 1 dose of PCV to all healthy children aged 24-59 months who are not completely vaccinated for their age.
- Administer PPSV to children aged ≥2 years with certain underlying medical conditions [see *MMWR*, 2000, 49(RR-9)], including a cochlear implant.

[6]**Influenza vaccine.** *(Minimum age: 6 months for trivalent inactivated influenza vaccine [TIV]; 2 years for live, attenuated influenza vaccine [LAIV])*

- Administer annually to children age 6 months through 18 years.
- For healthy nonpregnant persons (ie, those who do not have underlying medical conditions that predispose them to influenza complications) aged 2-49 years, either LAIV or TIV may be used.
- Children receiving TIV should receive 0.25 mL if age 6-35 months or 0.5 mL if age ≥3 years.
- Administer 2 doses (separated by ≥4 weeks) to children age <9 years who are receiving influenza vaccine for the first time or who were vaccinated for the first time during the previous influenza season but only received 1 dose.

[7]**Measles, mumps, and rubella vaccine (MMR).** *(Minimum age: 12 months)*

- Administer the second dose of MMR at age 4-6 years. However, the second dose may be administered before age 4, provided at least 28 days have elapsed since the first dose.

[8]**Varicella vaccine.** *(Minimum age: 12 months)*

- Administer the second dose at age 4-6 years. However, the second dose may be administered before age 4, provided at least 3 months have elapsed since the first dose.
- For children aged 12 months through 12 years the minimum interval between doses is 3 months. However, if the second dose was administered at least 28 days after the first dose, it can be accepted as valid.

[9]**Hepatitis A vaccine (HepA).** *(Minimum age: 12 months)*

- Administer to all children aged 1 year (ie, age 12-23 months). Administer the 2 doses in the series at least 6 months apart.
- Children not fully vaccinated by age 2 years can be vaccinated at subsequent visits.
- HepA also is recommended for children >1 year who live in areas where vaccination programs target older children or who are at increased risk of infection. See *MMWR*, 2006, 55(RR-7).

[10]**Meningococcal vaccine.** *(Minimum age: 2 years for meningococcal conjugate vaccine [MCV] and for meningococcal polysaccharide vaccine [MPSV])*

- Administer MCV to children aged 2-10 years with terminal complement component deficiency, anatomic or functional asplenia, and certain other high-risk groups. See *MMWR*, 2005, 54(RR-7).
- Persons who received MPSV ≥3 years previously and who remain at increased risk for meningococcal disease should be revaccinated with MCV.

The recommended immunization schedules for persons aged 0-18 years are approved by the Advisory Committee on Immunization Practices (**http://www.cdc.gov/vaccines/recs/acip**), the American Academy of Pediatrics (**http://www.aap.org**), and the American Academy of Family Physicians (**http://www.aafp.org**).

Recommended Immunization Schedule for Ages 7-18 Years United States, 2009

Vaccine ▼ / Age ▶	7-10 y	11-12 y	13-18 y
Tetanus, diphtheria, pertussis[1]	*See footnote 1*	Tdap	Tdap
Human papillomavirus[2]	*See footnote 2*	HPV (3 doses)	HPV series
Meningococcal[3]	MCV	MCV	MCV
Influenza[4]	Influenza (yearly)		
Pneumococcal[5]	PPSV		
Hepatitis A[6]	HepA series		
Hepatitis B[7]	HepB series		
Inactivated poliovirus[8]	IPV series		
Measles, mumps, rubella[9]	MMR series		
Varicella[10]	Varicella series		

Range of recommended ages | Catch-up immunization | Certain high-risk groups

Note: For those who fall behind or start late, see also the Catch-up Immunization Schedule table.

This schedule indicates the recommended ages for routine administration of currently licensed vaccines, as of December 17, 2008, for children aged 7-18 years. Any dose not administered at the recommended age should be administered at a subsequent visit, when indicated and feasible. Licensed combination vaccines may be used whenever any component of the combination is indicated and other components are not contraindicated and if approved by the Food and Drug Administration for that dose of the series. Providers should consult the relevant Advisory Committee on Immunization Practices statement for detailed recommendations, including **high-risk conditions: http://www.cdc.gov/vaccines/pubs/acip-list.htm**. Clinically significant adverse events that follow immunization should be reported to the Vaccine Adverse Event Reporting System (VAERS). Guidance about how to obtain and complete a VAERS form is available at **http://www.vaers.hhs.gov** or by telephone, 800-822-7967.

Footnotes to Recommended Immunization Schedule for Ages 7-18 Years

[1]**Tetanus and diphtheria toxoids and acellular pertussis vaccine (Tdap).** *(Minimum age: 10 years for Boostrix® and 11 years for Adacel®)*

- Administer at age 11 or 12 years for those who have completed the recommended childhood DTP/DTaP vaccination series and have not received a tetanus and diphtheria toxoid (Td) booster dose.
- Persons aged 13-18 years who have not received Tdap should receive a dose.
- A 5-year interval from the last Td dose is encouraged when Tdap is used as a booster dose; however, a shorter interval may be used if pertussis immunity is needed.

[2]**Human papillomavirus vaccine (HPV).** *(Minimum age: 9 years)*

- Administer the first dose to females at age 11 or 12 years.
- Administer the second dose 2 months after the first dose and the third dose 6 months after the first dose (at least 24 weeks after the first dose).
- Administer the series to females at age 13-18 years if not previously vaccinated.

[3]**Meningococcal conjugate vaccine.**

- Administer at age 11 or 12 years, or at age 13-18 years if not previously vaccinated.
- Administer to previously unvaccinated college freshmen living in a dormitory.
- MCV is recommended for children aged 2-10 years with terminal complement component deficiency, anatomic or functional asplenia, and certain other groups at high risk. See *MMWR*, 2005, 54(RR-7).
- Persons who received MPSV ≥5 years previously and remain at increased risk for meningococcal disease should be vaccinated with MCV.

[4]**Influenza vaccine.**

- Administer annually to children aged 6 months to 18 years.
- For healthy nonpregnant persons (ie, those who do not have underlying medical conditions that predispose them to influenza complications) aged 2-49 years, either LAIV or TIV may be used.

- Administer 2 doses (separated by ≥4 weeks) to children aged <9 years who are receiving influenza vaccine for the first time or who were vaccinated for the first time during the previous influenza season but only received 1 dose.

[5]Pneumococcal polysaccharide vaccine (PPSV).

- Administer to children with certain underlying medical conditions [see *MMWR*, 1997, 46(RR-8)], including a cochlear implant. A single revaccination should be administered to children with functional or anatomic asplenia or other immunocompromising condition after 5 years.

[6]Hepatitis A vaccine (HepA).

- Administer 2 doses at least 6 months apart.
- HepA is recommended for children >1 year who live in areas where vaccination programs target older children or who are at increased risk of infection. See *MMWR*, 2006, 55(RR-7).

[7]Hepatitis B vaccine (HepB).

- Administer the 3-dose series to those not previously vaccinated.
- A 2-dose series (separated by ≥4 months) of adult formulation Recombivax HB® is licensed for children aged 11-15 years.

[8]Inactivated poliovirus vaccine (IPV).

- For children who received an all-IPV or all-oral poliovirus (OPV) series, a fourth dose is not necessary if the third dose was administered at age ≥4 years.
- If both OPV and IPV were administered as part of a series, a total of 4 doses should be administered, regardless of the child's current age.

[9]Measles, mumps, and rubella vaccine (MMR).

- If not previously vaccinated, administer 2 doses or the second dose for those who have received only 1 dose, with ≥28 days between doses.

[10]Varicella vaccine.

- For persons aged 7-18 years without evidence of immunity [see *MMWR*, 2007, 56(RR-4)], administer 2 doses if not previously vaccinated or the second dose if they have received only 1 dose.
- For persons aged 7-12 years, the minimum interval between doses is 3 months. However, if the second dose was administered ≥28 days after the first dose, it can be accepted as valid.
- For persons aged ≥13 years, the minimum interval between doses is 28 days.

The recommended immunization schedules for persons age 0-18 years are approved by the Advisory Committee on Immunization Practices (**http://www.cdc.gov/vaccines/recs/acip**), the American Academy of Pediatrics (**http://www.aap.org**), and the American Academy of Family Physicians (**http://www.aafp.org**).

Catch-up Immunization Schedule for Persons Age 4 Months - 18 Years Who Start Late or Who Are >1 Month Behind - United States, 2009

The table below provides catch-up schedules and minimum intervals between doses for children whose vaccinations have been delayed. A vaccine series does not need to be restarted, regardless of the time that has elapsed between doses. Use the section appropriate for the child's age.

Vaccine (Minimum Age for Dose 1)	Minimum Interval Between Doses			
	Dose 1 to Dose 2	**Dose 2 to Dose 3**	**Dose 3 to Dose 4**	**Dose 4 to Dose 5**
Catch-up Schedule for Persons Age 4 Months – 6 Years				
Hepatitis B[1] (birth)	**4 weeks**	**8 weeks** (and ≥16 weeks after 1st dose)		
Rotavirus[2] (6 wk)	**4 weeks**	**4 weeks**[2]		
Diphtheria, tetanus, pertussis[3] (6 wk)	**4 weeks**	**4 weeks**	**6 months**	**6 months**[3]
Haemophilus influenzae type b[4] (6 wk)	**4 weeks** if 1st dose administered at age <12 months **8 weeks (as final dose)** if 1st dose administered at age 12-14 months **No further doses needed** if 1st dose administered at age ≥15 months	**4 weeks**[4] if current age <12 months **8 weeks (as final dose)**[4] if current age ≥12 months and 2nd dose administered at age <15 months **No further doses needed** if previous dose administered at age ≥15 months	**8 weeks (as final dose)** This dose only necessary for children age 12-59 months who received 3 doses before age 12 months	
Pneumococcal[5] (6 wk)	**4 weeks** if 1st dose administered at age <12 months **8 weeks (as final dose for healthy children)** if 1st dose administered at age ≥12 months or current age 24-59 months **No further doses needed** for healthy children if 1st dose administered at age ≥24 months	**4 weeks** if current age <12 months **8 weeks (as final dose for healthy children)** if current age ≥12 months **No further doses needed** for healthy children if previous dose administered at age ≥24 months	**8 weeks (as final dose)** This dose only necessary for children age 12-59 months who received 3 doses before age 12 months or for high-risk children who received 3 doses at any age	
Inactivated poliovirus[6] (6 wk)	**4 weeks**	**4 weeks**	**4 weeks**[6]	
Measles, mumps, rubella[7] (12 mo)	**4 weeks**			
Varicella[8] (12 mo)	**3 months**			
Hepatitits A[9] (12 mo)	**6 months**			
Catch-up Schedule for Persons Age 7-18 Years				
Tetanus, diphtheria/tetanus, diphtheria, pertussis[10] (7 y)	**4 weeks**	**4 weeks** if 1st dose administered at age <12 months **6 months** if 1st dose administered at age ≥12 months	**6 months** if 1st dose administered at age <12 months	
Human papillomavirus[11] (9 y)	**Routine dosing intervals are recommended**[11]			
Hepatitis A[9] (12 y)	**6 months**			
Hepatitis B[1] (birth)	**4 weeks**	**8 weeks** (and ≥16 weeks after 1st dose)		
Inactivated poliovirus[6] (6 wk)	**4 weeks**	**4 weeks**	**4 weeks**[6]	
Measles, mumps, rubella[7] (12 mo)	**4 weeks**			
Varicella[8] (12 mo)	**4 weeks** if the person is age ≥13 years **3 months** if the person is age <13 years			

Footnotes to Catch-up Immunization Schedule Table

[1]**Hepatitis B vaccine (HepB).**

- Administer the 3-dose series to those not previously vaccinated.
- A 2-dose series (separated by at least 4 months) of adult formulation of Recombivax HB® is licensed for children aged 11-15 years.

[2]**Rotavirus vaccine (RV).**

- The maximum age for the first dose is 14 weeks 6 days. Vaccination should not be initiated for infants aged ≥15 weeks (ie, ≥15 weeks 0 days).
- Administer the final dose in the series by age 8 months 0 days.
- If Rotarix® was administered for the first and second doses, a third dose is not indicated.

[3]**Diphtheria and tetanus toxoids and acellular pertussis vaccine (DTaP).**

- The fifth dose is not necessary if the fourth dose was administered at age ≥4 years.

[4] ***Haemophilus influenzae* type b conjugate (Hib).**

- Hib vaccine is not generally recommended for persons aged ≥5 years. No efficacy data are available on which to base a recommendation concerning use of Hib vaccine for older children and adults. However, studies suggest good immunogenicity in persons who have sickle cell disease, leukemia, or HIV infection, or who have had a splenectomy; administering 1 dose of Hib vaccine to these persons is not contraindicated.
- If the first 2 doses were PRP-OMP (PedvaxHIB® or ComVax®), and administered at age ≤11 months, the third (and final) dose should be administered at age 12-15 months and at least 8 weeks after the second dose.
- If first dose administered at age 7-11 months, administer 2 doses separated by 4 weeks and a final dose at age 12-15 months.

[5]**Pneumococcal vaccine.**

- Administer 1 dose of pneumococcal conjugate vaccine (PCV) to all healthy children aged 24-59 months who have not received at least 1 dose of PCV on or after age 12 months.
- For children aged 24-59 months with underlying medical conditions, administer 1 dose of PCV if 3 doses were received previously or administer 2 doses of PCV at least 8 weeks apart if <3 doses were received previously.
- Administer pneumococcal polysaccharide vaccine (PPSV) to children aged ≥2 years with certain underlying medical conditions (see *MMWR*, 2000, 49(RR-9)], including a cochlear implant, at ≥8 weeks after the last dose of PCV.

[6]**Inactivated poliovirus vaccine (IPV).**

- For children who received an all-IPV or all-oral poliovirus (OPV) series, a fourth dose is not necessary if third dose was administered at age ≥4 years.
- If both OPV and IPV were administered as part of a series, a total of 4 doses should be administered, regardless of the child's current age.

[7]**Measles, mumps, and rubella vaccine (MMR).**

- Administer the second dose at age 4-6 years. However, the second dose may be administered before age 4, provided ≥28 days have elapsed since the first dose.
- If not previously vaccinated, administer 2 doses with ≥28 days between the doses.

[8]**Varicella vaccine.**

- Administer the second dose at age 4-6 years. However, the second dose may be administered before age 4, provided ≥3 months have elapsed since the first dose.
- For persons aged 12 months through 12 years, the minimum interval between doses is 3 months. However, if the second dose was administered ≥28 days after the first dose, it can be accepted as valid.
- For persons aged ≥13 years, the minimum interval between doses is 28 days.

[9]**Hepatitis A vaccine (HepA).**

- HepA is recommended for children >1 year who live in areas where vaccination programs target older children or who are at increased risk of infection. See *MMWR*, 2006, 55(RR-7).

[10]**Tetanus and diphtheria toxoids vaccine (Td) and tetanus and diphtheria toxoids and acellular pertussis vaccine (Tdap).**

- Doses of DTaP are counted as part of the Td/Tdap series
- Tdap should be substituted for a single dose of Td in the catch-up series or as a booster for children aged 10-18 years; use Td for other doses.

[11]**Human papillomavirus (HPV).**

- Administer the series to females at age 13-18 years if not previously vaccinated.
- Use recommended routine dosing intervals for series catch-up (ie, the second and third doses should be administered at 2 and 6 months after the first dose). However, the minimum interval between the first and second doses is 4 weeks. The minimum interval between the second and third doses is 12 weeks, and the third dose should be given ≥24 weeks after the first dose.

Information about reporting reactions after immunization is available online at **http://www.vaers.hhs.gov** or by telephone, 800-822-7967. Suspected cases of vaccine-preventable diseases should be reported to the state or local health department. Additional information, including precautions and contraindications for immunization, is available from the National Center for Immunization and Respiratory Diseases at **http://www.cdc.gov/vaccines** or telephone, 800-CDC-INFO (800-232-4636).

Reference

"Recommended Immunization Schedules for Persons Aged 0-18 Years - United States, 2009," *MMWR*, 2008, 57(51&52):Q1-4.

Figure 1. Recommended Adult Immunization Schedule, by Vaccine and Age Group United States, 2009

Vaccine	Age Group (years) 19-26	27-49	50-59	66-64	≥65
Tetanus, diphtheria, pertussis (Td/Tdap)[1]*	Substitute 1-time dose of Tdap for Td booster; then boost with Td every 10 years				Td booster every 10 years
Human papillomavirus (HPV)[2]*	3 doses (females)				
Varicella[3]*	2 doses				
Zoster[4]				1 dose	
Measles, mumps, rubella (MMR)[5]*	1 or 2 doses		1 dose		
Influenza[6]*	1 dose annually		1 dose annually		
Pneumococcal (polysaccharide)[7,8]	1 or 2 doses				1 dose
Hepatitis A[9]*	2 doses				
Hepatitis B[10]*	3 doses				
Meningococcal[11]*	1 or more doses				

Figure 2. Vaccines That Might Be Indicated for Adults Based on Medical and Other Indications United States, 2009

Vaccine	Indication: Pregnancy	Immunocompromising conditions (excluding human immunodeficiency virus [HIV])[13]	HIV infection[3,12,13] CD4+ T lymphocyte count <200 cells/μL	HIV infection CD4+ T lymphocyte count ≥200 cells/μL	Diabetes, heart disease, chronic lung disease, chronic alcoholism	Asplenia[12] (including elective splenectomy and terminal complement component deficiencies)	Chronic liver disease	Kidney failure, end-stage renal disease, receipt of hemodialysis	Healthcare personnel
Tetanus, diphtheria, pertussis (Td/Tdap)[1]*	Td	Substitute 1-time dose of Tdap for Td booster; then boost with Td every 10 years							
Human papillomavirus (HPV)[2]*		3 doses for females through age 26 years							
Varicella[3]*	Contraindicated			2 doses					
Zoster[4]	Contraindicated				1 dose				
Measles, mumps, rubella (MMR)[5]*	Contraindicated			1 or 2 doses					
Influenza[6]*	1 dose TIV annually								1 dose TIV or LAIV annually
Pneumococcal (polysaccharide)[7,8]		1 or 2 doses							
Hepatitis A[9]*	2 doses								
Hepatitis B[10]*	3 doses								
Meningococcal[11]*	1 or more doses								

*Covered by the Vaccine Injury Compensation Program.

Note: These recommendations must be read along with the footnotes, which can be found following this schedule.

- For all persons in this category who meet the age requirements and who lack evidence of immunity (eg, lack documentation of vaccination or have no evidence of prior infection)
- Recommended if some other risk factor is present (eg, on the basis of medical, occupational, lifestyle, or other indications)
- No recommendation

Footnotes to Recommended Adult Immunization Schedule

[1]**Tetanus, diphtheria, and acellular pertussis (Td/Tdap) vaccination.**
Tdap should replace a single dose of Td for adults aged 19-64 years who have not received a dose of Tdap previously. Adults with uncertain or incomplete history of primary vaccination series with tetanus and diphtheria toxoid-containing vaccines should begin or complete a primary vaccination series. A primary series for adults is 3 doses of tetanus and diphtheria toxoid-containing vaccines; administer the first 2 doses ≥4 weeks apart and the third dose 6-12 months after the second. However, Tdap can substitute for any one of the doses of Td in the 3-dose primary series. The booster dose of tetanus and diphtheria toxoid-containing vaccine should be administered to adults who have completed a primary series and if the last vaccination was received ≥10 years previously. Tdap or Td vaccine may be used, as indicated.
If a woman is pregnant and received the last Td vaccination ≥10 years previously, administer Td during the second or third trimester. If the woman received the last Td vaccination <10 years previously, administer Tdap during the immediate postpartum period. A dose of Tdap is recommended for postpartum women, close contacts of infants aged <12 months, and all healthcare personnel with direct patient contact if they have not previously received Tdap. An interval as short as 2 years from the last Td is suggested; shorter intervals can be used. Td may be deferred during pregnancy and Tdap substituted in the immediate postpartum period, or Tdap can be administered instead of Td to a pregnant woman after an informed discussion with the woman.
Consult the ACIP statement for recommendations for administering Td as prophylaxis in wound management.

[2]**Human papillomavirus (HPV) vaccination.**
HPV vaccination is recommended for all females aged 11-26 years (and many begin at 9 years) who have not completed the vaccine series. History of genital warts, abnormal Papanicolaou test, or positive HPV DNA test is not evidence of prior infection with all vaccine HPV types; HPV vaccination is recommended for persons with such histories.
Ideally, vaccine should be administered before potential exposure to HPV through sexual activity; however, females who are sexually active should still be vaccinated consistent with age-based recommendations. Sexually active females who have not been infected with any of the four HPV vaccine types receive the full benefit of the vaccination. Vaccination is less beneficial for females who have already been infected with one or more of the HPV vaccine types.
A complete series consists of 3 doses. The second dose should be administered 2 months after the first dose; the third dose should be administered 6 months after the first dose.
HPV vaccination is not specifically recommended for females with the medical indications described in Figure 2, "Vaccines That Might Be Indicated for Adults Based on Medical and Other Indications." Because HPV vaccine is not a live-virus vaccine, it may be administered to persons with the medical indications described in Figure 2. However, the immune response and vaccine efficacy might be less for persons with the medical indications described in Figure 2 than in persons who do not have the medical indications described or who are immunocompetent. Healthcare personnel are not at increased risk because of occupational exposure, and should be vaccinated consistent with age-based recommendations.

[3]**Varicella vaccination.**
All adults without evidence of immunity to varicella should receive 2 doses of single-antigen varicella vaccine if not previously vaccinated or the second dose if they have received only one dose, unless they have a medical contraindication. Special consideration should be given to those who 1) have close contact with persons at high risk for severe disease (eg, healthcare personnel and family contacts of persons with immunocompromising conditions) or 2) are at high risk for exposure or transmission (eg, teachers; child care employees; residents and staff members of institutional settings, including correctional institutions; college students; military personnel; adolescents and adults living in households with children; nonpregnant women of childbearing age; and international travelers).
Evidence of immunity to varicella in adults includes any of the following: 1) documentation of 2 doses of varicella vaccine ≥4 weeks apart; 2) U.S.-born before 1980 (although for healthcare personnel and pregnant women, birth before 1980 should not be considered evidence of immunity); 3) history of varicella based on diagnosis or verification of varicella by a healthcare provider (for a patient reporting a history of or presenting with an atypical case, a mild case, or both, healthcare providers should seek either an epidemiologic link to a typical varicella case or to a laboratory-confirmed case or evidence of laboratory confirmation, if it was performed at the time of acute disease); 4) history of herpes zoster based on healthcare provider diagnosis or verification of herpes zoster by a healthcare provider; or 5) laboratory evidence of immunity or laboratory confirmation of disease.
Pregnant women should be assessed for evidence of varicella immunity. Women who do not have evidence of immunity should receive the first dose of varicella vaccine upon completion or termination of pregnancy and before discharge from the healthcare facility. The second dose should be administered 4-8 weeks after the first dose.

[4]**Herpes zoster vaccination.**
A single dose of zoster vaccine is recommended for adults aged ≥60 years regardless of whether they report a prior episode of herpes zoster. Persons with chronic medical conditions may be vaccinated unless their condition constitutes a contraindication.

[5]**Measles, mumps, rubella (MMR) vaccination.**
Measles component: Adults born before 1957 can be considered immune to measles. Adults born during or after 1957 should receive ≥1 dose of MMR unless they have a medical contraindication, documentation of ≥1 dose, history of measles based on healthcare provider diagnosis, or laboratory evidence of immunity.
A second dose of MMR is recommended for adults who 1) have been recently exposed to measles or are in an outbreak setting; 2) have been vaccinated previously with killed measles vaccine; 3) have been vaccinated with an unknown type of measles vaccine during 1963-1967; 4) are students in postsecondary educational institutions; 5) work in a healthcare facility; or 6) plan to travel internationally.
Mumps component: Adults born before 1957 can generally be considered immune to mumps. Adults born during or after 1957 should receive 1 dose of MMR unless they have a medical contraindication, history of mumps based on healthcare provider diagnosis, or laboratory evidence of immunity.
A second dose of MMR is recommended for adults who 1) live in a community experiencing a mumps outbreak and are in an affected age group; 2) are students in postsecondary educational institutions; 3) work in a healthcare facility; or 4) plan to travel internationally. For unvaccinated healthcare personnel born before 1957 who do not have other evidence of mumps immunity, administering 1 dose on a routine basis should be considered and administering a second dose during an outbreak should be strongly considered.
Rubella component: 1 dose of MMR vaccine is recommended for women whose rubella vaccination history is unreliable or who lack laboratory evidence of immunity. For women of childbearing age, regardless of birth year, rubella immunity should be

determined and women should be counseled regarding congenital rubella syndrome. Women who do not have evidence of immunity should receive MMR vaccine upon completion or termination of pregnancy and before discharge from the healthcare facility.

[6]**Influenza vaccination.**

Medical indications: Chronic disorders of the cardiovascular or pulmonary systems, including asthma; chronic metabolic diseases, including diabetes mellitus, renal or hepatic dysfunction, hemoglobinopathies, or immunocompromising conditions (including immunocompromising conditions caused by medications or human immunodeficiency virus [HIV]); any condition that compromises respiratory function or the handling of respiratory secretions or that can increase the risk of aspiration (eg, cognitive dysfunction, spinal cord injury, or seizure disorder or other neuromuscular disorder); and pregnancy during the influenza season. No data exist on the risk for severe or complicated influenza disease among persons with asplenia; however, influenza is a risk factor for secondary bacterial infections that can cause severe disease among persons with asplenia.

Occupational indications: Healthcare personnel, including those employed by long-term care and assisted living facilities, and caregivers of children <5 years old.

Other indications: Residents of nursing homes and other long-term care and assisted living facilities; persons likely to transmit influenza to persons at high risk (eg, in-home household contacts and caregivers of children age <5 years old, persons ≥65 years old, and persons of all ages with high-risk condition[s]); and anyone who would like to decrease their risk of getting influenza. Healthy, nonpregnant persons aged <50 years without high-risk medical conditions who are not contacts of severely immunocompromised persons in special care units can receive either intranasally administered live, attenuated influenza vaccine (FluMist®) or inactivated vaccine. Other persons should receive the inactivated vaccine.

[7]**Pneumococcal polysaccharide (PPSV) vaccination.**

Medical indications: Chronic lung disease (including asthma); chronic cardiovascular diseases; diabetes mellitus; chronic liver diseases, cirrhosis; chronic alcoholism, chronic renal failure or nephrotic syndrome; functional or anatomic asplenia (eg, sickle cell disease or splenectomy [if elective splenectomy is planned, vaccinate at least 2 weeks before surgery]); immunocompromising conditions; and cochlear implants and cerebrospinal fluid leaks. Vaccinate as close to HIV diagnosis as possible.

Other indications: Residents of nursing homes or other long-term care facilities and persons who smoke cigarettes. Routine use of PPSV is not recommended for Alaska Native or American Indian persons <65 years unless they have underlying medical conditions that are PPSV indications. However, public health authorities may consider recommending PPSV for Alaska Natives and American Indians aged 50-64 years who are living in areas in which the risk of invasive pneumococcal disease is increased.

[8]**Revaccination with PPSV.**

One-time revaccination after 5 years is recommended for persons with chronic renal failure or nephrotic syndrome; functional or anatomic asplenia (eg, sickle cell disease or splenectomy); and for persons with immunocompromising conditions. For persons aged ≥65 years, one-time revaccination if they were vaccinated ≥5 years previously and were aged <65 years at the time of primary vaccination.

[9]**Hepatitis A vaccination.**

Medical indications: Persons with chronic liver disease and persons who receive clotting factor concentrates.

Behavioral indications: Men who have sex with men and persons who use illegal drugs.

Occupational indications: Persons working with hepatitis A virus (HAV)-infected primates or with HAV in a research laboratory setting.

Other indications: Persons traveling to or working in countries that have high or intermediate endemicity of hepatitis A (a list of countries is available at http://www.cdc.gov/travel/contentdiseases.aspx) and any person seeking protection from HAV infection.

Single-antigen vaccine formulations should be administered in a 2-dose schedule at either 0 and 6-12 months (Havrix®), or 0 and 6-18 months (Vaqta®). If the combined hepatitis A and hepatitis B vaccine (Twinrix®) is used, administer 3 doses at 0, 1, and 6 months; alternatively, a 4-dose schedule, administered on days 0, 7, and 21-30 followed by a booster dose at month 12 may be used.

[10]**Hepatitis B vaccination.**

Medical indications: Persons with end-stage renal disease, including patients receiving hemodialysis; persons with HIV infection; and persons with chronic liver disease.

Occupational indications: Healthcare personnel and public-safety workers who are exposed to blood or other potentially infectious body fluids.

Behavioral indications: Sexually active persons who are not in a long-term, mutually monogamous relationship (eg, persons with more than one sex partner during the previous 6 months); persons seeking evaluation or treatment for a sexually transmitted disease (STD); current or recent injection-drug users; and men who have sex with men.

Other indications: Household contacts and sex partners of persons with chronic hepatitis B virus (HBV) infection; clients and staff members of institutions for persons with developmental disabilities; international travelers to countries with high or intermediate prevalence of chronic HBV infection (a list of countries is available at http://www.cdc.gov/travel/contentdiseases.-aspx); and any adult seeking protection from HBV infection.

Hepatitis B vaccination is recommended for all adults in the following settings: STD treatment facilities; HIV testing and treatment facilities; facilities providing drug-abuse treatment and prevention services; healthcare settings targeting services to injection-drug users or men who have sex with men; correctional facilities; end-stage renal disease programs and facilities for chronic hemodialysis patients; and institutions and nonresidential daycare facilities for persons with developmental disabilities. If the combined hepatitis A and hepatitis B vaccine (Twinrix®) is used, administer 3 doses at 0, 1, and 6 months; alternatively, a 4-dose schedule, administered on days 0, 7, and 21-30 followed by a booster dose at month 12 may be used.

Special formulation indications: For adult patients receiving hemodialysis and other immunocompromising conditions, 1 dose of 40 mcg/mL (Recombivax HB®) administered on a 3-dose schedule or 2 doses of 20 mcg/mL (Engerix-B®), administered simultaneously on a 4-dose schedule at 0, 1, 2, and 6 months.

[11]**Meningococcal vaccination.**

Medical indications: Adults with anatomic or functional asplenia, or terminal complement component deficiencies.

Other indications: First-year college students living in dormitories; microbiologists routinely exposed to isolates of *Neisseria meningitidis*; military recruits; and persons who travel to or live in countries in which meningococcal disease is hyperendemic or epidemic (eg, the "meningitis belt" of sub-Saharan Africa during the dry season [December-June]), particularly if their contact with local populations will be prolonged. Vaccination is required by the government of Saudi Arabia for all travelers to Mecca during the annual Hajj.

Meningococcal conjugate vaccine (MCV) is preferred for adults with any of the preceding indications who are aged ≤55 years, although meningococcal polysaccharide vaccine (MPSV) is an acceptable alternative. Revaccination with MCV after 5 years might be indicated for adults previously vaccinated with MPSV who remain at increased risk for infection (eg, persons residing in areas in which disease is epidemic).

[12] **Selected conditions for which *Haemophilus influenzae* type b (Hib) vaccine may be used.**

Hib vaccine generally is not recommended for persons aged ≥5 years. No efficacy data are available on which to base a recommendation concerning use of Hib vaccine for older children and adults. However, studies suggest good immunogenicity in patients who have sickle cell disease, leukemia, or HIV infection or who have had a splenectomy; administering 1 dose of vaccine to these patients is not contraindicated.

[13] **Immunocompromising conditions.**

Inactivated vaccines generally are acceptable (eg, pneumococcal, meningococcal, and influenza [trivalent inactivated influenza vaccine]) and live vaccines generally are avoided in persons with immune deficiencies or immunocompromising conditions. Information on specific conditions is available at http://www.cdc.gov/vaccines/pubs/acip-list.htm.

Reference

"Recommended Adult Immunization Schedule - United States, 2009," *MMWR*, 2009, 57(53):Q1-4.

These schedules indicate the recommended age groups and medical indications for which administration of currently licensed vaccines is commonly indicated for adults ages ≥19 years, as of January 1, 2009. Licensed combination vaccines may be used whenever any components of the combination are indicated and when the vaccine's other components are not contraindicated. For detailed recommendations on **all** vaccines, including those used primarily for travelers or that are issued during the year, consult the manufacturers' package inserts and the complete statements from the Advisory Committee on Immunization Practices (http://www.cdc.gov/vaccines/pubs/acip-list.htm).

Report all clinically significant postvaccination reactions to the Vaccine Adverse Event Reporting System (VAERS). Reporting forms and instructions on filing a VAERS report are available at http://www.vaers.hhs.gov or by telephone, 800-822-7967.

Information on how to file a Vaccine Injury Compensation Program claim is available at http://www.hrsa.gov/vaccinecompensation or by telephone, 800-338-2382. To file a claim for vaccine injury, contact the U.S. Court of Federal Claims, 717 Madison Place, NW, Washington, DC 20005; telephone, 202-357-6400.

Additional information about the vaccines in this schedule, extent of available data, and contraindications for vaccination is also available at http://www.cdc.gov/vaccines or from the CDC-INFO Contact Center at 800-CDC-INFO (800-232-4636) in English and Spanish, 24 hours a day, 7 days a week.

Use of trade names and commercial sources is for identification only and does not imply endorsement by the U.S. Department of Health and Human Services.

VACCINE INJURY TABLE

The Vaccine Injury Table makes it easier for some people to get compensation. The table lists and explains injuries/conditions that are presumed to be caused by vaccines. It also lists time periods in which the first symptom of these injuries/conditions must occur after receiving the vaccine. If the first symptom of these injuries/conditions occurs within the listed time periods, it is presumed that the vaccine was the cause of the injury or condition unless another cause is found. For example, if the patient received the tetanus vaccines and had a severe allergic reaction (anaphylaxis) within 4 hours after receiving the vaccine, then it is presumed that the tetanus vaccine caused the injury if no other cause is found.

If the injury/condition is not on the table or if the injury/condition did not occur within the time period on the table, it must be proven that the vaccine caused the injury/condition. Such proof must be based on medical records or opinion, which may include expert witness testimony.

National Childhood Vaccine Injury Act

Vaccine Injury Table

Vaccine	Adverse Event	Time Interval
Tetanus toxoid-containing vaccines (eg, DTaP, Tdap, DTP-Hib, DT, Td, TT)	A. Anaphylaxis or anaphylactic shock	0-4 hours
	B. Brachial neuritis	2-28 days
	C. Any acute complication or sequela (including death) of above events	Not applicable
Pertussis antigen-containing vaccines (eg, DTaP, Tdap, DTP, P, DTP-Hib)	A. Anaphylaxis or anaphylactic shock	0-4 hours
	B. Encephalopathy (or encephalitis)	0-72 hours
	C. Any acute complication or sequela (including death) of above events	Not applicable
Measles, mumps, and rubella virus-containing vaccines in any combination (eg, MMR, MR, M, R)	A. Anaphylaxis or anaphylactic shock	0-4 hours
	B. Encephalopathy (or encephalitis)	5-15 days
	C. Any acute complication or sequela (including death) of above events	Not applicable
Rubella virus-containing vaccines (eg, MMR, MR, R)	A. Chronic arthritis	7-42 days
	B. Any acute complication or sequela (including death) of above events	Not applicable
Measles virus-containing vaccines (eg, MMR, MR, M)	A. Thrombocytopenic purpura	7-30 days
	B. Vaccine-strain measles viral infection in an immunodeficient recipient	0-6 months
	C. Any acute complication or sequela (including death) of above events	Not applicable
Polio live virus-containing vaccines (OPV)	A. Paralytic polio	
	• In a nonimmunodeficient recipient	0-30 days
	• In an immunodeficient recipient	0-6 months
	• In a vaccine associated community case	Not applicable
	B. Vaccine-strain polio viral infection	
	• In a nonimmunodeficient recipient	0-30 days
	• In an immunodeficient recipient	0-6 months
	• In a vaccine associated community case	Not applicable
	C. Any acute complication or sequela (including death) of above events	Not applicable
Polio inactivated-virus containing vaccines (eg, IPV)	A. Anaphylaxis or anaphylactic shock	0-4 hours
	B. Any acute complication or sequela (including death) of above events	Not applicable
Hepatitis B antigen-containing vaccines	A. Anaphylaxis or anaphylactic shock	0-4 hours
	B. Any acute complication or sequela (including death) of above events	Not applicable
Hemophilus influenzae (type b polysaccharide conjugate vaccines)	A. No condition specified for compensation	Not applicable
Varicella vaccine	A. No condition specified for compensation	Not applicable
Rotavirus vaccine	A. No condition specified for compensation	Not applicable
Pneumococcal conjugate vaccines	A. No condition specified for compensation	Not applicable
Any new vaccine recommended by the Centers for Disease Control and Prevention for routine administration to children, after publication by Secretary, HHS of a notice of coverage[1,2]	A. No condition specified for compensation	Not applicable

Note: Effective date: November 1, 2008.

[1]As of December 1, 2004, hepatitis A vaccines have been added to the Vaccine Injury Table under this category. As of July 1, 2005, trivalent influenza vaccines have been added to the table under this category. Trivalent influenza vaccines are given annually during the flu season either by needle and syringe or in a nasal spray. All influenza vaccines routinely administered in the U.S. are trivalent vaccines covered under this category.

[2]As of February 1, 2007, meningococcal (conjugate and polysaccharide) and human papillomavirus (HPV) vaccines have been added to the table under this category.

See *News* on the VICP website for more information. Avaliable at: http://www.hrsa.gov/vaccinecompensation.

MANAGEMENT OF HEALTHCARE WORKER EXPOSURES TO HBV, HCV, AND HIV

Factors to Consider in Assessing the Need for Follow-up of Occupational Exposures

- **Type of exposure**
  - Percutaneous injury
  - Mucous membrane exposure
  - Nonintact skin exposure
  - Bites resulting in blood exposure to either person involved
- **Type and amount of fluid/tissue**
  - Blood
  - Fluids containing blood
  - Potentially infectious fluid or tissue (semen; vaginal secretions; and cerebrospinal, synovial, pleural, peritoneal, pericardial, and amniotic fluids)
  - Direct contact with concentrated virus
- **Infectious status of source**
  - Presence of HB_sAg
  - Presence of HCV antibody
  - Presence of HIV antibody
- **Susceptibility of exposed person**
  - Hepatitis B vaccine and vaccine response status
  - HBV, HCV, HIV immune status

Evaluation of Occupational Exposure Sources

Known sources

- Test known sources for HB_sAg, anti-HCV, and HIV antibody
  - Direct virus assays for routine screening of source patients are **not** recommended
  - Consider using a rapid HIV-antibody test
  - If the source person is **not** infected with a blood-borne pathogen, baseline testing or further follow-up of the exposed person is **not** necessary
- For sources whose infection status remains unknown (eg, the source person refuses testing), consider medical diagnoses, clinical symptoms, and history of risk behaviors
- Do not test discarded needles for blood-borne pathogens

Unknown sources

- For unknown sources, evaluate the likelihood of exposure to a source at high risk for infection
  - Consider the likelihood of blood-borne pathogen infection among patients in the exposure setting

Recommended Postexposure Prophylaxis for Exposure to Hepatitis B Virus

Vaccination and Antibody Response Status of Exposed Workers[1]	Treatment		
	Source HB_sAg[2]-Positive	Source HB_sAg[2] -Negative	Source Unknown or Not Available for Testing
Unvaccinated	HBIG[3] x 1 and initiate HB vaccine series[4]	Initiate HB vaccine series	Initiate HB vaccine series
Previously vaccinated			
Known responder[5]	No treatment	No treatment	No treatment
Known nonresponder[6]	HBIG[3] x 1 and initiate revaccination or HBIG x 2[7]	No treatment	If known high risk source, treat as if source was HB_sAg-positive
Antibody response unknown	Test exposed person for anti-HB_s[8] 1. If adequate,[5] no treatment is necessary 2. If inadequate,[6] administer HBIG[3] x 1 and vaccine booster	No treatment	Test exposed person for anti-HB_s 1. If adequate,[4] no treatment is necessary 2. If inadequate,[4] administer vaccine booster and recheck titer in 1-2 months

[1]Persons who have previously been infected with HBV are immune to reinfection and do not require postexposure prophylaxis.

[2]Hepatitis B surface antigen.

[3]Hepatitis B immune globulin; dose is 0.06 mL/kg intramuscularly.

[4]Hepatitis B vaccine.

[5]A responder is a person with adequate levels of serum antibody to HB_sAg (ie, anti-HB_s ≥10 mIU/mL).

[6]A nonresponder is a person with inadequate response to vaccination (ie, serum anti-HB_s <10 mIU/mL).

[7]The option of giving one dose of HBIG and reinitiating the vaccine series is preferred for nonresponders who have not completed a second 3-dose vaccine series. For persons who previously completed a second vaccine series but failed to respond, two doses of HBIG are preferred.

[8]Antibody to HB_sAg.

Recommended HIV Postexposure Prophylaxis (PEP) for Percutaneous Injuries

Exposure Type	Infection Status of Source				
	HIV-Positive Class 1[1]	HIV-Positive Class 2[1]	Source of Unknown HIV Status[2]	Unknown Source[3]	HIV-Negative
Less severe[4]	Recommend basic 2-drug PEP	Recommend expanded ≥3-drug PEP	Generally, no PEP warranted; however, consider basic 2-drug PEP[5] for source with HIV risk factors[6]	Generally, no PEP warranted; however, consider basic 2-drug PEP[5] in settings in which exposure to HIV-infected persons is likely	No PEP warranted
More severe[7]	Recommend expanded 3-drug PEP	Recommend expanded ≥3-drug PEP	Generally, no PEP warranted; however consider basic 2-drug PEP[5] for source with HIV risk factors[6]	Generally, no PEP warranted; however, consider basic 2-drug PEP[5] in settings in which exposure to HIV-infected persons is likely	No PEP warranted

[1]HIV-positive, class 1 - asymptomatic HIV infection or known low viral load (eg, <1500 ribonucleic acid copies/mL). HIV-positive, class 2 – symptomatic HIV infection, AIDS, acute seroconversion, or known high viral load. If drug resistance is a concern, obtain expert consultation. Initiation of PEP should not be delayed pending expert consultation, and, because expert consultation alone cannot substitute for face-to-face counseling, resources should be available to provide immediate evaluation and follow-up care for all exposures.

[2]For example, deceased source person with no samples available for HIV testing.

[3]For example, a needle from a sharps disposal container.

[4]For example, solid needle or superficial injury.

[5]The recommendation "consider PEP" indicates that PEP is optional; a decision to initiate PEP should be based on a discussion between the exposed person and the treating clinician regarding the risk versus benefits of PEP.

[6]If PEP is offered and administered and the source is later determined to be HIV-negative, PEP should be discontinued.

[7]For example, large-bore hollow needle, deep puncture, visible blood on device, or needle used in patient's artery or vein.

Recommended HIV Postexposure Prophylaxis (PEP) for Mucous Membrane Exposures and Nonintact Skin[1] Exposures

Exposure Type	Infection Status of Source				
	HIV-Positive Class 1[2]	**HIV-Positive Class 2[2]**	**Source of Unknown HIV Status[3]**	**Unknown Source[4]**	**HIV-Negative**
Small volume[5]	Consider basic 2-drug PEP[6]	Recommend basic 2-drug PEP	Generally, no PEP warranted[7]	Generally, no PEP warranted	No PEP warranted
Large volume[8]	Recommend basic 2-drug PEP	Recommend expanded ≥3-drug PEP	Generally, no PEP warranted; however consider basic 2-drug PEP[6] for source with HIV risk factors[7]	Generally, no PEP warranted; however, consider basic 2-drug PEP[6] in settings in which exposure to HIV-infected persons is likely	No PEP warranted

[1]For skin exposures, follow-up is indicated only if evidence exist of compromised skin integrity (eg, dermatitis, abrasion, or open wound).

[2]HIV-positive, class 1 – asymptomatic HIV infection or known low viral load (eg, <1500 ribonucleic acid copies/mL). HIV-positive, class 2 – symptomatic HIV infection, AIDS, acute seroconversion, or known high viral load. If drug resistance is a concern, obtain expert consultation. Initiation of PEP should not be delayed pending expert consultation, and, because expert consultation alone cannot substitute for face-to-face counseling, resources should be available to provide immediate evaluation and follow-up care for all exposures.

[3]For example, deceased source person with no samples available for HIV testing.

[4]For example, splash from inappropriately disposed blood.

[5]For example, a few drops.

[6]The recommendation "consider PEP" indicates that PEP is optional; a decision to initiate PEP should be based on a discussion between the exposed person and the treating clinician regarding the risks versus benefits of PEP.

[7]If PEP is offered and administered and the source is later determined to be HIV-negative, PEP should be discontinued.

[8]For example, a major blood splash.

Situations for Which Expert[1] Consultation for HIV Postexposure Prophylaxis Is Advised

- **Delayed (ie, later than 24-36 hours) exposure report**
  - The interval after which there is no benefit from postexposure prophylaxis (PEP) is undefined
- **Unknown source (eg, needle in sharps disposal container or laundry)**
  - Decide use of PEP on a case-by-case basis
  - Consider the severity of the exposure and the epidemiologic likelihood of HIV exposure
  - Do not test needles or sharp instruments for HIV
- **Known or suspected pregnancy in the exposed person**
  - Does not preclude the use of optimal PEP regimens
  - Do not deny PEP solely on the basis of pregnancy
- **Breast-feeding in the exposed person**
  - Use of optimal PEP regimen not precluded
  - PEP should not be denied solely on the basis of breast-feeding
- **Resistance of the source virus to antiretroviral agents**
  - Influence of drug resistance on transmission risk is unknown
  - Selection of drugs to which the source person's virus is unlikely to be resistant is recommended, if the source person's virus is unknown or suspected to be resistant to ≥1 of the drugs considered for the PEP regimen
  - Resistance testing of the source person's virus at the time of the exposure is not recommended
  - Initiation of PEP not to be delayed while awaiting results of resistance testing
- **Toxicity of the initial PEP regimen**
  - Adverse symptoms, such as nausea and diarrhea, are common with PEP
  - Symptoms can often be managed without changing the PEP regimen by prescribing antimotility and/or antiemetic agents
  - Modification of dose intervals (ie, administering a lower dose of drug more frequently throughout the day, as recommended by the manufacturer), in other situations, might help alleviate symptoms

[1]Local experts and/or the National Clinicians' Postexposure Prophylaxis Hotline (PEPline 1-888-448-4911).

Occupational Exposure Management Resources

National Clinicians' Postexposure Prophylaxis Hotline (PEPline) Run by University of California-San Francisco/San Francisco General Hospital staff; supported by the Health Resources and Services Administration Ryan White CARE Act, HIV/AIDS Bureau, AIDS Education and Training Centers, and CDC	Phone: (888) 448-4911 Internet: http://www.ucsf.edu/hivcntr
Needlestick! A website to help clinicians manage and document occupational blood and body fluid exposures. Developed and maintained by the University of California, Los Angeles (UCLA), Emergency Medicine Center, UCLA School of Medicine, and funded in part by CDC and the Agency for Healthcare Research and Quality.	Internet: http://www.needlestick.mednet.ucla.edu
Hepatitis Hotline	Phone: (888) 443-7232 Internet: http://www.cdc.gov/hepatitis
Reporting to CDC Occupationally acquired HIV infections and failures of PEP	Phone: (800) 893-0485
HIV Antiretroviral Pregnancy Registry	Phone: (800) 258-4263 Fax: (800) 800-1052 Address: 1410 Commonwealth Drive, Suite 215 Wilmington, NC 28405 Internet: http://www.glaxowellcome.com/preg_reg/antiretroviral
Food and Drug Administration Report unusual or severe toxicity to antiretroviral agents	Phone: (800) 332-1088 Address: MedWatch HF-2, FDA 5600 Fishers Lane Rockville, MD 20857 Internet: http://www.fda.gov/medwatch
HIV / AIDS Treatment Information Service	Internet: http://www.aidsinfo.nih.gov

Management of Occupational Blood Exposures

Provide immediate care to the exposure site

- Wash wounds and skin with soap and water
- Flush mucous membranes with water

Determine risk associated with exposure by:

- Type of fluid (eg, blood, visibly bloody fluid, other potentially infectious fluid or tissue, and concentrated virus)
- Type of exposure (ie, percutaneous injury, mucous membrane or nonintact skin exposure, and bites resulting in blood exposure)

Evaluate exposure source

- Assess the risk of infection using available information
- Test known sources for HB_sAg, anti-HCV, and HIV antibody (consider using rapid testing)
- For unknown sources, assess risk of exposure to HBV, HCV, or HIV infection
- Do not test discarded needle or syringes for virus contamination

Evaluate the exposed person

- Assess immune status for HBV infection (ie, by history of hepatitis B vaccination and vaccine response)

Give PEP for exposures posing risk of infection transmission

- HBV: See Recommended Postexposure Prophylaxis for Exposure to Hepatitis B Virus Table
- HCV: PEP not recommended
- HIV: See Recommended HIV Postexposure Prophylaxis for Percutaneous Injuries Table and Recommended HIV Postexposure Prophylaxis for Mucous Membrane Exposures and Nonintact Skin Exposures Table
  - Initiate PEP as soon as possible, preferably within hours of exposure
  - Offer pregnancy testing to all women of childbearing age not known to be pregnant
  - Seek expert consultation if viral resistance is suspected
  - Administer PEP for 4 weeks if tolerated

Perform follow-up testing and provide counseling

- Advise exposed persons to seek medical evaluation for any acute illness occurring during follow-up

HBV exposures

- Perform follow-up anti-HB_s testing in persons who receive hepatitis B vaccine
  - Test for anti-HB_s 1-2 months after last dose of vaccine
  - Anti-HB_s response to vaccine cannot be ascertained if HBIG was received in the previous 3-4 months

HCV exposures

- Perform baseline and follow-up testing for anti-HCV and alanine (ALT) 4-6 months after exposures
- Perform HCV RNA at 4-6 months if earlier diagnosis of HCV infection is desired
- Confirm repeatedly reactive anti-HCV enzyme immunoassays (EIAs) with supplemental tests

HIV exposures

- Perform HIV antibody testing for at least 6 months postexposure (eg, at baseline, 6 weeks, 3 months, and 6 months)
- Perform HIV antibody testing if illness compatible with an acute retroviral syndrome occurs
- Advise exposed persons to use precautions to prevent secondary transmission during the follow-up period
- Evaluate exposed persons taking PEP within 72 hours after exposure and monitor for drug toxicity for at least 2 weeks

Basic and Expanded HIV Postexposure Prophylaxis Regimens

BASIC REGIMENS

Zidovudine (Retrovir®; ZDV; AZT) + lamivudine (Epivir®; 3TC); available as Combivir®

Preferred dosing

- ZDV: 300 mg twice daily or 200 mg three times daily, with food; total: 600 mg daily
- 3TC: 300 mg once daily or 150 mg twice daily
- Combivir®: One tablet twice daily

Advantages

- ZDV associated with decreased risk for HIV transmission
- ZDV used more often than other drugs for PEP for healthcare personnel (HCP)
- Serious toxicity rare when used for PEP
- Side effects predictable and manageable with antimotility and antiemetic agents
- Can be used by pregnant HCP
- Can be given as a single tablet (Combivir®) twice daily

Disadvantages

- Side effects (especially nausea and fatigue) common and might result in low adherence
- Source-patient virus resistance to this regimen possible
- Potential for delayed toxicity (oncogenic/teratogenic) unknown

Zidovudine (Retrovir®; ZDV; AZT) + emtricitabine (Emtriva®; FTC)

Preferred dosing

- ZDV: 300 mg twice daily or 200 mg three times daily, with food; total: 600 mg/day, in 2-3 divided doses
- FTC: 200 mg (one capsule) once daily

Advantages

- ZDV: See above
- FTC
  - Convenient (once daily)
  - Well tolerated
  - Long intracellular half-life (~40 hours)

Disadvantages

- ZDV: See above
- FTC
  - Rash perhaps more frequent than with 3TC
  - No long-term experience with this drug
  - Cross resistance to 3TC
  - Hyperpigmentation among non-Caucasians with long-term use: 3%

Tenofovir DF (Viread®; TDF) + lamivudine (Epivir®; 3TC)

Preferred dosing

- TDF: 300 mg once daily
- 3TC: 300 mg once daily or 150 mg twice daily

Advantages

- 3TC: See above
- TDF
  - Convenient dosing (single pill once daily)
  - Resistance profile activity against certain thymidine analogue mutations
  - Well tolerated

Disadvantages

- TDF
  - Same class warnings as nucleoside reverse transcriptase inhibitors (NRTIs)
  - Drug interactions
  - Increased TDF concentrations among persons taking atazanavir and lopinavir/ritonavir; need to monitor patients for TDF-associated toxicities
- Preferred dosage of atazanavir if used with TDF: 300 mg + ritonavir 100 mg once daily + TDF 300 mg once daily

Tenofovir DF (Viread®; TDF) + emtricitabine (Emtriva®; FTC); available as Truvada®

Preferred dosing

- TDF: 300 mg once daily
- FTC: 200 mg once daily
- As Truvada®: One tablet daily

Advantages

- FTC: See above
- TDF
  - Convenient dosing (single pill once daily)
  - Resistance profile activity against certain thymidine analogue mutations
  - Well tolerated

Disadvantages

- TDF
  - Same class warnings as NRTIs
  - Drug interactions
  - Increased TDF concentrations among persons taking atazanavir and lopinavir/ritonavir; need to monitor patients for TDF-associated toxicities
  - Preferred dosing of atazanavir if used with TDF: 300 mg + ritonavir 100 mg once daily + TDF 300 mg once daily

ALTERNATE BASIC REGIMENS

Lamivudine (Epivir®; 3TC) + stavudine (Zerit®; d4T)

Preferred dosing

- 3TC: 300 mg once daily or 150 mg twice daily
- d4T: 40 mg twice daily (can use lower doses of 20-30 mg twice daily if toxicity occurs; equally effective but less toxic among HIV-infected patients with peripheral neuropathy); 30 mg twice daily if body weight is <60 kg

Advantages

- 3TC: See above
- d4T: Gastrointestinal (GI) side effects rare

Disadvantages

- Possibility that source-patient virus is resistant to this regimen
- Potential for delayed toxicity (oncogenic/teratogenic) unknown

Emtricitabine (Emtriva®; FTC) + stavudine (Zerit®; d4T)

Preferred dosing

- FTC: 200 mg daily
- d4T: 40 mg twice daily (can use lower doses of 20-30 mg twice daily if toxicity occurs; equally effective but less toxic among HIV-infected patients who developed peripheral neuropathy); if body weight is <60 kg, 30 mg twice daily

Advantages

- 3TC and FTC: See above; d4T's GI side effects rare

Disadvantages

- Potential that source-patient virus is resistant to this regimen
- Unknown potential for delayed toxicity (oncogenic/teratogenic) unknown

Lamivudine (Epivir®; 3TC) + didanosine (Videx®; ddl)

Preferred dosing

- 3TC: 300 mg once daily or 150 mg twice daily
- ddl: Videx® chewable/dispersible buffered tablets can be administered on an empty stomach as either 200 mg twice daily or 400 mg once daily. Patients must take at least two of the appropriate strength tablets at each dose to provide adequate buffering and prevent gastric acid degradation of ddl. Because of the need for adequate buffering, the 200 mg strength tablet should be used only as a component of a once-daily regimen. The dose is either 200 mg twice daily or 400 mg once daily for patients weighing >60 kg and 125 mg twice daily or 250 mg once daily for patients weighing <60 kg.

Advantages

- ddl: Once-daily dosing option
- 3TC: See above

Disadvantages

- Tolerability: Diarrhea more common with buffered preparation than with enteric-coated preparation
- Associated with toxicity: Peripheral neuropathy, pancreatitis, and lactic acidosis
- Must be taken on empty stomach except with TDF
- Drug interactions
- 3TC: See above

Emtricitabine (Emtriva®; FTC) + didanosine (Videx®; ddl)

Preferred dosing

- FTC: 200 mg once daily
- ddl: See above

Advantages

- ddl: See above
- FTC: See above

Disadvantages

- Tolerability: Diarrhea more common with buffered than with enteric-coated preparation
- Associated with toxicity: Peripheral neuropathy, pancreatitis, and lactic acidosis
- Must be taken on empty stomach except with TDF
- Drug interactions
- FTC: See above

PREFERRED EXPANDED REGIMEN

Basic regimen plus:

Lopinavir / Ritonavir (Kaletra®; LPV/RTV)

Preferred dosing

- LPV/RTV: 400 mg/100 mg = twice daily with food

Advantages

- Potent HIV protease inhibitor
- Generally well-tolerated

Disadvantages

- Potential for serious or life-threatening drug interactions
- Might accelerate clearance of certain drugs, including oral contraceptives (requiring alternative or additional contraceptive measures for women taking these drugs)
- Can cause severe hyperlipidemia, especially hypertriglyceridemia
- GI (eg, diarrhea) events common

ALTERNATE EXPANDED REGIMENS

Basic regimen plus one of the following:

Atazanavir (Reyataz®; ATV) ± ritonavir (Norvir®; RTV)

Preferred dosing

- ATV: 400 mg once daily, unless used in combination with TDF, in which case ATV should be boosted with RTV, preferred dosing of ATV 300 mg + RTV: 100 mg once daily

Advantages

- Potent HIV protease inhibitor
- Convenient dosing – once daily
- Generally well tolerated

Disadvantages

- Hyperbilirubinemia and jaundice common
- Potential for serious or life-threatening drug interactions
- Avoid coadministration with proton pump inhibitors
- Separate antacids and buffered medications by 2 hours and H_2-receptor antagonists by 12 hours to avoid decreasing ATV levels
- Caution should be used with ATV and products known to induce PR prolongation (eg, diltiazem)

Fosamprenavir (Lexiva™; FOSAPV) ± ritonavir (Norvir®; RTV)

Preferred dosing

- FOSAPV: 1400 mg twice daily (without RTV)
- FOSAPV: 1400 mg once daily + RTV 200 mg once daily
- FOSAPV: 700 mg twice daily + RTV 100 mg twice daily

Advantages

- Once daily dosing when given with ritonavir

Disadvantages

- Tolerability: GI side effects common
- Multiple drug interactions. Oral contraceptives decrease fosamprenavir concentrations
- Incidence of rash in healthy volunteers, especially when used with low doses of ritonavir. Differentiating between early drug-associated rash and acute seroconversion can be difficult and cause extraordinary concern for the exposed person.

Indinavir (Crixivan®; IDV) ± ritonavir (Norvir®; RTV)

Preferred dosing

- IDV 800 mg + RTV 100 mg twice daily without regard to food

Alternative dosing

- IDV: 800 mg every 8 hours, on an empty stomach

Advantages

- Potent HIV inhibitor

Disadvantages

- Potential for serious or life-threatening drug interactions
- Serious toxicity (eg, nephrolithiasis) possible; consumption of 8 glasses of fluid/day required
- Hyperbilirubinemia common; must avoid this drug during late pregnancy
- Requires acid for absorption and cannot be taken simultaneously with ddl, chewable/dispersible buffered tablet formulation (doses must be separated by ≥1 hour)

Saquinavir (Invirase®; SQV) + ritonavir (Norvir®; RTV)

Preferred dosing

- SQV: 1000 mg (given as Invirase®) + RTV 100 mg, twice daily
- SQV : Five capsules twice daily + RTV: One capsule twice daily

Advantages

- Generally well-tolerated, although GI events common

Disadvantages

- Potential for serious or life-threatening drug interactions
- Substantial pill burden

Nelfinavir (Viracept®; NFV)

Preferred dosing

- NFV: 1250 mg (2 x 625 mg or 5 x 250 mg tablets), twice daily with a meal

Advantages
- Generally well-tolerated

Disadvantages
- Diarrhea or other GI events common
- Potential for serious and/or life-threatening drug interactions

Efavirenz (Sustiva®; EFV)

Preferred dosing
- EFV: 600 mg daily, at bedtime

Advantages
- Does not require phosphorylation before activation and might be active earlier than other antiretroviral agents (a theoretic advantage of no demonstrated clinical benefit)
- Once daily dosing

Disadvantages
- Drug associated with rash (early onset) that can be severe and might rarely progress to Stevens-Johnson syndrome
- Differentiating between early drug-associated rash and acute seroconversion can be difficult and cause extraordinary concern for the exposed person
- Central nervous system side effects (eg, dizziness, somnolence, insomnia, or abnormal dreaming) common; severe psychiatric symptoms possible (dosing before bedtime might minimize these side effects)
- Teratogen; should not be used during pregnancy
- Potential for serious or life-threatening drug interactions

ANTIRETROVIRAL AGENTS GENERALLY NOT RECOMMENDED FOR USE AS PEP

Nevirapine (Viramune®; NVP)

Disadvantages
- Associated with severe hepatotoxicity (including at least one case of liver failure requiring liver transplantation in an exposed person taking PEP)
- Associated with rash (early onset) that can be severe and progress to Stevens-Johnson syndrome
- Differentiating between early drug-associated rash and acute seroconversion can be difficult and cause extraordinary concern for the exposed person
- Drug interactions: Can lower effectiveness of certain antiretroviral agents and other commonly used medicines

Delavirdine (Rescriptor®; DLV)

Disadvantages
- Drug associated with rash (early onset) that can be severe and progress to Stevens-Johnson syndrome
- Multiple drug interactions

Abacavir (Ziagen®; ABC)

Disadvantages
- Severe hypersensitivity reactions can occur, usually within the first 6 weeks
- Differentiating between early drug-associated rash/hypersensitivity and acute seroconversion can be difficult

Zalcitabine (Hivid®; ddC)

Disadvantages
- Three times a day dosing
- Tolerability
- Weakest antiretroviral agent

ANTIRETROVIRAL AGENT FOR USE AS PEP ONLY WITH EXPERT CONSULTATION

Enfuvirtide (Fuzeon™; T20)

Preferred dosing
- T20: 90 mg (1 mL) twice daily by subcutaneous injection

Advantages
- New class
- Unique viral target; to block cell entry
- Prevalence of resistance low

Disadvantages
- Twice-daily injection
- Safety profile: Local injection site reactions
- Never studied among antiretroviral-naive or HIV-negative patients
- False-positive EIA HIV antibody tests might result from formation of anti-T20 antibodies that cross-react with anti-gp41 antibodies

References

Centers for Disease Control and Prevention (CDC), "Notice to Readers: Updated Information Regarding Antiretroviral Agents Used as HIV Postexposure Prophylaxis for Occupational HIV Exposures," *MMWR Morb Mortal Wkly Rep*, 2007, 56(49):1291-2. Available at http://www.cdc.gov/mmwr/preview/mmwrhtml/mm5649a4.htm.

Panlilio AL, Cardo DM, Grohskopf LA, et al, "Updated U.S. Public Health Service Guidelines for the Management of Occupational Exposures to HIV and Recommendations for Postexposure Prophylaxis," *MMWR Recomm Rep*, 2005, 54(RR-9):1-17. Available at http://www.cdc.gov/mmwr/preview/mmwrhtml/rr5409a1.htm.

U.S. Public Health Service, "Updated U.S. Public Health Service Guidelines for the Management of Occupational Exposures to HBV, HCV, and HIV and Recommendations for Postexposure Prophylaxis," *MMWR Recomm Rep*, 2001, 50(RR-11):1-42. Available at http://www.cdc.gov/mmwr/preview/mmwrhtml/rr5011a1.htm.

PERINATAL HIV GUIDELINES

Antiretroviral agents are used during pregnancy for two reasons, the treatment of maternal human immunodeficiency virus (HIV) infection and to reduce the risk of perinatal HIV transmission. Recommendations for the use of antiretroviral drugs during pregnancy are updated regularly by the Department of Health and Human Services Panel on Treatment of HIV-Infected Pregnant Women and Prevention of Perinatal Transmission. The latest guidelines are available at http://AIDSinfo.nih.gov. With the use of highly active combination antiretroviral therapy (HAART), prenatal HIV counseling and testing, antiretroviral prophylaxis, scheduled cesarean delivery, and avoidance of breastfeeding, perinatal transmission of HIV infection has decreased to <2% in the United States. Health care professionals are encouraged to contact the antiretroviral pregnancy registry to monitor outcomes of pregnant women exposed to antiretroviral medications (1-800-258-4263 or www.APRegistry.com). The 2008 Panel recommendations include the following:

Preconception:

- Effective and appropriate contraception should be selected to avoid unintended pregnancy.
- Preconception counseling concerning safe sexual practices should be conducted.
- Choice of antiretroviral therapy should consider efficacy for maternal treatment the potential for teratogenicity if pregnancy should occur.
- Attaining a stable maximally suppressed viral load prior to conception is recommended for HIV infected women who wish to become pregnant.

Antepartum:

- Antiretroviral prophylaxis should be provided to all HIV-infected women, regardless of HIV RNA copy number.
- Resistance studies should be conducted prior to starting/modifying therapy if HIV RNA is detectable.
- Combination regimens are more effective than single drug regimens to reduce perinatal transmission.
- Prophylaxis for a longer duration (eg, starting at 28 weeks) is more effective than shorter duration (eg, starting at 36 weeks).
- If antiretroviral therapy is stopped electively during pregnancy, consider stopping nucleoside reverse transcriptase inhibitors (NRTIs) 7 days after stopping non-nucleoside reverse transcriptase inhibitors (NNRTIs); recommendation based on limited data. If therapy is stopped acutely for severe or life-threatening toxicity or severe pregnancy induced hyperemesis not responsive to antiemetics, stop all drugs at the same time and restart at the same time. If nevirapine is stopped and >2 weeks have passed, restart with the 2 week dose escalation period.
- Optimal adherence to antiretroviral medications is a key part of the strategy to reduce the development of resistance.
- Additional specific medication issues:
  - Zidovudine should be included in the regimen unless there is severe toxicity or documented resistance.
  - Efavirenz use should be avoided during the first trimester.
  - Nevirapine can be used as part of initial therapy in pregnant women with CD4 cell count <250 cells/mm^3. Use as initial therapy in pregnant women with a CD4 cell count >250 cells/mm^3 should only be done if the benefit outweighs the risk of hepatic toxicity. Nevirapine can be continued in pregnant women who are virologically suppressed and tolerating therapy regardless of CD4 count.
  - Protease inhibitors may require dosing adjustments during pregnancy.
  - Stavudine and didanosine in combination may cause lactic acidosis with prolonged use during pregnancy; use should be avoided.
  - NRTIs may be associated with lactic acidosis; monitor.

Intrapartum:

- Scheduled cesarean delivery at 38 weeks is recommended for women with suboptimal viral suppression near delivery (eg, >1000 copies/mL) or with unknown HIV RNA near the time of delivery.
- If antepartum antiretroviral drugs were not administered, intrapartum therapy combined with infant antiretroviral prophylaxis should be given.
- Stavudine should be discontinued during labor while zidovudine is being administered.
- Nevirapine use as a single dose is not recommended for women in the U.S. who are receiving standard antiretroviral prophylaxis regimens.

Postpartum:

- If antepartum or intrapartum antiretroviral drugs were not administered, postnatal infant prophylaxis is recommended.
- Breast-feeding is not recommended for HIV-infected women in the United States where safe, affordable, and feasible alternatives are available and culturally acceptable.

Special Situations

Hepatitis B virus coinfection:

- Screening for hepatitis B is recommended for all HIV-infected women not already screened during current pregnancy.
- Pregnant women with chronic hepatitis B virus (HBV) infection and HIV coinfection who require treatment for both diseases, a 3-drug regimen including a dual NRTI backbone of tenofovir plus lamivudine or emtricitabine is recommended. Consultation with an expert is advised for pregnant women needing treatment for HBV but not HIV and for pregnant women who do not require treatment for either HBV or HIV infection.
- Pregnant women with HBV and HIV coinfection and receiving antiretroviral medications should be monitored for liver toxicity.

Hepatitis C virus coinfection:

- Screening for hepatitis C is recommended for all HIV-infected women not already screened during current pregnancy.
- Pregnant women with chronic hepatitis C virus (HCV) infection and HIV coinfection should receive combination antiretroviral therapy with 3 drugs, regardless of CD4 count or viral load. If treatment for HIV infection is not needed for maternal health, it may be discontinued postpartum.
- Pregnant women with HCV and HIV coinfection and receiving antiretroviral medications should be monitored for liver toxicity.
- Decisions concerning mode of delivery should be based on HIV infection alone.

Clinical Scenarios and Recommendations for the Use of Antiretroviral Drugs to Reduce Perinatal HIV Transmission

SCENARIO #1

HIV-infected women receiving antiretroviral therapy during the current pregnancy

- Continue current HAART regimen if successfully suppressing viremia, except avoid the use of efavirenz or other potentially teratogenic drugs in the first trimester and avoid drugs with known adverse potential for the mother (combination stavudine and didanosine).
- Resistance testing is recommended if there is detectable viremia on therapy.
- In general, if a women requires treatment, antiretroviral medications should not be stopped during the first trimester.
- Continue HAART during the intrapartum period (give zidovudine as a continuous infusion and other antiretroviral medications orally).
- Scheduled cesarean delivery at 38 weeks is recommended for women with suboptimal viral suppression near delivery (eg, >1000 copies/mL).

SCENARIO #2

HIV-infected pregnant women who have not received prior antiretroviral therapy and have indications for antiretroviral therapy

- Resistance studies should be conducted prior to starting therapy.
- Initiate HAART regimen as soon as possible, even if during the first trimester. Avoid the use of efavirenz or other potentially teratogenic drugs in the first trimester and avoid drugs with known adverse potential for the mother (combination stavudine and didanosine).
- Zidovudine should be included in the regimen unless there is severe toxicity or documented resistance.
- Nevirapine can be used as part of initial therapy in pregnant women with CD4 cell count <250 cells/mm^3. Use as initial therapy in pregnant women with a CD4 cell count >250 cells/mm^3 should only be done if the benefit outweighs the risk of hepatic toxicity.
- Continue HAART during the intrapartum period (give zidovudine as a continuous infusion and other antiretroviral medications orally).
- Scheduled cesarean delivery at 38 weeks is recommended for women with suboptimal viral suppression near delivery (eg, >1000 copies/mL).

SCENARIO #3

HIV-infected pregnant women who have not received prior antiretroviral therapy and do NOT require treatment for their own health

- Resistance studies should be conducted prior to starting therapy.
- HAART is recommended for prophylaxis of perinatal transmission. Delaying treatment until after the first trimester may be considered.
- Avoid the use of efavirenz or other potentially teratogenic drugs in the first trimester and avoid drugs with known adverse potential for the mother (combination stavudine and didanosine).
- Zidovudine should be included in the regimen unless there is severe toxicity or documented resistance. The use of zidovudine alone is controversial, but may be considered if plasma HIV RNA levels are <1000 copies/mL on no therapy.
- Nevirapine can be used in pregnant women with CD4 cell count <250 cells/mm^3. Initial therapy in pregnant women with a CD4 cell count >250 cells/mm^3 should only be done if the benefit outweighs the risk of hepatic toxicity.
- Continue HAART during the intrapartum period (give zidovudine as a continuous infusion and other antiretroviral medications orally).

- Evaluate the need for continued therapy postpartum. Discontinue HAART unless there are indications for continued therapy. If regimen includes drug with long half-life, like NNRTI, consider stopping NRTIs 7 days after stopping NNRTI (recommendation based on limited data).
- Scheduled cesarean delivery at 38 weeks is recommended for women with suboptimal viral suppression near delivery (eg, >1000 copies/mL).

SCENARIO #4

HIV-infected woman who is antiretroviral experienced but not currently receiving antiretroviral medications

- Obtain full treatment history and evaluate the need for treatment for maternal health. Resistance studies should be conducted prior to starting therapy.
- Initiate HAART regimen. Avoid the use of efavirenz or other potentially teratogenic drugs in the first trimester and avoid drugs with known adverse potential for the mother (combination stavudine and didanosine).
- Zidovudine should be included in the regimen unless there is severe toxicity or documented resistance.
- Nevirapine can be used as part of initial therapy in pregnant women with CD4 cell count <250 cells/mm^3. Use as initial therapy in pregnant women with a CD4 cell count >250 cells/mm^3 should only be done if the benefit outweighs the risk of hepatic toxicity.
- Continue HAART during the intrapartum period (give zidovudine as a continuous infusion and other antiretroviral medications orally).
- Evaluate the need for continued therapy postpartum. Discontinue HAART unless there are indications for continued therapy. If regimen includes drug with long half-life, like NNRTI, consider stopping NRTIs 7 days after stopping NNRTI (recommendation based on limited data).
- Scheduled cesarean delivery at 38 weeks is recommended for women with suboptimal viral suppression near delivery (eg, >1000 copies/mL).

SCENARIO #5

HIV-infected women in labor who have had no prior therapy

Several regimens are available. These include:

- Zidovudine as an intravenous infusion during labor followed by 6 weeks of zidovudine for the newborn **OR**
- Zidovudine as an intravenous infusion during labor plus a single dose of nevirapine at the onset of labor. For the newborn, one dose of nevirapine plus zidovudine for 6 weeks **OR**
- Zidovudine as an intravenous infusion during labor. For the newborn, some clinicians may choose to use zidovudine in combination with additional medications, but appropriate dosing in neonates is not well defined.

If single-dose nevirapine is given to the mother, alone or in combination with zidovudine, consideration should be given to adding maternal zidovudine/lamivudine starting as soon as possible (intrapartum and postpartum) and continuing for 7 days, which may reduce development of nevirapine resistance. (Single dose nevirapine is not recommended for women in the U.S. who are receiving standard antiretroviral prophylaxis regimens.)

In the immediate postpartum period, the woman should have appropriate assessments (eg, CD4$^+$ count and HIV RNA copy number) to determine whether antiretroviral therapy is recommended for her own health.

SCENARIO #6

Infants born to HIV-infected mothers who have received no antiretroviral therapy during pregnancy or intrapartum

- Administer zidovudine for 6 weeks to the infant, beginning as soon as possible after birth.
- Some clinicians may choose to use zidovudine in combination with additional medications, but appropriate dosing in neonates is not well defined. Consultation with a pediatric HIV specialist is recommended.
- Evaluate the need for postpartum maternal therapy.

Clinical Scenarios and Recommendations Regarding Mode of Delivery to Reduce Perinatal HIV Transmission

SCENARIO A

Women presenting in late pregnancy (after about 36 weeks of gestation), known to be HIV-infected but not receiving antiretroviral therapy, and who have HIV RNA level and lymphocyte subsets pending but unlikely to be available before delivery.

Recommendations

Therapy options should be discussed in detail. The woman should be started on antiretroviral therapy. The woman should be counseled that scheduled cesarean section is likely to reduce the risk of transmission to her infant. She should also be informed of the increased risks to her of cesarean section, including increased rates of postoperative infection, anesthesia risks, and other surgical risks.

If cesarean section is chosen, the procedure should be scheduled at 38 weeks of gestation based on the best available clinical information. When scheduled cesarean section is performed, the woman should receive continuous intravenous zidovudine infusion beginning 3 hours before surgery and her infant should receive 6 weeks of zidovudine therapy after birth. Options for continuing or initiating combination antiretroviral therapy after delivery should be discussed with the woman as soon as her viral load and lymphocyte subset results are available.

SCENARIO B

HIV-infected women who initiated prenatal care early in the third trimester, are receiving highly active combination antiretroviral therapy, and have an initial virologic response, but have HIV RNA levels that remain substantially over 1000 copies/mL at 36 weeks of gestation.

Recommendations

The current combination antiretroviral regimen should be continued as the HIV RNA level is dropping appropriately. The woman should be counseled that although she is responding to the antiretroviral therapy, it is unlikely that her HIV RNA level will fall below 1000 copies/mL before delivery. Therefore, scheduled cesarean section may provide additional benefit in preventing intrapartum transmission of HIV. She should also be informed of the increased risks to her of cesarean section, including increased rates of postoperative infection, anesthesia risks, and surgical risks.

If she chooses scheduled cesarean section, it should be performed at 38 weeks' gestation according to the best available dating parameters, and intravenous zidovudine should begin at least 3 hours before surgery. Other antiretroviral medications should be continued on schedule as much as possible before and after surgery. The infant should receive oral zidovudine for 6 weeks after birth. The importance of adhering to therapy after delivery for her own health should be emphasized.

SCENARIO C

HIV-infected women on highly active combination antiretroviral therapy with an undetectable HIV RNA level at 36 weeks of gestation.

Recommendations

The woman should be counseled that her risk of perinatal transmission of HIV with a persistently undetectable HIV RNA level is low, probably 2% or less, even with vaginal delivery. There is currently no information to evaluate whether performing a scheduled cesarean section will lower her risk further.

Cesarean section has an increased risk of complications for the woman compared to vaginal delivery, and these risks must be balanced against the uncertain benefit of cesarean section in this case.

SCENARIO D

HIV-infected women who have elected scheduled cesarean section but present in early labor or shortly after rupture of membranes.

Recommendations

Intravenous zidovudine should be started immediately since the woman is in labor or has ruptured membranes.

If labor is progressing rapidly, the woman should be allowed to deliver vaginally. If cervical dilatation is minimal and a long period of labor is anticipated, some clinicians may choose to administer the loading dose of intravenous zidovudine and proceed with cesarean section to minimize the duration of membrane rupture and avoid vaginal delivery. Others might begin oxytocin augmentation to enhance contractions and potentially expedite delivery.

If the woman is allowed to labor, scalp electrodes and other invasive monitoring and operative delivery should be avoided if possible. The infant should be treated with 6 weeks of zidovudine therapy after birth.

Reference

Public Health Service Task Force, "Recommendations for Use of Antiretroviral Drugs in Pregnant HIV-Infected Women for Maternal Health and Interventions to Reduce Perinatal HIV Transmission in the United States," July 8, 2008. Available at: http://aidsinfo.nih.gov/contentfiles/PerinatalGL.pdf.

Recommended Antiretroviral Therapy in Pregnant HIV-Infected Women

Drug	Recommended	Alternative	Not Recommended	Insufficient Data	Rationale / Concerns
Nucleoside Reverse Transcriptase Inhibitors (NRTIs)					
Zidovudine	X				Preferred NRTI for use in **combination** antiretroviral regimens in pregnancy; include in regimens unless significant toxicity or stavudine use.
Lamivudine	X				Lamivudine plus zidovudine is the recommended dual NRTI backbone for pregnant women.
Didanosine		X			Cases of lactic acidosis; do not use with stavudine unless alternative regimens are not available.
Emtricitabine		X			No studies in pregnant women.
Stavudine		X			Lactic acidosis noted in pregnant women in combination with didanosine; avoid use with didanosine; do not use with zidovudine due to antagonism.
Abacavir		X			Triple NRTI regimens including abacavir have been less potent virologically compared to PI-based HAART regimens; use only when an NNRTI or PI based regimen cannot be used.
Tenofovir				X	Studies in children have shown bone demineralization with chronic use; clinical significance unknown. Because tenofovir significantly crosses the placenta and because there is a lack of data concerning use during human pregnancy, use only after careful consideration of alternatives.
Zalcitabine			X		No studies in pregnant women. No longer available in the United States.
Non-nucleoside Reverse Transcriptase Inhibitors (NNRTIs)					
Nevirapine	X				Possible increased risk of liver toxicity; use only if benefit outweighs risk with CD4 counts >250. Women who enter pregnancy on nevirapine regimens and are tolerating them well, may continue therapy regardless of CD4 count.
Efavirenz			X		No studies in pregnant women. Avoid use during the first trimester; use after the second trimester only if other alternatives are not available. Alternate regimens should be considered in women of childbearing potential.
Delavirdine			X		No pharmacokinetic studies in pregnant women; carcinogenic and teratogenic in animal studies.
Protease Inhibitors (PIs)					
Lopinavir/ritonavir	X				Teratogenic effects were not observed in phase I/II studies. Pharmacokinetic studies are not yet completed using the tablet formulation. Studies using the previously available capsule formulation showed that an increased dose may be needed during the third trimester. Until data is available for the tablet, standard dosing can be used, monitor virologic response and consider increasing the dose during the third trimester. Once daily administration is not recommended.
Saquinavir		X			No evidence of teratogenicity; well-tolerated and short-term safety demonstrated in mother and infant; use with ritonavir boosting. The softgel capsules are no longer available. Until additional pharmacokinetic studies are completed using the hard gel capsule or the tablet, saquinavir is considered an alternative PI for use during pregnancy.
Indinavir		X			Possible increased bilirubin levels; use with ritonavir boosting.
Ritonavir		X			Minimal experience in human pregnancy; recommended as part of boosted regimen.
Amprenavir				X	Oral solution contraindicated; insufficient safety/kinetic data available. No longer available in the United States.
Atazanavir				X	Possible increased bilirubin levels; insufficient safety/kinetic data available.
Darunavir				X	Insufficient safety/kinetic data available.
Fosamprenavir				X	Limited experience in human pregnancy; insufficient safety/kinetic data available.

Recommended Antiretroviral Therapy in Pregnant HIV-Infected Women *continued*

Drug	Recommended	Alternative	Not Recommended	Insufficient Data	Rationale / Concerns
Tipranavir				X	No experience in human pregnancy; insufficient safety/kinetic data available.
Nelfinavir		X			No evidence of teratogenicity; well-tolerated and short-term safety demonstrated in mother and infant. When used in nonpregnant adults, nelfinavir-based regimens had a lower rate of viral response than some alternative regimens. Therefore, use is recommended only as an alternative PI in pregnant women receiving HAART for perinatal prophylaxis. As of March 31, 2008, all Viracept® manufactured by Pfizer meets new limits of EMS content and may be prescribed as indicated to all patient populations (including pregnant women).
Entry Inhibitors					
Enfuvirtide				X	Minimal studies in pregnant women; insufficient safety/kinetic data available.
Maraviroc				X	Insufficient safety/kinetic data available.
Integrase Inhibitors					
Raltegravir				X	Insufficient safety/kinetic data available.

PREVENTION OF INFECTIVE ENDOCARDITIS

Recommendations by the American Heart Association

(*Circulation*, 2007, 116(15):1736-54.)

Consensus Process – The recommendations were formulated by a writing group under the auspices of the American Heart Association (AHA), and included representation from the Infectious Diseases Society of America (IDSA), the American Academy of Pediatrics (AAP), and the American Dental Association (ADA). Additionally, input was received from both national and international experts on infective endocarditis (IE). These guidelines are based on expert interpretation and review of scientific literature from 1950 through 2006. The consensus statement was subsequently reviewed by outside experts not affiliated with the writing group and by the Science Advisory and Coordinating Committee of the American Heart Association. These guidelines are meant to aid practitioners but are not intended as the standard of care or as a substitute for clinical judgment.

Significant change from the previous 1997 guidelines – The previously published guidelines identified a broad range of cardiac conditions thought to predispose patients to a higher risk of IE. The document stratified these conditions into high-, moderate-, and low-risk categories, based on the likelihood of developing IE. The subsequent recommendations for prophylaxis were based on this classification, in conjunction with specification of numerous invasive procedures which were assumed to confer a higher risk of bacteremia, and therefore a higher risk of endocarditis. However, it is the consensus of the current writing group that existing data fail to show a clear link between many of these procedures, preexisting cardiovascular condition and IE. In the case of dental procedures, it was determined that the cumulative lifetime risk of developing bacteremia as a result of normal hygiene measures (eg, teeth brushing, flossing) vastly exceeded the risk associated with many of the procedures for which prophylaxis was previously recommended. Similarly, the writing group estimated that the absolute risk of developing IE as a result of dental procedures in patients with preexisting cardiac conditions was quite low, and there was little evidence to support the value of prophylactic antimicrobial efficacy in these cases.

In a major departure from the former recommendations, the current guidelines have been greatly simplified to place a much greater emphasis on a very limited number of underlying cardiac conditions (see below). These specific conditions have been associated with the highest risk of adverse outcomes due to IE. Patients should receive IE prophylaxis only if they are undergoing certain invasive procedures (see Table 1) and have one of the underlying cardiovascular conditions specified below.

Common situations for which routine prophylaxis was previously, but no longer recommended, include mitral valve prolapse, general dental cleanings and local anesthetic administration (noninfected tissue), and bronchoscopy (see Table 1).

Specific cardiac conditions for which IE antibiotic prophylaxis is recommended:

- Previous infective endocarditis
- Prosthetic cardiac valve or prosthetic material used for cardiac valve repair
- Cardiac transplantation patients who develop valvulopathy
- Congenital heart disease (CHD), only under the following conditions:
  - Unrepaired cyanotic CHD, including palliative shunts and conduits
  - Completely repaired defects (with prosthetic materials/devices), regardless of method of repair, within the first 6 months after the procedure
  - Repaired CHD with residual defects at or adjacent to the site of repair

Table 1. Guidance for Use of Prophylactic Antibiotic Therapy Based on Procedure or Condition[1]

Location of Procedure	Prophylaxis Recommended	Prophylaxis NOT Recommended
Dental	All invasive manipulations of the gingival or periapical region or perforation of oral mucosa	Anesthetic injections (through noninfected tissue), radiographs, placement/adjustment/removal of prosthodontic/orthodontic appliances or brackets, shedding of deciduous teeth, trauma-induced bleeding from lips, gums, or oral mucosa
Respiratory tract	Biopsy/incision of respiratory mucosa (eg, tonsillectomy/adenoidectomy); drainage of abscess or empyema[2]	Bronchoscopy (unless incision of mucosa required)
Gastrointestinal (GI) or genitourinary (GU) tract	Established GI/GU infection or prevention of infectious sequelae[3]; elective cystoscopy or other urinary tract procedure with established enterococci infection/colonization[3,4]	Routine diagnostic procedures, including esophagogastroduodenoscopy or colonoscopy in the absence of active infection; vaginal delivery and hysterectomy
Skin, skin structure, or musculoskeletal	Any surgical procedure involving infected tissue	Procedures conducted in noninfected tissue; tattoos and ear/body piercing

[1]Patients should receive prophylactic antibiotic therapy if they meet the criteria for a specified procedure/condition in this table and they have a high-risk cardiovascular condition listed in the preceding text.

[2]If treating an infection of known staphylococcal origin, consider antistaphylococcal penicillin or cephalosporin, or vancomycin in beta-lactam-sensitive patients.

[3]Alternative agents with activity against enterococci to consider: Vancomycin (for beta-lactam-sensitive patients) or piperacillin.

[4]Eradication of enterococci from the urinary tract should be considered.

Table 2. Prophylactic Regimens for Oral / Dental, Respiratory Tract, Genitouinary Tract, or Esophageal Procedures

Situation	Agent	Regimen to Be Given 30-60 Minutes Before Procedure: Adults	Children[1]
Standard general prophylaxis	Amoxicillin	2 g P.O.	50 mg/kg P.O.
Unable to take oral medications	Ampicillin **or**	2 g I.M./I.V.	50 mg/kg I.M./I.V.
	Cefazolin or ceftriaxone	1 g I.M./I.V.	50 mg/kg I.M./I.V.
Allergic to penicillin	Clindamycin **or**	600 mg P.O.	20 mg/kg P.O.
	Cephalexin[2] or other dose-equivalent first/second generation cephalosporin **or**	2 g P.O	50 mg/kg P.O.
	Azithromycin or clarithromycin	500 mg P.O.	15 mg/kg P.O.
Allergic to penicillin and unable to take oral medications	Clindamycin **or**	600 mg I.V.	20 mg/kg I.V.
	Cefazolin or ceftriaxone[2]	1 g I.M./I.V.	50 mg/kg I.M./I.V.

[1]Total children's dose should not exceed adult dose.

[2]Cephalosporins should not be used in individuals with immediate-type hypersensitivity reaction (urticaria, angioedema, or anaphylaxis) to penicillins.

Reference

Wilson W, Taubert KA, Gewitz M, et al, "Prevention of Infective Endocarditis. Guidelines From the American Heart Association. A Guideline From the American Heart Association Rheumatic Fever, Endocarditis, and Kawasaki Disease Committee, Council on Cardiovascular Disease in the Young, and the Council on Clinical Cardiology, Council on Cardiovascular Surgery and Anesthesia, and the Quality of Care and Outcomes Research Interdisciplinary Working Group," *Circulation*, 2007, 116(15):1736-54.

PREVENTION OF WOUND INFECTION AND SEPSIS IN SURGICAL PATIENTS

Nature of Operation	Likely Pathogens	Recommended Drugs	Adult Dosage Before Surgery[1]
Cardiac	*S. aureus, S. epidermidis*	Cefazolin or cefuroxime or vancomycin[3]	1-2 g I.V.[2] 1.5 g I.V.[2] 1 g I.V.
Gastrointestinal			
Esophageal, gastroduodenal	Enteric gram-negative bacilli, gram-positive cocci	*High risk*[4] *only:* Cefazolin[5]	1-2 g I.V.
Biliary tract	Enteric gram-negative bacilli, enterococci, clostridia	*High risk*[6] *only:* Cefazolin[5]	1-2 g I.V.
Colorectal	Enteric gram-negative bacilli, anaerobes, enterococci	*Oral:* Neomycin + erythromycin base[7] or neomycin + metronidazole[7]	1 g of each x 3 doses 2 g of each x 2 doses
		Parenteral:	
		Cefoxitin[5] or cefazolin[5] + metronidazole[5]	1-2 g I.V. 1-2 g I.V. 0.5-1 g I.V.
Appendectomy, nonperforated	Enteric gram-negative bacilli, anaerobes, enterococci	Cefoxitin[5] or cefazolin[5] + metronidazole or ampicillin/sulbactam	1-2 g I.V. 1-2 g I.V. 0.5 g I.V. 3 g I.V.
Ruptured viscus	Enteric gram-negative bacilli, anaerobes, enterococci	Cefoxitin ± gentamicin [5,8]	1-2 g I.V. q6h 1.5 mg/kg I.V. q8h
Genitourinary	Enteric gram-negative bacilli, enterococci	*High risk*[9] *only:* Ciprofloxacin	500 mg P.O. or 400 mg I.V.
Gynecologic and Obstetric			
Vaginal, abdominal, or laparoscopic hysterectomy	Enteric gram-negative bacilli, anaerobes, group B streptococci, enterococci	Cefoxitin[5] or cefazolin[5] or ampicillin/sulbactam[5]	1-2 g I.V. 1-2 g I.V. 3 g I.V.
Cesarean section	Same as for hysterectomy	Cefazolin[5]	1-2 g I.V. after cord clamping
Abortion	Same as for hysterectomy	*First trimester, high-risk*[10]*:*	
		Aqueous penicillin G or doxycycline	2 mill units I.V. or 300 mg P.O.[11]
		Second trimester:	
		Cefazolin[5]	1-2 g I.V.
Head and Neck			
Incisions through oral or pharyngeal mucosa	Anaerobes, enteric gram-negative bacilli, *S. aureus*	Clindamycin + gentamicin or cefazolin	600-900 mg I.V. 1.5 mg/kg I.V. 1-2 g I.V.
Neurosurgery	*S. aureus, S. epidermidis*	Cefazolin or vancomycin[3]	1-2 g I.V. 1 g I.V.
Ophthalmic	*S. epidermidis, S. aureus*, streptococci, enteric gram-negative bacilli, *Pseudomonas*	Gentamicin, tobramycin, ciprofloxacin, levofloxacin, moxifloxacin, ofloxacin, or neomycin- gramicidin- polymyxin B	Multiple drops topically over 2-24 hours
		Cefazolin	100 mg subconjunctivally
Orthopedic	*S. aureus, S. epidermidis*	Cefazolin[12] or cefuroxime[12] or vancomycin[3,12]	1-2 g I.V. 1.5 g I.V. 1 g I.V.
Thoracic (Noncardiac)	*S. aureus, S. epidermidis*, streptococci, enteric gram-negative bacilli	Cefazolin or cefuroxime or vancomycin[3]	1-2 g I.V. 1.5 g I.V. 1 g I.V.

Nature of Operation	Likely Pathogens	Recommended Drugs	Adult Dosage Before Surgery[1]
Vascular			
Arterial surgery involving a prosthesis, the abdominal aorta, or a groin incision	*S. aureus*, *S. epidermidis*, enteric gram-negative bacilli	Cefazolin or vancomycin[3]	1-2 g I.V. 1 g I.V.
Lower extremity amputation for ischemia	*S. aureus*, *S. epidermidis*, enteric gram-negative bacilli, clostridia	Cefazolin or vancomycin[3]	1-2 g I.V. 1 g I.V.

[1]Parenteral prophylactic antimicrobials can be given as a single I.V. dose begun 60 minutes or less before the operation. For prolonged operations, additional intraoperative doses should be given at intervals 1-2 times the half-life of the drug for the duration of the procedure. If vancomycin or a fluoroquinolone is used, the infusion should be started 60-120 minutes before incision in order to minimize the possibility of an infusion reaction close to the time of induction of anesthesia and to have adequate tissue levels at the time of incision.

[2]Some consultants recommend an additional dose when patients are removed from bypass during open-heart surgery.

[3]For hospitals in which methicillin-resistant *S. aureus* and *S. epidermidis* are a frequent cause of postoperative wound infection, for patients previously colonized with MRSA, or for patients allergic to penicillins or cephalosporin. Rapid I.V. administration may cause hypotension, which could be especially dangerous during induction of anesthesia. Even if the drug is given over 60 minutes, hypotension may occur; treatment with diphenhydramine (Benadryl® and others) and further slowing of the infusion rate may be helpful. For procedures in which enteric gram-negative bacilli are likely pathogens, such as vascular surgery involving a groin incision, cefazolin or cefuroxime should be included in the prophylaxis regimen for patients not allergic to cephalosporins; ciprofloxacin, levofloxacin (750 mg), gentamicin, or aztreonam, each one in combination with vancomycin, can be used in patients who cannot tolerate a cephalosporin.

[4]Morbid obesity, esophageal obstruction, decreased gastric acidity, or gastrointestinal motility.

[5]For patients allergic to cephalosporins, clindamycin with either gentamicin, ciprofloxacin, levofloxacin (750 mg), or aztreonam is a reasonable alternative.

[6]Age >70 years, acute cholecystitis, nonfunctioning gallbladder, obstructive jaundice, or common duct stones.

[7]After appropriate diet and catharsis, 1 g of neomycin plus 1 g of erythromycin at 1 PM, 2 PM, and 11 PM the day before an 8 AM operation or 2 g of neomycin plus 2 g of metronidazole at 7 PM and 11 PM the day before an 8 AM operation.

[8]Therapy is often continued for about 5 days. Ruptured viscus in postoperative setting (dehiscence) requires antibacterials to include coverage of nosocomial pathogens.

[9]Urine culture positive or unavailable, preoperative catheter, transrectal prostatic biopsy, placement of prosthetic material.

[10]Patients with previous pelvic inflammatory disease, previous gonorrhea, or multiple sex partners.

[11]Divided into 100 mg 1 hour before the abortion and 200 mg 30 minutes after.

[12]If a tourniquet is to be used in the procedure, the entire dose of antibiotic must be infused prior to its inflation.

References

Adapted with permission from "Antimicrobial Prophylaxis for Surgery," *Treatment Guidelines From The Medical Letter®*, 2006, 4(52):83-8.

Bratzler DW, Houck PM, Surgical Infection Prevention Guidelines Writers Workgroup, et al, "Antimicrobial Prophylaxis for Surgery: An Advisory Statement From the National Surgical Infection Prevention Project," *Clin Infect Dis*, 2004, 38(12):1706-15.

GUIDELINES FOR THE PREVENTION OF OPPORTUNISTIC INFECTIONS IN HIV INFECTED PERSONS

Adapted from "2002 USPHS/IDSA Guidelines for the Prevention of Opportunistic Infections in Persons Infected With Human Immunodeficiency Virus. USPHS/IDSA Prevention of Opportunistic Infections Working Group" (www.aidsinfo.nih.gov)

DRUG REGIMENS FOR ADULTS AND ADOLESCENTS

Prophylaxis to Prevent First Episode of Opportunistic Disease in HIV-Infected Adults and Adolescents

Pathogen	Indication	Preventive Regimens	
		First Choice	Alternatives
I. Strongly Recommended as Standard of Care			
Pneumocystis jiroveci[1]	CD4[+] count <200/μL or oropharyngeal candidiasis	TMP-SMZ, 1 DS P.O. every day; TMP-SMZ, 1 SS P.O. every day	Dapsone, 50 mg P.O. twice daily *or* 100 mg P.O. every day; dapsone, 50 mg P.O. every day *plus* pyrimethamine, 50 mg P.O. weekly *plus* leucovorin, 25 mg P.O. weekly; dapsone, 200 mg P.O. *plus* pyrimethamine, 75 mg P.O. *plus* leucovorin, 25 mg P.O. weekly; aerosolized pentamidine, 300 mg monthly via Respirgard II™ nebulizer; atovaquone, 1500 mg P.O. every day; TMP-SMZ, 1 DS P.O. 3 times/week
Mycobacterium tuberculosis			
Isoniazid-sensitive[2]	TST reaction ≥5 mm *or* prior positive TST result without treatment or contact with case of active tuberculosis **regardless of TST result**	Isoniazid, 300 mg P.O. *plus* pyridoxine, 50 mg P.O. every day x 9 months or isoniazid, 900 mg P.O. *plus* pyridoxine, 100 mg P.O. twice a week x 9 months	Rifampin, 600 mg P.O. every day x 4 months or rifabutin, 300 mg P.O. every day x 4 months Pyrazinamide, 15-20 mg/kg P.O. every day x 2 months *plus* either rifampin, 600 mg P.O. every day x 2 months or rifabutin, 300 mg P.O. every day x 2 months
Isoniazid-resistant	Same as above; high probability of exposure to isoniazid-resistant tuberculosis	Rifampin, 600 mg P.O. or rifabutin, 300 mg P.O. every day x 4 months	Pyrazinamide, 15-20 mg/kg P.O. every day *plus* either rifampin, 600 mg P.O. or rifabutin, 300 mg P.O. every day x 2 months
Multidrug (isoniazid and rifampin)-resistant	Same as above; high probability of exposure to multidrug- resistant tuberculosis	Choice of drugs requires consultation with public health authorities. **Depends on susceptibility of isolate from source patient.**	None
Toxoplasma gondii[3]	IgG antibody to *Toxoplasma* and CD4[+] count <100/μL	TMP-SMZ, 1 DS P.O. every day	TMP-SMZ, 1 SS P.O. every day; dapsone, 50 mg P.O. every day *plus* pyrimethamine, 50 mg P.O. once weekly *plus* leucovorin, 25 mg P.O. weekly; dapsone, 200 mg P.O. *plus* pyrimethamine, 75 mg P.O. *plus* leucovorin, 25 mg P.O. weekly; atovaquone, 1500 mg P.O. every day with or without pyrimethamine, 25 mg P.O. every day *plus* leucovorin, 10 mg P.O. every day
Mycobacterium avium complex	CD4[+] count <50/μL	Azithromycin, 1200 mg P.O. weekly or clarithromycin,[4] 500 mg P.O. twice daily	Rifabutin, 300 mg P.O. every day; azithromycin, 1200 mg P.O. weekly *plus* rifabutin, 300 mg P.O. every day
Varicella zoster virus (VZV) **Note:** VZIG has been discontinued; an investigational product VariZIG™ is available under an IND. IRB approval required for access to product.	Significant exposure to chickenpox or shingles for patients who have no history of either condition or, if available, negative antibody to VZV	Varicella zoster immune globulin (VZIG), 5 vials (1.25 mL each) I.M., administered ≤96 hours after exposure, ideally within 48 hours	
II. Generally Recommended			
Streptococcus pneumoniae[5]	CD4[+] count ≥200/μL	23 valent polysaccharide vaccine, 0.5 mL I.M.	None
Hepatitis B virus[6,7]	All susceptible (anti-HB_c-negative) patients	Hepatitis B vaccine: 3 doses	None

Prophylaxis to Prevent First Episode of Opportunistic Disease in HIV-Infected Adults and Adolescents *(continued)*

Pathogen	Indication	Preventive Regimens	
		First Choice	Alternatives
Influenza virus[6,8]	All patients (annually, before influenza season)	Inactivated trivalent influenza virus vaccine: One annual dose (0.5 mL) I.M.	Oseltamivir, 75 mg P.O. every day (influenza A or B); while not formally endorsed in the guideline document, zanamivir 10 mg (2 inhalations) once daily for 10 days is indicated for treatment/prevention of influenza A and B
Hepatitis A virus[6,7]	All susceptible (anti-HAV-negative) patients at increased risk for HAV infection (eg, illicit drug users, men who have sex with men, hemophiliacs) or with chronic liver disease, including chronic hepatitis B or hepatitis C	Hepatitis A vaccine: 2 doses	None
III. Evidence for Efficacy but Not Routinely Indicated			
Bacteria	Neutropenia	Granulocyte-colony-stimulating factor (G-CSF), 5-10 mcg/kg SubQ every day x 2-4 weeks or granulocyte-macrophage colony-stimulating factor (GM-CSF), 250 mcg/m² SubQ, I.V. x 2-4 weeks	None
Cryptococcus neoformans	CD4⁺ count <50/µL	Fluconazole, 100-200 mg P.O. every day	Itraconazole capsule, 200 mg P.O. every day
Histoplasma capsulatum[9]	CD4⁺ count <100/µL, endemic geographic area	Itraconazole capsule, 200 mg P.O. every day	None
Cytomegalovirus (CMV)[10]	CD4⁺ count <50/µL and CMV antibody positivity	Oral ganciclovir, 1 g P.O. 3 times/day	None

Note: Information included in these guidelines may not represent Food and Drug Administration (FDA) approval or approved labeling for the particular products or indications in question. Specifically, the terms "safe" and "effective" may not be synonymous with the FDA-defined legal standards for product approval.

Abbreviations: Anti-HB_c = antibody to hepatitis B core antigen; CMV = cytomegalovirus; DS = double-strength tablet; HAART = highly active antiretroviral therapy; HAV = hepatitis A virus; SS = single-strength tablet; TMP-SMZ = trimethoprim-sulfamethoxazole; and TST = tuberculin skin test. The Respirgard II™ nebulizer is manufactured by Marquest, Englewood, CO.

[1]Prophylaxis should also be considered for persons with a CD4⁺ percentage <14%, for persons with a history of an AIDS-defining illness, and possibly for those with CD4⁺ count >200 but <250 cells/µL. TMP-SMZ also reduces the frequency of toxoplasmosis and some bacterial infections. Patients receiving dapsone should be tested for glucose-6-phosphate dehydrogenase deficiency. A dosage of 50 mg every day is probably less effective than 100 mg every day. The efficacy of parenteral pentamidine (eg, 4 mg/kg/month) is uncertain. Fansidar® (sulfadoxine-pyrimethamine) is rarely used because of severe hypersensitivity reactions. Patients who are being administered therapy for toxoplasmosis with sulfadiazine-pyrimethamine are protected against *Pneumocystis jiroveci* pneumonia and do not need additional prophylaxis against PCP.

[2]Directly observed therapy is recommended for isoniazid (eg, 900 mg twice weekly); INH regimens should include pyridoxine to prevent peripheral neuropathy. If rifampin or rifabutin are administered concurrently with protease inhibitors or non-nucleoside reverse transcriptase inhibitors, careful consideration should be given to potential pharmacokinetic interactions. There have been reports of fatal and severe liver injury associated with the treatment of latent TB infection in HIV-uninfected persons treated with the 2 month regimen of daily rifampin and pyrazinamide; therefore it may be prudent to use regimens that do not contain pyrazinamide in HIV-infected persons whose completion of treatment can be assured (CDC. "Update: Fatal and Severe Liver Injuries Associated with Rifampin and Pyrazinamide for Latent Tuberculosis Infection and Revisions in American Thoracic Society/CDC Recommendations, United States 2001," *MMWR*, 2001, 50(34). Exposure to multidrug-resistant tuberculosis might require prophylaxis with two drugs; consult public health authorities. Possible regimens include pyrazinamide plus either ethambutol or a fluoroquinolone.

[3]Protection against toxoplasmosis is provided by TMP-SMZ, dapsone plus pyrimethamine, and possibly by atovaquone. Atovaquone may be used with or without pyrimethamine. Pyrimethamine alone probably provides little, if any, protection.

[4]During pregnancy, azithromycin is preferred over clarithromycin because of the teratogenicity in animals of clarithromycin.

[5]Vaccination **may** be offered to persons who have a CD4⁺ T-lymphocyte count <200 cells/µL, although the efficacy **is likely to** be diminished. Revaccination 5 years after the first dose or sooner if the initial immunization was given when the CD4⁺ count was <200 cells/µL and if the CD4⁺ count has increased to >200 cells/µL on HAART is considered optional. Some authorities are concerned that immunizations may stimulate the replication of HIV.

[6]Although data demonstrating clinical benefit of these vaccines in HIV-infected persons are not available, it is logical to assume that those patients who develop antibody responses will derive some protection. Some authorities are concerned that immunizations may stimulate HIV replication, although for influenza vaccination, a large observational study of HIV-infected persons in clinical care showed no adverse effect of this vaccine, including multiple doses, on patient survival (J. Ward, CDC, personal communication). Also, this concern may be less relevant in the setting of HAART. However, because of the theoretical concern that increases in HIV plasma RNA following vaccination during pregnancy might increase the risk of perinatal transmission of HIV, providers may wish to defer vaccination for such patients until after HAART is initiated.

[7]Hepatitis B vaccine has been recommended for all children and adolescents and for all adults with risk factors for hepatitis B virus (HBV). For persons requiring vaccination against both hepatitis A and hepatitis B, a combination vaccine is now available. For additional information regarding vaccination against hepatitis A and B, see CDC, "Hepatitis B Virus: A Comprehensive Strategy for Eliminating Transmission in the United States Through Universal Childhood Vaccination. Recommendations of the Advisory Committee on Immunization Practices (ACIP)," *MMWR Morb Mortal Wkly Rep*, 1991, 40(RR13).

[8]Oseltamivir or zanamivir are appropriate during outbreaks of either influenza A or influenza B. The CDC announced in January, 2006, that rimantadine and amantadine are no longer recommended due to increased rates of resistance. Dosage reduction for antiviral chemoprophylaxis against influenza might be indicated for decreased renal or hepatic function, and for persons with seizure disorders. Physicians should consult the drug package inserts and the annual CDC influenza guidelines for more specific information about adverse effects and dosage adjustments. For additional information about vaccinations, antiviral chemoprophylaxis, and therapy against influenza, see CDC, "Prevention and Control of Influenza: Recommendations of the Advisory Committee on Immunization Practices (ACIP)," *MMWR Morb Mortal Wkly Rep*, 2001, 50(RR-4).

[9]In a few unusual occupational or other circumstances, prophylaxis should be considered; consult a specialist.

[10]Acyclovir is not protective against CMV. Valacyclovir is not recommended because of an unexplained trend toward increased mortality observed in persons with AIDS who were being administered this drug for prevention of CMV disease.

Prophylaxis to Prevent Recurrence of Opportunistic Disease (After Chemotherapy for Acute Disease) in HIV-Infected Adults and Adolescents

Pathogen	Indication	Preventive Regimens	
		First Choice	Alternatives
I. Recommended as Standard of Care			
Pneumocystis jiroveci	Prior *P. jiroveci* pneumonia	TMP-SMZ, 1 DS P.O. every day; TMP-SMZ, 1 SS P.O. every day	Dapsone, 50 mg P.O. twice daily or 100 mg P.O. every day; dapsone, 50 mg P.O. every day *plus* pyrimethamine, 50 mg P.O. weekly *plus* leucovorin, 25 mg P.O. weekly; dapsone, 200 mg P.O. *plus* pyrimethamine, 75 mg P.O. *plus* leucovorin, 25 mg P.O. weekly; aerosolized pentamidine, 300 mg monthly via Respirgard II™ nebulizer; atovaquone, 1500 mg P.O. every day; TMP-SMZ, 1 DS P.O. 3 times/week
Toxoplasma gondii[1]	Prior toxoplasmic encephalitis	Sulfadiazine, 500-1000 mg P.O. 4 times/day *plus* pyrimethamine 25-50 mg P.O. every day *plus* leucovorin, 10-25 mg P.O. every day	Clindamycin, 300-450 mg P.O. every 6-8 hours *plus* pyrimethamine, 25-50 mg P.O. every day *plus* leucovorin, 10-25 mg P.O. every day; atovaquone, 750 mg P.O. every 6-12 hours with or without pyrimethamine, 25 mg P.O. every day *plus* leucovorin 10 mg P.O. every day
Mycobacterium avium complex[2]	Documented disseminated disease	Clarithromycin,[2] 500 mg P.O. twice daily *plus* ethambutol, 15 mg/kg P.O. every day; with or without rifabutin, 300 mg P.O. every day	Azithromycin, 500 mg P.O. every day *plus* ethambutol, 15 mg/kg P.O. every day; with or without rifabutin, 300 mg P.O. every day
Cytomegalovirus	Prior end-organ disease	Ganciclovir, 5-6 mg/kg I.V. 5-7 days/week or 1000 mg P.O. 3 times/day; or foscarnet, 90-120 mg/kg I.V. every day; or (for retinitis) ganciclovir sustained-release implant, every 6-9 months *plus* ganciclovir, 1-1.5 g P.O. 3 times/day	Cidofovir, 5 mg/kg I.V. every other week with probenecid 2 g P.O. 3 hours before the dose followed by 1 g P.O. given 2 hours after the dose, and 1 g P.O. 8 hours after the dose (total of 4 g); fomivirsen [DSC], 1 vial (330 mcg) injected into the vitreous, then repeated every 2-4 weeks; valganciclovir 900 mg P.O. every day
Cryptococcus neoformans	Documented disease	Fluconazole, 200 mg P.O. every day	Amphotericin B, 0.6-1 mg/kg I.V. weekly to 3 times/week; itraconazole capsule, 200 mg P.O. every day
Histoplasma capsulatum	Documented disease	Itraconazole capsule, 200 mg P.O. twice daily	Amphotericin B, 1 mg/kg I.V. weekly
Coccidioides immitis	Documented disease	Fluconazole, 400 mg P.O. every day	Amphotericin B, 1 mg/kg I.V. weekly; itraconazole capsule, 200 mg P.O. twice daily
Salmonella species (non-*typhi*)[3]	Bacteremia	Ciprofloxacin, 500 mg P.O. twice daily for several months	Antibiotic chemoprophylaxis with another active agent
II. Recommended Only if Subsequent Episodes Are Frequent or Severe			
Herpes simplex virus	Frequent/severe recurrences	Acyclovir, 200 mg P.O. 3 times/day or 400 mg P.O. twice daily; famciclovir, 250 mg P.O. twice daily	Valacyclovir, 500 mg P.O. twice daily
Candida (oropharyngeal or vaginal)	Frequent/severe recurrences	Fluconazole, 100-200 mg P.O. every day	Itraconazole solution, 200 mg P.O. every day
Candida (esophageal)	Frequent/severe recurrences	Fluconazole, 100-200 mg P.O. every day	Itraconazole solution, 200 mg P.O. every day

Note: Information included in these guidelines may not represent Food and Drug Administration (FDA) approval or approved labeling for the particular products or indications in question. Specifically, the terms "safe" and "effective" may not be synonymous with the FDA-defined legal standards for product approval.

DS = double-strength tablet; SS = single-strength tablet; and TMP-SMZ = trimethoprim-sulfamethoxazole. The Respirgard II™ nebulizer is manufactured by Marquest, Englewood, CO.

[1]Pyrimethamine/sulfadiazine confers protection against PCP as well as toxoplasmosis; clindamycin-pyrimethamine does **not offer protection against PCP**.

[2]Many multiple-drug regimens are poorly tolerated. Drug interactions (eg, those seen with clarithromycin/rifabutin) can be problematic; rifabutin has been associated with uveitis, especially when administered at daily doses of >300 mg or concurrently with fluconazole or clarithromycin. **During pregnancy, azithromycin is recommended instead of clarithromycin because clarithromycin is teratogenic in animals**.

[3]Efficacy of eradication of *Salmonella* has been demonstrated only for ciprofloxacin.

Criteria for Starting, Discontinuing, and Restarting Opportunistic Infection Prophylaxis for Adult Patients With HIV Infection[1]

Opportunistic Illness	Criteria for Initiating Primary Prophylaxis	Criteria for Discontinuing Primary Prophylaxis	Criteria for Restarting Primary Prophylaxis	Criteria for Initiating Secondary Prophylaxis	Criteria for Discontinuing Secondary Prophylaxis	Criteria for Restarting Secondary Prophylaxis
Pneumocystis jiroveci pneumonia	$CD4^+$ <200 cells/μL or oropharyngeal candidiasis	$CD4^+$ >200 cells/μL for ≥3 months	$CD4^+$ <200 cells/μL	Prior *Pneumocystis jiroveci* pneumonia	$CD4^+$ >200 cells/μL for ≥3 months	$CD4^+$ <200 cells/μL
Toxoplasmosis	IgG antibody to *Toxoplasma* and $CD4^+$ <100 cells/μL	$CD4^+$ >200 cells/μL for ≥3 months	$CD4^+$ <100-200 cells/μL	Prior toxoplasmic encephalitis	$CD4^+$ >200 cells/μL sustained (eg, ≥6 months) and completed initial therapy, and asymptomatic for toxoplasmosis	$CD4^+$ <200 cells/μL
Disseminated *Mycobacterium avium* complex	$CD4^+$ <50 cells/μL	$CD4^+$ >100 cells/μL for ≥3 months	$CD4^+$ <50-100 cells/μL	Documented disseminated disease	$CD4^+$ >100 cells/μL sustained (eg, ≥6 months) and completed 12 months of MAC therapy, and asymptomatic for MAC	$CD4^+$ <100 cells/μL
Cryptococcosis	None	Not applicable	Not applicable	Documented disease	$CD4^+$ >100-200 cells/μL sustained (eg, ≥6 months) and completed initial therapy, and asymptomatic for cryptococcosis	$CD4^+$ <100-200 cells/μL
Histoplasmosis	None	Not applicable	Not applicable	Documented disease	No criteria recommended for stopping	Not applicable
Coccidioidomycosis	None	Not applicable	Not applicable	Documented disease	No criteria recommended for stopping	Not applicable
Cytomegalovirus retinitis	None	Not applicable	Not applicable	Documented end-organ disease	$CD4^+$ >100-150 cells/μL sustained (eg, ≥6 months) and no evidence of active disease, and regular ophthalmic examination	$CD4^+$ <100-150 cells/μL

[1]The safety of discontinuing prophylaxis in children whose $CD4^+$ counts have increased in response to HAART has not been studied.

DRUG REGIMENS FOR INFANTS AND CHILDREN

Prophylaxis to Prevent First Episode of Opportunistic Disease in HIV-Infected Infants and Children

Pathogen	Indication	Preventive Regimens	
		First Choice	Alternatives
I. Strongly Recommended as Standard of Care			
Pneumocystis jiroveci[1]	HIV-infected or HIV-indeterminate infants 1-12 mo of age HIV-infected children 1-5 y of age with $CD4^+$ count <500/μL or $CD4^+$ percentage <15% HIV-infected children 6-12 y of age with $CD4^+$ count <200/μL or $CD4^+$ percentage <15%	TMP-SMZ, 150/750 mg/m²/day in 2 divided doses P.O. 3 times/week on consecutive days Acceptable alternative dosage schedules: • Single dose P.O. 3 times/week on consecutive days • 2 divided doses P.O. every day; 2 divided doses P.O. 3 times/week on alternate days	Dapsone (children ≥1 mo), 2 mg/kg (max: 100 mg) P.O. every day or 4 mg/kg (max: 200 mg) P.O. once weekly) Aerosolized pentamidine (children ≥5 y), 300 mg/mo via Respirgard II™ nebulizer Atovaquone (1-3 mo and >24 mo, 30 mg/kg P.O. every day; 4-24 mo, 45 mg/kg P.O. every day)
Mycobacterium tuberculosis[2]			
Isoniazid-sensitive	TST reaction, ≥5 mm *or* prior positive TST result without treatment **or contact** with any case of active tuberculosis **regardless of TST result**	Isoniazid, 10-15 mg/kg (max: 300 mg) P.O. every day x 9 mo or 20-30 mg/kg (max: 900 mg) P.O. twice weekly x 9 mo	Rifampin, 10-20 mg/kg (max: 600 mg) P.O. every day x 4-6 mo
Isoniazid-resistant	Same as above; high probability of exposure to isoniazid-resistant tuberculosis	Rifampin, 10-20 mg/kg (max: 600 mg) P.O. every day x 4-6 mo	Uncertain
Multidrug (isoniazid and rifampin)-resistant	Same as above; high probability of exposure to multidrug-resistant tuberculosis	Choice of drug requires consultation with public health authorities and depends on susceptibility of isolate from source patient	
Mycobacterium avium complex[2]	For children ≥6 y, $CD4^+$ count <50/μL; 2-6 y, $CD4^+$ count <75/μL; 1-2 y, $CD4^+$ count <500/μL; <1 y, $CD4^+$ count <750/μL	Clarithromycin, 7.5 mg/kg (max: 500 mg) P.O. twice daily, or azithromycin, 20 mg/kg (max: 1200 mg) P.O. weekly	Azithromycin, 5 mg/kg (max: 250 mg) P.O. every day; children ≥6 y, rifabutin, 300 mg P.O. every day
Varicella zoster virus[3] **Note:** VZIG has been discontinued; an investigational product VariZIG™ is available under an IND. IRB approval required for access to product.	Significant exposure to varicella or shingles with no history of chickenpox or shingles	Varicella zoster immune globulin (VZIG), 1 vial (1.25 mL)/10 kg (max: 5 vials) I.M., administered ≤96 hours after exposure, ideally within 48 hours	None
Vaccine- preventable pathogens[4]	HIV exposure/infection	Routine immunizations	None
II. Generally Recommended			
Influenza virus	All patients (annually, before influenza season)	Inactivated split trivalent influenza vaccine	Oseltamivir (during outbreaks of influenza A or B) for children ≥13 y, 75 mg P.O. every day; while not formally endorsed in the guideline document, zanamivir 10 mg (2 inhalations) once daily for 10 days is indicated for treatment/prevention of influenza A and B in children ≥5 years
Varicella zoster virus	HIV-infected children who are asymptomatic and not immunosuppressed	Varicella zoster vaccine	None
Toxoplasma gondii[5]	IgG antibody to *Toxoplasma* and severe immunosuppression	TMP-SMZ, 150/750 mg/m²/d in 2 divided doses P.O. every day	Dapsone (≥1 mo of age), 2 mg/kg or 15 mg/m² (max: 25 mg) P.O. every day *plus* pyrimethamine, 1 mg/kg P.O. every day *plus* leucovorin, 5 mg P.O. every 3 days Atovaquone (aged 1-3 mo and >24 mo, 30 mg/kg P.O. every day; aged 14-24 mo, 45 mg/kg P.O. every day)

Prophylaxis to Prevent First Episode of Opportunistic Disease in HIV-Infected Infants and Children *(continued)*

Pathogen	Indication	Preventive Regimens	
		First Choice	Alternatives
III. Not Recommended for Most Children; Indicated for Use Only in Unusual Circumstances			
Invasive bacterial infections[6]	Hypogamma- globulinemia (ie, IgG <400 mg/dL)	IVIG (400 mg/kg every 2-4 weeks)	None
Cryptococcus neoformans	Severe immunosuppression	Fluconazole, 3-6 mg/kg P.O. every day	Itraconazole, 2-5 mg/kg P.O. every 12-24 hours
Histoplasma capsulatum	Severe immunosuppression, endemic geographic area	Itraconazole, 2-5 mg/kg P.O. every 12-24 hours	None
Cytomegalovirus (CMV)[7]	CMV antibody positivity and severe immunosuppression	Oral ganciclovir 30 mg/kg P.O. 3 times/day	None

Note: Information included in these guidelines may not represent FDA approval or approved labeling for the particular products or indications in question. Specifically, the terms "safe" and "effective" may not be synonymous with the FDA-defined legal standards for product approval. CMV = cytomegalovirus; IVIG = intravenous immune globulin; TMP-SMZ = trimethoprim-sulfamethoxazole; and VZIG = varicella zoster immune globulin. The Respirgard II™ nebulizer is manufactured by Marquest, Englewood, CO.

[1]Daily TMP-SMZ reduces frequency of some bacterial infections. TMP-SMZ, dapsone-pyrimethamine, and possibly atovaquone (with or without pyrimethamine) appear to protect against toxoplasmosis, although data have not been prospectively collected. When compared with weekly dapsone, daily dapsone is associated with lower incidence of *Pneumocystis jiroveci* pneumonia (PCP) but higher hematologic toxicity and mortality (McIntosh K, Cooper E, Xu J, et al, "Toxicity and Efficacy of Daily vs Weekly Dapsone for Prevention of *Pneumocystis carinii* Pneumonia in Children Infected With HIV," *Ped Infect Dis J* 1999, 18:432-9.). Efficacy of parenteral pentamidine (eg, 4 mg/kg/every 2-4 weeks) is controversial. Patients receiving therapy for toxoplasmosis with sulfadiazine-pyrimethamine are protected against PCP and do not need TMP-SMZ.

[2]Significant drug interactions may occur between rifamycins (rifampin and rifabutin) and protease inhibitors, and non-nucleoside reverse transcriptase inhibitors. Consult a specialist.

[3]Children routinely being administered intravenous immune globulin (IVIG) should receive VZIG if the last dose of IVIG was administered >21 days before exposure.

[4]HIV-infected and HIV-exposed children should be immunized according to the childhood immunization schedule, which has been adapted from the January-December 2001 schedule recommended for immunocompetent children by the Advisory Committee on Immunization Practices, the American Academy of Pediatrics, and the American Academy of Family Physicians. This schedule differs from that for immunocompetent children in that both the conjugate pneumococcal vaccine (PCV-7) and the pneumococcal polysaccharide vaccine (PPV-23) are recommended and vaccination against influenza should be offered. MMR should not be administered to severely immunocompromised children. Vaccination against varicella is indicated only for asymptomatic nonimmunosuppressed children. Once an HIV-exposed child is determined not to be HIV infected, the schedule for immunocompetent children applies.

[5]Protection against toxoplasmosis is provided by the preferred antipneumocystis regimens and possibly by atovaquone. Atovaquone may be used with or without pyrimethamine. Pyrimethamine alone probably provides little, if any, protection.

[6]If available, respiratory syncytial virus (RSV) IVIG (750 mg/kg), not monoclonal RSV antibody, may be substituted for IVIG during RSV season to provide broad anti-infective protection.

[7]Oral ganciclovir and perhaps valganciclovir results in reduced CMV shedding in CMV-infected children. Acyclovir is not protective against CMV.

Prophylaxis to Prevent Recurrence of Opportunistic Disease (After Chemotherapy for Acute Disease) in HIV-Infected Infants and Children

Pathogen	Indication	Preventive Regimens: First Choice	Preventive Regimens: Alternatives
I. Recommended for Life as Standard of Care			
Pneumocystis jiroveci	Prior *P. jiroveci* pneumonia	TMP-SMZ, 150/750 mg/m^2/d in 2 divided doses P.O. 3 times/week on consecutive days Acceptable alternative schedules for same dosage Single dose P.O. 3 times/week on consecutive days; 2 divided doses P.O. daily; 2 divided doses P.O. 3 times/week on alternate days	Dapsone (children ≥1 mo of age), 2 mg/kg (max: 100 mg) P.O. once daily *or* 4 mg/kg (max: 200 mg) P.O. weekly; aerosolized pentamidine (children ≥5 y of age), 300 mg monthly via Respirgard II™ nebulizer; atovaquone (children 1-3 mo and >24 mo of age, 30 mg/kg P.O. every day; children 4-24 mo, 45 mg/kg P.O. every day)
Toxoplasma gondii[1]	Prior toxoplasmic encephalitis	Sulfadiazine, 85-120 mg/kg/d in 2-4 divided doses P.O. daily *plus* pyrimethamine, 1 mg/kg *or* 15 mg/m^2 (max: 25 mg) P.O. every day *plus* leucovorin, 5 mg P.O. every 3 days	Clindamycin, 20-30 mg/kg/d in 4 divided doses P.O. every day *plus* pyrimethamine, 1 mg/kg P.O. every day *plus* leucovorin, 5 mg P.O. every 3 days
Mycobacterium avium complex[2]	Prior disease	Clarithromycin, 7.5 mg/kg (max: 500 mg) P.O. twice daily *plus* ethambutol, 15 mg/kg (max: 900 mg) P.O. every day; with or without rifabutin, 5 mg/kg (max: 300 mg) P.O. once daily	Azithromycin, 5 mg/kg (max: 250 mg) P.O. every day *plus* ethambutol, 15 mg/kg (max: 900 mg) P.O. every day; with or without rifabutin, 5 mg/kg (max: 300 mg) P.O. once daily
Cryptococcus neoformans	Documented disease	Fluconazole, 3-6 mg/kg P.O. every day	Amphotericin B, 0.5-1 mg/kg I.V. 1-3 times/week; itraconazole, 2-5 mg/kg P.O. every 12-24 hours
Histoplasma capsulatum	Documented disease	Itraconazole, 2-5 mg/kg P.O. every 12-48 hours	Amphotericin B, 1 mg/kg I.V. weekly
Coccidioides immitis	Documented disease	Fluconazole, 6 mg/kg P.O. every day	Amphotericin B, 1 mg/kg I.V. weekly; itraconazole, 2-5 mg/kg P.O. every 12-48 hours
Cytomegalovirus	Prior end-organ disease	Ganciclovir, 5 mg/kg I.V. every day, *or* foscarnet, 90-120 mg/kg I.V. every day	(For retinitis) — ganciclovir sustained-release implant, every 6-9 mo *plus* ganciclovir, 30 mg/kg P.O. 3 times/d
Salmonella species (non-*typhi*)[3]	Bacteremia	TMP-SMZ, 150/750 mg/m^2 in 2 divided doses P.O. every day for several months	Antibiotic chemoprophylaxis with another active agent
II. Recommended Only if Subsequent Episodes Are Frequent or Severe			
Invasive bacterial infections[4]	>2 infections in 1-year period	TMP-SMZ, 150/750 mg/m^2 in 2 divided doses P.O. every day; *or* IVIG, 400 mg/kg every 2-4 weeks	Antibiotic chemoprophylaxis with another active agent
Herpes simplex virus	Frequent/severe recurrences	Acyclovir, 80 mg/kg/d in 3-4 divided doses P.O. daily	
Candida (oropharyngeal)	Frequent/severe recurrences	Fluconazole, 3-6 mg/kg P.O. every day	
Candida (esophageal)	Frequent/severe recurrences	Fluconazole, 3-6 mg/kg P.O. every day	Itraconazole solution, 5 mg/kg P.O. every day; ketoconazole, 5-10 mg/kg P.O. every 12-24 hours

Note: Information included in these guidelines may not represent Food and Drug Administration (FDA) approval or approved labeling for the particular products or indications in question. Specifically, the terms "safe" and "effective" may not be synonymous with the FDA-defined legal standards for product approval. IVIG = intravenous immune globulin and TMP-SMZ = trimethoprim-sulfamethoxazole. The Respirgard II™ nebulizer is manufactured by Marquest, Englewood, CO.

[1]Only pyrimethamine plus sulfadiazine confers protection against PCP as well as toxoplasmosis. Although the clindamycin plus pyrimethamine regimen is the preferred alternative in adults, it has not been tested in children. However, these drugs are safe and are used for other infections.

[2]Significant drug interactions may occur between rifabutin and protease inhibitors and non-nucleoside reverse transcriptase inhibitors. Consult an expert.

[3]Drug should be determined by susceptibilities of the organism isolated. Alternatives to TMP-SMZ include ampicillin, chloramphenicol, or ciprofloxacin. However, ciprofloxacin is not approved for use in persons aged <18 years; therefore, it should be used in children with caution and only if no alternatives exist.

[4]Antimicrobial prophylaxis should be chosen based on the microorganism and antibiotic sensitivities. TMP-SMZ, if used, should be administered daily. Providers should be cautious about using antibiotics solely for this purpose because of the potential for development of drug-resistant microorganisms. IVIG may not provide additional benefit to children receiving daily TMP-SMZ, but may be considered for children who have recurrent bacterial infections despite TMP-SMZ prophylaxis. Choice of antibiotic prophylaxis vs IVIG should also involve consideration of adherence, ease of intravenous access, and cost. If IVIG is used, RSV-IVIG (750 mg/kg), not monoclonal RSV antibody, may be substituted for IVIG during the RSV season to provide broad anti-infective protection, if this product is available.

ANIMAL AND HUMAN BITES

Bite Wound Antibiotic Regimens

	Dog Bite	Cat Bite	Human Bite
Prophylactic Antibiotics			
Prophylaxis	No routine prophylaxis, consider if involves face or hand, or immunosuppressed or asplenic patients	Routine prophylaxis	Routine prophylaxis
Prophylactic antibiotic	Amoxicillin	Amoxicillin	Amoxicillin
Penicillin allergy	Doxycycline if >10 y or co-trimoxazole	Doxycycline if >10 y or co-trimoxazole	Doxycycline if >10 y or erythromycin and cephalexin[1]
Outpatient Oral Antibiotic Treatment (mild to moderate infection)			
Established infection	Amoxicillin and clavulanic acid	Amoxicillin and clavulanic acid	Amoxicillin and clavulanic acid
Penicillin allergy (mild infection only)	Doxycycline if >10 y	Doxycycline if >10 y	Cephalexin[1] or clindamycin
Outpatient Parenteral Antibiotic Treatment (moderate infections – single drug regimens)			
	Ceftriaxone	Ceftriaxone	Cefotetan
Inpatient Parenteral Antibiotic Treatment			
Established infection	Ampicillin + cefazolin	Ampicillin + cefazolin	Ampicillin + clindamycin
Penicillin allergy	Cefazolin[1]	Ceftriaxone[1]	Cefotetan[1] or imipenem
Duration of Prophylactic and Treatment Regimens			
Prophylaxis: 5 days			
Treatment: 10-14 days			

[1]Contraindicated if history of immediate hypersensitivity reaction (anaphylaxis) to penicillin.

ANTIBIOTIC TREATMENT OF ADULTS WITH INFECTIVE ENDOCARDITIS

Table 1. Suggested Regimens for Therapy of Native Valve Endocarditis Due to Penicillin-Susceptible Viridans Streptococci and *Streptococcus bovis* (Minimum Inhibitory Concentration ≤0.12 mcg/mL)[1]

Antibiotic	Dosage and Route	Duration (wk)	Comments
Aqueous crystalline penicillin G sodium **or**	12-18 million units/24 h I.V. either continuously or in 4-6 equally divided doses	4	Preferred in most patients older than 65 y and in those with impairment of the 8th cranial nerve or renal function
Ceftriaxone sodium	2 g once daily I.V. or I.M.[2]	4	
Either penicillin or ceftriaxone regimen above with gentamicin sulfate[3]	3 mg/kg/24 h I.M./I.V. as single daily dose	2	When using combination therapy, both β-lactam and aminoglycoside regimen duration is 2 weeks; 2-week regimen not intended if known cardiac or extracardiac abscess, Cl_{cr} <20 mL/min, 8th cranial nerve impairment or *Abiotrophia*, *Granulicatella*, or *Gemella* spp
Vancomycin hydrochloride[4]	30 mg/kg/24 h I.V. in 2 equally divided doses, not to exceed 2 g/24 h unless serum levels are monitored	4	Vancomycin therapy is recommended for patients allergic to β-lactams; peak serum concentrations of vancomycin should be obtained 1 h after completion of the infusion and should be in the range of 30-45 mcg/mL and trough of 10-15 mcg/mL for twice-daily dosing

[1]Dosages recommended are for patients with normal renal function. For nutritionally variant streptococci, see Table 3. I.V. indicates intravenous; I.M., intramuscular.

[2]Patients should be informed that I.M. injection of ceftriaxone is painful.

[3]Dosing of gentamicin on a mg/kg basis will produce higher serum concentrations in obese patients than in lean patients. Therefore, in obese patients, dosing should be based on ideal body weight. (Ideal body weight for men is 50 kg + 2.3 kg per inch over 5 feet, and ideal body weight for women is 45.5 kg + 2.3 kg per inch over 5 feet.) Relative contraindications to the use of gentamicin are age >65 years, renal impairment, or impairment of the eighth nerve. Other potentially nephrotoxic agents (eg, nonsteroidal anti-inflammatory drugs) should be used cautiously in patients receiving gentamicin.

[4]Vancomycin dosage should be reduced in patients with impaired renal function. Vancomycin given on a mg/kg basis will produce higher serum concentrations in obese patients than in lean patients. Therefore, in obese patients, dosing should be based on ideal body weight. Each dose of vancomycin should be infused over at least 1 hour to reduce the risk of the histamine-release "red man" syndrome.

Table 2. Therapy for Native Valve Endocarditis Due to Strains of Viridans Streptococci and *Streptococcus bovis* Relatively Resistant to Penicillin G (Minimum Inhibitory Concentration >0.12 mcg/mL and ≤0.5 mcg/mL)[1]

Antibiotic	Dosage and Route	Duration (wk)	Comments
Aqueous crystalline penicillin G sodium	24 million units/24 h I.V. either continuously or in 4-6 equally divided doses	4	Cefazolin or other first-generation cephalosporins may be substituted for penicillin in patients whose penicillin hypersensitivity is not of the immediate type.
With gentamicin sulfate[2]	3 mg/kg/24 h I.M./I.V. as single daily dose	2	
Ceftriaxone sodium	2 g once daily I.V. or I.M.[2]	4	
With gentamicin sulfate[2]	3 mg/kg/24 h I.M./I.V. as single daily dose	2	
Vancomycin hydrochloride[3]	30 mg/kg/24 h I.V. in 2 equally divided doses, not to exceed 2 g/24 h unless serum levels are monitored	4	Vancomycin therapy is recommended for patients allergic to β-lactams

[1]Dosages recommended are for patients with normal renal function. I.V. indicates intravenous; I.M., intramuscular.

[2]For specific dosing adjustment and issues concerning gentamicin (obese patients, relative contraindications), see Table 1 footnotes.

[3]For specific dosing adjustment and issues concerning vancomycin (obese patients, length of infusion), see Table 1 footnotes.

Table 3. Standard Therapy for Endocarditis Due to Enterococci[1]

Antibiotic	Dosage and Route	Duration (wk)	Comments
Aqueous crystalline penicillin G sodium	18-30 million units/24 h I.V. either continuously or in 6 equally divided doses	4-6	Native valve: 4-week therapy recommended for patients with symptoms ≤3 months in duration; 6-week therapy recommended for patients with symptoms >3 months in duration Prosthetic valve or other prosthetic material: 6-week minimum therapy recommended Target gentamicin peak concentration of 3-4 mcg/mL and trough of <1 mcg/mL
With gentamicin sulfate[2]	1 mg/kg I.M. or I.V. every 8 h	4-6	
Ampicillin sodium	12 g/24 h I.V. in 6 equally divided doses	4-6	
With gentamicin sulfate[2]	1 mg/kg I.M. or I.V. every 8 hours	4-6	
Vancomycin hydrochloride[2,3]	30 mg/kg/24 h I.V. in 2 equally divided doses, not to exceed 2 g/24 h unless serum levels are monitored	6	Vancomycin therapy is recommended for patients allergic to β-lactams; cephalosporins are not acceptable alternatives for patients allergic to penicillin
With gentamicin sulfate[2]	1 mg/kg I.M. or I.V. every 8 h	6	

[1]All enterococci causing endocarditis must be tested for antimicrobial susceptibility in order to select optimal therapy. This table is for endocarditis due to penicillin-, gentamicin-, and vancomycin-susceptible enterococci, viridans streptococci with a minimum inhibitory concentration of >0.5 mcg/mL, nutritionally variant viridans streptococci, or prosthetic valve endocarditis caused by viridans streptococci or *Streptococcus bovis*. If penicillin-resistant organisms, use vancomycin/gentamicin regimen above, or may use ampicillin/sulbactam (12 g/24 h in 4 divided doses) with gentamicin for 6 weeks. Antibiotic dosages are for patients with normal renal function. I.V. indicates intravenous; I.M., intramuscular.

[2]For specific dosing adjustment and issues concerning gentamicin (obese patients, relative contraindications), see Table 1 footnotes.

[3]For specific dosing adjustment and issues concerning vancomycin (obese patients, length of infusion), see Table 1 footnotes.

Table 4. Therapy for Native or Prosthetic Valve Endocarditis Due to Enterococci[1] Resistant to Vancomycin, Aminoglycosides, and Penicillin[2]

Antibiotic	Dosage and Route	Duration (wk)	Comments
E. faecium			
Linezolid	1200 mg/24 h P.O./I.V. in 2 divided doses	≥8	May cause severe, but reversible thrombocytopenia, particularly with extended therapy >2 weeks.
Quinupristin-dalfopristin	22.5 mg/kg/24 h I.V. in 3 divided doses	≥8	May cause severe myalgia; not effective against *E. faecalis*.
E. faecalis			
Imipenem/cilastatin	2 g/24 h I.V. in 4 divided doses	≥8	Limited patient experience with these regimens.
With ampicillin sodium	12 g/24 h in 6 divided doses	≥8	
or			
Ceftriaxone sodium	2 g/24 h I.V./I.M.[3] once daily	≥8	Limited patient experience with these regimens.
With ampicillin sodium	12 g/24 h in 6 divided doses	≥8	

[1]Endocarditis caused by the organisms should be treated in consultation with an infectious disease specialist; bacteriologic cure with antimicrobial therapy alone may be <50% and valve replacement may be required.

[2]Dosages recommended are for patients with normal renal function. I.V. = intravenous; I.M. = intramuscular.

[3]Patients should be informed that I.M. injection of ceftriaxone is painful.

Table 5. Therapy for Endocarditis Due to *Staphylococcus* in the Absence of Prosthetic Material[1]

Antibiotic	Dosage and Route	Duration	Comments
Methicillin-Susceptible Staphylococci			
Regimens for non-β-lactam-allergic patients			
Nafcillin sodium or oxacillin sodium	12 g/24 h I.V. in 4-6 divided doses	6 wk	Uncomplicated right side endocarditis may be treated for 2 weeks.
With optional addition of gentamicin sulfate[2]	3 mg/kg/24 h I.M./I.V. in 2-3 divided doses	3-5 d	Benefit of additional aminoglycosides has not been established.
Regimens for β-lactam-allergic patients (nonanaphylactic)			
Cefazolin (or other first-generation cephalosporins in equivalent dosages)	2 g I.V. every 8 h	6 wk	Cephalosporins should be avoided in patients with immediate-type hypersensitivity to penicillin; if penicillin-sensitive, vancomycin should be used.
With optional addition of gentamicin[2]	3 mg/kg/24 h I.M./I.V. in 2-3 divided doses	3-5 d	Benefit of additional aminoglycosides has not been established.
Methicillin-Resistant Staphylococci			
Vancomycin hydrochloride[3]	30 mg/kg/24 h I.V. in 2 equally divided doses; not to exceed 2 g/24 h unless serum levels are monitored	4-6 wk	Vancomycin therapy is recommended for patients allergic to β-lactams; peak serum concentrations of vancomycin should be obtained 1 h after completion of the infusion and should be in the range of 30-45 mcg/mL and trough of 10-15 mcg/mL for twice-daily dosing.

[1]For treatment of endocarditis due to penicillin-susceptible staphylococci (minimum inhibitory concentration ≤0.1 mcg/mL and non-beta-lactamase producing), aqueous crystalline penicillin G sodium 24 million units/24 h can be used instead of nafcillin or oxacillin. Shorter antibiotic courses have been effective in some drug addicts with right-sided endocarditis due to *Staphylococcus aureus*. I.V. indicates intravenous; I.M., intramuscular.

[2]For specific dosing adjustment and issues concerning gentamicin (obese patients, relative contraindications), see Table 1 footnotes.

[3]For specific dosing adjustment and issues concerning vancomycin (obese patients, length of infusion), see Table 1 footnotes.

Table 6. Treatment of Staphylococcal Endocarditis in the Presence of a Prosthetic Valve or Other Prosthetic Material[1]

Antibiotic	Dosage and Route	Duration (wk)	Comments
Methicillin-Susceptible Staphylococci			
Nafcillin sodium or oxacillin sodium[2]	12 g/24 h I.V. in 6 divided doses	≥6	First-generation cephalosporins or vancomycin should be used in patients allergic to β-lactam. Cephalosporins should be avoided in patients with immediate-type hypersensitivity to penicillin or with methicillin-resistant staphylococci.
With rifampin[3]	300 mg P.O./I.V. every 8 h	≥6	–
And with gentamicin sulfate[4,5]	3 mg/kg I.M./I.V. in 2-3 divided doses	2	Aminoglycoside should be administered in close proximity to vancomycin, nafcillin, or oxacillin.
Methicillin-Resistant Staphylococci			
Vancomycin hydrochloride[6]	30 mg/kg/24 h I.V. in 2 equally divided doses, not to exceed 2 g/24 h unless serum levels are monitored	≥6	–
With rifampin[3]	300 mg P.O./I.V. every 8 h	≥6	Rifampin increases the amount of warfarin sodium required for antithrombotic therapy.
And with gentamicin sulfate[4,5]	3 mg/kg I.M./I.V. in 2-3 divided doses	2	Aminoglycoside should be administered in close proximity to vancomycin, nafcillin, or oxacillin.

[1]Dosages recommended are for patients with normal renal function. I.V. = intravenous; I.M. = intramuscular.

[2]May use aqueous penicillin G 24 million units/24 h in 4-6 divided doses if strain is penicillin susceptible (MIC ≤0.1 mcg/mL and non-beta-lactamase producing).

[3]Rifampin plays a unique role in the eradication of staphylococcal infection involving prosthetic material; combination therapy is essential to prevent emergence of rifampin resistance.

[4]For a specific dosing adjustment and issues concerning gentamicin (obese patients, relative contraindications), see Table 1 footnotes.

[5]Use during initial 2 weeks.

[6]For specific dosing adjustment and issues concerning vancomycin (obese patients, relative contraindications), see Table 1 footnotes.

Table 7. Therapy for Native or Prosthetic Valve Endocarditis Due to HACEK Microorganisms (*Haemophilus parainfluenzae, Haemophilus aphrophilus, Actinobacillus actinomycetemcomitans, Cardiobacterium hominus, Eikenella corrodens,* and *Kingella kingae*)[1]

Antibiotic	Dosage and Route	Duration (wk)	Comments
Ceftriaxone sodium[2]	2 g once daily I.V. or I.M.[2]	4	Cefotaxime sodium or other third- or fourth-generation cephalosporins may be substituted.
Ampicillin/sulbactam[3]	12 g/24 h I.V. in 6 equally divided doses	4	
Ciprofloxacin	1000 mg/24 h orally or 800 mg/24 h I.V. in 2 divided doses	4	Use of fluoroquinolone recommended only if patient intolerant to ampicillin or cephalosporins; may substitute fluoroquinolone with equivalent coverage (eg, levofloxacin, moxifloxacin); if prosthetic material involved, treatment duration should be 6 weeks.

[1]Antibiotic dosages are for patients with normal renal function. I.V. indicates intravenous; I.M. intramuscular.

[2]Patients should be informed that I.M. injection of ceftriaxone is painful.

[3]Ampicillin should not be used if laboratory tests show β-lactamase production.

Reference

Baddour LM, Wilson WR, Bayer AS, et al, "Infective Endocarditis. Diagnosis, Antimicrobial Therapy, and Management of Complications. A Statement for Healthcare Professionals from the Committee on Rheumatic Fever, Endocarditis, and Kawasaki Disease, Council on Cardiovascular Disease in the Young, and the Councils on Clinical Cardiology, Stroke, and Cardiovascular Surgery and Anesthesia, American Heart Association," *Circulation*, 2005, 111(23):e394-434.

ANTIMICROBIAL DRUGS OF CHOICE

Empirical treatment of some common infecting organisms is listed below. These recommendations are based on results of susceptibility studies, clinical trials, and the opinions of *Medical Letter* consultants. The site and severity of the infection, pharmacokinetic characteristics of antibiotics, local resistance patterns, potential drug interactions, and specific patient factors should be taken into account in choosing an appropriate regimen.

Infecting Organism	Drug of First Choice	Alternative Drugs
GRAM-POSITIVE COCCI		
**Enterococcus*[1]		
endocarditis or other severe infection	Penicillin G or ampicillin + gentamicin or streptomycin[2]	Vancomycin + gentamicin or streptomycin[2]; linezolid; daptomycin[3]; quinupristin/dalfopristin[4]
uncomplicated urinary tract infection	Ampicillin or amoxicillin	Nitrofurantoin; a fluoroquinolone[5]; fosfomycin
**Staphylococcus aureus* or *epidermidis*		
methicillin-susceptible	A penicillinase- resistant penicillin[6]	A cephalosporin[7,8]; vancomycin; imipenem or meropenem; clindamycin; linezolid; daptomycin[3]; a fluoroquinolone[5]
methicillin-resistant[9]	Vancomycin ± gentamicin ± rifampin	Linezolid; daptomycin[3]; a fluoroquinolone[5]; quinupristin/dalfopristin; a tetracycline[10]; trimethoprim-sulfamethoxazole
Streptococcus pyogenes (group A[11]) and groups C and G	Penicillin G or V[12]	Clindamycin; erythromycin; a cephalosporin[7,8]; vancomycin; clarithromycin[13]; azithromycin; linezolid; daptomycin[3]
Streptococcus, group B	Penicillin G or ampicillin	A cephalosporin[7,8]; vancomycin; daptomycin[3]; erythromycin
**Streptococcus*, viridans group[1]	Penicillin G ± gentamicin	A cephalosporin[7,8]; vancomycin
Streptococcus bovis	Penicillin G	A cephalosporin[7,8]; vancomycin
Streptococcus, anaerobic or *Peptostreptococcus*	Penicillin G	Clindamycin; a cephalosporin[7,8]; vancomycin
**Streptococcus pneumoniae*[14] (pneumococcus)		
penicillin-susceptible (MIC <0.1 mcg/mL)	Penicillin G or V[12]; amoxicillin	A cephalosporin[7,8]; erythromycin; azithromycin; clarithromycin[13]; levofloxacin[5,16] or moxifloxacin[5,16]; meropenem; imipenem or ertapenem; trimethoprim-sulfamethoxazole; clindamycin; a tetracycline[10]; vancomycin
penicillin-intermediate resistance (MIC 0.1-≤2 mcg/mL)	Penicillin G I.V. (12 million units/day for adults); ceftriaxone or cefotaxime	Levofloxacin[5,16] or moxifloxacin[5,16]; vancomycin; clindamycin
penicillin-high level resistance (MIC >2 mcg/mL)	**Meningitis:** Vancomycin ± rifampin + ceftriaxone or cefotaxime	
	Other Infections: Vancomycin + ceftriaxone or cefotaxime; levofloxacin, gatifloxacin, or moxifloxacin[16]	Linezolid; quinupristin/dalfopristin
GRAM-NEGATIVE COCCI		
Moraxella (Branhamella) catarrhalis	Cefuroxime[7]; a fluoroquinolone[5]	Trimethoprim-sulfamethoxazole; amoxicillin/clavulanate; erythromycin; clarithromycin[13]; azithromycin; a tetracycline[10]; cefotaxime[7]; ceftizoxime[7]; ceftriaxone[7]; cefpodoxime[7]
**Neisseria gonorrhoeae* (gonococcus)[17]	Ceftriaxone[7]	Cefotaxime[7]; cefoxitin, cefixime, ceftizoxime, cefpodoxime
Neisseria meningitidis[18] (meningococcus)	Penicillin G	Cefotaxime[7]; ceftizoxime[7]; ceftriaxone[7]; chloramphenicol[19]; a sulfonamide[20]; a fluoroquinolone[15]
GRAM-POSITIVE BACILLI		
**Bacillus anthracis*[21] (anthrax)	Ciprofloxacin; a tetracycline[10]	Penicillin G, amoxicillin; erythromycin; imipenem; clindamycin; levofloxacin
Bacillus cereus, subtilis	Vancomycin	Imipenem or meropenem; clindamycin
Clostridium perfringens[22]	Penicillin G; clindamycin	Metronidazole; imipenem, meropenem, or ertapenem; chloramphenicol[19]
Clostridium tetani[23]	Metronidazole	Penicillin G; a tetracycline[10]
Clostridium difficile[24]	Metronidazole (oral)	Vancomycin (oral)
Corynebacterium diphtheriae[25]	Erythromycin	Penicillin G

Infecting Organism	Drug of First Choice	Alternative Drugs
Corynebacterium, JK group	Vancomycin	Penicillin G + gentamicin; erythromycin
**Erysipelothrix rhusiopathiae*	Penicillin G	Erythromycin, a cephalosporin[7,8]; a fluoroquinolone[16]
Listeria monocytogenes	Ampicillin ± gentamicin	Trimethoprim-sulfamethoxazole
ENTERIC GRAM-NEGATIVE BACILLI		
**Campylobacter fetus*	A third-generation cephalosporin[8]; gentamicin	Ampicillin; imipenem or meropenem
**Campylobacter jejuni*	Erythromycin or azithromycin	A fluoroquinolone[5,16]; a tetracycline[10]; gentamicin
**Citrobacter freundii*	Imipenem or meropenem[26]	A fluoroquinolone[5,16];ertapenem; amikacin; a tetracycline[10]; trimethoprim-sulfamethoxazole; cefotaxime[7,26]; ceftizoxime[7,26]; ceftriaxone[7,26]; cefepime[7,26] or ceftazidime[7,26]
**Enterobacter*	Imipenem or meropenem[26]; cefepime[7,26]	Gentamicin, tobramycin or amikacin; trimethoprim-sulfamethoxazole; ciprofloxacin[16]; ticarcillin/clavulanate[27] or piperacillin/sulbactam[27]; aztreonam[26]; cefotaxime, ceftizoxime, ceftriaxone, or ceftazidime[7,26]
**Escherichia coli*[28]	Cefotaxime, ceftriaxone, cefepime, or ceftazidime[7,26]	Ampicillin ± gentamicin, tobramycin or amikacin; gentamicin, tobramycin, or amikacin; amoxicillin/clavulanate[26]; ticarcillin/clavulanate[27]; piperacillin/tazobactam[27]; ampicillin/sulbactam[26]; trimethoprim-sulfamethoxazole; imipenem, meropenem, or ertapenem[26]; aztreonam[26]; a fluoroquinolone[5,16]; another cephalosporin[7,8]
**Klebsiella pneumoniae*[28]	Cefotaxime, ceftriaxone, cefepime, or ceftazidime[7,26]	Imipenem, meropenem, or ertapenem[26]; gentamicin, tobramycin or amikacin; amoxicillin/clavulanate[26]; ticarcillin/clavulanate[27]; piperacillin/tazobactam[27]; ampicillin/sulbactam[26]; trimethoprim-sulfamethoxazole; aztreonam[26]; a fluoroquinolone[5,16]; another cephalosporin[7,8]
**Proteus mirabilis*[28]	Ampicillin[29]	A cephalosporin[7,8,26]; ticarcillin/clavulanate or piperacillin/tazobactam[27]; gentamicin, tobramycin, or amikacin; trimethoprim-sulfamethoxazole; imipenem, meropenem, or ertapenem[26]; aztreonam[26]; a fluoroquinolone[5,16]; chloramphenicol[19]
**Proteus*, indole-positive (including *Providencia rettgeri, Morganella morganii*, and *Proteus vulgaris*)	Cefotaxime, ceftriaxone, cefepime, or ceftazidime[7,26]	Imipenem, meropenem, or ertapenem[28]; gentamicin, tobramycin, or amikacin; amoxicillin/clavulanate[26]; ticarcillin/clavulanate[27]; piperacillin/tazobactam[27]; ampicillin/sulbactam[26]; aztreonam[26]; trimethoprim-sulfamethoxazole; a fluoroquinolone[5,16]
**Providencia stuartii*	Cefotaxime, ceftriaxone, cefepime, or ceftazidime[7,26]	Imipenem, meropenem, or ertapenem[26]; ticarcillin/clavulanate[27]; piperacillin/tazobactam[27]; gentamicin, tobramycin, or amikacin; aztreonam[26]; trimethoprim-sulfamethoxazole; a fluoroquinolone[5,16]
**Salmonella typhi* (typhoid fever)[30]	A fluoroquinolone[16] or ceftriaxone[7]	Chloramphenicol[19]; trimethoprim-sulfamethoxazole; ampicillin; amoxicillin; azithromycin[31]
*Other *Salmonella*[32]	Cefotaxime[7] or ceftriaxone[7] or a fluoroquinolone[16]	Ampicillin or amoxicillin; trimethoprim-sulfamethoxazole; chloramphenicol[19]
**Serratia*	Imipenem or meropenem[26]	Gentamicin or amikacin; cefotaxime, ceftizoxime, ceftriaxone, cefepime, or ceftazidime[7,26]; aztreonam[26]; trimethoprim-sulfamethoxazole; a fluoroquinolone [5,16]
**Shigella*	A fluoroquinolone[16]	Azithromycin; trimethoprim-sulfamethoxazole; ampicillin; ceftriaxone[7]
**Yersinia enterocolitica*	Trimethoprim-sulfamethoxazole	A fluoroquinolone[16]; gentamicin, tobramycin, or amikacin; cefotaxime[7]
OTHER GRAM-NEGATIVE BACILLI		
**Acinetobacter*	Imipenem or meropenem[26]	An aminoglycoside; ciprofloxacin[16]; trimethoprim-sulfamethoxazole; ticarcillin/clavulanate,[27] or piperacillin/tazobactam[27]; ceftazidime[26]; minocycline[10]; doxycycline[10]; sulbactam[33]; polymyxin
**Aeromonas*	Trimethoprim-sulfamethoxazole	Gentamicin or tobramycin; imipenem; a fluoroquinolone[5]
**Bacteroides*	Metronidazole	Clindamycin; imipenem, meropenem or ertapenem; amoxicillin/clavulanate; ticarcillin/clavulanate; piperacillin/tazobactam or ampicillin/sulbactam; cefoxitin[7]; chloramphenicol[19]
Bartonella henselae or *quintana* (bacillary angiomatosis, trench fever)	Erythromycin	Azithromycin; doxycycline[10]
Bartonella henselae[34] (cat scratch bacillus)	Azithromycin	Erythromycin; ciprofloxacin[16]; trimethoprim-sulfamethoxazole; gentamicin; rifampin
Bordetella pertussis (whooping cough)	Erythromycin; clarithromycin[13]	Azithromycin; trimethoprim-sulfamethoxazole

Infecting Organism	Drug of First Choice	Alternative Drugs
**Brucella*	A tetracycline[10] + rifampin	A tetracycline[10] + streptomycin or gentamicin; chloramphenicol[19] ± streptomycin; trimethoprim-sulfamethoxazole ± gentamicin; ciprofloxacin[16] + rifampin
**Burkholderia cepacia*	Trimethoprim-sulfamethoxazole	Ceftazidime[7]; chloramphenicol[19]; imipenem
Burkholderia (Pseudomonas) mallei (glanders)	Streptomycin + a tetracycline[10]	Streptomycin + chloramphenicol[19]; imipenem
**Burkholderia (Pseudomonas) pseudomallei* (melioidosis)	Imipenem; ceftazidime[7]	Meropenem; chloramphenicol[19] + doxycycline[10] + trimethoprim-sulfamethoxazole; amoxicillin/clavulanate
Calymmatobacterium granulomatis (granuloma inguinale)	Trimethoprim-sulfamethoxazole	Doxycycline[10] or ciprofloxacin[16] ± gentamicin
Capnocytophaga canimorsus[35]	Penicillin G	Cefotaxime, ceftizoxime, or ceftriaxone[7]; imipenem or meropenem; vancomycin; a fluoroquinolone[16]; clindamycin
**Eikenella corrodens*	Ampicillin	Erythromycin; azithromycin; clarithromycin[13]; a tetracycline[10]; amoxicillin/clavulanate; ampicillin/sulbactam; ceftriaxone[7]
**Francisella tularensis* (tularemia)	Gentamicin or streptomycin either + a tetracycline[10]	Chloramphenicol[19]; ciprofloxacin[16]
**Fusobacterium*	Penicillin G; metronidazole	Clindamycin; cefoxitin[7]; chloramphenicol[19]
Gardnerella vaginalis (bacterial vaginosis)	Oral metronidazole[37]	Topical clindamycin or metronidazole; oral clindamycin
**Haemophilus ducreyi* (chancroid)	Azithromycin or ceftriaxone	Ciprofloxacin[16] or erythromycin
**Haemophilus influenzae*		
meningitis, epiglottitis, arthritis, and other serious infections	Cefotaxime or ceftriaxone[7]	Cefuroxime[7] (not for meningitis); chloramphenicol[19]; meropenem
upper respiratory infections and bronchitis	Trimethoprim-sulfamethoxazole	Cefuroxime[7]; amoxicillin/clavulanate; cefuroxime axetil[7]; cefpodoxime[7]; cefaclor[7]; cefotaxime[7]; ceftizoxime[7]; ceftriaxone[7]; cefixime[7]; a tetracycline[10]; clarithromycin[13]; azithromycin; a fluoroquinolone[5]; ampicillin or amoxicillin
**Helicobacter pylori*[38]	Proton pump inhibitor[39] + clarithromycin[13] + either amoxicillin or metronidazole	Bismuth subsalicylate + metronidazole + tetracycline HCl[10] + either a proton pump inhibitor[39] or H_2-blocker[39]
Legionella species	Azithromycin or a fluoroquinolone[5] ± rifampin	Doxycycline[10] ± rifampin; trimethoprim-sulfamethoxazole; erythromycin
Leptotrichia buccalis	Penicillin G	A tetracycline[10]; clindamycin; erythromycin
Pasteurella multocida	Penicillin G	A tetracycline[10]; a second- or third-generation cephalosporin[7,8]; amoxicillin/clavulanate; ampicillin/sulbactam
**Pseudomonas aeruginosa*		
urinary tract infection	Ciprofloxacin[5,16]	Levofloxacin[5,16]; ticarcillin/clavulanate or piperacillin/tazobactam; ceftazidime[7]; cefepime[7]; imipenem or meropenem; aztreonam; tobramycin; gentamicin or amikacin
other infections	Piperacillin/tazobactam or ticarcillin/clavulanate **each** + tobramycin, gentamicin, or amikacin[40]	Ceftazidime,[7] ciprofloxacin[5,16]; imipenem or meropenem, aztreonam, cefepime[7] **each** + tobramycin, gentamicin, or amikacin
Spirillum minus (rat bite fever)	Penicillin G	A tetracycline[10]; streptomycin
**Stenotrophomonas maltophilia*	Trimethoprim-sulfamethoxazole	Minocycline[10]; a fluoroquinolone[5,16]
Streptobacillus moniliformis (rat bite fever, Haverhill fever)	Penicillin G	A tetracycline[10]; streptomycin
Vibrio cholerae (cholera)[41]	A tetracycline[10]	A fluoroquinolone[5]; trimethoprim-sulfamethoxazole
Vibrio vulnificus	A tetracycline[10]	Cefotaxime[7]; ciprofloxacin[13]
Yersinia pestis (plague)	Streptomycin ± a tetracycline[10]	Chloramphenicol[19]; gentamicin; trimethoprim-sulfamethoxazole; ciprofloxacin[13]
ACID-FAST BACILLI		
**Mycobacterium tuberculosis*	Isoniazid + rifampin + pyrazinamide ± ethambutol or streptomycin[19]	A fluoroquinolone[5]; cycloserine[19]; capreomycin[19] or kanamycin[19] or amikacin[19]; ethionamide[19]; para-aminosalicylic acid[19]
**Mycobacterium kansasii*	Isoniazid + rifampin ± ethambutol or streptomycin[19]	Clarithromycin [13] or azithromycin; ethionamide[19]; cycloserine[19]

Infecting Organism	Drug of First Choice	Alternative Drugs
**Mycobacterium avium* complex		
treatment	Clarithromycin[13] or azithromycin + ethambutol ± rifabutin	Ciprofloxacin[16]; amikacin[19]
prophylaxis	Clarithromycin[13] or azithromycin ± rifabutin	
**Mycobacterium fortuitum/chelonae* complex	Amikacin + clarithromycin[13]	Cefoxitin[7]; rifampin; a sulfonamide; doxycycline[10]; ethambutol; linezolid
Mycobacterium marinum (balnei)[42]	Minocycline[10]	Trimethoprim-sulfamethoxazole; rifampin; clarithromycin[13]; doxycycline[10]
Mycobacterium leprae (leprosy)	Dapsone + rifampin ± clofazimine	Minocycline[10]; ofloxacin[16]; clarithromycin[13]
ACTINOMYCETES		
Actinomyces israelii (actinomycosis)	Penicillin G	A tetracycline[10]; erythromycin; clindamycin
Nocardia	Trimethoprim-sulfamethoxazole	Sulfisoxazole; amikacin[19]; a tetracycline[10]; ceftriaxone; imipenem or meropenem; cycloserine[19]; linezolid
**Rhodococcus equi*	Vancomycin ± a fluoroquinolone,[5] rifampin, imipenem, or meropenem; amikacin	Erythromycin
Tropheryma whippelii (Whipple's disease)	Trimethoprim-sulfamethoxazole	Penicillin G; a tetracycline[10]; ceftriaxone
CHLAMYDIAE		
Chlamydia trachomatis		
trachoma	Azithromycin	A tetracycline[10] (topical plus oral); a sulfonamide (topical plus oral)
inclusion conjunctivitis	Erythromycin (oral or I.V.)	A sulfonamide
pneumonia	Erythromycin	A sulfonamide
urethritis, cervicitis	Azithromycin or doxycycline[10]	Erythromycin; ofloxacin[16]; amoxicillin
lymphogranuloma venereum	A tetracycline[10]	Erythromycin
Chlamydophilia (formerly Chlamydia) pneumoniae (TWAR strain)	Erythromycin; a tetracycline[10]; clarithromycin[13] or azithromycin	A fluoroquinolone[5]
Chlamydophilia (formerly Chlamydia) psittaci (psittacosis, ornithosis)	A tetracycline[10]	Chloramphenicol[19]
EHRLICHIA		
Anaplasma phagocytophilum (formerly *Ehrlichia phagocytophila)*	Doxycycline[10]	Rifampin
Ehrlichia chaffeensis	Doxycycline[10]	Chloramphenicol[19]
Ehrlichia ewingii	Doxycycline[10]	
MYCOPLASMA		
Mycoplasma pneumoniae	Erythromycin; a tetracycline[10]; clarithromycin[13] or azithromycin	A fluoroquinolone[16]
Ureaplasma urealyticum	Azithromycin	Erythromycin; a tetracycline[10]; clarithromycin[13]; ofloxacin[16]
RICKETTSIOSES		
Coxiella burnetii (Q fever)	Doxycycline[10]	Chloramphenicol[19]; a fluoroquinolone[16]
Orientia tsutsugamushi (scrub typhus)	Doxycycline[10]	Chloramphenicol[19]; a fluoroquinolone[16]
Rickettsia prowazekii (epidemic typhus – l ouse-borne)	Doxycycline[10]	Chloramphenicol[19]; a fluoroquinolone[16]
Rickettsia rickettsii Rocky Mountain spotted fever)	Doxycycline[10]	Chloramphenicol[19]; a fluoroquinolone[16]
Rickettsia typhi (endemic typhus – murine)	Doxycycline[10]	Chloramphenicol[19]; a fluoroquinolone[16]
SPIROCHETES		
Borrelia burgdorferi (Lyme disease)[43]	Doxycycline[10]; amoxicillin; cefuroxime axetil[7]	Ceftriaxone[7]; cefotaxime[7]; penicillin G; azithromycin; clarithromycin[13]
Borrelia recurrentis (relapsing fever)	A tetracycline[10]	Penicillin G; erythromycin
Leptospira	Penicillin G	A tetracycline[10]; ceftriaxone[7,44]
Treponema pallidum (syphilis)	Penicillin G[12]	A tetracycline[10]; ceftriaxone[7]
Treponema pertenue (yaws)	Penicillin G	A tetracycline[10]

***Resistance may be a problem; susceptibility tests should be used to guide therapy.**

[1]Disk sensitivity testing may not provide adequate information; beta-lactamase assays, "E" tests, and dilution tests for susceptibility should be used in serious infections.

[2]Aminoglycoside resistance is increasingly common among enterococci; treatment options include ampicillin 2 g I.V. every 4 hours, continuous infusion of ampicillin, a combination of ampicillin plus a fluoroquinolone, or a combination of ampicillin, imipenem, and vancomycin.

[3]Daptomycin should not be used to treat pneumonia.

[4]Quinupristin/dalfopristin is not active against *Enterococcus faecalis*.

[5]Among the fluoroquinolones, levofloxacin, and moxifloxacin have excellent *in vitro* activity against *S. pneumoniae*, including penicillin- and cephalosporin-resistant strains. Levofloxacin and moxifloxacin also have good activity against many strains of *S. aureus*, but resistance has become frequent among methicillin-resistant strains. Ciprofloxacin has the greatest activity of the quinolones against *Pseudomonas aeruginosa*. For urinary tract infections, norfloxacin can be used. For tuberculosis, levofloxacin, ofloxacin, ciprofloxacin, or moxifloxacin could be used. Ciprofloxacin, levofloxacin, and moxifloxacin are available for intravenous use. None of these agents are generally recommended for use in pregnant women. Ciprofloxacin has FDA approval for use in children.

[6]For oral use against staphylococci, cloxacillin or dicloxacillin is preferred; for severe infections, a parenteral formulation of nafcillin or oxacillin should be used. Ampicillin, amoxicillin, carbenicillin, ticarcillin, and piperacillin are not effective against penicillinase-producing staphylococci. The combinations of clavulanate with amoxicillin or ticarcillin, sulbactam with ampicillin, and tazobactam with piperacillin may be active against these organisms.

[7]Cephalosporins have been used as alternatives to penicillins in patients allergic to penicillins, but such patients may also have allergic reactions to cephalosporins.

[8]For parenteral treatment of staphylococcal or nonenterococcal streptococcal infections, a first-generation cephalosporin such as cefazolin can be used. For oral therapy, cephalexin or cephradine can be used. The second-generation cephalosporins cefamandole, cefprozil, cefuroxime, cefotetan, and cefoxitin, are more active than the first-generation drugs against gram-negative bacteria. Cefuroxime is active against ampicillin-resistant strains of *H. influenzae*. Cefoxitin and cefotetan are the most active of the cephalosporins against *B. fragilis*, but cefotetan has been associated with prothrombin deficiency. The third-generation cephalosporins cefotaxime, cefoperazone, ceftizoxime, ceftriaxone, and ceftazidime, and the fourth-generation cefepime have greater activity than the second-generation drugs against enteric gram-negative bacilli. Ceftazidime has poor activity against many gram-positive cocci and anaerobes, and ceftizoxime has poor activity against penicillin-resistant *S. pneumoniae*. Cefepime has *in vitro* activity against gram-positive cocci similar to cefotaxime and ceftriaxone and somewhat greater activity against enteric gram-negative bacilli. The activity of cefepime against *Pseudomonas aeruginosa* is similar to that of ceftazidime. Cefixime, cefpodoxime, cefdinir, ceftibuten, and cefditoren are oral cephalosporins with more activity than second-generation cephalosporins against facultative gram-negative bacilli; they have no useful activity against anaerobes or *P. aeruginosa*, and cefixime and ceftibuten have no useful activity against staphylococci. With the exception of cefoperazone (which, like cefamandole, can cause bleeding), ceftazidime and cefepime, the activity of all currently available cephalosporins against *P. aeruginosa* is poor or inconsistent.

[9]Many strains of coagulase-positive and coagulase-negative staphylococci are resistant to penicillinase-resistant penicillins; these strains are also resistant to cephalosporins, imipenem, and meropenem, and are often resistant to fluoroquinolones, trimethoprim-sulfamethoxazole, and clindamycin. Community-acquired MRSA often is susceptible to clindamycin and trimethoprim-sulfamethoxazole.

[10]Tetracyclines are generally not recommended for pregnant women or children younger than 8 years of age.

[11]For serious soft-tissue infection due to group A streptococci, clindamycin may be more effective than penicillin. Group A streptococci may, however, be resistant to clindamycin; therefore, some *Medical Letter* consultants suggest using both clindamycin and penicillin, with or without I.V. immune globulin, to treat serious soft-tissue infections. Surgical debridement is usually needed for necrotizing soft tissue infections due to group A streptococci. Group A streptococci may also be resistant to erythromycin, azithromycin, and clarithromycin.

[12]Penicillin V (or amoxicillin) is preferred for oral treatment of infections caused by nonpenicillinase-producing streptococci. For initial therapy of severe infections, penicillin G, administered parenterally, is first choice. For somewhat longer action in less severe infections due to group A streptococci, pneumococci or *Treponema pallidum*, procaine penicillin G, an intramuscular formulation, can be given once or twice daily, but is seldom used now. Benzathine penicillin G, a slowly absorbed preparation, is usually given in a single monthly injection for prophylaxis of rheumatic fever, once for treatment of group A streptococcal pharyngitis and once or more for treatment of syphilis.

[13]Not recommended for use in pregnancy.

[14]Some strains of *S. pneumoniae* are resistant to erythromycin, clindamycin, trimethoprim-sulfamethoxazole, clarithromycin, azithromycin, and chloramphenicol, and resistance to the newer fluoroquinolones is rare but increasing (Davidson R, Cavalcanti R, Brunton JL, et al, "Resistance to Levofloxacin and Failure of Treatment of Pneumococcal Pneumonia," *N Engl J Med*, 2002, 346(10):747-50). Nearly all strains tested so far are susceptible to linezolid and quinupristin/dalfopristin *in vitro*.

[15]Fluoroquinolone-resistant strains of gonococcus are increasingly common (*MMWR*, 2002, 51:1041; Fenton KA, Ison C, Johnson AP, et al, "Ciprofloxacin Resistance in *Neisseria gonorrhoeae* in England and Wales in 2002," *Lancet*, 2003, 361(9372):1867-9). The CDC no longer recommends quinolones for empiric treatment of sexually-transmitted gonococcal disease ("Update to CDC's Sexually Transmitted Diseases Treatment Guidelines, 2006: Fluoroquinolones No Longer Recommended for Treatment of Gonococcal Infections," *MMWR*, 2007, 56(14):332-6).

[16]Usually not recommended for use in children or pregnant women.

[17]Patients with gonorrhea should be treated presumptively for coinfection with *C. trachomatis* with azithromycin or doxycycline.

[18]Rare strains of *N. meningitidis* are resistant or relatively resistant to penicillin. A fluoroquinolone or rifampin is recommended for prophylaxis after close contact with infected patients.

[19]Because of the possibility of serious adverse effects, this drug should be used only for severe infections when less hazardous drugs are ineffective.

[20]Sulfonamide-resistant strains are frequent in the U.S.A; sulfonamides should be used only when susceptibility is established by susceptibility tests.

[21]For postexposure prophylaxis, ciprofloxacin for 4 weeks if given with vaccination, and 60 days if not given with vaccination, might prevent disease; if the strain is susceptible, doxycycline is an alternative (Bartlett JG, Inglesby TV Jr, and Borio L, "Management of Anthrax," *Clin Infect Dis*, 2002, 35(7):851-8; *Medical Letter*, 2001, 43:87.

[22]Debridement is primary. Large doses of penicillin G are required. Hyperbaric oxygen therapy may be a useful adjunct to surgical debridement in management of the spreading, necrotizing type of infection.

[23]For prophylaxis, a tetanus toxoid booster and, for some patients, tetanus immune globulin (human) are required.

[24]In order to decrease the emergence of vancomycin-resistant enterococci in hospitals and to reduce costs, most clinicians now recommend use of metronidazole first in treatment of patients with *C. difficile* colitis, with oral vancomycin used only for seriously ill patients or those who do not respond to metronidazole.

[25]Antitoxin is primary; antimicrobials are used only to halt further toxin production and to prevent the carrier state.

[26]In severely ill patients, most *Medical Letter* consultants would add gentamicin, tobramycin, or amikacin.

[27]In severely ill patients, most *Medical Letter* consultants would add gentamicin, tobramycin, or amikacin (but see footnote 40).

[28]For an acute, uncomplicated urinary tract infection, before the infecting organism is known, the drug of first choice is trimethoprim-sulfamethoxazole.

[29]Large doses (6 g or more daily) are usually necessary for systemic infections. In severely ill patients, some *Medical Letter* consultants would add gentamicin, tobramycin, or amikacin.

[30]A fluoroquinolone or amoxicillin is the drug of choice for *S. typhi* carriers (Parry CM, Hien TT, Dougan G, "Typhoid Fever," *N Engl J Med*, 2002, 347 (22):1770-82).

[31]Frenck RW Jr, Nakhla I, Sultan Y, et al, "Azithromycin Versus Ceftriaxone for the Treatment of Uncomplicated Typhoid Fever in Children," *Clin Infect Dis*, 2000, 31(5):1134-8.

[32]Most cases of *Salmonella* gastroenteritis subside spontaneously without antimicrobial therapy. Immunosuppressed patients, young children, and the elderly may benefit the most from antibacterials.

[33]Sulbactam may be useful to treat multidrug resistant *Acinetobacter*. It is only available in combination with ampicillin as Unasyn®. *Medical Letter* consultants recommend 3 g I.V. every 4 hours (Urban C, Segal-Maurer S, and Rahal JJ, "Considerations in Control and Treatment of Nosocomial Infections Due to Multidrug-Resistant *Acinetobacter baumannii*," *Clin Infect Dis*, 2003, 36(10):1268-74; Levin AS, Levy CE, Manrique AE, et al, "Severe Nosocomial Infections With Imipenem-Resistant *Acinetobacter baumannii* Treated With Ampicillin/Sulbactam," *Int J Antimicrob Agents*, 2003, 21 (1):58-62.

[34]Role of antibiotics is not clear (Conrad DA, "Treatment of Cat-Scratch Disease," *Curr Opin Pediatr*, 2001, 13(1):56-9).

[35]Pers C, Gahrn-Hansen B, Frederiksen W, et al, " *Capnocytophaga canimorsus* Septicemia in Denmark, 1982-1995: Review of 39 Cases," *Clin Infect Dis*, 1996, 23(1):71-5.

[36]For postexposure prophylaxis, doxycycline, or ciprofloxacin begun during the incubation period and continued for 14 days might prevent disease (*Medical Letter*, 2001, 43:87).

[37]Metronidazole is effective for bacterial vaginosis even though it is not usually active *in vitro* against *Gardnerella*.

[38]Eradication of *H. pylori* with various antibacterial combinations, given concurrently with a proton pump inhibitor or H_2-blocker, has led to rapid healing of active peptic ulcers and low recurrence rates (Mégraud F and Marshall BJ, "How to Treat *Helicobacter pylori*. First-line, Second-line, and Future Therapies," *Gastroenterol Clin North Am*, 2000, 29(4):759-73; *Treatment Guidelines*, 2004, 2:9.).

[39]Proton pump inhibitors available in the U.S.A. are omeprazole (Prilosec®, and others) lansoprazole (Prevacid®), pantoprazole (Protonix®), esomeprazole (Nexium®), and rabeprazole (Aciphex®). Available H_2-blockers include cimetidine (Tagamet®, and others), famotidine (Pepcid®, and others), nizatidine (Axid®, and others), and ranitidine (Zantac®, and others).

[40]Neither gentamicin, tobramycin, netilmicin, or amikacin should be mixed in the same bottle with carbenicillin, ticarcillin, mezlocillin, or piperacillin for intravenous administration. When used in high doses or in patients with renal impairment, these penicillins may inactivate the aminoglycosides.

[41]Antibiotic therapy is an adjunct to and not a substitute for prompt fluid and electrolyte replacement.

[42]Most infections are self-limited without drug treatment.

[43]For treatment of erythema migrans, uncomplicated facial nerve palsy, mild cardiac disease, and arthritis, oral therapy is satisfactory; for other neurologic or more serious cardiac disease, parenteral therapy with ceftriaxone, cefotaxime, or penicillin G is recommended. For recurrent arthritis after an oral regimen, another course of oral therapy or a parenteral drug may be given (Wormser GP, Nadelman RB, Dattwyler RJ, et al, "Practice Guidelines for the Treatment of Lyme Disease. The Infectious Diseases Society of America," *Clin Infect Dis*, 2000, 31(Suppl 1):1-14).

[44]Vinetz JM, "A Mountain Out of a Molehill: Do We Treat Acute Leptospirosis, and if so, With What?" *Clin Infect Dis*, 2003, 36(12):1514-5; Panaphot T et al, *Clin Infect Dis*, 2003, 36:1507.

Adapted with permission from "Choice of Antibacterial Drugs," *Treatment Guidelines*, 2004, 2(19):18-23.

Adapted from "Update to CDC's Sexually Transmitted Diseases Treatment Guidelines, 2006: Fluoroquinolones No Longer Recommended for Treatment of Gonococcal Infections," *MMWR*, 2007, 56(14):332-6.

ANTIRETROVIRAL THERAPY FOR HIV INFECTION: ADULTS AND ADOLESCENTS

Adapted from the Panel on Antiretroviral Guidelines for Adult and Adolescents, "Guidelines for the Use of Antiretroviral Agents in HIV-1-Infected Adults and Adolescents," Department of Health and Human Services, November 3, 2008; 1-139. Available at http://www.aidsinfo.nih.gov/ContentFiles/AdultandAdolescentGL.pdf. Accessed January 26, 2009.

GOALS OF THERAPY

Goals of Therapy

- Maximal and durable suppression of viral load
- Restoration and/or preservation of immunologic function
- Improvement of quality of life
- Reduction of HIV-related morbidity and mortality
- Prevent vertical HIV transmission

Tools to Achieve Goals of Therapy

- Rational selection and sequencing of drugs
- Maximize adherence to the antiretroviral regimen
- Preservation of future treatment options
- Use of pretreatment drug resistance testing and therapeutic drug monitoring in selected clinical settings

Indications for Viral Load Assessment

Indications for Plasma HIV RNA Testing[1]

Clinical Indication	Information	Use
Syndrome consistent with acute HIV infection	Establishes diagnosis when HIV antibody test is negative or indeterminate	Diagnosis[2]
Initial evaluation of newly diagnosed HIV infection	Baseline viral load "set point"	Decision to start or defer therapy (in conjunction with $CD4^+$ T-cell counts)
Every 3-4 months in patients not on therapy	Changes in viral load	Decision to start therapy (in conjunction with $CD4^+$ T-cell counts)
2-4 weeks (preferably, but not more than 8 weeks) after initiation or change in antiretroviral therapy. Repeat at 4-8 week intervals until level falls below limit of detection	Initial assessment of drug efficacy	Decision to continue or change therapy
2-8 weeks after change in antiretroviral therapy due to drug toxicity or regimen simplification	Confirm potency of new regimen	Decision to continue or change therapy
Every 3-4 months in patients on stable therapy; some clinicians may extend interval to every 6 months in adherent patients who have viral suppression for >2-3 years and are clinically stable	Durability of antiretroviral effect	Decision to continue or change therapy
Clinical event or significant decline in $CD4^+$ T cells	Association with changing or stable viral load	Decision to continue, initiate, or change therapy

[1]Acute illness (eg, bacterial pneumonia, tuberculosis, HSV, PCP) and immunizations can cause increases in plasma HIV RNA for 2-4 weeks; viral load testing should not be performed during this time. Plasma HIV RNA results should usually be verified with a repeat determination before starting or making changes in therapy.

[2]Diagnosis of HIV infection determined by HIV RNA testing should be confirmed by standard methods (eg, Western blot serology) performed 2-4 months after the initial indeterminate or negative test.

WHEN TO TREAT

Criteria for Initiating Treatment

The optimal time to initiate therapy in asymptomatic individuals with >200 $CD4^+$ T cells is not known. This table provides general guidance rather than absolute recommendations for an individual patient. Recent literature suggests that a $CD4^+$ cell count may be a more important prognostic indicator than viral load and that a significantly increased risk of progression occurs when viral load exceeds 100,000 copies/mL. All decisions to initiate therapy should be based on prognosis as determined by the $CD4^+$ T-cell count and viral load, the potential benefits and risks of therapy, and the willingness of the patient to accept therapy.

Indications for the Initiation of Antiretroviral Therapy in the Chronically HIV-1 Infected Patient

Clinical Category and / or $CD4^+$ T Cell Count	Recommendation
History of AIDS defining illness[1]	Treat
$CD4^+$ T cells <200/mm^3	Treat[2]
$CD4^+$ T cells ≥200/mm^3 but ≤350/mm^3	Treat[3]
Pregnancy	Treat
HIV-associated nephropathy	Treat
Coinfection with hepatitis B (HBV, when treatment indicated)	Treat
$CD4^+$ T cells >350/mm^3	Assess benefit:risk of treatment initiation or deferring therapy[4]

[1]AIDS-defining illness per Centers for Disease Control, 1993. Severe symptoms include unexplained fever or diarrhea >2-4 weeks, oral candidiasis, or >10% unexplained weight loss.

[2]Randomized controlled trials strongly support initiation of therapy in patients with $CD4^+$ T cells <200/mm^3. Strong evidence from a prospective controlled study showed that treatment of symptomatic patients and patients with $CD4^+$ T cells <200/mm^3 improved survival and reduced disease progression.

[3]No randomized trial addresses the optimal time to initiate therapy in patients with CD4 T cells >200/mm^3. Recommendation to treat is based on several large, long-term observational cohort studies which collectively support use of ART in all patients with $CD4^+$ T cells>200/mm^3.

[4]Optimal time to initiate therapy in asymptomatic patients with $CD4^+$ T cells >350/mm^3 is not well defined.

Benefits and Risks of Early Treatment

Benefits and Risks of Early Treatment in the Asymptomatic HIV-Infected Patient (With $CD4^+$ T cells >350/mm^3)[1]

Benefits	Risks
• Higher $CD4^+$ T cell count maintenance and prevention of potentially irreversible immune system damage • Decreased risk for complications associated with HIV at $CD4^+$ T cells >350/mm^3 (eg, tuberculosis, non-Hodgkin's lymphoma, peripheral neuropathy) • Decreased risk of nonopportunistic conditions (eg, cardiovascular disease, renal/liver disease, non-AIDS associated malignancies/ infections) • Decreased risk of HIV transmission to others[2]	• Side effects/toxicities associated with treatment • Drug resistance occurring from lack of complete viral suppression leading to a loss of future treatment options • Less time to prepare patient with HIV education stressing need for adherence to therapy • Prematurely using therapy before possible development of more effective, less toxic agents, and additional studies using HIV antiretroviral combinations • Transmission of drug resistant virus in patients without full virologic suppression[2] • Disease progression

[1]See table, "Indications for the Initiation of Antiretroviral Therapy in the Chronically HIV-1 Infected Patient," for consensus recommendations regarding when to initiate therapy.

[2]Antiretroviral therapy cannot substitute for primary HIV prevention measures (eg, use of condoms and safer sex practices).

TREATMENT OPTIONS

Recommended Antiretroviral Agents for Initial Treatment of Established HIV Infection

The following tables provide a guide to treatment regimens for patients who have no previous experience with HIV therapy. Regimens should be individualized based on the advantages and disadvantages of each combination such as pill burden, dosing frequency, toxicities, drug-drug interactions, patient variables (such as pregnancy), comorbid conditions, and level of plasma HIV-RNA. Regimens are designated as "preferred" for use in treatment-naive patients when clinical trial data suggest optimal efficacy and durability with acceptable tolerability and ease of use. Alternative regimens are those in which clinical trial data show efficacy, but may be disadvantageous compared to the preferred regimens in terms of antiviral activity, demonstrated durable effect, tolerability, or ease of use. Based on individual patient characteristics, a regimen listed as an alternative may actually be the preferred regimen for a selected patient. Of note, the designation of preferred or alternative regimens may change as new safety and efficacy data emerge, which, in the opinion of the Panel, warrants reassignment of regimens in these categories. Revisions will be updated on an ongoing basis. Clinicians initiating antiretroviral regimens in pregnant women or pediatric patients should refer to the specific guidelines found at http://www.aidsinfo.nih.gov/guidelines. Additional guidelines are available for postexposure prophylaxis (occupational and nonoccupational) as well as management of opportunistic infections.

NNRTI-Based Regimens

Preferred Regimens	**Efavirenz + emtricitabine + tenofovir – except in 1st trimester pregnancy or women with high pregnancy potential[1]**
Alternative Regimens	Efavirenz + (lamivudine or emtricitabine) + (zidovudine or didanosine or abacavir[2] – except in 1st trimester pregnancy or women with high pregnancy potential[1]
	Nevirapine[3] + (lamivudine or emtricitabine) + (zidovudine or didanosine or abacavir or tenofovir). **Note:** Nevirapine should only be used if $CD4^+$ T-cell counts are ≤250 cells/mm^3 in women or ≤400 cells/mm^3 in men. Nevirapine in combination with tenofovir/emtricitabine (or lamivudine) should be used with caution; early virologic failure has been reported.

[1]Women with high pregnancy potential implies women who want to conceive or those who are not using effective contraception.

[2]To reduce the potential for abacavir-induced hypersensitivity, patients should not receive abacavir unless confirmed to be negative for the HLA-B*5701 genotype.

[3]High incidence (11%) of hepatotoxicity and skin reactions; close clinical monitoring advised, especially during first 18 months of therapy. Do not use in treatment-naïve patients with $CD4^+$ T-cell counts of >250 cells/mm^3 in women or >400 cells/mm^3 in men.

PI-Based Regimens

Preferred Regimens	**Lopinavir / ritonavir[1] (once or twice-daily regimen) + emtricitabine + tenofovir**
	Fosamprenavir and ritonavir[2] (twice-daily regimen) + emtricitabine + tenofovir
	Atazanavir and ritonavir[2,3] (once daily) + emtricitabine + tenofovir
	Darunavir and ritonavir[2] (once daily) + emtricitabine + tenofovir
Alternative Regimens	Fosamprenavir and ritonavir[2] (once-daily regimen) + (lamivudine or emtricitabine) + (zidovudine or abacavir[4] or tenofovir or didanosine)
	Fosamprenavir (twice daily) + (lamivudine or emtricitabine) + (zidovudine or abacavir[4] or tenofovir or didanosine)
	Atazanavir (once daily) + (lamivudine or emtricitabine) + (zidovudine or abacavir[4] or didanosine) **Note:** Do not use unboosted atazanavir in combination with didanosine + emtricitabine (or lamivudine)
	Lopinavir / ritonavir[1] (once-daily or twice-daily regimen) + (emtricitabine or lamivudine) + (abacavir[4] or didanosine or zidovudine)
	Fosamprenavir and ritonavir[2] (twice-daily regimen) + (lamivudine or emtricitabine) + (zidovudine or didanosine or abacavir[4])
	Atazanavir and ritonavir[2,3] (once daily) + (lamivudine or emtricitabine) + (zidovudine or abacavir[4] or didanosine)
	Saquinavir and ritonavir[2] (twice daily)+ (lamivudine or emtricitabine) + (zidovudine or abacavir[4] or tenofovir or didanosine)
	Darunavir + ritonavir[2] (once daily) + (lamivudine or emtricitabine) + (abacavir[4] or didanosine or zidovudine)

[1]Do not use lopinavir/ritonavir in pregnant women.

[2]Ritonavir "boosted" dosing (100-400 mg/day).

[3]Do not use atazanavir/ritonavir combination with high dose Proton Pump Inhibitor (PPI) therapy (>20 mg omeprazole equivalent/day); use caution with any other dose of PPI, H2 blockers, or antacids.

[4]To reduce the potential for abacavir-induced hypersensitivity, patients should not receive abacavir unless confirmed to be negative for the HLA-B*5701 genotype.

Triple NRTI Regimen

Only as alternative to NNRTI- or PI-based regimen – should not be used first-line	Abacavir[1] + lamivudine + zidovudine

[1]To reduce the potential for abacavir-induced hypersensitivity, patients should not receive abacavir unless confirmed to be negative for the HLA-B*5701 genotype.

TREATMENT LIMITATIONS

Antiretroviral Drugs Not Recommended as Initial Therapy

Drugs	Reasons for Not Recommending as Initial Therapy
Abacavir/lamivudine/zidovudine (coformulated) as triple-NRTI combination regimen	• Inferior virologic efficacy
Abacavir + didanosine	• Insufficient data in treatment-naïve patients
Abacavir + tenofovir	• Insufficient data in treatment-naïve patients
Darunavir (unboosted)	• Use without ritonavir has not been studied
Delavirdine	• Inferior virologic efficacy • Inconvenient dosing (3 times/day)
Didanosine + tenofovir	• High rate of early virological failure in combination with efavirenz or nevirapine • Rapid selection of resistant mutations • Potential for immunologic nonresponse
Enfuvirtide	• No clinical trial experience in treatment-naive patients • Requires twice-daily subcutaneous injections
Etravirine	• Insufficient data in treatment-naïve patients
Indinavir (ritonavir-boosted)	• High incidence of nephrolithiasis
Indinavir (unboosted)	• Inconvenient dosing (3 times/day with meal restrictions) • Fluid requirement
Maraviroc	• Insufficient data in treatment-naïve patients
Nelfinavir	• Inferior virologic efficacy
Raltegravir	• Insufficient data in treatment-naïve patients
Ritonavir as sole PI	• High pill burden • Gastrointestinal intolerance
Saquinavir (unboosted)	• High pill burden • Inferior virologic efficacy
Stavudine + lamivudine	• Significant toxicities
Tipranavir (ritonavir-boosted)	• Inferior virologic efficacy

Antiretroviral Drugs Not Recommended as Initial Therapy *(continued)*

Antiretroviral Regimens or Components That Should Not Be Offered at Any Time

	Rationale	Exception
Antiretroviral Regimens Not Recommended		
Monotherapy with NRTI or NNRTI	• Rapid development of resistance • Inferior antiretroviral activity when compared to combination with three or more antiretrovirals	Pregnant women with HIV-RNA <1000 copies/mL using zidovudine monotherapy for prevention of perinatal HIV transmission[1] and not for HIV treatment for the mother
Dual-NRTI drug combinations	• Rapid development of resistance • Inferior antiretroviral activity when compared to combination with three or more antiretrovirals	No exception
Triple-NRTI combinations	• High rate of early virologic nonresponse seen when this triple NRTI combination was used as initial regimen in treatment-naive patients	May consider (abacavir or possibly tenofovir) + zidovudine + lamivudine
Antiretroviral Components Not Recommended as Part of Antiretroviral Regimen		
Atazanavir + indinavir	• Potential additive hyperbilirubinemia	No exception
Didanosine + stavudine	• High incidence of toxicities – peripheral neuropathy, pancreatitis, and hyperlactatemia • Reports of serious, even fatal cases of lactic acidosis with hepatic steatosis with or without pancreatitis in pregnant women	When no other antiretroviral options are available and potential benefits outweigh the risks[1]
Dual-NNRTI combinations	• Efavirenz + nevirapine associated with higher incidence of adverse reactions • Efavirenz + nevirapine may induce metabolism leading to reduced drug exposure (shown with etravirine)	No exception
Efavirenz in 1st trimester pregnancy or in women with high pregnancy potential[2]	• Teratogenic in nonhuman primates	When no other antiretroviral options are available and potential benefits outweigh the risks[1]
Emtricitabine + lamivudine	• Similar resistance profile • No potential benefit	No exception
Etravirine + unboosted PI	• Etravirine may induce metabolism of these PIs, appropriate doses not yet established	No exception
Etravirine + ritonavir-boosted atazanavir, fosamprenavir, or tipranavir	• Etravirine may induce metabolism of these PIs, appropriate doses not yet established	No exception
Nevirapine initiation with $CD4^+$ T-cell count >250 cells/mm^3 in women or >400 cells/mm^3 in men	• Higher incidence of symptomatic (including serious or fatal) hepatic events	Only if benefit clearly outweighs risk
Saquinavir hard gel capsule (Invirase®) as **single** protease inhibitor	• Poor oral bioavailability (4%) • Inferior antiretroviral activity when compared to other protease inhibitors	No exception
Stavudine + zidovudine	• Antagonistic	No exception
Unboosted darunavir, saquinavir, or tipranavir	• Inadequate bioavailability	No exception

[1]When constructing an antiretroviral regimen for an HIV-infected pregnant woman, please consult "Public Health Service Task Force Recommendations for the Use of Antiretroviral Drugs in Pregnant HIV-1-Infected Women for Maternal Health and Interventions to Reduce Perinatal HIV-1 Transmission in the United States" in http://www.aidsinfo.nih.gov/guidelines.

[2]Women with high pregnancy potential implies women who want to conceive or those who are not using effective contraception.

SPECIAL CONSIDERATIONS

Resistance Testing

Viral drug resistance is generally determined by one of two methods: genotypic assays or phenotypic assays. Genotypic assays involve sequencing techniques to identify the presence of specific drug-resistant genes. While these assays produce relatively rapid results (1-2 weeks) they require knowledge of specific drug-resistance mutations for appropriate interpretation. Alternatively, phenotypic assays measure the ability of the patient's virus (as monitored by recombination with a reporter gene) to replicate in the presence of antiretroviral drugs. These assays can be more time-consuming and costly, and also suffer from the drawback that resistance level breakpoints are unknown.

Despite these methodological limitations, resistance testing can assist in designing an appropriate therapeutic regimen, by identifying, and thus avoiding less effective antiretroviral drugs in the setting of virologic failure. In addition, prior knowledge of specific drug-resistant viral phenotypes can guide selection of initial therapy which offers a greater likelihood of success.

The following table identifies the appropriate settings for the use of resistance testing.

Clinical Setting	Drug-Resistance Assay Recommendation[1]	Rationale
Virologic failure during combination antiretroviral therapy >1000 copies/mL. May consider testing in patients with levels >500 but <1000 copies/mL	Recommended	Determine the role of resistance in drug failure and maximize selection of active drugs. Test while on therapy or within 4 weeks of discontinuation.
Suboptimal suppression of viral load after antiretroviral therapy initiation	Recommended	Determine the role of resistance and maximize selection of active drugs.
Acute HIV infection regardless of whether therapy is initiated	Recommended	Determine if drug-resistant virus was transmitted to assist in designing initial regimen. If therapy deferred, testing will permit detection of resistance factors earlier in the course of infection; consider retesting when initiating antiretroviral treatment.
Chronic HIV, regardless of whether therapy is initiated	Recommended	Baseline resistance may be present in up to 16% of patients, leading to suboptimal virologic response. If therapy deferred, testing will permit detection of resistance factors earlier in the course of infection; consider retesting when initiating antiretroviral treatment.
Pregnancy, prior to initiation of therapy, or when entering pregnancy with detectable RNA levels	Recommended	Goal to achieve maximal viral suppression and prevent perinatal transmission.
After discontinuation of drugs (>4 weeks)	Not usually recommended	Assays may not detect minor drug-resistant species which may occur in the absence of selective drug pressure.
Plasma viral load <500 HIV RNA copies/mL	Not usually recommended	Assays may not reliably detect low numbers of viral RNA.

[1]Genotypic assays are recommended due to more rapid turnaround time.

Summary of Guidelines for Changing an Antiretroviral Regimen for Suspected Treatment Regimen Failure

Patient Assessment

- Review antiretroviral treatment history.
- Assess for evidence of clinical progression (eg, physical exam, laboratory and/or radiologic tests)
- Assess adherence, tolerability, and pharmacokinetic issues.
- Distinguish between limited, intermediate, and extensive prior therapy and drug resistance.
- Perform resistance testing while patient is taking therapy (or within 4 weeks after regimen discontinuation).
- Assess for virologic failure.
- Identify active drugs and drug classes to use in designing new regimen, taking into consideration importance of drug sequencing and cross-resistance issues.

Patient Management: Specific Clinical Scenarios

- **Prior treatment with no resistance identified:** Consider the timing of the drug resistance test (eg, was the patient off antiretroviral medications for >4 weeks?) and/or nonadherence. Consider resuming the same regimen or starting a new regimen and then repeating genotypic testing early (eg, 2-4 weeks) to determine if a resistant virus becomes evident. Consider intensifying with one drug (eg, tenofovir) or pharmacokinetic enhancement (ie, ritonavir boosting). If continuing the same treatment regimen, HIV RNA levels should be followed closely because ongoing viral replication will lead to accumulation of additional resistance mutations.
- **Limited Prior treatment and drug resistance:** The goal of treatment is to resuppress HIV RNA maximally (eg, <50 copies/mL). Consider changing regimens sooner, rather than later to minimize resistance selection. This is particularly important with evidence of NNRTI resistance. New regimens should include two, and preferably three fully active agents.
- **Extensive prior treatment and drug resistance:** In patients with active antiretroviral agents available (eg, an active ritonavir-boosted PI with enfuvirtide), the goal of therapy is suppression of viremia (<50 copies/mL). In patients without active antiretroviral agents available in which maximal viral suppression cannot be achieved, the goal of therapy is preservation of immune response and delay of clinical progression.
- **Cannot identify new regimen with at least 2 fully-active agents:** It is reasonable to continue the same antiretroviral regimen with observation if there are few or no treatment options. Evidence suggests that continued therapy in the presence of viremia and stable CD4 counts decreases the risk of disease progression. In general, avoid adding a single active drug because of the risk for the rapid development of resistance to that drug. In advanced HIV disease with a high likelihood of clinical progression (eg, $CD4^+$ cell count <100 cells/mm^3), adding a single drug may reduce the risk of immediate clinical progression. In this complicated scenario, expert advise should be sought.
- **Immunologic failure (or blunted $CD4^+$ response) with virologic suppression:** Immunologic failure (or blunted $CD4^+$ cell response) may not warrant a change in therapy in the setting of suppressed viremia. Factors to assess for immunologic failure include low baseline CD4 counts (<200/mm^3), older age, coinfection (eg, HCV), certain medication regimens (eg, tenofovir + ddI), persistent immune activation, and loss of immune system regenerative potential. In the setting of immunologic failure (or blunted $CD4^+$ response <200/mm^3), changing drug regimens is an unproven strategy, but should be considered if the regimen or a specific component is believed to be a contributing factor in the immunologic failure. Intensifying with additional antiretroviral drugs or the use of immune-based therapies (eg, interleukin-2) to improve immunologic responses remain unproven strategies and generally should not be offered.

Treatment Options Following Virologic Failure on Initial Recommended Therapy Regimens

Antiretroviral therapy regimens should be selected on the basis of treatment history and drug-resistance testing to optimize antiretroviral potency in the second regimen. This is particularly important in selecting NRTIS for an NNRTI-based regimen where drug resistance may occur rapidly to the NNRTI if the NRTIs are not sufficiently potent.

General Considerations

- Design new regimen with at least two, and preferably three, fully active drugs, based on history, resistance testing, and/or new mechanistic class. **Note:** A "new" drug that a patient has not yet been exposed to may not necessarily be fully-active. Class cross-resistance must be considered.
- Conduct resistance testing while patient is on the failing regimen, to better identify fully-active agents.
- Adding only a single, fully active drug to an existing regimen is typically not recommended due to potential for rapid resistance development. An exception would be in patients with a high risk for clinical progression and for whom limited drug options exist. In this setting, addition of a single agent may reduce risk of progression.
- Consider drug sequencing and potential for class-associated cross-resistance when designing new regimens. This is particularly evident with NNRTIs, in which mutations conferring resistance to one agent reduce the effectiveness of the others (except etravirine).
- New options for treatment-experienced patients exhibiting resistance and/or virologic failure include maraviroc, raltegravir, and etravirine.

Discontinuation or Interruption of Therapy

Short-term Interruption

- Planned or unplanned interruption of therapy may occur due to a number of situations including, but not limited to, adverse drug reactions, intercurrent illness, and surgical procedures. Generally, short-term therapy interruptions (as with elective surgery) can be managed by simultaneously stopping all drug therapy, as long as all components of the regimen exhibit similar half-lives. Accordingly, all drugs would be resumed simultaneously when clinically appropriate.
- However, in the event that the medication regimen includes drugs exhibiting different biological half-lives, there is a risk of inducing functional monotherapy when discontinuing all of the medications at once. There is no clear guidance on how best to address this situation. One option may involve discontinuing the drug with the longest half-life first (typically an NNRTI such as nevirapine or efavirenz), while continuing the other components of therapy, ideally for the duration of detectable plasma levels of the first drug. Given the polymorphic nature of drug metabolism, this "endpoint" is difficult to ascertain. Thus, some experts recommend substituting the NNRTI with a PI, and continuing with the other components of the regimen for approximately 4 weeks.
- In the event of a severe or life-threatening toxicity, all components of the drug regimen should be discontinued, regardless of half-life.

Long-term Discontinuation

- A number of strategies have been considered as a basis for treatment interruption. These include preservation of virologic response in patients with few treatment options, patients who have achieved virologic suppression, or who have maintained a CD4 count above recommended treatment initiation threshold levels. Additionally, planned discontinuation has been proposed as a method for reducing the overall costs, inconvenience, and/or toxicities of therapy. However, data are conflicting with respect to optimal discontinuation/reinitiation parameters and current clinical trials data have generally shown worsened outcomes in those who have experienced a planned interruption compared to patients on continuous therapy. Therefore, planned long-term treatment interruptions are **not** recommended under any circumstance outside of a controlled, clinical trial setting. Nevertheless, if discontinuation is going to be implemented, both the patient and physician must be aware of the potential complications or consequences of this action, including, but not limited to viral rebound, disease progression, and opportunistic infection.

Recommendations for Treatment of Hepatitis B (HBV) or Hepatitis C (HCV) Coinfection

HBV

- All patients should be advised to avoid alcohol and receive hepatitis A vaccine (if not previously immunized).
- Use more than one antiretroviral agent with activity against hepatitis B virus. Recommended first-line therapy should consist of tenofovir + lamivudine or tenofovir + emtricitabine as the NRTI backbone. Lamivudine, emtricitabine, or tenofovir should **not** be the sole agent with anti-HBV activity in an antiretroviral regimen due to the risk for resistance.
- Discontinuation of antiviral agents with activity against HBV has been associated with hepatocellular damage due to flare of HBV infection.
- HBV coinfection increases the risk of medication-related transaminase elevations. Generally, it is recommended to withhold the causative agent when ALT is ≥5-10 times ULN, but one should recognize that transaminase elevations may signify HB_eAg seroconversion.
- If treating HBV only: Peginterferon alfa may be used since it does not induce HIV or HBV resistance.

HCV

- All patients should be advised to avoid alcohol and receive hepatitis A and B vaccines (if not previously immunized).
- Initiate treatment according to standard guidelines, preferentially in patients with a higher CD4 count (>200 cells/mm^3); in those with lower CD4 counts, HCV treatment may be deferred in favor of antiretroviral therapy.
- Monitor closely for drug interactions.
- Growth factors may be necessary to manage HCV treatment-related anemia or neutropenia.

Therapeutic Drug Monitoring

As with other drug classes (eg, antibiotics, anticonvulsants), the goal of therapeutic drug monitoring (TDM) is to maximize therapeutic efficacy and minimize drug-related toxicities. The utility of TDM in the setting of antiretroviral drug therapy is supported by data showing considerable interpatient variability with respect to drug concentrations among patients taking similar doses, as well as data demonstrating concentration/effect and concentration/toxicity correlations.

However, limitations involving use of TDM include lack of prospective data showing improved outcomes due to TDM. Further, the optimal plasma concentrations of many antiretroviral drugs have yet to be determined (eg, NRTIs). At present, TDM is not recommended for routine use in the management of the HIV infected adult. Those drugs for which target trough levels are defined are shown below on next page.

Suggested Minimum Target Trough Concentrations for Persons With Wild-Type HIV-1

Drug	Concentration (ng/mL)
Amprenavir **or** Fosamprenavir	400 (concentration assayed as amprenavir)
Atazanavir	150
Indinavir	100
Lopinavir / ritonavir (Kaletra®)	1000
Nelfinavir[1]	800
Ritonavir[2]	2100
Saquinavir	100-250
Efavirenz	1000
Nevirapine	3400
Recommendations Applicable Only to Treatment-Experienced Persons Who Have Resistant HIV-1 Strains	
Maraviroc	>50
Tipranavir	20,500

[1]Measurable active M8 metabolite.

[2]Ritonavir given as a single PI.

Regimen Simplification

Regimen simplification involves a change in effective established therapy to reduce pill burden and dosing frequency, to enhance tolerability, or to decrease requirements involving food or fluid intake. The rationale behind simplification involves improving the patient's quality of life and adherence, decreasing the risk of virologic failure, and avoiding long-term drug toxicities.

Candidates for regimen simplification include:

- Patients without suspected drug-resistant virus. Patients on first or modified antiretroviral regimens without a history of treatment failure are less likely to harbor drug-resistant virus, particularly if a pretreatment genotype did not detect drug resistance, and are ideal candidates for regimen simplification.
- Patients with documented or suspected drug resistance. Simplification may be appropriate in certain selected patients whose virus is suppressed after having either documented or suspected drug resistance. Generally, these patients are on regimens that were selected at a time when there was limited understanding of the management of drug resistance, drug-drug interactions, and treatment options. Patients may be able to take advantage of newer agents which offer simplified regimens without sacrificing antiviral activity. However, simplifying regimens in patients with extensive treatment histories should be done only after an extensive review of treatment history, response and resistance tests, and after consideration given to seeking expert consultation.

Types of Treatment Simplification: Within-Class Simplifications and Out-of-Class Substitutions

Within-Class Simplifications	Appropriate Patient or Rationale
NRTI substitutions (eg, changing from zidovudine or stavudine to tenofovir or abacavir)	Patients without a history of viral resistance on a NRTI regimen. Create regimens with lower dosing frequency using coformulated agents which may avoid long-term toxicity
Switching of NNRTIs (eg, from nevirapine to efavirenz)	Reduce dosing frequency or use coformulated agents
Switching of PIs (eg, one PI or another, same PI at lower dosing frequency, or administration without ritonavir boosting)	Patients without a history of documented or suspected PI resistance; switching is not recommended in patients with a history of documented/suspected PI resistance (lack of convincing data in these patients)
Out-of-Class Substitutions	**Considerations**
Change from a PI-based to an NNRTI-based regimen	Consider potential for drug-resistant virus prior to attempting; high treatment failure has been observed in patients who had previous suboptimal response with either mono- or dual-NRTI therapy
Change involving utilization of novel drug class (eg, raltegravir and maraviroc)	Limited study information available
Reducing the number of active drugs in a currently suppressive regimen to a regimen with fewer active drugs	Not recommended in any patient at present

COMMUNITY-ACQUIRED PNEUMONIA IN ADULTS

Alternative methods exist to facilitate the objective rating of disease severity in community-acquired pneumonia patients in order to guide appropriate site of care and aggressiveness of treatment. The first option, the Pneumonia Severity Index (PSI) was derived from the Pneumonia Patient Outcomes Research Team (PORT). This is a well-validated instrument which stratifies patients based on risk of mortality; however, calculation of the patient's score requires assessment of 19 variables. The second method is referred to as the "Confusion, Uremia, Respiratory rate, Blood pressure, and age >65 years (CURB-65)" score. This system has fewer variables to evaluate and focuses more on assessment of disease severity, but is less well validated. In either case, these measures should not be used in exclusion to appropriate clinical judgement.

PNEUMONIA SEVERITY INDEX (PSI)

The initial site of treatment should be based on a 3-step process:

1. Assessment of pre-existing conditions that compromise safety of home care
2. Calculation of the Pneumonia Severity Index with recommendation for home care for risk classes I, II, and III, and
3. Clinical judgment

Algorithm

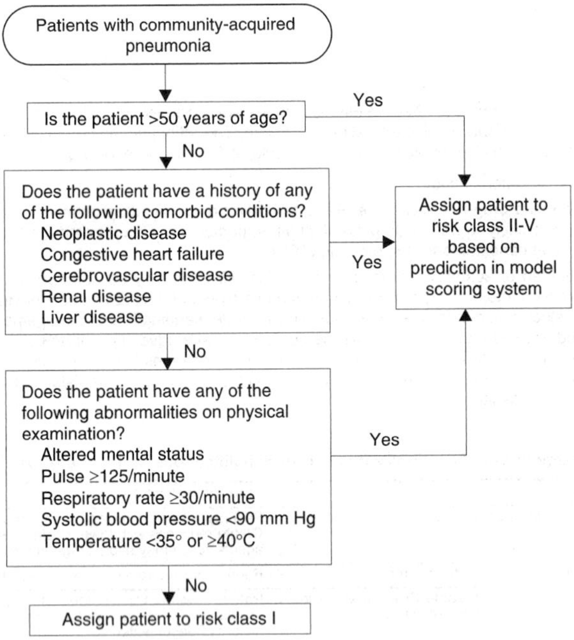

Stratification of Risk Score

Risk	Risk Class	Based on
Low	I	Algorithm
	II	≤70 total points
	III	71-90 total points
Moderate	IV	91-130 total points
High	V	>130 total points

Risk-Class Mortality Rates for Patients With Pneumonia

		Validation Cohort		
Risk Class	No. of Points	No. of Patients	Mortality (%)	Recommended Site of Care
I	No predictors	3034	0.1	Outpatient
II	≤70	5778	0.6	Outpatient
III	71-90	6790	2.8	Outpatient or brief inpatient
IV	91-130	13,104	8.2	Inpatient
V	>130	9333	29.2	Inpatient

Scoring System: Assignment to Risk Classes II-V

Patient Characteristic	Points Assigned[1]
Demographic factors	
Age	
Male	No. of years
Female	No. of years -10
Nursing home resident	+10
Comorbid illnesses	
Neoplastic disease[2]	+30
Liver disease[3]	+20
Congestive heart failure[4]	+10
Cerebrovascular disease[5]	+10
Renal disease[6]	+10
Physical examination findings	
Altered mental status[7]	+20
Respiratory rate >30 breaths/minute	+20
Systolic blood pressure <90 mm Hg	+20
Temperature <35°C or >40°C	+15
Pulse >125 beats/minute	+10
Laboratory or radiographic findings	
Arterial pH <7.35	+30
BUN >30 mg/dL	+20
Sodium <130 mEq/L	+20
Glucose >250 mg/dL	+10
Hematocrit <30%	+10
pO_2 <60 mm Hg[8]	+10
Pleural effusion	+10

[1]A total point score for a given patient is obtained by adding the patient's age in years (age -10, for females) and the points for each applicable patient characteristic.

[2]Any cancer, except basal or squamous cell cancer of the skin, that was active at the time of presentation or diagnosed within 1 year of presentation.

[3]A clinical or histologic diagnosis of cirrhosis or other form of chronic liver disease such as chronic active hepatitis.

[4]Systolic or diastolic ventricular dysfunction documented by history and physical examination, as well as chest radiography, echocardiography, Muga scanning, or left ventriculography.

[5]A clinical diagnosis of stroke, transient ischemic attack, or stroke documented by MRI or computed axial tomography.

[6]A history of chronic renal disease or abnormal blood urea nitrogen (BUN) and creatinine values documented in the medical record.

[7]Disorientation (to person, place, or time; not known to be chronic), stupor, or coma.

[8]In the Pneumonia Patient Outcome Research Team cohort study, an oxygen saturation value <90% on pulse oximetry or intubation before admission was also considered abnormal.

CONFUSION, UREMIA, RESPIRATORY RATE, BLOOD PRESSURE, AND AGE >65 YEARS (CURB-65)

Risk factors:

1. Presence of confusion (based on specific tests or noted disorientation to people, place, or time)
2. Blood urea nitrogen (BUN) of >7mmol/L (20 mg/dL)
3. Respiratory rate >30 breaths/minute
4. Systolic blood pressure <90 mmHg or diastolic <60 mmHg
5. Age >65 years

Number of Risk Factors	30-Day Mortality Risk (%)
0	0.7
1	2.1
2	9.2
3	14.5
4	40
5	57

Scoring:

0-1 risk factors: Treat as outpatient.

2 risk factors: Treat as inpatient.

3-5 risk factors: Treat as inpatient; likely requires more aggressive management, possibly ICU.

Epidemiological Conditions Related to Specific Pathogens in Patients With Selected Community-Acquired Pneumonia

Condition	Commonly Encountered Pathogens
Alcoholism	*Streptococcus pneumoniae*, anaerobes
COPD and/or smoker	*S. pneumoniae, Haemophilus influenzae, Moraxella catarrhalis, Legionella* species
Nursing home residency	*S. pneumoniae*, gram-negative bacilli, *H. influenzae, Staphylococcus aureus*, anaerobes, *Chlamydia pneumoniae*
Poor dental hygiene	Anaerobes
Epidemic Legionnaires' disease	*Legionella* species
Exposure to bats or soil enriched with bird droppings	*Histoplasma capsulatum*
Exposure to birds	*Chlamydia psittaci*
Exposure to rabbits	*Francisella tularensis*
HIV infection (early stage)	*S. pneumoniae, H. influenzae, Mycobacterium tuberculosis*
HIV infection (late stage)	Above plus *P. carinii, Cryptococcus, Histoplasma* species
Travel to southwestern United States	*Coccidioides* species
Exposure to farm animals or parturient cats	*Coxiella burnetii* (Q fever)
Influenza active in community	Influenza, *S. pneumoniae, S. aureus, Streptococcus pyogenes, H. influenzae*
Suspected large-volume aspiration	Anaerobes (chemical pneumonitis, obstruction)
Structural disease of the lung (bronchiectasis, cystic fibrosis, etc)	*Pseudomonas aeruginosa, Burkholderia (Pseudomonas) cepacia, S. aureus*
Injection drug use	*S. aureus*, anaerobes, *M. tuberculosis, S. pneumoniae*
Airway obstruction	Anaerobes, *S. pneumoniae, H. influenzae, S. aureus*

COPD = chronic obstructive pulmonary disease.

Initial Empiric Therapy for Suspected Bacterial Community-Acquired Pneumonia (CAP) in Immunocompetent Adults

Patient Variable	Preferred Treatment Options
Outpatient	
Previously healthy	
No recent antibiotic therapy or risk for DRSP	A macrolide[1] or doxycycline
Comorbidities[2]; recent antibiotic therapy[3]; risk factors for DRSP[4]	A respiratory fluoroquinolone[5] alone, or an advanced macrolide[6] plus high-dose amoxicillin,[7] high-dose amoxicillin-clavulanate,[8] cefpodoxime, ceftriaxone, or cefuroxime.
Suspected aspiration with infection	Amoxicillin-clavulanate or clindamycin
Influenza with bacterial superinfection	Antiviral agent oseltamivir or zanamivir, plus a cefotaxime or ceftriaxone or a respiratory fluoroquinolone[5]
Inpatient	
Non-ICU	A respiratory fluoroquinolone alone or macrolide plus a β-lactam[9]
ICU	
Pseudomonas infection is not an issue	Cefotaxime, ceftriaxone, or ampicillin-sulbactam plus either azithromycin or a respiratory fluoroquinolone[5]
Pseudomonas infection is not an issue but patient has a β-lactam allergy	A respiratory fluoroquinolone,[5] with aztreonam
Pseudomonas infection is an issue[10]	Either (1) an antipseudomonal agent[11] plus ciprofloxacin or levofloxacin, or (2) an antipseudomonal agent plus an aminoglycoside[12] plus a respiratory fluoroquinolone[5] or azithromycin
Pseudomonas infection is an issue but the patient has a β-lactam allergy	Substitute aztreonam for any β-lactam antipseudomonal agent[11]
Nursing home	
Receiving treatment in nursing home	A respiratory fluoroquinolone[5] alone or amoxicillin-clavulanate plus an advanced macrolide
Suspicion or MRSA	Add vancomycin or linezolid to any suggested regimens

DRSP = drug-resistant *Streptococcus pneumoniae*; ICU = intensive care unit.

[1]Erythromycin, azithromycin, or clarithromycin.

[2]Chronic heart, lung, liver, and/or renal disease, diabetes, malignancy, or immunosuppressive medication and/or conditions.

[3]That is, the patient was given a course of antibiotic(s) for treatment of any infection within the past 3 months, excluding the current episode of infection. Such treatment is a risk factor for drug-resistant *Streptococcus pneumoniae* and possibly for infection with gram-negative bacilli. Depending on the class of antibiotics recently given, one or other of the suggested options may be selected. Recent use of a fluoroquinolone should dictate selection of a nonfluoroquinolone regimen, and vice versa.

[4]Risk factors for β-lactam-resistant *S. pneumoniae* include age <2 or >65 years, recent antimicrobial therapy (within previous 3 months, and especially to repeated courses of same antibiotic class), alcoholism, comorbidities, immunosuppressive illness or therapy, and exposure to child care centers.

[5]Moxifloxacin, levofloxacin, or gemifloxacin.

[6]Azithromycin or clarithromycin.

[7]Dosage, 1 g P.O. 3 times/day.

[8]Dosage, 2 g P.O. twice daily.

[9]Cefotaxime, ceftriaxone, ampicillin (or ampicillin-sulbactam), or ertapenem; ertapenem was recently approved for such use (in once-daily parenteral treatment), but there is little experience thus far. **Note:** The 2007 CAP guidelines excluded ampicillin-sulbactam in favor of the single agent without the lactamase inhibitor. While this may be useful in specific situations, the prevalence of beta-lactamase-producing *H. influenzae* should be a concern, and thus the use of ampicillin-sulbactam may be more appropriate for empiric use.

[10]The antipseudomonal agents chosen reflect this concern. Risk factors for *Pseudomonas* infection include severe structural lung disease (eg, bronchiectasis), and recent antibiotic therapy or stay in hospital (especially in the ICU). For patients with CAP in the ICU, coverage for *S. pneumoniae* and *Legionella* species must always be assured. Piperacillin-tazobactam, imipenem, meropenem, and cefepime are excellent β-lactams and are adequate for most *S. pneumoniae* and *Haemophilus influenzae* infections. They may be preferred when there is concern for relatively unusual CAP pathogens, such as *Pseudomonas aeruginosa*, *Klebsiella* species, and other gram-negative bacteria.

[11]Piperacillin-tazobactam, imipenem, meropenem, or cefepime.

[12]Data suggest that elderly patients receiving aminoglycosides have worse outcomes.

References

Bartlett JG, Breiman RF, Mandell LA, et al, "Community-Acquired Pneumonia in Adults: Guidelines for Management. The Infectious Diseases Society of America," *Clin Infect Dis*, 1998, 26(4):811-38.

Mandell LA, Bartlett JG, Dowell SF, et al, "Update of Practice Guidelines for the Management of Community-Acquired Pneumonia in Immunocompetent Adults," *Clin Infect Dis*, 2003, 37(11):1405-33.

Mandell LA, Wunderink RG, Anzueto A, et al, "Infectious Diseases Society of America/American Thoracic Society Consensus Guidelines on the Management of Community-Acquired Pneumonia in Adults," *Clin Infect Dis*, 2007, 44(Suppl 2):S27-72.

MALARIA TREATMENT

Malaria Treatment

Recommended Drug	Adult Dose[1,8]	Pediatric Dose[1,8] *(Pediatric dose should NEVER exceed adult dose)*	Region Infection Acquired
Uncomplicated Malaria / *P. falciparum* or Species Not Identified (If "species not identified" is subsequently diagnosed as *P. vivax* or *P. ovale*, see *P. vivax* and *P. ovale* (below) regarding treatment with primaquine)			
Chloroquine phosphate (Aralen® and generics)	600 mg base (= 1000 mg salt) P.O. immediately, followed by 300 mg base (= 500 mg salt) P.O. at 6, 24, and 48 hours Total dose: 1500 mg base (= 2500 mg salt)	10 mg base/kg P.O. immediately, followed by 5 mg base/kg P.O. at 6, 24, and 48 hours Total dose: 25 mg base/kg	**Chloroquine-sensitive** (Central America west of Panama Canal; Haiti; the Dominican Republic; and most of the Middle East)
2nd line alternative for treatment: Hydroxychloroquine (Plaquenil® and generics)	620 mg base (= 800 mg salt) P.O. immediately, followed by 310 mg base (= 400 mg salt) P.O. at 6, 24, and 48 hours Total dose: 1550 mg base (= 2000 mg salt)	10 mg base/kg P.O. immediately, followed by 5 mg base/kg P.O. at 6, 24, and 48 hours Total dose: 25 mg base/kg	
A. Quinine sulfate[2] plus one of the following: Doxycycline, tetracycline, or clindamycin	**Quinine sulfate:** 542 mg base (= 650 mg salt)[3] P.O. tid x 3-7 days **Doxycycline:** 100 mg P.O. bid x 7 days **Tetracycline:** 250 mg P.O. qid x 7 days **Clindamycin:** 20 mg base/kg/day P.O. divided tid x 7 days	**Quinine sulfate:** 8.3 mg base/kg (= 10 mg salt/kg) P.O. tid x 3-7 days **Doxycycline[4]:** 2.2 mg/kg P.O. every 12 hours x 7 days **Tetracycline[4]:** 25 mg/kg/day P.O. divided qid x 7 days **Clindamycin:** 20 mg base/kg/day P.O. divided tid x 7 days	**Chloroquine-resistant or unknown resistance[1]** (All malarious regions except those specified as chloroquine-sensitive listed in the box above. Middle Eastern countries with chloroquine-resistant *P. falciparum* include Iran, Oman, Saudi Arabia, and Yemen. Of note, infections acquired in the Newly Independent States of the former Soviet Union and Korea to date have been uniformly caused by *P. vivax* and should therefore be treated as chloroquine-sensitive infections.)
B. Atovaquone-proguanil (Malarone®)[5]	**Adult tab = 250 mg atovaquone/100 mg proguanil** 4 adult tabs P.O. qd x 3 days	**Adult tab = 250 mg atovaquone/100 mg proguanil** **Peds tab = 62.5 mg atovaquone/25 mg proguanil** 5-8 kg: 2 peds tabs P.O. qd x 3 d 9-10 kg: 3 peds tabs P.O. qd x 3 d 11-20 kg: 1 adult tab P.O. qd x 3 d 21-30 kg: 2 adult tabs P.O. qd x 3 d 31-40 kg: 3 adult tabs P.O. qd x 3 d >40 kg: 4 adult tabs P.O. qd x 3 d	
C. Mefloquine (Lariam® and generics)[6]	684 mg base (= 750 mg salt) P.O. as initial dose, followed by 456 mg base (= 500 mg salt) P.O. given 6-12 hours after initial dose Total dose = 1250 mg salt	13.7 mg base/kg (= 15 mg salt/kg) P.O. as initial dose, followed by 9.1 mg base/kg (= 10 mg salt/kg) P.O. given 6-12 hours after initial dose Total dose = 25 mg salt/kg	
Uncomplicated Malaria / *P. malariae*			
Chloroquine phosphate	Treatment as above	Treatment as above	**All regions**
2nd line alternative for treatment: Hydroxychloroquine	Treatment as above	Treatment as above	
Uncomplicated Malaria / *P. vivax* or *P. ovale*			
Chloroquine phosphate plus primaquine phosphate[7]	**Chloroquine phosphate:** Treatment as above **Primaquine phosphate:** 30 mg base P.O. qd x 14 days	**Chloroquine phosphate:** Treatment as above **Primaquine phosphate:** 0.5 mg base/kg P.O. qd x 14 days	**All regions[8]** **Note:** For suspected chloroquine-resistant *P. vivax*, see row below
2nd line alternative for treatment: Hydroxychloroquine plus primaquine phosphate[7]	**Hydroxychloroquine:** Treatment as above **Primaquine phosphate:** 30 mg base P.O. qd x 14 days	**Hydroxychloroquine:** Treatment as above **Primaquine phosphate:** 30 mg base P.O. qd x 14 days	
Uncomplicated Malaria / *P. vivax*			
A. Quinine sulfate[2] plus either doxycycline or tetracycline plus primaquine phosphate[7]	**Quinine sulfate:** Treatment as above **Doxycycline or tetracycline:** Treatment as above **Primaquine phosphate:** Treatment as above	**Quinine sulfate:** Treatment as above **Doxycycline or tetracycline[4]:** Treatment as above **Primaquine phosphate:** Treatment as above	**Chloroquine-resistant[8]** (Papua New Guinea and Indonesia)
B. Mefloquine plus primaquine phosphate[7]	**Mefloquine:** Treatment as above **Primaquine phosphate:** Treatment as above	**Mefloquine:** Treatment as above **Primaquine phosphate:** Treatment as above	

Malaria Treatment *continued*

Recommended Drug	Adult Dose[1,8]	Pediatric Dose[1,8] ***(Pediatric dose should NEVER exceed adult dose)***	Region Infection Acquired
	Uncomplicated Malaria: Alternatives for Pregnant Women[9,10,11,12]		
Chloroquine phosphate	Treatment as above	Not applicable	**Chloroquine-sensitive**[12] (See uncomplicated malaria sections above for chloroquine-sensitive *Plasmodium* species by region)
2nd line alternative for treatment: Hydroxychloroquine	Treatment as above	Not applicable	
Quinine sulfate[2] plus clindamycin	**Quinine sulfate:** Treatment as above **Clindamycin:** Treatment as above	Not applicable	**Chloroquine resistant *P. falciparum***[9,10,11] (See uncomplicated malaria sections above for regions with known chloroquine-resistant *P. falciparum*)
Quinine sulfate	650 mg[3] salt P.O. tid x 7 days	Not applicable	**Chloroquine-resistant *P. vivax***[9,10,11,12] (See uncomplicated malaria sections above for regions with chloroquine-resistant *P. vivax*)
	Severe Malaria[13,14,15,16]		
Quinidine gluconate[14] plus one of the following: Doxycycline, tetracycline, or clindamycin	**Quinidine gluconate:** 6.25 mg base/kg (= 10 mg salt/kg) loading dose I.V. over 1-2 hours, then 0.0125 mg base/kg/min (= 0.02 mg salt/kg/min) continuous infusion for at least 24 hours. An alternative regimen is 15 mg base/kg (= 24 mg salt/kg) loading dose I.V. infused over 4 hours, followed by 7.5 mg base/kg (= 12 mg salt/kg) infused over 4 hours every 8 hours, starting 8 hours after the loading dose (see package insert). Once parasite density <1% and patient can take oral medication, complete treatment with oral quinine, dose as above. Quinidine/quinine course = 7 days in Southeast Asia; = 3 days in Africa or South America. **Doxycycline:** Treatment as above. If patient not able to take oral medication, give 100 mg I.V. every 12 hours and then switch to oral doxycycline (as above) as soon as patient can take oral medication. For I.V. use, avoid rapid administration. Treatment course = 7 days. **Tetracycline**: Treatment as above **Clindamycin:** Treatment as above. If patient not able to take oral medication, give 10 mg base/kg loading dose I.V. followed by 5 mg base/kg I.V. every 8 hours. Switch to oral clindamycin (oral dose as above) as soon as patient can take oral medication. For I.V. use, avoid rapid administration. Treatment course = 7 days.	**Quinidine gluconate:** Same mg/kg dosing and recommendations as for adults. **Doxycycline**[4]**:** Treatment as above. If patient not able to take oral medication, may give I.V. For children <45 kg, give 2.2 mg/kg I.V. every 12 hours and then switch to oral doxycycline (dose as above) as soon as patient can take oral medication. For children ≥45 kg, use same dosing as for adults. For I.V. use, avoid rapid administration. Treatment course = 7 days. **Tetracycline**[4]**:** Treatment as above **Clindamycin:** Treatment as above. If patient not able to take oral medication, give 10 mg base/kg loading dose I.V. followed by 5 mg base/kg I.V. every 8 hours. Switch to oral clindamycin (oral dose as above) as soon as patient can take oral medication. For I.V. use, avoid rapid administration. Treatment course = 7 days.	**All regions**

Source: http://www.cdc.gov/malaria/diagnosis_treatment/tx_clinicians.htm

[1]**Note:** There are three options (A, B, or C) available for treatment of uncomplicated malaria caused by chloroquine-resistant *P. falciparum*. Options A and B are equally recommended. Because of a higher rate of severe neuropsychiatric reactions seen at treatment doses, we do not recommend option C (mefloquine) unless options A and B cannot be used. For option A, because there is more data on the efficacy of quinine in combination with doxycycline or tetracycline, these treatment combinations are generally preferred to quinine in combination with clindamycin.

[2]For infections acquired in Southeast Asia, quinine treatment should continue for 7 days. For infections acquired in Africa and South America, quinine treatment should continue for 3 days.

[3]U.S. manufactured quinine sulfate capsule is in a 324 mg dosage; therefore 2 capsules should be sufficient for adult dosing.

[4]Doxycycline and tetracycline are not indicated for use in children <8 years old. For children <8 years old with chloroquine-resistant *P. falciparum*, quinine (given alone for 7 days or given in combination with clindamycin) and atovaquone-proguanil are recommended treatment options; mefloquine can be considered if no other options are available. For children <8 years old with chloroquine-resistant *P. vivax*, quinine (given alone for 7 days) or mefloquine are recommended treatment options. If none of these treatment options are available or are not being tolerated and if the treatment benefits outweigh the risks, doxycycline or tetracycline may be given to children <8 years old.

[5]Give atovaquone-proguanil with food. If patient vomits within 30 minutes of taking a dose, then they should repeat the dose.

[6]Treatment with mefloquine is not recommended in persons who have acquired infections from the Southeast Asian region of Burma, Thailand, and Cambodia due to resistant strains.

[7]Primaquine is used to eradicate any hypnozoite forms that may remain dormant in the liver, and thus prevent relapses, in *P. vivax* and *P. ovale* infections. Because primaquine can cause hemolytic anemia in persons with G6PD deficiency, patients must be screened for G6PD deficiency prior to starting treatment with primaquine. For persons with borderline G6PD deficiency or as an alternate to the above regimen, primaquine may be given 45 mg orally one time per week for 8 weeks; consultation with an expert in infectious disease and/or tropical medicine is advised if this alternative regimen is considered in G6PD-deficient persons. Primaquine must not be used during pregnancy.

[8]**Note:** There are two options (A or B) available for treatment of uncomplicated malaria caused by chloroquine-resistant *P. vivax*. High treatment failure rates due to chloroquine-resistant *P. vivax* have been well documented in Papua New Guinea and Indonesia. Rare case reports of chloroquine-resistant *P. vivax* have also been documented in Burma (Myanmar), India, and Central and South America. Persons acquiring *P. vivax* infections outside of Papua New Guinea or Indonesia should be started on chloroquine. If the patient does not respond, the treatment should be changed to a chloroquine-resistant *P. vivax* regimen and CDC should be notified (Malaria Hotline number: (770) 488-7788 Monday-Friday, 8 AM to 4:30 PM EST or (770) 488-7100 after hours, weekends, and holidays). For treatment of chloroquine-resistant *P. vivax* infections, options A and B are equally recommended.

[9]For pregnant women diagnosed with uncomplicated malaria caused by chloroquine-resistant *P. falciparum* or chloroquine-resistant *P. vivax* infection, treatment with doxycycline or tetracycline is generally not indicated. However, doxycycline or tetracycline may be used in combination with quinine (as recommended for nonpregnant adults) if other treatment options are not available or are not being tolerated, and the benefit is judged to outweigh the risks.

[10]Because there are no adequate, well-controlled studies of atovaquone and/or proguanil hydrochloride in pregnant women, atovaquone-proguanil is generally not recommended for use in pregnant women. For pregnant women diagnosed with uncomplicated malaria caused by chloroquine-resistant *P. falciparum* infection, atovaquone-proguanil may be used if other treatment options are not available or are not being tolerated, and if the potential benefit is judged to outweigh the potential risks. There are no data on the efficacy of atovaquone-proguanil in the treatment of chloroquine-resistant *P. vivax* infections.

[11]Because of a possible association with mefloquine treatment during pregnancy and an increase in stillbirths, mefloquine is generally not recommended for treatment in pregnant women. However, mefloquine may be used if it is the only treatment option available and if the potential benefit is judged to outweigh the potential risks.

[12]For *P. vivax* and *P. ovale* infections, primaquine phosphate for radical treatment of hypnozoites should not be given during pregnancy. Pregnant patients with *P. vivax* and *P. ovale* infections should be maintained on chloroquine prophylaxis for the duration of their pregnancy. The chemoprophylactic dose of chloroquine phosphate is 300 mg base (= 500 mg salt) orally once per week. After delivery, pregnant patients who do not have G6PD deficiency should be treated with primaquine.

[13]Persons with a positive blood smear **or** history of recent possible exposure and no other recognized pathology who have one or more of the following clinical criteria (impaired consciousness/coma, severe normocytic anemia, renal failure, pulmonary edema, acute respiratory distress syndrome, circulatory shock, disseminated intravascular coagulation, spontaneous bleeding, acidosis, hemoglobinuria, jaundice, repeated generalized convulsions, and/or parasitemia of >5%) are considered to have manifestations of more severe disease. Severe malaria is practically always due to *P. falciparum*.

[14]Patients diagnosed with severe malaria should be treated aggressively with parenteral antimalarial therapy. Treatment with I.V. quinidine should be initiated as soon as possible after the diagnosis has been made. Patients with severe malaria should be given an intravenous loading dose of quinidine unless they have received >40 mg/kg of quinine in the preceding 48 hours or if they have received mefloquine within the preceding 12 hours. Consultation with a cardiologist and a physician with experience treating malaria is advised when treating malaria patients with quinidine. During administration of quinidine, blood pressure monitoring (for hypotension) and cardiac monitoring (for widening of the QRS complex and/or lengthening of the QT_c interval) should be monitored continuously and blood glucose (for hypoglycemia) should be monitored periodically. Cardiac complications, if severe, may warrant temporary discontinuation of the drug or slowing of the intravenous infusion.

[15]Consider exchange transfusion if the parasite density (ie, parasitemia) is >10% **or** if the patient has altered mental status, nonvolume overload pulmonary edema, or renal complications. The parasite density can be estimated by examining a monolayer of red blood cells (RBCs) on the thin smear under oil immersion magnification. The slide should be examined where the RBCs are more or less touching (approximately 400 RBCs per field). The parasite density can then be estimated from the percentage of infected RBCs and should be monitored every 12 hours. Exchange transfusion should be continued until the parasite density is <1% (usually requires 8-10 units). I.V. quinidine administration should not be delayed for an exchange transfusion and can be given concurrently throughout the exchange transfusion.

[16]Pregnant women diagnosed with severe malaria should be treated aggressively with parenteral antimalarial therapy.

TREATMENT OF SEXUALLY TRANSMITTED INFECTIONS

Type or Stage	Drugs of Choice / Dosage	Alternatives
CHLAMYDIAL INFECTION AND RELATED CLINICAL SYNDROMES[1]		
Urethritis, cervicitis, conjunctivitis, or proctitis (except lymphogranuloma venereum)		
	Azithromycin 1 g oral once **or** Doxycycline[2,3] 100 mg oral bid x 7 d	Ofloxacin[3] 300 mg oral bid x 7 d **or** Levofloxacin[3] 500 mg oral once daily x 7 d **or** Erythromycin[4] 500 mg oral qid x 7 d
Infection in pregnancy		
	Azithromycin 1 g oral once **or** Amoxicillin 500 mg oral tid x 7 d	Erythromycin[4] 500 mg oral qid x 7 d
Neonatal ophthalmia or pneumonia		
	Azithromycin 20 mg/kg oral once daily x 3 d	Erythromycin 12.5 mg/kg oral qid x 14 d[5]
Lymphogranuloma venereum		
	Doxycycline[2,3] 100 mg oral bid x 21 d	Erythromycin[4] 500 mg oral qid x 21 d
EPIDIDYMITIS		
	Ceftriaxone 250 mg I.M. once **plus** doxycycline[2] 100 mg oral bid x 10 d	Only if negative for gonococcal organism: Ofloxacin 300 mg bid x 10 d **or** Levofloxacin 500 mg oral once daily x 10 d
GONORRHEA[6]		
Disseminated gonococcal infection		
	Ceftriaxone 1 g I.M. or I.V. q24h	Cefotaxime 1 g I.V. q8h **or** Ceftizoxime 1 g I.V. q8h **or** **For persons allergic to β-lactam drugs:** Ciprofloxacin 400 mg I.V. q12h **or** Levofloxacin 250 mg I.V. once daily **or** Ofloxacin 400 mg I.V. q12h **or** Spectinomycin 2 g I.M. q12h[7] All regimens should be continued for 24-48 hours after improvement begins, at which time therapy may be switched to one of the following regimens to complete a full week of antimicrobial therapy: Cefixime suspension 500 mg oral bid **or** Cefpodoxime 400 mg bid
Gonococcal meningitis and endocarditis		
	Ceftriaxone 1-2 g I.V. q12h	
Uncomplicated urethral, cervical, or rectal		
	Cefixime 400 mg oral once **or** Ceftriaxone 125 mg I.M. once	Cefpodoxime 400 mg or cefuroxime axetil 1 g orally once **or** Cefotaxime 500 mg I.M. **or** Ceftizoxime 500 mg I.M., **or** Cefoxitin 2 g I.M. (with 1 g probenecid orally) **or** Spectinomycin 2 g I.M. once[7]
Uncomplicated pharyngeal		
	Ceftriaxone 125 mg I.M. once	
PELVIC INFLAMMATORY DISEASE		
– parenteral	Cefoxitin 2 g I.V. q6h **plus** doxycycline[3] 100 mg oral or I.V. q12h, until improved **followed by** doxycycline[3] 100 mg oral bid to complete 14 d[10] **or** Clindamycin 900 mg I.V. q8h **plus** gentamicin 2 mg/kg I.V. once, then 1.5 mg/kg I.V. q8h,[11] until improved **followed by** doxycycline[3] 100 mg oral bid to complete 14 d[10]	Ampicillin/sulbactam 3 g I.V. q6h **plus** doxycycline[3] 100 mg oral or I.V. q12h; continue until improved, then doxycycline[3] 100 mg oral bid to complete 14 d[10]
– oral	Cefoxitin 2 g once **plus** probenecid 1 g oral once **plus** doxycycline[3,12] 100 mg bid ± metronidazole x 14 d **or** Ceftriaxone 250 mg I.M. once (or other parenteral 3rd generation cephalosporin) **plus** doxycycline[3,12] 100 mg bid ± metronidazole x 14 d	Ofloxacin[3] 400 mg bid x 14 d **or** Levofloxacin[3] 500 mg once daily x 14 d ± metronidazole[9] 500 mg bid x 14 d. **Note:** Only if community prevalence (of quinolone-resistant organisms) and individual patient risk is low and quinolone susceptibility can be established

TREATMENT OF SEXUALLY TRANSMITTED INFECTIONS

Type or Stage	Drugs of Choice / Dosage	Alternatives
TRICHOMONIASIS		
	Metronidazole 2 g oral once **or** Tinidazole 2 g oral once	Metronidazole 375 or 500 mg oral bid x 7 d
BACTERIAL VAGINOSIS		
	Metronidazole 500 mg oral bid x 7 d **or** Metronidazole gel 0.75%[14] 5 g intravaginally once or twice daily x 5 d **or** Clindamycin 2% cream[14] 5 g intravaginally qhs x 3-7 d	Metronidazole 2 g oral once[13] or Flagyl ER® 750 mg once daily x 7 d **or** Clindamycin 300 mg oral bid x 7 d **or** Clindamycin ovules[14] 100 mg intravaginally once daily x 3 d
VULVOVAGINAL CANDIDIASIS		
	Intravaginal butoconazole, clotrimazole, miconazole, terconazole, or tioconazole[15] **or** Fluconazole 150 mg oral once	Nystatin 100,000 unit vaginal tablet once daily x 14 d
SYPHILIS		
Early (primary, secondary, or latent <1 y)		
	Penicillin G benzathine 2.4 million units I.M. once[16]	Doxycycline[3] 100 mg oral bid x 14 d
Late (>1 year's duration, cardiovascular, gumma, late-latent)		
	Penicillin G benzathine 2.4 million units I.M. weekly x 3 wk	Doxycycline[3] 100 mg oral bid x 4 wk
Neurosyphilis[17]		
	Penicillin G 3-4 million units I.V. q4h or 24 million units continuous I.V. infusion x 10-14 d	Penicillin G procaine 2.4 million units I.M. daily **plus** probenecid 500 mg qid oral, both x 10-14 d **or** Ceftriaxone 2 g I.V. once daily x 10-14 d
Congenital		
	Penicillin G 50,000 units/kg I.V. q8-12h for 10-14 d **or** Penicillin G procaine 50,000 units/kg I.M. daily for 10-14 d	
CHANCROID[18]		
	Azithromycin 1 g oral once **or** Ceftriaxone 250 mg I.M. once	Ciprofloxacin[3] 500 mg oral bid x 3 d **or** Erythromycin[4] 500 mg oral qid x 7 d
GENITAL WARTS[19]		
	Trichloroacetic or bichloroacetic acid, or podophyllin[3] or liquid nitrogen 1-2 times/wk until resolved **or** Imiquimod 5% 3 times/wk x 16 wk **or** Podofilox 0.5% bid x 3 d, 4 days rest, then repeated up to 4 times	Surgical removal **or** Laser surgery **or** Intralesional interferon
GENITAL HERPES		
First episode		
	Acyclovir 400 mg oral tid x 7-10 d **or** Famciclovir 250 mg oral tid x 7-10 d **or** Valacyclovir 1 g oral bid x 7-10 d	Acyclovir 200 mg oral 5 times/d x 7-10 d
Severe (hospitalized patients)		
	Acyclovir 5-10 mg/kg I.V. q8h x 5-7 d	
Suppression of recurrences[20]		
	Acyclovir 400 mg oral bid **or** Famciclovir 250 mg oral bid **or** Valacyclovir 500 mg - 1 g once daily[21]	Acyclovir 200 mg oral, 2-5 times/d
Episodic treatment of recurrences[22]		
	Acyclovir 800 mg oral tid x 2 d or 400 mg oral tid x 3-5 d[23] **or** Famciclovir 125 mg oral bid x 3-5 d[23] **or** Valacyclovir 500 mg oral bid x 3 d	

Type or Stage	Drugs of Choice / Dosage	Alternatives
GRANULOMA INGUINALE		
	TMP-SMZ 1 double-strength tablet oral bid for a minimum of 3 wk **or** Doxycycline 100 oral bid for a minimum of 3 wk	Ciprofloxacin 750 mg oral bid for a minimum of 3 wk **or** Erythromycin base 500 mg oral qid for a minimum of 3 wk **or** Azithromycin 1 g oral once per week for a minimum of 3 weeks

[1]Related clinical syndromes include nonchlamydial nongonococcal urethritis and cervicitis.

[2]Or oral tetracycline 500 mg qid.

[3]Not recommended in pregnancy.

[4]Erythromycin ethylsuccinate 800 mg may be substituted for erythromycin base 500 mg; erythromycin estolate is contraindicated in pregnancy.

[5]Pyloric stenosis has been associated with use of erythromycin in newborns.

[6]All patients should also receive a course of treatment effective for *Chlamydia*.

[7]Not available in the United States.

[8]Recommended only for use during pregnancy in patients allergic to β-lactams.

[9]Some clinicians believe the addition of metronidazole is not required.

[10]Or clindamycin 450 mg oral qid to complete 14 days.

[11]A single daily dose of 3 mg/kg is likely to be effective, but has not been studied in pelvic inflammatory disease.

[12]Some experts would add metronidazole 500 mg bid.

[13]Higher relapse rate with single dose, but useful for patients who may not comply with multiple-dose therapy.

[14]In pregnancy, topical preparations have not been effective in preventing premature delivery; oral metronidazole has been effective in some studies.

[15]For preparations and dosage of topical products, see *Med Lett Drugs Ther*, 1994, 36:81; single-dose therapy is not recommended.

[16]Some experts recommend a repeat dose after 7 days, especially in patients with HIV infection or pregnant women.

[17]Patients allergic to penicillin should be desensitized and treated with penicillin.

[18]All regimens, especially single-dose ceftriaxone, are less effective in HIV-infected patients.

[19]Recommendations for external genital warts. Liquid nitrogen can also be used for vaginal, urethral, and oral warts. Podofilox or imiquimod can be used for urethral meatus warts. Trichloroacetic or bichloroacetic acid can be used for anal warts.

[20]Some Medical Letter consultants discontinue preventive treatment for 1-2 months once a year to reassess the frequency of recurrence.

[21]Use 500 mg once daily in patients with <10 recurrences per year and 500 mg bid or 1 g daily in patients with <10 recurrences per year.

[22]Antiviral therapy is variably effective for episodic treatment of recurrences; only effective if started early.

[23]No published data are available to support 3 days' use.

Adapted from "Sexually Transmitted Diseases Treatment Guidelines 2002," *MMWR Morb Mortal Wkly Rep*, 2002, 51(RR-6).

Adapted from "Drugs for Sexually Transmitted Infections," *Treatment Guidelines From The Medical Letter®*, 2004, 2(26):70-2.

Adapted from "Update to CDC's Sexually Transmitted Diseases Treatment Guidelines, 2006: Fluoroquinolones No Longer Recommended for Treatment of Gonococcal Infections," *MMWR*, 2007, 56(14):332-6.

TUBERCULOSIS

Tuberculin Skin Test Recommendations[1]

Children for whom immediate skin testing is indicated:

- Contacts of persons with confirmed or suspected infectious tuberculosis (TB) (contact investigation); this includes children identified as contacts of family members or associates in jail or prison in the last 5 years
- Children with radiographic or clinical findings suggesting tuberculosis
- Children immigrating from endemic countries (eg, Asia, Middle East, Africa, Latin America)
- Children with travel histories to endemic countries and/or significant contact with indigenous persons from such countries

Children who should be tested annually for tuberculosis[2]:

- Children infected with human immunodeficiency virus (HIV) or living in household with HIV-infected persons
- Incarcerated adolescents

Children who should be tested every 2-3 years[2]:

- Children exposed to the following individuals: HIV-infected, homeless, residents of nursing homes, institutionalized adolescents or adults, users of illicit drugs, incarcerated adolescents or adults, and migrant farm workers. Foster children with exposure to adults in the preceding high-risk groups are included.

Children who should be considered for tuberculin skin testing at ages 4-6 and 11-16 years:

- Children whose parents immigrated (with unknown tuberculin skin test status) from regions of the world with high prevalence of tuberculosis; continued potential exposure by travel to the endemic areas and/or household contact with persons from the endemic areas (with unknown tuberculin skin test status) should be an indication for repeat tuberculin skin testing
- Children without specific risk factors who reside in high-prevalence areas; in general, a high-risk neighborhood or community does not mean an entire city is at high risk; rates in any area of the city may vary by neighborhood, or even from block to block; physicians should be aware of these patterns in determining the likelihood of exposure; public health officials or local tuberculosis experts should help clinicians identify areas that have appreciable tuberculosis rates

Children at increased risk of progression of infection to disease: Those with other medical risk factors, including diabetes mellitus, chronic renal failure, malnutrition, and congenital or acquired immunodeficiencies deserve special consideration. Without recent exposure, these persons are not at increased risk of acquiring tuberculosis infection. Underlying immune deficiencies associated with these conditions theoretically would enhance the possibility for progression to severe disease. Initial histories of potential exposure to tuberculosis should be included on all of these patients. If these histories or local epidemiologic factors suggest a possibility of exposure, immediate and periodic tuberculin skin testing should be considered. An initial Mantoux tuberculin skin test should be performed before initiation of immunosuppressive therapy in any child with an underlying condition that necessitates immunosuppressive therapy.

Footnotes

[1]BCG immunization is not a contraindication to tuberculin skin testing.
[2]Initial tuberculin skin testing is at the time of diagnosis or circumstance, beginning as early as at age 3 months.
Adapted from "Report of the Committee on Infectious Diseases," *2003 Red Book®*, 26th ed, 646.

Table 1. Tuberculosis Prophylaxis Infection Without Disease
(Positive Tuberculin Test)[1]

Specific Circumstances / Organism	Comments	Regimen
Regardless of age (see INH Preventive Therapy)	Rx indicated	INH (5 mg/kg/d, maximum: 300 mg/d for adults, 10 mg/kg/d not to exceed 300 mg/d for children). Results with 6 months of treatment are nearly as effective as 12 months (65% vs 75% reduction in disease). *Am Thoracic Society* (6 months), *Am Acad Pediatrics*, 1991 (9 months). If CXR is abnormal, treat for 12 months. In HIV-positive patient, treatment for a minimum of 12 months, some suggest longer. Monitor transaminases monthly (*MMWR Morb Mortal Wkly Rep* 1989, 38:247).
Age <35 y	Rx indicated	Reanalysis of earlier studies favors INH prophylaxis for 6 months (if INH-related hepatitis case fatality rate is <1% and TB case fatality is ≥6.7%, which appears to be the case, monitor transaminases monthly (*Arch Int Med*, 1990, 150:2517).
INH-resistant organisms likely	Rx indicated	Data on efficacy of alternative regimens is currently lacking. Regimens include ETB + RIF daily for 6 months. PZA + RIF daily for 2 months, then INH + RIF daily until sensitivities from index case (if available) known, then if INH-CR, discontinue INH and continue RIF for 9 months, otherwise INH + RIF for 9 months (this latter is *Am Acad Pediatrics*, 1991 recommendation).
INH + RIF resistant organisms likely	Rx indicated	Efficacy of alternative regimens is unknown; PZA (25-30 mg/kg/d P.O.) + ETB (15-25 mg/kg/d P.O.) (at 25 mg/kg ETB, monitoring for retrobulbar neuritis required), for 6 months unless HIV-positive, then 12 months; PZA + ciprofloxacin (750 mg P.O. bid) or ofloxacin (400 mg P.O. bid) for 6-12 months *(MMWR Morb Mortal Wkly Rep*, 1992, 41(RR11):68).

INH = isoniazid; RIF = rifampin; KM = kanamycin; ETB = ethambutol; SM = streptomycin; PZA = pyrazinamide; CXR = chest x-ray; Rx = treatment.

See also guidelines for interpreting PPD in "Skin Testing for Delayed Hypersensitivity."

[1]Tuberculin test (TBnT). The standard is the Mantoux test, 5 TU PPD in 0.1 mL diluent stabilized with Tween 80. Read at 48-72 hours measuring maximum diameter of induration. A reaction ≥5 mm is defined as positive in the following: positive HIV or risk factors, recent close case contacts, CXR consistent with healed TBc. A reaction ≥10 mm is positive in foreign-born in countries of high prevalence, injection drug users, low income populations, nursing home residents, patients with medical conditions which increase risk (see above, preventive treatment). A reaction ≥15 mm is positive in all others (*Am Rev Resp Dis*, 1990, 142:725). Two-stage TBnT: Use in individuals to be tested regularly (ie, healthcare workers). TBn reactivity may decrease over time but be boosted by skin testing. If unrecognized, individual may be incorrectly diagnosed as recent converter. If first TBnT is reactive but <10 mm, repeat 5 TU in 1 week, if then ≥10 mm = positive, not recent conversion (*Am Rev Resp Dis*, 1979, 119:587).

Changes From Prior Recommendations on Tuberculin Testing and Treatment of Latent Tuberculosis Infection (LTBI)

Tuberculin Testing

- Emphasis on targeted tuberculin testing among persons at high risk for recent LTBI or with clinical conditions that increase the risk for TB, regardless of age; testing is discouraged among persons at lower risk
- For patients with organ transplants and other immunosuppressed patients (eg, persons receiving the equivalent of ≥15 mg/day prednisone for 1 month or more), 5 mm of induration rather than 10 mm of induration rather than 10 mm of induration as a cut-off level for tuberculin positivity
- A tuberculin skin test conversion is defined as in increase of ≥10 mm of induration within a 2-year period, regardless of age

Treatment of Latent Tuberculosis Infection

- For HIV-negative persons, isoniazid given for 9 months is preferred over 6-month regimens
- For HIV-positive persons and those with fibrotic lesions on chest x-ray consistent with previous TB, isoniazid should be given for 9 months instead of 12 months
- For HIV-negative and HIV-positive persons, rifampin and pyrazinamide should be given for 2 months
- For HIV-negative and HIV-positive persons, rifampin should be given for 4 months

Clinical and Laboratory Monitoring

- Routine baseline and follow-up laboratory monitoring can be eliminated in most persons with LTBI, except for those with HIV infection, pregnant women (or those in the immediate postpartum period), and persons with chronic liver disease or those who use alcohol regularly
- Emphasis on clinical monitoring for signs and symptoms of possible adverse effects, with prompt evaluation and changes in treatment, as indicated

Adapted from *MMWR*, 2000, 49(RR-6).

Table 2. Recommended Treatment Regimens for Drug-Susceptible Tuberculosis in Infants, Children, and Adolescents

Infection or Disease Category	Regimen	Remarks
Latent tuberculosis infection (positive tuberculin skin test, no disease):		
• Isoniazid-susceptible	9 months of isoniazid once a day	If daily therapy is not possible, directly observed therapy twice a week may be used for 9 months.
• Isoniazid-resistant	6 months of rifampin once a day	
• Isoniazid-rifampin-resistant[1]	Consult a tuberculosis specialist	
Pulmonary and extrapulmonary (except meningitis)	2 months of isoniazid, rifampin, and pyrazinamide daily, followed by 4 months of isoniazid and rifampin[2]	If possible drug resistance is a concern, another drug (ethambutol or aminoglycoside) is added to the initial 3-drug therapy until drug susceptibilities are determined. Directly observed therapy is highly desirable. If hilar adenopathy only, a 6-month course of isoniazid and rifampin is sufficient. Drugs can be given 2 or 3 times/week under directly observed therapy in the initial phase if nonadherence is likely.
Meningitis	2 months of isoniazid, rifampin, pyrazinamide, and aminoglycoside or ethionamide, once a day, followed by 7-10 months of isoniazid and rifampin once a day or twice a week (9-12 months total)	A fourth drug, usually an aminoglycoside, is given with initial therapy until drug susceptibility is known. For patients who may have acquired tuberculosis in geographic areas where resistance to streptomycin is common, capreomycin, kanamycin, or amikacin may be used instead of streptomycin.

[1]Duration of therapy is longer for human immunodeficiency virus (HIV)-infected people, and additional drugs may be indicated.

[2]Medications should be administered daily for the first 2 weeks to 2 months of treatment and then can be administered 2-3 times/week by directly observed therapy.

Adapted from "Report of the Committee on Infectious Diseases," *2003 Red Book®*, 26th ed, 649.

Table 3. Recommended Drug Regimens for Treatment of Latent Tuberculosis Infection in Children

Drug	Interval and Duration	Comments
Isoniazid	Daily for 9 mo Twice weekly for 9 mo	This includes treatment for any child <5 years of age who is exposed to household members or other close contacts who are potentially infectious even if skin test is negative
Rifampin	Daily for 4-9 mo	No controlled trials; only to be used in INH intolerant or resistant
Rifampin-pyrazinamide	Daily for 3 mo	No controlled trials; only to be used in INH intolerant or resistant

Modified from *MMWR*, 2000, 14(RR-6).

Table 4. Recommended Drug Regimens for Treatment of Latent Tuberculosis Infection in Adults

Drug	Interval and Duration	Comments	Rating[1] (Evidence)[2] HIV⁻	HIV⁺
Isoniazid	Daily for 9 mo[3,4]	In HIV-infected patients, isoniazid may be administered concurrently with nucleoside reverse transcriptase inhibitors (NRTIs), protease inhibitors (PIs), or non-nucleoside reverse transcriptase inhibitors (NNRTIs)	A (II)	A (II)
	Twice weekly for 9 mo[3,4]	Directly-observed therapy (DOT) must be used with twice-weekly dosing	B (II)	B (II)
Isoniazid	Daily for 6 mo[4]	Not indicated for HIV-infected persons, those with fibrotic lesions on chest radiographs, or children	B (I)	C (I)
	Twice weekly for 6 mo[4]	DOT must be used with twice-weekly dosing	B (II)	C (I)
Rifampin	Daily for 4 mo	For persons who cannot tolerate pyrazinamide	B (II)	B (III)
		For persons who are contacts of patients with isoniazid-resistant, rifampin-susceptible TB who cannot tolerate pyrazinamide		
Rifampin plus pyrazinamide	Daily for 2 mo	May also be offered to persons who are contacts of pyrazinamide patients with isoniazid-resistant, rifampin-susceptible TB	B (II)	A (I)
		In HIV-infected patients, protease inhibitors or NNRTIs should generally not be administered concurrently with rifampin. Rifabutin can be used as an alternative for patients treated with indinavir, nelfinavir, amprenavir, ritonavir, or efavirenz, and possibly with nevirapine or soft-gel saquinavir[5]		
	Twice weekly for 2-3 mo	DOT must be used with twice-weekly dosing	C (II)	C (I)

[1]Strength of recommendation: A = preferred; B = acceptable alternative; C = offer when A and B cannot be given.

[2]Quality of evidence: I = randomized clinical trial data; II = data from clinical trials that are not randomized or were conducted in other populations; III = expert opinion.

[3]Recommended regimen for children <18 years of age.

[4]Recommended regimens for pregnant women. Some experts would use rifampin and pyrazinamide for 2 months as an alternative regimen in HIV-infected pregnant women, although pyrazinamide should be avoided during the first trimester.

[5]Rifabutin should not be used with hard-gel saquinavir or delavirdine. When used with other protease inhibitors or NNRTIs, dose adjustment of rifabutin may be required.

Adapted from *MMWR Recomm Rep*, 2000, 49(RR6).

Table 5. TB Drugs in Special Situations

Drug	Pregnancy[1]	CNS TB Disease	Renal Insufficiency
Isoniazid	Safe	Good penetration	Normal clearance
Rifampin	Safe	Fair penetration Penetrates inflamed meninges (10% to 20%)	Normal clearance
Pyrazinamide	Avoid	Good penetration	Clearance reduced Decrease dose or prolong interval
Ethambutol	Safe	Penetrates inflamed meninges only (4% to 64%)	Clearance reduced Decrease dose or prolong interval
Streptomycin	Avoid	Penetrates inflamed meninges only	Clearance reduced Decrease dose or prolong interval
Capreomycin	Avoid	Penetrates inflamed meninges only	Clearance reduced Decrease dose or prolong interval
Kanamycin	Avoid	Penetrates inflamed meninges only	Clearance reduced Decrease dose or prolong interval
Ethionamide	Do not use	Good penetration	Normal clearance
Para-amino-salicylic acid	Safe	Penetrates inflamed meninges only (10% to 50%)	Incomplete data on clearance
Cycloserine	Avoid	Good penetration	Clearance reduced Decrease dose or prolong interval
Ciprofloxacin	Do not use	Fair penetration (5% to 10%) Penetrates inflamed meninges (50% to 90%)	Clearance reduced Decrease dose or prolong interval
Ofloxacin	Do not use	Fair penetration (5% to 10%) Penetrates inflamed meninges (50% to 90%)	Clearance reduced Decrease dose or prolong interval
Amikacin	Avoid	Penetrates inflamed meninges only	Clearance reduced Decrease dose or prolong interval
Clofazimine	Avoid	Penetration unknown	Clearance probably normal

[1]Safe = the drug has not been demonstrated to have teratogenic effects.

Avoid = data on the drug's safety are limited, or the drug is associated with mild malformations (as in the aminoglycosides).

Do not use = studies show an association between the drug and premature labor, congenital malformations, or teratogenicity.

Table 6. Recommendations for Coadministering Different Antiretroviral Drugs With the Antimycobacterial Drugs Rifabutin and Rifampin

Antiretroviral	Use in Combination with Rifabutin	Use in Combination with Rifampin	Comments
Saquinavir[1]			
Hard-gel capsules (HGC)	Possibly,[2] if antiretroviral regimen also includes ritonavir	Possibly, if antiretroviral regimen also includes ritonavir	Coadministration of saquinavir SGC with usual-dose rifabutin (300 mg/day or 2-3 times/week) is a possibility. However, the pharmacokinetic data and clinical experience for this combination are limited.
Soft-gel capsules (SGC)	Probably[3]	Possibly, if antiretroviral regimen also includes ritonavir	The combination of saquinavir SGC or saquinavir HGC and ritonavir, coadministered with 1) usual-dose rifampin (600 mg/day or 2-3 times/week), or 2) reduced-dose rifabutin (150 mg 2-3 times/week) is a possibility. However, the pharmacokinetic data and clinical experience for these combinations are limited. Coadministration of saquinavir or saquinavir SGC with rifampin is not recommended because rifampin markedly decreases concentrations of saquinavir.
Ritonavir	Probably	Probably	If the combination of ritonavir and rifabutin is used, then a substantially reduced-dose rifabutin regimen (150 mg 2-3 times/week) is recommended. Coadministration of ritonavir with usual-dose rifampin (600 mg/day or 2-3 times/week) is a possibility, though pharmacokinetic data and clinical experience are limited.
Indinavir	Yes	No	There is limited, but favorable, clinical experience with coadministration of indinavir[4] with a reduced daily dose of rifabutin (150 mg) or with the usual dose of rifabutin (300 mg 2-3 times/week). Coadministration of indinavir with rifampin is not recommended because rifampin markedly decreases concentrations of indinavir.
Nelfinavir	Yes	No	There is limited, but favorable, clinical experience with coadministration of nelfinavir[5] with a reduced daily dose of rifabutin (150 mg) or with the usual dose of rifabutin (300 mg 2-3 times/week). Coadministration of nelfinavir with rifampin is not recommended because rifampin markedly decreases concentrations of nelfinavir.
Amprenavir	Yes	No	Coadministration of amprenavir with a reduced daily dose of rifabutin (150 mg) or with the usual dose of rifabutin (300 mg 2-3 times/week) is a possibility, but there is no published clinical experience. Coadministration of amprenavir with rifampin is not recommended because rifampin markedly decreases concentrations of amprenavir.
Nevirapine	Yes	Possibly	Coadministration of nevirapine with usual-dose rifabutin (300 mg/day or 2-3 times/week) is a possibility based on pharmacokinetic study data. However, there is no published clinical experience for this combination. Data are insufficient to assess whether dose adjustments are necessary when rifampin is coadministered with nevirapine. Therefore, rifampin and nevirapine should be used only in combination if clearly indicated and with careful monitoring.
Delavirdine	No	No	Contraindicated because of the marked decrease in concentrations of delavirdine when administered with either rifabutin or rifampin.
Efavirenz	Probably	Probably	Coadministration of efavirenz with increased-dose rifabutin (450 mg/day or 600 mg/day, or 600 mg 2-3 times/week) is a possibility, though there is no published clinical experience. Coadministration of efavirenz[6] with usual-dose rifampin (600 mg/day or 2-3 times/week) is a possibility, though there is no published clinical experience.

[1]Usual recommended doses are 400 mg twice daily for each of these protease inhibitors and 400 mg of ritonavir.

[2]Despite limited data and clinical experience, the use of this combination is potentially successful.

[3]Based on available data and clinical experience, the successful use of this combination is likely.

[4] Usual recommended dose is 800 mg every 8 hours; some experts recommend increasing the indinavir dose to 1000 mg every 8 hours if indinavir is used in combination with rifabutin.

[5]Usual recommended dose is 750 mg 3 times/day or 1250 mg twice daily; some experts recommend increasing the nelfinavir dose to 1000 mg if the 3-times/day dosing is used and nelfinavir is used in combination with rifabutin.

[6]Usual recommended dose is 600 mg/day; some experts recommend increasing the efavirenz dose to 800 mg/day if efavirenz is used in combination with rifampin.

Updated March 2000 from www.aidsinfo.nih.gov - "Updated Guidelines for the Use of Rifabutin or Rifampin for the Treatment and Prevention of Tuberculosis Among HIV-Infected Patients Taking Protease Inhibitors or Non-nucleoside Reverse Transcriptase Inhibitors," *MMWR,* March 10, 2000, 49 (09):185-9.

Table 7. Criteria for Tuberculin Positivity, by Risk Group

Reaction ≥5 mm of Induration	Reaction ≥10 mm of Induration	Reaction ≥15 mm of Induration
HIV-positive persons	Recent immigrants (ie, within the last 5 years) from high prevalence countries	Persons with no risk factors for TB
Recent contacts of tuberculosis (TB) case patients	Injection drug users	
Fibrotic changes on chest radiograph consistent with prior TB	Residents and employees[1] of the following high risk congregate settings: prisons and jails, nursing homes and other long-term facilities for the elderly, hospitals and other healthcare facilities, residential facilities for patients with AIDS, and homeless shelters	
Patients with organ transplant and other immunosuppressed patients (receiving the equivalent of ≥15 mg/day of prednisone for 1 month)[2]	Mycobacteriology laboratory personnel Persons with the following clinical conditions that place them at high risk: Silicosis, diabetes mellitus, chronic renal failure, some hematologic disorders (eg, leukemias and lymphomas), other specific malignancies (eg, carcinoma of the head or neck and lung), weight loss of ≥10% of ideal body weight, gastrectomy, and jejunoileal bypass	
	Children <4 years of age or infants, children, and adolescents exposed to adults at high-risk	

[1]For persons who are otherwise at low risk and are tested at the start of employment, a reaction of ≥15 mm induration is considered positive.

[2]Risk of TB in patients treated with corticosteroids increases with higher dose and longer duration.

Modified from *MMWR Morb Mortal Wkly Rep*, 2000, 49(RR-6).

Table 8. Recommendations, Rankings, and Performance Indicators for Treatment of Patients With Tuberculosis (TB)

Recommendation	Ranking[1] (Evidence)[2]	Performance Indicator
Obtain bacteriologic confirmation and susceptibility testing for patients with TB or suspected of having TB	A (II)	90% of adults with or suspected of having TB have 3 cultures for mycobacteria obtained before initiation of antituberculosis therapy (50% of children 0-12 y)
Place persons with suspected or confirmed smear-positive pulmonary or laryngeal TB in respiratory isolation until noninfectious	A (II)	90% of persons with sputum smear-positive TB remain in respiratory isolation until smear converts to negative
Begin treatment of patients with confirmed or suspected TB disease with one of the following drug combinations, depending on local resistance patterns: INH + RIF + PZA **or** INH + RIF + PZA + EMB **or** INH + RIF + PZA + SM	A (III)	90% of all patients with TB are started on INH + RIF + PZA + EMB or SM in geographic areas where >4% of TB isolates are resistant to INH
Report each case of TB promptly to the local public health department	A (III)	100% of persons with active TB are reported to the local public health department within 1 week of diagnosis
Perform HIV testing for all patients with TB	A (III)	80% of all patients with TB have HIV status determined within 2 months of a diagnosis of TB
Treat patients with TB caused by a susceptible organism for 6 months, using an ATS/CDC-approved regimen	A (I)	90% of all patients with TB complete 6 months of therapy with 12 months of beginning treatment
Re-evaluate patients with TB who are smear positive at 3 months for possible nonadherence or infection with drug-resistant bacilli	A (III)	90% of all patients with TB who are smear positive at 3 months have sputum culture/susceptibility testing performed within 1 month of the 3-month visit
Add ≥2 new antituberculosis agents when TB treatment failure is suspected	A (II)	100% of patients with TB with suspected treatment failure are prescribed ≥2 new antituberculosis agents
Perform tuberculin skin testing on all patients with a history of ≥1 of the following: HIV infection, I.V. drug use, homelessness, incarceration, or contact with a person with pulmonary TB	A (II)	80% of persons in the indicated population groups receive tuberculin skin test and return for reading
Administer treatment for latent TB infection to all persons with latent TB infection, unless it can be documented that they received such treatment previously	A (I)	75% of patients with positive tuberculin skin tests who are candidates for treatment for latent TB infection complete a course of therapy within 12 months of initiation

Note: ATS/CDC = American Thoracic Society and Centers for Disease Control and Prevention; EMB = ethambutol; INH = isoniazid; PZA = pyrazinamide; RIF = rifampin; SM = streptomycin.

[1]Strength of recommendation: A = preferred; B = acceptable alternative; C = offer when A and B cannot be given.

[2]Quality of evidence: I = randomized clinical trial data; II = data from clinical trials that are not randomized or were conducted in other populations; III = expert opinion.

Adapted from the Infectious Diseases Society of America, *Clinical Infectious Diseases,* 2000, 31:633-9.

Table 9. Drug Regimens for Culture-Positive Pulmonary Tuberculosis Caused by Drug-Susceptible Organisms

Initial Phase			Continuation Phase			Range of Total Doses (minimal duration)	Rating[1] (Evidence)[2]	
Regimen	Drugs	Interval and Doses[3] (minimal duration)	Regimen	Drugs	Interval and Doses[3,4] (minimal duration)		HIV^-	HIV^+
1	INH RIF PZA EMB	Seven days per week for 56 doses (8 wk) or 5 d/wk for 40 doses (8 wk)[5]	1a	INH/RIF	Seven days per week for 126 doses (18 wk) or 5 d/wk for 90 doses (18 wk)[5]	182-130 (26 wk)	A (I)	A (II)
			1b	INH/RIF	Twice weekly for 36 doses (18 wk)	92-76 (26 wk)	A (I)	A (II)[6]
			1c[7]	INH/RPT	Once weekly for 18 doses (18 wk)	74-58 (26 wk)	B (I)	E (I)
2	INH RIF PZA EMB	Seven days per week for 14 doses (2 wk), then twice weekly for 12 doses (6 wk) or 5 d/wk for 10 doses (2 wk)[5], then twice weekly for 12 doses (6 wk)	2a	INH/RIF	Twice weekly for 36 doses (18 wk)	62-58 (26 wk)	A (II)	B (II)[6]
			2b[7]	INH/RPT	Once weekly for 18 doses (18 wk)	44-40 (26 wk)	B (I)	E (I)
3	INH RIF PZA EMB	Three times weekly for 24 doses (8 wk)	3a	INH/RIF	Three times weekly for 54 doses (18 wk)	78 (26 wk)	B (I)	B (II)
4	INH RIF EMB	Seven days per week for 56 doses (8 wk) or 5 d/wk for 40 doses (8 wk)[5]	4a	INH/RIF	Seven days per week for 217 doses (31 wk) or 5 d/wk for 155 doses (31 wk)[5]	273-195 (39 wk)	C (I)	C (II)
			4b	INH/RIF	Twice weekly for 62 doses (31 wk)	118-102 (39 wk)	C (I)	C (II)

Definition of abbreviations: EMB = ethambutol; INH = isoniazid; PZA = pyrazinamide; RIF = rifampin; RPT = rifapentine.

[1]Definitions of evidence ratings: A = preferred; B = acceptable alternative; C = offer when A and B cannot be given; E = should never be given.

[2]Definitions of evidence ratings: I = randomized clinical trial; II = data from clinical trials that were not randomized or were conducted in other populations; III = expert opinion.

[3]When directly observed therapy (DOT) is used, drugs may be given 5 days/week and the necessary number of doses adjusted accordingly. Although there are no studies that compare five with seven daily doses, extensive experience indicates this would be an effective practice.

[4]Patients with cavitation on initial chest radiograph and positive cultures at completion of 2 months of therapy should receive a 7-month (31-week; either 217 doses daily] or 62 doses [twice weekly]) continuation phase.

[5]Five-day/week administration is always given by DOT. Rating for 5 day/week regimens is AIII.

[6]Not recommended for HIV-infected patients with $CD4^+$ cell counts <100 cells/µL.

[7]Options 1c and 2b should be used only in HIV-negative patients who have negative sputum smears at the time of completion of 2 months of therapy and who do not have cavitation on initial chest radiograph. For patients started on this regimen and found to have a positive culture from the 2-month specimen, treatment should be extended an extra 3 months.

Adapted from *MMWR*, 2003, 52(RR11).

Table 10. Suggested Pyrazinamide Doses, Using Whole Tablets, for Adults Weighing 40-90 kg

	Weight (kg)[1]		
	40-55	**56-75**	**76-90**
Daily, mg (mg/kg)	1000 (18.2-25)	1500 (20-26.8)	2000[2] (22.2-26.3)
Thrice weekly, mg (mg/kg)	1500 (27.3-37.5)	2500 (33.3-44.6)	3000[2] (33.3-39.5)
Twice weekly, mg (mg/kg)	2000 (36.4-50)	3000 (40-53.6)	4000[2] (44.4-52.6)

[1]Based on estimated lean body weight

[2]Maximum dose regardless of weight.

Table 11. Suggested Ethambutol Doses, Using Whole Tablets, for Adults Weighing 40-90 kg

	Weight (kg)[1]		
	40-55	**56-75**	**76-90**
Daily, mg (mg/kg)	800 (14.5-20)	1200 (16-21.4)	1600[2] (17.8-21.1)
Thrice weekly, mg (mg/kg)	1200 (21.8-30)	2000 (26.7-35.7)	2400[2] (26.7-31.6)
Twice weekly, mg (mg/kg)	2000 (36.4-50)	2800 (37.3-50)	4000[2] (44.4-52.6)

[1]Based on estimated lean body weight

[2]Maximum dose regardless of weight.

CALCULATIONS FOR TOTAL PARENTERAL NUTRITION THERAPY – ADULT PATIENTS

Condition	Calorie Requirement (kcal/kg/d)	Protein Requirement (g/kg/d)
Resting state (adult medical patient)	20-30	0.8-1
Uncomplicated postop patients	25-35	1-1.3
Depleted patients	30-40	1.3-1.7
Hypermetabolic patients (trauma, sepsis, burns)	35-45	1.5-2

1 g protein yields 4 kcal/g
1 g fat yields 9 kcal/g
1 g dextrose yields 3.4 kcal/g
1 g nitrogen = 6.25 g protein

Electrolytes Required / Day

	mEq/d
Sodium	60-120
Potassium	60-120
Chloride	100-150
Magnesium	10-24
Calcium	10-20
Phosphate	20-50 mmol/d
Sulfate	10-24
Acetate	60-150
Bicarbonate	Should not be added

Estimated Fluid Requirements

30-35 mL/kg/d

or

mL/d = 1500 mL for first 20 kg of body weight + 20 mL/kg for body weight >20 kg

Estimated Energy Requirements

Basal energy expenditure (BEE)	
Harris Benedict equation	
male	BEE_{mal} = 66.67 + (13.75 x kg) + (5 x cm) - (6.76 x y)
female	BEE_{fem} = 665.1 + (9.56 x kg) + (1.85 x cm) - (4.68 x y)
Total daily energy expenditure (TDE)	**TDE = BEE x activity factor x injury factor**
Activity factor	Confined to bed = 1.2 Out of bed = 1.3
Injury factor	Surgery: Minor operations = 1-1.1 Major operations = 1.1-1.2
	Infection: Mild = 1-1.2 Moderate = 1.2-1.4 Severe = 1.4-1.6
	Skeletal trauma = 1.2-1.35
	Head injury (treated with corticosteroids) = 1.6
	Blunt trauma = 1.15-1.35
	Burns ≤20% body surface area (BSA) = 2 20%-30% BSA = 2-2.2 >30% BSA = 2.2

MEDIAN HEIGHTS AND WEIGHTS AND RECOMMENDED ENERGY INTAKE[1]

Age (y) or Condition	Weight (kg)	Weight (lb)	Height (cm)	Height (in)	REE[2] (kcal/d)	Average Energy Allowance (kcal)[3] Multiples of REE	/kg	/d[4]
Infants								
0-0.5	6	13	60	24	320		108	650
0.5-1	9	20	71	28	500		98	850
Children								
1-3	13	29	90	35	740		102	1300
4-6	20	44	112	44	950		90	1800
7-10	28	62	132	52	1130		70	2000
Male								
11-14	45	99	157	62	1440	1.70	55	2500
15-18	66	145	176	69	1760	1.67	45	3000
19-24	72	160	177	70	1780	1.67	40	2900
25-50	79	174	176	70	1800	1.60	37	2900
51+	77	170	173	68	1530	1.50	30	2300
Female								
11-14	46	101	157	62	1310	1.67	47	2200
15-18	55	120	163	64	1370	1.60	40	2200
19-24	58	128	164	65	1350	1.60	38	2200
25-50	63	138	163	64	1380	1.55	36	2200
51+	65	143	160	63	1280	1.50	30	1900
Pregnant								+0
1st trimester								+300
2nd trimester								+300
3rd trimester								+300
Lactating								
1st 6 months								+500
2nd 6 months								+500

[1]From *Recommended Dietary Allowances*, 10th ed, Washington, DC: National Academy Press, 1989.

[2]Calculation based on FAO equations, then rounded.

[3]In the range of light to moderate activity, the coefficient of variation is ±20%.

[4]Figure is rounded.

PEDIATRIC ALS ALGORITHMS

PALS Bradycardia Algorithm

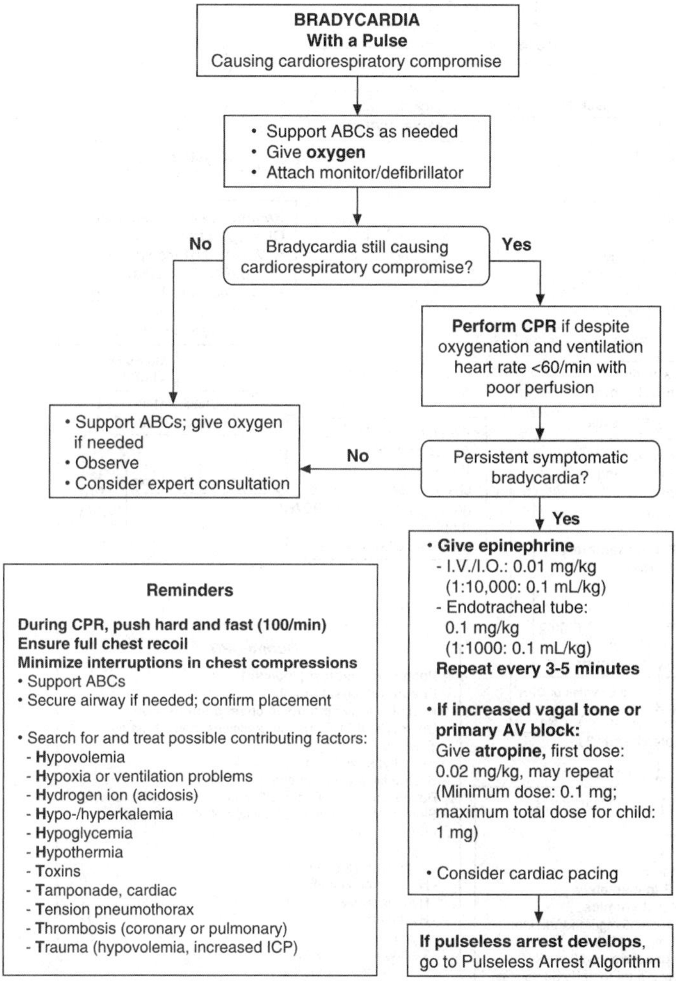

PALS Pulseless Arrest Algorithm

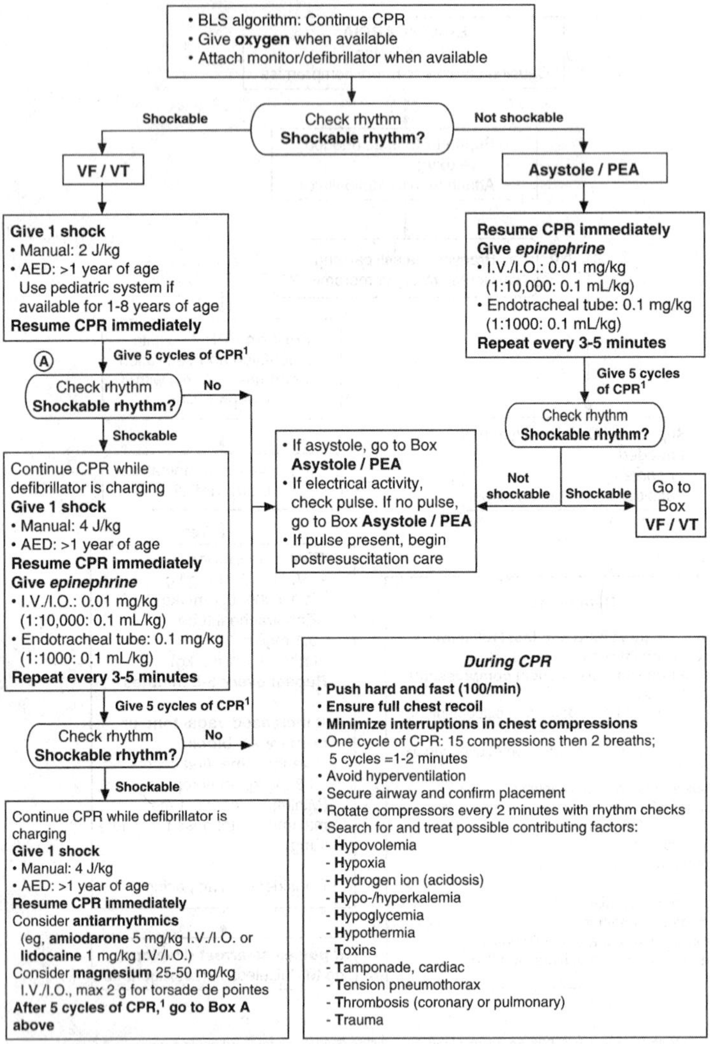

VF = ventricular fibrillation; VT = ventricular tachycardia; PEA = pulseless electrical activity; AED = automated external defibrillator.

[1]After an advanced airway is placed, rescuers no longer deliver "cycles" of CPR. Give continuous chest compressions without pauses for breaths. Give 8-10 breaths/min. Check rhythm every 2 minutes.

PALS Tachycardia Algorithm With Pulses and Poor Perfusion

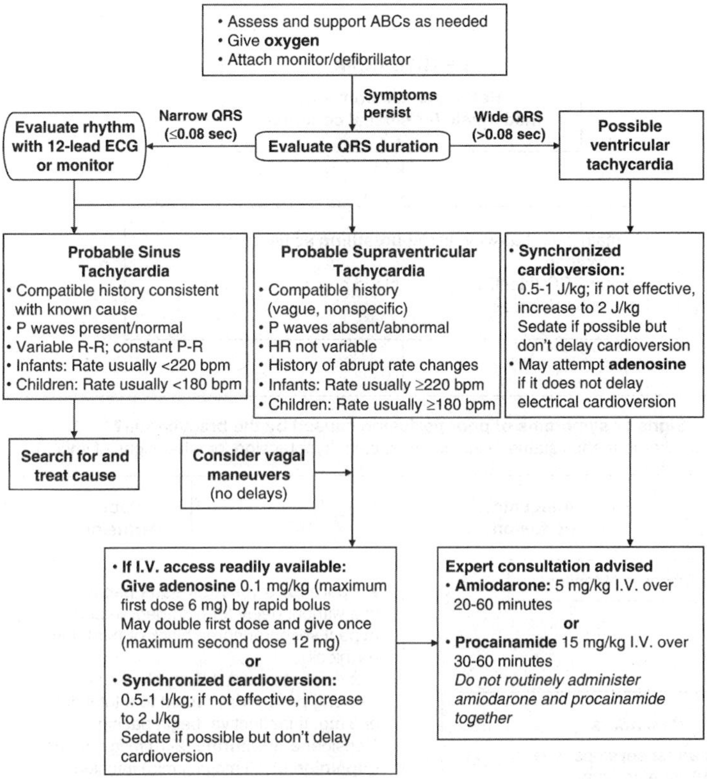

During Evaluation

- Secure, verify airway and vascular access when possible
- Consider expert consultation
- Prepare for cardioversion

Treat possible contributing factors:

- **H**ypovolemia
- **H**ypoxia
- **H**ydrogen ion (acidosis)
- **H**ypo-/hyperkalemia
- **H**ypoglycemia
- **H**ypothermia
- **T**oxins
- **T**amponade, cardiac
- **T**ension pneumothorax
- **T**hrombosis (coronary or pulmonary)
- **T**rauma (hypovolemia)

ADULT ACLS ALGORITHMS

Bradycardia Algorithm

BRADYCARDIA

Heart rate <60 bpm and inadequate for clinical condition

↓

- Maintain patent **airway**; assist **breathing** as needed
- Give **oxygen**
- Monitor ECG (identify rhythm), blood pressure, oximetry
- Establish I.V. access

↓

Signs or symptoms of poor perfusion caused by the bradycardia?
(eg, acute altered mental status, ongoing chest pain, hypotension, or other signs of shock)

Adequate Perfusion ↓

Observe / Monitor

Poor Perfusion ↓

- **Prepare for transcutaneous pacing;** use without delay for high-degree block (type II second-degree block or third-degree AV block)
- Consider **atropine** 0.5 mg I.V. while awaiting pacer. May repeat to a total dose of 3 mg. If ineffective, begin pacing.
- Consider **epinephrine** (2-10 mcg/min) or **dopamine** (2-10 mcg/kg/min) infusion while awaiting pacer or if pacing ineffective

↓

- Prepare for **transvenous pacing**
- Treat contributing causes
- Consider expert consultation

Reminders

- If pulseless arrest develops, *see* Pulseless Arrest Algorithm
- Search for and treat possible contributing factors:
  - **H**ypovolemia
  - **H**ypoxia
  - **H**ydrogen ion (acidosis)
  - **H**ypo-/hyperkalemia
  - **H**ypoglycemia
  - **H**ypothermia
  - **T**oxins
  - **T**amponade, cardiac
  - **T**ension pneumothorax
  - **T**hrombosis (coronary or pulmonary)
  - **T**rauma (hypovolemia, increased ICP)

ACLS Pulseless Arrest Algorithm

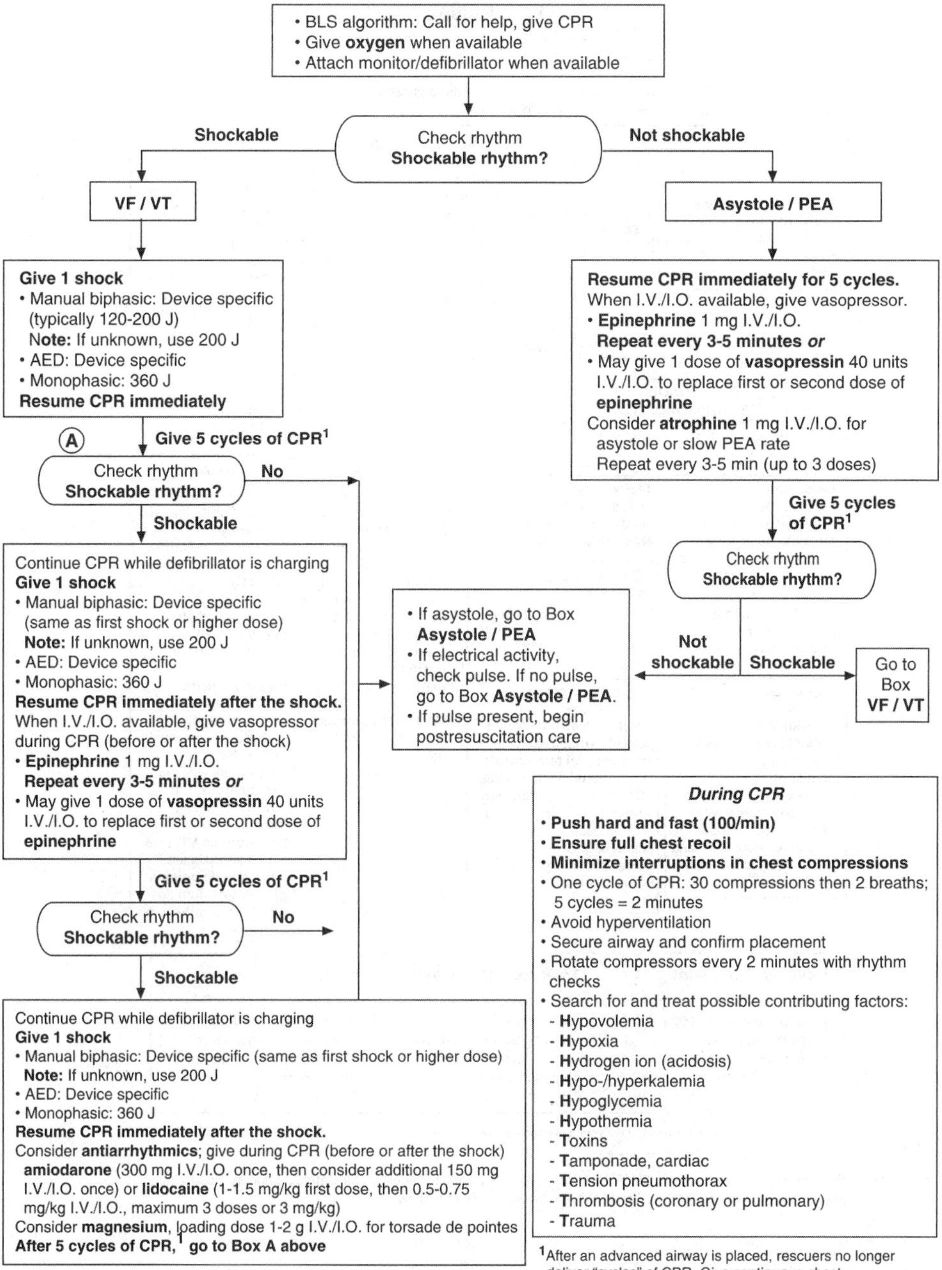

[1]After an advanced airway is placed, rescuers no longer deliver "cycles" of CPR. Give continuous chest compressions without pauses for breaths. Give 8-10 breaths/min. Check rhythm every 2 minutes.

VF = ventricular fibrillation; VT = ventricular tachycardia; PEA = pulseless electrical activity; AED = automated external defibrillator.

ACLS Tachycardia Algorithm With Pulses

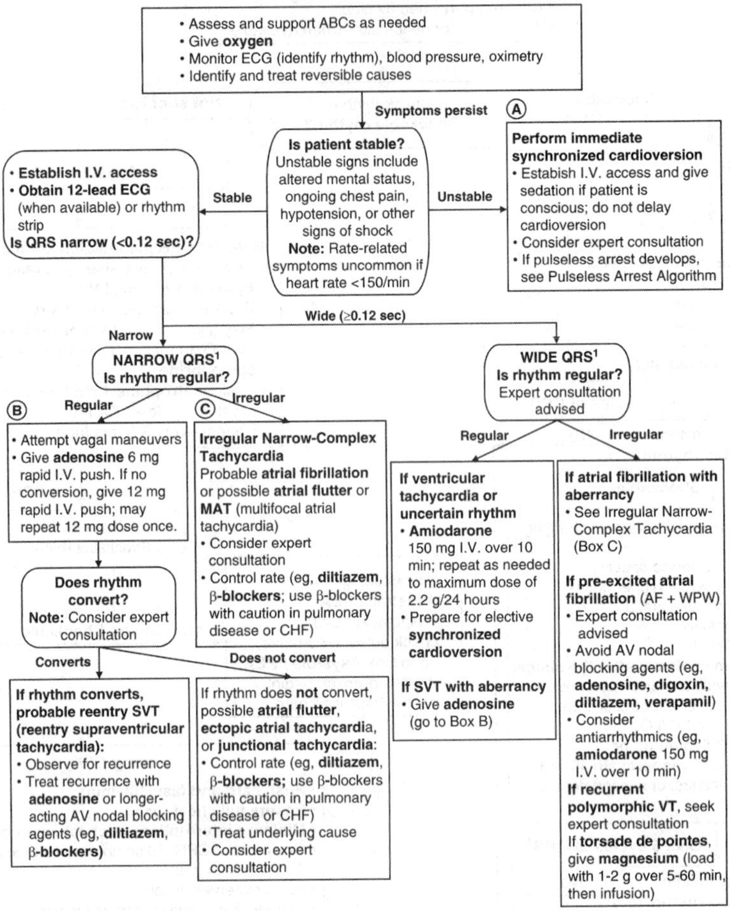

During Evaluation

- Secure, verify airway and vascular access when possible
- Consider expert consultation
- Prepare for cardioversion

Treat possible contributing factors:

- **H**ypovolemia
- **H**ypoxia
- **H**ydrogen ion (acidosis)
- **H**ypo-/hyperkalemia
- **H**ypoglycemia
- **H**ypothermia
- **T**oxins
- **T**amponade, cardiac
- **T**ension pneumothorax
- **T**hrombosis (coronary or pulmonary)
- **T**rauma (hypovolemia)

SVT = supraventricular tachycardia; VT = ventricular tachycardia.

[1]If patient becomes unstable, go to Box A.

ASTHMA

MANAGEMENT OF ASTHMA IN ADULTS AND CHILDREN

Goals of Asthma Treatment

- Prevent chronic and troublesome symptoms: Minimal or no chronic symptoms day or night
- No limitations on activities; no school/work missed
- Minimal use of inhaled short-acting $beta_2$-agonist (≤2days/week, <1 canister/month) (not including prevention of exercise induced asthma)
- Minimal or no adverse effects from medications
- Maintain (near) normal pulmonary function
- Prevent recurrent exacerbations (ie, trips to emergency department or hospitalizations)

All Patients

- Short-acting bronchodilator: **Inhaled $beta_2$-agonists** as needed for symptoms.
- Intensity of treatment will depend on severity of exacerbation; see "Management of Asthma Exacerbations".
- Use of short-acting inhaled $beta_2$-agonists on a daily basis, or increasing use, indicates the need to initiate or titrate long-term control therapy.

Education

- Teach self-management.
- Teach about controlling environmental factors (avoidance of allergens or other factors that contribute to asthma severity).
- Review administration technique and compliance with patient.
- Use a written action plan to help educate.

Stepwise Approach for Managing Asthma in Adults and Children ≥12 Years of Age

Symptoms	Lung Function	Daily Medications
	STEP 6: Severe Asthma	
Day: Throughout the day Night: Often 7 times/week SABA use: Several times/day	FEV_1 <60% predicted FEV_1/FVC reduced 5%	**Preferred:** High dose ICS plus LABA plus oral corticosteroid AND Consider: Omalizumab (in those with allergies)[1]
	STEP 5: Severe Asthma	
Day: Throughout the day Night: Often 7 times/week SABA use: Several times/day	FEV_1 <60% predicted FEV_1/FVC reduced 5%	**Preferred:** High dose ICS plus LABA AND Consider: Omalizumab (in those with allergies)[1]
	STEP 4: Severe Asthma	
Day: Throughout the day Night: Often 7 times/week SABA use: Several times/day	FEV_1 <60% predicted FEV_1/FVC reduced 5%	**Preferred:** Medium dose ICS plus LABA **Alternatives[2]:** Medium dose ICS plus either LTRA, theophylline, or zileuton[3]
	STEP 3: Moderate Asthma	
Day: Daily Night: >1 night/week (not nightly) SABA use: Daily	FEV_1 >60%, <80% predicted FEV_1/FVC reduced 5%	**Preferred:** Low dose ICS plus LABA OR Medium dose ICS **Alternatives[2]:** Low dose ICS plus either LTRA, theophylline, or zileuton[3]
	STEP 2: Mild Asthma	
Day: >2 days/week (not daily) Night: 3-4 times/month SABA use: >2 days/week, no more than once per day (not daily)	FEV_1 <80% FEV_1/FVC normal	**Preferred:** Low dose ICS **Alternatives[2]:** Cromolyn, LTRA, nedocromil, or theophylline
	STEP 1: Intermittent Asthma	
Day: ≤2 days/week Night: ≤2 nights/month SABA use: ≤2 days/week	FEV_1 normal between exacerbations FEV_1 >80% predicted FEV_1/FVC normal	Preferred: SABA as needed

Note: Treatment options within each step are listed in alphabetical order.

Steps 2-4: Consider subcutaneous allergen immunotherapy for patients with allergic asthma.[1]

Consult with asthma specialist if Step 4 or higher care is needed.

FEV_1 = forced expiratory volume in 1 second; FVC = forced vital capacity; ICS = inhaled corticosteroid; LABA = long-acting inhaled $beta_2$-agonist; SABA = short-acting inhaled $beta_2$-agonist; LTRA = leukotriene receptor antagonist.

[1]When using immunotherapy or omalizumab, clinicians should be prepared to identify and treat anaphylaxis in the event it occurs.

[2]If alternative treatment is used and response is inadequate, discontinue it and use preferred treatment before stepping up.

[3]Zileuton is less desirable alternative due to limited studies and need to monitor liver function.

Notes:

- **The stepwise approach presents general guidelines to assist clinical decision making; it is not intended to be a specific prescription. Asthma is highly variable; clinicians should tailor specific medication plans to the needs and circumstances of individual patients.**
- Gain control as quickly as possible; then decrease treatment to the least medication necessary to maintain control.
- A rescue course of systemic corticosteroids may be needed at any time and at any step.
- Some patients with intermittent asthma experience severe and life-threatening exacerbations separated by long periods of normal lung function and no symptoms. This may be especially common with exacerbations provoked by respiratory infections.
- At each step, patient education, environmental control, management of comorbidities emphasized.
- Antibiotics are not recommended for treatment of acute asthma exacerbations except where there is evidence or suspicion of bacterial infection.
- Consultation with an asthma specialist is recommended for moderate or severe persistent asthma.
- Peak flow monitoring for patients with moderate-severe persistent asthma and patients who have a history of severe exacerbations should be considered.

MANAGEMENT OF ASTHMA IN INFANTS AND YOUNG CHILDREN (<12 YEARS OF AGE)

Stepwise Approach for Managing Asthma in Children 0-4 Years of Age

Symptoms	Daily Medications[1]
STEP 6: Severe Asthma	
Day: Throughout the day Night: >1 time/week SABA use: Several times/day	**Preferred:** High dose ICS plus either LABA or montelukast Oral systemic corticosteroids
STEP 5: Severe Asthma	
Day: Throughout the day Night: >1 time/week SABA use: Daily	**Preferred:** High dose ICS plus either LABA or montelukast
STEP 4: Moderate Asthma	
Day: Daily Night: 3-4 times/month SABA use: Daily	**Preferred:** Medium dose ICS plus either LABA or montelukast
STEP 3: Moderate Asthma	
Day: Daily Night: 3-4 times/month SABA use: Daily	**Preferred:** Medium dose ICS
STEP 2: Mild Asthma	
Day: >2 days/week (not daily) Night: 1-2 times/month SABA use: >2 days/week, no more than once per day (not daily)	**Preferred:** Low dose ICS **Alternatives[2]:** Cromolyn, montelukast
STEP 1: Intermittent Asthma	
Day: ≤2 days/week Night: No symptoms SABA use: ≤2 days/week	SABA as needed

Consult with asthma specialist if Step 3 or higher care is needed.

FEV_1 = forced expiratory volume in 1 second; FVC = forced vital capacity; ICS = inhaled corticosteroid; LABA = long-acting inhaled $beta_2$-agonist; SABA = short-acting inhaled $beta_2$-agonist.

[1]Studies on children 0-4 years old are limited. Many recommendations are based on expert opinion and extrapolation from studies of older children.

[2]If alternative treatment is used and response is inadequate, discontinue it and use preferred treatment before stepping up.

Stepwise Approach for Managing Asthma in Children 5-11 Years

Symptoms	Lung Function	Daily Medications
STEP 6: Severe Asthma		
Day: Throughout the day Night: Often 7 times/week SABA use: Several times/day	FEV_1 <60% predicted FEV_1/FVC <75%	**Preferred:** High dose ICS plus LABA plus oral corticosteroid **Alternative[1]:** High dose ICS plus either LTRA or theophylline[2] plus oral systemic corticosteroid
STEP 5: Severe Asthma		
Day: Throughout the day Night: Often 7 times/week SABA use: Several times/day	FEV_1 <60% predicted FEV_1/FVC <75%	**Preferred:** High dose ICS plus LABA **Alternative[1]:** High dose ICS plus either LTRA or theophylline[2]
STEP 4: Severe Asthma		
Day: Throughout the day Night: Often 7 times/week SABA use: Several times/day	FEV_1 <60% predicted FEV_1/FVC <75%	**Preferred:** Medium dose ICS plus LABA **Alternative[1]:** Medium dose ICS plus either LTRA or theophylline[2]
STEP 3: Moderate Asthma		
Day: Daily Night: >1 time/week (not nightly) SABA use: Daily	FEV_1 60% to 80% predicted FEV_1/FVC 75% to 80%	**Preferred:** Low dose ICS plus either LABA, LTRA, or theophylline[2] OR Medium dose ICS
STEP 2: Mild Asthma		
Day: >2 days/week (not daily) Night: 3-4 times/month SABA use: >2 days/week, no more than once per day (not daily)	FEV_1 ≥80% predicted FEV_1/FVC >80%	**Preferred:** Low dose ICS **Alternatives[1]:** Cromolyn, LTRA, nedocromil, or theophylline[2]
STEP 1: Intermittent Asthma		
Day: ≤2 days/week Night: ≤2 times/month SABA use: ≤2 days/week	FEV_1 normal between exacerbations FEV_1 >80% predicted FEV_1/FVC >85%	SABA as needed

Steps 2-4: Consider subcutaneous allergen immunotherapy for patients with allergic asthma.[3]

Consult with asthma specialist if Step 4 or higher care is needed.

FEV_1 = forced expiratory volume in 1 second; FVC = forced vital capacity; ICS = inhaled corticosteroid; LABA = long-acting inhaled $beta_2$-agonist; SABA = short-acting inhaled $beta_2$-agonist; LTRA = leukotriene receptor antagonist.

[1]If alternative treatment is used and response is inadequate, discontinue it and use preferred treatment before stepping up.

[2]Theophylline is a less desirable alternative due monitoring required.

[3]When using immunotherapy, clinicians should be prepared to identify and treat anaphylaxis in the event it occurs.

Management of Asthma Exacerbations: Home Treatment

Assess Severity

- **Patients at high risk for a fatal attack require immediate medical attention after initial treatment.**
- Symptoms and signs suggestive of a more serious exacerbation such as marked breathlessness, inability to speak more than short phrases, use of accessory muscles, or drowsiness should result in initial treatment while immediately consulting with a clinician.
- If available, measure PEF—values of 50% to 79% predicted or personal best indicate the need for quick-relief mediation. Depending on the response to treatment, contact with a clinician may also be indicated. Values below 50% indicate the need for immediate medical care.

↓

Initial Treatment

- Inhaled SABA: Up to two treatments 20 minutes apart of 2–6 puffs by metered-dose inhaler (MDI) or nebulizer treatments.
- Note: Medication delivery is highly variable. Children and individuals who have exacerbations of lesser severity may need fewer puffs than suggested above.

↓

Good Response

No wheezing or dyspnea (assess tachypnea in young children).

PEF ≥80% predicted or personal best.

- Contact clinician for followup instructions and further management.
- May continue inhaled SABA every 3–4 hours for 24–48 hours.
- Consider short course of oral systemic corticosteroids.

Incomplete Response

Persistent wheezing and dyspnea (tachypnea).

PEF 50% to 79% predicted or personal best.

- Add oral systemic corticosteroid.
- Continue inhaled SABA.
- Contact clinician urgently (this day) for further instruction.

Poor Response

Marked wheezing and dyspnea.

PEF <50% predicted or personal best.

- Add oral systemic corticosteroid
- Repeat inhaled SABA immediately.
- If distress is severe and nonresponsive to initial treatment:
  - Call your doctor AND
  - **PROCEED TO EMERGENCY DEPARTMENT**;
  - Consider calling 911 (ambulance transport).

↓

- To emergency department.

MDI: Metered-dose inhaler; PEF: Peak expiratory flow; SABA: Short-acting $beta_2$-agonist (quick relief inhaler)

Management of Asthma Exacerbations: Emergency Department and Hospital-Based Care

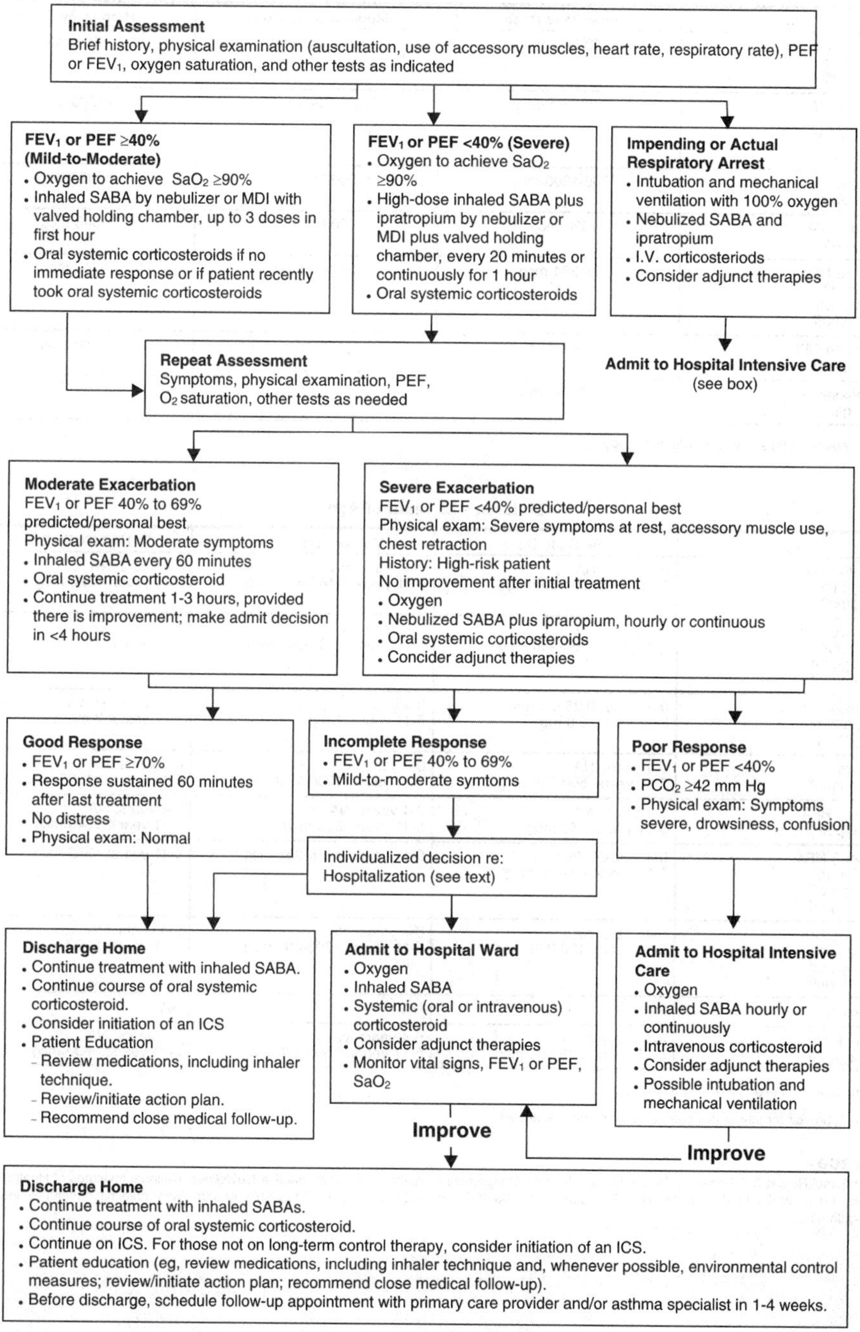

FEV$_1$ = forced expiratory volume in 1 second; ICS = inhaled corticosteroid; MDI = metered dose inhaler; PCO$_2$ = partial pressure carbon dioxide; PEF = peak expiratory flow; SABA = short-acting beta$_2$-agonist; SaO$_2$ = oxygen saturation

ESTIMATED COMPARATIVE DAILY DOSAGES FOR INHALED CORTICOSTEROIDS

Children ≥12 Years of Age and Adults

Drug	Low Daily Dose	Medium Daily Dose	High Daily Dose
Beclomethasone HFA 40 mcg/puff 80 mcg/puff	80-240 mcg	>240-480 mcg	>480 mcg
Budesonide DPI 90 mcg/puff 180 mcg/puff 200 mcg/puff	180-600 mcg	>600-1200 mcg	>1200 mcg
Flunisolide 250 mcg/puff	500-1000 mcg	>1000-2000 mcg	>2000 mcg
Flunisolide HFA 80 mcg/puff	320 mcg	>320-640 mcg	>640 mcg
Fluticasone HFA 44 mcg/puff 110 mcg/puff 220 mcg/puff	88-264 mcg	>264-440 mcg	>440 mcg
Mometasone DPI 220 mcg/puff	220 mcg	440 mcg	>440 mcg
Triamcinolone 100 mcg/puff	300-750 mcg	>750-1500 mcg	>1500 mcg

DPI = dry powder inhaler; HFA = hydrofluoroalkane.

Children <12 Years of Age

Drug	Low Daily Dose	Medium Daily Dose	High Daily Dose
Beclomethasone HFA 40 mcg/puff 80 mcg/puff	0-4 years: NA 5-11 years: 80-160 mcg	0-4 years: NA 5-11 years: >160-320 mcg	0-4 years: NA 5-11 years: >320 mcg
Budesonide DPI 90 mcg/puff 180 mcg/puff 200 mcg/puff	0-4 years: NA 5-11 years: 180-400 mcg	0-4 years: NA 5-11 years: >400-800 mcg	0-4 years: NA 5-11 years: >800 mcg
Budesonide nebulized 0.25 mg/2 mL 0.5 mg/2 mL	0-4 years: 0.25-0.5 mg 5-11 years: 0.5 mg	0-4 years: >0.5-1 mg 5-11 years: 1 mg	0-4 years: >1 mg 5-11 years: 2 mg
Flunisolide 250 mcg/puff	0-4 years: NA 5-11 years: 500-750 mcg	0-4 years: NA 5-11 years: 1000-1250 mcg	0-4 years: NA 5-11 years: >1250 mcg
Flunisolide HFA 80 mcg/puff	0-4 years: NA 5-11 years: 160 mcg	0-4 years: NA 5-11 years: 320 mcg	0-4 years: NA 5-11 years: ≥640 mcg
Fluticasone HFA 44 mcg/puff 110 mcg/puff 220 mcg/puff	0-4 years: 176 mcg 5-11 years: 88-176 mcg	0-11 years: >176-352 mcg	0-11 years: >352 mcg
Fluticasone DPI 50 mcg/puff 100 mcg/puff 250 mcg/puff	0-4 years: NA 5-11 years: 100-200 mcg	0-4 years: NA 5-11 years: >200-400 mcg	0-4 years: NA 5-11 years: >400 mcg
Mometasone	NA	NA	NA
Triamcinolone 100 mcg/puff	0-4 years: NA 5-11 years: 300-600 mcg	0-4 years: NA 5-11 years: >600-900 mcg	0-4 years: NA 5-11 years: >900 mcg

DPI = dry powder inhaler; HFA = hydrofluoroalkane.

NA = not approved for use in this age group or no data available.

Reference

Expert Panel Report 3, "Guidelines for the Diagnosis and Management of Asthma," *Clinical Practice Guidelines*, National Institutes of Health, National Heart, Lung, and Blood Institute, NIH Publication No. 08-4051, prepublication 2007. Available at http://www.nhlbi.nih.gov/guidelines/asthma/asthgdln.htm.

CONTRAST MEDIA REACTIONS, PREMEDICATION FOR PROPHYLAXIS

American College of Radiology Guidelines for Use of Nonionic Contrast Media

It is estimated that approximately 5% to 10% of patients will experience adverse reactions to administration of contrast dye (less for nonionic contrast). In approximately 1000-2000 administrations, a life-threatening reaction will occur.

A variety of premedication regimens have been proposed, both for pretreatment of "at risk" patients who require contrast media and before the routine administration of the intravenous high osmolar contrast media. Such regimens have been shown in clinical trials to decrease the frequency of all forms of contrast medium reactions. Pretreatment with a 2-dose regimen of methylprednisolone 32 mg, 12 and 2 hours prior to intravenous administration of HOCM (ionic), has been shown to decrease mild, moderate, and severe reactions in patients at increased risk and perhaps in patients without risk factors. Logistical and feasibility problems may preclude adequate premedication with this or any regimen for all patients. It is unclear at this time that steroid pretreatment prior to administration of ionic contrast media reduces the incidence of reactions to the same extent or less than that achieved with the use of nonionic contrast media alone. Information about the efficacy of nonionic contrast media combined with a premedication strategy, including steroids, is preliminary or not yet currently available. For high-risk patients (ie, previous contrast reactors), the combination of a pretreatment regimen with nonionic contrast media has empirical merit and may warrant consideration. Oral administration of steroids appears preferable to intravascular routes, and the drug may be prednisone or methylprednisolone. Supplemental administration of H_1 and H_2 antihistamine therapies, orally or intravenously, may reduce the frequency of urticaria, angioedema, and respiratory symptoms. Additionally, ephedrine administration has been suggested to decrease the frequency of contrast reactions, but caution is advised in patients with cardiac disease, hypertension, or hyperthyroidism. No premedication strategy should be a substitute for the ABC approach to preadministration preparedness listed above. Contrast reactions do occur despite any and all premedication prophylaxis. The incidence can be decreased, however, in some categories of "at risk" patients receiving high osmolar contrast media plus a medication regimen. For patients with previous contrast medium reactions, there is a slight chance that recurrence may be more severe or the same as the prior reaction, however, it is more likely that there will be no recurrence.

A general premedication regimen is

Methylprednisolone	32 mg orally 12 and 2 hours prior to procedure
Diphenhydramine	50 mg orally 1 hour prior to the procedure

An alternative premedication regimen is

Prednisone	50 mg orally 13, 7, and 1 hour before the procedure
Diphenhydramine	50 mg orally 1 hour before the procedure
Ephedrine	25 mg orally 1 hour before the procedure (except when contraindicated)

Unlabeled Use (Nephroprotective)

N-acetylcysteine, P.O.	600 mg orally twice daily on the day before and the day of the scan in addition to hydration with 0.45% saline intravenously

Indications for nonionic contrast are

- Previous reaction to contrast – premedicate[1]
- Known allergy to iodine or shellfish
- Asthma, especially if on medication
- Myocardial instability or CHF
- Risk for aspiration or severe nausea and vomiting
- Difficulty communicating or inability to give history
- Patients taking beta-blockers
- Small children at risk for electrolyte imbalance or extravasation
- Renal failure with diabetes, sickle cell disease, or myeloma
- At physician or patient request

[1]Life-threatening reactions (throat swelling, laryngeal edema, etc), consider omitting the intravenous contrast.

DEPRESSION

Medications That May Precipitate Depression

Anti-inflammatory & analgesic agents	Indomethacin, pentazocine, phenacetin, phenylbutazone
Antimicrobial agents	Cycloserine, ethambutol, sulfonamides, select gram-negative antibiotics
Cardiovascular/antihypertensive agents	Clonidine, digitalis, diuretics, guanethidine, hydralazine, indapamide, methyldopa, prazosin, procainamide, propranolol, reserpine
CNS-agents	Alcohol, amantadine, amphetamine & derivatives (withdrawal), barbiturates, benzodiazepines, chloral hydrate, carbamazepine, cocaine (withdrawal), haloperidol, L-dopa, phenothiazines, succinimide derivatives, levetiracetam
Hormonal agents	ACTH, corticosteroids, estrogen, melatonin, oral contraceptives, progesterone
Miscellaneous	Antineoplastic agents, cimetidine, disulfiram, organic pesticides, physostigmine, mercury

Medical Disorders and Psychiatric Disorders Associated With Depression

Endocrine diseases	Acromegaly, Addison's disease, Cushing's disease, diabetes mellitus, hyperparathyroidism, hypoparathyroidism, hyperthyroidism, hypothyroidism, insulinoma, pheochromocytoma, pituitary dysfunction
Deficiency states	Pellagra, pernicious anemia, severe anemia, Wernicke's encephalopathy
Infections	AIDS, encephalitis, fungal infections, meningitis, neurosyphilis, influenza, mononucleosis, pneumonia, toxoplasmosis, tuberculosis, viral hepatitis
Collagen disorders	Rheumatoid arthritis, systemic lupus erythematosus
Metabolic disorders	Electrolyte imbalance, hypokalemia, hyponatremia, hepatic encephalopathy, Pick's disease, uremia, Wilson's disease
Cardiovascular disease	Cerebral arteriosclerosis, chronic bronchitis, congestive heart failure, emphysema, myocardial infarction, paroxysmal dysrhythmias
Neurologic disorders	Alzheimer's disease, amyotrophic lateral sclerosis, brain tumors, chronic pain syndrome, complex partial seizures, Creutzfeldt-Jakob disease, Huntington's disease, multiple sclerosis, myasthenia gravis, Parkinson's disease, poststroke, sleep apnea, trauma (postconcussion)
Malignant disease	Breast, gastrointestinal, lung, pancreas, prostate
Psychiatric disorders	Alcoholism, anxiety disorders, eating disorders, schizophrenia

DIABETES MELLITUS MANAGEMENT, ADULTS

OVERVIEW

Diabetes represents a significant health care problem in the United States and worldwide. Of the nearly 23.6 million Americans with diabetes, the majority (90% to 95%) have type 2 diabetes. Of this number, nearly one-quarter are undiagnosed. The incidence of type 2 diabetes is increasing around the world. There is strong evidence to support an interaction between a genetic predisposition and behavioral or environmental factors, such as obesity and physical inactivity, in the development of this disease. In individuals at high risk of developing type 2 diabetes, it has been shown that the development of diabetes may be prevented or delayed by changes in lifestyle or pharmacologic intervention.

Within the United States, type 1 diabetes is estimated to comprise 5% to 10% of those with diabetes, and therefore represents the minority of individuals with diabetes. In addition to type 1 and type 2 diabetes, approximately 7% of pregnancies are complicated by the development of gestational diabetes. Gestational diabetes mellitus is defined as the first onset or recognition of glucose intolerance during pregnancy. Women who have had gestational diabetes are at an increased risk for later development of type 2 diabetes. In addition to the causes noted above, diabetes may result from genetic syndromes, surgery (pancreatectomy), chemicals and/or drugs, recurrent pancreatitis, malnutrition, and viral infections.

COMPLICATIONS OF DIABETES

Diabetes was listed as the seventh leading cause of death in the United States in 2006. Complications of diabetes are often contributing factors in the death of these patients; the most frequently reported diabetes complications on the death certificates of patients with diabetes in 2004 were heart disease and stroke, which were listed as contributing factors in 68% and 16% of diabetes-related deaths, respectively.

In addition to cardiovascular effects, diabetes is the leading cause of new blindness in people 20-74 years of age, and diabetic nephropathy is the most common cause of end-stage renal disease. Mild to severe forms of diabetic neuropathy are common. Neuropathy and circulatory insufficiency combine to make diabetes the most frequent cause of nontraumatic lower-limb amputations. The rate of impotence in diabetic males over 50 years of age has been estimated to be as high as 35% to 50%. Control of hyperglycemia may significantly decrease the rate at which diabetic complications develop, and provides compelling justification for early diagnosis and management of this disorder.

DIAGNOSIS

Diabetes

Diagnosis of diabetes is made by any of the three criteria described below. In the absence of unequivocal hyperglycemia with acute metabolic decompensation, these criteria should be confirmed by repeat testing on a different day. The use of Hb A_{1c} for diagnosis is not currently recommended. However, in 2008, a joint committee consisting of the American Diabetes Association (ADA), the European Association for the Study of Diabetes, and the International Diabetes Federation (IDF) was formed and will likely recommend that the Hb A_{1c} become the preferred diagnostic test (ADA, 2009). Screening should be considered in overweight adult patients (BMI ≥25 kg/m^2) who have at least one risk factor for diabetes (eg, physical inactivity, first-degree relative with diabetes, history of cardiovascular disease, etc). In patients without risk factors, testing should begin at age 45. Repeat testing should occur at least every 3 years in patients with normal test results.

Criteria for Diagnosis

1. Fasting plasma glucose (no caloric intake for at least 8 hours) ≥126 mg/dL (7 mmol/L)

   OR

2. Symptoms of hyperglycemia (polydipsia, polyuria, unexplained weight loss) plus casual plasma glucose concentration ≥200 mg/dL (11.1 mmol/L). **Note:** Casual plasma glucose is defined as any time of day without regard to time of last meal.

   OR

3. A 2-hour plasma glucose ≥200 mg/dL (11.1 mmol/L) during an oral glucose tolerance test (OGTT) as described by the World Health Organization (WHO) using a 75 gram anhydrous glucose load (or equivalent) dissolved in water. **Note:** OGTT is not recommended for routine clinical use.

Prediabetes

Patients with impaired fasting glucose (IFG) or impaired glucose tolerance (IGT) are considered to be in an intermediate group whose glucose levels do not meet the criteria for diabetes, yet are higher than normal. Patients with IFG or IGT are considered to be at high risk for developing diabetes and cardiovascular disease, and are referred to as having "prediabetes."

Prediabetes Categories using Fasting Plasma Glucose (FPG) or the Oral Glucose Tolerance Test (OGTT)

	FPG	OGTT[1]
Normal	<100 mg/dL (5.6 mmol/L)	<140 mg/dL (<7.8 mmol/L)
Impaired	100-125 mg/dL (5.6-6.9 mmol/L) [IFG]	≥140 mg/dL (≥7.8 mmol/L) and <200 mg/dL (<11.1 mmol/L) [IGT]

[1]Value corresponds to a 2-hour postload (75 g) glucose.

Gestational Diabetes Mellitus (GDM)

Assessment of risk should be undertaken at the first prenatal visit.

Low risk: Women who fulfill **all** of the following criteria are considered at lower risk for the development of GDM and do not require routine screening.

- <25 years of age
- normal body weight before pregnancy
- no family history of diabetes (ie, first-degree relatives)
- no history of abnormal glucose tolerance
- no history of poor obstetrical outcome
- not a member of an ethnic/racial group with a high prevalence of diabetes (Hispanic, Native American, Asian, African, Pacific Islander)

Average risk: Testing at 24-28 weeks gestation is recommended. Two approaches may be followed for GDM screening:

Two-step approach:

- Administer a 50 g oral glucose load and measure a serum or plasma glucose level 1 hour post-load (50 g).
- No further testing is required in patients with a serum or plasma glucose <130 m/dL
- In patients with a 1-hour post-load (50 g) serum or plasma glucose ≥130-140 mg/dL (depending on the desired threshold); perform a diagnostic 100 g OGTT on a separate day (see One-step approach).

One-step approach:

- Obtain a fasting plasma glucose following an overnight fast of at least 8 hours.
- Administer a 100 g oral glucose load and measure the plasma glucose levels at 1 hour, 2 hours, and 3 hours post-load (100 g).
- To make a diagnosis of GDM, **at least two** of the following plasma glucose values must be found:
  - Fasting ≥95 mg/dL
  - 1 hour: ≥180 mg/dL
  - 2 hour: ≥155 mg/dL
  - 3 hour: ≥140 mg/dL

High risk: The following are characteristics considered to be high risk for GDM. Women at high risk should be screened for diabetes as soon as feasible using standard diagnostic tests; repeat at 24-28 weeks gestation in patients not found to have GDM upon initial testing.

- severe obesity
- prior history of GDM or delivery of a large-for-gestational age infant
- glycosuria
- strong family history of type 2 diabetes
- diagnosis of polycystic ovary syndrome

Women with GDM should be screened for diabetes at 6-12 weeks postpartum using standard, nonpregnant diagnostic procedures.

GOALS

The goals of diabetes treatment include normalization of hyperglycemia, avoidance of hypoglycemia, and slowing the development of diabetic complications. The following is a summary of recommendations for adults with diabetes.

2008 ADA Summary of Recommendations for Adults With Diabetes

Glycemic control	
Hb A_{1c}	<7%[1]
Preprandial capillary plasma glucose	70-130 mg/dL
Peak postprandial capillary plasma glucose[2]	<180 mg/dL
Blood pressure	<130/80 mm Hg
Lipids[3]	
LDL[4]	<100 mg/dL
Triglycerides	<150 mg/dL
HDL	Male: >40 mg/dL Female: >50 mg/dL
Non-HDL chloesterol[5]	<130 mg/dL
Apolipoprotein B[6]	<90 mg/dL

[1]Referenced to a nondiabetic range of 4% to 6% using a DCCT-based assay. **Note:** The Hb A_{1c} goal for patients in general is <7%; even a lower goal may be appropriate for selected individuals (eg, short duration of diabetes, long life expectancy, and no significant cardiovascular disease) so long as a lower goal can be achieved without significant hypoglycemia or other adverse effects

[2]Postprandial glucose measurements should be made 1-2 hours after the beginning of the meal, generally peak levels in patients with diabetes.

[3]Current NCEP/ATP III guidelines suggest that in patients with triglycerides ≥200 mg/dL, the non-HDL cholesterol (total cholesterol minus HDL) be used. The goal is <130 mg/dL.

[4]In patients with overt CVD or cardiometabolic risk factors (eg, central obesity, insulin resistance, hypertension), a lower LDL goal of <70 mg/dL is an option.

[5]In patients with an LDL goal of <70 mg/dL, the non-HDL cholesterol goal is <100 mg/dL

[6]In patients on a statin with an LDL goal of <70 mg/dL or patients with cardiometabolic risk factors (eg, central obesity, insulin resistance, hypertension), the apolipoprotein B goal is <80 mg/dL

Key concepts in setting glycemic goals:

- Hb A_{1c} is the primary target for glycemic control.
- Goals should be individualized.
- Certain populations (children, pregnant women, and elderly) require special considerations.
- Less intensive glycemic goals may be indicated in patients with severe or frequent hypoglycemia.
- A lower glycemic goal (eg, Hb A_{1c} <6%) may further reduce the risk of microvascular complications at the cost of an increased risk of hypoglycemia (particularly in those with type 1 diabetes). However, recent studies (eg, ACCORD, ADVANCE, and VADT) have highlighted certain patient populations in which the risks of intensive glycemic control may outweigh the benefits, including patients with a very long duration of diabetes, history of severe hypoglycemia, advanced atherosclerosis, and advanced age or frailty.
- Postprandial glucose may be targeted if Hb A_{1c} goals are not met despite reaching preprandial glucose goals.

MANAGEMENT

Current American Diabetes Association (ADA) recommendations emphasize a multidisciplinary approach to the management of diabetes, with an emphasis on the participation of the patient and/or caregivers in the monitoring and management of the disease. Consultation with a diabetes educator and dietitian may help to prepare the patient to manage his/her disease and adjust to the necessary changes in diet and lifestyle. Patients must be educated about disease monitoring procedures, including blood glucose self-monitoring equipment and tests. Patients should be encouraged to wear or carry appropriate identification to inform health care providers of their disease in the event of an emergency. Issues related to possible complications (eg, foot care, eye care) should be addressed. It is extremely important to educate patients concerning the recognition and management of hypoglycemic symptoms. Weight management, which may include diet and exercise, is recommended for all overweight or obese patients. Bariatric surgery should be considered in adult patients with type 2 diabetes and a body mass index (BMI) ≥35 kg/m^2. Weight loss not only improves glycemic control, but decreases cardiovascular risk and can prevent development of type 2 diabetes. The management of diabetes is constantly adapting to new information, techniques, and technologies. For the most current information on diabetes diagnosis and management, visit the ADA website at http://diabetes.org.

Additional Management Issues

Recommendations by the ADA include glycemic control as well as the following:

1. In all patients with diabetes, cardiovascular risk factors should be assessed at least annually.
2. Use an ACEI or ARB in patients with diabetes who have hypertension and micro- or macroalbuminuria to slow the progression of nephropathy, unless contraindicated (eg, pregnancy); additional agents (eg, thiazide or loop diuretics) may be added as needed to achieve blood pressure goals.

3. Consider statin use in all patients with diabetes and cardiovascular disease or in patients with diabetes >40 years of age without cardiovascular disease but have at least one other cardiovascular disease risk factor, irrespective of lipoprotein levels (**Exception:** Statin use is contraindicated in pregnancy).
4. Immunize against pneumococcal disease and influenza.
5. Use aspirin (75-162 mg daily) for primary prevention in all patients with diabetes at increased cardiovascular risk, including those >40 years of age or who have additional risk factors (eg, hypertension, smoking, etc), unless contraindicated. In secondary prevention, all patients with a history of cardiovascular disease should receive aspirin (75-162 mg daily). Aspirin is not recommended in patients with diabetes <30 years of age, and is contraindicated in patients with diabetes <21 years of age. In patients unable to take aspirin (eg, documented allergy), the use of clopidogrel is considered a reasonable alternative.
6. Patients should be advised not to smoke.

DRUG TREATMENT

Insulin

Insulin therapy is required in type 1 diabetes, and may be necessary in some individuals with type 2 diabetes. The general objective of insulin replacement therapy is to approximate the physiologic pattern of insulin secretion which is characterized by two distinct phases. Phase 1 insulin secretion suppresses hepatic glucose production and phase 2 insulin secretion occurs in response to carbohydrate ingestion. This requires a basal level of insulin throughout the day (such as intermediate- or long-acting insulin or continuous insulin infusion administered via an external SubQ insulin infusion pump), supplemented by additional insulin at mealtimes (eg, short- or rapid-acting insulin).

Multiple daily doses guided by blood glucose monitoring are the standard of diabetes care. Combinations of insulin are commonly used. The number and size of daily doses, time of administration, and diet and exercise require continuous medical supervision. In addition, specific formulations may require distinct administration procedures/timing (refer to individual monographs).

There is solid scientific documentation of the benefit of tight glucose control, either by insulin pump or multiple daily injections (4-6 times daily). However, the benefits must be balanced against the risk of hypoglycemia, the patient's ability to adhere to the regimen, and other issues regarding the complexity of management. Diabetes self-management education (DSME) and medical nutrition therapy (MNT) are essential to maximize the effectiveness of therapy. In addition to the educational issues outlined above, patients should be instructed in insulin administration techniques, timing of administration, and sick-day management.

The initial dose of insulin in type 1 diabetes is typically 0.2-0.6 units/kg/day in divided doses. Conservative initial doses of 0.2-0.4 units/kg/day are often recommended to avoid the potential for hypoglycemia. Generally, one-half to three-fourths of the daily insulin dose is given as an intermediate- or long-acting form of insulin (in 1-2 daily injections). The remaining portion of the 24-hour insulin requirement is divided and administered as a rapid-acting or short-acting form of insulin. These may be given with meals (before or at the time of meals depending on the form of insulin) or at the same time as injections of intermediate forms (some premixed combinations are intended for this purpose).

Since combinations of agents are frequently used, dosage adjustment must address the individual component of the insulin regimen which most directly influences the blood glucose value in question, based on the known onset and duration of the insulin component (see table). The frequency of doses and monitoring must also be individualized in consideration of the patient's ability to manage therapy.

Types of Insulin	Onset (h)	Peak Glycemic Effect (h)	Duration (h)
Rapid-Acting			
Insulin lispro (Humalog®)	0.2-0.5	1.5-2.5	3-4
Insulin aspart (NovoLog®)	0.2-0.5	1-3	3-5
Insulin glulisine (Apidra™)	0.2-0.5	1.6-2.8	3-4
Short-Acting			
Insulin regular (Humulin® R, Novolin® R)	0.5	2.5-5	4-12
Intermediate-Acting			
Insulin NPH (isophane suspension) (Humulin® N, Novolin® N)	1-2	4-12	18-24
Intermediate- to Long-Acting			
Insulin detemir (Levemir®)	3-4	3-14	6-23
Long-Acting			
Insulin glargine (Lantus®)	3-4	*	≥24
Combinations			
Insulin aspart protamine suspension and insulin aspart (Novolog® Mix 70/30)	0.2	1-4	18-24
Insulin lispro protamine and insulin lispro (Humalog® Mix 75/25™)	0.2-0.5	2-12	18-24
Insulin NPH suspension and insulin regular solution (Novolin® 70/30)	0.5	2-12	18-24

*Insulin glargine has no pronounced peak.

Maintenance Dosing

Typical maintenance insulin doses are between 0.5 and 1.2 units/kg/day in divided doses. Adolescents may require ≤1.5 units/kg/day during growth spurts. Nonobese patients typically require 0.4-0.6 units/kg/day while obese patients may require 0.8-1.2 units/kg/day. In patients with renal impairment, insulin requirements may be reduced due to changes in insulin clearance and/or metabolism; insulin requirements may be <0.2 units/kg/day.

As stated above, the general objective of insulin replacement therapy is to approximate the physiologic pattern of insulin secretion. This requires a basal level of insulin throughout the day, supplemented by additional insulin at mealtimes. Combination regimens which exploit differences in the onset and duration of different insulin products are commonly used to approximate physiologic secretion. Frequently, split-mixed or basal-bolus regimens are used to approximate physiologic secretion.

Split-mixed regimens: In split-mixed regimens, an intermediate-acting insulin (such as NPH insulin) is administered once or twice daily and supplemented by short-acting (regular) or rapid-acting (lispro, aspart, or glulisine) insulin. Blood glucose measurements are completed several times daily. Dosages are adjusted emphasizing the individual component of the regimen which most directly influences the blood sugar in question (either the intermediate-acting component or the shorter-acting component). Fixed-ratio formulations (eg, 70/30 mix) may be used as twice daily injections in this scenario; however, the ability to titrate the dosage of an individual component is limited. An example of a "split-mixed" regimen would be 21 units of NPH plus 9 units of regular in the morning and an evening meal dose consisting of 14 units of NPH plus 6 units of regular insulin.

Basal-bolus regimens: Basal-bolus regimens are designed to more closely mimic physiologic secretion. These regimens employ intermediate- to long-acting insulins (eg, glargine, detemir) or a continuous insulin infusion administered via an external SubQ insulin infusion pump to simulate basal insulin secretion. The basal component is frequently administered at bedtime or in the early morning or as a continuous insulin infusion and then supplemented by multiple daily injections of very rapid-acting products (lispro, glulisine, or aspart) immediately prior to a meal; thereby, providing insulin at the time when nutrients are absorbed. An example of basal-bolus regimen would be 30 units of glargine at bedtime and 12 units of lispro insulin prior to each meal.

Adjustment of Insulin Dose

Dosage must be titrated to achieve glucose control and avoid hypoglycemia. In general, dosage is adjusted to maintain recommendations for glycemic control. Since combinations of agents are frequently used, dosage adjustment must address the individual component of the insulin regimen which most directly influences the blood glucose value in question, based on the known onset and duration of the insulin component. Individual insulin products have specific dosage recommendations.

Estimation of the effect per unit: A "Rule of 1500" has been frequently used as a means to estimate the change in blood sugar relative to each unit of insulin administered. In fact, the recommended values used in these calculations may vary from 1500-2200 (a value of at least 1800 is recommended for lispro). The higher values lead to more conservative estimates of the effect per unit of insulin, and therefore lead to more cautious adjustments. The effect per unit of insulin (aka, correction factor) is approximated by dividing the selected numerical value (eg, 1500-2200) by the number of units/day received by the patient. The correction factor may be used as a crude approximation of the patient's insulin sensitivity to determine the correction doses of insulin or adjust the current insulin regimen. Each additional unit of insulin added to the corresponding insulin dose may be expected to lower the blood glucose by the value of the correction factor.

To illustrate, in the "basal-bolus" regimen which includes 30 units of glargine at bedtime and 12 units of lispro insulin prior to each meal, the rule of 1800 would indicate an expected change of 27 mg/dL per unit of insulin (the total daily insulin dose is 66 units; using the formula: correction factor = 1800/66 = 27). A patient may be instructed to add additional insulin if the preprandial glucose is >125 mg/dL. For a prelunch glucose of 195 mg/dL (70 mg/dL higher than goal), this would mean the patient would administer the scheduled 12 units of lispro along with an additional "correction dose" of 3 units (70 divided by the correction factor of 27 derived from the formula) for a total of 15 units prior to the meal. If correction doses are required on a consistent basis, an adjustment of the patient's diet and/or scheduled insulin dose may be necessary.

Insulin Therapy in Type 2 Diabetes Mellitus

Insulin may be used in type 2 diabetes as a means to augment response to oral antidiabetic agents or as monotherapy in selected patients. According to a consensus statement developed by the ADA and the European Association for the Study of Diabetes, basal insulin (eg, glargine, detemir) should be considered in patients who have failed to achieve their glycemic goals following lifestyle interventions and the administration of the maximal tolerated dose of metformin (ADA, 2009). Furthermore, intensive insulin therapy (eg, basal-bolus regimens) should be considered in patients who have failed to achieve their glycemic goals with an optimized two- or three-drug regimen (ADA, 2009). Augmentation to control postprandial glucose may be accomplished with regular, glulisine, aspart, or lispro insulin. Dosage must be carefully adjusted.

When used as monotherapy, the requirements for insulin are highly variable. An empirically defined scheme for dosage estimation based on fasting plasma glucose and degree of obesity has been published with recommended doses ranging from 6-77 units/day (Holman, 1995). In the setting of glucose toxicity (loss of beta-cell sensitivity to glucose concentrations), insulin therapy may be used for short-term management to restore sensitivity of beta-cells; in these cases, the dose may need to be rapidly reduced/withdrawn when sensitivity is re-established.

Oral Agents

A large number of drugs for oral administration have become available for the management of type 2 diabetes. Oral antidiabetic agents include sulfonylureas, meglitinides, alpha-glucosidase inhibitors, biguanides, thiazolidinediones (TZDs), and dipeptidyl peptidase IV (DPP-IV) inhibitors. The drug classes vary in terms of their magnitude of effect on glycemic control, mechanism of action, and adverse effect profiles. In many cases, the adverse effect profile may influence the selection of a particular drug. The risk of hypoglycemia is higher for drugs which promote insulin secretion (particularly sulfonylureas or insulin secretagogues). Drug selection is based on patient-specific factors and anticipated tolerance of adverse effects.

At least two drugs have been withdrawn from the U.S. market due to toxicities. Phenformin, a biguanide, was removed many years ago after a number of cases of fatal lactic acidosis were reported. Metformin (also a biguanide) carries some risk of this reaction, but it is much lower than the risk associated with phenformin. Troglitazone, a prototype thiazolidinedione, was associated with hepatic failure and several deaths, and it was withdrawn shortly after introduction. Currently, marketed drugs from this class appear to have a lower risk of these reactions.

Combination therapy may be necessary to achieve glycemic goals. The risk of additive or additional adverse effects must be balanced with the desire to achieve goals of glycemic control as well as normalization of other metabolic parameters. In particular, weight gain and lipid disturbances may complicate drug treatment.

Oral Antidiabetic Agents for Type 2 Diabetes

Generic Name (Brand Name)	Expected Decrease (%) in Hb A_{1c} With Monotherapy	Key Adverse Effects
Alpha-Glucosidase Inhibitors		
Acarbose (Precose®)	0.5 to 0.8	GI distress, bloating, flatulence
Miglitol (Glyset®)		
Antilipemic Agent (Adjunct Therapy)		
Colesevelam (WelChol®)	0.5 to 1 (not for use as monotherapy	Constipation, dyspepsia
Biguanide		
Metformin (Fortamet™; Glucophage® XR; Glucophage®; Riomet™)	1 to 2	GI distress, lactic acidosis (rare)
Dipeptidyl Peptidase IV (DPP-IV) Inhibitors		
Sitagliptin (Januvia™)	0.5 to 0.8	Nasopharyngitis, upper respiratory tract infection, headache
Meglitinide Derivatives		
Nateglinide (Starlix®)	0.5 to 1.5	Hypoglycemia
Repaglinide (Prandin®)		
Sulfonylurea, 1st Generation		
Chlorpropamide (Diabinese®)	1 to 2	Dizziness, headache, GI distress, SIADH
Tolazamide		
Tolbutamide		
Sulfonylurea, 2nd Generation		
Glimepiride (Amaryl®)	1 to 2	Dizziness, headache, GI distress, SIADH
Glipizide (Glucotrol® XL; Glucotrol®)		
Glyburide (Diaβeta®; Glynase® PresTab®; Micronase®)		
Thiazolidinediones		
Pioglitazone (Actos®)	0.5 to 1.4	Hepatic dysfunction, hepatic failure, weight gain, edema, CHF, lipid changes
Rosiglitazone (Avandia®)		

Injectable Agents (Noninsulin)

In addition to insulin and oral agents, two injectable products are available for the management of diabetes. Exenatide (Byetta®) is FDA approved for the treatment of type 2 diabetes in patients previously treated with a sulfonylurea, metformin, thiazolidinedione, or a combination of these agents but still do not have adequate glycemic control. Exenatide increases insulin secretion, increases B-cell growth/replication, slows gastric emptying, and may decrease food intake.

Pramlintide (Symlin®) is FDA approved for the treatment of type 1 and type 2 diabetes. In type 1 diabetes, it is approved for use in patients who have failed to achieve glucose control despite optimal insulin therapy. When used for type 2 diabetes, pramlintide is approved for use in patients who have failed to achieve desired glucose control despite optimal insulin therapy, with or without concurrent sulfonylurea and/or metformin. Pramlintide is a synthetic analog of human amylin cosecreted with insulin by pancreatic beta cells. It reduces postprandial glucose increases by prolonging gastric emptying time, reducing postprandial glucagon secretion, and reducing caloric intake through centrally-mediated appetite suppression. It should be noted that the concentration of this product is in mcg/mL; patients and healthcare providers should exercise caution when administering this product to avoid inadvertent calculation of the dose based on "units," which could result in a sixfold overdose.

Injectable Agents (Non-Insulin) for Type 2 Diabetes

Generic Name (Brand Name)	Expected Decrease (%) in Hb A_{1c} With Monotherapy	Key Adverse Effects
Glucagon-Like Peptide 1 (GLP-1) Agonist		
Exenatide (Byetta®)	0.5 to 1	Nausea, vomiting, pancreatitis
Amylin Agonists		
Pramlintide (Symlin®)	0.5 to 1	Nausea, vomiting, hypoglycemia

References

Action to Control Cardiovascular Risk in Diabetes Study Group, "Effects of Intensive Glucose Lowering in Type 2 Diabetes," *N Engl J Med*, 2008, 358 (24):2545-59.
ADVANCE Collaborative Group, "Intensive Blood Glucose Control and Vascular Outcomes in Patients With Type 2 Diabetes," *N Engl J Med*, 2008, 358 (24):2560-72.
American Diabetes Association, "Diagnosis and Classification of Diabetes Mellitus," *Diabetes Care*, 2008, 31(Suppl 1):S55-60.
American Diabetes Association, "Standards of Medical Care in Diabetes - 2009," *Diabetes Care*, 2009, 32(Suppl 1):S13-61.
Brunzell JD, Davidson M, Furberg CD, et al, "Lipoprotein Management in Patients With Cardiometabolic Risk: Consensus Statement From the American Diabetes Association and the American College of Cardiology Foundation," *Diabetes Care*, 2008, 31(4):811-22.
Centers for Disease Control (CDC), "National Diabetes Fact Sheet: 2007 General Information," Available at: http://www.cdc.gov/diabetes/pubs/pdf/ndfs_2007.pdf. Accessed January 9, 2009.
Colhoun HM, Betteridge DJ, Durrington PN, et al, "Primary Prevention of Cardiovascular Disease With Atorvastatin in Type 2 Diabetes in the Collaborative Atorvastatin Diabetes Study (CARDS): Multicentre Randomised Placebo-Controlled Trial," *Lancet*, 2004, 364(9435):685-96.
Dailey G, "New Strategies for Basal Insulin Treatment in Type 2 Diabetes Mellitus," *Clin Ther*, 2004, 26(6):889-901.
DeFronzo RA, "Pharmacologic Therapy for Type 2 Diabetes Mellitus," *Ann Intern Med*, 2000, 133(1):73-4.
Duckworth W, Abraira C, Moritz T, et al, "Glucose Control and Vascular Complications in Veterans With Type 2 Diabetes," *N Engl J Med*, 2009, 360 (2):129-39.
Holman RR and Turner RC, "Insulin Therapy in Type II Diabetes," *Diabetes Res Clin Pract*, 1995, (28 Suppl):S179-84.
Joint Commission on Accreditation of Healthcare Organizations, "2005 National Patient Safety Goals," available at http://www.jcaho.org/accredited+organizations/patient+safety/05_npsg_guidelines.
Kitabchi AE, Umpierrez GE, Murphy MB, et al, "Hyperglycemic Crises in Diabetes," *Diabetes Care*, 2004, 27(Suppl 1):S94-102.
Nathan DM, Buse JB, Davidson MB, et al, "Medical Management of Hyperglycemia in Type 2 Diabetes: A Consensus Algorithm for the Initiation and Adjustment of Therapy: A Consensus Statement of the American Diabetes Association and the European Association for the Study of Diabetes," *Diabetes Care*, 2009, 32(1):193-203.
National Institute of Diabetes and Kigestive and Kidney Diseases, "Erectile Dysfunction," available at http://kidney.niddk.nih.gov/kudiseases/pubs/pdf/ErectileDysfunction.pdf. Accessed January 9, 2009.
Oiknine R, Bernbaum M, and Mooradian AD, "A Critical Appraisal of the Role of Insulin Analogues in the Management of Diabetes Mellitus," *Drugs*, 2005, 65(3):325-40.
Silverstein J, Klingensmith G, Copeland K, et al, "Care of Children and Adolescents With Type 1 Diabetes: A Statement of the American Diabetes Association," *Diabetes Care*, 2005, 28(1):186-212.
The Diabetes Control and Complications Trial Research Group, "The Effect of Intensive Treatment of Diabetes on the Development and Progression of Long-Term Complications in Insulin-dependent Diabetes Mellitus," *N Engl J Med*, 1993, 329(14):977-86.
Tuomilehto J, Lindstrom J, Eriksson JG, et al, "Prevention of Type 2 Diabetes Mellitus by Changes in Lifestyle Among Subjects With Impaired Glucose Tolerance," *N Engl J Med*, 2001, 344(18):1343-50.
UK Prospective Diabetes Study Group, " Intensive Blood Glucose Control With Sulphonylureas or Insulin Compared With Conventional Treatment and Risk of Complications in Patients With Type 2 Diabetes (UKPDS 33)," *Lancet*, 1998, 352(9131):837-53.

GLAUCOMA DRUG THERAPY

Ophthalmic Agent (Brand)	Reduces Aqueous Humor Production	Increases Aqueous Humor Outflow	Average Duration of Action	Strengths Available
Cholinesterase Inhibitors[1]				
Echothiophate (Phospholine Iodide®)	No data	Significant	2 wk	0.125%
Direct-Acting Cholinergic Miotics				
Carbachol	Some activity	Significant	8 h	0.75% to 3%
Pilocarpine (various)	Some activity	Significant	5 h	0.5%, 1%, 2%, 3%, 4%
Sympathomimetics				
Apraclonidine (Iopidine®)	Moderate	Moderate	4 h	0.5%, 1%
Brimonidine (Alphagan®, Alphagan® P)	Moderate	Moderate	12 h	0.1%, 0.15%
Dipivefrin (Propine®)	Some activity	Moderate	12 h	0.1%
Epinephrine	Some activity	Moderate	18 h	0.25% to 2%
Beta-Blockers				
Betaxolol (Betoptic® S)	Significant	Some activity	12 h	0.5%
Carteolol	Yes	No	12 h	1%
Levobunolol (Betagan®)	Significant	Some activity	18 h	0.5%
Metipranolol (OptiPranolol®)	Significant	Some activity	18 h	0.3%
Timolol (Betimol®, Timoptic®)	Significant	Some activity	18 h	0.25%, 0.5%
Carbonic Anhydrase Inhibitors				
Acetazolamide (Diamox®)	Significant	No data	10 h	125 mg tab, 250 mg tab; 500 mg cap
Brinzolamide (Azopt®)	Yes	No data	8 h	1%
Dorzolamide (Trusopt®)	Yes	No	8 h	2%
Methazolamide	Significant	No data	14 h	25 mg, 50 mg
Prostaglandin Agonists				
Bimatoprost (Lumigan®)		Yes	≥24 h	0.03%
Latanoprost (Xalatan®)		Yes	≥24 h	0.005%
Travoprost (Travatan®)		Yes	20 h	0.004%

[1]All miotic drugs significantly affect accommodation.

HEART FAILURE (SYSTOLIC)

INTRODUCTORY COMMENTS

This summarizes the pharmacotherapy of patients with systolic heart failure with respect to treating mild-moderate exacerbations and chronic therapy. A more detailed discussion is available at: www.acc.org/qualityandscience/clinical/guidelines/failure/update/index.pdf.

It should be recognized that the most common cause for exacerbations of patents' heart failure is poor adherence to therapy (medications and diet restriction). Healthcare providers need to educate patients about the importance of adherence to medical regimens.

For many years, therapy of heart failure focused on correcting the hemodynamic imbalances that occurred in heart failure. It is now recognized that heart failure triggers the release of several neurohormones that, in the short-run, help the patient; but, in the long-run, are detrimental. Newer pharmacotherapeutic approaches address counteracting the actions of these harmful neurohormones as well as address hemodynamic issues.

Diuretics

Although data have yet to demonstrate that diuretics reduce the mortality associated with heart failure, they relieve symptoms seen in heart failure. Diuretics should only be used in patients experiencing congestion with their heart failure. Although not usually the case, some patients do have heart failure without any congestion. In such rare instances, diuretic therapy is not indicated since they further stimulate the deleterious neurohormonal responses seen.

Although some heart failure patients with congestion can be controlled with thiazide diuretics, most will require the more potent loop diuretics, either because a strong diuretic effect is needed or the renal function of the patients is compromised (thus limiting the effectiveness of the thiazide diuretic). When patients with heart failure are discovered to have mild-moderate worsening congestion, they often can be controlled by adjusting their oral loop diuretic dose or, if applicable, initiating a loop diuretic regimen. If a more aggressive diuresis is indicated, especially if the patient is suffering from pulmonary congestion, intravenous loop diuretics would be indicated. When loop diuretics are given intravenously, before any diuretic effect occurs, they benefit the patient by dilating veins and reducing preload, thus relieving pulmonary congestion. Intravenous loop diuresis may also be considered in a patient where concerns exist about the ability of the patient to absorb the orally administered medication.

If already on an oral loop diuretic, the dosage should be increased (generally, 1.5-2 times their current regimen) in an effort for the patient to lose about 1-1.5 liters of fluid per day (about equivalent to 1-1.5 kg of weight per day). If the patient had yet to be started on a diuretic or was previously receiving a thiazide diuretic, initiating furosemide at 20-40 mg once or twice daily is a reasonable consideration. If the initial increase (or initiation) in dosage fails to induce a diuretic response, the dosage may be increased. If the initial increase (or initiation) does induce a diuretic response but the patient fails to lose weight or is not losing more fluids than taking in, the frequency of giving the loop diuretic can be increased. When an effective regimen is achieved, this regimen should be continued until the patient achieves a goal "dry" weight. Once this weight is attained, a decision needs to be made on how to continue the patient on diuretic therapy. If the patient had not been on a diuretic at home, continuation of the loop diuretic at a reduced dose is a worthy consideration. If the exacerbation was related to noncompliance with the diuretic or diet, the previous home dose might be continued with education on compliance. If the exacerbation was caused by an inadequate pharmacotherapeutic regimen (such as vasodilator was not being use), the previous home dose might be continued in conjunction with a more complete pharmacotherapeutic regimen. If the patient was compliant and on an acceptable pharmacotherapeutic regimen, the patient's original diuretic dose would be increased to some dosage greater than their home regimen, yet generally less than what was just used to achieve their dry weight.

The use of loop diuretics can lead to hypokalemia and/or hypomagnesemia. Electrolyte disturbances can predispose a patient to serious cardiac arrhythmias particularly if the patient is concurrently receiving digoxin. Fluid depletion, hypotension, and azotemia can also result from excessive use of diuretics. In contrast to thiazide diuretics, a loop diuretic can also lower serum calcium concentrations. For some patients, despite higher doses of loop diuretic treatment, an adequate diuretic response cannot be attained. Diuretic resistance can usually be overcome by intravenous administration (including continuous infusion), the use of 2 diuretics together (eg, furosemide and metolazone), or the use of a diuretic with a positive inotropic agent. When such combinations are used, serum electrolytes need to be monitored even more closely.

When loop diuretics are used in patients with renal dysfunction, to achieve the desired diuretic response, dosages typically will need to be greater than what is used in patients with normal renal function.

Due to its long existence and inexpensive price, furosemide tends to be the loop diuretic most commonly used. Bumetanide is now available as a generic and its use has been increasing consequently. The oral bioavailability of bumetanide and torsemide are nearly 100%; whereas, furosemide's oral bioavailability averages about 50%. A useful rule of thumb for conversion of intravenous loop diuretics is 40 mg of furosemide is equal to 1 mg bumetanide is equal to 15 mg torsemide. A few patients have allergies to diuretics because many contain a sulfur element. The only loop diuretic that lacks a sulfur element is ethacrynic acid.

Vasodilators

Vasodilator therapy, specifically the combination of hydralazine and isosorbide dinitrate, was the first pharmacotherapeutic treatment demonstrated to enhance survival of heart failure patients. The use of hydralazine 75 mg (which reduces afterload) and isosorbide dinitrate 40 mg four times a day (which reduces preload) demonstrated enhanced survival compared to placebo and prazosin. Unfortunately, many patients were unable to tolerate this regimen (primarily due to headaches and gastrointestinal disturbances) and the magnitude of benefit in survival dissipated with time.

Later, a series of investigations demonstrated that enalapril (which reduces both afterload and preload) enhances the survival of heart failure patients. Dosages used in these trials averaged about 10 mg twice daily. Since these trials, other ACE inhibitors were proven to benefit heart failure patients.

ACE Inhibitors

This led to the question, which is superior, ACE inhibitor or the combination of hydralazine and isosorbide dinitrate? In a comparative trial, using doses described above, enalapril was superior to the combination of hydralazine and isosorbide dinitrate, making an ACE inhibitor the vasodilator of choice in heart failure patients. An ACE inhibitor can alleviate symptoms, improve clinical status, and enhance a patient's quality of life. In addition an ACE inhibitor can reduce the risk of death and the combined risk of death or hospitalization.

Adverse effects associated with ACE inhibitors include hyperkalemia, rash, dysgeusia, dry cough, and (rarely) angioedema. Patients sometime develop renal dysfunction with the initiation of ACE inhibitors. This is not due to direct nephrotoxicity of the kidney but related to the ACE inhibitor dilating the efferent renal artery of the kidney, thus shunting blood away from being filtered in the glomerulus. The risk for renal dysfunction is increased when the ACE inhibitor is introduced to a patient who is hypovolemic, is being aggressively diuresed, is on an NSAID, or has bilateral renal artery stenosis (unilateral if only one kidney is present). Avoid NSAIDs in heart failure patients. ACE inhibitors should be avoided in patients with known renal artery stenosis. Monitor renal function and serum potassium within 1 to 2 weeks of initiation of therapy and routinely thereafter especially in patients with pre-existing hypotension, hyponatremia, diabetes, azotemia, or in those taking potassium supplements. Some patients will have an exaggerated hypotensive response following the initial doses (especially the first dose) of an ACE inhibitor.

A major limitation to using ACE inhibitors treatment in heart failure can be the dry cough that some patients develop. Lowering the ACE inhibitor dose sometimes can control it, but this may limit the effectiveness of the ACE inhibitor treatment. The development of angiotensin receptor blockers (ARBs) has helped address this issue. ARBs were demonstrated to enhance survival of heart failure patients. Although they are not the vasodilator of first choice in heart failure, they are a reasonable alternative in patients who cannot tolerate an ACE inhibitor due to the cough or some other adverse effect (with the exception of hyperkalemia and renal dysfunction; ARBs can induce as well). ARBs do not cause an accumulation of kinins as ACE inhibitors do.

Can ARBs can be used in patients who suffer angioedema with ACE inhibitors? Reports are available in the literature describing patients who experienced angioedema with both ACE inhibitors and ARBs. These cases do not indicate the safety of an ARB when used in a patient who has experienced an ACE inhibitor-induced angioedema. The CHARM-Alternative trial confirmed that only one of 39 patients (~2.6%) who experienced angioedema with an ACE inhibitors also experienced it with an ARB.

Concurrent Use of an ACE Inhibitor and an ARB

In Val-HeFT, valsartan added to conventional treatment (included ACE inhibitor treatment) did not impact survival but did reduce morbidity. Of note, a subgroup analysis of this trial suggested the combination of valsartan and an ACE inhibitor may be detrimental to patients also receiving a beta-blocker. In CHARM-Added, candesartan added to ACE inhibitor therapy was of benefit to heart failure patients (modest reduction in hospitalization; increased risk of hyperkalemia and renal dysfunction), even for those receiving a beta-blocker. As a result, the recently released ACC/AHA Practice Guidelines do not speak against using the combination of ACE inhibitors and ARBs. However, few patients in these trials were receiving an aldosterone blocker (such as spironolactone), which is now known to be of benefit to heart failure patients. Since there is enhanced risk for hyperkalemia and outcome data are currently unknown, the ACC/AHA Practice Guidelines for heart failure do not advocate the combined use of ACE inhibitors, ARBs, and an aldosterone inhibitor.

In summary, vasodilator therapy should initially consist of an ACE inhibitor. If such therapy cannot be tolerated due to renal failure or hyperkalemia, the combination of hydralazine and isosorbide dinitrate may be considered as ARBs can also cause renal failure and hyperkalemia. If the ACE inhibitor cannot be tolerated due to adverse effects such as dry cough, an ARB may be considered. If an ACE inhibitor and beta-blocker have been maximized yet heart failure symptoms persist, consider adding hydralazine and isosorbide dinitrate. This approach, in fact, has been demonstrated to enhance the survival of African-American patients with heart failure. Another approach may be to add an ARB to the ACE inhibitor; but caution should occur, due to the risk of hyperkalemia.

Beta-Blockers

Despite being negative inotropes, beta-blockers have been demonstrated to enhance the survival of systolic heart failure patients. Their benefit is attributed to their ability to protect the myocardium from the "bombardment" of catecholamines present in heart failure that can lead to ventricular remodeling. Bisoprolol, metoprolol succinate (extended release), and carvedilol have been demonstrated in trials to improve survival. At present, superiority of one agent over another has not been definitively demonstrated. For patients to be able to tolerate this therapy, beta-blocker treatment needs to be initiated at low doses and titrated slowly (generally, the dose is double every two weeks). Following the initiation of treatment and the increase in dosage, patients may feel that their disease is worsening but this should dissipate after a few days. If this ill feeling continues beyond a few days, consideration should be given to regimen adjustments. If the patient is congested, increase the diuretic dosage. If the patient's discomfort is related to hypotension, staggering the beta-blocker dose with the vasodilator dose and/or lowering the vasodilator dosage may be helpful. If these approaches are ineffective or cannot explain the patient's ill feeling, consideration should be given to lowering the beta-blocker dosage and attempt a dose titration increase later on. Sometimes, a patient may not be able to tolerate "goal" doses of both beta-blockers and concurrent vasodilator treatment due to hypotension. It is the consensus opinion that a reduced dose of each agent is better than a goal dose of just one agent. Beta-blockers are not necessarily contraindicated but need to be used cautiously in patients with bronchospastic disease, peripheral artery disease, or diabetes mellitus.

Aldosterone Blockers

Of the pharmacotherapeutic treatments of heart failure demonstrated to benefit patients, the use of aldosterone blockers is the newest. It has been demonstrated, especially in the more severe forms of heart failure, that spironolactone, at an average dose of 25 mg daily, enhances the survival of heart failure patients. In patients who suffer hyperkalemia at this relatively low dosage, lowering the dose to 25 mg every other day may be attempted. In patients who remain symptomatic with their heart failure and have maximized the other proven treatments of heart failure and whose potassium concentrations can tolerate increases, the spironolactone dose may be increased to 50 mg daily.

Obviously, hyperkalemia is a concern with this treatment, especially since patients generally will also be receiving an ACE inhibitor or ARB. It has been demonstrated that the number of emergency visits related to hyperkalemia in heart failure has increased with the introduction of aldosterone blocking therapy in treating heart failure. About 10% of patients will experience endocrinological effects with spironolactone. In men, breast tenderness and gynecomastic may occur. In women, menstrual irregularities may be seen. In such instances, the use of eplerenone may be considered. Eplerenone is less apt to induce endocrinological effects but it is more expensive. A typical dose is 25-50 mg daily. Eplerenone has been demonstrated to enhance survival of post-MI patients with reduced ejection fractions. Spironolactone has not been studied in this patient group.

These medications should not be started in patients with renal insufficiency. These medications should be avoided if the serum creatinine exceeds 2.5 mg/dL in men (2 mg/dL in women) or if baseline potassium ≥5 mEq/L.

Digoxin

The value of digoxin in heart failure has crossed the spectrum. In the late 1980s further investigation with digoxin suggested that indeed it may have a role in heart failure treatment, but the methods of these trials were not ideal (digoxin was taken away from stabilized patients to see if the condition of patients worsened – it did). Finally, digoxin was studied in a prospective manner where patients were on known optimal heart failure treatment at the time and randomized to placebo or digoxin. The digoxin dosage used resulted in digoxin steady-state concentrations of 1 mcg/L. This trial revealed that digoxin did not impact survival but reduced the number of patient hospitalizations, suggesting digoxin has a morbidity benefit. Many are of the opinion that digoxin's benefit is unrelated to its positive inotropic activity but related to inhibiting neurohormal activity. Healthcare providers may consider adding digoxin in patients with persistent heart failure symptoms as a fourth line agent.

Digoxin is primarily renally eliminated; therefore, renal function of patients should be closely monitored and the dose adjusted. Digoxin does become difficult to use in patients whose renal function is unstable. In the DIG trial, effective digoxin steady-state concentrations ranged between 0.7-1 mcg/L. Concentrations much beyond 1 mcg/L were associated with worsened outcomes, especially in women. Since digoxin's benefit is long-term, a loading dose is not necessary. When checking a digoxin serum concentration, the sample should not be obtained until 12 hours after a dose, especially if it was oral, since digoxin has a relatively long distribution phase. It should also be assured that the patient is at steady-state (recall that the half-life of digoxin in a patient with normal renal function is approximately 36 hours and that patients with heart failure generally have worsened renal function).

Hypokalemia, hypomagnesia, hypercalcemia, and hypothyroidism can precipitate digoxin toxicity in the presence of a therapeutic digoxin concentration. This toxicity can be alleviated by correcting the electrolyte abnormality. In acute digoxin overdoses, hyperkalemia can occur since digoxin inhibits the sodium-potassium ATPase pump. For this reason, one should not assume potassium is given to just **any** patient with digoxin toxicity. Digoxin toxicity can present as bradyarrhythmias, heart blocks, ventricular tachyarrhythmias, and atrial tachyarrhythmias (PAT with block is pathognomic). Other toxic manifestations include visual disturbances (including greenish-yellowish vision and halos around lights), gastrointestinal disturbances, anorexia, and altered mental status. Many medications elevate digoxin concentrations and a patient's regimen should be assessed for potential interactions.

Other Heart Failure Therapeutic Considerations

- If a calcium channel blocker is desired, amlodipine and felodipine are preferred choices.
- To treat arrhythmias, amiodarone and dofetilide are best documented to lack significant proarrhythmic propensity in heart failure patients.
- In heart failure patients with diabetes mellitus, metformin should not be used and "glitazones" should not be used in severe heart failure (NYHA III and IV) and used cautiously, if at all, in mild-moderate heart failure.
- The use of cilostazol, because it has type III phosphodiesterase-inhibiting properties, is contraindicated in heart failure. This is because the chronic use of oral milrinone and inamrinone, also type III phosphodiesterase inhibitors, resulted in enhanced mortality in heart failure patients (and therefore, these two agents were never FDA-approved for oral use).
- NSAID use should be avoided or used minimally as these agents antagonize the effects of diuretics and ACE inhibitors.
- Retrospective data suggests that daily aspirin may also negate the effects of ACE inhibitors but this has yet to be definitively proven in prospective trials. Using the lowest possible aspirin dose with the highest possible ACE inhibitor dose has been suggested as a way to best circumvent this issue.
- Routine intermittent infusions of positive inotropes are not recommended. Can be used as palliation in end-stage disease.

Dosing of ACE Inhibitors in Heart Failure[1]

ACEI	Initial Dose	Maximum Dose
Captopril	6.25 mg tid	50 mg tid
Enalapril	2.5 mg bid	10-20 mg bid
Fosinopril	5-10 mg daily	40 mg daily
Lisinopril	2.5-5 mg daily	20-40 mg daily
Perindopril	2 mg daily	8-16 mg daily
Quinapril	5 mg bid	20 mg bid
Ramipril	1.25-2.5 mg daily	10 mg daily
Trandolapril	1 mg daily	4 mg daily

[1]From ACC/AHA Guidelines.

Dosing of ARBs in Heart Failure[1]

ARB	Initial Dose	Maximum Dose
Candesartan	4-8 mg daily	32 mg daily
Losartan	25-50 mg daily	50-100 mg daily
Valsartan	20-40 mg bid	160 mg bid

[1]From ACC/AHA Guidelines.

Initial and Target Doses for Beta-Blocker Therapy in Heart Failure[1]

Beta-Blocker	Starting Dose	Target Dose	Comment
Bisoprolol	1.25 mg daily	10 mg daily	β_1-Selective blocker Inconvenient dosage forms for initial dose titration
Carvedilol	3.125 mg bid	25 mg bid (≤85 kg)	β-Nonselective blocker
		50 mg bid (>85 kg)	α-Blocking properties
Metoprolol succinate, extended release	12.5-25 mg daily	200 mg daily	β_1-Selective blocker

[1]From ACC/AHA Guidelines.

References

Brater DC, "Diuretic Therapy," *N Engl J Med*, 1998, 339(6):387-95.

Granger CB, McMurray JJ, Yusuf S, et al, "Effects of Candesartan in Patients With Chronic Heart Failure and Reduced Left-Ventricular Systolic Function Intolerant to Angiotensin-Converting-Enzyme Inhibitors: The CHARM-Alternative Trial," *Lancet*, 2003, 362(9386):772-6.

Hunt SA, Abraham WT, Chin MH, et al, "ACC/AHA 2005 Guideline Update for the Diagnosis and Management of Chronic Heart Failure in the Adult. A Report of the American College of Cardiology/American Heart Association Task Force on Practice Guidelines (Writing Committee to Update the 2001 Guidelines for the Evaluation and Management of Heart Failure)," *J Am Coll Cardiol*, 2005, 46(6):1116-43. Available online at www.acc.org.

McMurray JJ, Ostergren J, Swedberg K, et al, "Effects of Candesartan in Patients With Chronic Heart Failure and Reduced Left-Ventricular Systolic Function Taking Angiotensin-Converting-Enzyme Inhibitors: The CHARM-Added Trial," *Lancet*, 2003, 362(9386):767-71.

Taylor AL, Ziesche S, Yancy C, et al, "Combination of Isosorbide Dinitrate and Hydralazine in Blacks With Heart Failure," *N Engl J Med*, 2004, 351 (20):2049-57.

HELICOBACTER PYLORI TREATMENT

Multiple Drug Regimens for the Treatment of *H. pylori* Infection

Drug	Dosages	Duration of Therapy
H_2-receptor antagonist[1]	Any one given at appropriate dose	4 weeks
plus		
Bismuth subsalicylate	525 mg 4 times/day	2 weeks
plus		
Metronidazole	250 mg 4 times/day	2 weeks
plus		
Tetracycline	500 mg 4 times/day	2 weeks
Proton pump inhibitor[1]	Esomeprazole 40 mg once daily	10 days
plus		
Clarithromycin	500 mg twice daily	10 days
plus		
Amoxicillin	1000 mg twice daily	10 days
Proton pump inhibitor[1]	Lansoprazole 30 mg twice daily or Omeprazole 20 mg twice daily	10-14 days
plus		
Clarithromycin	500 mg twice daily	10-14 days
plus		
Amoxicillin	1000 mg twice daily	10-14 days
Proton pump inhibitor[1]	Rabeprazole 20 mg twice daily	7 days
plus		
Clarithromycin	500 mg twice daily	7 days
plus		
Amoxicillin	1000 mg twice daily	7 days
Proton pump inhibitor	Lansoprazole 30 mg twice daily or Omeprazole 20 mg twice daily	2 weeks
plus		
Clarithromycin	500 mg twice daily	2 weeks
plus		
Metronidazole	500 mg twice daily	2 weeks
Proton pump inhibitor	Lansoprazole 30 mg once daily or Omeprazole 20 mg once daily	2 weeks
plus		
Bismuth	525 mg 4 times/day	2 weeks
plus		
Metronidazole	500 mg 3 times/day	2 weeks
plus		
Tetracycline	500 mg 4 times/day	2 weeks

[1]FDA-approved regimen

Modified from Howden CS and Hunt RH, "Guidelines for the Management of *Helicobacter pylori* Infection," *AJG*, 1998, 93:2336.

HYPERGLYCEMIA- OR HYPOGLYCEMIA-CAUSING DRUGS

Hyperglycemia	Hypoglycemia	Hyperglycemia or Hypoglycemia
Caffeine Calcitonin Corticosteroids Diltiazem Estrogens Isoniazid Morphine Nicotine Nicotinic acid Nifedipine Oral contraceptives Phenytoin Sympathomimetic amines Theophylline Thiazide diuretics Thyroid products	ACE inhibitors Anabolic steroids Chloramphenicol Clofibrate Disopyramide MAO inhibitors Miconazole (oral form) Probenecid Pyridoxine Salicylates Sulfonamides Tetracycline Verapamil Warfarin	Alcohol Beta-blockers (also may mask symptoms of hypoglycemia) Fluoxetine Lithium Octreotide Phenothiazines Rifampin

Adapted from American Association of Diabetes Educators, A Core Curriculum for Diabetes Education, 3rd ed, Vol 10, Chicago, IL, 1998, 338-41.

HYPERLIPIDEMIA MANAGEMENT

MORTALITY

There is a strong link between serum cholesterol and cardiovascular mortality. This association becomes stronger in patients with established coronary artery disease. Lipid-lowering trials show that reductions in LDL cholesterol are followed by reductions in mortality. In general, each 1% fall in LDL cholesterol confers a 2% reduction in cardiovascular events. The aim of therapy for hyperlipidemia is to decrease cardiovascular morbidity and mortality by lowering cholesterol to a target level using safe and cost-effective treatment modalities. The target LDL cholesterol is determined by the number of patient risk factors (see the following Risk Factors and Goal LDL Cholesterol tables). The goal is achieved through diet, lifestyle modification, and drug therapy. The basis for these recommendations is provided by longitudinal interventional studies, demonstrating that lipid-lowering in patients with prior cardiovascular events (secondary prevention) and in patients with hyperlipidemia but no prior cardiac event (primary prevention) lowers the occurrence of future cardiovascular events, including stroke.

Major Risk Factors That Modify LDL Goals

Positive risk factors	Male ≥45 years
	Female ≥55 years
	Family history of premature coronary heart disease, defined as CHD in male first-degree relative <55 years; CHD in female first-degree relative <65 years
	Cigarette smoking
	Hypertension (blood pressure ≥140/90 mm Hg) or taking antihypertensive medication
	Low HDL (<40 mg/dL [1.03 mmol/L])
Negative risk factors	High HDL (≥60 mg/dL [1.6 mmol/L])[1]

[1]If HDL is ≥60 mg/dL, may subtract one positive risk factor.

Adult Treatment Panel (ATP) III LDL-C Goals and Cutpoints for Therapeutic Lifestyle Changes (TLC) and Drug Therapy in Different Risk Categories

Risk Category	LDL-C Goal	Initiate TLC	Consider Drug Therapy[1]
High risk: CHD[2] or CHD risk equivalents[3] (10-year risk >20%)	<100 mg/dL (optional goal: <70 mg/dL)[4]	≥100 mg/dL[5]	≥100 mg/dL[6] (<100 mg/dL: Consider drug options)[1]
Moderately high risk: ≥2 risk factors[7] (10-year risk 10% to 20%)[8]	<130 mg/dL[9]	≥130 mg/dL[5]	≥130 mg/dL (100-120 mg/dL: Consider drug options)[10]
Moderate risk: ≥2 risk factors[7] (10-year risk <10%)[8]	<130 mg/dL	≥130 mg/dL	≥160 mg/dL
Lower risk: 0-1 risk factor[11]	<160 mg/dL	≥160 mg/dL	≥190 mg/dL (160-189 mg/dL: LDL-lowering drug optional)

[1]When LDL-lowering drug therapy is employed, it is advised that intensity of therapy be sufficient to achieve at least a 30% to 40% reduction in LDL-C levels.

[2]CHD includes history of myocardial infarction, unstable angina, stable angina, coronary artery procedures (angioplasty or bypass surgery), or evidence of clinically significant myocardial ischemia.

[3]CHD risk equivalents include clinical manifestations of noncoronary forms of atherosclerotic disease (peripheral arterial disease, abdominal aortic aneurysm, and carotid artery disease [transient ischemic attacks or stroke of carotid origin or >50% obstruction of a carotid artery]), diabetes, and 2+ risk factors with 10-year risk for hard CHD >20%.

[4]Very high risk favors the optional LDL-C goal of <70 mg/dL, and in patients with high triglycerides, non-HDL-C <100 mg/dL.

[5]Any person at high risk or moderately high risk who has lifestyle-related risk factors (eg, obesity, physical inactivity, elevated triglyceride, low HDL-C, or metabolic syndrome) is a candidate for therapeutic lifestyle changes to modify these risk factors regardless of LDL-C level.

[6]If baseline LDL-C is <100 mg/dL, institution of an LDL-lowering drug is a therapeutic option on the basis of available clinical trial results. If a high-risk person has high triglycerides or low HDL-C, combining a fibrate or nicotinic acid with an LDL-lowering drug can be considered.

[7]Risk factors include cigarette smoking, hypertension (BP ≥140/90 mm Hg or on antihypertensive medication), low HDL cholesterol (<40 mg/dL), family history of premature CHD (CHD in male first-degree relative <55 years of age; CHD in female first-degree relative <65 years of age), and age (men ≥45 years; women ≥55 years).

[8]Electronic 10-year risk calculators are available at www.nhlbi.nih.gov/guidelines/cholesterol.

[9]Optional LDL-C goal <100 mg/dL.

[10]For moderately high-risk persons, when LDL-C level is 100-129 mg/dL, at baseline or on lifestyle therapy, initiation of an LDL-lowering drug to achieve an LDL-C level <100 mg/dL is a therapeutic option on the basis of available clinical trial results.

[11]Almost all people with zero or 1 risk factor have a 10-year risk <10%, and 10-year risk assessment in people with zero or 1 risk factor thus not necessary.

Any person with elevated LDL cholesterol or other form of hyperlipidemia should undergo evaluation to rule out secondary dyslipidemia. Causes of secondary dyslipidemia include diabetes, hypothyroidism, obstructive liver disease, chronic renal failure, and drugs that increase LDL and decrease HDL (progestins, anabolic steroids, corticosteroids).

Elevated Serum Triglyceride Levels

Elevated serum triglyceride levels may be an independent risk factor for coronary heart disease. Factors that contribute to hypertriglyceridemia include obesity, inactivity, cigarette smoking, excess alcohol intake, high carbohydrate diets (>60% of energy intake), type 2 diabetes, chronic renal failure, nephrotic syndrome, certain medications (corticosteroids, estrogens, retinoids, higher doses of beta-blockers), and genetic disorders. Non-HDL cholesterol (total cholesterol minus HDL cholesterol) is a secondary focus for clinicians treating patients with high serum triglyceride levels (≥200 mg/dL). The goal for non-HDL cholesterol in patients with high serum triglyceride levels can be set 30 mg/dL higher than usual LDL cholesterol goals. Patients with serum triglyceride levels <200 mg/dL should aim for the target LDL cholesterol goal.

ATP classification of serum triglyceride levels:

- Normal triglycerides: <150 mg/dL
- Borderline-high: 150-199 mg/dL
- High: 200-499 mg/dL
- Very high: ≥500 mg/dL

NONDRUG THERAPY

Dietary therapy and lifestyle modifications should be individualized for each patient. A total lifestyle change is recommended for all patients. Dietary and lifestyle modifications should be tried for 3 months, if deemed appropriate. Nondrug and drug therapy should be initiated simultaneously in patients with highly elevated cholesterol (see LDL Cholesterol Goals and Cutpoints for Therapeutic Lifestyle Changes and Drug Therapy in Different Risk Categories table). Increasing physical activity and smoking cessation will aid in the treatment of hyperlipidemia and improve cardiovascular health.

Note: Refer to the National Cholesterol Education Program reference for details concerning the calculation of 10-year risk of CHD using Framingham risk scoring. Risk assessment tool is available on-line at http://hin.nhlbi.nih.gov/atpiii/calculator.asp?usertype=prof, last accessed March 14, 2002.

Total Lifestyle Change (TLC) Diet

	Recommended Intake
Total fat	25%-35% of total calories
Saturated fat[1]	<7% of total calories
Polyunsaturated fat	≤10% of total calories
Monounsaturated fat	≤20% of total calories
Carbohydrates[2]	50%-60% of total calories
Fiber	20-30 g/day
Protein	~15% of total calories
Cholesterol	<200 mg/day
Total calories[3]	Balance energy intake and expenditure to maintain desirable body weight/prevent weight gain

[1]*Trans* fatty acids (partially hydrogenated oils) intake should be kept low. These are found in potato chips, other snack foods, margarines and shortenings, and fast-foods.

[2]Complex carbohydrates including grains (especially whole grains, fruits, and vegetables).

[3]Daily energy expenditure should include at least moderate physical activity.

DRUG THERAPY

Drug therapy should be selected based on the patient's lipid profile, concomitant disease states, and the cost of therapy. The following table lists specific advantages and disadvantages for various classes of lipid-lowering medications. The expected reduction in lipids with therapy is listed in the Lipid-Lowering Agents table. Refer to individual drug monographs for detailed information.

Advantages and Disadvantages of Specific Lipid-Lowering Therapies

	Advantages	Disadvantages
Bile acid sequestrants	Good choice for ↑ LDL, especially when combined with a statin (↓ LDL ≤50%); low potential for systemic side effects; good choice for younger patients	May increase triglycerides; higher incidence of adverse effects; moderately expensive; drug interactions; inconvenient dosing
Niacin	Good choice for almost any lipid abnormality; inexpensive; greatest increase in HDL	High incidence of adverse effects; may adversely affect NIDDM and gout; sustained release niacin may decrease the incidence of flushing and circumvent the need for multiple daily dosing; sustained release niacin may not increase HDL cholesterol or decrease triglycerides as well as immediate release niacin
HMG-CoA reductase inhibitors	Produces greatest ↓ in LDL; generally well-tolerated; convenient once-daily dosing; proven decrease in mortality	Expensive
Gemfibrozil	Good choice in patients with ↑ triglycerides where niacin is contraindicated or not well-tolerated; gemfibrozil is well tolerated	Variable effects on LDL
Ezetimibe	Additional cholesterol-lowering effects when combined with HMG-CoA reductase inhibitors	Effects similar to bile acid sequestrants

Lipid-Lowering Agents

Drug	Dose / Day	Effect on LDL (%)	Effect on HDL (%)	Effect on TG (%)
HMG-CoA Reductase Inhibitors				
Atorvastatin	10 mg	-39	+6	-19
	20 mg	-43	+9	-26
	40 mg	-50	+6	-29
	80 mg	-60	+5	-37
Fluvastatin	20 mg	-22	+3	-12
	40 mg	-25	+4	-14
	80 mg	-36	+6	-18
Lovastatin	10 mg	-21	+5	-10
	20 mg	-27	+6	-8
	40 mg	-31	+5	-8
	80 mg	-40	+9.5	-19
Pravastatin	10 mg	-22	+7	-15
	20 mg	-32	+2	-11
	40 mg	-34	+12	-24
	80 mg	-37	+3	-19
Rosuvastatin	5 mg	-45	+13	-35
	10 mg	-52	+14	-10
	20 mg	-55	+8	-23
	40 mg	-63	+10	-28
Simvastatin	5 mg	-26	+10	-12
	10 mg	-30	+12	-15
	20 mg	-38	+8	-19
	40 mg	-41	+13	-28
	80 mg	-47	+16	-33
Bile Acid Sequestrants				
Cholestyramine	4-24 g	-15 to -30	+3 to +5	+0 to +20
Colestipol	7-30 g	-15 to -30	+3 to +5	+0 to +20
Colesevelam	6 tablets	-15	+3	+10
	7 tablets	-18	+3	+9
Fibric Acid Derivatives				
Fenofibrate	67-200 mg	-20 to -25	+1 to +20	-30 to -50
Gemfibrozil	600 mg twice daily	-5 to -10[1]	+10 to +20	-40 to -60
Niacin	1.5-6 g	-21 to -27	+10 to +35	-10 to -50
2-Azetidinone				
Ezetimibe	10 mg	-18	+1	-8
Omega-3-Acid Ethyl Esters	4 g	+44.5	+9.1	-44.9
Combination Products				
Ezetimibe and fenofibrate	10/160 mg	-20	+19	-44
Ezetimibe and simvastatin	10/10 mg	-45	+8	-23
	10/20 mg	-52	+10	-24
	10/40 mg	-55	+6	-23
	10/80 mg	-60	+6	-31
Niacin and lovastatin	1000/20 mg	-30	+20	-32
	1000/40 mg	-36	+20	-39
	1500/40 mg	-37	+27	-44
	2000/40 mg	-42	+30	-44
Niacin and simvastatin	1000/20 mg	-12	+21	-27
	1000/40 mg	-7	+15	-23
	2000/20 mg	-14	+29	-38
	2000/40 mg	-5	+24	-32

[1]May increase LDL in some patients.

Recommended Liver Function Monitoring for HMG-CoA Reductase Inhibitors

Agent	Initial and After Elevation in Dose	6 Weeks[1]	12 Weeks[1]	Periodically
Atorvastatin (Lipitor®)	x		x	x
Fluvastatin (Lescol®)	x		x	x
Lovastatin (Mevacor®)	x	x	x	x
Pravastatin (Pravachol®)	x			x
Simvastatin (Zocor®)	x			x

[1]After initiation of therapy or any elevation in dose.

Progression of Drug Therapy in Primary Prevention

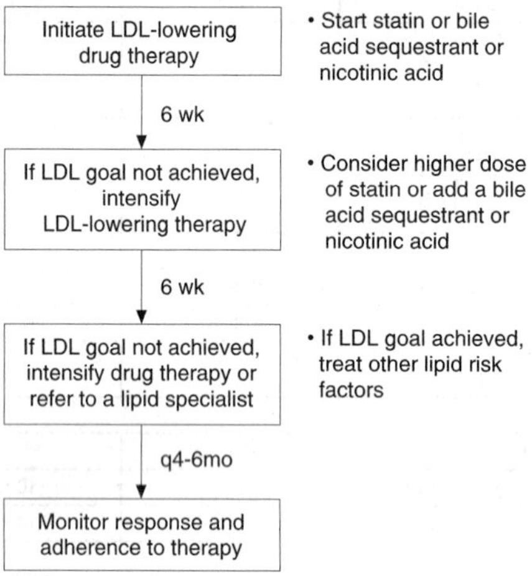

DRUG SELECTION

Lipid Profile	Monotherapy	Combination Therapies
Increased LDL with normal HDL and triglycerides (TG)	Resin Niacin[1] Statin	Resin plus niacin[1] or statin Statin plus niacin[1,2]
Increased LDL and increased TG (200-499 mg/dL)[2]	Intensify LDL-lowering therapy	Statin plus niacin[1,3] Statin plus fibrate[3]
Increased LDL and increased TG (≥500 mg/dL)[2]	Consider combination therapy (niacin,[1] fibrates, statin)	
Increased TG	Niacin[1] Fibrates	Niacin[1] plus fibrates
Increased LDL and low HDL	Niacin[1] Statin	Statin plus niacin[1,2]

[1]Avoid in diabetics.

[2]Emphasize weight reduction and increased physical activity.

[3]Risk of myopathy with combination.

Resins = bile acid sequestrants; statins = HMG-CoA reductase inhibitors; fibrates = fibric acid derivatives (eg, gemfibrozil, fenofibrate).

COMBINATION DRUG THERAPY

If after at least 6 weeks of therapy at the maximum recommended or tolerated dose, the patient's LDL cholesterol is not at target, consider optimizing nondrug measures, prescribing a higher dose of current lipid-lowering drug, or adding another lipid-lowering medication to the current therapy. Successful drug combinations include statin and niacin, statin and bile acid sequestrant, or niacin and bile acid sequestrant. At maximum recommended doses, LDL cholesterol may be decreased by 50% to 60% with combination therapy. This is the same reduction achieved by atorvastatin 40 mg twice daily. If a bile acid sequestrant is used with other lipid-lowering agents, space doses 1 hour before or 4 hours after the bile acid sequestrant administration. Statins combined with either fenofibrate, clofibrate, gemfibrozil, or niacin increase the risk of rhabdomyolysis. In this situation, patient education (muscle pain/weakness) and careful follow-up are warranted.

References

Guidelines

American Diabetes Association, "Standards of Medical Care in Diabetes - 2008," *Diabetes Care*, 2008, 31(Suppl 1):S12-54.

National Cholesterol Education Program, "Third Report of the Expert Panel on Detection, Evaluation, and Treatment of High Blood Cholesterol in Adults (Adult Treatment Panel III)," *JAMA*, 2001, 285(19):2486-97.

Grundy SM, Cleeman JI, Merz CN, et al, "Implications of Recent Clinical Trials for the National Cholesterol Education Program Adult Treatment Panel III Guidelines," *J Am Coll Cardiol*, 2004, 44(3):720-32.

Others

Berthold HK, Sudhop T, and von Bergmann K, "Effect of a Garlic Oil Preparation on Serum Lipoproteins and Cholesterol Metabolism: A Randomized Controlled Trial," *JAMA*, 1998, 279(23):1900-2.

Bertolini S, Bon GB, Campbell LM, et al, "Efficacy and Safety of Atorvastatin Compared to Pravastatin in Patients With Hypercholesterolemia," *Atherosclerosis*, 1997, 130(1-2):191-7.

Blankenhorn DH, Nessim SA, Johnson RL, et al, "Beneficial Effects of Combined Colestipol-Niacin Therapy on Coronary Atherosclerosis and Venous Bypass Grafts," *JAMA*, 1987, 257(23):3233-40.

Brown G, Albers JJ, Fisher LD, et al, "Regression of Coronary Artery Disease as a Result of Intensive Lipid-Lowering Therapy in Men With High Levels of Apolipoprotein B," *N Engl J Med*, 1990, 323(19):1289-98.

Capuzzi DM, Guyton JR, Morgan JM, et al, "Efficacy and Safety of an Extended-Release Niacin (Niaspan®): A Long-Term Study," *Am J Cardiol*, 1998, 82 (12A):74U-81U.

Coronary Drug Project Research Program, "Clofibrate and Niacin in Coronary Heart Disease," *JAMA*, 1975, 231(4):360-81.

Dart A, Jerums G, Nicholson G, et al, "A Multicenter, Double-Blind, One-Year Study Comparing Safety and Efficacy of Atorvastatin Versus Simvastatin in Patients With Hypercholesterolemia," *Am J Cardiol*, 1997, 80(1):39-44.

Davidson MH, Dillon MA, Gordon B, et al, "Colesevelam Hydrochloride (Cholestagel): A New Potent Bile Acid Sequestrant Associated With a Low Incidence of Gastrointestinal Side Effects," *Arch Intern Med*, 1999, 159(16):1893-900.

Davidson M, McKenney J, Stein E, et al, "Comparison of One-Year Efficacy and Safety of Atorvastatin Versus Lovastatin in Primary Hypercholesterolemia," *Am J Cardiol*, 1997, 79(11):1475-81.

Frick MH, Heinonen OP, Huttunen JK, et al, "Helsinki Heart Study: Primary-Prevention Trial With Gemfibrozil in Middle-Aged Men With Dyslipidemia," *N Engl J Med*, 1987, 317(20):1237-45.

Garber AM, Browner WS, and Hulley SB, "Clinical Guideline, Part 2: Cholesterol Screening in Asymptomatic Adults, Revisited," *Ann Intern Med*, 1995, 124(5):518-31.

Johannesson M, Jonsson B, Kjekshus J, et al, "Cost-Effectiveness of Simvastatin Treatment to Lower Cholesterol Levels in Patients With Coronary Heart Disease. Scandinavian Simvastatin Survival Study Group," *N Engl N Med*, 1997, 336(5):332-6.

Jones P, Kafonek S, Laurora I, et al, "Comparative Dose Efficacy Study of Atorvastatin Versus Simvastatin, Pravastatin, Lovastatin, and Fluvastatin in Patients With Hypercholesterolemia," *Am J Cardiol*, 1998, 81(5):582-7.

Kasiske BL, Ma JZ, Kalil RS, et al, "Effects of Antihypertensive Therapy on Serum Lipids," *Ann Intern Med*, 1995, 122(2):133-41.

Lipid Research Clinics Program, "The Lipid Research Clinics Coronary Primary Prevention Trial Results: I. Reduction in Incidence of Coronary Heart Disease," *JAMA*, 1984, 251(3):351-64.

Mauro VF and Tuckerman CE, "Ezetimibe for Management of Hypercholesterolemia," *Ann Pharmacother*, 2003, 37(6):839-48.

Multiple Risk Factor Intervention Trial Research Group, "Multiple Risk Factor Intervention Trial: Risk Factor Changes and Mortality Results," *JAMA*, 1982, 248(12):1465-77.

Pitt B, Waters D, Brown WV, et al, "Aggressive Lipid-Lowering Therapy Compared With Angioplasty in Stable Coronary Artery Disease. Atorvastatin Versus Revascularization Treatment Investigators," *N Engl J Med*, 1999, 341(2):70-6.

Ross SD, Allen IE, Connelly JE, et al, "Clinical Outcomes in Statin Treatment Trials: A Meta-Analysis," *Arch Intern Med*, 1999, 159(15):1793-802.

Sacks FM, Pfeffer MA, Moye LA, et al, "The Effect of Pravastatin on Coronary Events After Myocardial Infarction in Patients With Average Cholesterol Levels," *N Engl J Med*, 1996, 335(14):1001-9.

Scandinavian Simvastatin Survival Study, "Randomized Trial of Cholesterol Lowering in 4444 Patients With Coronary Heart Disease: The Scandinavian Simvastatin Survival Study (4S)," *Lancet*, 1994, 344(8934):1383-9.

Schrott HG, Bittner V, Vittinghoff E, et al, "Adherence to National Cholesterol Education Program Treatment Goals in Postmenopausal Women With Heart Disease. The Heart and Estrogen/Progestin Replacement Study (HERS)," *JAMA*, 1997, 277(16):1281-6.

Shepherd J, Cobbe SM, Ford I, et al, "Prevention of Coronary Heart Disease With Pravastatin in Men With Hypercholesterolemia, The West of Scotland Coronary Prevention Study Group," *N Engl J Med*, 1995, 333(20):1301-7.

Stein EA, Davidson MH, Dobs AS, et al, "Efficacy and Safety of Simvastatin 80 mg/day in Hypercholesterolemic Patients. The Expanded Dose Simvastatin U.S. Study Group," *Am J Cardiol*, 1998, 82(3):311-6.

HYPERTENSION

The optimal blood pressure for adults is <120/80 mm Hg. Consistent systolic pressure ≥140 mm Hg or a diastolic pressure ≥90 mm Hg, in the absence of a secondary cause, defines hypertension. Hypertension affects approximately 25% (50 million people) in the United States. Of those patients on antihypertensive medication, only one in three have their blood pressure controlled (<140/90 mm Hg).

Controlling systolic hypertension has been much more difficult than controlling diastolic hypertension. Educating patients in lifestyle management, cardiovascular risk reduction, and drug therapy aids in improving the morbidity and mortality of patients with hypertension.

The Seventh Report of the Joint National Committee (JNC VII) is an excellent reference and guide for the treatment of hypertension (Chobanian AV, Bakris GL, Black HR, et al, "The Seventh Report of the Joint National Committee on Prevention, Detection, Evaluation, and Treatment of High Blood Pressure: The JNC 7 Report," *JAMA*, 2003, 289(19):2560-71). For adults, hypertension is classified in stages (see following table).

Adult Classification of Blood Pressure

Category	Systolic (mm Hg)		Diastolic (mm Hg)
Normal	<120	and	<80
Prehypertension	120-139	or	80-89
Hypertension			
Stage 1	140-159	or	90-99
Stage 2	≥160	or	≥100

Adapted from Chobanian AV, Bakris GL, Black HR, et al, "The Seventh Report of the Joint National Committee on Prevention, Detection, Evaluation, and Treatment of High Blood Pressure: The JNC 7 Report," *JAMA*, 2003, 289(19):2560-71.

Normal Blood Pressure in Children

Age (y)	Girls' SBP / DBP (mm Hg)		Boys' SBP / DBP (mm Hg)	
	50th Percentile for Height	75th Percentile for Height	50th Percentile for Height	75th Percentile for Height
1	104/58	105/59	102/57	104/58
6	111/73	112/73	114/74	115/75
12	123/80	124/81	123/81	125/82
17	129/84	130/85	136/87	138/88

SBP = systolic blood pressure.

DBP = diastolic blood pressure.

Adapted from the report by the NHBPEP Working Group on Hypertension Control in Children and Adolescents, *Pediatrics*, 1996, 98(4 Pt 1):649-58.

PATIENT ASSESSMENT

- **Cardiovascular Risk Factors:** Hypertension, cigarette smoking, obesity (BMI ≥30), inactive lifestyle, dyslipidemia, diabetes mellitus, microalbuminuria or estimated GFR <60 mL/minute, age (>55 years for men, >65 years for women), family history of premature cardiovascular disease (men <55 years or women >65 years).

  Components of metabolic syndrome include hypertension, obesity, dyslipidemia, diabetes mellitus.
- Identify causes of high BP.
- Assess target-organ damage and CVD.

Target-Organ Disease

Organ System	Manifestation
Cardiac	Clinical, ECG, or radiologic evidence of coronary artery disease; prior MI, angina, post-CABG; left ventricular hypertrophy (LVH); left ventricular dysfunction or cardiac failure, prior coronary revascularization
Cerebrovascular	Transient ischemic attack or stroke
Peripheral vascular	Absence of pulses in extremities (except dorsalis pedis), claudication, aneurysm, peripheral arterial disease
Renal	Serum creatinine ≥130 µmol/L (1.5 mg/dL); proteinuria (≥1+); microalbuminuria, chronic kidney disease
Eye	Hemorrhages or exudates, with or without papilledema; retinopathy

Adapted from Chobanian AV, Bakris GL, Black HR, et al, "The Seventh Report of the Joint National Committee on Prevention, Detection, Evaluation, and Treatment of High Blood Pressure: The JNC 7 Report," *JAMA*, 2003, 289(19):2560-71.

BLOOD PRESSURE MEASUREMENT

At an office visit, patients should be seated quietly for ≥5 minutes in a chair with feet on the floor and arm supported at heart level. At least two measurements should be made. Patients should be given their results and their goal BP.

Ambulatory BP monitoring is useful in evaluating "white coat hypertension" (no end-organ damage), drug resistance, hypotensive symptoms, episodic hypertension, and autonomic dysfunction. Ambulatory BP monitoring correlates better with end-organ damage than office measurements.

Having patients monitor their own BP helps to improve compliance and provides information on response to therapeutic interventions.

Based on these initial assessments, treatment strategies for patients with hypertension are stratified based on their blood pressure and comorbidities (compelling indications).

Management of Blood Pressure

	Management: Based upon highest BP category		
BP Classification	**Lifestyle Modification**	**Initial Therapy Without Compelling Indication**	**Initial Therapy With Compelling Indication**[1]
Normal	Encourage	None	None
Prehypertensive	Yes	None	Treat patients with chronic kidney disease or diabetes to BP goal of <130/80 mm Hg
Hypertension			
Stage 1	Yes	Thiazide-type diuretic for most; consider ACEI, ARB, β-blocker, CCB, or combination	Drugs for the compelling indications; other antihypertensives as needed
Stage 2	Yes	Two drug combos (typically a thiazide-type diuretic and ACEI or ARB or β-blocker or CCB). Use combo cautiously in patients at risk for orthostasis.	Drugs for the compelling indications; other antihypertensives as needed

[1]Compelling Indication: Conditions for which specific classes of antihypertensive drugs have proven beneficial.

Adapted from Chobanian AV, Bakris GL, Black HR, et al, "The Seventh Report of the Joint National Committee on Prevention, Detection, Evaluation, and Treatment of High Blood Pressure: The JNC 7 Report," *JAMA*, 2003, 289(19):2560-71.

ACHIEVING BLOOD PRESSURE CONTROL

Treatment of hypertension should be individualized. Lower blood pressure (goal <130/80 mm Hg) should be achieved in patients with diabetes or chronic renal disease. The following Hypertension Treatment Algorithm may be used to select specific antihypertensives based on compelling indications.

Special consideration for starting combination therapy should be made in each patient.

Starting drug therapy at a low dose and titrating upward if blood pressure is not controlled is recommended.

Most patients with hypertension will require two or more drugs to achieve their BP goals.

Adding a second drug from a different class will help when a single drug at reasonable doses has failed to achieve the goal.

If the untreated BP is >20/10 mm Hg away from the goal, consider initiating therapy with two drugs. Use caution in those at risk for orthostasis (eg, diabetics, geriatrics, and those with autonomic dysfunction).

Low-dose aspirin therapy should be considered when BP is controlled; use in uncontrolled hypertension can increase the risk of hemorrhagic stroke.

Lifestyle modification and risk reduction should always be reviewed and reinforced.

MONITORING THERAPY

Generally, monthly follow-up is recommended until BP control is reached.

More frequent monitoring is required for those patients with Stage 2 hypertension or those with complications.

Serum potassium and serum creatinine should be monitored at least twice yearly.

When BP is at goal and stable, follow-up can be maintained every 3-6 months. Treat other cardiovascular risk factors if present.

Hypertension Treatment Algorithm

Begin or continue lifestyle modifications

↓

Not at goal blood pressure (<140/90 mm Hg or <130/80 mm Hg for patients with diabetes or chronic renal disease)

↓

Initial Drug Choice

Hypertension

Stage I
Thiazide-type diuretic for most.
Consider ACEI, ARB, β-blocker, CCB, or combo.

Stage 2
Two-drug combo for most (typically thiazide-type diuretic + ACEI or ARB or β-blocker or CCB)

Compelling Indications

Chronic kidney disease
- ACEI
- ARB

Diabetes mellitus
- ACEI
- ARB
- β-blocker
- CCB
- Diuretic

Heart failure
- ACEI
- Aldosterone blocker
- ARB
- β-blocker
- Diuretic

High coronary risk
- ACEI
- β-blocker
- CCB
- Diuretic

Myocardial infarction
- ACEI
- Aldosterone blocker
- β-blocker

Recurrent stroke prevention
- ACEI
- Diuretic

↓

Not at goal blood pressure

↓

Optimize dosages or add additional drugs until goal BP achieved.

Consider consultation with hypertension specialist.

Additional Considerations for Specific Therapies

Indication	Drug Therapy
Atrial tachyarrhythmias	β-blocker, CCB (non-DHP)
Chronic kidney disease	
Cl_{cr} <60 mL/min or albuminuria	ACEI or ARB
Cl_{cr} <30 mL/min	Increase loop diuretic
Diabetes	Thiazide diuretic, β-blocker, ACEI, ARB, CCB
Nephropathy	ACEI, ARB
Essential tremor	β-blocker (noncardioselective)
Heart failure	
Ventricular dysfunction (asymptomatic)	ACEI, β-blocker
Ventricular dysfunction (symptomatic)	ACEI, β-blocker, ARB, aldosterone blocker, loop diuretic
Hypertensive women who are pregnant	Methyldopa, β-blocker, vasodilator
Ischemic heart disease	
Angina	β-blocker, CCB (long-acting)
Acute coronary syndromes	β-blocker, ACEI
Migraine	β-blocker (noncardioselective), CCB (long-acting, non-DHP)
Osteoporosis	Thiazide diuretic
Perioperative hypertension	β-blocker
Prostatism (BPH)	Alpha-adrenergic blocking agent
Raynaud syndrome	CCB
Thyrotoxicosis	β-blocker

Note: ACEI = angiotensin-converting enzyme inhibitor; ARB = angiotensin receptor blocker; CCB = calcium channel blocker; DHP = dihydropyridine.

May Have Unfavorable Effects on Comorbid Conditions

Condition	Drug Therapy to Avoid
Angioedema	ACEI
Bronchospastic disease	β-blocker
Gout	Thiazide diuretic
Heart block (second or third degree)	β-blocker, CCB (non-DHP)
Hyponatremia	Thiazide diuretic
Potassium >5 mEq/L before treatment	Potassium sparing diuretic, aldosterone antagonist
Pregnancy or those likely to become pregnant	ACEI, ARB

Note: ACEI = angiotensin-converting enzyme inhibitor; ARB = angiotensin receptor blocker; CCB = calcium channel blocker; DHP = dihydropyridine.

HYPERTENSIVE EMERGENCIES AND URGENCIES

General Treatment Principles in the Treatment of Hypertensive Emergencies

Principle	Considerations
Admit the patient to the hospital, preferably in the ICU. Monitor vital signs appropriately.	Establish I.V. access and place patient on a cardiac monitor. Place a femoral intra-arterial line and pulmonary arterial catheter, if indicated, to assess cardiopulmonary function and intravascular volume status.
Perform rapid but thorough history and physical examination.	Determine cause of, or precipitating factors to, hypertensive crisis if possible (remember to obtain a medication history including Rx, OTC, and illicit drugs). Obtain details regarding any prior history of hypertension (severity, duration, treatment), as well as other coexisting illnesses. Assess the extent of hypertensive end organ damage. Determine if a hypertensive urgency or emergency exists.
Determine goal blood pressure based on premorbid level, duration, severity and rapidity of increase of blood pressure, concomitant medical conditions, race, and age.	Acute decreases in blood pressure to normal or subnormal levels during the initial treatment period may reduce perfusion to the brain, heart, and kidneys, and must be avoided except in specific instances (ie, dissecting aortic aneurysm). Gradually establish a normal (or reasonable) blood pressure over the next 1-2 weeks.
Select an appropriate antihypertensive regimen depending on the individual patient and clinical setting.	Initiate a controlled decrease in blood pressure. Avoid concomitant administration of multiple agents that may cause precipitous falls in blood pressure. Select the agent with the best hemodynamic profile based on the primary treatment goal. Avoid diuretics and sodium restriction during the initial treatment period unless there is a clear clinical indication (ie, CHF, pulmonary edema). Avoid sedating antihypertensives in patients with hypertensive encephalopathy, CVA, or other CNS disorders in whom mental status must be monitored. Use caution with direct vasodilating agents that induce reflex tachycardia or increase cardiac output in patients with coronary heart disease, history of angina or myocardial infarction, or dissecting aortic aneurysm. Preferably choose an agent that does not adversely affect glomerular filtration rate or renal blood flow and also agents that have favorable effects on cerebral blood flow and its autoregulation, especially for patients with hypertensive encephalopathy or CVAs. Select the most efficacious agent with the fewest adverse effects based on the underlying cause of the hypertensive crisis and other individual patient factors.
Initiate a chronic antihypertensive regimen after the patient's blood pressure is stabilized	Begin oral antihypertensive therapy once goal blood pressure is achieved before gradually tapering parenteral medications. Select the best oral regimen based on cost, ease of administration, adverse effect profile, and concomitant medical conditions.

Oral Agents Used in the Treatment of Hypertensive Urgencies

Drug	Dose	Onset	Cautions
Captopril[1]	P.O.: 25 mg, repeat as required	15-30 min	Hypotension, renal failure in bilateral renal artery stenosis
Clonidine	P.O.: 0.1-0.2 mg, repeated every hour as needed to a total dose of 0.6 mg	30-60 min	Hypotension, drowsiness, dry mouth
Labetalol	P.O.: 200-400 mg, repeat every 2-3 h	30 min to 2 h	Bronchoconstriction, heart block, orthostatic hypotension

[1]There is no clearly defined clinical advantage in the use of sublingual over oral routes of administration with these agents.

Recommendations for the Use of Intravenous Antihypertensive Drugs in Selected Hypertensive Emergencies

Condition	Agent(s) of Choice	Agent(s) to Avoid or Use With Caution	General Treatment Principles
Hypertensive encephalopathy	Nitroprusside, labetalol	Methyldopa, reserpine	Avoid drugs with CNS-sedating effects.
Acute intracranial or subarachnoid hemorrhage	Nicardipine,[1] nitroprusside	β-blocker	Careful titration with a short-acting agent.
Cerebral infarction	Nicardipine,[1] nitroprusside, labetalol	β-blocker, minoxidil	Careful titration with a short-acting agent. Avoid agents that may decrease cerebral blood flow.
Head trauma	Esmolol, labetalol	Methyldopa, reserpine, nitroprusside, nitroglycerin, hydralazine	Avoid drugs with CNS-sedating effects, or those that may increase intracranial pressure.
Acute myocardial infarction, myocardial ischemia	Nitroglycerin, nicardipine[1] (calcium channel blocker), labetalol	Hydralazine, minoxidil	Avoid drugs which cause reflex tachycardia and increased myocardial oxygen consumption.
Acute pulmonary edema	Nitroprusside, nitroglycerin, loop diuretics	β-blocker (labetalol), minoxidil, methyldopa	Avoid drugs which may cause sodium and water retention and edema exacerbation.
Renal dysfunction	Hydralazine, calcium channel blocker	Nitroprusside, ACE inhibitors, β-blocker (labetalol)	Avoid drugs with increased toxicity in renal failure and those that may cause decreased renal blood flow.
Eclampsia	Hydralazine, labetalol, nitroprusside[2]	Diuretics	Avoid drugs that may cause adverse fetal effects, compromise placental circulation, or decrease cardiac output.
Pheochromo- cytoma	Phentolamine, nitroprusside, β-blocker (eg, esmolol) only after alpha blockade (phentolamine)	β-blocker in the absence of alpha blockade, methyldopa, minoxidil	Use drugs of proven efficacy and specificity. Unopposed beta-blockade may exacerbate hypertension.
Dissecting aortic aneurysm	Nitroprusside and beta-blockade	Hydralazine, minoxidil	Avoid drugs which may increase cardiac output.
Postoperative hypertension	Nitroprusside, nicardipine,[1] labetalol, clevidipine		Avoid drugs which may exacerbate postoperative ileus.

[1]The use of nicardipine in these situations is by the recommendation of the author based on a review of the literature.

[2]Reserve nitroprusside for eclamptic patients with life-threatening hypertension unresponsive to other agents due to the potential risk to the fetus (cyanide and thiocyanate metabolites may cross the placenta).

Selected Intravenous Agents for Hypertensive Emergencies

Drug	Dose[1]	Onset of Action	Duration of Action	Adverse Effects[2]	Special Indications
Vasodilators					
Sodium nitroprusside	0.25-10 mcg/kg/min as I.V. infusion[3] (max: 10 min only)	Immediate	1-2 min	Nausea, vomiting, muscle twitching, sweating, thiocyanate and cyanide intoxication	Most hypertensive emergencies; caution with high intracranial pressure or azotemia
Nicardipine hydrochloride	5-15 mg/h I.V.	5-10 min	1-4 h	Tachycardia, headache, flushing, local phlebitis	Most hypertensive emergencies except acute heart failure; caution with coronary ischemia
Clevidipine butyrate	1-21 mg/h I.V.	2-4 min	5-15 min	Atrial fibrillation, nausea, insomnia, fever	Most hypertensive emergencies; caution with lipid disorder
Fenoldopam mesylate	0.1-0.3 mcg/kg/min as I.V. infusion	<5 min	30 min	Tachycardia, headache, nausea, flushing	Most hypertensive emergencies; caution with glaucoma
Nitroglycerin	5-100 mcg/min as I.V. infusion[3]	2-5 min	3-5 min	Headache, vomiting, methemoglobinemia, tolerance with prolonged use	Coronary ischemia
Enalaprilat	1.25-5 mg every 6 hours I.V.	15-30 min	6 h	Precipitous fall in pressure in high-renin states; response variable	Acute left ventricular failure; avoid in acute myocardial infarction
Hydralazine hydrochloride	10-20 mg I.V. 10-50 mg I.M.	10-20 min 20-30 min	3-8 h	Tachycardia, flushing, headache, vomiting, aggravation of angina	Eclampsia
Adrenergic Inhibitors					
Labetalol hydrochloride	20-80 mg I.V. bolus every 10 min; 0.5-2 mg/min as I.V. infusion	5-10 min	3-6 h	Vomiting, scalp tingling, burning in throat, dizziness, nausea, heart block, orthostatic hypotension	Most hypertensive emergencies except acute heart failure
Esmolol hydrochloride	250-500 mcg/kg/min for 1 min, then 50-100 mcg/kg/min for 4 min; may repeat	1-2 min	10-20 min	Hypotension, nausea	Aortic dissection, perioperative
Phentolamine	5-15 mg I.V.	1-2 min	3-10 min	Tachycardia, flushing, headache	Catecholamine excess

[1]These doses may vary from those in the *Physicians' Desk Reference* (51st edition).

[2]Hypotension may occur with all agents.

[3]Require special delivery system.

References

Guidelines

"1999 World Health Organization-International Society of Hypertension Guidelines for the Management of Hypertension. Guidelines Subcommittee," *J Hypertens*, 1999, 17(2):151-83.

Chobanian AV, Bakris GL, Black HR, et al, "The Seventh Report of the Joint National Committee on Prevention, Detection, Evaluation, and Treatment of High Blood Pressure: The JNC 7 Report," *JAMA*, 2003, 289(19):2560-72.

National High Blood Pressure Education Program Working Group on Hypertension Control in Children and Adolescents, "Update on the 1987 Task Force Report on High Blood Pressure in Children and Adolescents: A Working Group Report From the National High Blood Pressure Education Program," *Pediatrics*, 1996, 98(4 Pt 1):649-58.

National High Blood Pressure Education Program Working Group, "1995 Update of the Working Group Reports on Chronic Renal Failure and Renovascular Hypertension," *Arch Intern Med*, 1996, 156(17):1938-47.

"The Sixth Report of the National Committee on Detection, Evaluation, and Treatment of High Blood Pressure (JNC-VI)," *Arch Intern Med*, 1997, 157 (21):2413-46.

Others

Appel LJ, Moore TJ, Obarzanek E, et al, "A Clinical Trial of the Effect of Dietary Patterns on Blood Pressure. The DASH Collaborative Research Group," *N Engl J Med*, 1997, 336(16):1117-24.

Epstein M and Bakris G, "Newer Approaches to Antihypertensive Therapy: Use of Fixed-Dose Combination Therapy," *Arch Intern Med*, 1996, 156 (17):1969-78.

Estacio RO and Schrier RW, "Antihypertensive Therapy in Type II Diabetes: Implications of the Appropriate Blood Pressure Control in Diabetes (ABCD) Trial," *Am J Cardiol*, 1998, 82(9B):9R-14R.

Flack JM, Neaton J, Grimm RJ, et al, "Blood Pressure and Mortality Among Men With Prior Myocardial Infarction. The Multiple Risk Factor Intervention Trial Research Group," *Circulation*, 1995, 92(9):2437-45.

Frishman WH, Bryzinski BS, Coulson LR, et al, "A Multifactorial Trial Design to Assess Combination Therapy in Hypertension: Treatment With Bisoprolol and Hydrochlorothiazide," *Arch Intern Med*, 1994, 154(13):1461-8.

Furberg CD, Psaty BM, and Meyer JV, "Nifedipine: Dose-Related Increase in Mortality in Patients With Coronary Heart Disease," *Circulation*, 1995, 92 (5):1326-31.

Glynn RJ, Brock DB, Harris T, et al, "Use of Antihypertensive Drugs and Trends in Blood Pressure in the Elderly," *Arch Intern Med*, 1995, 155:1855-60.

Gradman AH, Cutler NR, Davis PJ, et al, "Combined Enalapril and Felodipine Extended Release (ER) for Systemic Hypertension. The Enalapril-Felodipine ER Factorial Study Group," *Am J Cardiol*, 1997, 79(4):431-5.

Grimm RH Jr, Flack JM, Grandits GA, et al, "Long-Term Effects on Plasma Lipids of Diet and Drugs to Treat Hypertension. The Treatment of Mild Hypertension Study (TOMHS) Research Group," *JAMA*, 1996, 275(20):1549-56.

Grimm RH Jr, Grandits GA, Cutler JA, et al, "Relationships of Quality-of-Life Measures to Long-Term Lifestyle and Drug Treatment in the Treatment of Mild Hypertension Study. The TOMHS Research Group," *Arch Intern Med*, 1997, 157(6):638-48.

Grossman E, Messerli FH, Grodzicki T, et al, "Should a Moratorium Be Placed on Sublingual Nifedipine Capsules Given for Hypertensive Emergencies and Pseudoemergencies?" *JAMA*, 1996, 276(16):1328-31.

Hansson L, Zanchetti A, Carruthers SG, et al, "Effects of Intensive Blood Pressure Lowering and Low-Dose Aspirin in Patients With Hypertension: Principal Results of the Hypertension Optimal Treatment (HOT) Randomized Trial. HOT Study Group," *Lancet*, 1998, 351(9118):1755-62.

Kaplan NM and Gifford RW Jr, "Choice of Initial Therapy for Hypertension," *JAMA*, 1996, 275(20):1577-80.

Kasiske BL, Ma JZ, Kalil RSN, et al, "Effects of Antihypertensive Therapy in Serum Lipids," *Ann Intern Med*, 1995, 122(2):133-41.

Kostis JB, Davis BR, Cutler J, et al, "Prevention of Heart Failure by Antihypertensive Drug Treatment in Older Persons With Isolated Systolic Hypertension. SHEP Cooperative Research Group," *JAMA*, 1997, 278(3):212-6.

Lazarus JM, Bourgoignie JJ, Buckalew VM, et al, "Achievement and Safety of a Low Blood Pressure Goal in Chronic Renal Disease: The Modification of Diet in Renal Disease Study Group," *Hypertension*, 1997, 29(2):641-50.

Lindheimer MD, "Hypertension in Pregnancy," *Hypertension*, 1993, 22(1):127-37.

Materson BJ, Reda DJ, Cushman WC, et al, "Single-Drug Therapy for Hypertension in Men: A Comparison of Six Antihypertensive Agents With Placebo. The Department of Veterans Affairs Cooperative Study Group on Antihypertensive Agents," *N Engl J Med*, 1993, 328(13):914-21.

Miller NH, Hill M, Kottke T, et al, "The Multi-Level Compliance Challenge: Recommendations for a Call to Action; A Statement for Healthcare Professionals," *Circulation*, 1997, 95(4):1085-90.

Neaton JD and Wentworth D, "Serum Cholesterol, Blood Pressure, Cigarette Smoking, and Death From Coronary Heart Disease: Overall Findings and Differences by Age for 316,099 White Men. The Multiple Risk Factor Intervention Trial Research Group," *Arch Intern Med*, 1992, 152(1):56-64.

Neaton JD, Grim RH, Prineas RJ, et al, "Treatment of Mild Hypertension Study. Final Results. Treatment of Mild Hypertension Study Research Group," *JAMA*, 1993, 270(6):713-24.

Oparil S, Levine JH, Zuschke CA, et al, "Effects of Candesartan Cilexetil in Patients With Severe Systemic Hypertension," *Am J Cardiol*, 1999, 84 (3):289-93.

Peacock WF, Varon J, Garrison N, et al, "I.V. Clevidipine for Hypertension: Safety, Efficacy, and Transition to Oral Therapy," *Ann Emerg Med*, 2007, 50(3 Suppl):S8-9.

Perloff D, Grim C, Flack J, et al, "Human Blood Pressure Determination by Sphygmomanometry," *Circulation*, 1993, 88(5 Pt 1):2460-7.

Perry HM Jr, Bingham S, Horney A, et al, "Antihypertensive Efficacy of Treatment Regimens Used in Veterans Administration Hypertension Clinics. Department of Veterans Affairs Cooperative Study Group on Antihypertensive Agents," *Hypertension*, 1998, 31(3):771-9.

Preston RA, Materson BJ, Reda DJ, et al, "Age-Race Subgroup Compared With Renin Profile as Predictors of Blood Pressure Response to Antihypertensive Therapy," *JAMA*, 1998, 280(13):1168-72.

Psaty BM, Smith NL, Siscovick DS, et al, "Health Outcomes Associated With Antihypertensive Therapies Used as First-Line Agents. A Systemic Review and Meta-analysis," *JAMA*, 1997, 277(9):739-45.

Radevski IV, Valtchanova SP, Candy GP, et al, "Comparison of Acebutolol With and Without Hydrochlorothiazide Versus Carvedilol With and Without Hydrochlorothiazide in Black Patients With Mild to Moderate Systemic Hypertension," *Am J Cardiol*, 1999, 84(1):70-5.

Setaro JF and Black HR, "Refractory Hypertension," *N Engl J Med*, 1992, 327(8):543-7.

SHEP Cooperative Research Group, "Prevention of Stroke by Antihypertensive Drug Treatment in Older Persons With Isolated Systolic Hypertension: Final Results of the Systolic Hypertension in the Elderly Program (SHEP)," *JAMA*, 1991, 265(24):3255-64.

Sibai BM, "Treatment of Hypertension in Pregnant Women," *N Engl J Med*, 1996, 335(4):257-65.

Singla N, Warltier DC, Gandhi SD, et al, "Treatment of Acute Postoperative Hypertension in Cardiac Surgery Patients: An Efficacy Study of Clevidipine Assessing Its Postoperative Antihypertensive Effect in Cardiac Surgery-2 (ESCAPE-2), a Randomized, Double-Blind, Placebo-Controlled Trial," *Anesth Analg*, 2008, 107(1):59-67.

Sowers JR, "Comorbidity of Hypertension and Diabetes: The Fosinopril Versus Amlodipine Cardiovascular Events Trial," *Am J Cardiol*, 1998, 82 (9B):15R-19R.

Sternberg H, Rosenthal T, Shamiss A, et al, "Altered Circadian Rhythm of Blood Pressure in Shift Workers," *J Hum Hypertens*, 1995, 9(5):349-53.

"The Hypertension Prevention Trial: Three-Year Effects of Dietary Changes on Blood Pressure. Hypertension Prevention Trial Research Group," *Arch Intern Med*, 1990, 150(1):153-62.

Trials of Hypertension Prevention Collaborative Research Group, "Effects of Weight Loss and Sodium Reduction Intervention on Blood Pressure and Hypertension Incidence in Overweight People With High-Normal Blood Pressure: The Trials of Hypertension Prevention, Phase II," *Arch Intern Med*, 1997, 157(6):657-67.

Tuomilehto J, Rastenyte D, Birkenhager WH, et al, "Effects of Calcium Channel Blockade in Older Patients With Diabetes and Systolic Hypertension," *N Engl J Med*, 1999, 340(9):677-84.

Veelken R and Schmieder RE, "Overview of Alpha-1 Adrenoceptor Antagonism and Recent Advances in Hypertensive Therapy," *Am J Hypertens*, 1996, 9(11):139S-49S.

White WB, Black HR, Weber MA, et al, "Comparison of Effects of Controlled Onset Extended Release Verapamil at Bedtime and Nifedipine Gastrointestinal Therapeutic System on Arising on Early Morning Blood Pressure, Heart Rate, and the Heart Rate-Blood Pressure Product," *Am J Cardiol*, 1998, 81(4):424-31.

OBESITY TREATMENT GUIDELINES FOR ADULTS

SUMMARY OF CLINICAL PRACTICE GUIDELINES

Note: Weight loss treatment for children and adolescents is not covered by these guidelines.

ASSESSMENT

Assessment of weight involves evaluating body mass index, waist circumference, and the patient's risk factors.

A. Body Mass Index (BMI)

1. BMI should be calculated for all adults (see table). Those with normal BMI should be reassessed in 2 years. A very muscular person may have a high BMI without the additional health risks. A BMI calculator is available through Lexi-CALC™.
2. Normal body weight is defined as a BMI of 18.5-24.9 kg/m^2. Overweight is defined as a BMI of 25-29.9 kg/m^2.
3. Obesity is defined as a BMI of ≥30 kg/m^2. There are 3 classes of obesity: Class I (BMI 30-34.9), Class II (BMI 35-39.9), Class III (BMI ≥40).

B. Abdominal Fat

1. Excess abdominal fat, not proportional to total body fat, is an independent predictor for risk and morbidity.
2. Waist circumference for men >40 inches or women >35 inches is an increased risk for those with a BMI of 25-34.9.

C. Risk Factors

1. Coronary heart disease, hypertension, stroke, or other atherosclerotic diseases, type 2 diabetes, gallbladder disease, osteoarthritis, sleep apnea, and other respiratory problems are associated with a very high risk of developing disease complications and higher mortality in an obese individual.
2. Obesity is also associated with complications of pregnancy, menstrual irregularities, stress incontinence, and psychological disorders (eg, depression).
3. **Cardiovascular Risk Factors:** Hypertension, cigarette smoking, obesity (BMI ≥30), inactive lifestyle, dyslipidemia, diabetes mellitus, microalbuminuria or estimated GFR <60 mL/minute, age (>55 years for men, >65 years for women), family history of premature cardiovascular disease (men <55 years or women >65 years).
Weight loss is recommended for those who are obese and for those who are classified as overweight or have a high waist circumference and increased disease risks.

Body Mass Index (BMI), kg/m^2

Height (feet, inches)

Weight (lb)	5'0"	5'3"	5'6"	5'9"	6'0"	6'3"
140	27	25	23	21	19	18
150	29	27	24	22	20	19
160	31	28	26	24	22	20
170	33	30	28	25	23	21
180	35	32	29	27	25	23
190	37	34	31	28	26	24
200	39	36	32	30	27	25
210	41	37	34	31	29	26
220	43	39	36	33	30	28
230	45	41	37	34	31	29
240	47	43	39	36	33	30
250	49	44	40	37	34	31

Note: For BMI calculations see "Body Mass Index."

TREATMENT

Patients who are overweight or obese, but are not candidates for weight loss (eg, those with serious psychiatric illness) or do not wish to lose weight, should be counseled to avoid further weight gain. Women who are overweight or obese at the onset of pregnancy are advised to gain less total weight during pregnancy.

A. Goals of Treatment

1. Prevent further weight gain.
2. Reduce body weight. The initial goal is to reduce body weight by 10% from baseline over the suggested time period of 6 months.
3. Maintain a lower body weight, long term.

B. Nonpharmacologic treatment should include:

1. An individually-planned diet which includes a decrease in fat as well as total calories.
2. An increase in physical activity. Physical activity should be gradually increased to a goal of 30 minutes per day of moderate-intensity activity.
3. Behavior therapy, which should include tools to help overcome individual barriers to weight loss.

C. Drug Therapy
In select patients with BMI ≥30, or BMI ≥27 with other risk factors (eg, hypertension, diabetes, dyslipidemia), who did not lose weight or maintain weight loss, drug therapy can be started along with dietary therapy and physical activity.

D. Surgery
Patients with severe clinical obesity, BMI ≥40 or BMI ≥35 with coexisting conditions, can be considered for weight loss surgery when other methods have failed. Lifelong surveillance after surgery is necessary.

Medications Approved for Long-Term Use in the Treatment of Obesity

Generic (Trade) Name	Therapeutic Category / Mechanism of Action	Usual Adult Dosage
Orlistat (Xenical®)	Lipase inhibitor; a reversible inhibitor of gastric and pancreatic lipases thus inhibiting absorption of dietary fats by 30% (at doses of 120 mg 3 times/day)	120 mg 3 times/day with each main meal containing fat (during or up to 1 hour after the meal); omit dose if meal is occasionally missed or contains no fat.
Sibutramine (Meridia®)	Anorexiant; blocks the neuronal uptake of norepinephrine and, to a lesser extent, serotonin and dopamine	Initial: 10 mg once daily; after 4 weeks may titrate up to 15 mg once daily as needed and tolerated

References

McTigue KM, Harris R, Hemphill B, et al, "Screening and Interventions for Obesity in Adults: Summary of the Evidence for the U.S. Preventive Services Task Force," *Ann Intern Med*, 2003, 139(11):933-49.

National Heart, Lung, and Blood Institute Obesity Education Initiative, "Clinical Guidelines on the Identification, Evaluation, and Treatment of Overweight and Obesity in Adults. The Evidence Report," NIH Publication No. 98-4083. Bethesda, MD: U.S. Department of Health and Human Services, Public Health Service, National Institutes of Health, National Heart, Lung, and Blood Institute, 1998.

Snow V, Barry P, Fitterman N, et al, "Pharmacologic and Surgical Management of Obesity in Primary Care: A Clinical Practice Guideline From the American College of Physicians," *Ann Intern Med*, 2005, 142(7):525-31.

STATUS EPILEPTICUS

CONVULSIVE STATUS EPILEPTICUS

Treatment Guidelines

Convulsive status epilepticus is an emergency that is associated with high morbidity and mortality. The outcome largely depends on etiology, but prompt and appropriate pharmacological therapy can reduce morbidity and mortality. Etiology varies in children and adults and reflects the distribution of disease in these age groups. Antiepileptic drug administration should be initiated whenever a seizure has lasted 5-10 minutes. Immediate concerns include supporting respiration, maintaining blood pressure, gaining intravenous access, and identifying and treating the underlying cause. Initial therapeutic and diagnostic measures are conducted simultaneously. The goal of therapy is rapid termination of clinical and electrical seizure activity; the longer a seizure continues, the greater the likelihood of an adverse outcome. Several drug protocols now in use will terminate status epilepticus. Common to all patients is the need for a clear plan, prompt administration of appropriate drugs in adequate doses, and attention to the possibility of apnea, hypoventilation, or other metabolic abnormalities.

Management of Status Epilepticus

Time Since Seizure Onset	Drug Treatment		Evaluations / Actions
	Adults	Children	
Prolonged Seizure: Premonitory Stage (Out-of-Hospital)			
5 min	Diazepam 10 mg rectally	Diazepam 0.5 mg/kg rectally	• Airway/breathing • Monitor vital signs • Establish I.V. access • Blood glucose determination
If seizures continue ↓ **Early Status Epilepticus: First Stage (Out-of-Hospital or Inpatient)**			
5-30 min	Lorazepam 4 mg I.V. bolus (≤2 mg/min) **or** Diazepam 5-10 mg I.V. (≤5 mg/min; maximum dose: 30 mg) May repeat dose after 5-10 minutes	Lorazepam 0.05-0.1 mg/kg I.V. (≤2 mg/min; maximum dose: 4 mg) **or** Diazepam 0.1-0.3 mg/kg I.V. (≤5 mg/min; maximum dose: 10 mg) May repeat dose after 5-10 minutes	• ABGs, oxygen/ventilation • CBC, electrolytes, renal/hepatic status • Cardiac monitoring, ECG • Neurologic assessment toxicology screen • Consider I.V. dextrose ± thiamine • AED concentrations
If seizures continue ↓ **Established Status Epilepticus: Second Stage**			
30-60 min	Fosphenytoin 15-20 mg PE/kg I.V. (maximum rate: 150 mg/min) **or** Phenytoin 15-20 mg/kg I.V. (maximum rate: 50 mg/min)	Fosphenytoin 15-20 mg PE/kg I.V. (maximum rate: 150 mg/min) **or** Phenytoin 20 mg/kg I.V. (maximum rate: 50 mg/min) **or** Phenobarbital 15-20 mg/kg I.V. (maximum rate: <100 mg/min[1])	• Intubation/mechanical ventilation • Cardiorespiratory function • Vasopressors if needed • Neurologic: CT, CSF, EEG
If seizures continue ↓ **Refractory Status Epilepticus: Third Stage**			
>60 min	Phenobarbital 10-20 mg/kg I.V. (maximum: 100 mg/min[1]) **or** Pentobarbital 10-20 mg/kg I.V. (maximum: 100 mg/min[1]), then 0.5-3 mg/kg/h **or** Midazolam 0.2 mg/kg bolus, then continuous infusion of 0.05-0.6 mg/kg/h **or** Propofol 1-2 mg/kg bolus, then continuous infusion of 1.5-10 mg/kg/h	Phenobarbital 15-20 mg/kg I.V. (maximum: <100 mg/min[1]) **or** Pentobarbital 5-15 mg/kg I.V., then 0.5-5 mg/kg/h[1] **or** Midazolam 0.15 mg/kg bolus, then continuous infusion of 0.06 mg/kg/h	• ICU admission • Anesthesia monitoring/hemodynamics • Therapeutic AED monitoring

AED = antiepileptic drug.

[1]May induce hypotension; consider alternative agents in hemodynamically unstable patients. Monitor closely and reduce rate if hypotension develops. Fluids and/or vasopressors may be necessary to control significant hypotension.

References

Hanhan UA, Fiallos MR, and Orlowski JP, "Status Epilepticus," *Pediatr Clin North Am*, 2001, 48(3):683-94.

Kälviäinen R, "Status Epilepticus Treatment Guidelines," *Epilepsia*, 2007, 48(Suppl 8):99-102.

Kälviäinen R, Eriksson K, and Parviainen I, "Refractory Generalised Convulsive Status Epilepticus: A Guide to Treatment," *CNS Drugs*, 2005, 19 (9):759-68.

Lowenstein DH, "Treatment Options for Status Epilepticus," *Curr Opin Pharmacol*, 2005, 5(3):334-9.

Meierkord H, Boon P, Engelsen B, et al, "EFNS Guideline on the Management of Status Epilepticus," *Eur J Neurol*, 2006, 13(5):445-50.

BREAST-FEEDING AND DRUGS

Breast-feeding is recommended for all infants unless specific contraindications exist. Human breast milk is superior to alternative products for both full-term and premature infants and exclusive breast-feeding provides sufficient nutrition for up to 6 months of life. Breast-feeding provides additional health benefits to the infant, such as decreased incidence of infection; some studies suggest breast-feeding may also decrease the risk of sudden infant death syndrome, type 1 or 2 diabetes mellitus, and increase neurodevelopment.

Breast-feeding is not recommended in the following situations:

- Infants with classic galactosemia (galactose 1-phosphate uridyltransferase deficiency)
- Mothers with untreated/active tuberculosis
- Mothers who are human t-cell lymphotropic virus type I or II positive
- Mothers exposed to radioactive materials (diagnostic or therapeutic; until they are cleared from breast milk)
- Mothers who are receiving chemotherapeutic agents or antimetabolites (until they are cleared from breast milk)
- Mothers using drugs of abuse
- Mothers with herpes simplex lesions on the breast (breasts clear of lesions may be used to breast-feed)
- Mothers who are HIV-infected and living in the United States (the benefits of breast-feeding may be greater than the risk of HIV transmission in other, underdeveloped countries where safe alternatives to breast-feeding are not as readily available as in the United States)

While breast-feeding is encouraged for all women (without specific contraindications), prior to recommending or prescribing medications to a lactating woman, the following should be considered:

- Is drug therapy necessary?
- Can drug exposure to the infant be minimized? (Using a different route of administration, timing of the dose in relation to breast-feeding, length of therapy, using breast milk stored prior to treatment, etc)
- The infant's age and health status (their own ability to metabolize the medication)
- The pharmacokinetics of the drug
- Will the drug interact with a medication the infant is prescribed?
- If medications must be used, pick the safest drug possible.
- In situations where the only drug available may have adverse effects in the nursing infant, consider measuring the infants blood levels.

The tables presented below have been adapted from the American Academy of Pediatrics Committee on Drugs report "Transfer of Drugs and Other Chemicals Into Human Milk," September 2001. It should not be inferred that if a medication is not in the tables it is considered safe for administration to a lactating woman; only that published reports concerning their use were not available at the time the report was published. Always consider the unique circumstances or a particular mother/child pair when making recommendations.

Table 1. Cytotoxic Drugs

Cyclophosphamide	Doxorubicin
Cyclosporine	Methotrexate

These are medications thought to interfere with cellular metabolism in the nursing infant. Immune suppression may be possible; effects on growth or carcinogenesis are not known. In addition, doxorubicin is concentrated in human milk; methotrexate and cyclophosphamide are associated with neutropenia in the nursing infant.

Table 2. Drugs of Abuse

Amphetamine	Marijuana
Cocaine	Phencyclidine
Heroin	

Drugs of abuse are not only dangerous to the nursing infant, but also to the mother. Women should be encouraged to avoid their use completely. Effects to the infant reported with amphetamine use in the mother include irritability and poor sleeping; it is also a substance that is concentrated in human milk. Cocaine may cause irritability, vomiting, diarrhea, tremors, or seizures in the infant. Heroin may also cause tremors as well as restlessness, vomiting, and poor feeding.

Nicotine, which was previously on this list, is associated with decreased milk production, decreased weight gain in the infant, and possible increased respiratory illness in the infant. Although there are still questions outstanding regarding smoking and breast-feeding, women should be counseled on the possible effects to their infants and offered aid to smoking cessation if appropriate.

Table 3. Radioactive Compounds That Require Temporary Cessation of Breast-Feeding

Drug	Recommended Time for Cessation of Breast-Feeding
Copper 64 (^{64}Cu)	Radioactivity in milk present at 50 h
Gallium 67 (^{67}Ga)	Radioactivity in milk present for 2 wk
Indium 111 (^{111}In)	Very small amount present at 20 h
Iodine 123 (^{123}I)	Radioactivity in milk present up to 36 h
Iodine 125 (^{125}I)	Radioactivity in milk present for 12 d
Iodine 131 (^{131}I)	Radioactivity in milk present 2-14 d, depending on study
Iodine^{131}	If used for thyroid cancer, high radioactivity may prolong exposure to infant
Radioactive sodium	Radioactivity in milk present 96 h
Technetium-99m (^{99m}Tc), ^{99m}Tc macroaggregates, ^{99m}Tc O4	Radioactivity in milk present 15 h to 3 d

Consider pumping and storing milk prior to study for use during the radioactive period. Pumping should continue after the study to maintain milk production; however, this milk should be discarded until radioactivity is gone. Notify nuclear medicine physician prior to study that the mother is breast-feeding; a short-acting radionuclide may be appropriate. Contact Radiology Department after testing is complete to screen milk samples before resuming feeding.

Table 4a. Psychotropic Drugs Whose Effect on Nursing Infants Is Unknown But May Be of Concern

Antianxiety	Antidepressant	Antipsychotic
Alprazolam	Amitriptyline	Chlorpromazine
Diazepam	Amoxapine	Clozapine[1]
Lorazepam	Bupropion	Haloperidol
Midazolam	Clomipramine	Mesoridazine
Perphenazine	Desipramine	Trifluoperazine
Quazepam	Doxepin	
Temazepam	Fluoxetine	
	Fluvoxamine	
	Imipramine	
	Nortriptyline	
	Paroxetine	
	Sertraline[1]	
	Trazodone	

[1]Drug is concentrated in human milk.

Psychotropic medications usually appear in the breast milk in low concentrations. Although adverse effects in the infant may be limited to a few case reports, the long half-life of these medications and their metabolites should be considered. In addition, measurable amounts may be found in the infants plasma and also brain tissue. Long-term effects are not known. Colic, irritability, feeding and sleep disorders, and slow weight gain are effects reported with fluoxetine. Chlorpromazine may cause galactorrhea in the mother, while drowsiness and lethargy have been reported in the nursing infant. A decline in developmental scores has been reported with chlorpromazine and haloperidol.

Table 4b. Additional Drugs Whose Effect on Nursing Infants Is Unknown But May Be of Concern

Drug	Reported Effect in Nursing Infant
Amiodarone	Hypothyroidism
Chloramphenicol	Idiosyncratic bone marrow suppression
Clofazimine	Increase in skin pigmentation; high transfer of mothers dose to infant is possible
Lamotrigine	Therapeutic serum concentrations in infant
Metoclopramide[1]	
Metronidazole	
Tinidazole	

[1]Drug is concentrated in human milk.

No adverse effects to the infant have been reported for metoclopramide; however, it should be recognized that it is a dopaminergic agent. Metronidazole and tinidazole are *in vitro* mutagenic agents; in cases where single dose therapy is appropriate for the mother, breast-feeding may be discontinued for 12-24 hours to allow excretion of the medication.

Table 5. Drugs That Have Been Associated With Significant Effects on Some Nursing Infants and Should Be Given to Nursing Mothers With Caution[1]

Drug	Reported Effect
Acebutolol	Hypotension, bradycardia, tachypnea
5-Aminosalicylic acid	Diarrhea (one case)
Atenolol	Cyanosis, bradycardia
Bromocriptine	Suppresses lactation; may be hazardous to the mother
Aspirin (salicylates)	Metabolic acidosis (one case)
Clemastine	Drowsiness, irritability, refusal to feed, high-pitched cry, neck stiffness (one case)
Ergotamine	Vomiting, diarrhea, convulsions (doses used in migraine medications)
Lithium	One-third to one-half therapeutic blood concentration in infants
Phenindone	Anticoagulant: increased prothrombin and partial thromboplastin time in one infant; not used in the United States
Phenobarbital	Sedation; infantile spasms after weaning from milk-containing phenobarbital, methemoglobinemia (one case)
Primidone	Sedation, feeding problems
Sulfasalazine (salicylazosulfapyridine)	Bloody diarrhea (one case)

[1]Blood concentration in the infant may be of clinical importance; measure when possible.

References

2006 Red Book: Report of the Committee on Infectious Diseases, 27th ed, Elk Grove Village, IL: American Academy of Pediatrics, 2006, 123-30.

American Academy of Pediatrics Committee on Drugs, "Transfer of Drugs and Other Chemicals Into Human Milk," *Pediatrics*, 2001, 108(3): 776-89.

Gartner LM, Morton J, Lawrence RA, et al, "Breastfeeding and the Use of Human Milk," *Pediatrics*, 2005, 115(2):496-506.

DISCOLORATION OF FECES DUE TO DRUGS

Black
Acetazolamide
Alcohols
Alkalies
Aluminum hydroxide
Aminophylline
Aminosalicylic acid
Amphetamine
Amphotericin
Antacids
Anticoagulants
Aspirin
Betamethasone
Bismuth
Charcoal
Chloramphenicol
Chlorpropamide
Clindamycin
Corticosteroids
Cortisone
Cyclophosphamide
Cytarabine
Dicumarol
Digitalis
Ethacrynic acid
Ferrous salts
Floxuridine
Fluorides
Fluorouracil
Halothane
Heparin
Hydralazine
Hydrocortisone
Ibuprofen
Indomethacin
Iodine drugs
Iron salts
Levarterenol
Levodopa
Manganese
Melphalan
Methylprednisolone
Methotrexate
Methylene blue
Oxyphenbutazone
Phenacetin
Phenolphthalein
Phenylbutazone
Phenylephrine
Phosphorous
Potassium salts
Prednisolone
Procarbazine
Pyrvinium
Reserpine
Salicylates
Sulfonamides
Tetracycline
Theophylline
Thiotepa
Triamcinolone
Warfarin

Blue
Chloramphenicol
Methylene blue

Dark Brown
Dexamethasone

Gray
Colchicine

Green
Indomethacin
Iron
Medroxyprogesterone

Greenish Gray
Oral antibiotics
Oxyphenbutazone
Phenylbutazone

Light Brown
Anticoagulants

Orange-Red
Phenazopyridine
Rifampin

Pink
Anticoagulants
Aspirin
Heparin
Oxyphenbutazone
Phenylbutazone
Salicylates

Red
Anticoagulants
Aspirin
Heparin
Oxyphenbutazone
Phenolphthalein
Phenylbutazone
Pyrvinium
Salicylates
Tetracycline syrup

Red-Brown
Oxyphenbutazone
Phenylbutazone
Rifampin

Tarry
Ergot preparations
Ibuprofen
Salicylates
Warfarin

White/Speckling
Aluminum hydroxide
Antibiotics (oral)
Indocyanine green

Yellow
Senna

Yellow-Green
Senna

Adapted from Drugdex® — Drug Consults, Micromedex, Vol 62, Denver, CO: Rocky Mountain Drug Consultation Center, 1998.

DISCOLORATION OF URINE DUE TO DRUGS

Black
Cascara
Cotrimoxazole
Ferrous salts
Iron dextran
Levodopa
Methocarbamol
Methyldopa
Naphthalene
Pamaquine
Phenacetin
Phenols
Quinine
Sulfonamides

Blue
Anthraquinone
DeWitt's pills
Indigo blue
Indigo carmine
Methocarbamol
Methylene blue
Mitoxantrone
Nitrofurans
Resorcinol
Triamterene

Blue-Green
Amitriptyline
Anthraquinone
DeWitt's pills
Doan's® pills
Indigo blue
Indigo carmine
Magnesium salicylate
Methylene blue
Resorcinol

Brown
Anthraquinone dyes
Cascara
Chloroquine
Hydroquinone
Levodopa
Methocarbamol
Methyldopa
Methocarbamol
Metronidazole
Nitrofurans
Nitrofurantoin
Pamaquine
Phenacetin
Phenols
Primaquine
Quinine
Rifabutin
Rifampin
Senna
Sodium diatrizoate
Sulfonamides

Brown-Black
Isosorbide mono- or dinitrate
Methyldopa
Metronidazole
Nitrates
Nitrofurans
Phenacetin
Povidone iodine
Quinine
Senna

Dark
p-Aminosalicylic acid
Cascara
Levodopa
Metronidazole
Nitrites
Phenacetin
Phenol
Primaquine
Quinine
Resorcinol
Riboflavin
Senna

Green
Amitriptyline
Anthraquinone
DeWitt's pills
Indigo blue
Indigo carmine
Indomethacin
Methocarbamol
Methylene blue
Nitrofurans
Phenols
Propofol
Resorcinol
Suprofen

Green-Yellow
DeWitt's pills
Methylene blue

Milky
Phosphates

Orange
Chlorzoxazone
Dihydroergotamine mesylate
Heparin sodium
Phenazopyridine
Phenindione
Rifabutin
Rifampin
Sulfasalazine
Warfarin

Orange-Red-Brown
Chlorzoxazone
Doxidan
Phenazopyridine
Rifampin
Warfarin

Orange-Yellow
Fluorescein sodium
Rifampin
Sulfasalazine

Pink
Aminopyrine
Anthraquinone dyes
Aspirin
Cascara
Danthron
Deferoxamine
Merbromin
Methyldopa
Phenazopyridone
Phenolphthalein
Phenothiazines
Phenytoin
Salicylates
Senna

Purple
Phenolphthalein

Red
Anthraquinone
Cascara
Chlorpromazine
Daunorubicin
Deferoxamine
Dihydroergotamine mesylate
Dimethyl sulfoxide
DMSO
Doxorubicin
Heparin
Ibuprofen
Methyldopa
Oxyphenbutazone
Phenacetin
Phenazopyridine
Phenolphthalein
Phenothiazines
Phensuximide
Phenylbutazone
Phenytoin
Rifampin
Senna

Red-Brown
Cascara
Deferoxamine
Methyldopa
Oxyphenbutazone
Pamaquine
Phenacetin
Phenazopyridine
Phenolphthalein
Phenothiazines
Phenylbutazone
Phenytoin
Quinine
Senna

Red-Purple
Chlorzoxazone
Ibuprofen
Phenacetin
Senna

Rust
Cascara
Chloroquine
Metronidazole
Nitrofurantoin
Pamaquine
Phenacetin
Quinacrine
Riboflavin
Senna
Sulfonamides

Yellow
Nitrofurantoin
Phenacetin
Quinacrine
Riboflavin
Sulfasalazine

Yellow-Brown
Aminosalicylate acid
Bismuth
Cascara
Chloroquine
DeWitt's pills
Methylene blue
Metronidazole
Nitrofurantoin
Pamaquine
Primaquine
Quinacrine
Senna
Sulfonamides

Yellow-Pink
Cascara
Senna

Adapted from Drugdex® — Drug Consults, Micromedex, Vol 62, Denver, CO: Rocky Mountain Drug Consultation Center, 1998.

FEVER DUE TO DRUGS

Most Common

Atropine
Amphotericin B
Asparaginase
Barbiturates
Bleomycin
Cephalosporins
Interferon
Methyldopa
Penicillins
Phenytoin
Procainamide
Quinidine
Salicylates (high doses)
Streptomycin
Sulfonamides

Less Common

Allopurinol
Antihistamines
Azathioprine
Carbamazepine
Cimetidine
Cisplatin
Colistimethate
Diazoxide
Folic acid
Hydralazine
Hydroxyurea
Imipenem
Iodides
Isoniazid
Mercaptopurine
Metoclopramide
Nifedipine
NSAIDs
Nitrofurantoin
Pentazocine
Procarbazine
Propylthiouracil
Rifampin
Streptokinase
Triamterene
Vancomycin

References

Cunha BA, "Antibiotic Side Effects," *Med Clin North Am*, 2001, 85(1):149-85.
Mackowiak PA and LeMaistre CF, "Drug Fever: A Critical Appraisal of Conventional Concepts. An Analysis of 51 Episodes in Two Dallas Hospitals and 97 Episodes Reported in the English Literature," *Ann Intern Med*, 1987, 106(5):728-33.
Tabor PA, "Drug-Induced Fever," *Drug Intell Clin Pharm*, 1986, 20(6):413-20.

HERB – DRUG INTERACTIONS / CAUTIONS

Herb	Drug Interaction / Caution
Acidophilus / bifidobacterium	Antibiotics (oral)
Activated charcoal	Vitamins or oral medications may be adsorbed
Alfalfa	Do not use with lupus due to amino acid L-canavanine; causes pancytopenia at high doses; warfarin (alfalfa contains a large amount of vitamin K)
Aloe vera	Caution in pregnancy, may cause uterine contractions; digoxin, diuretics (hypokalemia)
Ashwagandha	May cause sedation and other CNS effects
Asparagus root	Causes diuresis
Barberry	Normal metabolism of vitamin B may be altered with high doses
Birch	If taking a diuretic, drink plenty of fluids
Black cohosh	Estrogen-like component; pregnant and nursing women should probably avoid this herb; also women with estrogen-dependent cancer and women who are taking birth control pills or estrogen supplements after menopause; caution also in people taking sedatives or blood pressure medications
Black haw	Do not give to children <6 years of age (salicin content) with flu or chickenpox due to potential Reye's syndrome; do not take if allergic to aspirin
Black pepper (*Piper nigrum*)	Antiasthmatic drugs (decreases metabolism)
Black tea	May inhibit body's utilization of thiamine
Blessed thistle	Do not use with gastritis, ulcers, or hyperacidity since herb stimulates gastric juices
Blood root	Large doses can cause nausea, vomiting, CNS sedation, low BP, shock, coma, and death
Broom (*Cytisus scoparius*)	MAO inhibitors lead to sudden blood pressure changes
Bugleweed (*Lycopus virginicus*)	May interfere with nuclear imaging studies of the thyroid gland (thyroid uptake scan)
Cat's claw (*Uncaria tomentosa*)	Avoid in organ transplant patients or patients on ulcer medications, antiplatelet drugs, NSAIDs, anticoagulants, immunosuppressive therapy, intravenous immunoglobulin therapy
Chaste tree berry (*Vitex agnus-castus*)	Interferes with actions of oral contraceptives, HRT, and other endocrine therapies; may interfere with metabolism of dopamine-receptor antagonists
Chicory (*Cichorium intybus*)	Avoid with gallstones due to bile-stimulating properties
Chlorella (*Chlorella vulgaris*)	Contains significant amounts of vitamin K
Chromium picolinate	Picolinic acid causes notable changes in brain chemicals (serotonin, dopamine, norepinephrine); do not use if patient has behavioral disorders or diabetes
Cinnabar root (*Salviae multorrhizae*)	Warfarin (increases INR)
Deadly nightshade (*Atropa belladonna*)	Contains atropine
Dong quai	Warfarin (increases INR), estrogens, oral contraceptives, photosensitizing drugs, histamine replacement therapy, anticoagulants, antiplatelet drugs, antihypertensives
Echinacea	Caution with other immunosuppressive therapies; stimulates TNF and interferons
Evening primrose oil	May lower seizure threshold; do not combine with anticonvulsants or phenothiazines
Fennel	Do not use in women who have had breast cancer or who have been told not to take birth control pills
Fenugreek	Practice moderation in patients on diabetes drugs, MAO inhibitors, cardiovascular agents, hormonal medicines, or warfarin due to the many components of fenugreek
Feverfew	Antiplatelets, anticoagulants, NSAIDs
Forskolin, coleonol	This herb lowers blood pressure (vasodilator) and is a bronchodilator and increases the contractility of the heart, inhibits platelet aggregation, and increases gastric acid secretion
Foxglove	Digitalis-containing herb
Garlic	Blood sugar-lowering medications, warfarin, and aspirin at medicinal doses of garlic
Ginger	May inhibit platelet aggregation by inhibiting thromboxane synthetase at large doses; *in vitro* and animal studies indicate that ginger may interfere with diabetics; has anticoagulant effect, so avoid in medicinal amounts in patients on warfarin or heart medicines
Ginkgo biloba	Warfarin (ginkgo decreases blood clotting rate); NSAIDs, MAO inhibitors
Ginseng	Blood sugar-lowering medications (additive effects) and other stimulants
Ginseng (American, Korean)	Furosemide (decreases efficacy)
Ginseng (Siberian)	Digoxin (increases digoxin level)

Herb	Drug Interaction / Caution
Glucomannan	Diabetics (herb delays absorption of glucose from intestines, decreasing mean fasting sugar levels)
Goldenrod	Diuretics (additive properties)
Gymnema	Blood sugar-lowering medications (additive effects)
Hawthorn	Digoxin or other heart medications (herb dilates coronary vessels and other blood vessels, also inotropic)
Hibiscus	Chloroquine (reduced effectiveness of chloroquine)
Hops	Those with estrogen-dependent breast cancer should not take hops (contains estrogen-like chemicals); patients with depression (accentuate symptoms); alcohol or sedative (additive effects)
Horehound	May cause arrhythmias at high doses
Horseradish	In medicinal amounts with thyroid medications
Kava	CNS depressants (additive effects, eg, alcohol, barbiturates, etc); benzodiazepines
Kelp	Thyroid medications (additive effects or opposite effects by negative feedback); kelp contains a high amount of sodium
Labrador tea	Plant has narcotic properties, possible additive effects with other CNS depressants
Lemon balm	Do not use with Graves disease since it inhibits certain thyroid hormones
Licorice	Acts as a corticosteroid at high doses (about 1.5 lbs candy in 9 days) which can lead to hypertension, edema, hypernatremia, and hypokalemia (pseudoaldosteronism); do not use in persons with hypertension, glaucoma, diabetes, kidney or liver disease, or those on hormonal therapy; may interact with digitalis (due to hypokalemia)
Lobelia	Contains lobeline which has nicotinic activity; may mask withdrawal symptoms from nicotine; it can act as a polarizing neuromuscular blocker
Lovage	Is a diuretic
Ma huang	MAO inhibitors, digoxin, beta-blockers, methyldopa, caffeine, theophylline, decongestants (increases toxicity)
Marshmallow	May delay absorption of other drugs taken at the same time; may interfere with treatments of lowering blood sugar
Meadowsweet	Contains salicylates
Melatonin	Acts as contraceptive at high doses; antidepressants (decreases efficacy)
Mistletoe	May interfere with medications for blood pressure, depression, and heart disease
L-phenylalanine	MAO inhibitors
Pleurisy root	Digoxin (plant contains cardiac glycosides); also contains estrogen-like compounds; may alter amine concentrations in the brain and interact with antidepressants
Prickly ash (Northern)	Contains coumarin-like compounds
Prickly ash (Southern)	Contains neuromuscular blockers
Psyllium	Digoxin (decreases absorption)
Quassia	High doses may complicate heart or blood-thinning treatments (quassia may be inotropic)
Red clover	May have estrogen-like actions; avoid when taking birth control pills, HRT, people with heart disease or at risk for blood clots, patients who suffer from estrogen-dependent cancer; do not take with warfarin
Red pepper	May increase liver metabolism of other medications and may interfere with high blood pressure medications or MAO inhibitors
Rhubarb, Chinese	Do not use with digoxin (enhanced effects)
St John's wort	Indinavir, cyclosporine, SSRIs or any antidepressants, tetracycline (increases sun sensitivity); digoxin (decreases digoxin concentration); may also interact with diltiazem, nicardipine, verapamil, etoposide, paclitaxel, vinblastine, vincristine, glucocorticoids, cyclosporine, dextromethorphan, ephedrine, lithium, meperidine, pseudoephedrine, selegiline, yohimbine, ACE inhibitors (serotonin syndrome, hypertension, possible exacerbation of allergic reaction)
Saw palmetto	Acts an antiandrogen; do not take with prostate medicines or HRT
Squill	Digoxin or persons with potassium deficiency; also not with quinidine, calcium, laxatives, saluretics, prednisone (long-term)
Sweet woodruff	Contains coumarin
Tonka bean	Contains coumarin, interacts with warfarin
Vervain	Avoid large amounts of herb with blood pressure medications or HRT

Herb	Drug Interaction / Caution
Wild Oregon grape	High doses may alter metabolism of vitamin B
Wild yam	May interfere with hormone precursors
Wintergreen	Warfarin, increased bleeding
Yarrow	Interferes with anticoagulants and blood pressure medications
Yohimbe	Do not consume tyramine-rich foods; do not take with nasal decongestants, PPA-containing diet aids, antidepressants, or mood-altering drugs

LABORATORY DETECTION OF DRUGS

Agent	Time Detectable in Urine[1]
Alcohol	12-24 h
Amobarbital	2-4 d
Amphetamine	2-4 d
Butalbital	2-4 d
Cannabinoids	
Occasional use	2-7 d
Regular use	30 d
Cocaine (benzoylecgonine)	12-72 h
Codeine	2-4 d
Chlordiazepoxide	30 d
Diazepam	30 d
Dilaudid®	2-4 d
Ethanol	12-24 h
Heroin (morphine)	2-4 d
Hydromorphone	2-4 d
Librium®	30 d
Marijuana	
Occasional use	2-7 d
Regular use	30 d
Methamphetamine	2-4 d
Methaqualone	2-4 d
Morphine	2-4 d
Pentobarbital	2-4 d
Phencyclidine (PCP)	
Occasional use	2-7 d
Regular use	30 d
Phenobarbital	30 d
Quaalude®	2-4 d
Secobarbital	2-4 d
Valium®	30 d

[1]The periods of detection for the various abused drugs listed above should be taken as estimates since the actual figures will vary due to metabolism, user, laboratory, and excretion.

Chang JY, "Drug Testing and Interpretation of Results," *Pharmchem Newsletter*, 1989, 17:1.

ORAL DOSAGES THAT SHOULD NOT BE CRUSHED

There are a variety of reasons for crushing tablets or capsule contents prior to administering to the patient. Patients may have nasogastric tubes which do not permit the administration of tablets or capsules; an oral solution for a particular medication may not be available from the manufacturer or readily prepared by pharmacy; patients may have difficulty swallowing capsules or tablets; or mixing of powdered medication with food or drink may make the drug more palatable.

Generally, medications which should not be crushed fall into one of the following categories.

- **Extended-Release Products**. The formulation of some tablets is specialized as to allow the medication within it to be slowly released into the body. This is sometimes accomplished by centering the drug within the core of the tablet, with a subsequent shedding of multiple layers around the core. Wax melts in the GI tract. Slow-K® is an example of this. Capsules may contain beads which have multiple layers which are slowly dissolved with time.

  Common Abbreviations for Extended-Release Products

CD	Controlled dose
CR	Controlled release
CRT	Controlled-release tablet
LA	Long-acting
SR	Sustained release
TR	Timed release
TD	Time delay
SA	Sustained action
XL	Extended release
XR	Extended release

- **Medications Which Are Irritating to the Stomach**. Tablets which are irritating to the stomach may be enteric-coated which delays release of the drug until the time when it reaches the small intestine. Enteric-coated aspirin is an example of this.
- **Foul-Tasting Medication**. Some drugs are quite unpleasant to taste so the manufacturer coats the tablet in a sugar coating to increase its palatability. By crushing the tablet, this sugar coating is lost and the patient tastes the unpleasant tasting medication.
- **Sublingual Medication**. Medication intended for use under the tongue should not be crushed. While it appears to be obvious, it is not always easy to determine if a medication is to be used sublingually. Sublingual medications should indicate on the package that they are intended for sublingual use.
- **Effervescent Tablets**. These are tablets which, when dropped into a liquid, quickly dissolve to yield a solution. Many effervescent tablets, when crushed, lose their ability to quickly dissolve.

RECOMMENDATIONS

1. It is not advisable to crush certain medications.
2. Consult individual monographs prior to crushing capsule or tablet.
3. If crushing a tablet or capsule is contraindicated, consult with your pharmacist to determine whether an oral solution exists or can be compounded.
4. Refer to individual drug monograph for crushing information.

Summary of Drug Formulations That Preclude Crushing

Type	Reason(s) for the Formulation
Enteric-coated	Designed to pass through the stomach intact with drug released in the intestines to: • prevent destruction of drug by stomach acids • prevent stomach irritation • delay onset of action
Extended release	Designed to release drug over an extended period of time. Such products include: • multiple layered tablets releasing drug as each layer is dissolved • mixed release pellets that dissolve at different time intervals • special matrixes that are themselves inert but slowly release drug from the matrix
Sublingual buccal	Designed to dissolve quickly in oral fluids for rapid absorption by the abundant blood supply of the mouth
Miscellaneous	Drugs that: • produce oral mucosa irritation • are extremely bitter • contain dyes or inherently could stain teeth and mucosal tissue

TOP 200 PRESCRIBED DRUGS

Brand Name (if appropriate)	Generic Name	Rank
Abilify®	aripiprazole	79
Aciphex®	rabeprazole	54
Actonel®	risedronate	38
Actoplus Met™	pioglitazone and metformin	182
Actos®	pioglitazone	22
Adderall XR®	dextroamphetamine and amphetamine	36
Advair Diskus®	fluticasone and salmeterol	10
Aggrenox®	aspirin and dipyridamole	172
Aldara®	imiquimod	194
Allegra-D® 12 Hour	fexofenadine and pseudoephedrine	88
Allegra-D® 24 Hour	fexofenadine and pseudoephedrine	169
Alphagan® P	brimonidine	129
Altace®	ramipril	32
Ambien®	zolpidem	45
Ambien CR®	zolpidem	39
AndroGel®	testosterone	171
Apri®	ethinyl estradiol and desogestrel	116
Aricept®	donepezil	61
Arimidex®	anastrozole	149
Armour® Thyroid	thyroid, desiccated	101
Arthrotec®	diclofenac and misoprostol	196
Asacol®	mesalamine	155
Asmanex® Twisthaler®	mometasone	174
Astelin®	azelastine	102
Atacand®	candesartan	133
Avalide®	irbesartan and hydrochlorothiazide	80
Avandamet®	rosiglitazone and metformin	156
Avandia®	rosiglitazone	50
Avapro®	irbesartan	62
Avelox®	moxifloxacin	78
Aviane™	ethinyl estradiol and levonorgestrel	97
Avodart®	dutasteride	106
Bactroban®	mupirocin	160
Benicar®	olmesartan	59
Benicar HCT®	olmesartan and hydrochlorothiazide	60
BenzaClin®	clindamycin and benzoyl peroxide	153
Boniva®	ibandronate	76
Budeprion™ SR	bupropion	92
Budeprion® XL	bupropion	67
Byetta®	exenatide	121
Caduet®	amlodipine and atorvastatin	105
Catapres-TTS®	clonidine	187
Celebrex®	celecoxib	25
Ceron-DM	chlorpheniramine, phenylephrine, and dextromethorphan	198
Chantix®	varenicline	49
Cialis®	tadalafil	65
Ciprodex®	ciprofloxacin and dexamethasone	145

Brand Name (if appropriate)	Generic Name	Rank
Clarinex®	desloratadine	100
Combivent®	ipratropium and albuterol	66
Concerta®	methylphenidate	44
Coreg®	carvedilol	41
Coreg CR®	carvedilol	189
Cosopt®	dorzolamide and timolol	135
Coumadin® tablets	warfarin	83
Cozaar®	losartan	40
Crestor®	rosuvastatin	17
Cymbalta®	duloxetine	21
Depakote®	valproic acid and derivatives	93
Depakote® ER	valproic acid and derivatives	85
Detrol® LA	tolterodine	63
Differin®	adapalene	163
Digitek®	digoxin	47
Dilantin®	phenytoin	151
Diovan®	valsartan	14
Diovan HCT®	valsartan and hydrochlorothiazide	19
Effexor® XR	venlafaxine	12
Elidel®	pimecrolimus	200
Enablex®	darifenacin	185
Endocet®	oxycodone and acetaminophen	91
EpiPen®	epinephrine	181
Estrostep® Fe	ethinyl estradiol and norethindrone	177
EtheDent™	fluoride	199
Evista®	raloxifene	71
Flomax®	tamsulosin	26
Flovent® HFA	fluticasone	77
Fluzone®	influenza virus vaccine	152
Focalin® XR	dexmethylphenidate	140
Fosamax®	alendronate	15
Fosamax Plus D™	alendronate and cholecalciferol	120
Geodon®	ziprasidone	136
–	glipizide XL	124
GlycoLax®	polethylene glycol 3350	69
Guaifenex® PSE [DSC]	guaifenesin and pseudoephedrine	162
Humalog®	insulin lispro	89
Humulin® 70/30	insulin NPH and insulin regular	144
Humulin® N	insulin NPH	127
Hyzaar®	losartan and hydrochlorothiazide	55
Imitrex®	sumatriptan	70
Jantoven®	warfarin	186
Januvia™	sitagliptin	108
Junel™ Fe	ethinyl estradiol and norethindrone	188
Kariva™	ethinyl estradiol and desogestrel	109
Keppra®	levetiracetam	107
Klor-Con®	potassium chloride	20
Lamictal®	lamotrigine	51
Lanoxin®	digoxin	157
Lantus®	insulin glargine	31
Lescol® XL	fluvastatin	179

Brand Name (if appropriate)	Generic Name	Rank
Levaquin®	levofloxacin	18
Levitra®	vardenafil	112
Levora®	ethinyl estradiol and levonorgestrel	167
Levothroid®	levothyroxine	118
Levoxyl®	levothyroxine	35
Lexapro®	escitalopram	3
Lidoderm®	lidocaine	95
Lipitor®	atorvastatin	1
Loestrin® 24 Fe	ethinyl estradiol and norethindrone	117
Lotrel®	amlodipine and benazepril	37
Lovaza®	omega-3-acid ethyl esters	138
Low-Ogestrel®	ethinyl estradiol and norgestrel	114
Lumigan®	bimatoprost	128
Lunesta®	eszopiclone	58
Lyrica®	pregabalin	43
Methylin®	methylphenidate	170
Micardis®	telmisartan	137
Micardis® HCT	telmisartan and hydrochlorothiazide	139
Mirapex®	pramipexole	142
Namenda™	memantine	94
Nasacort® AQ	triamcinolone	86
Nasonex®	mometasone	29
Necon® 0.5/35	ethinyl estradiol and norethindrone	195
Necon® 1/35	ethinyl estradiol and norethindrone	119
Nexium®	esomeprazole	4
Niaspan®	niacin	74
Norvasc®	amlodipine	28
Novolin® 70/30	insulin NPH and insulin regular	180
NovoLog® Mix 70/30	insulin aspart protamine and insulin aspart	175
NuvaRing®	ethinyl estradiol and etonogestrel	72
Omnicef®	cefdinir	73
Ortho Evra®	ethinyl estradiol and norelgestromin	113
Ortho Tri-Cyclen®	ethinyl estradiol and norgestimate	190
Ortho Tri-Cyclen® Lo	ethinyl estradiol and norgestimate	52
–	oxycodone	183
OxyContin®	oxycodone	141
Patanol®	olopatadine	98
Paxil CR®	paroxetine	123
Plavix®	clopidogrel	6
Premarin® cream	estrogens (conjugated/equine)	164
Premarin® tablet	estrogens (conjugated/equine)	23
Prempro™	estrogens (conjugated/equine) and medroxyprogesterone	110
Prevacid®	lansoprazole	8
PrimaCare® One	vitamins (multiple/prenatal)	191
ProAir™ HFA	albuterol	24
Prometrium®	progesterone	143
Propecia®	finasteride	173
Protonix®	pantoprazole	13
Proventil® HFA	albuterol	99
Provigil®	modafinil	125

Brand Name (if appropriate)	Generic Name	Rank
Pseudovent™ 400 [DSC]	guaifenesin and pseudoephedrine	165
Pulmicort Respules®	budesonide	122
Relpax®	eletriptan	168
Requip®	ropinirole	81
Restasis®	cyclosporine	146
Rhinocort® Aqua®	budesonide	111
Risperdal®	risperidone	46
Rozerem®	ramelteon	184
Seroquel®	quetiapine	27
Singulair®	montelukast	2
Skelaxin®	metaxalone	87
Spiriva®	tiotropium	56
Sprintec™	ethinyl estradiol and norgestimate	150
Strattera®	atomoxetine	96
Suboxone®	buprenorphine and naloxone	147
Sular®	nisoldipine	178
Synthroid®	levothyroxine	5
Tamiflu®	oseltamivir	161
TobraDex®	tobramycin and dexamethasone	131
Topamax®	topiramate	48
Toprol-XL®	metoprolol	7
Travatan®	travoprost	158
TriCor®	fenofibrate	30
Trileptal®	oxcarbazepine	126
TriLyte®	polyethylene glycol-electrolyte solution	193
TriNessa™	ethinyl estradiol and norgestimate	64
Tri-Sprintec™	ethinyl estradiol and norgestimate	75
Trivora®	ethinyl estradiol and levonorgestrel	132
Tussionex®	hydrocodone and chlorpheniramine	104
Ultram® ER	tramadol	197
Uroxatral®	alfuzosin	176
Vagifem®	estradiol	166
Valtrex®	valacyclovir	42
VESIcare®	solifenacin	154
Viagra®	sildenafil	32
Vigamox™	moxifloxacin	90
Vivelle-Dot®	estradiol	115
Vytorin®	ezetimibe and simvastatin	9
Wellbutrin XL™	bupropion	57
Xalatan®	latanoprost	53
Xopenex®	levalbuterol	134
Xopenex HFA™	levalbuterol	130
Yasmin®	ethinyl estradiol and drospirenone	34
Yaz®	ethinyl estradiol and drospirenone	68
Zetia®	ezetimibe	16
Zoloft®	sertraline	159

Brand Name (if appropriate)	Generic Name	Rank
Zovirax® topical	acyclovir	192
Zymar®	gatifloxacin	148
Zyprexa®	olanzapine	84
Zyrtec-D 12 Hour® [DSC]	cetirizine and pseudoephedrine	103
Zyrtec® syrup	cetirizine	82
Zyrtec® tablets	cetirizine	11

"The Top 200 Drugs for 2007 by Prescriptions Dispensed," Available at: http://www.rxlist.com/script/main/hp.asp

TYRAMINE CONTENT OF FOODS

Food[1]	Allowed	Minimize Intake	Not Allowed
Beverages	Decaffeinated beverages (eg, coffee, tea, soda); milk, soy milk, chocolate beverage	Caffeine-containing drinks, clear spirits, wine, bottled/canned beers	**Tap** beer
Breads/cereals	All except those containing cheese	None	Cheese bread and crackers
Dairy products	Cottage cheese, farmers or pot cheese, cream cheese, ricotta cheese, all milk, eggs, ice cream, pudding, yogurt, sour cream, processed cheese, mozzarella	None	All other cheeses (**aged** cheese, American, Camembert, cheddar, Gouda, gruyere, parmesan, provolone, romano, Roquefort, stilton)
Meat, fish, and poultry	All fresh packaged or processed (eg, hot dogs, bologna), or frozen	Pepperoni	**Aged** chicken and beef liver, dried and pickled fish, shrimp paste, summer or dry sausage, dried meats (eg, salami, cacciatore), meat extracts, liverwurst
Starches — potatoes/rice	All	None	Soybean (including paste), tofu
Vegetables	All fresh, frozen, canned, or dried vegetable juices except those not allowed	Chili peppers, Chinese pea pods	Sauerkraut, broad or fava bean pods (not beans)
Fruit	Fresh, frozen, or canned fruits and fruit juices	Avocado, figs	Banana peel, avocado (over-ripened)
Soups	All soups not listed to limit or avoid	None	Soups which contain **aged** cheese, **tap** beer, any made with flavor cubes or meat extract, miso soup, broad or fava bean pods (not beans)
Fats	All except fermented	None	None
Sweets	Sugar, hard candy, honey, molasses, syrups, chocolate candy	None	None
Desserts	Cakes, cookies, gelatin, pastries, sherbets, sorbets, chocolate desserts	None	None
Miscellaneous	Salt, nuts, spices, herbs, flavorings, Worcestershire sauce, Brewer's or Baker's yeast, monosodium glutamate, vitamins with Brewer's yeast	Peanuts	Soy sauce, all aged and fermented products, marmite and other concentrated yeast extracts

[1]Freshness is of primary importance. Food that is spoiled or improperly stored should be avoided.

References:

Shulman KI and Walker SE, "A Reevaluation of Dietary Restrictions for Irreversible Monoamine Oxidase Inhibitors" *Psychiatr Ann*, 2001, 31(6):378-84.

Shulman KI and Walker SE, "Refining the MAOI Diet: Tyramine Content of Pizza and Soy Products," *J Clin Psychiatry*, 1999, 60(3):191-3.

Walker SE, Shulman KI, Tailor SAN, et al, "Tyramine Content of Previously Restricted Foods in Monoamine Oxidase Inhibitor Diets," *J Clin Psychopharmacol*, 1996, 16(5):383-8.

VITAMIN K CONTENT IN SELECTED FOODS

The following lists describe the relative amounts of vitamin K in selected foods. The abbreviations for vitamin K are "H" for high amounts, "M" for medium amounts, and "L" for low amounts.

Foods[1]	Portion Size[2]	Vitamin K Content
Coffee brewed	10 cups	L
Cola, regular and diet	3½ fl oz	L
Fruit juices, assorted types	3½ fl oz	L
Milk	3½ fl oz	L
Tea, black, brewed	3½ fl oz	L
Bread, assorted types	4 slices	L
Cereal, assorted types	3½ oz	L
Flour, assorted types	1 cup	L
Oatmeal, instant, dry	1 cup	L
Rice, white	½ cup	L
Spaghetti, dry	3½ oz	L
Butter	6 Tbsp	L
Cheddar cheese	3½ oz	L
Eggs	2 large	L
Margarine	7 Tbsp	M
Mayonnaise	7 Tbsp	H
Oils		
Canola, salad, soybean	7 Tbsp	H
Olive	7 Tbsp	M
Corn, peanut, safflower, sesame, sunflower	7 Tbsp	L
Sour cream	8 Tbsp	L
Yogurt	3½ oz	L
Apple	1 medium	L
Banana	1 medium	L
Blueberries	⅔ cup	L
Cantaloupe pieces	⅔ cup	L
Grapes	1 cup	L
Grapefruit	½ medium	L
Lemon	2 medium	L
Orange	1 medium	L
Peach	1 medium	L
Abalone	3½ oz	L
Beef, ground	3½ oz	L
Chicken	3½ oz	L
Mackerel	3½ oz	L
Meatloaf	3½ oz	L
Pork, meat	3½ oz	L
Tuna	3½ oz	L
Turkey, meat	3½ oz	L
Asparagus, raw	7 spears	M
Avocado, peeled	1 small	M
Beans, pod, raw	1 cup	M
Broccoli, raw and cooked	½ cup	H
Brussel sprout, sprout and top leaf	5 sprouts	H
Cabbage, raw	1½ cups shredded	H

VITAMIN K CONTENT IN SELECTED FOODS

Foods[1]	Portion Size[2]	Vitamin K Content
Cabbage, red, raw	1½ cups shredded	M
Carrot	⅔ cup	L
Cauliflower	1 cup	L
Celery	2½ stalks	L
Coleslaw	¾ cup	M
Collard greens	½ cup chopped	H
Cucumber peel, raw	1 cup	H
Cucumber, peel removed	1 cup	L
Eggplant	1¼ cups pieces	L
Endive, raw	2 cups chopped	H
Green scallion, raw	⅔ cup chopped	H
Kale, raw leaf	¾ cup	H
Lettuce, raw, heading, bib, red leaf	1¾ cups shredded	H
Mushroom	1½ cups	L
Mustard greens, raw	1½ cups	H
Onion, white	⅔ cup chopped	L
Parsley, raw and cooked	1½ cups chopped	H
Peas, green, cooked	⅔ cup	M
Pepper, green, raw	1 cup chopped	L
Potato	1 medium	L
Pumpkin	½ cup	L
Spinach, raw leaf	1½ cups	H
Tomato	1 medium	L
Turnip greens, raw	1½ cups chopped	H
Watercress, raw	3 cups chopped	H
Honey	5 Tbsp	L
Jell-O® Gelatin	⅓ cup	L
Peanut butter	6 Tbsp	L
Pickle, dill	1 medium	M
Sauerkraut	1 cup	M
Soybean, dry	½ cup	M

[1]This list is a partial listing of foods. For more complete information, refer to references 1-2.

[2]Portions in chart are calculated from estimated portions provided in reference 4.

References

Booth SL, Sadowski JA, Weihrauch JL, et al, "Vitamin K_1 (Phylloquinone) Content of Foods a Provisional Table," *J Food Comp Anal*, 1993, 6:109-20.
Ferland G, MacDonald DL, and Sadowski JA, "Development of a Diet Low in Vitamin K_1 (Phylloquinone)," *J Am Diet Assoc*, 1992, 92, 593-7.
Hogan RP, "Hemorrhagic Diathesis Caused by Drinking an Herbal Tea," *JAMA*, 1983, 249:2679-80.
Pennington JA, *Bowes and Church's Food Values of Portions Commonly Used*, 15th ed, JP Lippincott Co, 1985.

PHARMACOLOGIC CATEGORY INDEX

NOTES

NOTES

NOTES

NOTES

Other Products Offered by Lexi-Comp®

Lexi-Comp ON-HAND

Available for Palm OS®, Pocket PC,
BlackBerry®, iPhone™, and mobile devices

At Lexi-Comp, we take pride in creating and delivering timely, quality drug information for use at the point-of-care. Our content is not subject to third party recommendations or suggestions, but is based on the contributions of our respected authors, internal clinical team, and the thousands of professionals within the healthcare industry who constantly review and validate our data.

With Lexi-Comp® ON-HAND™ you can be confident you are accessing the most up-to-date information on the latest warnings and new drug information. All updates are included with your annual subscription.

Lexi-Comp ON-HAND databases include:

- Lexi-Drugs®
- Pediatric Lexi-Drugs®
- Lexi-Drugs® para Pediatría (Spanish Version)
- Lexi-Interact™
- Lexi-Natural Products™
- Lexi-Tox™
- Household Products
- Lexi-Infectious Diseases™
- Lexi-Lab & Diagnostic Procedures™
- Nursing Lexi-Drugs®
- Dental Lexi-Drugs®
- Lexi-Pharmacogenomics™
- Lexi-PALS™ (Patient Advisory Leaflets)
- Lexi-Drug ID™
- Lexi-CALC™
- Lexi-I.V. Compatibility™*
- Lexi-Companion Guides™
- Lexi-NBCA™ (Nuclear, Biological, & Chemical Agent) Exposures
- The 5-Minute Clinical Consult
- The 5-Minute Pediatric Consult
- AHFS Essentials
- Harrison's Practice
- Stedman's Medical Dictionary for the Health Professions and Nursing
- Medical Abbreviations by Neil Davis

* I.V. compatibility information © copyright King Guide Publications, Inc.

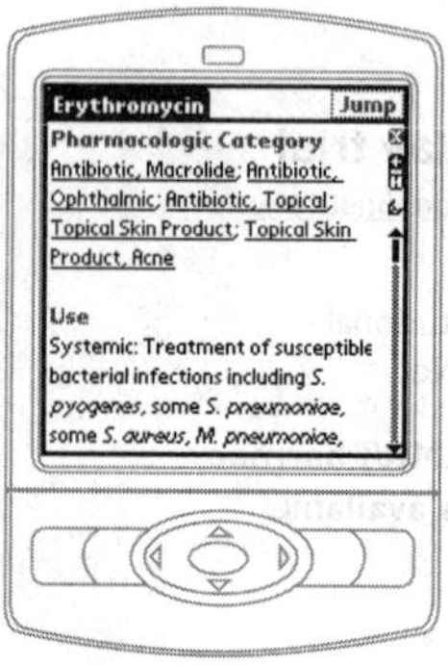

Go to www.lexi.com for more information on Lexi-Comp's products and packages.

See opposite page for clinical areas covered by the LEXI-COMP® Knowledge Solution™.

Available on the following platforms:

Palm OS® | Pocket PC | BlackBerry | iPhone™ | MOBILE

To order, call Customer Service at 1-866-397-3433 or visit www.lexi.com.
Outside of the U.S., call 330-650-6506 or visit www.lexi.com